McKee's

Pathology of the Skin

McKee's
Pathology of the Skin
WITH CLINICAL CORRELATIONS

Eduardo Calonje MD, DipRCPath
Director of Dermatopathology
Department of Dermatopathology
St John's Institute of Dermatology
St Thomas' Hospital
London, UK

CO-EDITORS

Thomas Brenn MD, PhD, FRCPath
Professor
Department of Pathology & Laboratory Medicine, Section of Anatomic Pathology
Department of Medicine, Section of Dermatology
Cumming School of Medicine
University of Calgary
Calgary Laboratory Services and Alberta Health Services
Calgary, AB, Canada

Alexander J. Lazar MD, PhD
Professor
Departments of Pathology, Genomic Medicine and Dermatology
Sections of Dermatopathology, Soft Tissue & Bone Pathology, and Clinical Genomics
Faculty, Sarcoma Research Center and Graduate School of Biomedical Science
The University of Texas M.D. Anderson Cancer Center Houston, Texas, USA

Steven D. Billings MD
Professor
Co-Director Dermatopathology Section
Department of Anatomic Pathology
Cleveland Clinic
Cleveland, OH, USA

For additional online content visit **ExpertConsult.com**

ELSEVIER

ELSEVIER

© 2020, Elsevier Limited. All rights reserved.
First edition 1989
Second edition 1996
Third edition 2005
Fourth edition 2012
Fifth edition 2020

The rights of Eduardo Calonje, Thomas Brenn, Alexander J. Lazar, Steven D. Billings to be identified as authors of this work has been asserted by them in accordance with the Copyright, Designs and Patents Act 1988.

Notices

ISBN: 978-0-7020-6983-3 (2 volume set)
eISBN: 978-0-7020-7552-0

Content Strategist: Michael J. Houston
Content Development Specialist: Louise Cook
Project Manager: Andrew Riley
Design: Renee Duenow
Illustration Manager: Nichole Beard
Marketing Manager: Melissa Fogarty

Printed in India
Last digit is the print number: 9   8   7   6   5   4

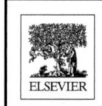

Contents

Preface to the fifth edition

It is unbelievable that it is more than 5 years since Phillip McKee announced that he was retiring and standing down as the editor of the textbook that he started as a solo author back in the early 1990s. This book, to which he devoted a large part of his life and career, became a household name many years ago and I am very lucky that he, with his boundless generosity, invited me to be part of it when the third edition was planned. Since then, "the book" has become an intrinsic part of my life and almost my whole existence since I became the main editor three years ago when Phillip retired. It is needless to say that Phillip is sorely missed not only as a teacher and friend, but also as somebody that for so many years devoted countless hours to something that can only be described as a labour of love. Thankfully we remain close friends and in communication. However, the void that he has left is difficult if not impossible to fill. I am eternally grateful to him for putting his trust in me and can only hope that I will not disappoint him.

Although for most of the 20th century, single author books were the norm and giants in the field of pathology and dermatology produced wonderful textbooks with little outside help, the amount of knowledge and information produced at an incredible rate in all fields make it impossible to perpetuate this trend and Phillip recognized this when the third edition was planned. Thomas Brenn and Alex Lazar continue to be associate editors of this textbook, as in the past, and their help has been as always invaluable, especially as the task is daunting when one has a full-time job to take care of. In this edition we have asked Steven Billings to join the team as a third co-editor and, although I never doubted the choice, he has surpassed expectations as somebody with incredible energy, knowledge and will to help in every possible way. Many of the previous contributors have been asked to contribute again and a few new ones have joined the effort with their knowledge and expertise. To all these contributors we are deeply indebted.

In the fourth edition we made the decision to provide the references online-only to allow us to expand the text and figures facilitating a more comprehensive textbook. Unfortunately, although following the same option this time, not much extra space is available and therefore the number of new images is limited. The editors, however, have been very generous in allowing extra text to keep up to date with new developments. They have also allowed us to include a new chapter entitled 'Animal Models of Skin Disease' by John P. Sundberg and colleagues which we believe is a valuable addition to the book.

A very esteemed and famous dermatopathologist has for many years started his lectures by predicting the demise of classical dermatopathology and its almost complete replacement by molecular techniques. In his view, it is a matter of a few years before this happens and light microscopy of sections stained with H&E will be a thing of the past or limited to places where newer techniques are not available. Although there is undoubtful truth in this, as clearly demonstrated in the fields of neoplasms and inherited diseases, it is also true that light microscopy remains the gold standard and that most of the diagnoses depend at least partially on the evaluation of sections stained in routine manner with the aid of special techniques. Our view is that all these techniques complement each other. Therefore, in the fifth edition we have tried to keep a balance between traditional diagnostic techniques and recent advances, particularly in the field of molecular diagnosis. It is difficult to keep up to date with the latest developments in the field as there has been an explosion of information as never before, particularly with regards to molecular mechanisms of disease. We have tried to reflect this in the book as accurate and as extensively as possible.

During the production of this book, I have been very lucky to work with two highly professional individuals that have gone out of their way to make my life easier. They are Louise Cook and Michael Houston. I had worked with both in the past and knew that every crisis no matter how big it seems, could be resolved with patience and resolution. For more than 2 years, I have had a weekly telephone conversation with Louise to sort out even the smallest problem. I will miss this. She has never let me down and I cannot thank her enough for her patience, her resilience and for just doing an amazing job.

This preface will not be complete if I did not acknowledge the person that has been unflinchingly there for me without asking for anything in return. My wife Claudia has given her love, her time, her patience and her understanding to help me complete this project. Having to share your marriage with a book is an unenviable task and she has done wonders.

EC
2018

List of contributors

The authors would like to acknowledge and offer grateful thanks for the input of all previous editions' contributors, without whom this new edition would not have been possible.

Josette André MD
Head of the Dermatology and Dermatopathology Department.
CHU Saint-Pierre - CHU Brugmann
Hôpital Universitaire des Enfants Reine Fabiola
Université Libre de Bruxelles
Brussels, Belgium

Boris C. Bastian MD, PhD
Professor of Dermatology and Pathology
University of California, San Francisco;
Gerson and Barbara Bass Baker Distinguished Professor in Cancer
    Research, UCSF
San Francisco, CA, USA

Marcus Bosenberg MD, PhD
Co-Leader of the Genomics, Genetics and Epigenetics Program
Yale Cancer Center;
Dermatopathologist, Departments of Dermatology and Pathology
Yale University School of Medicine
New Haven, CT, USA

Chris Bunker MA, MD, FRCP
Consultant Dermatologist
University College and Chelsea and Westminster Hospitals London;
Professor of Dermatology
University College London
London, UK

Alistair J. Cochran, MD
Distinguished Professor of Pathology and Laboratory
Medicine and Surgery
Department of Pathology and Laboratory Medicine
David Geffen School of Medicine at UCLA
Los Angeles, CA, USA

Antonio L. Cubilla MD
Instituto de Patología e Investigación
Asuncion, Paraguay

Vasileia Damaskou MD
Consultant Histopathologist
2nd Department of Pathological Anatomy
National and Kapodistrian University of Athens
School of Medicine,
Attikon University Hospital,
Athens, Greece

John Goodlad MD, FRCPath
Consultant Haematopathologist and Honorary
Senior Lecturer
Department of Pathology
Western General Hospital and University of Edinburgh,
    Edinburgh, UK

Wayne Grayson MBChB, PhD, FCPath(SA)
Consultant Anatomical Pathologist and Dermatopathologist
AMPATH National Laboratories;
Honorary Associate Professor
School of Pathology
University of the Witwatersrand, Johannesburg
Johannesburg, South Africa

Lloyd E. King Jr. MD, PhD
Professor of Medicine, Dermatology and Dermatopathology
Division of Dermatology, Department of Medicine
Vanderbilt University Medical Center
Nashville, TN, USA

Fiona Lewis MB ChB, MD, FRCP
Consultant Dermatologist
St John's Institute of Dermatology
Guy's and St Thomas' NHS Trust
London, UK

Qiaoli Li PhD
Department of Dermatology and Cutaneous Biology
Jefferson Institute of Molecular Medicine
Thomas Jefferson University
Philadelphia, PA, USA

Amy Y. Lin MD
Associate Professor of Pathology and Ophthalmology
University of Illinois College of Medicine
Chicago, IL, USA

Boštjan Luzar MD, PhD
Professor of Pathology
Consultant Pathologist
Institute of Pathology
Medical Faculty University of Ljubljana
Ljubljana, Slovenia

Diego Fernando Sánchez Martínez MD
Pathologist
Instituto de Patologia e Investigación
Asunción, Paraguay

John A. McGrath MD, FRCP, FMedSci
Mary Dunhill Chair in Cutaneous Medicine
St John's Institute of Dermatology
King's College London
Guy's Hospital
London, UK

Dieter Metze MD
Professor of Dermatology
Director, Dermatopathology Unit
Department of Dermatology
University Hospital Münster
Münster, Germany

Jeffrey P. North MD
Assistant Professor
Department of Dermatology
UCSF School of Medicine
San Francisco, CA, USA

Vinzenz Oji MD
Assistant Professor
Department of Dermatology
University Hospital Münster
Münster, Germany

C. Herbert Pratt PhD
Scientific Program Manager
Department of Research and Development
The Jackson Laboratory
Bar Harbor, ME, USA

Pratistadevi K. Ramdial MBChB, FCPath(SA)
Professor and Head
Department of Anatomical Pathology
Nelson R. Mandela School of Medicine
University of Kwazulu-Natal and the National Health
Laboratory Service
Durban, South Africa

Rodrigo Restrepo MD
Director, Dermatopathology Fellowship Program
Universidad CES
Professor of Dermatopathology
Universidad Pontificia Bolivariana
Director, Laboratory of Pathology
Clinica Medellin
Medellin, Colombia

Ursula Sass MD
Assistant Professor
Dermatology and Dermatopathology Department
CHU Saint-Pierre
Université Libre de Bruxelles
Brussels, Belgium

John P. Sundberg DVM, PhD
Principal Investigator
Research and Development Department
The Jackson Laboratory
Bar Harbor, ME, USA

Anne Theunis MD
Assistant Professor
Dermatopathology and Pathology Department
CHU Saint-Pierre and Institut Bordet
Université Libre de Bruxelles
Brussels, Belgium

Jouni Uitto MD, PhD
Professor of Dermatology and Cutaneous Biology, and Biochemistry
    and Molecular Biology;
Chair, Department of Dermatology and Cutaneous Biology
Jefferson Institute of Molecular Medicine
Thomas Jefferson University
Philadelphia, PA, USA

Steve L. Walker PhD, MRCP (UK), DTM&H
Consultant Dermatologist and Associate Professor
Department of Clinical Research
London School of Hygiene and Tropical Medicine
London, UK

Michael V. Wiles PhD
Senior Director
Department of Technology Evaluation and Development
The Jackson Laboratory
Bar Harbor, ME, USA

Sook-Bin Woo DMD, MMSc
Associate Professor
Department of Oral Medicine, Infection and Immunity
Harvard School of Dental Medicine, Boston, MA, USA
Attending Dentist and Consultant Pathologist
Brigham and Women's Hospital
Boston, MA, USA
Co-Director
Center for Oral Pathology Strata Pathology Services Inc.,
Lexington, MA, USA

Acknowledgments

All the editorial team, including Louise Cook, Michael Houston, Thomas Brenn, Alex Lazar and Steven Billings have been invaluable in helping to carry this work to fruition and I am forever grateful for their efforts and hard work. My wife Claudia has never deserted me and has endured so much for the sake of my well-being that my admiration and love for her knows no boundaries. My children Matteo and Isabella have always supported me through thick and thin and I am indebted to them for this. Many people including colleagues and friends have made my life easier during these years and have helped in any way they can in order for me to complete this work. Many especially visiting fellows have had to endure lots and they have been always there for me not only with words of support but also with their help. I especially want to thank Drs Adriana Garcia Herrera, Eduardo Rozas, Fiona Lewis, Zlatko Marusic, Chao-Kai Hsu, Giri Raj, Tawatchai Suttikoon, László Fónyad, Erica Ahn, Agnes Pekar-Lukacs and Yi-Gou Feng. I am also forever grateful to my friends Celmira Manzano and Patricia Otero.

EC

The path of life is determined by the people we meet. There are many ways in which certain individuals touch our hearts, steer us in the right direction and help us achieve goals which would have been unattainable otherwise. Words aren't ever enough to really show one's true appreciation for the generosity, support and motivation received over the years.

My wonderful, loving parents, Sonja and Walter, have always been there for me and supported my every move. My professional life could have gone very wrong indeed had it not been for the kindness and gracious support from these truly unique mentors and teachers Uta Francke, Heinz Furthmayr, Ramzi Cotran and Christopher Fletcher. There is so much I owe to these two wonderful individuals who have become very close friends, Phillip McKee and Eduardo Calonje. Tinka, Yäelle and Pippa, thank you for all the color and joy you bring to my life and for keeping me humble and (relatively) sane.

TB

Our decidedly cynical postmodern outlook gives short shrift and virtually no quarter to being earnest and sincere in demeanor. Nonetheless, I find I that I am truly and greatly honored to have worked with my exceedingly talented three co-editors and the distinguished cast of chapter authors who stayed this long strange journey with us. Numerous gracious individuals have and continue to inspire and influence me and help me to find my way in life from mentors to colleagues and friends to fellows and students of various sorts and types. I am loath to attempt to name this entire cast of characters lest I neglect to list anyone in particular. Suffice it to say, you know who you are and my many glaring faults are indeed my own and exist despite what you have all tried so hard to do for me! To the many fellows and students who have endured learning with me over the years, please know that you definitely taught me at least as much if not more than I ever managed to impart to you. Your quite reasonable demands for clear, concise and reproducible diagnostic criteria and intellectual curiosity spur me to be my very best and have ignited a numerous studies and publications over the years. Truly, whatever success I have achieved is the product of intense exposure to the generosity of so many wonderfully talented and stimulating people.

AJL

I was surprised, humbled and deeply honored to be included as an editor on the book I use every day in practice. I am very grateful to Eduardo, Alex, and Thomas for including me and to Phillip McKee for his incredible contributions that are still present throughout this book. I would never have had this opportunity without the help and support of many people in my life. Notably, my parents for their support of my somewhat wandering path and my wife and daughter, Beth and Maeve, for their unending patience during the many hours spent on this book. I can never thank you enough. I am also deeply indebted to a number of mentors who have influenced me throughout my career, including Lawrence Roth, Thomas Ulbright, Thomas Davis, John Eble, Jenny Cotton, Sharon Weiss, and Andrew Folpe. I especially thank Antoinette Hood and the late William "Joe" Moores for teaching me dermatopathology. The influence of their wisdom is felt every day. Finally, I would like to thank my colleagues, residents and fellows who always teach me so much and inspire me.

SB

Dedication

To my wife Claudia, the light of my life and a person that I greatly admire in every respect.

To my children Matteo and Isabella.

EC

To Filippa.

TB

To my exceedingly patient and supportive family, Victoria, Elliott, Abigail and Sara.

AJL

To Beth, Maeve, Richard, Sally, Diane and Richard.

SB

Glossary of abbreviations

5-ARD	5-a-reductase		DIMF	direct immunofluorescence
AA	alopecia areata		DLE	discoid lupus erythematosus
ACE	angiotensin converting enzyme [inhibitor]		DNCB	dinitrochlorobenzene
AgNORS	argyrophilic nucleolar organizer regions		DSAP	disseminated superficial actinic porokeratosis
AHNMD	associated clonal hematological non-mast cell lineage disease		Dsc	desmocollin
AIDS	acquired immunodeficiency syndrome		dsDNA	double-stranded DNA
AILD	angioimmunoblastic lymphadenopathy with dysproteinemia		Dsg	desmoglein
ALA	aminolevulinic acid		DSP	disseminated superficial porokeratosis
ALK	anaplastic lymphoma kinase		EB	epidermolysis bullosa
ALK1	activin-like receptor kinase 1		EBA	epidermolysis bullosa acquisita
ALM	acral lentiginous melanoma		EBS	epidermolysis bullosa simplex
AN	acanthosis nigricans		EBS-DM	epidermolysis bullosa simplex, Dowling–Meara
ANA	antinuclear antibodies		EBS-K	epidermolysis bullosa simplex, Koebner
ANCA	antineutrophil cytoplasmic antibodies		EBS-MD	epidermolysis bullosa simplex with muscular dystrophy
API2	apoptosis inhibitor-2		EBS-WC	epidermolysis bullosa simplex, Weber–Cockayne
ARC	AIDS-related complex		EBV	Epstein–Barr virus
ATF1	activating transcription factor 1		ECE	endothelin-converting enzyme
ATLL	adult T-cell leukemia/lymphoma		ECM	extracellular membrane
BANS	back, arm, neck and scalp [sites]		EDS	Ehlers–Danlos syndrome
BB	mid borderline leprosy		EGFR	endothelial growth factor receptor
BCC	basal cell carcinoma		ELAM	endothelial leukocyte adhesion molecule
BCG	bacille Calmette–Guérin		ELISA	enzyme-linked immunosorbent assay
B-FGF	basic fibroblast growth factor		EM	electron microscopy
BIDS	brittle sulfur-deficient hair, intellectual impairment, decreased fertility and short stature		EMA	epithelial membrane antigen
			ENA	extractable nuclear antigen
BL	borderline lepromatous leprosy		ENL	erythema nodosum leprosum
BLAISE	Blaschko linear acquired inflammatory skin eruption		EPPER	eosinophilic, polymorphic and pruritic eruption associated with radiotherapy
BMP	bone morphogenetic protein			
BP	bullous pemphigoid		EPPK	epidermolytic palmoplantar keratoderma
BPA	bullous pemphigoid antigen		EPS	extracellular polysaccharide substance
BSAP	B-cell-specific activator protein		ESR	erythrocyte sedimentation rate
BSLE	bullous systemic lupus erythematosus		ETA	exfoliative toxin A
BT	borderline tuberculoid leprosy		ETB	exfoliative toxin B
C3NeF	C3 nephritic factor		EV	epidermodysplasia verruciformis
CAD	chronic actinic dermatitis		EWSR1	Ewing's sarcoma [proto-oncogene]
cAMP	cyclic adenosine 3'-5'- monophosphate		FACE	facial Afro-Caribbean childhood eruption
c-ANCA	cytoplasmic-antineutrophil cytoplasmic antibodies		FADS	fetal akinesia deformation sequence
CDC	Centers for Disease Control and Prevention		FAMMM	familial atypical multiple mole melanoma [syndrome]
CEA	carcinoembryonic antigen		FAP	familial adenomatous polyposis
CGRP	calcitonin-gene-related polypeptide		FAPA	fever, aphthous stomatitis, pharyngitis, adenitis [syndrome]
CHILD	congenital hemidysplasia with ichthyosiform nevus and limb defects [syndrome]		FHIT	fragile histidine triad
			FIGURE	facial idiopathic granulomata with regressive evolution
CK	cytokeratin		FISH	fluorescent in situ hybridization
CLA	cutaneous lymphocyte antigen		GA	granuloma annulare
CLL	chronic lymphocytic leukemia		GABEB	generalized atrophic benign epidermolysis bullosa
CMG	capillary morphogenesis protein		GCDFP	gross cystic disease fluid protein
CNS	central nervous system		G-CSF	granulocyte-colony stimulating factor
CP	cicatricial pemphigoid (mucous membrane pemphigoid)		GFAP	glial fibrillary acidic protein
CRASP	complement regulator-acquiring surface protein		GM-CSF	granulocyte–macrophage colony stimulating factor
CREST	calcinosis, Raynaud's phenomenon, esophageal dysfunction, sclerodactyly, telangiectasis [syndrome]		GSE	gluten-sensitive enteropathy
			GVHD	graft-versus-host disease
CTCL	cutaneous T-cell lymphoma		HA	hyperandrogenism
dcSSc	diffuse cutaneous systemic sclerosis		HAART	highly active antiretroviral therapy
DDEB	dominant dystrophic epidermolysis bullosa		HAIR-AN	hyperandrogenism–insulin resistance–acanthosis nigricans [syndrome]
DEB	dystrophic epidermolysis bullosa			
DH	dermatitis herpetiformis		HBV	hepatitis B virus
DIC	disseminated intravascular coagulation		HDL	high density lipoprotein

HF	hemorrhagic fever
HG	herpes gestationis
HHV	human herpesvirus
HIT	heparin-induced thrombocytopenia [syndrome]
HIV	human immunodeficiency virus
HLA	human leukocyte antigen
HMFG	human milk fat globulin
HNPCC	hereditary non-polyposis colorectal carcinoma [syndrome]
HPF (hpf)	high power fields
HPL	hyperlipoproteinemia
HPV	human papillomavirus
HRF	histamine-releasing factor
HSP	heat shock protein
HSV	herpes simplex virus
HTLV	human T-cell lymphotropic virus
hTR	telomerase RNA
HUS	hemolytic uremic syndrome
IBIDS	ichthyosis and BIDS (see BIDS above)
ICAM	intercellular adhesion molecule
ICH	indeterminate cell histiocytosis
IDL	intermediate density lipoproteins
IEN	intraepidermal neutrophilic [IgA dermatosis variant]
IFAP	ichthyosis follicularis–alopecia–photophobia [syndrome]; intermediate filament associated protein
IFN	interferon
Ig	immunoglobulin
IIMF	indirect immunofluorescence
ILVEN	inflammatory linear verrucous epidermal nevus
IMF	immunofluorescence
IP	inducible protein; immunoprecipitation
IR	insulin resistance
ISSVD	International Society for the Study of Vulvovaginal Disease
JEB	junctional epidermolysis bullosa
JEB-H	junctional epidermolysis bullosa, Herlitz
JEB-nH	junctional epidermolysis bullosa, non-Herlitz
JEB-PA	junctional epidermolysis bullosa with pyloric atresia
KID	keratitis–ichthyosis–deafness [syndrome]
KOH	potassium hydroxide
KPAF	keratosis pilaris atrophicans faciei
L& H cells	lymphocytic and/or histiocytic Reed–Sternberg cell variants
LAD	linear IgA disease
LATS	long-acting thyroid stimulator
LCA	leukocyte common antigen
LCH	Langerhans' cell histiocytosis
lcSSc	limited cutaneous systemic sclerosis
LDL	low density lipoprotein
LE	lupus erythematosus
LFA	lymphocyte function-associated antigen
LH–RH	luteinizing hormone–releasing hormone
LL	lamina lucida; lepromatous leprosy
LP	lichen planus
LPP	lichen planus pemphigoides
LS	lichen sclerosus
LYVE	lymphatic vessel endothelial [hyaluronan receptor]
MAC	membrane attack complex
MAI	M. avium intracellulare
MALT	mucosa-associated lymphoid tissue
MART-1	melanoma antigen recognized by T-cells 1
MBP	myelin basic protein
MC1R	melanocortin-1 receptor
MCGN	mesangiocapillary glomerulonephritis
MCP	molecule chemoattractant protein
M-CSF	macrophage colony stimulating factor
MCTD	mixed connective tissue disease
MDR	multidrug resistance gene
Mel-CAM	melanoma cell adhesion molecule
MEN	multiple endocrine neoplasia [syndrome]

MFH	malignant fibrous histiocytoma
MGS/GRO	melanoma growth stimulatory activity
MHC	major histocompatibility complex
miH	minor histocompatibility complex
MITF	microphthalmia transcription factor
MMP	matrix metalloproteinase
MMR	mismatch repair
MSA	muscle-specific actin
MSI	microsatellite instability
NADH	nicotine adenine dinucleotide, reduced
nDNA	native [double-stranded] DNA
NEMO	nuclear factor [NF]-kappaB gene modulator
NF	necrotizing fasciitis
NFI	neurofibromatosis type I
NFII	neurofibromatosis type II
NFP	neurofilament protein
NIH	National Institutes of Health
NISH	non-isotopic in situ hybridization
NK	natural killer
NL	necrobiosis lipoidica
NRAMP1	natural resistance-associated macrophage protein 1
NSAIDs	non-steroidal anti-inflammatory drugs
NSE	neuron-specific enolase
OL-EDA- ID	osteopetrosis, lymphedema, anhidrotic ectodermal dysplasia, immunodeficiency [syndrome]
ORF	open reading frame
PAIN	perianal intraepithelial neoplasia
p-ANCA	perinuclear-antineutrophil cytoplasmic antibodies
PAPA	pyogenic sterile arthritis, pyoderma gangrenosum and acne [syndrome]
PAS	periodic acid–Schiff
PBG	porphobilinogen
PCNA	proliferating cell nuclear antigen
PCR	polymerase chain reaction
PDGFβ	platelet-derived growth factor β
PECAM	platelet endothelial cell adhesion molecule
PEComa	perivascular epithelioid cell tumor
PGL	phenolic glycolipid
PGP	protein gene product
PGWG	purely granulomatous
PI	protease inhibitor
PIBIDS	photosensitivity and IBIDS (see IBIDS above)
PILA	papillary intralymphatic angioendothelioma
PLEVA	pityriasis lichenoides et varioliformis acuta
PNET	primitive neuroectodermal tumor
POEMS	polyneuropathy, organomegaly, endocrinopathy, M-protein and skin changes [syndrome]
PPD	purified protein derivative
PPDL	pure and primitive diffuse leprosy
PPK	palmoplantar keratoderma
pRB	retinoblastoma protein
PSS	progressive systemic sclerosis
PTEN	phosphatase and tensin homolog
PUPPP	pruritic urticarial papules and plaques of pregnancy
PUVA	psoralen plus ultraviolet light of A [long] wavelength
r IL-2	recombinant interleukin 2
RBC	red blood cell
RDEB	recessive dystrophic epidermolysis bullosa
RDEB-HS	recessive dystrophic epidermolysis bullosa, Hallopeau–Siemens
RDEB- nHS	recessive dystrophic epidermolysis bullosa, non-Hallopeau–Siemens
RER	rough endoplasmic reticulum
RNP	ribonucleoprotein
RT-PCR	reverse transcription polymerase chain reaction

SA	syphilitic alopecia
SA1	slowly adapting type-1 [mechanoreceptor]
SALE	summertime actinic lichenoid eruption
SALT	skin-associated lymphoid tissue
SAPHO	synovitis, acne, pustulosis, hyperostosis, osteitis [syndrome]
SCC	squamous cell carcinoma
SCH	squamous cell hyperplasia
SCID	severe combined immunodeficiency
SCLE	subacute cutaneous lupus erythematosus
scRNP	small cytoplasmic ribonuclear protein
SEA	staphylococcal enterotoxin A
SEB	staphylococcal enterotoxin B
Shh	Sonic Hedgehog
SIBIDS	osteosclerosis and IBIDS (see IBIDS above)
SIL	squamous intraepithelial lesion
SLE	systemic lupus erythematosus
SLL	small lymphocytic lymphoma
SMA	smooth muscle actin
snRNP	small nuclear ribonuclear protein
SPD	subcorneal pustular dermatosis
SPRRs	small proline rich proteins/cornifins
SPTL	subcutaneous panniculitis-like T-cell lymphoma
SRP	signal recognition particle
ssDNA	single-stranded DNA
SSSS	staphylococcal scalded skin syndrome
STD	sexually transmitted disease
sub-LD	sub-lamina densa
TCR	T-cell receptor
TEN	toxic epidermal necrolysis
TFIIH	transcription/DNA repair factor IIH
TGF	transforming growth factor
thio-TEPA	triethylene thiophosphoramide
TIMP	tissue inhibitor of metalloproteinase
TNF	tumor necrosis factor
TORCH	toxoplasmosis, other infections, rubella, cytomegalovirus and herpes simplex [syndrome]
TRAPS	tumor necrosis factor receptor-associated periodic syndrome
TSST	toxic shock syndrome toxin
TT	tuberculoid leprosy
tTA	tetracycline transactivator [transcription factor]
TTF-1	thyroid-transcription factor 1
tTG	tissue transglutaminase
TTP	thrombotic thrombocytopenic purpura
UPS	undifferentiated pleomorphic sarcoma
URO	uroporphyrinogen
URO-D	uroporphyrinogen decarboxylase
URR	upstream regulatory region
UV	ultraviolet
UVA	ultraviolet A
UVB	ultraviolet B
UVL	ultraviolet light
VCAM	vascular cell adhesion molecule
VEGF	vascular endothelial growth factor
VEGFR	vascular endothelial growth factor receptor
VIN	vulval intraepithelial neoplasia
VIP	vasoactive intestinal peptide
VLDL	very low density lipoprotein
VZV	varicella-zoster virus
wrfr	wrinkle free [mouse model]
XP	xeroderma pigmentosum

McKEE'S

Pathology of the Skin

Human immunodeficiency virus (HIV) and acquired immunodeficiency syndrome (AIDS)-associated cutaneous diseases

Stephen L. Walker and Wayne Grayson

See
www.expertconsult.com
for references and
additional material

Introduction

UNAIDS estimates that globally 36.7 million people, including 2.1 million children, were living with human immunodeficiency virus (HIV) infection in 2016.[1] The number of people who acquired HIV infection in 2016 was 1.8 million. Since the start of the epidemic, 35 million people have died of acquired immune deficiency syndrome (AIDS)-related illnesses. Tuberculosis is still the leading cause of death in people living with HIV; however, deaths due to AIDS have fallen by 48% since their peak in 2005. Access to antiretroviral therapy (ART) is increasing, and an estimated 19.5 million people with HIV infection were receiving ART in 2016.[1]

HIV is an enveloped RNA virus belonging to the genus *Lentivirus* within the family *Retroviridae*. The disease-causing viruses are HIV-1 and HIV-2, which result in a decline in CD4 T lymphocytes.[2] HIV-2 is detected mainly in West Africa. Both HIV types cause a similar clinical disease profile. HIV-2, however, is associated with a reduced rate of transmissibility, more gradual decline in CD4 T lymphocytes, and clinical progression.[2] HIV enters cells via CD4 and the chemokine co-receptors CCR5 and CXCR4.[2] The lack of natural eliminatory mechanisms of HIV following primary infection and continued viral replication throughout the course of the disease are pivotal to the initiation, establishment, and propagation of HIV infection.

In a Danish population-based study, adults with both skin infections and 'skin diseases' were significantly more likely to be diagnosed with HIV infection in the subsequent 5 years compared to individuals without.[3] More than 90% of HIV-infected individuals will develop one or more dermatological disorders during the course of their illness, either as a result of AIDS or due to the effects of treatment.[4,5] Furthermore, cutaneous disease is often the first manifestation of undiagnosed HIV infection or AIDS.

Late diagnosis is significantly related to HIV associated morbidity and mortality in the UK. The British HIV Association and the US Centers for Disease Control and Prevention (CDC) recommend offering and encouraging patients to have an HIV test in a wide variety of clinical settings.[6,7]

A wide variety of skin diseases may arise in concert with or be modified by the progressively declining CD4 lymphocyte count. HIV infection should always be suspected when the clinical history reveals that a common skin disorder has presented with atypical clinical features, followed an abnormal clinical course, displayed greater clinical severity than anticipated, or failed to exhibit a satisfactory clinical response to standard therapy for that particular condition. The spectrum of cutaneous HIV disease includes AIDS-defining opportunistic infections and neoplasms (summarized at the end of the chapter and discussed in depth elsewhere in the book), drug-induced cutaneous manifestations, and a range of noninfectious dermatoses that may occur in all stages of HIV progression. This latter group comprises dermatoses peculiar to HIV infection (e.g., acute HIV exanthem, pruritic papular eruption), those occurring with greater frequency or modified by HIV/AIDS (e.g., seborrheic dermatitis, psoriasis), and a variety of less common conditions in which an association with HIV infection has been reported (e.g., cutaneous manifestations of reactive arthritis, pityriasis rubra pilaris). HIV-positive patients may present with more than one skin disorder, a fact of which the practicing histopathologist should always remain cognizant when examining skin biopsies in this clinical context.[8]

In resource-limited settings, malnutrition is commonly associated with HIV infection and is difficult to manage.[9] Noma (cancrum oris) has been reported in HIV-infected children and adults in Africa[10] and beyond.[11]

Immune reconstitution inflammatory syndrome (IRIS) may present with cutaneous manifestations of infections or inflammatory dermatoses.[12]

This chapter focuses on the acute exanthema of HIV, papulosquamous, photosensitivity, pruritic papular, vasculitic, and autoimmune bullous dermatoses that may be associated with HIV infection.

Acute HIV exanthem

Clinical features

Symptomatic primary or acute HIV infection, which occurs in more than 95% of HIV-infected patients,[1] is often heralded by a mononucleosis-like illness with fever, lymphadenopathy, sore throat, myalgia, arthralgia, malaise, and an exanthem.[1,2] The rash is of varied morphology and occurs in approximately 60% of patients.[1,2] It may be a macular exanthem with roseola-like features, or maculopapular with hemorrhagic and necrotic lesions (*Fig. 19.1*). There is a painful erosive enanthem in 25% of cases.[2] There may be vesicles, urticaria, alopecia, genital ulceration, and

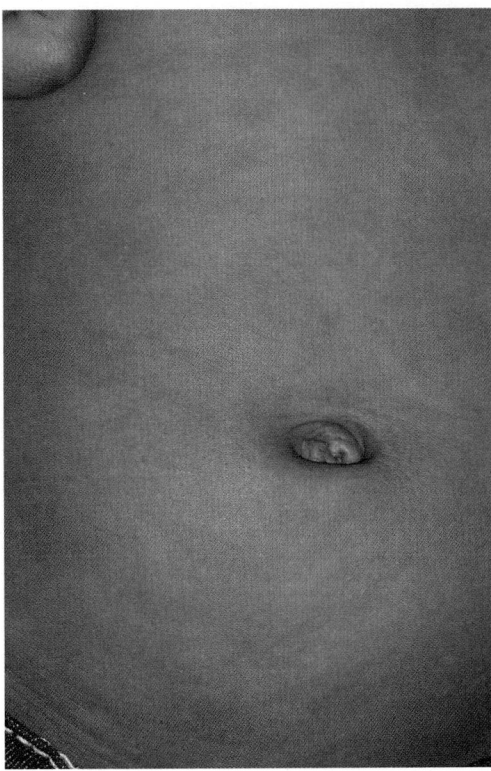

Fig. 19.1
Acute HIV exanthem: erythematous, edematous macules are present.

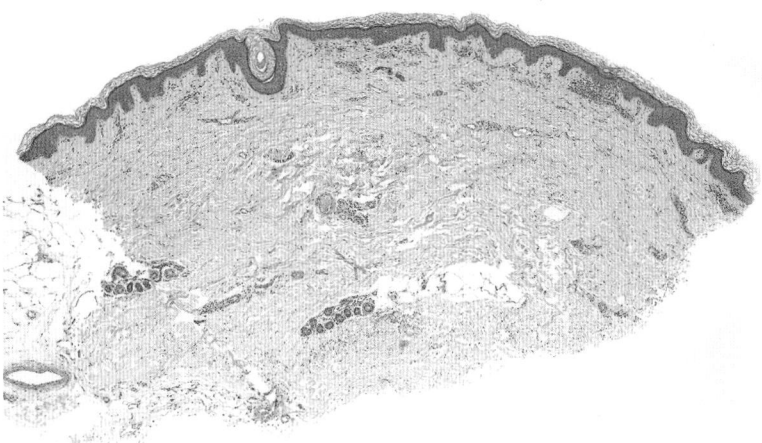

Fig. 19.2
Acute HIV exanthem: early lesion showing a superficial perivascular lymphocytic infiltrate.

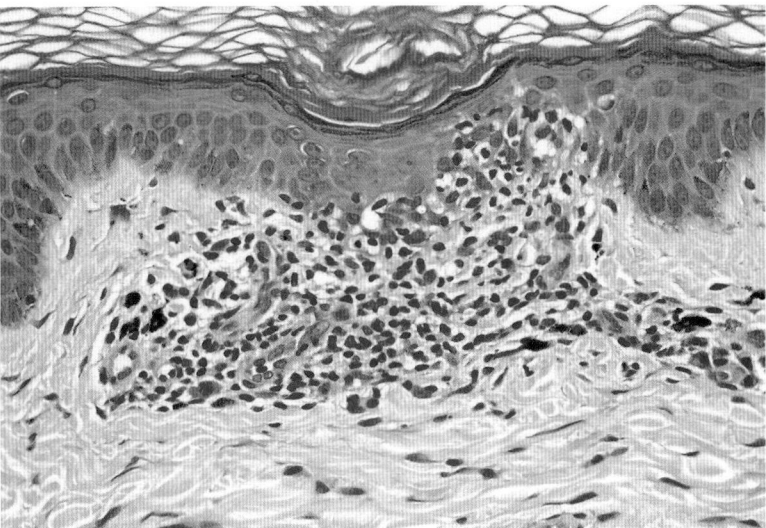

Fig. 19.3
Acute HIV exanthem: there is a tiny focus of lymphocytic exocytosis.

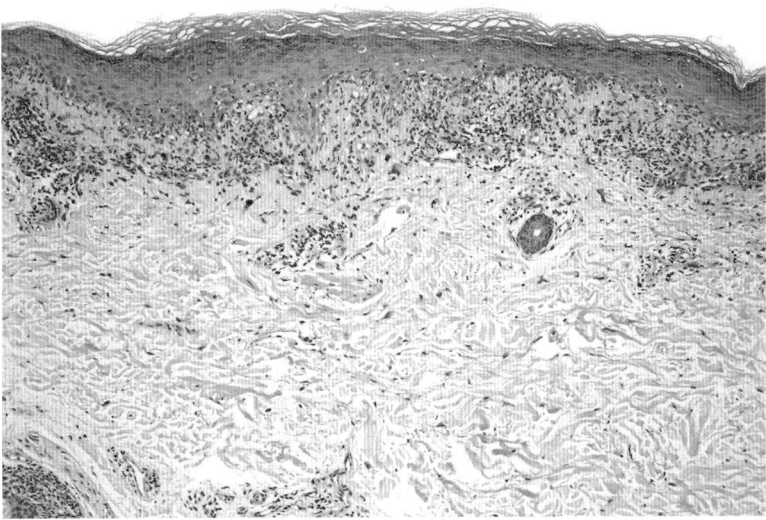

Fig. 19.4
Acute HIV exanthem: established lesion showing hyperkeratosis, irregular acanthosis, and interface change associated with an upper dermal bandlike infiltrate.

Stevens-Johnson syndrome.[3] The mean duration of symptoms is 10 days and resolves spontaneously.[1] The triad of a maculopapular rash with oral and genital ulcers should raise suspicion of acute HIV infection.

Pathogenesis and histologic features

CD1a intraepidermal Langerhans cells are significantly decreased. Individual Langerhans cells that express HIV-p24 antigen are seen in close apposition to cytotoxic T cells. Dendritic cells are the putative virus reservoir, and the skin is a major site of HIV replication during the course of the disease.

The histopathologic alterations are not specific. Early macular and papular lesions of HIV exanthem demonstrate dermal inflammatory changes without epidermal alterations (Figs 19.2 and 19.3).[4,5] With progression, there is confluent epidermal parakeratosis, as well as isolated and aggregated keratinocyte necrosis with associated satellite lymphocytes (Fig. 19.4). Basal layer vacuolar change, keratinocyte ballooning degeneration, exocytosis,

upper dermal colloid bodies, and pigmentary incontinence are variably present (Fig. 19.5).[4] A perivascular, periadnexal, and interstitial lympho-histiocytic inflammatory infiltrate, with a predominance of CD4-positive T lymphocytes, is present in the papillary and upper and mid-reticular dermis.[6] Similar changes may be seen in hair follicle epithelium. Advanced papular or papulovesicular lesions demonstrate spongiosis, intraepidermal vesicles, or ballooning degeneration.[4]

The history of a seroconversion illness is critical as the spectrum of histologic changes encountered in chronic HIV interface dermatitis induced by drugs and lichenoid HIV photoeruptions may overlap with that of acute HIV exanthem.[3]

HIV-associated papulosquamous dermatoses

HIV-associated seborrheic dermatitis

Clinical features

Seborrheic dermatitis is the most common cutaneous disease to affect HIV-infected patients and often occurs early on in HIV infection or it may reflect disease progression. It is seen in up to 85% of all HIV-infected

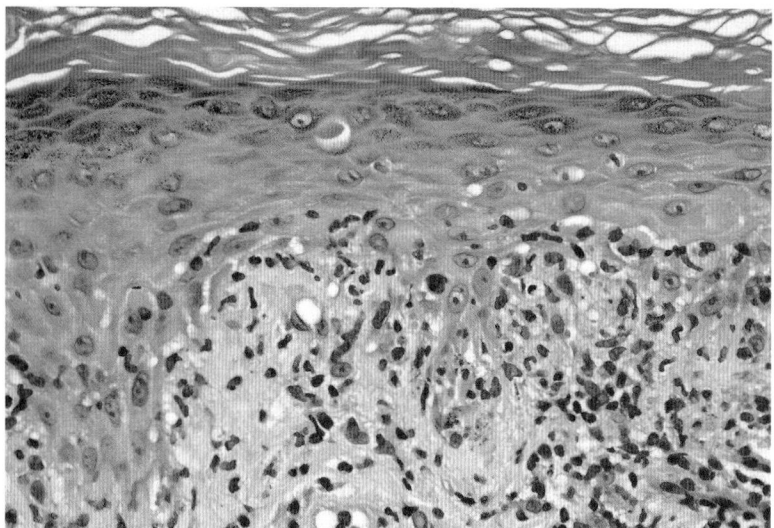

Fig. 19.5
Acute HIV exanthem: high-power view showing interface change and cytoid bodies with pigment incontinence.

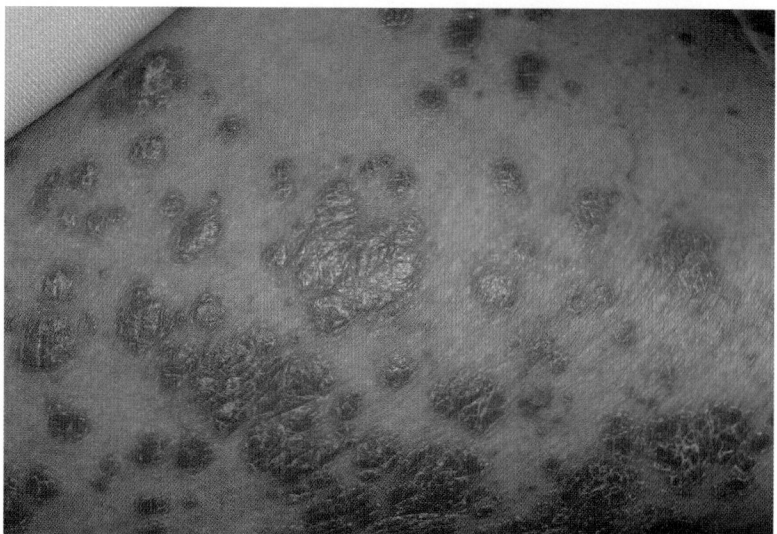

Fig. 19.6
HIV-associated psoriasis: there are numerous silver scaly plaques as seen in psoriasis vulgaris.

individuals at some stage during the course of their disease.[1,2] Although seborrheic dermatitis is characterized by erythema and greasy scaling of the nasolabial and postauricular areas, eyebrows, external ears, and scalp, as is seen in the general population, it can be more widespread, involving the chest, trunk, groin, and extremities with progression to erythroderma in those with HIV infection.[2,3] Other HIV-associated clues of seborrheic dermatitis include a predominance of inflammatory and hyperkeratotic lesions, papular and scaly plaquelike lesions resembling psoriasis, hypo- and hyperpigmentation, a 'cradle cap' appearance of the scalp, and a sudden onset or acute worsening of seborrheic dermatitis.[2]

Pathogenesis and histologic features

The exact pathogenesis of HIV-associated seborrheic dermatitis is not known. A relationship with AIDS-associated dementia and central nervous system disease has nevertheless been documented in 20% of AIDS patients and in HIV-negative patients with neurological diseases.[1] HIV-1 possesses neurotropic characteristics. It has therefore been proposed that the same mechanism promoting seborrheic dermatitis in neurological diseases occurs in HIV.[1] Seborrheic dermatitis is sometimes associated with *Malassezia furfur* infection, but the exact role has not been clarified.[4,5]

The histologic features include those seen in seborrheic dermatitis in HIV-negative patients, including hyperkeratosis, parakeratotic mounds localized particularly to the ostia of hair follicle infundibula, acanthosis with regular elongation of the rete ridges, and mild spongiosis with intraepidermal lymphocytes and neutrophils.[1,6] Features specific for AIDS-related seborrheic dermatitis include spotty keratinocyte necrosis, hyperkeratosis, leukocytic exocytosis, a perivascular plasma cell infiltrate in the dermis, and focal leukocytoclasis.[1]

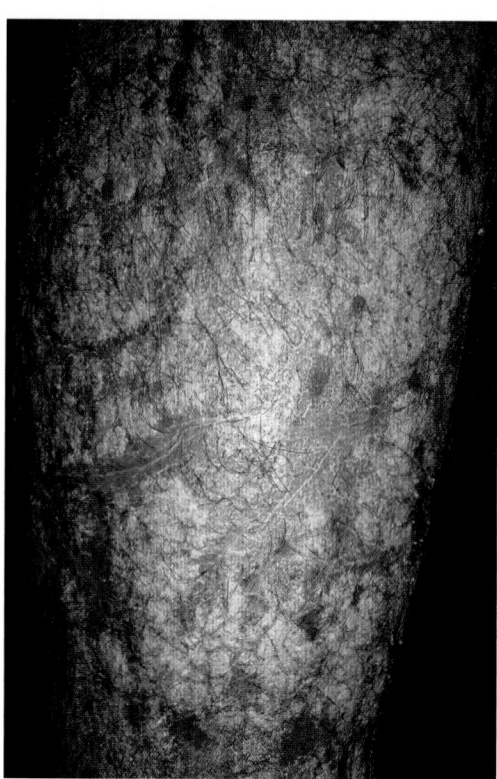

Fig. 19.7
HIV-associated psoriasis: in this patient, the lesions are much more extensive.

HIV-associated psoriasis

Clinical features

The overall incidence of HIV-associated psoriasis does not appear to exceed that of the general population.[1] Occurring in 1% to 3% of HIV-infected individuals, the spectrum of clinical manifestations may be similar to psoriasis in the non-HIV-exposed group. Psoriasis may be the first clue to HIV infection and may undergo remission with advanced disease.[1] Although all degrees of severity of psoriasis may occur at any stage of HIV infection, there may be deterioration with worsening immunosuppression. Pre-existing psoriasis may undergo severe exacerbation with HIV infection (*Figs 19.6* and *19.7*). Patients may present with classic signs of psoriasis, rupioid lesions, sebopsoriasis, erythrodermic psoriasis, or a combination of lesions of various morphologies.[1]

Pathogenesis and histologic features

The pathogenesis of HIV-induced psoriasis is complex. Psoriasis is considered to be a T-helper-1 dominant disease. The milieu of cytokines includes interleukin-17 produced by CD4+ T lymphocytes, which seems incongruous in the context of psoriasis in HIV.[2] Immune dysregulation is postulated to play a pivotal role in HIV-associated psoriasis. HLA-Cw6 is the most frequently described genetic factor in association with psoriasis. A significantly higher proportion of patients with HIV-associated psoriasis carry the HLA-Cw*0602 allele.[3] It has been suggested that immune dysregulation may activate microorganisms to trigger psoriasis in predisposed patients carrying the Cw*0602 allele. This allele is postulated to be a putative target for CD8+ T lymphocytes responding to processed peptides from microorganisms, via molecular mimicry. A study showed a significant association

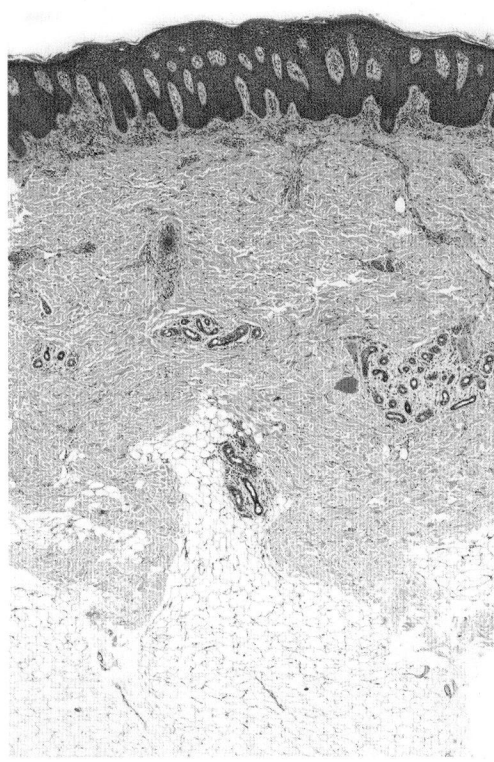

Fig. 19.8
HIV-associated psoriasis: low-power view showing parakeratosis. Psoriasiform hyperplasia with fused club-shaped rete ridges and an upper dermal perivascular inflammatory cell infiltrate.

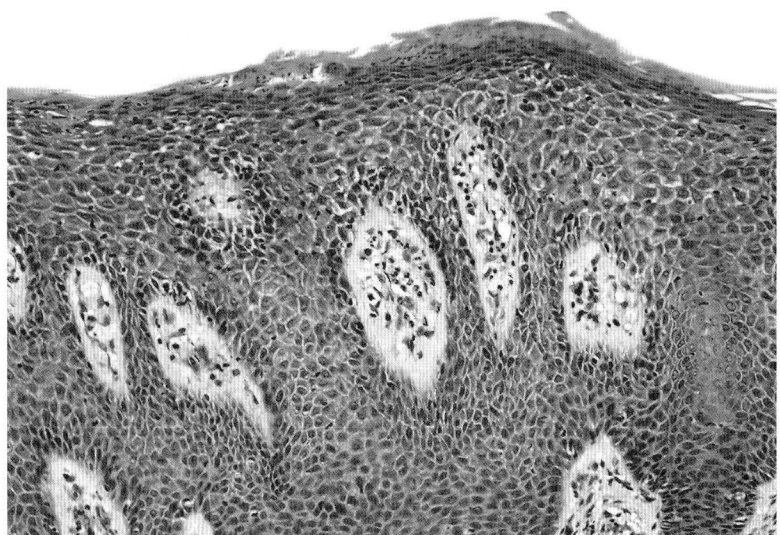

Fig. 19.9
HIV-associated psoriasis: a neutrophil Munro microabscess is present. There is mild spongiosis of the underlying dermis and vascular dilatation.

between a CD4 count of <200 × 10[6]/L and the evolution of psoriasis in HIV-positive patients.[4]

The histologic spectrum of HIV-associated psoriasis is similar to that of psoriasis vulgaris, but the dermal infiltrate contains fewer T lymphocytes and significantly more plasma cells (*Figs 19.8–19.10*).[1]

HIV-associated pityriasis rubra pilaris

Clinical features

HIV-associated pityriasis rubra pilaris (PRP), also referred to as pityriasis rubra pilaris type VI (PRP-VI), is characterized by cutaneous lesions of PRP,

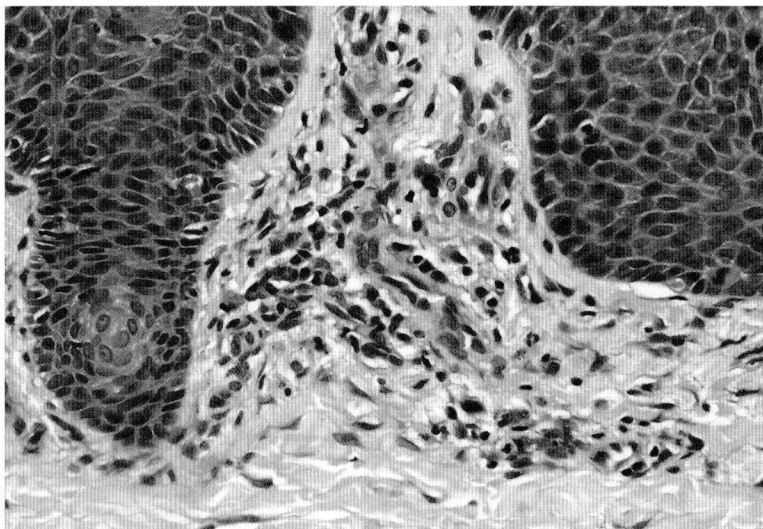

Fig. 19.10
HIV-associated psoriasis: the dermal infiltrate consists of lymphocytes and one or two plasma cells.

and variable association with acne conglobata, hidradenitis suppurativa, and lichen spinulosus.[1] Although PRP-VI is a disease usually encountered in young adults, children may be afflicted.[2] It occurs predominantly in males and may be the sentinel of HIV infection. Clinically, PRP-VI is characterized by pruritic, symmetrical, erythematous, desquamative follicular papules that tend to become confluent, frequently resulting in erythroderma. The eruption occurs mainly over the extensor surfaces. There is variable palm and sole keratoderma, scalp scaling, and nail hyperkeratosis.[1] The CD4 cell count is highly variable, ranging from values as low as 8 cells/mm[3] to > 1000 cells/mm[3]. Patients with higher CD4 counts (> 500 cells/mm[3]) may suffer fatal PRP complications. Improvement of PRP (and the associated hidradenitis suppurativa) following the institution of ART has been reported.[3,4]

Pathogenesis and histologic features

Although the association between HIV infection and PRP seems clear, the exact pathogenetic mechanisms involved are unknown. A direct role for HIV has been proposed because of the association with HIV and the response to ART.[5,6] Infection of the follicular hair bulge by HIV and secondary follicular inflammation have been suggested, as has precipitation of PRP in genetically predisposed individuals.[6] The coexistence of PRP, acne conglobata, and follicular plugging was a rare occurrence prior to HIV. The overlapping histologic features have heralded the possibility that the spectrum of clinicopathological features may be due to a single disorder of follicular keratinization. PRP-VI may therefore be part of a unique and distinctive disease, more appropriately placed under the wider rubric of HIV-associated follicular syndrome.[3,6–8]

Histologically, there is variable epidermal psoriasiform hyperplasia and lamellar hyperkeratosis, with alternating zones of vertical and horizontal parakeratosis and an intact granular cell layer (*Figs 19.11* and *19.12*). There is follicular hyperkeratosis and variable infundibular dilation with orthokeratotic and hyperkeratotic keratin.[9] A sparse mononuclear infiltrate is present around the superficial vascular plexus and hair follicles. Perifollicular mucinosis may be present.[10]

Xerosis

Clinical features

Xerosis is common in HIV infection, occurring at any time throughout disease progression but significantly associated with lower CD4 counts and the ART drug indinavir.[1,2] Xerosis is often pruritic but less so than other HIV associated dermatoses.[3] Xerotic dermatitis was reported by 42.1% of men and 51.5% of women infected with HIV in the FRAM study.[2] It is characterized by diffuse dryness of the skin with hyperpigmented scales and

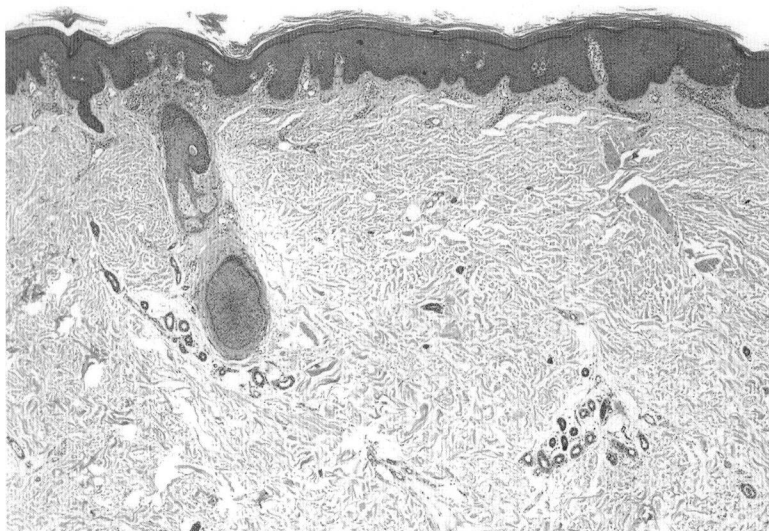

Fig. 19.11
HIV-associated pityriasis rubra pilaris: low-power view showing a thickened stratum corneum and psoriasiform hyperplasia.

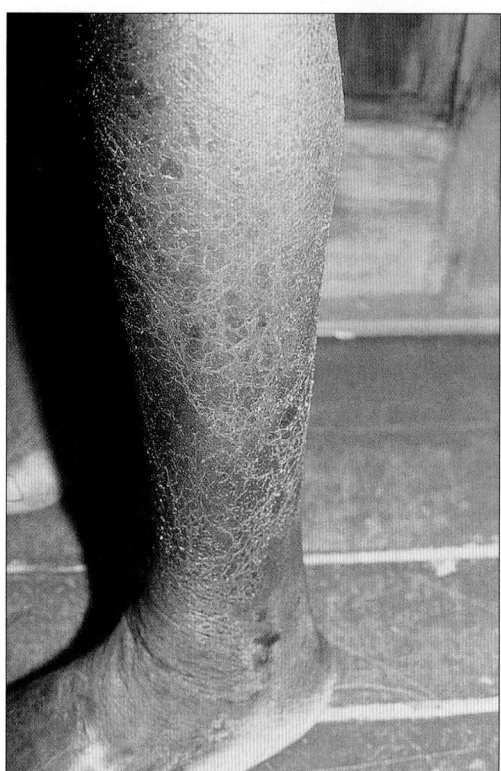

Fig. 19.13
HIV-associated xerosis: marked scaling has resulted in an eczema craquelé-like appearance. Dry skin is a common complaint in patients with HIV infection. By courtesy of C. Furlonge, MD, Port of Spain, Trinidad.

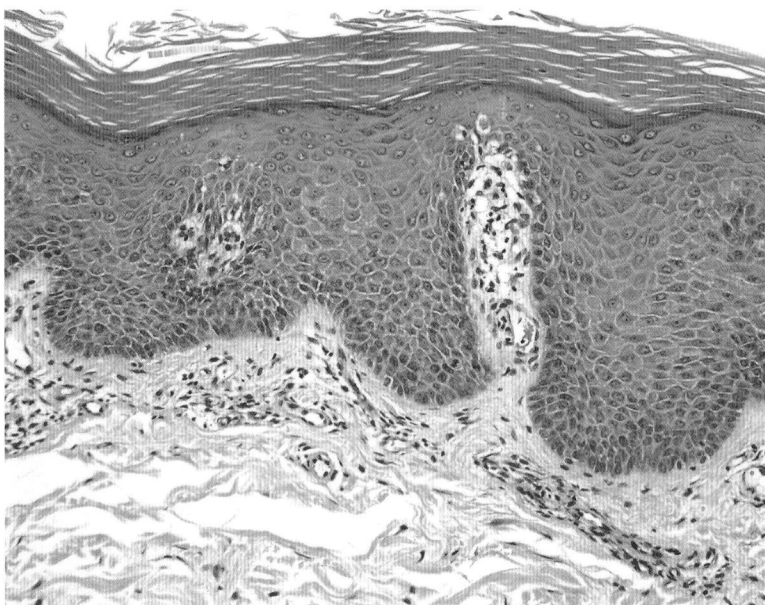

Fig. 19.12
HIV-associated pityriasis rubra pilaris: there is alternating orthohyperkeratosis and parakeratosis.

focal crusting (*Fig. 19.13*).[1,4] It is often prominent on the extremities and is worse in the winter months. Affected skin may fissure, leading to eczema craquelé and secondary infection in some patients. Occasionally, discrete thickened patches occur.[1]

Pathogenesis and histopathology

The pathogenesis of xerosis, although obscure, may be related to a range of factors, including cutaneous microcirculation and nutritional alterations, altered sweat or sebaceous gland activity, alterations in the composition of sweat, and changes in the cutaneous mast cell population. Decreased calcitonin gene-related peptide and substance P levels have been documented in HIV-associated xerosis.[5] Epidermal lipid content has been shown to be reduced in individuals with HIV.[6] These factors may result in decreased epidermal integrity, with a resultant reduction in the effectiveness of the epidermal barrier.[5]

Skin biopsies often demonstrate minimal superficial epidermal hyperkeratosis with parakeratosis, mild acanthosis, and focal spongiosis in the absence of microvesiculation (*Fig. 19.14*). The dermis demonstrates a minimal perivascular lymphocytic infiltrate. An inconsistent finding is the presence of

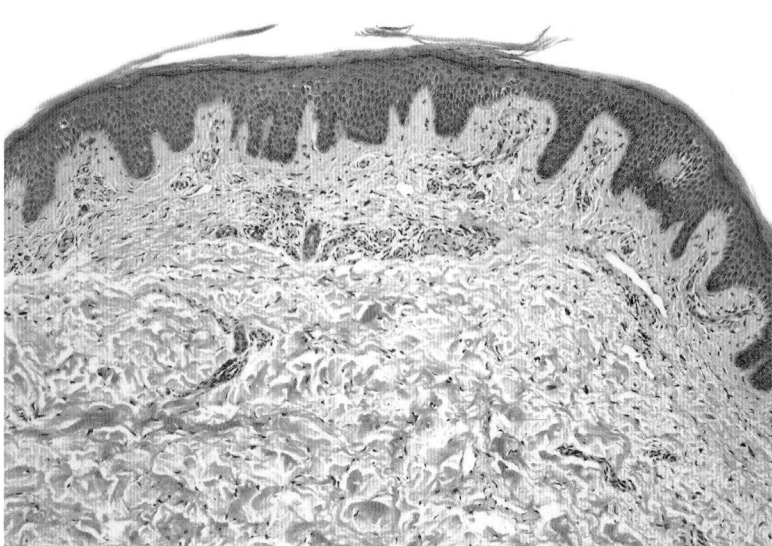

Fig. 19.14
HIV-associated xerosis: there is hyperorthokeratosis and parakeratosis associated with psoriasiform hyperplasia. There is only minimal spongiosis on the right side of the figure.

early alterations of acquired ichthyosis, characterized by dense orthokeratosis with a diminished granular cell layer and minimal inflammation. Other pruritic scaling dermatoses, such as scabies, dermatophytosis, and the 'flaky skin' appearance of kwashiorkor, are clinicopathological mimickers, as all of these conditions may occur in individuals with advanced HIV infection.[1]

HIV-associated photodistributed eruptions

Photosensitivity refers to an abnormal response to nonionizing radiation.[1] Photosensitivity is reported in more than 5% of individuals with HIV attending a specialized dermatology clinic.[1]

The spectrum of photodistributed eruptions in HIV-infected patients includes porphyria cutanea tarda (PCT), granuloma annulare, hypertrophic lichen planus, erythroderma, chronic actinic dermatitis (CAD), photodistributed hyperpigmentation, and lichenoid photoeruptions.[1–3] Some of the aforementioned conditions are discussed in further detail below.

HIV-associated lichenoid photoeruptions and chronic actinic dermatitis

Clinical features

Lichenoid photoeruptions are frequently seen as the CD4 cell count decreases and may be related to potentially photosensitizing drugs.[1] The cutaneous disease may be persistent and extend to involve nonexposed areas and become generalized.[1] Lower lip involvement may be present, but oral involvement is typically absent.[1] CAD is associated with advanced HIV disease.[2] Monochromator phototesting elicits reproducible sensitivity in the UVB range (290–320 nm).[2] Vitiligo-like depigmentation may be encountered in some cases.[3,4]

Pathogenesis and histologic features

CAD is characterized by subacute dermatitis with variable psoriasiform dermatitis and an atypical lymphocytic infiltrate.[2,5] The pathogenesis of CAD is unclear, but a delayed-type immune mechanism is postulated. The immune response in CAD appears regulated by CD8-positive T lymphocytes, which are thought to be reacting to a photoinduced antigen of endogenous origin.[5] The role of HIV in this is unclear.

Histologically, lichenoid photoeruptions are characterized by marked hyperkeratosis, focal parakeratosis, acanthosis, papillomatosis, hydropic degeneration, and pigmentary incontinence (Figs 19.15 and 19.16). There is variable keratinocyte necrosis with involvement of the upper half of the epidermis, a superficial perivascular infiltrate with a lichenoid pattern, and a mid to deep dermal infiltrate of mononuclear cells (including plasma cells) and eosinophils. Occasional features include a diffuse dermal infiltrate, wedge-shaped hypergranulosis, and a microscopic subepidermal blister.

It has been postulated that the vitiligo-like depigmentation observed in some cases is potentiated by cytotoxic destruction of basal melanocytes by CD8+ lymphocytes.[6]

HIV-associated granuloma annulare

Clinical features

HIV infection is associated with atypical forms of granuloma annulare (GA), including oral, perforating, and generalized forms (Fig. 19.17).[1–5] The generalized form occurs most frequently in HIV-infected patients.[6] HIV-associated GA (HAGA) occurs predominantly in males, usually men who have sex with men, with an age range of 25 to 58 years.[3] HAGA is characterized by a transient or chronic course and a more frequent occurrence on the extremities. A photodistributed generalized form of HAGA may occur.[1]

Pathogenesis and histologic features

The exact pathogenesis of HAGA is uncertain. Polymerase chain reaction investigation and in situ hybridization have failed to confirm Epstein-Barr virus (EBV) as a causative agent. A type IV cell-mediated hypersensitivity reaction to an unknown antigen causing degenerative change has been proposed. The release of cytokines from activated fibroblasts and macrophages

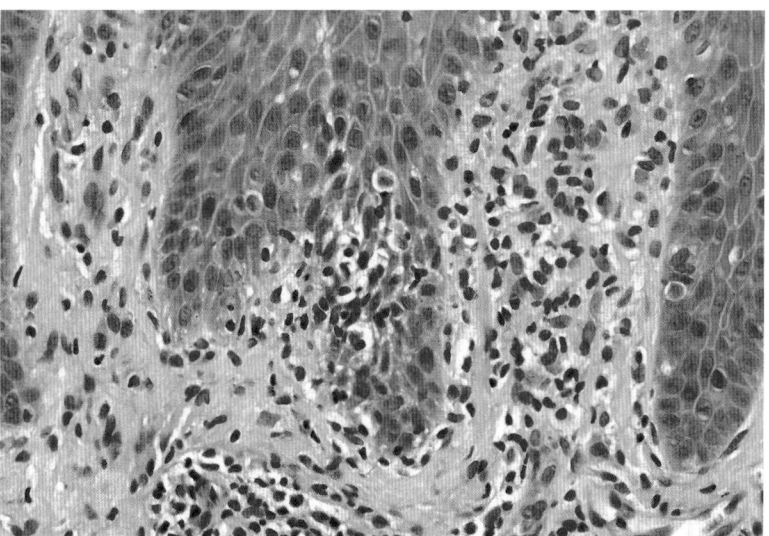

Fig. 19.16
HIV-associated lichenoid photoeruption: high-power view showing interface change, lymphocytic exocytosis, and a dense infiltrate in the papillary dermis. There is pigment incontinence.

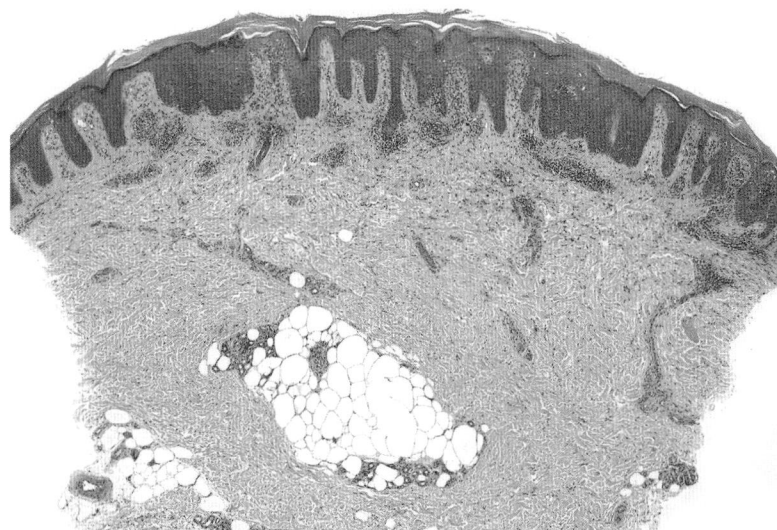

Fig. 19.15
HIV-associated lichenoid photoeruption: there is marked hyperkeratosis with psoriasiform hyperplasia. A dense interstitial and perivascular chronic inflammatory cell infiltrate is present in the upper dermis.

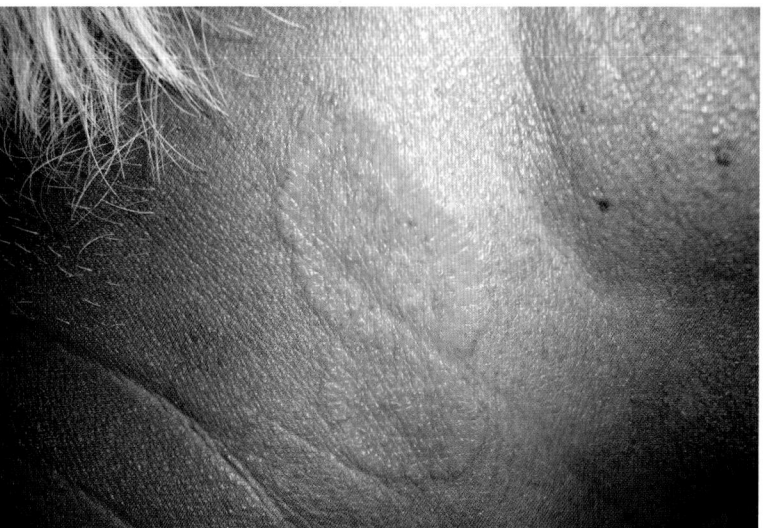

Fig. 19.17
HIV-associated granuloma annulare: note the irregular annular lesion with raised border. This lesion could be easily clinically misdiagnosed as a dermatophyte infection.

in GA has been proposed as the cause of degeneration of elastic tissue and collagen.[3,4] Although immunophenotypic analyzes have demonstrated a CD4-positive T-helper cell response in most cases, similar to that in GA in HIV-negative patients, a predominant CD8-positive lymphocytic infiltrate may be present.[2,4]

The histopathological picture is one of a necrobiotic granulomatous pattern that may be interstitial, palisaded, or mixed, similar to that in HIV-negative patients.[7] Increased amounts of interstitial mucin can be demonstrated by Alcian blue or colloidal iron staining. The histologic changes in the incomplete (or interstitial) form of GA are often subtle.[8]

HIV-associated porphyria cutanea tarda

Clinical features

Porphyria cutanea tarda (PCT) has been reported with increased frequency in HIV-infected patients; however, it is possible that this may be due to co-infection with hepatitis C virus (HCV).[1,2] A study from Spain demonstrated that treatment of HCV in co-infected individuals resulted in resolution of PCT.[2] The clinical signs of type 1 PCT, the sporadic form in which there is an acquired deficiency of uroporphyrinogen decarboxylase, are confined to the skin. Features include pruritic, fluid-filled vesicles, and bullae that develop in sun-exposed sites, including the face, dorsa of hands, and forearms. Additional findings include hyperpigmentation, hypertrichosis, and scarring.[3-6]

Pathogenesis and histologic features

The involvement of HIV in the pathogenesis of PCT is unclear because porphyrinogenic factors other than HIV such as alcohol use, drug therapy, and HCV infection have been identified in the majority of reported cases.[7-14] The deposition of iron in the liver in patients consuming alcohol may be responsible for triggering PCT through direct inhibition of uroporphyrinogen decarboxylase activity.[5] HIV may alter porphyrin metabolism through interference with the hepatic oxidase system or by creating ineffective erythropoiesis, which results in increased iron deposition. The altered steroid metabolism in patients with HIV infection could increase endogenous estrogen production, causing disruption of heme synthesis.[6] Concomitant HIV and HCV infection increases HCV RNA levels, promoting clinical manifestations of PCT.[10-12] The coexistent use of drugs may trigger PCT in the setting of HIV infection.[15]

The histologic features are identical to those encountered in HIV-negative patients. Bullous lesions are characteristically cell-poor, with rigid papillary dermal capillary walls thickened by eosinophilic, PAS-positive material. The diagnosis of PCT in a young patient should prompt further investigation for underlying HIV and HCV infection.

HIV-associated pruritic papular eruptions

HIV-associated pruritic papular eruption

Clinical features

Pruritic papular eruption (PPE) is a unique manifestation of HIV disease characterized by chronic, pruritic, symmetrical, 3- to 5-mm diameter, firm, discrete, erythematous urticarial papules (Fig. 19.18).[1] Clinically similar cutaneous lesions, however, may be encountered in eosinophilic folliculitis and suppurative folliculitis in HIV-positive patients.[2] The condition is said to occur in 10% to 50% of HIV-infected patients and is associated with advanced disease. The odds of having PPE increase with increasing pre-ART viral loads.[2] It occurs in adults and children.[1] Some studies confirm a roughly equal sex distribution, while others have shown a striking female predominance.[1,2] The distribution of the disease may be localized or generalized, occurring mainly on the extremities. The lesions tend to heal with hyperpigmentation, and prurigo nodularis-like lesions may develop. An increase in the absolute eosinophil count and relative peripheral eosinophilia are common.

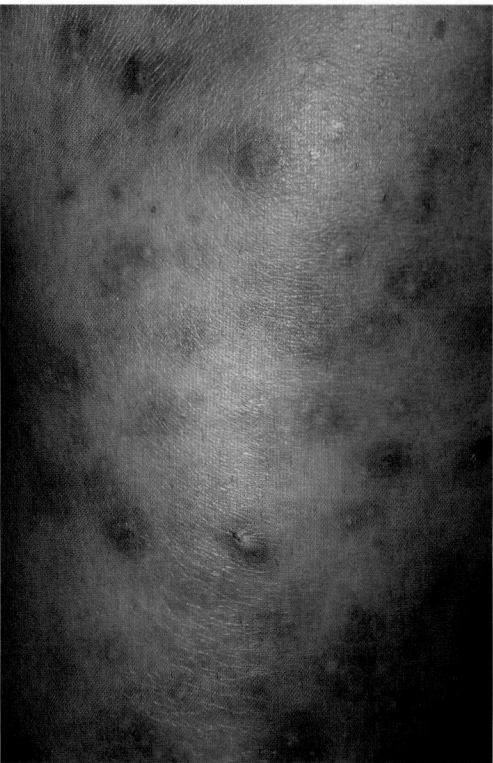

Fig. 19.18
HIV-associated pruritic papular eruption: there are numerous small erythematous papules.

Pathogenesis and histologic features

Whether PPE is a distinct entity or whether it is part of the spectrum of eosinophilic folliculitis remains controversial. Unproven pathogenetic theories include the role of infections (*Staphylococcus aureus*, *Demodex folliculorum*, and *Sarcoptes scabiei*), drug eruptions, a direct HIV effect, pemphigoid-like autoimmunity,[3] and a primary abnormality of the pilosebaceous unit. The relationship between mosquito bites and PPE is complex. Proposed mechanisms include the hypothesis that the individual lesions in PPE represent mosquito bites, or that the eruption represents a generalized hypersensitivity reaction to mosquito saliva, similar to papular urticaria.[2,4] A study has highlighted the role of arthropod bites, mainly those of the mosquito, in the pathogenesis of PPE, emphasizing that PPE represents an exaggerated immune response to arthropod antigens in predisposed HIV-infected patients.[4] Increased concentrations of interleukin-2, interleukin-12, δ-interferon, and interleukin-5, in association with a decreased CD4-positive T-lymphocyte count in the blood and increased CD8-positive T lymphocytes in lesional skin, are hypothesized to explain the occurrence of a mixed Th1/Th2 or Th0 pattern, leading to cytokine production and an influx of eosinophils in the cutaneous infiltrate.[5,6]

The histologic features vary, depending on whether older, scarred, and excoriated nodules or new lesions are biopsied. The early lesions demonstrate a moderately dense to dense, superficial, and deep, perivascular, perifollicular, perieccrine, and interstitial infiltrate of lymphocytes and eosinophils, with variable extension into the subcutis, and epidermal hyperplasia (Figs 19.19 and 19.20).[4] There is a predominance of CD8-positive T lymphocytes. Healed lesions demonstrate variable scarring and postinflammatory hyperpigmentation.[1,2,4] Long-standing nodular lesions that are the result of chronic pruritus and excoriation show histologic features of prurigo nodularis.

Differential diagnosis

The histologic differential diagnoses include folliculitis (suppurative or eosinophilic), scabies, secondary syphilis, and a drug eruption. Against folliculitis and scabies are the absence of a dominant folliculocentric localization of the pathology and the absence of mite parts of *S. scabiei* or mite's feces,

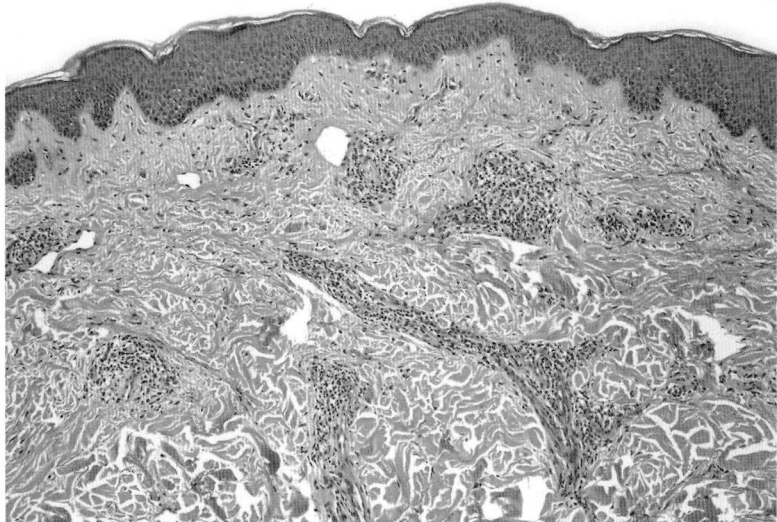

Fig. 19.19
HIV-associated pruritic papular eruption: there is focal mild acanthosis. Within the dermis is a dense perivascular infiltrate, and vessels are dilated.

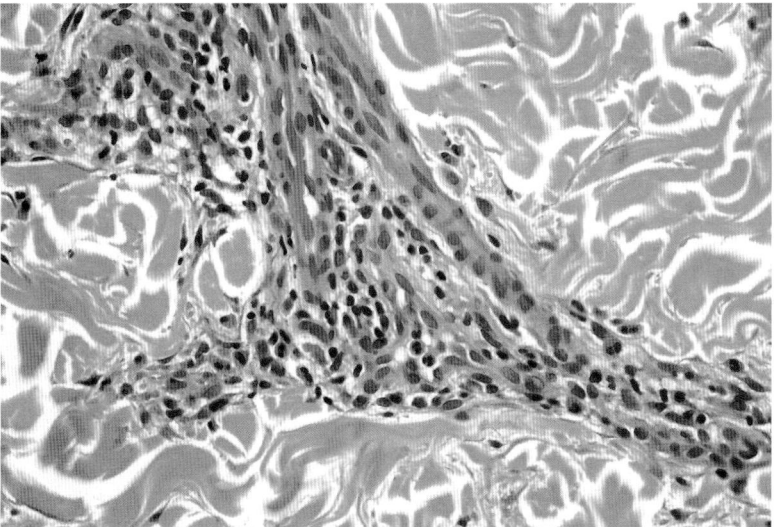

Fig. 19.20
HIV-associated pruritic papular eruption: the infiltrate consists of lymphocytes and numerous eosinophils.

respectively. Examination of multiple serial sections is required to exclude the aforementioned conditions.[7] A drug eruption may resemble PPE, but the inflammatory infiltrate in this setting usually does not extend into the subcutis and is not as dense as that seen in PPE.[4] A lichenoid interface reaction pattern and the presence of a dominant infiltrate of histiocytes and plasma cells in the cellular infiltrate distinguishes secondary syphilis from PPE.

HIV-associated eosinophilic folliculitis

Clinical features

HIV-associated eosinophilic folliculitis (HIV-EF) is a distinctive, chronic pruritic skin eruption characterized by discrete, urticarial follicular papules scattered on the trunk, the head and neck, and the proximal extremities.[1-5] Excoriation and crusting are frequent. Less commonly, small pustules are noted atop the papules.[1] There may be significant clinical overlap with other HIV-related papular and/or follicular eruptions such as HIV-associated PPE or suppurative folliculitis.[3] Increased absolute or relative peripheral eosinophil counts and elevated serum IgE levels have been documented. HIV-EF is associated with advanced HIV disease and may be a manifestation of IRIS. Although the disease is encountered almost exclusively in adults, rare cases have been documented in infancy and childhood.[6]

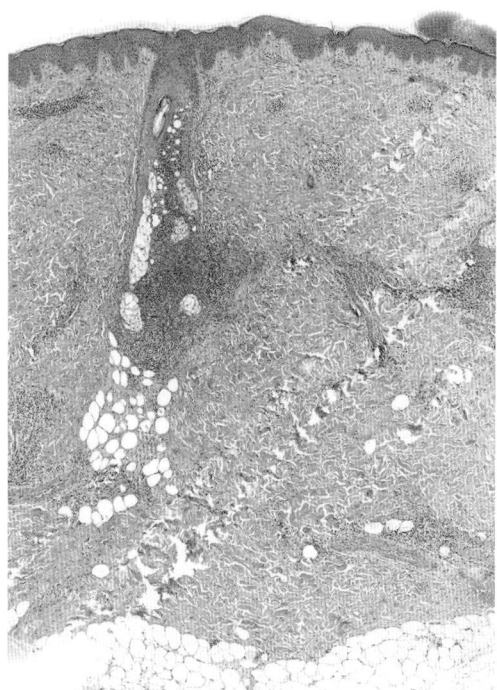

Fig. 19.21
HIV-associated eosinophilic folliculitis: there is a dense follicular infiltrate. Perivascular inflammatory cells are also evident.

Pathogenesis and histologic features

The exact etiology and pathogenesis of HIV-EF remain unestablished. Fungal (*Pityrosporum ovale*), parasitic (*D. folliculorum*), and bacterial (*Leptotrichia, Mycobacterium, Staphylococcus*) organisms have been the focus of several theories, but these infective agents are rarely found in association with HIV-EF, evoking a possible bystander role.[1-5,7-13] A lipid-soluble chemotactic factor for eosinophils and neutrophils has been proposed as a causative factor; eotaxin has been shown to be upregulated in sebocytes.[14] Follicular disruption and exposure of the sebaceous antigen are implicated in the stimulation of an inflammatory process involving lymphocytes, cytokines, and eosinophils.[2-5,7-13] The presence of mast cells and evidence of their degranulation have implicated a role for mast cells in the evolution of HIV-EF.[1]

The histopathological features are those of follicular disruption and infiltration by eosinophils, with the surrounding dermis showing perivascular and interstitial infiltration by lymphocytes, eosinophils, and mast cells (*Figs 19.21* and *19.22*). Occasionally, elaborated *D. folliculorum* mites are observed in the perifollicular dermis when intradermal rupture of an involved, distended follicle has occurred.[3]

Differential diagnosis

The main histologic differential diagnoses are eosinophilic pustular folliculitis (Ofuji disease) and PPE. Follicular eosinophil accumulation is common to both HIV-EF and Ofuji disease. The latter condition is more prevalent in the East and occurs in healthy individuals, with an increased peripheral leukocyte count, pruritus in <50% of patients, and coalescence of papulopustular plaques, with central clearing and postinflammatory hyperpigmentation. A similar histologic reaction pattern may sometimes be triggered by fungal infections of the hair shaft.[15] PPE shares many of the clinical features of HIV-associated PPE. The follicular involvement by eosinophils, however, serves as the main distinguishing feature.[1,3,16] To this end, examination of multiple serial sections is advised to assess the presence of folliculitis, and some authors have advocated the use of CD15 immunohistochemistry.[3,17]

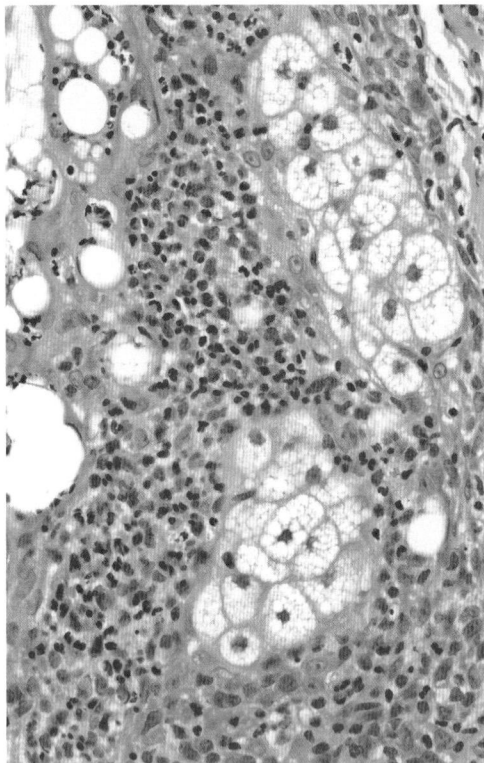

Fig. 19.22
HIV-associated eosinophilic folliculitis: high-power view showing a dense eosinophilic infiltrate.

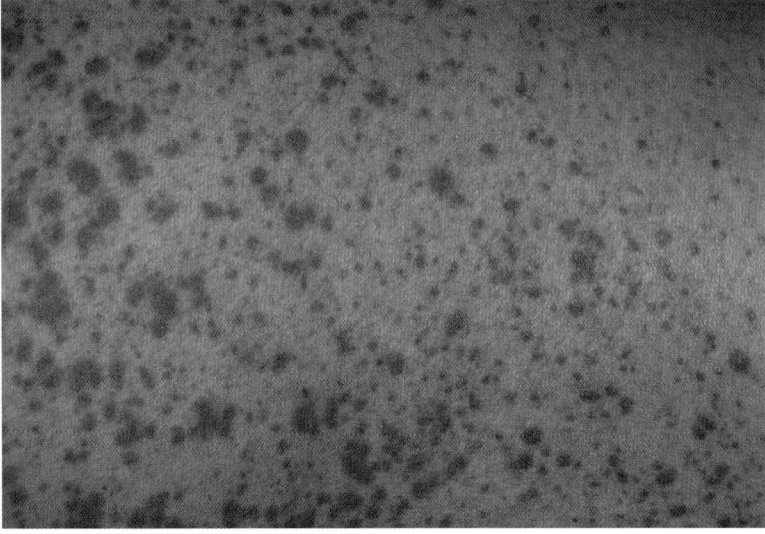

Fig. 19.23
HIV-associated leukocytoclastic vasculitis: numerous erythematous papules are present.

HIV-associated vasculitic disorders

Excluding drug-related hypersensitivity reactions, vasculitic syndromes are not common in HIV-positive patients.[1-3] Small, medium, and large vessel vasculitis has been reported at all stages of HIV infection.[2]

Hypersensitivity reactions to drugs are common in HIV-positive patients.[3,4] Hypersensitivity reactions have been reported with almost all the HIV antiretroviral medications, typically involving small vessels, producing a lymphocytic or leukocytoclastic vasculitis (*Fig. 19.23*).

The mechanisms underlying HIV-associated vasculitis are unclear and are largely inferential, based on the absence of a defined etiology, a disproportionate number of rare illnesses among HIV-positive patients, and unusual presentations that do not fit prior defined clinical diseases.[3]

Erythema elevatum diutinum

Clinical features

Erythema elevatum diutinum (EED), a rare chronic disease of unknown etiology, is part of the spectrum of cutaneous leukocytoclastic vasculitis.[1] The disease is characterized by symmetrical, persistent, and raised erythematous plaques and nodules over the extensor surfaces of the extremities. There is a predilection for involvement of skin overlying the elbow, knee, ankle, and interphalangeal joints.[1-5] Bulla formation has been reported.[5] Early lesions are soft and yellow and may contain petechiae or exhibit purpura. The duration of the disease is typified by a chronic course, varying between 1 and 39 years. The lesions of EED are usually asymptomatic, but may be pruritic or painful. Later lesions are doughy to firm and of red to purple color. EED has been reported in the context of IRIS.[4]

Pathogenesis and histologic features

The leukocytoclastic vasculitis is the result of ongoing immune complex-mediated, neutrophil-induced, dermal small vessel damage. Antigen-antibody complexes from hepatitis B, C, and D viruses and HIV have been implicated.[1]

Histopathologically, the early lesions demonstrate leukocytoclastic vasculitis and capillary proliferation.[3] This is followed by a fascicular proliferation of spindle cells and macrophages in the background of leukocytoclastic vasculitis.[2] Late lesions demonstrate homogenization and fibrosis of the dermis. Serial sectioning may be required to identify foci of leukocytoclastic vasculitis. The fibrosis may assume an acellular, laminated appearance, with a parallel, wavy orientation of collagen with respect to the overlying epidermis. Capillaries are oriented vertically. Skin biopsy is essential to differentiate EED from a range of clinically similar HIV-associated lesions, including Kaposi sarcoma (KS) and bacillary angiomatosis. Stains to exclude infective causes for the fibrovascular and cellular alterations may be required.

Microscopic polyangiitis-like and polyarteritis nodosa-like illnesses

Clinical features

Polyarteritis nodosa (PAN) is the most common HIV-associated vasculitis and is not associated with hepatitis B virus infection.[1-3] Patient age ranges from 29 to 72 years.[3] In contrast to HIV-negative patients, fever, cutaneous, renal, cardiac, and gastrointestinal manifestations are encountered less frequently in HIV-infected individuals. The most common presentation is that of peripheral neuropathy and muscle atrophy.[1] In addition, the waxing and waning of classic PAN is absent.[4] Recognition of these HIV-associated vasculitides is important because of the clinical cutaneous and serological response to ART, leading to healing of skin lesions with postinflammatory pigmentation, and improvement in HIV surrogate markers such as viral load and CD4 cell counts.[4]

Pathogenesis and histologic features

Whether or not HIV or other agents such as hepatitis C virus and cytomegalovirus are directly involved in the vascular injury remains unestablished.[2,5,6] An immune complex deposition process, similar to that proposed in hepatitis B-associated PAN, has been suggested because of the demonstration of vascular deposits of HIV antigens, immunoglobulins, and complement components.[2,3,5]

The histologic features mirror those of classic PAN, with focal and segmental vasculitis of medium-sized arterioles and arteries, fibrinoid necrosis of vessel walls, and a transmural inflammatory cell infiltrate[4] (*Figs 19.24* and *19.25*).

HIV-associated Kawasaki-like syndrome

Clinical features

The diagnosis of Kawasaki-like syndrome (K-LS) is complex due to the potential for adverse drug reactions in the face of HIV-associated polypharmacy

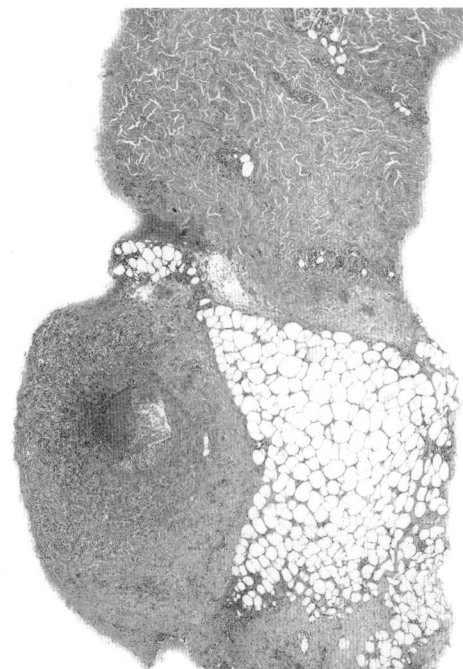

Fig. 19.24
HIV-associated polyarteritis nodosa: there are marked inflammatory changes in a large muscular artery in the subcutaneous fat.

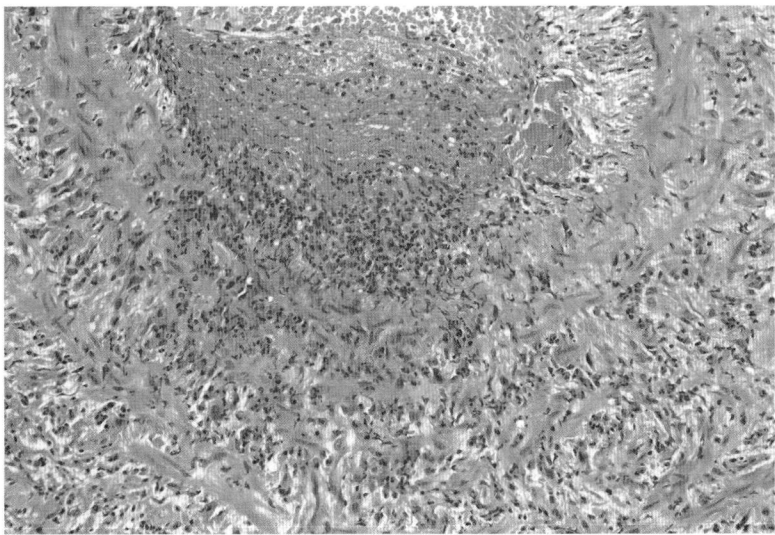

Fig. 19.25
HIV-associated polyarteritis nodosa: the vessel is thrombosed and numerous eosinophils are present.

and possible opportunistic infections in HIV-positive patients.[1,2] Patients usually have moderate to severe immune dysfunction. While Kawasaki disease (KD) usually occurs in children <5 years of age, K-LS occur mainly in HIV-infected adults. Recently Johnson et al. have argued that the two conditions are likely to be the same entity.[3]

KD is diagnosed by a history of fever of 5 days' duration, plus four of the following five features[4]:
• bilateral non-purulent conjunctivitis,
• changes of the oropharynx, including an injected pharynx, injected and/ or dry fissured lips, and/or strawberry tongue,
• changes of the peripheral extremities, including edema and/or erythema of the hands and the feet (usually followed by desquamation),
• a nonvesicular, polymorphous, erythematous exanthema,
• cervical lymphadenopathy with lymph nodes measuring ≥1.5 cm in diameter.

Other infectious or noninfectious causes must be excluded prior to the diagnosis of K-LS.[5] Gastrointestinal symptoms are common, and cervical lymphadenopathy is less pronounced.[6]

Pathogenesis and histologic features

It has been hypothesized that compromised cellular immunity, resistance to intracellular pathogens, and reactivation or infection by an intracellular infectious agent are responsible for K-LS.[1,2,5,6]

Skin biopsies reveal an infiltrate of lymphocytes, neutrophils, and IgA-positive plasma cells surrounding the superficial papillary vascular plexus, accompanied by necrotizing vasculitis. Coronary artery histology demonstrates marked infiltration of the vessel wall by IgA-positive plasma cells, in a similar manner to that described in KD.[1,2]

HIV-associated autoimmune bullous diseases

Clinical features

A spectrum of autoimmune bullous diseases occurs in HIV-infected patients. Conditions include bullous pemphigoid, epidermolysis bullosa acquisita, pemphigus herpetiformis, pemphigus vegetans, mucocutaneous pemphigus vulgaris, pemphigus foliaceus, antiepiligrin mucous membrane pemphigoid, IgA dermatosis, dermatitis herpetiformis, intraepidermal neutrophilic IgA dermatosis, and endemic pemphigus foliaceus.[1–14] While pemphigus vegetans is typified by vegetating plaques, pemphigus herpetiformis is characterized by arcuate, erythematous lesions and tense vesicles.[1,8] Intraepidermal neutrophilic IgA dermatosis demonstrates superficial scaling, vesicles, or pustules. Bullous pemphigoid in HIV-infected patients is characterized by pruritic, excoriated, erythematous papules, 3–10 mm in diameter, or tense blisters with scarring. Antiepiligrin mucous membrane pemphigoid, similar clinically to that occurring in HIV-negative patients, has been described. These autoimmune bullous disorders may occur in the absence of any other HIV-related clinical conditions.

Pathogenesis and histologic features

The development of autoimmune disease in HIV-infected individuals is well documented.[1–14] Low titers of pemphigus antibodies have been detected in 65% of HIV-positive patients with no manifestations of vesiculobullous disease.[6] While biological autoimmune abnormalities of unknown significance are frequently observed in HIV-seropositive patients, true autoimmune diseases are rare. A fortuitous association between HIV infection and autoimmune diseases remains a possibility. Although the exact mechanism is not known, several theories have been proposed. There is structural homology between HIV env proteins and molecules that are responsible for self-tolerance. Antigen presentation of HIV env proteins may therefore induce the production of autoantibodies.[15] A second theory proposes that HIV-infected macrophages produce increased amounts of IL-1 and IL-6, leading to non-specific stimulation of B lymphocytes and the resultant activation of autoantigen clones and production of autoantibodies. HIV is postulated to precipitate the onset of the bullous disease.[7]

Pemphigus vulgaris is caused by the production of autoantibodies to desmoglein 3, a transmembrane protein involved in cell adhesion, being present in greatest concentration in the stratum spinosum. Binding of autoantibodies results in skin fragility. The histologic and immunofluorescence findings of pemphigus vulgaris are similar to those encountered in HIV-negative patients. Pemphigus vegetans is characterized by papillomatous epidermal hyperplasia, suprabasal acantholytic clefts, and intraepidermal collections of neutrophils and eosinophils with foci of spongiosis. Endemic pemphigus foliaceus (fogo selvagem) is characterized by spontaneous intraepidermal blisters and epidermis-specific autoantibodies, predominantly of the IgA4 subclass, which recognize the epidermal antigen, desmoglein 1.[4] Pemphigus herpetiformis demonstrates spongiosis and epidermal infiltration with eosinophils rather than acantholysis. Intraepidermal acantholytic pustules with neutrophils are a hallmark of intraepidermal neutrophilic IgA dermatosis. Direct immunofluorescence in the latter condition reveals IgA deposits around keratinocytes.

The histologic and direct immunofluorescence findings of bullous pemphigoid are similar to those observed in HIV-negative patients. Antiepiligrin mucous membrane pemphigoid is characterized by circulating autoantibodies to laminin.[9,10] Dermatitis herpetiformis and epidermolysis bullosa acquisita have also been reported in HIV-infected patients; the histologic features are identical to those encountered in HIV-negative subjects.[3,5,12]

HIV-associated cutaneous mucinoses

Clinical features

A range of conditions associated with cutaneous mucin deposition has been documented in HIV-infected patients.[1] These disorders include papular mucinosis (lichen myxedematosus), reticular erythematous mucinosis (REM), scleredema, follicular mucinosis, eccrine ductal mucinosis, granuloma annulare, and an atypical PRP-like eruption.[1–7]

Papular mucinosis is the most common form of cutaneous mucinosis occurring in HIV-infected patients.[5] While papular mucinosis occurs with equal frequency in both sexes in the general population, HIV-associated papular mucinosis occurs almost exclusively in men, mainly in the fourth decade of life. The trunk and limbs are characteristically involved by multiple, smooth, skin-colored papules 1–3 mm in diameter.[3] Hypergammaglobulinemia and paraproteinemia are known associations, with the former being more common.[5] Papular mucinosis occurs more commonly in patients with a CD4 cell count $<100/mm^3$. Pruritus is uncommon. Visceral mucin deposition and an association with drugs have not been documented.[3] Papular mucinosis may resolve spontaneously or improve with ART.[8]

HIV-associated REM manifests with numerous isolated or coalescing erythematous plaques on the chest and back.[1,5] HIV-associated follicular mucinosis is characterized by the presence of erythematous, papular lesions on the head, chest, and limbs.[9] HIV-associated eccrine ductal mucinosis is a pruritic papular and erythematous eruption that involves the trunk and extremities.[1]

Pathogenesis and histologic features

The exact pathogenesis of HIV-associated papular mucinosis is not known. It has, however, been suggested that direct fibroblastic stimulation by HIV, immunoglobulins related to non-specific HIV-induced B-lymphocyte stimulation, or several upregulated serum cytokines (in particular, interleukin 1, interleukin 6, epidermal growth factor, and tumor necrosis factor [TNF]-α and TNF-β) may serve as factors promoting heightened glycosaminoglycan production by dermal fibroblasts.[3,5] HIV-associated papular mucinosis is characterized by dermal expansion, thickening, and a fenestrated appearance with broad collagen bundles separated by Alcian blue (pH 2.5) and colloidal iron positive interstitial mucin. Inflammatory cells are absent. Eczematous changes may be encountered in the overlying epidermis.

A heightened predisposition of HIV-infected patients to photosensitivity has been proposed as a potential mechanism for the evolution of REM. REM is typified by dermal vascular dilatation and a sparse perivascular lymphocytic infiltrate around the upper and mid-dermal vascular plexuses (*Figs 19.26–19.28*).[5] Mucin may be evident with special stains (*Fig. 19.29*).

Direct or indirect stimulation of eccrine ductal or follicular epithelium by inflammatory cells, especially T lymphocytes and eosinophils, has been proposed as the pathogenetic mechanism for mucin deposition in follicular mucinosis and eccrine ductal mucinosis.[1] Follicular mucinosis is characterized by the presence of a follicular infundibular inflammatory infiltrate consisting of mononuclear cells, neutrophils, eosinophils, and deposition of Alcian blue-positive mucin between the follicular epithelial cells (*Figs 19.30 and 19.31*).[9] Eccrine ductal mucinosis is identified by the presence of granular, basophilic mucinous material in eccrine ducts, limited to the straight intradermal portion and acrosyringium. There is expansion of the outer cell layer, accompanied by a perivascular and interstitial inflammatory infiltrate of lymphocytes and eosinophils in the superficial and deep dermis.[1] Follicular mucinosis may occur in association with eccrine ductal mucinosis.

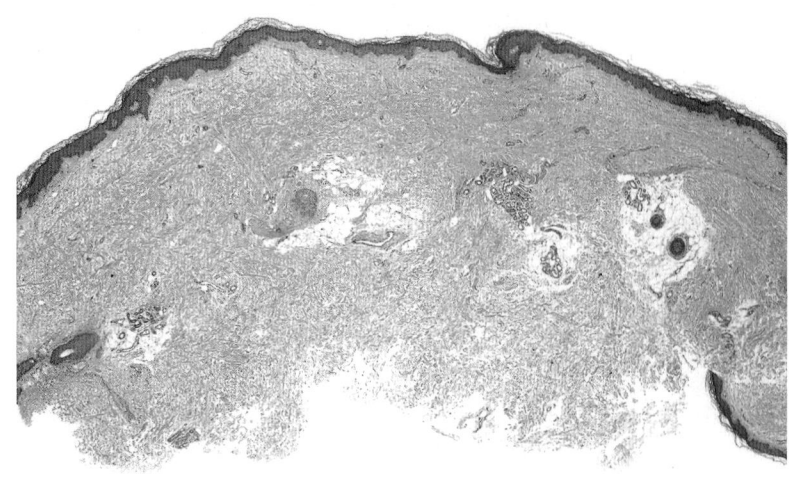

Fig. 19.26
HIV-associated reticular erythematous mucinosis: low-power view showing a patchy perivascular light chronic inflammatory cell infiltrate.

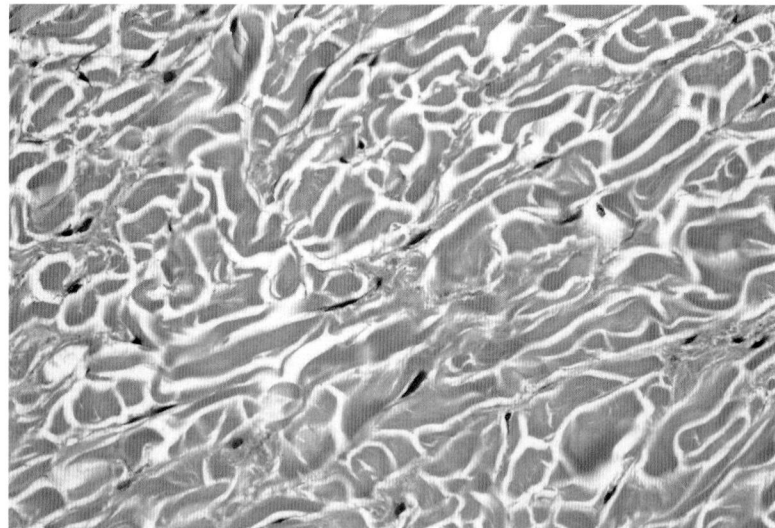

Fig. 19.27
HIV-associated reticular erythematous mucinosis: the collagen bundles appear slightly thickened and are separated by delicate mucinous strands.

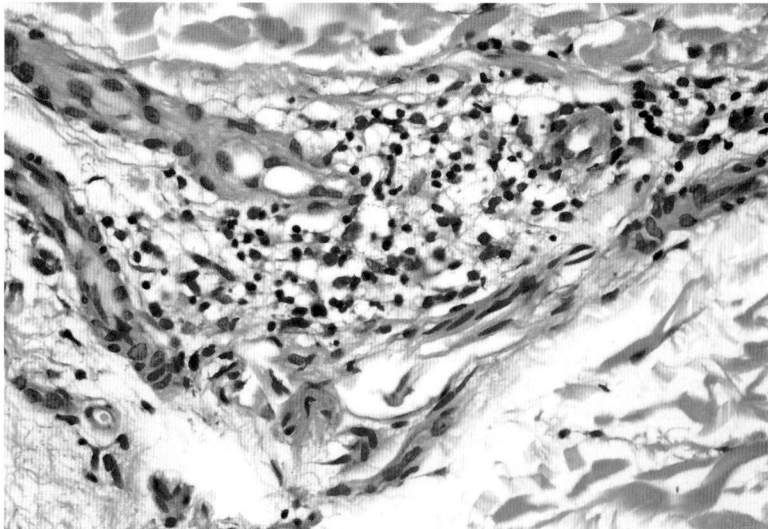

Fig. 19.28
HIV-associated reticular erythematous mucinosis: the vessels are surrounded by a light lymphocytic infiltrate.

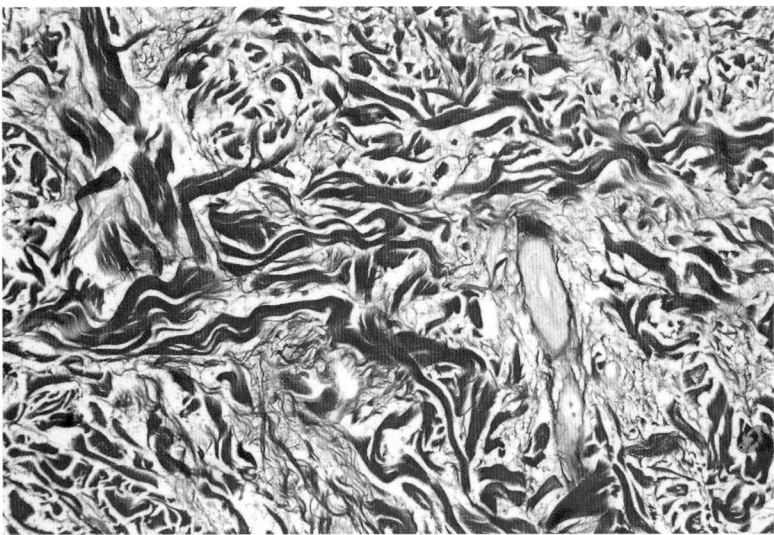

Fig. 19.29
HIV-associated reticular erythematous mucinosis: Alcian blue highlights the excessive dermal mucin.

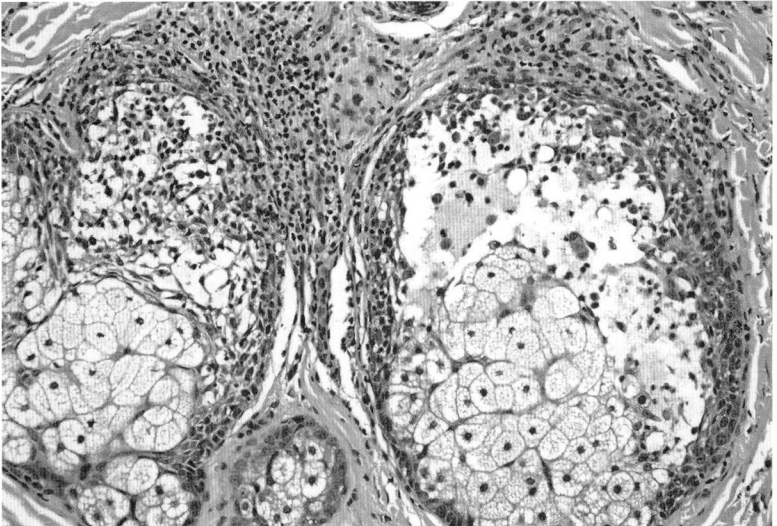

Fig. 19.30
HIV-associated follicular mucinosis: there is extensive intrafollicular mucin deposition and lymphocytic infiltration.

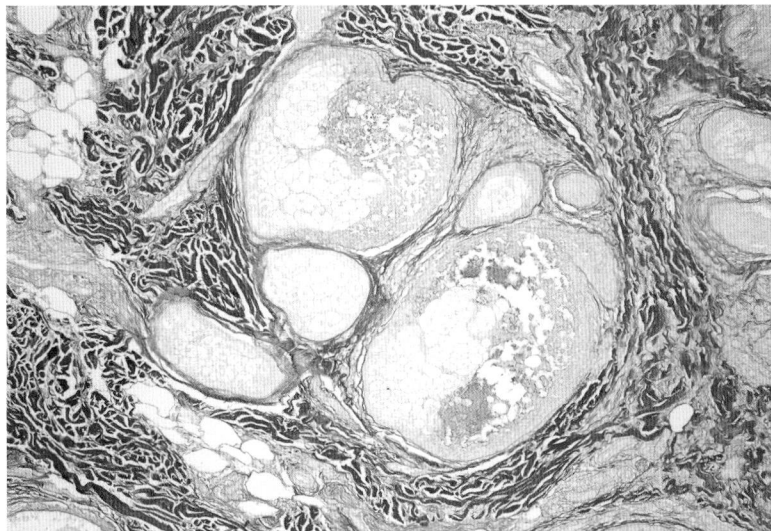

Fig. 19.31
HIV-associated follicular mucinosis: the Alcian blue stain highlights the mucin deposition.

Lichenoid reactions in HIV

Clinical features

Although certain diseases such as psoriasis may be triggered or aggravated by HIV infection, classic lichen planus is very rarely associated with HIV infection.[1-4] A rare association with hypertrophic lichen planus, sometimes with photosensitivity, has been described.[2-4] Patients with HIV infection may develop lichenoid eruptions, but these are usually associated with photosensitivity and may be triggered by drugs including nonsteroidal anti-inflammatory drugs and trimethoprim-sulfamethoxazole.[5] The majority of patients in this US study were black and had advanced HIV disease.

Lichenoid lesions have also been described both in skin and in the oral mucosa of individuals co-infected with HIV and HCV during antiviral treatment with interferon alpha, ribavirin, and tenofovir.[6,7]

Histologic features

Histologically, patients with a lichenoid photoeruption display acanthosis with hyperkeratosis and may have focal parakeratosis, variable spongiosis, high epidermal necrotic keratinocytes, and a dermal infiltrate that is composed of lymphocytes and may have variable numbers of eosinophils. Very rarely, the lichenoid photoeruption has histologic features of lichen nitidus.[5]

HIV interface dermatitis

The issue of AIDS interface dermatitis is a potential source of controversy.[1,2] An association between HIV infection and interface dermatitis was first recognized in the 1980s.[3,4] Many of these patients, however, had one or more opportunistic infections (e.g., herpes), and nearly all had been receiving one or more medications prior to the onset of the eruption.[3] It is therefore likely that the 'condition' represents a reaction pattern triggered by a variety of infective and/or pharmacological etiologies rather than a discrete clinicopathological entity.[1] The need for careful clinicopathological correlation is emphasized by the fact that interface dermatitis is a characteristic histologic feature of acute HIV exanthem and is an invariable finding in morbilliform drug eruptions. Interface dermatitis is nevertheless encountered occasionally as an incidental finding in a skin biopsy performed for another reason, such as confirmation of a clinical diagnosis of KS (*Fig. 19.32*). In cases like these, there is sometimes no significant drug history.[1]

Other HIV-associated dermatoses

Other dermatoses including acanthosis nigricans, atopic-like eczema, anetoderma, erythroderma, reactive arthritis, acquired acrodermatitis enteropathica, and coagulation disorders such as acquired protein S deficiency have all been described in HIV-infected patients.[1-5] While HIV infection is the common factor in these patients, underlying systemic illnesses unrelated to the HIV status may be responsible for the disease presentation in many cases. Concomitant drug ingestion, including antiretroviral agents, may contribute to the clinical picture in some instances.

Cutaneous infections

The cutaneous infections that occur in people with HIV infection are outlined below and discussed in greater detail in Chapter 18.

Bacterial infections

Individuals with HIV have high a higher rate of skin and soft tissues infections (SSTIs).[1] Group A streptococci and *S. aureus* may be causative organisms in cellulitis, impetigo, necrotizing folliculitis, furunculosis, pyoderma, and erysipelas. *S. aureus* is the most common bacterial pathogen in patients with HIV. It may present as botryomycosis.[2] Bacterial folliculitis can also be a feature of HIV infection. It presents as an acneiform eruption affecting the face, back, chest, and buttocks or else as a relapsing condition in the axillae.[3] Histologically, bacterial folliculitis is characterized by a purulent exudate within the follicular epithelium accompanied by a surrounding lymphohistiocytic infiltrate.[3] Plasma cells and eosinophils may also be evident.

The incidence of community-associated methicillin-resistant *Staphylococcus aureus* (MRSA) is increased in individuals with HIV infection and is a risk factor for recurrent SSTIs.[4] *S. aureus* strains in HIV infected individuals often carry the Panton-Valentine leukocidin, which is associated with severe necrotizing infections.[5,6]

Bacillary angiomatosis is a vasoproliferative lesion induced by infection with either *Bartonella henselae* or *B. quintana*.[7] Patients with CD4 lymphocyte counts of less than 100 cells/mm^3 are at risk.[8]

HIV-infected individuals with *Mycobacterium tuberculosis* infections may have varied features on histology from noncaseating granulomata to caseating granulomata to an absence of granulomata.[9] In infection with the nontuberculous mycobacteria *Mycobacterium avium* complex (MAC), the features may be granulomatous, but more commonly consist of a nongranulomatous infiltrate of neutrophils, numerous foamy macrophages, lymphocytes, plasma cells, and eosinophils (*Figs 19.33–19.37*).[9] Skin lesions due to MAC are rare and usually represent disseminated disease.[9] *Mycobacterium kansasii* infection may result in a spindle cell 'proliferative' lesion reminiscent of the histoid variant of lepromatous leprosy.[10] The presence of more typical foamy macrophages is a useful diagnostic discriminant.

Syphilis is associated with increased acquisition of HIV. Data from the CDC in 2014 showed that approximately 40% of individuals diagnosed with syphilis were HIV infected.[11] False-negative RPR/VDRL tests due to the prozone phenomenon and delayed seroreactivity may be more common in HIV-infected individuals.[12]

Ecthyma gangrenosum secondary to *Pseudomonas aeruginosa* has been associated with HIV.[13]

Viral infections

HPV-induced lesions such as verruca vulgaris and condylomata acuminata are common (*Fig. 19.38*). Plane warts and epidermodysplasia verruciformis-like lesions are seen in children and adolescents with HIV.[1–3]

HPV-associated cervical, vulvar, anal, penile carcinoma in situ, and invasive squamous cell carcinomas are a significant and potentially vaccine-preventable problem.[4–6]

Cytomegalovirus is the most common viral pathogen seen in advanced AIDS, evidence for which is found in 93% of autopsies. It is responsible for retinitis, colitis, pneumonitis, encephalitis, and generalized wasting.[7] Skin involvement, however, is very rare. Molluscum contagiosum (*Fig. 19.39*) and reactivation of varicella zoster virus is common.

Oral, genital, digital, and perianal herpes simplex (reactivation) are very common in severe infections in patients with AIDS (*Figs 19.40 and 19.41*).[7] Perianal lesions may present as very extensive, painful, necrotic, nonhealing ulcers with a circinate border.[8]

Oral hairy leukoplakia, which is due to Epstein-Barr virus (EBV), is seen as a usually asymptomatic, white, poorly demarcated, raised plaque most often on the lateral border of the tongue (*Fig. 19.42*).[8] The ventral and dorsal surfaces, buccal mucosa, palate, and floor of the mouth may also be affected.[9] Although *Candida* is often found in the lesions, they do not respond to anticandidal therapy. There are fine projections of keratin from the surface said to resemble hairs. Alternatively, there may be vertical white lines running across the edge of the tongue. Balloon cells with pyknotic nuclei are seen in the superficial epithelium as well as marked parakeratosis and epithelial hyperplasia.[10] Electron microscopy has revealed both papilloma and herpes-type virus.[11] EBV replication has been demonstrated within the epithelial cells of hairy leukoplakia.[12]

EBV-positive mucocutaneous ulcer of the oral cavity has been reported in association with HIV.[13]

Fungal infections

Oral candidiasis is often a sign of progression of HIV infection. Angular cheilitis and onychomycosis are frequent manifestations of candidiasis in patients with severe HIV-induced immunosuppression.[1]

Dermatophyte infections (e.g., tinea pedis, tinea cruris, and tinea capitis) and onychomycosis often become very severe and extensive. Disseminated mycoses caused by *Cryptococcus neoformans*, *Histoplasma capsulatum*, *Coccidioides* species, and *Talaromyces (Penicillium) marneffei* and pneumonia due to *Pneumocystis jirovecii* are indicator conditions of advanced HIV disease.[2] Other fungi causing systemic or cutaneous infection in association with HIV include *Paracoccidioides brasiliensis*, *Aspergillus* species, and *Mucor* species *Sporothrix schenckii*.[3,4]

An interesting and unusual observation has been the identification of *P. jirovecii* in middle ear infections presenting as polyps within the external auditory meatus in a patient who subsequently developed pulmonary involvement.[5] Histologically, these lesions showed features similar to those seen in pulmonary lesions.

Other infections and infestations

Toxoplasma gondii is a common cause of morbidity in HIV, but cutaneous disease is very rare.[1] Individuals with HIV are at risk of developing crusted scabies.[2] Unusual forms such as localized crusted lesions and head and neck involvement may occur.

HIV is reported to result in more severe disease in cutaneous leishmaniasis and may even lead to visceral disease.[3]

Prototheocosis that responded to itraconazole has been reported in a man with HIV.[4]

Lipodystrophy in HIV

This acquired variant is characterized by loss of fat from the face, gluteal region, and the extremities with deposition around the neck, abdomen, and trunk, and predisposes to cardiovascular disease (*Fig. 19.43*).[1] There is associated insulin resistance with glucose intolerance, diabetes mellitus, hypertriglyceridemia, and low serum high density lipoprotein cholesterol levels.[2]

Lipoatrophy is associated with the use of thymidine analogue drugs particularly stavudine and, to a lesser extent, zidovudine.[2] Protease inhibitors are linked to lipohypertrophy and, to a lesser, extent lipoatrophy. In the latter case, it is not clear whether this effect is a result of interactions with other classes of ART drugs.[3] Other risk factors include age, gender, nadir CD4 count, viral load, older age, and overt disease.[4] HIV-positive patients with lipodystrophy frequently have associated intramuscular fat accumulation.[5]

Histologic features

HIV-associated partial lipodystrophy has been variably characterized by loss of subcutaneous fat without any other recognizable histologic abnormality.[6,7]

Neoplasia

Individuals with HIV have a higher incidence of nonmelanoma skin cancer and melanoma.[1,2] Melanoma mortality is increased in people with HIV.[1] Individuals with a CD4 count below 200 cells/mm^3 or a lack of sustained viral suppression have an increased the risk of oropharyngeal squamous cell carcinoma.[3] The prevalence of Merkel cell polyomavirus DNA in the skin is increased in men with HIV and is thought to be the cause of the increased incidence of Merkel cell carcinoma in people with HIV.[4,5]

AIDS defining malignancies (ADMs) include invasive cervical carcinoma, Kaposi sarcoma (KS), and non-Hodgkin lymphomas (NHLs). The incidence of these has declined in well-resourced settings with accessibility to effective ART, although the incidence of non-ADMs did not.[6] However, in Africa, KS is an increasing public health problem.[7]

The most common presentation of KS is multifocal macules or nodules. Extracutaneous KS occurs in 50% and can occur in the absence of skin disease.[8] KS is associated with infection with human herpesvirus-8 (HHV-8). Other HHV-8 associated neoplasms are primary effusion lymphoma, a B cell lymphoma and plasmablastic lymphoma. Multicentric Castleman disease (MCD) is associated with HHV-8, and untreated patients are at high risk of developing large B-cell lymphoma (LBCL).[9]

AIDS-associated NHLs are predominantly of B-cell type. The spectrum includes diffuse LBCL, Burkitt lymphoma, and plasmablastic lymphoma.[10] Primary skin involvement is rare, but secondary cutaneous dissemination from a nodal or visceral NHL occurs.[11,12]

Surprisingly, mycosis fungoides (MF) may rarely develop in patients with HIV and should be distinguished from the uncommon benign epidermotropic CD8+ T-cell infiltrate that has been reported in HIV.[13] The latter condition may mimic MF clinically and pathologically.[14]

Immune reconstitution inflammatory syndrome

The paradoxical worsening of a partially treated condition or unmasking of an unrecognized or latent infection or other condition following the initiation of ART is referred to as IRIS. The risk of IRIS increases with lower CD4 cell count nadir. The onset may be weeks or months after starting ART.[1] *Table 19.1* lists conditions with skin involvement that have been associated with IRIS.

Acknowledgments

The author and editors would like to thank Pratista Ramdial for her contribution to the previous edition.

Access **ExpertConsult.com** for the complete list of references

Table 19.1
IRIS-associated infections and noninfectious pathologies of the skin

IRIS-associated infections	IRIS-associated noninfectious
Bacillary angiomatosis	Alopecia universalis
Blastomycosis	Acne
Cryptococcus	Eosinophilic folliculitis
Cytomegalovirus	Erythema elevatum diutinum
Crusted scabies	Lupus erythematosus –
Dermatophytosis	systemic and discoid
Epidermodysplasia verruciformis	Mid-dermal elastolysis
Fusariosis	Non-Hodgkin lymphoma
Herpes simplex	Papular pruritic eruption
Herpes zoster	Psoriasis
Histoplasmosis	Pyoderma gangrenosum
Kaposi sarcoma	Reactive arthritis
Leishmaniasis	Sarcoidosis
Leprosy	Seborrheic dermatitis
Molluscum contagiosum	Sweet syndrome
Mycobacterium avium complex	Urticaria
Paracoccidioidomycosis	
Pityriasis versicolor	
Secondary syphilis	
Sporotrichosis	
Strongyloidiasis – pruritus, rash	
Talaromycosis	
Tuberculosis – scrofuloderma	
Warts	

Adapted from Nelson, Manabe and Lucas.[1]

CHAPTER

20

Disorders of pigmentation

See
www.expertconsult.com
for references and
additional material

DISORDERS OF HYPOPIGMENTATION

Vitiligo

Clinical features

Vitiligo is a common acquired disease of unknown etiology characterized by loss of melanocytes resulting in macular areas of leukoderma that progressively enlarge and often become confluent.[1–4] The incidence has been calculated as between 1% and 2% of the population.[5,6] It affects all races but appears to be more common in people with dark skin. However, the latter may represent an overestimate, as the disease tends to be more noticeable in patients with darker skin. The sex incidence is equal, with a peak incidence between the ages of 10 and 30 years (up to 50% of cases). The disease is also seen in the very young and the elderly.[7–10] In children, the mean age of onset is 6 years and there appears to be a slight predilection for females.[9] Between 25% and 40% of patients have a positive family history of the disease; inheritance is non-mendelian, multifactorial, and polygenic.[6,11,12] In patients with a positive family history the disease usually appears earlier in life.[6] The frequency of the disease in siblings of affected patients is about 18 times that encountered in the general population.[6] Vitiligo affects monozygotic twins concordantly in about 23% of cases.[6]

The progression of vitiligo is slow and it is common for lesions to start on sun-exposed skin and usually with a symmetrical distribution (*Figs 20.1* and *20.2*).[13,14] Stress has been suggested as a precipitating event in vitiligo in a number of patients.[15] In a minority of cases involvement is unilateral. Segmental vitiligo refers to a variant of the disease presenting with linear or block-like distribution and erroneously described in the past as dermatomal.[16–18] The distribution of lesions in this type of vitiligo is more suggestive of mosaicism and presentation is in the first decades of life, with predilection for the face, early leukotrichia, and rapid progression followed by stabilization.[16] Generalized disease may be associated with segmental involvement in what is referred to as mixed pattern vitiligo and the latter is more commonly associated with halo nevi and leukotrichia.[19,20] Focal vitiligo is defined as a nonsegmental isolated lesion usually several centimeters in diameter.[16–18] Mucosal vitiligo is restricted to oral mucosa and genitals. In vitiligo, the skin over bony prominences is commonly affected, suggesting that repeated trauma may play a role. Involvement of flexural areas, genitalia, and the skin around the eyes and mouth is also frequently seen (*Fig. 20.3*). Premature graying of the hair is a common event and occurs even in children. Affected areas are prone to sunburn and the Koebner phenomenon may be seen (*Fig. 20.4*). Early lesions can have an erythematous 'inflammatory' border and in a minority of cases focal peripheral hyperpigmentation is a feature. Some patients describe mild pruritus in the early stages of the disease. The hairs within affected areas tend to remain pigmented but may lose the pigment in late stages (*Fig. 20.5*). A tanned zone between pigmented and completely nonpigmented skin is detected in some patients with darker skin. Known as trichrome vitiligo,[21,22] it tends to indicate the presence of active disease.[21] Activity is also indicated by inflammatory and confetti-like lesions. An unusual variant of inflammatory, figurate papulosquamous vitiligo has been documented.[23] Vitiligo can also develop in individuals exposed to phenolic compounds, particularly in cleaning solutions.[24] Patients may develop halo nevi (see *Fig. 20.4*) or vitiligo may develop after the development of halo nevi.[25,26] Generalized complete depigmentation is exceptional. Spontaneous repigmentation may be seen but it is patchy and tends to concentrate in perifollicular skin (*Fig. 20.6*). A case of repigmentation of

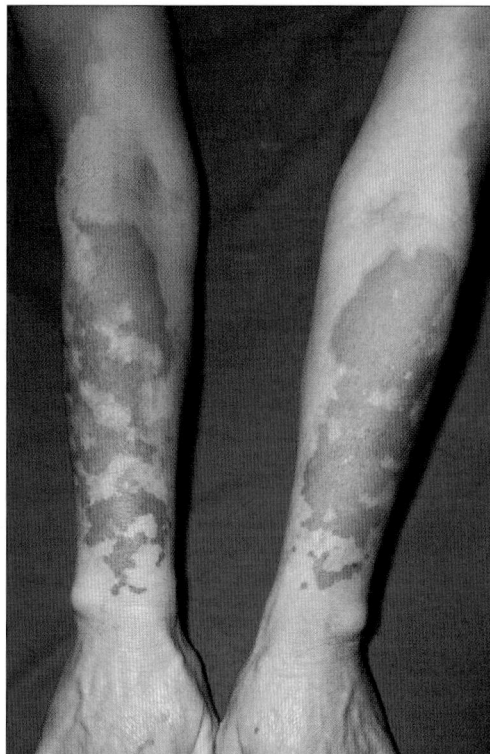

Fig. 20.1
Vitiligo: symmetrical involvement of the upper limbs. By courtesy of the Institute of Dermatology, London, UK.

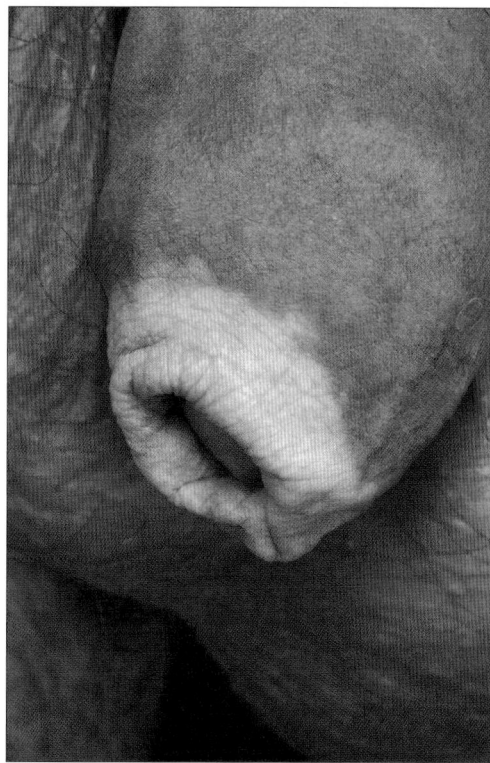

Fig. 20.3
Vitiligo: genital involvement is often seen in vitiligo. By courtesy of the Institute of Dermatology, London, UK.

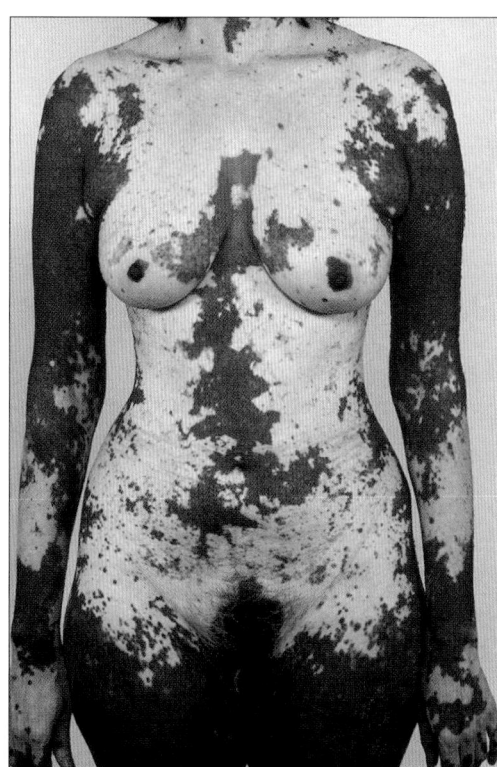

Fig. 20.2
Vitiligo: symmetrical involvement of the body. Note patchy repigmentation secondary to PUVA treatment. By courtesy of the Institute of Dermatology, London, UK.

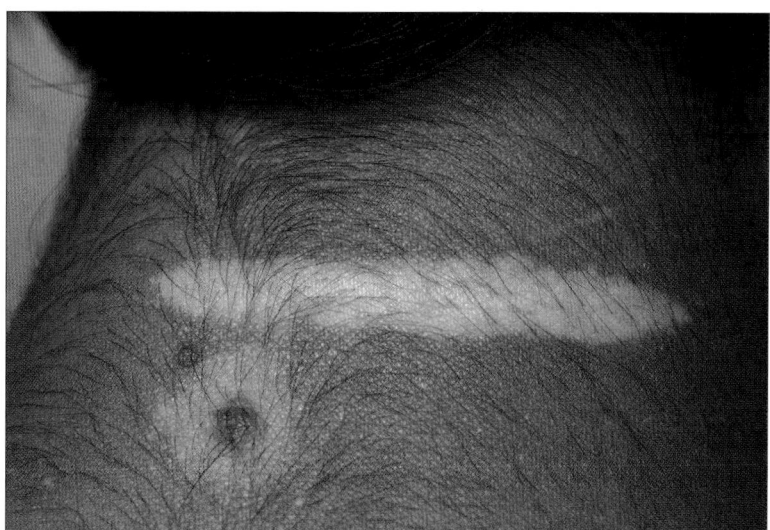

Fig. 20.4
Vitiligo: area of hypopigmentation due to the Koebner phenomenon and the presence of a halo nevus. These are frequent findings in vitiligo. By courtesy of the Institute of Dermatology, London, UK.

vitiligo after a beetle dermatitis has been documented.[27] Patients with the disease occasionally have uveitis, and an association with deafness has also been reported.[28,29]

Some patients with vitiligo develop actinic keratoses and squamous cell carcinomas on sun-exposed areas affected by the disease.[30,31] This occurrence is, however, not as high as might be expected and may be due to inadequate sun protection. Patients treated with psoralen plus ultraviolet light of A [long] wavelength (PUVA) may be more prone to develop skin cancer in the involved skin.[32]

Polymorphic light eruption lesions limited to areas of skin involved by vitiligo has been described.[33] Allergic contact dermatitis may exceptionally present as vitiligo.[34]

Vitiligo can be associated with numerous diseases, particularly (but not exclusively) those with a clear or suspected autoimmune basis. Autoimmune diseases may be seen in up to a third of patients with vitiligo. Patients with generalized vitiligo are more likely to have autoimmune disease. The latter associations include thyroid disease (hypo- and hyperthyroidism and Hashimoto disease), diabetes mellitus, Addison disease, and (much less commonly) alopecia areata, acanthosis nigricans, dermatitis

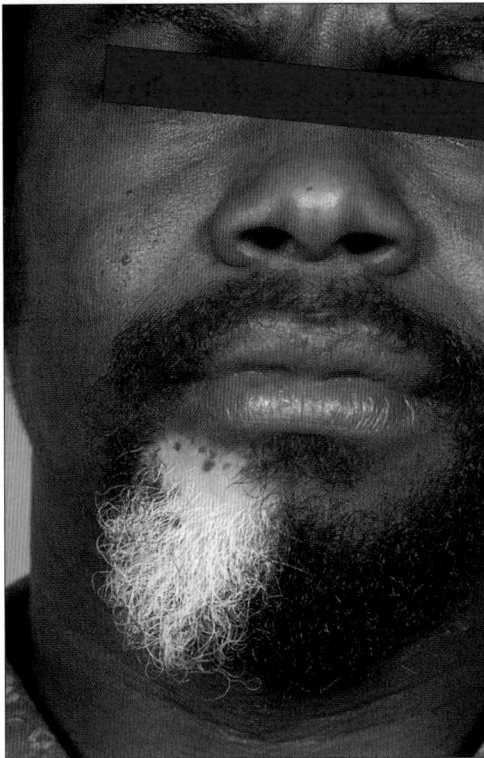

Fig. 20.5
Vitiligo: development of gray hair in a longstanding patch of vitiligo. By courtesy of the Institute of Dermatology, London, UK.

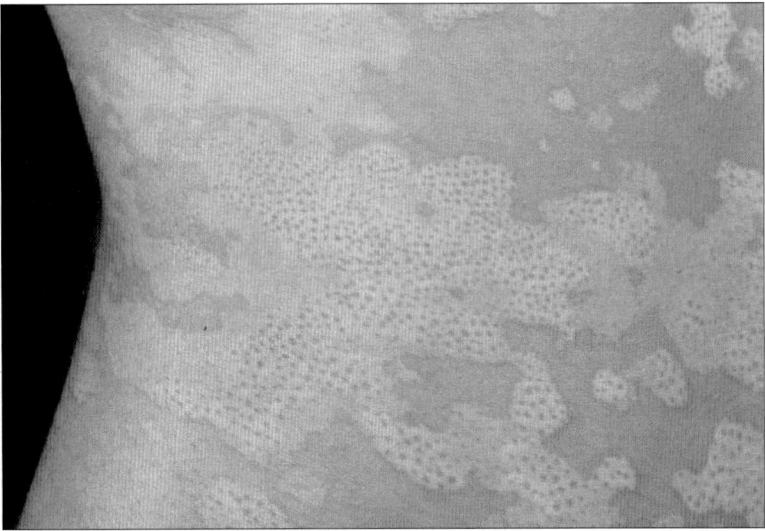

Fig. 20.6
Vitiligo: repigmentation in vitiligo frequently has a perifollicular distribution. By courtesy of the Institute of Dermatology, London, UK.

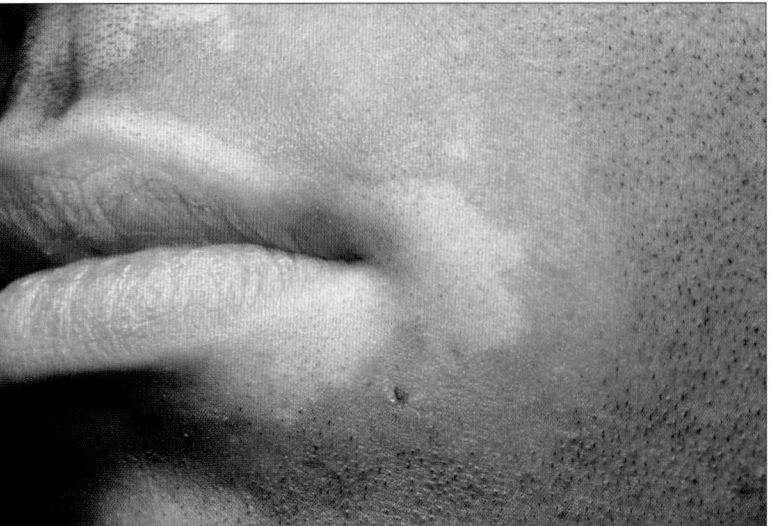

Fig. 20.7
Vitiligo: coexistence of vitiligo and alopecia areata. By courtesy of the Institute of Dermatology, London, UK.

herpetiformis, pernicious anemia, spondyloarthritis, and pemphigus vulgaris (*Fig. 20.7*).[35–45] The most frequent associations are with thyroid autoimmune disease, autoimmune gastritis, and alopecia areata.[46] Patients with Grave disease or Hashimoto thyroiditis have a risk of more than 10-fold of developing vitiligo.[47] Other reported associations of vitiligo include sarcoidosis, Crohn disease, morphea, lichen sclerosus, actinic granuloma, chronic mucocutaneous candidiasis, 20-nail dystrophy, chronic actinic dermatitis, psoriasis, lepromatous leprosy, AIDS, MELAS (mitochondrial encephalomyopathy, lactic acidosis and stroke-like episodes syndrome), frontoethmoidal meningoencephalocele, dysgammaglobulinemia, phakomatosis pigmentovascularis type IIa, and idiopathic CD4+ T-cell lymphocytopenia.[43,48–64] Unilateral involvement in association with trigeminal autonomic cephalalgia has also been described.[65] The vitiligo-spasticity syndrome seems to be a distinctive syndrome, mainly described in Arab patients but also documented in a patient of North European extraction.[66] Vitiligo may rarely occur at the site of radiotherapy.[67,68] A single case of Baboon syndrome (systemic contact dermatitis as a result of inhalation of mercury vapor) with segmental vitiligo has been reported.[69] Patients with melanoma rarely develop areas of leukoderma, not only around the tumor but also away from it and in association with metastasis.[70–74] Poliosis may also occur. Of note, it has been suggested that the prognosis is better in patients with leukoderma and melanoma.[72] It is controversial whether the depigmentation seen in patients with melanoma represents vitiligo.[71]

Rarely, a number of drugs have been associated with vitiligo. These include chloroquine, ganciclovir, interferon-alpha (IFN-α), tolcapone, levodopa, PUVA, and imiquimod.[72–83] Vitiligo has also occurred following narrow-band TL-01 phototherapy for psoriasis, at a site of allergic contact dermatitis to nickel, and after intense pulsed light treatment.[84–86] The disease has also been induced by a lymphocyte infusion in a patient with relapsed leukemia and there is a report of an exceptional case of transfer of vitiligo after allogeneic bone marrow transplantation.[87,88]

Pathogenesis

The pathogenesis of vitiligo remains obscure and there are a number of theories as to why the epidermal melanocytes are destroyed. It is likely that the disease is multifactorial, has an autoimmune basis, and in a number of cases, involves a genetic predisposition. Environmental factors may also be associated with the causation of the disease. Several of the mechanisms proposed are probably involved simultaneously.[89,90] They are likely to be interrelated and often, genetic predisposition plays a role. The inheritance is polygenic. Around 50 gene loci have been identified in association with vitiligo risk in genome-wide association and genetic linkage studies. The genes are associated with innate immunity or adaptive immunity, or are only related to melanocytes.[17,91,92]

The autoimmune hypothesis is based on the observation that patients with vitiligo have an associated autoimmune disease in 15% to 30% of cases.[15,35] Affected patients are also frequently found to have autoantibodies to gastric parietal, thyroid, and adrenal cells.[93] Antibodies to normal melanocytes have been reported in patients with vitiligo.[94–96] The level of these antibodies in the serum appears to correlate with disease activity.[95,97] Important links have been shown between generalized vitiligo and single-nucleotide polymorphisms at several loci associated with autoimmune diseases.[97] Interestingly, one of these associations is with a locus containing TYR, which encodes tyrosinase. A mutually exclusive relationship between the tendency to develop vitiligo and susceptibility to melanoma has been suggested.[98] Both antibody-dependent, cell-mediated cytotoxicity and direct destruction of melanocytes by antibodies have been proposed as mechanisms.[95,99] Although it was initially suggested that the antibodies

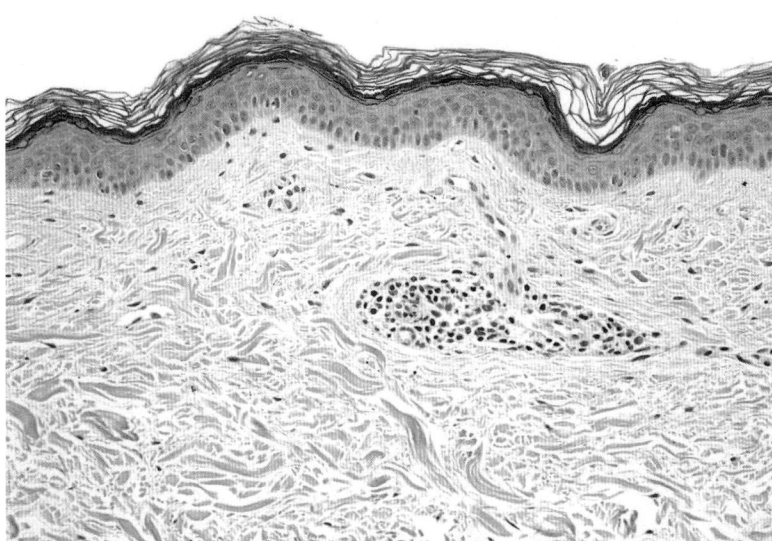

Fig. 20.8
Vitiligo: skin biopsy from lesional skin stained with hematoxylin and eosin. There is complete absence of melanocytes and melanin pigment. There is a light perivascular chronic inflammatory cell infiltrate.

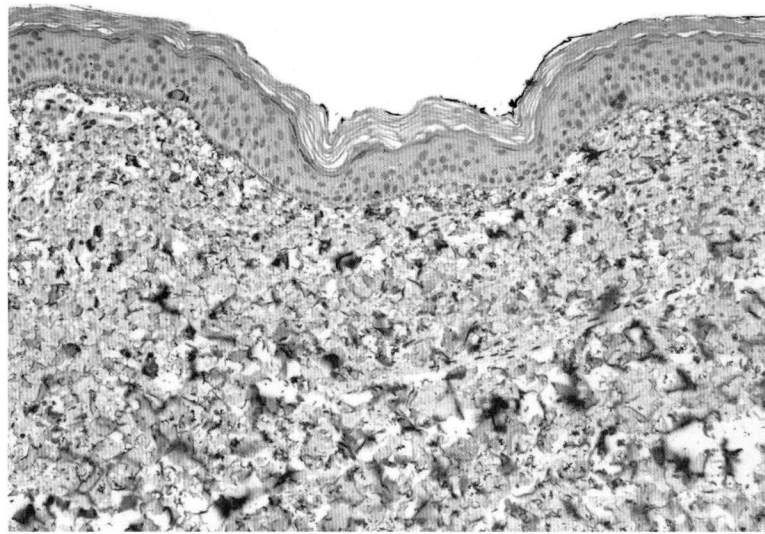

Fig. 20.9
Vitiligo: skin biopsy from lesional skin stained with S-100 protein. A single residual positive cell is present.

in the serum of patients are directed against tyrosinase, this view has been challenged.[100–103] The activation of natural killer (NK) cells by antibodies does not seem to play an important role in some studies.[104,105]

An important theory in the pathogenesis of vitiligo is referred to as the self-destruction theory.[106] This proposes that melanocytes are destroyed not only by toxic melanin precursors, such as free radicals, but also by melanin itself in predisposed individuals.[107] It is not clear, however, why these toxic melanin precursors and melanin affect the melanocytes in some individuals and not in others, but it may be that the mechanism for their disposal is faulty in patients who develop vitiligo. Experimental evidence is based on the fact that a number of chemicals, including phenols like monobenzyl ether of hydroquinone, induce pigmentary changes indistinguishable from vitiligo.[108] It has also been demonstrated that death of melanocytes in vitiligo results from increased sensitivity to oxidative stress.[109] The group of enzymes known as glutathione transferases is involved in protecting cells against toxic chemicals. Interestingly, it has been shown in a Chinese population that patients with GSTT1 and GSTM1-null genotypes have increased risk of developing vitiligo as compared to those that exhibit GSTP1 polymorphisms.[110] It has been proposed that an alteration in the membrane lipids of vitiligo cells after stress leads to mitochondrial damage and production of reactive oxygen species.[111] Thioredoxin domain containing 5 (TXNDC5) polymorphisms has been associated with the development of nonsegmental vitiligo in Korean patients.[112] TXNDC5 is a member of the thioredoxin family and its function resides in protein folding and chaperone activity against endoplasmic reticulum stress induced by oxidative stress. It is likely that affected cells activate inflammatory signals leading to the triggering of innate immunity by dendritic cells and NK cells, the former of which present melanocytic antigens to T cells. Melanocyte-specific CD8-positive T cells play a very active role in the destruction of melanocytes.[17,113,114] IFN-gamma seems to play a crucial role in the recruitment of CD8-positive T cells through the induction of CXCL10 and its receptor CXCR3.[115–117]

Histologic features

Microscopic examination of involved skin in vitiligo shows complete absence of melanocytes in association with total loss of epidermal pigmentation (Fig. 20.8). Biopsies from the periphery of lesions with a clinically inflammatory border show lymphocytes and histiocytes in the papillary dermis. Some inflammatory cells may also be found at the periphery, even in the absence of a clinically inflamed border. A prominent mononuclear inflammatory cell infiltrate is exceptional.[118] Degenerative changes have been documented in keratinocytes and melanocytes, not only from the border of lesions, but also from adjacent skin.[119,120] Degenerative changes in nerves and sweat glands have also been documented.[121] Absence of Merkel cells in lesional

skin was found in one study.[122] Other reported changes include increased numbers of Langerhans cells, epidermal vacuolization, and thickening of the basal membrane.[123] The loss of pigment and melanocytes in the epidermis is highlighted by a Masson-Fontana stain and by immunohistochemistry (Fig. 20.9). To avoid confusion with Langerhans cells (which are also S-100+) other melanocyte markers such as Melan-A and particularly microphthalmia transcription factor 1 (MITF1) or SOX10 (both expressed in the nuclei of melanocytes) may be used. Although both CD4- and CD8-positive cells are found within the infiltrate in active lesions, CD8-positive cells seem to predominate, appear to be associated with the damage at the dermal–epidermal junction, and are associated with the severity of the disease.[124,125] This has been shown both in generalized and segmental vitiligo.

Differential diagnosis

Distinction from guttate hypomelanosis is based on clinical presentation and on the complete absence of melanocytes in vitiligo, and the persistence of at least some melanocytes in the former. Distinction from postinflammatory hypopigmentation is based on the preservation of melanocytes with only loss of pigment in the latter. In the inflammatory stages of vitiligo, changes may mimic cutaneous T-cell lymphoma and distinction can be very difficult without close clinicopathological correlation.

Vogt-Koyanagi-Harada disease

Clinical features

Vogt-Koyanagi-Harada (VKH) (uveoencephalitis) disease is characterized by bilateral uveitis, poliosis, vitiligo, alopecia, dysacousia, and aseptic meningitis.[1–5] It is more common in females (2:1), particularly from Latin America, Asia, and Africa, and in Native Americans. It shows a predilection for adults, occurring only rarely in children. The initial phase of the disease usually starts with neurological symptoms and this is followed by ocular manifestations. In the acute phase, exudative retinal detachment is quite specific.[6] As the disease progresses, patients develop cutaneous manifestations with focal or diffuse alopecia areata, vitiligo (mainly head and trunk), and poliosis (eyebrows, lashes, and hair) in the chronic stage of the disease. In the latter phase, sunset glow fundus is often found.[6] It has been suggested that VKH disease is part of the spectrum of vitiligo with manifestations in other melanocyte-containing organs.[1] Not every patient displays all the manifestations of the syndrome. Ocular complications consist mainly of glaucoma and cataracts.[2,3] Rarely, the patches of depigmentation have an inflammatory edge.[7,8] The disease is exceptionally preceded by erythroderma.[9]

VKH disease has been described in association with diabetes, hypothyroidism, melanoma, ulcerative colitis, Graves disease, psoriasis, brainstem encephalitis, tuberculosis, bacille Calmette-Guérin (BCG) and influenza vaccination, and seronegative rheumatoid arthritis.[10–18] A possible association with combination therapy with IFN-α 2b/ribavirin and with ipilimumab and pembrolizumab for metastatic melanoma have been documented.[19–21]

Pathogenesis and histologic features

As with vitiligo, the pathogenesis of the disease remains unknown. An autoimmune etiology in which melanocytes are targeted is favored;[22] however, it is likely that the etiology is multifactorial. This is based on the occurrence of the disease in identical twins and after cutaneous injury.[23,24] An infectious etiology – particularly a virus – has been suggested in the past and this is supported by the simultaneous onset of the syndrome in a group of six patients living and working together.[25] An association with human leukocyte antigen (HLA)-DR53, HLA-DQ4, HLA-DR1, HLA-DR *0405 in Saudi Arabian patients, and HLA-DR4 in Brazilian patients suggests a genetic predisposition.[26,27] A study has raised the possibility that the disease is triggered by synergistic hyporesponsiveness of NK cells and cytotoxic T lymphocytes resulting in failure to mount an effective immune response as a result of a viral infection in genetically susceptible individuals (e.g., HLA-DR4 carriers).[28] A similar disease has been induced in rats by tyrosinase-related proteins TRP1 and TRP2, suggesting a role in the pathogenesis of the disease.[29] Increased susceptibility to the disease has been suggested in Han Chinese as a result of hypermethylation of GATA3 and transforming growth factor (TGF)-ß.[30] Susceptibility loci have been identified at chromosomes 1p31.2 and 10q21.3.[31]

The histopathology of the areas of cutaneous depigmentation is identical to that seen in vitiligo. In a single case report of a patient presenting with inflammatory vitiligo, filamentous masses and amyloid were described.[8] The histologic findings in areas of alopecia are identical to those seen in alopecia areata.[32] However, more prominent release of melanin has been described, suggesting that the prime targets are the melanocytes within the hair follicle rather than the keratinocytes, as in classic alopecia areata.[32]

Idiopathic guttate hypomelanosis

Clinical features

Idiopathic guttate hypomelanosis is a common asymptomatic dermatosis first described in 1951.[1] It is characterized by a few to numerous white macules developing on sun-exposed skin, particularly the extensor surfaces of forearms and legs of middle aged to elderly patients, with no sex predilection (Fig. 20.10).[2–4] Presentation in early life is exceptional and only rarely do lesions occur on the face and trunk.[5,6] Most lesions are 5 mm or less in diameter. The condition affects all races and there is some suggestion of an increased familial incidence.[7] Spontaneous repigmentation does not tend to occur. Lesions identical to those seen in this disease may also be a feature of Darier disease and develop following PUVA therapy.[8,9]

Pathogenesis and histologic features

The exact pathogenesis of idiopathic guttate hypomelanosis remains unknown. It is likely that the cause of the disease is multifactorial. Factors that have been involved in its causation include inheritance, ultraviolet (UV) light, and loss of melanocytes due to aging in addition to autoimmunity.[4–7,10–12] An association with HLA-DQ3 was found in a group of renal transplant patients with the disease while a similar group of renal transplant patients without the disease had HLA-DR8, suggesting that the latter may have a protective effect.[13]

The main histologic feature consists of variable loss of melanin granules in epidermal keratinocytes. This is sometimes associated with epidermal atrophy and flattening of the rete ridges. Orthokeratotic hyperkeratosis in a basket-weave pattern has also been documented.[7] A Masson-Fontana stain is useful to highlight the loss of epidermal melanin, and a dopa oxidase reaction reveals a patchy reduction in the number of melanocytes.[2] However, complete loss of melanocytes is not a feature. Hypopigmented keratosis

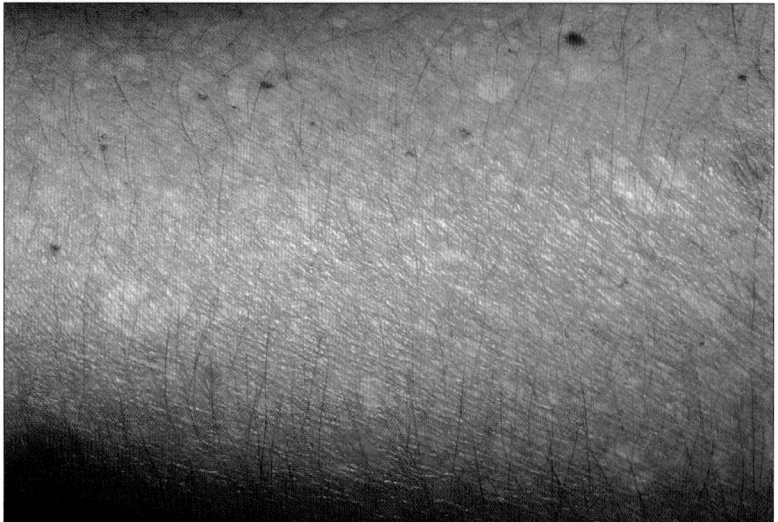

Fig. 20.10
Guttate hypomelanosis: multiple small hypopigmented macules in sun-exposed skin. By courtesy of O. Dueñas, MD, Bogotá, Colombia.

has been proposed as a variant of guttate hypomelanosis with prominent hyperkeratosis.[14]

Electron microscopy studies confirm the reduction in the number of melanocytes. Changes described in melanocytes include cytoplasmic vacuolization and decrease or loss of mature melanosomes.[5,6,11,15] Although the number of Langerhans cells is normal, a reduction in the number of Birbeck granules has been documented.[10]

Differential diagnosis

The clinical differential diagnosis is very wide and includes lichen sclerosus, hypopigmented mycosis fungoides, atrophie blanche, vitiligo, pityriasis versicolor, leprosy, and the hypopigmented lesions seen in tuberous sclerosis. Most of these entities are easy to exclude histologically except for vitiligo. In the latter, there is complete absence of melanocytes and this can be confirmed with a melanocyte-specific immunostain such as Melan-A, since S-100 also stains Langerhans cells.

Oculocutaneous albinism

The term 'albinism' is used to refer to a heterogeneous group of autosomal recessive conditions resulting from diverse genetic abnormalities that cause absent or reduced production of melanin pigment but no reduction in the total number of melanocytes (Fig. 20.11).[1,2] The genetic abnormality may result in eye involvement only (ocular albinism) or may combine involvement of the eyes, hair, and skin (oculocutaneous albinism). Here, only the different types of oculocutaneous albinism will be discussed.

At least 15 different gene mutations leading to different types of albinism have been identified.[3] The prevalence of oculocutaneous albinism is around 1:17 000.[4] The clinical manifestations of oculocutaneous albinism depend on the type of biochemical abnormality. In all types of albinism, the lack of melanin in the developing eye results in hypoplasia of the fovea and abnormal routing of the optic nerves. As a result, all patients have variable strabismus, nystagmus, and reduced visual acuity.[4] Affected patients often have an increased risk of skin cancer (Figs 20.12 and 20.13). Based on clinical features alone, it is not always possible to separate the different types of oculocutaneous albinism.

The most common types of albinism are oculocutaneous albinism types IA and II. Most types are inherited in an autosomal recessive manner and affect all races.[5,6] Prenatal diagnosis of oculocutaneous albinism is possible.[7,8] Rare variants of albinism are associated with systemic manifestations and include the Hermansky-Pudlak and the Chédiak-Higashi syndromes (see below). The different types of oculocutaneous albinism and the histopathology of all variants are discussed briefly.

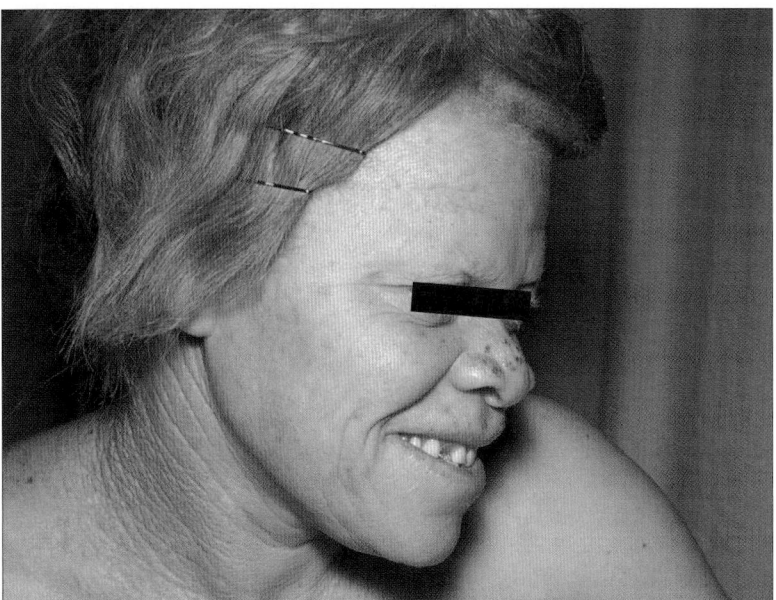

Fig. 20.11
Oculocutaneous albinism: the hair is red and there is complete loss of skin pigmentation with some freckling and actinic damage. By courtesy of the Institute of Dermatology, London, UK.

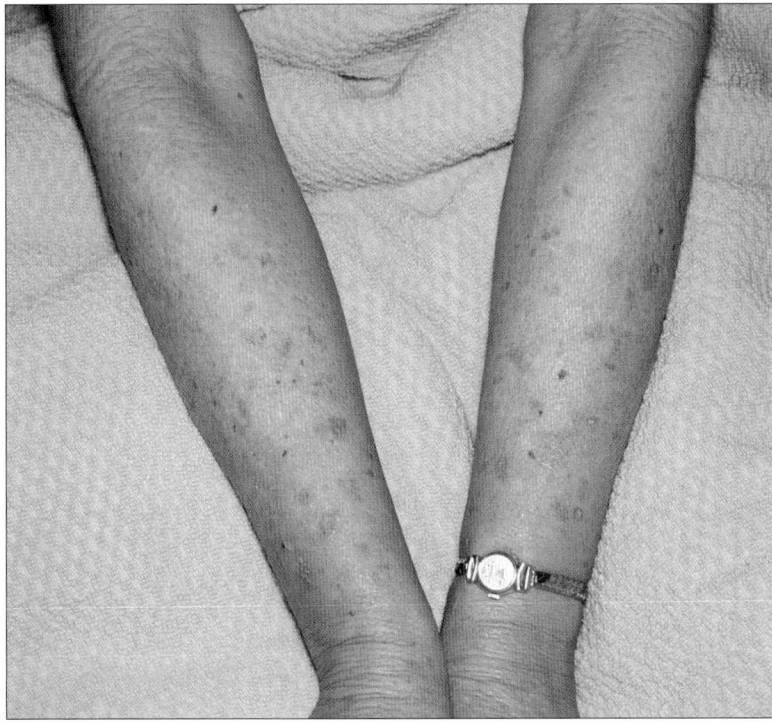

Fig. 20.12
Oculocutaneous albinism: numerous actinic keratoses on sun-exposed skin. By courtesy of the Institute of Dermatology, London, UK.

Oculocutaneous albinism type IA

Type IA oculocutaneous albinism is the most severe variant and is characterized by complete absence of tyrosinase activity in melanocytes. It is seen in all races, but it is very rare in blacks. The prevalence is 1 in 40 000. At birth, patients have white hair, white or pink skin, and blue or gray eyes. Visual acuity is severely reduced. Patients usually do not have nevi or, if present, they are amelanotic and with sun exposure develop dark-brown freckles. Sun exposure leads to severe skin damage with an increased risk of skin cancer, including basal cell carcinoma, squamous cell carcinoma, and (rarely) melanoma.[9–13] A case of leukodystrophy and oculocutaneous albinism type IA has been documented.[14]

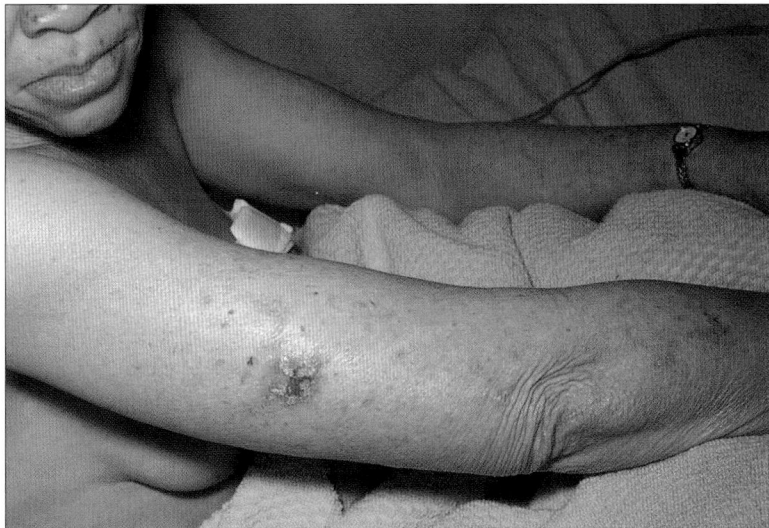

Fig. 20.13
Oculocutaneous albinism: an early squamous cell carcinoma on sun-exposed skin. By courtesy of the Institute of Dermatology, London, UK.

Pathogenesis

In all variants of albinism melanocytes and melanosomes are normal. The reduction or absence of melanin results from a biochemical abnormality in the synthesis of the pigment. The gene for tyrosinase has been cloned to chromosome 11q14.3. Numerous different mutations in the gene lead to absence of tyrosinase activity and the manifestations of the disease.[4,15–18]

Oculocutaneous albinism type IB

Oculocutaneous albinism type IB (yellow mutant) is uncommon and characterized by greatly reduced tyrosinase activity. It appears to be more common in Amish communities living in the United States.[19] The hair of affected patients is white at birth and becomes yellow after a few months and light brown by the end of the second decade. The skin is milky white and becomes slightly tanned after sun exposure. The irises are gray. Visual acuity is better than in type IA disease and there is a lower incidence of skin cancer.

Pathogenesis

The changes are the result of markedly reduced synthesis of melanin due to mutations in the tyrosinase gene located in chromosome 11q14.3.

Type I variants

Other type I variants of oculocutaneous albinism include type I (temperature sensitive) and type I (minimal pigment). Each of these variants is thought to result from different mutant alleles at the tyrosinase locus.[20]

Type II oculocutaneous albinism

Type II oculocutaneous albinism (tyrosinase positive) is the most common type of oculocutaneous albinism. The color of the hair varies according to the race of the individual. All races have pale skin but in black patients, skin is brown and the irises are gray. The hair in Caucasian individuals is white or light yellow at birth and turns dark yellow during the first two decades of life.[5] In individuals of African origin, the hair is yellow at birth and becomes dark yellow in the first two decades. Patients often develop nevi, lentigines, and freckles, which are particularly prominent on sun-exposed skin.

Pathogenesis

Oculocutaneous albinism type II is caused by mutations in the gene OCA2 (previously known as P-gene), which has been mapped to chromosome 15q11-q12.[21–24] The OCA2 protein is important in the formation of melanosomes and in transport of melanosomal proteins TYR and TYRP1.[24] It has been demonstrated that mutations in the melanocortin-1 receptor (MC1R) gene modify the classic phenotype seen in oculocutaneous albinism type II.[25]

Type III oculocutaneous albinism

Type III oculocutaneous albinism (rufous albinism) is also referred to as red oculocutaneous albinism. It is mainly seen in patients from Africa and New Guinea and exceptionally in patients from Pakistan.[26] A single Caucasian patient has been reported.[27] It results in red or ginger hair and red/brown skin.[28,29] Visual anomalies are not always present.

Pathogenesis

Affected individuals are tyrosinase positive. The disease is caused by mutations in the tyrosinase-related protein 1 (TRP1), an important enzyme in melanin synthesis.[30] The mutation results in delayed maturation and early degradation of tyrosinase. Electron microscopy examination reveals smaller melanosomes, aggregates of melanosomes within keratinocytes, and increase in pheomelanin synthesis.[31]

Oculocutaneous albinism type IV

Oculocutaneous albinism type IV (brown) is a very rare variant of oculocutaneous albinism and is mainly seen in patients of African or Japanese origin.[5,32] It is very rare in Europeans. Clinically, it is not possible to distinguish it from oculocutaneous albinism type II. Lentigines and freckles are rare. The hair is light brown and there is slight increase in pigmentation with age.

Pathogenesis

Oculocutaneous albinism type IV is caused by mutations in the membrane-associated transporter protein (MATP) gene in chromosome 5p13.3.[33,34] The function of the protein is unknown, but it probably acts as a membrane transporter in melanosomes.[34]

Oculocutaneous albinism type V

Oculocutaneous albinism type V was described in a family from Pakistan with golden hair.

Pathogenesis

A locus has been mapped to chromosome 4q24, but the specific gene has not yet been identified.[35,36]

Oculocutaneous albinism type VI

Oculocutaneous albinism type VI is a recently described variant in which patients present with variable skin color ranging from white to light brown to blond.[37,38] Some patients display nevi. It has been described in various ethnic groups.

Pathogenesis

This variant of oculocutaneous albinism is associated with mutations in SLC24A5 located on chromosome 15q21.1 and encoding a protein that appears to play a role in the maturation of melanosomes.[37,38]

Oculocutaneous albinism type VII

Oculocutaneous albinism type VII is a recently described variant in which patients present with light skin and prominent eye symptoms.[36,38] It was originally described in individuals from the Faroe Islands and latterly in a patient from Lithuania.[39]

Pathogenesis

This variant of oculocutaneous albinism is associated with mutations in C10orf11 located on chromosome 10.[38,39] Its function is unknown.

Chédiak-Higashi syndrome and Hermansky-Pudlak syndrome are described below.

Histologic features (in all types of oculocutaneous albinism)

Skin biopsies from individuals with oculocutaneous albinism show reduced or complete absence of melanin in the epidermis and hair follicles, depending on the type of oculocutaneous albinism. The melanocytes are normal.

Ultrastructural studies show no defects in either melanocytes or melanosomes.

Hermansky-Pudlak syndrome

Clinical features

Hermansky-Pudlak syndrome is a very rare heterogeneous disorder inherited in an autosomal recessive manner. It is characterized by partial tyrosinase positive oculocutaneous albinism, platelet storage deficiency with bleeding diathesis, and the accumulation of ceroid in the cytoplasm of macrophages.[1-6] These macrophages are found in various organs including the skin and lung; pulmonary fibrosis is a frequent complication and leads to death.[1,2] Additional manifestations include frequent infections, granulomatous colitis, and (more rarely) renal involvement leading to renal failure.[2-7] Other cutaneous features include trichomegaly, dysplastic nevi, actinic keratoses, basal cell carcinomas, and lesions resembling acanthosis nigricans.[8] The phenotypic range of the disease is wide. The disease has mainly been described in Puerto Rico and people of Ashkenazi Jewish heritage and is exceptional in Europe.

Pathogenesis and histologic features

There are eight variants of the disease involving the following genes: HPS1, AP3B1 (HPS2), HPS3, HPS4, HPS5, HPS6, DTNBP1 (HPS7), and BLOC1S3 (HPS8). Mutations in these genes give rise to the HPS subtypes 1 to 8, respectively.[9-11] A further type associated with mutations in AP3D1 and presenting with immunodeficiency and seizures has been described.[12] The syndrome is thought to be due to abnormal trafficking to lysosomes and related organelles, including melanosomes and platelet dense granules. It also affects T cells, neutrophils, and lung type II epithelial cells. Some variants of the disease are due to mutations in the adaptor-related code complex (AP-3) subunits.[13] The role of the latter is to facilitate transport of vesicles from the Golgi apparatus and endosomal compartments. It has been demonstrated that the gene defects causing the disease in mice block melanosome biogenesis.[14] The mechanisms of hypopigmentation demonstrated in mice consist of:

- exocytosis of immature hypopigmented melanosomes from melanocytes with subsequent keratinocyte uptake,
- decreased intramelanocyte steady-state number of melanosomes available for transfer to keratinocytes,
- an accumulation of melanosomes within melanocytes.[14]

The histologic features are similar to those of other forms of oculocutaneous albinism, with reduction in the amount of melanin in the epidermis and hair follicles.

Chédiak-Higashi syndrome

Clinical features

Chédiak-Higashi syndrome is an uncommon autosomal recessive multisystem disorder characterized by partial oculocutaneous albinism, severe immunological dysfunction resulting in recurrent bacterial infections, a bleeding tendency, progressive neurological dysfunction, particularly peripheral neuropathy, and severe periodontitis.[1-9] Characteristically, many cells (including melanocytes, myeloid cells, and lymphocytes) contain peroxidase-positive giant granules. The majority of patients die early in childhood as a result of either bacterial infection or an accelerated phase characterized by diffuse infiltration of organs (e.g., liver, spleen), lymph nodes, and bone marrow by lymphocytes and histiocytes.[1,3] The accelerated phase is only rarely the first manifestation of the disease.[10]

Hemophagocytosis is common, as are hepatosplenomegaly, anemia, thrombocytopenia, and neutropenia. About 10% of patients survive into adulthood but usually succumb to progressive neurological disease. Bone marrow transplant has a dramatic effect in preventing recurrent infections; it also prevents the accelerated phase of the disease but not the progressive neurological deterioration.[11]

The defect in pigmentation may affect skin, hair, and eyes. Affected individuals usually have light silvery hair, and speckled hyper- and hypopigmentation of exposed areas may be seen.[12] Patches of hyperpigmentation mainly seen in sun-exposed areas are, however, rare.[13]

Pathogenesis and histologic features

The tendency to develop recurrent infections is due to impaired chemotaxis and abnormal NK-cell function. Chédiak-Higashi syndrome and Hermansky-Pudlak syndrome (see above) are regarded as disorders of vesicle formation and trafficking.[3,4,14-16] The gene for Chédiak-Higashi syndrome has been mapped to chromosome 1 and has been designated CHS1/LYST. The gene encodes a cytosolic protein of 430 kD. The exact function of this protein in vesicle trafficking is as yet unknown.[3,4]

A biopsy from involved skin shows marked reduction in the amount of melanin present in the epidermis and hair follicles. Giant melanosomes may be seen. These – and the giant granules found in other cells – are the result of giant lysosomes formed during fusion and phagocytosis.[14,17]

Giant melanosomes and smaller granules can be demonstrated in melanocytes by electron microscopy. Giant cytoplasmic granules have also been documented in Langerhans cells.[18]

Griscelli syndrome

Clinical features

Griscelli syndrome is a rare disease inherited in an autosomal recessive fashion and characterized by skin hypopigmentation, silver-gray hair, neurological abnormalities, and recurrent infections secondary to immunodeficiency (*Fig. 20.14*).[1-3] Other features include hepatosplenomegaly, pancytopenia, hypoproteinemia, hypofibrinogenemia, and hypertriglyceridemia. Patients with neurological manifestations but no immunological problems are classified as Griscelli syndrome type 1. Many of the manifestations of the disease are secondary to the presence of hemophagocytic lymphohistiocytosis and severe immunodeficiency – these patients are classified as Griscelli syndrome type 2.[1,4,5] The two phenotypes of the disease correlate with the type of genetic mutation (see below). A third type of the syndrome presents only with hypopigmentation: Griscelli syndrome type 3.[6,7] All patients with any subtype of the disease share the presence of hypopigmentation and silver-gray hair. Examination of hair shafts reveals prominent accumulation of melanin. An association with myelodysplastic syndrome has also been documented. Most clinical manifestations occur between the age of 4 months and 4 years. Unless bone marrow transplant is performed early in the course of the disease in patients with Griscelli syndrome type 2, death invariably occurs.[8]

Pathogenesis and histologic features

The gene maps to chromosome 15q21 and mutations in two genes located in this region – MYO5a (myosin-Va gene) (Griscelli syndrome type 1) and RAB27A (GTP-binding protein) (Griscelli syndrome type 2) – have been described.[9] RAB27A protein appears to be involved in the control of the immune system as patients with mutations of this protein (but not those with mutations of myosin-Va gene) develop hemophagocytic lymphohistiocytosis.[9] T cells deficient in this protein also show decrease in cytotoxic activity. In Griscelli syndrome type 3 there are mutations of either the melanophilin gene (MLPH) or deletions of MYO5A F-exon.[7] Although, in general, there is correlation between genotype and phenotype, a number of cases display genotypic-phenotypic disparity.[10,11]

A skin biopsy from affected skin reveals that melanin is present in basal melanocytes but absent in keratinocytes. Examination of involved hair shafts reveals irregular clumps of melanin, particularly in the medulla of the hair shaft (*Fig. 20.15*). Cutaneous granulomas due to the immunodeficiency have been reported in Griscelli type 2.[12]

Differential diagnosis

Distinction between Griscelli and Chédiak-Higashi syndromes is possible with the use of polarized light to examine hair shafts. In both conditions, larger than normal melanin granules are seen.[13] However, in the latter disease, the granules are evenly distributed with bright and polychromatic appearance under polarized light. In Griscelli syndrome, granules are larger and more irregular, tend to aggregate near the medulla, and have a white appearance under polarized light.

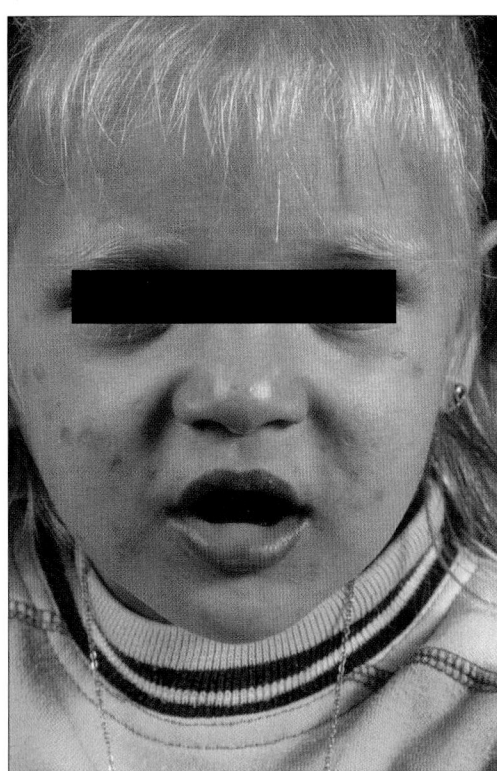

Fig. 20.14
Griscelli syndrome: cutaneous hypopigmentation and silvery hair. By courtesy of M. Canningavan, MD, University of Utrecht, the Netherlands.

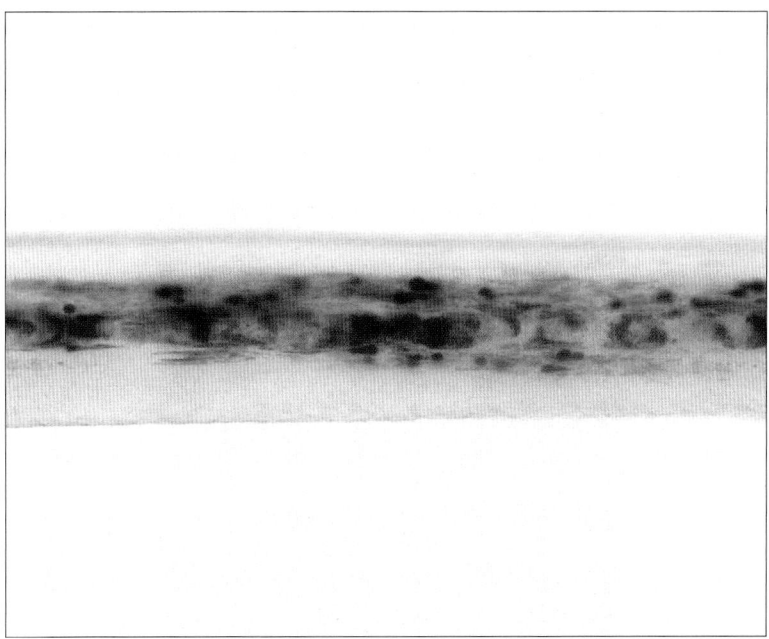

Fig. 20.15
Griscelli syndrome: clumps of melanin within hair shafts. By courtesy of M. Canningavan, MD, University of Utrecht, the Netherlands.

Elejalde syndrome

Elejalde syndrome (also known as neuroectodermal melanolysosomal syndrome) is an autosomal recessive disease presenting in infancy. It probably represents a variant of Griscelli syndrome type 1 and is characterized by skin hypopigmentation, silvery hair, bronze skin color after sun exposure and severe neurological impairment with seizures, severe hypotonia, and mental retardation.[1–4] It differs from Griscelli syndrome in that patients have no immunological abnormalities.

Histology of involved hair and skin shows features similar to those seen in Griscelli syndrome (see above).

Piebaldism

Clinical features

Piebaldism is a rare congenital disorder inherited in an autosomal dominant manner. In the past, the name 'partial albinism' was used as a synonym but this term is no longer accepted, as piebaldism is not considered to be a variant of albinism.[1] It is characterized by localized macular areas of hypopigmentation and affects all races, with the same sex incidence.[2,3] The central area of the forehead, the anterior trunk, and the mid areas of the extremities are characteristically affected (Figs 20.16 and 20.17). There may be involvement of the eyelashes and of the medial aspect of the eyebrows but the hands, feet, and back are usually spared. In 90% of cases there is a white forelock in the frontal mid scalp (Fig. 20.18); this may be the only manifestation of the disease. Poliosis circumscripta refers the absence of pigment in a circumscribed hairy area and, although more frequently seen on the scalp, it can affect many areas of the body, including the eyebrows and eyelashes. Poliosis is not specific of piebaldism and can be associated with other genetic conditions, including Waardenburg syndrome, neoplastic conditions, and even medications. The macular areas of hypopigmentation vary in size from 1 cm to several centimeters. They are usually stable and show no progression, but rarely contraction, expansion of lesions, or exceptionally complete regression has been documented.[4,5] Areas of hyperpigmentation may be seen either within the patches of hypopigmentation or in normally pigmented skin. Café-au-lait spots are a frequent finding and intertriginous freckling may also be seen. An association with neurofibromatosis

type 1 has been documented and in an affected family a p.Gly610Asp mutation in the KIT gene was found; however, this relationship has been doubted, as the reported patients had no neurofibromas and the current consensus is that they are not related.[6–11] Piebaldism has been described in association with Hirschsprung disease and with dyserythropoietic anemia type II.[12–14]

Pathogenesis and histologic features

Point mutations and deletions in the kit proto-oncogene have been demonstrated in most patients with piebaldism.[15–23] These different point mutations and deletions are responsible for the range of phenotypes seen in affected patients. The KIT gene encodes a cell-surface transmembrane receptor – tyrosine kinase – for the stem/mast cell growth factor. The gene has been mapped to chromosome 4q11-q12. The different severity of presentation is

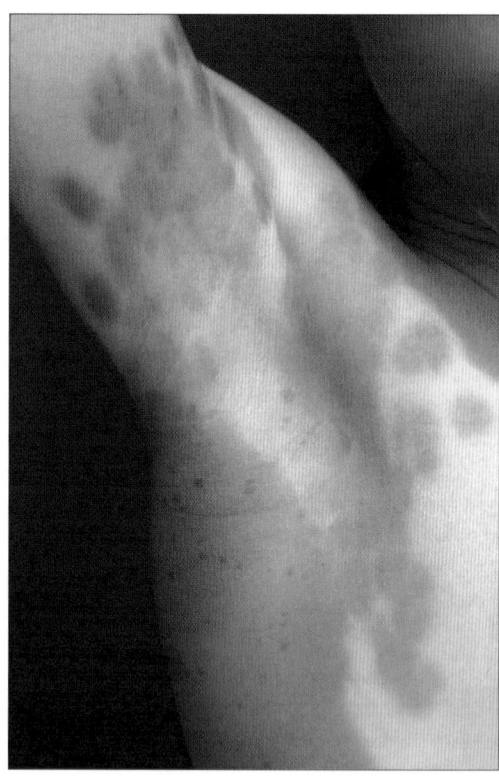

Fig. 20.17
Piebaldism: hypopigmentation of the trunk and proximal limbs. By courtesy of the Institute of Dermatology, London, UK.

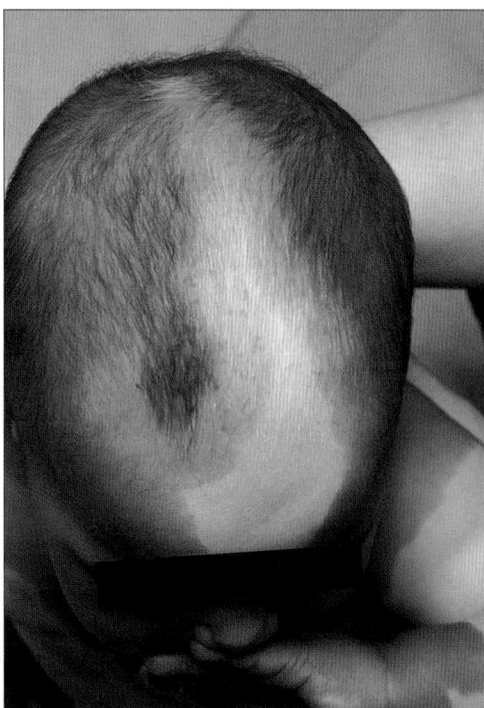

Fig. 20.16
Piebaldism: patchy hypopigmentation of the scalp. By courtesy of the Institute of Dermatology, London, UK.

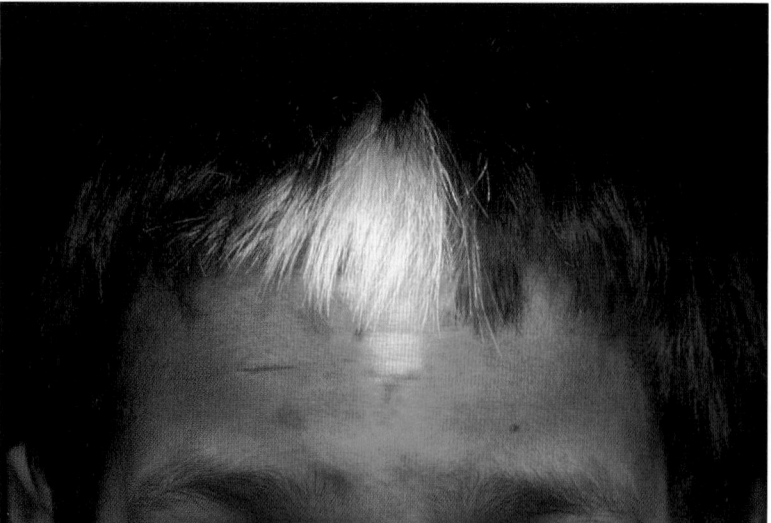

Fig. 20.18
Piebaldism: typical white forelock. By courtesy of the Institute of Dermatology, London, UK.

associated with truncated mutations in the tyrosine kinase domain resulting in haploinsufficiency or a dominant-negative effect.[24]

In some patients in whom KIT mutations are not demonstrated, deletion of the SLUG gene, mapped to chromosome 8, has been documented.[25] SLUG is a zinc-finger neural crest transcription factor, which is critical for the development of hematopoietic stem cells, melanoblasts, and germ cells in the mouse.

Histologic examination of affected skin usually shows complete absence of melanocytes, and this is confirmed by ultrastructural studies.[1,26] Abnormal melanocytes may be seen in areas of transition between involved and normal skin.

Waardenburg syndrome

Clinical features

Waardenburg syndrome is a rare heterogeneous, often but not always autosomal dominant condition characterized by a white forelock and areas of cutaneous hypopigmentation (piebaldism), congenital sensorineural deafness, partial or total iris heterochromia, confluent eyebrows, a broad nasal root, and dystopia canthorum (increase in the distance between the inner angles of the eyelids).[1,2] The patches of hypopigmentation are seen in about 20% of patients, are present at birth, involve the face, neck, anterior chest, abdomen, and limbs, and tend to remain stationary throughout life. Hyperpigmented patches are exceptional.[3] Some patients lack the white forelock and in a percentage of these there is premature graying of the hair in early adulthood. An association with Hirschsprung disease has been described.[4,5] The incidence of clinical manifestations varies in different patients and, based on this, four variants of the syndrome have been described:

- Waardenburg syndrome I,
- Waardenburg syndrome II,
- Waardenburg syndrome III (Klein-Waardenburg),
- Waardenburg syndrome IV (Shah-Waardenburg).

The difference between types I and II is based on the absence of dystopia canthorum in type II. In the latter, neurological abnormalities may also be found.[6] Deafness tends to be more common in the latter. In type III the manifestations are similar to type I but in addition there are congenital musculoskeletal abnormalities of the upper limbs including flexion contractures and muscle hypoplasia. In type IV there is absence of dystopia canthorum and an association with Hirschsprung disease.[7] In a number of patients with type IV disease there are associated neurological abnormalities including peripheral neuropathy, cerebellar ataxia, mental retardation, and spasticity.[8] A subtype of type IV disease is known as PCHW (peripheral demyelinating neuropathy, central dysmyelinating leukodystrophy, Waardenburg syndrome, Hirschsprung disease).

Pathogenesis and histologic features

Mutations in the PAX-3 gene located on chromosome 2q37 have been reported in Waardenburg syndrome types I and III.[9–11] Mutations in the MITF gene located on chromosome 3p14.1-p12.3 and SOX10 are responsible for about 30% of cases of the cases of Waardenburg syndrome type II.[12,13] EDNRB (endothelin receptor type B) mutations are found in the heterozygous state in between 5% to 6% of cases. In the rest, a specific mutation has not been identified.[13,14] Type IV syndrome is associated with mutations in the endothelin 3 gene and in the endothelin receptor type 3.[15] Cases with neurological disease also show mutations in SOX10 and the latter has been associated with type II syndrome with or without neurological symptoms.[6,16]

Histologically, the patches of hypopigmentation in all variants of the disease show absence or reduction in the number of epidermal melanocytes.

Nevus anemicus

Clinical features

Nevus anemicus is a congenital anomaly characterized by an asymptomatic, ill-defined patch of slightly hypopigmented skin with predilection for the trunk.[1–3] Some cases involve the face or extremities. The area of hypopigmented skin usually measures several centimeters and may contain small patches of normal skin. A case of generalized nevus anemicus has been documented.[4] Nevus anemicus is often associated with port-wine stain, nevus spilus, lymphedema, phakomatosis pigmentovascularis, tuberous sclerosis, and capillary malformation-arteriovenous malformation syndrome.[5–10] It has also been recently reported as a newly noted manifestation of neurofibromatosis type 1.[11,12] Lesions are more frequently noted in younger patients.[13] Nevus oligemicus has been described as a variant of nevus anemicus.[14,15]

Pathogenesis and histologic features

The pathogenesis of nevus anemicus is not clear. It has been suggested that the anomaly is a form of capillary malformation and may result from localized vasoconstriction due to increased levels of catecholamines.[3,4,16,17] A recent study demonstrated that the vessels in nevus anemicus do not respond normally to proinflammatory cytokines.[18]

Histopathology of involved skin appears unremarkable.

Nevus depigmentosus

Clinical features

Nevus depigmentosus (also known as nevus achromicus) is a common nevoid abnormality present in 0.5% to 1.25% of neonates or develops in the first few years of life.[1–3] A single, well-defined, macular, rounded hypopigmented patch, ranging in size from less than 1 cm to several centimeters, is characteristically seen.[4,5] In rare cases the distribution may be segmental or systematized along Blaschko lines (Fig. 20.19).[6–8] In the latter setting the lesion resembles hypomelanosis of Ito. There is predilection for the trunk and proximal extremities. In one case, involvement of the iris was seen.[9] Rare associations include pes cavus, mental retardation, hemihypertrophy, inflammatory linear verrucous epidermal nevus, lentiginosis (unilateral or segmental), congenital linear punctate keratoderma, Becker nevus, nevus flammeus, nevus spilus, and eccrine angiomatous nevus.[6,10–17] In rare cases, melanocytic nevi or lentigines may develop within lesions of nevus depigmentosus, in one case lentigines developed after UVB therapy, and in a further case a nevus depigmentosus with lentigines was associated with underlying breast hypoplasia.[18–23]

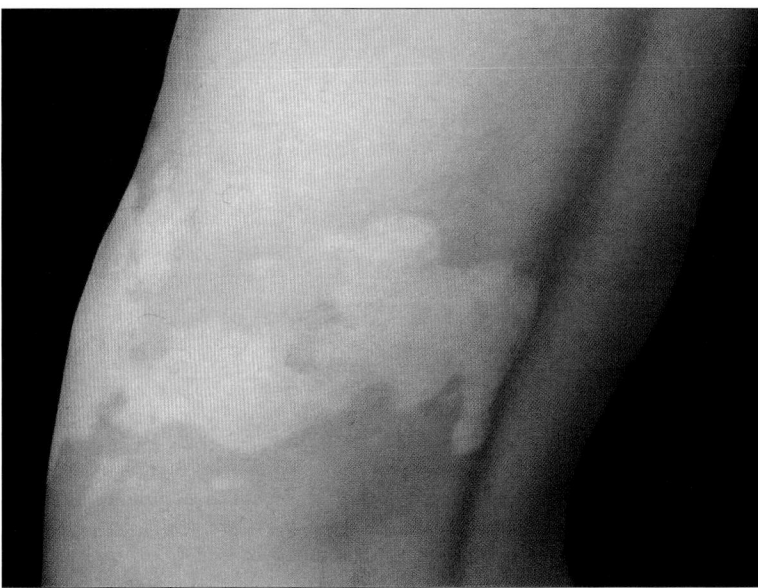

Fig. 20.19
Nevus depigmentosus: segmental distribution. By courtesy of the Institute of Dermatology, London, UK.

Pathogenesis and histologic features

The etiology of nevus depigmentosus is as yet unknown but in cases with a systematized distribution it has been suggested that the lesion is the result of a somatic mutation.[7]

Histology has been reported as showing a normal or reduced number of melanocytes.[3] More recently, however, it has been suggested that there is decreased pigmentation but a normal number of melanocytes.[3] Electron microscopy studies suggest that there may be a defect in the transfer of melanosomes, and aggregates of melanosomes have been observed in keratinocytes.[3,6]

Progressive macular hypomelanosis

Clinical features

Progressive macular hypomelanosis is a relatively common type of acquired patchy hypopigmentation presenting on the central trunk, mainly the back, of young adults, with predilection for females.[1-4] It can affect all races, has a worldwide distribution being rare in Caucasians, and with most reported cases occurring in the Caribbean.[1,5] In some Caribbean islands the disease is known as Creole dyschromia.[1] The areas of hypopigmentation are well defined and vary in size but tend to be symmetrical. Over many years, lesions usually regress spontaneously.[6] They are often clinically confused with pityriasis versicolor and pityriasis alba. Treatment is very difficult, but the disease is self-limiting, usually lasting no more than 3–4 years.[2] A single case of a probably fortuitous association with toxic nodular goiter and another with congenital ichthyosiform erythroderma have been reported.[7,8]

Pathogenesis and histologic features

Propionibacterium acnes may have a role in the pathogenesis of the disease.[3] Follicular red fluorescence of the involved skin suggests porphyrin production by bacteria. Biopsies from involved skin have demonstrated Gram-positive bacteria in the pilosebaceous ducts with a mild perifollicular lymphocytic infiltrate. Cultures demonstrate the presence of *P. acnes* in lesional skin.[9] However, the latter is not always present and patients with acne do not usually have progressive macular hypomelanosis. A study has demonstrated the presence of bacteria of the genus *Propionibacterium* but of a different as yet unidentified species than *P. acnes*.[10] A further study, however, found an increased number of *P. acnes* in lesional skin by real-time polymerase chain reaction (PCR) in comparison to normal skin.[11] Further reports have identified the strain *P. acnes* phylogenetic type III as the most commonly associated with the condition.[12,13] An exceptional association with the use of antiretrovirals in HIV has been reported.[14]

Histology of involved skin usually shows loss of melanin in the basal cell layer of the epidermis, but the melanocytes appear normal.[2,3,15]

Ultrastructurally, there seems to be an increase in immature melanosomes in involved skin compared to normal skin.[4] There is a switch from stage IV (negroid) melanosomes to small type I–III aggregated melanosomes (caucasoid).[2]

Hypomelanosis of Ito

Clinical features

Although described here as a single entity, it is now clear that this represents pigmentary mosaicism in the setting of different diseases (see below). Hypomelanosis of Ito (also known as incontinentia pigmenti achromians) presents at birth or less commonly during infancy (about 25% of cases), with well-defined areas of macular linear or whorled hypopigmentation involving the trunk and limbs and usually (but not always or exclusively) following the lines of Blaschko (*Figs 20.20* and *20.21*).[1,2] The hypopigmentation can be bilateral or unilateral. The areas of hypopigmentation may progress during infancy and undergo some pigmentation later in life. There is slight predilection for females, and a family history of the disease is elicited in some patients.[3] The disease also occurs exceptionally in twins.[4] A case associated with whorled hyperpigmentation has been described.[5]

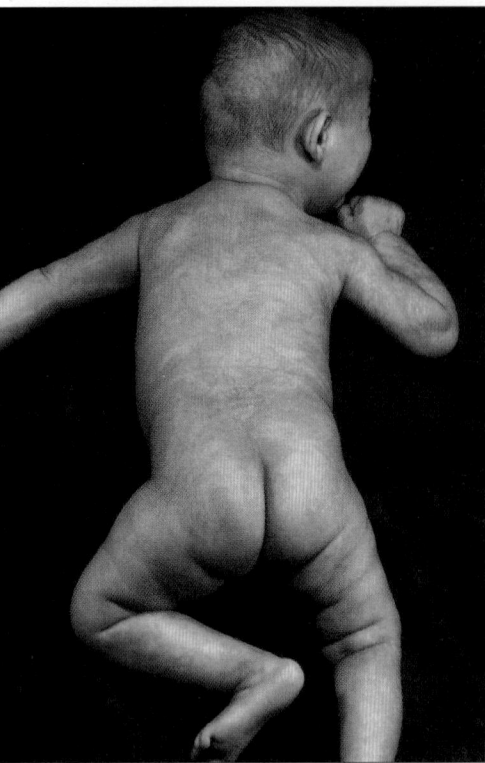

Fig. 20.20
Hypomelanosis of Ito: whorled hypopigmentation on trunk and limbs. By courtesy of the Institute of Dermatology, London, UK.

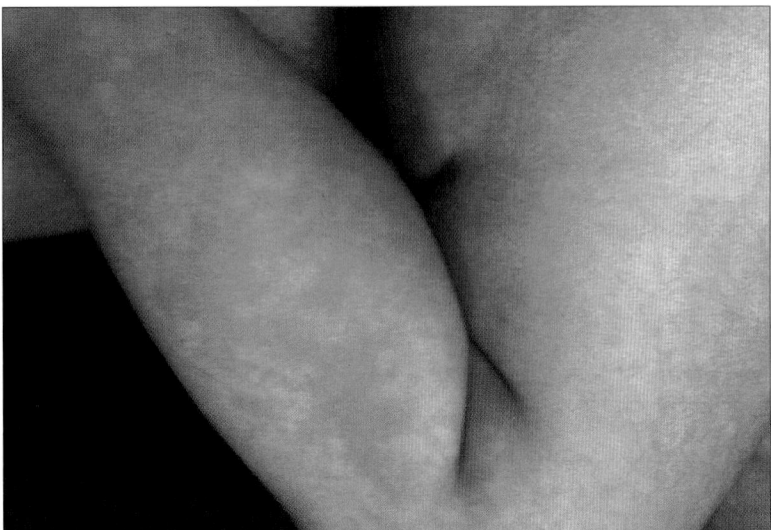

Fig. 20.21
Hypomelanosis of Ito: detail of whorled hypopigmentation in a limb. By courtesy of the Institute of Dermatology, London, UK.

Neurological and/or musculoskeletal anomalies are often associated with the disease. These include mental retardation, autism, epilepsy, seizures, macrocephaly, microcephaly, hypotonia, pes valgus, genu valgus, cerebellar hypoplasia, an intracranial arteriovenous malformation, distal spinal muscular atrophy, and hemi-overgrowth.[6-8] Other more uncommon manifestations include deafness, syndactyly, clinodactyly, skeletal abnormalities, asymmetry of the facies, body or extremities, cleft palate, vesicoureteral reflux, segmental dilation of the colon, gynecomastia, cryptorchidism, inguinal hernia, short stature, oral abnormalities, congenital cardiopathies, ileal atresia, precocious puberty, and glomerulocystic disease of the kidney.[6-14] Neoplasms, including neuroblastoma and coroid plexus papilloma, have also rarely been documented.[15,16] An association with Moyamoya disease has been described.[17]

Pathogenesis and histologic features

Various chromosomal abnormalities have been detected in lymphocytes and/or skin fibroblasts including X;17 translocation and trisomy 18, trisomy 7, trisomy 2, and trisomy 13 mosaicisms.[18–22]

In view of the wide variety of anomalies associated with the cutaneous hypopigmentation and the variable chromosomal abnormalities, it is now believed that hypomelanosis of Ito does not represent a single disease entity but is a cutaneous sign of a group of heterogeneous disorders resulting from genetic mosaicism or chimerism.[23–25]

Histologically, there is reduction in the amount of melanin in the basal cell layer of the epidermis. The decrease in pigment occurs both in keratinocytes and melanocytes and the change is easy to evaluate in biopsies stained by Masson-Fontana. Decrease in the number of melanocytes does not seem to be a feature but has been reported occasionally. Ultrastructurally, melanocytes may show vacuolization and decrease in size and in the number of dendrites.[26,27] Increased numbers of epidermal Langerhans cells have been documented.[28]

Differential diagnosis

Distinction from incontinentia pigmenti is based on the absence of melanophages in the papillary dermis in hypomelanosis of Ito.

Pityriasis alba

Clinical features

Pityriasis alba is one of the most common localized disorders of hypopigmentation in children. The incidence varies between 1.9% and 5.2%.[1] Young adults may also be affected. It characteristically presents as ill-defined, slightly scaly macules of hypopigmentation on the face with predilection for the cheeks (*Fig. 20.22*).[2–8] Involvement of the neck, trunk, and limbs may also be seen and a variant with lesions restricted to the knees has been documented.[9] Patients often (but not always) have an atopic diathesis. Pityriasis alba tends to be slightly more common in males and in patients with darker skin. A case associated with the antiepileptic drug Zonisamide has been reported.[10]

A possible variant of the disease has been described as 'pigmenting pityriasis alba', in which there is facial involvement only, with macules displaying a central area of bluish hyperpigmentation surrounded by a halo of hypopigmentation.[11] Interestingly, affected patients had an associated dermatophyte infection in 65% of cases. This variant is more commonly seen in patients with pigmented skin.[1]

An extensive variant of pityriasis alba has been described but it is not clear whether this represents an example of progressive macular hypomelanosis.[12–14]

Pathogenesis and histologic features

The pathogenesis of the disease is not well understood but there is a clear link to atopic eczema, and some regard it as a form of postinflammatory hypopigmentation secondary to eczema. One large study found a higher incidence of the disease in association with higher sun exposure and personal hygiene (long and frequent baths and mechanical exfoliation) in atopic individuals.[1,15] Low copper levels have been demonstrated in patients with the disease.[1]

Histologically, the changes are often subtle and consist of mild hyperkeratosis, focal parakeratosis, minimal spongiosis, and variable exocytosis of lymphocytes.[16] This is associated with mild loss of melanin in basal keratinocytes but not in the number of melanocytes.[6] In the dermis there is mild pigment incontinence and a sparse superficial, perivascular lymphohistiocytic inflammatory cell infiltrate. A histologic study of pityriasis alba in non-atopic patients found predominantly follicular pathology with infundibular spongiosis, follicular plugging, and atrophic sebaceous glands.[17]

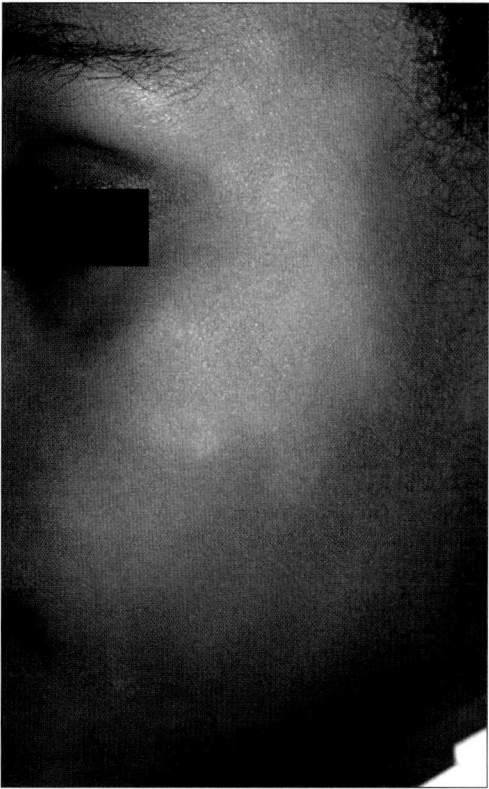

Fig. 20.22
Pityriasis alba: ill-defined patches of hypopigmentation on the face. By courtesy of the Institute of Dermatology, London, UK.

Ultrastructurally, the melanocytes display degenerative changes and keratinocytes show a reduced number of melanosomes.[6]

Postinflammatory hypopigmentation

Clinical features

Postinflammatory hypopigmentation is relatively common and is often a cosmetic nuisance in patients with darker skin.[1,2] Almost any inflammatory dermatosis may result in areas of hypopigmentation and these are not infrequently combined with areas of hyperpigmentation. Hypopigmentation in eczema, psoriasis, blistering disorders, lichen sclerosus, scleroderma, morphea, and pityriasis lichenoides is not rare, and some diseases (including infections) characteristically present with hypopigmentation. These include pityriasis versicolor, indeterminate and tuberculoid leprosy, post-Kala-azar dermal leishmaniasis, pinta, and pityriasis alba.[1–4] Loss of pigment may also occur in sarcoidosis, syphilis, and graft-versus-host disease.[2,5] Interface dermatoses (i.e., lupus erythematosus lichen planus) are more often associated with hyperpigmentation. Postinflammatory hypopigmentation is also seen after cryotherapy and dermabrasion and less commonly associated with the use of various lasers.[5]

Pathogenesis and histologic features

The pathogenesis of postinflammatory hypopigmentation is not entirely clear but it probably involves alterations in the transfer of melanin from melanocytes to keratinocytes.[1] The number of melanocytes usually remains within the normal range.

Histologically, there is focal reduction in pigmentation in the basal cell layer of the epidermis.

DISORDERS OF HYPERPIGMENTATION

Melasma

Clinical features

Melasma is a common, usually symmetric, acquired hypermelanosis characterized by irregular light- to dark-brown confluent or speckled macules with sharply demarcated margins involving sun-exposed skin; there is a marked predilection for the face (*Fig. 20.23*).[1] A useful clinical sign not entirely specific of melasma but present within most large of lesions consists of a confetti-like macular area of regular pigmentation.[2] Mild erythema is sometimes seen. Women (particularly Hispanic or Indian) are more commonly affected than men. In the latter, melasma has been reported due to estrogen therapy for prostatic cancer.[3] The most common patterns are centrofacial and malar but mandibular involvement may also be seen.[1,4] Presentation in other sites such as the upper limbs is uncommon and is more often described in older patients, particularly postmenopausal women on estrogen replacement therapy.[5–9] It usually develops in association with oral contraceptives and pregnancy and it is triggered and worsened by sun exposure. An association has also been documented with cosmetics, phototoxic drugs, isotretinoin, anticonvulsants, and clomipramine.[10] A melasma-like pigmentation has been described with imatinib.[11] Exogenous ochronosis occurring in skin affected by melasma after hydroquinone use has been reported.[12]

Pathogenesis and histologic features

The exact pathogenesis of melasma remains unknown but there is a clear etiological link to female hormones (oral contraceptives, hormone replacement therapy, and pregnancy), UV light exposure, and family history.[13,14] The hormonal relationship is further supported by the fact that men with melasma have higher circulating luteinizing hormone (LH) and low testosterone.[15] Etiological mechanisms independent of sun exposure have been suggested in some studies as relevant in the pathogenesis of melasma. The latter include downregulation of the H19 gene (which encodes a 2.3-kb noncoding mRNA that plays a role in limiting body weight and cell proliferation) and reduced WIF-1 expression all resulting in stimulation of hyperpigmentation.[16–18] Upregulation of PDZK1 (insulin promoter factor 1) in estrogen-induced melasma has also been regarded as an important factor.[19]

Histologically, two main patterns have been described: epidermal and mixed. In the former, there is an increase in the content of melanin in keratinocytes in all levels of the epidermis.[20–24] In the latter, there is pigmentation

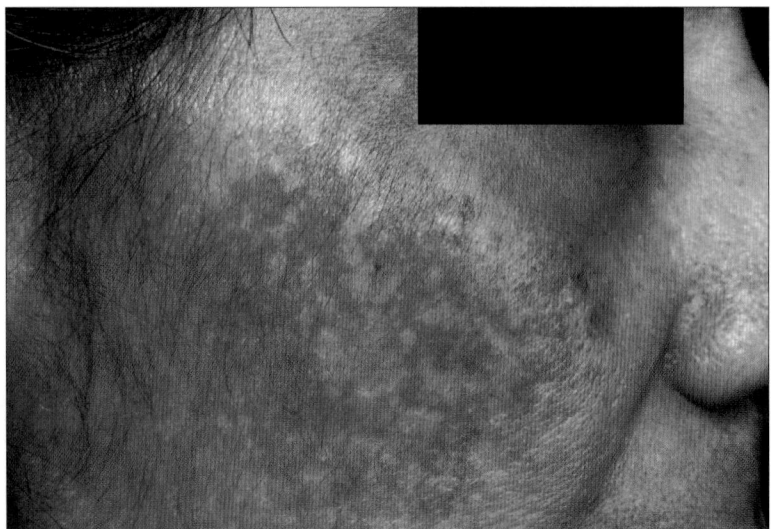

Fig. 20.23
Melasma: dark-brown macular pigmentation. By courtesy of the Institute of Dermatology, London, UK.

of the epidermis and also melanin deposition in the superficial dermis. The type of melasma can be determined by reflectance confocal microscopy – determination of the type is important for treatment purposes. Interestingly, the elimination of melanin through the stratum corneum appears to remain the same as in normal skin.[25] It is not clear whether epidermal melanocytes are increased in number, as the results of different publications are contradictory.[20–26] In the dermis there is increased solar elastosis and mast cells compared to normal skin and in the papillary dermis there are often melanophages but their numbers are variable.[27] Increase in the number of dermal vascular channels has also been described.[28] Two very unusual cases have been reported. In one, epidermal melanocytes protruded into the dermis, and in the other, there were superficial dermal melanocytes mimicking a dermal melanocytosis.[25] Prominent melanocytes protruding into the papillary dermis have been described as pendulous cells.[29,30] It has been suggested that these cells are characteristic of melasma and this change may be explained by increased MMP2 expression leading to loosening of the basement membrane.[30]

Electron microscopy demonstrates an increase in the number of melanosomes, which are more widely dispersed in keratinocytes.[21] The melanocytes show an increase in mitochondria, Golgi apparatus, rough endoplasmic reticulum, and ribosomes.

Laugier-Hunziker syndrome

Clinical features

Laugier-Hunziker syndrome (idiopathic lenticular mucocutaneous pigmentation) is an acquired disorder characterized by macular pigmentation of the lips, oral cavity (mainly hard palate and less commonly buccal mucosa, soft palate, and gums), and, less frequently, fingers and palms (*Fig. 20.24*).[1–6] Longitudinal melanonychia is seen in up to 50% of patients.[1,7] Pigmentation of the proximal nail fold resulting in a pseudo-Hutchinson sign may be seen. Genital and conjunctival pigmentation is very rare (*Fig. 20.25*).[4,8] The sex incidence is similar and most patients are Caucasian and middle aged. The pigmented macules are not associated with any systemic disease. Familial occurrence is exceptional.[9] A case with esophageal melanocytosis has been documented.[10] A patient with coexistent actinic lichen planus has also been reported.[11] In a further patient, macular pigmentation developed at the sites of irritant contact dermatitis and viral warts.[12] Hyperpigmentation identical to that seen in Laugier-Hunziker syndrome may occur in association with chemotherapy for cancer and, in one case, after levodopa therapy.[13,14] A melanoma has been reported in a mucosal lesion.[15]

The dermoscopic appearance of the pigmented lesions has been described.[16–18] Macular pigmented lesions on oral mucosa and genital skin show a parallel pattern; lesions of melanonychia show longitudinal brown and gray lines and bands with ill-defined margins in the lesions of melanonychia. Acral macular lesions show a parallel furrow pattern.

Pathogenesis and histologic features

The pathogenesis of the pigmentation is not yet known.

Histologically, there is hyperpigmentation of basal keratinocytes and pigment incontinence with melanophages in the papillary dermis. Recently, it has been suggested that there is an increase in the number of basal dendritic melanocytes and the term 'mucocutaneous lentiginosis' of Laugier and Hunziker has been proposed.[19]

Ultrastructural studies show the presence of increased mature melanosomes in the cytoplasm of keratinocytes.[2]

Differential diagnosis

Distinction from Peutz-Jeghers syndrome cannot be made based on histologic examination alone, and close clinicopathological correlation is therefore required.[20] Primary adrenocortical insufficiency may clinically simulate Laugier-Hunziker syndrome.[21]

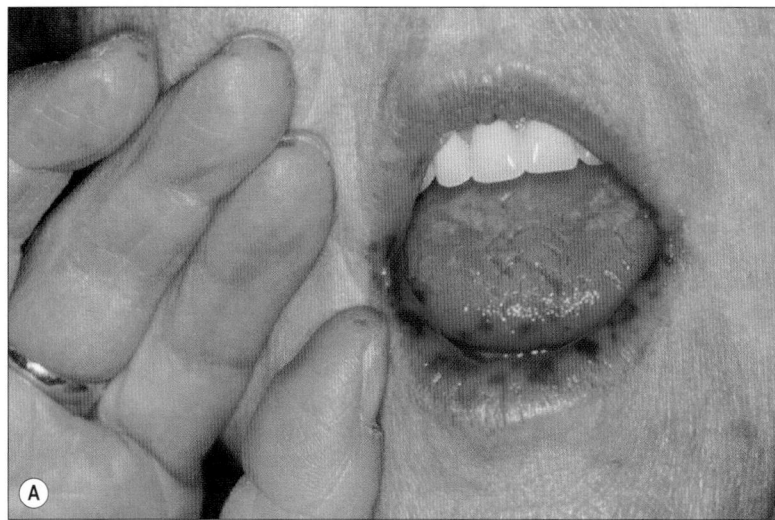

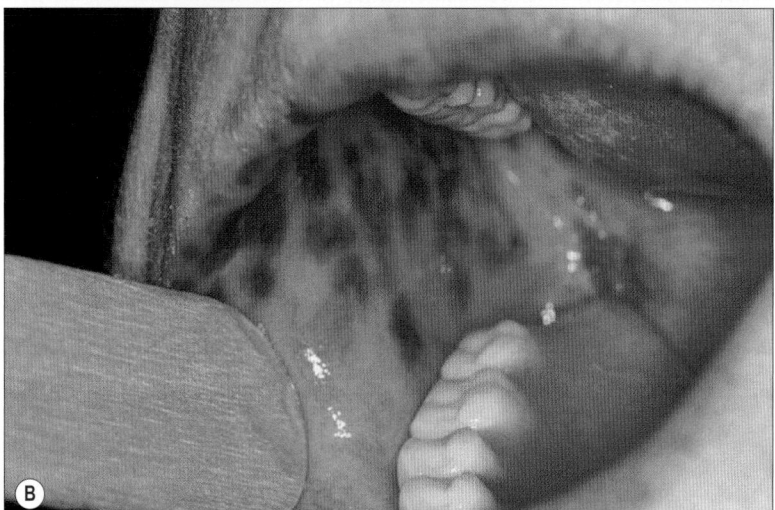

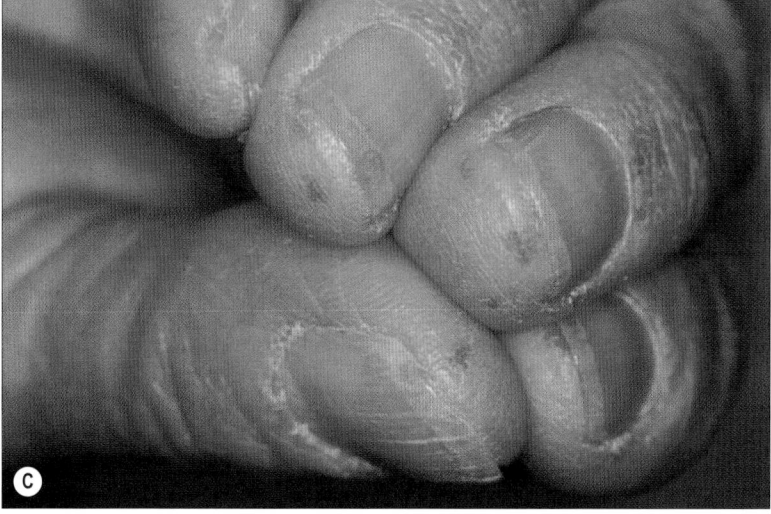

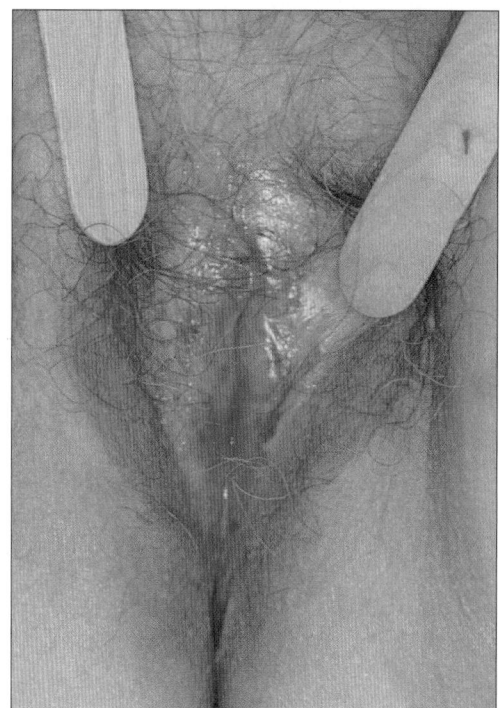

Fig. 20.25
Laugier-Hunziker syndrome: pigmented macules on the vulva. By courtesy of I. Viana, MD, Lisbon, Portugal.

Fig. 20.24
Laugier-Hunziker syndrome: pigmented macules on (**A**) the lips, (**B**) the buccal mucosa, and (**C**) the fingers. By courtesy of I. Viana, MD, Lisbon, Portugal.

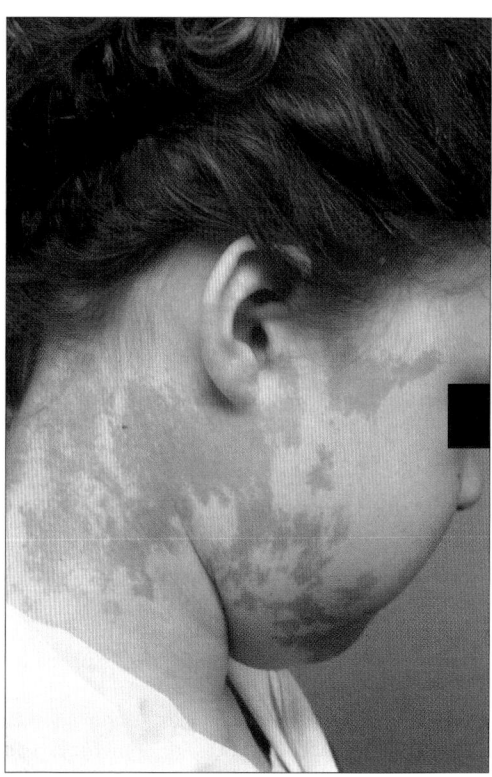

Fig. 20.26
McCune-Albright syndrome: light-brown pigmented macular lesions with an irregular margin. By courtesy of the Institute of Dermatology, London, UK.

McCune-Albright syndrome

Clinical features

McCune-Albright syndrome (also known as Albright disease or polyostotic fibrous dysplasia) is a rare disease initially characterized by café-au-lait macules, polyostotic fibrous dysplasia, and sexual precocity (mainly in females).[1,2] The disease can be diagnosed in the presence of two of the three major features. Other rare manifestations include hyperthyroidism, liver disease, growth hormone hypersecretion, anemia, hyperprolactinemia, Cushing disease, renal phosphate wasting with or without rickets/osteomalacia, and hepatic and cardiac involvement.[3,4] It mainly affects females. Osteomas and calcifications in the skin and soft tissues may be seen.[5,6] Cutaneous café-au-lait spots are asymmetrical and develop during the first 2 years of life or more infrequently are present at birth.[7] They mainly involve the trunk and proximal lower limbs and less commonly the face and neck (*Fig. 20.26*). It has been proposed that the pigmented macules

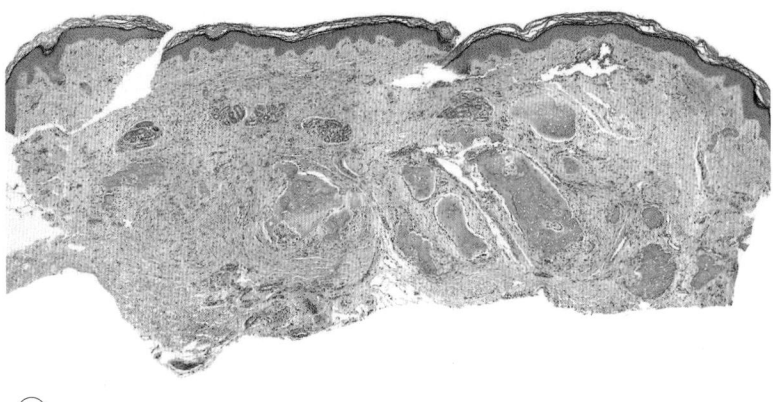

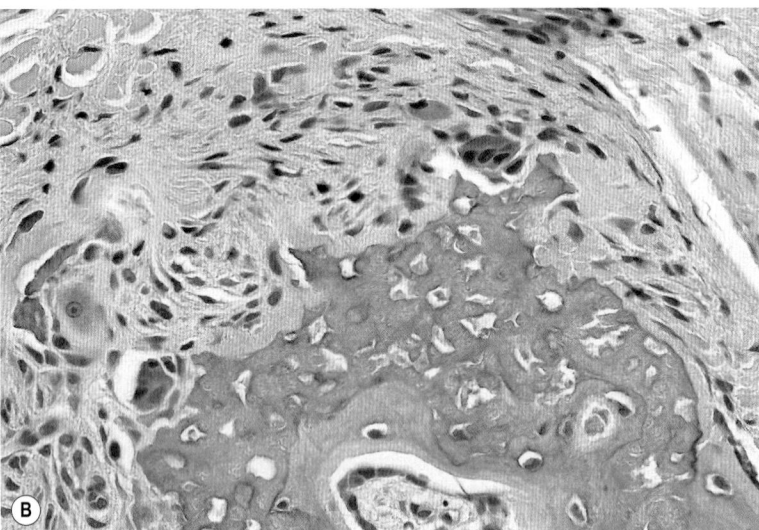

Fig. 20.27
McCune-Albright syndrome: osteoid is present in the dermis (**A**); high-power view (**B**).

in McCune-Albright syndrome may be distinguished from the lesions seen in neurofibromatosis by a smoother margin in the café-au-lait spots in the latter. However, this is not always the case and differential diagnosis may be very difficult.

Pathogenesis and histologic features

A noninherited postzygotic activating mutation in the Gs alpha protein encoded by the GNAS gene has been described in the syndrome.[4,8–10] The Gs alpha protein is a component of the G-protein complex that binds hormone receptors to adenylate cyclase. The activation of this protein results in over-production of different proteins.

A skin biopsy from a pigmented macular lesion shows hyperpigmentation of basal cells. Giant melanosomes are sometimes seen but are not as frequent as in the café-au-lait spots of neurofibromatosis type I. In the dermis and subcutaneous tissue, plaquelike osteomas may be seen (*Fig. 20.27*). Rarely, other lesions have been described in skin and soft tissues including nevi with osteoid, calcifying aponeurotic fibroma-like lesions, and calcinosis circumscripta-like lesions.[6]

Reticulate pigmented anomaly of the flexures (Dowling-Degos disease)

Clinical features

This rare condition (also known as Dowling-Degos disease, DD disease) has an autosomal dominant mode of inheritance. It presents with a progressive evolution of small (1–2 mm) hyperpigmented macules in a reticulate or confluent distribution, showing a predilection for the flexural regions including axillae, antecubital fossae, inframammary regions, neck, and groins (*Fig. 20.28*).[1–8] Involvement of the vulva (sometimes as an exclusive manifestation) and (more rarely) the scalp may also be seen.[9–11] Small, pigmented comedone-like lesions (dark dot follicles), pigmented, follicular hyperkeratotic papules (see *Fig. 20.28A*), and perioral pitted acneiform scars are also features.[3]

Hypopigmented or achromic macules are sometimes seen.[12,13] A case with extensive generalized hyperpigmentation and hypopigmented macules has been reported.[14] Presentation is usually in adolescence or early adulthood.[15] Females are more frequently affected.[4] The disease may occasionally be aggravated by heat.[16] Rare patients have had associated mental retardation. Described associations of the disease include, hidradenitis suppurativa, multiple epidermoid and trichilemmal cysts, arthritis, multiple keratoacanthomas, multiple seborrheic keratoses, and squamous cell carcinoma.[2,3,17–22] A case of squamous cell carcinoma arising in an area of pigmentation has been documented.[23] A likely coincidental presentation of DD disease and Darier disease in the same patient has been described.[24]

Increasing evidence over the years suggests a range of different phenotypic presentations in DD disease including Galli-Galli disease (see below). In Galli-Galli disease, the presentation is identical to that of classic DD disease but histologically there is suprabasal nondyskeratotic acantholysis.[25–28] A variant of Galli-Galli disease lacking reticulate hyperpigmentation and presenting with erythematous scaly plaques and lentigo-like macules of the trunk and lower limbs has been described.[29]

Pathogenesis and histologic features

The phenotypic spectrum of DD disease can be attributed to loss-of-function mutations in three genes that are pivotal in melanin transport. These are *KRT5* (encoding keratin 5), *POFUT1* (encoding protein O-fucosyltransferase), and *POGLUT1* (encoding protein O-glucosyltransferase).[30–34] These mutations likely result in alteration in the distribution of melanosomes within keratinocytes. Mutations in *KRT5* result mainly in flexural disease appearing in young adults.[35] Mutations in *POFUT1* result a similar but more generalized disease with involvement not only of the flexures, but also the trunk, abdomen, neck, and acral sites.[35] Palmar pits and interrupted dermatoglyphs may also be seen. Mutations in *POGLUT1* result in a disease that may be expressed early or later in life and is associated mainly with involvement of non-flexural areas, including trunk and extremities, and skin biopsies may display focal acantholysis.[35,36] A variant of DD disease presenting with hidradenitis suppurativa (acne inversa) is associated with mutations in the gamma-secretase subunit-encoding *PSENEN* (encoding presenilin enhancer protein 2).[37]

The features are reminiscent of an adenoid seborrheic keratosis. There is hyperkeratosis overlying an epidermis of normal or reduced thickness. Thin, filiform, pigmented, interconnecting epithelial strands grow down from the epidermis and walls of hair follicles into the superficial dermis (*Fig. 20.29*).[15,38] The infundibular portion of the hair follicles appears dilated. Occasional small horn cysts may be present. Inflammation is not usually a feature but a lichenoid tissue reaction may be present. In Galli-Galli disease, focal acantholysis is seen (*Fig. 20.30*)

Ultrastructural studies have shown a normal number of melanocytes with increased numbers of partially and fully melanized melanosomes.[38,39] The keratinocytes contain dispersed single melanosomes in contrast to the compound aggregates usually seen in white skin.[38,39]

Differential diagnosis

Distinction from an adenoid seborrheic keratosis may be difficult but the filiform epithelial strands seen in DD disease are very closely related to the infundibular portion of the hair follicles. The clinical background is very helpful in reaching a diagnosis.

The histologic changes are quite distinctive but not specific of the disease. Haber syndrome is characterized by a facial rosacea-like eruption, pitted scars, and seborrheic keratoses-like lesions on the trunk and flexures.[40–44] Additional reported features include palmoplantar keratoderma and prominent nail cuticles.[45] Although it has been suggested that Haber syndrome is

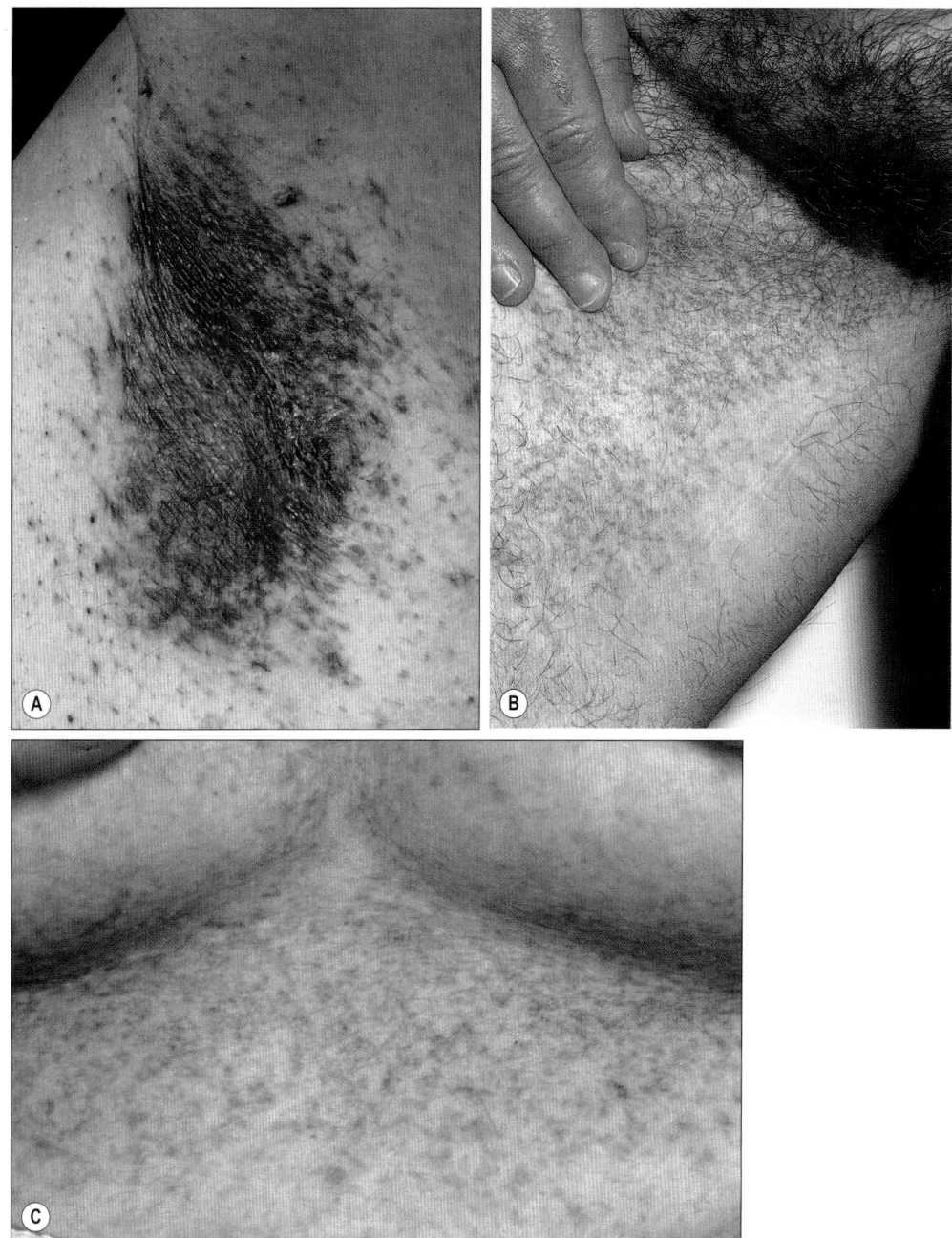

Fig. 20.28
Dowling-Degos disease: pigmented reticulate macules on (**A**) the axilla, (**B**) the groin, and (**C**) the inframammary area. Note also follicular pigmented hyperkeratotic papules on the axilla. (**A**, **C**) By courtesy of the Institute of Dermatology, London, UK; (**B**) by courtesy of E. Wilson Jones, MD, Institute of Dermatology, London, UK.

a variant of DD disease, the clinical presentation is different and mutations in keratin 5 have not been found so far.[46]

Reticulate acropigmentation of Kitamura

Clinical features

Reticulate acropigmentation of Kitamura (RAPK) is a rare inherited pigmentary disorder, with an autosomal dominant pattern of transmission with high penetrance. For many years it was regarded as part of the spectrum of DD disease.[1–7] This view, however, has recently been challenged based on the identification in patients with RAPK of mutations in *ADAM10*, a gene unrelated to those associated with DD disease (see below).[8] The disease presents in the first two decades of life, and patients have reticulate, slightly depressed macular pigmented lesions on the dorsum of the hands and feet that progress to involve the proximal limbs and trunk. Other features include facial pits, breaks in dermatoglyphics, partial alopecia, and, in rare

cases, plantar keratoderma (*Figs 20.31* and *20.32A & B*).[2,8,9] Progression of the disease stops in middle age.

Pathogenesis and histologic features

Recently, a mutation in *ADAM10*, a gene that encodes a zinc metalloprotease, a desintegrin, and metalloprotease domain-containing protein 10, has been identified. Mutations on *KRT5*, associated with DD disease, have not been identified.[8,10]

Histologically, lesions show mild elongation of rete ridges with pigmentation at their tips, slight hyperkeratosis, minimal inflammation, and absence of pigment incontinence.[8,11] Melanocytes appear mildly increased and giant melanosomes and melanosome complexes are identified in melanocytes and keratinocytes.[11–13]

Differential diagnosis

Distinction from DD disease is not only based on the differences in genetic abnormalities, but also on clinical and histologic findings.[8,14] The

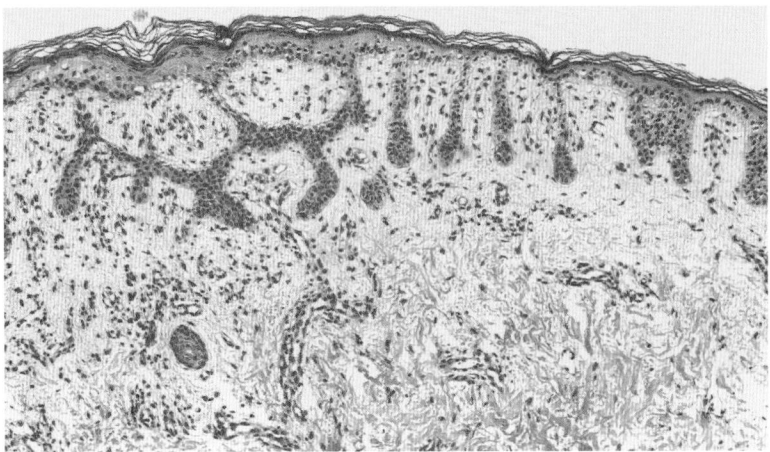

Fig. 20.29
Dowling-Degos disease: note the hyperpigmented thin epidermal strands. By courtesy of E. Wilson Jones, MD, Institute of Dermatology, London, UK.

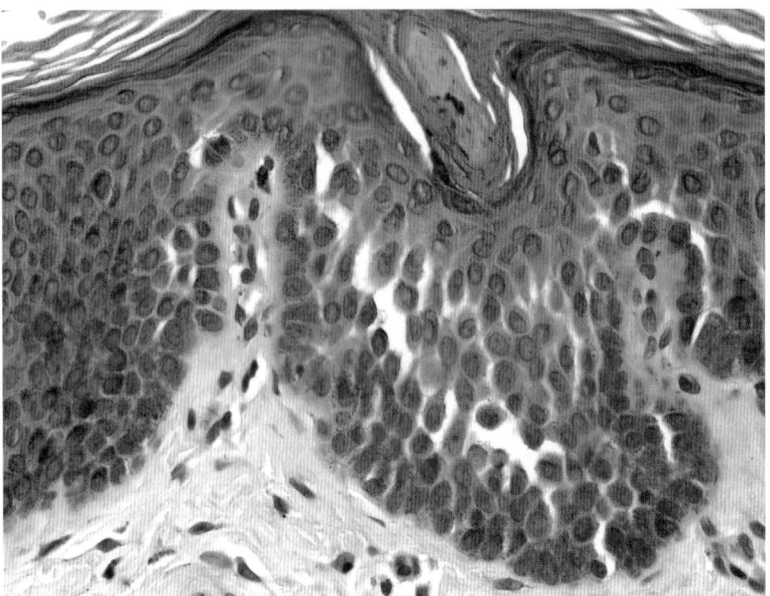

Fig. 20.30
Galli-Galli variant of Dowling-Degos disease: focal nondyskeratotic acantholysis is seen.

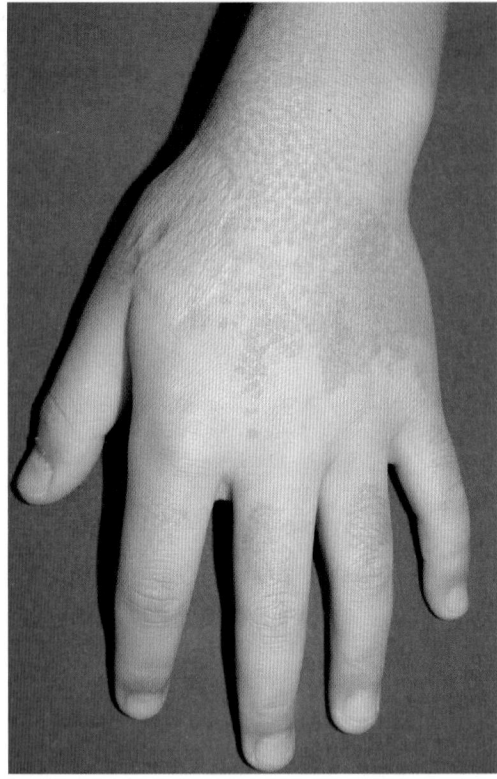

Fig. 20.31
Reticulate acropigmentation of Kitamura (macular reticulate pigmentation). By courtesy of Dr. Chao Sheau-Chiou, Tainan, Taiwan.

lesions in the former are more variable in color and histologically, the rete ridges appear more pigmented and elongated with involvement of hair follicles. In RAPK, the changes are more subtle, with mild elongation of rete ridges, more focal pigmentation, and absence of involvement of hair follicles.

Naegeli-Franceschetti-Jadassohn syndrome

Clinical features

Naegeli-Franceschetti-Jadassohn syndrome is a very rare genetic variant of ectodermal dysplasia with an autosomal dominant form of transmission. It is characterized by cutaneous reticulate patchy and mottled hyperpigmentation of the neck, trunk, and limbs, absence of dermatoglyphics, diffuse and/or punctate palmoplantar keratoderma, nail dystrophy, teeth abnormalities, and hypohidrosis resulting in heat intolerance (Fig. 20.33).[1,2] The reticulate hyperpigmentation tends to be more pronounced around the neck, fades after puberty, and may disappear completely in old age.[2,3] Tooth involvement is usually severe and may lead to complete loss early in life. The

punctate keratoses may be linear or can be accentuated along the creases. Malalignment of the toenails (predominantly the great toenails) has also been documented in some patients (Fig. 20.34).[2] Rare patients present with an incomplete form of the disease and additional clinical features such as short stature and milia.[4,5] A segmental variant due to mosaicism has also been described.[6]

Pathogenesis and histologic features

The gene for this syndrome has been mapped to a 6 cM interval on chromosome 17q21 in a region that contains the type I keratin gene cluster and other genes expressed in epithelia.[7,8] Mutations in keratin 14 occur in both variants and these conditions may be part of the same spectrum. The diseases are regarded as variants of allelic ectodermal dysplasia.[9,10] It has been proposed that keratin 14 haploinsufficiency leads to increased susceptibility of keratinocytes to tumor necrosis factor (TNF)-alpha-induced apoptosis and this causes the disease.[11] However, this theory has more recently been challenged.[12]

Biopsies from the pigmented areas show non-specific findings consisting of hyperpigmentation of basal cells and pigment incontinence in the papillary dermis with scattered melanophages.

Dermatopathia pigmentosa reticularis

Clinical features

Dermatopathia pigmentosa reticularis is a very rare inherited disorder characterized by the triad of reticulate hyperpigmentation, noncicatricial alopecia, and onychodystrophy.[1-5] The reticulate hyperpigmentation may be present at birth or in the first years of life. The hair of eyebrows, axillae, and pubis is sparse. Other associated features include dark nipples, adermatoglyphia (absence of fingertip and toetip prints), hypo- or hyperhidrosis, hypopigmented macules, and palmoplantar hyperkeratosis. Additionally, nonscarring blisters on the dorsum of the feet and hands have been documented.[4] In another patient, there were two neurofibromas but no other

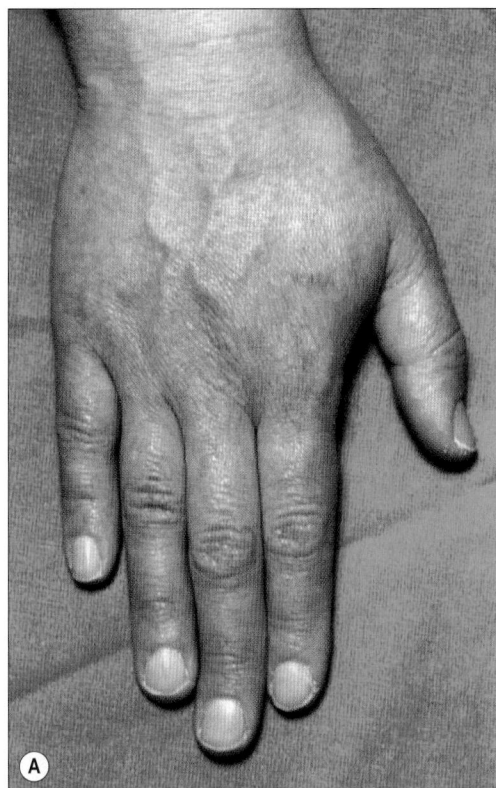

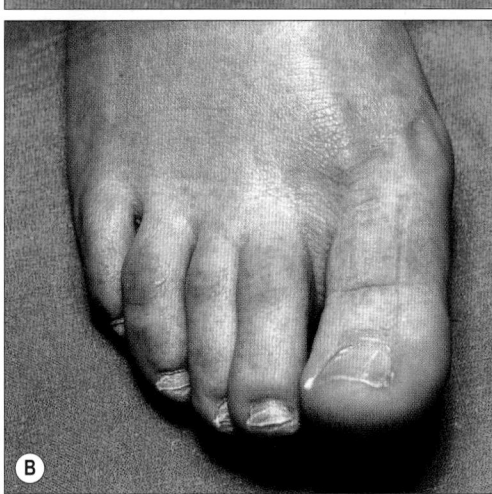

Fig. 20.32
Reticulate acropigmentation of Kitamura (macular reticulate pigmentation). By courtesy of the Institute of Dermatology, London, UK.

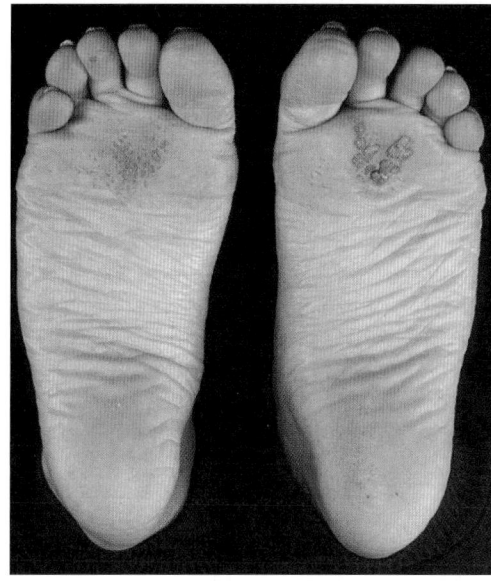

Fig. 20.33
Naegeli-Franceschetti-Jadassohn syndrome: palmoplantar keratoderma is often seen. By courtesy of the Institute of Dermatology, London, UK.

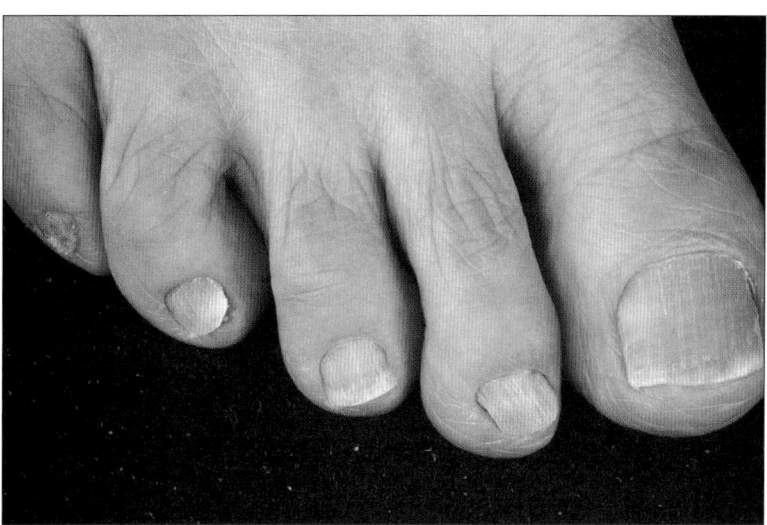

Fig. 20.34
Naegeli-Franceschetti-Jadassohn syndrome: misalignment of the toenails is seen in some cases. By courtesy of the Institute of Dermatology, London, UK.

evidence of neurofibromatosis type I was found.[2] In a further patient, there was wiry hair on the scalp and digital fibromatosis, and in another there was early-onset gastric carcinoma.[6,7] A report of a familial case suggested autosomal dominant inheritance.[3] Most cases of the disease have been reported in Europe.

Pathogenesis and histologic features

Genetic studies in a family with the disease have suggested that the responsible gene may map to the same chromosomal region as that for the Naegeli-Franceschetti-Jadassohn syndrome on chromosome 17q21.[8] Mutations in keratin 14 occur in both, and these conditions may be part of the same spectrum.[9] The diseases are regarded as variants of allelic ectodermal dysplasia.[10,11]

The histologic features have not been described in detail. Pigment incontinence and melanophages are conspicuous but the epidermis appears normal.[1] Transmission electron microscopy of hair shafts in two affected siblings revealed no abnormalities.[12]

Dyschromatosis symmetrica hereditaria

Clinical features

Dyschromatosis symmetrica hereditaria (DSH) (symmetrical dyschromatosis of the extremities, reticulate acropigmentation of Dohi) is a rare condition with an autosomal dominant or (more rarely) a recessive pattern of inheritance.[1–6] It is characterized by pigmented and hypopigmented macules on the extremities presenting in a reticulate pattern, developing during infancy and childhood, and persisting for life. Lesions occur particularly on the dorsum of the hands, forearms, and feet. Involvement of the face may be seen. The disease occurs mainly in Oriental patients (mainly Japanese and Chinese) but has also been reported in Europeans, Indians, Afro-Caribbeans, and Middle Eastern populations.[3] In some patients there are associated neurological abnormalities, including brain calcification, seizures, autism, mental deterioration, and dystonia.[7] Neurological changes are only described in Aicardi-Goutières syndrome 6, also caused by mutations in the same gene as DSH (see below). As some patients present with skin changes and neurological abnormalities, it has been proposed that both conditions are phenotypic variants of the same disease.[8] A case associated with intracranial hemangiomas and a further case with acral hypertrophy have been described.[9,10]

Pathogenesis and histologic features

Mutations of the double-stranded RNA-specific adenosine deaminase gene (ADAR1 gene) in chromosome 1q21–22 have been found in patients with the disease.[11–16] More than 100 mutations have been described.[17] The mechanism of pigmentation is unknown.

Biopsies from hypopigmented macules reveal absence of melanin and this correlates with abnormal melanocytes on electron microscopy.[2] Histology of hyperpigmented areas shows an increase in the deposition of basal melanin and this is reflected by an increase in the number of melanocytes on electron microscopy.[2]

Peutz-Jeghers syndrome

Clinical features

Peutz-Jeghers syndrome is an autosomal dominant disease characterized by gastrointestinal polyposis and pigmented macules with involvement of perioral skin, lips, buccal mucosa, and hands and feet – particularly palms, soles, fingers, and toes (Figs 20.35 and 20.36).[1–3] They may rarely occur on the nose and cheeks. Pigmentation of the umbilicus has been reported in one case.[4] Lesions are brown or black and usually measure less than 5 mm in diameter, although acral lesions may be larger. Cutaneous macules can be congenital or appear very early in life, usually before the age of 2 years. Skin lesions may fade at puberty but mucosal lesions tend to persist. The clinical appearance is almost identical to that of lentigines. Interestingly, pigmented macules have been reported in psoriatic plaques.[5,6] Males and females are equally affected. Patients presenting without a family history are likely to have developed the disease as a result of a spontaneous mutation.

Identification of cutaneous lesions is important because they usually precede the clinical manifestations of the gastrointestinal polyps. The polyps seem to have low potential for malignant transformation. They are associated with acute or chronic bleeding, often resulting in anemia, and may also be complicated by intestinal obstruction and intussusception.[7] Polyps occur mainly in the jejunum and ileum, followed by the stomach, duodenum, and colon.

The disease is also associated with an increase in the incidence of malignancies involving the small intestine, stomach, pancreas, breast, esophagus, cervix, testicles (Sertoli cell tumors), and ovaries (sex cord tumors).[8]

Some patients present only with pigmented macules and no polyps, and these have been described as isolated mucocutaneous melanotic pigmentation.[9] Female patients with this presentation do seem to be at increased risk of developing breast and gynecological malignancy.[9]

Pathogenesis and histologic features

The disease has been cloned to chromosome 19p13.3. It is caused by germline mutations in LKB1 (STK11) responsible for encoding a serine/threonine kinase that acts as a tumor suppressor gene.[10–12] Mutations in LKB1 are found in up to 80% of patients with the disease.[13] Rare cases have been cloned to chromosome 19p13.4.[14] The LKB1 protein is present in both the nuclei and the cytoplasm and translocates to the mitochondria during apoptosis.[15] It associates with p53 and regulates specific p53-dependent apoptosis.[15] The gastrointestinal polyps in Peutz-Jeghers syndrome do not stain for LKB1 whereas this protein is highly expressed in pyknotic nuclei of neighboring intestinal cells. This suggests that the polyps are formed as a result of a deficiency in apoptosis and may also explain the development of cancer in this syndrome.[15] It has been suggested that the LKB1 mutations lead to the activation of the Wnt/beta-catenin pathway and this is a contributor to the neoplastic predisposition in the syndrome.[16,17] Interestingly, in some families with Peutz-Jeghers syndrome germline mutations in LKB1 are not found, suggesting that mutations in an unidentified gene may cause the disease in this group of patients.[18,19]

Histologically, the skin lesions show increased pigmentation of basal cells but there appears to be no increase in the number of basal melanocytes. The latter allows distinction from a lentigo. Histologic distinction from a freckle is not possible.

The intestinal polyps do not have any specific features that allow distinction from other polyps. In some cases, misplacement of the epithelium in the polyps into the submucosa, muscularis propria, or subserosa has been documented and this may be confused with malignancy.[20]

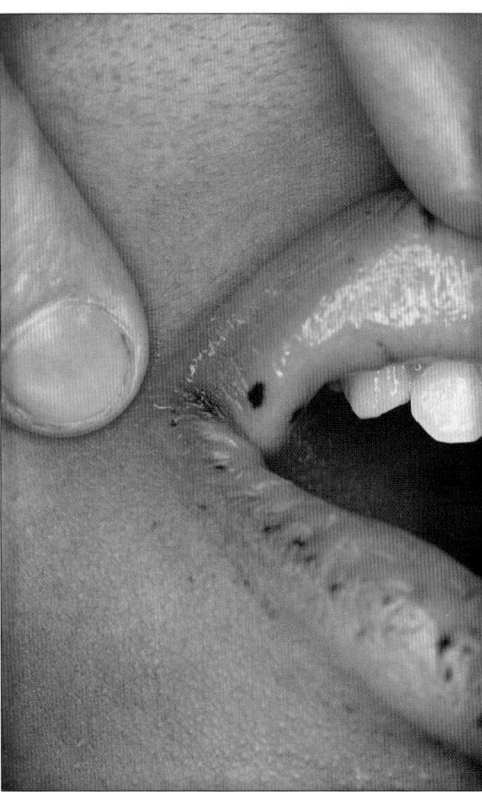

Fig. 20.35
Peutz-Jeghers syndrome: darkly pigmented macular lesion on the lips. By courtesy of the Institute of Dermatology, London, UK.

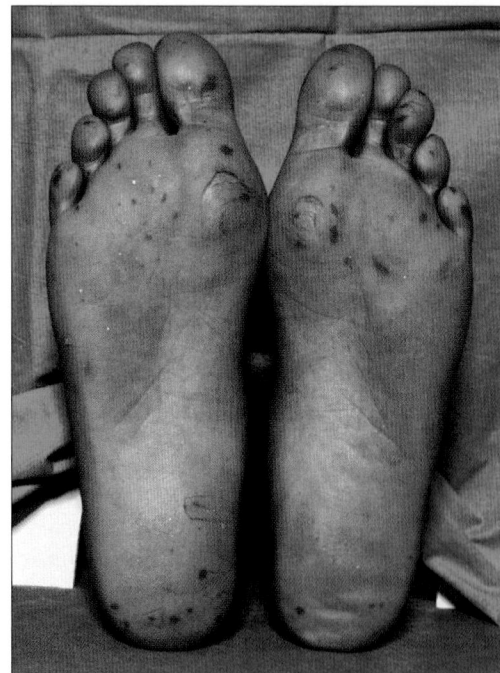

Fig. 20.36
Peutz-Jeghers syndrome: multiple darkly pigmented larger macular lesions on the soles. By courtesy of the Institute of Dermatology, London, UK.

Bannayan-Riley-Ruvalcaba syndrome

Clinical features

Bannayan-Riley-Ruvalcaba syndrome is also known as Ruvalcaba-Myhre-Smith syndrome, Riley-Smith syndrome, and Bannayan-Zonana syndrome.[1-4] It is transmitted in an autosomal dominant fashion and is characterized by macrocephaly, hamartomatous intestinal polyps, and pigmented macules on the glans penis and vulva.[1-3] Additional findings include Hashimoto thyroiditis, multiple subcutaneous lipomas, acanthosis nigricans, warty and papular lesions, cutaneous and central nervous system vascular malformations, macrocephaly, mental retardation, skeletal abnormalities, and occasionally epidermal nevi.[5,6]

Pathogenesis and histologic features

It has been suggested that this syndrome may represent a variant of Cowden syndrome.[4,5,7] Both conditions show mutations in the tumor suppressor gene PTEN (phosphatase and tensin homologue) and it appears that the syndromes are age-related manifestations of the same entity and are classified under the PTEN hamartoma tumor syndrome.[8-11]

- Biopsies of the cutaneous warty lesions show the features of a papilloma or a trichilemmoma.
- Biopsies of the papules show the features of a syringoma.[5]
- Biopsies of the pigmented macules show increased melanin in basal cells and a slight increase in the number of basal melanocytes.[5]

Cronkhite-Canada syndrome

Clinical features

Cronkhite-Canada syndrome is a rare disorder that presents mainly in middle aged to elderly patients and is characterized by gastrointestinal polyposis, diarrhea, and malabsorption. Mortality may be high, particularly in elderly patients, due to malabsorption, malnutrition, intussusceptions, and infection. A possible association with gastrointestinal cancers, particularly gastric cancer, has been suggested.[1-3] Skin changes include alopecia, nail dystrophy (in up to 98% of patients), and pigmentation, which may be diffuse or localized and macular, and predominantly involves the hands.[4-7] Focal vitiligo may be seen. The nail changes consist mainly of a thin and soft triangular area in the proximal half of the nail surrounded by a thick nail plate.[8] Onycholysis, onychoschizia, and onychomadesis may also be seen.[8]

Pathogenesis and histologic features

The pathogenesis of the syndrome is unknown. Autoimmunity has been proposed as a contributing factor and some cases are associated with hypothyroidism.[5,9] It has been suggested that the cutaneous signs are secondary to malabsorption, but the nail and hair changes may precede the diarrhea.[4]

A report of the histology from a macular area of hyperpigmentation showed increased melanin granules in keratinocytes, an increased number of melanosomes in melanocytes, and areas with an increased number of melanocytes.[10]

Histology of the alopecia in one case showed loss of follicular units, miniaturization of hair shafts, and deposition of glycosaminoglycans in the reticular dermis.[11] A further report of two cases described diffuse anagen-telogen conversion with no inflammation or miniaturization suggesting acute telogen effluvium.[12] A recent single case report suggested that the hair loss is the result of alopecia areata incognita with telogen shift and miniaturization of hair follicles.[13]

Carney complex

Clinical features

This syndrome was reported at the beginning of the 1980s under the acronyms NAME (nevi, atrial myxomas, myxoid neurofibromas and ephelides) and LAMB (lentigines, atrial myxoma, mucocutaneous myxomas and blue nevi) and was delineated in 1985 by Carney in a large series of patients.[1-3]

The disease had, however, been reported earlier in the literature.[4] It is a multiple neoplasia syndrome. Carney complex is transmitted as an autosomal dominant trait with rare sporadic cases.[5] It is characterized by cutaneous and cardiac (atrial) myxomas, multiple lentigines, blue nevi, endocrine overactivity, and osteochondromyxomas.[6-12] The endocrine activity may manifest as Cushing syndrome (due to primary pigmented nodular adrenocortical disease), acromegaly (due to a growth hormone-producing pituitary adenoma), and sexual precocity (caused by a large-cell calcifying Sertoli cell tumor). Male infertility not related to testicular neoplasms may be seen.[13] Other types of endocrine tumors can occur including thyroid hyperplasia or follicular or papillary carcinoma.[14,15] Intraductal papillary mucinous tumor of the pancreas is exceptional.[16] A distinctive type of schwannoma initially described as psammomatous melanotic schwannoma (occasionally nonpsamommatous) and now regarded as malignant and renamed as malignant melanotic schwannian tumor that also occurs in a sporadic setting is seen rarely, may be multiple, and affects the sympathetic nerve chains, the gastrointestinal tract, and (exceptionally) the skin.[7,17-22] The label of malignant is because prediction of behavior is not possible based on histologic features; metastasis of some tumors may result in death.[17,18] Ovarian cysts may also occur.[18] A rare case of intrathyroidal ectopic thymus, two with intracranial aneurysms, and very rarely hepatocellular carcinoma have been reported.[23-26] In a pediatric patient, the syndrome presented with a maxillary sinus melanoma.[27]

Atrial myxomas may affect any chamber of the heart and are a very important cause of mortality, causing death in up to 25% of patients.[28] Removal is essential to avoid death.[28] Fortunately, the cutaneous markers of the disease often allow early diagnosis and treatment of the cardiac lesions.

The cutaneous myxomas are identical to sporadic superficial angiomyxomas and may present anywhere, involve the dermis and/or subcutis, have a predilection for the eyelids, external ear, and nipples, and may occur in up to 31% of patients (*Fig. 20.37*).[29,30] They have a tendency to recur locally.[6] Intraoral myxomas are exceptional.[29] The lentigines affect mainly the center of the face (including the lips and conjunctiva) and occur in up to 75% or more of patients (*Figs 20.38* and *20.39*).[31] Intraoral pigmented macules are rare (*Fig. 20.40*).[5] Vulval lentigines are exceptional but have been documented.[32] Blue nevi may occur in up to 50% of patients and are commonly seen on the trunk, face, and limbs (except for the hands and feet). They comprise ordinary blue nevi and lesions described as epithelioid blue nevi.[28,33] The latter lesions are histologically identical to sporadic proliferations initially described as animal type melanoma and pigment synthesizing melanoma and more recently classified under the umbrella term pigmented epithelioid melanocytoma. These tumors are regarded as low-grade malignant with relatively frequent regional lymph node metastases but indolent clinical behavior.[34] Banal nevi may also be seen.

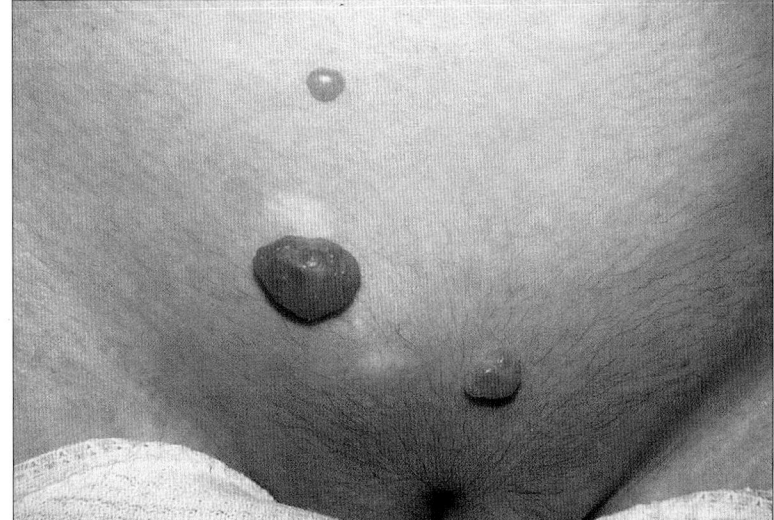

Fig. 20.37
Carney complex: multiple soft tumor nodules are evident on the lower trunk. By courtesy of M. Walsh, MD, Royal Victoria Hospital, Belfast, UK.

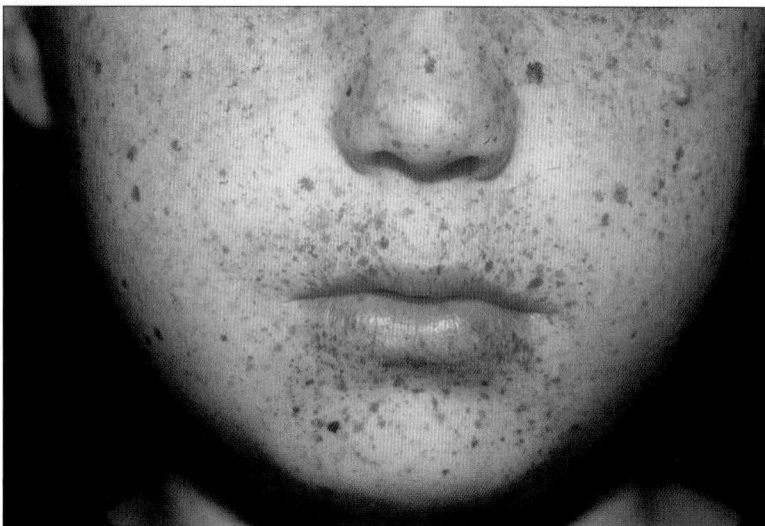

Fig. 20.38
Carney complex: numerous lentigines on the central face. By courtesy of M. Walsh, MD, Royal Victoria Hospital, Belfast, UK.

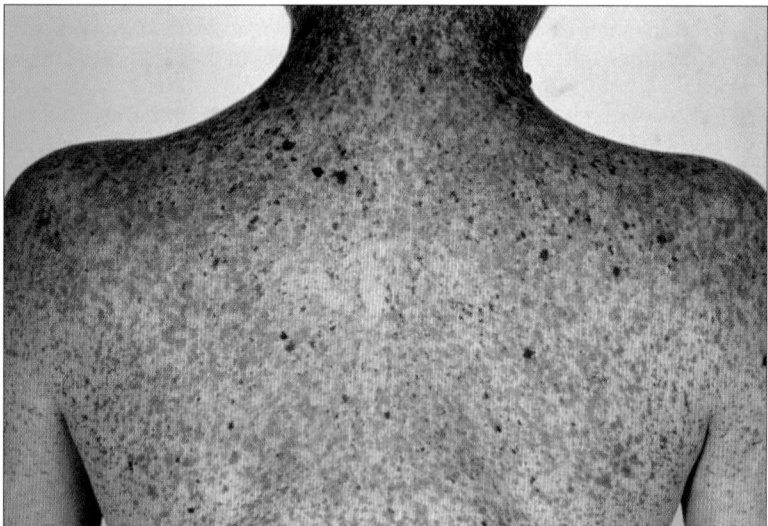

Fig. 20.39
Carney complex: multiple lentigines and scattered banal nevi and blue nevi on the trunk. By courtesy of D. Atherton, MD, St John's Institute of Dermatology, London, UK.

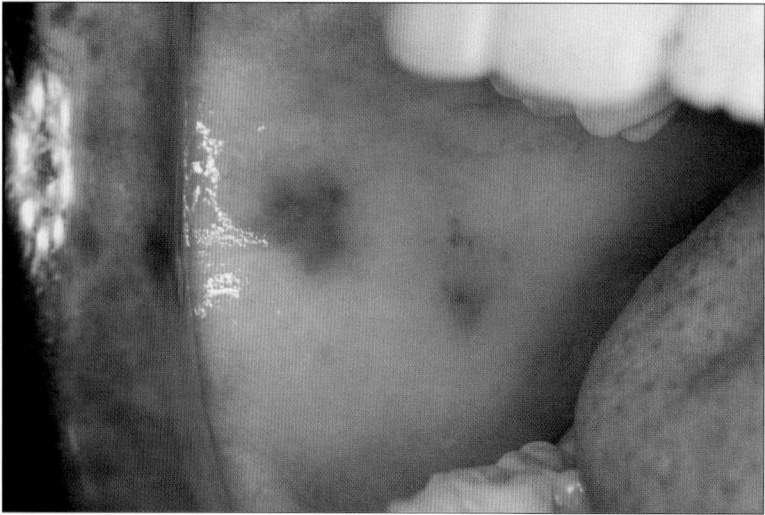

Fig. 20.40
Carney complex: pigmented macules in the oral cavity are rare. By courtesy of the Institute of Dermatology, London, UK.

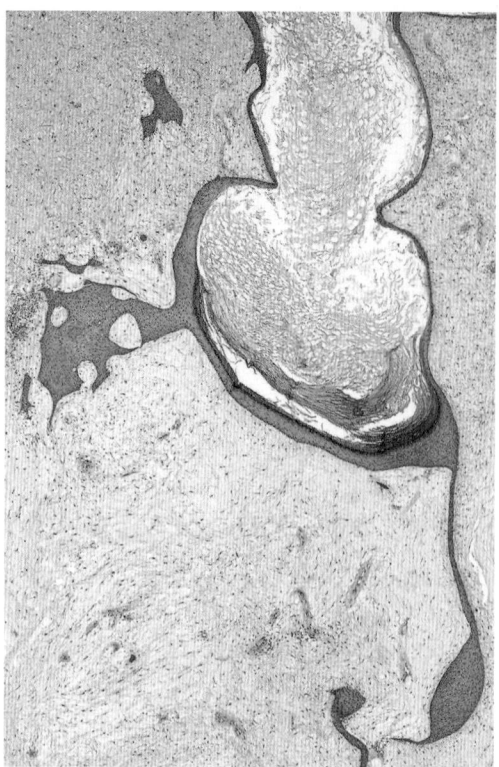

Fig. 20.41
Cutaneous angiomyxoma: dermal poorly cellular angiomyxoma with cystically dilated follicular structure.

Skin involvement was the predominant finding in four generations of a reported kindred and it has been suggested that, in these cases, the presence of a pilonidal sinus is an associated feature of the disease.[35]

Parenchymal breast lesions include myxoid fibroadenoma and (rarely) ductal adenoma.[36,37]

Pathogenesis and histologic features

Carney complex is a genetically heterogeneous disease. So far, the genes responsible for the syndrome have been mapped to chromosomes 17q22-q24 and 2p16.[38-41] In up to 65% of the affected patients investigated there were heterozygous inactivating mutations in the tumor suppressor gene PRKAR1A that maps to 17q and codes for the type Iα regulatory subunit of protein kinase A. This protein is an essential component of many cellular signaling systems and it appears to be important in cardiac function and myxogenesis.[42] A pituitary-specific knockout of the PRKAR1A model in mice induced tumors in the gland.[43] Tumors from affected individuals have shown decreased basal activity of protein kinase A but an increase in the cAMP-stimulated activity, which may lead to tumorigenesis.[44-46] Missense mutations in PRKAR1A are very unusual.[47] Patients with no PRKAR1A gene defects identified by sequencing may have large PRKAR1A deletions in the germline.[48]

The cardiac myxomas have features that are indistinguishable from other cardiac myxomas and present as sessile or polypoid mobile masses. Histologically, there is an abundant myxoid matrix, variable vascularity, and scattered tumor cells. These cells are bland and may be elongated or stellate. Exceptionally, ossification and extramedullary hematopoiesis have been reported.[49]

Endocrine and testicular tumors are identical to their counterparts occurring in a nonfamilial setting and will not be described here.

Cutaneous myxomas are identical to sporadic cutaneous angiomyxomas except for the fact that the latter tend to be more ill defined. The tumor is well circumscribed and hypocellular, with prominent myxoid change and abundant small thin-walled vascular channels (*Fig. 20.41*).[7] The cells within the lesion are bland, short, spindle-shaped or stellate, with vesicular nuclei (*Fig. 20.42*). Mitotic figures are rare. An epithelial component – probably

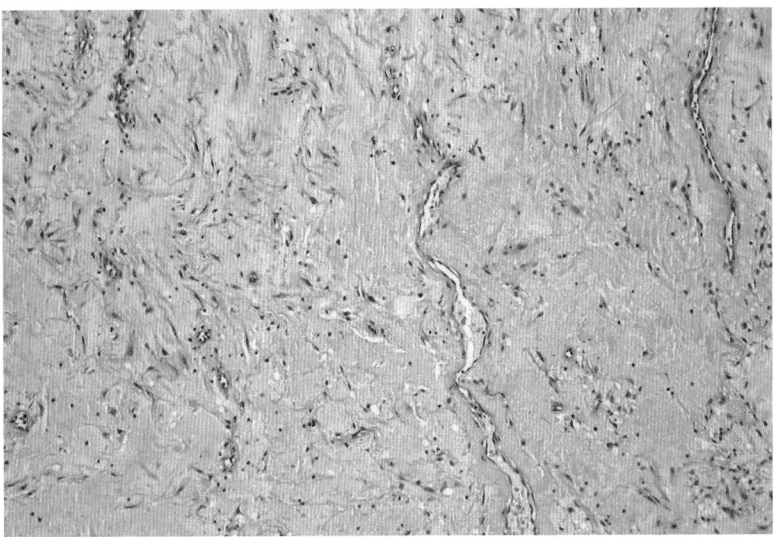

Fig. 20.42
Cutaneous angiomyxoma: bland stellate and short spindle-shaped cells in a myxoid stroma with prominent small blood vessels.

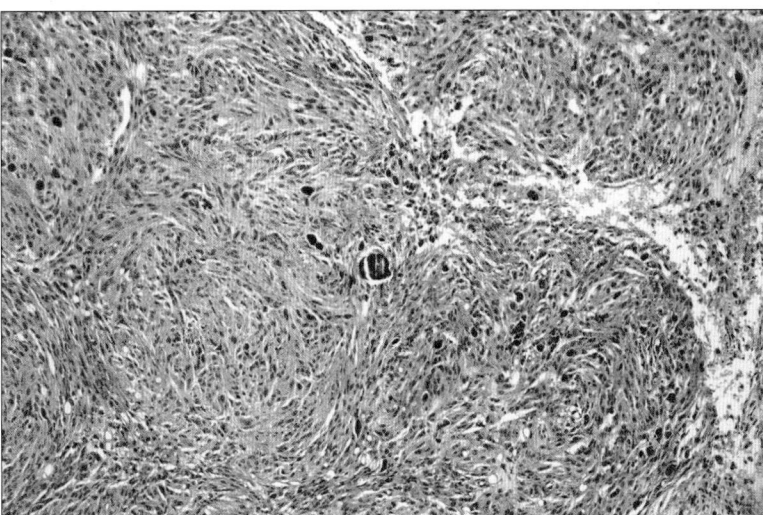

Fig. 20.44
Psammomatous melanotic schwannoma: pigmented spindle-shaped cells. There is a psammoma body in the center.

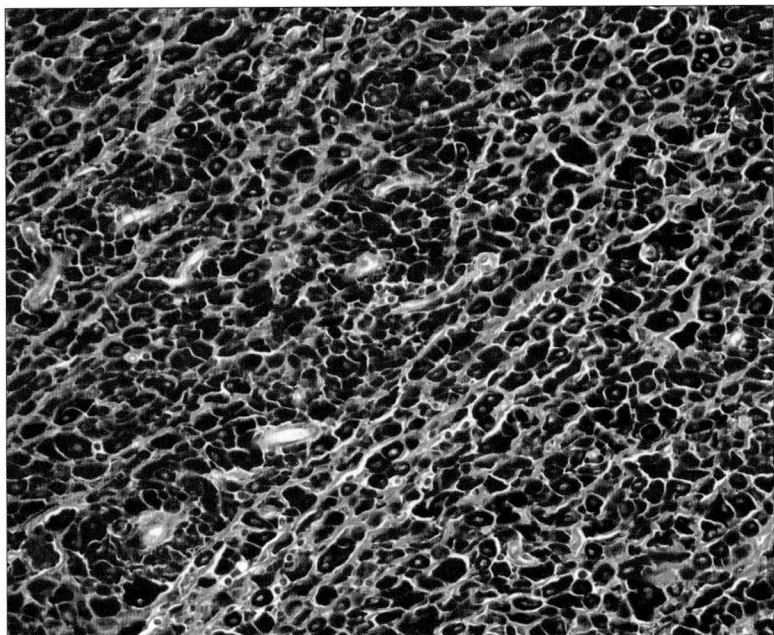

Fig. 20.43
Epithelioid blue nevus (pigmented epithelioid melanocytoma): deeply pigmented epithelioid melanocytes.

representing entrapped follicular structures with cystic change or focal basaloid buds – is often seen (see *Fig. 20.41*).[27]

The lentigines show histologic features indistinguishable from ordinary lentigines.

Epithelioid blue nevi (pigmented epithelioid melanocytomas) are located in the dermis, lack a junctional component, and are composed of epithelioid, polygonal pigmented melanocytes interspersed with short spindled pigmented melanocytes (*Fig. 20.43*). Melanophages are seen throughout the tumor.[17] Cytological atypia is mild and mitotic figures are rare. These tumors are identical to those occurring in a sporadic setting. As mentioned before, these proliferations have been classified within the spectrum of the so-called pigmented epithelioid melanocytoma, a term that includes pigment synthetizing melanoma (animal-type melanoma), a lesion that occurs sporadically and is regarded as of low-grade malignant potential.[34] Loss of expression of protein kinase A regulatory subunit type alpha and recurrent alterations in PRKAR1A and PRKCA genes have been found in some of these lesions but not in other melanocytic tumors.[50,51]

Lesions previously described as psammomatous melanotic schwannoma are now classified along with the identical sporadic counterpart as malignant melanotic schwannian tumors as they all have potential for malignant behavior regardless of the histologic features.[51] These tumors are very rare in the skin and tend to be fairly circumscribed but not encapsulated containing a mixture of spindled and epithelioid melanocytes with variable pigmentation and often, but not always, psammoma bodies (*Fig. 20.44*). The bundles of melanocytes may show whorling and there is focal nuclear palisading. Cytological atypia may be mild and prediction of behavior cannot be made based on histologic features.[16,17,52]

LEOPARD syndrome

Clinical features

LEOPARD syndrome is a rare congenital syndrome inherited in an autosomal dominant manner with variable expression. It is characterized by lentiginosis, electrocardiographic conduction abnormalities (due to hypertrophic cardiomyopathy), ocular hypertelorism, pulmonary valve stenosis, abnormalities of the genitalia (particularly cryptorchidism and hypospadias), growth retardation (in up to 50% of individuals), and sensorineural deafness (*Fig. 20.45*).[1-6] Lentigines may rarely be absent. When present, they appear after the first 4 or 5 years of life and by adolescence patients have perhaps developed hundreds of lesions.[7] Lentigines have a predilection for the upper trunk and neck but can occur anywhere in the skin (including genitalia, palms, and soles) and sclera sparing other mucosal surfaces. Additional findings include mild mental retardation, involvement of aortic and mitral valves, focal hypopigmentation, axillary freckling, café-au-lait spots (in up to 80% of patients and usually preceding the lentigines), interdigital webs, onychodystrophy, dermatoglyphics, hyperelasticity of the skin, and steatocystoma multiplex.[3,4-12] Corneal choristomas, granular cell tumors, morphea, and acro-osteolysis have also been documented.[5,12,13] Rare associations include Werner syndrome and Chiari malformation.[14,15] Occasional associations with hematological malignancies and multiple granular cell tumors have been reported.[16-18] It has been demonstrated that LEOPARD syndrome and Noonan syndrome (facial dysmorphology, congenital cardiac defects, and short stature) are allelic disorders.[19,20] Generalized lentiginosis has been documented in patients with no other evidence of LEOPARD syndrome and it is not clear whether these patients are part of the spectrum of the disease.[21] Males appear to be more affected than females.

Pathogenesis and histologic features

Mutations in the PTPN11 (tyrosine phosphatase SHP2) gene located on chromosome 12q24 have been found in up to 90% of patients with

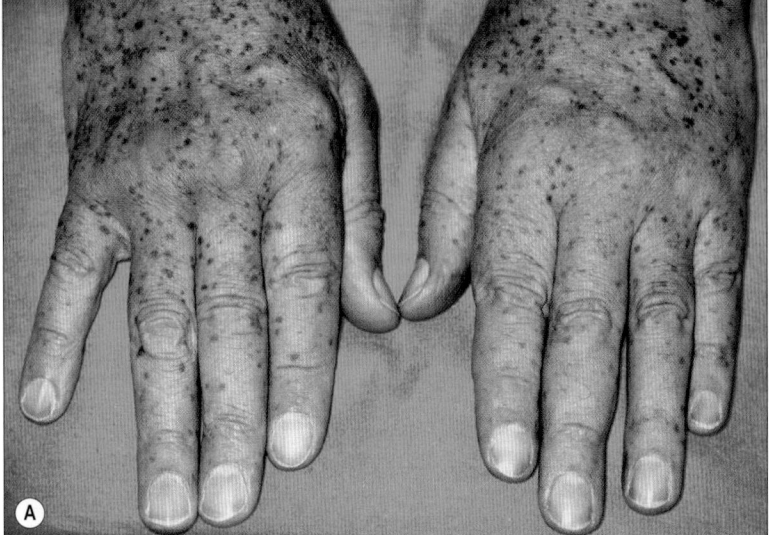

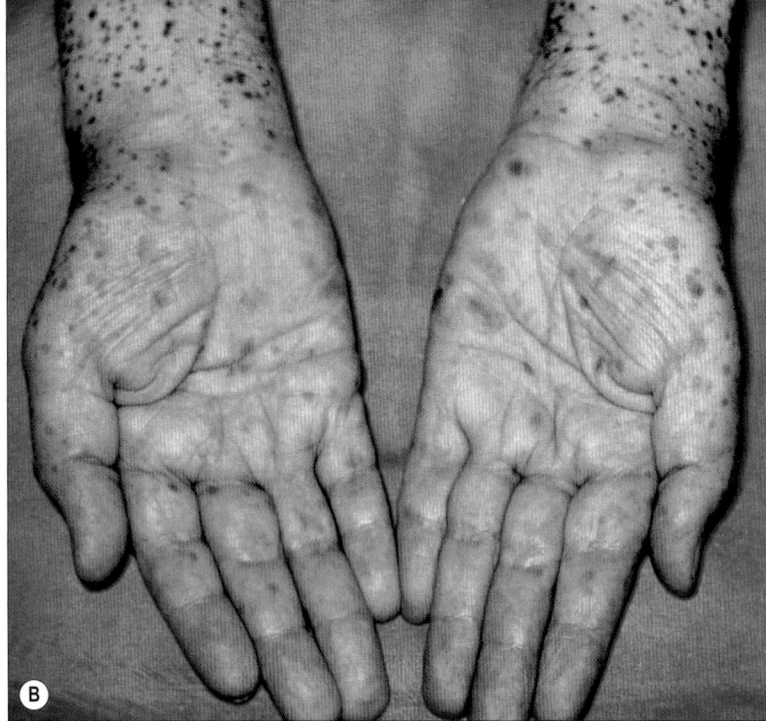

Fig. 20.45
LEOPARD syndrome: prominent lentigines on (**A**) the dorsum and (**B**) the palms
of the hands. By courtesy of the Institute of Dermatology, London, UK.

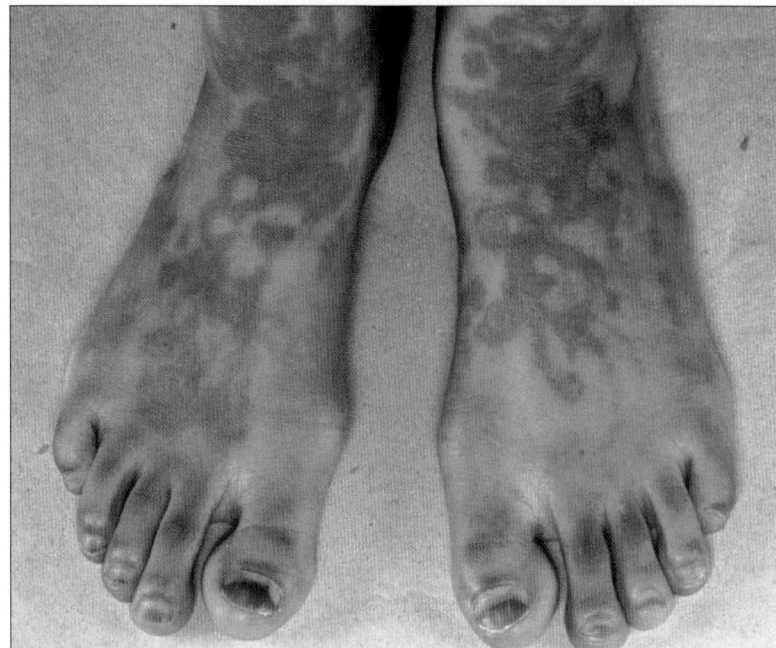

Fig. 20.46
Postinflammatory hyperpigmentation: prominent hyperpigmentation after the
application of henna for cosmetic purposes. By courtesy of the Institute of
Dermatology, London, UK.

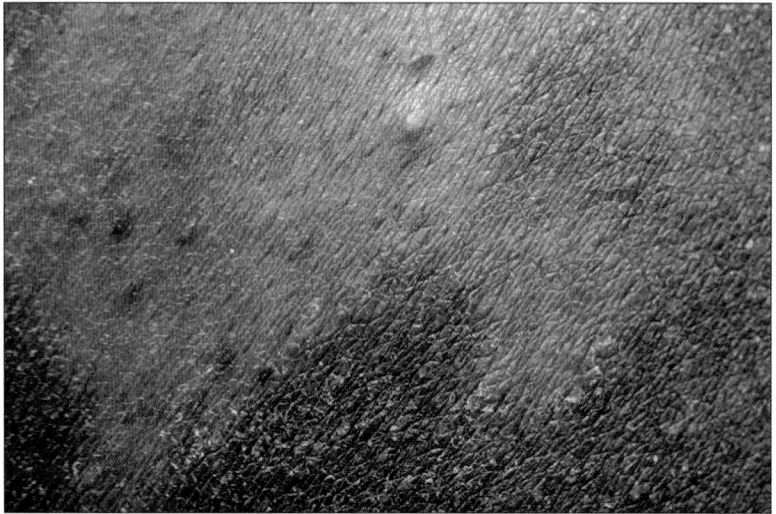

Fig. 20.47
Postinflammatory hyperpigmentation: marked hyperpigmentation after resolution
of lichen planus. By courtesy of the Institute of Dermatology, London, UK.

LEOPARD syndrome,[20-22] the same gene identified in patients with Noonan
syndrome. However, in LEOPARD syndrome different mutations (the
most common being T468M and Y279C mutations) have been found in
the PTPN11 gene.[22-24] PTPN11 is the gene encoding the nonreceptor-type
protein phosphatase SHP-2. It has been suggested that some PTPN11
mutations are associated with typical Noonan syndrome and other mutations, including the Y279C mutation, are associated with a Noonan syndrome phenotype plus multiple lentigines and café-au-lait spots.[22] This
group of autosomal dominant syndromes are now referred to as RASopa-
thies as they are caused by germline mutations in the RAS/RAF/MEK/ERK
mitogen-activated protein kinases (MAPKs) pathway.[25] PTPN11 mutations
can cause epidermal growth factor-induced phosphoinositide 3-kinase/AKT/
glycogen synthase kinase 3beta signaling which may be of importance in the
pathogenesis of the syndrome.[26] Missense mutations in the RAF1 gene have
been found in patients with no PTPN11 mutations.[27] RAF1 gene encodes a
serine-threonine kinase that activates MEK1 and MEK2 (mitogen-activated
protein kinases). This mutation is particularly associated with hypertrophic

cardiomyopathy. In a few cases, no mutations of PTPN11 or RAF1 are
present. BRAF mutations have also rarely been described.[28]

The lentigines and café-au-lait spots in LEOPARD syndrome are identical histologically to ordinary lentigines and café-au-lait spots. Giant melanosomes are seen in keratinocytes and melanocytes in lesional skin.[29] It
has been proposed that the lentigines are caused by increased melanin production induced by the SPH2 mutations with contribution by activation of
AKT/mTOR signaling.[29]

Postinflammatory hyperpigmentation

Clinical features

Postinflammatory hyperpigmentation is relatively common and may occur
following almost any inflammatory dermatosis and after the application of
exogenous substances (*Figs 20.46* and *20.47*).[1,2] Hyperpigmentation is also
commonly seen after trauma to the skin and may occur following cosmetic

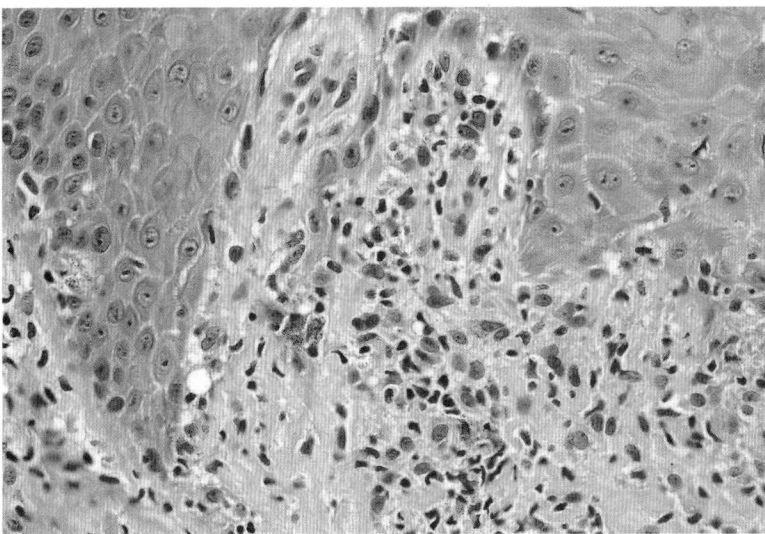

Fig. 20.48
Postinflammatory hyperpigmentation: focal pigment incontinence in a case of lichen planus.

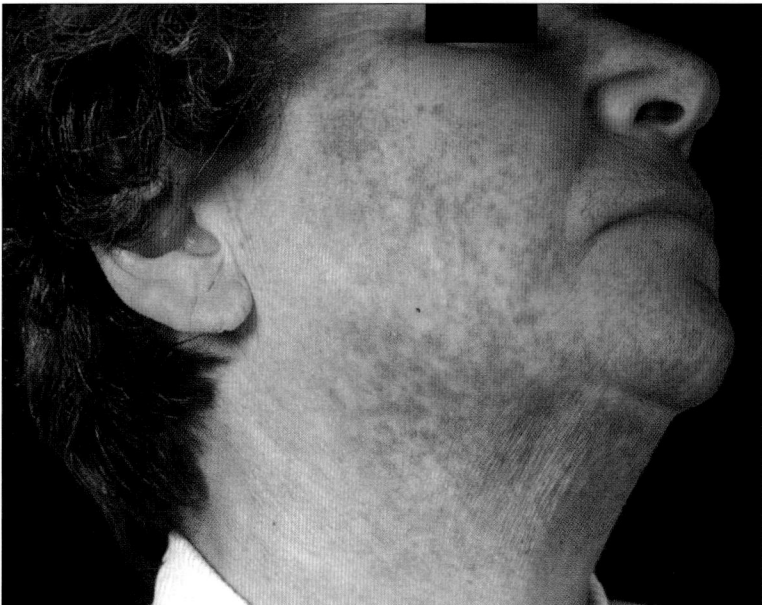

Fig. 20.49
Riehl melanosis: prominent patchy hyperpigmentation of the face. By courtesy of the Institute of Dermatology, London, UK.

procedures such as chemical peeling. The changes are seen in all races but are more common and noticeable in people with dark skin.[1,2] Dermatoses such as lichen planus, lichenoid drug eruptions, fixed drug eruptions, and lupus erythematosus (where there is usually prominent damage of basal cells) are more often associated with pigmentary changes. Hypo- and hyperpigmentation not uncommonly occur in the same patient. Hyperpigmentation of some areas of the skin, for example the periorbital area, is more common than involvement of other parts of the skin and multiple exogenous and endogenous etiologies have been associated with it.[3] In some instances, patients present with established hyperpigmentation and cannot recall an episode of skin inflammation. Spontaneous resolution of the pigmentation is usually partial at best and treatment is frequently disappointing.

Pathogenesis and histologic features

The pathogenesis of postinflammatory hyperpigmentation may be explained by the damage to keratinocytes and melanocytes with resulting pigment incontinence and phagocytosis of the melanin by macrophages (melanophages) (Fig. 20.48). In vitro studies have demonstrated that normal human epidermal melanocytes become swollen and more dendritic with an increase in the amount of immunoreactive tyrosinase when they are cultured for several days with arachidonic acid metabolites, including prostaglandin D2, leukotriene B4, C4, D4, thromboxane B2, and eicosatetraenoic acid.[4–8] The effect of leukotriene C4 appears to be particularly intense. These findings suggest an important role of melanocytes in the induction of postinflammatory hyperpigmentation. A further proposal suggests that fibroblast-derived growth factors, particularly keratinocyte growth factor, on its own or in association with interleukin-1alpha, may play a role in inducing the hyperpigmentation.[9]

Histologically, two histopathologic patterns have been described: epidermal and dermal. In the former, there is increase in pigmentation of basal cells within the epidermis. In the latter, there is pigmentation in the upper dermis with melanophages and decreased pigmentation in basal cells.[10] Interestingly, a study on exogenous hyperpigmentation has found an increase in the number of basal melanocytes in affected areas as compared to normal skin.[11] In some cases, colloid bodies are seen at the dermal–epidermal junction suggesting a pre-existing interphase tissue reaction.

Acquired brachial cutaneous dyschromatosis

Clinical features

Acquired brachial cutaneous dyschromatosis appears to be related to poikiloderma of Civatte.[1] It presents as asymptomatic, gray-brown patches with geographic borders and occasional focal hypopigmented macules on the dorsum of the forearms.[1] Most cases are bilateral and there is predilection for postmenopausal females. Very rare cases may occur in males.[2]

Pathogenesis and histologic features

The changes do not appear to be associated with estrogens, pregnancy, or hormone replacement therapy and although the initial report found no clear relationship with sun exposure, it has recently been proposed that it may be associated with chronic sun damage.[1–3] An association with hypertension and/or antihypertensive drugs has been suggested.[1]

Histologically, epidermal atrophy, basal hyperpigmentation, elastosis, and telangiectasia are described.

Riehl melanosis

Clinical features

Riehl melanosis, first described in 1917, consists of prominent hyperpigmentation of the face with involvement of the forehead and the zygomatic and/or temporal regions (Fig. 20.49).[1] The condition has been reported in both Caucasians and patients with darker skin. Women are mainly affected.

Pathogenesis and histologic features

Riehl proposed that the changes were secondary to some food items used during the First World War. However, more recently, the condition has been regarded as a variant of pigment contact dermatitis. The most common allergens involved are cosmetics, including fragrances.[2] Riehl melanosis has rarely been reported in association with Sjögren syndrome and lichen planus.[3,4]

Dermoscopic findings include a pseudonetwork, gray dots/granules, telangiectasia, mild scaliness, follicular keratotic plugs, and perifollicular whitish halos.[5]

Histologically, there is prominent pigment incontinence and melanophages in the papillary dermis. Other described features include telangiectasia, dilated hair follicles, and hyperkeratosis of the infundibula of hair follicles.[5] Colloid bodies are often seen and formation of amyloid has been documented. The latter, however, is demonstrated only by electron microscopy as it tends to be negative for amyloid stains including thioflavin T and Congo red.[6]

Notalgia paresthetica

Clinical features

Notalgia paresthetica is a common sensory neuropathy characterized by pruritus on the back involving an area innervated by the dorsal spinal nerves 2–6.[1-5] In one case, the condition was attributed to cervical spinal stenosis and in a further case it was associated with neuralgic amyotrophy.[6,7] Additional symptoms include burning and dysesthesia. A study has found that females tend to present more severe symptoms, patients with higher body mass index have longer disease duration, and the affected site is associated with the prevailing sleep position.[8] Interestingly, lesions in women tend to be more common in the subscapular area and in men in the interscapular area. This may be due to the differences between the length of the arm in males and females.[9] Notalgia paresthetica mainly occurs in elderly patients and presents with well-defined areas of macular hyperpigmentation. The disease probably represents the same entity that has been described as macular posterior pigmentary incontinence.[9-11] The lesions are also similar to macular amyloidosis, and amyloid is often found in biopsies taken from involved sites (see below).[10] Symptoms tend to be persistent and treatment is difficult.[12] An association with multiple endocrine neoplasia syndrome 2A has been reported.[13] A case of inverse notalgia paresthetica with involvement of the parasternal area, probably associated with the patient's trade as a painter, has been documented.[14]

Pathogenesis and histologic features

The cause of the disease is unknown but in many cases the symptoms may be triggered by musculoskeletal compression of spinal nerves secondary to arthrosis or spinal static disequilibrium.[15-17] This theory is supported by improvement of the symptoms after nerve decompression.[18] An increase in dermal innervation has also been suggested as a likely cause and an increase in the number of intradermal nerves may be seen (dermal hyperneury).[19,20] However, an immunohistochemical study of a fairly large number of biopsies using neural markers failed to show any significant neural abnormalities in biopsies from involved skin.[21]

The clinical lesions are likely to be the results of chronic rubbing, which may also explain the presence of amyloid derived from epidermal keratinocytes.

The epidermis usually appears unremarkable but mild acanthosis, scattered apoptotic keratinocytes, and focal hyperpigmentation of basal cells are sometimes seen. In the papillary dermis there are melanophages. Focal amyloid deposition in the papillary dermis is often demonstrated.

Differential diagnosis

Notalgia paresthetica and macular amyloid have identical histologic features in cases in which amyloid is detected in the papillary dermis. Close clinicopathological correlation is therefore essential to establish the correct diagnosis, as macular amyloid does not follow the distribution of the innervation of dorsal nerves.

Diffuse melanosis associated with metastatic melanoma

Clinical features

Diffuse (generalized) melanosis is a very rare phenomenon that occurs in patients with metastatic melanoma as a gray or blue diffuse pigmentation of the skin.[1-8] The mean time from the diagnosis of melanoma to development is 11.48 months as calculated from a systematic review of the literature.[9] Most patients have liver metastases and it is associated with very poor prognosis with a median survival between 4 and 6 months.[9-11] However, the survival appears to increase in patients with BRAF (V600E) mutation treated with targeted therapy.[12] The phenomenon has also been reported as the first manifestation of dermal micrometastasis of melanoma.[13] The pigmentation tends to be more prominent in sun-exposed areas. Pigmentation of nail beds, mucosal surfaces, and internal organs is also a feature. This phenomenon has been reported not only in metastatic primary cutaneous melanoma, but also in melanoma arising from mucosal surfaces.[14-16] A case of vulval melanoma in a pregnant woman presenting with melanosis and placental metastases has been reported and in a further case presentation heralded recurrence of a melanoma removed 26 years before.[17,18] Melanuria and melanoptysis may also occur.[19] Melanuria on its own is more common, presenting in up to 15% of cases of metastatic melanoma.[10] A localized variant of melanosis has been documented and one case responded to treatment with Imiquimod in the absence of metastatic disease at the site of pigmentation.[20,21]

Pathogenesis and histologic features

The exact pathogenesis is not known but the favored hypothesis is that it results from massive dissemination of melanin or a melanin precursor produced by tumor cells through the bloodstream into the skin and internal organs with deposition in macrophages.[6,7,22-24] Rare melanoma cells are detected in areas of pigmentation.[6,7] Melanosomes are not usually identified.

Histology typically reveals collections of macrophages with prominent cytoplasmic melanin in a predominant perivascular distribution throughout the dermis.[6,7] Mononuclear inflammatory cells are rare.

Access **ExpertConsult.com** for a complete list of all references

Disease of collagen
and elastic tissue

CHAPTER
21

See
www.expertconsult.com
for references and
additional material

Introduction

Improved and detailed understanding of the molecular basis of many of the diseases in this chapter continues to progress. While Ehlers-Danlos has been well understood for many years, our understanding has further expanded and a new classification scheme systematizes by both clinical presentation and pathogenesis into multiple categories. In other diseases, we have gone from virtually no knowledge or only speculation regarding their molecular determinates to identification of specific genetic mutations that drive their pathogenesis. Although the precise mechanistic details remain a work in progress, this expansion of knowledge has several important implications. The identification of the genetic origin of these diseases:

• permits better diagnosis and prognosis, including prenatal evaluation when relevant,
• informs our classification schemes,
• provides insight into pathogenesis and normal biology,
• enables rational, precision medicine for therapeutic interventions.

DISEASES OF COLLAGEN: GENERALIZED DISORDERS

Ehlers-Danlos syndrome

Clinical features

The earlier Berlin and Villefranche classification systems have been very recently replaced by that of the 2017 international classification of Ehlers-Danlos syndrome (EDS), in which the clinical variants are subtyped by molecular mechanisms (*Table 21.1*).[1-6] Thirteen major types are recognized. Most show autosomal dominant inheritance, but autosomal recessive variants are also recognized.[6-8] This classification is not perfect, but represents the most current and mature consensus understanding of the disease. It classifies the EDS spectrum of diseases in two ways: into 13 clinical entities which correspond in large degree to the prior Berlin and Villefranche systems, with some expansion for additional defined variants (see *Table 21.1*), and also into 6 genetic and pathogenetic groupings that are helpful in understanding the various molecular mechanisms of the disease (see *Table 21.2*). It also removes several conditions from the EDS spectrum that were included in the prior classification schemes.[6]

EDS is one of the most common inherited disorders, the incidence estimated being 1 : 5000 individuals.[9,10] The disease spectrum includes both relatively common and rare types.[11]

The clinical manifestations include[12-15]:
• hyperextensible skin (*Figs 21.1* and *21.2*),
• hypermobility of joints (*Figs 21.3* and *21.4*),
• atrophic, paper-thin scars (*Figs 21.5* and *21.6*),
• a tendency to easy bruising,
• connective tissue fragility,
• variable internal organ involvement.

Trauma, with resultant hematoma formation and scarring, may give rise to so-called molluscoid pseudotumors (*Fig. 21.7*). Patients also develop hard, discrete, mobile (sometimes calcified) fibrous nodules (spheroids) in the subcutaneous fat of the extremities. Redundant skin (acquired cutis laxa) may develop over the elbows and knees, particularly in elderly patients.[12,13]

Ocular manifestations include blue sclera, keratoconus, lens subluxation, and retinal detachments; dental involvement may present with severe periodontitis.

Table 21.1

The 2017 International Classification of Ehlers-Danlos syndromes

	2017 International	Villefranche	Berlin	Inheritance	Clinical features
1	Classical EDS (cEDS)	Classical type	Types I and II	AD	Soft hyperextensible skin Mesomorphic build Cigarette-paper scarring Molluscoid pseudotumors Spheroids
2	Classical-like EDS (clEDS)			AR	Velverty hyperextensible skin No atrophic scarring Generalized joint hypermobility Easy bruising
3	Cardiac-valvular EDS (cvEDS)			AR	Cardiac valve dysfunction Hyperextensible skin Atrophic scars and bruising
4	Vascular EDS (vEDS)	Vascular type	Type IV	AD	Bruising Thin translucent skin Aneurysms, vascular rupture, bowel rupture
5	Hypermobile EDS (hEDS)	Hypermobility type	Type III	AD	Marked joint hypermobility
6	Arthrochalasia EDS (aEDS)	Arthrochalasia type	Types VIIA and VIIB	AD	Short stature Extreme joint laxity Congenital dislocation of the hip
7	Dermatosparaxis EDS (dEDS)	Dermatosparaxis type	Type VIIC	AR	Skin fragility Cutis laxa
8	Kyphoscoliotic EDS (kEDS)	Kyphoscoliosis type	Type VI	AR	Neonatal muscle hypotonia Joint hyperextensibility Kyphoscoliosis Ocular lesions
9	Brittle Cornea syndrome (BCS)			AR	Thin cornea +/- rupture Early progressive ketaoconus / keratoglobus Blue sclerae
10	Spondylodysplastic EDS (spEDS)	EDS Progerioid type		AR	Short stature from childhood Muscle hypotonia Limbs bowing
11	Musculocontractural EDS (mcEDS)			AR	Multiple congenital contractures Characteristic congenital facies Skin hyperextensibility, brusing, atrophic scars
12	Myopathic EDS (mEDS)			AD or AR	Early muscle hypotonia/atrophy, improves with age Distal joint hypermobility Proximal joint contractures
13	Periodontal EDS (pEDS)	EDS periodontis	Type VIII	AD	Hyperextensible skin Mucosal fragility Periodontitis
No longer included in EDS spectrum					
X-linked EDS with muscle hematoma		Other	Type V	X-linked recessive	
Fibronectin-deficient		Other	Type X	Unknown	
Occiptal horn syndrome			Type IX	X-linked recessive	
Familial articular hypermobility		Other	Type XI	AD	

Modified from Beighton, P. et al. (1998) *Am J Med Genet*, 77, 31–37 & Malfait, F. et al. (2017) *Am J Med Genet C Semin Med Genet*, 175(1),8–26.

Gastrointestinal involvement presents as hematemesis, melena, and colonic rupture, and vascular lesions include arterial rupture and aortic or other major vessel aneurysms. Complications in pregnancy can occur.[16,17] Underlying coagulopathies, dysphonia, and tongue hypermobility have been described.[18–20] Mild to moderate neuromuscular symptoms including muscle weakness, myalgia, and decreased vibration sense can also be seen.[21]

The following briefly summarizes the salient clinical features of the 13 EDS disease subtypes of the 2017 international classification where each type is defined with major and minor criteria as well as causative genetics.[6] *Table 21.1* also summarizes the nomenclature of the prior Berlin and Villefranche systems and indicates where these overlap with the new system. The new system was created in response to the expanded understanding of the

genetics of EDS, leading to new and sometimes rare forms not well addressed under the prior systems. It also responds to the need to strictly define the clinical cohorts to provide appropriate management guidelines as the manifestations and complications of the disease vary between subtypes.[11,22]

1. Classical EDS

As in the 1997 Villefranche classification (*Table 21.1*), classic (autosomal dominant) EDS includes types I (gravis) and II (mitis) from the Berlin classification, as their difference is merely one of severity of involvement. Patients suffer from soft hyperextensible skin with a tendency to split over bony eminences.[8,23,24] A broad mesomorphic physique with wide hands and feet is characteristic. Extensive tissue paper scarring (said to resemble

Table 21.2
EDS groupings by pathogenetic mechanisms

	2017 International classification	Locus	Gene	Protein	Inheritance
Group A: Disorders of collagen primary structure and processing					
1	Classical EDS (cEDS)	9q34.3	COL5A1	Type V collagen	AD
		2q32.2	COL5A2	Type V collagen	
		17q21.33	COL1A1	Type I collagen	
4	Vascular EDS (vEDS)	2q32.2	COL3A1	Type III collagen	AD
		17q21.33	COL1A1	Type I collagen	
6	Arthrochalasia EDS (aEDS)	17q21.33	COL1A1	Type I collagen	AD
		7q21.3	COL1A2	Type I collagen	
7	Dermatospraxis EDS (dEDS)	5q35.3	ADAMTS2	A disintegrin-like and metalloproteinase with thrombospondin type 1 motif 2	AR
3	Cardiac-valvular EDS (CVEDS)	7q21.3	COL1A2	Type I collagen	AR
Group B: Defects in collagen folding and cross-linking					
8	Kyphoscoliotic EDS (kEDS-PLOD1)	1p36.22	PLOD1	Procollagen-lysin, 2-oxoglutarate 5-dioxygenase 1 (lysylhydroxylase 1)	AR
8	Kyphoscoliotic EDS (kEDS-FKBP14)	7p14.3	FKBP14	FK506-binding protein 14	AR
Group C: Defects in structure and function of myomatrix (interface of muscle and extracellular matrix)					
2	Classical-like EDS (clEDS)	6p21.33-p21.32	TNXB	Tenascin XB	AR
12	Myopathic EDS (mEDS)	6q13-q14	COL12A1	Collagen XII	AD / AR
Group D: Defects in glycosaminoglycan biosynthesis					
10	Spondylodysplastic EDS (spEDS-B4GALT7)	5q35.3	B4GALT7	Galactosyltransferase I β4GalT7	AR
10	Spondylodysplastic EDS (spEDS-B3GALT6)	1p36.33	B3GALT6	Galactosyltransferase II β3GalT6	AR
11	Musculocontractural EDS (mcEDS-CHST14)	15q15.1	CHST14	Dermatan-4 sulfotransferase-1	AR
11	Musculocontractural EDS (mcEDS-DSE)	6q22.1	DSE	Dermatan sulfate epimerase-1	AR
Group E: Defects in complement pathway					
13	Periodontal EDS (pEDS)	12p13.31	C1R	Complement C1r subcomponent	AD
		12p13.31	C1S	Complement C1s subcomponent	
Group F: Disorders of intracellular processes					
10	Spondylodysplastic EDS (spEDS-SLC39A13)	11p11.2	SLC39A13	Zinc transporter ZIP13	AR
9	Brittle Cornea Syndrome (BCS)	16q24	ZNF469	Zinc finger protein 469	AR
		4q27	PRDM5	PR domain zinc finger protein 5	AR
Unresolved forms of EDS					
5	Hypermobile EDS (hEDS)	?	?	?	AD

Modified from Malfait, F. et al. (2017) *Am J Med Genet C Semin Med Genet*, 175(1),8–26. Additional references.100–110

a fish's mouth) over the knees and shins is usually present and molluscoid pseudotumors are common, with the cutaneous findings more prominent than in hypermobility types.[12,25] Additional features may include epicanthic folds, mitral valve prolapse, cutaneous varicosities, myopia, and late-onset osteoarthrosis.[13] Complications in pregnancy include premature rupture of membranes, increasing perineal skin tearing, and prolapsing uterus and bladder.[25] Breast calcification has been reported as a complication from screening mammography.[26] Mutations involve multiple structural collagen genes including *COL5A1*, *COL5A2*, and *COL1A1*.[22]

2. Classical-like EDS

This subtype explicitly recognizes the autosomal recessive inheritance patterns seen in some cases with symptoms similar to classical EDS. A common feature is skin hyperextensibility with velvety texture, but not atrophic scarring. Generalized joint hypermobility can be seen both in the absence and presence of recurrent dislocations, mostly in the ankle and shoulder. Skin is easily bruised, often with spontaneous ecchymoses.[27] Other features such as foot deformities, leg edema, mild muscle weakness, and rectal and gynecological prolapse can be seen. Defects in *TNXB*, the gene encoding tenascin X, result in abnormally clumped elastic fibers and are responsible for autosomal recessive forms of EDS that phenotypically mimic the autosomal dominant classical subtype.[28–31] Tenascin X, an extracellular matrix glycoprotein that binds to and regulates collagen fibril arrangement and possibly

remodeling in the dermis can be affected. This and the cardiac-valvular subtype discussed below are newly defined within the 2017 international EDS classification, as are subtypes 9–12.[6]

3. Cardiac–valvular EDS

This autosomal recessive form of EDS is associated with severe and progressive deterioration of cardiac valve integrity and function.[32] Skin is thin and hyperextensible with atrophic scars and ready bruising. Inguinal hernias, joint dislocations, and various foot deformities can be encountered.[33,34]

4. Vascular EDS

Vascular EDS (vEDS), autosomal dominant, is of particular importance because it is associated with the most severe vascular involvement.[35–37] While vascular phonotypes can be seen in other EDS subtypes, they are particularly prominent here.[38,39] Patients manifest ecchymotic lesions on the knees, shins, and elbows, and features of acrogeria are often present.[13,40,41] The skin is characteristically thin and translucent. Additional cutaneous manifestations include short stature, keloidal or elastotic scars, elastosis perforans serpiginosa, large eyes, lobeless ears, tooth loss, a Madonna-like facies, acro-osteolysis, diffuse scalp alopecia, and orthopedic manifestations including congenital dislocation of the hip.[13,42–47] Aneurysms can arise in the aorta or other major vessels, and arteriovenous fistulae and arterial dissection may be complications.[13,48] Blood vessel walls are notoriously

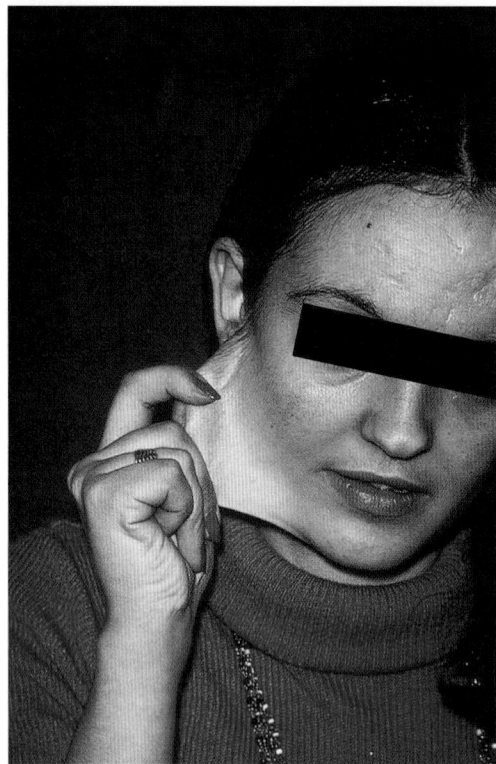

Fig. 21.1
Ehlers-Danlos syndrome: this female shows hyperelastic skin, hypertelorism, and a widened nasal bridge. By courtesy of R.A. Marsden, MD, St George's Hospital, London, UK.

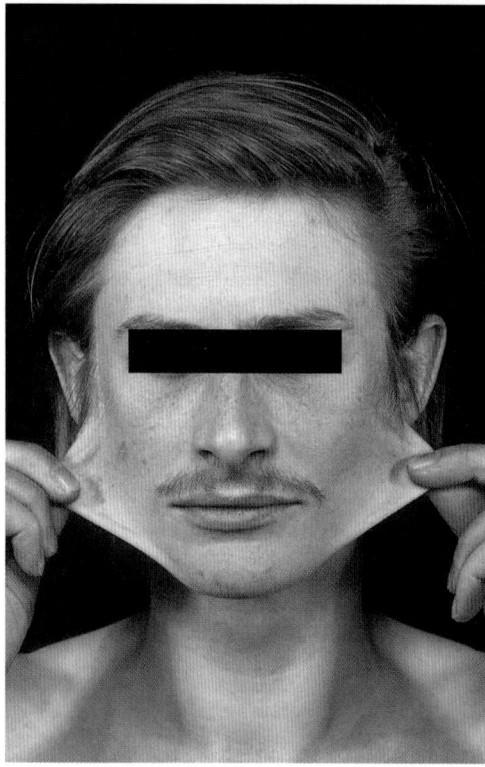

Fig. 21.2
Ehlers-Danlos syndrome: marked hyperelasticity of the skin which, in the younger patient, springs back on release is characteristic. By courtesy of the Institute of Dermatology, London, UK.

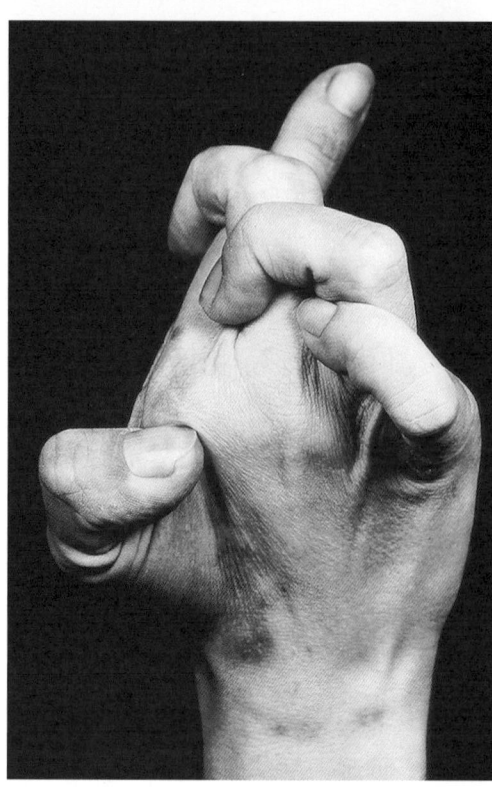

Fig. 21.3
Ehlers-Danlos syndrome: typical hyperextensible joints. By courtesy of F.M. Pope, MD, Northwick Park Hospital, London, UK.

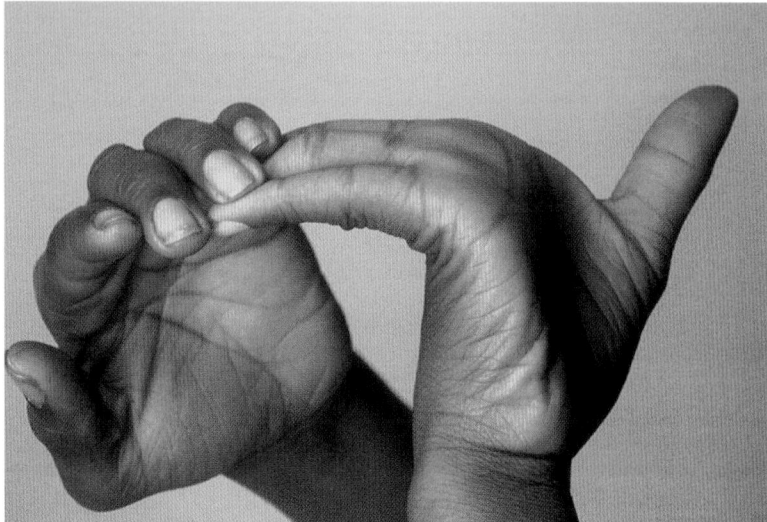

Fig. 21.4
Ehlers-Danlos syndrome: joints may be extremely lax. By courtesy of the Institute of Dermatology, London, UK.

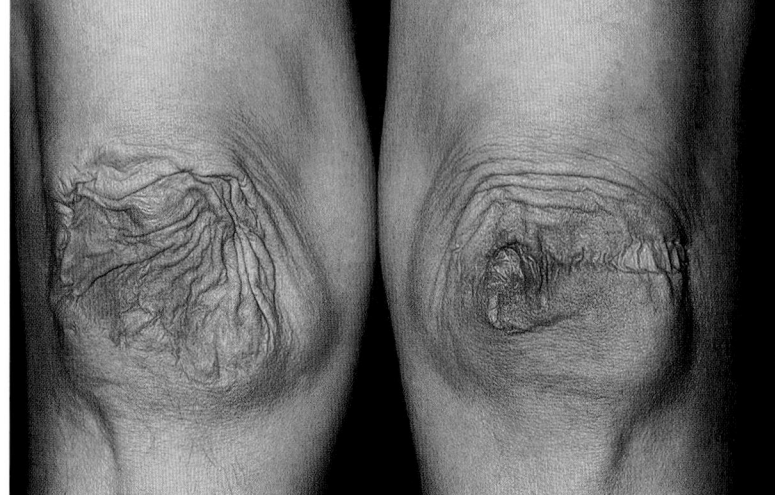

Fig. 21.5
Ehlers-Danlos syndrome: characteristic scarring involving the knees. By courtesy of F.M. Pope, MD, Northwick Park Hospital, London, UK.

fragile, complicating surgical correction and contributing to the very high mortality associated with this variant.[36,40] Fistulas of the carotid-cavernous sinus and bowel, pleuroperitoneal, and uterine rupture are also sometimes seen.[40–42,49]

5. Hypermobile EDS

Hypermobile (autosomal dominant) patients have minimal cutaneous manifestations, their presentation being limited to symptomatic joint laxity with hypermobility.[50] This is the most common subtype of EDS, representing 80–90% of all cases, and might represent the most common human connective tissue disease with an estimated prevalence of up to 10 million cases in the United States alone.[51] The stricter definitions of hypermobile EDS over prior criteria could reduce these higher prevalence estimates. Muscular pain both with and without activity is common. Additional uncommon findings in one study included dysphonia, Arnold-Chiari type I malformation, and dolichocolon.[52] This type is difficult to diagnose given the more limited spectrum of findings; many authors believe this is identical to the benign joint hypermobility syndrome.[51,53–55] The lack of established genetic causes suggests complexities such as polygenic disease, nonpenetrance, sex-linked penetrance, and multifactorial environmental influences.

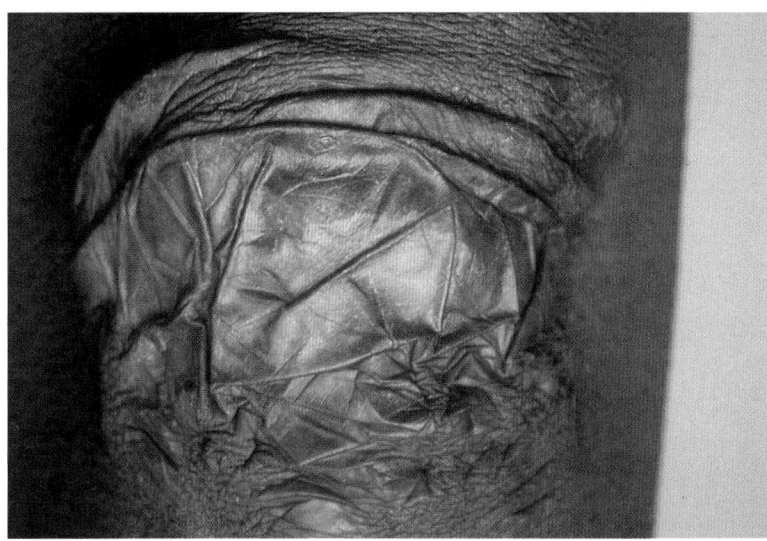

Fig. 21.6
Ehlers-Danlos syndrome: close-up view of the knee of a different patient. By courtesy of the Institute of Dermatology, London, UK.

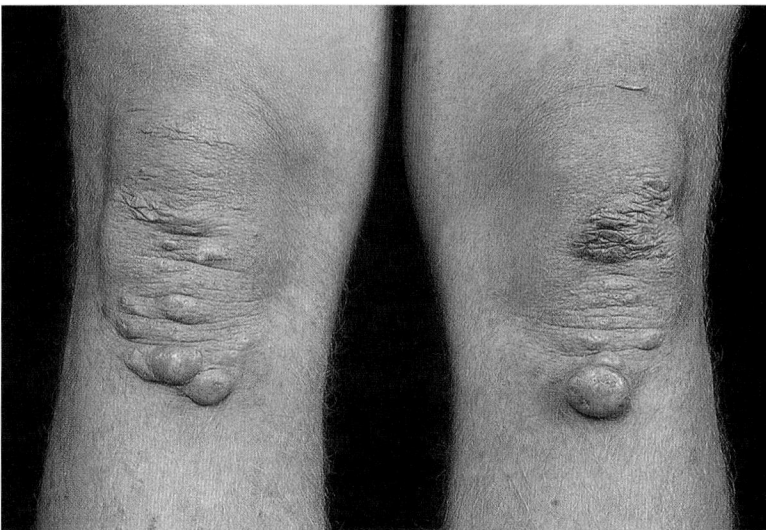

Fig. 21.7
Ehlers-Danlos syndrome: trauma to the subcutaneous tissues around the knees has resulted in these 'pseudotumors'. By courtesy of R.A. Marsden, MD, St George's Hospital, London, UK.

6. Arthrochalasia EDS

Arthrochalasia EDS, autosomal dominant, presents with bilateral congenital dislocation of the hips, severe widespread hypermobility and other joint dislocations, muscular hypotonia, and hyperextensible skin with fragility.[56,57]

7. Dermatosparaxis EDS

Dermatosparaxis EDS, autosomal recessive, named after a condition initially described in cows and sheep, is characterized by skin fragility with tearing and joint hypermobility (Gr. *sparagmos*, a tearing), is extremely rare, with only a handful of cases reported.[58–62] Mutations in *ADAMTS2* encoding procollagen I amino-peptidase are characteristic.[58,60] Patients present with marked skin fragility and laxity with redundant skin folds, blue sclerae, increased bruisability, micrognathia, large fontanelles, umbilical hernia, and growth retardation.[11,59,60,62–64]

8. Kyphoscoliosis EDS

Kyphoscoliosis EDS, autosomal recessive, presents with neonatal muscle hypotonia associated with generalized joint laxity, kyphoscoliosis, cystic malformation of the meninges, and cutaneous and ocular fragility with retinal detachment.[13,65–68] This type has been further bifurcated into those with deficiency of lysylhydroxylase (*PLOD1* mutations) and a second form which have normal levels of lysyl oxides, but harbor inactivating mutations in *FKBP14*.[69,70]

9. Brittle cornea syndrome

This autosomal recessive form is evidenced primarily with eye symptoms as the name brittle cornea syndrome implies.[71] Major features include thin cornea that can result in rupture, early onset of progressive keratoconus or keratoglobus, and bluish discoloration of the sclerae.[72] Hypermobility of distal joints can be seen and retinal detachment and deafness are also sometimes seen.[73] Mutations in *ZNF469* or *PRDM5* are seen.[74–76]

10. Spondylodysplastic EDS

Short stature, bowing of the limbs, and muscle hypotonia are important criteria. Skin hyperextensibility and osteopenia can be seen. Other features vary based on the which of three genes are involved in this autosomal recessive disorder: *SLC39A13*, *B3GALT6*, or *B4GALT7*.[77–81]

11. Musculocontractural EDS

This autosomal recessive subtype shows multiple flexural contractures that can be accompanied with clubfoot (talipes equinovarus), characteristic craniofacial dysmorphism, and skin with hyperextensibility, easy bruising, fagility with atrophic scars, and distinctly wrinkled palms.[82–84] Other complications include recurrent dislocations, pneumothorax, colonic diverticula, and spinal deformities.[85,86]

12. Myopathic EDS

Both autosomal dominant and autosomal recessive mechanisms of inheritance are described for musculocontractural EDS.[87,88] Early muscle hypotonia and/or atrophy improves with age. There is hypermobility of distal joint with contractures at the larger proximal joints such as the knees, hips, and elbows. Soft dough skin and atrophic scarring can be seen.[6]

13. Periodontal EDS

This autosomal dominant subtype features severe periodontitis with early onset, lack of attached gingiva, and pretibial plaques.[89–92] Because of the strong penetrance, a family history is often documented.[93,94] The usual EDS spectrum features of skin hyperextensibility, fragility and scarring with easy bruising, and hypermobile distal joints can also be seen.[95]

Other disease no longer considered to be within the EDS spectrum

- Berlin type V EDS resembles classic EDS with muscle hematomas, but has an X-linked transmission. Its existence as a separate entity has long been questioned.[12]
- Berlin type IX is currently classified in the cutis laxa spectrum (occipital horn syndrome).
- Berlin type X EDS is exceedingly rare and associated with fibronectin deficiency and abnormal platelet aggregation. It is uncertain whether this separation as a distinctive variant is justified.[12]
- Berlin type XI EDS is now considered to be a separate entity, familial joint laxity syndrome.

Pathogenesis and histologic features

EDS represents a heterogeneous group of related genetic disorders characterized not only by abnormal fibrillar collagen synthesis but also by abnormalities in proteins that interreact with collagen. The 2017 international classification also structures the 13 subtypes by pathogenic mechanism into the six groupings below (see *Table 21.2*)[22,96]:

- Group A: disorders of collagen structure and processing
- Group B: defects in collagen folding and crosslinking
- Group C: defects in structure and function of myomatrix (interface of muscle and extracellular matrix)
- Group D: defects in glycosaminoglycan biosynthesis
- Group E: defects in complement pathway
- Group F: disorders of intracellular processes

The known genetic defects of all 13 types recognized under the 2017 international classification are summarized in *Table 21.2*. Only the genetic details of the most common subtype, hypermobile EDS, is completely unknown. For many of the rarer subtypes, molecular testing is considered necessary to firmly establish the diagnosis.[6]

Generally, histologic examination of skin biopsies from patients with EDS is unrewarding.[97] While there may appear to be a diminution in the number and thickness of the collagen fibers, the range is so wide in normal skin that histopathological examination really has little to offer; diagnosis is essentially molecular now that the genetic basis of most EDS subtypes is understood.[6,89]

Ultrastructural observations are also of limited value. In the classic variant, the resultant abnormal collagen fibrils are 25% greater in diameter, disorganized, and there are characteristic composite fibrils with a cauliflower-like appearance.[12,13,63] Tenascin-X deficient fibrils are imperfectly aligned.[63] In the vascular type, collagen fibrils are disorganized, irregular, fragmented, frayed, and show a variable diameter.[13] Hyaluronic acid globules, amorphous matrix, microcalcifications, elastic-like fibers, and microcavities are also present.[98] Similar ultrastructural findings are seen in defects in type I collagen.[99] The fibrils in the arthrochalasia type are angular, whereas in the dermatosparaxis type they have a hieroglyphics-like appearance.[12]

Aplasia cutis congenita

Clinical features

Aplasia cutis congenita (congenital absence of the skin) presents as a focal or widespread loss of skin, subcutaneous fat, and sometimes deeper tissues.[1-4] The incidence is approximately 3:20000 live births.[1] The vast majority involve the scalp, but the extremities and trunk can be involved.[5-9] It represents a heterogeneous group of conditions of varied etiologies, which since 1986 has been usefully subdivided into nine groups based on associated features, etiological factors, distribution of lesions, and patterns of inheritance.[2] Usually, localized aplasia cutis is an isolated phenomenon (group 1), but in a significant proportion of patients it may signify a serious underlying congenital systemic disease.[10]

- Group 1 patients are prototypic. This can be an autosomal dominant condition or sporadic in nature.[11,12] Lesions are congenital and present as single or multiple, variably shaped (punched out, round, oval, linear, or stellate), crusted or ulcerated areas measuring 1–2 cm in diameter, usually situated over the posterior aspect of the scalp in close relationship to the parietal hair whorl (*Fig. 21.8*).[2,13,14] Sometimes they are accompanied by conspicuous dilated veins.[2] Bullous lesions are occasionally encountered.[15] Healing is by scarring that is sometimes hypertrophic.[7] In up to 20–30% of cases, these scalp lesions are associated with underlying defects of the skull, meninges, and, less commonly, brain.[1,10,16-20] Some patients have additional congenital defects such as cleft lip and palate.[1,5,21,22] Rare cases with large defects including the underlying bone have been reported.[5,19] Many of these cases are susceptible to infectious complications and hemorrhage, which rarely can be fatal.[19,20] Thrombosis can complicate larger lesions.[23] Unlike smaller defects that heal spontaneously, these require surgical intervention.[19]

- Group 2 patients have scalp defects associated with transverse terminal limb defects, of which hypoplasia or aplasia of the distal phalanges is the most common.[1] This was initially described to be an autosomal dominant condition (Adams-Oliver syndrome), but autosomal recessive cases are reported.[24-33] Some other features include syndactyly, eye defects, nail dystrophy, vascular defects including cutis marmorata telangiectatica congenita, cardiac defects, abdominal wall defects, and pulmonary and central nervous system abnormalities.[26,34-37] Cases of congenital heart defects and aplasia cutaneous cutis without limb defects have been reported and proposed by some as a form of Adams-Oliver syndrome.[38] Multiple genes have now been reported in classic Adams-Oliver syndrome including: *ARHGAP31*, *DLL4*, *DOCK6*, *EOGT*, *RBPJ*, and *NOTCH1*.[33,39-45] Some of the disease features correlate with particular gene defects.[33] Non-familial probands tend to have higher incidence of additional

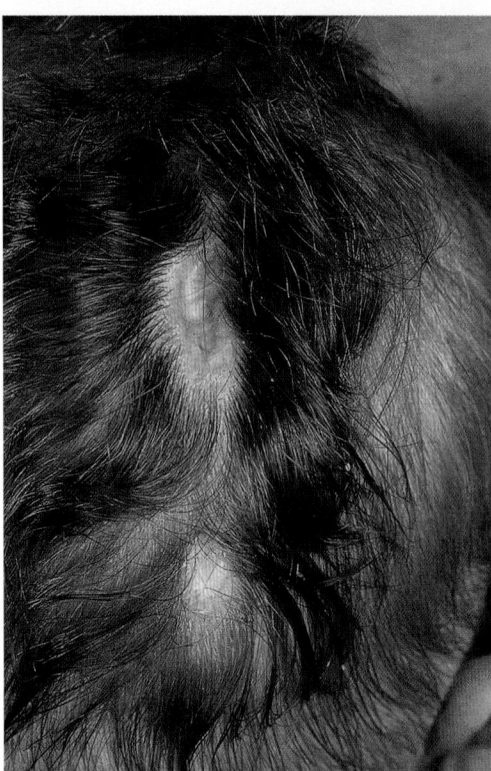

Fig. 21.8
Aplasia cutis: characteristic scarring with alopecia on the back of the head. By courtesy of D. Atherton, MD, Institute of Dermatology and Children's Hospital at Great Ormond Street, London, UK.

anomalies relative to familial probands.[33] *ARHGAP31* and *DOCK6* function in the cdc42/rac1 pathway while the remaining four are involved in the NOTCH signaling pathway.[33,46] *DOCK6* and *EOGT* are associated with the autosomal recessive form of the disease, while the other four genes show automosomal dominant inheritance.[37,47]

- Group 3 represents the combination of scalp aplasia with organoid (epidermal and sebaceous) nevi.[1,48-51] Patients may also have ophthalmological abnormalities including corneal opacities, scleral dermoids, and eyelid colobomata.[52-55] Occasionally, psychomotor retardation is evident.[52] SCALP syndrome has been described as nevus sebaceous syndrome, central nervous system malformation, aplasia cutis congenita, limbal dermoid, and pigmented nevus (giant congenital melanocytic nevus) with neurocutaneous melanosis and could be related.[51,56]

- Group 4 constitutes the association of aplasia cutis with an underlying maldevelopment of the brain or spinal cord (e.g., porencephaly, meningomyelocele, split cord).[1,5,57,58] Association with faun tail nevus (excessive lumbar hypertrichosis) has been noted.[58,59] Co-occurrence of both faun tail nevus and fetus papyraceus has been described, suggesting potential overlap with group 5.[60]

- Group 5 represents the association of truncal and limb aplasia cutis with fetus papyraceus or placental infarcts.[61-65]

- Group 6 defines aplasia cutis as a manifestation of epidermolysis bullosa (Bart syndrome). Patients present with skin defects accompanied by blistering on the trunk and extremities (*Figs 21.9* and *21.10*). This is a heterogeneous group which requires identification and classification of the underlying bullous dermatosis.[66-75]

- Group 7 patients have skin defects of the distal limbs unassociated with blistering. Autosomal dominant and recessive variants have been described.[1,12,76]

- Group 8 constitutes the development of aplasia cutis as a consequence of intrauterine infection (e.g., herpes simplex/varicella-zoster) or a teratogenic drug (e.g., methimazole, misoprostol).[77-85]

- Group 9 represents aplasia cutis developing against a background of malformation syndromes and ectodermal dysplasias (e.g., trisomy 13, 4p- syndrome, and focal dermal hypoplasia [FDH]).[86,87]

It is important that aplasia cutis is not mistaken for birth-related trauma with resultant medicolegal considerations.[88] Rare, fatal cases with systemic aplasia cutis congenita have been described.[89,90]

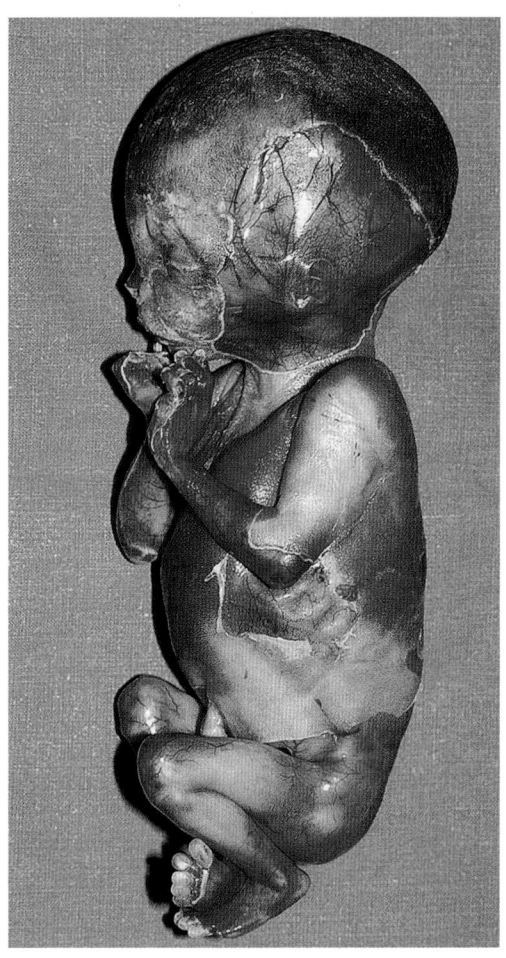

Fig. 21.9
Aplasia cutis: in this example, the widespread loss of the skin is a manifestation of epidermolysis bullosa (Bart syndrome).

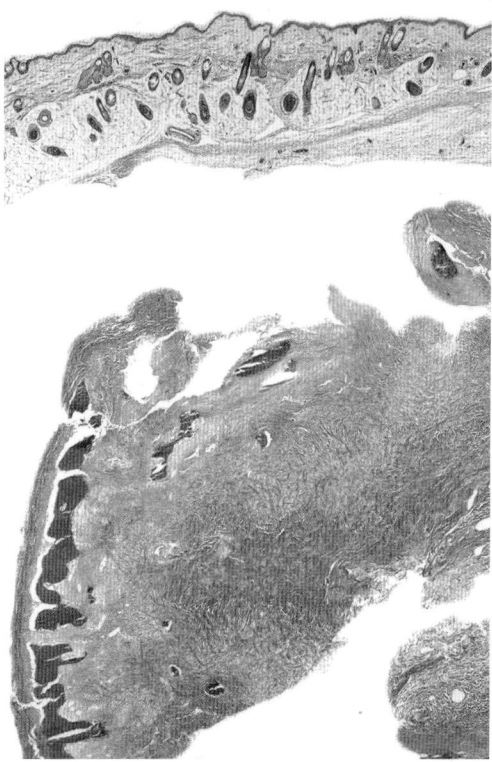

Fig. 21.11
Aplasia cutis: scanning view showing scarring and bone formation.

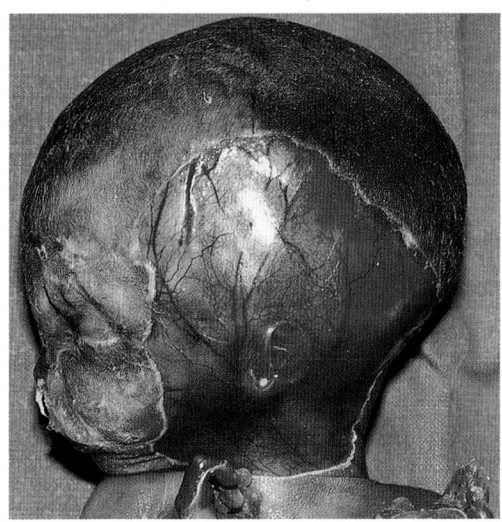

Fig. 21.10
Aplasia cutis: close-up view of Fig. 21.9.

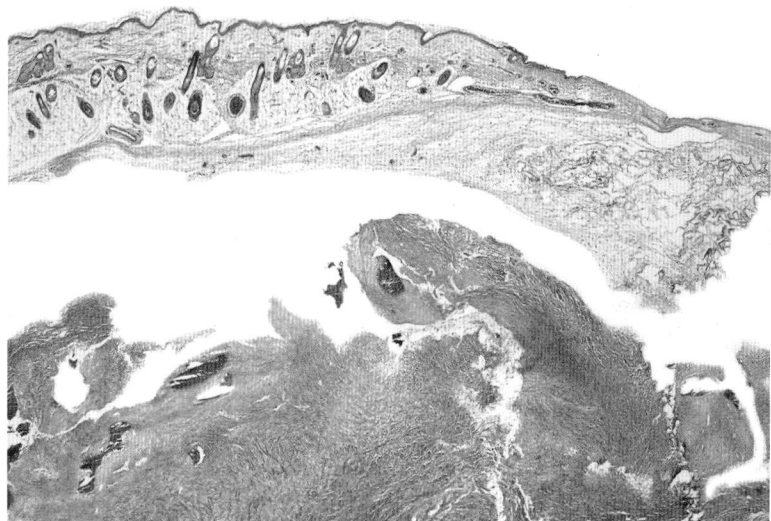

Fig. 21.12
Aplasia cutis: note the loss of appendages on the right side of the field.

Histologic features

Histologic examination typically reveals an ulcer bed deep to which granulation tissue may be evident (Figs 21.11–21.13). The appendages are absent. If a healed lesion is examined, re-epithelialization of the defect may be seen. There is associated scarring of the dermis.

Focal dermal hypoplasia syndrome

Clinical features

FDH (Goltz syndrome) is a rare X-link autosomal dominant disorder involving lesions of both ectoderm and mesoderm and is found almost exclusively in females.[1–6] Sporadic variants are frequently encountered, and a small number of affected males have been reported, possibly from postzygotic mutations; the male homozygous state appears to be lethal.[3–5,7–14] FDH syndrome is associated with cutaneous, skeletal, ocular, oral, dental, aural, and soft tissue defects.[1,2,4,15]

PORCN (Xp11.23) encodes an O-acetyltransferase that facilitates secretion of ligands for the Wnt pathway, and a variety of inactivating mutations including nonsense, missense, splicing, and frameshift (insertions and deletions, including microdeletions) are associated with FDH.[5,12,13,16–23] Sporadic cases tend to have point mutations and small deletions while familial cases show larger deletions.[11,24,25] The Wnt pathway is critical for embryological development of a number of tissues including skin, fibrous, adipose, muscle, bone, teeth, nervous system, and limb patterning.[21,26] A transgenic mouse model with a conditional PORCN mutant allele can recapitulate various features of the human disease including FDH.[27–29] The variability in phenotype has been attributed to mosaicism and lyonization.[5,11,30,31] Diagnosis has been proposed to include at least three characteristic skin findings and one or more limb malformations. Using such operational criteria, the vast majority of patients exhibit detectable PORCN mutations.[24] Prenatal diagnosis is an option where appropriate.[32]

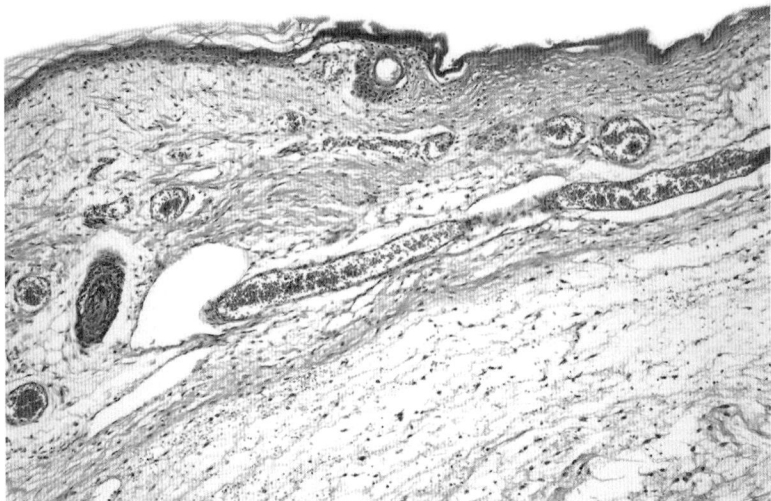

Fig. 21.13
Aplasia cutis: there is ulceration.

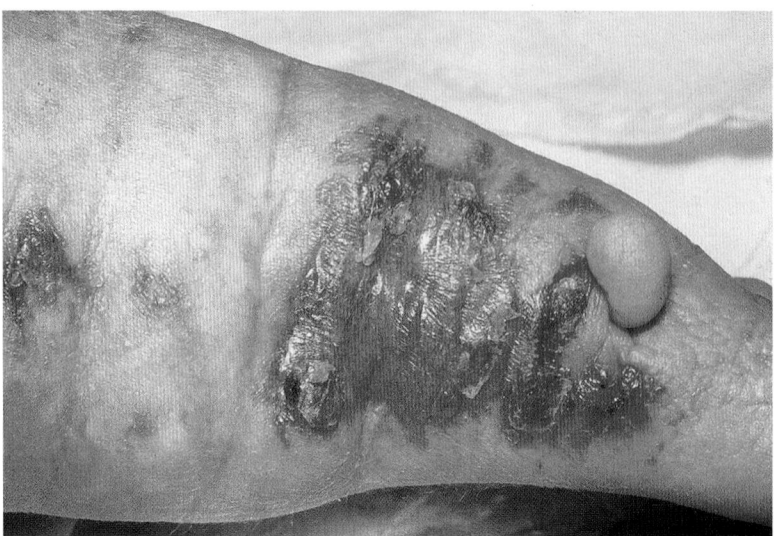

Fig. 21.15
Focal dermal hypoplasia: in addition to aplasia cutis there is a polypoid fatty tumor. By courtesy of D. Atherton, MD, Institute of Dermatology and Children's Hospital at Great Ormond Street, London, UK.

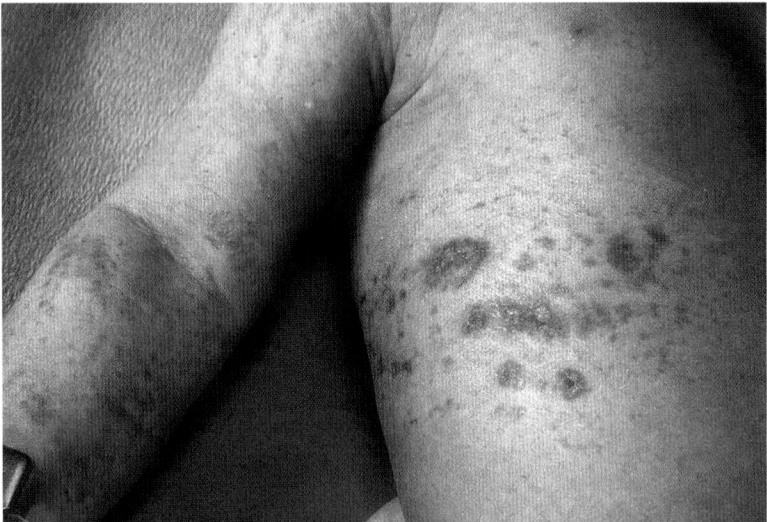

Fig. 21.14
Focal dermal hypoplasia: the early lesions have an inflammatory nature and a somewhat linear distribution. By courtesy of D. Atherton, MD, Institute of Dermatology and Children's Hospital at Great Ormond Street, London, UK.

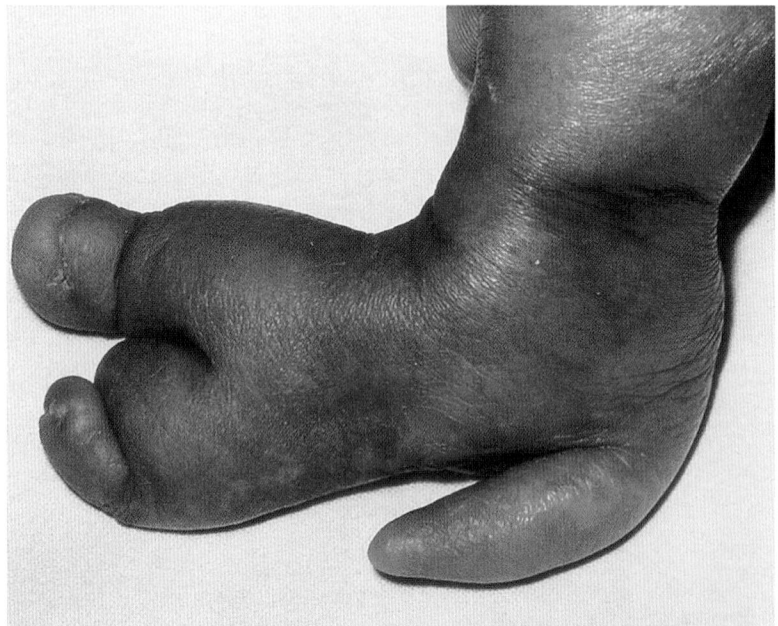

Fig. 21.16
Focal dermal hypoplasia: skeletal manifestations are an important feature. By courtesy of D. Atherton, MD, Institute of Dermatology and Children's Hospital at Great Ormond Street, London, UK.

Cutaneous defects

Cutaneous lesions, which are almost invariably present from birth, include areas of hypoplastic skin (such as aplasia cutis) which present clinically as depressed and atrophic cribriform and reticulated lesions, linear (Fig. 21.14) or reticular areas of erythema, hyper- or hypopigmentation, fatty tumors (most often on the limbs) (Fig. 21.15), and raspberry-like papillomatous or verrucous growths, particularly around the ostia of the body.[4,33–37] Telangiectasia is a frequent manifestation.[24,33] Linear lesions follow Blaschko lines and are most often seen on the limbs and cheeks.[4,33,38,39] Nail dystrophy, anonychia, and focal alopecia can be present.[4,33,37,40–42]

Skeletal defects

Skeletal manifestations, including hypoplasia or aplasia of the digits, 'lobster claw hand', syndactyly, and polydactyly, are seen in 60–70% of patients (Fig. 21.16).[4,33,43] Facial, trunk, or limb asymmetry is seen in 30%.[33] Linear, vertically oriented, radiopaque striations in the metaphyses of long bones (osteopathia striata) are characteristic (Fig. 21.17).[4,38] Bone weakness and early osteoporosis have been reported.[37] Microcrania, sometimes with mental retardation, scoliosis, kyphosis, and spina bifida occulta have also been described.[33]

Ocular, oral, dental, and aural defects

Ocular findings include hypertelorism, microphthalmia, anophthalmia, aniridia, strabismus, nystagmus, glaucoma, retinal detachment, and colobomata of the iris, retina, choroid, and optic nerve.[35,44,45] Oral and dental lesions involving tooth maldevelopment (dysplasia), partial agenesis, anodontia, malocclusion, and poor enamel and papillary gingival hyperplasia may occur in up to 40% of patients.[33,40,41,46–51] Aural involvement may result in both sensorineural and conduction deafness.[40] A history of tonsillectomy for obstructive sleep apnea was described in almost 90% in a series of 18 patients.[24]

Soft tissue and other defects

Soft tissue involvement can lead to striking facial asymmetry.[52] The facial characteristics include prominent narrow ears, pointed chin, and nasal changes of a narrow bridge and broadened tip.[33] Cleft lip and palate can occur.[5,6,48] Genitourinary, cardiac, abdominal wall defects, and mental retardation have also been reported.[17,48]

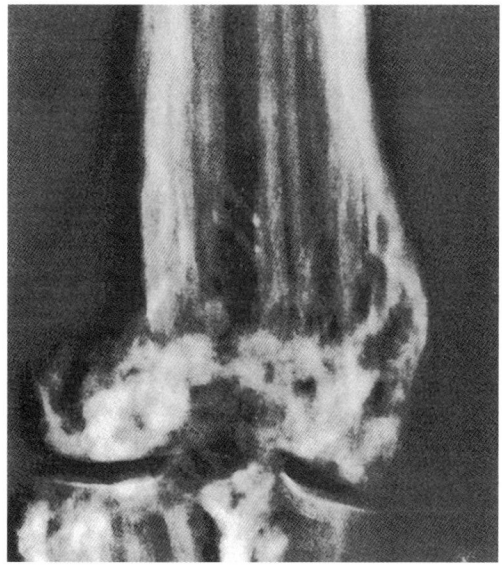

Fig. 21.17
Focal dermal hypoplasia: radiograph showing characteristic axially oriented dense striations of osteopathia striata of the lower femur of a 35-year-old man. Reproduced with permission from Bullough P.G. (1992) Atlas of Orthopedic Pathology, 2nd edn. New York: Gower Medical Publishing.

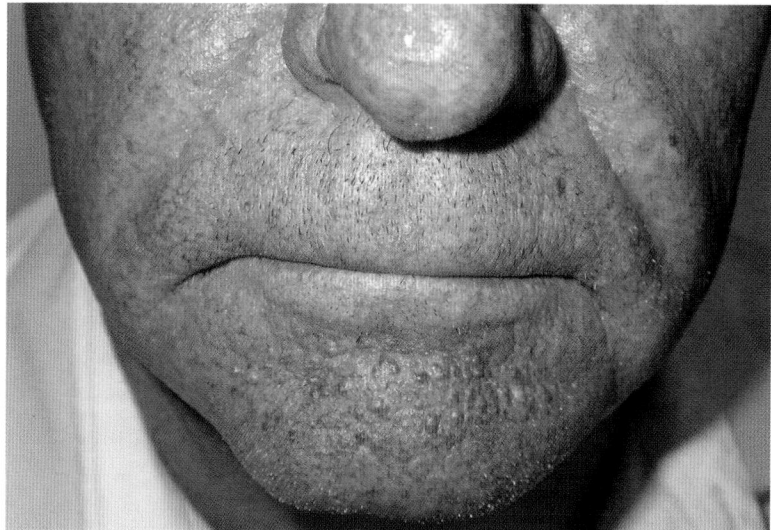

Fig. 21.18
Tuberous sclerosis: the lesions of adenoma sebaceum consist of numerous papules on the nose, cheeks, and chin. By courtesy of J.C. Pascual, MD, Alicante, Spain.

Histologic features

The fatty tumors show a markedly hypoplastic dermis with diminished, thinned collagen bundles and reduced elastic tissue accompanied by fatty replacement.[1,3,10,53,54] Adipocytes can be clearly seen approaching or even involving the papillary dermis.[4,48] Identical histologic appearances are seen in nevus lipomatosus superficialis.[55] Adnexa appear to be structurally normal, but may be reduced in number and situated abnormally superficial in the dermis.[48,56] The conventional view that fatty infiltration of the dermis represents mechanical herniation has been challenged and perhaps represents a heterotopic phenomenon (i.e., an adipocytic nevus).[34,47,48] The histologic appearances of the verrucous and papillomatous lesions include hyperkeratosis with epidermal hyperplasia and marked papillomatosis. The dermis is thinned, with fine collagen fibers and increased vascularity, especially in the papillary dermis.[3,57,58] The atrophic areas show dermal thinning with sparse attenuated collagen bundles and fatty replacement.[48,57] Elastic fibers may be increased and thickened.[3,48] The hyperpigmented foci are characterized by acanthosis with club-shaped rete ridges and increased melanin pigmentation. Melanophages are present in the papillary dermis.[48,57] By electron microscopy, collagen bundles are found loosely arranged in the extracellular matrix with smaller fibroblasts and irregular thickening of the nuclear lamina.[48]

Angiofibromas (adenoma sebaceum) and tuberous sclerosis

Clinical features

Tuberous sclerosis (epiloia, Bourneville disease) is a rare inherited systemic illness with an estimated incidence ranging broadly from 1:5800 to 1:300 000 and may affect up to 2 million people worldwide.[1-5] Although an autosomal dominant mode of inheritance is sometimes seen, many – if not most cases (up to 80%) – appear to arise by spontaneous mutation.[1-3,6-8] It comprises a constellation of cutaneous lesions as well as cerebral, ocular, cardiac, renal, pulmonary, and skeletal involvement.[4] The sex incidence is equal and there is no racial or ethnic predilection.[2]

Most characteristic of tuberous sclerosis are facial angiofibromas (adenoma sebaceum), which, while occasionally present at birth, more often appear during early childhood.[9-11] These were initially thought to be pathognomonic, but can also be seen in multiple endocrine neoplasia type I.[3,12,13] They are present in up to 90% of the adults with tuberous sclerosis and consist of smooth, dome-shaped, pink or reddish-brown papules and nodules (sometimes with associated telangiectases), bilaterally and symmetrically distributed, particularly in the butterfly area on the nose and cheeks and often extending to the chin, but sparing the upper lip (Fig. 21.18).[3,6,10] Rarely, the lesions can extend to the oral mucosa.[14] Occasionally, the lesions are very extensive and develop into large cauliflower-like masses.[15] Soft

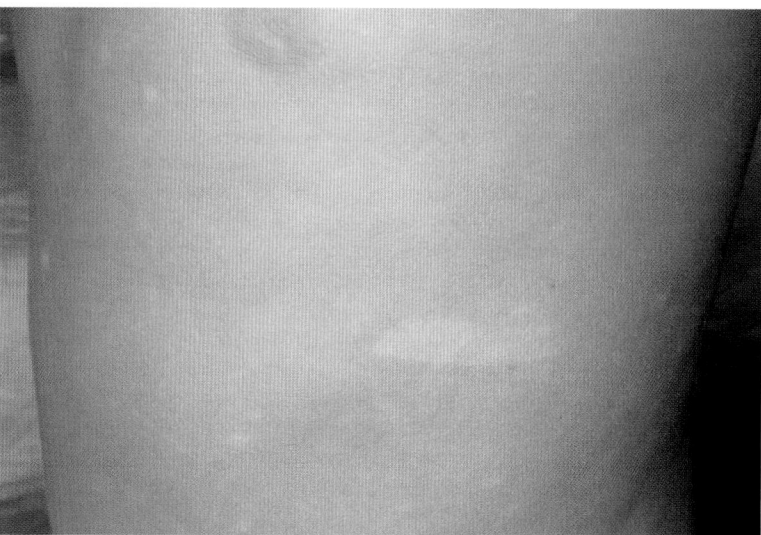

Fig. 21.19
Tuberous sclerosis: note the shagreen patch and typical 'ash-leaf' leukoderma. By courtesy of J.C. Pascual, MD, Alicante, Spain.

fibromas are also found about the face and scalp. Smooth, yellow or red fibrous plaques on the forehead may appear in infancy and be a presenting sign of tuberous sclerosis.[3,16,17] Unilateral facial angiofibromas have been noted and could represent segmental expression.[18] Multiple facial angiofibromas without any known genetic disorder have been described.[19]

White macular lesions, which may be single or multiple, are a very frequent initial cutaneous manifestation of tuberous sclerosis.[7,10,20-23] They are best appreciated when the skin is viewed with a Wood's lamp[3] and have been classified into three types[20]:
- The most common variant consists of polygonal 0.5–2.0-cm white lesions resembling a thumbprint.
- 'Ash leaf' variegate macules of leukoderma measuring approximately 1–3 cm in diameter are a particular feature of the second variant of tuberous sclerosis (Fig. 21.19).[3,9,12]
- The third variant consists of guttate scattered 1–3-mm white macules (so-called 'confetti lesions').[3,6,12]

These macular lesions are said to be present in 70% of patients with tuberous sclerosis.[2,10] They are evident at birth or develop in the neonatal period.[9] Hypopigmented patches may also affect the hair (poliosis), eyebrows, eyelashes, and occasionally the iris.[7,9,16,20,21,24-26]

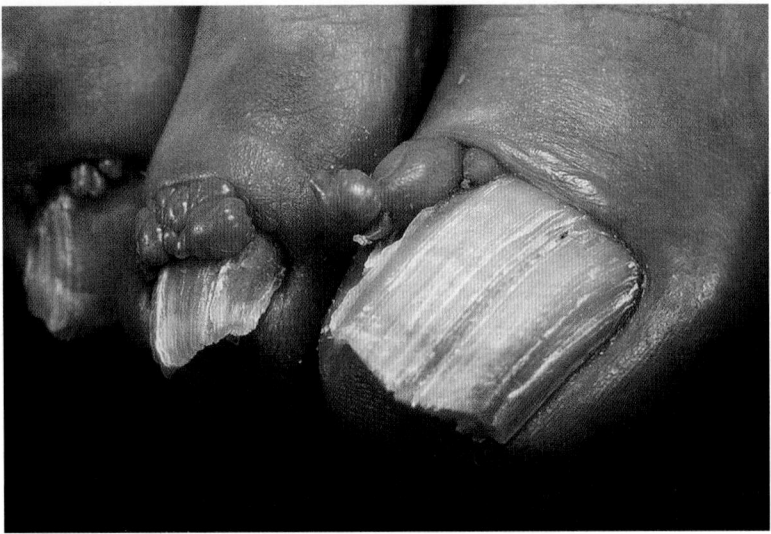

Fig. 21.20
Tuberous sclerosis: periungual fibromas are characteristic. By courtesy of the Institute of Dermatology, London, UK.

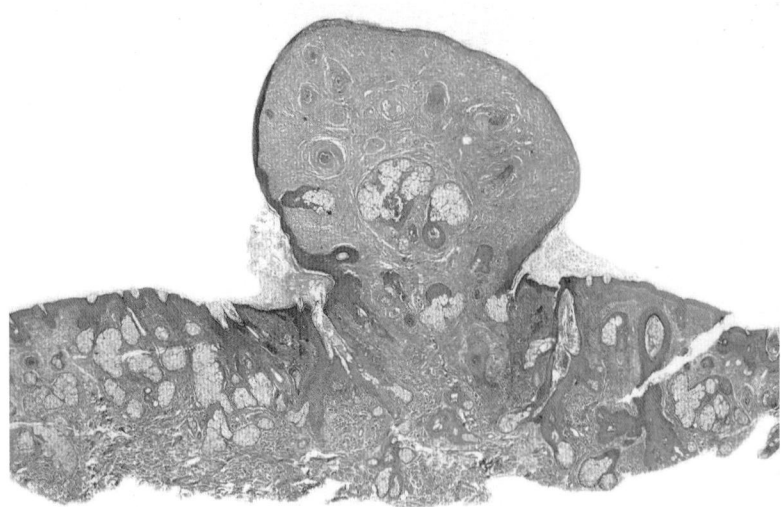

Fig. 21.21
Tuberous sclerosis: scanning view of a small polypoid lesion showing diminution of appendage structures and marked fibrosis.

Frequently seen is the shagreen patch – peau de chagrin (skin like grainy leather) – mildly yellow lesion found particularly on the lower back (see *Fig. 21.19*).[1–3,6,7,9,12,27–30] This is a connective tissue nevus, usually presenting in early childhood or around puberty.[7] Large patches in association with spina bifida occulta have been reported.[31] Skin tags are often present, sometimes in large numbers.[9] Other cutaneous lesions include flesh-colored sub- and periungual fibromas (*Fig. 21.20*).[3,29] These are found in up to 50% of patients with tuberous sclerosis and usually develop at or around puberty.[2,6,9] Café-au-lait macules may sometimes be present.[2,3,9,12,29,32] Oral and eyelid angiofibromas with blepharoptosis, enamel teeth pitting, and gingival fibromas can be seen.[3,33–35]

Involvement of the central nervous system usually, but not invariably, results in mental retardation, which is sometimes severe (50–82% of patients).[2,3,7,36] Epilepsy is a common manifestation (80–93% of patients) and often is the presenting symptom.[2,7,37] Patients may develop focal or generalized tonic-clonic fits or they can suffer from infantile spasms.[7] The term 'epiloia' was coined to define the triad of adenoma sebaceum, mental retardation, and epilepsy.[12] Calcification, particularly of the basal ganglia, is radiologically detected in up to 76% of cases.[38] Ophthalmological investigation reveals the presence of retinal 'tumors' or phakomata in up to 53% of cases, although similar lesions can be seen in neurofibromatosis.[2,39,40] Occasionally these are calcified. Subependymal nodules and subependymal giant cell astrocytomas are also common.[41,42]

Cardiac manifestations include murmurs, electrocardiographic abnormalities, heart failure, and sudden death.[43] Pulmonary lesions, although rare, may result in exertional dyspnea, cor pulmonale, and pneumothorax. Affected patients are usually female, often of normal intelligence, and seem less often to suffer from epilepsy.[21] The prognosis is poor.

Radiological examination of the hands and feet often reveals bone cysts, focal sclerosis, and periosteal thickening.[7,44]

Pathogenesis and histologic features

Tuberous sclerosis results from inactivating mutations including deletion, nonsense, missense, and frameshift of two separate genes: *TSC1* (9q34) and *TSC2* (16p13).[3,12,45–47] These encode the tumor suppressor proteins hamartin and tuberin, respectively. These two proteins heterodimerize and are important regulators of cell proliferation and survival. Loss of TSC1 or TSC2 function in the mTOR (mammalian target of rapamycin) pathway withdraws inhibition with numerous effects in the cells. The ensuing dysregulation of the downstream mTORC1 signaling complex (as opposed to mTORC2) impacts both directly and indirectly on a variety of signaling pathways including Akt in the phosphatidylinositol-3-kinase (PI3K) pathway, extracellular-regulated kinase (ERK), β-catenin, transforming

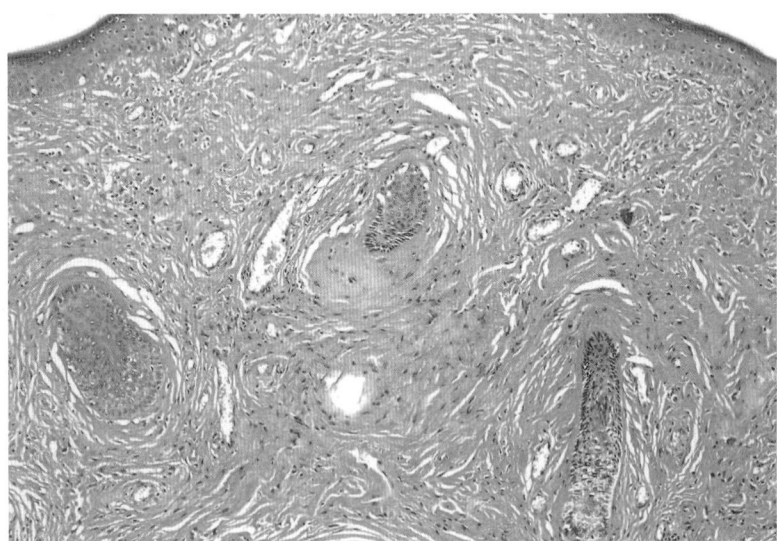

Fig. 21.22
Tuberous sclerosis: there is perifollicular scarring and vascular ectasia.

growth factor-β (TGF-β), protein kinase C alpha (PKCα), and p27.[3,12,29,47–60] mTORC1 impinges on a variety of processes including cell growth, autophagy, cell survival, angiogenesis, lymphangiogenesis, cellular differentiation, and inflammation/immune function.[61,62] The variety of associated tumors have very low mutational loads relative to carcinomas, but a subset can harbor large chromosomal aberrations.[63]

The previously applied term 'adenoma sebaceum' is, in fact, a misnomer, the histologic features being those of a fibrovascular hamartomatous proliferation with concomitant atrophy and compression of the skin adnexae. Although often described as an angiofibroma, connective tissue nevus is a more appropriate designation. The lesion consists of an irregular proliferation of fibrous tissue and blood vessels (*Figs 21.21* and *21.22*). Occasionally, the adnexae become surrounded and compressed by concentric lamellae of collagen (*Fig. 21.23*).

The shagreen patch is a collagenoma, the dermis being replaced by broad bundles of fibrous tissue with diminished or absent elastica (*Figs 21.24* and *21.25*). Similarly, the sub- and periungual fibromas are fibrous tissue hamartomas.

The hypopigmented macules may show normal or reduced numbers of melanocytes. Ultrastructurally, they show impaired melanogenesis (diminished numbers of small, immature melanosomes).[9,20] This appears to be due

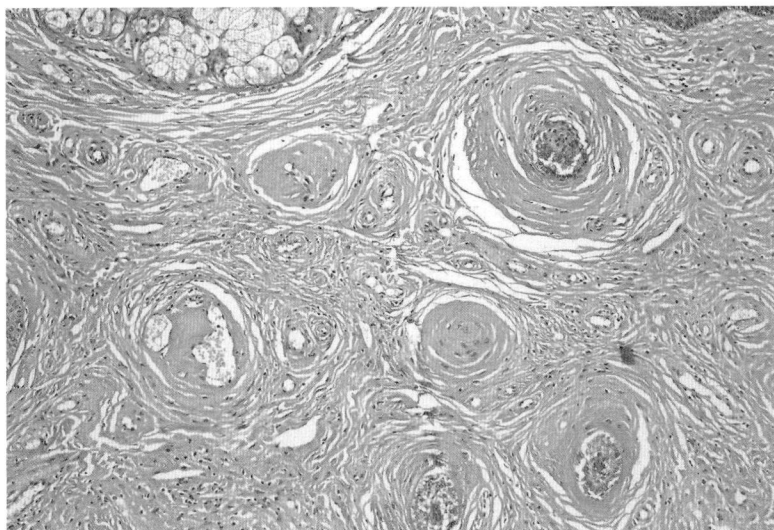

Fig. 21.23
Tuberous sclerosis: this view highlights the concentric perifollicular fibrosis.

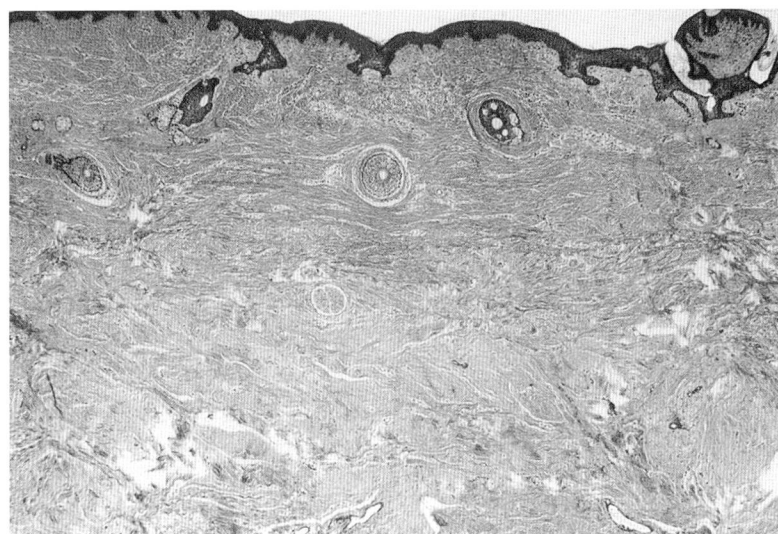

Fig. 21.24
Tuberous sclerosis: shagreen patch. The dermis is replaced by dense, relatively acellular collagen which extends down to the subcutaneous fat.

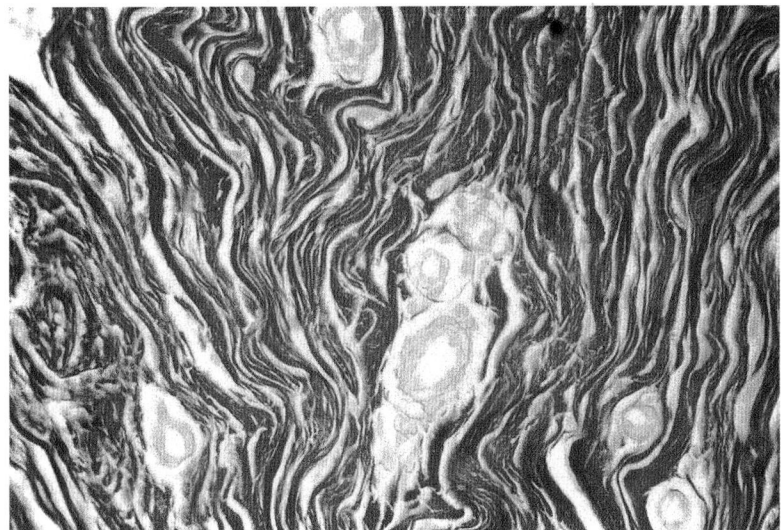

Fig. 21.25
Tuberous sclerosis: shagreen patch showing the complete absence of elastic tissue (elastic van Gieson).

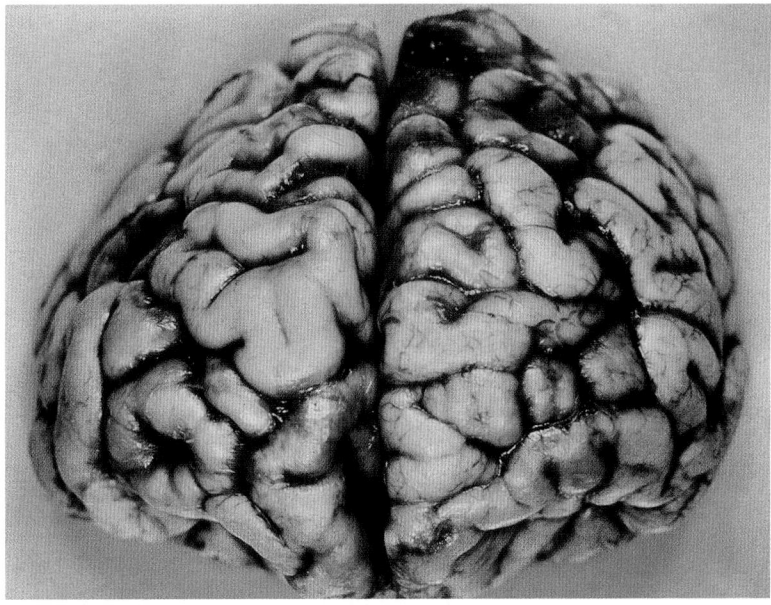

Fig. 21.26
Tuberous sclerosis: the brain is reduced in size and the gyri are markedly broadened. By courtesy of I. Allen, MD, Royal Victoria Hospital, Belfast, UK.

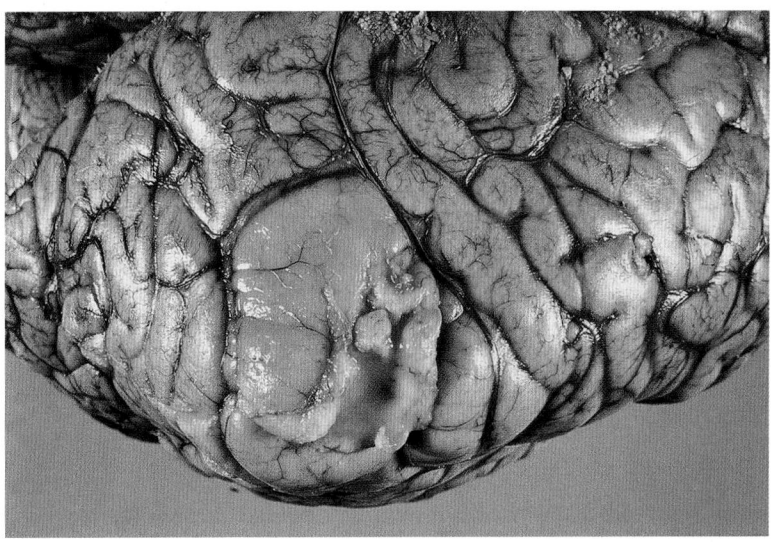

Fig. 21.27
Tuberous sclerosis: a typical 'tuber' on the cortex (lower midfield). By courtesy of I. Allen, MD, Royal Victoria Hospital, Belfast, UK.

to disrupted melanogenesis and is melanocyte mediated by constitutive activation of mTORC1 that occurs with loss of TSC1 or TCS2 function.[64,65]

The brain in tuberous sclerosis may be normal or diminished in size (Fig. 21.26). The neuropathology includes cortical tubers, subcortical heterotopic nodules, and subependymal giant cell astrocytomas (Figs 21.27–19.30).[66–68]

The cardiac manifestations are due to intramyocardial rhabdomyomas, composed of large vacuolated (glycogen-filled) muscle cells.[68–71] Spontaneous regression is well documented.[70,72]

The kidneys contain angiomyolipomata (often bilaterally and multiple) in up to 60% of patients and occasionally show infantile polycystic disease.[7,38,73–75] Interestingly, cutaneous angiomyolipomas not associated with tuberous sclerosis are negative for MART-1 and HMB-45.[76–78] Renal cell carcinoma (which may present in infancy or childhood) is also sometimes encountered.[62,79,80] A few patients with tuberous sclerosis complex also have mutations in the nearby PKD1 gene, resulting in autosomal dominant polycystic kidney disease.[47,81]

Multiple cysts (lymphangiomyomatosis) are the most important pulmonary manifestation.[3,82–86] Females are predominantly affected.[84,87] Angiomyolipoma at this site is exceptional.[88,89]

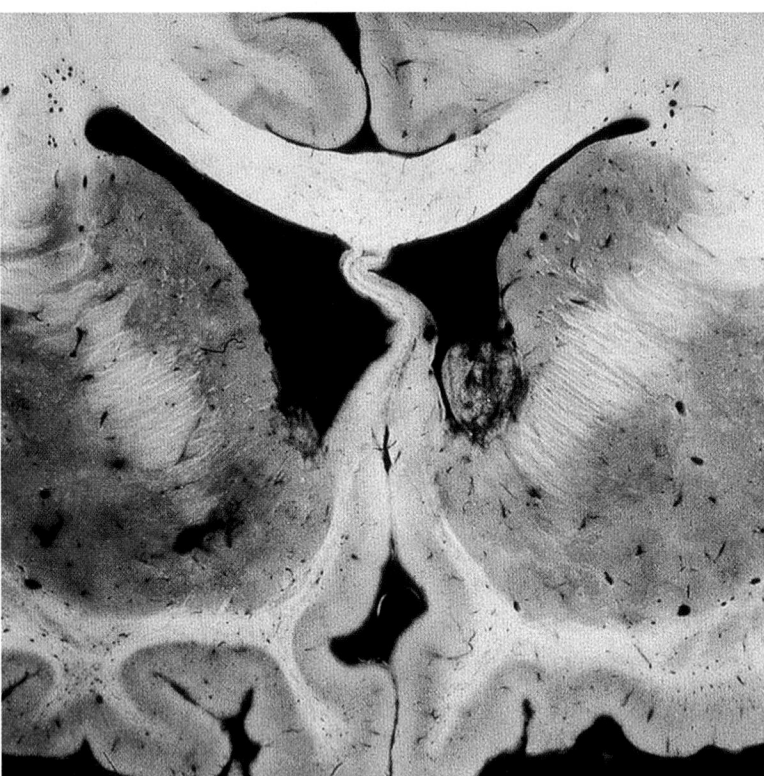

Fig. 21.28
Tuberous sclerosis: a small subependymal glial deposit projects into the right lateral ventricle. By courtesy of I. Allen, MD, Royal Victoria Hospital, Belfast, UK.

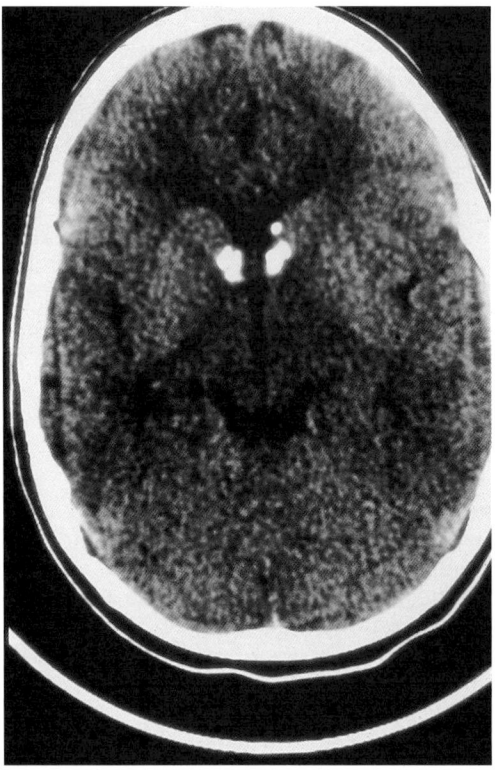

Fig. 21.29
Tuberous sclerosis: CT scan through the foramina of Monro shows the multiple periventricular calcific deposits characteristic of this disorder. By courtesy of the Division of Neuroradiology, University Health Center of Pittsburgh, USA.

There may be an association with neuroendocrine (parathyroid, pituitary, and pancreatic) tumors.[90–92]

In general, tuberous sclerosis is associated with a poor prognosis, but partial or mosaic expression of the disease is not uncommon and such patients may enjoy a normal life span.[62] Treatment with mTOR inhibitors is transforming the clinical management of some of the more devastating manifestations of this disease.[42,87,93–97]

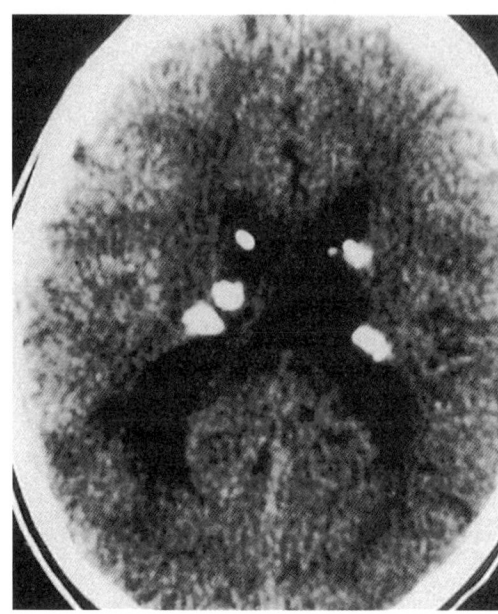

Fig. 21.30
Tuberous sclerosis: close-up view. By courtesy of the Division of Neuroradiology, University Health Center of Pittsburgh, USA.

Nephrogenic systemic fibrosis

Clinical features

Nephrogenic systemic fibrosis (formerly known as nephrogenic fibrosing dermopathy) is a multiorgan disease that can have a scleroderma-like dermatosis and is associated with renal failure often combined with exposure to gadolinium.[1–26]

Although it was initially thought to develop only in individuals undergoing hemodialysis, subsequent publications documenting its occurrence in patients being treated with peritoneal dialysis, or following transplantation, or solely with renal failure, broadened the definition.[1–3,27–31] Most patients have chronic kidney disease with the vast majority having stage 5 disease (estimated glomerular filtration rate [GFR] <15 mL/min/1.73 m^2). Disease course can parallel renal function.[32,33] Some patients with acute renal disease have also been reported to develop this condition.[34–38] Although the vast majority of documented patients are adults, presentation in children with renal insufficiency has been seen.[39–45] While several large studies have demonstrated an association with gadolinium exposure and renal failure, clearly not all patients with these conditions develop nephrogenic fibrosis.[20,46–55] Some of this variability may be due to the type of gadolinium contrast used.[24,25,56–58] The macrocyclic chelate bonds are more stable than linear bonds and thus considered to confer less risk in patients with compromised kidney function as defined by GFR guidelines.[23] Additional reported risk factors include cumulative exposure to gadolinium, erythropoietin exposure, and elevated ionized calcium and phosphate serum concentrations.[59,60] A mouse model of the disease suggests that changes in systemic iron mobilization may play a role as well.[61]

Although previously considered primarily a cutaneous disease, it is now known to affect other organs, as documented in several autopsy cases.[62–67] Extracutaneous findings can be seen, including in the deep soft tissue, blood vessels, thyroid, heart, kidney, dura, and lung.[62–66,68,69] In the skin, the condition is characterized by rapidly growing, symmetrical skin-colored or erythematous papules and nodules that coalesce to form erythematous or hyperpigmented progressive, brawny plaques, sometimes with a peau d'orange appearance (*Figs 21.31* and *21.32*).[3,5,12,34,70,71] These lesions on the breast sometimes mimic inflammatory breast cancer.[72,73] The plaques have an irregular border and islands of sparing are sometimes described.[30,71] The limbs and trunk are predominantly affected. The face is usually uninvolved, although there are a number of cases with yellow scleral plaques.[28,39,71] The skin is markedly thickened, hard, and has a wooden texture.[3,71,74] Lesions may be pruritic, painful, or associated with a burning sensation.[30] Flexion contractures are a common complication, often resulting in considerable immobility.[3] As a consequence, morbidity is high.[5] Occasionally, patients

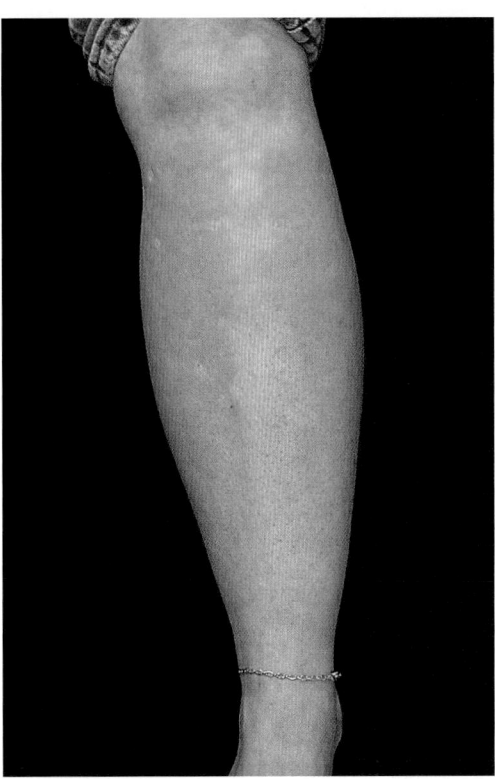

Fig. 21.31
Nephrogenic fibrosing nephropathy: note the swelling and erythema. By courtesy of S.E. Cowper, MD, Yale University, New Haven, USA.

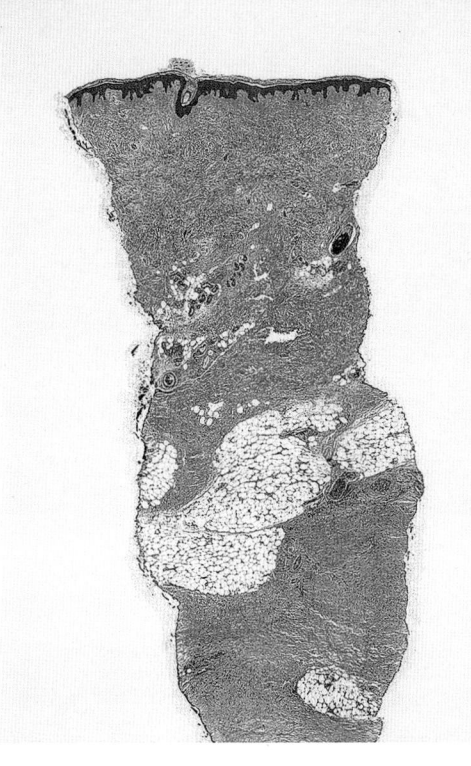

Fig. 21.33
Nephrogenic fibrosing dermopathy: there is diffuse fibrosis involving the full thickness of the dermis and extending into the septa of the subcutaneous fat.

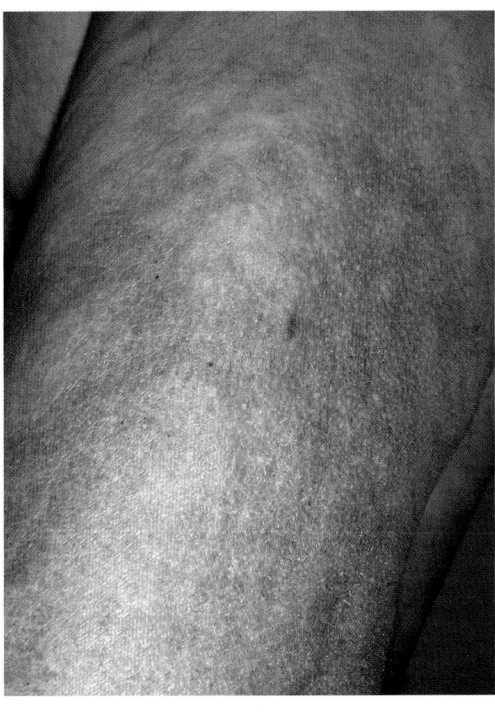

Fig. 21.32
Nephrogenic fibrosing nephropathy: this view shows an extensive brawny plaque with a peau d'orange appearance. By courtesy of S.E. Cowper, MD, Yale University, New Haven, USA.

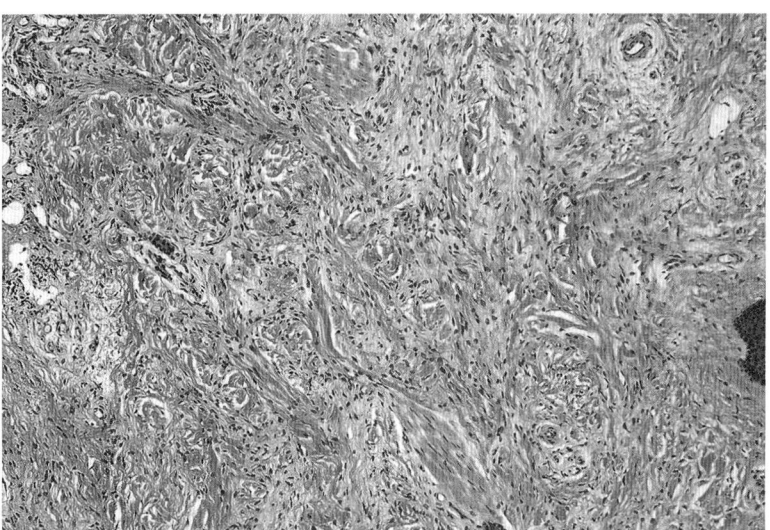

Fig. 21.34
Nephrogenic fibrosing dermopathy: there is a conspicuous spindle cell population.

may develop redundant skin similar to cutis laxa and generalized elastolysis.[75,76] Mortality can occur due to thromboembolism.[62]

Pathogenesis and histologic features

The exact mechanism of nephrogenic systemic fibrosis is still being unraveled.[77] The presence of high levels of gadolinium due to renal failure is thought to result in transmetallation, where various serum ions can interact with the gadolinium contrast complex, releasing free gadolinium.[22,78] Free gadolinium is toxic in animal studies and can be detected in tissue specimens from patients with nephrogenic systemic fibrosis.[4,16–18] In vitro studies have shown gadolinium to be profibrotic and proinflammatory, eliciting growth factors from monocytes.[79–83]

Histologically, early lesions are characterized by a subtle proliferation of fibroblasts and variable numbers of large epithelioid and stellate cells

(Figs 21.33–21.35).[2,84,85] In an established plaque, there are conspicuous CD34+ dermal dendritic cells with admixed CD68+ macrophages and factor XIIIa-positive cells (Figs 21.36–21.38).[2,39,84,86] Multinucleate forms are present and can show an osteoclast-like morphology.[87,88] There are numerous fibroblasts associated with irregularly distributed thickened collagen bundles and increased numbers of elastic fibers.[85] Sclerotic bodies or elastocollagenous balls, irregularly shaped paucicellular areas of collagen which can ossify, have been described.[89,90] Cleftlike spaces are typically present, and there is increased dermal stromal mucin. Progression of the lesion is accompanied by capillary proliferation. During the earlier stages of the illness myofibroblasts have also been identified, but they are typically absent in more chronic lesions. Osseous metaplasia and dystrophic calcification is sometimes evident.[2,28,84,87,91–94] Calciphylaxis has been documented in several cases.[92,95–97]

Nephrogenic systemic fibrosis is usually devoid of a significant inflammatory cell infiltrate, although occasionally a light superficial and deep perivascular lymphocytic infiltrate may be evident. Granulomatous inflammation has been rarely described.[98]

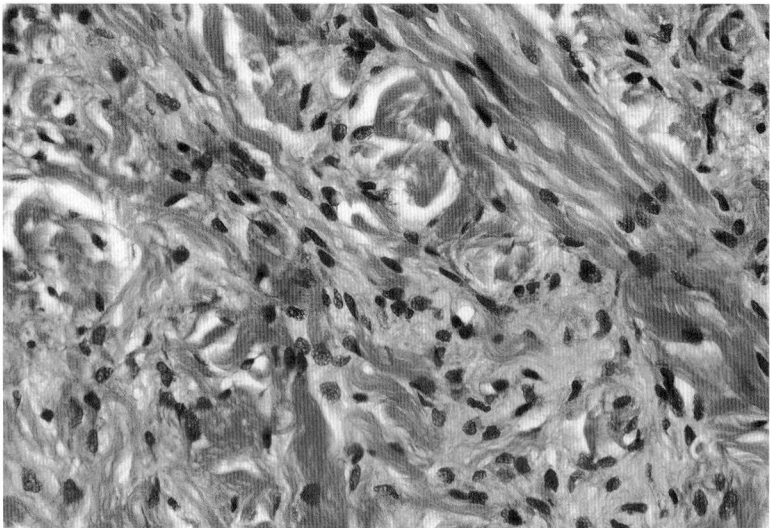

Fig. 21.35
Nephrogenic fibrosing dermopathy: high-power view.

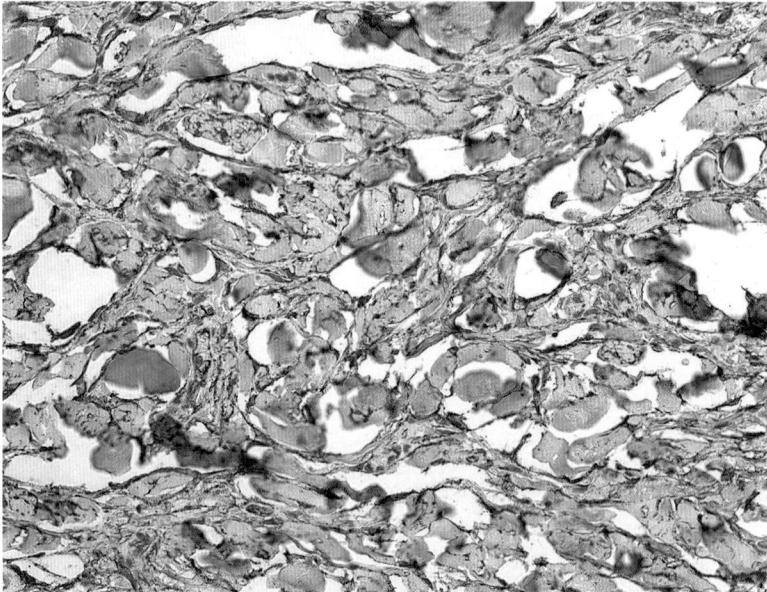

Fig. 21.36
Nephrogenic fibrosing dermopathy: there is diffuse expression of CD34. By courtesy of S.E. Cowper, MD, Yale University, New Haven, USA.

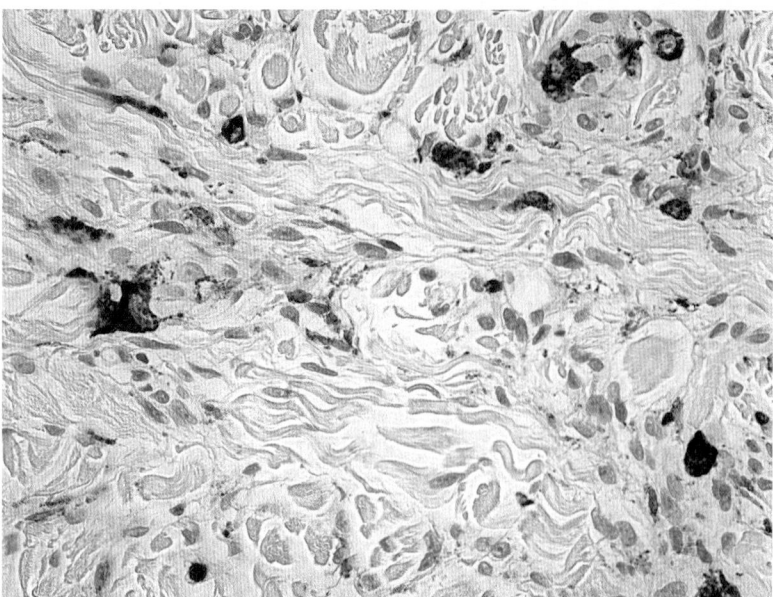

Fig. 21.37
Nephrogenic fibrosing dermopathy: scattered CD68+ cells are present. By courtesy of S.E. Cowper, MD, Yale University, New Haven, USA.

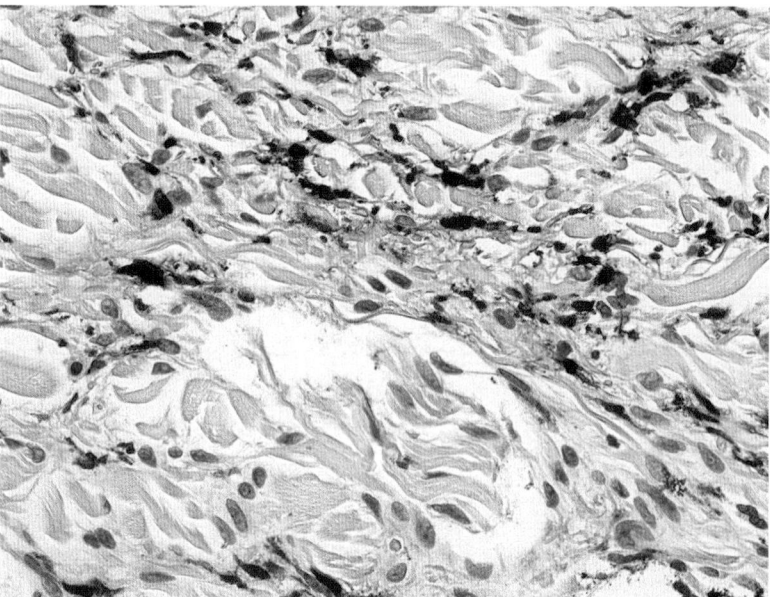

Fig. 21.38
Nephrogenic fibrosing dermopathy: factor XIIIa-positive cells are conspicuous. By courtesy of S.E. Cowper, MD, Yale University, New Haven, USA.

Differential diagnosis

Nephrogenic systemic fibrosis shows particular histologic overlap with scleromyxedema.[38,74,94,99] Mucin is generally more abundant in the latter condition and inflammatory cells (including plasma cells) are often conspicuous, but these findings are not always reliable to distinguish the two entities. Clinically, the two conditions are quite different: scleromyxedema characteristically affects the face, is commonly associated with systemic involvement, and is accompanied by paraproteinemia in most patients.

Restrictive dermopathy

Clinical features

Restrictive dermopathy is a very rare predominantly autosomal recessive condition that is classified within the group of lethal congenital contracture syndromes and presents with intrauterine (fetal) akinesia or hypokinesia deformation sequence (FADS).[1-8] Less than 75 cases have been reported.[9,10] It is invariably fatal, the average survival time after birth being less than 1 week.[5]

Affected infants are born prematurely at approximately 31 weeks and die from pulmonary hypoplasia and respiratory insufficiency.[1,3,8,11] Spontaneous complete chorioamniotic membrane separation can occur.[12,13] The clinical manifestations include a rigid, taut, adherent skin with erosions, ulcers, and a tendency to tear easily, generalized contractures, a dysmorphic facies with micrognathia, and a mouth fixed in an 'O' shape.[1-10,14,15] Additional features may include blepharophimosis, absent eyelashes, dilatation of the ascending aorta, dextrocardia, dysplasia of the clavicles, and enlarged fontanelles with wide cranial sutures.[1-9,14-16]

Pathogenesis and histologic features

The majority of restrictive dermopathy is caused by null autosomal recessive mutations in *ZMPSTE24* (*FACE-1*), encoding a zinc metalloprotease which modifies prelamin A to lamin A, with a minority of patients harboring autosomal dominant mutations in *LMNA*.[9,15,17-23] Defects in *ZMPSTE24* result in accumulation in farensylated prelamin A along the nuclear membrane; the degree of protease dysfunction can correlate with disease severity.[24,25]

Mutations in *LMNA* are also involved in Hutchinson-Gilford progeria syndrome and result in truncated lamin A precursors.[9,26–29] Prelamin A, the precursor to lamin A, plays both a structural role in forming the nuclear lamina and functional roles in nuclear chromatin remodeling and nuclear protein transport.[30–32] The accumulation of prelamin A results in altering of nuclear contours, is toxic to cells, and can disrupt DNA repair mechanisms.[8,33–38] Increased oxidative stress could play a role in cell damage.[39,40] A transgenic mouse model indicates that disruption of lamin A inhibits normal skin development in the infant.[41] The discovery of these defects has enabled prenatal diagnosis.[9,14,42,43]

Histologically, the epidermis appears normal to slightly thickened, although it is flattened with loss of the rete ridges and a straight lower border.[7,15,42] The dermis is thinned and the reticular collagen appears compact and oriented parallel to the surface.[2,6,7,9,15] Elastic tissue is reduced, and the dermal appendages are poorly developed.[7,9,44] The subcutaneous fat may appear increased in thickness.[6,8,15]

DISEASES OF COLLAGEN: LOCALIZED DISORDERS

White fibrous papulosis

Clinical features

This uncommon condition was initially described in a series of Japanese patients.[1,2] There was a marked predilection for males (4:1), and most patients were elderly (range, 39–79 years; mean, 62 years). Over the years, scattered reports have emerged from around the world including Europe, North and South America, China and other parts of Asia, and the Middle East showing a striking preponderance of females, all elderly.[3–18] The back and the sides of the neck are most often affected.[4,5,12,13,15,19] Very occasionally, lesions extend to the back or anterior upper chest, or upper arms.[7,10,20] Patients present with multiple (sometimes hundreds) round to oval sharply circumscribed, white, firm, asymptomatic 2–3 mm papules.[2] Lesions typically show no tendency to coalesce and are unrelated to hair follicles. They tend to temporally increase in number and do not regress.[16] One unusual case noted coalescing papules which involved axilla, forearms, and the supraclavicular region.[21] There are no systemic associations.

Histologic features

The precise nature of this lesion is uncertain. It could be a form of intrinsic aging.[9] The histologic changes are seen in the papillary and upper reticular dermis and consist of a fairly sharply delineated zone of thickened collagen bundles.[19] The elastic tissue may appear normal or slightly diminished in amount.[1,2,16] Ultrastructural studies show increased collagen fibril diameter and conspicuous fibroblasts with abundant rough endoplasmic reticulum.[2]

Differential diagnosis

Some authors have emphasized an overlap between white fibrous papulosis and pseudoxanthoma elasticum-like papillary dermal elastolysis, suggesting that both conditions represent a manifestation of aging and proposing the term fibroelastolytic papulosis of the neck to combine the two entities, a terminology that is increasingly used in the literature.[12,22–24] Unlike white fibrous papulosis, pseudoxanthoma elasticum lacks the thickened collagen bundles and typically displays calcifications.[12,25]

Collagenoma

Collagenoma is a collagenous connective tissue nevus. Familial and acquired variants are recognized.[1,2] The former tend to be multiple, while the latter can be fewer or even single lesions.

Familial cutaneous collagenoma

Clinical features

Familial cutaneous collagenoma is very rare and shows autosomal dominant inheritance.[3–9] Patients present, usually in the second decade, with multiple, symmetrical, flesh-colored papules and plaques measuring from 0.5 to 3.0 cm in diameter.[6] A peau d'orange appearance has sometimes been documented.[5] The trunk (particularly the back) and the upper arms are sites of predilection.[6–8] Lesions are generally asymptomatic although occasionally mild pruritus may be experienced. They increase in number with age and during pregnancy.[4] Some suggest that hormones may influence the development of this condition, although prepubertal cases have been reported.[7]

There are a number of associated conditions although their significance is uncertain in view of the small number of documented cases. These include various cardiovascular disorders including cardiomyopathy, atrioseptal defect, aortic insufficiency, and conduction defects, hypogonadism, congenital exophthalmos, learning disabilities, hypertrichosis, nystagmus, café-au-lait macules, and acanthosis nigricans.[3,5–8]

Histologic features

The lesion is characterized by a markedly thickened dermis due to broad bundles of haphazardly arranged or homogenized collagen bundles.[3–6,8–10] Elastic tissue may appear normal or abnormal, fragmented, and diminished in amount.[8,10,11] Ultrastructural studies have shown variation in collagen fibril diameter and abnormal elastic fibrils characterized by irregularity, branching, and a reduced microfibrillar component.[6]

Differential diagnosis

Other inherited conditions with multiple collagenous connective tissue nevi should be considered. Familial cutaneous collagenoma is most likely to be confused with Buschke-Ollendorf syndrome, an autosomal dominant disease associated with *LEMD3* mutations; some authors have noted a phenotypic overlap.[12] The latter, however, is characterized by the presence of multiple cutaneous elastomas and osteopoikilosis.[13] Tuberous sclerosis patients have other characteristic findings, as discussed above.

Eruptive collagenoma

Clinical features

Eruptive collagenoma is more common than the familial variant described above.[1–7] Similar to the familial variant, patients with eruptive collagenoma develop multiple 0.2–2.0-cm asymptomatic, skin-colored or white papules, nodules, or plaques predominantly affecting the trunk and proximal limbs.[6] Lesions in the Japanese, however, may be more generalized.[6] A case of eruptive collagenoma of the ears has been reported.[8] Very similar lesions were described to involve the esophagus and intestine in a single case report.[9] There is a predilection for males in Caucasians; however, in the Japanese literature, the sex distribution is equal.[6] Although a wide age range may be affected (5–78 years), the majority of patients present in their third decade.[10] A case has been reported with a pregnancy.[11] Multiple collagenomas have been reported in some, but not all, studies of patients with multiple endocrine neoplasia type I.[12–15] These findings suggest that hormones may play a role in some collagenomas.

Histologic features

The lesion is characterized by excess collagen. Some describe coarse, thickened collagen while other describe fine and dispersed collagen fibers.[16–18] A reduction in the dermal elastic tissue is universally noted.[6] Fragmentation of elastic fibers is sometimes encountered.[5]

Differential diagnosis

Eruptive collagenoma shows considerable overlap with white fibrous papulosis; however, in the latter condition, there is a predilection for females (in Europeans) and lesions predominantly affect the back and the sides of the neck.

Nevus anelasticus is also included in the differential diagnosis, but presents as perifollicular papules. Elastic fibers are degenerated or reduced.[16,17] Papular elastorrhexis is morphologically similar, with reduced elastic fibers that can be fragmented. However, collagen fibers appear normal.[16,19] Some have proposed that nevus anelasticus, papular elastorrhexis, and eruptive collagenoma may be related lesions.[17,18] The term 'eruptive papular collageno-elastopathy' has been proposed as a unifying term for eruptive collagenomas and papular elastorrhexis.[20]

Isolated collagenoma

Clinical features

Isolated collagenoma (solitary collagenoma) presents as a slowly growing, painless, flesh-colored or pink nodule or plaque, usually evident from childhood.[1–5] The lesions can become large with time.[6,7] While any region of the body may be affected, there is a predilection for the trunk and extremities (Fig. 21.39).[8] A subset affects the palms or soles and occasionally these are associated with cerebriform hyperplasia of the overlying skin.[9–12] These are of particular interest as they are considered one of the major skin manifestations, previously even considered pathognomonic, of Proteus syndrome.[13] However, patients with isolated plantar collagenomas lacking any other criteria for Proteus syndrome are seen.[14–16]

Variations exist including papulolinear arrangement involving the hands or back along Blaschko lines that can sometimes be arranged in an arborizing pattern with hypopigmentation.[17] One case involved the scalp, manifesting as cutis verticis gyrata.[18]

Isolated collagenoma has been associated with both Down syndrome and type III EDS.[19,20] The latter was a large plaque covering the posterior aspect of the shoulder, the left back, and extending down to the elbow.

Athlete's nodules and acquired knuckle pads are sometimes regarded as related lesions. They present on the dorsum of the feet, knees, and knuckles

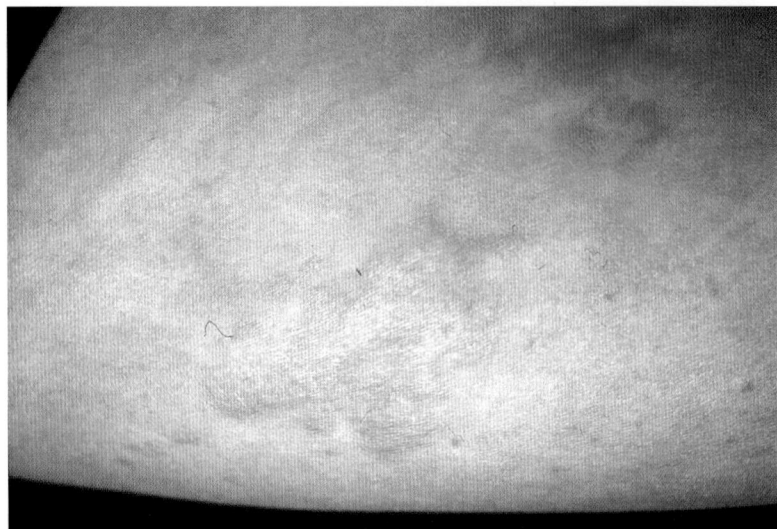

Fig. 21.39
Connective tissue nevus (collagenoma): there is a large erythematous plaque. By courtesy of the Institute of Dermatology, London, UK.

as a consequence of chronic friction or trauma.[21–23] They would be better classified as a reactive collagenous hyperplasia.

Histologic features

Although the pathogenesis is generally unknown, in one cerebriform variant, diminished collagenase production was suggested as being of etiological importance.[4] Isolated collagenoma is characterized by irregularly distributed and thick collagen bundles that can sometimes be associated with loss of elastic tissue.[5,15–18,24]

DISEASES OF ELASTIC TISSUE

Cutis laxa

Clinical features

The umbrella term cutis laxa (generalized elastolysis) covers a broad group of extremely rare systemic diseases of elastic tissue with both familial and acquired variants (the latter often present with localized lesions) (Figs 21.40–21.42).[1,2] It can occur in association with other inherited and sporadic genetic disorders including hereditary gelsolin amyloidosis, Kubuki make-up syndrome, Keutel syndrome, geroderma osteodysplastica, tranadolase deficiency, familial amyloid polyneuropathy, Wilson disease, Lenz-Majewski syndrome, Mounier-Kuhn syndrome (tracheobronchomegaly), Sotos syndrome, Leigh-like syndrome, cranioectodermal dysplasia, cardiofaciocutaneous syndrome, and Costello syndrome.[3–18]

Familial (inherited) variants

This group includes diseases where cutis laxa is the prodominant features and also syndromes where cutis laxa is a feature. The classification of this family is evolving from the historical clinical type scheme to a genetically based system. We present the most important familial variants below. With the assistance of genetics, more than 12 inherited variants are currently recognized, most of which show autosomal recessive inheritance.[19] Autosomal dominant and X-linked recessive variants have also been documented. Autosomal recessive variants are generally more severe.[2,3,20–24] Historically, type 1 disease was considered prototypical and includes cutaneous, pulmonary, and vascular lesions with diverticula (see below).[21,22,25,26] Hypothyroidism has been rarely described.[24] Type 1 likely includes cases from multiple of the genetic groupings, both autosomal dominant and recessive.[27] Gene names will be used here to help distinguish the different disease groups. The function and pathogenesis of the genetic deficits is briefly discussed further below.

Autosomal dominant disease is genetically heterogeneous and can have several causative genes. Autosomal dominant cutis laxa is generally mild but rarely can show systemic involvement, sometimes serious, of the lungs, gastrointestinal tract, and vessels.[22,25,28–32] Herniation and prolapse of genitals is also seen. Causative genes discovered so far include *ELN* (7q11.23), *FBLN5* (14q32.12), and *ALDH18A1* (10q24.1).[33–37]

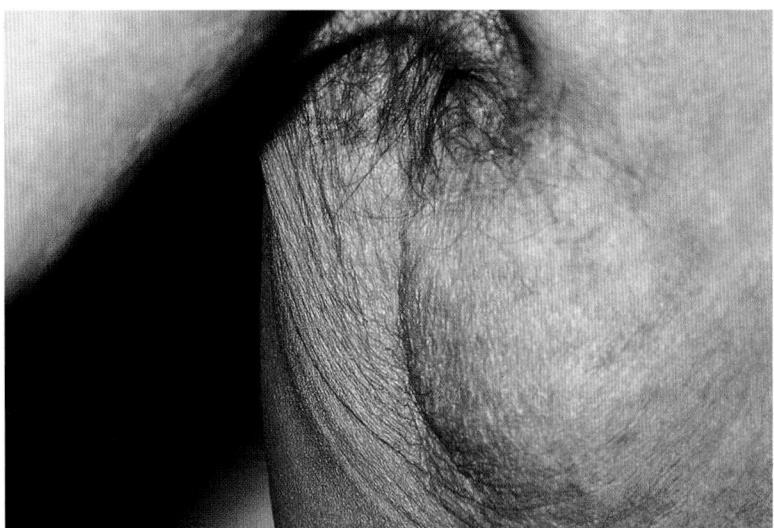

Fig. 21.40
Cutis laxa: there are conspicuous skin folds in the axilla. The patient had an exceedingly unusual acquired variant complicating cutaneous amyloid deposition, resulting in destruction of the elastica. By courtesy of J. Newton Bishop, MD, St James's University Hospital, Leeds, UK.

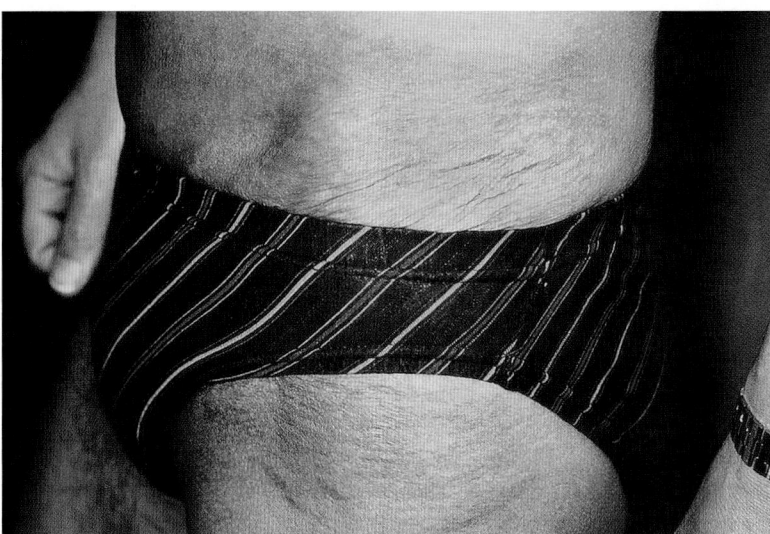

Fig. 21.41
Cutis laxa: the same patient as in Fig. 19.34 also has loose skin in the areas of the lower flank and upper thigh. By courtesy of J. Newton Bishop, MD, St James's University Hospital, Leeds, UK.

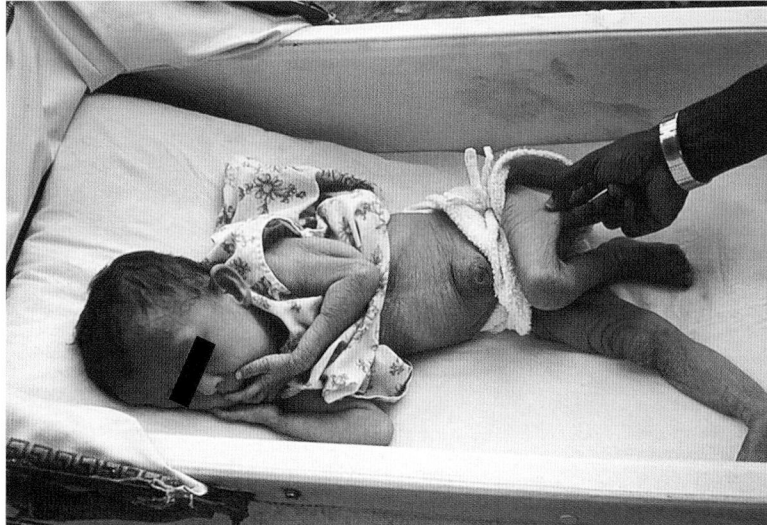

Fig. 21.42
Cutis laxa: this infant has very slack skin which, when stretched and released, does not return to its former position. Note the umbilical hernia. By courtesy of R.A. Marsden, MD, St George's Hospital, London, UK.

Autosomal recessive cutis laxa has a number of genetic causes including: *FBLN5* (14q32.12), *EFEMP2* (11q13.1), *LTBP4* (19q13.2), *PYCR1* (17q25.3), *ATP6V0A2* (12q24.31), *ATP6V1E1* (22q11.21), *ATP6V1A* (3q13.31), and *ALDH18A1* (10q24.1).[35–47] Two of these genes, *FBLN5* and *ALDH18A1*, overlap with the autosomal dominant forms above.[41,48] When inherited in autosomal recessive fashion, the expression of disease is usually more severe. Historically, two forms of autosomal recessive disease have been singled out for unique clinical features. Type 2, also known as Debre type, is characterized by cutis laxa features with associated bone dystrophy, congenital hip dislocation, and mental retardation.[21,22,49–52] Blue sclera is a rare association.[3,53] These cases show *ATP6V0A2* mutations.[40,44,54] Type 3 (also known as the De Barsy syndrome) combines cutis laxa with progeria, corneal clouding, athetosis, and mental retardation with brain dysgenesis, described by some as cobblestone-like.[22,25–61] Such cases show mutations in *ALDH18A1*.[37] *LTBP4* mutated cases are also known as Urban-Rifkin-Davis syndrome and can show severe defects in multiple systems beyond the skin including pulmonary, gastrointestinal, urinary, craniofacial, and musculoskeletal.[27,43] Wrinkly skin syndrome is the clinically less severe variant of the autosomal recessive form of cutis laxa (specifically type 2, Debre syndrome) with *ATP6V0A2* mutation.[40,44,54,62,63] Two other related syndromes

bear mention. MACS syndrome, which is characterized by macrocephaly, alopecia, cutis laxa, and scoliosis, is associated with autosomal recessive mutations in *RIN2* (20p11.23).[64–66] Geroderma osteodysplastica (Walt Disney dwarfism) has autosomal recessive mutations in *GORAB* (1q24.2) and loose skin on the hands feet, stomach, and face along with characteristic facies and joint laxity.[67–69] Many consider these latter two syndromes to fall within the broad spectrum of the cutis laxa family.[70,71] An apparently novel form of autosomal recessive cutis laxa with cleft palate, joint laxity, mental retardation, emphysema, and facial dysmorphism has been reported.[72] Another unique presentation with intellectual disability, abnormal fat distribution, cardiomyopathy, and cataracts with uncertain inheritance pattern has also been reported as a unique expression of the disease.[73] More study is needed in both cases to determine whether these two disease expressions fall within the known genetic groups.

X-linked recessive cutis laxa (occipital horn syndrome) shows mutations in *ATP7A* (Xq21.1).[74,75] Its features include hyperextensible joints, impaired wound healing, bladder diverticula, and mild mental retardation in addition to lax skin.[21,22,76–79] This variant was previously classified as type IX EDS and is now known to be allelic to Menkes disease, a disorder characterized by a defect in copper transport.[3,74,79–81] The term occipital horn derives from the characteristic bony horns that present bilaterally at the foramen magnum in this syndrome.[21,22] Some consider this condition to be an independent disease outside of the specific cutis laxa spectrum.[82]

Manifestations are present at birth or soon thereafter, and affected infants have coarse, loose, redundant folds of skin in the dependent regions of the body.[20,83] The skin is completely devoid of elastic recoil. Facial involvement may give rise to a 'bloodhound facies'.[3,20,22,84] Systemic lesions include pulmonary emphysema and bronchiectasis, vascular lesions (particularly aneurysms and valvular incompetence), and gastrointestinal manifestations including diverticula and multiple hernias (umbilical, inguinal, and diaphragmatic).[30,31,77,78,83,85] Aneurysms, dilatations, and stenosis are sometimes seen in blood vessels.[31,83,86] Gastrointestinal diverticula may be an additional feature.[87] Involvement of the urinary tract therefore results in vesicle diverticula with concomitant infections.[83] The vocal cords are affected, causing a coarsening and deepening of the voice. Ectropion is a typical feature.[88]

Inherited cutis laxa (particularly the recessive variant) is a serious illness which may lead to death due to cardiac and respiratory complications.[2]

Acquired variants

There are several clinical variants of acquired cutis laxa.

- Postinflammatory elastolysis and cutis laxa (Marshall syndrome) is seen in children presenting with urticarial or annular erythematous papular eruption associated with elastic tissue destruction and subsequent skin laxity.[85,87,89–92] Sweet syndrome can precipitate this in both adults and children, including neonates.[90,93–97] Other associations include infections, antibiotic exposure, leukocytosis with eosinophilia, and other non-specified generalized dermatoses.[91,98]

- Adult generalized acquired cutis laxa, disease involving multiple body regions or sometimes virtually the entire body, is less frequently encountered than the congenital form and is generally also associated with pulmonary and cardiovascular involvement and diverticula.[91,99,100] It may develop de novo or follow a variety of dermatoses including erythema, urticaria, eczema, erythema multiforme, and dermatitis herpetiformis.[100–108] The condition can complicate penicillamine, isoniazid, and penicillin sensitivity, cutaneous hypersensitivity to selective serotonin reuptake inhibitor therapy, multiple myeloma, both light and heavy chain deposition disease, angiocentric T-cell lymphoma, cutaneous mastocytosis, amyloidosis, monoclonal gammopathy, nephrotic syndrome, *Borrelia* infection, celiac disease, lupus profundus, and systemic lupus erythematosus.[91,100,109–127] While there is a predilection for adults, children can be affected.[91]

- Localized cutis laxa, involvement limited to a single body region, may follow syphilis, sarcoidosis, varicose veins, necrobiosis lipoidica, papular urticaria, multiple myeloma and amyloidosis, B-cell lymphoma, childbirth, Cesarian section, and rheumatoid arthritis.[105,128–136] There is a small number of reports describing acquired localized cutis laxa affecting the face, fingers, and toes.[1,91,128,135,137–141] A case of a child with urticaria pigmentosa and acquired cutis laxa has been described.[142] Sometimes no systemic disease or dermatosis is identified as a precursor.[140]

The features of acquired cutis laxa are variable, ranging from a localized or generalized purely cutaneous condition to a serious, potentially life-threatening condition with systemic involvement.[2,28,91,100]

Pathogenesis and histologic features

The molecular mechanisms in many of the inherited variants are increasingly well understood.[20] The cutis laxa family of disease should be understood as a broad complex of diseases of elastin including Marfan syndrome, Weill-Marchesani syndrome, Loeys-Dietz syndrome, pseudoxanthoma elasticum, some forms of Ehler-Danlos, and Williams syndrome.[143] All of these diseases have specific genetic deficits that impinge on the structure, production, processing, or stability of elastic fibers. The production of the elastic fiber macromolecule is complex and requires numerous molecular and cellular processes. In cutis laxa, elastin fibers are affected and compromised at multiple levels. Autosomal dominant cutis laxa is associated with a mutation in the *ELN* (7q11.23) gene encoding elastin in some patients.[30,31,72,84,144–146] Elastin comprises approximately 90% of the mature elastic fibers. Compromise of elastin can cause both quantitative and functional deficits in elastin. Mutation of one allele can act as a dominant negative and cause disease.[32,33] Various mutations can cause different functional deficits in the compromised elastic fibers and correlate to a degree with specific disease symptoms.[147] Rare cases of defects in *ELN* have been reported in the autosomal recessive variant with more severe disease expression.[148] Fibulins are important regulators of elastic fiber construction. Some autosomal recessive variants show mutations in the fibulin-5 (*FBLN5*) gene and fibulin-4 (*EFEMP2*).[39,41] Fibulin-4 is involved in elastin crosslinking cooperating with the *LOX* encoded lysyl oxidase, while fibulin-5 directs elastin interaction with microfibrils.[149–153] *LTBP4* mutations most often result in nonsense-mediated decay with no protein production.[38] LTBP4 is involved in preparing microfibrils for assembly with elastin and other components of the elastic fiber.[149] Lack of this protein leads to thickened and wavy microfibrils with compromised function. Defects in H+-ATPase activity encoded by *ATP6VOA2* is involved in vesicular acidification and appears to disrupt vesicular transport and secretion, perhaps in part through alteration of glycosylation.[154] The end result is disruption in the secretion of the properly formed structural elements used to form elastic fibers. Different mutated alleles may determine the phenotypic expression of autosomal recessive cutis laxa versus the less severe wrinkly skin syndrome.[83,155–161] Mutations in *ATP6V1E1* (22q11.21), *ATP6V1A* (both autosomal recessive), and *ATP7A* (X-linked recessive) also disrupt this the assembly or stability of the proton pump.[3,47,84,162–171] ATP7A is also involved with copper transport, particularly relevant in the Menkes form of the disease where treatment with copper can help alleviate symptoms and restore protein function.[172,173] The position and type of mutation in *ATP7A* correlates with the severity and expression of disease.[79] *GORAB* is also involved in vesicular transport and *RIN2* is involved with vesicular docking to the cell membrane for secretion to the extracellular environment.[174,175] Two related mitochondrial metabolic enzymes encoded by *ALDH18A1* (encoding pyrroline-5-carboxylate synthase) and *PYCR1* (encoding pyrroline-5-carbosylate reductase 1) resulting in autosomal recessive inheritance have also been reported in autosomal recessive cutis laxa and cause similar disease expression.[148,176–179] Dominant negative mutations in *ALDH18A1* can confer autosomal dominance.[177,180,181] Mutations appear to dysregulate the oxidative metabolic pathways as well as ornithine and proline biosynthesis; this may also help explain the broader progeroid and neurodegenerative effects of these mutations.[37,154,182–184]

The pathogenesis of the acquired form is uncertain but is likely related to local excess production of elastases, particularly in postinflammatory patients.[91,185,186] One patient with acquired cutis laxa was found to be heterozygotic for *FBLN5* and *ELN* defects, suggesting some patients are more susceptible to develop this disorder following an inflammatory skin disease.[187] Missense alleles in *ELN* alone may predispose to acquired cutis laxa by making the elastin more susceptible to inflammatory damage.[188] Some patients with sporadic cutis laxa have missense mutations in one *FBLN5* allele as well.[167] Absence of inhibitors such as α_1-antitrypsin has

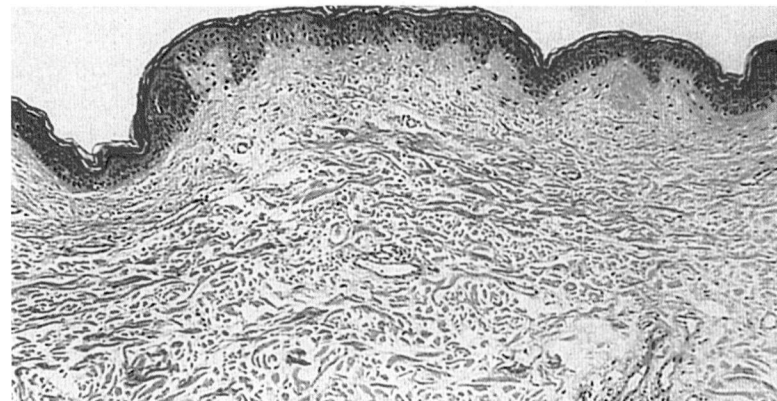

Fig. 21.43
Cutis laxa: with hematoxylin and eosin stained sections, the histologic features are quite unremarkable, consisting of a mild perivascular lymphocytic infiltrate.

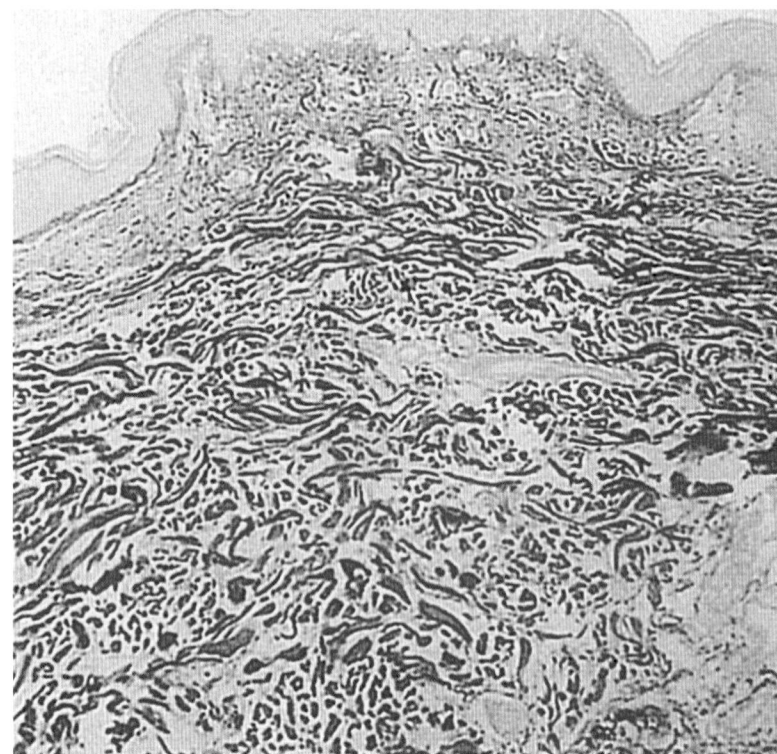

Fig. 21.44
Cutis laxa: there is widespread loss of the reticular dermal elastic tissue. The papillary dermis is relatively spared.

been documented.[91,94] More elastolytic activity and decreased elastin expression have been reported in the affected dermis.[91] A role of serum copper and lysyl oxidase has been suggested and is not unsuspected given the known mechanisms of the heritable forms.[71,91] The association with adverse drug reactions and the finding of immunoglobulin deposition on elastic fibers raises the possibility of an immune disorder in a subset of cases.[91,113,117] Some have proposed that postinflammatory cutis laxa may be secondary to an exuberant arthropod assault reaction or a reaction to some other environmental exposure including ultraviolet (UV) light and plants.[91]

The disease is characterized by a reduction in the number of elastic fibers and associated degenerative changes (*Figs 21.43* and *21.44*).[71,189] Fibers may be deficient in the papillary dermis, reticular dermis, or both; those present in the reticular dermis are usually shortened, tapered, and degenerate.[83,190] Similar changes in the elastic tissue may occur in the alveolar walls, blood vessels, and elsewhere.[2,169]

In postinflammatory cutis laxa, there may be a heavy dermal acute inflammatory cell infiltrate (including neutrophils and eosinophils) in addition to the changes in elastic tissue, and palisading of neutrophils around the elastic fibers has been described.[1,91,113] Vasculitis and granulomatous dermatitis are sometimes noted.[131,191]

Ultrastructurally, in unaffected skin, the elastic fibers appear morphologically normal.[113] In lesional specimens. the elastic fibers are fragmented, branched, electron dense, and degenerate, but lack the calcification seen in pseudoxanthoma elasticum.[144,190,192] Elastophagocytosis by histiocytes may be evident.[113] In one ultrastructural study of cutis laxa developing in association with Sweet disease, the elastic tissue appeared to be composed almost exclusively of elastin with minimal fibrillar component. As the complex genetics and multiple environmental causes demonstrate, cutis laxa is a very heterogeneous condition with many etiologies. Ultrastructural studies in a recessive variant have shown morphologically abnormal elastic fibers composed of fibril-free globular bodies of elastin surrounded by the microfibrillar component and sometimes abnormal adjacent collagen can be demonstrated as well.[152,190,193] Some syndromes such as the Debre type can show very subtle features by electron microscopy, but evaluation requires specific expertise as the findings will vary depending on the genotype underlying the defect.[40]

Immunohistochemistry or special stains can confirm loss of elastin in some forms of cutis laxa; sometimes defects can be visualized with light microscopy on hematoxylin and eosin (H&E) slides.[144,154] Increasingly, molecular diagnostics using single expected genes or a panel of cutis laxa genes with or without genes signifying other related syndromes with compromised elastin is used to confirm the heritable cases.[2] This provides a means for appropriate genetic counseling for other family members.

Pseudoxanthoma elasticum

Clinical features

Pseudoxanthoma elasticum (Grönblad-Strandberg syndrome) is a generalized degenerative disease of elastic tissue showing autosomal dominant inheritance, first described by Darier in 1896.[1-11] Prevalence estimates vary, but some are as high as 1:50000–70000.[4,12,13] All races may be affected, and there is a slight female predominance.[4,5] Onset is most often in the second decade although presentation in childhood, typically with skin manifestations first, has been documented.[4,14-19] The three major organ systems affected include skin, eye, and cardiovascular system.[4,20-22] There is, however, a striking variation in phenotypic expression.[3,5,24] Some families present with widespread disease involving the skin, eyes, and vasculature, whereas in others only one organ system may be affected such that the condition is not recognized until a severely involved descendant is encountered.[11,25,26]

The skin lesions consist of yellow papules, giving a pebbled appearance, and preferentially involve the flexural regions, the neck, axillae, umbilicus, groins, wrists, and antecubital and popliteal fossae (*Figs 21.45–21.47*).[4,5,11,27,28] The lesions may be accompanied by skin laxity in cases with extensive involvement, resulting in redundant folds reminiscent of a turkey's wattle.[4,29-31] Exceptionally, reticulate hyperpigmentation is a feature, and a patient with conspicuous comedo lesions has been documented.[32,33] Lesions have also been described about the nasolabial folds and on the soft palate, inner lip, rectum, and vagina.[4,14,28,34-36] A positive Koebner-like phenomenon is characteristic. It should be noted, however, that patients may occasionally be encountered in whom cutaneous lesions are completely absent, where the initial diagnosis is based on the recognition of angioid streaks or other manifestations.[37,38] At times, perforating lesions are encountered and are commonly reported in a periumbilical distribution (*Fig. 21.48*).[28,31,39-41]

A variety of ocular changes may occur with resulting loss of visual acuity and rarely blindness, but the best recognized ocular findings are angioid streaks (*Figs 21.49 and 21.50*).[4,21,28,42-46] These are irregular, usually bilateral gray to red, jagged radiating lines in the perimacular region of the retina.[3] All patients will eventually develop angioid streaks by their thirties if not before.[4,5,47] Ophthalmoscopic investigation reveals hemorrhages, mottled pigmentation (peau d'orange), peripapillary atrophy with gliosis, subretinal neovascularization, and optic disc drusen.[3,22,48,48] Trauma can worsen the condition.[4] A case complicated by glaucoma has been described.[49] Angioid streaks slowly grow over time and new ones can form.[5] Angioid streaks can

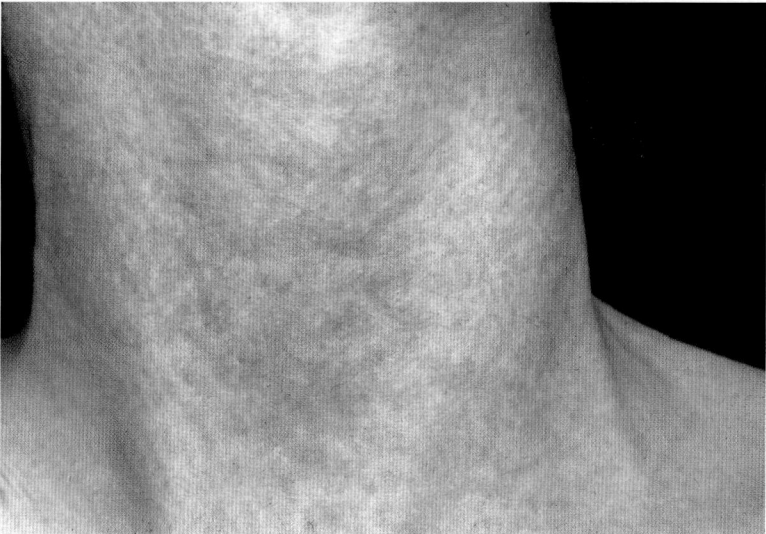

Fig. 21.45
Pseudoxanthoma elasticum: there are small, widely dispersed, yellow papules on this patient's neck. From the collection of the late N.P. Smith, MD, the Institute of Dermatology, London, UK.

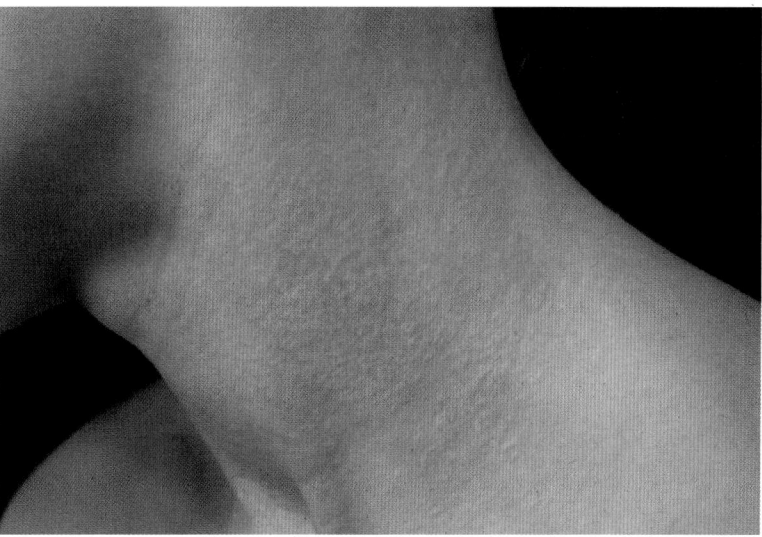

Fig. 21.46
Pseudoxanthoma elasticum: in this view, the appearances are more subtle. From the collection of the late N.P. Smith, MD, the Institute of Dermatology, London, UK.

rarely present without recognized skin involvement and hint at the diagnosis.[46] It is important to note that although angioid streaks are most commonly associated with pseudoxanthoma elasticum, they are not diagnostic, having been described in a wide range of other conditions including Paget disease of bone, EDS, hyperphosphatemia, hemoglobinopathies (see below), and lead poisoning.[3,4,21,46,50]

Involvement of the vascular system may lead to angina, restrictive cardiomyopathy, myocardial infarction, hypertension, intermittent claudication, decreased peripheral pulse, peripheral vascular disease, mitral incompetence and stenosis, aortic incompetence, aneurysm, and intracerebral hemorrhage.[4,5,13,26,28,51-58] Male erectile dysfunction has also been reported.[59] Rare cases of children presenting with coronary artery disease have been documented.[17,60,61] Cases of carotid rete mirabile and Moyamoya disease (progressive occlusive disease of cerebral vasculature, particularly the circle of Willis) with pseudoxanthoma elasticum has been reported.[62-64]

Gastrointestinal lesions result in hematemesis or melena.[4,65,66] Findings similar to the skin can be seen in the gastrointestinal tract, most frequently the stomach.[67] Massive bleeding may prove fatal.[68,69]

Pregnant patients may have an increased risk of cardiovascular problems, and gastric and uterine bleeding, but not necessarily an increased risk

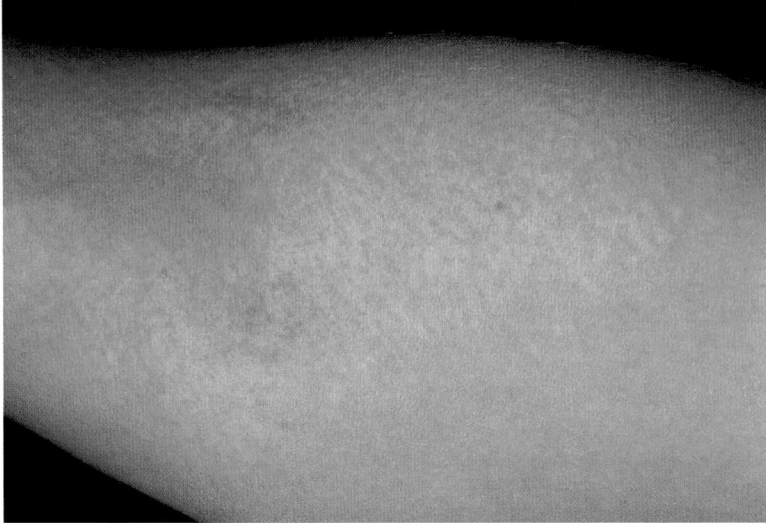

Fig. 21.47
Pseudoxanthoma elasticum: similar lesions are evident in the antecubital fossa extending onto the upper arm. By courtesy of the Institute of Dermatology, London, UK.

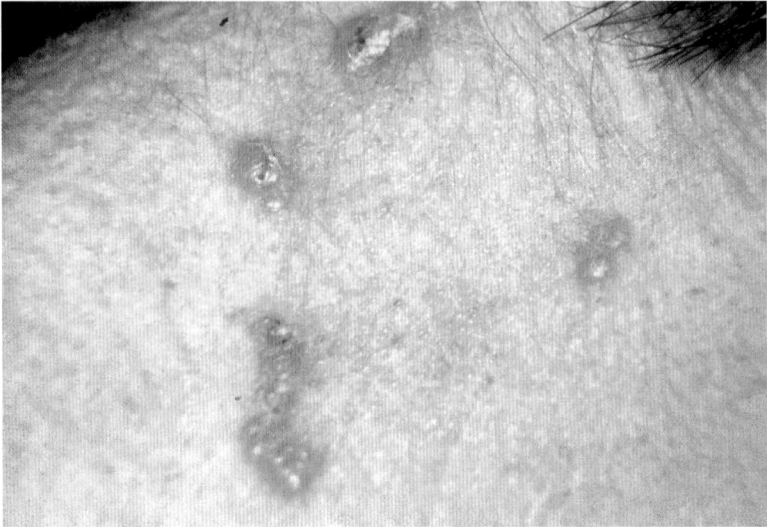

Fig. 21.48
Pseudoxanthoma elasticum: crusted papules representing transepidermal elimination of degenerate elastic tissue are present in a background of typical papules. By courtesy of the Institute of Dermatology, London, UK.

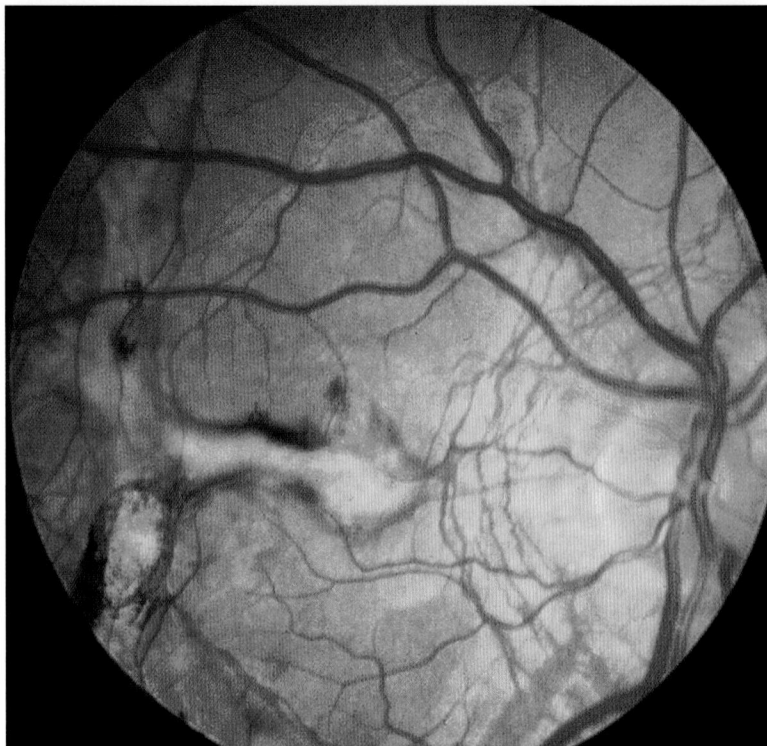

Fig. 21.49
Pseudoxanthoma elasticum: ocular fundus showing advanced angioid streaks with macular destruction from disciform degeneration and subretinal fibrosis.

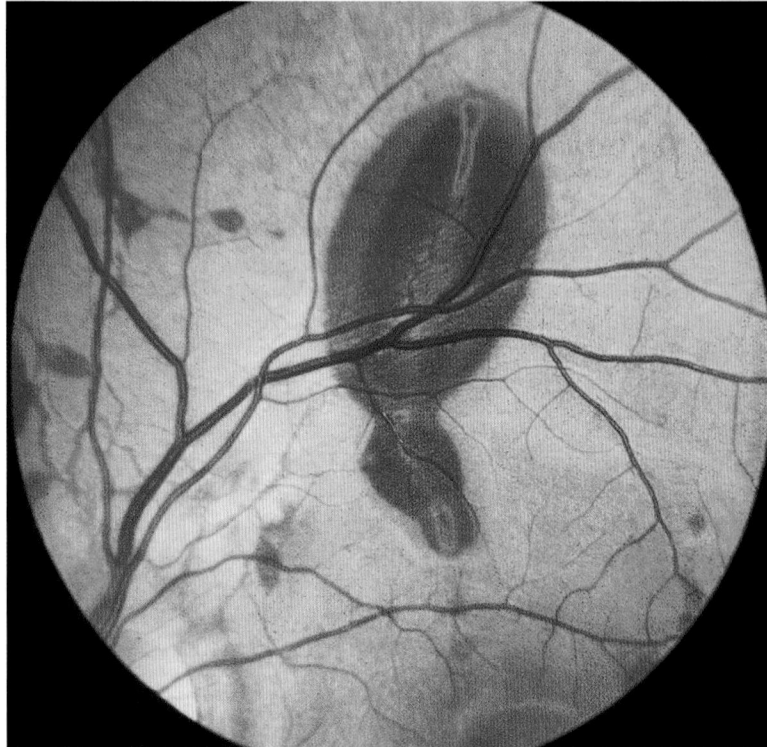

Fig. 21.50
Pseudoxanthoma elasticum: ocular fundus showing angioid streaks adjacent to the optic disc (far left) with a large area of subretinal hemorrhage.

of fetal loss.[4,70–74] Also in pregnancy, the placenta is often mineralized but often without significant consequence.[4,75] Skin changes can be more pronounced in pregnancy.[5]

Calcifications can also be seen in the liver, kidney, spleen, and testicles.[76–78]

Pathogenesis and histologic features

Mutations in the *ABCC6* gene (16p13.1) have been identified in pseudoxanthoma elasticum in humans with similar findings in multiple animal models; inheritance is usually autosomal recessive.[4,12,79–93] Mutations in *ABCC6* are also associated with the rare syndrome, generalized arterial calcification of infancy (GACI), although mutations in *ENPP1* are more canonical.[94–96] Rarely, *ENPP1* autosomal dominant mutations can show a phenotype that is most like pseudoxanthoma elasticum, further supporting the overlap of these syndromes and likely their pathogenic mechanisms.[97–100] Some report overlapping features in these two syndromes.[101] The *ABCC6* gene encodes a transmembrane ATP-binding cassette transporter ABCC6 (also known as multidrug resistance-associated protein 6) that is expressed predominantly in the liver and kidneys and has multiple functional protein domains and might be a mitochondrial protein.[3,102–104] Its exact function and physiological

substrate specificity are not known, but some evidence points to lipid and biliary secretion compounds that may be involved in mineralization.[105–107] More than 750 mutations (including missense, nonsense, and frameshift mutations) have been reported, and various mutations and mutation types are predominant in series from multiple regions of the world, including Asia, the Americas, and Europe.[3,4,12,18,46,108–110] However, a strict genotype-phenotype association model has not yet emerged. Some ABCC6 mutations affect its structure and ability to act as a transporter, others seem to prevent its assembly, while in others production of the protein is entirely halted.[111] The exact mechanism of *ABCC6* involvement is unknown, but two theories are predominant. The metabolic hypothesis proposes that due to mutations in *ABCC6*, there is a lack of circulating serum antimineralization factors such as matrix GLA protein and fetuin-A, the latter secreted by the liver, that normally prevent aberrant deposition of calcium and phosphate on the elastic tissue.[4,12,85,105,112–119] Alternative methodologies such as imaging mass spectrometry suggest that the calcification may affect more proteins than currently recognized.[120] Gamma glutamyl carboxylase, which activates of matrix GLA protein, is decreased, likely due to vitamin K cofactor deficiency resulting from reduced transport by mutant *ABCC6*, although it is unclear that this protein actually transports vitamin K specifically.[12,68,121–125] However, while supplemental vitamin K relieved hypermineralization in a zebrafish model, it was ineffective in multiple studies of mouse models.[126–131] Most recently, attention has focused on the involvement of ABCC6 in regulating plasma inorganic pyrophosphate levels, particularly in the liver; mutations led to lower levels of both circulating pyrophosphate itself and reduced ratios of pyrophosphate to phosphate.[106,132] This reduced ratio correlates closely with ectopic mineralization of elastic rich tissues. Some evidence suggests that ABCC6 could be an efflux transporter to adenosine triphosphate (ATP) in the liver and kidney.[133,134] A few studies suggest that dietary changes and supplementation could alter disease expression.[135] The pyrophosphate regulation angle is further supported by the involvement of four other genes involved in phosphate and pyrophosphate metabolism being associated with hypermineralization syndrome: *ENPP1* (generalized arterial calcification of infancy), *NT5E* (arterial calcification due to deficiency of CD73), *ALPL* (infantile and adult hypophosphatemia), and *ANKH* (calcium pyrophosphate deposition disease).[97,136–140] However, an *Abcc*^−/− mouse model indicates that plasma pyrophosphate, while a dominant mechanism, is not the only mechanism of ectopic mineralization.[141] An alternative mechanism, the 'PXE cell hypothesis', maintains that mutations in *ABCC6* may alter cell proliferation, cell–cell and cell–matrix relationship with increased expression of metalloproteinases and increased elastin and glycosaminoglycan production.[4,12,142,143] Patients with pseudoxanthoma elasticum also have increased serum levels of matrix metalloproteinases (MMP)-2 and MMP-9, intercellular adhesion molecule-1 (ICAM-1), xylosyltransferase I, desmosines, and P-selectins.[144–147] While these factors likely play a contributing role as well, the metabolic explanation is more widely explored presently. It is likely that both contribute to disease expression and could well be interdependent. Phenotypic heterogeneity is present even in patients with the same homozygous mutations, suggesting other involved factors such as increased oxidative stress, diet, environment, and/or other modifier genes.[4,5,109,148–157] Recently reported modifier genes include *ALP*, *ENPP1*, and *ANKH*; interestingly, all are also involved in cellular pyrophosphate metabolism.[158] Transcriptional regulation and polymorphism in the *ABCC6* promoter may also play a role in pathogenesis.[159–162]

While other areas can be involved, the particularly elastin-rich tissues of the skin, eyes, and blood vessels are particularly vulnerable and correlate with the characteristic expression of the disease.[99,163] Pseudoxanthoma elasticum is characterized by degenerative changes affecting the elastic fibers of the mid-dermis. The papillary and deep reticular dermis is unaffected.[164] In contrast to normal skin, the elastic fibers are readily identifiable with H&E staining and are rather basophilic and irregular, appearing as widely dispersed granular material amidst normal collagen fibers (*Figs 21.51* and *21.52*). Individual fibers are thickened, fragmented, and may adopt bizarre appearances reminiscent of a bishop's crook, best visualized using an elastic tissue stain (*Fig. 21.53*). Fibers stain positively with the von Kossa technique, confirming the presence of phosphates or carbonates (*Fig. 21.54*).[5,12,28,165–167] Calcium may be identified by the Alizarin red stain.[12,28] Increased dermal mucins are sometimes evident, and abnormal distribution of other dermal matrix constituents, including vitronectin and fibronectin, have been described.[28,165,168–170] There are exceptional reports of associated dermal milia-like calcinosis and osteoma cutis.[171–174] Calcium deposits may be extruded from the skin and termed by some as perforating pseudoxanthoma elasticum.[28]

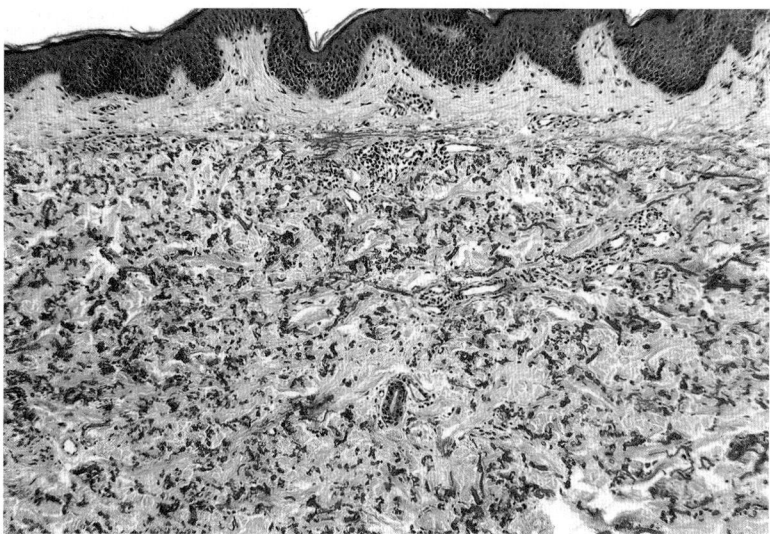

Fig. 21.51
Pseudoxanthoma elasticum: there is a broad band of intensely eosinophilic granular material occupying the middle and lower dermis.

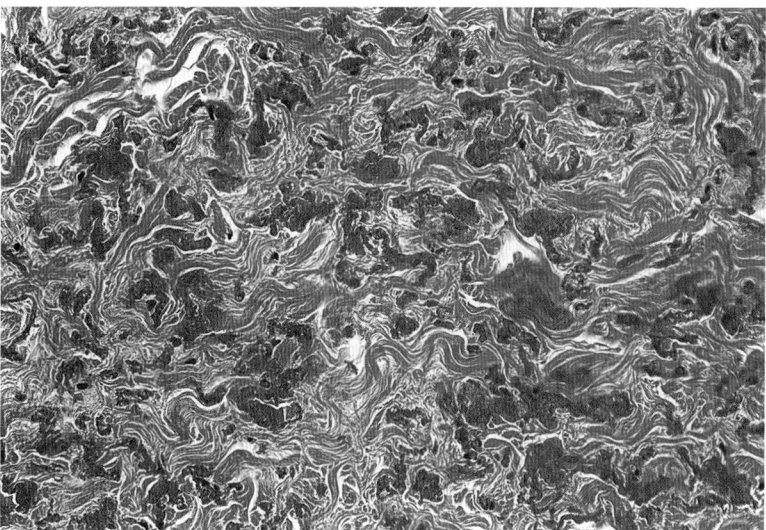

Fig. 21.52
Pseudoxanthoma elasticum: the elastic fibers are irregular, thickened, fragmented, and haphazard in orientation.

In one study, typical histologic features were sometimes identified in clinically normal skin and in traumatic scars of patients with noncutaneous manifestations, the latter perhaps related to the Koebner-like phenomenon.[42] A more recent study found that some patients with pseudoxanthoma elasticum had histologic features in clinically normal axillary skin, but these patients had classic clinical features elsewhere.[175] The skin of unaffected heterozygous carriers appears to be normal upon biopsy.[176]

Calcification of Bruch membrane, which separates the choroid from the pigment epithelium of the retina (*Fig. 21.55*), results in the development of angioid streaks and hemorrhage with resultant scarring and retinal detachment (*Fig. 21.56*).[46,177,178]

Vascular involvement consists of fragmentation and degenerative changes of the internal and external elastic laminae, accompanied by intimal fibrosis and thickening, resulting in weakness of the vessel wall and a tendency toward rupture and aneurysm formation.[51,68,167,179] The heart shows endocardial fibroelastotic thickening and calcification.[167]

Ultrastructurally, in earlier lesions calcification may be seen as a central area of increased electron density surrounded by morphologically normal elastin and microfibrils (*Fig. 21.57*).[165,170,180,181] In more advanced cases, the entire fiber is calcified and often fragmented. Sometimes, electron-lucent areas may be evident (*Fig. 21.58*).

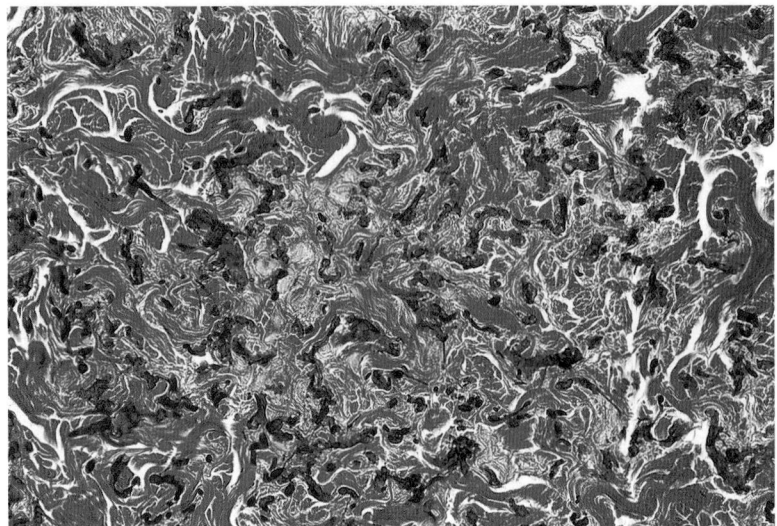

Fig. 21.53
Pseudoxanthoma elasticum: close-up view.

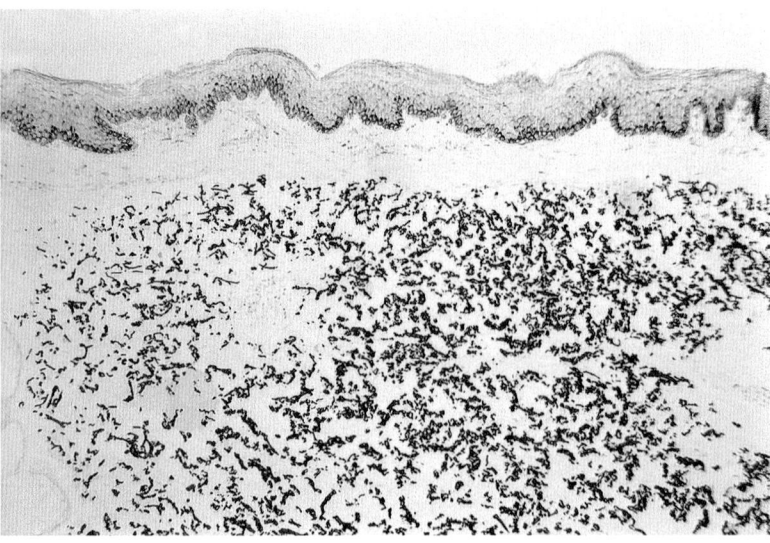

Fig. 21.54
Pseudoxanthoma elasticum: they are strongly von Kossa positive.

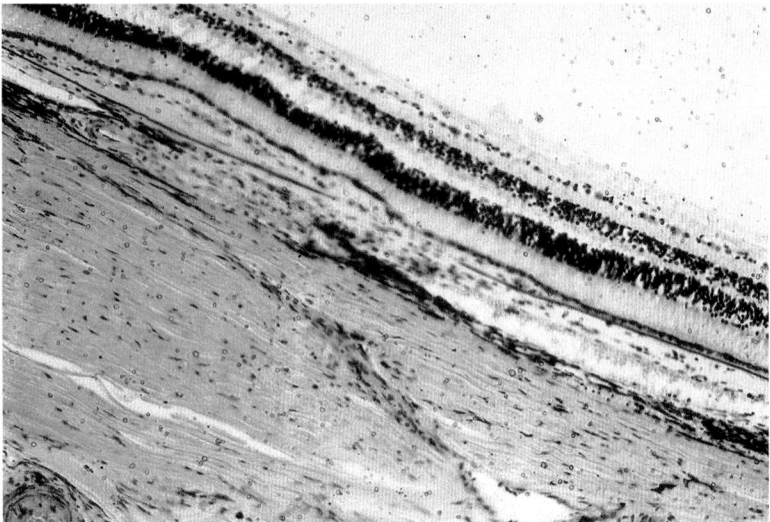

Fig. 21.55
Pseudoxanthoma elasticum: note the calcification and fragmentation of Bruch membrane. By courtesy of D. Archer, MD, Royal Victoria Hospital, Belfast, UK.

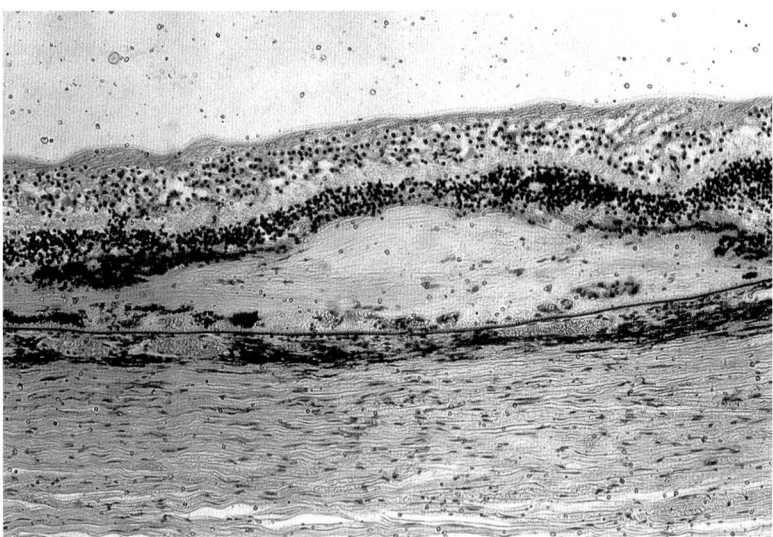

Fig. 21.56
Pseudoxanthoma elasticum: there is dense fibrosis on the inner aspect of Bruch membrane deep to the retina. By courtesy of D. Archer, Royal Victoria Hospital, Belfast, UK.

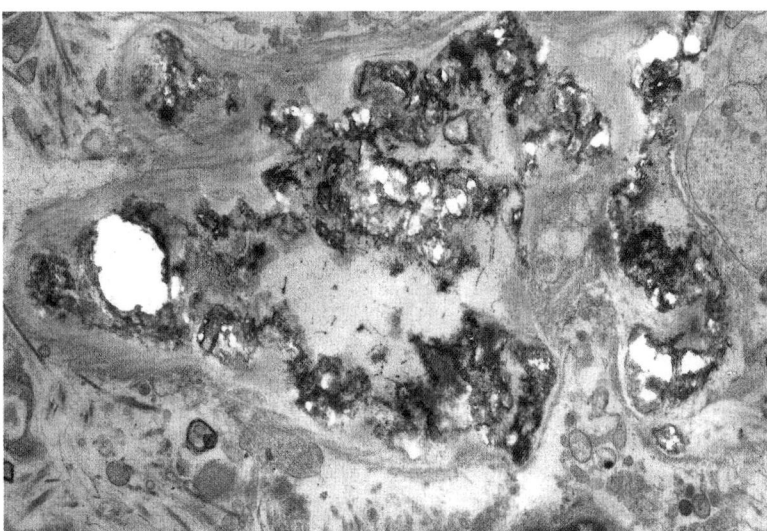

Fig. 21.57
Pseudoxanthoma elasticum: electron micrograph showing a distorted and bizarre elastic fiber. There is marked calcification.

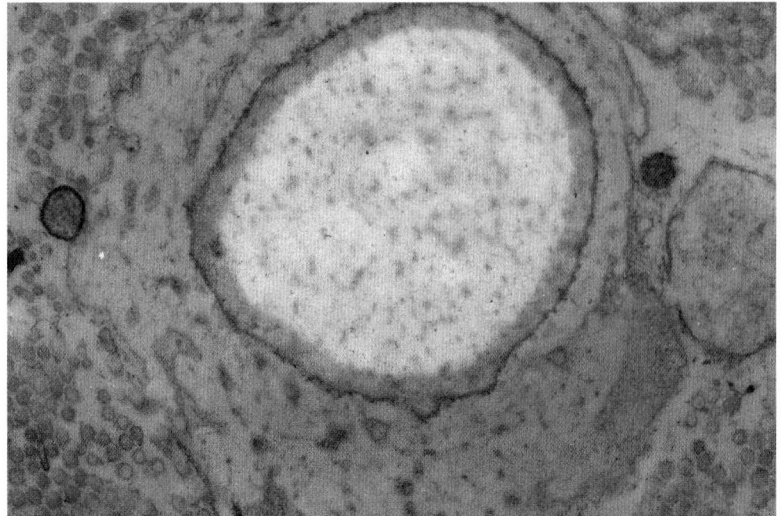

Fig. 21.58
Pseudoxanthoma elasticum: electron-lucent zones within the center of calcified foci are common findings.

Molecular diagnostic techniques based on next-generation sequencing are increasingly utilized in confirmation of disease and genetic counseling as well as evaluating for the involvement of novel genes.[182,183]

Differential diagnosis

Pseudoxanthoma elasticum may be confused clinically with pseudoxanthoma elasticum-like papillary dermal elastolysis and late-onset dermal elastosis (see below).

Penicillamine therapy may result in cutaneous lesions similar to pseudoxanthoma elasticum, but histologically the abnormal fibers are generally not calcified.[184-188] The fibers may have a serrated appearance.[184,185] The cutaneous clinical manifestations may be identical to pseudoxanthoma elasticum, but in some patients other manifestations of penicillamine therapy such as elastosis perforans serpiginosa and collagen defects may be evident.[186,187,189-191] Similarly, saltpeter (potassium nitrate) has been associated with dermal changes histologically and is electron microscopically indistinguishable from pseudoxanthoma elasticum.[192,193] Pseudoxanthoma elasticum-like features have been identified in association with calciphylaxis.[194,195] Pseudoxanthoma-like elastic fibers can also be seen in a variety of inflammatory conditions including lipodermatosclerosis, granuloma annulare, lichen sclerosus, morphea profunda, ertyhema nodosum, septal panniculitis, basal cell carcinoma, nephrogenic systemic fibrosis, tumefactive lipedema, and topical exposure to certain fertilizers.[12,196-199] Some of these patients may be heterozygous for mutations in ABCC6.[197] Pseudoxanthoma-like lesions are also seen in gamma-glutamyl carboxylase syndrome associated with GGCX (2p11.2) mutations.[200]

Identical histologic features associated with perforation are characteristic of so-called periumbilical perforating pseudoxanthoma elasticum (perforating calcific elastosis) (see below).

Pseudoxanthoma elasticum and inherited hemolytic and other syndromes

Manifestations of pseudoxanthoma elasticum, including cutaneous lesions, angioid streaks, and vascular calcification, have been identified in a number of hemolytic conditions including β-thalassemia, sickle cell disease, and hereditary spherocytosis.[1-17] The changes have been confirmed histologically and by electron microscopy.[2] There are also reports of a similar association with sickle thalassemia.[4,9,13] Angioid streaks have been reported in sickle cell anemia, β-thalassemia (hemoglobin H disease, AC hemoglobinopathy), β-thalassemia minor, and β-δ thalassemia, and types I and II congenital dyserythropoetic anemia.[4,18-20] Cardiac and arterial complications have also been reported.[21-23] The exact mechanism is not known but some have suggested increased oxidative damage to the elastic tissue via free iron and/or denatured free hemoglobin and heme.[11,24] Patients with β-thalassemia major tend to have more serious lesions, further suggesting that iron could contribute to the pathogenesis.[11] The condition does not appear to be associated with the ABCC6 gene mutation as in the inherited form (see above).[8-10] Interestingly, however, a mouse model of β-thalassemia shows downregulation of ABCC6 expression in the liver.[25] The frequency of pseudoxanthoma elasticum in patients with hemolytic disorders appears to be increasing due to their current prolonged survival.[9,10]

PXE-like changes are sometimes described in the setting of vitamin K-dependent factor deficiencies and hemochromatosis. The association with vitamin K-dependent factor deficiencies lends credence to the theory that vitamin K cofactor may be involved in inherited pseudoxanthoma elasticum.[24,26-29] Of note, inherited pseudoxanthoma elasticum is made worse by warfarin use, which affects the vitamin K-dependent synthesis of calcium-dependent clotting factors, as demonstrated by surveying a subset of the 4000 patients in the PXE International database.[30] A mouse model confirmed this association.[30]

Periumbilical pseudoxanthoma elasticum

Clinical features

Although originally thought to represent an association with elastosis perforans serpiginosa, periumbilical pseudoxanthoma elasticum (perforating calcific elastosis, localized acquired cutaneous pseudoxanthoma elasticum) is now recognized as a generally perforating variant of pseudoxanthoma elasticum.[1-15] In the majority of cases, disease is localized to the umbilicus in the absence of systemic involvement.[2] There are, however, occasional cases in which – in addition to the periumbilical lesion – patients have had angioid streaks and cardiovascular involvement.[6,10]

Patients are usually middle-aged to elderly, multiparous, and obese black females, although cases have been described in Indian, Asian, and Caucasian patients.[2,4,8,11] The condition presents as a periumbilical hyperpigmented, hyperkeratotic plaque with keratotic papules at the periphery.[10]

Pathogenesis and histologic features

Whether the condition represents an acquired and localized variant of pseudoxanthoma elasticum or a separate, distinct entity is uncertain.[10] Given the heterogeneity of clinical manifestations in the inherited condition, the former would seem quite likely. Localization to the periumbilical region may be a result of trauma. In addition to obesity and a multiparous state, the condition has also been associated with ascites, surgery, and renal failure.[10]

The histologic features are identical to those of the hereditary variant. Transepidermal elimination of altered elastic tissue is common.

Late-onset focal dermal elastosis

Clinical features

This is a recently described disorder in which patients present with yellow papules on the neck and in the flexures, clinically mimicking pseudoxanthoma elasticum.[1-7] It generally presents in the elderly, although a single report documents a case in a female teenager with acrogeria.[8] A potentially familial case involving two sisters was described.[9] No other stigmata of pseudoxanthoma elasticum are evident.

Pathogenesis and histologic features

The etiology and pathogenesis of this condition are unknown although an aging phenomenon has been proposed as has mechanical forces contributing accelerated turnover at the characteristic sites.[1,8]

Histologically, the papules are characterized by increased morphologically normal elastic fibers in the mid and deep dermis. There is no evidence of calcification. This clearly distinguishes this lesion from pseudoxanthoma elasticum, which it can mimic clinically.[6,10]

Anetoderma

Clinical features

Anetoderma (Gr. anetos, slack) is an acquired, purely cutaneous disorder characterized by numerous 0.5–3.0-cm foci of atrophic or wrinkled, flaccid skin, due to loss of elastic fibers, which may be accompanied by herniation into the subcutaneous fat (Figs 21.59 and 21.60).[1,2] Lesions, which are most common in young adults, particularly affect the upper trunk and proximal arms, although they may be more widespread.[3] One case was reported to have a granuloma annulare-like pattern.[4] An unusual linear form has been described.[5] There is a female predominance, and most patients range in age from 20 to 40 but all ages are affected.[2,3,6,7]

Although traditionally it has been divided into two subtypes – an erythematous inflammatory variant (Jadassohn-Pellizzari), in which inflammation with erythema or urticaria precedes the development of the more typical wrinkled lesions, and a more common clinically noninflammatory type (Schweninger-Buzzi) – the distinction is of little consequence since both types may histologically show an inflammatory stage.[1,2,8] Anetoderma is also classified into primary and secondary variants. Primary anetoderma arises in previously normal skin while the secondary form develops at the site of previous skin lesions.

Primary anetoderma

Primary anetoderma is associated with diseases of autoimmunity including antiphospholipid antibody, antiphospholipid syndrome, systemic lupus

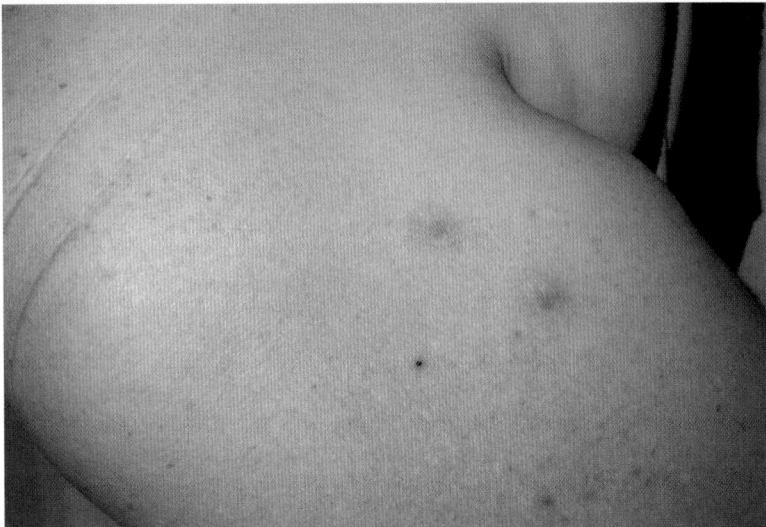

Fig. 21.59
Primary anetoderma: atrophic lesions with a wrinkled appearance. Courtesy of J.C. Pascual, MD, Alicante, Spain.

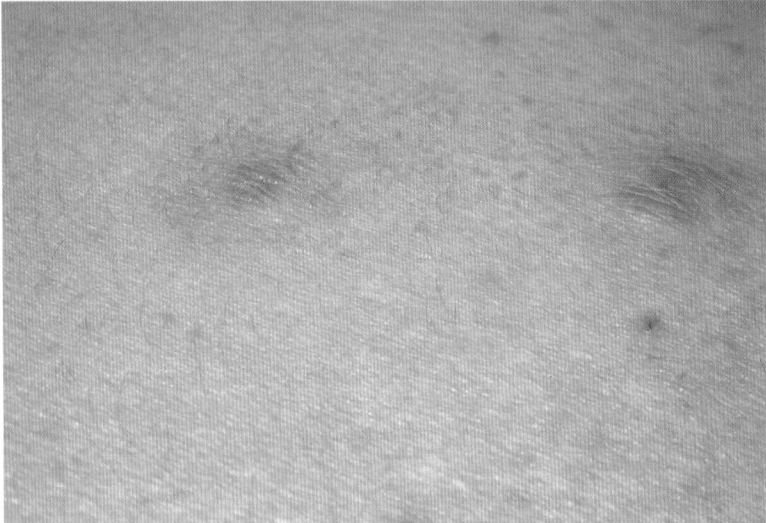

Fig. 21.60
Primary anetoderma: close-up view. Courtesy of J.C. Pascual, MD, Alicante, Spain.

erythematosus, discoid lupus erythematosus, systemic sclerosis, Sjögren syndrome, vitiligo, alopecia areata, autoimmune hemolytic anemia, prematurity, pregnancy, decreased alpha-1-antitrypsin, Hashimoto thyroiditis, Graves disease, and primary Addison disease.[3,7,8–27] The most significant association is with antiphospholipid antibodies (lupus anticoagulant and anticardiolipin antibodies).[9–13,28,29] In patients with systemic lupus erythematosus, it is those who have associated antiphospholipid antibodies who develop anetoderma, including a few patients with lupus panniculitis.[23,30] Rarely, anetoderma may proceed the appearance of antiphospholipid antibodies.[31] Similarly, human immunodeficiency virus (HIV)-positive patients who develop anetoderma have anticardiolipin antibodies.[32]

Secondary anetoderma

Secondary anetoderma has numerous associations: syphilis, tuberculosis, leprosy, varicella, molluscum contagiosum, Borrelia burgdorferi, HIV infection, pityriasis versicolor, perifolliculitis, Takayasu disease, hepatitis B vaccination, granuloma annulare, acne vulgaris, nodular prurigo, sarcoidosis, drugs (e.g., penicillamine), homocysteinemia, Wilson disease, terminal osseous dysplasia with pigmentary defects (TODPD, a rare X-linked syndrome), Reed syndrome (familial leiomyomatosis of skin and uterus) and tumors such as urticaria pigmentosa, pilomatrixoma, EBV-associated classical Hodgkin disease, and various B-cell lymphomas including cutaneous

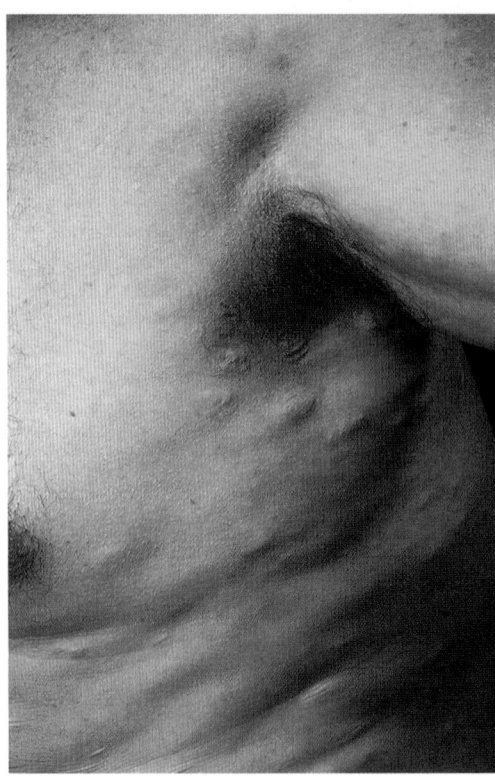

Fig. 21.61
Secondary anetoderma: in this case, the eruption developed after a syphilitic infection. By courtesy of R. Cerio, MD, The Royal London Hospital Trust, London, UK.

follicular center cell lymphoma and cutaneous marginal zone lymphoma (Fig. 21.61).[2,3,33–64] Some patients with lymphoma-associated anetoderma may have antiphospholipid antibodies.[65] Rarely, familial variants may be encountered.[66,67] Anetoderma has also been described in premature infants, possibly related to the sites of monitoring leads or the use of adhesive tape (anetoderma of prematurity).[68–71]

Pathogenesis and histologic features

The precise pathogenesis is unknown but is likely due to increased destruction of elastic tissue or diminished production. In favor of the former, an imbalance in metalloproteinases (such as gelatinase A, MMP-2, and MMP-9) and their tissue inhibitors (tissue inhibitor of metalloproteinase 1 [TIMP-1] and TIMP-2) has been demonstrated in lesional explants in tissue culture.[2,72–74] The strong association of primary anetoderma with autoimmune disease suggests that a primary immunological mechanism may sometimes be in play. Although antiphospholipid antibodies are associated with increased tendency for thrombosis, surprisingly, microthrombi are rarely – if ever – a feature of anetoderma. Antibodies against dermal elastic tissue components have not been identified.

Histologically, anetoderma is characterized by complete elastolysis or fragmented and sparse elastic fibers, particularly in the papillary and mid-reticular dermis (Figs 21.62–21.64).[1,2,74,75] Early inflammatory lesions may show a perivascular and periadnexal mononuclear or acute inflammatory cell component. Occasionally, plasma cells, histiocytes, giant cells, and ill-formed granulomata may be evident, and phagocytosis of elastic fibers has been described.[2,75,76] A case with underlying lobular granulomatous panniculitis has been reported.[23] The histologic appearances in clinically inflammatory and apparently noninflammatory types are identical.

Ultrastructural studies have confirmed the absence of elastic fibers. Small numbers of thin fibers composed of fibrils with little or no elastin are present.[77] Fragmented and fissured elastic fibers can be seen with granular degeneration while collagen fibers appear unaffected.[78] Immunofluorescence studies have shown granular Ig and C3 at the basement membrane region indistinguishable from lupus erythematosus.[11,79] Immunoreactants outlining the superficial vasculature and fibrillar deposits on elastic fibers have also been described.[11,80] Indirect studies are negative.[79]

Differential diagnosis

Anetoderma must be distinguished from cutis laxa, pseudoxanthoma elasticum-like papillary dermal elastolysis, mid-dermal elastolysis, and

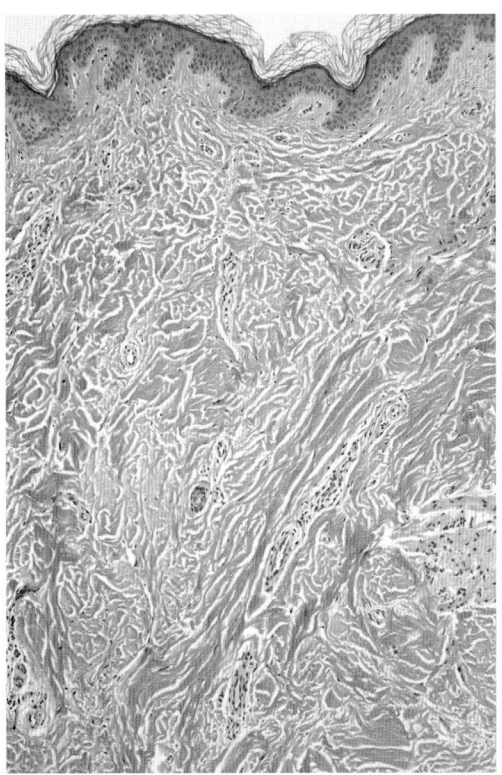

Fig. 21.62
Anetoderma: if inflammatory changes are absent, as in this example, it would be all too easy to dismiss the specimen as normal skin without adequate clinical information. By courtesy of Vince Liu, MD, University of Iowa, Iowa City, USA.

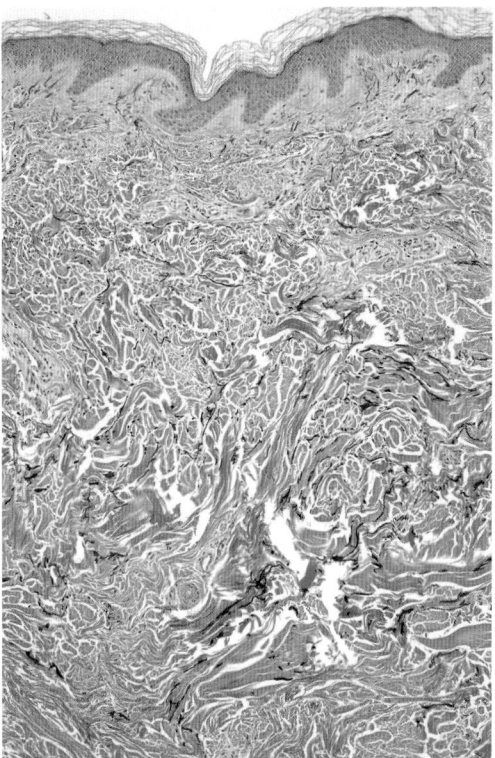

Fig. 21.63
Anetoderma: the elastic tissue stain shows a marked reduction in the number of fibers in both the papillary and reticular dermis. By courtesy of Vince Liu, MD., University of Iowa, Iowa City, USA.

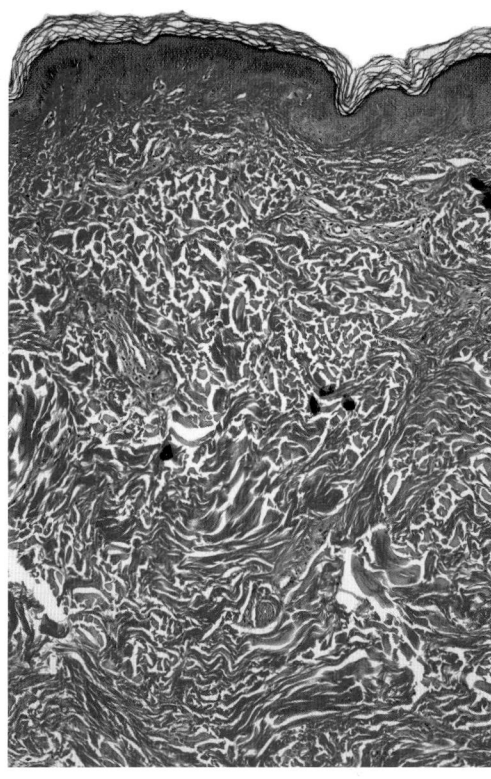

Fig. 21.64
Anetoderma: in contrast, the collagen appears normal in this trichrome-stained section. By courtesy of Vince Liu, MD., University of Iowa, Iowa City, USA.

perifollicular elastolysis. Atrophying tinea versicolor and mycosis fungoides can also clinically mimic anetoderma.[81,82]

Perifollicular elastolysis, anetoderma-like scars, and papular acne scars

Clinical features

Perifollicular elastolysis was the name applied to a condition in which small (2–4 mm) round or oval gray-white wrinkled lesions with a central hair follicle developed around the head, arms, and upper trunk of three female patients.[1] Anetoderma-like bulging was evident in some lesions. It was initially thought to represent a noninflammatory condition, and the authors postulated that it resulted from an elastase-producing strain of *Staphylococcus epidermidis*. It has now been described in the setting of atopic dermatitis and also Behçet disease.[2,3]

The term anetoderma-like scars was applied to a similar condition described in patients with acne vulgaris.[4]

More recently, it has been suggested that these lesions are probably identical and that, for the main, they represent post-acne papular scars.[5] The authors stress that although larger lesions can be soft, wrinkled, and resemble anetoderma, they lack the compressibility of the latter disorder.

Histologic features

Histologically, perifollicular elastolysis and acne-related anetoderma-like scars are characterized by loss of elastic tissue centered on a morphologically normal hair (*Fig. 21.65*).[6] Mid-dermal elastolysis can exhibit perifollicular accentuation of elastin loss, but it is not exclusively centered around hair follicles.[7]

Papular acne scars also show perifollicular elastolysis, but the collagen fibers are said to be thinned and abnormally distributed, as would be expected in a scar.

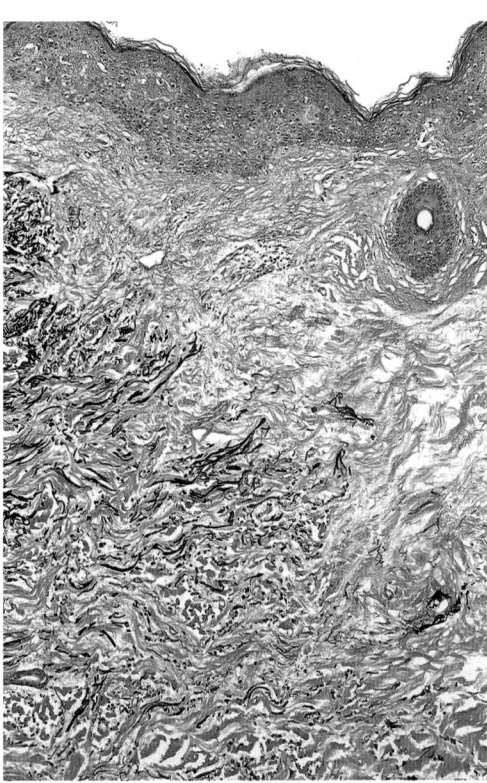

Fig. 21.65
Perifollicular elastolysis: this elastic tissue stain shows a dramatic loss of the perifollicular fibers. By courtesy of T. Quinn, MD, Pathology Services Incorporated, Boston, USA.

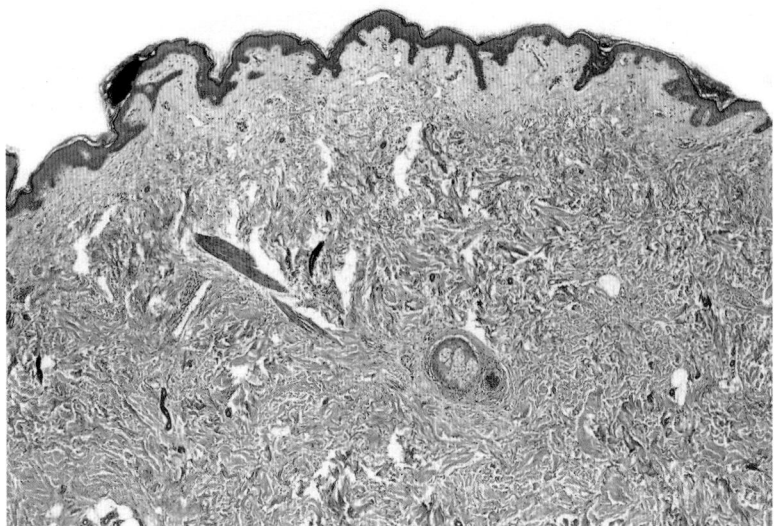

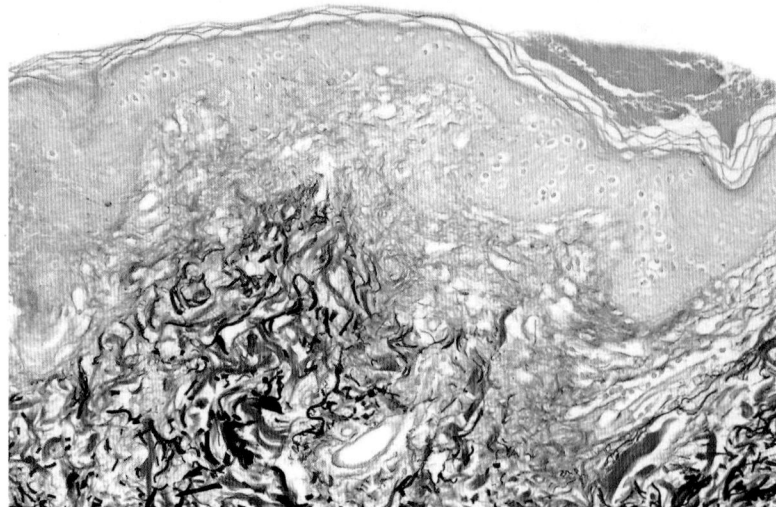

Fig. 21.66
Papillary dermal elastolysis: hematoxylin and eosin-stained sections generally show no significant features.

Fig. 21.67
Papillary dermal elastolysis: there is complete absence of thin elastic fibers in the papillary dermis.

Pseudoxanthoma elasticum-like papillary dermal elastolysis

Clinical features

Pseudoxanthoma elasticum-like papillary dermal elastolysis (age-related fibroelastolytic syndrome, fibroelastolytic papulosis of the neck) is a rare condition with less than 50 cases reported that appears to be primarily limited to elderly females, with rare reports in younger women and exceptional males.[1–16] A solitary familial occurrence has been documented.[17] Patients present with asymptomatic or mildly pruritic, 2–4-mm, yellowish, symmetrical, nonfollicular soft papules on the sides of the neck and the supraclavicular fossae.[8] The flexor aspect of the forearms, axillae, and the lower abdomen may also be affected.[2,4,5] Lesions often coalesce to form cobblestone plaques reminiscent of pseudoxanthoma elasticum. Systemic lesions are absent.

Pathogenesis and histologic features

The pathogenesis of papillary dermal elastolysis is unknown. Usually, no history of excessive prior sun exposure, urticarial reaction, or inflammatory dermatosis is elicited.[8,18,19] Although abnormal elastogenesis has been suggested as being of importance, it has been proposed that this condition represents an intrinsic aging phenomenon.[7]

Histologically, the epidermis may appear flattened.[7] The papules are characterized by partial or complete elastolysis involving the papillary dermis (*Figs 21.66* and *21.67*).[16] There may also be a slight reduction in the elastic tissue in the reticular dermis.[1,7,20] Irregular, variably thickened, and distorted elastic fibers in the reticular dermis have also been described.[3] Calcification is typically absent.[21] The collagen fibers are normal.

Ultrastructural studies confirm the absence of elastic fibers in the papillary dermis. Within the upper reticular dermis are immature elastic fibers and fibroblasts with dilated cisternae within their rough endoplasmic reticulum.[4,17] Rarefaction and disintegration of the elastin may also be present.[7]

Immunohistochemistry demonstrates loss of both elastin and fibrillin-1 in the papillary dermis.[18,22,23] Normal elderly skin is deficient in fibrillin-1 but not elastin.

Differential diagnosis

Pseudoxanthoma elasticum-like papillary dermal elastolysis shares some common histologic features with nonphotodamaged elderly skin. The latter and white fibrous papulosis have therefore been proposed as representing a variation of the intrinsic aging process.[7] This does not, however, explain the apparent predilection for females.

Distinction between pseudoxanthoma elasticum-like papillary dermal elastolysis and white fibrous papulosis of the neck may not be easy since there is considerable overlap.[7,24] Both affect the elderly and share the neck as the typical site of presentation. White fibrous papulosis differs by the finding of thickened collagen in the papillary and upper dermis. Loss of elastic tissue, however, is also commonly present.[7] As a consequence, Rongioletti and Rebora have proposed the name age-related fibroelastolytic syndrome[7] whereas Balus and coworkers have suggested the term fibroelastolytic papulosis of the neck to encompass the two conditions.[12,20,24,]

A likely related lesion was described as 'papillary dermal elastosis', although the description is more focused on abnormal rather than absence of elastin fibers in the papillary dermis.[25,26]

Mid-dermal elastolysis

Clinical features

Mid-dermal elastolysis is an uncommon acquired disorder with multiple presentations: most commonly as slowly progressive, asymptomatic plaques of fine wrinkling usually following Blaschko lines (type 1), and less often as either perifollicular papules (type 2) or reticular erythema and wrinkling (type 3).[1–22] Type 2 may give rise to a peau d'orange appearance.[11,18,20] Initially, these lesions were described as noninflammatory, but recent studies report that about half of these patients have a history of preceding or associated erythema, urticaria, or various inflammatory conditions.[9] There is a strong predilection for females (8:1), and most patients are young adults or middle-aged Caucasians.[10–12,17,18,23] Lesions particularly affect the trunk, neck, and arms.[12,18] The face and hands are almost invariably spared.[11,14] Lesions vary from only 1 or 2 cm in diameter to involvement of extensive areas of the trunk.[14] A reticular presentation has been described.[24] Rarely, the lesions can be generalized. There is no evidence of a familial incidence.[11,13]

There is a history of intense sun exposure in the majority of patients, and many also report using a sunbed or UVB phototherapy.[4,9,14,18,25] Mid-dermal elastolysis has been described in association with numerous conditions including Hashimoto thyroiditis, rheumatoid arthritis, lupus, positive ANA serology, silicone mammoplasty, urticaria, solar urticaria, atopic dermatitis, pityriasis rosacea, phototoxic dermatitis, Keutel syndrome (autosomal dominant with abnormal calcification of cartilage), chronic hemodialysis, protein S deficiency, uterine carcinoma, HIV, asthma, pacemaker placement, annular elastolytic giant cell granuloma, granuloma annulare, and a neutrophilic dermatosis.[1,10,11,14–19,26–34]

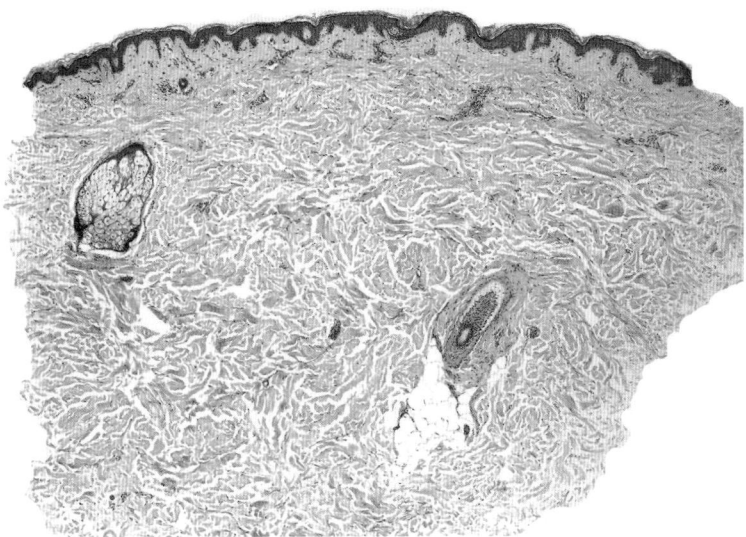

Fig. 21.68
Mid-dermal elastolysis: on low-power examination, there is a very light superficial perivascular chronic inflammatory cell infiltrate.

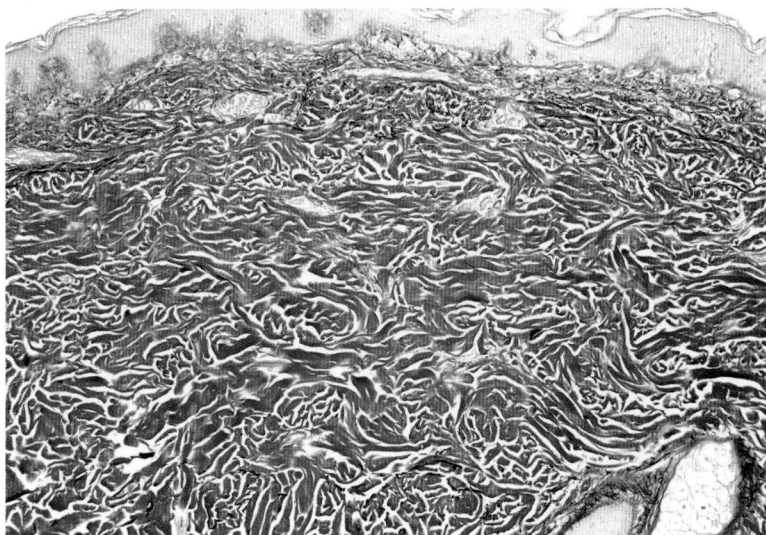

Fig. 21.70
Mid-dermal elastolysis: high-power view.

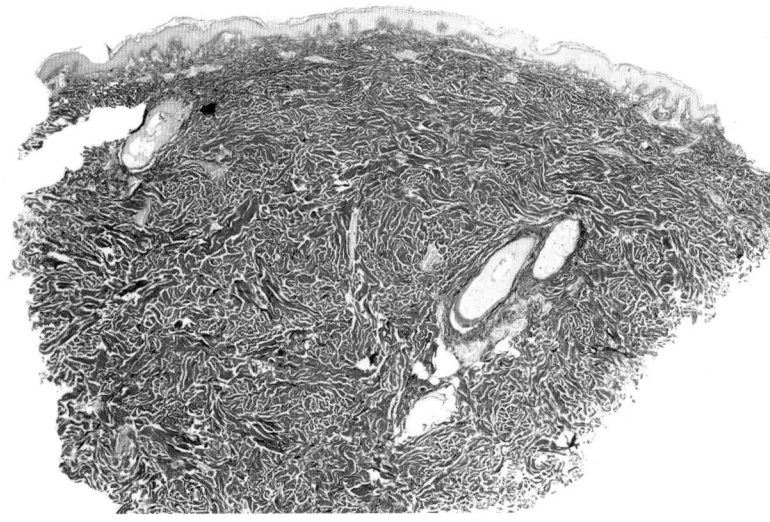

Fig. 21.69
Mid-dermal elastolysis: there is a marked reduction in staining for elastic fibers in the mid-dermis.

Pathogenesis and histologic features

It is unlikely that mid-dermal elastolysis represents a homogenous entity. Many cases appear to be related to UV light exposure although the clinical distribution is somewhat atypical since the face and backs of the hands are spared and gross solar elastosis is not usually a feature.[11] Other patients, however, give no such history, and alternative hypotheses have included postinflammatory elastolysis and autoimmunity.[3,11,16] Serology for *B. burgdorferi* is negative.[11] There is an increased incidence of cigarette smoking.[14] The loss of mid-dermal elastic tissue seen in this condition appears to be mediated at least in part by increased levels of dermal elastase, cathepsin G, and metalloproteinase.[9,11,14,17,26,35]

In early lesions there is a mid-dermal perivascular and, to a lesser extent, interstitial infiltrate of lymphocytes and histiocytes.[14,18] Multinucleate giant cells are occasionally seen and elastophagocytosis is sometimes present.[9,14,17,18] Granulomata have occasionally been described.[11] An elastic tissue stain shows diminution or complete absence of the elastic tissue in the mid-reticular dermis, while usually sparing the papillary, lower reticular, and perifollicular elastic fibers (*Figs 21.68–21.70*).[17] Obtaining a normal skin sample for comparison can be helpful to demonstrate elastic fiber loss.[36] Solar elastosis is generally absent or not prominent.[11] Older lesions

are characterized by absence of the inflammatory cell infiltrate and slightly thickened dermal collagen oriented parallel to the epidermis.[14]

Ultrastructurally, there is fragmentation of the elastic fibers which have a moth-eaten appearance due to loss of elastin.[9] Elastophagocytosis may be seen.[9,14,17] Immunohistochemistry demonstrates that the infiltrate consists of slightly increased CD3+, CD4+ T-helper cells admixed with CD68+ histiocytes.[14,18,37,38] CD34+ dermal dendritic cells are also conspicuous.[35] There is loss of elastin but not fibrillin.[14,18] Other studies reveal fibulin-5 to be unaffected in the upper and mid-dermis in both erythematous and wrinkled lesions, while in the deep dermis, fibulin-5 as well as fibulin-4 were found to be faint in the erythematous lesions and conglomerated in the wrinkled lesions.[38,39] Decreased lysyl oxidase-like 2 expression, involved in elastin fibril production, has been described.[40,41] Increased levels of MMP1 and MMP9 and reduced levels of TIMP-1 have been documented in fibroblast-like dermal multinucleate cells.[14,37,42] Additional reports demonstrate increased histiocytes and giant multinucleated cells expressing MMP9 and CD68 in erythematous lesions with fewer such cells in the wrinkled lesions.[38] Decorin expression, which identifies a microfibril component, is normal.[37]

Differential diagnosis

Mid-dermal elastolysis must be distinguished from anetoderma, postinflammatory elastolysis and cutis laxa, acquired cutis laxa, elastolytic giant cell granuloma, and pseudoxanthoma-like papillary dermal elastolysis.[11,15,17,18,21]

Linear focal elastosis

Clinical features

Linear focal elastosis (elastotic striae) is an uncommon disorder in which asymptomatic, palpable, symmetrical, horizontal, yellow striae develop on the mid and lower back.[1] The legs may also be affected.[2,3] Although originally described in elderly white males, the condition has been reported in females, children, and both Asians and blacks.[4–18] The lesions are more common in males. In some patients, the condition has been noticed since childhood.[8] Two separate possible familial examples have been documented.[5,19] There is a single report of simultaneous presentation of linear focal dermal elastosis and pseudoxanthoma elasticum-like papillary dermal elastolysis.[20]

There are occasional instances of patients with both focal elastosis and striae distensae; these may well be coincidental since the latter condition is relatively common.[7,10,21] In any event, in the majority of cases striae distensae are absent and patients do not give a history of recent weight change, hormonal imbalance, pregnancy, or steroid treatment, although exercise and growth spurt have been reported as an association.[1,5,9,22,23]

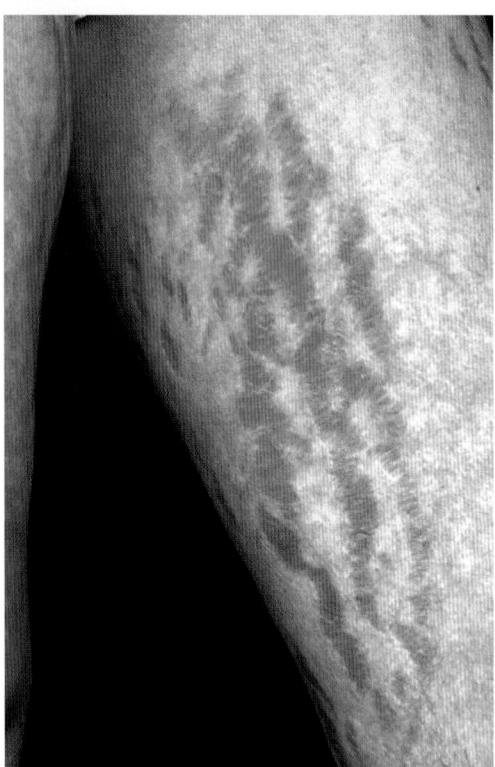

Fig. 21.71
Striae distensae: striae rubra (early lesions) in a characteristic distribution. By courtesy of the Institute of Dermatology, London, UK.

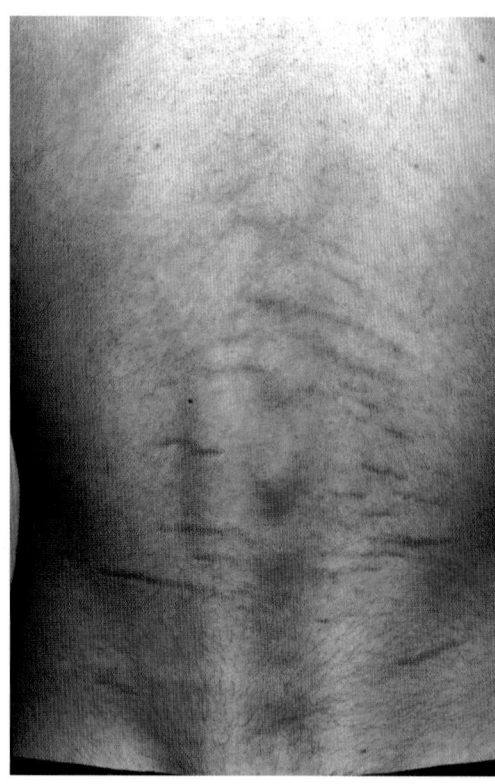

Fig. 21.72
Striae distensae: older lesions have a gray or white coloration. By courtesy of the Institute of Dermatology, London.

Pathogenesis and histologic features

The etiology of this condition is unknown, although some have proposed that it might represent a variant of striae distensae, a hamartoma, an inherited disorder, or a form of premature aging of elastic tissue.[5,9,12,22] The condition does not develop on exposed sites and there is no history of excessive sun exposure. Cycles of elastolysis and elastogenesis have been suggested to produce dermal accumulations of abnormal elastotic material.[16]

Histologically, linear focal elastosis is characterized by the presence of increased elastic tissue throughout the reticular dermis.[1,22] The fibers appear fragmented, wavy, or amorphous. There is no evidence of calcification.[1,12] Collagen is normal. The epidermis shows no abnormality. Special elastin stains highlight the abnormal accumulations which can be hard to discern on an H&E stain.

Ultrastructural studies have shown variable features including elastic fiber fragmentation, short, irregular, and branching elastic fibers with peripheral electron dense material, and evidence of active elastogenesis.[1,4,5,9]

Striae distensae

Clinical features

Striae distensae (stretch marks) are a common cosmetic problem and develop as a result of overstretching the skin as may be seen in obesity, pregnancy, puberty (striae gravidarium), breast augmentation, Marfan syndrome, febrile illness, and as a result of excess corticosteroids including Cushing syndrome.[1–15] They may also be a feature of weight loss and are therefore seen in anorexia nervosa.[16,17] Associations with medications include steroids and both cytotoxic and targeted (particularly bevacizumab) chemotherapy.[18–23] Females are affected more often than males. The early stage (striae rubra) presents as symmetrical linear red or violaceous lesions following the lines of cleavage (Fig. 21.71).[3,24] As they mature they become white, atrophic, and appear wrinkled (striae alba) (Fig. 21.72).[3,24] Involvement in darker individuals can produce striae nigra. Bullous or edematous forms can be encountered rarely.[25–27] Striae can precipitate koebnerization of psoriasis, lichen planus, systemic lupus erythematosus, vitiligo, and possibly graft-versus-host disease.[28–32]

Pathogenesis and histologic features

The pathogenesis of striae is uncertain, but the changes which most resemble a scar affect the dermal collagen, elastic tissue, and ground substance. The early stages are said to be characterized by mast cell degranulation, elastolysis, and elastophagocytosis by activated macrophages.[33] Responses to mechanical stress appears to play a role.[34]

In established striae, the epidermis appears atrophic with variable attenuation of the rete ridges. The thickness of the dermis is reduced and the collagen bundles are oriented in a horizontal plane.[35] Elastic fibers are diminished in the papillary dermis, while in the reticular dermis they are arranged parallel to the epidermis.[36] With chronicity they become thickened.[35,37] An excess of dermal glycosaminoglycans has been described.[36] A recent genome-wide association study suggested a linkage of single nucleotide polymorphisms in the regulatory elements of genes related to elastic microfibril production.[38]

Elastoma, elastic tissue nevus, and Buschke-Ollendorf syndrome

Clinical features

Elastoma (elastic tissue nevus, nevus elasticus) is a rare hamartomatous condition characterized by increased dermal elastic tissue (Figs 21.73 and 21.74). It may present as a solitary lesion or as a disseminated variant (juvenile elastoma) that is often familial and associated with osteopoikilosis, multiple foci of osteosclerosis, which together are known as Buschke-Ollendorf syndrome (Figs 21.75–21.77).[1–10]

Lesions present mainly on the trunk and limbs as 1–2-cm diameter, flesh-colored, white or yellow, smooth, asymptomatic disks, papules, plaques, and nodules. In some patients, lesions coalesce to cover large areas of the body.

Buschke-Ollendorf syndrome shows autosomal dominant inheritance.[5,11] It has a high penetrance with variable expression and affects 1 in 20 000 of the population.[2,12] Although in the majority of patients the two components of the syndrome are both present, in a given kindred either component may be present on its own.[13] The cutaneous manifestations vary

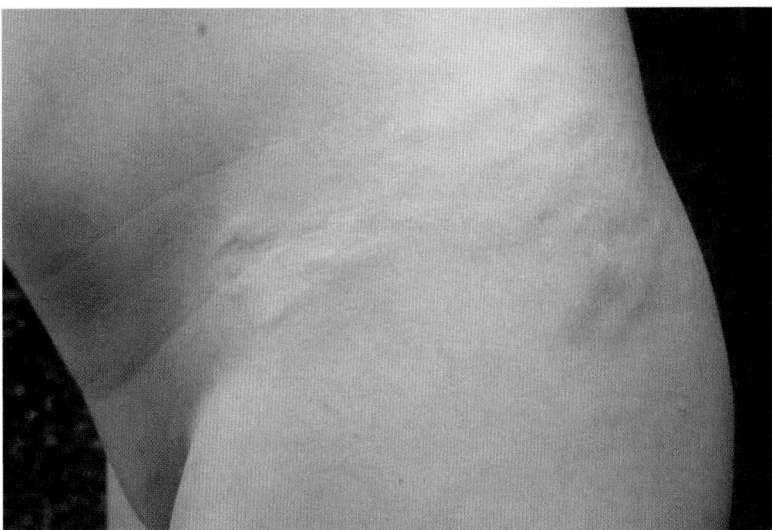

Fig. 21.73
Elastic tissue nevus: a flesh-colored plaque is present on the flank. By courtesy of the Institute of Dermatology, London, UK.

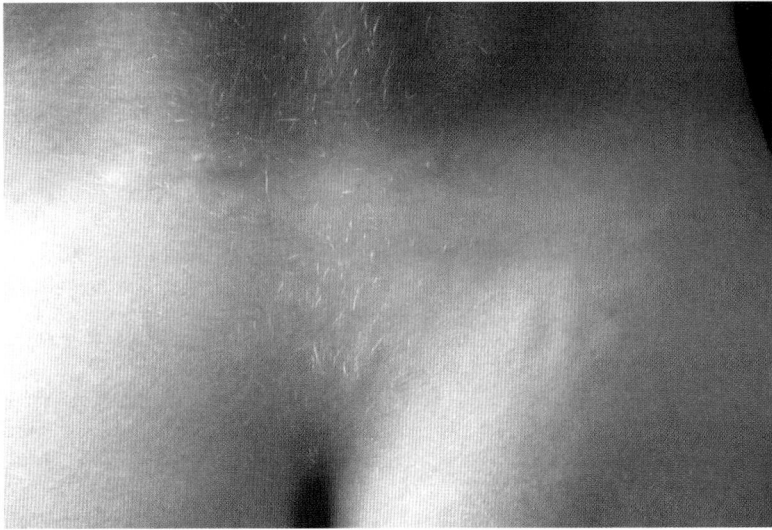

Fig. 21.74
Elastic tissue nevus: it extends onto the buttock. By courtesy of the Institute of Dermatology, London, UK.

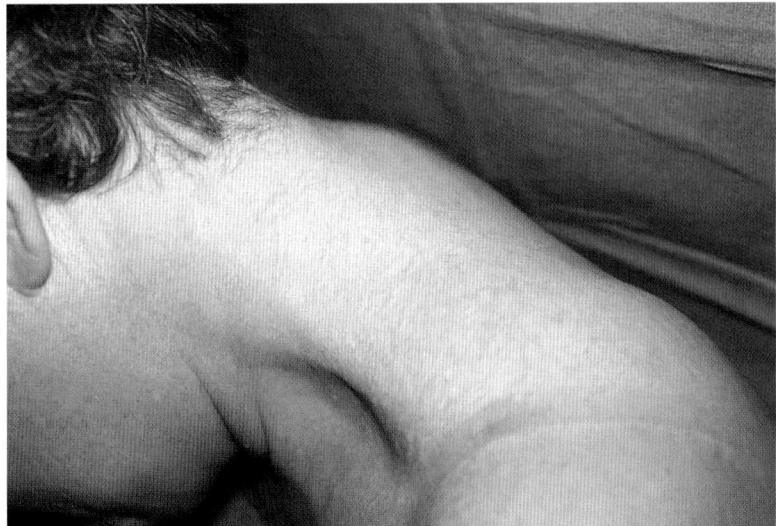

Fig. 21.75
Juvenile elastoma: multiple flesh-colored papules are present on the neck. By courtesy of N. Flanagan, MD, St James's Hospital, Dublin, Republic of Ireland.

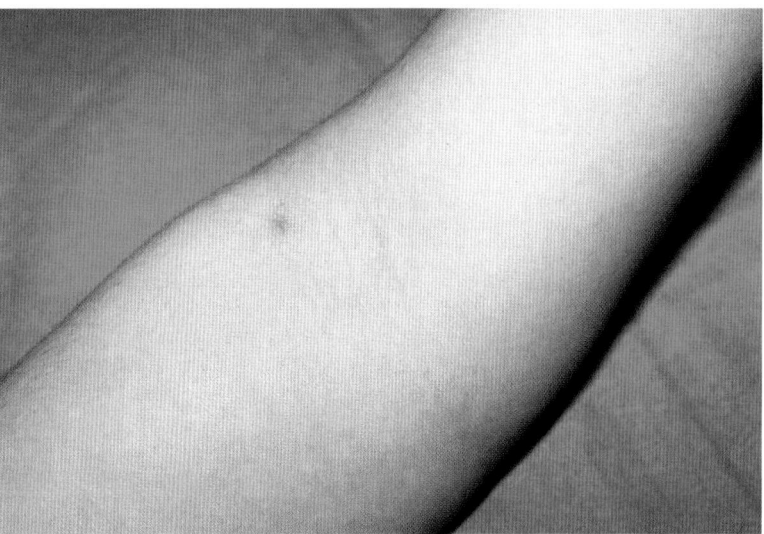

Fig. 21.76
Juvenile elastoma: the antecubital fossa is involved. By courtesy of N. Flanagan, MD, St James's Hospital, Dublin, Republic of Ireland.

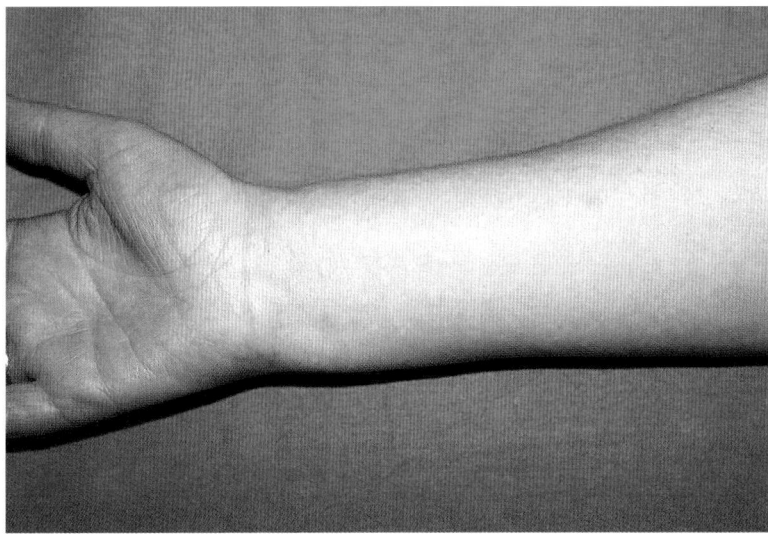

Fig. 21.77
Juvenile elastoma: the front of the forearm is affected. By courtesy of N. Flanagan, MD, St James's Hospital, Dublin, Republic of Ireland.

from asymmetrically distributed elastic-rich juvenile elastomas described earlier, to a symmetrical distribution of lichenoid collagen-rich papules, also known as dermatofibrosis lenticularis disseminata.[5,14–16] The skin manifestations generally present in the first or second decade and are occasionally evident at birth.[17] Osteopoikilosis is a usually asymptomatic, often incidental finding of little consequence discovered on X-ray examination.[1] It presents as 0.1–1.0-cm round radiopaque lesions in the epiphysis and metaphysis of the long bones, the pelvis, and the bones of the hands and feet.[3,17] The condition is not usually evident until the mid teens or later.[3,18] Other reported associations include craniosynostosis, cataracts, gastric ulcers, congenital spinal stenosis, otosclerosis, melorheostosis, muscle contractures, short stature, supernumerary ribs/vertebrae, mental retardation, diabetes, defects in teeth, neuropathy, and cryptorchidism.[5,19–21] A case was recently reported with osteopoikilosis and late-onset generalized morphea as a novel syndromic variant.[22]

Pathogenesis and histologic features

Although lesions with excess collagen or reduced and/or fragmented elastic tissue have been described in Buschke-Ollendorf syndrome, the majority of authors report an excess of elastic tissue.[4,5,9,12–14,17–19,23–26]

Loss-of-function mutations in *LEMD3* (also known as *MAN1*) have been described in patients with Buschke-Ollendorf syndrome and

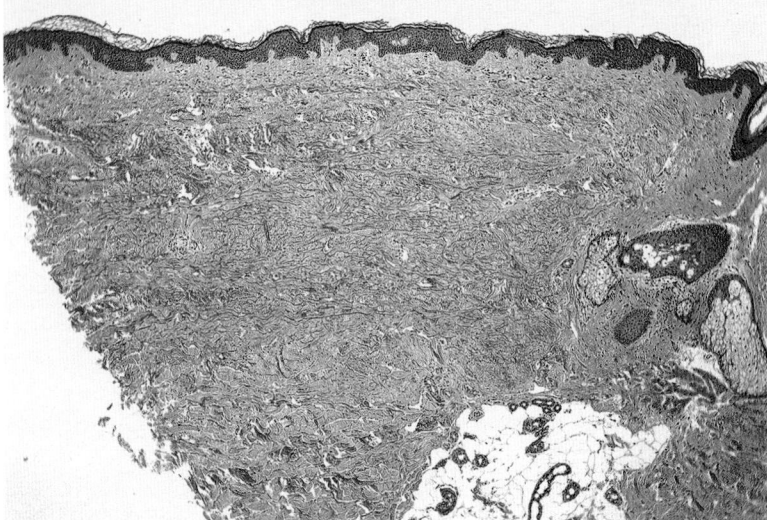

Fig. 21.78
Buschke-Ollendorf syndrome: in this example, the collagen fibers appear thickened. Broad elastic fibers are also apparent.

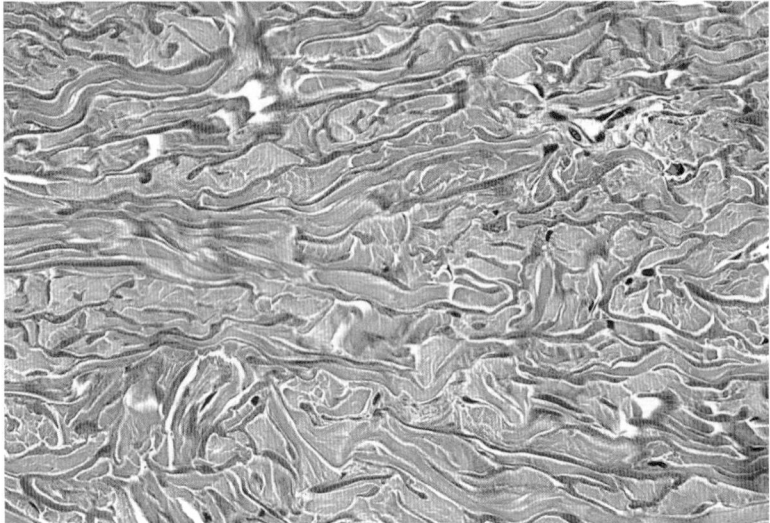

Fig. 21.79
Buschke-Ollendorf syndrome: the elastic tissue compartmentalizes the dermal collagen.

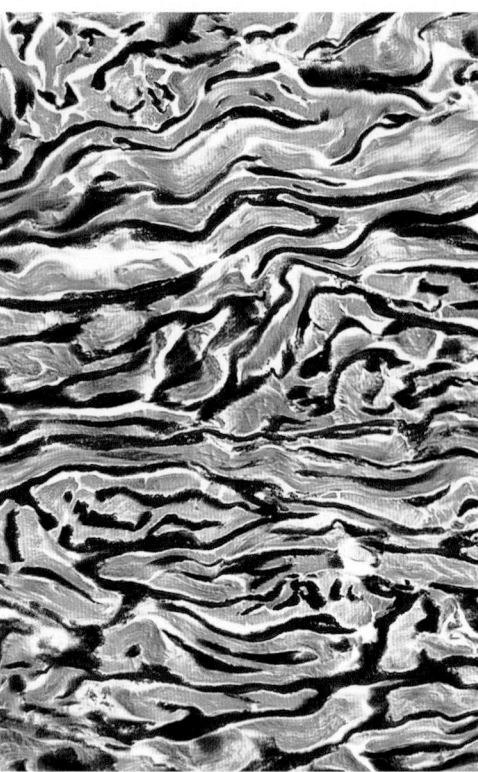

Fig. 21.80
Buschke-Ollendorf syndrome: the features are highlighted with an elastic tissue stain.

osteopoikilosis.[5,15,18,22,27–33] LEMD3 is an inner nuclear membrane protein that negatively regulates TGF-β and BMP (bone morphogenetic protein) using receptor-activated SMAD proteins. However, one family with classic features lacked detectable LEMD3 exonic mutations, suggesting alternative mutations or that other genes may be involved.[5,7] Patients with 12q14 microdeletion syndrome (which includes LEMD3) can also have both the skin and bone findings of Buskche-Ollendorf in addition to low birth weight, failure to thrive, and growth and mental retardation. In such cases, the additionally deleted HMGA2 on the 12q14 interval is thought to be important in regulating stature.[34–38] Silver-Russell syndrome, a heterogeneous disorder with growth restriction, hypoglycemia, macrocephaly, characteristic facies, and other dysmorphisms, can also delete LEMD3 and HMGA2 in a subset of cases.[39–41]

The histologic features are variable. Elastic tissue nevi may present as an irregular and sometimes compact aggregate of increased elastic tissue in the reticular dermis.[8,42–46] In Buschke-Ollendorf syndrome the features are often distinctive, consisting of thickened elastic fibers appearing to encircle and compartmentalize the dermal collagen (Figs 21.78–21.80).[5,13,16–19,25,47–49] Fragmentation is generally not a feature. In some patients with Buschke-Ollendorf syndrome, however, this distinctive pattern is not present.[3] Increased glycosaminoglycans is an occasional feature.[5,13,18,42,50]

Collagen bundles are variably described as normal or thickened.[1,42] The epidermis is normal or atrophic with loss of the rete ridges.[42]

Osteopoikilosis is characterized by irregular, dense, thickened bony trabeculae.[42]

Ultrastructurally, the elastic fibers show a variety of features including electron-lucent central defects in the elastin component, diminished microfibrils, granular deposits, and a branched, irregular morphology.[3,4,17,46] Calcification is not a feature. Collagen fibers may appear normal, homogenized, or show considerable variation in fiber diameter, with cauliflower forms.[2,17,43] Fibroblasts show dilated rough endoplasmic reticulum, sometimes containing fine granular material.[17,46]

A verrucous scrotal lesion characterized by massive dermal elastin deposits has been described in an isolated report as an exophytic elastoma.[51]

Some have proposed that papular elastorrhexis could be a variant of Buschke-Ollendorf syndrome without osteopoikilosis, but molecular genetics investigation of LEMD3 has not been presented. Papular elastorrhexis has loss and fragmentation of elastic fiber in contrast to elastomas.[52] However, skin lesions in Buschke-Ollendorf syndrome do not always show a clear increase in elastic fibers.[6,53–55]

Papular elastorrhexis

Clinical features

This is a rarely documented condition (less than 50 cases reported) in which children or adolescents present with asymptomatic, nonfollicular, 1- to 5-mm firm white papules on the trunk and extremities, with head and neck involvement less common.[1–7] More restricted and even solitary lesions have been reported.[8,9] There is no evidence of osteopoikilosis.[5] In the small number of cases documented, there appears to be a predilection for females (approximately 4:1). Although most examples have described sporadic cases, there is one report of familial occurrence.[3,10]

Pathogenesis and histologic features

The pathogenesis of papular elastorrhexis is unknown. It has been variably regarded as an example of nevus anelasticus and a form of connective tissue nevus.[1–3] Some suggest that papular elastorrhexis could be an incomplete form of Buschke-Ollendorff syndrome.[11,12] Evaluation of the LEMD3 gene associated with Buschke-Ollendorff has not been reported in papular elastorrhexis, but could provide insight.[13,14]

The lesions are characterized by homogenization of collagen and fragmentation and loss to absence of elastic tissue.[1–5] The epidermis is normal or slightly thickened. Conspicuous fibroblasts and a lymphohistiocytic infiltrate surrounding the superficial and deep plexuses have been described in one series.[5]

Ultrastructural studies have confirmed the loss of elastic tissue. Residual fibers have displayed relative preservation of the fibrillar component.[3] The collagen fibers appear normal.[3]

Differential diagnosis

Papular elastorrhexis should be distinguished from juvenile elastoma including Buschke-Ollendorf syndrome and papular acne scars.[5,15] The lesions of juvenile elastoma are characterized by increased elastic tissue rather than fragmentation and loss as seen in papular elastorrhexis. In addition, osteopoikilosis is a feature of Buschke-Ollendorf syndrome.

Papular acne scars are characterized by perifollicular scarring with loss of elastic tissue, and lesions predominantly affect the upper trunk. Papular elastorrhexis does not generally show an inflammatory phase and patients deny a history of preceding acne.[3,5]

A similar and also exceedingly rare lesion has been termed eruptive collagenoma.[16,17] Some find this to be identical to papular elastorrhexis and have suggested the unifying term of 'eruptive papular collageno-elastopathy'.[18] Eruptive collagenoma shows a predilection for males in Caucasians, and adults are predominantly affected.[19]

Cutaneous effects of chronic sun damage and chronological aging

Clinical features

Chronic sun exposure, in addition to its association with a number of cutaneous malignancies including basal cell carcinoma, squamous cell carcinoma, melanoma, and precursor lesions such as actinic keratosis, is responsible for aging of the skin (dermatoheliosis). Photoaging is to be distinguished from intrinsic (chronological) aging.[1–3] There is considerable individual variability in skin aging attesting to the complex multivariable nature of the process.[4]

Intrinsic aging is age-associated changes that occur in the skin due to the natural aging process without the superimposed effects of sun damage.[5] Consequently, it is most easily detected on non-sun-exposed skin and presents as thin, inelastic skin associated with fine, temporary wrinkles.[1,2] The latter, by definition, disappear on stretching the skin. Due to loss of elasticity, pendulous skin folds may also develop. Additional features include Campbell de Morgan spots and venous lakes.[6] Senile sebaceous hyperplasia and alopecia are also common. Rongioletti and Rebora also think that pseudoxanthoma elasticum-like papillary dermal elastolysis, white fibrous papulosis, and some cases of mid-dermal elastolysis represent aging phenomena.[7]

In contrast, photoaging (extrinsic aging) is characterized by diffusely thickened, leathery, inelastic skin with permanent coarse wrinkles. Actinic lentigines are common as is telangiectasia.[5,8] A variety of other clinical cutaneous manifestations due to the presence of large deposits of elastotic material (solar elastosis) in the superficial dermis have been described. These include cutis rhomboidalis nuchae, elastotic nodules of the ear, collagenous and elastotic plaques of the hands, keratoelastoidosis marginalis, solar elastotic bands of the forearm (Raimer bands), actinic comedonal plaque, bullous solar elastosis, adult colloid milium (papular elastosis), actinic granuloma, cutaneous nodular elastoidosis with cysts and comedones (Favre-Racouchot syndrome), linear focal elastosis, and poikiloderma of Civatte.[5–7,9–13] Many of these represent case reports and are simply variations on the theme.

- Favre-Racouchot syndrome preferentially occurs in older Caucasian males (fifth to seventh decades) with prolonged sun exposure. Patients have multiple cysts and open comedones involving the face, especially in the malar region, lateral canthus, temple, cheek, neck, and posterior auricular skin.[5,12,14,15]

- Cutis rhomboidalis nuchae represents an exaggeration of solar damage. Patients present with extremely leathery skin on the back of the neck associated with deep furrows dividing the skin into geometric shapes. It is associated with Favre-Racouchot syndrome.[5,12,16]

- Elastotic nodules of the ear present as pale gray, translucent, white or pink nodules.[12,17,18] Although the antihelix is preferentially affected, lesions may also develop on the helix where they can be mistaken for chondrodermatitis nodularis helicis.[12,18]

- Keratoelastoidosis marginalis (collagenous and elastotic marginal plaques of the hands, digital papular calcific elastosis, degenerative collagenous plaques of the hand) are characterized by hyperkeratotic, linear translucent papules and plaques and calcified dermal elastotic masses along the radial border of the hands.[12,19–21] They are thought to be related to chronic pressure in addition to the effect of ultraviolet radiation.[19] Keratoelastoidosis marginalis in which lesions develop along the borders of the hands and feet in association with ultraviolet light and manual labor is a related condition.[12,22]

- Solar elastotic bands of the forearm (Raimer bands) present on the forearm as a cordlike band of soft, flesh-colored or yellow papules and nodules at the junction between dorsal skin showing severe solar elastosis and relatively unaffected ventral skin.[10,12,23] Lesions are sometimes bilateral.[10]

- Actinic comedonal plaque presents on the forearms as erythematous to bluish confluent nodules and plaques associated with comedones.[5,24,25] This represents a variant of nodular elastoidosis with comedones and cysts (Favre-Racouchot syndrome).[5,12,15,25]

- Bullous lesions in solar elastosis are exceedingly rare. They present as asymptomatic to pruritic plaques and papules with tense bullae and most commonly on the forearms. Whether they are trauma related or develop as a consequence of a degenerative phenomenon is unknown.[4,7,26]

- Adult colloid milia present multiple papules consisting of amorphous degenerated elastin which affects the extremities (hands typically) and face.[12,27] These can sometimes be confused histologically with nodular amyloidosis.

Pathogenesis and histologic features

The mechanisms of intrinsic aging continue to be elaborated. Currently, it is thought to occur due to telomere shortening and accumulated DNA damage, both eventually triggering cellular senescence.[28,29] Examination of progeroid syndromes may also provide further insight.[28,30–33] Histologically, chronological aging is characterized by flattening of the epidermis, diminished numbers of epidermal melanocytes and Langerhans cells, and reduced pigmentation.[34–37] There is also reduced epidermal turnover with decreased proliferation, and less dermal cellularity.[38] Reduced numbers of thinner elastic fibers are present in the papillary dermis. The reticular dermal collagen bundles may appear coarser and disorganized.[35] Elastic fibers are reduced in the reticular dermis.[34] In temporary wrinkles, the vertically oriented elastic fibers of the papillary dermis are absent.[7,39]

Several mechanisms of photoaging have been suggested. UV induction of free oxygen radicals is known to trigger several intracellular pathways which results in reduction of collagen expression and TGF-β receptors, while also increasing matrix metalloproteinase production. Collagen damaged by UV could inhibit further collagen synthesis while continual accumulation of oxidized proteins inhibits cellular proteosomes thereby disrupting cellular functions.[3] UV insults to mitochondrial DNA results in accumulation of free radicals and disrupting cellular energy metabolism.[3,40] UV-induced telomere damage can result in cellular senescence and apoptosis.[3,41] Recruited neutrophils with their proteolytic enzymes and UV-induced keratinocytes may also play a role.[3,40] Infrared A radiation is associated with increased metalloproteinase expression.[42] Transcriptome analysis of UV-A irradiated cultured human fibroblastics revealed significant expression changes in more than 600 genes across many pathways and functional groups attesting to the initial complexity of this process.[43] Some changes can be induced within a week.[44] Another gene expression profiling study of both age- and photo-induced changes in the skin of the face and forearm in Caucasian women over 6 decades revealed progressive changes in gene sets enriched for oxidative stress, cellular senescence, energy metabolism, and epidermal barrier.[45] Animal models are also being created and evaluated.[46,47]

The histologic features of UVB radiation of the skin include epidermal and dermal changes.[48] In established lesions 24–72 hours after exposure, the epidermis contains damaged keratinocytes (sunburn cells) and shows intercellular edema and exocytosis of inflammatory cells. There are diminished numbers of Langerhans cells. The dermal changes include endothelial cell swelling and perivenular edema with a predominantly mononuclear intradermal chronic inflammatory cell infiltrate.[48] Chronic exposure, particularly in fair-skinned individuals, may be associated with the development of elastosis, lentigines, keratoses, and a variety of malignant tumors including basal cell carcinoma, squamous carcinoma, and melanoma. In some patients, nodular elastosis is present, often in association with cysts and comedones. This is usually seen on the face, particularly the cheek (Favre-Racouchot syndrome).[49]

UVA-induced cutaneous erythema is characterized by keratinocyte swelling and vacuolation accompanied by intercellular edema and diminished numbers of Langerhans cells. Sunburn cells are not a feature.[48] In the dermis, there is a mixed inflammatory cell infiltrate consisting of polymorphs, lymphocytes, and occasional basophils and eosinophils. Endothelial cell swelling is also evident.

Despite the ubiquitous presence of solar elastosis in Caucasians who experience any significant degree of sun exposure, its precise nature and mode of development remains a mystery.[50] Current evidence indicates that it is composed predominantly of elastic tissue although there is probably also a collagenous component. Whether it represents a degenerative phenomenon of elastic tissue or results from active synthesis (or both) remains uncertain.

Histologically, solar elastosis is composed of basophilic fibrillar material dispersed diffusely throughout the upper dermis and sometimes arranged in large nodules as in milia. The fibers are thick, irregular, and branched or reduced to an amorphous mass. They are positive with elastic tissue stains.[12] Cysts or open comedones can be present (Favre-Racouchot syndrome).[5] Bastian and coworkers have developed a practical scale for assessing the degree of solar damage based primarily on elastosis that has predictive value for melanoma genotypes and is discussed more fully in Chapter 26.[51–53]

Immunohistochemistry has demonstrated that the elastotic material contains elastin and fibronectin but not fibrillin.[54,55] There is considerably less collagen.[54]

Additional features which may develop in sun-damaged skin include epidermal atrophy or mild acanthosis, loss of rete ridges, hyperpigmentation, pigmentary incontinence and mild melanocytic nuclear irregularity, and hyperchromatism with a cytoplasmic retraction artifact.[36] In contrast to in situ melanoma, there is no significant increase in nuclear size, nucleoli are not a feature, and nuclear crowding or distinct palisades are absent. Spread of melanocytes along the adnexae is also not a feature of the photoaging process. Dermal collagen is reduced in amount.

Glucocorticoid-related cutaneous atrophy

Local glucocorticoid therapy may be associated with a variety of cutaneous side effects including atrophy of skin and subcutaneous tissue and hyper- and hypopigmentation (*Fig. 21.81*).[1–3] Ecchymoses are common.[4] Most of the effects are magnified over both by time and by the strength of the corticosteroid preparation. These cutaneous findings can be seen in Cushing syndrome of varying etiology.[5] Occasionally, linear atrophic lesions may develop after intralesional or intra-articular injections following the pathway of the local lymphatics.[6,7] In addition to diminishing dermal glycosaminoglycans content, local steroid injections are rapidly followed by reduced synthesis of collagen types I and III.[8–12]

Histologically, steroid atrophy is characterized by a diminished stratum corneum, epidermal thinning, and loss of the epidermal ridge pattern.[8,13,14] The dermal collagen initially appears compacted but, with progression, becomes thinned and the bundles separated. Pigment incontinence and vascular ectasia may also be evident.

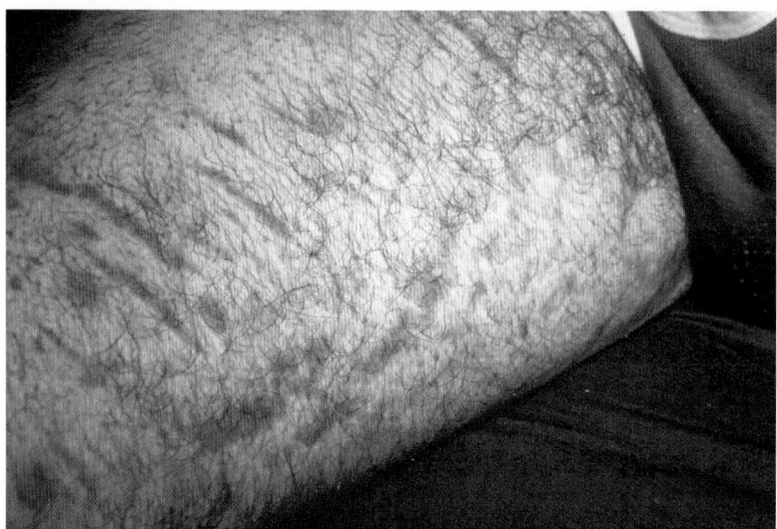

Fig. 21.81
Steroid striae: these striae developed following the use of a fluorinated steroid cream.

Hutchinson-Gilford syndrome

Clinical features

Hutchinson-Gilford syndrome (progeria) (Gr. *geriaos*, old age) is the prototype of the premature aging syndromes.[1–5] An incidence of 1 in 4 million is estimated.[6] In contrast to Werner syndrome which presents in adults, patients with Hutchinson-Gilford syndrome are invariably children. Exceptionally, the disease has been recognized in the neonate.[7] The skin, bones, joints, and cardiovascular systems are predominantly involved. It is invariably associated with premature death, with patients succumbing in the second decade.[1,8,9] Children present with failure to thrive and growth retardation.[1,10]

Dermatological manifestations have been extensively reviewed.[2,11–16] Common features include the clinical impression of a child looking radically aged, craniofacial disproportion, micrognathia with crowding of excessive teeth, scalp alopecia and conspicuous scalp veins, prominent eyes, absence of subcutaneous fat, nail dystrophy, generalized hypotrichosis, loose wrinkled skin affecting the fingers and toes, and impaired sweating.[1,15,17] Scleroderma-like changes are common, and there are rare reports of keloidal nodules affecting the extremities.[18–21]

Bone changes include osteoporosis, osteolysis, skeletal dysplasia, avascular necrosis of the hip, congenital dislocation of the hip, and impaired bone healing.[1] Radiology may show resorption of the distal ends of the clavicles, phalangeal sclerosis, diffuse osteopenia, and fish mouth vertebral bodies.[19,22] The major vascular lesion is accelerated atherosclerosis and patients commonly die from myocardial infarction and cerebrovascular effects.[1,13] Early-onset malignancies can be encountered.[6]

Despite such severe manifestations affecting multiple systems, other organs are unimpaired. For example, there is no evidence of cerebral involvement and intelligence is normal.[13] Similarly, the immune system shows no obvious disturbance.[1]

Pathogenesis and histologic features

The pathogenesis of this disease is unknown. Inheritance appears to be sporadic and autosomal dominant.[1] Hutchinson-Gilford syndrome has recently been shown to be associated with mutations in *LMNA* which disrupt the post-translational processing of the encoded protein, nuclear lamin A.[23,24] A C-terminal farnesyl group is abnormally retained, blocking proper function of the protein in the nuclear membrane. Lamin A plays a structural role by contributing to nuclear shape and mechanotransduction, but is also involved in nuclear assembly and trafficking, chromatin organization, and transcription.[25–27] This aberrant farnesyl moiety has been presumed to be the major pathogenetic factor, and farnesyl transferase inhibitors are available clinically.[28–31] Inhibition of farnesylation can restore some normal cellular properties such as nuclear shape, distribution of type A lamin, and DNA double-strand break repair.[32–35] Blocking farnesylation in a mouse model ameliorated major progeroid symptoms.[34] Clinical trials in humans have demonstrated benefits in growth and cardiovascular function.[36–38] A family of disparate diseases including forms of muscular dystrophy, lipodystrophy, cardiomyopathy, and premature aging are associated with mutations in various nuclear lamin genes now referred to as 'laminopathies'.[39–42] Also included is restrictive dermopathy. Current research also focuses on defective DNA damage response as the driver of premature aging.[43–45] Global histone modifications appear to drive changes in gene expression.[46] There appears to be an important connection between the mechanotransductive properties of lamin A and regulation of chromatin structure and thus gene regulation.[47]

The skin in Hutchinson-Gilford syndrome may be hyperkeratotic, atrophic, and hyperpigmented.[15,48] Basal cell hydropic degeneration has been documented.[21] The dermal collagen is thickened and hyalinized.[48,49] Elastic tissue is increased.[1] Skin appendages and blood vessels may be normal, reduced, or absent.[15,48] The subcutaneous fat is diminished or virtually absent. The dermal nodules are composed predominantly of type IV collagen.[20]

Werner syndrome

Clinical features

Werner syndrome is an adult form of progeria and is usually recognized by the third decade.[1–3] It is inherited as an autosomal recessive disorder. Clinical manifestations include short stature, low weight, a dysmorphic facies with a bird-like beaked nose and protuberant eyes, and distal sclerodermoid features.[1,4–9] There is an increased incidence of atherosclerosis (an important cause of death), heart block, cardiomyopathy, myocardial infarction, diabetes, and cancer.[1,10,11] Additional features include poor wound healing, cataracts, gray hair, osteoporosis, spondylitis, sclerodactyly, high-pitched voice, hypogonadism, mottled pigmentation, freckling, telangiectasia, and alopecia.[1,6,10,12] Despite the appearances of premature aging, the central nervous system is unaffected and there is no increase in incidence of Alzheimer disease.[1]

Up to 10% of patients develop malignancy, both cutaneous and visceral. Skin tumors include basal cell carcinoma and melanoma.[13–17] Systemic tumors include soft tissue sarcomas, bone osteosarcoma, thyroid neoplasms, leukemia, lung cancer, and meningioma.[12,16,18–24]

Pathogenesis and histologic features

Werner syndrome is due to inactivating mutation of the WRN gene in the RecQ family of DNA helicases.[1,25–29] The WRN protein, which has exonuclease in addition to helicase activity, is involved in genome integrity by regulating DNA double-strand break repair and telomere maintenance.[30–34] Mutation is associated with genomic instability and chromosomal abnormalities partially due to inability to repair UV-induced DNA damage through oxidative stress.[2,30,31,35,36] Epigenetic aging with progressive changes in DNA methylation causes aging of stem cell populations, perhaps through premature senescence.[37–41]

The cutaneous features are characterized by hyperkeratosis, epidermal atrophy, hyperpigmentation, and dermal fibrosis with hyalinization.[6] The fibrosis can appear similar to scleroderma.[42–45] The appendages are atrophic and the subcutaneous fat is thinned.[6]

Radiation dermatitis

Clinical features

Radiation dermatitis may be acute or chronic and follows either therapeutic or accidental overexposure.[1–3] The clinical and pathological features of cutaneous damage are variable and depend on the type of ionizing radiation, the dosage, and individual sensitivity.[4–6] Acute radiation dermatitis (that occurring within the first 6 months of exposure) is characterized by

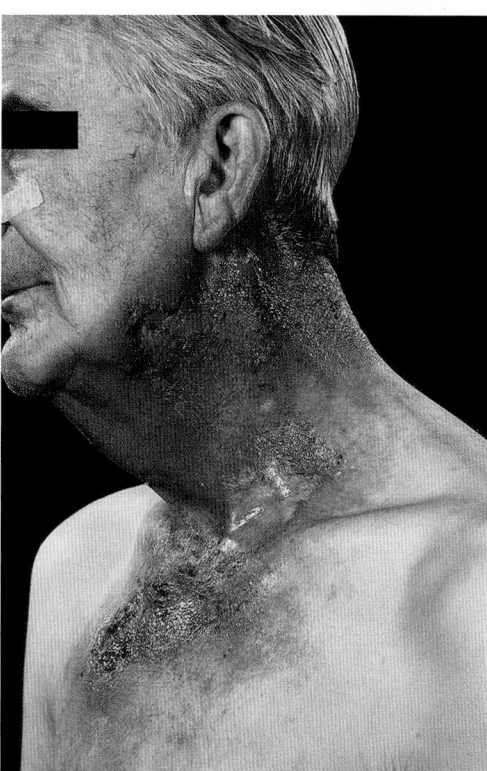

Fig. 21.82
Radiation dermatitis: this patient shows very severe radiation damage. Note the erythema, ulceration, and crusting. With the advent of modern techniques in radiotherapy, complications such as these are no longer seen. Archival material. By courtesy of A. Timothy, MD, St Thomas' Hospital, London, UK.

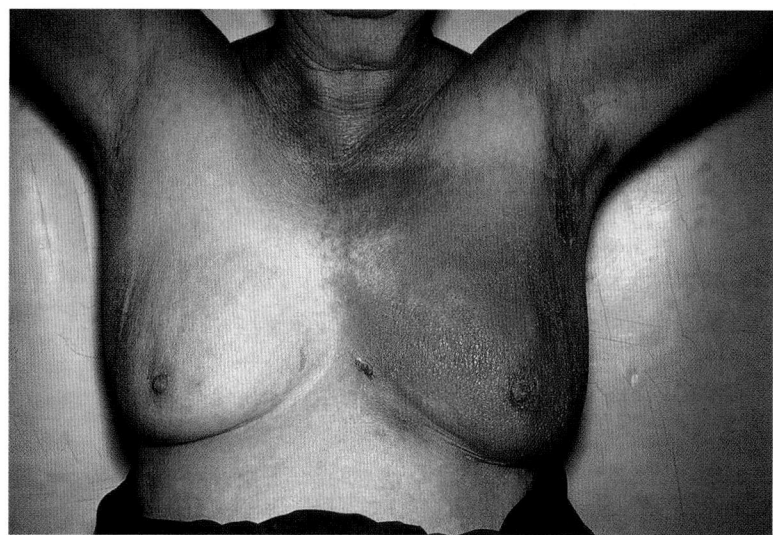

Fig. 21.83
Radiation dermatitis: there is widespread intense erythema and edema. Archival material. By courtesy of A. Timothy, MD, St Thomas' Hospital, London, UK.

a variable interplay of features including redness and swelling, hair loss, blistering (moist desquamation), and sometimes, particularly in severe cases, ulceration (Figs 21.82 and 21.83).[7–9] The disease burden has increased with accelerated radiation fractions currently used to obtain shorter treatment regimens and superior local control in many malignant tumors.[10] At least some degree of significant radiation dermatitis is seen in the great majority of treated patients, depending on the site, and the incidence is accentuated when combined with chemotherapy.[11–14]

As with burns, lesions are graded but into five categories rather than three, depending on the extent of damage. The National Cancer Institute of the United States (NCI) has developed common terminology criteria specifically for adverse events in radiation dermatitis for which modifications have been proposed over the years.[15,16] These are included in the NCI Common Terminology Criteria for Adverse Events (CTCAE), currently in version 4 with version 5 in draft form. The criteria are often used for assessing adverse events in clinical trials. Other systems to assess skin insults rely more on the self-reported subjective experience of patients and may be complementary.[17] The NCI-CTCAE v4.0 grading system for radiation dermatisis is as follows:

- Grade 1: faint erythema or dry desquamation
- Grade 2: moderate to brisk erythema; patchy moist desquamation, mostly confined to skin folds and creases; moderate edema
- Grade 3: moist desquamation in areas other than skin folds and creases; bleeding induced by minor trauma or abrasion
- Grade 4: life-threatening consequences; skin necrosis or ulceration of full thickness dermis; spontaneous bleeding from site; skin graft indicated
- Grade 5: Death

Adapted from Common Terminology Criteria for Adverse Events (CTCAE), Version 4.0, June 2010, National Institutes of Health, National Cancer Institute. Available at: http://evs.nci.nih.gov/ftp1/CTCAE/CTCAE_4.03_2010-06-14_QuickReference_5x7.pdf (accessed 1 January 2018).

More widespread eruptions extending outside of the radiation field have been described and include morbilliform, papular, annular, and bullous lesions, which can show mucous membrane involvement.[18] An erythema multiforme-like dermatosis is an important, albeit rare, complication of radiotherapy, particularly if accompanied by adjuvant chemotherapy.[19,20] Bullous pemphigoid and lichen sclerosus have also been described following radiation.[21,22]

Chronic radiation dermatitis (by convention, developing later than 6 months after radiation therapy) is insidious in onset and usually presents many years after exposure.[3] It used to be a complication of X-ray therapy for various dermatoses, including acne vulgaris and ringworm. The cutaneous manifestations include atrophy and scaling, variable hypo- and hyperpigmentation (poikiloderma), telangiectasia, and often alopecia (Figs 21.84–21.86). Ulceration is sometimes a feature. Morphea has rarely been noted.[23] Chronic radiation dermatitis can be complicated by the development of a variety of neoplasms, including basal cell and squamous cell carcinoma (often of the spindle cell pseudosarcomatous variant), Pinkus tumor, Merkel cell carcinoma, sebaceous carcinoma, and melanoma. Basal cell carcinoma is the most common on facial sites and tends to be multiple.[24,25] Atypical fibroxanthoma and angiosarcoma are well recognized as complications of radiation damage, and cutaneous osteosarcoma has occasionally been encountered. Atypical vascular proliferations can be encountered longer term in irradiated skin and are particularly noted following radiation for breast cancer.[26–30] These are benign, but can be mistaken for angiosarcoma, which is also seen after radiation for breast cancer. In rare cases of atypical vascular proliferations after radiotherapy, there is progression to angiosarcoma.

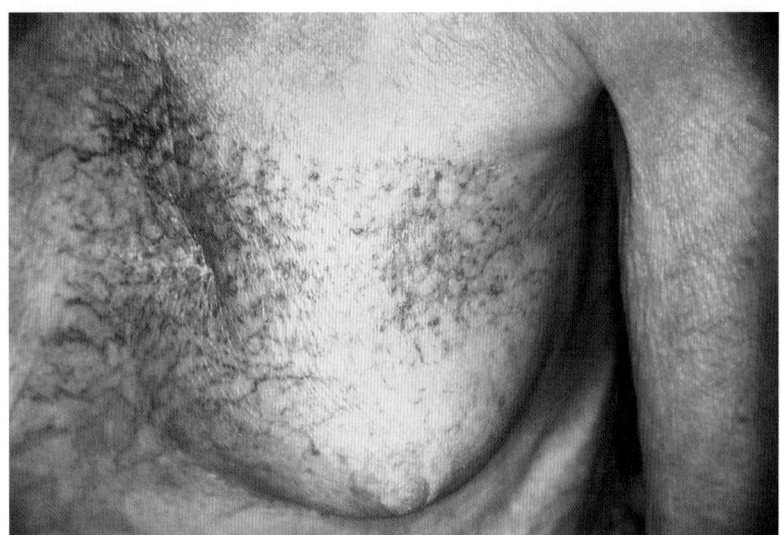

Fig. 21.85
Radiation dermatitis: note the chronic changes of atrophy, hypopigmentation, and telangiectasia–poikiloderma. Archival material. By courtesy of A. Timothy, MD, St Thomas' Hospital, London, UK.

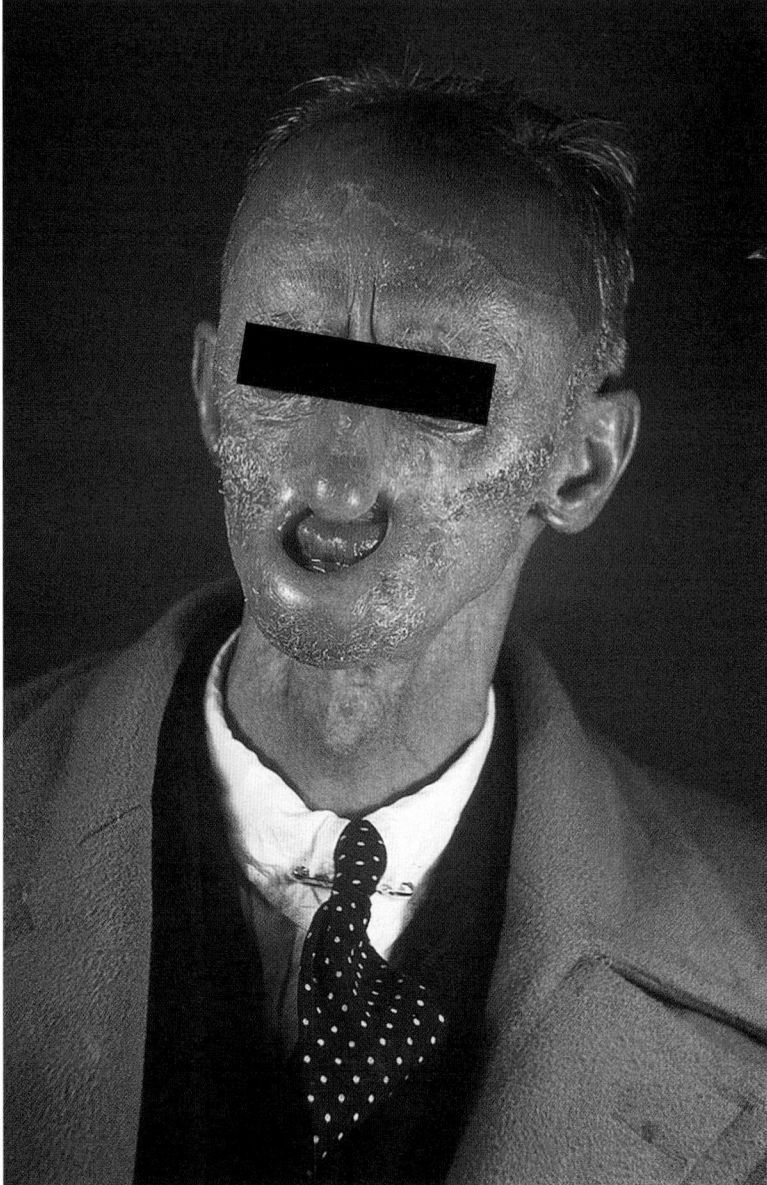

Fig. 21.86
Radiation dermatitis: a patient with radiation damage showing scarring and mutilation. By courtesy of the Institute of Dermatology, London, UK.

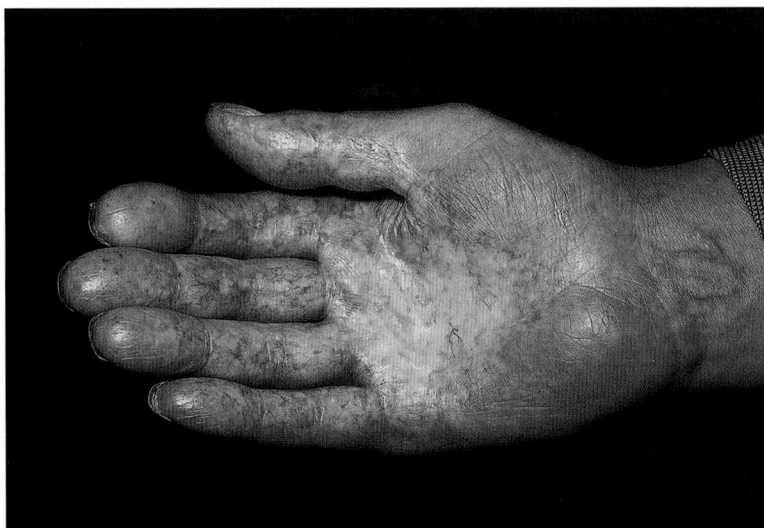

Fig. 21.84
Radiation dermatitis: there are marked pigmentary changes, telangiectasia, atrophy, and scarring. By courtesy of M.M. Black, MD, Institute of Dermatology, London, UK.

The acute clinical effects of cutaneous radiation with UVB include erythema, edema, heat, pain, and pruritus.[31] In more severe cases, vesication may occur.

The risk of developing cutaneous neoplasia (squamous cell carcinoma) following the use of Grenz rays (ultrasoft X-rays) is believed to be negligible.[32] Grenz rays have photon energies between those of conventional X-rays and ultraviolet light. Proton therapy, particularly when delivered as intensity-modulated fractions, could also have less skin effects and post-radiation malignancy.[33,34]

Recently, it has been noted that the combination of systemic epidermal growth factor receptor (EGFR) inhibitors and irradiation used in head and neck and other cancer patients can accentuate the severity of radiation dermatitis.[15,35–37] The majority of the drugs are used in chemotherapy, particularly nonselective cytotoxic agents such as docetaxel or doxorubicin, but targeted inhibitors are also implicated to a lesser degree.[38–40] Radiation recall dermatitis can also be induced by both cytotoxic and target chemotherapeutic agents.[41–51]

There do appear to be genetic determinates of radiation injury to the skin. A variety of polymorphisms in pathway genes involved in inflammation, DNA repair, cell cycle, apoptosis, oxidation, and stress response pathways have been implicated.[52] Such studies provide insights into the mechanism of skin damage and may lead eventually to better risk mitigation and treatments.

Histologic features

The histology of acute radiation damage to the skin is now rarely seen as severe lesions are uncommon and the condition itself is rarely biopsied. The features involve both the epidermis and its adnexae and the underlying dermis.[7] The epithelium may be necrotic and accompanied by both spongiosis and intracellular edema. Hydropic degeneration of the basal layer of the epidermis may be conspicuous, and sometimes subepidermal vesication is a feature. The dermis is edematous and may show fibrin deposition. An inflammatory cell infiltrate consisting of macrophages, eosinophils, plasma cells, and lymphocytes is present in the dermis. In the early stages vascular thrombosis is a feature, but later telangiectasia develops.

In chronic radiation dermatitis, the epidermis is hyperkeratotic and may show foci of parakeratosis. The epithelium is variable, showing either acanthosis or atrophy with attenuation of the ridge pattern (*Figs 21.87* and *21.88*). There may be spongiosis or basal cell liquefactive degeneration. Areas with cytological atypia and dyskeratosis may be evident. Sometimes subepidermal vesication is present. The dermis, which is densely fibrosed

and elastotic, often shows a deep fibrinous exudate. A typical feature of chronic radiation damage is the presence of scattered bizarre (radiation) fibroblasts which, if present in sufficient numbers, may suggest a neoplastic process to the unwary (*Fig. 21.89*).[53] They are characterized by abundant polydendritic basophilic cytoplasm and have large hyperchromatic or vesicular nuclei. These are virtually always scattered as single cells through the dermis and do not appear in clusters or sheets as expected in neoplastic processes. Similar cells may be seen in a variety of conditions including chronic lichen simplex, pressure ulcers, and pleomorphic fibroma.[54]

Blood vessel walls are often thickened, and fibrointimal hyperplasia is characteristic. Alternatively, telangiectatic vessels may be present. Loss of appendages, particularly hair follicles, is commonly seen. On occasions, examination of foci of radiation damage may reveal epidermal dysplasia, or squamous or basal cell carcinoma.

Differential diagnosis

It has been stressed that the response to acute radiation exposure may result in histologic appearances highly suggestive of acute graft-versus-host disease including interface dermatitis with conspicuous satellite cell necrosis.[4] This is obviously of great importance and should be considered in the assessment of all post-bone marrow transplant patients who develop cutaneous lesions. The presence of pleomorphism (particularly in dermal fibroblasts), disorderly

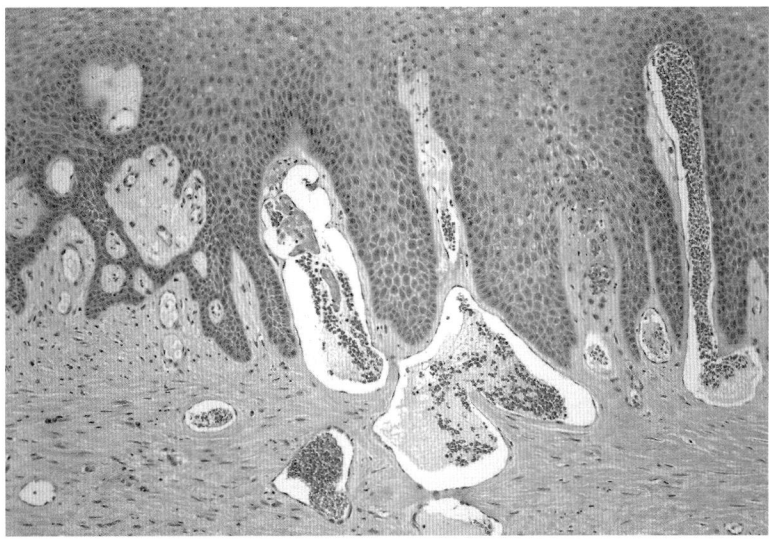

Fig. 21.88
Radiation dermatitis: higher-power view showing the ectatic vessels.

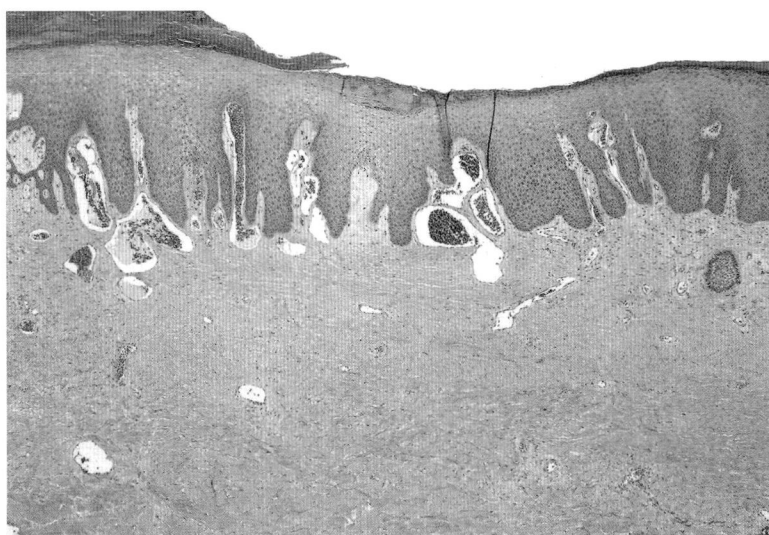

Fig. 21.87
Radiation dermatitis: there is hyperkeratosis, parakeratosis, and epidermal hyperplasia. The dermis is chronically inflamed and hyalinized in its deeper aspect. A small focus of basal cell carcinoma is evident at the edge of the specimen. Note the ectatic vessels.

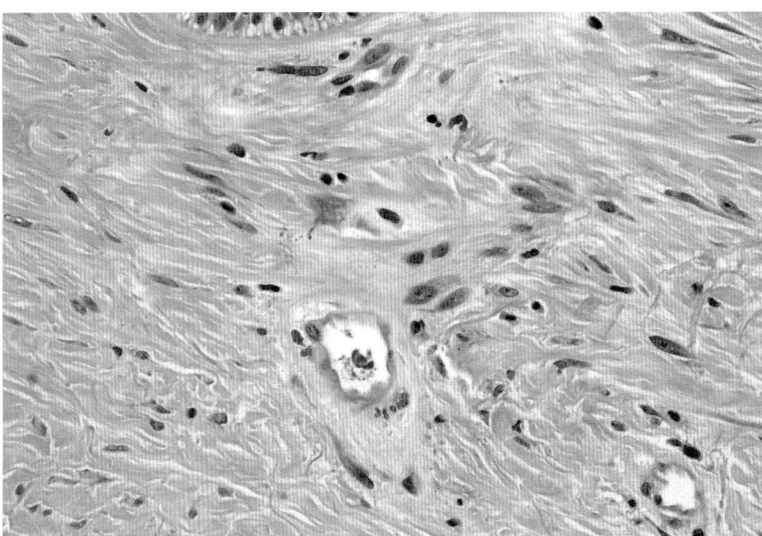

Fig. 21.89
Radiation dermatitis: high-power view highlighting atypical myofibroblasts.

maturation, and mitotic figures are aids to establishing a radiation-related pathogenesis although these features may also represent an adverse drug reaction.[4]

Proteus syndrome

Clinical features

Proteus syndrome was initially described in 1979 and is a rare congenital hamartomatous disease associated with a variable number of abnormalities.[1-9] Cases are usually sporadic. The variation in clinical presentation is probably due to mosaicism. Frequent manifestations include macrocephaly, macrodactyly, asymmetry of the limbs, verrucous epidermal nevi, subcutaneous and deep soft tissue hamartomas, long bone overgrowth, cranial exostoses of the ear canals, nasal bridge and alveolar ridge, and scoliosis.[1-5,9,10] Hypertrophy of the hands and feet often results in a cerebriform appearance. The subcutaneous lesions consist of lipomas, hemangiomas, lymphangiomas, and benign spindle cell tumors with no specific line of differentiation ('fibromas').[11] Additional vascular anomalies include multiple port wine stains and varicose veins.[12-14] Ocular manifestations include strabismus, nystagmus, myopia, epibulbar tumors, blue sclerae, telecanthus, epiblepharon, and retinal pigmentary abnormalities.[15-17] Neurological manifestations are epilepsy, hydrocephalus, and mental retardation.[18,19] An exceptional association with immunodeficiency has been documented.[20] Internal neoplasms are rare; however, papillary carcinoma of the thyroid and mesothelioma have been described.[21,22] Malignancy is usually not associated with Proteus syndrome.[23] Localized variants of this syndrome with involvement restricted to a hand exceptionally occur.[24,25] The term Proteus-like syndrome is reserved for cases that exhibit some features of Proteus syndrome, but do not meet formal diagnostic criteria.[9,23]

Although most of the manifestations are due to overgrowth of tissues, partial lipohypoplasia and patchy dermal hypoplasia have been documented as a frequent finding in the disease.[26-28]

Pathogenesis and histologic features

The exact molecular mechanism of the disease is unknown, but the main hypothesis is of a postzygotic somatic mutation of a gene leading to a mosaic effect.[29,30] In the absence of mosaicism the mutation will be lethal.

The mutated gene may be responsible for control of cell proliferation and/or may influence the mechanism of action of growth factors. In the past, up to 20% of cases of Proteus (and Proteus-like) syndrome have been thought to harbor mutations in the phosphatase and tensin homolog gene (PTEN) on chromosome 10q23.3. PTEN encodes a lipid phosphatase that modulates the phosphoinositol-3-kinase/Akt pathway and influences cell cycle progression and survival.[31,32] Germline mutations in PTEN have also been frequently found in Cowden syndrome, Bannayan-Riley-Ruvalcaba syndrome, and Proteus-like syndrome, defining a spectrum of PTEN hamartoma tumor syndromes.[23,28,31-34] The location and type of PTEN gene mutation can influence the spectrum of disease manifestation.[35] However, more recent research calls this association with PTEN mutation into doubt, as multiple landmark papers using strictly defined Proteus syndrome cases show mosaic activating mutations in AKT1 and much less commonly, PIK3CA rather than PTEN.[9,36-39] Rather than mosaic loss of the PTEN tumor suppressor, this disease is caused by mosaic mutations in two proto-oncogenes in the same pathway; physiologically PTEN dephosphorylates the signaling lipid produces by PIK3CA and prevents AKT activation.[37] Mosaic activating mutations in PIK3CA are also associated with the related spectrum such as CLOVE (congenital lipomatous overgrowth, vascular malformations, and epidermal nevi) syndrome or fibroadipose hyperplasia or overgrowth (FAO) syndrome designated as within the PIK3CA-related overgrowth spectrum (PROS).[40-42] Proteus syndrome is probably better considered in this PROS group rather than the upstream (though still related) PTEN hamartoma tumor syndrome group.[37]

Histopathology of the verrucous epidermal nevi, lipomas, port wine stains, and vascular malformations is identical to that seen in the same lesions in patients without Proteus syndrome.[27] Some of the soft tissue tumors are composed of a proliferation of bland spindle-shaped fibroblast-like cells that are CD34 positive.

Molecular testing can be helpful in sorting out these related syndromes, but expert clinical correlation is needed as the syndromes overlap and can have mutations in the same genes.[37] Broad exome characterization by next-generation sequencing will hopefully increase our understanding of the causative genetics of Proteus and related syndromes which are still incompletely understood.

Access **ExpertConsult.com** for the complete list of references

See
www.expertconsult.com
for references and
additional material

Diseases of the hair

CHAPTER

22

Rodrigo Restrepo and Eduardo Calonje

Introduction

A distinctive phenomenon of the human evolutionary process is the loss of a great proportion of the body hair. Vestiges of hair remain in areas such as the scalp, axillae, genital areas, and face. Among the many species of primates, only humans are almost hairless. The time and cause of this remarkable transformation remains an enigma.[1,2] Whatever the explanation for the loss of hair in the evolutionary process may be, the truth is that the protective function of the hair layer has been lost in great part.

Paradoxically, the little hair that still remains has acquired an unmeasurable importance in the realm of social interaction. Alterations in the quantity or the quality of hair often have great impact on the behavior and well-being of the individual.[3,4]

The study of hair pathology has always been challenging due to the anatomical and functional complexity of the hair follicle. It consists of two major compartments: epithelial and dermal, each of which interacts both jointly and independently in a cyclical manner, under the control of a complex network of growth factors, cytokines, and hormones.[5] Analysis and study of the hair follicle growth cycle is extremely informative, because it represents a miniature model for studying the complex physiological mechanisms controlling cell proliferation and growth. The hair follicle is capable of sustaining a permanent cycle of growth and degeneration due to the presence of adult stem cells that are maintained throughout our life span.[6,7] The hair follicle acts as an immunoprivileged site proliferating in a cyclical manner during anagen and regressing in catagen.[8]

Hair analysis can provide important information in forensic medicine through the study of nuclear and mitochondrial DNA.[9] The analysis of the hair is also useful in tracing various poisons such as arsenic, mercury, and trace element poisoning.[10,11] In the same way, analysis of hair follicles is a valuable tool in the diagnosis of many congenital diseases, metabolic disorders, and malformations.[12]

In this chapter, emphasis is given to histologic diagnosis of diseases of the hair follicles by evaluation of horizontal and vertical sections.

Diagnosis, history and laboratory tests

The majority of dermatopathologists perceive that the diagnosis and evaluation of patients presenting with hair disease is a difficult and tedious task, apparently lacking meaning. The latter occurs because they frequently forget that, as in the case of other dermatological disorders, an exhaustive clinical history and complete physical examination are essential to reach an accurate diagnosis. Equally important is the need to carefully determine the number of biopsies and sites from which these samples are to be taken. The pathologist not only needs to have an in-depth knowledge of the complex tridimensional anatomy, physiology, and pathology of the hair follicle but also has to be able to determine the type of sections needed – vertical, horizontal, or both.

History and physical examination

Family history is often of great importance, mostly concerning the type of hair loss present in first-degree family relatives, if any, age of onset, hirsutism, menopause, and menstrual and pregnancy history, particularly in patients with androgenetic alopecia. Likewise, it is a must to ask about history of major illnesses or other types of stress, autoimmune disease, thyroid abnormalities, past and current medications, and dietary history in patients with telogen effluvium. It is also critical to evaluate the grooming habits of the patient, especially with regard to use of hair cosmetics and chemical products (bleaching, permanent waving). The latter may cause considerable damage to the hair and lead to different types of hair loss, for example, tight braiding can result in traction alopecia.[1,2]

Physical examination provides important information about the pattern of hair loss and whether it is nonscarring and potentially reversible (visible follicular openings) or scarring and irreversible (no visible follicular openings). Whether the hair loss is due to increased shedding or increased thinning, this must be adequately investigated. Hair loss can be patterned as in androgenetic alopecia, diffuse and uniform as in telogen effluvium, or patchy with surrounding normal scalp as is typical of alopecia areata. The presence or absence of active inflammation, erythema, drainage, or scaling provides important clues about the nature of the process and extent of the damage.[3]

Laboratory tests

When evaluating a patient with hair disease, the approach to the investigation should concentrate on a very detailed history and a thorough clinical examination.

A suspected infectious etiology usually requires microbiological studies including direct examination and culture. If bacteria are suspected, a Gram stain may be performed, but usually a culture is more rewarding. In the case of a suspected fungal infection, examination of a hair sample with potassium hydroxide and culture are important. Serology is often necessary if syphilis is considered in the differential diagnosis.

Metabolic studies are sometimes essential to the investigation of hair loss. Thyroid function tests, for example, are often valuable in patients with telogen effluvium. Decreased ferritin and serum iron levels may be found in females with telogen effluvium and other types of alopecia. Hyperandrogenism is also sometimes responsible for hair loss in women.[4] In alopecia related to autoimmune disease, particularly lupus erythematosus, investigations should include screening for autoantibodies. Direct immunofluorescence may also be rewarding in patients with scarring alopecia, particularly lupus erythematosus and lichen planus.

Other diagnostic procedures frequently performed in the evaluation of hair diseases are the hair pluck (trichogram), the hair pull, daily hair shedding count, hair window, hair shaft microscopy, trichoscan, dermoscopy, and a scalp biopsy.

Hair-pluck test (trichogram)

The hair-pluck test is useful to evaluate the ratio of telogen to anagen hairs. With an adequate technique, approximately 50 hairs are forcibly plucked from the scalp with a clamp or needle holder. An increment of the hairs in telogen suggests telogen effluvium.[5]

Hair-pull test

The hair-pull test is an easy and rapid technique which allows an accurate estimate of the amount of hair loss that the patient is experiencing. The patient must not wash his/her hair in the preceding 24 hours before the pull test. The physician grabs 20–30 hairs between the fingers and gently pulls them. Normally, with gentle traction, no more than 10%, or two to three hairs shafts, are obtained, and these by definition are in telogen. When more than three hair shafts are obtained from each pull, this is usually indicative of hair disease (telogen effluvium).[6] Normally, follicles in anagen are not

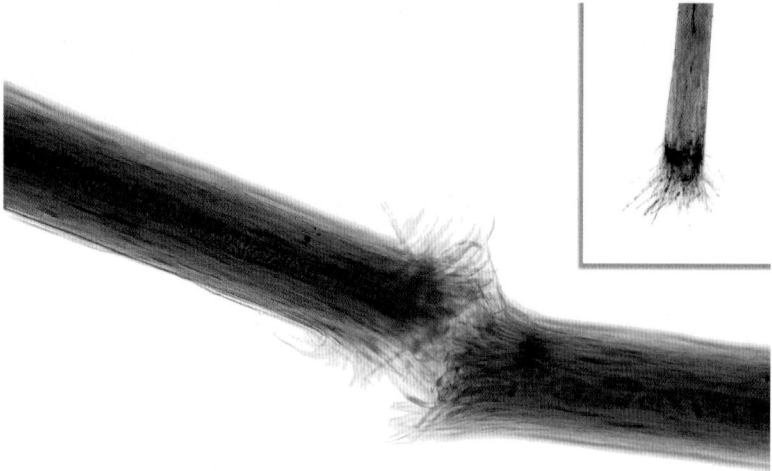

Fig. 22.1
Hair shaft sample. Trichorrhexis nodosa. The sample must not be taken using pull traction but rather by cutting it proximally. Otherwise, the sample will only show the distal end as shown in the upper right-hand corner. Courtesy of J.C. Garcés, MD, Hospital Luis Vernaza, Guayaquil, Ecuador.

obtained, except in children, because the attachment to the scalp is more loose.[7]

Daily hair shedding count

Patients are asked to collect all the hair they shed in the shower or sink, and to brush their hair and collect the hair daily for 7 days. Commonly, between 50 and 100 telogen hairs per day are lost in a normal individual.[8]

Hair window

The hair-growth window technique is used in the diagnosis of trichotillomania (described under trichotillomania).

Microscopic examination

The purpose of the microscopic examination of the hair is to carefully examine the shaft or the bulb for abnormalities. Hairs that have been obtained using the hair-pull test or trichogram may be used as samples for this test.

Hair shaft examination. To establish the correct diagnosis in cases of suspected hair shaft disease, the hair samples must be obtained from involved and uninvolved areas. This should be done preferably by gentle traction or by cutting the hair shaft proximally. It is crucial to avoid trauma to the hair shaft. Frequently, when trying to pull the hair shaft out, it breaks at the weakest point, which is generally the area of the defect (*Fig. 22.1*). This leads to loss or distortion of the abnormal area and the diagnosis is often missed [9,10].

The hair samples obtained should be placed on a glass slide and fixed to the surface with transparent adhesive tape.[11,12] As an alternative, the hairs can also be mounted as for routine microscopic sections with a coverslip. This method is excellent for obtaining photomicrographs, although air may obscure some details of the cuticle (*Fig. 22.2*). The slide preparation must be done with great care, without exerting undue pressure, to avoid artifact.[13]

It is important to examine both the proximal and distal ends of the hair shaft because the more specific changes are usually found in the proximal segment. Polarized light microscopy must be used in cases of children with alopecia characterized by short and fragile hairs (*Fig. 22.3*). This technique is particularly crucial in the differential diagnosis of trichothiodystrophy (TTD), as it shows the hair shafts with alternating light and dark transverse bands (tiger tail pattern). In loose anagen hair syndrome, special stains such as toluidine blue or elastic van Gieson must be performed to adequately visualize the internal root sheath.[14]

Additional examination with scanning electron microscopy allows a good evaluation of all the components of the hair shaft including the cuticle and cortex. With this method, tridimensional images may be obtained.

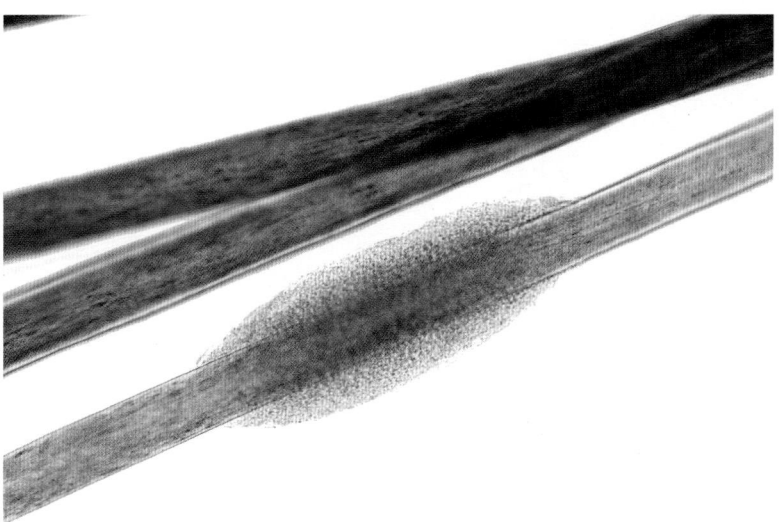

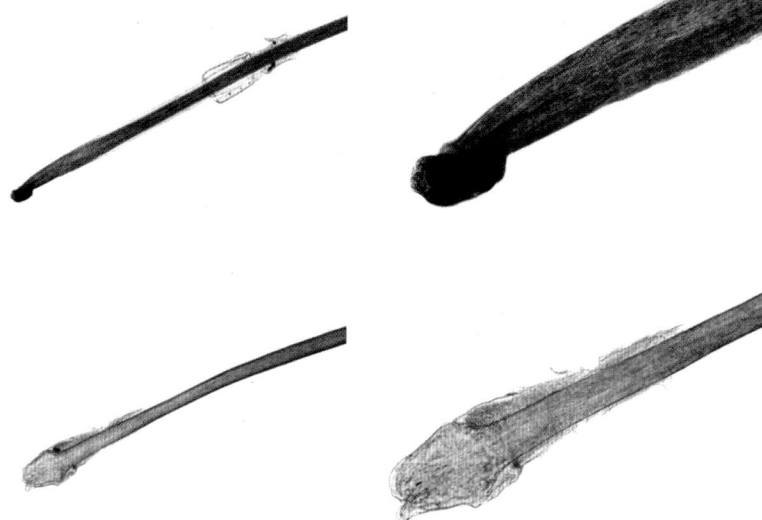

Fig. 22.2
Hair shaft examination. A better result is obtained if the hair shaft is examined by using a mounting medium and a coverslip rather than using transparent tape. An example of white stone in which the arthroconidia nodule and its relation to the hair shaft surface is clearly observed.

Fig. 22.4
Anagen and telogen hair shafts obtained by traction. Note differences in shape and pigmentation between the anagen hair (*top*) and the telogen club hair (*bottom*).

studies to compare the different efficiency of various hair growth-promoting substances.[15]

Dermoscopy

Dermoscopy is a technique that has recently been successful in the study of hair diseases. With the use of a dermatoscope, this noninvasive method enables identification of useful diagnostic structures for the majority of hair diseases of the scalp and identifies the best sites for a biopsy (*Table 22.1*).[16-18]

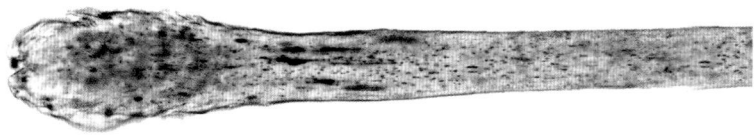

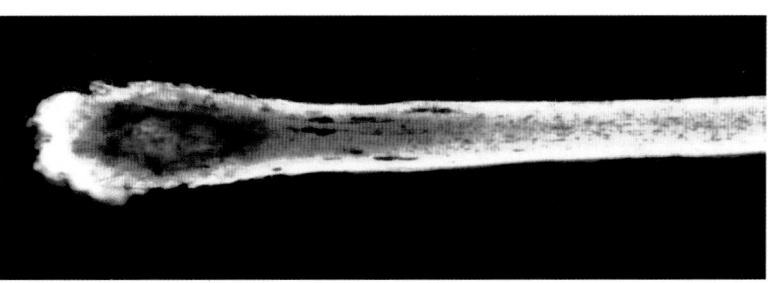

Fig. 22.3
Polarized light microscopy. Normal architecture of the hair shaft and the bulb in telogen is observed with normal light (*above*) and polarized light (*below*).

The hair shafts can be examined for irregularities, hair breakage, or extraneous matter. The hairs can also be examined under 20% potassium hydroxide and cultured in Sabouraud agar to rule out a fungal infection.

The hair tips should be examined to see whether they are tapered or broken. The distal segment is more prone to secondary changes due to wear and tear or secondary to hair shaft anomalies.

Hair bulb examination. The hair bulbs present the following characteristics:

- anagen bulb: pigment in bulb, dark keratogenous zone, medulla, inner root sheath, and outer root sheath,
- telogen bulb: club-shaped, without hair shaft pigment, keratogenous zone, inner or outer root sheath (*Fig. 22.4*),
- the rare hairs in catagen observed are vaguely similar to hairs in telogen with a sac of keratin and a short tail of clear semitransparent tissue.

Trichoscan

The trichoscan may be considered as a noninvasive modification of the trichogram which combines epiluminescence microscopy with automatic digital image analysis for the measurement of human hair. It can be used in clinical

Scalp biopsy and biopsy report

Scalp biopsy is a very valuable tool in the diagnosis of hair loss. Ideally, two deep punch biopsies 4 mm in diameter should be obtained for comparison from different sites: one should be taken from the affected area and the second from the periphery where there is healthy scalp. An alternative is to take the two biopsies from different involved areas (e.g., in cases of scarring alopecia). Sometimes a single biopsy is enough to make an accurate diagnosis, but this depends on the level of experience of the clinician and the pathologist. It is highly recommended to verify that the internal diameter of the punch which is to be used really measures 4 mm (12.6 mm²), as this measure varies from one company to another.[1] The biopsy is taken following the direction of the hair follicles with the intention of minimizing tangential sections. It should include epidermis, dermis, and a very generous amount of subcutaneous tissue. The obtained specimen must be delicately handled, avoiding any crushing by the forceps, and quickly placed in 10% neutral buffered formaldehyde.

The sections can be vertical, transversal (horizontal), or both, depending on the experience of the laboratory with one or the other particular section, with the type of alopecia being studied, and the number of biopsies taken.

For the transverse sections, the sample should be divided 2 mm away from the epidermis and serial sections obtained from both parts toward the surface and the deep layers of the specimen. In this way, the sections obtained from the upper portion will sequentially approach the surface epithelium and those derived from the lower portion will sequentially approach the deep dermis and subcutaneous fat (*Fig. 22.5*). Afterwards, the basic stainings are performed with hematoxylin and eosin and electively with toluidine blue, periodic acid-Schiff (PAS), Masson trichrome, and elastic tissue stain. The best sections to evaluate terminal anagen hair follicles/vellus hair and hair follicles in anagen, catagen, and telogen are those obtained at the limit between the upper and lower segment of the hair follicle (at level of the bulge).

Table 22.1
Key trichoscopic findings of Non-Scarrin and Scarring Alopecias*

Non-Scarring Alopecia	Trichoscopic characteristics[1-4]
Androgenetic alopecia	Hair shaft thickness heterogeneity more than 20 % Yellow dots Perifollicular brown discoloration or halo (peripilar sign) Increased proportion of vellus hairs Follicular units with only 1 emerging hair shaft
Telogen effluvium	Diagnosis of exclusion, limited diagnostic value Multiple short upright regrowing hairs Follicular units empty or with only 1 emerging hair shaft
Alopecia areata	Yellow dots and black dots Exclamation mark hairs, broken hairs, vellus hairs Active disease: black dots, exclamation mark hairs, broken hairs Disease severity and inactive disease: yellow dots, vellus hairs
Tinea capitis	Corkscrew hairs, comma hairs Black dots with scaling
Trichotillomania	Multiple hair shaft abnormalities with no significant changes in the perifollicular area Hairs broken at different lengths, short hairs with trichoptilosis, coiled hairs, exclamation mark hairs Black dots
Congenital triangular alopecia	Normal follicular openings with vellus hairs surrounded by normal terminal hair
Scarring alopecia	**Trichoscopic characteristics[1-3]**
General findings in scarring alopecia	Lack of black dots and yellow dots Milky red areas
Lichen planopilaris	Tubular perifollicular scaling Blue-grey dots with a target distribution Active disease: elongated linear blood vessels in concentric arrangement and violaceous inter or perifollicular violaceous areas Inactive end stage-disease: small, irregularly shaped, whitish areas lacking follicular openings
Frontal fibrosing alopecia	Lonely hairs, surrounded by areas of fibrosis Lack of follicular openings Perifollicular erythema and minor perifollicular scaling
Discoid lupus erythematosus	Large yellow-brownish dots Long-lasting disease: arborizing vessels Good prognostic factor: follicular red dots
Folliculitis decalvans	Hair tufts that contain 5 to 20 hair shafts Yellowish tubular perifollicular scaling Follicular pustules
Dissecting cellulitis	Early disease: empty follicular openings, black dots, yellow dots Advancing disease: yellow structureless areas and yellow dots with 3-dimensional structure imposed over dystrophic hair shafts End-stage fibrotic lesions: confluent ivory-white areas

1. Mubki T, Rudnicka L, Olszewska M, Shapiro J.Evaluation and diagnosis of the hair loss patient: part II. Trichoscopic and laboratory evaluations.J Am Acad Dermatol. 2014;71(3):431.e1-431.e11.
2. Jain N, Doshi B, Khopkar U. Trichoscopy in alopecias: diagnosis simplified.Int J Trichology. 2013;5(4):170-8.
3. Tosti A, Torres F.Dermoscopy in the diagnosis of hair and scalp disorders.Actas Dermosifiliogr. 2009;100 Suppl 1:114-9.
4. Ferrándiz L, Moreno D, Peral F, Camacho FM. Tricoscopia. Piel. 2011;26(7):323-29

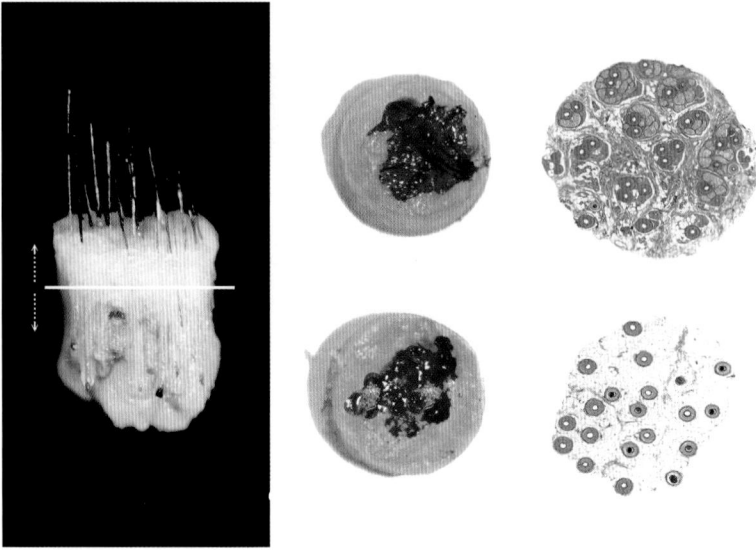

Fig. 22.5
Sections of a normal scalp biopsy: horizontal sections are cut through the middle of the punch biopsy specimen. Each half is stained with red ink to help with the orientation. The upper half progressively displays the more superficial structures while the deeper structures are displayed in the lower half. On the right note, the microscopic sections stained with hematoxylin and eosin. The top section is at the level of the isthmus and the bottom section is at the level of the subcutaneous fat. The hair follicles are of uniform size.

Although transverse sections of scalp skin have been studied for more than 100 years, it was not until 1984 that Headington carried out the first systematic studies of scalp biopsies using serial sections.[2,3] This method represented a significant advance in the diagnosis and understanding of diseases of the hair. The Headington technique demonstrated that transverse sections of biopsies obtained with a 4-mm punch provided excellent histologic material for morphometric and quantitative analysis, including the different phases of the normal hair growth cycle.[4,5] This technique has been modified over the years, and multiple horizontal sections throughout the sample are evaluated, enabling the pathologists to correctly evaluate most types of alopecia including chronic telogen effluvium, male androgenetic alopecia, alopecia areata, and the various types of scarring alopecia, and to perform digital image studies in cases of nonscarring alopecias.[6-13] It is also a very useful method to evaluate the effects on the hairs after the administration of a given drug.[14]

The biggest advantage of this type of technique is that all the hair follicles present in the biopsy may be counted and examined at different levels. An accurate count of all the hair follicles present in a specimen may be done by conventional microscopy or by computer-assisted techniques. Its principal limitation is the little representation of the dermal–epidermal junction (Fig. 22.6).

Vertical sections were exclusively used for many years and they provide a panoramic view from the epidermis to the hypodermis, more familiar to the general pathologist and to the dermatopathologist. These allow clear differentiation of all compartments of the skin, especially the dermal–epidermal junction and superficial dermis. This is particularly useful in the diagnosis of scarring alopecias which involve the epidermis and the interface such as discoid lupus erythematosus, folliculitis decalvans, and psoriasis (Fig. 22.7). However, only very few hair follicles are visualized with vertical sections (at best 10–15% of the total in a single section), and often these are sectioned transversely or obliquely (Fig. 22.8).[3] It is not an adequate technique for quantitative studies or for establishing the ratios between the different phases of the hair follicles (anagen/telogen ratio, terminal/vellus hair ratio), hence its use is very limited in the diagnosis of androgenic-type alopecias and those of chronic telogen effluvium. It is universally accepted that both techniques present obvious advantages and disadvantages, and if two biopsies are available the best option is to use one for the transverse sections and the other for the vertical sections (Fig. 22.9), hence using the second half

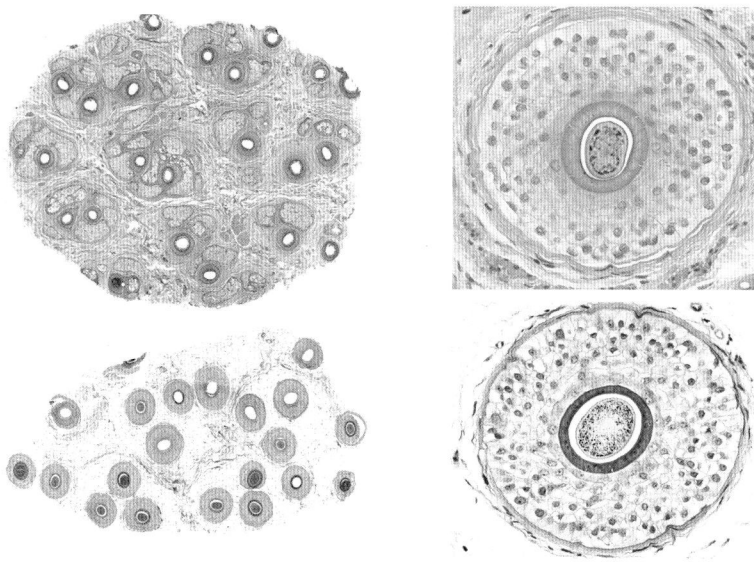

Fig. 22.6
Normal hair biopsy: horizontal section. On the left, all the hair follicles are visible at scanning magnification. On the right, all components of the hair follicle are seen in horizontal sections stained with H&E and toluidine blue.

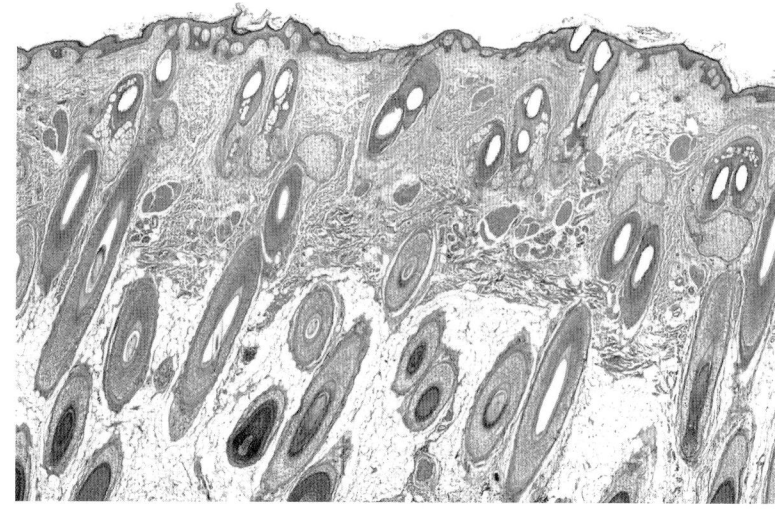

Fig. 22.8
Scalp biopsy: in this vertical section, no whole hair follicles are seen. Since they are all incomplete, additional sections are required to obtain an acceptable three-dimensional reconstruction.

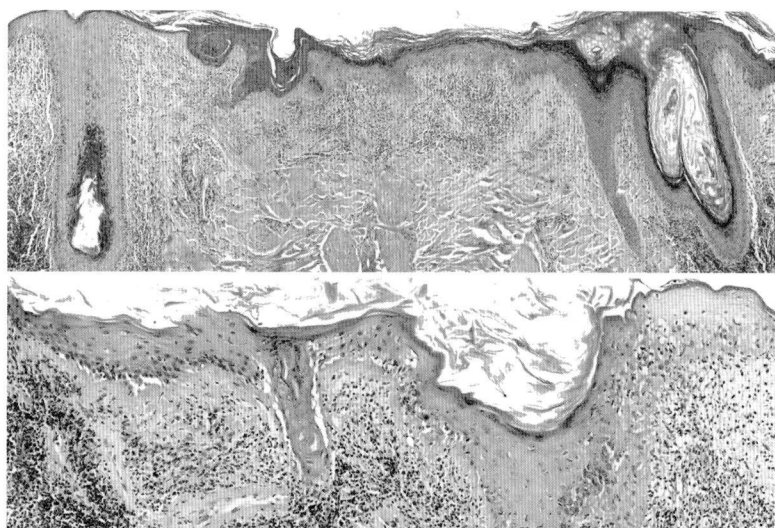

Fig. 22.7
Scalp biopsy, vertical section. Discoid lupus erythematosus: the section follows the plane of the hair follicles. The thickened basement membrane at the dermal–epidermal junction is clearly seen, as well as the distribution of the inflammatory cell infiltrate.

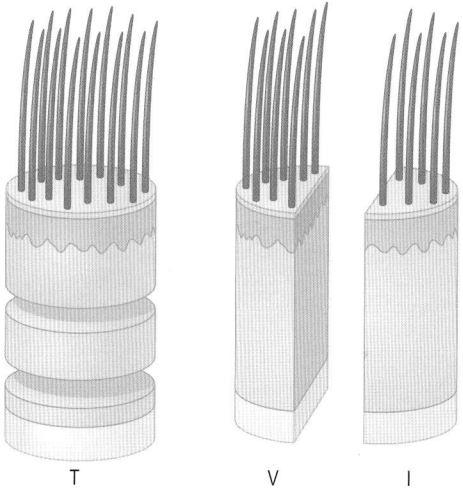

Fig. 22.9
Hair biopsy, transversal (T) and vertical (V) sections: ideally, two biopsies should be obtained. One of them is sectioned horizontally at different levels and the second can be vertically divided in two halves, one for routine histology and the other for immunofluorescence (I), electron microscopy, cultures and other techniques. Vertical sections are useful in cases that do not require comparison or follicle quantification; for example, in scarring alopecias. This type of sections must not be used in nonscarring alopecias, electron microscopy, cultures and other techniques. Vertical sections are useful in cases that do not require comparison or follicle quantification; for example, in scarring alopecias. This type of sections must not be used in nonscarring alopecias.

of the latter one for complementary studies (cultures, immunofluorescence, electron microscopy).[15-17]

There are other known methods to interpret scalp biopsies such as the HoVert (horizontal and vertical) and Tyler techniques.[18,19] In the former, the specimen is sectioned horizontally at a distance of 1 mm from the epidermal surface. The lower half is processed using horizontal sections and the upper part containing the epidermis is processed using vertical sections. In the Tyler technique, the specimen is divided vertically into two halves. One half is used for vertical sections and the other half for horizontal sections.

Regardless of the type of sections being chosen, it is important to remember that to reach a reliable histopathological diagnosis, it is of the utmost importance to carefully select and plan the site of the biopsy. Likewise, it is important to bear in mind that as the alopecia becomes more chronic, particularly in the scarring type, the findings in the biopsy will become less specific.

Hair biopsy report

It is crucial that all quantifiable data are included in the histology report. This often allows for an accurate diagnosis when the pathological findings are correlated with the clinical information (Box 22.1).

Even though the microscopic features, chemical composition, and molecular structure are very similar in different ethnic groups, significant differences in conformation, mechanical properties, and capacity to absorb water according to ethnic origin have been described.[20-22] Especially important are the striking differences in hair density and relative proportion of hair follicles in anagen/telogen and terminal/vellus hairs in blacks, Asians, and Caucasians, which should be always taken into consideration when interpreting scalp biopsies (Table 22.2).[23-28]

Embryology and anatomy of the normal hair follicle

Embryology

Embryologically, each follicle is composed of epithelial and mesenchymal components. Epithelial invaginations (placodes) derive from the fetal epidermis and project downward at regularly spaced intervals, proliferating under the influence of the underlying connective tissue cells which form the mesenchymal condensation of the hair peg. This occurs around the 10th week of gestation (*Fig. 22.10*). This dermal condensate will eventually mature into the dermal papilla. The hair follicle does not develop in the absence of this mesenchymal influence. Afterwards, the hair follicle elongates into a lace of epithelial cells and the deeper component forms the bulbous and the matrix cells, which give origin to the hair shaft and inner root sheath. The outer root sheath forms three bulges. The upper one will give origin, in the follicles located in the anogenital region, axillae, areolae, periumbilical region, eyelids, and external ear canals, to the apocrine glands. The middle bulge will give origin to the sebaceous gland. The lowermost bulge corresponds to the location of the epithelial stem cells. This is also the attachment site of the arrector pili muscle.[1]

The first follicles develop in the scalp, and from there they extend downwards to populate the rest of the body. Initially, they are observed as fine thin nonpigmented hairs, known as lanugo hair. These fall off at the end of the gestation period, although some remain until after birth. The majority are replaced by terminal hairs, present in the scalp, eyelashes, and eyebrows of the newborn and vellus hairs on the rest of the body. No new hair follicles form after birth. At puberty the vellus hairs present on genital skin and axilla in females and on the legs, torso, and the chin in males transform into terminal hairs under the influence of sexual hormones. Paradoxically, in individuals with androgenic alopecia the terminal hairs in the scalp transform into miniaturized hair follicles in those individuals who are susceptible. Hair follicles will eventually be found on all body surfaces except for the palms, soles, and mucous membranes.

The genes and molecules that participate in the development of the hair follicle have been extensively studied. Different positive and negative regulators which are expressed at variable time during the development of hair follicles have been identified.[2,3] Some of the most relevant of these regulators are described in *Table 22.3*.

Box 22.1

Hair biopsy report: basic information to be evaluated and included in a histology report of a 4.0 mm punch biopsy.

Total number of hair follicles in the biopsy (terminal + vellus, in anagen, catagen, and telogen)
Total number of hair follicles per square millimeter (total/12.6)
Number of terminal hair follicles
Number of vellus hairs (vellus + miniaturized hairs)
Number of undetermined follicles
Terminal:vellus hair ratio (T:V): terminal hair follicles / vellus
Number of terminal hair follicles in anagen
Number of terminal hair follicles in telogen
Number of terminal hair follicles in catagen
Telogen count: terminal telogen hairs (telogen + catagen) / terminal hair follicles.
Presence, type and localization of inflammatory cell infiltrate
Presence or absence of scar tissue
Presence or absence of pigmented casts

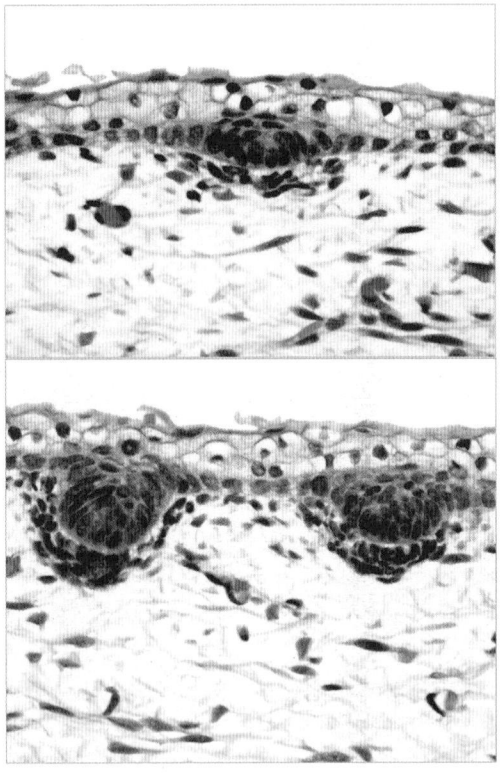

Fig. 22.10
Fetal hair follicle, upper and lower panel: epidermal precursor and primary hair germ with underlying connective tissue cells (dermal condensate).

Table 22.2

Comparison of Hair Density of Taiwanese, Koreans, Iranians, American Caucasians, and African Americans*

Characteristic	Asia			America		
Race	Taiwanese, *n* = 31	Korean, *n* = 35	Iranian, *n* = 30	Caucasian, *n* = 22	African American, *n* = 22	
Author	*Present study*	*Lee et al[6]*	*Aslani[8]*	*Whiting[2]*	*Sperling[3]*	p-*Value**
Age, mean ± SD	37.0 ± 15.3	33.1 ± 10.0	35.5 ± 14.7	43 ± 3.5	31.7 ± 8.5	.04
Number of terminal hairs, mean ± SD	20.5 ± 4.6	14.9 ± 3.2	34 ± 6.4	35 ± 2.1	18.4 ± 5.0	<.001
Number of vellus hairs, mean ± SD	0.8 ± 1.0	1.1 ± 1.3	2.4 ± 1.2	5 ± 0.6	3.0 ± 2.1	<.001
Number of total hairs, mean ± SD	21.3 ± 4.8	16.1 ± 3.6	36.3 ± 7.2	40 ± 2.2	21.5 ± 5.0	<.001
Number of follicular units, mean ± SD	9.4 ± 1.9	7.8 ± 1.7	ND	14 ± 0.5	ND	<.001
Anagen: telogen ratio,%	91.6:8.4	93.6:6.4	93.7:6.3	93.5:6.5	93.9:6.1	.47
Terminal: vellus ratio	25.3:1	13.5:1	17.4:1	7:1	6.1:1	<.001
Density of hair follicles/mm²	1.69 ± 0.4	1.2 ± 0.3	2.89 ± 0.6	3.1 ± 0.8	1.65 ± 0.4	<.001
Density of follicular units/mm²	0.75 ± 0.2	0.62 ± 0.1	ND	1.11 ± 0.04	ND	<.001

*Analysis of variance.
SD, standard deviation; ND, no data.
*Ko J.H., Huang Y.H., Kuo T.T. Hair counts from normal scalp biopsy in Taiwan. Dermatol Surg. 2012. 38, Sep;1516-20.

Table 22.3

Summary of the best defined molecular regulators of hair follicle morphogenesis.

Hair Follicle Morphogenesis Step	Gene Product
Outer root sheath	Sox9, Shh/Smo
Inner root sheath	*GATA3*, *Cut1 (CDP)*, BMPs/BMPR1a, Shh/ Smo, Notch1/Jagged/ Delta/RBP-Jk for IRS fate maintenance
Hair shaft	B-catenin, Wnt's and Lef-1, VDR (Vitamin D receptor)(only in postnatal hair cycle), BMPs/ BMPR1a, Shh/Smo, *msx1 and 2*, *FoxN1/Nude*, *HoxC13*, Notch1/Jagged/Delta/RBP-Jk (only in postnatal hair cycle)
Polarity, shaping and bending	Shh (asymmetric, polarized expression pattern in hair matrix), Igfbp5, Eda A1, *Krox-20*, *FoxE1*, *Runx3*, *Sox18*
Innervation	B-catenin, NCAM
Pigmentation	*FoxN1/Nude*, SCF/c-kit, Notch
Bulge region/hair stem cell maintenance	BMPs/BMPR1a, *Lhx2*, *Sox9*, *NFATc1*, *p63*, *Tcf3* (w/o Wnt activity), Rac1, integrins a3b1 and a6b4

Note: Transcription factors in Italics
Modified from Schneider MR, Schmidt-Ullrich R, Paus R. The hair follicle as a dynamic miniorgan. Curr Biol. 19, 2009;R132-42.

Anatomy

To correctly evaluate a scalp biopsy, it is important for the pathologist to be well versed not only in the histology of the different types of alopecias but also in the complex and changing anatomy of the healthy hair follicle and its features in both vertical and horizontal sections. There are important morphological variations related to the normal follicular cycle and to the miniaturization of the terminal follicles in susceptible individuals. In the following section, these aspects will be individually reviewed.

Horizontal sections of the upper segment of the hair follicle show that hair follicles in the scalp are grouped, forming anatomic structures known as follicular units, which are composed of terminal and vellus hairs, sebaceous glands, and arrector pili muscles. The distribution of hair follicles in follicular units is better appreciated at the level of the infundibulum and isthmus. The connective tissue surrounding the outer root sheath tends to condense around discrete units comprising three to six hair follicles, one or two of which represent vellus hairs (*Fig. 22.11* and also see *Fig. 22.6*).

Terminal hair follicles are easy to recognize in horizontal sections because they are much larger than vellus hairs (*Fig. 22.12*). These follicles are thick, pigmented, and usually descend to the subcutaneous fat (see *Fig. 22.8*). They contain a hair shaft, the diameter of which is greater than the thickness of the inner root sheath, and generally measures in excess of 0.06 mm (*Fig. 22.13* and also see *Fig. 22.6*).

True vellus hairs are thin, short, and nonpigmented, and are characterized by a hair bulb that only extends to the upper or mid-reticular dermis (*Fig. 22.14*). The arrector pili muscle is usually undetected. The hair shaft diameter is equal to or less than the thickness of the inner root sheath (*Fig. 22.15*). It is typically less than 0.03 mm.

Vellus-like hairs (miniaturized hairs) are very similar to vellus hairs. They correspond to terminal hair follicles that have miniaturized owing to the effect of androgens. They may be very difficult to differentiate from true vellus hairs, except for the fact that the miniaturized follicles leave a trail of stellate collapsed fibrous tissue, the follicular stellae. In a scalp biopsy, when reference is made to vellus hairs without qualifying its origin, it refers by convention to both miniaturized and to true vellus hairs.

Indeterminate hairs have an intermediate morphology between that of terminal and vellus hairs and are considered an intermediate step in the process of miniaturization. The diameter of an indeterminate hair shaft is between 0.03 and 0.06 mm. There is no clear consensus as to which group

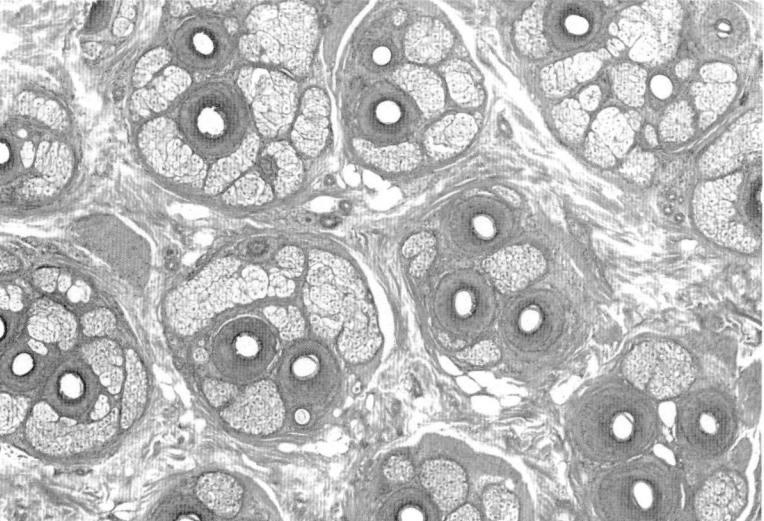

Fig. 22.11
Hair biopsy, horizontal section: the follicular units are clearly delineated by condensation of the adventitial collagen (Masson trichrome stain).

of hair follicles do indeterminate follicles belong to. We concur with the suggestion of some authors who recommend assigning half of these hairs to terminal hair follicles and the other half to vellus hairs.[4]

The hair shaft and the inner root sheath are easily identified in vertical and horizontal sections at the level of the stem, immediately below the bulge, with conventional staining procedures including hematoxylin and eosin, toluidine blue, and elastic stains (*Fig. 22.15* and see *Fig. 22.13*). The ratio between terminal and vellus hairs is approximately 7 : 1. Distinguishing between terminal and vellus hair follicles is critical for the diagnosis of androgenetic and temporal triangular alopecia. A ratio of 4 : 1 or less is suggestive of androgenetic alopecia. By definition, hair follicles and vellus hairs do not reach the subcutaneous tissue; therefore, to determine the final number of hair follicles and in particular vellus hair, superficial sections must be done at the level of the isthmus. For this reason, the quantification of follicles in deep and superficial sections is different. Superficial sections may reveal five to six more follicles than those counted in deep sections. As previously mentioned, the ratio of terminal follicles to vellus hairs may vary between different ethnic groups (*Table 22.2*).[5] It is important to bear in mind that the hair shaft is frequently lost during the biopsy process. In these cases, its size may be extrapolated from the diameter of the empty space delimited by the inner root sheath.

The hair follicle can be anatomically and functionally divided into two distinct segments. Differences between these two elements are explained by the fact that the upper portion of the hair follicle is very stable and not affected by maturation and shedding of the hair. The lower portion of the hair follicle is actively involved in hair growth and undergoes considerable morphological change according to its stage in the hair cycle.

The upper segment of the hair follicle consists of the follicular ostium, the infundibulum, and the isthmus (*Fig. 22.16*). The ostium is the physical orifice through which hair stems usually emerge in groups of two or three. The loss of it is clinically observed in scarring alopecias. The infundibulum extends from the ostium downwards to the opening of the sebaceous gland duct. It is cone shaped, its walls formed by the epidermis, and normally, around it there is mild concentric fibrosis and an inflammatory lymphocyte infiltrate, particularly seen in people of African descent. This phenomenon may cause confusion when evaluating inflammatory scarring alopecias (*Fig. 22.17*). [6]

The isthmus continues from the opening of the sebaceous gland duct to the site of attachment of the arrector pili muscle at the hair bulge (*Fig. 22.18*). The arrector pili muscle attaches to the bulge area through elastic tendons and extends to its upper attachment in the adjacent papillary dermis.

The lower segment extends from the arrector pili insertion to the lower part of the hair bulb and has two components: the stem (suprabulbar zone)

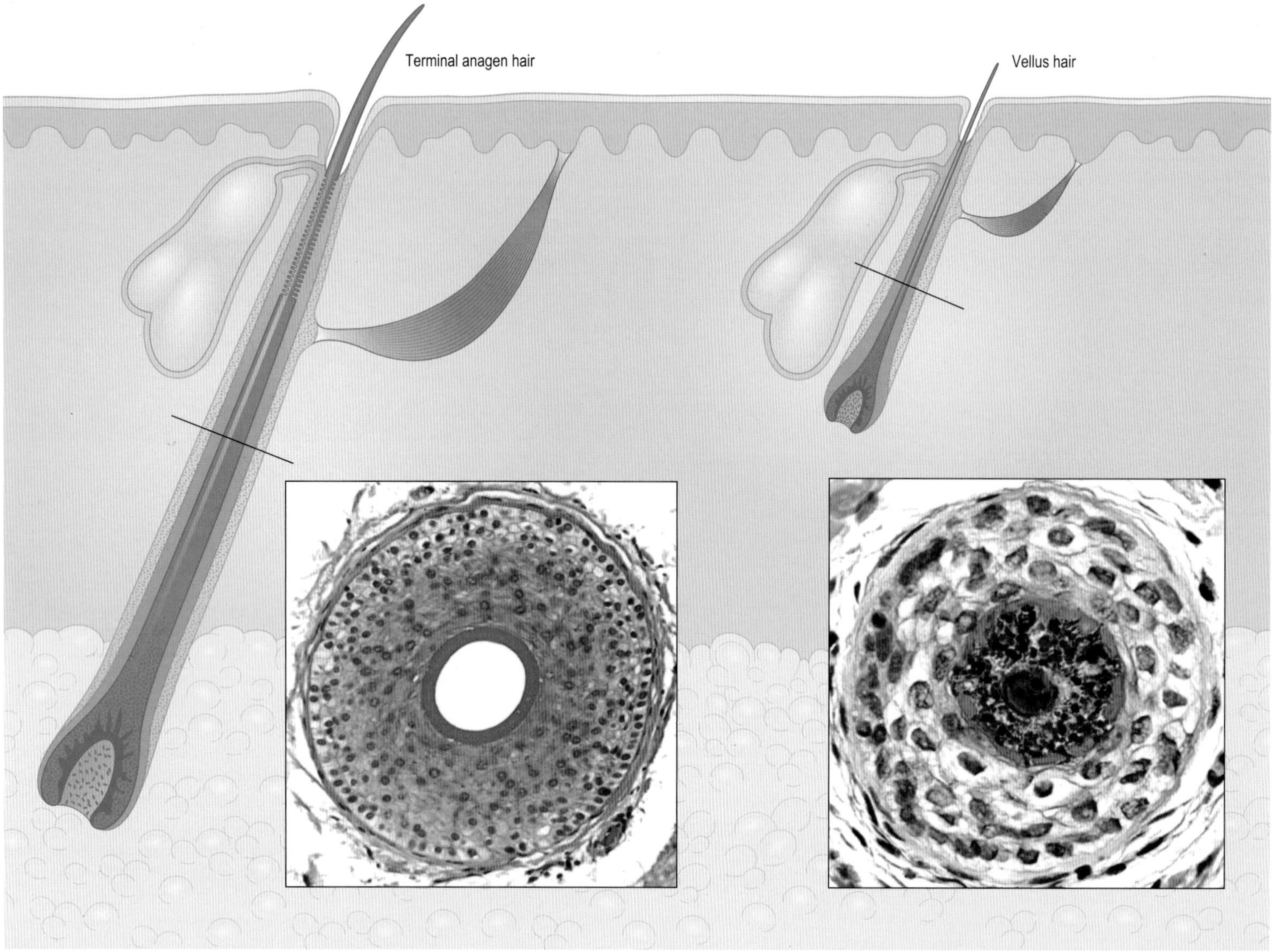

Terminal anagen hair

Vellus hair

Fig. 22.12
Terminal anagen and vellus hair, vertical and horizontal sections: the terminal hair follicles reach the fat and are deeply embedded within it. The vellus hairs and miniaturized follicles are located within the dermis. Note the differences between the relative size of the hair shaft and the inner root sheath in terminal and vellus hairs. Courtesy of M. Mejia, MD, Universidad Pontificia Bolivariana, Medellín, Colombia.

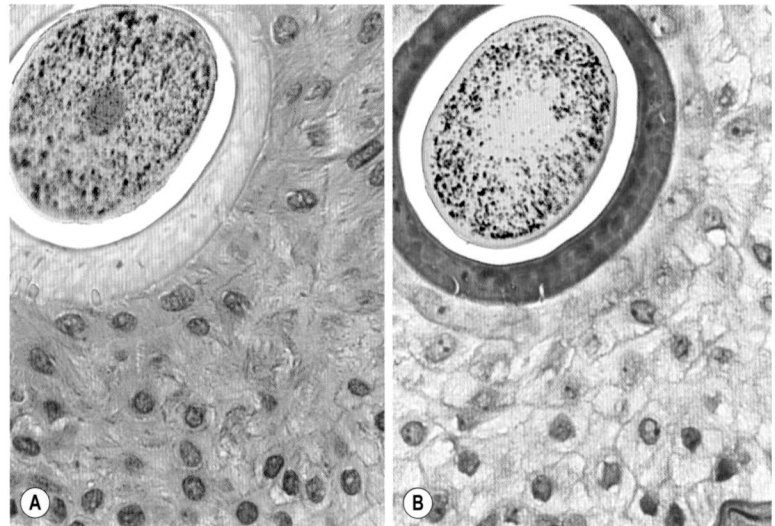

Fig. 22.13
Terminal anagen hair, horizontal section: compare the diameter of the hair shaft with the thickness of the thin internal root sheath (**A**) in pink with hematoxylin and eosin and in (**B**) dark blue with the toluidine blue stain.

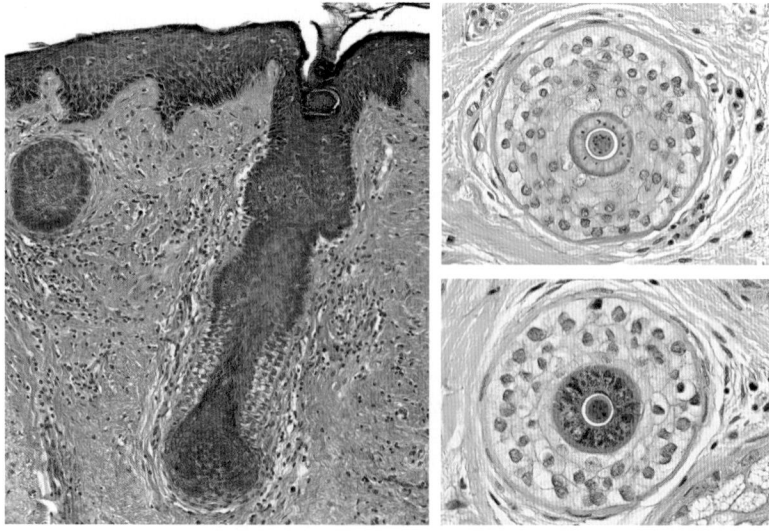

Fig. 22.14
Vellus hair, vertical and horizontal sections: short vellus hairs are located in the superficial dermis. In the horizontal sections, the diameter of the hair shaft is the same as or thinner than the inner root sheath.

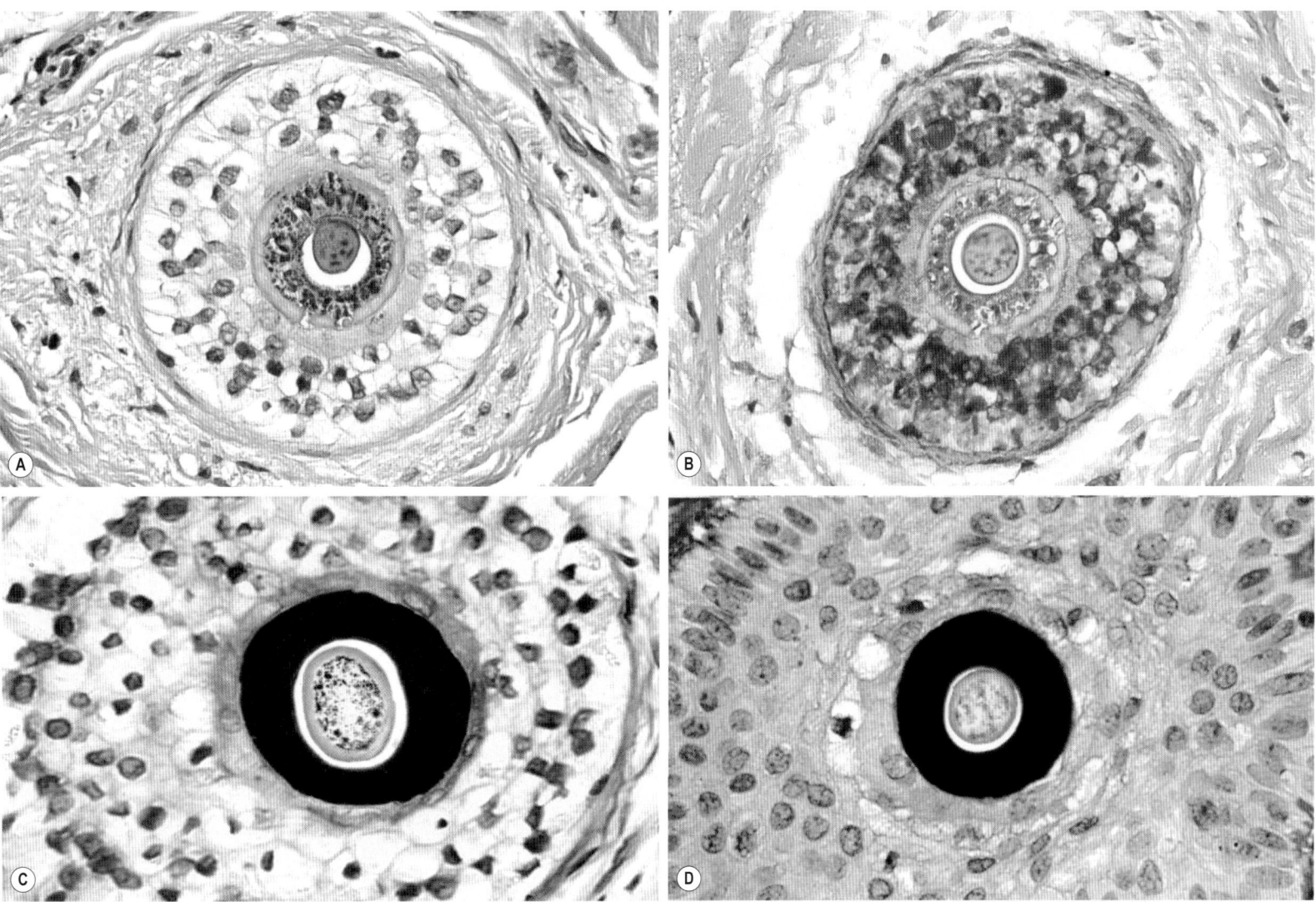

Fig. 22.15
Vellus hair, horizontal section: note the caliber of the hair shaft compared to the inner root sheath in: (**A**) pink, hematoxylin and eosin; (**B**) gray, PAS; (**C**) blue, toluidine blue; and (**D**) black, elastic tissue stain.

that extends from the arrector pili insertion to the Adamson fringe and the lower portion called the bulb (*Figs 22.19* and *22.20*). In a hair follicle in anagen, the stem is the longest structure in the hair follicle with a clearly differentiated internal and external radicular sheath clearly (*Fig. 22.21*). The bulb comprises the matrix cells and the basal melanocytes that surround the dermal papilla (*Fig. 22.22*).[7–9]

A hair shaft is composed of three layers: the medulla, the cortex, and the cuticle. The medulla, which represents the central region of the hair shaft, is not consistently present in humans, but it is often an important component of hair in other animals (*Fig. 22.23*). The cortex is the thickest layer and is responsible for the strength of the shaft. It is composed of intermediate filaments of hard keratin that are arranged in microfibrils, which intertwine to form cable-like structures called macrofibrils. The cuticle, which constitutes the outer part of the shaft, is responsible for the resistance to the wear and tear produced by the environment. It consists of scales orientated at right angles to the epidermis. These interlock with the cuticle of the internal root sheath maintaining integrity and in the bulbar zone appears as a single layer (*Fig. 22.24* and see *Fig. 22.21*). The linear or curved shape of the hair is determined by the curved or linear shape of the internal radicular sheath. In horizontal sections, the hair in individuals of African descent is curved, elliptical, and eccentrically located within the follicular channel. In Caucasian individuals the hair is circular and centrally located within the follicular channel. In horizontal sections of a terminal anagen hair follicle, different layers can be identified in the suprabulbar area. From the center to the periphery these comprise:

- Hair shaft (including the medulla, the cortex, and the cuticle of the hair),
- Inner root sheath (including the cuticular layer of the inner root sheath, Huxley layer, Henle layer, and companion layer),
- Outer root sheath,
- Vitreous and external fibrous layer (perifollicular connective tissue sheath) (*Fig. 22.24*).

These layers change noticeably depending on the level of the microscopic section. The cuticle of the hair shaft and all layers of the internal root sheath at the bulb level undergo trichohyaline keratinization. At the bulge, the inner root sheath starts to disappear and in the isthmus is replaced with trichilemmal keratin derived from the external root sheath (see *Fig. 22.18*).[10]

The external root sheath is continuous with the epidermis at the infundibulum and where it forms a granular layer with a basket weave arrangement of the epidermal keratin (see *Fig. 22.17*). Toward the bulb, the cells of the outer root sheath cells contain abundant glycogen (*Fig. 22.21* and see *Fig. 22.24*).

Hair cycle

The hair growth cycle, whether terminal or vellus, is divided into three stages: active growth (anagen), involution (catagen), a period of rest (telogen), and, as an extension of this last stage, two additional stages: hair shaft-extrusion (exogen) and empty hair follicle (kenogen) (*Fig. 22.25*). The duration of the anagen phase determines the length of the hair stem. Human beings

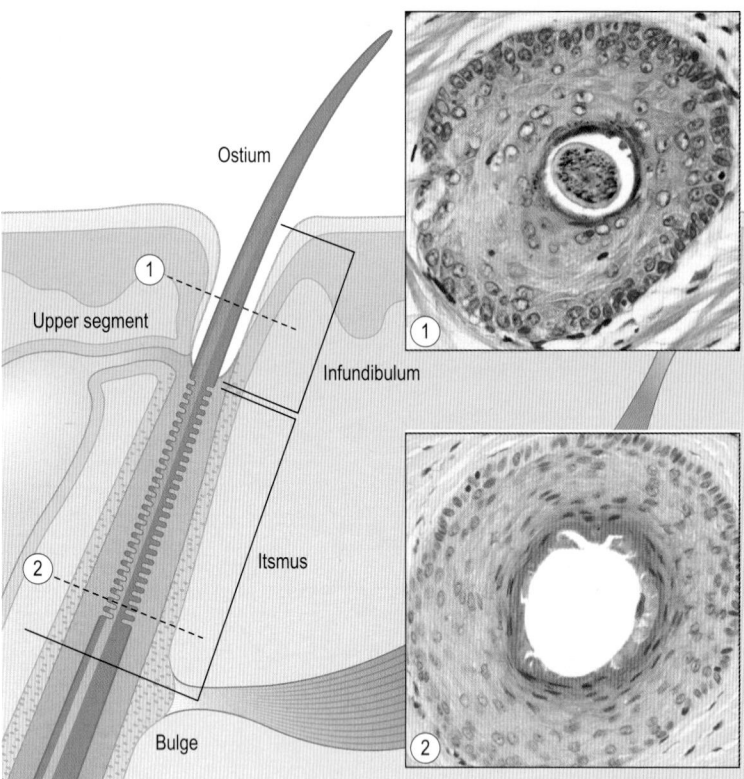

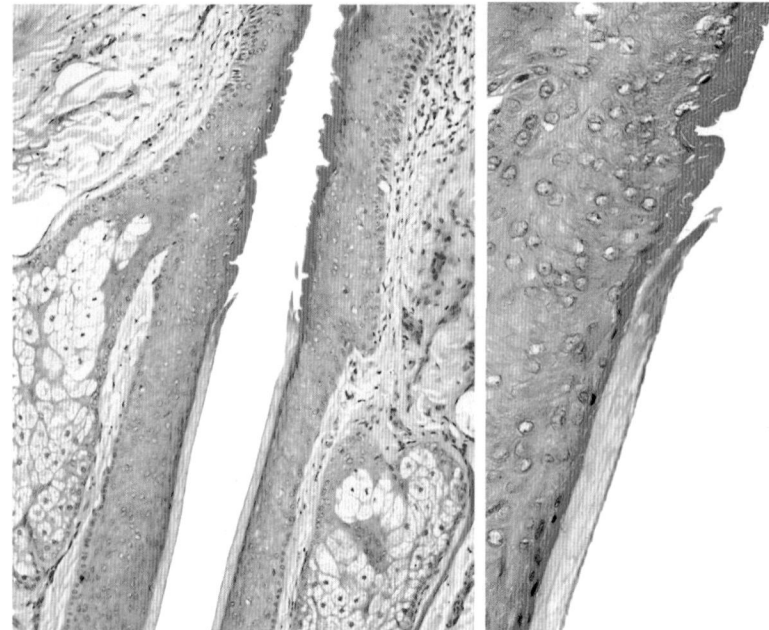

Fig. 22.16
Terminal anagen hair, vertical and horizontal sections of the upper segment: note the ostium, infundibulum and isthmus. The insets show horizontal sections through (1) the infundibulum and (2) the isthmus. The outer root sheath of the infundibulum is composed of squamous epithelium similar to the epidermis. Courtesy of M. Mejia, MD, Universidad Pontificia Bolivariana, Medellín, Colombia.

Fig. 22.18
Isthmus and lower segment, vertical sections: note the isthmus and the outer root sheath which keratinizes in the absence of a granular cell layer. Its silhouette is wavy and intensely eosinophilic (trichilemmal). At the junction between the isthmus and lower segment is a small bulge that protrudes from the outer sheath toward the dermis. At this site, the inner root sheath is shed. On the right-hand side, note the proximity between the upper and lower segments with the normal shedding site of the inner root sheath.

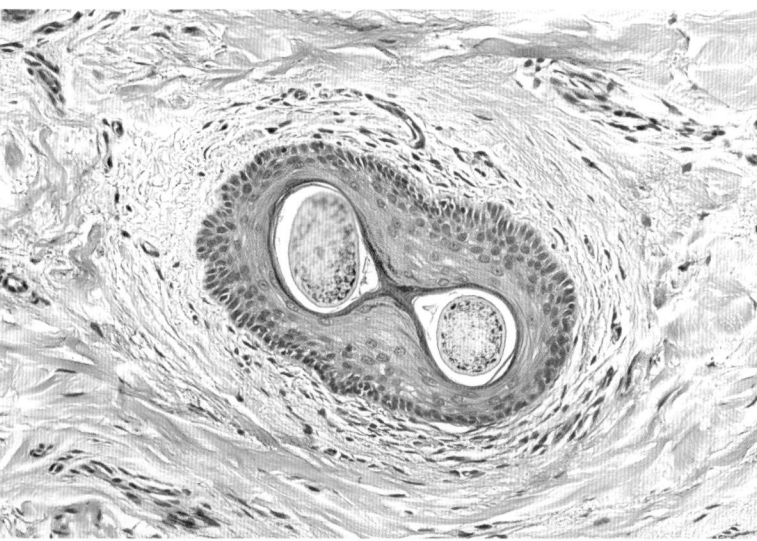

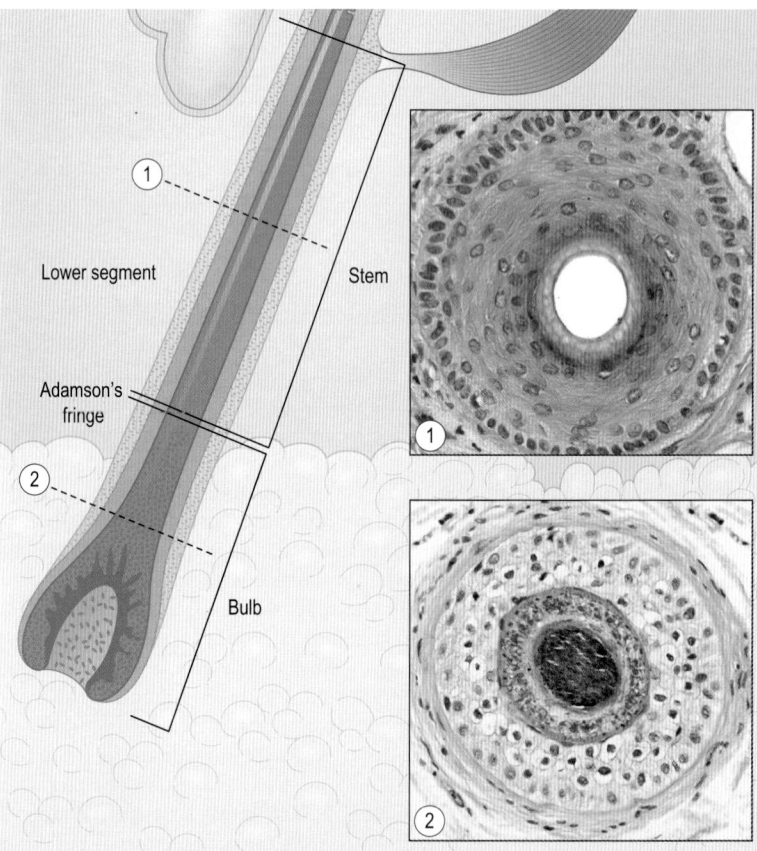

Fig. 22.17
Infundibulum. Horizontal section. The wall is made up of squamous stratified keratinized epithelium. The surrounding dermis is infiltrated by some lymphocytes. There are two hair shafts emerging from a single ostium.

Fig. 22.19
Terminal anagen hair, vertical and horizontal sections of the lower segment: note the shaft and the hair bulb deep to Adamson fringe. The horizontal sections show (1) the stem and (2) the upper part of the bulb. Note the loss of nuclei in the hair shaft and the inner root sheath. Courtesy of M. Mejia, MD, Universidad Pontificia Bolivariana, Medellín, Colombia.

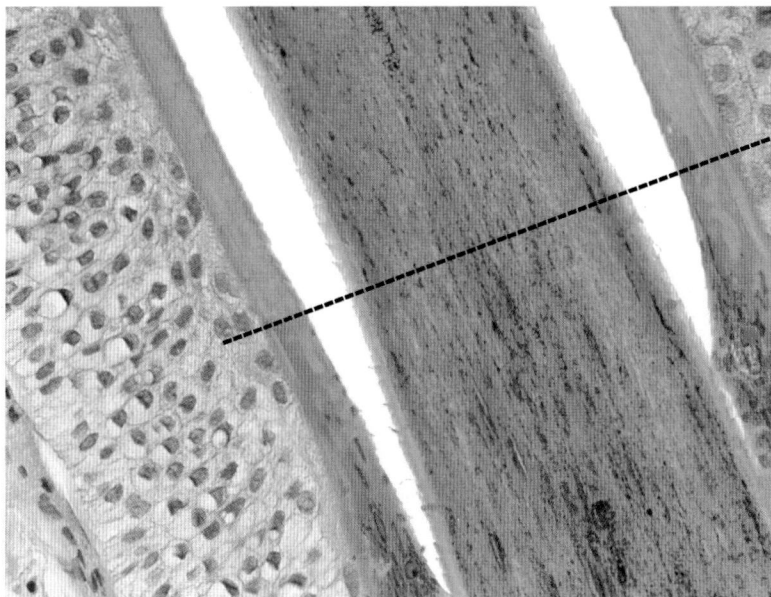

Fig. 22.20
Terminal anagen hair section showing Adamson fringe: there is loss of trichohyalin granules and nuclei in the inner root sheath and the hair shaft at the junction of the stem (*above*) and the bulb (*below*). Above this level, the inner root sheath keratinizes completely.

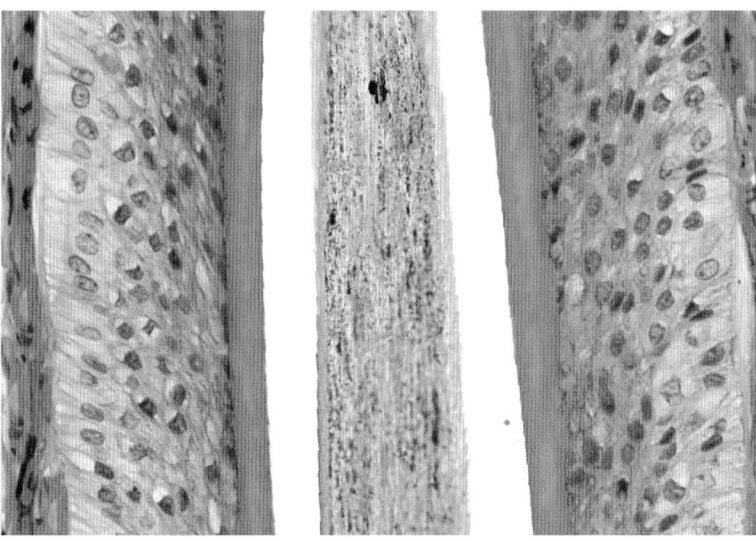

Fig. 22.21
Terminal anagen hair, lower segment: the pink inner root sheath (anucleated) clearly contrasts with the outer root sheath (nucleated) in this vertical section. The cuticle has a serrated border orientated in the opposite direction to that of the inner root sheath. The cells of the outer root sheath have clear cytoplasm due to prominent intracytoplasmic glycogen at this level.

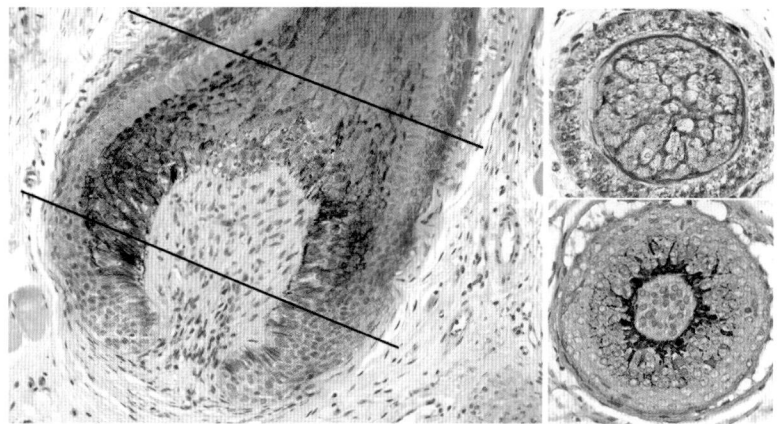

Fig. 22.22
Terminal anagen hair: hair bulb and hair follicle pigmentary unit, vertical and horizontal sections. In the vertical and horizontal sections, note the supramatricial cells with intracytoplasmic pigmentation transferred from the dendritic melanocytes that surround the dermal papilla. The latter is composed of connective tissue and blood vessels.

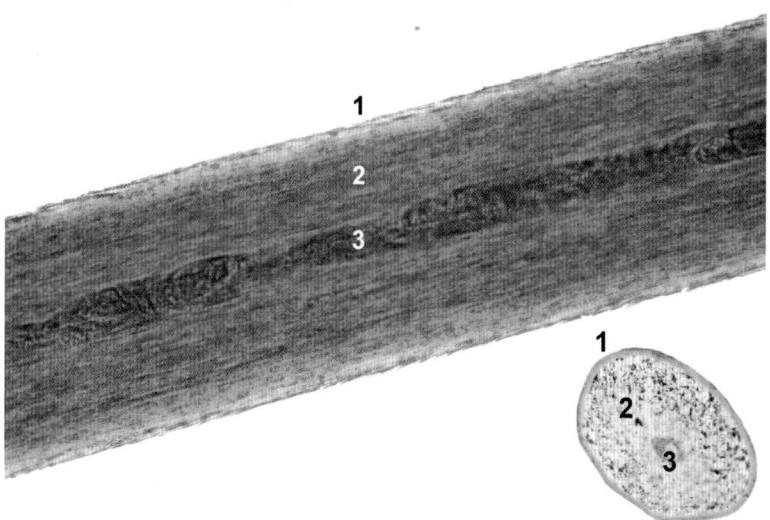

Fig. 22.23
Hair shaft: Note the cortex (2) and the cuticle (1). Sometimes, the medulla is easily visualized (3).

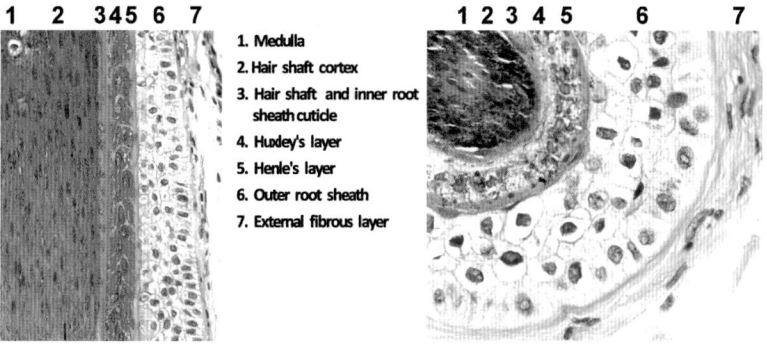

1. Medulla
2. Hair shaft cortex
3. Hair shaft and inner root sheath cuticle
4. Huxley's layer
5. Henle's layer
6. Outer root sheath
7. External fibrous layer

Fig. 22.24
Terminal anagen hair follicles: horizontal and vertical sections immediately below the Adamson fringe. Note the different layers of the hair follicle. (1) Medulla, (2) cortex, (3) cuticle of the hair and cuticle of the inner root sheath, (4) Huxley layer, (5) Henle layer, (6) outer root sheath, and (7) vitreous and external fibrous layer (perifollicular connective tissue sheath).

differ from other mammals in that these stages occur continuously rather than synchronously. There is no periodic change of the hair covering the body. The duration and relative proportion of each stage is variable: anagen 2–7 years (85–100%), catagen 2–3 weeks (0–1%), and telogen 100 days (0–15%). The cycles of miniaturized hair follicles and vellus hairs cycles are much faster, thus shortening the anagen phase.

The interaction of numerous growth factors, cytokines, hormones, neurotransmitters, and their receptors are important in the development and cycling of normal hair follicles. It appears that the driving force of cycling, the 'hair cycle clock', is located in the hair follicle itself, in the immediate niche and in the dermal microenvironment. However, no single growth factor appears to exert ultimate control over these processes.[1–4]

Anagen lasts from 2 to 7 years and is characterized by continuous growth, giving origin to a long and pigmented pilar stem, which is easily visible. It

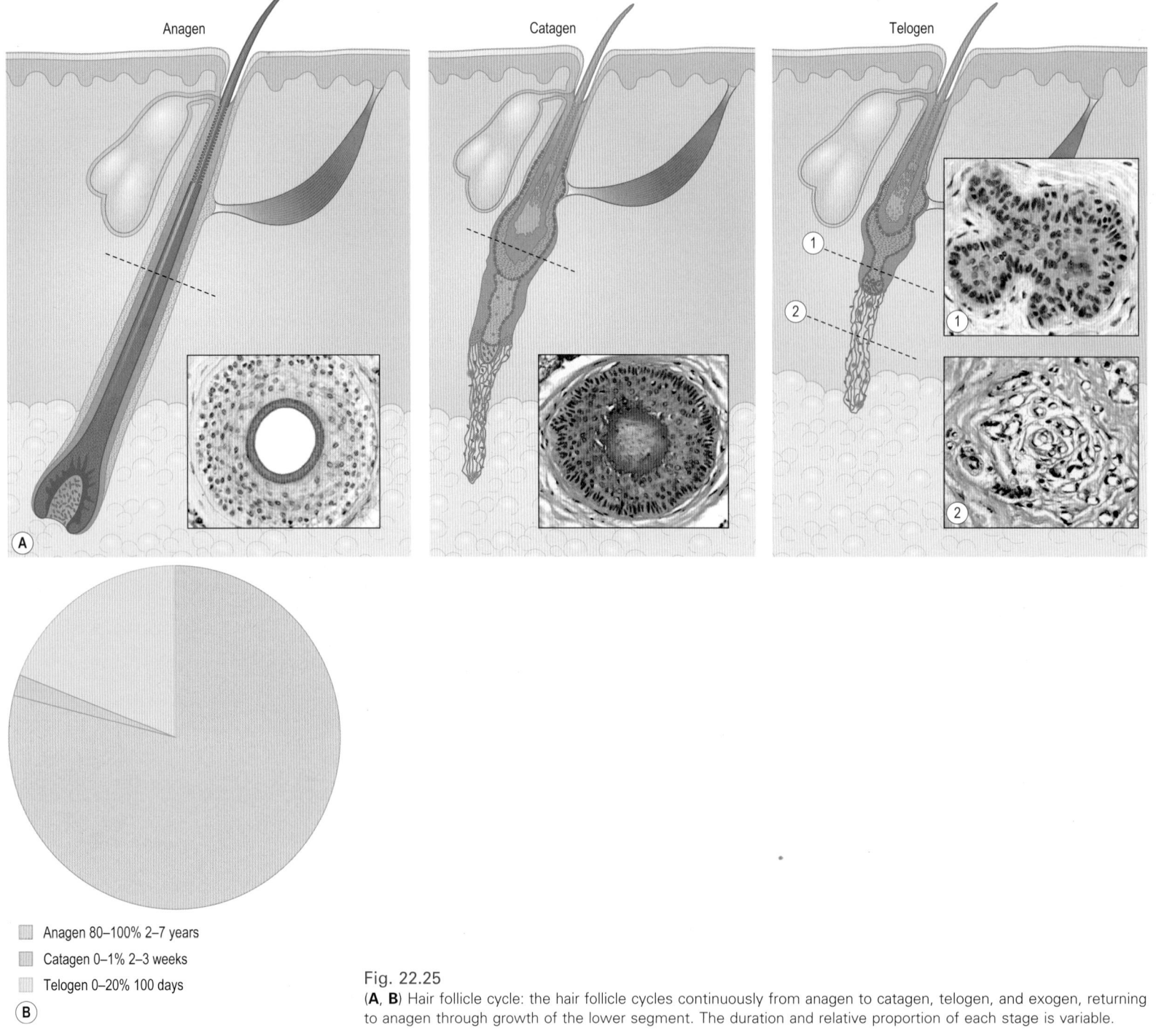

Fig. 22.25
(**A**, **B**) Hair follicle cycle: the hair follicle cycles continuously from anagen to catagen, telogen, and exogen, returning to anagen through growth of the lower segment. The duration and relative proportion of each stage is variable.

Anagen

Catagen

Telogen

Anagen 80–100% 2–7 years
Catagen 0–1% 2–3 weeks
Telogen 0–20% 100 days

is the phase that determines the length of the hair and the phase that varies the most depending on the body location. Morphologically, it corresponds to the already mentioned terminal hair follicles deeply situated in the subcutaneous fat (see *Fig. 22.19*). The pilar bulb of the follicles in anagen shows abundant melanin production and intense mitotic activity, resulting in the hair growing approximately 1.0 cm per month. At any particular moment, between 85% and 100% of the hair follicles are in anagen. As this is the phase with the highest mitotic activity, melanogenesis, and DNA synthesis, it is the most vulnerable to hormonal changes, drugs, and different toxins.

Pigmentation of the hair only occurs in anagen, and it is induced by interactions between bulbar melanocytes, keratinocytes, and dermal papilla fibroblasts (hair follicle pigmentary unit) (see *Fig. 22.22*).[5] The coupling of hair follicle melanogenesis to the anagen phase distinguishes follicular melanogenesis from the continuous melanogenesis of the epidermis. Cyclic reconstruction of the hair follicle pigmentary unit occurs optimally during

only the first 10 hair cycles, i.e., until approximately 40 years of age.[6] It is not clear if hair graying is a consequence of functional loss, or a selective melanocyte depletion of human hair.[7]

Catagen precedes telogen and during this phase, the inferior segment of the follicle undergoes massive apoptosis, reducing its size. It is the shortest phase and lasts from 2 to 3 weeks. Only 1% to 2% of the follicles are in catagen, and it is rare to find them in normal scalp biopsies. Horizontal sections are characterized by diffuse apoptosis and an absence of mitotic and pigmentary activity. Apoptotic cells have intensely eosinophilic cytoplasm and have a dark pyknotic nucleus (*Figs 22.26* and *22.27*). As the follicle retracts, the vitreous membrane collapses and appears thickened and corrugated (*Fig. 22.28*). It is important not to confuse this phenomenon with the thickening of the basal membrane observed in discoid lupus. The inner root sheath disappears and the outer root sheath appears morphologically similar to the epithelium of the isthmus, surrounding a club-shaped hair

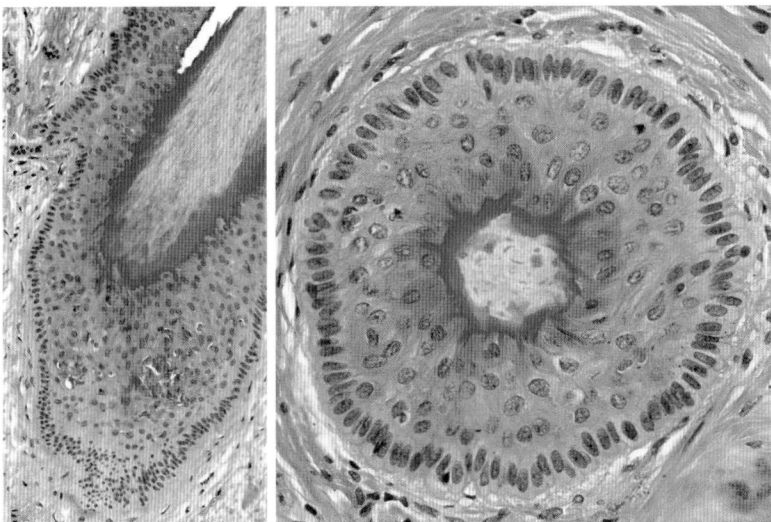

Fig. 22.26
Terminal hair follicle in catagen, vertical and horizontal sections: note the involution of the follicle and the deep red trichilemmal keratinization around the club-shaped hair shaft. The outer root sheath shows marked apoptosis. At the deepest part of the follicle, there is a hint of secondary germ formation.

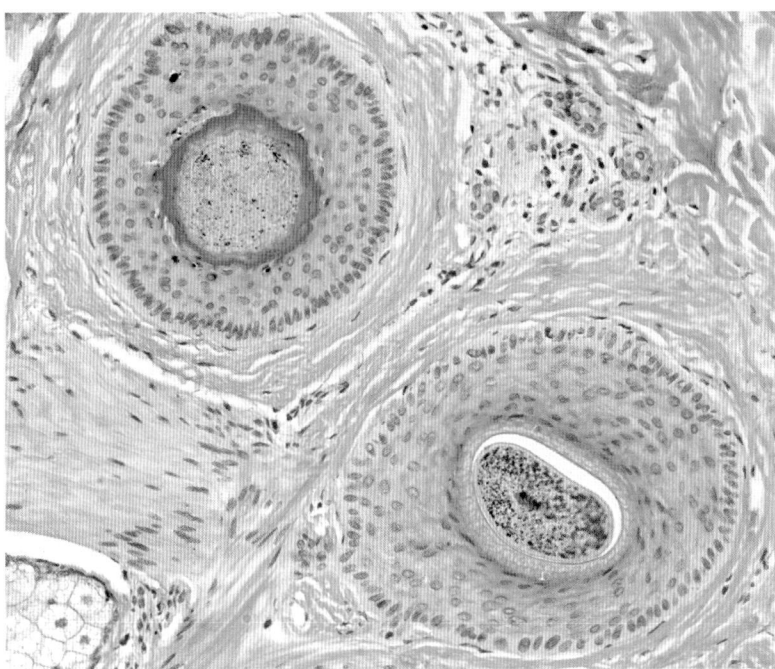

Fig. 22.27
Terminal hair follicles in catagen and anagen, horizontal sections: note the differences between a catagen follicle (*top left*) with trichilemmal keratin surrounding the hair shaft, apoptotic cells and loss of melanin and an anagen, heavily pigmented terminal follicle (inferior).

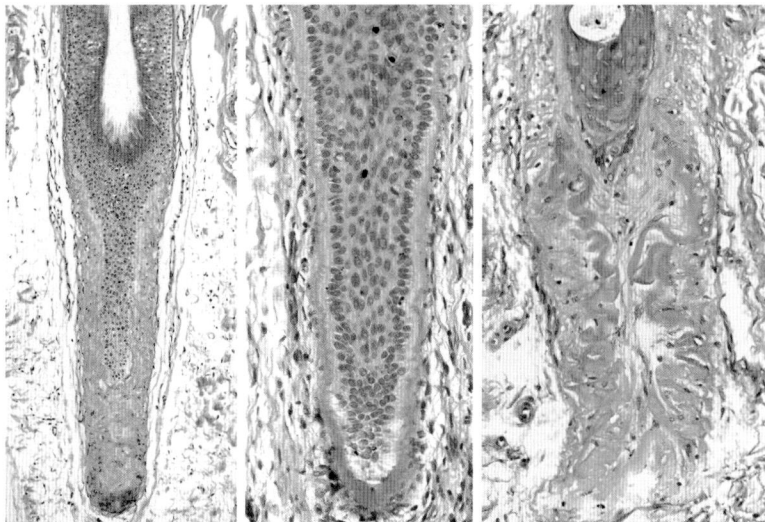

Fig. 22.28
Terminal hair follicles in catagen and telogen, vertical sections: the involution of the hair follicle leaves behind a thickened basement membrane.

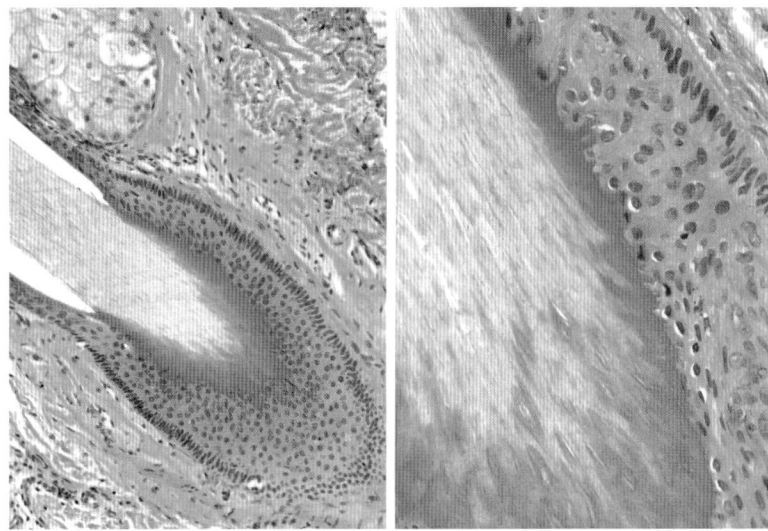

Fig. 22.29
Terminal hair follicles in late catagen: the outer root sheath has been lost and the keratinization is of trichilemmal type.

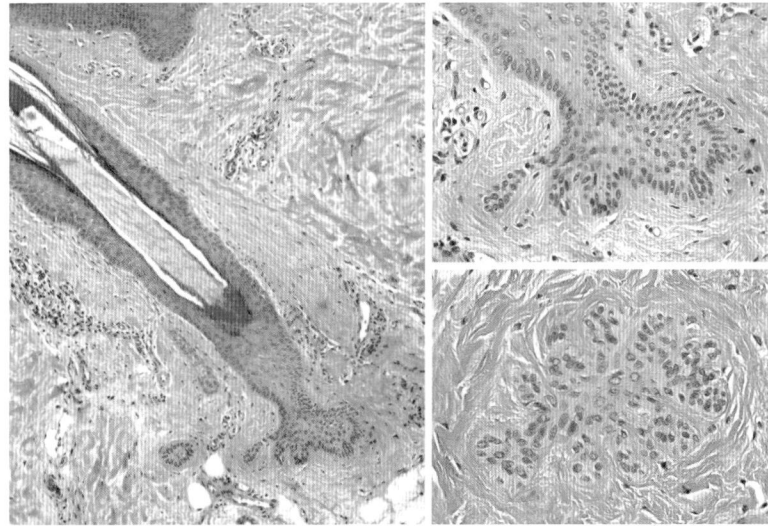

Fig. 22.30
Terminal hair follicle in telogen, secondary germ: note the condensation of basaloid cells in an asterisk or daisy shape in a horizontal section.

shaft and keratinizing in a trichilemmal manner (*Fig. 22.29*). Catagen follicles are frequent in trichotillomania.

Because of the brevity of the catagen phase which quickly follows the telogen phase, for quantifying purposes both the catagen and telogen follicles are counted together. Telogen lasts 100 days. Approximately 10–15% of the total number of hairs are in telogen phase at any given time and around 100 telogen hairs are shed per day. A hair follicle in telogen represents the final stage of involution of the lower segment. The hair papilla is present under the area of insertion of the arrector pili muscle and in a horizontal section appears as an aggregate of basaloid cells (the secondary germ: telogen germinal unit) (*Figs 22.30* and *22.31*). In the past, it was thought that the hair follicle stem cells were located in the telogen germinal unit. However, true stem cells are located in the bulge, in the insertion point

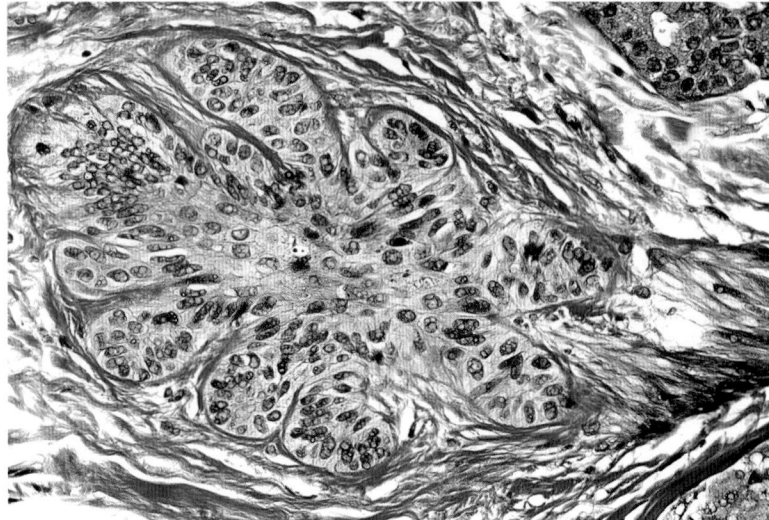

Fig. 22.31
Terminal hair follicle in telogen, secondary germ: horizontal section stained with Masson trichrome.

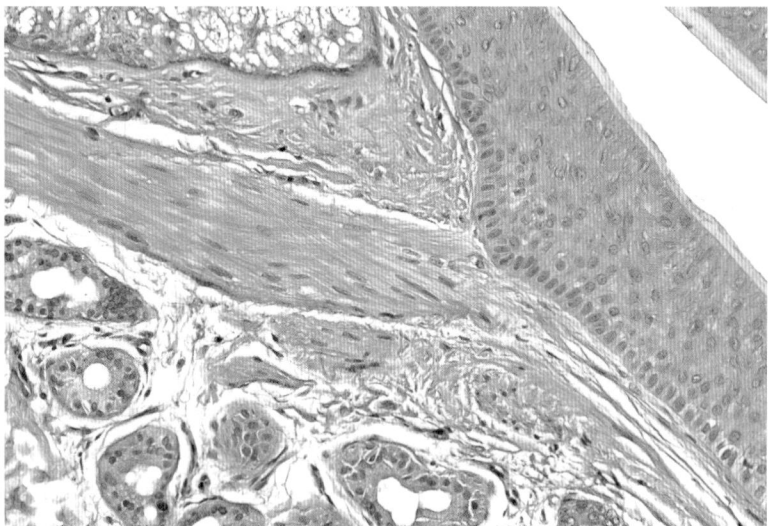

Fig. 22.32
Bulge and arrector pili muscle. In this vertical section, note the insertion of the arrector pili muscle erector in the bulge.

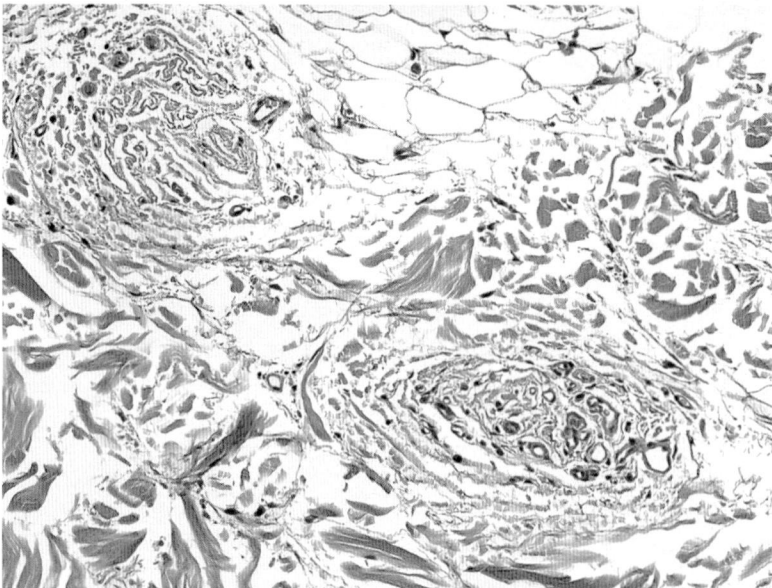

Fig. 22.33
Follicular stella, horizontal section: note the small blood vessels mixed with concentrically arranged connective tissue.

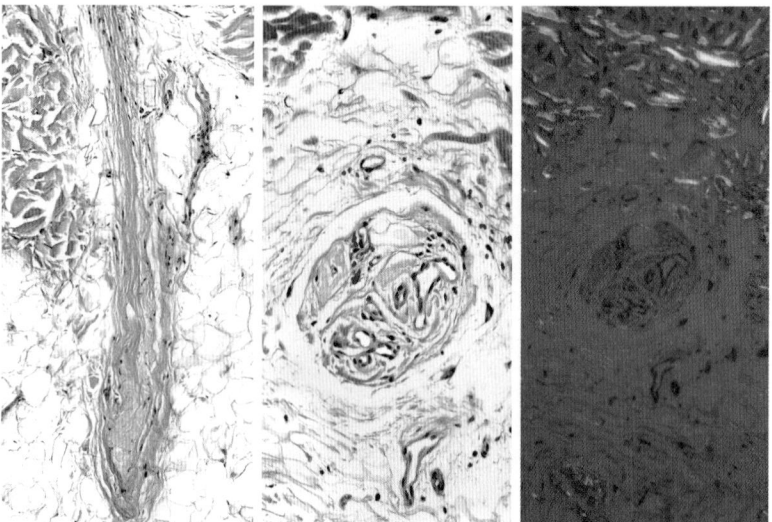

Fig. 22.34
Follicular stella: note the fibrovascular stella composed of collagen fibers, fibroblasts, and blood vessels in vertical and horizontal sections. The elastotic material is apparent between the collagen fibers. With polarized light, there is no birefringence of the follicular stellae.

of the arrector pili muscle; these cells are responsible for regenerating not only hair follicles but also sebaceous glands and epidermis[8,9] (*Fig. 22.32*). In the human hair follicle, the bulge is rarely visible, thus its detection requires the use of immunohistochemistry (cytokeratin 15). Loss of bulge stem cells leads to the cicatricial types of alopecia.

The lower segment of the hair follicle involutes completely, leaving only a structure called a follicular stella (follicular streamer, fibrous streamer), which indicates the position in which the retracted follicle was formerly located (*Fig. 22.33*). The follicular stella is not specific of the telogen phase as it is also observed as a consequence of the miniaturization of the terminal hair follicles in androgenetic alopecia. These follicular stella as opposed to those found in scarring alopecias are not birefringent under polarized light (*Fig. 22.34*).[10]

Two other phases are considered final components of the telogen stage:

- Exogen (teloptosis) represents a telogen club which has lost the adhesion between cells of the club hair and those of its epithelial envelope, apparently by a proteolytic mechanism activating an active shedding process.[11] This corresponds to the 100 hairs that are lost daily.
- Kenogen refers to an empty follicle after the follicle in telogen has been shed.[12] Follicles in exogen and kenogen are not easy to classify histologically.

Hair follicles also contain sebaceous glands that, with their secretion, lubricate the hair channel and skin surface. They are numerous and are easily identified in sections at the superior segment level. An early phenomenon in scarring alopecias is the loss of sebaceous glands. Apocrine glands are also associated with hair follicles in specific areas such as axillae, genital zone, medial abdomen, and areola.

Hair follicle immune privilege

The hair follicle immune system has distinctive configurations that maintain an area of relative immune privilege in the anagen stage of hair follicle cycle. The epithelium of the proximal hair follicle (the inner root sheath and hair matrix) is characterized by very low level of expression of major histocompatibility complex class Ia antigens, local production of immunosuppressive agents (transforming growth factor [TGF]-beta 1, alpha-melanocyte-stimulating hormone), and inhibition of natural killer (NK) cell activities. A collapse of this immune privilege is likely to play an important role in the pathogenesis of alopecia areata and possibly in some scarring alopecias.[13–15]

CLASSIFICATION OF ALOPECIA

Classification of alopecia is often difficult, both from a clinical perspective and in terms of etiology. Commonly, the cause cannot be identified, and there is considerable clinical and histologic overlap in the different types of alopecia. Many classifications have been proposed, and the most widely accepted divides alopecia into those that are patterned and those that diffusely involve the scalp and into cicatricial and noncicatricial (scarring and nonscarring) variants. Nonscarring alopecia is reversible whereas scarring alopecia is permanent. The follicular loss in the latter may result from the scarring process or develop independently.

The main problem with this classification is that there is a great degree of overlap, and clear-cut distinction is frequently not possible. In addition, some variants of alopecia (e.g., alopecia areata, trichotillomania, and traction alopecia) have a biphasic pattern: they are initially nonscarring but may become permanent (scarring) with time.

Scarring alopecias are classified into primary and secondary variants. Primary scarring alopecias are those in which the hair follicle is principally involved, as occurs in lichen planopilaris and lupus erythematosus. In the other variants, the hair follicle is not the main target of the inflammatory process and is destroyed as a secondary phenomenon. Examples of the latter include physical causes such as irradiation, infiltration of the scalp by tumor, inflammatory diseases including morphea, and infectious processes as may occur with fungi.[1–4]

Nonscarring alopecias

Androgenetic alopecia

Clinical features

Androgenetic alopecia is also known as common baldness and male and female pattern hair loss.[1] It is caused by androgens in genetically susceptible men, the role of androgens being less clear in women.[1,2] Typically, there is progressive miniaturization of hairs in the scalp between the ages of 12 and 40 years.

Androgens are the main regulator of normal human hair growth. After puberty, they promote transformation of vellus hair follicles into large pigmented terminal hairs. However, androgens may also reverse this process, resulting in the gradual replacement of terminal hairs with vellus hairs and the onset of androgenetic alopecia.[3]

Androgenetic alopecia is a very common disorder and is the most frequent type of hair loss in adults, affecting at least 50% of the male population by the age of 50, and about 40% of the female population by the age of 70.[4,5] The prevalence of vertex and full-blown androgenetic alopecia increases with age in males between 40 and 70 years, but the proportion of males with disease restricted to the frontal region remains fairly constant.[6]

Patients with androgenetic alopecia usually have a familial history of baldness. The absence of such a history reduces the risk but does not exclude the possibility of developing the condition. Rarely, it is associated with hyperandrogenism, and this is accompanied by other manifestations of excess androgens.[7,8]

In males, the condition usually starts early after puberty, mainly affecting the crown, vertex, frontal, central, and temporal areas of the scalp. There is usually no involvement of the occipital and lower parietal regions (Fig. 22.35). Some cases present in adolescence and in childhood, usually associated with a strong genetic predisposition.[9,10] It has been proposed that patients who develop hair loss before the end of the third decade may have a higher risk of coronary artery disease than nonaffected males.[11] However, other studies have restricted such association to alopecia localized to the vertex and some authors have totally discarded this association.[12–14]

An association with insulin resistance-linked diseases and with higher mortality for diabetes and cardiovascular disease has been noted in older patients with androgenetic alopecia.[15,16]

The condition also appears to be a risk factor for prostate cancer and benign prostatic hyperplasia.[17–19]

Androgenetic alopecia is more frequent in whites than in black men.[20] Association of androgenetic alopecia with smoking has been observed among Asian men.[21] The frequency appears to be increasing in this ethnic group.[22] Androgenetic alopecia appears to be more common in males with X-linked recessive ichthyosis.[23] Male-pattern baldness has been also associated with a susceptibility locus at chromosome 20p11.22.[24] Some patients may also have associated trichodynia.[25]

In females, the hair loss is patterned and characterized by progressive thinning over the frontal/parietal scalp, retention of the frontal hairline, and the presence of miniaturized hairs. The process is noted as widening of the central part of the scalp (Fig. 22.36). Female pattern hair loss is much less frequent than in men, and complete baldness very rarely ensues. The hair loss often starts around the onset of the menopause, although occasionally

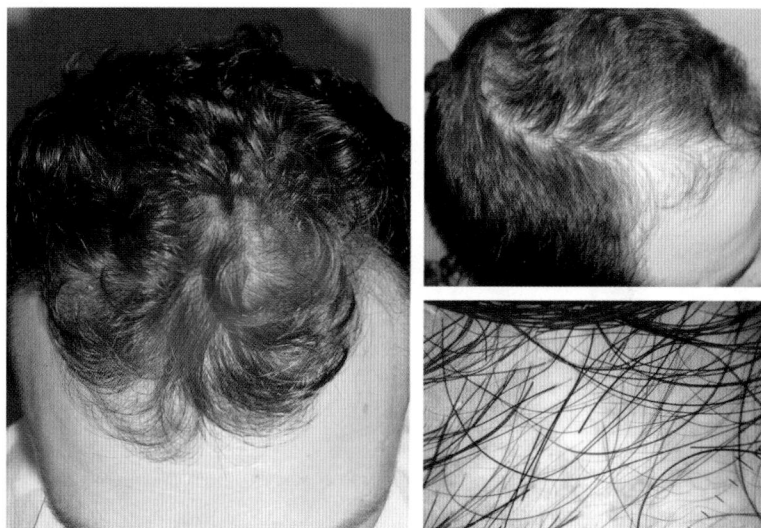

Fig. 22.35
Male androgenetic alopecia: this patient shows well-established male pattern baldness with bifrontal hair line recession and hair loss on the scalp vertex. In the dermoscopic image on the right, note the difference in caliber between hair follicles. Courtesy of L.M. Gómez, MD, UPB, Medellín, Colombia.

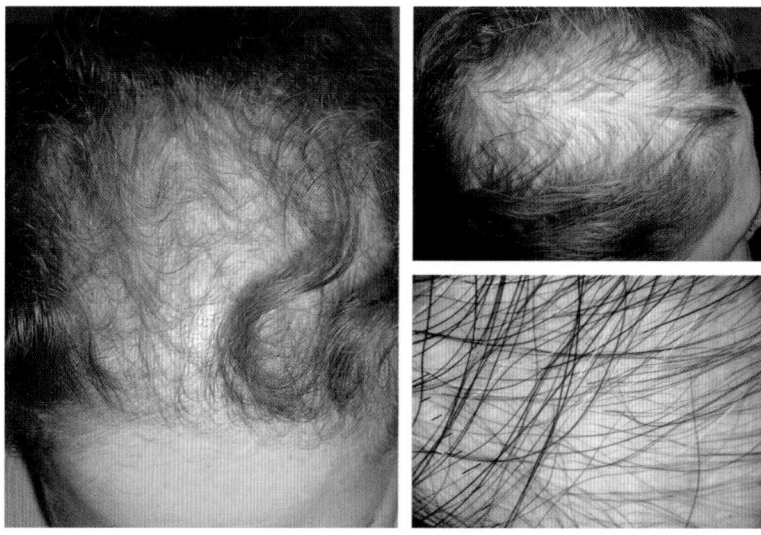

Fig. 22.36
Female pattern hair loss: this example shows a typical example with parietal and posterior frontal hair loss. Note the sparing of the frontal hairline. In the dermoscopic image on the right lower panel, note the hair loss due to extensive miniaturization on a noninflammatory background. Courtesy of L.M. Gómez, MD, UPB, Medellín, Colombia.

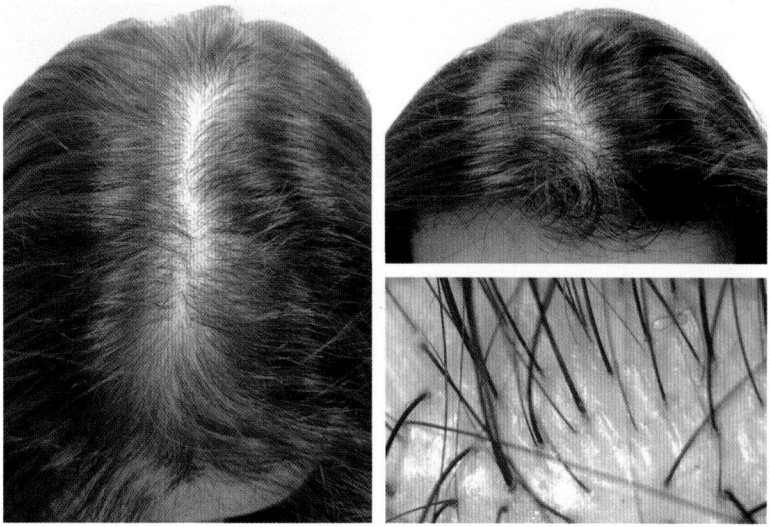

Fig. 22.37
Female pattern hair loss in a girl: early hair loss is observed with widening of the interparietal line. In the dermoscopic image on the right lower panel, note a tendency to miniaturization with hair follicles of different calibers. Courtesy of L.M. Gómez, MD, UPB, Medellín, Colombia.

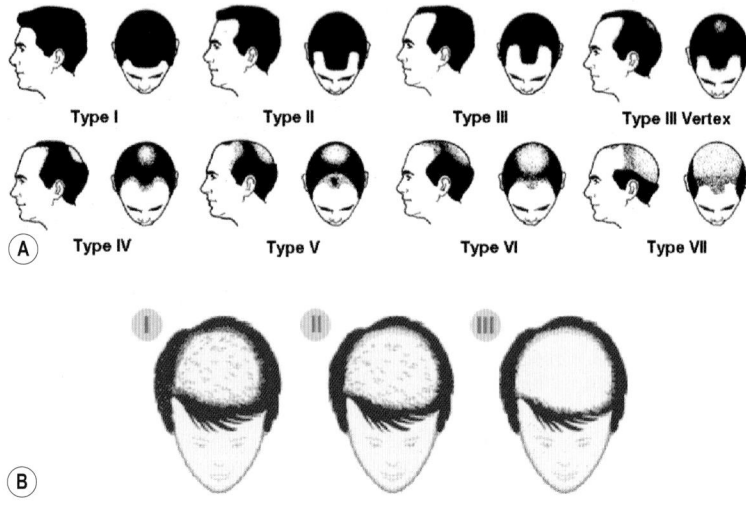

Fig. 22.38
(**A**) Hamilton-Norwood classification of male pattern androgenetic alopecia (*top*). Reproduced with permission from Norwood, O.T. (1984) Hair transplant surgery. Springfield: Charles C. Thomas, p 6. (**B**) Ludwig patterns of female pattern hair loss (*bottom*). Reproduced with permission from Ludwig, E. (1977) Classification of the types of androgenetic alopecia occurring in the female sex. British Journal of Dermatology, 97;247–254.

it develops much earlier (*Fig. 22.37*). Female pattern hair loss has been associated with hyperprolactinemia.[26]

The two patterns of hair loss in androgenetic alopecia are sometimes known as Hamilton-Norwood 'male pattern' and Ludwig 'female pattern' (*Fig. 22.38*).[27,28] However, there is considerable overlap. Some women present with male pattern and vice versa. Korean men tend to have a more 'female pattern' of hair thinning than Caucasians.[29] These types of inverse presentation do not define the hormonal state of the individual; a woman with a masculine pattern of alopecia does not necessarily present with hyperandrogenism.

The different clinical presentations and the fact that the occipital scalp is generally respected is a consequence of the different embryological origins of the dermis in the different areas of the scalp. The dermis of the frontal/parietal scalp is of neural crest origin, whereas the dermis of the occipital scalp is of mesodermal origin.[30]

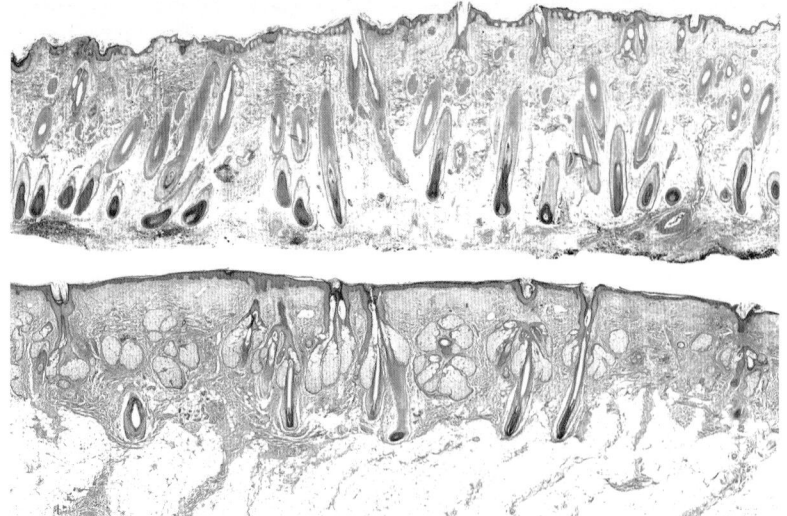

Fig. 22.39
Androgenetic alopecia. Vertical sections. In the top panel normal scalp with numerous terminal hair follicles extending into the deep subcutaneous fat. In the lower panel, note a scalp biopsy from a patient with advanced androgenic alopecia. Barely visible, are a few thin follicles which only just reach the limit between the dermis and the subcutaneous tissue.

Dermoscopy and videodermoscopy of hair and scalp show important differences in hair shaft diameter, with a mixture of indeterminate and terminal hairs. Its use has enabled both the clinical diagnosis and the monitoring of the response to treatment to be more accurate. The site most affected by the alopecia is easily located and consequently will be the best site to biopsy (see *Figs 22.35–22.37*).[31–33]

Men suffering from androgenetic alopecia do not usually require laboratory investigations. The decision to perform laboratory tests in affected females depends on a variety of factors including family history, clinical presentation, evolution, and age at onset of the disease. A woman with menstrual irregularities, a history of infertility, polycystic ovaries, or physical signs suggesting hyperandrogenism (hirsutism, cystic acne unresponsive to treatment, acanthosis nigricans, virilization, or galactorrhea) should have further investigations including free and total testosterone levels. If these are high the source should be determined, especially with respect to the presence of an ovarian tumor or adrenal hyperplasia. In women with androgenetic alopecia without a family history or physical signs suggestive of hyperandrogenism, it is not usually necessary to perform any laboratory tests.[30]

In androgenetic alopecia, a gentle hair pull is normal. Only a few hairs are obtained, and these are all in telogen phase. Hair pluck can give misleading results due to an apparent higher count of hair in telogen in the affected areas. This occurs because, in the early stages, hair follicles more frequently enter telogen as a result of shortening of the anagen phase. Confusion with telogen effluvium is possible but distinction is easy, based on the fact that telogen effluvium is generalized and androgenetic alopecia is localized.

Pathogenesis and histologic features

Androgenetic alopecia results from a progressive decrease in the size of hair follicles and their transformation into vellus forms (*Fig. 22.39* and see *Figs 22.12* and *22.14*). However, it has also been observed that this miniaturization may occur suddenly within only a few cycles.[34] This phenomenon is the direct result of 5α-reductase type II activity, which is mainly found in the external root sheath and the hair bulb papilla. The enzyme converts testosterone into dihydrotestosterone, which has a great affinity for the androgen receptors in the outer root sheath and follicular papilla of the hair follicle.[35] The hormone receptor complex activates the genes responsible for the gradual transformation of large terminal hairs into miniaturized hair follicles. Young women and men with this condition have higher levels of 5α-reductase and androgen receptor in frontal hair follicles when compared with occipital follicles.[34] Finasteride inhibits 5α-reductase type-2 isozyme, lowering the levels of dihydrotestosterone and promoting hair growth in men.

However, the role of androgens in the female pattern hair loss variant is not fully established. Scalp hair loss is a feature of hyperandrogenism in females but many women with female pattern hair loss have no other clinical or biochemical evidence of androgen excess. Female pattern hair loss is probably a multifactorial, genetically determined trait and it is possible that both androgen-dependent and androgen-independent mechanisms contribute to the phenotype.[36–38] Other enzymes that modulate the effect of the androgens and estrogens and serve as protecting factors against androgenetic alopecia are cytochrome p450 aromatase and 17β-hydroxysteroid dehydrogenase. These lead to increase in the level of local estrogen in the hair follicle with variations in relation to sex, age, and location of the hair follicles.[39]

In both, male and female pattern hair loss there is a decline in anagen duration, increase in the percentage of hair follicles in telogen, and a higher frequency and prolongation of the kenogen phase, particularly in cases of high miniaturization of the hair follicles. It would seem that the telogen hair follicle follows an alternative route, one not followed by a new early anagen phase but rather remaining for a prolonged period as an empty follicle. The final result is nonpigmented hair shafts, which progressively become thinner and smaller, and this finally results in empty follicles without stems (teloptosis). Some follicles could fade away and be replaced by fibrous tracts.[40–42]

For the microscopic study of androgenetic alopecia, two 4-mm punch biopsies should be obtained: a control from healthy scalp in the occipital region and the other from the affected area. Both biopsies must be sectioned horizontally from the lower part of the infundibulum for comparative quantification purposes. The ratio between terminal and vellus hairs is approximately 7:1. A ratio of 4:1 or less is suggestive of androgenetic alopecia.

The histologic features are different in the early and late stages of the disease. Terminal, indeterminate, and vellus hairs should be counted. It is easier to appreciate the miniaturization of hair follicles and dropping out of follicular units when a comparison is made with the biopsy of normal scalp taken from the occipital area (*Fig. 22.40*). This process does not present in a uniform manner as initially it can be focal and may even only affect some of the follicles within a follicular unit (*Fig. 22.41*). A toluidine blue stain is particularly useful to highlight the outer and inner root sheaths in contrast to the pale staining of the hair shaft (*Fig. 22.42* and see *Fig. 22.15*).[43,44]

Histologically, terminal hairs progressively transform to vellus hairs (*Figs 22.43* and *22.44*). There is a decrease in the size of the dermal papilla and bulb.[34] The diameter of the hair shaft also decreases and varies noticeably from one follicle to another. This histologic feature is closely related to the miniaturization observed clinically (*Fig. 22.45*).[45]

Although the total hair count is normal, it will appear reduced if the count is taken at the junction of the dermis and subcutaneous fat, since by definition terminal hairs are diminished in number. Even though these changes may also be seen in vertical sections (see *Fig. 22.39*), they are more difficult to interpret and quantify.

Along with these changes, there is a reduction in the duration of the hair follicle cycle at the expense of the anagen phase. Therefore, in patients with evolving or fully established androgenetic alopecia, it is very common to find an increment in the number of catagen and telogen follicles in the miniaturized follicles component.[46] The histologic picture of the female variant is identical.

A mild to moderate T lymphocytic inflammatory cell infiltrate frequently surrounds the upper third of the hair follicle, associated with discrete perifollicular concentric fibrosis particularly in patients of African descent (*Fig. 22.46* and see *Fig. 22.17*).[47,48] The significance of this phenomenon has yet to be ascertained as, unlike primary scarring alopecias, there is no loss of hair follicle stem cells. However, there does seem to be a decrease in the conversion of stem cells to progenitor cells.[49]

The miniaturization of hair follicles affects the whole of the hair follicle including, in late stages, the arrector pili muscle and the sebaceous gland. The degeneration and replacement of the arrector pili muscle by fat tissue and the loss of contact with the bulge occurring in the miniaturized follicle seems to be a critical factor in defining whether an androgenetic alopecia will respond to treatment. The persistence of the union between these two structures is a sign of the reversibility in alopecia as it appears to protect the integrity of the stem cells in the bulge even in the advanced stages of

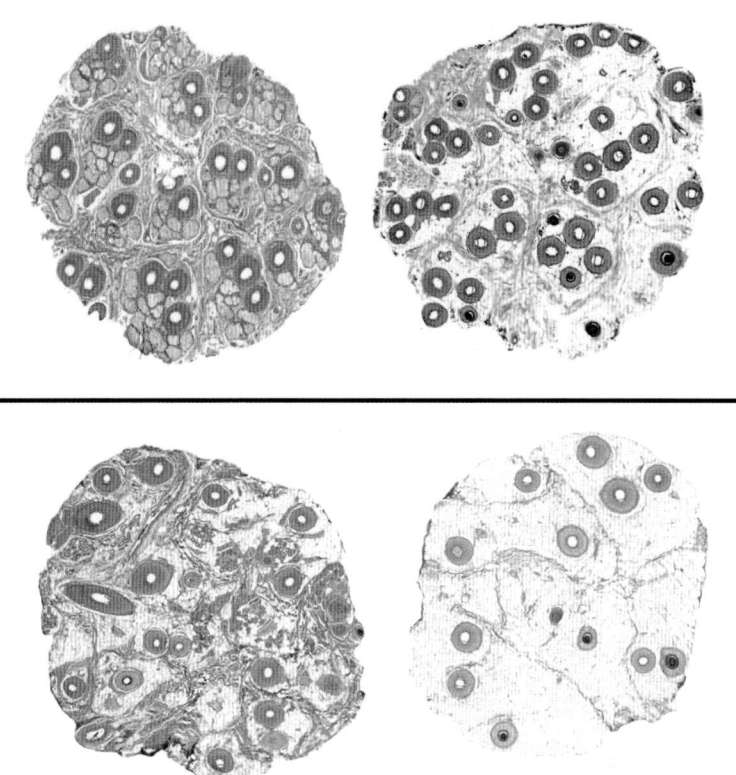

Fig. 22.40
Androgenetic alopecia, horizontal sections: in the upper panel, a biopsy of normal scalp taken from the occipital area. There are numerous follicular units formed by follicles of uniform size. Below are sections from an area of frontal alopecia with more than half of the follicles miniaturized (vellus) or in the process of miniaturization. The follicular units have disappeared and in the subcutaneous fat there are numerous stellae.

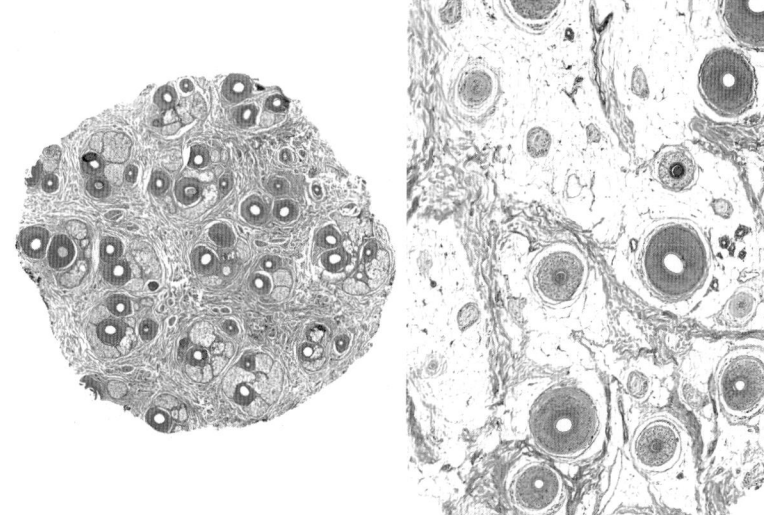

Fig. 22.41
Androgenetic alopecia, horizontal sections. This image highlights how the miniaturization phenomenon is not uniform but affects focal areas leaving normal areas in between. A section at a deeper level is shown in the right panel.

the process.[50] The sebaceous glands remain normal, but in androgenetic alopecias of long evolution hyperplasia of the eccrine glands may be observed and sometimes form syringoma-like structures (*Fig. 22.47*).[51,52]

In deeper sections, hair bulbs are present at different depths, and they may be completely absent focally, with only follicular stellae remaining. These stellae are seen in a variety of conditions and reflect either miniaturized

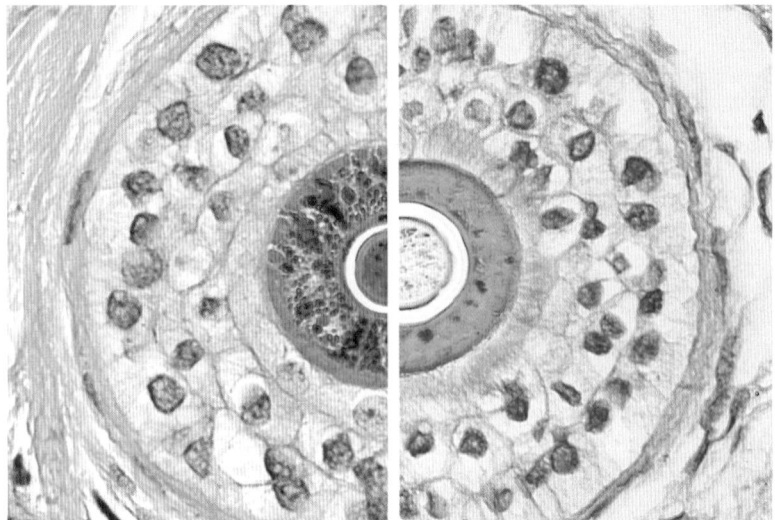

Fig. 22.42
Miniaturized hair follicle. Compare the staining of the inner root sheath on the left (red with hematoxylin and eosin) with the one on the right (blue with toluidine blue).

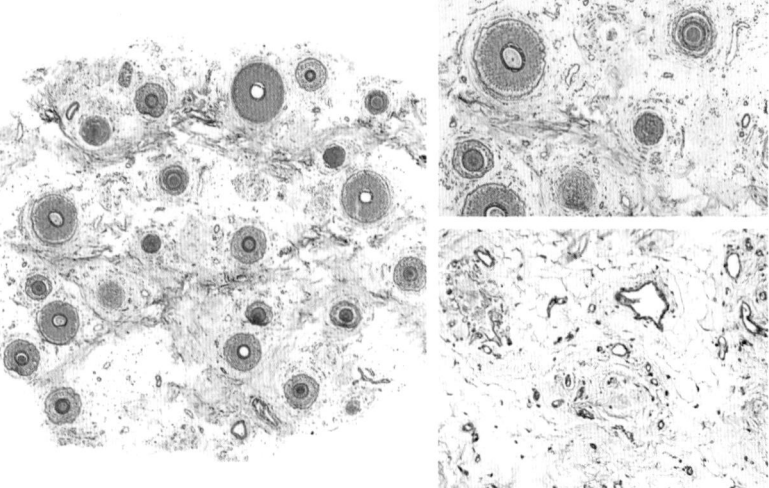

Fig. 22.44
Androgenetic alopecia: in this more advanced example, the follicular density is greatly reduced with many miniaturized hair follicles (*left*) and numerous stellae (*right*). Toluidine blue stain.

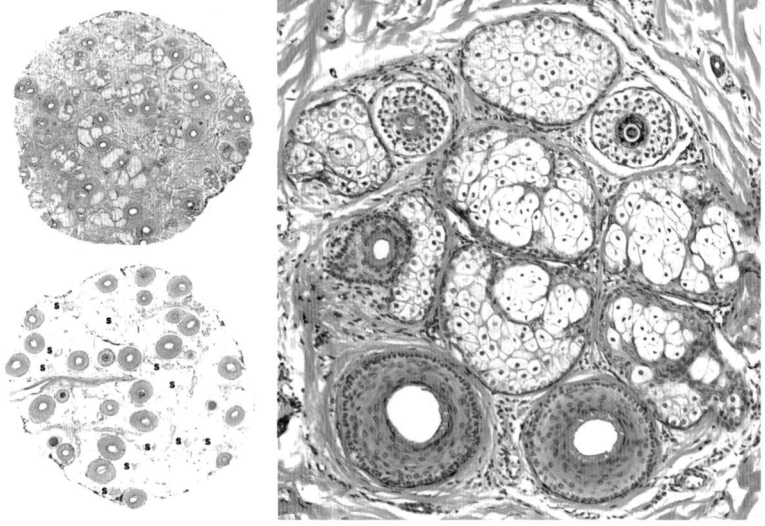

Fig. 22.43
Androgenetic alopecia, horizontal sections: (*left*) this is a scalp biopsy taken from the interparietal area. In the superficial section (*top*), there are numerous miniaturized hair follicles. In the section at the level of the subcutaneous tissue (*bottom*), many of the follicles have been replaced by follicular stellae (S); (*right*) follicular units with two terminal follicles at the bottom and three miniaturized follicles at the top.

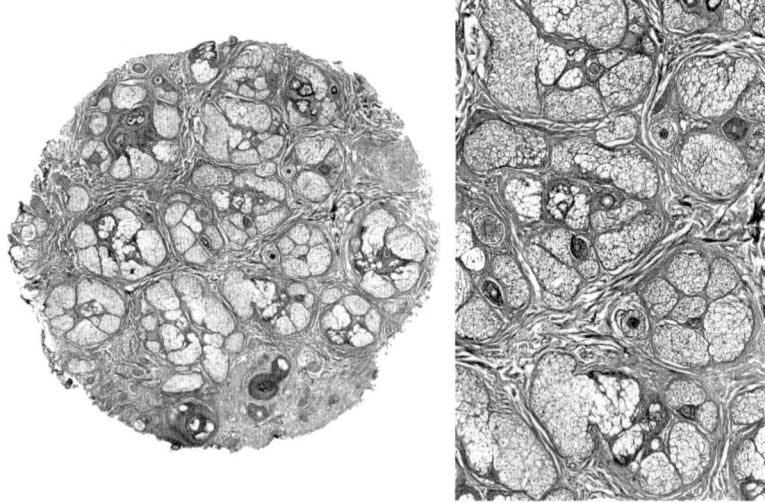

Fig. 22.45
Androgenetic alopecia: almost all hair follicles are miniaturized and the sebaceous glands appear prominent. The hair shafts are barely visible. Masson trichrome stain.

follicles or else follicles that have entered catagen or telogen stage (*Fig. 22.48*). As the stellae mature, they become less vascularized, presenting as fibrous scars with a blue-gray hue, which corresponds to condensations of elastic tissue known as Arao-Perkins bodies (*Fig. 22.49*).[53,54] In late androgenic alopecia, the stellae become abnormally thick and could impede the growth of the follicle.

The terminal/vellus hair ratio (7:1) is much reduced and varies from 1:1 or even 1:2. Although initially the number of hair follicles is normal, in longstanding disease there can be a real reduction. A biopsy may therefore show a decrease in hair follicle density in addition to diminution in size of the individual hair follicles. Sometimes the appearances may be more suggestive of a scarring alopecia (*Fig. 22.50*).

Differential diagnosis

The most important differential diagnosis is with diseases which present with diffuse nonscarring alopecia including chronic telogen effluvium,

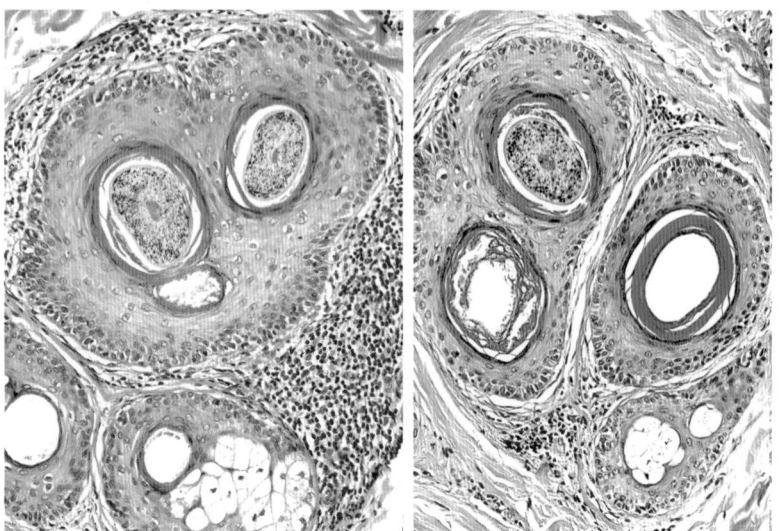

Fig. 22.46
Compound hair infundibulum surrounded by a lymphocytic infiltrate and mild concentric fibrosis in a patient with androgenetic alopecia.

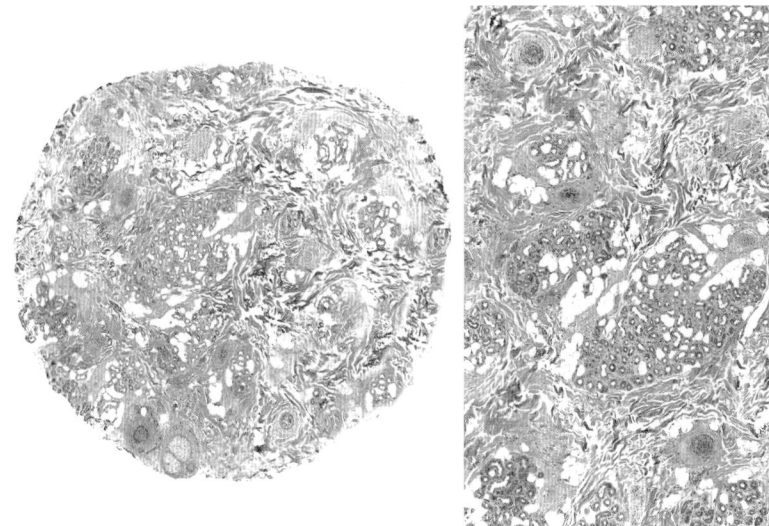

Fig. 22.47
Sweat gland duct proliferation. Case of advanced androgenetic alopecia with follicular structures replaced by lobules of hyperplastic sweat glands and ducts.

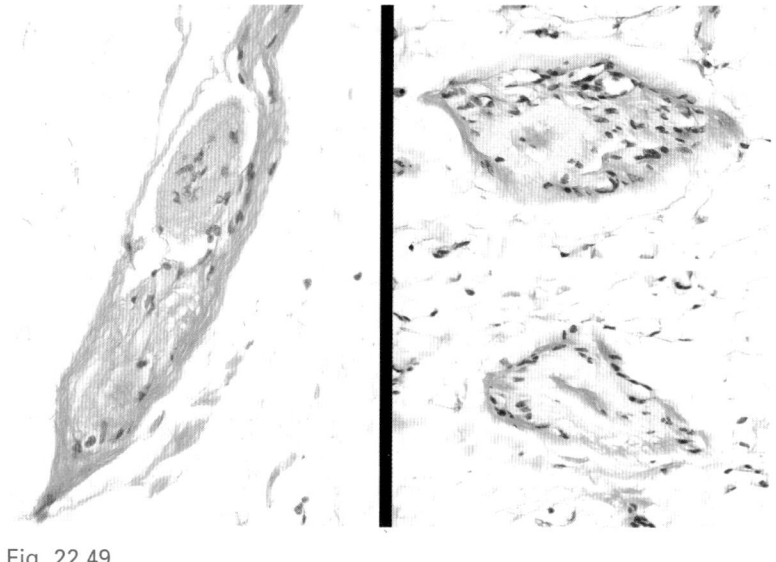

Fig. 22.49
Arao-Perkins bodies, in vertical (*left*) and horizontal (*right*) sections. Note the collagenous and elastotic material deposited in the center of the follicular stellae.

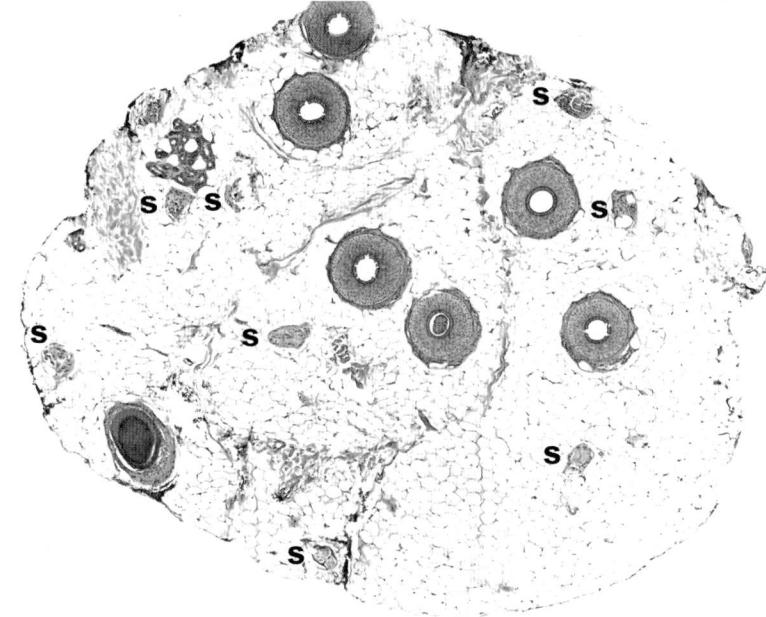

Fig. 22.48
Androgenetic alopecia, follicular stellae; as the follicles undergo miniaturization they leave behind numerous follicular stellae (S).

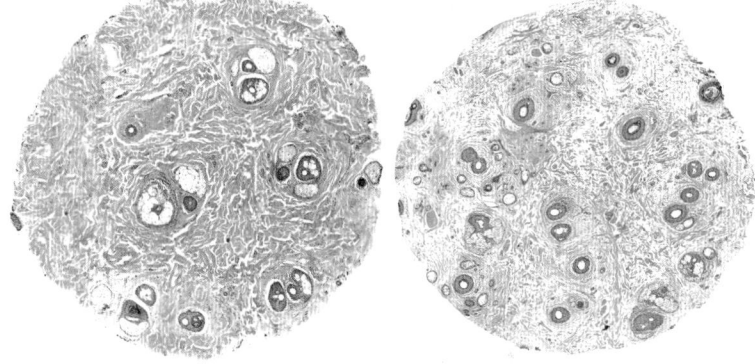

Fig. 22.50
Androgenetic alopecia, final stage: follicular units and miniaturized hair follicles are rare. In this advanced stage, connective tissue has almost completely replaced follicular structures and the appearance resembles a scarring alopecia. In the section on the right, upper part, a syringoma-like proliferation of sweat ducts is observed.

alopecia areata, and fibrosing alopecia in a pattern distribution. In such cases, a biopsy is crucial to reach an accurate diagnosis.

Although androgenetic alopecia may show increased numbers of telogen hairs, telogen effluvium is clinically more diffuse and there are no miniaturized hair follicles. The biopsy from the occipital region is of great value in order to record whether or not the follicular involvement is diffuse. It is important, however, to note that both diseases may present simultaneously and that chronic telogen effluvium may uncover occult androgenetic alopecia.

Alopecia areata may show miniaturized hair follicles, particularly in its diffuse form and in very chronic cases. Characteristically, however, there is a prominent increase in the number of hair follicles in catagen and telogen, and usually a sparse peribulbar lymphocytic infiltrate is present, sometimes accompanied by eosinophils. Without adequate clinical information, however, distinction may be impossible.

In fibrosing alopecia in pattern distribution (*Fig. 22.51*) the lymphocytic inflammatory cell infiltrate affects the infundibulum and the follicular isthmus and there is epithelial and bulge cell destruction. Additionally,

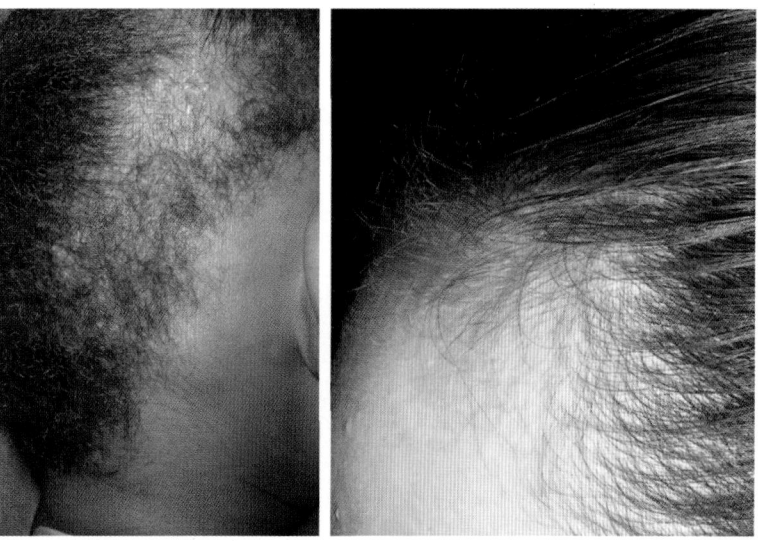

Fig. 22.51
Traction alopecia, ophiasis and frontal fibrosing alopecia pattern of hair loss. The patient on the left with the ophiasis pattern also has a superimposed tinea.
Courtesy of L.M. Gómez, MD, UPB, Medellín, Colombia.

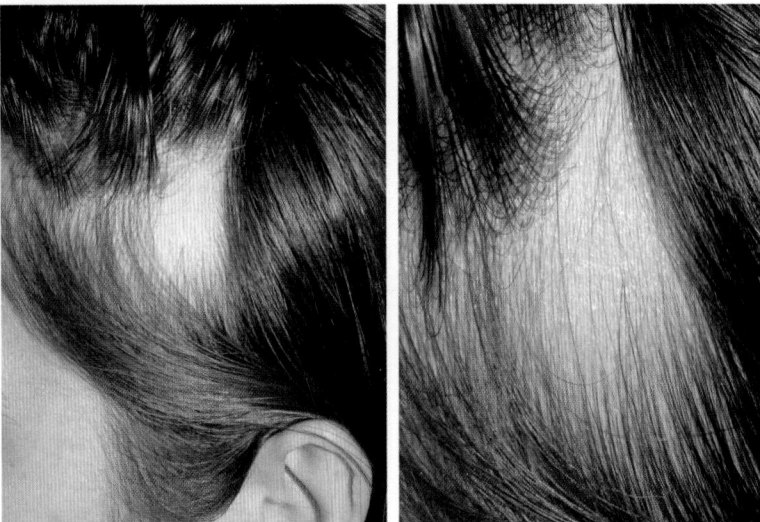

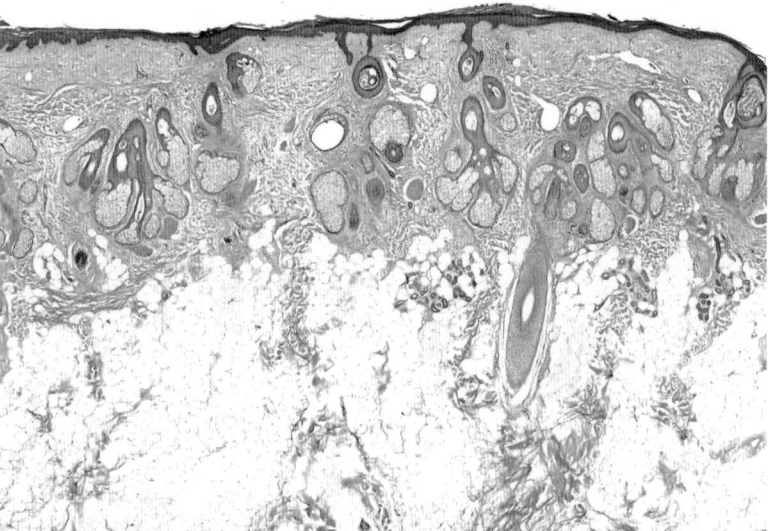

Fig. 22.52
Triangular alopecia: note the characteristic triangular patch of alopecia. In the right panel, a close-up view shows absence of inflammatory changes. Courtesy of A.M. Aristizábal, MD, CES, Medellín, Colombia.

Fig. 22.53
Triangular alopecia: this biopsy is taken from the edge of a lesion. One terminal hair follicle is present on the right side of the field (unaffected scalp). There are no stellae or inflammatory cells.

there are apoptotic bodies, perifollicular fibrosis, and early loss of sebaceous glands.[55–57]

Temporal triangular alopecia

Clinical features

Temporal triangular alopecia (congenital triangular alopecia, Brauer nevus)[1] was described by Saboreau in 1905.[2] Although it usually appears in the early years of life rather than at birth, congenital cases are not rare.[3–5] Familial cases rarely occur.[6] Occasionally, the disease presents in adults.[7,8] In the general population, the estimated incidence is 0.11%.[9]

It involves one side of the scalp and characteristically presents as a single patch of alopecia with its base directed toward the frontotemporal area.[5] Occasionally, other areas are affected and, exceptionally, patients show bilateral involvement.[8] Clinical examination reveals vellus hairs in the almost complete absence of terminal hairs and inflammatory changes (Fig. 22.52).

Temporal triangular alopecia has been described in association with aplasia cutis, phakomatosis pigmentovascularis, Down syndrome, Klippel-Trénaunay syndrome, mental retardation and epilepsy, in a mother and daughter, leopard syndrome, and congenital heart disease with renal and genital abnormalities.[9,10–16]

Pathogenesis and histologic features

The genetic basis of the disease is uncertain, but a paradominant trait has been suggested.[14–17]

The diagnosis of temporal triangular alopecia is generally based on clinical features. A biopsy is only taken when the diagnosis is in doubt. Horizontal sections may be performed, paying particular attention to the most superficial sections at the level of the infundibulum.

The epidermis and dermis are normal, but there are almost no terminal hairs and the number of vellus hairs is increased. The sebaceous and eccrine glands are normal. Fibrous stellae and inflammation are absent (Fig. 22.53). In general, the histologic appearance is very similar to that of a normal skin biopsy.[18]

Differential diagnosis

The differential diagnosis includes other causes of circumscribed nonscarring alopecia, particularly alopecia areata, tinea capitis, and trichotillomania. In the former, the bulbs of anagen follicles are surrounded and infiltrated by lymphocytes and there are terminal and miniaturized hair follicles cycling to catagen and telogen. In tinea capitis, the demonstration of fungal organisms

by hydroxide potassium (KOH) or PAS and/or culture of the hair shaft are sufficient to establish a diagnosis. Clinical examination in trichotillomania reveals broken hairs. Histologically, besides pigmentary casts, terminal hair follicles – many of them in catagen and telogen – may be seen.[19–21]

Alopecia areata

Clinical features

Alopecia areata is quite common, affecting up to 1% of the population. The frequency of a family history is very high, ranging from 10% up to 42% of cases. It is more common in individuals between 15 and 40 years of age, and about 60% of cases occur before the age of 20.[1] The disease is very rare in newborns and young children.[2] Exceptionally, however, congenital cases may occur.[3]

The degree of involvement is very variable and can range from very mild disease where the hair loss is difficult to detect through to very severe cases with diffuse hair loss affecting the entire scalp or even the whole body (Fig. 22.54). Any hair-bearing surface may be affected. A typical patient presents with an abrupt development of patches of nonscarring alopecia in different patterns: circumscribed, bandlike in the temporo-occipital region (ophiasic), bandlike in the frontoparietal region in a 'sisaipho' pattern (ophiasis inversus) (Fig. 22.55),[4] and reticular. When the patches extend and become confluent, involving the entire scalp, the appearance is known as alopecia totalis (Fig. 22.56). If there is hair loss on the entire body, the condition is referred to as alopecia universalis.[5,6] Even in the most severe forms of alopecia totalis and universalis, one can observe isolated small groups of unaffected hair follicles. Alopecia areata may occasionally present with a pattern mimicking acute telogen effluvium, a positive pull test, and trichodynia (alopecia areata incognita).[7] The proportion of patients who eventually develop alopecia totalis and universalis varies but is around 7%.[8] Alopecia totalis is more frequent in children.[9]

Examination of the involved scalp generally reveals that except for the absence of hair, the skin appears normal, follicular openings are preserved, and there is no evidence of scarring (Fig. 22.57). In occasional cases, however, edema and erythema are observed.

Hair color may appear normal or it may show mild lightening and loss of sheen. In the periphery of the patches of alopecia, one typically finds exclamation mark hairs, which are short and become thinner as they gradually approach the scalp. They are a very characteristic feature but may also be seen in trichotillomania.[10] Sometimes, the damage to the hair follicles in

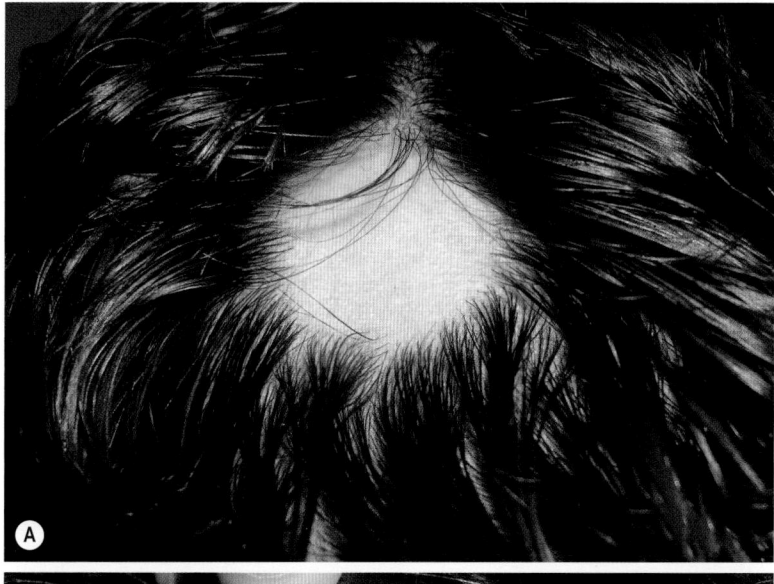

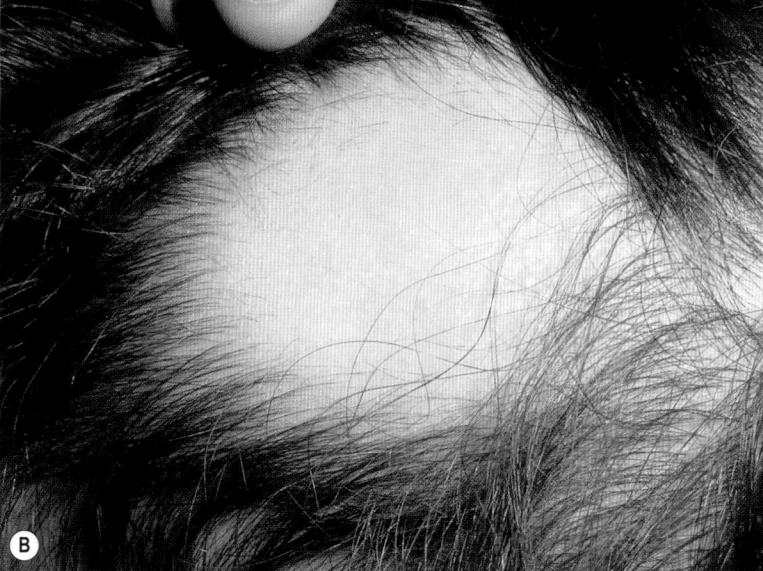

Fig. 22.54
(**A**, **B**) Alopecia areata: typical annular noninflammatory areas of alopecia. Courtesy of L.M. Gómez, MD, UPB, Colombia.

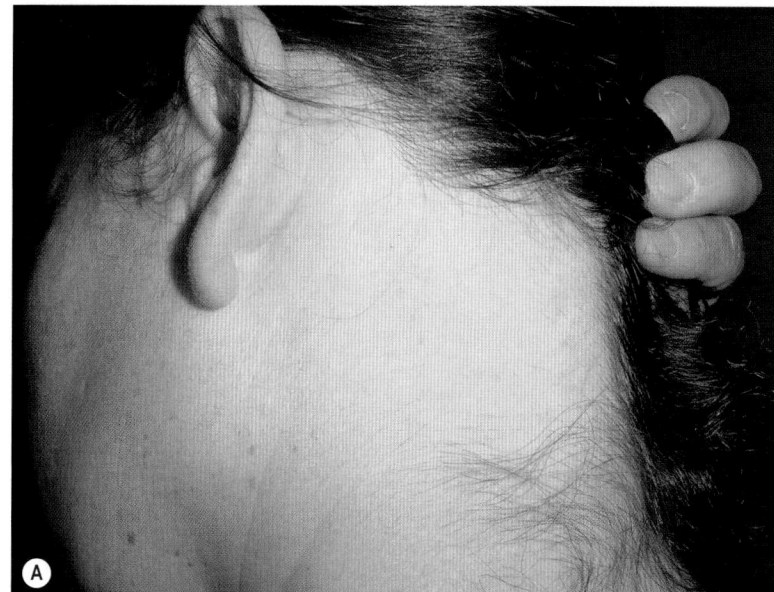

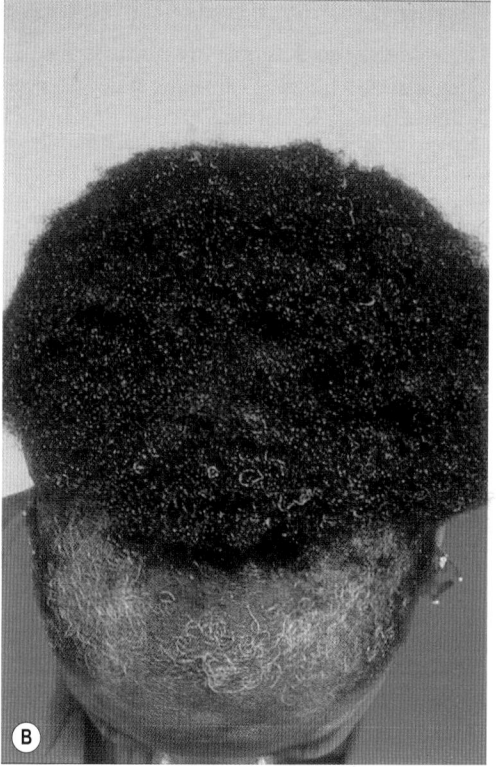

Fig. 22.55
Alopecia areata: (**A**) this broad band of alopecia in the occipital region is known as ophiasis. (**B**) A similar pattern in the frontoparietal region it is known as ophiasis inversus, or a 'sisaipho' pattern. Courtesy of the Institute of Dermatology, London, UK.

anagen is so intense that the hairs break as soon as they emerge from the scalp. A dermoscopy finding consist of yellow dots, found in 95% of cases of the disease.[11] The process usually affects pigmented hairs. Nonpigmented hairs appear to be more resistant, at least temporarily. This phenomenon of selective black hair loss where the gray hair is spared may give the impression of speedy graying (Marie Antoinette syndrome).[12] When the hair grows back, it is often white or light brown and slowly recovers its normal color. Exceptionally, persistent white hair is a feature.

Alopecia areata sparing a congenital nevus of the eyebrow and a nevus flammeus has been called Renbök phenomenon (inverse Koebner phenomenon) and interpreted as a localized form of genetic resistance.[13,14]

Nail changes may be present in patients with alopecia areata and include pitting, spotted lunula, and red lunula. Changes may be seen in one, several, or all of the nails (*Fig. 22.58*). Trachyonychia (twenty-nail dystrophy) occurs in up to 3% of patients.[15–19] The dystrophy may precede, coincide with, or occur after resolution of the episode of alopecia.[20]

Alopecia areata has been associated with many other diseases. Some of these have an autoimmune etiology such as Hashimoto thyroiditis, type I (insulin-dependent) diabetes, Addison disease, vitiligo, hereditary thrombocytopenia (pseudo-von Willebrand disease), myasthenia gravis, polymorphism in the interleukin (IL)-1 receptor antagonist gene, lupus erythematosus, autoimmune polyendocrinopathy-candidiasis-ectodermal dysplasia syndrome (autoimmune polyglandular syndrome-1), common variable immunodeficiency, relapsing polychondritis, kidney-pancreas transplant recipients taking ciclosporine and after allogeneic bone marrow transplantation.[21–35] Other associations include lichen planus, atopy, human immunodeficiency virus (HIV) infection, twenty-nail dystrophy, Down syndrome, cytomegalovirus and Epstein-Barr virus infection, celiac disease in children, chemotherapy, interferon-alpha (IFN-α), ribavirin, ciclosporine A, rifampicin, borderline tuberculoid leprosy, and ocular alterations (keratoconus, symptomless punctate lens opacities).[22,36–48] It has also been observed in Clozapine-induced hypereosinophilia, narcolepsy type 1, and as recurrent disease after vaccination.[49–51] Several biological agents such as etanercept, infliximab, and adalimumab are associated with the appearance or worsening of the illness.[52–54] It has also developed in a patient with pili annulati.[55] Patients with severe alopecia areata appear to have an increased incidence of nuchal nevus flammeus.[56]

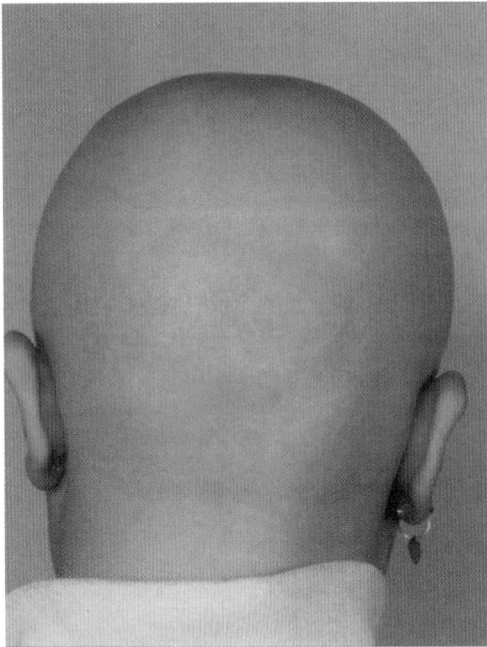

Fig. 22.56
Alopecia areata totalis: in this patient, there is complete loss of scalp hair.
Courtesy of the Institute of Dermatology, London, UK.

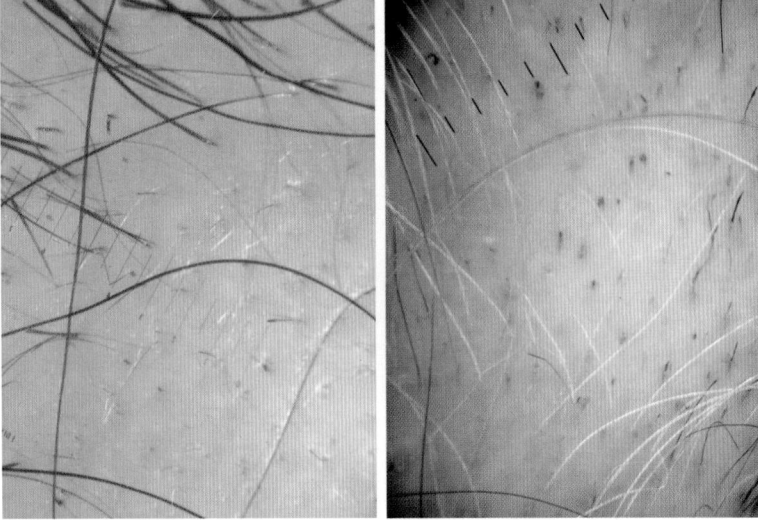

Fig. 22.57
Alopecia areata dermoscopy: note that the follicular density is normal and the
opening of the follicles have not been lost. There are some miniaturized hair
follicles and an exclamation mark hair. On the right panel, yellow dots are
observed. The gray hairs have persisted despite the loss of the pigmented hair.
There are also some exclamation mark hairs. Courtesy of L.M. Gómez, MD, UPB,
Medellín, Colombia.

Prognosis in alopecia areata is variable and not very predictable in the
individual patient.[57] Nevertheless, it has been observed that the prognosis tends to be good in patients who have experienced hair growth with
long-lasting remissions between episodes. Spontaneous remission can be
expected in 34–50% of patients within 1 year, although almost all will
experience more than one episode of the disease.[58] Contrariwise, those who
have had persistent hair loss or brief or incomplete remissions have a poor
prognosis. The severity of alopecia areata at the time of first consultation
and response to therapy is an important prognostic factor.[59] The outlook is
particularly poor in those patients with onset of the disease before puberty,
those with a family history of the disease (present in 25% of cases), and
those with alopecia totalis and alopecia universalis.[7] Atopic patients appear
to suffer a more severe form of alopecia areata.

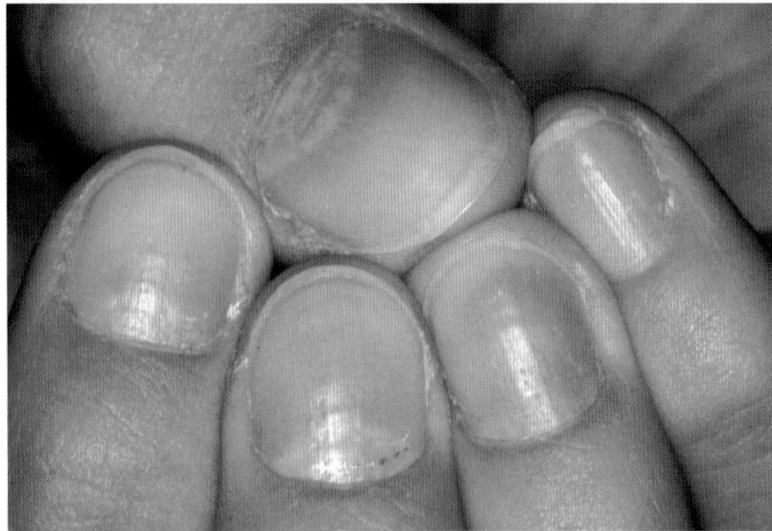

Fig. 22.58
Alopecia areata: in this patient, there is severe involvement of the nails
(trachyonychia). Courtesy of P. Reygagne, MD, Centre Sabouraud, Paris, France.

Pathogenesis and histologic features

Experimental studies have shown that alopecia areata is basically an
organ-specific autoimmune disease thought to result from a collapse of
hair follicle immune privilege, driven by cellular immunity with autoantibody production representing a secondary phenomenon.[60–62] Autoantibodies
to a diverse range of antigens including smooth muscle cells, gastric parietal cells, thyroid cells, and components of anagen hair follicles have been
described.[62–65]

It is unknown whether induction of the disease results from exposure to
exogenous or endogenous antigens and whether it represents a consequence
of an immune reaction to normal or aberrant epitopes. However, research
suggests that the pathogenesis involves at least four events:

- failure of the anagen hair follicle to maintain its privileged immunity
  (the inner root sheath and hair matrix do not express, or express
  very low level of, major histocompatibility complex class Ia antigens
  and maintains an active NK cell suppression) resulting in exposure of
  epitopes, which initiate an immune response,[66,67]
- antigen presentation, activation, and response of the lymphocyte to
  antigen-presenting cells,
- migration of activated inflammatory cells and infiltration of hair
  follicles,
- damage to the hair follicle by the inflammatory cell infiltrate.[68]

It has been proposed that neurotrophins play a role in the pathogenesis
of the disease. Since neurotrophins and their receptors are differentially
expressed in subsets of immune cells in alopecia areata, a role for these
proteins in the pathogenesis appears likely.[69]

The increased frequency of alopecia areata in genetically related individuals suggests that there is a genetic link to the disease. Among the general
population the condition does not display a mendelian pattern of expression
since the resulting phenotype demonstrates variable degrees of hair loss. It
has been proposed that expression of alopecia areata involves a complex
interaction of multiple genes, in which major genes control susceptibility to
the disease while other minor ones modify the phenotype.[70]

Many illnesses with an autoimmune basis have been associated with specific human leukocytic antigens (HLA). Alopecia areata has been studied in
association with both HLA class I and class II. The most relevant associations have been found with the HLA class II antigens (HLA-DR, -DQ, -DP).
The molecular basis of this genetic association is supported by the fact that
HLA binds and presents peptides derived from self and foreign protein antigens to the immune system for recognition and activation. More than 80%
of all cases evaluated in one study were positive for the antigen DQB1*03
(DQ3), suggesting that this antigen is a marker for susceptibility. Furthermore, in patients with alopecia totalis and universalis, the frequency of the

antigens DRB1*0401 and DBQ1*0301 (DR4 and DQ7) is significantly increased.[71-73] HLA-DR5 has been linked to the early-onset and severe form of alopecia areata. Other HLA genes associated are NOTCH4 and MICA. Non-HLA genes associated with the disease are PTPN22 and AIRE.[74]

In the last genome study supported by the genetic database of the national registry of alopecia areata in the United States, 139 nucleotides with polymorphism and significantly associated with alopecia areata were identified.[64] There were eight different associated regions. One of such regions corresponds to the already well-known HLA complex. Seven loci genomes were also found. Five of them are expressed in the immunological system and two of them in the hair follicle. Interestingly, these genes were more related to illnesses such as diabetes type I, multiple sclerosis, rheumatoid arthritis, and celiac disease, rather than to psoriasis and vitiligo diseases to which they were initially thought to be associated.[75-77] These diseases present a unifying mechanism known as ULBP3, which is the enhancement of the regulation of the danger signal in the target organ. Under normal circumstances, ULBP3 is not found in hair follicles, but in the affected hair follicles of alopecia areata it is prominent. These proteins attract the killer cells marked by the receptor NKG2D.[78]

The effect of stress on the pathogenesis is unclear and controversial, although it has been suggested that it can trigger the disease. It has been observed that substance P and nerve growth factor could be acting as key mediators of stress-induced hair growth-inhibitory effects, through keratinocyte apoptosis, inhibition of hair follicle proliferation, and catagen induction.[79,80]

Laboratory tests are not usually necessary for the diagnosis, but they may be of value in detecting associated conditions, particularly autoimmune disease. The hair-pull and hair-pluck tests show an increase in the number of telogen and dystrophic anagen hairs. The remaining anagen hairs are dystrophic because the continuous inflammatory process results in premature transformation into catagen and telogen phase. This abbreviated growth cycle results in many terminal follicles with poorly keratinized short stems that break readily (exclamation mark hairs).[81]

Histologically, alopecia areata is characterized by four basic features:

- normal numbers of follicular units and hair follicles in the initial stages with loss of follicles in the recalcitrant and most chronic phases,
- an increase in the number of catagen and telogen hair follicles,
- a lymphocytic infiltrate of variable severity affecting the bulbs of the anagen hair follicles and the catagen and telogen follicular stellae,
- a tendency for hair follicles to become miniaturized in the more chronic and recalcitrants forms of the disease.

It is important to remember that the histopathological features depend on the stage of the disease.[82]

The best site to take biopsies from is the periphery of an active lesion. The extraction (hair-pull tests) and dermoscopy are useful when it comes to selecting the most active areas as one can observe exclamation point hairs, yellow dots, or black dots.[81]

All the changes in alopecia areata described in vertical sections are better observed in horizontal sections (Fig. 22.59).[83] This is particularly true of hair bulb lymphocytic infiltration. Nevertheless, the inflammatory infiltrate is not always visible. The frequency with which this and other histologic changes are observed depends on the stage of the illness when the biopsy is performed.

Early stages

In the early stages of the disease, the peribulbar inflammatory infiltrate is intense (Fig. 22.60). However, the infiltrate gradually decreases and there

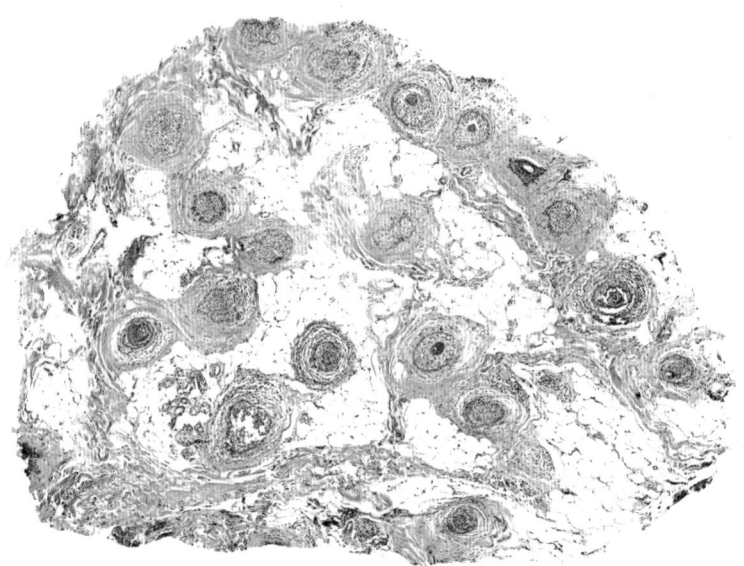

Fig. 22.59
Alopecia areata: Horizontal section displays a near normal density of hair follicles; some of the follicles on the left upper side are in catagen and telogen. Courtesy of J.C. Perez, MD, HPTU, Medellín, Colombia.

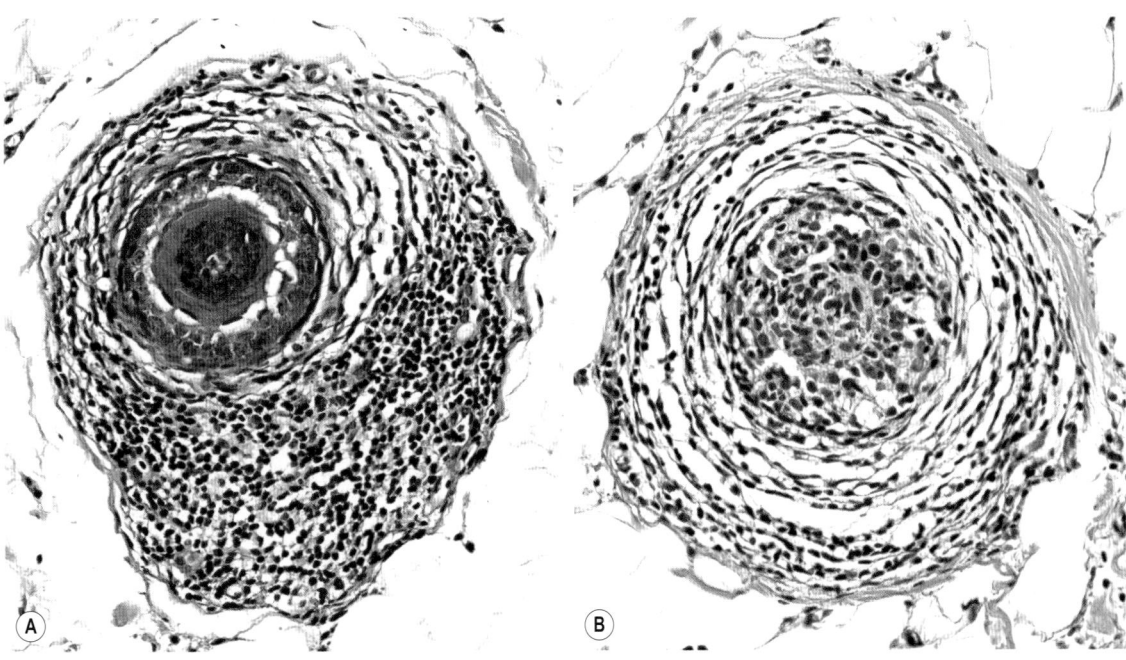

Fig. 22.60
(A, B) Alopecia areata: high-power view of the peribulbar lymphocytic infiltrate, which is sometimes referred to as 'swarm of bees'. Note (from left to right) that as the pili bulb disappears the inflammatory infiltrate becomes less dense.

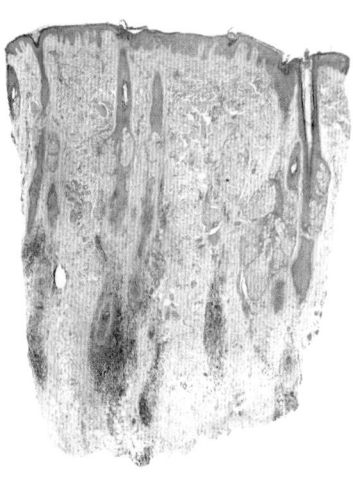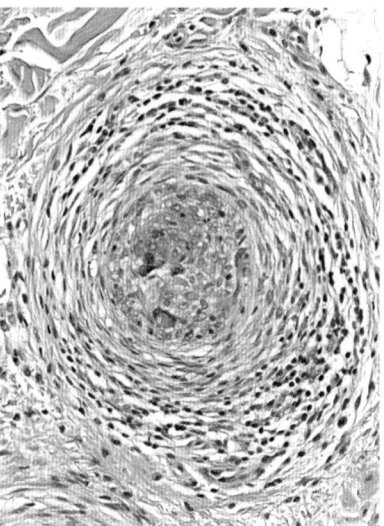

Fig. 22.61
Alopecia areata: vertical and horizontal sections of catagen-telogen hair bulbs. The inflammatory infiltrate is still present in the telogen remnants.

is an increase in the number of catagen and telogen hair follicles. Telogen counts may exceed those seen in telogen effluvium (*Fig. 22.61*). The follicles show a variable inflammatory lymphocytic infiltrate in the peribulbar region (*Figs 22.60 and 22.62*). This may occasionally be very mild, even in more active lesions. The latter feature is particularly noticeable in the atypical, incognita, and ophiasic forms of the disease (*Fig. 22.63*). The presence of eosinophils in the stellae and within the hair bulbs has been described as an early and typical feature.[84] The earliest follicular changes consist of loss of structural integrity of the centrally located supramatrical upper bulbar region and shrinkage of hair bulbs.[85] The hair matrix is infiltrated by lymphocytes, and there is also pigment incontinence, matrix cell necrosis, and vacuolar damage. The inflammatory infiltrate is especially prominent in terminal hair follicles, the bulbs of which are located in the subcutaneous tissue (*Fig. 22.64*). Pigment incontinence may be very conspicuous and lead to the formation of clumps of melanin pigment (pigment casts) in the distorted hair bulb and follicular streamer (*Fig. 22.65*).[86] The infiltrate is composed of an admixture of CD4+ and CD8+ T lymphocytes (*Fig. 22.66*).[87]

In the upper part of the hair follicle within the epidermis, one can observe dilated infundibulae filled with keratin which correspond to the yellow dots seen clinically (*Fig. 22.67* and see *Fig. 22.57*). Those in horizontal sections could display a swiss cheese pattern.[88]

Immunofluorescence studies have shown deposits of C3, IgG, and IgM along the basement membrane of the inferior part of the hair follicle.[89] Once the follicle enters catagen stage and progresses to telogen, the inflammatory cell infiltrate decreases.[90]

Follicular lymphocytic infiltration is accompanied by progression to catagen and telogen. After this, the hair follicle rapidly returns to anagen and the cycle starts again. Because of this continuous cycle and the accompanying inflammatory process, the follicles go through two important morphological changes:

- trichomalacia characterized by short, incompletely keratined (pencil-point) hairs which are susceptible to trauma,
- miniaturization of some anagen follicles.

Late stage

In the late stage of the disease, the inflammation decreases and numerous miniaturized hair follicles and telogen follicles are present. The number of miniaturized follicles increases with chronicity, and these may simulate hair follicles in late anagen stage. Such hairs are found in the middle or upper dermis and have been described as nanogen. They represent an intermediate stage between vellus and terminal anagen hair follicles. In horizontal sections there is generally no hair shaft production, although occasionally a very thin incompletely keratinized form is produced, correlating with the empty infundibula observed on the scalp. In vertical sections the proximal

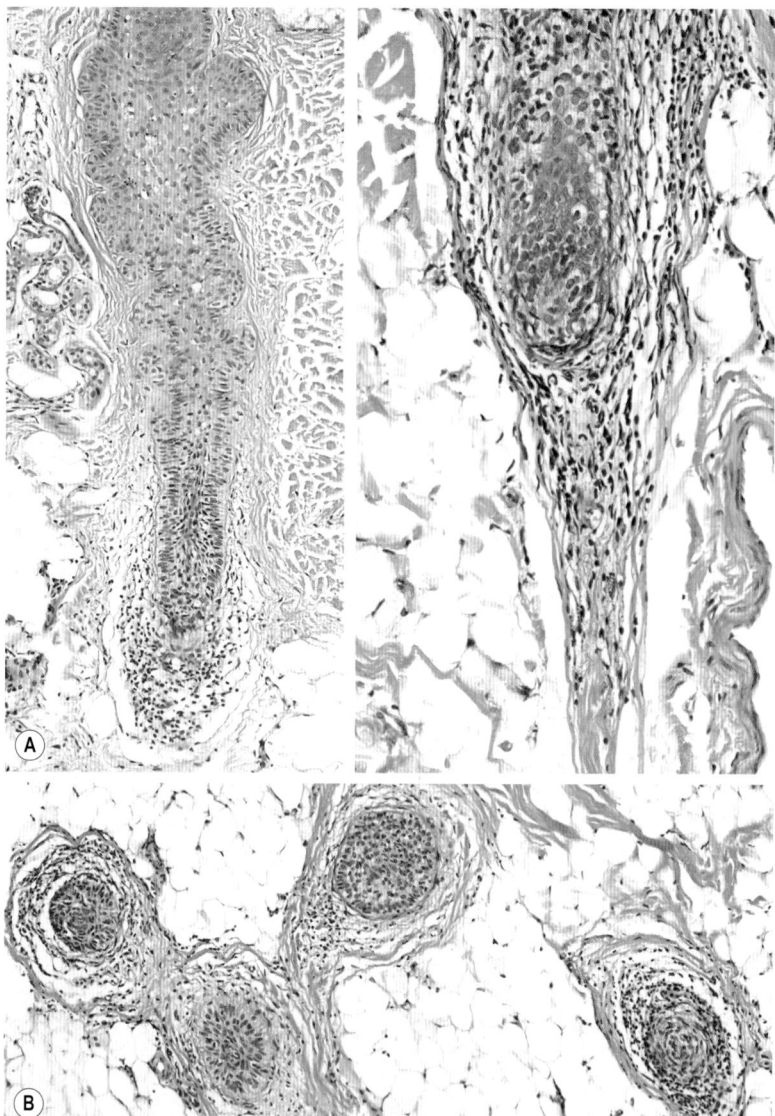

Fig. 22.62
Alopecia areata: hair follicle in involution. (**A**) Vertical section. In the follicle on the right there is a hair bulb lymphocytic infiltrate which also involves the follicular stella. (**B**) Horizontal section. Hair follicles in the subcutaneous tissue with a lymphocyte infiltrate of variable intensity.

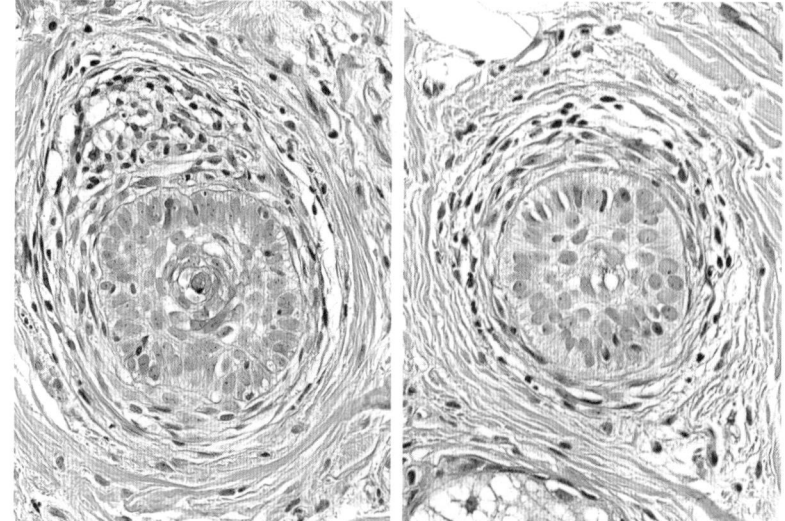

Fig. 22.63
Alopecia areata incognita: follicles in telogen. The hair follicle on the right displays features of a follicle in nanogen. There is a lymphocytic infiltrate associated with eosinophils and masts cells.

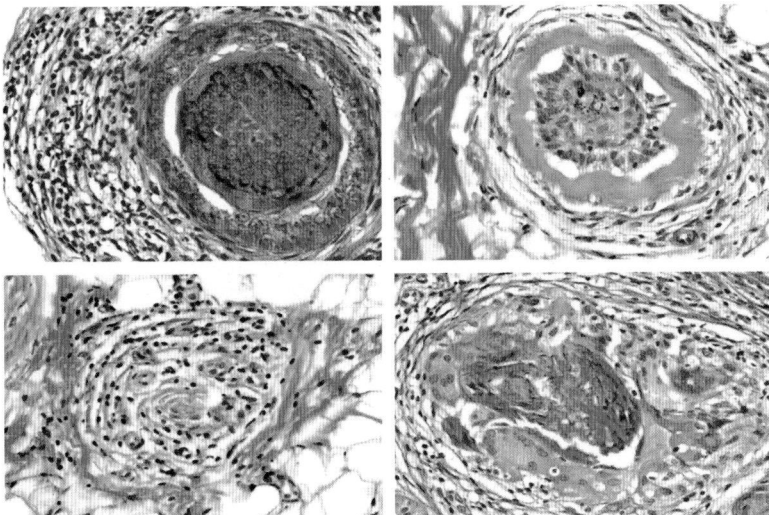

Fig. 22.64
Alopecia areata: in the top panel, the hair bulb is infiltrated by lymphocytes and progresses into a catagen hair follicle with a thick eosinophilic basement membrane. The lower panel shows follicular stellae with a lymphocytic infiltrate and destruction of the follicle by a granulomatous inflammatory cell infiltrate composed of epithelioid histiocytes and giant cells. The images shown here are at the level of the subcutaneous tissue.

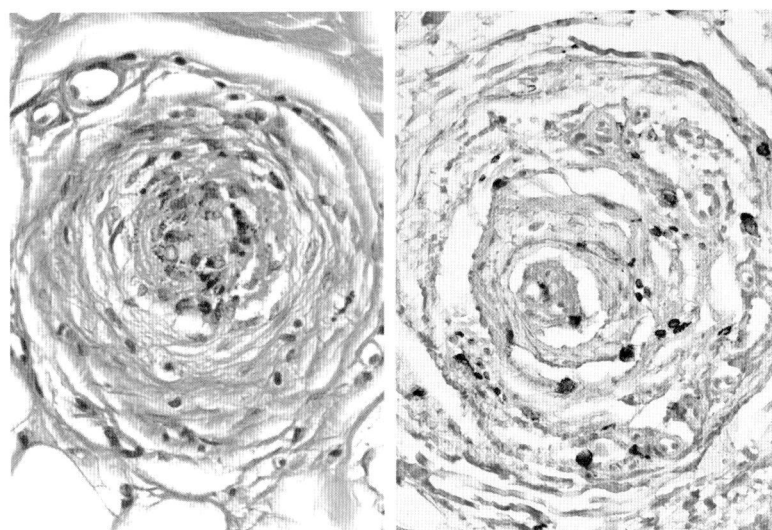

Fig. 22.65
Alopecia areata, follicular stella: note the sparse inflammatory cell infiltrate with numerous melanophages.

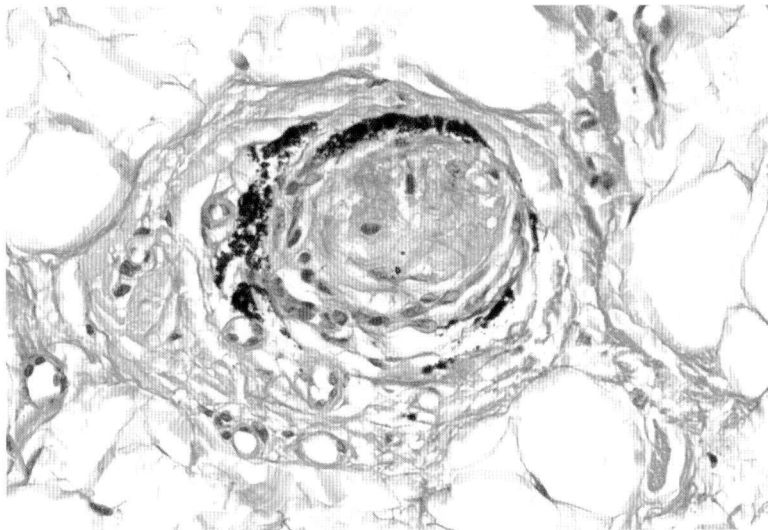

Fig. 22.66
Alopecia areata, follicular stella. The lymphocytes are highlighted by immunohistochemistry (CD3).

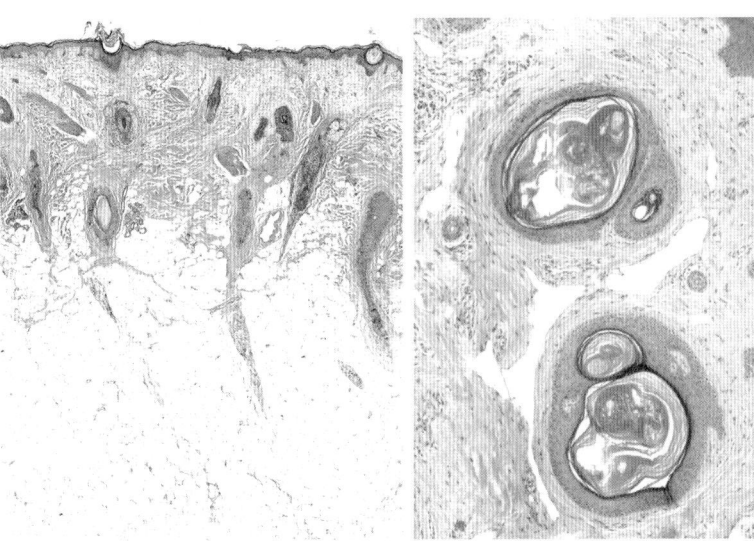

Fig. 22.67
Alopecia areata, dilated infundibulae. On the left vertical sections and on the right horizontal sections showing a swiss cheese appearance due to dilated follicles. These correspond to the yellow dots seen clinically.

end of the hair shaft acquires a ragged appearance instead of the normal club shape. These hair follicles can sometimes display histologic features of the anagen, catagen, and telogen phases simultaneously with evidence of growth and involution in the form of mitotic activity and apoptosis (*Fig. 22.68*).

In longstanding alopecia areata, the majority of the hair follicles are in catagen and telogen. Since the inflammatory infiltrate does not affect hair follicles in these growth phases, inflammation may be absent in the subcutaneous tissue (*Fig. 22.69*).[82,91]

Inactive alopecia areata can resemble androgenetic alopecia with many miniaturized hair follicles (*Fig. 22.70*).

Numerous stellae are present in the deep dermis and the subcutaneous tissue, and these may be accompanied by an inflammatory cell infiltrate and melanin pigment (*Fig. 22.71*). In some cases, there may be destruction of the hair follicle by the inflammatory cell infiltrate and this is associated with histiocytes and giant cells (see *Fig. 22.64*).

In patients presenting with trachyonychia, a nail biopsy usually shows a lymphocytic infiltrate with exocytosis and spongiosis involving the proximal nail fold, nail matrix, nail bed, and hyponychium.[18] Rarely, the histology is indistinguishable from lichen planus.

Differential diagnosis

The differential diagnosis of alopecia areata varies depending on whether the clinical pattern of hair loss is localized or diffuse.

In cases with localized areas of hair loss, the differential diagnosis includes trichotillomania, triangular temporal alopecia, syphilis, discoid lupus erythematosus, lichen planopilaris, frontal fibrosing alopecia, pseudopélade, tinea capitis, and psoriatic alopecia.

Trichotillomania may closely simulate alopecia areata but microscopic examination in the former condition shows more pigmented casts, an absence of miniaturized hairs, and minimal inflammatory infiltrate. Triangular temporal alopecia shows no clinical or histologic evidence of inflammation and there is no excess of hair follicles in telogen or catagen. Alopecia syphilitica may be very similar but clinically the plaques rarely show complete absence of hairs. Histologic examination can also be problematical since both conditions show a peribulbar inflammatory cell infiltrate. Eosinophils are not frequent in syphilis but plasma cells tend to be prominent. Serology is often essential in difficult cases.

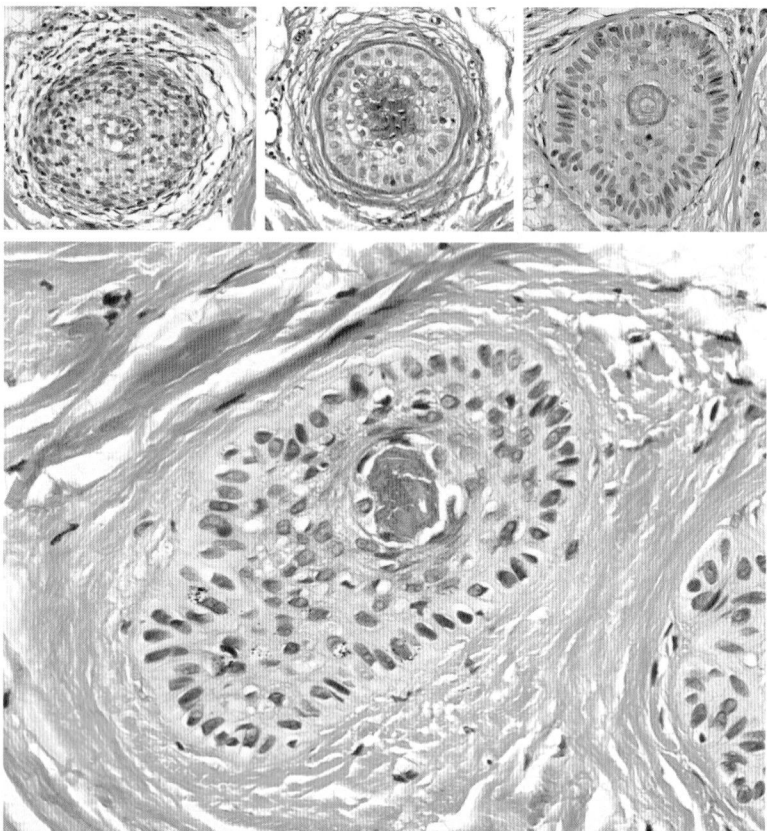

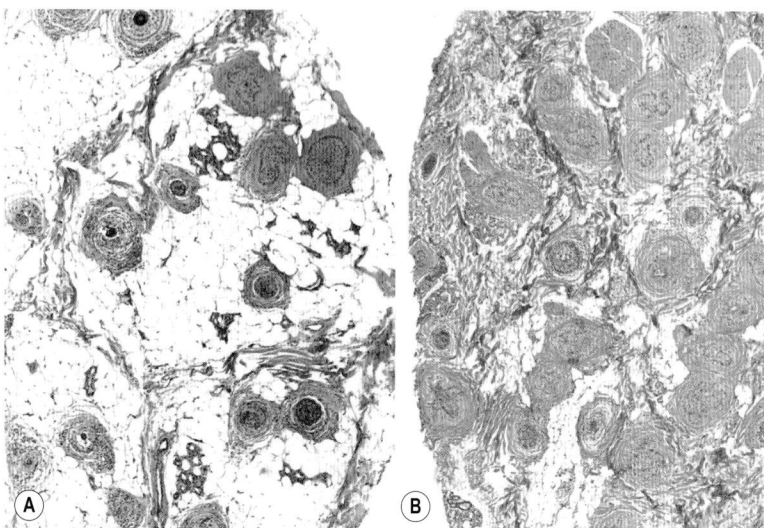

Fig. 22.68
Alopecia areata, nanogen hair: the hair follicle shows a decrease in the thickness of the epithelial component with fusion of the internal and external root sheaths. In place of a hair shaft, note detritus of amorphous keratin. The central and right top images display a follicle in telogen with a radicular internal root sheath and a malformed hair follicle.

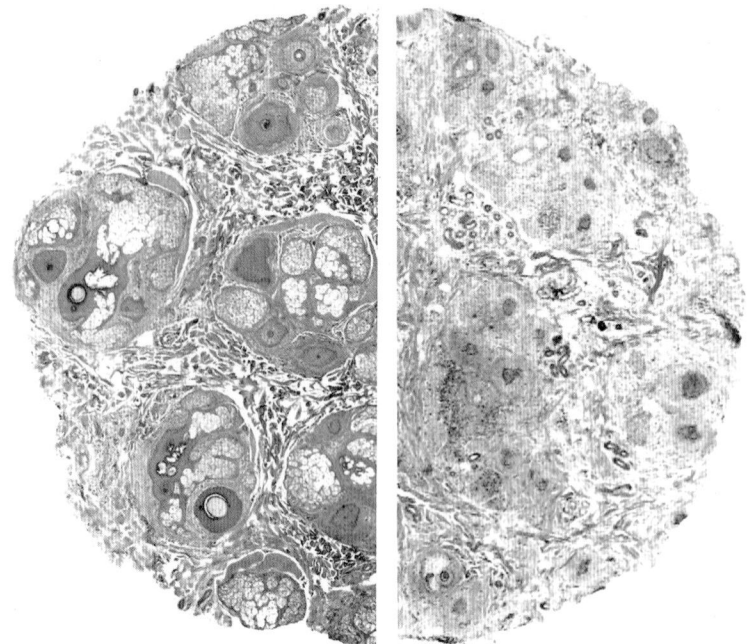

Fig. 22.70
Alopecia areata: left panel, early phase of alopecia areata; right panel, late stage. All follicles are miniaturized and the great majority are in telogen. Compare with the image on the left.

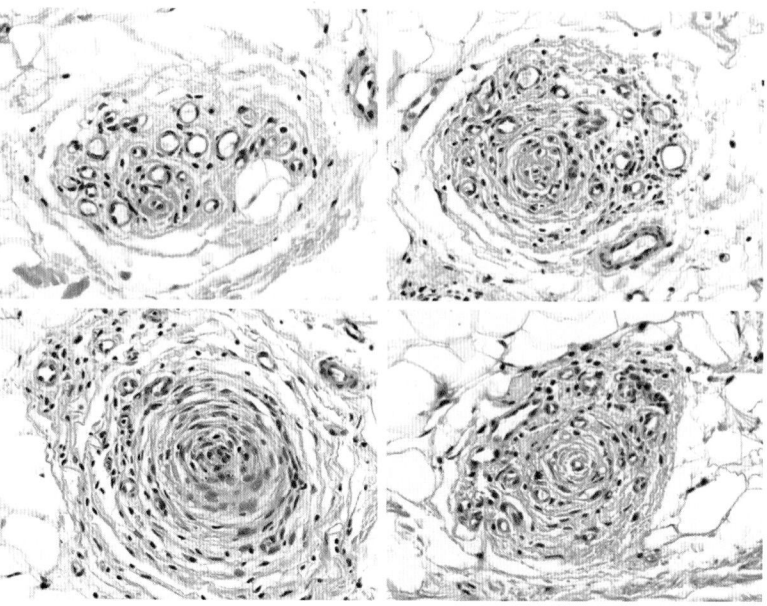

Fig. 22.71
Alopecia areata: different images of follicular stellae infiltrated by lymphocytes.

Fig. 22.69
(**A**, **B**) Alopecia areata, late stage: there is a remarkable increase in catagen/telogen follicles, and a sparse peribulbar lymphocytic infiltrate with formation of stellae.

Discoid lupus erythematosus, lichen planopilaris, and frontal fibrosing alopecia display more prominent inflammation in the upper segment of the follicle, around the bulge, and result in scarring alopecia with interface change and permanent loss of terminal hair follicles.[92] Direct immunofluorescence is useful to confirm the diagnosis in the first two conditions. Equally, the presence of dermal mucin is a diagnostic clue in discoid and systemic lupus. It is important however, to keep in mind that both entities may coexist. The incidence of alopecia areata in patients with lupus erythematosus may even reach 10%.[93] Cases of lupus panniculitis clinically simulating alopecia areata have also been described.[94] In pseudopélade, there is extensive scarring, with loss of terminal hair follicles and a mild inflammatory cell infiltrate localized to the upper segment of the follicle. Tinea capitis also shows an inflammatory infiltrate in the upper segment of the hair follicle with neutrophils, lymphocytes, and histiocytes. The fungi are usually easily found in association to the hair shaft with a PAS stain and may be grown in Sabouraud agar. Psoriatic alopecia may be distinguished by the presence of typical changes of psoriasis in the interfollicular epidermis and the atrophy of the sebaceous glands. It is important to highlight that there is a type of psoriatic alopecia/alopecia areata-like reaction secondary to antitumor necrosis factor-α therapy with simultaneous histologic changes of alopecia areata and psoriatic alopecia associated with an inflammatory cell infiltrate of plasma cells and eosinophils.[95,96]

The differential diagnosis of diffuse alopecia areata is mainly telogen effluvium and androgenetic alopecia. Clinically, telogen effluvium and androgenetic alopecia never produce such extensive hair loss as that seen in the most severe variants of alopecia areata including alopecia totalis and alopecia universalis. In the less severe cases, histologically, telogen effluvium lacks inflammation and there is only an increase in the number of telogen hair follicles. In androgenetic alopecia, the histologic presentation may be very similar to that of chronic areata alopecia as in the former the miniaturization of hairs may be very extensive. However, the lack of lymphocytic infiltration and the different clinical picture are aids in the differential diagnosis.

Alopecia areata incognita may be particularly difficult to differentiate from chronic telogen effluvium as both share a large number of hair follicles in telogen.[7,97] However, dermoscopy in the former shows the presence of a larger number of yellow dots; furthermore, there may be a greater tendency to miniaturization.[88] Recently, with the use of immunohistochemistry there has also been an emphasis in the detection of high levels of UL16 binding protein-3 (ULBP3) as an aid in the diagnosis of alopecia areata incognita[88,98]

Psoriatic alopecia

Clinical features

Psoriatic alopecia was first described in 1972 by Shuster.[1] Between 50% and 80% of patients with psoriasis will develop scalp involvement at different stages during the course of the disease.[2,3] Psoriatic alopecia may be caused by psoriasis itself, by systemic or topical therapy, or may be associated with other autoimmune diseases particularly alopecia areata.[4] The most common form of presentation is involvement of skin already affected by psoriasis (*Fig. 22.72*). Another way in which psoriasis may cause hair loss is through effluvium telogen particularly in the course of erythrodermic or generalized pustular psoriasis.[5]

The majority of the patients with psoriatic alopecia present with a reversible nonscarring alopecia. Only a small percentage of patients will develop scarring alopecia secondary to psoriasis. This seems to be related to the duration and intensity of the inflammatory process.[6–8] However, it is not always clear which patients will develop a reversible nonscarring alopecia or scarring alopecia.[3]

An association has been found between psoriatic alopecia, alopecia areata, and Renböck phenomenon.[9,10] Drugs that have been associated with psoriatic alopecia include methotrexate, hydroxyurea, retinoids, lithium, and carbamezapine[11–16] The use of tumor necrosis factor-alpha inhibitors, particularly infliximab and adalimumab, in patients with Crohn disease has also been linked with the disease.[17,18]

Pathogenesis and histologic features

The mechanism leading to atrophy and loss of sebaceous glands in psoriasis is unknown. An explanation could be that some of the numerous cytokines secreted in psoriasis are responsible for the damage to the sebaceous glands or that they are lost because of the inflammation around the superior segment of the hair follicle.[3]

Histologic changes in both scarring alopecia and nonscarring psoriatic alopecia include typical features of psoriasis in the interfollicular epithelium, namely, psoriasiform hyperplasia of the epidermis, hyper- and parakeratosis with hypogranulosis, and exocytosis of neutrophils to the areas of parakeratosis. The infundibulum becomes dilated and there is a noticeable increase in the number of catagen and telogen hair follicles, pronounced atrophy and eventual loss of sebaceous glands, and a perifollicular lymphocyte inflammatory cell infiltrate in the superior and inferior segments of the hair follicle, including the hair bulb. There may be some miniaturization. The inflammation may lead to a granulomatous foreign body reaction with follicular destruction. At a later stage perifollicular fibrosis and fibrous tracts with inflammation may be observed (*Fig. 22.73*). Sometimes the changes in the superficial epidermis closely simulate those seen in seborrheic dermatitis (*Fig. 22.74*).[3,4,7,19] Psoriatic alopecia associated with tumor necrosis factor-alpha inhibitors is histologically very similar to conventional psoriatic alopecia but more severe with a more prominent inflammatory cell infiltrate including plasma cells and eosinophils.

Differential diagnosis

The most important histologic differential diagnosis is with alopecia areata. In alopecia areata, there are no epidermal changes of psoriasis and there is no loss of sebaceous glands.

Traumatic alopecias

Traumatic alopecias are caused by physical agents that act on the scalp, inducing hair loss of variable degree that range from transitory to permanent alopecia. This section will review those traumatic alopecias in which a biopsy may be useful to establish a diagnosis. These include trichotillomania, pressure alopecia, and traction alopecia.

Trichotillomania

Clinical features

Trichotillomania was described in 1889 by Hallopeau.[1] It is a variant of traumatic alopecia caused by traction and pulling of hair.[2] It mainly affects

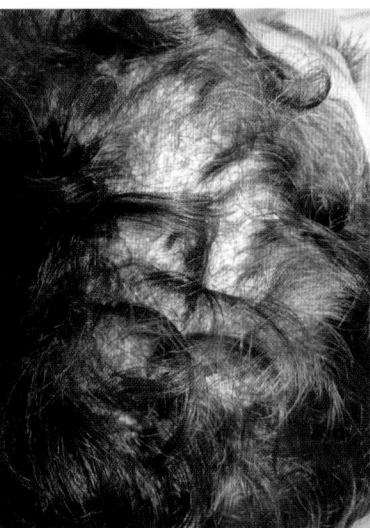
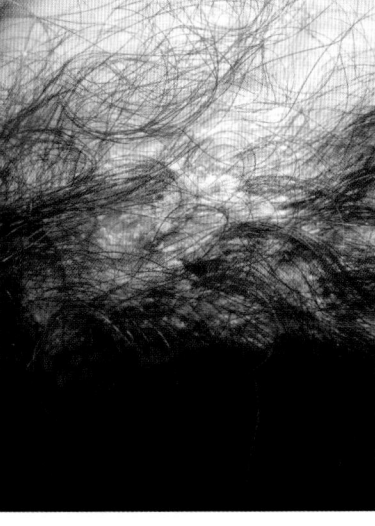

Fig. 22.72
Psoriasis. Note a thick scale covering an area of alopecia simulating tinea capitis. Courtesy of C. Velázquez, MD, CES, Medellín, Colombia.

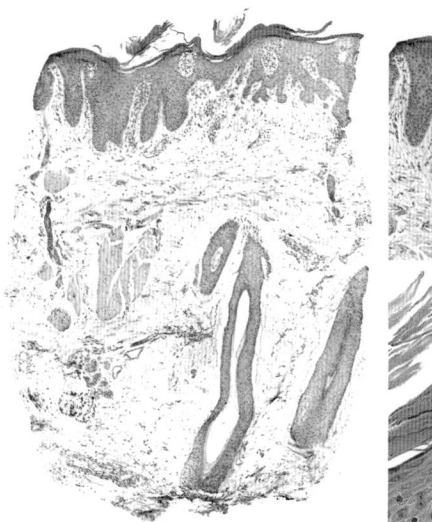
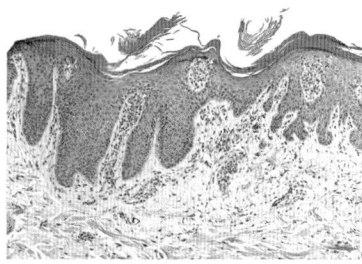
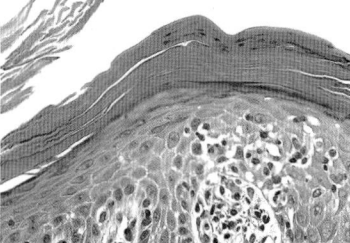

Fig. 22.73
Psoriasis. On the left the loss of sebaceous glands and follicular units is evident. On the right panel epidermal psoriatic changes including elongation of the rete ridges, hyperkeratosis, parakeratosis, hypogranulosis and corneal neutrophils.

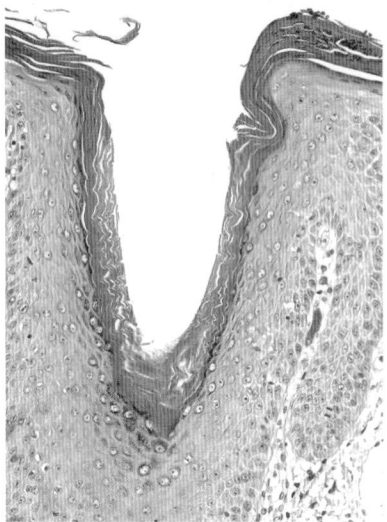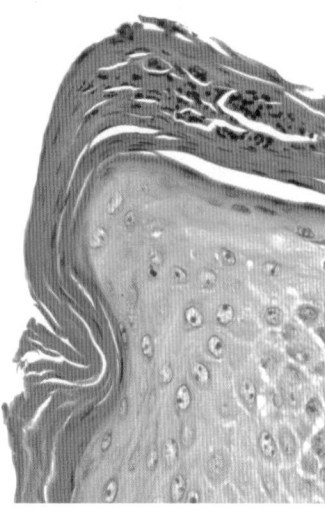

Fig. 22.74
Psoriasis of the scalp with changes simulating of seborrheic dermatitis. There is hyperkeratosis and parakeratosis with collections of neutrophils, more pronounced at the lip of the follicular ostium.

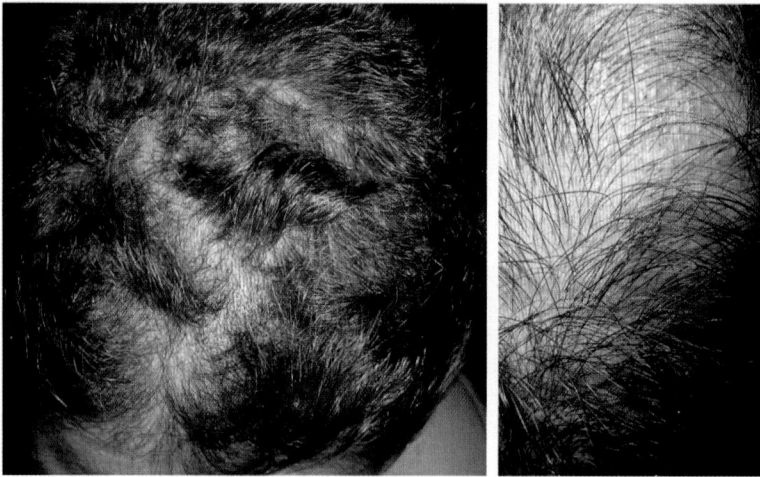

Fig. 22.75
Trichotillomania: mild involvement with very patchy hair loss. Courtesy of L.M. Gómez, MD, UPB, Medellín, Colombia.

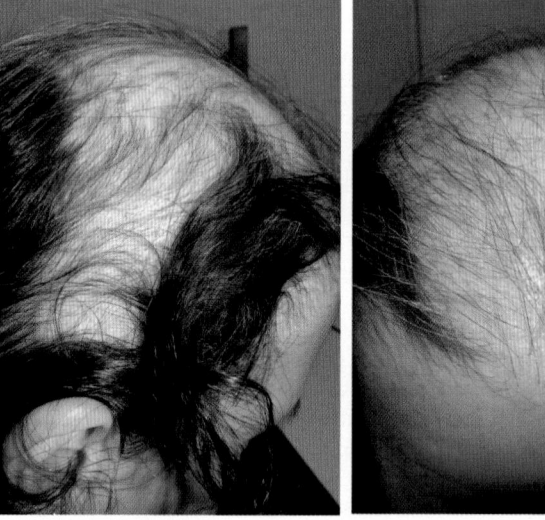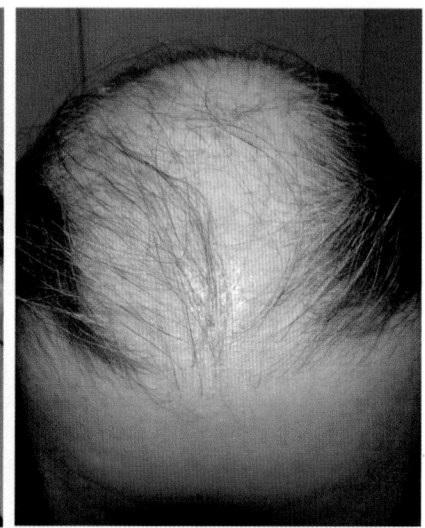

Fig. 22.76
Trichotillomania: severely affected young patient, with much more obvious and extensive hair loss with a bizarre pattern. Courtesy of C. Velázquez, MD, CES, Medellín, Colombia.

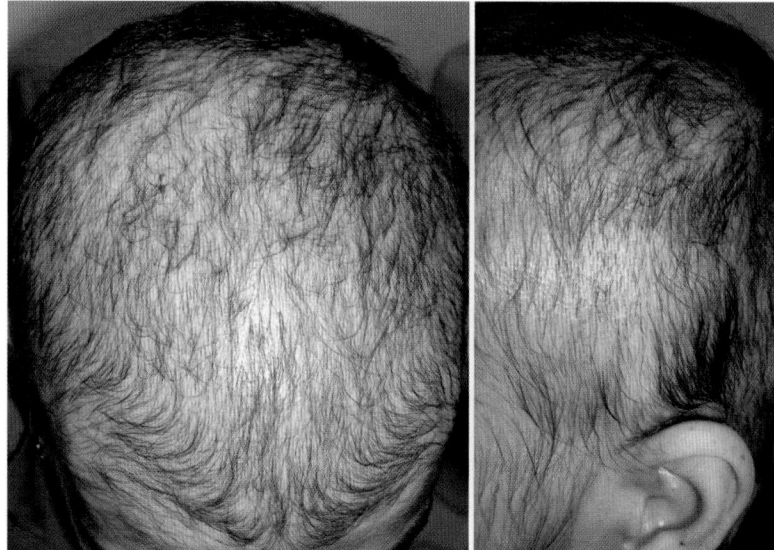

Fig. 22.77
Trichotillomania: note excoriations on the left side. Courtesy of L.M. Gómez, MD, UPB, Medellín, Colombia.

young women but can also be found in older adults and children, including toddlers.[3–5] Although some patients admit to pulling their hair, in our experience the great majority emphatically deny this. For this reason, a thorough interview and detailed psychiatric history are usually required.

Trichotillomania constitutes a chronic mental illness, of variable intensity and presentation, which can lead to severe emotional and social limitations to the patient's life. Trichotillomania shares some characteristics with obsessive-compulsive disorder.[6] In the most severe cases, it can be associated with deeper personality disorders such as self-harming, trichophagia, and trichobezoar (Rapunzel syndrome).[7,8] Occasionally, the compulsion to pull hair is not limited to the scalp but can involve other body sites including the pubis, the eyebrows, the eyelashes, and even the nostrils.[9–11]

Trichotillomania may be as common as obsessive-compulsive disorder and affect as many as 3% of the US population. Subclinical forms are also quite common, possibly affecting 1 in 10 Americans.[12–14]

There are two patterns of chronic hair pulling. The most severe and disfiguring is that in which patients pull off large amounts of hair during a brief period, and this is triggered by negative affective states. The least severe pattern is that of patients who engage in hair pulling during sedentary and social activities, such as reading, watching television, or talking on the telephone.[15]

The pattern of hair loss in trichotillomania is very variable, ranging from involvement of an isolated area (the 'friar Tuck sign') through to multiple geometric zones that may affect practically the entire scalp (Figs 22.75 and 22.76). In contrast to alopecia areata, the hair loss is typically incomplete. In every individual affected area there is hair loss, but this is not total, as the use of a magnifying glass shows residual small, broken, nonpigmented hairs. Sometimes there is evidence of erythema, pustule formation, or traumatic excoriations (Fig. 22.77). It is not infrequent to find other hair-bearing areas affected (Fig. 22.78).

Owing to the shortness of the hairs in this form of alopecia, it is usually not possible to obtain hairs by the hair-pull or hair-pluck techniques. Hairs evaluated by these techniques at the edges of the areas of alopecia are normal.

The hair-growth window technique is very useful in the diagnosis of trichotillomania. It involves shaving an area of 2.0 cm² on the scalp such that the patient cannot pull hairs from this site (back of the head). If possible, this area should be chosen so that adjacent hairs may hide the shaved area (Fig. 22.79). A diagnosis of trichotillomania is confirmed if, by the end of a week, hairs are developing normally. Hair growth is evaluated after a period of 1 week only because at this stage normal hairs are still very short and the patient cannot reach them. The hair grows by about 1.0 cm per month, and in 1 week the length of the hair should average

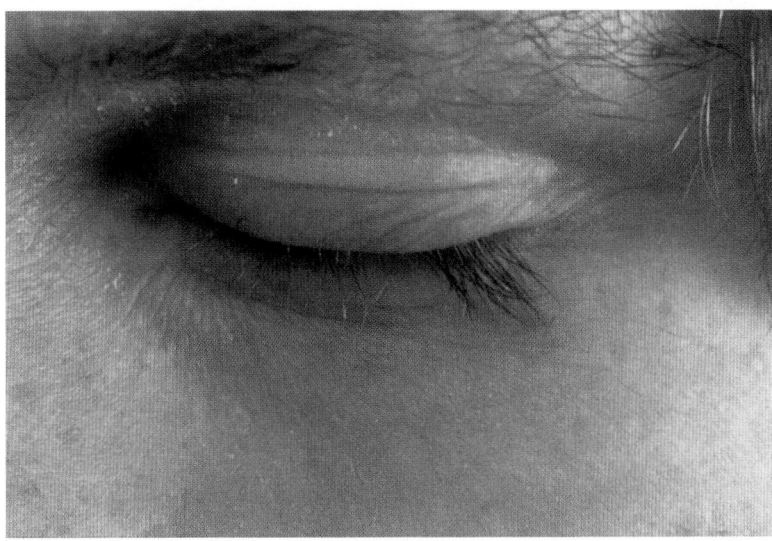

Fig. 22.78
Trichotillomania: many of the eyelashes have been pulled out. Courtesy of the Institute of Dermatology, London, UK.

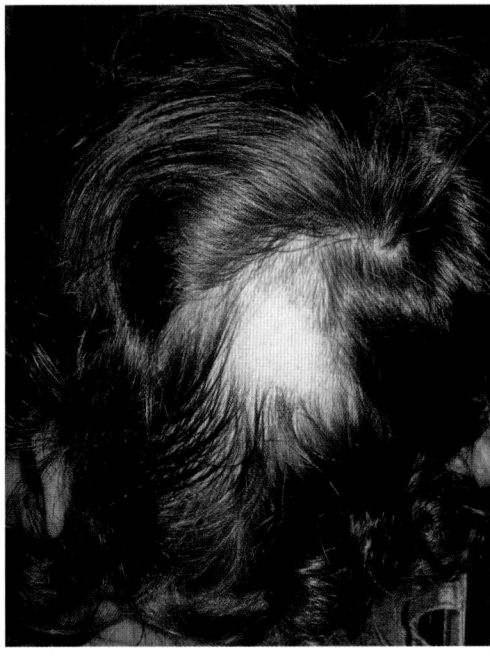

Fig. 22.79
Hair window: a small area of 1.5 × 1.5 cm of the scalp is shaved and then evaluated after a week to observe if there has been hair growth. Courtesy of M.S. Aluma, MD, Medellín, Colombia.

2.5 mm. However, the individual hair growth rate may be heterogeneous on the scalp.[16,17]

In rare patients with extensive trichotillomania, a moth-eaten appearance is seen such that it may be necessary to exclude syphilis by serology.[18]

Histologic features

The histologic features of trichotillomania are quite distinct and, with clinical correlation, enable the diagnosis to be made in the majority of cases.[19] In horizontal and vertical sections it is fairly easy to observe the most important histologic components, which only affect terminal follicles. The miniaturized vellus and follicles are protected from being pulled out because of their short length. The most important histologic alterations are catagen follicles, pigmented casts, and traumatized and distorted hair follicles.

The best biopsies are obtained in the first 2 months after the hairs have been pulled. Many sections should be examined because only a few sections may show the characteristic changes.[20]

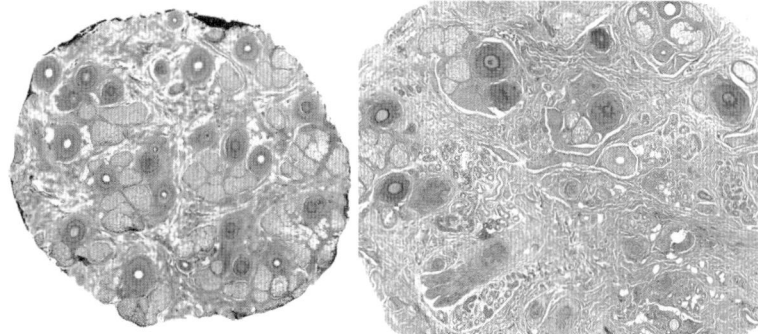

Fig. 22.80
Trichotillomania: in addition to residual anagen and telogen follicles, there are conspicuous catagen follicles with a bright eosinophilic center. No significant inflammation is seen.

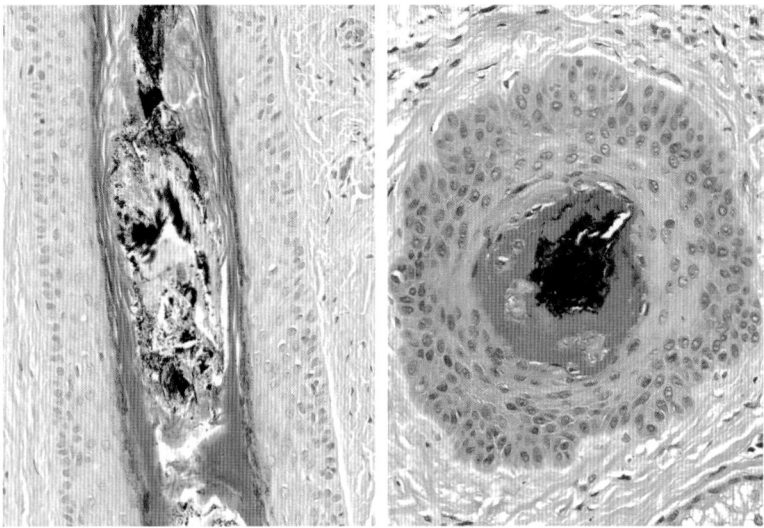

Fig. 22.81
Trichotillomania: note infundibular dilation with a pigment cast.

At scanning magnification, the most salient features consist of very high percentage of catagen or telogen hair follicles, a number of normal hair follicles, and absence of inflammation (Fig. 22.80). The affected hair follicles are easily recognized because they contain dark-red keratin and the external root sheath displays extensive apoptosis (see Figs 22.26 and 22.29).

Pigment casts correspond to pigmented cells in the hair matrix and cortex, which due to traction are dislodged and become displaced to the hair canal, outer root sheath, fibrous streamers, and the dermal papilla.

In trichotillomania, pigment casts are seen at every level of the hair canal, mainly in the infundibulum and in the ostium, and are associated with hyperkeratosis (Figs 22.81 and 22.82). These casts are occasionally observed in alopecia areata, chemotherapy-induced alopecia, and pressure induced alopecia.[20] They may be difficult to detect in poorly pigmented blond or red-haired individuals.[21] Another morphological alteration observed has been the presence of a vertically oriented split within the hair shafts. This split defect is full of proteinaceous material and erythrocytes. The histologic image is reminiscent of a hamburger within a bun (the 'hamburger sign') (Fig. 22.83).[22] Sometimes, the pigmented material takes other shapes similar to a zipper or a button and its buttonhole.[20]

Traumatized and distorted hair follicles represent follicular structures that display different alterations. The most frequent changes consist of collapse of the inner root sheath, inter- and intrafollicular hemorrhage, and trichomalacia. The latter refers to distorted, small, and incompletely keratinized hair follicles with walls of uneven thickness (Fig. 22.84). They may show irregular pigmentation.[23] Despite the extensive anatomical and physiological alteration of the hair follicles in trichotillomania, inflammation is minimal.[24] Additional histologic findings include pigmented follicular stellae (Fig. 22.85).

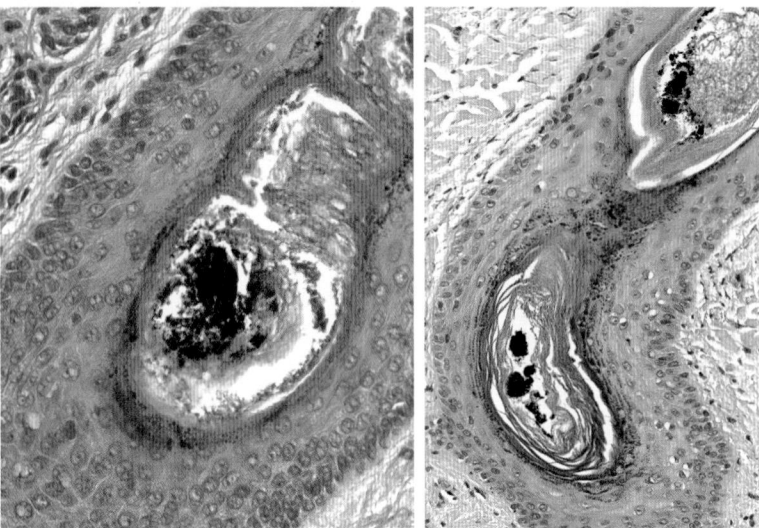

Fig. 22.82
Trichotillomania: there is infundibular dilatation, irregularity in the thickness of the inner root sheath, marked hyperkeratosis, and a pigmented cast.

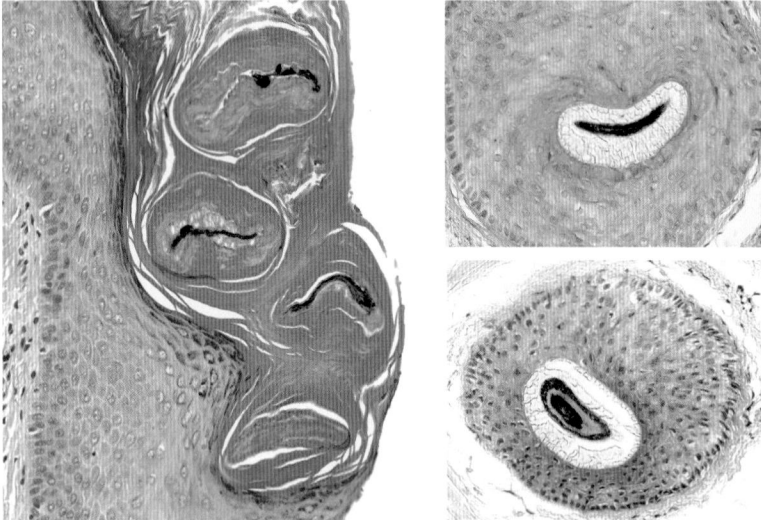

Fig. 22.83
Trichotillomania: hamburger sign. Left panel, note pigment aggregates within the hair shaft. On the right side, for comparison, note the pigment aggregates in a partially collapsed follicular channel.

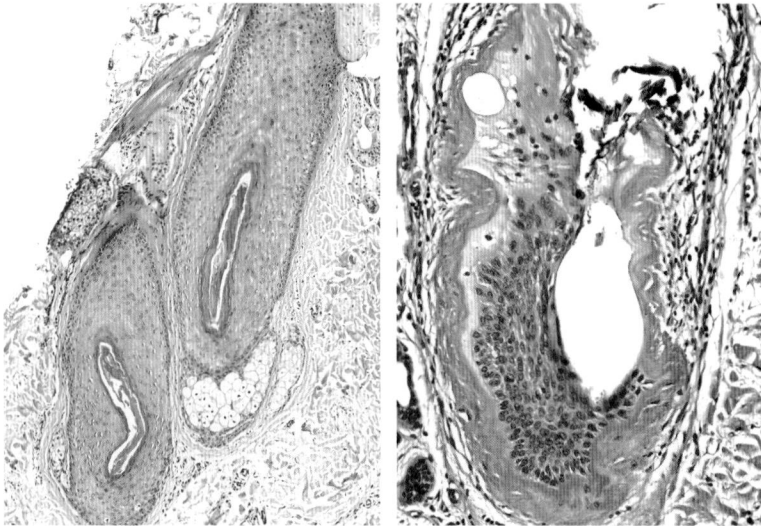

Fig. 22.84
Trichomalacia: left panel, note a hair follicle showing irregularities in the thickness of its wall. Right panel, this hair follicle has almost lost all its structural integrity. Courtesy of the L.E. Muñoz, Cali, Colombia.

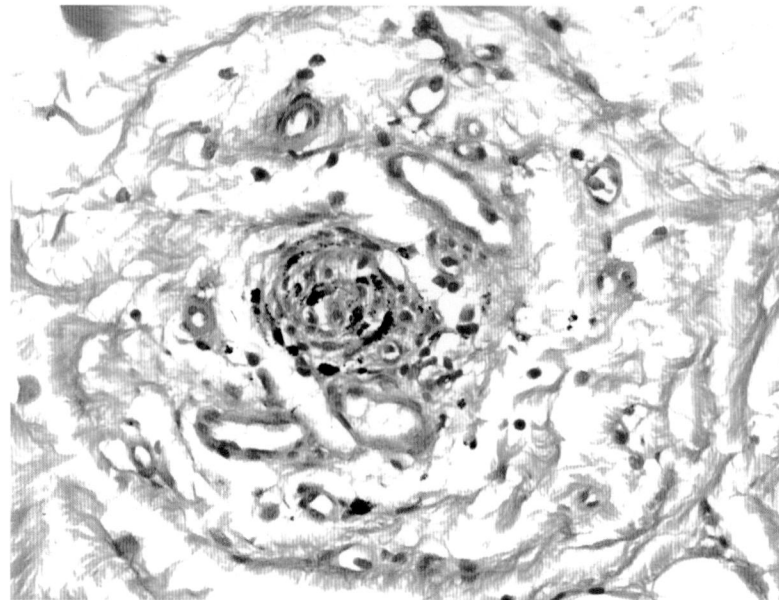

Fig. 22.85
Trichotillomania: pigmented follicular stellae. Compare with *Figs 22.64* and *22.65*.

Differential diagnosis

The most important clinical and histologic differential diagnosis of traumatic alopecia, particularly trichotillomania, is alopecia areata. In the latter, one can also occasionally find pigmented casts and trichomalacia. However, in alopecia areata the latter component is minimal and there are telogen follicles, small anagen follicles, miniaturized hairs, and a peribulbar inflammatory cell infiltrate.[25] Syphilitic alopecia may also resemble trichotillomania clinically, but the pigmented casts, trichomalacia, and absence of an inflammatory cell infiltrate in the latter condition usually afford their easy distinction. In difficult cases, however, serology is sometimes necessary.

Two other conditions that must be kept in mind in the differential diagnosis are trichotemnomania, an obsessive-compulsive habit to cut the hair with scissors or with a razor, and trichoteiromania, which results from perpetual rubbing of the scalp with fracturing of the hair shafts. Related to the latter is the appearance of frictional hair loss due to continuous pressure from items of clothing such as socks and trousers or the bed. The latter entities have no diagnostic histopathological features and show normal histology.[26–28]

Pressure alopecia

Clinical features

Abel and Lewis first described postoperative (supine or pressure) alopecia in 1960.[1] Pressure alopecia is an uncommon complication of surgery and is reported mainly in adults who undergo anesthesia, typically affecting the occiput and resulting from head immobilization during prolonged periods of unconsciousness. The pressure induces tissue hypoxia and ischemia. Most alopecia is temporary, but rare cases are permanent. Pressure alopecia was first described after long-lasting gynecological operations.[1] It has also been reported after cardiac, gynecological, abdominal, esthetic, and breast reconstruction surgery. Further associations include numerous surgical and therapeutic procedures, and occurrence in severely ill or comatose patients.[2–6] It is more frequent after cardiovascular surgery, prolonged endotracheal intubation, prolonged head immobilization, and the intraoperative use of the Trendelenburg position.[7–10]

Patients with this condition typically complain of occipitoparietal pain and tenderness within 24 hours of surgery. Hair loss is usually complete within 3–28 days after surgery. Most cases are self-limiting with regrowth occurring within 12 weeks. However, there are reported cases of permanent alopecia.[11]

Histologic features

The histopathology in early stages shows vascular thrombosis and necrosis of the dermis and subcutaneous tissue. Later, the microscopic findings include features in common with trichotillomania, including the presence of pigment casts, abundant catagen and telogen follicles, melanophages, and apoptotic bodies.[12–14]

Differential diagnosis

Distinction from other causes of localized hair loss is usually easy and can be done on clinical grounds alone. However, the differential diagnosis with chronic radiodermatitis after intraoperative fluoroscopic imaging may be problematic. In these cases, the antecedent of having been exposed to radiation and the location of the bald patches along the scalp margins with an ophiasis pattern is an important clue. The latter pattern occurs because this is the area of the scalp that receives the highest dose of radiation during fluoroscopy.[15,16]

Traction alopecia

Clinical features

Traction alopecia is another form of traumatic alopecia secondary to the application of tensile forces to the hair of the scalp with a histologic pattern similar to that of trichotillomania. It is a reversible form of alopecia which presents in adults and children.[1] It may become a permanent alopecia and result in a scarring alopecia if the traction is intense and sustained. Its causes are varied and often related to cultural and cosmetic practices. The most important are secondary to grooming styles such as excessive brushing, hair weaves, tight braiding, ponytails/pigtails, buns (chignon alopecia), cornrows, or wearing elastic hair bands.[2] Traction alopecia is particularly frequent in individuals of African descent (ancestry) (Fig. 22.86).[3,4] Other variants of traction alopecia may occur in nurses as a result of the use of a cap and among Sikh males from wearing a turban.[5,6] It has also been reported from hair extensions and a recognized feature as a sequel of torture.[7,8]

The hair loss usually occurs in the frontal and temporal areas but depends on the hairstyle used, and it is particularly noticeable at the margin of the tightly styled hair, leading over time to a widening of the parting lines, with retained hairs along the frontal and temporal rim called the 'fringe' sign (Fig. 22.87).[9,10]

A recent observation with potential therapeutic implications is the finding that the piloerection induced by α1-AR agonists makes hair extraction difficult and this indirectly protects against the development of alopecia.[11]

Histologic features

The biopsy should be processed in short horizontal sections as this may provide more information, particularly when the traction details are not very clear.[12]

The microscopic features are biphasic and depend on the time at which the biopsy is taken. In the early phases, there is a normal number of terminal hair follicles, some inflammation, abundant hair follicles in telogen and catagen, and trichomalacia (Fig. 22.88). As the process evolves, the terminal hair follicles disappear and only miniaturized follicles mixed with fibrous tracts are left. The number of sebaceous glands may be diminished.[10,13]

Differential diagnosis

The differential diagnosis is mainly with those alopecias that show a bandlike pattern of hair loss, such as alopecia areata in an ofiasic pattern and frontal fibrosing alopecia especially when the clinical history is not very clear (Fig. 22.51). Nevertheless, the clinical findings of preservation of ostium follicles and histologic findings of a peribulbar inflammatory cell infiltrate are enough to allow the diagnosis of alopecia areata to be made. In fibrosing frontal alopecia, there is clinical evidence of erythema and perifollicular scaling and histologic features of an interphase lymphocytic inflammatory cell infiltrate in the upper segment.[13–15]

Late traction alopecia is often indistinguishable on histology grounds from end-stage cicatricial alopecia. In difficult cases, clinicopathological correlation is essential.[10,13]

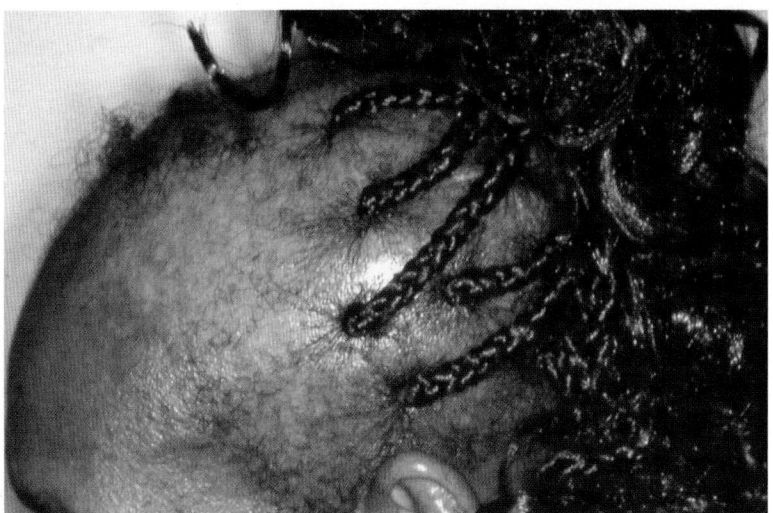

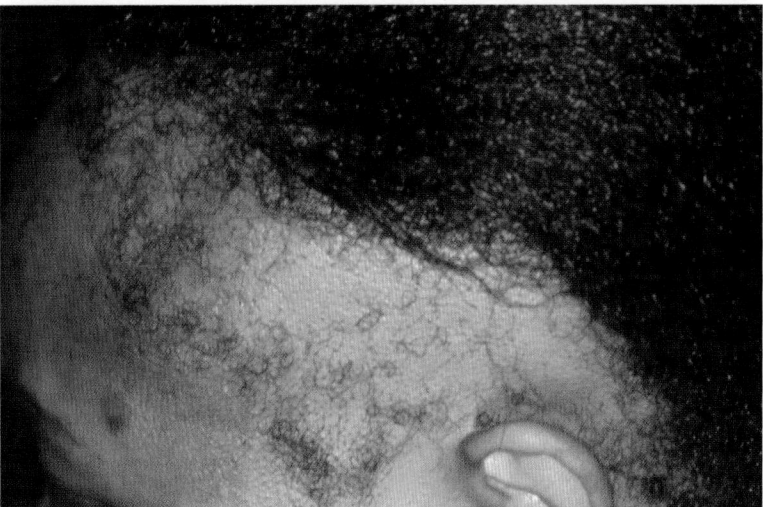

Fig. 22.86
Traction alopecia: prolonged traction for extended periods of time results in severe frontal hair loss. Pronounced changes are observed. Courtesy of P. Reygagne, MD, Centre Sabouraud, Paris, France.

Senescent alopecia

Clinical features

Senescent (senile, involutional) alopecia most probably represents a physiological event, as the majority of elderly people develop loss of hair pigment (canities), and there is a diffuse decrease in the density and thickness of the hair in the scalp, axillary, and pubic regions (Fig. 22.89).[1–3] Typically, patients with senile alopecia are older than 50, although the predictive value of age in total hair count has been found to be limited.[4] Patients have no relevant family history of alopecia. In some animal models, such as female squirrel monkeys (Saimiri boliviensis), age-related alopecia has been observed.[5]

The hair-pull/hair-pluck tests are normal with no increase in the number of telogen hairs.

Histologic features

Senescent alopecia is a controversial concept. It has characteristics that defined it as an entity and probably related to accumulative oxidative stress directly related to age; yet, sometimes the separation from androgenic alopecia or telogen effluvium is not clear.[6–9]

Horizontal sections are very useful in the diagnosis of senile alopecia, particularly if the biopsies are from two different sites, because they allow a comparative evaluation in relation to the diffuse or localized nature of the process allowing distinction from other types of alopecia.[1]

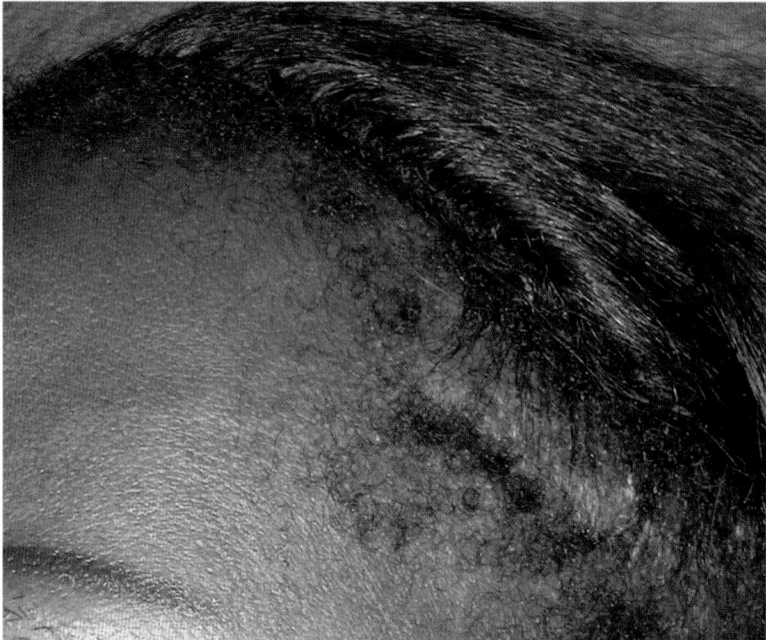

Fig. 22.87
Fringe sign: note the retained hairs along the frontal and temporal rim. Courtesy of J. Cadavid, MD, Clínica Medellín, Medellín, Colombia.

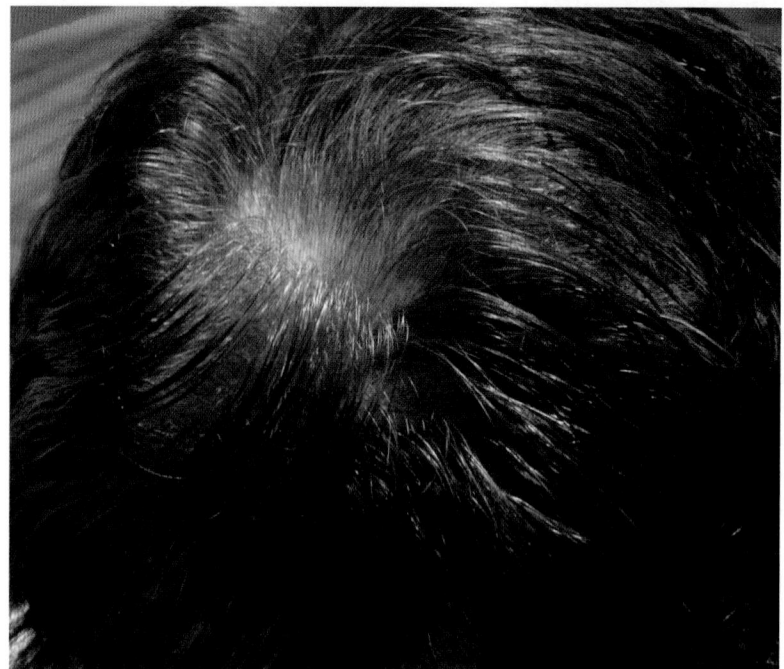

Fig. 22.89
Senescent alopecia: the reduction in the hair density is evident in the lighter areas of the scalp.

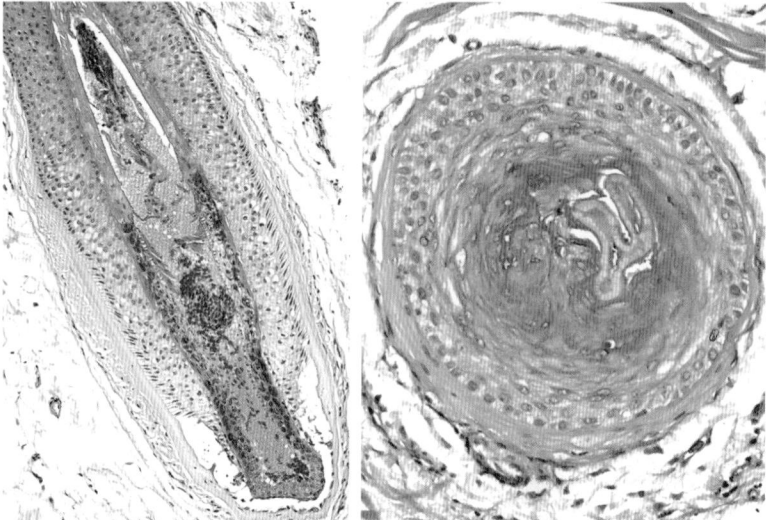

Fig. 22.88
Traction alopecia, early stage: vertical and horizontal sections of a hair follicle showing marked damage to the inner root sheath.

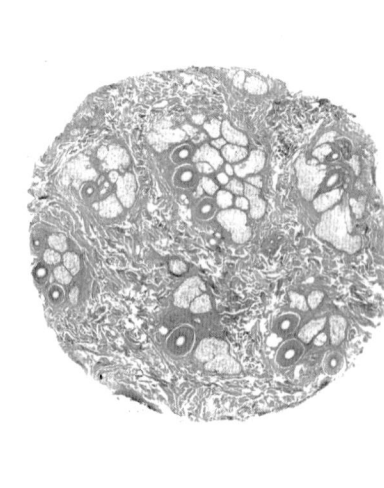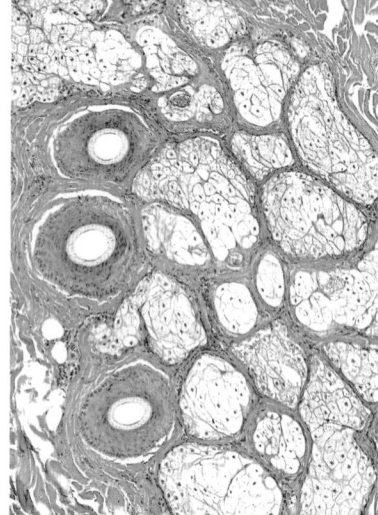

Fig. 22.90
Senile alopecia: there is a subtle decrease in the number of hair follicles and follicular units with preservation of the ratios between the number of terminal and vellus hair follicles and the hair follicles in anagen and telogen. There is an apparent increase in the amount of connective tissue between the follicular units which should not be confused with a scarring alopecia.

Histologically, there is a slight decrease in the number of follicular units and terminal hair follicles, with a normal ratio between terminal and vellus hair follicles and between anagen and telogen hair follicles (*Fig. 22.90*).

Differential diagnosis

Distinction from telogen effluvium and from androgenetic alopecia may be difficult but the pattern of diffuse involvement, without an increase in the percentage of telogen hairs or an increase in the number of vellus hairs, is very suggestive of senile alopecia.[10]

Telogen effluvium

Clinical features

Telogen effluvium is one of the most frequent forms of diffuse hair loss in women. In general, the term is applicable to those cases in which there is

an early end to anagen stage with progression of many hairs to catagen and subsequently to telogen.[1]

Telogen effluvium was first described by Kligman in 1961 to refer to a phenomenon of increased loss of telogen hairs in different processes without making any reference to a particular disease.[2] Telogen effluvium is characterized by diffuse hair shedding. There are two clinical presentations: an acute self-limiting presentation, lasting less than 6 months, generally precipitated by a recognizable event, and a chronic presentation of longer duration and unknown etiology.

Acute telogen effluvium may be precipitated by an extensive range of events and diseases, such as:

- physiological processes such as telogen effluvium in the newborn and postpartum, severe psychological stress, crash diets,

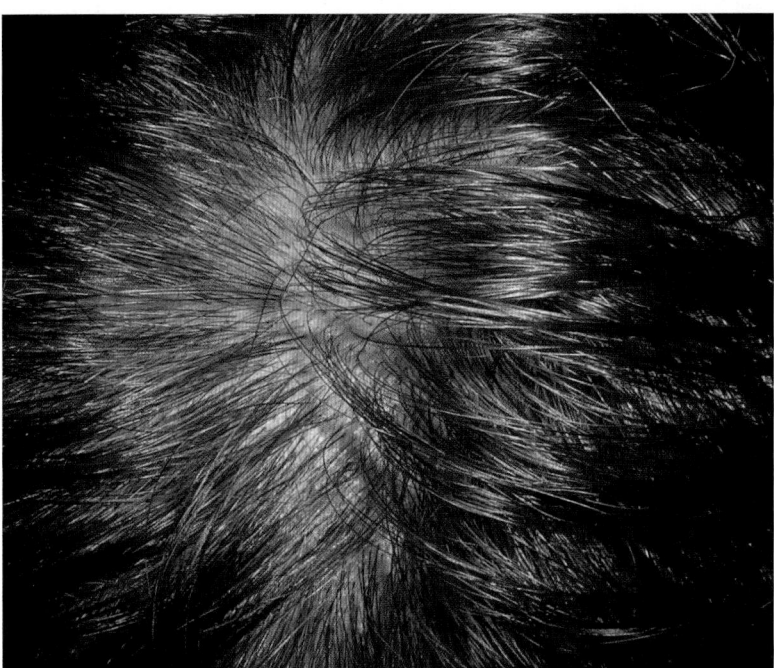

Fig. 22.91
Telogen effluvium: note diffuse hair loss without inflammation.

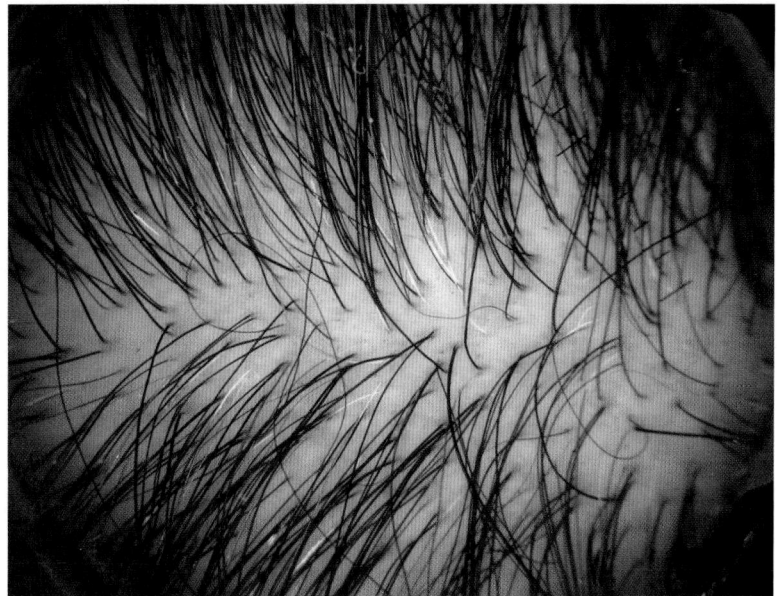

Fig. 22.92
Dermoscopy of telogen effluvium: the follicular density is lower than usual, without inflammation or loss of follicular ostia. Courtesy of L.M. Gómez, MD, UPB, Medellín, Colombia.

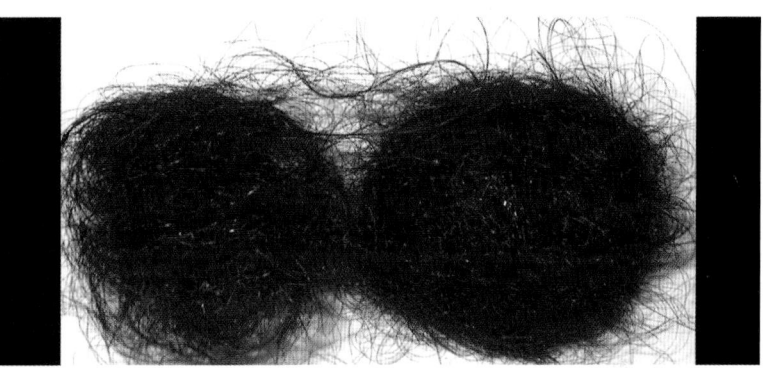

Fig. 22.93
Telogen effluvium; daily hair shedding count: during 10 days the patient has collected the hair she has shed. Despite the amount of hair loss there are no localized areas of hair loss. Courtesy of J. Cadavid, MD, Clínica Medellín, Medellín, Colombia.

- pathological events including spinal cord injury, intense fever (malaria, yellow and typhoid fevers), severe systemic illnesses, major surgery, anesthesia, septicemia, HIV-1 infection, after orthognathic surgery, early androgenetic alopecia, hypothyroidism, hyperthyroidism, iron-deficiency anemia, eosinophilia-myalgia syndrome, Hodgkin lymphoma, contact dermatitis of the scalp, and eating disorders.[3–16]

A number of drugs have also been implicated. The most relevant include antihyperlipidemic agents, retinoids, anticoagulants, antithyroid medications, anticonvulsants, heavy metals, propranolol, nadolol, metoprolol, minoxidil, oral contraceptives, heparin, clofibrate, salicylates, gentamicin, nicotinic acid, nitrofurantoin, vitamin A, albendazole, IFN-α2b, imiquimod, and the dopamine agonist pramipexole.[2,17–24] The list of drugs associated with telogen effluvium is continuously increasing and may be consulted in specialized references. Drug-induced hair loss is often reversible and may present in various forms such as telogen effluvium, anagen effluvium, or both.[25,26]

A seasonal increased hair loss (seasonal alopecia) has been observed in clinical practice.[27]

Most patients are adults, mainly women, but the process also occurs fairly commonly in children and adolescents.[28] Associated trichodynia has been documented.[29]

On examination, patients show diffuse noninflammatory hair loss involving the entire scalp (*Figs 22.91* and *22.92*). The loss of hair begins approximately 3–4 months after the precipitating event and, although it can be significantly noticeable, baldness is never observed (*Fig. 22.93*). Telogen effluvium can overlap with androgenetic alopecia.

The hair-pull test and trichogram show a net increase in the number of telogen hairs (see *Figs 22.3* and *22.4*). The number of telogen hairs varies from individual to individual and also according to the stage of evolution of the disease. In the initial stages the telogen hair count in trichogram is high, but by the end of the process almost normal counts may be found. The upper normal limit of telogen hairs is considered to be 15% of terminal hairs. Between 15% and 20% is suggestive of effluvium telogen, yet this count is the most frequently found in chronic effluvium telogen. More than 20% is a determinant of the disease. The hair-pull test is positive in all areas of the scalp (*Fig. 22.94*).

Owing to the great number of diseases that may present as telogen effluvium, a thorough clinical history is necessary. Diagnostic tests to identify the etiology and cause of the disease are also required. It is often prudent to carry out laboratory tests to exclude or confirm a subclinical illness such as hypothyroidism, systemic lupus erythematosus (SLE), or syphilis.

Some studies have found decreased ferritin and serum iron levels in females with telogen effluvium, androgenetic alopecia, and alopecia areata. The clinical and therapeutical significance of these findings is still unclear, as other studies have not found any relationship between iron deficiency and hair loss. Currently, in the absence of a clinical setting suggestive of anemia (menstruating women, vegetarians, and women with a history of anemia), there is insufficient evidence to recommend universal screening for iron deficiency in patients with hair loss.[30–32]

Some patients, particularly middle-aged postmenopausal women, may present with a chronic form of telogen effluvium that lasts more than 6 months, is of unknown etiology, has a fluctuating course, and is characterized by a diffuse pattern of hair thinning and hair loss, often associated with bitemporal recession (chronic telogen effluvium). The biopsy generally shows borderline findings between a biopsy with no alterations and a telogen effluvium of low intensity. Baldness does not develop because lost hairs are quickly replaced.[33–36] The disease appears to be self-limiting, but some patients continue to experience chronic diffuse telogen hair shedding without tendency toward spontaneous improvement or development of female pattern hair loss.[37] An exceptional case has been documented in a man.[38]

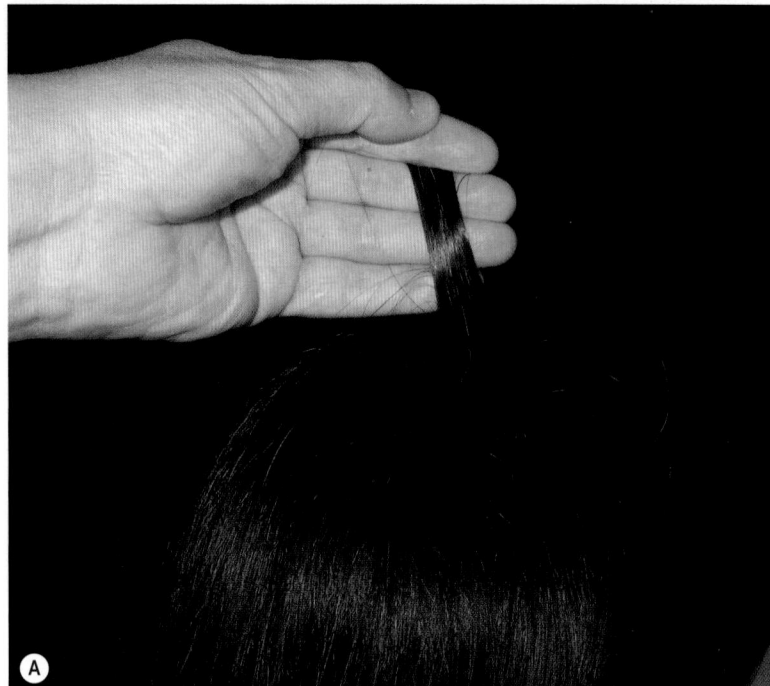

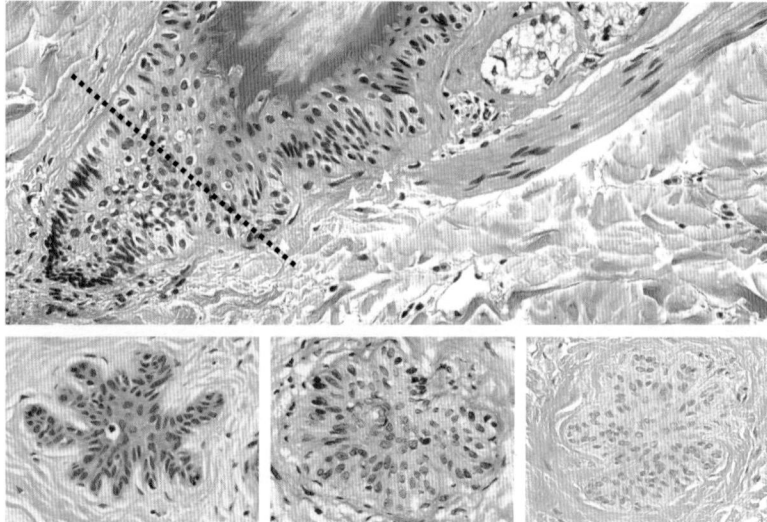

Fig. 22.95
Telogen germinal units (secondary germ): the top panel is a vertical section of a hair follicle in telogen with retraction of the lower segment at the level of the arrector pili muscle. Next to this structure is the telogen germinal unit. Bottom panel, note transverse sections of 3 telogen germinal units.

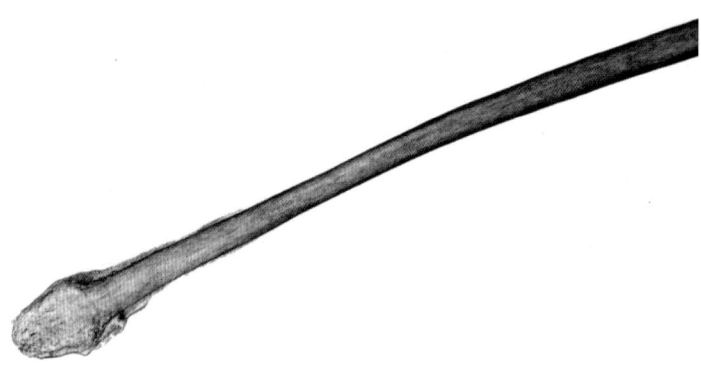

Fig. 22.94
Hair-pull test: (**A**) Take 20 to 30 hairs between the fingers and gently pull. The only hairs one should obtain are those in telogen; usually 10% of the total hairs, or 2 or 3 of the 30 pulled. Those that are in anagen remain adhered to the scalp. When more hair shafts are obtained from each pull, this suggests hair disease (telogen effluvium). (**B**) The hairs in telogen are usually recognizable because of their club shape.

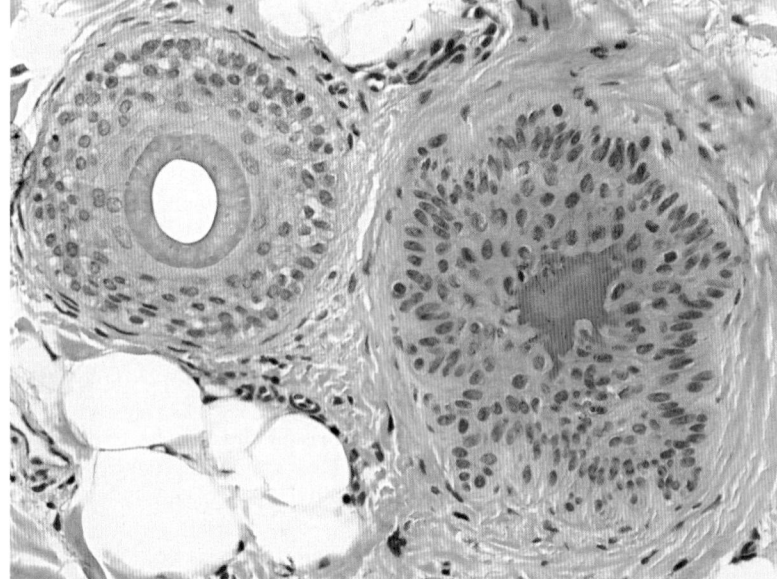

Fig. 22.96
Telogen follicle: on the left there is a terminal follicle in anagen and on the right a hair follicle in telogen with its center displaying prominent trichilemmal bright red keratin.

Pathogenesis and histologic features

Telogen effluvium is caused by a disturbance of the hair cycle which results in telogen shedding. It has been proposed that telogen effluvium develops as a result of five different functional changes in the hair follicle:[39,40]

- immediate anagen release (episode of fever, stress or medication),
- delayed anagen release (postpartum),
- short anagen syndrome (chronic telogen effluvium),
- immediate telogen release (topical minoxidil therapy, seasonal alopecia),
- delayed telogen release (a theoretical possibility).

These different mechanisms are precipitated by the different stimuli and processes mentioned above. The underlying molecular mechanisms controlling these processes are unknown. Interestingly, however, it has been shown that inducible transgenic mice, which display a reversible hair loss phenotype, express high levels of the transcription factor tTA (tetracycline transactivator) and reporter luciferase gene.[41] This results in a decreased number of anagen hair follicles and an increase in the number of telogen hair follicles.

Although the diagnosis can be made on clinical grounds, when the clinical presentation is unclear, a biopsy may be necessary. Ideally, two biopsies should be taken from different sites and processed with horizontal sections to verify the diffuse nature of the process and to produce an exact count of the number of hair follicles in telogen, catagen, and anagen and the number of miniaturized hair follicles. The histologic findings in telogen effluvium are subtle, the only finding being an increase in the number of telogen germinal units (*Fig. 22.95*, and see *Figs 22.29–22.31*), telogen hair follicles (*Fig. 22.96*), and follicular stellae (*Fig. 22.97*) in the deep layers, with a normal number of hair follicles and absence of a significant inflammatory infiltrate or follicular miniaturization. The follicular stellae are identical to those observed in androgenic alopecia.[42,43] These changes are better observed when the illness is active, as in the resolution state the number of follicles

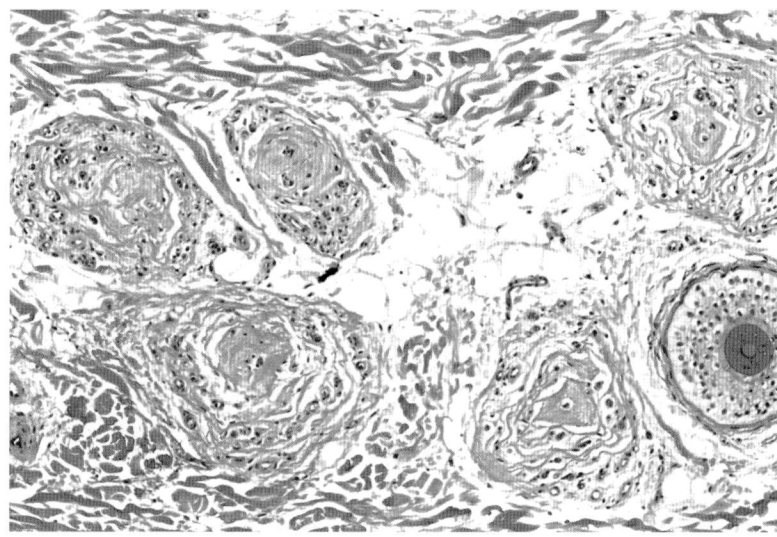

Fig. 22.97
Follicular stellae: five stellae corresponding to telogen follicles that have involuted. To the right a miniaturized hair follicle.

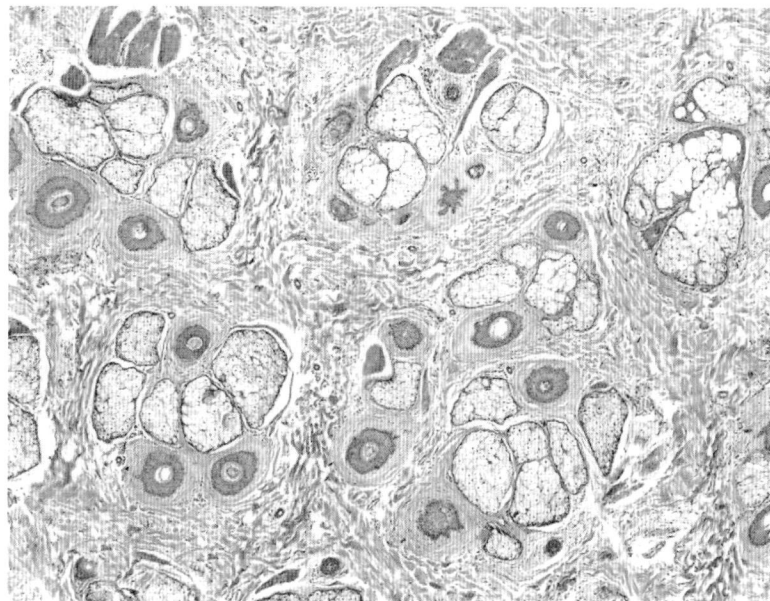

Fig. 22.98
Telogen effluvium and androgenetic alopecia: normal numbers of follicular units and hair follicles are present with increased numbers of telogen and miniaturized hair follicles.

in telogen may be normal. It is very important to bear in mind this fact, as normally this is the moment in which the patient notices the shedding and consults the dermatologist. Many scalp biopsies that appear 'normal' or 'supernormal' (all terminal follicles in anagen) belong to patients with the clinical diagnosis of telogen effluvium.[44,45] The percentage of telogen terminal hair follicles is generally greater than 20%; however, this figure should not be taken as a rigid definition since lower counts are occasionally found in patients with chronic disease as discussed before.

Differential diagnosis

The differential diagnosis of telogen effluvium is mainly with diffuse non-scarring alopecias, including androgenetic alopecia, alopecia areata incognito, and loose anagen hair syndrome.[40]

In androgenetic alopecia, the main histologic feature consists of a zonal pattern of hair loss with miniaturization of hairs. In addition, the gentle hair pull is normal. Hair pluck can be puzzling due to a higher count of hairs in telogen. It is important to remember, however, that in the early stages of androgenetic alopecia, hair follicles more frequently enter telogen. Nevertheless, in telogen effluvium the ratio between terminal hair follicles and vellus hairs remains within the normal range of greater than 7:1 and there is no inflammation.[46] In cases when there is overlap with androgenetic alopecia, it is very useful to biopsy two different sites to correlate the findings (focal changes in androgenetic alopecia versus diffuse changes in telogen effluvium) and establish a precise diagnosis. However, it is also important to remember that the two conditions may coexist and that chronic telogen effluvium may uncover occult androgenetic alopecia (*Fig. 22.98*).[45,47–49]

Alopecia areata incognito displays many yellow dots (dilated infundibular openings), numerous hair follicles in telogen, and increased number of miniaturized hairs. Lymphoid infiltration of the hair bulbs is sometimes observed. In contrast, telogen effluvium lacks histologic evidence of inflammation and dilated infundibular openings.[50]

Loose anagen hair syndrome which may occasionally affect adults without a family history can be confused with telogen effluvium. The differential diagnosis is easy, with the hair-pull test showing the majority of the hairs in anagen and the extracted hairs lacking external and internal root sheaths. Short anagen syndrome presents also in blonde girls with short hair; the difference is that the hair that is obtained in the pull test is telogen.[51] Additionally, the patients with short anagen do not improve with age.[52]

Another condition that may present with an excess of telogen hair follicles, (with number counts near 50% or more) is trichotillomania. Nevertheless, in this latter disorder, the stellae and telogen germinal units present melanin debris, in addition to the other findings such as pigmented casts and trichomalacia (*Fig. 22.99*).

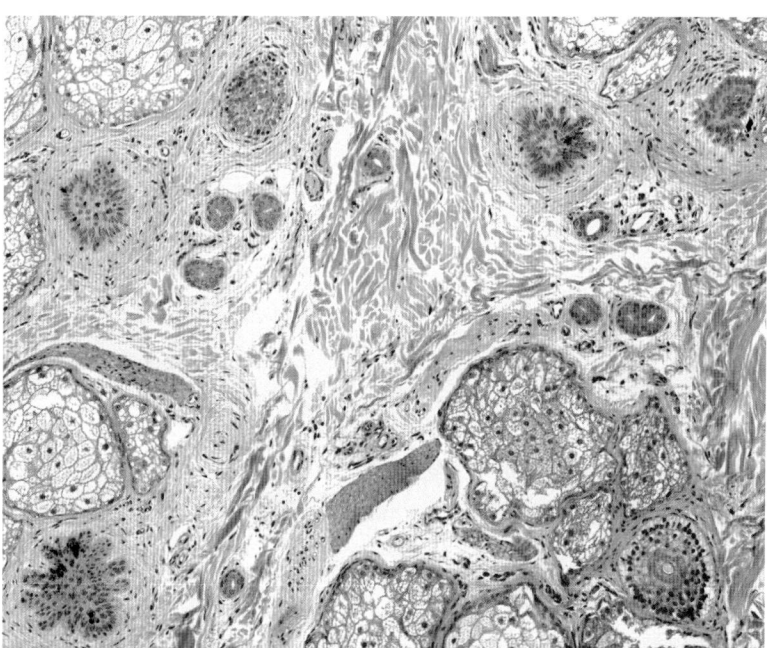

Fig. 22.99
Trichotillomania, pigmented telogen germinal units: in this biopsy there are five follicular structures, and four are telogen germinal units with melanin pigment related to the traumatic extraction of the hairs. Courtesy of A. Ruiz, MD, CES, Medellín, Colombia.

Anagen effluvium

Anagen effluvium usually refers to extensive shedding of anagen hairs due to abrupt interruption of mitotic activity in hair matrix cells.[1] It generally presents in a diffuse manner although with diverse patterned hair loss.[2,3]

It is typically induced by the administration of antineoplastic drugs, particularly alkylating agents, and low-dose radiation exposure, but has also been documented with some toxins (boric acid, copper, cadmium, mercury, bismuth, thallium), seeds of the selenium-rich plant *Lecythis ollaria* (coco de mono), and in inflammatory diseases such as alopecia areata and pemphigus vulgaris.[4–7] The hair loss occurs in the second or third week during which the drug has been administered. It presents as broken off rather than shed hairs and may affect other hair areas such as the beard, eyebrows, eyelashes, axillae, and pubic hair. Once the medication is stopped, the loss is usually reversible, although permanent alopecia after high busulfan therapy in recipients of bone marrow transplantation, taxanes for breast cancer, and cisplatin and etoposide for lung cancer has been reported.[8,9] Not all drugs produce anagen effluvium; nevertheless, some like retinoids, 5-fluorouracil and methotrexate trigger telogen effluvium.[10]

Histologic features

The diagnosis is commonly established on the basis of clinical correlation. There are no large histologic studies of the acute phase of anagen effluvium related to chemotherapy. There are only limited studies of patients with permanent alopecia postchemotherapy. The biopsy does not show characteristic changes, and the histologic picture may closely simulate a nonscarring alopecia, an advanced androgenetic alopecia, or a late alopecia areata without an inflammatory cell infiltrate. The utility of the biopsy lies in the differential diagnosis with the aforementioned entities, but more often than not, it may be impossible to reach a correct diagnosis if an appropriate clinical history is lacking.[8,11]

Loose anagen hair syndrome

Clinical features

Loose hair syndrome or loose anagen hair is a noninflammatory, nonscarring form of hair loss. It was first described in 1984 by Zaun as a variant of hair dysplasia in which hair can be easily pulled out.[1] The actual name was introduced simultaneously by Hamm and Price in 1989.[2,3]

The disease, which usually presents in female children between the ages of 2 and 5 years, is characterized by very fine hair that can be removed without pain. The hair does not grow and therefore does not need to be cut.[4] In the majority of patients, the disease develops spontaneously and improves with age. In a minority of cases, an autosomal dominant mode of inheritance has been described with variable expression and incomplete penetrance. Affected females characteristically have blond hair (*Fig. 22.100*). The disease has also been documented in boys with black hair of Egyptian, Indian, or African descent.[5–8]

If the hair is pulled out, regrowth may be normal or very slow. Washing and light brushing induce shedding. There is no involvement of the hair of the eyebrows, eyelashes, or on any other part of the body. The disease

improves with age as the hair increases in caliber, density, and length. However, a tendency to anagen hair loss persists indefinitely.[3] The phenotype is heterogeneous, and in some patients with no family history the onset of the disease is in adult life. Such cases are often misdiagnosed as telogen effluvium.[9] There are three phenotypes: type A, which shows decreased hair density; type B, which is characterized by unruly and curly hair; and type C, which has normal hair density.[10] Types A and B occur in children, possibly evolving into the type C phenotype around the age of 8 years.[11]

Diagnosis is relatively easy with a hair-pull test or a trichogram.[12] The hairs loosen without any effort, just by soft traction. The diagnosis is confirmed by microscopic examination, demonstrating that the majority (more than 70%), if not all, the hairs are in anagen. Adherence to the follicle is so poor that the extracted hairs lack inner and outer root sheaths. The hair cuticle shows some folding (ruffled cuticle) (*Figs 22.101 and 22.102*).[13]

It is important to bear in mind that the hair-pull test varies according to the age of the patient, and in children aged 10 years or under it is quite normal to find a high percentage of anagen hairs. However, in loose anagen hair syndrome the percentage is much higher and the hairs have absent inner and outer root sheaths.[14] One also must bear in mind that the number of hairs in anagen obtained with the hair-pull test may vary over time; hence, a single negative hair-pull test does not exclude the diagnosis.[15]

Loose anagen hair syndrome has been associated with Noonan syndrome, Moyamoya disease, epidermolysis bullosa simplex, Dowling-Meara type, trichotillomania, alopecia areata, hypohidrotic ectodermal dysplasia, ocular colobomata, macular dystrophy, spun-glass hair, and woolly hair.[9,16–26]

Pathogenesis and histologic features

The cause of loose anagen hair syndrome appears to be a mutation of keratins K6HF and K6IRS. K6HF is a type II cytokeratin found solely in the companion layer associated to Henle layer. K6IRS is specific for the inner root sheath of the hair follicle. The mutations lead to premature keratinization of the inner root sheath and poor adhesion of the cuticle of the hair shaft to the cuticle of the internal root sheath, resulting in premature cessation of the anagen phase.[27–30]

Histologic examination reveals no consistent morphological abnormalities except for fragmentation of the inner root sheath, with clefts between the inner root sheath and hair shafts and between the inner and outer root

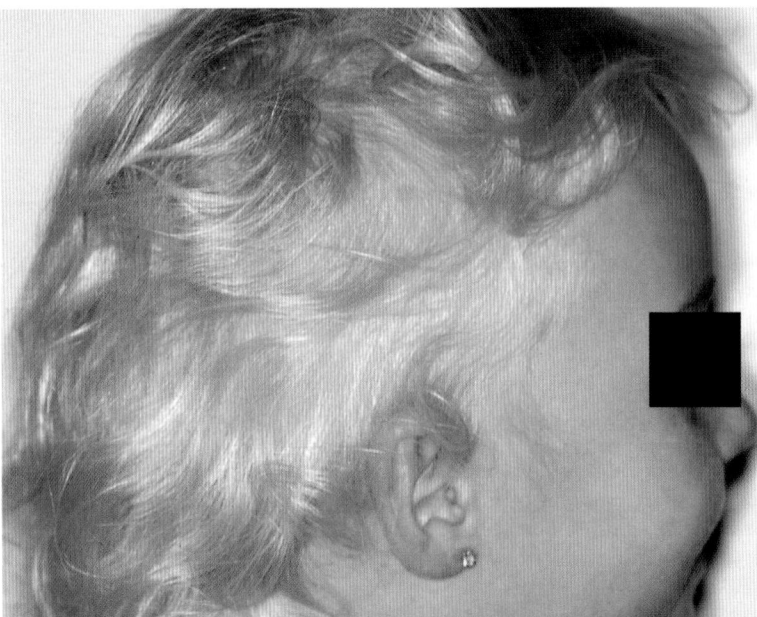

Fig. 22.100
Loose anagen hair syndrome: the hair is fine and is easily pulled out. Note the pattern of nonscarring, noninflammatory diffuse alopecia. Courtesy of P. Reygagne, MD, Centre Sabouraud, Paris, France.

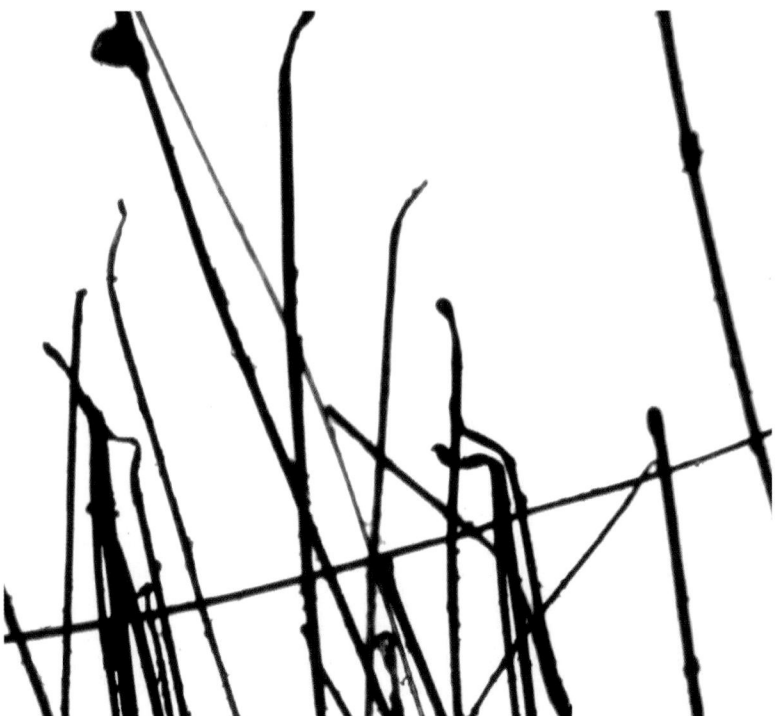

Fig. 22.101
Loose anagen hair syndrome, trichogram: the majority of plucked hairs are anagen hairs devoid of root sheaths. Courtesy of P. Reygagne, MD, Centre Sabouraud, Paris, France.

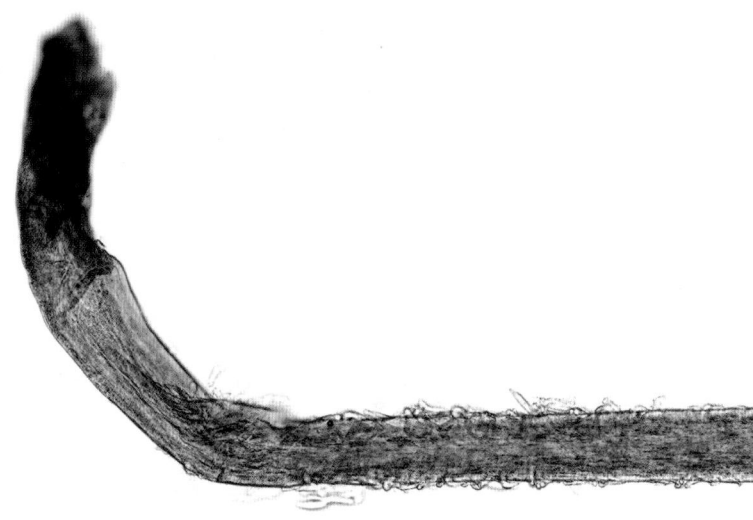

Fig. 22.102
Loose anagen hair syndrome, hair-pull test: note the anagen hair with ruffled cuticle and lacking a root sheath. Courtesy of A. Aristizábal, MD, CES, Medellín, Colombia.

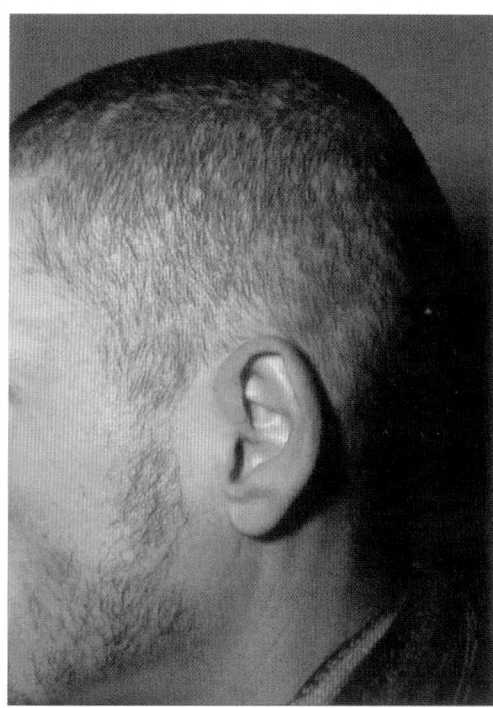

Fig. 22.103
Syphilitic alopecia: typical 'moth-eaten' pattern of alopecia. Courtesy of P. Reygagne, MD, Centre Sabouraud, Paris, France.

sheath probably as a result of the abnormal composition and keratinization of the inner root sheath with loss of its anchoring properties.[9,30,31] However, this histologic feature may also be seen in biopsies from normal patients without alopecia as a consequence of processing artifact.[32]

Differential diagnosis

The differential diagnosis of loose anagen hair syndrome is mainly with diffuse nonscarring alopecias such as diffuse alopecia areata, telogen effluvium, and short anagen hair syndrome. This is usually an easy task and can be done on clinical grounds alone or with the aid of a gentle hair-pull test or a biopsy.[33] Alopecia areata may be confused with loose anagen hair syndrome due to the presence in the trichogram of numerous dystrophic anagen hairs. In these cases, a biopsy may be useful to show the presence of lymphocytes in the hair bulbs in alopecia areata. Histologically, loose anagen hair syndrome lacks inflammation.[34] Distinction from telogen effluvium is easy if a gentle hair-pull test shows only hairs in telogen. In short anagen syndrome, the pull test and trichogram only show short telogen hairs.[35]

Short anagen syndrome

Clinical features

Short anagen syndrome was described by Kersey in 1987 in a patient with trichodental syndrome.[1,2] It is a congenital disease characterized by short fine hair from birth due to a decrease in the duration of anagen. In the most frequent presentation, the hair does not grow longer than the neck and never needs cutting.[3,4] The majority of the cases have been described in Caucasian women with blonde hair.[5,6] Some cases of short anagen have been described in African-American patients and Caucasian patients with brown hair and one in an Asian patient.[1,7,8] Short anagen syndrome has been associated with trichodental syndrome and congenital hypotrichosis.[1,9]

As the anagen phase is shortened, there is an increase in the number of hair follicles in telogen. Family groupings have been described suggesting an autosomal dominant hereditary pattern.[10] Clinically, the hair is normal but there is an increase in the number of hairs obtained in a pull test.

Pathogenesis and histologic features

Short anagen syndrome is a form of hair growth defect due to a shortened anagen phase; consequently, there is an increase in the hair follicles that enter telogen phase.[1,2,10] The cause of this phenomenon is unknown.

A diagnosis is usually easy to make based on clinical features and a trichogram or pull test. The trichogram reveals a reduction in the ratio of anagen/telogen hairs due to a decrease of the follicles in anagen. The pull test is positive for hair in telogen.[9] Usually, it is not necessary to perform a biopsy as the findings are unspecific.

Differential diagnosis

The most important differential diagnosis is with loose anagen syndrome. This also presents in blonde girls with short hair that does not grow. The most important difference is that the hairs obtained in the pull test are in telogen, not in anagen.[10] Furthermore, patients with loose anagen syndrome improve with age, whereas in those with short anagen the abnormality persists.[9]

Syphilitic alopecia

Clinical features

Syphilitic alopecia is a nonscarring variant of alopecia that has resurfaced in recent years, particularly in association with HIV infection.[1–3]

The clinical manifestations of syphilitic alopecia were divided into two groups by McCarthy in 1940:

- Symptomatic syphilitic alopecia, which is associated with other manifestations of secondary syphilis, is the rarest form of alopecia. The hair loss may affect the scalp or any other hair-bearing area of the body. It can present in a diffuse or localized pattern (*Figs 22.103* and *22.104*).
- Essential syphilitic alopecia with no other features of secondary syphilis. This may also be diffuse or localized and represents a variant of latent syphilis.[4] Three clinical forms have been described: moth eaten, which is the most frequent and presents usually in the occipital zone, diffuse, which corresponds to telogen effluvium as a reactive phenomenon and a mixed form.[5]

Patients with symptomatic syphilitic alopecia have other manifestations of secondary syphilis and the diagnosis is usually easy. Patients with essential syphilitic alopecia are asymptomatic, and a high degree of suspicion is essential to achieve a correct diagnosis. Alopecia as a manifestation of secondary or latent syphilis has been reported to occur with an incidence varying between 2.9% and 12.5%.[6-9] Therefore, a serological test for syphilis should be considered when there is hair loss for which a satisfactory explanation is not apparent.[10]

It is important to bear in mind that syphilitic alopecia can involve the whole body and also occasionally present as localized disease at sites away from the scalp.[11] Alopecia syphilitica has been described in a neonate with congenital syphilis and in accelerated form as a complication of the Jarisch-Herxheimer reaction.[12,13]

Clinically, symptomatic and essential syphilitic alopecia are very similar and can only be differentiated by the presence of papulosquamous lesions on the scalp or other areas of the body in the symptomatic variant. In both forms, the patches of alopecia present with a characteristic 'moth-eaten' appearance.

The clinical differential diagnosis of syphilitic alopecia is very broad, and the 'moth-eaten' alopecia pattern can be confused with trichotillomania, traction alopecia, or alopecia areata. The diffuse variant may be confused with telogen effluvium and a diffuse type of alopecia areata.[14,15]

The trichogram and the hair-pull test show an increase in the number of telogen hairs in the affected areas.

Histologic features

The histologic findings in the lesions of symptomatic syphilitic alopecia are similar to those of secondary syphilis occurring elsewhere. In the papulosquamous lesion, there is psoriasiform hyperplasia of the epidermis, spongiosis and exocytosis of neutrophils, and focal interface change with hydropic degeneration of basal cells. Lymphocytes and plasma cells are present at the dermal–epidermal junction. In the dermis, there is a superficial and deep perivascular and periadnexal lymphohistiocytic inflammatory cell infiltrate with a variable number of plasma cells and occasionally a granulomatous infiltrate in the upper dermis (Fig. 22.105).[16]

Essential syphilitic alopecia is characterized by less prominent epidermal changes, reduced anagen hairs, increased telogen and catagen hairs, and a bulbar, peribulbar, and peri-isthmic lymphocytic infiltrate with a variable number of plasma cells. Fibrous tracts may also show lymphocyte infiltration. Identification of *Treponema pallidum* in sections of tissue in biopsies of patients with syphilitic alopecia yields variable results. Immunohistochemistry is more reliable and sensitive than a silver stain (Fig. 22.105C).[14,17-19] Molecular studies with the polymerase chain reaction may also be useful.

Differential diagnosis

In essential syphilitic alopecia, the histologic features are very similar to those of alopecia areata. The presence of plasma cells and the tendency of the infiltrate to spare the hair bulb and involve the external root sheath at a higher level without eosinophils are helpful diagnostic pointers.[4]

Essential syphilis may also present as a telogen effluvium, and distinction between both these conditions on histologic grounds can be impossible, making serological screening for syphilis essential.

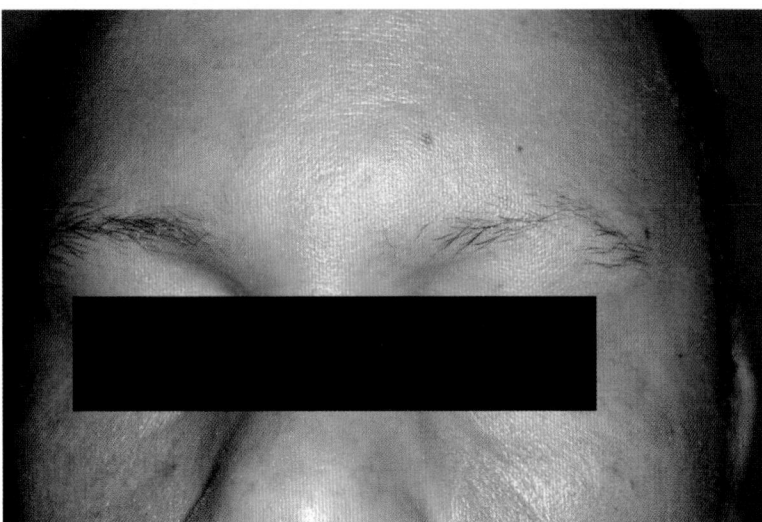

Fig. 22.104
Syphilitic alopecia: loss of eyebrows is not uncommon. Courtesy of L.M. Gómez, MD, UPB, Medellín, Colombia.

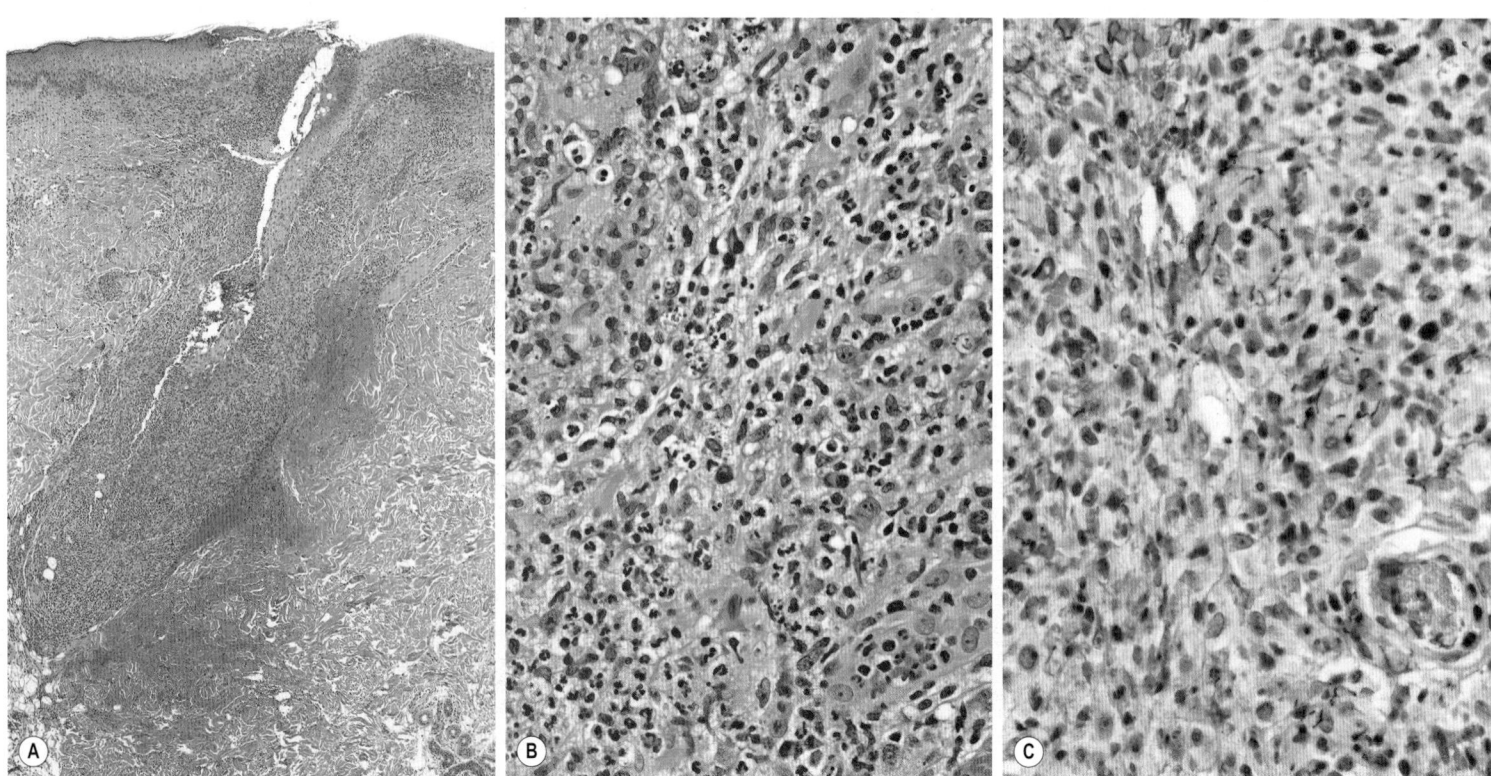

Fig. 22.105
Syphilitic alopecia: (**A**) there is follicular destruction and an intense inflammatory cell infiltrate; (**B**) the infiltrate consists of neutrophils, lymphocytes, histiocytes, and plasma cells; (**C**) numerous spirochetes are present (immunoperoxidase). (The case was kindly supplied by Nooshin Brinster.)

Lipedematous alopecia and lipedematous scalp

Clinical features

Lipedematous scalp was described by Cornbleet in 1935 as scalp swelling in a black woman without hair loss.[1] The term lipedematous alopecia was first mentioned by Coskey et al. in 1961, in two women of African descent.[2] It is also known as spongy scalp syndrome.[3] It is a very rare form of noninflammatory and nonscarring alopecia of unknown etiology characterized by thickening and swelling of the scalp with diffuse hair loss and typically presents in adult black women with predilection for the vertex and the occipital regions. The disease may have a slowly progressive course. It has been associated with other medical conditions such as skin and joint hyperelasticity, discoid lupus erythematosus, diabetes mellitus, renal failure, Sjögren syndrome, hyperlipidemia, androgenic alopecia, hypertension, nevus lipomatosus, scalp psoriasis, obesity, and with the use of a special tight head covering called 'Mandil'.[1,4–15] A congenital form may also occur. Other cases have been described in a child, white females, Orientals, males, and in a Maori girl.[8,16–23]

Occasionally, patients present with edema and bogginess of the scalp in the absence of hair loss (lipedematous scalp).[24] It is not clear whether this condition is part of the spectrum of lipedematous alopecia or a different entity altogether, as patients with lipedematous scalp do not seem to develop hair loss.

The clinical appearance of lipedematous alopecia is characteristic. The hairs are thin, short, broken, and of less than 2 cm in length. A boggy and spongy thickened scalp is more evident on palpation than visually (Fig. 22.106). There may be pain and pruritus in the affected area. The diagnosis can be established by magnetic resonance imaging (MRI), computed tomography (CT) scan, and head ultrasound by demonstrating the irregular thickening of the subcutaneous tissue. The normal scalp thickness varies with age, between 4.8 ± 0.12 mm in women 20 to 39 years of age and 5.6 ± 0.15 mm in women 40 to 69 years of age.[25] In lipedematous alopecia, the scalp thickness varied between 10 and 15 mm.[16] With videodermoscopy, lipedematous scalp shows linear areas of telangiectasia within the scalp creases.[9]

Pathogenesis and histologic features

There has been speculation with regard to the role played by thickened adipose tissue, edema, and dilated lymphatic vessels in the development of hair loss. It has been speculated that obesity and hormonal factors may play a role as the majority of patients are women. Leptin may also play a role in the distribution of the fat tissue.[26] At present, the exact pathogenesis of the disease is unknown.[7,17]

The scalp biopsy must be deep and include the whole thickness of the subcutaneous tissue, reaching the galea, as superficial biopsies may give a false impression of normality. The specimen must be processed with serial vertical sections. The histologic features consist of an increase of almost double the thickness of the scalp, with tissue edema, expansion of the subcutaneous fat, and infiltration of fat into the dermis (Fig. 22.107). In some cases, dilated lymphatic vessels have been observed.[21] Mucin deposition is

minimal or absent. Scarring is not present. Electron microscopy demonstrates localized edema with disruption and degeneration of the subcutaneous tissue.[27] In patients with alopecia, there is a mild decrease in the number of hair follicles but, there is no associated inflammation or scarring.[13]

Differential diagnosis

The differential diagnosis includes cutis verticis gyrata and lipoma. Primary cutis verticis gyrata is characterized by redundant skin on the scalp that exhibits typically symmetrical deep furrows, oriented in an anteroposterior direction and with a cerebriform pattern (Fig. 22.108). In contrast to lipedematous alopecia, primary cutis verticis gyrata usually starts after puberty in men and most commonly affects the crown and back of the head. A skin biopsy of the affected area can be normal or display thick connective tissue. Secondary cutis verticis gyrata appears at any age and has been associated with many diseases including inflammatory processes, systemic illnesses, acromegaly, idiopathic hypertrophic osteoarthropathy, benign and malignant tumors including nevi, and chromosomal abnormalities. In these cases, the histology is that of the underlying process.[28] A lipoma of the scalp is a well-circumscribed nodule that grows under the skin. It is surrounded by a capsule and may occur anywhere. It is not associated with alopecia and it does not contain hair follicles.[26,29]

Scarring alopecias

A wide variety of follicular and nonfollicular scalp conditions including hereditary, developmental, and acquired disorders may result in scarring or permanent alopecia as a secondary phenomenon (Fig. 22.109).[1] Permanent alopecia may also take place in the late stages of some nonscarring alopecias such as androgenetic alopecia, alopecia areata, psoriatic alopecia, and traction alopecia ('transitional scarring or biphasic pattern' alopecias).[2,3]

In this section, only those diseases that primarily affect the scalp or involve it secondarily with distinctive clinicopathological features will be described.

Scarring alopecia constitutes one of the most difficult and complex areas in the study of hair disease. It includes a wide variety of nosological entities

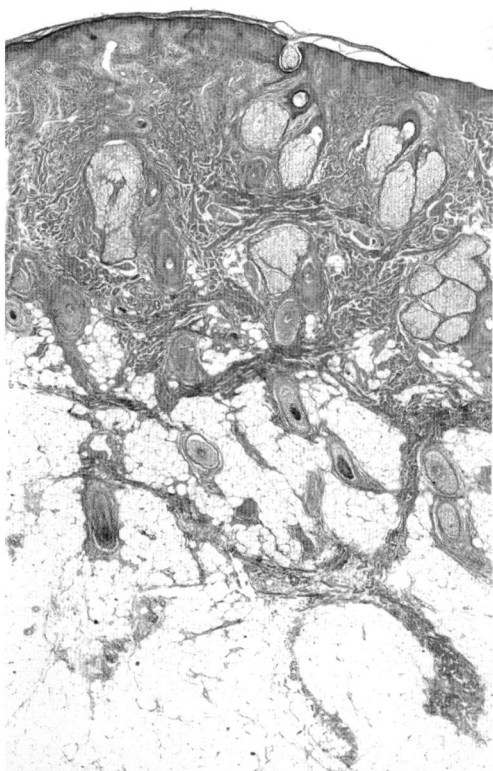

Fig. 22.107
Lipedematous alopecia. The subcutaneous tissue is thickened, in the absence of mucin deposition.

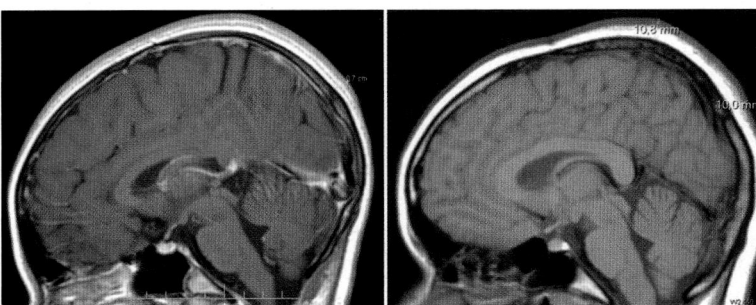

Fig. 22.106
Lipedematous alopecia: note the difference between the normal thickness of the scalp on the left and the increased thickness of the scalp on the right in a case of lipedematous alopecia. Courtesy of T. González, MD, CES, Medellín, Colombia.

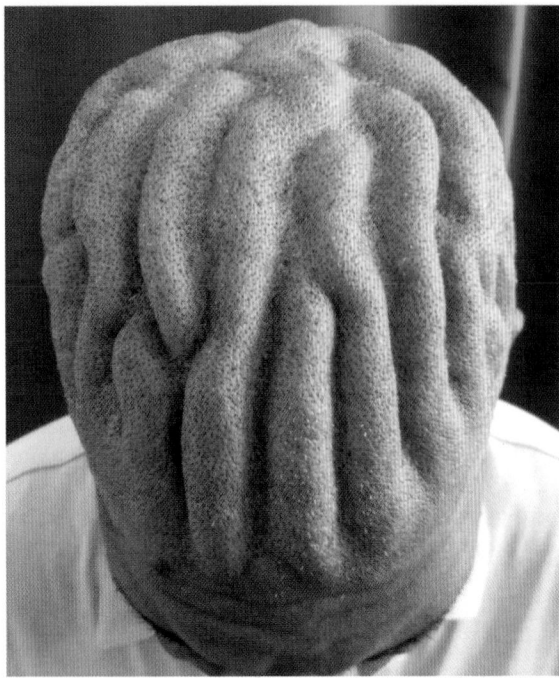

Fig. 22.108
Cutis verticis gyratum. Convoluted folds and furrows formed from thickened skin of the scalp in a cerebriform pattern. Courtesy of N. Valderrama, MD, Cali, Colombia.

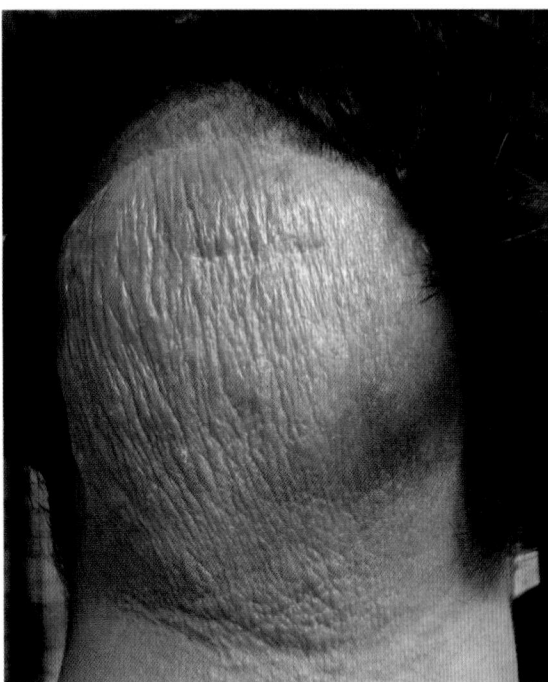

Fig. 22.109
Scarring alopecia secondary to folliculotropic mycosis fungoides. There is total loss of hair in the occipital and posterior parietal regions. Courtesy of Y. Corredoira Salum, MD, Universidad de Chile, Santiago, Chile.

with different etiologies and distinctive clinical features. However, the characteristic findings are usually only evident in the early stages, and as the disease progresses the clinical and pathological features of different diseases overlap, making categorization often impossible.

Scarring alopecias are characterized by irreversible loss and destruction of hair follicles and hair shafts. There is frequently, but not always, associated dermal fibrosis. Clinical examination reveals absence of follicular ostia (usually in a focal distribution), induration or atrophy of the skin, pigmentary alterations, follicular plugging, and occasionally, follicular pustules

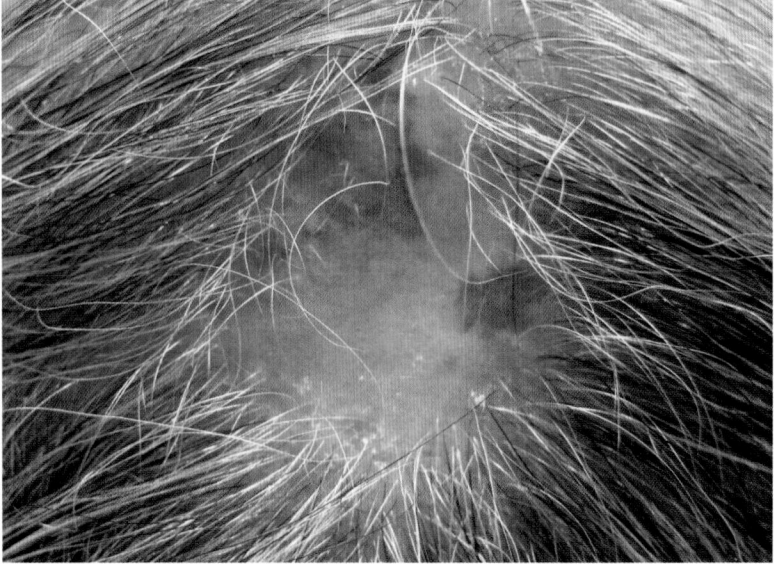

Fig. 22.110
Scarring alopecia, lichen planopilaris: there is a plaque of alopecia with hyper- and hypopigmentation, loss of follicular ostia, and follicular hyperkeratosis at the periphery. Courtesy of J. Gutiérrez, MD, Instituto de Ciencias de la Salud, Medellín, Colombia.

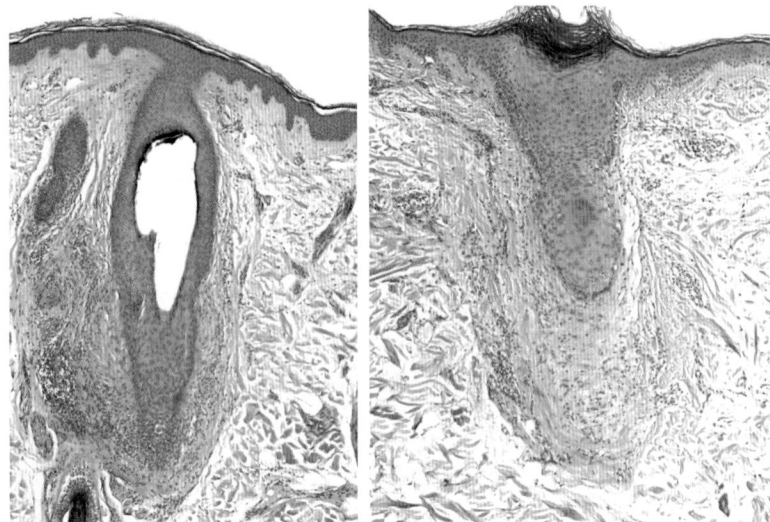

Fig. 22.111
Scarring alopecia, lichen planopilaris. Note the inflammatory infiltrate around the isthmus. There is perifollicular fibrosis, perifollicular mucin deposition and complete loss of sebaceous glands.

(Fig. 22.110). The histopathological hallmark is usually the presence of an inflammatory infiltrate surrounding the bulge and isthmus and loss of sebaceous glands, later followed by the formation of a scar with the hair follicle being replaced by follicular fibrous tracts (Figs 22.111 and 22.112). These fibrous tracts clearly represent scarring and are different to the follicular stellae seen in androgenic alopecia and telogen effluvium. They extend from the epidermis to the deep dermis. They are easy to identify using polarized light (Fig. 22.113 and see Fig. 22.34).[4] Histochemical stains including elastic stain and trichrome are useful to define the scarring areas and in the differential diagnosis with discoid lupus erythematosus, lichen planopilaris, and pseudopélade of Brocq (Fig. 22.114).[1] Sometimes the only structure left of the hair follicle is the arrector pili muscle (Fig. 22.115).

From the point of view of clinical management, scarring alopecia represents a real 'trichologic emergency' because in a short period of time the hair follicles may be permanently destroyed.[5] The resulting alopecia is irreversible and has a significant psychological impact. As the treatment is guided by the histopathologic findings, a scalp biopsy should be the first step in management.[5,6]

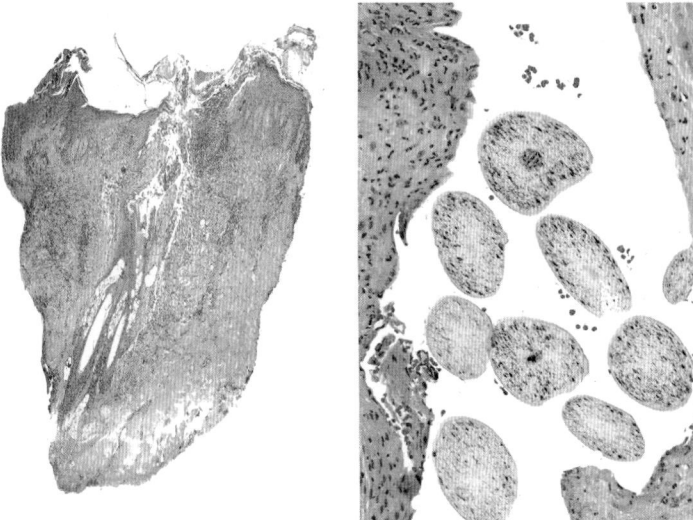

Fig. 22.112
Scarring alopecia, folliculitis decalvans. Vertical and horizontal sections. The destruction of hair follicles and sebaceous glands is associated with peri and interfollicular fibrosis. On the right side, fusion of follicles with numerous hair shafts associated with a single infundibulum (tufted folliculitis).

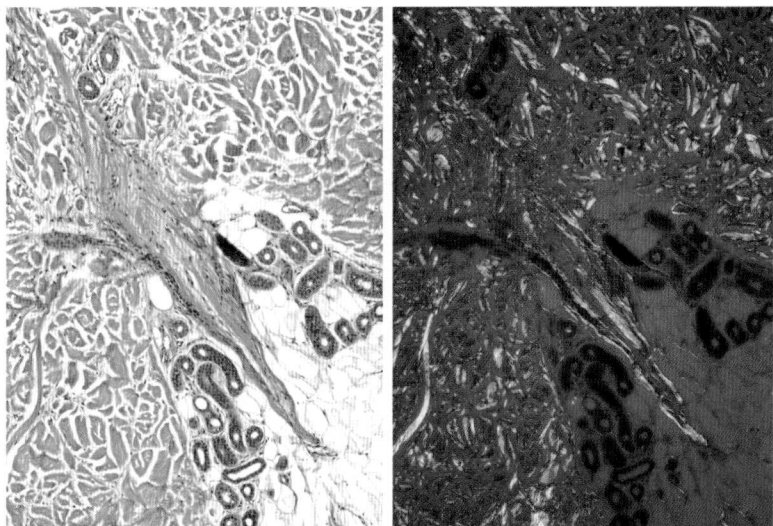

Fig. 22.113
Scarring alopecia, lichen planopilaris, follicular tracts. Note the birefringence of the collagen in the fibrous tract with polarized light.

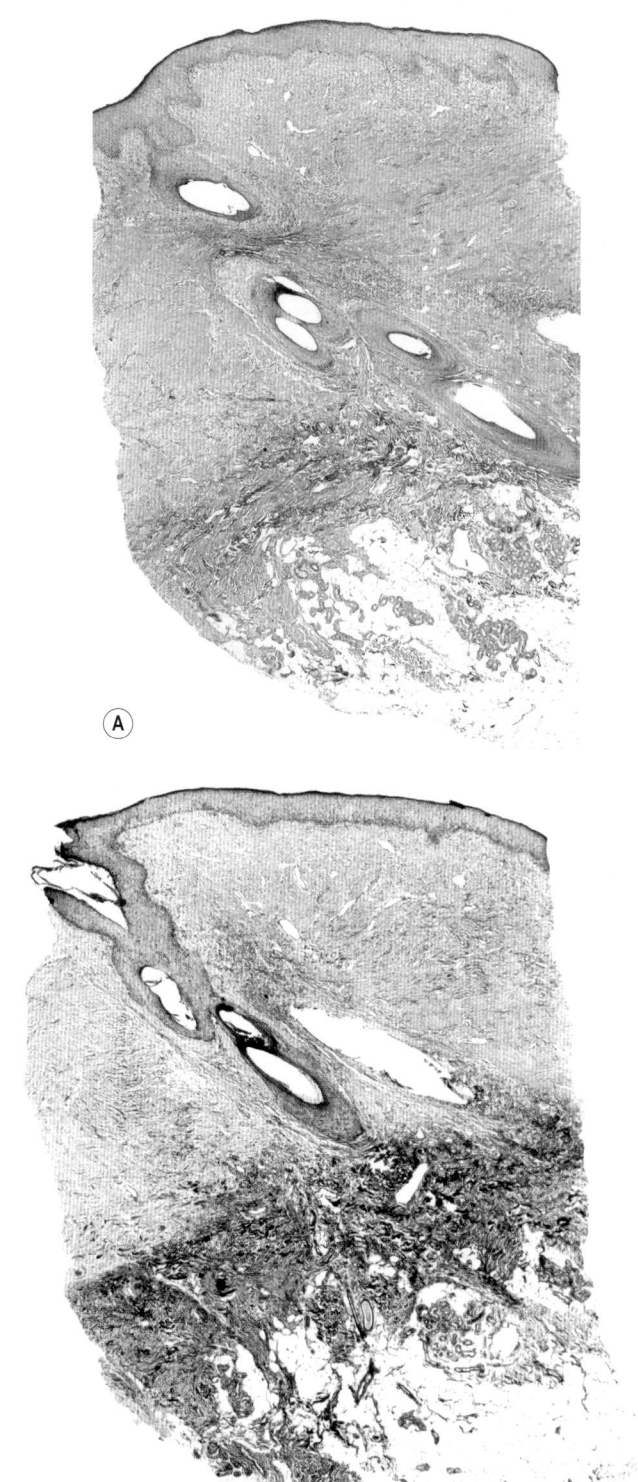

Fig. 22.114
Scarring alopecia, end-stage lupus erythematosus. (**A**) There are several fused follicles with an inflammatory cell infiltrate and absent sebaceous glands. (**B**) Elastic stain shows absence of staining in the dermis that surrounds the upper part of the hair follicle due to extensive loss of elastic fibers and scarring.

Scalp biopsies in cicatricial alopecia

Scalp biopsy is the most important test to achieve the diagnosis in all cases of primary scarring alopecia. These should be taken from the active border. Multiple biopsies may be necessary to reach a definitive diagnosis. Ideally, vertical and horizontal sections should be examined stained with hematoxylin and eosin, PAS, and elastic tissue stains. The use of horizontal and vertical sections yields the higher results as it enables the pathologist to evaluate the type and location of the inflammatory infiltrate, the presence or absence of fibrosis, the morphology of the hair follicles, and their stage in the cycle (*Fig. 22.116*; see *Fig. 22.112*).[7-9] In advanced cases in which only a scar without inflammatory infiltrate or hair follicles is present, direct immunofluorescence evaluation may be of great help in the differential diagnosis between discoid lupus erythematosus, lichen planopilaris, and pseudopélade of Brocq. For immunofluorescence studies, the second half of the punch biopsy submitted for vertical sections may be used (see *Fig. 22.9*).[7,10,11]

It is important not to forget that the evaluation of patients with scarring alopecia requires very close clinicopathological correlation, detailed clinical history, and laboratory tests including serology for syphilis, direct Gram and PAS stains, and culture of the lesions.

Pathogenesis

The pathophysiology of scarring is unclear and varies according to the different processes that result in permanent hair loss. However, some unifying generalizations concerning alterations on the stem cell-rich region in the bulge, the sebaceous gland, and the outer root sheath have emerged.[12,13]

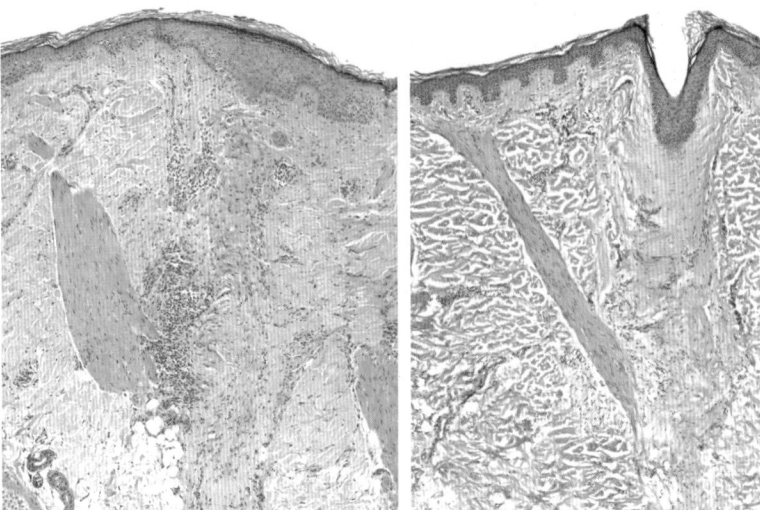

Fig. 22.115
Scarring alopecia, lichen planopilaris: the hair follicles have disappeared and been replaced by two vertical fibrous scars in which an arrector pili muscle is inserted.

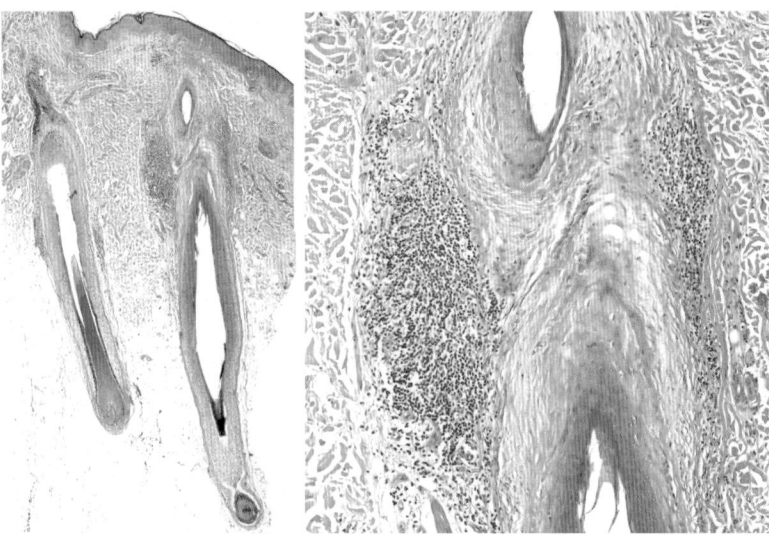

Fig. 22.117
Scarring alopecia, lichen planopilaris: note the lymphocytic infiltrate in the upper segment and in the area of insertion of the arrector pili muscle. In the figure on the right, note the loss of sebaceous glands and the premature shedding of the internal root sheath.

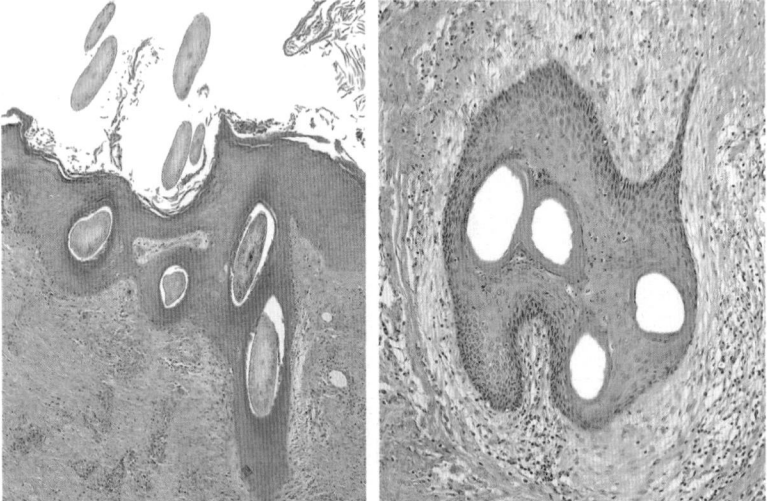

Fig. 22.116
Scarring alopecia, vertical and horizontal sections: this biopsy has been cut in two planes allowing a complementary view of tufted folliculitis (polytrichia) with hair follicle fusion into a single follicular structure which contains multiple hair shafts emerging at the surface through a single ostium.

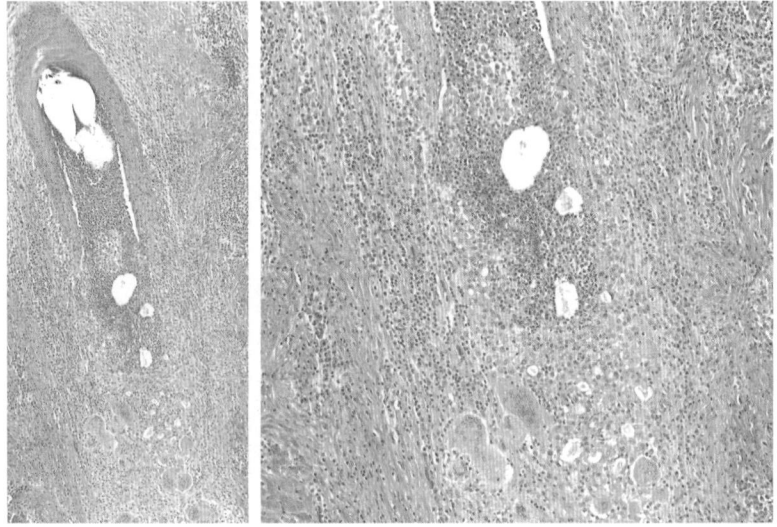

Fig. 22.118
Folliculitis decalvans: the hair follicle has ruptured and the intrafollicular neutrophils spill into the dermis inducing a strong granulomatous inflammatory response.

In many of the diseases that cause scarring alopecia, the inflammatory infiltrate is concentrated around the upper part of the hair follicle, involving the bulge and, as a consequence, the stem cells (*Fig. 22.117*, see *Fig. 22.111* and *22.112*). This damages the regenerative capacity of the hair follicle. The damage may be physical or by inhibition of the function resulting in interference in the interaction between hair follicle mesenchymal cells and the bulge epithelium. The hair follicle cycle is abolished.[14–16] The retained hair shaft bursts the bulb and lies free in the dermis, inducing a strong granulomatous inflammatory response with scarring (*Figs 22.118* and *22.119*). The only case in which the inflammatory infiltrate surrounds the bulge is in dissecting cellulitis of the scalp (perifolliculitis capitis abscedens et suffodiens), where the infiltrate is very deep at the limit between the dermis and the subcutaneous tissue.

Another common associated marker of scarring alopecia is early loss of sebaceous glands. This observation has been extensively studied in the asedia variant of mutant mice that lacks a gene to make sebum, has hypoplastic glands, and rapidly develops scarring alopecia.[17–19] It appears therefore that the localization of the infiltrate at the upper part of the hair follicle, including the bulge, is crucial to the development of permanent damage.[20,21,12]

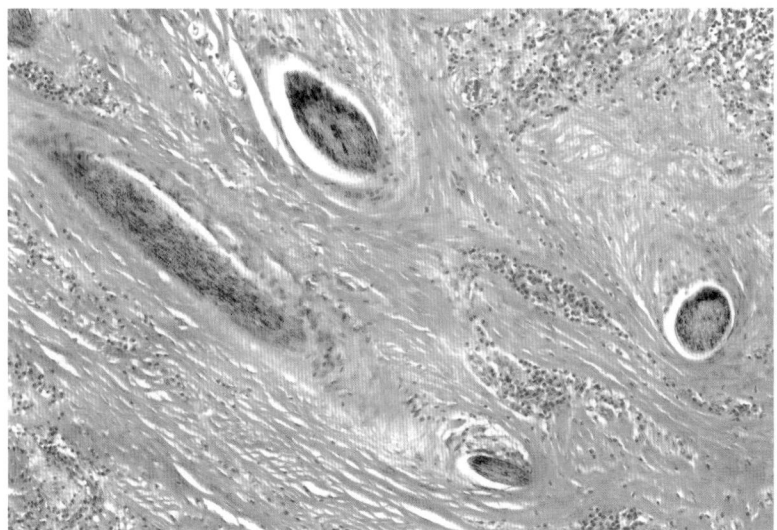

Fig. 22.119
Acne keloidalis nuchae. Multiple free hair shafts in the dermis surrounded by dense scarring.

Table 22.4

Proposed NAHRS working classification of primary cicatricial alopecia*

Lymphocytic
Chronic cutaneous lupus erythematosus
Lichen planopilaris
Classic lichen planopilaris
Frontal fibrosing alopecia
Graham-Little syndrome
Classic pseudopelade (Brocq)
Central centrifugal cicatricial alopecia
Alopecia mucinosa
Keratosis follicularis spinulosa decalvans
Neutrophilic
Folliculitis decalvans
Dissecting cellulitis/folliculitis (perifolliculitis capitis abscedens et suffodiens)
Mixed
Folliculitis (acne) keloidalis
Folliculitis (acne) necrotica
Erosive pustular dermatosis
Nonspecific

*Olsen, E.A., Bergfeld, W.F., Cotsarelis, G. et al. (2003). Workshop on Cicatricial Alopecia. Summary of North American Hair Research Society (NAHRS)-sponsored Workshop on Cicatricial Alopecia. *J Am Acad Dermatol*, **48**, 103–110.

Classification of scarring alopecias

There are as many classifications of scarring alopecias as there are authors who have written about the subject.[22]

In view of the fact that many primary scarring alopecias have clinical and histologic features in common, distinction between different clinical variants is often very difficult. Due to this, it has been proposed that primary cicatricial alopecia be separated in groups (lymphocytic, neutrophilic, mixed, and non-specific), based on the type of infiltrate that predominates within and around the affected hair follicles (*Table 22.4*).[8]

This classification was proposed at the first consensus meeting on cicatricial alopecia held at Duke University in North Carolina (2001) by the North American Hair Research Society (NAHRS). It has gained wide acceptance and thus, it will be taken as the basis for this chapter.[2,5,8,12,23–27]

Lymphocyte-associated primary cicatricial alopecias

This group of scarring alopecias is characterized by a lymphocyte infiltrate that always affects the superior segment of the follicle around the bulge. In general, the infiltrate does not change unless the follicle ruptures, giving place to a granulomatous reaction. There is loss of the sebaceous glands and fusion of hair follicles in numbers of two to a maximum of three. This fusion must be differentiated from that frequently observed in normal hair follicles at the infundibular level, hence the evaluation of a scarring alopecia must be done at the level of the isthmus or deeper (*Fig. 22.120*; see also *Figs 22.17* and *22.46*).[1,2]

Chronic cutaneous lupus erythematosus (discoid lupus erythematosus)

Clinical features

About 30–50% of patients with discoid lupus erythematosus present with scalp involvement.[1,2] Women are more frequently affected than men, and the disease rarely progresses to SLE.[3] Patients with SLE have cutaneous involvement in approximately 70% of cases. Of these, a high percentage show some degree of scalp involvement with alopecia during the course of the illness.[4–6]

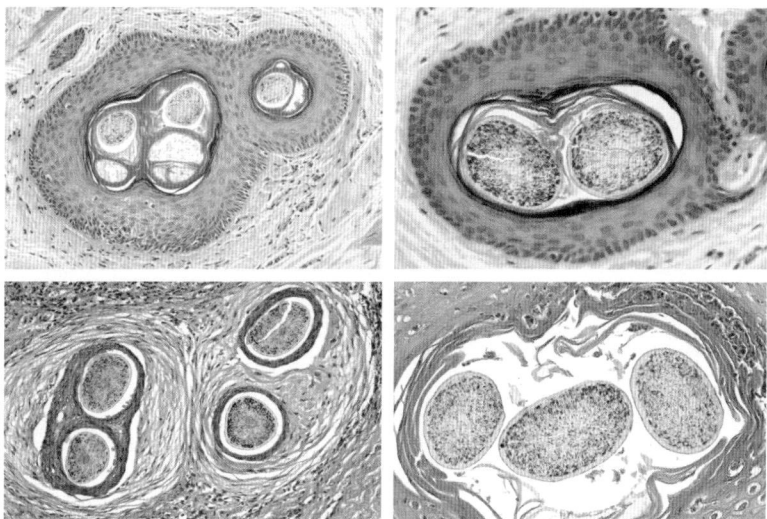

Fig. 22.120
Compound follicles. Upper panel, compound normal follicles transversally cut at the level of the infundibulum. Note the granular cell layer and discrete perifollicular fibrotic layer and minimal lymphocytic infiltrate. Lower panel, compound follicles in scarring alopecia. Horizontal sections at the level of the isthmus. There is extensive perifollicular fibrosis and an inflammatory infiltrate. The follicles on the left lower panel are from a case of acne keloidalis nuchae and those on the right panel from a case of folliculitis decalvans.

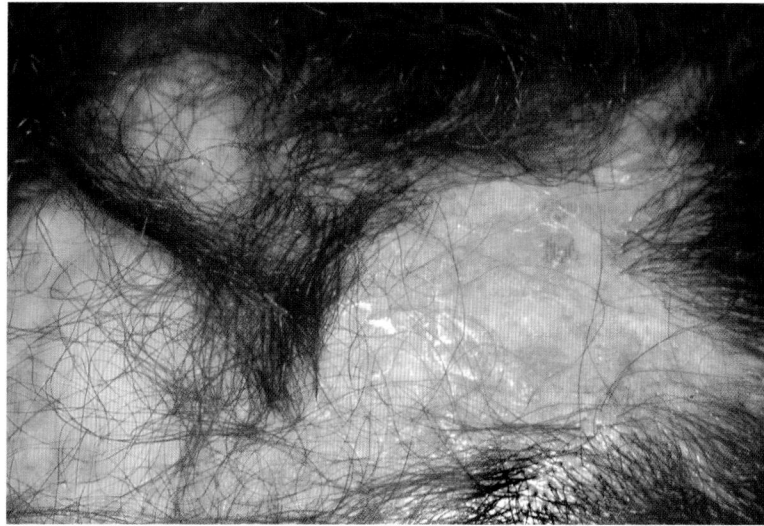

Fig. 22.121
Discoid lupus erythematosus: note the erythema, scaling, follicular plugging and scarring alopecia. Courtesy of P. Reygagne, MD, Centre Sabouraud, Paris, France.

The alopecia associated with lupus erythematosus may manifest as nonscarring and scarring forms. The nonscarring form has two variants: the first shows clinical and histologic features similar to those of common telogen effluvium,[7] whereas the second presents with patchy areas of hair loss that can simulate alopecia areata or syphilitic alopecia and occurs in patients who usually have severe SLE.[6,8] Clinically, erythema and edema in the involved areas are sometimes evident. These two nonscarring variants of alopecia are reversible when the primary illness is treated. The scarring form of lupus erythematosus-associated alopecia is typically seen in patients with the discoid variant and frequently occurs in adults, particularly women. Although it may also occur in SLE, this is infrequent. Scalp involvement is similar to that seen at other sites and consists of erythema, atrophy, follicular plugging, hyper- and hypopigmentation, and hair loss (*Fig. 22.121*). Contrary to other types of scarring alopecia, these changes are observed in both the periphery and the center of the lesion (*Fig. 22.122*).[9] The lesions, which can be solitary or multiple, small or confluent large plaques, may progressively affect extensive areas of the scalp (*Fig. 22.123*).

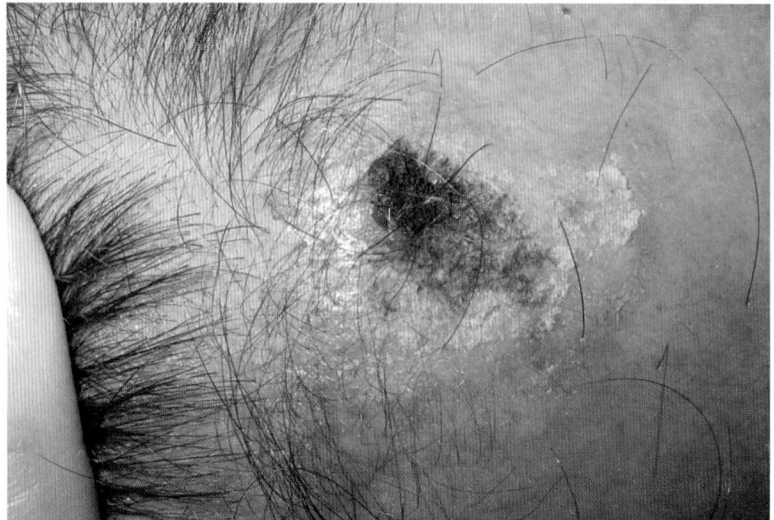

Fig. 22.122
Discoid lupus erythematosus. In this plaque, of alopecia, inflammatory activity is present at the periphery as well as in the center and there is crusting and erythema. Courtesy of L.M. Gómez, MD, UPB, Medellín, Colombia.

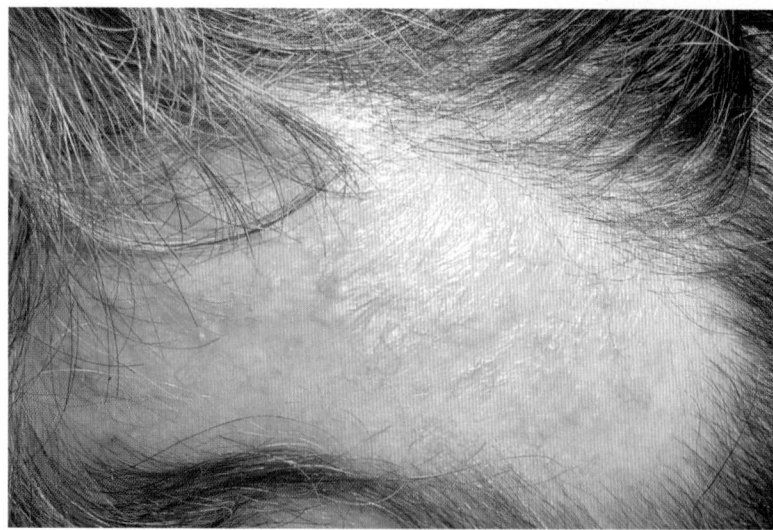

Fig. 22.124
Discoid lupus erythematosus: atrophic plaque with scarring, and loss of hair. Courtesy of A. Londoño, MD, CES, Medellín, Colombia.

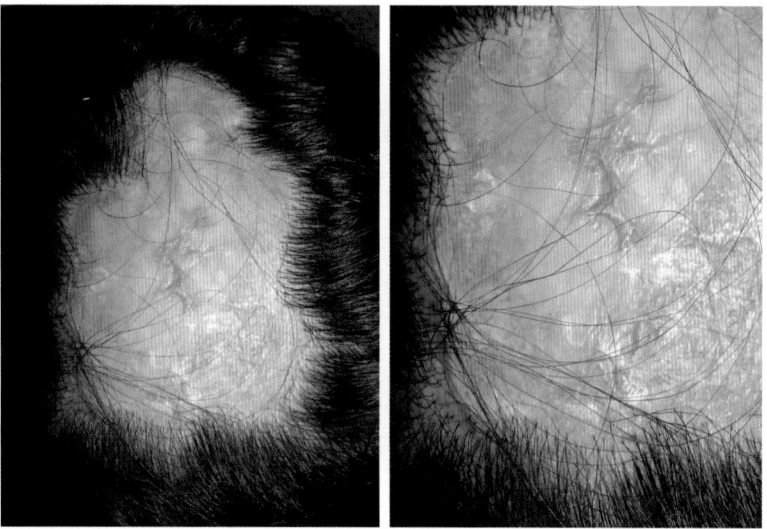

Fig. 22.123
Discoid lupus erythematosus: large erythematous plaque with telangiectasia, scarring, atrophy, and loss of hair, in the interparietal area. Courtesy of C. Velázquez, MD, CES, Medellín, Colombia.

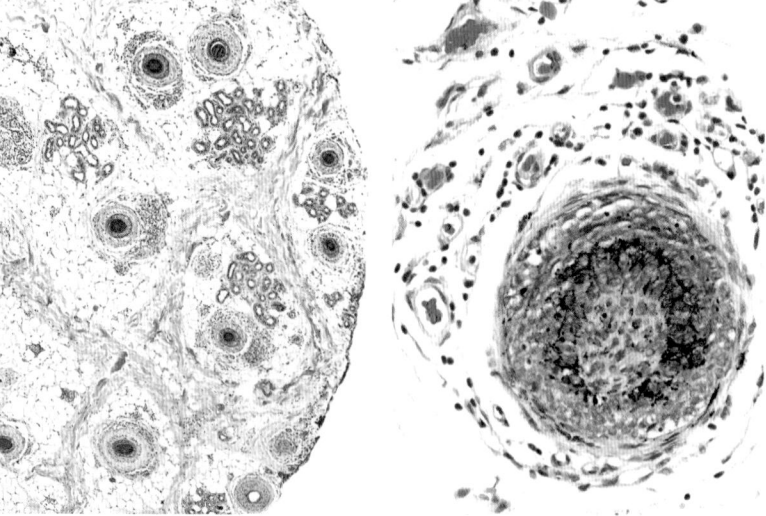

Fig. 22.125
Discoid lupus erythematosus: focal alopecia variant. The inflammatory infiltrate surrounding hair follicles is prominent. Note the similarity with alopecia areata or syphilitic alopecia.

As the illness progresses, the similarity to pseudopélade of Brocq and lichen planopilaris becomes more pronounced (*Fig. 22.124*). Discoid lupus erythematosus may present with loss of the eyebrows or eyelashes (madarosis) in the absence of involvement of the scalp.[10,11] In patients with discoid lupus erythematosus the incidence of alopecia areata is increased and, in longstanding disease, squamous cell carcinoma may rarely ensue.[12,13]

A rare form of lupus panniculitis with involvement of the lower part of the hair follicle and a transitory form of alopecia similar to alopecia areata have been documented.[14] Another rare form of linear alopecia related to lupus erythematosus profundus following the lines of Blaschko has been recognized.[15] Lipedematous alopecia has been associated with discoid lupus erythematosus.[16] The disease has also been associated with chronic granulomatous disease, frontal fibrosing alopecia, Parry-Romberg syndrome, and cutaneous horns.[17–20]

Pathogenesis and histologic features

The pathogenesis of lupus affecting the scalp is identical to that occurring at other sites of the body. The most appropriate site for the biopsy is best selected through dermoscopy of the affected areas of the scalp.[21]

Scalp involvement by lupus erythematosus equally affects the hair follicle and the epidermis at the dermal–epidermal junction. For this reason, vertical sections are preferred in the histologic study of the condition. However, if two biopsies can be obtained, a combination of vertical and horizontal sections for histologic interpretation and direct immunofluorescence is ideal.[22]

The histologic appearances of alopecia in lupus erythematosus are as varied as the clinical forms.

In the nonscarring variants, the chronic telogen effluvium-like form shows features identical to common telogen effluvium. The biopsy and trichogram both show a net increase in the number of telogen hair follicles.

In the variant with patchy alopecia, the histologic findings are very similar to those seen in alopecia areata and syphilitic alopecia except that the inflammatory infiltrate is generally more prominent and deep in lupus erythematosus (*Fig. 22.125*). Furthermore, other findings more typical of lupus erythematosus, including dermal mucin deposition and focal hydropic degeneration of the follicular epithelium, are often present.[23,24] The diagnosis in patients with systemic disease is generally straightforward, as symptoms and signs of systemic disease and typical laboratory findings are usually evident.

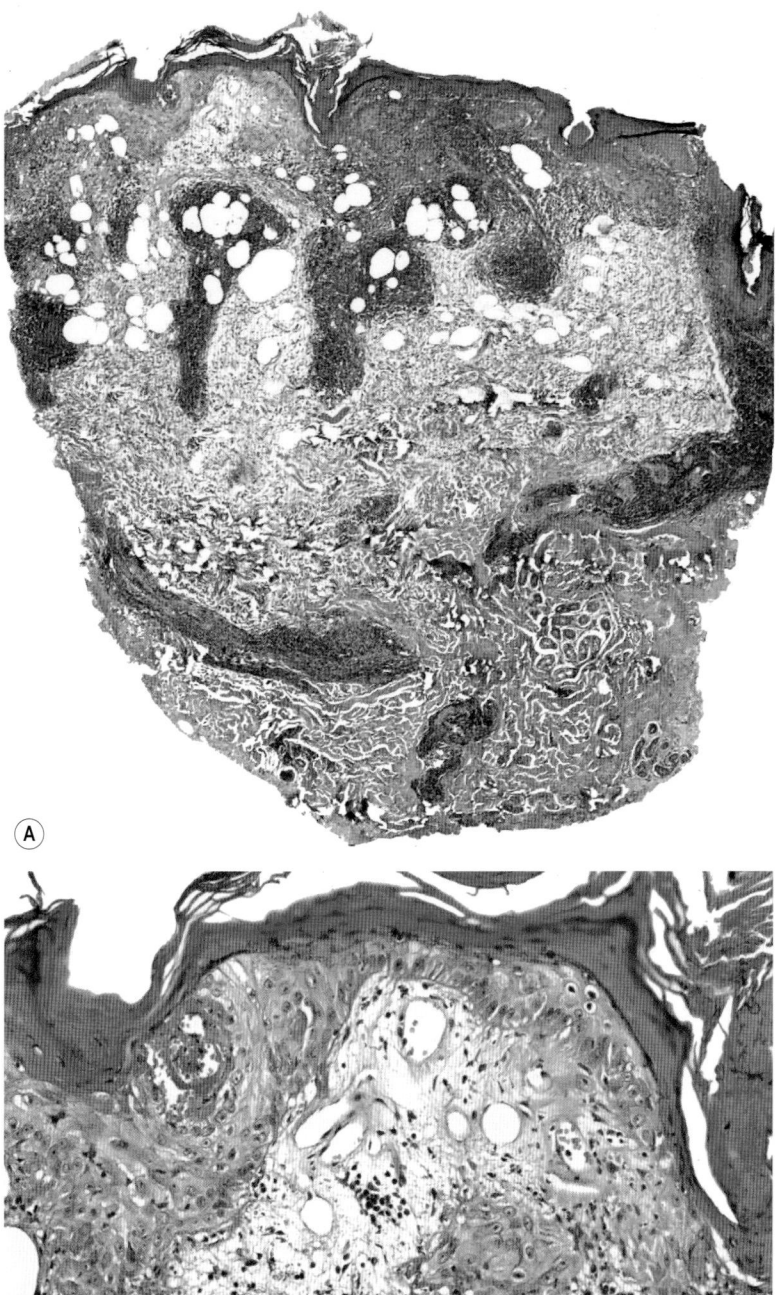

(A)

(B)

Fig. 22.126
Discoid lupus erythematosus: (**A**) there is loss of all the hair follicles and sebaceous glands with an intense lymphocytic infiltrate around superficial and deep blood vessels; (**B**) the epidermis shows dilated follicular infundibula with keratinous debris, hyperkeratosis. Also note epidermal atrophy, dermal edema, and telangiectasia.

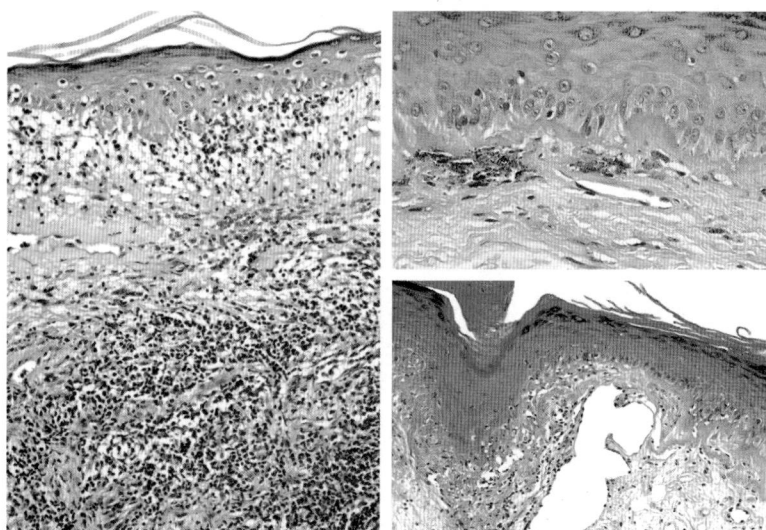

Fig. 22.127
Discoid lupus erythematosus. This image shows the typical histologic features of lupus erythematosus. Note the marked interface change and vacuolar degeneration of basal keratinocytes. In the dermis, there is a mononuclear inflammatory infiltrate with edema. The basement membrane is thickened.

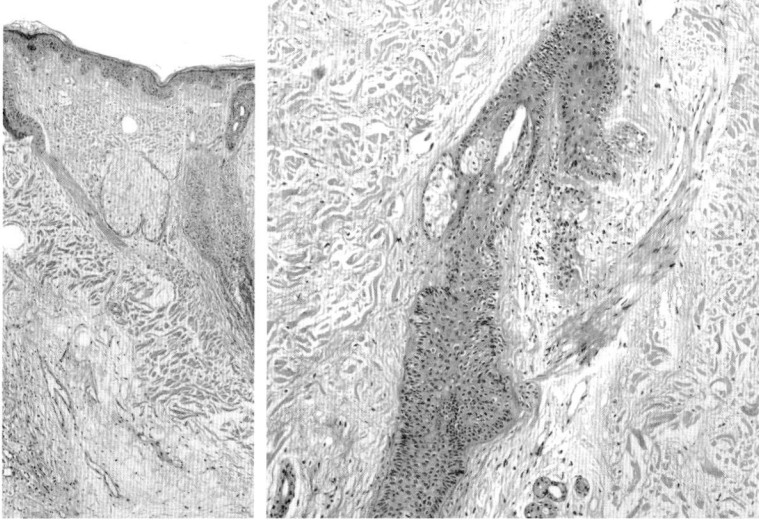

Fig. 22.128
Tumid lupus erythematosus: view of the dermis showing abundant mucin in this case with scalp involvement.

In the scarring variant, the microscopic findings differ little from those found in cutaneous discoid lupus presenting elsewhere. The degree of perifollicular inflammation, however, tends to be more intense than that seen in discoid lesions at other cutaneous sites (*Fig. 22.126*, see *Fig. 22.7*). In some cases, there may be intense hydropic degeneration of basal cells with minimal inflammation, whereas in others the features are those of a typical lichenoid dermatitis (*Fig. 22.127*). Colloid bodies are often present but they are less abundant than in lichen planopilaris. The presence of mucin and an infiltrate of plasma cells in a perivascular or periadnexal location are strong pointers toward a diagnosis of discoid lupus erythematosus (*Fig. 22.128*). Other histologic features that may also be seen include epidermal atrophy with hyperkeratosis and follicular plugging, thickening of the basement membrane, highlighted with the PAS stain with or without diastase, telangiectasia, and edema (*Fig. 22.129*). An inflammatory infiltrate within the fibrous stellae deep to the hair follicles may sometimes be present simulating alopecia areata and syphilitic alopecia.

As is typical of other scarring alopecias, the inflammatory cell infiltrate in discoid lupus is particularly prominent around the mid portion of the hair follicle at the level of the sebaceous glands, which eventually disappear (*Fig. 22.130*). The location is important because of the resulting reduction in the number of stem cells. Nevertheless, in longstanding lesions the inflammatory cell infiltrate may almost completely disappear, leaving only fibrosis and atrophy (*Fig. 22.131*).[25] In these cases, staining for elastic fibers will underscore the loss of elastic tissue within the broad scarred areas of the dermis and destruction of the elastic sheath surrounding the fibrous tracts (see *Fig. 22.114*).[26]

Differential diagnosis

The two most important differential diagnoses include lichen planopilaris and pseudopélade of Brocq.

Clinically, in lichen planopilaris hyperkeratotic lesions are located at the periphery of the areas of alopecia as opposed to lupus erythematosus where

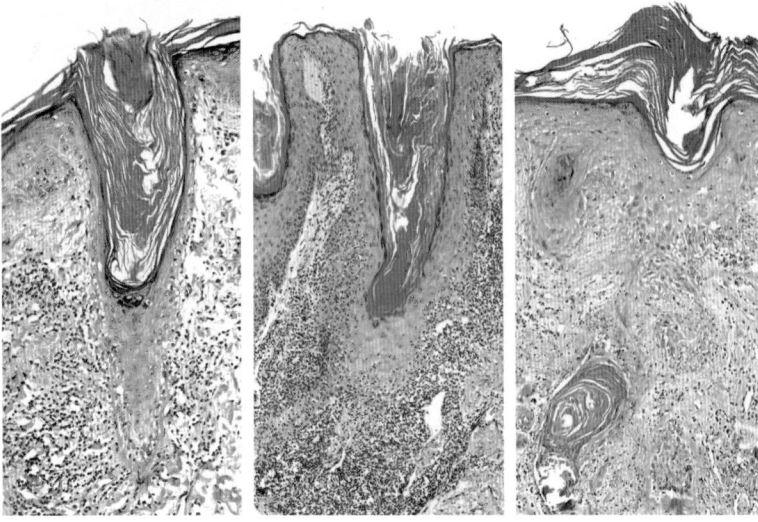

Fig. 22.129
Discoid lupus erythematosus: follicular plugging with almost complete involution of the hair follicles. There is sclerosis of the papillary and upper reticular dermis.

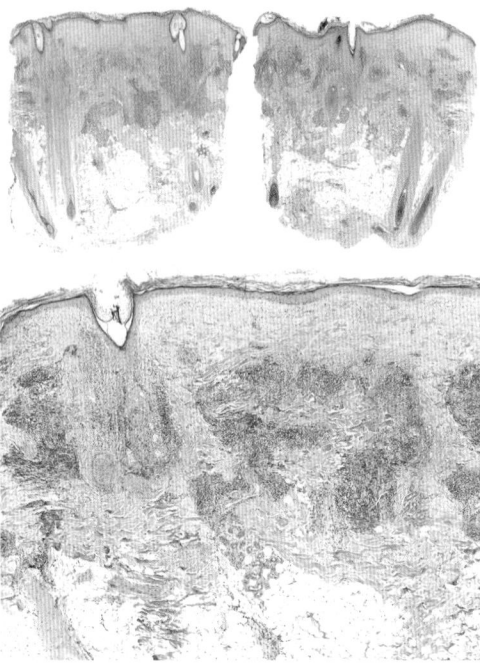

Fig. 22.130
Discoid lupus erythematosus: Prominent inflammatory cell infiltrate located around the upper segment of the hair follicles and also in a perivascular location.

the follicular hyperkeratosis is constantly present in the central part of the bald patches.[9,27] Histologically, the dermal–epidermal interface change in discoid lupus erythematosus is usually pronounced and of vacuolar type, whereas in lichen planopilaris lichenoid features (i.e., a more bandlike inflammatory cell infiltrate) predominate around the hair follicle. Additional histologic features that help in the diagnosis of lupus erythematosus are the more prominent perivascular infiltrate, the presence of dermal mucin, and plasma cells.[28]

The histologic diagnosis distinction from pseudopélade of Brocq is based on the absence of marked inflammation, significant follicular plugging, thickened basement membrane, and basal vacuolar degeneration in lupus erythematosus. Pseudopélade of Brocq is characterized by white-ivory colored patches of alopecia limited to the scalp, with a 'footprints in the snow' appearance.[29]

In histopathologically inconclusive cases, direct immunofluorescence is an important tool in the differential diagnosis of discoid lupus erythematosus.[30] A positive lupus band test is seen in up to 83% of cases and

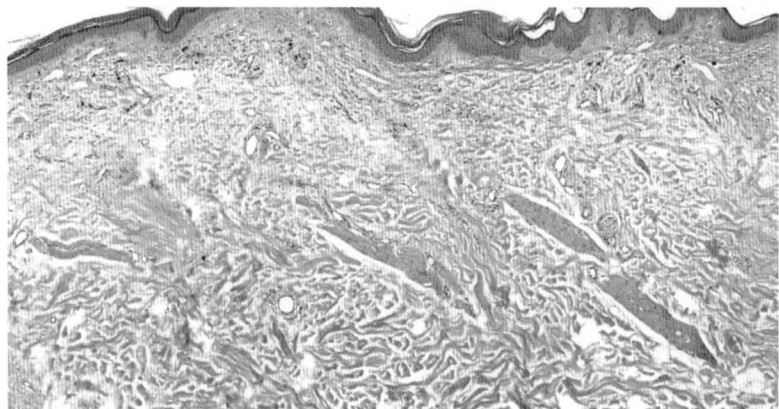

Fig. 22.131
Discoid lupus erythematosus, late stage: the hair follicles have completely disappeared, leaving follicular stellae and arrector pili muscles. In the papillary dermis, there are melanophages, and telangiectasia is evident. The inflammatory cell infiltrate is minimal.

consists of granular deposits of IgG, C3, and C1q at the level of the basement membrane, both at the dermal–epidermal junction and at the junction between the follicular epithelium and the dermis.[31] A negative result does not completely exclude the possibility of discoid lupus erythematosus.[32] In lichen planopilaris, direct immunofluorescence shows globular deposition, particularly of IgM at the junction between the follicular epithelium and the dermis, highlighting apoptotic bodies. Linear deposition of Ig along the follicular basement membrane region, however, may also be seen. Direct immunofluorescence in pseudopélade of Brocq is usually negative. It seldom shows finely granular IgM deposition along the follicular infundibular basement membrane.[33,34] Finally, another recent important finding that may help in the differential diagnosis is the presence of groups of CD123+ plasmocytoid dendritic cells (defined as clusters of at least five cells) in discoid lupus whereas in lichen planopilaris these cells are arranged as single interstitial cells.[35,36]

Lichen planopilaris

Lichen planopilaris includes several variants with similar clinical, histopathological, and immunohistopathological features: classic lichen planopilaris, frontal fibrosing alopecia, fibrosing alopecia in a pattern distribution, and Graham-Little syndrome.

Clinical features
Classic lichen planopilaris
Classic lichen planopilaris is a very common form of scarring alopecia first described by Pringle in 1895.[1] It is characterized by a variable clinical course resulting in patchy areas of hair loss accompanied by follicular inflammation. It is more frequent in women (70%) and has an average age of onset of 51 years.[2] It has occasionally been reported in children.[3] Approximately 50% of the patients have typical lesions of lichen planus elsewhere on the skin at one time or another.[2] Typical lichen planus associated with lichen planopilaris of the scalp is rarely observed.[4] However, involvement of the nails and oral/vulval mucosae may also be seen.[5,6]

Common clinical symptoms include itching, scaling, tenderness, and burning sensation. Physical examination shows variable changes depending on the stage of clinical evolution. The lesions may be single or multiple and usually involve the parietal and vertex areas of the scalp. In general, the findings result from a mixture of inflammatory changes and scarring. The inflammation is characterized by follicular keratotic papules, scaling, and perifollicular erythema (see Fig. 22.110). The scarring results in hair loss with dilated follicular ostia containing keratotic debris (Fig. 22.132). Several hair shafts may emerge through these dilated ostia, generally in a number lower than 3.[7] If examination of the scalp is performed at a late stage of the disease, overlap with other scarring alopecias is common, particularly pseudopélade of Brocq. The resemblance is such that some authors claim that these two entities represent the same illness.[8]

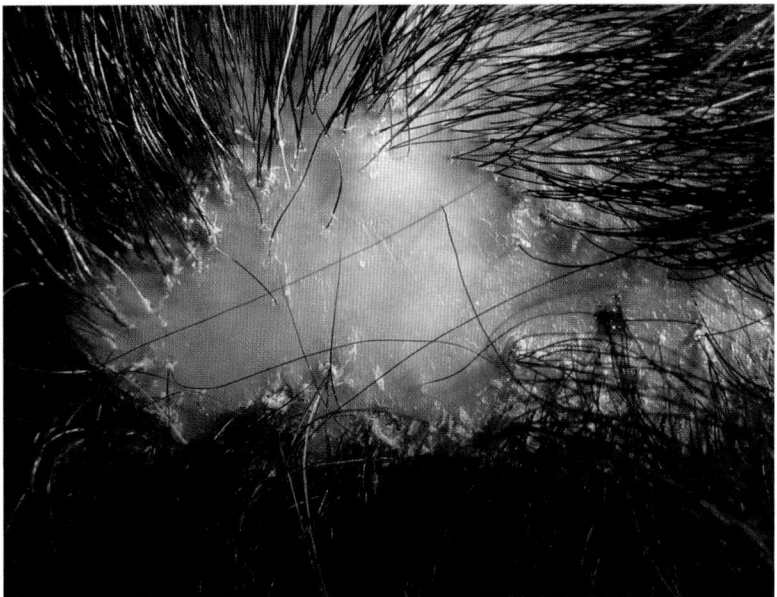

Fig. 22.132
Lichen planopilaris: atrophic patch with loss of follicular orifices, perifollicular erythema, and scaling. Courtesy of L.M. Gómez, MD, UPB, Medellín, Colombia.

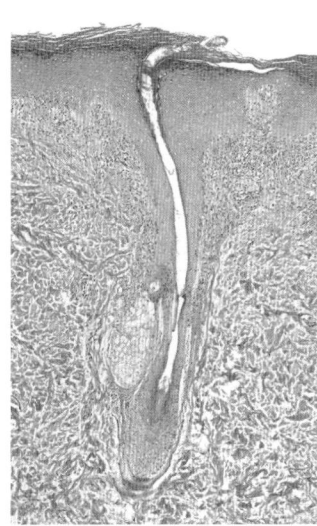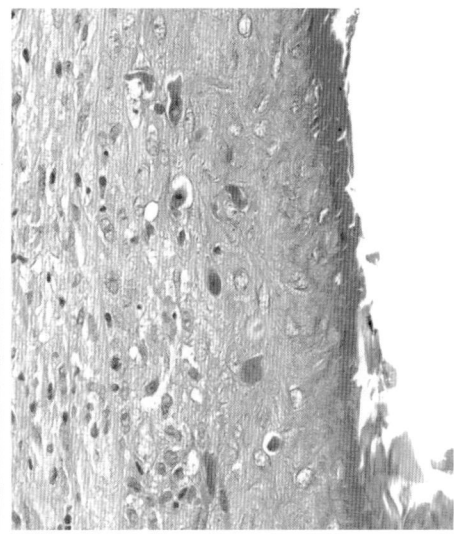

Fig. 22.133
Lichen planopilaris, vertical sections. *Left*: the inflammatory cell infiltrate surrounds the superior segment without involving the inferior segment. There is complete loss of sebaceous glands. In these cases, an infrequent finding is the subepidermal bandlike inflammatory cell infiltrate. *Right*: numerous apoptotic bodies are seen in the outer root sheath. There is shedding of the internal root sheath.

In the active stages, the hair-pull and hair-pluck tests show an increase in the number of anagen hairs.[9] The most useful laboratory tests other than biopsy include direct immunofluorescence and antibody screening to exclude discoid and SLE.

Occasionally, lichen planopilaris may present in areas such as the extremities, trunk, and vulva, without involvement of the scalp.[10,11] Exceptionally, a facial and truncal linear distribution has been documented, following Blaschko lines.[12,13] Another variant of lichen planus that may affect the adnexal structures is lichen planus poritis (lichen planus of the eccrine glands), which involves the acrosyringium and proximal eccrine ducts in the superficial part of the dermis.[14]

Lichen planopilaris has been associated with exposure to gold, autoimmune thyroiditis, psoriasis, scleroderma en coup de sabre, dermatitis herpetiformis, erythema dyschromicum perstans, scalp trauma, and break dancing.[15–23] The disease has also been reported restricted to an epidermal nevus, in association with etanercept and imiquimod treatment, following whole brain irradiation and after hair transplantation and facial cosmetic surgery.[23–30]

Pathogenesis and histologic features

Although the pathogenesis of lichen planopilaris is similar to that of lichen planus occurring elsewhere, several differences have been reported.[31]

Lichen planopilaris is considered a hair-specific autoimmune disease in which activated T lymphocytes target follicular antigens, mainly the epithelium of the infundibulo-isthmic region (the bulge area). In the majority of cases it does not affect the hair bulb or the dermal–epidermal interface. The antigen targeted in this response is unknown. Lichen planopilaris has been associated with an increased frequency of HLA DRB1*11 and DQB1*03 alleles.[32]

Some studies have shown an increment in the number of CD8+ T cells compared with the CD4+ T-cell population and a decrease in proliferative bulge stem cells. The latter favors a cell-mediated cytotoxic immune response in the pathogenesis of the disease.[33] Nevertheless, a further study has shown low numbers of CD8+ T cells in 'early' active stages of the disease and in the late 'fibrotic' phase, preservation of the bulge stem cells. This suggests that the irreversible loss of hair follicles bulge cells is not necessarily a consequence of T cell-mediated destruction.[34] A further significant finding in the etiopathogenesis of lichen planopilaris has been the observation of an altered distribution of integrins in the affected follicular keratinocytes, facilitating loss of adhesion of follicular keratinocytes to the stroma.[35] This could also explain the artifactual clefts observed in histologic

studies and the phenomenon of easy plucking of the hair in the more active lesions of the disease.

Lichen planopilaris is considered a true trichologic emergency in which treatment should be instituted promptly to avoid irreversible hair loss. In this context, the biopsy is an essential component of the diagnostic work-up.[36,37] It is very important to take an adequate biopsy from an active lesion, preferably from an area that is erythematous and scaly and in which there are still hair follicles that could be easily plucked, with anagen-like hair roots.[9] This affords the best opportunity of identifying the diagnostic features. A biopsy of a nonactive or burned-out area usually does not offer much information and leads to a diagnosis of end-stage scarring alopecia of undetermined etiology.

The histologic study should include an examination of horizontal and vertical sections, (*Fig. 22.133*).[38] However, horizontal sections provide particularly valuable information, as the infiltrate is limited mainly to the infundibulum and isthmic region of the hair follicle. Typical findings consist of a lichenoid tissue reaction with formation of apoptotic bodies within the follicular epithelium but with little involvement of the intervening epidermis. Perifollicular fibrosis facilitates a tendency for the follicles to fuse creating an 'owl eye' appearance (*Fig. 22.134* and see *Fig. 22.117*). The lower portion of the hair follicle and the bulb are usually not affected, but in severe cases the inferior segment and the suprabulbar zone may be involved These changes are uneven according to disease progression and provide more information in the active and early-stage disease process. Lichen planopilaris does not usually show the classic bandlike infiltrate seen in ordinary lichen planus.

The interface changes are characterized by focal loss of attachment between the follicular epithelium and the surrounding dermis. As a result, artifactual clefts are sometimes apparent and colloid bodies are often found. An associated mononuclear inflammatory cell infiltrate is present within the perifollicular connective tissue sheath, which is usually thickened (*Fig. 22.135*). Basal follicular keratinocytes in the involved area become squamotized with larger size, prominent eosinophilic cytoplasm, and cytoplasmic angulation (*Fig. 22.136*). Although mucinous perifollicular fibroplasia may be observed around the follicle, there is no accumulation of dermal mucin (*Fig. 22.137*, see *Fig. 22.111*).[36]

In the late stages, the hair follicle is completely destroyed and replaced by a sclerotic collagenous follicular scar with loss of sebaceous glands. The only structures left are the arrector pili muscles (see *Fig. 22.115*). On occasions, the predominant pattern is that of foreign body granulomas distributed around the free hair shafts (*Fig. 22.138*).[39,40] Other forms of

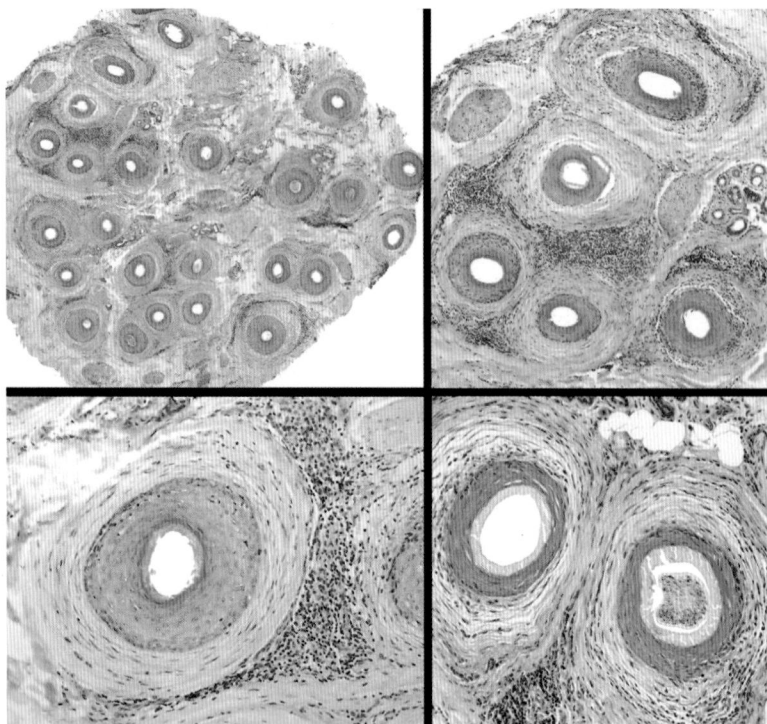

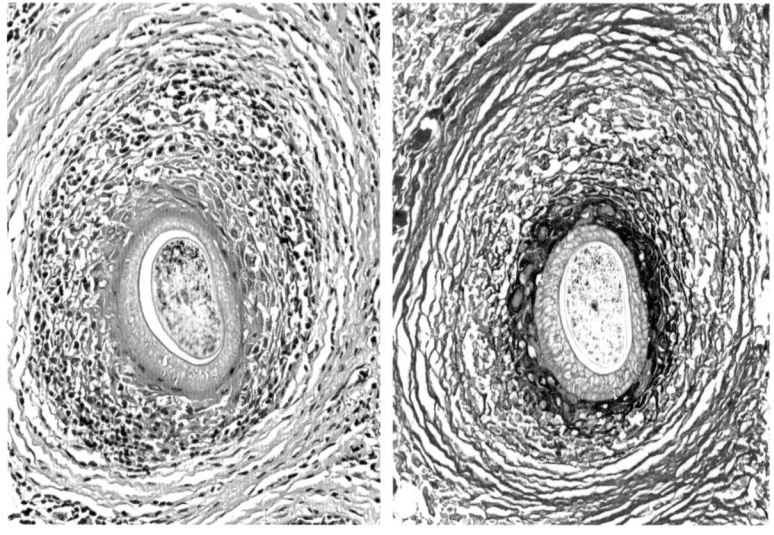

Fig. 22.134
Lichen planopilaris, horizontal sections: in this biopsy, there are no sebaceous glands and all the follicles show a perifollicular mononuclear inflammatory cell infiltrate. Most hair follicles show lamellar fibroplasia separating the lymphocytic infiltrate from the outer root sheath. In the right panel, upper and lower images, an 'owl eye' appearance is appreciated.

Fig. 22.135
Lichen planopilaris, frontal fibrosing alopecia type: horizontal sections. *Left*: the destruction of the outer root sheath is evident with interface change, fibrosis and lymphocytic inflammation. *Right*: with the Mason trichrome staining, the lamellar fibrosis around the mononuclear cell infiltrate is apparent.

scarring alopecia (including pseudopélade of Brocq and discoid lupus erythematosus) share this end-stage histologic appearance. In order to highlight the presence of scarring tissue, special stains to delineate elastic fibers are particularly useful. They allow distinction between normal dermis and scarred areas, as the latter lack elastic fibers. A perifollicular and superficial wedge-shaped scar with loss of the elastic sheath surrounding fibrous tracts is identified, although occasionally it may be seen in other scarring alopecias (*Fig. 22.139*).[41–43]

Immunofluorescence studies show staining of colloid bodies with IgM and IgA and linear deposits of fibrin along the basement membrane of the

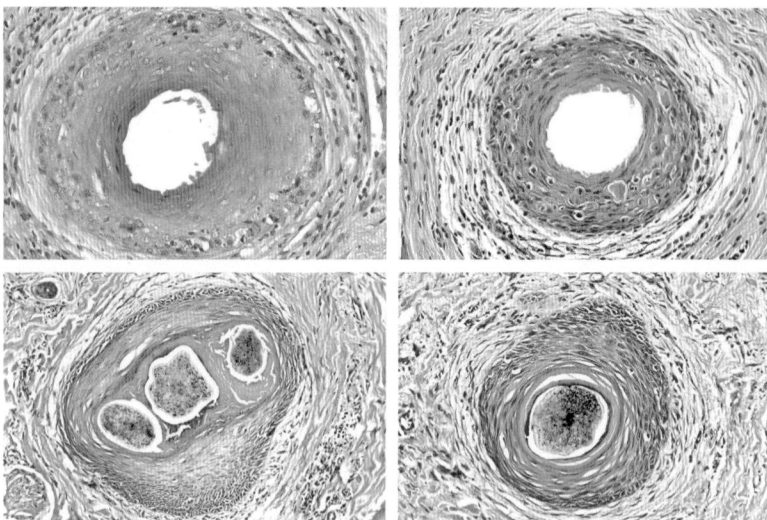

Fig. 22.136
Lichen planopilaris, horizontal sections: photographic composition of the typical changes. (*Top*) Initial changes with apoptosis and loss of internal root sheath. (*Bottom*) Advanced changes with fusion of follicles and thinning of the outer root sheath.

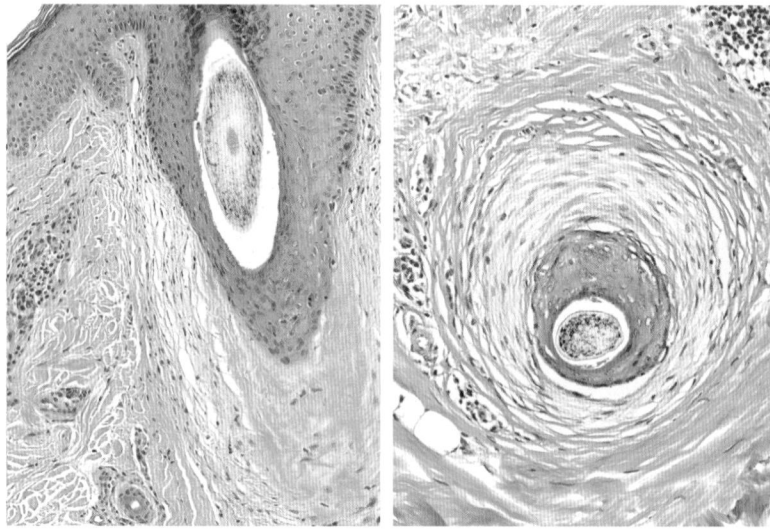

Fig. 22.137
Lichen planopilaris, vertical and horizontal sections: there is mucinous perifollicular fibroplasia.

infundibular portion of the hair follicle.[4] Linear deposition of immunoglobulin (usually IgG or IgA) restricted to the follicular epithelium has also been described.[44] However, these immunofluorescence findings are not specific to lichen planopilaris and they may also be observed in other diseases with interface change and damage to the basal cell layer. Increased birefringence within the fibrous tracts is a frequent finding in lichen planopilaris but may occasionally be found in other scarring and nonscarring alopecias (see *Fig. 22.113*).[45,46]

Differential diagnosis

The correct diagnosis may be reached in the majority of the cases by careful correlation of histopathological, clinical, and immunohistopathological findings. The most important entities to consider in the differential diagnosis are discoid lupus erythematosus and pseudopélade of Brocq.

In discoid lupus erythematosus, the typical findings include a superficial and deep perivascular lymphohistiocytic infiltrate, dermal mucin, and vacuolar interphase change affecting not only the follicles but also the intervening dermal–epidermal junction. In lichen planopilaris, the infiltrate is mainly seen around hair follicles, and interface change of the interfollicular epidermis is rarely present.

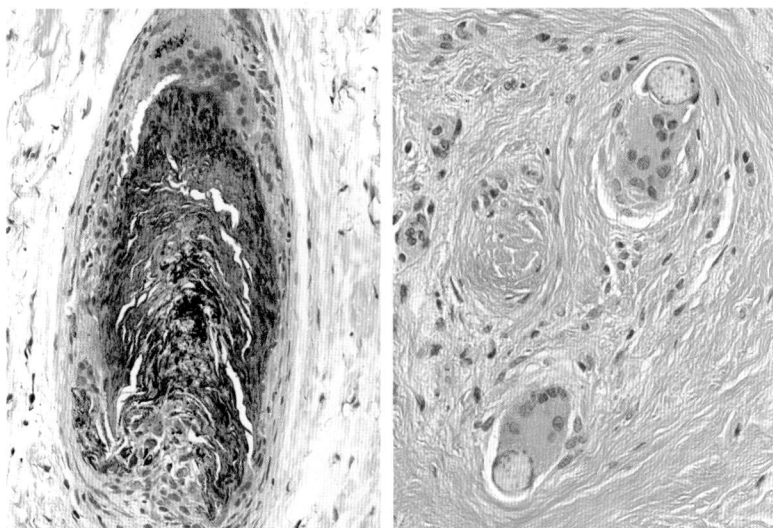

Fig. 22.138
Lichen planopilaris: there are numerous giant and epithelioid cells surrounding the free hair shafts in the dermis.

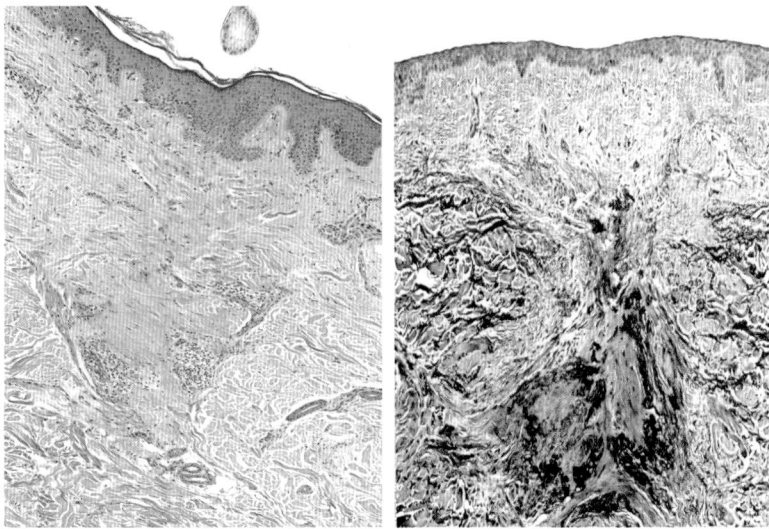

Fig. 22.139
Lichen planopilaris. *Left*: follicular scar extending from the epidermis to the deep dermis. *Right*: With the elastic stain loss of elastic fibers in triangular shape with the base toward the epidermis is observed. The follicular scarring shows condensation of elastic fibers with a vertical orientation.

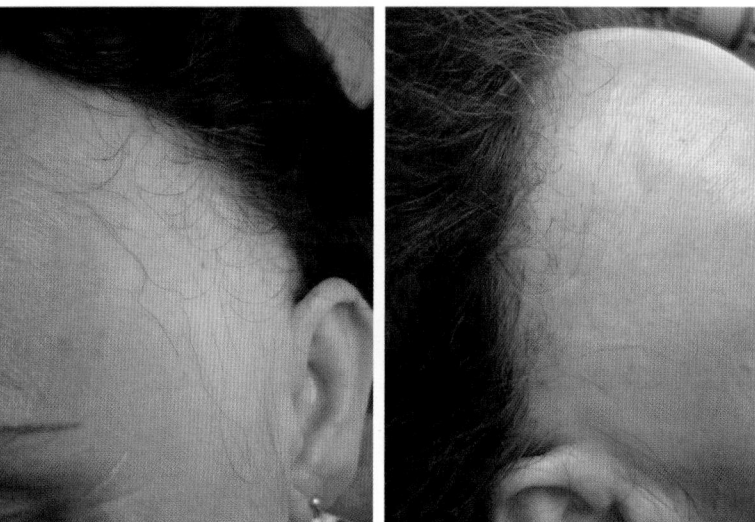

Fig. 22.140
Frontal fibrosing alopecia: bandlike recession of the frontotemporal hairline associated with lateral eyebrow thinning. Note the solitary hairs in the frontal scalp. Courtesy of L.M. Gómez, MD, Universidad Pontificia Bolivariana, Medellín, Colombia.

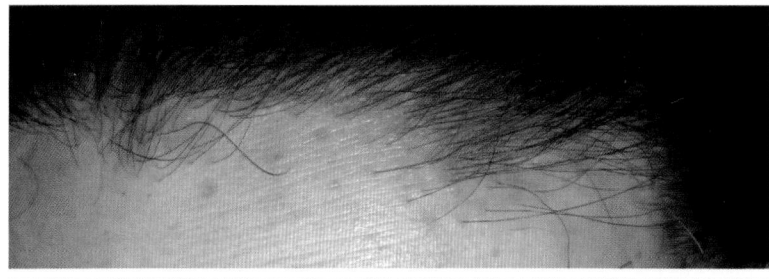

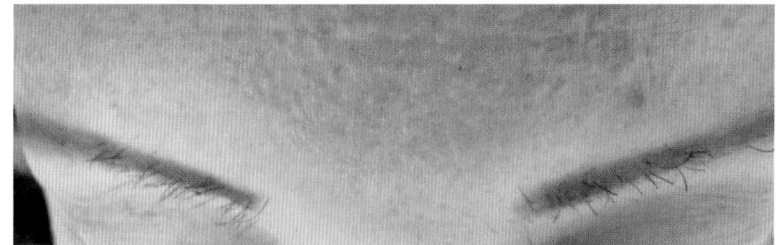

Fig. 22.141
Frontal fibrosing alopecia. *Above*: there is hair loss on the frontal scalp. The skin shows perifollicular erythema. *Below*: the skin appears mildly scarred with prominence of the follicles and inflammation. There is almost total absence of eyebrows.

Pseudopélade of Brocq presents as progressive patches of scarring alopecia, and histologically the changes are essentially those of marked scarring with no interface change. It is possible that pseudopélade of Brocq represents a late stage of various forms of scarring alopecia, including lichen planopilaris.

In the end stages of the disease, it may be impossible to differentiate lichen planopilaris from pseudopélade of Brocq and discoid lupus erythematosus. The presence of a band of fibrosis in the papillary dermis accompanied by fibrous tracts in the reticular dermis following the path of destroyed follicles appears to be a valuable pointer toward 'burn-out' lesions of lichen planopilaris.[47]

Clinical features
Frontal fibrosing alopecia
Kossard first described frontal fibrosing alopecia in 1994 as a variant of scarring alopecia closely related to lichen planus and affecting mainly postmenopausal women (postmenopausal frontal fibrosing alopecia).[1,2] However, some cases have been reported in premenopausal women as well as on the sideburns and beard in males and in patients of African descent.[3–10] Furthermore, some cases in children and adolescents have also been described.[11,12]

It presents with progressive and symmetric recession of the frontal hairline associated with smooth and pale skin. Sometimes perifollicular erythema, follicular keratinization, and extension onto the temporal and parietal zones may be observed (*Fig. 22.140*). In addition, there is loss or reduction of the hair follicles of the eyebrows, the rest of the face, and also of the extremities, axillae, trunk, and pubis (*Fig. 22.141*). [13,14] Eyebrow alopecia is thought to precede the scalp alopecia.[15]

Progression is unpredictable, but the disease becomes stable in almost all patients.[16] Clinically, the disease does not present with the multifocal areas of hair loss typically seen in lichen planus or pseudopélade of Brocq. There are usually no manifestations of lichen planus elsewhere although isolated cases have shown typical lichen planus in the skin or mucosae, particularly in pigmented lichen planus.[17–21] In some patients, diffuse hair loss has been described. [7,22]

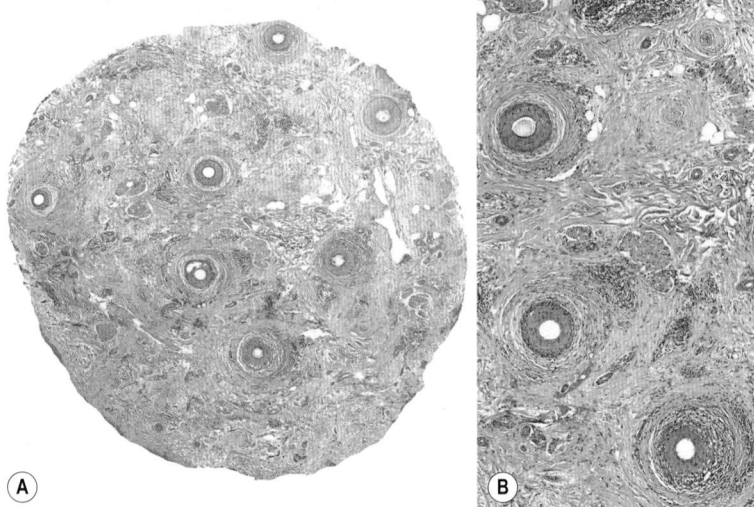

Fig. 22.142
Frontal fibrosing alopecia, horizontal section. (**A**) In this scanning magnification, there is absence of sebaceous glands, loss of hair follicles, and perifollicular fibrosis. (**B**) Lichenoid interface dermatitis of the outer root sheath, with vacuolar change, lymphocytic inflammation and perifollicular lamellar fibrosis.

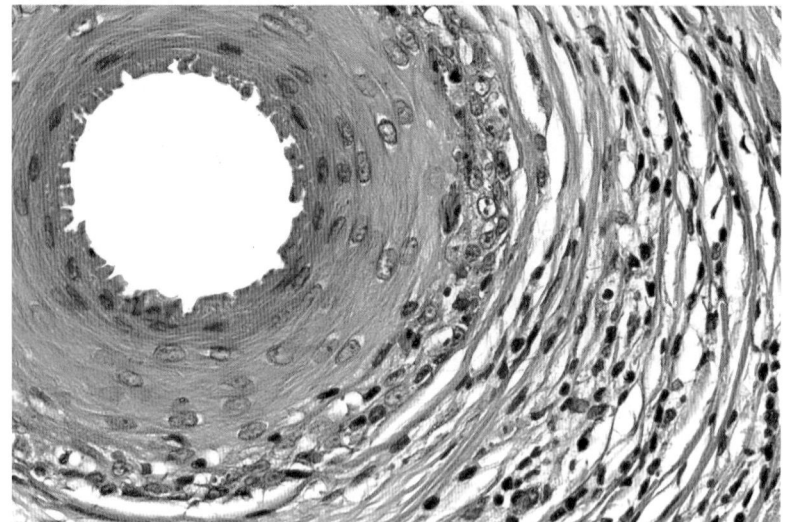

Fig. 22.143
Frontal fibrosing alopecia, horizontal section. The destruction of the outer root sheath is evident with interface change, numerous apoptotic bodies, fibrosis, and lymphocytic inflammation.

Other cases have been associated with some components of Piccardi-Lassueur-Graham-Little syndrome, Sjögren syndrome, bilateral oophorectomy, hair repigmentation close to a patch of frontal fibrosing alopecia, hair transplantation for androgenetic alopecia, increased scalp sweating, and scalp vitiligo.[23–29]

Pathogenesis and histologic features

The pathogenesis of frontal fibrosing alopecia is unknown.[30] Some cases of family groupings that share HLA-D have been observed, but it is not a consistent finding.[31–34] The disease is considered a frontal variant of lichen planopilaris since the histologic findings are similar.[25,35–41] Nevertheless, other studies have found differences in respect to the type of hair follicles affected, emphasizing the selective compromise of vellus-like and indeterminate hair follicles in this disease.[42,43] Similar to lichen planopilaris, the histologic changes are not necessarily restricted to the scalp but may be observed on the eyebrows, face, and upper limbs even in asymptomatic patients.[44–47]

The best biopsies to diagnose fibrous frontal alopecia are those that have been taken guided by dermoscopy and interpreted with horizontal sections. The histologic study shows a decrease in the number of hair follicles, which are replaced by fibrous tracts. There is a lymphocytic infiltrate in a lichenoid pattern, accompanied by perifollicular lamellar fibrosis (*Fig. 22.142*). The disease in its initial state shows a tendency to simultaneously affect terminal, indeterminate, and vellus hair follicles in all phases of the cycle including telogen. As the disease progresses, the involvement is more restricted to terminal hair follicles.[44,48] Sometimes, apoptosis is prominent (*Fig. 22.143*, see *Fig. 22.135*). The interfollicular epidermis is not involved.[40] The immunofluorescence pattern is similar to that of other more conventional variants of lichen planus.

Differential diagnosis

The differential diagnoses include female pattern hair loss, androgenetic alopecia, alopecia areata in a 'sisaipho' pattern (ophiasis inversus), and marginal traction alopecia.

Female pattern hair loss and androgenetic alopecia are not associated with perifollicular erythema, and female pattern hair loss is not related to frontal hair recession. In alopecia areata, a noninflammatory alopecic band with preservation of follicular orifices and presence of exclamation mark hairs is observed. Dermoscopy could be a helpful diagnostic tool as the yellow dots typically seen in alopecia areata are absent in frontal fibrosing alopecia.[49] Histologically, in frontal fibrosing alopecia the infiltrate is found around the isthmus and in alopecia areata the infiltrate is seen around the peribulbar area.[50] In cases of female pattern hair loss and androgenetic

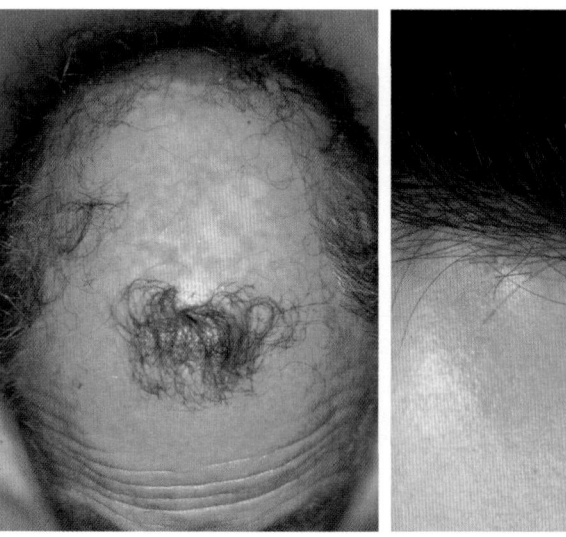

Fig. 22.144
Lichen planopilaris, fibrosing alopecia in a pattern distribution. *Left*: note the absence of follicular orifices with pigment alteration in the pattern of androgenetic alopecia. *Right*: a male patient with androgenetic alopecia and follicular inflammation. Courtesy of P. Reygagne, MD, Centre Sabouraud, Paris, France.

alopecia, the inflammatory infiltrate is minimal and the histologic picture is dominated by follicular miniaturization. Traction alopecia can be easily differentiated on the basis of physical examination and history of hair traction.

Finally, without adequate clinical information, distinction from conventional lichen planopilaris is not possible.

Clinical features
Fibrosing alopecia in a pattern distribution

Fibrosing alopecia in a pattern distribution was described by Zinkernagel and Trüeb as a form of alopecia that shares similar characteristics with androgenic alopecia and lichen planopilaris. It affects both women and men.[1–3] It is clinically characterized by progressive miniaturization of the hairs of the central scalp, perifollicular erythema, and follicular hyperkeratosis leading to complete loss of follicular ostia and scarring (*Fig. 22.144*).[1–3]

Pathogenesis and histologic features

The pathogenesis of fibrosing alopecia in a pattern distribution is unknown. Histologic features consist of hair follicle miniaturization with a lymphocytic

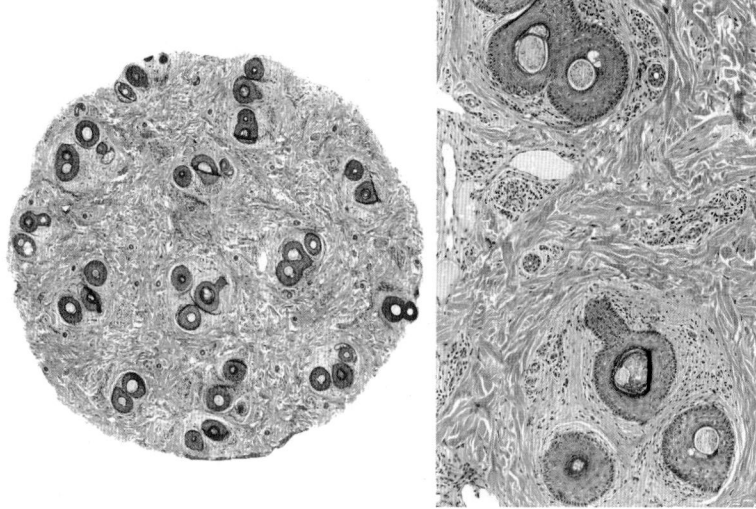

Fig. 22.145
Lichen planopilaris, fibrosing alopecia in a pattern distribution: horizontal section. Extensive miniaturization with loss of sebaceous glands, discrete fibrosis and perifollicular lymphocyte inflammation. Courtesy of Y. Corredoira Salum, MD, Universidad de Chile, Santiago, Chile.

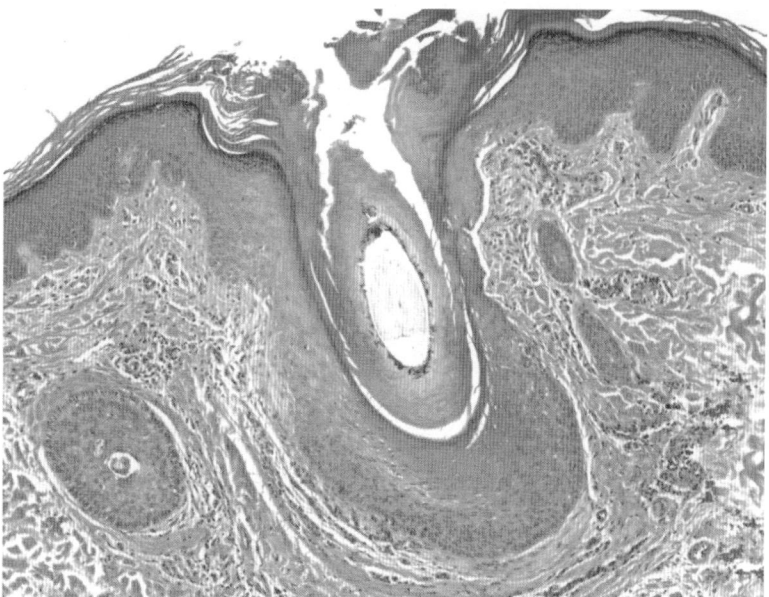

Fig. 22.146
Graham-Little syndrome: dilated infundibulum with hyperkeratosis, mild perifollicular inflammation and fibrosis.

inflammatory cell infiltrate in the region of the isthmus and the infundibulum (*Fig. 22.145*). Late lesions are characterized by perifollicular lamellar fibrosis and fibrous follicular tracts.

Differential diagnosis

The differential diagnosis includes androgenetic alopecia, lichen planopilaris, and frontal fibrosing alopecia. Although in androgenetic alopecia a peri-infundibular lymphocytic inflammatory cell infiltrate may be seen (see *Figs 22.17* and *Fig. 22.46*), this infiltrate does not concentrate around the isthmus and there is no apoptosis, loss of sebaceous glands, or lamellar fibrosis. Lichen planus is associated with all the latter features, but there is no involvement of vellus hairs by inflammation and there is a lack of miniaturization of hair follicles. In the initial stages of frontal fibrosing alopecia, there may be a predominant involvement of vellus hairs. In these cases, close clinicopathological correlation is necessary.

Clinical features

Graham-Little syndrome

The clinical triad of scarring alopecia of the scalp, noncicatricial alopecia of pubic and axillary hair, and the development of keratosis pilaris on multiple hairy areas was originally described in 1914 by Piccardi and in 1915 by Graham-Little in two patients, one of them studied by Lassueur (Lassueur-Graham-Little-Piccardi syndrome).[1–3] The disease is very rare and presents more frequently in middle-aged women, and the scarring alopecia frequently precedes the other components of the syndrome by months to years.[4,5]

Graham-Little syndrome has been associated with classic lichen planus, frontal fibrosing alopecia, erosive lichen planus, complete androgen insensitivity syndrome (testicular feminization syndrome), hepatitis B vaccination, and HLA-DR1 type in a mother and her daughter.[3,6–11]

Pathogenesis and histologic features

The etiology is unknown. Recently, an autoimmune response against the INCENP centromere protein has been reported.[12] Graham-Little syndrome has usually been considered a variant of lichen planopilaris. However the clinical features differ from ordinary lichen planopilaris and the microscopic appearance is variable, including the presence of a lichenoid tissue reaction and follicular hyperkeratosis (*Fig. 22.146*).[13]

Differential diagnosis

The most important differential diagnosis is keratosis follicularis spinulosa decalvans. However, the clinical picture of the latter is distinctly different. Keratosis follicularis is frequently familial, starting in infancy and affects atopic individuals. It is characterized by patchy alopecia of the scalp, eyebrows, and eyelashes. The clinical course is unpredictable: some cases regress during puberty and others progress with variable intensity.

Pseudopélade of Brocq

Clinical features

In 1885, Brocq described a form of progressive, idiopathic, noninflammatory scarring alopecia, which he named pseudopélade.[1] This is a very controversial entity that has been the subject of heated debate for more than 100 years.[2] At present, many of the cases described as pseudopélade are considered to represent final stages of diverse scarring alopecias including discoid lupus erythematosus, lichen planopilaris, and central centrifugal scarring alopecia.[3,4] The term pseudopélade of Brocq should be restricted to those patients in whom exhaustive clinical and histologic examination and pertinent laboratory tests have excluded all other forms of scarring alopecia.[5,6]

Patients are generally white adult females with no previous symptoms who present with discrete asymptomatic areas of alopecia. These vary in shape and location and tend not to involve the peripheral hairline region of the scalp (*Fig. 22.147*). Lesions progress slowly with alternating periods of inactivity and exacerbation. When the disease stabilizes, confluent plaques of alopecia with a shiny white porcelain-like surface are seen (*Fig. 22.148*). There is loss of follicular ostia but a few follicles sometimes survive within the plaque. Mild erythema may be detected but in general there is little or no inflammation. Some lesions are hypopigmented and even depressed. Frequently, they are irregular and have a geometric form. Such foci have been classically described as 'footprints in the snow', implying that the atrophy is visualized as a focal depression within the plaque.[7] However, many cases of pseudopélade of Brocq do not show atrophy or the 'footprints in the snow' sign.[8] No cases involving individuals of black African descent have been reported so far in the literature.

The diagnosis of pseudopélade is one of exclusion since an identical clinical and histologic picture may be seen in the end stages of other forms of scarring alopecia. In general, inflammation is minimal and, if prominent, the disease is most unlikely to represent pseudopélade.[9] Cases particularly affecting the crown or vertex that are thought to represent pseudopélade are probably best classified as central centrifugal scarring alopecia.

Although pseudopélade classically affects the scalp, a case with concomitant involvement of the beard area has been documented.[10] While the

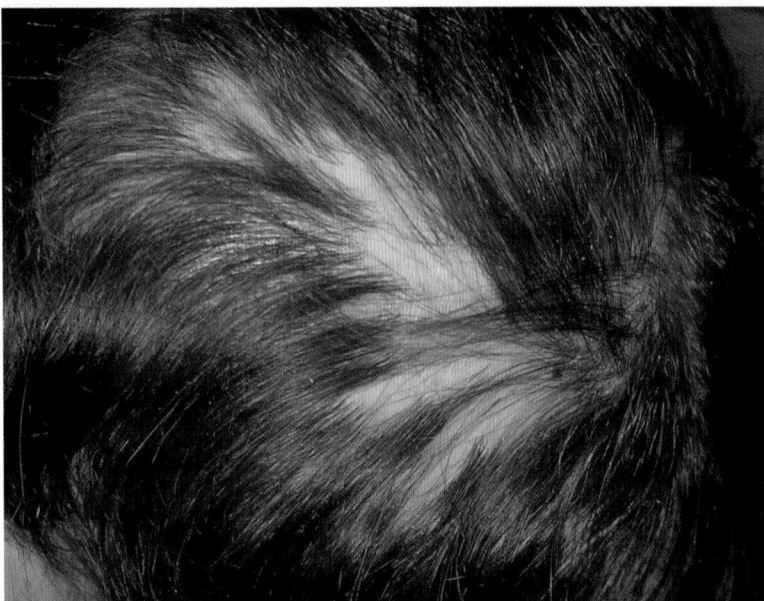

Fig. 22.147
Pseudopélade of Brocq: there are multiple foci of small atrophic patches containing isolated, scattered residual hairs. Courtesy of P. Reygagne, MD, Centre Sabouraud, Paris, France.

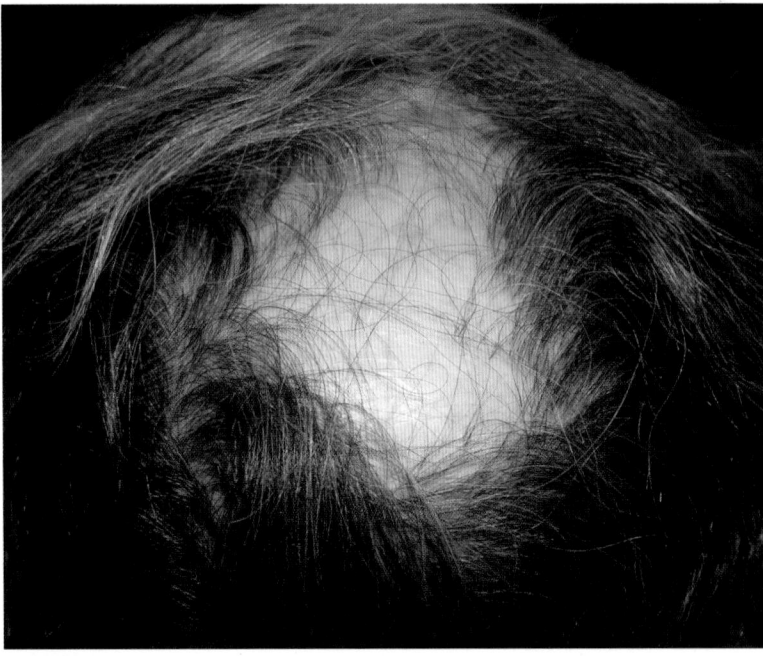

Fig. 22.148
Pseudopélade of Brocq, late lesion: this example shows the characteristic porcelain-white hypopigmented plaque. Courtesy of A.M. Aristizábal, MD, Instituto de Ciencias de la Salud, Medellín, Colombia.

disease is more frequent in adult women, there are isolated cases reported in children.[11] It has also been described in several families including in two brothers and in a mother and her son.[12–15]

Pathogenesis and histologic features

The precise mechanism whereby hair loss and scarring develop is unknown. *Borrelia burgdorferi* has been detected within the scarred plaques of a number of patients, suggesting that it may be of etiological importance in at least a subset of cases.[16] Specific genes, such as MMP11, TNFSF13B, and APOL2, have been identified with significant differential expression in association with lichen planopilaris and pseudopelade of Brocq, suggesting that they may represent two different diseases and not simply lichen planopilaris in its late phase.[17]

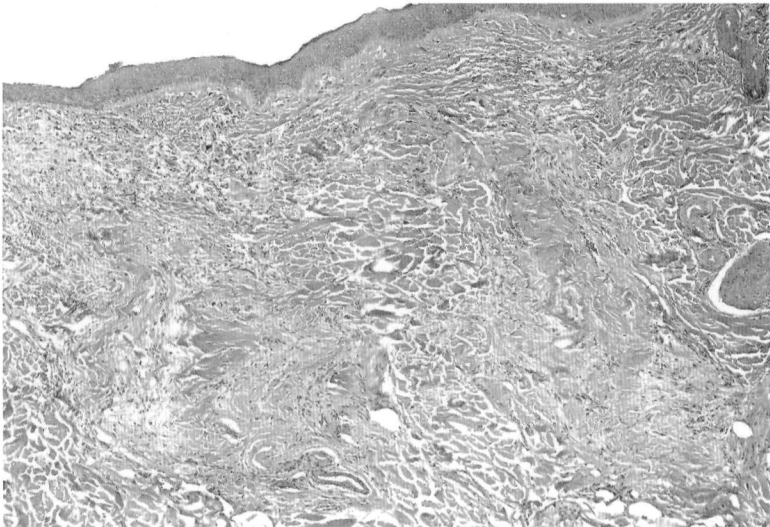

Fig. 22.149
Pseudopélade of Brocq: there is a dense fibrous scar, devoid of an inflammatory cell infiltrate. Two follicular stellae are visible. Note the absence of sebaceous glands.

Many conditions progress to scarring alopecia with irreversible loss of hair follicles as a final event. The minimal inflammatory cell infiltrate which is present in pseudopélade is particularly located around the follicular bulge. This is believed to lead to irreversible damage to the hair follicle with eventual complete destruction and subsequent scarring (*Fig. 22.149*).[18]

As mentioned above, a histologic diagnosis of pseudopélade of Brocq is one of exclusion. No pathognomonic pathological features of pseudopélade have been described, and an accurate diagnosis depends on an adequate biopsy.[19] The best specimens are those taken from the periphery of a lesion. Biopsies from the central sclerotic area are likely to be identical irrespective of whether they come from a patient with pseudopélade, discoid lupus erythematosus, or lichen planopilaris. The most important characteristic to bear in mind at the moment of choosing the place to take the biopsy is the presence of inflammation in the scalp. Thus, any area with redness, perifollicular erythema, or scaliness must be preferred over others and submitted for biopsy.[20]

When pseudopélade is suspected, at least two biopsies should be taken: one for conventional staining for horizontal sections and the other for vertical sections and other studies including direct immunofluorescence, microbiological cultures, and Gram staining.[21]

The diagnosis is based on the presence of a scarring alopecia in the absence of other features which would allow a more specific diagnosis to be made. Pseudopélade has a very mild or absent mononuclear inflammatory cell infiltrate at the level of the follicular infundibulum and follicular fibrous tracts (*Figs 22.150* and *22.151*). Interface changes are not observed. The sebaceous glands are reduced or absent.

In the end stage, there is extensive fibrosis and bands of fibrous tissue containing elastic fibers replace the hair follicles. In contrast to the follicular stellae normally present underneath telogen follicles, in pseudopélade these bands of fibrosis extend above and below the insertion of the arrector pili muscle (*Fig. 22.152*). In spite of the prominent scarring, the arrector pili muscles are resistant to the process and remain until the final stages of the disease (see *Fig.22.150* and *Fig. 22.152*).

Direct immunofluorescence is usually negative although occasionally deposits of IgM are found along the basement membrane region.[22,23]

Differential diagnosis

Pseudopélade of Brocq often represents the final phase of a wide range of scarring alopecias. Systematic examination of a biopsy often shows that cases clinically suspected of representing pseudopélade actually represent examples of central centrifugal scarring alopecia, lichen planopilaris, discoid lupus erythematosus, or any other type of alopecia that can lead to prominent scarring.[24–26] With an adequate biopsy, clinical correlation, and

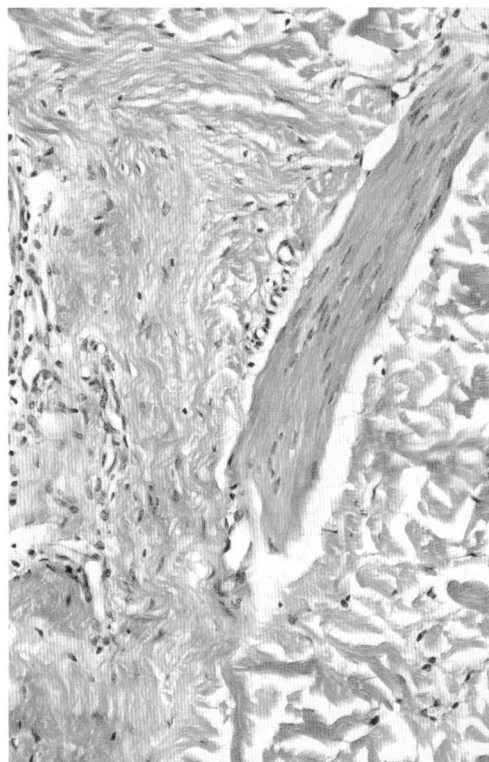

Fig. 22.150
Pseudopélade of Brocq: note the insertion of the arrector pili muscle into a fibrotic scar. There is a sparse inflammatory cell infiltrate.

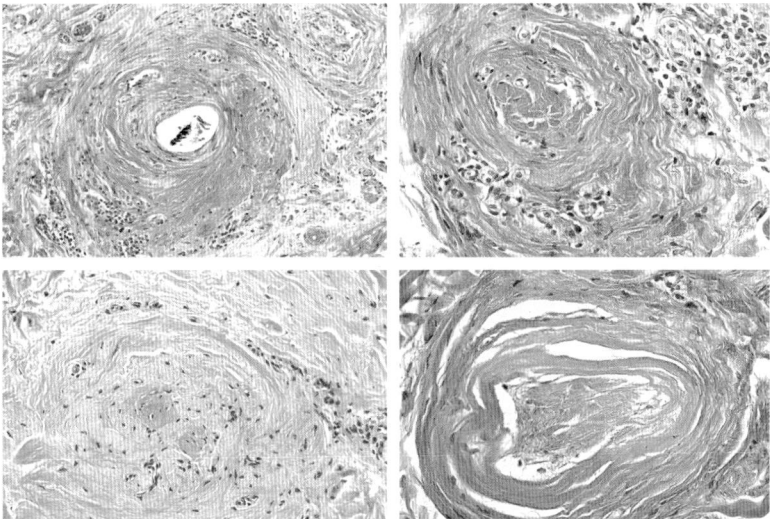

Fig. 22.151
Pseudopélade of Brocq. Follicular scars. In the top right-hand image, a residual lymphocyte inflammatory cell infiltrate is observed.

immunopathological approach, most of these entities can be excluded.[27,28] Clinically, pseudopélade of Brocq may also be confused with alopecia areata; nevertheless, the histologic study easily sets aside the latter as inflammatory peribulbar inflammation is seen.[29]

Central centrifugal cicatricial alopecia

Clinical features

The term central centrifugal cicatricial alopecia is now used to refer specifically to a type of alopecia starting in the central scalp that progresses centrifugally.[1-3] It is seen predominantly in black women and encompasses other entities previously referred to as follicular degeneration syndrome and hot comb alopecia.[4-6]

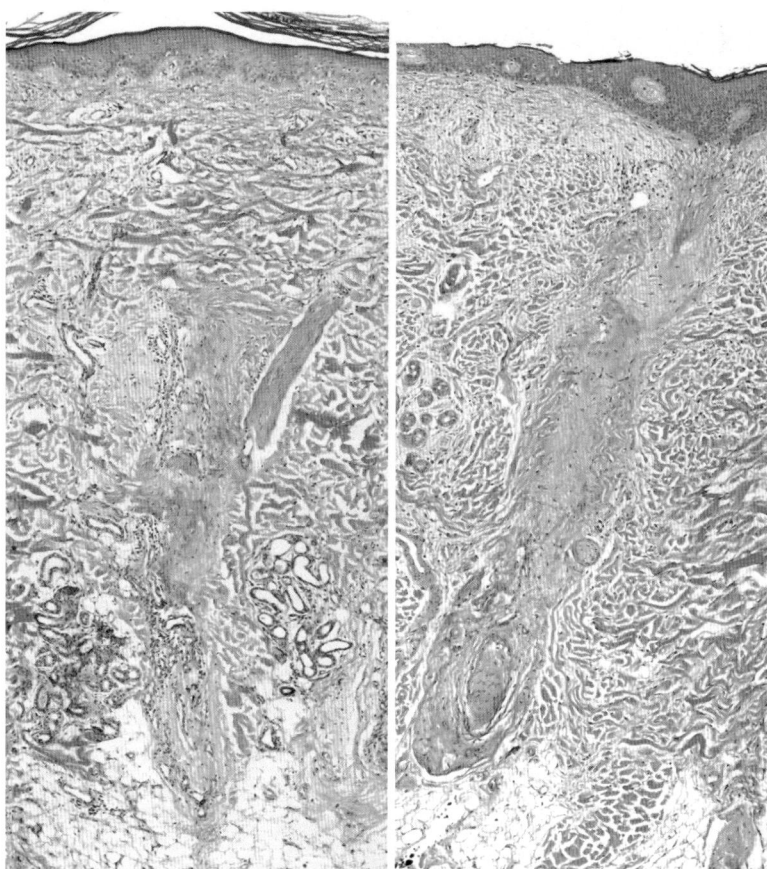

Fig. 22.152
Pseudopélade of Brocq: scarring of the hair follicles extends above and below the insertion of the arrector pili muscle.

The condition is characterized by alopecia localized primarily to the vertex and crown, a chronic and progressive course (which gradually stabilizes), and symmetric expansion with inflammatory activity at the periphery of the lesions.[7] The disease is usually asymptomatic. The presence of pruritus may indicate a fungal infection.[8]

The inflammatory component has variable expression. In some patients, it is mild and only evident after careful inspection. Other patients have a more progressive course with scaling, crusting, intense erythema, and pustules. Such variability may reflect superimposed bacterial infection and differences in the inflammatory reaction to follicular damage.

The condition can present with multiple small, solitary lesions measuring a few centimeters in diameter that gradually become confluent, or it may affect the whole vertex of the scalp. Isolated areas of alopecia show partial or complete loss of hair follicles and the degree of inflammation is variable (Fig. 22.153). In old scarred lesions, polytrichia (tufting) may be a feature.

Central centrifugal scarring alopecia is the most common variant of scarring alopecia in patients of African heritage. The majority of the patients are adult women, and almost all of them have a history of using chemical products to straighten and style their hair.[9] It has also been described in men but in this group the use of chemical products is not usually a feature.[10] There are no identified cases of central centrifugal cicatricial alopecia in children.[11]

Pathogenesis and histologic features

The cause of central centrifugal cicatricial alopecia is unknown and probably multifactorial, including factors such as hair care practices and a racial genetic predisposition. Several cases have been reported in families.[5,12-14] It is not yet clear whether central centrifugal cicatricial alopecia is a single disease or multiple entities that predominantly affect adult women and have similar histology.[15,16]

A biopsy is useful to rule out other causes of scarring alopecia. It must be obtained from a still active peripheral area containing remnants of hair follicles.[17] The histologic features vary slightly from one case to another,

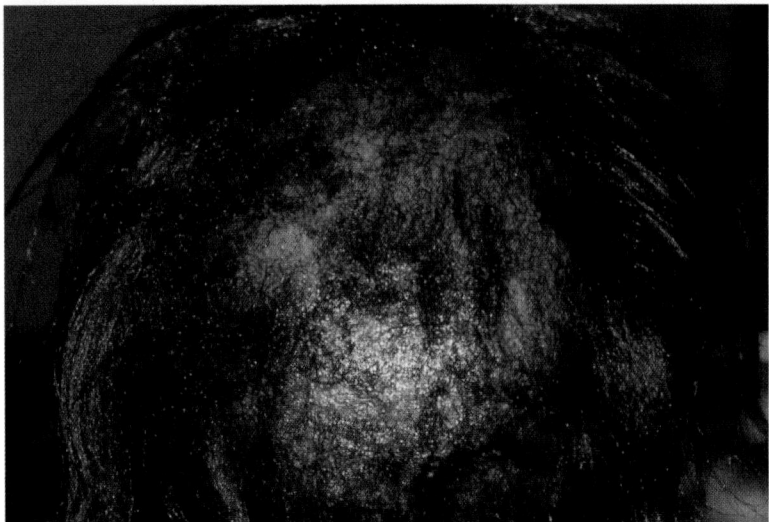

Fig. 22.153
Central centrifugal cicatricial alopecia: 40-year-old African woman with a patch of permanent hair loss with centrifuge extension from the vertex. By courtesy of P. Reygagne. Centre Sabouraud. Paris. France.

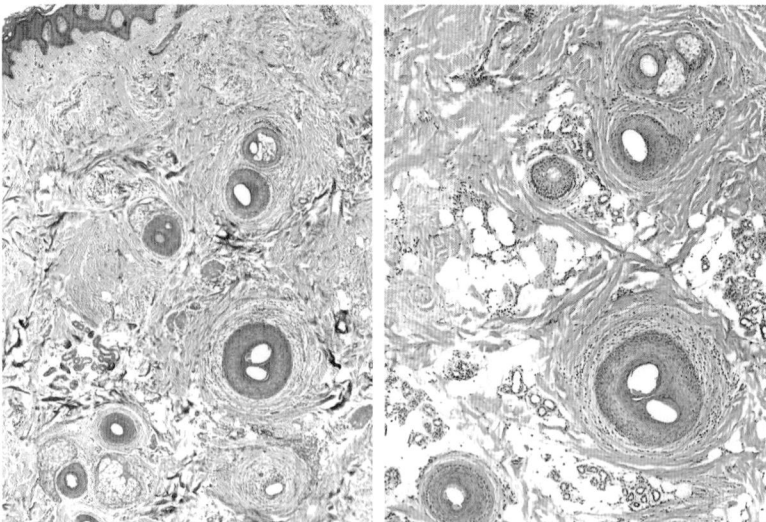

Fig. 22.155
Central centrifugal cicatricial alopecia. In this end-stage example, there is lamellar fibroplasia surrounding the hair follicle. Some follicles have fused forming 'goggles' with a single outer root sheath. Masson trichrome and hematoxylin and eosin stain.

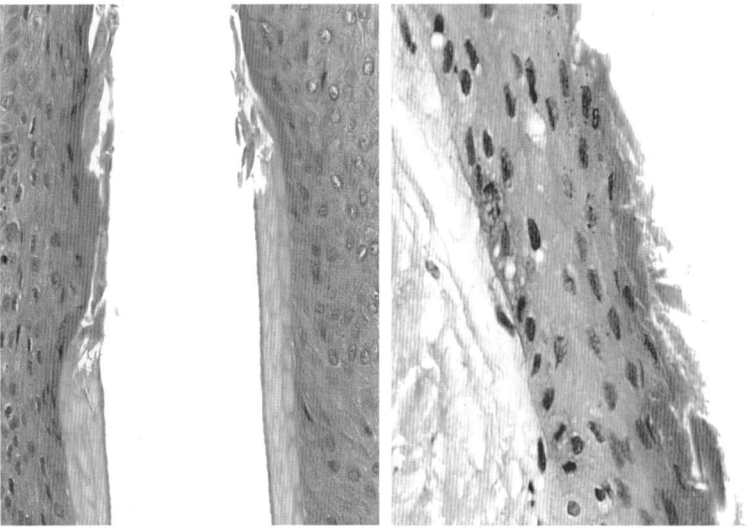

Fig. 22.154
Central centrifugal cicatricial alopecia: note the degeneration and desquamation of the inner root sheath that takes place before it reaches the isthmus.

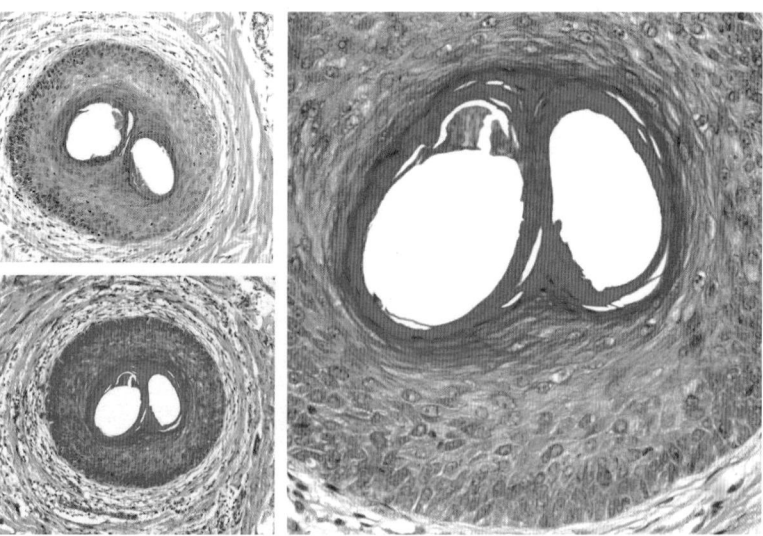

Fig. 22.156
Central centrifugal cicatricial alopecia. The outer root sheath has fused and the inner root sheath shows premature desquamation. There is discrete lamellar fibrosis and lymphocyte inflammation. There are no clefts between the outer root sheath and the perifollicular fibrosis. Top left hematoxylin and eosin stain. Bottom left and right Masson trichrome stain.

most probably reflecting different stages in the evolution of the disease, host response, and effects of secondary infection. The most relevant histologic findings are follicular miniaturization, premature desquamation of the internal root sheath (follicular degeneration syndrome), and focal preservation of the sebaceous glands.[18] Normally, the internal root sheath persists up until the level of the isthmus and then disappears (see *Fig. 22.18*). Desquamation in central centrifugal cicatricial alopecia takes place deep to the isthmus and may be observed along the whole length of the suprabulbar portion of the hair follicle (*Fig. 22.154*). Although desquamation may be observed in hair follicles in many other inflammatory diseases, in follicular degeneration syndrome it is a very extensive and constant phenomenon. It is also observed in hair follicles that appear clinically uninvolved.[7,19]

In more advanced stages, premature desquamation of the internal root sheath is associated with damage to the external root sheath manifesting as thinning of the outer root sheath and eccentric atrophy. The hair follicle becomes deformed and protrudes into the dermis. Subsequent features include concentric lamellar fibroplasia and a lymphocytic inflammatory cell infiltrate in the upper portion of the hair follicle with partial loss of associated sebaceous glands.[20] With progression, the infiltrate becomes more intense, and neutrophils, plasma cells, and histiocytes are also apparent. In late lesions, naked hair shafts in fibrous streamers are frequent and the

few remaining hair follicles fuse together to form aggregates resembling 'goggles' (*Figs 22.155* and *22.156*; see *Fig. 22.134*).[21] Sometimes, foreign body multinucleate giant cells surround hair shaft fragments. If there is secondary infection at the level of the follicular ostium, this is associated with hyperkeratosis, parakeratosis, scale crust formation, and numerous bacteria with neutrophils and cellular debris. The elastic stain shows fibrous tracts surrounded by elastic fibers and, in the dermis, thickened ('hypertrophic') elastic fibers.[22] Direct immunofluorescence is typically negative.[23]

Differential diagnosis

The differential diagnosis may be difficult as central centrifugal cicatricial alopecia shares similar clinical and histologic features with other types of scarring alopecias and nonscarring alopecias including pseudopélade of Brocq, androgenetic alopecia, traction alopecia, and trichotillomania. In classic pseudopélade of Brocq, histologic distinction may be impossible in scarring lesions with only a mild inflammatory component, and close clinicopathological correlation is required to reach a diagnosis.[24] It is important to remember that cases of classical pseudopélade of Brocq in individuals of black African descent have not been reported. Androgenetic alopecia is characterized by hair thinning. The follicular ostia are preserved and the biopsy is useful as it shows a nonscarring alopecia with miniaturization of the hair follicles. In traction alopecia and trichotillomania, the clinical history of traction and particularly the biopsy with findings of numerous hair follicles in catagen and telogen besides the presence of pigmented casts allows the diagnosis.

In lesions with prominent inflammation and an active border, the differential diagnosis includes dissecting cellulitis, mycotic and bacterial infections, lichen planopilaris, and discoid lupus erythematosus. Dissecting cellulitis is characterized by fluctuating nodules with a purulent discharge. Histologically, there is a prominent neutrophilic inflammatory cell infiltrate associated with fistulous tracts. In central centrifugal cicatricial alopecia the inflammatory component is superficial and fistulous tracts are not a feature. Biopsy, cultures, and special stains for microorganisms may exclude infectious processes involving the scalp, although an association between central centrifugal cicatricial alopecia and fungal infection has been reported.[8] Histologic distinction from lichen planopilaris is based on the presence in the latter of interface dermatitis at the junction between the hair follicle and the dermis and in the association with more colloid bodies.

Alopecia mucinosa

This disorder, also known as follicular mucinosis, is discussed under pathology of cutaneous lymphoproliferative diseases and related disorders (Chapter 18).

Keratosis follicularis spinulosa decalvans

This disorder is discussed under pathology of disorders of keratinization (Chapter 3).

Neutrophilic-associated primary scarring alopecias

Neutrophilic-associated primary scarring alopecias are clinically characterized by suppuration with edema and induration. In the late phase, the acute inflammatory process decreases and a loss of follicular orifices and scarring is observed. Histologically, there is an inflammatory infiltrate of neutrophils that may affect both the upper and deepest segments of the hair follicle (dissecting cellulitis of the scalp). In one single structure containing several hair shafts, there is loss of sebaceous glands and prominent destruction and fusion of the infundibular portion of the hair follicles. The fibrosis is more extensive than that seen in the lymphocyte-associated primary scarring alopecias involving not only the perifollicular fibrous layer but also the surrounding dermis. With time, the inflammatory cell infiltrate becomes mixed with the presence of mononuclear cells, plasma cells, and giant cells around the free hair shafts. In the later phases, it may be difficult to reach a precise histologic diagnosis without clinical correlation.[1–3]

Folliculitis decalvans

Clinical features

Quinquaud originally described folliculitis decalvans in 1888.[1] It is presently considered a form of scarring alopecia with a prominent inflammatory component characterized by pustules at the periphery of the lesions, perifollicular erythema, and follicular tufting (*Figs 22.157* and *22.158*). In its initial phase it is very symptomatic with pain, pruritus, and a burning sensation in the scalp. It is more frequent in young and middle-aged adult men. Occipital and vertex areas are the main areas affected.[2–4] Bad prognostic factors include early onset of the disease before 25 years of age and presence of pustules within the patch of alopecia.[5]

Folliculitis decalvans may involve the beard area (lupoid sycosis), the face, and the nape of the neck.[6] It has been associated with Darier disease, human T-cell lymphotropic virus type I-associated myelopathy/tropical spastic paraparesis, squamous cell carcinoma, and micronychia. It also has

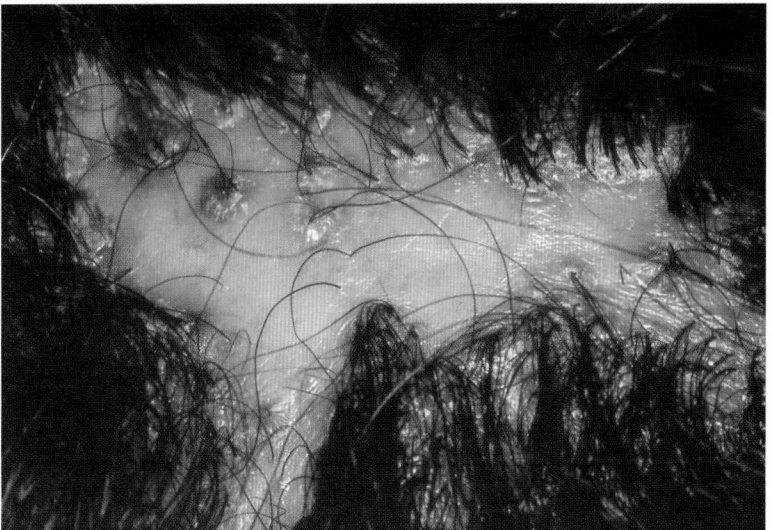

Fig. 22.157
Folliculitis decalvans: this patient shows tufted folliculitis. Courtesy of P. Reygagne, MD, Centre Sabouraud, Paris, France.

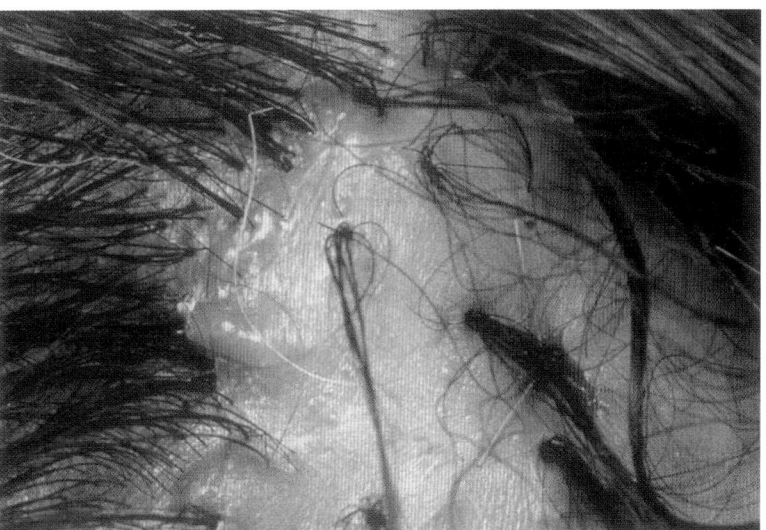

Fig. 22.158
Folliculitis decalvans, tufted folliculitis: multiple hair shafts can be clearly seen exiting from the follicular ostia. Courtesy of the Institute of Dermatology, London, UK.

occurred simultaneously in two pairs of identical twins.[6–11] There are also reports of a case associated with multiple cutaneous osteomas and a further case preceding a cutaneous adenoid cystic carcinoma.[12,13] Finally, there are isolated reports associated with the use of Erlotinib and the appearance of the disease 20 years after hair restoration surgery by punch grafts.[14,15]

Pathogenesis and histologic features

The pathogenesis of folliculitis decalvans is unknown. Although *Staphylococcus aureus* can be isolated in the majority of the patients it is thought that the pustules are the result of secondary bacterial colonization and not the cause of the illness. In nonpustular areas, the clinical picture is very similar to that of central centrifugal cicatricial alopecia. An immunity defect based on genetics and race has been considered.[3,16] In early lesions, an infiltration of activated T-helper cells has been observed. Infiltration by neutrophils and fibrosis can be explained as the result of secretion of IL-8 and intercellular adhesion molecule (ICAM)-1 in the acute phase, and by basic fibroblast growth factor (B-FGF) and TGF-beta in the late phase, respectively.[17]

Biopsy should be taken of an active lesion for conventional histologic study and direct immunofluorescence. Vertical or horizontal sections may

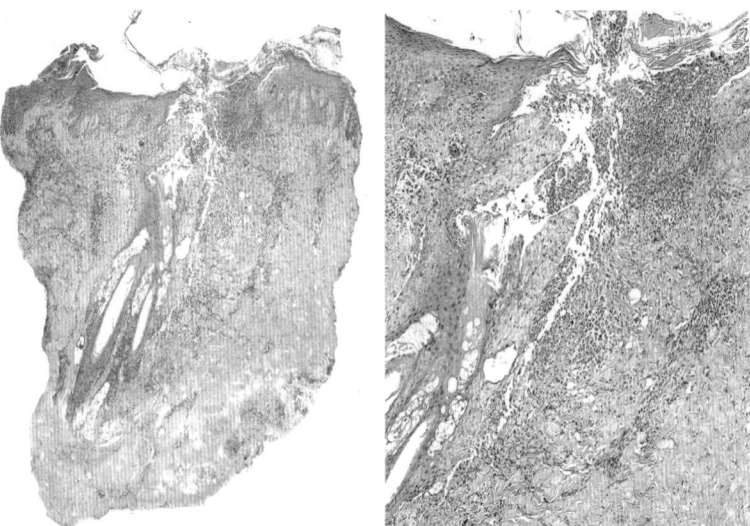

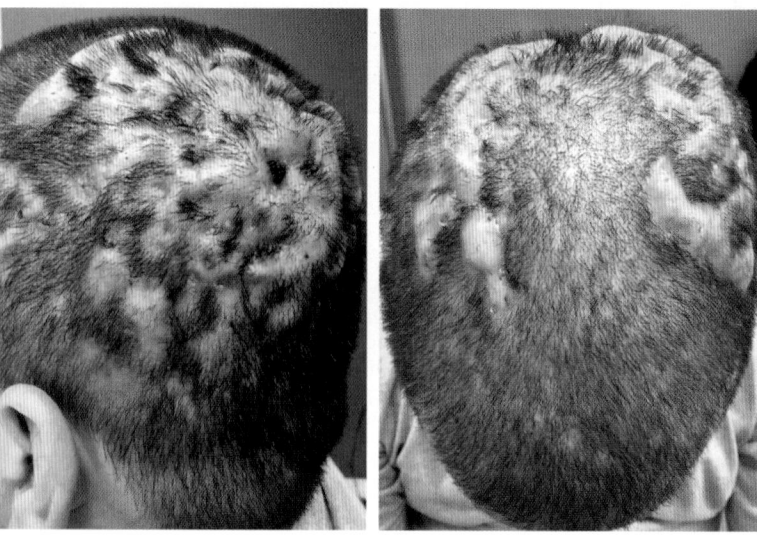

Fig. 22.159
Folliculitis decalvans: in this composite image, there is a superficial squamous crust containing neutrophils surrounding the opening of some hair follicles. In the dermis there is fusion of hair follicles (*right*).

Fig. 22.161
Dissecting cellulitis of the scalp: there are nodules and sinuses with suppuration, and scarring alopecia. Courtesy of E.Peña, MD, Clínica Medellín. Medellín, Colombia.

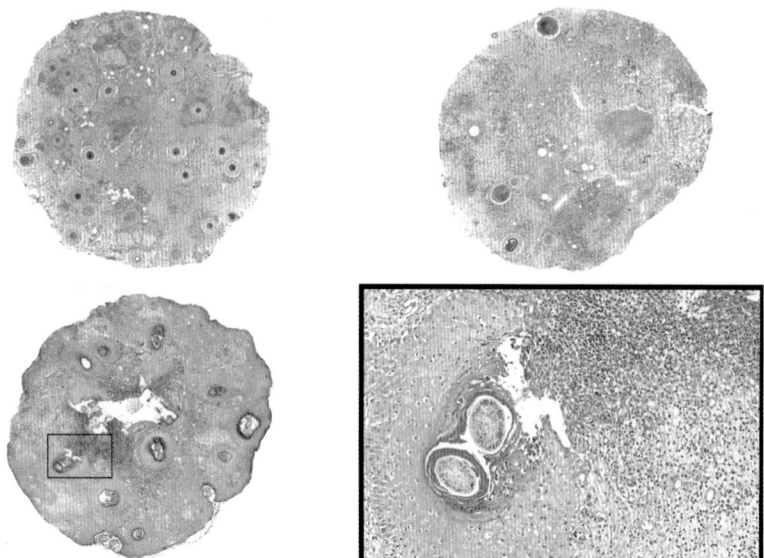

Fig. 22.160
Folliculitis decalvans, horizontal sections. In this compound image, successive sections from the middle of the follicle (*upper left*) to the superficial portion of the infundibulum (*lower left*). In the right hand insert note abscess formation and destruction of the wall of the follicle by a neutrophilic inflammatory cell infiltrate.

Differential diagnosis

The differential diagnosis of folliculitis decalvans includes perifolliculitis capitis abscendens et suffodiens and infectious processes. Perifolliculitis capitis abscedens et suffodiens is characterized by sinus tracts lined by squamous epithelium. Bacterial or fungal folliculitis have to be excluded by the use of cultures and special stains.[18,19]

As previously mentioned, end-stage lesions may be impossible to differentiate from a central centrifugal cicatricial alopecia or classic pseudopélade of Brocq.[20,21]

Dissecting cellulitis of the scalp

Clinical features

Dissecting cellulitis of the scalp (dissecting folliculitis) was described in 1908 by Hoffman with the name perifolliculitis capitis abscedens et suffodiens.[1–4]

It is a rare disease that mainly affects young men of African heritage, although recently more cases in white men are described. It predominantly affects the crown and vertex. The typical presentation consists of fluctuating, interconnecting nodules which progressively become confluent, rupture, and drain pus (*Fig. 22.161*). Due to the extensive and wide interconnection of the nodules in the scalp, the discharge of purulent material at a distant site when a nodule is pinched is a characteristic clinical finding (*Fig. 22.162*). Patients fundamentally complain of hair loss and purulent discharge. The lesions are practically asymptomatic, with no pain or pruritus.[5] Despite this clinical picture, cultures for bacteria and fungi are almost always negative. The course of the illness is chronic and is characterized by long periods of exacerbations and remissions. Lesions at different stages of evolution may be seen at any given moment during the course of the disease.[6] End-stage lesions show dermal fibrosis with hypertrophic scarring and prominent alopecia.

Chronic lesions can involve the skull, and secondary bacterial infection sometimes leads to pyogenic osteomyelitis. In very long-standing lesions, squamous cell carcinoma has been described.[7,8] Dissecting cellulitis can rarely occur in girls, and it has also been observed in white men and in an Aboriginal Canadian patient.[9–12] A familial case has been reported.[13] Associations with multiple muscle, bone, and articular disorders have been described. These include osteomuscular diseases, arthropathies, sternocostoclavicular hyperostosis, and spondylarthropathy.[14–17] Other associations have been marginal keratitis and dissecting cellulitis of the scalp triggered by a traumatic event.[18,19]

Acne conglobata, hidradenitis suppurativa, and dissecting cellulitis form the follicular occlusion triad. In 1975, some authors proposed the inclusion

be obtained, although the best option is a combination of both. PAS is particularly useful to rule out a fungal infection. Bacterial cultures must always be performed to identify colonization by *S. aureus*.

In the active lesions, folliculitis decalvans is histologically characterized by a neutrophilic inflammatory infiltrate principally affecting the upper portions of the hair follicle. Neutrophils accumulate in the dilated infundibula and the surrounding dermis (*Figs 22.159* and *22.160*) The sebaceous glands are destroyed by the inflammatory infiltrate. It is common to observe between 5 to 20 hair shafts surrounded by a single external radicular sheath corresponding to the clinical image of folliculitis in plume (see *Fig. 22.112*). The lower part of the hair follicle shows a lymphoplasmacytic inflammatory cell infiltrate. In the later phases of the disease, the inflammatory infiltrate becomes mixed with neutrophils, lymphocytes, and plasma cells. There is destruction and phagocytosis of the hair shafts by foreign body giant cells and macrophages (see *Fig. 22.118*). Later, the scarring process is made more evident with complete loss of pilosebaceous units, interfollicular dermal fibrosis, and loss of elastic tissue, visible with an elastic tissue stain.[2]

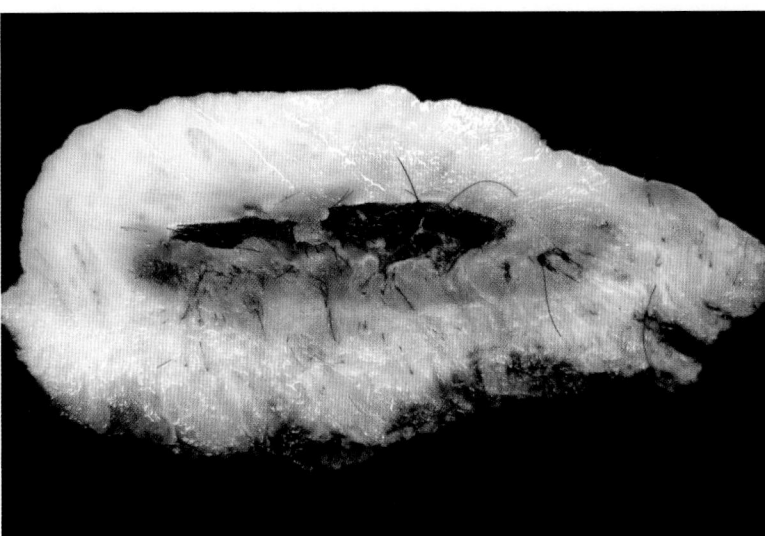

Fig. 22.162
Dissecting cellulitis of the scalp. Surgical specimen with fistulous tracts containing hair shafts and surrounded by extensive scarring and edematous granulation tissue.

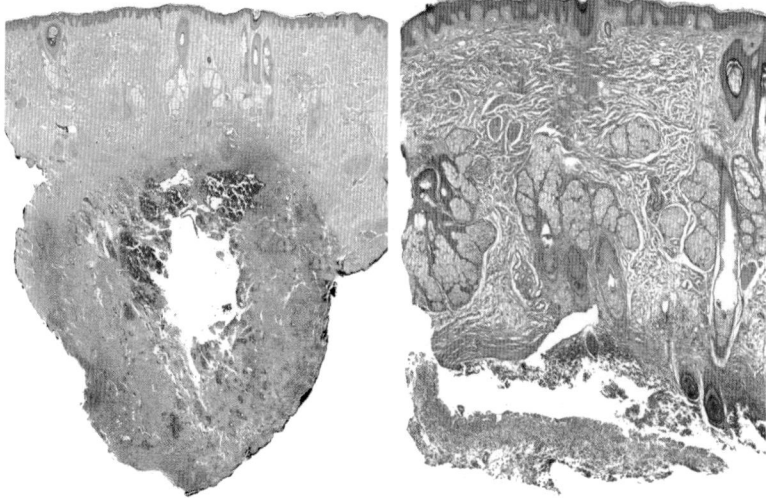

Fig. 22.163
Dissecting cellulitis of the scalp. There is a sinus partially lined by stratified squamous epithelium in the deep dermis. The mid and superficial dermis and the epidermis are unaffected.

of pilonidal cysts to form a tetrad.[3,20,21] There are some contradictory aspects in this association as dissecting cellulitis is more frequent in adult men than in women, whereas suppurative hidradenitis is more frequent in young women[22]. The follicular occlusion syndrome has been associated with pityriasis rubra pilaris, pyoderma vegetans, pyoderma gangrenosum, spondyloarthritis, and squamous cell carcinoma.[23-27]

Pathogenesis and histologic features

Dissecting cellulitis represents a variant of deep folliculitis apparently caused by obstruction at the level of the ostium or follicular infundibulum similar to hidradenitis suppurativa and acne conglobata.[28] The mechanism that triggers this phenomenon is unknown.

Dissecting cellulitis is best studied histologically with vertical sections as these allow adequate visualization of the deep dermis and of the subcutaneous tissue. Early histologic changes consist of the presence of dilatation of the follicular infundibulum with follicular clogging, neutrophils in the ostium, and a deep lymphocytic inflammatory cell infiltrate around the hair follicles.[29,30] This progressively extends into the wall of the hair follicle, leading eventually to its destruction. Free hair shafts in the dermis are associated with a heavy mixed inflammatory cell infiltrate consisting of neutrophils, lymphocytes, plasma cells, and histiocytes.[31] Epithelioid and foreign body giant cells with formation of granulomata are commonly present, and suppurative granulomata may also be a feature. As the process evolves, multiple abscesses and fistulous tracts lined by stratified squamous epithelium develop (*Fig. 22.163*).[32] Additional features include granulation tissue and stromal edema. Active lesions persist as long as there are residual hair follicles. In the final stages, hair follicles and sebaceous glands are completely destroyed and replaced by fibrous tissue. Cultures and special stains for bacteria may show microorganisms in the dilated follicular ostium, but generally microorganisms are not found within the fistulous tracts or dermal abscesses.

Differential diagnosis

The differential diagnosis of dissecting cellulitis includes folliculitis decalvans, aseptic nodules of the scalp (pseudocyst of the scalp), and infectious processes.

The fluctuating suppurative nodules with fistulous tracts typical of dissecting cellulitis are not a feature of folliculitis decalvans. Histologically, the latter condition is characterized by a neutrophilic inflammatory infiltrate predominantly affecting the upper part of the hair follicle, and a lymphocytic infiltrate with focal foreign body granulomata to hair shafts. The aseptic nodule of the scalp consists of a solitary nodular lesion that drains purulent material leaving a cystic cavity. Contrary to dissecting cellulitis, the alopecia is reversible and the prognosis excellent.[22,33,34]

Inflammatory tinea capitis (kerion celsi) and other infections of the scalp may present with deep involvement and simulate dissecting cellulitis.[35-38] The problem is further compounded by the presence of neutrophilic abscesses and granulomata. It is therefore important to always perform special stains for microorganisms to exclude bacteria, fungi, and mycobacteria.

Finally, folliculotropic mycosis fungoides with large-cell transformation has presented with a clinical picture similar to that of dissecting cellulitis of the scalp.[39]

Mixed primary cicatricial alopecias

This is a group of scarring alopecias that may not be easily fit in any of the latter groups Stop Presentation is with alopecia displaying extensive follicular destruction and fibrosis with a variable inflammatory cell infiltrate that may change over time. The rupture of the hair follicles initially evoke inflammation of an acute nature which later mixes with a mononuclear lymphocytic infiltrate and a granulomatous reaction.

Acne keloidalis nuchae

Clinical features

Acne keloidalis nuchae (folliculitis keloidalis nuchae) is the commonest form of scarring alopecia occurring in African males. It involves the nape of the neck, with a 20:1 male-to-female predominance.[1-3]

The denomination acne keloidalis is incorrect as the disease is not associated with acne lesions, or keloidal collagen in the histologic study.[4]

The disease begins as localized follicular papules that progressively increase in size and become confluent, forming keloidal plaques with subsequent loss of hair (*Fig. 22.164*). It has also been described in women of African and Latin American heritage and has been associated with keratosis follicularis spinulosa decalvans, tufted hair folliculitis, acanthosis nigricans, renal transplant patients on tacrolimus and sirolimus, ciclosporine A (in both white and African-heritage patients), lithium carbonate, antiepileptic medications, and the use of football helmets.[5-17]

Pathogenesis and histologic features

The cause is unknown. It most probably reflects a response to a local irritative phenomenon complicated by secondary bacterial infection.[18] Curly hairs that have been cut too short and grow back into the skin, inducing an inflammatory reaction, are thought to represent a likely cause. Although this same phenomenon has been postulated in the pathogenesis of pseudofolliculitis barbae there is no relationship between the two diseases.[1,19] It

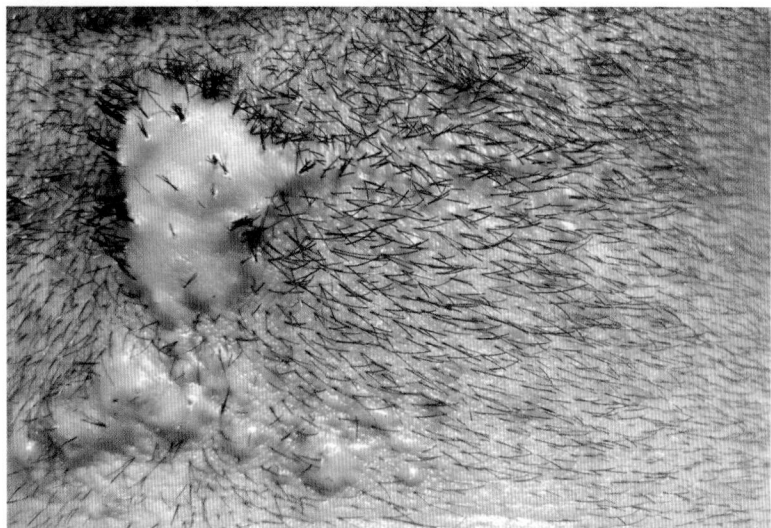

Fig. 22.164
Acne keloidales nuchae: papules have coalesced forming a keloidal plaque.
Pustules are also seen. Courtesy of C. Velázquez, MD, CES, Medellín, Colombia.

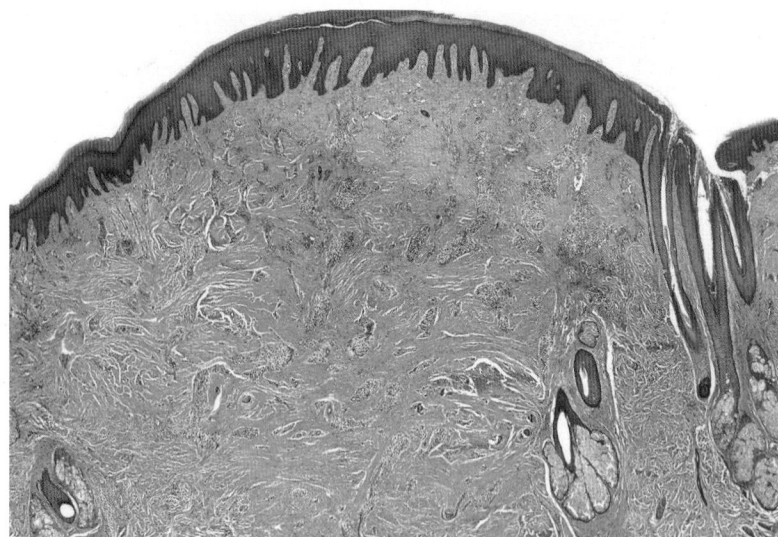

Fig. 22.166
Acne keloidales nuchae: scanning magnification showing dermal scarring and
multiple free hair shaft fragments.

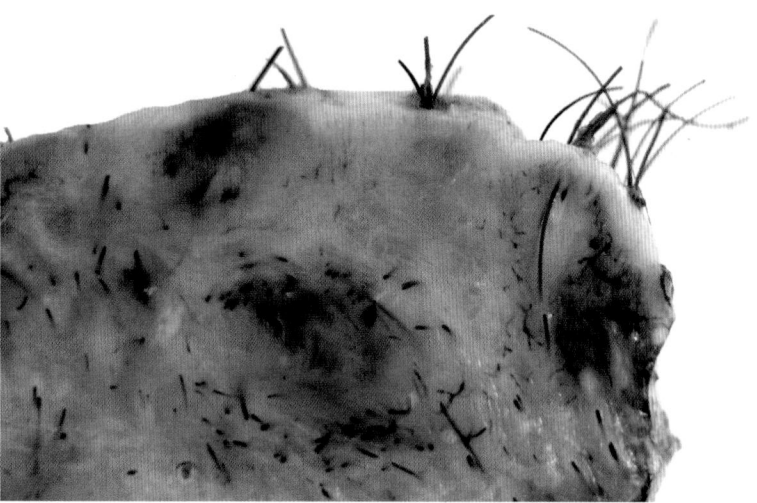

Fig. 22.165
Acne keloidales nuchae: surgical specimen showing intense fibrosis of the dermis
with distortion of the orientation of the hair follicles. The epidermal surface shows
some tufted follicles.

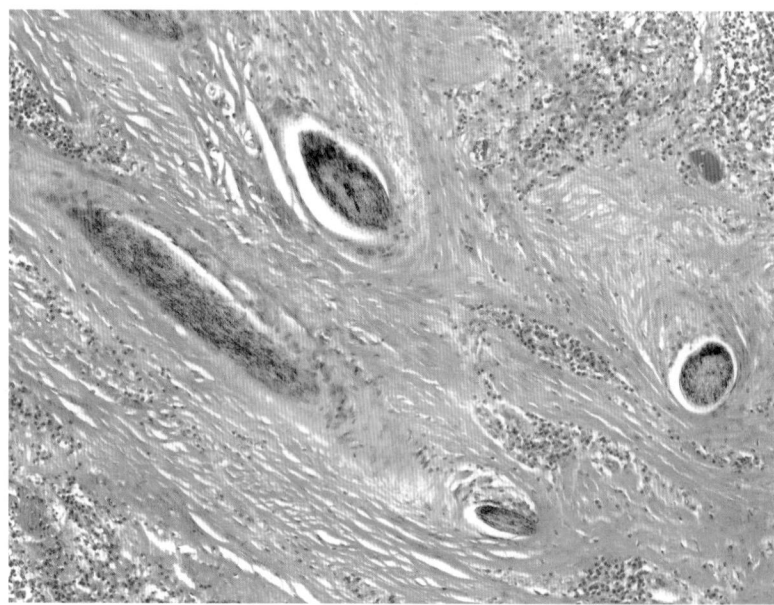

Fig. 22.167
Acne keloidales nuchae: high-power view of hair shaft fragments surrounded by
dense fibrosis.

has also been considered a disorder of transepidermal elimination.[1,20] Associations include high levels of testosterone, seborrheic dermatitis, and an increased density of mast cells in the nape of the neck.[21]

The best way to evaluate acne keloidalis is with vertical sections (*Fig. 22.165*). Histologically, the initial lesion is similar to that of folliculitis decalvans with a neutrophilic infiltrate in the isthmus and around sebaceous glands which eventually disappear. The infundibulum is dilated. Later, there are thick bands of compact collagen admixed with a variable lymphoplasmacytic inflammatory cell infiltrate centered mainly on the follicular infundibulum and isthmus (*Fig. 22.166*). As previously mentioned, true keloidal collagen is not observed.[22] There is associated thinning of the external root sheath with lamellar fibroplasia (see *Fig. 22.120*), and eventually follicular destruction results in free hair shafts within the dermis where they elicit an intense inflammatory cell reaction (*Fig. 22.167*).[23] Abscesses and fistulous tracts similar to those observed in dissecting cellulitis may sometimes be encountered. The hair follicles lose their sebaceous glands, and multiple follicles may fuse together to form a single follicular ostium containing multiple hair shafts (polytrichia).[24]

Biopsies of clinically normal skin from the vicinity of abnormal lesions may show evidence of follicular destruction and fibrosis.[23]

Differential diagnosis

Central centrifugal scarring alopecia represents the main differential diagnosis. Although the clinical presentation and sites of involvement are very different, there is considerable histologic overlap. A case of tinea capitis mimicking acne keloidalis has also been reported in a female patient.[25,26]

Acne necrotica

Clinical features

Acne necrotica (necrotizing lymphocytic folliculitis, acne necrotica varioliformis, acne frontalis, acne pilaris) is a rare disease characterized by chronic recurrent crops of variably pruritic or tender pea-sized erythematous follicular papules which undergo central ulceration and heal with the formation of disfiguring varioliform scars.[1-3] Comedones are not a feature and the disease must not be considered a variant of acne vulgaris. It usually involves the anterior hairline and temporal region of the scalp, seborrheic areas, nose, cheek, upper chest, and interscapular area.[1,4,5] There is a slight predilection for males and most patients are in the fourth and fifth decades.[3]

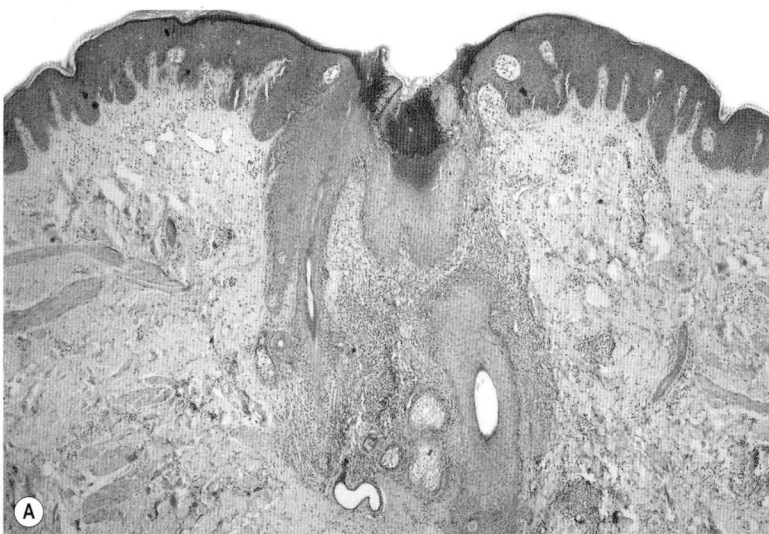

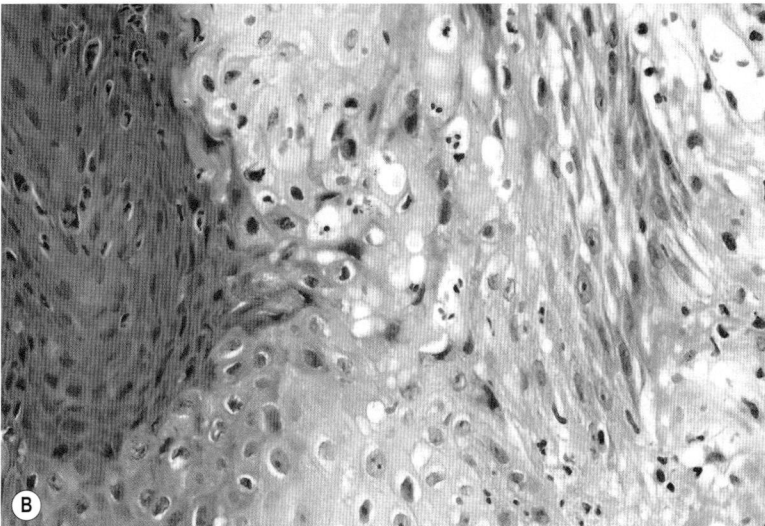

Fig. 22.168
(**A**, **B**) Acne necrotica. Note necrosis of the hair follicle.

A nonscarring pruritic superficial variant predominantly affecting the scalp may also be encountered (acne necrotica miliaris).[1]

Pathogenesis and histologic features

Both *S. aureus* and *Propionibacterium acnes* have been implicated in the etiology of acne necrotica, and at least a subset of patients respond to antibiotic therapy.[3-7] However, the latter response may well be the result of the anti-inflammatory action of antibiotics. Stress and manipulation have also been suggested as possible factors as have rosacea and seborrheic dermatitis.[1,6,8]

Early lesions are characterized by dermal edema and a superficial to mid-dermal perivascular and perifollicular lymphocytic infiltrate associated with spongiosis and apoptosis of the external root sheath, adjacent epidermis, and sebaceous gland.[1] Eosinophils may also be present but neutrophils are not a feature. With progression, there is necrosis of the whole follicle and overlying epidermis (*Fig. 22.168*). A neutrophil-rich crust overlies the lesion and bacterial colonies may be prominent.[1] Granulomatous inflammation is not a feature.[1] Chronic lesions are characterized by loss of follicles and vertically oriented dermal scars.[3]

Differential diagnosis

Differential diagnosis includes neurotic excoriations, eczema herpeticum, and conventional folliculitis. Lesions in neurotic excoriations are superficial and are not limited to the anterior part of the scalp. Eczema herpeticum may be differentiated with a biopsy or a Tzank test which will show the characteristic viral inclusions.[5] Early varioliform necrotic acne may be

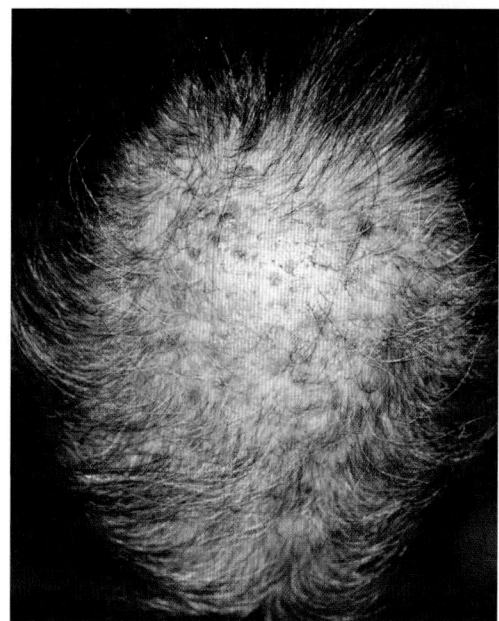

Fig. 22.169
Erosive pustular dermatosis: note the eroded and edematous appearance as a consequence of surgery. Courtesy of P. Reygagne, MD, Centre Sabouraud, Paris, France.

differentiated by the extensive damage of the hair follicles present in the latter.[1]

Erosive pustular dermatosis

Clinical features

Erosive pustular dermatosis of the scalp was first described by Pye in 1979 as a chronic, noninfectious dermatosis principally affecting elderly women, and there is a frequent history of trauma to the scalp.[1-3] Some cases outside the scalp have been reported, particularly on the legs and in areas of cutaneous atrophy and venous insufficiency.[4-7] Isolated cases affecting the mucosal surfaces and in a child with Klippel-Feil syndrome have also been described. [8,9] Associations described include exogenous factors such as contusions, erosions, solar burns, perinatal scalp injury, cochlear implant, surgery, after skin grafts, hair transplant, radiation, synthetic fiber implantations, cryotherapy, CO_2 laser treatment, and photodynamic therapy.[2,10-26] Trauma may antedate the disease by days or years.[2] The disease may also develop after herpes zoster. Its onset after treatment with topical, imiquimod, latanoprost, imiquimod, gefitinib, minoxidil, tacrolimus, and ingenol mebutate has also been described. Association with systemic diseases associated include rheumatoid arthritis, myasthenia gravis, and myelodysplastic syndrome.[27-36] It has also been associated with basal cell carcinoma.[37]

Early lesions are asymptomatic and edematous, with well-defined borders characterized by a scaly scab that upon removal leaves a lesion with pustules (*Fig. 22.169*). Late lesions develop scarring alopecia. There may be secondary bacterial or fungal colonization.[2]

Pathogenesis and histologic features

The pathogenesis is unknown. Due to the high incidence in elderly patients, there has been speculation as to the role that chronic actinic damage, immunosuppression, and autoimmune disease may have in the pathogenesis of the disease.[2,38] Laboratory data and bacteriological and mycological investigations are usually non-contributory.[39]

The histopathological picture is not specific.[40] Erosion of the superficial epidermis with acanthosis, focal atrophy, parakeratosis, and subcorneal pustules is seen. In the dermis, there is a mixed inflammatory cell infiltrate composed of lymphocytes, neutrophils, and some giant cells. The hair follicles are progressively affected and disappear.[41]

Differential diagnosis

The differential diagnosis is wide and includes many suppurative nonmicrobial diseases such as amicrobial pustulosis associated with autoimmune disease, pustular ulcerative dermatosis of the scalp, inflammatory tinea capitis (kerion celsi), folliculitis decalvans, sterile eosinophilic pustulosis of Ofuji, pustular psoriasis vulgaris, dissecting cellulitis, pemphigus vulgaris, mucous membrane pemphigoid, gangrenous pyoderma, bacterial folliculitis, and ischemic diseases such as temporal arteritis.[42] From this list, only the first three will be discussed.

Amicrobial pustulosis associated with autoimmune disease principally affects young women; however, it shares many clinical and histologic features with erosive pustular dermatosis.[43–45] Pustular ulcerative dermatosis of the scalp affects mainly young men of African origin with severe malnutrition.[46] Inflammatory tinea capitis may closely simulate an erosive pustular dermatosis of the scalp, requiring a direct scrape for KOH and culture. PAS or silver stains are also useful to confirm the diagnosis.[47,48]

Non-specific cicatricial alopecias

This category includes idiopathic scarring alopecias with inconclusive clinical and histopathological findings. Many inflammatory cicatricial alopecias, such as lichen planopilaris and folliculitis decalvans, are part of this group when the patient presents in late stages.[1]

HAIR SHAFT DISEASES

Hair shaft disorders refer to the spectrum of hair shaft alterations varying from changes secondary to normal weathering to primary conditions presenting with hair shaft changes. As a consequence of the latter, the hair is more susceptible to injury by chemical and physical agents. Primary hair shaft disorders are frequently hereditary and until recently, many of the genes causing hair shaft defects had not been identified (Table 22.5).[1]

Since the hair shafts in these conditions are very fragile, alopecia is a common mode of presentation. Alterations can also be seen in other hair-bearing sites including the eyebrows, eyelashes, and beard area.[2,3] Scalp manifestations vary from mild to severe. In the latter setting, the hair is dark, fragile, and easy to break, with areas of focal or generalized alopecia.[4] According to the particular entity, various other clinical manifestations and associated metabolic disorders are present.

Hair samples must be carefully evaluated to see whether the hair shafts are narrowed or broken (see hair examination at the beginning of the chapter).

Hair shaft defects are classified according to three parameters: whether the alopecia is diffuse or localized, the presence or absence of hair shaft fragility, and the morphology of the hair.

From the histopathological point of view, morphology is of particular importance, and changes to be evaluated include hair shaft fractures, irregularities, coiling or twisting abnormalities, and extraneous matter on the hair shaft (Box 22.2). Many of these basic morphological alterations are present in a single disorder and this makes characterization of individual conditions difficult (Fig. 22.170).[5,6]

Fractures of the hair shaft

Trichorrhexis nodosa

Clinical features

Trichorrhexis nodosa is the most common hair shaft defect. It is mainly found in patients who complain of fragile and easily breakable hair, and it is not a specific disease. The defect arises from trauma imposed on the hair shaft either congenitally or by acquired disorders. The genetic type is related to genodermatoses and metabolic disorders and the traumatic type to damage by mechanical and chemical trauma.[1]

The condition presents with beaded thickening of the proximal or distal end of the hair shaft. These changes resemble minute spheres or dust particles adherent to the hair shaft and represent fractures (Fig. 22.171).[2]

Table 22.5

Single gene mutations affecting human hair growth*

Disease	Affected gene	Role of encoded protein	Hair phenotype
Monilethrix	hHb6 or hHb	Hair keratin (structure protein)	Thin fragile hair with a beaded appearance under light microscope
Netherton's syndrome	SPINK5	Serine protease inhibitor LEK1	Defective hair shart differentiation ('bamboo hair')
Generalized atrichia with papular lesions	Hairless (HR)	Putative transcription factor	Failure of first postnatal hair growth cycle
Human nude	WHN	Transcription factor	Hair shafts fail to emerge from skin
X-linked hypohidrotic ectodermal dysplasia	Ectodysplasin (EDN)	Intercellular signaline molecule	Sparse hair
Autosomal hypohidrotic ectodermal dysplasia	Ectodysplasin receptor (EDN)	Receptor for ectodysplasin	Sparse hair
Ectodermal dysplasia/familial incontinentia pigmenti	IKK-gamma (NEMO)	Kinase required for activation of the transcription factor NF-kB	Sparse hair
Naxos disease	Plakoglobin	Adhesion molecule	Woolly hair
Ectodermal dysplasia/skin fragility syndrome	Plakoglobin 1	Desmosomal adhesion molecule	Sparse hair
Menke's disease	ATP7a	Copper-transporting P-type ATPase	Hair loss; abnormal hair texture
Tricho-rhino-phalangeal syndrome type I	TRPS I	Zinc finger protein, putative transcription factor	Sparse and unruly scalp hair
X-linked dominant chondrodysplasia puntata	EBP	$\Delta(8)$, $\Delta(7)$ sterol isomerase emopamil-binding protein	Coarse hair, alopecia
Giant axonal neuropathy	Gigaxonin (GAN)	Unknown	Curly or kinky hairs

*Cheng, A.S., Bayliss, S.J. (2008). The genetics of hair shaft disorders. J Am Acad Dermatol, 59, 1–22.

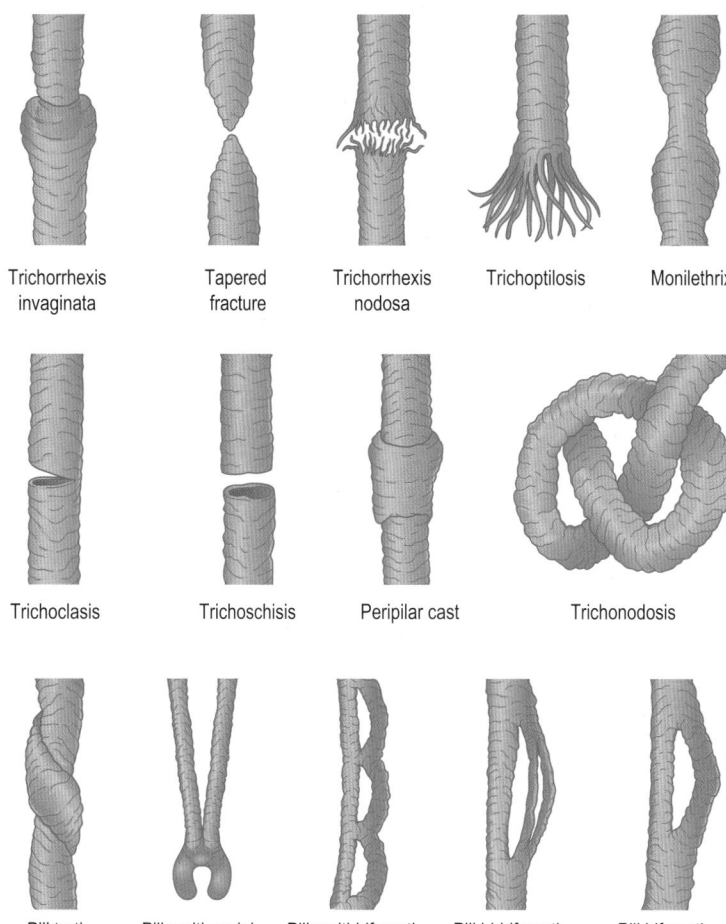

Fig. 22.170
Hair shaft defects.

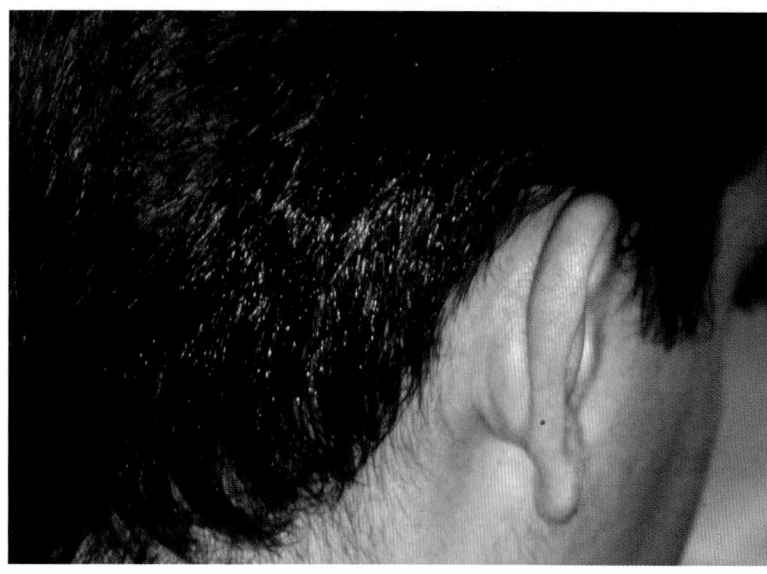

Fig. 22.171
Trichorrhexis nodosa: example from a localized form. Courtesy of P. Reygagne, MD, Centre Sabouraud, Paris, France.

Box 22.2
Hair shaft diseases

Fractures of the hair shaft
Trichorrhexis nodosa
Trichothiodystrophy
Trichoschisis and trichoclasis
Trichorrhexis invaginata
Tapered fracture
Trichoptilosis

Irregularities of the hair shaft
Uncombable hair syndrome
Pili bifurcati
Pili multigemini
Trichostasis spinulosa
Pili annulati
Monilethrix
Bubble hair

Hair shaft coiling and twisting
Pili torti
Woolly hair
Acquired progressive kinking of the hair
Trichonodosis
Circled and rolled hair

Extraneous matter on the hair shaft
Hair casts

The distal form of the condition is very common and often results from general weathering of the hair. It presents in all races, especially in people with long hair.

There are two types of proximal trichorrhexis nodosa: one variant is restricted to patients of African heritage and presents as plaques of alopecia on the scalp, moustache, beard area, or pubis. It is generally associated with other wear-and-tear changes such as split ends (trichoptilosis).

The second variant is much less frequent and includes congenital and hereditary defects of the hair shaft, the most important of which is TTD (see below). The abnormal hair in these patients, which is highly susceptible to daily wear and mild trauma, fractures easily. Other abnormalities of the hair shaft are also commonly present. The hair breaks so easily that even people with short hair develop areas of alopecia. Trichorrhexis nodosa has been associated with ectodermal defects and multiple genetic syndromes including Netherton, Basex-Dupré-Christol, Menkes, Kabuki, and Tay syndromes. Metabolic disorders associated with trichorrhexis nodosa are anomalies of the urea cycle such as argininosuccinic aciduria and citrullinemia. Other reported metabolic disorders are acquired deficiencies or congenital deficiencies in biotin and zinc metabolism. Trichorrhexis nodosa has also been associated with many other conditions including untreatable infant diarrhea, tricho-hepato-enteric syndrome, mitochondrial diseases, trichorrhexis invaginata, monilethrix, pseudomonilethrix, pili torti, pili annulati, ectodermal dysplasia, giant axonal neuropathy, hypothyroidism, adrenoleukodystrophy, improper use of ceramic flat irons, combing habits, hair transplantation, and after tumor necrosis factor-α inhibitor therapy.[3–22]

Pathogenesis and histologic features

Microscopic study shows a normal hair shaft except for the beaded areas where the cortex has herniated through the cuticular cells (see *Fig. 22.1*). The latter are fragmented and in many cases totally absent. In specimens with good preservation, where the hair has not broken up completely, the appearances are reminiscent of two worn-out paintbrushes joined by their hairs (*Figs 22.172* and *22.173*).[23,24]

Differential diagnosis

Hair shaft fractures may be seen in a variety of other conditions including trichoschisis, trichoclasis, trichorrhexis invaginata, tapered fracture, and trichoptilosis. Extensive clinical and laboratory studies are often required to establish the correct diagnosis. Distal forms can simulate dandruff, peripilar casts, and pediculosis. The differential diagnosis in these cases can be easily made by microscopic examination of the hair.

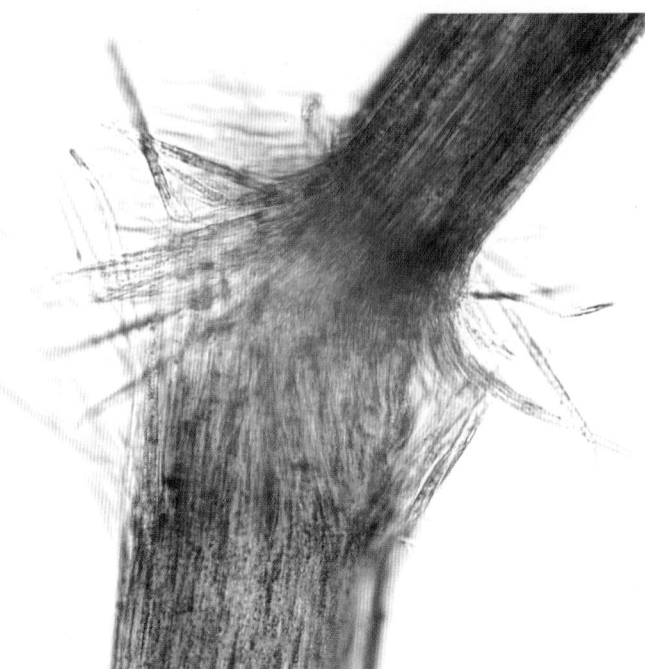

Fig. 22.172
Trichorrhexis nodosa: typical node as a result of fracture of cortical fibers protruding through a broken cuticle.

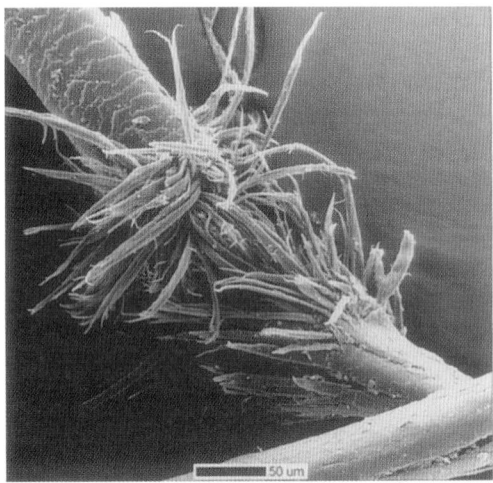

Fig. 22.173
Trichorrhexis nodosa: the features are likened to dried paintbrushes joined by their hair. The condition is commonly the result of trauma. Reproduced with permission from Hordinsky, M.E., Sawaya, M.E., Scher, R.K. (eds) (2000) Atlas of hair and nails. Philadelphia: Saunders.

Trichothiodystrophy

Clinical features

Pollit and colleagues described TTD in 1968 as a rare group of autosomal recessive disorders presenting in children and characterized by short, fragile, brittle hair associated with a variety of other hair shaft abnormalities.[1,2] Clinically, it is a heterogeneous condition with frequent systemic manifestations predominantly affecting organs derived from the neuroectoderm. Hairs, which have low sulfur content, break easily with resultant hair loss. Changes of trichorrhexis nodosa are usually evident in the proximal portion of the hair shaft.

TTD is a feature of many syndromes including BIDS (brittle sulfur-deficient hair, intellectual impairment, decreased fertility and short stature), IBIDS (ichthyosis and BIDS), PIBIDS (photosensitivity and IBIDS), SIBIDS (otosclerosis and IBIDS), ONMR (onychotrichodysplasia, chronic

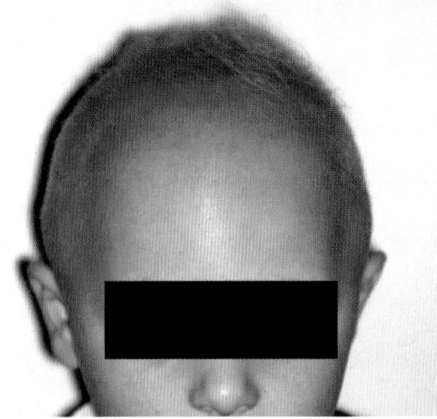

Fig. 22.174
Trichothiodystrophy: note the sparse, short, and fragmented hairs. Courtesy of P. Reygagne, MD, Centre Sabouraud, Paris, France.

neutropenia, and mental retardation) and Tay (ichthyosiform erythroderma, hair shaft abnormalities, mental and physical retardation) Sabinas, and Pollitt syndromes.[3–7]

Sporadic cases of patients with TTD without any associated neuroectodermal defects have also been documented.[8,9] The condition may also present with urological malformations and primary hypercalciuria, sideroblastic anemia, hypereosinophilic syndrome, congenital heart disease, and beta-thalassemia.[10–14]

Pathogenesis and histologic features

Patients with TTD and photosensitivity have a defect in the DNA nucleotide excision repair (NER) mechanism. The NER pathway involves at least 28 genes and is linked to DNA repair and transcription.[15,16] Three NER genes are part of the basal transcription factor, TFIIH.

Three autosomal recessive syndromes are associated with NER defects: the photosensitive form of TTD, xeroderma pigmentosum (XP), and Cockayne syndrome. TTD results from mutation in the XPB, XPD, or TTD-A genes. These three genes encode for proteins that are part of the basal transcriptor factor TFIIH, including XPB and XPD, helicases that excise and repair DNA.

It is thought that the clinical features of XP are linked to mutations in the repair function of NER genes, while mutations affecting the transcription-related function of NER genes result in the TTD phenotype. Patients with TTD do not have an increased risk in cancer susceptibility, as seen in XP patients (1000-fold increase risk).[17,18]

The diagnosis of TTD can be confirmed by demonstrating DNA repair defects after exposure to ultraviolet light. Abnormalities in excision repair of ultraviolet-damaged DNA are recognized in about half of the patients.

The hair of patients with TTD, which shows loss of sulfur bonds, is characterized by a significant decrease in the concentration of cystine.[19] The sulfur and cystine content of the hair is reduced in the order of 50%.[3] The cuticular cells become weak, fracturing readily with formation of trichorrhectic nodules (Fig. 22.174).[20] The hair shafts appear flattened, with trichoschisis and absence or deficiency of the cuticle.[21,22] Examination with polarized light is essential to visualize the typical alternating dark and light band pattern resulting from the undulation of cortical pilar fibers. The appearance resembles a tiger's tail (Fig. 22.175).[23,24]

TTD may be diagnosed in utero by a fetal eyebrow biopsy or from amniotic fluid trophoblasts by identifying defects in the DNA repair capacity.[25–27]

Trichoschisis and trichoclasis

Trichoschisis means a clean transverse fracture across the hair shaft involving both the cuticle and the cortex (Fig. 22.176).[1] It develops as a consequence of loss of cuticular cells and is frequently associated with TTD.[2,3] It has also been observed in patients with normal hair.[4]

Trichoclasis refers to a greenstick fracture of the hair shaft. It is therefore an oblique or transverse incomplete fracture involving the cortex but

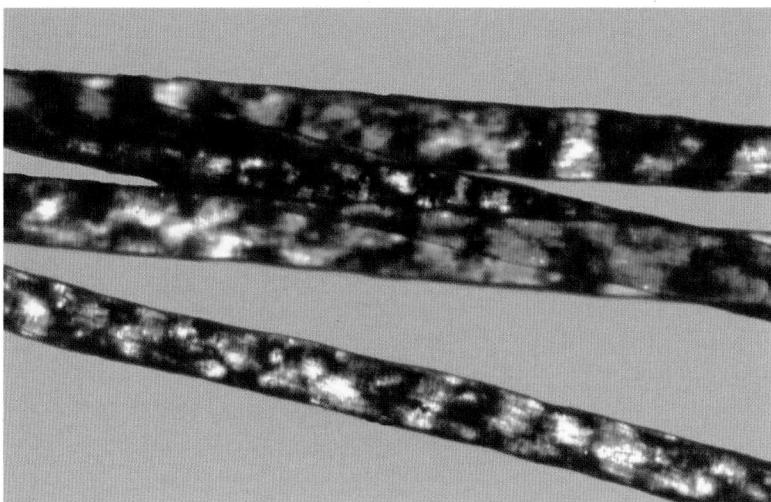

Fig. 22.175
Trichothiodystrophy: typical tiger tail appearance in hair shafts under polarized light. Courtesy of P. Reygagne, MD, Centre Sabouraud, Paris, France.

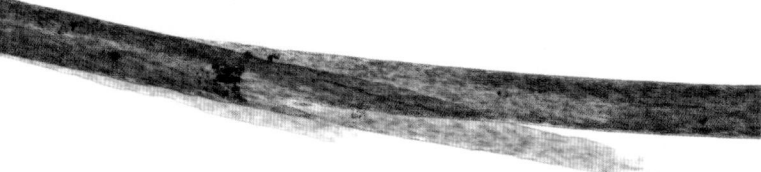

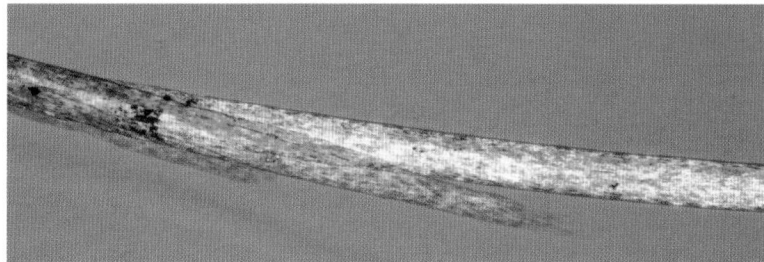

Fig. 22.177
Trichoclasis 'Greenstick' fracture of the hair shaft, consisting of an oblique fracture splinted by an intact cuticle, easily visible with polarized light (*bottom*).

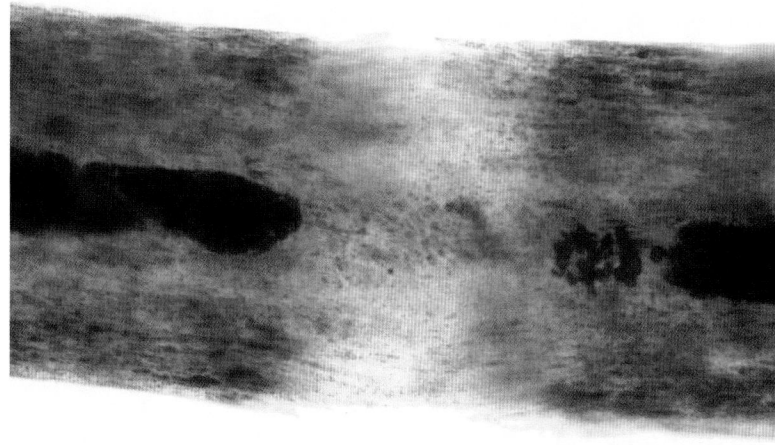

Fig. 22.176
Trichoschisis: note a crack in the cuticle that is perpendicular to the axis of the hair fiber; the cortical fibers do not protrude.

leaving the cuticle intact.[1] The sulfur content in the cuticle and the cortex is normal. It is not a specific sign and can be seen associated with a wide range of hair shaft disorders (*Fig. 22.177*).

Trichorrhexis invaginata

Clinical features

Trichorrhexis invaginata (bamboo hair) represents an alteration of the hair shaft characterized by development of small nodules at variable intervals along the length of the hair shaft, giving it a bamboo cane-like appearance. This results in very fragile hair that breaks readily, leaving it short and thin. The hair of the eyebrows and eyelashes may also be affected.

Trichorrhexis invaginata is typical of Netherton syndrome, which was described in 1958. This is an autosomal recessive disorder with variable penetrance, characterized by trichorrhexis invaginata, ichthyosis linearis circumflexa or ichthyosis vulgaris, and atopic dermatitis. The latter occurs in about 75% of patients.[1] The presence of trichorrhexis invaginata is necessary for the diagnosis of Netherton syndrome.

The degree of hair involvement varies in severity but tends to be more pronounced in girls. This is apparently due to girls wearing their hair longer, which is then more susceptible to trauma. The clinical manifestations of Netherton syndrome generally appear in the first weeks of life and are characterized by a generalized desquamative erythroderma. The defects of the hair shaft appear early in life and involve all the hairs in the body. In a minority of patients the manifestations are very mild. In typical cases, however, the hair is short, dry, dull, and breakable. Eyelashes and eyebrows are scarce or absent. The eyebrows are more commonly and severely affected than the scalp and therefore represent the site of choice for a biopsy.[2] Although Netherton syndrome has been associated with aminoaciduria, this is not a constant finding.

Other clinical features that have been reported are neurological defects, mental retardation, short stature, delayed growth, recurrent infections, and hypo- or hypergammaglobulinemia.[3,4]

Pathogenesis and histologic features

Netherton syndrome is caused by a mutation in the SPINK5 gene at chromosome 5q32, which encodes an inhibitor of serine protease called LEKT1 (lymphoepithelial Kazal-type related inhibitor), a new type of serine protease inhibitor involved in the regulation of skin barrier formation and immunity. It is thought that the alteration in the epidermal expression of LEKT1 leads to the premature activation of proteolytic enzymes in the stratum corneum with separation of corneocytes.[5–7] SPINK5 testing can be performed as an aid in the diagnosis of Netherton syndrome by immunohistochemistry of a skin biopsy with an antibody against LETK1.[8]

Histologically, the hair shaft shows a dome-shaped expansion at the proximal end. This results from invagination of the distal segment into the proximal segment. The resulting deformity resembles a joint or a 'cup and ball' (*Fig. 22.178*). The nodules are very fragile and the hair sample must be taken with great care so that they remain intact. If the sample is obtained by traction, only the distal ends of the hair shaft will be obtained, and these are not suitable for diagnosis. When only the proximal half of the invagination with its dome-shaped morphology is observed, its appearance is characteristic and described as 'golf-tee' hair or a tulip.[9]

The morphological features of trichorrhexis invaginata result from mechanical factors acting upon the hair shaft while it is still within the follicle. It is thought that invagination occurs because the proximal end of the hair follicle is impacted into the distal segment.

Ultrastructural findings are suppression of cornification, with absence of keratohyalin granules and decrease of keratin filaments. In some cases, the pathological findings are more prominent in vellus hairs than in terminal hairs.[3]

Differential diagnosis

Although trichorrhexis invaginata is characteristic of Netherton syndrome, it can occasionally be observed as a consequence of trauma or in association with other hair shaft disorders.[10]

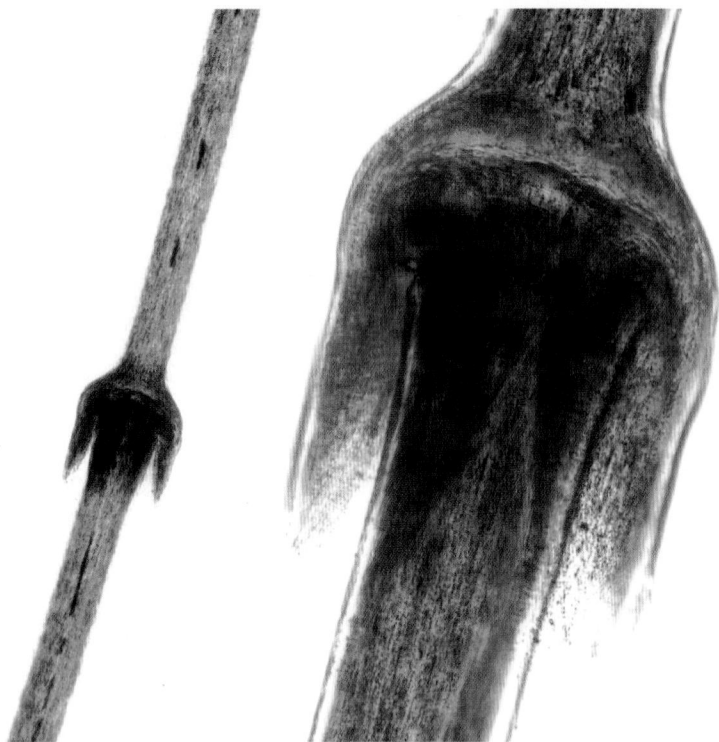

Fig. 22.178
Trichorrhexis invaginata: this is pathognomonic of Netherton disease. It represents impaction of the lower element of the hair shaft on the upper segment. This occurs within the hair follicle. Courtesy of N. Valderrama, MD, Cali, Colombia.

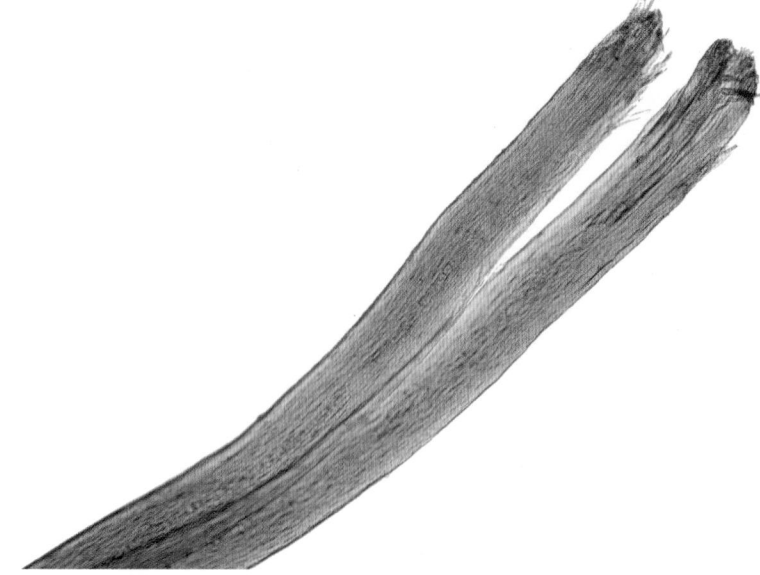

Fig. 22.179
Trichoptilosis: typical split ends commonly seen in long normal hairs. The hair tip is more vulnerable to trauma than more proximal areas.

Tapered fracture

Clinical features

The development of tapered hairs is associated with any process that suddenly inhibits cellular division in the hair matrix such as that which follows use of cytotoxic agents or intense radiotherapy while simultaneously precipitating anagen effluvium. However, it has recently been reported that cytotoxic drugs act on the hairs, inducing tapering of the proximal hair shaft and premature entry of the follicle into telogen, conflicting with the conventional view that affected hair follicles continue in anagen.[1] The resulting hair, in this defect, becomes progressively thinner and flattened, is very susceptible to fracture, and a 'pencil pointing' appearance is characteristic.[2]

Tapered hairs are seen in alopecia areata and occasionally in a background of normal hair. Another cause of tapered hairs, or hairs with a bayonet appearance, is intoxication with thallium.[3,4] Various hair shaft abnormalities may be associated with tapered hairs.

Trichoptilosis

Clinical features

Trichoptilosis (split ends) is one of the acquired structural abnormalities of the hair shaft. It is very frequent and defined as a longitudinal fracture, splitting or fraying of the distal end of the hair. It is observed more commonly in women and children with long and poorly groomed hair as a result of the cumulative effects of chemical and physical trauma. It has also been observed in numerous hair shaft disorders including monilethrix, TTD, Netherton syndrome, and pili torti. Trichoptilosis is often seen with trichorrhexis nodosa and trichoclasis. Selenium shampoo, ketoconazole 2% shampoo, and hair gels have been regarded as contributing factors.[1]

Pathogenesis and histologic features

The pathogenesis is loss of cuticular cells due to wear of the distal portion of the shaft leaving the cortex exposed, resulting in a split. The distal part of the hair separates longitudinally into two or more divisions that extend

2.0–3.0 cm or occasionally longer (*Fig. 22.179*). Central trichoptilosis has also been observed as a longitudinal split in the hair shaft without involvement of the proximal and distal ends of the split.[2,3]

Differential diagnosis

Trichoptilosis must be differentiated from pili bifurcati. In the latter condition, each hair division produces two separate parallel branches that subsequently fuse to form a single hair shaft. In contrast to trichoptilosis, in pili bifurcati, a cuticle covers each branch.[4]

Irregularities of the hair shaft

Uncombable hair syndrome

Clinical features

Uncombable hair syndrome (pili canaliculi et trianguli, cheveux incoiffables, spun glass hair) is a disorder of the hair shaft first described by Dupré, Rochiccioli, and Bonafé in 1973.[1] It is sporadic or inherited as a monogenic autosomal dominant disorder with variable penetrance.[2]

The condition is restricted to the scalp and is characterized by hair that is unruly and impossible to comb flat (*Fig. 22.180*).[3] It is frequently seen in children and presents between the ages of 3 months and 3 years. The quantity of hair is usually normal, but it appears dry, dull, frizzy, short, and light in color. It can also be observed in dark hair, but it is usually not as perceptible. The hair is described as unmanageable. Hair fragility is not usually a feature. Partial forms have also been documented in which a localized area of uncombable hair is seen in the frontal and occipital areas.[2] The condition tends to improve with time.[4,5]

Usually, uncombable hair syndrome occurs in isolation without an associated syndrome. However, it has been described with ectodermal dysplasia, retinal dysplasia/pigmentary dystrophy, juvenile cataracts, abnormalities of the digits, tooth enamel anomalies, oligodontia, phalangoepiphyseal dysplasia, angel-shaped phalangoepiphyseal dysplasia, loose anagen syndrome, neurofibromatosis type I, Wilson disease, alopecia areata, lichen sclerosus, anagen hair syndrome, and in a pre-menarche girl with a yolk sac tumor (endodermal sinus tumor). [6–15]

Pathogenesis and histologic features

The pathogenesis is unknown. It has been hypothesized that the disease results from premature keratinization of a triangular-shaped internal root sheath, the latter resulting from an abnormally shaped dermal papilla.[4]

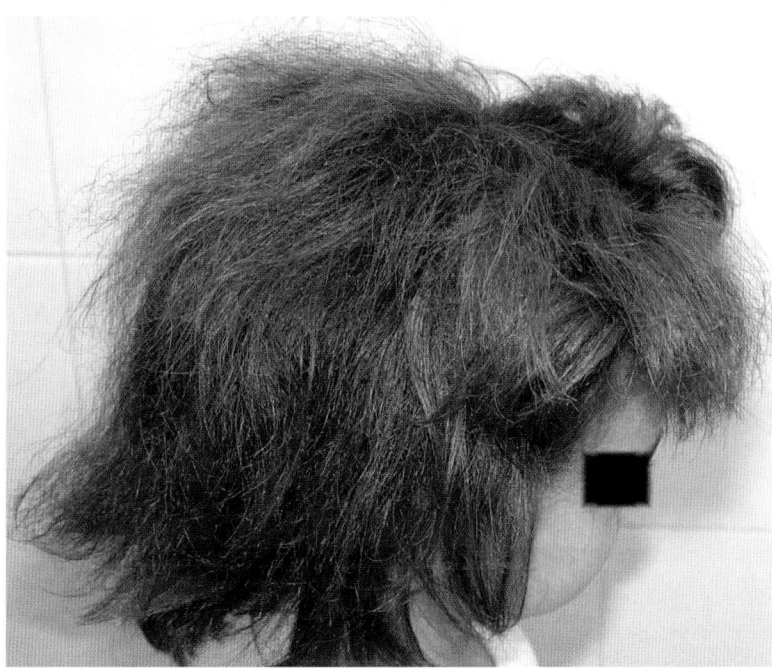

Fig. 22.180
Uncombable hair syndrome: in this condition, the hair resembles spun glass. The condition only affects the scalp. Courtesy of A.M. Aristizábal, MD, CES, Medellín, Colombia.

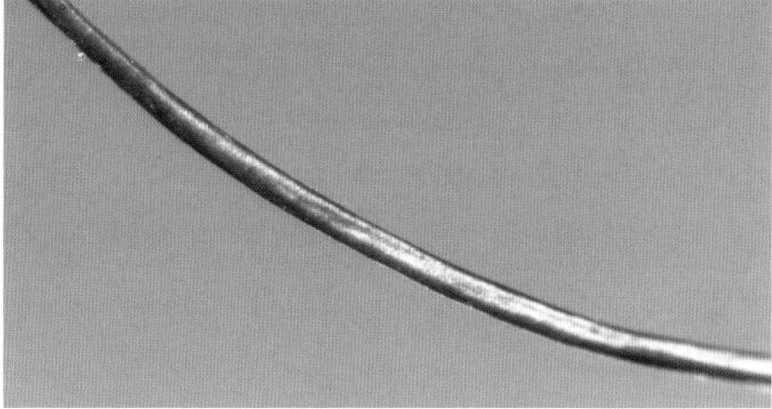

Fig. 22.181
Uncombable hair syndrome (pili canaliculi): there is a longitudinal grooving within the hair (pili canaliculi) which contributes to the structural rigidity and clinical appearance. Courtesy of A.M. Aristizábal, MD, CES, Medellín, Colombia.

Under light microscopy, the hair shafts may initially seem normal but when horizontal sections are examined the hair follicles and shafts are triangular, kidney- or heart-shaped. The hair shafts may also have a longitudinal canalicular dent or a prominent longitudinal groove along the long axis of the hair (*Fig. 22.181*). In some cases, the internal root sheath forms an angle which results in hair follicle deformity. The best method to observe the triangular hair configuration and canalicular dent is with scanning electron microscopy. More than 50% of the hairs from an individual with this syndrome will have this characteristic appearance, compared to less than 5% in the general population.[4,16–18]

Differential diagnosis

The differential diagnosis includes pili torti, monilethrix, woolly hair, and acquired progressive kinking of the hair. Overall, the clinical features are typical and the differential diagnosis is usually straightforward.[19]

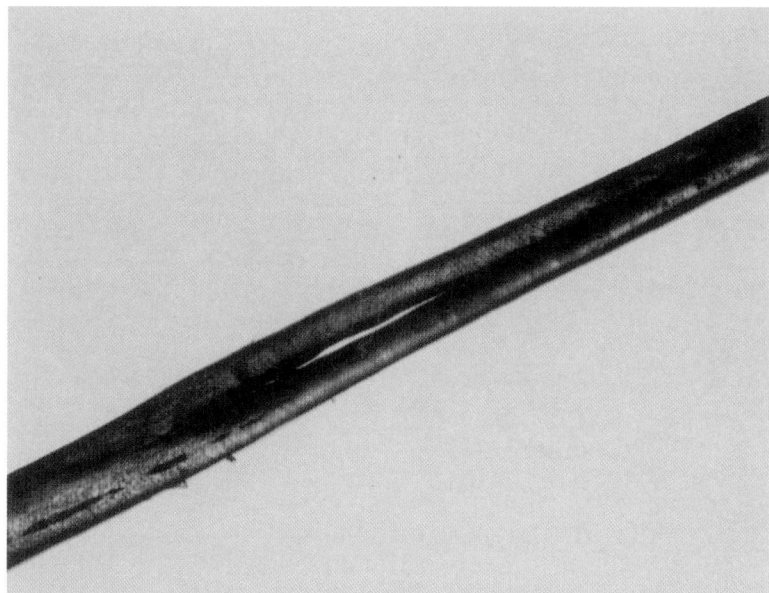

Fig. 22.182
Pili bifurcati: the hair is split within the longitudinal mid-zone and then rejoins. Courtesy of David de Berker, MD, Bristol Royal Infirmary, Bristol, UK.

Pili bifurcati

Clinical features

Pili bifurcati is a very common hair shaft disorder characterized by focal bifurcation of the hair shaft which, after a short distance, fuses to reform a single hair (*Fig. 22.182*). Each branch of the bifurcation is covered by its own cuticle. Pili bifurcati has been associated with mosaic trisomy 8 syndrome.[1,2]

Differential diagnosis

Pili bifurcati can be distinguished from trichoptilosis because in the latter condition the bifurcations are not surrounded by a complete cuticle and are generally present in the distal segment of the hair shaft. In some cases, the bifurcation occurs in the proximal segment. Pili bifurcati should also be differentiated from pili multigemini in which multiple hair shafts emerge from a single follicular channel.[1,3]

Pili multigemini

Clinical features

Pili multigemini (multi hair) was first described by Flemming in 1883 and Giovanni in 1892. It is a hair shaft developmental abnormality, which occurs mostly on the face, particularly the beard area and the scalp in children, but has also been described with involvement of the entire body. Several hair shafts emerge from a single follicular ostium.[1]

The condition is usually asymptomatic, but it may be associated with erythema and recurrent follicular inflammation leading to scarring. In some cases, the abnormality follows Blaschko lines. An association with cleidocranial dysostosis has been documented.[2,3]

Most cases of pili multigemini have been found incidentally. A recent study showed that all the Europeans randomly chosen had the condition. Because of this finding, it has been concluded that, rather than a rare development defect of hair, it should be considered as a varying vestige of evolution.[4]

Histologic features

Pili multigemini is characterized by several hair shafts within a single follicular canal (from two to eight), each of which originates from an individual matrix and papilla (*Fig. 22.183*). The hair may have a flattened or

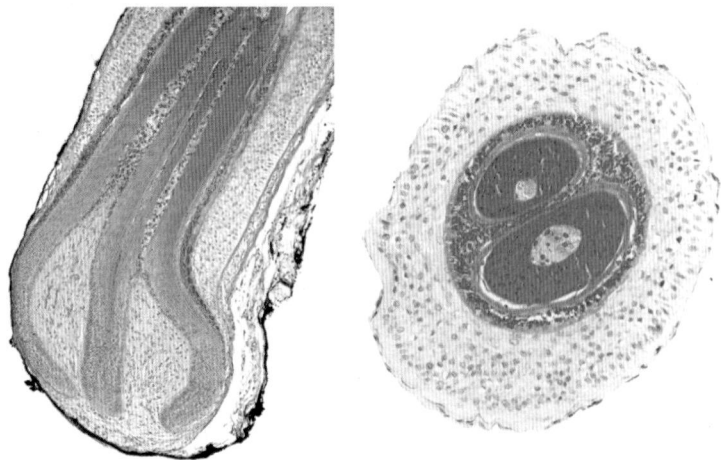

Fig. 22.183
Pili multigemini: in these vertical and horizontal sections, note the two hair shafts within a single follicular canal. The hairs have all the components of a normal follicle and a common external root sheath.

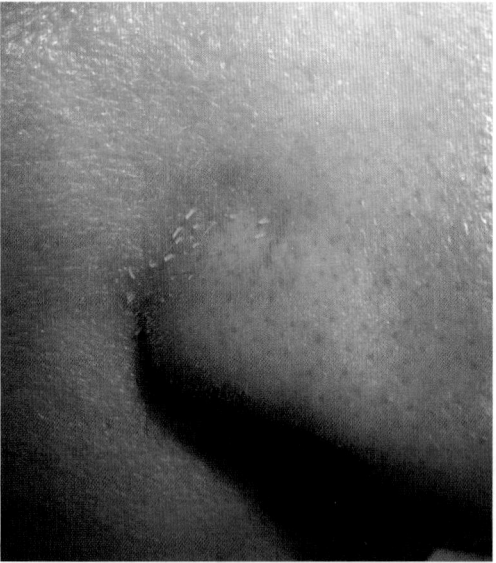

Fig. 22.184
Trichostasis spinulosa: note the follicular prominence on the nasal fold. Courtesy of L.M. Gómez, MD, UPB, Medellín, Colombia.

triangular shape and has all the components of a normal follicle except that there is a common external root sheath.[2]

Differential diagnosis

The condition must be distinguished from tufted folliculitis. In the latter condition, fusion of hair follicles occurs in the upper segment of the follicle as a result of inflammation, and each hair is surrounded by its own external root sheath.

Trichostasis spinulosa

Clinical features

Trichostasis spinulosa is a very frequent alteration of the hair follicle characterized by dilated vellus hair follicles with retention of successive telogen hairs that protrude from a single dilated ostium. The disorder was first recognized by Felix Franke in 1901, who named it 'Das Pinselhaar Thysonatrix' (paintbrush hair). The term trichostasis spinulosa was coined by Noble in 1913.[1]

Lesions present as multiple hyperkeratotic follicular papules that usually resemble comedones, but close examination may reveal a tuft of hairs. It has predilection for areas with abundant pilosebaceous units, including the face, neck, chest, upper arms, and interscapular area (*Fig. 22.184*). The defect is seen after adolescence in males and females, but it is more commonly seen in elderly patients.

There are two variants: a classic nonpruritic form that presents on the face (particularly on the nose of middle-aged to elderly individuals as a solitary comedo-like lesion) and a pruritic variant that especially involves the limbs and trunk of young adults.[2-4] It has also been classified as primary trichostasis spinulosa when it is seen as an isolated finding or as secondary trichostasis spinulosa when it is described within pre-existing skin lesions.

Pathogenesis and histologic features

The pathogenesis is unknown although some studies have suggested that *Pityrosporum* and/or *P. acnes* may be responsible for induction of follicular hyperkeratosis with vellus hair retention.[5] Follicles may also contain *Malassezia furfur* yeasts. Difusse trichostasis spinulosa has been reported in prolonged use of topical corticosteroids and chronic renal failure.[1,6]

Histology reveals a dilated hair follicle in which a keratin plug surrounds multiple hair shafts derived from a single matrix and papilla (*Fig. 22.185*). Dermoscopy may help identify the characteristic hair tuft.[7]

Trichostasis spinulosa has been described as an associated finding in intradermal melanocytic nevi, seborrheic keratoses, syringomas, and nodular basal cell carcinomas.[8-11]

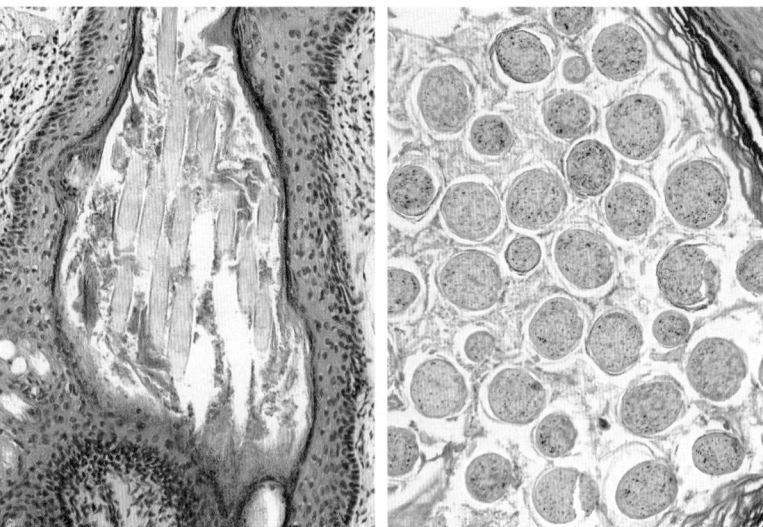

Fig. 22.185
Trichostasis spinulosa: vertical and horizontal sections. Numerous nonpigmented hair shafts in a single hair follicle.

Differential diagnosis

Conditions presenting as keratotic follicular papules may be considered in the differential diagnosis. These include keratosis pilaris, ichthyosis follicularis, hypovitaminosis A and C, eruptive vellus hair cysts, and Darier disease. It also has to be differentiated from entities such as comedonal acne and Favre-Racouchot syndrome.[1]

Pili annulati

Clinical features

Pili annulati (ringed hair) usually presents as a rare autosomal dominant disorder with high penetrance, although very occasionally sporadic cases are seen. Alternate light and dark bands are present along the length of the hair shaft, giving it a spangled and sandy appearance best observed under a bright light and microscopic examination. It is most obvious in patients with light-colored hair. However, it has also been reported in patients of African heritage.[1] The condition usually presents in children, and mild fragility of the hair shaft is sometimes a feature. Other hair-bearing areas are occasionally affected. The growth of the scalp hair is usually normal.[2]

Pili annulati has been associated with alopecia areata and, interestingly, the clinical manifestations sometimes disappear when the hair regrows.[3–6] Microscopic examination, however, shows that the banding persists although it is less frequent.[5] A simultaneous association with alopecia areata, autoimmune thyroid disease, and primary IgA deficiency simultaneously has also been reported. However, some authors have regarded this association as a coincidence. [7,8]

Pathogenesis and histologic features

The pathogenesis of pili annulati is unknown. It has been suggested that the alterations result from a disorder of protein metabolism in which malfunction of cytoplasmic ribosomes results in formation of defective cortical keratins, not yet identified.[9,10] Another hypothesis states that the genetic defect may be a mutation in proteins involved in the signaling and regulation of formation and degradation of the lamina densa and sublamina densa region, resulting in abnormal assembly or remodeling of the basement membrane zone.[11] Recently, a locus for pili annulati was mapped to chromosome 12q24.32–24.33, but as yet the gene or genes responsible have not been completely identified.[12–14]

Light microscopic examination reveals alternating dark and light bands that become less frequent in the distal part of the hair shaft. The light bands represent air-filled spaces between the macrofibrillar units within the cortex of the hair shaft.[15] An unknown defect in the formation of the micro-/macrofibrillar matrix complex is considered to be the cause. The medullary portion of the hair shaft is not affected.[10,16] It has also been observed that the cystine content of hair is lower than normal, while the level of lysine is elevated compared to normal controls.[17]

With scanning electron microscopy, the air-filled cavities are seen within cortical cells or in larger cavities replacing these cells. Occasional hair shafts show an unusual weathering pattern. This may consist of minor surface abnormalities at regular intervals in areas overlying the abnormal spaces or else it presents as marked damage to the cuticle with exposure and even cracking of the underlying cortex.[18]

Differential diagnosis

Pseudopili annulati has been described when normal hairs show a similar banding pattern to that seen in pili annulati as a result of flattening or twisting of the hair.[19,20] This has no clinical implications.

Monilethrix

Clinical features

Monilethrix (beaded hair) is a hair shaft disorder mostly transmitted as an autosomal dominant disorder with incomplete penetrance and variable expressivity.[1] It was first described in 1879 by Walter Smith.[2] In this disease, the hairs are easily fractured due to areas of narrowing. This results in short, fragile, and easily breakable hairs that result in partial or diffuse alopecia.

The hair shaft resembles a rosary due to the presence of ellipsoidal nodules interrupted by narrow zones. After emerging from the follicle, the hair breaks at the latter sites with resultant hair loss. The alopecia is initially localized to the occipital area, and progressively extends, causing almost total alopecia in those who are severely affected. Involvement of other hair-bearing areas may be seen. The phenotypic expression is variable and the condition sometimes improves with age and pregnancy. Follicular abnormalities range from subtle perifollicular erythema to papules and hyperkeratosis, which are almost invariable concomitant findings.[3,4]

Other reported abnormalities associated with monilethrix are mostly of ectodermal origin, and include juvenile cataracts, cutis laxa, dermal abnormalities, nail disorders, syndactyly, mental deficiency, epilepsy, spinocerebellar ataxia, schizophrenia, argininosuccinic aciduria, growth retardation, holt-oram syndrome, and hereditary unilateral external auditory canal atresia.[5–7]

The condition may be diagnosed prenatally by biopsy of chorionic villi.[8]

Pathogenesis and histologic features

Monilethrix is a disease of the hair cortex. The mutation has been mapped to chromosome 12q11-q13, which contains the genes that encode three type II hair keratins expressed in the hair cortex: HB1 (KRT81), HB6 (KRT86), and HB3 (KRT83). The main defect is in HB6.[1,8–12] The mutations in HB1 produce a less severe phenotype and have been associated with nail dystrophy.[13]

Histologically, the nodal areas represent the normal hair and the narrowed areas represent affected hair. In the latter areas, there is a reduction in the thickness of the cortex and an absence of the medulla. The fractures occur within these foci, and in some patients, other hair shaft abnormalities are present.

Electron microscopy studies have confirmed that the internodal region is the site of the pathology.[14] The appearances of the nodes and the distance between them vary considerably, not only in different hairs but also within the same hair.[15]

Differential diagnosis

Pseudomonilethrix has been classified into three types[1]: familiar pseudomonilethrix of Bentley-Phillips (autosomal dominant inheritance), acquired pseudomonilethrix in dysplastic disorders with hair fragility, and iatrogenic pseudominolethrix that represents an artifact, rather than a true abnormality of the hair shaft, induced by compression of hairs between glass slides during preparation of the specimen.[2,16,17]

Histologically, there are rosary-like nodular thickenings of the hair shaft alternating with thin areas, in a more irregular fashion than in monilethrix.[2,17]

Bubble hair

Described by Brown et al. in 1986, bubble hair refers to an acquired hair shaft abnormality, primarily in young females, characterized by bubbles within the hair shaft, particularly the medullary region.[1,2]

Bubble hair develops as a result of heat-induced gas accumulation within the hair shaft. The condition is often due to the use of hair dryers or of any other instrument that heats the hair.[3–5] It can also be associated with environmental factors such as swimming in chlorinated pools and exposure to the sun and wind. The bubbles are formed by rapid evaporation of the water within the hair shaft. It is unclear whether the bubble itself is enough to break the hair or if concomitant weathering is also required. Examination under light microscopy reveals vacuolization within the hair shafts. The vacuoles vary in size and appear to distend the shafts. Electron microscopy reveals loss of cortical cells and medulla, with large cavities in some areas and reticulated 'Swiss cheeselike' loss of cells in others.[6]

The differential diagnosis of bubble hair includes pili annulati, fungal infections, and thallium intoxication.[7]

Hair shaft coiling and twisting

Pili torti

Clinical features

Pili torti represents one of the coiling and twisting abnormalities of the hair shaft. Four main variants have been identified.[1,2] In the classic early-onset Ronchese type of pili torti, the hair from the entire scalp, eyebrows, and eyelashes looks dry, short, and fragile from the first 2 years of life. It initially presents in the occipital area in early infancy and extends gradually. The hair is fragile and usually breaks within the first few centimeters. In the light, the hair appears to be adorned with sequins. Inheritance patterns are variable, and the underlying genetic defect has not been identified.[2] Late-onset Beare type is an autosomal dominant disorder which typically presents with breakage of the hairs of the eyebrows and eyelashes in white patients. The onset of this disorder is in childhood or after puberty.

In patients with Menkes syndrome, the main hair finding is fragility due to pili torti. Menkes syndrome is an X-linked recessive disorder of copper metabolism. After birth, hairs gradually become sparse, short, fragile, brittle, and depigmented, resembling steel wool.[3-5] In a number of patients, sensorineural loss of hearing has been reported associated with clinical hair changes of pili torti, which is known as Björnstad syndrome. Moreover, when these two findings appear with hypogonadism, the condition is called Crandall syndrome. The former has an autosomal recessive pattern of inheritance caused by mutations of the gene BCS1L mapped to chromosome 2q34-q36.[6-10]

Pili torti has also been associated with ectodermal disorders such as pachyonychia congenita type 2 (with particular involvement of the eyebrows and facial hair), hypohidrotic ectodermal dysplasia, Bazex-Dupré-Christol syndrome (follicular atrophoderma, multiple basal cell carcinomas and hypotrichosis), Marie-Unna hereditary congenital hypotrichosis, Rapp-Hodgkin ectodermal dysplasia syndrome, ectrodactyly-ectodermal dysplasia-clefting syndrome, onychodysplasia, and hyperkeratosis palmoplantaris striata.[11-18]

Acquired pili torti is due to trauma. It can be associated with diverse forms of alopecia. Pili torti has also been reported with acquired structural defects of the hair similar to those observed in pseudopélade, suggesting that the disorder may be due to a dysfunctional hair papilla secondary to fibrosis.[19] Other associations reported include: mitochondrial diseases, synthetic retinoids, citrullinemia, argininosuccinic aciduria, juvenile macular dystrophy, anorexia nervosa, and Netherton syndrome. Pili torti has been described on the abdomen of hirsute men and women.[20-28]

Pathogenesis and histologic features

The twisting and abnormal molding of the hair shaft is likely due to alterations of the inner root sheath, probably due to mitochondrial dysfunction.[29,30]

Histologic examination shows flat hairs that are twisted 180° on their axes at irregular intervals. The twisting may rarely occur at different angles varying from 90° to 360°. At the torsion sites, the hair is fragile and breaks easily, resulting in trichoptilosis. The phenomenon of many hairs twisted in a double spiral is called corkscrew hair.

The sequin-like clinical appearance is due to the irregular reflection of light on the twisted surface.

Differential diagnosis

Pili torti is frequently confused with monilethrix because of similar light microscopic appearances. Scanning electron microscopy readily affords their distinction.

Woolly hair

Clinical features

The term woolly hair refers to prominent curly or coiled hair involving the scalp in a focal or diffuse manner that affects persons of non-African ancestry. Woolly hair can appear as a symptom of some systemic diseases, or without associated findings. When it is not syndromic, it can be classified as: a diffuse autosomal dominant variant, a diffuse autosomal recessive variant, or a localized, circumscribed variant.

Hereditary dominant woolly hair usually occurs unaccompanied by other diseases and affects the whole scalp. It appears within the first months of life. The underlying associated genetic defect has not been identified.[1]

In the autosomal recessive variant, hair is short and fragile with a light, pale color at birth. The genetic defect of autosomal recessive woolly hair has been found in chromosome 13q14.2–14.3, gene P2RY5, which encodes a G protein-coupled receptor. P2RY5 is expressed in both Henle and Huxley layers of the inner root sheath. Another mutation has been described in the lipase H gene (LIPH) found in chromosome 3q27. Both mutations have been related to autosomal recessive hypotrichosis, a rare hair disorder characterized by sparse hair on scalp and the body of affected individuals.[2-7]

The localized circumscribed variant presents at birth or early infancy and is known as woolly hair nevus. This is an uncommon disease that affects a localized area where the hair tends to be lighter and thinner than in the rest of the scalp (*Fig. 22.186*). Up to 50% of cases are associated with an epidermal nevus in the skin adjacent to the woolly hair nevus or elsewhere

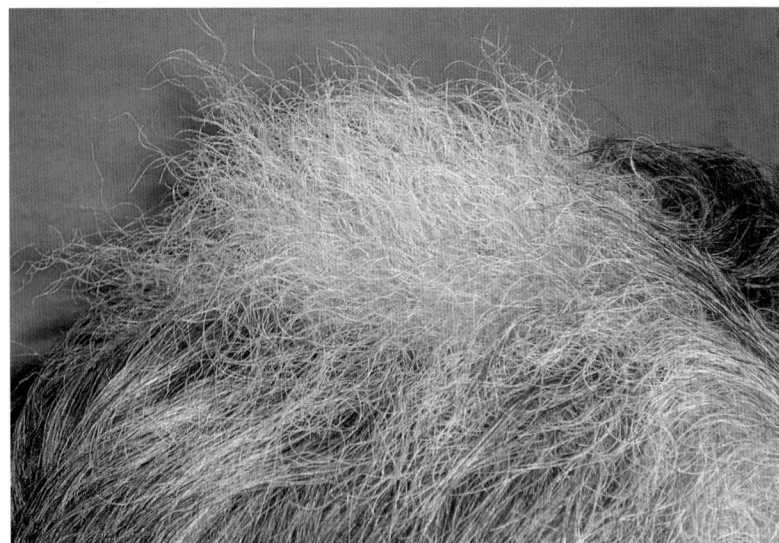

Fig. 22.186
Woolly hair: note the tightly coiled golden hair. Courtesy of A.M. Aristizábal, MD, CES, Medellín, Colombia.

in the skin.[1,8-10] Woolly hair nevus has been associated with epidermal nevus syndrome and precocious puberty, persistent pupillary membrane, verrucous epidermal nevus, systematized linear epidermal nevus, loose anagen hair syndrome, intractable infant diarrhea, osteoma cutis with multiple café-au-lait spots, pachyonychia congenita, ectodermal dysplasia-skin fragility syndrome, Pallister-Killian syndrome, ichthyosis, familial keratosis follicular spinulosa decalvans, and ulerythema ophryogenes.[11-25] In some cases, a woolly hair nevus can follow Blaschko lines, suggesting a mosaic disorder. The underlying genetic defect has not been identified.

Woolly hair has also been described in association with cardiac abnormalities such as Naxos disease, Carvajal syndrome, and Naxos-like disease.[26] The first condition, an autosomal recessive disorder which affected multiple families on the Greek island of Naxos, was first described in 1986.[27] Since then, it has also been documented in other countries.

Patients are born with woolly hair, and around the first year of life develop palmoplantar keratoderma. Naxos disease (palmoplantar keratoderma with arrhythmogenic right ventricular cardiomyopathy and woolly hair) manifests in adolescence with 100% penetrance. The initial symptoms are characterized by syncope, ventricular tachycardia, or sudden death. Symptoms of right heart failure appear during the end stages of the disease.[28-30] The cause is mutations in the genes encoding the desmosomal proteins plakoglobin and desmoplakin.[31-34] Defects in the linking sites of these proteins can interrupt the cell adhesion causing cell death, progressive loss of myocardium, and fibrofatty replacement. The disease locus has been mapped to chromosome 17q21.[35-39] Other genes encoding different components of the desmosome have been reported.[40]

Carvajal syndrome is a more severe variant of Naxos disease. The cardiomyopathy manifests at an earlier age and involves mainly the left ventricle, although if may affect both. Similar to Naxos disease, it is characterized by woolly hair and palmoplantar keratoderma. It is also caused by a recessive mutation in desmoplakin. Most cases have been described in Ecuador and in India.[41-43] The clinical diagnosis must be confirmed by a myocardial biopsy showing fibrofatty replacement.

Another cardiac manifestation described with woolly hair is mitral valve regurgitation, associated with subcapsular cataracts.[44]

Histologic features

The changes are variable and range from completely normal hair with a normal hair growth rate to hairs with wide twists over several millimeters along their longitudinal axis. Hair shafts have oval, flattened, triangular, and irregular shape or are of reduced diameter.[45,46] The hair composition of keratin and amino acids is normal.

Acquired progressive kinking of the hair

Clinical features

Acquired progressive kinking of the hair is a rare disease first described by Wise and Sulzberger in 1932. The condition predominantly affects the vertex, frontal, and temporal areas of the scalp including the supra- and postauricular margins. It is characterized by onset around puberty and presents with localized, curly, and lusterless hair. The affected scalp hairs with time acquire an appearance similar to that of the pubic hair, both in color and texture.[1] The hair growth rate can be either normal or delayed. This condition has been described in both men and women.[2] The disease has been described following use of sodium valproate.[3]

Pathogenesis and histologic features

The exact etiology and pathogenesis remains unknown. It has been proposed that acquired progressive kinking hair is a variant of androgenetic alopecia. This is based on several observations including the frequent family history of androgenetic alopecia, the same affected areas as those seen in male pattern baldness, the presence of an increased scalp concentration of dihydrotestosterone, and a decreased anagen/telogen ratio. It has also been noted that in some patients the condition evolves into androgenetic alopecia.[4,5]

Whisker hair is considered a variant of acquired progressive kinking. It frequently affects the regions around the ears. This condition can also progress to androgenetic alopecia.[6]

The histologic changes are similar to those seen in androgenetic alopecia.[4,7] The hair shafts show flattening and longitudinal channels.[8]

Trichonodosis (knotted hair)

Clinical features

Trichonodosis was first described by McCarthy.[1] It is a fairly frequent incidental finding, particularly in people with curly hair.[2,3] Generally, only a few hairs are affected. The knot induces weakness in the cortex and the cuticle (*Fig. 22.187*). One or multiple knots are seen, and as a result of trauma the hairs may break at the site of the knot. The knots are usually located on the outer third of the hair shaft.[1]

Trichonodosis may also be observed in pubic hair and other areas of the body, and a variant with multiple large knots has been documented.[4] The condition has been described in association with zinc deficiency and trichoschisis.[1,5]

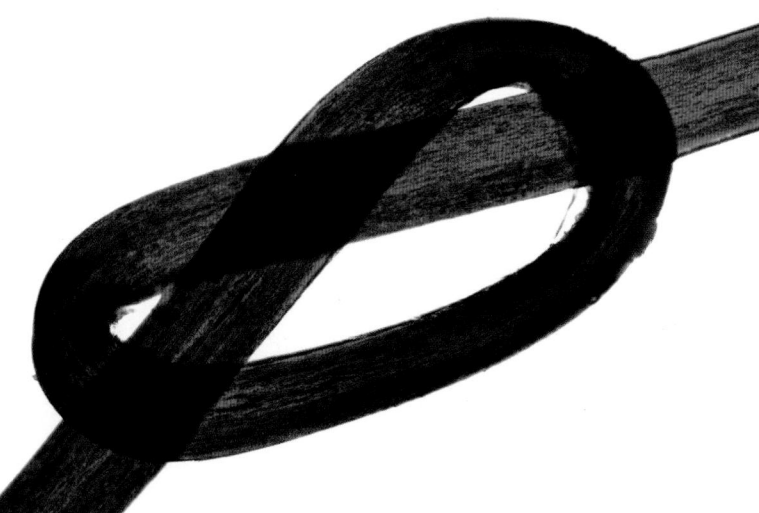

Fig. 22.187
Trichonodosis: the knots are readily seen by light microscopy.

Histologic features

The knots are readily seen by light microscopy. Scanning electron microscopy shows longitudinal fissures in the cuticle and fractures.

Circled and rolled hair

Circled and rolled hairs present as black wavy circles located under the stratum corneum next to hair follicles. They are found particularly on the abdomen, thigh, and back of middle-aged men. It is not associated with any follicular abnormality and there is no inflammation. It is believed to be a variant of ingrown hairs.[1]

They have been described in patients following renal transplantation and treatment with corticosteroids and ciclosporine.[2] The condition has also been documented in patients with juvenile hypothyroidism.[3] It has also been associated with pili multigemini.[4]

Extraneous matter on the hair shaft

Hair casts

Hair casts (peripilar keratin casts, pseudo-nits) are common, small tubular formations of amorphous material of variable shape that surround the hair shaft.[1] Their proximal ends are conical and their distal ends are funnel shaped. They appear as yellow/whitish material adherent to the hair. The condition is predominantly observed in women but has occasionally been described in children.[2] Kligman described them for the first time in 1957 as scalp pseudoparasites.[3]

Two variants have been described: primary, which particularly occurs in girls with no other associated disease and sometimes affects families,[4–6] and secondary, which develops as a consequence of inflammatory diseases accompanied by intense parakeratosis of the scalp such as psoriasis, seborrheic dermatitis, or pityriasis capitis.[7,8]

Pathogenesis and histologic features

A significant number of patients with the primary variant wear their hair in ponytails or pigtails.[6] Repeated traction of the scalp or mild trichotillomania may lead to hair casts.[9]

In the secondary variant, the hair casts are composed of parakeratotic debris derived from the external root sheath and most probably originating in the follicular infundibulum and external root sheath.[10]

A number of transmission and scanning electron microscopic studies have shown that the typical cast is composed of two concentric layers of keratinized cells: the internal layer originates from Huxley layer while the outer derives from Henle layer.[11] Other studies, however, have shown three layers: two emerging from the internal root sheath and an external layer originating from the external root sheath.[10] Energy dispersive X-ray microanalysis has shown that the casts contain silica, aluminum, and molybdenum.[6]

The histologic appearance is quite characteristic. The material surrounds and adheres to the cuticle without affecting the hair structure (*Fig. 22.188*).

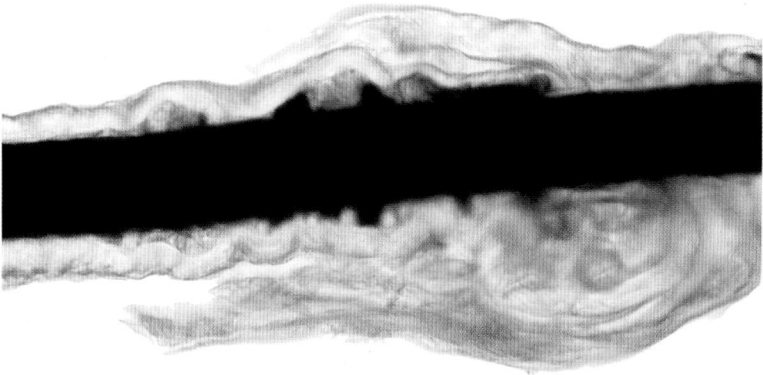

Fig. 22.188
Hair casts: amorphous material surrounds the hair shaft. Courtesy of J.C. Garcés, MD, Hospital Luis Vernaza, Guayaquil, Ecuador.

Differential diagnosis

The differential diagnoses include pediculosis capitis, tinea alba, trichorrhexis nodosa, and deposits of extraneous material.[12,13] Hair casts may be distinguished since peripilar casts are circumferential rather than eccentric matter and can be easily moved up and down the hair shaft. Hair casts stain blue with toluidine blue due to the presence of the internal root sheath.[14]

Deposits of extraneous material

Foreign material such as lacquer, paint, glue, and hair spray may adhere to the hair shaft and cause diagnostic difficulties.

The diagnosis is easy with a thorough clinical history and by paying close attention to the focal nature of the deposits. Deposits of extraneous material can be distinguished from hair casts as they cannot be moved up and down the hair shaft.[1–3]

MISCELLANEOUS FOLLICULAR DERMATOSES

Acne vulgaris

Clinical features

Acne vulgaris is an extremely common dermatological disorder, predominantly affecting teenagers and adolescents (85%), or 15% of the general population.[1,2] It shows no racial predilection and has a worldwide distribution, although clinical presentation can be different in patients with white and black skin.[3–5] The sex incidence is equal, although it is often more severe in males than in females, presumably reflecting androgen levels. It is a cosmetically serious and disfiguring condition, which may be associated with considerable scarring, and often causes important psychological effects.[6,7] Acne is associated with seasonal variation, worsening in winter and improving in summer.

Acne vulgaris is primarily a disorder of the sebaceous follicle, and it particularly involves the face, the nose and forehead, back, and chest (*Fig. 22.189*).[1] Sebaceous follicles have widely dilated follicular channels, fine vellus hairs, and numerous associated sebaceous glands. The distribution of the lesions of acne vulgaris reflects that of sebaceous glands and there is a close relationship between the amount of sebum produced and the severity of the disease.

Patients present with comedones (see below), which in many patients are accompanied by abscess formation, nodules, 'cysts', and scarring (*Fig. 22.190*). In the most seriously affected patients, groups of nodules joined by multiple sinuses may be present (acne conglobata). In patients of African descent and Africans, the disease is typically milder than in the white population. Postinflammatory hyperpigmentation is, however, a common problem. Nodulocystic disease is rare but, when it does occur, keloidal scarring is a significant problem (*Fig. 22.191*).[4,5,8]

Pathogenesis and histologic features

The pathogenesis of acne vulgaris is complex and includes: production of androgens, excessive sebum production, abnormal desquamation of the follicular epithelium in the sebaceous gland duct and hyperkeratosis of the sebaceous duct, proliferation of *P. acnes* with subsequent inflammatory changes, and inflammatory and immunological responses.[9–12]

The process is mediated by production of IL-1α and tumor necrosis factor-alpha by keratinocytes and T lymphocytes with resultant increased proliferation of keratinocytes, diminished apoptosis, and consequent hypergranulosis.[10] As a result, the sebaceous follicle becomes blocked with dense, compact keratin to form a microcomedone.

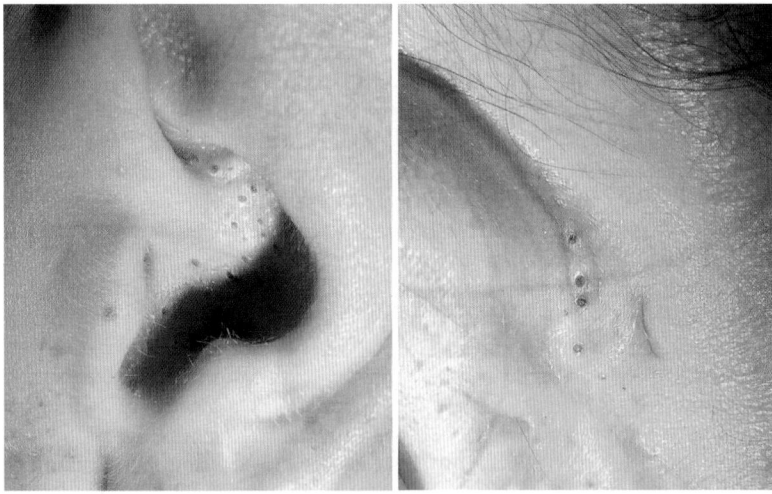

Fig. 22.190
Acne vulgaris: there are prominent blackheads which develop as a result of blockage of the pilosebaceous duct by keratotic debris. By courtesy of L.M. Gómez, MD, UPB, Medellín, Colombia.

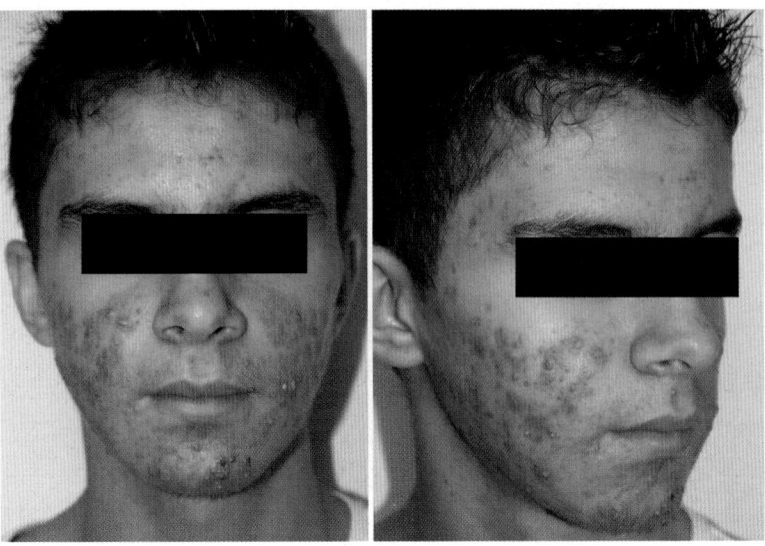

Fig. 22.189
Acne vulgaris: note the numerous papules and pustules. By courtesy of J. Cadavid, MD, Clinica Medellín, Medellín, Colombia.

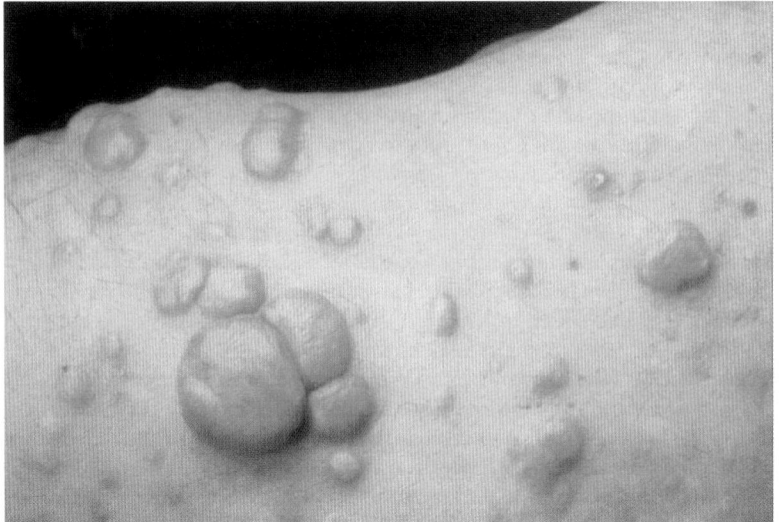

Fig. 22.191
Acne vulgaris: multiple keloids have complicated areas of previous acneiform scarring. By courtesy of the Institute of Dermatology, London, UK.

Acne can be classified into noninflammatory (purely comedonal) and inflammatory (mild papular, scarring papular, pustules and nodular or scarring acne). A severity grade (mild, moderate, or severe) is based on the approximate lesion count. A noninflammatory comedone is a consequence of impaired sebum secretion followed by subsequent dilatation of the follicle. Closed comedones are known as whiteheads; open comedones are called blackheads because the contents of the comedone oxidizes upon exposure to the air. Subsequent further overgrowth of *P. acnes* (a habitual follicular resident) results in inflammatory changes and damage to the follicular epithelium with eventual rupture and scarring.[2] It is likely that hypersensitivity to *P. acnes* plays a role in the pathogenesis of the inflammatory response.[13] This is associated with a foreign body reaction and the development of pustules, inflammatory cysts, nodules, and scarring. In addition to activating both the classic and indirect complement cascades, *P. acnes* also promotes neutrophil chemotaxis. Subsequent release of hydrolytic enzymes damages the follicular epithelium.[2,14]

Circulating androgens are also of importance in acne vulgaris, the development of the disease at puberty coinciding with a rise in the levels of circulating androgens.[15] Androgens directly stimulate sebum secretion and also hair growth.[2,16] Hypersecretion of androgens or increased 5-α-reductase (5-ARD) activity may play an etiopathogenetic role.[16] It is uncertain, however, whether acne necessarily develops as a result of excess circulating androgens or because increased 5-ARD activity results in enhanced sensitivity of the pilosebaceous unit to normal levels of serum androgens. Increased androgen levels have been demonstrated in women with polycystic ovaries and in cases of adrenal hypersecretion, but increased target organ responsiveness may be responsible in some patients. Androgen receptors have been shown to be present in the nuclei of epidermal basal keratinocytes, the sebaceous glandular epithelium, the outer root sheath of hair follicles, and in the eccrine sweat glands. They are also present in the nuclei of fibroblasts, smooth muscle cells, and endothelium.[16] What role they may play in the development of acne vulgaris is as yet unknown.

Drugs – in particular the progestin-only contraceptives, anticonvulsants, lithium, isoniazid, corticosteroids, ciclosporine A, and anabolic steroids – may exacerbate acne.[2,17] Topical medicaments such as coal tar, hair oil (pomade acne), and mineral oil (engine oil) are also of importance (*Fig. 22.192*).[18] Cosmetics may have a similar effect (so-called acne cosmetica).[19] Cosmetics may directly promote the development of comedones but, also by virtue of chemical irritation, they can cause folliculitis with resultant pustules and papules. Hemodialysis has been associated with development of nodulocystic acne.[20]

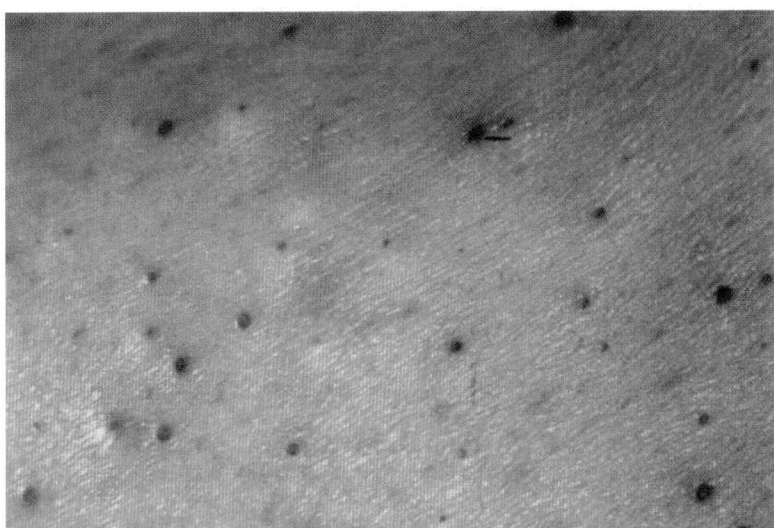

Fig. 22.192
Oil acne: these lesions follow use of hair oil or exposure to mineral oil. By courtesy of the Institute of Dermatology, London, UK.

Patients in whom the clinical history or physical examination suggests hyperandrogenism should have endocrinological testing. Acne has been associated with disorders such as Alpert syndrome, polycystic ovarian syndrome, and Cushing syndrome.[2,21]

Early comedones show a cystically dilated hair follicle with either a narrow or a wide opening associated with infundibular hyperkeratosis (*Fig. 22.193*). Later, due to rupture, an acute dermal inflammatory response develops, which may be complicated by a foreign body granulomatous reaction (*Fig. 22.194*). In severe cases, abscesses are frequently present and cysts and sinuses often form. Dense dermal scarring (sometimes with keloidal change) is an important long-term sequel.[22] Occasionally, dystrophic calcification with bone formation is a feature.[23]

Differential diagnosis

The granulomatous reaction may be difficult to distinguish from other granulomatous disorders, and the presence of fragments of hair or keratin may be helpful diagnostic pointers. Often, the clinical information as to the location of the lesions and the age of the patient is useful.

Chloracne

Clinical features

Chloracne (halogen acne) was first described by Herxheimer in 1899.[1] It is a cutaneous manifestation of systemic poisoning by dioxin (2,3,7,8-tetra chlorodibenzo-*p*-dioxin) known as TCDD.[2] It is characterized by follicular hyperkeratosis with the formation of open comedones in the absence of a significant inflammatory component. Exposure is usually due to accidental industrial release of chloracnegens (e.g., as the ICMESA plant explosion in Seveso, Italy in 1976; Yusho, Kyushu Island, Japan in 1968; and Yu-Cheng, Taiwan in 1979), contamination of material sprayed into the atmosphere (e.g., agent orange in Vietnam) or as a deliberate poisoning method.[3-9]

The characteristic cutaneous manifestations of chloracne include open comedones (blackheads), milia, and epidermoid inclusion cysts.[3,4] Lesions are predominantly found on the malar crescent, the crow's foot region, the postauricular region, the penis, scrotum, and axillae (*Fig. 22.195*). Nasal involvement is characteristically absent.[10] In severe cases, lesions may be more widespread (shoulders, chest, and back) and inflammatory features may be evident. The meibomian glands are typically affected (ophthalmic chloracne).[11] Other cutaneous manifestations have included solar elastosis, severe xerosis, facial gray pigmentation, conjunctivitis, follicular hyperkeratosis, and erythema confined to exposed areas.[10,12,8] Palmoplantar hyperhidrosis has also been described.[10]

Systemic involvement may present as hepatotoxicity, peripheral neuropathy, central nervous system manifestations (headache, fatigue, irritability, insomnia and impotence), chronic obstructive pulmonary disease, hypertriglyceridemia, diabetes, hypertension, cardiovascular disease, and, rarely, hepatic porphyria (porphyria cutanea tarda).[10,6,13] There is a significant risk of carcinogenesis related to lymphatic/hematopoietic tissue neoplasms, breast cancer, and soft tissue sarcomas.[14-17] A form of chloracne has been associated with smoking which permanently activates the AhR signaling pathway in the skin.[18,19] It has equally been reported associated to the use of sorafenib.[20,21]

Pathogenesis and histologic features

Dioxin accumulates in the sebum leading to dysregulation of sebaceous gland homeostasis, and to apoptosis of sebocytes.[2]

The primary histopathological lesion in chloracne is noninflammatory and comprises follicular infundibular dilatation and plugging (hyperkeratosis) with comedone formation in association with stimulation of the outer root sheath and sebaceous duct epithelium. Inflammatory changes are minimal. Squamous metaplasia of the sebaceous glands results in milia formation and eventual epidermoid cysts with disappearance of sebaceous glands.[22]

The final diagnosis of chloracne should always be confirmed in serum and tissues by direct chemical analysis or a biological assay.[3,23]

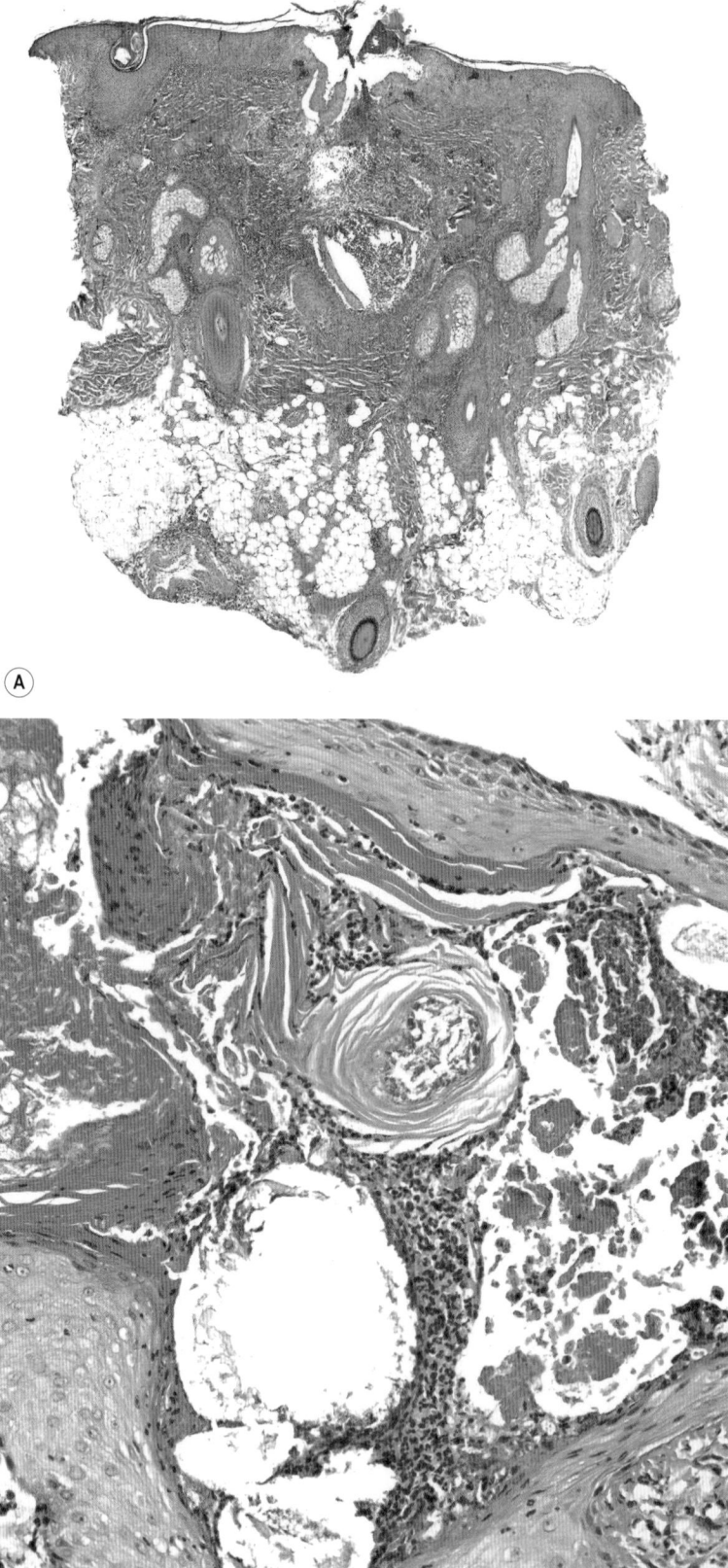

Fig. 22.193
(**A**, **B**) Acne vulgaris: rupture of a comedone releases keratin into the dermis with a resultant intense inflammatory reaction.

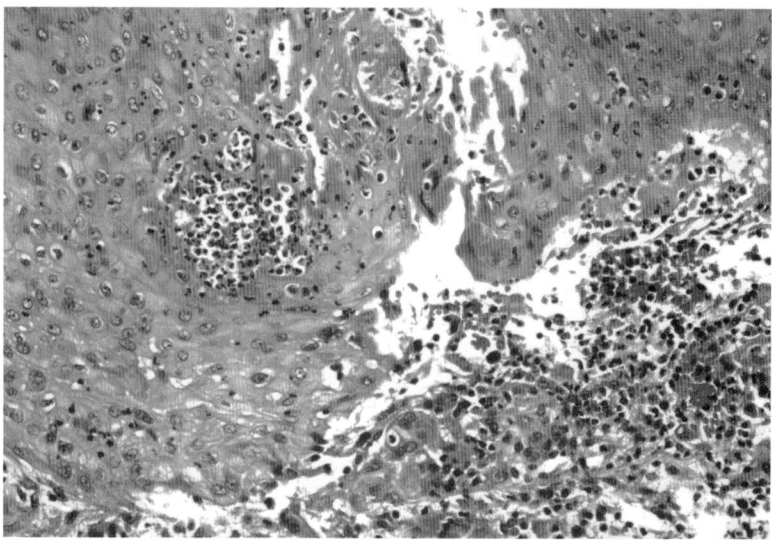

Fig. 22.194
Acne vulgaris: intense foreign body granulomatous reaction is present.

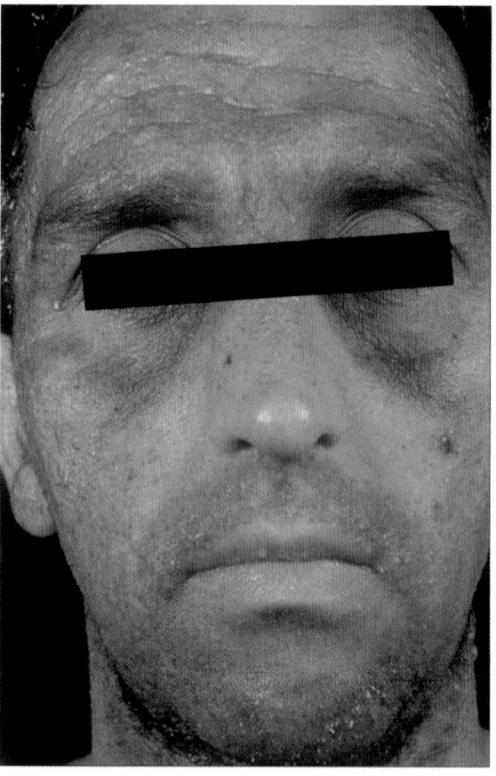

Fig. 22.195
Chloracne: there is a diffuse grayish discoloration. Comedones, milia, and cysts are present. By courtesy of the Institute of Dermatology, London, UK.

Acne fulminans

Clinical features

Acne fulminans was originally described in 1959 as acne conglobata with septicemia by Burns and Colville.[1] It is an exceedingly rare systemic disease which is generally restricted to young teenage males. Very occasionally, however, females are affected.[2] Patients – who usually have a background of acne vulgaris – present with a sudden onset of multiple tender inflammatory nodules and plaques on the face, neck, upper chest, and back. These are soon replaced by extensive areas of liquefying necrosis which ulcerate and slowly heal with severe scarring (*Fig. 22.196*).[3] The condition is generally self-remitting.

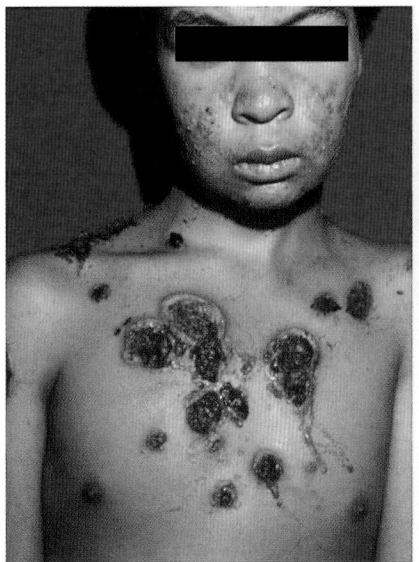
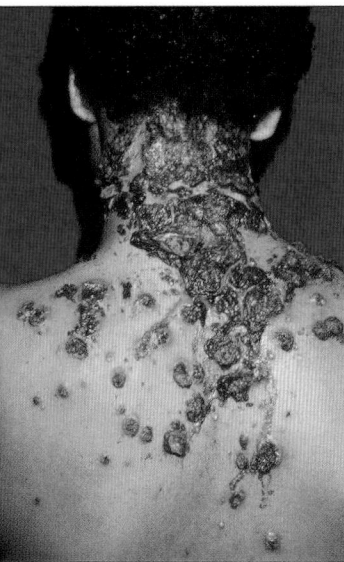

Fig. 22.196
Acne fulminans: note comedones joining together with associated ulceration and crusting. By courtesy of Department of Dermatology, Universidad de Antioquia, Medellín, Colombia.

Systemic manifestations may include arthralgia, myalgia, and hepatosplenomegaly. In addition, there is fever, malaise, anemia, headaches, weight loss, leukocytosis (sometimes with a leukemoid reaction), raised C-reactive protein, increased liver enzymes, and a raised erythrocyte sedimentation rate, although there is a subset of patients without systemic involvement.[4-6] Joint swelling (particularly affecting the iliosacral, iliac, and knee joints) and osteolytic bone lesions predominantly involving the sternum and clavicle may also be present.[3,5,7-9] Erythema nodosum is sometimes a feature.[4,10] Acne fulminans has been associated with Marfan syndrome, hemophagocytosis, late-onset congenital adrenal hyperplasia, and following measles infection.[11-14] Exceptionally, posterior scleritis and a pyoderma gangrenosum-like eruption have been associated.[15] Acne fulminans can also be the dermatological manifestation of the synovitis-acne-pustulosis-hyperostosis-osteitis (SAPHO) syndrome.[16,17]

Pathogenesis and histologic features

Acne fulminans is of unknown etiology. The restriction to males suggests a hormonal influence. The condition has been reported in monozygotic twins, and occasionally in siblings with identical HLA phenotypes.[3,7,18] Factors which may be of importance include infections, abnormal immune responses to *P. acnes*, immune complex deposition, adverse drug reactions, and after treatment with isotretinoin.[3,19-22] Bacterial cultures, however, are negative.[3,8] An association with Crohn disease has been documented.[23]

Histologically, follicular and sebaceous gland destruction with abscess formation is followed by epidermal necrosis and ulceration. Thrombosed hyalinized vessels are seen deep to the ulcer, and hemorrhage is present.[3] The surrounding dermis is infiltrated by neutrophils, eosinophils, histiocytes, plasma cells, and giant cells. Lymphocytic vasculitis has been described in early lesions.[15] The late stages are characterized by dermal scarring.

Linear IgM and fibrin deposition at the basement membrane region accompanied by fibrin around the sebaceous gland has occasionally been described.[3]

Bone lesions are characterized by abscess formation with granulation tissue.[24]

Acne aestivalis

Clinical features

Acne aestivalis (Mallorcan acne, actinic folliculitis) is a UVA-related dermatosis in which patients develop papules or pustules on the cheeks, sides of neck, shoulders, and upper arms.[1,2]

Table 22.6
Subtypes and variants of rosacea and their characteristics*

Characteristics	
Subtype	
Erythematotelangiectatic	Flushing and persistent central facial erythema with or without telangiectasia.
Papulopustular	Persistent central facial erythema with transient, central facial papules or pustules or both.
Phymatous	Thickening skin, irregular surface nodularities and enlargement. May occur on the nose, chin, forehead, cheeks, or ears.
Ocular	Foreign body sensation in the eye, burning or stinging, dryness, Itching, ocular photosensitivity, blurred vision, telangiectasia of the sclera or other parts of the eye, or periorbital edema.
Variant	
Granulomatous	Noninflammatory; hard; brown, yellow, or red cutaneous papules; or nodules of uniform size.

*Wilkin, J., Dahl, M., Detmar, M. et al (2002) Standard classification of rosacea: Report of the National Rosacea Society Expert Committee on the Classification and Staging of Rosacea. *J Am Acad Dermatol*, **46**, 584–587.

Table 22.7
Severity grading of rosacea papules and pustules*

Severity	Papules/pustules	Plaques
Mild	Few	None
Moderate	Several	None
Severe	Many	Present

*Wilkin, J, Dahl., M, Detmar, M. et al (2004) National Rosacea Society Expert Committee. Standard grading system for rosacea: report of the National Rosacea Society Expert Committee on the Classification and Staging of Rosacea. *J Am Acad Dermatol*, **50**, 907–912.

Recurrences are common. The term was initially applied to Scandinavians vacationing in Mallorca.[3]

Histologic features

The histologic features are those of a neutrophil-rich folliculitis, followed by necrosis of the follicular epithelium. Abscess formation and comedones are later secondary lesions.[1,4]

Acne aestivalis should be differentiated from acne vulgaris aggravated by sunlight. With adequate clinical information, it is easy to reach a correct diagnosis.[5]

Rosacea

Clinical features

Rosacea is a cutaneous reaction that presents with 'flushing', a transient redness of the convexities of the central face, which may extend to other parts of the body, usually the trunk and epigastrium.[1-3] The National Rosacea Society's Expert Committee on the Classification and Staging of Rosacea identified four subtypes of rosacea and three severity grading systems. This committee does not accept that stages of the disease evolve from one stage to another and recognize only one variant (granulomatous rosacea) (*Tables 22.6* and *22.7*).[4-7]

Rosacea most often presents in the fourth to sixth decades but may be seen in the late teens or early twenties. Exceptionally, children are affected.[8] The condition is characterized by episodes of remission and recurrence. It is a common disease, accounting for 0.5–1.0% of all cases seen in a

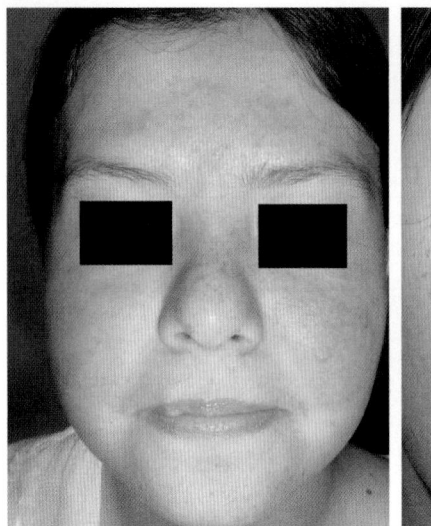
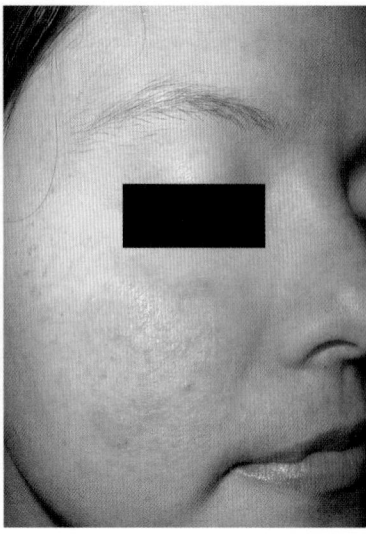

Fig. 22.197
Rosacea erythematotelangiectatic subtype: there is diffuse erythema of the face with malar telangiectasia. By courtesy of L.M. Gómez, MD, UPB, Medellín, Colombia.

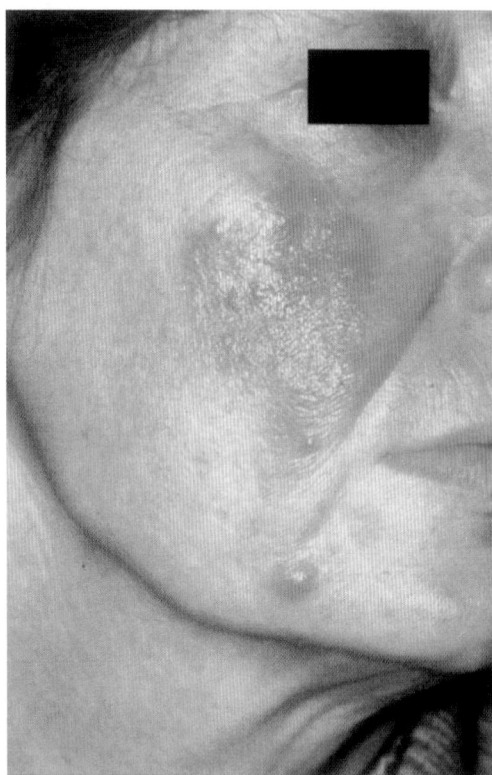

Fig. 22.198
Rosacea papulopustular subtype: note the papules and pustules on the cheek. By courtesy of the Institute of Dermatology, London, UK.

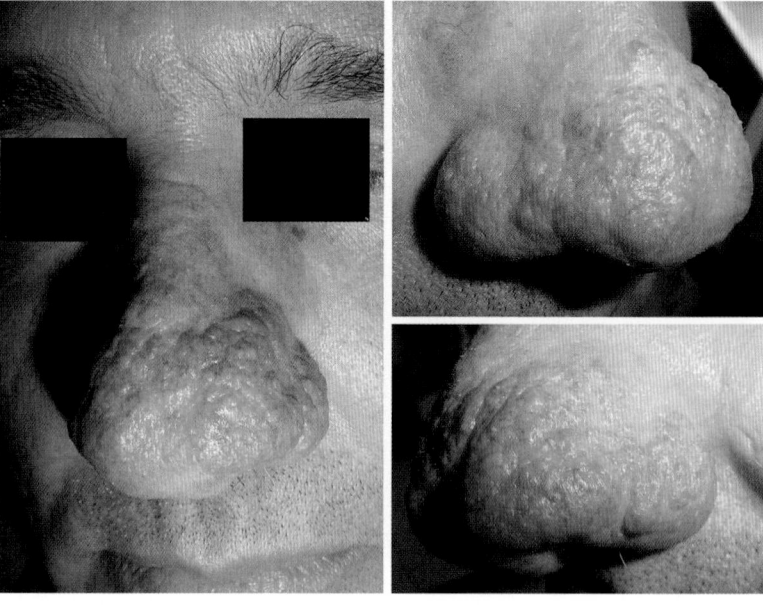

Fig. 22.199
Rosacea phymatous subtype: this is the typical appearance of rhinophyma. Note the irregular surface nodularities and enlargement of the nose. Courtesy of L.M. Gómez, MD, Universidad Pontificia Bolivariana, Medellín, Colombia.

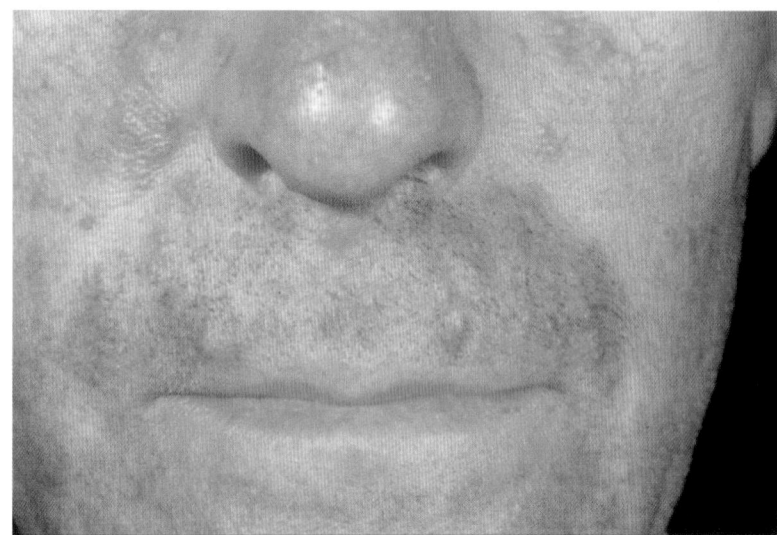

Fig. 22.200
Granulomatous rosacea variant: note the papules which have arisen against a background of rosacea. By courtesy of the Institute of Dermatology, London, UK.

dermatology outpatient department. There is a predilection for females (2–3:1), and those with fair skin and a Northern European ancestry are most often affected.[9]

In the erythematotelangiectatic subtype of rosacea, the erythema may last from hours to days.[1] Pruritus is not a feature. Telangiectasia can be coarse or fine. It develops on the cheeks, nasolabial folds, and nose (*Fig. 22.197*).[5]

In the papulopustular subtype, crops of papules and (less commonly) pustules are present over the forehead, malar areas, nose, and chin (*Fig. 22. 198*). The papules are not tender and are not associated with scarring[5]

Vascular changes tend to be more common in women. In men, 'phymatous' change may occur on the chin (gnatophyma), forehead (metophyma), ears (otophyma), eyelids, malar areas, and the nose, culminating in the formation of rhinophyma of the nose (*Fig. 22.199*).[5,10,11] This disfiguring enlargement of the nose is the most common phyma. It is caused by both persistent lymphedema and hypertrophy of the sebaceous glands and surrounding connective tissue. The follicles appear prominent and are often plugged with grumous material.

The eye is frequently involved in rosacea, particularly in children.[8] Patients complain most often of a foreign body sensation or burning; clinically, superficial punctate erosions or blepharitis (often with meibomianitis) may be present.[12] Chalazia and sties are commonly found. Less frequently, corneal ulceration, scarring, thinning, and vascularization occur. Rosacea keratitis comprises a triangular tongue-like vascularization of the margin of the cornea.[5]

Rarely, extrafacial rosacea occurs in a papular or vascular form involving the buttocks, limbs, and/or the presternal area (disseminated rosacea).[7,13]

The granulomatous rosacea variant is characterized by periorificial cutaneous papules or nodules that can lead to scarring (*Fig. 22.200*). Patients often do not have persistent facial erythema or other signs of rosacea.[5,7]

Pathogenesis and histologic features

The pathogenesis of rosacea is largely unknown, and current research is particularly directed toward the role of cytokines and other inflammatory mediators.[14] Many studies have shown that patients with rosacea experience much stronger and more frequent 'flushing reactions' when provoked by psychological and physical agents than a control population. It has recently been suggested that this may be due to an underlying vascular disorder. Lesional blood flow is three to four times the normal rate.[7] This may, however, be a consequence rather than a cause of the condition. Rosacea has also been associated with sunlight, menstruation, pregnancy, hypertension, medications, oral contraceptive pills, facial cosmetics, occupational heat, alcohol, spicy food, and lifestyle.[3,15] The mite *Demodex folliculorum* has also been implicated. *D. folliculorum* is present, particularly within the hair follicles of the nasolabial folds, nose, and eyelids.[16,17] Migraine is often an associated feature.[18] There is no evidence of an HLA predisposition. An association with upper gastrointestinal *Helicobacter pylori* infection has been proposed although the more recent literature offers little support for this hypothesis.[19,20]

Many of the histopathological findings are non-specific.[21] In the erythematotelangiectatic subtype of rosacea, there is a non-specific lymphohistiocytic inflammatory infiltrate in the dermis, often in a perivascular and perifollicular distribution with associated edema and telangiectasia (*Fig. 22.201*).

Examination of papules or pustules in the papulopustular subtype reveals neutrophils aggregated in the follicle, with a surrounding non-specific chronic inflammatory cell infiltrate. Some papules show evidence of granulomatous inflammation (granulomatous rosacea) associated with damaged follicles, and the mite *D. folliculorum* may be identified (*Figs 22.202 and 22.203*). Solar elastosis is often a feature, but this may be coincidental.

In rhinophyma, the sebaceous glands are increased in size and number. The follicular infundibula may be dilated and filled with keratinous debris. The upper dermis contains a chronic inflammatory cell infiltrate and there is dilatation of the capillaries. Increased dermal connective tissue is sometimes present, and in the later stages this may predominate, with loss of the sebaceous glands.[22]

The histologic diagnosis of granulomatous rosacea is often extremely difficult because foreign body granulomata reacting to *D. folliculorum*, keratin, sebum, and ruptured cysts are very common on the face; the diagnosis should therefore be restricted to lesions that show clearly defined granulomata in an interfollicular distribution and in the appropriate clinical setting.[23,24]

Differential diagnosis

Rosacea is distinguished from acne vulgaris by the absence of comedones and the presence of telangiectasia and a history of flushing episodes.

A rosacea-like dermatosis characterized by erythema, papules, and pustules may follow excessive use of topical steroids and has been reported to occur with prolonged use of only 1% topical hydrocortisone (*Fig. 22.204*).[24] There are three types of steroid-induced rosacea-like dermatitis based on the location of the eruption: perioral, centrofacial, and diffuse.[25] The erythema involves the whole of the area of application and is usually associated with atrophy.

Acne agminata (lupus miliaris disseminatus faciei) is of unknown etiology although it most probably represents a granulomatous reaction to ruptured hair follicles (*Fig. 22.205*). It presents as yellow-brown papules on the central face with a predilection for the periorbital region. Diascopy may reveal apple-jelly nodules. It is not associated with flushing episodes or telangiectasia and does not represent a variant of rosacea although there is considerable histologic overlap with the granulomatous form. The lesions frequently progress to deep scars. Acne agminata can be differentiated into four histopathology groups: epithelioid cell granuloma with necrosis, epithelioid cell granuloma without necrosis, epithelioid cell granuloma with abscesses, and nongranulomatous non-specific inflammatory cell infiltrates.[26,27] Special stains to exclude fungal and mycobacterial infections are often necessary in those cases where there is marked granulomatous inflammation.

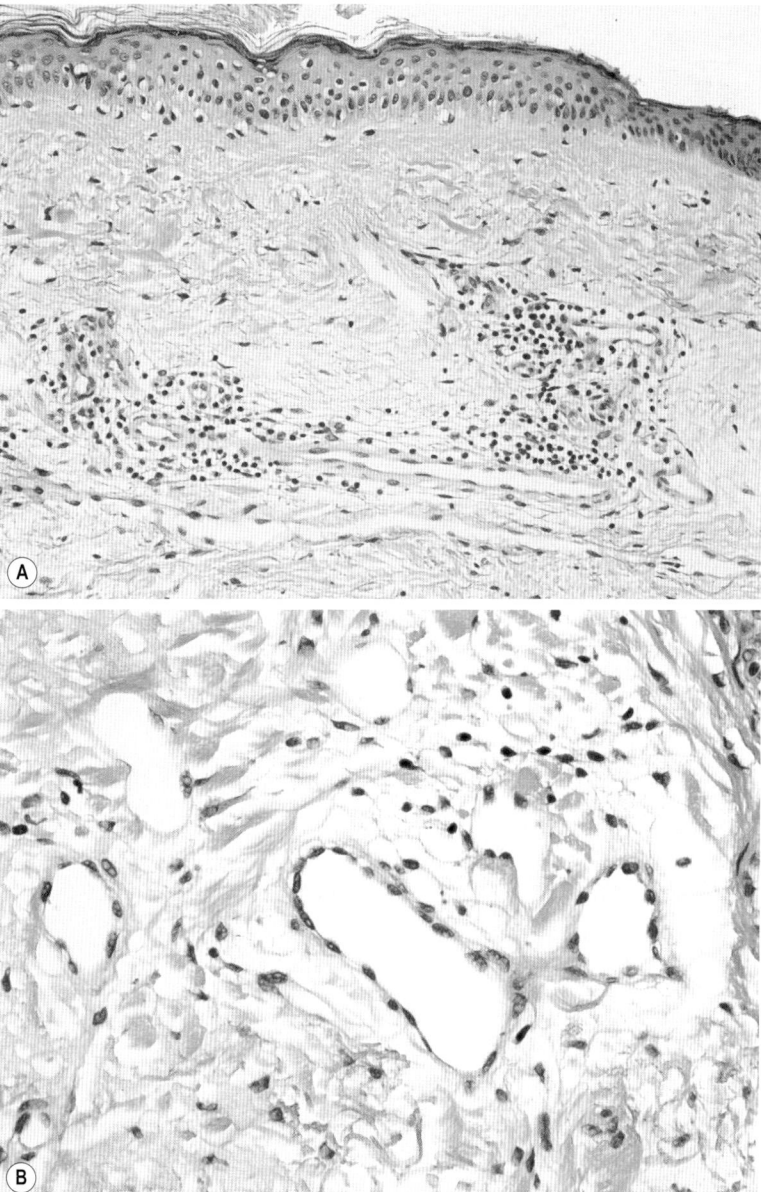

Fig. 22.201
(**A**, **B**) Rosacea erythematotelangiectatic subtype: there is edema, telangiectasia, and a mild lymphohistiocytic inflammatory cell infiltrate.

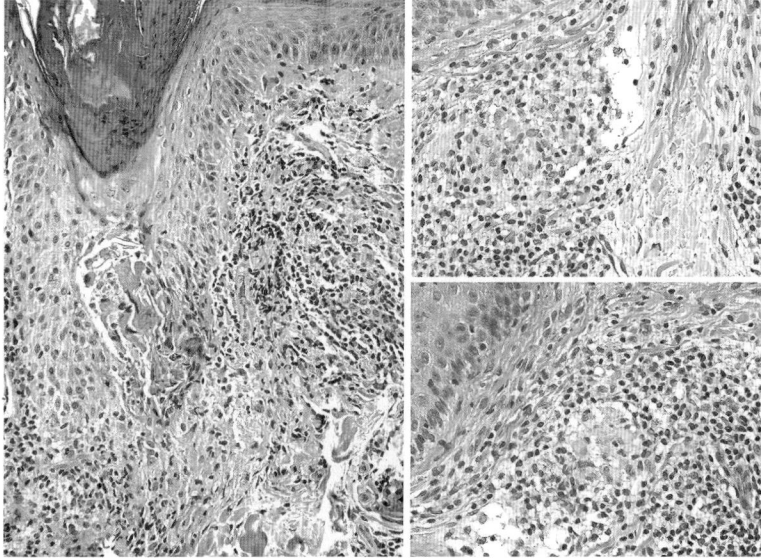

Fig. 22.202
Granulomatous rosacea: note the perifollicular noncaseating granulomata.

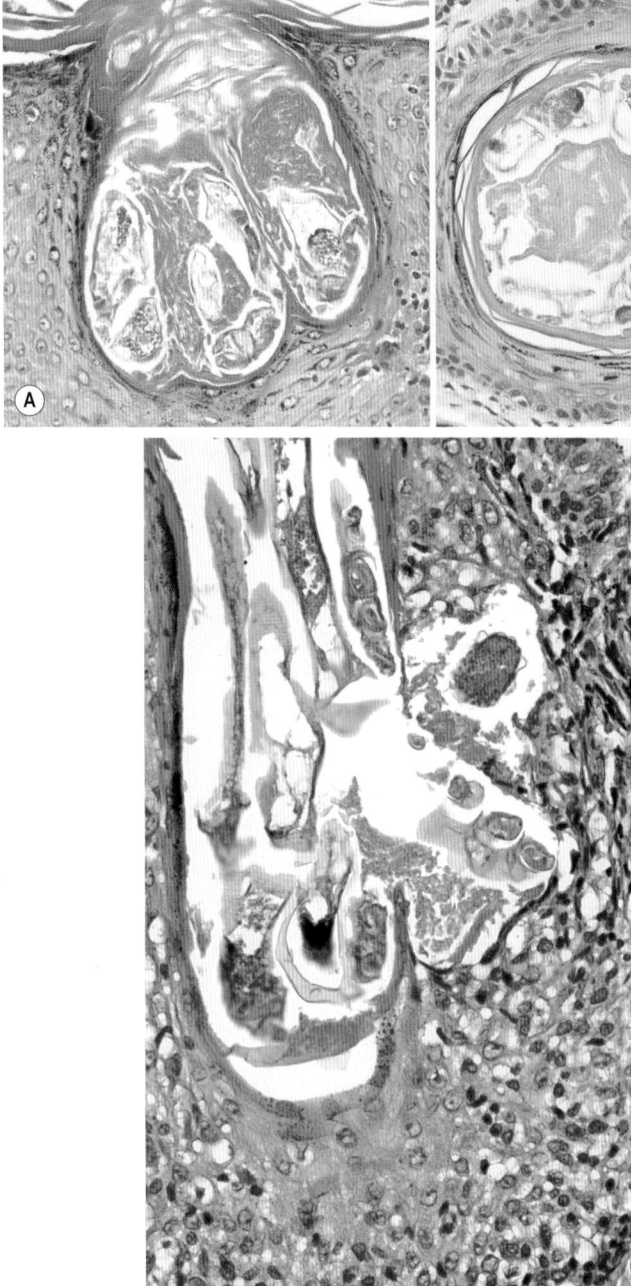

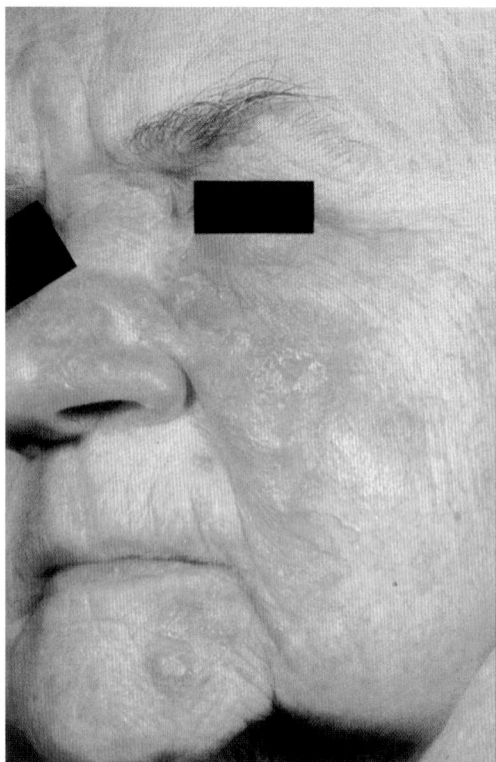

Fig. 22.204
Topical steroid-related rosacea: prolonged topical steroid therapy has resulted in erythema, telangiectasia, and atrophy. By courtesy of R.A. Marsden, MD, St George's Hospital, London, UK.

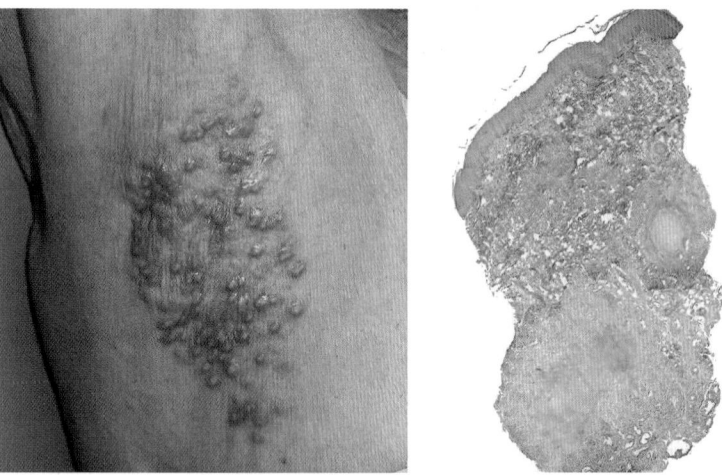

Fig. 22.205
Acne agminata: note some flesh-colored papules and nodules on the axillae (*left*), and caseating granulomatous inflammation (*right*). Courtesy of J.E. Arroyave, MD, Hospital Pablo Tobón Uribe, Medellín, Colombia.

Fig. 22.203
Rosacea: (**A**) *Demodex folliculorum* mite (class Arachnida, order Acarina) within this infundibulum in vertical and horizontal sections. (**B**) Some *D. folliculorum* mites exiting through a nearby ruptured hair follicle. Note the lymphocytic infiltrate.

Perioral dermatitis is sometimes regarded as a variant of rosacea although it differs clinically.[28,29] Patients (particularly young women and children) present with variably pruritic, erythematous microvesicles, scaling, papules, micronodules, and pustules affecting the chin, nasolabial folds, and the periocular region (*Fig. 22.206*).[5,28] Histologically, it is similar to rosacea with spongiotic changes.

Severe *D. folliculorum* infection (demodicosis) may present with rosacea-like features.[30,31] Flushing and telangiectasia are absent.

Histologically, the condition is characterized by follicular cysts with a granulomatous inflammatory reaction and numerous mites (*Fig. 22.207*).[30]

Rhinophyma may also be associated with other causes of flushing, such as carcinoid syndrome and alcohol abuse.[32]

Rosacea fulminans

Clinical features

Rosacea fulminans (pyoderma faciale) is very rare and presents with a sudden onset of papulopustules, cysts, and innumerable conglobate nodular lesions predominantly affecting the face or a single region on the face.[1–4] Sinuses

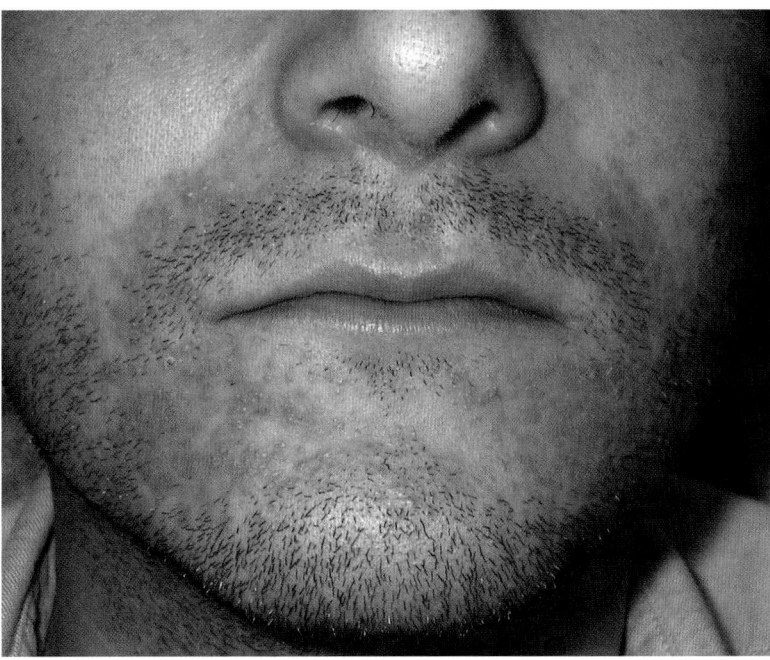

Fig. 22.206
Perioral dermatitis: grouped follicular reddish papules and papulovesicles on an eczematous and erythematous base.

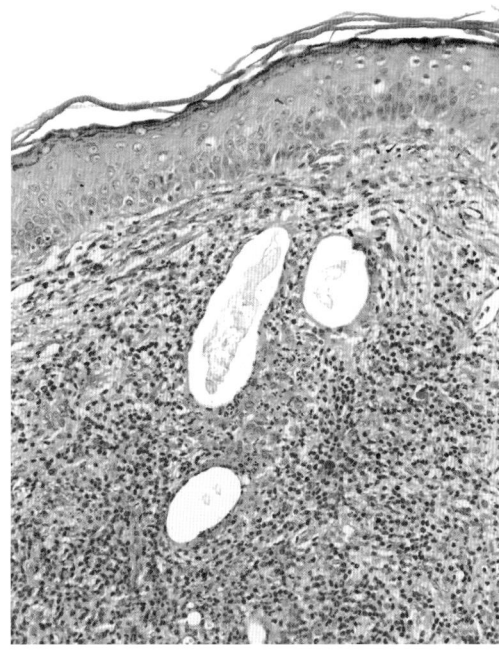

Fig. 22.207
Demodicosis: note some *Demodex folliculorum* mites free in the dermis, surrounded by an inflammatory cell infiltrate.

are also often present, and the surrounding skin appears erythematous and cyanotic. Telangiectasia is sometimes evident.[4,5] Occasionally, extrafacial involvement is encountered.[5,6] The condition is usually self-limiting. Resolution is often accompanied by scarring.[1] Although young women in their 20s and 30s are most often affected, there are rare reports of male and childhood involvement.[7,8] A history of episodes of flushing and seborrhea is common.[4] Comedones are not a feature and, in contrast to rosacea, ocular involvement does not occur.[1,4]

There are occasional reports of associated inflammatory bowel disease (ulcerative colitis more often than Crohn disease), erythema nodosum, and pegylated IFN alpha-2B and ribavirin therapy.[4,9–11]

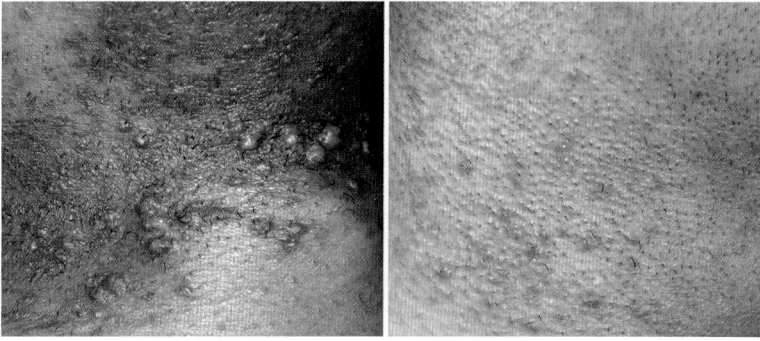

Fig. 22.208
Pseudofolliculitis: predominantly seen in patients of African or Hispanic ancestry. Numerous papules and curved hairs in the beard area.

Pathogenesis and histologic features

The pathogenesis is largely unknown although pregnancy, the contraceptive pill, and hormonal influences are likely since the condition is restricted to females.[12–14] A case associated with high-dosage vitamin B supplements has been documented.[15] Cultures are invariably negative for pathogenic bacteria.

The histologic features include dermal edema and follicular abscesses accompanied by a mixed perivascular and perifollicular inflammatory cell infiltrate including lymphocytes, histiocytes, neutrophils, and eosinophils, sometimes with an epithelioid or foreign body granulomatous component.[5,7,15–17] Lobular and septal panniculitis have also been described.[2]

Neutrophilic sebaceous adenitis

Clinical features

Neutrophilic sebaceous adenitis is a very rare condition presenting as erythematous circinate plaques with a raised edge with predilection for the face and upper chest.[1,2] Papules and pustules may be seen. There is no sex predilection, and lesions may rarely present on vulva.[3] Spontaneous regression tends to occur.

Pathogenesis and histologic features

The pathogenesis is unknown, and light and Demodex have been suggested as possibly linked with the etiology of the process but there is limited evidence to support this.[4,5]

Histologically, there is a mixed infiltrate with predominance of neutrophils and centered around the sebaceous gland is identified. Neutrophils infiltrate the sebaceous lobules and ducts, and necrosis of sebocytes may be seen.

Pseudofolliculitis

Clinical features

Pseudofolliculitis (sycosis barbae, pili incarnati, shaving bumps) is an exceedingly common condition which may affect anyone with curly hair, although black males are most often involved (45–83%).[1–3] The incidence is also high in Hispanics.[4] It develops as a consequence of growth of curved hairs and faulty shaving techniques.[1] In this disease, shaving can be a very difficult task.[5]

Patients present with firm skin-colored or erythematous inflammatory papules and nodules in the shaving areas of the face, often associated with postinflammatory hyperpigmentation (*Fig. 22.208*).[2] Pustule formation generally results from secondary bacterial infection. Hair shafts can sometimes be visible just under the skin surface. The use of epiluminescence dermoscopy can be very useful for visualization of the ingrowing hairs at the sites of individual papules.[6] The mustache region is generally spared.[1] Scalp shaving may also result in the condition.[2] Black and particularly hirsute females may also be affected, and then the axillae and pubic regions are especially involved.[4] Hair waxing and pulling with tweezers can have a similar effect.[4]

Pseudofolliculitis has been associated with ciclosporine and renal transplant recipients.[7]

Pathogenesis and histologic features

Pseudofolliculitis develops as a result of two mechanisms: curly or kinky hair in black individuals tends to curve back directly into the adjacent skin (extrafollicular penetration).[1] It continues to grow through the epidermis into the dermis where it may reach a length of 2–3 mm. As it grows longer, it tends to 'spring back' out of the skin.[8] Shaving techniques that stretch the skin can result in the cut hair end retracting under the epidermis when the skin is released (transfollicular penetration).[2]

Dry shaving worsens the condition.[2] The shaft penetrates directly through the adjacent follicular epithelium into the superficial dermis. Hair in individuals with black skin is elliptical in shape and, when cut, often has a sharp pointed end.[1] In addition, the majority of these individuals have helical or spiral hair and as the follicles are curved in the dermis with the hair shaft leaving the skin at an oblique angle, the risk of hair reentering the skin after close shaving is very high.[9]

Early lesions are characterized by a neutrophilic response, and intraepidermal abscesses are sometimes seen.[8] This is later replaced by a foreign body granulomatous reaction to hair shafts. In those lesions that have developed following a transepidermal route, the hair may be ensheathed by an epidermal downgrowth. Chronic lesions are scarred and keloid formation is not uncommon. Scar-associated noncaseating granulomata in a patient with sarcoidosis have been documented.[10]

Gram-negative folliculitis

Clinical features

This is an uncommon complication of long-term broad-spectrum antibiotic therapy for acne or rosacea.[1-6] Growth of Gram-negative organisms in the anterior nasal region has been observed to occur in 85% of patients. Up to 4% of such patients may present with suppurative folliculitis, either as papules and pustules emanating from the anterior nasal region or, less often, with acne conglobata-like nodules.[1,3,4] The former most commonly are due to *Enterobacter*, *Klebsiella*, or *Escherichia coli*, whereas the latter results from *Proteus* infection.[7]

Pathogenesis and histologic features

Long-term antibiotic therapy results in bacterial colonization of the anterior nostrils.[1-4] The presence of low serum IgM and α_1-antitrypsin levels and raised serum IgE suggests that immune abnormalities may also be of importance.[8]

Diagnosis is often difficult as bacteria may be scanty and multiple cultures are often necessary.[1,4]

Access **ExpertConsult.com** for the complete list of references

See
www.expertconsult.com
for references and
additional material

Diseases of the nails

Josette André, Ursula Sass and Anne Theunis

INTRODUCTION

Nail histopathology requires a sound knowledge of the anatomy of the nail apparatus and excellent clinical-pathological correlation.[1] The first major challenge for the nail histopathologist is to obtain interpretable biopsies, i.e., specimens that are correctly sampled by the nail surgeon, but also that are correctly handled and processed in the pathology laboratory. This requires input from the physician, who is expected to provide high-quality clinical information. A drawing showing the lesion and the type of biopsy performed is helpful. A standardized form with a nail sketch should always be sent with the clinical information.

Almost any skin disease may affect the nail apparatus. The diseases that are most often biopsied, restricted to the nail apparatus, and those that show different histologic features when they are located in the nail apparatus, will be considered in this chapter.

Anatomy and physiology of the nail apparatus

The nail plate, also abbreviated as 'nail', is a semihard keratin plate, slightly convex in the longitudinal and transverse axes. It is set in the soft tissues of the dorsal digital extremity from which it is separated by the periungual grooves (proximal, lateral, and distal). It stems from the nail matrix located in the proximal part of the nail apparatus. The nail plate and matrix are proximally covered by a skin fold called the proximal nail fold (PNF). The lunula, also known as 'half-moon', is a whitish crescent, distally convex, visible at the proximal part of some nails and more specifically those of the thumbs and the big toes. It corresponds to the distal part of the matrix. From the latter, the nail plate grows toward the distal region, sliding along the nail bed to which it adheres closely. The nail bed is the major area seen through the nail plate. The nail plate only separates from the nail bed at its distal part called the hyponychium (*Fig. 23.1*).[2]

The upper surface of the nail plate is smooth while the under surface is corrugated with parallel longitudinal grooves that interdigitate with opposing ones on the nail bed surface, enhancing adhesion of the nail plate to the nail bed.

The nail grows continuously. In 1 month, fingernails grow about 3 mm and toenails about 1 mm.

The origin of the nail plate proper remains debatable. Most studies agree and show that at least 80% of the nail plate is produced by the matrix. It should be added that the main source of nail plate production is the proximal part of the matrix. This probably explains why distal matrix surgery or nail bed surgery has a low potential for scarring as compared to proximal matrix surgery.[3] Some studies suggest that the nail bed produces 20% of the nail plate, whereas others suggest that the nail bed hardly participates in the making of the nail plate.

The nail plays an important role in everyday life. It protects the distal phalanx from trauma and provides counterpressure to the pulp, which is essential for tactile sensation involving the fingers. The nail allows scratching as a reaction to itch and can be used as a means for attack or defense. Finally, the esthetic importance of the nail should not be forgotten.[2]

Nail biopsy

The main indications for nail biopsies are inflammatory nail disorders restricted to the nails, longitudinal melanonychia, and nail tumors. Different types of biopsies can be performed (*Fig. 23.2*).[4,5]

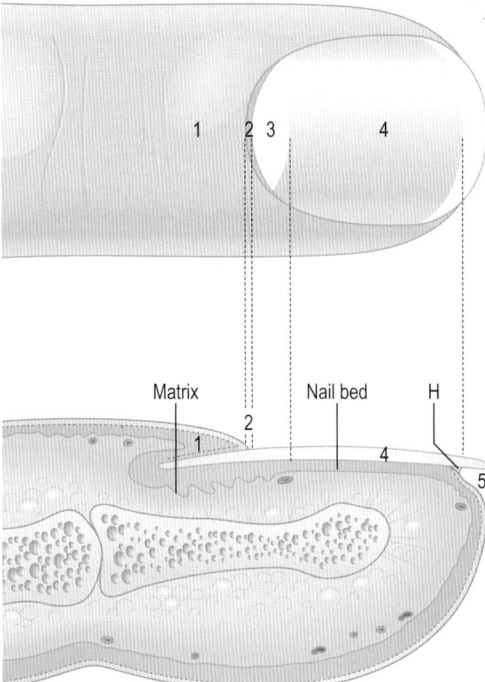

Fig. 23.1

Normal nail: proximal nail fold (*1*), cuticle (*2*), lunula (*3*), nail plate (*4*), distal nail groove (*5*), hyponychium (*H*). The small dots represent the stratum granulosum.

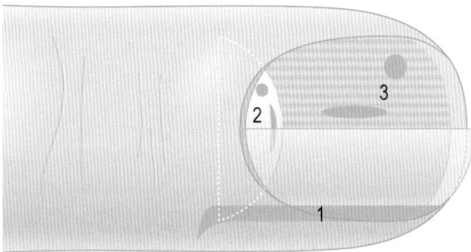

Fig. 23.2

Nail biopsies: lateral-longitudinal biopsy (*1*), punch and transverse crescentic matrix biopsies (*2*), punch and longitudinal elliptic nail bed biopsies (*3*).

- The longitudinal nail biopsy allows examination of all the nail apparatus components, but leaves a slightly narrowed nail (*Fig. 23.3*).
- Matrix biopsies should preferably be taken after partial nail plate avulsion. A 3-mm punch biopsy is the most frequently used. Transverse crescentic biopsies are also sometimes obtained. The more recently described matrix shave biopsy is mainly used for longitudinal melanonychia.[6,7]
- In the nail bed, a 3- to 4-mm punch biopsy or a longitudinal elliptic biopsy are the most frequently employed.
- Distal nail plate samples, which are easily obtained with nail clippers, can be used for the diagnosis of onychomycosis.[8]

In the laboratory, nail biopsies should be handled by dedicated technicians and read by a dermatopathologist with particular expertise in nails. It should be appreciated that nail dermatopathology is time consuming, even for experienced people.

- Inking small nail biopsies must be exacting because China ink may be responsible for pigment artifacts which can make histologic examination more difficult.
- If the nail plate is still attached, the keratin in the nail plate can be too hard for ready cutting with a microtome, so some softening method may be required.[1] Our method is to use Mollifex Gurr (VWR Int Ltd). Paraffin blocks are dipped in the Mollifex Gurr before cutting. The length of time (2–12 hours) is dependent on the thickness of the nail plate. Omura places the formalin fixed specimen in a 3 molar solution of potassium hydroxide (KOH) for 1 hour, before paraffin embedding.

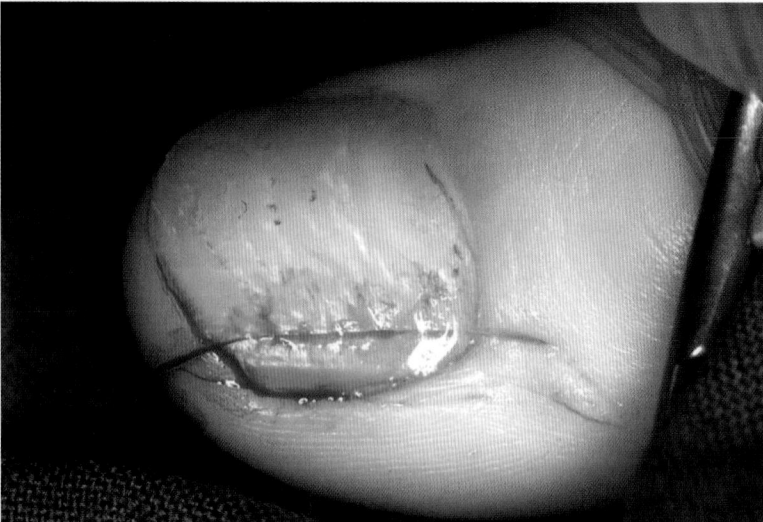

Fig. 23.3

Nail: lateral longitudinal biopsy. Courtesy of B. Richert, MD, PhD, Université Libre de Bruxelles, Belgium.

Prior to cutting, the blocks are placed in KOH for 30 minutes and in a solution of detergent and ammonia for 20 minutes.[1] Five percent trichloroacetic acid in 10% formalin, 5% trichloroacetic acid with a modification of the water-soluble Carbowax embedding method, 'chitin softening solution', and softening in cedar oil have also been suggested.[1]

- The sample needs to be correctly oriented. We usually try to perform sections parallel to the longitudinal axis of the nail. Lateral longitudinal biopsies are cut, starting from the central part of the nail and progressing toward the skin side. Three- to four-millimeter punch biopsies are embedded as such (without having been previously cut in two). A few sections are first made. If they are correctly oriented, other sections are performed. For nail biopsies, multiple sections are systematically performed.
- Special stainings and immunohistochemistry are often necessary.

Histology of the normal nail

Nail folds

The lateral nail folds are comparable to normal skin. Hyperkeratosis related to chronic trauma may be observed.

The PNF has a dorsal surface, which is in continuity with, and similar to, the epidermis of the digit. The ventral surface of the PNF is a flat and rather thin squamous epithelium that keratinizes with a stratum granulosum and a stratum corneum. At the angle between its dorsal and ventral parts, the PNF produces a thick stratum corneum called the cuticle. The latter acts as a seal between the nail plate and the PNF, thus protecting the ungual cul-de-sac (*Figs 23.4* and *23.5*).

Nail matrix and nail bed

Both structures are located under the nail plate and are typically devoid of a stratum granulosum. The boundary between the nail matrix and nail bed is barely visible on histologic examination (*Fig. 23.6*).

- The nail matrix is a multilayered epithelium with three different compartments: basaloid, prekeratogenous, and keratogenous (*Fig. 23.7*). The latter is characterized by an eosinophilic onychogenous band, devoid of keratohyaline granules (*Fig. 23.8*). It gives rise to the nail plate: the proximal part of the matrix contributes to its dorsal aspect and the distal part of the matrix gives rise to its ventral aspect. The nail matrix epithelium is the sole site of hard keratin synthesis.[3,9] In the midline of the nail unit, the matrix epithelium is thick with long, oblique rete ridges, distally oriented. Laterally, the matrix rete ridges are less marked. Distally, near the nail bed, the matrix epithelium is thinner and its onychogenous band markedly reduced.

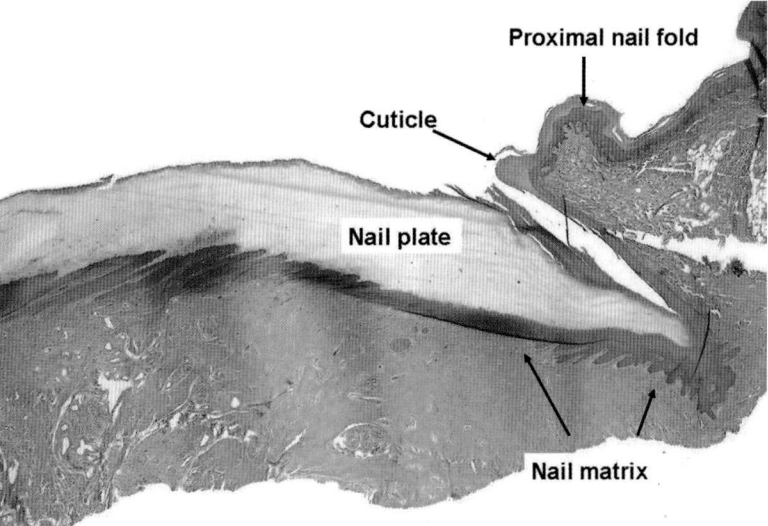

Proximal nail fold

Cuticle

Nail plate

Nail matrix

Fig. 23.4
Normal nail: scanning view of the proximal part of the nail apparatus.

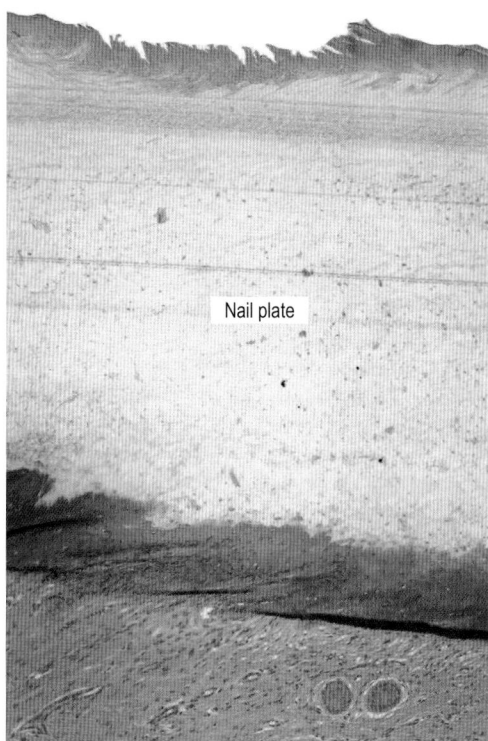

Nail plate

Fig. 23.6
Normal nail, around the junction between the nail matrix and nail bed: medium-power view of nail plate and underlying epithelium.

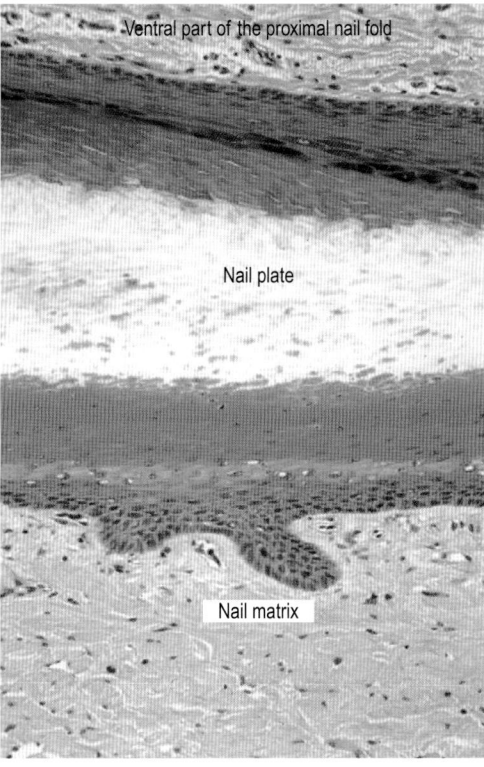

Ventral part of the proximal nail fold

Nail plate

Nail matrix

Fig. 23.5
Normal nail: high-power view of the ventral part of the proximal nail fold and the nail plate with underlying matrix.

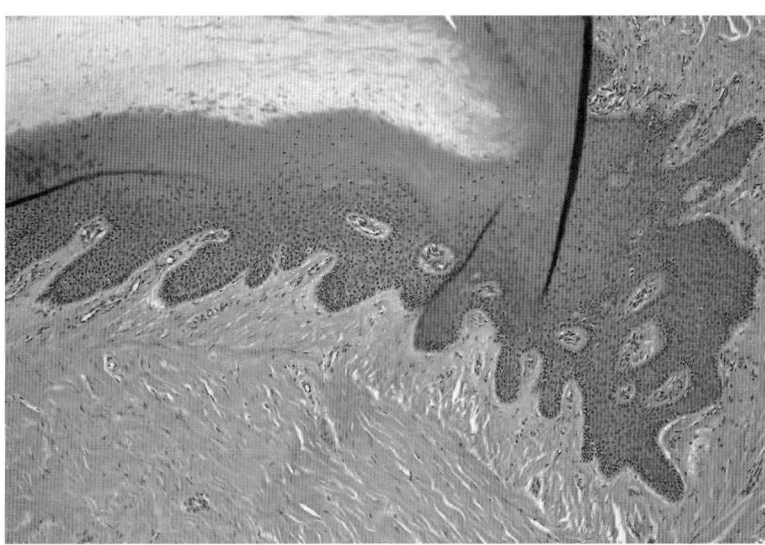

Fig. 23.7
Normal nail: low-power view showing the proximal nail matrix.

- Over the bulk of its area, the nail bed epithelium is thin, reduced to a few cellular layers. In longitudinal sections, it appears flat while in transverse sections, pronounced rete ridges are observed, parallel to the longitudinal axis of the nail. The keratinization is abrupt with no granular cell layer. The nail isthmus designates a transitional zone between the most distal part of the nail bed and the hyponychium, preventing onycholysis.[3,10] The stratum granulosum reappears only at the hyponychium, which represents the distal thickened part of the nail bed and is bordered by the distal groove and the digital pulp (*Fig. 23.9*).
- The basement membrane of the nail apparatus is almost identical to that of the skin.[11]
- The nail matrix and nail bed dermis do not contain pilosebaceous appendages. In the matrix, the dermis comprises two parts: a thin papillary dermis and a relatively thick reticular dermis. The nail bed comprises a single, relatively homogeneous compartment.[12] Eccrine sweat glands are usually absent. However, sweat ducts have been observed by in vivo microscopic examination, near the distal end of the nail bed.[13] Glomus bodies, which are specialized arteriovenous anastomoses involved in temperature regulation, can also be observed in the dermis.
- No genuine hypodermis is present in the nail, but a cushion-like layer of adipocytes can be observed in the matrix.[12]

Nail plate

The nail plate is made up of parallel layers of keratinized, flat, and completely differentiated cells called onychocytes. The latter are firmly adherent and not desquamated, in contrast to corneocytes. Remnants of nuclei are frequently observed in the proximal, ventral part of the nail plate.

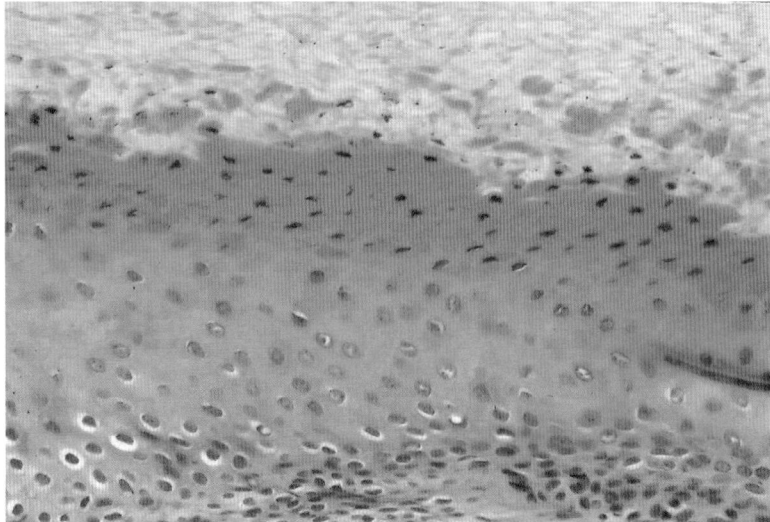

Fig. 23.8
Normal nail: high-power view of the matrix showing the onychogenous band.

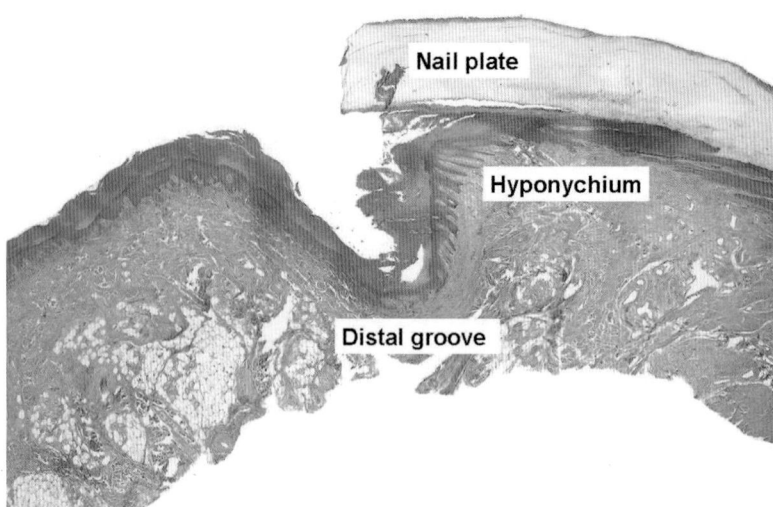

Fig. 23.9
Normal nail: scanning view of the distal part of the nail apparatus.

Microscopic examination of the distal part of the nail, which can easily be sampled with nail clippers, is useful in clinical practice for the diagnosis of onychomycosis. In transverse sections, three zones (characterized by different staining affinities) can be identified at the distal part of the nail: the upper (or dorsal) nail plate, which makes up approximately one-third of the nail; the lower (or ventral) nail plate, which makes up two-thirds of the nail; and the subungual keratin.[14]

INFECTIOUS DISEASES OF THE NAIL

Onychomycosis

Epidemiology and clinical features

Onychomycosis is the most frequent cause of nail abnormality representing 18% to 50% of nail diseases.[1,2] In the United Kingdom, North America, and Australia, nail mycoses affect 2% to 3% of the general population and up to 15% of older people.[3] Six types of onychomycosis are now recognized: distal and lateral subungual onychomycosis (DLSO) (Fig. 23.10), superficial onychomycosis (SO), proximal subungual onychomycosis (PSO), endonyx onychomycosis (EO), total dystrophic onychomycosis (TDO), and mixed pattern onychomycosis (MPO).[4] DLSO is the most common form with invasion of fungal hyphae that begins at the hyponychium and spreads along the nail bed proximally, resulting in discoloration, thickening of the nail,

subungual hyperkeratosis, and onycholysis.[5] SO develops as an invasion of the dorsal surface of the nail plate, appearing as a white or, more rarely, black powdery and patchy discoloration. PSO is characterized by fungal invasion of the PNF followed by a deeper infection of the nail plate. It may be associated with paronychia. EO is characterized by direct invasion of distal nail plate and absence of nail bed invasion, resulting in a characteristic pattern with lamellar splitting and discoloration of the nail plate. In TDO, there is complete dystrophy of the nail plate. It can be secondary, resulting from complete progression of any of the different types previously mentioned, or primary, affecting immunocompromised patients, especially those suffering from chronic mucocutaneous candidiasis. MPO associates different types of onychomycosis, more frequently PSO and SO or DLSO and SO.

Pathogenesis and histologic features

Onychomycoses may be caused by three groups of pathogens[3]:
- dermatophytes,
- yeasts,
- nondermatophyte molds.

Dermatophytes are by far the most commonly encountered, responsible for up to 80% of cases of onychomycosis in Central Europe.[6] Trichophyton rubrum is isolated in 60% to 70% of cases followed by Trichophyton mentagrophytes var. interdigitale.[7] Yeasts will grow in about 5% to 17% of cases,[8] and in 7 out of 10 cases the responsible agent is Candida albicans in the fingernails and Candida parapsilosis in the toenails. Pathogenic molds (Scytalydium, Aspergillus, Fusarium, Acremonium, and Onychocola canadensis) are found in fewer than 5% of cases.[9] The clinical classification of onychomycosis and their most frequent causative organisms are shown in Table 23.1.[10]

Onychomycosis is usually diagnosed by direct examination and culture. Histologic examination of a nail sample stained with periodic acid-Schiff (PAS) is a useful complementary technique, especially when there is strong clinical suspicion, but negative results have resulted from fungal culture and KOH preparation.[11,12] It enables one to:
- confirm the diagnosis of onychomycosis,
- specify the extent of nail plate invasion (subungual, superficial or total onychomycosis),
- suggest the nature of the infecting agent (dermatophyte, yeast, mold),

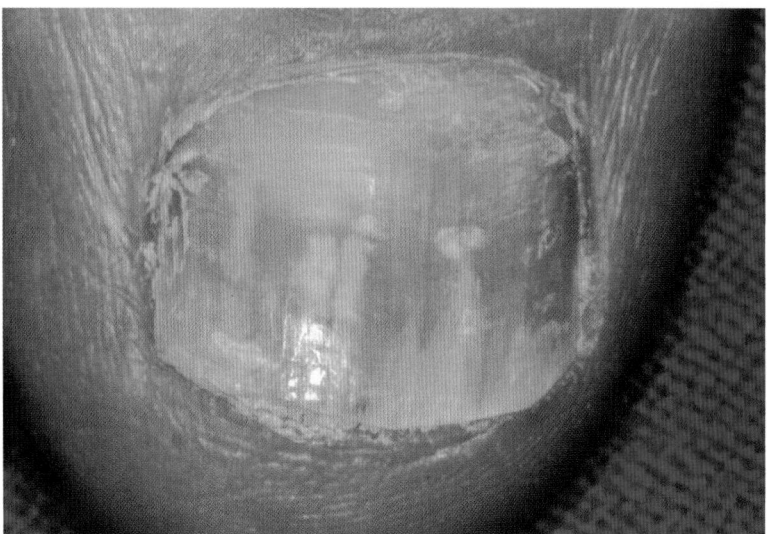

Fig. 23.10
Onychomycosis: this is an example of distal lateral subungual involvement.

Table 23.1

Clinical classification of onychomycosis and their most frequent causative organisms

Clinical type of onychomycosis	Main causative organisms[10]
Distal and lateral subungual onychomycosis	*Trichophyton rubrum* Less frequently: *Trichophyton mentagrophytes* var. *interdigitale* Rarely: *Epidermophyton floccosum*
Superficial white onychomycosis	*Trichophyton mentagrophytes* var. *interdigitale* Rarely: *Trichophyton rubrum* *Aspergillus terreus, Fusarium oxysporum, Acremonium* spp. in tropical and subtropical environments *Candida albicans* in children
Proximal subungual onychomycosis	*Trichophyton rubrum* Exceptionally: *Trichophyton megninii, Trichophyton schoenleinii, Epidermophyton floccosum*
Proximal subungual onychomycosis with paronychia	*Candida* spp. *Fusarium, Scopulariopsis brevicaulis, Aspergillus niger*
Endonyx onychomycosis	*Trichophyton soudanense* *Trichophyton violaceum*

- store the histopathological slides for possible re-evaluation.[3]
- In the absence of onychomycosis, histologic examination of a nail plate sampling may disclose an alternative diagnosis especially psoriasis.

More and more studies indicate that staining with PAS is the most sensitive method for diagnosing onychomycosis.[13–16] Others, however, consider that it is no more valuable than direct examination.[3] This is probably dependent on the sampling technique used.[17] In rare cases, histologic examination is the only investigation which confirms the clinical diagnosis of onychomycosis.[3]

In subungual onychomycosis, the fungi are located in the subungual keratin from where they involve the ventral nail plate. In SO, they are usually restricted to the superficial part of the nail plate. However, they can also invade deeper.[18,19] In total onychomycosis, the hyphae invade the entire nail plate and subungual keratin. Histologic examination does not allow precise identification of the infecting agent. This requires fungal culture or polymerase chain reaction (PCR). However, regular, straight, septate hyphae that tend to run parallel to the nail surface speak in favor of a dermatophytic infection while small round, yeast forms, some of them budding, pseudohyphae, and/or short filaments are observed in yeast onychomycosis (*Fig. 23.11*). Spores without pseudohyphae can be contaminants and do not allow a diagnosis of onychomycosis. Truncated spores and irregular hyphae from which arise thin perforating filaments represent a mold infection (*Fig. 23.12*).

Longitudinal nail biopsies are usually not performed in onychomycosis, except when another diagnosis such as psoriasis or lichen planus is clinically suspected. The histology is often psoriasiform with hyperplasia of the nail bed epithelium and exocytosis of neutrophils. Spongiosis is frequently present. The subungual keratin and nail plate may be thickened or thinned. They contain parakeratotic foci with neutrophil mounds.[20] PAS staining allows the correct diagnosis to be made (*Figs 23.13–23.15*).

Periungual warts and other nail infections

Numerous infections can affect the nail apparatus, particularly the periungual folds. Lesions are generally only biopsied when:

- the clinical appearances are atypical (e.g., an extensive herpetic whitlow in a human immunodeficiency virus [HIV]-positive patient, or a paronychia-like cutaneous leishmaniasis),[1]
- if excision constitutes a treatment modality (e.g., excision of subungual tungiasis (*Figs 23.16* and *23.17*),
- to exclude a malignant tumor.

The histologic appearances of these infections are similar to those observed in the skin.

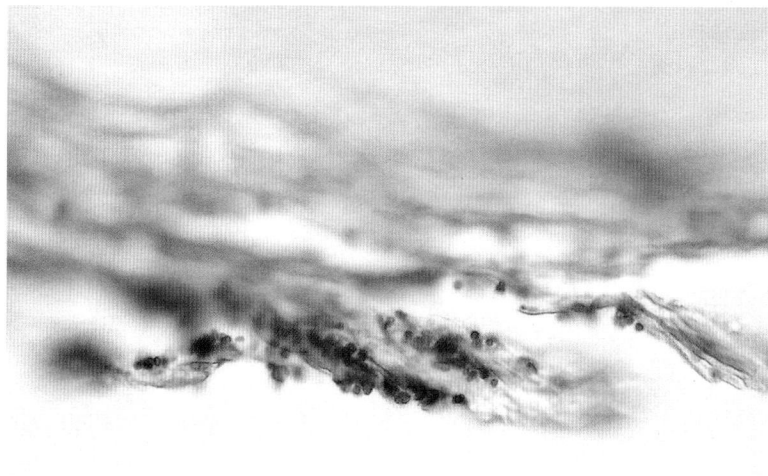

Fig. 23.11
Onychomycosis: this example is caused by uniform yeasts (periodic acid-Schiff).

Fig. 23.12
Onychomycosis: an example of mold infection. Note the vertically orientated thin perforating hyphae invading the nail plate.

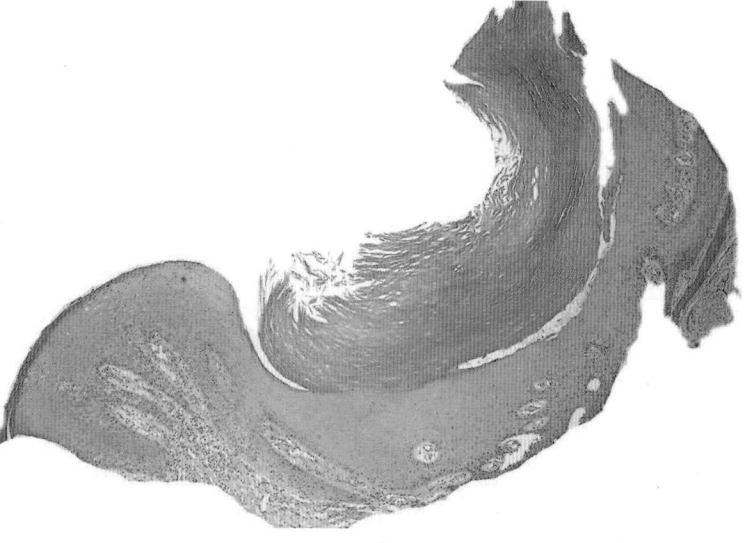

Fig. 23.13
Onychomycosis: this example caused by a dermatophyte infection has resulted in a psoriasiform appearance. Scanning view.

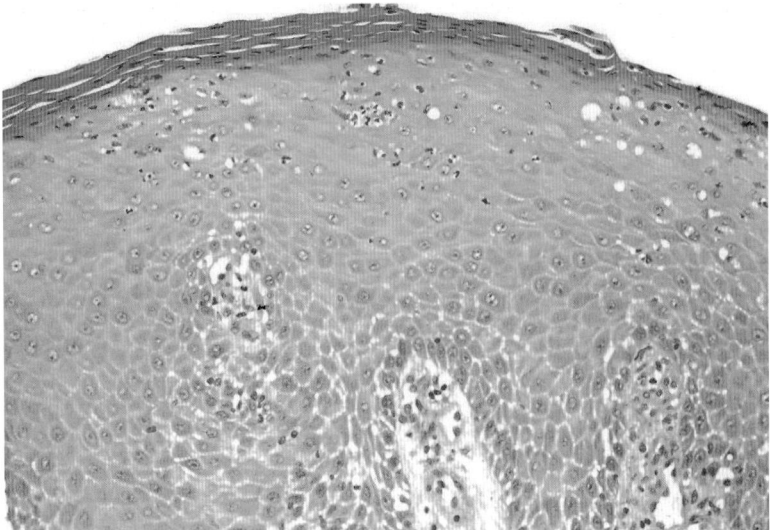

Fig. 23.14
Onychomycosis: note the parakeratosis and neutrophil microabscesses.

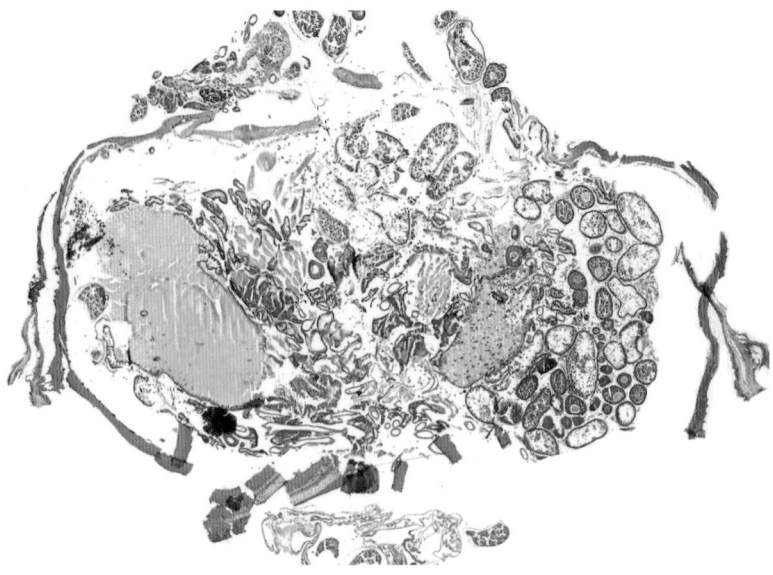

Fig. 23.17
Tungiasis: scanning view showing fragmented tegument and numerous eggs on the right side.

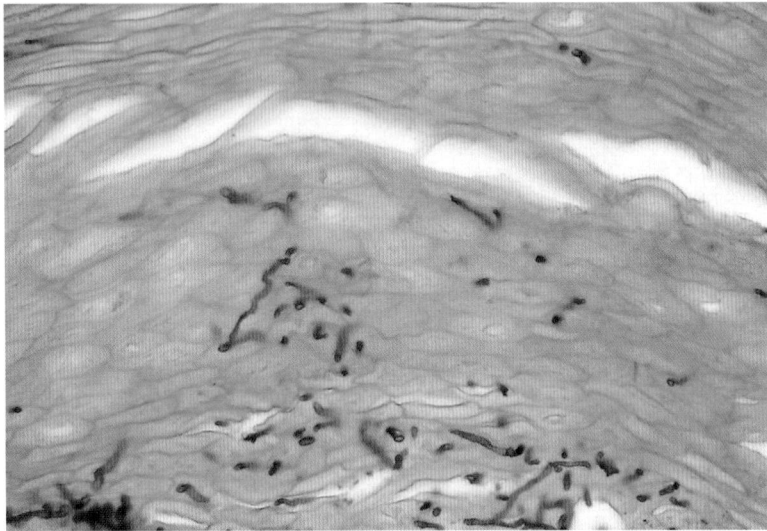

Fig. 23.15
Onychomycosis: numerous hyphae are present (periodic acid-Schiff).

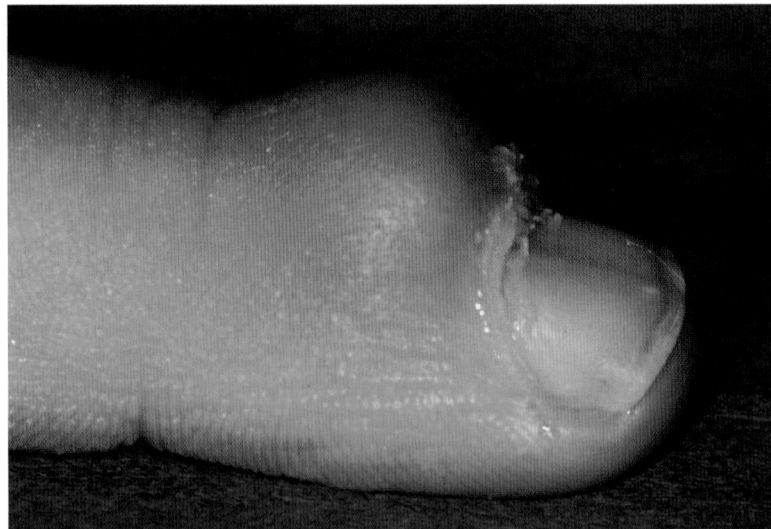

Fig. 23.18
Viral wart: note the white papillary processes just protruding at the proximal nail fold.

Clinical features[2]

Periungual warts are frequently seen in children and young adults. They are mainly located around the nail, leaving the nail plate generally unaffected. They present as firm, keratotic papules with sizes ranging from a few millimeters to several centimeters in diameter. Subungual warts generally involve the hyponychium, located in the distal nail bed, and cause subungual hyperkeratosis, or onycholysis. Presentation under the PNF is rare, although the clinical appearance is typical, with a paronychia-like inflammatory reaction and distal wart papillae emerging from under the cuticle (*Fig. 23.18*).[3]

The diagnosis of a periungual wart is generally made from the clinical appearances. However, resistant periungual warts in adults require a biopsy, particularly when only one finger is involved, in order to exclude Bowen disease or an amelanotic melanoma.

Pathogenesis and histologic features

Periungual warts are benign epithelial tumors caused by the human papillomavirus (HPV), usually HPV 2 and 4. The histologic appearances include acanthosis, papillomatosis, parakeratosis, and koilocytes in the most superficial layers. In cases of HPV 1-induced infection (myrmecia), the keratinocytes contain numerous inclusions resembling eosinophilic coarse-grained keratohyaline.

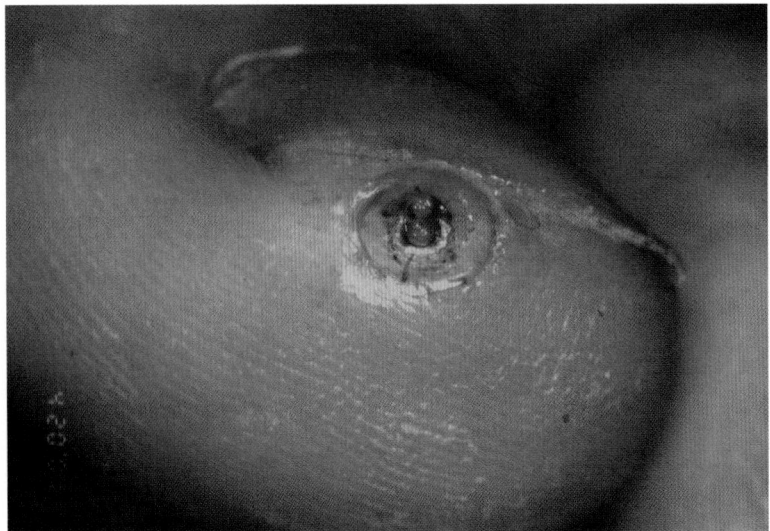

Fig. 23.16
Tungiasis: a typical site. The flea is partially visible.

INFLAMMATORY DISEASES OF THE NAIL

The nail has a limited repertoire of clinical manifestations. This is why nail biopsies are often necessary to reach an accurate diagnosis, especially when there is no associated skin or hair involvement.

The interpretation of nail biopsies is difficult because punch biopsies, rather than longitudinal nail biopsies, are often performed and because in almost all specimens a degree of parakeratosis, spongiosis, and rare neutrophils are present.

Psoriasis

Clinical features

Nail involvement is frequent in psoriasis, occurring in 10% to 50% of patients.[1] It is estimated that over a lifetime, between 80% and 90% of psoriatic patients will suffer nail disease.[2] Fingernails are more frequently affected than toenails. Several nails are usually affected, but involvement of a single nail can sometimes be seen.

The clinical appearance depends upon the part of the nail involved. Matrix involvement results in pitting, leukonychia, nail plate thickening or thinning, onychorrhexis, and crumbling (Fig. 23.19). Nail bed involvement gives rise to the 'oil drop' or 'salmon patch' signs, splinter hemorrhages, subungual hyperkeratosis, and onycholysis. PNF involvement can mimic chronic paronychia. Pitting, onycholysis, discoloration, and subungual hyperkeratosis are the most common symptoms.[1,3,4]

Pustular psoriasis of the nail, also known as Hallopeau acrodermatitis continua, is mainly observed in middle-aged females and has a chronic, relapsing course. It generally affects a single digit and is usually not associated with other manifestations of pustular psoriasis. Involvement of the nail bed with pustules, scale crusts, and onycholysis is seen.[5,6]

Parakeratosis pustulosa typically affects a single fingernail (thumb or index) in girls younger than 7 years. It is a chronic condition not regarded as a specific disease but as a manifestation of atopic dermatitis, contact dermatitis, and psoriasis. It is characterized by erythematosquamous paronychia accompanied by intermittent vesicles and pustules, onycholysis, mild distal or lateral hyperkeratosis, and nail plate deformities.[7–9] Although the disease generally resolves after a few years, some children develop psoriasis.[9]

Histologic features

Precise descriptions of the histologic changes associated with the different clinical manifestations of nail psoriasis were first described by Zaias in 1969[1] and were reviewed in 2007.[3] Histologic changes are rarely typical but often show similarity with those seen in the skin.[10] However, nail psoriasis also displays some distinctive features. As with volar psoriasis, spongiosis is frequently present. The hyponychium loses its normally present granular cell layer, while, in contrast, the nail matrix and nail bed may develop a granular cell layer.[11] The matrix hypergranulosis is analogous to epidermal parakeratosis.[12] Mounds of parakeratosis with neutrophils and focal accumulation of proteinaceous serum-like material, in the nail plate or subungual keratin, are a good clue to the diagnosis.[13] For Grover, hyperkeratosis with parakeratosis and a neutrophilic infiltrate (dermal or epidermal) were the most common findings (Fig. 23.20). However, a definite diagnosis of psoriasis was possible in only 54% of the cases.[10] The best results are obtained with longitudinal biopsies.[10] Nail bed punch biopsies are useful in subungual hyperkeratosis, but rarely in onycholysis.[14] Nail clippings showing severe parakeratosis with neutrophils, pits, or microscopic hemorrhage may suggest psoriasis, if onychomycosis has been ruled out.[15,16]

In pustular psoriasis, true spongiform pustules can be observed in the nail bed. They may coalesce to form intraepidermal or subcorneal macropustules (Figs 23.21 and 23.22).[5]

In parakeratosis pustulosa, histology may show spongiotic or psoriasiform changes.[9,17]

Differential diagnosis

A PAS stain should always be performed to exclude onychomycosis because the latter may clinically and histologically mimic nail psoriasis and because a mycotic superinfection or colonization is observed in 13% to 27% of cases of nail psoriasis.[18,19]

Lichen planus

Clinical features

Nails are affected in 1% to 10% of patients with lichen planus and permanent damage of at least one nail occurs in up to 4% of patients.[1,2]

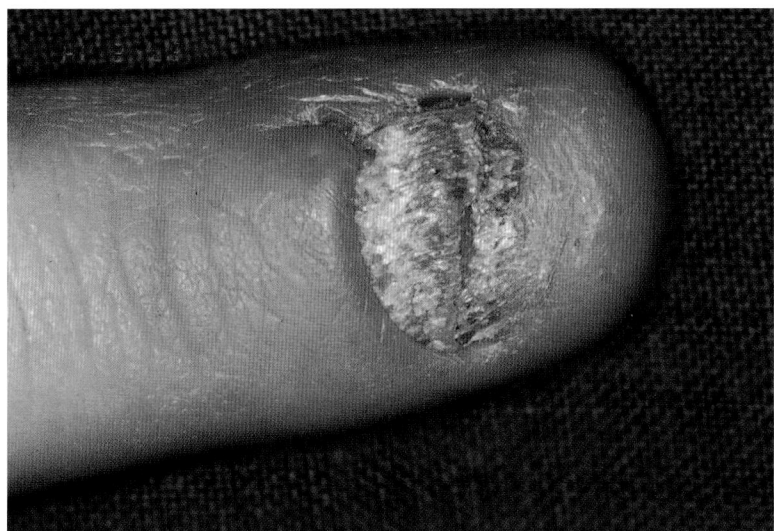

Fig. 23.19
Psoriasis: note the scar from the prior lateral-longitudinal biopsy. The nail plate is dystrophic and thickened. Courtesy of B. Richert, MD, PhD, Université Libre de Bruxelles, Belgium.

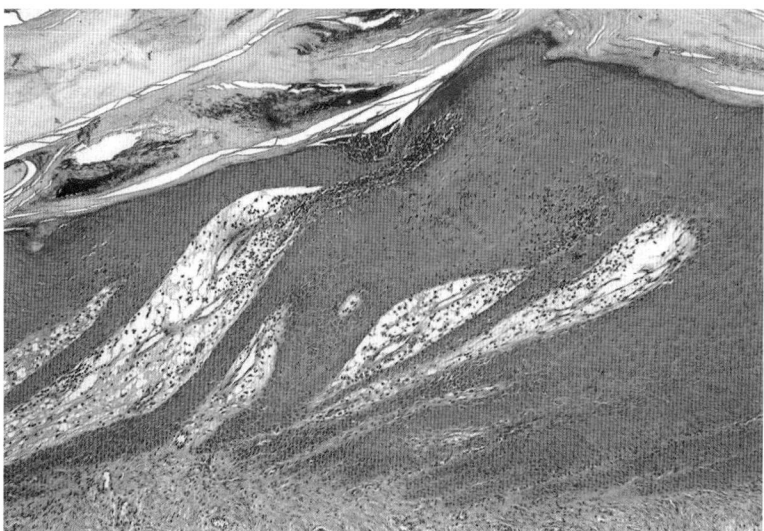

Fig. 23.20
Psoriasis: distal matrix involvement. Note the psoriasiform hyperplasia, neutrophil exocytosis, and subungual hyper- and parakeratosis. There is edema in the superficial dermis with vasodilatation.

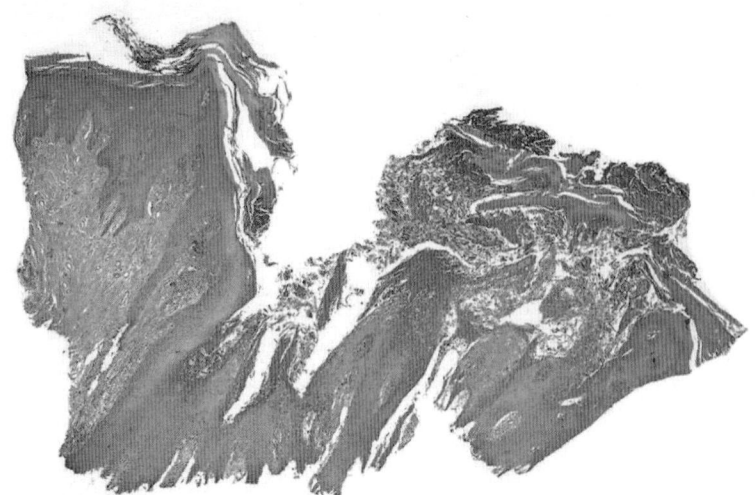

Fig. 23.21
Pustular psoriasis: there is crusting, parakeratosis, and a macropustule.

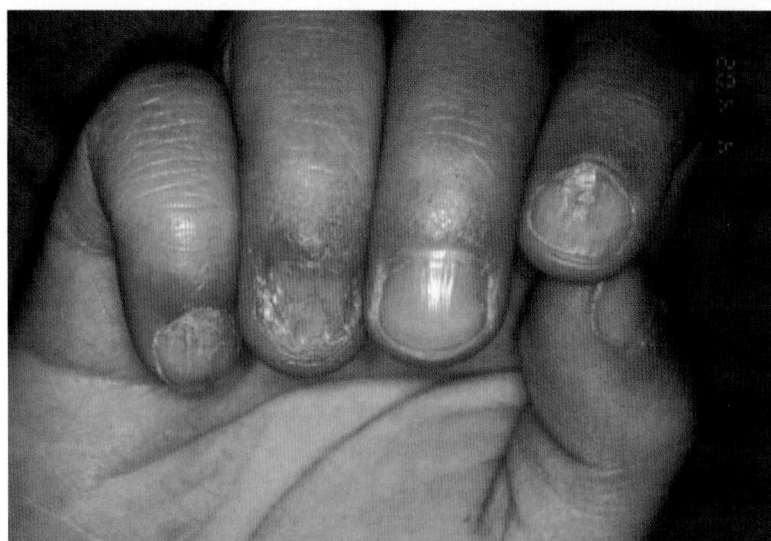

Fig. 23.23
Lichen planus: typical nail changes in a 3.5-year-old boy.

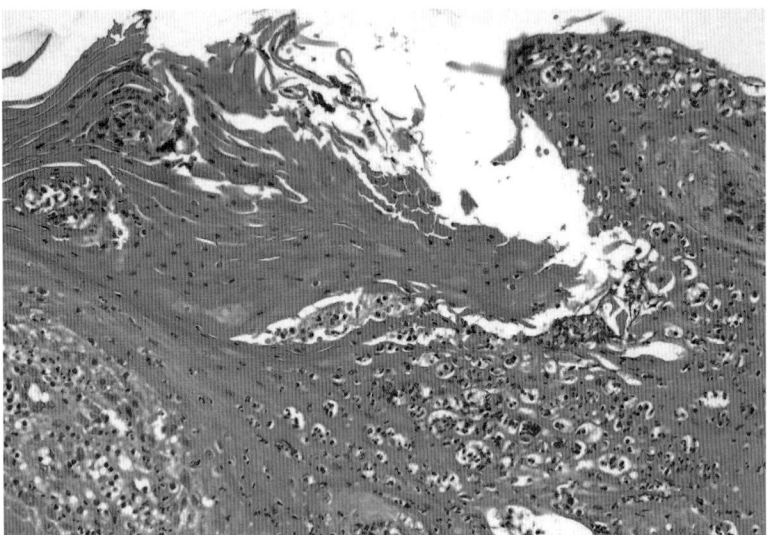

Fig. 23.22
Pustular psoriasis: high-power view showing conspicuous spongiform pustules. Cases such as this should always be examined for the presence of fungi.

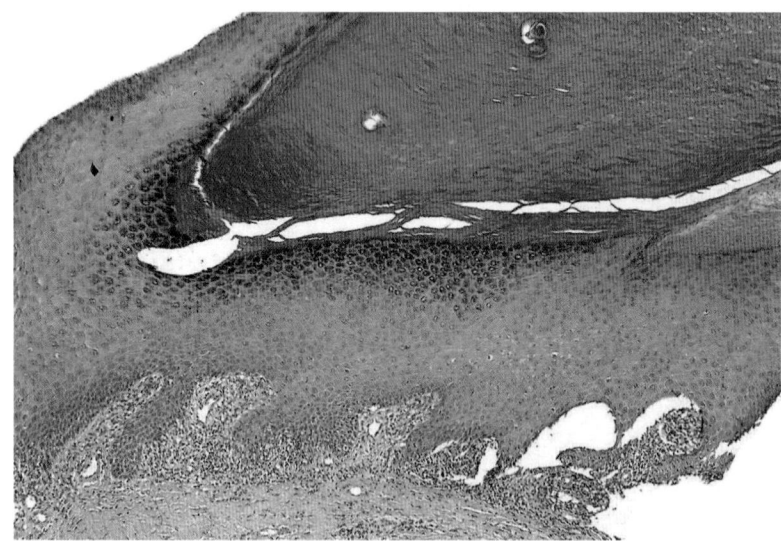

Fig. 23.24
Lichen planus: this is a biopsy of the proximal nail matrix. Note the hypergranulosis, hypertrophic acanthosis, and superficial bandlike infiltrate.

Approximately 25% of patients with nail lichen planus have clinical lesions at other sites before or after the onset of nail lesions.[3] Fingernails are more frequently affected than toenails. Nail changes are not pathognomonic. However, a diagnosis should be considered when multiple nails are affected by lichenoid nail changes:

- longitudinal ridges and splitting,
- thinning of the nail plate, with or without dorsal pterygium (dorsal expansion of the PNF resulting from the fusion of the ventral aspect of the PNF with the underlying nail matrix and nail bed),
- erythematous patches in the lunula and longitudinal melanonychia (less frequent).

All these features are caused by matrix involvement, the most frequent region affected. Involvement of the nail bed is also possible and results in subungual hyperkeratosis and onycholysis. Complete involvement of the nail matrix and the nail bed leads to a total loss of the nail plate with permanent atrophy of the nail area.[1] Rarer presentations include erosive nail lichen planus, yellow nail syndrome-like features,[4,5] onychopapilloma,[6] and nail degloving.[7] In children, nail lichen planus has three different presentations: typical nail lesions as above (*Fig. 23.23*), trachyonychia, and idiopathic atrophy of nails.[8] Nail biopsies are frequently performed due to the risk of permanent nail destruction and because treatment often necessitates systemic corticosteroid therapy.

Histologic features

Histologic features of nail lichen planus were first described by Zaias.[1] He observed that it can involve each of the nail unit constituents separately or together. The matrix is more frequently affected than the nail bed and PNF.[3] Punch biopsies confirmed the diagnosis in 85.5% to 100% of the cases.[9] Indeed, histologic changes are usually typical showing acanthosis, hypergranulosis, liquefactive degeneration of the basal cell layer with apoptotic cells, and a bandlike superficial lymphocytic inflammatory infiltrate in the superficial dermis (*Figs 23.24–23.26*). In the matrix and nail bed, a compact horny layer replaces the normal nail plate above the zones of hypergranulosis. Spongiosis can be prominent.[10] Numerous plasma cells in the infiltrate have been described.[11]

Differential diagnosis

Matrix hypergranulosis is a major feature of nail lichen planus. However, it has also been observed in spongiotic trachyonychia, psoriasis, and pustular psoriasis.[12] Nail lichen planus is indistinguishable from the nail changes seen in graft-versus-host disease[13,14] and lichenoid drug reactions. In lupus erythematosus, the infiltrate is usually more perivascular, with thickening of the capillary wall.[15] Lichenoid nail changes have been described in systemic amyloidosis and can be the first sign of the disease. Histology reveals typical amyloid deposits in the superficial dermis of the matrix.[16–18]

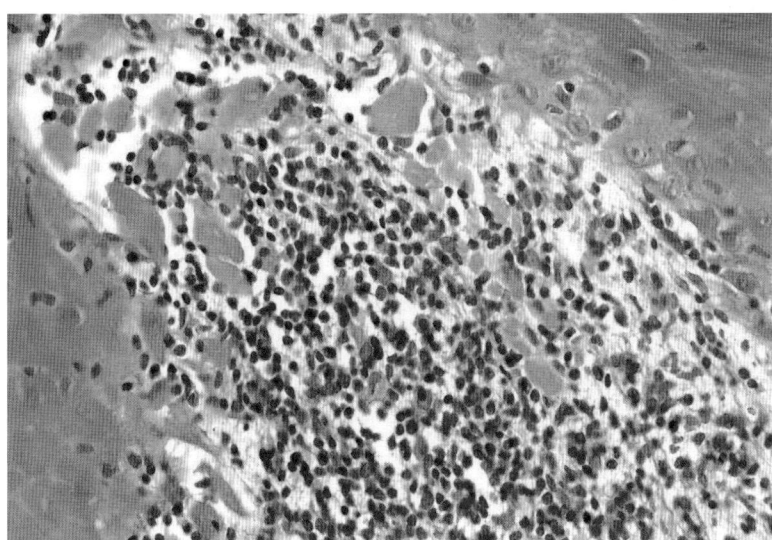

Fig. 23.25
Lichen planus: high-power view showing conspicuous cytoid bodies.

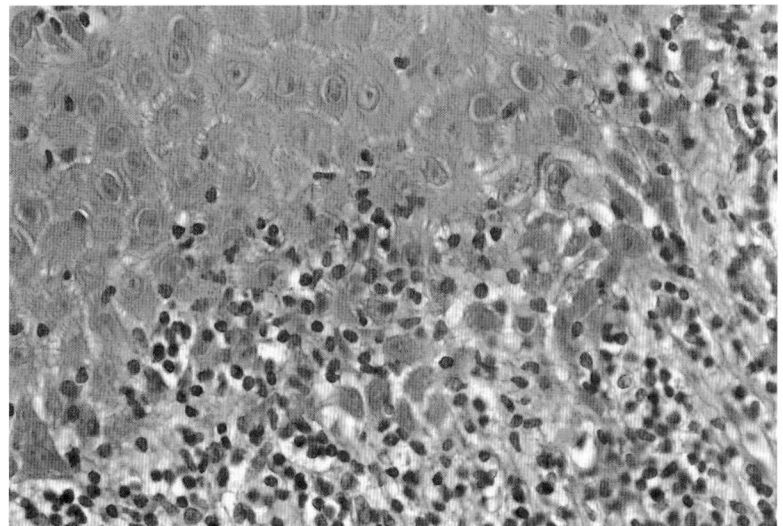

Fig. 23.26
Lichen planus: high-power view showing interface change and lymphocytic infiltration.

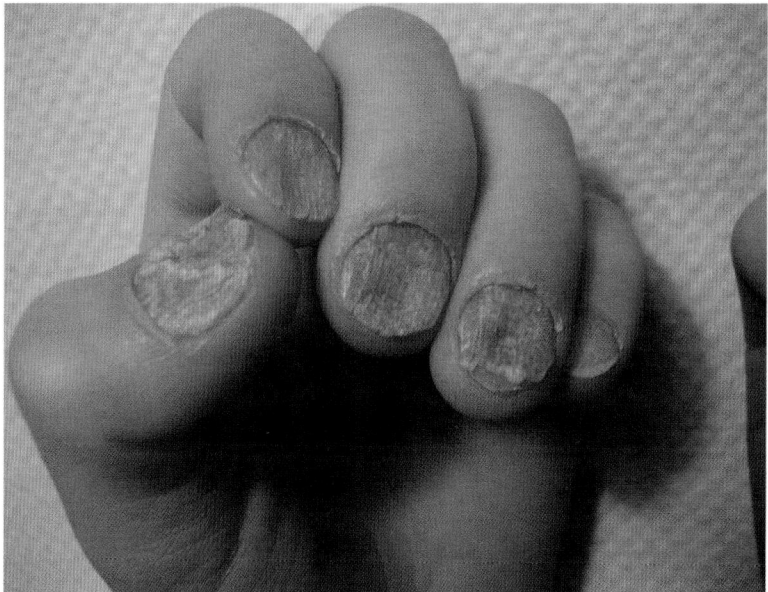

Fig. 23.27
Trachyonychia: there is loss of translucency and the nails appear rough and jagged at their distal borders. The cuticles are hyperplastic and ragged. Courtesy of B. Richert, MD, PhD, Université Libre de Bruxelles, Belgium.

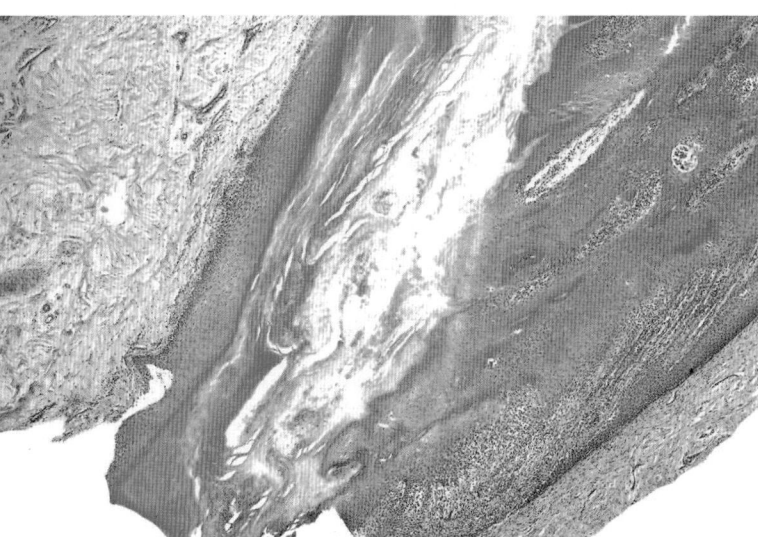

Fig. 23.28
Trachyonychia: there is florid spongiosis with lymphocytic exocytosis.

Trachyonychia

Clinical features

Trachyonychia means rough nail. The nail is opaque and covered with thin scales (*Fig. 23.27*). It shows excessive superficial longitudinal ridging. Thinning of the nail plate is responsible for brittleness, which may be associated with koilonychia (spoon nail deformation) and splitting at the free edge. The cuticles are often hyperplastic and ragged. Baran et al. described another form of trachyonychia, called the shiny type, characterized by multiple punctuate depressions that reflect light.[1] Trachyonychia may affect one, several, or all 20 nails (twenty-nail dystrophy syndrome). Trachyonychia is mainly observed in three dermatological diseases: lichen planus, psoriasis, and alopecia areata. In alopecia areata, trachyonychia is observed in 12% of the cases in children[2] and 3% in adults.[3] The incidence of trachyonychia in psoriasis and lichen planus is unknown. Trachyonychia has also been described in association with atopic dermatitis, ichthyosis vulgaris, IgA deficiency, incontinentia pigmenti, pemphigus, and vitiligo.[4] Idiopathic trachyonychia, i.e., without any concomitant skin or hair disease, has been reported mostly in children and males.[5] Total resolution or marked improvement is observed within the first 6 years in 50% of cases. A nail biopsy is not routinely recommended.[6,7]

Histologic features

Trachyonychia is best investigated with longitudinal biopsies. Trachyonychia associated with alopecia areata usually shows a mild to moderate lymphocytic infiltrate in the superficial dermis, exocytosis of lymphocytes, and mild to moderate spongiosis, without vacuolar degeneration of the basal cell layer (*Figs 23.28* and *23.29*). The changes predominantly affect the ventral PNF, the proximal matrix, and the hyponychium.[5] In so-called idiopathic trachyonychia, spongiotic alterations were observed in 83% of the cases, a psoriatic pattern in 13%, while 4% of cases were due to lichen planus.[8] In another series, the proportion was different, with spongiotic dermatitis occurring in 45%, psoriasis in 26%, lichen planus in 18.5%, and non-specific changes in 10%.[9] The results yielded in a third study cannot be compared, as 65.6% of cases were not idiopathic but associated with different known dermatoses.[10]

Differential diagnosis

The possibility that idiopathic spongiotic trachyonychia is actually a variant of alopecia areata limited to nails has been suggested.[3] However, the exact significance of spongiosis is not fully understood. Spongiosis is frequently

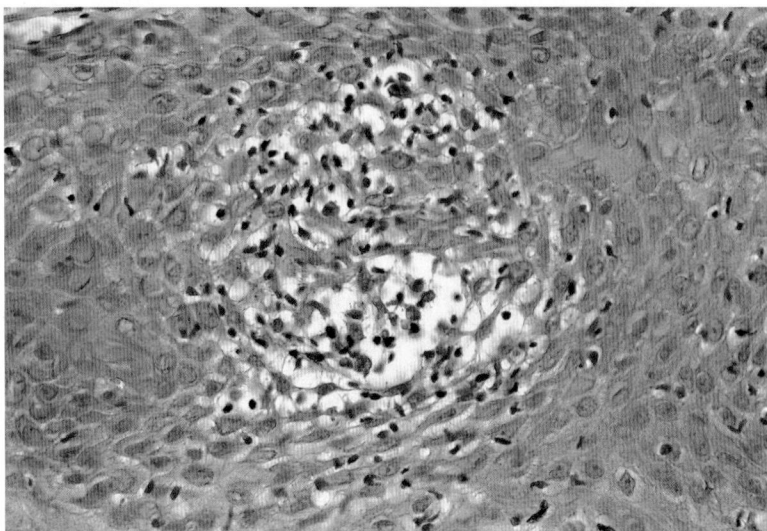

Fig. 23.29
Trachyonychia: high-power view of a spongiotic vesicle.

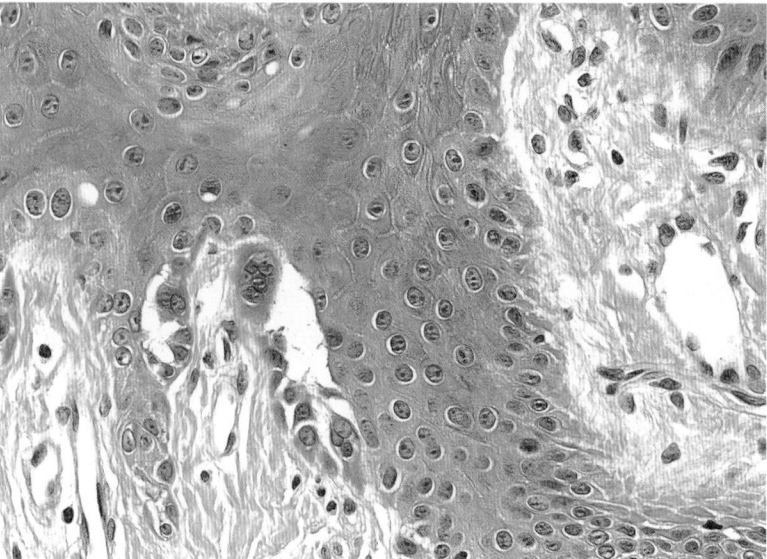

Fig. 23.31
Darier-White disease: suprabasal acantholysis with multinucleated cells.

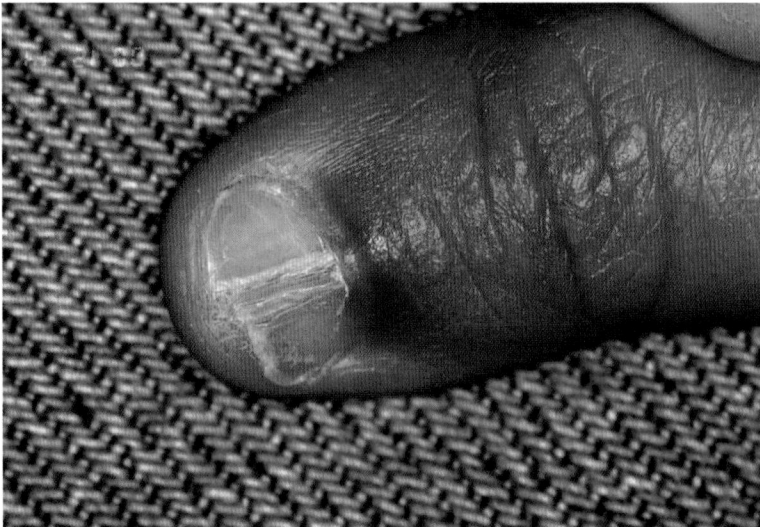

Fig. 23.30
Lichen striatus: there is a median, longitudinal, lichenoid nail involvement.
Discrete flesh-colored linear papules are present on the dorsum of the finger. The
patient is a 2-year-old boy.

observed with more specific changes in many nail disorders such as psoriasis
and lichen planus. Typical spongiotic changes may also be associated with
contact dermatitis, atopic dermatitis, and dyshidrosis. In all of these, the
spongiosis usually extends to involve the periungual tissues. This is not seen
in alopecia areata.

Lichen striatus

Clinical features

Nail lichen striatus is rare but probably under-reported. It has mainly been
described in children and young adults and usually affects a single digit. It
is characterized by a median or asymmetrical, longitudinal, lichenoid nail
plate dystrophy (*Fig. 23.30*).[1] Upper limbs are more frequently affected than
the lower limbs. When the typical cutaneous involvement characterized by
small, flesh-colored papules in a linear distribution is present, diagnosis is
easy. However, the nail dystrophy may appear before the skin involvement[2]
or can be isolated. Spontaneous regression after a median duration of 22.6
months is the rule.[1]

Histologic features

A longitudinal nail biopsy from two cases of lichen striatus restricted to a
nail showed a moderately dense bandlike lymphohistiocytic inflammatory
cell infiltrate affecting the PNF, the nail bed, and the dermis of the nail
matrix.[1] It was associated with exocytosis, slight spongiosis, focal hypergranulosis, and dyskeratotic cells in the nail matrix epithelium and with
slight focal spongiosis and exocytosis in the ventral PNF, nail bed, and
hyponychium. Dyskeratotic cells surrounded by lymphocytes were also
present in the nail bed.[1]

Darier-white disease

Clinical features

Nails are affected in 92% of patients with Darier-White disease,[1] and
involvement may also be seen in the absence of any other evidence of the
disease.[2] The number of abnormal nails ranges from two or three, to all
nails in a minority of patients.[1] The fingernails are more severely affected.
Characteristic features are longitudinal red and white streaks associated
with distal wedge-shaped subungual keratosis.[2]

Histologic features

Each component of the nail apparatus may be affected, but the most dramatic changes are seen in the nail bed.[2,3] White longitudinal streaks and
subungual keratosis are characterized by epithelial hyperplasia with marked
parakeratosis and numerous multinucleated (from 2 to more than 20 nuclei)
epithelial cells (*Fig. 23.31*). The longitudinal red streaks are due to mild
epithelial hyperplasia and vasodilatation. The histologic findings in the nail
bed of Darier disease differ from those of the skin: presence of multinucleate
epithelial giant cells and near-absence of inflammatory infiltrate. The matrix
may be completely spared. However, if the distal nail matrix is affected,
typical changes of Darier disease may be observed. The proximal matrix is
rarely affected.

Differential diagnosis

Multinucleate giant cells in the nail bed epithelium were thought to be specific to Darier disease. In fact, they may also be observed in several unrelated
nail conditions such as onychopapilloma[4,5] (see erythronychia) and Bowen
disease. A case of focal subungual warty dyskeratoma and three cases of
acantholytic dyskeratotic acanthomas of the nail have been described.[6,7]
Clinically, they presented as median longitudinal erythronychia with distal
onycholysis. Histologically, they were characterized by suprabasal clefts,
acantholytic cells, grains and corps ronds.

Pemphigus vulgaris

Clinical features

Nail changes in pemphigus vulgaris may be more frequent than previously thought. Nail changes were present in 30 of 64 (47%) affected patients. Sixteen patients had onychomycosis and 14 had nail changes due to pemphigus, confirmed by nail biopsy.[1] No correlation was found between duration or severity of the skin disease and nail involvement. Nail involvement may either be an isolated primary manifestation or, more frequently, it may accompany the initial mucocutaneous presentation. It may also occur just before or concurrent with a flare-up of a pre-existing disease.[2] Nail symptoms are varied with chronic paronychia and proximal separation of the nail plate from the nail matrix and/or the nail bed, with subsequent nail shedding (onychomadesis) being the most common.[2,3] Several nails are usually affected, mainly fingernails. Rare cases of chronic nail involvement restricted to one toenail may lead to permanent loss of nail.[4,5] Nail biopsies are only performed when chronic paronychia or onychomadesis precede the mucocutaneous lesions or when only one nail is affected. In this instance, a subungual tumor (*Fig. 23.32*) or herpetic whitlow must be excluded.[6]

Histologic features

Suprabasal clefting and acantholysis, typical of pemphigus vulgaris, are observed in nail matrix, nail bed, and PNFs, as well as are intercellular deposits of IgG and C3 on direct immunofluorescence.[2]

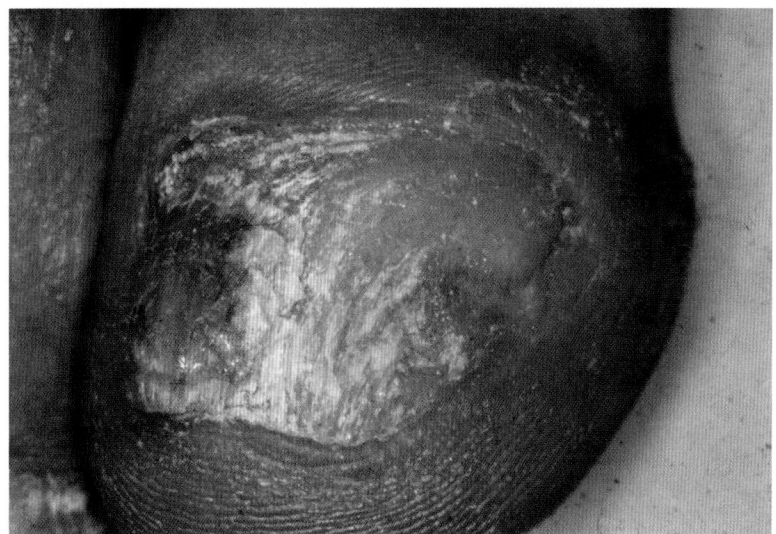

Fig. 23.32
Pemphigus: this example has presented as a subungual destructive tumor of the nail bed. Courtesy of P. Gheeraert MD, Université Libre de Bruxelles.

MELANOCYTIC LESIONS OF THE NAIL APPARATUS

Melanocytes in the nail unit

There are fundamental differences between the nail and skin melanocytic populations.

The number of melanocytes is much lower in the nail than in the skin. Nail matrix melanocytes are about 200/mm² compared with around 1150/mm² in the epidermis. They also differ by their usual quiescence. In the proximal matrix, most melanocytes are dormant and do not produce any pigment, while in the distal matrix 50% are dormant and 50% are active. In the nail bed, melanocytes are even rarer (approximately 50/mm²) and they are dormant.[1]

Melanocytes in a suprabasal position are physiological in the matrix. In the proximal matrix, melanocytes are located within the lower two to four germinative cell layers, while in the distal matrix, they are located in the first and second layers.[1]

The melanocyte density can be routinely measured as the number of intraepithelial melanocytes over a stretch of 1 mm epithelial-dermal junction of the nail matrix and/or nail bed. In normal nails, the density ranges from 4 to 9 melanocytes (mean: 7.7) per 1 mm of nail matrix epithelium.[2,3] Melanocytes are small; some have dendritic process. Immunostainings with HMB-45 and Mart-1 (Melan A) are useful to better visualize the epithelial nail melanocytes. Immunostaining with S100 protein should not be used, at least alone, as many nail epithelial melanocytes do not express this antigen.[4]

Longitudinal melanonychia (melanonychia striata)

Definition

Most melanocytic lesions of the nail apparatus present as a longitudinal or a total melanonychia. A longitudinal melanonychia is a longitudinal pigmented band extending from the matrix up to the distal part of the nail plate, caused by the presence of melanin in the nail plate (*Fig. 23.33*). In total melanonychia, the whole nail plate is pigmented. The melanosomes originate from matrix melanocytes and are transferred via their dendrites to differentiating matrix cells and will be incorporated in the nail plate. Longitudinal melanonychia may be the first sign of a nail apparatus melanoma, especially when it involves a single digit. This is why biopsies are

generally performed. Lateral longitudinal excision (for lateral lesions) and matrix biopsies can be performed.

Histologic features

If the nail plate is available for histologic examination, brown melanin granules can be observed in the onychocytes. They appear black with the Fontana-Masson staining. In most examples, the pigment is located in the ventral nail plate, arising from the distal matrix. The pigment location in the nail plate is used to guide the matrix biopsy and to anticipate postsurgical sequelae, as a biopsy performed on the distal matrix carries a much lower risk of postsurgical dystrophy than a proximal matrix biopsy. Nowadays, the location of the pigment can also be determined by dermoscopic examination of the free edge of the nail plate.[1] Moreover, it is recommended

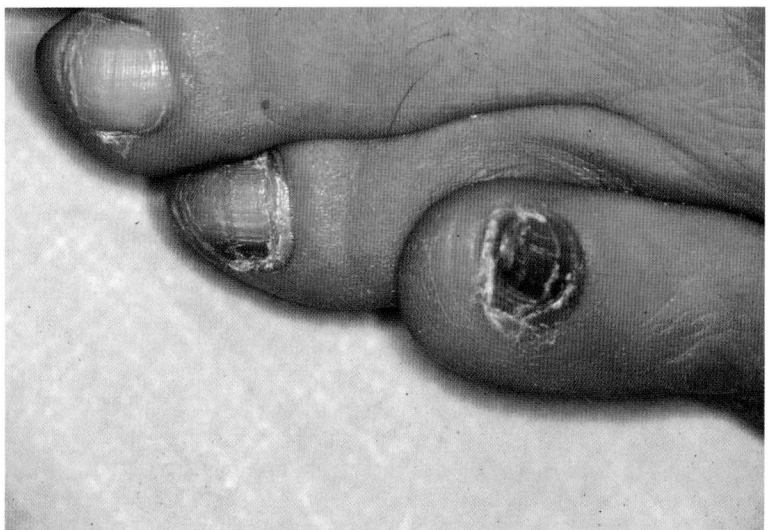

Fig. 23.33
Longitudinal melanonychia: there is involvement of the fourth toenail and complete melanonychia of the fifth toenail. This has resulted from melanocytic activation due to repeated friction from ill-fitting shoes.

to perform the matrix biopsy after proximal nail avulsion and direct visualization of the pigmented area in the matrix.

Histologic examination of the nail matrix allows the identification of two broad groups of longitudinal melanonychia: melanocytic activation and melanocytic proliferation, frequently designated as melanocytic hyperplasia. Their relative incidence is completely different in adults and in children: 73% of single-digit lesions in adults are due to melanocytic activation, while 75% of single-digit lesions in children are due to benign melanocytic hyperplasia, mainly nevi.[2,3]

- In melanocytic activation, melanotic pigmentation of the matrix epithelium is seen, without any increase in the density of melanocytes.
- Melanocytic hyperplasia is defined as an increased number of matrix melanocytes. Benign melanocytic hyperplasia can be subdivided into lentigo when benign melanocytes remain arranged in individual units or nevus when at least one nest is present. The proliferation of melanocytes may also be malignant, corresponding to in situ or invasive melanoma.

Although a number of clinical and dermatoscopic features can help in the distinction between benign melanonychia and melanoma, accurate diagnosis requires histologic examination.

Differential diagnosis

A longitudinal pigmented band extending from the matrix but stopping at the distal part of the nail bed, and leaving the free edge of the nail plate unpigmented, has been described. It is due to a pigmented cornified acanthoma of the nail bed. This can be considered as the equivalent of a pigmented seborrheic keratosis.[4] Melanin should not be confused with other chromogens that are not stained with the Fontana-Masson reaction. In the absence of melanin, subungual hematoma is the main differential diagnosis. It is characterized by degrading red blood cells. Perls reaction is always negative in the nail plate, as iron requires macrophage processing to be transformed into hemosiderin.

Melanocytic activation

Clinical features

Longitudinal melanonychia due to melanocytic activation or stimulation is also called hypermelanosis, functional melanonychia, or melanotic macule.[1] The etiologies are multiple and can be classified as physiological, local and regional, dermatological, systemic, and iatrogenic. Laugier-Hunziker syndrome as well as Peutz-Jeghers and Touraine syndrome can be added to this list.[2,3] Melanocytic activation is more frequent in patients with darker phototypes and increases with age.[4] The pigmented bands frequently involve several nails, but melanocytic activation is also responsible for 73% of single-digit longitudinal melanonychia in adults.[5] Dermatoscopic examination reveals a grayish background usually associated with thin regular gray lines.[6]

Histologic features

By definition, there is no increase in the density of melanocytes. Only some melanocytes with pigmented dendrites and pigmented keratinocytes are observed (Figs 23.34 and 23.35). If the pigment is barely visible, a Fontana-Masson stain should be performed. A few melanophages are frequently present in the superficial dermis.

Differential diagnosis

The pathologist can only diagnose melanocytic activation, but cannot determine its precise cause except in pigmented onychomycosis or pigmented Bowen disease.

Longitudinal melanonychia due to fungal infections may show melanin pigmentation of the matrix and nail plate together with nonpigmented fungus in the nail plate. It may also reveal brown-colored hyphae as in onychomycosis caused by the dematiaceous family.

In cases due to pigmented Bowen disease, typical features of Bowen disease are observed (see below) together with melanin pigmentation of the epithelium.

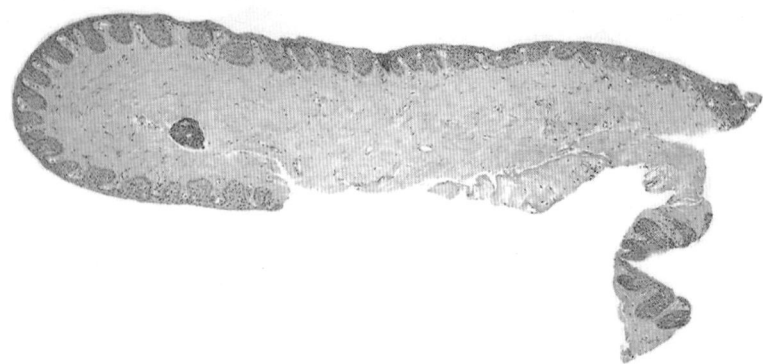

Fig. 23.34
Melanocytic activation: scanning view of nail matrix.

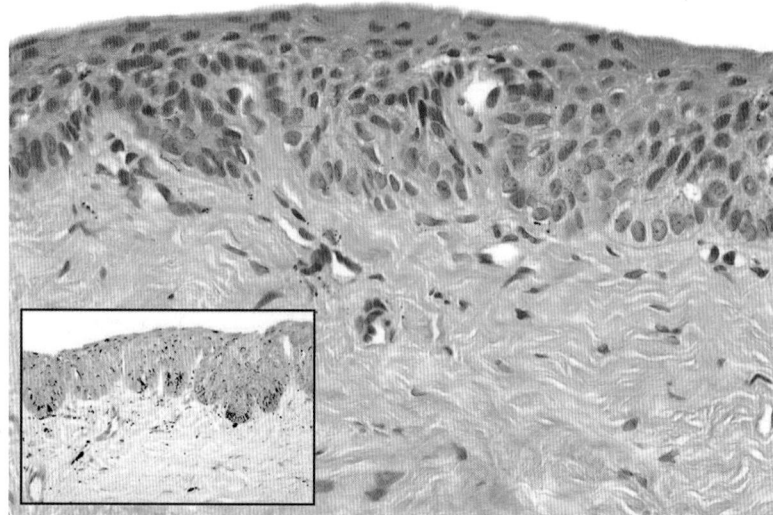

Fig. 23.35
Melanocytic activation: high-power view showing increased pigmentation within the epithelium and melanophages in the dermis (inset: Masson-Fontana stain).

Melanocytic activation is sometimes difficult to differentiate from a lentigo with a slight increase in the melanocyte density.[7] Immunostainings with HMB-45 and Mart-1 may be helpful. This, however, is of little therapeutic consequence, as both entities are benign.

Lentigo and nevus

Clinical features

Lentigo is frequently considered together with melanocytic activation and nevus. In a series of 15 'subungual melanotic macules', 6 lesions showed increased pigmentation only (melanocytic activation) while 9 lesions proved to be a lentigo with an increased density of melanocytes.[1] The clinical appearances are indistinguishable from a nevus.[2] Lentigo has been reported to account for 9% of single-digit longitudinal melanonychia in adults[3] and for 30% in children.[2]

A nevus was observed in 12% of single-digit longitudinal melanonychia in adults but in almost 50% in children. Nevi can be congenital or acquired. Longitudinal melanonychia due to nevi prevails on the fingers, mainly the thumb. Their width measures 3 mm or more, in half of the cases (Fig. 23.36). A brown-black coloration is observed in two-thirds of the cases, periungual pigmentation (benign pseudo-Hutchinson sign) in one-third.[2] However, nail matrix nevi can also present as scarcely pigmented bands. The only clinical feature that suggests a diagnosis of nail matrix nevus is onset during childhood. However, nevus can also appear after puberty.[3] Dermatoscopic examination of a nevus reveals a brown coloration of the background and regular parallel longitudinal brown lines.[4]

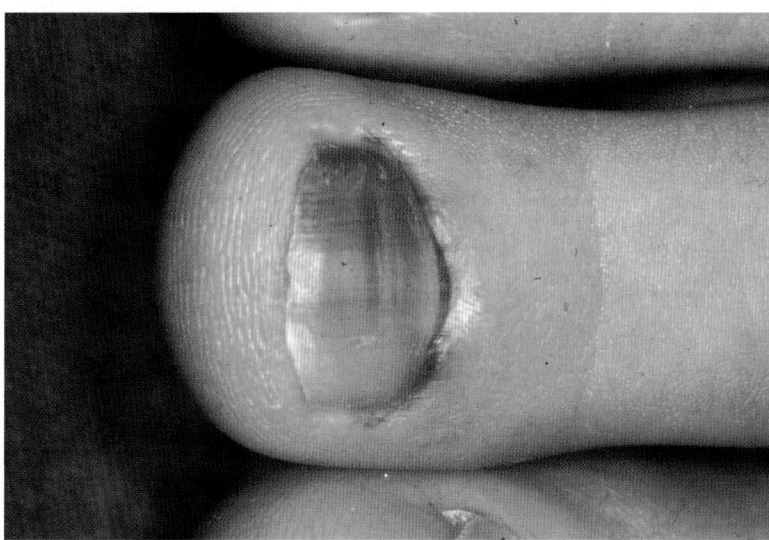

Fig. 23.36
Melanocytic nevus: this example presenting as total melanonychia occurred in a 10-year-old boy. (Courtesy of B. Richert, MD, PhD, Université Libre de Bruxelles, Belgium.)

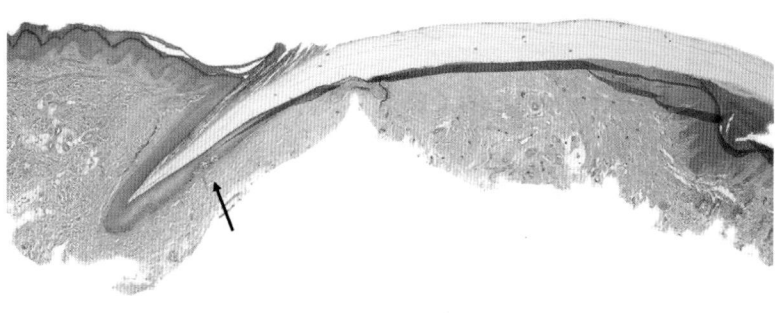

Fig. 23.37
Junctional melanocytic nevus: scanning view showing two junctional nests in the nail matrix (*arrowed*).

Histologic features

Lentigo is characterized by a mild to moderate increase in the number of matrix melanocytes (10 to 31 cells per mm).[1] The melanocytes remain in individual units, without confluence. The epidermal rete ridges are often less prominent than in cutaneous lentigo. Cytological atypia is absent or mild. Pagetoid spread can be observed but it is rare or focal. Pigmentation is usually limited to the lower third of the nail epithelium but can be observed throughout its full thickness. Scattered melanophages are frequently observed in the superficial dermis.[1,2]

In nevi, nests are located in the matrix, and sometimes also in the ventral part of the PNF and/or the hyponychium. The latter are only visible on longitudinal biopsy. Nests are not usually observed in the nail bed. The vast majority of ungual nevi are junctional.[2,3] In compound nevi, dermal nests are most often observed in the hyponychium. Symmetry is not a useful feature in ungual nevi because biopsies are often partial and small in size. Moreover, nevi are asymmetrical in longitudinal biopsies because of the nail architecture.[3] Also, margins cannot usually be evaluated. Nests tend to be scarce, but rare cases display intense melanocytic hyperplasia with confluent nests often consisting of large epithelioid melanocytes (*Figs 23.37* and *23.38*). The presence of some melanocytes with nuclear atypia can be seen in 15% of lesions and a mild degree of melanocytic upward migration in

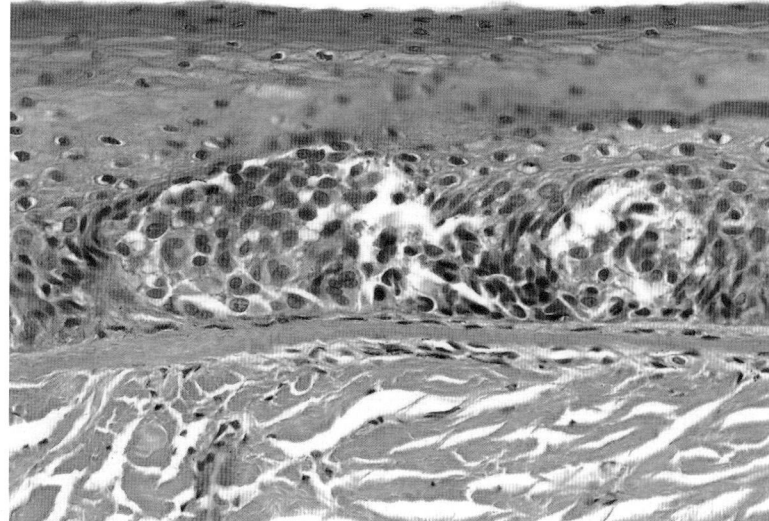

Fig. 23.38
Junctional melanocytic nevus: the nevus cells are uniform. There is no atypia or mitotic activity.

20% of cases.[2] Small numbers of melanophages are commonly scattered throughout the superficial dermis.

Differential diagnosis

In situ melanoma is associated with a higher melanocyte density and confluence compared with lentigo.[1,5] The pagetoid spread is usually multifocal and can reach the upper epithelial layers. Atypia characterized by angular hyperchromatic nuclei is present. In children, the diagnosis of in situ melanoma should be made cautiously[6] and only when there is a severe increase in melanocyte density together with both atypical hyperchromatic nuclei and an obvious pagetoid migration reaching the onychogenous band. Clinical-pathological correlation is also useful: childhood longitudinal melanonychia present for more than 2 years with continuous widening and darkening, and the appearance of periungual pigmentation or nail plate dystrophy is of concern, as is a stable lesion present since childhood that starts to change in adulthood.[7] In adults, if the melanocytic hyperplasia is atypical and the biopsy only partial, an early in situ melanoma cannot be excluded and complete excision of the nail apparatus is advisable, especially if the clinical presentation is worrying.

Blue nevus

Clinical features

Ten cases of well-documented blue nevus in the nail apparatus have been published. Three cases were congenital, the others presented in adults aged 20 to 64 years. Their clinical characteristic are summarized in *Table 23.2*.[1–10]

Histologic features

Common blue nevus was observed in seven cases, cellular blue nevus in two cases, atypical blue nevus in one case, and a combined blue nevus in two cases (*Table 23.2*).

Differential diagnosis

Rarely, partially regressed subungual melanoma may mimic a cellular blue nevus in partial biopsies.[11]

Melanoma

Clinical features

Nail apparatus melanoma, also called subungual melanoma, is rare, accounting for only 1.4% to 2.8% of all cutaneous melanomas in the United Kingdom.[1,2] Its incidence is higher in African-Americans (15–20%)[3]

Table 23.2

Blue nevus of the nail apparatus: clinical data and pathological diagnosis. (A, acquired; C, congenital; F, female; M, male)

		Location	Sex	Age (years)	Onset	Clinical presentation	Pathology
1	Soyer and Kerl[1]	Left, Toe 1	F	4	C	Well circumscribed, blue-black, 1.2 × 0.4 cm lesion on the proximal nail fold with minute satellite lesions	Combined nevus
2	Vidal et al.[2]	Right, Toe 1	M	20	C	0.9 cm in diameter, bluish nodule in the distal nail bed and hyponychium	Common blue nevus
3	Duhard[3]	Left, Finger 1	F	50		Bluish macule in the matrix with distal fissuring of the nail plate	Atypical blue nevus
4	Causeret et al.[4]	Right, Toe 1	F	42	A	Ovoid-shaped blue spot, in the distal matrix associated with ethnic longitudinal melanonychia on several nails	Cellular blue nevus
5	Smith et al.[5]	Right, Finger 3	M	61	A	Wide (almost total) heterogeneous brown-black melanonychia	Common blue nevus
6	Moulonguet-Michau, Abimelec[3]	Right, Finger 1	M	42	A	Triangular blue-black macule in the lateral part of the lunula, with longitudinal groove in the nail plate	Common blue nevus
7	Moulonguet-Michau, Abimelec[3]	Left, Toe 1	F	32	A	Blue macule in the lateral part of the lunula	Common blue nevus
8	Kim et al.[6]	Right, Finger 1	F	44	A	Longitudinal melanonychia and bluish discoloration of the lunula	Common blue nevus
9	Dalle et al.[7]	Right, Finger 2	F	34	A	Blue-gray, well-limited, semicircular spot in the middle of the lunula, with superficial linear erosion of the nail plate	Common blue nevus
10	Naylor et al.[8]	Left, Finger 4	F	40	A (during childhood)	Semicircular dark blue discoloration of the proximal nailbed and matrix, with pseudo clubbing	Combined blue nevus
11	Gershtenson et al.[9]	Right, Toe 2	F	21	C	1.7 × 2.3 cm irregularly shaped, sharply delineated, blue black plaque on the proximal and lateral nail folds, with longitudinal melanonychia	Cellular blue nevus
12	Lee et al.[10]	Right, Finger 3	F	64	A	Black longitudinal melanonychia (?)	Common blue nevus

and also in Japanese (up to 23%).[4] The incidence, however, is actually the same across racial groups but, as nonacral skin melanoma is less frequently seen in pigmented people, their proportion of subungual lesions is higher.[5] Nail melanoma is known to be associated with a poor prognosis, mainly because of late diagnosis.[6–8] One study found that 52% of cases had been misdiagnosed by the first clinician to see the patient. This was responsible for an 18 months median delay in diagnosis.[9]

Melanoma and longitudinal melanonychia

Melanoma was observed in 6% of single-digit longitudinal melanonychia cases in adults.[10] It is extremely rare in children with only about 14 reported cases.[11–14] In a series of 44 subungual melanomas, 30% presented as longitudinal melanonychia, 36% as total melanonychia, and 5% presented as a tumor with residual longitudinal melanonychia, meaning that about 70% of nail melanomas actually started with a longitudinal melanonychia.[15] One should be particularly careful with longitudinal melanonychia appearing on a single digit in a patient older than 60 years, especially if the lesion is located on the thumb or big toe. In a pigmented population, longitudinal melanonychia caused by a melanoma can be associated with racial longitudinal melanonychia on other nails.[16]

The ABCDE rule for cutaneous melanoma also applies to the longitudinal pigmented band. Thus, if it is:

- **A**symmetrical,
- has **B**lurred borders,
- has a heterogeneous **C**olor,
- has a **D**iameter of greater than 6 mm,
- and if the lesion is **E**volving, the probability of a melanoma is high.

Periungual pigmentation (Hutchinson sign) or nail plate dystrophy are also clues to the diagnosis of nail melanoma (*Fig. 23.39*). An ABCDEF rule for subungual melanoma has also been suggested which includes a family or personal history of dysplastic nevi or melanoma.[17]

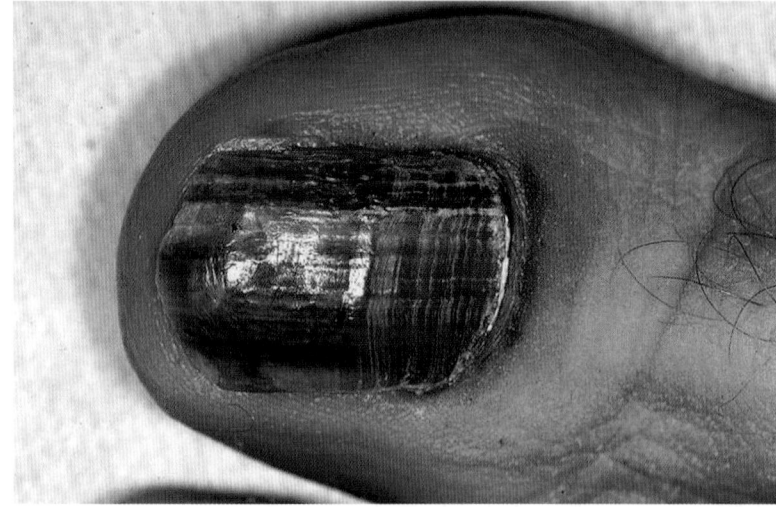

Fig. 23.39

Invasive melanoma: this tumor presented with total melanonychia. Note the Hutchinson sign – pigmentation spreading to the adjacent skin.

Dermatoscopic examination of longitudinal melanonychia due to melanoma reveals a brown color in the background and irregular brown longitudinal lines with disruption of parallelism.[18] A pigmented band involving more than two-thirds of the nail plate, gray or black color together with irregular brown pigmentation, granular pigmentation, nail dystrophy, dots, and globules are also suggestive of melanoma.[19–21]

A mass below the nail, loss of the nail, and ulceration of the nail bed are observed in later stages.[22] Rarely, nail melanoma may present as a brown-black spot in the distal nail bed.[23]

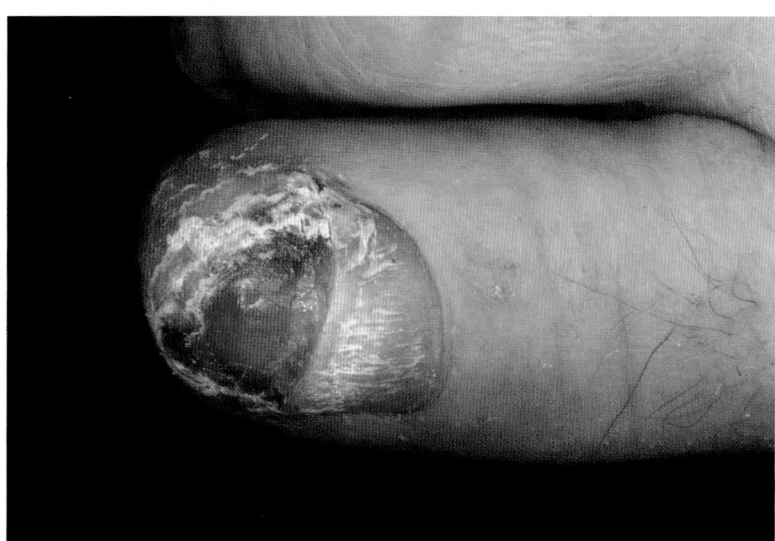

Fig. 23.40
Invasive melanoma: this example is amelanotic. Courtesy of J. Van Geertruyden, MD, Hôpital Erasme, Université Libre de Bruxelles, Belgium.

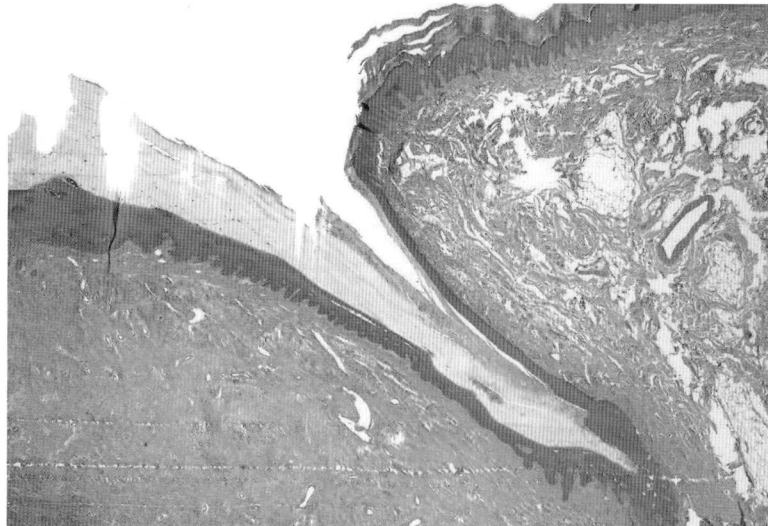

Fig. 23.41
In situ melanoma: scanning view showing nail matrix.

Amelanotic melanoma

Amelanotic melanoma of the nail apparatus represents 20% to 30% of lesions compared with less than 7% in other cutaneous melanomas.[24] It usually presents as a chronic paronychia, a torpid granulomatous ulceration, a wartlike keratotic tumor, or a pyogenic granuloma-like lesion (*Fig. 23.40*). Clinical misdiagnosis is particularly common in amelanotic melanoma.[25] Four cases of in situ amelanotic melanoma have been described: three presented as lichenoid nail alterations and one as an erythronychia. [26,27]

Pathogenesis and histologic features

There is no demonstrable link between the development of subungual melanoma and excessive exposure to ultraviolet light. Although trauma is commonly reported in patients with these tumors, its role in pathogenesis has not been conclusively established.[8]

In situ melanoma

In situ melanoma usually arises in the nail matrix from where it can extend to the ventral part of the PNF or to the nail bed. It is characterized by an increased number of melanocytes in the basal cell layer. In a study published in 2008, the mean number of melanocytes was 58.9 per 1 mm stretch of epithelial-stromal junction (range, 39–136) compared with 15.3 (range, 5–31) for benign melanocytic hyperplasia.[28] Because of the distribution of matrix melanocytes, nail apparatus melanoma may also arise from suprabasal melanocytes with atypical melanocytes predominating in the lower third of the matrix epithelium and contrasting with sparse basal melanocytes.[29] In in situ melanoma, single melanocytes predominate over nests in most fields but rare small nests are often present.[22,28,30] Nuclear atypia is evident, as is pagetoid spread (*Figs 23.41* and *23.42*). In early lesions, the atypia is often focal and moderate, as is the pagetoid spread.

Scattered atypical melanocytes with hyperchromatic nuclei are a clue to the diagnosis.[31] In more advanced lesions, a confluence of single cells is observed, nuclear atypia is more marked, and pagetoid spread can be florid. Most cases are diagnosed as acral lentiginous melanoma. Elongation of the rete ridges is usually less marked than in similar lesions on the palms and soles. Melanocytes are both spindled and epithelioid, and some have long pigmented dendrites.[32] 'Tumor-infiltrating lymphocytes' have been described as a clue to the diagnosis,[8] but this is not confirmed by other authors.[31,33]

Hutchinson sign

Hutchinson sign corresponds to the lateral extension of a nail melanoma onto the periungual tissue (PNF, hyponychium, and digital pulp or lateral nail folds). It is malignant by definition.[34] Although it is tempting for the clinician to take the biopsy from the periungual skin, this is unwise since the histologic appearances can be falsely reassuring. In this lateral part of

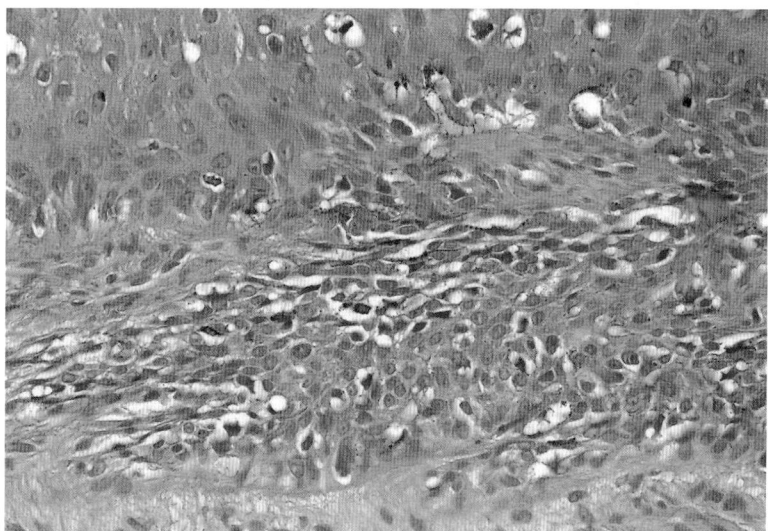

Fig. 23.42
In situ melanoma: basally and suprabasally located atypical melanocytes with surrounding halo are present. The crowded appearance in the lower field results from tangentional sectioning.

the melanoma, histologic alterations frequently only consist of mild atypical melanocytic hyperplasia with rare melanocytic pagetoid spread. It sometimes only reveals epidermal hyperpigmentation.

Invasive melanoma

Invasive melanoma is characterized by atypical melanocytes infiltrating the dermis (*Figs 23.43–23.45*). Even if in situ melanoma starts in the nail matrix, dermal invasion tends to occur first in the nail bed dermis.[35,36] Subungual melanoma with an intraepithelial component is often diagnosed as an acral lentiginous variant but many cases show overlapping features with superficial spreading melanoma.[8] Indeed, marked acanthosis, elongation of the rete ridges, and lentiginous proliferation of atypical melanocytes typical of acral lentiginous melanoma are usually observed in thin subungual lesions. With increasing thickness, junctional tumor cell nests develop, with pagetoid spread of individual melanocytes and sometimes also nests of tumor cells.[37]

In nodular melanoma, the gross appearance varies from a large fungating mass to rather small inconspicuous lesions.[38] By definition, there is no intraepithelial growth of tumor cells beyond the adjacent lateral three rete ridges.

In nail apparatus melanoma, the histogenic type, Clark level, and Breslow thickness are more difficult to assess than in comparable skin lesions because the biopsies are often partial and because of the unique nail

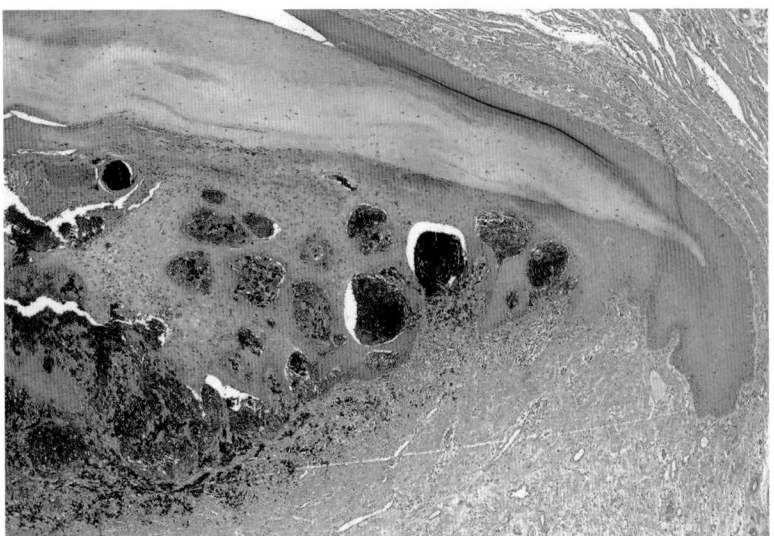

Fig. 23.43
Invasive melanoma: low-power view showing large pigmented nests within the epithelium. Note the lymphocytic infiltrate in the underlying dermis (a useful diagnostic clue) and the conspicuous melanophages.

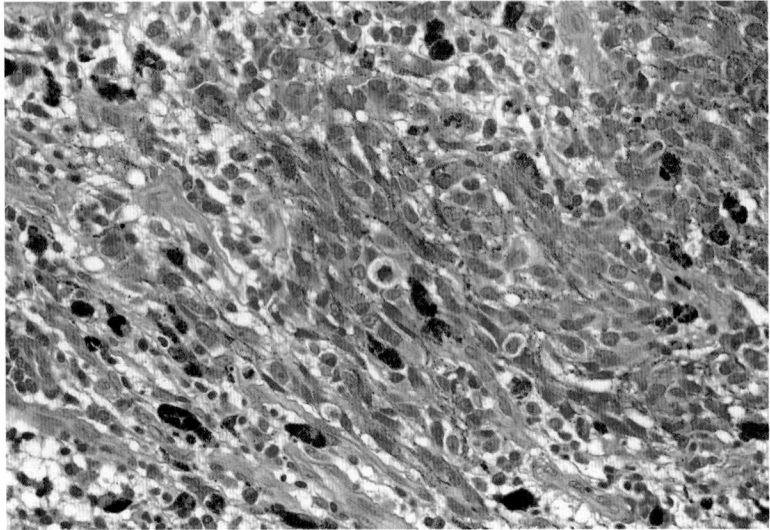

Fig. 23.44
Invasive melanoma: high-power view of the invasive component showing spindled cells and a central mitotic figure.

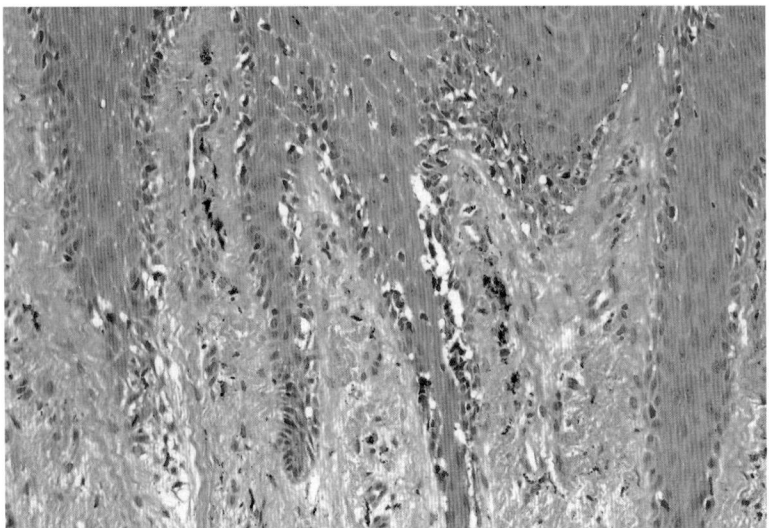

Fig. 23.45
Invasive melanoma: in situ changes are evident in the adjacent epithelium.

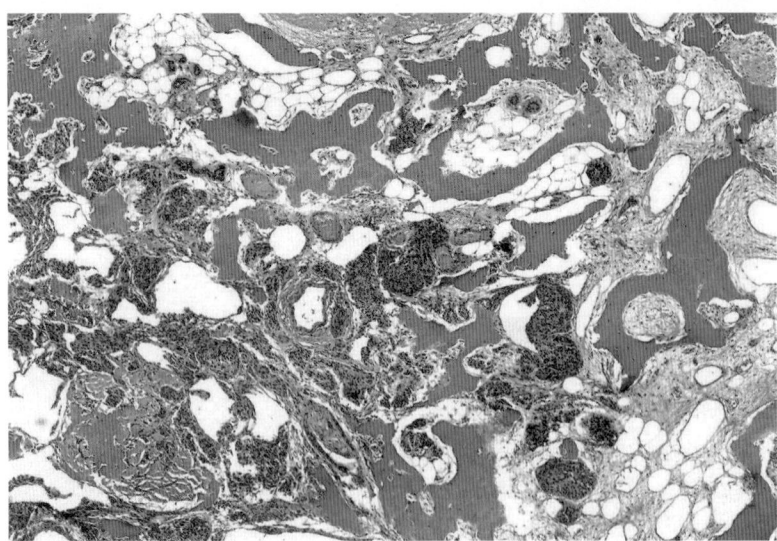

Fig. 23.46
Metaplastic melanoma: this example shows extensive malignant osteoid. Courtesy of Z. Tannous, MD, Massachusetts General Hospital, Boston, USA.

anatomy. Equally, the accurate definition of the junction between papillary and reticular dermis can be problematical. In addition, in most cases there is no adipose tissue between the nail bed and periosteum.[39] This is why it has been suggested that melanoma extending to the periosteum or invading the underlying bone should be classified as Clark level V.[8,38] Concerning Breslow thickness, there is usually no granular layer in the nail matrix and nail bed. The epithelium is often markedly acanthotic, thereby giving a false measurement of tumor thickness.[38] A simple classification of Breslow thickness of ≤2.5 or >2.5 mm has produced different survival curves.[8] In an English series of 105 patients, the mean Breslow thickness was 4.8 mm. The 5-year survival was 88% for Breslow thickness of 2.5 mm or less, and 40% for melanomas greater than 2.5 mm.[1] Other clinicopathological features that have been found to correlate with adverse prognosis in subungual melanoma include advanced age at diagnosis, high number of dermal mitoses, tumor-associated ulceration, amelanotic tumors, and higher stage of disease.[8] In a large Australian retrospective study published in 2007, 9% of cases were in situ acral lentiginous melanoma, the commonest histogenic subtype of invasive melanoma was acral lentiginous (67%), followed by nodular (25%) and desmoplastic (7%).[8] The majority of tumors were locally advanced at presentation with 79% being Clark level IV or V. The median Breslow thickness was 3.2 mm. The median mitotic rate was 3 per mm² and 33% of cases demonstrated tumor ulceration.[8] In this study, the AJCC (American Joint Committee on Cancer melanoma staging system) staging[40] at diagnosis was the most significant predictor of survival to the exclusion of all other variables. Sentinel lymph node biopsy has been reported to be positive in 17% to 24% of patients.[8,41]

Fifteen cases of melanoma with osteocartilaginous differentiation (metaplastic melanoma) have been reported (*Fig. 23.46*), 53% of which were subungual melanomas.[42]

Immunohistochemistry

Limited data have been published about the role of immunohistochemistry in nail apparatus melanoma. In an in situ lesion, HMB-45 has been shown to be the best method for detecting nail apparatus melanocytes.[43] Similarly, in another study of nine cases of in situ acral lentiginous melanoma including four subungual lesions, strong positive staining with HMB-45 was seen while S100 protein was only weakly positive or even negative in the atypical melanocytes.[32]

In our experience of nail melanocytic lesions, immunochemistry is particularly useful for the diagnosis of early melanomas and for the determination of the margins in acral lentiginous tumors. When dealing with intraepithelial melanocytes, the sensitivity is better with HMB-45 than with Mart-1 (Melan A). S100 protein is the least valuable. However, in invasive subungual melanoma, S100 protein is the most sensitive and was the only positive marker in cases of desmoplastic melanoma and in foci of chondroid differentiation.[44] Nuclear markers such as microphtalmia transcription factor and Sox-10 give a more precise quantification of melanocytes as the dendrites are not highlighted and can be more helpful in determining localization of the melanocyte within the matrix.[45]

Genetics

In acral melanoma, mutations in BRAF occur in only 15% of the cases. Activating mutations or amplifications of wild type KIT are found in 15% to 40% and approximately 15% have NRAS mutations. A unique feature is the high frequency of gene amplifications throughout the genome, with amplifications already present in the early phases of the disease.[46] A recent fluorescent in situ hybridization (FISH) analysis of seven cases of nail melanoma shows multiple abnormalities, including gain of RREB1, CCND1, and MYC. Loss of CDKN2A appears less common.[47]

Differential diagnosis

Firm diagnosis of melanoma is often problematic in nail biopsy specimens because the tissue fragment(s) are often tiny. In addition, nail apparatus melanoma is rare and few pathologists have significant experience in this field. Moreover, absolute criteria for the diagnosis in early lesions have not been agreed upon.[24]

It is often a difficult challenge to differentiate very early melanoma from benign conditions.[29] Criteria to differentiate in situ melanoma from lentigo have recently been suggested but require validation. Features include high melanocyte density, melanocyte multinucleation, multifocal pagetoid spread, cytological atypia, and/or the presence of a moderately dense lichenoid inflammatory infiltrate. It is equally important, however, not to overinterpret focal pagetoid spread as this is commonly seen in benign nail lesions.[28] In nevi, nests usually predominate over single melanocytes, while the reverse is true for in situ melanoma. If the intraepithelial component of the melanoma is lacking, immunohistochemistry may be necessary to differentiate an amelanotic melanoma, and especially a desmoplastic variant,[48] from epithelial or mesenchymal tumors.

When assessing small biopsies, the possibility of nonrepresentative sampling should always be considered and should be clearly stated in the report. A further biopsy should always be considered if clinically appropriate.[8]

NONMELANOCYTIC TUMORS OF THE NAIL APPARATUS

Epithelial tumors

Subungual epidermoid cysts

There are two main types of subungual epidermoid cysts[1]:
- *Epidermoid implantation cyst* is usually secondary to heavy or penetrating trauma with implantation of epidermis into the subcutaneous tissue, or even into the bone with associated osteolysis. It may be observed after inadequate wedge excision for ingrowing nails and implantation of matrix epithelium. Histopathology shows a simple epidermoid and/or 'onycholemmal' (matrix) cyst filled with orthokeratin and lined by a thin epithelium.[2]
- *Subungual epidermoid inclusion cysts* are mainly observed in the thumb or great toenail. Histologically, they are similar to implantation epidermoid cyst but are microscopic in size and usually an incidental histologic finding in a nail presenting with subungual hyperkeratosis and a shortened dystrophic nail plate. They have also been observed in pincer nails, clubbed nails, and even in normal nails. Subungual epidermoid inclusions frequently occur in the nail bed or distal nail matrix and result from bulbous proliferation of the rete ridges with cyst formation (*Fig. 23.47*). They contain homogeneous keratin without a granular layer.[3] Calcification may sometimes be observed. These cysts represent a benign, probably reactive, process.[1, 4, 5]

Onychopapilloma

Clinical features

Onychopapilloma is a frequent benign neoplasm of the nail bed and distal matrix. The lesion prevails on fingers; most patients are middle-aged. It presents as a longitudinal discoloration (longitudinal erythronychia or leukonychia or melanonychia) with splinter hemorrhages, distal onycholysis, or fissuring overlying a subungual hyperkeratosis. In a recent paper, the most common clinical presentation was longitudinal erythronychia ($n = 25$); longitudinal leukonychia ($n = 7$); longitudinal melanonychia ($n = 4$); long splinter hemorrhages without erythronychia, leukonychia, or melanonychia ($n = 8$); and short splinter hemorrhages without erythronychia, leukonychia or melanonychia ($n = 3$), with subungual mass ($n = 47$) and distal fissuring ($n = 11$) (*Fig. 23.48*).[1]

Dermoscopy of the free edge of the nail plate shows a small subungual keratotic mass where the band reaches the nail plate margin, which represents a useful clue to the diagnosis.[1]

Pathological features

The etiology of onychopapilloma is unknown, but possible relevant factors include local trauma and/or true benign neoplastic process.[2]

Pathology reveals papillomatous acanthosis arising from the distal part of the matrix and spreading to the distal part of the nail bed, longitudinal canaliform deformity of the ventral nail plate, matrix-like metaplasia of the nail bed, and distal subungual hyperkeratosis (*Fig. 23.49*).[3]

Multinucleated epithelial cells with 2 to 20 nuclei may be observed. Onychopapilloma with multinucleated cells was originally described as 'localized multinucleate distal subungual keratosis'.[4]

Differential diagnosis

The diagnosis of onychopapilloma may be difficult when the nail plate had been avulsed and put back in place during the surgical longitudinal excision, with most of the lesion remaining attached to the nail plate.[5]

Pathological examination of localized (isolated) longitudinal erythronychia may reveal onychopapilloma but also a glomus tumor.[6] More rarely, warty dyskeratoma,[7] benign vascular proliferations, lichen planus,[8]

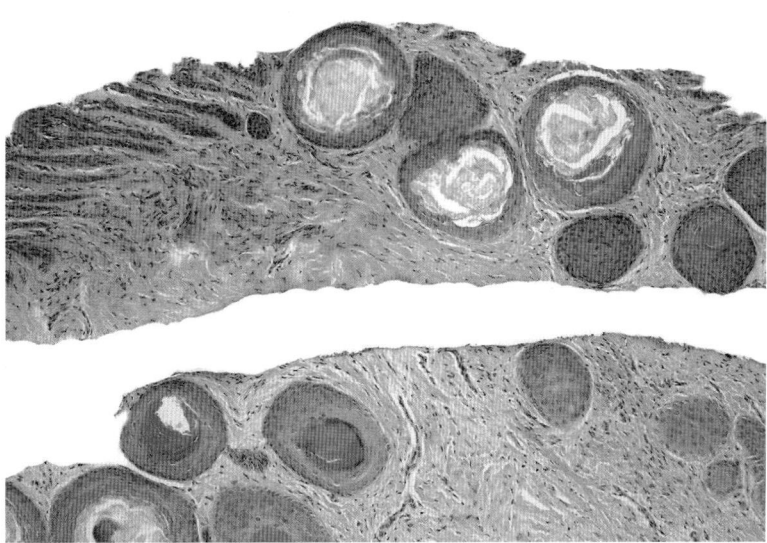

Fig. 23.47
Subungual epidermoid inclusions: numerous small inclusion cysts are present.

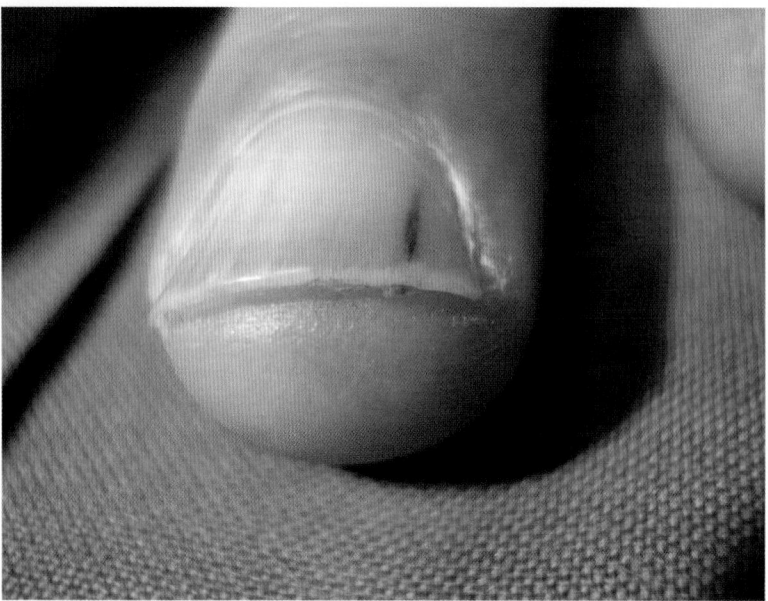

Fig. 23.48
Onychopapilloma: long splinter hemorrhages and distal subungual hyperkeratosis.
Courtesy of B. Richert, MD, PhD, Université Libre de Bruxelles, Belgium.

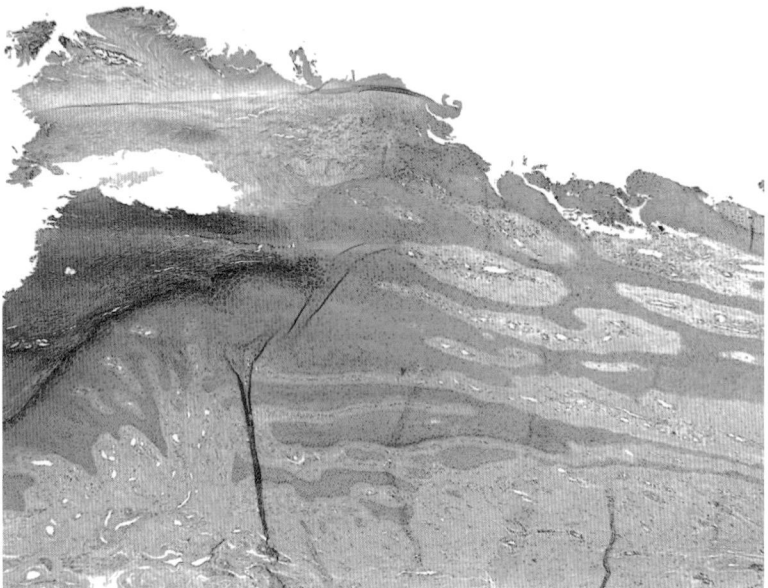

Fig. 23.49
Onychopapilloma: distal subungual hyperkeratosis and marked nail bed papillomatosis. The nail plate had been avulsed during surgery.

amelanotic melanoma,[9] or basal cell carcinoma[10] causing longitudinal erythronychia have been reported.[11,12]

Nail matrix and nail bed acanthoma

Ten cases of onychocytic matricoma (acanthoma of the nail matrix producing onychocytes)[1–3] and rarer cases of acanthoma of the distal matrix and nail bed have been described (pigmented cornified acanthoma of the nail bed or ungual seborrheic keratosis).[4–8]

It presents as a localized longitudinal band characterized by black pigmentation or yellow discoloration. In onychocytic matricoma, the nail plate is also slightly thickened.

On pathological examination, onychocytic matricoma resembles an irritated seborrheic keratosis, with an endophytic proliferation of primarily basaloid cells and several zones displaying squamous eddies. However, the squamous eddies are composed of larger pale pink cells arranged in

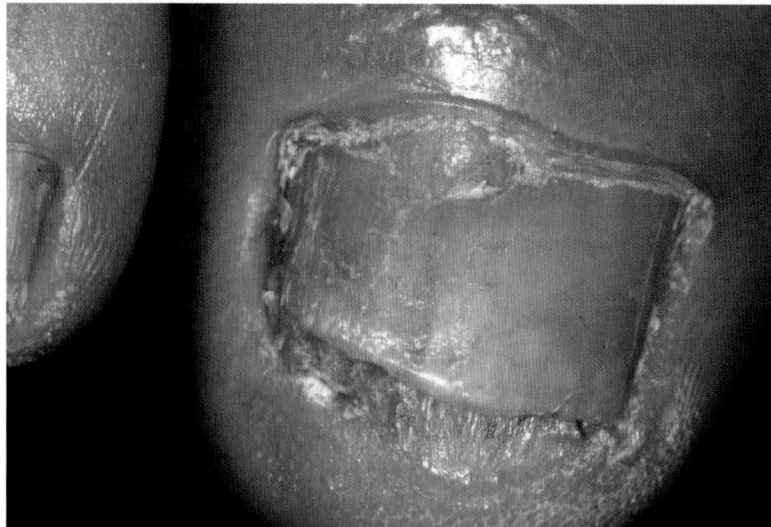

Fig. 23.50
Keratoacanthoma: the tumor is located in the proximal part of the nail apparatus. There is painful paronychia and focal nail plate destruction.

an onion ring fashion, representing the matrix prekeratogenous zone, with central eosinophilic collections representing the matrix keratogenous zone. There are only minimal dermal changes. In nail bed acanthoma, the pathological appearance is very close to an acanthotic seborrheic keratosis with or without horn cysts.

Subungual (distal digital) keratoacanthoma

Clinical features

Subungual keratoacanthoma is a rare variant of keratoacanthoma. It has a predilection for the thumb, index, and middle fingers. It is more frequently observed in males with an age range of 28–76 years.[1] Characteristically, it is a rapidly growing tumor (within a period of weeks), always painful and located in the distal part of the nail bed. Partial onycholysis precedes the appearance of a keratotic crusted nodule. The distal digit is sometimes erythematous and edematous. More rarely, the lesion affects the PNF and may cause a painful paronychia (Fig. 23.50).[1] Radiological examination reveals a well-circumscribed osteolytic area, with no sclerosis or periosteal reaction. It results from pressure erosion. Spontaneous regression is uncommon. Multiple subungual keratoacanthomas have been described as a late manifestation of incontinentia pigmenti in which case they present almost exclusively in females. These are also named subungual tumors of incontinentia pigmenti.[2,3]

Pathogenesis and pathological features

The pathogenesis of subungual keratoacanthoma is poorly understood. The role of trauma, oncogenic HPV, and exposure to steel wool has been inconclusively reported.[1,4,5] The presence of many dyskeratotic cells in the subungual tumors of incontinentia pigmenti may result from increased apoptosis. Interestingly, incontinentia pigmenti is due to mutations in the NEMO gene involved in the regulation of apoptosis.[3]

Microscopic examination shows a squamoproliferative lesion with a focal crateriform growth pattern and overlying hyperkeratosis with ortho- and parakeratosis (Fig. 23.51). It is characterized by lobules of squamous epithelium composed of large keratinocytes with copious 'glassy' eosinophilic cytoplasm and numerous dyskeratotic cells (Fig. 23.52). A peripheral rim of basophilic keratinocytes is present. Cellular atypia and mitotic figures are rare. An infiltrative growth pattern is absent.[6] Onycholemmal keratinization (without a granular cell layer) is frequently seen in the center of the lobules. The histologic features have the same general configuration as keratoacanthoma elsewhere, but tend to be more vertically oriented and exhibit more dyskeratotic cells, fewer neutrophils and eosinophils, and little or no fibrosis at their base.[7]

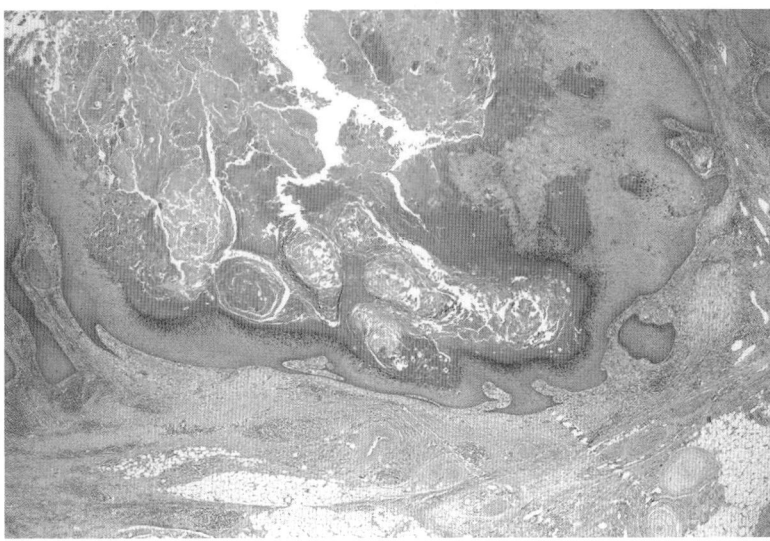

Fig. 23.51
Keratoacanthoma: scanning view. Note the keratin-filled crater.

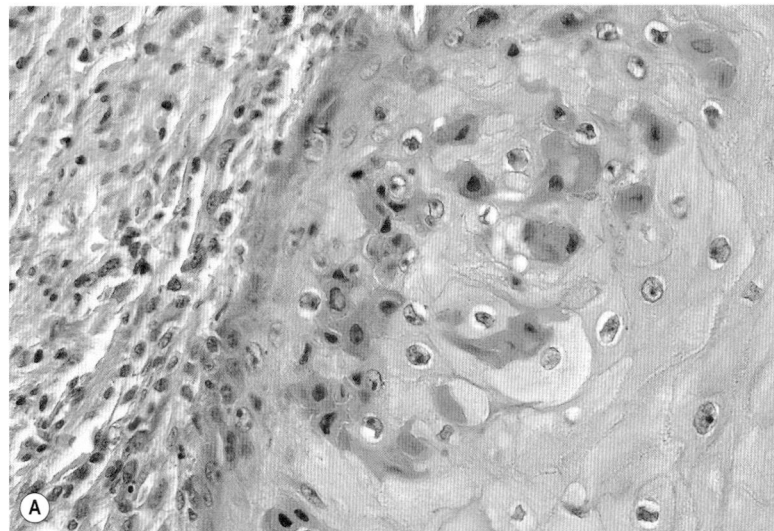

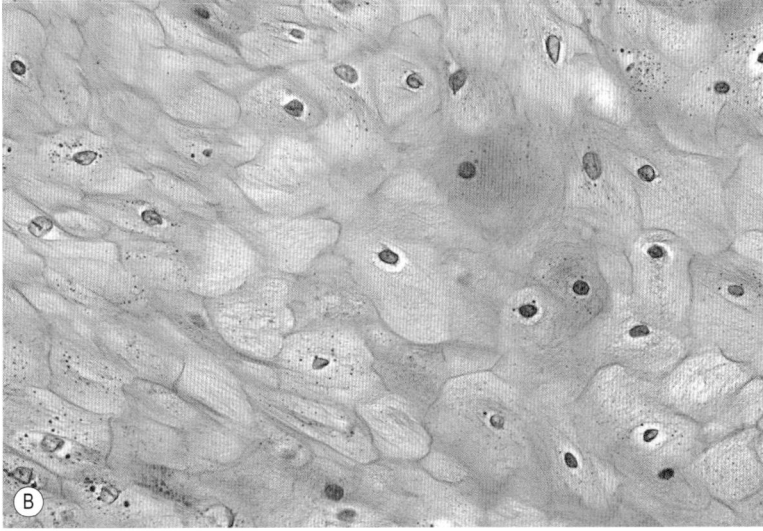

Fig. 23.52
(**A**, **B**) Keratoacanthoma: high-power view of differentiated squamous epithelium. There is no cytological atypia. Dyskeratotic cells are conspicuous.

Differential diagnosis

The diagnosis of subungual keratoacanthoma should be based on correlation between clinical, radiological, and pathological findings. Subungual keratoacanthoma must be differentiated from invasive subungual squamous cell carcinoma (SCC) and verrucous carcinoma in order to avoid unnecessary amputation (see below).

Basal cell carcinoma

Clinical features

Basal cell carcinoma arising in the nail unit is very rare, with fewer than 25 cases reported.[1] Average age at diagnosis is 66.3 years. The lesion occurs almost three times as often on the fingers, mainly the thumb, than on the toes.[2] It has a slight predilection for males.[3] Nail plate involvement (including two cases with longitudinal melanonychia) was observed in about 50% of cases. Involvement of the periungual folds and ulceration are common findings. The tumor may clinically mimic chronic paronychia, pyogenic granuloma, SCC, amelanotic melanoma, trauma, mycotic or bacterial infection, and eczema. Duration prior to diagnosis has ranged from 1 to 40 years.[1] Correct diagnosis requires a biopsy.

Histologic features

Basal cell carcinoma of the nail unit has histologic features identical to those of skin lesions occurring elsewhere. Superficial, nodular, cystic, pigmented, and infiltrative variants have been reported.[1]

Squamous cell or epidermoid carcinoma of the nail apparatus

Clinical features

In situ SCC (Bowen disease) and invasive SCC are the most common neoplasms of the nail apparatus.[1]

SCC has been reported in individuals between 13 and 90 years, the incidence being highest in the 50–69 year range.[2,3] There is a male predominance (ratio 2:1).[4] Fingernails, particularly right index and right long fingers, are significantly more frequently affected than toenails.[4] The tumor grows slowly and the duration from onset to the time of diagnosis varies from several months to 30 years.[3] In a large recent series, the commonest clinical signs were subungual hyperkeratosis, onycholysis, oozing, and nail plate destruction (*Fig. 23.53*). Most cases were of the warty type.[4] These misleading clinical appearances are frequently responsible for delayed diagnosis.

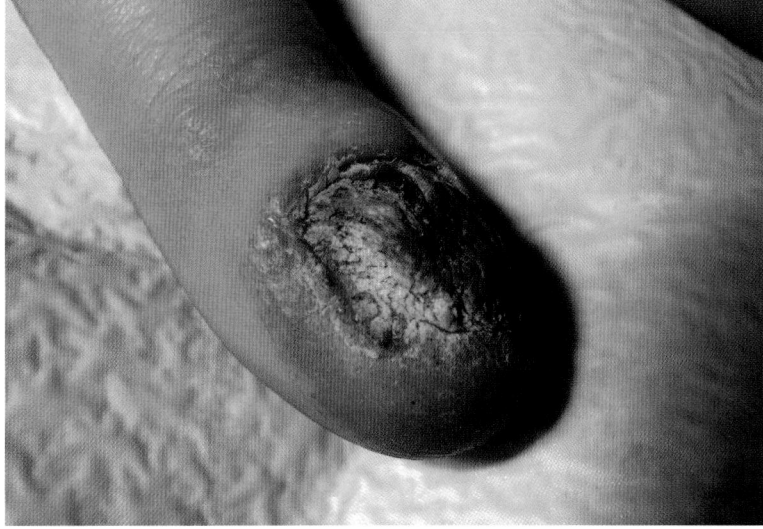

Fig. 23.53
In situ squamous cell carcinoma: the nail has been replaced by a warty lesion.

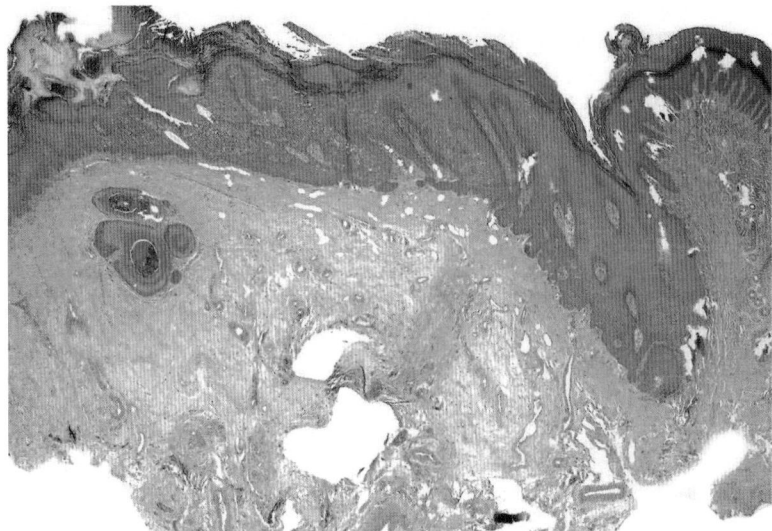

Fig. 23.54
In situ squamous cell carcinoma: the epithelium is thickened and even at this magnification there is obvious atypia.

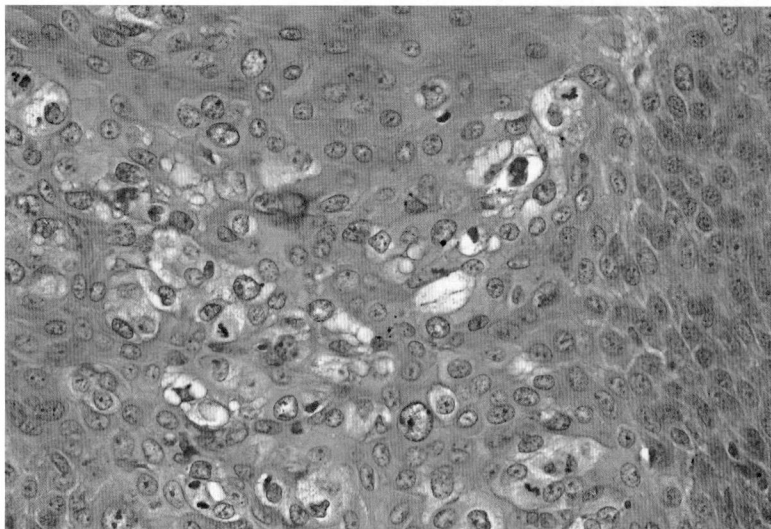

Fig. 23.55
In situ squamous cell carcinoma: high-power view showing pleomorphism and mitotic activity.

Over the past years, in situ SSC of the nail apparatus has become the focus of interest for several reasons[3]:

- increasing awareness of its frequency and of its potential polydactylous involvement,[1,5]
- identification of new clinical presentations such as longitudinal melanonychia,[6] fibrokeratoma-like growth,[2,7,8] longitudinal erythronychia,[9] and pigmented onychomatricoma-like features,[10]
- the discovery of genital oncogenic HPV as an etiological factor.

Although the presence of ulceration, bleeding, or nodule formation usually indicates that the carcinoma is invasive,[11] in situ and invasive epidermoid carcinomas of the nail unit are often difficult to differentiate clinically. Localized pain may be noted[11] but is usually absent.[12] Bone involvement is seen in less than 20% of patients[3] with invasive SCC of the nail apparatus and is characterized by periosteal thickening and reactive sclerosis of the underlying bone, due to a protracted course.[13] Metastases are rare.[4,6,14]

In a series published in 2007, SCC was suspected at first medical examination in only 29% of cases. Onychomycosis and warts were the most frequent causes of diagnoses. When mycological cultures were made, they were found positive in one-third of cases, adding to the confusion.[12] The key to diagnosis is histologic examination, which requires an appropriate surgical biopsy.

Pathogenesis and histologic features

Oncogenic genital HPVs (mainly HPV 16) have been reported in about 60% to 80% of in situ or invasive SCC of the nail apparatus.[3,6,14] The possibility of genital-digital transmission has been suggested. X-rays, arsenic, trauma, chronic paronychia, and dyskeratosis congenita are other etiological factors.[3]

The histologic features of Bowen disease of the nail unit are identical to those of Bowen diseases of the skin. Depending on the clinical presentation, the lesion may be located in the nail matrix, the nail bed, and the periungual grooves and folds. Histologic changes frequently extend beyond the area clinically involved, and specimen margins are often involved. The epithelium is irregularly thickened and disorganized, and shows impaired maturation. Dyskeratotic cells, atypical keratinocytes with large, irregularly shaped nuclei, and necrotic keratinocytes are observed as well as scattered mitotic figures (Figs 23.54 and 23.55). Koilocytes may be observed. Histologic diagnosis is usually easy, but early lesions with only slight architectural disorganization, rare dyskeratotic cells, and mild to moderate atypia may be challenging.

Although SCC in situ has a greater likelihood to become invasive in the nail unit than at other skin sites, invasive nail carcinoma is less likely to metastasize.[15] Invasive SCC of the nail apparatus has identical features to that seen in the skin elsewhere but is rarely extensively described (Figs 23.56

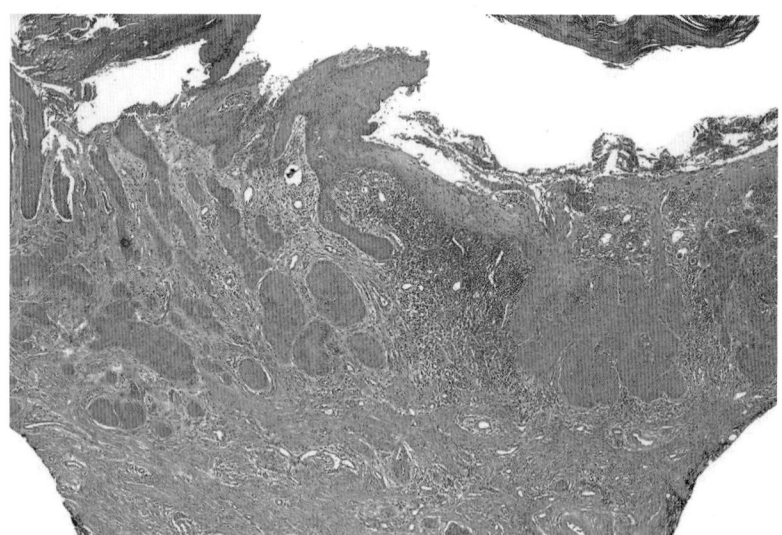

Fig. 23.56
Invasive squamous cell carcinoma: low-power view.

and 23.57).[16] Most appear to arise in pre-existing Bowen disease, which may explain their relatively good prognosis.[11] The depth of invasion, as defined by the distance from the basal layer to the deepest carcinoma cell, ranged from 0.3 to 2.6 mm (mean, 1.1 mm).[12]

Differential diagnosis

Invasive SCC of the nail apparatus should not be confused with subungual epidermoid inclusions, subungual keratoacanthoma, verrucous carcinoma, and malignant onycholemmal tumors. Porocarcinoma[17,18] and metastases[19,20] may also enter the differential diagnosis.

Subungual keratoacanthoma should be diagnosed based on its clinical, radiological, and pathological features (see above). Use of p53 and Ki-67 immunohistochemistry can help distinguish subungual keratoacanthoma from subungual squamous carcinoma. In subungual keratoacanthoma, expression of p53 is rare and, if present, weak, contrasting with the strong diffuse staining in subungual carcinoma. Moreover, in subungual keratoacanthoma, expression of Ki-67 is restricted to the basal and suprabasal layer. In squamous carcinoma, the staining pattern is more diffuse, throughout the tumor mass.[21,22] The nuclear factor kappa B1, which is amplified in keratoacanthoma, could also be used as an aid in diagnosis.[22]

Verrucous carcinoma (carcinoma cuniculatum) is a rare, highly keratinizing, low-grade variant of SCC (Fig. 23.58). Eighteen cases have been

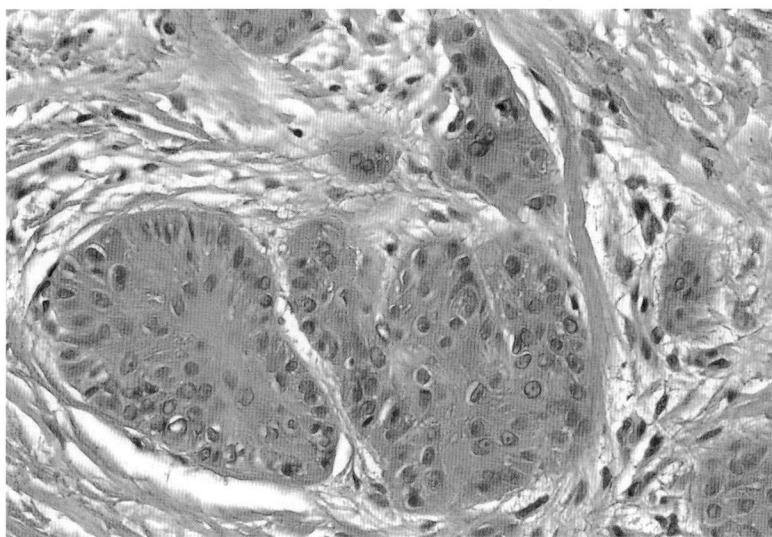

Fig. 23.57
Invasive squamous cell carcinoma: nests of well-differentiated squamous cell carcinoma are present deep in the dermis.

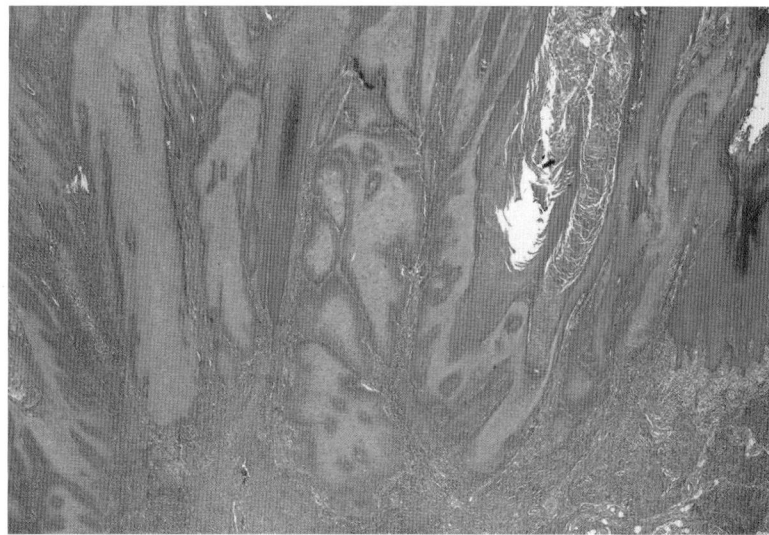

Fig. 23.59
Verrucous carcinoma: low-power view showing the deeply penetrating broad bulbous growth pattern. Courtesy of C. Deprez, MD, Hôpital Brugmann, Université Libre de Bruxelles, Belgium.

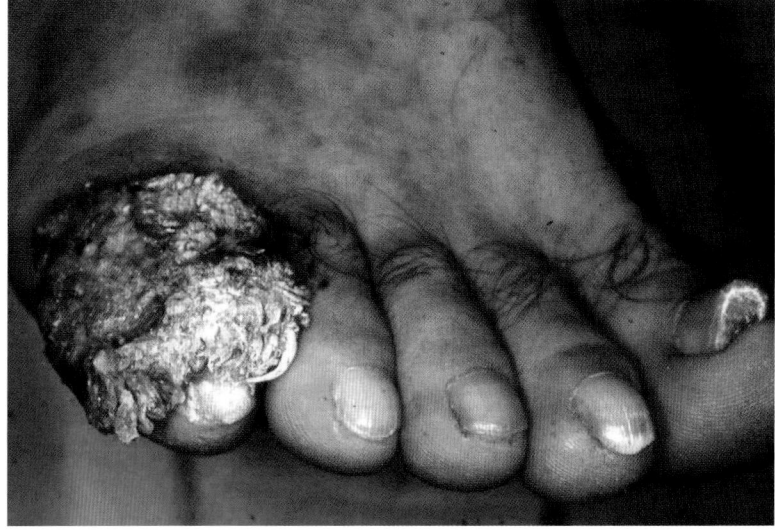

Fig. 23.58
Verrucous carcinoma: typical example showing the warty, hyperkeratotic surface. Courtesy of P. Gheeraert, MD, Hôpital Brugmann, Université Libre de Bruxelles, Belgium.

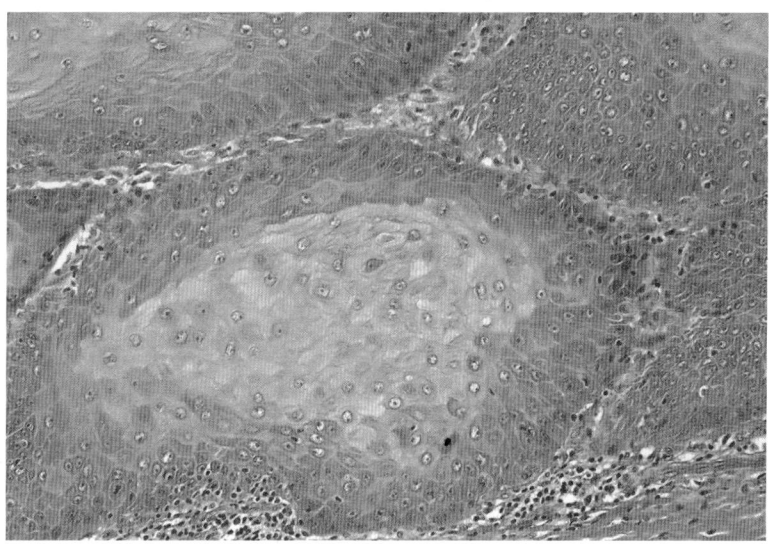

Fig. 23.60
Verrucous carcinoma: high-power view showing typical ground-glass epithelium. Note that there is no cytological atypia. Courtesy of C. Deprez, MD, Hôpital Brugmann, Université Libre de Bruxelles, Belgium.

reported in the nail apparatus.[21-31] The tumor has both exophytic and endophytic components. The epithelium is markedly hyperkeratotic and hypertrophic, with broad bulbous processes extending into the deep dermis (Fig. 23.59). It is composed of large, well-differentiated keratinocytes with ground-glass cytoplasm (Fig. 23.60). Occasional dyskeratotic cells may be seen. Mitoses are few in number and confined to the basal layers.[32]

Eleven cases of malignant subungual onycholemmal tumor have been described, characterized by abrupt (without a granular cell layer) onycholemmal keratinization.[16,33-35] Based on the relative number of onycholemmal cysts and solid lobules of atypical cells, they have been classified as malignant onycholemmal proliferating cyst[33] or onycholemmal carcinoma, respectively.[16,34] The tumors are observed in elderly people and have a long evolution time, with an infiltrative growth pattern. Small squamous pearls and cells exhibiting individual keratinization are lacking[35]. Genuine bone invasion is rare. These tumors may represent an unusual variant of SCC originating from the nail bed epithelium, more precisely the nail isthmus.[16,35]

In subungual metastasis, the most frequent sites of primary tumor are the lung and the genitourinary tract.[19,20]

Fibroepithelial tumors

Onychomatricoma

Clinical features

Onychomatricoma is a rare benign matrix tumor, with distinct clinical and histologic features, first described in 1992 by R. Baran.[1] Similar tumors of the nail matrix have also been reported as 'onychoblastoma', 'unguioblastoma', and 'unguioblastic fibroma'.[2,3] It mainly occurs on fingers, less frequently on toes, with no sex predilection. It usually occurs in Caucasian middle-aged and elderly patients.[4] The lesion is solitary, rarely multiple.[5,6] It is characterized by thickening of the nail plate with pronounced longitudinal ridging, yellow discoloration (xanthonychia) along the entire length of the nail plate, multiple splinter hemorrhages, and a tendency towards transverse overcurvature of the nail (Fig. 23.61). Unusual clinical presentations such as longitudinal melanonychia or pterygium have also been described.[7,8] Surgical excision is the recommended treatment. Recurrence may be observed. Association of onychomatricoma with onychomycosis is not infrequent.[5.]

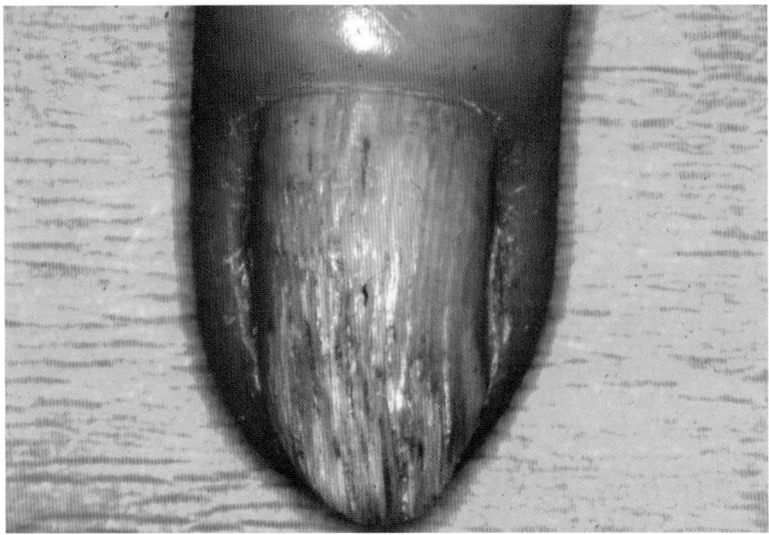

Fig. 23.61
Onychomatricoma: note the thickening of the nail plate with longitudinal ridging, yellow discoloration, and excessive curvature.

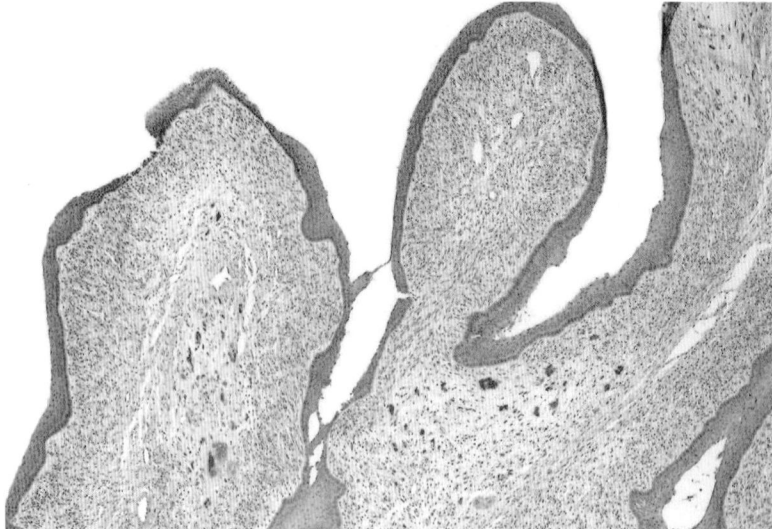

Fig. 23.63
Onychomatricoma: scanning view showing the 'glove finger' papillary projections covered by matrix type epithelium.

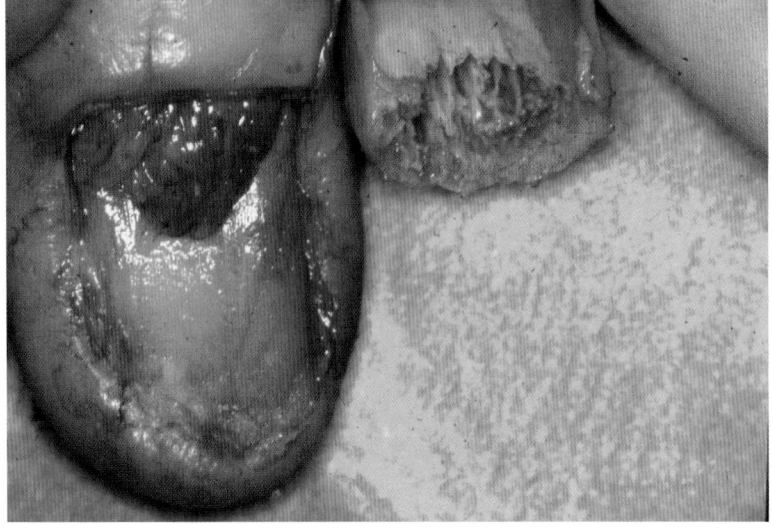

Fig. 23.62
Onychomatricoma: the typical gross appearances are seen after avulsion of the nail plate.

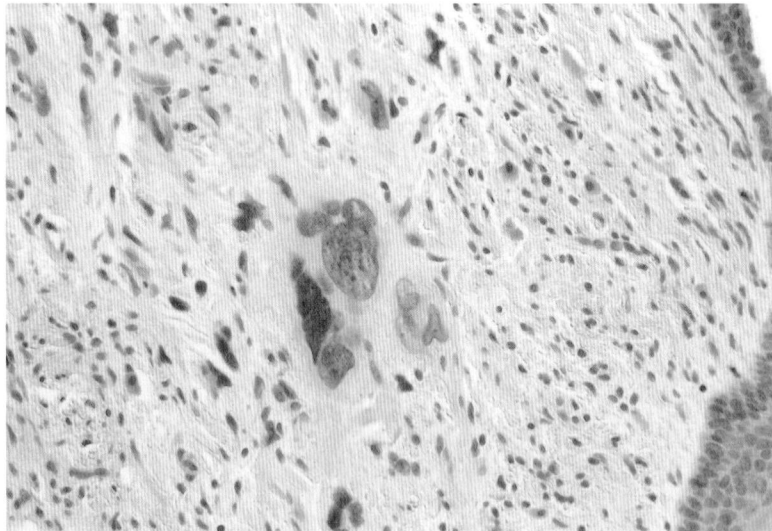

Fig. 23.64
Onychomatricoma: the stroma is highly cellular with marked nuclear pleomorphism. Note the conspicuous mast cells.

Histologic features

Nail avulsion discloses a pedunculated villous tumor of the matrix with characteristic distal digitations extending into multiples holes in the proximal nail plate (*Fig. 23.62*).[9] This results in the thickened funnel-shaped nail plate. Distal nail plate clipping, showing multiple lacunar spaces may be a clue to the diagnosis.[10]

This fibroepithelial tumor has the configuration of an 'anemone', and the histologic features are quite different in the distal and proximal zones of the tumor.

The distal zone is characterized by multiple 'glove finger' papillary projections covered by a matrix-type epithelium which is devoid of stratum granulosum and keratinizes through an eosinophilic keratogenous zone (*Fig. 23.63*).[6,9] The proximal zone, corresponding to the peduncle, is dome-shaped in transverse sections. It is lined by a papillomatous matrix-type epithelium, with vertically oriented deep invaginations into the stroma. These invaginations surround optically empty cavities in a characteristic V-shaped configuration. The recognition of matrix-type epithelium with V-shaped depressions is crucial to make the diagnosis of onychomatricoma on fragmented or incomplete specimens which lack the 'glove finger' papillary projections. The stroma is moderately to highly cellular, composed of CD34

positive fibroblastic cells with random orientation and increased numbers of mast cells. In some cases, cells with bizarre hyperchromatic and pleomorphic nuclei and multinucleated giant cells have been reported (*Fig. 23.64*).[3] The matrix is collagenous, myxocollagenous, or myxoid. In the deeper part of the lesion, the stroma is usually less cellular with thicker collagen bundles oriented around the same horizontal axis. Stromal cells express CD34. In very few cases, CD10, a marker of the onychodermis, was tested and reported diffusely expressed in the stroma.[11–14]

Differential diagnosis

The differential diagnosis includes fibrokeratoma and fibroma of the nail matrix.[15] Both are characterized by the absence of multiple papillary projections and the presence of a granular layer and hyperkeratosis. According to Perrin, the papillomatous type of onychocytic matricoma may mimic onychomatricoma, but displays smaller holes in the nail plate, more basaloid cells and lacks the typical fibrous stroma of onychomatricoma.[16]

Onychomatricoma, especially its proximal part, can also be confused with superficial acral fibromyxoma (AFM; acral fibromyxoma); however, the latter lacks the matrix-type epithelium with characteristic V-shaped invaginations.

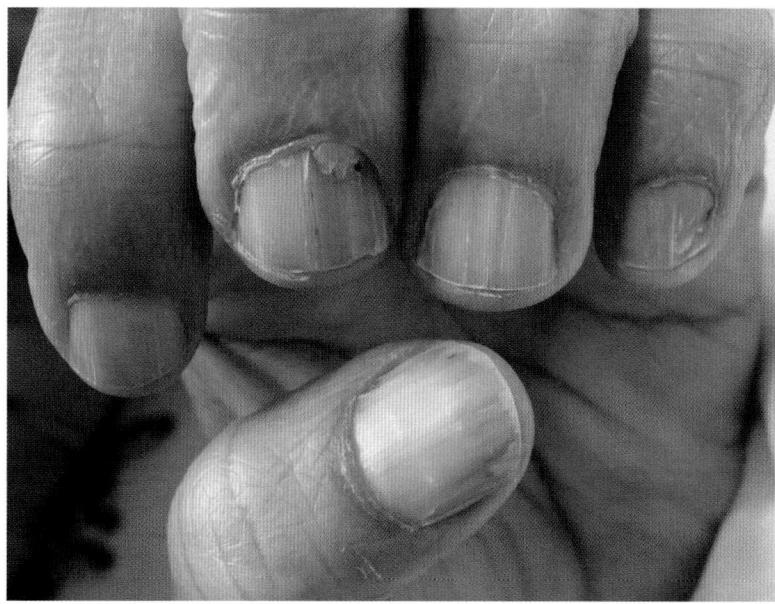

Fig. 23.65
Koenen tumors (tuberous sclerosis): typical lesion emerging from the proximal nail fold of the fourth finger and multiple longitudinal depressions in the fingernails. Courtesy of B. Richert, MD, PhD, Université Libre de Bruxelles, Belgium.

Ungual fibrokeratoma and fibroma

Clinical features

Ungual fibrokeratoma (acquired ungual fibrokeratoma) is mainly observed in males over 50 years of age. It presents as a slowly growing, elongated or oval, flesh-colored lesion with distal hyperkeratosis. It generally measures less than 1 cm. The tumor usually emerges from the ventral part of the PNF, causing a longitudinal depression in the nail plate. Some lesions originate from the matrix, growing therefore into the nail plate. Others originate from the nail bed, leading to onycholysis.[1]

Multiple lesions are usually associated with tuberous sclerosis and are designated as sub- and periungual fibromas or Koenen tumors (*Fig. 23.65*). They can be considered a variant of fibrokeratoma.[1,2,3] They occur in about 50% of the patients with tuberous sclerosis and usually start to grow around puberty or in early adulthood. They progressively increase in number and size, and they are more common on toenails than fingernails.[1,4,5] They rarely present the only clinical manifestation of tuberous sclerosis.[4]

Histologic features

Histologically, no significant difference has been found between isolated ungual fibrokeratoma and Koenen tumors.[2,6]

They are pedunculated fibroepithelial lesions (*Figs 23.66* and *23.67*). The epidermis is hyperkeratotic and acanthotic with thickened, often branching rete ridges. The core of the lesions is composed of fibroblasts and dense collagen fibers, often with vertical orientation. The vascular component is sometimes prominent.

Differential diagnosis

Pleomorphic fibroma has been described at a subungual location. It is characterized by hyperchromatic spindled, pleomorphic, and floret-like giant cells embedded in a collagenous or myxocollagenous matrix.[7,8]

Soft tissue and bone tumors

Superficial acral fibromyxoma

Clinical features

Superficial acral fibromyxoma (SAFM), also called digital fibromyxoma, is a distinct clinicopathological entity, described by Fetsch et al. in 2001.[1]

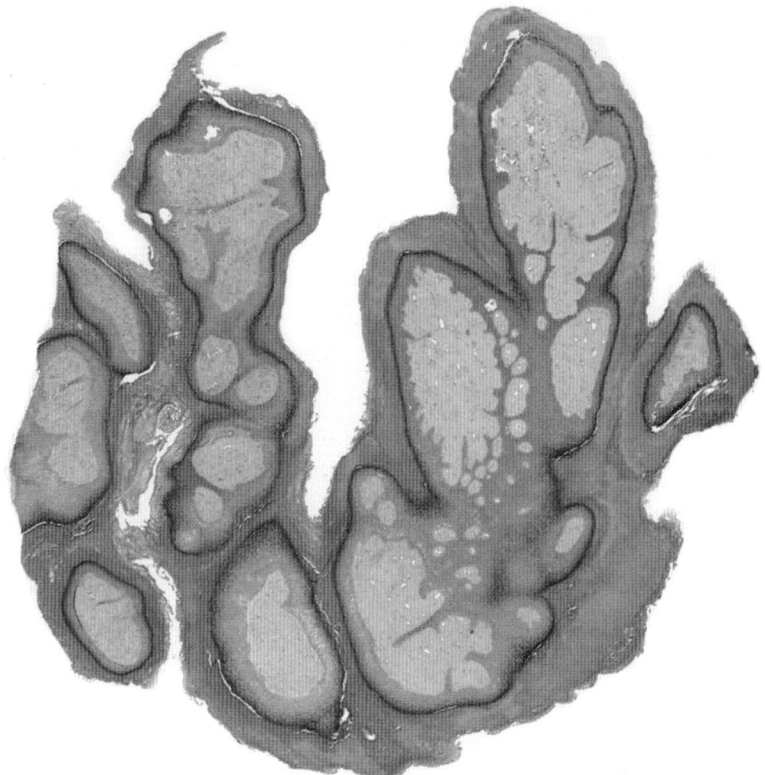

Fig. 23.66
Koenen tumor: scanning view of a hyperkeratotic papillary tumor.

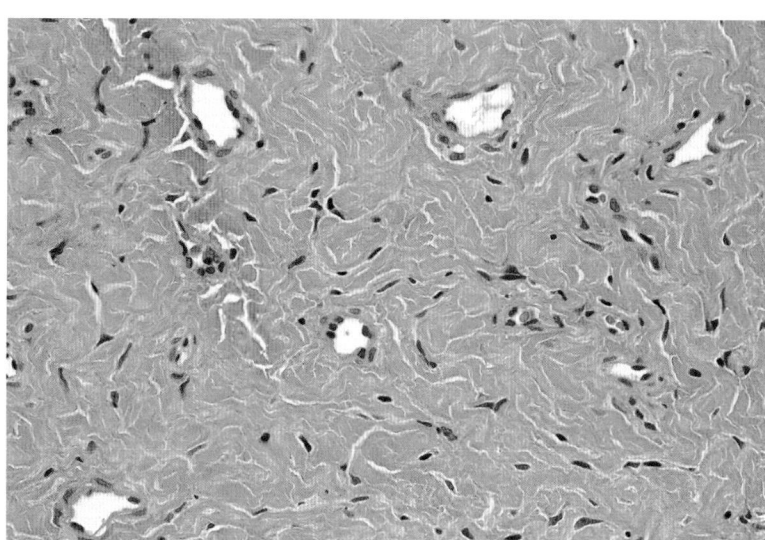

Fig. 23.67
Koenen tumor: high-power view showing the collagenous stroma and spindled tumor cells.

Similar tumors of the nail bed have also been reported as 'cellular digital fibromas'.[2,3]

This neoplasm has a wide age range with a peak incidence in middle-aged adults. It shows a predilection for males and occurs mainly on the fingers and toes, with more than 50% of cases involving the nail bed (*Fig. 23.68*).[4,5] The lesion presents as a solitary, slow-growing, and painless tumor. Erosion of the underlying bone is present in 3% of the cases.

SAFM is a benign tumor, but local recurrences are observed in 24% of the cases with positive margins on initial biopsy. Occasional cases with atypical histologic features (see below) are reported, but this is not associated with aggressive behavior.[6] To date, no tumor has metastasized.[6] Complete excision and follow-up are recommended.

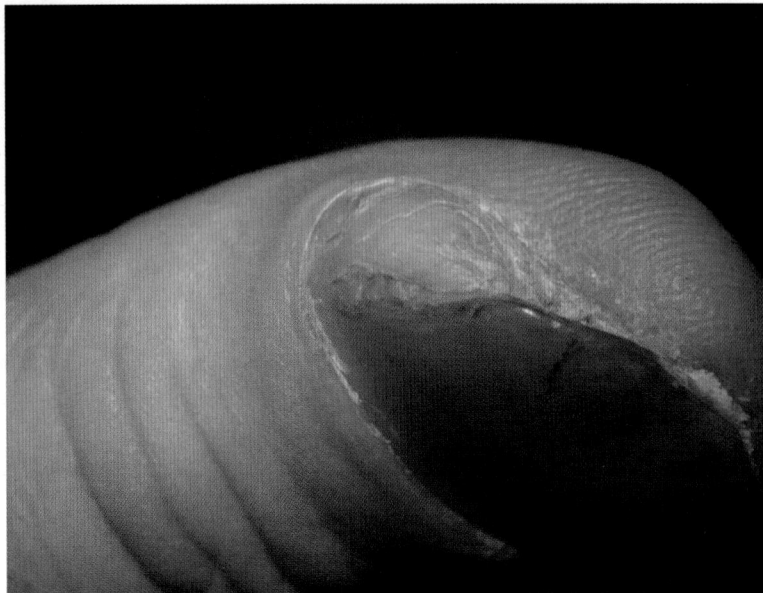

Fig. 23.68
Superficial acral fibromyxoma: lateral subungual tumor, lifting up the nail plate. Courtesy of B. Richert, MD, PhD, Université Libre de Bruxelles, Belgium.

Fig. 23.69
Superficial acral fibromyxoma: fibrous dermal tumor with spindled cells and numerous capillaries.

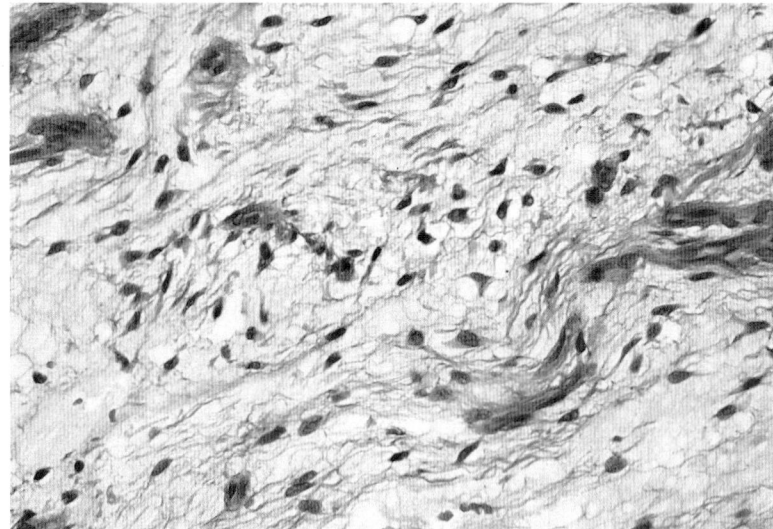

Fig. 23.70
Superficial acral fibromyxoma: high-power view of a sparse population of spindle cells in a myxoid stroma. Courtesy of B. Cavellier-Balloy, MD. Paris, France.

Histologic features

Tumors are dermal and/or subcutaneous, with only rare bone involvement. Lesions can be circumscribed but not encapsulated or ill defined.[1,6] Some tumors have a collarette or are polypoid. A 'grenz zone' is often seen separating the epidermis from the tumor. Lesions are moderately cellular, composed of stellate and spindled cells with pale eosinophilic cytoplasm with random, loose storiform, or fascicular growth patterns. The cells are embedded in a myxoid, myxocollagenous, or collagenous matrix, often with accentuated vasculature and increased numbers of mast cells (*Figs 23.69* and *23.70*). Occasional multinucleated cells can be present, and a lipomatous component has been described in one case that probably represents a spindle cell lipoma.[7] Cartilaginous or osseous metaplasia rarely occurs. Occasional cases present scattered cells with atypical features such as enlarged, irregular, and hyperchromatic nuclei ('degenerative change'). No necrosis, lymphovascular, or perineural invasion is seen.[6]

SAFM appears to be of fibroblastic origin. Immunohistochemically, most of the cases express CD34. CD10 is often positive.[7] CD99 and epithelial membrane antigen (EMA) are rarely expressed. Recently, loss of Rb1 immunoexpression and Rb1 deletion confirmed by FISH have been reported in a few tumors.[8]

Differential diagnosis

The differential diagnosis of SAFM encompasses benign and malignant myxoid and spindle cell tumors showing a predilection for the distal extremities. Myxoid neurofibroma is rare at acral sites and is consistently positive for S100 protein. Sclerosing perineurioma is composed of spindled and epithelioid cells arranged in a whorling pattern within a hyalinized collagenous stroma.[9] It is positive for EMA and sometimes CD34. Superficial angiomyxoma is lobulated and composed of spindled or stellate cells usually admixed with neutrophils in a myxoid matrix with prominent small blood vessels in the background.[10] Myxoid dermatofibrosarcoma protuberans is exceedingly uncommon and almost never occurs on the toes and fingers.[11] It is more infiltrative, usually negative for EMA, and is associated with the t(17;22) translocation. Low-grade fibromyxoid sarcoma does not usually involve the fingers and toes and is characterized by curvilinear vessels, and long fascicles of spindle-shaped cells with mild cytological atypia. The tumor is associated with t(7;16) or t(11;16) translocations[12] and MUC4 is positive in tumor cells, and this is a highly sensitive and relatively specific marker. Myxoinflammatory fibroblastic sarcoma, which has a predilection for subcutaneous soft tissue of the extremities, shows a prominent inflammatory infiltrate and characteristic bizarre tumor cells with vesicular nuclei and inclusion-like nucleoli.[13] The proximal part of onychomatricoma, corresponding to the peduncle, is dome-shaped and its stroma can be very similar to superficial acral fibromyxoma, but onychomatricoma is covered by a characteristic hyperplastic onychogenic epithelium.[14] A rare variant of synovial sarcoma described as minute synovial sarcoma is an important differential diagnosis.[15] These rare lesions of less than 1 cm have a predilection for the hands and feet and may involve the digits but do not tend to involve the nail. Myxoid monophasic examples may be similar to SAFM. However, the former often displays calcifications and tumor cells are usually negative for CD34 and positive not only for EMA but also for keratin and CD99. Cytogenetic analysis demonstrates the t(X;18) translocation.

Myxoid pseudocyst

Clinical features

Myxoid pseudocyst (digital mucous cyst) was initially thought to represent focal myxoid degeneration of connective tissue. However, there is now some evidence to suggest that it results from escape of synovial fluid through a breach in the synovial capsule.[1] It is usually located in the PNF and occurs in middle-aged or elderly patients.[2] It is about 10 times more frequent on the fingers than on the toes. The lesion starts as an asymptomatic swelling which slowly enlarges up to 2 cm. The cyst contains clear viscous fluid. It characteristically causes a longitudinal depression in the nail plate. Lesions can be solitary or multiple and can be job related.[3–5] Subungual location associated with transverse overcurvature of the nail plate has also been reported.[6] Recurrence after incomplete excision is not uncommon.

Histologic features

Myxoid pseudocyst is well circumscribed but unencapsulated dermal and devoid of any lining epithelium. It consists of a large mucin-filled space containing spindle-shaped and stellate fibroblasts without atypia. The mucin contains mucopolysaccharides, which stain positively with Alcian blue and colloidal iron.[7]

Differential diagnosis

Ganglion cyst is usually subcutaneous, and occasionally a connection between the cyst and the underlying joint cavity can be demonstrated.[7] It consists of myxoid spaces incompletely lined by flattened synovial cells and surrounded by a fibrous wall.[8]

Superficial angiomyxoma is larger, lobulated, and characterized by more abundant spindled-shaped and stellate cells, frequent small blood vessels, and collections of neutrophils.[9]

Lobular capillary hemangioma (pyogenic granuloma)

Clinical features

Lobular capillary hemangioma (pyogenic granuloma) is common in ingrowing toenails, where it is thought to be induced by the interaction of the nail plate and the lateral nail fold. Nail plate alterations are sometimes present. It is mostly seen in the early decades and presents as a rapidly growing, painful, ulcerated and bleeding, exophytic tumor.[1] Subungual location has also been reported.[2] There may be local recurrences after excision. Multiple periungual pyogenic granuloma-like lesions may be induced by systemic drugs such as retinoids, ciclosporine, chemotherapeutic agents, and antiretroviral therapies.[3–7]

Histologic features

In many cases, histology reveals a mass of exuberant small vascular channels. The epidermis is hyperplasic and frequently ulcerated. There is a proliferation of capillaries associated with a prominent mixed inflammatory cell infiltrate in the dermis. Neutrophils and plasma cells are usually predominant. The stroma can be loose and edematous or fibrotic in the late stages. Rarely, ungual lesions are polypoid and show a well-developed lobular architecture. The lobules are composed of aggregates of capillaries and venules with or without discernible lumina, lined by plump endothelial cells, and surrounded by a layer of smooth-muscle actin positive pericytes.[8]

Differential diagnosis

In elderly patients or patients with acquired immunodeficiency syndrome, the differential diagnosis encompasses nodular Kaposi sarcoma, which is characterized by a prominent spindle cell component and positivity for human herpesvirus 8.

Glomus tumor

Clinical features

Glomus tumor arises in young adults and is usually located in the distal extremities, with a predilection for the fingers. The single most common site is the subungual region,[1] where a female predominance is observed.[2]

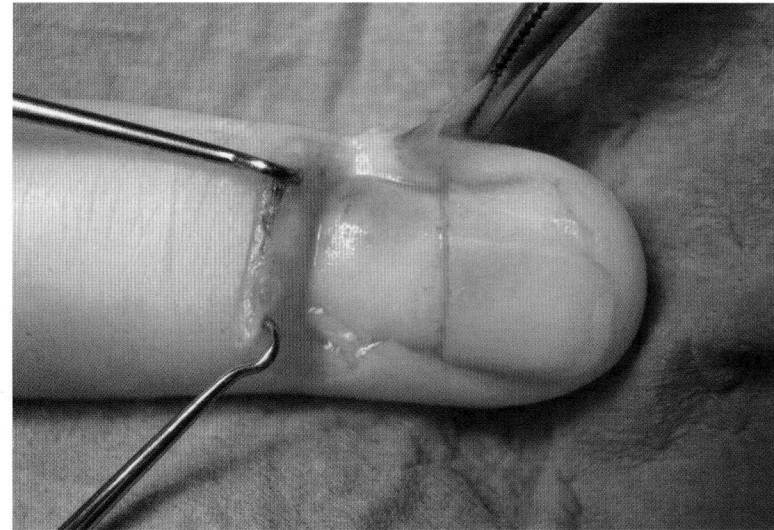

Fig. 23.71
Glomus tumor: there is an ill-defined bluish tumor deep to the proximal nail plate. Courtesy of B. Richert, MD, Université de Liège, Belgium.

The tumors are small (usually less than 1 cm) flesh-colored or red-blue nodules (*Fig. 23.71*), often associated with paroxysmal pain in relation to minor tactile stimulation or cold exposure.[3,4] Nail deformity and osseous defect can be present.[5] The recommended treatment is complete surgical excision. Recurrences are rare.[2]

Pathogenesis and histologic features

Glomus tumor arises from modified smooth muscle cells located in glomus bodies. Multiple familial glomus tumors with an autosomal dominant pattern of inheritance have been linked to inactivating mutations in the glomulin gene.[6,7] In these 'familial glomangioma', the tumors rarely occur in the subungual region[1]. An association between subungual glomus tumors and neurofibromatosis type I has been reported (with *NF1* inactivation or chromosomes copy number change).[8–11] *MIR143-NOTCH* fusions have been described in a series of benign and malignant glomus tumors encompassing some acral lesions.[12] The translocation t(1;5) has been reported in only one case of sporadic tumor.[13]

Glomus tumors are composed of glomus cells, vessels, and smooth muscle cells. According to the relative proportions of these components, they are divided into three groups: 'solid glomus tumor', 'glomangioma', and 'glomangiomyoma'.[11]

Glomus tumor is usually well circumscribed, but some clusters of cells can be observed around vessels outside the main tumor mass. Solid glomus tumor is composed of sheets of glomus cells surrounding capillaries. Glomus cells are uniform and round, with pale eosinophilic cytoplasm and a centrally located round nucleus (*Fig. 23.72*). A basal lamina, highlighted by PAS, surrounds each cell. In glomangioma, the vascular component is prominent and composed of numerous dilated vascular spaces. Glomangiomyoma is characterized by gradual transition from glomus cell to elongated cells resembling mature smooth muscle cells. Glomus tumors are positive for smooth muscle actin and type IV collagen. h-Caldesmon, desmin, and CD34 may also be positive.[4]

Malignant glomus tumors and glomus tumor of uncertain malignant potential are usually not encountered in a subungual location (see Glomus tumor, Chapter 35). Nevertheless, symplastic glomus tumor has been described in the nail apparatus. This benign variant is characterized by high-grade nuclear atypia in the absence of any other malignant features. The atypia is thought to represent a degenerative phenomenon.[14]

Differential diagnosis

The differential diagnosis encompasses eccrine spiradenoma and hidradenoma. Both are characterized by focal ductal differentiation and positivity for epithelial markers.

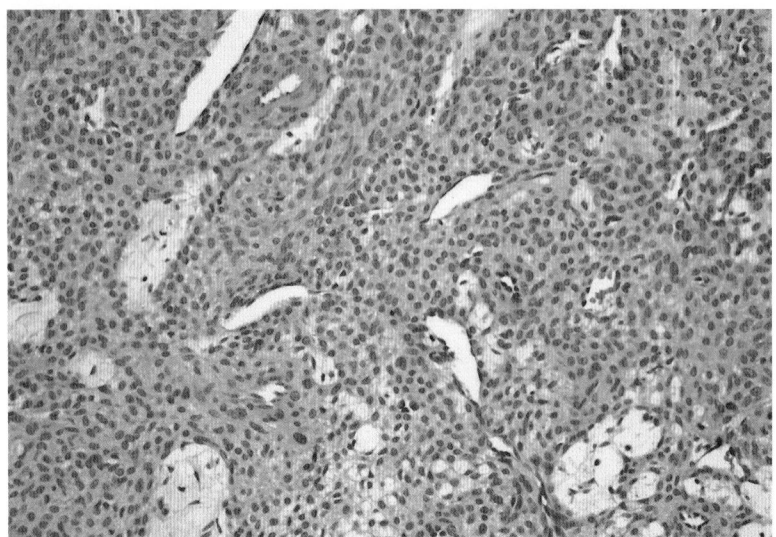

Fig. 23.72
Glomus tumor: medium-power view showing thin-walled dilated vessels surrounded by typical glomus cells.

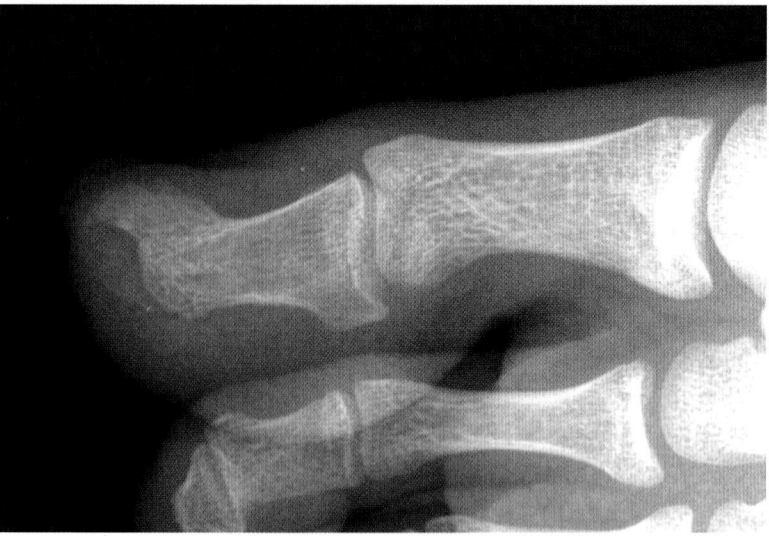

Fig. 23.74
Subungual exostosis: there is an irregular bony tumor deep to the nail plate. Courtesy of B. Richert, MD, PhD, Université Libre de Bruxelles, Belgium.

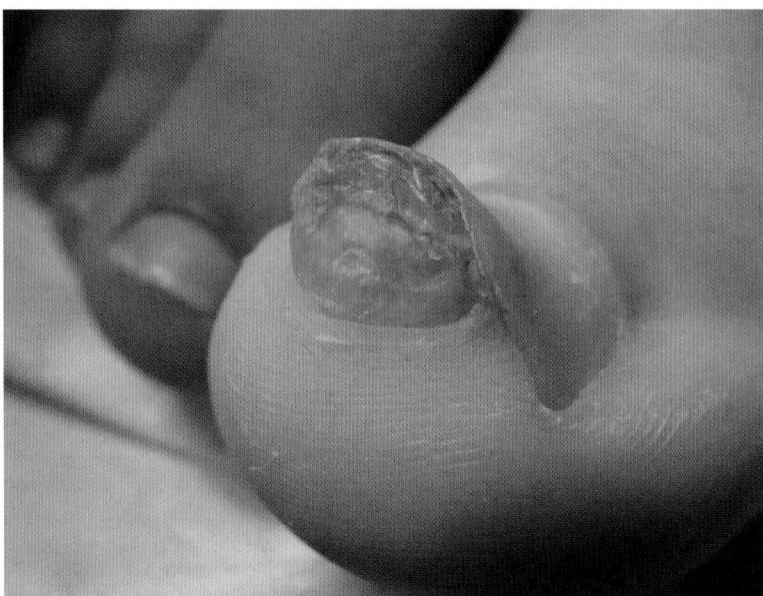

Fig. 23.73
Subungual exostosis: hyperkeratotic tumor lifting up the distal nail plate. Courtesy of B. Richert, MD, PhD, Université Libre de Bruxelles, Belgium.

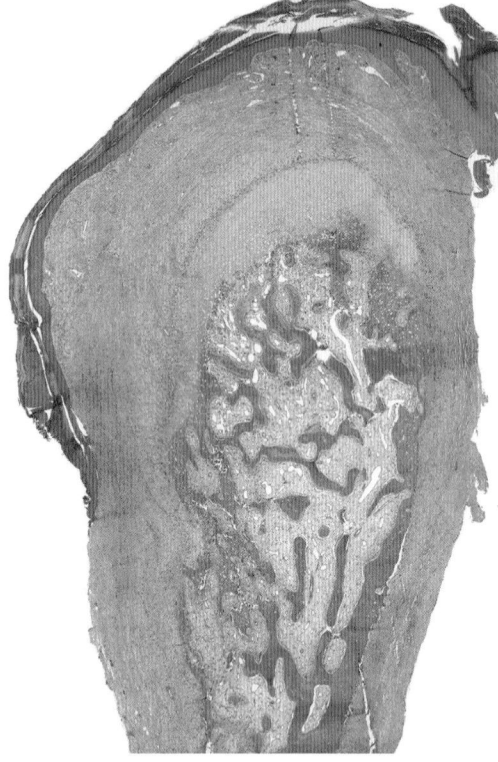

Fig. 23.75
Subungual exostosis: scanning view of an oval bony stalk covered by a cartilaginous cap with overlying thin, hyperkeratotic epidermis.

Subungual exostosis

Clinical features

Subungual exostosis is a benign lesion that occurs exclusively in the nail region. It presents as a slowly growing, flesh-colored or erythematous, tender nodule under the nail plate. Subungual hyperkeratosis, onycholysis, nail deformity, superficial erosion, or ulceration may be observed (Fig. 23.73).

The lesion usually occurs in the second and third decades of life. There is a strong predilection for the toes, especially the great toes. Involvement of the fingers is rare.[1] An X-ray scan shows a mineralizing tumor attached to the distal phalanx in the absence of cortical and medullary continuity between the tumor and the underlying bone (Fig. 23.74).[2] Complete excision is the recommended treatment.

Pathogenesis and histologic features

Subungual exostosis was thought to be a reactive process; however, recent genetic data suggest that these are probably true neoplasms. The tumors contain a t(X;6) translocation.[3–6] The lesion is typically composed of a bony stalk lined by osteoblasts and covered by a cartilaginous cap (Figs 23.75 and 23.76). There is a spindle cell proliferation that matures into cartilage. The cartilage, which appears proliferative with increased cellularity and binucleate forms, in turn, matures into trabecular bone. The intertrabecular spaces contain adipocytes and loosely arranged spindle cells.[6]

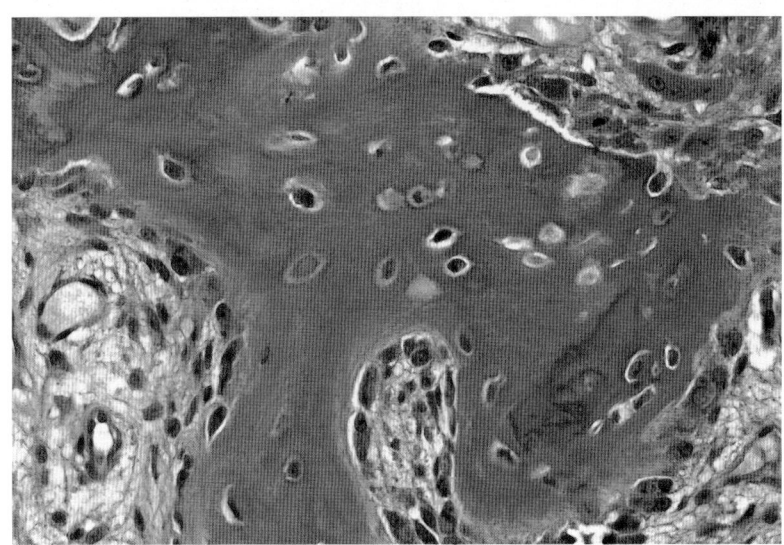

Fig. 23.76
Subungual exostosis: high-power view of the bony stalk.

Differential diagnosis

Osteochondroma, the most common benign bone tumor, usually arises in the femur, humerus, and tibia. It is extremely unusual in a subungual location. It is a projection from the surface of the bone, with its cortex and spongiosa continuous with the cortex and the spongiosa of the underlying bone. Subungual exostosis is attached to the distal phalanx but shows no such continuity. Osteochondroma is a bony projection capped by hyaline cartilage. It lacks the spindle cell proliferation which matures into cartilage, encountered in subungual exostosis.

Enchondroma and periosteal chondroma are cartilaginous neoplasms that do not form bone.[5]

Access **ExpertConsult.com** for the complete list of references

CHAPTER

24

See
www.expertconsult.com
for references and
additional material

Tumors of the surface epithelium

Epidermal nevi

Clinical features

Epidermal nevi are of the following three subtypes, which are histologically identical and differ only in the degree of clinical involvement:
- nevus verrucosus,
- nevus unius lateris,
- ichthyosis hystrix (this has no relationship to ichthyosis).[1–4]

Lesions, which may be present at birth or develop during childhood, are usually yellowish-brown warty papules or plaques with irregular margins. They commonly affect the trunk or limbs and vary from trivial small lesions to very extensive areas of involvement that may cause the patient great cosmetic embarrassment (*Fig. 24.1*).[5,6] They can follow a Blaschkoid distribution.[7] The sex incidence is equal and there is no racial predilection. Familial cases may rarely be seen and are transmitted in an autosomal dominant fashion.[7,8]

Nevus verrucosus refers to solitary or multiple localized lesions, nevus unius lateris refers to a more severe unilateral linear distribution, and ichthyosis hystrix refers to the most extreme example with a bilateral or generalized distribution (*Figs 24.2 and 24.3*). Rare but important complications are development of basal cell and squamous cell carcinoma in addition to keratoacanthoma, eccrine syringofibroadenoma, syringocystadenoma papilliferum, and clear cell acanthoma.[9–22] Unusual presentations include onset in adulthood; involvement of the maxilla, palm, or oral mucosa; and a bilateral symmetric distribution.[23–29] Association with a number of diseases and syndromes has been reported including KID (keratitis-ichthyosis-deafness) syndrome, CHILD (congenital hemidysplasia with ichthyosiform nevus and limb defects) syndrome, CLOVE (congenital lipomatous overgrowth, vascular malformations, and epidermal nevi) syndrome, SCALP (nevus sebaceous, central nervous system malformations, aplasia cutis congenital, limbal dermoid and pigmented nevus) syndrome, Gardner syndrome, Rubinstein-Taybi syndrome, precocious puberty, hypophosphatemic vitamin D-resistant rickets, digital constrictions, divided fingers, localized cranial defects, hemimegalencephaly, temporal lobe enlargement, vascular anomalies and malformations, renal artery stenosis, polyostotic fibrous dysplasia, choristomas, hypermelanosis and chronic hyponatremia, segmental hypermelanosis, trichilemmal and proliferating trichilemmal cysts, central nervous system (CNS) lipomas, mandibular ameloblastoma, chondroblastoma, rhabdomyosarcoma, transitional cell carcinoma, multiple apocrine adenomas, and malignant eccrine poroma.[30–69] Epidermal nevi may also present together with nevus sebaceous, woolly hair nevus, and nevus comedonicus.[17,70–77] They may also rarely be complicated by a dermatitis such as psoriasis.[74,78]

Patients with the epidermal nevus syndrome show a variety of systemic manifestations. They also have an increased incidence of café-au-lait macules, congenital hypopigmented macules, congenital as well as Spitz melanocytic nevi, and a range of vascular malformations. Visceral features particularly affect the skeletal, ocular, and central nervous systems.[1,2,9,79–81] These include kyphoscoliosis, bone cysts, genu valgum, skull abnormalities, limb reduction defects, strabismus, mental retardation, delayed motor milestones, cranial nerve palsies and nonfebrile seizures.[1,2,9,82] Patients with the epidermal nevus syndrome may have an increased incidence of systemic malignancy.[1] More

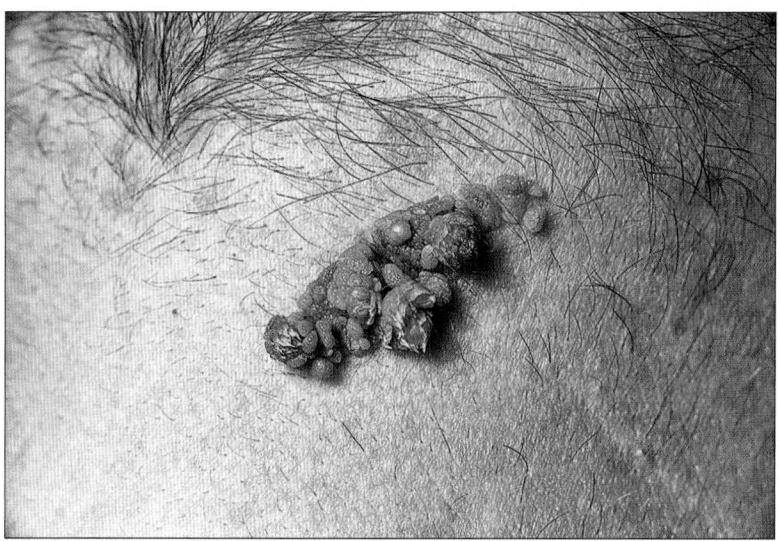

Fig. 24.1
Epidermal nevus: this fairly typical lesion presented on the chest of a young male. By courtesy of R.A. Marsden, MD, St George's Hospital, London, UK.

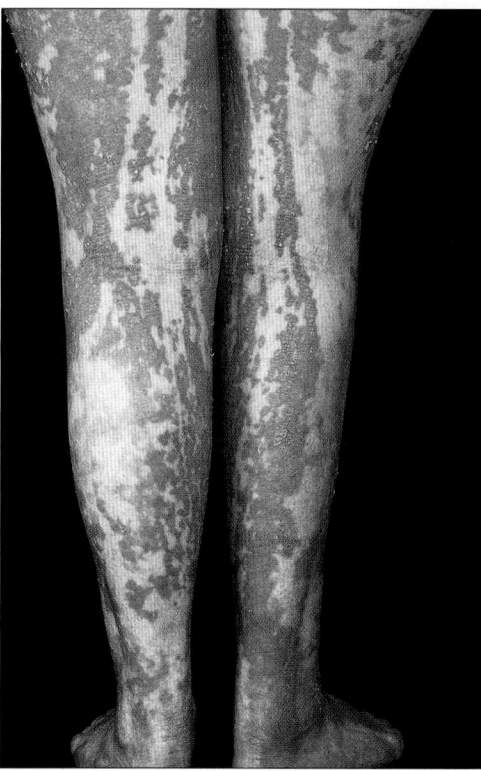

Fig. 24.3
Ichthyosis hystrix: in this variant there is extensive and bilateral involvement. By courtesy of R.A. Marsden, MD, St George's Hospital, London, UK.

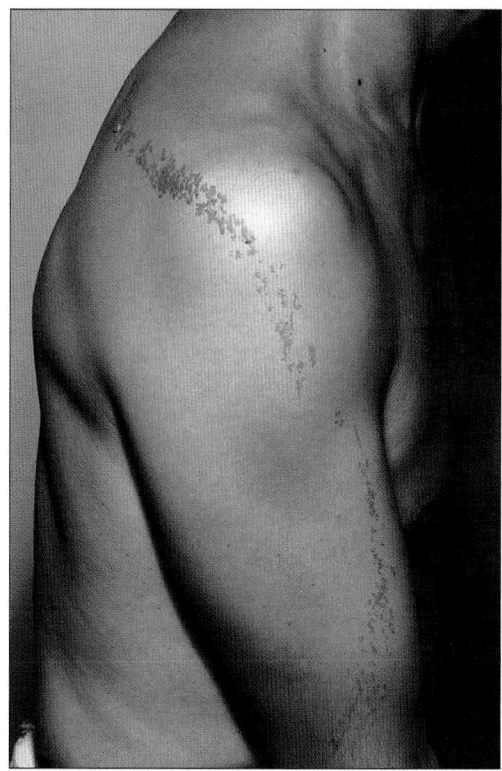

Fig. 24.2
Linear epidermal nevus: this is a more extensive lesion involving the scapular region, shoulder, and upper arm. By courtesy of R.A. Marsden, MD, St George's Hospital, London, UK.

- pigmented hairy epidermal nevus syndrome (Becker nevus syndrome),
- angora hair nevus syndrome,
- Proteus syndrome,
- type 2 segmental Cowden disease,
- FGFR3 epidermal nevus syndrome,
- CHILD syndrome,
- porokeratotic adnexal ostial nevus,
- phakomatosis pigmentokeratotica,
- inflammatory linear verrucous epidermal nevus syndrome,
- cutaneous-skeletal hypophosphatemia syndrome.

Schimmelpenning syndrome

Schimmelpenning syndrome (Schimmelpenning-Feuerstein-Mims syndrome, organoid nevus phakomatosis) is characterized by unilateral nevus sebaceous of the head and neck in combination with cerebral, ocular, cardiac, vascular, and skeletal abnormalities.[83,84,100–109] It is believed to represent a lethal autosomal inherited condition with survival dependent upon a mosaic state.[83] It appears to be driven by postzygotic activating mutations in either *HRAS*, *KRAS*, or *NRAS* recently coined as "mosaic RASopathy."[90,91,110,111] A dominant variant presenting in one of two monozygotic twins is compatible with de novo postzygotic mosaicism.[102] Neurological abnormalities include mental retardation, convulsions, hemiparesis, cranial asymmetry, and hydrocephalus.[112,113] Oral involvement has also been documented. Patients may present with gingival papillomata, hemihypertrophy of the tongue, bone cysts, aplasia of teeth, and hypoplastic or absent enamel as well as pigmented malformed teeth, multiple odontomas, bilateral maxillary fibro-osseous lesions, recurrent central giant cell granulomas of the jaw, and adenomatoid odontogenic tumor.[109,114,115] Ocular manifestations take the form of microphthalmos, eyelid coloboma, nystagmus, ptosis, dermoids, and teratomas of the conjunctiva.[66,73,116] Skeletal abnormalities include skull asymmetry, exostoses, and scoliosis.[73]

Nevus comedonicus syndrome

The nevus comedonicus syndrome consists of nevus comedonicus, cataract, and skeletal defects.[117]

recent studies suggest that the epidermal nevus syndrome is a heterogeneous group of disorders that can be separated by clinical and pathological as well as genetic criteria.[4,83,84] Happle has suggested nine distinct syndromic entities, each associated with distinct epithelial nevi.[7,59,60,84–89] Others have recently suggested largely overlapping but not identical groupings.[4,7]

This is a rapidly evolving area and increased discovery of mosaic mutational genotypes is informing the definition of discrete entities. It is increasingly recognized that many epidermal nevi are manifestations of mosaic RASopathy as will be discussed further below.[90–97] Other genes such as *FGFR3*, *PTEN*, *AKT1*, *PIK3CA*, *PTEN* and others can also be involved in mosaic fashion.[7,98,99] We briefly present some of the distinguishing features of 12 relatively well-defined syndromes with prominent epidermal nevi:

- Schimmelpenning syndrome (nevus sebaceous syndrome),
- nevus comedonicus syndrome,

Pigmented hairy epidermal nevus syndrome

The pigmented hairy epidermal nevus syndrome comprises Becker nevus in association with ipsilateral hypoplasia of the breast and other cutaneous as well as skeletal anomalies.[84,118]

Angora hair nevus syndrome

The exceedingly rare angora hair nevus syndrome (Schauder syndrome) shows a nevus with prominent soft white hair that occurs along Blaschko lines.[89,119,120] Associated cerebral and ocular malformations and dysfunctions can occur along with skeletal deformations and facial features.[119] The white hair and lack of breast hypoplasia distinguishes it from Becker nevus syndrome.

Proteus syndrome

Proteus syndrome is an exceedingly rare hamartomatous condition that can be very disfiguring and is associated with an increased risk of malignancy. It is sporadic and is thought to result from mosaicism for a mutation that is lethal in the nonmosaic state.[121,122] Males are more frequently affected than females and the syndrome is associated with an increased risk of premature death.[123] A subset has been linked to PTEN mutations, thereby displaying genetic in addition to clinical overlap with other hamartomatous conditions including Cowden syndrome and Bannayan-Riley-Ruvalcaba syndrome.[122,124–128] This group is now termed the PTEN hamartoma tumor syndromes.[129] Recent mutational analyses of patients with 'bona fide' Proteus syndrome, however, failed to detect mutation in the PTEN gene and the contribution of PTEN mutations remains an issue of ongoing debate.[130,131] Rather than PTEN, very recent data suggest constitutive and mosaic activating mutations in PIK3CA and AKT1, encoding critical kinases in the PTEN/PIK3CA/AKT signaling pathway.[132–136] It is now considered to be part of the PIK3CA-related overgrowth syndrome (PROS) group rather than the related PTEN hamartoma tumor syndromes.[137] Proteus syndrome is a complex disorder comprising malformations and overgrowth of multiple tissues in addition to epidermal nevi. The latter are flat, soft, and of nonorganoid type and are present in about two-thirds of cases.[7,83,138–143] They are associated with other cutaneous anomalies such as connective tissue nevi, cystic lymphangiomas, hemangiomas, lipomas, and fibromas.[144–148] Cerebriform hyperplasia of the plantar connective tissue (moccasin lesion) is a characteristic finding.[83,146,149] A hallmark of Proteus syndrome is asymmetrical hypertrophy affecting the face, limbs, and trunk including macrocephaly and hemihypertrophy of the body.[121,122,150] Macrodactyly is thought to be characteristic.[139,151]

Other noncutaneous manifestations include bony exostoses, kyphoscoliosis, spinal canal stenosis, hydrocephalus, hemimegancephaly, CNS cysts, seizures, epibulbar tumors, enlargement of the eye, cataract and strabismus, paraovarian endometrioid cystic tumors, genitourinary abnormalities, and nephrogenic diabetes insipidus.[99,132,139,152–154] Patients are at increased risk for a number of tumors including testicular papillary adenocarcinoma, ovarian cystadenoma, meningioma, parotid monomorphic adenoma, astrocytoma, optic nerve tumor, leiomyoma, and endometrial carcinoma.[106,130,155]

Type 2 segmental Cowden disease

Linear Cowden nevus syndrome is associated with non-organoid epidermal nevus that is soft and thick with distinctly papillomatous features.[89,156] This occurs in the setting of PTEN loss of function mutation heterozygote that undergoes embryonal loss of heterozygosity. It lacks the cerebriform hyperplasia of the palms and soles seen in Proteus syndrome.

Two patients from families with Cowden syndrome have been described with a unique phenotype related to bi-allelic inactivation of PTEN. These patients showed classic features of Cowden syndrome in addition to segmental overgrowth, lipomatosis, arteriovenous malformation, and linear epidermal nevus for which the term SOLAMEN syndrome has been proposed.[157] These are likely identical to type 2 segmental Cowen disease. It is possible that biallelic PTEN loss might result in levels of PIK3CA and

AKT activity that resemble that seen from the direct mutation activation of these genes in Proteus syndrome and thus partially phenocopy Proteus syndrome. A small subset of Cowden patients are also reported to harbor activating PIK3CA and AKT1 mutations instead of the characteristic inactivating PTEN mutations.[158]

FGFR3 epidermal nevus syndrome

A mosaic FGFR3 mutation was detected in a patient with epidermal nevus syndrome with cerebral involvement.[159] Underlying neurological and structural deficits can be seen in this syndrome.[160] FGFR3 epidermal nevus syndrome (Garcia-Hafner-Happle syndrome) shows a soft velvety epidermal nevus specifically driven by mosaic activating mutations in FGFR3 (usually R284C).[161,162] This same activating mutation is seen in up to one-third of keratinocytic nevi that are nonepidermolytic in type as well as some sporadic seborrheic keratoses.[89,163–166] FGFR3 and PIK3CA activating mutations are also seen in familial seborrheic keratosis.[167]

CHILD syndrome

CHILD syndrome is an X-linked dominant disorder almost exclusively affecting females and is characterized by a unique epidermal nevus involving one side of the body in addition to ipsilateral defects of the limbs and internal organs.[168,169] Mutations in the NSDHL (NADPH steroid dehydrogenase-like protein) gene, which is located on Xq28 and is involved in the cholesterol synthesis pathway, have been identified in this syndrome.[170–175] The CHILD nevus is a unilateral, circumscribed, inflammatory, ichthyosiform nevus typically presenting at birth. It is erythematous and covered by yellow, waxy scales.[67,176,177] Frequently, the body folds are affected. It may be linear and follow the lines of Blaschko. Disease presentation can be mild and familial, affecting multiple generations.[7,178]

Histologically, the cutaneous manifestations are characterized by psoriasiform epidermal hyperplasia, and features reminiscent of verruciform xanthoma may be present. Ultrastructural data suggest that the formation of the cutaneous lesion may be due to abnormal lipid metabolism.[179] Although CHILD nevus has a distinctive presentation there is considerable overlap with inflammatory linear verrucous nevus (ILVEN).[176,177] Other clinical findings in CHILD syndrome include ipsilateral hypoplasia or aplasia of limbs and other skeletal structures. Neurological defects may include hypoplasia of a cerebral hemisphere or cranial nerve but mental development is typically unimpaired. Cardiovascular, renal, and pulmonary anomalies may be present.[84] Development of a cutaneous squamous cell carcinoma has been reported.[180]

Phakomatosis pigmentokeratotica

This syndrome is characterized by the presence of a nevus sebaceous following the lines of Blaschko in addition to a speckled lentiginous nevus (nevus spilus) typically in a segmental distribution with a checkerboard pattern.[4,88,99,181–184] Extracutaneous manifestations are typically but not invariably present.[99,185,186] They comprise predominantly skeletal, neurological, and ocular abnormalities and the most consistent extracutaneous finding is hemiatrophy.[88,89,181–184] Neurological findings include hyperpathia, dysesthesia, hyperhidrosis, seizures, deafness, ptosis, strabismus, and mild mental retardation.[88,99,181–184,187] Other associations include hypophosphatemic vitamin D-resistant rickets, hemihypertrophy, linear connective tissue nevus, juvenile onset hypertension, aortic stenosis, scoliosis, dermoid cysts, nephroblastoma, pheochromocytoma, and rhabdomyosarcoma.[188–196] A melanoma arising in a nevus spilus has been documented and the organoid nevus may be complicated by the development of multiple basal cell carcinomas.[189,197,198] This syndrome is also a mosaic RASpathy.[199]

Inflammatory linear verrucous epidermal nevus syndrome

Inflammatory linear verrucous epidermal nevus (ILVEN) syndrome shows a linear verucous nevus with a distinct inflammatory characteristics usually

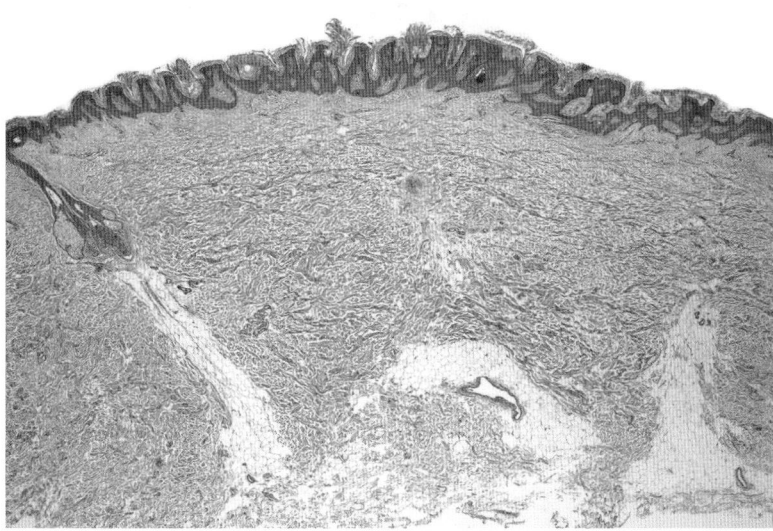

Fig. 24.4
Epidermal nevus: scanning view; note the hyperkeratosis, papillomatosis, and acanthosis.

described as eczematous or psoriasiform.[200–202] Some have likened it to the rare linear form of psoriasis in presentation.[78,203,204] While some have suggested that an ILVEN syndrome exists with various additional malformations, others do not consider this to be a well-defined association.[4,200] A single case of ILVEN was associated with a *GJA1* mutation, encoding a gap junction protein, though this is probably best considered as a postzygotic and mosaic form of erythrokeratoderma variabilis et progressiva which is normally autosomal dominant.[205,206] There is an entire family of autosomal dominant and recessive syndromes with mutations in *GJA1* and other gap junction and connexin encoding genes.[207,208] It has also been suggested that ILVEN is a primary inflammatory condition rather than an epidermal nevus.[209] It also shares features with the lesions seen in CHILD syndrome.[210]

Cutaneous skeletal hypophosphatemia syndrome

This mosaic RASopathy shows epidermal nevi with a profound hypophosphatemia that is not present at birth, but has a later onset and leads to osteomalacia.[94,95] Other skeletal defects can also be seen and are not usually correlated with overlying epidermal nevi.[4,211]

Histologic features

Epidermal nevi represent developmental abnormalities limited to proliferation of the epidermis, sometimes accompanied by anomalous terminal differentiation. Although they are related to sebaceous (organoid) nevi and frequently coexist, it is convenient to consider them separately. Commonly, they show the features of a sharply demarcated simple squamous cell papilloma (*Fig. 24.4*). They, therefore, manifest hyperkeratosis, papillomatosis, acanthosis, and elongation of the rete ridges (*Fig. 24.5*).[160,212] The histologic features are often subtle and occasionally resemble acanthosis nigricans or a seborrheic keratosis.[213] Rarely, the lesions show focal acantholytic dyskeratosis, acrokeratosis verruciformis-like features, cornoid lamellae formation, epidermolytic hyperkeratosis, an associated lichenoid tissue reaction or cutaneous horn formation.[214–219] Acantholytic dyskeratosis in epidermal nevi is thought by some authors to represent zosteriform Darier disease.[220–222] The presence of epidermolytic hyperkeratosis may be indicative of mosaicism for bullous ichthyosiform erythroderma as further supported by the identification of keratin 1 and 10 mutations.[223–227]

Epidermal nevi in Proteus syndrome are characterized by hyperorthokeratosis, acanthosis and papillomatosis in the absence of adnexal hyperplasia or epidermolytic hyperkeratosis.[83]

The CHILD nevus is characterized histologically by marked acanthosis with overlying parakeratosis admixed with areas of hyperorthokeratosis.

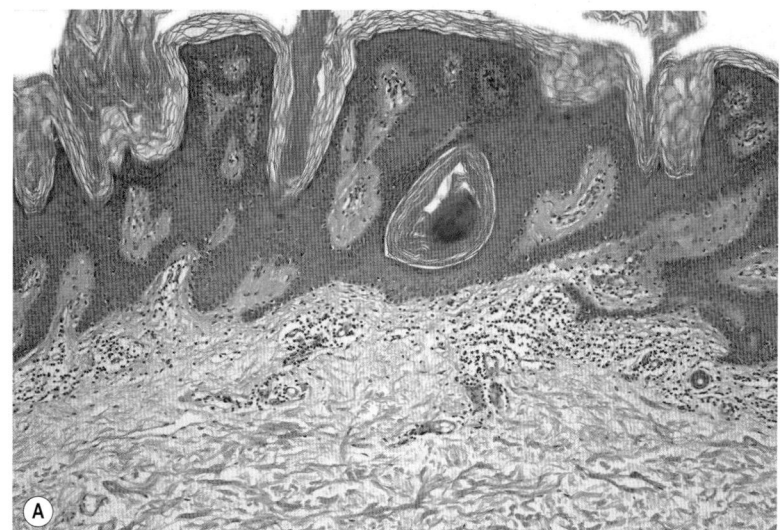

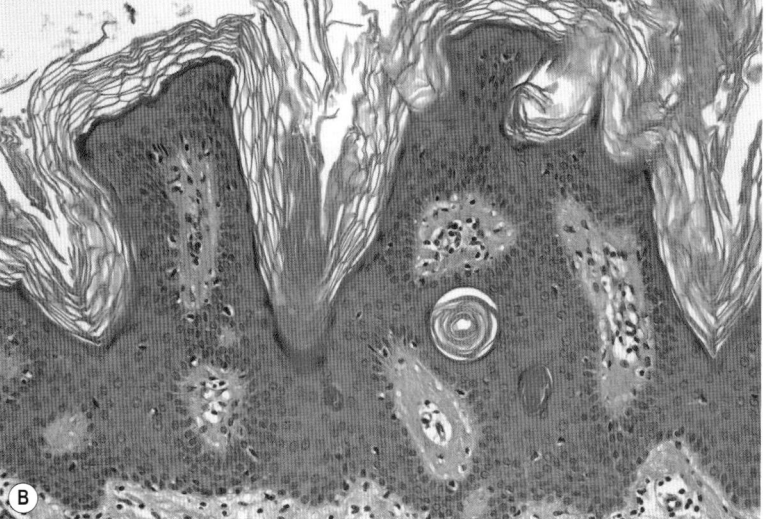

Fig. 24.5
Epidermal nevus: (**A**) medium-power view; (**B**) the features are reminiscent of seborrheic keratosis. Note the keratin-filled pseudocysts. Scattered lymphocytes are present in the superficial dermis.

Intraepidermal neutrophils, also forming aggregates similar to Munro abscesses, are sometimes present. The dermis shows a lymphohistiocytic infiltrate. Dermal papillae may be filled with foamy histiocytes reminiscent of verruciform xanthoma.[177,228]

ILVEN show epidermal psoriasiform hyperplasia with hyperkeratosis, parakeratosis and sometimes Muro abscesses.[209,229] A prominent mixed perivascular dermal inflammatory infiltrate is present associated with dilated capillaries.[230] There is considerable overlap with the lesions of CHILD syndrome, but ILVEN lacks the *NSDHL* mutations and X-linked dominant inheritance of CHILD syndrome.[7]

Cornu cutaneum

Cornu cutaneum (cutaneous horn) is a clinical diagnosis based upon the presence of a large protuberant mass of keratin (*Fig. 24.6*). They can occur at virtually any body site, but are typical on the sun-exposed areas of the face and head, and can also involve other upper torso and extremity sites.[1–12] It may complicate a variety of conditions and accurate diagnosis depends upon histologic examination of tissue from the base of the lesion. Cutaneous horns may complicate solar keratosis, viral wart, seborrheic keratosis, squamous cell carcinoma, keratoacanthoma, lichenoid keratosis, and basal cell carcinoma.[3,13–16] It has been noted that these horns are considerably more likely to arise from benign or premalignant lesions (more than 80%) rather than invasive malignancies (less than 20%).[5,17]

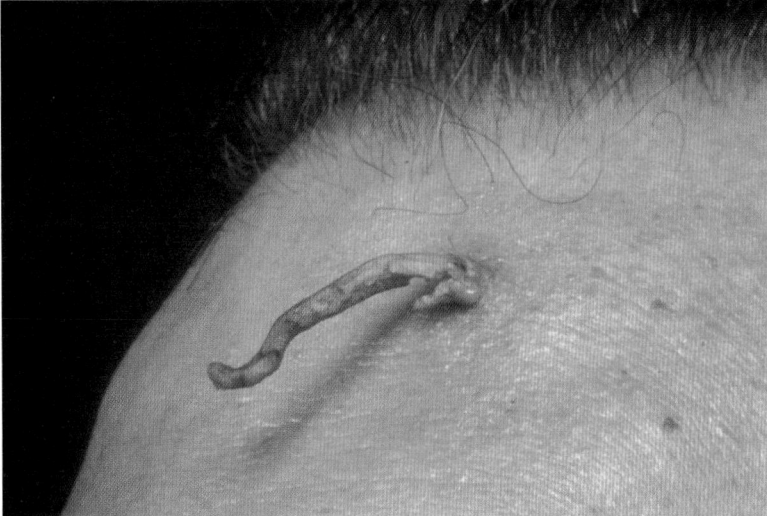

Fig. 24.6
Cutaneous horn: a rather dramatic example. The base of the keratin horn must be sampled to determine the nature of the underlying lesion. By courtesy of The Institute of Dermatology, London, UK.

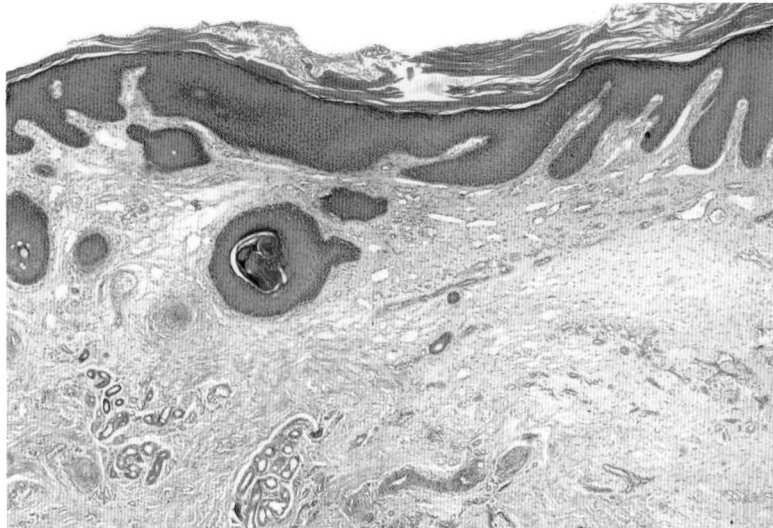

Fig. 24.8
Spectacle frame acanthoma: this field is taken from the edge of the fissure. The features are non-specific and comprise hyperkeratosis, irregular acanthosis, and marked dermal scarring with chronic inflammatory changes. The major importance of a biopsy of this lesion is to exclude a basal cell or squamous cell carcinoma.

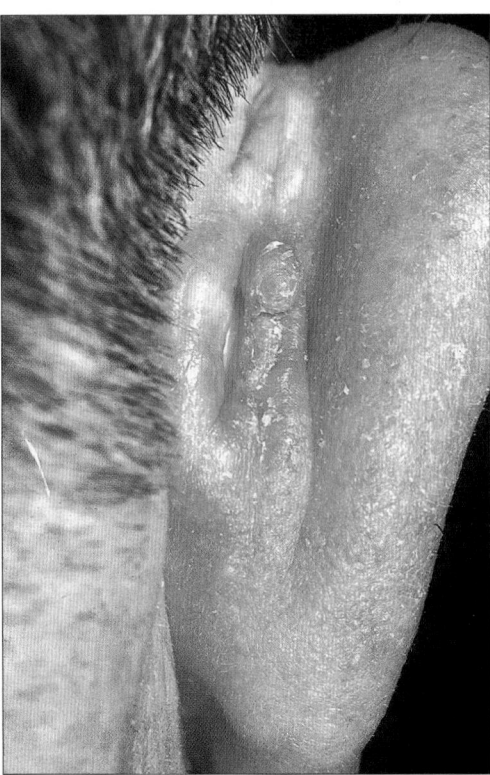

Fig. 24.7
Spectacle frame acanthoma: a 'tumor' behind the ear of a middle-aged male. Note the characteristic central groove or furrow. By courtesy of the late N. Smith, MD, The Institute of Dermatology, London, UK.

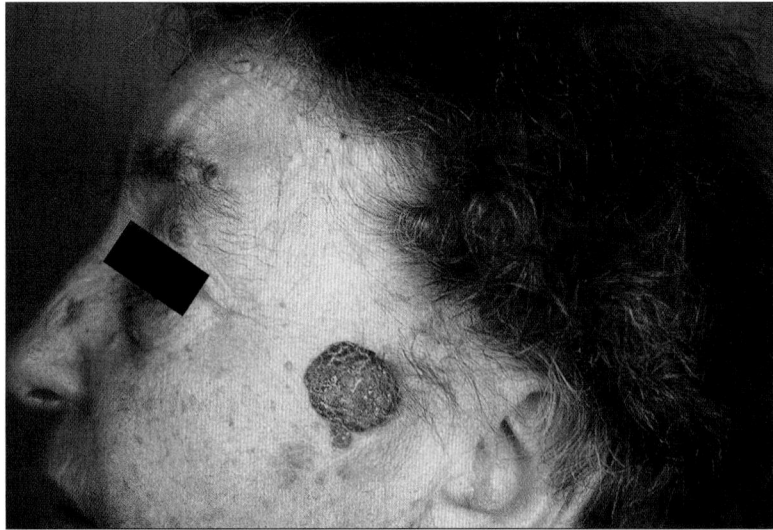

Fig. 24.9
Seborrheic keratosis: multiple lesions on an elderly female. By courtesy of the late M. Beare, MD, Royal Victoria Hospital, Belfast, N. Ireland.

Histologic features

The histopathology is not specific, diagnosis being dependent upon knowledge of the clinical history. Its features usually include acanthosis (sometimes amounting to pseudoepitheliomatous hyperplasia) with hyperkeratosis and patchy parakeratosis, particularly at the edges of the fissure (*Fig. 24.8*).[9] The underlying dermis is edematous, fibrosed, and hyalinized. A chronic inflammatory cell infiltrate of variable severity is commonly present.

Seborrheic keratosis

Clinical features

Seborrheic keratoses are very common lesions, developing in the middle aged and elderly. They are frequently numerous and appear as sharply delineated, round or oval, flesh-colored or brown-black warty plaques with a rather greasy texture (*Figs 24.9 and 24.10*).[1,2] Sometimes they are dome-shaped with a smooth surface and occasionally they may show an inflammatory halo or eczema-like features (Meyerson phenomenon).[3–6] Although they may

Acanthoma fissuratum

Clinical features

Acanthoma fissuratum (spectacle frame acanthoma) is a benign epidermal 'tumor' which develops as a result of chronic irritation from spectacles.[1–5] It presents as an erythematous or flesh-colored, sometimes tender, nodule situated on the bridge of the nose or behind the ears (*Fig. 24.7*).[1–5] Typically, the center of the lesion shows a linear groove. The importance of this entity is that it is clinically frequently misdiagnosed as a basal cell or squamous cell carcinoma. An analogous lesion termed granuloma (epulis) fissuratum has been described in the mouth as a result of poorly fitting dentures.[6] An exceptional case involved the penis with tight fitting undergarments.[7] What is described as "vulvar granuloma fissuratum" is a fissuring process that complicates a variety of vulvar dermatoses with dyspareunia and other discomforts. This seems to represent a different lesion altogether.[8]

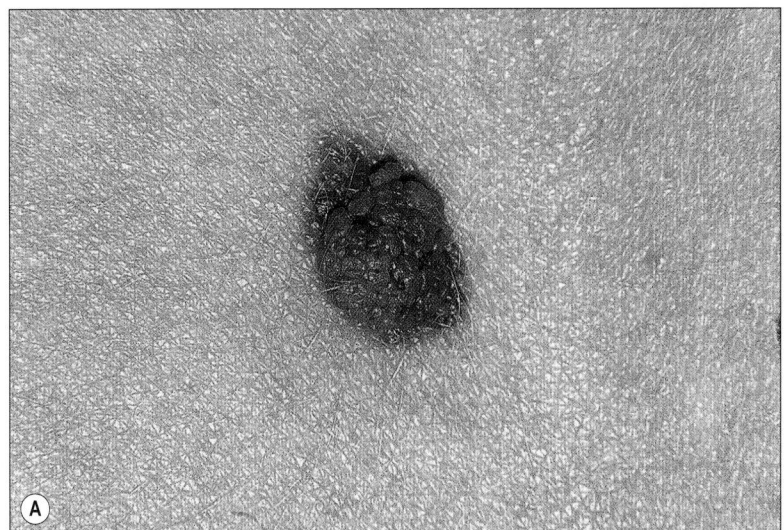

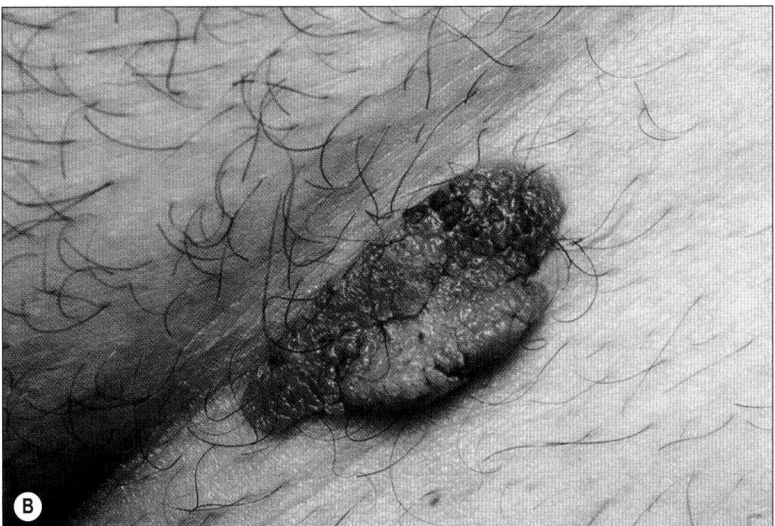

Fig. 24.10
Seborrheic keratosis: (**A**) close-up view showing the warty surface; (**B**) pigmented variants may be mistaken for malignant melanoma. (A) By courtesy of the late M. Beare, MD, Royal Victoria Hospital, Belfast, N. Ireland; (B) by courtesy of the Institute of Dermatology, London, UK.

be found anywhere on the body (except for the palms and soles), they are particularly common on the face, chest, and back.[1] The conjunctiva may also be involved.[7,8]

Other unusual clinical presentations include distribution along skin cleavages,[9] involvement of the areola[10,11] or the back of elderly patients (raindrop seborrheic keratosis), as well as a distribution along the lines of Blaschko.[12,13] Occasionally, deeply pigmented or traumatized lesions are mistaken clinically for melanoma.[14] The irritated seborrheic keratosis (inverted follicular keratosis) presents as a small warty papulonodule (*Fig. 24.11*). It commonly affects middle-aged or elderly males and shows a predilection for the face.[15] Multiple inverted follicular keratoses have been reported as a presenting sign in a patient with Cowden syndrome.[16]

Sudden onset of numerous seborrheic keratoses (Leser-Trélat sign) has been reported in association with internal malignancy, most commonly adenocarcinoma of the stomach. Other tumors which may be present include lymphoma (particularly mucosis fungoides and Sézary syndrome), leukemia, metastatic melanoma, malignant solitary fibrous tumor, bronchial and breast carcinoma, cholangiocarcinoma, carcinoma of the ampulla of Vater, the pancreas and the esophagus, adenocarcinoma of the rectum, renal cell carcinoma, endometrial adenocarcinoma, transitional cell carcinoma, and anaplastic ependymoma (*Fig. 24.12*).[17–40] Leser-Trélat sign has also been described after treatment with chemotherapy, as well as in association with a benign Leydig cell tumor.[35,41,42] The relationship of seborrheic keratosis and malignancy, however, has been questioned.[43,44] Although neoplasia and

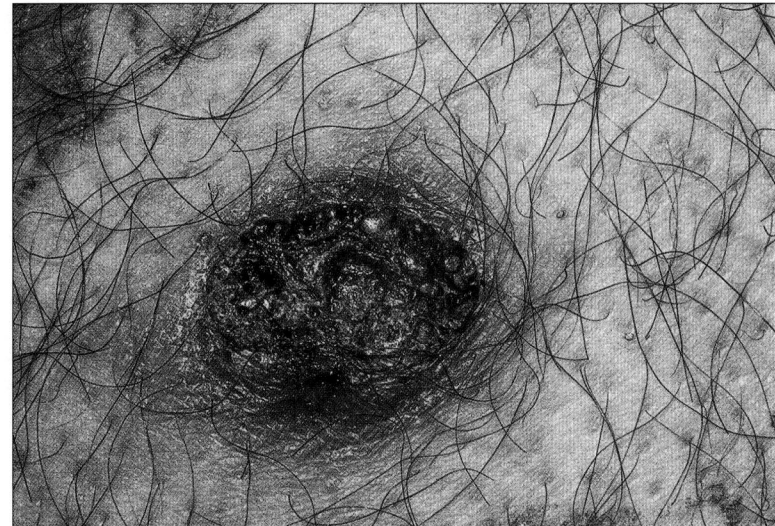

Fig. 24.11
Irritated seborrheic keratosis: the lesion has a characteristic dark coloration and there is surrounding erythema. By courtesy of R.A. Marsden, MD, St George's Hospital, London, UK.

seborrheic warts are both common in the elderly, we believe that a sudden eruption of the latter should still warrant careful investigation. Spontaneous regression of multiple seborrheic keratoses has also been reported in association with malignancy.[45] Multiple eruptive seborrheic keratoses have been observed in a background of erythroderma, at a postoperative site, and with leprosy.[46–49] Eruptive seborrheic keratosis has been reported with the use of the hepatitis C virus protease inhibitor telaprevir and also rarely with adalimumab anti-tumor necrosis factor (TNF)-α therapy for rheumatoid arthritis.[50,51] In some cases, no underlying cause is found despite exhaustive clinical investigation.

Disappearance or fading of pigmented seborrheic keratoses has been reported with use of immune checkpoint inhibitor therapy (PD-1 inhibitor) for metastatic melanoma.[52]

Pathogenic and histologic features

This benign epidermal tumor is definitely monoclonal in nature and represents a true neoplasm rather than epidermal hyperplasia.[53] It has become clear that a subset of seborrheic harbor activating mutations oncogenes. The first noted was *FGFR3* (usually R284C or S249C).[54–57] The rates of *FGFR3* mutations in patients with multiple to many seborrheic keratosis ranges from about 25% of lesions to almost 90%. Multiple oncogenic mutations were seen in different lesions from the same patients. These few patients had many seborrheic keratoses occurring in the genetic background of the rare anaphoric dysplasia and severe achondroplasia with developmental delay and acanthosis nigricans syndrome.[58] There is increased incidence of these mutations with older patient age and location in head and neck region.[59] Activating *PIK3CA* somatic mutations have also been noted (usually E542K or E454K).[60,61] In a small subset of cases, both PIK3CA and FGFR3 mutations are encountered simultaneously.[61] Either *FGFR3* or *PIK3CA* mutation has been seen limited to the lesions in the setting of familial seborrheic keratoses.[62] Interestingly, studies of human skin explants into mice indicate that *FGFR3* is insufficient to drive seborrheic keratosis tumor formation in that model and other data suggest that *FGFR3* signaling in keratinocytes provides more of a senescence than oncogenic impetus.[63–65] Other model systems indicate *FGFR3* mutation is associated with increased proliferation and reduced apoptosis in keratinocytes with little effect on senescence.[66] Examining broader panels of genes have reviewed rare mutations in additional oncogenes including *KRAS*, *HRAS*, *EGFR* and *AKT1*.[67–69] Mutational signatures suggest ultraviolet (UV) exposure and very recently *TERT* and *DPH3* promoter mutations have been noted in older patients in lesions from the head and neck region.[70] More work is needed to understand how these various drivers work in these neoplasms that so rarely progress to malignancy.[68,71]

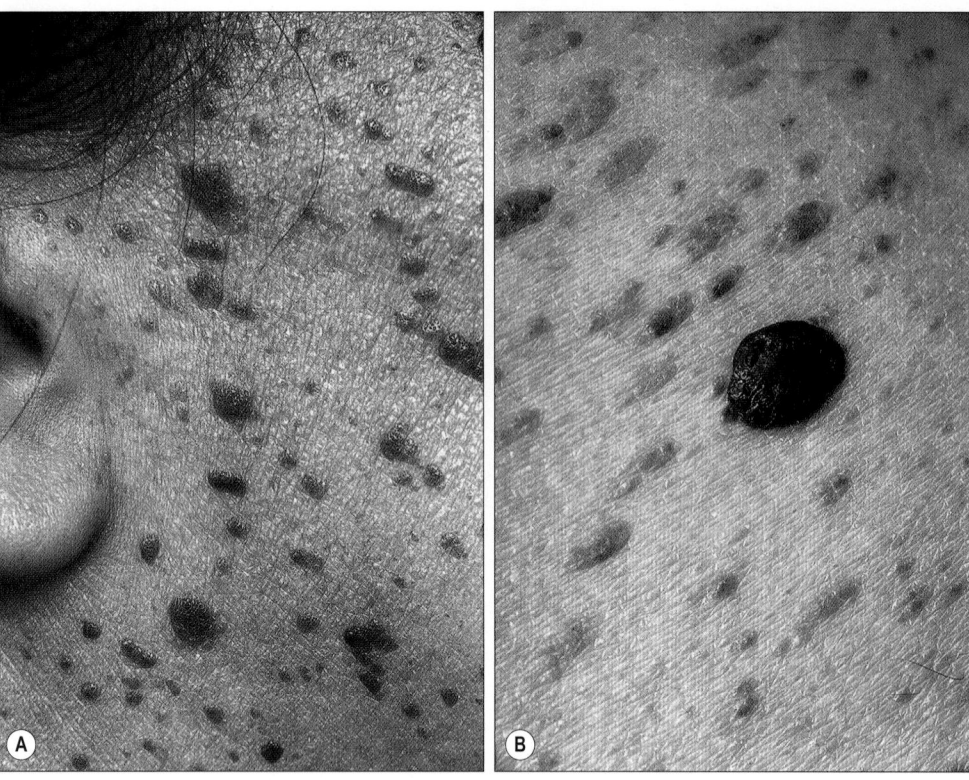

Fig. 24.12

(**A**, **B**) Leser-Trélat sign: the sudden onset of numerous seborrheic keratoses may indicate an underlying malignant visceral neoplasm. By courtesy of M.M. Black, MD, Institute of Dermatology, London, UK.

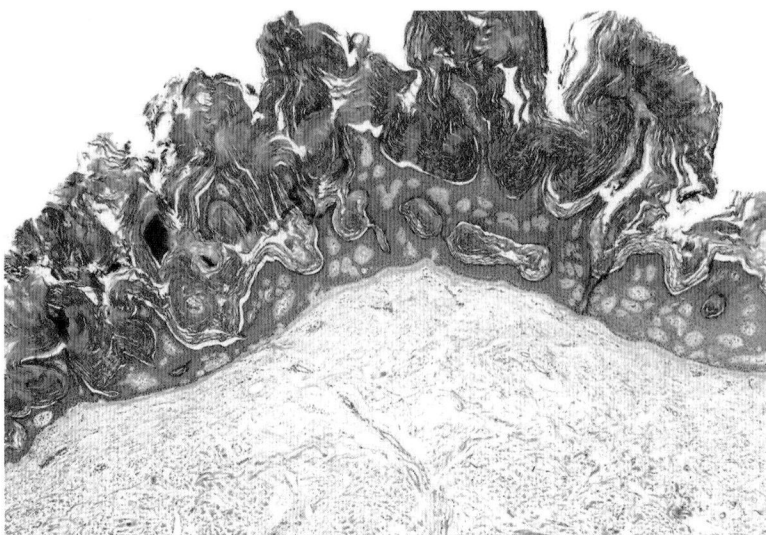

Fig. 24.13

Papillomatous seborrheic keratosis: there is massive hyperkeratosis and papillomatosis.

Seborrheic keratosis is characterized by proliferation of basaloid cells with a variable degree of squamoid differentiation.[1,72] There is a range of histopathological patterns, including: hyperkeratotic (papillomatous), adenoid or reticulated variants, acanthotic or solid keratosis, clonal or nested, inflamed, and irritated seborrheic keratosis (inverted follicular keratosis).[2,73–75]

- The keratotic (papillomatous) variant has a verrucous appearance with variable proliferation of basaloid and squamoid cells (*Fig. 24.13*). The lesion shows acanthosis, papillomatosis, and hyperkeratosis, often with the development of pseudohorn cysts (*Fig. 24.14*).[76,77]
- In the adenoid type of seborrheic keratosis, the lesion is typified by thin proliferating strands of basaloid cells arising from the epidermis (*Fig. 24.15*).[78] These lesions may be highly pigmented and pseudohorn cysts are less often evident.
- In the acanthotic variant, the surface of the tumor is hyperkeratotic, rounded, and smooth (*Figs 24.16 and 24.17*).[78] Melanocytic proliferation is not uncommon.[79] When marked, the designation

melanoacanthoma is sometimes applied (*Fig. 24.18*).[1] Pigmentation in seborrheic keratosis has been linked to increased expression of keratinocyte-derived endothelin 1 mediated by TNF-alpha and endothelin-converting enzyme 1 alpha (ECE1 alpha).[80]

Many seborrheic keratoses show a mixture of the patterns described above. Occasionally, intraepithelial nesting gives rise to the Borst-Jadassohn appearance (so-called clonal seborrheic keratosis) and some variants barely protrude above the adjacent epidermis (flat seborrheic keratosis) (*Figs 24.19–24.21*).[78,81–83] Rare patterns include the adamantinoid variant characterized by intercellular mucin and pseudorosette formation due to a radial arrangement of basal keratinocytes around central small empty spaces.[84] Bowenoid seborrheic keratosis has a predilection for sun-exposed areas, has intraepidermal atypia, and is seen in only about 1% of excised cases.[2,85] Some have reported an association with human papillomavirus (HPV) with Bowenoid transformation.[86] The presence of numerous basal cells with abundant clear cytoplasm is a rare finding and may lead to an erroneous diagnosis of melanoma in situ within a seborrheic keratosis on H&E-stained sections.[87] By immunohistochemistry, these basal clear cells are, however, positive for cytokeratins and negative for markers of melanocytic differentiation, confirming their epithelial nature.[87] The etiology of marked clear cell change is unclear but appears unrelated to glycogen deposition. A desmoplastic variant is characterized by nests and strands of bland-appearing basaloid epithelium within a dense desmoplastic stromal response. Analogous to desmoplastic trichilemmoma, the tumor shows an exophytic growth pattern, is well-demarcated, and lacks cytological atypia.[88] Stromal amyloid deposition may occasionally be evident, and an accumulation of xanthomatized histiocytes within dermal papillae reminiscent of verruciform xanthoma has been reported.[53,89]

Seborrheic keratosis is sometimes characterized by an intradermal or 'inverted' type of proliferation known as inverted follicular keratosis (*Fig. 24.22*).[15,72] In this variant, characteristic whorls of maturing squamous epithelium (squamous eddies) are particularly evident (*Figs 24.23 and 24.24*). These tumors are usually seen arising close to a hair follicle ostium and squamous eddies have been shown to be related to follicular units.[90] Mitotic figures are sometimes conspicuous, but are invariably normal.[15] Some of the lesions contain large numbers of horn cysts and are frequently accompanied by an intense chronic inflammatory cell infiltrate, hence its alternative designation, 'irritated seborrheic keratosis.' Conspicuous apoptosis is sometimes present in areas of squamous differentiation.[91]

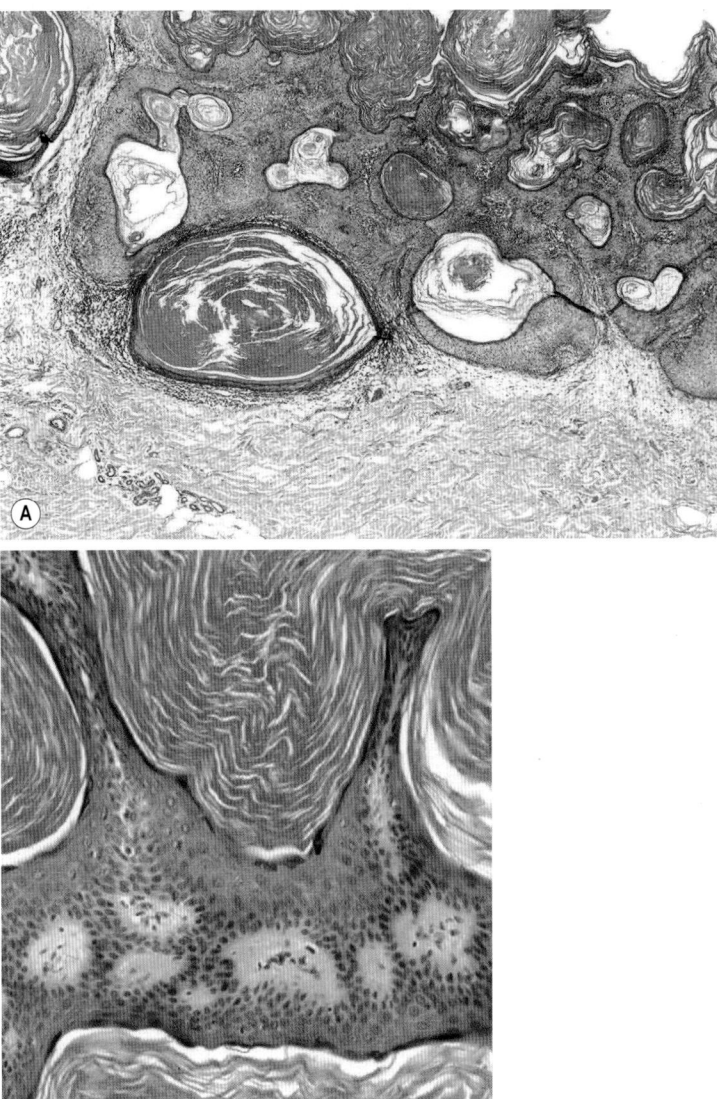

Fig. 24.14
Papillomatous seborrheic keratosis: (**A**) in addition to hyperkeratosis and papillomatosis, horn cysts are conspicuous; (**B**) close-up view.

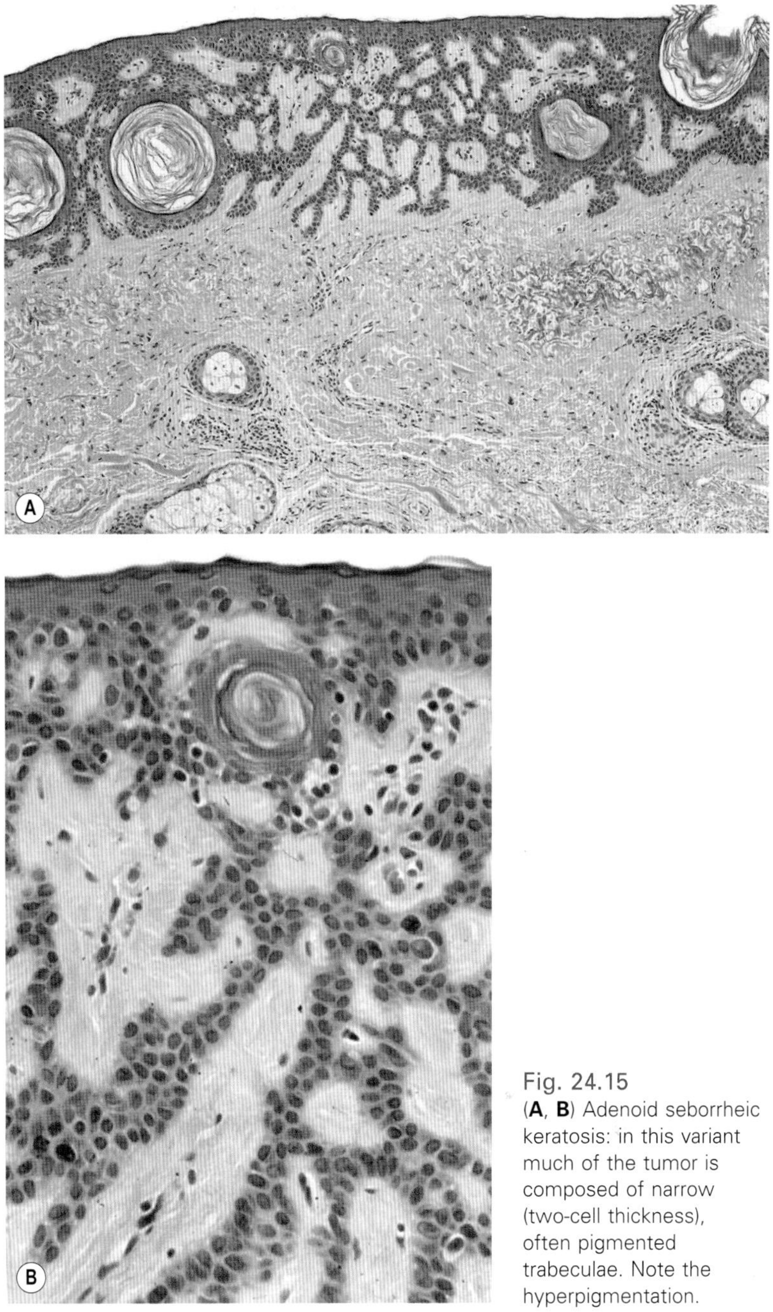

Fig. 24.15
(**A**, **B**) Adenoid seborrheic keratosis: in this variant much of the tumor is composed of narrow (two-cell thickness), often pigmented trabeculae. Note the hyperpigmentation.

Acantholysis is not uncommon in seborrheic keratoses, particularly in the 'irritated' variant.[92,93]

Malignant change within a seborrheic keratosis is very rare, but has occasionally been documented.[85,94–96] Usually this represents an in situ change, but basal cell carcinoma and squamous cell carcinoma have also been reported.[97–101] Both elevated UV exposure and immunosuppression can play a role in malignant transformation.[102,103] More frequently (in up to 5% of tumors) other neoplasms arise in association with seborrheic keratoses, sometimes referred to as collision tumors.[104] The most frequent association is with superficial basal cell carcinoma but squamous cell carcinoma and melanoma have also been reported.[97,105–113] Unusual combined tumors that have very occasionally been documented include cutaneous ganglioneuroma, melanocytic nevi, sebaceoma, eccrine poroma, and trichilemmoma in addition to adenocarcinoma.[114–122]

In contrast to nongenital lesions, seborrheic keratoses arising on genital skin are frequently (in approximately 70%) related to HPV.[123–127] These HPV-positive lesions are probably better regarded as condyloma acuminatum rather than true seborrheic keratoses.[128]

Dermatosis papulosa nigra

Clinical features

Dermatosis papulosa nigra is an extremely common condition in which adults of Afro-Caribbean origin develop multiple, small, darkly pigmented papules, predominantly on the face, particularly the cheek.[1,2] The neck, chest, and upper back may also be involved.[3–7] There is a female preponderance of 2:1, and a family predisposition has been identified in the majority of patients.[4,8,9] Very rarely, children may be affected and exceptionally the disorder presents in the white races.[5,6,10–12] An eruptive presentation has been reported in a patient with a colonic adenocarcinoma analogous to eruptive seborrheic keratoses associated with internal malignancy (Leser-Trélat sign).[13]

Pathogenesis and histologic features

The lesions are indistinguishable from seborrheic keratoses (*Fig. 24.25*). Like seborrheic keratoses, activating mutations in both *FGFR3* and *PIK3CA*

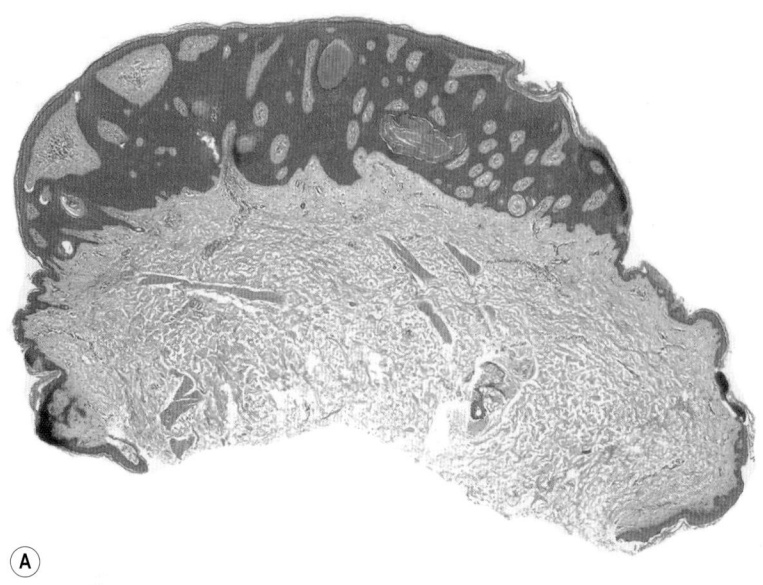

(A)

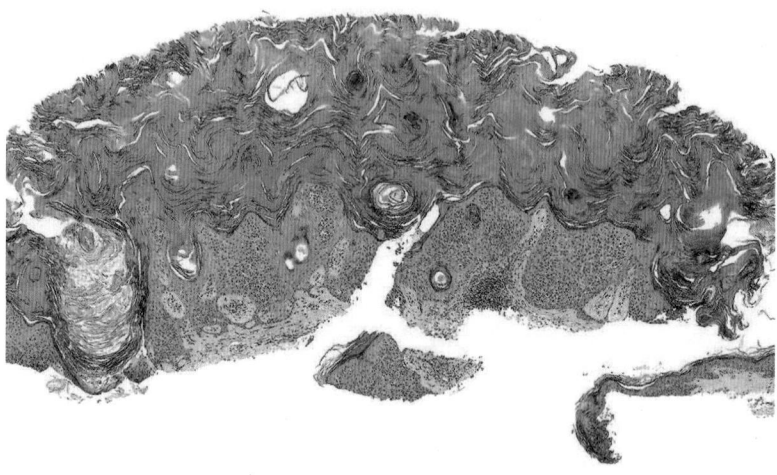

Fig. 24.18
Pigmented seborrheic keratosis: abundant melanin is present in this variant. Some authors classify this lesion as a melanoacanthoma.

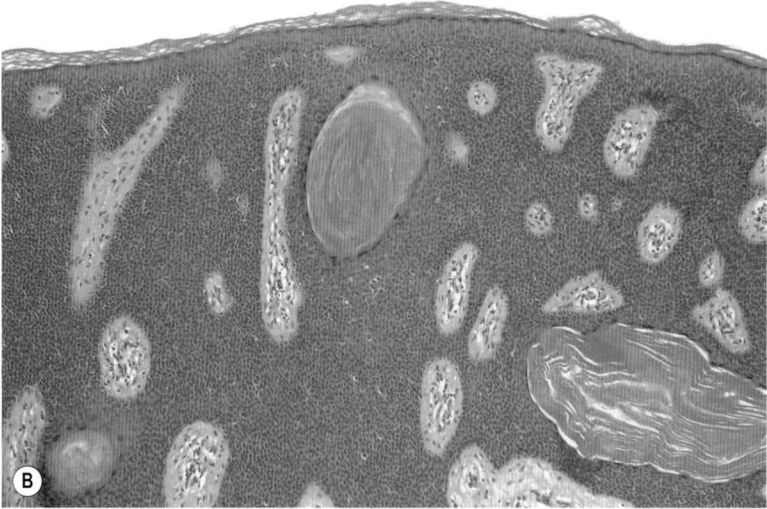

(B)

Fig. 24.16
Acanthotic seborrheic keratosis: (A) in this variant the surface is smooth and rounded and there is much more obvious acanthosis; (B) note the horn cysts and basaloid cell population.

Fig. 24.19
Clonal seborrheic keratosis: in this variant, tumor cells present as tightly aggregated intraepidermal 'nodules.'

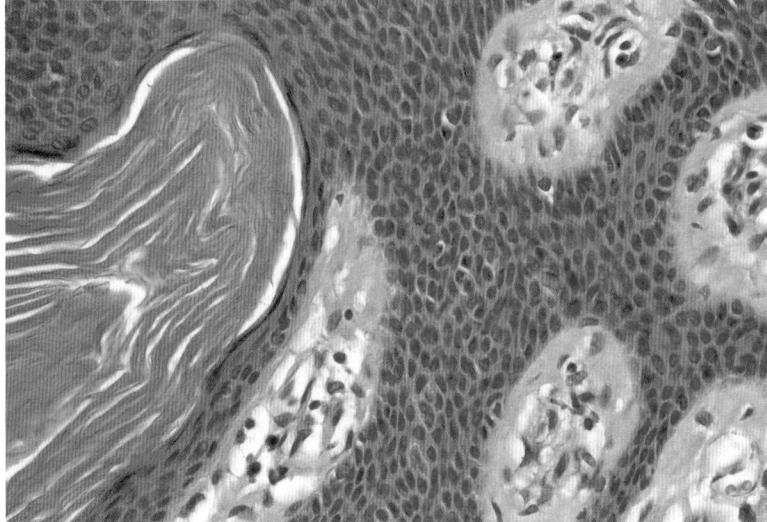

Fig. 24.17
Acanthotic seborrheic keratosis: high-power view showing basaloid cell population. Note that there is no cytological atypia.

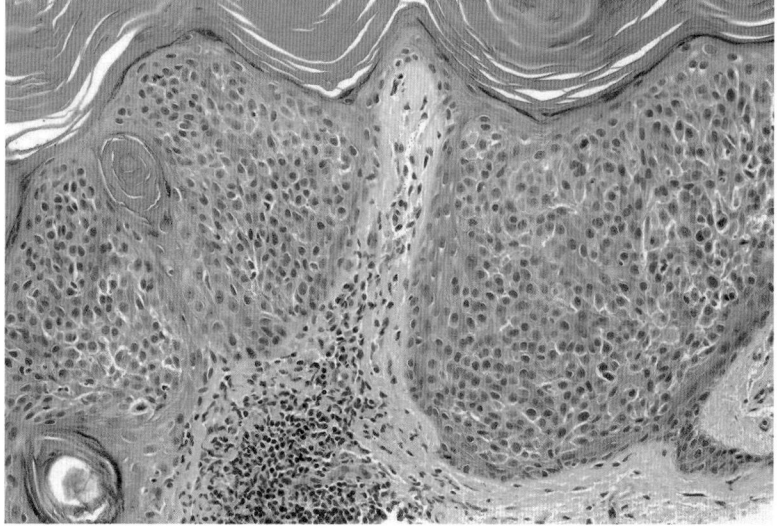

Fig. 24.20
Clonal seborrheic keratosis: in this view, the circumscribed collections of basaloid cells are clearly seen.

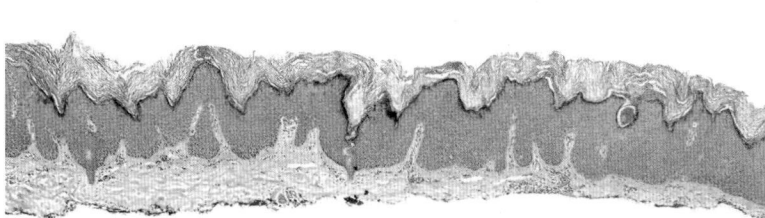

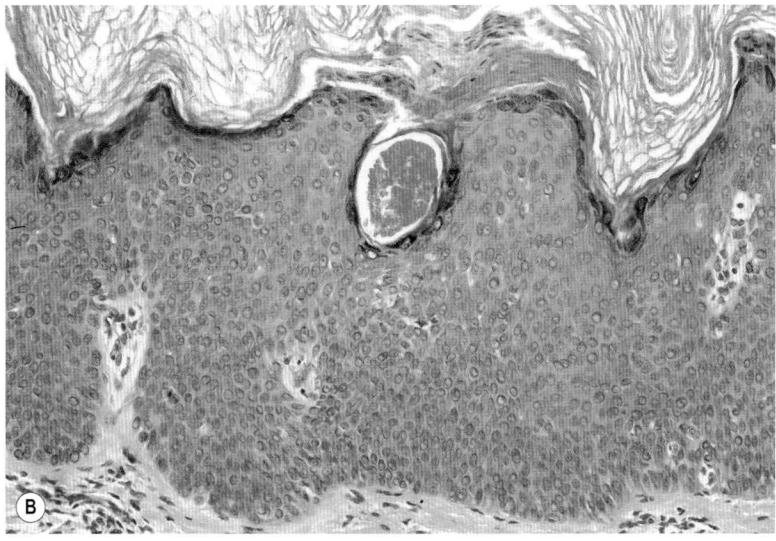

Fig. 24.21
(**A**, **B**) Flat seborrheic keratosis: this variant may clinically be mistaken for Bowen disease.

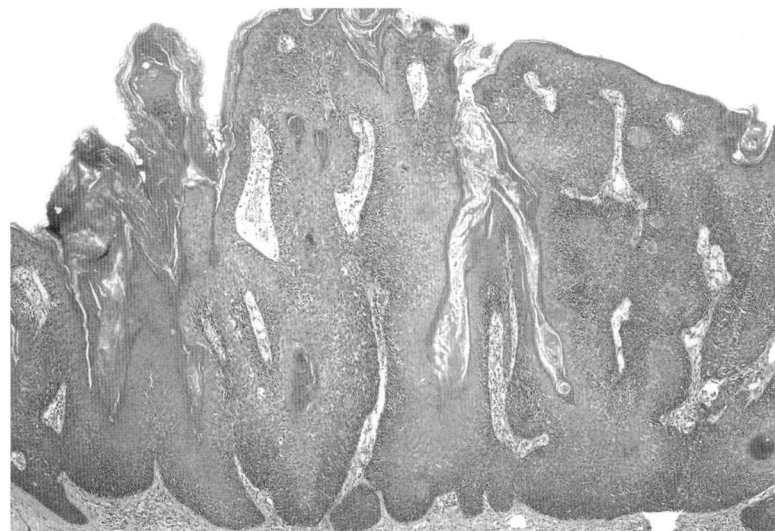

Fig. 24.22
Irritated seborrheic keratosis: low-power view showing pseudohorn cysts, squamous eddies, and patchy chronic inflammation.

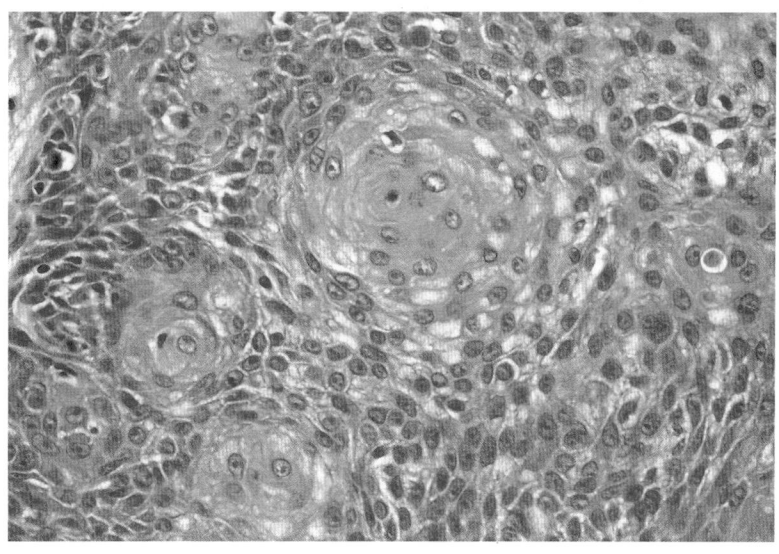

Fig. 24.23
Irritated seborrheic keratosis: high-power view of squamous eddies.

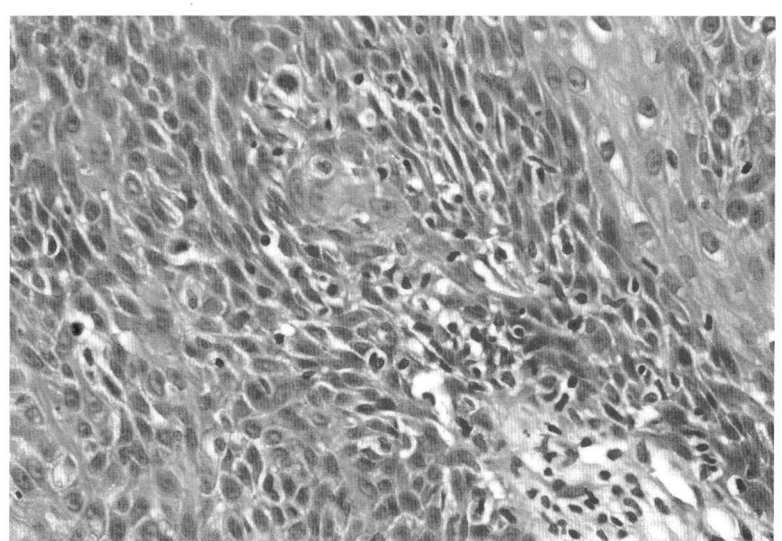

Fig. 24.24
Irritated seborrheic keratosis: there is a light lymphocytic infiltrate with focal spongiosis and exocytosis.

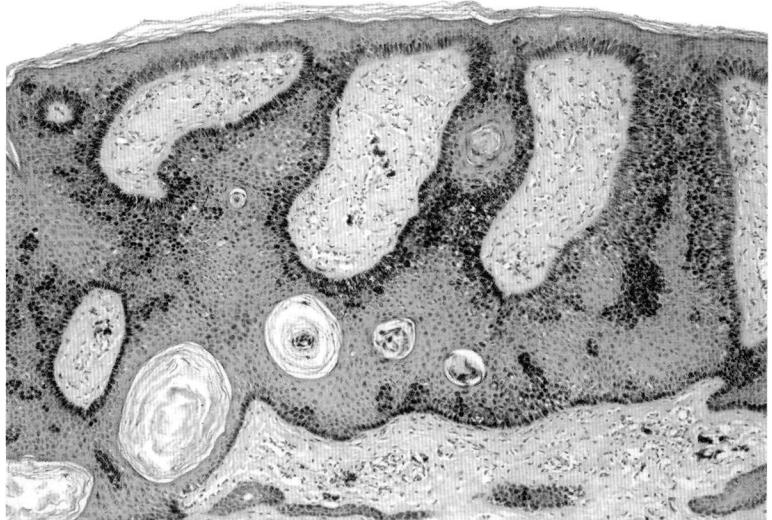

Fig. 24.25
Dermatosis papulosa nigra: there is acanthosis and marked melanin pigmentation. Horn pseudocysts are conspicuous.

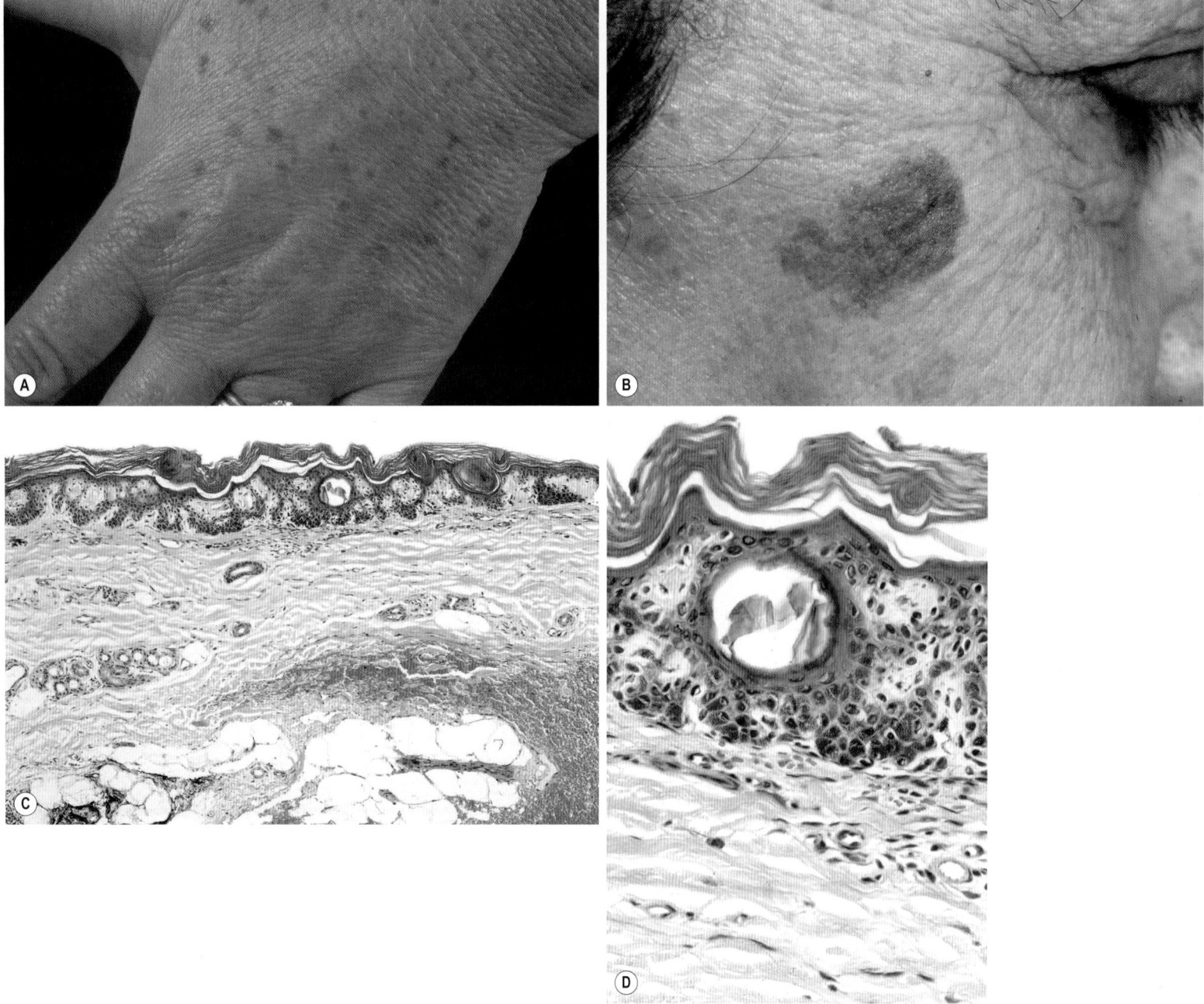

Fig. 24.26
(**A**) Actinic lentigo: there are large numbers of pale brown, variably sized macules on the dorsal aspect of the hand of this middle-aged woman. There was a history of excessive exposure to sunlight. By courtesy of R.A. Marsden, MD, St George's Hospital, London, UK. (**B**) Actinic lentigo: the face is commonly affected. Biopsy is usually necessary to exclude lentigo maligna. From the collection of the late N.P. Smith, MD, the Institute of Dermatology, London, UK. (**C**) Actinic lentigo: note the hyperkeratosis and hypergranulosis with extension of the epidermal ridges forming clublike processes. (**D**) Actinic lentigo: there is increased epidermal melanin and occasional melanophages are present in the papillary dermis (pigmentary incontinence).

have been documented.[14] There is hyperkeratosis, acanthosis with a reticulated pattern, and 'horn cyst' formation.[3] The epithelium shows abundant melanin pigmentation. A chronic inflammatory cell infiltrate may be present in the superficial dermis.

Actinic lentigo

Clinical features

Actinic lentigines (also known as lentigo senilis, solar lentigo, senile freckle, senile lentigo, liver spot) are benign, irregular, macular lesions that commonly develop on sun-damaged skin of the middle aged and elderly people, and are therefore most numerous on the face and dorsal aspects of hands and forearms (*Figs 24.26A and 24.26B*).[1–3] Both acute and chronic sun exposure have been implicated in their pathogenesis.[4] An increased incidence in

the setting of type 2 diabetes has recently been noted.[5] It has been proposed that actinic lentigines, especially those that are large, irregularly sized, and located on the upper back and shoulders, serve as a clinical marker of past severe sunburn.[6,7]

Actinic lentigines measure 0.1–1.0 cm or more in diameter, have a tendency to coalesce, and vary from light to dark brown.[8] Caucasians are particularly affected.[8] The lesions may be clinically mistaken for lentigo maligna.[9]

Unstable solar lentigo is a variant of solar lentigo, often presenting as a solitary irregularly pigmented macule and is usually darker and larger than classical solar lentigines.[10] It has been hypothesized that unstable solar lentigo could be a precursor lesion to lentigo maligna.[10]

Histologic features

Actinic lentigo usually develops against a background of solar elastosis. There may be slight hyperkeratosis. The epidermis shows extension of the rete ridges to form budlike processes expanding into the papillary dermis (see *Fig. 24.26C*). The inter-ridge epithelium is often atrophic. The melanocytes may be normal or slightly increased in number, but appear to be functionally hyperactive because there is a marked increase in the amount of melanin production (see *Fig. 24.26D*). A pivotal role for fibroblast-derived growth factors in regulating hyperpigmentation has recently been suggested.[11] Mild nuclear hyperchromatism and nuclear irregularity are sometimes seen as a reflection of the chronic actinic exposure. Similar changes may be evident in apparently normal skin from sun-exposed sites. Vacuolar degeneration of basal keratinocytes has also been reported to be a fairly consistent histologic abnormality.[12] Unstable solar lentigo is characterized by melanocytic hyperplasia not extending beyond the confines of the lesion.[10] Although melanocytes may be somewhat larger, they nevertheless lack nuclear atypia and hyperchromasia.[10]

In some examples, epidermal proliferation may lead to a reticular pattern due to the formation of anastomoses between adjacent attenuated ridges.[13] Occasionally, formation of small horn cysts can result in histologic overlap with seborrheic keratosis. Interestingly, similar genetic alterations, namely activating mutations in both *FGFR3* and *PIK3CA* pathways, have been demonstrated in both actinic lentigo and seborrheic keratosis, suggesting a possible relationship at the molecular level.[14,15] Altered fibroblasts in the underlying dermis may also trigger changes in keratinocytes.[16,17] Local cytokine and keratinocyte functional dysregulation likely also contribute.[18–20] Gene expression studies support the primary keratinocytic nature of these lesions.[21] Genome-wide association studies suggest a role for the immunoregulatory pathways as well as melanocytic pigmentation function as predisposition factors.[22] Actinic lentigo is increasingly viewed primarily as a keratinocytic lesion and it is therefore included in this chapter.

Actinic lentigo is sometimes associated with a slight increase in collagen within the papillary dermis. Pigmentary incontinence is often evident and a slight chronic inflammatory cell infiltrate is usually seen in the adjacent dermis. Dermal melanophages are also often seen.[12] A study demonstrated significant increase in dermal vessel density.[23] Some (but not all) authors believe that actinic lentigo may evolve into large cell acanthoma (see tumors of the surface epithelium)[24,25] or that the latter represents a variant of solar lentigo with cellular hypertrophy.[26]

Ultrastructurally, the melanocytes contain increased numbers of morphologically normal melanosomes.[26]

Large cell acanthoma

Clinical features

Large cell acanthoma presents as a discrete scaly papule or plaque up to 1 cm or more in diameter and is most commonly found on the head, arms, trunk, and lower limbs in decreasing order of frequency (*Fig. 24.27*).[1–5] Conjunctival involvement is rarely described.[6,7] Lesions, which are sharply demarcated, are often single, but multiple acanthomas have occasionally been documented.[1,8] The papules are commonly hyperpigmented or flesh colored, although achromic lesions have also been described.[9] The sex incidence is equal and patients are usually elderly. Large cell acanthoma does not therefore have distinctive clinical features, most examples being submitted as seborrheic keratoses, actinic keratoses or actinic lentigines.[2]

Pathogenesis and histologic features

The precise nature of this curious lesion is unknown. It has been variably described as a distinct entity, a variant of actinic keratosis or Bowen disease, a form of stucco keratosis, or a subtype of solar lentigo; we favor the latter interpretation.[1,2,5,10] The recent finding of aneuploidy in this clinically benign acanthoma suggests that it merits separate classification.[3,11,12] HPV type 6 has been identified from lesional skin in one patient with multiple disseminated large cell acanthomata.[13] Characterization for *FGFR3* or *PIK3CA* mutations as seen in some seborrheic keratoses is of interest, but not yet reported.

Histologically, large cell acanthoma is composed of keratinocytes measuring about twice normal size (*Fig. 24.28*).[14–16] Hyperkeratosis is usual and not associated with parakeratosis and the acanthotic epithelium shows bulbous

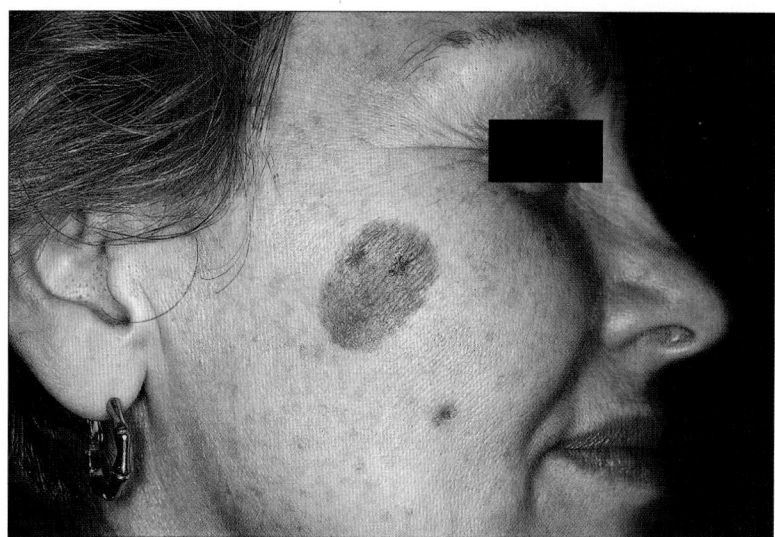

Fig. 24.27
Large cell acanthoma: this pigmented lesion could be mistaken for lentigo maligna. By courtesy of D. Santa Cruz, MD, St John's Mercy Medical Center, St Louis, USA.

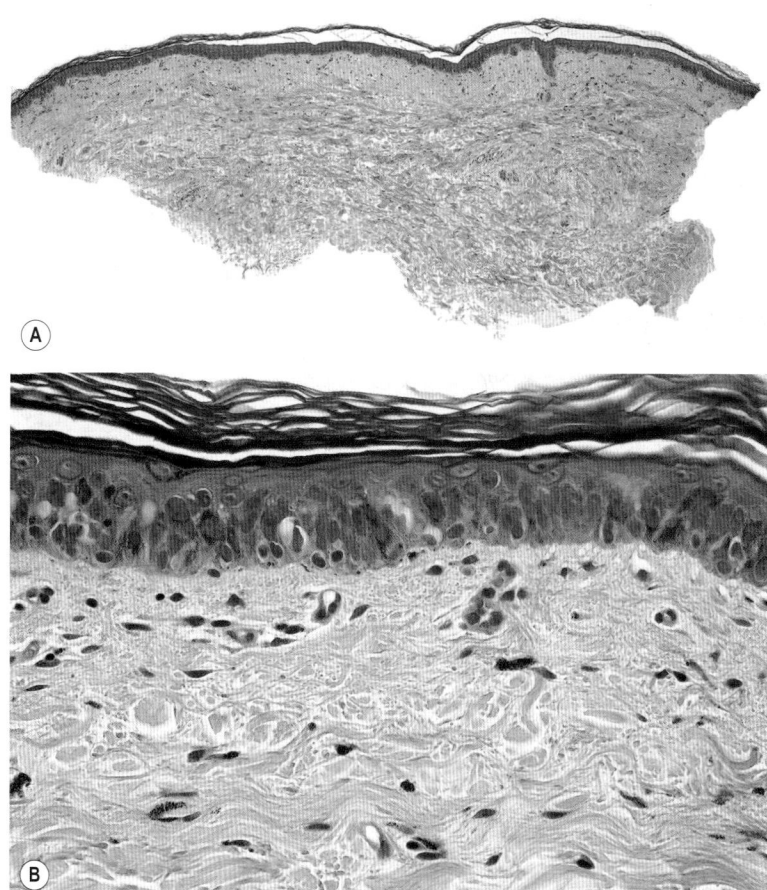

Fig. 24.28
Large cell acanthoma: (**A**) scanning view showing a rather flat featureless epidermis in this example; (**B**) the keratinocytes are enlarged but devoid of atypia. Note the hyperpigmentation.

epidermal ridges. Keratinocytes contain enlarged and rounded nuclei and the cytoplasm is abundant. Cytological atypia is not a feature and mitotic activity is limited to basal keratinocytes. Lesions may be hyperpigmented, normally pigmented, or achromic. Verrucous variants reminiscent of stucco keratoses have also been described.[1] Some large cell acanthomas can recede in the form of benign lichenoid keratoses.[17]

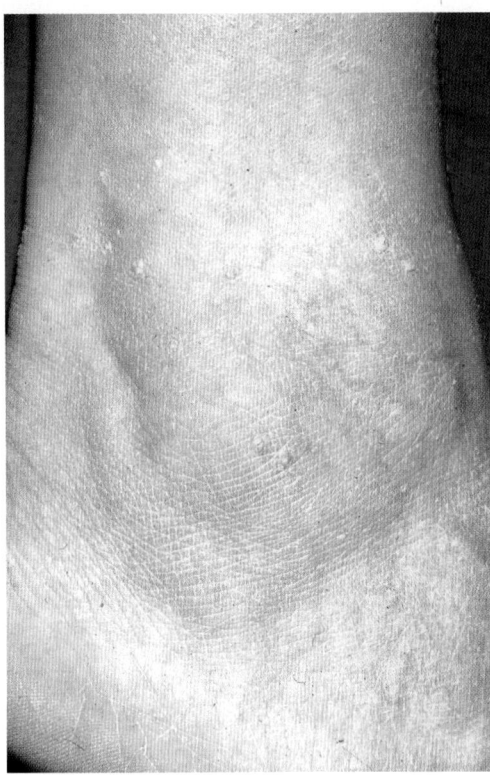

Fig. 24.29
Stucco keratosis: typical clinical appearance of multiple small warty lesions on the ankle of an elderly male. By courtesy of A. du Vivier, MD, King's College Hospital, London, UK.

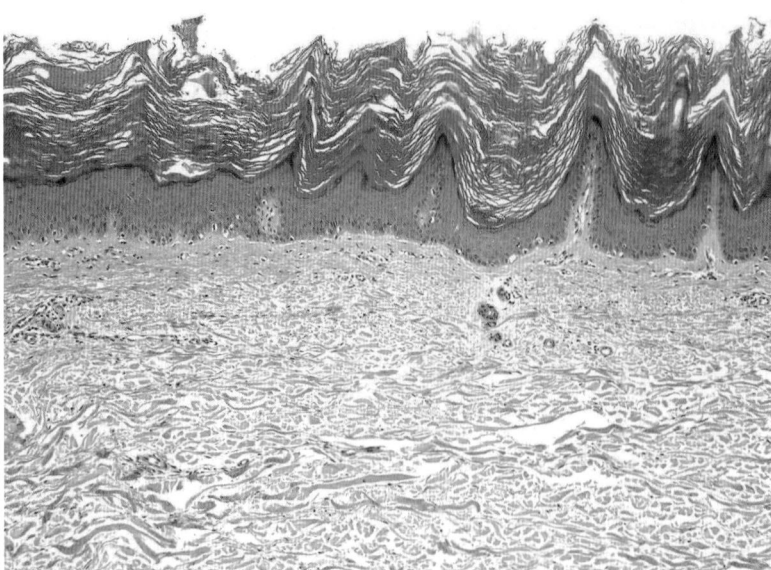

Fig. 24.30
Stucco keratosis: there is marked hyperkeratosis. The acanthotic epidermis has the typical church-spire appearance.

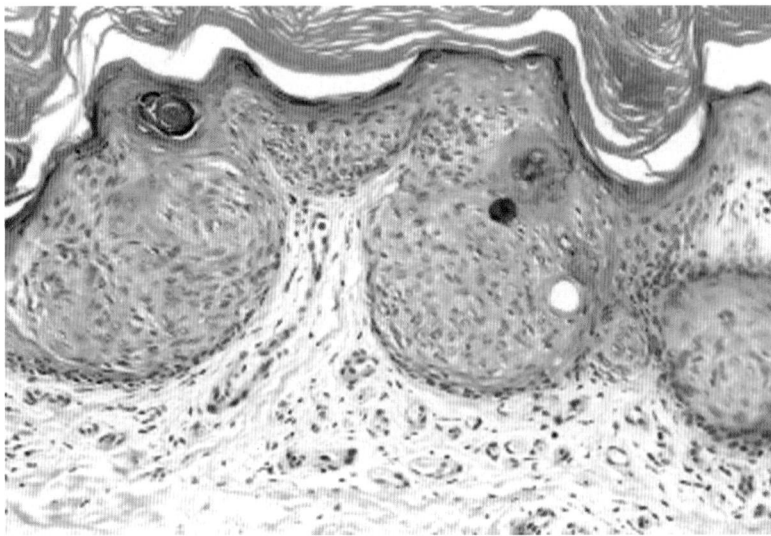

Fig. 24.31
Intraepidermal (Borst-Jadassohn) epithelioma: this example represents a clonal seborrheic keratosis.

Differential diagnosis

When pigmented, large cell acanthoma may be confused with actinic lentigo. However, actinic lentigo is composed of small basaloid cells aggregated within narrow, elongated epidermal ridges.[1]

Stucco keratoses

Clinical features

Stucco keratoses are warty lesions found on the extremities of elderly people and are more common in males than in females.[1–4] They are small (1–2 mm), sharply defined, round or oval verrucous papules of gray or brown coloration, commonly located around the foot, ankle, and dorsum of the hand (Fig. 24.29).[2,3,5] The extensor surface of the forearm is also often affected. The lesions are typically numerous, often in excess of 100. The papules appear stuck to the underlying skin but can be easily scratched off, leaving an intact undersurface with a scaly collarette.[2] Xerosis is often present and patients may also show scattered seborrheic keratoses. An eruptive case associated with esophageal cancer has been reported.[6]

Pathogenesis and histologic features

Ultrastructural studies have shown normal epidermal differentiation without evidence of intracellular viral particles.[7] Two patients with disseminated eruptive lesions demonstrated HPV DNA.[8,9] Activating mutations in *FGFR3* and *PIK3CA* have been documented, suggesting a pathogenetic relationship with seborrheic keratosis.[10]

The lesions are typified by dense orthokeratosis and 'peaked' or church-spire acanthosis (Fig. 24.30).[2,3] Basaloid cell proliferation and horn cyst formation as seen in seborrheic keratosis are characteristically absent.[3] There are no significant inflammatory changes.

Differential diagnosis

The histology of stucco keratosis is indistinguishable from acrokeratosis verruciformis. In contrast to the latter condition, stucco keratoses are not associated with Darier disease.

Intraepidermal epithelioma of Borst-Jadassohn

The Borst-Jadassohn epithelioma refers to a histopathological appearance rather than a precise clinicopathological entity.[1] It had initially been regarded as a distinctive clinicopathological entity.[2] The histologic findings, however, are seen in a number of lesions of different etiology such as Bowen disease, actinic keratosis, hidroacanthoma simplex, and seborrheic keratosis; it is therefore preferable to regard this as a histologic pattern rather than a distinct entity.[3–5] Histologically, it is characterized by nests of neoplastic cells situated within and surrounded by normal keratinocytes (Fig. 24.31).

Porokeratoma

Clinical features

Porokeratoma is an entity characterized by histologic features of porokeratosis presenting as a solitary lesion. It shows a marked male predominance and affects adults with a mean age of 57 years.[1] One case showed an association with HPV type 16.[2] The clinical presentation is of a hyperkeratotic plaque or nodule that may appear verrucous. A wide range of anatomic sites is affected but there is a predilection for distal extremities.[1] There is no underlying or associated porokeratosis and behavior is benign.

Histologic features

Histologically, porokeratoma is well circumscribed and characterized by marked epidermal hyperplasia and papillomatosis showing prominent distinct or broad and confluent cornoid lamella formation with dyskeratosis and loss of the granular cell layer.[1,3] There is an abrupt transition with areas of adjacent hyperorthokeratosis. The dermis shows a non-specific chronic inflammatory infiltrate and mild vascular dilatation.

Psoriasiform keratosis

Clinical features

Psoriasiform keratosis typically presents as solitary and occasionally multiple erythematous scaly papules or plaques measuring between 0.5 and 3 cm.[1,2] The anatomic distribution is wide and there is a predilection for the extremities. Adults are affected, with a mean age at presentation of 66 years.[1,2] The gender distribution is roughly equal and there is no history of psoriasis. Behavior is benign. HPV type 6 was identified in a single case.[3]

Histologic features

The histologic findings are at least somewhat reminiscent of psoriasis. There is sharp lesional circumscription and marked irregular, verrucous epidermal acanthosis with overlying hyperparakeratosis.[1,2,4] Focal to confluent mounds of parakeratosis contain collections of neutrophils and there is an absence or diminution of the granular cell layer in these areas.[1,2] Prominent and dilated vessels are present within the papillary dermis, accompanied by a chronic inflammatory infiltrate predominantly containing lymphocytes. A fungal etiology is excluded by PAS staining.

Granular parakeratotic acanthoma

Clinical findings

This solitary keratosis presents in adulthood with a median age of 59 years. Trunk and extremities are mainly affected and, based on the limited information available, there is a slight female bias.[1]

Histologic features

The histologic hallmark is the presence of keratinocytes showing conspicuous granular parakeratosis as observed in granular parakeratosis.[1,2] The lesion is otherwise circumscribed, with an endophytic growth pattern reminiscent of the adenoid pattern in seborrheic keratosis showing infundibular pseudocyst formation.[1] There is a florid accompanying chronic inflammatory infiltrate within the superficial dermis and lichenoid features may be present. Eosinophils and histiocytes are admixed.

Clear cell acanthoma

Clinical features

Clear cell acanthoma (of Degos) is an uncommon, usually solitary, tumor occurring in the middle aged or elderly but which may rarely present in younger patients.[1–3] Occasional multiple or disseminated eruptive variants have been described.[4–15] It is most commonly found on the lower limbs and presents as a circumscribed pink to bright red or brown oval-shaped papule or nodule measuring 1–4 cm in diameter (*Fig. 24.32*).[16] Rarely, lesions have been described at other sites including the face, forearm, hand, finger, trunk, inguinal region, scrotum, buttocks, hallux, and nipple.[16–23]

Occasionally, clear cell acanthoma presents as a polypoid lesion and large variants measuring up to 6 cm have been reported.[18,24–30] Rare pigmented variants are also recognized.[22,31,32] It often shows a collarette of scale, and erythematous puncta that bleed with minor trauma are commonly present on the surface.[6] Clinically, it may resemble a lobular capillary hemangioma

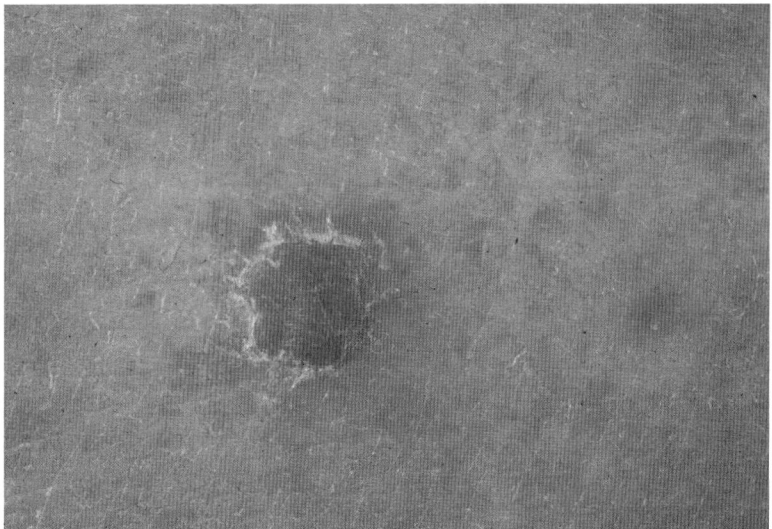

Fig. 24.32
Clear cell acanthoma: typical lesion on the shin of an elderly female. By courtesy of the Institute of Dermatology, London, UK.

(pyogenic granuloma) or an eccrine poroma. Individual case reports describe clear cell acanthoma arising within an epidermal nevus, in association with a melanocytic nevus, in a split-thickness skin graft and within a psoriatic plaque.[28,29,31,33–35] Multiple lesions have been reported in association with ichthyosis.[36] A case of Cowden syndrome associated with multiple clear cell acanthomas has been reported.[37]

Pathogenesis and histologic features

The precise nature of the clear cell acanthoma is unknown. Although variably regarded as an inflammatory epithelial hyperplasia, a hamartoma, or a variant of a seborrheic keratosis, most authors believe it to be a benign neoplasm, although the cell of origin is subject to dispute.[15,38] Derivation from epidermal, sebaceous, and sweat gland epithelium have all been proposed. The high glycogen content coupled with keratin and involucrin positivity and carcinoembryonic antigen (CEA) negativity has led some authors to suggest an origin from the follicular outer root sheath.[38] However, considering the characteristic follicular sparing this seems an unlikely hypothesis. The presence of striking epithelial membrane antigen (EMA) expression could suggest an eccrine acrosyringeal derivation.[39,40] However, immunohistochemical studies on cytokeratin, involucrin, and filaggrin expression support an epidermal derivation and raise the possibility that clear cell acanthoma could represent an inflammatory dermatosis rather than a true neoplasm.[41–43] This hypothesis is further supported by studies suggesting that, similar to psoriasis, keratinocyte growth factor (KGF) upregulation may be responsible for keratinocyte hyperproliferation in clear cell acanthoma.[44]

Clear cell acanthoma is composed of markedly acanthotic (often psoriasiform) epithelium, which has a characteristically clearly demarcated lateral border (*Fig. 24.33*). The epidermal ridges are commonly fused. Individual cells have clear cytoplasm due to the presence of abundant glycogen, best demonstrated with a periodic acid-Schiff (PAS) reaction (*Fig. 24.34*). Variably pigmented, dendritic melanocytes are sometimes present, both along the basal epithelial layer and also intermingled with keratinocytes in the upper layers of the lesion.[22,31,32,45] This latter feature appears to be more common in patients of Mediterranean ancestry.[46] In cases where pigmentation is clinically apparent, the confusing term clear cell melanoacanthoma (cf. seborrheic keratosis)[47] or pigmented clear cell acanthoma has sometimes been applied.[31,48,49] Typically, the intraepidermal portions of the adnexae are spared. Intralesional neutrophils are characteristic and are often evident within an overlying parakeratotic scale. The underlying dermal papillae commonly contain dilated capillaries, and an inflammatory cell infiltrate with a predominance of neutrophils is often present. These latter features show considerable overlap with psoriasis.

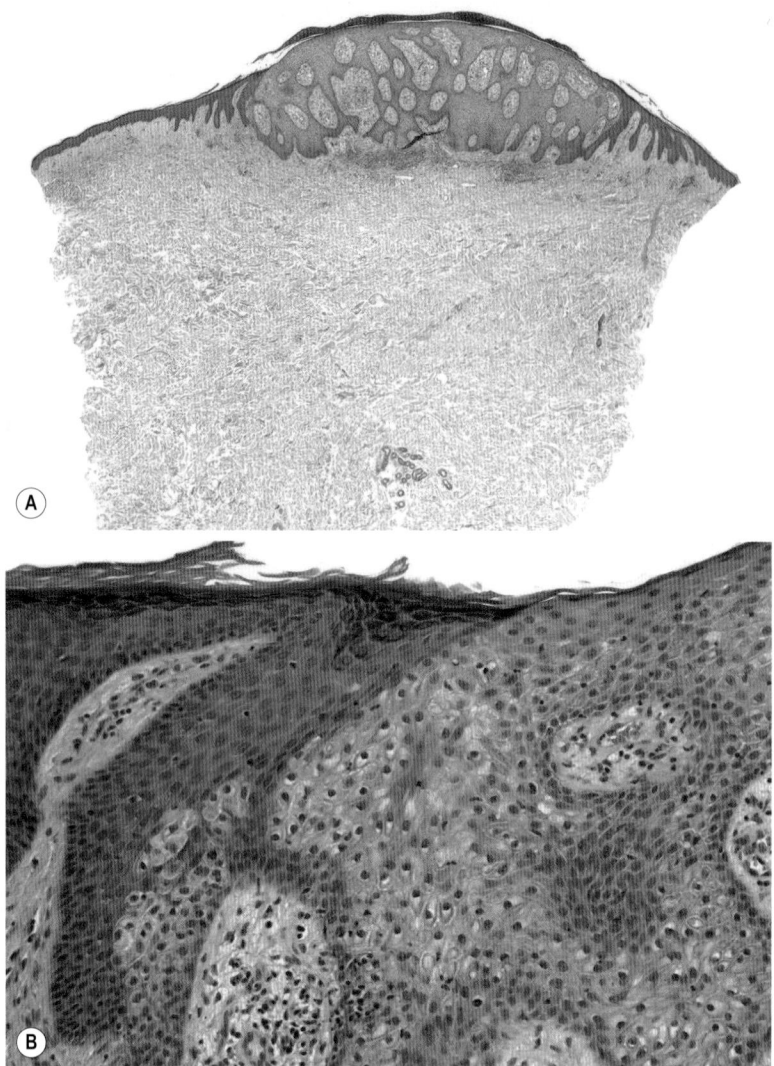

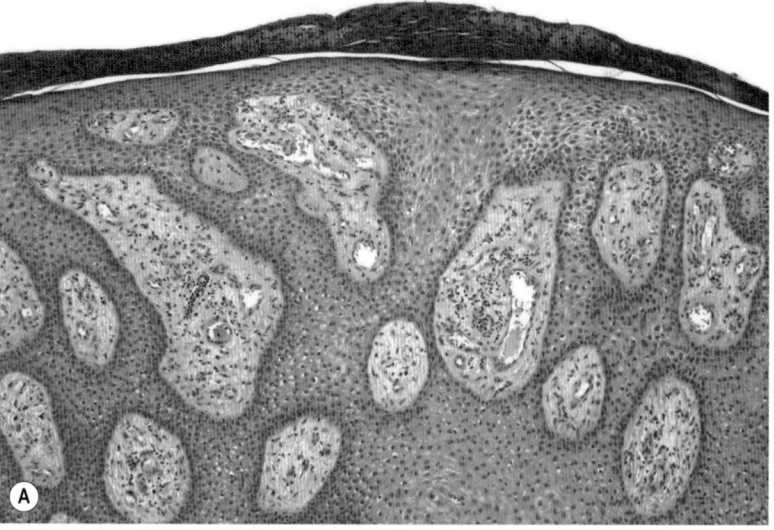

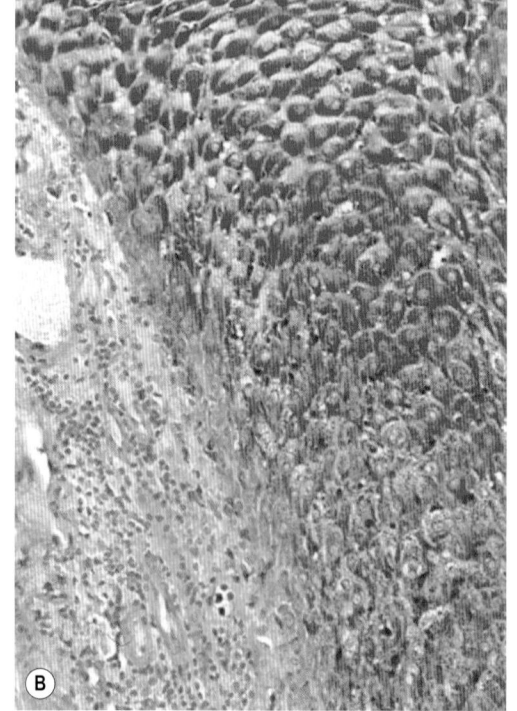

Fig. 24.33
Clear cell acanthoma: (**A**) the lesion, which is sharply demarcated, shows striking hyperplasia; (**B**) although the basal epithelial cells retain their normal tinctorial properties, most of the epithelium shows marked pallor.

Fig. 24.34
Clear cell acanthoma: (**A**) neutrophils in transit and within the crust on the surface of the lesion are characteristic; (**B**) the keratinocyte pallor is due to massive glycogen deposition as seen in this periodic acid-Schiff reaction.

Rarely, so-called atypical or malignant clear cell acanthoma has been documented in which cellular pleomorphism and mitotic activities are features.[50,51] Whether, in reality, this represents a true variant is uncertain.

Pseudoepitheliomatous hyperplasia

Clinical features

Pseudoepitheliomatous (pseudocarcinomatous) hyperplasia represents an extreme degree of acanthosis, which histologically mimics squamous cell carcinoma.[1] It may be seen in association with:
- chronic venous stasis,
- ulceration,
- chronic inflammatory conditions, such as pyoderma gangrenosum, lupus vulgaris, syphilis and fungal infections (e.g., blastomycosis), hypertrophic lichen planus, insect bite granuloma and bromoderma.[1–3]
- CD30 positive lymphoproliferative disorders and more rarely in reactive conditions rich in CD30 positive cells.[4]

It is occasionally found in the epithelium overlying neoplasms such as granular cell tumor and fibrous histiocytoma.[5–7]

Histologic features

The histologic features of pseudoepitheliomatous hyperplasia vary from a marked degree of irregular acanthosis to changes highly suggestive of

squamous cell carcinoma (*Fig. 24.35*).[8] In such instances, distinction from the latter can be very difficult. The diagnosis of this entity depends on awareness of the condition and on a careful survey of the surrounding dermis to find a predisposing lesion.

Basal cell carcinoma

Clinical features

Nonmelanoma skin cancer – consisting predominantly of basal cell carcinoma (BCC) and squamous cell carcinoma (SCC) – is the most prevalent cutaneous malignant neoplasm in the United States with an estimated incidence broadly ranging from 600,000 to 2,800,000 persons affected per year.[1–4] However, since basal cell carcinoma is not a reportable disease in the United States, reliable estimates are challenging to obtain and differ based on methodology.[3] Basal cell carcinoma constitutes well over 70% of skin cancers and one-third of all cancers in the United States,and its incidence outnumbers melanoma by a factor of approximately 20-40. Thus while not as deadly as melanoma, it constitutes a huge public health concern and population screening remains a priority.[5,6] Basal cell carcinoma (epithelioma) is

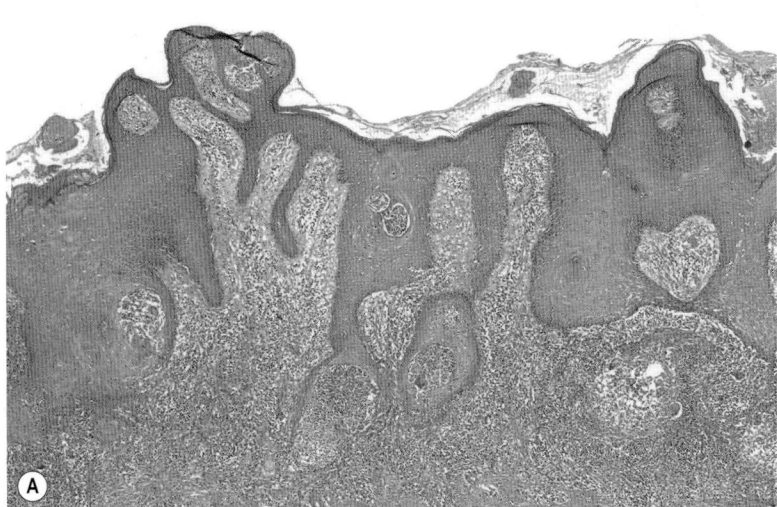

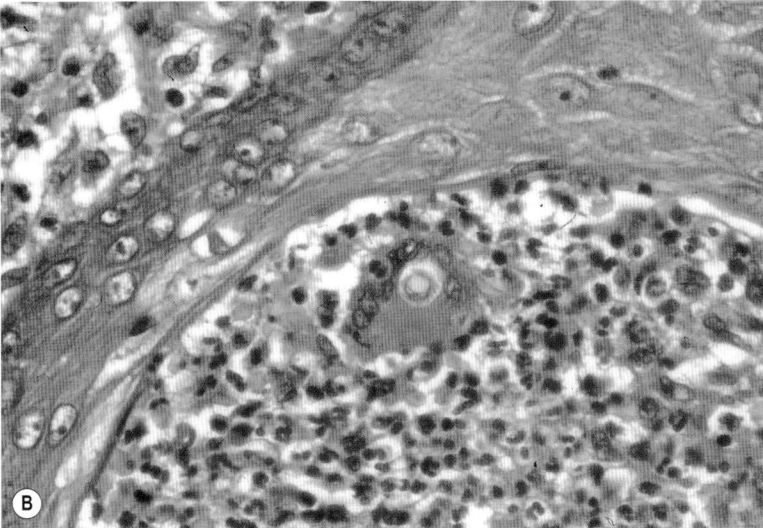

Fig. 24.35
Pseudoepitheliomatous hyperplasia: (**A**) there is very marked irregular acanthosis extending deeply into the reticular dermis. Note the inflammation; (**B**) this is a case of blastomycosis. A yeast form is present in the multinucleate giant cell.

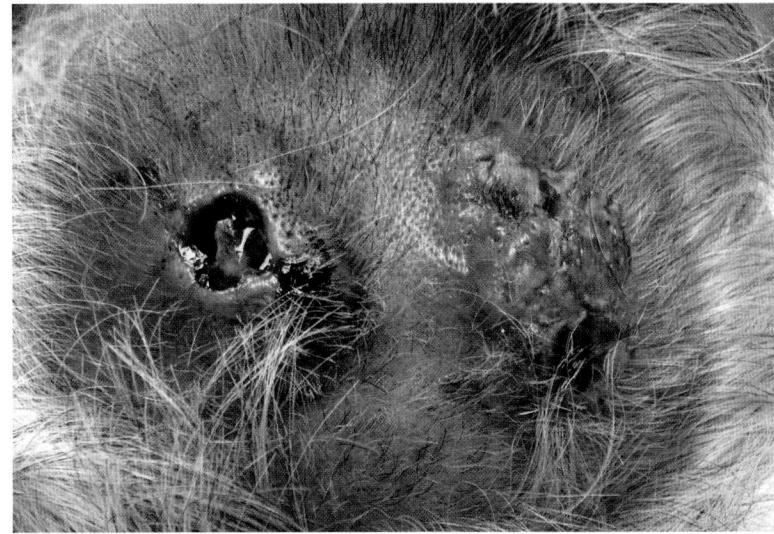

Fig. 24.36
Basal cell carcinoma: multiple ulcerated lesions are present on this patient's scalp. By courtesy of J. Dayrit, MD, Manila, The Philippines.

the most common cutaneous malignant neoplasm, being four to five times more frequent than squamous cell carcinoma, and the incidence appears to be rising at a rate of 3–10% annually.[1,7–10] Accurate current data are not available, but the incidence of basal cell carcinoma in the United States in 1977–78 was approximately 180 per 100,000 of the population and estimated at 191 per 100,000 in 1990.[11] Based on a study from 1994, the estimated incidence of basal cell carcinoma in the United States was as high as 407 per 100,000 for men and 212 per 100,000 for women.[2,12,13] Estimated differently based on procedure data, the total burden of non-melanoma skin cancer in the United States is suggested to be as high 5.4 million cases and 3.3 million patients per year.[14] There is marked regional variation in incidence.[15] A slightly lower figure has been reported in Northern Europe in contrast to a drastically increased incidence in Australia.[16–21] Basal cell carcinoma is slightly more common in men than in women and it is very rare in blacks.[9,15,22–26] Basal cell carcinoma in the Oriental population is frequently pigmented (55–75% of BCC), while this phenomenon is much less prevalent in India (around 20%).[27–29] The term carcinoma is preferred to epithelioma because, although these tumors metastasize exceptionally rarely, locally advanced cases are capable of gross tissue destruction, particularly those lesions arising on the head, which may erode the nose or orbital contents and even extend into the brain (*Fig. 24.36*).[4,30–35]

In less sunny climates, basal cell carcinoma represents a tumor of the elderly, commonly presenting in patients in their sixth decade or older.[9] Exceptions to this include those with xeroderma pigmentosum, albinism,

the nevoid basal cell carcinoma syndrome, and Bazex syndrome. In sunny climates, presentation may be at a much younger age, and even children without associated genetic disorders may be affected.[36–44] Basal cell carcinoma presenting at an early age has been thought to behave more aggressively, a view that has recently been challenged.[45,46] Tumors are often multiple; a recent study from Australia demonstrated that 46% of patients with an initial diagnosis of basal cell carcinoma suffered from more than one tumor over a 10-year period.[47] Data from the United States are similar.[14]

Although the face is most commonly involved, the tumors being particularly related to excessive sunlight, lesions are not usually seen on the dorsal aspects of the hands.[48] Less often, basal cell carcinoma presents on the neck, trunk, and proximal extremities. Lesions affecting the lower leg are rare and have been suggested to ulcerate more frequently.[49–51] Other unusual and rare locations include the vulva, penis, scrotum, perineum, buttock, nipple, areola, umbilicus, subungual region, soles, palms, axilla, conchal bowl, caruncle, lacrimal duct, and the oral mucosa.[52–91] Lesions of the scrotum are of particular importance because of an associated high rate of metastasis (13%) (*Fig. 24.37*).[60,92–95] Occasionally, basal cell carcinoma may complicate venous stasis ulcers.[96,97] These are particularly significant as they may mimic granulation tissue.[98,99] The rolled margin, however, is the diagnostic clue. Basal cell carcinoma has also been reported to arise in scars of variable etiology, such as surgical, burn, and postvaccination, in addition to scars which have followed healed infectious diseases such as leishmania and chickenpox.[6,100–115] An increased risk for the development of basal cell carcinoma has also been documented at the site of prior radiation therapy with potential for more aggressive behavior and higher local recurrence as well as distant metastasis rates.[116–120] Basal cell carcinoma that has been described in association with nevus sebaceous and dermatofibroma are better regarded as variants of trichoblastoma.

Basal cell carcinoma may also arise in association with melanoma either in the form of a collision tumor or as a melanoma metastasis to a basal cell carcinoma.[121–134] The intimate association of melanoma cells and basaloid epithelial proliferations has recently been reported as 'basomelanocytic tumor'.[134–137] Whether this truly represents a distinct entity rather than colonization of basal cell carcinoma by melanoma cells is a topic of current debate and awaits further study.[138]

Basal cell carcinoma may also complicate other lesions such as dilated pore of Winer, port-wine stain, Marjolin ulcer, arteriovenous malformation, rhinophyma, pilonidal sinus, lupus vulgaris, multiple trichoepitheliomas, and hair and skin graft transplantation sites.[139–156] Basal cell carcinoma may also show involvement by underlying systemic disorders such as chronic lymphocytic leukemia.[157–160] An increased incidence of basal cell carcinoma has been reported in young females who smoke and use tanning beds and

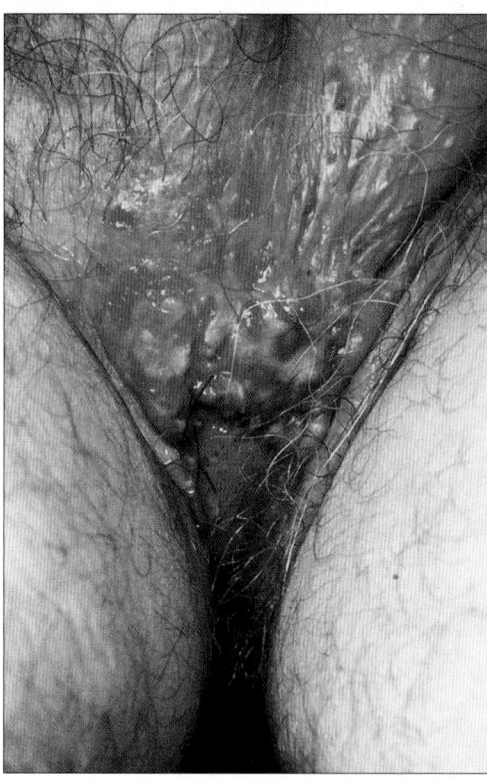

Fig. 24.37
Basal cell carcinoma: scrotal tumors are extremely rare but are of particular importance because of their high recurrence and metastasis rates. The mortality is high. By courtesy of the Institute of Dermatology, London, UK.

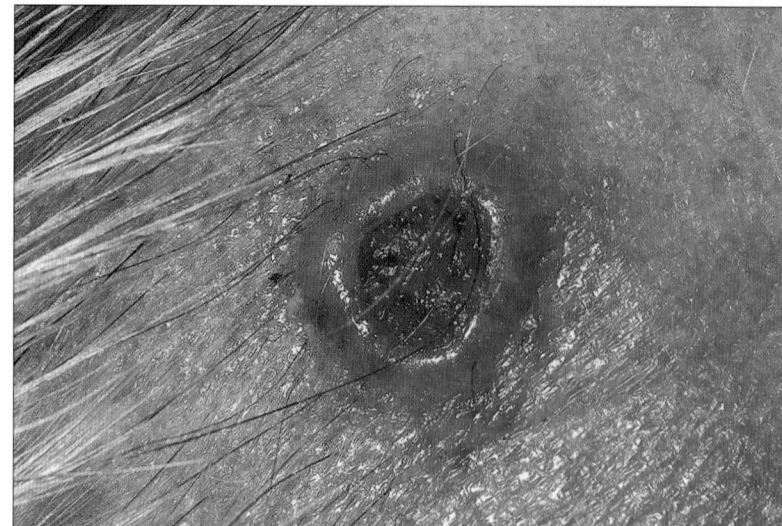

Fig. 24.38
Ulcerative basal cell carcinoma: note the central ulceration and characteristic rolled border. By courtesy of R.A. Marsden, MD, St George's Hospital, London, UK.

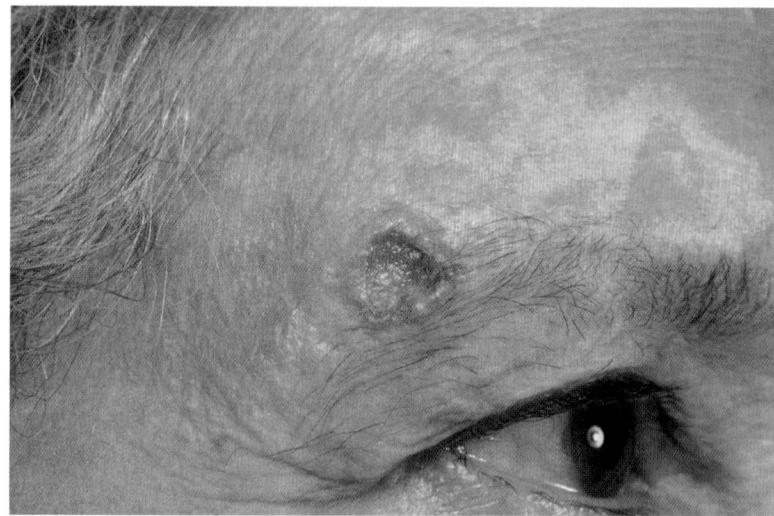

Fig. 24.39
Ulcerative basal cell carcinoma: the rolled border is well developed in this example. By courtesy of the Institute of Dermatology, London, UK.

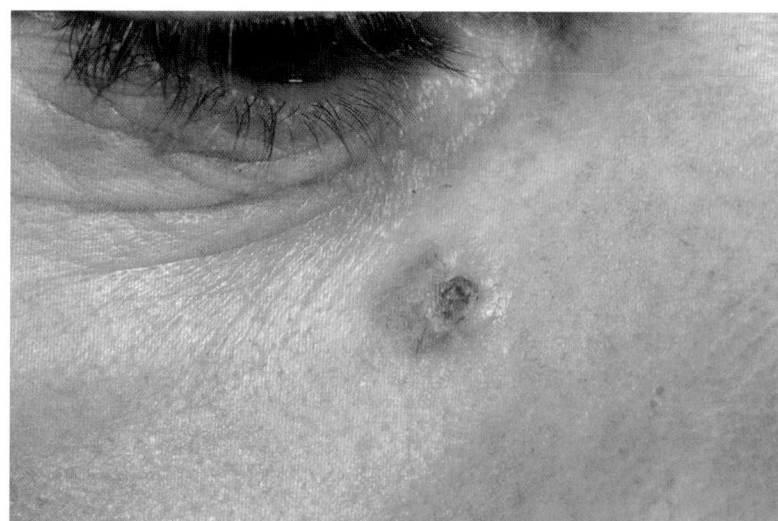

Fig. 24.40
Ulcerative basal cell carcinoma: typical lesion on the upper cheek. By courtesy of the Institute of Dermatology, London, UK.

there appears to be a similar sex predilection for tumors arising on the upper lip.[161-164]

It is convenient to divide basal cell carcinoma into five main clinical subtypes, which to some extent correlate with their general growth pattern and treatment. Nodular and morpheaform basal cell carcinomas are most frequently located in the head and neck area whereas those lesions on the trunk are predominantly of the superficial subtype.[165]

- nodular/ulcerative (45–60%),
- diffuse (infiltrating and morpheaform) (4–17%),
- superficial (15–35%),
- pigmented (1–7%),
- fibroepithelioma of Pinkus.[166-173]

Ulcerative variant

Ulcerative basal cell carcinoma (rodent ulcer) commences life as a small translucent papule, which may be yellow or pink or have a pearly appearance. The epidermis is thinned and is stretched over the surface of the tumor and often a few telangiectatic vessels are evident. As the lesion enlarges, central erosion or ulceration develops (Figs 24.38–24.44). A history of an ulcer that never quite heals is characteristic. An established rodent ulcer is sharply demarcated and typically has a rolled margin.

Nodulocystic variant

The nodulocystic variant is lobulated and usually does not ulcerate; it may therefore be mistaken for a simple cutaneous cyst. The tumor may grow quite large, measuring 2 cm or more in diameter, and presents as a smooth pearly nodule that is frequently associated with telangiectatic vessels (Figs 24.45 and 24.46).

Diffuse variant

The diffuse type comprises several patterns, all of which are associated with a poorly demarcated clinical margin. The prototype is the morpheaform or sclerosing basal cell carcinoma. This is a flat, whitish-pink plaque, which feels indurated and tethered and slowly enlarges over the course of several years (Fig. 24.47). In contrast to the noduloulcerative tumors, the morpheaform variant is not usually associated with obvious translucency.

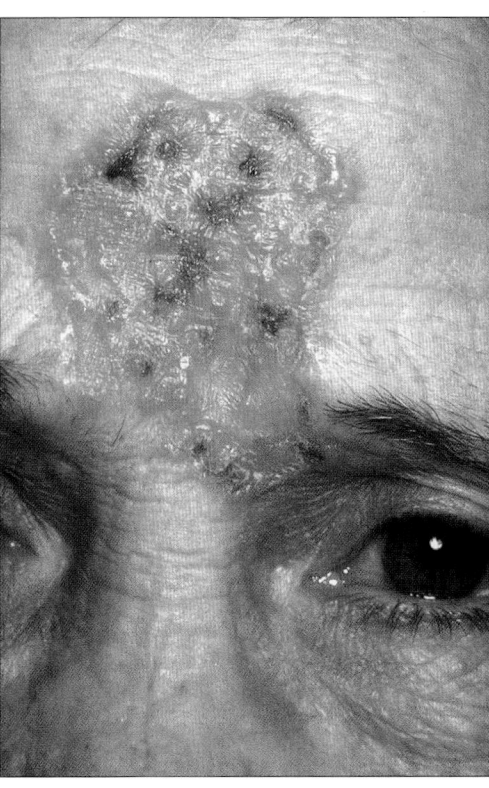

Fig. 24.41
Ulcerative basal cell carcinoma: a rather more extensive lesion showing partial central healing. By courtesy of R.A. Marsden, MD, St George's Hospital, London, UK.

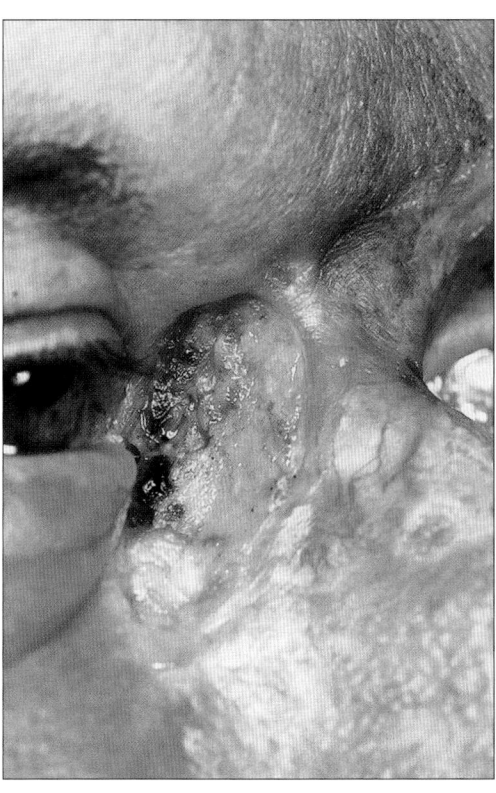

Fig. 24.42
Ulcerative basal cell carcinoma: this example shows very extensive nasal destruction. By courtesy of the Institute of Dermatology, London, UK.

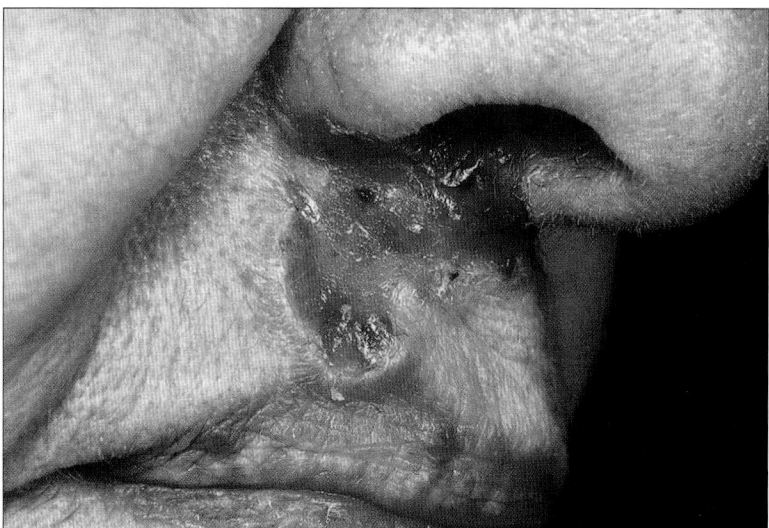

Fig. 24.43
Ulcerative basal cell carcinoma: it is particularly important with this variant to exclude perineural infiltration which in part accounts for the very high recurrence rate. By courtesy of the Institute of Dermatology, London, UK.

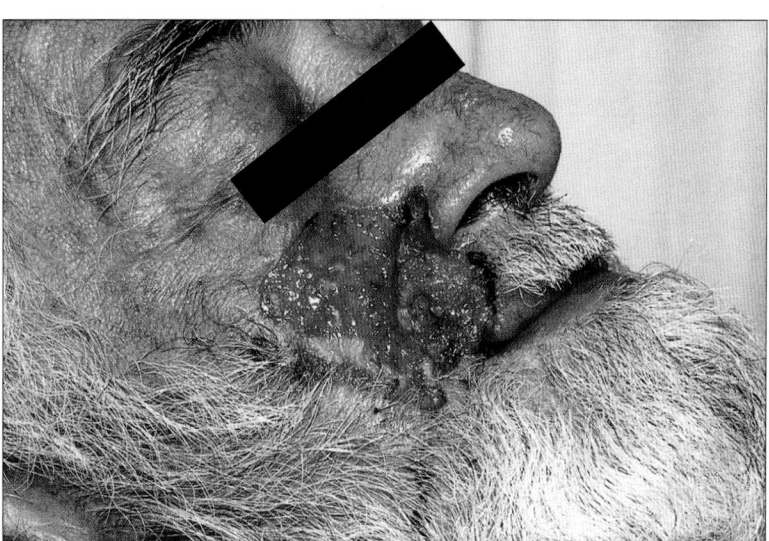

Fig. 24.44
Ulcerative basal cell carcinoma: this patient shows very extensive facial involvement. By courtesy of N. Saxe, MD, University of Cape Town and Groote Schuur Hospital, Cape Town, South Africa.

Sometimes, however, in examples where the fibrous component is less dense, some translucency may be present and is best highlighted by stretching the skin under a good light. Erosions, crusting, or ulceration are common, with the center of the lesion showing either a cicatrized or healed regressed area. Morpheaform basal cell carcinomas are notoriously difficult to treat, the pathological extent of the tumor often being greatly in excess of the clinical impression.

Superficial variant

Superficial basal cell carcinoma presents mainly on the trunk as a slowly enlarging, scaly red patch that has usually been present for years (*Fig.*

24.48). Lesions, particularly when multiple, may be clinically confused with psoriasis. The surface in the center of the lesion may occasionally be eroded, but more often it is intact. Careful examination sometimes reveals a delicate rolled thin translucent border that greatly facilitates establishing the diagnosis. Multiple superficial basal cell carcinomas are a known complication of arsenic ingestion (and also actinic keratosis and Bowen disease).

Pigmented variant

Both superficial and localized basal cell carcinomas may contain pigment, which is distributed patchily or evenly and may therefore cause clinical confusion with melanoma – pigmented basal cell carcinoma (*Figs 24.49–24.51*).[174,175]

Giant basal cell carcinoma

Giant basal cell carcinoma, by definition measuring 10 cm or more in diameter, is preferentially found on the trunk (*Fig. 24.52*). It is thought to be a high-grade variant with a high metastasis rate (30%) and significant mortality,

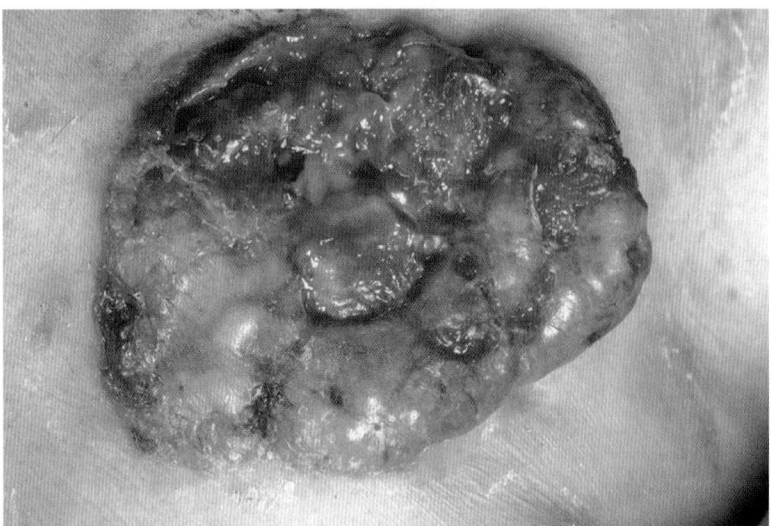

Fig. 24.45
Ulcerative basal cell carcinoma: this is a very large multinodular lesion showing focal ulceration. Lesions as large as this example are uncommon in Western societies. By courtesy of the Institute of Dermatology, London, UK.

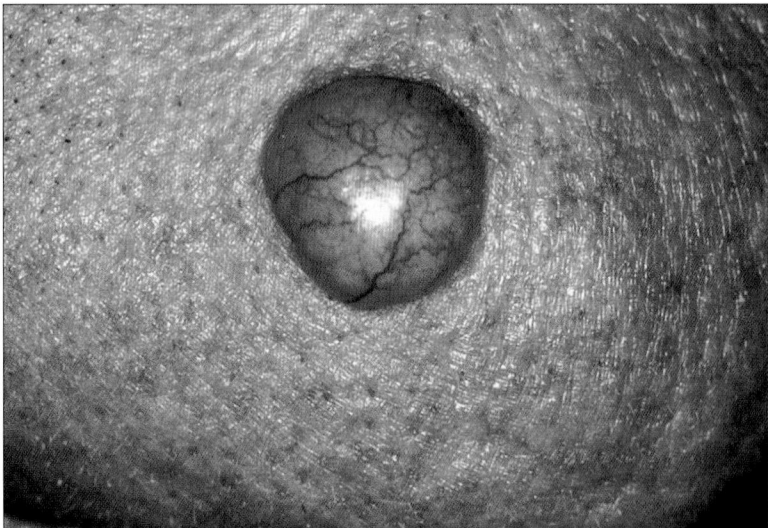

Fig. 24.46
Nodular basal cell carcinoma: note the characteristic telangiectatic vessels coursing over the surface. By courtesy of R.A. Marsden, MD, St George's Hospital, London, UK.

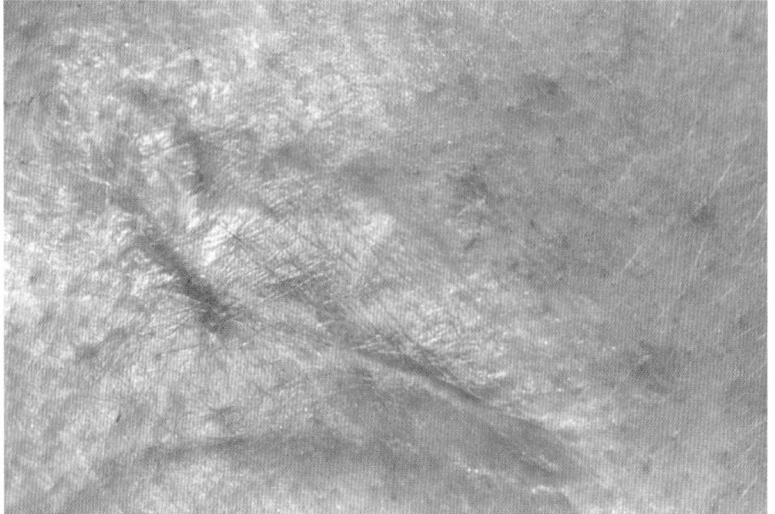

Fig. 24.47
Morpheaform basal cell carcinoma: this ill-defined white–pink, flat lesion is characteristic. By courtesy of the Institute of Dermatology, London, UK.

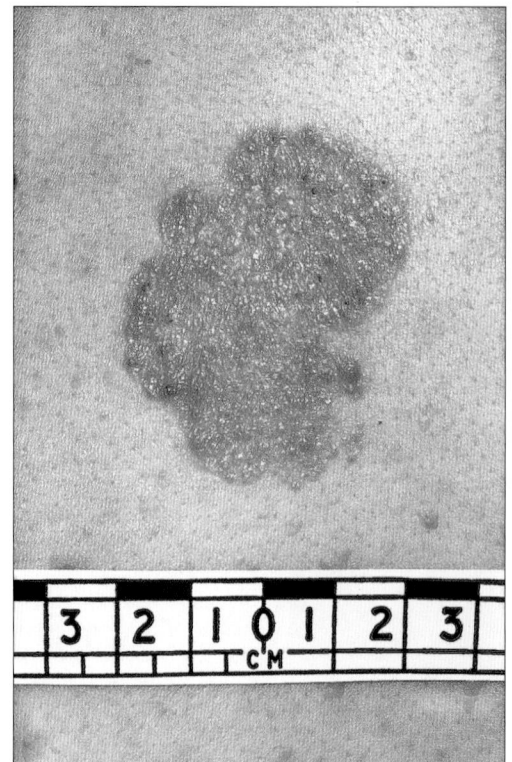

Fig. 24.48
Superficial basal cell carcinoma: note the erythema and scaling. This variant may be clinically mistaken for eczema or psoriasis. It is notoriously difficult to identify the radial border of this lesion. By courtesy of R.A. Marsden, MD, St George's Hospital, London, UK.

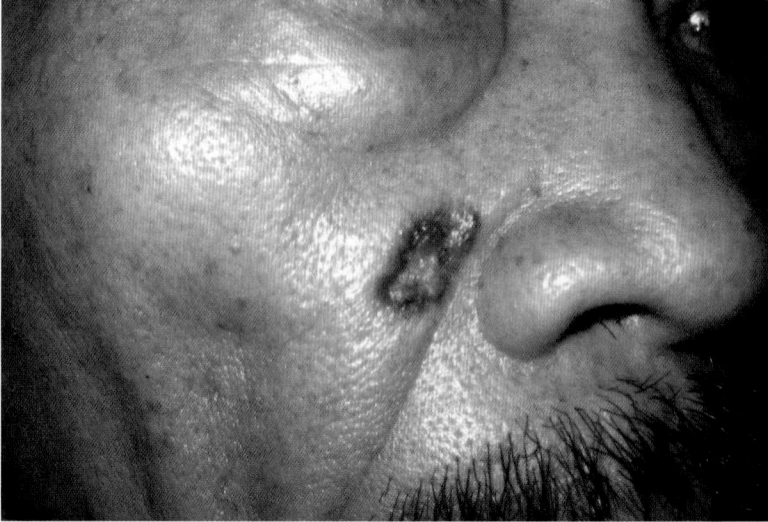

Fig. 24.49
Pigmented basal cell carcinoma: the pigmented nature of this variant sometimes causes clinical confusion with malignant melanoma. By courtesy of J. Dayrit, MD, Manila, The Philippines.

although some studies do not detect any evidence of metastasis.[176-180] It is usually associated with neglect.[181] There is a high incidence of alcoholism as well as cigarette smoking.[177,182]

Other less frequent clinical presentations include linear as well as unilateral basal cell carcinoma, polypoid basal cell carcinoma, and pedunculated basal cell carcinoma.

- Linear basal cell carcinoma presents predominantly on the neck, eyelid, and medial canthus in the elderly as an ill-defined linear lesion.[153,183–185]
- Polypoid basal cell carcinoma has been described recently and presents in the elderly as an exophytic, polypoid lesion connected by a stalk. The most prevalent sites are the scalp, ear, and genital area but only limited data are available.[186–189] A patient with multiple infundibulocystic basal cell carcinomas in a unilateral distribution around the mouth and with indolent clinical behavior has also been reported.[190]

The reported recurrence rates are very variable (1–8.7%) and depend upon the location, size, histologic subtype and form, and adequacy of primary

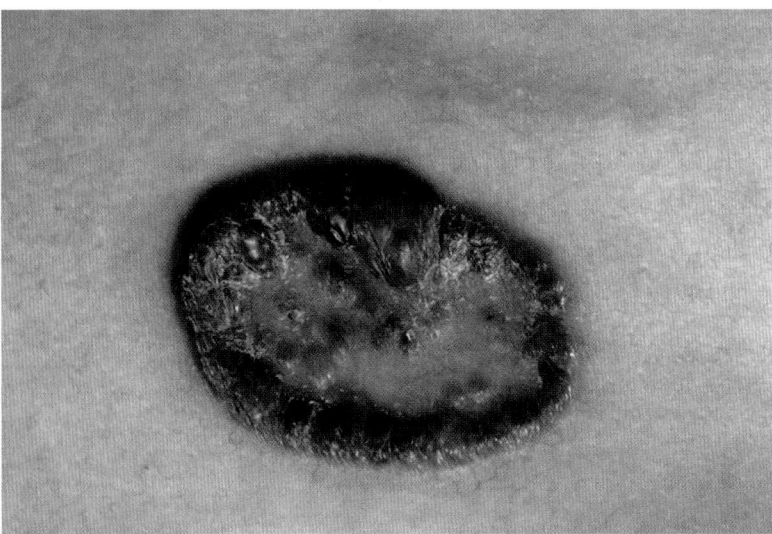

Fig. 24.50
Pigmented basal cell carcinoma: this extensively pigmented example could easily be mistaken for a melanoma with central regression. By courtesy of the Institute of Dermatology, London, UK.

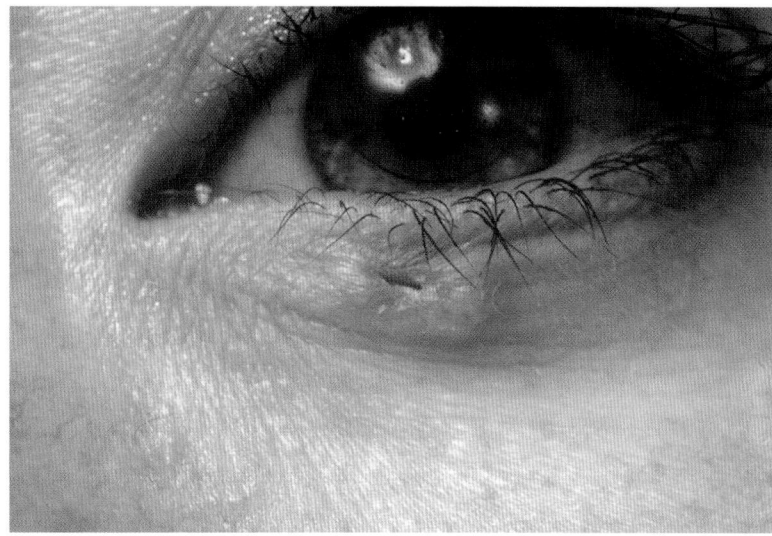

Fig. 24.53
Basal cell carcinoma: tumors involving the periocular tissues are notoriously difficult to treat and have a high recurrence rate. By courtesy of the Institute of Dermatology, London, UK.

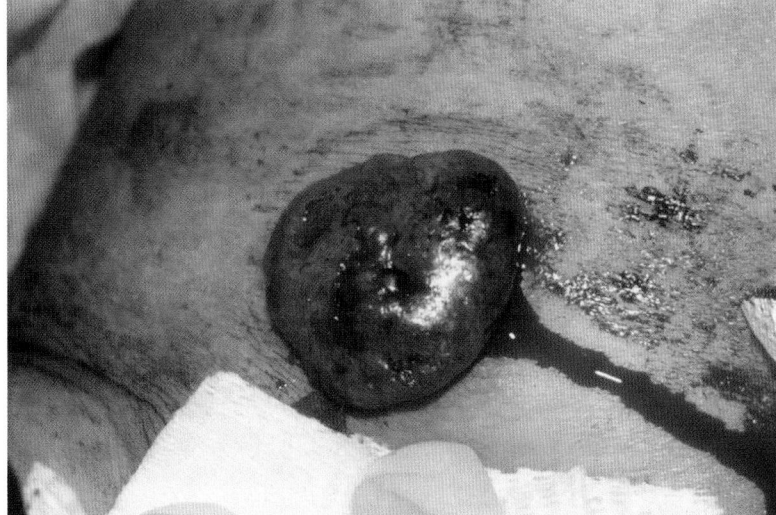

Fig. 24.51
Pigmented basal cell carcinoma: this is an unusually large nodular pigmented variant. By courtesy of the Institute of Dermatology, London, UK.

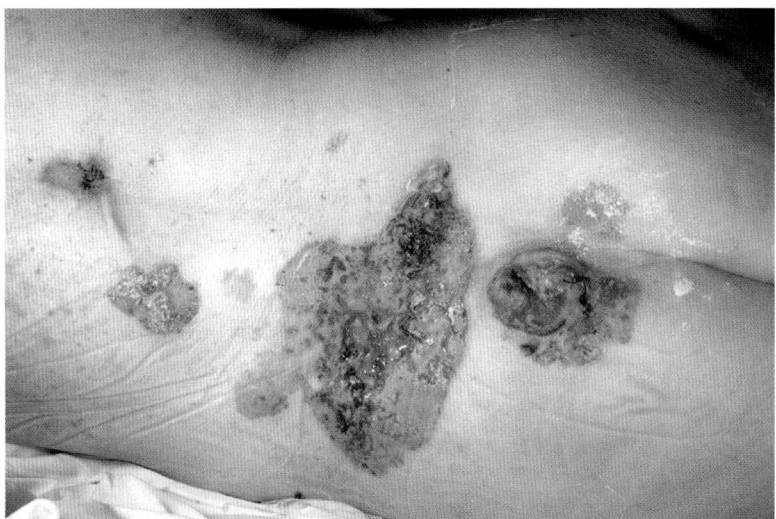

Fig. 24.52
Giant basal cell carcinoma: multiple superficial and nodular variants are present including a giant lesion. By courtesy of the Institute of Dermatology, London, UK.

therapy.[9,166,176,191–208] Facial tumors, especially those around the nose, eye, lip, and ear, are most likely to recur, particularly when greater than 2 cm in diameter (Fig. 24.53).[9,167,168] Morpheaform, metatypical, and infiltrative variants have the highest recurrence rates.[9,167,208,209] Superficial basal cell carcinoma is also associated with a high risk of recurrence due to difficulty in assessing the anatomical limits of the tumor. Patients with chronic lymphocytic leukemia appear to have a higher risk for local recurrence following Mohs surgery independent of other prognostic factors such as tumor type and thickness.[159,210]

Systemic spread of basal cell carcinoma is rare, quoted incidences having ranged from 0.0028% to 0.55%.[208,211,212] Metastases are more common in men and average age at presentation is younger (45 years) than that of nonmetastatic tumors (61 years).[9] Most tumors have arisen on the scalp, ear, and neck and there may be a past history of antecedent radiotherapy for an unrelated dermatosis or unsuccessful previous radiation treatment for the neoplasm.[211,213] The majority of tumors are large and often deeply invasive and may show evidence of lymphovascular invasion.[214,215] The most common sites of metastasis include lymph nodes (65%), lung (34%), bone (18.5%), and skin (18.5%).[211,216–220] Other sites of metastasis include the parotid gland,[221] liver,[222] oral cavity, and auditory meatus.[223] Secondary amyloidosis has been reported to occur in the setting of metastatic basal cell carcinoma.[224,225] The prognosis has been very poor, but targeted therapies that address the driving pathogenic mechanism of basal cell carcinoma are now available.[226–228]

Pathogenesis and histologic features

A basal cell carcinoma consists of a dual population of a fibrous stroma surrounding islands of dependent cells that resemble those of the basal layer of the epidermis and hair follicle. The tumor is believed to be derived from an undifferentiated pluripotent epithelial germ cell. These cells arise from interfollicular basal cells or from germ cells in hair follicles or sebaceous glands and immunohistochemically and ultrastructurally share many features with follicular matrix cells.[229,230] Because of the stromal dependence and the capacity of basal cell carcinomas for differentiation towards any skin appendage, their pathogenetic mechanism possibly represents flawed rehearsal of embryological differentiation. Animal dermal–epidermal recombination experiments show that dermis from a given site is responsible at a given time-window for the presence or absence of appendage development in heterotopic epidermis. Basal cell carcinomas have developed over the fibrosis of venous stasis, and it seems likely, though unproven, that dermal damage with secondary induction of basaloid epidermal changes is the mechanism of development of many basal cell carcinomas.

Overexposure to UV radiation and the inadequate protection provided by fair skin correlates best, though not completely, with the distribution of up to 80% of tumors on the head and neck.[166,231–234] The relationship to sunlight, however, is complex and incompletely understood.[235,236] Basal cell carcinoma correlates particularly with the degree of freckling and a positive history of severe sunburn in childhood, in addition to excessive recreational exposure in the first two decades of life.[7,237,238] This last is particularly evident in children who tend to burn rather than tan.[7] The relationship to cumulative and occupational sun exposure and adult recreational sun exposure is less certain.[7,75,239] Red hair is associated with an increased incidence of basal cell carcinoma whereas Southern European ancestry has a protective effect.[7,237,240,241] Similar to squamous cell carcinoma, basal cell carcinoma may also be a complication of psoralen plus UV light of A wavelength (PUVA) therapy.[242,243]

Skin damage from irradiation, grenz rays, burns, tattoos, and other forms of physical injury has also been incriminated.[244–250] Basal cell carcinoma is sometimes a complication of chronic arsenic ingestion or exposure to coal tar derivatives. Immunosuppressed patients following organ transplantation, with human immunodeficiency virus (HIV) infection or leukemia/lymphoma have a higher incidence of basal cell carcinoma.[251–262] Although the tumor has been described as a complication of nevus sebaceous, this is more likely in most instances to represent a trichoblastoma.[109,263,264] Rarely, it may develop within a linear epidermal nevus.[265–267]

Basal cell carcinoma is driven by mutations that activate the hedgehog (HH) pathway, involved in embryonic patterning and development.[268] Genetic studies on patients with the nevoid basal cell carcinoma syndrome (Gorlin-Goltz syndrome) who present with multiple basal cell carcinomas at an early age have identified germline mutations in PTCH1 (9q22.32), PTCH2 (1p34.1), and SUFU (10q24.32), all in the HH pathway as underlying defects.[269–273] Mutations in PTCH1 or PTCH2 have also been identified in about two-thirds of sporadic basal cell carcinomas with SUFU mutations being more rare (2-5%).[273–276] Another gene in this pathway, SMO (9q32.1), was mutated in 10% of sporadic cases and can be linked to inherited basal cell carcinoma susceptibility independently of Gorlin-Goltz syndrome.[277,278] All mutations are inactivating, confirming that each is indeed a tumor suppressor gene. PTCH1 is a transmembrane protein, as is the much less mutated homolog PTCH2, and serves as a receptor for sonic hedgehog (SHH) ligand.[279,280] PTCH forms a receptor complex with smoothened (SMO), a seven-span transmembrane protein.[281,282] Upon ligand binding of SHH, the inhibitory function of PTCH1 upon SMO is released which leads to subsequent activation of the zinc-finger transcription factor GLI1. In the HH pathway, PTCH inhibits SMO which inhibits SUFU which inhibits GLI1.[268] Overall, at least 85% of basal cell carcinomas have a relevant mutation in the an SHH pathway member.[283]

As an indicator of the importance of the HH pathway, GLI1 has been found to be overexpressed in virtually all sporadic basal cell carcinomas examined.[284] Its homolog GLI2 also promotes epidermal proliferation and tumorigenesis.[285,286] Transgenic mice with loss of one Ptch1 gene develop basal cell carcinomas after UV irradiation.[287–289] In contrast, epidermal proliferations resembling basal cell carcinoma can be induced by overexpression of Shh or Smo in transgenic mice and overexpression of Gli1 results in several skin tumors including hair follicular tumors as well as basal cell carcinoma.[277,278,290]

The sonic hedgehog pathway has been linked to the Wnt signaling cascade. Activation of this pathway leads to nuclear translocation of beta-catenin, which then functions as a transcription factor. Nuclear localization of beta-catenin was observed in over 50% of basal cell carcinomas analyzed.[291] More recent data confirm that Wnt/beta-catenin signaling is induced by constitutively active SHH signaling and that this is a requirement for tumor formation in basal cell carcinoma.[292,293] Epigenetic gene silencing also helps to coordinate these two pathways in tumor development.[294]

An additional pathway involved in the tumorigenesis of basal cell carcinoma involves mutations in the tumor suppressor gene TP53.[295] Mutations in TP53 are observed in a multitude of human cancers including squamous cell, basal cell carcinomas, and less frequently in melanoma. In basal cell carcinomas, TP53 mutations have been detected in nearly two-thirds of cases.[283] Signatures of UVB irradiation are common in TP53, and seen

across all subtypes. Patients with basal cell carcinoma appear to have a reduced capacity to repair UV-induced DNA damage.[296,297] These findings provide further molecular evidence linking development of basal cell carcinoma to UV irradiation. In contrast, the UV signature has been reported in only 40% of PTCH1 mutations in sporadic basal cell carcinoma. This lower incidence of UV signature mutations implies that there are mutagenic events other than solely UV irradiation.[298] Characteristic mutations in the TERT gene promoter conferring increased expression and thus promoting tumorigenesis by preventing the senescence that can be invoked by increased cell proliferation has been described.[299–301] These mutations are also linked to UV exposure. Recent genomic profiling of a large cohort of almost 300 basal cell carcinomas revealed mutations in the RAS and MYC pathways as well as many other oncogenes and tumor suppressors seen across many other forms of cancer.[283]

Gene expression microarray data demonstrate that basal cell carcinoma shows distinctive gene expression patterns compared to surrounding epidermal basal cell keratinocytes and that histologic variants associated with more aggressive disease (i.e., morpheaform basal cell carcinoma) display a gene expression profile distinctly different from more indolent variants such as nodular and superficial basal cell carcinoma.[302,303] Recently, use of inhibitors of SMO have been helpful in the rare cases of basal cell carcinoma not amenable to a surgical approach, though developmental resistance remains an issue.[304–307]

Basal cell carcinomas frequently show an origin from the overlying epidermis (Fig. 24.54). They are composed of small cells with uniform round or oval darkly staining nuclei and minimal cytoplasm (Fig. 24.55). Intercellular bridges are not evident. Mitoses and apoptosis are commonly seen (Figs 24.56 and 24.57).

A variety of histologic subtypes are recognized, as follows.[308]

Nodulocystic basal cell carcinoma

Approximately 75% of all basal cell carcinomas fall into the nodulocystic category in which large basaloid lobules of varying shape and size form a relatively circumscribed mass (Figs 24.58–24.60). A peripheral palisade is typically present around the rim of the lobule, which may be solid or show central cystic dilatation (Figs 24.61–24.64). The stroma surrounding these lobules varies in quality and quantity, but is usually loose and rich in mucin, predominantly hyaluronic acid. Fixation often results in mucin shrinkage; the resultant separation of the tumor lobules from their associated stroma is

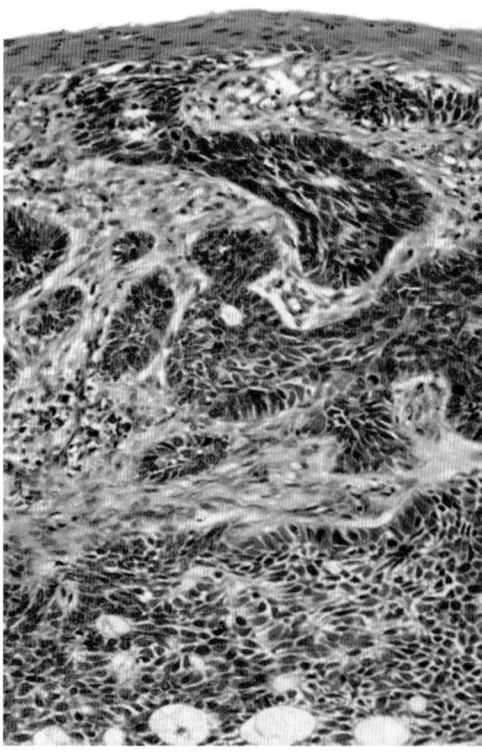

Fig. 24.54
Basal cell carcinoma: an origin from the epidermis is clearly seen.

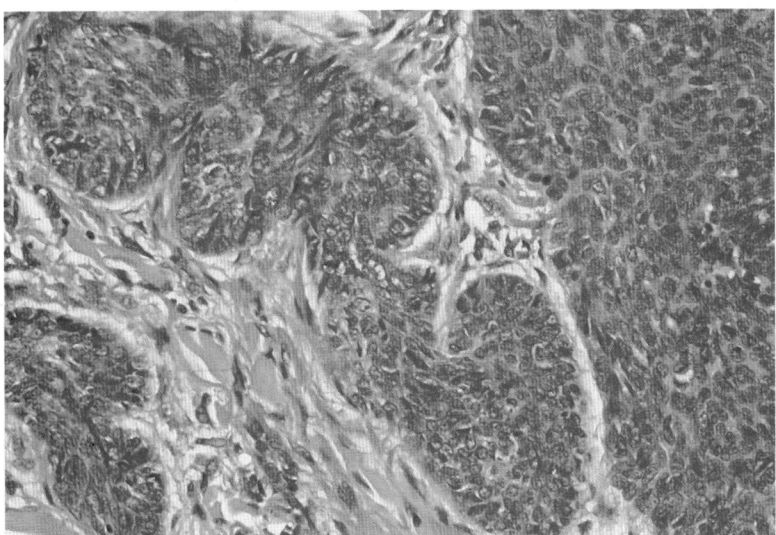

Fig. 24.55
Basal cell carcinoma: the tumor cells have indistinct cytoplasmic borders and oval basophilic vesicular nuclei. Note the retraction artifact.

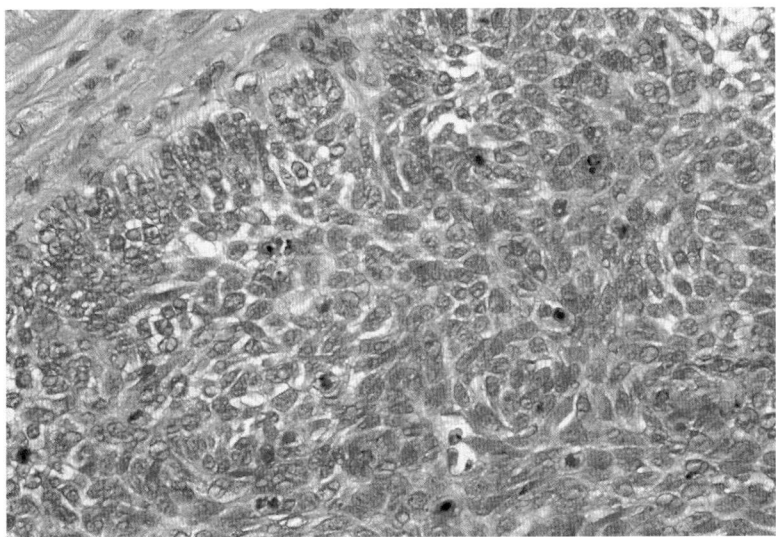

Fig. 24.56
Basal cell carcinoma: mitoses are often numerous.

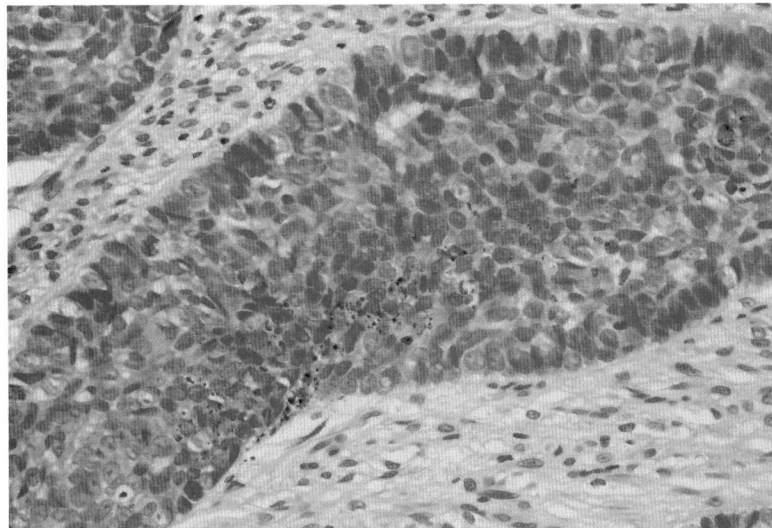

Fig. 24.57
Basal cell carcinoma: apoptosis is sometimes conspicuous, accounting for the slow growth of many tumors despite abundant mitoses.

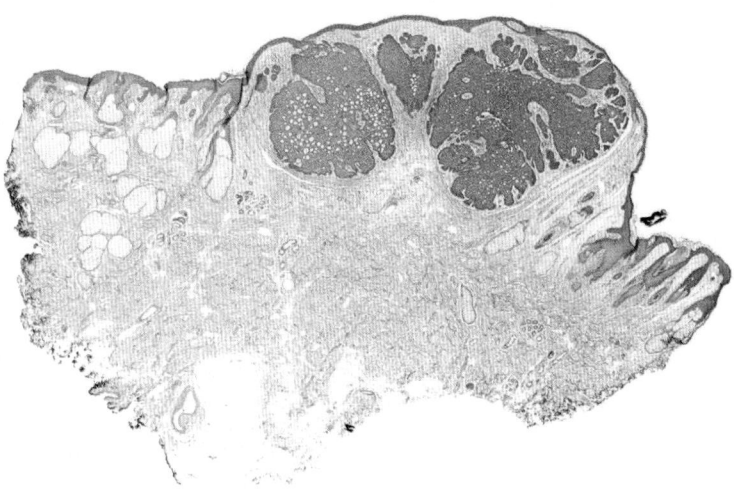

Fig. 24.58
Nodular basal cell carcinoma: scanning view of a typical lesion from the eyelid.

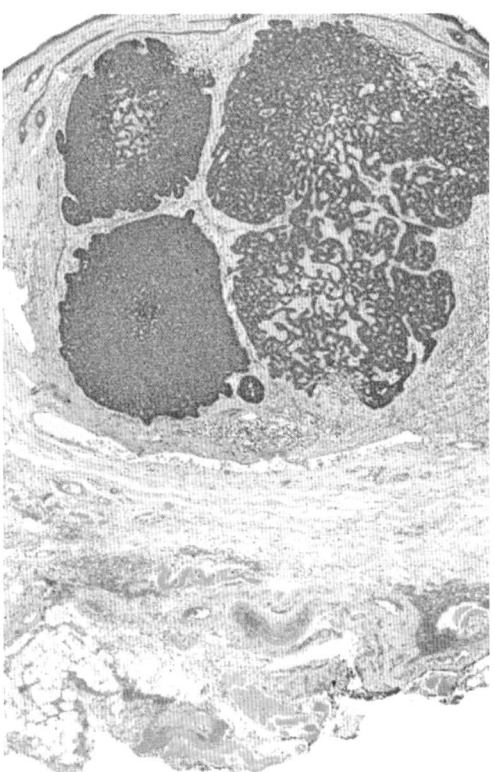

Fig. 24.59
Nodular basal cell carcinoma: note the well-circumscribed tumor lobules.

characteristic of this tumor. Retraction, however, is also related to basement membrane abnormalities of adhesion, including diminished expression of bullous pemphigoid antigen and reduced numbers of hemidesmosomes and anchoring fibrils.[309-311]

Amyloid may be present in the stroma in from 66% to 75% of basal cell carcinomas, usually at the advancing edge (*Fig. 24.65*).[312] It may be found in all subtypes and is probably formed from keratin as a consequence of apoptosis.[313] Rarely, metaplastic bone formation is observed.[314,315]

Adenoid basal cell carcinoma

A reticulate pattern of basaloid cells may combine with an almost pure mucinous stroma to form the adenoid variant of basal cell carcinoma, which on occasion mimics glandular formation (*Fig. 24.66*).

Micronodular basal cell carcinoma

The micronodular variant is characterized by a basaloid cellular proliferation arranged in small nests (*Figs 24.67 and 24.68*). Peripheral palisading

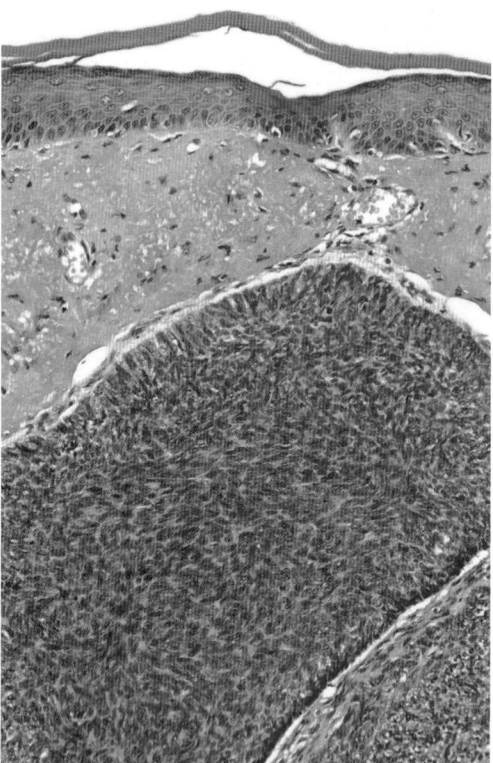

Fig. 24.60
Nodular basal cell carcinoma: marked solar elastosis is present. Note the peripheral palisading.

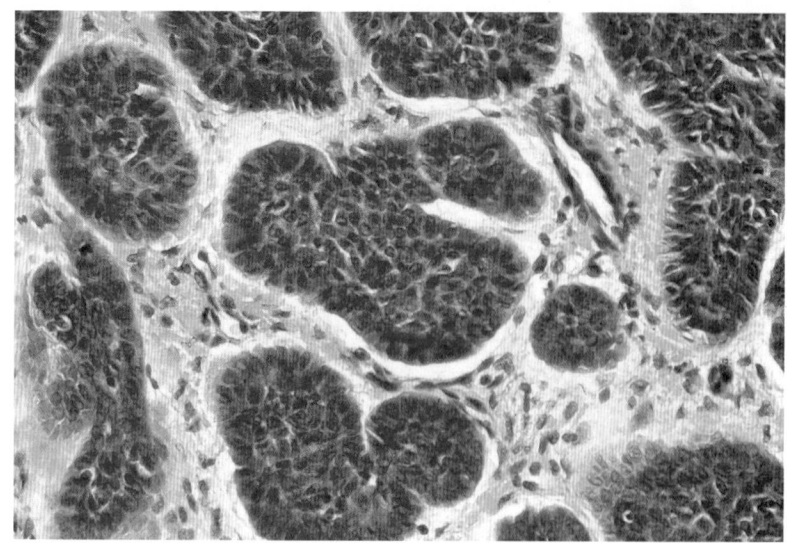

Fig. 24.62
Nodular basal cell carcinoma: high-power view showing the retraction artifact.

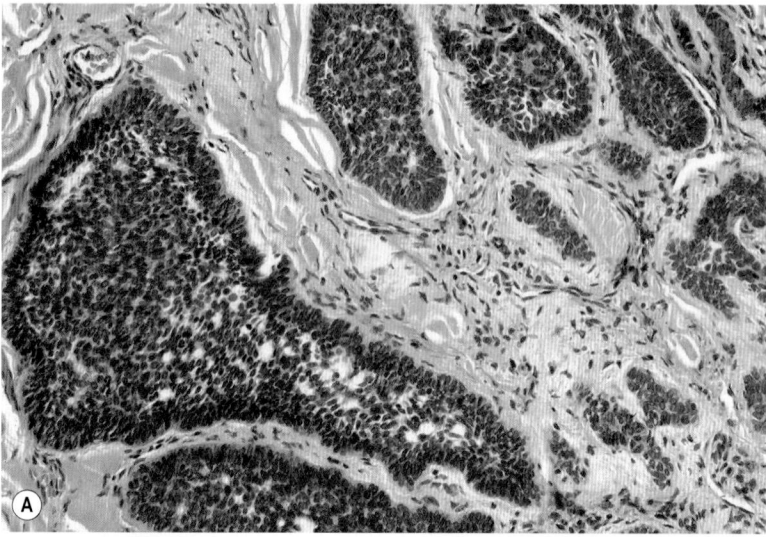

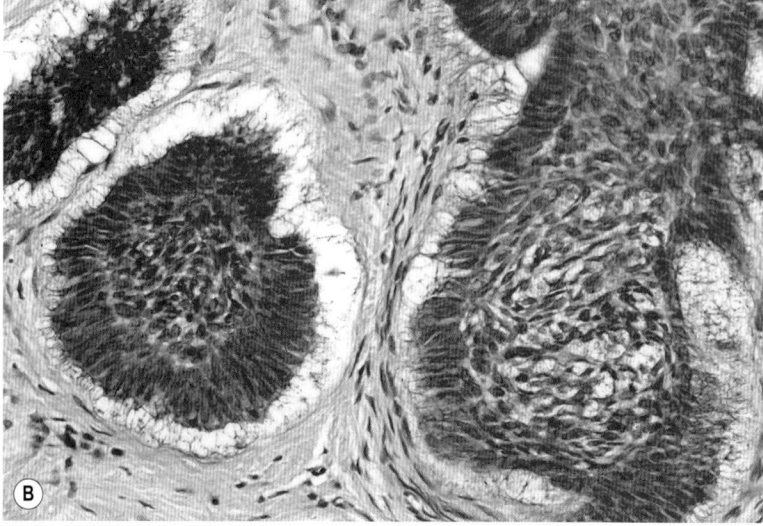

Fig. 24.61
Nodular basal cell carcinoma: (A) a peripheral palisade is typically present; (B) the retraction artifact as seen in this field is a characteristic feature.

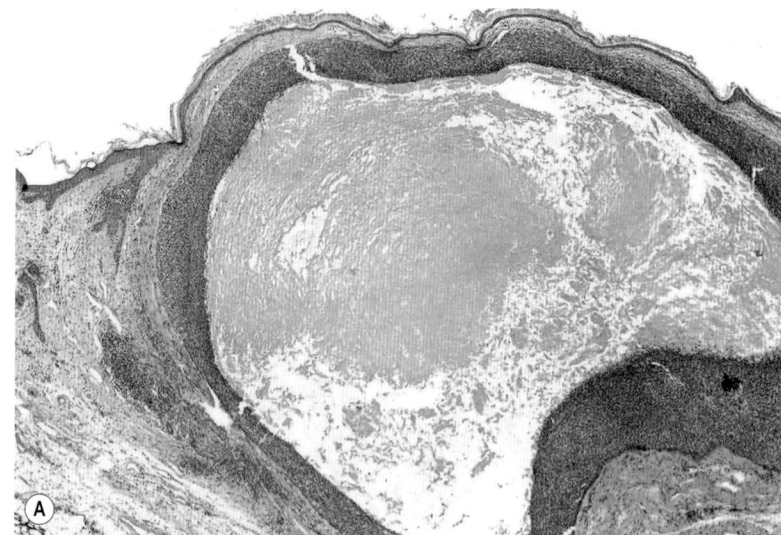

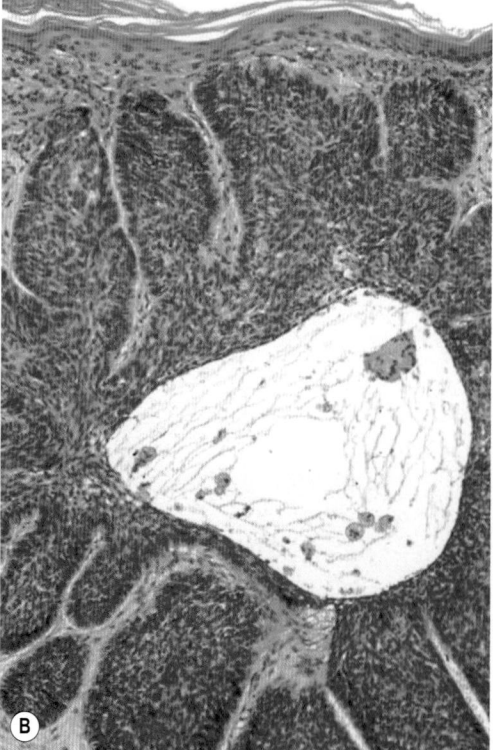

Fig. 24.63
Nodulocystic basal cell carcinoma: (A) scanning view of a typical lesion; (B) the cysts contain abundant stromal mucin.

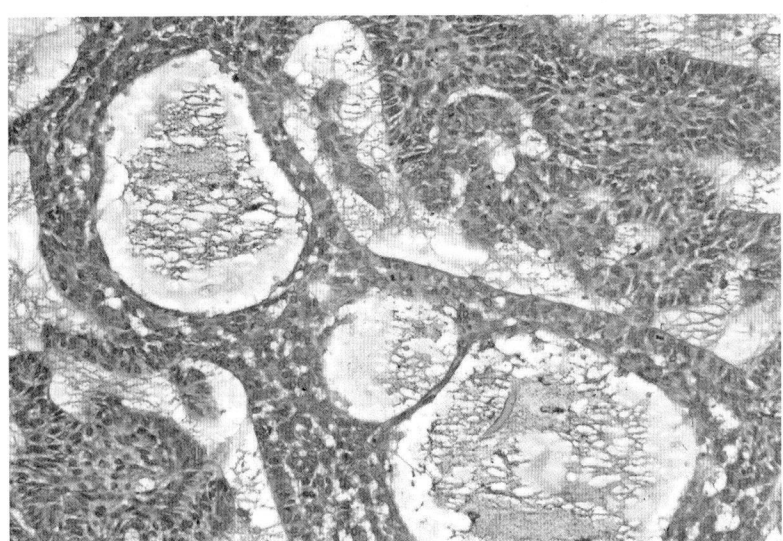

Fig. 24.64
Nodulocystic basal cell carcinoma: the mucin is Alcian blue (pH 2.5) positive.

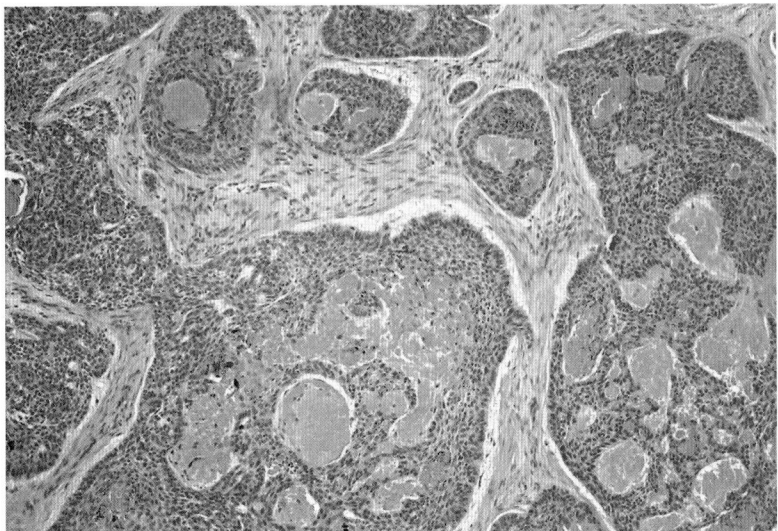

Fig. 24.65
Basal cell carcinoma: amyloid deposits as seen in this field are common. Their presence is of no clinical significance.

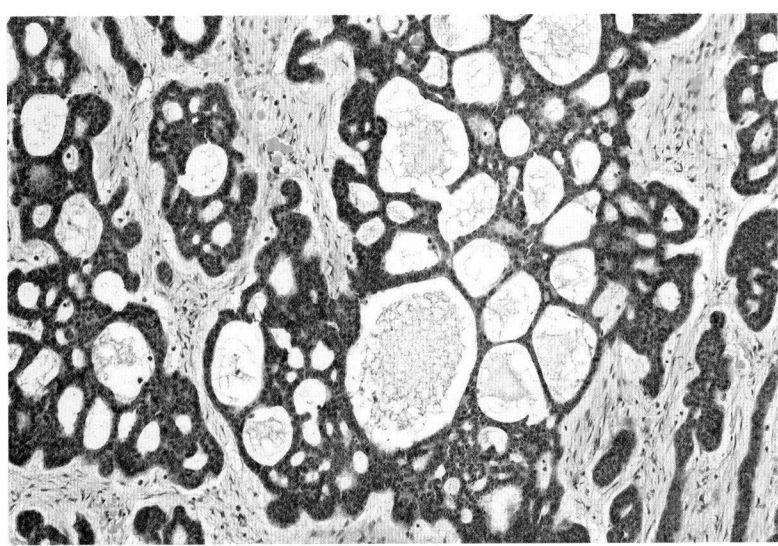

Fig. 24.66
Adenoid basal cell carcinoma: this pseudoglandular appearance is characteristic.

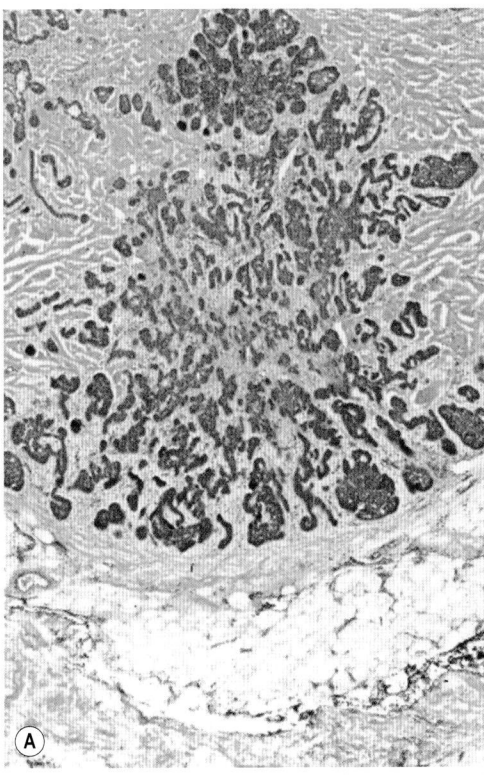

Fig. 24.67
Micronodular basal cell carcinoma: (A) low-power view showing the small size and relative uniformity of the tumor nodules; (B) absence of a retraction artifact is typical of this variant. Brisk mitotic activity and apoptosis aid in distinction from trichoepithelioma.

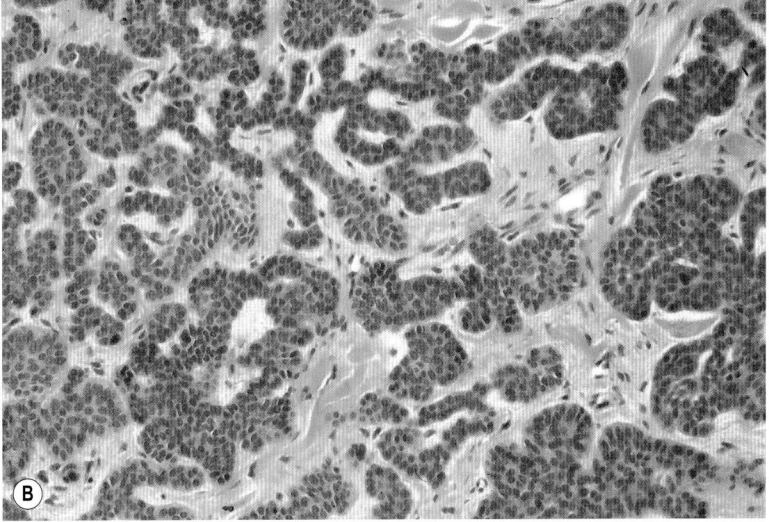

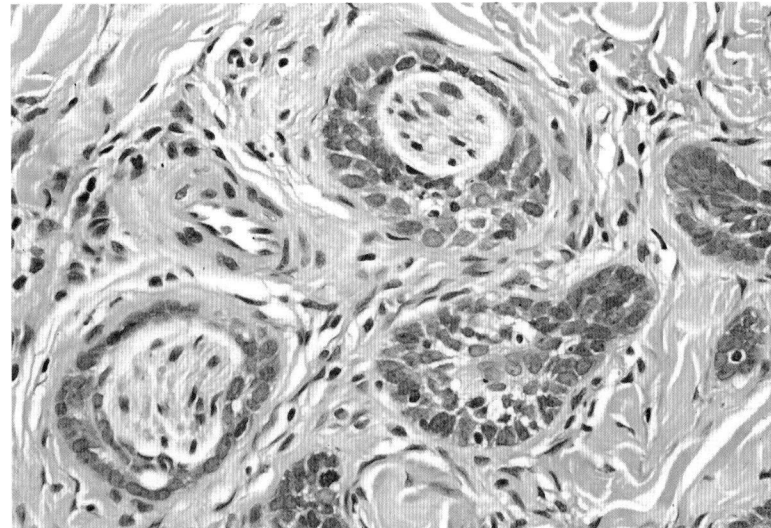

Fig. 24.68
Micronodular basal cell carcinoma: perineural infiltration.

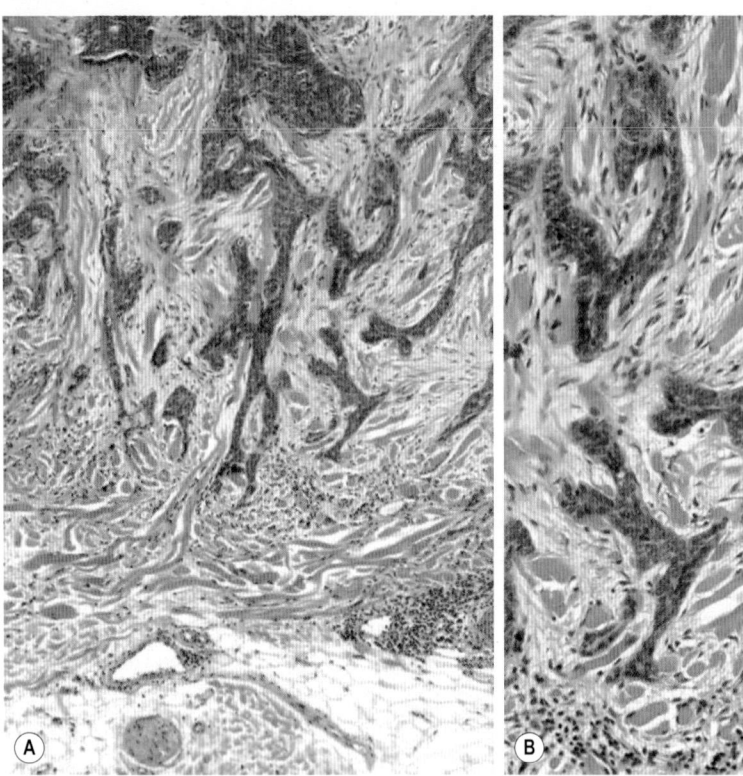

Fig. 24.69
Infiltrative basal cell carcinoma: (**A**) the tumor cells are present as narrow strands surrounded by a mucin-rich stroma; (**B**) close-up view.

is frequently less prominent than in the nodulocystic type and a retraction artifact is usually absent. This variant may often diffusely infiltrate the dermis and extend into the subcutis. It is therefore associated with a higher local recurrence rate.[316–318]

Infiltrative basal cell carcinoma

The infiltrative basal cell carcinoma is characterized by small irregular clumps of basaloid cells with a jagged border and limited peripheral palisading (*Fig. 24.69*).[168,209,319] In contrast to the morpheaform variant, the stroma often appears rather loose and mucin may be prominent. The tumor usually shows extensive spread, and involvement of the perineural space is not uncommon.[169] An infiltrative component may also be a feature of noduloulcerative variants.

Morpheaform (sclerosing) basal cell carcinoma

Similar to the infiltrating type, morpheaform basal cell carcinoma is composed of thin strands and nests of basaloid cell showing only limited peripheral palisading. The surrounding stroma is dense and sclerotic, giving rise to the indurated appearance clinically resembling morphea (*Fig. 24.70*).[320,321] Extensive spread and perineural infiltration are not infrequent.[322]

Keratotic basal cell carcinoma

Keratinization is a rare feature of basal cell carcinoma, presenting horn cyst formation (*Fig. 24.71*). The keratotic variant of basal cell carcinoma may be indistinguishable from a familial trichoepithelioma.[323,324] Where doubt exists, particularly in the elderly, it is advisable to treat the lesion as basal cell carcinoma.

Basosquamous (metatypical) basal cell carcinoma

When foci of neoplastic squamous differentiation occur, the tumors are labeled basosquamous or 'metatypical' and, because of their usual infiltrative growth pattern, are associated with a poorer outlook including increased risk of distant metastasis (*Fig. 24.72*).[325–332]

Pigmented basal cell carcinoma

Pigmentation in basal cell carcinomas may be present in both dendritic melanocytes and stromal macrophages (*Fig. 24.73*).[169] Its only significance lies in the clinical misinterpretation of the tumor as melanoma. Hemosiderin may also sometimes be evident. The mechanism for increased pigmentation

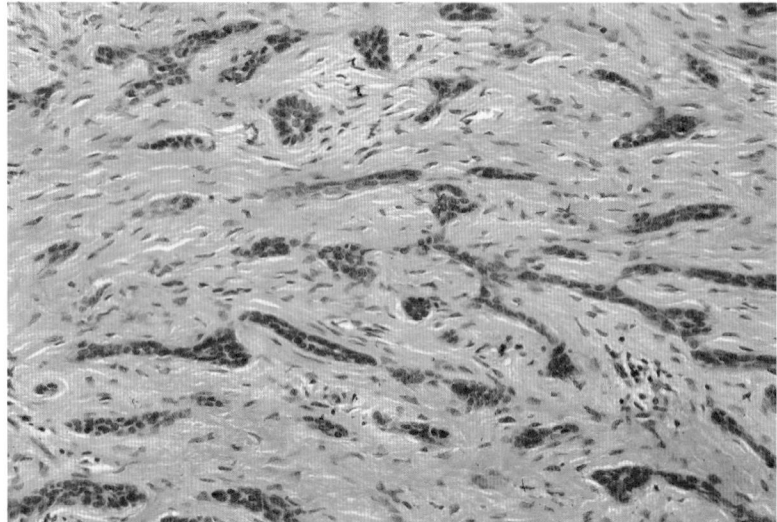

Fig. 24.70
Morpheaform basal cell carcinoma: this variant is characterized by narrow epithelial strands compressed by a dense fibrous stroma. Mucin is absent.

is unclear but it has been correlated with the endothelin pathway and in particular with increased expression of endothelin-1.[333]

Superficial basal cell carcinoma

Superficial basal cell carcinoma (erroneously referred to as multifocal basal cell carcinoma) appears as apparently isolated basaloid lobules projecting from the lower margin of the epidermis (*Fig. 24.74*). The lobules, however, are in fact interconnected and do not usually differentiate, but they may become invasive. It is often quite difficult to determine the lateral limits of this variant and therefore recurrences are quite common.

Ulcerative basal cell carcinoma

Ulcerative basal cell carcinomas may show a highly infiltrative growth pattern or less commonly be based upon the nodulocystic variant.

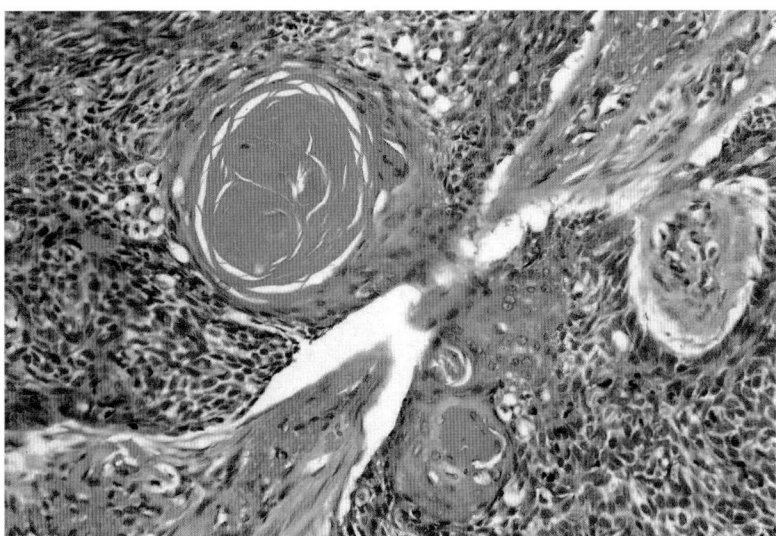

Fig. 24.71
Keratotic basal cell carcinoma: this rare variant is characterized by the presence of keratocysts.

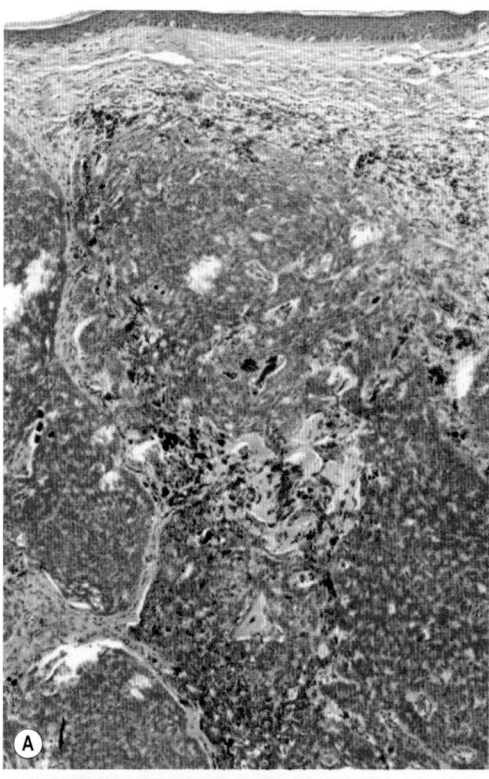

Fig. 24.73
(**A**, **B**) Pigmented basal cell carcinoma: in this example, melanin is present both within tumor cells and in stromal macrophages.

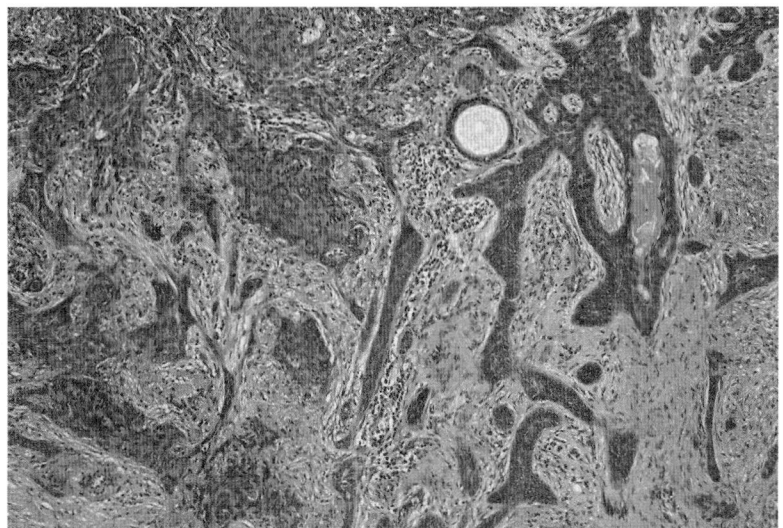

Fig. 24.72
Metatypical basal cell carcinoma: on the left side of the field the features are those of squamous differentiation.

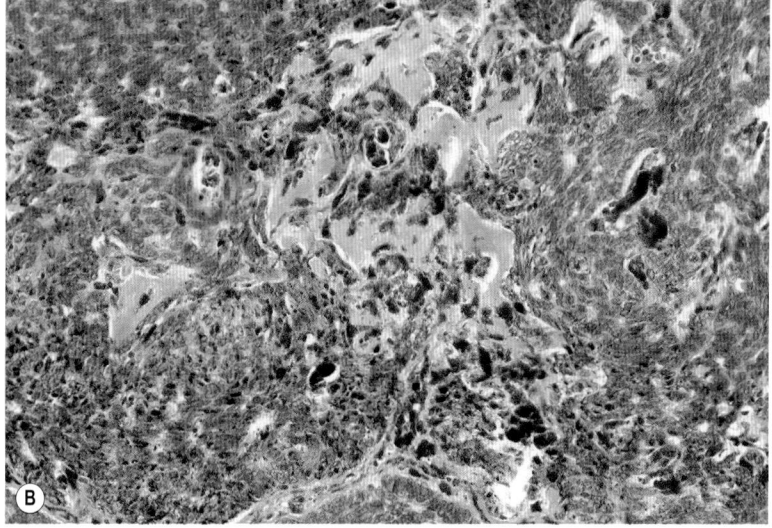

Rare variants

Rare and unusual variants of basal cell carcinoma are listed below.

Pleomorphic (giant cell, with monster cells) basal cell carcinoma

Mitotic activity, apoptosis, cellular pleomorphism, and giant cell formation are frequent observations in basal cell carcinoma, but have no prognostic significance (*Fig. 24.75*).[334,335] Pleomorphic basal cell carcinoma is an uncommon variant in which large numbers of extremely large mononuclear and multinucleate giant cells are evident. Intranuclear cytoplasmic invaginations may be present and intracytoplasmic basophilic and eosinophilic inclusions are sometimes a feature.[335,336] In addition, stromal giant cells are also sometimes seen.[337] Pleomorphism does not appear to influence the behavior of the tumor.[338]

Clear cell basal cell carcinoma

Occasional tumors show focal clear cell change with clear to finely granular eosinophilic cytoplasm (*Fig. 24.76*). This change may be due to accumulation of lysosomes rather than glycogen and represents a degenerative phenomenon.[339-342] Clear cell change may be seen focally only or, in

rare cases, may affect most of the lesion. Peripheral palisading is usually preserved.

Signet ring cell basal cell carcinoma

A variant which is characterized by compressed and laterally displaced nuclei is referred to as signet ring cell basal cell carcinoma (*Fig. 24.77*). In contrast to clear cell basal cell carcinoma, this is not regarded as a degenerative event. Instead, the cytoplasm contains hyaline inclusions composed of aggregates of intermediate filaments representing aberrant keratinization. In addition, signet ring cells may also stain positive for S100 protein, glial fibrillary acidic protein, and smooth muscle actin, suggesting myoepithelial differentiation;[343–350] it has also been referred to as basal cell carcinoma with myoepithelial differentiation. The term rhabdoid basal cell carcinoma would be equally applicable.

Granular basal cell carcinoma

Infrequently, some, if not all, neoplastic cells may have abundant granular eosinophilic cytoplasm due to membrane-bound lysosome-like granules (*Fig. 24.78*).[351–359] This variant may be related to clear cell basal cell carcinoma and also probably represents a degenerative phenomenon.

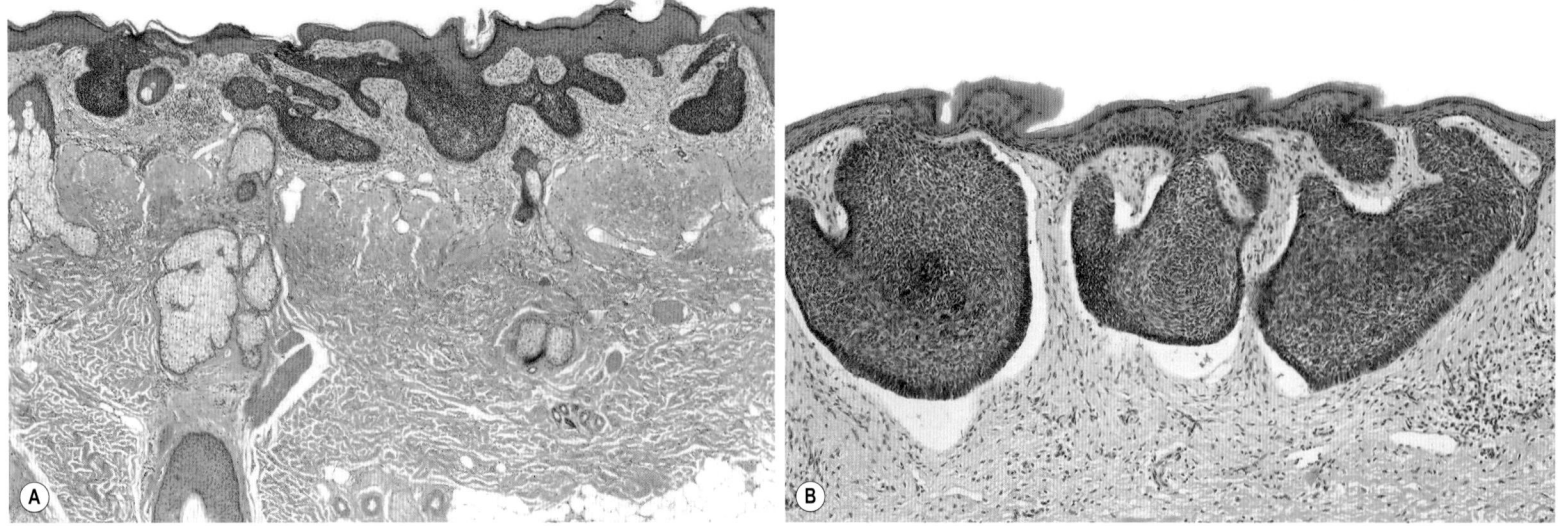

Fig. 24.74
(**A**, **B**) Superficial basal cell carcinoma: the tumor islands appear suspended from the epidermis. The presence of dermal scarring and chronic inflammation is a consistent feature.

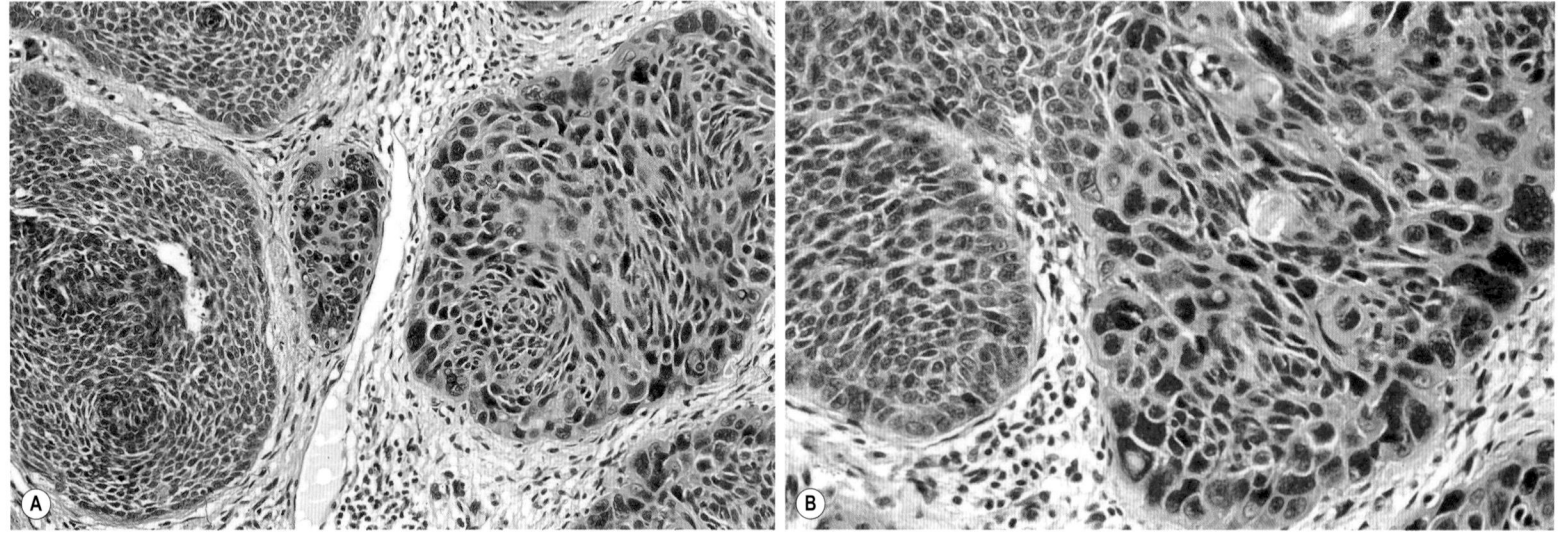

Fig. 24.75
(**A**, **B**) Pleomorphic basal cell carcinoma: the more typical tumor nodules on the left side of each image contrast with the marked pleomorphism and hyperchromatism seen on the right.

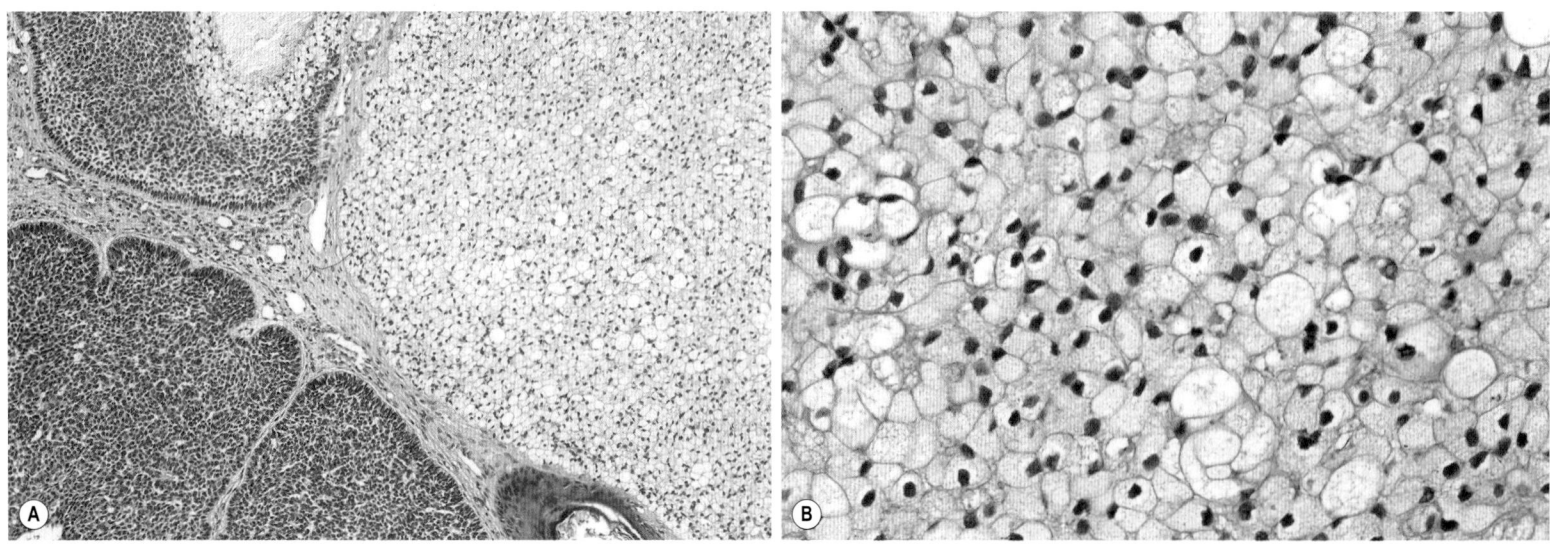

Fig. 24.76
Clear cell basal cell carcinoma: (**A**) residual typical nodular basal cell carcinoma is present on the left; (**B**) note the striking cytoplasmic vacuolation.

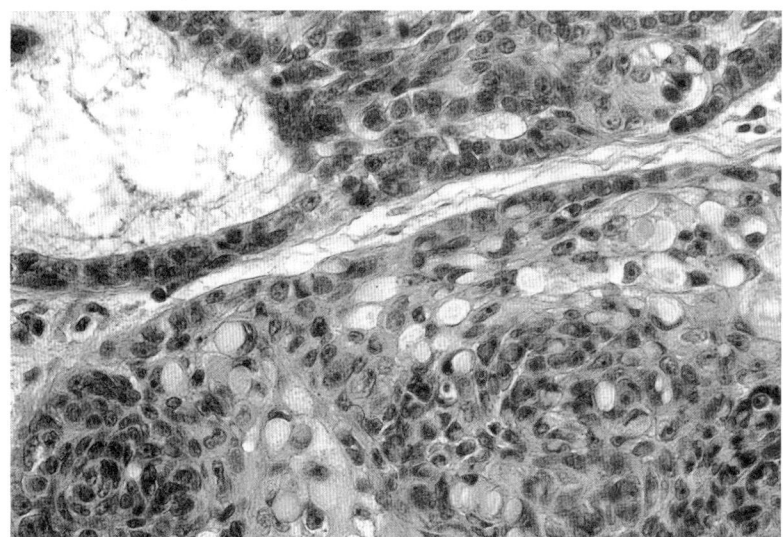

Fig. 24.77
Signet ring cell basal cell carcinoma: cytoplasmic inclusions which compress the nucleus to the edge of the cell result in this variant.

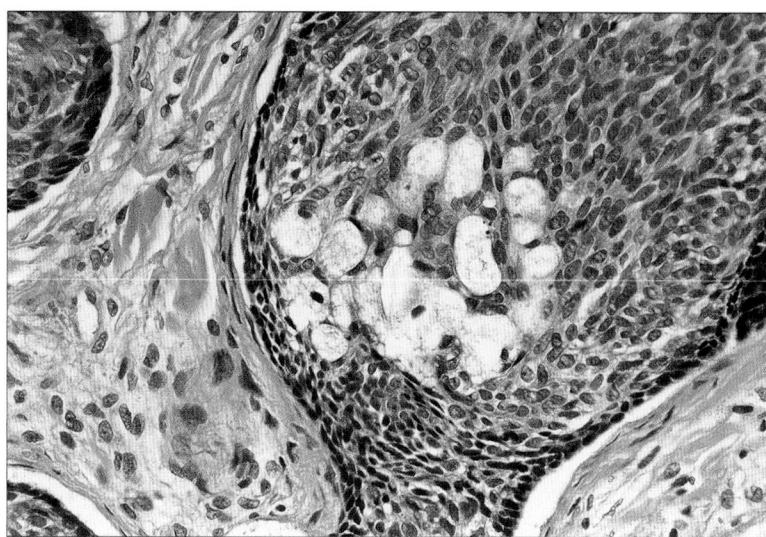

Fig. 24.79
Basal cell carcinoma: the enlarged, pale-staining, foamy cells are indicative of sebaceous differentiation.

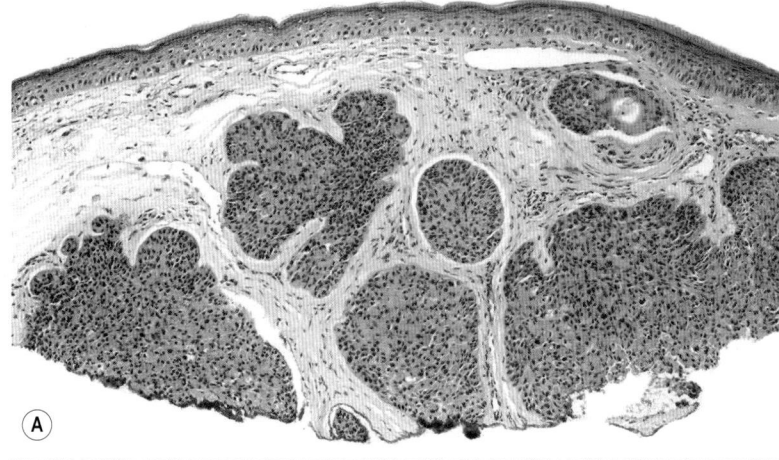

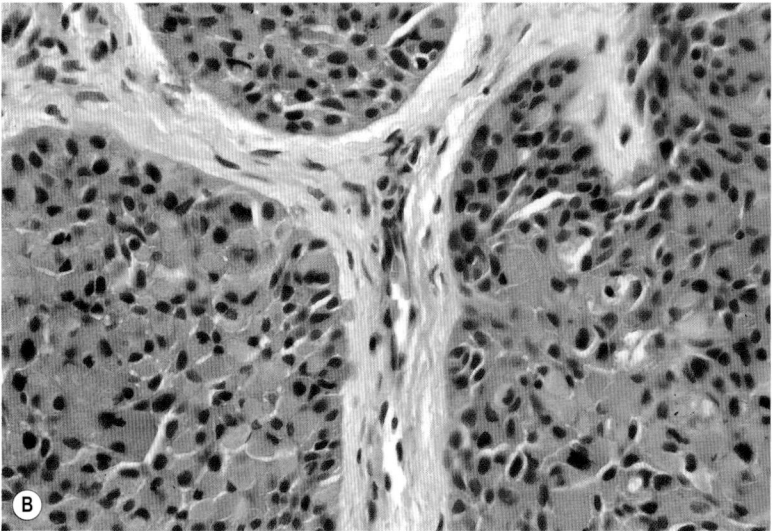

Fig. 24.78
(A, B) Granular cell basal cell carcinoma: in this variant, the cytoplasm is granular and strikingly eosinophilic. By courtesy of R. Margolis, MD, St Elizabeth's Hospital, Boston, USA.

Basal cell carcinoma with differentiation towards adnexal structures

Rarely, differentiation appears to be directed towards sebaceous, follicular, eccrine, or apocrine structures (*Figs 24.79 and 24.80*).[360–369]

Infundibulocystic basal cell carcinoma

This variant typically presents on the face of the elderly and was originally referred to as basal cell carcinoma with follicular differentiation.[362,370,371] It presents as a well-circumscribed, small, symmetrical, superficial dermal proliferation of basaloid cells arranged in anastomosing cords and strands. Peripheral palisading is present but the stroma is typically scanty. Small infundibular cysts are present. This lesion should be distinguished from basaloid follicular hamartoma and trichoepithelioma.[372] A germline mutation in *SUFU* has been reported in a patient with multiple hereditary infundibulocystic basal cell carcinoma syndrome.[373]

Metaplastic basal cell carcinoma

Extremely rarely, basal cell carcinoma may show stromal malignant metaplastic features (carcinosarcoma) (*Figs 24.81–24.84*).[374,375]

Basal cell carcinoma with matrical differentiation (shadow cell basal cell carcinoma)

An exceedingly rare variant of basal cell carcinoma shows differentiation towards matrical cells of the hair follicle displaying shadow cells (*Fig. 24.85*). A differential diagnosis from benign and malignant pilomatrixoma has to be considered.[376–383]

Keloidal basal cell carcinoma

Thick, sclerotic collagen bundles may be prominent within the tumor stroma (*Fig. 24.86*). These lesions may clinically be mistaken for keloids.[366,384,385] This keloidal change is due to collagen 1 deposition and may be found in different histologic subtypes of basal cell carcinoma. It is frequently associated with morpheic features, ulceration, and tumor necrosis and occurs more frequently on the ear.[386] Some find designation of this as a distinctive clinicopathologic entity dubious.[387,388]

Basal cell carcinoma with thickened basement membrane

A variant characterized by thickened basement membrane surrounding the tumor lobules can be mistaken for benign adnexal neoplasms.[389]

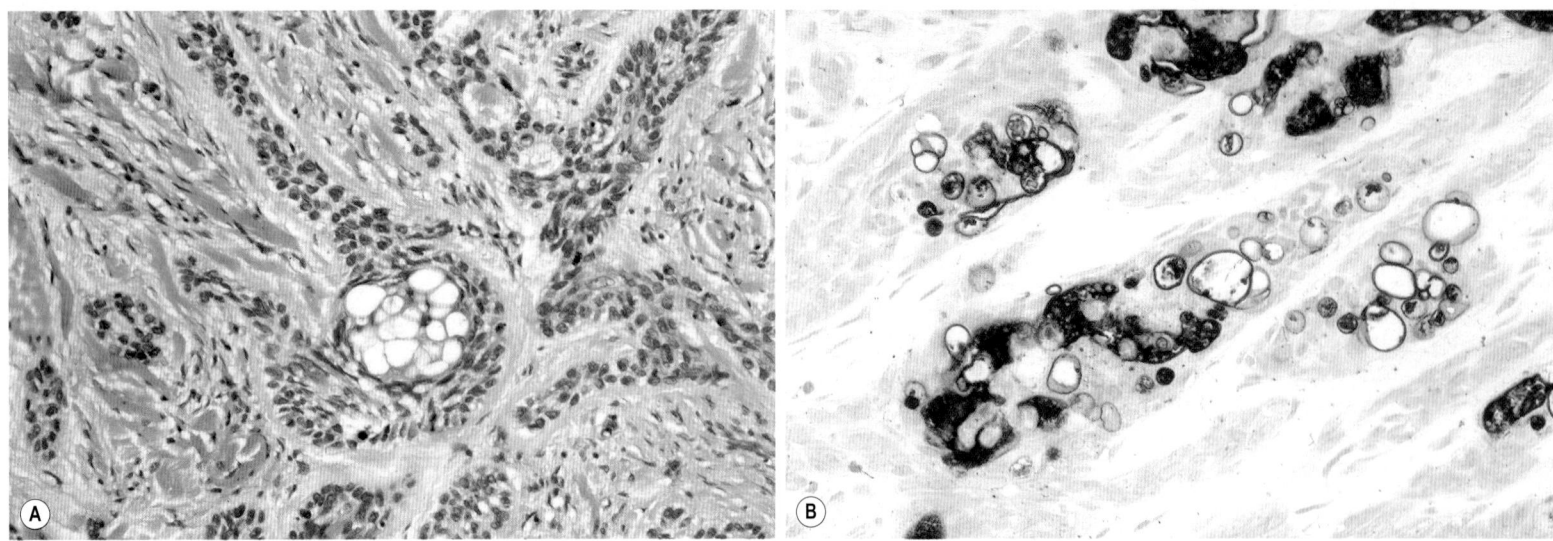

Fig. 24.80
Basal cell carcinoma with ductal differentiation: (**A**) infiltrating variant showing well-developed intracytoplasmic lumina; (**B**) the presence of ductal differentiation is confirmed with CEA immunohistochemistry.

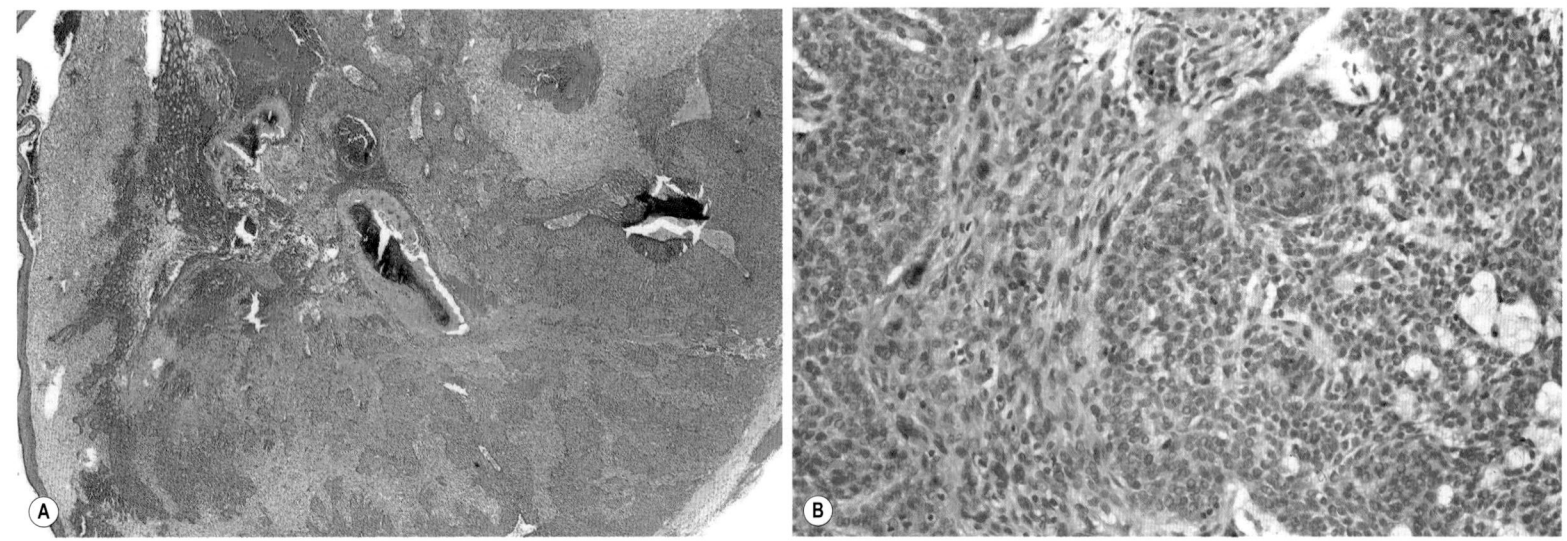

Fig. 24.81
Metaplastic basal cell carcinoma: (**A**) tumor from the scalp showing bone formation; (**B**) focal adenoid features are present.

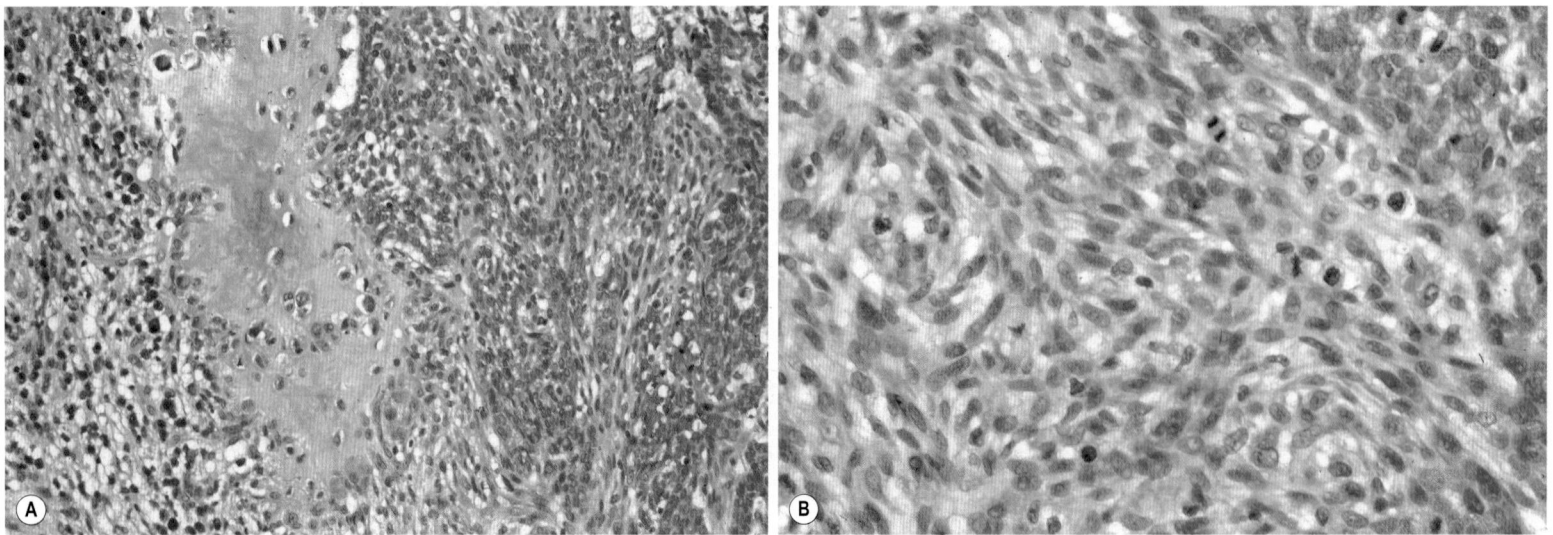

Fig. 24.82
Metaplastic basal cell carcinoma: (**A**) higher-power view of osteoid; (**B**) focally, the stroma shows superficial MFH-like features. Note the mitotic figures.

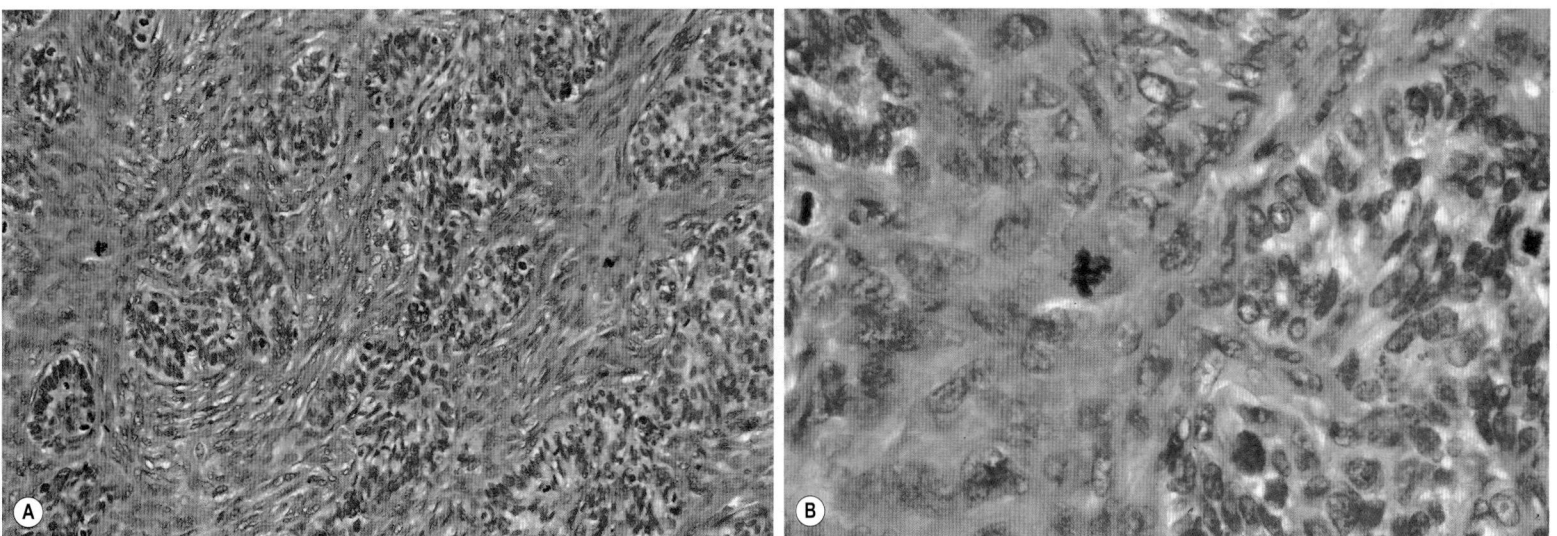

Fig. 24.83
Metaplastic basal cell carcinoma: (A) typical tumor nodules are dispersed in a dense spindle cell stroma; (B) the spindle cells have eosinophilic cytoplasm and show marked mitotic activity.

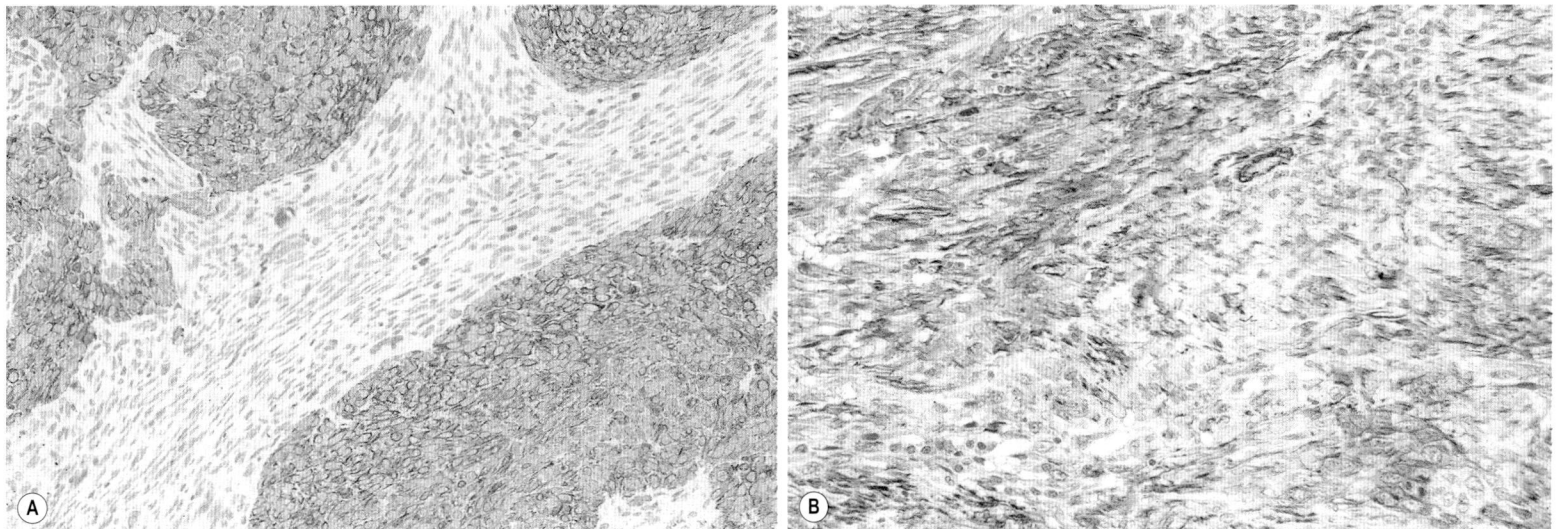

Fig. 24.84
Metaplastic basal cell carcinoma: (A) the epithelial component expresses pankeratin; (B) the spindle cells express desmin, indicating smooth muscle differentiation.

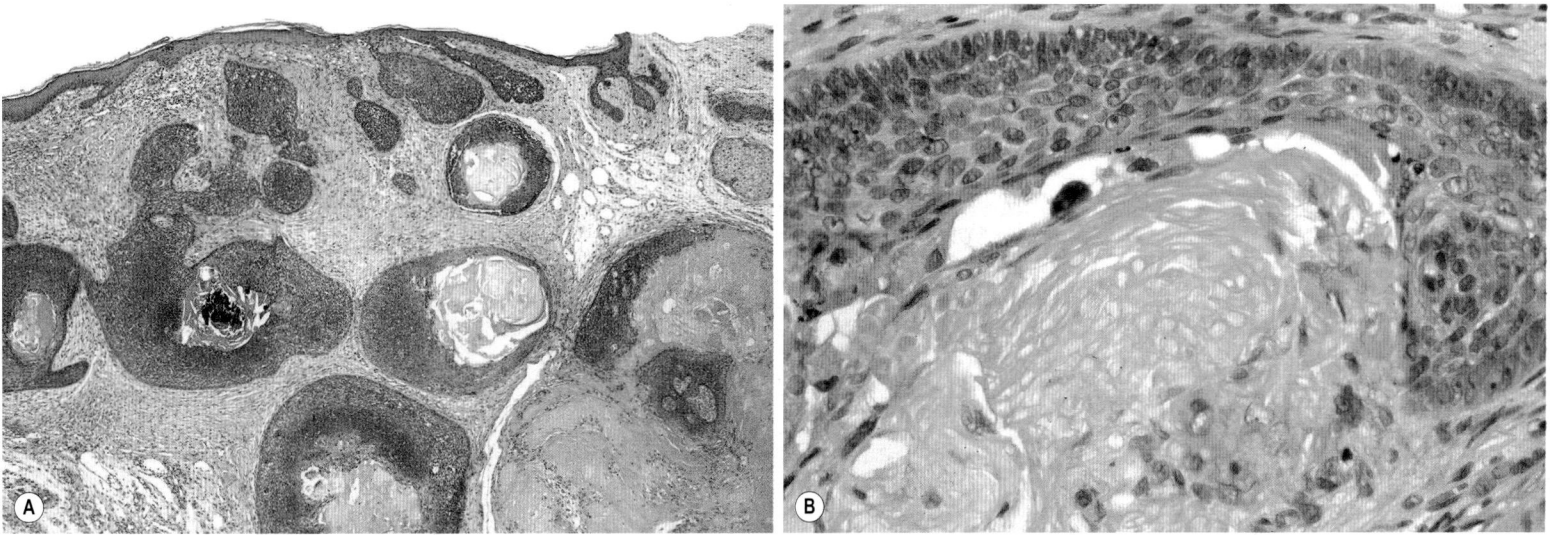

Fig. 24.85
Basal cell carcinoma with matrical differentiation: (A) at low power, the typical features of nodular basal cell carcinoma are present; (B) high-power view showing eosinophilic ghost cells.

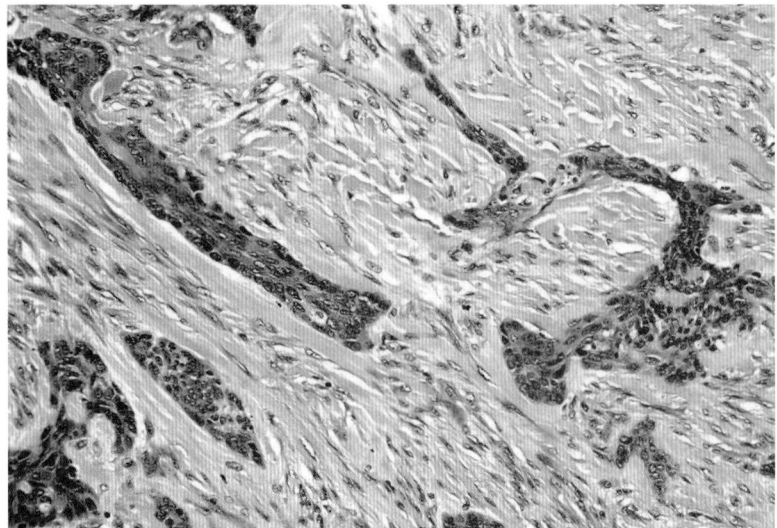

Fig. 24.86
Keloidal basal cell carcinoma: this is a variant of morpheaform basal cell carcinoma in which the stroma is replaced by broad bundles of eosinophilic keloidal collagen. The prognosis of this variant is poor.

Basal cell carcinoma with neuroid-type nuclear palisading

Very few reports describe prominent central nuclear palisading reminiscent of that seen in schwannoma. Staining for S100 protein is negative but strong positive staining for keratin is present. Adjacent foci of conventional basal cell carcinoma are typically identified.[390,391]

Regression is sometimes a feature, and therefore loss of appendages, remodeled collagen, foci of calcification, or a plasma cell-rich infiltrate should prompt examination of further sections to detect residual tumor.

By immunohistochemistry, basal cell carcinoma shows a cytokeratin expression profile analogous to that of follicular epithelium in the hair bulge.[392-394] In contrast to Merkel cell carcinoma, basal cell carcinoma does not stain with antibodies against cytokeratin 20 and only a subset are positive for cytokeratin 7.[395] Tumors express BerEP4 as well as bcl-2, CD10, SOX9, and p53, but are largely negative for EMA.[395-401] Increased actin expression is observed in more aggressive subtypes but has been found to be decreased in metastatic tumors.[402]

Nevoid basal cell carcinoma syndrome

Clinical features

Nevoid basal cell carcinoma syndrome (Gorlin-Goltz syndrome), which affects the sexes equally, is defined by multiple basal cell carcinomas presenting at an early age, odontogenic keratocysts of the jaw, skeletal abnormalities, ectopic calcification, and pits of the hands and feet.[1-5] It is inherited in an autosomal dominant fashion with complete penetrance and variable expressivity.[3,6] Spontaneous germ cell mutations also account for a significant proportion of cases.[7] Gorlin syndrome has been mapped to three tumor suppressor genes in the sonic hedgehog (SHH) pathway—*PTCH1* (9q22.32) and much less commonly *PTCH2* (1p34.1) and *SUFU* (10q24.32).[8-14] Homozygous inactivation of the gene results in basal cell carcinomas whereas hemizygous germline mutations cause the numerous congenital abnormalities.[8] A wide spectrum of mutations has been identified in the PTCH gene in patients with Gorlin syndrome, the majority of which are predicted to result in premature protein truncation.[15-19] The patched gene is part of the sonic hedgehog (SHH) signaling pathway. This pathway is involved in control of cell proliferation as well as the embryological patterning and development of neural tube, pharyngeal pouches, somites, and limb buds in vertebrates.[20,21] The combination of developmental abnormalities are consistent with the developmental roles of the SHH pathway.

Basal cell carcinomas usually develop in adolescence, although they have been recorded in early childhood.[3] They have a variable appearance, some

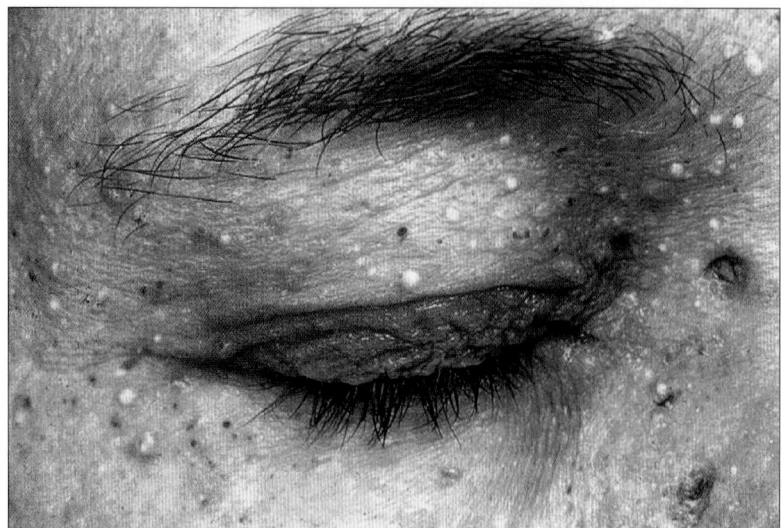

Fig. 24.87
Gorlin syndrome: multiple basal cell carcinomas are present on the nose of this young patient. By courtesy of the Institute of Dermatology, London, UK.

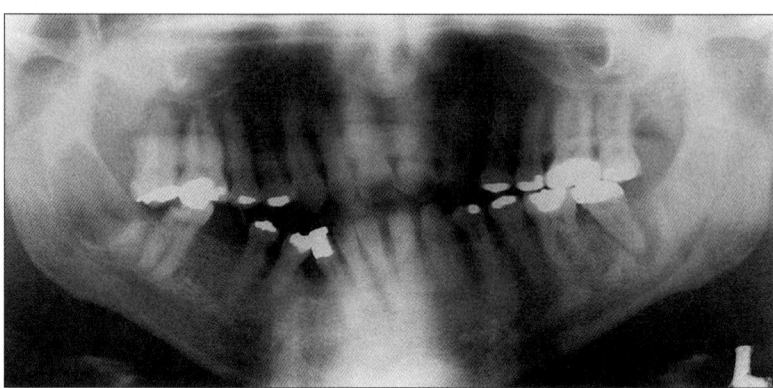

Fig. 24.88
Gorlin syndrome: note the radiolucent cyst at the angle of the right mandible. By courtesy of J. Newton, MD, St James's University Hospital, Leeds, UK.

being small flesh-colored or brown dome-shaped papules, while others are soft and nodular or flat plaques measuring up to 1 cm in diameter. Frequently, numerous milia are also evident. The larger tumors are usually pigmented, often ulcerate, and typically behave in an aggressive fashion. Both exposed and covered sites are affected. The central part of the face is commonly the first area to be involved, followed by the chest, back, and scalp and then other exposed sites (*Fig. 24.87*). Unusual anatomical sites include the vulva and the buccal mucosa.[22,23] Patients may harbor up to thousands of basal cell carcinomas, but about 10% of adult patients do not manifest skin tumors.[3] Rarely, the tumors have a unilateral distribution. Multiple large epidermoid cysts are also often evident on the trunk and limbs.[24,25]

Odontogenic keratocysts of the jaws occur in up to 90% of patients, usually presenting in childhood or adolescence.[26] They are commonly multiple and show a predilection for the premolar area and are associated with tooth displacement, pain, and swelling of the jaws (*Fig. 24.88*). Recurrence following surgical treatment is common.[3]

Skeletal abnormalities, which are present in up to 75% of cases, include generalized overgrowth, macrocephaly, bridging of the sella turcica, high-arched palate, vertebral abnormalities, splayed, fused, missing or bifid ribs, kyphoscoliosis, spina bifida occulta, hyperplasia of the mandibular coronoid processes, and bone cysts (*Fig. 24.89*).[3,27] A rather 'dished' facial appearance due to frontal and biparietal bossing, broadening of the nasal root, and ocular hypertelorism is characteristic.

Ectopic lamellar calcification of the falx cerebri (85–90%) and also of the diaphragma sellae (60–80%), tentorium cerebelli (40%), and petroclinoid ligaments (20%) are frequent manifestations.[3] Craniocerebral manifestations may be evident in utero.[28] Epilepsy is an occasional complication.[29]

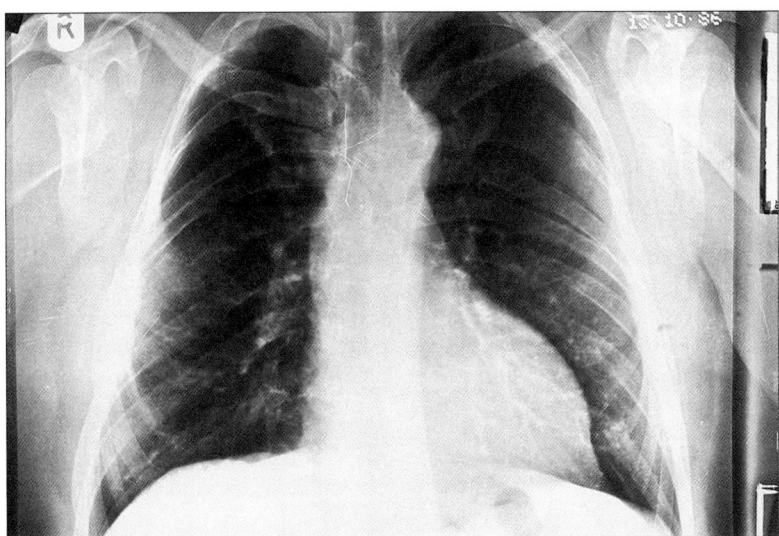

Fig. 24.89
Gorlin syndrome: note the splaying of the left third rib. By courtesy of J. Newton, MD, St James's University Hospital, Leeds, UK.

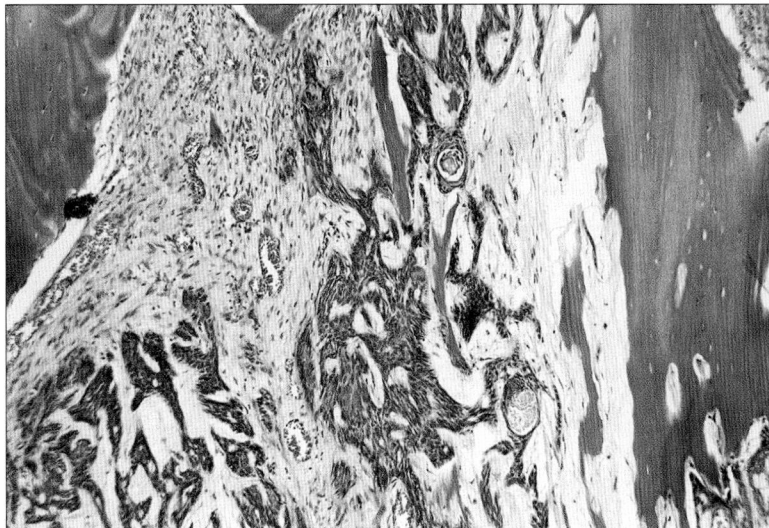

Fig. 24.91
Gorlin syndrome: this tumor originally presented as an ulcerated tumor on the scalp. Following radiotherapy, infiltration of the skull rapidly ensued and eventually metastases developed.

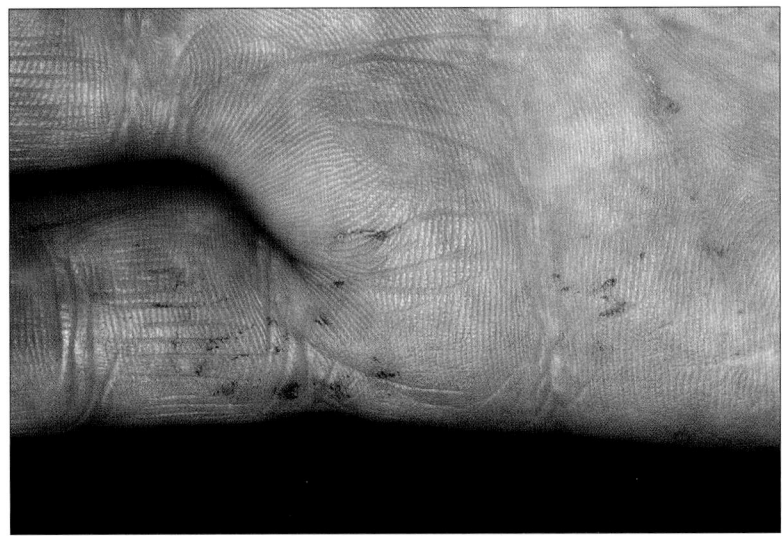

Fig. 24.90
Gorlin syndrome: note the tiny palmar pits. By courtesy of J. Newton, MD, St James's University Hospital, Leeds, UK.

The shallow pits of the palms and soles are pathognomonic and are present in approximately 65–80% patients, appearing in the second decade of life (*Fig. 24.90*).[3,30] They are asymptomatic, 1–3 mm deep and 2–3 mm across, and may be present in the hundreds. Occasionally, patients develop basal cell carcinoma on the palms or soles.

Patients with the nevoid basal cell carcinoma syndrome may have many other abnormalities, including dystopia canthorum and congenital blindness, hypogonadism, ovarian fibromas (75% of females), cardiac fibromas, and an increased incidence of central nervous system tumors, including medulloblastoma and meningiomas.[1,31–33] Rare associations include eosinophilic pustular folliculitis, nevus sebaceous, microphthalmia, ulcerative colitis, unilateral renal agenesis, multiple acrochorda, ameloblastoma, thyroid neoplasia, prenatal chylothorax, hepatic mesenchymal tumor, fetal rhabdomyoma, lymphomatoid papulosis, primary ovarian leiomyosarcoma, rhabdomyosarcoma, and Wilms tumor as well as undifferentiated sinonasal carcinoma.[34–49]

Histologic features

All variants of basal cell carcinoma may be seen, but the solid and superficial types are most common.[6] Morpheaform tumors are rare and only one carcinosarcoma has been documented.[50] There are no particular distinguishing

features by which they might be distinguished from ordinary basal cell carcinoma.

The jaw cysts are lined by stratified squamous epithelium with a thick fibrous capsule and may be associated with the development of spindle cell squamous carcinoma, myxoma, ameloblastoma, and fibrosarcoma.[51,52]

The palmar and plantar pits show a diminution or loss of the keratin and granular layers, associated with a thinned underlying Malpighian layer.[3] Electron microscopic examination reveals incompletely discharged Odland bodies. The pits are therefore believed to develop as a result of reduced 'intralamellar cement' resulting in diminished adherence between the keratin lamellae. The rete ridge pattern is irregular in size and shape and some pits may show basaloid proliferation. Although these pits only rarely progress into basal cell carcinomas, ionizing radiation has converted some into highly aggressive tumors. This sensitivity to radiation is also seen elsewhere, indicating a specific contraindication to this mode of treatment (*Fig. 24.91*).[1]

Differential diagnosis

The nevoid basal cell carcinoma syndrome should be distinguished from the linear unilateral basal cell nevus (Carney) syndrome, which comprises an extensive unilateral lesion consisting of basaloid follicular hamartomas in addition to comedones, epidermoid cysts, and areas of epidermal atrophy.[53,54] Patients may also have scoliosis, but there are no other significant internal abnormalities. A number of other specific genodermatoses can be associated with basal cell carcinoma as well, but lack the structural stigmata of Gorlin syndrome.[55]

Bazex-Dupré-Christol and Rombo syndromes

Clinical features

Bazex-Dupré-Christol syndrome is a rare genodermatosis initially described in 1964.[1] It is associated with development of multiple basal cell carcinomas at an early age (second to third decades), although not as young as in the nevoid basal cell carcinoma syndrome.[2–7] Most tumors are located around the face.[2] It is thought to have an X-linked dominant mode of inheritance[2] and more recently the gene has been mapped to chromosome Xq24~q27 and appears to involve the *ACTRT1* gene whose encoded protein directly binds the *GLI1* promoter, a downstream activator of the hedgehog pathway.[8,9] Mutations appear to involve both the coding and non-coding regulatory elements of this gene.[9]

Follicular atrophoderma (85%), presenting as prominent follicular ostia (resembling orange peel) on the backs of the hand, the face, the extensor surfaces of the limbs, and the back, is the most consistent finding.[2] Congenital and permanent hypotrichosis (85%), shown by very sparse scalp and body hair including eyebrows and eyelashes, is also present.[2] Milia (66%) and hypohidrosis (27%) complete the clinical picture.[10] Rare documented associations include multiple genital trichoepitheliomas as well as scarring folliculitis of the scalp.[11–13]

Only a single patient with a clinical picture resembling Bazex-Dupré-Christol syndrome has been reported without a family history, possibly representing sporadic presentation of this syndrome.[14]

Rombo syndrome, which is an exceedingly rare autosomal dominant condition, is similar, but does not feature follicular atrophoderma or absent sweating.[7,15–17] Patients present with vermiculate atrophoderma, facial milia, hypotrichosis, with loss of eyelashes, and both trichoepitheliomas and basal cell carcinomas, as well as peripheral vasodilatation with cyanosis.

Histologic features

Follicular atrophoderma is characterized by follicular dilatation and plugging associated with malformed, poorly developed or absent follicular structures.[2,5]

Basal cell carcinomas, trichoepitheliomas, and possibly basaloid follicular hamartomas may all feature histologically, and therefore the condition must be distinguished from the nevoid basal cell carcinoma syndrome and multiple familial trichoepitheliomas.

Fibroepithelioma of Pinkus

Clinical features

Fibroepithelioma of Pinkus is an uncommon tumor that is seen most commonly on the trunk and thigh, and clinically often resembles a fibroepithelial polyp (*Fig. 24.92*).[1,2] Pigmentation is rare.[3] Multiple nodular plaques or polypoid lesions, which are firm, erythematous or skin-colored and without translucency, may develop on the lower back in patients who have had radiotherapy (*Fig. 24.93*). Single cases have been reported to occur overlying a breast cancer, on the penis, and in association with a dermoid cyst.[4-6] Pigmented forms have been reported.[7–9] Some suggest that fibroepithelioma of Pinkus might be regarded as a form of trichoblastoma, yet it has been described in continuity with classic basal cell carcinoma.[9–12] A recent large series of 49 cases suggested a possibly correlation with gastrointestinal cancer (18% showed such an association), but additional study is needed.[13]

Histologic features

The tumor is characterized by basaloid epithelial strands, two to three cells thick, arising from many foci along the epidermis and anastomosing to compartmentalize the fibrous stroma (*Figs 24.94 and 24.95*). Cyst formation and primitive hair germ maturation may be additional features.[14,15] Rarely, a more typical invasive basal cell carcinoma develops within a Pinkus tumor. It has been postulated that these distinctive histologic features might be a consequence of tumor spread along pre-existent dermal eccrine ducts.[16] The presence of pleomorphic giant cells has been reported in a single case. These are speculated to represent senescence rather than malignant change based on DNA ploidy analysis.[17]

By immunohistochemistry, fibroepithelioma of Pinkus has a low mib-1 proliferative index and shows only low-level expression of p53. Cytokeratin 20 staining reveals retention of intratumoral Merkel cells analogous to trichoblastoma.[2] This raises the possibility that fibroepithelioma of Pinkus is a variant of trichoblastoma. The majority of tumors, however, express androgen receptors similar to basal cell carcinoma.[18]

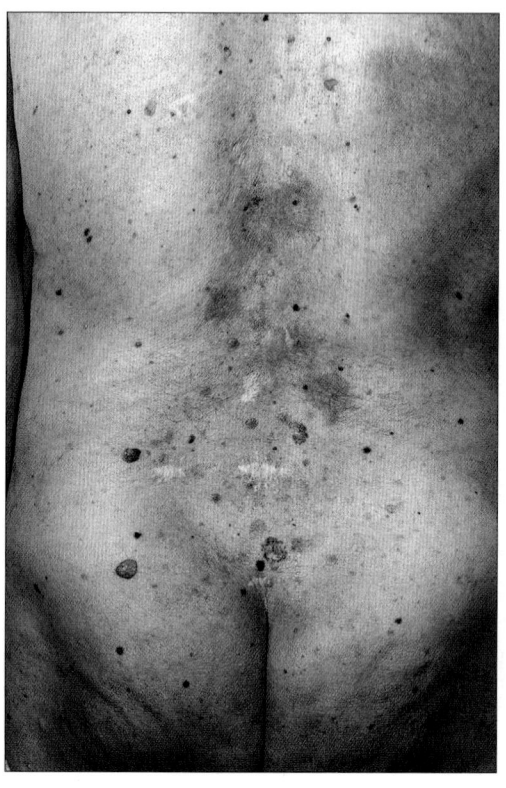

Fig. 24.93
Fibroepithelial tumor of Pinkus: multiple lesions are present on the back of this patient who was previously treated with radiotherapy. Note the scars representing excised basal cell carcinomas. By courtesy of R.A. Marsden, MD, St George's Hospital, London, UK.

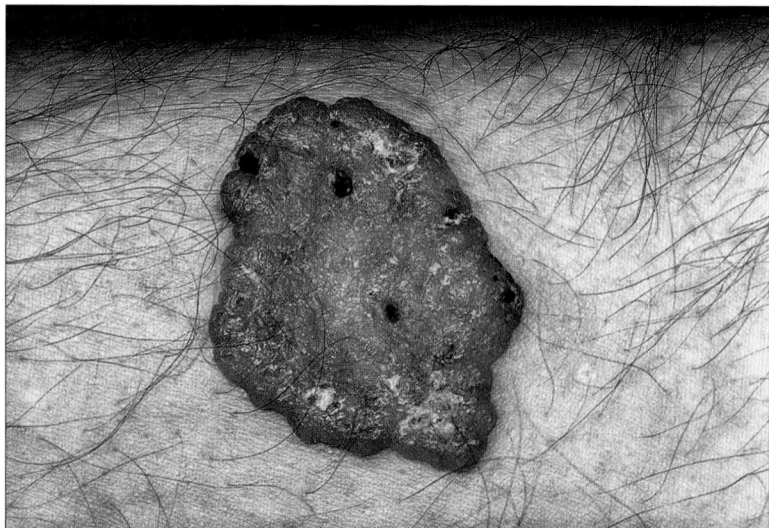

Fig. 24.92
Fibroepithelial tumor of Pinkus: erythematous lesion at a characteristic location on the thigh. By courtesy of R.A. Marsden, MD, St George's Hospital, London, UK.

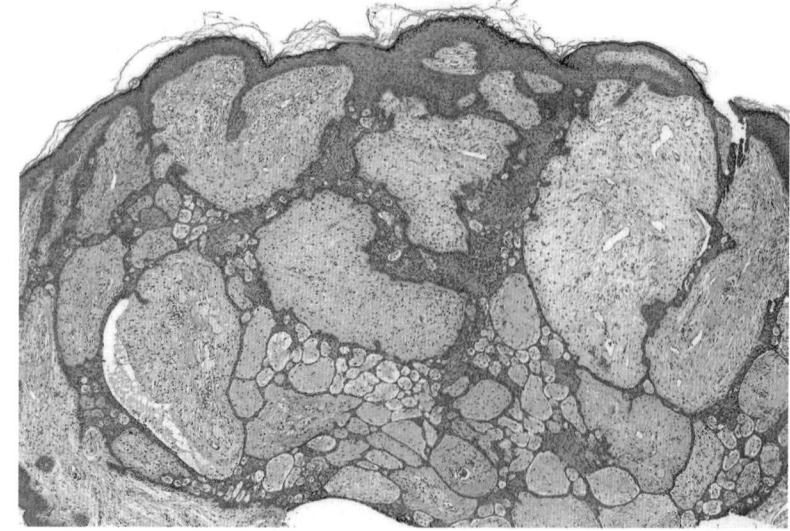

Fig. 24.94
Fibroepithelial tumor of Pinkus: low-power view showing delicate interconnecting epithelial strands.

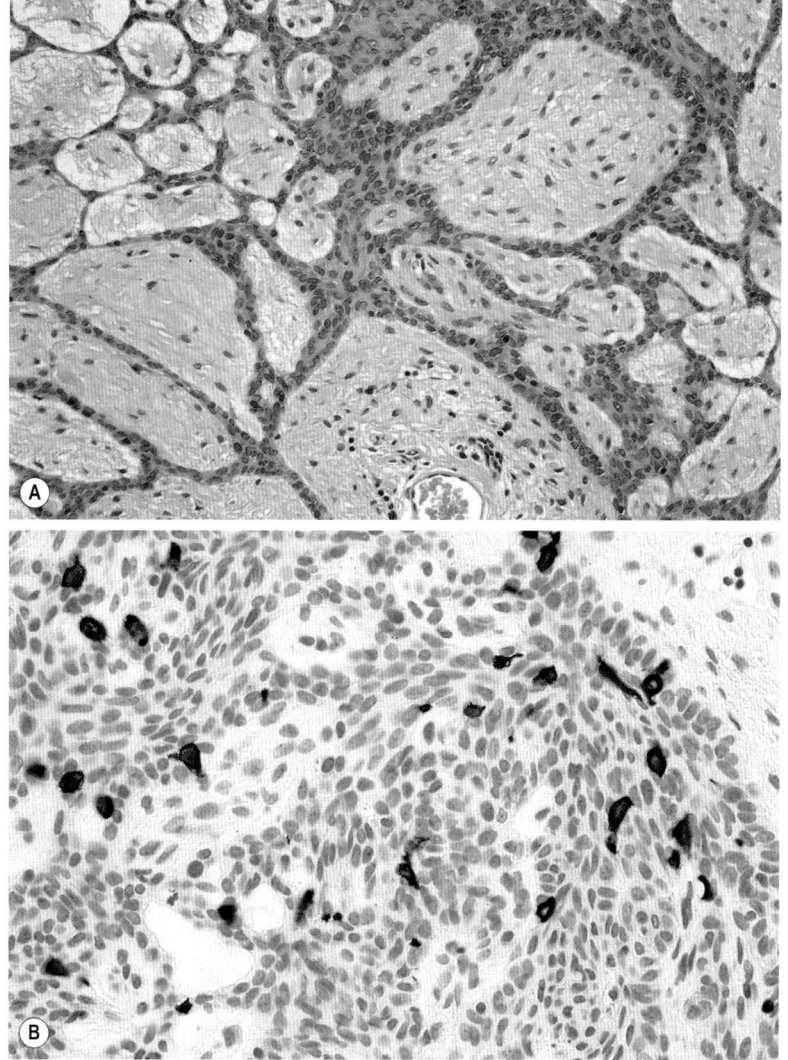

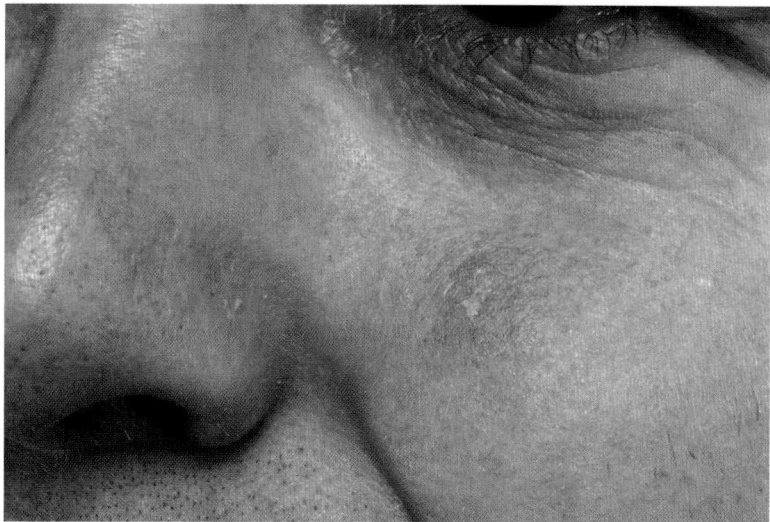

Fig. 24.96
Actinic keratosis: this is a typical lesion characterized by yellow scales overlying an erythematous base. By courtesy of the Institute of Dermatology, London, UK.

Fig. 24.95
Fibroepithelial tumor of Pinkus: (**A**) the epithelial cells have hyperchromatic cytoplasm and minimal eosinophilic cytoplasm; (**B**) numerous CK20-positive Merkel cells are present.

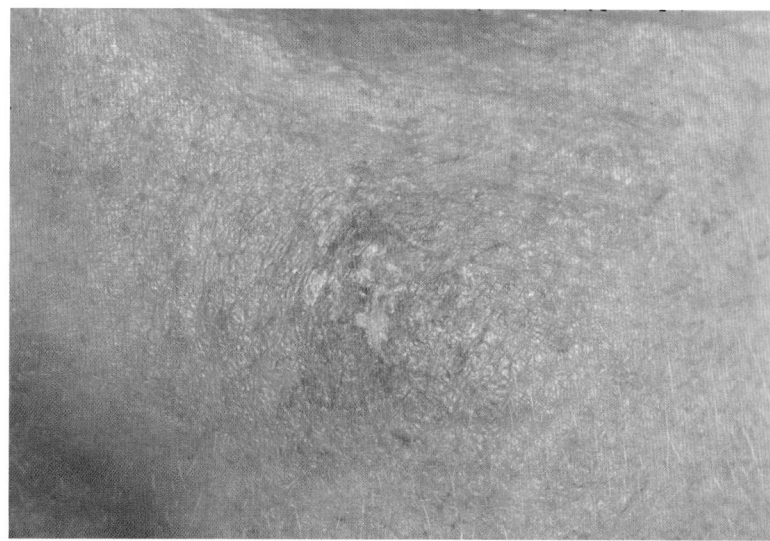

Fig. 24.97
Actinic keratosis: close-up view. By courtesy of the Institute of Dermatology, London, UK.

Actinic keratoses

Clinical features

Actinic (solar, senile) keratoses are common, usually presenting as multiple, erythematous, or yellow-brown, dry, scaly lesions in the middle aged or elderly. Heavily pigmented variants that may be clinically mistaken for lentigo maligna are occasionally encountered.[1,2] Actinic keratoses may also coexist with lentigo maligna, thereby adding to problems in the differential diagnosis. They are more common in males than in females and especially in those with fair complexions who burn rather than tan following sun exposure.[3–6] They usually measure 1 cm in diameter or less.[3] The surrounding skin frequently shows additional features of sun damage including atrophy, pigmentary changes, and telangiectasia. Actinic keratoses are of particular importance because they are a sensitive indicator of exposure to UV light and strongly predict the likelihood of developing cutaneous squamous cell carcinoma.[7,8]

Despite the publication of many large series (mostly from Australia), the prevalence of actinic keratosis is uncertain. Histologic confirmation has been uniformly absent in these reports and variation in the populations studied and lack of consistency of clinical diagnostic criteria make accurate assessment and comparison difficult.[3,6,9] Nevertheless, actinic keratoses are markedly influenced by latitude, with the quoted prevalence ranging from approximately 10% of the adult population in Galway, Ireland, to 40% in Queensland, and in excess of 60% in Victoria, Australia.[10–13]

Because these hyperkeratotic skin lesions occur on sun-damaged skin, the sites of involvement are usually the face and neck and the dorsal aspects of the hands and forearms (*Figs 24.96 and 24.97*). Oral lesions (chronic actinic cheilitis) tend to affect the middle of the lower lip and present as burning or painful scaly lesions. Eyelid and conjunctival involvement have also been described.[14,15] Hyperkeratosis is sometimes marked and the lesion may present as a cutaneous horn. Actinic keratoses may rarely be associated with Kindler syndrome,[16] and an eruptive presentation has been reported after heart transplantation.[17] Organ transplant recipients show increased incidence of actinic keratoses that can resolve with adjustment of immunosuppressive regimens.[18–20] Sun-exposed lesions of vitiligo may also be affected.[21]

Although only a small proportion of actinic keratoses appear to develop into an invasive squamous cell carcinoma, patients usually have multiple and often numerous lesions for many years and so have a much higher risk of ultimately developing squamous carcinoma. Only an estimated 0.1–10% of actinic keratoses (with the low end of this range likely being most relevant) are thought to progress to invasive squamous cell carcinoma.[6,22–26] Nonetheless, the presence of these keratoses reflects the total actinic damage to the skin and serves as an indicator to identify a high-risk population for the development of sun damage-related disease such as squamous cell

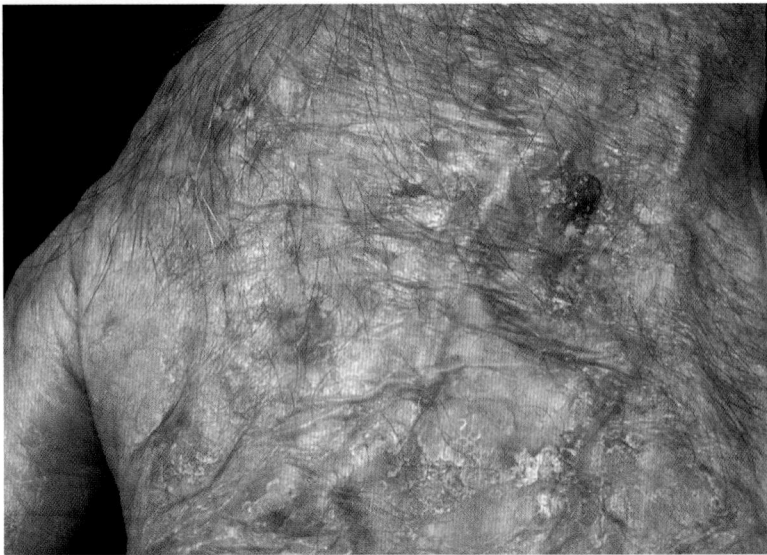

Fig. 24.98
Squamous cell carcinoma: this tumor arose within a pre-existent actinic keratosis. Note the background skin atrophy and multiple keratoses. By courtesy of the Institute of Dermatology, London, UK.

carcinoma, basal cell carcinoma, and, to a lesser extent, melanoma at other sites.[7,27–29] A recent study suggested a relative risk of skin cancer at 4.52 in patients with a previous diagnosis of actinic keratosis.[30] The cumulative probability of development of invasive squamous cell carcinoma in patients with 10 or more actinic keratoses has been estimated at 14% in a 5-year period.[31] In general, increasing number and severity of actinic keratoses is associated with increasing risk of squamous cell carcinoma.[32] Actinic keratoses may be contiguous with an invasive squamous cell carcinoma in 44% of cases with metastasis.[33] Metastases, however, are rare except for those arising on the ear and lip, which are often associated with more aggressive behavior.[22] A higher rate of malignant transformation is also observed in hyperkeratotic lesions located on the dorsum of hands, wrists, or forearms (Fig. 24.98).[34] Other proposed clinical parameters that may be associated with increased risk for the development of invasive tumors include induration, inflammation, diameter greater than 1 cm, rapid growth, bleeding, erythema, and ulceration.[35] Sometimes actinic keratoses appear to regress, presumably as a consequence of immune mechanisms.[23,36] Radiation keratoses may resemble solar-induced lesions.

Diffuse epidermal and periadnexal squamous cell carcinoma in situ refers to an unusual presentation in which actinic keratoses cover a large area of skin. There is a strong predilection for sun-exposed areas of the head of males. The clinical characteristics are large areas of erythema, hyperkeratosis, and ulceration. They are rarely pigmented. Due to extensive involvement of skin adnexal structures, topical treatment may be ineffective and there is a rate of local recurrence. Most importantly, the condition shows a strong association with development of invasive nonmelanoma skin cancer.[37]

Pathogenesis and histologic features

Actinic keratoses arise in white-skinned populations as a consequence of the effects of excessive exposure to UV radiation, particularly UVB. Owing to the protective effects of a higher epidermal melanin concentration, they are much less common in dark-skinned races.[3] In addition to the total dosage and possibly the rate of exposure, inherent susceptibility is probably important in determining the extent of skin damage.[38] Actinic keratoses are common in individuals with an increased sensitivity to the effects of UV radiation such as occurs in albinism and xeroderma pigmentosum.[3] Outdoor workers or those who devote a considerable proportion of their leisure time to sunbathing have a much higher risk. It has also been suggested that sun exposure in childhood is particularly important.[39] Treatment with hydroxyurea has been implicated in the development of multiple actinic keratoses.[40] Although the keratosis is objective evidence of skin damage, it should be noted that perilesional skin frequently shows evidence of a 'field effect' of

minor cellular damage such as nuclear hyperchromatism, cytoplasmic and nuclear pleomorphism, slight architectural disarray, and increased uptake of [³H] thymidine.[41] Adjacent morphologically normal epidermis often overexpresses p53 protein.[42] Spontaneous regression of actinic keratoses has been reported.[23,43]

Genetically, actinic keratoses show a high rate of aneuploidy in addition to clonal karyotypic abnormalities and frequent loss of heterozygosity of 17p, 17q, 9p, and 9q in addition to microsatellite instability as well as mutations in CDKN2A and TP53.[44–47] The p53 mutations are observed in most actinic keratoses in Caucasians (75–80%) but are present to a significantly lesser extent in Asians (30–40%).[48,49] Recently, it has been noted that actinic keratoses can arise in the setting of what have been termed 'p53 immunopositive patches' (PIPs) that are small accumulations of skin cells (usually less than 3,000 total) that carry many of the same mutations described in the subsequent section as common in squamous cell carcinoma, including HRAS, KRAS, TP53, NOTCH1, NOTCH2, CDKN2A, and others.[50,51] Expression of CD95 (Fas) appears to be reduced in actinic keratoses compared to sun-damaged nondysplastic skin, and patients with a glutathione-S-transferase M1 null phenotype are at increased risk of developing actinic keratoses.[52,53] The direct link of UV light to the development of actinic keratosis has been established in an animal model. Actinic keratoses have been induced in human skin maintained in severe combined immunodeficient (SCID) mice exposed to UVB and specific UV signature mutations identified in the tp53 gene.[54] The role of HPV infection in sporadic actinic keratoses continues to be debated; it may have increased importance in the immunosuppressed organ transplant setting.[55–59]

Squamous cell carcinoma frequently develops in a background and in association with actinic keratoses (more than 80%).[60–62] Certain events may play a role in the progression of actinic keratoses to squamous cell carcinoma including deletion of chromosome 9p21 encoding the p16 tumor suppressor gene, activation of RAS genes, and loss of the inflammatory cell infiltrate when invasion occurs.[47,63–66] Overexpression of p16ink4 appears to be more associated with in situ squamous cell carcinoma than actinic keratosis.[67–69]

UV-induced immunosuppression is also probably of importance, but the precise mechanisms are uncertain. Immunosuppressed renal transplant patients have an increased risk of developing actinic keratoses in addition to squamous cell carcinomas.[3] There is no evidence of a pathogenetic role for either Epstein-Barr virus or herpesvirus 8.[70,71] However, a wide spectrum of HPV has been identified in a significant subset of actinic keratoses from both immunocompetent and immunosuppressed patients.[55–59,72–74] The virus appears to be present predominantly in the outer, more superficial layers of the epidermis.[75]

Although a variety of quite distinct histopathological variants of actinic keratoses may be recognized, many examples display a spectrum of patterns, manifesting epithelial dysplasia from mild changes through to carcinoma in situ and commonly accompanied by parakeratosis (Fig. 24.99).[76–78] A grading of epidermal dysplasia as keratinocytic intraepidermal neoplasia analogous to that applied to squamous dysplasia of the cervix uteri has been proposed.[79,80] While intraobserver variability in grading dysplasia in a three-tiered system was found to be relatively low, its significance is uncertain as no classical tumor progression model exists for epidermal dysplasia and the formation of squamous cell carcinoma in situ is not a necessary step for the development of dermal invasion.[81,82]

A frequently seen subtype is the hyperkeratotic/hyperplastic actinic keratosis (Fig. 24.100). This lesion is characterized by alternating bands of hyperkeratosis and parakeratosis. The latter covers areas of dysplastic epithelium, whereas the former overlies the uninvolved epithelia of the follicular ostia and sweat gland orifices (Freudenthal funnel) (Fig. 24.101). Actinic keratoses are typified by varying degrees of epidermal dysplasia involving the interadnexal epidermis. Sometimes this is limited to the basal layers only; in other examples the lesion appears as budding of atypical epithelium into the papillary dermis (proliferative actinic keratosis) (Figs 24.102 and 24.103).[83] In occasional keratoses the atypical cells form a mantle around the outer aspects of the cutaneous adnexae (Fig. 24.104).

Characteristically, the edges of these lesions are angulated with their broader aspects occupying the base. Sometimes actinic keratoses are

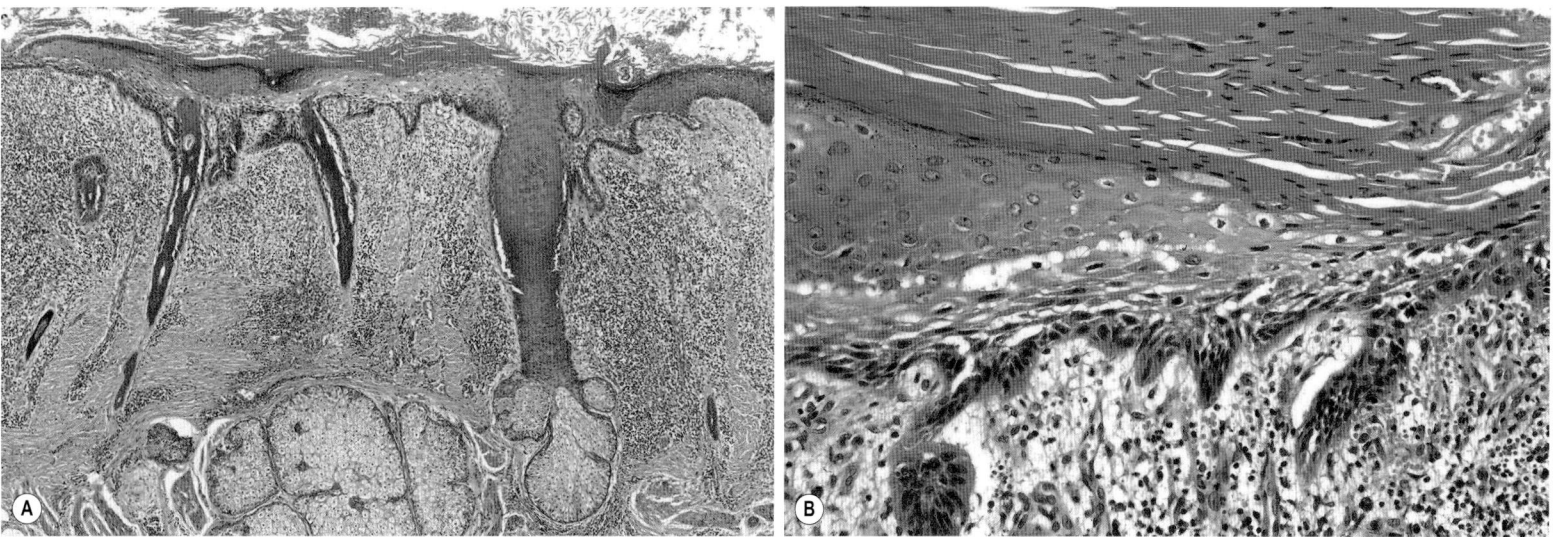

Fig. 24.99

(**A**, **B**) Actinic keratosis: there is parakeratosis overlying a thickened epidermis. Basal cell atypia presenting as cells with enlarged, irregular, hyperchromatic nuclei is present. There is involvement of the straight dermal sweat ducts.

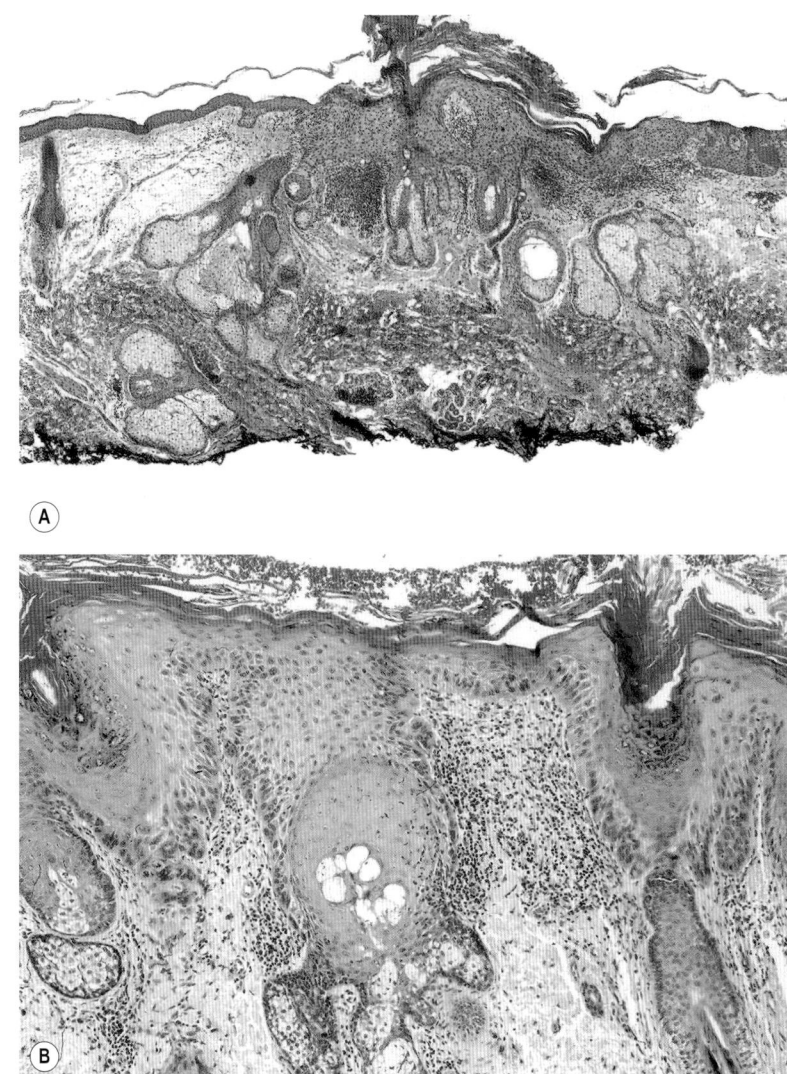

Fig. 24.100

Hyperkeratotic actinic keratosis: (**A**) scanning view showing parakeratotic scale overlying an acanthotic lesion; (**B**) the atypia predominantly affects the basal epithelium.

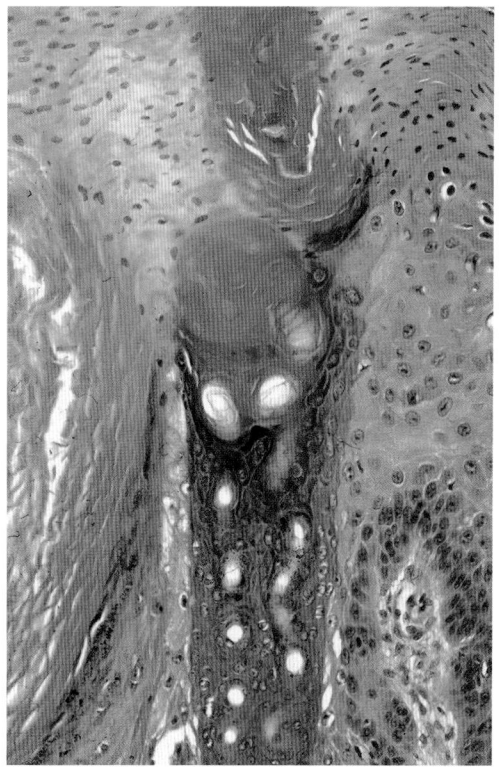

Fig. 24.101

Actinic keratosis: note the parakeratosis overlying the dysplastic epithelium. There is hyperkeratosis over the sweat duct ostium.

atrophic and occasionally, due to marked acantholysis, an acantholytic or pseudoglandular pattern results, which may show a marked resemblance to lesions of Darier disease (acantholytic actinic keratoses) (*Figs 24.105 and 24.106*).[84] Some actinic keratoses are typified by full-thickness dysplasia (squamous cell carcinoma in situ – Bowenoid actinic keratoses) (*Fig. 24.107*). Bowenoid actinic keratosis is associated with a loss of desmosomes as well as hemidesmosomes, and it has been postulated that this correlates with more aggressive behavior compared to acantholytic actinic keratoses.[85] Clear cell change due to an excess of cytoplasmic glycogen is sometimes evident and occasionally the features of epidermolytic hyperkeratosis or a keratin horn may be superimposed (*Fig. 24.108*). The dermis underlying and adjacent to the keratosis usually shows solar elastosis and vascular ectasia. A lymphohistiocytic infiltrate is commonly evident and sometimes this is associated with the features of an interface dermatitis including basal cell liquefactive degeneration and apoptosis (lichenoid actinic keratosis).

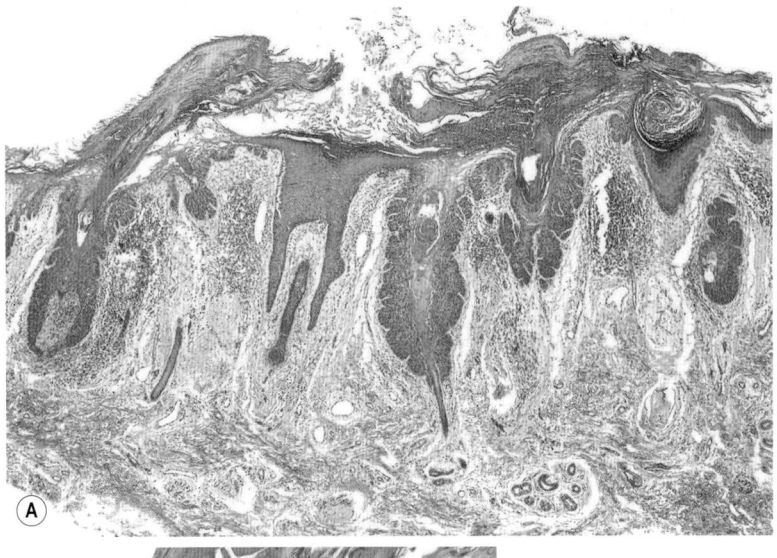

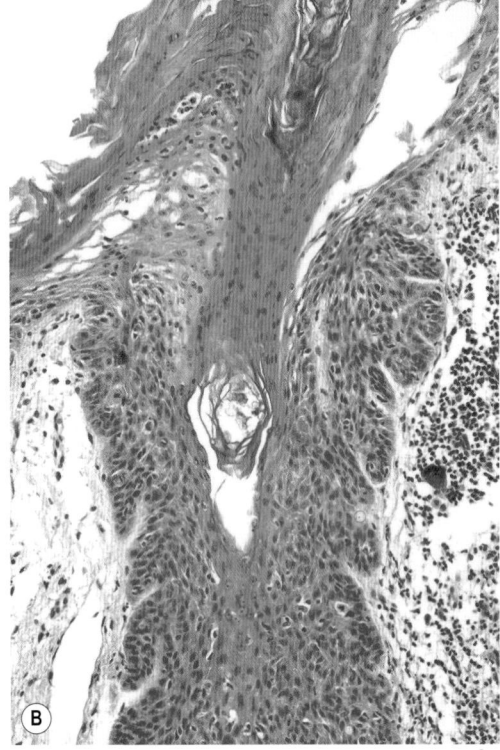

Fig. 24.102
Proliferative actinic keratosis: (**A**) in this example the dysplastic epithelium is proliferating in budlike downgrowths into the papillary dermis, there is a dense overlying scale, and marked chronic inflammatory changes are present; (**B**) the dysplastic changes are seen predominantly within the basal epidermal layers. The nuclei are intensely hyperchromatic.

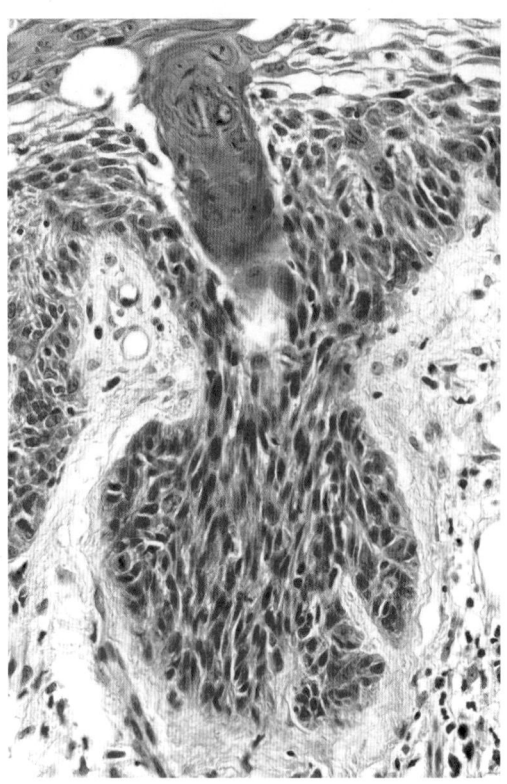

Fig. 24.103
Proliferative actinic keratosis: the presence of buds at the base of the lesion should not be mistaken for squamous cell carcinoma.

This variant is reminiscent of lichenoid keratoses but may be distinguished from it by the presence of nuclear atypia. The Pagetoid variant is rare and most frequently observed in squamous cell carcinoma in situ. It is characterized by dysplastic keratinocytes arranged singly or in small nests throughout the epidermis closely resembling extramammary Paget disease from which it must be distinguished.[86]

Actinic keratoses may be pigmented, showing increased melanin pigment in the lower epidermis within keratinocytes as well as in melanocytes and dermal macrophages. This variant has been referred to as spreading pigmented actinic keratosis.[87,88] On occasion, difficulty may be experienced in distinguishing this lesion from in situ melanoma (lentigo maligna). In such cases the use of immunohistochemistry to exclude a melanocytic lesion is often helpful.[89] Immunohistochemical results need to be interpreted with care as especially Melan A expression may also be observed in keratinocytes and nonmelanocytic cells.[90] Therefore, melanocytic markers that display nuclear staining, including MITF and SOX10, are preferred over the latter. Actinic keratoses arising in immunosuppressed patients are more often hyperkeratotic with confluent parakeratosis and more prominent mitotic figures. They occur in younger and predominantly male patients.[91]

The intensity of immunohistochemical expression of tenascin has been found to correlate with the degree of dysplasia in actinic keratosis.[92,93]

Differential diagnosis

A common problem is the histologic differentiation between proliferating actinic keratosis and early squamous cell carcinoma. Although this is a somewhat artificial distinction because both conditions form part of a continuum, the presence of atypical keratinocytes, either singly or in groups, detached from the main lesion or often associated with a stromal reaction, are features that imply dermal invasion. Thickness of the keratosis is irrelevant and whether the tumor cells are present in the reticular as well as the papillary dermis has little bearing in distinguishing between the two lesions. At some sites where the prognosis of squamous carcinoma is known to be poor, it is wise to err on the side of the hawks rather than the doves.[94] In general, however, the distinction between a proliferating solar keratosis and a 'microinvasive' squamous carcinoma is of little clinical significance because both lesions will have an identical outcome provided excision is complete.

The distinction of actinic keratoses from superficial basal cell carcinoma may sometimes be problematic. In these circumstances, immunohistochemistry for bcl-2 and Ber-EP4, both of which stain positively in basal cell carcinoma and are negative in actinic keratoses, can be helpful.[95,96]

Squamous carcinoma in situ (Bowen disease)

Clinical features

Squamous carcinoma in situ (Bowen disease) predominantly affects white-skinned races and is most common in the middle aged or elderly. It is a rare disease in blacks and young patients.[1-3] It may affect any part of the integument, mucous membranes, or nail bed and therefore involves both sun-exposed and non–sun-exposed skin.[4-7] The sex incidence appears to be variable. For example, in Northern Ireland the male:female ratio is 1:2.8, but in the United States the sexes are affected equally.[8]

Lesions may be single or multiple and are slow growing, persistent, discrete, irregular in shape, and measure from a few millimeters to several centimeters in diameter (*Figs 24.109 and 24.110*).[5] Occasionally, the disease may be extensive.[9] Bowen disease is erythematous and scaly or crusted, often clinically resembling psoriasis or dermatitis. Indeed, presentation as a non–steroid-responsive dermatosis is a classic clinical history. Pigmented variants are very rare but may be confused with melanoma (*Fig. 24.111*).[10-15] Most of such examples have been described in the anogenital region.[16,17]

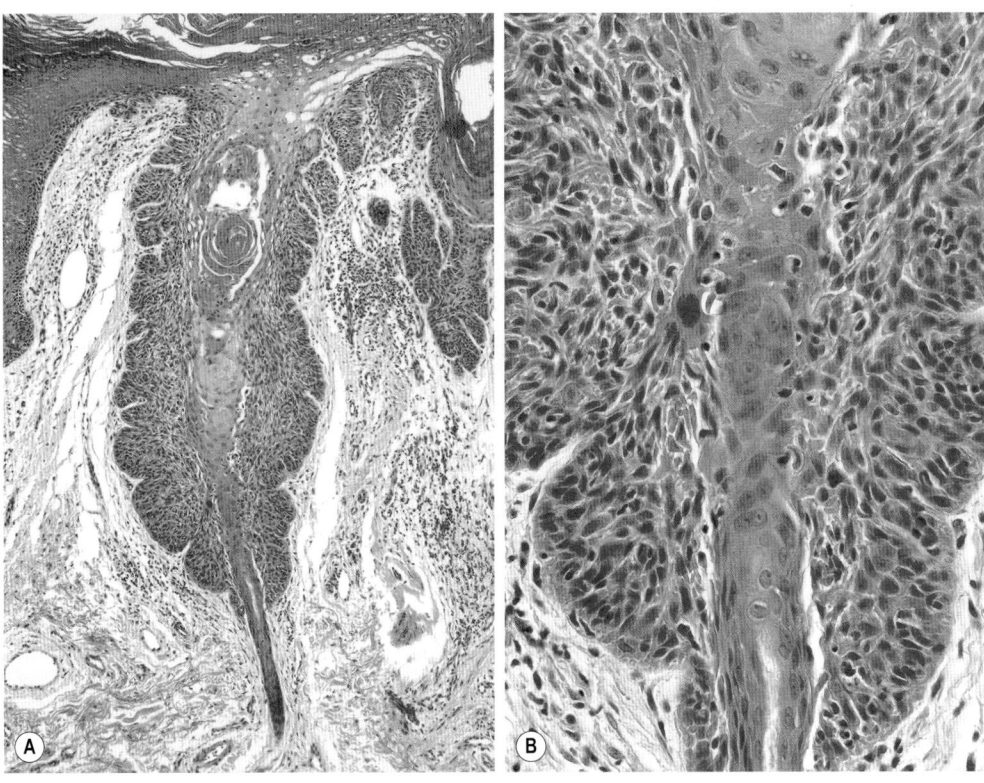

Fig. 24.104
(**A**, **B**) Proliferative actinic keratosis: atypical epithelium ensheaths the dermal sweat duct.

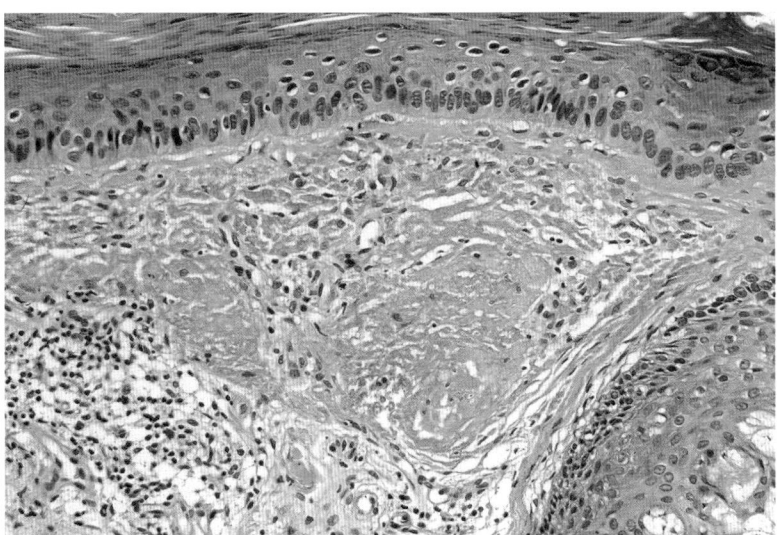

Fig. 24.105
Atrophic actinic keratosis: there is parakeratosis, epidermal atrophy, and basal nuclear atypia. Note the gross actinic elastosis.

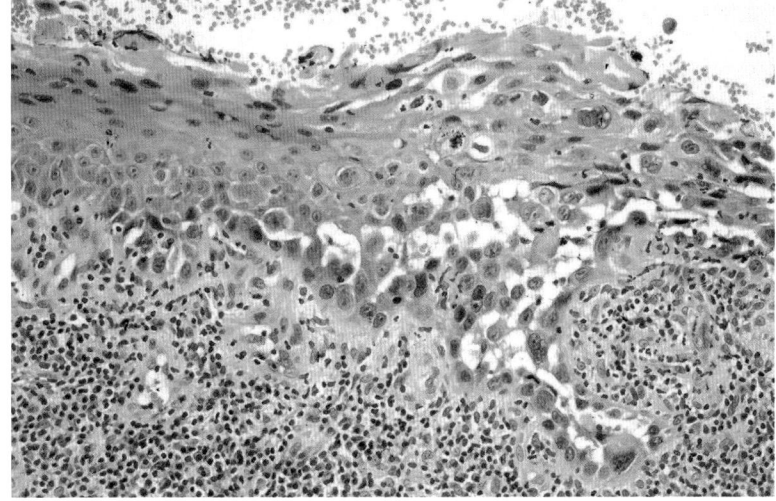

Fig. 24.106
Acantholytic actinic keratosis: the dysplastic epithelium is accompanied by extensive acantholysis. Note the nuclear pleomorphism.

Bowen disease commonly presents on the head, trunk, extremities, and genitalia.[6,18,19] While there appears to be a predilection for cheeks and lower limbs in women, the scalp and ears are the most frequently affected sites in men.[20] Unusual sites of involvement include the palm, sole, eyelid, conjunctiva, external auditory canal, nail, nipple, and umbilicus.[21–31] Approximately 5% of cases develop an invasive component and of these roughly 30% have metastatic potential.[32] Partial or complete spontaneous regression has been documented but is exceedingly rare.[33–35]

Immunocompromised patients are at increased risk of developing Bowen disease. Patients are younger at presentation and tumors are often multiple, showing more aggressive behavior with higher recurrence rates compared to immunocompetent patients.[36–38] Tumor size may be extensive, as documented in an HIV-positive patient, and a symmetrical bilateral distribution has been described in a patient with chronic lymphocytic leukemia.[39–41]

In young adults, lesions tend to be located predominantly about the genitalia. Bowen disease of the penis is also known as erythroplasia of Queyrat.[42,43] Patients present with slightly scaly, erythematous, velvety plaques.[5,42] The disease may arise in association with Zoon balanitis and may be complicated by urethral involvement.[44–48] In a series of 100 such cases, 22% recurred, 8% progressed to invasive tumor, and 2% metastasized.[49]

Perianal Bowen disease presents as raised, irregular, brownish-red, itchy, and sometimes bleeding plaques.[50–52] It is more common in females than in males. Progression towards invasive carcinoma appears to be relatively uncommon, occurring in 2–6% of patients. Following adequate surgery, recurrences are unusual.

Involvement of multiple fingers as well as multicentricity in the setting of Fanconi anemia has been reported.[53,54] Rarely, Bowen disease may present as longitudinal erythronychia and distal subungual keratoses, longitudinal melanonychia, a pigmented pseudofibrokeratoma, or a viral wart.[55–60]

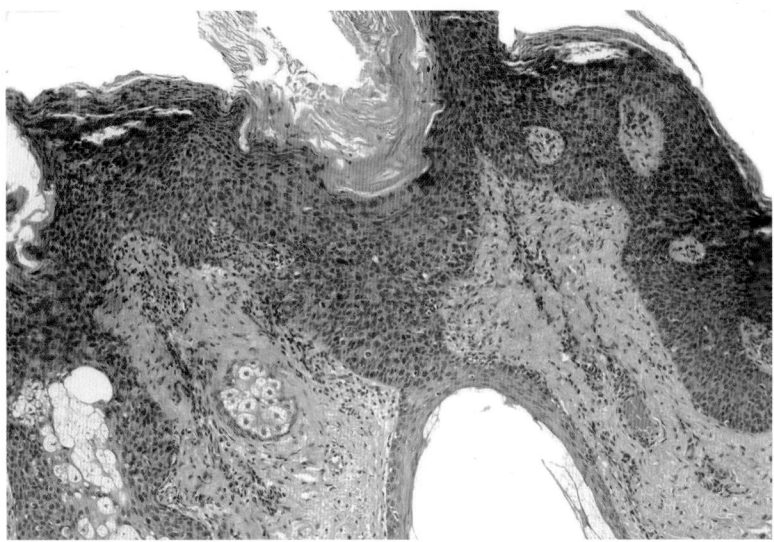

Fig. 24.107
Bowenoid actinic keratosis: the epidermis is acanthotic and shows full-thickness dysplasia (squamous cell carcinoma in situ).

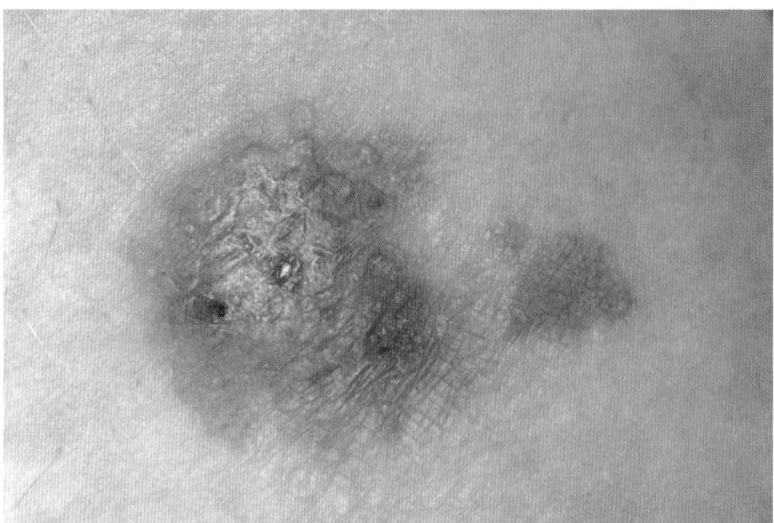

Fig. 24.109
Bowen disease (squamous cell carcinoma in situ): characteristic erythematous scaly plaque with erosions and multiple foci of ulceration. By courtesy of the Institute of Dermatology, London, UK.

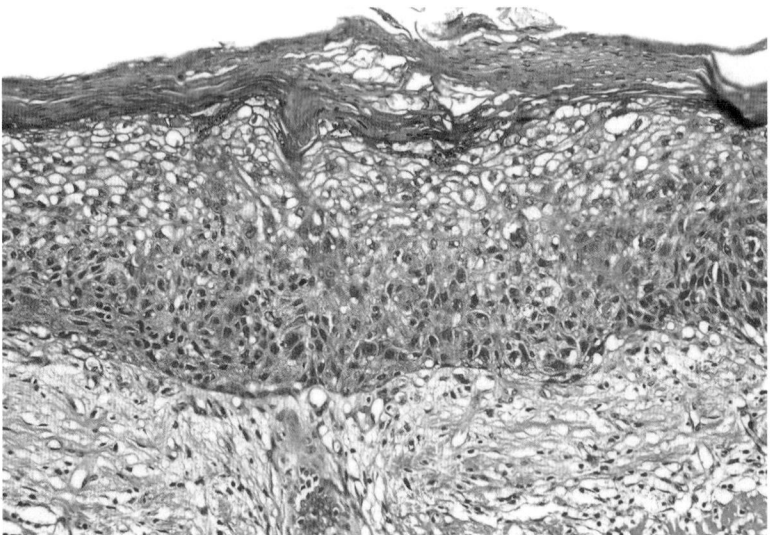

Fig. 24.108
Clear cell actinic keratosis: this lesion shows full-thickness dysplasia (carcinoma in situ) accompanied by extensive cytoplasmic vacuolization. The clear cell change is due to excessive glycogen accumulation and therefore this lesion is often periodic acid-Schiff positive.

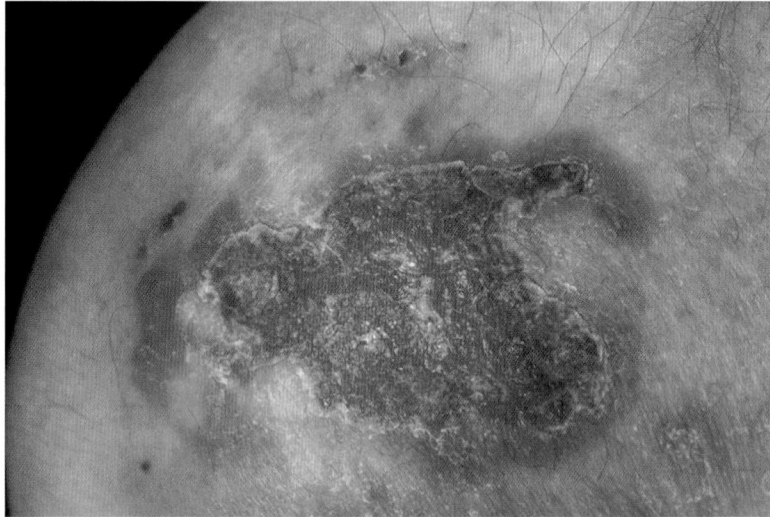

Fig. 24.110
Bowen disease (squamous cell carcinoma in situ): this large ulcerated example shows a pigmented irregular border. Invasive tumor is likely. By courtesy of the Institute of Dermatology, London, UK.

It may complicate porokeratosis and coexist with extramammary Paget disease, skin adnexal carcinoma, and Merkel cell carcinoma or develop within the setting of erythema ab igne, a pre-existent seborrheic wart, scar or Becker nevus.[61–76]

In the past, Bowen disease on covered skin was believed by some to be associated with an increased risk of subsequent internal malignancy.[7,77,78] Subsequently, in particular the meta-analysis study of Lycka, suggests that a significant association between the two conditions is unlikely.[79–82] In general, it is therefore unnecessary to subject patients with cutaneous Bowen disease to rigorous investigation to reveal an internal neoplasm.[83] Rarely, however, the cutaneous lesions reflect a systemic carcinogen (e.g., arsenic) and an underlying malignancy would then not be unexpected.[81]

The clinical differential diagnosis of Bowen disease includes psoriasis, eczema, superficial basal cell carcinoma, and cutaneous Paget disease.[5]

Pathogenesis and histologic features

The etiology of in situ squamous carcinoma is probably multifactorial and includes UV light and chemicals such as arsenic. Arsenic used to be found in a number of medications, including bromide solution for epilepsy and

Fowler's solution for psoriasis, but it is now used in a variety of insecticides, fungicides, and weedkillers and may also contaminate natural water supplies.[4,84] Evidence of HPV infection has been detected in a significant number of patients, particularly in periungual and anogenital lesions.[85–89] More recent reports have detected HPV in Bowen disease at a number of extragenital locations.[90] Although HPV 16 is the most prevalent HPV, other virus strains including 2, 18, 31, 33, 54, 56, 58, 61, 62, and 73 have also been identified.[87,91–101] At a molecular level, the lesions of Bowen disease show a high incidence of aneuploidy[102–104] and DNA instability.[105]

Histologically, the epidermis shows full-thickness dysplasia (carcinoma in situ), which characteristically involves the entire epidermis including the intraepidermal portions of the cutaneous adnexae (Fig. 24.112). Parakeratosis is usually present. There is marked acanthosis with complete disorganization of the epidermal architecture, loss of maturation, and lack of polarity of cells. The latter are large and contain prominent irregular, often hyperchromatic, nuclei with conspicuous nucleoli and abundant cytoplasm (Figs 24.113–24.115). The keratinocytes are sometimes vacuolated due to glycogen deposition, in which instance they may be strongly PAS positive (Fig. 24.116). This may result in striking clear cell change (clear cell variant).[106]

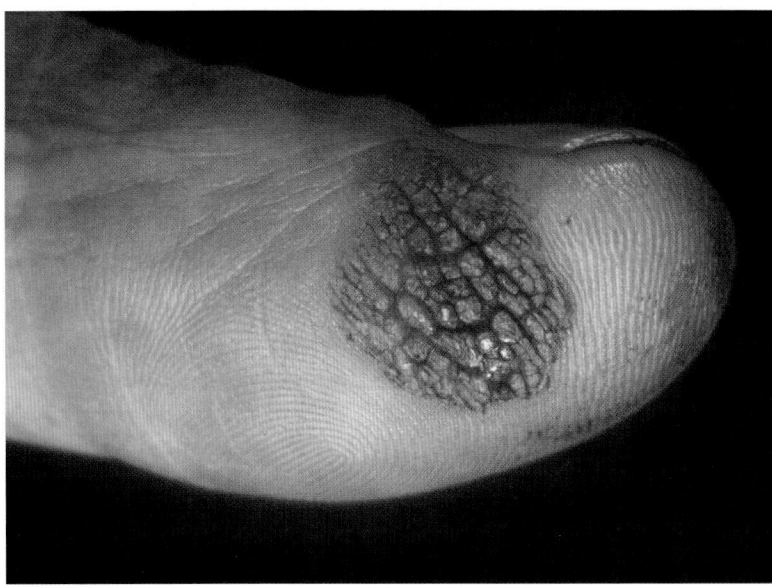

Fig. 24.111
Bowen disease (squamous cell carcinoma in situ): the thumb is an uncommon site of presentation. The hyperpigmentation may result in clinical confusion with a melanocytic lesion. By courtesy of the Institute of Dermatology, London, UK.

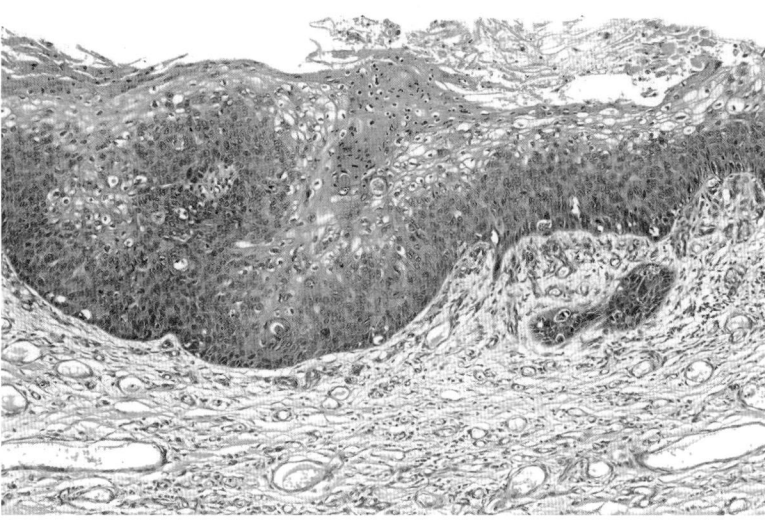

Fig. 24.113
Squamous cell carcinoma in situ: there is full-thickness cytological atypia; in addition, superficial clear cell change is apparent.

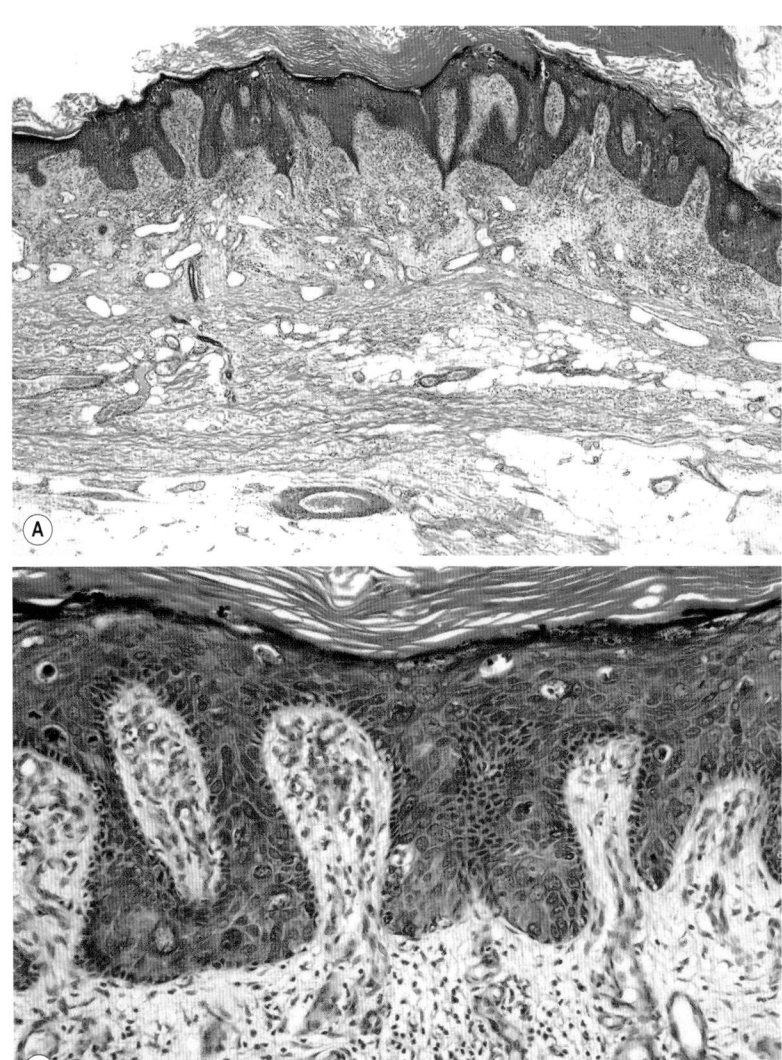

Fig. 24.112
Squamous cell carcinoma in situ: (A) this low-power view shows gross hyperkeratosis with parakeratosis overlying a thickened dysplastic epidermis; (B) note the atypical mitoses.

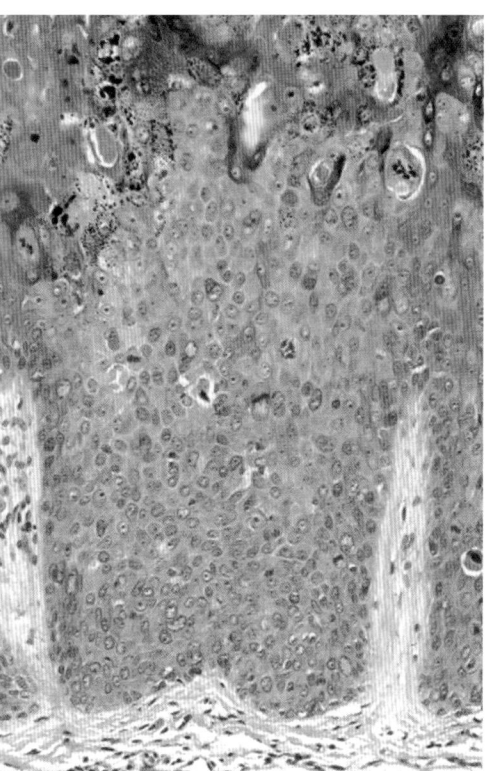

Fig. 24.114
Squamous cell carcinoma in situ: in this example there is complete loss of maturation; suprabasal mitoses are present.

Occasional individually keratinized cells are seen. Koilocytosis is commonly evident in genital lesions. Frequent mitoses, including abnormal forms, may be seen in abundance in all layers of the epidermis. Acantholytic variants and foci of epidermolytic hyperkeratosis are very occasionally encountered (*Figs 24.117 and 24.118*). In some lesions, particularly those affecting the genital mucosae, the lack of maturation combined with epithelial disorganization are the predominant features, with cellular atypia being relatively inconspicuous – so-called basaloid variant of vulvar intraepithelial neoplasia.[107] The tumor cells are:
- pankeratin positive, variably EMA positive,
- CAM 5.2, CEA, S100 protein and HMB-45 negative.

The dermis is infiltrated by numerous chronic inflammatory cells including lymphocytes, histiocytes, and plasma cells. Sometimes the infiltrate adopts a lichenoid distribution and is associated with basal cell hydropic degeneration and apoptosis, thereby simulating a lichenoid keratosis. The infiltrate is composed mainly of T lymphocytes, with the T-helper subset

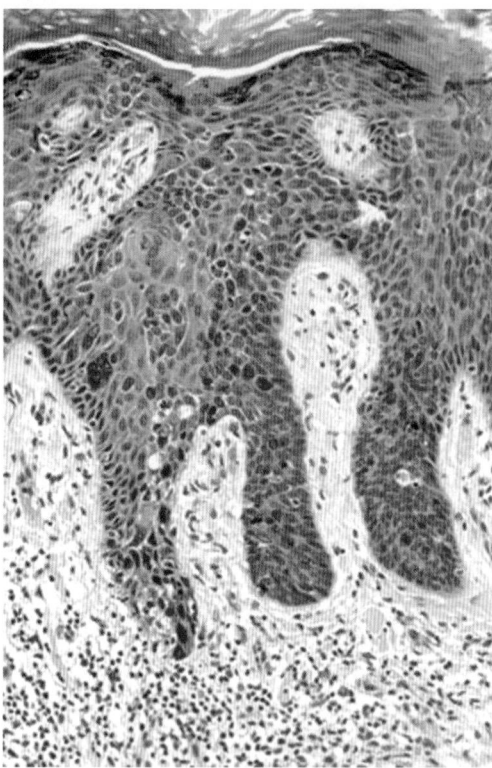

Fig. 24.115
Squamous cell carcinoma in situ: in this example there is marked nuclear pleomorphism.

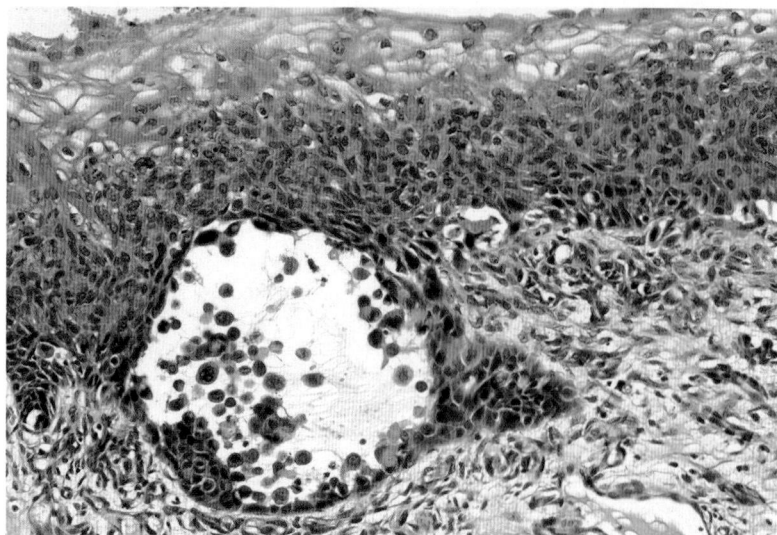

Fig. 24.117
Acantholytic squamous cell carcinoma in situ: there is marked acantholysis. This is a not uncommon finding and has no prognostic significance.

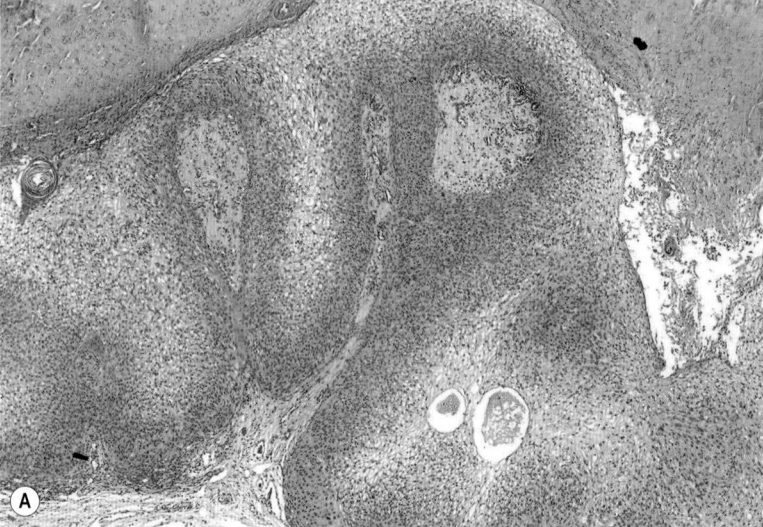

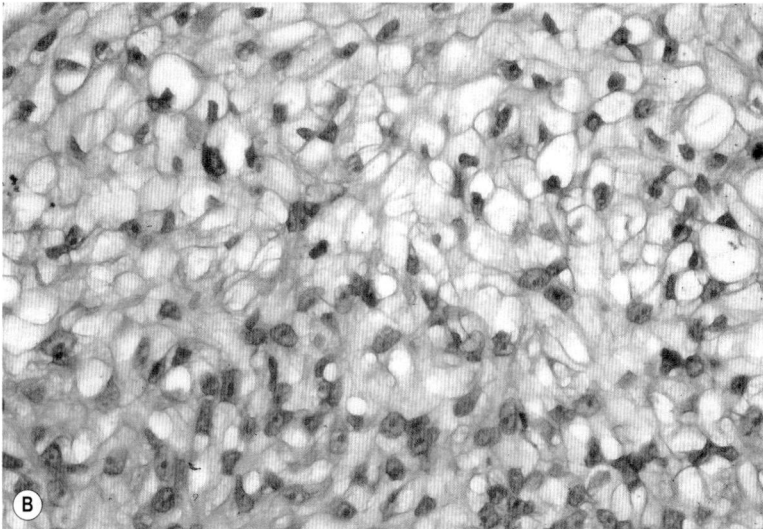

Fig. 24.116
(**A**, **B**) Clear cell squamous cell carcinoma in situ: there is very marked cytoplasmic vacuolation affecting the upper layers of the epithelium.

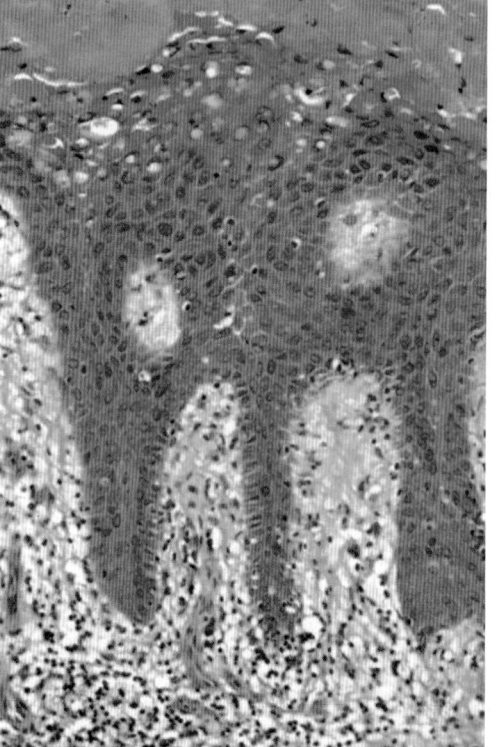

Fig. 24.118
Epidermolytic squamous cell carcinoma in situ: there is superficial cytoplasmic vacuolation with eosinophilic globular keratin aggregates. These features are of no clinical importance.

predominating.[108] Occasionally, vascular proliferation in the superficial dermis is conspicuous.[107]

Bowen disease may show a variety of morphological subtypes. Psoriasiform, atrophic, verrucous hyperkeratotic, papillated, and irregular variants have been delineated.[107]

- The psoriasiform lesion shows parakeratosis and regular, marked acanthosis with broad and sometimes fused epidermal ridges.
- The atrophic type is similar to the atrophic actinic keratosis, except that the atypia and lack of maturation is full thickness and involves the intraepidermal adnexal structures.
- Verrucous hyperkeratotic bowenoid plaques are highly irregular and often show hyperkeratosis and church-spire papillomatosis in addition to characteristic pit-like invaginations.[107]
- The papillated variant is sharply demarcated, showing a verrucous and papillomatous exo- and endophytic growth pattern. There is

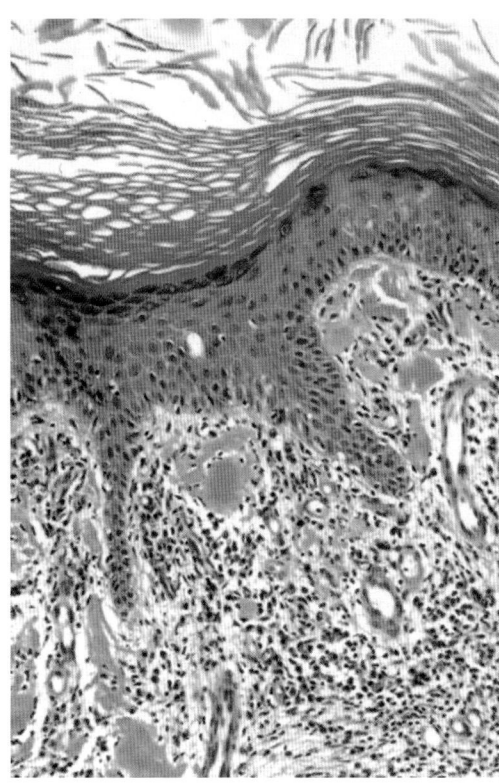

Fig. 24.119
Squamous cell carcinoma in situ: dense eosinophilic deposits of amyloid are present in the dermis of the perilesional skin.

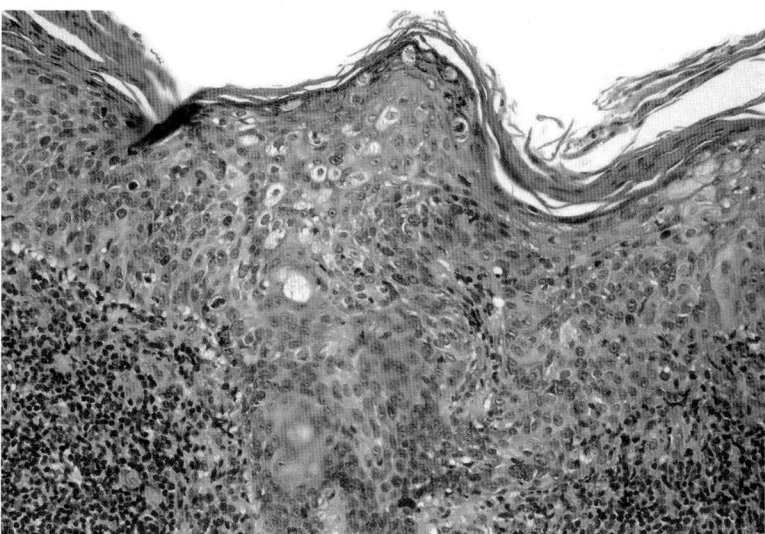

Fig. 24.120
Pagetoid squamous cell carcinoma in situ: within the thickened epidermis are small, discrete nests of pale cells. Special stains for epithelial mucin and immunohistochemistry for S100 protein, CEA, and CAM 5.2 were negative. Pankeratin was positive.

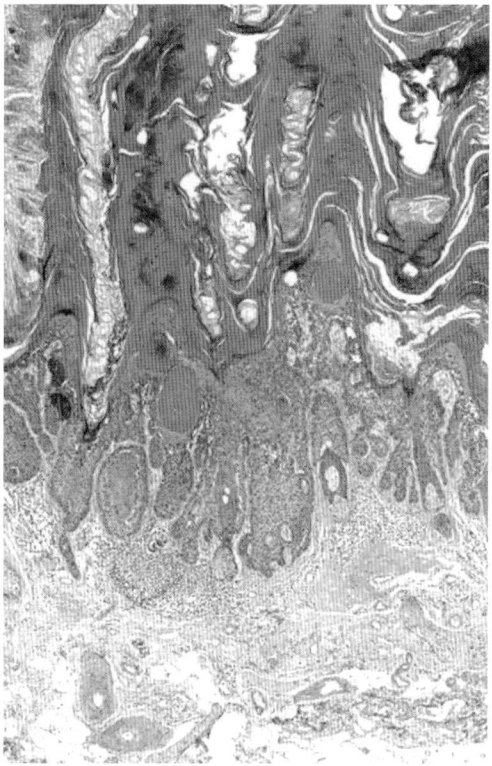

Fig. 24.121
Squamous cell carcinoma in situ: this patient presented with a keratin horn.

full-thickness epidermal dysplasia with prominent koilocytic change. Despite the cytological characteristics, HPV was not demonstrable by routine methods.[109]

- The irregular variant, which is commonly highly pleomorphic, shows variable acanthosis, often in the absence of either hyperkeratosis or parakeratosis.

Not surprisingly, many plaques of Bowen disease show an admixture of these histologic variants. It is unlikely that this subclassification serves any useful purpose other than recognition of the full histologic spectrum of this disease.

Squamous cell carcinoma in situ has also been described in association with stromal amyloid deposition and mucinous or sebaceous metaplasia (Fig. 24.119).[110,111] Rarely, it may be seen in the epidermis overlying or adjacent to a cutaneous neuroendocrine carcinoma.[112]

Occasionally, the lesions are characterized by a tendency to intraepithelial nesting, one variant of the so-called Borst-Jadassohn intraepidermal epithelioma.[113] This feature, combined with cytoplasmic pallor, may result in histologic confusion with cutaneous and mucosal Paget disease (Fig. 24.120). Bowenoid features may also be seen in radiation and arsenical keratoses and occasionally at the base of a keratin horn (Fig. 24.121). Bowenoid actinic keratosis may be histologically indistinguishable from Bowen disease. It is doubtful whether there is any value in trying to differentiate between the two.

Differential diagnosis

Bowen disease may rarely be confused with Paget disease (both mammary and extramammary variants) and, occasionally, with superficial spreading melanoma.[114-117] Immunohistochemistry and special stains for mucin should resolve any diagnostic difficulties in the majority of cases.

Before accepting a diagnosis of anogenital Bowen disease, it is essential that the patient be carefully questioned about previous therapeutic measures. The treatment of condyloma acuminatum by podophyllin may result in the development of bowenoid histology, an unfortunate catch for the unwary. Conspicuous cells in metaphase are a clue to podophyllin therapy. Distinction from seborrheic keratosis showing atypia depends upon the recognition of the pre-existent benign element. It is always advisable to assess multiple areas from a plaque of Bowen disease to exclude any evidence of invasion.

PUVA keratosis

Clinical features

PUVA phototherapy is associated with an increased risk of nonmelanoma skin cancer, especially squamous cell carcinoma.[1,2] Follow-up studies of patients receiving PUVA therapy have also revealed development of multiple keratoses presenting at non–sun-exposed skin, predominantly trunk and thigh, after prolonged PUVA exposure (Fig. 24.122). Clinically, these lesions present as warty hyperkeratotic and scaly papules with a broad base measuring several millimeters up to 1 cm.[3,4] Although it is unclear whether such keratoses represent a significant precursor lesion, their presence indicates a higher risk for the development of nonmelanoma skin cancer at other sites.[3]

Recently, a pattern of keratoses has been described involving the lateral aspects of hands and feet.[5]

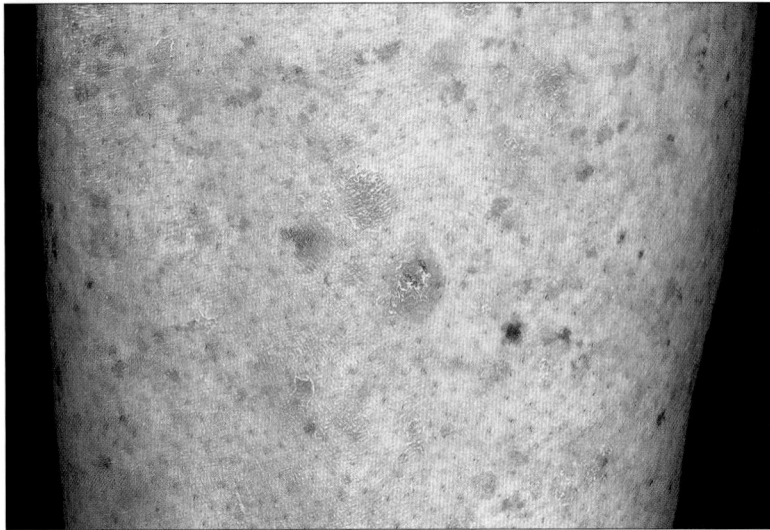

Fig. 24.122
PUVA keratosis: there are numerous small scaly lesions. Many lentigines are also present. By courtesy of C.M. Proby, MD, the Institute of Dermatology, London, UK.

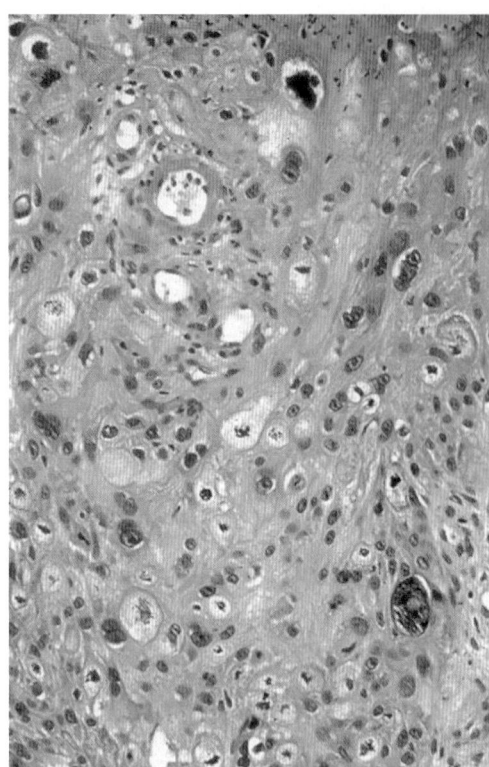

Fig. 24.124
Arsenical keratosis: in this example, there is marked nuclear pleomorphism and mitoses are numerous.

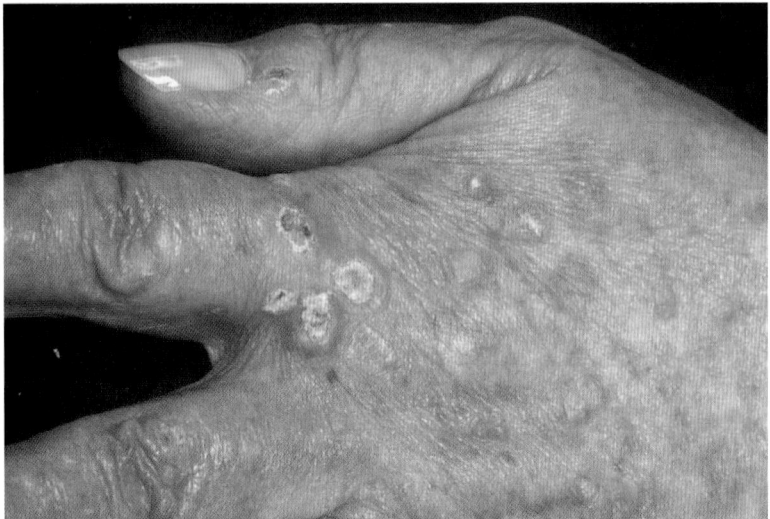

Fig. 24.123
Arsenical keratosis: multiple scaly lesions are present. By courtesy of the Institute of Dermatology, London, UK.

Histologic features

The majority of PUVA keratoses are associated with mutations in *TP53* and *HRAS*, which are predominantly of the ultraviolet signature type.[6]

PUVA keratoses are characterized histologically by acanthosis, papillomatosis, hyperkeratosis, and focal parakeratosis.[3,4] Nuclear atypia is observed in about 50% but is usually only mild. The lesions are typically well circumscribed.

Arsenical keratoses

Clinical features

Arsenical keratoses are multiple horny lesions on the extremities, particularly the palms and soles (*Fig. 24.123*).[1–4] Exposure to arsenic may be occupational, therapeutic, dietary or even as poisoning, and has occurred in patients exposed to ore smelting and refining, insecticides, cattle and sheep dip, contamination of water in places such as Bangladesh, and various medications.[3–13] Patients may also have generalized pigmentation, characteristic 'rain drop' pigmentation predominantly on the trunk, Bowen disease on other sites, multiple basal cell carcinomas, and an increased risk of

internal malignancy.[6,7] An increased incidence of Dupuytren contracture has been described.[14] Neuroendocrine carcinoma has also been documented in a patient with chronic arsenic poisoning, although whether this is coincidental is uncertain.[15]

Histologic features

The histologic features vary from areas of hyperkeratosis and acanthosis through to dysplastic lesions and squamous carcinoma in situ (*Fig. 24.124*). Some cases are characterized by striking vacuolation of the epithelial cells, and keratin horn formation is an occasional feature.

Squamous cell carcinoma

Clinical features

Squamous cell carcinoma of the skin is the second commonest cutaneous malignancy (basal cell carcinoma being the most frequent).[1,2] The majority develop as a consequence of exposure to excessive UVB and therefore occur mainly on sun-exposed surfaces of the body, especially the face, neck, arms, and hands (*Fig. 24.125*). Concomitant actinic keratoses are often evident and the majority of squamous cell carcinomas arise in actinic keratoses.[3,4]

Cutaneous squamous cell carcinoma is more common in men than in women, in older age groups, and in those with fair skin and light hair. It is rare in children and adolescents and is then mainly associated with other disorders such as xeroderma pigmentosum, epidermolysis bullosa, or pansclerotic morphea of childhood.[5–13] Although the incidence of cutaneous lesions is low in dark-skinned races, cutaneous squamous cell carcinoma is nevertheless the most common skin cancer in African-Americans.[14] Lesions usually arise on non–sun-exposed skin and are commonly associated with a poor prognosis.[15] People who work outdoors or who spend a lot of leisure time in the sun are particularly at risk. Susceptibility is increased in those who burn easily or show a prolonged erythema following sun exposure (skin types I and II).[1,2] In addition, poor tanning, excessive freckling, and a Celtic ancestry are significant risk factors.[1] Familial clustering is also observed.[16] Sites of particular importance include the lips and ears, because in these regions the lesions behave rather more aggressively (*Figs 24.126 and 24.127*).[17–19] Rare sites of involvement include a subungual location, the external auditory canal, and the eyelid.[19–27]

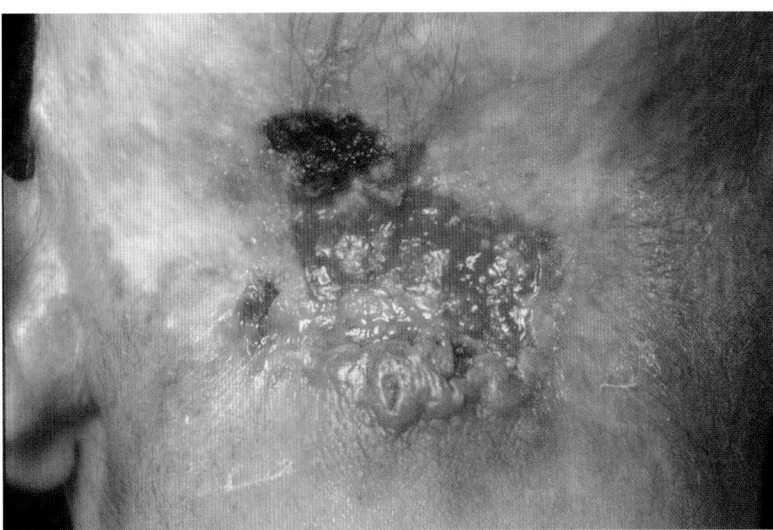

Fig. 24.125
Squamous cell carcinoma: sun-exposed skin is commonly affected, as seen in this large scalp tumor. By courtesy of the Institute of Dermatology, London, UK.

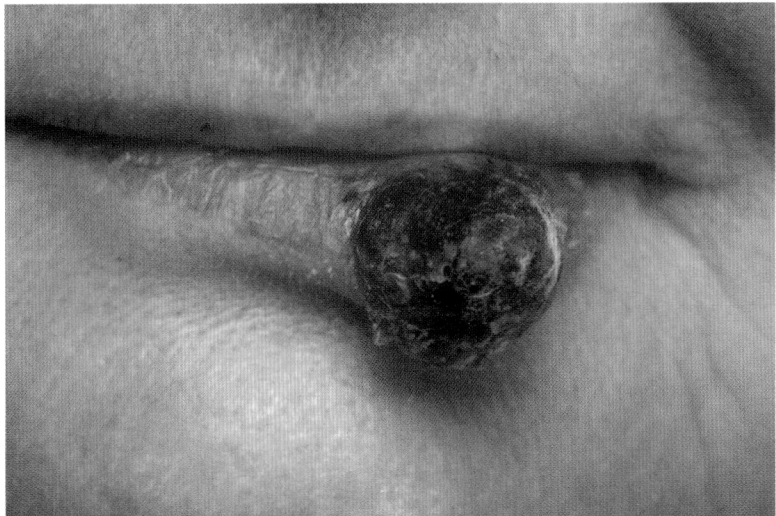

Fig. 24.126
Squamous cell carcinoma: tumors on the lip may be associated with a poor prognosis. By courtesy of the Institute of Dermatology, London, UK.

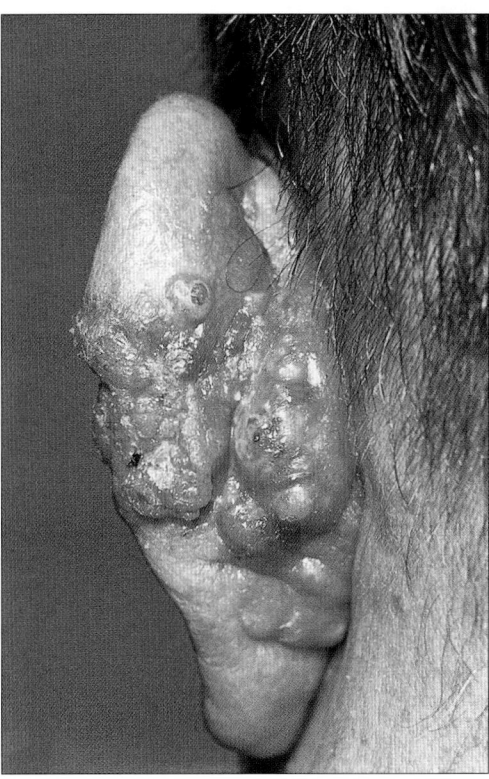

Fig. 24.127
Squamous cell carcinoma: tumors on the ear are often high grade. By courtesy of the Institute of Dermatology, London, UK.

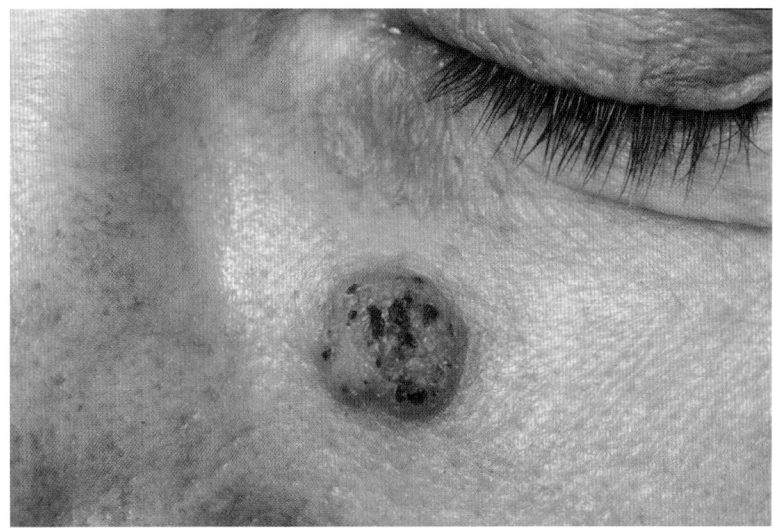

Fig. 24.128
Squamous cell carcinoma: nodular tumor on the cheek. Note the adjacent scarring. By courtesy of the Institute of Dermatology, London, UK.

The reported annual incidence is variable, but appears to be increasing in the United States by more than 250% during the intervals of 1976–1984 and 2000–2010 per a detailed study in Minnesota.[28] The precise incidence is challenging to track in the United States because squamous cell carcinoma of the skin is not tracked in national tumor registries. While basal cell carcinoma has traditionally been more common, in the U.S. Medicare fee-for-service population, basal cell and squamous cell carcinomas are now of roughly equal recorded incidence.[29] Estimates range from 81 to 136 for men and from 26 to 59 for women per 100,000 of the population in the United States[30] to 1,332 (men) and 755 (women) per 100,000 of the population in Townsville, Australia.[31,32] Overall, European rates are similar to those in the United States.[33–35] There is considerable evidence to show that the incidence is progressively rising due to increased sun exposure and increased life expectancy, and sun-related skin cancer is now said to be the commonest form of malignancy in developed countries.[30,36,37]

Other important sites of cutaneous squamous cell carcinoma include the perianal region, the external genitalia, and around the nail bed. These all appear to be HPV associated. Periungual lesions are particularly important because they are commonly clinically misdiagnosed as chronic verruca vulgaris or paronychia.[38,39] Although the recurrence rate is high at this site (30% in one series), metastases are very rare.[39]

Most commonly cutaneous squamous cell carcinoma presents as an indurated slow-growing tumor, which is often painless and may be nodular, ulcerated, plaque-like or verrucous (Figs 24.128–24.135). Tumors are rarely pigmented.[40,41]

Squamous cell carcinoma can complicate other lesions and has been described in association with lichen planus, prurigo nodularis, necrobiosis lipoidica, nonbullous ichthyosiform erythroderma, pilonidal sinus, acne conglobata, smallpox vaccination, burn scars, chronic lymphedema, port-wine stain, hidradenitis suppurativa, necrobiosis lipoidica, factitial dermatitis, folliculitis decalvans, chronic osteomyelitis, lupus vulgaris, leprosy, cutaneous leishmaniasis, epidermal nevi, nevus sebaceous, pityriasis rubra pilaris, discoid lupus erythematosus, generalized vitiligo, porokeratosis, porokeratotic eccrine ostial and dermal duct nevus, Rothmund-Thomson syndrome, Hailey-Hailey disease, skin flap, Netherton syndrome, a psoriatic nail bed, epidermoid cysts, eccrine syringofibroadenoma, tattoos, and venous ulcers.[42–88] Squamous cell carcinoma may also coexist with invasive melanoma and lentigo maligna.[89–91]

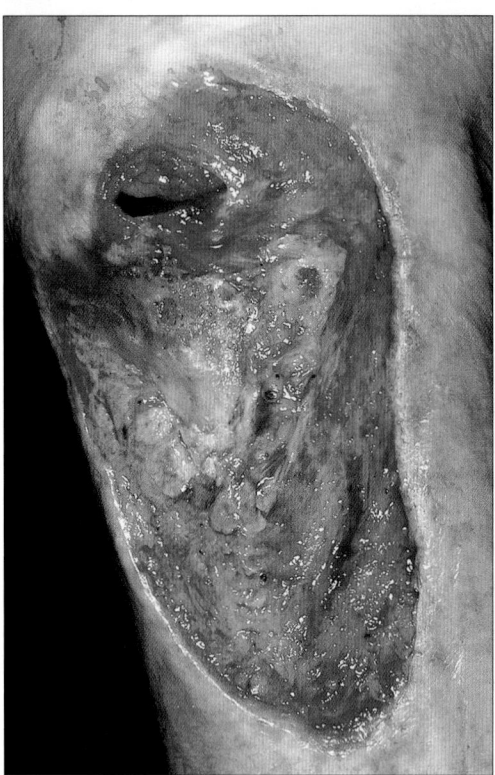

Fig. 24.129
Squamous cell carcinoma: this longstanding ulcer showed histological evidence of squamous cell carcinoma. By courtesy of R.A. Marsden, MD, St George's Hospital, London, UK.

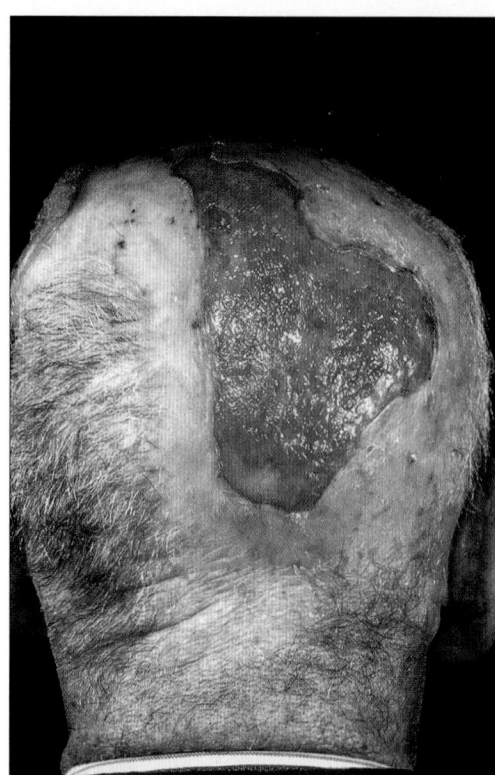

Fig. 24.131
Squamous cell carcinoma: this ulcerated tumor complicated previous radiotherapy for an unknown scalp dermatosis. By courtesy of the Institute of Dermatology, London, UK.

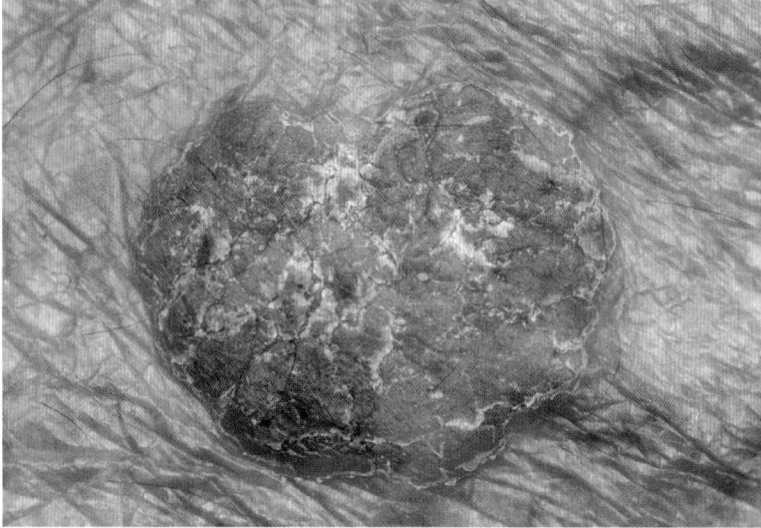

Fig. 24.130
Squamous cell carcinoma: scaly nodular tumor arising on the skin of the back of the hand. By courtesy of the Institute of Dermatology, London, UK.

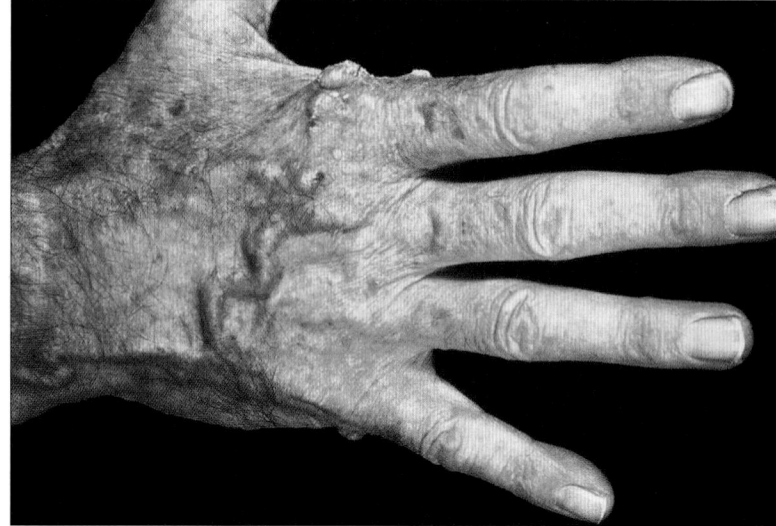

Fig. 24.132
Renal transplantation-associated neoplasia: widespread keratoses are evident in this patient. By courtesy of M. Glover, MD, Royal London Hospital Trust, London, UK.

The recurrence and metastasis rates quoted in the literature are very variable.[1] Metastatic rates appear to be increasing along with the incidence of primary disease.[92] In a meta-analyses combining results from major documented series, the overall recurrence rate was 3.7–10% depending upon the form of treatment.[93,94] However, important regional variation was identified, with tumors of the lip and ear faring particularly badly with recurrence rates of 10.5% and 18.7%, respectively. Although the overall 5-year metastasis rate was 5.2%, tumors of the ear and lip again had a much poorer prognosis with respective metastasis rates of 11% and 13.7%. Other factors associated with an increased risk of recurrence and metastasis included tumors larger than 2 cm in diameter or 0.4 cm thick, neurotropism, immunosuppression, and recurrent lesions.[93] Poorly differentiated tumors generally have a poorer prognosis, but many well-differentiated tumors may be associated with metastatic spread.

The etiology of the lesion is also of some prognostic importance. Squamous cell carcinomas developing as a consequence of burns, radiation, and scarring or complicating chronic ulceration are high-risk tumors, which commonly metastasize (18–40%).[94-96] In addition to regional lymph nodes, the liver, lungs, bones, and brain are most often affected.[1] Despite a marked increase in incidence over the past decades, the overall mortality has been steadily declining, presumably as a consequence of earlier recognition and improved treatment.[97] Squamous cell carcinomas of the penis, scrotum, and anus are also associated with a high risk of metastases.[98,99] Over 25% of patients with scrotal tumors have inguinal node involvement at presentation.[100,101]

Pathogenesis and histologic features

The etiology of squamous carcinoma is multifactorial and is summarized in *Table 24.1*. Chronic actinic damage is the most important factor, particularly in pale-skinned races. UVB is of greatest significance, since most UVC is filtered out by the ozone layer. The likelihood of an individual developing

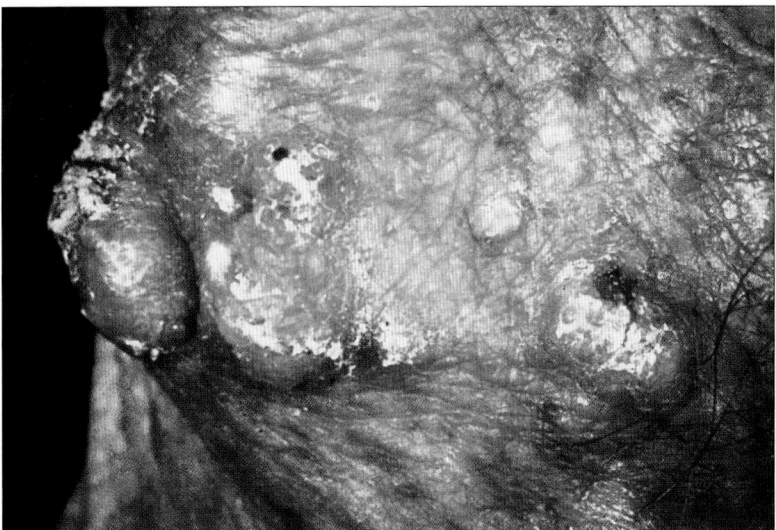

Fig. 24.133
Renal transplantation-associated neoplasia: several squamous cell carcinomas are evident in addition to numerous keratoses. By courtesy of M. Glover, MD, Royal London Hospital Trust, London, UK.

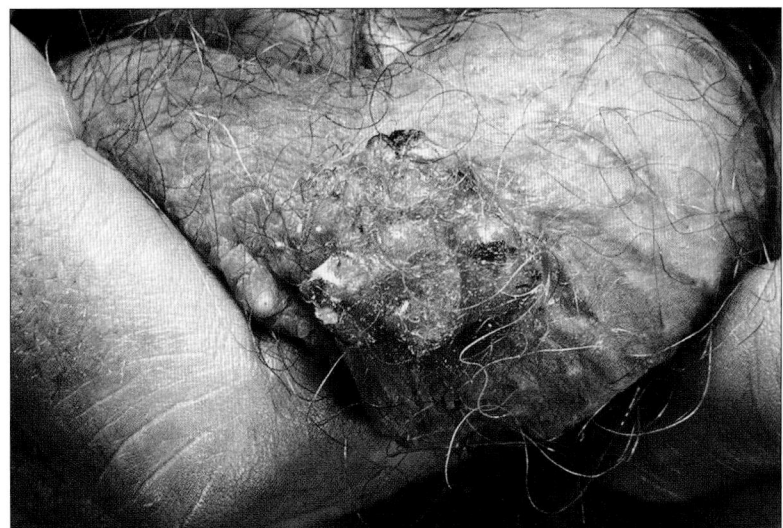

Fig. 24.134
Scrotal squamous cell carcinoma: tumors at this site are sometimes seen complicating PUVA therapy and coal tar treatment for psoriasis. By courtesy of the Institute of Dermatology, London, UK.

keratoses or squamous cell carcinoma is particularly related to the cumulative total lifetime exposure to sunlight.[4,90]

Radiation

UVA on its own does not appear to be mutagenic in humans, but when combined with photosensitizers, such as in PUVA therapy, it is associated with a dose-dependent increased risk of both keratoses and invasive squamous carcinoma, which particularly involves the genitalia in males.[102-105] It appears, however, that PUVA-associated tumors usually have a good prognosis with a low rate of metastasis.[98]

UVB is known to induce skin cancer in experimental animals. It has major effects on both DNA repair mechanisms and cell-mediated immunity, and functions as both an initiator and promoter of cutaneous carcinogenesis.[1] UV irradiation is associated with the formation of free radicals and the induction of thymidine dimer photoproducts. The latter are of particular significance in patients with xeroderma pigmentosum in whom excision-repair mechanisms are defective. This autosomal recessive disorder which commonly presents in the first decade is associated with a 1,000-fold increased risk of skin cancer.[11,95] Patients with actinic keratoses have also

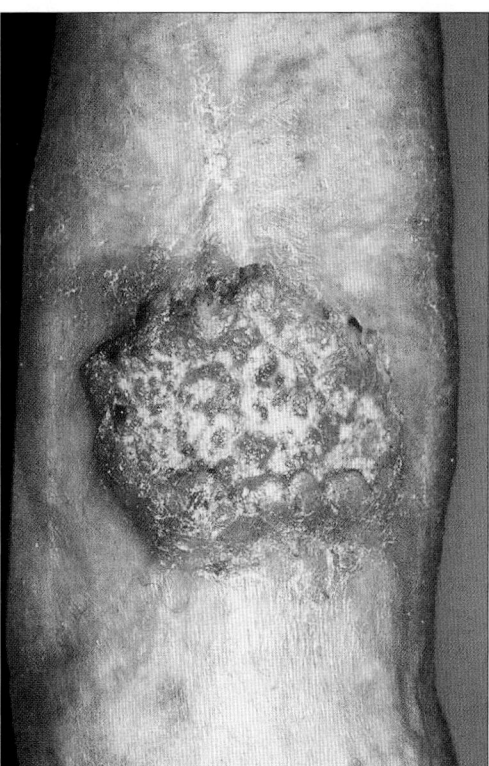

Fig. 24.135
Squamous cell carcinoma: this large ulcerated tumor has arisen at the site of a previous burn (Marjolin ulcer). By courtesy of R.A. Marsden, MD, St George's Hospital, London, UK.

been shown to have slightly diminished levels of unscheduled DNA synthesis, but whether this is of pathogenetic significance is unknown.[106] Oculocutaneous albinism is also characterized by an increased incidence of UVB-induced squamous carcinoma. This is particularly well demonstrated in African albino patients. In a series of 111 people with albinism from the black population of Johannesburg, approximately 23% developed skin tumors, mainly squamous cell carcinoma, particularly of the head.[107]

UVB causes specific distinctive mutations including C–T transitions at dipyrimidine sites and in particular the formation of CC–TT double base changes.[106] These alterations, which constitute a fingerprint for UV damage, are present in the TP53 tumor suppressor gene in human cutaneous squamous cell carcinoma.[108-110] Other consequences of UV irradiation include production of cytosine photohydrates, purine photoproducts, single-strand DNA breaks and (6–4) photoproducts.[106] The latter appear to be of particular significance in UV-induced mutagenesis.[106]

Activation of cellular proto-oncogenes by point mutations, amplifications, and rearrangements induced by UV irradiation are also important in cutaneous neoplastic transformation.[106,111] Cutaneous squamous cell carcinoma carries more mutations than most other malignancies—about 4 times more than melanoma which is itself heavily mutated—with some exomes carrying more than 10 000 mutations.[112] The vast majority of these mutations are not functional for driving pathogenesis.[2,112] Functionally important mutations in a number of oncogenes have been seen in cutaneous squamous cell carcinoma including NOTCH1, PTCH1, TP53, CDKN2A, BRCA2, HRAS, ATM, ERBB4, NF1, TERT promoter and many others with a prevalence of at least 5%.[111-119] This raises the possibility that these oncogenes contribute to the pathogenesis of at least some cutaneous squamous cell carcinomas. Codetection of HPV DNA in a significant proportion of cancers suggests that neoplastic transformation may sometimes develop as a consequence of activation of cellular proto-oncogenes by HPV, but the precise role and relevance is uncertain.[120,121] Apoptosis is a key mechanism in the elimination of genetically damaged cells. Fas (CD95) mediated apoptosis appears to be a crucial pathway for homeostasis of human epidermis.[122] CD95 is upregulated in actinically damaged skin but is significantly decreased in actinic keratoses as well as invasive squamous cell carcinoma resulting in a defective defense mechanism against genetically damaged keratinocytes.[123] Furthermore, two tumor suppressor genes involved in the p53 and retinoblastoma pathways, p16^{INK4} and p14^{ARF} (both encoded by CDKN2A), have frequently been found to be inactivated in squamous cell carcinoma.[124-126]

Table 24.1

Etiology of squamous cell carcinoma

Radiation	Genetic syndromes
UVB	Albinism
PUVA	Xeroderma pigmentosum
X-rays	Dystrophic epidermolysis bullosa
Grenz rays	Rothmund-Thomson syndrome
	Epidermodysplasia verruciformis

HPV	
Anogenital – type 16/18	
Periungual – type 16/18	
Verrucous carcinoma	
Epidermodysplasia verruciformis type 5	

Immunosuppression	
Iatrogenic	
Solid organ transplantation	
HIV	
Systemic disease (e.g., rheumatoid arthritis)	
Malignancy (e.g., lymphoproliferative disorders)	

Chemical carcinogen	
Arsenic	
Hydrocarbons	

Chronic inflammation	
Burns	
Chronic osteomyelitis	
Varicose ulcers	
Lichen planus	
Discoid lupus erythematosus	
Hidradenitis suppurativa	
Acne conglobata	
Oral/hypertrophic lichen planus	
Lichen sclerosus	
Erythema ab igne	

Chronic infection	
Lupus vulgaris	
Leprosy	
Cutaneous syphilis	
Lymphogranuloma venereum	
Granuloma inguinale	

This oversimplified diagram emphasizes the early pathogenetic steps in the development of squamous cell carcinoma and their convergence on the retinoblastoma (Rb) and p53 gene pathways. Ultraviolet (UV) light damage directly results in UV-signature mutations of the *TP53* gene leading to inhibition of cell cycle control and apoptosis. The p53 pathway is also compromised through altered p14ARF gene signaling either directly due to mutations in the p14ARF gene itself or indirectly through UV-related mutations in the ras gene. Mutations in the p16INK4a gene lead to increased phosphorylation of the Rb gene through interactions between cyclin dependent kinase 4 (CDK4) and cyclin D1 with subsequent cellular proliferation. Viral oncoproteins exert their effects through functional inactivation of the p53 and Rb gene alike. (Adapted from Tsai K and Tsao H (2004) *Am J Med Genet C*, 131C, 82–92.)

HPV, human papillomavirus; PUVA, psoralen plus UV light of A wavelength; UVB, ultraviolet light of B wavelength.

Tumor invasion is a complex process and involves degradation of the basement membrane and tumor cell migration. This process is mediated in part by the action of matrix metalloproteinase (MMP) produced by tumor as well as stromal cells. In squamous cell carcinoma, matrilysin (MMP-7) and stromelysin-1 (MMP-3) are expressed by tumor as well as stromal cells at the stromal interface but are not detected in normal epidermis.[127,128]

Ionizing radiation is associated with a variety of genetic abnormalities including point mutations, chromosomal aberrations, DNA strand breaks, deletions, and gene rearrangements.[129] Although less common nowadays, skin cancer complicating the therapeutic use of X-rays occasionally developed in staff as a consequence of occupational exposure and in patients following its use for a variety of conditions including dermatitis, acne, tinea capitis, and skin tumors.[95,130]

Nonmelanoma skin cancer, both squamous and basal cell, may rarely follow the therapeutic use of grenz rays.[131]

Abnormalities of cell-mediated immunity, which develop as a consequence of UV radiation, are likely to be of pathogenetic significance. Alterations including diminished numbers of circulating T cells, reduced T-helper/suppressor ratios and impaired delayed hypersensitivity reactions have been documented.[98,132] A fundamental effect is loss of epidermal dendritic Langerhans cells and their replacement by a CD1–, DR+ population of antigen-presenting cells, which preferentially activate T-suppressor cells.[133] The effect of this appears to be the development of a state of tolerance to UV-induced neoantigens and the subsequent promotion of epidermal neoplasms. Similarly, UVB-irradiated mice show reduced contact

hypersensitivity reactions, diminished numbers of Langerhans cells, and a T-suppressor cell-mediated inability to reject syngeneic transplanted cutaneous tumors.[134]

Epidermodysplasia verruciformis is associated with impaired cell-mediated immunity and an increased risk of cutaneous neoplasia. Squamous carcinoma develops in up to 30% of patients, typically on sun-exposed skin.[135,136] The face is particularly affected and tumors commonly present in the third and fourth decades.[98] Squamous carcinoma is an important cause of mortality; in a series of patients with advanced tumors, over 50% proved fatal.

Immunosuppressive agents

An integral component of transplantation therapy is a long-term requirement for immunosuppressive agents. Patients have an increased risk of a variety of cutaneous complications, including bacterial, fungal, and viral infections such as those due to tinea versicolor, onychomycosis, dermatophytosis, candidiasis, herpes simplex, and HPV.[137] Persistent viral warts are very common and are often present in large numbers.[138,139] There is an increased incidence of a variety of neoplasms including systemic lymphoma and Kaposi sarcoma. In addition, patients have also been found to be susceptible to a variety of UVB-induced cutaneous tumors including actinic keratosis, squamous cell carcinoma, basal cell carcinoma, keratoacanthoma, melanoma, and occasionally epidermodysplasia verruciformis-like lesions.[138–145] The incidence of these tumors is variable, but with sufficient follow up may occur in as many as 50% of transplanted patients.[145,146] Although some associations may be fortuitous, the risk of developing actinic keratoses, keratoacanthoma, and squamous cell carcinoma is a very real and serious problem. Estimations of the risk factor for immunosuppressed renal transplant patients developing keratinocyte-derived neoplasms range from 4 to 20 times the incidence in the normal population.[138] In general, the tumors develop at a much earlier age compared to those in normal, nonimmunosuppressed individuals.[147] In the past the implicated immunosuppressive therapy included prednisolone and azathioprine; more recently ciclosporin has also been incriminated.[148-150]

The presence of a polymorphism in the methylenetetrahydrofolate reductase gene (*MTHFR* C677T) has been associated with a significantly increased risk for the development of squamous cell carcinoma in renal transplant recipients, thereby implicating folate-sensitive pathways in the pathogenesis of squamous cell carcinoma in the immunosuppressed state.[151] Furthermore, increased telomere length has also been associated with increased risk for squamous cell carcinoma in this patient population.[152,153]

The tumors, which are commonly multiple, develop on sun-exposed skin, but correlation with skin type is poor.[144,145,147] The usual ratio of basal cell:squamous cell carcinoma of up to 4:1 is reversed as is their distribution, with a greater proportion of lesions presenting on the hands and forearms compared with the usual propensity for the face.[95,154] However, their incidence shows a positive correlation with diminishing latitude, being highest in Australia and New Zealand.[145] The presence of tumors has been shown to be directly related to the duration and level of immunosuppressive chemotherapy.[137,138,155,156] HPV infection can also drive tumors in this setting.[157]

Behavior of these tumors is variable: some authors relate a somewhat nonaggressive pattern, while others (including more recent studies) describe a more aggressive behavior with significant incidence of metastasis and even fatal outcome.[145,158-161] The behavior appears to be worse in patients with increased sun exposure early in life.[162] Patients from the Australian continent appear to fare worst. HLA compatibility also seems to be important, the prevalence being particularly high in recipients of HLA-B mismatched transplants.[155] It has also been shown that the absence of HLA-A11 and presence of HLA-DR homozygosity in the recipient also correlate with the development of skin cancer. Immunosuppressed female patients have an increased risk of cervical intraepithelial neoplasia.[143]

The incidence of cutaneous squamous cell carcinoma also appears to be increased in nontransplant patients receiving immunosuppressive therapy (e.g., for rheumatoid arthritis)[163,164] and in patients with immunosuppression associated with systemic lymphoma,[165] and chronic or acute myelogenous leukemia.[166-168] Tumors in this latter group are high grade with aggressive clinical behavior and poor outlook. Squamous cell carcinomas developing in HIV-infected patients present at an earlier age and behave in a more aggressive fashion.[169,170]

Human papillomavirus

There is now considerable evidence to suggest an etiological role for HPV in anogenital squamous carcinoma and its precursor lesions.[171,172] The relationship with cutaneous lesions is, however, less well defined.[173] Transfection with HPV is associated with transformation of both human fibroblasts and keratinocytes and both episomal and integrated viral DNA have been identified in mucosal and occasionally cutaneous tumors.[171,174] HPV 16 has been detected in many cases of both Bowen disease and invasive squamous carcinoma of the vulva, penis, and perianal region.[175-178] In addition, HPV 18 may sometimes be identified.[179] HPV 16 as well as HPV 73 and HPV 26 also often appear to be present in periungual Bowen disease and in invasive carcinoma, suggesting possible venereal transmission.[120,174,177,180-183] These patients frequently have genital lesions containing the same HPV type. HPV-related digital lesions are characterized by a higher recurrence but not metastatic rate compared to ordinary squamous cell carcinomas.[184-186] Not uncommonly, several subtypes are demonstrable in any one tumor.[120] There is a proposed link with human beta-papillomavirus species 2 and the development of squamous cell carcinoma on sun-exposed skin.[187-189] HPV DNA sequences, particularly HPV 5, are regularly detected in in situ and invasive carcinomas in patients with epidermodysplasia verruciformis.[189,190] The observation that black patients with epidermodysplasia verruciformis seldom develop squamous carcinoma suggests that UVB may be an important cocarcinogen.[95] HPV DNA has also been reported in tumors arising in immunosuppressed patients following organ transplantation.[120,157,191-194]

However, conflicting results using the polymerase chain reaction (PCR) have been reported.[145,195] Inactivation of tumor suppressor genes by HPV has also been implicated in the development of squamous carcinoma. The E6/E7 oncoproteins of HPV 16 and 18 bind both TP53 and RB1 proteins, which may render them nonfunctional.[173]

The role of HPV in sunlight-induced malignancies is uncertain.[196] Some authors have found an almost complete absence of HPV DNA sequences while others have detected HPV 16 in up to 60% of tumors.[173,197]

Chemical carcinogens

Chemical carcinogens are important in a small number of cases. In addition to arsenic (present in some insecticides, medications, and occasionally contaminating natural water supplies), a wide range of substances, especially hydrocarbons, have been incriminated.[1,198-200] Hydrocarbons are now derived predominantly from combustion and distillation of carbon-containing compounds, and are particularly found in the coal and petroleum industries.[95] They are present in a wide range of products, including coal tar, pitch, paraffin oil, fuel oil, and creosote.[95]

In the past, chemical carcinogens were of particular importance in the pathogenesis of scrotal cancer. In addition to contamination from chimney soot (Pott cancer), there were many at-risk occupations including tar workers, paraffin and shale oil workers, machine operators in engineering and screw making, and cotton mule spinners.[100,201] Nowadays, scrotal cancer seems to be particularly related to past arsenic or coal tar therapy for psoriasis and HPV infection.[100] Treatment with PUVA has already been mentioned.

Chronic inflammation and chronic infection

Tumors complicating chronic infective and inflammatory (particularly scarring) conditions are now rare in developed countries.[202] In developing countries, however, postinfective tumors are still important: in a series from Thailand, it has been estimated that among patients with severe leprosy there is an approximately 1% incidence of squamous carcinoma, commonly affecting the foot.[203] Postburn lesions, so-called Marjolin ulcer, which usually develop after a very long delay period (sometimes spanning decades), commonly recur and metastasize, despite being histologically well differentiated.[204-207] They have a very high mortality: in one series of patients, 60% developed metastases and all died within 2 years of primary treatment.[208] Interestingly, squamous carcinoma developing in a background of dense scarring in patients with recessive dystrophic epidermolysis bullosa is also generally well differentiated and similarly has a high morbidity and mortality – in fact, metastatic disease is the leading cause of death in the majority of patients with severe involvement.[10,12,96,209-215] Less commonly, squamous carcinoma has been reported in patients with junctional and generalized atrophic benign epidermolysis bullosa or epidermolysis bullosa acquisita.[12,216,217]

Association with BRAF inhibitors

Squamous proliferations associated with the use of BRAF inhibitors in the treatment of melanoma have been noted.[218-221] These range from warty proliferations to actinic keratoses to invasive squamous cell carcinomas.[222] These are often driven by paradoxical activation of the ERK pathway; activating mutations in *RAS*, mainly *HRAS*, are also frequently encountered.[223,224] Viral involvement by HPV may play a role as well.[225] The combination of BRAF and MEK inhibition, common in melanoma treatment, is associated with a reduced incidence of these tumors.[226,227] Regression of the tumors can occur with cessation of BRAF inhibitor treatment or the addition of MEK inhibitor.[228] Some consider at least a subset of these lesions to represent keratoacanthomas.[229,230]

Differentiation of squamous cell carcinoma

Squamous carcinoma is a malignant tumor of keratinocytes and must be distinguished from premalignant lesions such as Bowen disease and actinic keratosis. The tumor often, but not invariably, arises from an epithelium with features of dysplasia and appears as infiltrating sheets and islands of variably differentiated squamous epithelium with a greater or lesser degree of mitotic activity. Differentiation is towards keratinization; it is therefore convenient to classify such tumors into well-differentiated, moderately differentiated, and poorly differentiated variants. Alternatively, the Broders system of classification has been used. This includes four grades of differentiation:

- grade 1 – 75% or more of the lesion is well differentiated,
- grade 2 – 50% or more is well differentiated,
- grade 3 – 25–50% is well differentiated,
- grade 4 – less than 25% is well differentiated.

Although this latter system has often been used in the past, it is unnecessarily complicated and too subjective (particularly the middle two categories) to be of value. It is also important to remember that the tumor should be classified according to its most poorly differentiated region.

- Well-differentiated tumors are characterized by squamous epithelium that frequently shows easily recognizable and often abundant keratinization (*Figs 24.136–24.138*). The epithelium is obviously squamous and intercellular bridges (prickles) are readily apparent. The tumors display minimal pleomorphism and mitotic figures are mainly basally located.
- Moderately differentiated tumors show rather more structural disorganization in which the squamous epithelial derivation is less obvious (*Fig. 24.139*). Nuclear and cytoplasmic pleomorphism is more pronounced and mitotic figures (including abnormal forms) are much more commonly seen. Usually, less keratin formation is evident, often being limited to the formation of keratin 'pearls' (concentric laminated whorls of keratinized squames), horn cysts, and scattered individually keratinized cells.
- In the poorly differentiated variants it may be difficult to establish the true nature of the lesion unless intercellular bridges are identified or small foci of keratinization found (*Fig. 24.140*).

Rarely, the tumor is completely anaplastic and an origin from an overlying dysplastic epidermis may be the only clue to the diagnosis. In such instances, examination of multiple sections of tumor is frequently necessary to elicit the correct diagnosis. The immunohistochemical demonstration of keratin expression is often of value (*Figs 24.141 and 24.142*). The use of antibodies against high-molecular-weight keratin or those with a broad specificity is more likely to be helpful than antibodies against low-molecular-weight filaments (e.g., CAM 5.2), which are often negative.[231] Increased immunohistochemical expression of p53 appears to correlate well with advanced tumor stage, and p53 as well as MIB-1 expression correlates inversely with the degree of tumor differentiation.[232,233] Furthermore, expression of CD44v6 and MMP-1 positively correlate with depth of invasion.[233] The use of antibodies to vimentin as an aid to differential diagnosis is unhelpful because many poorly differentiated squamous carcinomas express this intermediate filament, particularly spindle cell and acantholytic variants.[234] If tissue is available for electron microscopy, the presence of desmosomes and tonofilaments may be sought. Rhabdoid morphology is a rare finding but when present it is assumed to be associated with a more aggressive behavior.[235,236] Similar to melanoma, erythrophagocytosis of tumor cells may be identified in squamous cell carcinoma.[237]

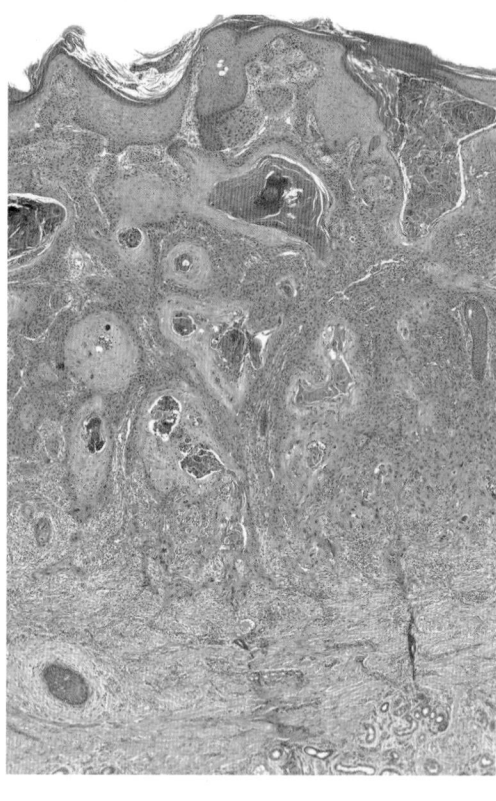

Fig. 24.136
Well-differentiated squamous cell carcinoma: scanning view showing an obviously keratinizing tumor infiltrating deep into the reticular dermis.

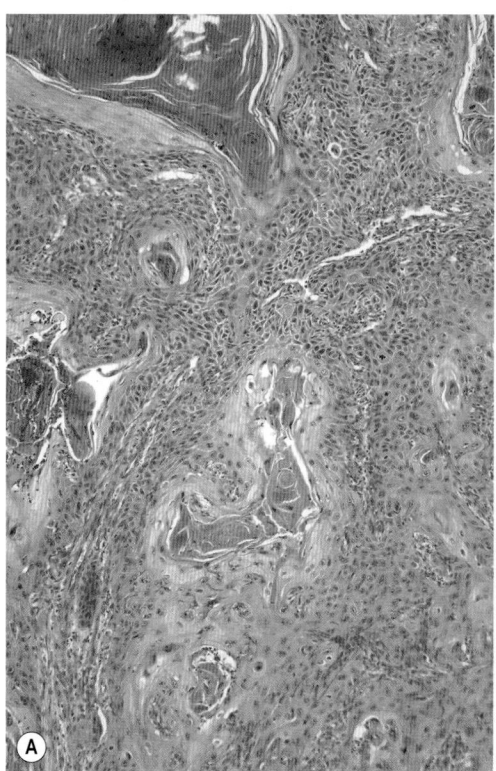
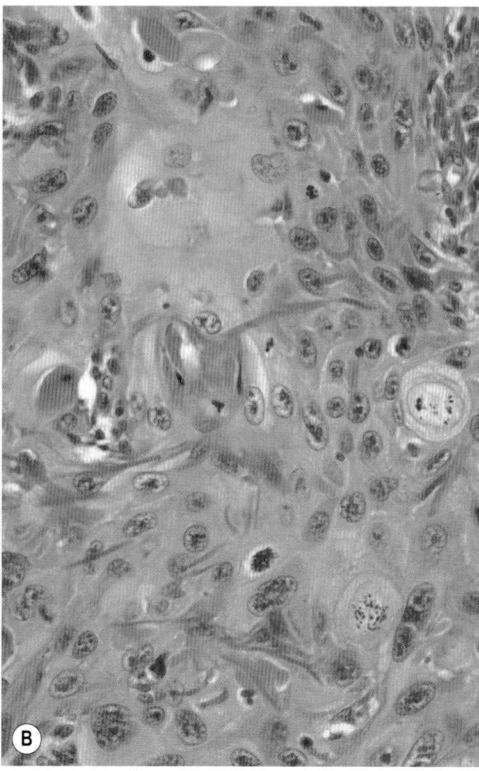

Fig. 24.137
(**A, B**) Well-differentiated squamous cell carcinoma: in addition to marked keratinizing the tumor cells show only mild pleomorphism. Note the mitotic activity.

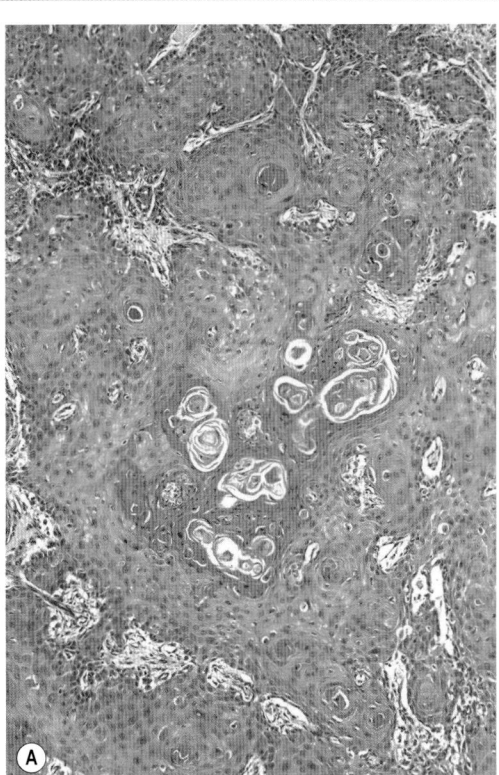
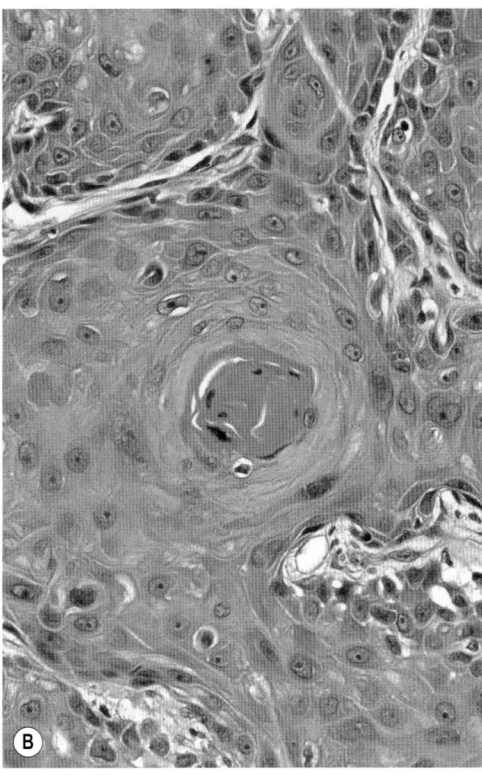

Fig. 24.138
(**A**, **B**) Well-differentiated squamous cell carcinoma: in these variants, the epithelium shows minimal nuclear pleomorphism and mitoses are often sparse. There is conspicuous keratinization.

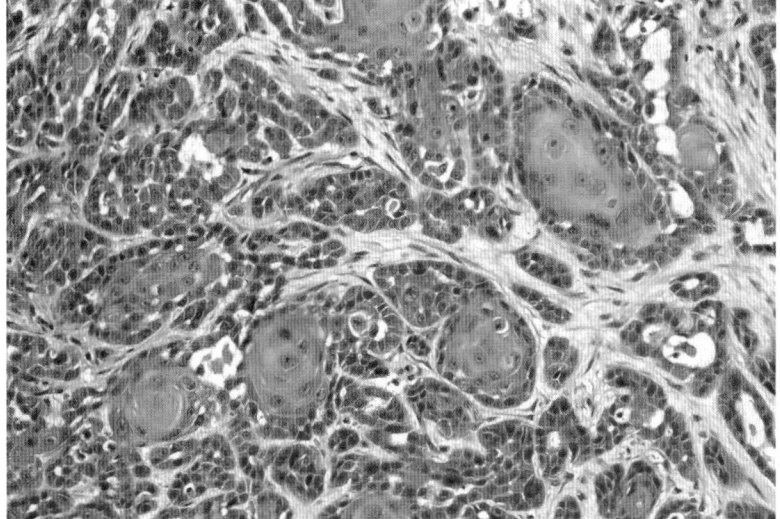

Fig. 24.139
Moderately differentiated squamous cell carcinoma: there is much more obvious pleomorphism. Nevertheless, the squamous nature of the tumors is still readily apparent.

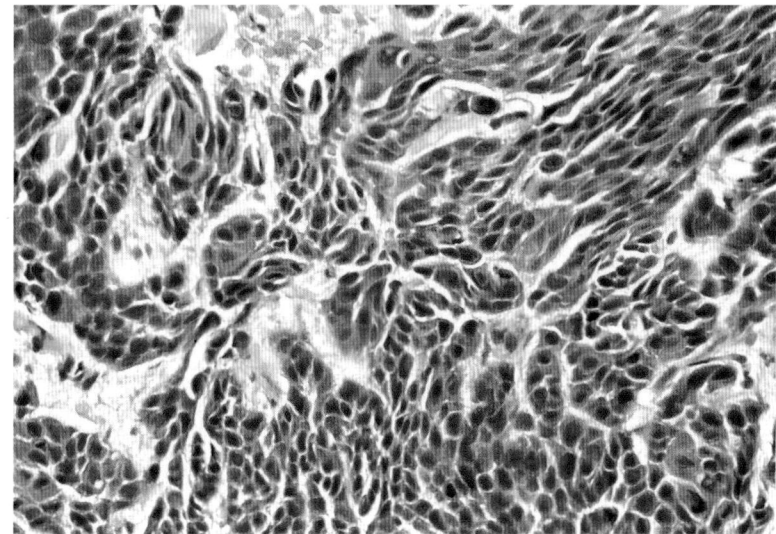

Fig. 24.140
Poorly differentiated squamous cell carcinoma: there is marked nuclear pleomorphism but no keratinization.

It is important to note that a tumor should be graded on the least differentiated element even if this constitutes only a minor component of the neoplasm.

The tumors are often accompanied by a heavy chronic inflammatory cell infiltrate in which T lymphocytes are predominant. Natural killer cells, mast cells, B lymphocytes, plasma cells, macrophages, and Langerhans cells are often present.[98] The infiltrate may resemble a lymphoepithelial lesion but no clonality of either B or T cells has been identified nor is there evidence of Epstein-Barr virus infection. This phenomenon likely represents a local immune response to the tumor.[238] Sometimes eosinophils are conspicuous. The infiltrate, however, is often much less prominent in the more extensive, deeply invasive tumors.[95] The adjacent dermis frequently shows solar elastosis. Rarely, tumors may be accompanied by a histiocytic infiltrate composed of epithelioid histiocytes and osteoclast-like multinucleate giant cells.[239,240]

The giant cells represent multinucleated CD68-positive histiocytes rather than tumor giant cells as seen in sarcomatoid transformation.

A rare variant of squamous cell carcinoma is characterized by exophytic growth, papillary architecture, and a fibrovascular stalk.[241-244] These tumors are typically only superficially invasive and clinical outcome appears to be favorable. No association with HPV has been detected.

In addition to reporting the histologic subtype (see below) and degree of differentiation, a record of tumor maximum diameter and depth of invasion (measured from the granular cell layer of the surface epithelium if present) should be made. Tumors larger than 2 cm in diameter have double the recurrence rate and triple the metastasis rate of tumors less than 2 cm in diameter (15.7% vs. 5.8% and 23.4% vs. 7.6%, respectively).[93,95,245-247] Tumor thickness is also a useful prognostic indicator.[248] No metastasis was identified in tumors with a thickness of less than 2.0 mm as documented

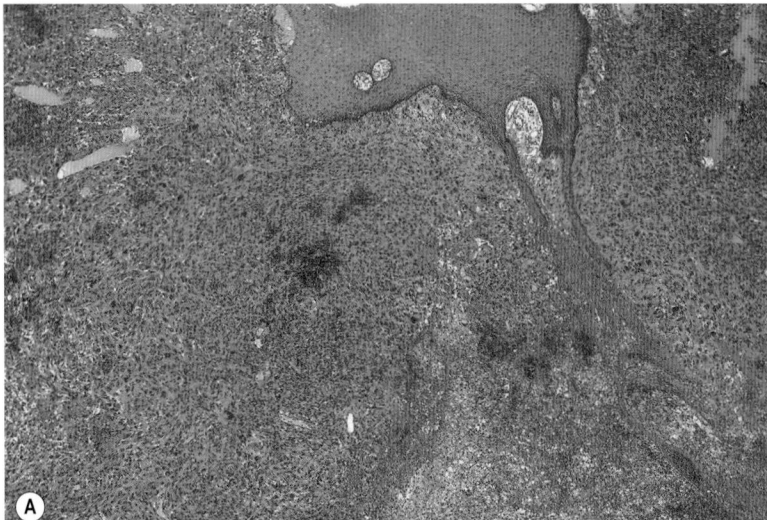

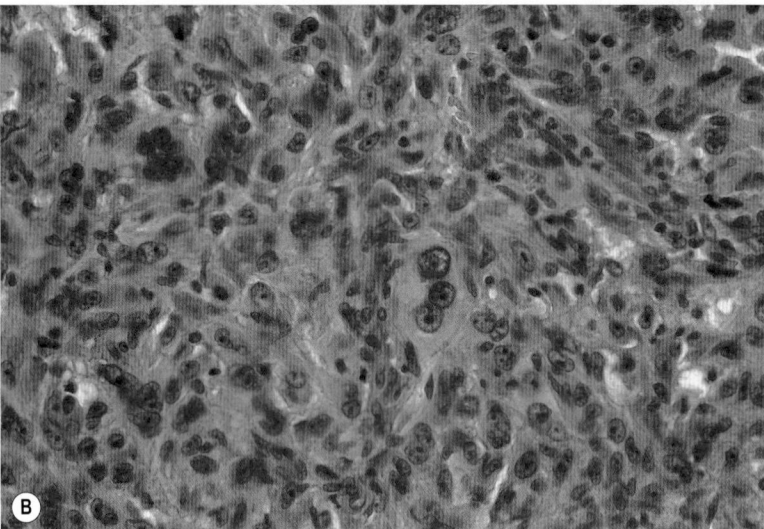

Fig. 24.141
(**A**, **B**) Anaplastic squamous cell carcinoma: this example shows no evidence of keratinization. Diagnosis is ultimately dependent on immunohistochemistry.

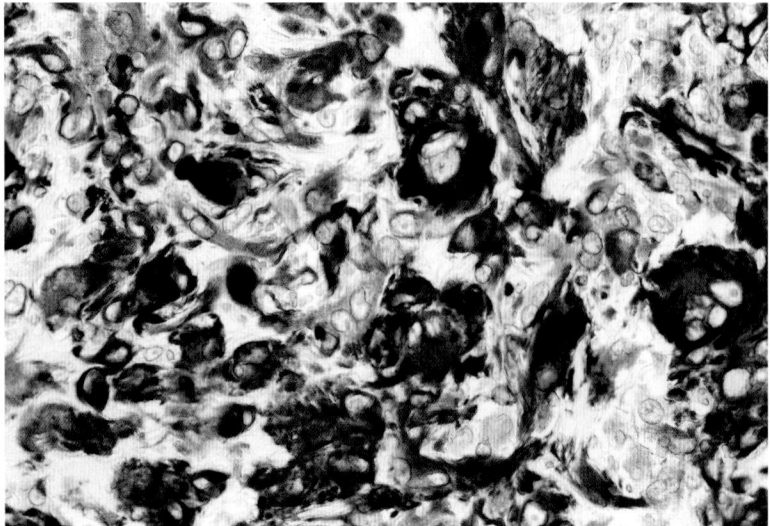

Fig. 24.142
Anaplastic squamous cell carcinoma: the tumor cells show uniform, strong labeling with MNF116.

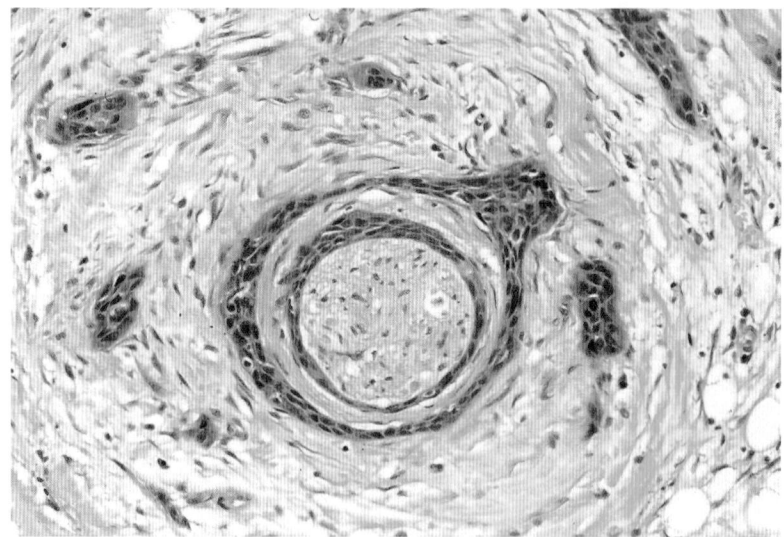

Fig. 24.143
Squamous cell carcinoma: neurotropism is an important prognostic indicator correlating with a high recurrence rate and aggressive local growth.

in two large studies.[249–251] However, the risk for metastasis increased with tumor thickness and was 4% for tumor thickness of 2.1 to 6 mm, and 16% for tumors greater than 6 mm in thickness.[250,252] The level of invasion is also of prognostic importance. The likelihood of recurrence and metastasis increases significantly with invasion beyond the reticular dermis.[95]

In general, poorly differentiated tumors recur and metastasize more frequently than well-differentiated variants and the presence of stromal desmoplasia is a risk factor for metastasis.[248,250,251] Neurotropism is associated with high recurrence and metastasis rates (*Fig. 24.143*). Perineural spread is particularly common in tumors arising on the head and neck, especially the mid face and lip. In a large series of such cases, 14% of tumors showed involvement of the perineural space, particularly spindle cell and acantholytic variants.[253] The presence or absence of lymphatic and vascular involvement should be documented (*Fig. 24.144*).

Local recurrence is a poor prognostic sign; recurrent tumors are associated with a 25–45% metastasis rate, depending upon the site.[93]

Staging criteria for primary cutaneous squamous cell carcinoma were adjusted in the 2017 8th Edition of the *AJCC Staging Manual* (chapter for head and neck tumors).[254] This staging system became effective on January 1, 2018. The elements for primary staging are presented in *Table 24.2*. Since metastases (both regional and distant) are rare, these staging elements are not presented here. For the T (tumor) element, relevant cutoffs for greatest dimension (in any orientation) are 2 and 4 cm; however, upstaging can occur with perineural invasion or deep invasion. The latter is defined as going through the subcutis to involve deeper soft tissue or bone or simply invasion greater than 6 mm as measured by the criteria of the Breslow assessment for melanoma. It is important to highlight that these staging criteria only apply to tumors presenting on the head and neck.

Differential diagnosis

Despite the wide variety of differential diagnoses, establishing the correct diagnosis is not usually a problem (*Table 24.3*). However, occasionally it is extremely difficult to make the correct diagnosis, especially if an adequate clinical history is not available. Of particular importance is the distinction between squamous cell carcinoma and keratoacanthoma, discussed later in the chapter.

Differentiation of squamous cell carcinoma from its precursor lesions depends upon examining sufficient numbers of sections to confirm the intraepidermal location of the latter conditions. Pseudoepitheliomatous hyperplasia may show all the features of a squamous cell carcinoma. In these cases, the correct diagnosis can only be made after careful examination of the surrounding tissues.

Occasionally, squamous cell carcinoma may be confused with eccrine porocarcinoma, particularly as the latter may show bowenoid features. The

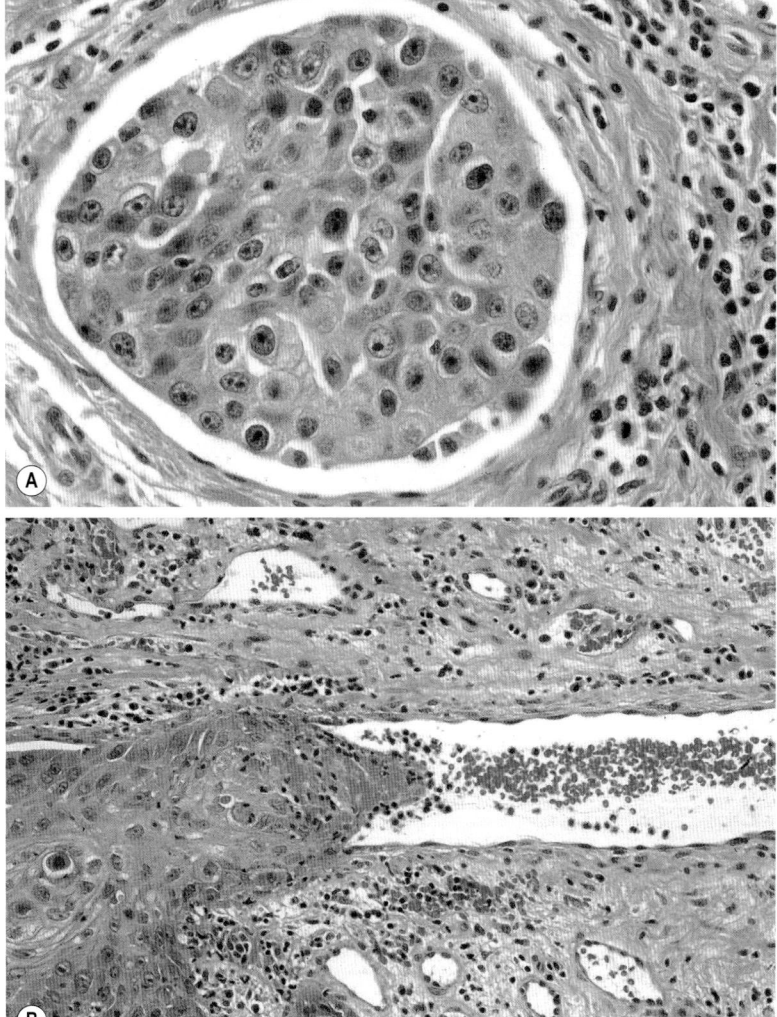

Fig. 24.144
(**A**, **B**) Squamous cell carcinoma: lymphovascular invasion also signifies a likely poor prognosis.

Table 24.2
Definition of primary tumor (T)

T category	T criteria
TX	Primary tumor cannot be assessed
Tis	Carcinoma *in situ*
TI	Tumor smaller than or equal to 2 cm in greatest dimension
T2	Tumor larger than 2 cm. but smaller than or equal to 4 cm in greatest dimension
T3	Tumor larger than 4 cm in maximum dimension or minor bone erosion or perineural invasion or deep invasion*
T4	Tumor with gross cortical bone/marrow, skull base invasion and/or skull base foramen invasion
T4a	Tumor with gross cortical bone/marrow invasion
T4b	Tumor with skull base invasion and/or skull base foramen involvement

*Deep invasion is defined as invasion beyond the subcutaneous fat or >6 mm (as measured from the granular layer of adjacent normal epidermis to the base of the tumor): perineural invasion for T3 classification is defined as tumor cells within the nerve sheath of a nerve lying deeper than the dermis or measuring 0.1 mm or larger in caliber. or presenting with clinical or radiographic involvement of named nerves without skull base invasion or transgression.
Kalifano JA, Lydiatt WM, Nehal KS, et al. Cutaneous Carcinoma of the Head and Neck. In: Amin MB, Edge SB, Greene FL, et al, eds. AJCC Cancer Staging Manual. 8th ed. New York: Springer International Publishing; 2017:171-181.Used with permission.

Table 24.3
Squamous cell carcinoma: differential diagnosis

SCC variant	Differential diagnosis
Classic	Eccrine porocarcinoma Hidradenocarcinoma Inverted follicular keratosis Desmoplastic trichilemmoma Keratoacanthoma Pseudoepitheliomatous hyperplasia Basi-squamous (metatypical) carcinoma Pilar tumor
Acantholytic	Adenocarcinoma Angiosarcoma
Verrucous	Viral wart
Clear cell	Sebaceous carcinoma Clear cell porocarcinoma Clear cell pilar tumor Clear cell hidradenocarcinoma Trichilemmal carcinoma Clear cell metastases (kidney, lung) Balloon cell melanoma
Spindled cell	Spindle cell melanoma Dermatofibrosarcoma protuberans Leiomyosarcoma Metastatic spindled cell carcinoma Atypical fibroxanthoma Metastatic sarcoma

SCC, squamous cell carcinoma.

demonstration of ductal differentiation or intracytoplasmic lumina by the diastase-PAS reaction or immunohistochemically with EMA or CEA usually resolves any difficulty.

Microcystic adnexal carcinoma may be mistaken for an abundantly keratinizing squamous cell carcinoma, particularly if ductal differentiation is not obvious and especially if only shave or punch biopsy specimens are available.

Variants of squamous cell carcinoma

A number of variants of squamous cell carcinoma are of sufficient importance to merit individual attention. These include the clear cell, spindle cell, desmoplastic, acantholytic, pseudovascular, adenosquamous/mucoepidermoid, verrucous, and metaplastic squamous cell carcinoma in addition to keratoacanthoma.

Clear cell and signet ring cell squamous carcinoma

Clinical features

Clear cell squamous carcinoma is a rare tumor that occurs primarily on the head and neck.[1,2] It is usually seen in the elderly, particularly males, and is often associated with exposure to sunlight; there is sometimes an antecedent history of multiple skin tumors.

Histologic features

Clear cells may appear as foci in otherwise typical squamous tumors, but occasionally they occupy the bulk of the lesion (*Figs 24.145 and 24.146*).[1,3] Although the clear cells are usually the result of glycogen accumulation, they can be due to hydropic degeneration. Signet ring cell change showing compressed crescent-shaped and laterally displaced nuclei due to cytosolic glycogen accumulation is an exceedingly rare finding and this variant is also referred to as signet ring squamous cell carcinoma (*Fig. 24.147*).[4,5]

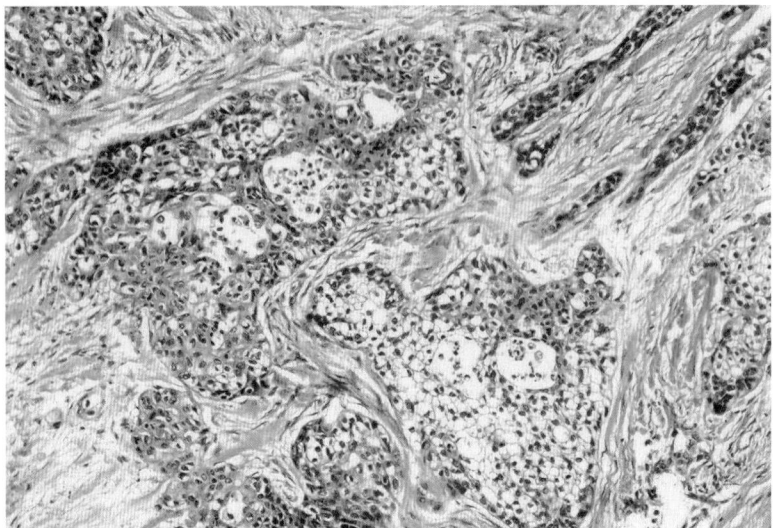

Fig. 24.145
Clear cell squamous carcinoma: in this field the entire tumor is composed of vacuolated cells due to intense glycogen accumulation.

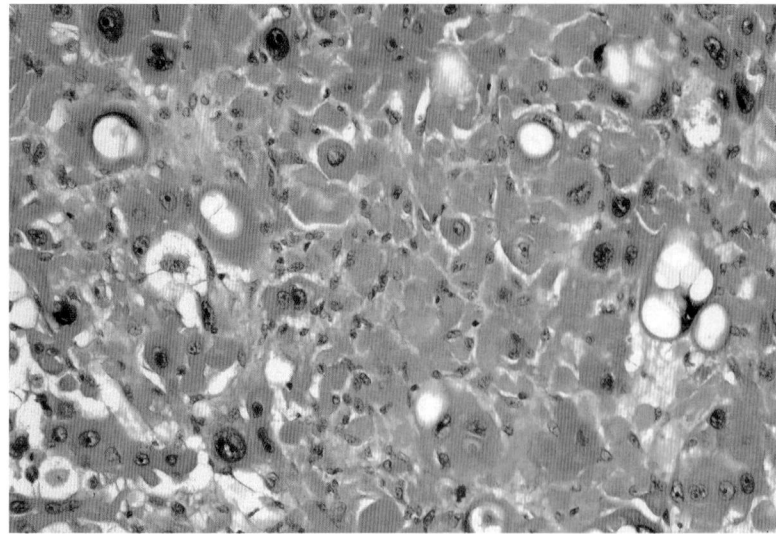

Fig. 24.147
Signet ring cell squamous cell carcinoma: signet ring cells are extremely rarely seen in squamous cell carcinoma. Immunohistochemistry should always be performed to exclude intracytoplasmic lumen formation (EMA and CEA) as would be seen in a sweat gland carcinoma. Diastase-PAS staining may also be useful.

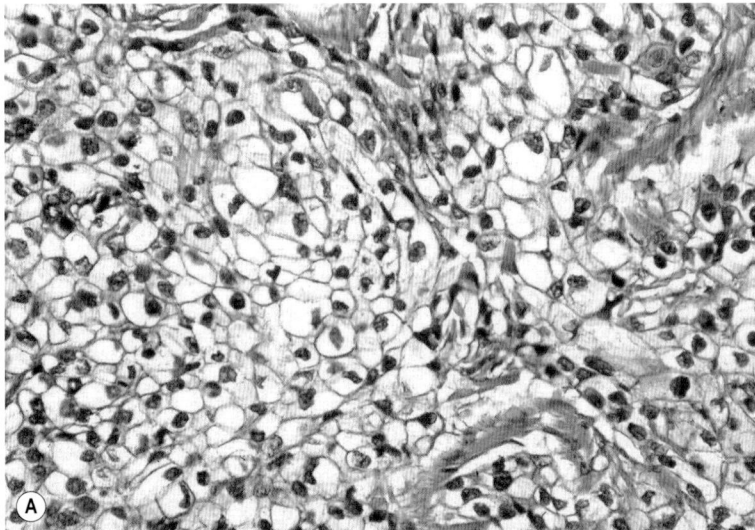

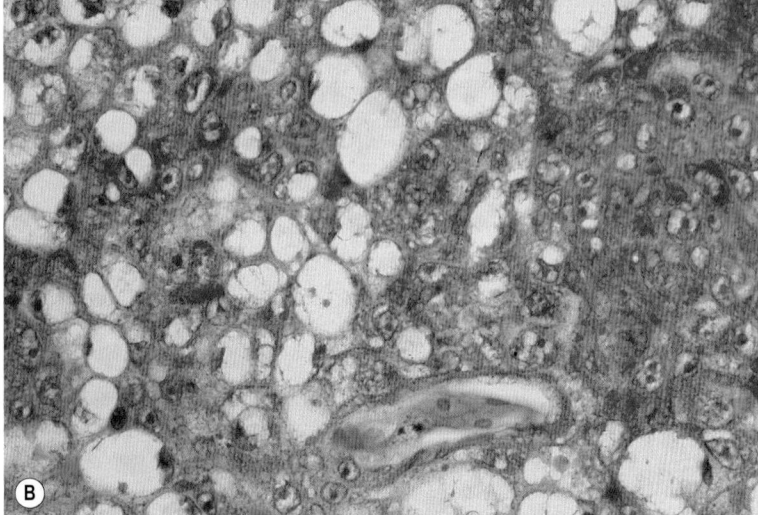

Fig. 24.146
(A, B) Clear cell squamous carcinoma: high-power views showing cytoplasmic vacuolation and striking periodic acid-Schiff positivity.

Differential diagnosis

The differential diagnosis includes clear cell basal cell carcinoma, sebaceous carcinoma, trichilemmal carcinoma, clear cell hidradenocarcinoma (and porocarcinoma), amelanotic melanoma, clear cell atypical fibroxanthoma, and metastases from clear cell tumors elsewhere.

- Clear cell basal cell carcinoma can be differentiated by the presence of areas of typical basal cell carcinoma and peripheral palisading.
- In sebaceous carcinoma the cytoplasm of the cells tends to be much more obviously bubbly with indentation of the nucleus.
- Trichilemmal carcinoma shows peripheral palisading in addition to pilar keratinization. This distinction may be difficult but is of clinical significance since trichilemmal carcinomas tend to behave in a less aggressive fashion.[6]
- Separation from clear cell hidradenocarcinoma/porocarcinoma relies on the identification of ductal structures, which can be highlighted by immunohistochemistry for EMA and CEA.
- Distinction from amelanotic clear cell melanoma can be difficult; numerous levels may have to be examined to find foci of more obvious squamous differentiation. If doubt remains, immunohistochemistry should readily establish the correct diagnosis.
- Clear cell atypical fibroxanthoma does not show cytokeratin or epithelial membrane antigen expression by immunohistochemistry and lacks squamous differentiation on morphology.[7]
- Metastases from clear cell tumors elsewhere (e.g., the kidney and lung) enter into the differential diagnosis, but kidney clear cell tumor cells characteristically contain both glycogen and lipid while those from the lung contain mucopolysaccharides in addition to glycogen.

Spindle cell squamous carcinoma

Clinical features

Spindle cell squamous carcinoma is a not uncommon subtype of which there are two distinct biological variants. More commonly, these tumors are actinically derived, present on the exposed surfaces (particularly the scalp and face), and are associated with a good prognosis, recurring infrequently and metastasizing rarely. This lesion usually presents as a 1–2 cm discrete and often ulcerated nodule.[1,2] Rare sites of involvement are the conjunctiva and the external auditory meatus.[3–5]

Less often, spindle cell squamous carcinoma follows exposure to ionizing radiation or trauma, including burns, and is of high grade with

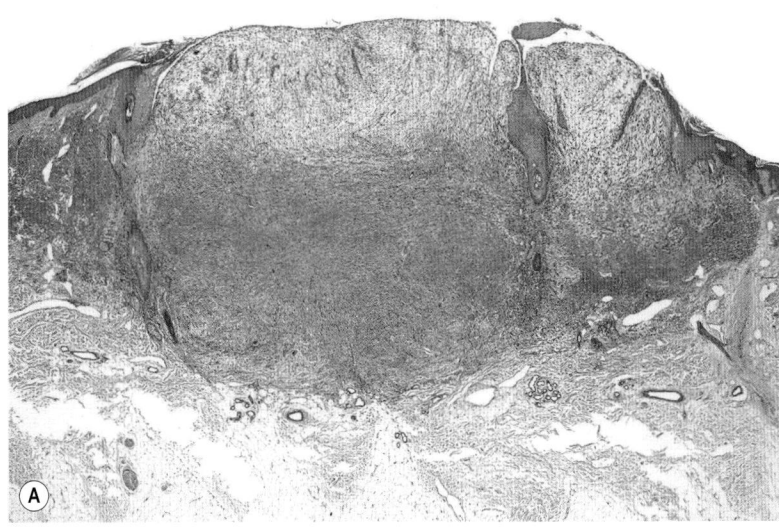

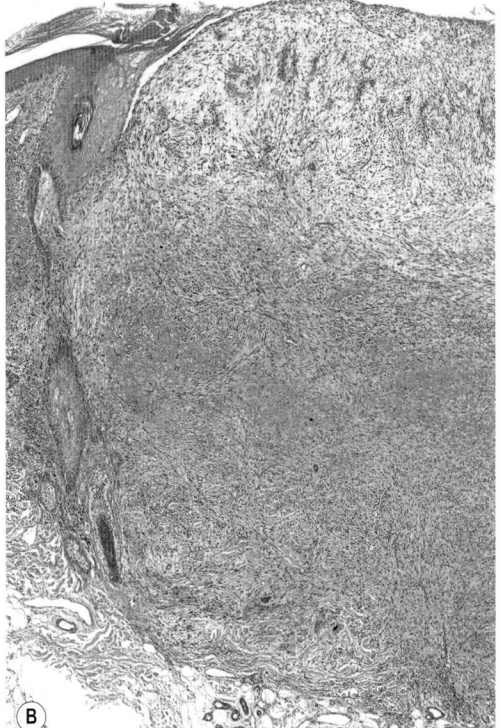

Fig. 24.148
Spindle cell squamous carcinoma: (A) this spindle cell tumor arose on the head of an elderly male; (B) no evidence of an epidermal origin is visible. Diagnosis in lesions such as this is often one of exclusion, and immunohistochemistry is frequently essential.

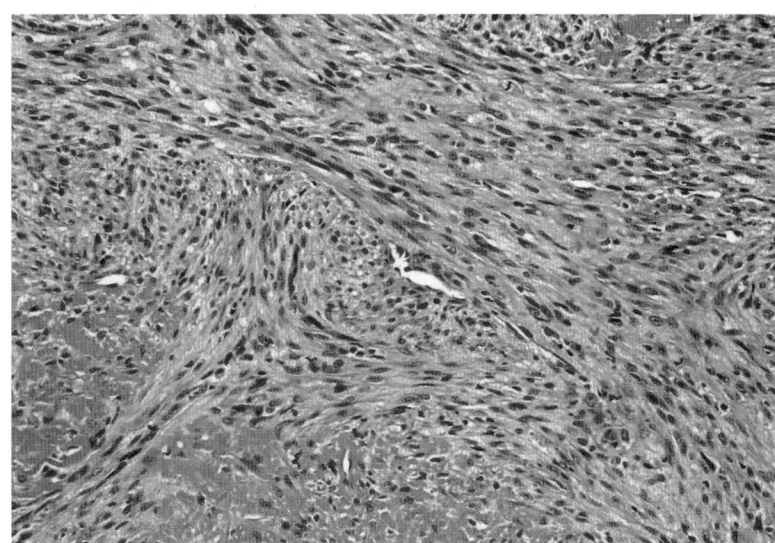

Fig. 24.149
Spindle cell squamous carcinoma: the spindled cells have fusiform pleomorphic, hyperchromatic nuclei.

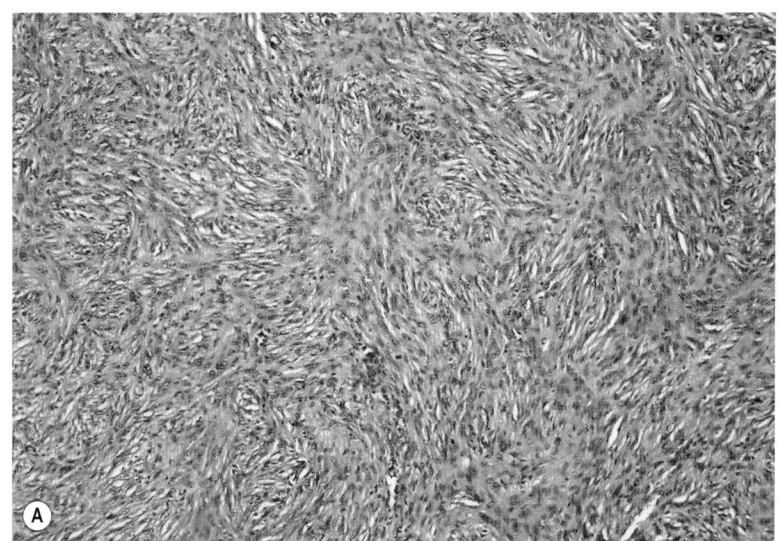

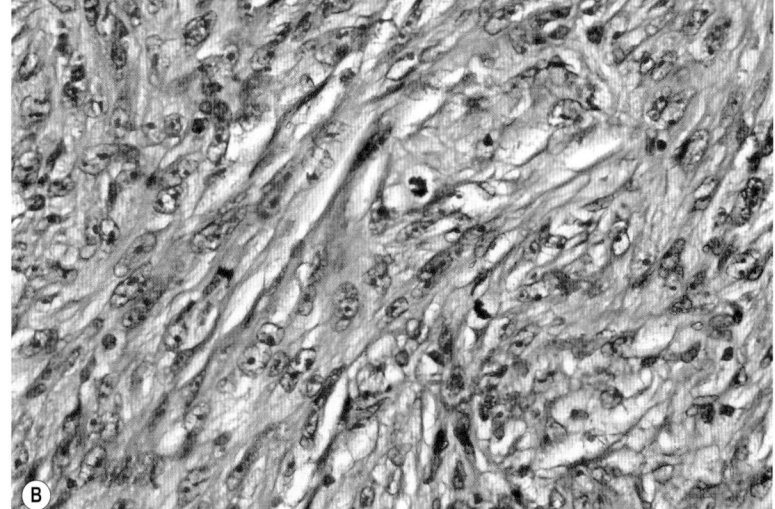

Fig. 24.150
Spindle cell squamous carcinoma: (A) this example shows a storiform growth pattern; (B) numerous mitoses are present.

frequent recurrences and metastases and associated with a significant mortality. Spindle cell squamous cell carcinoma with poor prognosis has also been reported in immunosuppressed patients following solid organ transplantation.[6]

Pathogenesis and histologic features

In the past, a spindled cell component in squamous carcinoma was thought to represent a pseudosarcomatous element or imply the presence of a collision tumor. On the basis of both immunohistochemistry and ultrastructural findings, this tumor is now recognized as squamous cell carcinoma showing fibroblastic and myofibroblastic differentiation.[1,7–11]

Histologically, spindle cell squamous carcinoma may present as spindled cell areas in an otherwise readily recognizable squamous tumor. More commonly, however, it consists entirely of a pleomorphic spindled cell population showing no evidence of epidermal derivation or squamous differentiation (*Figs 24.148 and 24.149*). The latter variant always constitutes a diagnosis of exclusion dependent upon careful interpretation of immunohistochemical findings and occasionally ultrastructural observations. Very occasionally, a storiform growth pattern may result in confusion with dermatofibrosarcoma protuberans (*Fig. 24.150*). Helpful diagnostic pointers

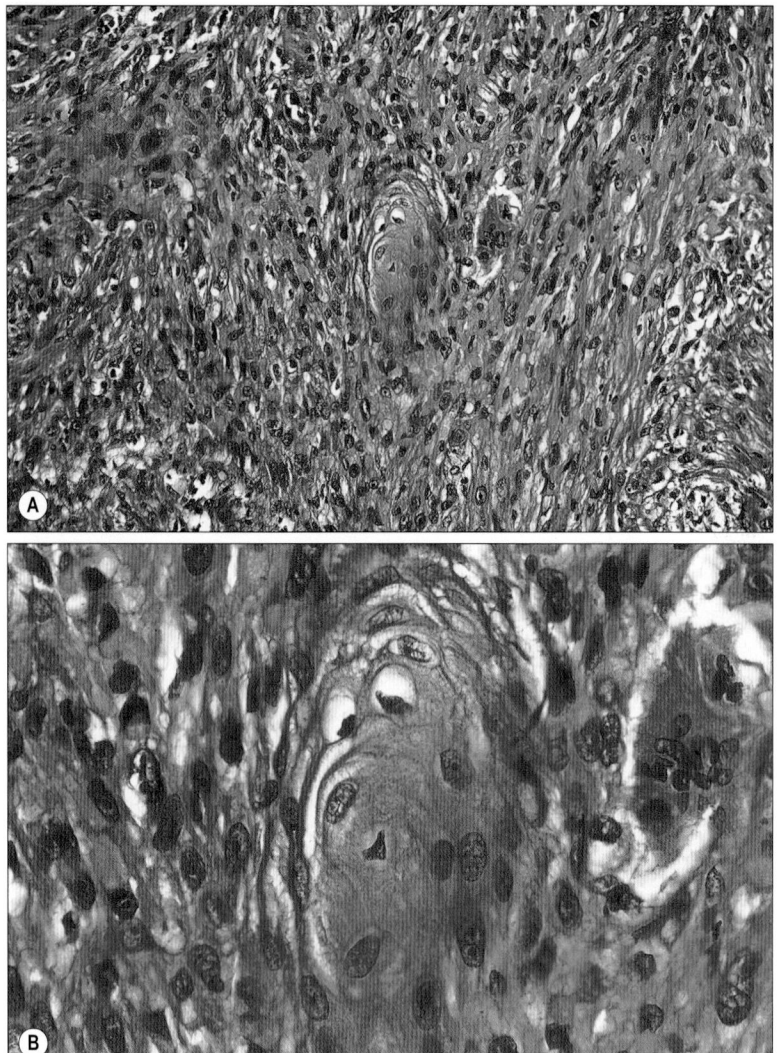

Fig. 24.151
Spindle cell squamous cell carcinoma: (**A**) arising from an actinic keratosis is a spindle cell carcinoma; (**B**) the spindle cells have eosinophilic cytoplasm and fusiform hyperchromatic nuclei. Note the mitoses.

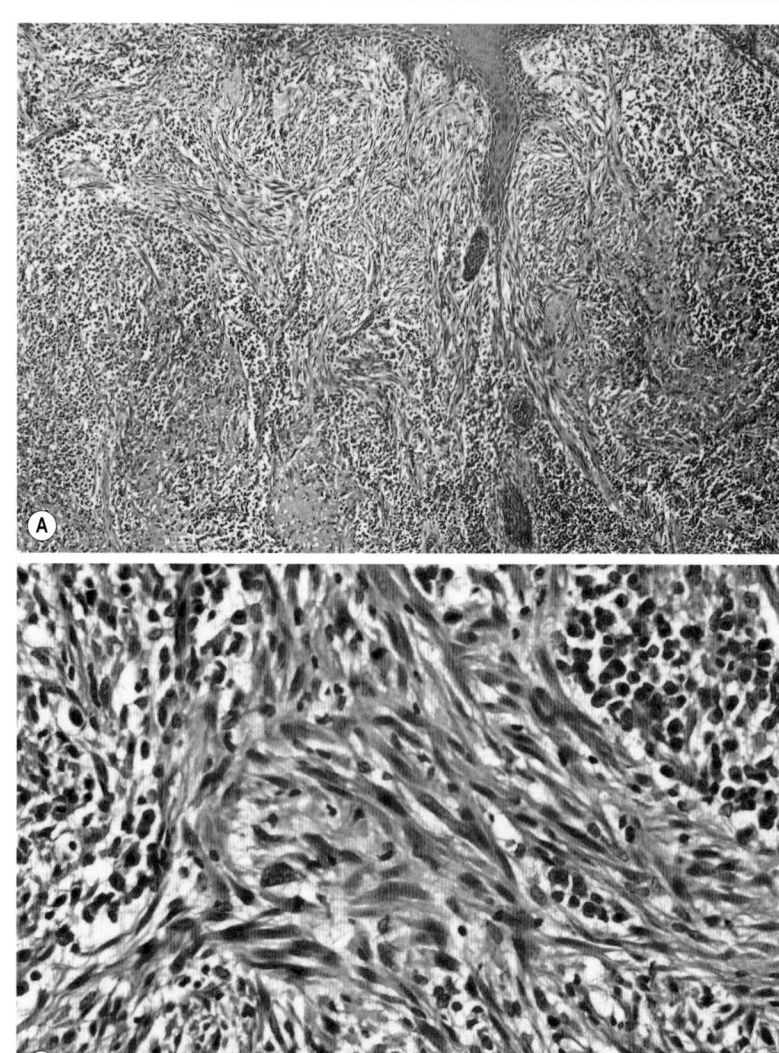

Fig. 24.152
(**A**, **B**) Spindle cell squamous carcinoma: in this example, there are very occasional small foci of residual squamous differentiation thus obviating any need for immunohistochemistry.

include an origin in grossly sun-damaged skin and the presence of actinic keratosis in the adjacent nonulcerated epidermis (*Fig. 24.151*). Sometimes there is evidence of direct transition from epithelial to spindled cell morphology and a careful search for dyskeratosis or intercellular bridges may be rewarding (*Figs 24.151 and 24.152*).

Immunohistochemical studies usually disclose keratin positivity and often EMA is at least focally present (*Fig. 24.153*).[12,13] Pancytokeratin antibodies (MNF116) and high-molecular-weight cytokeratins (34betaE12) in addition to staining for p63 can be particularly useful.[14–16] Focal positivity for muscle-specific actin is sometimes seen.[7,16] In contrast to conventional squamous cell carcinoma, HER2 and epidermal growth factor receptor (EGFR) expression is unusual in the spindle cell variant.[17]

Ultrastructural studies occasionally reveal tonofilament-desmosomal complexes in addition to evidence of fibroblastic differentiation (abundant rough endoplasmic reticulum and/or intracellular collagen synthesis) and myofibroblastic differentiation (abundant cytoplasmic glycogen and microfilaments with dense bodies).[7]

Differential diagnosis

Spindle cell squamous carcinoma must be distinguished from spindle cell melanoma, cutaneous leiomyosarcoma, sarcomatous and pseudosarcomatous (carcinomatous) metastases, and atypical fibroxanthoma.[2,12,13,18,19]

Often, the diagnosis of spindle cell squamous carcinoma can be arrived at by careful evaluation of immunohistochemistry using a panel of antibodies reactive against keratin, S100 protein, HMB-45, muscle-specific

actin, and desmin.[20] The presence of vimentin is of lesser value because poorly differentiated and spindle cell squamous carcinomas, tumors of mesenchymal derivation, and melanoma frequently express this intermediate filament.[21]

Desmoplastic squamous cell carcinoma

Clinical features

Desmoplastic squamous cell carcinoma is a rare but clinically significant variant.[1] It accounts for approximately 7% of invasive tumors and is characterized by an increased risk of local recurrence (27.3%) as well as metastasis (22.7%). It affects the elderly with a marked male predominance and presents on sun-exposed skin with a predilection for the head and neck. The ear is most often affected while the incidence on the lip is less frequent when compared with other subtypes of squamous carcinoma.[2,3] Tumors tend to present as more advanced and thicker lesions and tumor thickness >5 mm is an indicator of poor outcome.[4–7]

Pathogenesis and histologic features

Histologically, this variant is characterized by tumor aggregates arranged in nests and strands surrounded by an intense desmoplastic stromal reaction (*Figs 24.154–24.156*). By definition, this pattern comprises more than one-third of the squamous cell carcinoma invasive component. Cellular pleomorphism and perineural invasion are frequent features.[4,5]

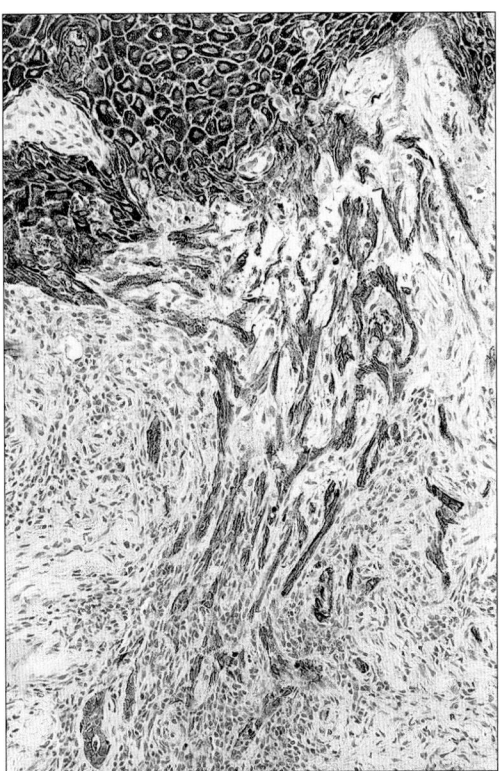

Fig. 24.153
Spindle cell squamous carcinoma: the spindle cells are positive for keratin (same case as Fig. 24.152).

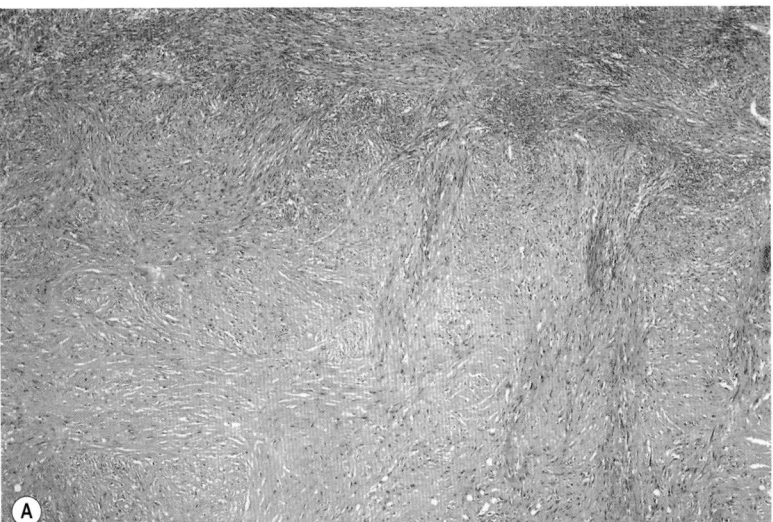

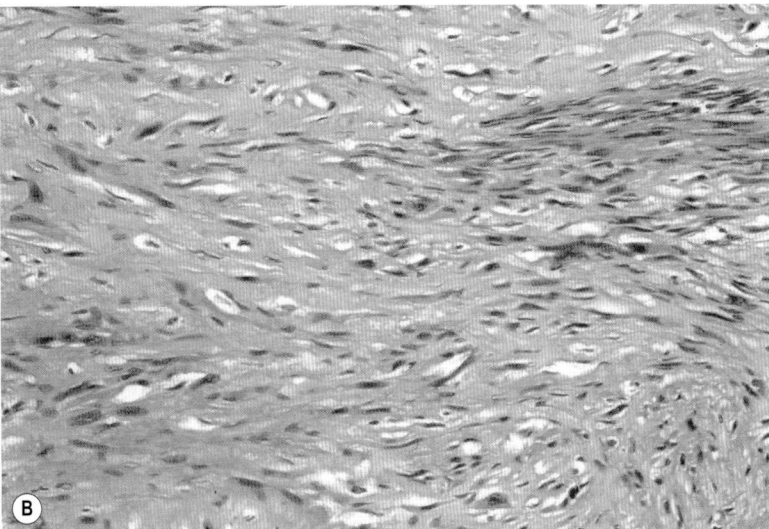

Fig. 24.154
(A, B) Desmoplastic squamous cell carcinoma: the tumor is paucicellular and associated with a hyalinized stroma.

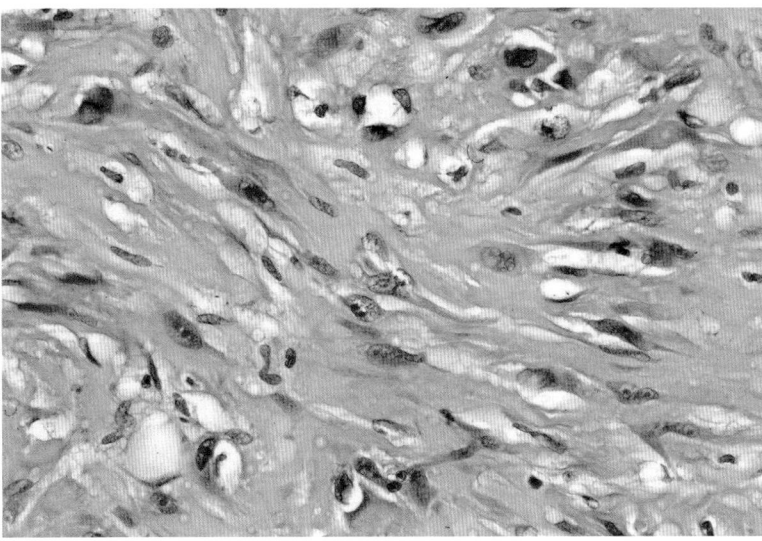

Fig. 24.155
Desmoplastic squamous cell carcinoma: nuclei are variably hyperchromatic and vesicular. Nucleoli are prominent.

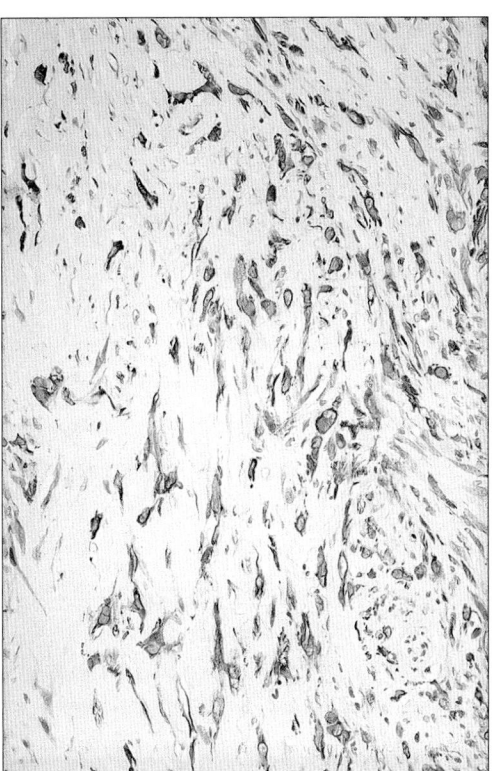

Fig. 24.156
Desmoplastic squamous cell carcinoma: the tumor cells express pankeratin.

Differential diagnosis

Desmoplastic squamous cell carcinoma can be distinguished from sclerosing basal cell carcinoma, microcystic adnexal carcinoma, desmoplastic tricho-epithelioma, and metatypical basal cell carcinoma by the presence of foci of obvious squamous differentiation including single-cell keratinization and the presence of squamous pearls, the coexistence of a component of more typical squamous cell carcinoma, as well as absence of basaloid areas with peripheral palisading and microcysts or evidence of ductal differentiation.

Acantholytic squamous cell carcinoma

Clinical features

Acantholytic squamous carcinoma is an uncommon tumor. It is frequently ulcerated, flesh-colored, and nodular and largely confined to the head and neck.[1-3] Occasionally, however, it may present at a variety of other sites

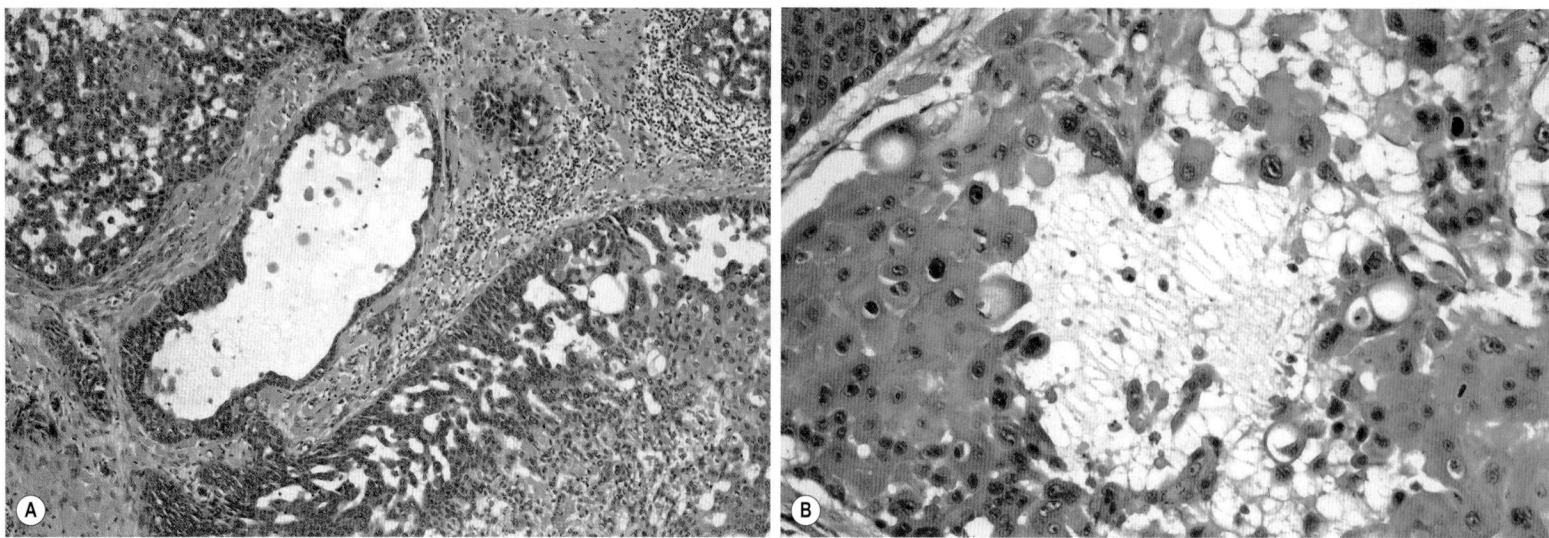

Fig. 24.157
(**A**, **B**) Acantholytic squamous cell carcinoma: in these fields, cystic spaces are evident, which in the absence of keratinization might raise the possibility of glandular differentiation.

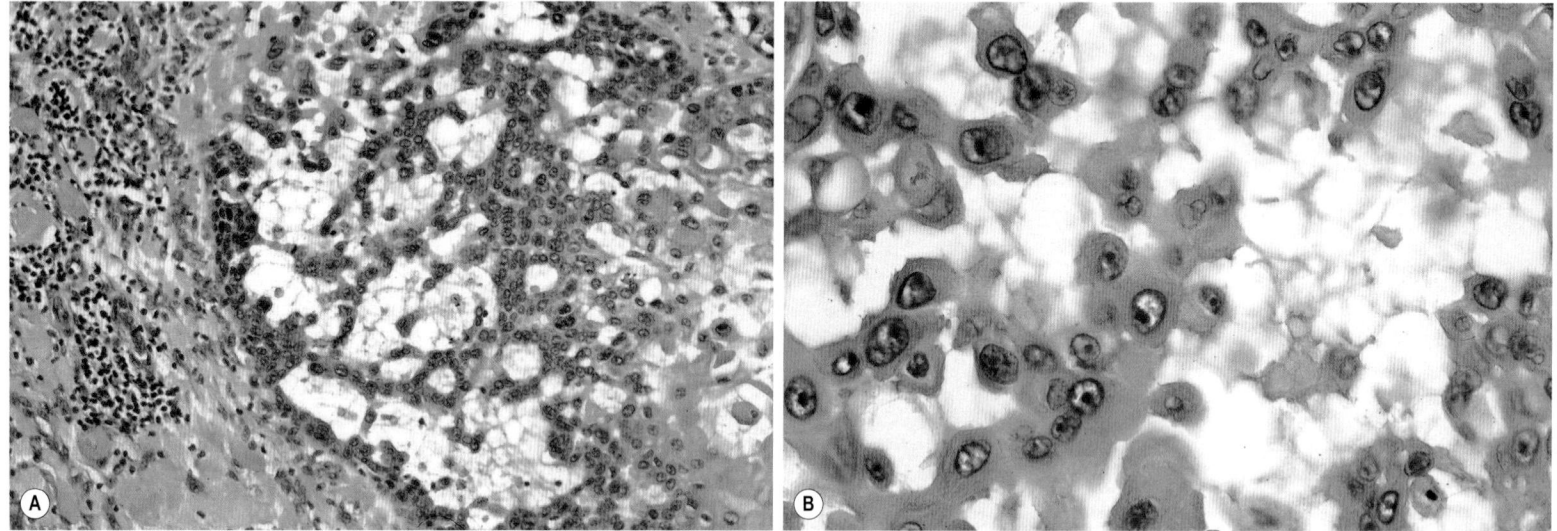

Fig. 24.158
(**A**, **B**) Acantholytic squamous cell carcinoma: acantholytic change seen on the left side of the tumor merges with more obvious squamous differentiation on the right and shown in higher power in (**B**).

including the hand, arm, leg, foot, breast, penis, and vulva and has been documented to arise in areas of pre-existing scarring and in patients with chronic lymphocytic leukemia.[3-8] Intraoral presentation has also been described.[9,10] It is often cup-shaped and may appear to have arisen in an acantholytic solar keratosis.[1] Although originally thought to have a good prognosis, it has been suggested that it might be associated with high morbidity and mortality.[3,4] In a series of 55 patients, 19% died of recurrent or metastatic disease.[3] However, a recent series of 115 cases did not find that this variant conferred aggressive behavior with no deaths reported.[11] Size appears to be of particular importance: in all these fatalities, the tumor was larger than 1.5 cm in diameter.

Pathogenesis and histologic features

Histologically, the tumor appears as a squamous carcinoma in which a pseudoglandular component is conspicuous (*Figs 24.157 and 24.158*). Careful examination of the 'glandular foci' reveals that their presence is due to the development of marked acantholysis. Epithelial mucin production is consistently absent. A peculiar feature in some tumors is sweat duct epithelium atypia, which can make the diagnosis even more difficult (*Fig. 24.159*). A recent study suggested frequent involvement of the follicular epithelium.[11] Acantholytic squamous cell carcinoma labels positively for pankeratin and

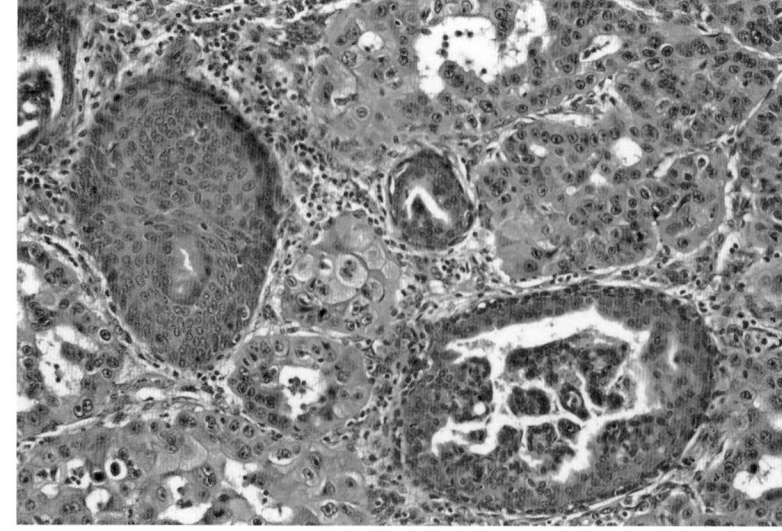

Fig. 24.159
Acantholytic squamous cell carcinoma: hyperplasia of the sweat duct lining epithelium is marked in this example (same case as Fig. 24.157).

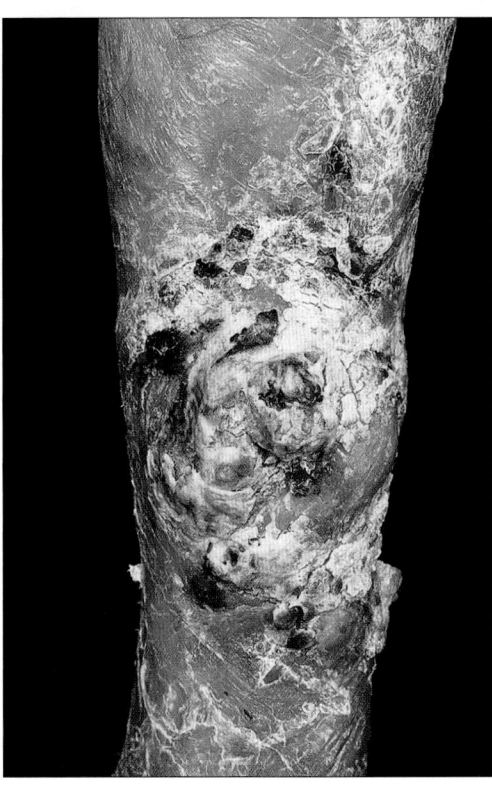

Fig. 24.160
Pseudovascular squamous cell carcinoma: this patient suffers from recessive dystrophic epidermolysis bullosa. The tumor arose against a background of dense dermal scarring. By courtesy of R.A.J. Eady, MD, Institute of Dermatology, London, UK.

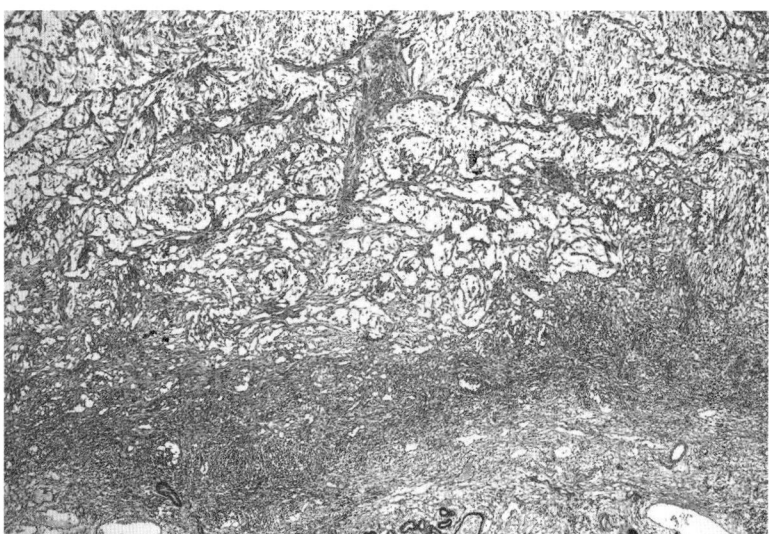

Fig. 24.161
Pseudovascular squamous cell carcinoma: the tumor is composed of numerous variably sized, cystic spaces containing pale-staining fluid. There is red cell extravasation.

EMA, but is invariably negative for CEA. Some examples have also been shown to coexpress vimentin.[12] It is thought that this is a consequence of diminished cell–cell contact and reduced expression of cell adhesion molecules, in particular syndecan-1, has been reported.[13,14] The diastase–PAS reaction is negative, but occasional foci of Alcian blue positivity may be seen due to stromal mucin production.

Differential diagnosis

Acantholytic squamous carcinoma must be distinguished from metastatic carcinoma and adenosquamous (mucoepidermoid) carcinoma of the skin. The latter more commonly presents in the salivary gland and bronchus, is extremely rare, and consists of a moderate to poorly differentiated squamous component admixed with a mucus-secreting glandular element.[15] The glandular component strongly expresses CEA and the mucin is sialidase sensitive. From the small number of cases reported so far, mucoepidermoid carcinoma of the skin appears to be a high-grade neoplasm commonly associated with nodal and systemic spread.[16] Similarly, acantholytic squamous carcinoma should not be confused with squamous carcinoma showing mucinous metaplasia. The latter presents as an admixture of mucin-containing signet ring cells in an otherwise typical squamous carcinoma.[16,17]

Pseudovascular squamous cell carcinoma

Clinical features

So-called pseudoangiosarcomatous or pseudovascular squamous cell carcinoma is an exceedingly rare subtype of acantholytic squamous cell carcinoma. Acantholysis in these tumors is extreme and it mimics a vascular tumor.[1-4] This variant is more often a systemic neoplasm seen particularly in the breast and thyroid. In series reported on the skin, almost all the patients are male and the majority of tumors present on sun-exposed areas of the head and neck as discrete, solitary, tan–pink nodules or ulcerated lesions, quite unlike cutaneous angiosarcoma (*Fig. 24.160*). Involvement of the oral cavity as well as the genital area of both vulva and penis has also been documented.[5-8] One recent case was reported to arise in a burn scar.[9] Recurrences and metastases are high with a mortality of at least 30%.[1-4,10]

Pathogenesis and histologic features

Histologically, extreme acantholysis is accompanied by the development of pseudovascular channels and cystic spaces often lined by atypical plump epithelial cells containing vesicular or hyperchromatic nuclei and sometimes showing a hobnail appearance (*Figs 24.161–24.163*).[1-4] The lumina may contain erythrocytes, but often faintly basophilic granular material showing hyaluronidase-sensitive Alcian blue pH 2.5 positivity (hyaluronic acid) is present.[1] More solid nests and cords of polygonal tumor cells may be evident in the surrounding tissues. Additional features that heighten the resemblance to a vascular tumor include collagen dissection by tumor cells, pseudovascular intracytoplasmic lumina (containing stromal mucin), and the presence of epithelium-covered fibrovascular tufts protruding into the pseudovascular spaces. A careful search may sometimes show an origin from the surface epithelium or reveal foci of more obvious squamous differentiation. Multifocality, a feature typically seen in cutaneous angiosarcoma, is not present in pseudovascular squamous cell carcinoma, and the endothelial cells lining the stromal vessels are invariably normal.

Immunohistochemistry reveals keratin positivity and the majority of cells are outlined by epithelial membrane antigen (*Fig. 24.164*). In contrast to cutaneous angiosarcoma (particularly the epithelioid variant with which this tumor may sometimes be confused), pseudovascular squamous carcinoma is invariably negative for the endothelial cell markers factor VIII-related antigen, CD31, and CD34,[1-4] as well as a recently described vascular marker Fli-1, which displays nuclear staining of endothelial cells.[11] The lectin *Ulex europaeus* agglutinin is of no value in the differential diagnosis because positive labeling is commonly seen in normal squamous epithelium, many conventional squamous cell carcinomas, and tumors of endothelial derivation.[12]

Ultrastructural studies may also be of value because both desmosomes and tonofibrils are consistently present.[1,3] Endothelial cell features, in particular the formation of Weibel-Palade bodies, are not evident.

Adenosquamous carcinoma/mucoepidermoid carcinoma of skin

Clinical features

Primary cutaneous squamous cell carcinoma with glandular differentiation is a rare but aggressive neoplasm that has been variably referred to as adenosquamous or mucoepidermoid carcinoma when resembling its counterpart in salivary gland.[1-10] Clinically it presents as an elevated plaque ranging from 0.5 to 6.0 cm in the elderly without sex predilection.[3,11] Presentation in childhood is exceptional.[12] The head and neck area is almost exclusively affected and the central face is the single most common site.[3] Rare reports describe involvement of the hand, finger, axilla, and penis and the tumor has been reported to arise within a pre-existing nevus sebaceous.[3,6,13-16] A case of

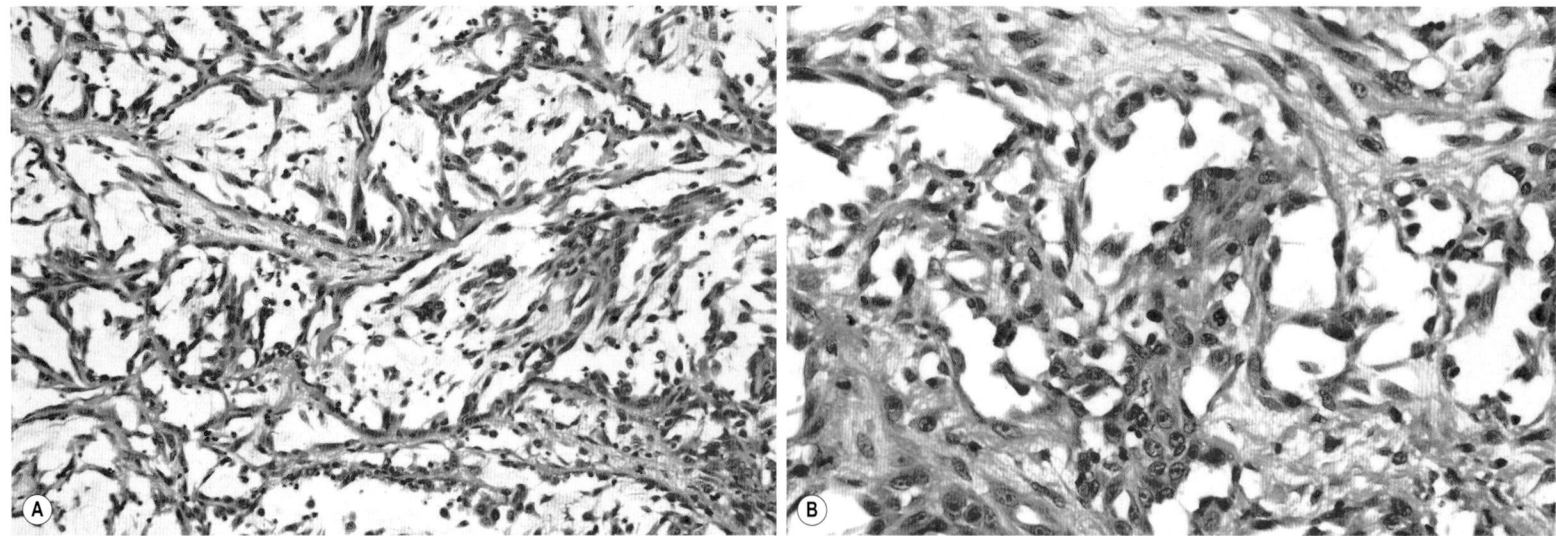

Fig. 24.162
Pseudovascular squamous cell carcinoma: (**A**) the spaces are 'lined' by spindle cells with vesicular nuclei containing prominent nucleoli; (**B**) mitoses are conspicuous.

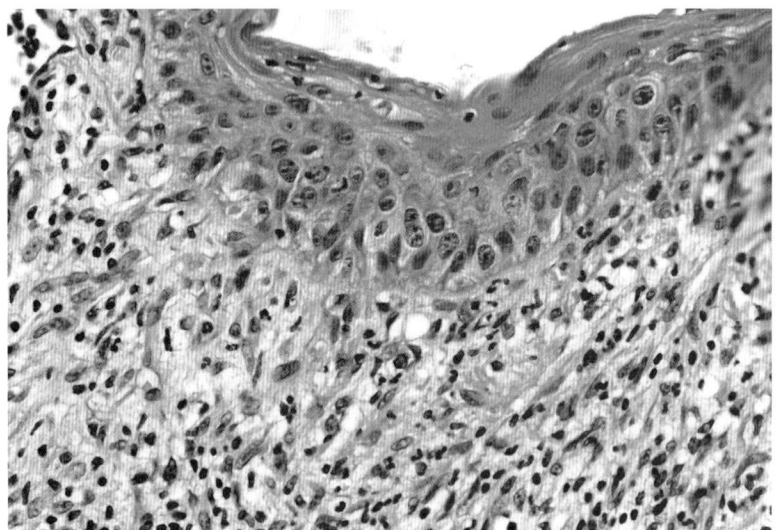

Fig. 24.163
Pseudovascular squamous cell carcinoma: the overlying epidermis is severely dysplastic.

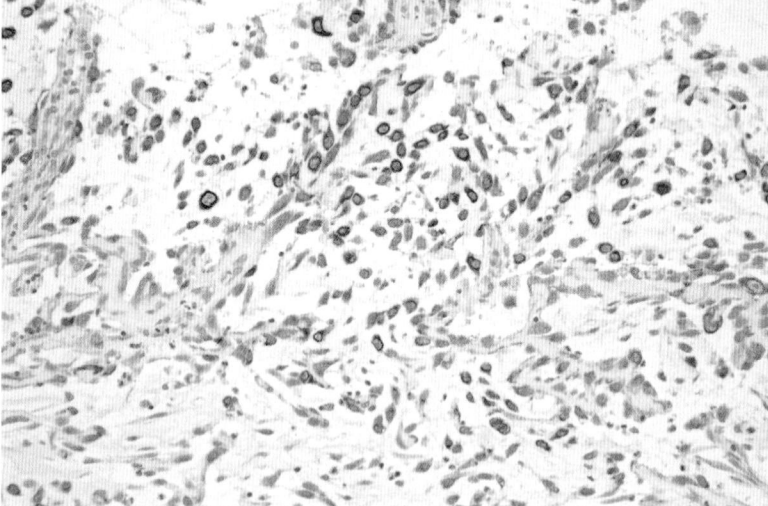

Fig. 24.164
Pseudovascular squamous cell carcinoma: the spindle cells are keratin positive. Endothelial cell markers were negative.

adenosquamous carcinoma of the vulva did not clearly separate this tumor from acantholytic squamous cell carcinoma.[17] Adenosquamous carcinomas of the skin have potential for aggressive behavior with locally destructive disease and lymph node as well as distant metastases.

Pathogenesis and histologic features

Histologically, adenosquamous carcinomas of skin are characterized by areas of conventional invasive squamous cell carcinoma arising often multifocally from the overlying epidermis. Glandular differentiation is appreciated as intracytoplasmic vacuoles, which coalesce to form luminal spaces. These lumina may be lined by an eosinophilic cuticle or by layers of flattened cells and may contain eosinophilic material. Glandular differentiation is more common in the deeper reaches and may be focal or widespread within the tumors (*Fig. 24.165*). Nuclear pleomorphism and mitotic figures are frequent features in both the squamous as well as glandular areas. These tumors are often deeply invasive and perineural infiltration is frequently evident. Additional features include superficial keratocysts and overlying ulceration. Special stains for mucin including mucicarmine or Alcian blue and immunohistochemistry for CEA highlight areas of glandular differentiation.[3] Cutaneous squamous cell carcinoma with areas showing signet ring

cell differentiation has also been referred to as cutaneous squamous cell carcinoma with mucinous metaplasia.[18]

The histogenesis as well as terminology of adenosquamous/mucoepidermoid carcinoma of the skin is uncertain. While an adnexal origin has to be considered, most authors regard this tumor as a variant of squamous cell carcinoma with divergent differentiation.[3,5] In addition, there is dispute in regard to the appropriate terminology. Adenosquamous carcinoma has been suggested for all squamous cell carcinomas showing glandular differentiation while the term mucoepidermoid carcinoma be reserved for tumors of salivary gland origin.[1,3,8] Some authors feel that the term mucoepidermoid carcinoma should be applied to the low-grade end of the spectrum of adenosquamous carcinoma.[7]

Differential diagnosis

Adenosquamous carcinoma of the skin can be distinguished from acantholytic or pseudovascular squamous cell carcinoma by the presence of mucin. Microcystic adnexal carcinoma enters the differential diagnosis but typically lacks marked cytological atypia, and mitoses are often sparse. Extension or metastases from mucoepidermoid carcinoma of salivary gland origin has to be excluded on clinical grounds.[19,20]

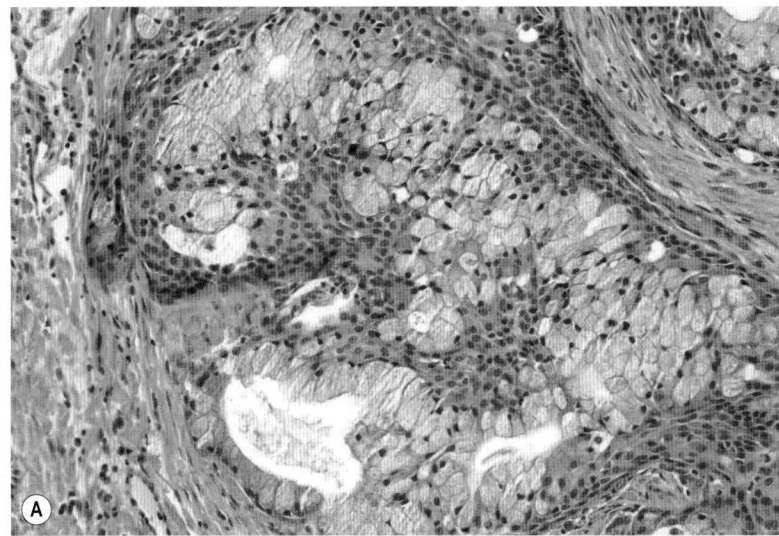
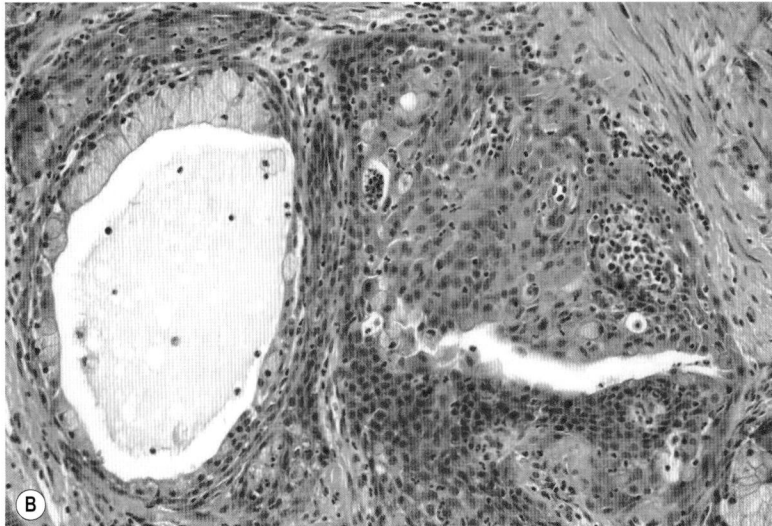

Fig. 24.165
(**A**, **B**) Mucoepidermoid carcinoma: the tumor comprises an admixture of squamous and mucus-secreting elements. The possibility that this represents skin involvement by an underlying salivary gland tumor cannot be excluded. By courtesy of W. Grayson, MD, Johannesburg, South Africa

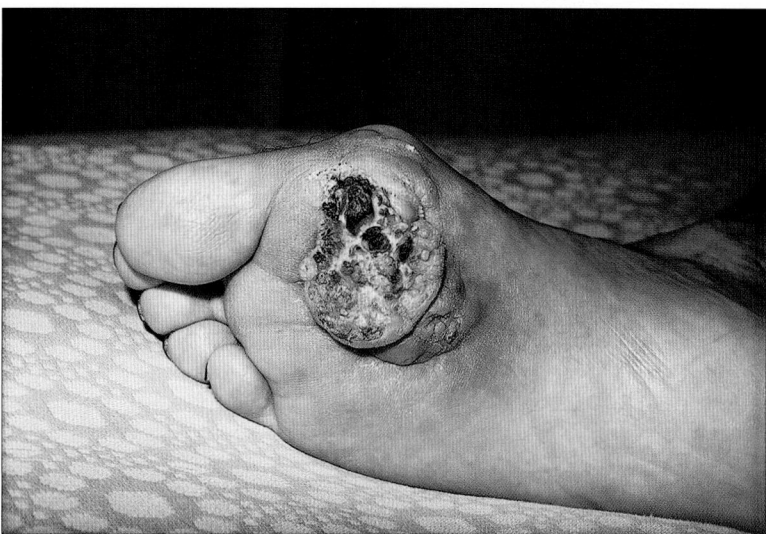

Fig. 24.166
Verrucous carcinoma: typical plantar lesion, so-called carcinoma cuniculatum, is warty, crusted, and penetrated by sinus tracts. Reproduced with permission from McKee, P.H., Wilkinson, J.D., Black, M.M., Whimster, I.W. (1981) Histopathology, 5, 425–436, with permission from Blackwell Publishing.

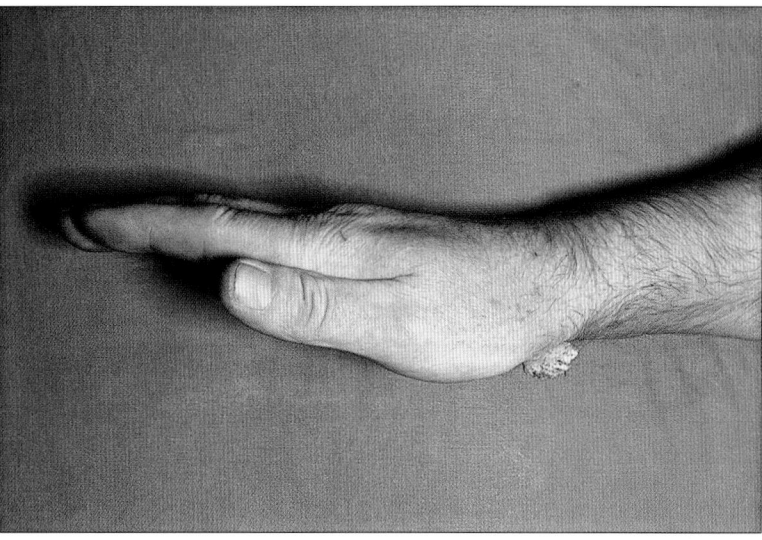

Fig. 24.167
Verrucous carcinoma: tumors arising at non–weight bearing sites often have a more substantial exophytic component. By courtesy of the Institute of Dermatology, London, UK.

Verrucous carcinoma

Clinical features

Verrucous carcinoma was originally described as a variant of well-differentiated squamous carcinoma arising in the oral cavity, but is now equally applied to oral florid papillomatosis, cutaneous lesions (carcinoma cuniculatum), and anogenital variants (Buschke-Löwenstein tumor).[1–9] It is controversial whether Buschke-Löwenstein tumor represents a variant of verrucous carcinoma or whether it is indeed a giant condyloma acuminatum. This controversy is reflected in various chapters of this book. Most authors favor it being a variant of verrucous carcinoma. Its significance is that recurrences are common, but metastases are rare.[10–13]

Cutaneous verrucous carcinoma presents most commonly on the sole of the foot, but lesions at a wide variety of sites, including the wrists, fingers, nail bed, ear, nose, eyelid, scalp, buttocks, shoulder, axilla, abdominal wall, and lip, have also been documented (*Figs 24.166–24.167*).[14–26] Tumors are rarely multicentric and they present as hyperkeratotic warty growths, often associated with the development of keratin-filled sinuses.[1,2,27] The latter appearance leads to the alternative designation 'epithelioma cuniculatum' because of the fanciful resemblance of the tumor growth to a rabbit warren. Although this endophytic aspect is particularly well developed in plantar lesions and may be accentuated by mechanical effects, sinus formation has

also been documented at extrapedal sites.[1] Chronic lesions may be associated with considerable bony destruction (*Fig. 24.168*). Tumors are most often found in middle-aged men and usually evolve over a considerable period of time. Presentation in childhood is rare and the development of verrucous carcinoma within a syringocystadenoma papilliferum is exceptional.[28–30]

Anogenital lesions are clinically similar, but the exophytic aspect is usually more pronounced. They often appear to have arisen from pre-existent condyloma acuminatum. The development of fistulae with abscess formation is common, particularly in lesions arising in the perianal region (*Fig. 24.169*).[11,31] Penile tumors most commonly arise on or around the prepuce, but the shaft may sometimes be affected.[6,7,11,32,33] Tumors of the female genital tract involve the vulva, vagina, and rarely the cervix.[34–38] They may arise in association with lichen sclerosus, lichen simplex chronicus, or conventional squamous cell carcinoma and are rarely multicentric.[37,39]

Verrucous carcinoma is associated with considerable morbidity. Anal and perianal lesions have a recurrence rate of approximately 70% and mortality (as a consequence of the effects of local spread) ranges between 20% and

30%.[31,40-42] Metastases from cutaneous lesions have rarely been documented (*Fig. 24.170*).[43-46]

Pathogenesis and histologic features

Many cutaneous (particularly plantar) lesions can be confused both clinically and microscopically with viral warts and, indeed, it is likely that many have arisen within a pre-existent viral wart (*Fig. 24.171*).[47] Further evidence in support of a viral etiology has been the localization of HPV genome, including subtypes 1, 2, 11, 16, and 18, by in situ hybridization.[48-53] Another potential etiological factor is scarring and chronic inflammation.

Verrucous carcinomas occasionally arise in the sinuses of chronic osteomyelitis, at the site of chronic cutaneous tuberculosis, as a complication of ulcerative leprosy, in association with psoriasis or lichen planus, areas of scarring, dystrophic epidermolysis bullosa, chronic pressure ulcers, and hypospadiasis.[39,54-60]

The etiology of the anogenital lesions is probably variable, but in many instances is thought to be related to HPV infection. Tumors sometimes appear to arise within pre-existent condyloma acuminatum and often show koilocytosis of the superficial epithelium. HPV types 6 and 11 are most often implicated, but cases in which types 1-4 have been identified are also documented.[5,18,61] Penile verrucous carcinoma has also been associated with chronic infection, chronic phimosis, trauma, and poor hygiene.[7] Patients are usually uncircumcised.

Verrucous carcinomas have similar histologic appearances irrespective of site.[1-3] They are characterized by both exophytic and endophytic components:

- The exophytic component consists of acanthotic papillary processes usually showing massive hyperkeratosis and often parakeratosis (*Figs 24.172 and 24.173*).
- The endophytic component is composed of well-differentiated squamous epithelium growing down into the underlying tissues as

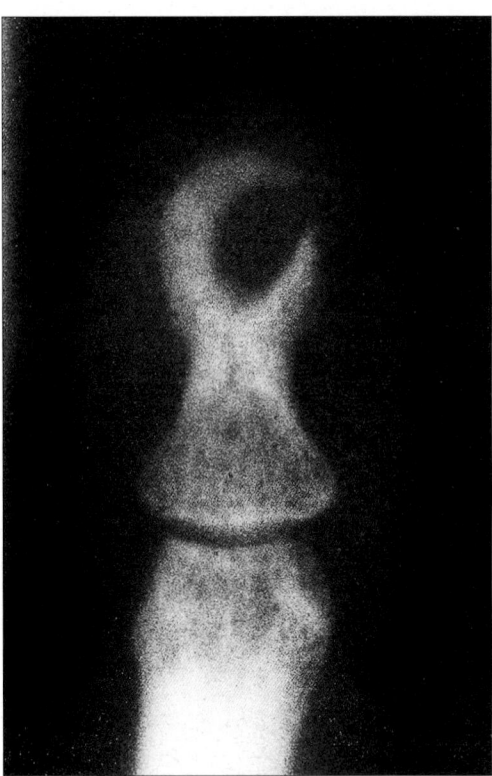

Fig. 24.168
Verrucous carcinoma: this radiograph of a digital lesion shows gross osteolytic change. By courtesy of R.A. Marsden, MD, St George's Hospital, London, UK.

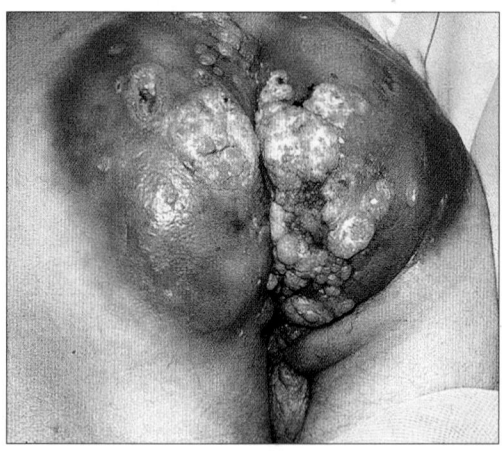

Fig. 24.169
Verrucous carcinoma: Buschke-Löwenstein variant showing massive infiltration of the buttocks and perineum with numerous sinuses. By courtesy of A. Grassegger, MD, University of Innsbruck, Austria.

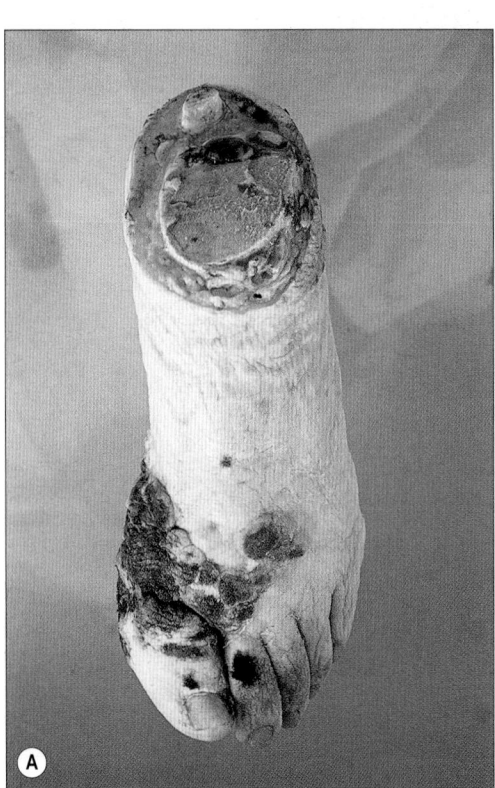

(A)

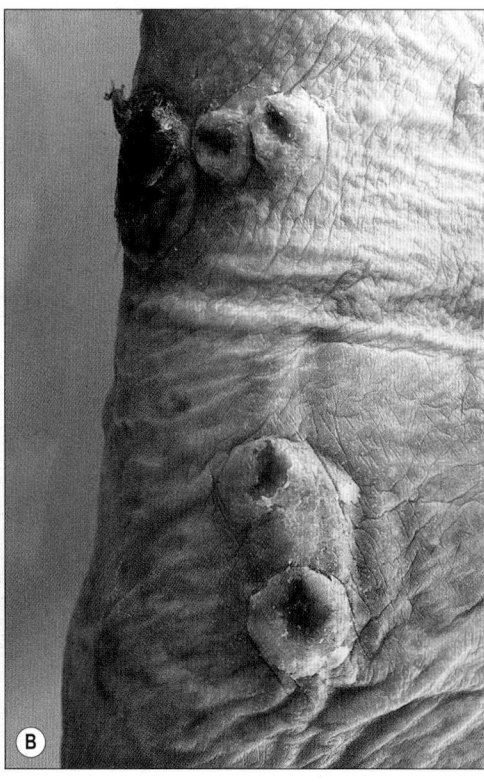

(B)

Fig. 24.170
Verrucous carcinoma: (**A**) this tumor, which arose on the sole of the foot, penetrated through to the dorsal surface and (**B**) metastasized to the skin of the shin. The popliteal lymph nodes were also affected. Reproduced with permission from McKee, P.H., Wilkinson, J.D., Corbett, M.F. et al (1981) Clinical and Experimental Dermatology, 6, 613–618, with permission from Blackwell Publishing.

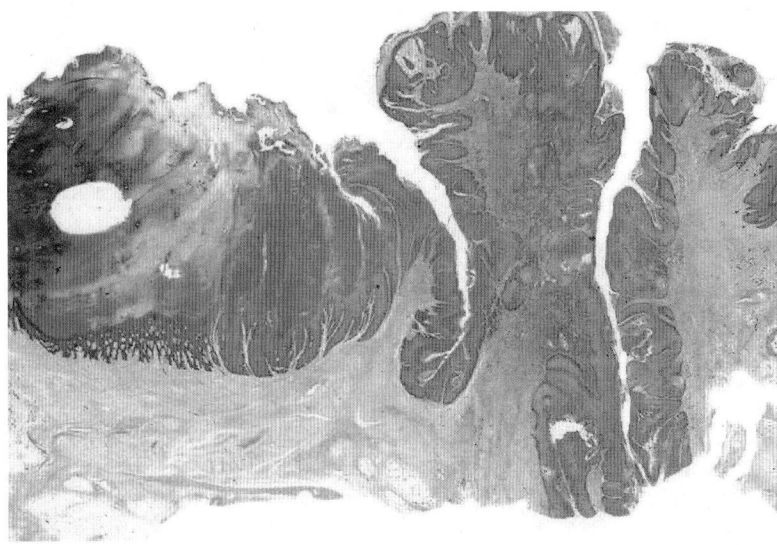

Fig. 24.171
Verrucous carcinoma with coexistent viral wart: a typical plantar wart is present on the left. Arising adjacent to it is a verrucous carcinoma. Reproduced with permission from Wilkinson, J.D., McKee, P.H., Black, M.M. et al (1981) Clinical and Experimental Dermatology, 6, 619–623, with permission from Blackwell Publishing.

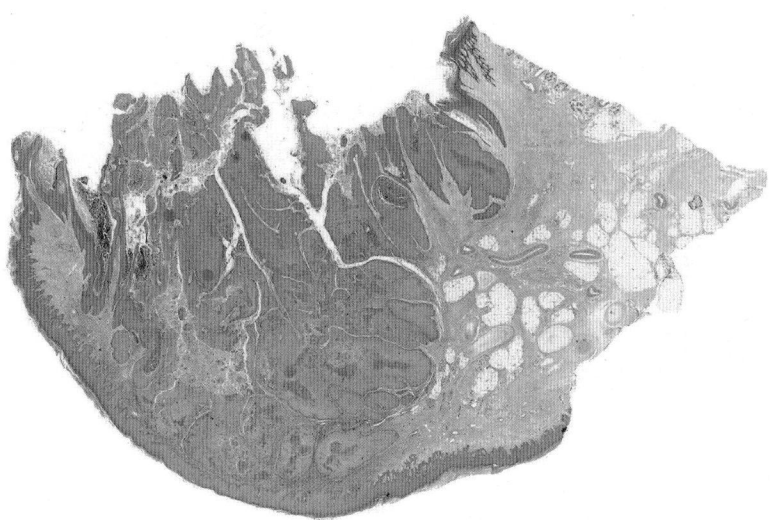

Fig. 24.172
Verrucous carcinoma: this specimen shows the typical features of a verrucous carcinoma. Note the 'pushing' lower border.

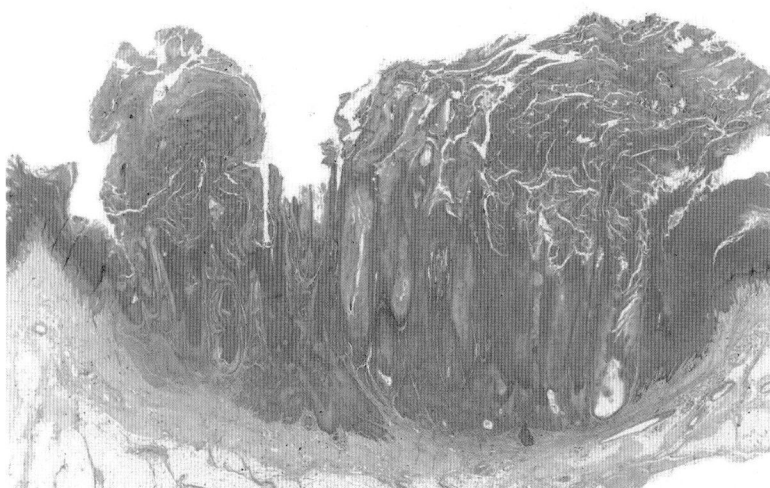

Fig. 24.173
Verrucous carcinoma: this tumor arose on the shin. There is a largely exophytic growth pattern.

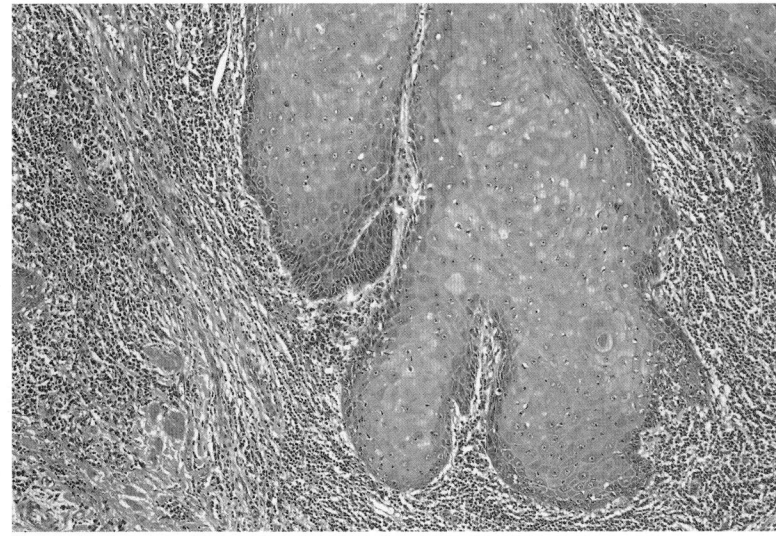

Fig. 24.174
Verrucous carcinoma: the invasive component of the tumor consists of broad bulbous processes composed of extensively keratinized, well-differentiated squamous epithelium.

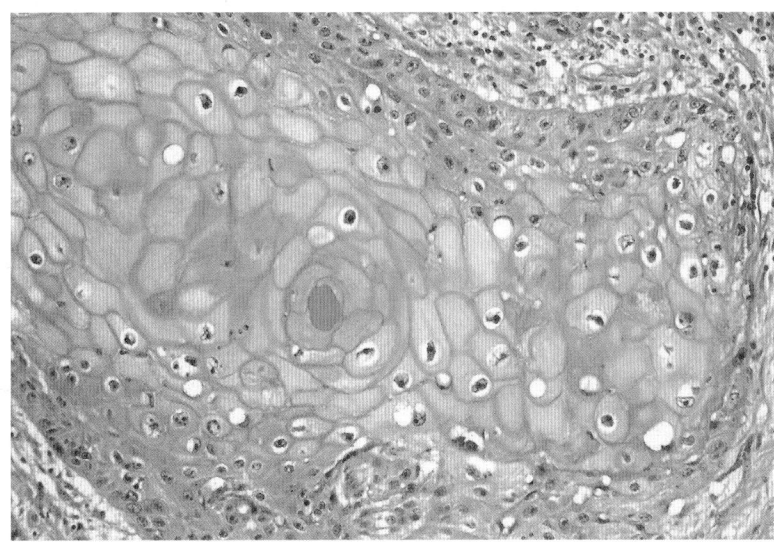

Fig. 24.175
Verrucous carcinoma: close-up view.

deeply penetrating, bulbous processes showing a characteristic 'pushing' margin in contrast to the infiltrative border of an ordinary squamous cell carcinoma.

Keratinization is usually massive and when accompanied by necrosis gives rise to the sinuses so characteristic of this tumor. Pleomorphism is minimal, as is mitotic activity, which is usually related predominantly to the basal layers of the epithelium. Intercellular bridges are invariably conspicuous, and a feature of many verrucous carcinomas is the presence of marked intracellular edema giving the cytoplasm a watery, glassy appearance (*Figs 24.174–24.176*). Intraepithelial abscesses are common and a heavy chronic inflammatory cell infiltrate is often evident in the adjacent lamina propria or dermis.

Differential diagnosis

Distinguishing between viral warts and verrucous carcinoma can sometimes be difficult, if not impossible, particularly when only superficial specimens or extremely fragmented tissues are available for study. The problem is worsened in those lesions that appear to have arisen within pre-existent viral warts or condylomata when typical koilocytosis may be evident. In cases of doubt, repeated deeper biopsies are essential. Examination of these reveals

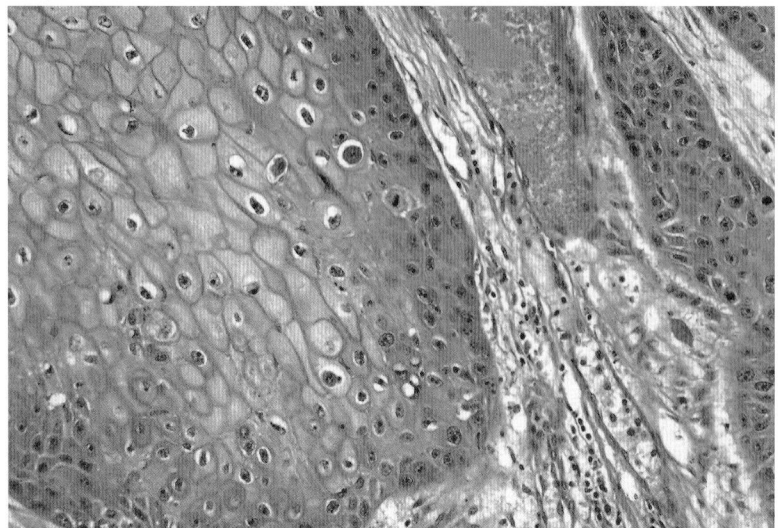

Fig. 24.176
Verrucous carcinoma: the tumor is composed of well-differentiated epithelium. Mitoses are usually inconspicuous and basally located.

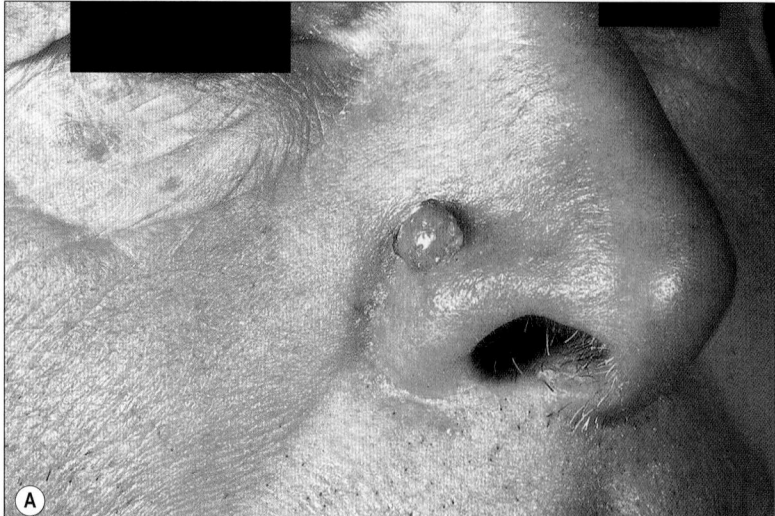

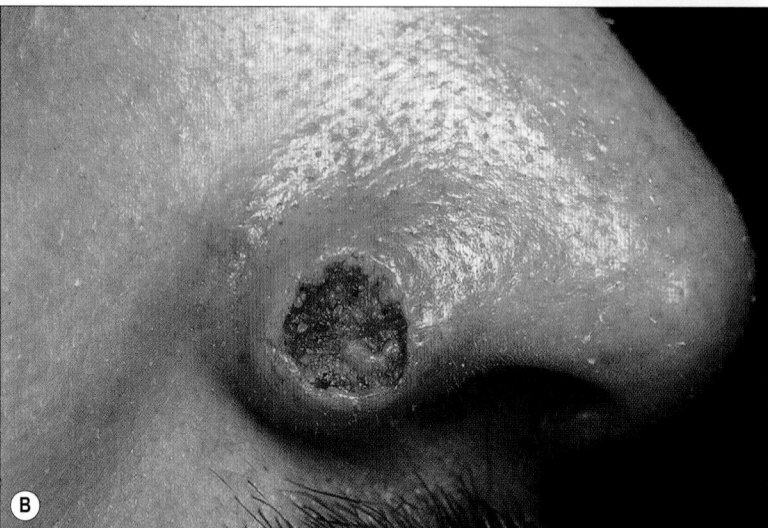

Fig. 24.177
Keratoacanthoma: (**A**) typical dome-shaped lesion on the nose, a commonly affected site; (**B**) in this example, the central crater is particularly well developed. By courtesy of the Institute of Dermatology, London, UK.

infiltration of the underlying tissues in verrucous carcinomas, whereas warts and condylomata have typically exophytic growth patterns.

Cutaneous verrucous carcinoma can be distinguished from keratoacanthoma by the clinical history, architectural differences, and the depth of infiltration. Keratoacanthoma characteristically does not extend beyond the depth of the eccrine sweat glands in contrast to verrucous carcinoma, which commonly involves the subcutaneous fat and beyond.

It is important to restrict the diagnosis of verrucous carcinoma to tumors that are entirely well differentiated and lack pleomorphism or an infiltrative growth pattern. If foci of the latter are evident it is more appropriate to diagnose the tumor as a conventional squamous cell carcinoma.

Keratoacanthoma

Keratoacanthoma (molluscum sebaceum) is a rapidly growing skin tumor arising predominantly on the exposed surfaces of the body.[1-3] Although believed to be of follicular infundibular derivation and, therefore, not strictly speaking a tumor of the epidermis, it is included in this section because of its histologic similarities to squamous cell carcinoma.[4,5]

Few entities in dermatology have been responsible for as much controversy as keratoacanthoma.[6] It has been variously described as a benign tumor, a pseudomalignancy, a regressing malignancy, and as a variant of squamous cell carcinoma.[7-9] Cited examples have documented persistent[10] and recurrent tumors, perineural infiltration, vascular involvement, and metastatic spread.[8,11-16] Despite the presence of perineural infiltration these lesions are said not to show metastatic spread or recurrence.[15] In contrast, however, there are cases that apparently fulfill both the clinical features and 'diagnostic histologic criteria' of keratoacanthoma and yet behave in a malignant fashion.[17-19] Although regarded by many as a variant of squamous cells carcinoma, this view is controversial and not universally accepted.

Clinical features

A variety of subtypes have been recognized.[7,20,21] Most common is the solitary keratoacanthoma. This is predominantly a tumor of the white-skinned races, Asians and Afro-Caribbeans rarely being affected.[22] Usually it appears to be related to excessive exposure to UVB and therefore lesions are most commonly found on sun-damaged skin, particularly of the face (*Fig. 24.177*), forearms, wrists, and backs of the hands.[20,23-25] Conjunctival lesions have also been very rarely described, predominantly in middle-aged males.[26-30] Other infrequently affected sites include the tongue, penis, vulva, oral mucosa, lip, sole, perianal skin, and anal canal.[26,31-40] The lesions may be multiple.[27,41] Intersex variation is evident: lesions on the calves are not uncommon in females but are rare in males, while the dorsum of the hand is a common site in males but not in females.[3] Keratoacanthoma is diagnosed

more often in males than in females (2–3:1) and increases in incidence with age, most patients being in their sixth or seventh decade.[20,42] Presentation in children is rare.[43] Although it is not uncommon in colder, temperate climates, the incidence increases dramatically with diminishing latitude.[42] Typical squamous cell carcinoma occurs at least three times more often than keratoacanthoma.[20,44]

Clinically, solitary keratoacanthoma presents as a smooth, hemispherical papule that rapidly enlarges over the course of a few weeks to produce a 1- to 2-cm diameter, discrete, round or oval, often flesh-colored umbilicated nodule with a central keratin-filled crater (*Figs 24.178 and 24.179*).[20] Pigmentation is exceedingly rare.[45] Lesions larger than 3 cm in diameter are sometimes known as giant keratoacanthoma (*Fig. 24.180*).[46-50] Occasionally, multiple lesions are present.[43,51-55] Usually, involution then occurs with tumor resorption and loss of the keratin plug, to leave a depressed, hypopigmented scar.[7] The lifespan of a typical keratoacanthoma is 4–6 months. Recurrence following surgical intervention may occur in up to 8% of patients.[3]

Agglomerate keratoacanthoma consists of several lesions coalescing to form a single large plaque, which may persist for up to 6 months and then undergo regression.[20]

Keratoacanthoma centrifugum marginatum (multinodular keratoacanthoma) is extremely rare and is characterized by marked peripheral expansion; lesions up to 20 cm in diameter have been recorded.[55-64] The central area heals as the tumor expands, but often resolution takes longer (6–12

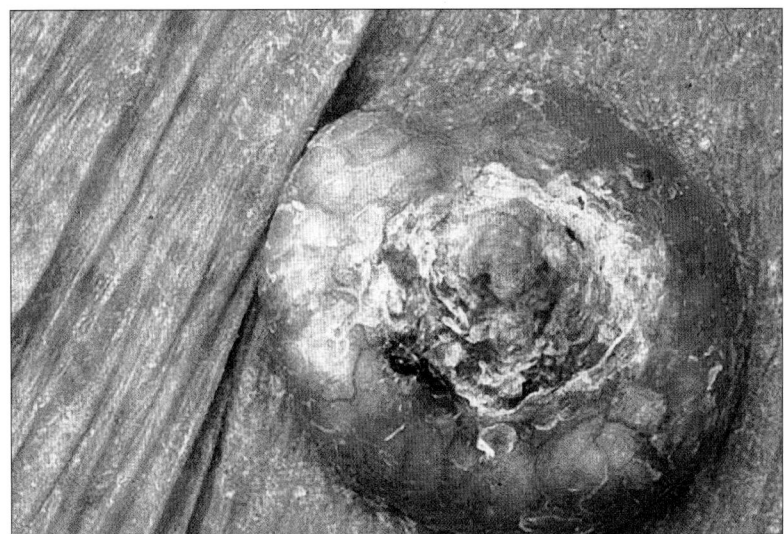

Fig. 24.178
Keratoacanthoma: close-up view of keratotic plug. By courtesy of the Institute of Dermatology, London, UK.

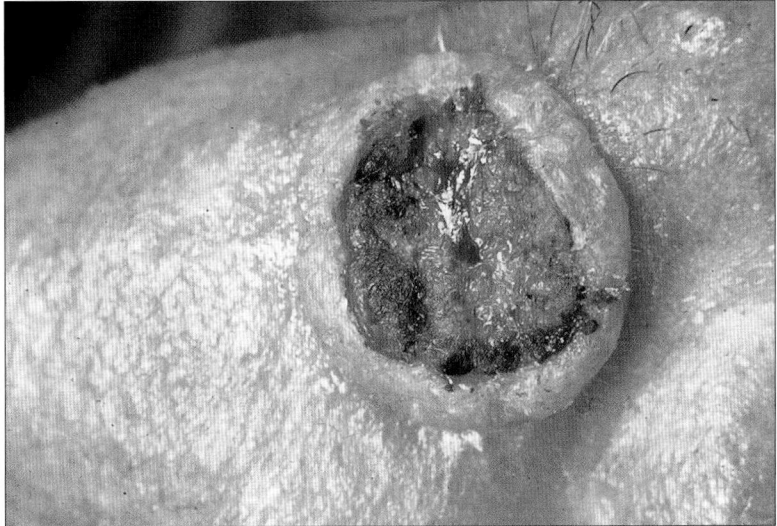

Fig. 24.179
Keratoacanthoma: the crater border is clearly seen in this example. By courtesy of the Institute of Dermatology, London, UK.

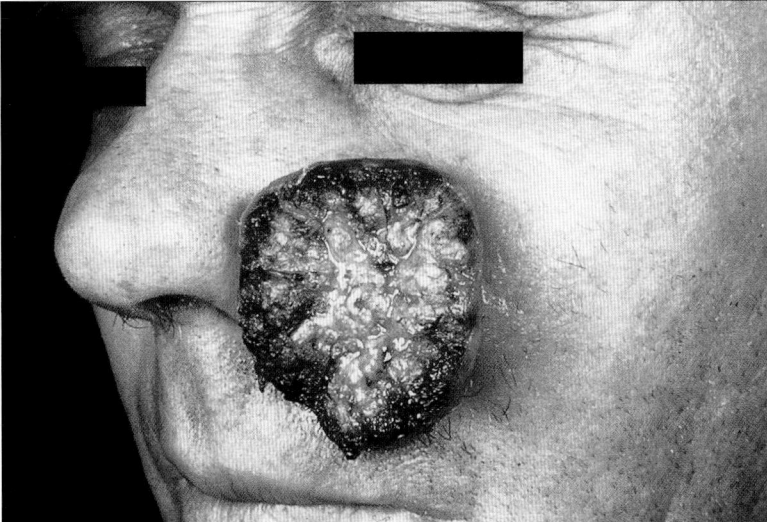

Fig. 24.180
Giant keratoacanthoma: massive variants, such as seen here, are associated with considerable tissue damage and scarring. By courtesy of the Institute of Dermatology, London, UK.

months) than that of the more conventional variant. Multiple lesions may rarely be encountered.[55,58–60,65] Some examples have persisted for many years, shown no tendency for spontaneous resolution, and have been associated with considerable tissue destruction.[56] It would be particularly appropriate to regard these latter as low-grade squamous cell carcinomas.

A peculiar rare tumor known as subungual keratoacanthoma has also been delineated.[66–77] Although histologically similar to the cutaneous type, its apparent derivation from the nail matrix rather than the follicular infundibulum suggests a different histogenesis, and it appears to behave in a more destructive fashion than ordinary keratoacanthoma.[71–73] Lesions predominantly affect the thumb and forefinger and present with pain, swelling, and erythema[67] and may mimic chronic paronychia.[78] Radiological studies reveal a characteristic cup-shaped area of osteolysis with absent periosteal reaction or reactive new bone formation. The tumor appears to respond well to curettage, the recurrence rate being only 14%.[69] These lesions are identical to the subungual tumors of incontinentia pigmenti.[79,80] An association with steel wool has been postulated[81] and a familial case has been reported to occur in association with ectodermal dysplasia.[82]

Keratoacanthoma may rarely develop within a pre-existent nevus sebaceous or represent a manifestation of the Muir-Torre syndrome.[83–86]

A variety of extremely rare syndromes have been described in which patients present with large numbers of keratoacanthomas:

- Familial primary self-healing squamous epitheliomata of the skin (Fergusson-Smith syndrome) has been documented, largely in a Scottish kindred, and is a rare, but distinct, clinical entity with an autosomal dominant mode of inheritance.[87] It is three times more common in males than in females.[20] Patients, usually in childhood or early adulthood, develop multiple (sometimes hundreds) recurrent tumors (Fig. 24.181). Although sun-exposed skin is predominantly affected, lesions may also be found on the external genitalia and scalp and are sometimes trauma induced.[20,88] The lesions are much slower to resolve and may be associated with greater tissue damage and scarring than with the more commonly encountered variant.

- In eruptive keratoacanthoma (Grzybowski syndrome), patients develop enormous numbers (hundreds to thousands) of follicular papules 1–5 mm in diameter.[89–102] The sex incidence is equal.[20] The lesions, which are often pruritic and sometimes painful, often present on sun-exposed skin, but may become generalized. Ectropion is a distressing complication. Koebnerization is occasionally evident.

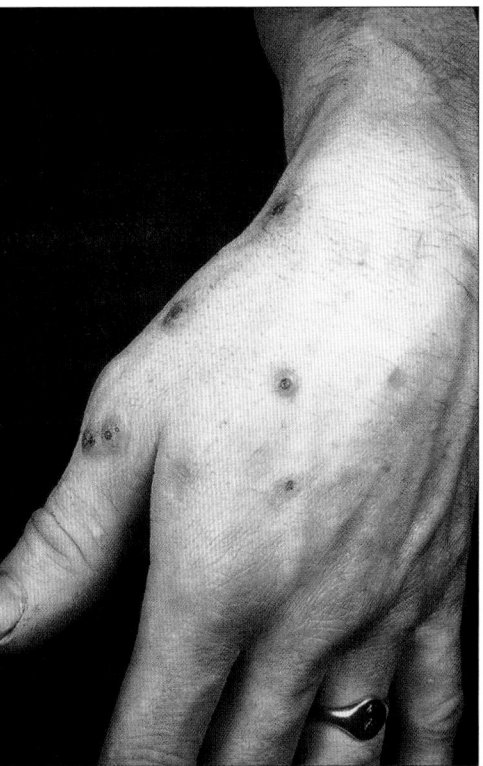

Fig. 24.181
Fergusson-Smith syndrome: numerous small, but otherwise typical, lesions are evident. By courtesy of the Institute of Dermatology, London, UK.

Similar keratotic squamoproliferative lesions may develop in the mouth, pharynx, and larynx.[89] Long-term follow up of patients with this variant has not disclosed any evidence of metastatic potential.[90,91] Eruptive lesions may also develop in the immunosuppressed.[103] Associations of eruptive keratoacanthomas have also been noted with pembrolizumab, laser resurfacing, skin grafting, photodynamic therapy, leflunomide, tattoos, ruxolitinib, quizartinib, imiquimod, and sorafenib.[104–113] These lesions however, are not related to eruptive keratoacanthomas of Grzybowski type.

- A mixed syndrome (Witten and Zak syndrome) combining the features of the above two variants has also been documented.[56,114,115]

There is no evidence that solitary keratoacanthoma is associated with an increased incidence of internal malignancy.[3]

Pathogenesis and histologic features

Keratoacanthoma may be induced in a variety of experimental animals by painting the skin with coal tar derivatives.[116] Although now rare, a human counterpart has been described in people who had prolonged contact with pitch and tar.[1] More recently, keratoacanthoma has occasionally been described in patients receiving coal tar preparations to treat psoriasis.

Keratoacanthomas have been shown to be clonal and numerous chromosomal abnormalities have since been identified including trisomy 7, gains of 1p, 8q, 9q and deletions of 3p, 9p, 19p, 19q, and a translocation involving chromosomes 2 and 8.[117–120] RAS mutations (HRAS and NRAS) have been noted.[121] Microsatellite instability has been observed in some lesions.[86,122,123] Most tumors, however, appear to have a UVB-mediated pathogenesis.[23,26] The great majority arise on sun-exposed skin and signs of actinic damage are usually evident. There is an increased incidence in xeroderma pigmentosum and in those who are chronically immunosuppressed, particularly following renal transplantation.[20,42,124,125] Concurrent UVB-induced epidermal lesions, such as actinic keratoses and basal cell and squamous cell carcinoma, are commonly present.[3]

While most lesions are negative,[126,127] HPV DNA has been demonstrated in a small number of lesions.[121,128–132] Subtypes that have been identified include HPV types 5, 9, 10, 14, 16, 19, 20, 21, 25, 37, 38, 49, and 80.[133] HPV is identified more frequently in tumors from immunosuppressed rather than immunocompetent patients.[133]

Rarely, keratoacanthoma may develop at the site of scarring due to prior trauma, radiation or skin grafting, or in association with inflammatory dermatoses, such as lichen planus, hypertrophic lichen planus, vitiligo, discoid lupus erythematosus, atopic eczema, and psoriasis.[3,134–152] It has also been reported to complicate lesions such as linear epidermal nevus, nevus sebaceous, a pigmented patch in incontinentia pigmenti, pseudoxanthoma elasticum, stasis dermatitis, and sites of treatment for, as well as within, lesions of psoriasis.[153–160] Keratoacanthoma may also be associated with Dowling-Degos disease, hidradenitis suppurativa, suramin therapy, PUVA therapy, and radiotherapy.[161–165]

An accurate diagnosis of keratoacanthoma is totally dependent upon an adequate clinical history. In the absence of this or when only tissue fragments are available for histologic interpretation, it is most inadvisable to make this diagnosis.

The histologic diagnosis depends upon the identification of the typical crateriform architecture.[25] Excisional or deep incisional biopsies across the center of the lesion are therefore required. An established tumor is symmetrical and has both exophytic and endophytic components (Figs 24.182 and 24.183). It consists of an often large central keratin plug (sometimes showing continuity with dilated follicular infundibula) accompanied by marked squamous epithelial proliferation. The epidermis on either side of the lesion is thrown up into a well-formed collarette.

Although the epithelium may occasionally appear mildly pleomorphic, typical keratoacanthoma is characterized by well-differentiated, often pale-staining, eosinophilic, glassy cytoplasm showing a striking tendency towards keratinization (Fig. 24.184). Intracytoplasmic glycogen is often abundant. Necrosis may be evident and microabscesses containing neutrophils are frequently present (Fig. 24.185). Entrapped elastic fibers, particularly when associated with marked solar elastosis, are said to be characteristic.[166,167] The presence of these does not necessarily discriminate

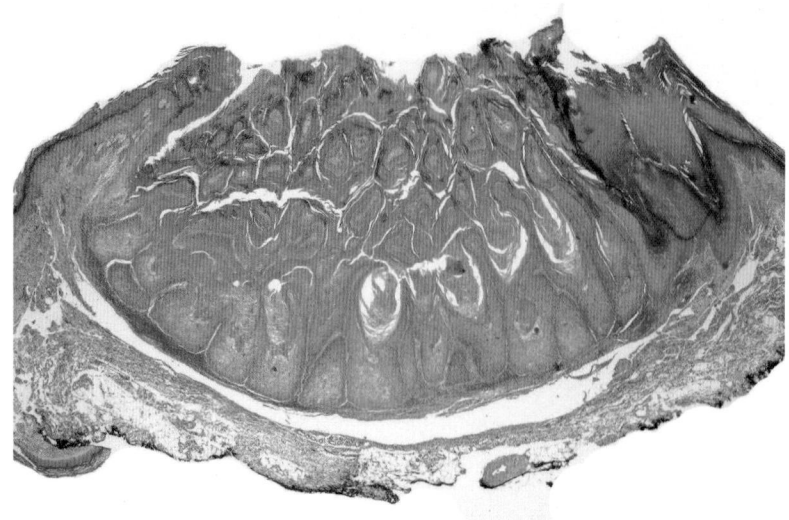

Fig. 24.182
Keratoacanthoma: scanning view of a typical keratoacanthoma showing a well-developed collarette.

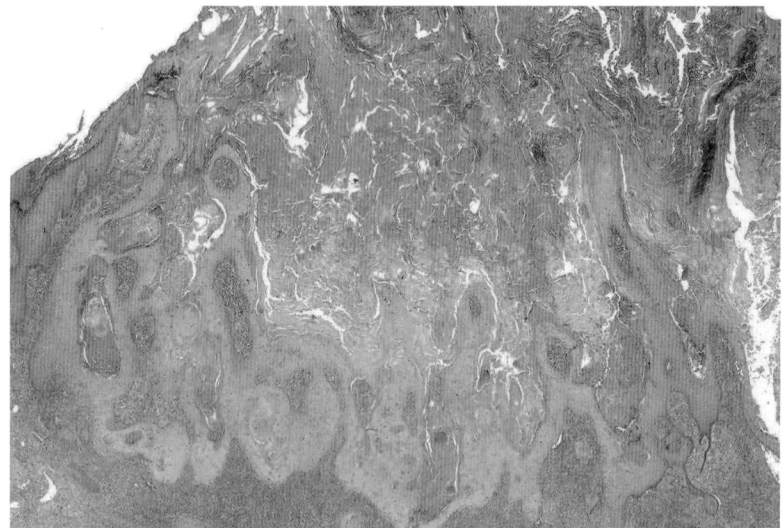

Fig. 24.183
Keratoacanthoma: this example shows the lateral collarette, keratin plug, and underlying proliferating well-differentiated squamous epithelium.

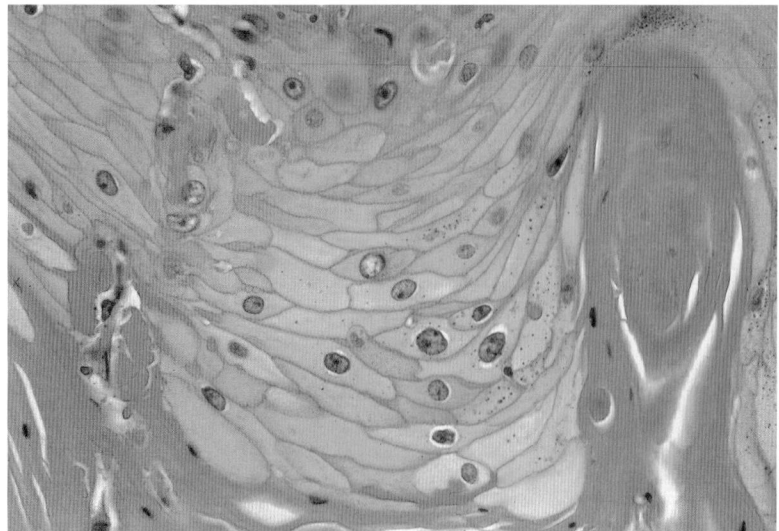

Fig. 24.184
Keratoacanthoma: the proliferating epithelium is well differentiated. The epithelial pallor is characteristic.

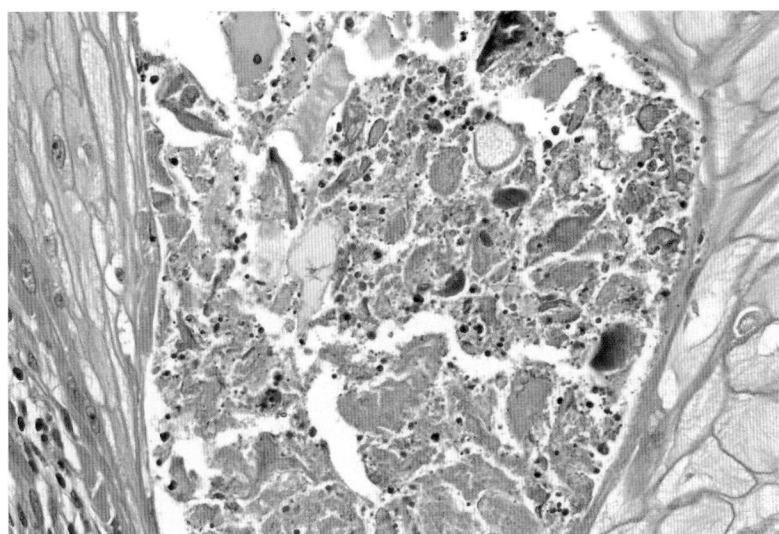

Fig. 24.185
Keratoacanthoma: intraepithelial abscesses as seen in this field are a common finding.

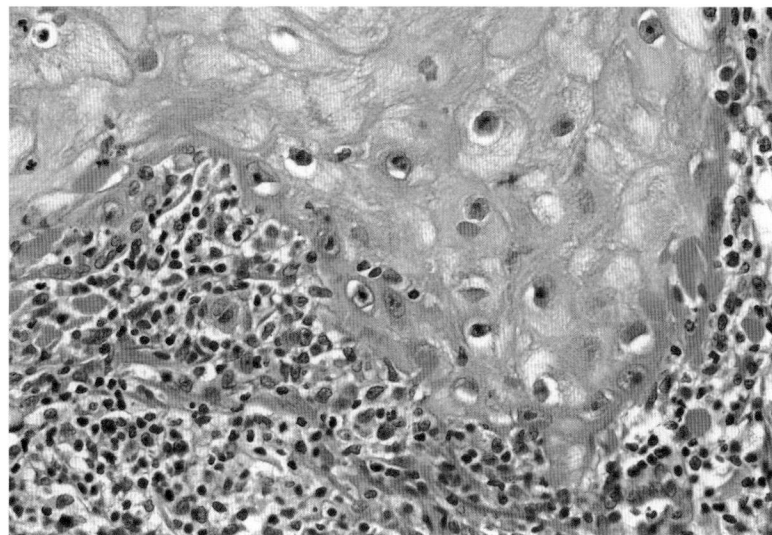

Fig. 24.187
Keratoacanthoma: the tumor is commonly associated with a mixed chronic inflammatory cell infiltrate.

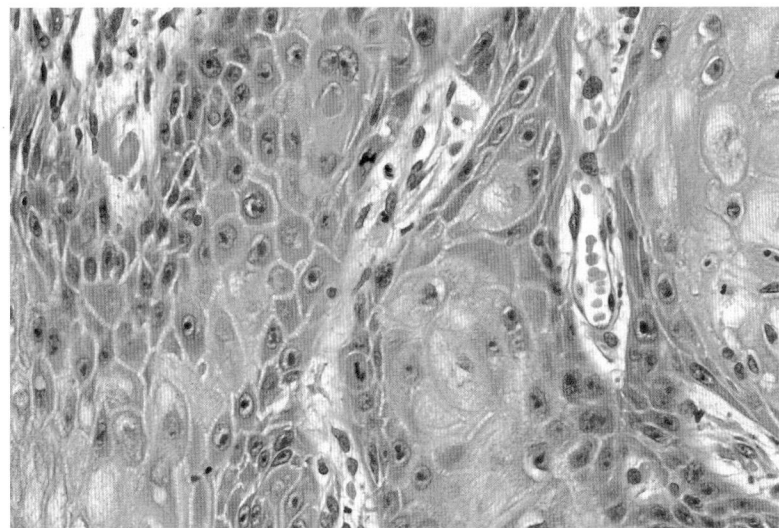

Fig. 24.186
Keratoacanthoma: mitoses are generally limited to the basal epithelial layer.

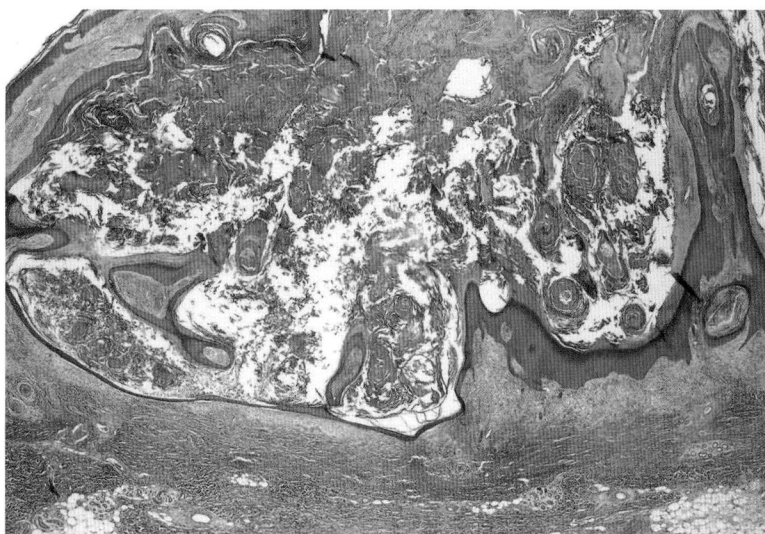

Fig. 24.188
Regressing keratoacanthoma: the keratin plug is still present, but epithelial proliferation is markedly diminished and the floor of the lesion is beginning to flatten. Note the collarette on either side.

between keratoacanthoma and frank squamous cell carcinoma. However, their identification within foci of differentiating epithelium in the center of the lesion and/or their disposal by transepidermal elimination appears to correlate well with a diagnosis of keratoacanthoma.[129] Rarely, acantholysis is a feature.[20] The tumor may show conspicuous mitotic figures, but these are almost invariably normal and are found predominantly within the proliferative epithelium at the periphery of the tumor lobules (*Fig. 24.186*). Growth of the lesion rarely extends beyond the depth of the sweat glands and is frequently accompanied by a vascular stroma, often heavily infiltrated by lymphocytes, histiocytes, plasma cells, neutrophils, and variable numbers of eosinophils (*Fig. 24.187*).[20]

With progressive aging (and regression) of the lesion, the keratin horn is lost and the proliferating epithelium tends to flatten out, leaving a somewhat papillomatous base with underlying chronic inflammation and fibrosis (*Figs 24.188 and 24.189*).[168] The infiltrate sometimes adopts a lichenoid distribution and is composed predominantly of cytotoxic T cells that may play a role in lesion regression (*Fig. 24.190*).[20,169,170] At the edges a residual collarette may sometimes be evident. Not infrequently, regressing keratoacanthoma is accompanied by a foreign body giant cell reaction to released keratin. The mechanism of regression is uncertain. Although immunological factors are likely to be of significance, it has been suggested that apoptosis may be particularly important.[20]

Analysis of keratin and filaggrin expression points to differentiation towards the outer root sheath in keratoacanthoma.[171]

Unusual histologic features include atypical sweat duct hyperplasia and glandular proliferation, as well as coexistence with basal cell carcinoma and melanoma in situ.[172-175]

Classic squamous cell carcinoma arising from typical keratoacanthomas is a rare phenomenon seen in the elderly.[176]

So-called subungual keratoacanthoma arises from the nail matrix and presents as a keratin-filled cystic cavity lined by abundant, well-differentiated squamous epithelium showing marked dyskeratosis.[67] Mitoses are few and basally located. Because the diagnosis invariably follows surgical treatment, the biological behavior of this tumor is uncertain. Regression has not been documented. Despite some histologic overlap with verrucous carcinoma, the absence of frequent recurrences argues against this diagnosis.

Differential diagnosis

There are marked similarities between keratoacanthoma and squamous cell carcinoma and occasionally it may be impossible to distinguish the two on clinical, let alone histologic, grounds though many exert great effort to do so.[25,177,178]

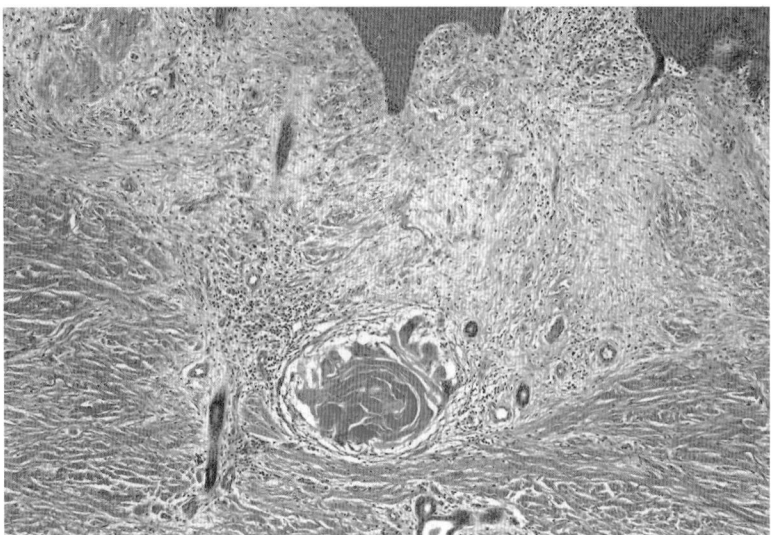

Fig. 24.189
Regressing keratoacanthoma: a prominent giant cell reaction to free keratin is often present at the base of the lesion with adjacent scarring.

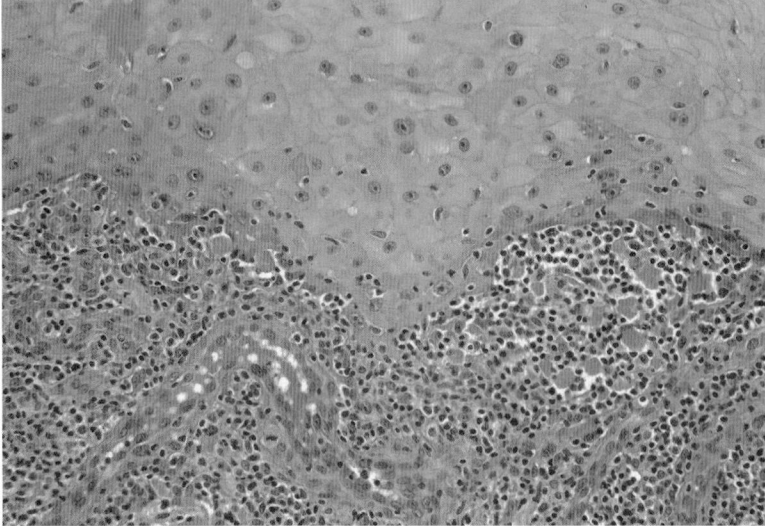

Fig. 24.190
Keratoacanthoma: in this example there are marked interface changes with conspicuous cytoid bodies.

Keratoacanthomas showing a deeply infiltrative growth pattern, perineural invasion, and vascular (venous) involvement have occasionally been reported. Such lesions commonly affect the head, particularly the lips and the nose. Despite the apparent absence of metastases, it is difficult to reconcile such features with a biologically benign condition.[12] Personal experience (EC) suggests that they do not have a more aggressive behavior. Just as with conventional squamous cell carcinoma, such histologic changes do not necessarily always correlate with an aggressive clinical outcome. Nevertheless, the presence of these traditionally malignant features in an otherwise clinically and histologically typical lesion adds considerable weight to the concept that keratoacanthoma represents a variant of squamous cell carcinoma. Perhaps keratoacanthoma constitutes the most benign end of a spectrum with intermediate more aggressive stages finally merging with overt squamous cell carcinoma. Progression is likely to be dependent on genetic, environmental, and immunological factors.

While earlier studies failed to identify significant differences in H-ras activation, p53 expression, nucleolar organizer region enumeration, cyclins, cyclin-dependent kinases and Ki-67 (MIB-1) proliferation fractions in classical solitary keratoacanthoma, regressing keratoacanthoma and variably differentiated squamous cell carcinomas, data suggest significant differences in the expression of bcl-xL, TP53, and COX-2 as well as telomerase activity

and the cytolytic receptor P2X7.[179–192] Expression of TP53 and MIB-1 may also differ in subungual keratoacanthomas compared to subungual squamous cell carcinoma.[193] Flow cytometric analysis of proliferation indices and S-phase fractions, however, fail to discriminate between these two lesions and studies on proteins related to tumor invasion such as matrix metalloproteinases, E-cadherin, catenins, and syndecan-1 also revealed only subtle differences in the staining pattern between keratoacanthoma and invasive squamous cell carcinoma.[194–196] There is some evidence to suggest that vascular cell adhesion molecule (VCAM) and intercellular adhesion molecule (ICAM) expression may be of some value in distinguishing between keratoacanthoma and more typical well-differentiated squamous cell carcinoma.[197] All of these are only relative guides and distinction requires careful observation and clinical correlation.

Usually, the clinical history and histopathological features allow a diagnosis of keratoacanthoma and predict a trouble-free outcome, but if there is any doubt about the potential biological behavior of a lesion, complete surgical excision, as for squamous cell carcinoma, is recommended.

Metaplastic carcinoma of the skin (carcinosarcoma, carcinoma with heterologous differentiation)

Clinical features

Metaplastic carcinoma of the skin is an exceedingly rare malignant cutaneous neoplasm with only a few cases reported in the literature.[1–13] It typically arises on sun-damaged skin as a nodular lesion ranging in size from 1 to 15 cm and often showing ulceration. The duration of these tumors ranges from several months to many years, frequently presenting with recent change. The most commonly affected sites include the face and scalp.[1–7,14,15] Although it presents in a wide age range, metaplastic carcinoma is predominantly a tumor of the elderly. Clinically, there are no distinguishing features and the differential diagnosis is broad. Metaplastic carcinoma of skin has also been reported in patients with nevoid basal cell carcinoma syndrome and Brooke-Spiegler syndrome.[16,17] In contrast to its counterparts in visceral organs, cutaneous metaplastic carcinoma does not appear to be necessarily associated with a high mortality rate.[14] Based on the few reported cases in the literature with albeit limited follow-up intervals (median: 19 months), the overall recurrence and metastasis rate is 22% with a mortality of 11%.[1–7,15] Data from a recent meta-analysis indicate that younger age at presentation, a history of recent growth in a long-standing tumor, as well as size greater than 2 cm correlate with poor prognosis.[18] This analysis further suggests that 'epidermal derived' tumors, in which the epithelial component represents either squamous cell carcinoma or basal cell carcinoma, are associated with a better prognosis and a 5-year disease-free survival of 70% compared to 'adnexal derived' tumors that are associated with a malignant skin adnexal epithelial component. These tumors are characterized by poor 5-year disease-free survival of 25%.[18] While 'epidermal derived' metaplastic carcinoma is largely a tumor of sun-exposed sites of the head and neck with a strong predilection for elderly males, those associated with a skin adnexal component are often characterized by a long-standing mass and younger age at presentation.[18]

Pathogenesis and histologic features

Although metaplastic carcinoma has been described at multiple sites other than the skin, little is known about their histogenesis. Possible explanations include the development of separate neoplasms at the same site, so-called collision tumors, although this appears to be an exceedingly rare phenomenon. Alternatively, epithelial tumors may (by as yet unknown mechanisms) induce sarcomatous change in the adjacent stroma.[19] Currently favored, however, is the hypothesis that epithelial tumors undergo further genetic change, enabling metaplastic differentiation towards other epithelial as well as mesenchymal components. This theory is favored by the identification of a single monoclonal population of both epithelial and mesenchymal elements in such tumors from various sites including uterus, gastrointestinal tract, lung, breast, soft tissue, and bladder.[20] Recent genomic profiling of cutaneous carcinosarcoma cases suggests that TP53 mutations are common and other perturbations such as inactivating mutations in CDKN2A or

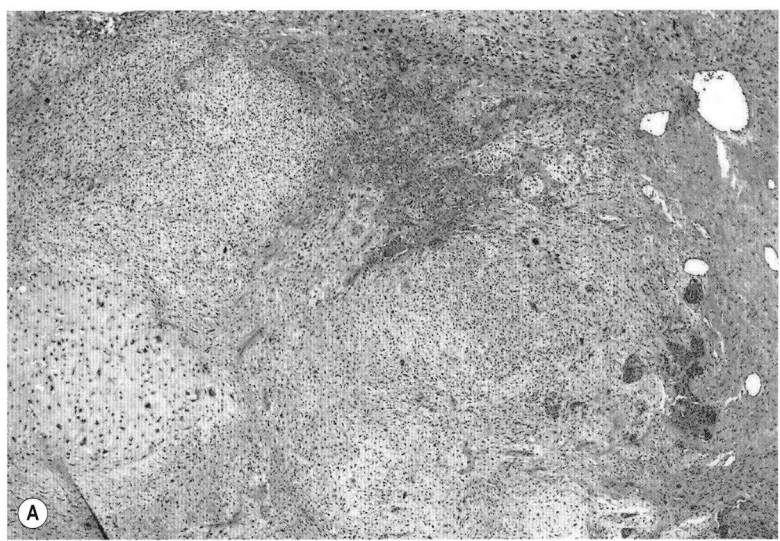

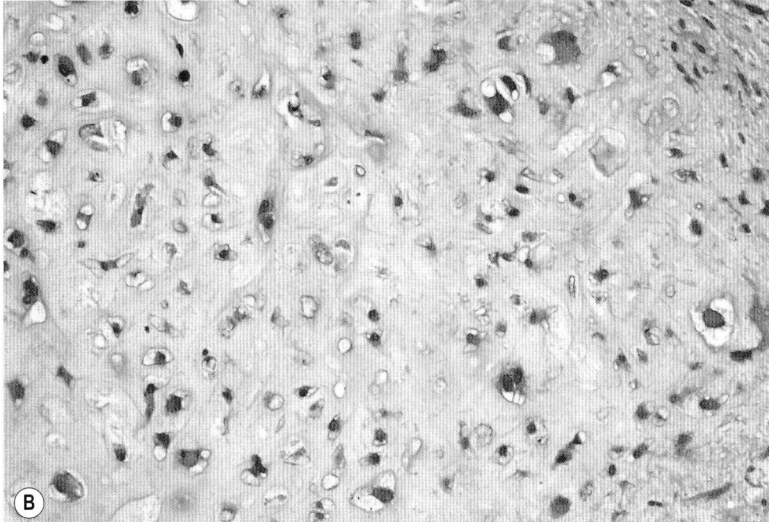

Fig. 24.191
(**A, B**) Metaplastic squamous cell carcinoma: this example displays chondroid differentiation in addition to squamous elements, hence its alternative designation of carcinosarcoma.

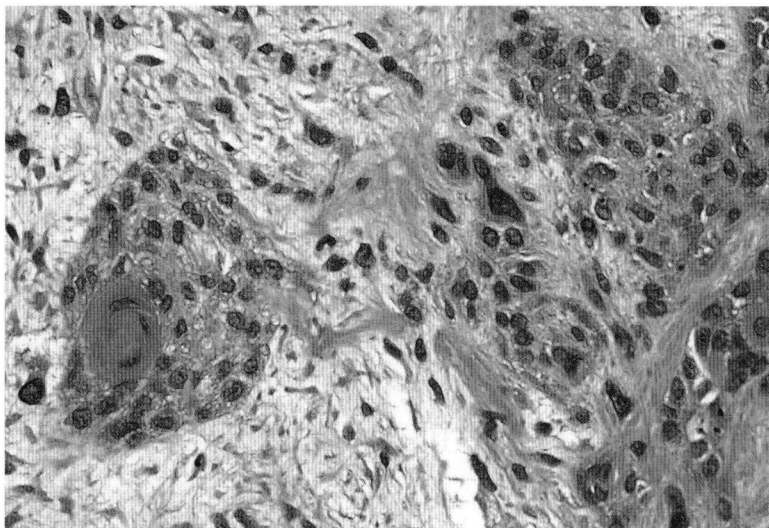

Fig. 24.192
Metaplastic squamous cell carcinoma: high-power view of squamous component.

The osteoblastic and chondroblastic components are readily identified on hematoxylin and eosin stained sections while skeletal and smooth muscle differentiation can be confirmed with immunohistochemistry for smooth muscle actin, desmin, or myogenin.

Differential diagnosis

Since metaplastic carcinoma of the skin is a rare tumor, the diagnosis may be difficult and includes a broad differential. The mesenchymal component must be distinguished from reactive or desmoplastic stroma as well as from atypical fibroxanthoma or spindle cell squamous cell carcinoma. Cutaneous sarcomas such as dermatofibrosarcoma protuberans or leiomyosarcoma may also enter the differential diagnosis. Cutaneous metastases from high-grade sarcomas of bone and soft tissues are infrequent, and only very few cases of primary cutaneous osteosarcoma have been reported in the literature.[43,44] It is imperative to recognize the biphasic nature of this neoplasm, i.e., the presence of both the malignant epithelial as well as the malignant mesenchymal components, and careful sampling of the tissue is essential. Metastasis from metaplastic carcinoma of visceral origin constitutes the main differential diagnosis. This is of great importance since metastatic lesions are associated with a much poorer prognosis than primary cutaneous tumors.

Squamous cell carcinoma with chronic lymphocytic leukemia

Very occasionally, in patients with chronic lymphocytic leukemia, primary cutaneous tumors (notably squamous cell carcinoma and basal cell carcinoma) may be accompanied by a dense population of monomorphic tumor lymphocytes (*Fig. 24.193*).[1-4] It has been thought that this is of no prognostic significance.[1] A recent series of 42 patients chronic lymphocytic leukemia and cutaneous squamous cell carcinoma suggests that the carcinomas may behave more aggressively; however, this may not be related to colonization of the carcinoma by neoplastic lymphocytes, but rather immunosuppression or some other systemic effect associated with the chronic lymphocytic leukemia.[5]

Xeroderma pigmentosum

Xeroderma pigmentosum (XP; first described by Kaposi) is an autosomal recessive condition with an incidence of approximately 1 : 250 000.[1,2] The sexes are affected equally. There is a high frequency of parental consanguinity.[3] It is a heterogeneous disorder, characterized by an inability to repair DNA damage induced by UV irradiation through the nucleotide excision repair pathway.[4-9] One of the effects of this radiation (wavelength 280–320 nm) is the induction of potentially mutagenic dimers between adjacent pyrimidines (e.g., thymine) on a single strand of DNA. In normal

oncogenic mutations in *PIK3CA* are present in both the malignant epithelial and mesenchymal components.[21,22] Carcinosarcomas with a basal cell carcinoma epithelial element show the same mutations in *PTCH1* characteristic of classic basal cell carcinoma.[23]

Metaplastic carcinoma of the skin is a biphasic tumor composed of malignant epithelial and heterologous mesenchymal components similar to its counterpart in visceral organs including uterus, ovary, lung, bladder, breast, and larynx. The malignant epithelial component in cutaneous tumors comprises squamous cell carcinoma, basal cell carcinoma, and malignant adnexal neoplasms including malignant pilomatrixoma, spiradenocarcinoma, and eccrine porocarcinoma as well as malignant trichoblastoma and Merkel cell tumor.[1-7,14,18,24-37] The mesenchymal component shows histologic features of malignancy and consists of spindled and pleomorphic cells showing marked nuclear atypia, necrosis, and numerous as well as atypical mitotic figures. Osteoblastic differentiation is the most commonly identified heterologous element, followed by chondroblastic differentiation (*Figs 24.191 and 24.192*). Only rare examples showing skeletal, smooth muscle, myofibroblastic, fibrosarcomatous, or angiosarcomatous differentiation have been reported.[29,32,38-41] The mesenchymal component is scattered throughout the tumor and sometimes focally merges with the epithelial proliferation.[1-7,24] The pleomorphic spindled cell population may infrequently express cytokeratin but is usually negative for most immunohistochemical markers except vimentin. Expression of p63 may be retained at the transition between epithelial and sarcomatoid components of the tumor.[42]

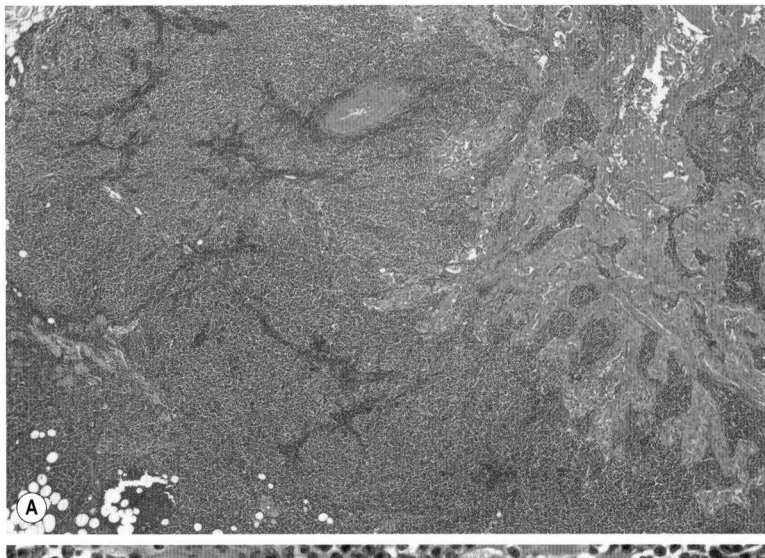

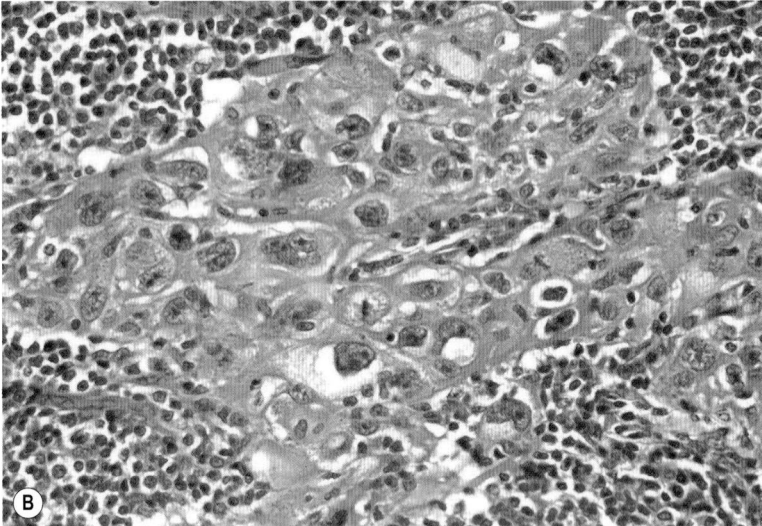

Fig. 24.193
(**A**, **B**) Squamous cell carcinoma with chronic lymphocytic leukemia: this tumor presented on the face of an elderly male patient. The squamous component is surrounded by a dense infiltrate of monotonous lymphocytes with darkly staining nuclei.

individuals, the nucleotide excision repair process ensures that such dimers are excised and replaced, and that there is restoration of correct DNA structure, using specific endonucleases and exonucleases. Persistence of such dimers blocks transcription of messenger RNA and inhibits the development of DNA replication forks, therefore preventing cell division.[9-12] The inability to repair dimers has a critical effect on the germinative basal cells of the epidermis, resulting in an exaggeration of the effects of sunlight, including the expression of mutant genes and subsequent development of cutaneous (and ocular) neoplasms.[13,14]

The impaired excision-repair process can be studied using fibroblast culture techniques. Fibroblasts are irradiated with UV light, incubated with tritiated thymidine, and the amount of the latter incorporated (therefore monitoring DNA repair) evaluated using autoradiography. Patients with xeroderma pigmentosum take up less tritiated thymidine than normal controls.

XP is not a single disease entity.[15] By using fibroblast fusion techniques and assessing DNA repair, at least seven complementation groups (groups A to G) plus an excision-proficient variant group have been discovered.[16-18] Groups H and I have been subsequently reassigned to groups D and C, respectively.[1,16] If fusion of fibroblasts from two patients results in an improvement towards normal uptake of tritiated thymidine following UV irradiation, the patients are genotypically different and belong to different complementation groups. If no increase occurs, then the patients can be

regarded as belonging to the same group. The majority of these complementation groups are associated with enzyme deficiencies in the initial incision stage of the DNA nucleotide excision -repair mechanism.[10]

- XP complementation group A, which is one of the most serious variants, accounting for approximately 25% of cases of this disease, results from mutations in the *XPA* gene localized to 9q34.1.[10,19] *XPA* encodes a zinc finger protein involved in photoproduct recognition and DNA binding by recognition of helical kinks.
- The gene responsible for XP complementation group B *ERCC3* (also known as *XPB*) belongs to the family of DNA helicases and has been localized to chromosome 2 (2q21).
- The *XPC* gene encodes a DNA-binding protein essential for repair of non-transcribed regions of the genome and is localized to chromosome 3p25.1.[20]
- The *ERCC2* gene (also known as *XPD*) represents another helicase located on chromosome 19q13.2.[10,16,21]
- *DDB2* (also termed *XPE*) gene mutations typically result in a mild phenotype. *DDB2* is located on chromosome 11p11.12 and encodes damaged DNA binding protein 2. DBB2 together with DBB1 forms a heterodimer, the DBB complex, which is involved in recognition of damaged DNA.[22-24]
- The *ERCC4* gene (also known as *XPF*) is located on chromosome 16p13.3. This is a rare group and is most commonly seen in Japan.[25]
- The XPG group is rare and patients are severely affected. The causative *ECCR5* gene is located on chromosome 13q32~33.[26]
- Between 80% and 90% of patients with XP have defective excision – repair mechanisms; the residual 10–20% shows no defect of the excision – repair mechanism and is defective in daughter strand repair. The excision proficient XP variant is caused by mutations in the *POLH* gene, a translesion DNA polymerase located at 6p21.1.[2,27-30]

Activated oncogenes (*NRAS*, *HRAS*, *MYC*, etc.) have been demonstrated in skin tumors from patients with XP.[31] This is related to UV-induced DNA damage.[32] Defects of nucleotide excision repair mechanisms may not completely explain the pathogenesis in all cases. Not all patients with serious nucleotide excision repair defects are at risk of developing cutaneous malignancy. Other mechanisms currently under investigation, which could prove to be of importance, include the effects of background skin pigmentation, total UV exposure, and abnormalities of immune surveillance mechanisms.[10,33]

Clinical features

Patients show extreme photosensitivity, which may manifest as a blistering rash on exposure to sunlight, but also may include development of numerous freckles, mainly on sun-exposed parts, accompanied by hypopigmented and atrophic lesions, xerosis, areas of telangiectasia, scarring, and actinic keratoses (*Fig. 24.194*).[1] Patients show a reduced minimal erythema dose of UV light and delayed maximum reaction time.[16] Sooner or later in the course of the disease, patients develop multiple and often widespread tumors, including squamous cell carcinoma, basal cell carcinoma, basisquamous carcinoma, keratoacanthoma, and melanoma as well as, albeit less frequently, atypical fibroxanthoma and cutaneous angiosarcoma.[3,34-42] Patients with xeroderma pigmentosum have a 1000-fold higher incidence of cutaneous neoplasia when compared with a normal population.[43] The face, neck, and head are predominantly affected.[44] The median age for tumor development is 8 years.[44] As the development of these lesions appears to be directly associated with the level of DNA repair capacity,[16] patients with a lower capacity develop larger numbers of tumors at an earlier age.[16,34] Patients with XP also appear to have an increased incidence of internal malignancy.[16,45]

Ocular manifestations, which are varied, develop on areas exposed to UV light and include conjunctivitis with photophobia, loss of eyelashes, corneal ulceration, scarring and perforation, ectropion, entropion, and neoplasms, including squamous cell and basal cell carcinomas of the eyelids, conjunctivae, and cornea.[3,44] Patients with XP complementation group A are at particular risk.[16] Oral lesions, including stenosis and neoplasia, have also been described.[44]

About one patient in five develops neurological symptomatology due to progressive neuronal loss.[1,3] A wide variety of mild to severe abnormalities

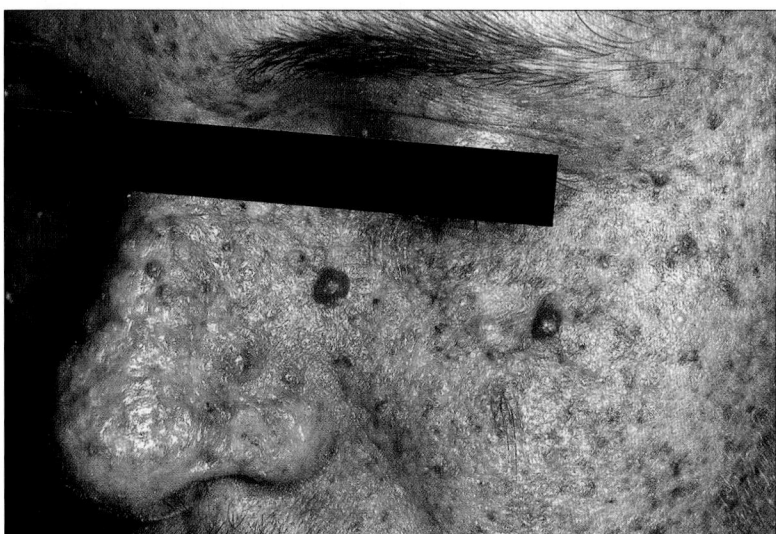

Fig. 24.194
Xeroderma pigmentosum: there are gross changes including marked freckly hyperpigmentation, atrophy, and numerous warty and nodular growths. Telangiectatic vessels are evident. By courtesy of R.A. Marsden, MD, St George's Hospital, London, UK.

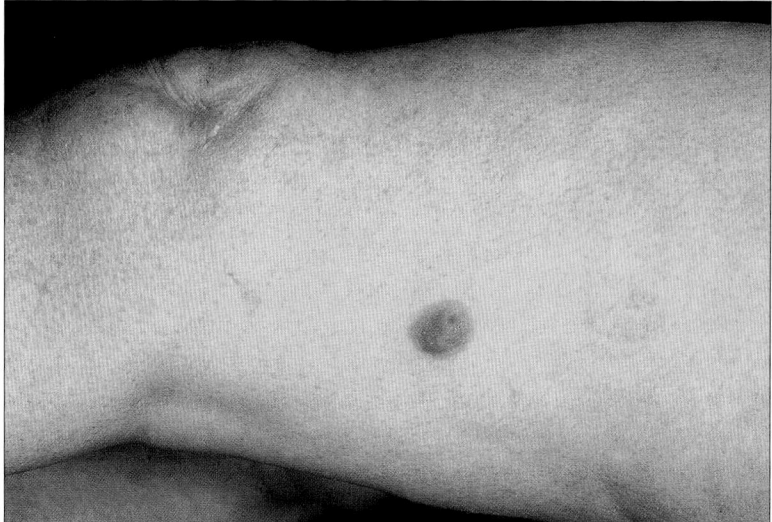

Fig. 24.195
Cutaneous neuroendocrine carcinoma: this tumor presented as a pigmented nodule on the thigh. By courtesy of M. Judge, MD, Institute of Dermatology, London, UK.

may be detected.[46,47] Those more frequently encountered include microcephaly, mental deficiency, electroencephalographic abnormalities, and basal ganglia and cerebellar abnormalities. The most severe neurological symptoms are features of the rare De Sanctis-Cacchione syndrome (group A), consisting of the usual skin lesions accompanied by microcephaly and progressive mental deficiency, retarded growth and sexual development, hearing loss, choreoathetosis, cerebellar ataxia, convulsions and quadriparesis with shortening of the Achilles tendon.[47,48] Patients with complementation groups C and E and the XP variant do not develop neurological disease but concomitant autism and hypoglycinemia have been reported in a patient with complementation group C.[1,49] Patients with combined features of XP and Cockayne syndrome or trichothiodystrophy have also been documented.[50–52] Laboratory studies may disclose an impaired T-cell–mediated immune response.[25,53]

Histologic features

The significant histopathological lesions in XP include evidence of actinic damage, hyperkeratosis with epidermal atrophy, pigmentary incontinence, telangiectasia, actinic keratoses, and the various neoplasms mentioned above. Solar elastosis is seen in older patients with the disease.

In those with neurological involvement, the pathological changes are not specific, consisting of loss of cortical Betz cells and cerebellar Purkinje cells, and a reduction in the number of neurons of the nuclei of the basal ganglia and cerebellum. There is no associated gliosis.[46]

Merkel cell carcinoma

Clinical features

Merkel cell carcinoma (neuroendocrine carcinoma of the skin; trabecular carcinoma) is a rare but highly aggressive tumor, which shows a propensity for sun-damaged skin.[1–9] The commonest sites affected are the head and neck (50%), particularly the eyelid and periorbital region, and the extremities (40%). Primary tumors of the trunk (10%) are uncommon and only occasional cases have been reported on sun-protected sites such as the oral and nasal mucosa, ear canal, vulva, or penis.[2,3,10–21] Caucasians are predominantly affected, with an estimated annual incidence of 0.23 per 100,000, whereas only rare cases presenting in black skin have been reported, with an estimated incidence of 0.01 per 100,000.[22–26] Recent studies show a male predilection and a wide age range may be involved (7–104 years), but most patients are in their seventh decade or older and only 5% of all reported patients are below the age of 50.[5,11,22,25–29] Presentation in children

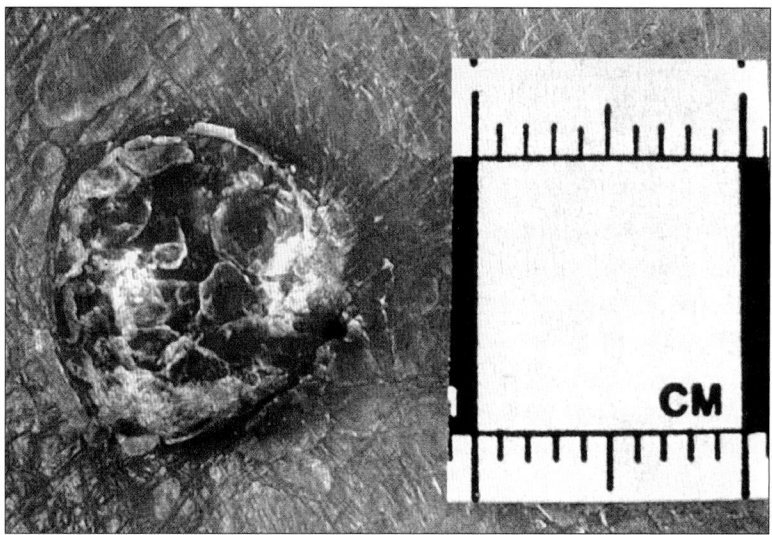

Fig. 24.196
Cutaneous neuroendocrine carcinoma: this example presented as an exophytic nodule. By courtesy of the Institute of Dermatology, London, UK.

is exceptional.[30,31] Cases can arise in the setting of immunosuppression such as following solid organ transplantation.[32]

The tumor has no distinctive clinical features and presents as a firm raised painless nodule that usually measures 2 cm or less in diameter and slowly increases in size (*Figs 24.195 and 24.196*).[11,33–36] Giant variants have also been reported measuring up to 23 cm.[37,38] The overlying skin may be erythematous, violaceous or purple. Ulceration is uncommon. Occasional patients present with multiple tumors.[39] Regression of the primary cutaneous tumor rarely occurs.[40–48] This, however, may explain lymph node involvement in the absence of cutaneous lesions.[49] It is important to note that Merkel cell carcinoma can also present as a primary neoplasm involving lymph nodes or visceral locations.[38,50–54] The recurrence rate of cutaneous Merkel cell carcinoma is approximately 40%.[1,55] Regional spread, primarily to lymph nodes, occurs in 55% of patients and distant metastases occur in about 35% of patients and particularly affect the liver, bone, lung, and skin (*Fig. 24.197*).[1,5,56] Rare metastatic sites include brain, leptomeninges, bladder, heart, pancreas, the gastrointestinal tract, oropharynx, larynx, and gingiva, and leukemic dissemination is unusual.[57–66] Originally, the tumor was believed to behave in a rather indolent fashion, but with more adequate clinical information it is now appreciated that the mortality is high.[67] Data derived from a large comprehensive review many cases have show survival

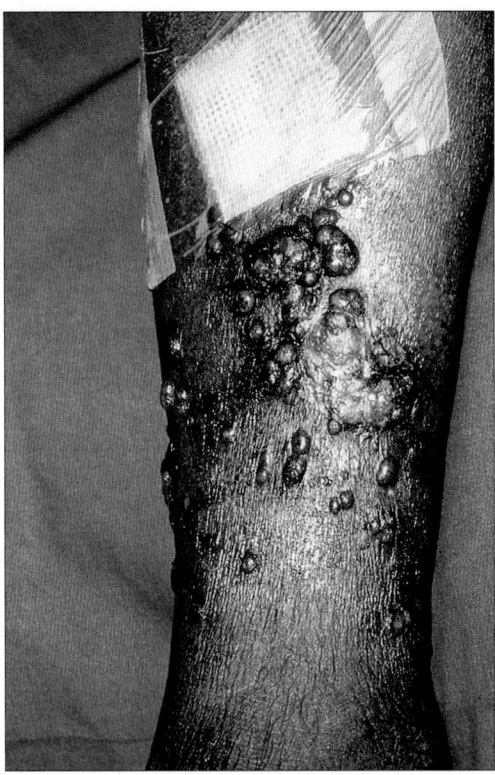

Fig. 24.197
Cutaneous
neuroendocrine
carcinoma: this patient
presented with numerous
cutaneous metastases. By
courtesy of R.A. Marsden,
MD, St George's Hospital,
London, UK.

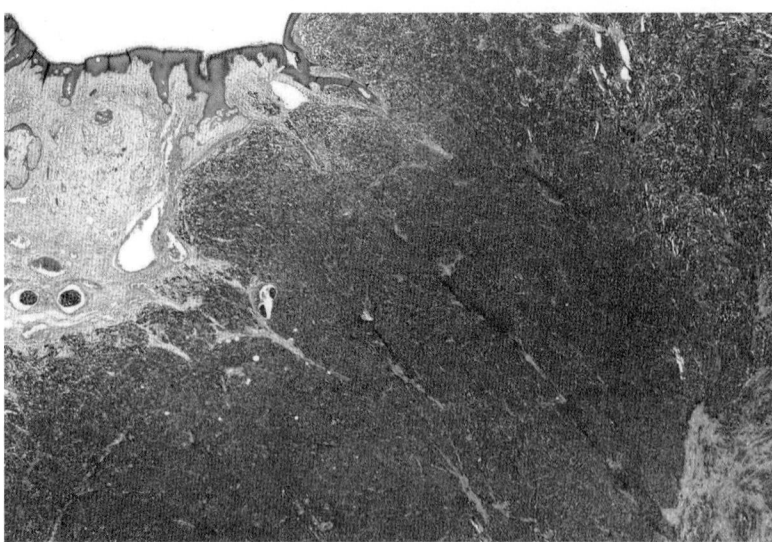

Fig. 24.198
Cutaneous neuroendocrine carcinoma: typical low-power view of a small blue cell tumor extending deeply into the subcutaneous fat.

rates of 88% at 1 year, 72% at 2 years, and 55% at 3 years.[1,68] Five-year survival for distant disease is particularly poor at 14–25% compared with 59% for regional and 75% for localized disease.[5,55,69] Favorable prognostic factors appear to be primary tumor location in the limbs, tumor size ≤2 cm, localized disease, younger age at presentation and female sex.[1,5,26,70–75] Wide local excision combined with adjuvant radiotherapy may improve locoregional control of the disease as well as relapse-free survival.[76,77] Immunotherapy with checkpoint inhibitors has also emerged as a significant treatment avenue.[6,29,78,79] Based on the high rate of lymph node metastasis, sentinel lymph node mapping is currently a frequently performed procedure in therapy and staging of this tumor, and the finding of positive sentinel lymph nodes is a strong predictor of short-term risk of recurrence and/or metastasis.[56,80–86] Multidisciplinary care is critical to achieve superior outcomes in this disease.[87] Immunohistochemistry for cytokeratin 20 (CK20) may be useful in identifying lymph node micrometastases not discernible on routinely stained sections.[88,89]

Pathogenesis and histologic features

The precise histogenesis of neuroendocrine carcinoma of the skin is uncertain. Whether it is derived from epidermal Merkel cells, dermal neuroendocrine cells, or pluripotent epidermal stem cells is the subject of considerable debate.[90] The immunocytochemical profile and ultrastructural findings seem to favor the first option as the most reasonable line of differentiation.

The integration of viral DNA from Merkel cell polyomavirus (MCV or MCPyV), a previously unknown polyomavirus, into the genome of tumor cells in a significant subset of Merkel cell carcinomas has identified an infectious etiology.[91–96] Evidence of viral infection is reported in up to 90% of cases.[8,9,97] Merkel cell carcinoma is also related to sun exposure and UV light irradiation.[22] A 100-fold increased incidence has been reported in patients receiving PUVA treatment for psoriasis.[98] UVB-induced mutations in the TP53 gene have been described in individual cases of Merkel cell carcinoma, similar to those seen in squamous and basal cell carcinoma, and this tumor frequently arises in association with synchronous or metachronous squamous cell carcinoma.[23,33,99–105] These two mechanisms are related as clonal integration of the MCV leads to sequestration of retinoblastoma protein with subsequent loss of cell cycle control while UV associated cases harbor TP53 mutations with Rb1 loss of function through various mutations or hypermethylation of the encoding gene RB1.[9,106–114] Basically, there appear to be two pathogenic mechanisms for Merkel cell carcinoma.

In the Northern hemisphere, the most common is viral associated with a low mutational load and then a much smaller subset is UV-damage driven and has a high mutational load, including TP53 mutations.[6,7,110] In geographies with chronic, high UV exposure, the UV-damage driven form is often predominant.[7,8] Both forms are immunogenic and thus immunotherapy has shown success in both.[78,79,115] Also, patients with Merkel cell carcinoma are at increased risk for developing a second malignancy (in up to 25% of patients), which includes hematologic malignancies, as well as breast and ovarian carcinomas in addition to the above mentioned cutaneous squamous cell carcinomas.[103]

Altered immune status is also associated with a higher incidence of cutaneous neuroendocrine carcinoma in patients following organ transplantation (including renal, cardiac, as well as bone marrow), receiving immunosuppressive therapy for rheumatoid arthritis and with aplastic anemia or lymphoma.[32,116–133] In addition, there is an increased incidence in patients with HIV infection (relative risk: 134 compared to the general population) and chronic lymphocytic leukemia.[134–144] Similar to cutaneous squamous cell carcinoma, an association between Merkel cell carcinoma and arsenic ingestion has been postulated.[145–148] Development of this tumor after radiation therapy, however, is infrequent.[149] Rarely, neuroendocrine carcinoma may be accompanied by paraneoplastic presentations such as myasthenia (Eaton-Lambert syndrome) or hyponatremia due to ACTH production of the tumor analogous to other neuroendocrine tumors such as small cell carcinoma of the lung.[150,151]

From a cytogenetic point of view, Merkel cell carcinoma shows multiple chromosomal abnormalities including the deletion of the short arm of chromosome 1 (1p36), an additional isochromosome i(1)(q10), trisomy 6, and loss of heterozygosity of chromosome 13, the latter being the site of the RB1 gene.[108,152–158]

Histologically, the tumor is commonly located primarily in the dermis and often there is extension into the subcutaneous fat (Fig. 24.198). In up to 10% of cases, however, there is intraepidermal spread, including Pautrier-like microabscess formation, and therefore cutaneous T-cell lymphoma and superficial spreading melanoma enter the differential diagnosis (Fig. 24.199).[10,159–163] Rare cases with only intraepidermal components have been described.[164–167] Occasionally, the epidermis shows coexistent actinic keratosis and squamous carcinoma in situ and rarely there is associated squamous cell or basal cell carcinoma or atypical fibroxanthoma (Figs 24.200–24.202).[10,23,160,168–178] Rarely, transitional forms have been documented.[179] Merkel cell carcinoma with associated squamous cell carcinoma correlates with an increased risk of recurrence, although metastasis rates and overall survival figures are not affected.[169]

A variety of histologic subtypes are recognized.[9,10] These include trabecular, intermediate, and small cell variants.[8,171]

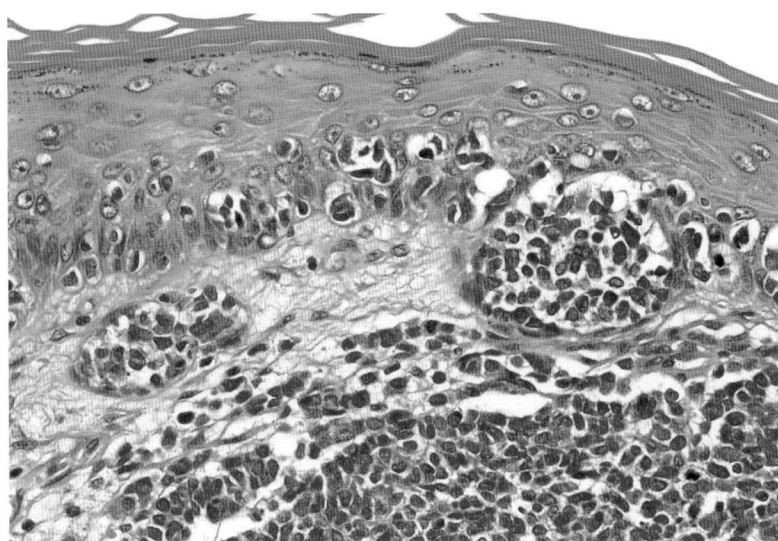

Fig. 24.199
Cutaneous neuroendocrine carcinoma: in this example, there is extensive intraepidermal spread.

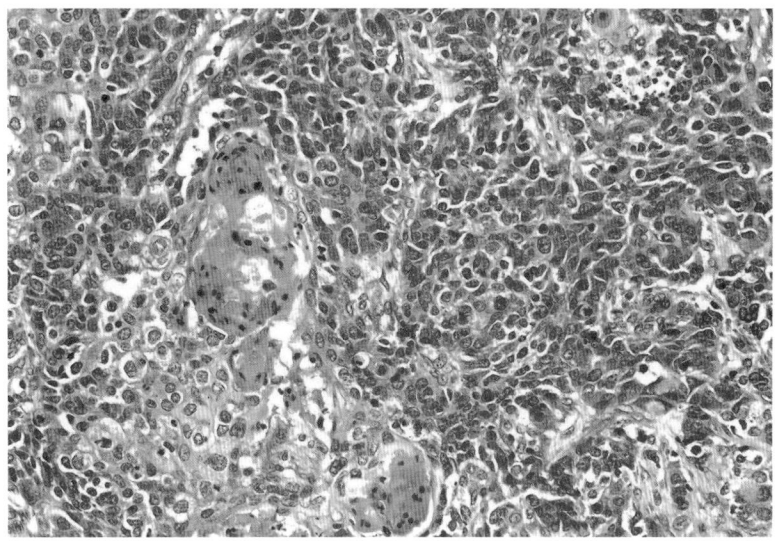

Fig. 24.201
Cutaneous neuroendocrine carcinoma: high-power view of squamous component.

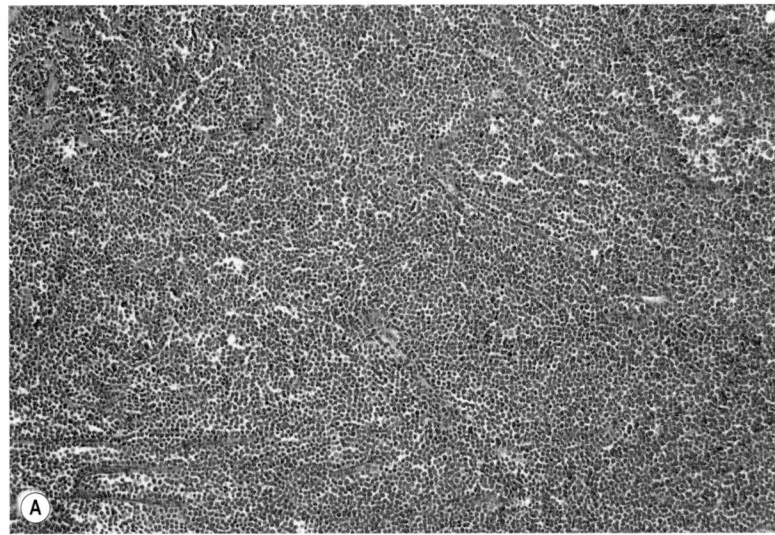

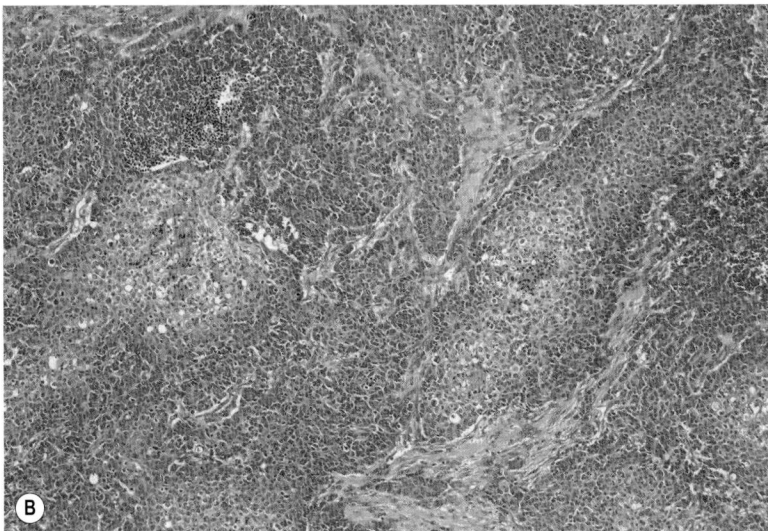

Fig. 24.200
(A, B) Cutaneous neuroendocrine carcinoma: this example shows extensive squamous differentiation.

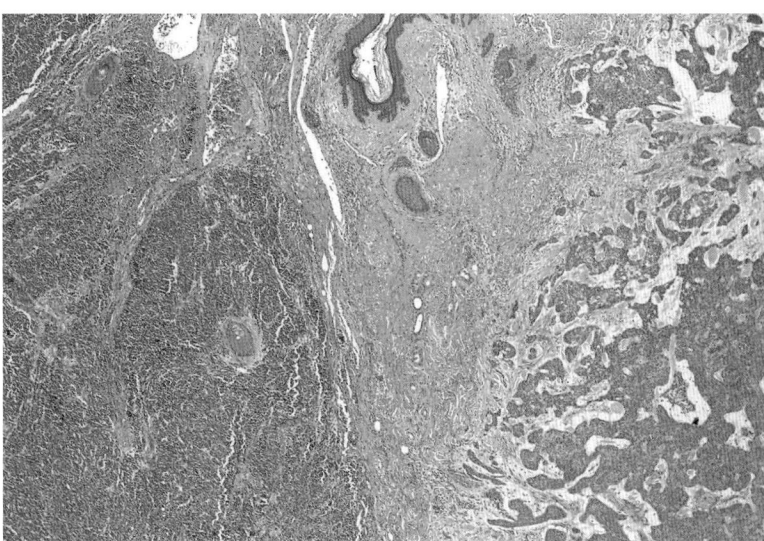

Fig. 24.202
Cutaneous neuroendocrine carcinoma: this tumor, which presented on the scalp, shows combined neuroendocrine carcinoma and basal cell carcinoma. By courtesy of M. Seywright, MD, Western Infirmary, Glasgow, UK.

- The trabecular pattern is the least common and consists of delicate ribbons of uniform cells, which often show nuclear molding (parallel alignment of nuclear membranes) (Figs 24.203–24.205).
- The intermediate variant is the most common and is composed of nodules and diffuse sheets of basophilic tumor cells with vesicular, often watery, nuclei containing small nucleoli (Fig. 24.206). Cytoplasm is often inconspicuous. Dissection of collagen and nuclear molding are frequently present. Foci of necrosis are commonly present and often there is widespread apoptosis.
- The small cell variant is composed of a hyperchromatic 'oat cell–like' infiltrate, which often shows a marked crush artifact (Fig. 24.207).[168]

Rarely, ductal or eccrine as well as sarcomatous and melanocytic differentiation has been documented (Fig. 24.208). The sarcomatous component may be reminiscent of atypical fibroxanthoma but divergent rhabdomyosarcomatous, leiomyosarcomatous, fibrosarcomatous as well as ganglion cell differentiation may be observed.[180–184] Lymphoepithelioma-like features or prominent microcystic features mimicking eccrine carcinoma are unusual.[10,173,179,185–197]

In some tumors, the cells adopt spindled cell characteristics (Fig. 24.209). There is commonly an admixture of intermediate cells with paler staining vesicular nuclei. Mitotic activity is often marked (Fig. 24.210). Lymphatic and vascular infiltration are common and important prognostic indicators

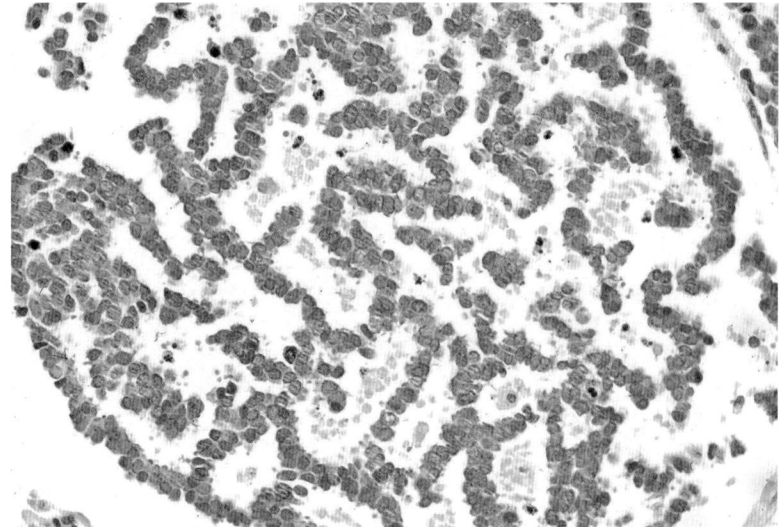

Fig. 24.203
Cutaneous neuroendocrine carcinoma: although this tumor is often known as trabecular carcinoma, such a pattern is uncommon. Note the delicate strands of small basophilic cells.

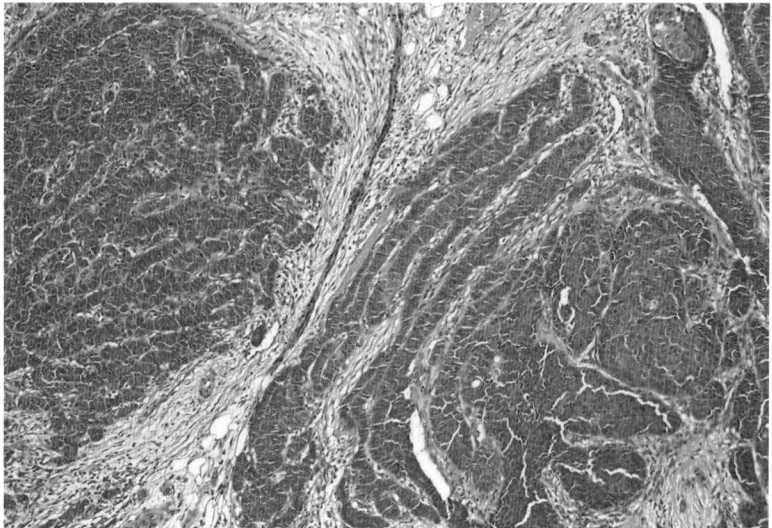

Fig. 24.204
Cutaneous neuroendocrine carcinoma: in this field, the trabecular growth pattern imparts a carcinoid-like appearance.

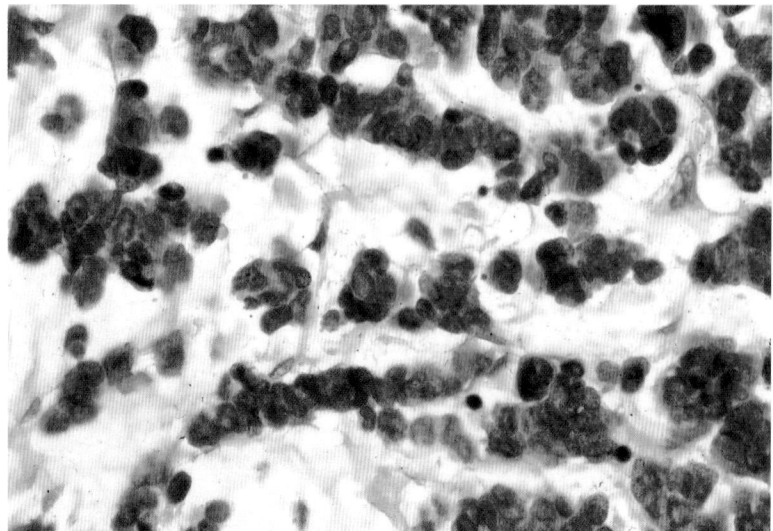

Fig. 24.205
Cutaneous neuroendocrine carcinoma: this field shows characteristic nuclear molding.

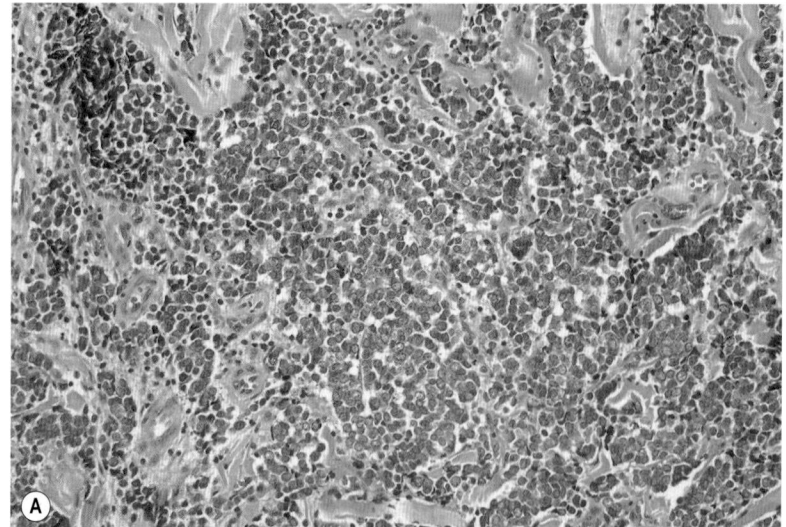

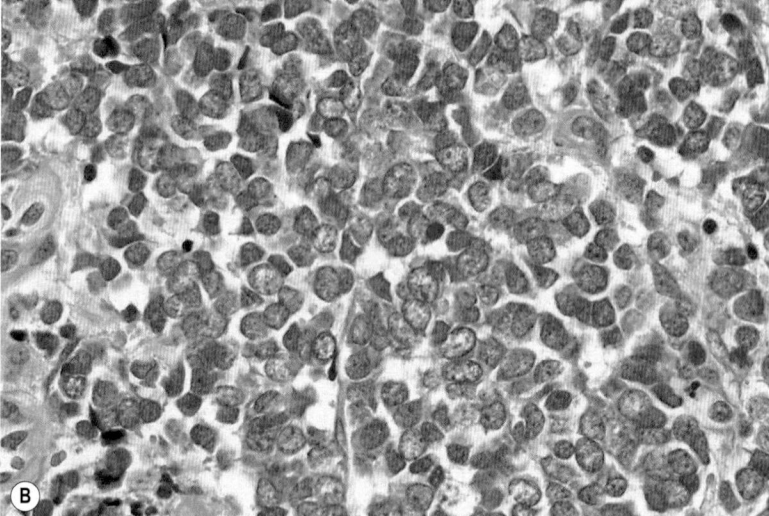

Fig. 24.206
(**A, B**) Cutaneous neuroendocrine carcinoma: the tumor nuclei in this intermediate variant are large and pale staining and contain tiny nucleoli. This watery appearance is pathognomonic.

(*Fig. 24.211*).[198] Merkel cell carcinoma may rarely be accompanied by amyloid deposition, desmoplasia, and a florid vascular proliferation characterized by glomeruloid vascular tufts and long cords of vessels.[199-202] Occasionally, the tumor is accompanied by a heavy lymphoid infiltrate with formation of lymphoid follicles.[203] Tumors with features of both squamous cell carcinoma and Merkel cell carcinoma tend to be negative for MCV and while long considered to be a variant of Merkel cell carcinoma, recently genomic studies suggest these may be different and these have been provisionally termed cutaneous squamous and neuroendocrine carcinoma by some.[204] Other types of divergent differentiation including adnexal, glandular, and sarcomatous components also tend to be negative for MCV.[182,205,206]

Histologic features indicative of adverse outcome include tumor size >5 mm, tumor thickness >5 mm, diffuse infiltrative growth pattern, invasion of subcutis and deeper structures, and lymphovascular invasion.[28,198] The presence of a heavy lymphocytic infiltrate was found to be an adverse prognostic factor in one study while the presence of tumor-infiltrating lymphocytes was associated with superior survival in subsequent studies.[28,198,207] Currently, immunotherapy is a commonly employed therapeutic option suggesting that tumor infiltrating lymphocytes can certainly have anti-tumor properties.[208] Other findings that may be associated with adverse outcome include increased intratumoral mast cells and increased vascularity.[209,210]

An unusual phenomenon is the development of Merkel cell carcinoma in association with trichilemmal or follicular cysts.[211-213]

Merkel cell carcinoma often exhibits a positive argyrophil (Grimelius) reaction, but the tumors are uniformly argentaffin negative.[10,214] They

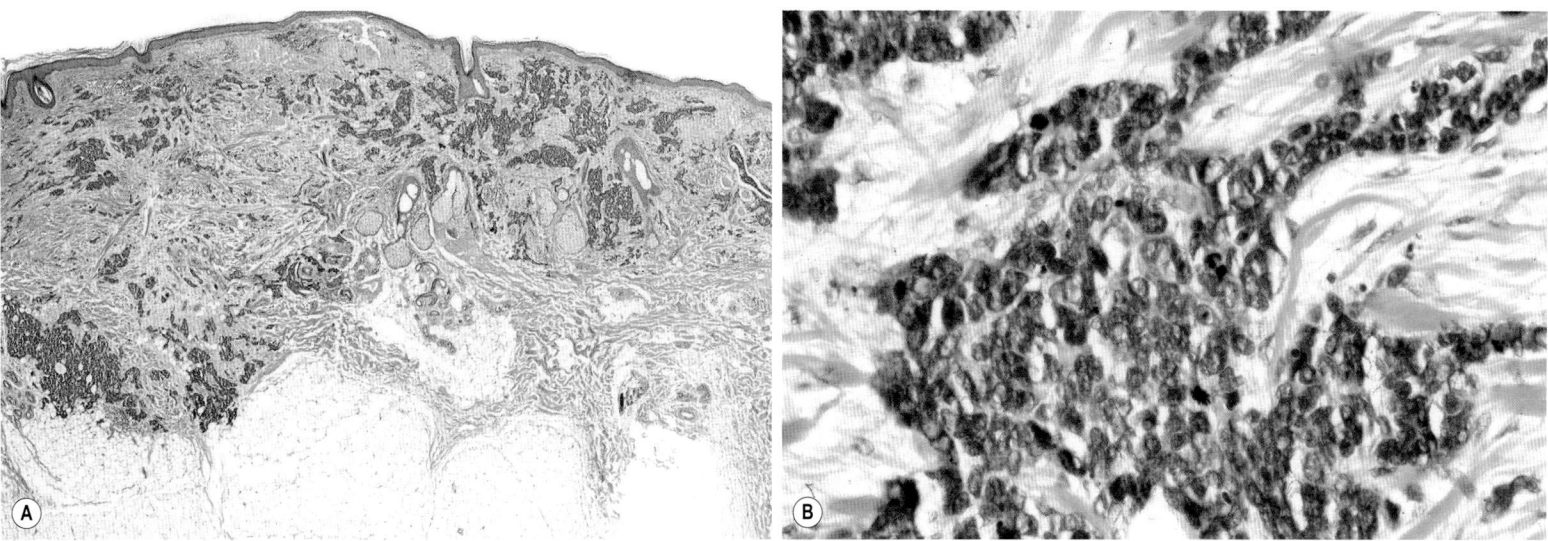

Fig. 24.207
(**A**, **B**) Cutaneous neuroendocrine carcinoma: an example of a small cell variant. The features are indistinguishable from metastatic neuroendocrine carcinoma.

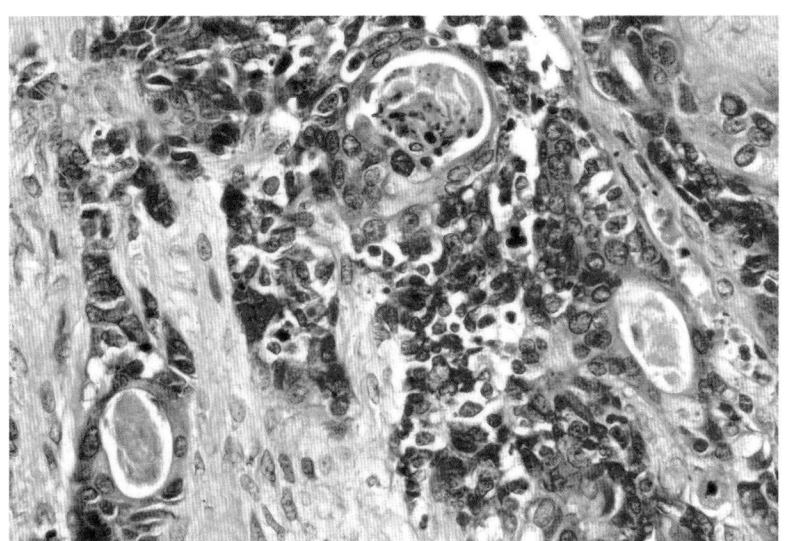

Fig. 24.208
Cutaneous neuroendocrine carcinoma: rarely, glandular differentiation is a feature.

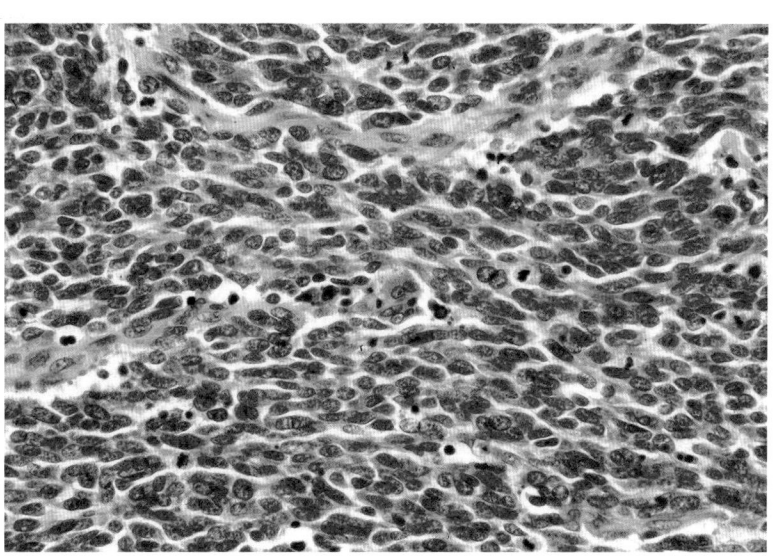

Fig. 24.209
Cutaneous neuroendocrine carcinoma: exceptionally, spindle cell morphology is apparent.

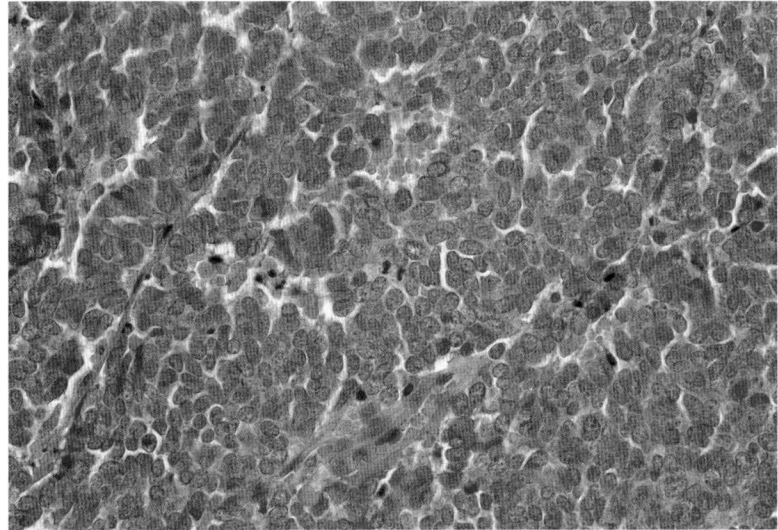

Fig. 24.210
Cutaneous neuroendocrine carcinoma: in this example there is marked mitotic activity.

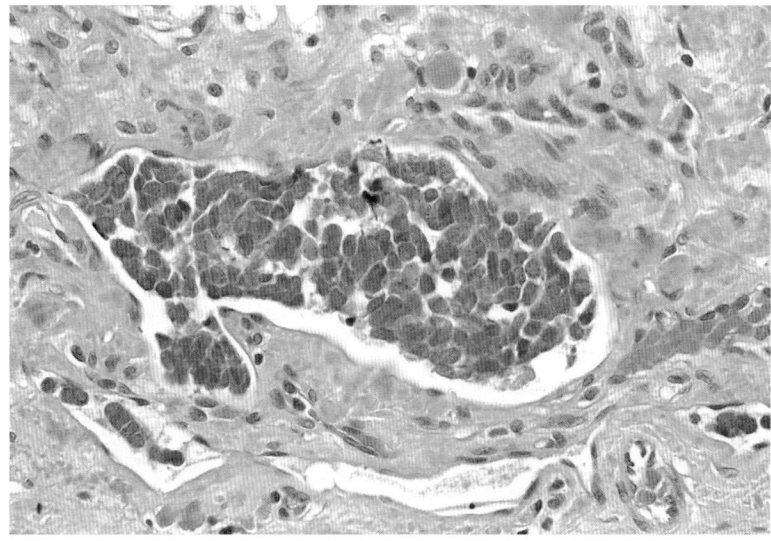

Fig. 24.211
Cutaneous neuroendocrine carcinoma: lymphovascular invasion, as seen in this field, is an almost constant histological finding.

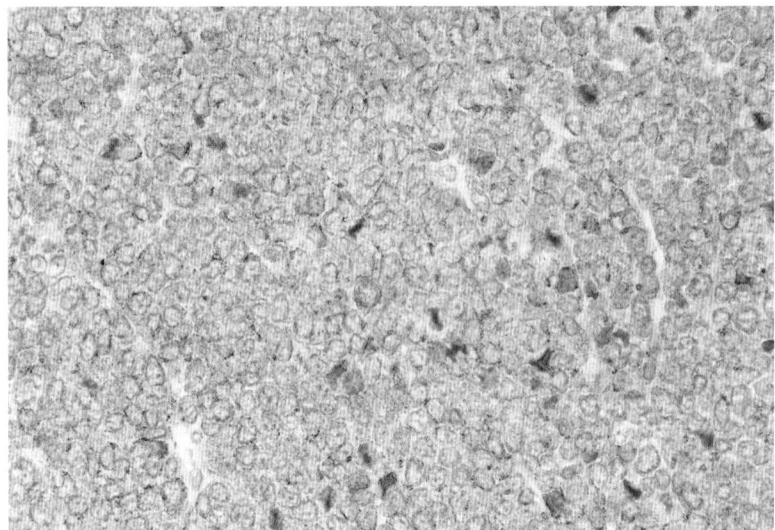

Fig. 24.212
Cutaneous neuroendocrine carcinoma: in this example the tumor cells express chromogranin.

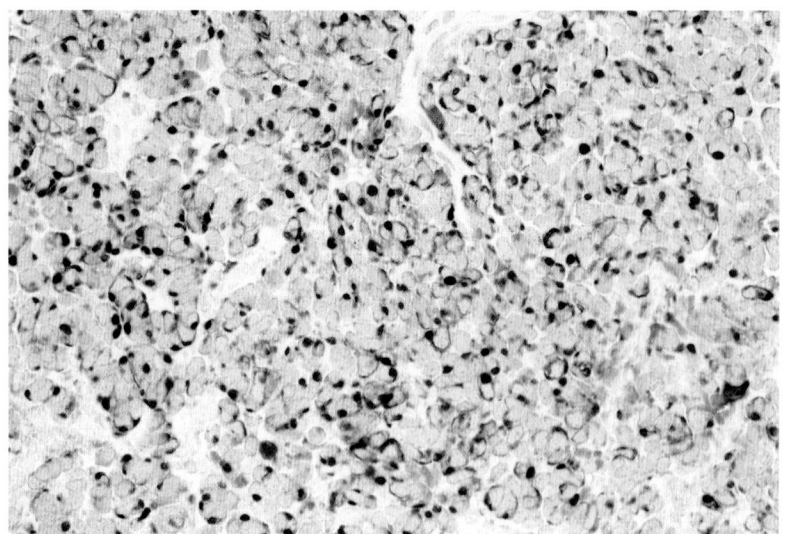

Fig. 24.214
Cutaneous neuroendocrine carcinoma: cutaneous lesions characteristically express CK20 as shown here; they are CK7 negative.

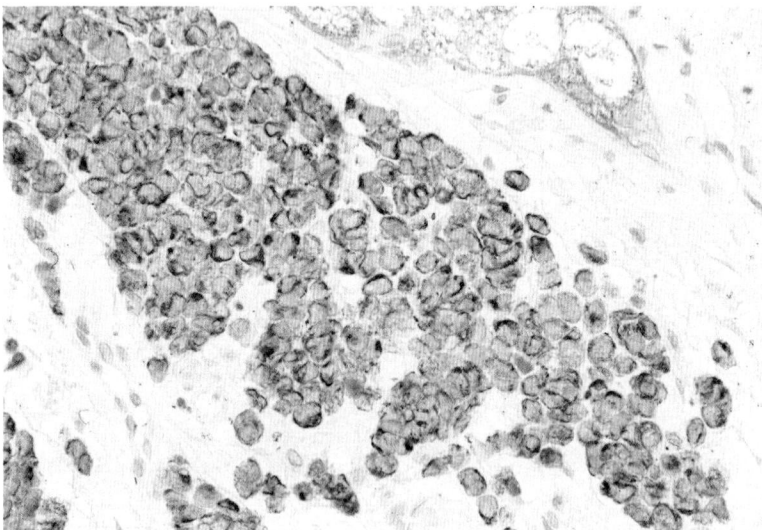

Fig. 24.213
Cutaneous neuroendocrine carcinoma: the tumor cells commonly express CAM 5.2. Note the dotlike positivity.

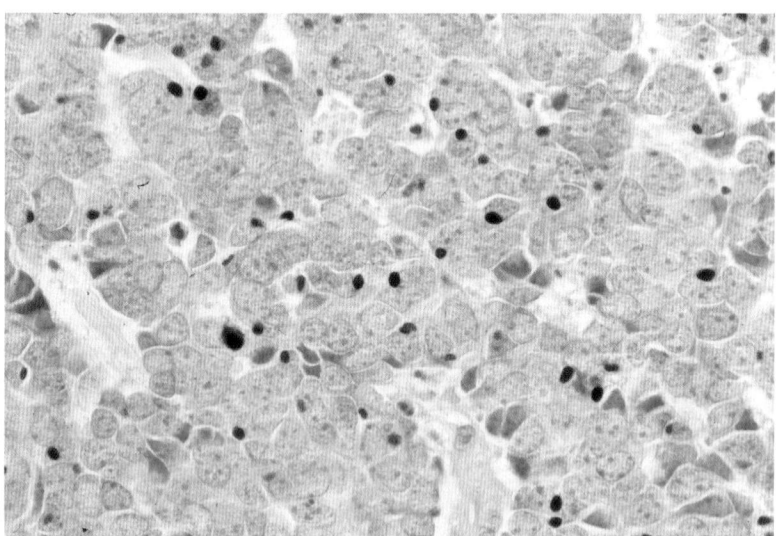

Fig. 24.215
Cutaneous neuroendocrine carcinoma: neurofilament dot-positivity helps to distinguish this tumor from bronchial tumors which do not express this protein.

commonly contain a variety of neuropeptides including chromogranin, calcitonin, vasoactive intestinal peptide, metenkephalin, somatostatin, calcitonin, and synaptophysin (Fig. 24.212).[10,67,215–217]

With immunohistochemistry, the tumor cells express epithelial antigens in addition to showing neuroendocrine features. Most characteristic of neuroendocrine carcinoma of the skin is low molecular weight (CAM 5.2) keratin and more specifically cytokeratin 20 expression, which is often evident as a paranuclear globule (Figs 24.213 and 24.214).[67,214,218–226] Cytokeratin 7, MASH-1, and thyroid transcription factor 1 (TTF-1), which are typically negative, aid in distinguishing primary lesions from cutaneous metastases from bronchial small cell carcinoma.[227–230] It is, however, important to remember that cytokeratin 7 or TTF-1 expression may be a feature and rare cases may express cytokeratin 7 but not cytokeratin 20.[231] Cytokeratin 20 negative cases might be less commonly associated with MCV.[232,233] Neurofilament protein is frequently expressed in cutaneous tumors, again in a paranuclear dot-like distribution (Fig. 24.215).[224,234,235] Tumor cells also commonly express neuron-specific enolase (NSE), chromogranin A, synaptophysin, CD56, CD57, and EMA, but are vimentin and S100 protein negative (Figs 24.216 and 24.217).[236–241] Ber-EP4 expression has also been documented,[185] and tumors are frequently positive for bcl-2, Fli-1, CD99, and microtubule-associated protein-2 (MAP-2).[242–245] PAX-5, an otherwise B-cell specific transcription factor, is expressed in most cases of Merkel cell

carcinoma and small cell carcinoma of the lung and is therefore not useful in this distinction.[246] Expression of CD117 has also been reported.[247,248] There is, however, no evidence that there are gain of function mutations in the KIT receptor, and such findings should not prompt treatment attempts with tyrosine kinase inhibitors such as imatinib mesylate.[249,250] Tumors stain positively for survivin and expression of p63 is observed in a subset of Merkel cell carcinoma. Nuclear localization of survivin and p63 staining may be indicative of more aggressive clinical behavior.[251,252] Evidence of MCV can be readily detected in Merkel cell carcinoma using PCR based methods, but this is not frequently performed in routine clinical practice.[253–255] Immunohistochemistry to detect MCV large T antigen has not been routinely employed.[256]

Ultrastructurally, the tumor cells closely resemble Merkel cells.[257] They have a vesicular, indented or lobulated nucleus containing a small nucleolus, and membrane-bound neurosecretory granules are present in the cytoplasm, usually peripherally located along the plasma membrane and within dendritic processes.[34,218,258,259] The granules resist the effects of poor fixation and of routine paraffin processing and can therefore be demonstrated even in material reprocessed from paraffin-embedded tissue (Fig. 24.218). The Golgi is prominent and primitive junctions are often present. Typical of neuroendocrine carcinoma of the skin is the presence of a paranuclear aggregate (fibrous bundle) of intermediate keratin filaments corresponding to the globules noted on immunohistochemistry.

Differential diagnosis

Merkel cell carcinoma may be confused with lymphomatous deposits, small cell melanoma, and metastatic small cell carcinoma, primarily of bronchial origin (*Table 24.4*). The first two can readily be excluded by the absence of leukocyte common antigen (LCA) or S100 protein expression.[260] Systemic neuroendocrine tumors not uncommonly metastasize to the skin and on occasion this may be the presenting feature.[261] In an immunohistochemical comparative study, the presence of bombesin, leucine enkephalin, methionine enkephalin, and β-endorphin expression were shown to favor the diagnosis of secondary rather than primary neuroendocrine carcinoma.[262] Also, as mentioned above, expression of cytokeratin 20 and neurofilament protein in a paranuclear dotlike pattern favors the diagnosis of a primary skin tumor over metastatic bronchial small cell carcinoma, especially in the absence of cytokeratin 7, MASH-1, and TTF-1 expression.[218–230,234,235,263]

Lymphoepithelioma-like carcinoma of the skin

Clinical features

Lymphoepithelioma-like carcinoma of the skin is an exceedingly rare tumor. Morphologically, this tumor closely resembles undifferentiated nasopharyngeal carcinoma (lymphoepithelioma). Lymphoepithelioma-like carcinomas have been described in multiple sites including salivary glands, stomach, lung, thymus, and rarely in the larynx, uterine cervix, and urinary bladder.[1] In the skin, it was first reported in 1988 and subsequently less than 70 cases have been described in the literature.[2–31]

Clinically, the tumor presents as a solitary nodule in the elderly (range: 39–96 years; median: 70 years) without sex predilection.[18] The head and neck area is almost exclusively affected with only rare reports at other sites including the shoulder, forearm, or vulva.[11,18,22] Cases with identical histologic features are rarely reported at other sites including stomach salivary

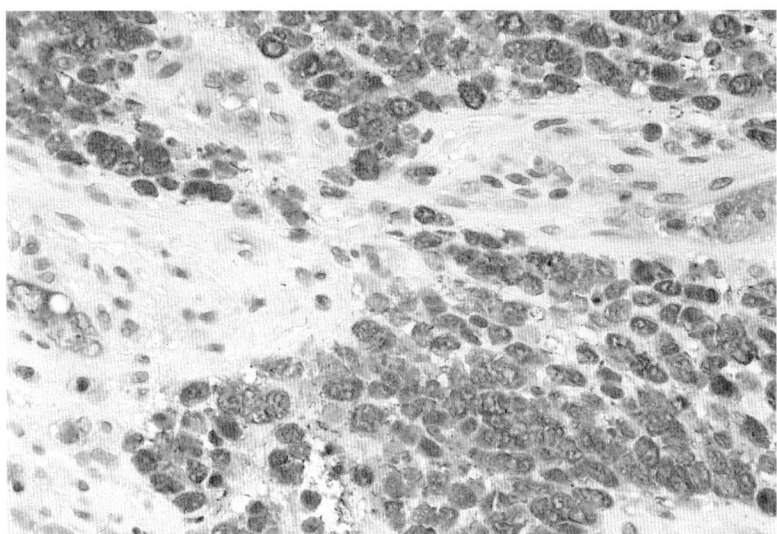

Fig. 24.216
Cutaneous neuroendocrine carcinoma: neuron-specific enolase expression is commonly present.

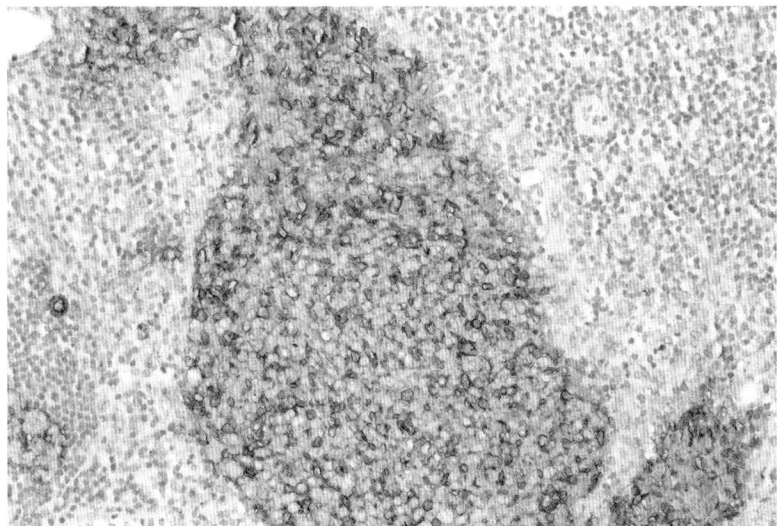

Fig. 24.217
Cutaneous neuroendocrine carcinoma: this tumor showed quite striking EMA expression.

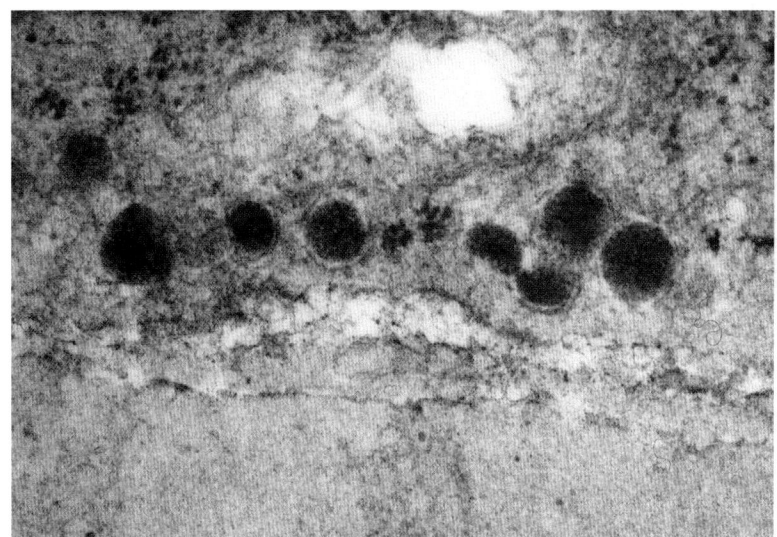

Fig. 24.218
Cutaneous neuroendocrine carcinoma: membrane-bound granules may be identified in reprocessed formalin-fixed, paraffin-embedded material.

Table 24.4
Differential diagnosis of cutaneous neuroendocrine carcinoma by immunohistochemistry

Tumor	CK20	CK7	NSE	NFP	S100	LCA	CD99	TTF-1
Merkel cell carcinoma	90%	few cases	80%	50%	0%	0%	19% Cyt	Exceptionally focally positive
Small cell carcinoma	3%	40%	64%	0%	0%	0%	12% Cyt	91%
Lymphoma	0%	0%	11%	0%	6%	98%	7%	
PNET/Ewing's sarcoma			50%	19%	50%	0%	92% Mem	
Small cell melanoma	0%	0%	71%	0%	97%	0%	8%	0%

CK, cytokeratin; Cyt, cytoplasmic; LCA, leukocyte common antigen; Mem, membranous; NFP, neurofilament protein; NSE, neuron-specific enolase; PNET, primitive neuroectodermal tumor; TTF-1, thyroid-transcription factor 1.

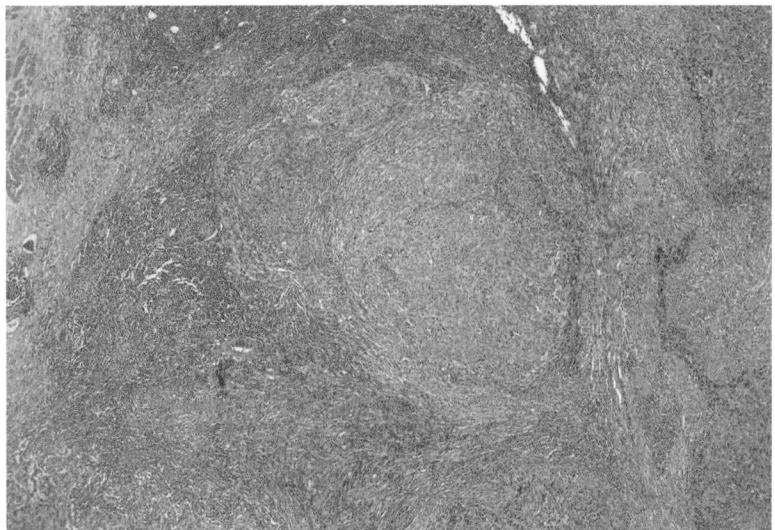

Fig. 24.219
Lymphoepithelioma-like carcinoma: low-power view showing a tumor nodule associated with a dense lymphocytic infiltrate.

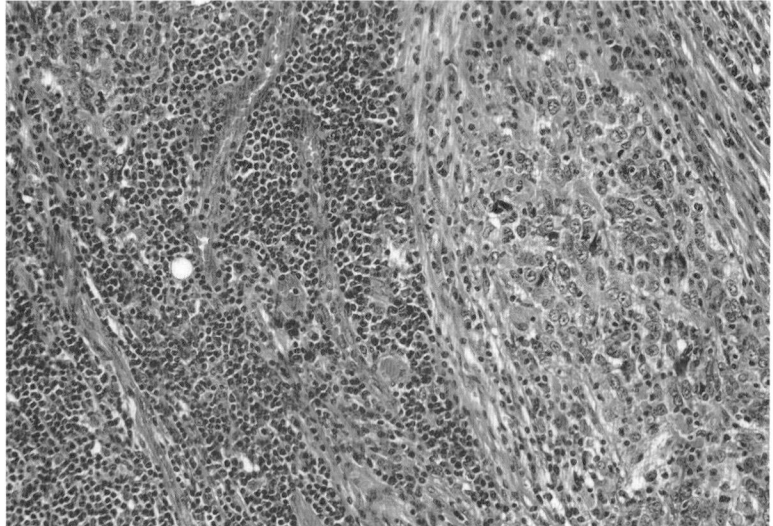

Fig. 24.220
Lymphoepithelioma-like carcinoma: higher-power view.

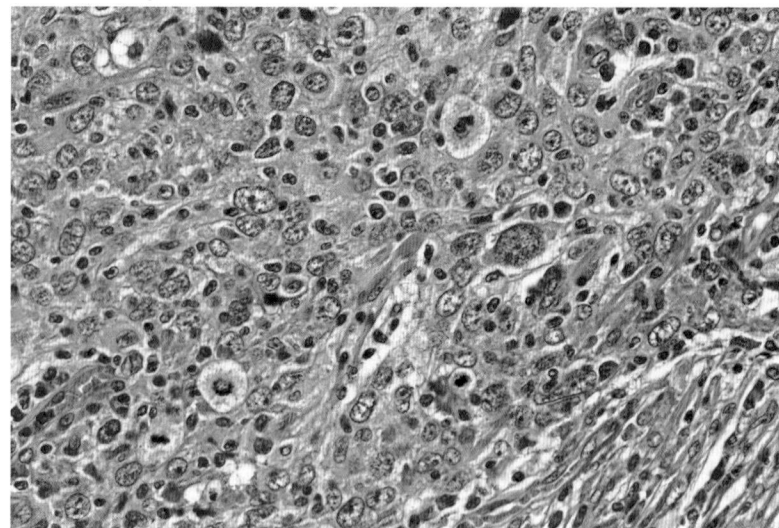

Fig. 24.221
Lymphoepithelioma-like carcinoma: the tumor cells have large watery nuclei with prominent nucleoli. Mitotic activity is conspicuous. There are admixed lymphocytes and plasma cells.

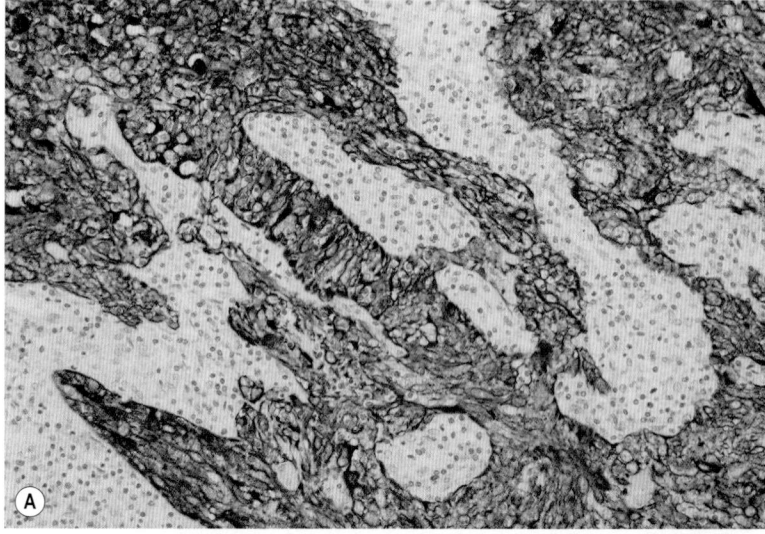

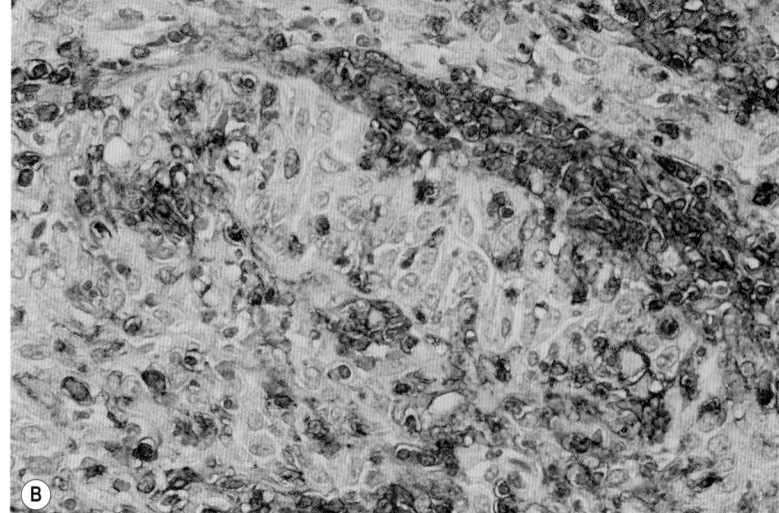

Fig. 24.222
Lymphoepithelioma-like carcinoma: (**A**) the tumor cells express AE1/AE3; (**B**) CD45 highlights the lymphocytes. The tumor cells are negative.

gland, thymus, lung, breast, gynecologic tract organs, and bladder.[32,33] A case in the anal canal was recently reported to harbor high risk HPV type 16.[32] Although no comprehensive follow-up studies are available, the prognosis for this tumor appears to be relatively good.[18] Most patients are cured by local excision. Local occurrence and regional metastasis are rare and only one reported patient has died from widespread metastatic disease.[2,23]

Pathogenesis and histologic features

Lymphoepithelioma-like carcinoma of the skin presents as a lobulated, well-circumscribed tumor involving the dermis and subcutaneous tissue without epidermal connection (*Fig. 24.219*). It is composed of large cohesive epithelioid cells with poorly defined eosinophilic cytoplasm containing vesicular nuclei and prominent nucleoli arranged in lobules, nests, cords, and strands (*Figs 24.220 and 24.221*). Mitoses are frequent. There is an intense lymphoplasmacytic infiltrate closely associated with tumor cells, which is composed of a mixed B- and T-cell population.[19] Squamous differentiation is not a feature but rarely this tumor may show adnexal differentiation towards follicular, eccrine glandular, and sebaceous structures.[4,8,21] Spindle cell differentiation is a rare finding.[20] Perineural invasion has been noted.[34] A condensation of factor XIII-positive dendritic cells has been observed around tumor lobules.[6,18] By immunohistochemistry, tumor cells stain positive for cytokeratin and EMA (*Fig. 24.222*).[35] Ultrastructural analysis reveals the presence of tonofilaments and desmosomes.[14,35] While undifferentiated nasopharyngeal carcinoma is invariably associated with Epstein-Barr virus (EBV), lymphoepithelioma-like carcinoma of some other sites such as salivary glands, lung, thymus, and stomach may also be linked to EBV, especially in the Asian population.[1,6,13,18,34,36] In contrast, EBV has never been detected in tumors confined to the skin even in patients of Asian descent.[14,24,37] Traditionally, this tumor has been classified as a variant of squamous cell carcinoma but at this time the histogenesis remains uncertain.[38] The general lack of epidermal origin and absence of true squamous differentiation as well as the ability to show differentiation towards adnexal structures suggests an adnexal origin.[4,8] In contrast, findings such as overlying epidermal dysplasia and a single report of epidermal involvement raise the possibility of an epidermal origin.[14,17]

Differential diagnosis

The main differential diagnosis includes metastatic spread from undifferentiated nasopharyngeal carcinoma or lymphoepithelioma-like carcinoma from other sites. Clinical work-up for primary carcinoma at other sites as well as detection of EBV are helpful means in differentiating primary cutaneous tumors from metastases. Poorly differentiated squamous cell carcinoma with a heavy lymphocytic infiltrate usually shows an epidermal origin and epidermal dysplasia.[39] Merkel cell carcinoma shows characteristic staining for cytokeratin 20 and neuroendocrine markers; melanoma and lymphoma can be differentiated using immunohistochemistry for S100 protein or lymphoid markers, respectively. Separation from cutaneous lymphadenoma may be difficult as this tumor is also characterized by an epithelial proliferation containing a lymphocytic infiltrate. In contrast to lymphoepithelioma-like carcinoma, it shows no cytological atypia or mitoses and the epithelial nests display peripheral palisading. Cases can mimic cutaneous lymphoma, but characteristic lymphoid markers of such cases are lacking.[40]

Access **ExpertConsult.com** for the complete list of references

Melanocytic nevi

Boštjan Luzar, Boris C. Bastian, Jeffrey P. North and
Eduardo Calonje

See
www.expertconsult.com
for references and
additional material

Ephelide

Clinical features

Ephelides (freckles) are extremely common lesions that present as clusters of small (approximately 2.0 mm in diameter), uniformly pigmented macules (*Fig. 25.1*).[1-5] They are directly related to exposure to sunlight and are much more conspicuous in summer than in winter. Sites of predilection therefore include the nose, cheeks, shoulders, and dorsal aspects of the hands and arms.[2] Although virtually everyone shows some degree of freckling, ephelides are particularly common and numerous in individuals with red hair and blue eyes, where there is probably an autosomal mode of inheritance.[5] Ephelides present in childhood, increasing in frequency in adults and typically regressing in the elderly.[2,5] There is a predilection for females. High levels of freckling may indicate a raised susceptibility to the later development of melanoma.[6] Similarly, increasing numbers of freckles correlate with a higher frequency of acquired melanocytic nevi.[7] Otherwise, although a cosmetic nuisance, they are of no clinical importance. A recent study demonstrated two independent risk factors associated with history of freckle formation; frequent and constant sunburns and the presence of *melanocortin-1 receptor gene* polymorphism with major variants being associated with more freckling.[8]

Histologic features

Ephelides are characterized by excessive keratinocyte pigmentation associated with normal or even diminished numbers of melanocytes (*Fig. 25.2*).[9,10] The epidermal architecture is normal. Solar elastosis is not a feature of ephelides.

Ultrastructurally, the melanocytes contain enlarged spherical granular melanosomes in contrast to the striated ellipsoid forms seen in normal white skin.[11]

Lentigo simplex

Clinical features

Lentigo simplex is a very common melanocytic lesion. Lesions – which are small (1–5 mm), uniformly pigmented, brown to black, sharply circumscribed macules – may be found anywhere on the integument, the conjunctivae, and mucocutaneous orifices (*Fig. 25.3*).[1,2] They often develop in

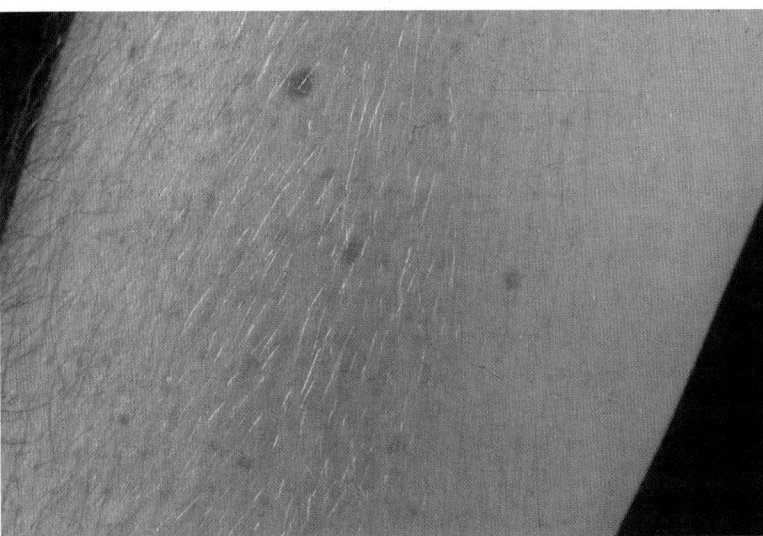

Fig. 25.1
Ephelides: these present as small pigmented macules that darken on exposure to sunlight.

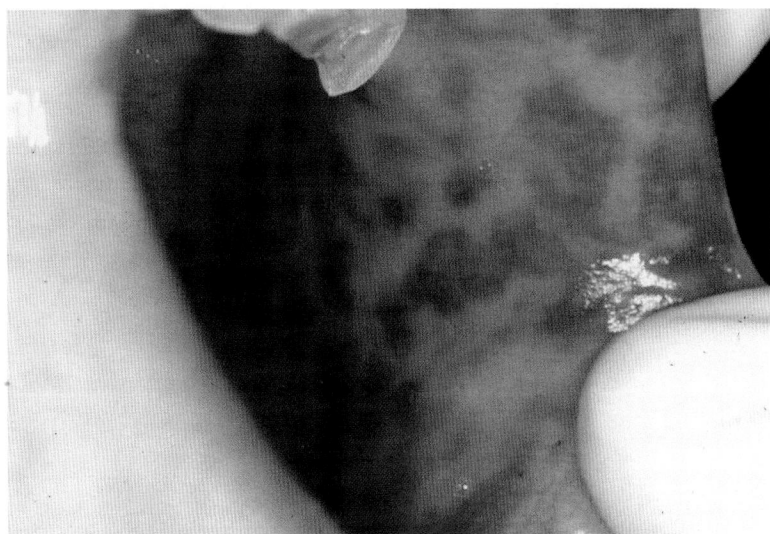

Fig. 25.4
Laugier-Hunziker syndrome: oral melanotic macules. By courtesy of S.-B. Woo, MD, Harvard Medical School, Boston, USA.

childhood (juvenile lentigo) and become more conspicuous during pregnancy. Rarely, numerous lentigines may develop following an infection or an exanthem, and exceptionally they are generalized (generalized lentigines, lentigines profusa).[1,3] Segmental lentigines have also been documented.[4] Development of simple lentigines limited to areas treated with tacrolimus has been reported in children with atopic dermatitis.[5] Simple lentigines have also been described in association with type I hereditary punctate palmoplantar keratoderma.[6] Hyperpigmentation and increased numbers of lentigines are features of Addison disease. Simple lentigines have no malignant potential and, in contrast to ephelides, have no connection with sunlight.

Lentigines assume a particular importance when their presence is associated with a variety of inherited systemic conditions, including Peutz-Jeghers, LEOPARD (multiple lentigines), and Carney syndromes, centrofacial lentiginosis, and Laugier-Hunziker syndrome (idiopathic lenticular mucocutaneous pigmentation). The last is characterized by oral melanotic macules and longitudinal pigmentation of the nails (Figs 25.4 and 25.5). An association between somatic mutation in keratin 10 (KRT10) gene and development of numerous simple lentigos, linear epidermolytic nevus, and epidermolytic nevus comedonicus has also been reported.[7]

Histologic features

The histologic features are those of slight to moderate elongation of the epidermal ridges associated with an increased number of basally located melanocytes (Figs 25.6 and 25.7).[1,2] Generally, no atypia of melanocytes is seen. There is no junctional activity and pigmentation is increased, both within the epidermis and within melanophages in the papillary dermis. Rarely, giant melanosomes (macromelanosomes) may be identified (Fig. 25.8). A superficial dermal lymphohistiocytic infiltrate is often present. Not uncommonly, lentigo and junctional nevus may coexist – lentiginous junctional nevus (Fig. 25.9).

Interestingly, a recent study failed to demonstrate the presence of $BRAF^{V600E}$ mutations in simple lentigo.[8] However, $BRAF^{V600E}$ mutations have been demonstrated in 17% of lentiginous/junctional nevi, in 55% of compound nevi, and in 78% of intradermal nevi.[8]

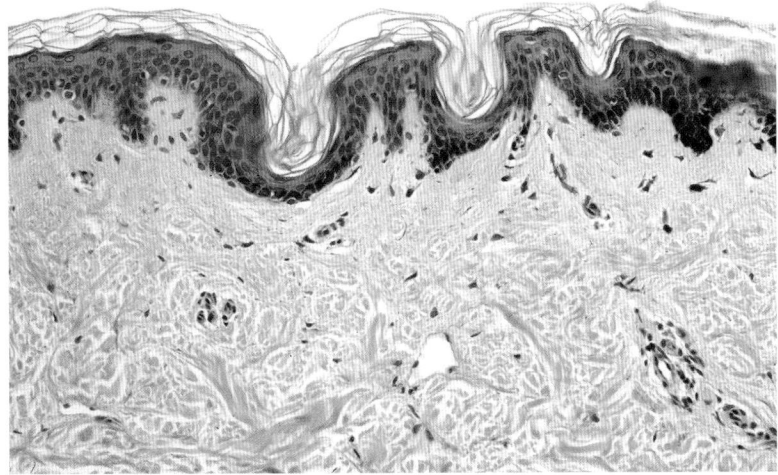

Fig. 25.2
Ephelis: note the hyperpigmentation of the basal layer of the epidermis. The number of melanocytes is within normal limits and there is no evidence of junctional activity.

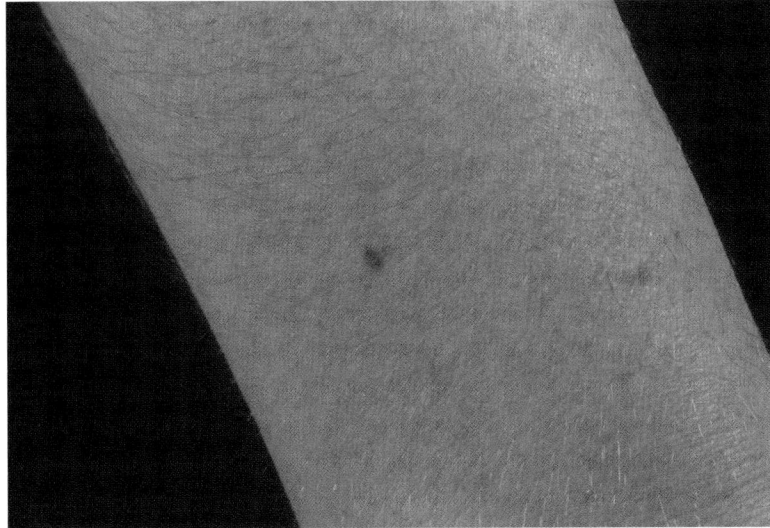

Fig. 25.3
Lentigo simplex: this is a small, uniformly pigmented macule clinically indistinguishable from an ephelide. It is unrelated to sun exposure.

Labial melanotic macule and labial lentigo

This disorder, also known as oral melanotic macule and mucosal melanosis, is discussed under pathology of the oral cavity.

Laugier-Hunziker syndrome

This disorder, also known as idiopathic lenticular mucocutaneous pigmentation, is discussed under disorders of pigmentation.

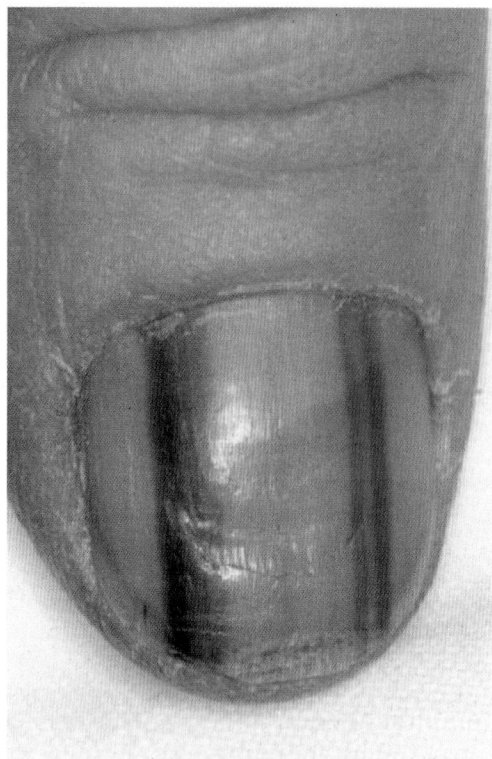

Fig. 25.5
Laugier-Hunziker syndrome: longitudinal pigmented bands in the nails. By courtesy of S.-B. Woo, MD, Harvard Medical School, Boston, USA.

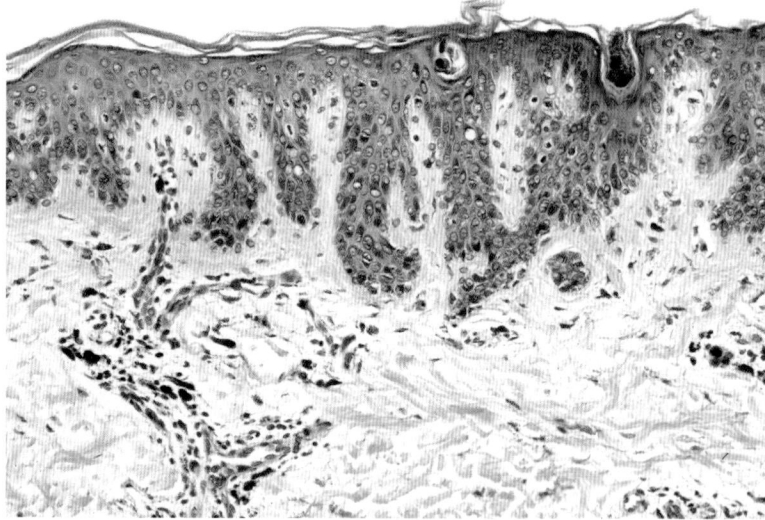

Fig. 25.6
Lentigo simplex: there is acanthosis with elongation of the epidermal ridges. Basally located melanocytes are increased in number. There is excessive pigmentation of the epidermis, but no junctional activity is present.

Oral melanoacanthoma

This disorder, also known as melanoacanthosis, is discussed under pathology of the oral cavity.

Cutaneous melanoacanthoma

This disorder is discussed under tumors of the surface epithelium.

Peutz-Jeghers syndrome

This disorder is discussed under disorders of pigmentation.

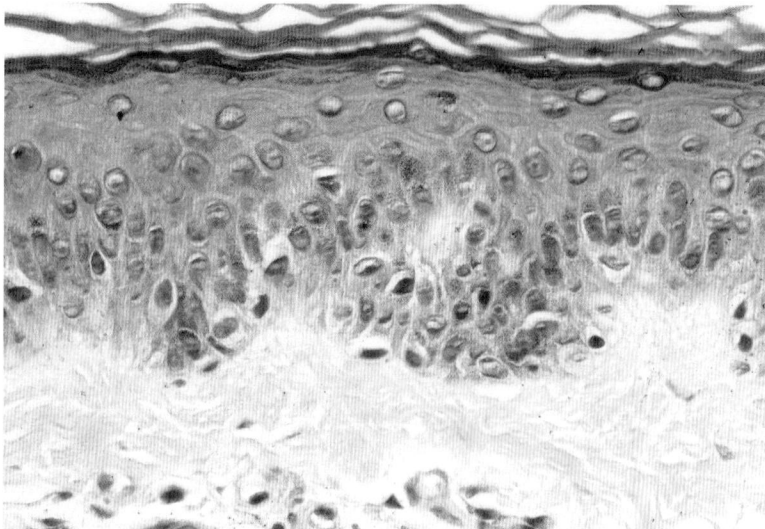

Fig. 25.7
Lentigo simplex: close-up view showing increased numbers of melanocytes.

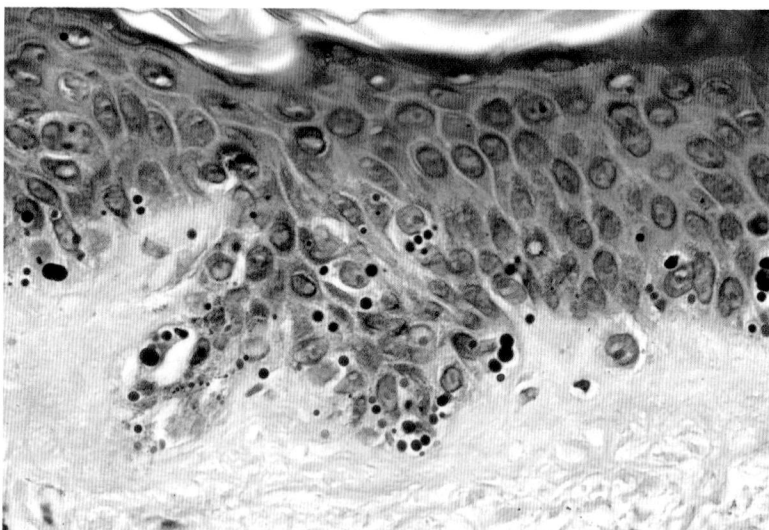

Fig. 25.8
Lentigo simplex: note the presence of macromelanosomes.

Genital lentiginosis

This disorder, also known as penile lentigo, penile lentiginosis, atypical penile lentigo, vulval lentigo, penile melanosis, and vulval melanosis, is discussed under pathology of the external genitalia.

Acral lentigo

Clinical features

Acral lentigines are small, 1–5 mm diameter, circumscribed pigmented macules that present on the palms and soles.[1,2] They are seen more often in blacks than in whites. Eruptive acral lentigines have been reported in patients with AIDS, and also in patients with diffuse large cell lymphoma, breast cancer, gastric adenocarcinoma, and advanced stage melanoma.[3–5] Acral lentigines are devoid of sinister potential.

Histologic features

Acral lentigines are histologically identical to lentigo simplex (*Fig. 25.10*).

Multiple lentigines syndrome

This disorder is discussed under disorders of pigmentation.

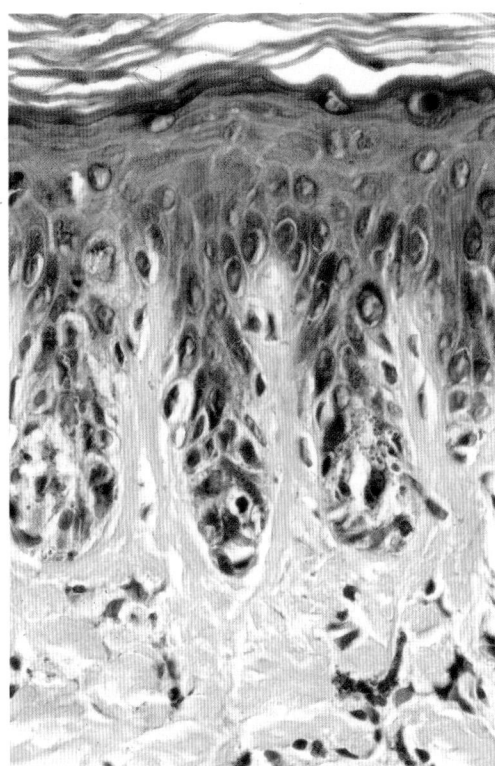

Fig. 25.9
Lentiginous junctional nevus: the rete ridges are elongated, and increased numbers of melanocytes are present as nests at the tips of the rete ridges and single cells distributed along the sides.

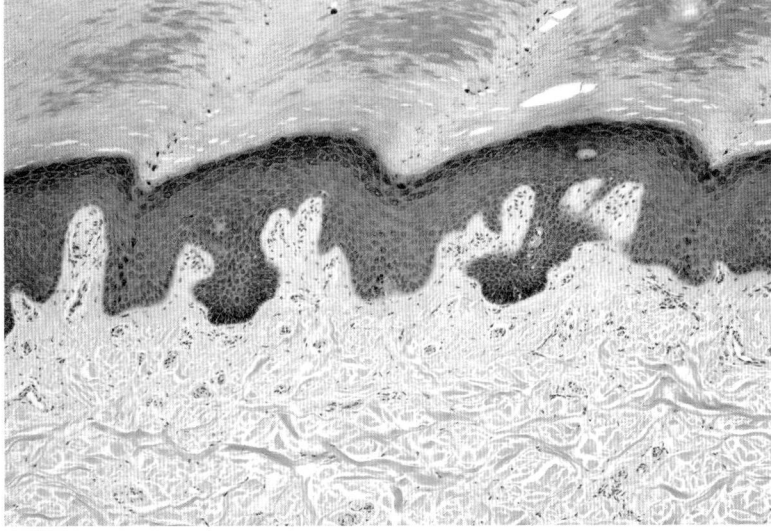

Fig. 25.10
Acral lentigo: there is marked basal cell hyperpigmentation.

Carney complex

Lentigines are a feature of Carney complex (*Fig. 25.11*). This topic is discussed under disorders of pigmentation, epithelioid blue nevus, and superficial angiomyxoma.

Centrofacial lentiginosis

Clinical features

Centrofacial lentiginosis is a rare autosomal dominant condition in which patients develop a characteristic zone of pigmented macules, particularly about the central region of the face (*Fig. 25.12*).[1-3] They may also have a variety of skeletal abnormalities including high arched palate, dental

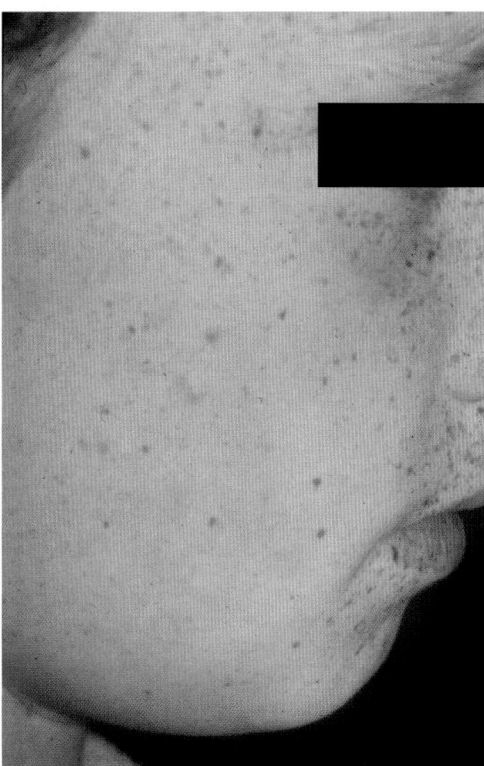

Fig. 25.11
Carney syndrome: in addition to lentiginosis, patients may manifest cutaneous and cardiac myxomas and develop endocrine abnormalities. By courtesy of M. Walsh, MD, The Royal Victoria Hospital, Belfast, N. Ireland.

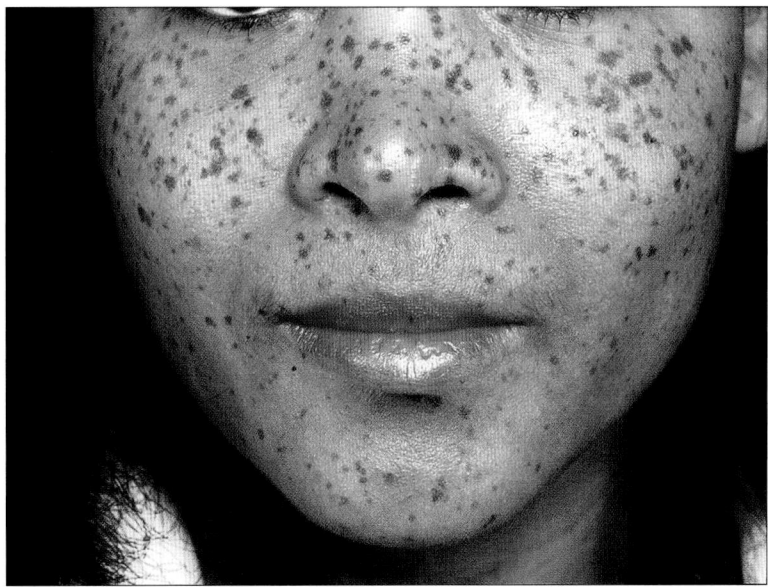

Fig. 25.12
Centrofacial lentiginosis: innumerable lentigines are present on the face of this young girl. By courtesy of the Institute of Dermatology, London, UK.

malpositions, cervical or cervicothoracic kyphosis, funnel chest, winged scapulae, spina bifida, hammer toes, bilateral pes cavus, and sacral dehiscence.[3] They can also suffer from neuropsychiatric disturbances including mental retardation, behavioral disturbances, and epilepsy.[3] Endocrine dysfunction, including goiter, hypothyroidism, and calcium metabolism abnormalities, has occasionally been documented.[3] An association of centrofacial lentiginosis and giant nevus spilus developing on the left side of the upper back in a dermatomal distribution has been reported in a child.[4]

Histologic features

The histologic features of the pigmented macules have not been described.

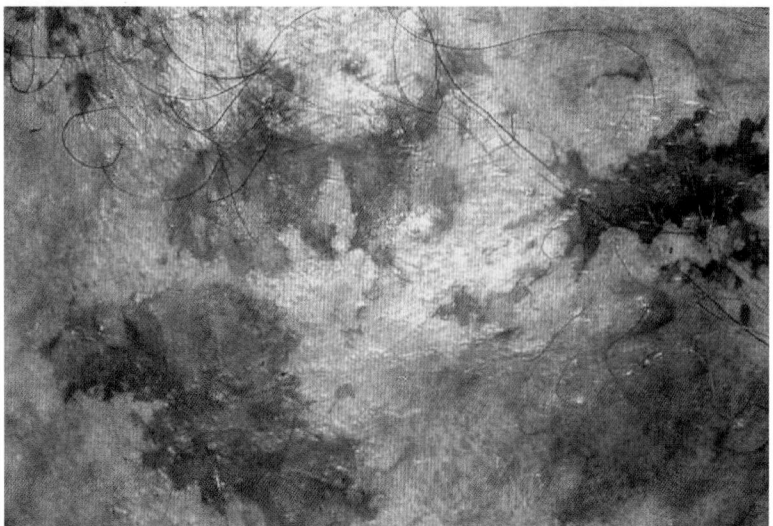

Fig. 25.13
PUVA lentigines: multiple lentigines are evident against a background of variable hypo- and hyperpigmentation. By courtesy of the Institute of Dermatology, London, UK.

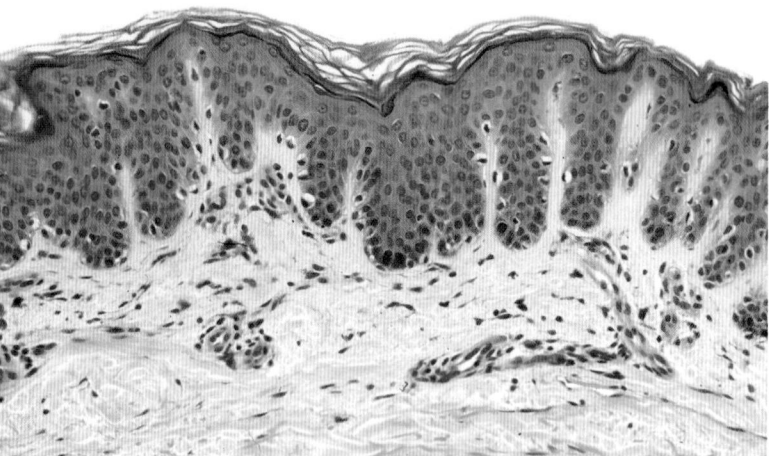

Fig. 25.14
PUVA lentigo: the features are indistinguishable from a lentigo simplex.

PUVA and sunbed lentigines

Clinical features

Long-term psoralen photochemotherapy (PUVA) may be complicated by a variety of cutaneous pigmentary changes including variable hyper- and hypopigmentation, vitiligo-like features, and multiple lentigines.[1-5] PUVA lentigines are dose-dependent, irregular, small, brown-black macules that are particularly seen on the shoulders, upper back, and limbs (Fig. 25.13).[3,4] They are commonly numerous. Males are more often affected than females, and skin types I and II are particularly at risk. Similar lesions have occasionally been described in patients, including one with systemic lupus erythematosus, following the use of sunbeds for artificial tanning.[6-8] Lesions tend to regress after therapy is discontinued.[4] Development of PUVA lentigines has been reported at the sites of mycosis fungoides lesions, as well as in normal and vitiliginous skin.[9,10] Furthermore, narrow band ultraviolet (UV) B used in patients with early-stage mycosis fungoides induce development of lentigines in both involved and non-involved skin much earlier and at lower cumulative dose than those developing after PUVA treatment. However, lentigines develop less frequently than those presenting after PUVA treatment.[11]

Pathogenesis and histologic features

The presence of T1799 BRAF mutations has been demonstrated in 33% of PUVA lentigines.[12]

Histologically, PUVA lentigines show a variety of features.[1-5,13,14] In some, there is increase in basal cell pigmentation with no increase in melanocyte numbers, reminiscent of an ephelis, whereas others resemble lentigines with pronounced rete ridge elongation and increased numbers of melanocytes (Fig. 25.14). Melanocytic nuclear atypia including enlargement, pleomorphism, and hyperchromasia, multinucleation, and giant melanosomes has been described.[13,14] There does not appear to be any link between PUVA lentigines and development of melanoma.[5]

Epidermal abnormalities, including dyskeratosis and actinic keratosis-like features, may also sometimes be observed.[15]

Ink spot lentigo

Clinical features

Ink spot lentigo (reticulated black solar lentigo, reticular lentigo, acquired reticulated lentigo, reticulated melanotic macule) is a rare variant of lentigo; it is particularly important because clinically it may be confused with melanoma. It affects fair-skinned individuals with red to blond hair and blue

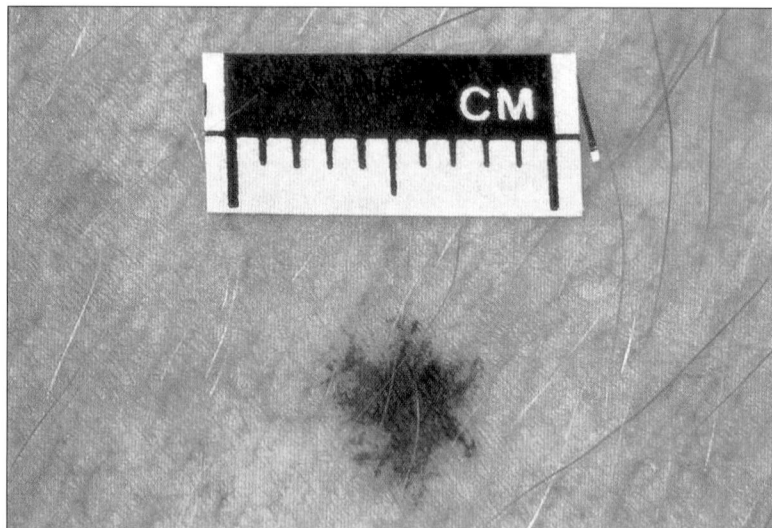

Fig. 25.15
Ink spot lentigo: this is a typical extremely irregular pigmented macule. By courtesy of the Institute of Dermatology, London, UK.

eyes (skin types I and II) and presents on a background of solar-damaged skin as a usually solitary, irregular, reticulated black macule with a wiry or beaded appearance (reminiscent of an ink spot) (Fig. 25.15).[1-3] Although the features may be clinically worrying, the lesion is completely benign. Ink spot lentigo can exceptionally develop in the background of a nevus spilus.[4]

Histologic features

Ink spot lentigo shows lentiginous hyperplasia with very marked basal cell hyperpigmentation, rete-tip accentuation, and characteristic achromic skip areas (Fig. 25.16).[1-3] Melanocytes may be normal or slightly increased in number, but there is no cytological atypia or junctional activity. Pigmentary incontinence is usually evident, and a perivascular chronic inflammatory cell infiltrate is commonly present.

Becker nevus

Clinical features

Becker nevus (pigmented hairy epidermal nevus, Becker melanosis, melanosis neviformis Becker) is an androgen-dependent organoid lesion that becomes more prominent after puberty.[1] It is uncommon and probably shows an equal sex distribution, although lesions in females are said to be

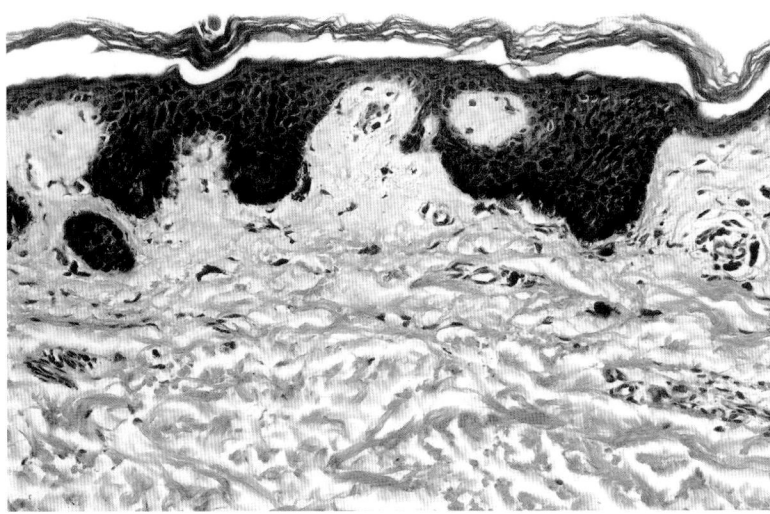

Fig. 25.16
Ink spot lentigo: there is massive basal cell hyperpigmentation.

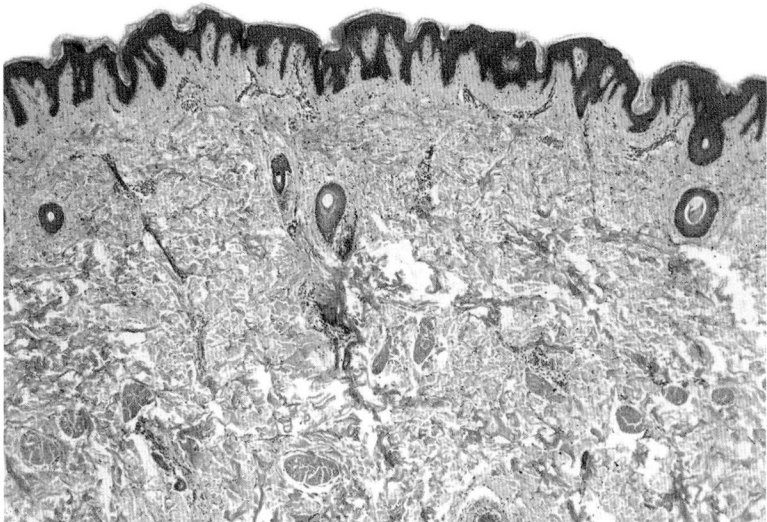

Fig. 25.18
Becker nevus: at scanning magnification, the changes are subtle and comprise slight hyperkeratosis and accentuation of the epidermal ridge pattern. A very slight chronic inflammatory cell infiltrate surrounds the vessels of the papillary dermis.

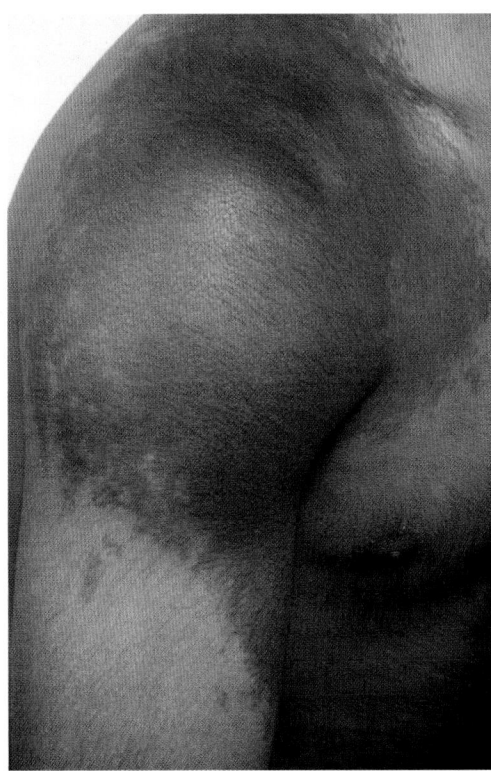

Fig. 25.17
Becker nevus: this example shows a characteristic distribution around the shoulder region. From the collection of the late N.P. Smith, MD, the Institute of Dermatology, London, UK.

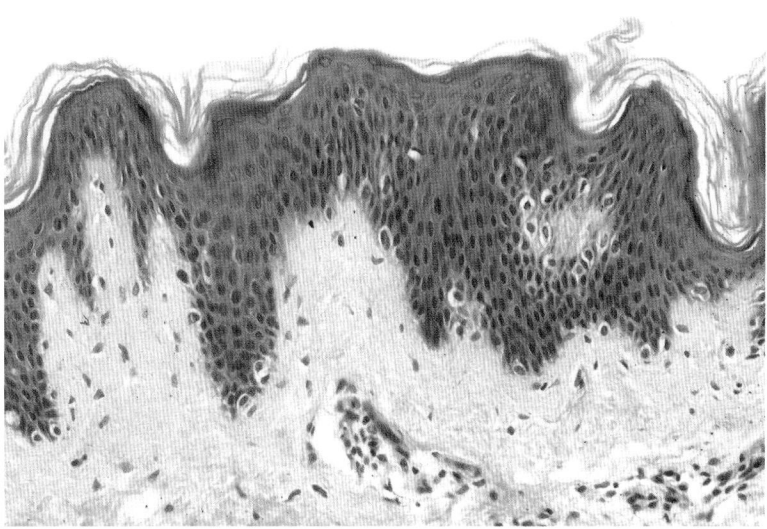

Fig. 25.19
Becker nevus: there is mild acanthosis and increased numbers of basal melanocytes are present. In addition, there is obvious hyperpigmentation, but no junctional activity.

more difficult to appreciate than in males.[1] While all races may be affected, there appears to be a predilection for non-whites.[2] It usually presents in the second decade, initially as a light to dark brown enlarging macular lesion, which subsequently shows hypertrichosis (*Fig. 25.17*).[1,3–6] Although most frequently the chest, shoulder, or upper arm are involved, examples have occurred everywhere on the skin surface. Lesions on the scalp or face can be associated with asymmetrical growth of scalp hair or beard.[7,8] Sometimes they are multiple, and familial examples have been recorded.[9] Rarely, Becker nevus may be congenital.[10] Linear distribution of congenital Becker nevus following Blaschko lines, giant bilateral Becker nevus over the back, chest and upper arms, as well as symmetrical bilateral Becker nevus on the anterior chest and back have also been reported.[11–14] Involvement of oral mucosa in a case with segmental distribution on the face has also been

described.[15] Of particular importance is the occasional association of Becker nevus with developmental anomalies, including cutaneous, muscular, and skeletal anomalies – the so-called pigmented hairy epidermal nevus syndrome (e.g., breast and limb hypoplasia, pectus excavatum, spina bifida, scoliosis, and hypoplasia of subcutaneous fatty tissue, to mention just the most common conditions).[1,3,6,16–20] A case in which a scalp lesion occurred with underlying loss of cranium has been documented.[21]

Becker nevus is thought to be the consequence of an early postzygotic mutational event representing a genetic mosaicism.[22]

Histologic features

The features are subtle, comprising slight hyperkeratosis, variable acanthosis, and elongation of the epidermal ridges, accompanied by increased pigmentation in the basal region (*Figs 25.18–25.20*). Additional changes can include flattening of the epidermis, keratotic plugging, and fusion of two or three neighboring elongated rete ridges.[23] In contrast to uninvolved epidermis, the epidermis of Becker nevus shows increased expression of androgen receptors.[23] Melanocytes often appear increased in number, but there is no evidence of proliferative activity.[24] The superficial dermis may contain

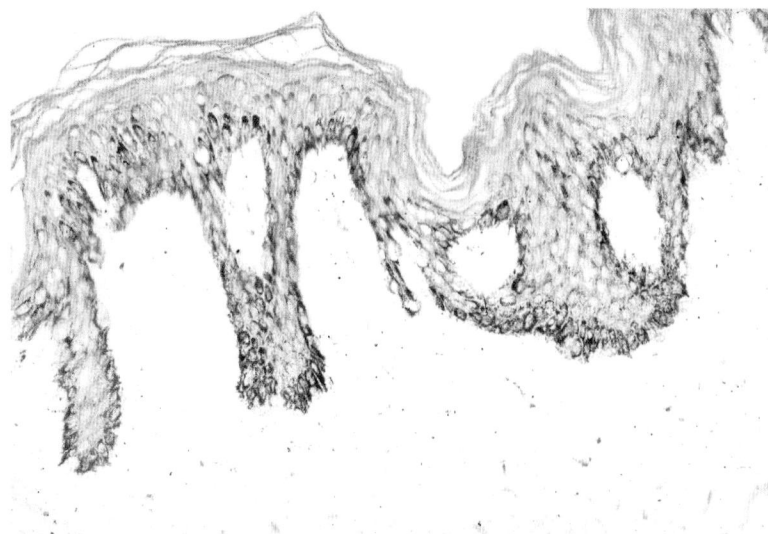

Fig. 25.20
Becker nevus: the increased pigmentation may be accentuated by the Masson-Fontana reaction.

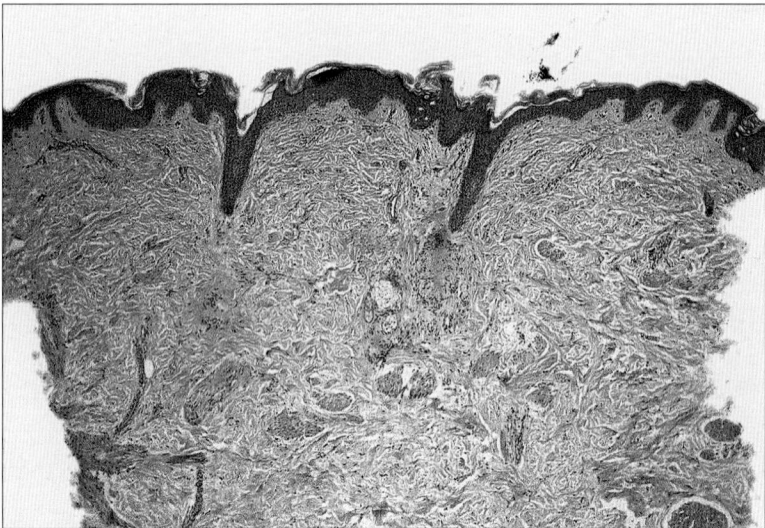

Fig. 25.21
Becker nevus: in this example, hamartomatous aggregates of smooth muscle cells are widely distributed throughout the dermis.

melanophages, and a mild perivascular chronic inflammatory cell infiltrate is sometimes present.

In occasional lesions, the reticular dermis contains large numbers of hamartomatous, irregular, enlarged smooth muscle fibers (*Fig. 25.21*).[25–28] Associated dermal fibrosis, sebaceous hyperplasia, neves sebaceous, localized acneiform lesions, solitary plexiform neurofibroma, neurofibromatosis type I, basal cell carcinoma, compound melanocytic nevus, pigmented epithelioid melanocytoma, nevus anemicus, lichen planus, pityriasis versicolor, a psoriasiform dermatitis suggestive of an inflammatory linear verrucous epidermal nevus, and hyperkeratosis with focal diminution of granular cell layer (e.g., ichthyotic changes) have also been documented.[3,28–38]

Ultrastructural studies have revealed an increased number and size of compound melanosomes within basal keratinocytes.[3] An increase in the number of melanosomes per complex may also be evident.

Pseudomelanocytic nests

Clinical features

Pseudomelanocytic nests are aggregates of nonmelanocytic cells, or cell fragments within the epidermis mimicking a melanocytic proliferation on histologic examination.[1–7] These nests usually develop in the setting of lichenoid

tissue reactions, for example, fixed drug eruptions, phototoxic reactions, lichen planus pigmentosus, lupus erythematosus, or pigmented lichenoid keratosis.[1–3]

Patients are usually adults in their sixth decade of life with equal gender distribution.[5] The lesions are either solitary or multiple and of recent onset. Interestingly, pseudomelanocytic nests have also been reported in the oral mucosa.[5] Clinicopathological correlation is essential for correct recognition of these lesions.

Histologic features

Pseudomelanocytic nests represent irregularly sized and usually dyscohesive collections of keratinocytes, macrophages, and lymphocytes along the dermal–epidermal junction.[1,2] In addition, isolated melanocytes can also be present within the nests, but they generally do not exceed two cells.[3] Nonmelanocytic cells within the nests frequently contain cytoplasmic melanin pigment. The epidermis can display irregular acanthosis with effacement of the rete ridges, but it is more frequently atrophic. A variably dense lichenoid inflammatory cell infiltrate including melanophages is also seen. Solar elastosis is commonly seen on sun-exposed sites.

By immunohistochemistry, nonmelanocytic cells within the nests can express Melan-A/MART-1 positivity, but are usually S100, tyrosinase, and HMB-45 negative.[1–3] It is believed that Melan-A/MART-1 positivity is the result of non-specific staining of melanosomes within the cytoplasm of cells other than melanocytes, thus representing a potential diagnostic pitfall that may lead to a misdiagnosis of a melanocytic proliferation, in particular, melanoma in situ.

Differential diagnosis

Pseudomelanocytic nests should be distinguished from melanoma in situ. The latter is typically associated with lentiginous, nested, and pagetoid proliferation of atypical melanocytes. A combination of melanocytic markers, including S100, SOX-10, microphthalmia transcription factor, and tyrosinase, should aid in distinction in dubious cases. Clinicopathological correlation is essential.

Melanocytic nevus

Melanocytic nevus (banal nevus) is a benign tumor that usually presents in childhood and adolescence. The sex distribution is equal. An average white individual can expect to develop 15–40 such lesions during life, reaching the maximum number in the third decade before regression to virtual disappearance by the eighth and ninth decades.[1–5]

In addition to those derived from hair-bearing skin, melanocytic nevi may develop on glabrous skin, beneath fingernails and toenails, within the conjunctivae and uveal tract, and mucosae (*Fig. 25.22*). They have an ordered and histologically defined natural history, which may, to some extent, be predicted from their clinical appearance. Their existence commences as a focus of melanocytic proliferation (junctional activity) within the lower reaches of the epithelium, the so-called junctional nevus. This progresses to the presence of melanocytes within both the epidermis and the dermis, which is the compound nevus. Further development results in a completely intradermal lesion called the dermal nevus.[6]

While there is unquestionable malignant transformation on occasions in these lesions, such events are rare; therefore, there is no indication for widespread prophylactic excision of otherwise typical melanocytic nevi (*Figs 25.23* and *25.24*). It has been estimated that the likelihood of any one nevus evolving into melanoma is roughly 1/100 000.[7] Subsequent mortality is of the order of 1/500 000 original nevi. However, the prevalence of nevi is of major epidemiological importance, increased numbers correlating with a greater risk of subsequent development of melanoma, of superficial spreading and nodular subtypes.[8–10] Lentigo maligna melanoma does not derive from pre-existent nevi and is not related to their prevalence. In young children and adolescents in whom these lesions are at an early stage of development, increased pigmentation is to be anticipated. However, in adults, evidence of junctional activity is to be viewed with caution; it is those nevi with increasingly marked pigmentation, or appearing de novo in the older age groups, which are often excised for histologic evaluation.

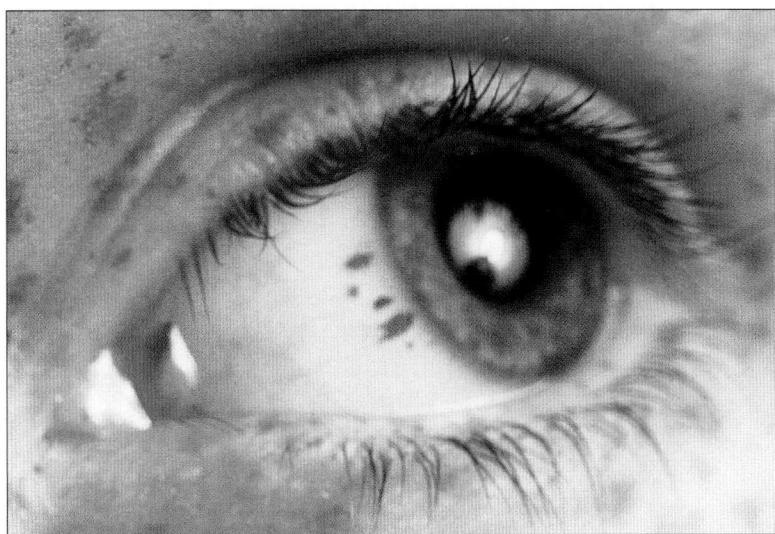

Fig. 25.22
Conjunctival junctional melanocytic nevus: there is uniform pigmentation and a regular border. By courtesy of the late M. Beare, MD, Royal Victoria Hospital, Belfast, N. Ireland.

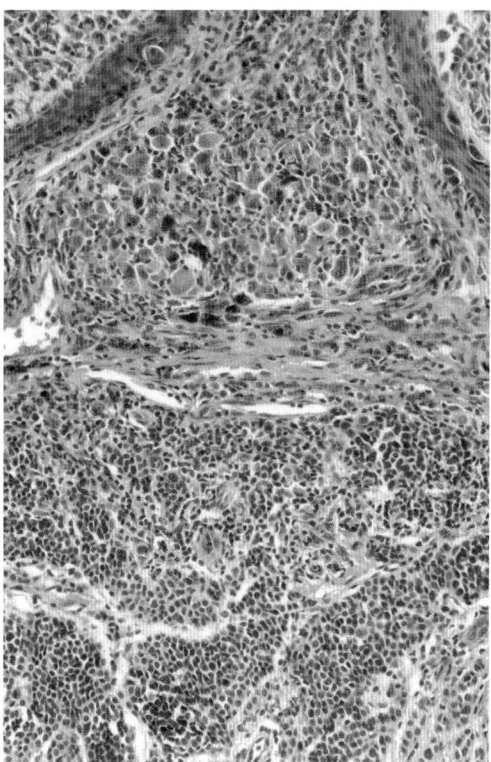

Fig. 25.24
Melanoma: high-power view of *Fig. 25.23*.

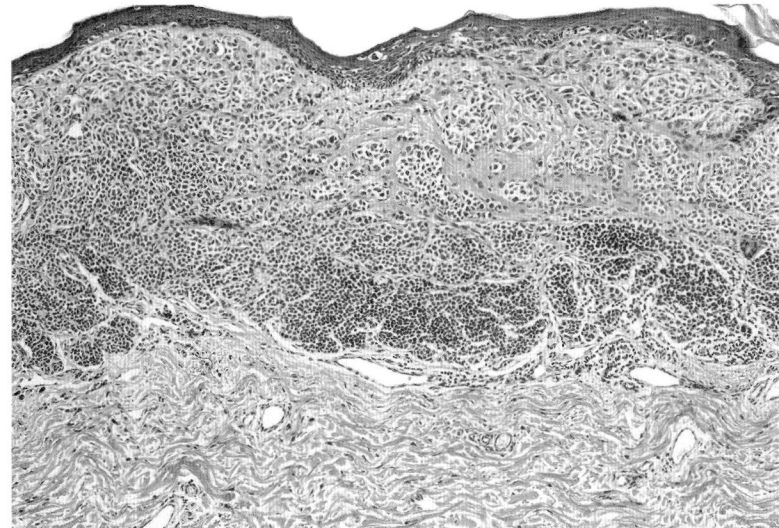

Fig. 25.23
Melanoma: this lesion has arisen within a pre-existent compound melanocytic nevus. The residual benign component is present in the lower field. Compare the pleomorphism of the melanoma with the uniform nevus population.

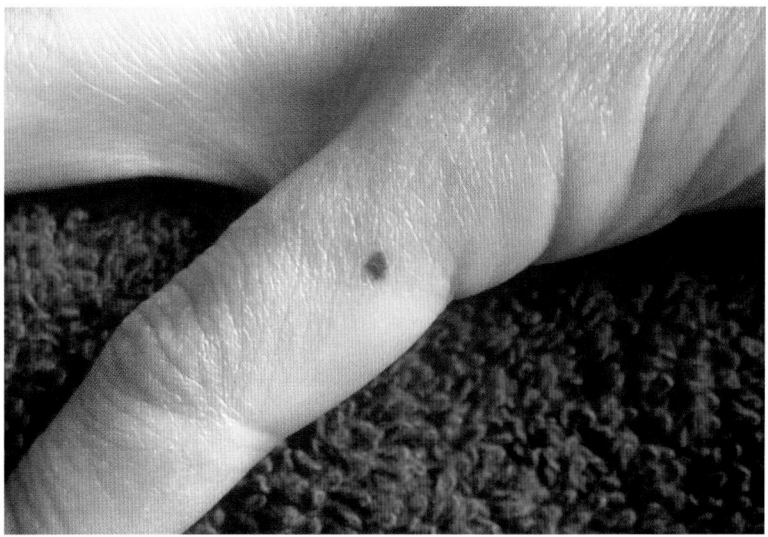

Fig. 25.25
Junctional melanocytic nevus: the lesion is small. Note the uniform coloration. By courtesy of M. Liang, MD, The Children's Hospital, Boston, USA.

Clinical features

Melanocytic nevi first appear in early childhood and increase in number during the second and third decades.[5,6,11–13] In males, the head, neck, and trunk are particularly affected, whereas in females the upper and lower limbs are more often involved.[5,12,14,15] Distribution of acquired melanocytic nevi in an agminate (grouped) pattern can occasionally be seen.[16] Melanocytic nevi involute during middle age, and most have completely regressed in the elderly. They are more common in individuals with pale skin and light-colored eyes.[10,17] Melanocytic nevi are much less frequently seen in Asians and Afro-Caribbeans.[10] In these races, the acral sites are particularly affected.[1] Dark brown or black hair correlates with increasing numbers of nevi, whereas red hair appears to protect.[8,10] Development of melanocytic nevi is related to the extent of sun exposure during the first two decades of life.[17–19] Intermittent intense sunlight is of greater importance than chronic exposure.[12] In fact, chronic sun exposure correlates with low levels of nevi (i.e., it appears to be protective).[14] Increasing nevus counts are found in individuals who tend to sunburn rather than tan following sun exposure and correlate with the degree of freckling.[10,20,21] As these factors are also

important in the etiology of melanoma, high levels of freckles and nevi at an early age may be of predictive value.

Melanocytic nevi present a variety of features depending on their stage of evolution. Junctional nevi are usually macular or slightly raised, up to 0.5 cm in diameter and from light to dark brown in color (*Figs 25.25–25.27*). They are well circumscribed with a regular border and are usually uniformly pigmented, but sometimes the central area is darker. Typically, the skin lines can be clearly discerned on the surface of the lesion.

The compound nevus is raised, sometimes dome-shaped or warty, and often still deeply pigmented (*Figs 25.28* and *25.29*). Occasionally, there are coarse hairs projecting from its surface; plucking these hairs may traumatize the dermal component of the hair follicle, resulting in granulomatous inflammation, which may cause concern to both the patient and clinician as to the possibility of malignant transformation.[8,19]

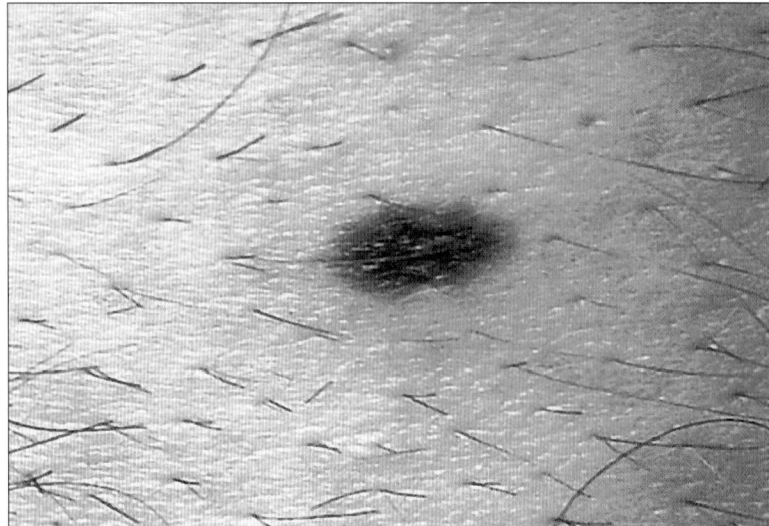

Fig. 25.26
Junctional melanocytic nevus: banal nevi are typically sharply circumscribed. By courtesy of M. Liang, MD, The Children's Hospital, Boston, USA.

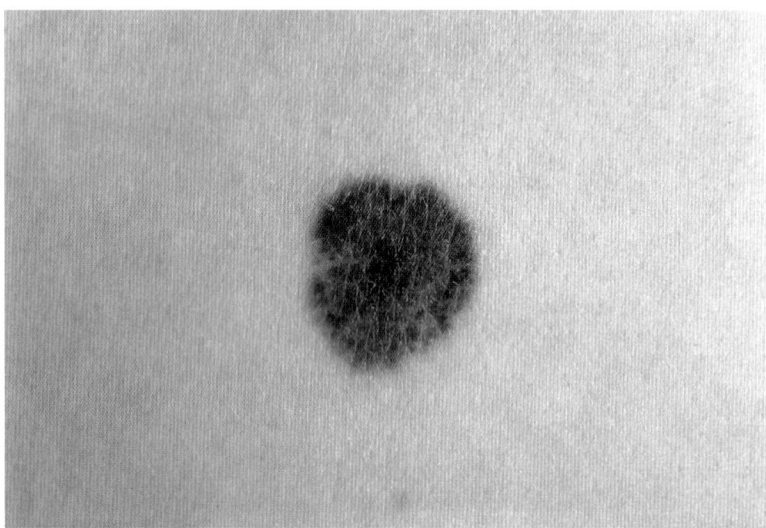

Fig. 25.27
Junctional nevus: the skin markings overlying the nevus are typically present, in contrast to melanoma when they are usually lost. By courtesy of the Institute of Dermatology, London, UK.

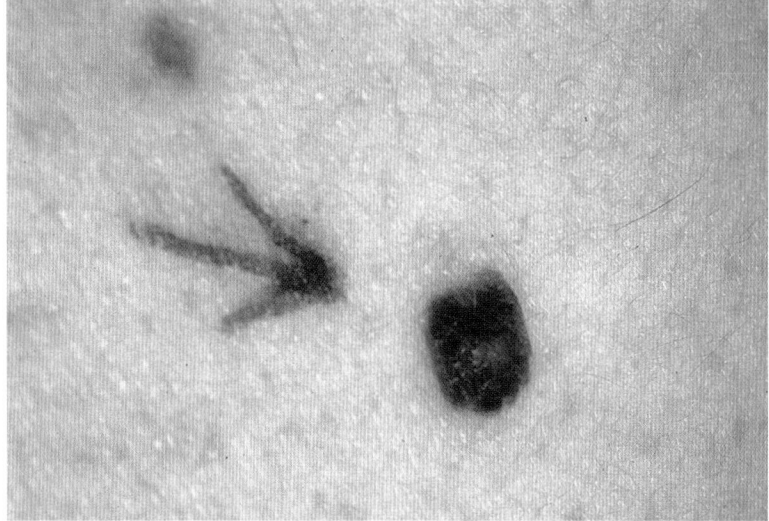

Fig. 25.28
Compound nevus: the nevus has a central raised dome-shaped component. Color is uniform, and the margin is sharply defined. By courtesy of the Institute of Dermatology, London, UK.

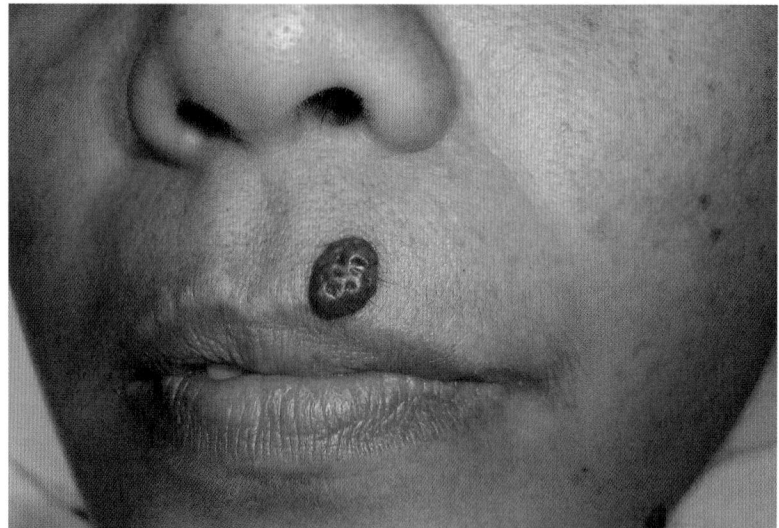

Fig. 25.29
Compound nevus: this is a heavily pigmented example. The sharply defined border is a clue to its benign nature. By courtesy of J. Dayrit, MD, Manila, The Philippines.

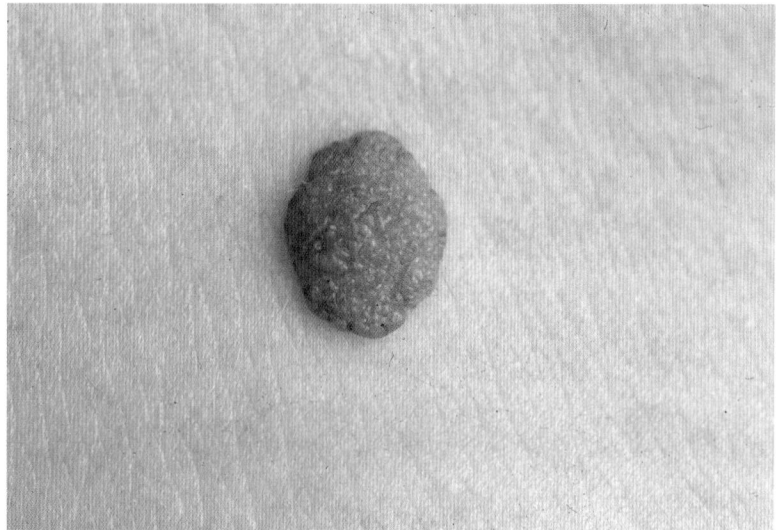

Fig. 25.30
Dermal melanocytic nevus: presentation as a pale, raised, dermal warty, nodule is a common finding. From the collection of the late N.P. Smith, MD, the Institute of Dermatology, London, UK.

The intradermal nevus is often devoid of pigment and may present as a dome-shaped nodule, a papillomatous lesion, or a pedunculated skin tag (*Figs 25.30* and *25.31*).

Nevi may become more highly pigmented under the influence of pregnancy or the oral contraceptive pill.[22] There is, however, no evidence that pregnancy in any significant way stimulates their development or alters the biological potential of pre-existent nevi.[5]

Histologic features

There is considerable confusion about the nature of the nevocyte and its distinction from a melanocyte. A nevocyte is merely a melanocyte that has multiplied to form a melanocytic nevus. It has the same electron microscopic appearance as a melanocyte, and identical organelles and enzyme systems; the only significant differences are that the dermal component lacks dendritic processes and with increasing depth melanin synthesis is arrested.

In the earliest stage of development, junctional nests of melanocytes appear in the lower aspect of the epidermis (confined by the basement membrane), usually within the tips or, less often, sides of sometimes broadened and elongated epidermal ridges (lentiginous junctional nevus) (*Figs 25.32* and *25.33*). The melanocytes may be polygonal and epithelioid, or more

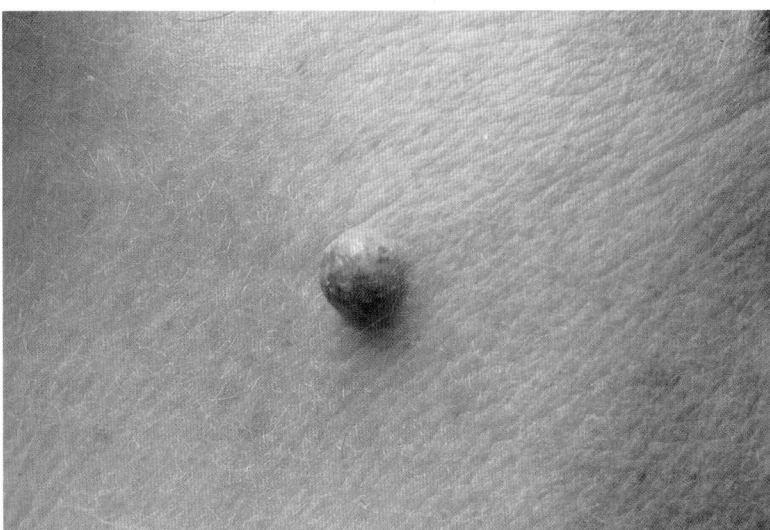

Fig. 25.31
Dermal melanocytic nevus: this example presents a dome-shaped appearance. There is focal residual pigmentation. From the collection of the late N.P. Smith, MD, the Institute of Dermatology, London, UK.

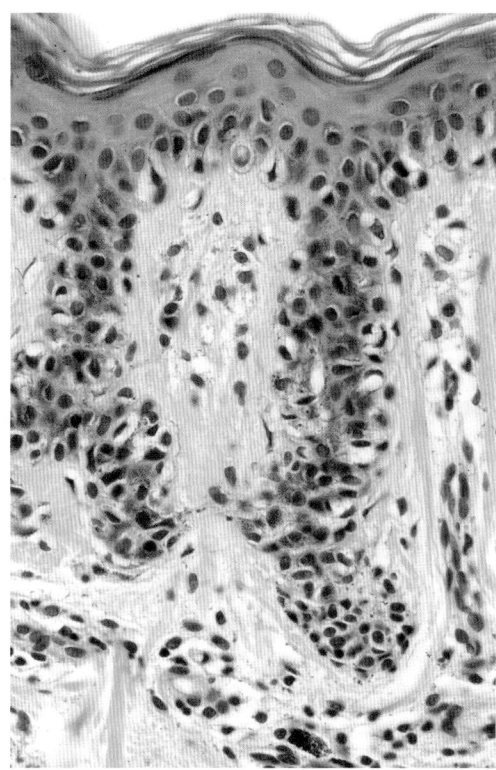

Fig. 25.33
Lentiginous junctional nevus: in this field, nevus cells are distributed as a palisade outlining the margins of the rete. Note the pigment incontinence.

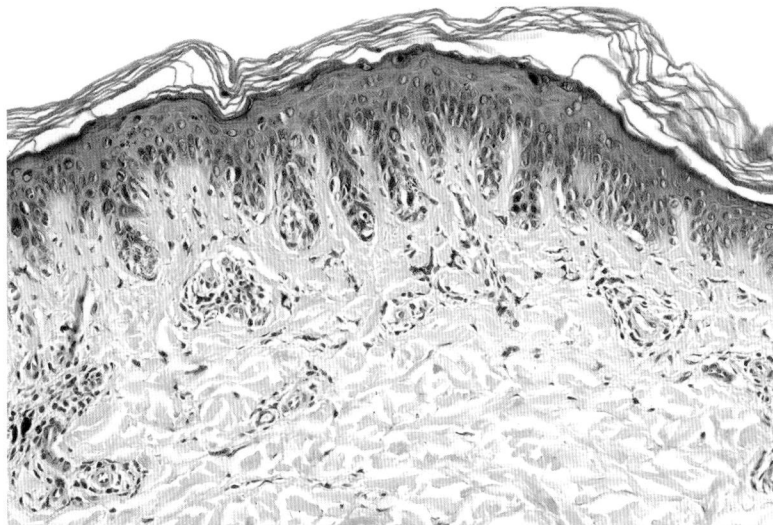

Fig. 25.32
Lentiginous junctional nevus: note the marked elongation of the rete ridges. The junctional nests are present at their tips, a characteristic location in banal nevi.

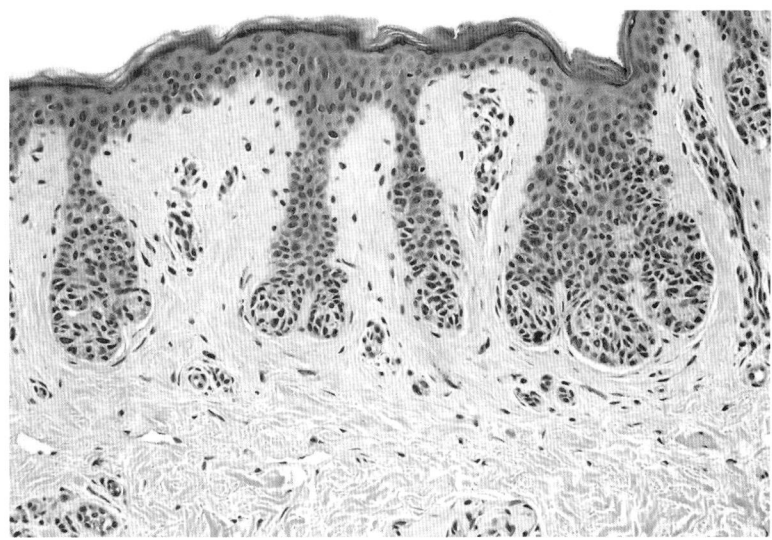

Fig. 25.34
Junctional nevus: in this example, the nests of melanocytes are located at the tips of the rete ridges (compare with dysplastic nevi in which nests are often seen along the sides of the rete and overlying the tips of the dermal papillae).

rarely spindled with clear to pale staining or lightly eosinophilic cytoplasm, and contain uniform round to oval small nuclei with prominent nucleoli (type A nevus cells) (*Figs 25.34* and *25.35*). The cytoplasm typically contains sparse, evenly distributed, delicate melanin granules. In benign junctional nevi, growth is towards dermal involvement. Any tendency for melanocytes to spread towards the upper reaches of the epidermis (pagetoid spread) is suggestive of malignant change and should be viewed with caution. However, upward migration of melanocytes on its own is not diagnostic of malignancy as this feature may be seen in variants of nevi-like lesions occurring at some special sites (see below). Melanocytes between epidermal ridges may sometimes appear increased in number.[2] By definition, junctional nevi are solely intraepidermal; however, in heavily pigmented variants, melanin is typically present in macrophages (melanophages) within the papillary dermis (pigmentary incontinence).

In addition to junctional activity, compound nevi show nests and strands of nevus cells within both the papillary and the superficial reticular dermis (*Figs 25.36–25.39*). Compound banal nevi are usually fairly well circumscribed and symmetrical. The junctional component does not typically extend beyond the dermal component, i.e., a shoulder is absent in the majority of banal nevi (compare with dysplastic nevus). It should,

however, be noted that a shoulder can sometimes be present in a banal compound nevus, i.e., the presence of a shoulder in itself does not make a nevus dysplastic. Compound nevi may sometimes be associated with marked hyperkeratosis, acanthosis with keratinous pseudocyst formation, and papillomatosis (reminiscent of a seborrheic keratosis), accounting for a warty clinical appearance – the so-called papillomatous (verrucous) melanocytic nevus or keratotic melanocytic nevus (*Fig. 25.40*).[23–25] These nevi are more often found in females, and the trunk is the commonest site affected. The change may be related to estrogens as the nevus cells express pS2.[25]

The cells of the more superficial component of the dermal lesion may retain cytological characteristics similar to the junctional nevus. The cells in the deeper aspect are much smaller with less cytoplasm and have dense,

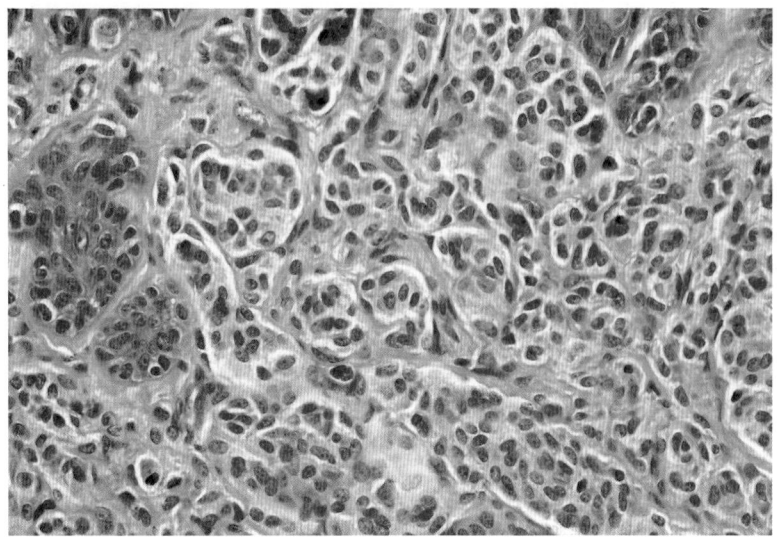

Fig. 25.35
Type A nevus cells: the cytoplasm is pale staining, and nuclei are vesicular and uniform. Nucleoli when visible are typically small.

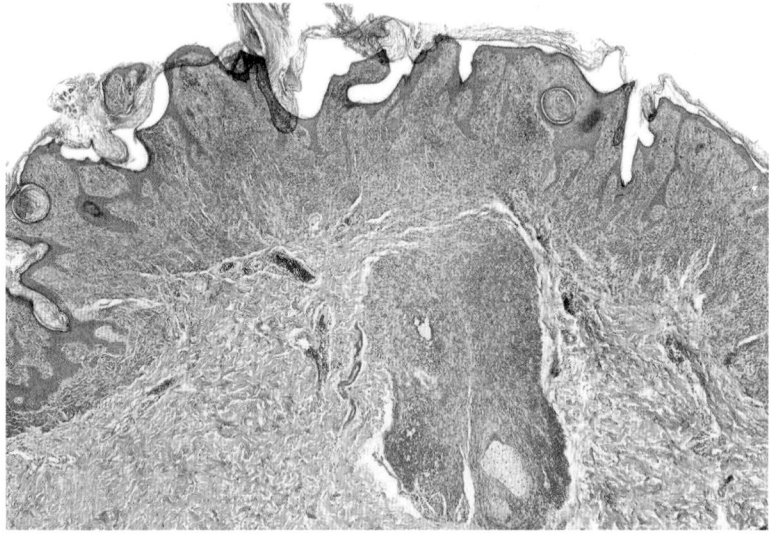

Fig. 25.36
Compound nevus: ensheathing of the hair follicle as shown in this field is more often a feature of congenital lesions, but can sometimes be seen in acquired melanocytic nevi.

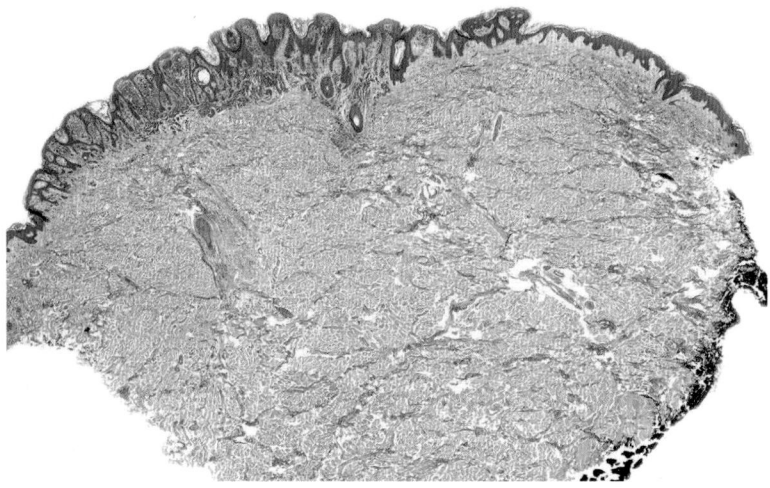

Fig. 25.37
Compound nevus: lesions often have a verrucous or warty appearance.

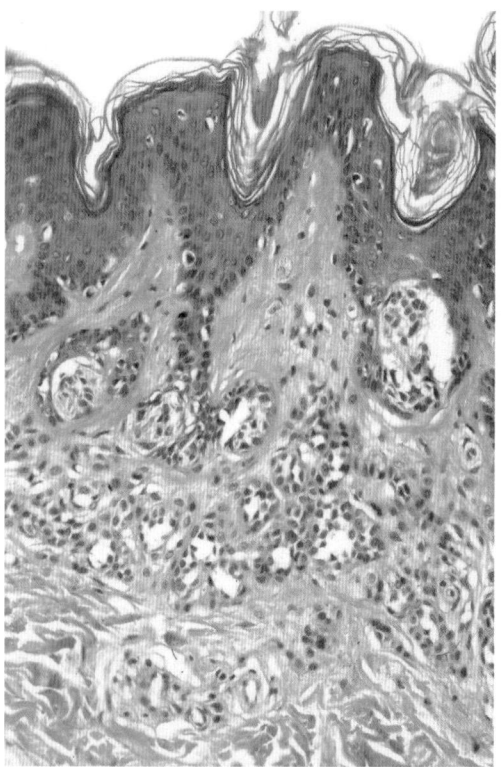

Fig. 25.38
Compound nevus: both junctional and dermal components are present.

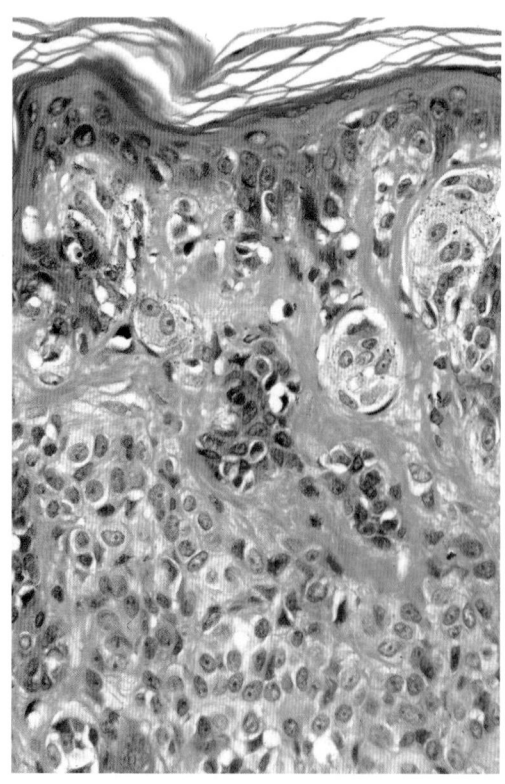

Fig. 25.39
Compound nevus: high-power view of type A nevus cells. The nuclei are uniform and many contain small nucleoli.

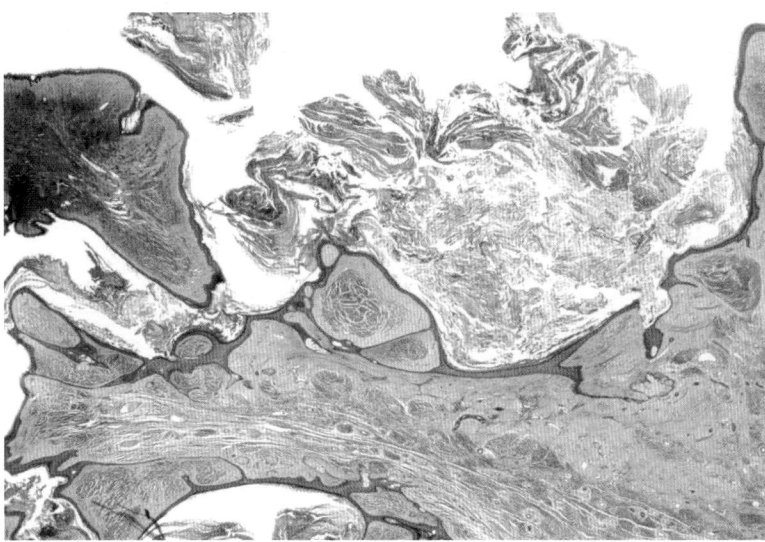

Fig. 25.40
Verrucous compound nevus: this variant shows gross papillomatosis and very marked hyperkeratosis.

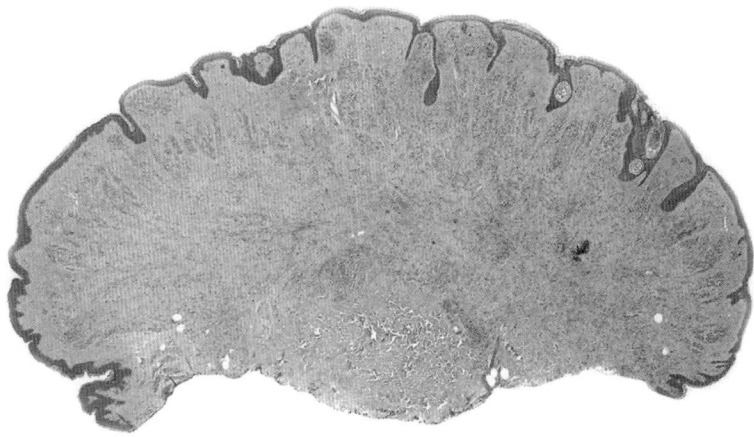

Fig. 25.41
Dermal nevus: at scanning magnification, these lesions typically have a dome-shaped or verrucous morphology.

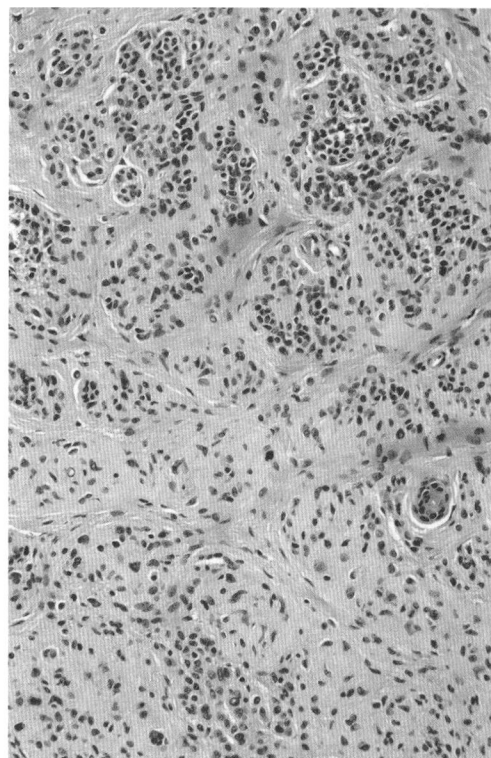

Fig. 25.42
Dermal nevus: the darkly staining superficial nevus cells are type B cells. In the deeper reaches, spindled forms are evident, a feature of maturation.

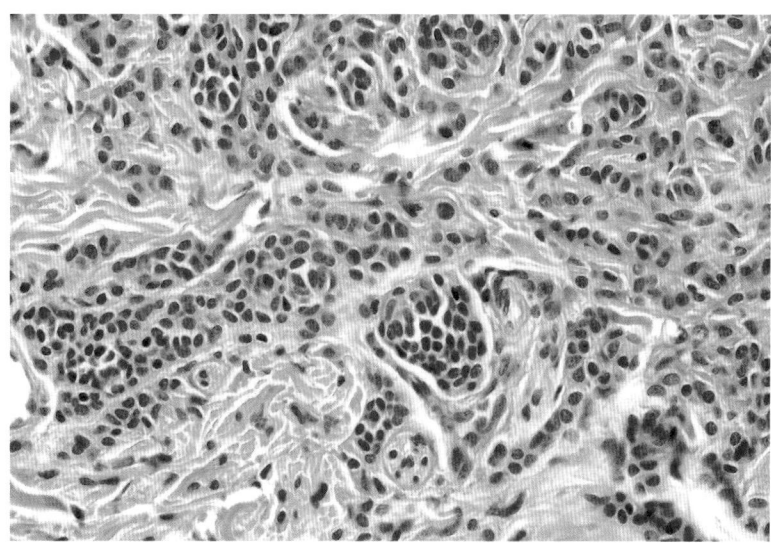

Fig. 25.43
Dermal nevus: type B cells have uniform hyperchromatic nuclei with little cytoplasm.

more darkly staining nuclei resembling lymphocytes (type B nevus cells) (*Figs 25.41–25.43*). Mitotic activity can occasionally be seen in the dermal component of an acquired melanocytic nevus (see differential diagnosis). Mitotic activity may also be increased in melanocytic nevi in pregnancy. An analysis of dermal mitoses in otherwise banal compound melanocytic nevi has demonstrated the mean number of 0.024 dermal mitoses/mm².[26] Mitoses are normal and never atypical, evenly distributed, usually located in the upper half of the dermis, and do not appear in clusters.[26] Although isolated regular mitoses can also be seen in the deep dermal melanocytic component, they are about three times less frequent than mitoses in the upper half of the dermis.[26] Importantly, banal nevi with dermal mitoses are significantly more common in younger age groups (e.g., between 0 and 20 years of age).[26] Therefore, more than an occasional dermal mitosis in older patients should be viewed with caution.

The dermal nevus, the 'end stage' of the melanocytic nevus, is typified by progressively less pigmentation with atrophy (so-called nevus maturation) (*Fig. 25.44*). This is usually accompanied by the accumulation of loose fibrous tissue. Rarely, dense fibrosis may develop, resulting in separation of individual residual melanocytes (desmoplastic nevus) (see below). In some dermal nevi, there may be worrying nuclear pleomorphism and hyperchromatism. The latter, however, appears smudged, and the nuclei are devoid of nucleoli and mitotic activity (ancient nevus, nevus with senescent atypia).[27]

In dermal nevi, the melanocytes often develop spindled cell and Schwann cell-like characteristics (neurotization), such as a fibrillar appearance with pale eosinophilic cytoplasm and wavy nuclei (type C nevus cells) (*Fig. 25.45*). Cholinesterase positivity may be present, and often Meissner corpuscle-like structures are found (*Figs 25.46 and 25.47*). The cells are nevertheless still truly melanocytic: ultrastructurally, they contain melanosomes. In addition, they are S100 and dopa positive and do not show Schwann cell morphology, nor do they react with antibodies to myelin basic protein.[27] Occasionally, intradermal nevi take on truly neurofibromatous appearances (*Fig. 25.48*). Other features of 'maturation'/senescence in dermal nevi include giant cell formation, mucinous degeneration, xanthomatization, and fat accumulation (*Figs 25.49–25.51*).[3] More rarely, changes include calcification and bone formation (usually based on a degenerate hair follicle) (*Fig. 25.52*). Lesions with bone formation are known as osteonevus of Nanta. A not uncommon observation is the presence of pseudovascular spaces imparting an angiomatous-like appearance (*Figs 25.53 and 25.54*).

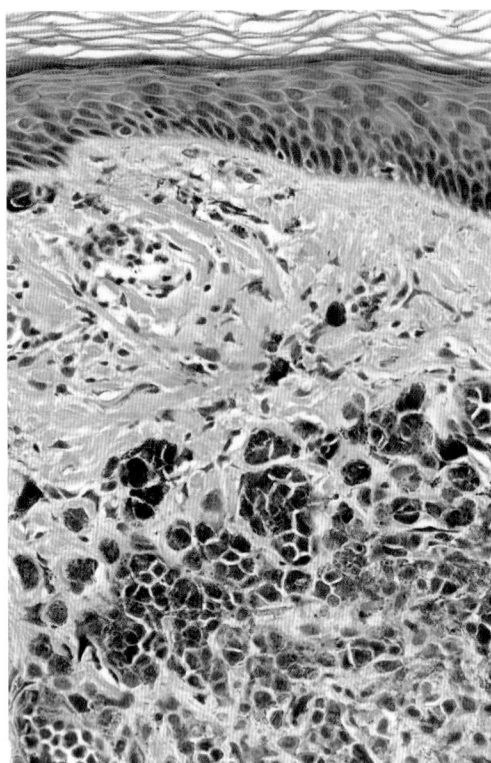

Fig. 25.44
Dermal nevus: melanin pigmentation typically diminishes with depth.

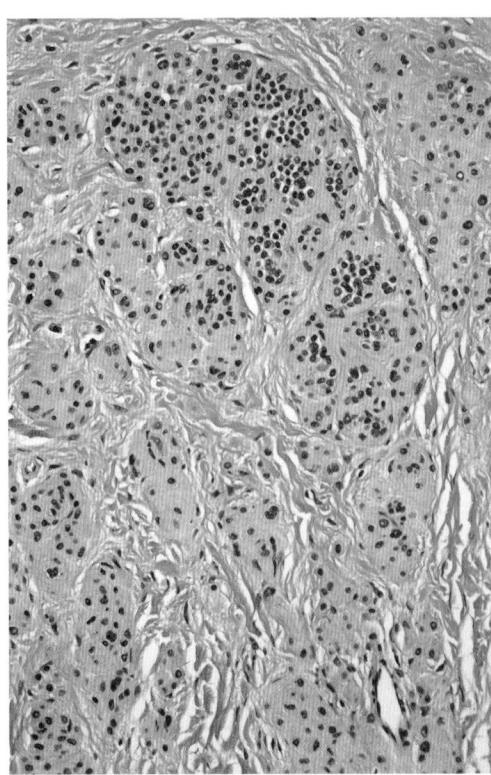

Fig. 25.45
Dermal nevus: this view shows maturation with spindle-shaped type C cells at the base. Nuclei at the top of the lesion are larger than those at the base (maturation). Nests, when present, also diminish in size with depth.

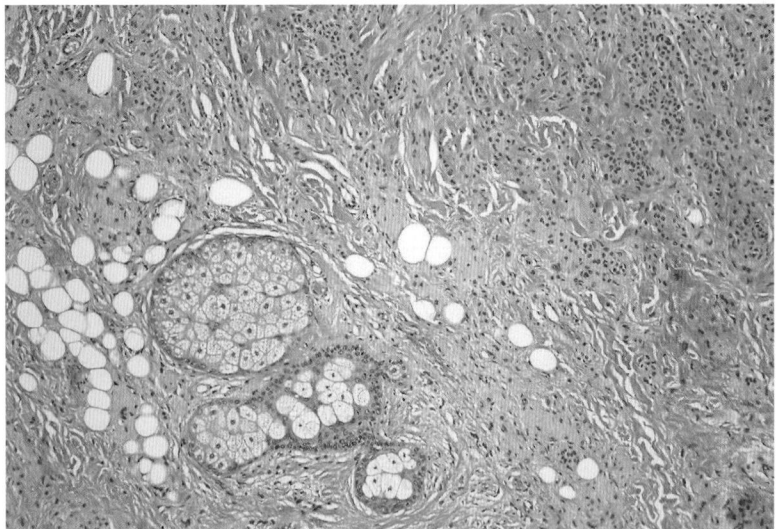

Fig. 25.46
Dermal nevus: neurotization is often accompanied by formation of typically lamellated, Meisner corpuscle-like structures.

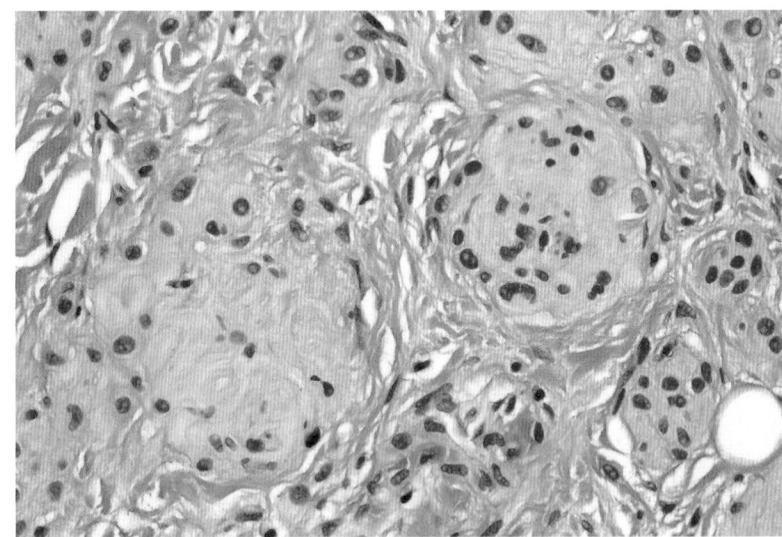

Fig. 25.47
Dermal nevus: high-power view of Meisner corpuscle-like structure.

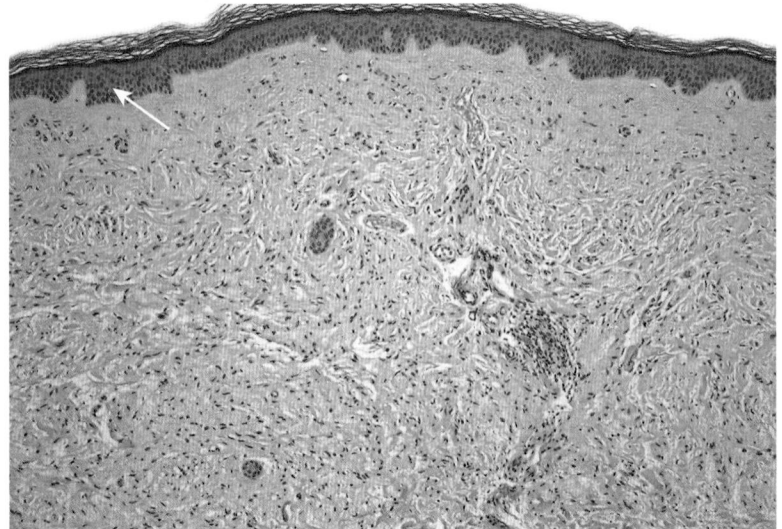

Fig. 25.48
Dermal nevus: this example has undergone extensive neurotization, making it indistinguishable from a neurofibroma. One or two residual nests of nevus cells are evident in the top-left corner of the field (*arrowed*).

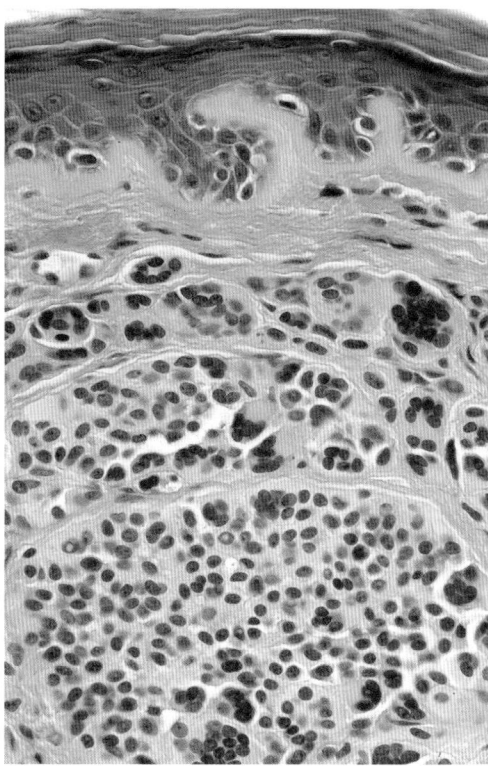

Fig. 25.49
Dermal nevus: multinucleated giant cells often with smudged chromatin are commonly found and are of no significance.

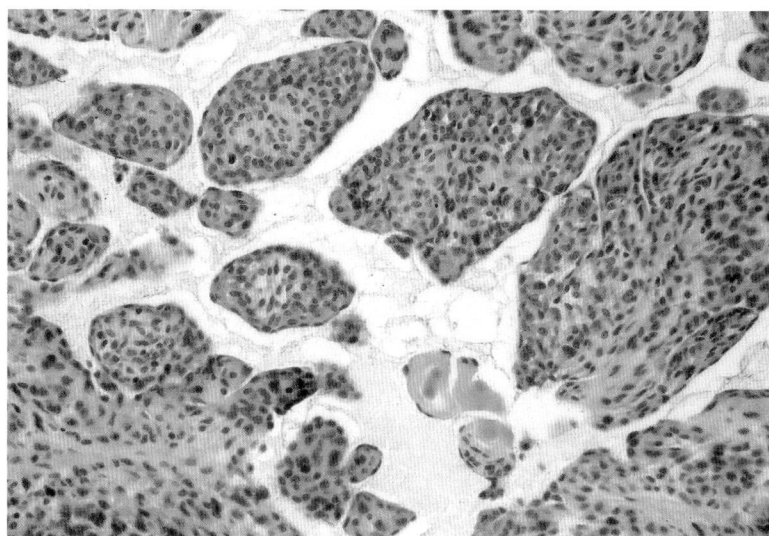

Fig. 25.51
Dermal nevus: high-power view of *Fig. 25.57*. Note the delicate wisps of mucin.

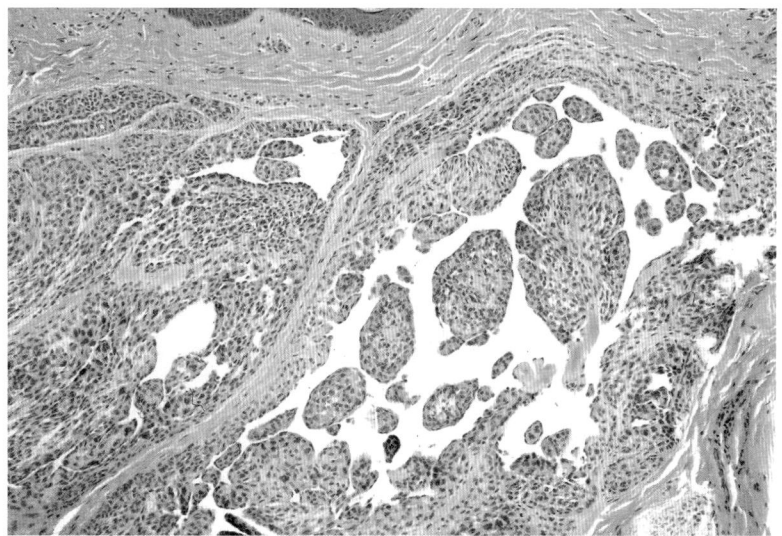

Fig. 25.50
Dermal nevus: very occasionally excessive stromal mucin deposition results in lakes. In extreme cases, this is sometimes known as a myxoid nevus.

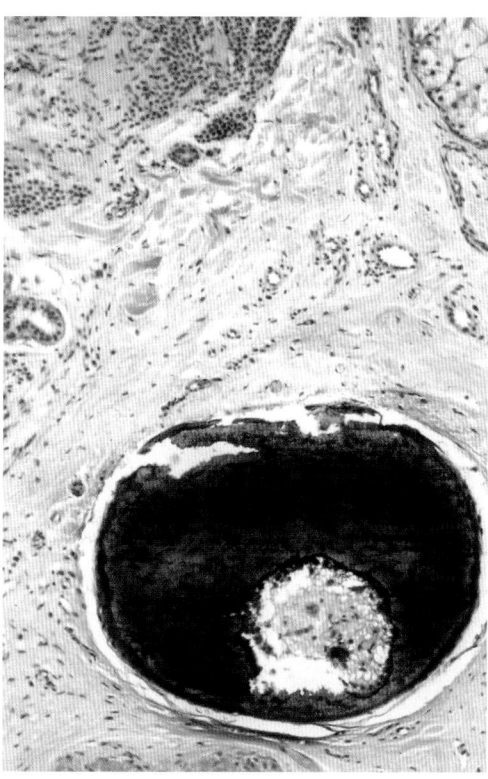

Fig. 25.52
Dermal nevus: focal calcification and even bone formation are not uncommon and usually represent a destroyed hair follicle.

The cause of this change is unknown, although it is probably artifactual and may relate to the effect of a local anesthetic. Immunohistochemical studies using endothelial cell markers are invariably negative.[28,29] The cells lining the spaces are of melanocytic derivation and label positively with S100 protein. Amyloid may rarely be identified within a nevus.[30] Exceptionally, a nevus may be accompanied by proliferation of the sweat gland epithelium; coexistence of nevus and desmoplastic trichoepithelioma is occasionally encountered.[31–33] Melanocytic nevus has also been reported in association with a trichoadenoma.[34]

The presence of intravascular melanocytes or evidence of lymphatic involvement is a very disturbing finding and should prompt a thorough search for other features of melanoma. Herniation of a nevus nest into the lumen of a vessel should not be confused with vascular invasion. The distinction can be made by finding a layer of endothelium covering the protruding nevus cells in the benign lesion (*Fig. 25.55*).

Differential diagnosis

Distinction between a banal nevus and melanoma in the majority of cases is straightforward. Low-power examination of melanoma may reveal obvious intralesional transformation, i.e., the malignant cells stand out as an expansile and often circumscribed nest, nodule, or plaque that is cytologically different from the adjacent nevus cells. Additional distinguishing features include the presence of dense pigmentation, lack of maturation, nuclear pleomorphism, mitotic activity, apoptosis, lymphocytic infiltration, and a deep nested growth pattern, which are commonly evident in melanoma but not in intradermal nevi. Upward, intraepidermal, or pagetoid spread of melanocytes is an additional feature seen in many melanomas. Caution,

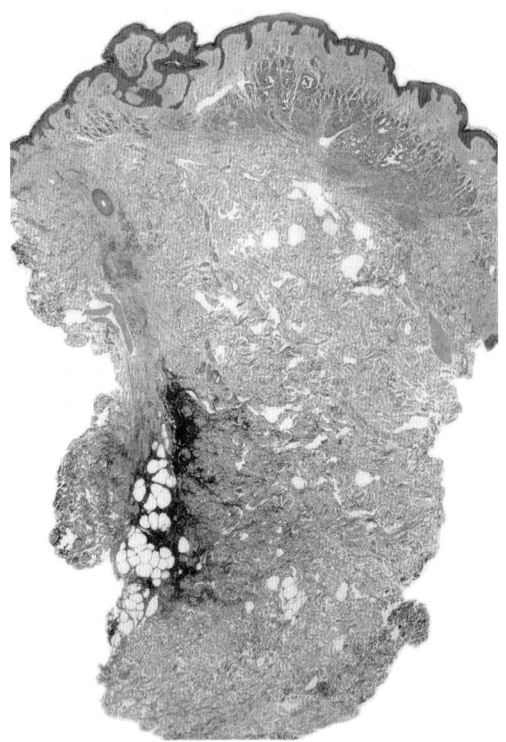

Fig. 25.53
Dermal nevus: the formation of pseudovascular spaces as shown in this example is a common artifact.

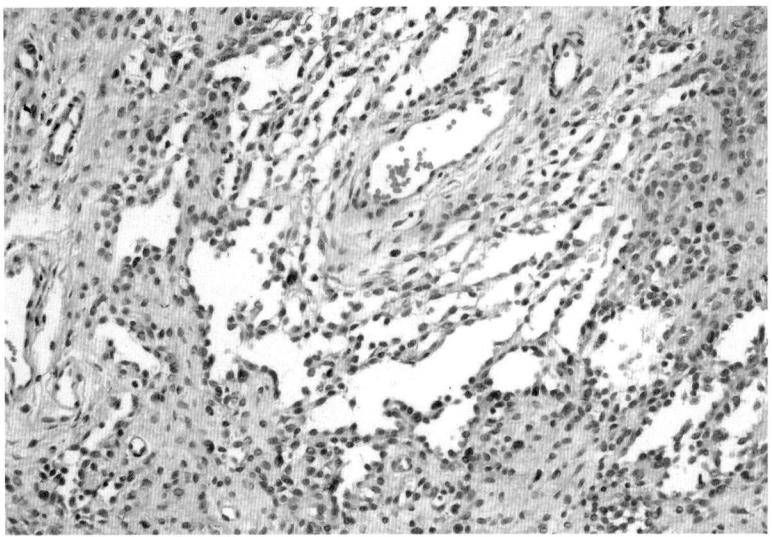

Fig. 25.54
Dermal nevus: the pseudovascular spaces are lined by nevus cells and are negative for vascular markers.

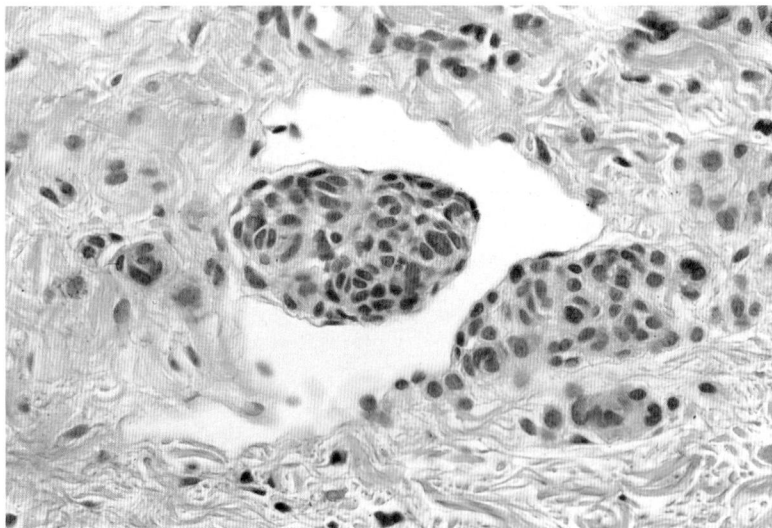

Fig. 25.55
Dermal nevus: invagination of nevus cells into the lumen of a vessel should not be confused with true vascular invasion. Distinction depends on identification of a layer of endothelial cells covering the surface of the nevoid aggregate, as shown in this example.

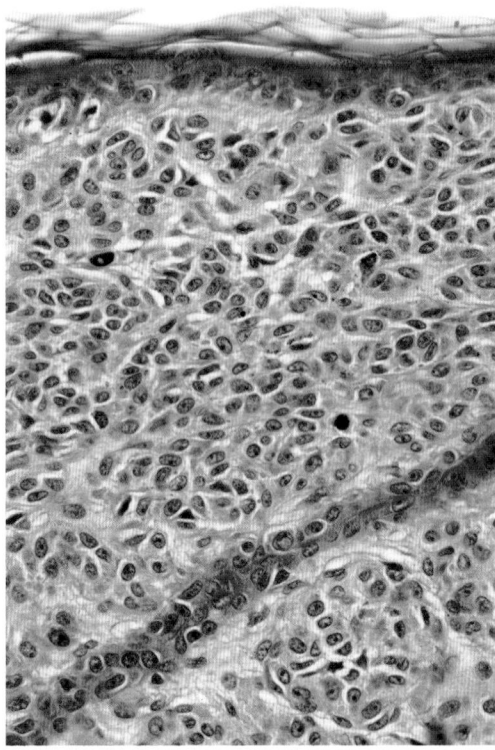

Fig. 25.56
Banal nevus: identification of one or two dermal mitotic figures is not always synonymous with melanoma. Their presence, however, should be viewed with considerable concern and other mitoses or additional features indicative of melanoma sought.

however, is advised when viewing sections from neonatal and even childhood nevi when nests and occasionally single cells, sometimes showing mild or even severe cytological atypia, may be identified within the upper reaches of the epidermis (see neonatal nevus).[35] Similarly, pagetoid spread may be a feature of acral and genital nevi (see below). Reticulin fibers outline nests of melanoma cells whereas they tend to surround individual nevus cells.

Dermal nevus cells may rarely show mitotic activity (*Fig. 25.56*). Their presence should therefore be viewed with caution and other features suggestive of malignancy sought. Nevoid melanoma may be cytologically similar at a casual glance. Careful inspection, however, reveals asymmetry and lack of circumscription, multiple dermal mitoses, subtle lack of maturation, and nucleolar prominence (see nevoid melanoma).

Small cell melanoma cells, although often of a similar size to type B nevus cells, usually have prominent eosinophilic nucleoli, and mitoses are invariably present (see small cell melanoma).

Difficulties are sometimes experienced in differentiating invasive melanoma (particularly the nevoid and small cell variants) from residual benign intradermal nevus cells. The latter is particularly important when assessing tumor thickness or the level of invasion. Immunohistochemistry may be of value in making this distinction. HMB-45 expression is often positive in superficial dermal nevus but is lost with depth (*Figs 25.57* and *25.58*).[36] In

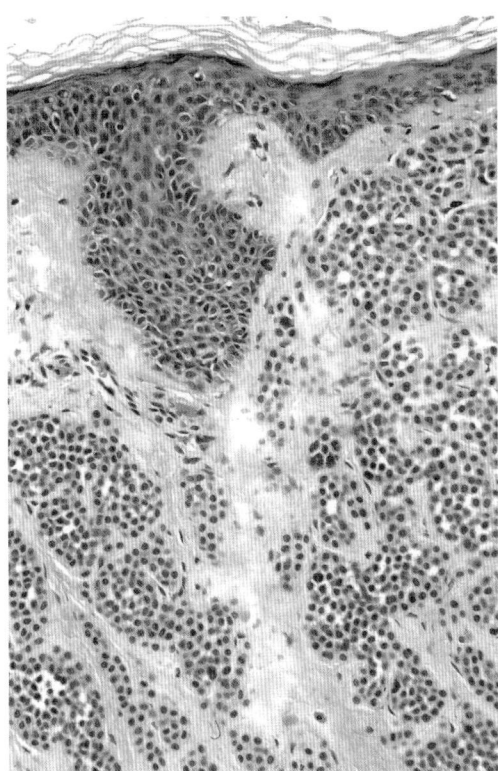

Fig. 25.57
Dermal nevus: medium-power view of banal nevus cells.

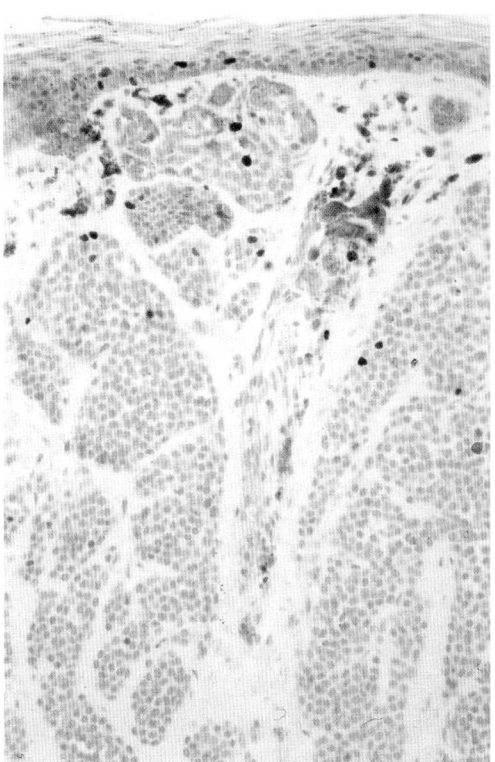

Fig. 25.59
Dermal nevus: only one or two nevus cells express MIB-1.

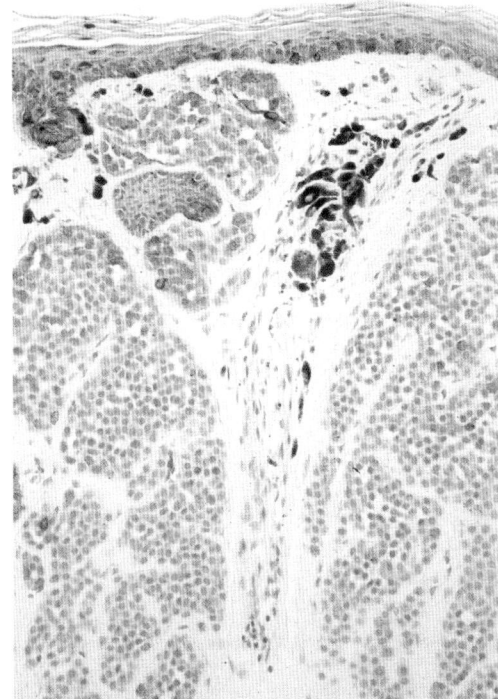

Fig. 25.58
Dermal nevus: the superficial component expresses HMB-45 but this is lost with depth.

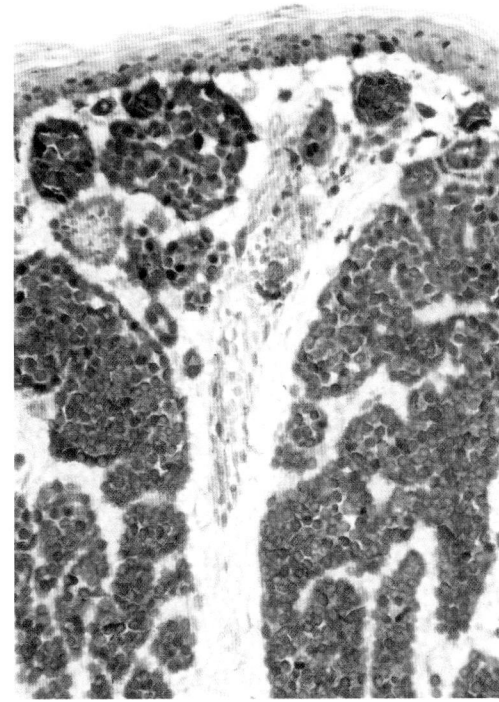

Fig. 25.60
Dermal nevus: very occasional superficial nevus cells express cyclin D1. Note that only the nuclear staining is significant.

melanoma, in contrast, the tumor cells are often positive throughout the lesion. p53 protein is not expressed in banal dermal nevi. In contrast, it is frequently present in melanoma.[37] In banal nevi, small numbers of Ki-67 and cyclin D1 positive cells may be seen in the more superficial dermal component (*Figs 25.59* and *25.60*). In melanoma, they are usually much more numerous, and often they are present throughout the thickness of the

lesion.[38] The pattern of cyclin D1 staining, however, should not be relied on in the distinction between benign and malignant.

Banal nevi may show some histologic overlap with dysplastic nevi. Thus they are often lentiginous and sometimes show shoulder formation, eosin-ophilic or lamellar fibrosis around the elongated epidermal ridges. In con-trast, architectural disorder (i.e., nests of nevus cells scattered irregularly

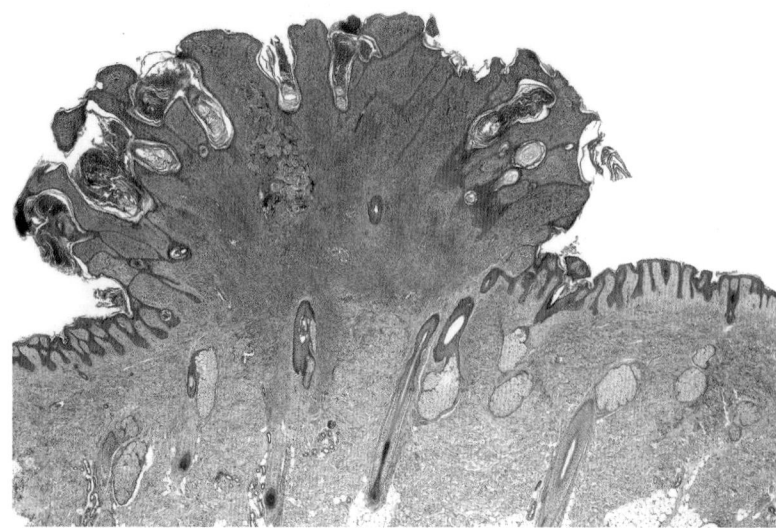

Fig. 25.61
Clonal nevus: this is a banal compound nevus. Note the distinct nodule in the deeper dermis surrounded by pigment-laden melanophages. By courtesy of W. Grayson, MD, National Health Laboratory Service, Johannesburg, South Africa.

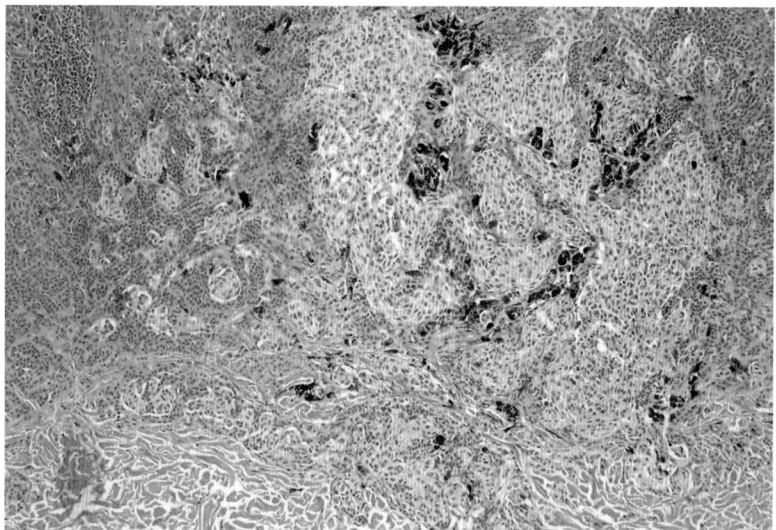

Fig. 25.62
Clonal nevus: medium-power view contrasting the nests of type A cells with the type B cells. There is abundant melanin pigment within macrophages. By courtesy of W. Grayson, MD, National Health Laboratory Service, Johannesburg, South Africa.

throughout the epidermis) and bridging are not seen. In addition, cytological atypia is not a feature of banal nevi.

Clonal nevus

Clinical features

Many so-called clonal nevi (inverted type A nevi) are clinically unremarkable. Those that are recognized are characterized by a recent change, usually in color, in an otherwise typical banal or (less commonly) congenital nevus.[1,2] Alternatively, they may exhibit darker pigmentation in the background of an otherwise uniformly pigmented nevus.[3]

On dermoscopy, clonal nevi are characterized by a uniform globular/cobblestone pattern typically containing an eccentric fairly uniform blue gray blotch.[4,5]

Histologic features

This variant of nevus is characterized by the presence of a usually circumscribed nest or collection of nests in the superficial dermis distinct from the background nevoid population (*Figs 25.61–25.64*). The melanocytes are typically epithelioid, with often abundant, heavily or finely pigmented cytoplasm and irregular nuclei containing small nucleoli.[1,2] Melanophages are usually numerous in the adjacent dermis, but a lymphocytic response is absent. Mitoses are absent or extremely rare. The nests stand out against the background population of type B nevus cells – hence the designation inverted type A nevus.

Differential diagnosis

The vast majority of clonal nevi most likely represent combined or deep penetrating nevi. Melanocytic nevi with a focal atypical epithelioid component (clonal nevus) share similar age, anatomic distribution, and cytological features with the deep penetrating nevus, but lack the deep extension of melanocytes.[6]

Eccrine centered nevus

Clinical features

Eccrine centered nevus (spotted grouped pigmented nevus) is a rare variant of melanocytic nevus, and has been mainly described in the Japanese.[1–4] Lesions, which are typically congenital, consist of a brown plaque covered by numerous dark brown to black 1–3 mm diameter papules or macules. The trunk and thigh are most commonly affected.[1,3]

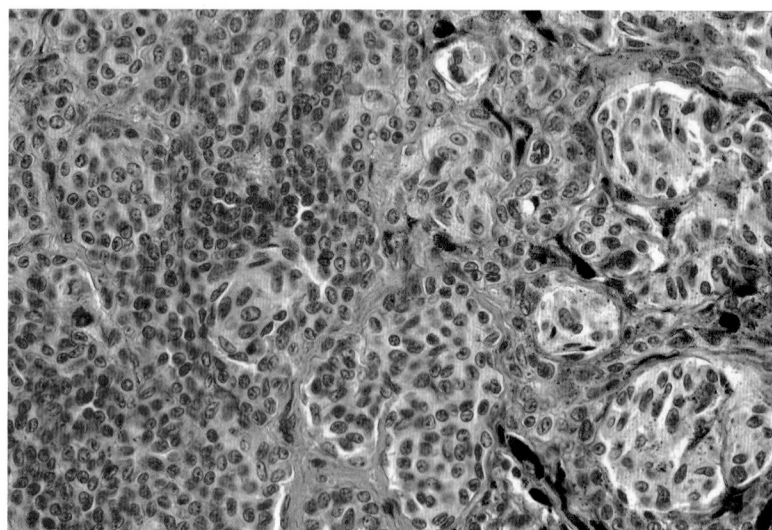

Fig. 25.63
Clonal nevus: high-power view of type A nevus cells with fine pigmentation. By courtesy of W. Grayson, MD, National Health Laboratory Service, Johannesburg, South Africa.

Histologic features

The nevus is characterized by a striking syringocentric distribution. The sweat duct epithelium may be involved but the secretory unit is typically unaffected. The overlying and adjacent epidermis shows features of a lentigo.

Melanocytic nevi at special sites

Nevi at special sites usually show histologic features identical to nevi seen elsewhere. However, a subset of nevi at special sites displays worrying histologic features that can simulate melanoma. The latter include architectural as well as cytological abnormalities not correlated with an aggressive clinical behavior.

Nevi on the scalp

Clinical features

Nevi on the scalp occur most frequently on the occipital region, followed by left parietal region, right parietal region, and frontal region (*Fig. 25.65*).[1]

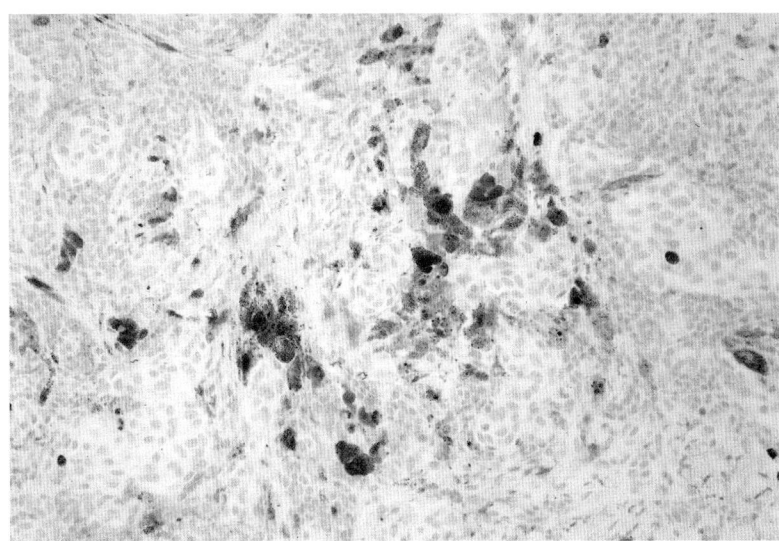

Fig. 25.64
Clonal nevus: the nevus cells do not express MIB-1. By courtesy of W. Grayson, MD, National Health Laboratory Service, Johannesburg, South Africa.

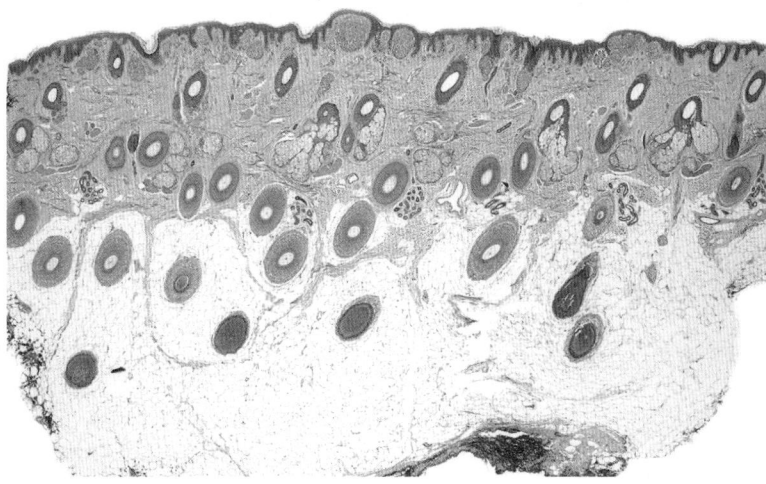

Fig. 25.66
Scalp nevus: even at low-power magnification, large expansile junctional nests can be appreciated.

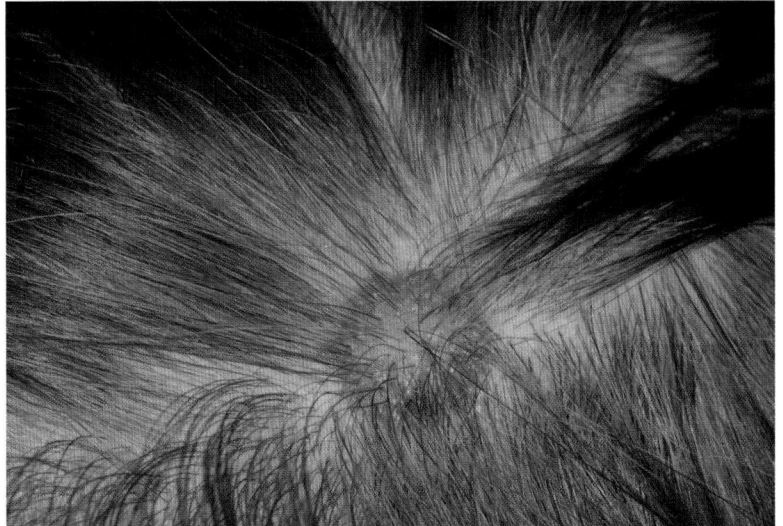

Fig. 25.65
Scalp nevus: lesions at this site may on occasions show cytological features that can raise concern for a diagnosis of melanoma by the unwary. Note the central pallor with a rim of hyperpigmentation.

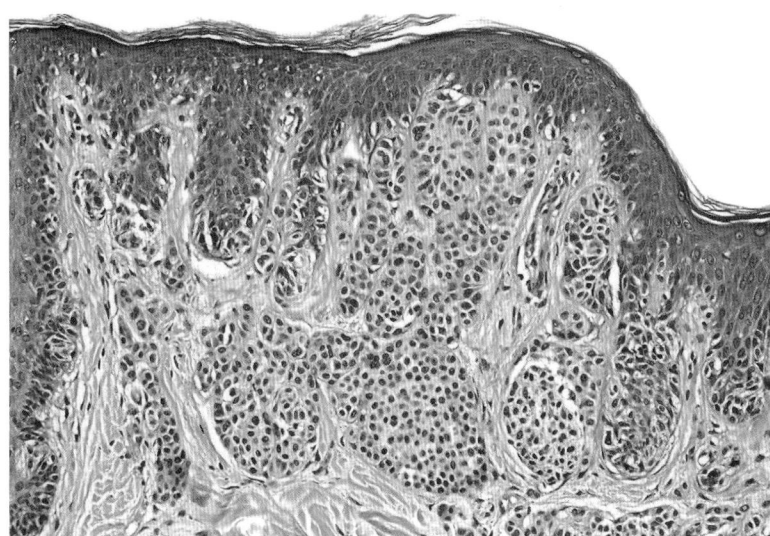

Fig. 25.67
Scalp nevus: the dermal nests are larger than the junctional ones, a feature which always results in concern.

Their number is related to the number of total body nevi and are most common in the fourth decade of life (mean age, 35 years).[1] Nevi on the scalp show male predominance.

About 10% of nevi on the scalp show disturbing histologic features.[2] Such nevi are usually seen in adolescents and young adults.[2,3] They have histologic features similar to those found on lesions in the mammary line, genital area, and flexural sites.

Histologic features

Two main morphological patterns of atypical melanocytic nevi can usually be appreciated at this site: a large nested pattern and a pattern mimicking a dysplastic nevus.[2,3] In general, atypical nevi on the scalp are characterized by asymmetry and poor lateral circumscription (*Figs 25.66–25.70*).[2] The nested pattern of proliferation consists of large nests of melanocytes located at the tips and sides of rete ridges and randomly scattered along the dermal–epidermal junction. In addition, melanocytic nests show variation in shape, with frequent bizarre forms and discohesion of tumor cells within them. Involvement of skin adnexa can be seen and may be prominent.[3] Focal lentiginous proliferation along the dermal–epidermal junction is frequently present. Melanocytic atypia is usually mild (although occasionally severe

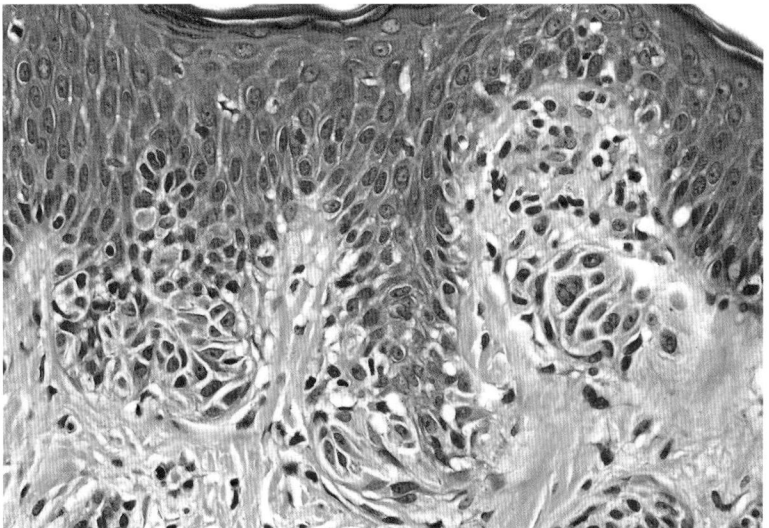

Fig. 25.68
Scalp nevus: in this field, the junctional nevus cells show moderate to severe cytological atypia.

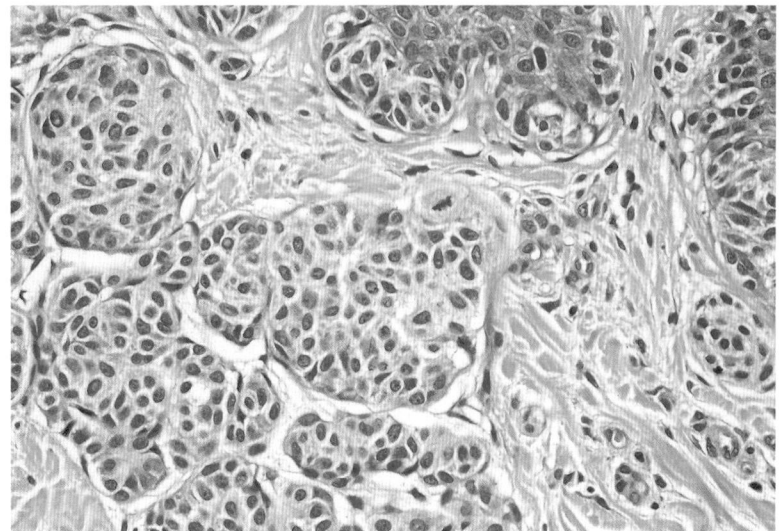

Fig. 25.69
Scalp nevus: note the mitotic figure in the superficial dermal component.

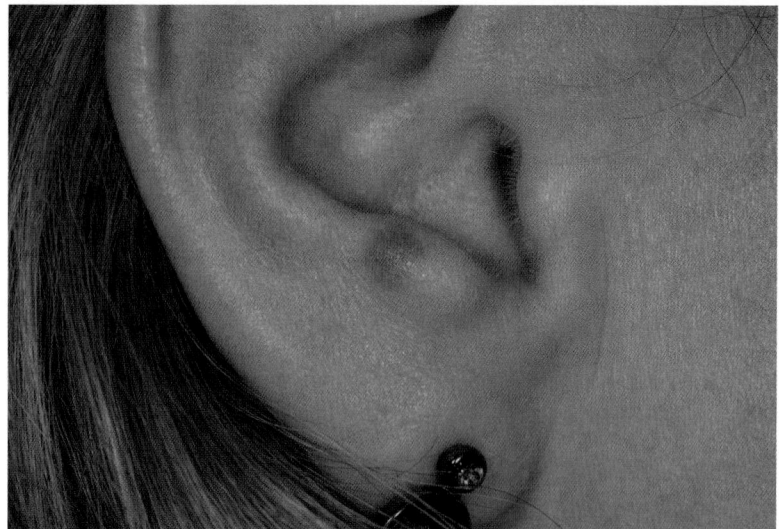

Fig. 25.71
Nevus of ear: note the ill-defined pigmented, macular lesion.

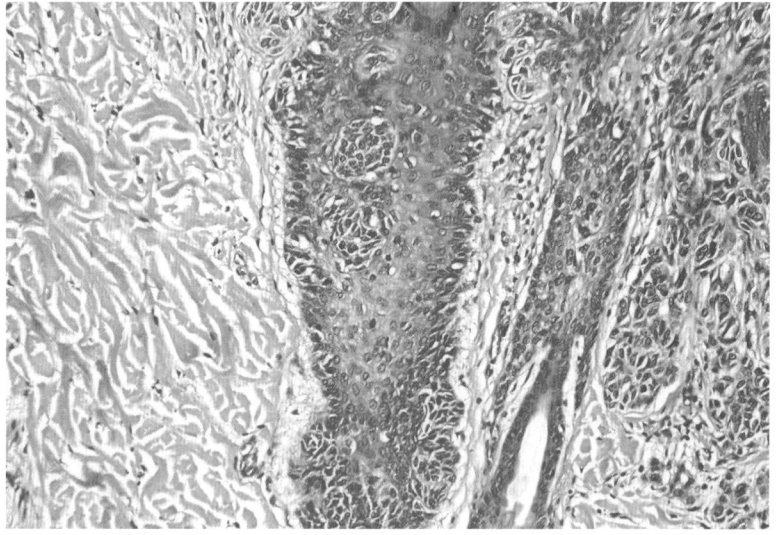

Fig. 25.70
Scalp nevus: there is follicular involvement accounting for the significant recurrence rate for these lesions.

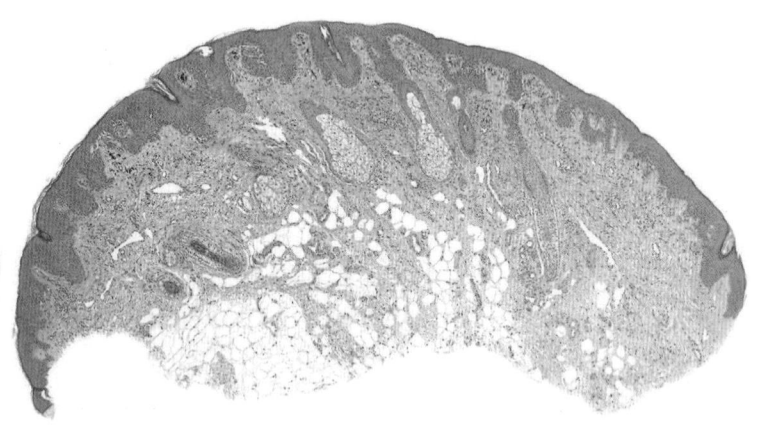

Fig. 25.72
Nevus of ear: scanning view of a largely junctional lesion.

cytological atypia is present) and random, and consists of hyperchromatic nuclei and indistinct nucleoli. Upward migration of isolated melanocytes can sometimes be seen in the central part of the lesion. The dysplastic nevus-like pattern is characterized by bridging of the rete ridges, extension of the junctional component past the dermal component, and papillary dermal fibroplasia.[3] The dermal melanocytic component is usually unremarkable, although occasionally superficial mitotic activity can be seen.

Nevi in and around the ear

Nevi in and around the skin of the ear demonstrating disturbing histologic features are usually indistinguishable from banal nevi on clinical grounds (*Fig. 25.71*).[1] Such lesions are most frequently found in the fourth and fifth decades of life (mean age, 45 years).[1,2,3] Although a slight male predominance was found in one study,[2] the most recent analysis of melanocytic nevi in the external auditory canal and auricle demonstrated predilection for females.[3]

Histologic features

Nevi in and around the ear can demonstrate architectural disarray including poor circumscription, shouldering, bridging, and elongation of rete ridges (*Figs 25.72–25.74*).[1,2] Nests of melanocytes show variation in size and

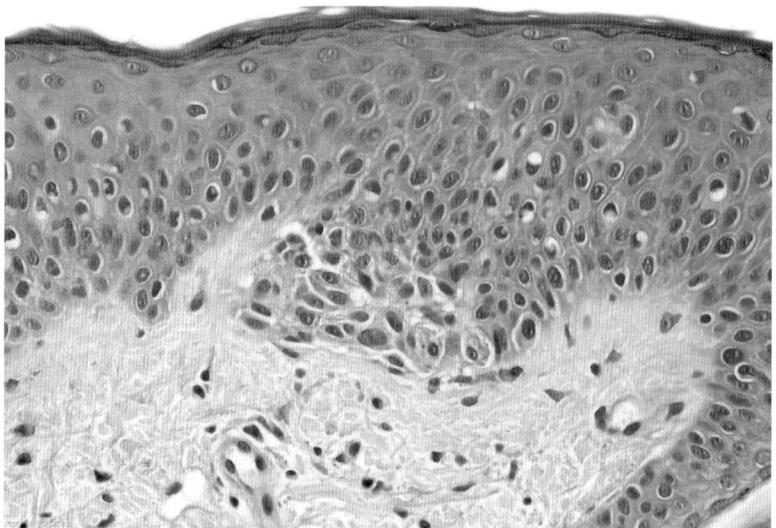

Fig. 25.73
Nevus of ear: the junctional nevus cells show severe cytological atypia.

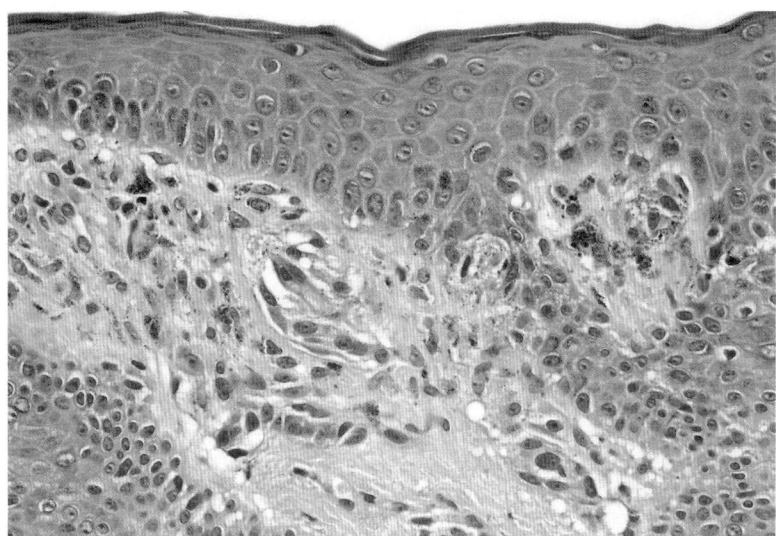

Fig. 25.74
Nevus of ear: note the cytological atypia in the dermal component.

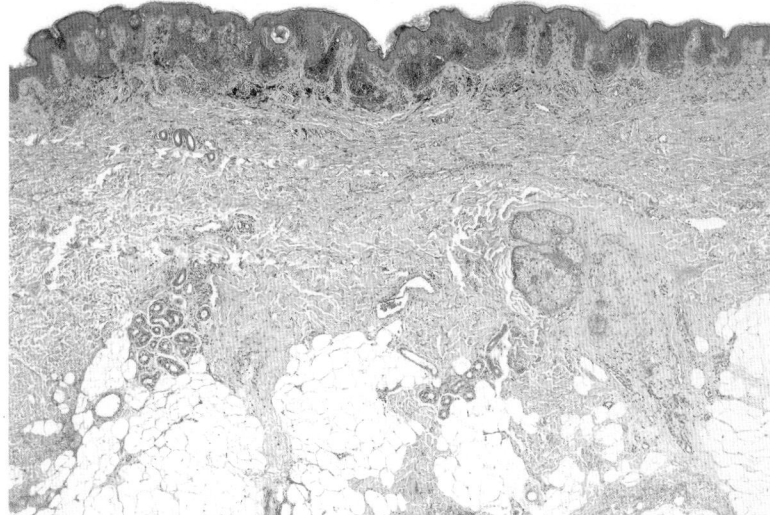

Fig. 25.75
Nevus of breast: there is architectural disorder, pigment incontinence, and a superficial perivascular lymphocytic infiltrate.

shape.[1] Particularly in young patients, junctional melanocytes can display epithelioid morphology with prominent vesicular nuclei, a single basophilic nucleolus, and pink cytoplasm. These lesions often have a Spitz-like appearance. Cytological atypia is sometimes present. Upward migration of single melanocytes into the lower third of the epidermis can be seen.[2]

The dermal melanocytic component can also show epithelioid or short spindled cell morphology. Although maturation is generally present and mitotic figures are absent, on occasions there may be atypia of the superficial dermal component particularly in lesions with Spitz-like morphology.

Nevi of the breast

Nevi can occur anywhere on the breast, including in and around the nipple. Unusual histologic features appear to be more common in young adults than in elderly patients.[1]

Histologic features

An analysis of 101 nevi of the breast demonstrated that in comparison to 97 nevi at conventional sites, nevi of the breast more frequently display limited upward migration of melanocytes above the basal layer, presence of random melanocytic cytological atypia, and dermal fibroplasia.[1,2] Histologic features of nevi of breast are similar in both genders (Figs 25.75–25.78)[2] Nests of melanocytes along the dermal–epidermal junction are variably sized.[1] Confluence of nests which are sometimes dyscohesive can be seen. Melanocytes are enlarged with clear to dusty cytoplasm, and dendritic forms may sometimes be seen. Random cytological atypia is frequent and can also be observed in the melanocytes of the papillary dermis.[1] The deeper dermal component shows maturation and is generally unremarkable with lack of mitosis activity.

Nevi of flexural skin

Flexural sites are defined as sites with cutaneous folds, including axilla, mammary folds, popliteal and antecubital fossae, umbilicus, pubis, scrotum, and perianal skin, but also folds on the neck and abdomen.[1,2] Nevi at flexural sites have predilection for umbilicus and axilla, show equal gender distribution, and have an average size of less than 1 cm. They are well circumscribed and symmetrical.[1] Interestingly, development of agminated flexural melanocytic nevi, involving most commonly the inguinal area and axilla, has been reported in children with a history of Langerhans cell histiocytosis.[3–5]

Histologic features

The peculiar histologic features of nevi at flexural sites include enlarged junctional nests, variation in the size and shape of nests, confluence of

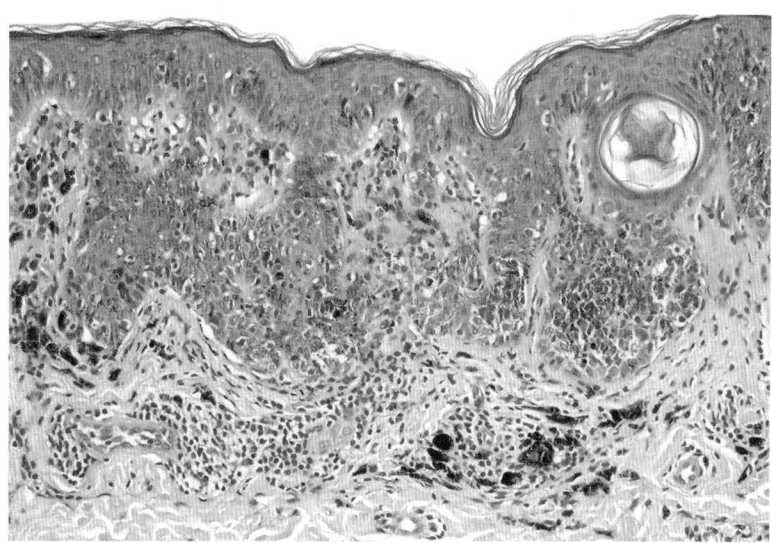

Fig. 25.76
Nevus of breast: note the heavily pigmented lentiginous and nested junctional component.

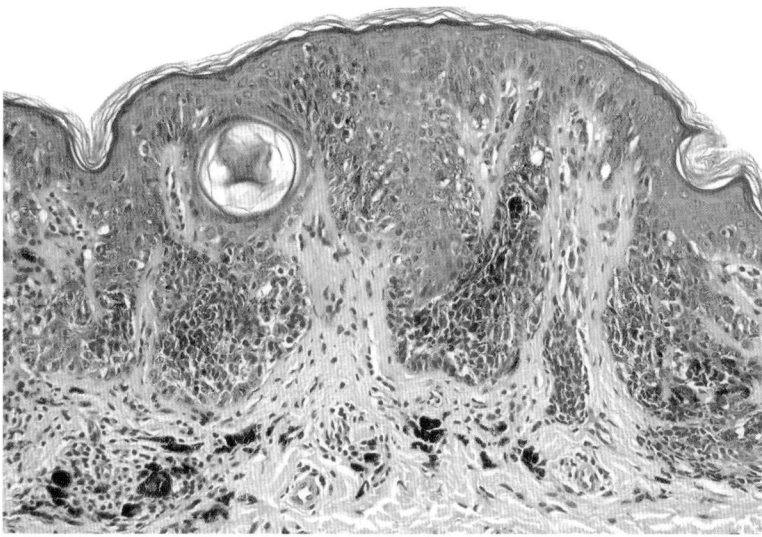

Fig. 25.77
Nevus of breast: the nests are large and dyscohesive.

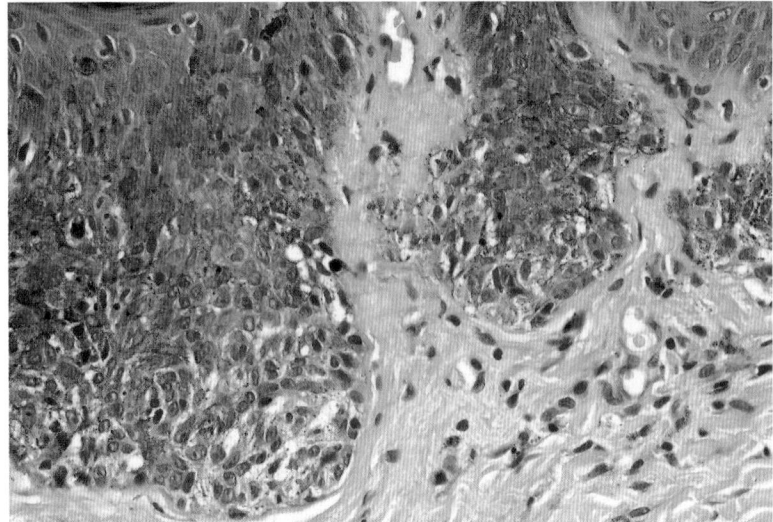

Fig. 25.78
Nevus of breast: scattered severely atypical nevus cells are present with large vesicular nuclei and prominent nucleoli. There is also a conspicuous dendritic cell population.

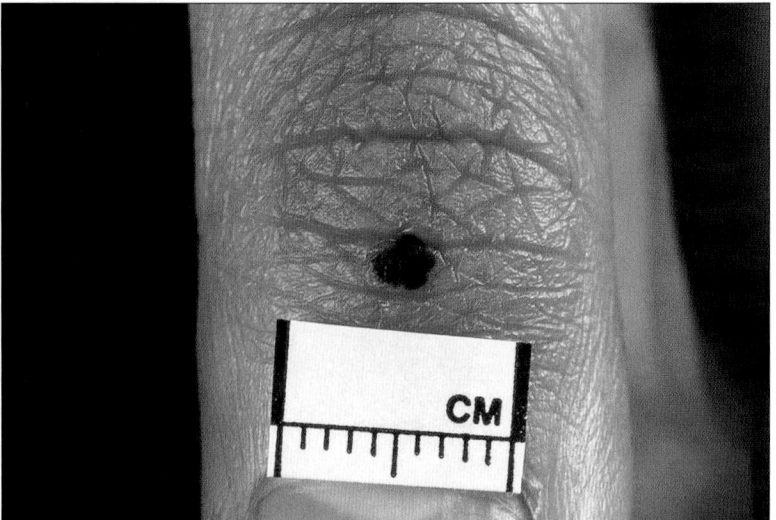

Fig. 25.79
Acral nevus: note the intense pigmentation and irregular border. By courtesy of the Institute of Dermatology, London, UK.

nests, and diminished cohesion of melanocytes within the nests – a so-called nested and dyshesive pattern of melanocytic proliferation.[1] The nests are localized at the tips and sides of the rete ridges. Involvement of skin adnexa is not uncommon. Some degree of nuclear atypia is invariably present. Focal fibrosis at the tips of the rete ridges, often of the lamellar type, can be seen.

A further subset of melanocytic nevi in the umbilicus is characterized by more extensive lentiginous proliferation of melanocytes displaying moderate degree of cytological atypia, focal and limited upward migration, as well as prominent lamellar fibrosis, often extending into the reticular dermis.[6] This peculiar type of lamellar fibrosis frequently contains entrapped melanocytic nests displaying mild cytological atypia, with either horizontal or irregular arrangement of the collagen bundles.[6]

The dermal melanocytic component is unremarkable, maturation is retained, and dermal mitoses are usually absent.

Genital nevi

Genital melanocytic nevi are Chapter 12.

Nevi of the lower leg/ankle

Atypical nevi of the lower leg/ankle have been reported.[1] They are generally small lesions, measuring between 2 and 4 mm (mean diameter, 3 mm), and show female predominance with a ratio of 4:1.

Histologic features

Atypical nevi of the lower leg/ankle can be junctional or compound. The lesions may be asymmetrical, lack lateral circumscription, and display single cell proliferation, especially at the lateral aspects.[1] Although focal upward migration into the lower layers of the epidermis may be seen, pagetoid spread into the upper layers is generally not seen. Cytological atypia is usually mild to moderate in degree.

The dermal component, when present, is thin and unremarkable. A mild nonbrisk inflammatory cell infiltrate can be seen. Usually, no dermal fibrosis is identified.

Differential diagnosis

Distinction from dysplastic nevus is made by the absence of the stromal response, typically seen in dysplastic nevi, including lamellar or concentric fibrosis and vascular proliferation. However, it has been suggested that at least some atypical nevi of the lower leg/ankle might actually represent an early dysplastic nevus.

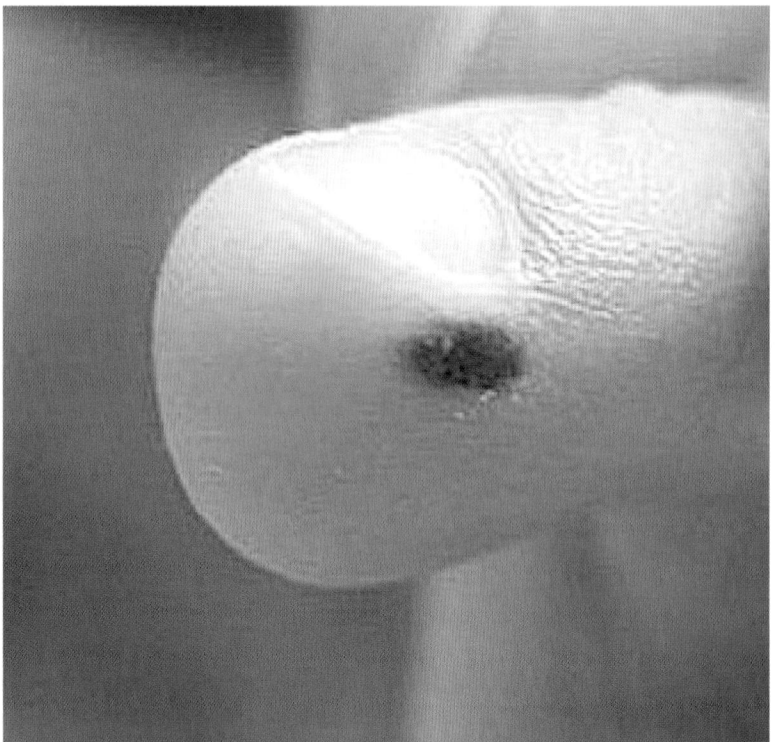

Fig. 25.80
Acral nevus: Note irregular outline. Courtesy of Yi-Guo Feng, Xi'an, China.

Acral nevus

Clinical features

Acral palmar and plantar nevi may be symmetrical, well circumscribed, and identical to banal melanocytic or congenital nevi as seen at any other site, or they may be asymmetrical, poorly circumscribed, and a source of diagnostic difficulty, both clinically and pathologically.[1-5] Acral nevi are more common in skin-of-color patients and patients with darker Fitzpatrick types than in whites.[6]

The second category (acral nevus), also sometimes known as atypical acral nevus, usually is not distinctive clinically, presenting as a less than 1.0-cm uniformly pigmented dark brown to black macule or papule with irregular and sometimes indistinct margins (Figs 25.79 and 25.80).[1,5,7] Similar lesions may also be found on the dorsal surfaces of the hands, feet, and digits, under the nails, and on the knees and elbows.[5] Development of

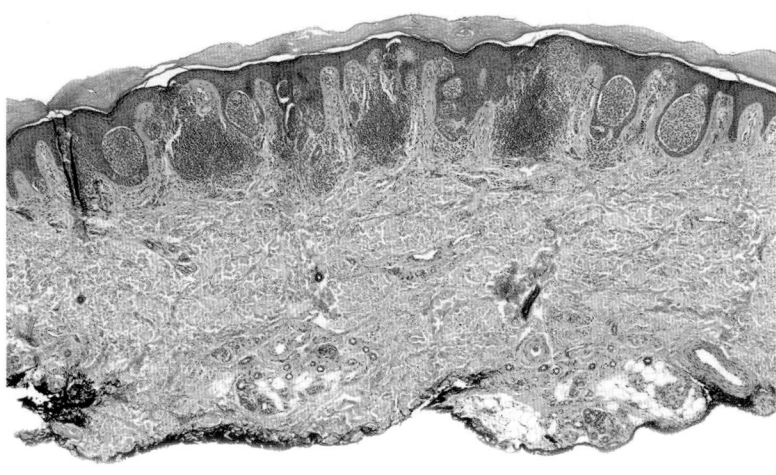

Fig. 25.81
Acral nevus: compound nevus showing vertically oriented junctional nests surrounded by a retraction artifact.

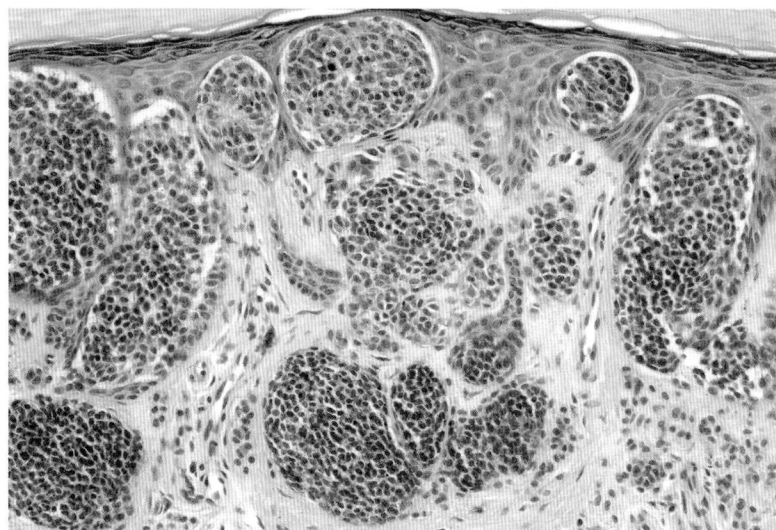

Fig. 25.82
Acral nevus: close-up view showing intraepidermal nests.

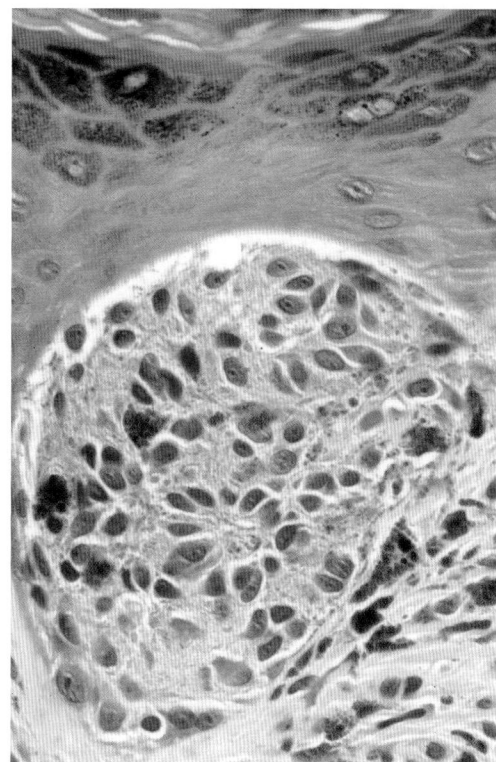

Fig. 25.83
Acral nevus: note the cytological atypia.

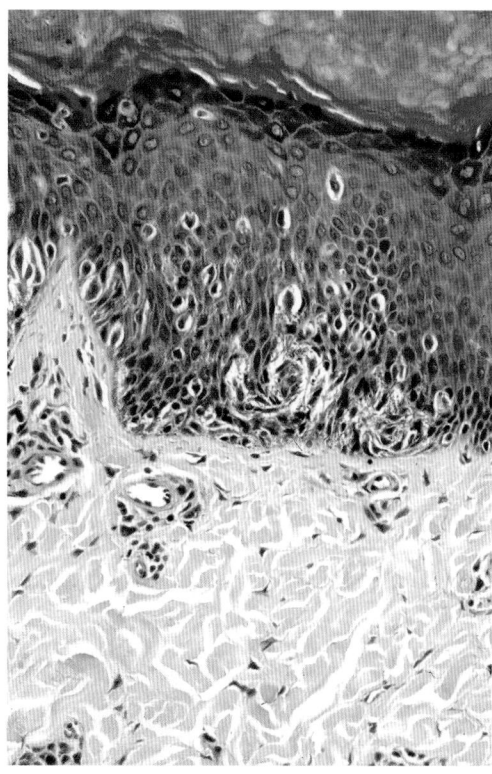

Fig. 25.84
Acral nevus: pagetoid spread (particularly over the center of the lesion) is common and should not be misinterpreted as implying malignancy. Note the dendritic cell population.

eruptive acral nevi on the sole of the foot has been reported in children following chemotherapy for acute lymphoblastic leukemia.[8,9]

Acral nevi have distinctive features on dermoscopy, which are influenced by their anatomic position.[9-12] The most common dermoscopic feature represents the parallel furrow pattern and is seen in the majority of acral nevi occurring on non-arch and non weight-bearing parts of the foot.[9,13] In contrast, acral nevi on the arch of the foot typically display lattice-like pattern, while those on weight-bearing surfaces depict fibrillary or filamentous patterns.[9-12]

Histologic features

Acral (atypical) nevus is characterized by a circumscribed and usually symmetrical, lentiginous and nested, often continuous, melanocytic proliferation along the dermal–epidermal junction (*Figs 25.81* and *25.82*).[4,5,7,14-17] The nests are commonly variable in size and often vertically oriented. A retraction artifact separating them from the adjacent keratinocytes is a characteristic feature. The rete ridges may be elongated and narrowed. The nevus cells have conspicuous pale-staining cytoplasm and hyperchromatic to vesicular nuclei, sometimes showing cytological atypia (usually mild) (*Fig. 25.83*). Nucleoli may be conspicuous. Mild to moderate pagetoid spread is not uncommonly present, particularly in the center of the nevus. Sometimes pagetoid spread can be very marked and involve almost the entire lesion – such melanocytic proliferation is generally referred to as a melanocytic acral

nevus with intraepidermal ascent of cells (MANIAC) (*Fig. 25.84*).[5,7,15] As a result, spotty pigmentation is frequently evident in the stratum corneum.[18] In addition, melanocytes along the dermal–epidermal junction frequently display dendritic morphology. A characteristic feature of acral nevus is transepidermal elimination of nests.[4,15] Involvement of eccrine ducts by nests of melanocytes is not infrequent, but is usually limited to upper portions of the ducts.[19] Pigmentary incontinence is generally present, and there may be mild

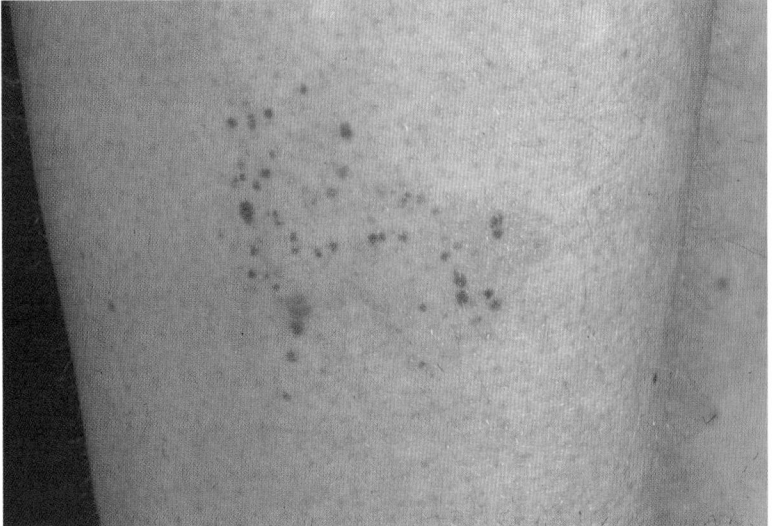

Fig. 25.85
Nevus spilus: heavily pigmented macules are present within a background circumscribed paler lesion. From the collection of the late N.P. Smith, MD, the Institute of Dermatology, London, UK.

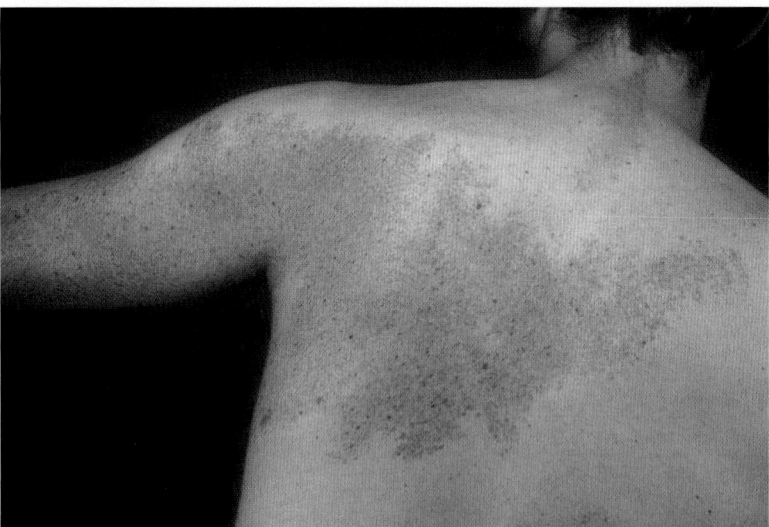

Fig. 25.86
Nevus spilus: in this patient, the lesion has a segmental distribution. This type of lesion is associated with an increased risk of developing melanoma. By courtesy of the Institute of Dermatology, London, UK.

fibrosis, rarely accompanied by a sparse lymphocytic infiltrate. Superficial dermal fibrosis is more prominent in lesions from weight-bearing areas such as the soles and should not be interpreted as regression. The dermal component matures with depth and lacks mitotic activity.

Differential diagnosis

Atypical acral nevus may be distinguished from an acral dysplastic nevus by the absence of a shoulder, dusty pigmentation, and bridging, in addition to lamellar and eosinophilic fibrosis. A host inflammatory response is generally absent in acral nevi. It differs from acral lentiginous melanoma by the absence of irregular epidermal acanthosis, severe cytological atypia, mitotic activity, and by maturation of the dermal component when present.[16] The presence of a dense lymphocytic infiltrate is highly suspicious for melanoma and should prompt careful examination of additional sections for confirmatory features.[4]

Nevus spilus

Clinical features

Nevus spilus (speckled lentiginous nevus) may be congenital but more often it presents in the first year of life. The sexes are involved equally, and there is a predilection for Caucasians. Up to 2% of the population is affected.[1] It consists of an aggregate of numerous tiny, pigmented macules and papules arising on a lightly tanned or brown macular background (*Figs 25.85* and *25.86*).[2-4] Nevus spilus ranges in size from less than 1 cm to more than 10 cm and most commonly arises on the trunk and extremities.[5] Hypertrichosis has rarely been reported in nevus spilus.[6] Lesions are usually solitary. Extensive unilateral (giant) and zosteriform variants have rarely been documented.[7-9] Nevus spilus has a tendency to grow along Blaschko lines.[10] It may coexist with a plaque blue nevus, bilateral nevus of Ito, or centrofacial lentiginosis and has also been described in association with a nevus sebaceous.[11-14] Exceptionally, nevus spilus has also been reported in the oral mucosa.[15] Melanoma can, on occasion, develop within a nevus spilus.[12,16-25] In such cases, women are particularly affected and the back is most often involved. A speckled lentiginous nevus syndrome has been recognized and consists of a speckled lentiginous nevus in combination with ipsilateral neurological abnormalities such as hyperhidrosis, muscle weakness, and dysesthesia.[26] A medial nerve paresis is a recent addition to the syndrome.[27]

Histologic features

The darkly pigmented speckled areas are characterized by junctional, compound, or dermal nevi. Less often, Spitz nevi and blue nevi also in an agminate pattern may be seen.[28-33] The intervening background skin may be

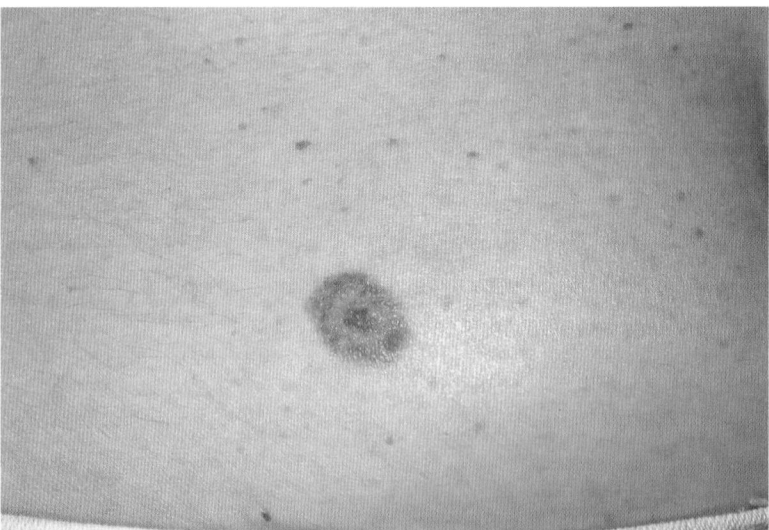

Fig. 25.87
Cockarde nevus: note the characteristic targetoid appearance. By courtesy of J.C. Pascual, MD, Alicante, Spain.

normal, nevoid, or show lentigo simplex-like features.[2-4] Cytological atypia may sometimes be encountered.[16] Such lesions with worrying features should be carefully monitored for the subsequent development of melanoma.

Nevus spilus has been demonstrated to harbor activating *HRAS* point mutations.[34,35]

Cockarde nevus

Clinical features

The Cockarde (Cockade, rosette-like, target-like) nevus is a very rare variant of banal nevus. It presents as a central pigmented papule separated by an intervening border of normal or flesh-colored skin from a hyperpigmented border (*Fig. 25.87*).[1-3] Multiple nevi have been associated with meningomyelocele and vertebral dysplasia.[4]

Histologic features

The central pigmented papule in the Cockarde nevus consists of a compound melanocytic lesion, whereas the peripheral aspect is composed of a junctional nevus.[1] The nonpigmented middle zone lacks melanocytes.

Combined nevus (melanocytic nevus with phenotypic heterogeneity)

Combined nevus is characterized by the occurrence of two or more different populations of melanocytes, i.e., different melanocytic nevus variants within the single lesion.[1-4] Combined nevi can thus be composed of any combination of common nevi (common acquired nevus, dysplastic nevus, congenital nevus), Spitz nevus, and blue nevus.[4-8] The most frequent combination represents a common acquired nevus and a deep penetrating nevus.[5] A combined $BRAF^{V600E}/BAP^{loss}$ melanocytic nevus (Wiesner nevus) and ordinary (conventional) melanocytic nevus has gained increasing attention in the recent literature.[9] It has been demonstrated that a subset of a so-called atypical Spitz tumors is characterized genetically by the presence of $BAP1$ and $BRAF^{V600E}$ mutation occurring in either familial or sporadic setting, the former being associated with development of diverse malignancies, thus representing a cutaneous marker of a cancer syndrome (see corresponding section).[10]

Clinical features

Combined nevi may be a source of concern because of variegate pigmentation and frequent asymmetry. They show an equal sex distribution and have predilection for children and young adults, developing most frequently on the trunk, followed by head and neck, upper extremity, lower extremity, perineum, and buttocks in decreasing order of frequency.[5] Combined nevi have also been documented in mucosal sites, including the conjunctiva.[11]

Histologic features

Different types of melanocytes may be admixed or relatively well separated from each other (Figs 25.88–25.90).

The term malignant combined nevus was used to describe an example of in situ melanoma that complicated a banal and cellular blue nevus.[12]

Differential diagnosis

Combined melanocytic nevus can be distinguished from melanoma by the absence of melanoma in situ in the junctional component, lack of pleomorphism including a prominent nucleolus in tumor cells and expansile growth pattern in the dermal component, and by the absence of or only very occasional normal mitoses in combined nevus.

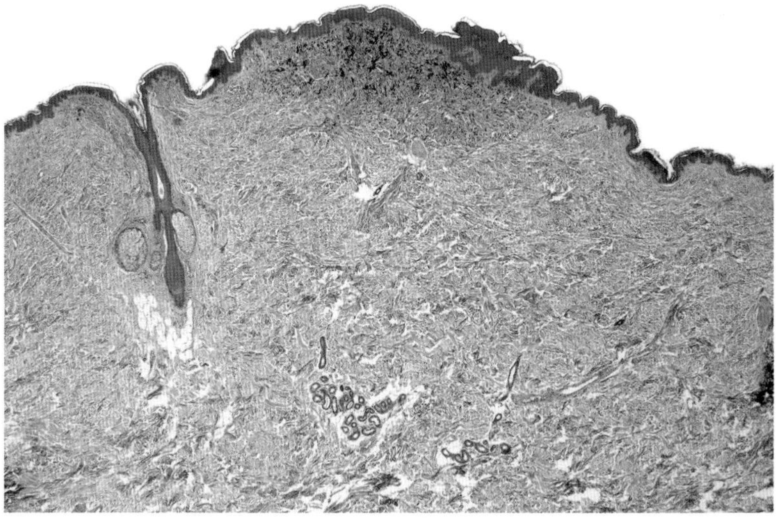

Recurrent and sclerosing nevus

Clinical features

Recurrent nevus (pseudomelanoma) refers to the development of an atypical melanocytic lesion following inadequate excision of a previous benign melanocytic nevus.[1-4] It most commonly follows a shave biopsy. Similar changes can also occur after trauma, laser treatment, and local application of topical agents.[5,6] Recurrent nevus presents as an asymmetrical, irregular, variably pigmented macular lesion, often with stippled black areas restricted to the area of the scar (Fig. 25.91).[1] In contrast, recurrent Spitz and blue nevi are frequently papular or nodular lesions that extend beyond the confines of the scar.[7-9] Furthermore, recurrent Spitz nevus can exceptionally present with multiple satellite nodules in the area of previous excision.[10] In general, recurrences most commonly develop within 6 months following the initial procedure, show female predominance, and most frequently occur on the back.[11]

On dermoscopy, helpful clues for recurrent/persistent melanocytic nevus include symmetry of the proliferation, the presence of radial lines, and centrifugal growth.[12] In contrast, the single most important parameter

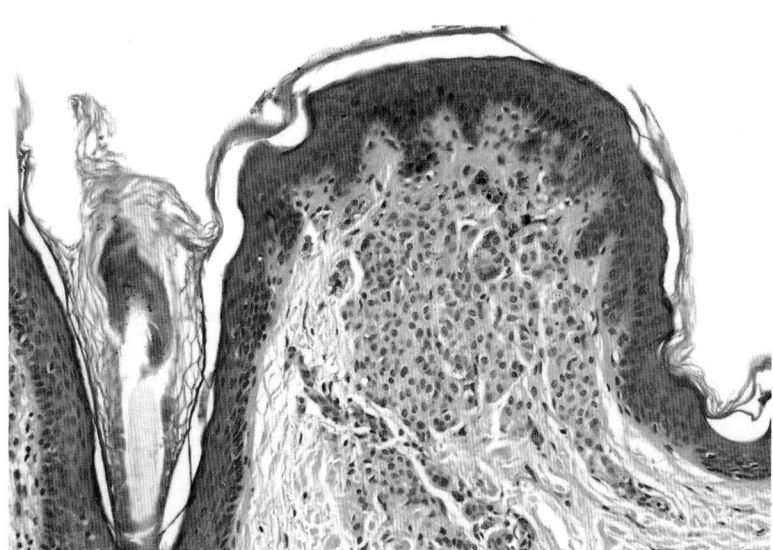

Fig. 25.89
Combined nevus: high-power view of perifollicular banal nevus cells.

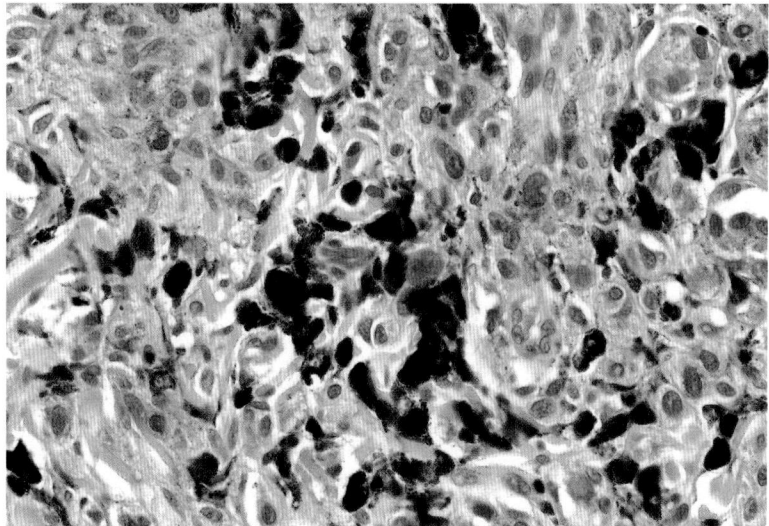

Fig. 25.90
Combined nevus: high-power view of admixed banal and dendritic cells with conspicuous melanophages.

Fig. 25.88
Combined nevus: low-power view showing banal nevus adjacent to the hair follicle and an admixture of banal and blue nevus cells in the center of the field.

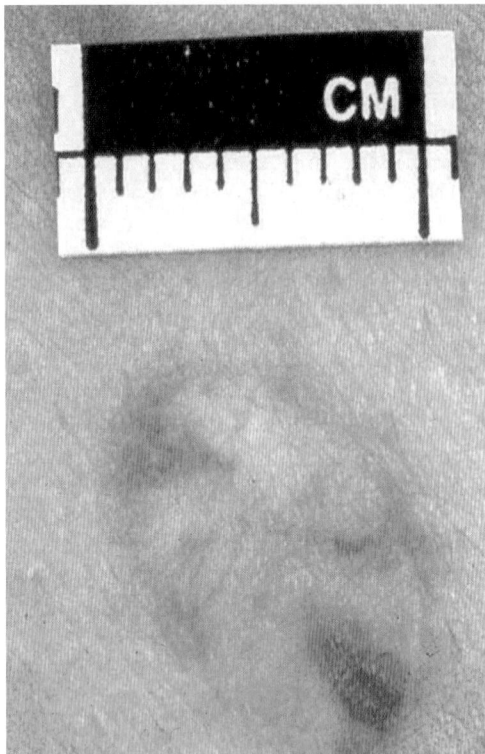

Fig. 25.91
Recurrent nevus: there are multiple irregular foci of pigmentation contrasting with background pallor representing superficial dermal scarring. By courtesy of the Institute of Dermatology, London, UK.

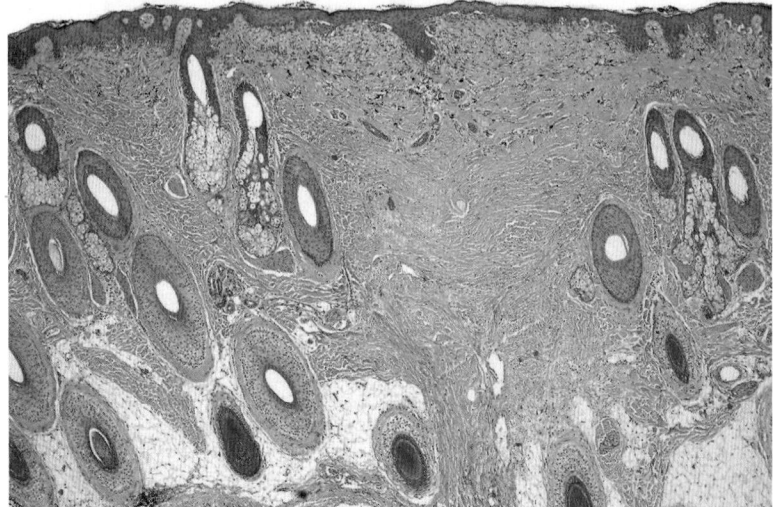

Fig. 25.92
Recurrent nevus: there is dense dermal scarring with an overlying predominantly junctional melanocytic proliferation. Dermal melanophages are conspicuous.

suggestive of melanoma was found to be pigmentation beyond the confines of the scar.[12]

Histologic features

Remnants of the previously excised nevus are often evident in the superficial dermis accompanied by dermal scarring; a superficial perivascular chronic inflammatory cell infiltrate is commonly present (*Fig. 25.92*). Melanophages are usually conspicuous.

The significant histologic features, however, are present in the epidermis. The junctional component is sharply delineated and characteristically does not extend beyond the area of scarring. Recurrent nevus consists of atypical melanocytes, both singly and in clusters, usually in the lower epidermis and sometimes showing mild or moderate nuclear pleomorphism and

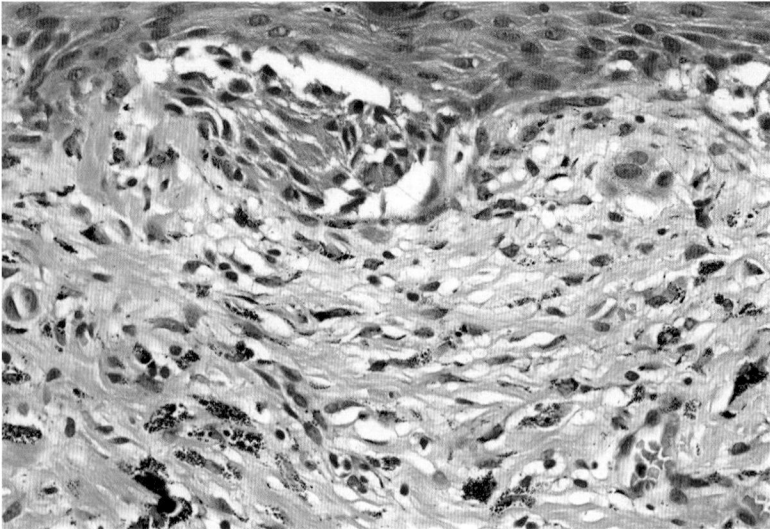

Fig. 25.93
Recurrent nevus: high-power view of junctional component showing a dyscohesive nest of atypical nevus cells. Scattered nevus cells with admixed melanophages are present in the superficial dermis.

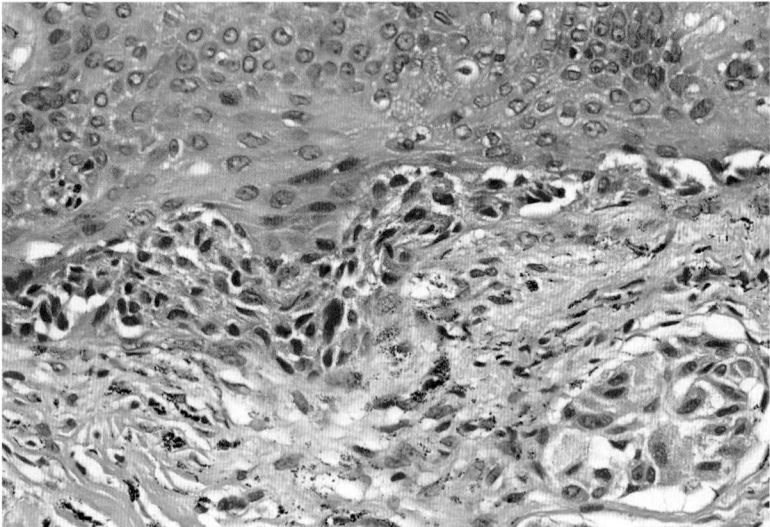

Fig. 25.94
Recurrent nevus: there is bridging, and cytological atypia is present in both junctional and dermal components. In cases of doubt, review of the previously excised lesion is advised.

hyperchromatism (*Fig. 25.93*).[1] An epithelioid morphology of melanocytes usually predominates.[11] Slight pagetoid spread is sometimes evident. Mitotic figures are not usually present, and apoptosis is not a feature. The rete ridge pattern overlying the scar is frequently effaced. On occasions, however, epidermal hyperplasia in a retiform pattern confined to the area of the scar can be seen.[11] Cytological atypia is sometimes evident in the superficial dermal component associated with scar (when present) (*Fig. 25.94*). In some cases, a residual ordinary component of the nevus is seen in the area underlying the scar. Dermal mitoses are generally absent although, exceptionally, careful scrutiny may reveal an occasional normal mitosis.

Differential diagnosis

In the absence of clinical information, melanoma may be suspected initially. Histologic points of distinction include the characteristic circumscription, the sharp restriction of the junctional component to the area immediately overlying the scar, the lack of mitotic activity and apoptosis, and the presence of dense reactive scarring.[1]

Clinicopathological correlation is essential. It should also be borne in mind that residual dysplastic nevi may be associated with a recurrent nevus phenomenon, and incompletely excised melanoma in situ may mimic a recurrent nevus. Review of previous pathological material is essential in difficult cases.

The pseudomelanoma phenomenon has also been reported in a subset of melanocytic nevi, the so-called sclerosing nevi.[13] These are characterized histologically by a central area of scarring, not related to previous procedure or trauma, accompanied by remnants of a nevus at the periphery of the scar. Similar to the pseudomelanoma phenomenon in recurrent nevi, the epidermal component in sclerosing nevus consists of irregularly sized and confluent nests of melanocytes with occasional upward extension of melanocytes, confined to the area above the scar. Sclerosing nevi typically display an orderly pattern of fibrosis, characterized by homogeneous bundles of eosinophilic collagen fibers arranged parallel to the epidermis. Areas of fibrosis/sclerosis contain irregular nests of melanocytes.[13] No significant atypia of melanocytes is seen in either the epidermal melanocytic component or in entrapped melanocytic nests within sclerotic areas, and mitoses are absent or scarce. These changes are thought to be related to partial regression of the lesion.

Balloon cell nevus

Clinical features

Balloon cell nevus is a rare variant of melanocytic nevus and is believed to represent a degenerative change due to accumulation of melanin precursors in premelanosomes with resultant vacuolation of the cytoplasm.[1-5] This phenomenon is present in less than 2% of common nevi.[2] Although balloon cell nevus may present at any age, about 80% are diagnosed in the first three decades of life. The incidence is equal in men and women, and there is a predilection for the head and neck, followed by trunk and extremities. The lesion displays no particular distinguishing clinical features, and usually presents as a smooth, dome-shaped, red or brown papule or nodule.[2] Balloon cell nevi have also been reported at mucosal sites, conjunctiva, and iris.[5-11]

On dermoscopy, balloon cell nests correspond to areas of white and yellow globules/clods within the nevus.[12,13]

Histologic features

The nevus may be compound or intradermal and, by definition, must show a predominance (greater than 50%) of balloon cells (primary phenomenon), since the occasional typical melanocytic nevus may contain a few scattered balloon cells (secondary phenomenon) (Fig. 25.95).[1,2] The latter are round or oval and variably sized, with abundant foamy pale-staining or clear cytoplasm. They contain a central rather hyperchromatic or vesicular nucleus with a conspicuous nucleolus (Fig. 25.96). Not uncommonly, affected cells display a striking resemblance to adipocytes. Multinucleate giant cells may be a feature. Mitotic activity is absent. Pigmentation is variable, ranging from lesions with abundant melanin to completely amelanotic examples. More obvious melanocytic features are sometimes evident at the periphery of the nevus (Fig. 25.97).

Balloon cell change has also been reported in proliferative nodules developing in the background of a large congenital melanocytic nevus.[14]

Differential diagnosis

Balloon cell change has also been documented in Spitz nevi, dysplastic nevi, cellular blue nevi, combined nevi, and melanoma (including metastatic tumors).[15-18] The last may be distinguished by the presence of nuclear pleomorphism, nucleolar prominence, and mitotic activity.

It should be noted that balloon cell melanoma can, on occasion, appear deceptively bland (similar to nevoid melanoma) and, as a result, balloon cell nevi should always be carefully scrutinized at multiple levels to exclude a melanoma.

Halo nevus

Clinical features

Halo nevus (Sutton nevus, leukoderma acquisitum centrifugum) presents clinically as a pigmented melanocytic nevus surrounded by a hypopigmented

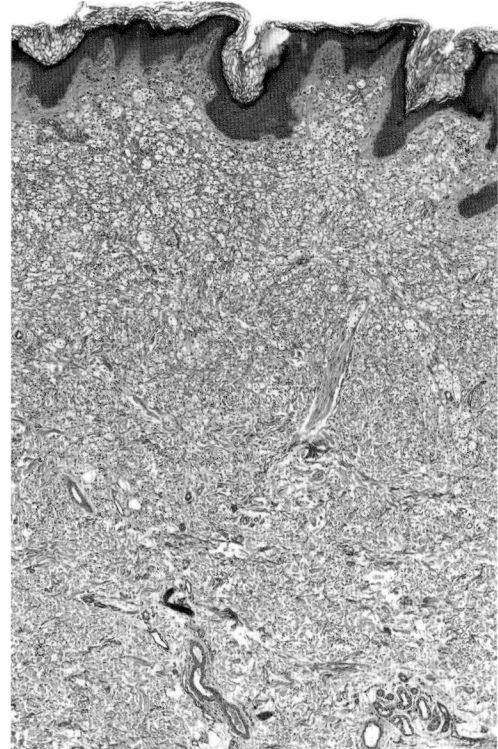

Fig. 25.95
Balloon cell nevus: scanning view showing a dermal nodule composed of pale-staining cells.

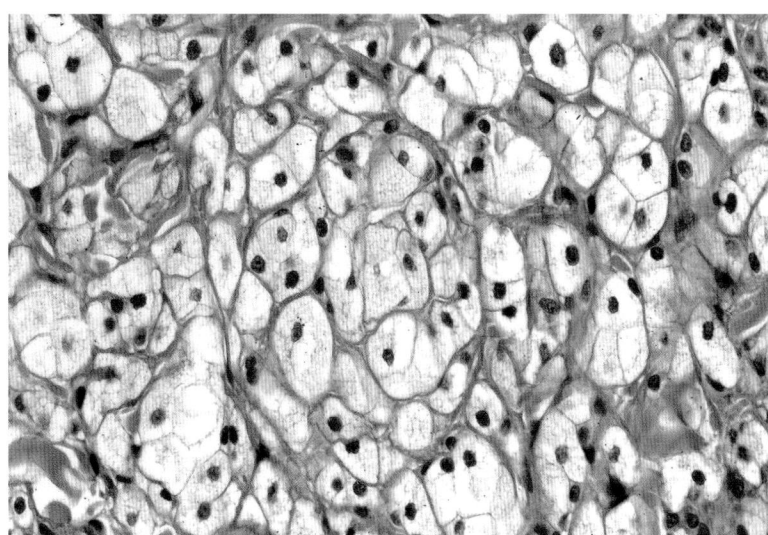

Fig. 25.96
Balloon cell nevus: the nevus cells have pale, slightly foamy cytoplasm and central hyperchromatic nuclei.

border and is usually associated with regression.[1,2] Rarely, development of a halo phenomenon in a melanocytic nevus can be predated, especially in children, by a preceding elevated or verrucous and crusted surface.[3] Occasionally, a halo may be seen around a congenital melanocytic nevus, blue nevus, Spitz nevus, dysplastic nevus, or even melanoma.[4-8]

Typically, halo nevus presents as a small pigmented macule surrounded by a narrow border of hypopigmentation (Figs 25.98–25.100). The incidence is equal in men and women. It arises most frequently in the second decade, usually on the trunk, particularly the back. The developing of a melanocytic lesion with a halo in an old adult should be viewed with suspicion. Halo nevi are sometimes multiple and occasionally exhibit a familial tendency; there is an increased incidence of associated intralesional and extralesional vitiligo.[5,9-12] Halo nevi are up to 10 times more frequent in patients with

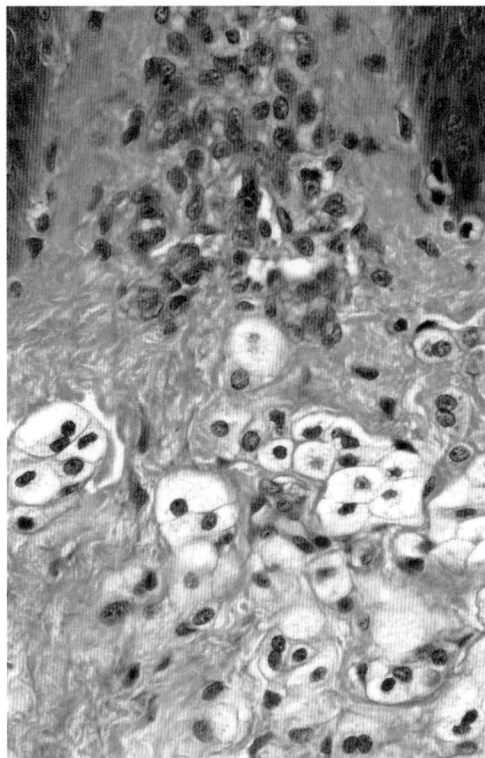

Fig. 25.97
Balloon cell nevus: diagnosis is facilitated by the identification of more typical nevus cells.

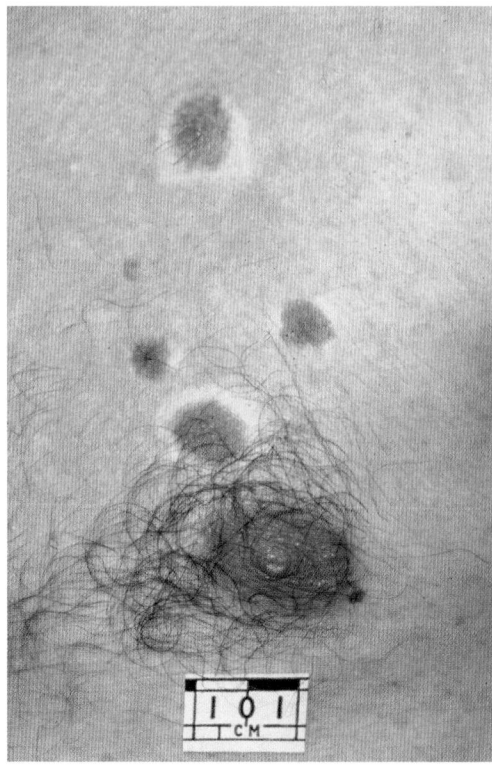

Fig. 25.98
Halo nevus: these nevi are surrounded by typical haloes. By courtesy of R.A. Marsden, MD, St George's Hospital, London, UK.

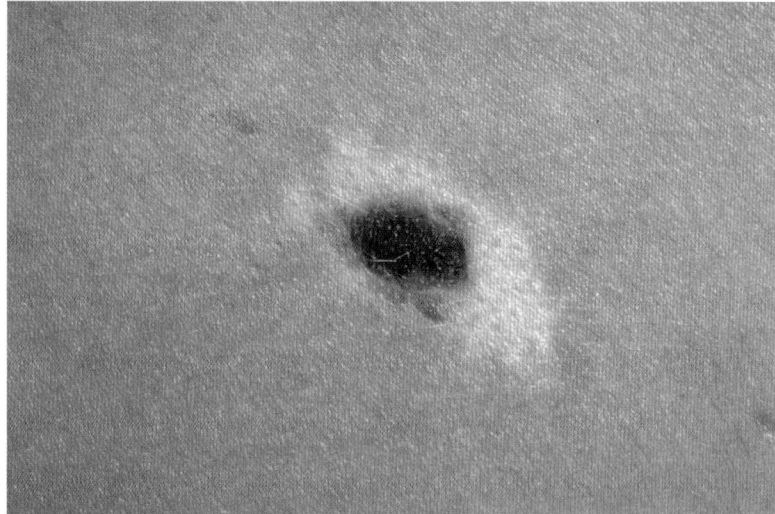

Fig. 25.99
Halo nevus: close-up view showing a heavily pigmented central nodule with a pale-staining halo. By courtesy of the Institute of Dermatology, London, UK.

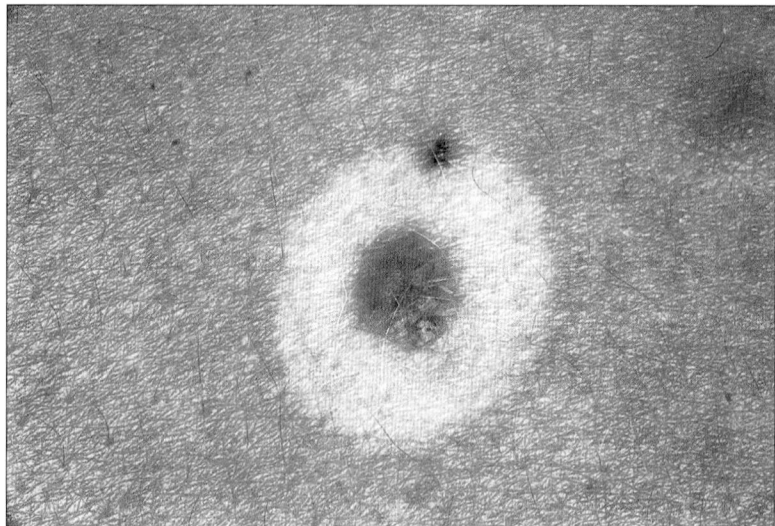

Fig. 25.100
Halo nevus: this is an 'end-stage' lesion in which the central nevus has largely disappeared. By courtesy of the Institute of Dermatology, London, UK.

vitiligo than in the general population.[13] In addition, children with halo nevi and vitiligo are more likely to develop generalized than segmental or focal vitiligo.[13] Development of multiple halo nevi has also been reported following treatment with infliximab, imatinib, and interferon beta-1a.[14–16] Furthermore, a short period of sunbathing has also been associated with the development of multiple halo nevi.[17] Patients with halo nevi very often have circulating antibodies to cytoplasmic antigen(s) in melanoma cells. These antibodies disappear after excision or spontaneous resolution of the central lesion.[18] Patients with Turner syndrome have an increased prevalence of halo nevi compared with the general population (18% vs. 1%).[19] An association of multiple halo nevi with carcinoid tumor of the ileum has been described.[20] Mycosis fungoides superimposed on a melanocytic nevus can present clinically with a halo phenomenon.[21]

The natural history of halo nevi is usually associated with persistence for years, often even more than a decade, frequently without complete regression.[22]

Histologic features

The lesion consists of a raised dermal nodule associated with an acanthotic and frequently hyperkeratotic epidermis (*Fig. 25.101*). The nevus is usually compound and infiltrated extensively by lymphocytes and histiocytes with occasional mast and plasma cells (*Figs 25.102* and *25.103*). The lymphocytes are predominantly of suppressor/cytotoxic T-cell phenotype, admixed with a minor population of CD4-positive T-helper cells, B lymphocytes, macrophages, and Langerhans cells.[23–25] Epithelioid granulomata can occasionally be found within the inflammatory cell infiltrate.[26] With progressive apoptosis, the nevus cells may become increasingly more difficult to identify, and their numbers are replaced by pigment-containing macrophages.

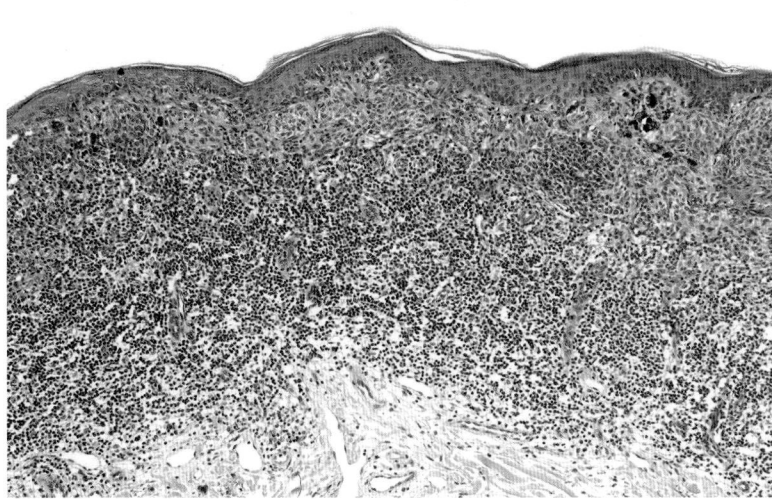

Fig. 25.101
Halo nevus: there are residual junctional nests deep to which is a dense, bandlike lymphohistiocytic infiltrate.

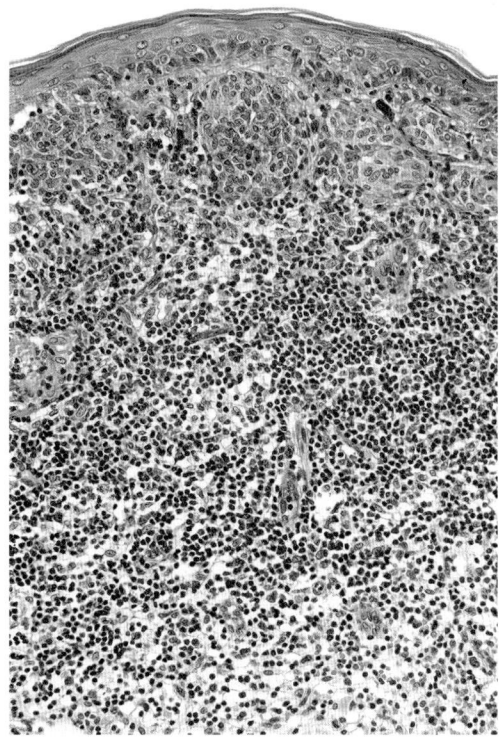

Fig. 25.102
Halo nevus: higher-power view of *Fig. 25.101*.

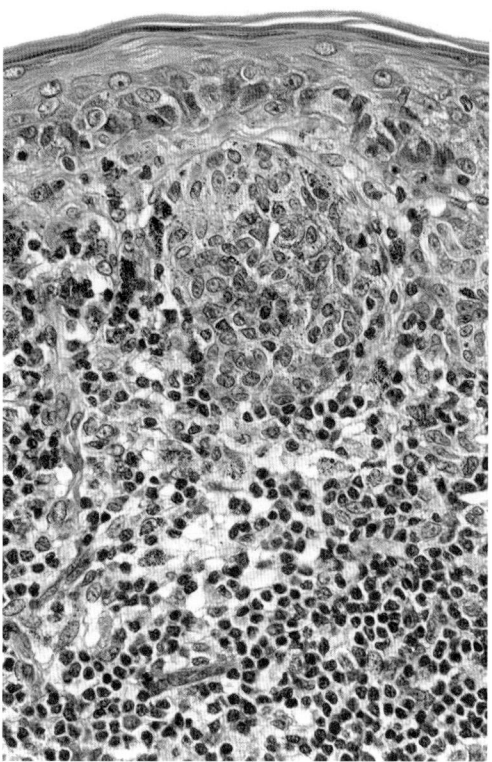

Fig. 25.103
Halo nevus: close-up view. Note the pigment incontinence.

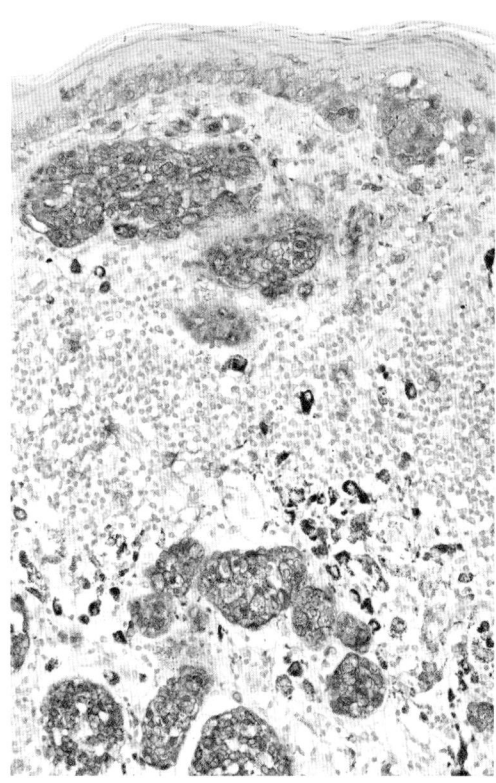

Fig. 25.104
Halo nevus: S100 protein immunohistochemistry highlights the residual nests in the dermis.

Degenerative cytological atypia may be seen. Mitotic activity is not a feature. However, inflammatory cells are often mitotic, and this is often a challenge. An accurate evaluation of the proliferation rate in the melanocytes population is aided by immunohistochemistry for Ki-67 counterstained with a melanocytes marker such as Melan-A using two different colors. Maturation is very difficult to evaluate during the evolution of the lesion, particularly in late stages due to the prominent inflammation. Residual nevus cells may be highlighted with immunohistochemistry using a melanocytic marker like S100 protein (*Fig. 25.104*). Since the latter often stains variable numbers of reactive dendritic cells, a marker such as MART-1/Melan-A may be used, remembering that the latter may sometimes label macrophages. It is at the late stages that the lesion may be histologically mistaken for melanoma. In the center of the lesion, blood vessels may sometimes be conspicuous. Rarely, halo nevi may develop in the absence of an inflammatory cell infiltrate.[27] Some lesions display identical histologic features to those seen in halo nevi, but a halo is not noticed clinically. Such lesions are described as showing a halo phenomenon.

The depigmented halo shows a complete absence of melanin pigment accompanied by a negative dopa reaction. Often, complete absence of melanocytes is also seen. The epidermis, however, contains increased numbers of Langerhans cells.

The resolved nevus is characterized by epidermal hypopigmentation accompanied by scattered dermal melanophages. Mild scarring may sometimes be evident.

Differential diagnosis

The halo nevus must be distinguished from melanoma. Typically, mitotic activity and nuclear and cytoplasmic pleomorphism (except the degenerative changes mentioned before) are not features, except in those that represent regressing melanoma or dysplastic nevi. Evaluation of mitotic activity in the melanocytes of halo nevi is often difficult because inflammatory cells are mitotically active. Double staining with Ki-67 and a melanocytic marker such as Melan-A is useful in identifying the proliferating population of cells. Also, the cellular infiltrate accompanying melanoma is usually more monomorphic and often hugs the base of the tumor rather than actively infiltrating it, except in those undergoing regression.

Meyerson nevus

Clinical features

Meyerson nevus represents an annular dermatitis (eczema) superimposed upon an acquired benign melanocytic nevus, usually a compound nevus, and is of unknown etiology (*Fig. 25.105*).[1-4] This phenomenon has also been reported in congenital melanocytic nevi, dysplastic nevi, common acquired nevi, Spitz nevi, melanoma in situ, and in invasive melanoma.[5-9]

Meyerson nevus presents with a sometimes pruritic, erythematous, scaly border measuring up to 1.0 cm in width.[2] Lesions, which are often multiple, appear most often on the trunk and proximal extremities, show a male predominance, and are most commonly seen in the third decade. Following resolution of the dermatitis, the nevus appears unchanged.[1,2] The evolution of a Meyerson nevus into a halo nevus and coexistence of the two types of nevi in the same patient have been reported.[10,11]

Histologic features

The histologic features are those of parakeratosis, acanthosis, and spongiosis associated with a superficial perivascular chronic inflammatory cell infiltrate (*Figs 25.106–25.108*). The spongiotic process is occasionally so prominent that the background melanocytic proliferation is obscured and may be missed.[9] In addition, spongiosis can be associated with significant distortion of the morphology of intraepidermal melanocytes, including the appearance of more epithelioid melanocytes and limited upward migration of tumor cells.[9] This is usually associated with mild cytological atypia.[9]

The inflammatory cell infiltrate consists predominantly of CD4+ lymphocytes.[5,12] Eosinophils are often seen and may be conspicuous, and

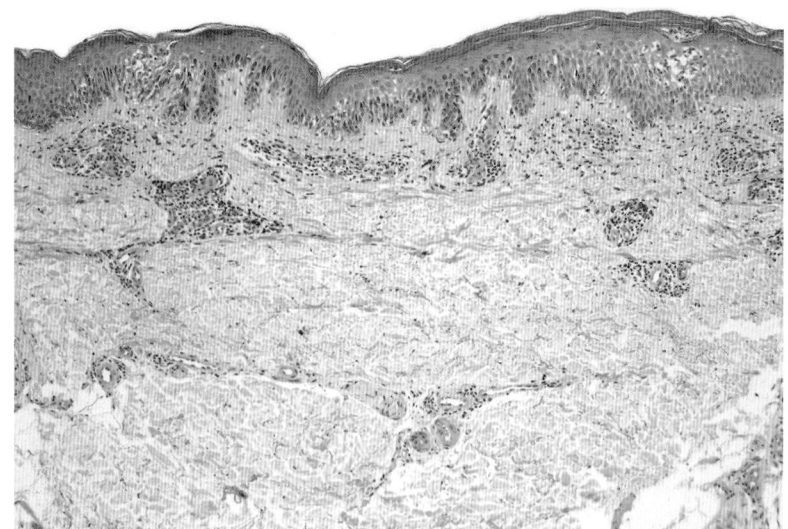

Fig. 25.106
Meyerson nevus: several junctional nests are evident in a background of spongiotic dermatitis.

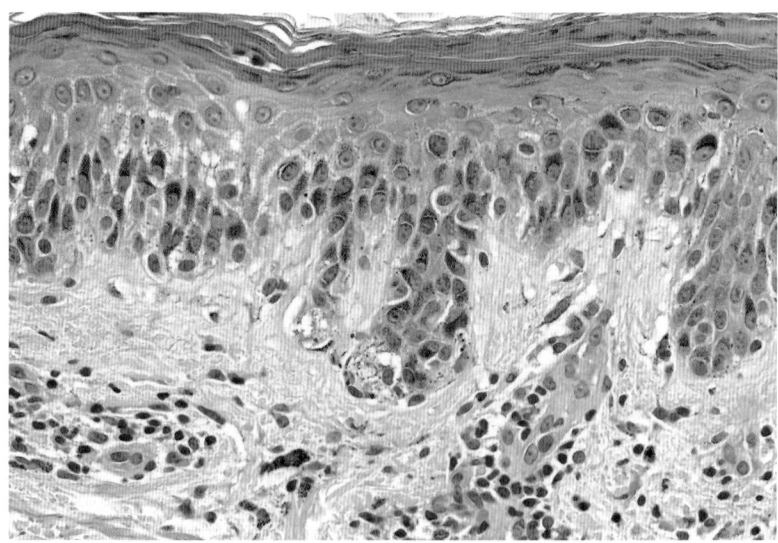

Fig. 25.107
Meyerson nevus: high-power view of *Fig. 25.106*.

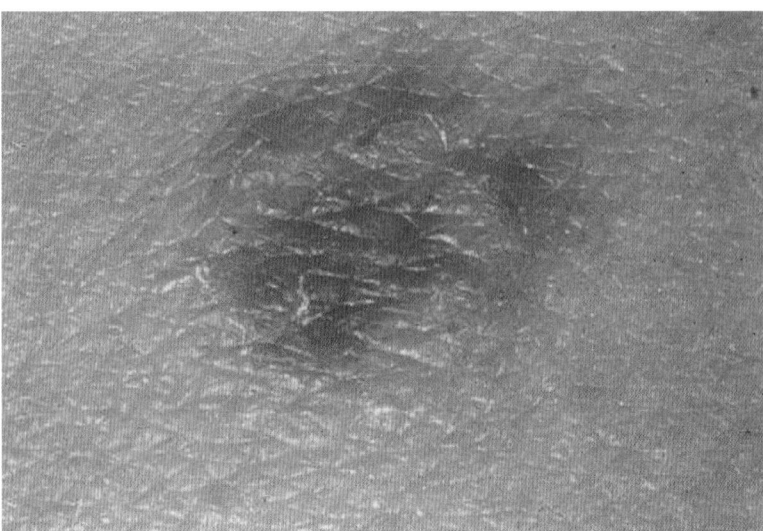

Fig. 25.105
Meyerson nevus: there is intense erythema surrounding this banal dermal nevus. By courtesy of the Institute of Dermatology, London, UK.

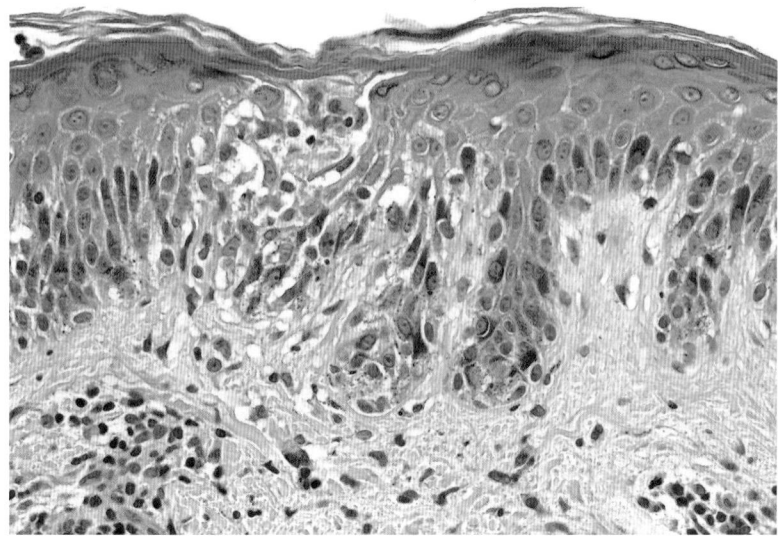

Fig. 25.108
Meyerson nevus: there is spongiosis with a microvesicle.

eosinophilic spongiosis is sometimes identified.[2] There is no histologic evidence of regression.[2]

Similar changes surrounding a wide range of lesions, including seborrheic keratosis, stucco keratoses, keloid, nevus flammeus, and squamous cell carcinoma, have rarely been described.[13,14]

Spitz nevus, atypical Spitz nevus and spitzoid melanoma

Spitz nevus (Spitz tumor, juvenile melanoma, spindle and epithelioid cell nevus) is of particular importance because, although biologically benign and associated with a good prognosis, it may be histologically misdiagnosed as a melanoma.[1–4] Similarly, melanoma may be mistaken for a Spitz nevus with disastrous consequences. Indeed, since its original description by Sophie Spitz in 1948, this lesion has been at the center of controversy relating to both histologic diagnosis and appropriate therapy.

The problem has been made considerably more complex by the recognition of malignant variants (spitzoid melanoma, malignant Spitz nevus, melanoma with spitzoid features) and histologically borderline lesions, the so-called atypical Spitz nevus (spitzoid tumor of uncertain biological potential).[5,6] It is also worth noting that one of the 'benign juvenile melanomas' in the original report metastasized.

Clinical features

Spitz nevus is uncommon, accounting for only approximately 1% of all nevi in children.[2] It is a usually solitary lesion that most often develops in children and adolescents.[2] In a series of 202 cases, 79% arose in patients younger than 20 years.[7] Nevertheless, a more recent study analyzing 247 cases found 66% of patients to be older than 20 years, with just over 15% being older than 40 years.[8] In a further report including 349 cases, only 6% of patients were older than 45 years.[9] Occasional lesions have been present at birth.[10] Exceptionally, it has been diagnosed in the elderly.[11] Extreme caution is advised before accepting such a diagnosis in patients in the fourth decade or older in which a spitzoid lesion is much more likely to be a melanoma than a benign nevus. A second opinion from an expert in melanocytic pathology is often critical to prevent misdiagnosis and undertreatment of a melanoma. Females are affected slightly more often than males.[2] Lesions are only very rarely encountered in blacks.[12]

Clinically, Spitz nevus typically presents as a solitary rapidly growing asymptomatic, pink or reddish brown, dome-shaped papule or nodule (*Figs 25.109–25.111*). Less often, lesions are macular (particularly early evolving lesions), polypoid, pedunculated, or verrucous.[2,13] Ulceration is rarely seen. Older lesions are often less pigmented and present as skin-colored firm papules reminiscent of dermatofibroma. Most frequently, the nevus is situated on the head or neck (particularly the cheek) or the extremities. The latter, especially the legs, are more commonly involved in females and adults.[7,14] The trunk is also a site of predilection. In a documented Hispanic population, the most common site was the lower extremities, irrespective of sex and age.[15] Examples have, however, been described at virtually any site on the body, including locations as diverse as genital mucosa, oral mucosa, tongue, glans penis, penile shaft, subungual area, perianal skin, and the sole of the foot.[13,16–24] Spitz nevi can exceptionally be painful. The lesion is usually less than 1 cm in diameter and is often vascular; it may therefore be clinically mistaken for a lobular capillary hemangioma (pyogenic granuloma).[23]

In contrast to solitary Spitz nevus, multiple Spitz nevi are exceedingly rare. In a review of 20 large series on Spitz nevi, multiple lesions were detected in 0.1% of patients.[25] They have been reported as either grouped (agminated) or widespread (widely disseminated, eruptive) and can develop in the background of normal skin, but also in hypopigmented or hyperpigmented skin (e.g., in speckled lentiginous nevus or café-au-lait macule).[25–38] While the agminated type predominates in children and frequently occurs on congenital hyperpigmented patches or plaques, the widespread type is usually seen in adults.[33] Agminated Spitz nevi can also have zosteriform, dermatome-like, and bilateral distribution.[29–32] A peculiar

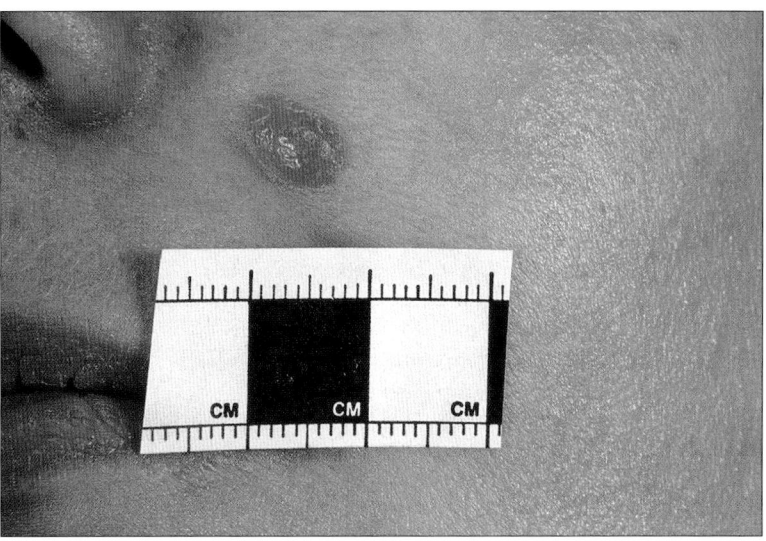

Fig. 25.110
Spitz nevus: the cheek is a commonly affected site. By courtesy of the Institute of Dermatology, London, UK.

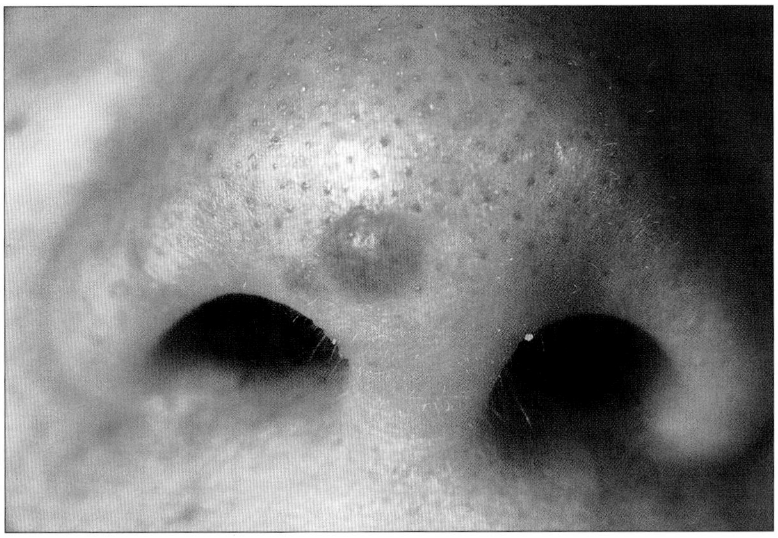

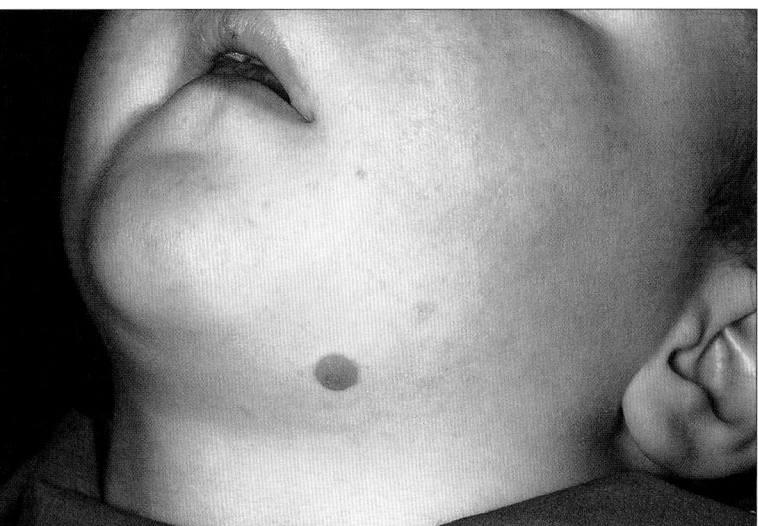

Fig. 25.109
Spitz nevus: dome-shaped nodule on the tip of the nose in a young child. Dilated vessels are apparent. By courtesy of the Institute of Dermatology, London, UK.

Fig. 25.111
Spitz nevus: pigmented variants overlap with pigmented spindle cell nevus of Reed. By courtesy of R.A. Marsden, MD, St George's Hospital, London, UK.

chemotherapy-induced agminated Spitz nevus developing in the background of nevus spilus has been reported.[34] The widespread type is characterized by numerous Spitz nevi, generally sparing palms, soles, and mucous membranes. They may on occasion be relapsing.[39] Rarely, Spitz nevus can be associated with a 'halo' phenomenon.[40,41] Gradual involution, similar to that observed in common melanocytic nevi, has also been reported in Spitz nevus.[42,43]

Frankly 'malignant Spitz nevus' (spitzoid melanoma) as proven by metastatic spread are exceptionally rare, and the majority represents cases seen in consultation.[44–47] Because of the difficulty in distinguishing between atypical Spitz nevi and spitzoid melanoma, many authors have used metastasis or death as the defining criterion.[47] Most cases have arisen in females, generally in the second decade.[48] There is no site predilection. In children, spitzoid melanoma is most frequently encountered on the extremities, followed by the trunk, and has similar sex distribution.[48] In general, although features highly reminiscent of Spitz nevus are present, in the vast majority of problematical cases or where there is diagnostic uncertainty, careful examination of multiple sections and the use of immunohistochemistry leaves a diagnosis of melanoma in no doubt (PHM, personal observation).

A subgroup of spitzoid melanoma has been described in which spread appears to be restricted to drainage lymph nodes although the number of cases is low and further documentation is lacking.[46,47]

On dermoscopy, nonpigmented Spitz nevi are characterized by dotted vascular pattern. In contrast, a starburst pattern is typically observed in pigmented spindle cell nevus of Reed.[49]

Histologic features

Spitz nevus shows the basic architecture common to all melanocytic nevi. Therefore, although compound lesions predominate, both junctional and intradermal variants may also be encountered (*Fig. 25.112*).[11,50,51]

The typical compound tumor is dome-shaped and often has a wedge-shaped outline with the base uppermost (*Fig. 25.113*). It shows lateral circumscription and striking symmetry, features that may be of value in distinguishing it from melanoma, which usually has a disorganized growth pattern and irregular lateral borders (*Figs 25.114* and *25.115*). Symmetry applies to depth of involvement in addition to the lateral aspects of the lesion; nests and single cells at an equivalent level of infiltration are morphologically similar, and maturation with depth is characteristically evident (*Figs 25.116–25.121*). Consumption of the epidermis, defined as thinning of the epidermis with attenuation of basal and suprabasal layers and loss of rete ridges in areas of melanocytic proliferation, is generally not a feature of Spitz nevus.[52] To the contrary, Spitz nevus commonly shows hyperkeratosis with acanthosis, sometimes amounting to pseudoepitheliomatous hyperplasia. Occasionally, the latter forms a collarette at the lateral border.[11]

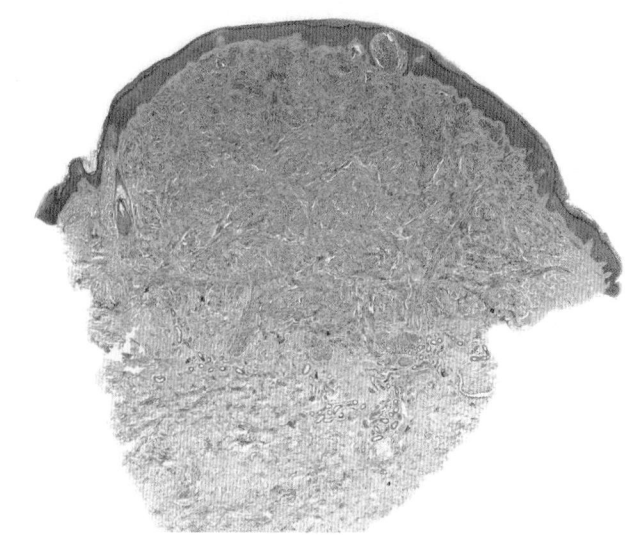

Fig. 25.113
Spitz nevus: this lesion is dome-shaped, symmetrical, and there is a wedge-shaped growth pattern.

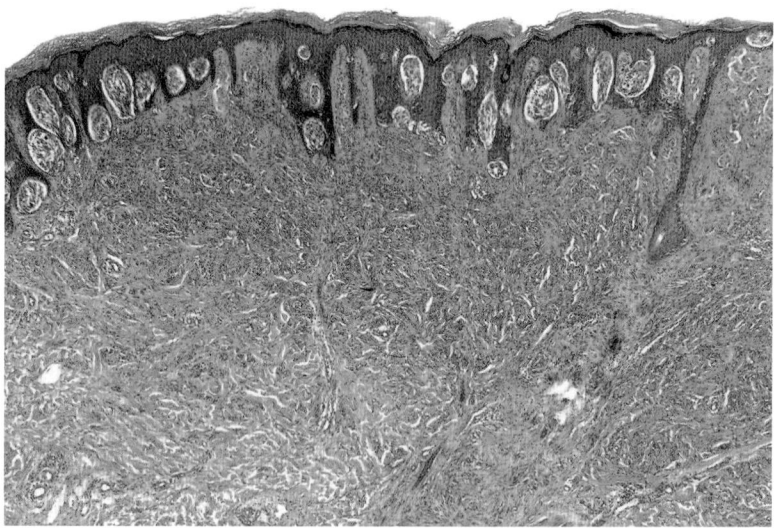

Fig. 25.114
Spitz nevus: this example shows the characteristic wedge-shaped dermal component.

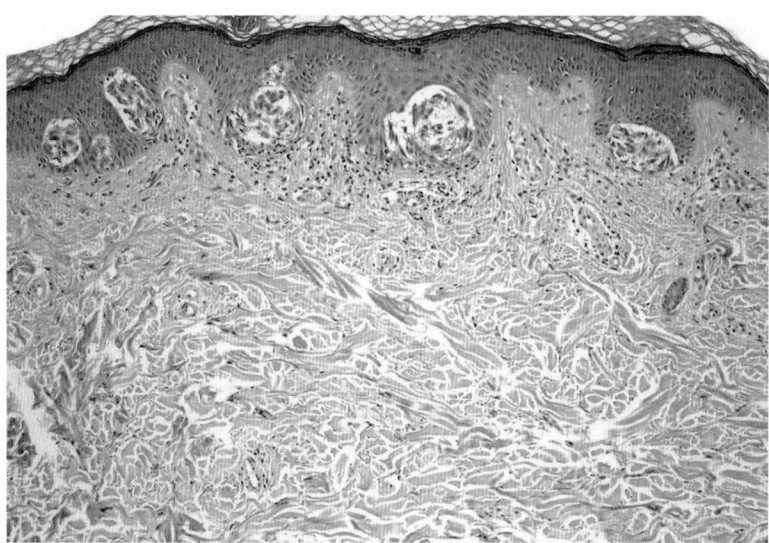

Fig. 25.112
Spitz nevus: this early lesion is characterized by a wholly junctional nested population. A typical retraction artifact surrounds each nest.

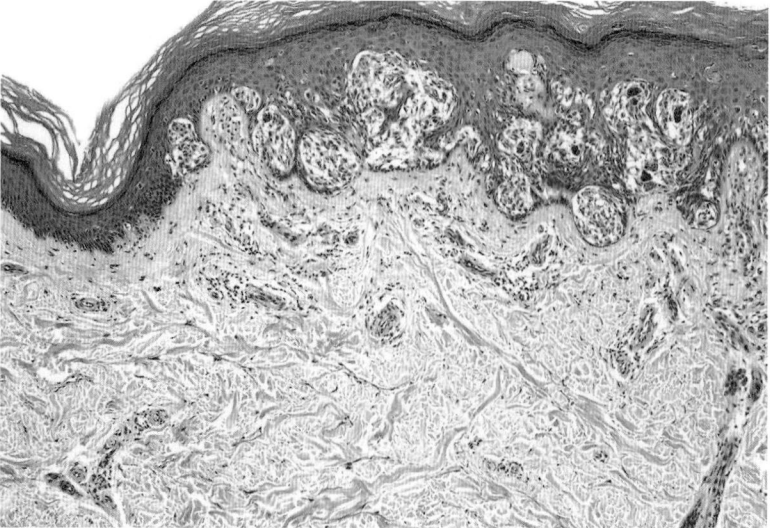

Fig. 25.115
Spitz nevus: the lateral border is sharply circumscribed. As a general rule, lesions which begin and end in a nest are benign. Same case as *Fig. 25.114*.

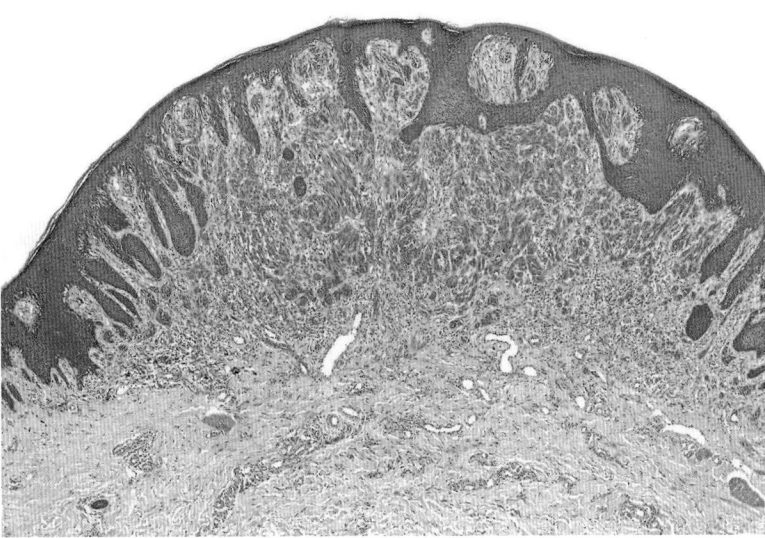

Fig. 25.116
Spitz nevus: low-power view showing vertical and horizontal symmetry.

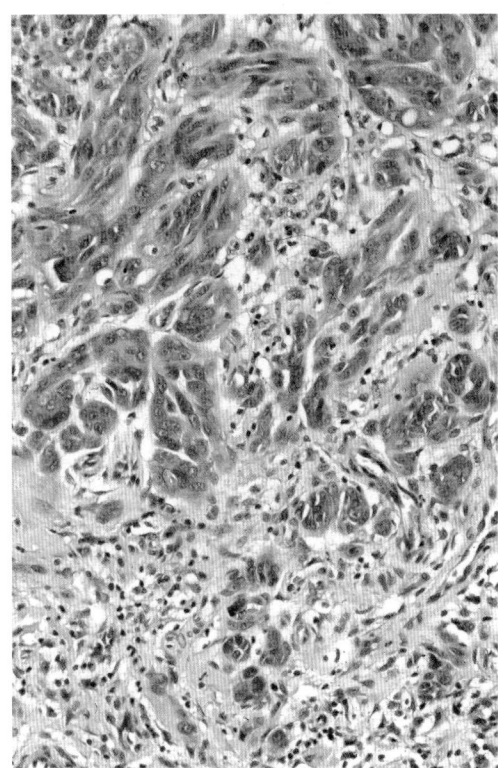

Fig. 25.118
Spitz nevus: deep component of lesion shown in *Fig. 25.117*.

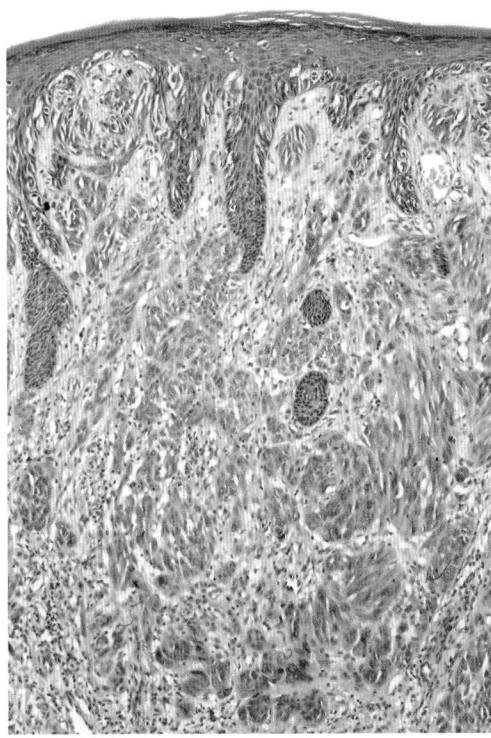

Fig. 25.117
Spitz nevus: nests and nevus cells diminish in size with depth (superficial aspect).

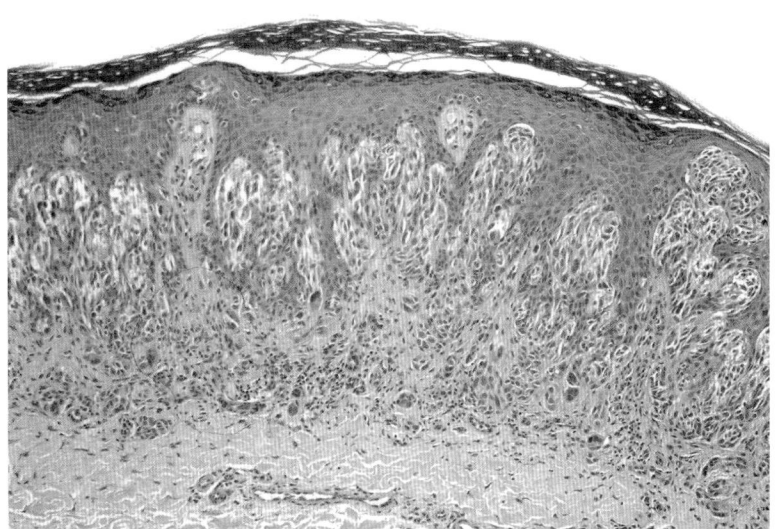

Fig. 25.119
Spitz nevus: medium-power view of a compound lesion.

Pseudoepitheliomatous hyperplasia can be prominent in Spitz nevi developing at mucosal sites, e.g., the oral cavity.[19] Edema of the upper dermis is also often present, and superficial telangiectatic vessels are a characteristic feature.

Spitz nevus is composed of spindled cells, epithelioid cells, or a mixture of both.[11,46] Pleomorphism is regularly present but, in contrast to melanoma, it tends to involve all of the cells to a similar degree. Single intraepithelial dendritic melanocytes, mainly oriented perpendicularly to the epidermis, can frequently be seen outside the junctional nests.[53]

In the spindled cell variant, the tumor cells (which are often arranged in fascicles) are large with abundant eosinophilic cytoplasm, and typically contain a single vesicular nucleus with a conspicuous (albeit small) eosinophilic nucleolus (*Fig. 25.122*).

In contrast, the epithelioid cells are frequently multinucleate, often adopt bizarre shapes, and although they may be arranged in nests and clusters,

they frequently lack cellular cohesion (*Figs 25.123* and *25.124*).[11,51,54] The cytoplasm sometimes has a ground-glass appearance. Intranuclear cytoplasmic pseudoinclusions are commonly seen but do not discriminate between Spitz nevus and melanoma. Nucleoli, which may be multiple, are eosinophilic and frequently large and inclusion-like. In the deeper reaches of the lesion, however, they often have a blue color. Mitotic activity is sometimes brisk, particularly in young people, but is limited to the more superficial aspect of the tumor and by definition is never atypical (*Fig. 25.125*). Mitoses in the deeper levels and atypical forms should prompt a search for other features of melanoma. The cytoplasm may be amelanotic or hypopigmented, but occasionally heavily pigmented variants overlapping with the pigmented epithelioid cell nevus and the spindle cell nevus (Reed) are encountered (see below).

The junctional component of compound lesions (and purely junctional variants) is characterized by usually large and often vertically oriented nests,

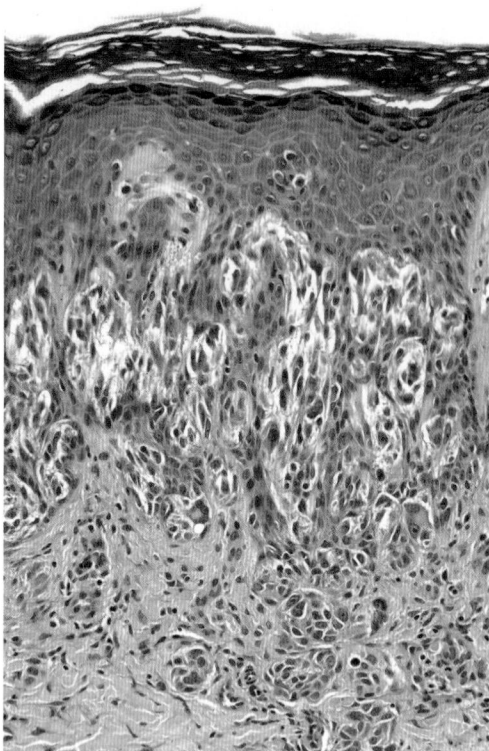

Fig. 25.120
Spitz nevus: the nests in the dermis are smaller than the junctional ones, another clue to the benign nature of the lesion.

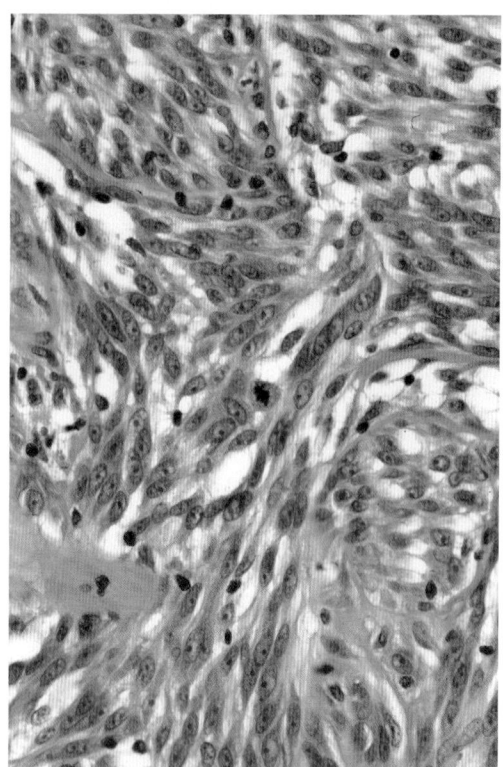

Fig. 25.122
Spitz nevus: spindled cell variant. The nevus cells are arranged in well-developed fascicles. The nuclei are vesicular and uniform, and contain small nucleoli. Note the mitotic figure.

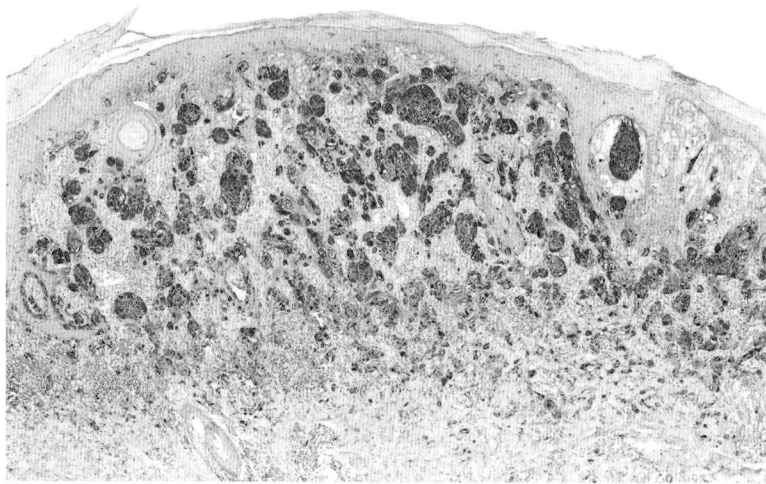

Fig. 25.121
Spitz nevus: S100 protein immunohistochemistry is a useful technique to demonstrate maturation with depth.

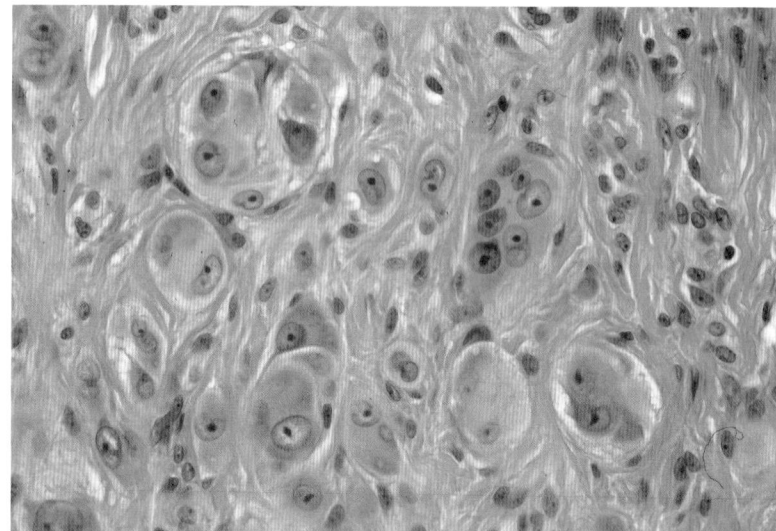

Fig. 25.123
Spitz nevus: epithelioid variant. The nevus cells have abundant eosinophilic cytoplasm with large vesicular nuclei and conspicuous eosinophilic nucleoli. 'Uniform' pleomorphism is characteristic of Spitz nevus.

typically surrounded by a prominent fixation retraction artifact (*Figs 25.126* and *25.127*). This may also be seen around the more superficial dermal nests and, in addition, is frequently found between individual tumor cells (*Fig. 25.128*). Its presence may be of help in differentiation from melanoma, in which such a feature is rare. Although there may be occasional single cells in the upper layers of the epidermis, pagetoid spread as is seen with in situ melanoma is not usually a feature, however, limited intraepidermal spread may sometimes be present in the center of the lesion (*Fig. 25.129*). Acral lesions, however, may be characterized by much more extensive involvement of the upper epidermal reaches.[55]

Traumatized Spitz nevi may show worrying intraepidermal spread. The presence of parakeratosis, crusting, fibrin, and hemorrhage are reassuring features.[55] Nests and more infrequently single cells are, however, sometimes present in the superficial epidermis and/or stratum corneum and in this context should not be taken to imply sinister biological potential.

A common feature of Spitz nevi is the presence, often in aggregates, of pale eosinophilic, periodic acid-Schiff-positive hyaline globules with scalloped borders (Kamino bodies) at the dermal–epidermal interface (*Fig. 25.130*).[56,57] Similar bodies are much less obvious in melanoma where they are usually solitary. They are composed of laminin, type IV collagen, and fibronectin and therefore do not represent apoptotic or cytoid bodies.[58–61]

The dermal component shows maturation with increasing depth of the lesion. The nests and single cells are smaller and rounder and have progressively less cytoplasm. Nuclei and nucleoli are also similarly affected. Towards the deeper dermis, the nests and fascicles of nevus cells become

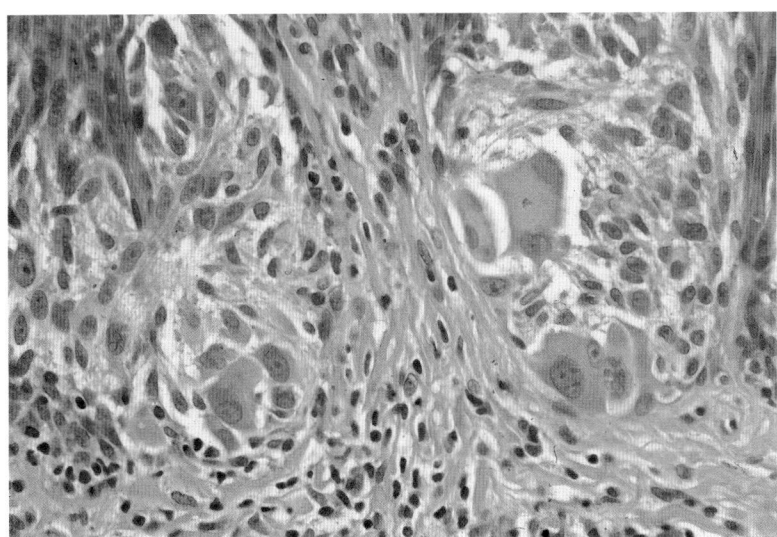

Fig. 25.124
Spitz nevus: epithelioid variant showing multinucleated giant cells.

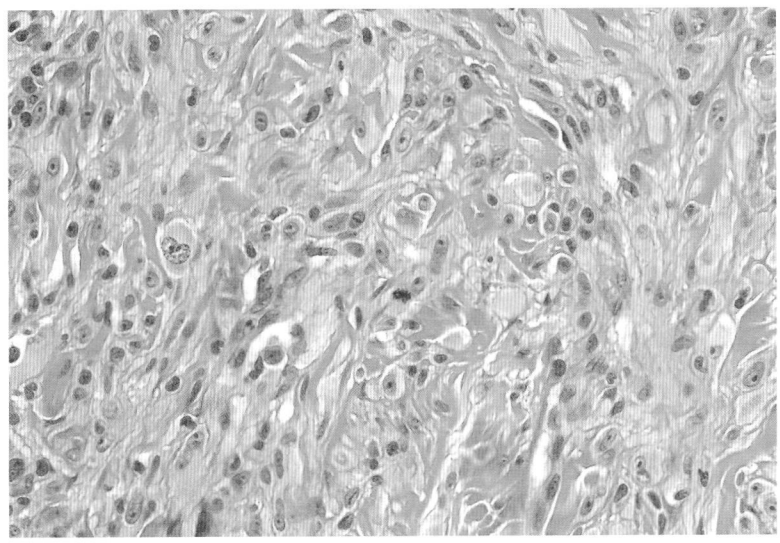

Fig. 25.125
Spitz nevus: epithelioid cell variant showing a centrally located mitotic figure.

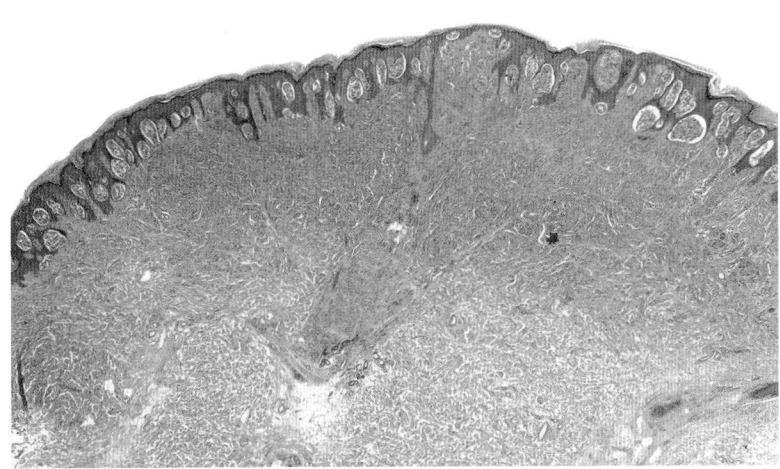

Fig. 25.126
Spitz nevus: the retraction artifact surrounding the junctional nests is clearly demonstrated.

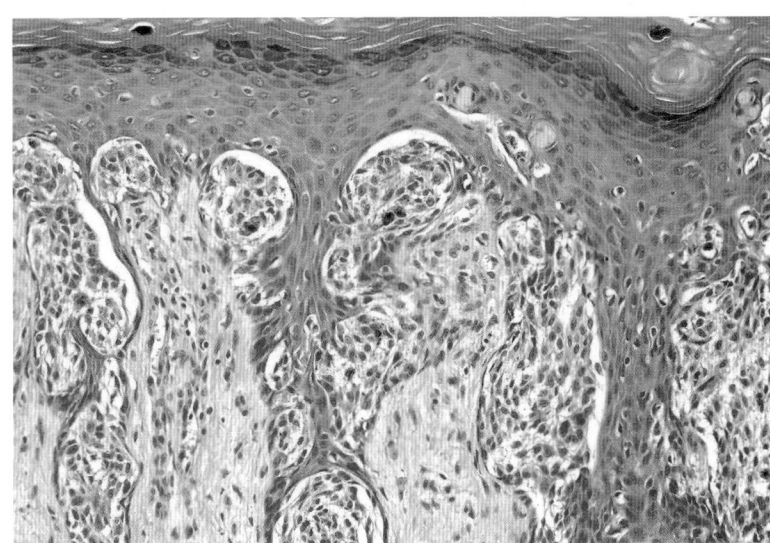

Fig. 25.127
Spitz nevus: high-power view of *Fig. 25.126*.

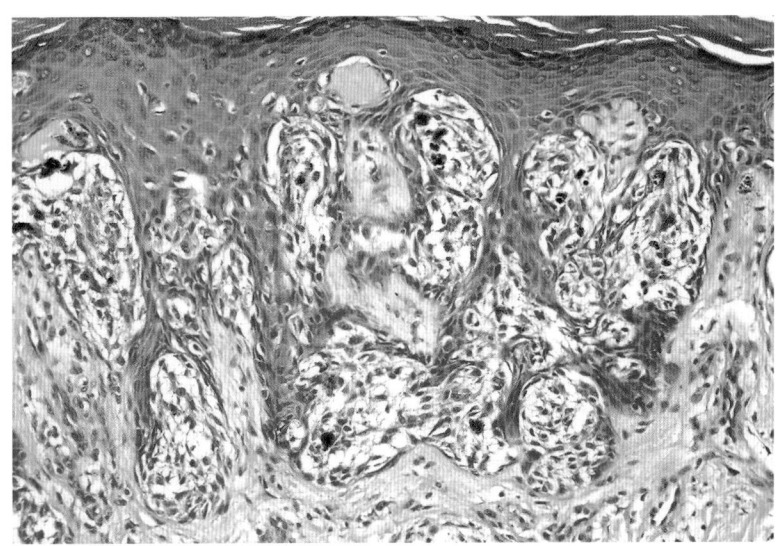

Fig. 25.128
Spitz nevus: dyscohesive junctional nests are characteristic.

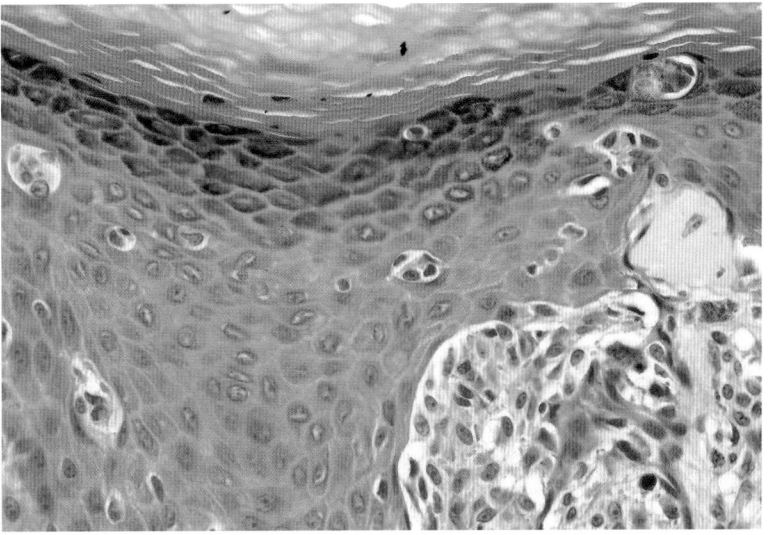

Fig. 25.129
Spitz nevus: pagetoid spread over the center of the lesion should not be misinterpreted as evidence of malignancy.

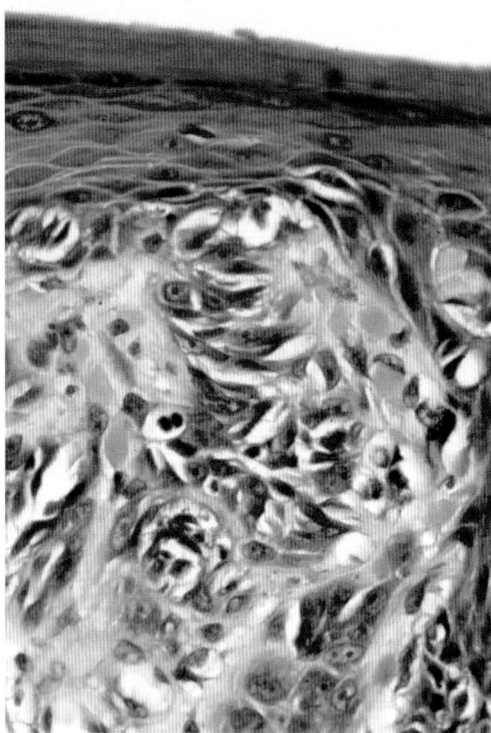

Fig. 25.130
Spitz nevus: multiple eosinophilic Kamino bodies are present.

replaced by a single-cell infiltrating pattern, which often shows an Indian-file distribution between adjacent collagen bundles at the base of the lesion. Progressive fibrosis is commonly evident, particularly in lesions where the dermal component predominates. Rarely, dense fibrous tissue may surround and isolate individual dermal nevus cells – the desmoplastic Spitz nevus (see below). Spitz nevi often have an associated perivascular lymphocytic infiltrate at the base of the lesion. In evolving lesions, however, a bandlike distribution is sometimes present.

Although lymphovascular spread has been documented in apparent Spitz nevi, its presence should be viewed with extreme suspicion and other features of malignancy sought.[62]

Several histologic variants of Spitz nevi have been reported, and include combined, pagetoid, desmoplastic, hyalinized, angiomatoid, halo-associated, pigmented, plexiform, tubular, rosette-like, Spitz nevus with Touton-like giant cells, pseudogranulomatous Spitz nevus, verrucous Spitz nevus, lipoblastoid/signet ring Spitz nevus, and recurrent Spitz nevus. Most recently, a subset of Spitzoid proliferations has been described with distinctive morphological features harboring *BAP1* mutations occurring in either familial or sporadic setting (see Fig. 25.71). Furthermore, an important percentage of Spitz nevi can now be classified according to the type of protein kinase fusion mutations (see corresponding section). Combined Spitz nevus is composed of banal, dysplastic, congenital, or blue nevus with focal Spitz features, or Spitz nevus with deep penetrating nevus.[63] Spitz nevus with halo nevus features consists of a typically symmetrical and diffuse infiltrate of lymphocytes, histiocytes with rare plasma cells, and eosinophils associated with degenerate nevus cells.[40,41] Impaired nevus maturation has been documented. The halo reaction pattern appears to be a particular feature of combined lesions but may also be seen in pure Spitz nevus.[41] Distinction of Spitz nevus with halo reaction from melanoma with halo reaction depends on the presence of symmetry and the absence of deep nodules, deep mitoses, and atypical mitoses. The angiomatoid variant is characterized by distinctive fibrovascular stroma, and represents a subset of desmoplastic Spitz nevus (see desmoplastic Spitz nevus).[64–67] Blood vessels have thin to mildly thickened walls and are lined by plump endothelial cells. The presence of CD34 and CD10 positive spindled mesenchymal cells corresponding to fibroblast dispersed among melanocytes and blood vessels throughout the lesion has been reported.[67] The myxoid variant is delineated by marked extracellular mucin deposition

within epidermal clefts as well as between melanocytes.[68] Spitz nevus with rosette-like structures is a variant consisting of eccentrically located or palisaded nuclei with centrally located cytoplasm, albeit without lumina formation.[69] The presence of S100 and MART-1-positive Touton-like giant cells has been noted in a single case of Spitz nevus.[70] Exceptionally, a tubular variant and a plexiform growth pattern have been described.[71,72] Pseudogranulomatous Spitz nevus is characterized by arrangements of epithelioid melanocytes into nodular aggregates embedded in a dense lymphocytic infiltrate mimicking thereby sarcoid granulomas.[73] Verrucous Spitz nevus is typically associated with papillomatosis, hyperkeratosis, acanthosis, and formation of horn cysts.[74,75] Lipoblastoid/signet-ring Spitz nevus is another addition to the group, delineated by remarkable vacuolization of the cytoplasm of melanocytes imparting a lipoblastoid or signet ringlike appearance of the cells.[76]

Recurrent Spitz nevus is often difficult to diagnose on histologic grounds.[77] The epidermal component displays pagetoid spread as seen in other types of pseudomelanoma.[77] The dermal component can show a residual lesion with features similar to those of an ordinary Spitz including a desmoplastic pattern. It may also show a nodular growth pattern within the scar mimicking melanoma. However, maturation is usually seen, and mitotic activity is very low. As with other types of pseudomelanoma, review of the original biopsy is of extreme importance.

Interesting examples of chronic leukocytoclastic vasculitis and glomovenous malformation occurring in the background of a Spitz nevus have recently been reported.[78,79]

Differential diagnosis

In addition to the anticipated S100 protein and neuron-specific enolase positivity, Spitz nevus commonly expresses HMB-45 antigen although this last is usually only present in the more superficial reaches of the dermal component and therefore full-thickness expression may be a diagnostic pointer for melanoma.[80,81] All Spitz nevi show diffuse and strong S100A6 positivity in both the epidermal and the dermal component, while only one-third of melanomas show patchy and weak staining with this antibody in the dermal component and absent or weak staining in the epidermal component.[82]

In contrast to melanoma, in which the tumor population is aneuploid, the majority of Spitz nevi are characterized by a diploid cell population.[83–85] Comparative genomic hybridization (CGH) studies have shown that, in general, there is no evidence of chromosomal abnormalities although a small subset show a gain of 11p.[86] Interstitial deletion of chromosome 9p has been identified in only a minority of tumors (loss of chromosome 9p is the commonest chromosomal abnormality in melanoma).[87] Spitz nevi have, however, been shown to be monoclonal proliferations.[86] It is worth mentioning that a subset of Spitz nevi are polyploid, a phenomenon rarely encountered in melanomas.[88] Additional immunohistochemical studies may prove invaluable in difficult cases including:

- MIB-1 expression is usually limited to small numbers (less than 5%) of cells in the superficial part of the dermal component of Spitz nevus compared with melanoma in which positive cells are often identified throughout the lesion.[89–91]
- Bcl-2 is frequently negative or only weakly positive in Spitz nevus, whereas in melanoma the majority of tumors are strongly positive.[92]
- Cyclin D1 is overexpressed in melanoma throughout the tumor. Contrariwise, in Spitz nevus, although the superficial aspect may be strongly positive, there is a progressive diminution in labeling with depth, mirroring the histologic feature of maturation.[93,94]
- p53 is typically absent in Spitz nevus but is positive in many nodular melanomas.[93]
- p21 has been found to be overexpressed in Spitz nevus compared to melanoma, while survivin and topoisomerase II alpha, in contrast, are overexpressed in melanoma.[91,95]
- Decreased nuclear immunoreactivity for p16 in the dermal melanocytic component is present in melanoma as compared with Spitz nevus.[96] Loss of both cytoplasmic and nuclear p16 immunoreactivity seems to be more specific for melanoma than loss of nuclear reactivity alone.[96] Such tumors have shown increased desmoplasia and pleomorphism with a distinct infiltrating lower border; however, these features do not appear to correlate with worsening biological behavior.

- CD40 is not expressed by Spitz nevus but is present in the dermal component of up to 40% of melanomas.[97]
- CD44 expression is maintained in Spitz nevus, in contrast to melanoma in which it is decreased.[98]
- Cdc7, a serine-threonine kinase is overexpressed in atypical Spitz nevus and melanoma, as compared to Spitz nevi.[99]
- No differences in the expression of c-kit (CD117) between Spitz nevus and melanoma has been detected by immunohistochemistry in one study.[100]
- CD99 staining has been detected in 56% of spitzoid melanomas and only 5% of Spitz nevi. While staining in melanomas is frequently diffuse and strong, such a pattern is not observed in Spitz nevi.[101]

None of these immunohistochemical stains is entirely reliable, and challenging lesions often produce equivocal results. Therefore, most of these immunostains, except MIB-1 and p16, are not used on a regular basis in daily practice. The final diagnosis as always will depend on close clinicopathological correlation, and interpretation of the sections stained with hematoxylin and eosin remains the gold standard.

The majority of Spitz nevi fulfills the histologic criteria described above, lack significant cytological atypia, and behave in a predictably benign fashion. They can be histologically recognized as such and should be diagnosed as Spitz nevi. Rare variants have been described which appear to deviate from the prototypic features and yet appear to fall short of the requirements for frank vertical growth-phase melanoma. Exceptionally, Spitz nevi have been documented which appear to be histologically typical, recur, and metastasize.[44–46] Some of these seem to have a propensity for nodal metastases only, whereas others behave in a truly malignant fashion with systemic dissemination. It should be noted that such publications are generally present in the older literature but are continuously quoted. As a result, the more recent literature is replete with reports discussing the differential diagnosis of this lesion and recommending various imprecise terminologies including atypical Spitz nevus, Spitz tumor, minimal deviation melanoma (Spitz nevus type), and melanocytic neoplasm of indeterminate malignant potential (Spitz nevus type).[102–106] While the last is probably the most appropriate, highlighting our basic ignorance of likely behavior, it is too cumbersome for general use. The term atypical Spitz nevus/tumor – implying deviation in some degree from the prototype and associated with a variable risk of malignant potential – has the merit of fairly common usage (*Figs 25.131–25.134*). It also signifies the need for particular care by the clinician in the patient's follow-up. An alternative designation of spitzoid tumor of uncertain biological potential would be equally appropriate.

The inherent risk of such a potentially wastepaper basket category is that too few tumors will be classified as typical Spitz nevus or frank melanoma, and the majority will therefore be included in the atypical Spitz tumor group for 'safety's sake'. If the term is to be used at all, it should only be as a last resort after appropriate immunohistochemistry, molecular genetic techniques (fluorescent in situ hybridization [FISH], CGH, next-generation sequencing), and seeking consultation with expert(s) in the field. The diagnosis benefits no one, least of all the patient. The problem has been exacerbated in recent decades by the use of shave and punch biopsy techniques with resulting incomplete specimens which render the pathologist unable to issue a definitive diagnosis since some of the features of malignancy such as deep mitoses and lack of maturation cannot be assessed. In addition, the term is associated with the attendant risk of overtreatment. Sentinel lymph node biopsy has become almost mandatory for all vertical growth-phase melanomas of 1.0 mm or greater. This investigative technique is increasingly being used for larger numbers of so-called atypical Spitz nevi or Spitz tumors of uncertain malignant potential, sometimes after correlation with cytogenetic studies (see end of the chapter).[107,108]

In general, these 'atypical' lesions are clinically no different from typical Spitz nevi, although there is some evidence that size may be a potential clue. Increasing age makes a diagnosis of Spitz nevus less likely. Lesions on the back in adult males and on the leg in adult females should be studied with great care to exclude a diagnosis of melanoma.

Although no one single histologic feature is necessarily diagnostic of malignancy, potentially worrying histologic features include lack of symmetry, poor lateral demarcation, ulceration, involvement of deep dermis or

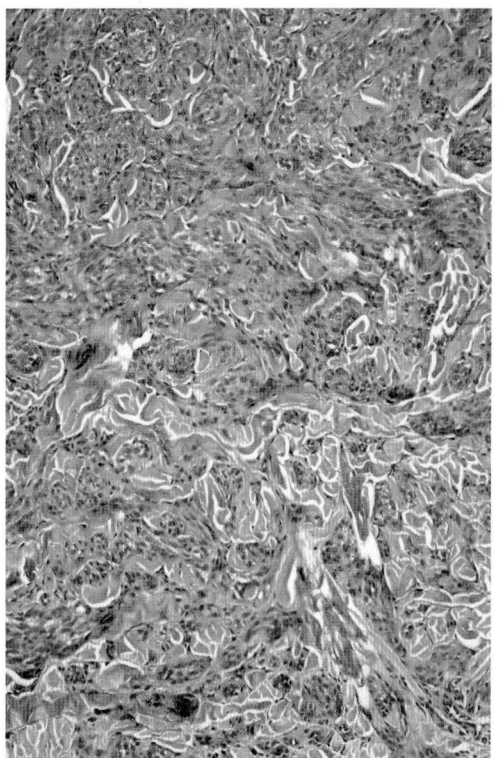

Fig. 25.131
Atypical Spitz nevus: medium-power view of the dermal component.

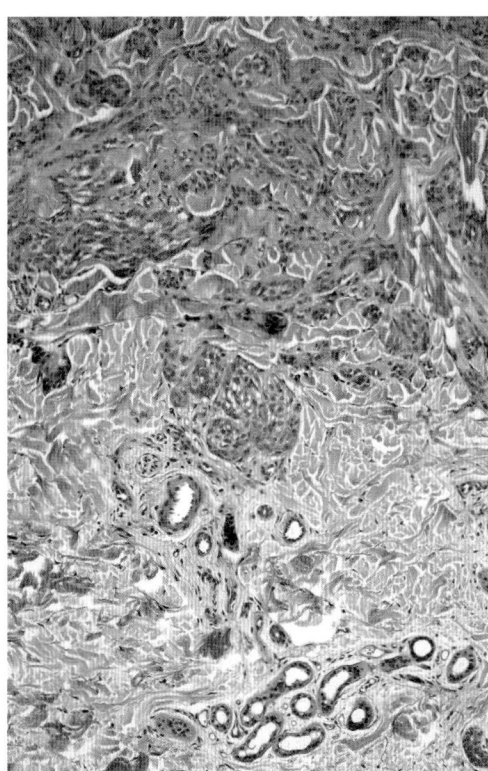

Fig. 25.132
Atypical Spitz nevus: low-power view showing impaired maturation with large nests persisting at the base.

subcutaneous fat, impaired maturation, excessive intraepidermal or pagetoid spread, nuclear hyperchromatism, high nuclear cytoplasmic ratio, absence of Kamino bodies, large expansile dermal nests, pushing deep margin, deep pigmentation, necrosis, increased dermal mitoses, deep dermal mitoses, and atypical dermal mitoses.[62]

The majority of the proliferations designated as atypical Spitz nevus/ tumor have good overall prognosis despite frequent involvement of the

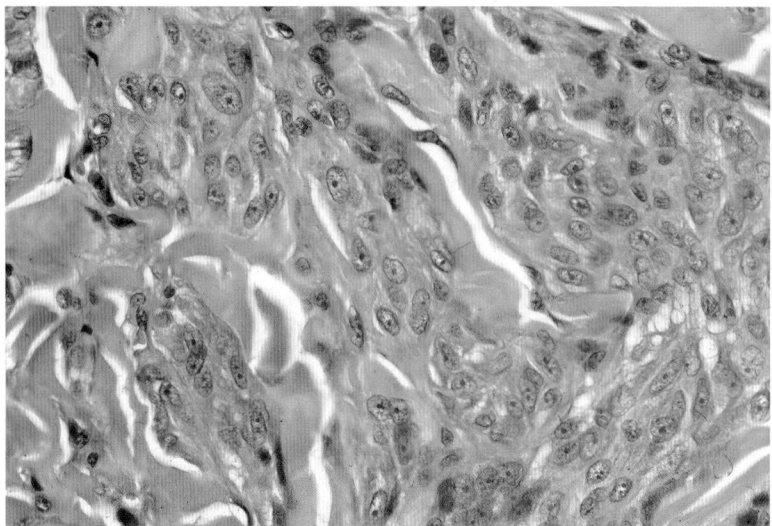

Fig. 25.133
Atypical Spitz nevus: high-power view of deep margin.

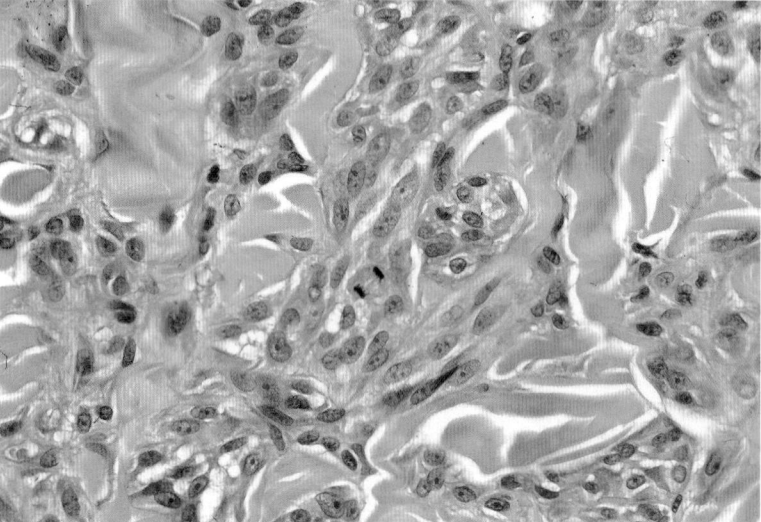

Fig. 25.134
Atypical Spitz nevus: note the mitosis at the deep margin. On the basis of lack of maturation extending to the base of the lesion and the presence of deep mitotic activity, this lesion is almost certainly malignant.

sentinel lymph node(s) (from 30% to 50%), and only a small proportion of patients develop distant metastases and die of disease.[109-114] Up to 99% of these patients were found to be alive at the mean follow-up of 5 years, which is significantly higher than those for comparable conventional melanomas.[110] The histologic features that were found to be associated with progression to lymph node(s) include asymmetry, high-grade cytological atypia, frequent mitoses, deep mitoses, and ulceration.[115] It has in addition been proven that having a positive sentinel lymph node does not seem to predict poorer outcome in patients with atypical Spitz nevi/tumors.[110]

A grading system for dividing atypical Spitz nevi into low-, medium-, and high-risk categories (of being frankly malignant) has been devised.[116] This is based on age, diameter, involvement of subcutaneous fat, presence or absence of ulceration, and mitotic rate but has yet to be validated in larger series of cases.

Pigmented epithelioid cell nevus

Clinical features

This uncommon variant of Spitz nevus has received scant attention in the literature. It presents as a small, darkly pigmented papule in children or

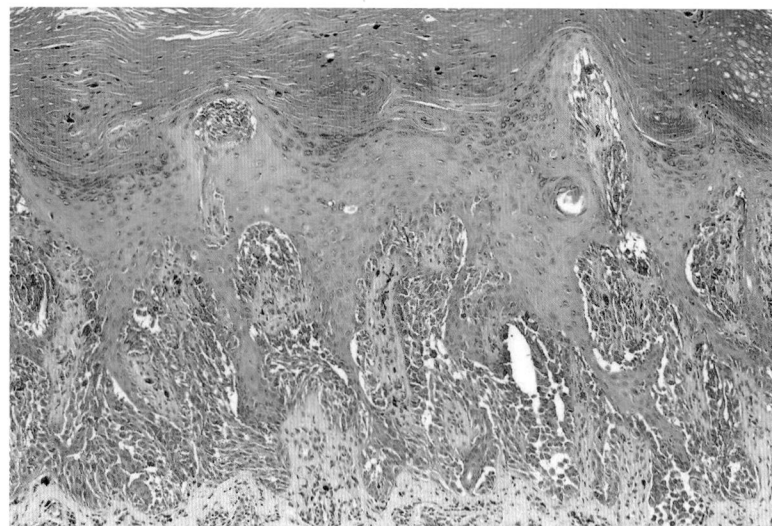

Fig. 25.135
Pigmented epithelioid nevus: this lesion overlaps Spitz and Reed nevi. The nevus consists of intensely pigmented epithelioid and spindled melanocytes. There are numerous melanophages in the underlying dermis.

young adults.[1,2] Pigmented epithelioid cell nevus shows predilection for the skin of the head and neck area.[1,2]

Histologic features

Histologically, it overlaps typical Spitz nevus and pigmented spindle cell tumor of Reed. It is composed of a symmetrical and circumscribed, intensely pigmented, epithelioid nested population affecting the epidermis and papillary dermis (*Fig. 25.135*). The cytoplasm is abundant and the nuclei vesicular with prominent eosinophilic nucleoli. Intraepidermal spread is minimal, and mitoses are very scant or absent.[1] The epidermis overlying the melanocytic proliferation generally shows prominent hyperplasia and hyperkeratosis.[2]

Differential diagnosis

The main differential diagnosis is with epithelioid blue nevus and pigment synthesizing melanoma (now classified within the spectrum of pigmented epithelioid melanocytoma). Epithelioid blue nevus usually lacks a junctional melanocytic component. In the dermis, dendritic melanocytes are typically found intermixed with heavily pigmented epithelioid melanocytes displaying a small basophilic nucleolus. Pigment synthesizing melanoma is an asymmetrical and poorly circumscribed predominantly, but not always dermal, proliferation of dendritic melanocytes. The latter display a prominent eosinophilic nucleolus, tend to be fairly regular, lack maturation, and show low but discernible mitotic activity.

Pagetoid Spitz nevus

Clinical features

Pagetoid Spitz nevus is a relatively rare variant of Spitz nevus. It much more common in females, shows striking predilection for extremities (with only a handful of the cases reported outside extremities), and typically presents as a light to dark brown macule measuring less than 6 mm in diameter.[1-6] Although a seminal paper by Busam and Barnhill suggested an exclusive occurrence in children and adolescents,[1] a recent large study on pagetoid Spitz nevi demonstrated much broader age distribution (from 15 to 57 years; average age, 34 years).[6] Pagetoid Spitz nevus usually presents as a solitary lesion.[1-6] Nevertheless, an exceptional example of multiple pagetoid Spitz nevi occurring in a single patient, initially misdiagnosed as multiple melanoma in situ, has also been reported.[7]

Histologic features

Histologically, Spitz nevus in its early stages of evolution is characterized by a wholly intraepidermal melanocytic proliferation which can be

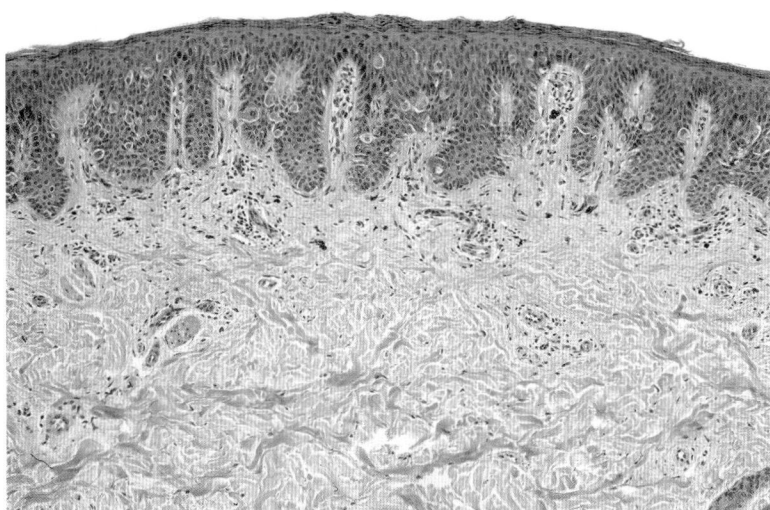

Fig. 25.136
Pagetoid Spitz nevus: low-power view showing a largely basally located epithelioid nevus population. This biopsy was taken from a 5-year-old child.

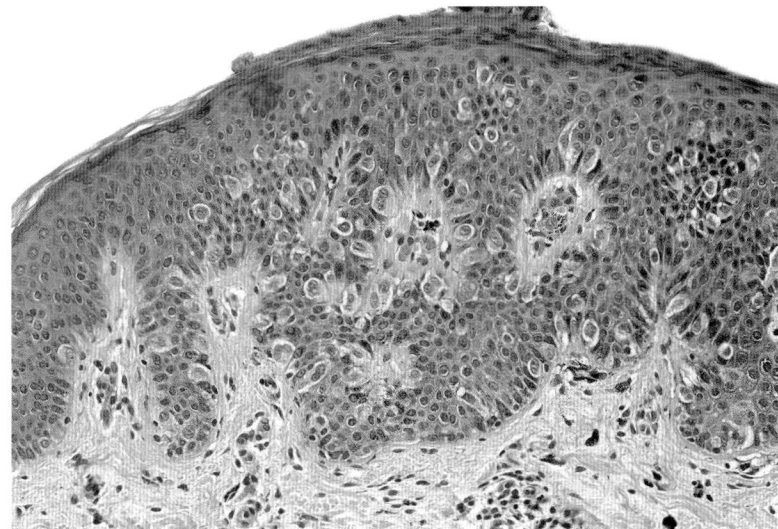

Fig. 25.137
Pagetoid Spitz nevus: there is central pagetoid spread.

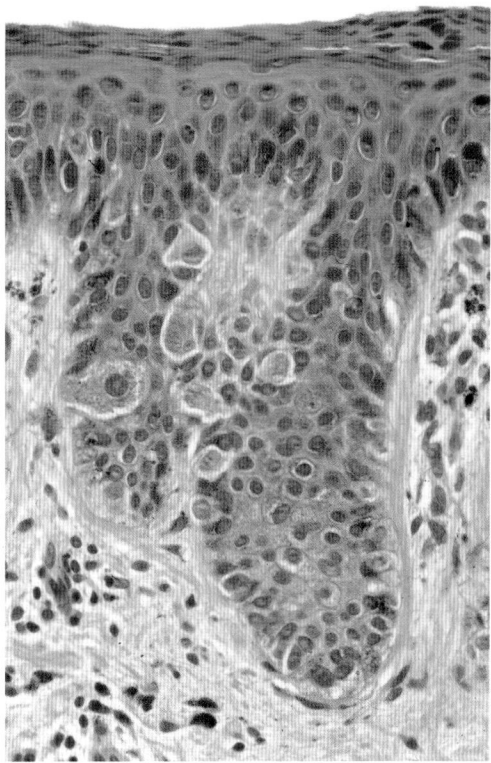

Fig. 25.138
Pagetoid Spitz nevus: the nevus cells have abundant eosinophilic cytoplasm and uniform vesicular nuclei with prominent nucleoli.

re-excision to ensure complete removal is advised.[4] In addition, fluorescence in situ hybridization assay can be performed to detect aberrations on chromosome 6 (6p25, 6q23, and Cep6) and chromosome 11 (11q13), their presence being suggestive of malignant melanocytic proliferations.[8,9]

Desmoplastic nevus

Clinical features

Several variants of desmoplastic nevus have been reported – they include a variant with spitzoid cytomorphology (desmoplastic Spitz nevus, hyalinizing spindle and epithelioid nevus), a variant with blue nevus-like morphology, desmoplastic nevus on chronic sun-damaged skin, congenital melanocytic nevus with desmoplasia, and ordinary/common melanocytic nevus with desmoplasia.[1–6] Recognition of a desmoplastic nevus is particularly important because it may be confused with a desmoplastic melanoma by the unwary.[1–4] Desmoplastic nevus is an entirely benign condition.

Desmoplastic Spitz nevus typically presents as a sometimes scaly, erythematous, or red-brown papulonodule that most often affects the extremities. Although a wide range of age groups may be affected, most patients are in their third decade. Lesions are often of several years' duration. Desmoplastic melanocytic nevus on chronic sun-damaged skin displays female predominance (70%), most commonly develops on the extremities, and typically presents in the sixth decade of life as a flesh-colored macule or papule.[6]

Histologic features

There is usually hyperkeratosis and the epidermis often shows acanthosis but sometimes appears normal (Fig. 25.139). The nevus is centered in the papillary dermis but commonly extends into the reticular dermis (Fig. 25.140).[2] It consists of a wedge-shaped infiltrate of somewhat pleomorphic cells with abundant eosinophilic cytoplasm containing darkly stained or vesicular nuclei with conspicuous nucleoli (Fig. 25.141).[1] Occasionally, residual nests of nevus cells showing spitzoid features are present in the superficial dermis (Fig. 25.142). Intranuclear cytoplasmic pseudoinclusions (invaginations) are often prominent, and sometimes ganglion-like cells are evident (Figs 25.143 and 25.144).[2] The nevus characteristically matures

confused histologically with in situ melanoma. In the pagetoid variant of intraepidermal Spitz nevus, increased numbers of uniform, enlarged, epithelioid melanocytes with abundant eosinophilic cytoplasm present as a small circumscribed and symmetrical lesion usually associated with mild to moderate acanthosis (Figs 25.136–25.138).[1] Typically, each nevus cell is separated from adjacent cells by a well-developed retraction artifact. Intraepidermal spread is usually limited to the lower half of the epidermis, but full-thickness involvement can occur. The nevus cells are oval or polygonal with ground-glass cytoplasm and round to oval uniform vesicular nuclei containing prominent eosinophilic nucleoli.[1] Tumor cells display an angulated cytoplasmic outline. Apoptotic forms are usually present, but mitoses are not seen. In some lesions, there may be an associated junctional nested component, generally representing a minor component of the proliferation (less than 30% of the total melanocytic population).[6] A perivascular lymphohistiocytic infiltrate is present in the superficial dermis, frequently associated with melanophages.[6]

Differential diagnosis

An irregular growth pattern and lack of uniformity of the nevus population accompanied by significant cytological atypia make a diagnosis of pagetoid Spitz nevus untenable. Fine melanin pigmentation and mitotic activity also favor a diagnosis of melanoma. If the diagnosis is in doubt, a modest

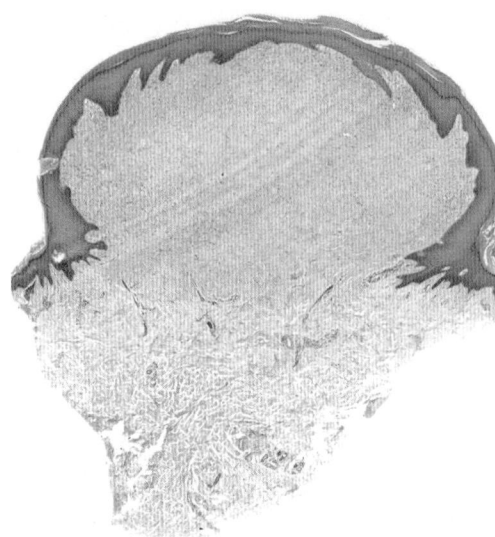

Fig. 25.139
Desmoplastic Spitz nevus: scanning view showing hyperkeratosis, acanthosis, and a well-developed collarette. The nevus predominantly involves an expanded papillary dermis.

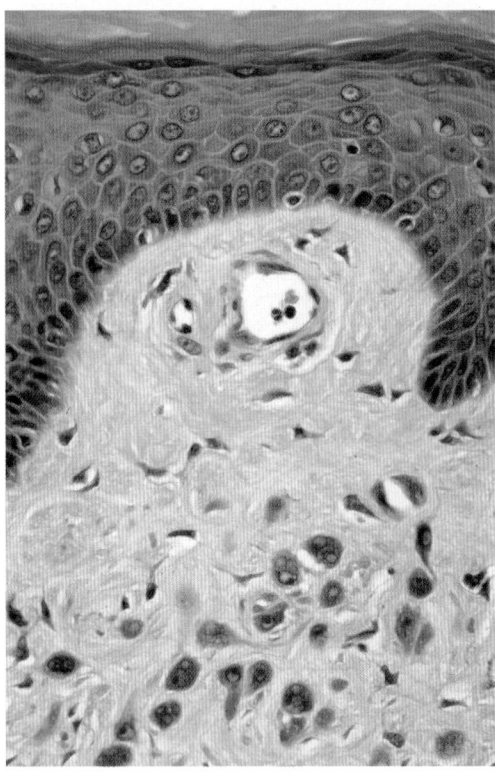

Fig. 25.141
Desmoplastic Spitz nevus: in this example, nevus cells are sparsely distributed in a desmoplastic stroma.

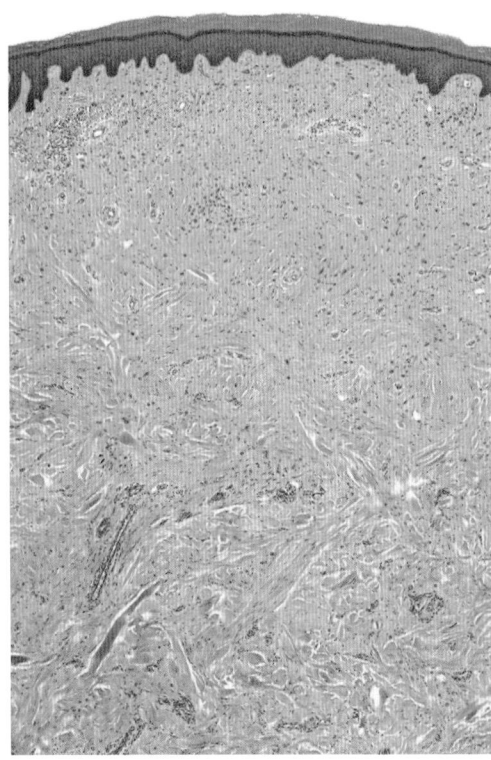

Fig. 25.140
Desmoplastic Spitz nevus: this field shows the full extent of the lesion. There is clear maturation with depth.

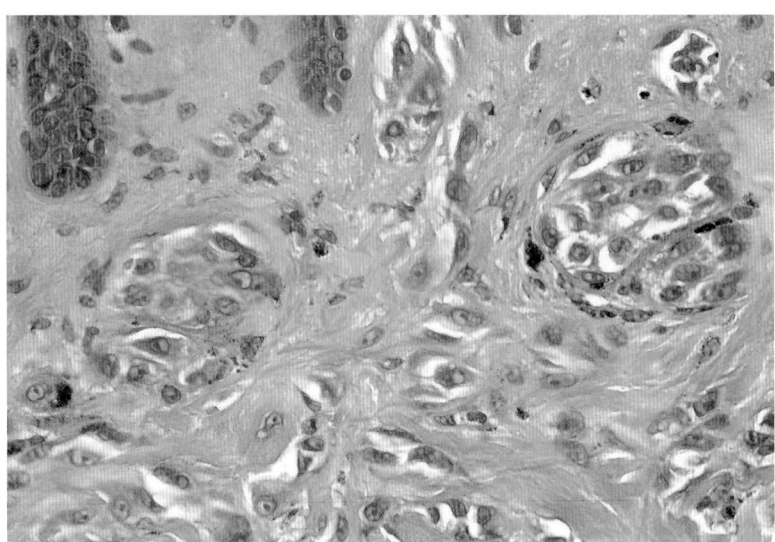

Fig. 25.142
Desmoplastic Spitz nevus: in some examples, the superficial dermal component shows obvious residual, more conventional spitzoid features.

with depth (*Fig. 25.145*). Spindled cell, round, and epithelioid forms may all be present (*Figs 25.146* and *25.147*). Melanin pigment is sometimes seen, but is usually sparse. Mitoses are very infrequent or absent. Occasionally, giant cells with a peripheral 'wreath-like' distribution of nuclei are seen.[1] The stroma is characteristically extremely dense and often isolates individual nevus cells (*Fig. 25.148*). Occasionally, there is striking hyalinization – so-called hyalinizing spindle and epithelioid cell nevus.[7,8]

Junctional activity is sometimes present, but is usually sparse and there is never significant intraepidermal or pagetoid spread. Residual well-formed dermal nests of nevus cells are not often a feature although they may be present in some lesions. Rarely, the nevus may be accompanied by conspicuous vasculature extending throughout the lesion – the so-called angiomatoid Spitz nevus.[9–11] The pathogenesis of the desmoplasia is unknown.

A minority of desmoplastic nevi can feature prominent inflammatory cell aggregates in the mid- or deep dermis composed of lymphocytes and rare plasma cells,[6] usually at the periphery of desmoplastic proliferation.[6]

Differential diagnosis

Desmoplastic Spitz nevus is commonly confused with epithelioid fibrous histiocytoma. Junctional activity, melanin pigment, and intranuclear inclusions are not features of epithelioid histiocytoma. In addition, although fibrosis is common, it does not show the extreme degree with often widespread separation of individual tumor cells characteristic of desmoplastic nevus. Desmoplastic nevi are S100 and often HMB-45 positive (*Fig. 25.149*). Epithelioid

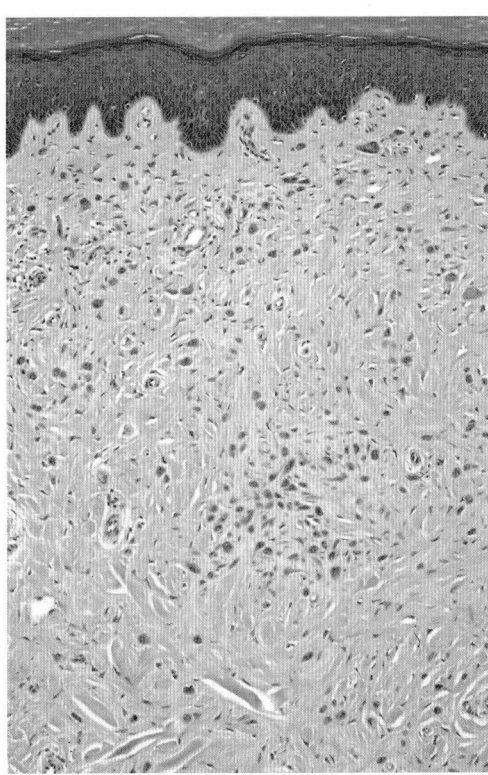

Fig. 25.143
Desmoplastic Spitz nevus: in this more characteristic lesion, the nevus cells are large and have abundant eosinophilic cytoplasm with associated desmoplastic stroma.

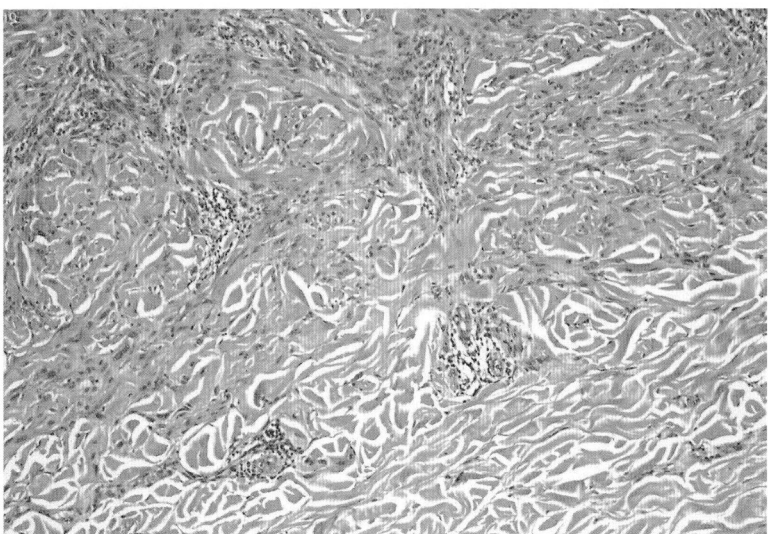

Fig. 25.145
Desmoplastic Spitz nevus: towards the deeper reaches, there is evidence of maturation, as seen by the greatly diminished cell size.

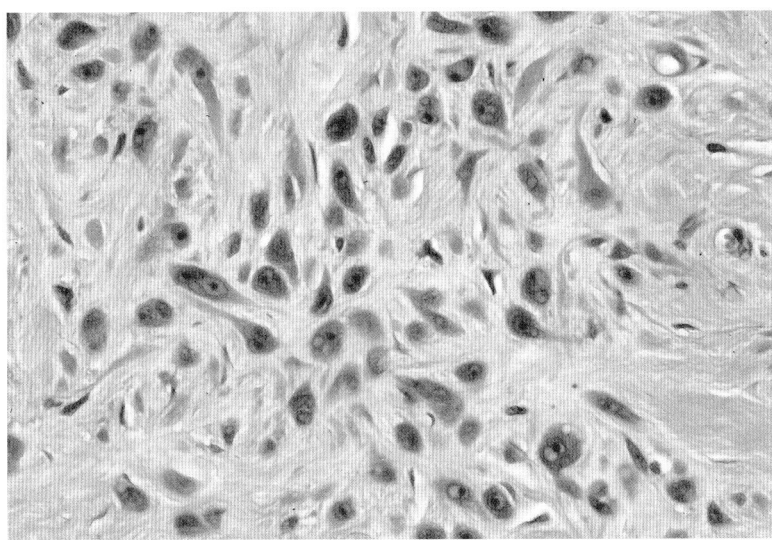

Fig. 25.144
Desmoplastic Spitz nevus: nuclei are vesicular. Cytoplasmic intranuclear pseudoinclusions are prominent.

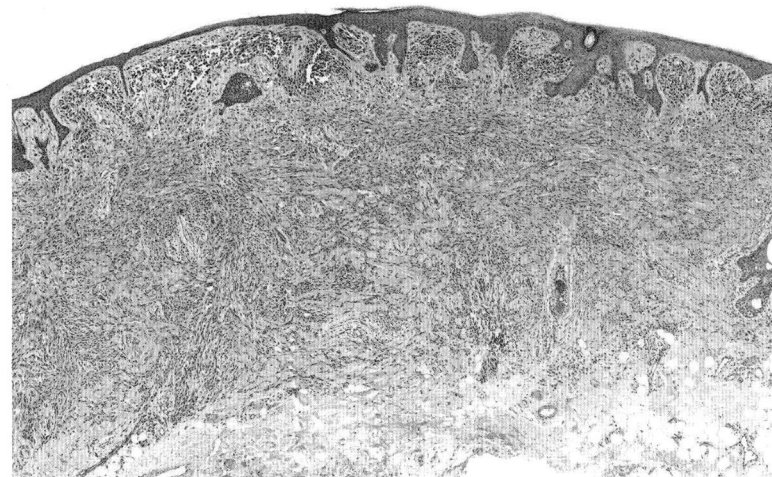

Fig. 25.146
Desmoplastic nevus: low-power view of a spindled cell variant. In this example, the lesion involves the full thickness of the dermis.

fibrous histiocytoma expresses often positive for ALK-1, and may be focally positive for EMA and smooth muscle actin.

Desmoplastic nevus must also be distinguished from desmoplastic melanoma.[12] The latter may show an in situ component (nevertheless, in situ component is absent in about 20–30% of desmoplastic melanomas)[6] and is characterized by spindled cells usually distributed in variably sized fascicles and characterized by nuclear basophilia and hyperchromatism. Furthermore, in contrast to desmoplastic nevus, desmoplastic melanoma is usually asymmetrical and frequently extends infiltratively into subcutis.[6] Mitotic activity, perineural infiltration, and lymphoid aggregates are also discriminating features and helpful features (see desmoplastic melanoma); however, all of these features can also be found in desmoplastic nevus.

p16 immunohistochemistry can be used as an ancillary method for separating desmoplastic melanoma from desmoplastic nevus. While the majority of desmoplastic melanomas lack or show only weak staining for p16, desmoplastic Spitz nevus consistently displays moderate to strong positivity for this marker.[13] Furthermore, p75 immunohistochemistry is usually strongly positive in the majority of desmoplastic melanomas and absent or weak in about 50% of desmoplastic nevi.[5]

Pigmented spindle cell tumor of Reed

Pigmented spindle cell tumor of Reed is not uncommon and probably represents a variant of Spitz nevus.[1] It is particularly important because it may easily be mistaken for melanoma, both clinically and histologically.[2–6]

Clinical features

The tumor presents as a dark brown or black macular or papular, often dome-shaped, lesion (Figs 25.150 and 25.151).[3,6] It is most often seen in the first four decades and shows a female preponderance (2:1).[1] The lower limbs, upper limbs, trunk, head, and neck are affected in decreasing order of frequency.[2] It is usually small (less than 1.0 cm in diameter),

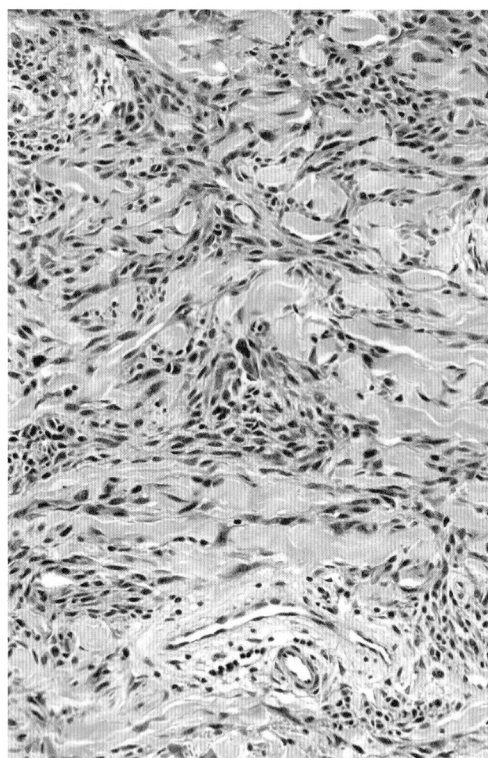

Fig. 25.147
Desmoplastic nevus: the spindled cells are uniform and devoid of significant cytological atypia. Mitoses are absent.

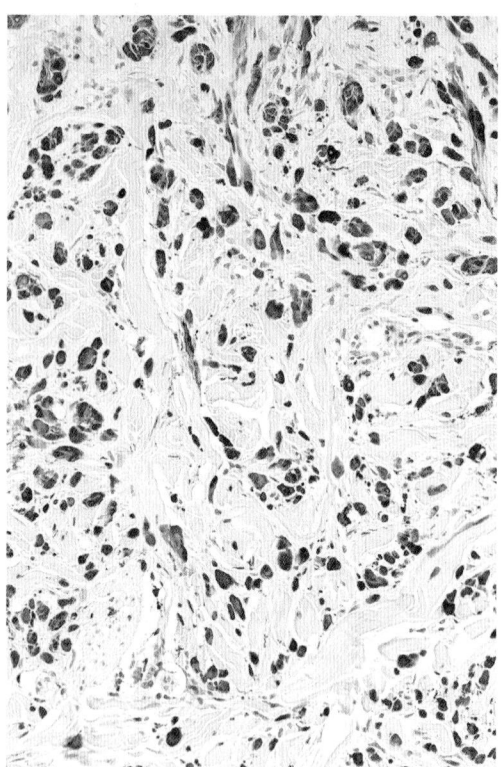

Fig. 25.149
Desmoplastic nevus: S100 protein immunohistochemistry may be helpful in cases where the diagnosis is in doubt.

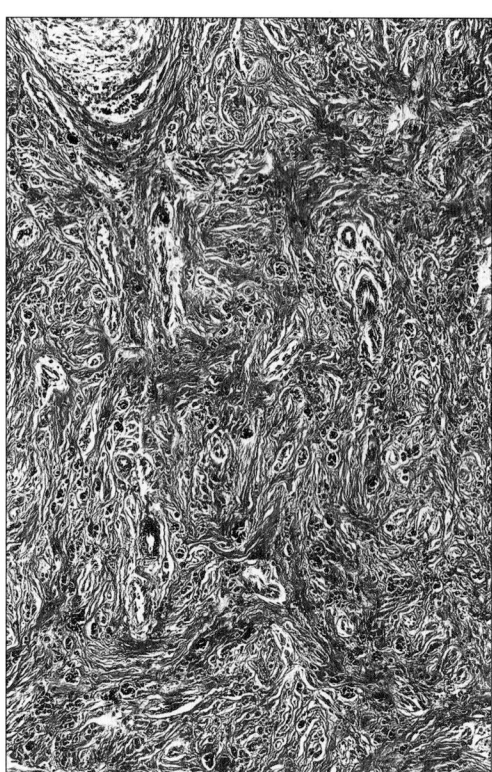

Fig. 25.148
Desmoplastic nevus: the collagenous stroma is highlighted by the Masson trichrome stain.

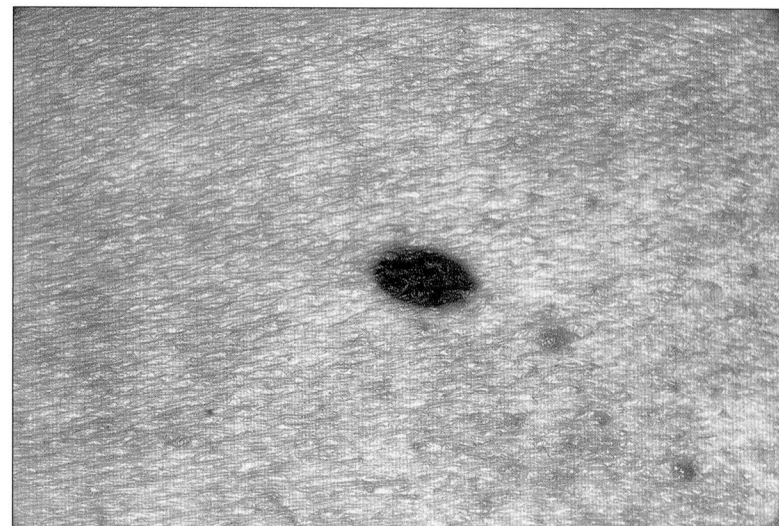

Fig. 25.150
Pigmented spindle cell tumor of Reed: this heavily pigmented lesion may be clinically mistaken for melanoma. Clues to the diagnosis include the sharp border and uniform pigmentation. By courtesy of the Institute of Dermatology, London, UK.

Histologic features

Recently, it has been demonstrated that the lesion is the result of genomic fusions and the most commonly involved aberration consist of an NTRK3 fusion.[8]

This lesion may be junctional or compound, involving the papillary dermis, but is never solely dermal in location (*Figs 25.152* and *25.153*). It is highly symmetrical and typically sharply demarcated at its lateral and deep borders.[2] The depth of dermal involvement is often strikingly uniform, and the lower border therefore appears parallel to the surface epithelium (*Fig. 25.154*). Hyperkeratosis is frequently present, and the epidermis is acanthotic with hyperplasia and elongation of the ridges. The junctional nests have a characteristic pear-shaped configuration and are composed predominantly

characteristically smooth surfaced, and sharply demarcated from the surrounding normal skin. Ulceration is not a feature.

On dermoscopy, early Reed nevus is characterized by a globular pattern, progressing to a typical starburst pattern consisting of structureless center with circumferential radial lines or pseudopods, eventually developing into a reticular pattern in late stage lesions.[7]

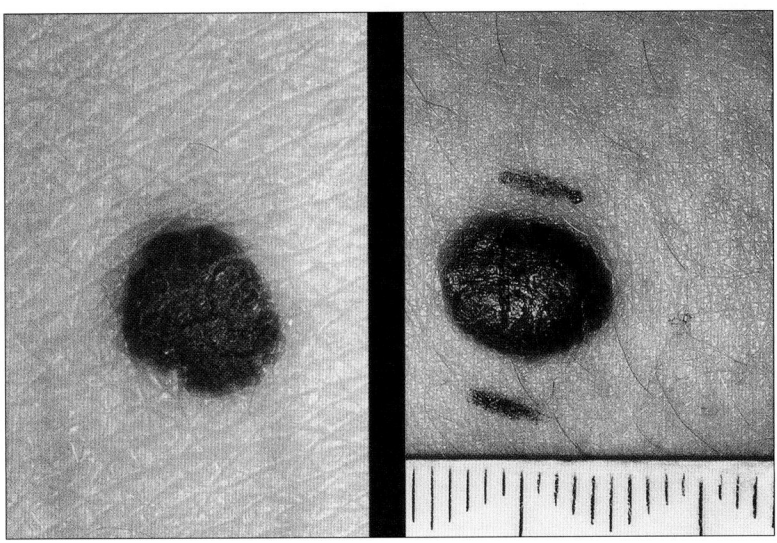

Fig. 25.151
Pigmented spindle cell tumor of Reed: these lesions most often present as small, darkly pigmented circumscribed macules or papules. The thigh is a characteristic site and females are affected more often than males. By courtesy of the late N.P. Smith, MD, St John's Dermatology Centre, St Thomas' Hospital, London, UK.

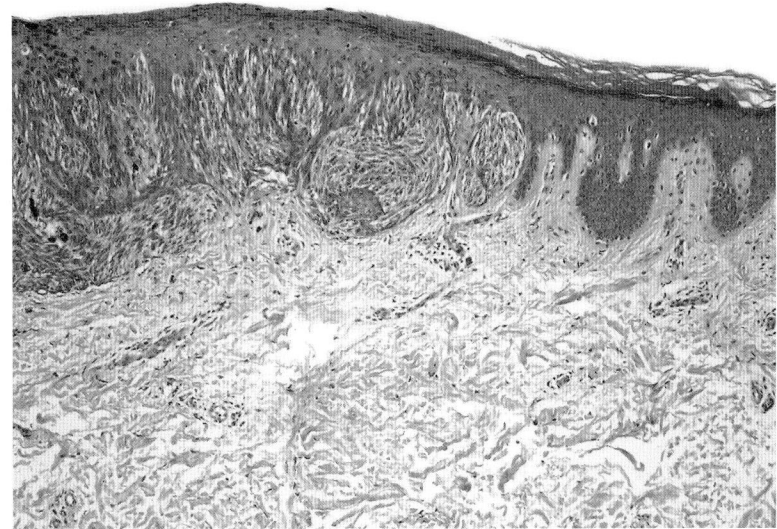

Fig. 25.153
Pigmented spindle cell tumor of Reed: the lower border is sharply defined. Pigmentation is very marked and is present in the stratum corneum. Dermal melanophages are conspicuous.

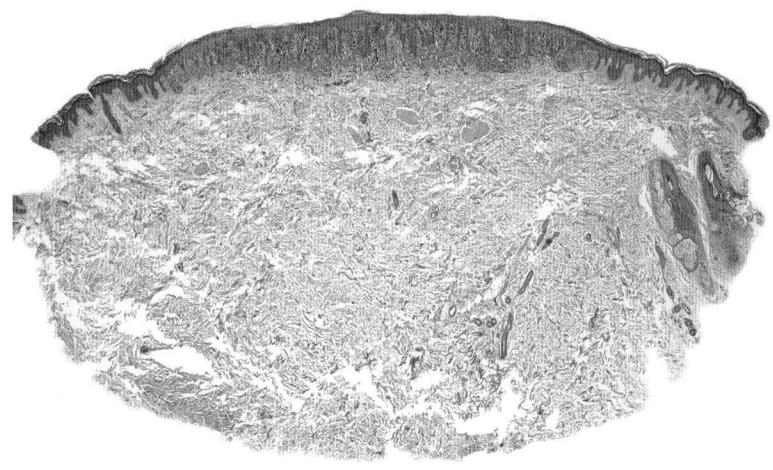

Fig. 25.152
Pigmented spindle cell tumor of Reed: this is a junctional variant. Note the very distinct horizontal lower border. The nevus begins and ends with a nest. Melanophages are conspicuous.

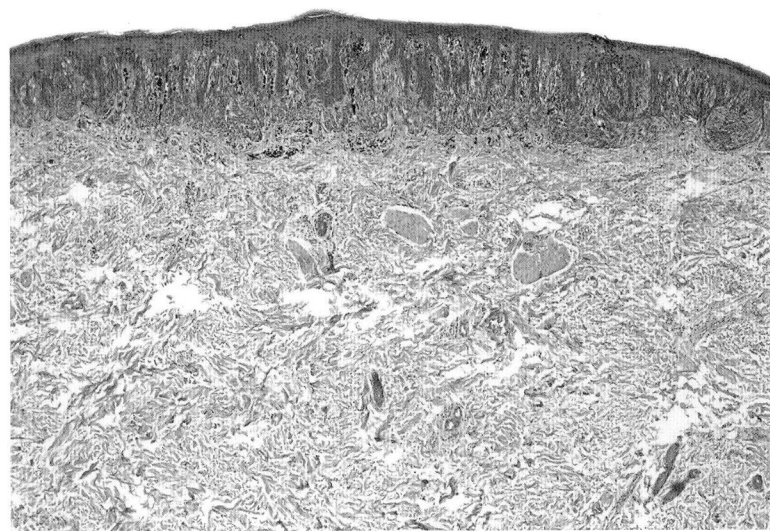

Fig. 25.154
Pigmented spindle cell tumor of Reed: the lateral border is sharply demarcated and the lower border appears parallel to the epidermis.

of clusters of plump spindled cells with oval or elongated vesicular nuclei, which often contain small nucleoli (*Figs 25.155* and *25.156*). Pleomorphism is usually not marked. Epithelioid cells are sometimes evident, and the very occasional presence of giant cells may result in overlap with Spitz nevus. Pigmentation is typically conspicuous and presents as fine cytoplasmic granules. Upward epidermal migration (pagetoid spread) into the lower epidermis in continuity with junctional nests may occasionally be seen.[1] In some lesions, involvement of the adnexa is a feature.[2] Compound lesions are as a rule very superficial and may show maturation (a decrease in cell size and quantity of cytoplasm) with depth. Mitoses are not uncommon, but when present are found within the lower aspect of the junctional nests and usually in small numbers (*Fig. 25.157*). A not infrequent finding is the presence of scattered eosinophilic hyaline globules (Kamino bodies).[8] Occasionally, a perivascular lymphocytic infiltrate is present. Dermal melanophages are often conspicuous.

Not infrequently, pigmented spindle cell tumors show atypical features, which may heighten confusion with melanoma. The presence of mild nuclear atypia (pleomorphism and prominent nucleoli), increased numbers of (invariably normal) mitotic figures, and focal pagetoid spread may be a source of alarm. Similarly, focal lentiginous hyperplasia at the lateral border

is occasionally present. The overall symmetry, relative uniformity of the infiltrate, and evidence of maturation with depth, however, strongly point towards a benign rather than a malignant process.[9]

Very occasionally, hypopigmented or amelanotic variants are encountered overlapping with Spitz nevus (*Figs 25.158–25.160*).[10]

Differential diagnosis

Many dysplastic nevi show spindled cell nests, which cause confusion with spindle cell nevus. The presence of architectural disorder and cytological atypia elsewhere in the specimen should make the distinction easy in the majority of cases (see dysplastic nevus).

Deep penetrating nevus

Deep penetrating nevus is a distinctive melanocytic nevus initially described by Seab et al. in 1989.[1] A plexiform spindle cell nevus subsequently reported by Barnhill et al. has essentially the same histologic characteristics.[2,3] Although the term 'deep penetrating nevus' implies extension into the deep dermis or subcutis, it is rather the combination of growth and cell morphology that define the entity. A superficial variant of the deep penetrating nevus, designated as melanocytic nevus with focal epithelioid component (clonal nevus), was reported in 1994.[4] This variant shares similar age,

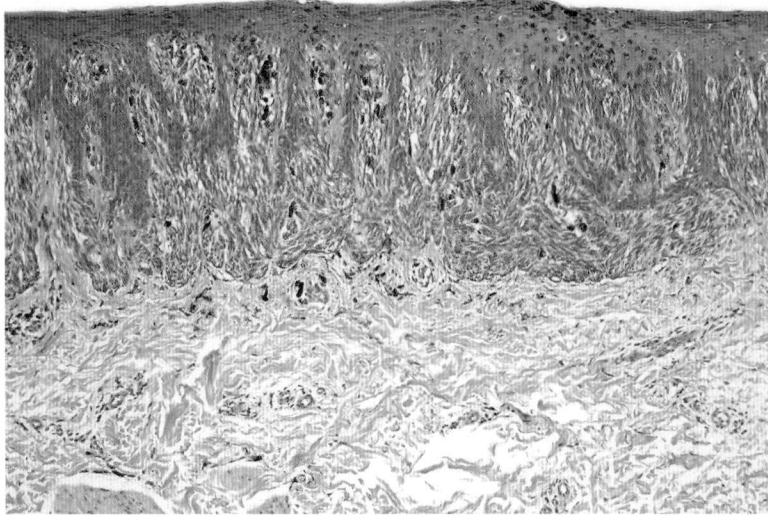

Fig. 25.155
Pigmented spindle cell tumor of Reed: the dermal papillae are distended by junctional nests of spindle cells. The presence of occasional nevus cells in the upper epidermis, particularly in the center of the lesion, is not uncommon and when taken in the context of the overall appearances of the lesion should not be a source of alarm..

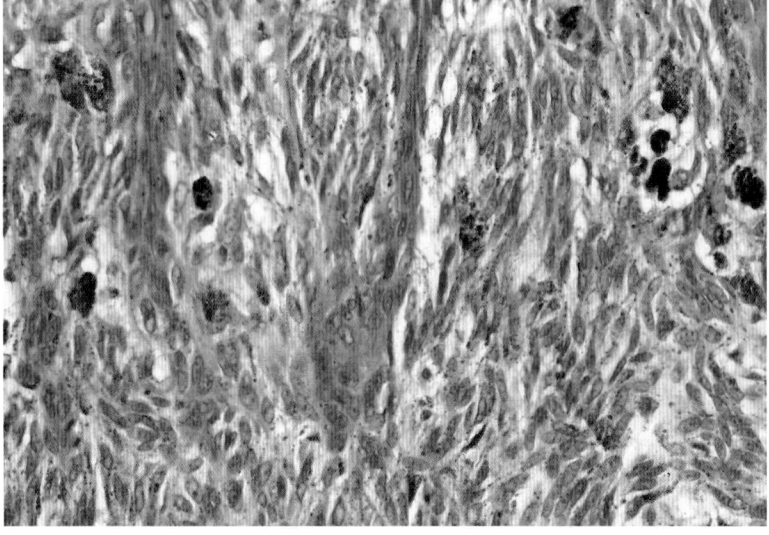

Fig. 25.156
Pigmented spindle cell tumor of Reed: the nevus cells have tapered vesicular nuclei with small nucleoli. Note the lack of pleomorphism. Heavily pigmented melanophages are also evident.

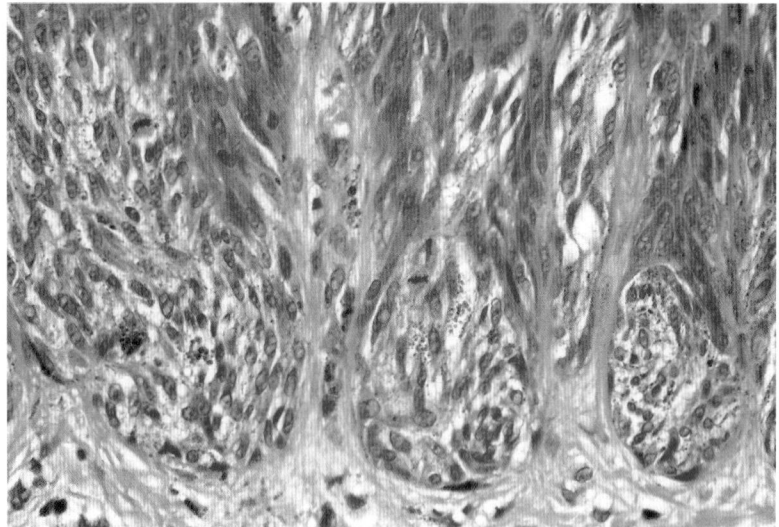

Fig. 25.157
Pigmented spindle cell tumor of Reed: junctional mitotic figures, as seen in this field, are not uncommon and should not necessarily be a source of concern unless numerous or atypical.

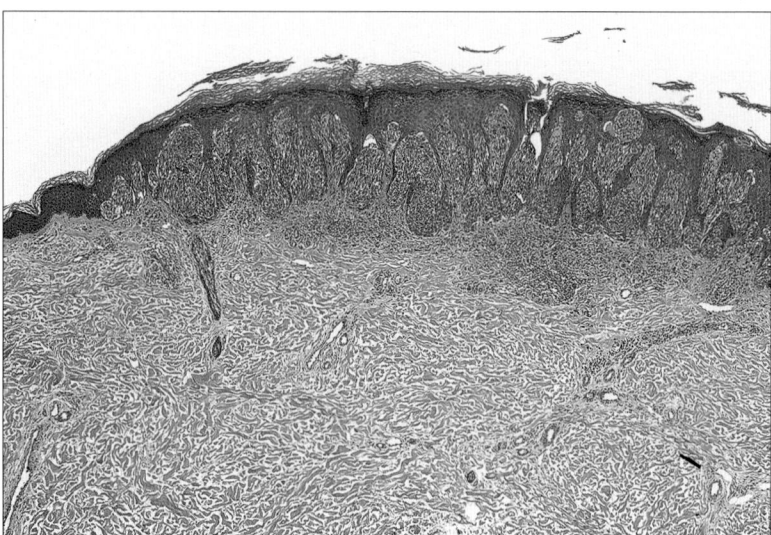

Fig. 25.158
Spindle cell tumor of Reed: low-power view of an amelanotic example. There is obvious overlap with Spitz nevus.

anatomic distribution, and cytological features with deep penetrating nevus, but lacks deep extension of melanocytes.[5]

Deep penetrating nevus is difficult to categorize. While in some cases it appears to represent an entity sui generis, in other instances it represents a variant of combined nevus. The presence of dendritic cells in a significant number of cases suggests that many examples might be better classified within the blue nevus spectrum.

Clinical features

Deep penetrating nevus is uncommon and of particular importance because it may be clinically and histologically mistaken for a melanoma. The age at presentation is quite broad (0–77 years), but less than 5% of deep penetrating nevi have been reported beyond the age of 50 years.[1,2,5–10] Patients are most often in their second or third decade and present with a solitary, circumscribed, usually less than 1 cm diameter, dome-shaped, blue or black papule or nodule.[1,2,5–9,11,12] Pigmentation can be variegated, from light brown to black, but most lesions are darkly pigmented. Especially if part of a combined melanocytic nevus, the lesion may appear asymmetrical and unevenly pigmented, thus raising clinical suspicion of melanoma. The face, upper trunk, or proximal extremities are particularly affected (Fig. 25.161).[1,2,5–9,11,12] A single case of a deep penetrating nevus has recently been reported on the sole of the foot.[13] A unique case of linear distribution of multiple deep penetrating nevi in the preauricular skin has also been published.[14] Deep penetrating nevus shows a slight female predominance (1.3:1).[1,2,5–9]

Histologic features

A distinctive morphological feature of deep penetrating nevus at scanning magnification is its symmetrical, wedge-shaped, and sharply circumscribed configuration with the broad base uppermost, parallel to the surface epithelium (Fig. 25.162).[1,9] The deep tapered component typically extends into the lower reticular dermis or even the subcutaneous fat.[6,12] One or more such extensions along the skin adnexa or neurovascular bundles are frequently seen.

A junctional component is present in 60% to 85% of deep penetrating nevi, usually limited to a few small nests.[1,2,5–8] Upward extension of melanocytes and pagetoid spread are not features of this lesion. In between one-third to two-thirds of cases, however, deep penetrating nevus presents as a combined lesion with banal or Spitz features as the superficial

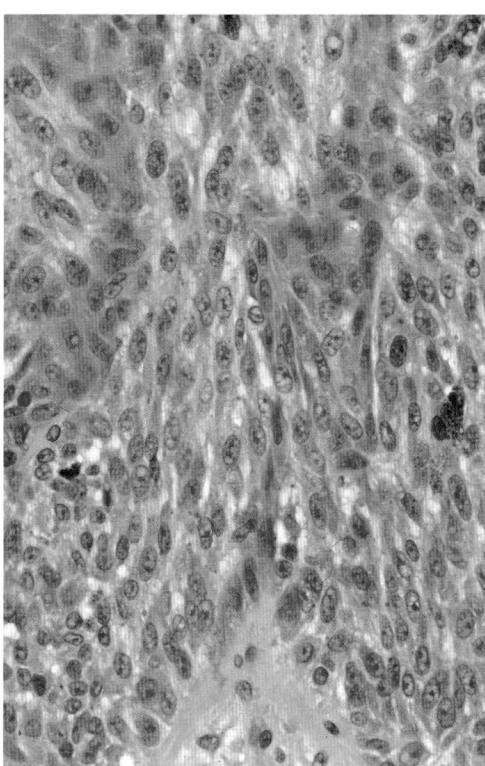

Fig. 25.159
Spindle cell tumor of Reed: careful search usually reveals small foci of melanin pigment. The nuclei are very uniform.

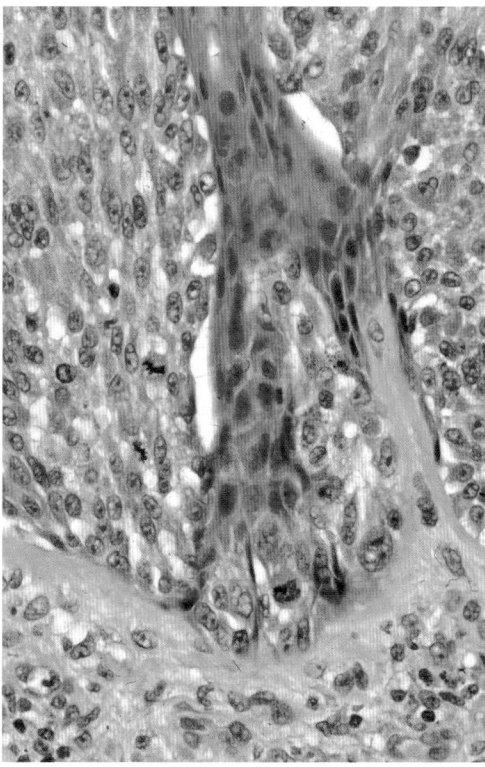

Fig. 25.160
Spindle cell tumor of Reed: note the mitotic figures.

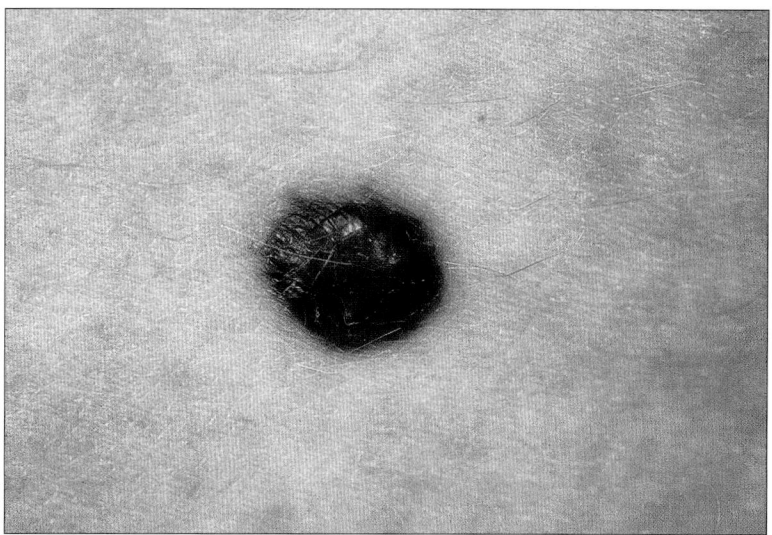

Fig. 25.161
Deep penetrating nevus: the nevus is intensely pigmented and sharply circumscribed. By courtesy of the Institute of Dermatology, London, UK.

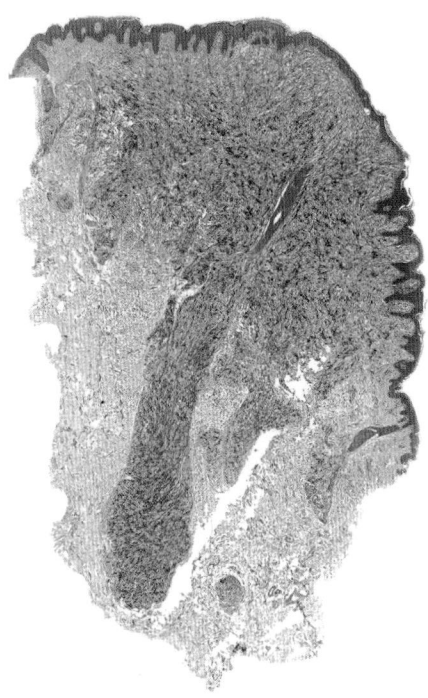

Fig. 25.162
Deep penetrating nevus: the nevus is wedge shaped with the broad base uppermost and a deeply penetrating lower border.

component (*Figs 25.163* and *25.164*).[15] The papillary dermis is frequently uninvolved, especially in lesions that have an exclusive deep penetrating nevus component. The dermal component is typically sharply delineated and follows neurovascular bundles and adnexal structures, often presenting a fascicular or plexiform outline (*Fig. 25.165*), hence its alternative designation, plexiform spindle cell nevus.[2,6] The dermal melanocytic component consists of loose nests and vertically oriented fascicles of epithelioid- and spindled-shaped melanocytes. Epithelioid melanocytes are more frequent in the more superficial parts of the lesion, and foci of clear cells are often present (*Figs 25.166* and *25.167*). Spindled cell melanocytes generally predominate toward the deeper reaches (*Fig. 25.168*). A confluence of nests may be seen, especially in the upper dermis and central areas of the lesion, but this is generally a focal phenomenon. Discohesion of melanocytes can be present at the periphery and base of the lesion. Perineural extension and infiltration of arrector pili muscle are common. No obvious maturation of melanocytes is seen. Mild nuclear pleomorphism is frequent, and nuclear hyperchromatism may be a feature. Moderate nuclear pleomorphism can also be evident, but is usually focal and random. This is not usually associated with an increase in mitotic activity. Variation in the size of the nuclei can be present within individual melanocytic nests or bundles. Nucleoli are small- to medium-sized and eosinophilic. However, mitoses are either very sparse or, more often, absent (*Fig. 25.169*). The number of mitosis ranges

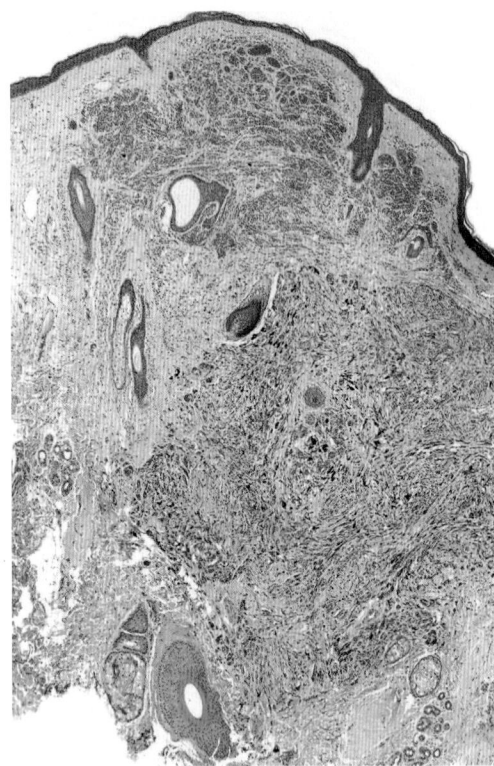

Fig. 25.163
Deep penetrating nevus: this example is a combined variant with a banal dermal component overlying the deep penetrating nevus.

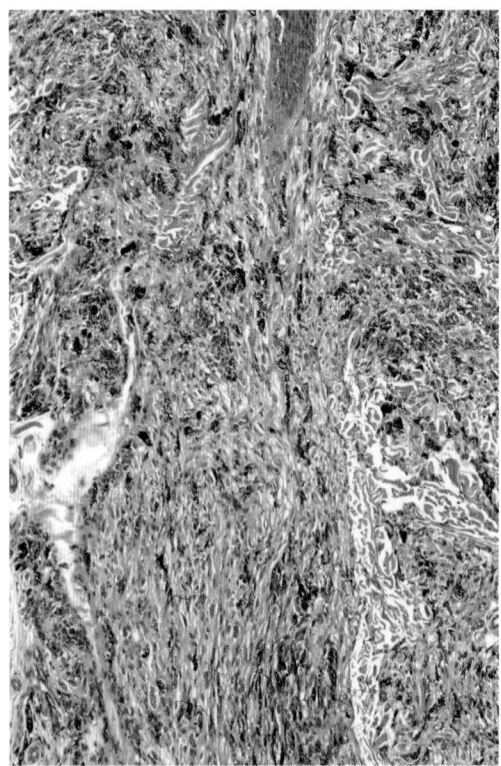

Fig. 25.165
Deep penetrating nevus: the deep extension typically follows the hair follicles and neurovascular bundles.

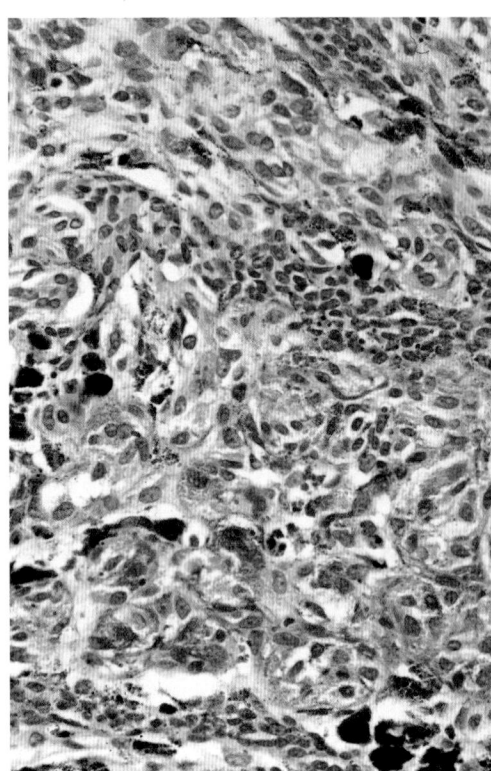

Fig. 25.164
Deep penetrating nevus: high-power view of *Fig. 25.163*.

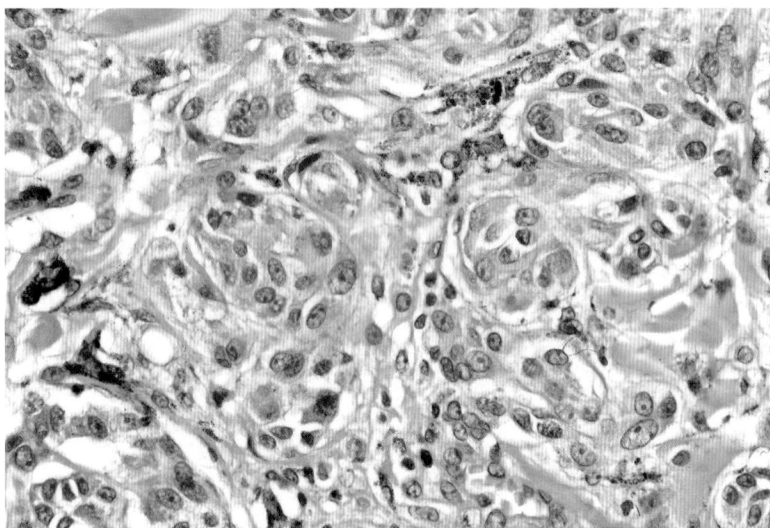

Fig. 25.166
Deep penetrating nevus: superficially, the nevus consists of epithelioid melanocytes with pale-staining or finely pigmented cytoplasm and vesicular nuclei, often with small eosinophilic nucleoli.

accompanies the nevus. There is usually minimal stromal reaction. Melanophages are a constant finding in deep penetrating nevi. They can be sparse and focal or abundant and dispersed throughout the lesion. They usually surround individual nests and bundles of melanocytes and can be especially prominent at the periphery of the lesion.

The melanocytes are consistently S100 and HMB-45 positive.[12] Proliferating cell nuclear antigen (PCNA) is typically expressed by less than 5% of cells.[12] While *HRAS* mutations have been detected in 2 of 32 deep penetrating nevi, none of them demonstrated *GNAQ* or *GNA11* mutations (commonly observed in blue nevi), suggesting possible relationship with spitzoid melanocytic proliferations.[16]

It has recently been demonstrated that the lesions are caused by combined activation of MAP-kinase pathway and beta catenin signaling and expression of B-catenin is retained throughout the tumor.[17]

from 0 to 1.2/mm².[6,8] The presence of more than an occasional mitosis is a worrying feature, however, and should raise suspicion on either atypical deep penetrating nevus (see below) or melanoma with features of deep penetrating nevus. Atypical mitoses are not found in deep penetrating nevus. Intranuclear pseudoinclusions are frequently seen. The cytoplasm of melanocytes is pale pink to amphophilic. Occasional dendritic melanocytes are frequently present. A variable reactive chronic inflammatory cell infiltrate

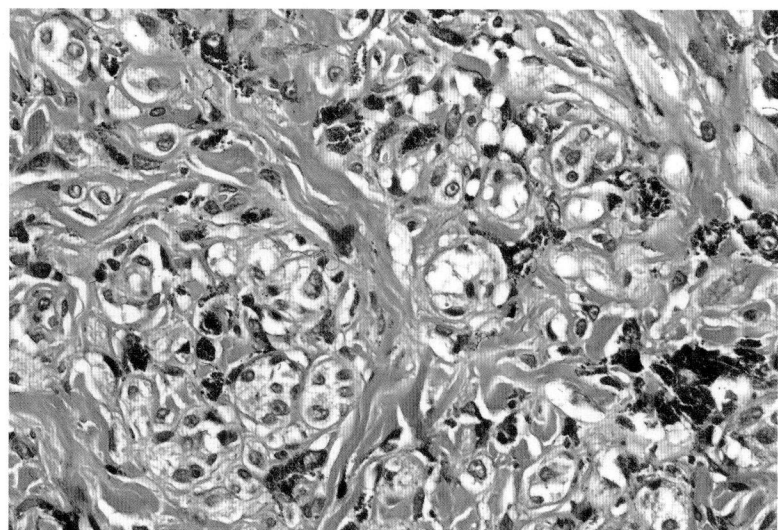

Fig. 25.167
Deep penetrating nevus: clear cells are commonly present.

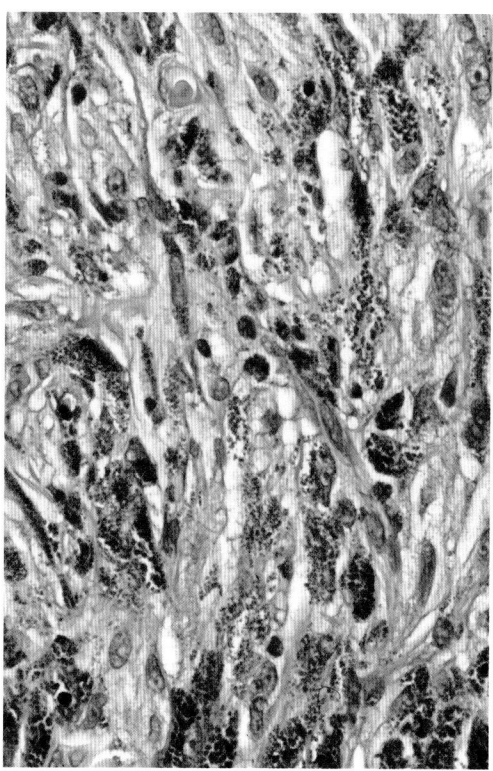

Fig. 25.169
Deep penetrating nevus: very occasional mitoses may be found but they are never numerous or abnormal.

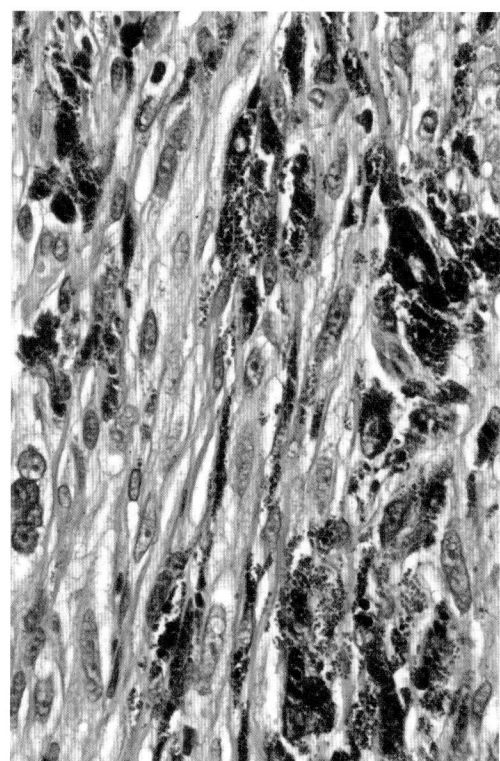

Fig. 25.168
Deep penetrating nevus: in the deeper reaches, spindled cell forms predominate and heavily pigmented melanophages are often conspicuous.

Deep penetrating nevus is a benign melanocytic proliferation. Local recurrences are most uncommon and are usually associated with incomplete or marginal excision.[5,8,12]

Differential diagnosis

The main differential diagnosis includes melanoma, which may rarely present with a deep penetrating growth pattern. Points of distinction include absence of atypical junctional melanocytic component, non-random cytological atypia of dermal melanocytes, more severe pleomorphism, nucleolar prominence, excessive mitoses (including abnormal forms), and impaired maturation (*Figs 25.170–25.173*).

A concept of atypical (or high grade) deep penetrating nevus has been proposed for proliferations fulfilling one or more of the following histologic features: lesional diameter greater than 5 mm, asymmetry, poor circumscription, involvement of subcutis, increased cellularity, nodular or

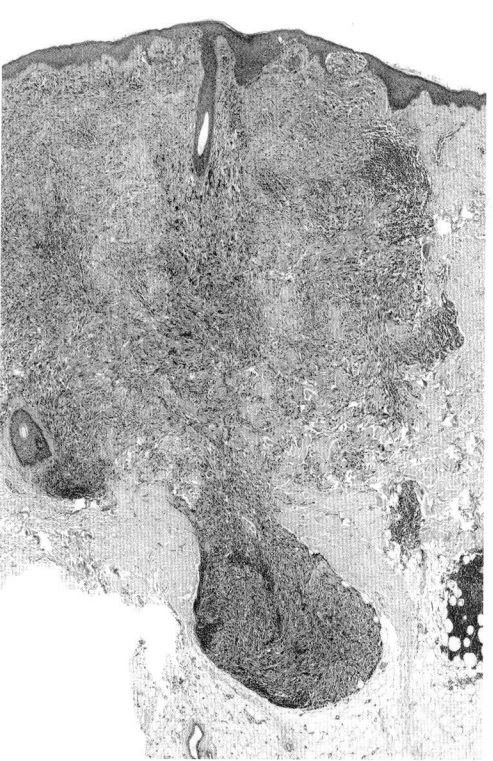

Fig. 25.170
Melanoma with deep penetrating growth pattern: at low-power magnification, this lesion shows a deep penetrating growth pattern.

sheetlike growth, moderate to severe cytological atypia, and mitotic activity greater than 2/mm².[18] Limited available data on atypical deep penetrating nevi suggest possible development of lymph-node deposits in a subset of the lesions, yet the outcome may not be unfavorable, drawing the parallels with the so-called atypical Spitz tumors.[18–20] Furthermore, atypical deep

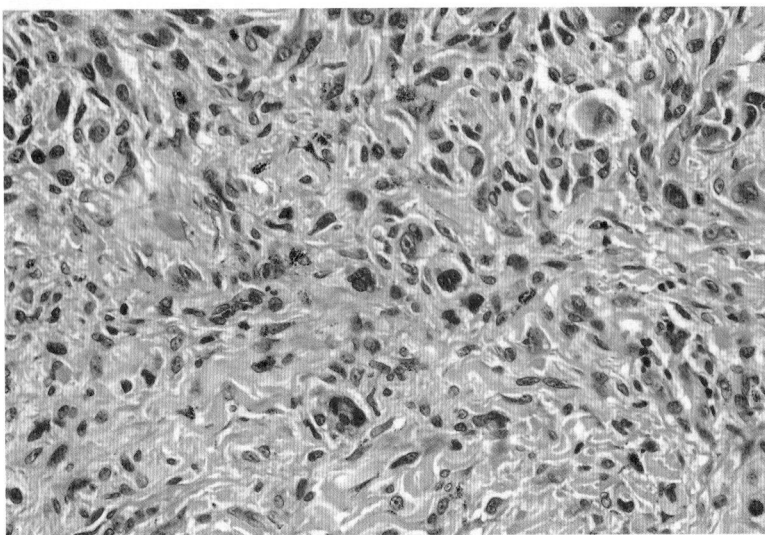

Fig. 25.171
Melanoma with deep penetrating growth pattern: at high-power magnification, however, there is marked nuclear pleomorphism and hyperchromatism.

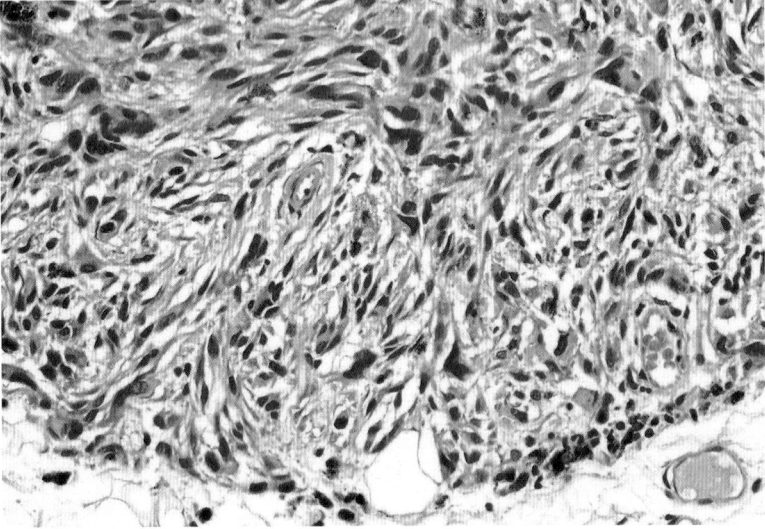

Fig. 25.172
Melanoma with deep penetrating growth pattern: there is no evidence of maturation.

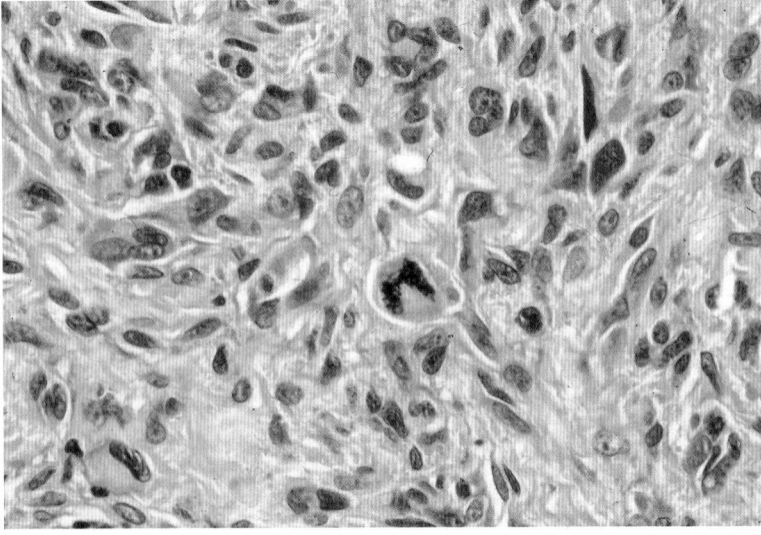

Fig. 25.173
Melanoma with deep penetrating growth pattern: mitoses including abnormal forms were present at all levels of the lesion.

penetrating nevi generally lack copy number aberrations typical of melanoma by either FISH or CGH.[19,20]

Benign melanocytic lesions that should be distinguished from deep penetrating nevus include common and cellular blue nevi.[21] While common blue nevi consist of pigmented spindled-shaped and dendritic melanocytes within a sclerotic stroma, cellular blue nevi are composed of nests and fascicles of poorly pigmented melanocytes with ovoid nuclei, inconspicuous nucleoli, and clear cytoplasm.

Dysplastic nevus syndrome and dysplastic nevi

Dysplastic nevus syndrome (familial atypical multiple mole melanoma [FAMMM] syndrome) and dysplastic nevi have been the source of considerable controversy since their original descriptions.[1,2] Debate has been particularly focused on nomenclature, defining histologic criteria and their reproducibility.[3–8] Numerous publications have documented varying degrees of interobserver reliability, ranging from poor when non-specialist pathologists review series of nevi to excellent when experts performed similar studies.[9–19] Nevertheless, criteria by which such nevi can be recognized clinically and diagnosed histologically in the majority of cases are now well established in the literature.

It is important, however, to note that not all clinically atypical nevi are dysplastic. Thus flexural and acral nevi, for example, may be clinically and histologically atypical and of concern to both the dermatologist and the pathologist but, as defined below, they are not dysplastic. Recurrent nevi may also be disturbing to the clinician but should be readily recognized by the pathologist as of little consequence. Equally well, histologic features of dysplasia may be occasionally found in clinically 'typical' banal nevi and the reverse is also sometimes true, although to some extent this may be a reflection of clinical inexperience and lack of clinicopathological correlation.

The importance of the dysplastic nevus syndrome is that it identifies an at-risk population group for the subsequent development of melanoma.[20–23] Although originally described as a familial condition, sporadic cases and isolated solitary lesions may also occur. The last two categories are by far the more common, with an estimated frequency of 1.8% to 17% of the population.[24] The association of dysplastic nevi and familial melanoma was originally termed the 'B-K mole syndrome' from the initials of two of the families in the original series.[1] It was also reported as FAMMM syndrome.[2] Numerous synonyms have since been recommended, of which 'dysplastic nevus syndrome' has gained most support. The syndrome consists essentially of a tendency for the affected individual to develop large numbers of clinically atypical nevi, which histologically show dysplastic features and are associated with an increased incidence of melanoma. The histologic finding of dysplastic nevi adjacent to invasive tumor in as many as 36% of melanomas supports the hypothesis that these lesions may progress to melanoma, at least in patients with the familial variants.[25] Similarly, a meta-analysis of sporadic dysplastic nevi has demonstrated a relative risk of 10.49 for melanoma developing in the presence of five dysplastic nevi.[26] An even higher relative risk for melanoma development of 46.1 in patients with five or more atypical nevi was detected in a recent Dutch cohort of sporadic atypical nevi patients. However, about 7% of these sporadic atypical nevus patients were reclassified to the familial variant during the subsequent follow-up.[27] Patients with dysplastic nevi have been subdivided into a variety of clinical categories (*Table 25.1*).[25] Patients in category D2 have a 100% incidence of melanoma.[28] Patients with dysplastic nevus syndrome have increased risk of developing other malignancies, particularly pancreatic cancer.[29–32]

Clinical features

While apparently normal at birth, affected individuals develop large numbers of morphologically normal nevi in early childhood. These become more numerous and acquire atypical clinical features at or around puberty.[33] New lesions continue to develop throughout life; numbers of lesions per patient range from a few to hundreds (*Figs 25.174* and *25.175*).[33]

Sites of predilection include the trunk, face, and arms, but covered sites, such as the buttocks, genitalia, breasts of females, and scalp, may also be affected. Local clustering of dysplastic nevi, i.e., agminated dysplastic nevus, has also been described.[34] The nevi are usually large (6 mm or more in

Table 25.1
Classification of dysplastic melanocytic nevi (DMN)

1. Hereditary melanoma
   a. Individuals with DMN phenotype* and at least one blood relative with melanoma (D_1)
   b. Individuals with DMN phenotype and at least two blood relatives with melanoma (D_2)
2. Familial DMN
   Individual with blood relatives having DMN phenotype but not melanoma
3. Personal history of melanoma
   Individuals with both DMN phenotype and personal history of melanoma
4. Sporadic DMN
   Individuals with DMN phenotype but no personal or family history of melanoma or a family history of DMN

*The minimum criteria for this phenotype have not been quantified. The classic presentation is one of increased numbers of both typical and clinically atypical nevi. Reproduced with permission from Elder, D.E. et al (1982) American Journal of Dermatopathology, 4, 455–460.

diameter) and irregularly shaped, frequently with an uneven or ill-defined border (*Figs 25.176* and *25.177*). Coloration is variable, often showing a mixture of pale and dark brown, and pink. Dysplastic nevi are sometimes surrounded by an erythematous macule (the shoulder phenomenon). The skin creases are frequently unaffected.

Clinically, these nevi tend to show marked variability both within and between patients. Although the lesions are generally macular, central nodules may develop, raising the possibility of malignancy. As patients with this syndrome, particularly those with a family history of melanoma, have an increased risk of developing melanoma, careful and frequent clinical follow-up examinations with photographic records are mandatory (*Figs 25.178* and *25.179*).[35] Features suggestive of malignant transformation include the acquisition of contour asymmetry, excessive pigment variegation, and the development of black foci or the presence of a gray coloration suggestive of regression. The malignancies occur at a somewhat younger age than usual (mid-thirties), are sometimes multiple, and are usually located on the trunk. All relatives of patients with the dysplastic nevus syndrome should be carefully examined, because at least 50% will be found to have evidence of clinical involvement.

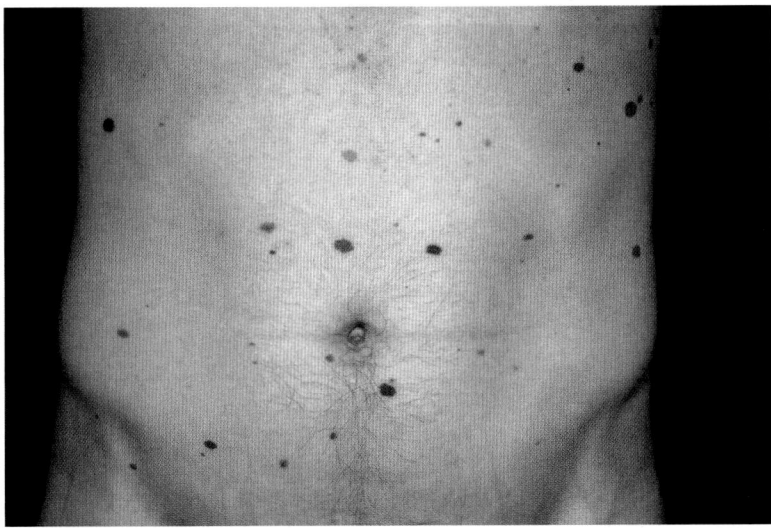

Fig. 25.174
Dysplastic nevus syndrome: numerous atypical nevi are commonly present. Note the large size and irregular borders. By courtesy of the late N.P. Smith, MD, the Institute of Dermatology, London, UK.

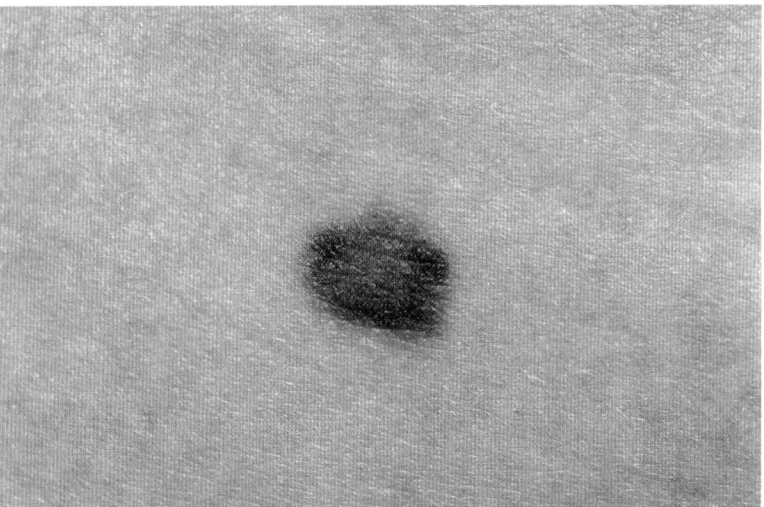

Fig. 25.176
Dysplastic nevus: nevi are often greater than 6 mm in diameter. Borders are typically irregular. From the collection of the late N.P. Smith, MD, the Institute of Dermatology, London, UK.

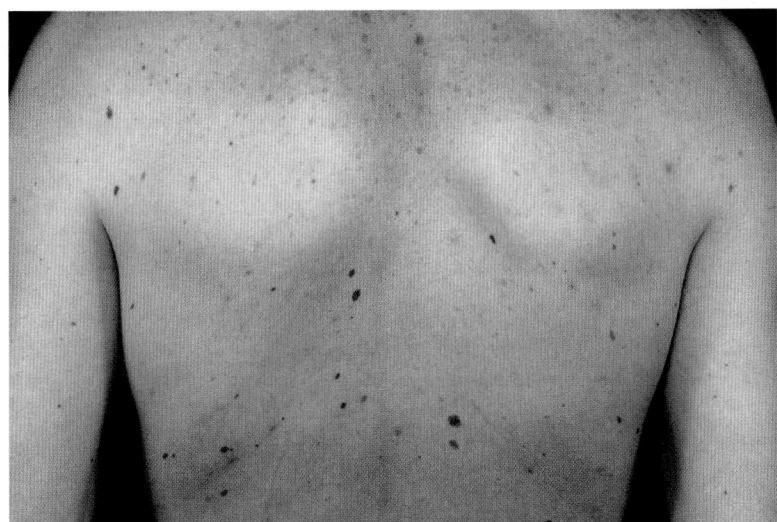

Fig. 25.175
Dysplastic nevus syndrome: the back was similarly involved. By courtesy of the late N.P. Smith, MD, the Institute of Dermatology, London, UK.

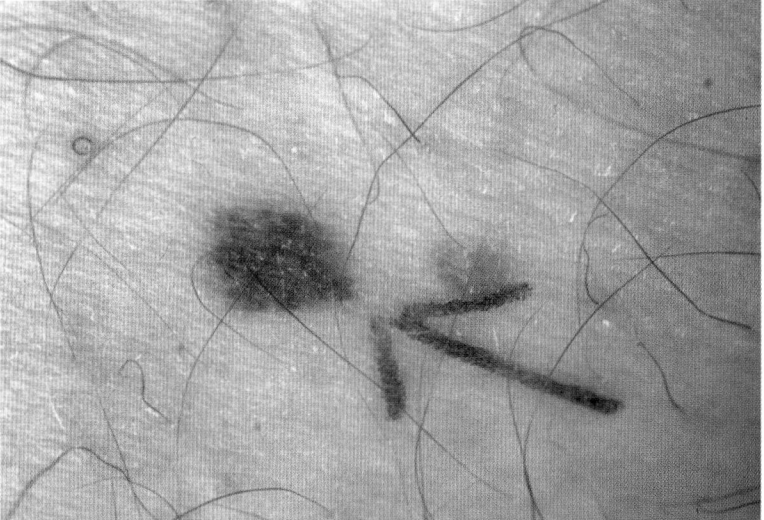

Fig. 25.177
Dysplastic nevus: there is variable pigmentation in this irregular lesion. From the collection of the late N.P. Smith, MD, the Institute of Dermatology, London, UK.

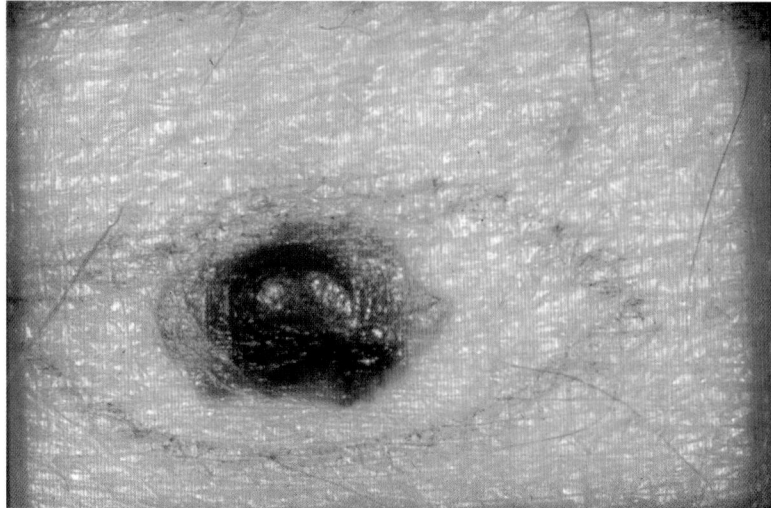

Fig. 25.178
Melanoma arising in a dysplastic nevus: note the heavily pigmented nodule. The border is highly irregular. By courtesy of J. Newton Bishop, MD, St James's University Hospital, Leeds, UK.

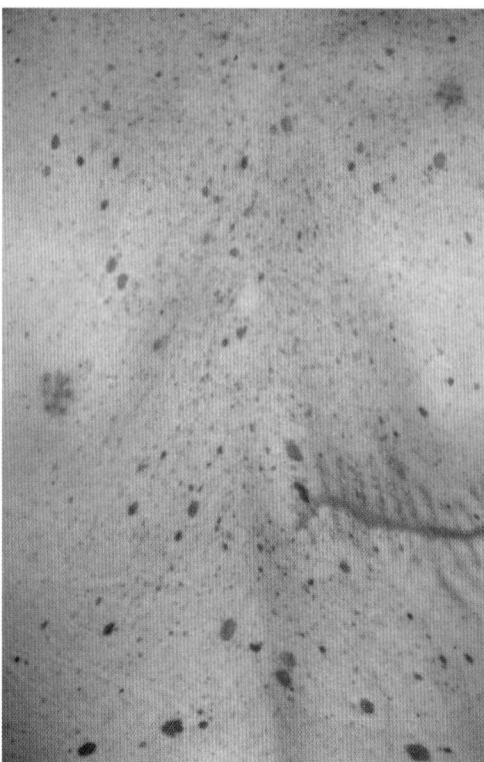

Fig. 25.179
Dysplastic nevus syndrome: there are numerous large, irregular nevi. The scar marks the site of a previously excised melanoma. By courtesy of R. Mackie, MD, University of Glasgow, UK.

A recent study demonstrated a low clinical recurrence rate of 3.6% for incompletely excised dysplastic nevi with mild to moderate dysplasia.[35] A 5-mm tumor-free margin is, however, recommended for dysplastic nevi with severe atypia.[36] Nevertheless, a recent study with a long-term follow-up (median, 11.9 years) of incompletely excised dysplastic nevi with severe atypia failed to detect any melanoma development at the site of previous procedure, suggesting that re-excision of previously completely excised dysplastic nevi with severe atypia may not be necessary.[37]

Development of clinically atypical melanocytic nevi, frequently in eruptive pattern, has been reported following chemotherapy, treatment with vemurafenib and nilotinib, administration of melanotropic peptides for tanning, but also in patients with myotonic dystrophy type I.[38–41]

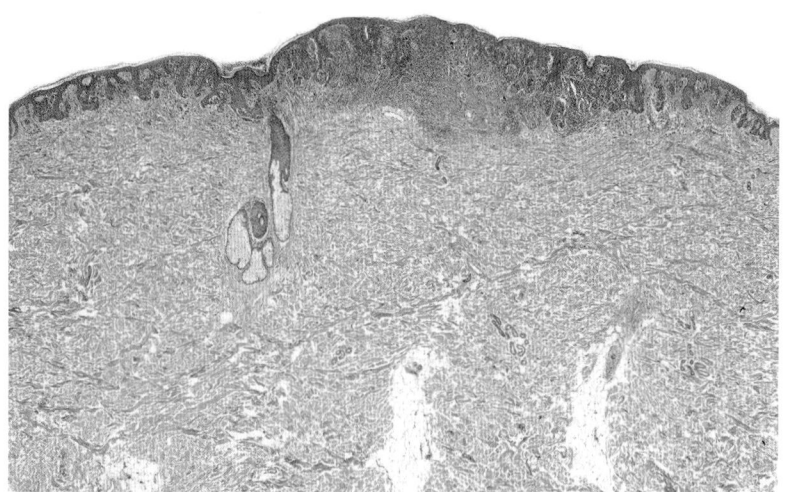

Fig. 25.180
Dysplastic nevus: compound lesion with a well-developed shoulder on either side.

Dysplastic nevus frequently reveals diverse morphological features on dermoscopy. Nevertheless, a classical example will feature a reticular pattern with thin lines, occasionally coupled with peripheral dots and clods.[42] While patterns are arranged symmetrically, color variegation can be prominent.[42] Most commonly, dysplastic nevus is characterized by central hyperpigmentation and uniform brown periphery.[42]

Pathogenesis and histologic features

Familial cutaneous melanoma (dysplastic nevus syndrome) is inherited as an autosomal dominant with incomplete penetrance. It is associated with mutations of the *CDKN2A* gene on 9p21–22 in approximately 40% of families. *CDKN2A* encodes the tumor suppresser gene products p14ARF and p16INK4a.[43–52] A novel atypical nevus susceptibility gene has recently been identified on 7q21.3, containing a candidate gene, *CDK6*.[53] Loss of heterozygosity of p16INK4a and p53 genes has been demonstrated in sporadic dysplastic nevi.[54,55] A dysplastic nevus syndrome associated with an inactivating germline *BAP1* mutation has been reported in a proband and his son.[56] Namely, in this novel kindred, the father developed multiple dysplastic nevi, *BAP*-deficient tumors, and conventional superficial spreading melanomas.[56]

Dysplastic nevi, whether familial or sporadic, show identical histologic features.[57–59] The changes can be divided into architectural, cytological, and host responses. Dysplastic nevi by definition should display melanocytic proliferative changes, the latter showing cytological atypia (dysplasia) not amounting to melanoma in situ. Some authors, however, recognize dysplastic nevi on the basis of architectural changes in the absence of cytological atypia; however, they are in the minority. Such a practice is unfortunate and should be discouraged as it blurs the distinction between banal and dysplastic nevi to such an extent that it renders the concept somewhat meaningless!

Dysplastic nevi may be junctional or compound. In compound lesions, the epidermal component frequently extends beyond the lateral border of the dermal nevus cells. This is sometimes referred to as the 'shoulder' phenomenon (*Figs 25.180* and *25.181*).

The dysplastic nevus is characterized by lentiginous hyperplasia. The epidermis – which is usually of normal thickness, although it may sometimes be slightly acanthotic – typically shows marked elongation of the rete ridges. Effacement of the rete ridges and attenuation of the epidermis overlying melanocytic proliferation, e.g., consumption of the epidermis, are features generally not seen in dysplastic nevus and suggest melanoma.[60] The nevus cells are distributed both singly along the basal layer of the epidermis (lentiginous hyperplasia) and also as nests (*Figs 25.182–25.184*). The latter are irregular in both shape and distribution and are not confined to the tips of the epidermal ridges, as is characteristic of the banal nevus. They therefore may be present along the sides of the rete ridges or at the tips of the dermal papillae. Bridging between adjacent nests is commonly seen

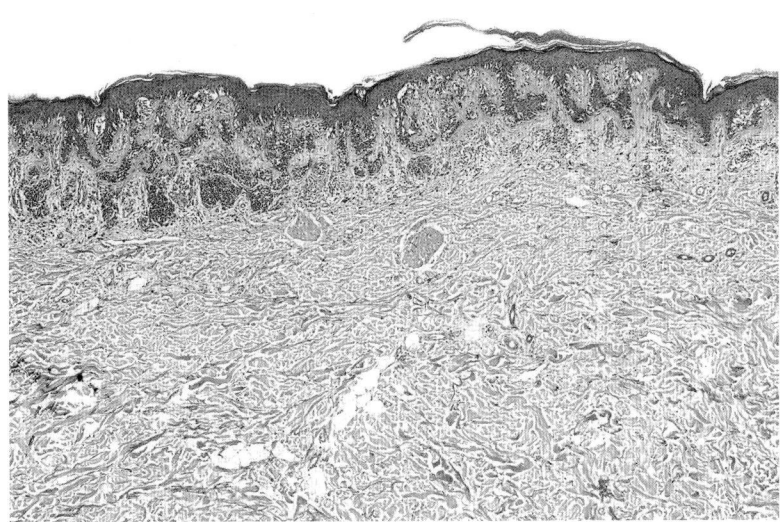

Fig. 25.181
Dysplastic nevus: medium-power view showing the typical architectural features of a dysplastic nevus. The rete ridges are elongated, junctional nests are randomly distributed, and the shoulder is clearly seen.

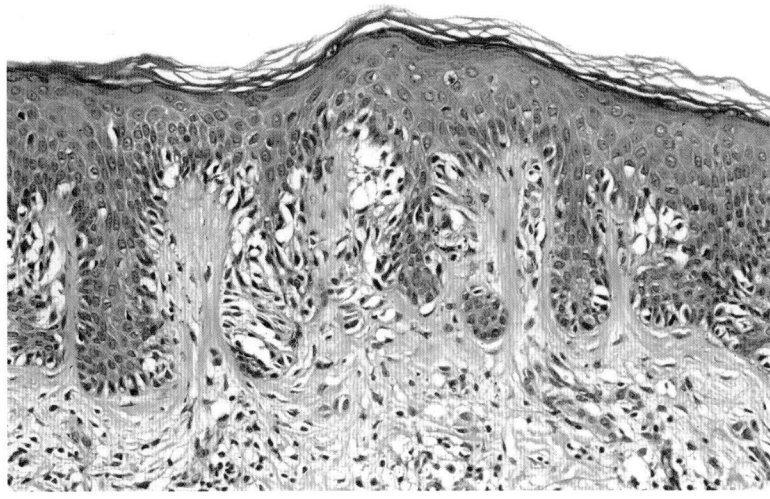

Fig. 25.183
Dysplastic nevus: the nuclei are hyperchromatic, spindled, and surrounded by a retraction artifact.

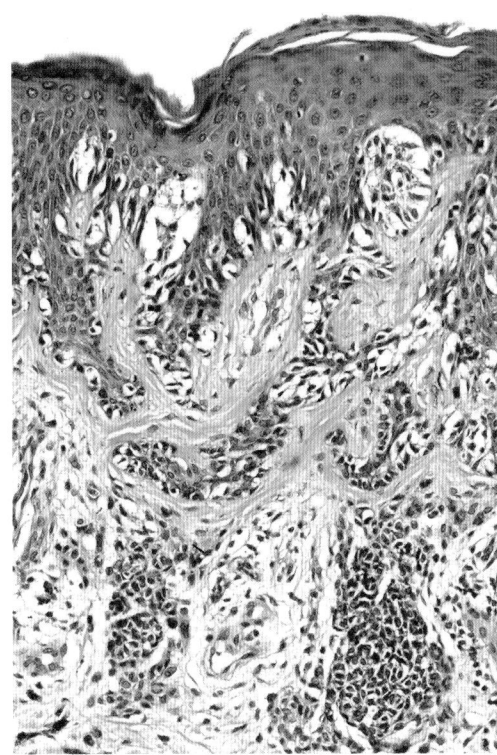

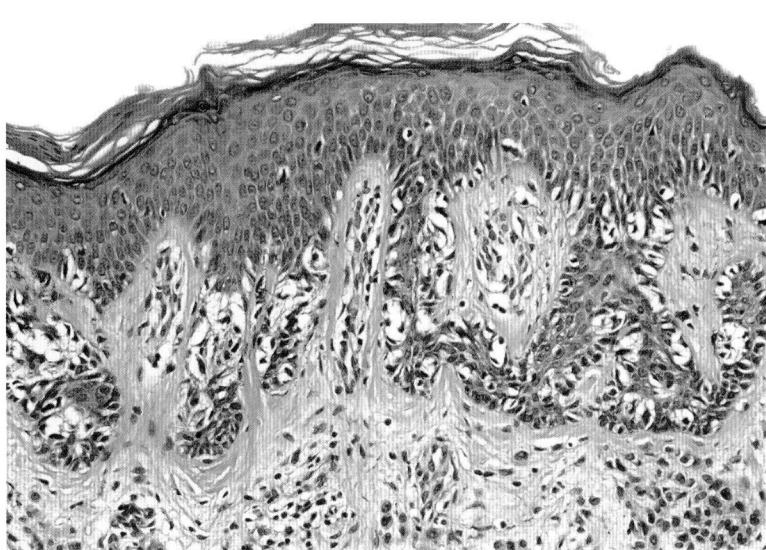

Fig. 25.184
Dysplastic nevus: in addition to nests, single cells are dispersed along the sides of the rete ridges.

Fig. 25.182
Dysplastic nevus: high-power view of the nevus shown in *Fig. 25.181*. Note the lentiginous growth pattern and the abnormal location of the junctional nests along the sides of the rete and over the tips of the dermal papillae.

(*Fig. 25.185*). Occasionally, spindle cell nests may appear expansile, compressing the dermal papillae and resulting in a superficial resemblance to spindle cell nevus of Reed.

Cytological atypia is characterized by increased nuclear size, nuclear membrane irregularity, prominent nucleoli, nuclear and cytoplasmic pleomorphism, and variable hyperchromatism. Dusty pigmentation giving rise to an olive green coloration is characteristically present (*Fig. 25.186*). The atypical melanocytes may be present singly or in small clusters and characteristically appear to sit within a lacuna due to a marked fixation retraction artifact. Typically, in any one nevus there is an admixture of normal and atypical nevus cells, i.e., the cytological atypia is random. Confluent

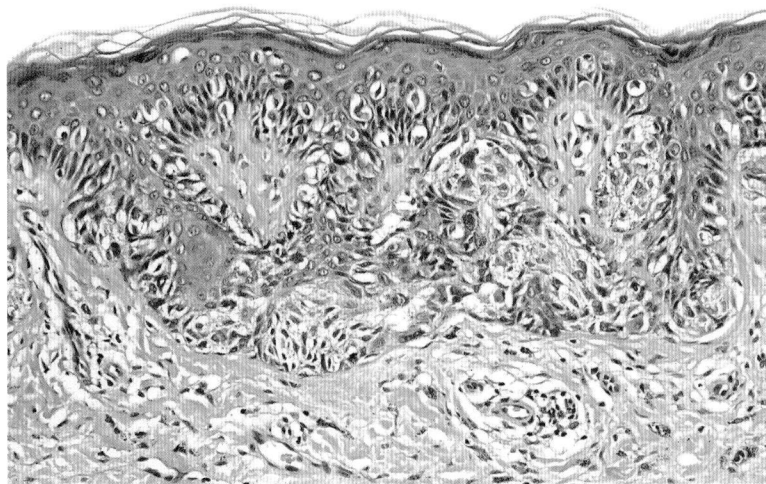

Fig. 25.185
Dysplastic nevus: bridging of melanocytic nests between adjacent rete is a common finding.

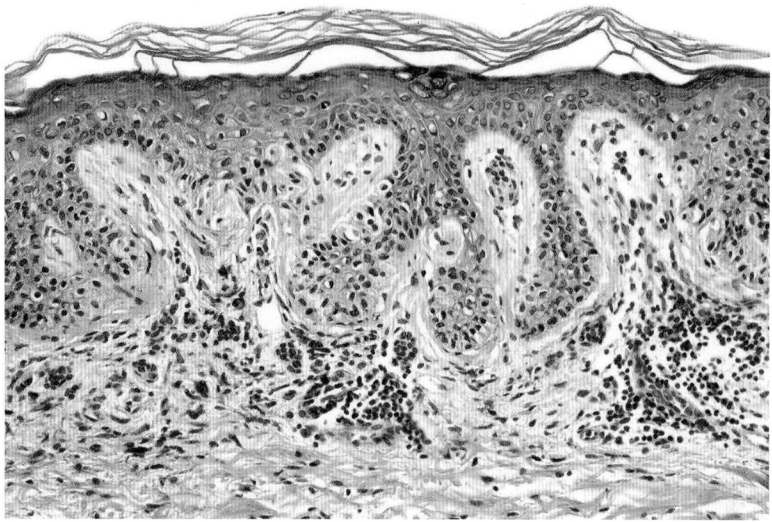

Fig. 25.186
Dysplastic nevus: dusty pigmentation often gives rise to an olive green coloration of the nevus cells.

Table 25.2
Grading criteria for dysplastic nevi

Parameter	Mild	Moderate	Severe
Nuclear size	Approximate size of keratinocyte nucleus	1–2 × keratinocyte nucleus	2 × or greater keratinocyte nucleus
Nuclear pleomorphism	Mild	Moderate	Severe
Chromatin	Hyperchromatic	Hyperchromatic or vesicular	Vesicular
Nucleolus	Absent or small	Absent or small	Prominent and enlarged
Cytoplasm	Usually little but sometimes abundant with dusty pigmentation	Usually little but sometimes abundant with dusty pigmentation	Often abundant

Modified from Weinstock, M.A. et al (1997) Archives of Dermatology, 133, 953–958.

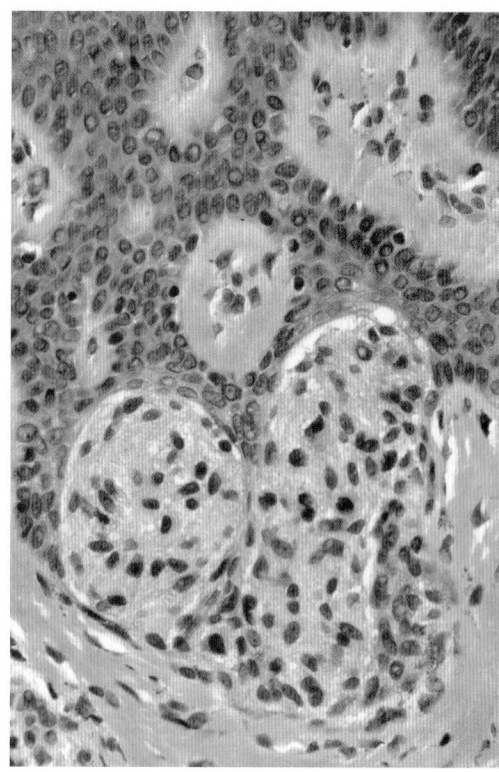

Fig. 25.187
Dysplastic nevus, mild cytological atypia: nuclei are of a similar size to the keratinocyte nuclei. They are hyperchromatic and have an irregular border. Note the fine pigmentation.

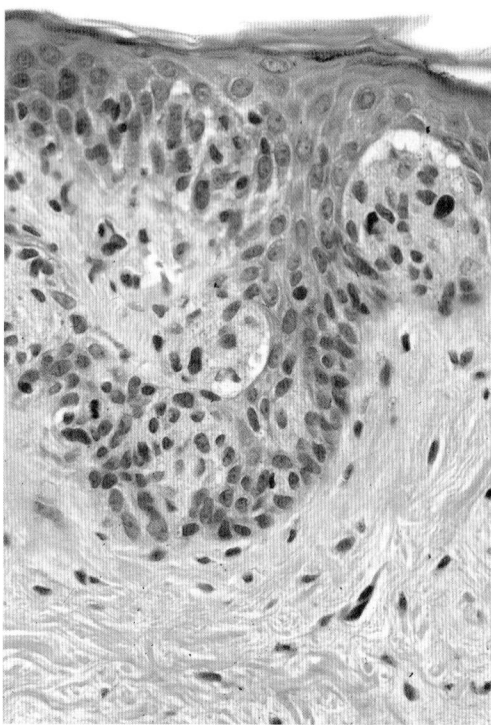

Fig. 25.188
Dysplastic nevus, moderate cytological atypia: the nuclei are variable in size. Some are larger than those of the adjacent keratinocytes. Note the mitosis.

cytological atypia should raise concern for in situ melanoma. Mitotic figures, though uncommon, are occasionally a feature. Although one or two cells may be seen in the suprabasal epidermis, any significant degree of pagetoid spread should be taken as evidence of evolving in situ melanoma. The dermal component, if present, often appears cytologically banal although in some nevi it shows superficial cytological atypia comparable to the junctional component. Sebocyte-like melanocytes, characterized by multivacuolated cytoplasm and scalloped nuclei, can exceptionally be observed in the dermal component of a dysplastic nevus.[61]

Cytological atypia may be classified into three grades: mild, moderate, and severe (Table 25.2; Figs 25.187–25.190).[18,19] A simplification into high and low grades also has merit.[62] Two studies have clearly demonstrated that the probability of melanoma development correlates with increasing grade of dysplasia, being the highest for severe dysplasia.[63,64] Grading, in addition, has the benefit of drawing the clinicians' attention to those lesions which cause pathologists most concern. It should not, however, be forgotten that on occasion one may encounter melanoma arising in a background of a dysplastic nevus with apparently only mild cytological atypia (Figs 25.191–25.193).

A recent study demonstrated site-specific and gender-related differences in histopathology of dysplastic nevi.[65] Dysplastic nevi on lower extremities were smaller and more likely displayed focal pagetoid spread than dysplastic nevi on the back. While dysplastic nevi on lower extremities in females were predominantly junctional, showed more prominent pagetoid spread, and were associated with deposition of melanin in the dermis, dysplastic nevi in males were predominantly compound nevi with little or no pagetoid spread.

A controversial entity, described as a 'de novo intraepidermal epithelioid melanocytic dysplasia', has been reported to be a marker of the dysplastic

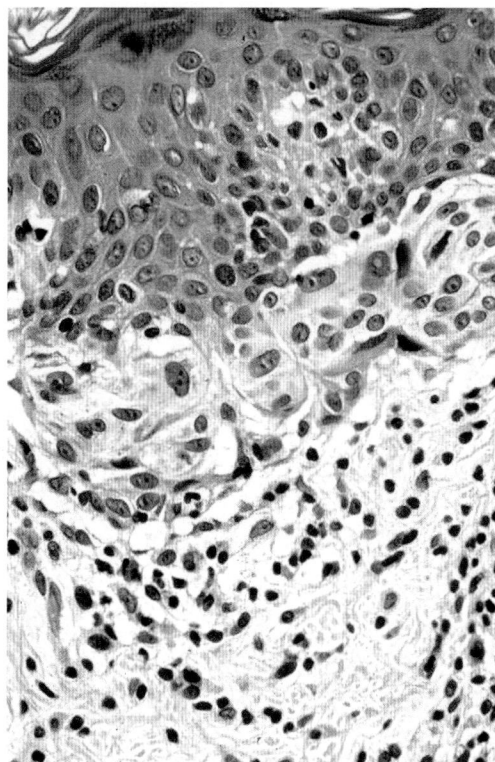

Fig. 25.189
Dysplastic nevus, severe cytological atypia: some of the nuclei are up to twice the size of keratinocyte nuclei. Nucleoli are prominent.

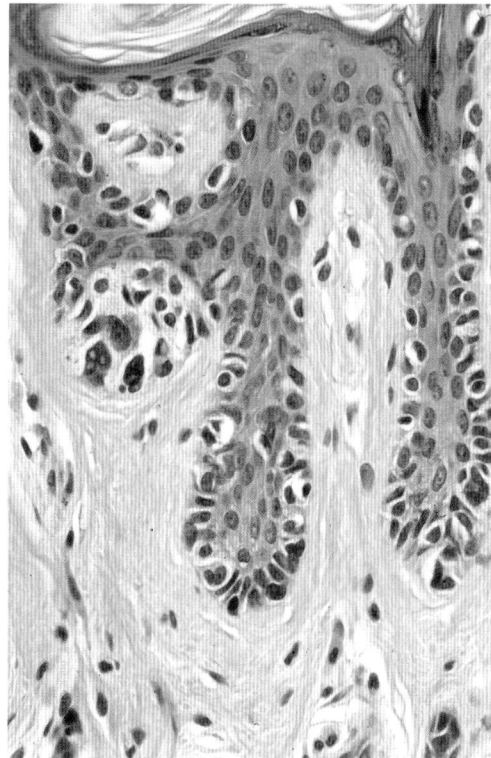

Fig. 25.190
Dysplastic nevus, severe cytological atypia: note the nuclear hyperchromatism.

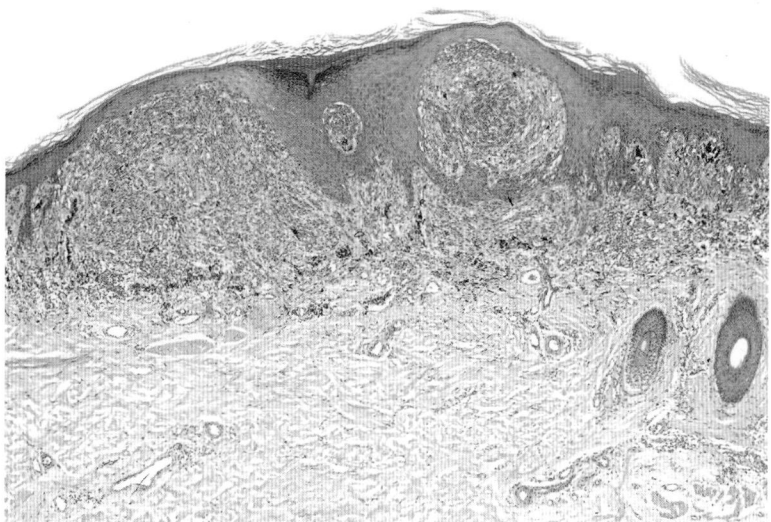

Fig. 25.191
Melanoma arising in a dysplastic nevus: invasive tumor with nevoid features.

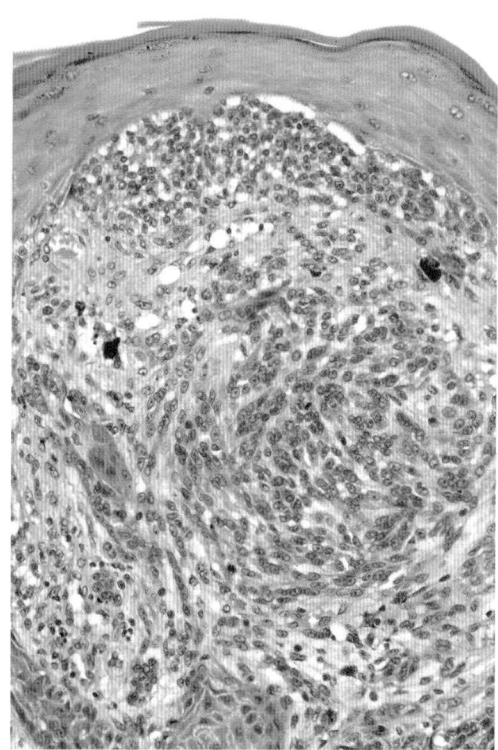

Fig. 25.192
Melanoma arising in a dysplastic nevus: close-up view of the center of the lesion.

nevus syndrome and to correlate with a familial or personal history of melanoma.[66] Histologically, it is characterized by poorly circumscribed lentiginous and pagetoid proliferation of moderately to severely atypical epithelioid melanocytes within the epidermis, and may represent a precursor lesion to melanoma in situ. Distinction from melanoma in situ is difficult, and there appears to be an overlap between the two entities.

The stromal changes include an eosinophilic or more characteristic lamellar fibroblastic response; patchily distributed lymphocytes and melanophages are often evident (*Figs 25.194–25.196*). A subacute spongiotic dermatitis, e.g., Meyerson phenomenon, may be an accompanying phenomenon of a dysplastic nevus.[67] A peculiar feature, reported in four dysplastic nevi from the same patient, was a prominent neutrophilic infiltrate within both the epidermal and dermal melanocytic components.[68] The vasculature sometimes appears accentuated.

All dysplastic nevi must be carefully scrutinized to exclude the coexistence of melanoma, which is most often of the superficial spreading subtype.

It should be noted, however, that some nevi from patients with the dysplastic nevus syndrome may appear architecturally and cytologically banal.

Differential diagnosis

Although any one of the above features (excluding cytological atypia) may be seen in a banal nevus, it is the combination of these features and the

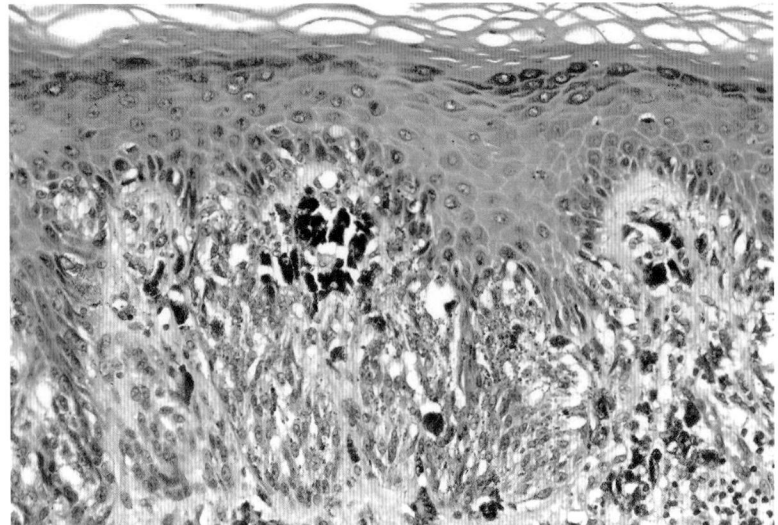

Fig. 25.193
Melanoma arising in a dysplastic nevus: the adjacent epidermis shows a junctional dysplastic lesion. Cytological atypia is mild. The patient has a long history of a dysplastic nevus that subsequently developed a nodule.

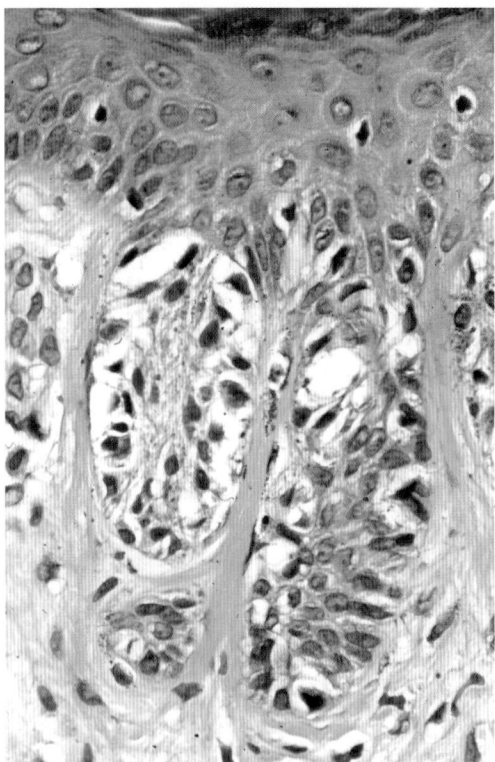

Fig. 25.195
Dysplastic nevus: note the lamellar fibroplasia.

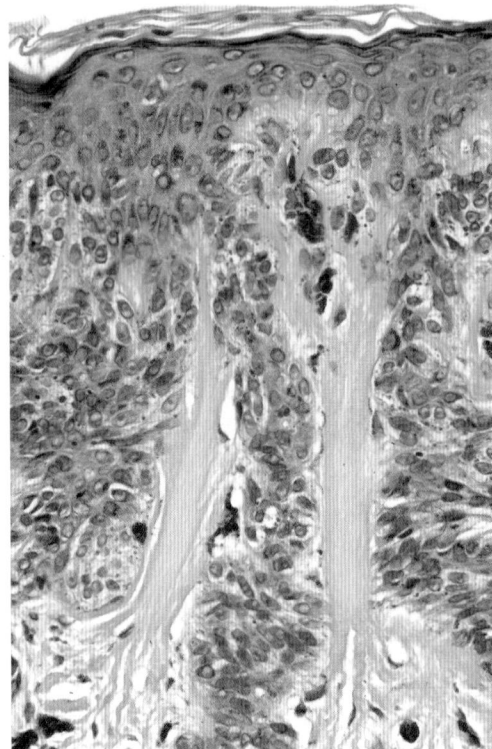

Fig. 25.194
Dysplastic nevus: there is striking eosinophilic fibroplasia.

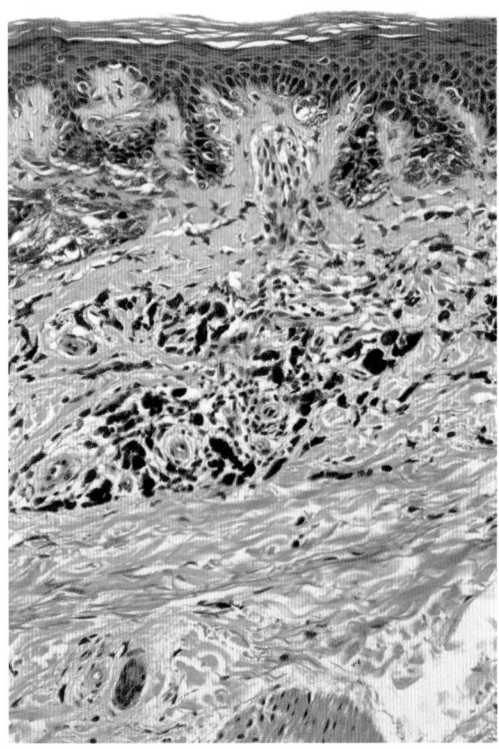

Fig. 25.196
Dysplastic nevus: in this example, pigment-laden macrophages are conspicuous.

invariable presence of cytological atypia that is essential for the diagnosis of a dysplastic nevus.

Lentiginous dysplastic nevus must be distinguished from lentiginous junctional nevus and lentigo maligna. In short, the former may show minor architectural anomalies and fibroplasia but by definition, cytological atypia is absent. The clinical setting of lentigo maligna (in situ melanoma) is quite different, and the lesion is associated with epidermal atrophy rather than epidermal hyperplasia with elongation of rete ridges; solar elastosis is characteristically present. Furthermore, lentigo maligna displays non-random cytological atypia distributed throughout the lesion.[69] Distinction between dysplastic nevus and lentigo maligna can be particularly challenging in small or partial biopsies.

Dysplastic nevus must be distinguished from radial growth-phase (in situ) superficial spreading melanoma. The difference, however, is subjective and usually one of degree. Severely dysplastic nevi show a continuum with early melanoma. Although most cases are readily classified, it must be acknowledged that they form a histologic (if not biological) spectrum. Reliable morphological criteria for their distinction do not exist. Since a diagnosis of either in situ melanoma or severely dysplastic nevus generally leads to the same therapy, such distinction is of little practical importance.

Atypical (dysplastic) lentiginous nevus of the elderly

Clinical features

The prevalence of an atypical (dysplastic) lentiginous nevus of the elderly (also known as pigmented lentiginous nevus with atypia, early or evolving melanoma in situ) increases particularly in individuals over the age of 60 years, although younger patients with chronic sun-damaged skin can also be affected.[1-3] The lesion presents as a solitary asymmetrical macule, or a few macules of variegated color measuring from 0.3 to 1 cm in diameter. It shows predilection for the back in males and for lower extremities in females. It is frequently associated with transition to melanoma in situ, usually of the lentiginous type.[1-4]

Histologic features

The rete ridges show variation in size and shape, and are unevenly spaced. Bridging of rete ridges can also be seen. Lentiginous proliferation of single melanocytes is present along the dermal–epidermal junction. Focal confluence of single melanocytes over the suprapapillary plates is sometimes present, but is not prominent. Nests of melanocytes vary in size and shape and are usually located at the tips of several rete ridges and also but less frequently, between rete ridges. Upward migration of melanocytes is generally not a feature. Melanocytes display mild to moderate cytological atypia with irregular hyperchromatic nuclei.[5] In the papillary dermis, focal fibrosis, pigment incontinence, and a lymphohistiocytic inflammatory cell infiltrate are evident.

Differential diagnosis

Junctional lentiginous nevus is typically a small lesion measuring less than 5 mm in diameter. It is characterized histologically by regular elongation of rete ridges. Nests of melanocytes are uniform and situated at the tips of the rete ridges. Cytological atypia is absent. Dermal fibrosis is generally absent.

Lesions must be distinguished from melanoma in situ, although it is important to remember that the latter can evolve within these lesions. Melanoma in situ is characterized by a variably elongated irregular rete ridge pattern. Continuous proliferation of melanocytes either as nests or single cells is present over a broad area of the epidermis.[4] Melanocytes display cytological atypia, which is non-random and is frequently confluent. Pagetoid spread of melanocytes is also present.

Congenital nevus

Clinical features

Congenital nevi are common, being found in 0.6% to 1.6% of the population.[1] They often have histologic features sufficiently characteristic to be distinguished readily from their acquired counterparts.[2,3] Because of the risk of developing melanoma, this is more than a mere academic exercise. It is difficult to give a precise figure, but the incidence of malignant change in large congenital nevi has been documented as ranging from 3.8% to 18%.[4,5] A retrospective analysis from the Netherlands demonstrated higher risk of melanoma development in females than males (14.1 vs. 6.4).[6] Medium and small congenital nevi may also be a potential source of concern, but the risk of melanoma in these is exceedingly low.[4,5,7–11]

The lesions are present at birth and are often multiple. In general, they show predilection for trunk and legs, followed by head and neck, feet, and hands.[12] By convention, they are classified into three subtypes: small (measuring up to 1.5 cm in diameter), medium (from 1.5 to 20 cm in diameter), and large (measuring over 20 cm in diameter). The last often cover a limb or large area of the trunk and are typically classified separately as giant or bathing-trunk congenital melanocytic nevi (see below). The majority of melanocytic nevi greater than 1.5 cm in diameter are most likely congenital.[13] Initially, congenital nevi are flat and often pale brown, reminiscent of café-au-lait macules. Occasionally, they become more heavily pigmented, thicker, and hairy.[14] They may also develop a warty surface with discrete small nodular projections (*Fig. 25.197*). Congenital nevi are widely distributed, and those occurring over the vertebral column are sometimes

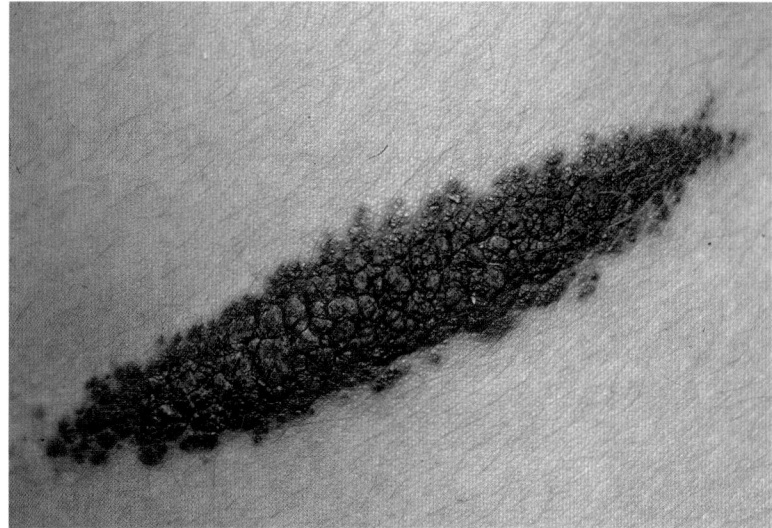

Fig. 25.197
Congenital melanocytic nevus: solitary large lesion showing hyperpigmentation and a verrucous surface. By courtesy of the Institute of Dermatology, London, UK.

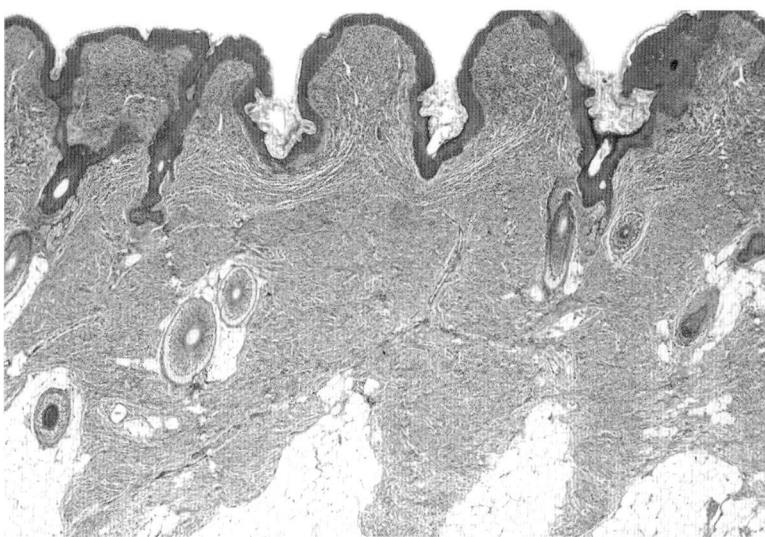

Fig. 25.198
Congenital melanocytic nevus: melanocytic proliferation extends from the superficial dermis to the septa of the subcutaneous fat. Such extensive cutaneous involvement is not a feature of an acquired melanocytic nevus.

associated with leptomeningeal melanocytosis, hydrocephalus, spina bifida, or meningomyelocele.[14] Annular dermatitis (eczema) can occasionally be superimposed upon congenital nevi.[15]

Histologic features

Congenital nevi have variable appearances. Some (particularly small lesions) are indistinguishable from conventional acquired variants.[16-18] Others, especially large examples, show a constellation of changes, which in the majority of cases enables an accurate assessment (*Figs 25.198–25.201*).[19,20] The reliable diagnosis of a congenital nevus, aside from the obvious clinical information, depends on the sum of the histologic changes rather than on any one feature in particular.

The epidermis, as with acquired nevi, often participates in the process. Frequently, there is hyperkeratosis, acanthosis, and papillomatosis, although occasionally the epidermis is atrophic. Sometimes the epithelium has a lentiginous pattern. Distinction may be made between those nevi examined in neonates and young children (see below) and those examined at a later stage.

A variety of histologic features are seen in congenital nevi.[21-23] Most important is the depth of the lesion. Usually, the nevus consists of a diffuse

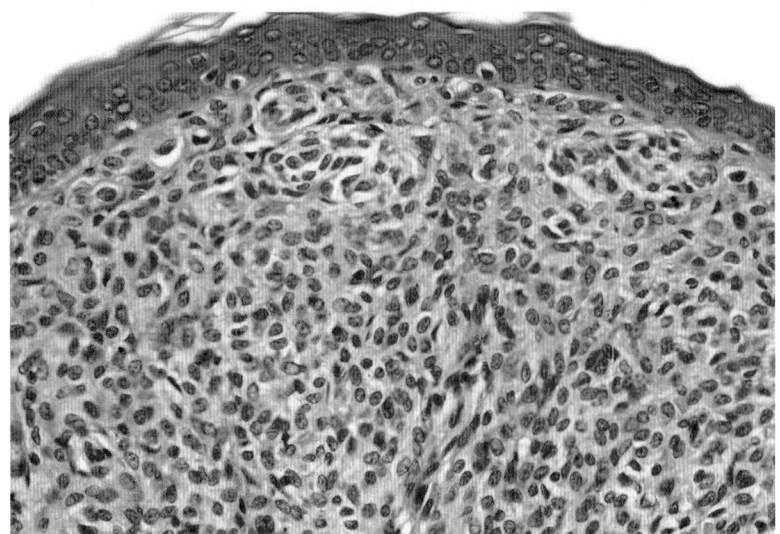

Fig. 25.199
Congenital melanocytic nevus: high-power view showing a uniform population of type A nevus cells.

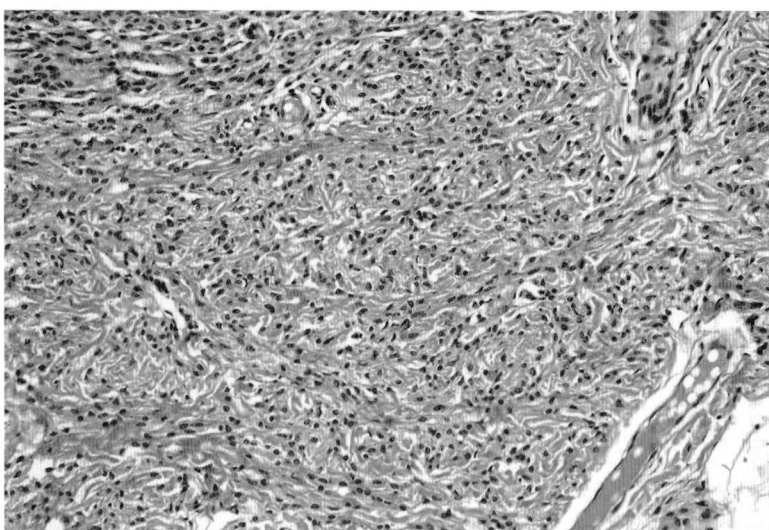

Fig. 25.202
Congenital melanocytic nevus: the nevus cells in the dermal component dissect between the collagen fibers.

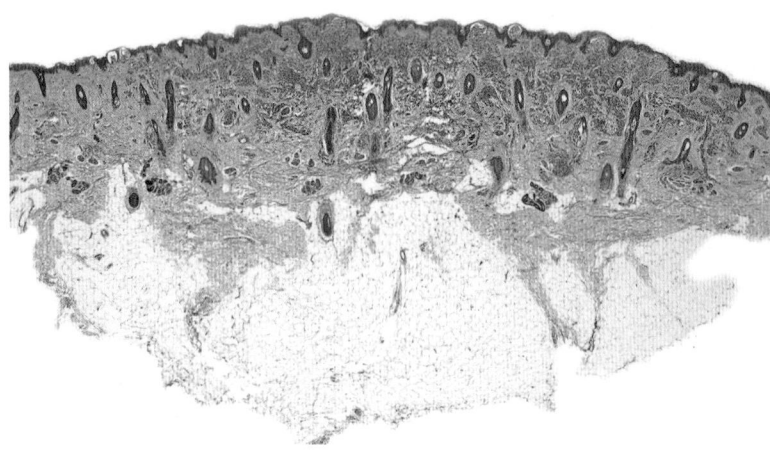

Fig. 25.200
Congenital melanocytic nevus: scanning view of a scalp lesion.

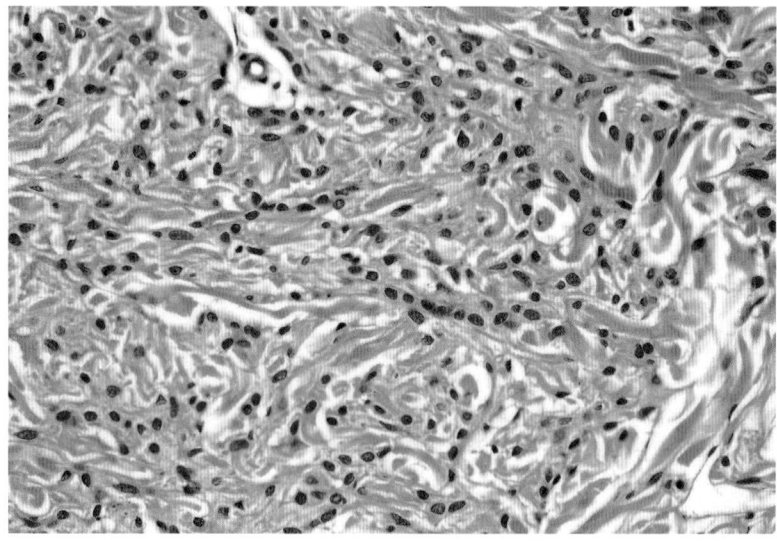

Fig. 25.203
Congenital melanocytic nevus: in this field, there is a characteristic Indian-file pattern.

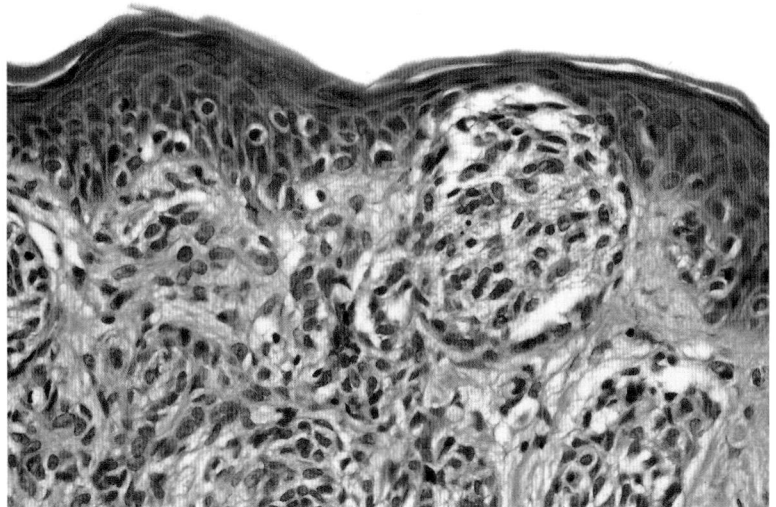

Fig. 25.201
Congenital melanocytic nevus: focal junctional activity is present.

infiltrate of melanocytes spreading from the papillary dermis into the deep reticular dermis and frequently involving the fibrous septa of the subcutaneous fat (*Figs 25.202–25.204*). Unlike acquired melanocytic nevi, there is little tendency to form discrete nests, except at the junctional zone and within the superficial papillary dermis. Not uncommonly, a grenz zone separates the nevus cells from the overlying epidermis.

Also, although an acquired nevus tends to have a well-developed fibrous stroma, congenital nevi depend on indigenous connective tissue as their supporting framework. Pigmentation is variable, being most conspicuous at the superficial aspect of the lesion. Nevus cells characteristically ensheath the epidermal appendages and very often actively involve them. Nevus cells may therefore be found within arrector pili muscles, hair follicles, sebaceous glands, and the walls of eccrine sweat ducts (*Figs 25.205* and *25.206*). A common finding is involvement of the perineural space and infiltration of the walls of lymphatic and blood vessels. In the context of a congenital nevus, the latter features should not necessarily be regarded as sinister. An occasional normal mitotic figure may be identified in the papillary dermal component of the tumor (*Fig. 25.207*).[24] Acquired nevi may occasionally involve an appendage structure, but the finding of nevus cells within multiple epidermal appendages is more suggestive of congenital nevi.[25]

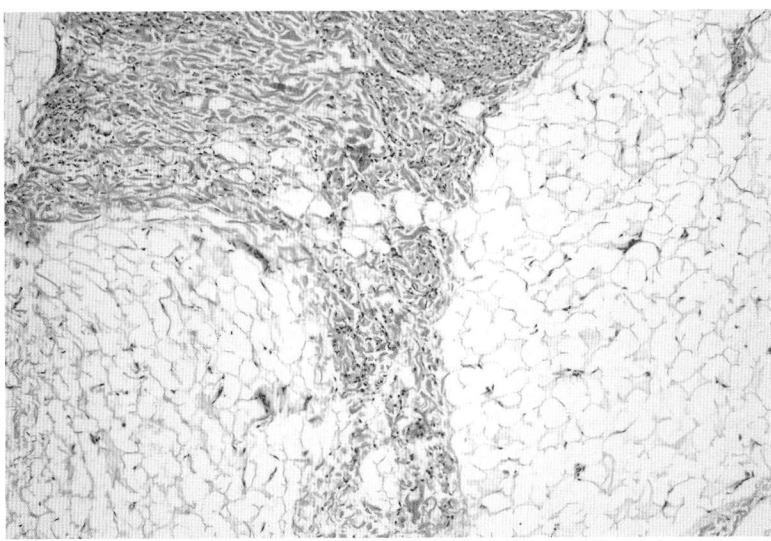

Fig. 25.204
Congenital melanocytic nevus: there is involvement of a septum of the
subcutaneous fat, a typical feature.

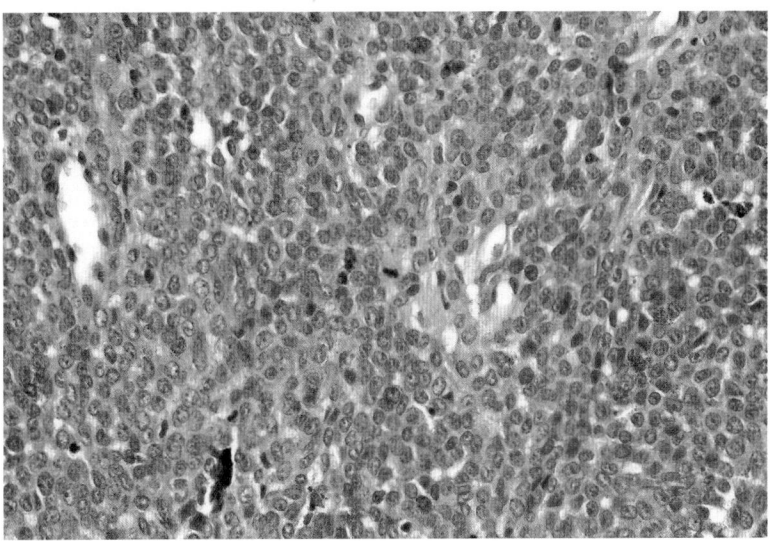

Fig. 25.207
Congenital melanocytic nevus: normal mitotic figures may be found in the
superficial component, particularly in young patients. In the absence of abnormal
forms and of nuclear or cytoplasmic pleomorphism, they do not imply malignancy.

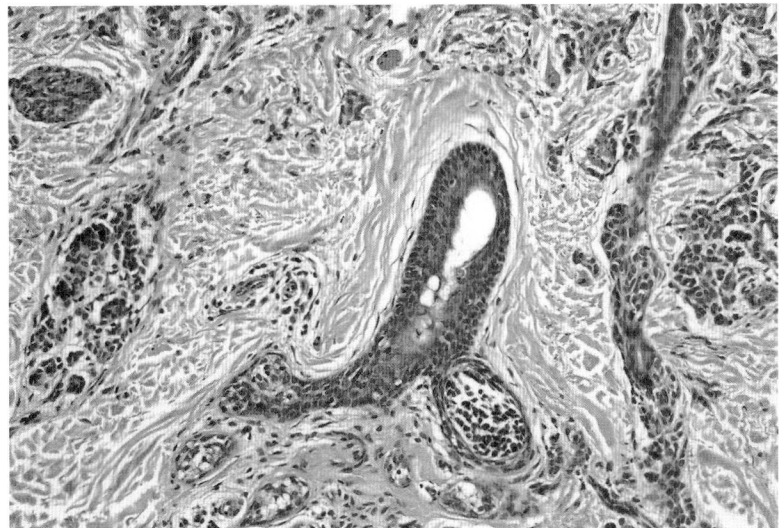

Fig. 25.205
Congenital melanocytic nevus: appendageal involvement is frequently present.

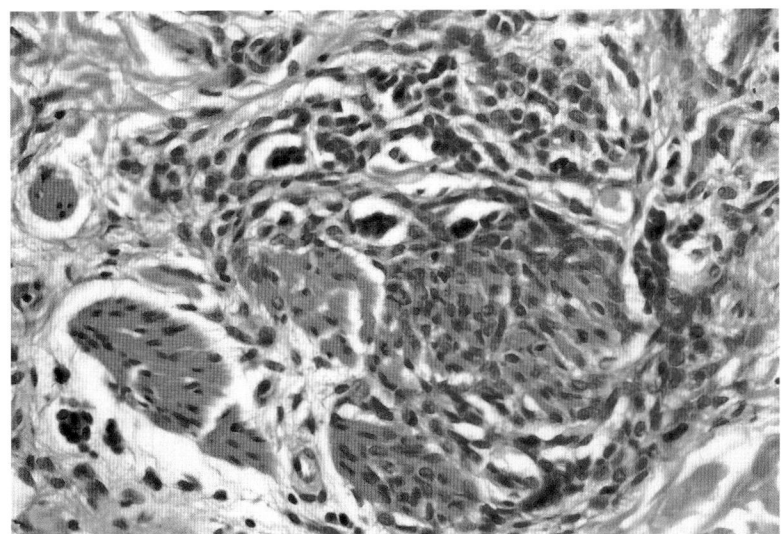

Fig. 25.206
Congenital melanocytic nevus: nevus cells are evident within this arrector pili
muscle.

With increasing depth, the nevus cells adopt a single-cell array and
Indian-file pattern, which are particularly evident in the reticular dermis
and subcutaneous fat.

The development of neuroid features is characteristic of both congenital
and acquired nevi. In congenital lesions, however, the process is often
patchy and remains cellular, in contrast to the relative hypocellularity of the
neuroid foci within acquired nevi.

Of the many differences between these two types of nevi, the single most
important diagnostic marker of congenital nevi is permeation of single nevus
cells between the collagen fibers of the deep reticular dermis and septa of
the subcutaneous fat.

Congenital nevi in neonates and young children

Congenital nevi in neonates and young children can be junctional, compound (the majority), or dermal. Pattern and depth of involvement are
related to the size of the nevus.[1] Superficial dermal, perivascular, and periadnexal distribution is more often seen in small nevi, whereas diffuse infiltration and extension into the subcutaneous fat is typical of the larger and
bathing-trunk variants. Maturation of the dermal component is invariably
present.

Occasionally, however, congenital nevi in neonates and young children
may display worrying histologic features that can be a source of concern
to the pathologist, particularly if the age of the patient is unknown, which
must not be confused with melanoma.[1–6] These changes include large
and abnormally located junctional nests, pagetoid spread either as single
nevoid melanocytes or small nests, cytological atypia and mitotic activity
in both junctional and dermal component, impaired maturation, uneven
pigmentation, and marked involvement of skin appendages. Although the
junctional component is usually composed of a fairly uniform population of basally located cells, sometimes dyscohesive nests and single cells
are dispersed throughout the epidermis, mimicking pagetoid spread (*Figs
25.208–25.210*).[3] This is most commonly present at the periphery of the
lesion, and should not be mistaken for melanoma in situ.[7] Cytological
atypia may be observed in up to 30% of cases, and rarely this may be
severe.[1] Variation in the amount of melanin pigment within dermal melanocytes is common.[7] Involvement of the adnexal epithelium is often seen.[2,3]
When dermal mitotic activity is apparent, the features can be alarming. Melanoma arising within a congenital nevus in a neonate is exceptional. It is
important that dermal melanocytic proliferation nodules are not mistaken
for intralesional transformation of melanoma (see below).

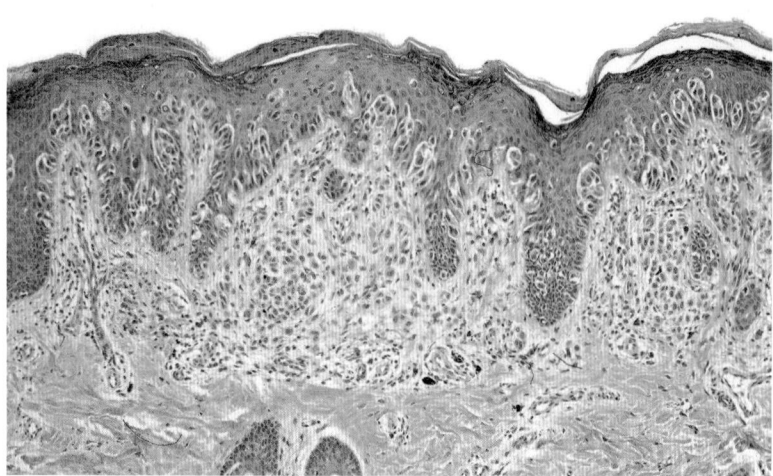

Fig. 25.208
Neonatal nevus: there is florid junctional activity with pagetoid spread.

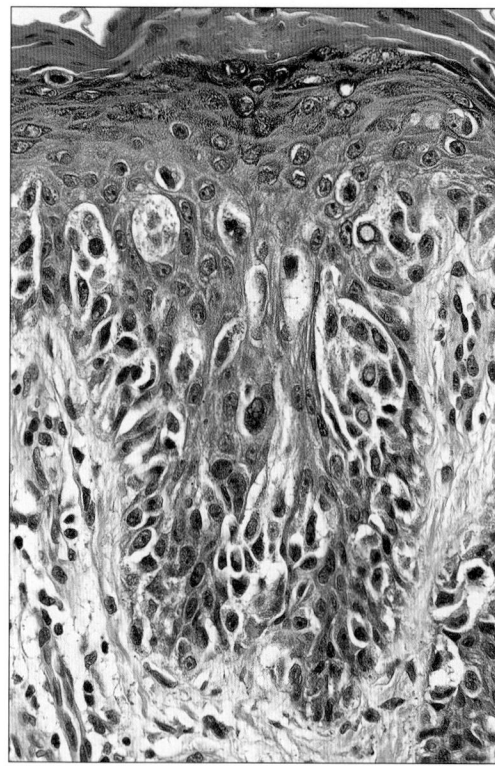

Fig. 25.210
Neonatal nevus: high-power view showing nuclear pleomorphism and pagetoid spread.

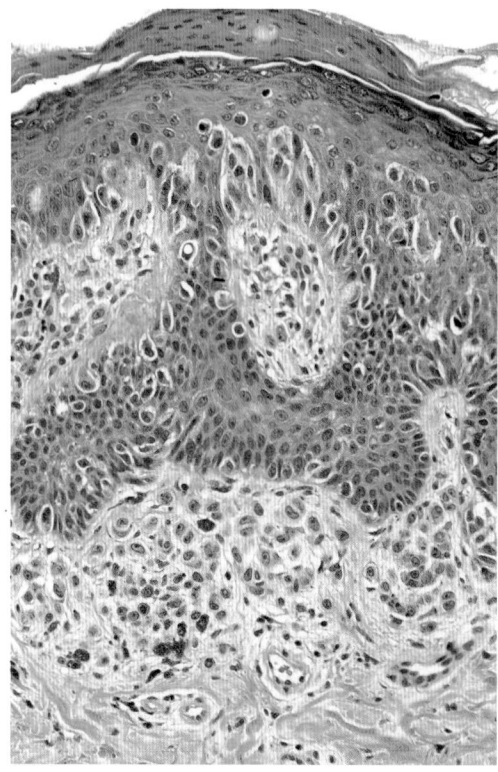

Fig. 25.209
Neonatal nevus: the nevus cells are epithelioid with abundant pale eosinophilic cytoplasm and vesicular nuclei containing prominent nucleoli.

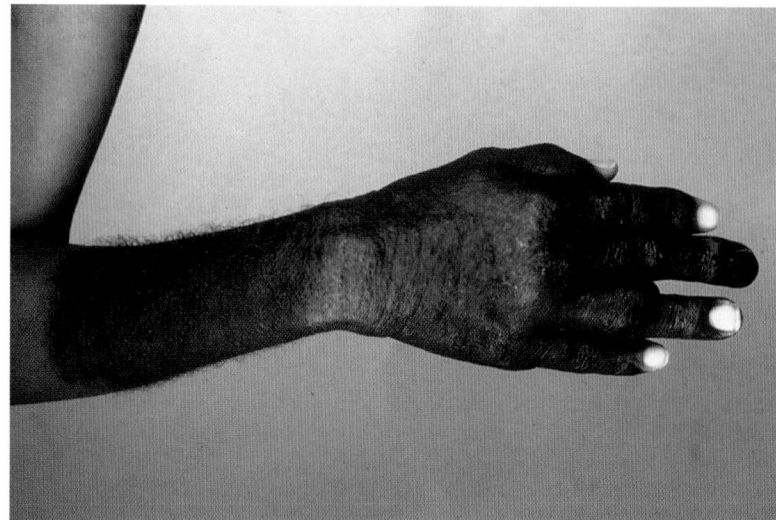

Fig. 25.211
Giant congenital melanocytic nevus: in this example, the nevus has a glove distribution. By courtesy of the Institute of Dermatology, London, UK.

Giant hairy 'bathing-trunk' nevi

Clinical features

Giant hairy 'bathing-trunk' nevi are defined as congenital melanocytic nevi measuring 20 cm or more in diameter.[1–6] In neonates, melanocytic nevi measuring more than 6 cm on the body and more than 9 cm on the head are considered as giant.[7] Giant nevi occur in about 1:20 000 neonates.[8] They affect the sexes equally and the majority present on the head, neck, and trunk.[6] Depending on their exact location, these nevi have been described as 'bathing-trunk', 'vest', 'shoulder-sleeve', 'stocking', or 'glove' nevi (*Figs 25.211–25.213*). Satellite lesions are frequently present.[4] Giant hairy nevi show variation in color from dark brown to black. Although their color can brighten a few weeks after birth, in most examples, however, it remains unchanged for life.[9] Spontaneous regression of giant nevi is exceptional.

Familial occurrence of giant hairy nevi is rare and is possibly linked to polygenic paradominant inheritance.[10]

A desmoplastic hairless hypopigmented nevus is a variant of giant nevus, characterized by hard consistency, absence of hair, and progressive loss of pigmentation.[9,11,12] Cerebriform giant congenital nevus is delineated by cerebriform or gyrate surface pattern of the lesion, and shows predilection for parietal and occipital areas of the scalp.[13–15]

Giant nevi are, fortunately, extremely rare, since in addition to the disfigurement and psychological trauma they may induce, there is an associated significant risk (3.8–18%) of developing a melanoma.[4,6,16] Malignant change usually takes place before puberty and has been reported to be present at birth. There is a striking predilection for axial lesions.[6] Giant congenital nevi presenting over the scalp, neck, and posterior midline may have associated leptomeningeal involvement (leptomeningeal or neurocutaneous

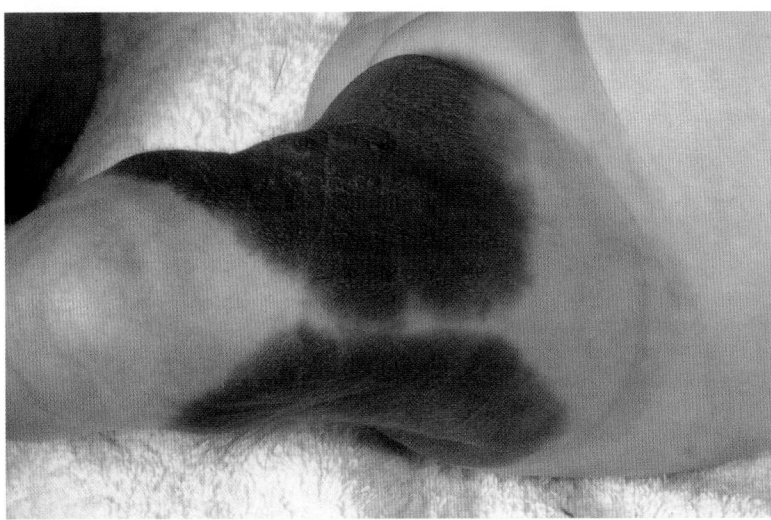

Fig. 25.212
Giant congenital melanocytic nevus: these lesions are very disfiguring and often a source of great concern to the parents. By courtesy of the Institute of Dermatology, London, UK.

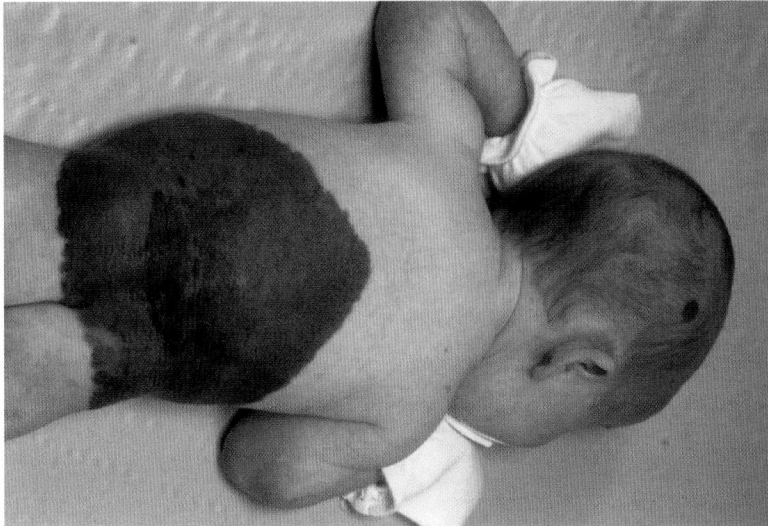

Fig. 25.213
Giant congenital melanocytic nevus: in addition to being of cosmetic importance, lesions such as this have a significant risk of malignant change. By courtesy of the Institute of Dermatology, London, UK.

melanocytosis).[17–23] Neurocutaneos melanosis has been found in 3% to 15% of patients with giant melanocytic nevi.[24–26] The risk for neurocutaneous melanosis is associated with the size of large cutaneous melanocytic nevi and the frequency of satellite nevi.[26] Although neurocutaneous melanosis may be asymptomatic, there is a significant risk of hydrocephalus or intracranial primary melanoma.[17,27,28] Symptomatic neurocutaneous melanosis has been associated with poor prognosis – there is over 50% mortality within the first 3 years of the diagnosis.[29] Giant nevi on extremities can be associated with hypotrophy of the affected limb.[1] Association with infantile hemangioma, vitiligo, hepatic melanin deposition, hypophosphatemic rickets, and lissencephaly with absent corpus callosum has also been reported.[30–34] SCALP syndrome is characterized by synchronous occurrence of nevus sebaceous, central nervous system malformations, aplasia cutis congenita, limbal dermoid, and pigmented nevus (e.g., giant congenital melanocytic nevus) together with neurocutaneous melanosis.[35]

Histologic features

The histologic features are similar to those of the more typical congenital pigmented nevus, but the development of neuroid features is often more marked. 'Bathing-trunk' nevi may also show neurofibroma-like changes and foci of blue nevus formation (reminiscent of or perhaps identical to

neurocristic hamartoma) or even Spitz nevus-like areas.[6,36] A coexistent subcutaneous ependymoma has been described.[37] Desmoplastic hairless hypopigmented nevus is delineated by prominent dermal fibrosis, progressive disappearance of lesional melanocytes, and hypotrophic or absent hair follicles and sebaceous glands.[9]

Malignant transformation particularly occurs in the dermal component of the nevus and, in addition to showing a typical melanomatous morphology, tumors may show malignant nerve-sheath tumorlike and anaplastic features.[38]

Small cell variants and heterologous foci, including rhabdomyosarcomatous and liposarcomatous differentiation, have also been described.[6]

Proliferation nodule within a congenital nevus

Clinical features

The proliferation nodule is a rarely encountered, benign lesion that develops within a congenital melanocytic nevus, usually but not invariably of the giant type, which both clinically and histologically may result in suspicion for melanoma. The frequency of proliferation nodules in giant congenital melanocytic nevi has been reported to be from 2.9% to 19%.[1–3] Lesions generally present at birth as a smooth-surfaced brown to black papule or nodule, most often measuring less than 1.0 cm in diameter although larger variants may also be encountered.[4–12] On occasion, they become ulcerated.[12] Although typical lesions are solitary, occasionally satellites or multifocal lesions are encountered. In some examples, ulceration or hemorrhage heightens the clinical concern for melanoma. The natural history of proliferation nodules is one of spontaneous gradual regression. Alternatively, they remain stable over prolonged period of time, or exhibit enlargement and hyperpigmentation.[6]

Histologic features

Several morphological patterns of proliferation can be present in proliferation nodules, the most common being expansile nodule with epithelioid (or sometimes more spitzoid) melanocytes (see below).[13] Additional morphological patterns in proliferation nodules include blue nevus-like pattern with increased pigmentation of melanocytes, nevoid melanoma-like pattern, small round blue cell tumorlike pattern, and complex pattern characterized by two or more melanocytic populations.[13]

In a classical example, a proliferation nodule is characterized by increased cellularity and larger melanocytes than in the background melanocytic component. Although distinctive and superficially appearing fairly well circumscribed, the nodule often blends imperceptibly at its margin with the adjacent melanocytes. However, a lack of blending with sharp circumscription is not uncommon (Fig. 25.214).[12] The lesion is composed of large epithelioid or spindled cell melanocytes with abundant cytoplasm and mildly pleomorphic nuclei (Fig. 25.215). Nucleoli are small and not prominent. Intranuclear pseudoinclusions are frequently present. Mitoses are typically rare and by definition do not usually exceed 1/mm² (Fig. 25.216). No atypical mitoses are seen. Maturation of melanocytes with depth may or may not be seen. Necrosis is not a feature. Occasionally, greater nuclear pleomorphism and macronucleoli can be observed in proliferation nodule, which is not associated with increased mitotic activity.[12] A mild to moderate mononuclear inflammatory cell infiltrate composed of lymphocytes, confined to proliferation nodule can sometimes be present.[12] Epidermal involvement is rare.[12] However, no pagetoid spread is seen. Areas of mesenchymal differentiation, including myofibroblastic, chondroid, and osteoid, can occasionally be seen within a proliferative nodule.

Proliferation nodules with high mitotic activity have increasingly been recognized.[9,11,14] Brisk mitotic activity (up to 30/mm²) is usually coupled with primitive cytology of the lesional cells, frequently with features of small blue round cell tumors displaying high nucleo-cytoplasmic ratio.[14] These morphological features are not associated with a sinister biological behavior. Nevertheless, atypical mitoses, necroses, and expansile border are typically absent.[9,11,14]

Proliferation nodules can on occasion also demonstrate infiltrative yet nondestructive growth, preserving hair follicles and eccrine ducts.[12]

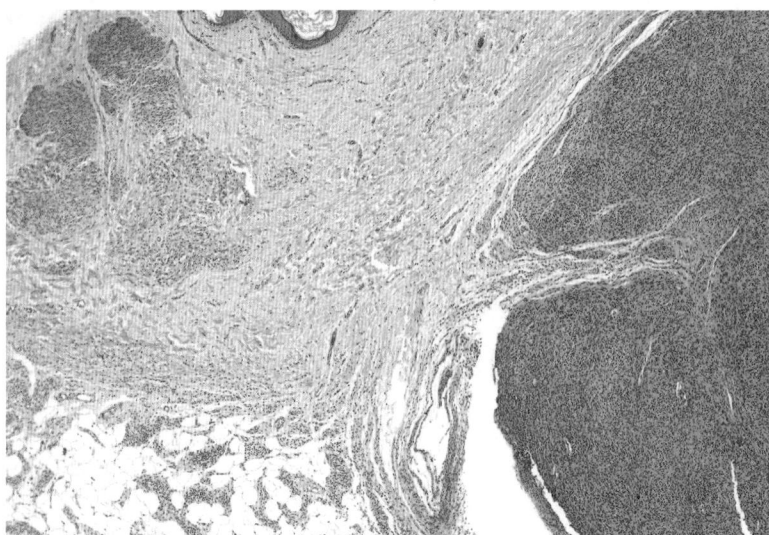

Fig. 25.214
Proliferation nodule: the congenital nevus present on the left contrasts with the hypercellular proliferation nodule of the right.

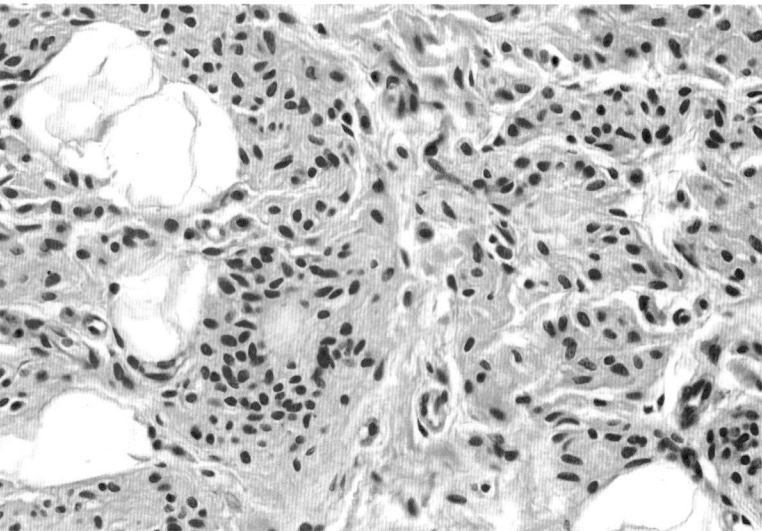

Fig. 25.215
Proliferation nodule: high-power view of the congenital nevus.

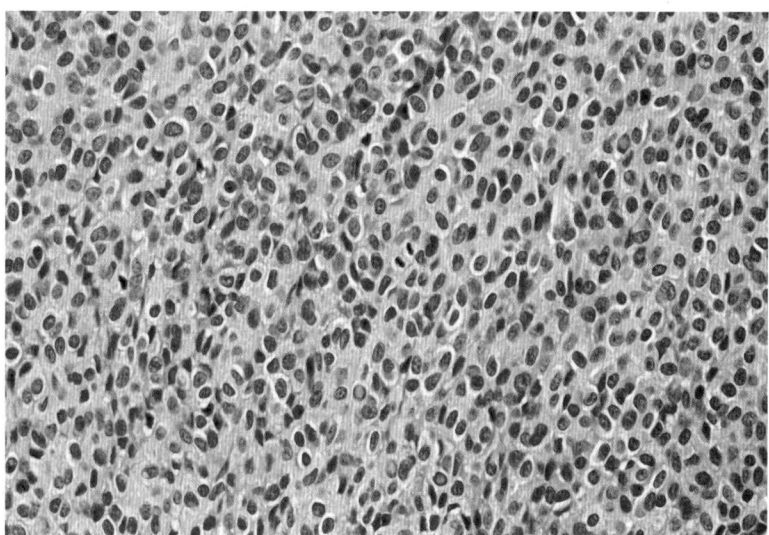

Fig. 25.216
Proliferation nodule: the nodule is composed of a uniform population of nevus cells. Note the central mitotic figure.

Differential diagnosis

Although exceedingly rare, dermal proliferation nodules must be distinguished from neonatal melanoma. Features, which should arouse suspicion for the latter, include marked pleomorphism, excessive mitotic activity, abnormal mitoses, and necrosis. A sharply delineated nodule, which does not merge with the adjacent nevus, is also a worrying feature (however, see above).

Distinction between proliferation nodule and neonatal melanoma can, however, be highly challenging, if not impossible on morphological grounds alone, in particular in lesions with brisk mitotic activity. A recent study detected the usefulness of H3K27me3 (an epigenetic gene silencer) immunohistochemistry in distinguishing between proliferative nodules and nodular melanomas developing in the background of congenital melanocytic nevi in childhood.[15] Namely, while all 20 cases of proliferative nodules and background congenital melanocytic nevi retained homogeneous expression of H3K27me3, 80% of melanomas (4 out of 5) revealed a significant loss of nuclear H3K27me3 staining ranging from 50% to as much as over 80% of tumor cells.[15] Furthermore, molecular diagnostic techniques including fluorescence in situ hybridization and CGH have increasingly been used to aid in this distinction. While proliferation nodules either display no detectable cytogenetic aberrations or show whole chromosomal copy number changes (gains or losses), melanoma on the other hand generally harbors more complex chromosomal aberrations including partial copy number gains and losses.[15–17]

Dermal melanocytic lesions (dermal melanocytoses)

Mongolian spot

Clinical features

Mongolian spots present as relatively uniform slate blue areas of non-blanching discoloration with a wavy border and irregular shape, most often situated over the sacral region (*Fig. 25.217*). Much less often, they are more

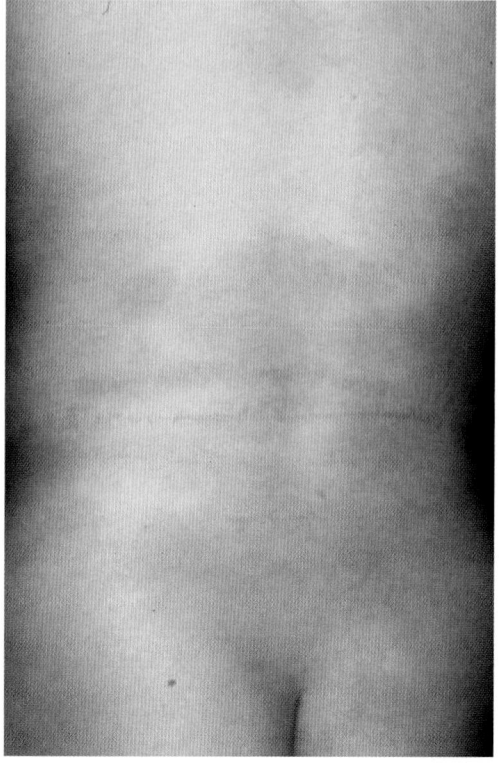

Fig. 25.217
Mongolian blue spot: there is extensive pale blue discoloration on this child's trunk and buttocks. By courtesy of S. Bleehen, MD, Royal Hallamshire Hospital, Sheffield, UK.

widely distributed, for example, over the posterior thighs, legs, back, and shoulders.[1,2] They usually present at birth or soon after and are most commonly seen in Japanese, Chinese, and pigmented races.[3] Mongolian spots are slightly more common in males. The lesions may be quite large, measuring up to 10 cm in diameter.[4] They can, on occasion, be superimposed upon another Mongolian spot.[5]

Mongolian spots are often associated with different comorbidities, including inherited disorders of metabolism, vascular birthmarks, and occult spinal dysraphism.[6] The most common underlying storage diseases are Hurler syndrome (mucopolysaccharidosis type II), GM1 type I gangliosidosis, and mucolipidosis type II, followed by Niemann-Pick disease and mannosidosis.[6-11] Coexisting Mongolian spot(s) and vascular birthmark(s), for example, nevus flammeus, have generally been referred to as phakomatosis pigmentovascularis. In addition, Mongolian spot(s) have also been reported in conjunction with noninvoluting congenital hemangioma, Sturge-Weber syndrome, Klippel-Trenaunay syndrome, cutis marmorata telangiectatica congenita, Sjögren-Larsson syndrome, and segmental café-au-lait macules.[12-20]

Most Mongolian spots undergo spontaneous regression during infancy or childhood, and generally disappear by puberty.[1,2] Persistence of the lesion into adulthood is, however, rare and has been usually linked to extrasacral locations.[1,21] Those associated with inheritable storage diseases usually do not show signs of resolution and can become even more pigmented with time.[9,10] Mongolian spot associated with a halo nevus-like appearance has been documented.[22]

Histologic features

Mongolian spot and other primary dermal melanocytic lesions (dermal melanocytoses) are believed to represent arrested transdermal migration of melanocytes from the neural crest to the epidermis. The lesion is therefore characterized by a sparse population of intradermal dendritic, variably pigmented melanocytes, which tend to be oriented parallel to the skin surface and situated predominantly in the deep reticular dermis (*Figs 25.218* and *25.219*). The overlying epithelium is normal.

Although Mongolian spot represents a benign dendritic cell proliferation, comorbidities generally define prognosis.

Nevus of Ota

Clinical features

Nevus of Ota (oculodermal melanosis, nevus fuscoceruleus ophthalmo-maxillaris) is not uncommon in the Japanese, but is only occasionally seen in Caucasians and pigmented races. It is an ill-defined slate blue, usually

unilateral lesion situated in the distribution of the ophthalmic and maxillary divisions of the trigeminal cranial nerve (*Fig. 25.220*).[1-3] Presentation in the form of bilateral multiple lentigines, e.g., agminated lentigines, has also been reported.[4] Nevus of Ota shows bilateral distribution in 5% of cases. In about 60% of patients, the sclera and conjunctiva are involved; occasionally, the mucous membranes of the nose and oral cavity are also affected.[1,2,5,6-8] Rarely, a similar discoloration involves the leptomeninges. Over 50% of these lesions are present at birth and most of the remainder appear at around puberty. It shows female predominance. Exceptional cases of familial occurrence have been documented.[5,9-11] Papules and nodules may also be seen, indicating blue nevus and cellular blue nevus components. In contrast to the Mongolian blue spot, the nevus of Ota is permanent.[2] A combined nevus of Ota with nevus spilus occurring in the same area has recently been reported.[12]

Only very rarely has malignant transformation occurred in nevus of Ota (see malignant blue nevus), predominantly in Caucasians.[13] Melanoma has been documented in the skin, iris, choroid, orbit, and meninges.[4-6,9-10,13-23] Additional tumors, described in association with this nevus, include meningeal melanocytoma and melanotic schwannoma.[24-26] Association of bilateral nevus of Ota with glaucoma and Klippel-Trenaunay syndrome has also been described.[5,27]

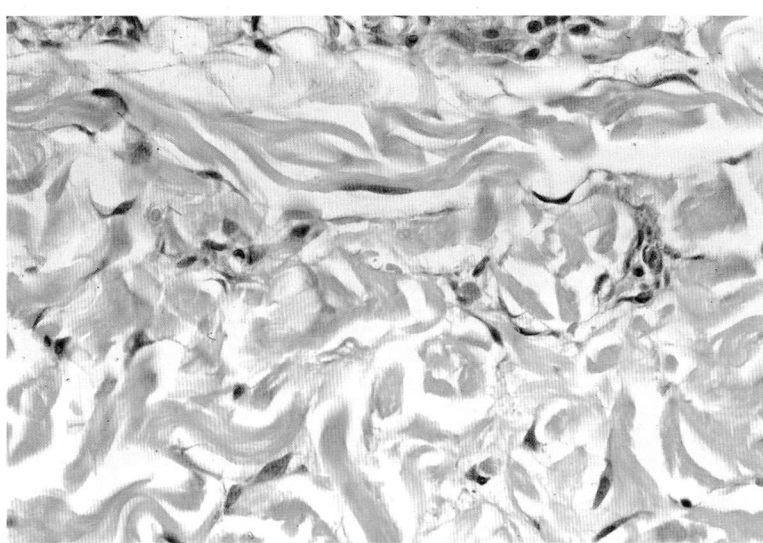

Fig. 25.219
Mongolian blue spot: scattered bipolar and dendritic cells are present.

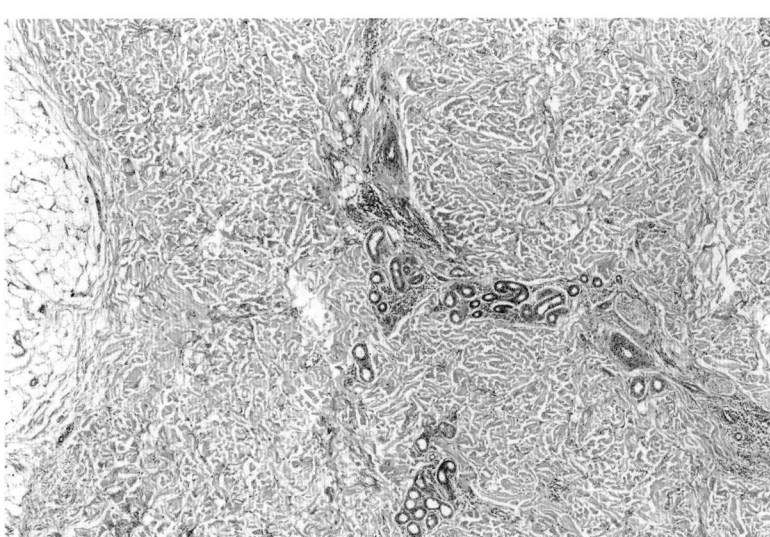

Fig. 25.218
Mongolian blue spot: at low-power examination, the features are subtle, comprising increased cellularity in the deeper dermis.

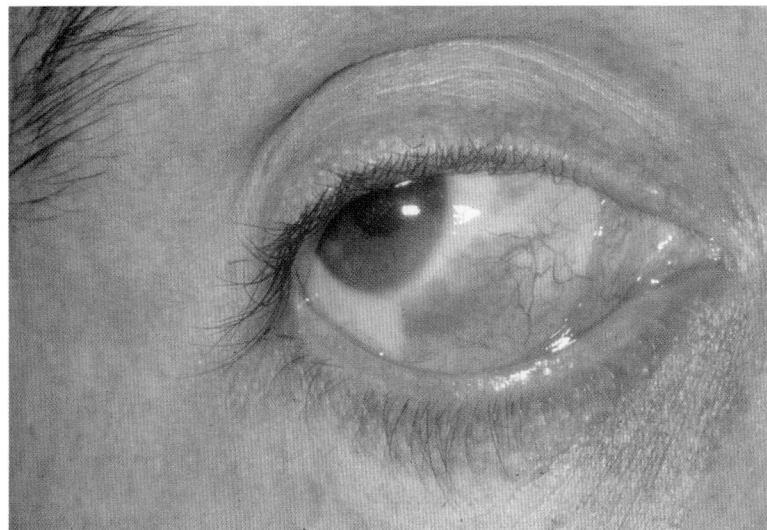

Fig. 25.220
Nevus of Ota: there is scleral involvement and a periocular bluish discoloration is evident. By courtesy of the Institute of Dermatology, London, UK.

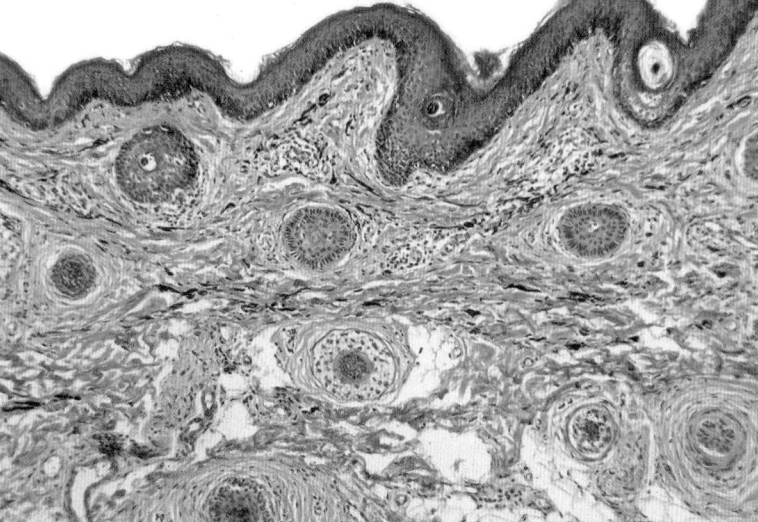

Fig. 25.221
Nevus of Ota: small numbers of bipolar and dendritic cells are present (hematoxylin and eosin and Masson-Fontana stain).

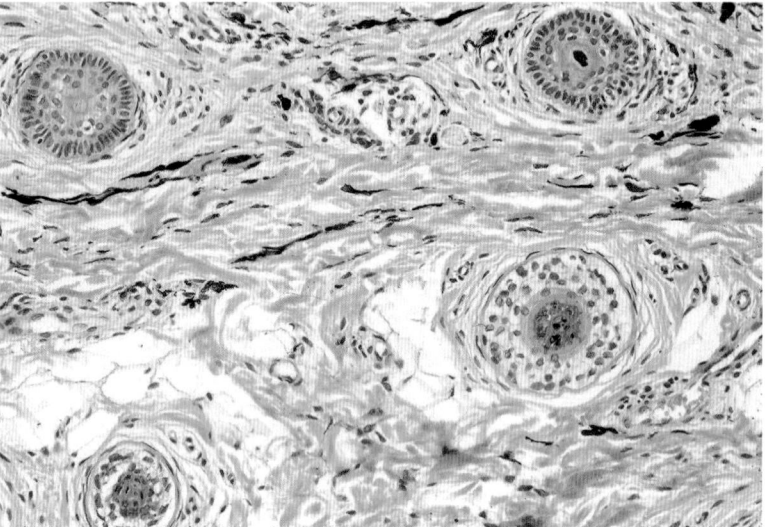

Fig. 25.222
Nevus of Ota: high-power view.

Histologic features

The epidermis may show hyperpigmentation and increased numbers of melanocytes, but there is no junctional activity. Situated within the upper and mid-dermis are collections of heavily pigmented, spindle-shaped, bipolar, or dendritic melanocytes (Figs 25.221 and 25.222).[1,3] Most are oriented parallel to the skin surface, but they may sometimes be seen encircling epidermal appendages.[1] There is a minimal fibroblastic component.

Nevus of Ota is associated with GNAQ and GNA11 mutations in a subset of the lesions.[28–30] BRAF mutations have also been reported, albeit less frequently.[31]

Nevus of Ito

Clinical features

Nevus of Ito is a very rare condition characterized by unilateral slate blue macular pigmentation in the region supplied by the posterior supraclavicular and lateral brachial cutaneous nerves (Fig. 25.223).[1] There may occasionally be a coexistent nevus of Ota[2–4,5] hypopigmentations along Blaschko lines (nevus depigmentosus), and associated Sturge-Weber syndrome.[6,7] Exceptionally, malignant transformation has been documented (see malignant blue nevus).[8–10]

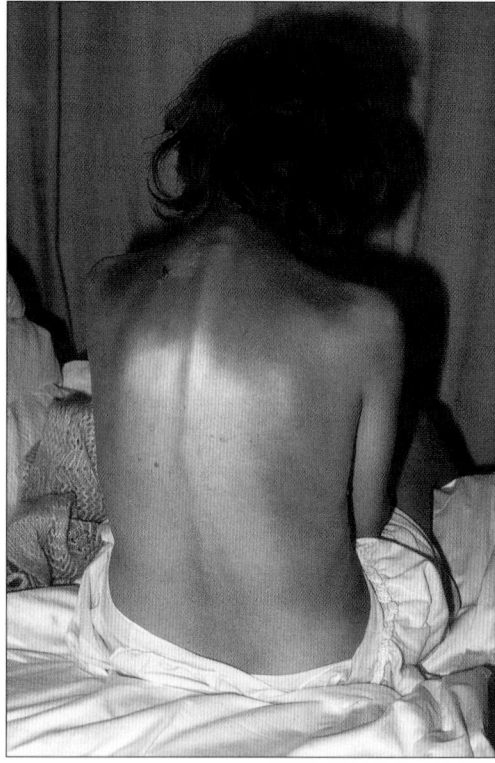

Fig. 25.223
Nevus of Ito: characteristic discoloration involving the shoulder and scapular regions. By courtesy of M.M. Black, MD, St Thomas' Hospital, London, UK.

The blue clinical appearances of nevus of Ito, the two previously mentioned lesions, and the blue nevus (see below) are artifacts due to the scattering of light during its passage through the relatively turbid dermis with absorption of all other spectral components.

Histologic features

The lesion is indistinguishable from the nevus of Ota.

Melanoma developing in the background of a nevus of Ito reported recently harbored mutations of the GNAQ and BAP1 gene.[10]

Sun nevus

Clinical features

Sun nevus is an acquired nevus of Ota (nevus of Ota acquisita) and has been described in Chinese and Japanese patients.[1–3]

Histologic features

The features are identical to those of nevus of Ota.

Hori nevus

Clinical features

Hori nevus (nevus fuscoceruleus zygomaticus, acquired dermal melanocytosis of the face and extremities, acquired bilateral nevus of Ota-like macules) is a rare acquired bilateral dermal melanocytosis, which predominantly affects Asian females.[1–5] Patients are mostly in the third and fourth decades. Early lesions are characterized by discrete brown macules which become more confluent and slate gray in color with time.[4] No spontaneous regression of the lesions is generally seen. Hori nevus shows predilection for the malar region of the cheek, followed by the forehead, upper eyelids, temples, and root/alae of the nose.[3,4,6] Lesions can also develop at extrafacial locations.[7,8] In males, the most common site of occurrence is forehead, and the incidence of additional extrafacial lesions is high.[5] Although most commonly triggered by sun exposure and pregnancy, additional factors include hormonal medications, stress, and trauma.[4] A recent prospective study has demonstrated a positive family history in the first-degree relatives in 42% of patients.[4] Hori nevus has also been reported at sites of refractory eczema and treated psoriasis.[9,10] Mucosal involvement has been reported in a single patient.[11]

Histologic features

The features are those of a superficial dermal dendritic melanocytosis. Bipolar dendritic melanocytes are dispersed throughout the upper dermis, frequently in parallel with the epidermis and in perivascular distribution.[5]

Dermal melanocytic hamartoma

This term has been applied to a congenital dermal melanocytosis in a dermatomal distribution, otherwise indistinguishable from the nevi of Ito and Ota.[1]

Common blue nevus

Clinical features

The common blue nevus is a relatively frequently encountered lesion and, like the Mongolian blue spot and nevi of Ota and Ito, it represents arrested melanocytic migration.[1,2] Although it may present anywhere on the integument, there is a predilection for the dorsal aspects of the hands and feet, the buttocks, scalp, and face.[3,4] Lesions presenting elsewhere, including the penis and subungual area, are very rare. The nevus is typically a solitary, well-demarcated, dome-shaped, blue or blue-black lesion, usually about 1.0 cm in diameter (Figs 25.224–25.226). Rarely, eruptive and plaque-type giant congenital variants have been documented (see below).[5–8] A common blue nevus with satellite lesions is a peculiar variant that can clinically simulate a melanoma.[9–11] Blue nevi show a female predominance (2:1) and have a very wide age distribution.[4] Although typically a tumor of the integument, examples have been reported at a variety of extracutaneous sites, including, oral mucosa, palate, maxillary sinus, conjunctiva, sclera, orbit, lymph nodes, breast, cervix, vagina, prostate, spermatic cord, and pulmonary hilus.[7,12–17] Exceptionally, a common blue nevus has been associated with development of melanoma (see malignant blue nevus).[18–21] Multiple common blue nevi are rare and can occur in a familial setting.[22]

On dermoscopy, common blue nevus is characterized by typical steel-blue homogeneous coloration due to the presence of abundant pigment in the dermis.[11]

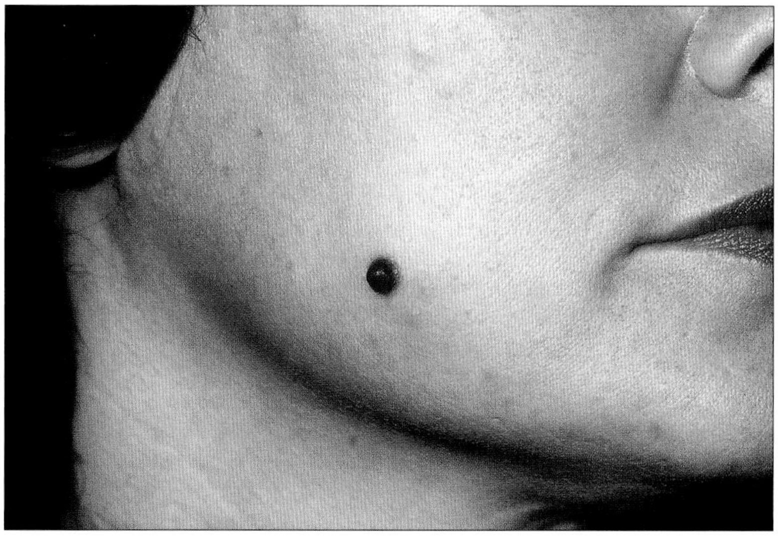

Histologic features

Common blue nevus typically lies within the deeper aspect of the reticular dermis, but occasionally may present in the superficial dermis or extend from the papillary dermis to the subcutaneous fat (Fig. 25.227). Although the overlying epidermis is usually normal, coexistent junctional activity (or a banal intradermal component) is sometimes present – the combined nevus (see above).[23] There is a population of frequently heavily pigmented, bipolar, dendritic spindled cells, associated with a host-derived dense fibroblastic and collagenous spindled cell response, and commonly accompanied by heavily pigmented melanophages (Figs 25.228 and 25.229).[4] Mitotic figures are rarely found, and there is no pleomorphism. The melanocytes frequently form aggregates around cutaneous appendages, blood vessels, and nerves, and are often oriented parallel to the surface epithelium. In general, the infiltrate of the common blue nevus is much denser than that of the nevi of Ito or Ota. Rare examples of smooth muscle hyperplasia within common/combined blue nevus have been reported.[24]

In nodal blue nevi, the pigmented spindled and dendritic cells are found within the perinodal fat, capsule, and septa but not within the lymph node parenchyma.[16,18,25]

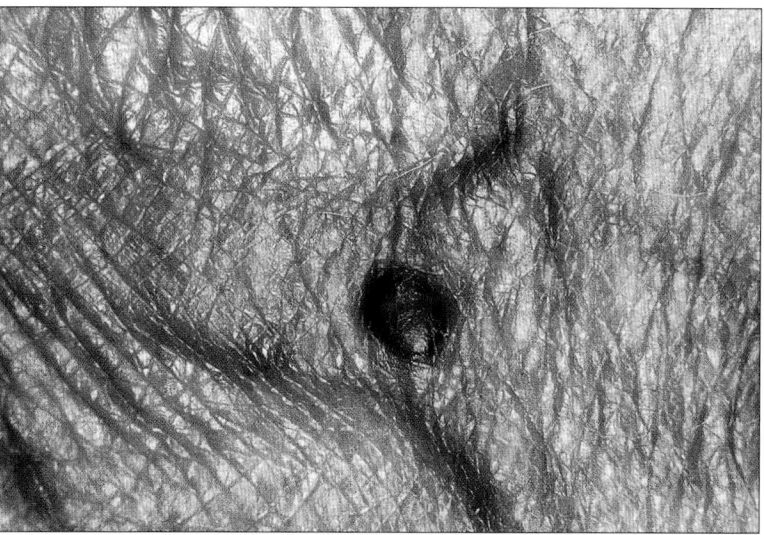

Fig. 25.225
Common blue nevus: the hand is a commonly affected site. By courtesy of A. du Vivier, MD, King's College Hospital, London, UK.

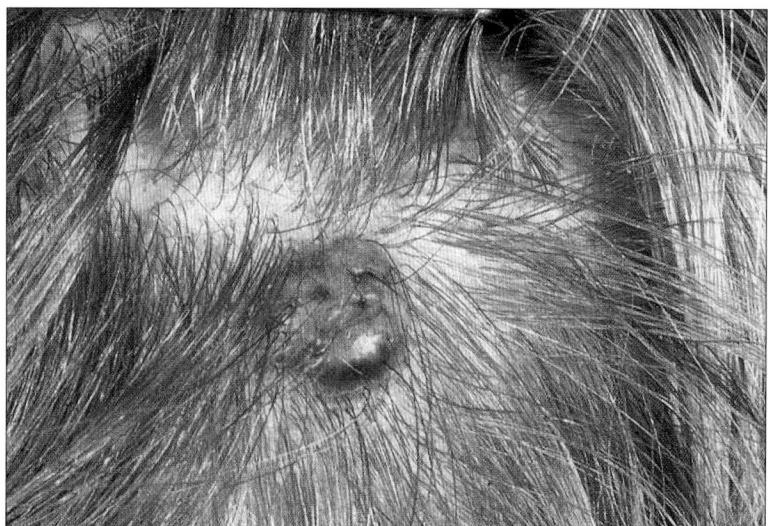

Fig. 25.226
Common blue nevus: the scalp is also frequently affected. By courtesy of the Institute of Dermatology, London, UK.

Fig. 25.224
Common blue nevus: typical dome-shaped lesion showing dark blue-black coloration. By courtesy of R.A. Marsden, MD, St George's Hospital, London, UK.

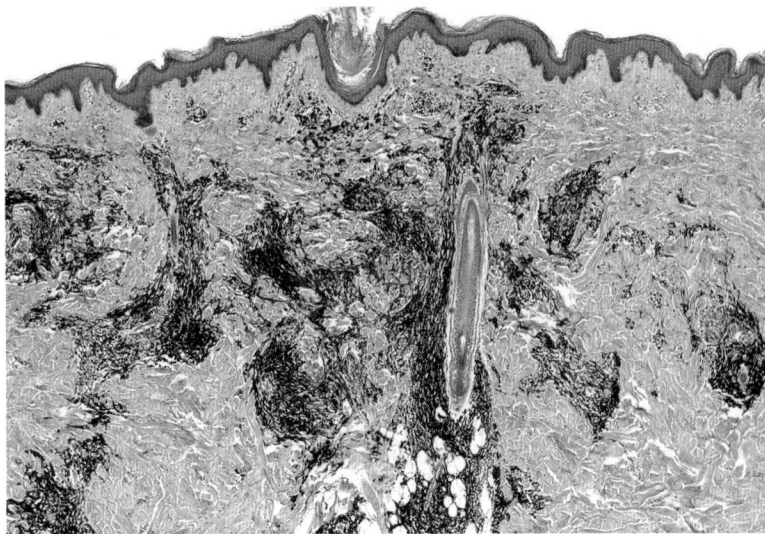

Fig. 25.227
Common blue nevus: this highly pigmented spindled cell neoplasm extensively involves the reticular dermis.

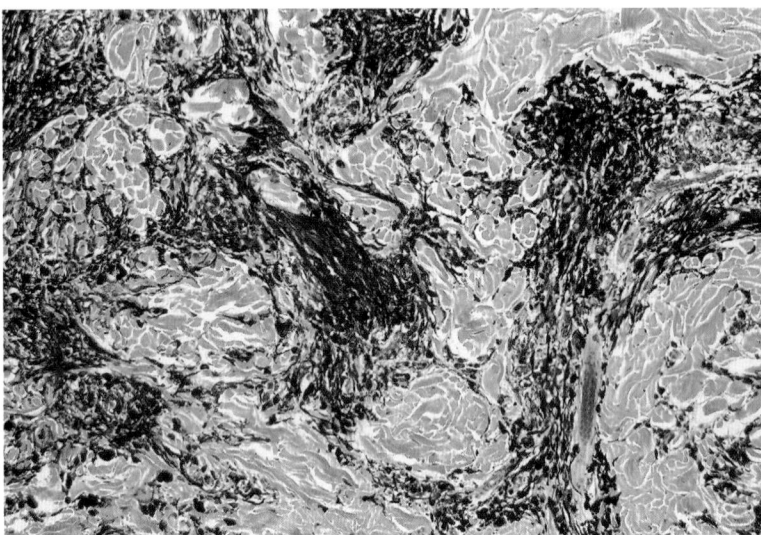

Fig. 25.228
Common blue nevus: medium-power view.

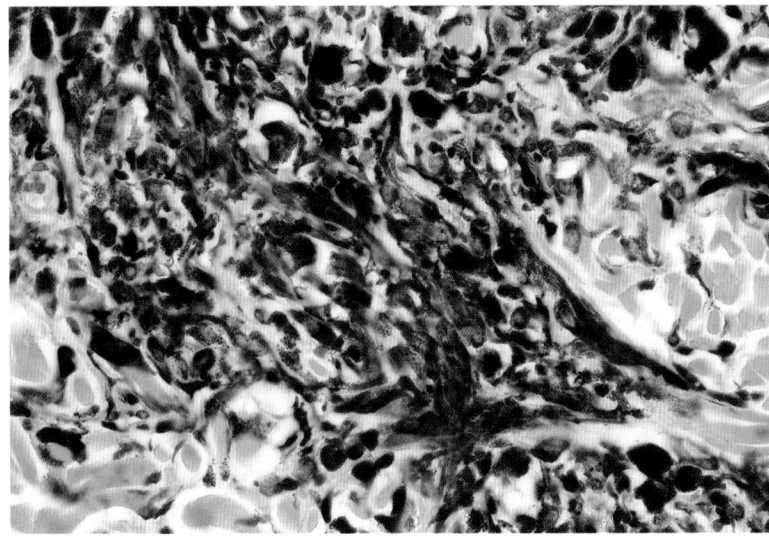

Fig. 25.229
Common blue nevus: high-power view of dendritic cells.

Patch-like blue nevus

Patch-like blue nevus refers to an acquired bilateral facial cutaneous dendritic melanocytosis with histologic features overlapping nevus of Ota and Mongolian blue spot.[1,2] A similar lesion has also been reported on the scalp and was associated with the development of local areas of vitiligo.[3]

Target blue nevus

Clinical features

Target blue nevus refers to an exceedingly rarely documented variant that presents as a dome-shaped blue nodule surrounded by a hypopigmented or flesh-colored rim which is further bordered by a blue zone, giving rise to a targetoid appearance. Lesions may be congenital or acquired, and the dorsal surface of the foot is affected.[1]

Pathogenesis and histologic features

The central nodule may be either a common or a cellular blue nevus in which the stroma is particularly sclerotic. The hypopigmented zone consists of dense collagen containing few dendritic cells, and the outer border is again rich in pigmented dendritic nevus cells.[1] The etiology of this variant is unknown, although trauma may be an important factor.[1]

Plaquelike blue nevus

Clinical features

Plaquelike blue nevus (papular plaque-type blue nevus, eruptive blue nevi, agminate blue nevi) is a rare variant, which may present at birth or develop in children or adults.[1–12] It shows a predilection for the trunk but has been described at a variety of sites including the cheek, forearm, breast, foot, scalp, and oral cavity. Clinically, it presents as a usually large (1.3–24 cm) bluish plaque containing multiple darker macules or blue-black papules or nodules. Plaquelike blue nevus has exceptionally been found in association with speckled lentiginous nevus, congenital melanocytic nevus, and atypical Spitz tumor.[13]

Histologic features

Histologically, the plaque-type blue nevus shows variable features. Most commonly, the papules and nodules represent common blue nevi and the intervening macular component shows features reminiscent of a Mongolian blue spot or a nevus of Ota (Figs 25.230 and 25.231). Less often, there are

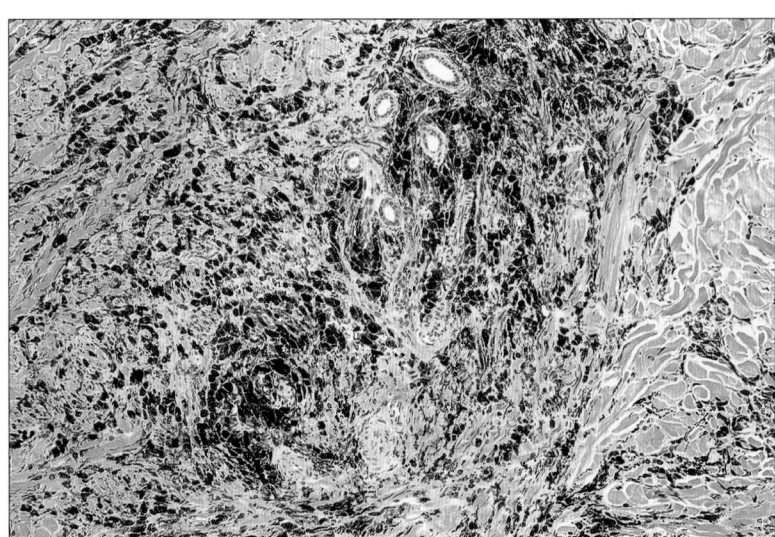

Fig. 25.230
Plaquelike blue nevus: this example shows features of a common blue nevus. By courtesy of K. Busam, MD, Memorial Sloan-Kettering Cancer Center, New York, USA.

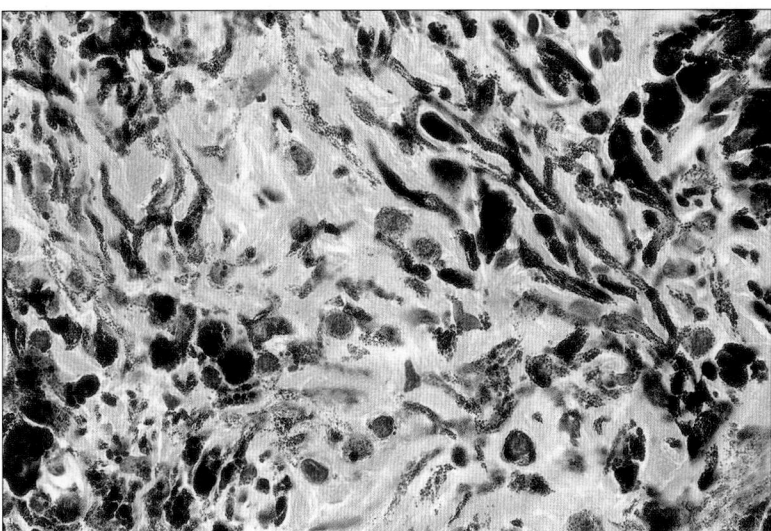

Fig. 25.231
Plaquelike blue nevus: note the heavily pigmented dendritic cells. By courtesy of K. Busam, MD, Memorial Sloan-Kettering Cancer Center, New York, USA.

cellular blue nevus-like features or foci of neurocristic hamartoma.[9–12,14,15] Lentiginous hyperplasia affecting the overlying epithelium has also been documented.[4]

Rare examples of malignant change with features of malignant blue nevus/pigment synthesizing melanoma have been documented.[12,16] However, malignant change within plaquelike blue nevus may be difficult to diagnose on morphological grounds alone and further molecular tests including CGH and fluorescence in situ hybridization are indicated to confirm melanoma-associated genomic aberrations.[16]

Compound blue nevus

Clinical features

Compound blue nevus (superficial blue nevus with prominent intraepidermal dendritic melanocytes) is a rarely documented variant of blue nevus that presents as blue-gray to blue or black papules or nodules measuring from 2 to 4 mm in greatest dimension.[1–3] Compound blue nevus shows predilection for the trunk, followed by extremities and head and neck area.[1–3] The lesion shows female predominance.

Histologic features

Histologically, the compound blue nevus is a symmetrical, well-delineated, and dome-shaped proliferation combining the features of a common blue nevus with epidermal hyperpigmentation and an intraepidermal dendritic cell population (*Fig. 25.232*).[1] Junctional nesting is usually absent.

Sclerosing (desmoplastic) blue nevus

Sclerosing blue nevus represents an uncommon atrophic variant of common blue nevus. It is characterized by a paucicellular pigmented dendritic melanocytic and melanophage population embedded in dense and often hyalinized stroma. The entity shows considerable overlap with, and is probably identical to, hypopigmented blue nevus (see below).

Hypopigmented common blue nevus

Clinical features

Hypopigmented common blue nevus (amelanotic blue nevus) is a rare and recently described variant of common blue nevus, which presents at a similar age and is seen most often on the extremities and buttocks.[1–4] Due to the lack or paucity of melanin pigment, it is usually thought to represent a banal nevus or a dermatofibroma (fibrous histiocytoma) clinically.

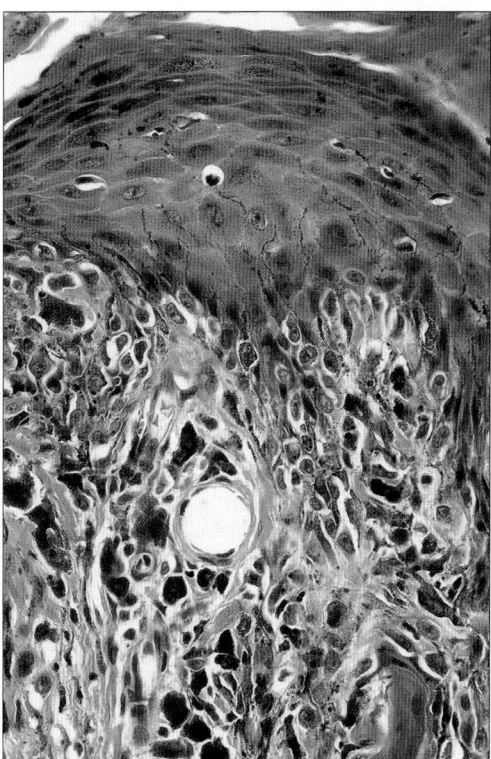

Fig. 25.232
Compound blue nevus: in addition to a dermal component, dendritic cells are apparent in the epidermis.

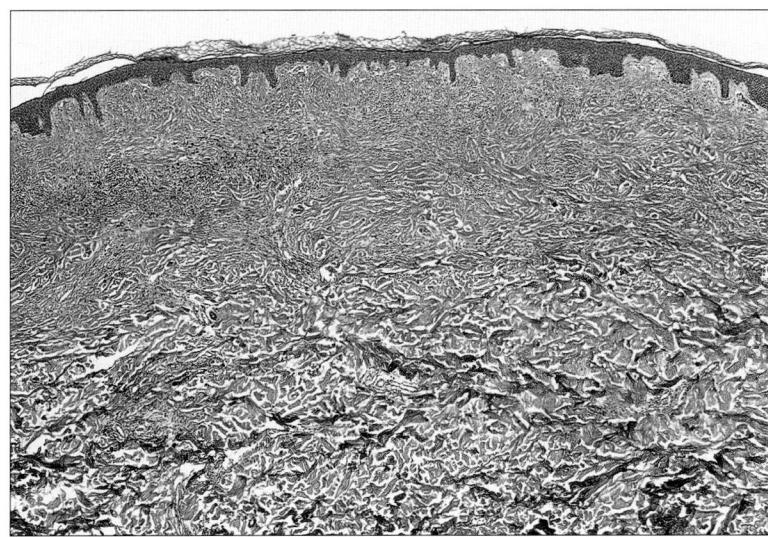

Fig. 25.233
Hypopigmented blue nevus: residual pigmentation is seen on the left side of the field. On the right, there is a paucicellular sclerosing component.

Histologic features

As with its more typical counterpart, the hypopigmented variant presents as an ill-defined infiltrating intradermal tumor. It is composed of bipolar and dendritic melanocytes dispersed in a dense collagenous stroma (*Figs 25.233 and 25.234*).[1] A storiform distribution may also sometimes be seen. The cells have indistinct eosinophilic cytoplasm and fusiform hyperchromatic nuclei often containing small nucleoli. Intranuclear cytoplasmic pseudoinclusions are occasionally evident. Melanocytes with multivacuolated cytoplasm and scalloped nuclei resembling sebocytes can exceptionally be seen.[5] Mitoses are not present. Although melanin pigment may be seen in a very small proportion of cells, it is mostly absent. Occasionally, however, it is relatively conspicuous at the edge of the lesion.[2]

Immunohistochemistry for S100 protein or HMB-45 is of value in demonstrating the bipolar and dendritic nature of the nevoid population.[1]

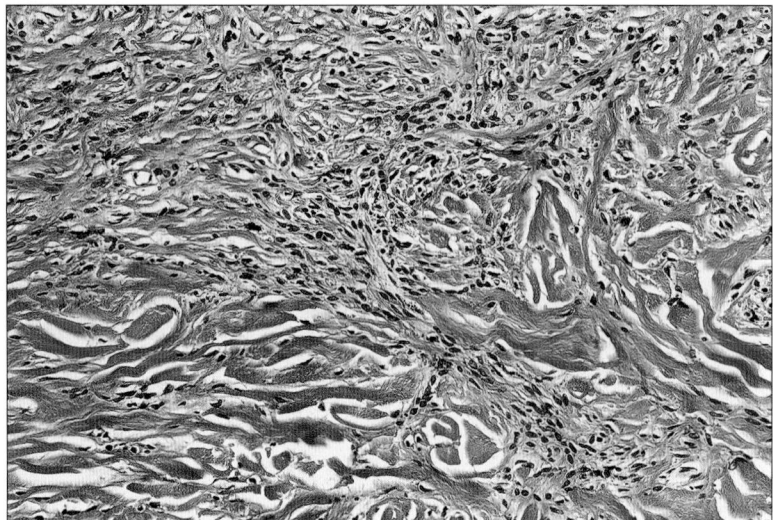

Fig. 25.234
Hypopigmented blue nevus: residual pigmentation is present. Note the nonpigmented spindle cells.

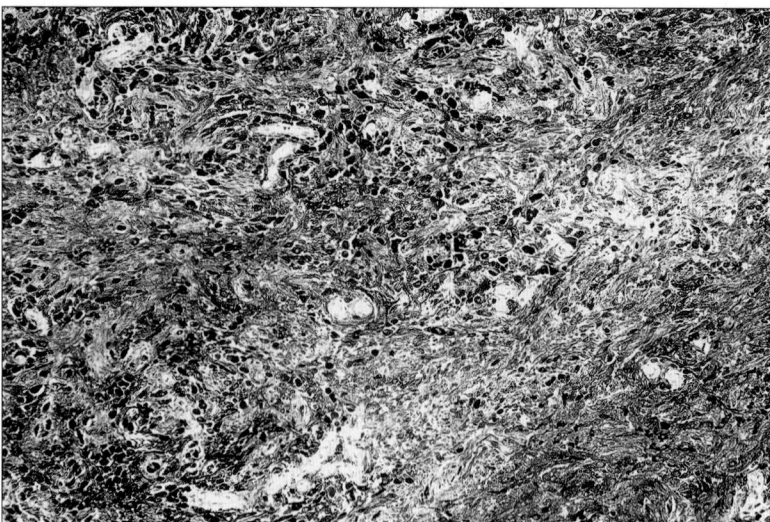

Fig. 25.235
Epithelioid blue nevus: heavily pigmented epithelioid cells are dispersed among dendritic cells and melanophages. By courtesy of C.D.M. Fletcher, MD, Brigham and Women's Hospital and Harvard Medical School, Boston, USA.

Differential diagnosis

Hypopigmented common blue nevus shows considerable overlap and is probably identical to sclerosing (common) blue nevus (see above).

Most commonly, it is confused with dermatofibroma (fibrous histiocytoma). There may, in fact, be considerable histologic overlap, and in those examples where no pigment is visible, immunohistochemical staining with S100 protein may be necessary to establish the correct diagnosis.

Occasionally, the sclerosis adopts a concentric or laminated distribution resembling so-called storiform collagenoma.[3] Immunohistochemistry may again be necessary to afford the distinction.

Epithelioid blue nevus

Clinical features

Epithelioid blue nevus is a rare variant of blue nevus that has been described most often in patients with Carney complex.[1,2] Small numbers of similar tumors presenting in the absence of Carney complex have also been documented.[3-7] Epithelioid blue nevus has also been described in the setting of a giant congenital melanocytic nevus.[8] Carney complex is an autosomal dominant condition in which patients suffer from a variety of lesions including cutaneous lentigines and blue nevi, cutaneous, mammary and cardiac myxomas, Cushing syndrome due to primary pigmented nodular adrenal hyperplasia, acromegaly due to pituitary adenoma, and sexual precocity as a result of a large cell calcifying Sertoli cell tumor. Malignant melanotic schwannian tumors (previously known as psammomatous melanotic schwannoma) is also a characteristic feature.

Epithelioid blue nevi present as blue to black or purple often dome-shaped lesions, which are most often encountered on the extremities and trunk and typically measure up to 1.0 cm in diameter.[2] Mucosal (oral and genital) involvement has been described.[9,10] Sometimes, multiple lesions may be encountered. An example of a generalized congenital variant has also been reported in an infant presenting with over 1000 epithelioid blue nevi.[11] Sporadic lesions are morphologically similar. They are biologically benign.

Some authors regard epithelioid blue nevus (both sporadic and in the context of Carney complex) and pigment synthesizing (animal-type) melanoma as part of a clinical and pathological spectrum, and use the term pigmented epithelioid melanocytoma in this context.[12,13] Lesions designated as pigmented epithelioid melanocytoma seem to have a low-grade malignant potential with frequent regional lymph node metastases (up to 60%), infrequent distant metastases, and a favorable long-term clinical course.[12,13] The term pigmented epithelioid melanocytoma is, however, controversial, and other authors suggest using the term pigment synthesizing melanoma to refer to such lesions.[14] Further long-term studies are necessary.

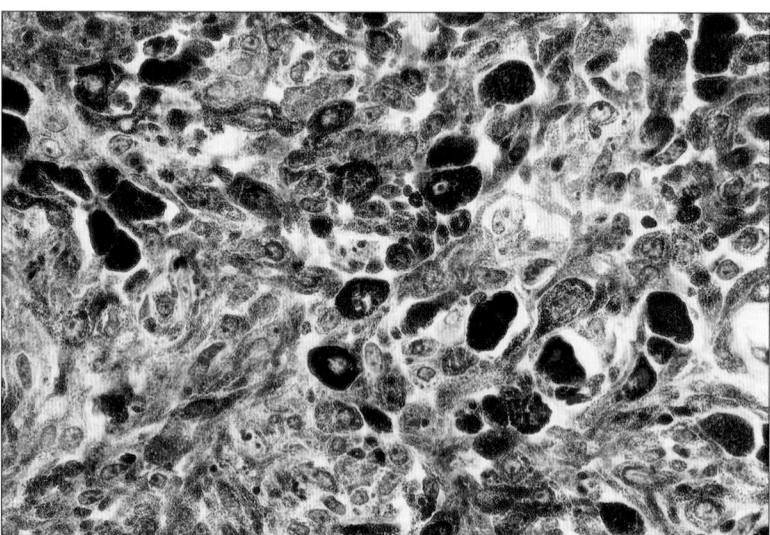

Fig. 25.236
Epithelioid blue nevus: the epithelioid cells are heavily pigmented and have vesicular nuclei with prominent nucleoli. By courtesy of C.D.M. Fletcher, MD, Brigham and Women's Hospital and Harvard Medical School, Boston, USA.

Histologic features

Epithelioid blue nevus is a poorly circumscribed, often dome-shaped, oval to spherical or wedge-shaped mass within the dermis and sometimes extending into the subcutaneous fat (*Fig. 25.235*).[2] Occasionally, combined lesions may be encountered.[4] It consists of an admixture of variably sized and heavily pigmented globular cells with small vesicular nuclei and distinct eosinophilic nucleoli and polygonal cells with only lightly pigmented cytoplasm, vesicular nuclei, and single large eosinophilic nucleoli (*Fig. 25.236*).[2] The cells are distributed interstitially, singly, in short rows, and sometimes as fascicles between the dermal collagen bundles. The adnexae are typically involved. Sparsely distributed mitotic figures may sometimes be identified. There is a background lesser population of spindled and dendritic cells. Fibrosis is not a feature of this lesion.

The globular cells express CD68 and CD163; the epithelioid forms express S100 protein and HMB-45 but not CD68.[2]

Sporadic epithelioid blue nevi are morphologically identical. Epithelioid combined nevus is associated with features of desmoplastic Spitz, deep penetrating, or banal nevus.[15]

Differential diagnosis

Epithelioid blue nevus should be distinguished from pigment synthesizing (animal-type, equine) melanoma. Cytological atypia, mitotic activity, and epidermal involvement favor the latter diagnosis.

Epithelioid and fusiform blue nevus of chronically sun-damaged skin

Clinical features

This recently described entity represents a subtype of blue nevus with predilection for sun-damaged skin of the head and neck and extremities.[1] Epithelioid and fusiform blue nevus shows female predominance (about 1.7 : 1), and most frequently presents in the seventh decade of life (from 40 to 84 years; average, 63 years) as a solitary variegated macule or papule measuring up to 1 cm in diameter. Epithelioid and fusiform blue nevus is not related to Carney complex.

The lesion is entirely benign, and recurrences following complete excision have not been reported. However, due to occurrence on sun-damaged skin coupled with mild cellular pleomorphism, nuclear atypia, and rare mitotic activity in a subset of these lesions, epithelioid and fusiform blue nevus can be mistaken for melanoma.

Histologic features

The melanocytic proliferation is typically centered in the superficial dermis and consists of plexiform growth of epithelioid and fusiform melanocytes with abundant melanin-filled cytoplasm. A second melanocytic component, a conventional blue nevus can also be identified. Solar elastotic bundles are characteristically seen admixed within epithelioid/fusiform melanocytic proliferation. No significant atypia of melanocytes is seen, and mitotic activity is usually absent. Maturation of the epithelioid component is typically preserved. However, focal moderate to high grade nuclear atypia associated with nuclear enlargement, hyperchromasia, prominent nucleoli, and occasional mitotic activity (less than 1 mitosis/mm²) can be observed in a subset of these proliferations.

Differential diagnosis

A plexiform growth pattern, lack of confluent high-grade atypia, low mitotic activity, and absence of atypical mitoses should aid in distinction from melanoma.

Neurocristic hamartoma

Clinical features

Neurocristic hamartoma (cutaneous neurocristic hamartoma, pilar neurocristic hamartoma) is an extremely rare developmental, complex hamartomatous lesion of neural crest derivation showing variable differentiation including melanocytic (nevoid, spindled cell, and dendritic components), neurosustentacular (Schwann and perineural cell), and mesenchymal fibrogenic elements.[1–11] The skin and superficial soft tissues are affected. Although the majority of these lesions are congenital, acquired variants have rarely been documented.[6] Clinically, it generally presents as a localized collection of often folliculocentric, brown, blue or black keratotic macules, papules, and nodules, sometimes with associated alopecia.[1,2,6,12] Lesions have been described on the scalp, face, neck, buttock, back, chest wall, and upper extremity.[1,2,6,12–14] Some authors have likened the condition to equine melanotic disease.[1,3] Occasional reports of melanoma complicating neurocristic hamartoma have been documented.[4,5,15] This is often a very late development.[15] Such tumors may be relatively indolent and characterized by multiple recurrences over many years or even decades.[15] Ultimately, however, metastases develop (particularly affecting the lung) in the majority of cases. Some malignant variants are characterized by very heavy pigmentation and have been described under the rubric pigment synthesizing (animal-type, equine) melanoma.[16] Neurocristic hamartoma developing in the background of a giant congenital melanocytic nevus has been reported.[17]

Histologic features

Superficially, pilar neurocristic hamartoma may show collections of banal intradermal nevus cells and common blue nevus-like features. In the reticular dermis, however, pigmented spindled cells surround the inferior segments of hair follicles and adjacent eccrine sweat glands (pilar neurocristic hamartoma) (Figs 25.237 and 25.238).[1] The hair follicles may be reduced in number or appear dystrophic.[2,16] The interfollicular dermis contains scattered heavily pigmented spindled cells and dendritic cells reminiscent of a Mongolian blue spot arising in a background of neurofibroma-like nonpigmented spindled cells containing sharply circumscribed Schwann cell nodules, sometimes associated with Meissner tactoid body-like structures.[2,6,18] Floret-like giant cells have been described.[2] There is no cytological atypia, and mitoses are absent. The overlying epidermis may be hyperpigmented and show

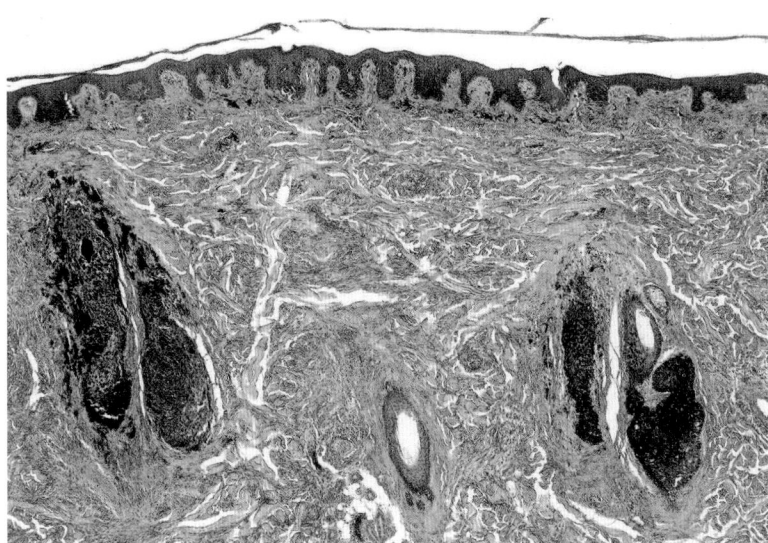

Fig. 25.237
Pilar neurocristic hamartoma: this example shows a strikingly folliculocentric lesion. The sweat glands were also involved.

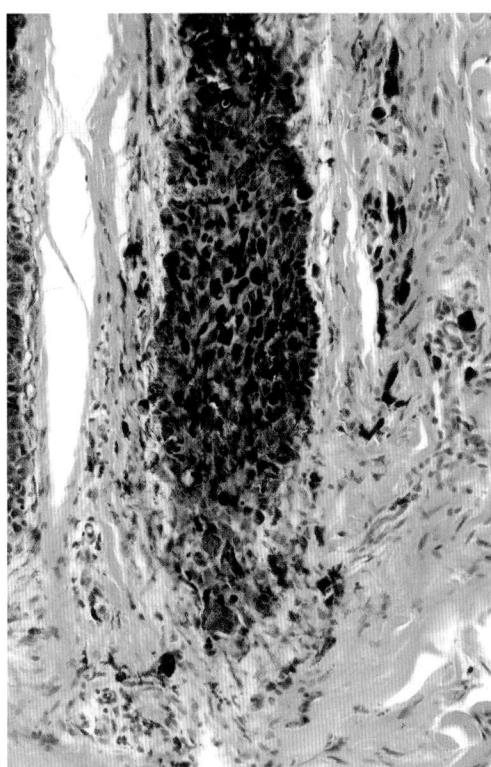

Fig. 25.238
Pilar neurocristic hamartoma: high-power view.

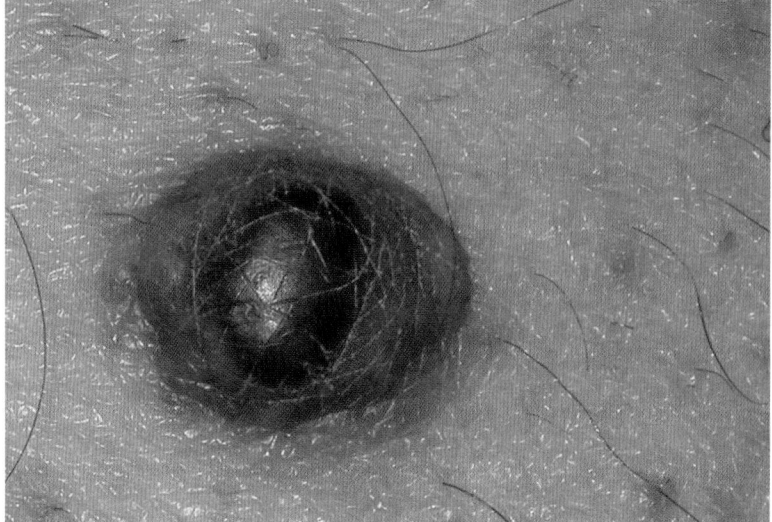

Fig. 25.239
Cellular blue nevus: large dome-shaped lesion with central blue nodule. By courtesy of J.C. Pascual, MD, Alicante, Spain.

seborrheic keratosis-like features.[1] Neurocristic hamartoma has also been described in a background of congenital nevus-like features.[15]

Deep local extension into the skeletal muscle or underlying bone, such as occipital bone with infiltration of bone marrow spaces, can exceptionally be seen in an otherwise ordinary neurocristic hamartoma.[14,19]

The melanocytic elements express both S100 protein and HMB-45. The Schwann cell nodules express S100 protein and Leu 7 but are HMB-45 negative. They are surrounded by epithelial membrane antigen (EMA)-positive perineural cells and embedded in them are CD34-positive sustentacular cells.[2]

Cellular blue nevus

The cellular blue nevus is a rare dermal neoplasm that is particularly important because it may be confused both clinically and histologically with melanoma. The recognition of benign 'metastasizing' variants is critical to prevent unnecessary potentially mutilating surgical treatment.[1,2]

Clinical features

Cellular blue nevi are uncommon lesions and occur much more often in Caucasians than in dark-skinned races. They show a female predominance (2:1).[1] Presentation is usually in the second, third, or fourth decade, but occasionally they are evident at birth.[1] Although they may arise at a wide variety of sites (scalp, face, trunk, and extremities), over 50% develop over the sacrococcygeal region and buttocks (*Fig. 25.239*).[1,3] The distal extremities are also sites of predilection.[3] Typically, they are slowly growing, grayish blue, blue-black or black, dome-shaped papules or nodules 1–2 cm or more in diameter, which may rarely ulcerate or become painful. Giant cellular blue nevi measuring in excess of 10 cm in diameter have rarely been reported.[4] Cellular blue nevus with satellitosis is characterized clinically by development of macules around a central papule or nodule, and may thus mimic a melanoma.[5] These nevi have been described at a variety of other sites including the cervix, vagina, spermatic cord, and breast.[1] Intraocular, conjunctival, and intraoral variants have also been documented.[3,6,7]

Histologic features

The cellular blue nevus is a large, often well-circumscribed nodular mass that fills the dermis and may occasionally involve the subcutaneous fat, giving the tumor a dumbbell morphology (*Fig. 25.240*).[1,3] The epidermis is normal unless the features of a combined nevus (i.e., junctional activity) are present.

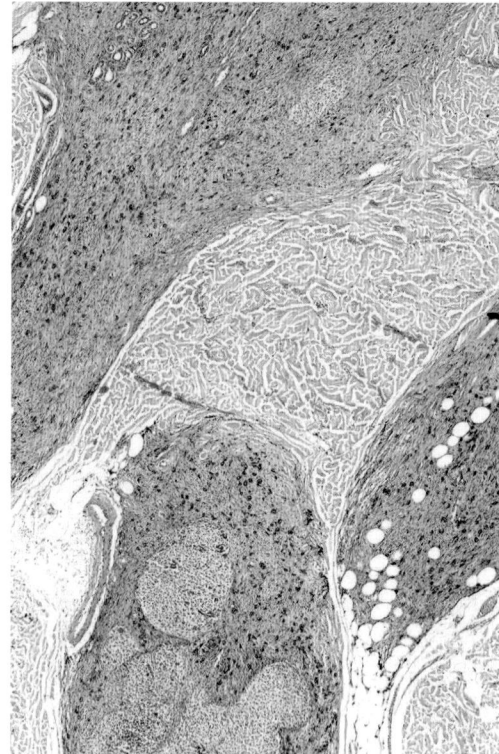

Fig. 25.240
Cellular blue nevus: this is the prototype. There is a typical dumbbell appearance.

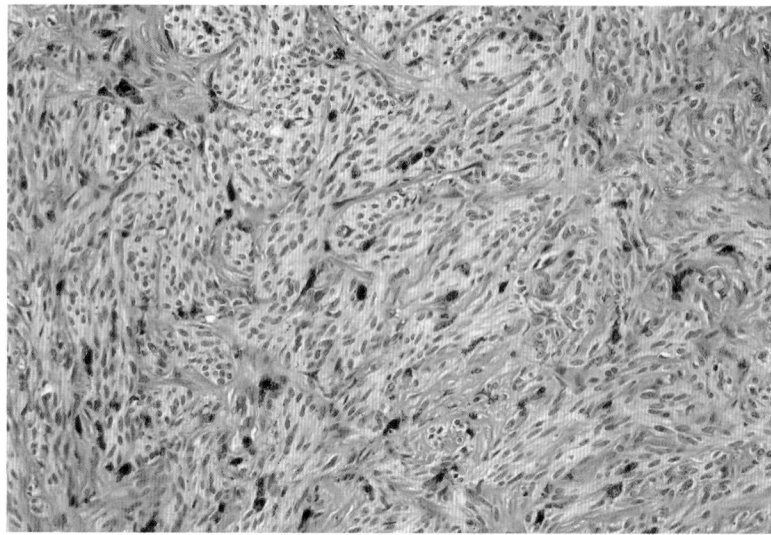

Fig. 25.241
Cellular blue nevus: the tumor is composed of a dual cell population consisting of large numbers of spindled and epithelioid cells admixed with heavily pigmented cells often arranged in an alveolar pattern, as in this example.

A number of histologic variants are recognized.[3] Most tumors show a biphasic pattern consisting of an admixture of:
- plump spindled cells with pale cytoplasm and round or oval vesicular nuclei containing small inconspicuous nucleoli,
- elongated bipolar or dendritic melanocytes containing variable quantities of fine melanin pigment indistinguishable from those seen in the common blue nevus (*Figs 25.241–25.243*).[1]

Heavily pigmented melanophages are commonly present, and the intervening stroma is frequently sclerotic. Necrosis is not a feature and mitoses are usually absent or very sparse (less than one mitosis per mm[2]) (*Fig. 25.244*).[3] Cyst formation with stromal myxoid change and vascular hyalinization – features reminiscent of ancient schwannoma – are sometimes present.[8–11]

Many tumors show an alveolar pattern characterized by nodules of plump or spindle-shaped nonpigmented or clear melanocytes surrounded by

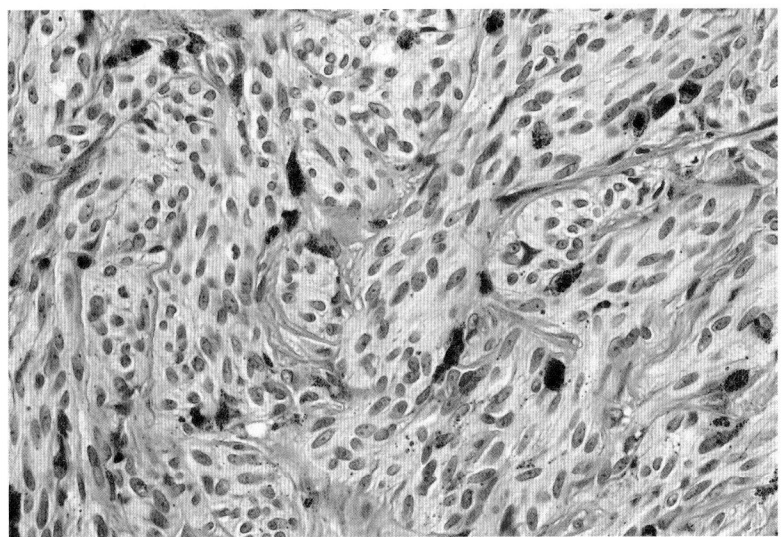

Fig. 25.242
Cellular blue nevus: high-power view. Nests of nevus cells are surrounded by fibrous septa.

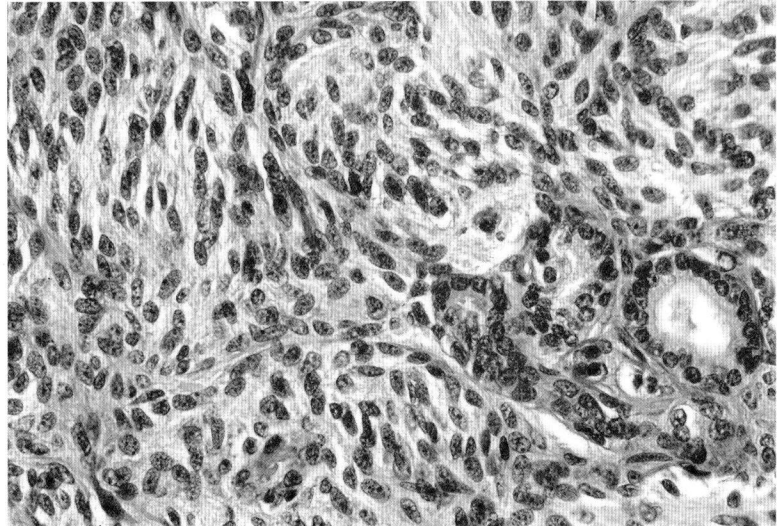

Fig. 25.243
Cellular blue nevus: there are elongated spindled cells with large oval vesicular nuclei containing prominent eosinophilic nucleoli.

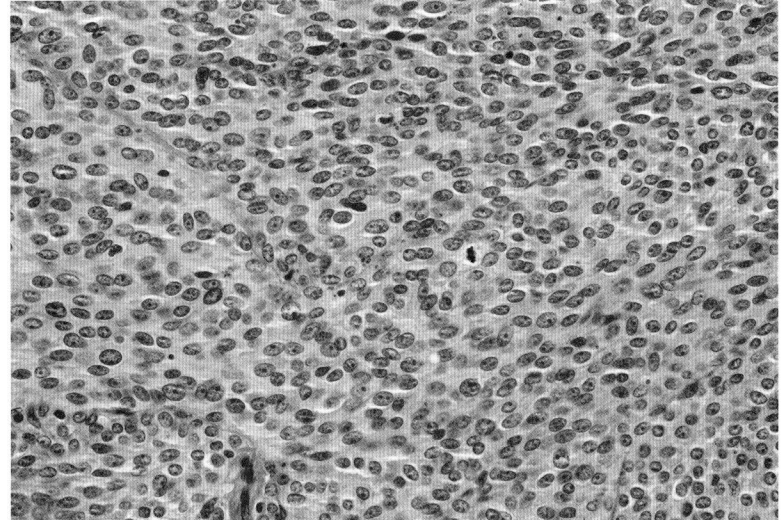

Fig. 25.244
Cellular blue nevus: mitotic figures, as seen in the center of the field, are uncommon. Atypical forms are never present.

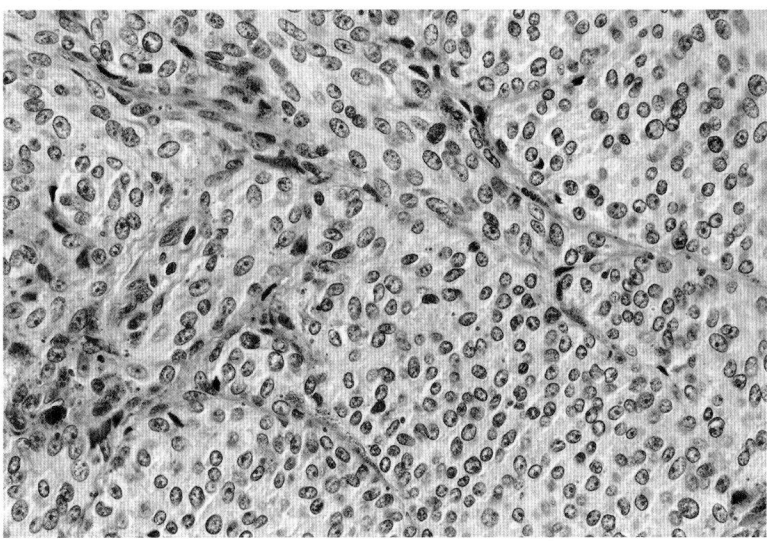

Fig. 25.245
Cellular blue nevus: an alveolar form, as shown in this field, is characteristic.

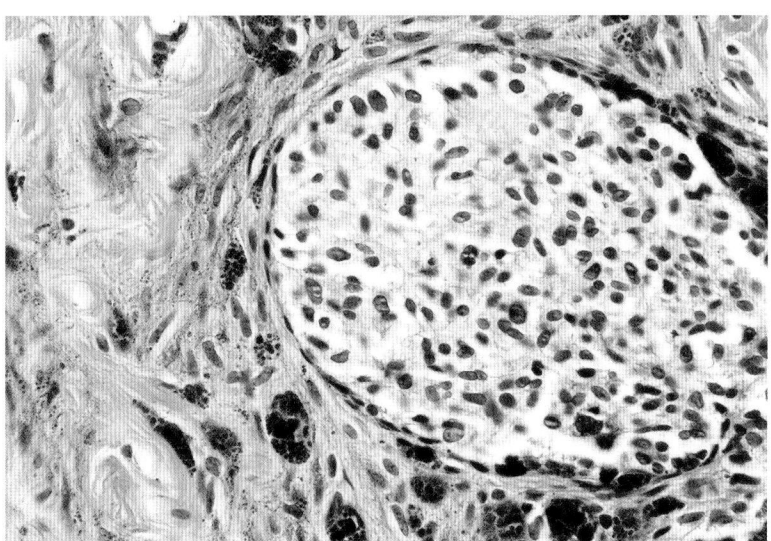

Fig. 25.246
Cellular blue nevus: note the clear cell population with surrounding spindle cells and melanophages.

dense collagenous septa containing dendritic and spindled melanocytes and often prominent pigmented macrophages (*Figs 25.245* and *25.246*). Multinucleated giant cells may be evident (*Fig. 25.247*). Necrosis is not a feature of benign cellular blue nevi. Mixed/biphasic (patternless) and fascicular/neuronevoid variants may also be encountered (*Figs 25.248–25.250*). Intralesional perineural extension is common. Combined nevi, including an overlying junctional melanocytic nevus, are occasionally seen. Balloon cell, amelanotic, and desmoplastic variants have been documented (*Figs 25.251–25.254*).[12–17] Occasionally, the margin of the cellular blue nevus infiltrates adjacent nerve trunks.[1,18]

Exceptionally, small deposits of nevus cells are found in the subcapsular sinuses and within the parenchyma of the drainage lymph nodes.[16,19] They are histologically identical to the spindled cells of the parent lesion, show no pleomorphism or mitotic activity, and do not appear to represent true metastases because they do not alter the prognosis of this benign lesion in any way.

Differential diagnosis

Cellular blue nevus must be distinguished from malignant blue nevus. Features in favor of the latter diagnosis include tumor necrosis, pleomorphism, and mitotic rate in excess of $1/mm^2$.[2,13]

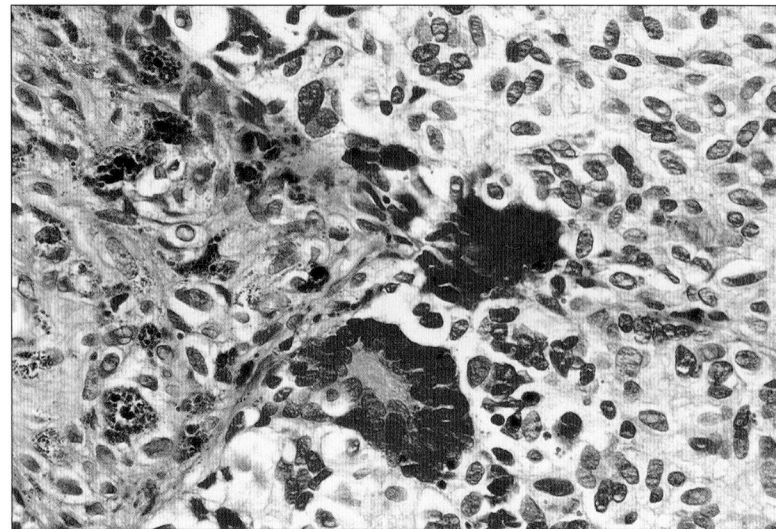

Fig. 25.247
Cellular blue nevus: multinucleated giant cells are sometimes present.

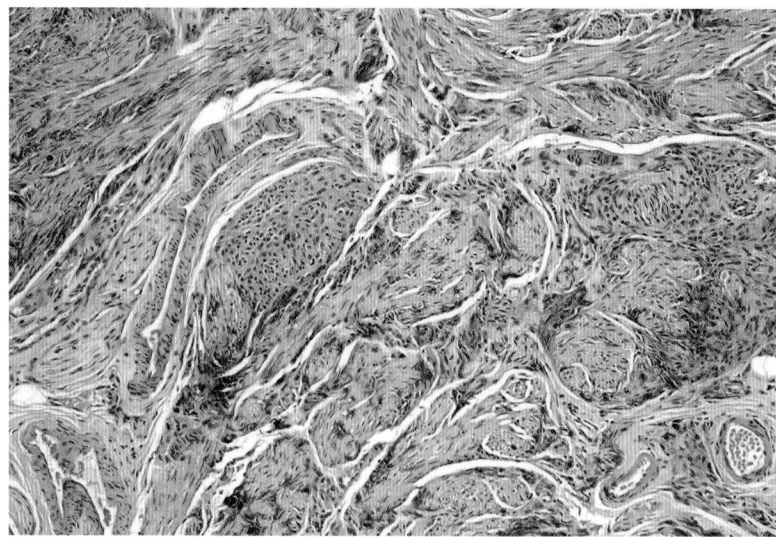

Fig. 25.250
Cellular blue nevus: this example shows a fascicular growth pattern.

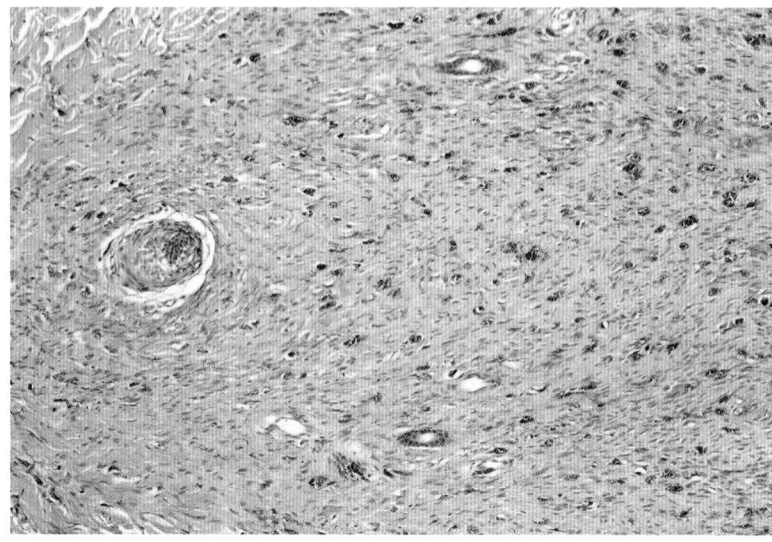

Fig. 25.248
Cellular blue nevus: low-power view of neuronevoid variant.

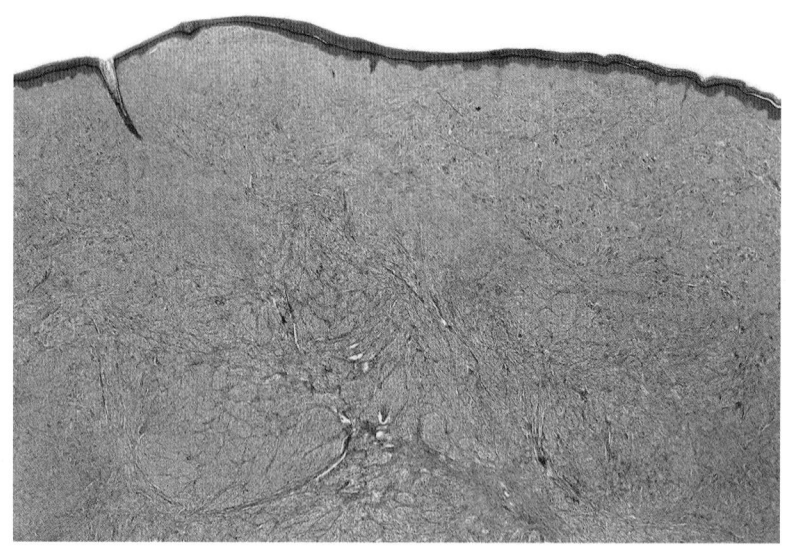

Fig. 25.251
Cellular blue nevus: low-power view of amelanotic variant.

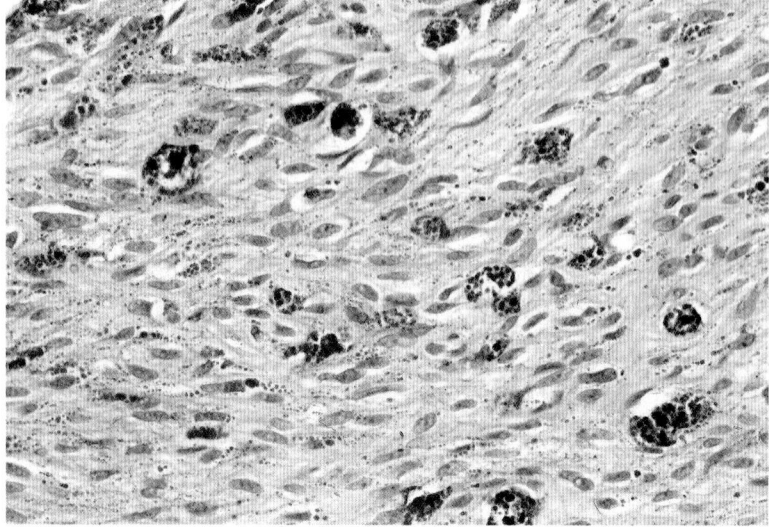

Fig. 25.249
Cellular blue nevus: the nevus cells have small twisted nuclei and pale indistinct cytoplasm in the neuronevoid variant.

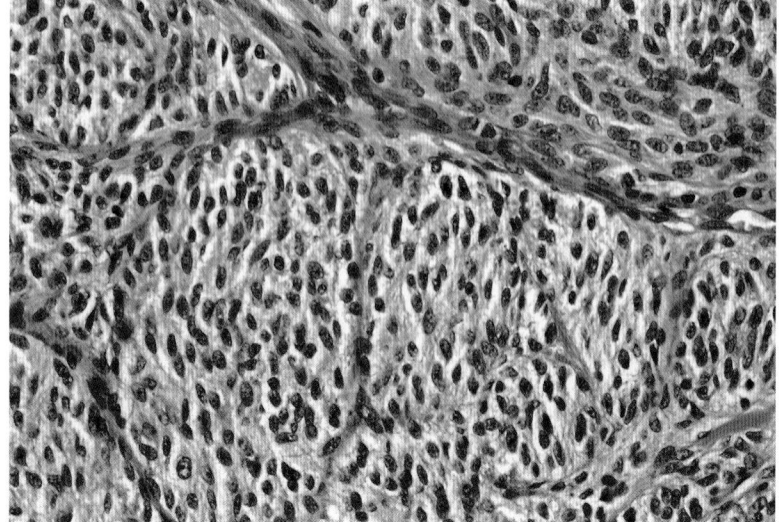

Fig. 25.252
Cellular blue nevus: this variant is composed of spindle cells with pale cytoplasm.

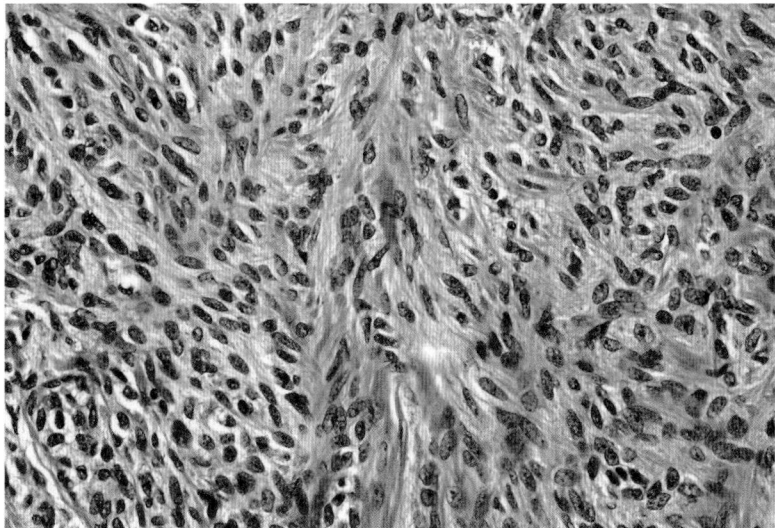

Fig. 25.253
Cellular blue nevus: careful inspection almost invariably discloses foci of pigmented cells.

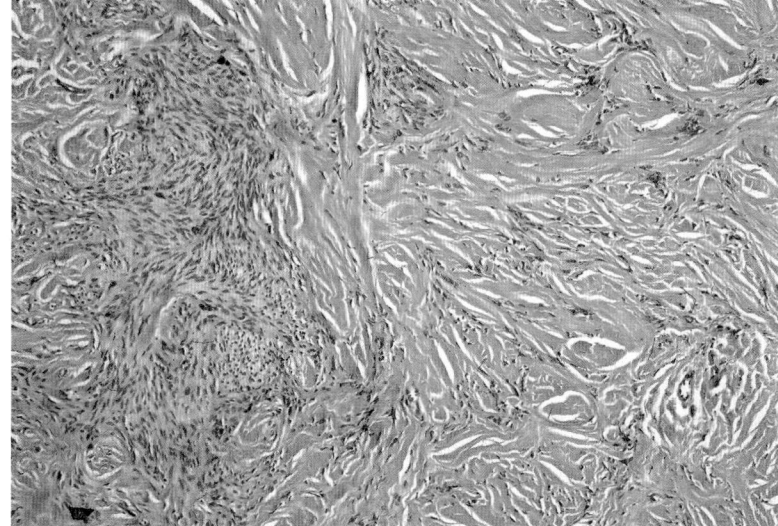

Fig. 25.254
Cellular blue nevus: desmoplastic cellular blue nevus showing residual, more typical tumor on the left side.

Locally invasive cellular blue nevus

Clinical features

This very rarely documented variant of cellular blue nevus presents in the scalp as a deeply infiltrating tumor which may involve the skull, meninges, and brain with resultant neurological abnormalities.[1,2] In the two cases described in the literature, one patient was alive and free from neurological abnormalities 13 months after surgery.[1] In another, widespread metastatic melanoma developed 3 years after incomplete surgery.[2] No further follow-up was recorded.

Histologic features

Extensive involvement of the skull, dura, and brain is characteristic of this tumor. Although no overt histologic features of frank malignancy were identified in either of the two cases documented, the very deeply infiltrating growth pattern combined with evidence of metastatic disease in one case suggests that this entity would be better regarded as a malignant rather than a locally aggressive variant of cellular blue nevus.

Atypical cellular blue nevus

Clinical features

Atypical cellular blue nevus is an extremely rare variant which occupies a position midway between cellular blue nevus and malignant blue nevus.[1-7] It presents more often in females than in males and affects the buttocks, scalp, and extremities. The age at presentation is wide, ranging from 4 to 78 years. Lesions, which are diagnosed clinically as blue nevi, seborrheic keratoses, hemangiomas or nevi, present as blue to blue-black nodules measuring up to 6 cm in diameter.

Although the documented cases have been followed by a benign course, these lesions show considerable overlap with malignant blue nevi. They are therefore best treated by complete excision with at least 1.0 cm margins and very careful follow-up. Nevertheless, a subset of atypical cellular blue nevi is associated with sentinel lymph node deposits, yet this is generally not associated with adverse biological behavior.[7]

Histologic features

Atypical blue nevus shows considerable histologic overlap with malignant blue nevus, differences being one of degree rather than any particular specific feature. Thus, atypical blue nevus presents as a biphasic multilobular lesion within the mid and deep dermis, sometimes extending into the subcutaneous fat. A background of common blue nevus is almost invariably present. The lower border of the lesion typically shows an infiltrative margin. The main bulk of the lesion consists of nests and fascicles of spindled and epithelioid cells showing mild cytological atypia: nuclear hyperchromatism, pleomorphism, and low mitotic activity of less than mitoses/mm². Heavily pigmented macrophages are an inevitable accompaniment. Abnormal mitoses are never present, and necrosis is not a feature. The atypia is centered in the lower aspect of the nevus. Perineural and periadnexal infiltration is typically present. A perivascular lymphocytic infiltrate is often seen at the edge of the lesion.

Differential diagnosis

Although the difference is one of degree only, frankly malignant blue nevus shows more cytological atypia, greater mitotic activity, abnormal mitoses, and necrosis. In cases where there is any doubt, a diagnosis of malignancy is advised.

Superficial atypical melanocytic proliferations of unknown significance

Superficial atypical melanocytic proliferations of unknown significance (SAMPUS) is a proposed designation for lesions that are difficult to separate from melanoma in situ or minimally invasive melanoma in the radial growth phase.[1,2] Defined as such, lesions designated as SAMUPS have limited, if any, capability for giving rise to metastatic disease since they lack a tumorigenic growth phase. Lesions designated as SAMPUS are generally cured by local excision with safe margins of 3–5 mm.[1]

Histologic features

The epidermal melanocytic component consists of a focal continuous lentiginous proliferation of melanocytes with random mild to moderate cytological atypia and limited upward migration of isolated melanocytes or individual nests.[1] Importantly, however, these changes are focal in nature and do not extend across the entire lesion. There is no severe cytological atypia. Furthermore, uniform nuclear atypia and mitoses are generally lacking. In the dermis, a few atypical melanocytes without mitotic activity can be observed.[2]

In the background, the histologic features of a junctional or compound dysplastic nevus, pigmented spindle cell nevus of Reed, or Spitz nevus are sometimes seen.

Comment

It seems unlikely that this represents a truly homogenous entity and that examination of additional sections and deeper levels will allow a more precise categorization in the overwhelming majority of cases. In such diffi-cult cases, the opinion of experts in the field should also be sought. We do not recommend use of this diagnostic category. It has the inherent danger of becoming a wastepaper basket diagnosis for any difficult melanocytic lesion that does not appear to readily fit into a specific category. It most certainly is of little use to the clinician or the patient!

Melanocytic tumors of uncertain malignant potential

The term 'melanocytic tumors of uncertain malignant potential' (MELTUMP) is a rather controversial expression and does not, in reality, represent a spe-cific entity in its own right (e.g., entity sui generis). MELTUMP has been proposed for lesions that defy proper categorization as clearly benign or clearly malignant. As such, MELTUMP reflects our inabilities and uncer-tainties in classification and interpretation of a subset of melanocytic lesions. MELTUMP has been used for entities such as atypical Spitz tumor and atypical blue nevus, but also for atypical epithelioid melanocytic prolif-erations of uncertain malignant potential, subsets of deep penetrating nevi, and dermal-based borderline melanocytic tumors.[1–6]

Thus, MELTUMP encompasses a group of melanocytic proliferations that share in common their propensity for locoregional lymph node metas-tases and rarity of distant metastases. Lesions designated as MELTUMP have been regarded as low-grade malignant melanocytic tumors, and it is thought that this might be due to inherent biological characteristics different from conventional melanoma.

Clinical features

Lesions designated as MELTUMP have been reported at diverse clinical sites, but show predilection for trunk and extremities, followed by shoulder, buttocks, foot, scalp, and face.[1,4] The lesions are slightly more common in females and exhibit wide age distribution (from 1 to 75 years; mean, 29 years). They are thick lesions with a mean Breslow thickness of 3.86 mm.[1] Approximately 50% of lesions are symmetrical.

Histologic features

Lesions designated as MELTUMP are characterized by deep dermal mela-nocytic component with epithelioid and/or spindled cell morphology. In addition, a number of disturbing histologic features within epidermal and particularly intradermal melanocytic components, either individually or in combination, can be seen, and include surface ulceration, consumption of the epidermis, asymmetry, lack of lateral circumscription, pagetoid spread, expansile growth, absence of maturation, atypia of melanocytes, mitotic activity including mitoses at the base of the lesion, and an inflammatory host response.[1–5] Lymphatic invasion has been associated with increased risk for melanoma metastases and melanoma associated death in a recent study on 32 cases with provisional diagnosis of MELTUMP.[7]

Biological behavior

Lesions designated as MELTUMP have been stratified as those with favorable and those with unfavorable behavior.[1] The presence of mitoses, their loca-tion near the base of the lesion, and inflammatory cell infiltrate within the lesion are histologic features that are more frequently found in MELTUMP with unfavorable prognosis. MELTUMP with unfavorable outcome were found to be associated with significantly higher frequency of tumor-related death and/or large metastatic deposits in the lymph nodes and/or visceral metastases.[1] In contrast, no evidence of metastatic disease after more than 5 years of follow-up was observed in MELTUMP with favorable behavior.[1]

Comment

Use of the term MELTUMP implies diagnostic uncertainty on behalf of the pathologist. As with 'atypical Spitz nevus', it must be composed of an admixture of benign and malignant lesions. It is highly likely that the overwhelming majority of such lesions can be more appropriately classified by the examination of extra sections, deeper levels, the appropriate use of immunohistochemistry, molecular genetic techniques, and the opinion(s) of expert(s) in the field sought unless only a partial biopsy specimen has been received. Although one should try and avoid using this diagnostic category

whenever possible, there are cases when its use is unavoidable. We do not recommend use of this diagnostic category.

The molecular pathology of melanocytic nevi

Melanocytic nevi are benign melanocytic neoplasms that arise from limited clonal expansion of genetically altered cells.[1] Nevi and melanomas fre-quently show somatic mutations in similar oncogenes, indicating that such oncogenic alterations are not sufficient for malignant transformation. To date, point mutations in the oncogenes BRAF, NRAS, HRAS, GNA11, and GNAQ have been identified in melanocytic nevi.[2,3] Oncogenes may also be activated through chromosomal translocations resulting in constitutively active kinase fusion proteins. Mutated oncogenes and kinase fusion events activate critical growth and survival-promoting pathways such as:

- the mitogen-activated protein kinase (MAP-kinase) pathway,
- the phosphatidyl-inositol-3-phosphate kinase (PI3-kinase) pathway.

The mutations and fusions lead to constitutive activation of downstream signaling pathways and as a consequence uncouple the cells from external growth-promoting stimuli. In nevi as well as melanoma, there is a striking association between types of oncogenes that are activated and the histomor-phology and clinical features of the lesions (Table 25.3):

- BRAF mutations are very common in acquired nevi of various types.[2]
- NRAS mutations occur in the majority of giant congenital nevi.[4]
- GNAQ or GNA11 is mutated in the majority of blue nevi.[3]
- HRAS mutations are found in 10% to 20% of Spitz nevi.[5]
- Kinase fusions of ROS1, ALK, NTRK1, NTRK3, RET, MET, or BRAF are found in approximately 50% of Spitz nevi.[6]

Genetic alterations in Spitz nevi

As noted above, HRAS mutations occur in a minority of Spitz nevi. HRAS mutant Spitz nevi frequently have gains of the HRAS gene at chromosome 11p and are associated with an intradermal desmoplastic and infiltrative growth pattern.[5] Approximately 50% of Spitz nevi harbor chromosomal translocations resulting in protein fusions containing the kinase domain of ROS1, NTRK1, NTRK3, ALK, BRAF, RET, or MET.[6–8] These kinase fusions form through translocations which decouple the 5′ regulatory portion of the proteins from the 3′ kinase domain, thereby leading to unrestrained kinase activity. The 5′ fusion partners are variable. When present in melanocytic tumors, these kinase fusion events produce tumors with spitzoid cytologi-cal features, with some additional distinguishing histopathological features associated with particular kinases. Tumors with ALK fusions are usually amelanotic and have plump, spindled melanocytes with prominent clefting and radially oriented, fusiform nests (Figs 25.255 and 25.256).[9] Vertically oriented, interweaving fascicles are often present in the reticular dermis, with an infiltrative growth pattern at the periphery that can be highlighted by ALK immunostaining (Figs 25.257A & B). Tumors with NTRK1 fusions have shorter fascicles and frequent extension along hair follicles and eccrine ducts. NTRK3 tumors have epithelioid or spindled melanocytes that form large nodular nests in the dermis.[8]

Mutation or loss of the BRCA1-associated protein 1 (BAP1) tumor sup-pressor gene in nevi with BRAF mutations can result in spitzoid tumors as well. Families with germline BAP1 mutations are predisposed to uveal and cutaneous melanoma, renal cell carcinoma, mesothelioma, and amelanotic, spitzoid tumors with nodular collections of epithelioid to plasmacytoid mela-nocytes with pale eosinophilic cytoplasm.[10] These spitzoid tumors are typi-cally dermal, often have multinucleated cells, and lack the typical epidermal hyperplasia and Kamino bodies associated with Spitz nevi. As they typically arise from common acquired nevi, they present in biphasic fashion with a component of small melanocytes adjacent to the spitzoid component (Fig. 25.258). A lymphohistiocytic inflammatory cell infiltrate of variable inten-sity may be seen. Mitotic activity is usually low. Both types of melanocytes frequently harbor BRAF mutations, while the spitzoid component alone has a BAP1 mutation. Immunostaining for BAP1 in areas of conventional nevus shows normal positive nuclear staining, while the spitzoid component exhibits no nuclear staining (Fig. 25.259A & B). Sometimes cytoplasmic staining is evident in the spitzoid component because some BAP1 mutations

Table 25.3
Oncogenic drivers in melanocytic nevi

Gene	Aberration	Cellular Pathway	Nevus type(s)	Histopathological features
BRAF	Point mutation	MAP kinase	Acquired nevi	-Nested pattern
BRAF	Rearrangement	MAP kinase	Congenital nevi, Spitz nevi	
NRAS	Point mutation	MAP kinase, PI3 kinase	Congenital nevi	
HRAS	Point mutation, copy number gain	MAP kinase, PI3 kinase	Spitz nevi	-Intradermal, desmoplastic, infiltrative architecture
BAP1	Truncating non- and missense mutation, deletion	BRCA1; chromatin remodeling	BAP1-inactivated spitzoid nevi	-Epithelioid, plasmacytoid melanocytes -Amelanotic, intradermal tumor -Multinucleated cells
GNAQ/GNA11	Point mutation	PKC, MAP kinase	Blue nevi, Nevi of Ota and Ito, melanocytomas, uveal nevi	-Hyperpigmented, dendritic dermal melanocytes
ALK	Rearrangement	MAP kinase, PI3 kinase, STAT3	Spitz nevi	-Fusiform melanocytes with prominent clefting -Interconnecting fascicular nesting pattern
NTRK1	Rearrangement	MAP kinase, PI3 kinase, PLCγ1, STAT3	Spitz nevi	-Fusiform nests with short fascicles -Adnexal extension
NTRK3	Rearrangement	MAP kinase, PI3 kinase, STAT3	Spitz nevi	-Epithelioid or fusiform -Large dermal nodules/nests
MET	Rearrangement	MAP kinase, PI3 kinase, STAT3	Spitz nevi	
RET	Rearrangement	MAP kinase, PI3 kinase, PLCγ1, STAT3	Spitz nevi	
ROS1	Rearrangement	MAP kinase, PI3 kinase, STAT3	Spitz nevi	

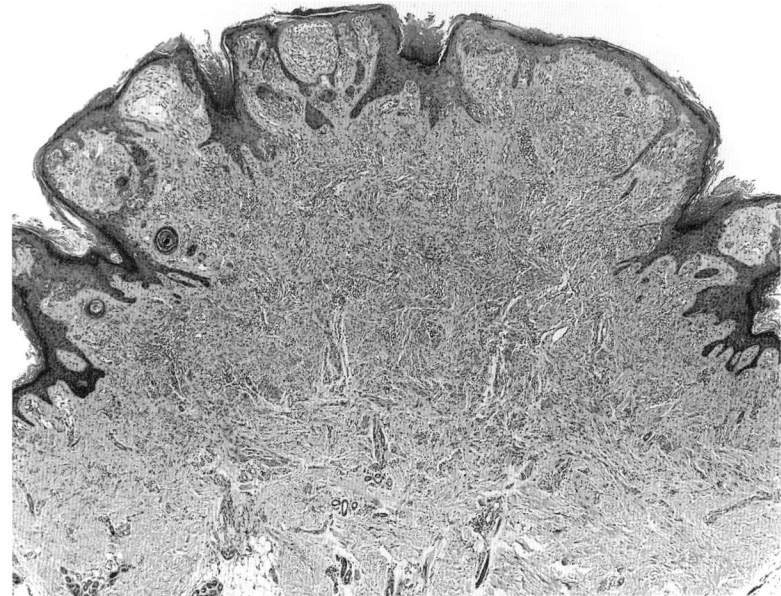

Fig. 25.255
Compound Spitz nevus with an ALK fusion: nests of melanocytes with clefts are present below an irregularly hyperplastic epidermis. Nests and fascicles of melanocytes stream from the junction into the reticular dermis with diminution of nest size in the deep portion.

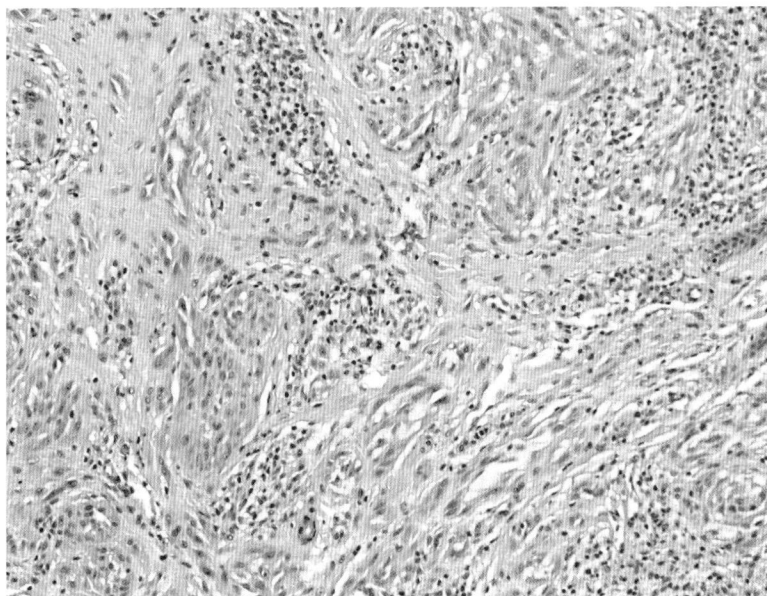

Fig. 25.256
Spitz nevus with an ALK fusion: fascicles of epithelioid and spindled melanocytes with prominent clefting in vertical orientation in the reticular dermis.

corrupt the nuclear localization sequence at the carboxy-terminus of the protein.[10] Loss of the remaining wild type *BAP1* allele typically occurs by deletion of the portion of chromosome 3p where *BAP1* resides, loss of the entire chromosome 3, or by copy number neutral loss of heterozygosity. These tumors with both *BAP1* and *BRAF* mutations represent intermediate neoplasms in which a second clonal expansion has occurred within a BRAF mutant nevus as a consequence of bi-allelic inactivation of *BAP1*.[10] Preliminary data suggest they have minimal metastatic potential at this stage of progression.[11] Patients with germline *BAP1* mutations typically have multiple of these lesions. Sporadic tumors with these histopathological features

have somatic inactivation of both *BAP1* alleles, and are not associated with germline mutations of *BAP1*.

The presence of identical oncogenic mutations in melanoma and nevi indicates that these mutations arise early during the malignant transformation of melanocytes. While they can induce a transient proliferation of cells, they are not sufficient for full transformation, which requires additional cooperating genetic alterations. This notion is supported by in vitro experiments in which the introduction of activated oncogenes such as RAS family members or the downstream kinase BRAF are insufficient by themselves to transform normal human cells.[12,13] Robust cellular safeguard mechanisms exist to restrict the proliferation of cells that acquire mutations due to repetitive exposure to UV radiation, exogenous mutagens, and reactive oxygen

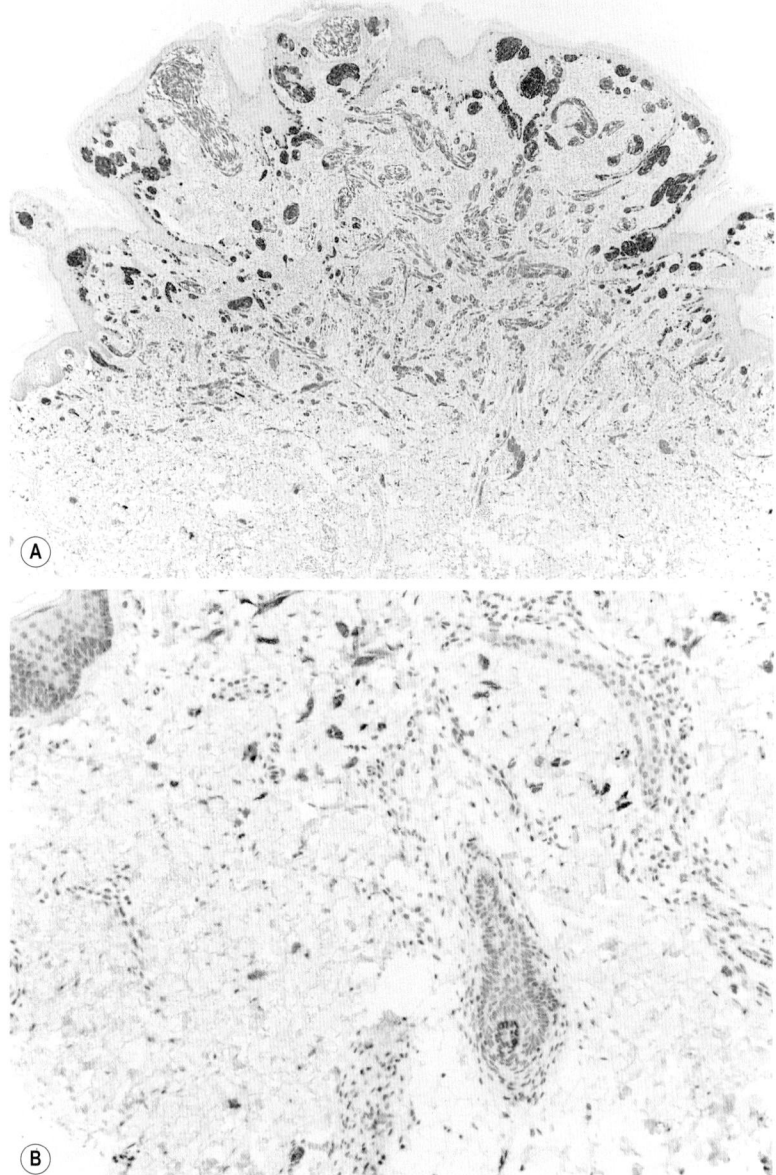

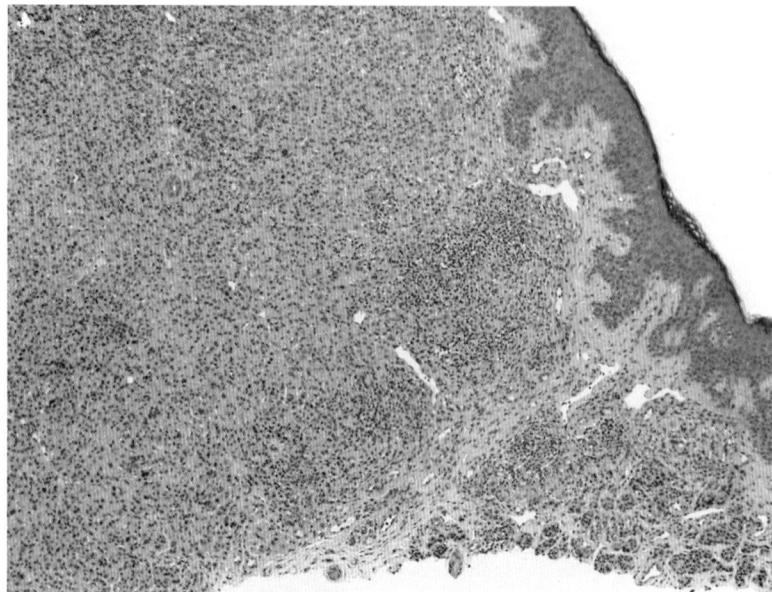

Fig. 25.258
BAP1-inactivated spitzoid tumor: adjacent to the large nodular collection of spitzoid cells, there are nests of small, round melanocytes representing a remnant population of the precursor nevus that retains a functional BAP1 protein (positive nuclear BAP1 staining).

Fig. 25.257
(**A**) Spitz nevus with an ALK fusion: ALK immunostaining highlights the entire neoplasm, including an infiltrative pattern at the periphery, with single positive melanocytes extending far from the main portion of the neoplasm (**B** or inset).

species. For instance, constitutive activation of signaling pathways such as the MAP-kinase pathway by mutations in signaling components results in abnormally high constitutive signaling flux that differs from the signaling pattern induced by exposure to a growth factor.[14] Under physiological conditions, growth signals attenuate rapidly through complex feedback mechanisms that dampen the input signal by, for example, receptor internalization and upregulation of inhibitory factors of critical signaling components (*Fig. 25.260A*). By contrast, excessive pathway activation by oncogenic mutations is thought to trigger similar and perhaps additional feedback mechanisms that counteract the growth-promoting effects (*Fig. 25.260B*). This involves the induction of cell cycle inhibitors such as p16 and p21 as well as other sensors of 'oncogenic stress' such as p14/ARF.[15] Whereas p16 and p21 are inhibitors of cyclin-dependent kinases which inactivate the RB tumor suppressor, p14/ARF acts upstream of p53 and blocks its degradation.[16] Oncogene activation engages the RB and p53 pathways which restrains proliferation. Expression of the above cell cycle inhibitory proteins can be detected in most nevi. Remarkably, however, the pattern of, for example, p16 expression within a nevus can be patchy, with some neoplastic melanocytes expressing robust levels, whereas others do not.[17] This could indicate that not all cells within a lesion rely on the same factor or mechanism to

stop proliferation. Furthermore, some cell cycle inhibitors are also found to be expressed in varying degrees in melanoma, indicating that the cells may have become resistant against their effects.[18,19] The *CDKN2A* gene, which encodes p16 and p14, appears to play a particularly important role in melanocytic neoplasia. Chromosome 9p21, where *CDKN2A* resides, is the most frequent area of chromosomal loss in melanoma, and a recent study has shown that homozygous loss of *CDKN2A* occurs frequently during the transition from nevus to invasive melanoma.[20]

According to this concept of 'oncogene-induced senescence', the growth arrest of a cell that has acquired an oncogenic mutation presents itself as a relatively acute phenomenon. However, the cell cycle arrest found in nevi appears to occur with considerable latency. In order to be clinically detectable, nevi must consist of thousands of cells produced from a considerable number of cell divisions from a progenitor cell. Oncogenic mutations in genes such as *BRAF* are found in the majority of nevus cells, indicating that these cells must have proliferated in the presence of the mutation and propagated it through the population.[21] The mechanism of oncogene-induced senescence outlined above, which relies on detecting oncogene activation by immediately triggering growth arrest in the form of a tripped fuse, does not explain this latency. It is possible that this immediate-type senescence exists in vivo, but as cells with oncogenic mutations would be arrested either immediately or after just a few rounds of divisions, the ensuing lesions would be clinically undetectable. This raises the intriguing possibility that in patients with a propensity to develop many nevi, oncogene-induced senescence may not be fully functional. Additional mechanisms of senescence appear to come into play if one of the barriers fails. For example, patients who are homozygous for loss-of-function mutations in the *CDKN2A* gene still develop nevi, although these nevi are typically large in size.[22] Different mechanisms outside the p16/p14 pathways are responsible for growth arrest in such nevi.

An alternative mechanism in the growth arrest of nevi is replicative or telomere-induced senescence (*Fig. 25.260C*). Telomeres are complex structures at chromosome ends that sequester the open ends of the DNA by forming a lariat structure with tandem DNA repeats protected by a matrix of nucleoproteins.[23] In most somatic cells, telomeres shorten with each cell division and after 60–70 divisions reach a critical length that exposes the open end of the DNA and triggers a DNA damage signal that permanently arrests the cell.[24] If this critical signal cascade is impaired, cells can continue to replicate and form end-to-end fusions of open telomeres between sister chromatids resulting in bicentric chromosomes. This leads to chromosome

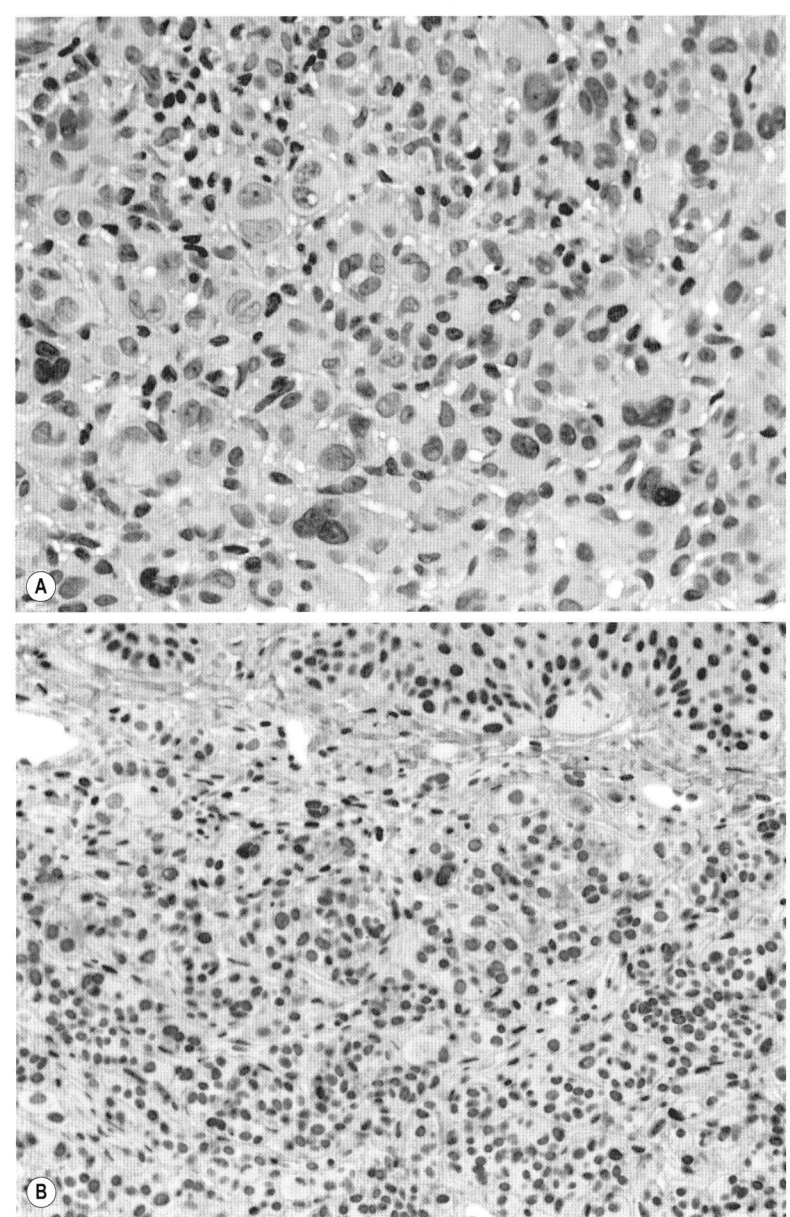

Fig. 25.259
(**A**) BAP1-inactivated spitzoid tumor: large epithelioid melanocytes with abundant pale cytoplasm form nodules in the dermis. Numerous multinucleated melanocytes are present. (**B**, inset) BAP1 stain showing intact nuclear staining of overlying epidermal keratinocytes and loss of nuclear staining in epithelioid melanocytes.

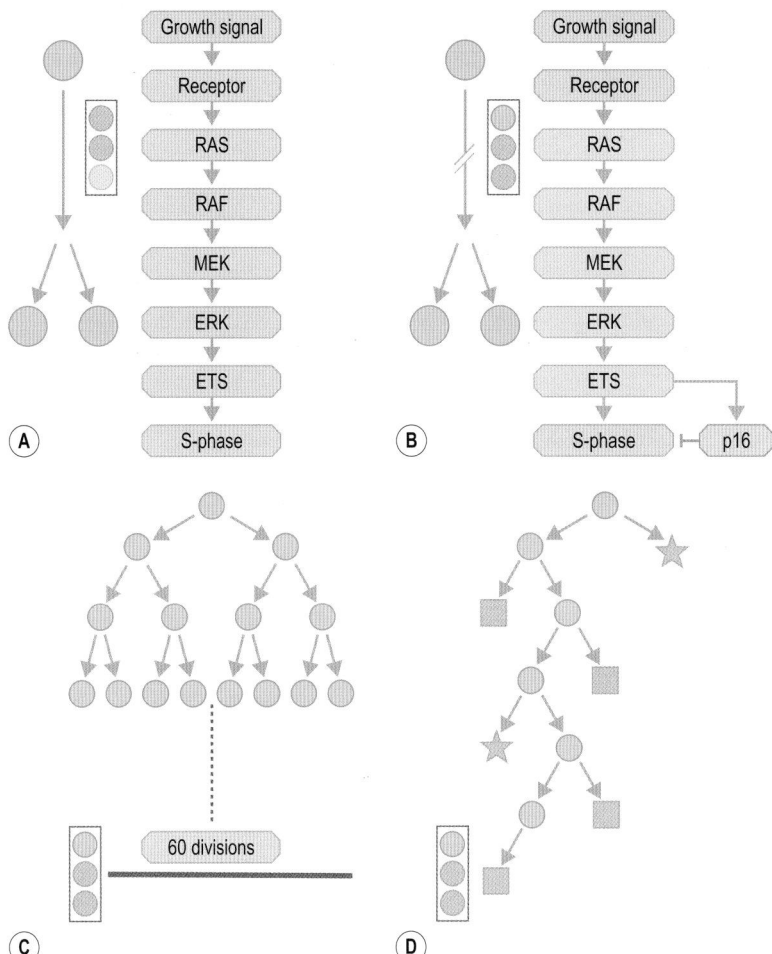

Fig. 25.260
Examples of mechanisms of senescence. (**A**) Under physiological circumstances, a growth signal is relayed down the MAP-kinase pathway and in the absence of inhibitory signals results in cell division. (**B**) If the pathway is hyperactivated, for example, by a mutation at the level of RAS, mediators of senescence such as p16 become induced and inhibit cell cycle entry. (**C**) Replicative senescence ensues when a population of cells continues to divide and exhausts its replicative potential due to telomere erosion. (**D**) DNA damaged-induced senescence is caused by random genetic alterations during the cell cycle with subsequent permanent growth arrest or apoptosis.

breakage/fusion/bridge cycles causing chromosomal gains and deletions. The ensuing genomic chaos results in a high frequency of cell death and is termed crisis.[25] Crisis, on one hand, acts as a tumor preventative mechanism for cells that have become genetically unfit because they have suffered too many genetic alterations to be compatible with viability.[24] On the other hand, it produces new genetic variants, some of which may have acquired increased proliferative capacity. The emergence of transformed clones occurs from rare cells that succeed in escaping crisis by acquiring the ability of restabilizing their telomeres, e.g., by activation of telomerase, an enzyme which extends telomeres using its own RNA template.[26] Mutations in the *TERT* promoter can facilitate production of telomerase to overcome telomere-induced senescence and are found in numerous cancers, including melanoma.[27] Recent study has shown that *TERT* promoter mutations are detectable already in intermediate-stage melanocytic neoplasms including dysplastic nevi, before full malignant transformation into melanoma has occurred.[20] The presence of TERT activation this early in the evolution of melanocytic neoplasia indicates that the cells of nevi may continue to divide to the point which their telomeres are exhausted. Most nevi are

composed of comparatively small numbers of cells, estimated to be between 10^5 and 10^6 cells, much lower than the number expected at a replicative limit of 60 cell divisions. This marked discrepancy between the expected and observed number indicates very significant attritional factors that must eliminate many of the cells in the nevus. Elimination of cells by the immune system and/or cell-autonomous mechanisms such as apoptosis are likely candidates.

Such a dynamic scenario of nevus formation and maintenance, as opposed to that of a stable population of senescent cells, would explain the changes in nevus appearance in longitudinal studies of nevus appearance.[28] It would also explain why nevi tend to fade after the age of 30. Once cells have reached their replicative life span, the balance between proliferation and attrition would tip in favor of attrition. Only lesions that have overcome this barrier by mutating the *TERT* promoter would be able to continue to proliferate (and acquire additional mutations to evolve towards melanoma).

Replicative life span is linked to nevus phenotype. Nevi acquired after birth typically do not exceed a size of 2 cm, whereas nevi that develop in utero when telomeres are longer can reach significantly larger sizes. This suggests that telomere size in the initiating melanocyte impacts the maximum size of the ensuing nevus,[29] and studies on nevus size and density have found an association with telomere length.[30] Additional mechanisms of senescence have been shown in nevi and colon adenomas that rely on an oncogene-induced inflammatory response involving interleukins 6 and 8.[31]

The link between senescence and inflammation is interesting, because many nevi, in particular dysplastic nevi, show a chronic inflammatory infiltrate.

DNA damage can also trigger growth arrest. Mutations in oncogenes such as RAS family members lead to increased DNA replication errors resulting in DNA damage.[32] Misfiring of replication origins results in abnormal DNA structures that trigger critical checkpoints, typically in a p53-dependent manner, which arrest the cells and permanently stop proliferation if the issue cannot be resolved by DNA repair mechanisms (see *Fig. 25.260*). If the problem cannot be repaired, the cells undergo a permanent growth arrest. This type of senescence has been termed *DNA damaged-induced senescence*.[33,34] The mechanism has been demonstrated in several types of precancerous lesions, including melanocytic nevi.[33] The scenario of DNA damage-induced senescence implies that a nevus can harbor cells with genetic alterations beyond simple point mutations, which arose from replication errors or missegregation of chromosomes. However, the induction of senescence in these cells restricts them from clonal expansion (*Fig. 25.261A*). By contrast, in melanoma these checkpoints are lost, allowing the proliferation of melanocytes with an abnormal genome from which clones with a favorable genomic constellation become selected

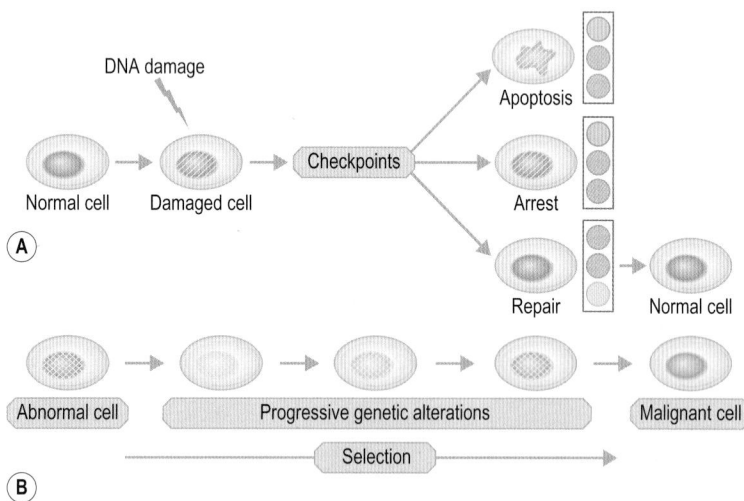

Fig. 25.261
Barriers that restrict expansion of genetically altered cells (**A**) and their failure in cancer (**B**): (**A**) If checkpoints of DNA damage are intact, any cells that acquire DNA damage are transiently arrested to give time to repair the defect. If the defect cannot be repaired, cells are permanently arrested or routed to a death pathway. (**B**) If these checkpoints fail, cells with acquired genetic alterations can clonally expand and acquire additional genetic alterations. Over time, variants with mutations that further promote growth and survival will be selected.

(*Fig. 25.261B*). This scenario would explain why clonal chromosomal aberrations are mostly absent in nevi but are very common in melanoma (*Fig. 25.262*).

In summary, current evidence strongly suggests that several independent mechanisms restrain the proliferation of melanocytes that have been initiated by activating mutations in potent oncogenes and, in concert, provide a robust barrier to cancer formation. Even if one mechanism fails, backup mechanisms can prevent malignant transformation. This concept would explain why individuals with loss-of-function alleles of *CDKN2A* can still develop nevi, albeit of larger sizes. However, if one of the senescence mechanisms is impaired, an increased risk for melanoma could ensue, explaining why inherited mutations in *CDKN2A* are a strong risk factor for melanoma.

Malignant transformation of melanocytes

The progression of melanocyte to melanocytic nevus to dysplastic nevus to melanoma in situ and finally to invasive melanoma has served as a logical model for melanoma genesis. While this step-by-step progression occurs in some melanomas, a subset of melanomas arises without an associated nevus or in situ component (e.g., primary dermal melanoma, blue nevus-like melanoma). The number of genetic alterations necessary for melanoma formation varies depending on an individual's inherent genetic susceptibility and the sequence and combination of genetic alterations that develop. In vitro studies using defined genetic elements indicate that as little as three different mutations are sufficient to induce melanoma-like lesions in human skin grafted on mice.[12] As opposed to experimental settings, genetic alterations in real cancers typically arise sequentially. Mutations in genes driving proliferation such as BRAF, NRAS, and GNAQ/11 drive clonal expansion of melanocytes. If such initiating mutations occur in cells with intact senescence pathways, dysregulated growth triggers protective tumor suppressor checkpoints to limit proliferation and a melanocytic nevus is formed. When those proliferation-inducing mutations occur in cells harboring genetic defects that have disabled such checkpoint mechanisms, stages in the stepwise progression model can be bypassed. This is illustrated in patients with germline *CDKN2A* mutations who have an inherent defect in one tumor suppressor pathway. As opposed to most individuals without this mutation, these individuals develop large atypical nevi, seemingly bypassing the first benign nevus stage in which only a single pathogenic mutation (e.g., $BRAF^{V600E}$) is present. It could therefore be expected that if a cell already harboring inactivated tumor suppressor pathway(s) subsequently acquired a proliferation-inducing mutation, 'de novo' melanoma could ensue, bypassing any phenotypically visible precursor stage.[35] The combination of genetic aberrations dictates the stage of malignant transformation, with some combinations having more transforming consequences than others. For example, the combination of BRAF and BAP1 mutations appears to have low malignant potential,[11] whereas combining GNAQ/11 with BAP1 mutations generates tumors with high metastatic potential.[36,37]

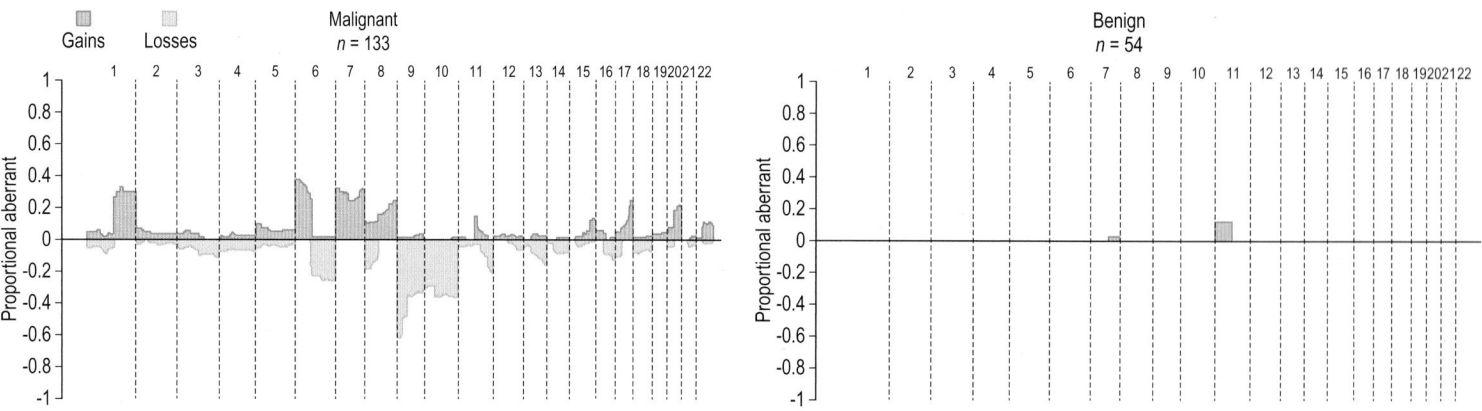

Fig. 25.262
Comparative genomic hybridization of melanoma (malignant) and nevi (benign): on the left, melanomas (*n* = 133) are associated with multiple copy number gains and losses that cluster. In contrast, the nevi (*n* = 54) on the right show minimal changes with the exception of the 11p copy number increase or amplification in Spitz nevi which includes the *HRAS* gene. These differences can be exploited using multiplexed FISH assays to support the diagnosis of melanoma or nevus in challenging cases.

Intermediate tumors (dysplastic/atypical nevi)

The existence of an intermediate category between the spectrum of nevus and melanoma has been controversial. Diagnostic discordance in tumors with mixed histopathological features has been documented in numerous studies, indicative of a histopathological gray zone but not necessarily a biological one. A recent investigation into the genetic events associated with melanoma progression has characterized the genetic profile of such intermediate lesions with intermediate histopathological characteristics.[20] Unequivocal nevi, defined in the study by diagnostic concordance among multiple dermatopathologists, were found to have a single driver mutation, typically $BRAF^{V600E}$. By contrast, intermediate lesions with more atypical histopathological features also had activating mutations in the MAP-kinase pathway, but these were enriched for other types of $BRAF$ mutations and $NRAS$ mutations. Intermediate lesions typically also had additional mutations such as $TERT$ promoter and/or hemizygous $CDKN2A$ mutations, supporting the existence of a genetically distinct intermediate category in which multiple genetic aberrations have accrued rather than the solitary pathogenic mutations found in unequivocal benign nevi. The transition to invasive melanoma is characterized by further genetic aberrations and includes mutations in genes such as $PTEN$, $TP53$, $ARID1/2$, and homozygous $CDKN2A$ mutations. Indications of intermediate stages have also been found in neoplasms with a cellular blue nevus phenotype[38] and atypical Spitz tumors.[39,40]

Striking differences exist in the number of genetic aberrations such as chromosomal gains and losses between nevi and melanomas. While the vast majority of melanomas show chromosomal aberrations, they are infrequent in nevi (see *Fig. 25.262*).[41] These chromosomal aberrations in melanomas are clonal in nature, i.e., aberrations that are found in the majority of the constituent melanocytes.[42] This can be demonstrated by techniques such as CGH, which measures the average DNA copy number of a population of cells across the entire genome.[43] Additionally, the pattern of chromosomal gains and losses is not random, but preferentially selects for specific chromosomal regions that harbor critical genes that inhibit progression (and therefore are decreased in copy number) or promote melanoma growth (and therefore are increased in copy number). For example, chromosome 9p21, which harbors the $CDKN2A$ gene mentioned above, is lost in more than 60% of melanomas, whereas chromosome 7q31, where $BRAF$ is located, is commonly gained, in particular in melanomas with $BRAF$ mutations.

Genetic biomarkers to assist diagnosis

The existence of multiple mechanisms that help deter malignant transformation in genetically damaged melanocytes limits the use of biomarkers to help distinguish benign from malignant lesions. Specifically, the redundant nature of the various senescence mechanisms makes it difficult to establish a lesion as malignant just because one barrier is dysfunctional. Assessment of cell proliferation also does not determine whether such proliferative activity within a given lesion is temporary, i.e., pre-senescent, or unrestricted.

The ability to detect clonal populations of cells with chromosomal aberrations represents a diagnostic parameter to assess the aftermath of barrier failure. CGH studies of benign nevi of various types show that the vast majority have no detectable copy number changes.[41] This finding does not exclude the possibility that chromosomal aberrations exist in individual melanocytes of nevi or that random aberrations are present in many of the cells. This finding indicates that any such cells have not undergone significant clonal expansion. Only a few categories of benign nevi studied by CGH have registered copy number changes. These include gains of chromosome 11p in $HRAS$ mutant Spitz nevi[44] and gains or losses of entire chromosomes in atypical nodular proliferations (proliferative nodules) arising in giant congenital nevi.[45] Copy number increases of chromosome 11p are not found in melanoma, and the aberrations in atypical nodular proliferation also have distinctive features. The latter frequently show gains or losses of entire chromosomes including loss of chromosome 7, which if altered in melanoma is gained, and chromosome 10 gain, which shows reciprocal copy number changes in melanoma. In contrast to the whole chromosomal gains and losses of proliferative nodules, most melanomas have losses or gains involving partial chromosomes. The most common aberrations in melanoma in decreasing order of frequency include losses of chromosomes 9p, 10q, 9q, 6q, 8p, and 11q and gains of chromosome 6p, 7, 1q, 8q, 17q, and 20 (*Fig. 25.262*). Therefore, both detection of aberrations and the pattern of aberrations help distinguish between nevi and melanomas.

The recurrent pattern of chromosomal aberrations in melanoma allows for assessment of such aberrations by more focused methods such as FISH. FISH can be applied to fixed tissue and allows a faster turnaround time and analysis of smaller samples than CGH, including entirely intraepidermal lesions. Multiple studies have shown the combination of probes targeted to chromosomes 6p, 6 centromere, 6q, and 11q can distinguish melanomas from nevi with a high specificity (approximately 95%) and acceptable sensitivity (approximately 85%).[46–49] The sensitivity and specificity in histopathologically ambiguous tumors is more difficult to assess given the limited number of such cases with long-term follow-up data. Of particular interest are spitzoid tumors, which are particularly prone to diagnostic uncertainty. The limited available data on such tumors that eventuated in metastatic disease and death suggest that homozygous $CDKN2A$ loss and $TERT$ promoter mutation are associated with metastatic potential.[40,50] A second set of FISH probes targeting chromosomes 6p, 8q, 9p, and 11q has been adopted by some to better target spitzoid tumors.[51] The use of tailored probe sets for specific differential diagnostic situations could help raise the sensitivity of FISH-based assays in the future.

Access **ExpertConsult.com** for the complete list of references

CHAPTER

26

See
www.expertconsult.com
for references and
additional material

Melanoma

Jeffrey P. North, Boris C. Bastian and Alexander J. Lazar

MELANOMA

Clinical features

Over the last several decades, the conspicuous increasing incidence of this malignant neoplasm has made this disease more prominent, linked to some rise in morbidity and mortality.[1-7] While roughly half of the major cancers in the United States showed decreasing incidence trends from 2009 to 2013, melanoma incidence continued to significantly increase over this period just as it had done previously in both men and women.[8,9] At present it accounts for approximately 4% and 6% of all new malignancies in females and males, respectively.[5] This has made melanoma the fifth and sixth most common cancers in the United States in terms of estimated new cases in 2017.[10] However, the number of deaths from this disease places it well outside the top 10 causes of cancer-related deaths for both sexes at 9730 annually.[10] Mortality for this disease is still increasing in males, but has leveled off and appears to be decreasing in females, according to present data.[6] Currently, the average rate of increasing incidence is of the order of 4–6% per year.[7,11-13] The estimated number of new cases of melanoma per year is in excess of 87,000 in the United States.[6,10,14] Current projections for non-Hispanic white individuals in the United States estimate that 1 person in 28 males and 1 in 44 females will ultimately develop melanoma.[10,15] Men are 1.6 times more likely to suffer from melanoma, but 2.4 times more likely to die of the disease.[10]

Although melanoma is seen predominantly in adults, it occasionally presents in children.[10,16-23] The latter often have an associated risk factor, such as xeroderma pigmentosum, congenital bathing-trunk nevus, familial dysplastic nevus syndrome or familial melanoma, and possibly immunosuppression. Pediatric melanoma accounts for 1–3% of all childhood malignancies, amounting to less than 500 cases per year in the United States.[24-26] Its biological behavior is more variable and difficult to predict than melanoma in adults, especially in patients less than 10 years of age; however, metastasis rates of 36–39% and overall mortality of 10–29% after 5 years or more follow-up have been documented.[20,27,28] Transplacental spread with resultant congenital melanoma has been documented exceptionally rarely.[29]

Melanoma may:
- develop within a pre-existent benign (congenital or acquired) melanocytic nevus,[30-36]
- complicate a dysplastic nevus,
- arise de novo,
- very rarely, evolve within a cellular blue nevus or other dermal dendrocytosis (see malignant blue nevus).

Precise figures are not available, but considering that the average adult has approximately 15–40 acquired melanocytic nevi and that the incidence of melanoma in the United States is roughly 30 per 100,000 of the population per annum, then the likelihood of any one benign acquired melanocytic nevus undergoing malignant transformation is markedly remote.[2,37] On the other hand, at least 35% of nodular and superficial spreading melanomas arise within a background of melanocytic nevi (congenital, acquired or dysplastic).[3,30,36,38-42] Only very rarely do the more typical (small) congenital nevi develop melanomatous features. Giant 'bathing-trunk' variants, however, are a greater cause for concern, with approximately 3–18% undergoing malignant transformation.[22,43-45] Lentigo maligna melanoma is not associated with pre-existent benign or dysplastic nevi.

While the etiology is multifactorial, including genetic and racial factors, by far the most important known predisposing environmental agent in the majority of tumors (with the exception of acral lentiginous and mucosal variants) is excessive exposure to ultraviolet (UV) light.[46-49] Surprisingly, the contribution of the UV is modest, with an estimated 1.7-fold increase in risk.[50] Although traditionally UVB has been regarded as the causative agent, more recent evidence implicates UVA, at least in some patients.[51-55] This association is complex and recent compelling work also stresses the importance of moderate, non-burning sun exposure for overall human health including vitamin D production and other benefits—including prevention of skin cancer.[56-58] Melanin pigment protects against the effects of solar irradiation and therefore cutaneous melanoma is rare in dark-skinned races, except for albinos and at those sites where pigment is absent (e.g., nail beds, palms, soles, and mucous membranes). UV irradiation, possibly by inducing free-radical formation, results in the development of dimers between adjacent pyrimidine molecules. Patients who lack the necessary endonucleases for repairing such damage, such as those with xeroderma pigmentosum, have a greatly increased risk of developing cutaneous neoplasms, including melanoma.[59]

Melanoma is particularly common in those individuals who are most susceptible to the effects of excessive sunlight (e.g., Celts with red hair, blue eyes, and fair complexions who tan poorly and tend towards sunburn and excessive freckling, i.e., skin types I and II). It is noteworthy that the incidence of superficial spreading melanoma is more closely related to sporadic intensive exposure to sunlight, particularly isolated episodes of severe sunburn in childhood, rather than to chronic lifelong exposure as with lentigo maligna melanoma.[47,53,60-62] It is more common in those who sporadically sunbathe than in long-term outdoor workers. The relationship between melanoma and sunlight is further highlighted by the increasing incidence towards the equator where UV radiation is most intense.[49,63]

Patients who already have one melanoma have an increased risk of developing a second independent primary tumor. The reported incidence varies from 1% to 8% of cases, with the upper end of this range being seen in the setting of familial melanoma.[64-67] It should be noted, however, that much of the literature referring to multiple melanomas does not take epidermotropic metastatic disease into account and therefore the true incidence is likely to be towards the lower figure. The incidence of other cancers is increased in melanoma survivors as well.[68]

There is a lack of convincing evidence that pregnancy strongly influences the outcome and prognosis of melanoma.[69-71] Although earlier studies indicated that the mean thickness of pregnancy-associated tumors was significantly greater than that of nonpregnancy-associated melanomas, later studies have not, and the clinical outcome parallels that of nonpregnant female patients of the same age and tumor characteristics, though dissenting meta-analyses remain.[72-84] Similarly, there is no clearly acceptable proof that the use of oral contraceptives by females increases the risk of developing melanoma.[69,74,85]

Familial melanoma accounts for between 8% and 14% of affected patients.[86,87] Genes that have been implicated include CDKN2A (9p21) (the majority), and very occasionally CDK4 (12q14). The former encodes p16, which normally functions to inhibit CDK4 activity.[88,89] Approximately 20–30% of patients with familial melanoma have germline mutations in CDKN2A.[86,90,91] Genetic variants in MC1R encoding the melanocortin 1 receptor and associated with red hair appears to increase the penetrance of melanoma in CDKN2A and CDK4 germline families.[92,93] BAP1 germline deficits are associated with familial ocular melanoma.[94-96] Researchers are focusing on other predisposition genes as well, such as EBF3, though additional work is needed.[97] Familial melanoma patients are often younger than those who develop sporadic melanoma and tumors are frequently multiple. Dysplastic nevi can be present.[98]

Melanoma shows a male preponderance (3:2) and males have a higher mortality.[6,10,37] This probably relates at least in part to later presentation. Females generally have thinner tumors than males at first examination. The leg (particularly the calf) is the site of predilection in females, whereas the back is most often affected in males.[37] Melanoma arising on the head and neck is also more common in males than in females.[37]

The prognosis of melanoma is to some extent site dependent. Tumors arising on the BANS sites (upper back, posterior arm, posterior neck, and posterior scalp) behave less favorably than those on the extremities.[37,99]

The majority of melanomas arise de novo and as such, at least in their radial (in situ) growth phase, they clinically present as flat lesions. The most important signs for newly acquired potentially early melanoma include[100]:

- a size of 6.0 mm diameter or greater,
- irregularity of the border of the lesion, usually with scalloping,
- irregular and variable pigmentation,
- asymmetry,
- recent and rapid change in a pre-existing lesion.

Irritation and bleeding are also a source of concern. The development of ulceration, which often relates to a rapidly evolving tumor, is important and is regarded as an indication of a potentially poor prognosis. Clinical evidence of nodule formation by definition implies that the tumor has entered the vertical growth phase. In contrast to benign melanocytic nevi, the skin lines are usually absent over the surface of a melanoma.

Lesions on the integument have traditionally been classified into four major clinicopathological subtypes although in the more recent literature the validity of such subdivision has been questioned, and classification into more genetically oriented groups may offer advantages.[101-103] Gene profiling and the results of other high-throughput technologies will also likely aid in revising our traditional classification scheme so that clinically and therapeutically relevant subsets can be identified.[104,105] An evolving molecular classification is presented in the final section of this chapter. The currently accepted subdivision is particularly based on perceived differences in prognosis and etiology and the genomic features of these groups largely bear this out. Although any variation in biological behavior relates more to tumor thickness than histogenetic subtype, there are certainly histologic differences that make the distinction possible in the majority of cases. Contrariwise, in some melanomas, it is not possible to effect a precise classification and, in such instances, an unqualified diagnosis of melanoma is quite sufficient. For the moment, however, subtyping melanoma is firmly entrenched in both the literature and pathology dogma.[106] Four major subtypes of cutaneous melanoma are currently recognized:[29,107-113]

- lentigo maligna melanoma (melanoma arising within a pre-existent lentigo maligna),
- superficial spreading melanoma,
- acral lentiginous melanoma,
- nodular melanoma.

The majority of melanomas have a radial (in situ) growth phase before the development of invasive tumor.[114] The radial growth phase is greatest in lentigo maligna, of shorter duration in superficial spreading melanoma and acral lentiginous melanoma, and, by definition, absent in nodular melanoma.

Our understanding of melanoma has been radically transformed through research of the genomics and tumor biology of this disease. These topics are discussed in the final section of this chapter, under the molecular classification of melanoma. A number of efficacious targeted treatments are available for melanoma such as those inhibiting the constitutively activated signaling proteins produced by mutated BRAF and KIT genes. In addition, the current ability to unleash the patient's own immune system through the application of immune checkpoint inhibitor therapy is providing treatment for many patients for whom there was little to offer in the past. Such therapies are transforming the treatment landscape for patients with metastatic disease and much research is ongoing to test such approaches in lower stage disease with adjuvant approaches. Much research is ongoing to identify which subsets of patients will benefit from immuno-oncological approaches and why some patients respond while others do not. Many factors including tumoral mutational load, tumor-infiltrating lymphocytes, serum lactate dehydrogenase (LDH) levels, oncogenic signaling pathways, gut microbiome, and immune checkpoint protein expression, to name a few, have been correlated with responses. However, a full understanding of exactly how and why these agents work in some patients and not others has yet to emerge and our ability to predict is currently limited. Discoveries are proceeding at an incredible rate in this area and thus are not addressed in greater detail in this chapter.

Lentigo maligna and lentigo maligna melanoma

Lentigo maligna (Hutchinson melanotic freckle) is a relatively uncommon variant of melanoma and typically develops on chronic sun-damaged skin of the elderly.[115-117] In the United States, it is estimated to account for 4% of all cases of cutaneous melanoma.[118] It is characterized by a positive correlation

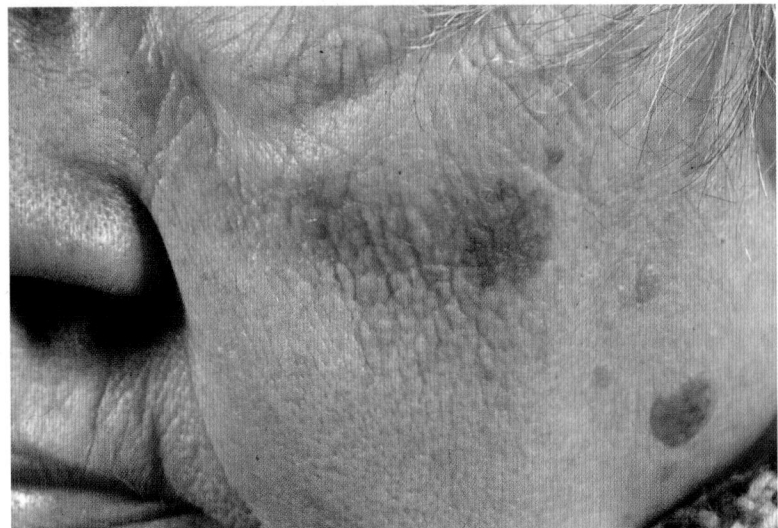

Fig. 26.1
Lentigo maligna: this variably pigmented lesion was present for many years. There is no invasive component. From the collection of the late N.P. Smith MD, the Institute of Dermatology, London, UK.

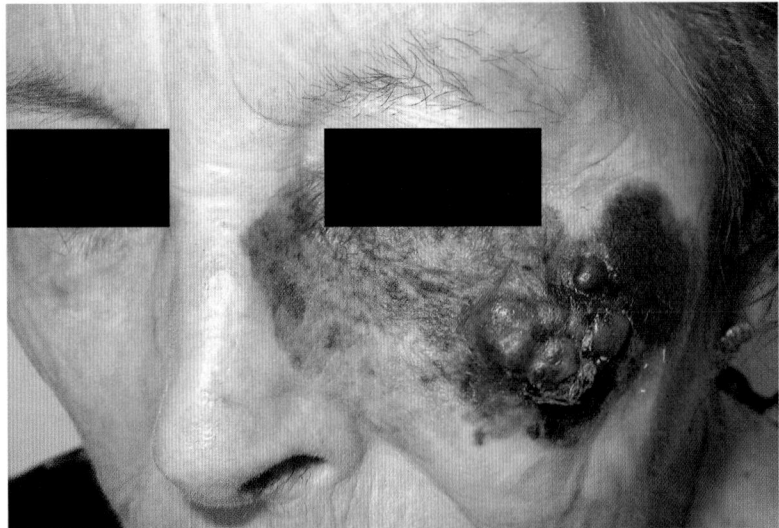

Fig. 26.3
Lentigo maligna melanoma: this is a very advanced lesion with a multinodular invasive component. By courtesy of J.C. Pascual, MD, Alicante, Spain.

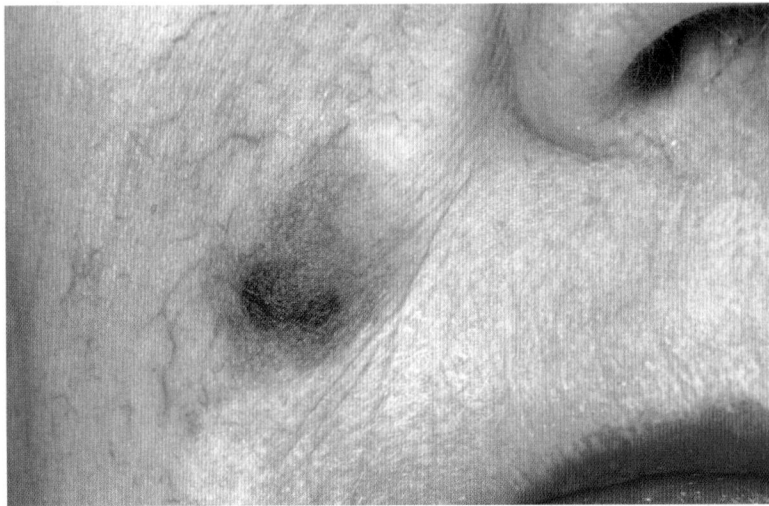

Fig. 26.2
Lentigo maligna: a dark black nodule of invasive tumor is surrounded by typical lentigo maligna. From the collection of the late N.P. Smith MD, the Institute of Dermatology, London, UK.

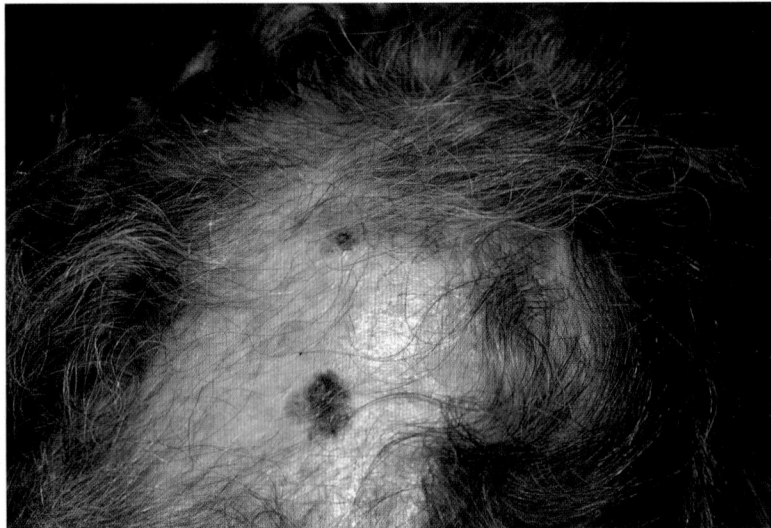

Fig. 26.4
Lentigo maligna: the sun-damaged skin of the bald scalp is at risk for developing this tumor. A concomitant ulcerated basal cell carcinoma is also evident above the melanoma. From the collection of the late N.P. Smith MD, the Institute of Dermatology, London, UK.

with increasing age.[119,120] Sites of predilection are the malar region, nose, temple, and forehead; much less frequently acral sites, such as the dorsum of the hands, may be involved (Figs 26.1–26.5). The tumor presents most often in the sixth and seventh decades as a variably pigmented, gradually enlarging, irregular, flat macule. It may be brown or black and usually shows areas of hypopigmentation representing areas of regression. The in situ lesion is often present for 10–15 years before invasive tumor develops. Lentigo maligna melanoma is a term used to denote to lentigo maligna that has progressed to dermal invasion.[121]

Superficial spreading melanoma

Superficial spreading melanoma is the most common variant and shows an equal sex incidence.[122] The sites most frequently affected are the leg (especially in females) and the back (particularly in males). The lesion initially presents as a flat scaly macule or plaque, which after a variable period of time develops a blue or blue-black nodule of invasive melanoma (Fig. 26.6). Hypopigmented or amelanotic variants are erythematous or flesh colored. The initial plaque is irregular, often 1–2 cm in diameter, and shows much greater variation in color than a banal or dysplastic nevus. Scalloping of the

border of the lesion is characteristic, and hypopigmented areas of regression are also a frequent finding. Ulceration is an important diagnostic (and prognostic) clue.

Acral lentiginous melanoma

Acral lentiginous melanoma accounts for approximately 8–10% of all melanomas in Caucasians.[123,124] It is, however, the predominant subtype affecting Afro-Caribbeans and Asians.[125–127] The tumor is particularly found on the digits (especially beneath the nails) and on weight-bearing sites; plantar tumors are the most common, with the heel being the most frequently affected region (Figs 26.7 and 26.8).[128,129] Subungual variants, which most commonly affect the great toe and the thumb, are rare tumors, accounting for only 2% of all cutaneous melanomas. They show a female preponderance and present most often in the elderly.[123] In addition to acral lentiginous lesions, subungual melanoma can also present as superficial spreading and nodular histologic variants.[130–132]

Acral lentiginous tumors usually present as irregular, gradually enlarging, and variably pigmented macules. With progression to vertical growth phase,

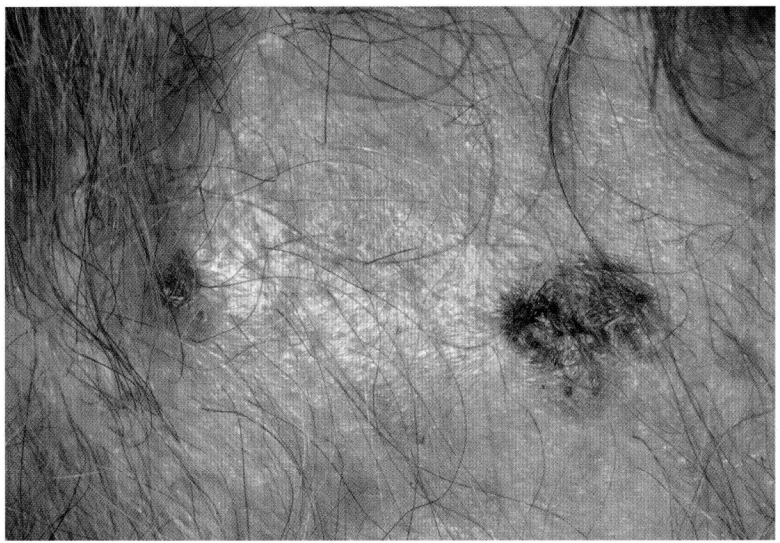

Fig. 26.5
Lentigo maligna: close-up view. From the collection of the late N.P. Smith MD, the Institute of Dermatology, London, UK.

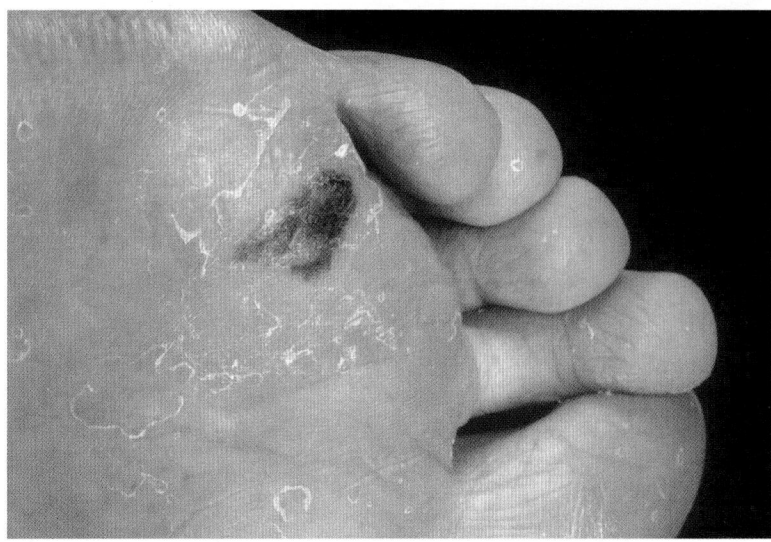

Fig. 26.7
Acral lentiginous melanoma: this variant arises on the non–sun-damaged skin of the palms, soles, and under the nails. From the collection of the late N.P. Smith MD, the Institute of Dermatology, London, UK.

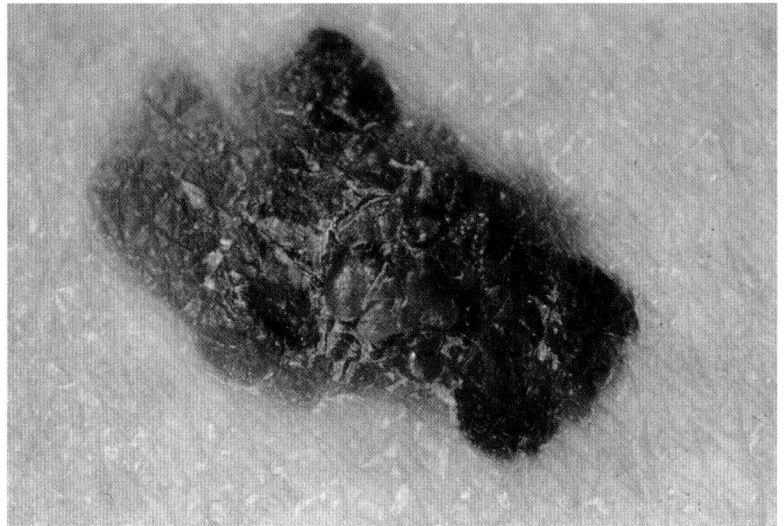

Fig. 26.6
Superficial spreading melanoma: there is a large nodule of invasive melanoma with a surrounding macular component. From the collection of the late N.P. Smith MD, the Institute of Dermatology, London, UK.

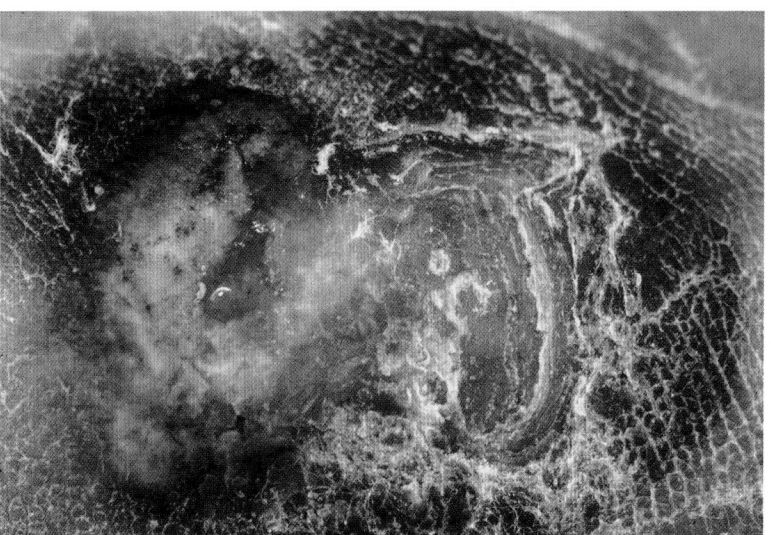

Fig. 26.8
Acral lentiginous melanoma: this ulcerated tumor had extended deeply into the underlying tissues. From the collection of the late N.P. Smith MD, the Institute of Dermatology, London, UK.

frequently ulcerated, blue or black nodular lesions are encountered. In Caucasians, acral lentiginous melanoma presents most often in the seventh decade, has an equal incidence in both sexes, and is generally associated with a poor prognosis since tumors are generally thick by the time of diagnosis. Mucosal melanomas are often classified within the acral lentiginous spectrum, given certain partial morphological overlap. These two types of melanoma are distinct clinically, although genomic characterization does indicate shared features.[103,133,134]

Nodular melanoma

Nodular melanoma (3–4%) has no radial growth phase and therefore may be distinguished clinically from nodules of invasive tumor that have arisen in lesions associated with a pre-existent radial growth phase.[135] It has a poor prognosis (the majority being thick tumors by the time of excision), affects more males than females (2:1), and generally arises in the fifth or sixth decade.[136] The trunk and limbs are most commonly involved. The tumor, which may be nodular or polypoid (polypoid melanoma), is often ulcerated and, when lacking pigment (amelanotic melanoma), is frequently mistaken

for a vascular tumor, such as lobular capillary hemangioma (pyogenic granuloma) (*Figs 26.9* and *26.10*).

Melanoma arising at noncutaneous (primarily mucosal) sites

Melanoma may arise at a diverse range of sites other than the skin, including the orbit, the oral cavity and nasal cavities, the external genitalia, vagina, urethra, and anus.[137–139] In general, mucosal tumors are associated with aggressive behavior and a poor prognosis.[138,140–143] This relates particularly to delayed presentation. Rare sites for primary melanoma also include the meninges, esophagus, stomach, uterus, cervix, breast, biliary system, bronchus, and adrenal gland.

Histologic features

Central to our understanding of the histologic classification of cutaneous melanoma is the concept of radial (horizontal) growth phase and vertical (invasive) growth phase.[33,108,114,144,145] By current definition, the radial

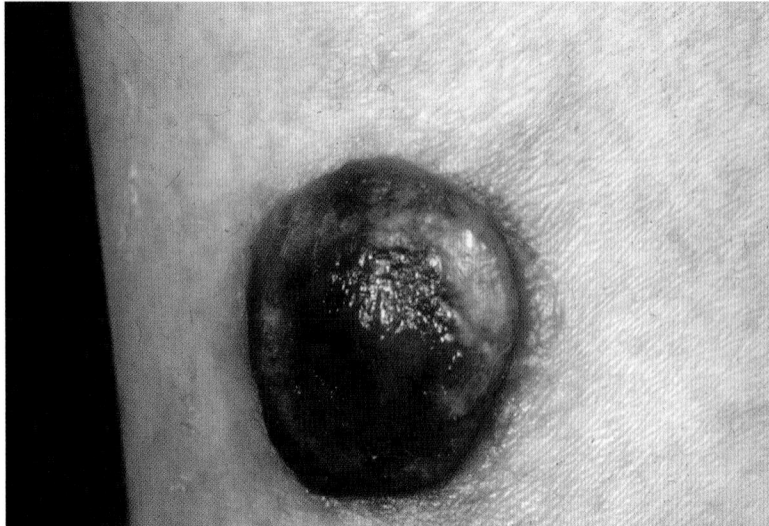

Fig. 26.9
Nodular melanoma: this heavily pigmented, dome-shaped nodule has no adjacent macular component. From the collection of the late N.P. Smith MD, the Institute of Dermatology, London, UK.

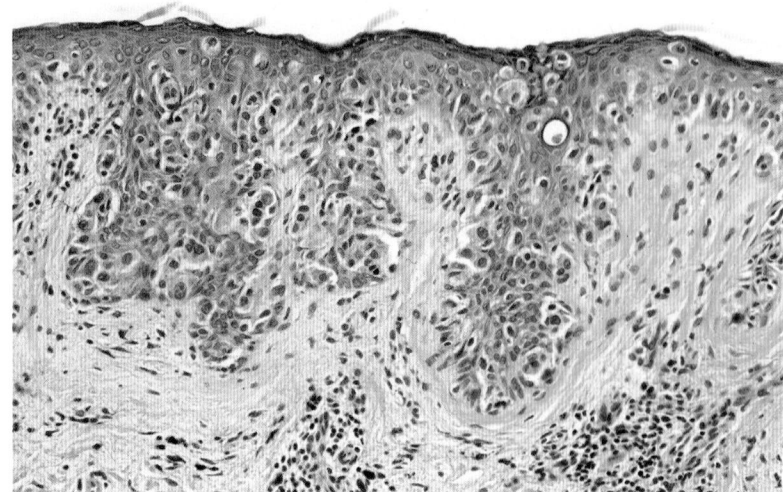

Fig. 26.11
Melanoma: radial growth phase. The tumor is wholly intraepidermal (in situ melanoma). Intraepidermal tumor cells at all levels are present (pagetoid spread).

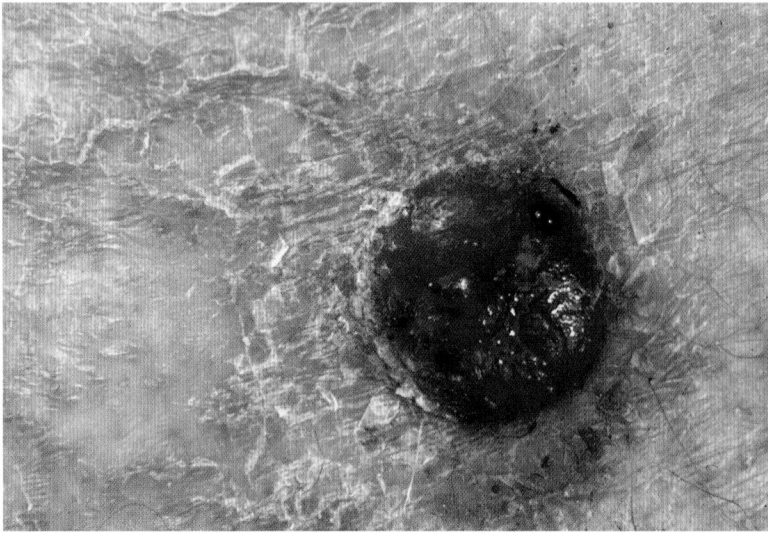

Fig. 26.10
Nodular melanoma: amelanotic tumors as shown here are often a source of clinical (and histological) diagnostic difficulty. From the collection of the late N.P. Smith MD, the Institute of Dermatology, London, UK.

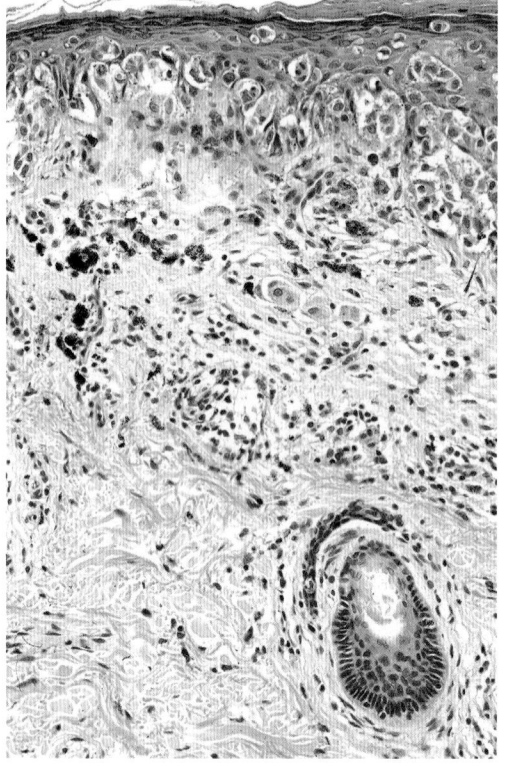

Fig. 26.12
Melanoma: microinvasive radial growth phase. In addition to in situ tumor, small numbers of single tumor cells are present in the papillary dermis.

growth phase may include (in addition to a wholly in situ, intraepidermal component) evidence of microinvasion into the papillary dermis (microinvasive radial growth phase), often accompanied by features of regression (*Figs 26.11* and *26.12*). The microinvasive stage of melanoma is believed to lack significant metastatic potential and as a consequence is associated with an excellent prognosis.[146–149] Indeed, in a large series of patients discussed by Clark and coworkers, no tumors in the radial growth phase were associated with metastatic spread.[109]

Histologically, the microinvasive radial growth phase tumor is characterized by single cells or small aggregates of melanoma cells, histologically similar to their intraepidermal counterparts and invariably forming tumor nests smaller than those present within the overlying epidermis.[33] A lymphohistiocytic infiltrate is usually present. Mitotic figures are absent by definition. The last feature is of particular importance; multiple levels should therefore be carefully examined before making a diagnosis of microinvasive radial growth phase melanoma (*Fig. 26.13*).[150]

Vertical growth phase melanoma is composed of cohesive nests, nodules, or plaques larger than those present within the epidermis and consisting of tumor cells that are cytologically different from those in the radial growth

phase (*Fig. 26.14*).[33,145,151] Mitotic figures are common.[33] Features of regression may be seen but are usually absent at the base of the tumor. The tumor cells in the vertical growth phase are pleomorphic and apoptosis is often present. Vertical growth phase implies an alteration in biological potential with a capacity for lymphovascular invasion and metastatic spread.[33,145,146]

A subset of melanocytic tumors can be challenging to definitively assess as either benign or malignant and are described under various names to indicate their uncertain malignant potential. Such cases often have some, but not all or fully developed features of the malignant phenotype histologically. Experts often disagree on the designation of malignancy in this group of exceedingly challenging lesions.[152–155] Multi-probe fluorescence in situ hybridization (FISH) and genomic hybridization can assist diagnostically, but in some cases the biological potential of these equivocal lesions remains uncertain.[156] Proposals have suggested that in such cases, grouping the lesions into classes linked to the type or extent of excision needed increases agreement and aids in communication of the clinical care needed despite the uncertainty in the diagnosis.[157]

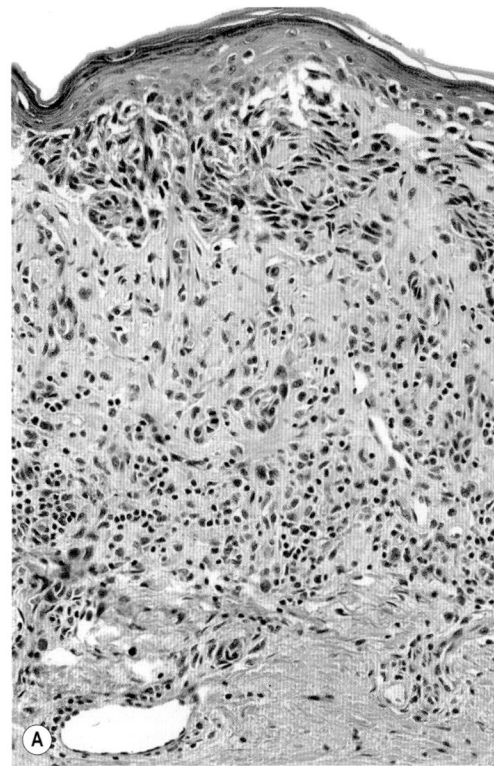

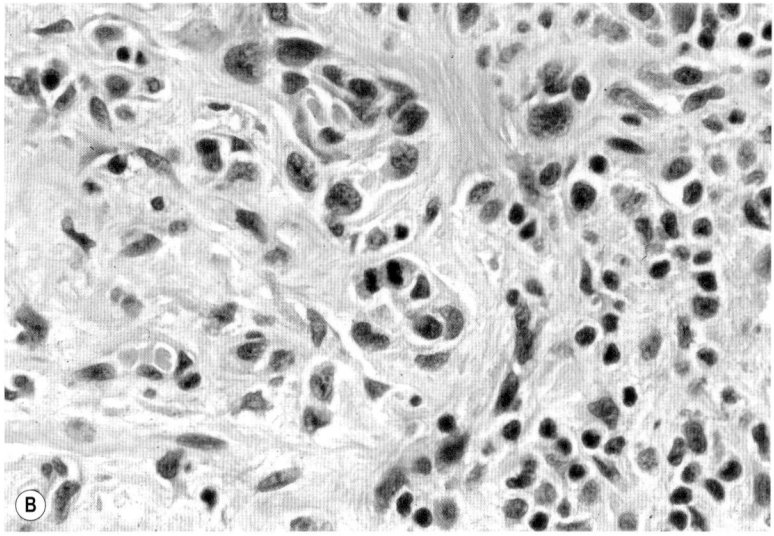

Fig. 26.13
(**A**, **B**) Melanoma: lentigo maligna melanoma. This tumor was incorrectly diagnosed as a microinvasive radial growth phase lesion on the grounds that only single cells were present in the dermis and there were no nests. Dermal mitoses were, however, present (**B**). The patient developed cerebral metastases.

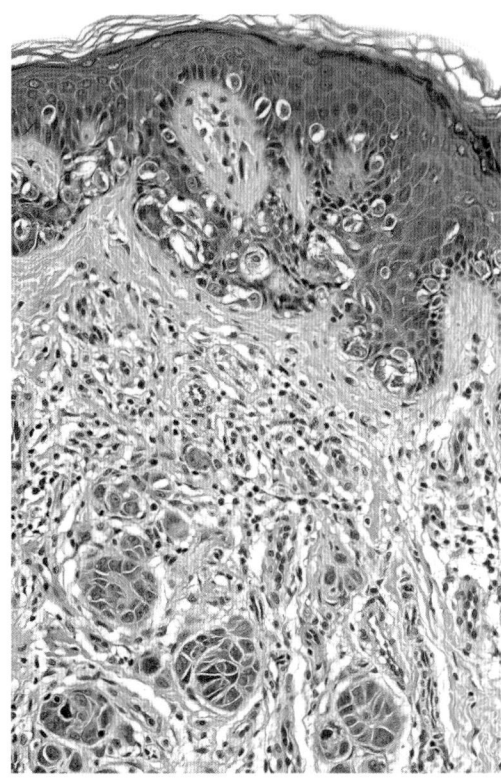

Fig. 26.14
Melanoma: vertical growth phase. In addition to in situ (radial growth phase) tumor, there are multiple nests in the dermis. These are larger than the epidermal ones.

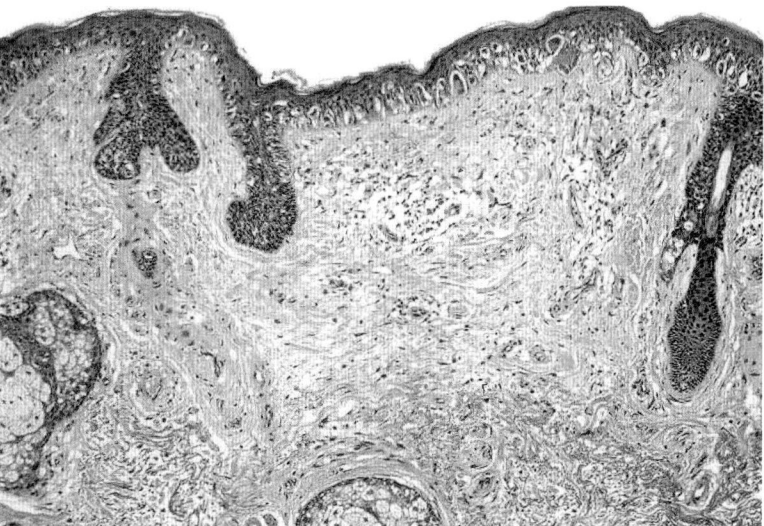

Fig. 26.15
Lentigo maligna: the epidermis is atrophic and flattened. Atypical melanocytes are basally located and the superficial dermis shows marked solar elastosis.

Lentigo maligna and lentigo maligna melanoma

Lentigo maligna is characterized by proliferation of atypical melanocytes predominantly located along the dermal–epidermal junction (*Figs 26.15 and 26.16*).[158] Chronic sun damage evidenced as extensive solar elastosis is often prominent, particularly in cases from the head and neck region.[159] The tumor cells often show a conspicuous cytoplasmic fixation retraction artifact and contain pleomorphic irregular hyperchromatic, sometimes angular, nuclei. The cells are frequently orientated perpendicular to the surface, and involvement of hair follicles and sweat duct epithelium is a characteristic finding (*Fig. 26.17*). This may sometimes result in difficulties in assessing

tumor thickness, particularly if obliquely cut sections are examined, when the relationship of the tumor cells to the adnexal epithelium may not be clear. In more advanced lesions, junctional nests are apparent and multinucleate tumor giant cells are commonly seen (*Figs 26.18–26.20*). Pigmentation is variable, but is often abundant, sometimes involving the full thickness of the epidermis, including the stratum corneum. The very occasional presence of marked intraepidermal (pagetoid) spread may result in histologic overlap with superficial spreading melanoma, though junctional nesting is usually less prominent in lentigo maligna. Assessing excision margins for residual atypical melanocytes in this variant is often fraught with difficulty. To avoid unnecessary surgery it is important not to confuse actinically damaged nuclei from residual lentigo maligna (*Fig. 26.21*), though molecular studies suggest that this may not be possible on strictly morphological grounds given the field effect of genomic aberration present in even morphologically normal melanocytes.[160] This likely underlies the elevated risk of local recurrence in

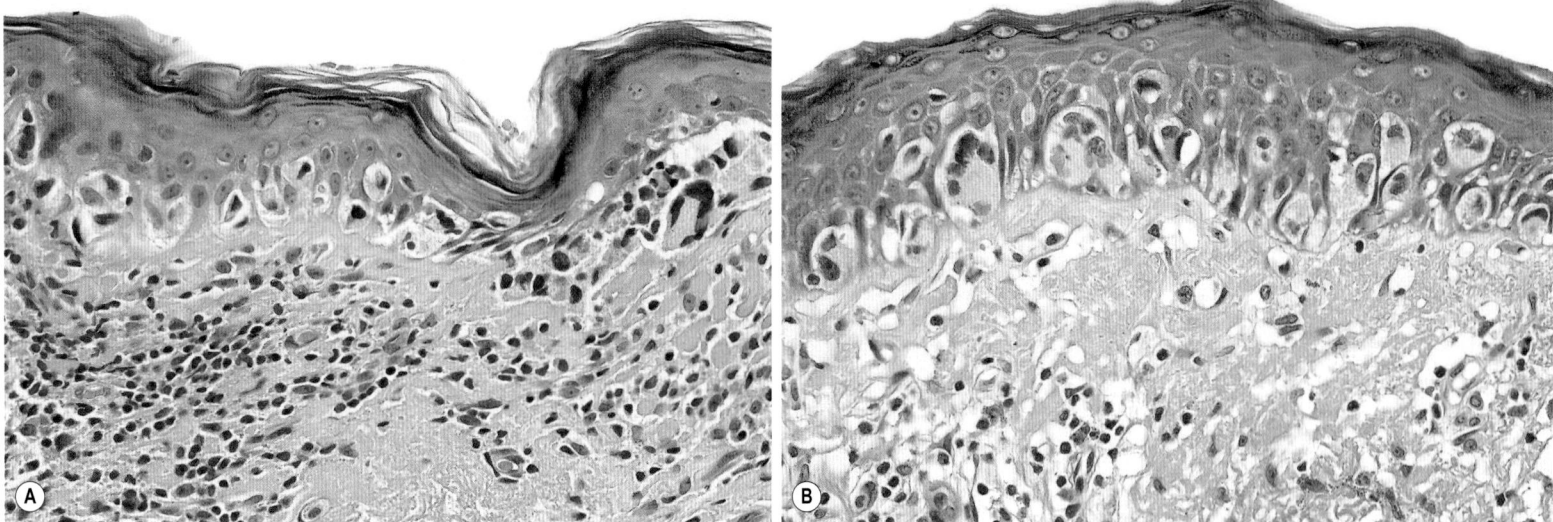

Fig. 26.16
Lentigo maligna: (**A**) viewed with higher power, the melanocytes demonstrate a prominent fixation artifact. The nuclei are irregular, angular, and hyperchromatic; (**B**) in this example, the tumor cells have abundant eosinophilic cytoplasm and there is early pagetoid spread.

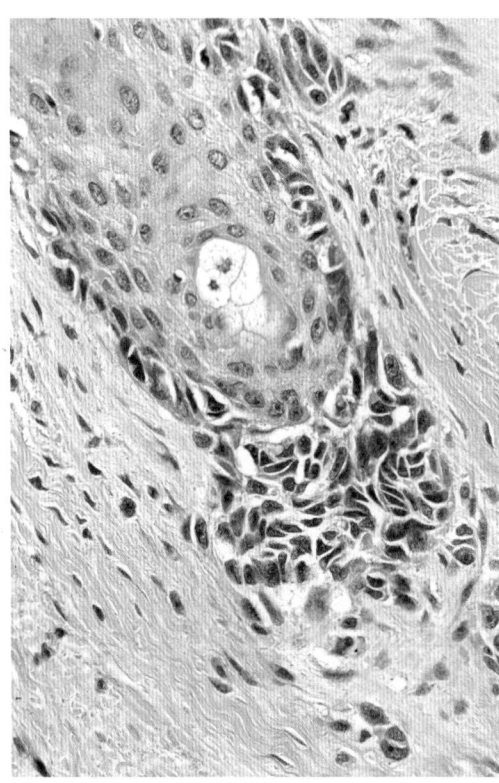

Fig. 26.17
Lentigo maligna: note the presence of atypical melanocytes within the outer aspect of a hair follicle. Shave biopsy of such lesions is accompanied by a high recurrence rate.

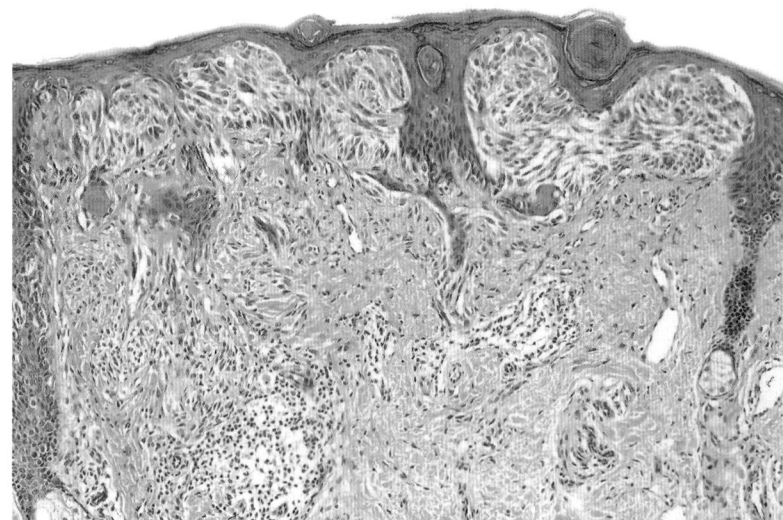

Fig. 26.18
Lentigo maligna: in this example there are conspicuous junctional nests. The tumor cells have a spindled morphology.

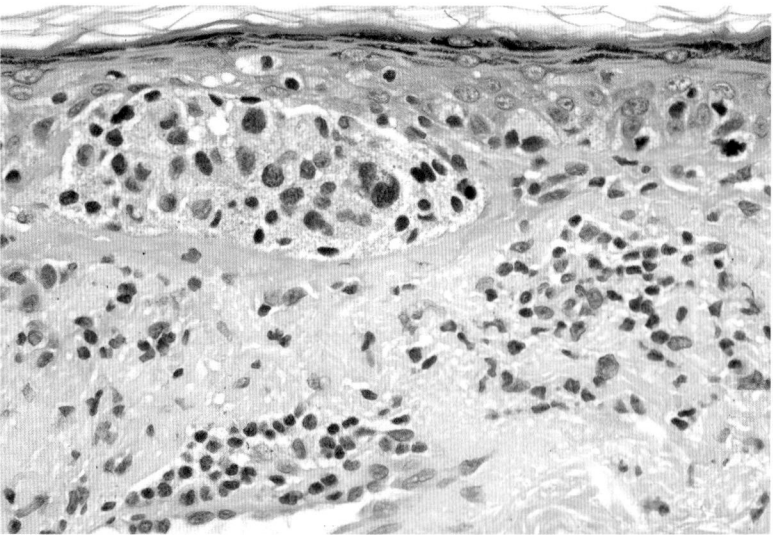

Fig. 26.19
Lentigo maligna: the tumor cells are pleomorphic and show very marked nuclear hyperchromatism.

these lesions. Evaluation of the extent of epidermal involvement in difficult cases or small samples can be done by immunohistochemistry ideally with markers that highlight nuclei including MITF and SOX10.

Lentigo maligna arises at sites showing actinic damage; the epidermis is therefore typically atrophic and the dermis shows solar elastosis. Usually the papillary dermis contains melanophages and scattered chronic inflammatory cells. The finding of the latter, particularly when present in large numbers, is often associated with invasion and should therefore prompt careful examination of multiple levels of the specimen. Invasive tumor (lentigo maligna melanoma) can be multifocal and is usually of the spindled cell type (*Figs 26.22–26.24*). Due to the extensive involvement of neighboring hair follicles and cross-sectioning, determining the presence or absence of early invasion can be very challenging and occasionally, impossible. Desmoplasia, often with neurotropism, is present in a significant percentage of cases. Very occasionally, a storiform growth pattern is evident and if the tumor is amelanotic there may be confusion with dermatofibrosarcoma protuberans, particularly

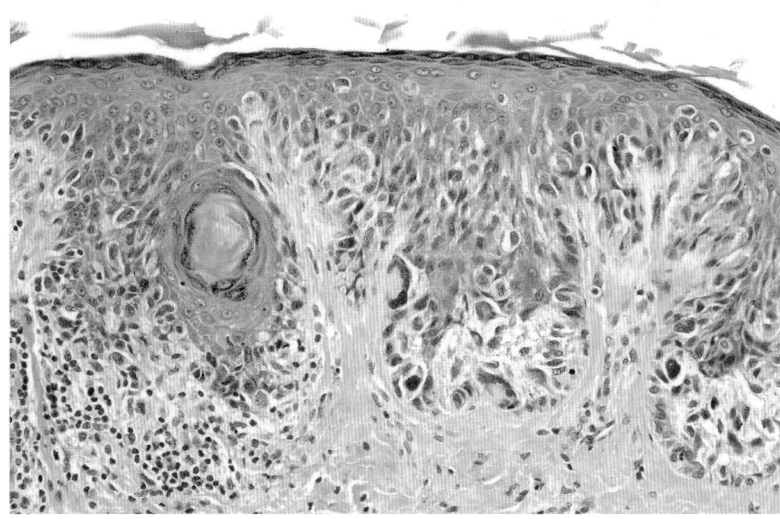

Fig. 26.20
Lentigo maligna: multinucleate tumor cells as shown in this example are a common feature and a useful diagnostic clue.

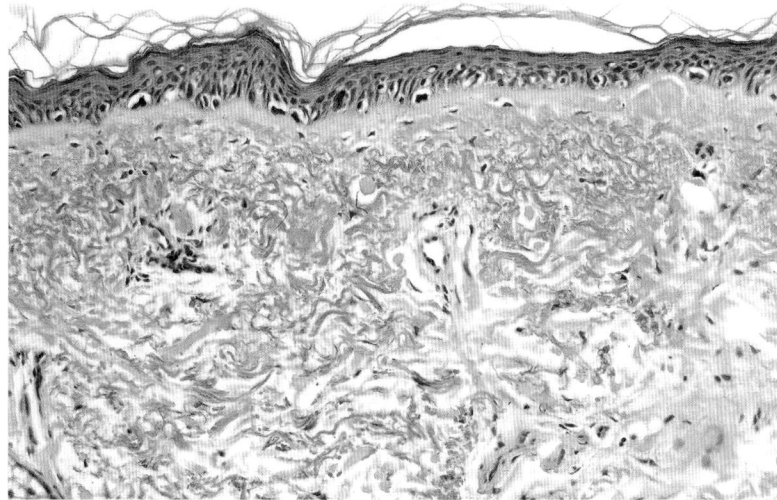

Fig. 26.21
Actinic nuclear atypia: sometimes distinguishing between the former and residual tumor cells as shown in this field can be a real problem. The former, however, show little nuclear enlargement and nucleoli are absent. In addition, such cells do not form nuclear palisades as is typical of lentigo maligna.

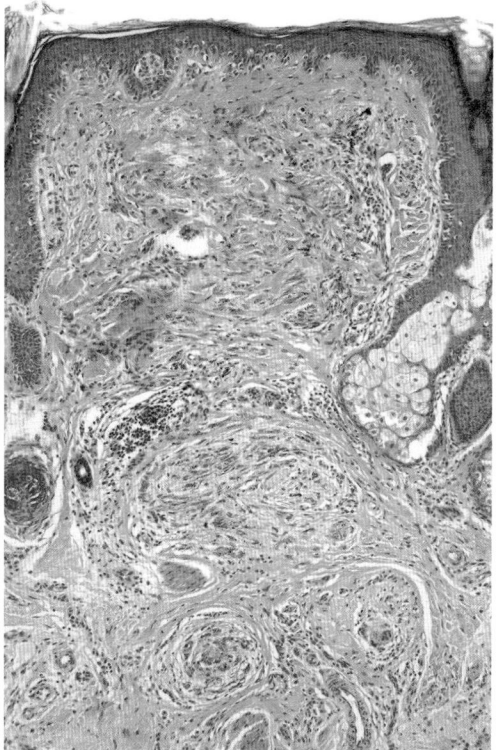

Fig. 26.22
Lentigo maligna melanoma: in this variant of melanoma, the invasive component is often of the spindle cell type.

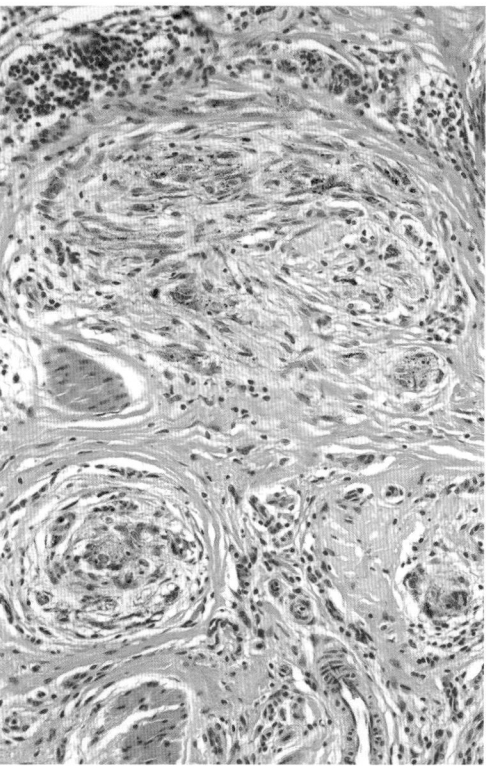

Fig. 26.23
Lentigo maligna melanoma: higher-power view.

in small biopsies (*Fig. 26.25*). More often, the associated melanoma is desmoplastic with subtle spindle cells and can be mistaken for fibrosis or scar rather than invasive tumor.

Exceptionally, lentigo maligna and lentigo maligna melanoma present as amelanotic lesions (amelanotic lentigo maligna and amelanotic lentigo maligna melanoma), both clinically and histologically.[161–164] Clinically, these appear as erythematous scaly lesions resembling actinic keratoses, squamous cell carcinoma in situ or eczema.[162] Immunocytochemistry may therefore be necessary to arrive at the correct diagnosis (*Fig. 26.26*).[165]

Superficial spreading melanoma (pagetoid melanoma)

The radial growth phase of superficial spreading melanoma is now encountered more commonly, largely as a consequence of public awareness of melanoma with the consequent removal of an increasing percentage of thin early lesions. It is typified by an asymmetrical proliferation of atypical nondendritic melanocytes scattered singly and in clusters throughout all levels of the epithelium (buckshot scatter), giving an appearance reminiscent of Paget disease (*Figs 26.27* and *26.28*). The melanoma cells involve all layers

of the epithelium while the cells of Paget disease tend to be superficial to the basal cell layer. The individual cells are epithelioid with abundant cytoplasm, often showing fine or dusty melanin pigmentation, and contain pleomorphic vesicular nuclei with prominent eosinophilic nucleoli; scattered mitotic figures including atypical forms may be evident. Characteristic of this variant is tumor growth in continuity from one rete ridge to another (a pattern not usually seen in acquired junctional or compound nevi). In contrast to lentigo maligna, there is often minimal visible evidence of actinic damage.[159] The epidermis often shows acanthosis with partial or complete effacement of the ridge pattern. Invasive tumor is mostly of the epithelioid type (*Figs 26.29–26.32*). Desmoplasia and/or neurotropism are uncommon.

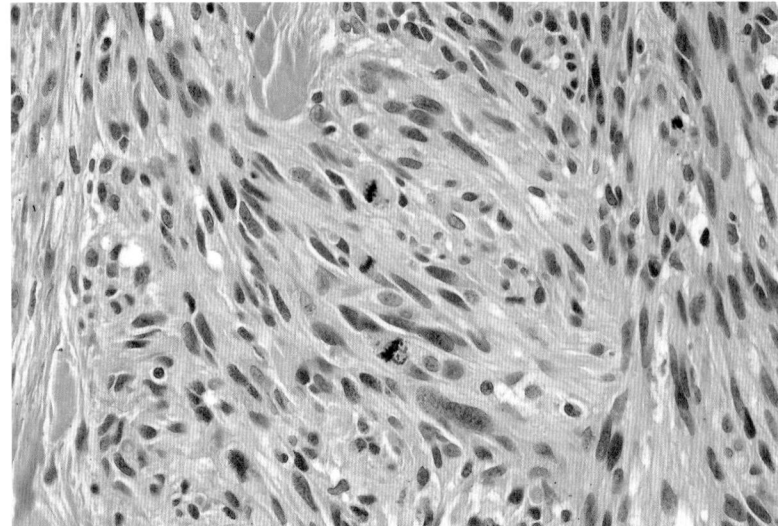

Fig. 26.24
Lentigo maligna melanoma: in this example, mitotic figures are conspicuous. Note the nuclear hyperchromatism.

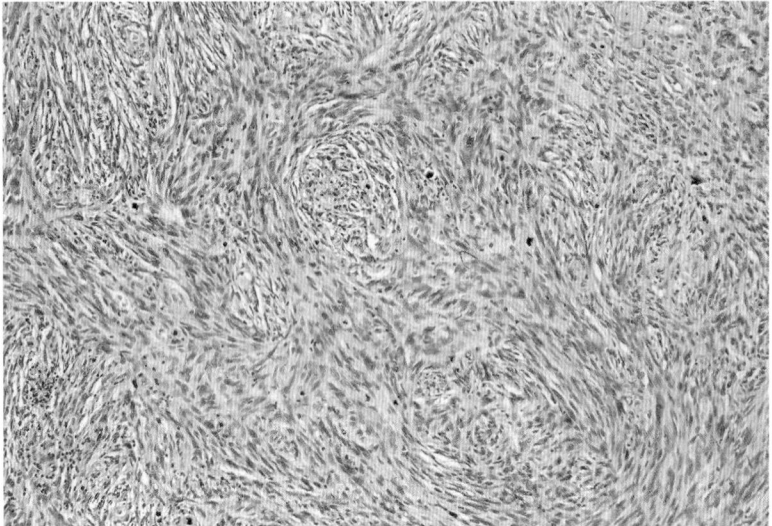

Fig. 26.25
Lentigo maligna melanoma: occasionally the tumor adopts a storiform pattern. When amelanotic, this may be confused with dermatofibrosarcoma protuberans or spindle cell squamous carcinoma.

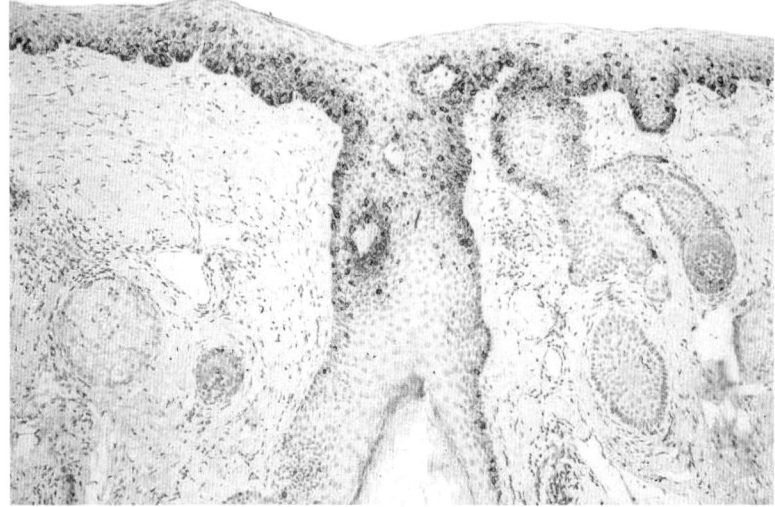

Fig. 26.26
Lentigo maligna: occasionally it is difficult to distinguish between actinic keratosis and lentigo maligna. In such cases, immunohistochemistry using a red chromogen (in this case alkaline phosphatase) can make the distinction easy.

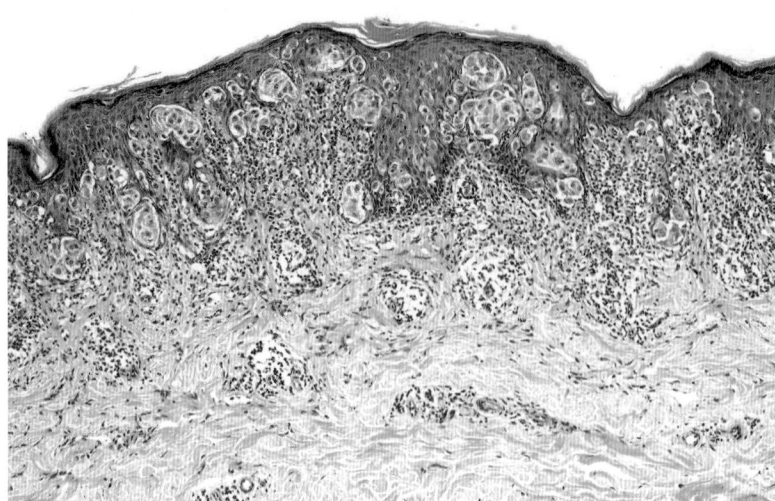

Fig. 26.27
Superficial spreading melanoma: there is prominent junctional activity and atypical melanocytes are widely scattered throughout the epidermis.

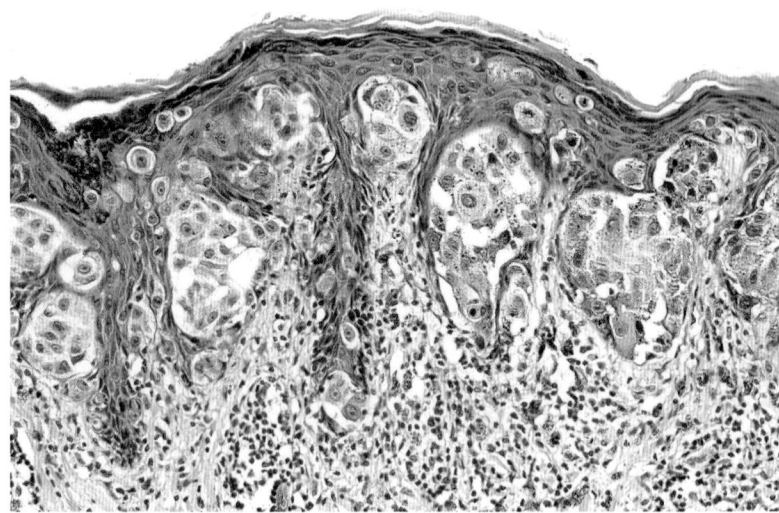

Fig. 26.28
Superficial spreading melanoma: the melanocytes have abundant eosinophilic cytoplasm and pleomorphic vesicular nuclei. Nucleoli are conspicuous.

Acral lentiginous melanoma

In the early stages of the radial growth phase of acral lentiginous melanoma the changes may be quite subtle, consisting of irregular epidermal hyperplasia and scattered, basally located, atypical melanocytes.[166–170] The established lesion shows acanthosis with marked elongation of the epidermal ridges and obvious melanocytic atypia (*Figs 26.33* and *26.34*). The lower reaches of the epidermis are infiltrated by large numbers of atypical melanocytes characterized by nuclear pleomorphism and hyperchromatism, and showing a cytoplasmic fixation retraction artifact. Nucleoli are conspicuous and mitotic figures may be identified. Although spindled forms are most often encountered, epithelioid and giant cells are sometimes evident. Scattered foci of junctional nests may also be detected, usually at the tips of the epidermal ridges (*Fig. 26.35*). A heavy bandlike chronic inflammatory cell infiltrate is frequently present. The invasive tumor is often a spindled cell in type and may elicit a desmoplastic reaction (*Fig. 26.36*). Deep extension along the sweat gland epithelium is common and neurotropism may be evident in a subset of cases. Cross-sectioning of involved sweat glands may lead to the erroneous interpretation of invasion. Occasionally, acral tumors may show a superficial spreading in situ component or represent de novo nodular melanoma with absent radial growth phase.

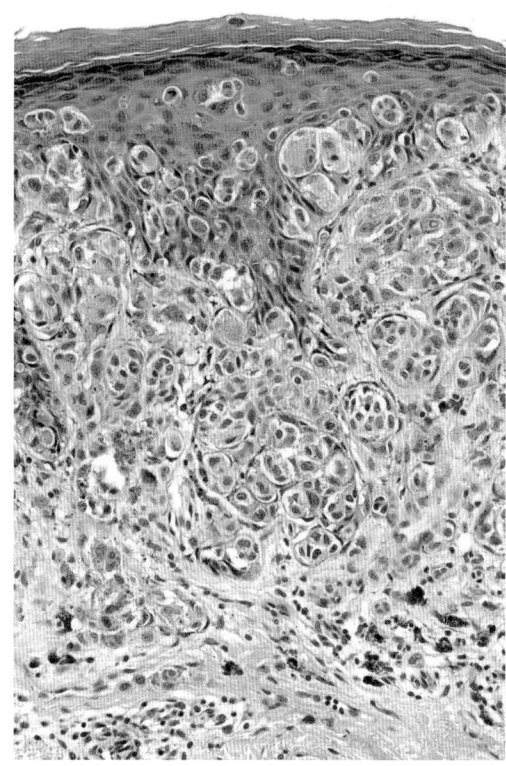

Fig. 26.29
Superficial spreading melanoma: invasive tumor is usually of the epithelioid type as shown in this field. Note the abundant cytoplasm, nuclear pleomorphism, and prominent nucleoli.

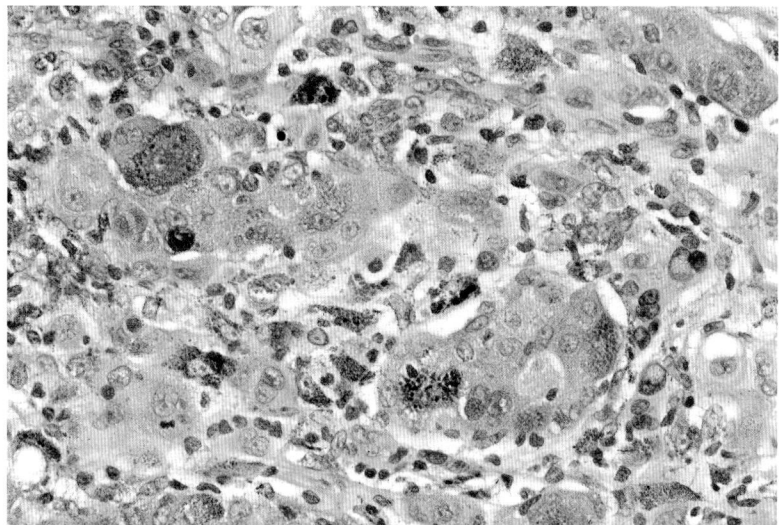

Fig. 26.30
Superficial spreading melanoma: in this example there is heavy melanin pigmentation.

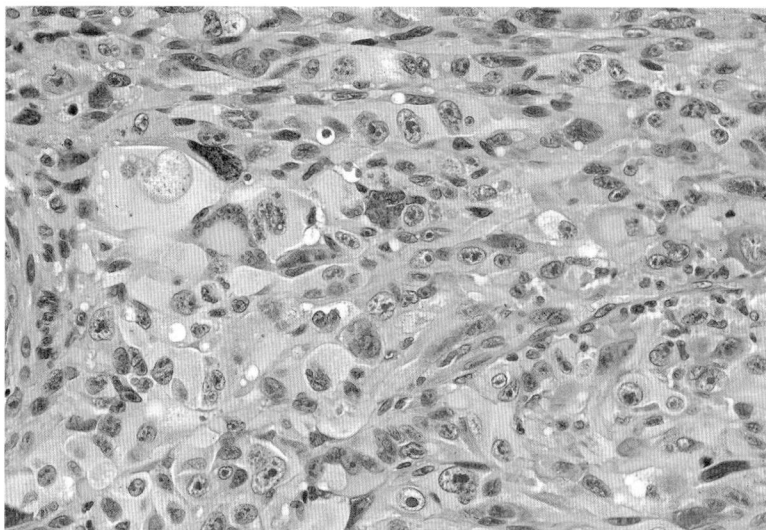

Fig. 26.31
Superficial spreading melanoma: diagnosis of amelanotic tumors, particularly when very pleomorphic as in this example, often depends upon immunohistochemistry if a junctional component is not evident.

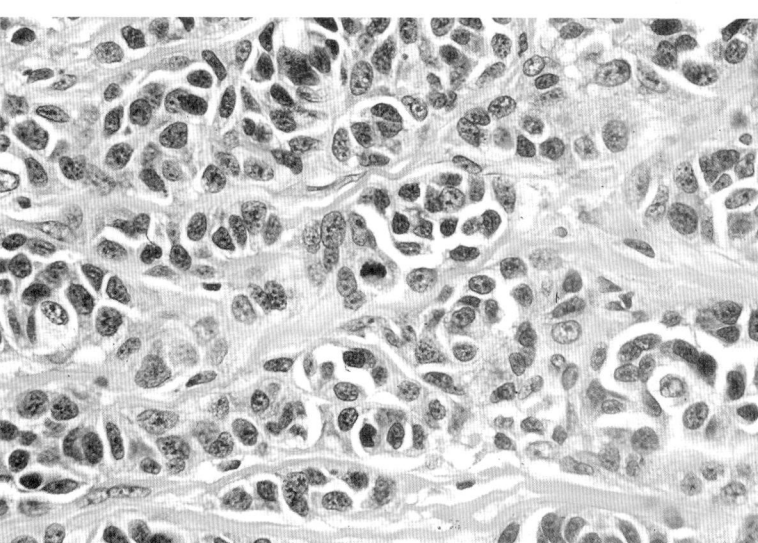

Fig. 26.32
Superficial spreading melanoma: this example shows a mitotic figure in the center of the field.

Nodular melanoma

By definition, nodular melanoma has no evident preceding radial growth phase, its growth pattern appearing vertical from inception. Such a tumor, therefore, does not show an intraepidermal melanocytic proliferation beyond three epidermal ridges on either side of the tumor mass (*Figs 26.37 and 26.38*). This histologic pattern is usually, but not always, seen in the same anatomic distribution as superficial spreading melanoma; these have overlapping genomic features, but some regard them as distinct entities.[135]

Cell types

Although many invasive tumors show a mixed pattern, melanoma cells are typically divided into two major types: epithelioid and spindled cell. Epithelioid cells most often arise within superficial spreading melanoma and nodular melanoma, while spindled cells are more commonly seen in lentigo maligna melanoma and acral lentiginous melanoma.

Epithelioid cells

Epithelioid melanoma cells are large and rounded with abundant, often eosinophilic, cytoplasm and contain prominent pleomorphic vesicular nuclei with conspicuous eosinophilic nucleoli. Mitotic figures may be either scant or numerous and sometimes abnormal. Pigmentation is variable and can be abundant or minimal. When minimal, Masson-Fontana silver staining is useful to reveal small quantities of pigment not detectable with conventional hematoxylin and eosin stained sections. Alternatively, immunohistochemistry may be necessary to establish the diagnosis (*Fig. 26.39*).

Spindled cells

The spindled cell variant is characterized by cells with elongated, narrow, tapering, cytoplasmic processes, which in nonpigmented variants may be confused with cells of mesenchymal derivation and therefore misdiagnosed as a variety of soft tissue neoplasms.

Occasional melanomas are exceedingly pleomorphic, containing tumor giant cells with enlarged nucleoli and conspicuous, frequently abnormal, mitotic figures; these variants must sometimes be distinguished from metastatic tumors, including pleomorphic secondary carcinoma, sarcomas, and even anaplastic CD30+ anaplastic large cell lymphoma (*Figs 26.40–26.42*).

Prognostic indicators

While the vast majority of thin melanomas do not metastasize, between 1% and 2% are known to do so. Conversely, occasional thick melanomas fail to disseminate. With this in mind, there has been intensive research in an effort to define those tumors that have the capacity for spread with

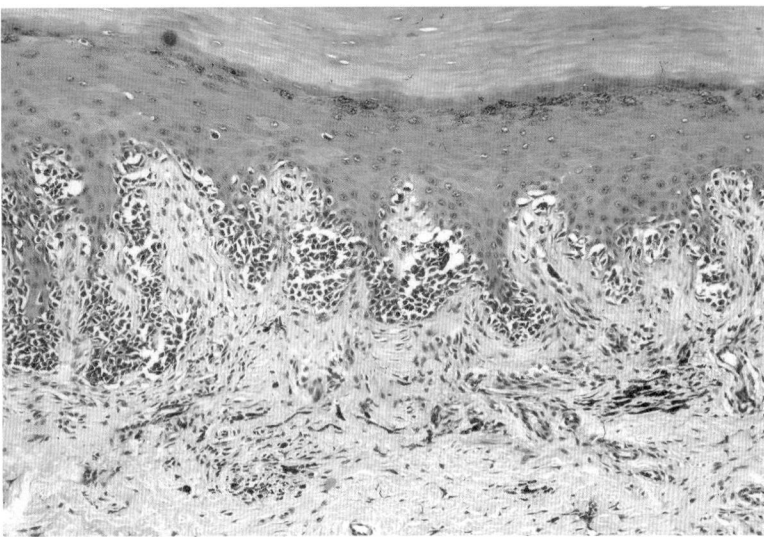

Fig. 26.33
Acral lentiginous melanoma: in this in situ lesion, there is irregular acanthosis, hypergranulosis, and hyperkeratosis. Tumor cells are hyperchromatic and distributed in a lentiginous and nested pattern. The dermis is scarred and there are conspicuous melanophages and chronic inflammatory cells.

resultant death, in the hope that adjuvant chemotherapy, immunotherapy, or other forms of treatment might eventually benefit significant numbers of patients. Prognostic indicators include clinical parameters, morphological observations, and measurements in addition to immunohistochemical markers of cell proliferation, cell regulation, and so on. Many of the morphological observations are tried and tested, but the search for the elusive immunohistochemical marker of metastatic potential has not yet been fruitful. Genomic biomarkers are also being explored, in particular limited gene expression panels.[171–173]

Clinical prognostic indicators include age, sex, and site of the primary tumor.[174–180] Older patients fare worse than younger ones, and males have a poorer outlook than females.[7,176,177,181–184] The latter is independent of tumor thickness and site.[176] Particularly high-risk sites include the back, upper arm, neck, and scalp (BANS).[185] The acral sites are also thought to be associated with a poorer prognosis.[186]

When reporting melanoma, it is generally accepted as essential worldwide to record and comment on the following variables:[176,187–193]

- tumor thickness (Breslow method),
- level of invasion (Clark method),
- growth phase (vertical or radial),
- mitotic rate,
- ulceration,
- lymphovascular invasion,
- perineural infiltration,
- regression,
- microsatellitosis,
- tumor infiltrating lymphocytes.

Growth phase is also noted although it should be emphasized that great care must be taken before allocating a melanoma to the microinvasive category of radial (horizontal) growth phase. Dermal mitoses automatically place a tumor in the vertical growth phase (see *Fig. 26.14*). These elements have become critical for proper staging and prognostic assignment of patients, but unfortunately even in countries with a high incidence and acute awareness of cutaneous melanoma, many of the above elements are absent from routine reports.[194]

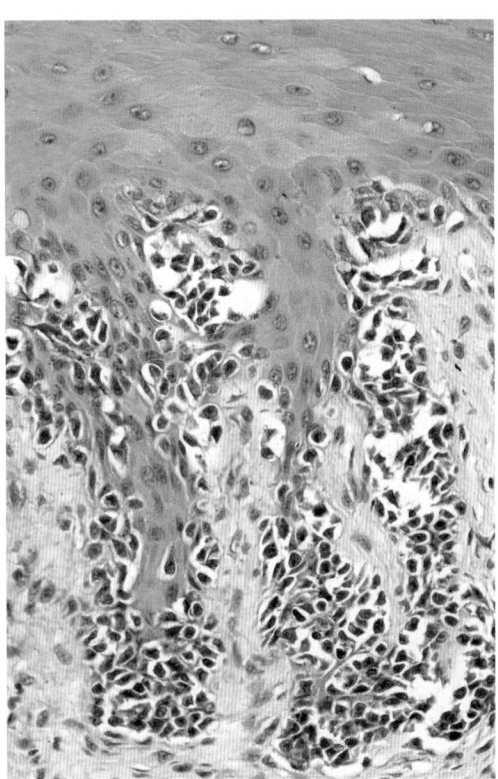

Fig. 26.34
Acral lentiginous melanoma: there is conspicuous cytoplasmic retraction, hyperchromatism, and nuclear atypia.

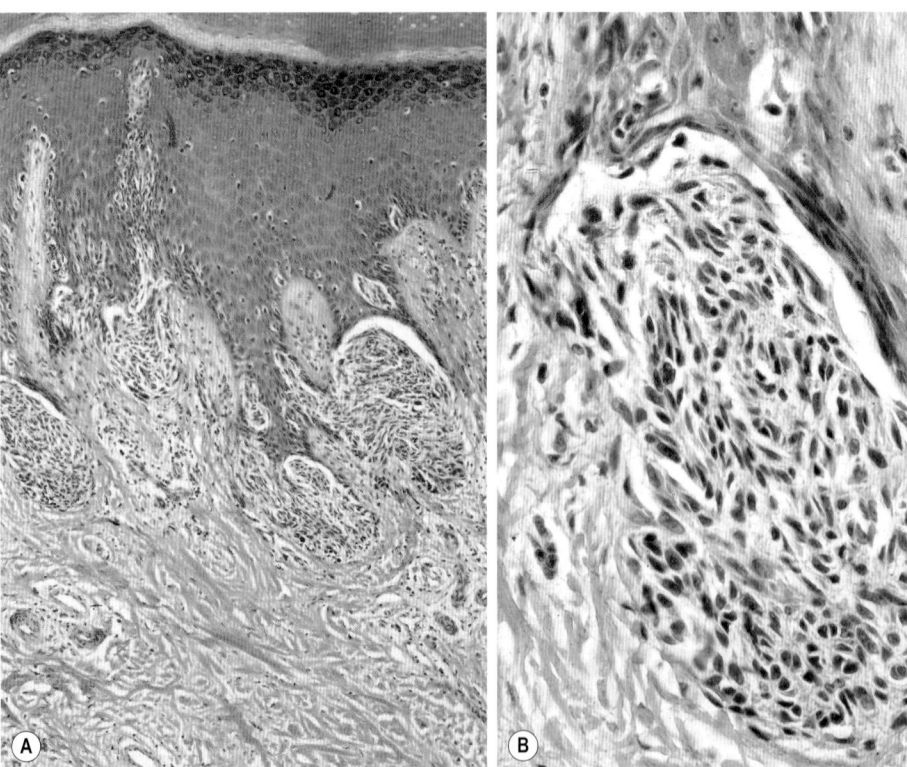

Fig. 26.35
(**A**, **B**) Acral lentiginous melanoma: large junctional nests are present at the tips of the rete.

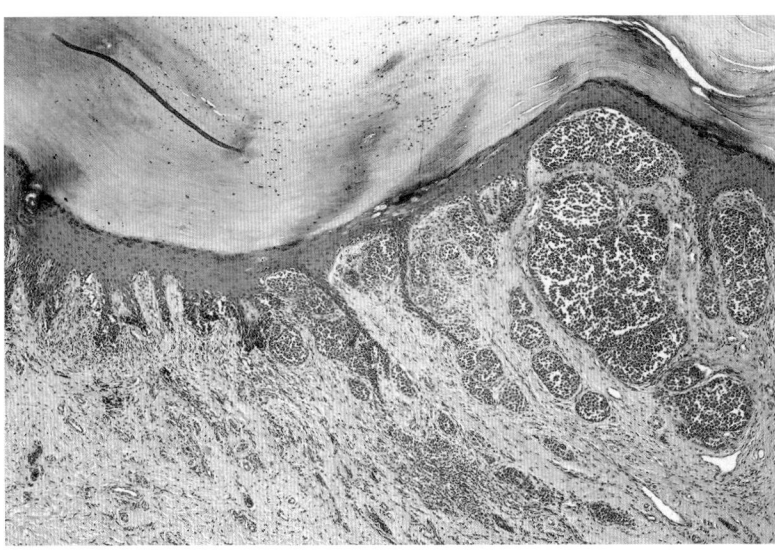

Fig. 26.36
Acral lentiginous melanoma: in this example, the invasive component is mixed epithelioid, spindled cell, and desmoplastic.

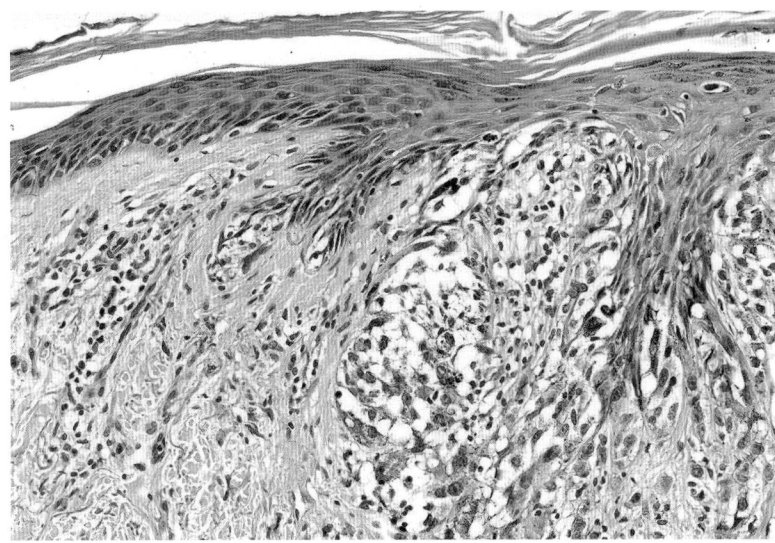

Fig. 26.38
Nodular melanoma: by definition, there is no melanocytic proliferative activity in the adjacent epidermis.

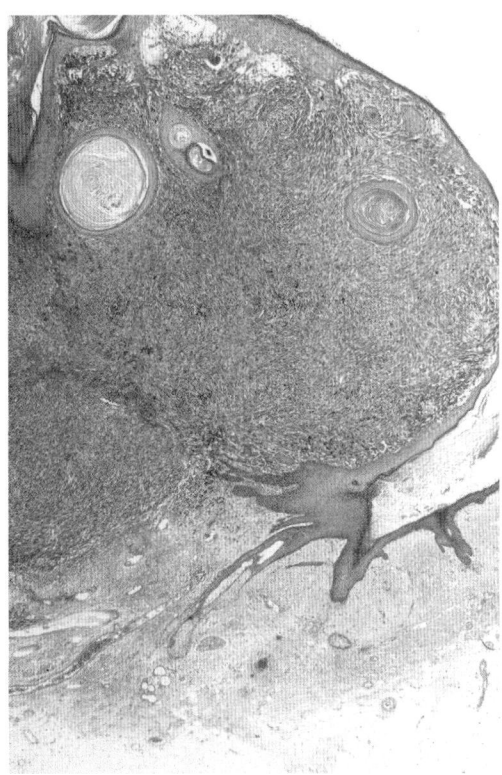

Fig. 26.37
Nodular melanoma: this variant is typically sharply circumscribed.

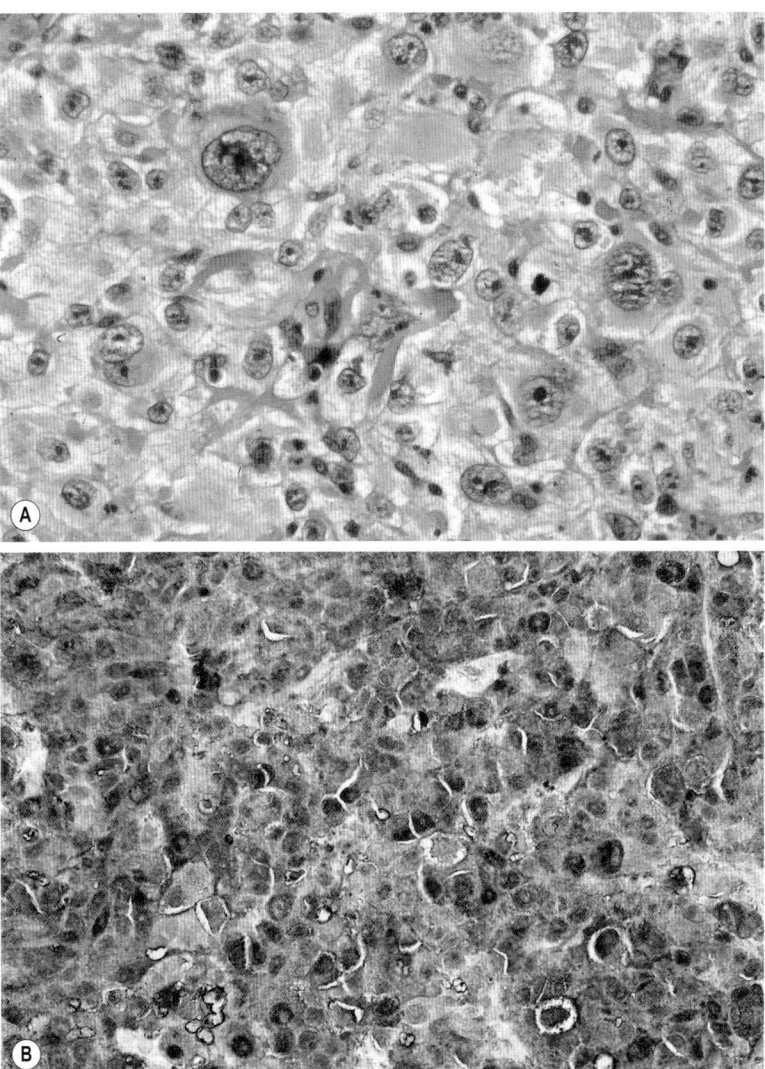

Fig. 26.39
Amelanotic melanoma: (**A**) the tumor cells are very pleomorphic with large vesicular nuclei and prominent nucleoli; (**B**) there is diffuse S100 expression. MART-1 was also positive. It is always of value to use at least two markers for melanoma as very occasionally S100 protein negative variants may be encountered.

Breslow tumor thickness is the single most important single prognostic indicator for primary cutaneous melanoma.[195,196] It is measured from the most superficial aspect of the granular cell layer to the deepest point of invasion of the tumor. In ulcerated tumors, the measurement should be from the base of the ulcer. The significance of periadnexal extension is less clear. If the latter is greater than the conventional Breslow thickness, the information should also be documented in addition to the traditional Breslow measurement (*Fig. 26.43*). Polypoid tumors should be treated no differently, and should be measured through the thickest region.[197] Tumor volume, therefore, is a most important factor influencing outcome in vertical growth phase melanoma. Careful evaluation of the greatest tumor thickness provides very useful prognostic guidance.[198–201] In the latest (8th) edition of the American Joint Committee on Cancer (AJCC) staging system (2017, effective in 2018), the thickness thresholds have been maintained as in the 7th Edition at 1.0, 2.0, and 4.0 mm, though the T1 group is subdivided 0.8 mm as well (*Table 26.1*).[196,202–206] The 7th edition staging is still

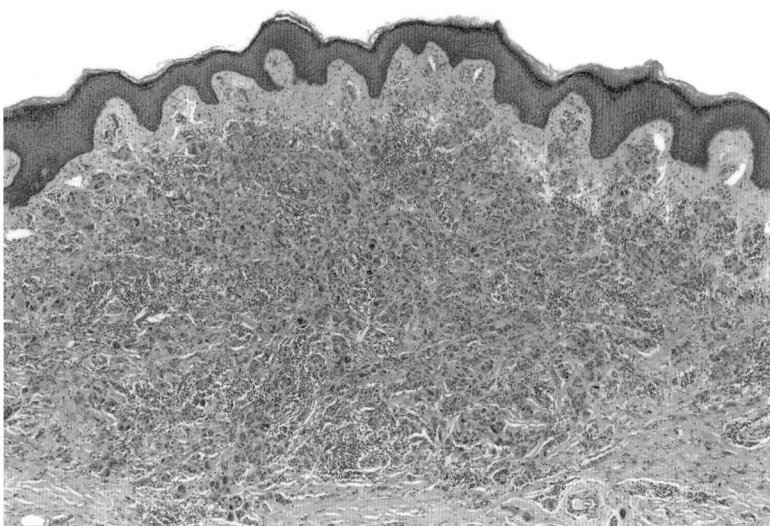

Fig. 26.40
Giant cell melanoma: within the dermis is a deposit of metastatic melanoma.

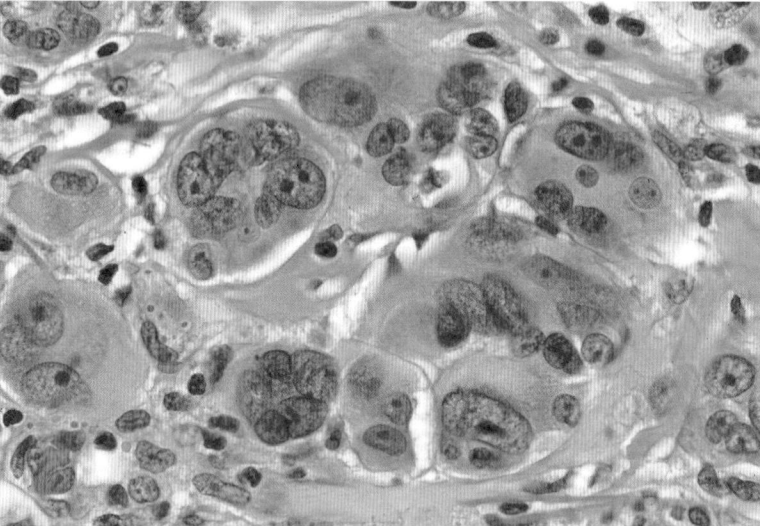

Fig. 26.41
Giant cell melanoma: the tumor cells are multinucleate and very pleomorphic with abundant cytoplasm and large vesicular nuclei containing prominent eosinophilic nucleoli.

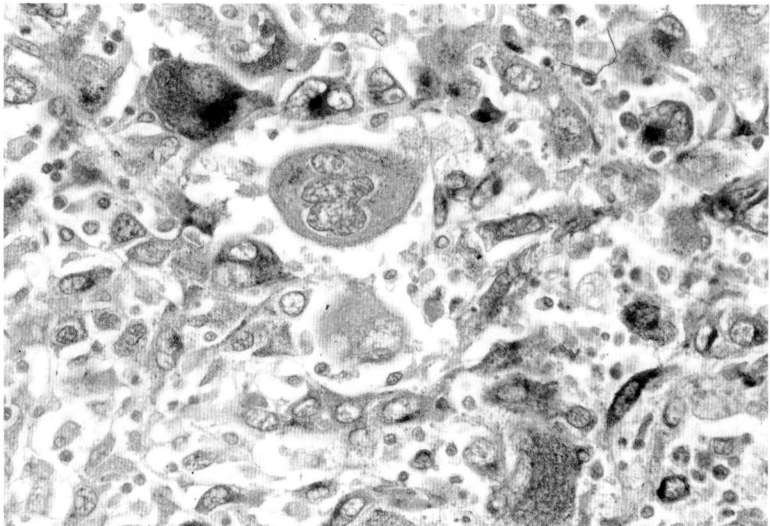

Fig. 26.42
Giant cell melanoma: the tumor cells are HMB-45 positive. The patient had a melanoma excised several years earlier.

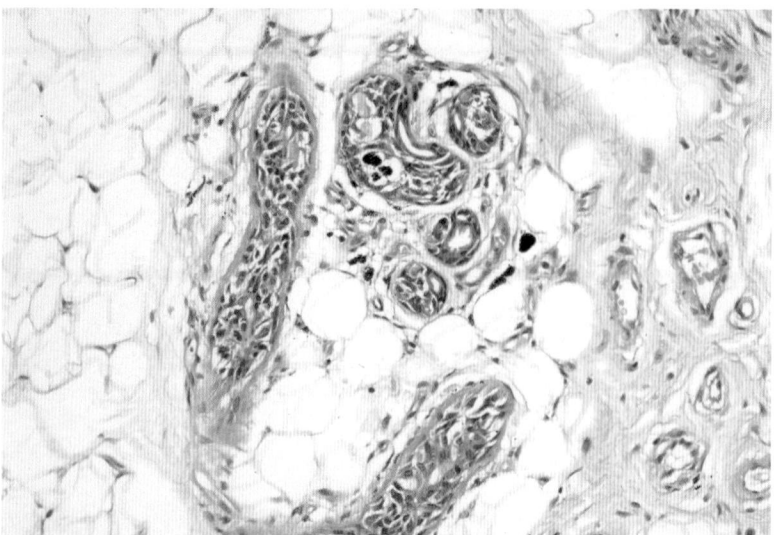

Fig. 26.43
Melanoma: periadnexal extension is of uncertain biological significance except that it is a potential source for recurrence of inadequately excised tumors. In this example, there is deep involvement of the eccrine sweat glands.

Major changes and clarifications of the 2017 AJCC melanoma staging system

- Database completely derived from patients of known sentinel lymph node status thus creating more homogeneous stage groups
- T0 designates no evidence of primary tumor; Tis designates *in situ* disease; TX designates tumor thickness that cannot be determined
- T categories maintained, but T1 with new 0.8 mm threshold
- Tumor thickness now reported only to nearest 0.1 mm
- Mitoses in primary tumor are recorded for prognosis, but no longer used for staging
- Clark level no longer used for staging primary
- For regional lymph node involvement, "microscopic" is now termed "clinically occult" and "macroscopic" termed "clinically detected" for clarity
- Sentinel lymph node is disease burden is prognostic and thus to be recorded, but not currently used for staging
- N category now has 4 subgroups rather than three
- Status of the primary (Breslow thickness and ulceration) extensively modifies stage III groupings
- In transit, satellite and microsatellite metastases are now categorized as N1c, N2c, N3c based on how many other regional nodes are involved (if any)
- Given the rapidly evolving systemic therapy landscape, Stage IV is no longer subdivided; metastatic site designation and LDH elevation are used solely to define clinically relevant patient groupings

provided here for purposes of comparison (*Table 26.2*). A pleasant feature of the new staging system is that Breslow thickness is now only reported to one significant digit after the decimal point, simplifying measurement with the micrometer. While certainly not perfect, clinical and particularly micro-pathological staging in melanoma is exceedingly powerful and serves as a model for other cancers.

The level of tumor invasion when classified according to Clark levels is as follows:

- Level I: in situ melanoma,
- Level II: invasion of the papillary dermis by single cells or small nests,
- Level III: invasive tumor usually as an expansile nodule abutting on the reticular dermal interface,
- Level IV: invasion of the reticular dermis,
- Level V: invasion of the subcutaneous fat.

The dermal interface may be identified by the site of the superficial capillary plexus. It also corresponds to the zone of transformation of the horizontally orientated reticular dermis elastic fibers to the vertically aligned ones of the papillary dermis. The distinction between Clark level II and III and perhaps

Table 26.1

AJCC 2017 (8th Edition) revised melanoma pathological staging system (effective, January 2018)

Stage group	Histological features/TNM designation	Disease specific survival[1]	
		5 years (%)	10 years (%)
0	Intraepithelial/in situ melanoma[2] (TisN0M0)	100	100
IA	<0.8 mm primary[3] without ulceration (T1aN0M0)	99	98
	<0.8 mm primary with ulceration (T1bN0M0)	99	98
	0.8-1.0 mm primary without ulceration (T1bN0M0)	99	96
IB	> 1.0-2.0 mm primary without ulceration (T2aN0M0)	97	94
IIA	> 1.0–2 mm primary without ulceration (T2bN0M0)	94	88
	2.0–4.0 mm primary without ulceration (T3aN0M0)	93	88
		94	88
IIB	2.0–4.0 mm with ulceration (T3bN0M0)	87	82
	> 4 mm without ulceration (T4aN0M0)	86	81
		90	83
IIC	> 4 mm with ulceration (T4bN0M0)	82	75
IIIA	Single regional node, clinically occult[4] (T1–2aN1aM0)	93	88
	2–3 regional nodes, clinically occult (T1–2aN2aM0)		
IIIB	Single regional node, clinically detected[5] (T1–T3aN1bM0)	83	77
	No regional node, in-transit / satellite disease (T1-2aN1cM0)		
	2–3 regional nodes, at least 1clinically detected (T1–2aN2bM0)		
	Single regional node, clinically occult (T2b–3aN1aM0)		
	Single regional node, clinically detected (T2b–T3aN1bM0)		
	No regional node, in-transit / satellite disease (T2b-3aN1cM0)		
	2–3 regional nodes, clinically occult (T2b–3aN2aM0)		
	2–3 regional nodes, at least 1clinically detected (T2b–3aN2bM0)		
	No evidence of primary tumor (T0N1b-1cM0)		
IIIC	Single regional node, occult or clinically detected; +/- in-transit / satellite disease (T1a-3aN2cM0)	69	60
	4 or more regional nodes, clinically occult (T1a-3aN3aM0)		
	4 or more regional nodes, at least 1 clinically detected (T1a-3aN3bM0)		
	2 or more regional nodes clinically occult or detected and/or matted nodes; 2+ regional nodes +/- in-transit / satellite disease (T1a-3aN3cM0)		
	Any regional node status greater than N1 (T3b-4aN2a-3cM0)		
	Any regional node status less than N3 (T4bN1a-2cM0)		
	No evidence of primary tumor (T0N2b-2c,3b-3cM0)		
IIID	Any N3 (T4bN3a-3cM0)	32	24
IV	Distant metastasis (T1a-4bN1a-3cM1)		
	M1a = distant metastasis to skin, soft tissue or nonregional node		
	M1b = distant metastasis to lung +/- M1a site(s)		
	M1c = distant metastasis to viscera (non-CNS) +/- M1a or M1b site(s)		
	M1d = distant metastasis to CNS +/- M1a, M1b or M1c site(s)		
	(0) = LDH normal / not elevated		
	(1) = LDH elevated		

[1]Five and 10 year disease specific survival provided for overall stage groups as well as individually defined cohorts that comprise the stage group where available.
[2]The underlined portion of the TNM designation is defined by the histologic features for each group.
[3]Breslow thickness is defined as the thickness of the lesion using an ocular micrometer to measure the total vertical height of the melanoma from the top of the granular layer to the area of deepest penetration (and reported to the nearest 0.1 mm). If the entire overlying epithelial surface is ulcerated, measure from the base of the ulcer to the depthest point of invasion.
[4]Clinically occult (previously termed microscopic) metastasis is defined as following pathologic assessment of sentinel lymph node and/or lymphadenectomy specimen. There is no minimum size lesion for metastasis. Immunohistochemistry can be used to screen for micrometastases, but should include at least one 'melanoma-specific' marker (i.e., HMB-45, MART1, MelanA).
[5]Clinically detected (previously termed macroscopic) metastasis is clinically evident nodal disease known prior to pathologic examination.
Adapted from AJCC Cancer Staging Manual, 8th Edition (2017) Eds: Amin MB, et al. Melanoma of the Skin, pp.563–585. Springer-Verlag, New York. © and Gershenwald, J. E., Scolyer, R. A. Hess, K. R., et al. (2017) Melanoma staging: Evidence-based changes in the American Joint Committee on Cancer eighth edition cancer staging manual. *CA Cancer J Clin*, 67;472–492.

more so between III and IV is somewhat difficult to apply in practice and is observer dependent.[207] Clark level was believed to provide independent prognostic information for thin tumors (1.0 mm or less in thickness) but not for thicker melanomas.[208,209] The latest data indicate that if mitotic rate is assessable in thin melanomas, then Clark level no longer provides additional prognostic information. The 2017 (8th) AJCC staging system no longer recommends the use of the Clark level, even for thin melanomas, as in the previous edition.[196,203,204,206] Mitotic rate in the primary melanoma correlates with sentinel lymph node positivity for metastasis.[210]

The presence or absence of ulceration and the width of the ulcer are independent prognostic indicators and should be recorded.[175,211] Ulceration is defined as 'the absence of an intact epidermis overlying a major portion of the primary melanoma based on microscopic examination of the histologic sections'.[203] Trauma and artifactual loss of the epidermis must be excluded. Ulceration is associated with a very significant increased risk of metastasis and was first included as a second determinant in the T classification in the AJCC 6th Edition and retained in the current 8th Edition.[196,203,206,208,209,212]

Tumor-infiltrating lymphocytes are an important independent prognostic variable and should be recorded as brisk, nonbrisk, or absent (*Figs 26.44–26.46*).[145,206,213–215] The brisk category implies lymphocytes present throughout the whole vertical growth phase or extending across its entire base. Nonbrisk tumor infiltrating lymphocytes implies focal infiltration

Table 26.2
AJCC 7th Edition Staging – For historical comparison only, no longer in clinical use

Stage	Histological features/TNM classification	Overall survival 1 year (%)	5 years (%)	10 years (%)
0	Intraepithelial/in situ melanoma (TisN0M0)		100	100
IA	≤ 1 mm without ulceration and mitoses <1/mm² * (T1aN0M0)		97	93
IB	≤ 1 mm with ulceration or level IV/V (T1bN0M0) 1.01–2 mm without ulceration (T2aN0M0)		94 91	87 83
IIA	1.01–2 mm with ulceration (T2bN0M0) 2.01–4 mm without ulceration (T3aN0M0)		82 79	67 66
IIB	2.01–4 mm with ulceration (T3bN0M0) > 4 mm without ulceration (T4aN0M0)		68 71	55 57
IIC	> 4 mm with ulceration (T4bN0M0)		53	39
IIIA	Single regional nodal micrometastasis**, nonulcerated primary (T1–4aN1aM0) 2–3 microscopic regional nodes, nonulcerated primary (T1–4aN2aM0)		78	68
IIIB	Single regional nodal micrometastasis, ulcerated primary (T1–4bN1aM0) 2–3 microscopic regional nodes, ulcerated primary (T1–4bN2aM0) Single regional nodal macrometastasis***, nonulcerated primary (T1–4aN1bM0) 2–3 macroscopic regional nodes, nonulcerated primary (T1–4aN2bM0) In-transit metastasis(es)/satellite lesion(s) without metastatic lymph nodes (T1–4a/bN2cM0)		59	43
IIIC	Single microscopic regional node, ulcerated primary (T1–4bN1bM0) 2–3 macroscopic regional nodes, ulcerated primary (T1–4bN2bM0) In-transit metastasis(es)/satellite lesion(s) without metastatic lymph nodes, ulcerated primary(T1–4bN2cM0) 4 or more metastatic nodes, matted nodes/gross extracapsular extension, or in-transit metastasis(es)/satellite(s) and metastatic nodes (anyTN3M0)		40	24
IV	Distant skin, subcutaneous, or nodal metastasis with normal LDH (any T any NM1a) Lung metastasis with normal LDH (any T any NM1b) All other visceral metastasis with normal LDH or any distant metastasis with increased LDH(any T any NM1c)	62 53 33		

Breslow thickness is defined as the thickness of the lesion using an ocular micrometer to measure the total vertical height of the melanoma from the top of the granular layer to the area of deepest penetration. The Clark level refers to levels of invasion according to depth of penetration of the dermis.
*Clark level is now only used when mitotic rate is not available in a T1 tumor. Level IV or V invasion would meet criterion for T1b.
**Micrometastases are defined as following pathological assessment of sentinel lymph node and/or lymphadenectomy specimen. There is no longer a minimum size lesion for metastasis. Immunohistochemistry may be used to screen for micrometastases, but must include at least one 'melanoma-specific' marker (i.e., HMB-45, MART1, MelanA).
***Macrometastasis is clinically detectable with pathological confirmation or gross extracapsular extension on pathological examination.Adapted with permission from AJCC Cancer Staging Manual, 7th Edition (2009) Eds: Edge SB, et al. Melanoma of the Skin, pp.325–344. Springer-Verlag, New York. © and Balch, C. M., Gershenwald, J. E., Soong, S. J. et al. (2009) Final Version of 2009 AJCC Melanoma Staging and Classification. *J Clin Oncol*, 27; 6199–6206.

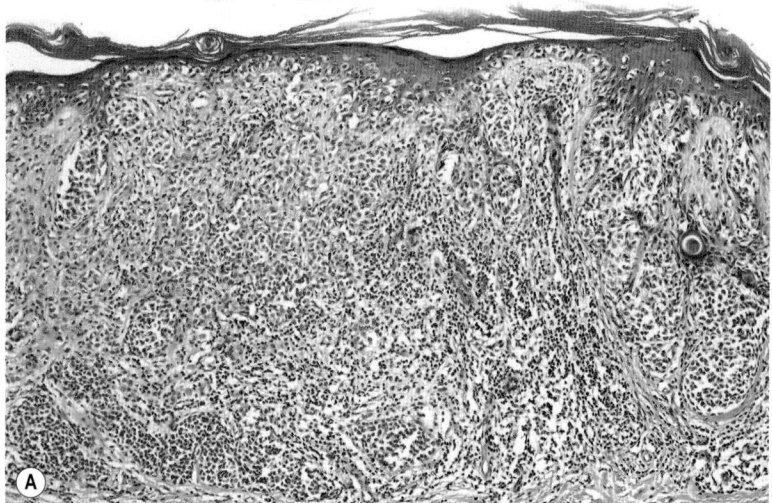
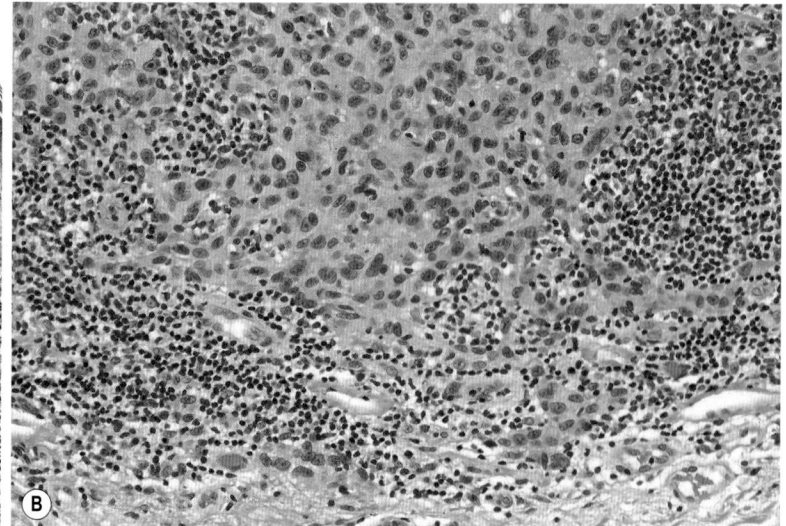

Fig. 26.44
(**A**, **B**) Melanoma: tumor infiltrating lymphocytes. Category A – Brisk: the lymphocytes infiltrate the tumor and extend along the whole of the base of the lesion.

only. Absent includes two categories: either no lymphocytes at all or lymphocytes are present but do not infiltrate the melanoma. Brisk lymphocytic responses tend to be a feature of thin melanomas whereas absence of a lymphocytic response is generally seen in thick melanomas.[200,214] In a study of 285 vertical growth phase tumors, the 10-year survival rates for brisk, nonbrisk, and absent tumor-infiltrating lymphocytes were 55%, 45%, and 27%, respectively.[214] Recently, it has been suggested that tumor-infiltrating lymphocytes are influenced by sex and sentinel lymph node status only correlated in men and not in women.[216] Not surprisingly, the absence of tumor-infiltrating lymphocytes also correlated with metastasis to sentinel lymph nodes as a surrogate marker of melanoma risk in a cohort of 887 patients with full multivariate analysis.[215] Image analysis and feature

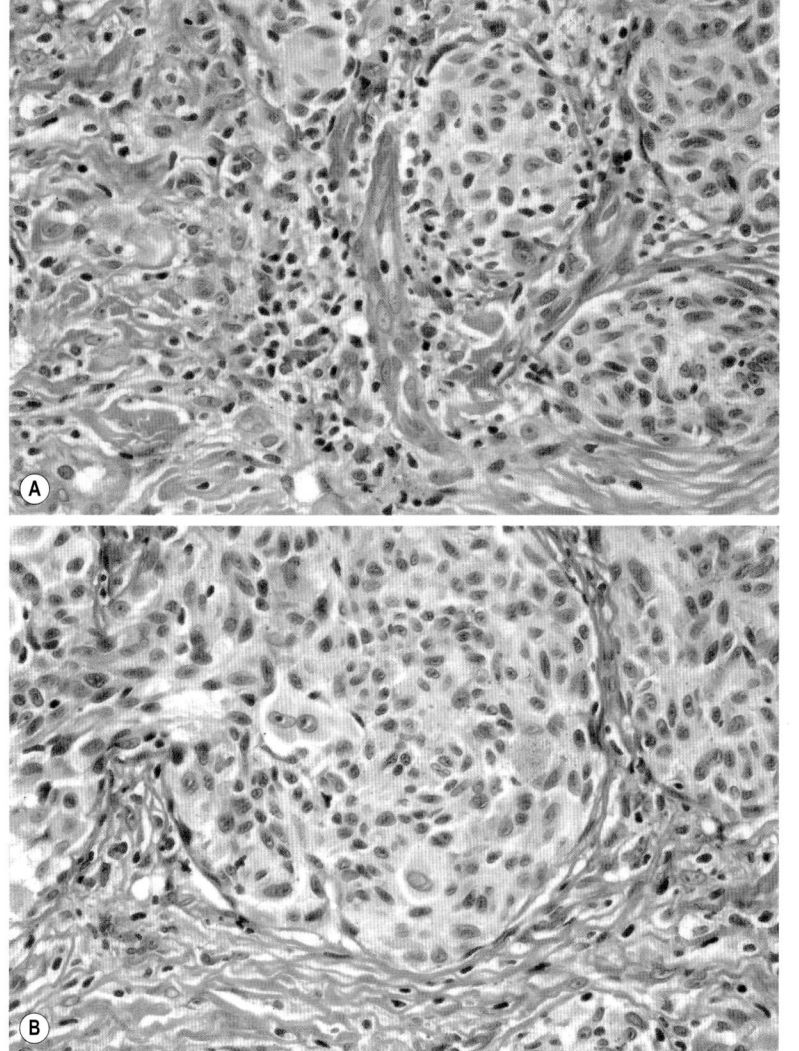

Fig. 26.45

(**A**, **B**) Melanoma: tumor infiltrating lymphocytes. Category B – Nonbrisk: the lymphocytes infiltrate only part of the tumor.

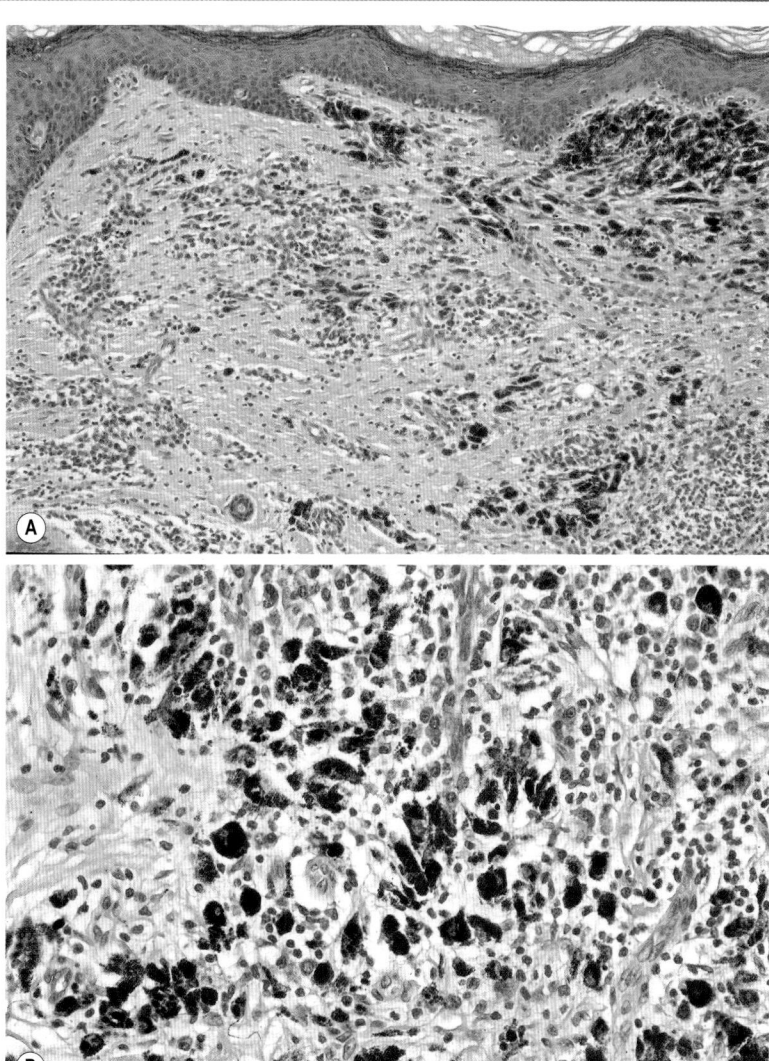

Fig. 26.47

(**A**, **B**) Regression: no residual epidermal component is present. Note the lymphocytic infiltrate, plasma cells, abundant melanin-containing macrophages, scarring, and conspicuous vasculature.

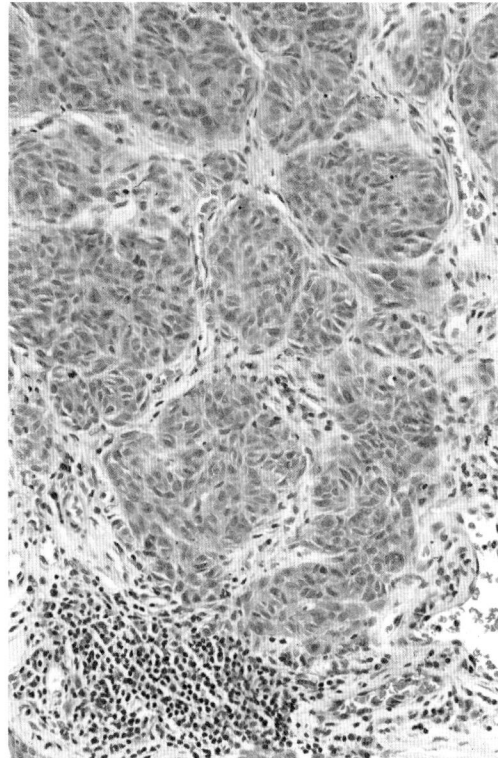

Fig. 26.46

Melanoma: tumor infiltrating lymphocytes. Category C – Absent: lymphocytes are present but they do not invade the tumor. The category also includes complete absence of lymphocytes.

extraction have been used to assess tumor-infiltrating lymphocytes with salutary results.[217] Assessing tumor-infiltrating lymphocytes in lymph node metastases also has predictive value.[218,219]

In thin melanoma it is important to recognize the features of regression, which may be particularly evident in the dermal component (*Figs 26.47* and *26.48*).[145,220] These include absence or reduced numbers of malignant melanocytes, degenerate (apoptotic) forms, and a chronic inflammatory cell infiltrate (*Fig. 26.49*).[221-223] Melanophages, horizontal scarring, isolated tumor islands, and telangiectatic vessels are also commonly present in the later stage. Clinically, regression presents as macular gray, white, or pink areas.

Although the importance of regression as a determinant of biological behavior has been the subject of considerable argument in the literature, a number of authors believe that, in thin tumors, it correlates with an impaired prognosis, though this contribution may be minor relative to other factors in many cases.[223-232] Complete regression of an undiagnosed primary melanoma may be the explanation for patients presenting with metastatic tumor of unknown primary (*Fig. 26.50*).[233] Some authors recommend sentinel node biopsy for thin melanomas if there is evidence of extensive (>50%) regression, while other series do not show an association between regression and nodal status.[176,234]

Mitotic rate is determined by the number of mitotic figures/1 mm^2 of tumor in the most mitotically active area. It has become clear that tumors displaying a high mitotic rate are associated with a poorer prognosis and that mitoses are a more robust predictor of outcome than ulceration and thus mitotic rate was incorporated into the 7th AJCC staging system.[145,204,235-240] While mitoses are still recognized as a prognostic factor, the current 8th

AJCC staging system relies on ulceration rather than mitoses due to stage group stability.[196,206] Despite earlier contrary evidence and the complex interrelations of tumor thickness, ulceration, and mitotic rate, mitotic rate appears to carry prognostic information independent of both of the other factors.[176,241,242]

The presence of a microscopic satellite is defined by a distinct tumor nodule of any size at any distance discontinuous from the main primary tumor mass separated by normal tissue (no scarring, fibrosis or extensive inflammation).[206] It is found in thicker tumors and is associated with an increased risk of local recurrence, regional lymph node metastases, and diminished survival.[243–246] The presence of microsatellites results in upstaging to N1c if there is no regional lymph node involvement, and upstaging to N2c or N3c with one or more than one lymph nodes involved, respectively, in the 2017 AJCC melanoma staging system.[206]

The presence of lymphatic invasion correlates with the development of in-transit metastases (Fig. 26.51).[247] Lymphovascular invasion has been shown to represent a predictor of diminished survival in melanoma in a number of studies.[215,248–253] The use of immunohistochemistry for D2-40 significantly increases the sensitivity for detection of lymphatic invasion and also correlates with lymph node metastasis and survival.[254–257] More study and a prospective trial is needed to validate the application and interpretation of the technique. Contrariwise, absence of vascular involvement in thick melanomas correlates with increased survival in a number of studies.[258,259] Perineural and intraneural infiltration are most often encountered in desmoplastic variants, thereby accounting, in part, for the increased risk of local recurrence (Fig. 26.52). In this context, CD57 immunohistochemistry can be helpful in identifying residual nerve (Fig. 26.53).

Angiogenesis, which is defined as the increasing development of new blood vessels at the base of the melanoma, parallels increases in tumor

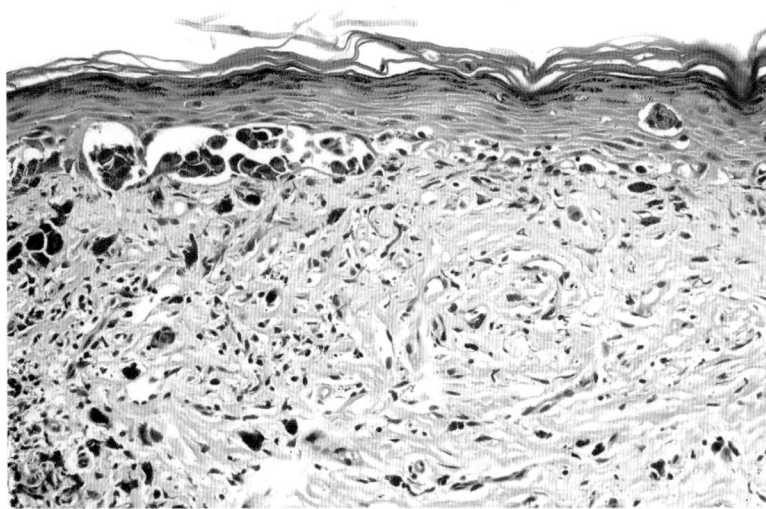

Fig. 26.48
Partial regression: in this variant, the junctional component is still present. Its significance is less certain.

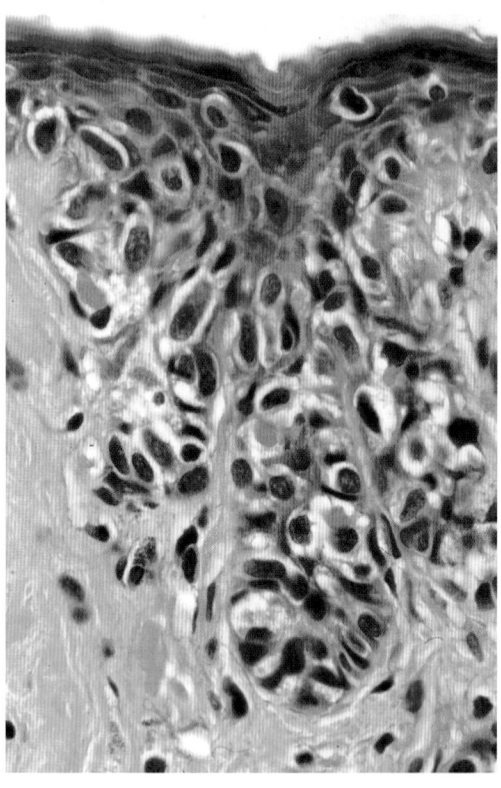

Fig. 26.49
Regression: in this example, there is conspicuous apoptosis. Note the eosinophilic bodies.

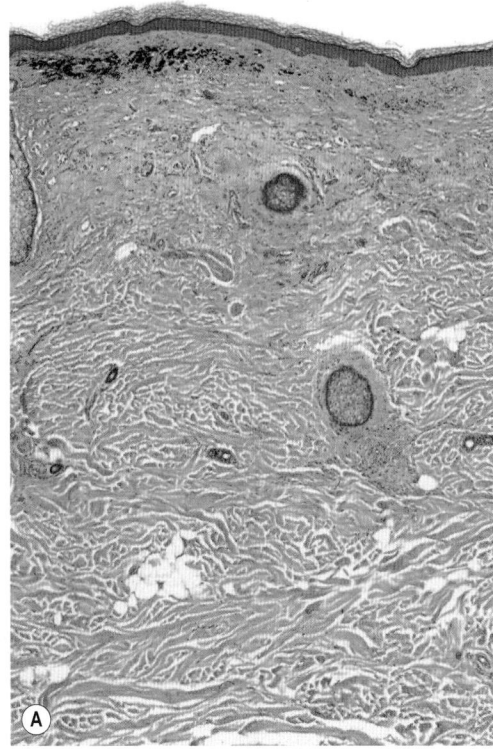

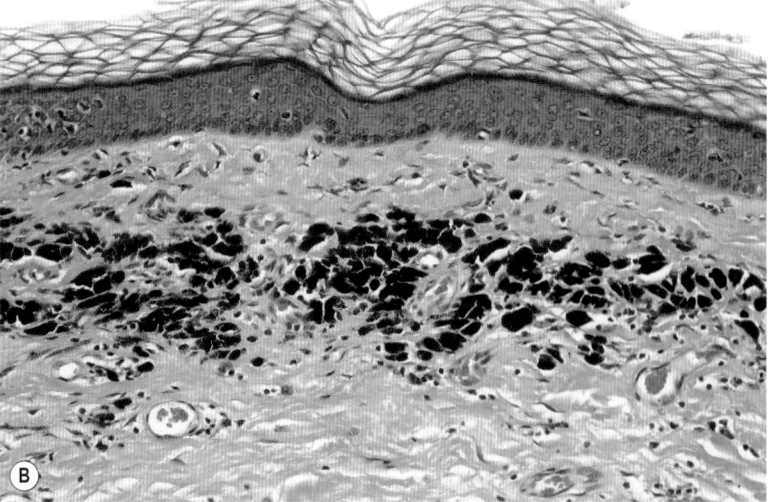

Fig. 26.50
(A, B) Regression: in this example, there is no residual tumor. The dermis is scarred and there is abundant melanin pigment. The patient presented with an unknown primary. By courtesy of M. Forder, MD, St Anne's Medical Center, Pietermaritzburg, South Africa.

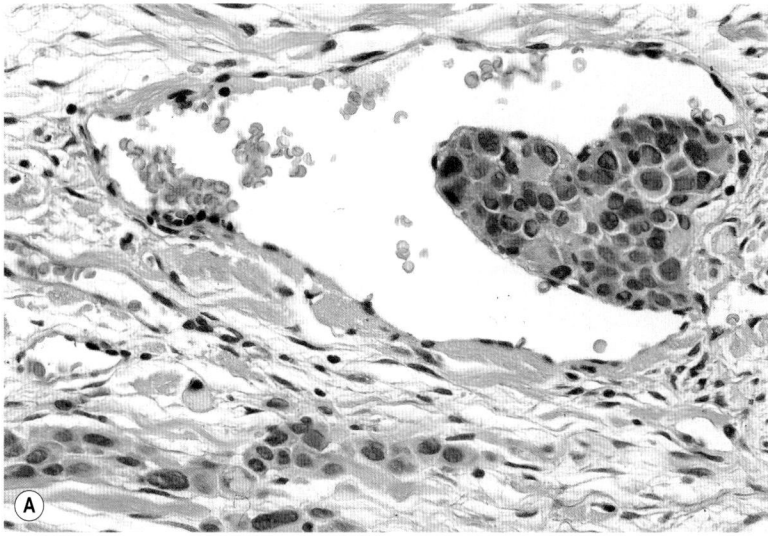

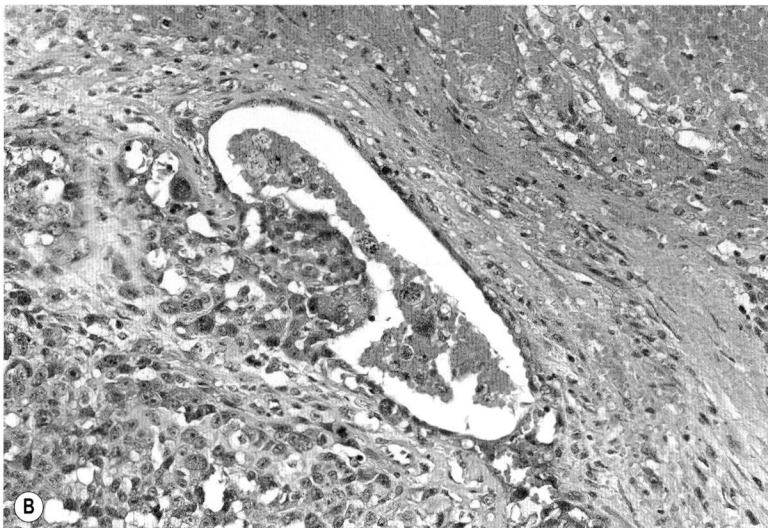

Fig. 26.51
Melanoma: vascular invasion: (**A**) pleomorphic tumor cells are adherent to the endothelium; (**B**) tumor cells are growing into the lumen.

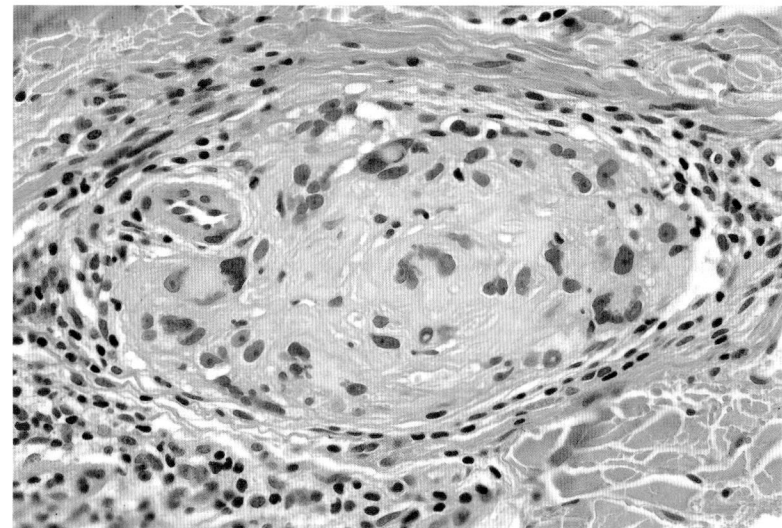

Fig. 26.52
Melanoma: intraneural invasion. Note the pleomorphic tumor nuclei within this nerve trunk.

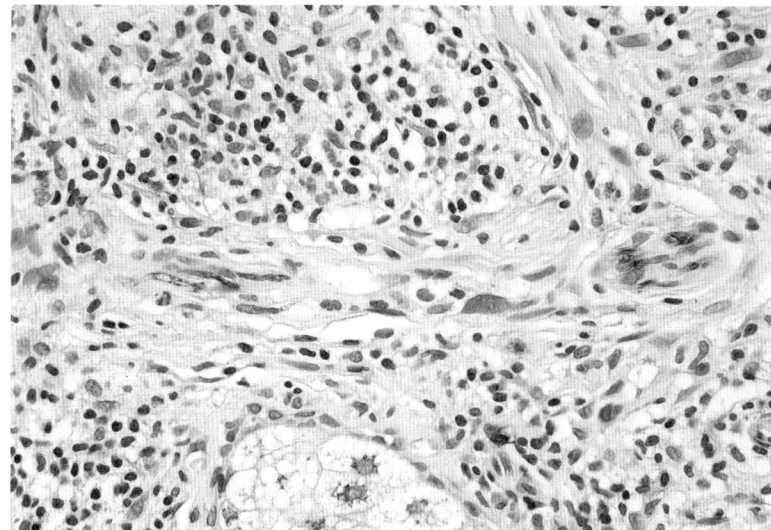

Fig. 26.53
Melanoma: CD57 immunohistochemistry may be particularly valuable when tumor growth has largely destroyed the nerve.

thickness.[260–265] Increasing angiogenesis therefore correlates with thick tumors, ulceration, relapse, and tumor-associated death.[263,266] Perhaps related to the likelihood of lymphovascular invasion, increased intratumoral and peritumoral lymphangiogenesis as measured by D2-40 or VEGF-C also correlates with metastasis to sentinel lymph nodes and reduced disease-specific survival.[267,268]

Sentinel node biopsy also adds extremely valuable prognostic information.[269–273] It has been shown to represent the most important factor in determining likelihood of tumor recurrence and patient survival in stage I and stage II disease.[270] Completion lymph node dissection for positive sentinel lymph nodes is expected to become less common with the MSLT-II trial failing to show a survival benefit of the completion procedure.[274,275] The latest AJCC staging system requires incorporation of sentinel lymph node data in cases where it would inform management, as this procedure significantly increases the accuracy and discriminatory power of the stage groups.[204,206] Lymph nodes are bivalved or serially sectioned along their long axis and in addition to the examination of hematoxylin and eosin stained sections, immunohistochemistry – such as S100 protein, HMB-45, and/or MART-1 (melanoma antigen recognized by T cells 1) – should invariably be performed in those cases where the initial sections are negative. Detection of single or tiny groups of cells using an antibody against a 'melanoma-specific' antigen such as HMB-45 or MART1 is now incorporated into the AJCC staging system. More recently, molecular techniques including reverse transcriptase polymerase chain reaction for tyrosinase messenger RNA have been proposed.[276,277] A major disadvantage of such procedures is the likelihood of false-positive results due to the common presence of banal capsular nevi, though the use of markers more specific to melanoma over nevus cells could potentially alleviate this problem.[278]

Sentinel node biopsy is currently recommended for all tumors measuring 1.00 mm or more in thickness. Other possible indications include ulcerated tumors, tumors with 50% or more regression, tumors having achieved the vertical growth phase, and those lesions which have been biopsied and involve the deep margin.[176,272,279,280] The procedure should also be considered for tumors that are less than 1.00 mm thick but display conspicuous mitotic activity.[281]

Differential diagnosis

Amelanotic spindled cell melanoma may be histologically indistinguishable from other cutaneous spindled cell tumors including leiomyosarcoma, spindled cell squamous carcinoma, atypical fibroxanthoma, and even dermatofibrosarcoma protuberans. In such cases, the use of an appropriate panel of immunohistochemical reagents, including antibodies to S100 protein, SOX10, HMB-45 or MART-1, pan-cytokeratin, AE1/AE3, smooth muscle actin (SMA), and CD34, is often essential. Similarly, highly pleomorphic, amelanotic epithelioid melanoma sometimes has to be distinguished from anaplastic carcinoma and occasionally anaplastic lymphoma. The use of antibodies to keratins, epithelial membrane antigen (EMA), carcinoembryonic antigen (CEA), leukocyte common antigen (LCA), T- and B-cell antigens, and CD30 may be necessary to achieve a definitive diagnosis.

Immunohistochemistry of melanoma

Immunohistochemistry is a valuable adjunct to histology in the diagnosis of melanoma, particularly in amelanotic, epithelioid, and spindled cell variants and their distinction from undifferentiated carcinomas and mesenchymal tumors.[1–3] Owing to problems of specificity and sensitivity, it is prudent to use two or even three 'melanoma markers' in such problematical cases. Using these markers as part of a panel looking at multiple lines of differentiation is also of practical use, such as inclusion of keratins to exclude epithelial tumors. In morphologically challenging cases, a panel of stains that supports the ultimate diagnosis by their pattern of reactivity or nonreactivity is very helpful. The role of immunohistochemistry is to provide supportive data. It should rarely if ever be used as the sole criterion by which a diagnosis of melanoma is achieved.

S100 protein remains the yardstick in the immunohistochemical diagnosis of melanoma.[4–6] Although there are now substantial numbers of new markers available, none as yet, in isolation, measures up to S100 protein. However, S100 protein lacks specificity and there are very exceptional S100 protein-negative melanomas, virtually all metastatic.[7,8] In cases where the diagnosis remains in doubt, use of a battery of immunohistochemical markers may be of great value.[1]

S100 protein is a calcium binding F-band protein, isolated from brain. It is variably positive in 94–100% of primary and metastatic melanomas.[1,2] In addition to melanocytes, Schwann cells, myoepithelial cells, adipocytes, chondrocytes, macrophages, Langerhans cells, and tumors derived thereof, express S100 protein. Staining of Langerhans cells can sometimes be a problem, particularly when assessing the extent of intraepidermal melanocyte spread. In such instances, the addition of MITF, SOX10, HMB-45, or MART-1 may be helpful. S100 protein may also be expressed in a number of breast carcinomas and undifferentiated carcinomas.[5,6] The most commonly employed antibody against S100 is a purified rabbit polyclonal antibody against S100 protein purified from bovine brain. More than 20 members of this family exist and monoclonal antibodies are available for many of them. While not well established in large series, there may be some selectivity of the isoforms between melanoma and other traditionally S100 protein reactive neoplasms in the differential diagnosis.[9]

HMB-45 reacts with the cytoplasmic premelanosome glycoprotein gp100 and is less sensitive than S100 protein.[9] It is expressed by 80–86% of metastatic melanomas and between 90% and 100% of primary tumors.[1,4,9] However, expression is often more focal than with S100. Sensitivity diminishes in spindled cell variants and it is usually negative in desmoplastic melanoma (see below).[10,11] The junctional and superficial dermal components of banal nevi also react with HMB-45 but the deeper dermal nevus cells are generally negative. This differential staining pattern may be of value in confirmation of pre-existent banal nevus cells associated with a melanoma and in particular their distinction from small cell and nevoid melanoma, which are typically positive in a patchy fashion in the deepest nests of cells (*Fig. 26.54*). It is very important to remember that this pattern is lost in cases where melanocytes are pigmented as the latter are positive for HMB-45. Dysplastic nevi are similarly labeled. Blue nevi and deep penetrating nevi are also HMB-45 positive.[1] Spitz nevi are often HMB-45 positive in the superficial aspect of the lesion and this is usually, but by no means always, lost with depth. This finding may be of value in its distinction from spitzoid melanoma in which staining is typically present throughout the tumor. Although it is more specific than S100 protein, HMB-45 also reacts with the group of perivascular epithelioid cell tumors (PEComas) including angiomyolipoma, lymphangiomyomatosis, and clear cell sugar tumor of the lung.[12,13]

MART-1 (Melan-A) is a melanosomal differentiation antigen recognized by autologous cytotoxic T cells.[14–20] Some antibodies raised to this protein (e.g., A103) label a variety of lesions including adrenocortical, Leydig cell,

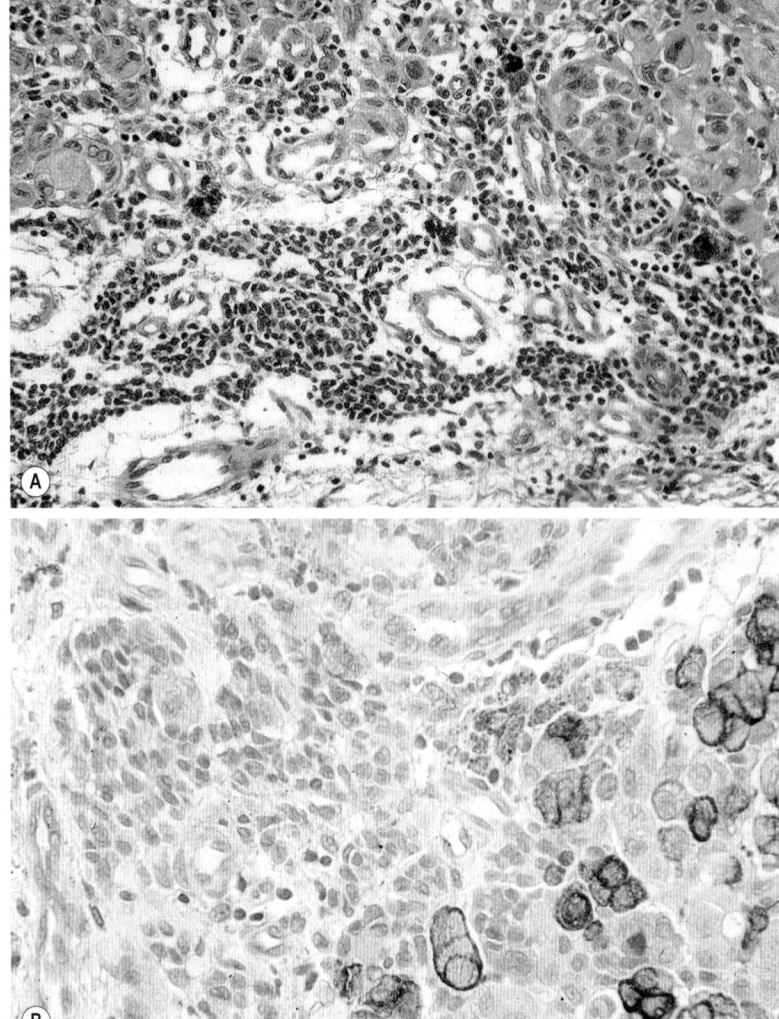

Fig. 26.54
Melanoma: this tumor has arisen in a background of a banal nevus. (**A**) Compare the eosinophilic, pleomorphic tumor cells with the small basophilic nevus cells; (**B**) the melanoma cells are HMB-45 positive; the nevus cells are negative.

Sertoli cell, and granulosa cell tumors, and tumors in the PEComa group of lesions including angiomyolipoma, lymphangiomyomatosis, and clear cell sugar tumors of the lung in addition to melanoma.[18,19] It has a similar sensitivity to S100 protein in epithelioid melanomas but is less sensitive in spindled cell tumors and is not usually expressed in the desmoplastic variant. A study has shown evidence that diminished MART-1 expression correlates with increasing tumor thickness, reduced disease-free interval, and increased patient mortality.[18] MART-1 expression has also been demonstrated in compound, dermal nevi and Spitz nevi with the exception of neurotized variants.[15–17]

Antityrosinase antibody (e.g., T311) appears to be less sensitive than either S100 protein, HMB-45, or Melan-A (A103).[21–26] It does not appear to label desmoplastic melanoma. Cocktails of HMB-45, MART-1, and antityrosinase antibodies are used by some to increase sensitivity for detection of melanocytic differentiation.[27]

Microphthalmia transcription factor (MITF) is a transcriptional regulator important for tyrosinase expression.[28] It is strongly positive in nevi and epithelioid melanoma.[29–31] Sensitivity is reduced in spindled cell and desmoplastic variants.[32] Spitz nevi and neurotized banal nevi show diminished expression. The specificity of MITF is low and this limits its use in the differential diagnosis of mimickers of melanocytic lesions. Its main use is in the evaluation of intraepidermal melanocytes as the staining is nuclear and other cells that reside in the epidermis are not positive for this marker.

The monoclonal antibody, SM5-1, was created by a subtractive immunization protocol using human melanoma samples and binds a variant of fibronectin.[33,34] Initial reports indicated that its sensitivity is similar to S100 protein with improved specificity for other traditionally S100 protein reactive, but the antibody also reacts with hepatocellular carcinoma and breast cancer cells.[26,35] This antibody is not widely used for clinical diagnosis.

SOX10 is a transcription factor that is a critical regulator of melanocytes.[36–38] Antibodies raised against it represent another marker of melanocytic and Schwann cells and tumors derived from the neural crest.[39] While it lacks specificity and stains other cells it is equally sensitive and more specific than S100 protein in relevant differential diagnoses with soft tissue neoplasms.[40,41] It is also useful in desmoplastic melanoma, though expression has also been noted in scars.[42–44] It has gained widespread use as a sensitive marker for melanoma, often used in combination with other melanocytic markers.[45] It has been suggested to be more specific than other melanocytic markers in the setting of determining melanocytic density in chronically sun-damaged skin where misleading false-positive rates are noted with other markers.[46] A role has also been suggested in evaluation of sentinel lymph nodes.[47]

The bar is high for inclusion of new markers as standards for melanoma in clinical practice. All antibodies have a natural history of decreasing specificity with study of additional tumor types and new antibodies are not as far down this curve as older antibodies, creating potential for misinterpretation if the new reagents are used alone.

Melanoma cells can express epithelial markers including keratins, EMA, and CEA.[2,48–50] Keratin, particularly those of low molecular weight, may be identified in as many as 10% of melanomas, both on frozen and on paraffin-embedded sections.[2] CEA is commonly encountered if polyclonal antibodies are utilized.[49,50] Metastatic disease more often shows such aberrant staining patterns than primary tumors. Diagnostic difficulties are unlikely to be encountered provided S100 protein and/or other melanoma markers have been included in the antibody panel. SMA and desmin are very rarely expressed in melanoma with the exception of the desmoplastic variant where, as in most spindle cell tumors, SMA can be detected to varying degrees.[51] One study with dual labeling for S100 protein and SMA in desmoplastic melanoma indicates that the SMA reactivity may be in accompanying stromal myofibroblasts.[52]

Melanoma cells can express histiocytic markers such as CD68 (KP1) in 80% or more of tumors.[53,54] Mac 387 and α_1-antitrypsin may also be positive. This is of particular significance since the distinction between tumor cells and histiocytes, particularly in sentinel lymph node specimens, can sometimes be problematical. In addition, distinguishing between balloon cell melanocytic lesions and xanthomatous infiltrates may require immunohistochemical confirmation, particularly if no residual recognizable melanocytic component is visible. In such circumstances, positive melanocytic markers are obviously of major diagnostic importance.

There is an ever-expanding range of reputed immunohistochemical prognostic markers.[55–57] Most of these lack appropriately powered full multivariate analysis linking the marker with specific outcome such as melanoma-specific mortality supplemented by hazard ratios and do not fully describe the methods utilized as recommended by the REMARK (Reporting recommendation for tumor MARKer prognostic studies) guidelines of the NCI-EORTC or AJCC precision medicine reporting recommendations for tumor marker prognostic studies.[58–62] The more useful of these are very briefly discussed below. Few of these are validated to the level necessary for routine application to clinical samples; virtually all are reported in retrospective cohorts with referral and other biases. Use of multiple markers and application of rigorous methods of quantification have efficacy, distinguishing different prognostic groups.[63] The markers discussed below are primarily used to help support a diagnosis of melanoma or nevus in the relatively small subset of cases where this determination is challenging on purely histologic grounds.

Ki-67 (MIB-1) is a particularly valuable adjunct in the distinction between benign melanocytic nevi (including Spitz nevi) and melanoma.[64,65] In nevi, less than 5% of nuclei are positive (and these are usually located in the most superficial aspect of the dermal component) whereas in melanoma 25% or more of cells are labeled (*Figs 26.55* and *26.56*). Its role in predicting biological behavior is controversial; thus although in earlier studies increased expression in thick tumors was thought to correlate with

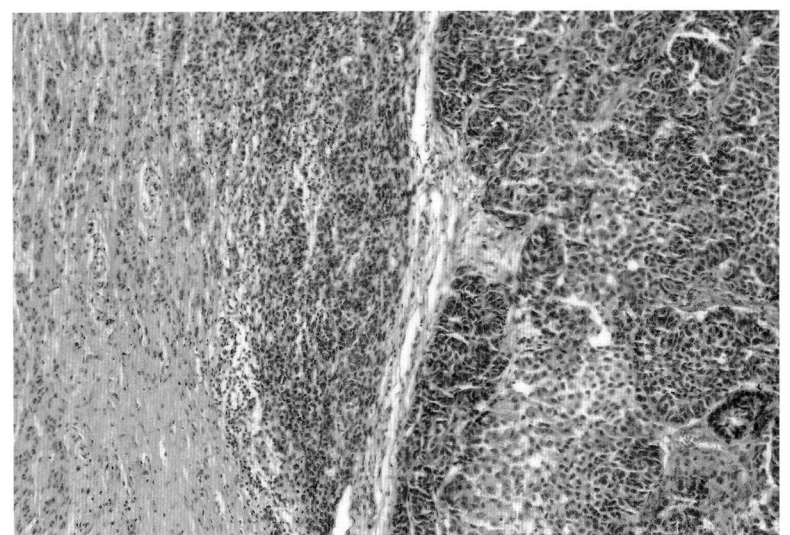

Fig. 26.55
Melanoma: this tumor (right side of field) has arisen in a background of a congenital nevus (left side of field).

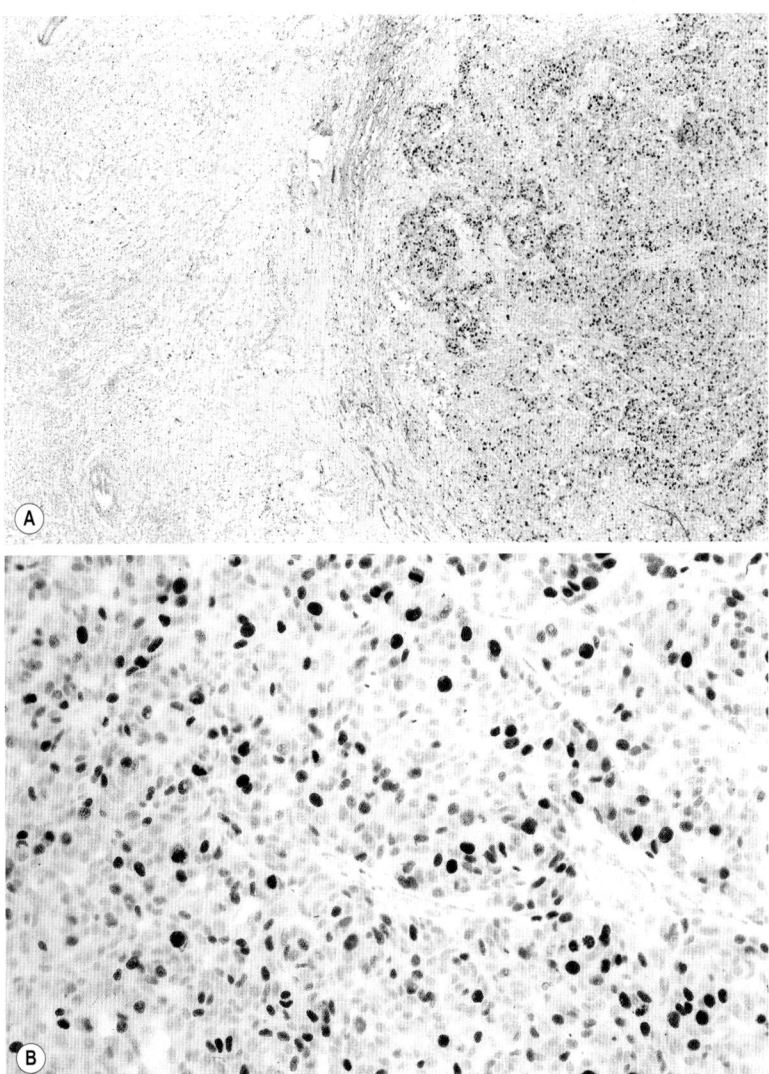

Fig. 26.56
(**A**, **B**) Melanoma: the melanoma shows very brisk MIB-1 expression, and the nevus is completely negative.

poor survival, more recently it has been claimed that increased expression in thin tumors (<1.5 mm) is of greater significance.[66–69] A further study indicates that increased MIB-1 reactivity is a poor prognostic factor in terms of disease-specific survival independent of tumor thickness.[70] Obviously, there is a proportional, though not exact, relationship between degree of nuclear MIB-1 reactivity and mitotic rate. Mitotic rate is an important determinate of melanoma outcome, though it no longer drives groupings in the 8th Edition of the AJCC staging system.[71] How to correlate Ki-67 reactivity with mitotic rates is evolving. Increased Ki-67 expression also correlates with overexpression of p53 protein and loss of p16 (see below).[68,70]

Phosphohistone H3 (PHH3) recognizes mitotic figures directly rather than cell cycle like MIB-1 and can assist in more objectively determining mitotic rates which do correlate with outcome.[72–79] Care must be taken when increasing the sensitivity of mitotic rate detection since the majority of the data is derived using the less sensitive, but currently gold standard microscopic detection on H&E stains, as inappropriate inflation of prognosis can occur.

Bcl-2 is strongly expressed in normal melanocytes and in a variety of nevi including banal, congenital, Spitz, blue, and dysplastic variants.[80–83] Although there is some variability of results in the literature, diminished expression has been said to correlate with melanoma, particularly metastatic lesions. Similarly, in problematical spitzoid lesions, strong expression may favor a diagnosis of benignancy.[84] Bcl-2 downregulation has been correlated with melanoma progression.[85–87] High bcl-2 was associated with improved disease-specific outcome when assessed in either primary or metastatic lesions using automated assessment of immunofluorescent immunohistochemistry.[88] From our own experience, however, bcl-2 is as often positive in melanoma as it is in banal nevi and it is therefore of little value in difficult cases.

Cyclin D1 may be of help in differentiating between a banal nevus and a nevoid melanoma or a nevic component within a melanoma. Its expression throughout the full thickness of a melanoma has been reported in up to 60% of cases, whereas staining may be absent or limited to only occasional cells in the superficial aspect of a nevus.[89,90] Increased cyclin D1 reactivity may correlate with amplification of its encoding genetic locus.[91–93] High levels of cyclin D3 in superficial melanoma have been found to correlate with early relapse and decreased survival.[94] This finding regarding cyclin D3 needs further confirmation.[90] Interestingly, cyclin D1 may interact more with CDK4 while cyclin D3 interacts more readily with CDK6, suggesting different functions for these two cyclin D isoforms.[95]

Loss of p16 protein expression correlates with invasive and metastatic melanoma.[96–99] It has also been shown to correlate with increased Ki-67 immunolabeling and independently to predict a poor prognosis.[70,98] P16 may also be helpful in differentiating capsular nevus from metastatic melanoma in sentinel lymph nodes.[100,101]

Although mutation of the *TP53* gene is relatively uncommon in melanoma at around 20%, overexpression of p53 protein may be identified in up to 40% of cases of invasive and metastatic melanoma, perhaps indicating disruption of this pathway.[102–107] It may therefore be of value in distinguishing between nevi (banal and Spitz) and melanoma. The former show virtually no positive cells whereas in the nodular and to a lesser extent superficial spreading melanoma they may be conspicuous. Expression of p53 also appears to be an independent predictor of poor prognosis.[68,106,108]

Immunohistochemistry for the BRAF V600E mutation using the VE1 clone is a highly sensitive and specific means of determining the mutational status of melanoma, usually applied in the metastatic setting.[109–111] It does not reliably detect common alternative BRAF V600 variants such as V600K that constitute 15–20% of BRAF mutations in some series.[112,113] This can be helpful in the rapid assessment for eligibility for BRAF inhibitor therapy, but DNA sequencing is still the gold standard for determining *BRAF* mutational status. A similar approach can detect a subset of the common NRAS mutant proteins Q61R and Q61L in melanoma with two separate antibody clones, but is not widely adopted.[110,114–118]

In the setting of immunotherapy, membranous expression of PD-L1 (programmed death-ligand 1) can influence the choice of immuno-oncological agents, but is not required to use such approaches.[119–122] A number of antibodies are available against PD-L1 for use in routine clinical immunohistochemistry, including some that are U.S. FDA-approved companion diagnostics, but such testing is not currently required to use immune checkpoint inhibitor therapy in melanoma.[123] Indeed, melanomas can respond to PD-1 (CD247/programmed cell death protein 1) inhibitors even if they completely lack membranous PD-L1 expression.[124] Most PD-L1 antibodies have very similar staining profiles in melanoma and other tumors as well.[125,126] Specific scoring approaches have been suggested and used for clinical trials and in routine practice. Staining for CD8-positive T-cells in melanoma can also be performed and higher levels are associated with increased likelihood of response to immuno-oncological therapy. Approaches for scoring these infiltrates have been suggested, but are not widely employed in routine clinical practice.[127–130] These biomarker approaches are used primarily in metastatic disease and their correlation with response is not perfect.[131,132] This is an active area of research and a number of genomic and other patient factors have also been associated with patient response. Companion immunohistochemical approaches are not currently used in clinical practice for CTLA-4 (CD152) inhibitors in melanoma. Anti-CTLA-4 therapy is sometimes used in combination with PD-1 inhibitors. PD-L1 expression can inform whether PD-1 monotherapy or combination approaches are employed in melanoma.[124] Additional work in this area is likely to produce more associated biomarkers as immuno-oncology expands to a number of emerging novel agents such as inhibitors of IDO1, LAG-3, and others where expression of the protein targets might be associated with treatment efficacy.[133,134]

Histologic variants of melanoma

Quite a range of histologic variants have been described.[1–3] With the exception of desmoplastic melanoma, these are of limited prognostic significance but are of importance because they may easily be mistaken for other tumors, with potentially serious consequences. In addition, some of the types are more or less likely to have mutations such as BRAF V600E that represent a therapeutic target, though the genotype histology correlation is not enough for treatment in most cases and direct molecular testing is required.[4,5]

Nested melanoma

This is a rare, recently described distinctive type of melanoma described as a variant of superficial spreading melanoma.[1,2] It presents in middle-aged to elderly adults with the same sex incidence. Although the clinical features are usually suspicious of melanoma, the histologic appearances are misleading. Tumors are in-situ or invasive and the junctional component is distinctively nested with little or no proliferation of melanocytes between the nests. The latter may be confluent and are located at the tips or less commonly, the slopes of the rete-ridges. Mitotic activity tends to be low within the nests and cytologic atypia varies from moderate to severe. Multiple chromosomal abnormalities are demonstrated by cytogenetic analysis.

Minimal deviation melanoma

The concept of minimal deviation melanoma was introduced to define a subset of invasive melanoma that showed minimal histologic deviation from banal nevi and therefore lacked the pleomorphism seen in classic melanoma. It was further postulated that such tumors appeared to have a better prognosis than classic melanoma.[1–8] Over the last decade, use of this nomenclature has precipitously declined and it is now presented primarily for historical interest.

As defined, two subtypes were recognized[6]:
- borderline minimal deviation melanoma where the dermal component is confined to the papillary dermis (Clark level 3),
- minimal deviation melanoma where there is infiltration into the reticular dermis or beyond (Clark level 4 or 5).

Minimal deviation melanoma is characterized by the presence of an expansile nodule showing only mild to moderate cytological atypia. It lacks the disorderly, more marked pleomorphism of conventional epithelioid or spindled cell melanoma. The spectrum includes epithelioid variants composed of cells resembling those of a compound melanocytic nevus, spitzoid forms, spindled cell variants, and halo nevus-like lesions.[1]

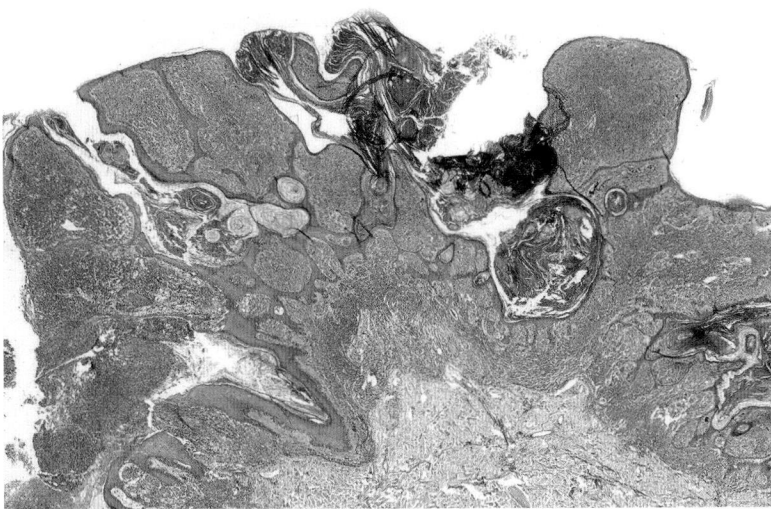

Fig. 26.57
Verrucous nevoid melanoma: verrucous nevoid lesions in the elderly should be viewed with suspicion.

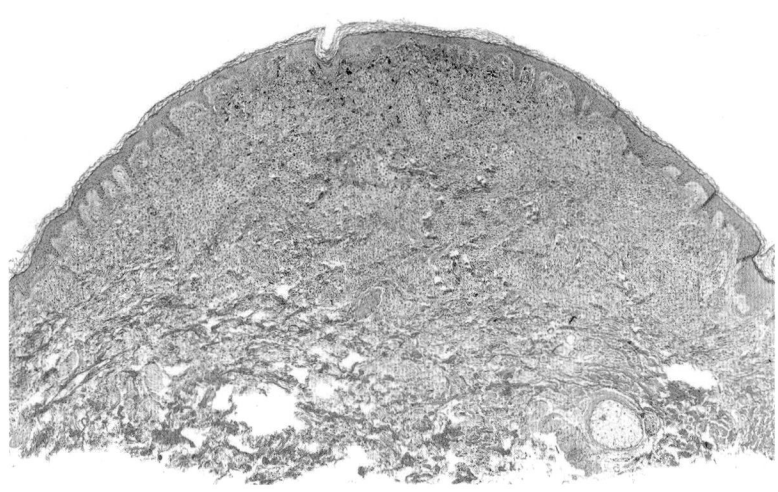

Fig. 26.58
Nodular nevoid melanoma: the diagnosis of nodular nevoid melanoma depends upon careful scrutiny of all 'nevi.' Inspection at scanning magnification will ensure misdiagnosis as a banal nevus!

Although widely publicized, the concept has not gained general acceptance.[1] This relates particularly to a lack of precise definitions combined with the well-known unpredictable behavior of many melanomas. Patients with apparently high-grade and thick tumors sometimes survive for many years, or even decades, while the converse may also be true. The postulated good behavior of these lesions has been challenged on the basis that those that neither recurred nor metastasized may have been benign nevi and those that metastasized and/or proved fatal were obviously malignant at the outset.

In our view, although there are histologic variants of melanoma that show only limited morphological deviation from banal nevi, the evidence relating to biological behavior suggests that these tumors fare no better than classical melanoma and should be treated in exactly the same way. Subtypes that could be included within this category of 'minimal deviation' are nevoid melanoma, small cell melanoma, and spitzoid melanoma. We prefer these categories for histologic classification and these three are dealt with below.

Nevoid melanoma

Nevoid melanoma is a rare histologic subtype of vertical growth phase melanoma, which on low-power inspection may be (and often is) confused with a banal melanocytic nevus.[1-5] It can be equally challenging to recognize clinically on patient skin examinations as well.[6] Diagnosis depends on a high index of suspicion and careful attention to cytological detail including a thorough search for dermal mitotic activity. A practical or functional definition of nevoid melanoma is the 'diagnosis of a nevus which one later regrets'.

Because nevoid melanoma is commonly misdiagnosed as a banal nevus, subsequent delay in appropriate treatment is common, with potentially devastating consequences.[1,2,7-12] Confusion with a banal nevus is most probably a reflection of too cursory an inspection of a 'nevus,' frequently at scanning magnification. Grossly, there are no particular distinguishing features, most lesions being clinically described as verrucous to dome-shaped variably pigmented nevi or non-specific papules or nodules. Follow-up information indicates a recurrence rate of 50%, a metastasis rate of 25–50%, and a mortality rate of at least 25%.[12]

Histologically, on low-power examination nevoid melanoma may present as a warty/verrucous or dome-shaped lesion (the former pattern in an elderly patient is itself a clue to the diagnosis, as nevi in the elderly are more often dome-shaped papulonodules) (Figs 26.57 and 26.58).

The verrucous variant has a rather characteristic histologic appearance presenting as an often asymmetrical, poorly circumscribed, warty lesion

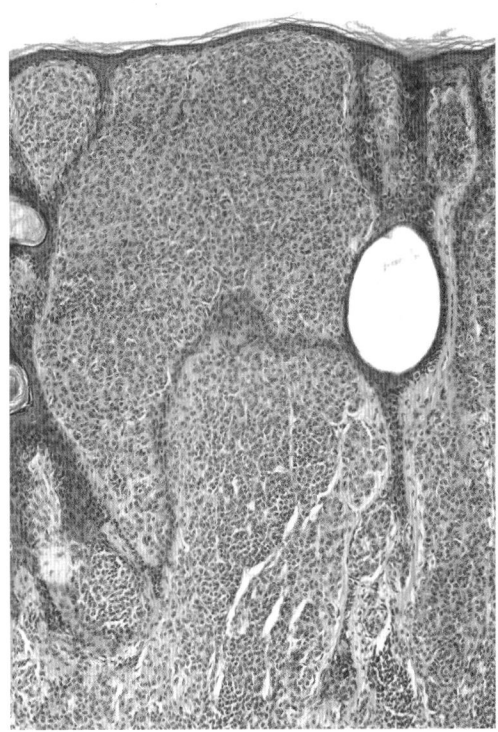

Fig. 26.59
Nevoid melanoma: expansion of the papillary dermis by a diffuse nevoid population with stretching and thinning of the associated epidermis may be a clue to the diagnosis.

with hyperkeratosis and marked papillomatosis. The epidermis frequently appears attenuated with loss of the rete-ridge pattern. In nodular tumors, the epidermis is similarly thin and stretched directly over the surface of a dense dome-shaped tumor cell population. Junctional activity in either variant is often minimal and limited to atypical cells distributed predominantly along the basal layer of the epidermis. Very occasionally, more obvious in situ melanoma may be seen.

At medium-power examination, diffuse and, less often, nested growth patterns may be encountered (Figs 26.59 and 26.60). In the latter there is often considerable variation in nest size accompanied by little tendency for diminution in nest size with depth.

The infiltrating tumor cells are small, epithelioid melanocytes (reminiscent of type-A nevus cells) with pale staining or eosinophilic cytoplasm and round to oval vesicular nuclei with small eosinophilic nucleoli. Although the low-power impression may suggest maturation with depth, closer inspection

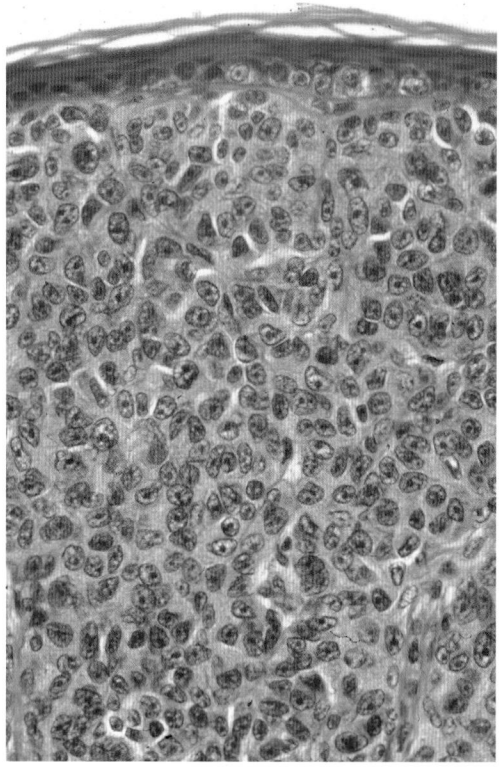

Fig. 26.60
Nevoid melanoma: the tumor cells are very uniform. Nuclei are vesicular and nucleoli prominent. A small number of tumor cells are evident in the overlying epidermis.

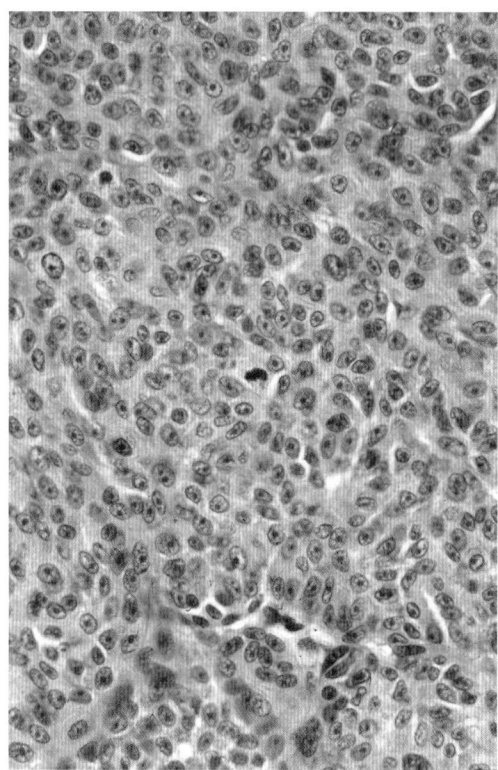

Fig. 26.61
Nevoid melanoma: there may sometimes be a suggestion of maturation with depth. Note the mitosis. This field is taken from the deep aspect of the lesion shown in Figure 26.58.

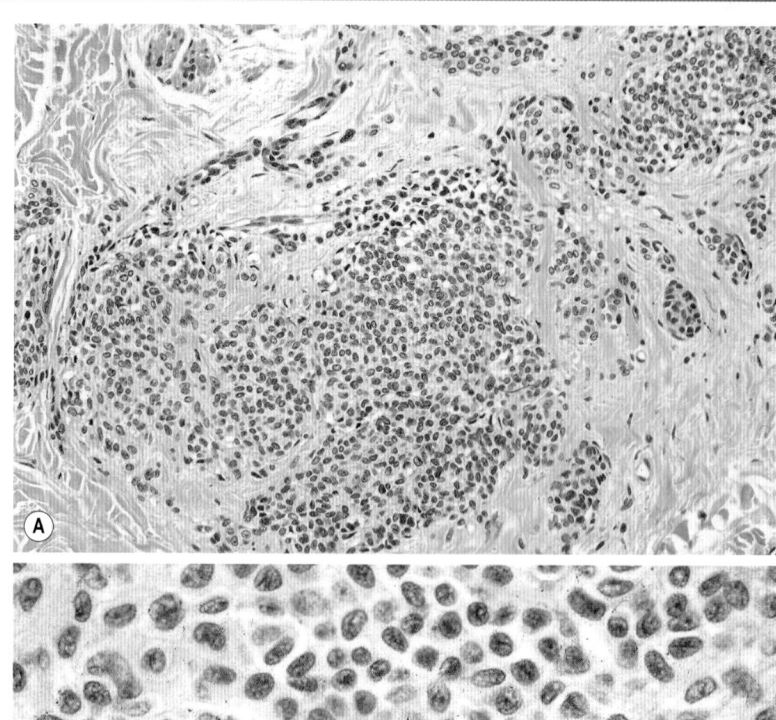

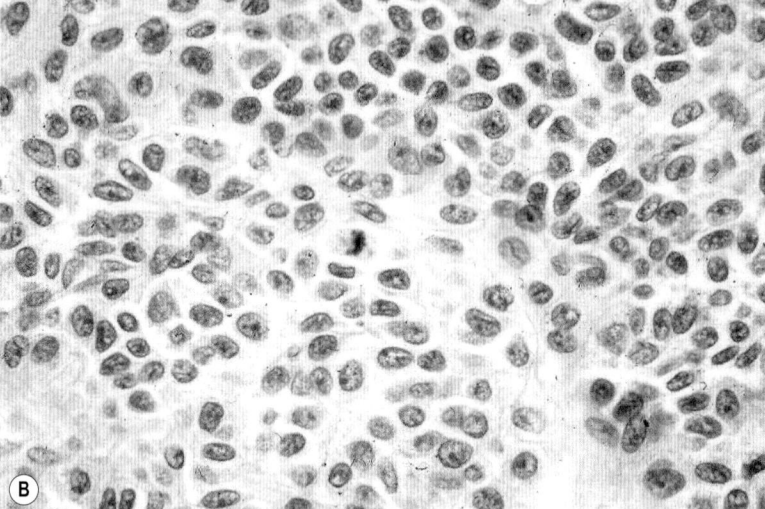

Fig. 26.62
(**A**, **B**) Nevoid melanoma: this lesion at low power is suggestive of a congenital nevus. At high-power magnification, multiple mitoses were present.

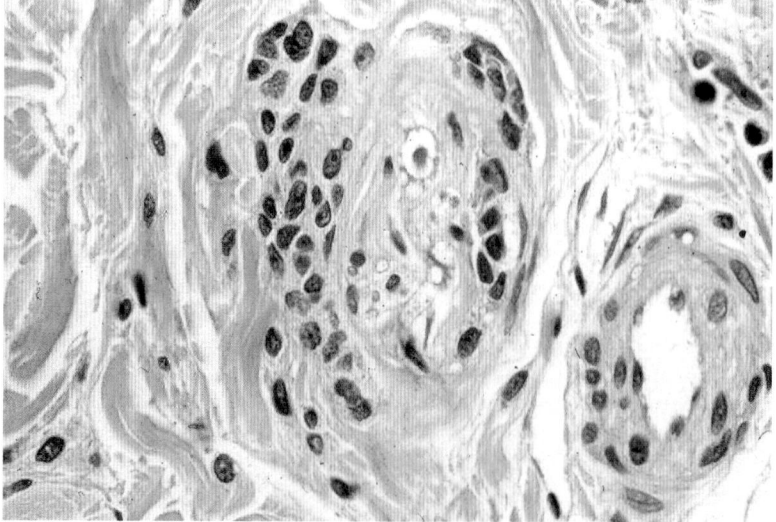

Fig. 26.63
Nevoid melanoma: note the perineural infiltration (same tumor as Fig. 26.64).

invariably shows this to be false (*Fig. 26.61*).[13] Pleomorphism, while subtle, is typically present and mitoses (frequently multiple) can invariably be identified, often within the deeper aspect of the tumor. Pigmentation, although variable, is sometimes seen in the deeper reaches of the dermal component and in a minority of cases, tumor-infiltrating lymphocytes are present. Occasionally, perineural infiltration is present (*Figs 26.62* and *26.63*). A single report describes a case with Homer-Wright type rosettes.[14]

Verrucous variants must be distinguished from keratotic melanocytic nevi, the most important histologic discriminants being the lack of maturation, subtle pleomorphism, and mitotic activity.[15] Others have termed

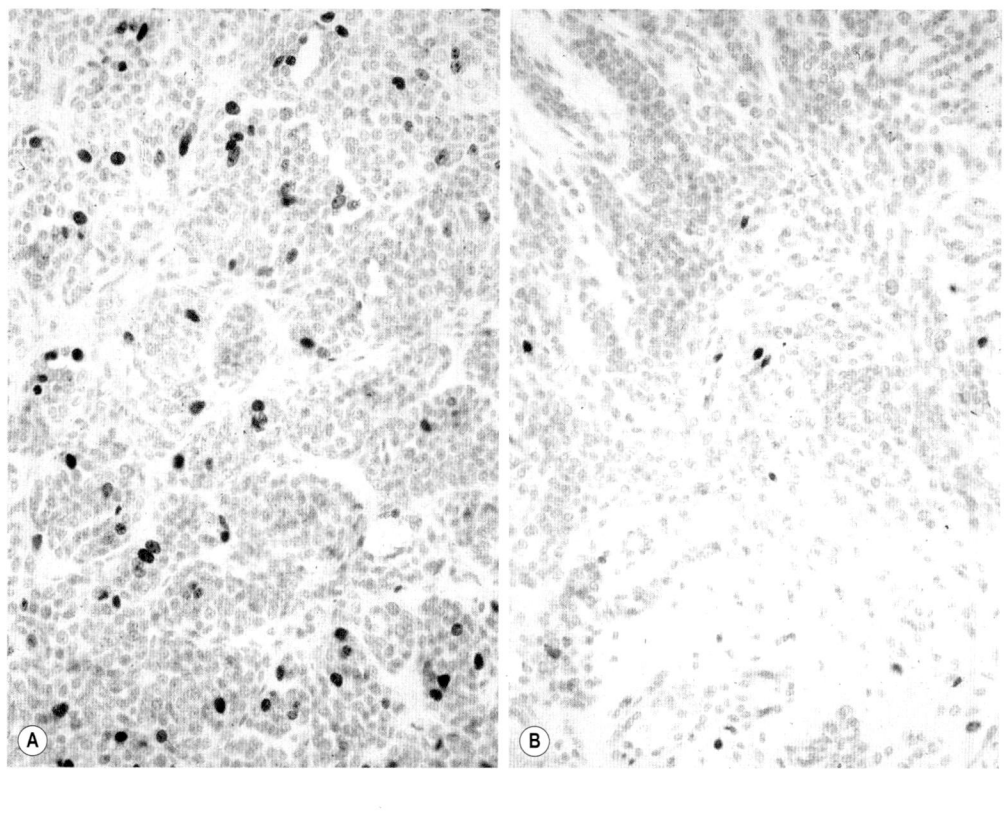

Fig. 26.64
Nevoid melanoma: MIB-1 expression is usually brisk and positively staining nuclei are commonly seen at all levels of the tumor compared with banal nevi in which only very rare positive cells are seen. (**A**) Nevoid melanoma; (**B**) banal dermal nevus.

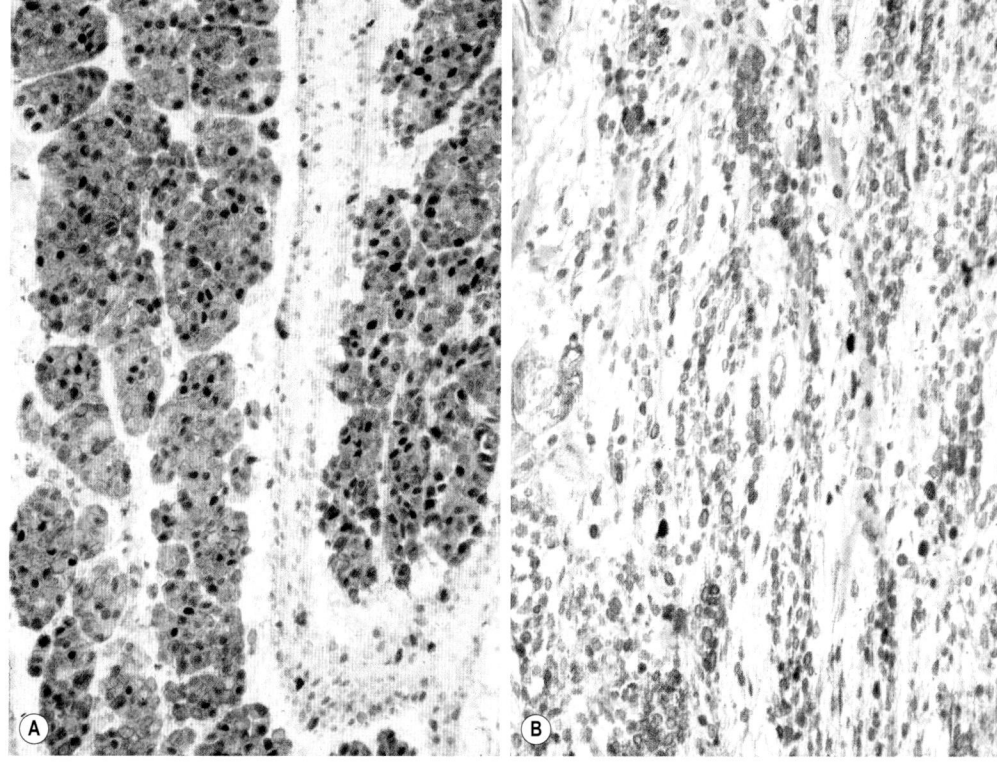

Fig. 26.65
Nevoid melanoma: nuclear cyclin D1 expression is typically brisk and present throughout the depth of the tumor compared to a banal nevus where only scattered cells are positive. (**A**) Nevoid melanoma; (**B**) banal nevus.

very similar lesions 'papillomatous nevoid' melanoma.[16] Very occasionally, melanoma metastatic to the skin from another cutaneous site can present with a nevoid appearance.[17]

Immunohistochemistry may be of help in distinguishing between nevoid melanoma and a banal nevus.[18] In our experience, demonstration of elevated proliferative activity using MIB-1 and sometimes cyclin D1 can be particularly valuable (*Figs 26.64* and *26.65*). Banal nevi show only very scattered positive cells in the superficial part of the dermal component, whereas in melanoma they may be numerous and present throughout the thickness of the lesion. It is important not to confuse positive lymphocytes

with melanoma cells when viewing MIB-1 stained sections. Double or dual staining with MIB-1 and a melanocytic marker such as MART-1 can be particularly valuable. Correlation with the hematoxylin and eosin stained section is always advised. HMB-45 can also sometimes be useful. Dermal nevi are only positive in the most superficial part of the nevus as a counterpart to morphological maturation, whereas in melanoma positive cells may be identified throughout the depth of the tumor.

FISH and comparative genomic hybridization (CGH) studies will often show findings similar to conventional melanoma and thus are frequently helpful in the diagnosis of nevoid melanoma.[5,19]

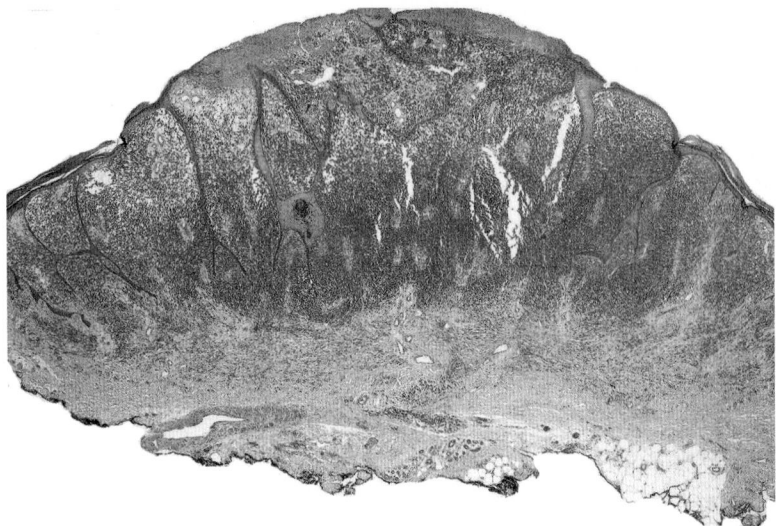

Fig. 26.66
Small cell melanoma: this variant of melanoma simulates type-B nevus cells at low-power magnification, the tumor cells being small and deeply basophilic.

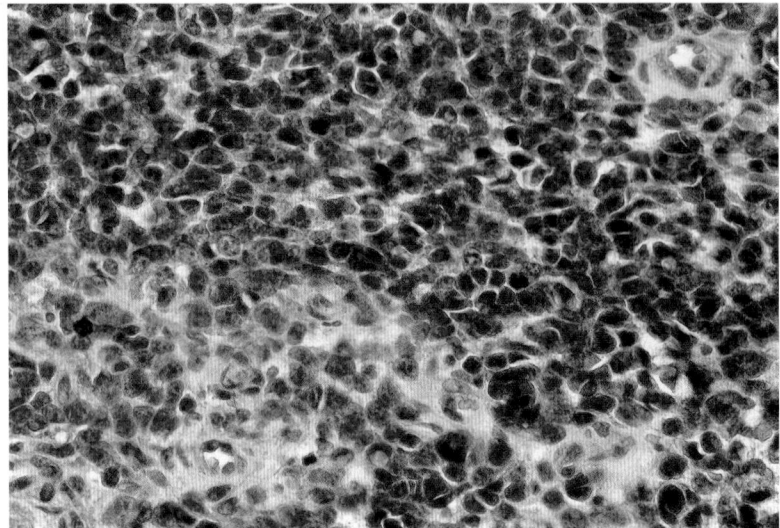

Fig. 26.67
Small cell melanoma: high-power view. The tumor is commonly mistaken for a lymphoma or neuroendocrine carcinoma if melanin pigment or junctional activity is absent.

While one must always be wary of missing nevoid melanoma, it is also important not to overdiagnose melanoma in nevi. This diagnostic reversal can also have untoward clinical and medicolegal consequences.[20]

Small cell melanoma

The term 'small cell melanoma' is often a source of confusion.[1–3] In the literature it has been applied to a variety of different lesions. It has been used as a synonym for nevoid melanoma as defined above.[4,5] It has also been utilized in the context of a high-grade variant of childhood melanoma. Such tumors, which present on the scalp or developing in a congenital nevus, are highly aggressive.[6,7] Other authors have employed the term to describe a tumor occurring in adults, which mimics lymphoma, cutaneous neuroendocrine carcinoma, or metastatic undifferentiated carcinoma.[8–11] It has been used in the Australian and UK literature to describe a low-grade variant of melanoma arising on the sun-damaged skin of middle-aged males.[12,13] A recent study indicates that a small cell component in cutaneous melanoma is a independent poor prognostic indicator.[14]

In our view, small cell melanoma should be distinguished from nevoid melanoma. We reserve the term for a high-grade melanoma, presenting as a small blue cell tumor reminiscent of type-B nevus cells. It is characterized by a monotonous population of cells with minimal cytoplasm and round to oval hyperchromatic nuclei, often containing prominent nucleoli (*Figs 26.66 and 26.67*). Mitoses are frequently conspicuous and karyorrhexis is common. The tumor cells are sometimes aggregated into elongated expansile nests but may also present as a diffusely sheeted infiltrate.[15] Maturation with depth is not apparent. A pseudorosette pattern has been documented.[15]

In recurrent tumors where junctional activity is no longer apparent, and in metastatic disease, small cell melanoma can be easily confused with a poorly differentiated carcinoma, a lymphomatous infiltrate, and neuroendocrine carcinoma.[8–10,16] Appropriate immunocytochemistry should readily solve the problem.

Spitzoid melanoma

The diagnosis of Spitz nevus, and in particular its distinction from melanoma, is one of the most difficult areas in dermatopathology.[1–3] Spitz nevus is predominantly a lesion of children and young adults, whereas melanoma occurs most often in the middle aged and elderly. There is therefore a tendency when encountering a spitzoid lesion in a child to automatically try to categorize it in the benign group merely on the basis of the age.[4] Overreliance on age is a dangerous practice, since although rare, melanoma occurring in childhood and showing spitzoid features has been well documented in the literature. This being said, age is a revealing variable with most Spitz-like features in young children being benign, but the same features in adults, particularly older adults, are much more likely to be associated with malignancy.[5,6] There have thus been a number of papers describing melanomas with features reminiscent of Spitz nevus (spitzoid melanoma, malignant Spitz nevus) and diagnostic criteria to afford their distinction have been proposed and extensively discussed.[7–20] Agreement between expert dermatopathologists in assessing malignancy in atypical spitzoid melanocytic tumors is quite poor.[21] Agreement on what should be considered spitzoid or Spitz-like is also suboptimal.[22] Given this uncertainty, treatment recommendations from pathologists can show considerable variance.[22]

Features that may favor a diagnosis of spitzoid melanoma include large size, deep dermal penetration, parakeratosis, epidermal atrophy (as opposed to the marked hyperplasia typical of Spitz nevus), asymmetry and lack of circumscription, pagetoid spread at the edge of the lesion (pagetoid spread in the center of the nevus is quite common in a Spitz nevus), absence of Kamino (eosinophilic) bodies, dusty pigmentation, dermal nests larger than the junctional ones, a diffuse (non-nested) dermal component, an expansile rather than infiltrating lower border, lack of maturation, nuclear pleomorphism and hyperchromatism, conspicuous mitoses, deep mitoses, and atypical mitoses (*Figs 26.68–26.70*).[7,9,15,23] In a meta-analysis, Walsh and coworkers[15] found the following to be the most useful and consistently applied criteria:

- symmetry,
- uniformity of nests from side to side,
- Kamino bodies,
- brisk mitotic rate,
- mitoses close to the base of the lesion,
- abnormal mitoses.

A recent study by 13 experts of 75 cases confirmed the usefulness of all these factors excepting Kamino bodies and adding ulceration as a feature favoring malignancy.[21] Thus the presence of the first three and absence of the second three argue for a diagnosis of Spitz nevus and vice versa. Spatz and coworkers[16] have devised a grading system for dividing atypical Spitz nevi into low-, medium-, and high-risk categories (of being frankly malignant). This is based on age, diameter, involvement of subcutaneous fat, presence or absence of ulceration, and mitotic rate. The category of atypical Spitz with uncertain biological (or malignant) potential has also been much discussed.[24,25] This concept is often applied to spitzoid lesions as many diagnosticians find these tumors challenging to definitively categorize as wholly benign or malignant in a subset of cases. Cases in this category may not represent neoplasms with the full biological potential of standard melanoma; however, this category

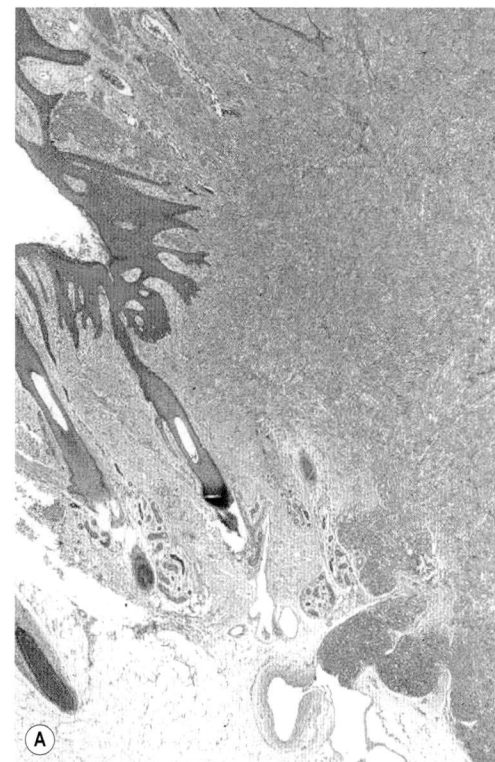

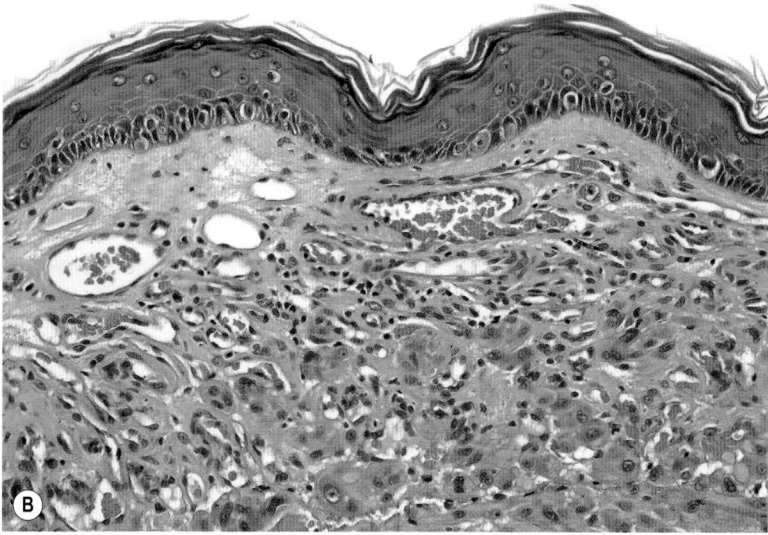

Fig. 26.68
Spitzoid melanoma: (**A**) low-power view showing deep extension into the subcutaneous fat; (**B**) the presence of ectatic vessels in the superficial dermis is reminiscent of Spitz nevus.

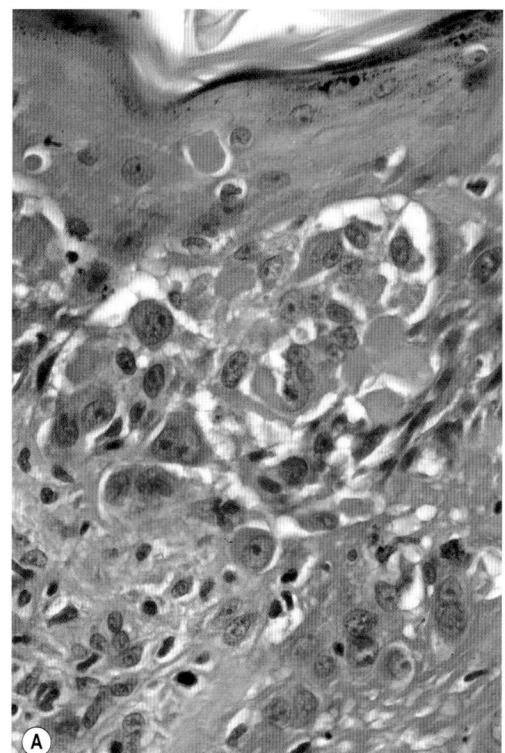

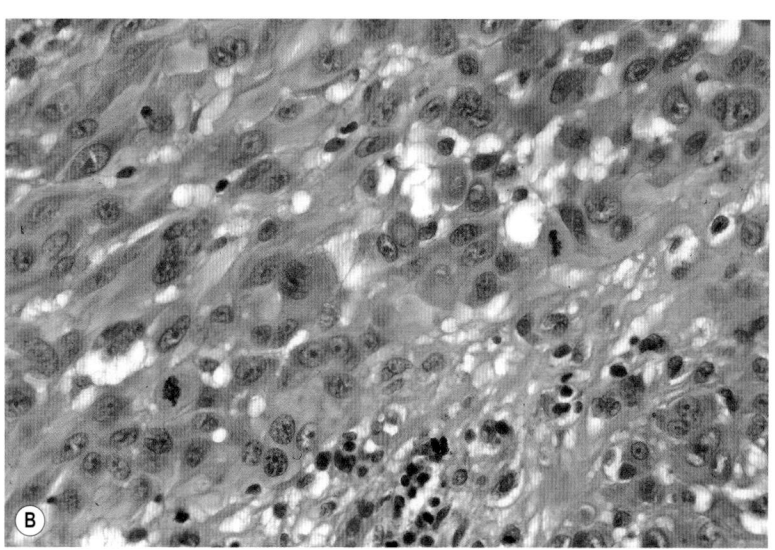

Fig. 26.69
Spitzoid melanoma: (**A**) multiple Kamino bodies may also mislead the unwary; (**B**) multiple mitoses, however, should raise a high index of suspicion.

may be tainted with Spitz nevi containing unusual features. The descriptions in the literature and use of these categories highlight the diagnostic difficulties presented by Spitz nevi and spitzoid melanoma.

Mones and Ackerman[20] have emphasized involvement of the deep dermis or subcutaneous fat by a vertically orientated tumor showing only mild asymmetry on scanning magnification. Other clues include uneven melanin distribution, often at the base of the tumor, variability in size and shape of the dermal nests and fascicles, confluence of nests and fascicles to form diffuse sheets of tumor cells, and diminution or loss of adnexae. They also make the point that the superficial features can be virtually indistinguishable from Spitz nevus. Consumption of the overlying epidermis is a helpful

feature pointing to melanoma as opposed to Spitz nevus when present, though some question its usefulness.[21,26,27] It is important to emphasize that this feature is useful when the thinning of the epidermis is continuous but usually not when it is focal.

Immunohistochemistry may be of value. Thus 50% or more of tumor cells in spitzoid melanoma may express proliferating cell nuclear antigen (PCNA) whereas in Spitz nevus, usually less than 5% of cells are positive.[28] A similar staining pattern is noted with MIB-1 where less than 2% strongly favors nevus and greater than 10% strongly favors melanoma with others factors impinging more strongly between these two thresholds.[29,30] HMB-45 expression in the deep dermal component would favor a diagnosis

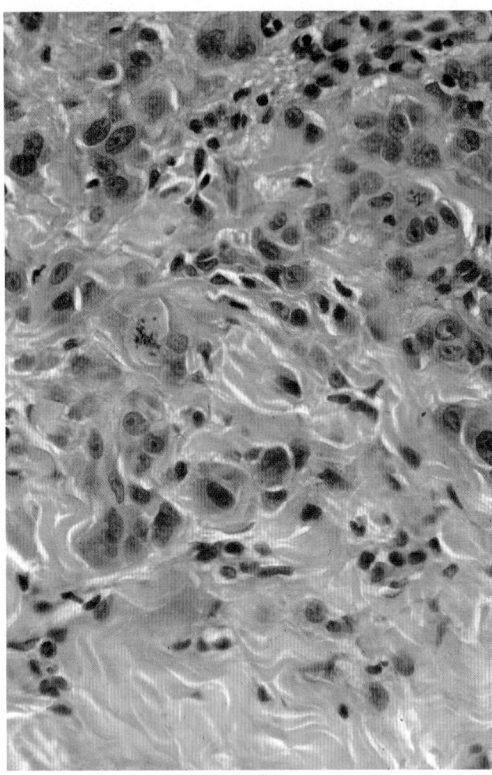

Fig. 26.70
Spitzoid melanoma: deep or abnormal forms are important diagnostic features and are absolute indicators of an unequivocal diagnosis of melanoma. Note that there is no evidence of maturation.

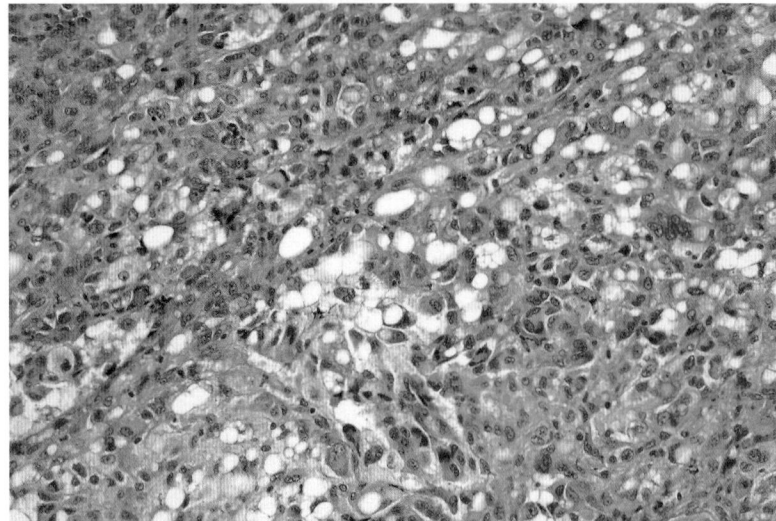

Fig. 26.71
Signet ring cell melanoma: very occasional signet ring melanoma cells are not uncommonly seen in epithelioid melanomas; exceptionally, however, they can constitute the majority of the tumor.

of spitzoid melanoma.[29,31] Amplification of the p-arm of chromosome 11 where the *HRAS* oncogene resides is seen in a subset of Spitz nevi; this change is not encountered in melanoma and thus this finding may be helpful in distinguishing Spitz nevi and melanoma.[32–35] Comparative genomic hybridization and FISH assays can be used to make this determination. The distinction between Spitz tumor and atypical Spitz tumor is not always well informed by such assays, but can be helpful when characteristic melanoma deficits are present.[36,37] As for spitzoid melanoma, 6p25 and/or 11q13 gains or 9p21 deletions on FISH favor malignancy while no FISH abnormality or 6q23 deletions are associated with less aggressive behavior or benignancy.[38] Spitzoid melanomas generally lack mutations in genes such as *BRAF* and *NRAS* common in some other melanoma subtypes in some studies, but not others.[39,40] This may illustrate the difficulty in histologically defining what amounts to a spitzoid melanoma versus a standard melanoma. Spitz lesions can also show inactivation of the tumor suppressor *BAP1* (*BRAF* V600 mutations can also be seen with *BAP1* loss) as well as rearrangements in *ALK*, *RET*, *ROS*, *BRAF*, *NTRK1*, and *RET*. These features can be seen in both benign and malignant Spitz tumors.[38,41–48]

Although Smith and coworkers[10] suggested that malignant Spitz nevus might represent a tumor that rarely spread beyond the draining lymph nodes, subsequent papers have suggested that the tumor is often no different from any other melanoma and therefore has the same risk of systemic spread and an identical mortality.[15,28,49] Spitz-like lesions that metastasize to lymph nodes in children do appear to be less aggressive than traditional melanoma in children and adults. Metastasis of Spitzoid lesions in adults appears to bear the same prognosis as that of other metastasizing melanoma. Some authors recommend sentinel lymph node biopsy in problematical spitzoid lesions to help establish a diagnosis of melanoma in addition to adding prognostic information, though this approach is not without controversy.[19,50–56] Patients younger than 11 years of age with spitzoid melanoma may have a better prognosis than older adolescents and adults, but this finding has not been universal.[49,56]

Signet ring cell melanoma

Signet ring cell melanoma is a very rare histologic variant, which shows considerable overlap with rhabdoid variants (see below). It has been mostly described in metastatic tumors. There are also reports of signet ring cell

change in recurrent and primary disease. The phenomenon does not have prognostic significance.[1–15]

Signet ring cell change is characterized by a large pale or eosinophilic cytoplasmic globular inclusion or vacuole, which compresses the nucleus to the edge of the cell (*Fig. 26.71*). This appearance may affect a melanoma in part or constitute the whole of the lesion. The periodic acid-Schiff (PAS) stain is variably weakly positive (diastase resistant) but an Alcian blue reaction is consistently negative.[1,2,11] The nature of the PAS-positive material is unknown. The signet ring appearance is due to excess intermediate filament presenting as an intracytoplasmic 'mass' or vacuole.

The signet ring cells contain vimentin and may express S100 protein and HMB-45 although the latter two can be patchily distributed and occasionally absent altogether.[2,4,16] Diagnosis in such a case is then dependent upon finding more typical melanoma cells with appropriate immunocytochemistry elsewhere in the specimen. Signet ring cell melanoma must be distinguished from other signet ring cell tumors, particularly mucin-containing adenocarcinoma and lymphoma. To this end, antibodies to LCA, keratin, EMA, and CEA should invariably be included in the immunocytochemistry panel.

Cytological diagnosis of signet ring cell melanoma (by fine needle aspiration and from a peritoneal effusion) has been documented.[8,10]

Signet ring cells have also exceptionally been described in banal and Spitz melanocytic nevi.[6,17,18]

Rhabdoid melanoma

Rhabdoid melanoma shows considerable overlap with signet ring cell melanoma.[1]

The term 'rhabdoid tumor' was originally coined to describe an aggressive childhood renal tumor, which was thought to represent a rhabdomyosarcomatous variant of nephroblastoma.[2] It was characterized by the presence of eosinophilic hyaline intracytoplasmic inclusions, later identified ultrastructurally as whorls of intermediate filaments. Extrarenal rhabdoid tumors have been identified at a wide range of sites including soft tissues, skin, brain, orbit, uterus, bladder, prostate, and liver. A rhabdoid phenotype was first described in metastatic melanoma.[3–10] More recently, small numbers of primary tumors showing rhabdoid features have been documented.[11–17] At present, there are too few cases documented to determine whether the rhabdoid phenotype in melanoma has any prognostic significance.

The rhabdoid phenotype is characterized by the presence of large epithelioid cells with abundant cytoplasm containing a large round eosinophilic hyaline inclusion (*Fig. 26.72*). The nuclei are typically vesicular and nucleoli are eosinophilic and conspicuous. Extrarenal rhabdoid tumors are not a

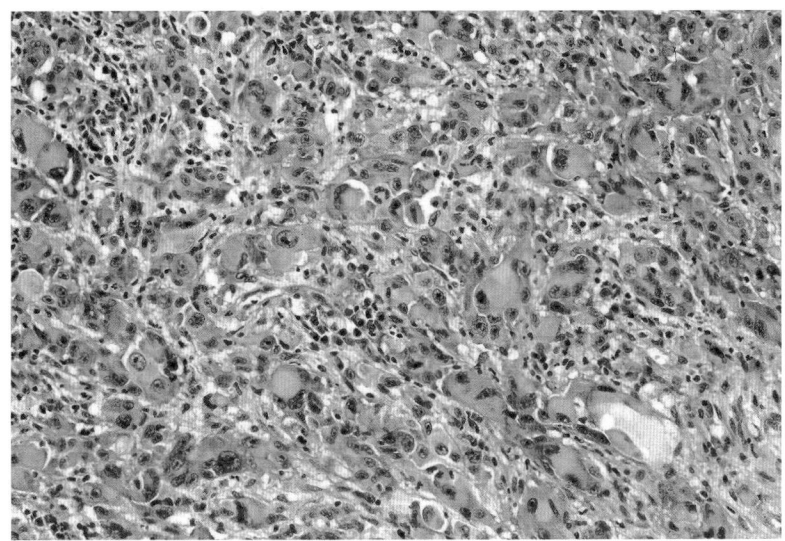

Fig. 26.72
Rhabdoid melanoma: this variant often causes diagnostic difficulty since lesions are commonly amelanotic. Note the vesicular nuclei, prominent nucleoli, and large eosinophilic cytoplasmic inclusions.

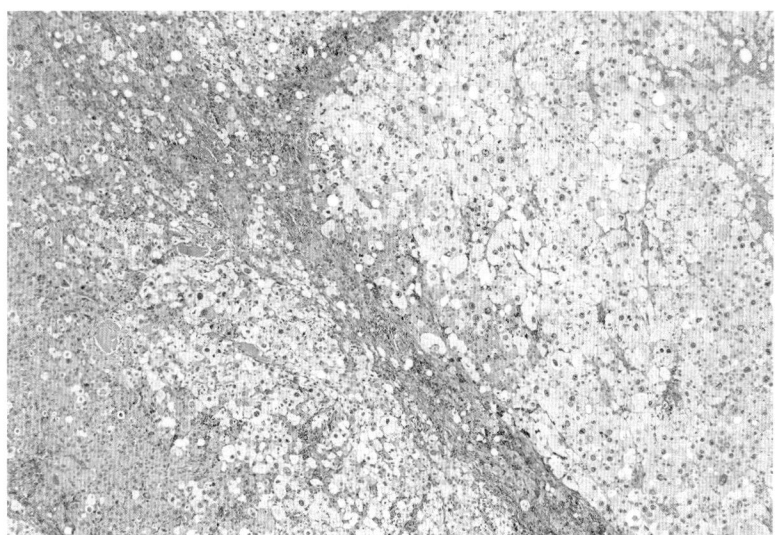

Fig. 26.74
Balloon cell melanoma: the tumor cells have clear or faintly granular cytoplasm. This example is amelanotic and could easily be mistaken for a xanthomatous lesion.

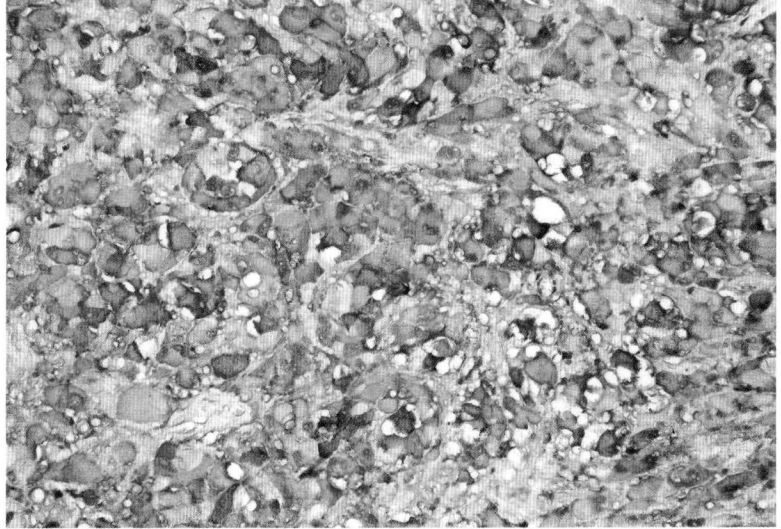

Fig. 26.73
Rhabdoid melanoma: in the absence of a known history of melanoma, the diagnosis commonly depends upon immunohistochemistry (S100 protein).

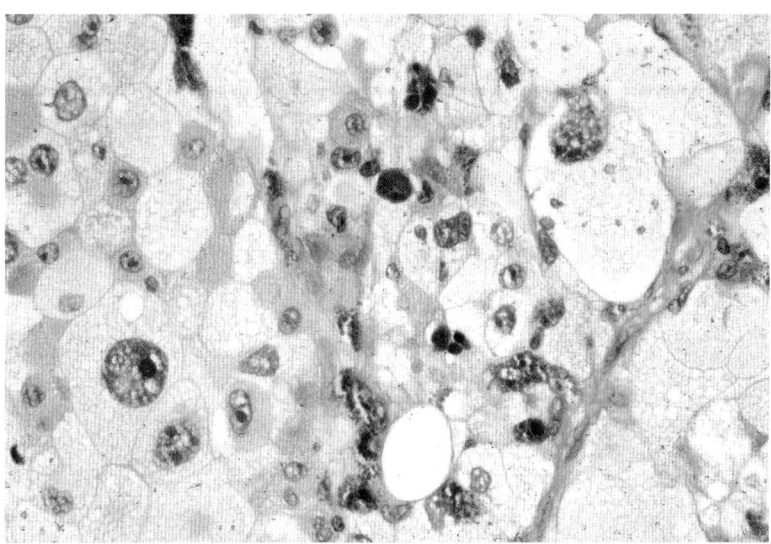

Fig. 26.75
Balloon cell melanoma: high-power view.

homogeneous entity; most often rhabdoid features are seen focally in an otherwise recognizable and classifiable lesion, i.e., rhabdoid change represents a morphological endpoint in dedifferentiation.

The results of immunocytochemistry are variable. Some tumors are characterized by S100 protein, SOX10, and HMB-45 expression (*Fig. 26.73*).[11,12] Mart-1 is also often expressed by tumor cells. In a number of tumors, however, the rhabdoid cells fail to show any of the above and the inclusions contain keratin, smooth muscle actin, or desmin.[3,12] Rare examples of melanoma with rhabdoid morphology display rhabdomyosarcomatous differentiation with expression of desmin, myogenin, and MYOD1.

Ultrastructurally, the inclusions have usually been found to consist of aggregates of intermediate filaments. In one series of metastatic melanoma, the rhabdoid inclusions were composed of tubular inclusions within dilated rough endoplasmic reticulum and mitochondria.[5]

Balloon and clear cell melanoma

Balloon cell melanoma is a very rare vertical growth phase variant with less than 20 cases well documented in the medical literature.[1–5] There are no particular distinguishing clinical features except that a polypoid configuration

is more commonly seen than in classic melanoma.[2] Prognosis is usually poor but this relates to the tumor thickness at presentation rather than any feature specific to this unusual melanoma variant. Balloon cell change appears to be more common in nevi than melanoma.[6]

Balloon cells have abundant eosinophilic or clear cytoplasm showing fine granularity or vacuolation (*Figs 26.74* and *26.75*). The tumor cells are typically S100 protein, Mart-1, SOX10, and HMB-45 positive. They contain PAS-positive, diastase-resistant granules. These are also iron hematoxylin positive, hyaluronidase resistant. Sensitivity to ribonuclease indicates that the granules are composed of ribonucleoprotein.[2] The cause of the vacuolation is uncertain but is believed to represent either abnormal melanosome metabolism or else a melanosome degenerative phenomenon.

Balloon cell melanoma can be distinguished from balloon cell nevus by the absence of nuclear pleomorphism and mitotic activity in the latter.[7] Balloon cell melanoma may also be confused with sebaceous and xanthomatous tumors. Sebaceous lesions have a characteristic 'bubbly' cytoplasm and often the nucleus is crenated. In addition, sebaceous tumors express epithelial membrane antigen as well as adipophylin and are S100 protein and HMB-45 negative. Xanthomatous lesions contain lipid, express CD68, and are S100 protein negative.[7–10]

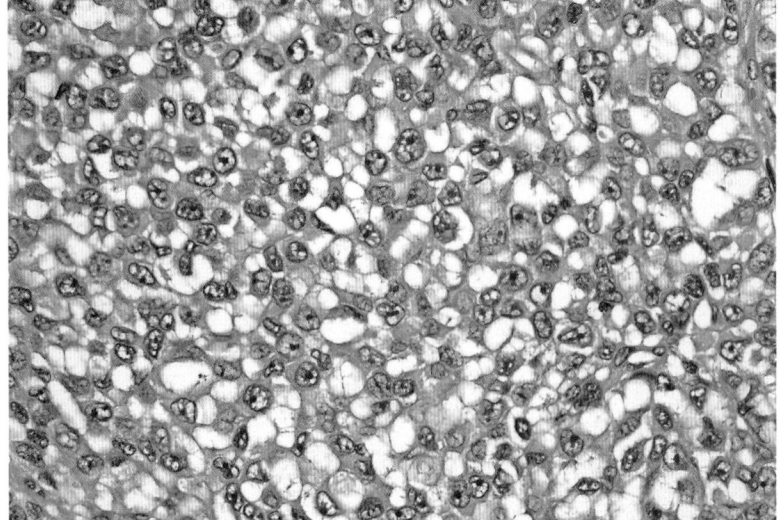

Fig. 26.76
Clear cell melanoma: this is an exceedingly rare variant of melanoma. In the absence of a known history of melanoma or visible melanin pigment, the diagnosis depends upon immunohistochemistry.

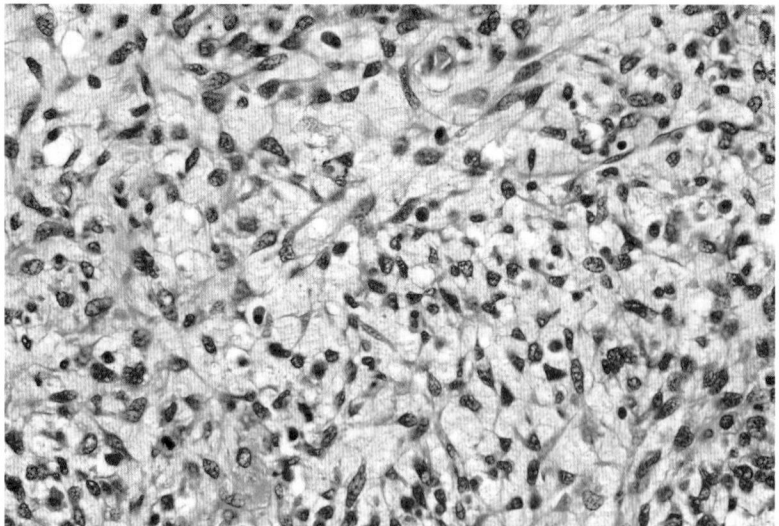

Fig. 26.77
Myxoid melanoma: this rare variant can be a source of considerable diagnostic difficulty. Note the 'undifferentiated' irregular cells associated with an abundant myxoid stroma.

Pure clear cell variants due to intracytoplasmic glycogen deposition are very rare and may be encountered in primary tumors or metastatic deposits (Fig. 26.76).[5,11–16] They may be confused with clear cell carcinomas, including clear cell squamous carcinoma, clear cell hidradenocarcinoma, and clear cell metastases such as from clear cell carcinoma of the kidney. In cases where there is real diagnostic difficulty, the use of immunocytochemistry for melanocytic and keratin expression will resolve the issue.

Exceptionally, multiple small intracytoplasmic vacuoles can give rise to a pseudolipoblast appearance with conspicuous nuclear scalloping.

Myxoid melanoma

Myxoid stromal change in melanoma is very rare and may be seen in primary, recurrent, and metastatic disease.[1–11] It is of no prognostic significance.[4,8]

Myxoid change is a feature of vertical growth phase melanoma. It may be evident as a minor component of the tumor or be present throughout. Tumors showing the latter can be a source of considerable diagnostic difficulty with epithelioid cases suggesting carcinoma and spindle cell cases mimicking sarcoma. It has been described as a reactive change after phototherapy.[12,13] Typically, the tumor cells are smaller than those present in nonmyxoid areas and may be epithelioid, spindled, or stellate in appearance (Fig. 26.77). Melanin pigmentation is variable. The mucin, which presents as basophilic 'stringy' material, is usually PAS negative, colloidal iron and Alcian blue positive, and sensitive to hyaluronidase (consistent with stromal mucin).[8] Often the melanoma cells are present as discohesive clumps, cords, and strands such that a pseudoglandular or 'acantholytic' appearance may sometimes result (Figs 26.78 and 26.79). Occasionally, pseudoacinar differentiation and intercellular molding reminiscent of adenocarcinoma are features.[8]

Immunohistochemistry is typical for melanoma, the tumor cells being invariably positive for S100 protein and usually positive for HMB-45.[8] HMB-45 negativity has, however, been documented.[5]

Myxoid change may sometimes be seen in the stroma of desmoplastic melanoma, but other areas more typical of conventional desmoplastic melanoma are usually present.

Myxoid melanoma may be confused with mucus-secreting adenocarcinoma and myxoid malignant peripheral nerve sheath tumor (MPNST) or other sarcomas. The former may be excluded on the basis of negative keratin immunocytochemistry and absence of PAS-positive mucin. Myxoid malignant peripheral nerve sheath tumor usually shows much less strong and only focal S100 protein expression, and HMB-45 is negative. In addition, MPNST limited to the dermis is exceedingly rare.

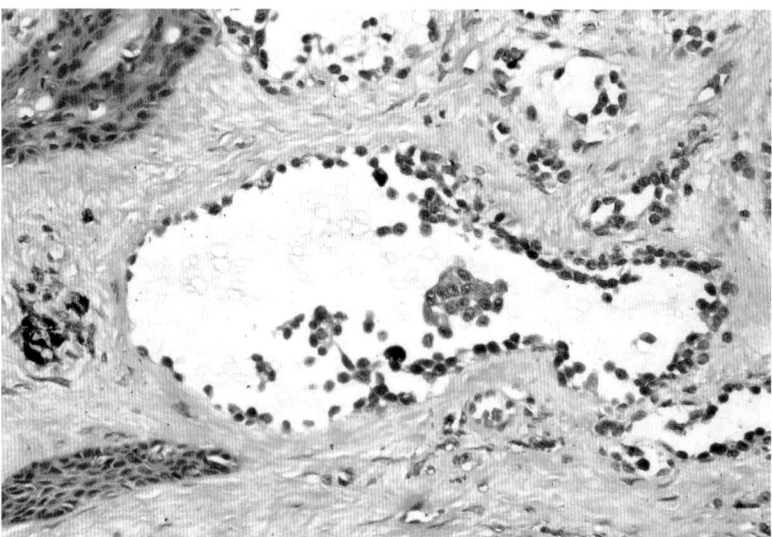

Fig. 26.78
Adenoid (pseudoglandular) melanoma: this variant also associated with excess mucin deposition may easily be misdiagnosed as an acantholytic squamous carcinoma or adenocarcinoma if a junctional component or pigment is absent. Diagnosis often depends upon immunohistochemistry. By courtesy of R. Margolis, MD, St Elizabeth's Medical Center, Boston, USA.

Melanoma with neuroendocrine differentiation

Neuroendocrine differentiation has been rarely described in melanoma cases and sometimes in non-cutaneous cases.[1–4] Mixed melanocytic and neuroendocrine tumors have also been described in the lung, thymus, and thyroid and challenge current classification schemes.[5] Immunohistochemical expression of chromogranin and synaptophysin, along with neurofilament protein, has been noted as has expression of CD56.[3] Less specific markers of neuroendocrine differentiation such as neuron-specific enolase and perhaps CD56 expressed in isolation should be interpreted with caution when seen in melanoma as they may not imply such differentiation. Characteristic melanocytic markers remain intact. While not clearly associated with any difference in natural history, neuroendocrine differentiation can be associated with diagnostic confusion, especially with presentation at sites where other neuroendocrine tumors can be seen such as in the sinonasal region.[6] Further complicating the distinction is that melanoma exhibiting

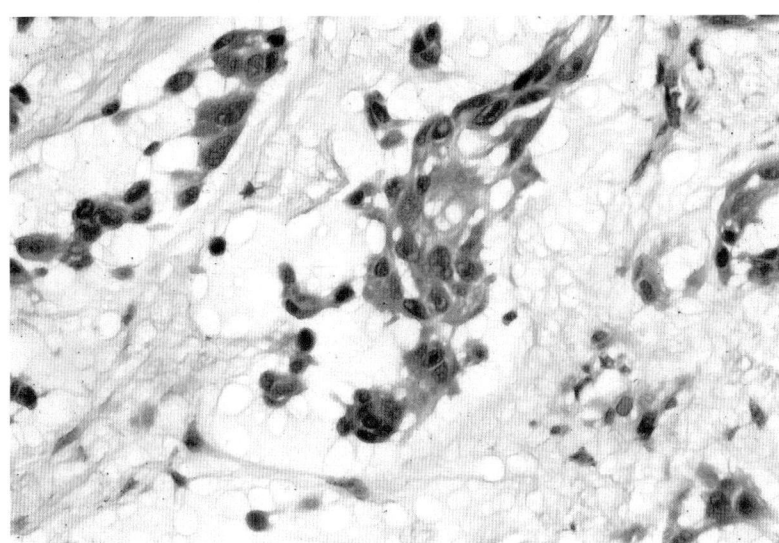

Fig. 26.79
Adenoid (pseudoglandular) melanoma: high-power view showing undifferentiated tumor cells dispersed within abundant mucin. By courtesy of R. Margolis, MD, St Elizabeth's Medical Center, Boston, USA.

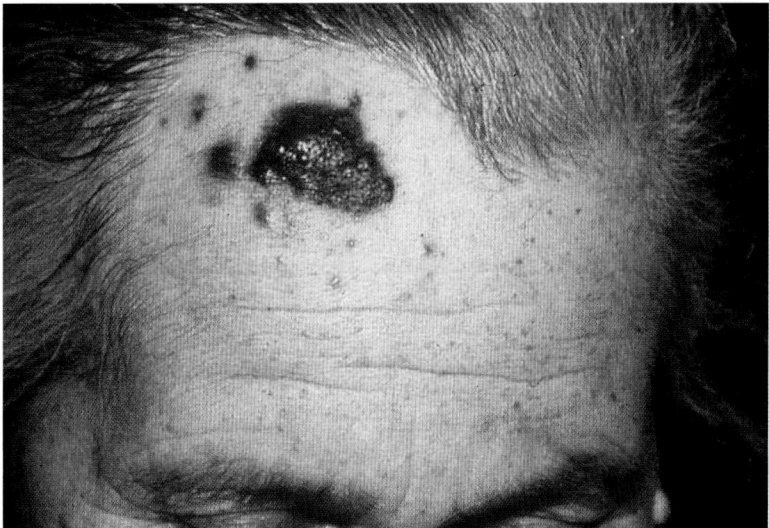

Fig. 26.80
Malignant blue nevus: note the heavily pigmented primary tumor associated with multiple satellite lesions on this elderly patient's forehead. By courtesy of the Institute of Dermatology, London, UK.

neuroendocrine differentiation appears to show small cell morphology. Interestingly, carcinoid-like trabecular and pseudorosette patterns have been noted in melanoma as well, but these cases lacked neuroendocrine markers.[7,8]

Adenoid and pseudopapillary melanoma

This rare variant shows considerable overlap with myxoid melanoma. Primary or metastatic deposits show extreme discohesion such that pseudoglandular spaces sometimes with papillary architecture are formed and sometimes these can be filled with mucin.[1,2] Occasionally 'intraluminal' papillary processes and 'mucin'-filled lakes are formed, heightening the resemblance to adenocarcinoma.[3] A possibly related form has been described as discohesive melanoma.[4,5] In the latter, melanomas showed striking discohesion of cells both in the intraepidermal and invasive component closely mimicking an acantholytic disease.

Blue nevus-like melanoma (malignant blue nevus)

This term covers a variety of lesions including melanoma arising in a background of cellular blue nevus and to a lesser extent common blue nevus or showing morphological overlap with blue nevus.[1-5] Variants have also been documented complicating nevi of Ito and Ota and pilar neurocristic hamartoma.[6-8] It also includes cases of melanoma that show histologic overlap with cellular blue nevi but which are devoid of a precursor lesion (de novo variants).[9-13] Pigmented epithelioid melanocytoma (previously termed animal-type or pigment-synthesizing melanoma; see below) can have a highly similar morphological spectrum but are distinct from blue nevus-like melanoma at the genomic level.[14]

Clinical features

Malignant blue nevi are often very slowly growing lesions that commonly present as a consequence of a sudden onset of growth and show a predilection for the scalp (Fig. 26.80). Males are affected more often than females. No age group is immune and exceptionally children are affected. This is a high-grade lesion with outcome similar to stage-matched cases of traditional melanoma cases.[15,16] The lung, liver, and lymph nodes are most commonly affected by metastatic disease.

Histologic features

Tumors that arise in a background of pre-existent blue nevus typically show an abrupt transition from a benign precursor lesion to obvious melanoma (Figs 26.81 and 26.82). The latter presents as one or more nodules of

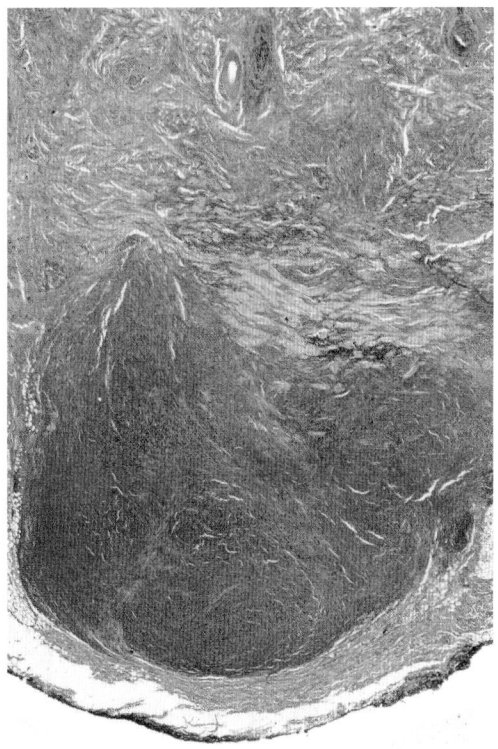

Fig. 26.81
Malignant blue nevus: this tumor arose on the scalp. There is a dense expansile tumor nodule which has extended into the subcutaneous fat.

epithelioid or spindled melanocytes showing a diffuse growth pattern and obvious cytological features of malignancy (Figs 26.83 and 26.84).

Tumors that mimic cellular blue nevus, but in which no precursor lesion can be identified, commonly show an expansile growth pattern with usually pushing borders extending into the subcutaneous fat (Fig. 26.85). Occasionally a dumbbell scanning morphology may be evident and rarely an alveolar growth pattern is seen.[11] Typically, at low-power magnification, a diagnosis of benign cellular nevus is anticipated. The tumor cells most often have spindled cell morphology but epithelioid and mixed variants are sometimes encountered. High-power detail, however, shows an increased nuclear-to-cytoplasmic ratio, mild to moderate nuclear pleomorphism, hyperchromatism, nucleolar prominence, and increased mitotic activity (Figs 26.86 and 26.87). Necrosis, sometimes exhibiting a geographic pattern, may also be present and perineural infiltration is an occasional feature.

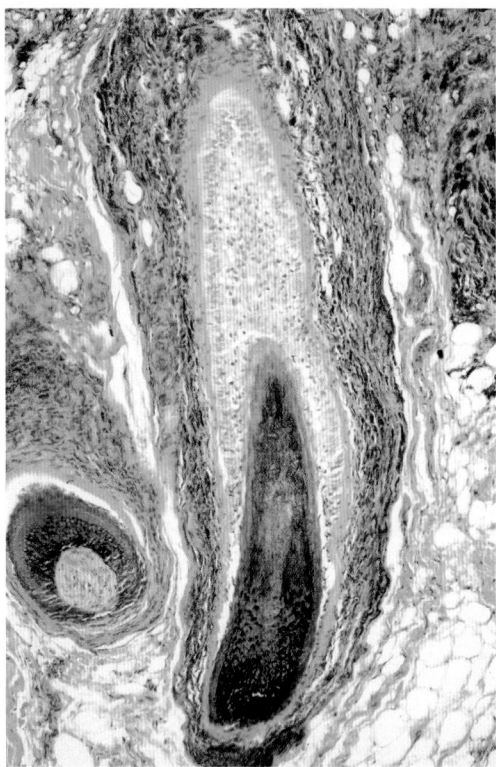

Fig. 26.82
Malignant blue nevus: a pilar blue nevus was evident in the adjacent skin.

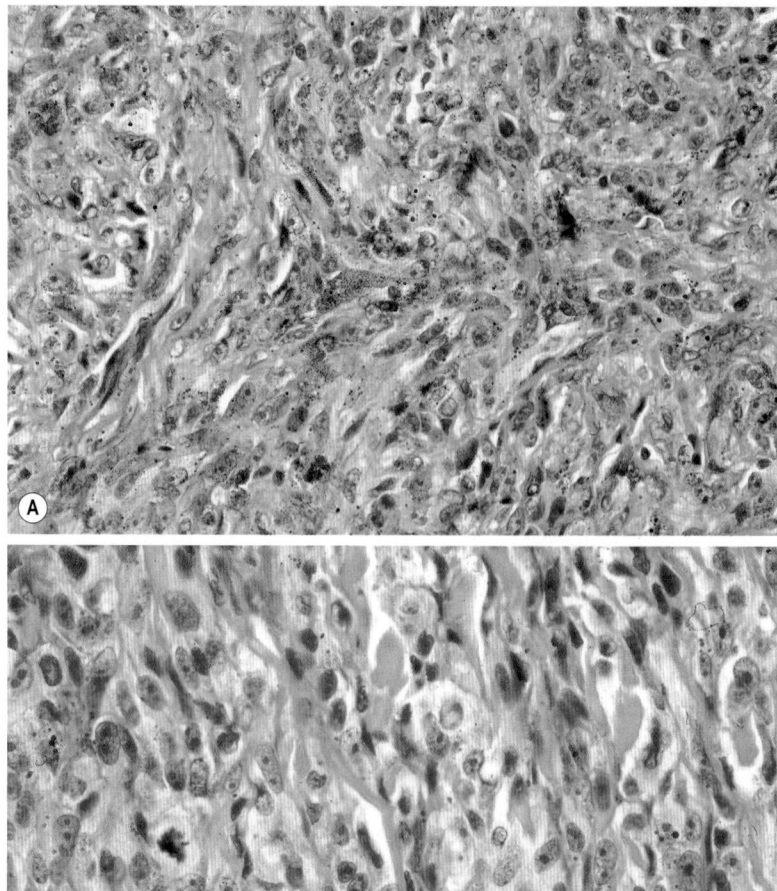

Fig. 26.84
Malignant blue nevus: (**A**) there are multiple dendritic cells; (**B**) note the two mitoses.

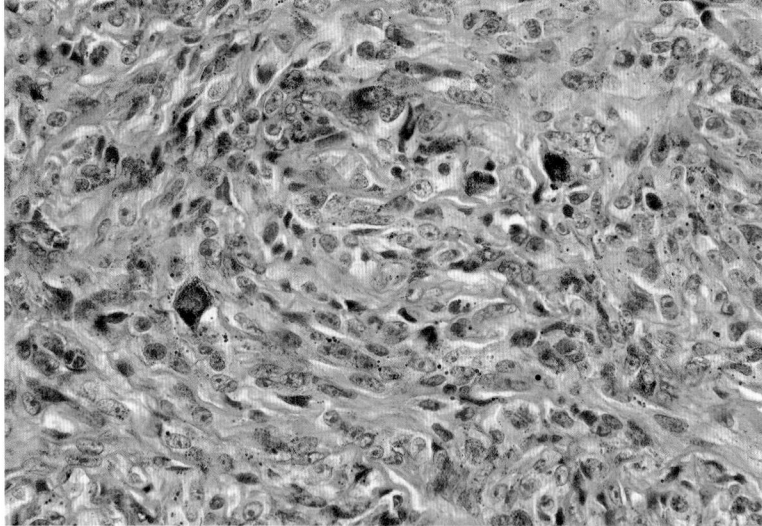

Fig. 26.83
Malignant blue nevus: the tumor cells have vesicular nuclei with prominent nucleoli.

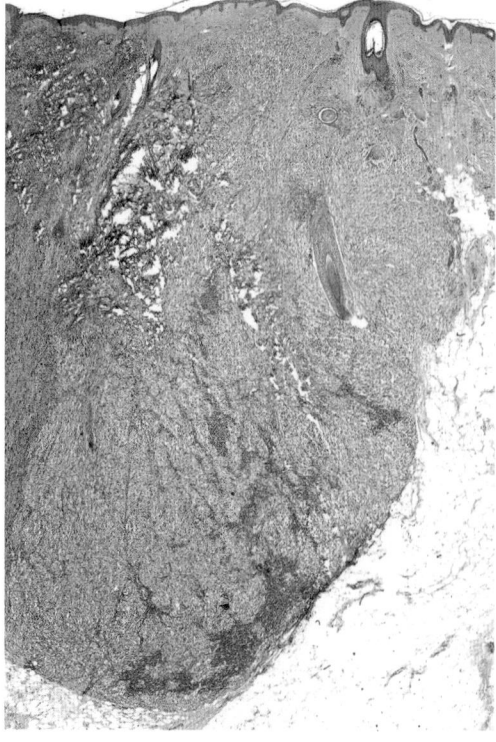

Fig. 26.85
Malignant blue nevus: a precursor lesion was not identified in this case.

Scattered dendritic cells are often present in this second variant. Whether this represents a residual benign precursor lesion or indicates malignant dendritic cells is problematical. In favor of the latter possibility is the presence of dendritic cells in metastases (*Fig. 26.88*).

A subset of melanocytic proliferations is difficult to classify definitively as benign or malignant. These have been referred to as atypical cellular blue nevi or cellular blue melanocytic proliferation of uncertain malignant potential.[1,17] There appears to be a lack of consensus regarding diagnostic criteria for malignancy across the blue nevus spectrum.[18]

Both blue nevus and blue nevus-like melanoma are associated with mutation in *GNAQ* or less commonly *GNA11*, encoding the alpha subunit of a heterotrimeric G-protein.[14,19] Similar to ocular melanoma, mutations in *BAP1*, *SF3B1*, and *EIF1AX* are commonly encountered in blue nevus-like melanoma and their presence may help to establish malignancy.[14,20] The standard multi-probe FISH assay can be helpful in distinguishing blue

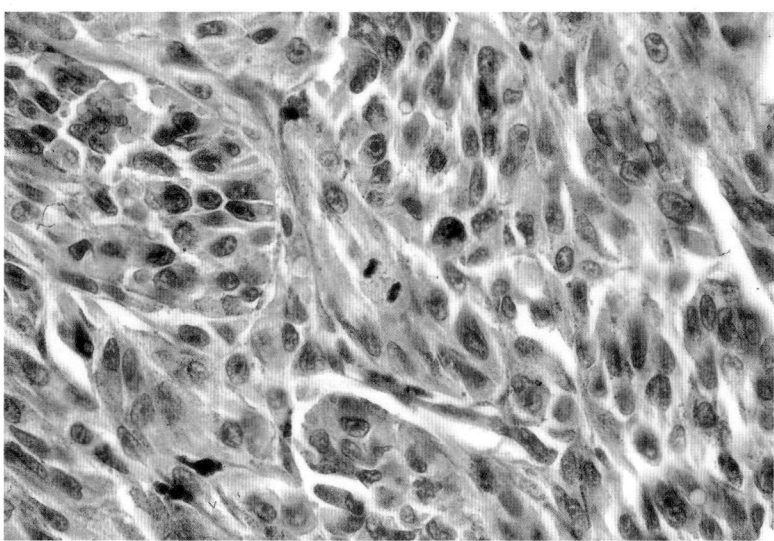

Fig. 26.86
Malignant blue nevus: note the central mitotic figure.

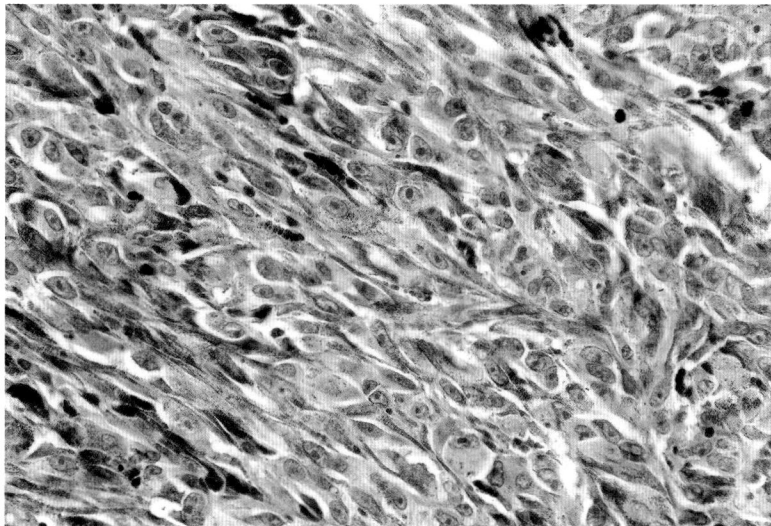

Fig. 26.87
Malignant blue nevus: dendritic cells are conspicuous in this field.

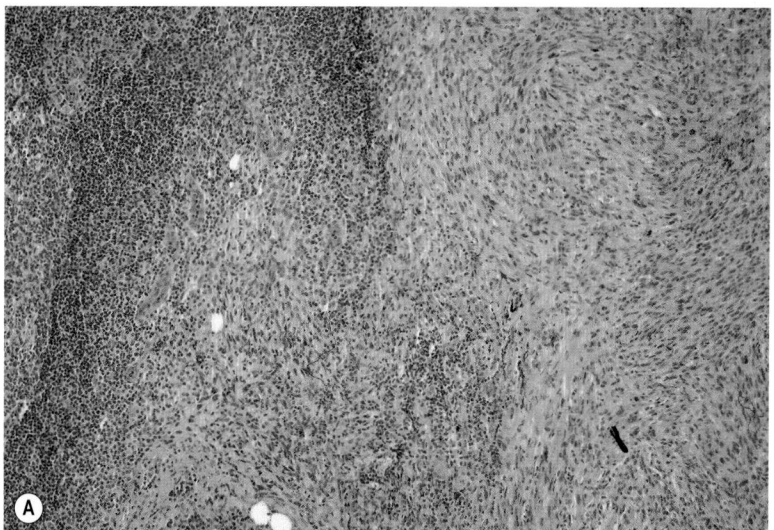

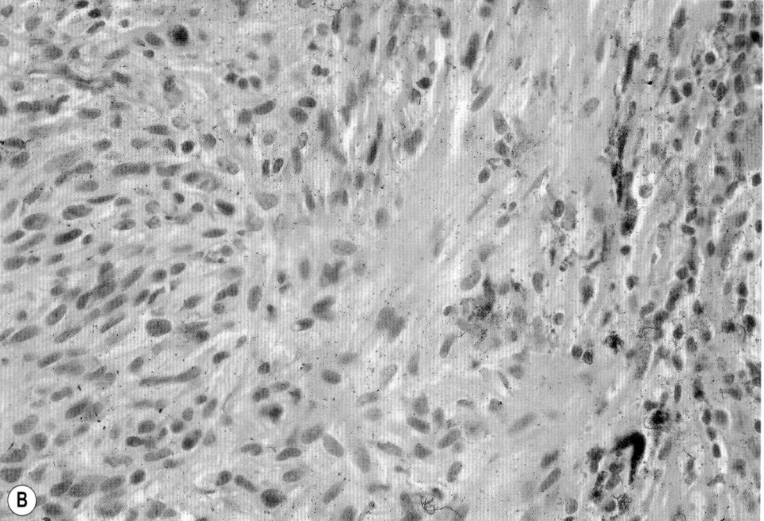

Fig. 26.88
(**A**, **B**) Malignant blue nevus: the sentinel node contained metastatic melanoma. A small number of dendritic cells are present. This is the same case as illustrated in *Figures 26.81–26.84*.

nevus-like melanoma from atypical forms of cellular blue nevus, but limited data are available.[21,22]

Angiotropic and angiomatoid (pseudovascular) melanoma

Angiotropism has been described in only a few cases of vertical growth phase melanoma.[1–5]

Histologically, this rare manifestation of melanoma is characterized by the growth of melanoma cells within or along the walls of vessels, principally veins, but usually without showing evidence of intravascular invasion.[1,6] While a relatively rare occurrence, interobserver concordance is high when standardized diagnostic criteria are applied.[7] More recently, this phenomenon has been suggested as a type of vascular invasion and shown to be associated with a poor prognosis, perhaps even brain metastases in some cases.[8,9] It is also independently correlated with the presence of microsatellites in primary cutaneous melanoma.[10] Some contend that this pericytic association may represent an extravascular mechanism for local or regional metastasis.[11,12] Angiotropism has also been described in epidermotropic and other metastatic melanomas.[13] A recent mouse model study indicated that inflammation induced by UV exposure can promote angiotropism and proposed this as a means of metastasis also relevant to humans in some

cases.[14,15] Angiotropism can also be seen in nevi, particularly congenital melanocytic nevi.[16]

Exceptionally, melanoma may show blood-filled dilated spaces lined by endothelium-like tumor cells reminiscent of angiosarcoma (angiomatoid melanoma).[17–22] Intraluminal tufting may result in pseudoglomeruloid structures.[18]

Metaplastic melanoma (melanoma with heterologous differentiation)

Exceptionally, melanoma is associated with heterologous metaplastic elements, including bone and cartilage.[1–6] Mostly, these have complicated acral lentiginous lesions (particularly arising in a subungual location) although examples have also been described in primary desmoplastic melanoma, mucosal melanoma, and melanoma arising in a congenital nevus.[6,7] It can also be seen in metastatic melanoma, both with or without being present in the cognate primary lesion.[8,9] From the limited available literature, these tumors are high grade (due to thickness at presentation) with frequent metastases and considerable mortality. Histologically, they usually present as sarcomatoid lesions with osteoid and to a lesser extent chondroblastic differentiation (*Figs 26.89* and *26.90*). A number of these cases represent osteosarcomatous differentiation, i.e., osteoid deposition in association with malignant cells, and/or chondrosarcomatous differentiation.[10,11] Too few cases have been reported to be certain whether heterologous differentiation

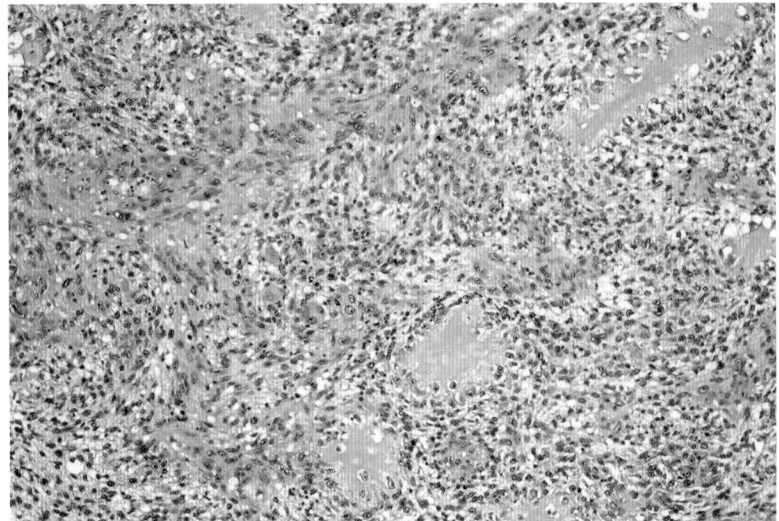

Fig. 26.89
Metaplastic melanoma: multiple deposits of osteoid are present in association with malignant cells in this amelanotic melanoma.

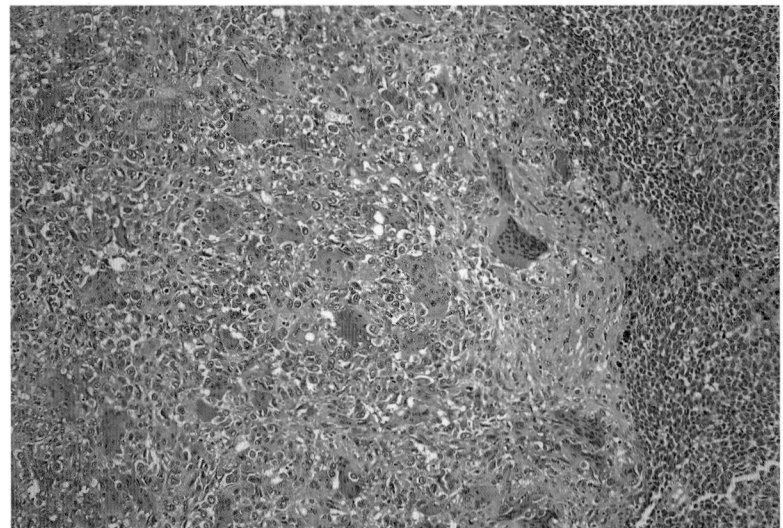

Fig. 26.91
Metaplastic melanoma: this melanoma was associated with an intense osteoclast-like giant cell infiltrate.

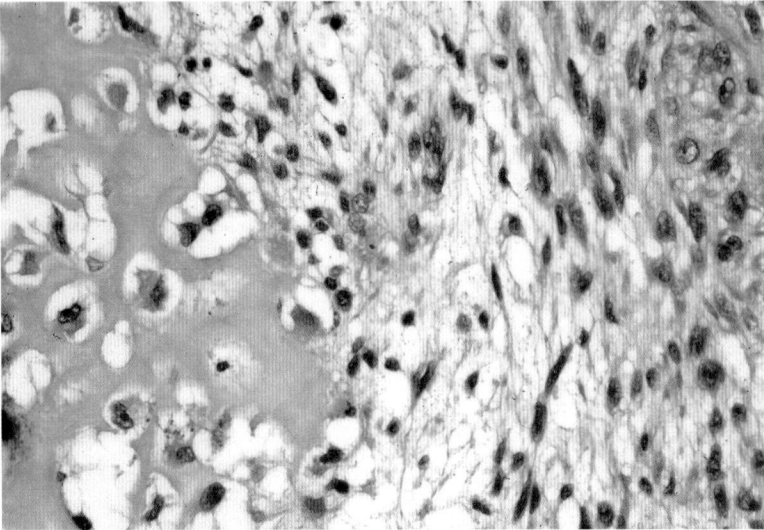

Fig. 26.90
Metaplastic melanoma: high-power view.

influences prognosis. Certain properties of mesenchymal stem or precursor cells suggest a pluripotency that includes neural crest, osteogenic, and chondrogenic potential and may help explain the existence of this melanoma variant.[12] Some cases have been shown to express immunohistochemical markers of master regulatory genes for osseous and cartilaginous differentiation such as SATB2 and SOX9.[6,9]

Unusually, melanoma may undergo smooth muscle and rhabdomyoblastic differentiation.[13–16] Case reports of melanoma showing ganglionic and ganglioneuroblastic differentiation have been documented.[17–19]

There are very occasional reports of conventional and desmoplastic melanoma containing osteoclast-like giant cells (*Fig. 26.91*).[20–25]

Rhabdomyosarcoma has been documented in a congenital nevus, including a giant form.[26–28]

Pigmented epithelioid melanocytoma (pigment synthesizing melanoma; animal-type melanoma)

An enigmatic lesion with many names, including pigment synthesizing melanoma, animal-type melanoma, melanoma with prominent pigment synthesis, equine type melanoma, and low-grade hypermelanotic dermal melanoma, this exceedingly rare variant of melanoma is now recognized by the WHO

under the name of pigmented epithelioid melanocytoma. There is certainly morphological overlap with malignant blue nevus, but genomically these two entities are distinct and we believe that they represent independent histologic entities based on this and differences in their natural history. The original term of animal-type melanoma was coined to reflect the similarity of these tumors to melanocytic lesions occurring in horses and a variety of experimental animal models – so-called equine melanotic disease.[1,2] This is a condition in which aging gray horses lose their pigmentation and develop melanocytic tumors particularly around the external genitalia, undersurface of tail, breast, and lip mucosa. Subsequent development of melanoma in these animals is an important complication.

Clinical features

Around 200 cases of this seemingly rare tumor have been documented, mostly as single case reports.[3] Although the age range is quite wide, the majority of lesions have arisen in patients in the second to fourth decades.[4–7] There is no recognized sex or site predilection. Most present as 1.0 cm or more diameter, brown, blue-black or black nodules or plaques clinically thought to represent melanoma.[8] These tumors can occur sporadically or as part of the autosomal dominant Carney complex where these tumors have traditionally been termed epithelioid blue nevus.[9] Carney complex consists of spotty skin pigmentation, and a variety of unusual endocrine and non-endocrine tumors such as myxomas, pigmented nodular adrenocortical disease, calcifying Sertoli cell tumor and psammomatous melanotic schwannomas. This complex is associated with germline inactivating mutations in the protein kinase A regulatory subunit, *PRKAR1A* on chromosome 17q.[10,11] The unrelated Carney triad is a distinct condition comprised of gastrointestinal stromal tumor, pulmonary chondroma, and extra-adrenal paraganglioma driven by succinate dehydrogenase (SDH) definiciency.[12,13]

Prognosis seems to be better than that of an ordinary melanoma of equivalent thickness and it has been proposed that it may be regarded as a low-grade variant of melanoma. A recent meta-analysis of around 190 cases seems to confirm this notion, but that study was hampered by limited follow-up for the reported cases and the lack of uniform diagnostic criteria.[3] Nonetheless, this study showed that with a median Breslow thickness of 3.8 mm and 16% ulceration, there were only six patients with distant metastases and five patient deaths. Sentinel lymph node positivity rates were notable at 41% of the 78 patients undergoing this procedure, but subsequent progression was uncommon. Thus this tumor has a markedly superior prognosis to conventional melanoma.

Histologic features

Pigmented epithelioid melanocytoma is characterized histologically by a very dense infiltrate of heavily pigmented melanocytes, typically filling the

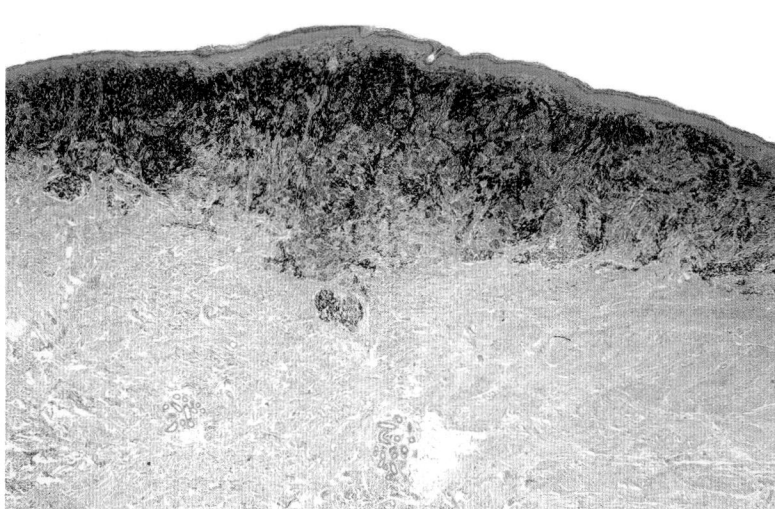

Fig. 26.92
Pigment synthesizing melanoma: this low-power view shows the intense pigmentation typical of this variant.

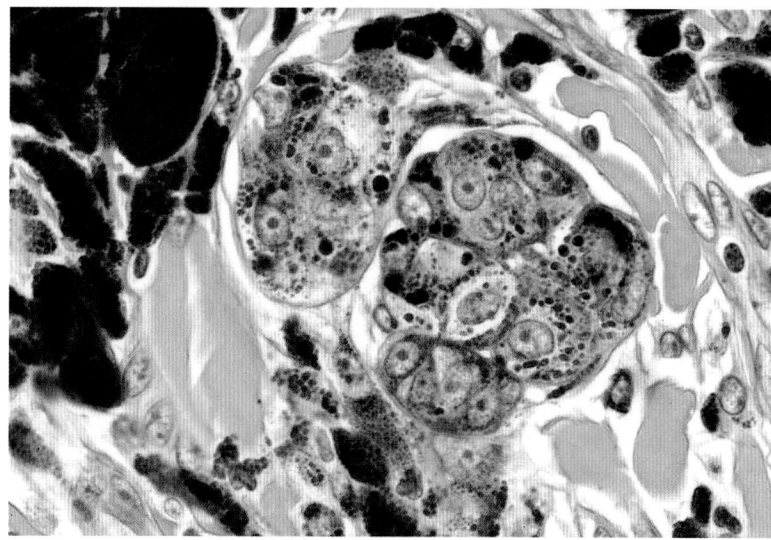

Fig. 26.94
Pigment synthesizing melanoma: the tumor cells are uniform with large vesicular nuclei and prominent eosinophilic nucleoli. Abundant pigment-laden macrophages are present.

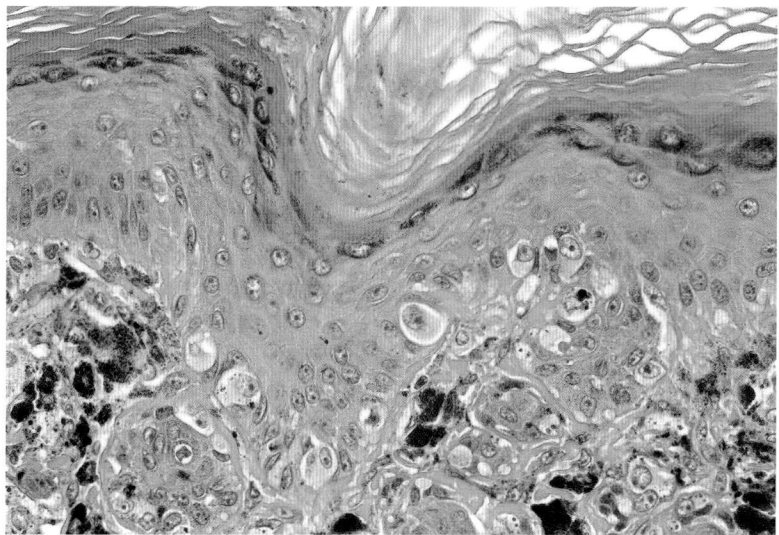

Fig. 26.93
Pigment synthesizing melanoma: scattered tumor cells are present in the lower epidermis.

papillary and reticular dermis and often spilling over into the subcutaneous fat (*Fig. 26.92*). The epidermis may be atrophic or hyperplastic. A small number of cases are not purely intradermal but display a junctional component (*Fig. 26.93*). In cases with a junctional component, tumor cells are plump and dendritic and do not tend to exhibit pagetoid spread. Tumor cells are spindled, polygonal, or rounded and are distributed in a fascicular or nodular growth pattern, sometimes displaying a focal storiform appearance.[6] Dendritic processes may be identified. The tumor cell cytoplasm typically contains abundant fine to coarse melanin granules, which commonly obscure the nuclear morphology. Examination of bleached sections can be helpful. The cytoplasm of tumor cells is pale, and nuclei appear enlarged and sometimes hyperchromatic. A single prominent basophilic nucleolus is often seen. Although there is cytological atypia, tumor cells display little variation throughout the tumor (*Fig. 26.94*).[6] Mitoses are typically sparse. The latter and the uniformity of tumor cells allow distinction from malignant blue nevus. Perineural infiltration may be present but lymphovascular invasion has not been described.

This is an unusual tumor, which shows some histologic overlap with other dermal dendrocytoses and blue nevus-like melanoma. These lesions form part of the spectrum of pigmented epithelioid melanocytoma, which includes the epithelioid blue nevus associated with the Carney complex and

tumors previously termed pigment synthesizing melanoma.[14–16] While these lesions appear to have metastatic potential to involve lymph nodes, their outcome is favorable compared to stage-matched cases of traditional melanoma.[3] More and longer-term study of this entity and the above-mentioned spectrum will be insightful.

Loss-of-function mutations in *PRKAR1A* are common. Gene fusions with *PRKCA* encoding protein kinase Cα can also be seen in pure melanoma.[17] In cases of combined nevi with conventional features and an area resembling pigmented epithelioid melanoma, *BRAF* V600 mutations can be seen with the *PRKAR1A* mutations. Cases with characteristic activating *GNAQ* or *GNA11* mutations would be better regarded as blue nevus or blue nevus-like melanoma rather than pigmented epithelioid melanocytoma. Use of the standard multi-color FISH assay to assess for malignancy in pigmented epithelioid melanocytoma has been reported as helpful in a few cases, but should be interpreted with caution given the alternative genetics of this tumor.[18,19]

Epidermotropic metastatic melanoma

Metastatic melanoma is common and, in the majority of cases, causes little diagnostic difficulty. Rarely, however, cutaneous deposits are accompanied by epidermal involvement such that distinction from a second or third primary tumor can be extremely difficult, if not impossible, particularly if clinical information is not available (*Figs 26.95* and *26.96*).[1–9] Traditionally, the features in favor of epidermotropic metastatic disease have included a well-circumscribed dermal nodule, widespread lymphovascular invasion, and filling of the papillary dermis by melanoma cells with atrophy of the overlying epidermis.[1,10] Typically, the epidermal component is equal in width to, or is less than, the dermal component. A lateral epidermal collarette may sometimes be present. Exceptionally, patients have presented with showers of metastases which, due to extensive lateral spread of the epidermal component beyond the dermal mass or even wholly intraepidermal disease, have histologically been indistinguishable from a primary tumor. In such instances, clinicopathological correlation is essential in establishing a diagnosis of metastatic disease.[2,3] A recent study with molecular testing suggests that the genetic relationship of primary melanomas and their potential epidermotropic metastases is complex, with certain cases showing divergent loss of heterozygosity and X-chromosome inactivation patterns consistent with either complex divergent clones or possibly new primaries.[11] Additional study is essential as the distinction has important staging implications. Epidermotropic melanoma is a satellite lesion that results in stage III groupings under the 8th edition AJCC, whereas a second primary would be individually staged.[12]

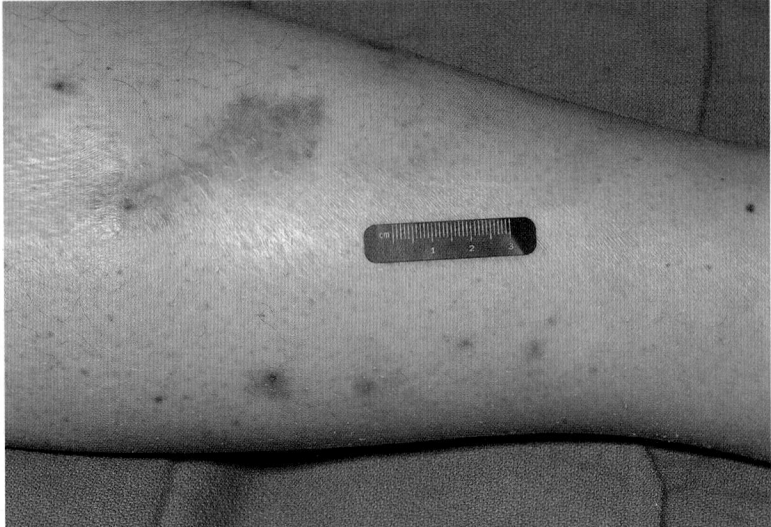

Fig. 26.95
Epidermotropic metastatic melanoma: numerous tiny blue tumor deposits are present in association with the scar from a previously excised melanoma. By courtesy of J. Gershewald, MD, MD Anderson Cancer Center, Houston, Texas, USA.

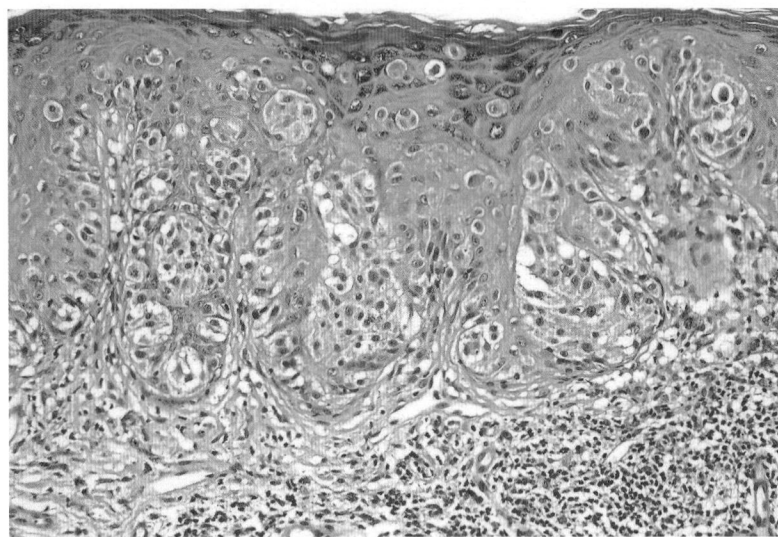

Fig. 26.96
Epidermotropic metastatic melanoma: this metastatic deposit is wholly intraepidermal and is indistinguishable from in situ superficial spreading melanoma. Diagnosis is entirely dependent upon the clinical history.

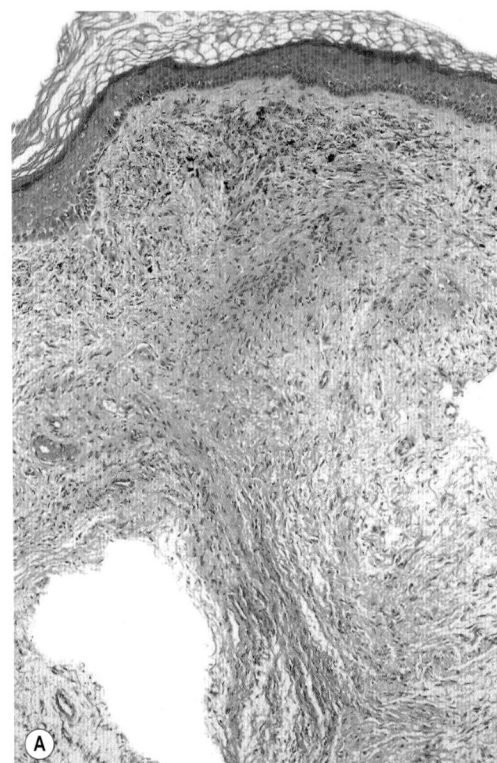

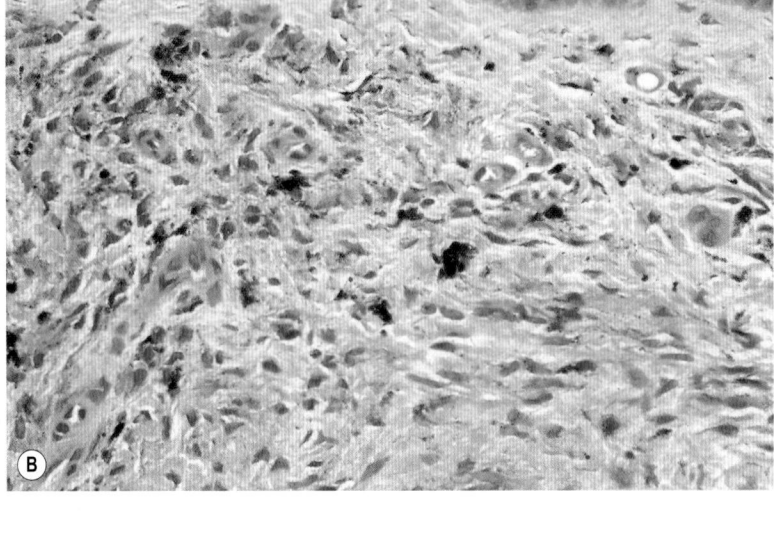

Fig. 26.97
Blue nevus-like metastatic melanoma: (**A**) at low-power examination, the features could easily be mistaken for a common blue nevus; (**B**) in addition to pigment-laden melanophages and dendritic cells, there are scattered melanoma cells. Note the multinucleate form with vesicular nuclei and prominent nucleoli. The patient had a melanoma previously excised at this site.

Blue nevus-like metastatic melanoma

Blue nevus-like metastatic melanoma is rare but represents a very serious source of misdiagnosis.[1-3] One or multiple lesions may be seen and they usually, but not always, develop at sites close to the primary tumor. Very rarely, lesions may be distant. They resemble a blue nevus clinically and histologically. They are often small and microscopically are characterized by dendritic, deeply pigmented melanocytes. Cytological atypia can be very subtle and this is further compounded by the prominent pigmentation (*Fig. 26.97*). Bleaching can therefore be useful. Resemblance to ordinary blue nevus or epithelioid blue nevus may be seen. Clues to the diagnosis of malignancy reside in the presence of cytological atypia, mitotic figures, and inflammation mainly at the periphery of the lesion. Histologic diagnosis is extremely difficult and close clinicopathological correlation is crucial.

Cytogenetic studies by FISH may be of help in establishing the distinction. In a study comparing epithelioid blue nevi with blue nevus-like cutaneous metastasis, it was shown that most of the latter had important copy number changes in chromosomes 6p25, 11q13, and centromere 6 while the former lacked cytogenetic changes.[2] Uveal melanoma can also give rise to blue nevus-like melanoma which can be detected by detection of genetic events such as monosomy for chromosome 3 resulting in loss of *BAP1*.[4] Detection of the *GNAS* or *GNA11* mutation of uveal melanoma is not helpful alone in this context since these mutations can also be seen in blue nevi.

Desmoplastic and neurotropic melanoma

Desmoplastic and neurotropic variants of spindled cell melanoma are inter-related high-grade tumors that are commonly associated with histologic

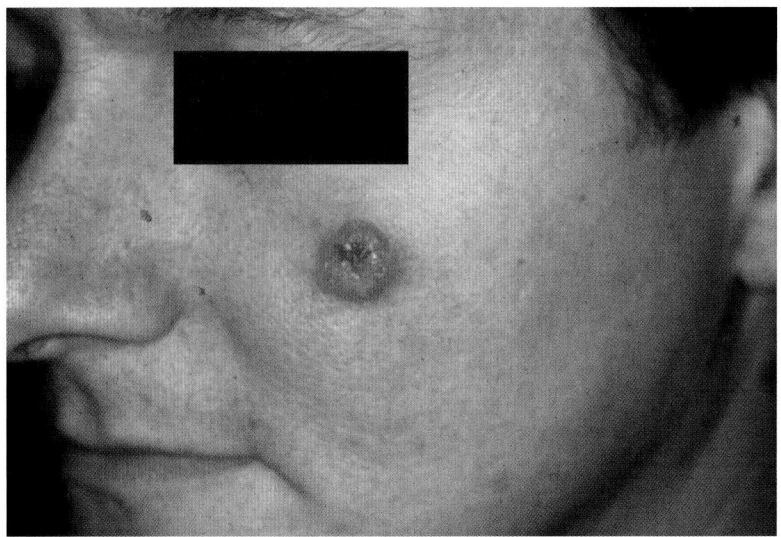

Fig. 26.98
Desmoplastic melanoma: these tumors are frequently amelanotic, as seen in this patient. By courtesy E. Wilson Jones, MD, Institute of Dermatology, London, UK.

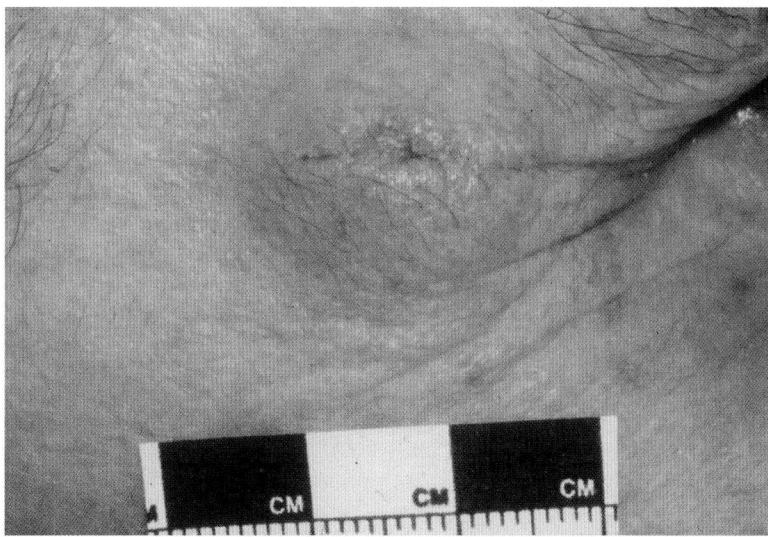

Fig. 26.99
Desmoplastic melanoma: this tumor was initially thought to represent a cyst. By courtesy of E. Wilson Jones, MD, Institute of Dermatology, London, UK.

diagnostic difficulty.[1-7] A history of a mistaken diagnosis of reactive fibroblastic proliferative lesion is common and relates particularly to the usual absence of melanin pigment and the relative infrequency of obvious epidermal melanocytic involvement, particularly in recurrent lesions. Desmoplastic melanoma represents an extreme degree of fibroblastic or myofibroblastic metaplasia accompanied by abundant collagen synthesis. In the neurotropic variant, the metaplasia may be towards Schwann cell-type differentiation. Although not all desmoplastic melanomas are neurotropic and not all neurotropic melanomas are desmoplastic, many authors regard them as variations on a theme.[8] These tumors are in general associated with a high incidence of recurrence and metastasis and a poor prognosis.

Clinical features

Although the tumor may present at any age, the majority arise in the elderly (mean age 61 years) and show a male preponderance (as high as 2.7:1), which is particularly evident with the frankly neurotropic lesions.[3,9-17] The head and neck are most frequently affected, but examples have been documented at a wide range of sites, including the trunk and upper or lower limbs.[9,18] The leg is particularly involved in females.[3] Although the majority of these neoplasms arise on sun-damaged skin in a background of lentigo maligna (melanoma), superficial spreading and acral lentiginous melanomas, including subungual variants, have occasionally been documented.[12,13] Desmoplastic melanoma has also been described on the palate, gingiva, lip, vulva, anus, and conjunctiva.[19] Although a superimposed pigmented lesion of lentigo maligna may draw attention to this tumor, more often they present as amelanotic, flesh-colored or erythematous nodules or indurated plaques (Figs 26.98 and 26.99). These tumors are notoriously deeply infiltrative and commonly have extended widely by the time of diagnosis. In addition to contributing to the high incidence of recurrence, neurotropism may result in peripheral and cranial neuropathy. Spread along the cranial nerves into the base of the skull with eventual meningeal involvement is a rare but important complication with an almost 100% mortality.[18,20] Although most desmoplastic melanomas arise in a background of severe sun damage, previous irradiation (therapeutic or otherwise) is occasionally of etiological importance.[9] Rarely, examples have complicated congenital melanocytic nevi and even chronic burns scarring.[21,22]

Recurrence is common (range 22–77%, mean 46%) and metastasis (particularly to the lungs) frequently supervenes (range 11–56%, mean of approximately 30%).[10,15] Local control in the head and neck region, where many of these tumors arise, is particularly problematic.[23] Careful evaluation of surgical margins is critical for local control.[17] Surprisingly, nodal spread has been documented very infrequently such that sentinel lymph node biopsy is not regarded by some as an effective staging tool in this

disease.[3,24-30] Others have not observed this phenomenon as starkly, but this could be due to differences in diagnostic criteria.[31-34] In this regard it is important to define desmoplastic melanoma carefully with the pure desmoplastic pattern being the predominant one, as cases showing a significant component (greater than 10%) of traditional melanoma show the more characteristic metastasis to lymph node.[35-37] Pure desmoplastic melanoma appears to behave more like a sarcoma in terms of local recurrence and metastatic pattern with the lung being the most common initial site rather than regional lymph nodes. In regard to disease-specific survival, desmoplastic melanoma may behave similarly to classic melanoma, the poor prognosis reflecting an increased thickness of greater than 1.5 mm at presentation in the vast majority of patients.[3,38] Others have found that disease-specific survival for desmoplastic melanoma is superior to conventional melanoma.[28] Pure and mixed variants of desmoplastic melanoma are reported by some to have similar survival.[39] There is some debate on this topic, with some data that indicate an improved outcome for desmoplastic melanoma patients.[28,40-42] Poor prognostic indicators are high mitotic rate, tumor thickness, ulceration, and inadequate excision margins (<1.0 cm).[3,17,23,43] The 5-year survival rate is of the order of 70–80%, and the overall mortality varies from 11% to 66%.[3,15,23]

Histologic features

Desmoplastic melanoma is characterized by a diffusely infiltrative, sometimes paucicellular, malignant spindle cell tumor with marked interstitial fibrosis and collagenization (Figs 26.100 and 26.101).[1,2,9,19,44,45] It is to be distinguished from the more common spindled cell melanoma unassociated with significant desmoplasia.

The infiltrate often leaves the immediate subepidermal papillary dermis unaffected, but frequently is found to extend into the subcutaneous fat or beyond at the time of diagnosis. Involvement of skeletal muscle or underlying bone is not uncommon. The tumor cytology is variable, the cells resembling fibroblasts, smooth muscle cells, or Schwann cells. They are typically elongated and have eosinophilic or more commonly basophilic cytoplasm (Fig. 26.102). Nuclei may be tapered and hyperchromatic or cigar-shaped and vesicular with prominent eosinophilic nucleoli (Figs 26.103 and 26.104). Mitoses are scanty but may be conspicuous, and sometimes abnormal forms are present (Fig. 26.105). Most commonly, the tumor has a distinctly fascicular arrangement, but focal storiform areas are occasionally evident, which can result in a mistaken diagnosis of dermatofibroma or dermatofibrosarcoma protuberans. Foci of myxoid change, giving the tumor a feathery appearance, are sometimes seen. Recurrent tumors are frequently paucicellular and are easily taken for scar tissue (Figs 26.106 and 26.107). Tumor giant cells are an infrequent manifestation. Lymphocytic infiltrates,

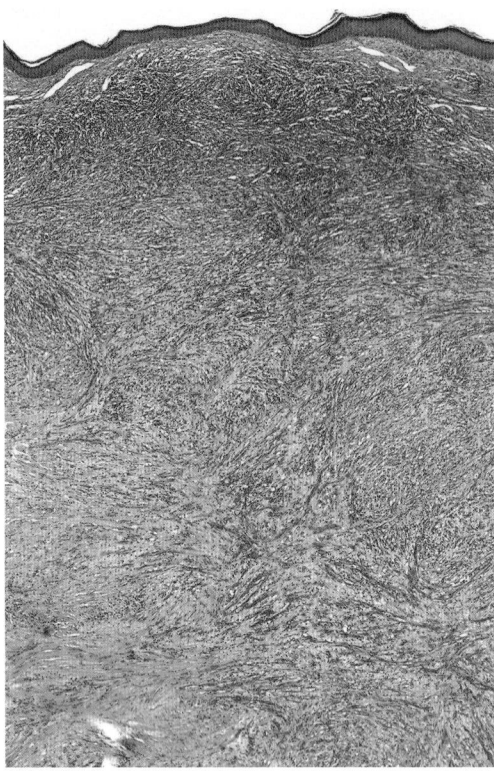

Fig. 26.100
Desmoplastic melanoma: low-power view showing a spindle cell tumor extending throughout the full thickness of the dermis and associated with superficial lymphoid infiltrates.

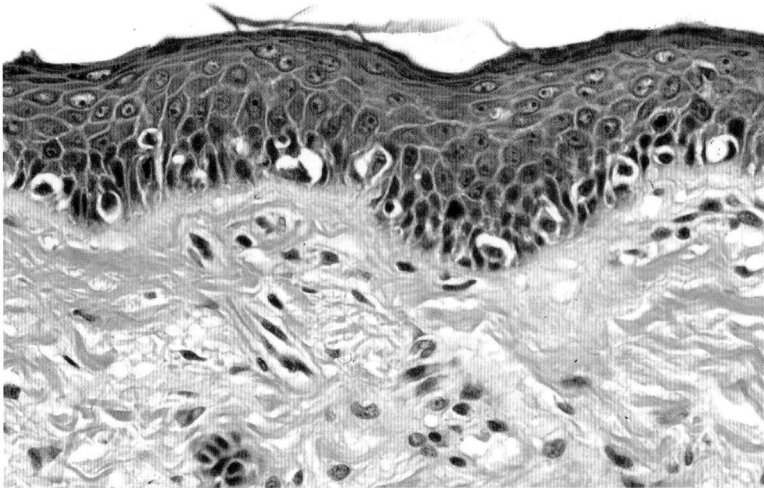

Fig. 26.101
Desmoplastic melanoma: the overlying epidermis shows an atypical lentiginous melanocytic proliferation.

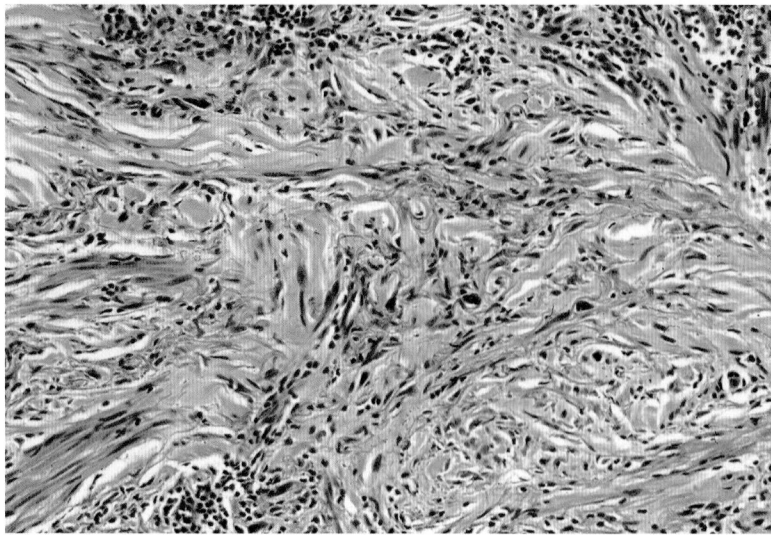

Fig. 26.102
Desmoplastic melanoma: the tumor cells have basophilic cytoplasm and are dispersed in a densely collagenous stroma.

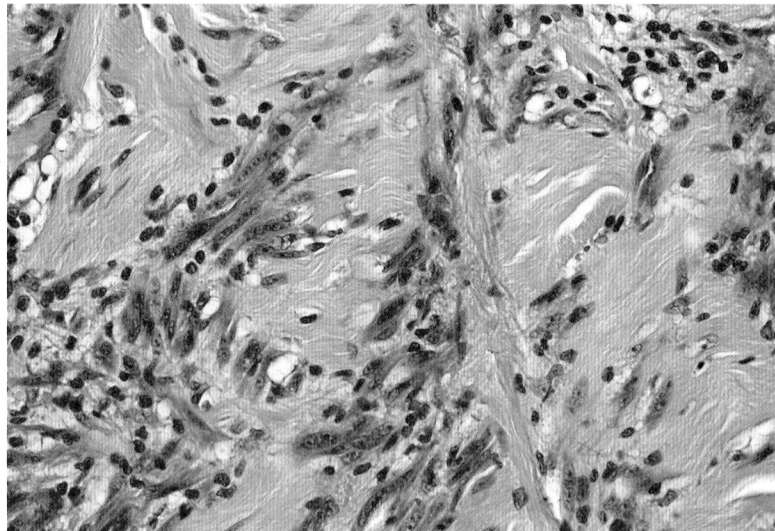

Fig. 26.103
Desmoplastic melanoma: nuclei are vesicular and nucleoli are prominent.

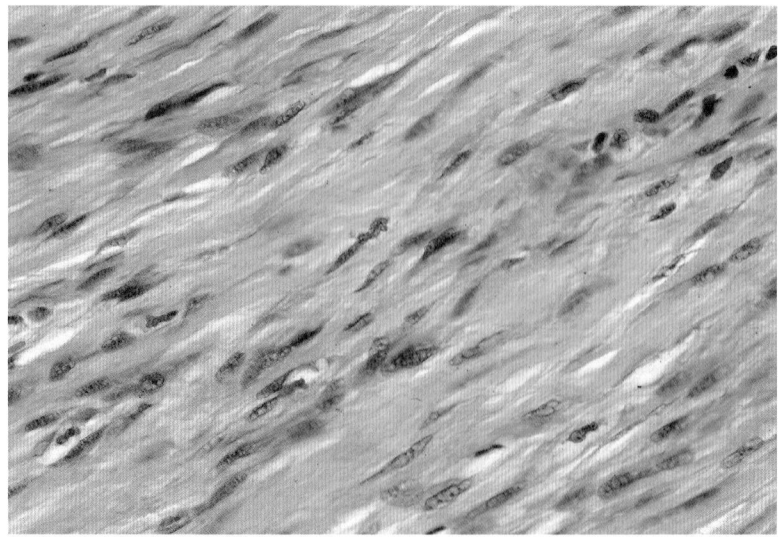

Fig. 26.104
Desmoplastic melanoma: the tumor cells are compressed by the adjacent sclerotic fibrous stroma.

often evident as nodular aggregates, are a characteristic (but not diagnostic) feature (*Fig. 26.108*). They are, however, a useful histologic pointer in early lesions.[46,47] Vascular invasion is sometimes present.

Careful scrutiny of the overlying epidermis not uncommonly shows features of atypical melanocytic hyperplasia, most often of the lentigo maligna pattern.[9] Very occasionally, the changes of superficial spreading melanoma are present. In a significant proportion of cases no such in situ change is detected (the so-called de novo variant) (*Fig. 26.109*). Whether this represents regression, inadequate sampling, a de novo dermal tumor, or a previously treated in situ component is uncertain. In most examples, the invasive tumor cell population is amelanotic.[9]

Vascular changes including hemangiopericytomatous features and glomeruloid vascular lesions may rarely be encountered.[48]

The neurotropic variant of melanoma may show a range of manifestations.[2,9,19,48] Microscopic perineural or endoneural involvement is common

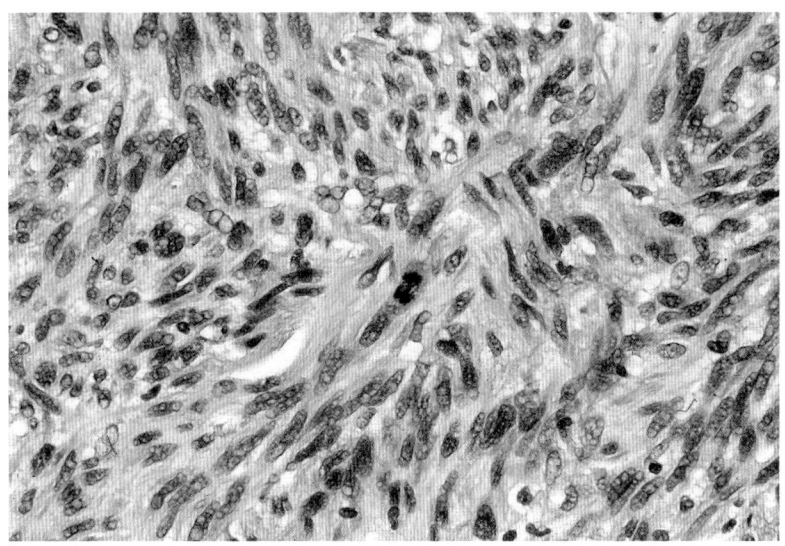

Fig. 26.105
Desmoplastic melanoma: note the central mitotic figure.

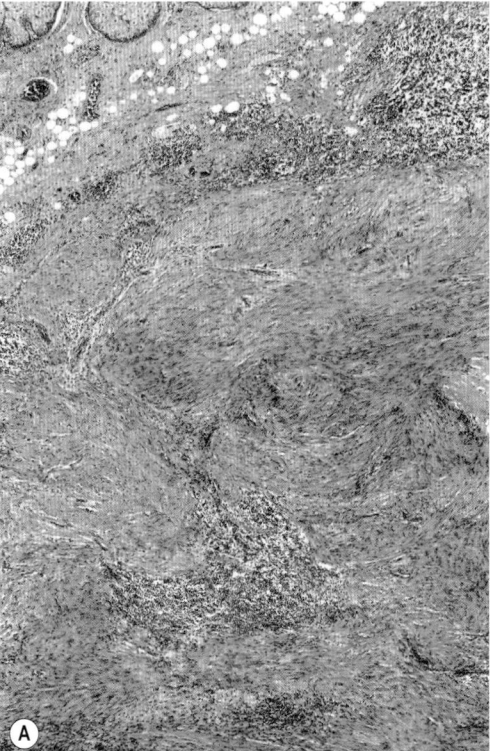

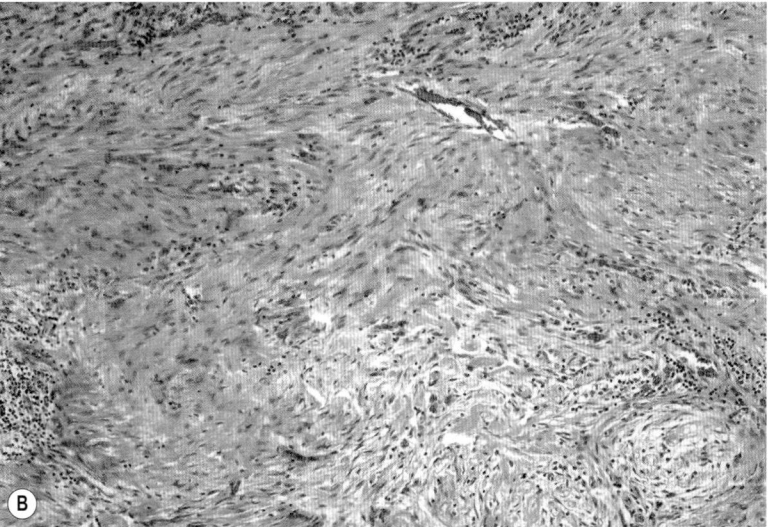

Fig. 26.106
(A, B) Desmoplastic melanoma: this example represents recurrent tumor following a previous excision. Melanoma can easily be mistaken for scar tissue, particularly if the clinical history is not available. The lymphoid aggregates should raise the suspicion of desmoplastic melanoma.

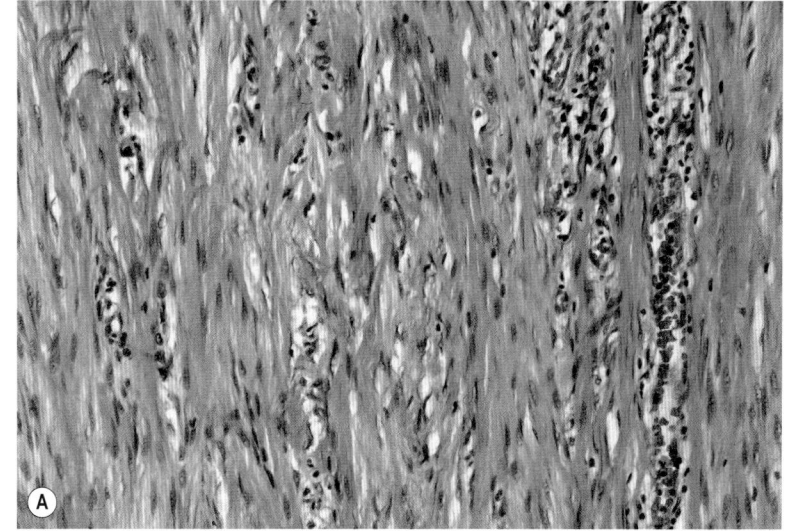

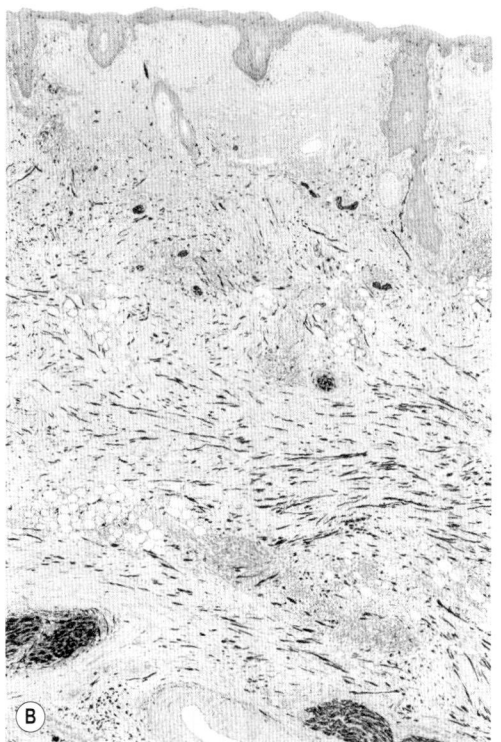

Fig. 26.107
Desmoplastic melanoma: (A) high-power view of tumor shown in Figure 26.106; (B) immunohistochemistry for S100 protein highlights the considerable tumor cell population.

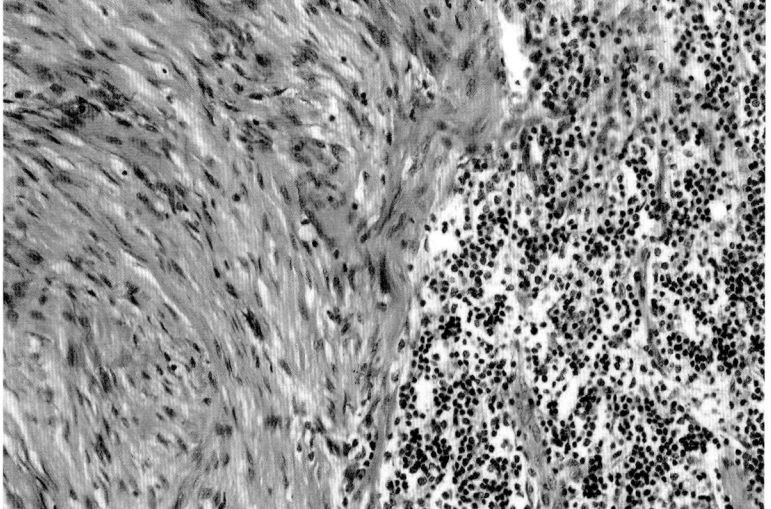

Fig. 26.108
Desmoplastic melanoma: nodular aggregates of lymphocytes are a useful diagnostic clue.

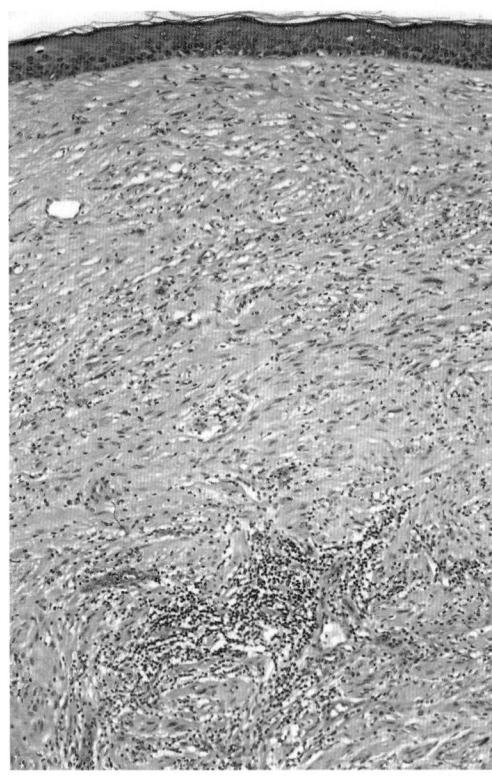

Fig. 26.109
Desmoplastic melanoma: in this example, the overlying epidermis shows no evidence of a pre-existent atypical melanocytic proliferative lesion (the so-called de novo variant).

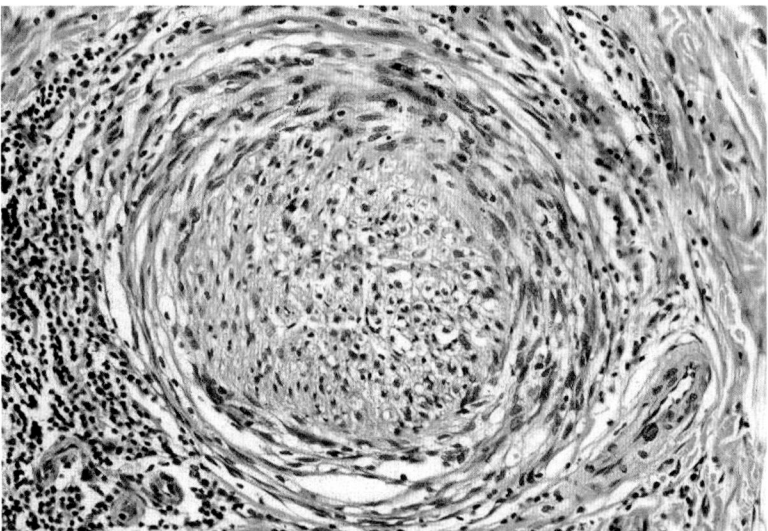

Fig. 26.110
Desmoplastic melanoma: perineural infiltration is very commonly present, accounting in part for the high recurrence rate of this tumor.

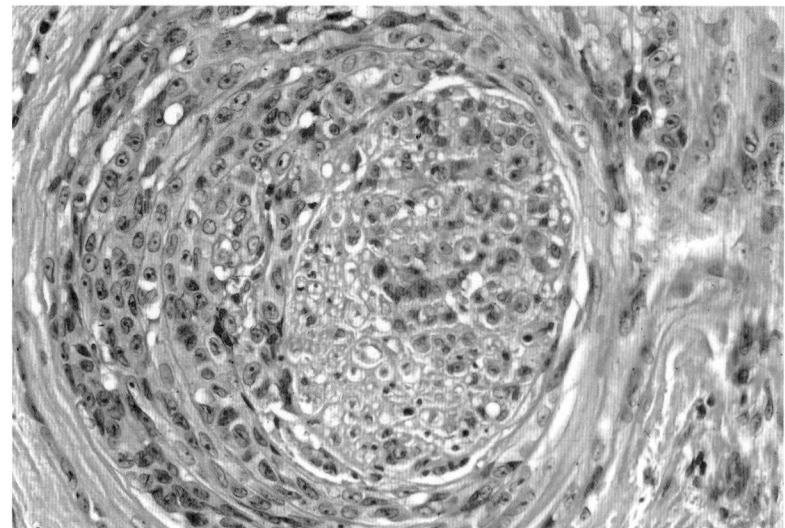

Fig. 26.111
Desmoplastic melanoma: epithelioid cells are sometimes encountered within the tumor. This example shows extensive peri- and intraneural spread.

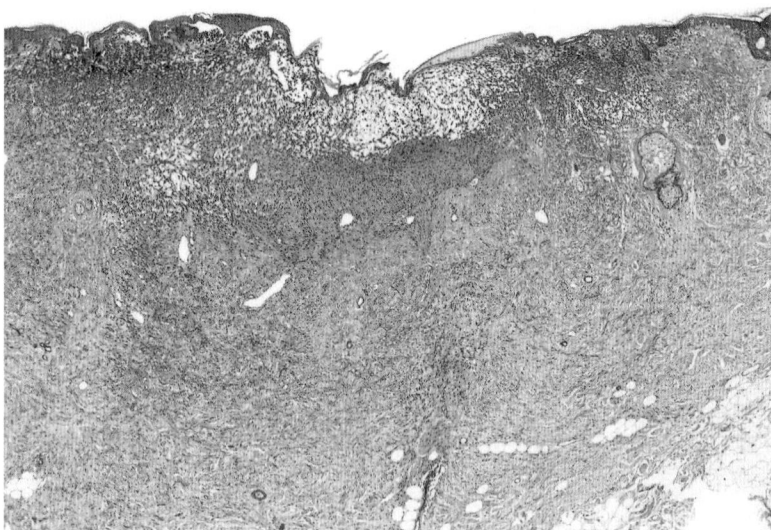

Fig. 26.112
Desmoplastic melanoma (neural transformation): low-power view of a tumor which has infiltrated through the full thickness of the dermis.

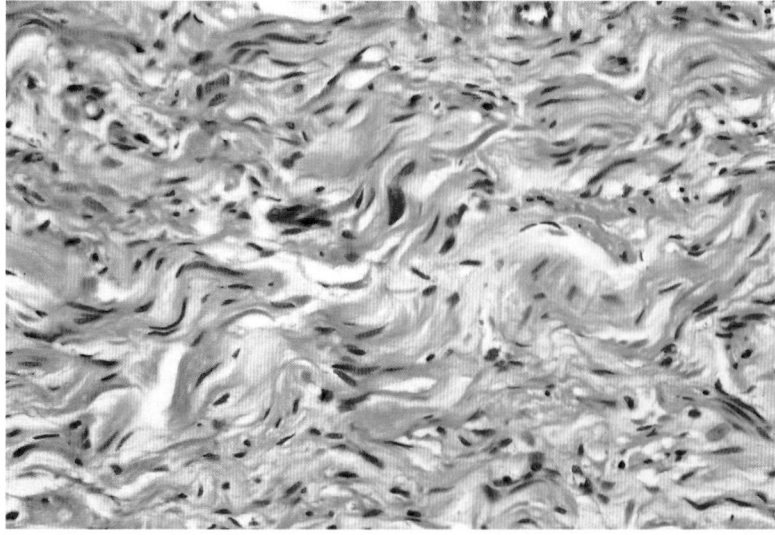

Fig. 26.113
Desmoplastic melanoma (neural transformation): the tumor cells have small, twisted, and comma-shaped nuclei with ill-defined eosinophilic cytoplasm reminiscent of peripheral nerve sheath tumor. Note the nuclear hyperchromatism.

in many desmoplastic melanomas (*Figs 26.110* and *26.111*). The term neurotropic, however, is often reserved for lesions where nerve involvement is very marked or more particularly when it results in clinical evidence of nerve irregularity and thickening. In rare examples, the tumor appears to be limited to a nerve trunk with no discernible spread to the adjacent tissues.[9] Occasionally, the spindled cell population displays histologic features reminiscent of neurofibroma, schwannoma, or malignant nerve sheath tumor (sometimes known as neural transformation) (*Figs 26.112–26.114*).[18,49] These latter features often comprise smaller cells, with pale eosinophilic cytoplasm and irregular wavy nuclei separated by variable amounts of collagen and ground substance and sometimes giving the tumor a loose myxoid appearance. Mitotic activity is variable and therefore these variants can sometimes be very deceptive, resulting in a mistaken diagnosis of benign nerve sheath tumor. Recently, neurotropic melanoma associated with profound vascular infiltration (so-called angiotropic melanoma) has

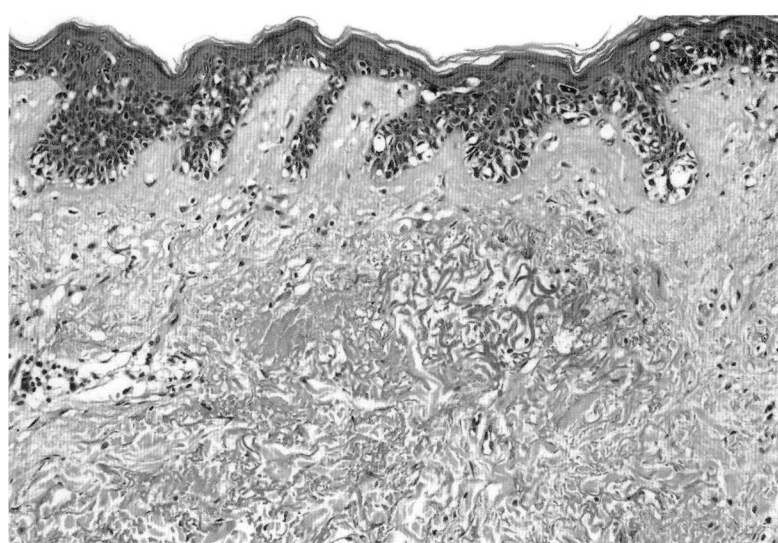

Fig. 26.114
Desmoplastic melanoma: the adjacent epidermis shows atypical melanocytic lentiginous hyperplasia.

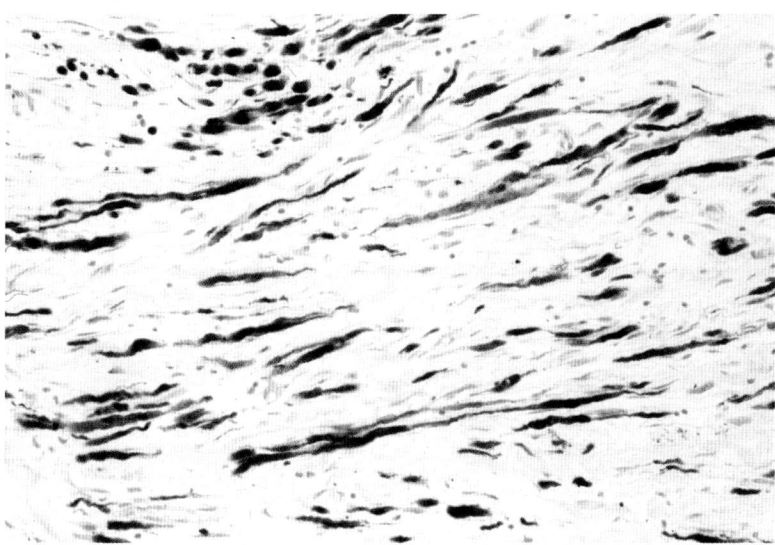

Fig. 26.115
Desmoplastic melanoma: the tumor cells are strongly S100 protein positive.

been documented.[50] Metaplastic bone formation has been described albeit rarely.[51] Sarcomatoid dedifferentiation is also rarely noted.[49]

Immunohistochemically, desmoplastic melanoma expresses S100 protein (94–100%), neuron-specific enolase, and vimentin (*Fig. 26.115*).[3,36–38,40,41] HMB-45 (gp100) may be positive in the superficial papillary dermal tumor cells but more often is totally negative.[52–57] The results with MART-1 (melan-A) are variable (24–60% positive), and tyrosinase does not appear to be present in desmoplastic melanoma.[58–60] Microphthalmia transcription factor (D5) is of limited value, expression having been documented in from only 35% to 55% of cases.[61,62] A relatively new marker, SOX10, is reactive in melanoma, desmoplastic melanoma, and peripheral nerve sheath tumors and can be a very useful marker.[63–66] Members of the S100 protein family such as S100A6 may have efficacy in distinguishing desmoplastic melanoma from malignant peripheral nerve sheath tumors, but the diffuse pattern of traditional polyclonal S100 protein expression in melanoma is usually sufficient in this regard.[67] Melanoma cell adhesion molecule may be more useful, 82% of tumors in a series of 17 tumors having shown strong expression.[68] EMA may be present in up to 43% of tumors but keratin, leu 7, CD31, and CD34 are uniformly negative.[48,55,56,68] Smooth muscle actin is often positive, reflecting the myofibroblastic population.[55,56,69] Although occasional desmin

positivity was documented in the earlier literature, more recent studies have not confirmed this observation.[70,71] Loss of p16 reactivity can be useful in distinguishing desmoplastic melanoma from desmoplastic nevus when this differential diagnosis arises in small biopsies, but not all desmoplastic cases show loss.[72,73] P75 nerve growth factor receptor, WT1, and nestin immunohistochemical markers have also been suggested to have clinical utility.[74–76] Desmoplastic melanoma has been described to MPNST. Loss of H3K27 nuclear staining characteristic of MPNST is not helpful for distinguishing MPNST from melanoma, desmoplastic, or otherwise, as a subset of melanomas also show nuclear loss of this histone trimethylation marker.[77]

Evaluation of scar versus desmoplastic melanoma can be difficult as the degree of fibrosis in desmoplastic melanoma can be extensive with only scattered melanoma cells. This same problem complicates the assessment of margins. Use of polyclonal S100 protein immunohistochemistry in the setting of re-excision can be complex given the focal S100 reactivity present in many scars due to scattered macrophages and other cells showing Schwannian differentiation.[78] Careful assessment of the degree of nuclear hyperchromasia in these spindled cells is paramount in evaluating these situations.[79]

Metastases may be desmoplastic, neuroid, or more obviously melanocytic. Although some authors have suggested that the desmoplasia is a consequence of reactive stromal fibroblast hyperplasia, it is now generally accepted that these features are of melanocytic derivation.

Ultrastructural studies have shown that the tumor spindled cells may rarely contain premelanosomes and melanosomes.[1,2] Fibroblastic, myofibroblastic, and Schwann cell differentiation, particularly in neurotropic variants (including elongated and interdigitating cellular processes sometimes encircling collagen fibers reminiscent of mesaxon formation, discontinuous basal lamina, and intercellular junctions) have also been documented.[19,71,80–83]

The genome of desmoplastic melanoma harbors approximately an order of magnitude more mutations than that seen in conventional cutaneous melanoma.[84] Most of these are UV-linked. Exome sequencing revealed recurrent *NFKBIE* promoter mutations, and activation of the MAP kinase and PI-3 kinase pathways through mutations in genes such as *NF1*, *MAP2K1*, *MAP3K1*, *EGFR*, *MET*, *RAC1*, and *PIK3CA*.[84–88] Mutations in *BRAF* V600 and *NRAS* G61 were not seen. *TERT* promoter mutations are common as well.[89] Standard multi-probe FISH can be useful to demonstrate desmoplastic melanoma over other mimics.[90]

Differential diagnosis

The diagnosis of desmoplastic melanoma is frequently missed, particularly if only superficial biopsies are available for study. The lesion is commonly misdiagnosed as a reactive process, such as scarring and superficial nodular fasciitis, and deeper lesions may be mistaken for a fibromatosis or even fibrosarcoma. Examples showing storiform morphology have sometimes been confused with atypical fibrous histiocytoma and dermatofibrosarcoma protuberans. Scar tissue may be a particular problem, especially in recurrent lesions.[91,92] Pointers towards the latter include horizontal orientation of the fibroblast population, absence of adnexae, loss of the rete-ridge pattern, and vertically orientated dermal blood vessels. Immature scar tissue, however, can be much more problematical and, in the case of re-excision specimens or recurrences, the features may represent an admixture of both.[92] Recurrent lesions following surgery may sometimes be associated with marked nerve proliferation in addition to scar tissue. SOX10 and S100 may display positivity in scars and although this positivity can be strong it is usually restricted to a small number of cells.[93]

Diagnosis is dependent upon an awareness of the condition and often requires the inclusion of a battery of immunohistochemical markers to establish the histogenesis of the tumor infiltrate. In many instances, however, careful scrutiny of the epidermis to detect atypical melanocytic hyperplasia combined with the use of antibodies to S100 protein and pankeratin (to exclude desmoplastic spindled cell squamous carcinoma) will be sufficient to establish the correct diagnosis. Occasionally, in recurrent disease, proliferating neural elements may be admixed with scar and residual tumor with resultant increased diagnostic difficulty. Neurofilament protein, which is expressed by the neural elements but not the melanomatous component, can often be of discriminatory value.

Melanoma in children

Clinical features

Melanoma is extremely rare in children; less than 1% of all melanomas present in childhood.[1-20] Historically, many so-called examples have likely represented misdiagnosed Spitz nevi.[13] As a consequence, pathologists and clinicians are extremely reluctant to make the diagnosis, with resultant delay in treatment and potentially devastating consequences. Although exceptionally the tumor may develop in utero (complicating a large congenital nevus or arising de novo) or be acquired transplacentally (from a maternal melanoma), the majority are acquired and may be related to sun exposure during childhood.[4,14,21] Predisposing conditions include xeroderma pigmentosum, dysplastic nevi, familial melanoma, melanoma-pancreatic cancer syndrome, giant congenital nevi, neurocutaneous melanosis (leptomeningeal melanoma), prior irradiation, Li-Fraumeni syndrome, and immunodeficiency.[3,4,14,22-27] Melanoma arises in up to 12% of giant congenital nevi (i.e., those that measure 20 cm or more in diameter) and this can occur during childhood or later adult life.[28-30] It has been suggested that childhood melanoma can be segregated into three distinct categories based on the age of diagnosis: congenital melanoma which occurs in utero up to birth; infantile melanoma that presents after birth up to 1 year of age; and childhood melanoma that occurs after 1 year of age to puberty.[31] Some include in the childhood melanoma category patients up to the age of 18, but such upper age ranges are clearly arbitrary.[32]

The sexes are affected equally and tumors are more common in the second than the first decade.[9] The majority of childhood melanomas have developed in Caucasians.[7] Lesions arise on the trunk and extremities, with only 20% affecting the head and neck.[5] Many childhood melanomas are not easily recognized clinically.[13,33] Sometimes, however, clinical features similar to those described in adults – including increase in size, change in color, and onset of bleeding – may be encountered.[14,17]

Some earlier reports suggested that the prognosis of melanoma in children might be favorable.[34] In our experience, however, childhood tumors behave no differently from adult ones with the possible exception of spitzoid melanomas in very young patients as discussed further below. This is also generally borne out in the more recent literature.[4-6,13,18,35-37] Overall, childhood melanoma should therefore be treated in much the same way as adult tumors and, when appropriate, sentinel lymph node mapping and biopsy are recommended.[4,6,13,38-40] The majority of children present with stage 1 disease with a 5-year disease-free survival rate of 77%.[4,7] Crude survival figures for the largest series reported to date are 71% overall, 64% males, 81% females.[9] Some, but clearly not all or even most in some series, melanomas of childhood exhibit Spitz-like histology.[41] These cases may have a more favorable outcome than in adults, particularly in patients aged 11 or less, but this finding is not universal.[41-44] This could be due to inappropriate assignment of Spitz nevi, albeit atypical, to the melanoma group; however, even such tumors metastatic to lymph nodes appear to have a better prognosis.[45,46] Clearly, more study is required. Nonetheless, mortality is encountered within this age group. Spitzoid melanoma is discussed in more detail in the section above.

Histologic features

Melanoma in children may arise within the context of a precursor lesion such as a banal, congenital, or dysplastic nevus or it may present de novo. Melanoma arising within a giant congenital nevus presents most often as a dermal, sharply delineated nodule composed of tumor cells showing obvious cytological features of malignancy (Figs 26.116–26.118).[30] Although all the common subtypes may be encountered, superficial spreading and nodular melanoma variants are most frequently seen (Figs 26.119–26.123). Particular subtypes that often cause diagnostic difficulty include small cell melanoma, spitzoid melanoma, and malignant blue nevus.[7,11,47] These are all described under variants of melanoma (see above).

Cytogenetic features detected by FISH are similar to those seen in adult superficial spreading melanoma.[48] BRAF mutations can be seen in freestanding cases while NRAS mutations are seen in the cases associated with congenital nevi.[49,50] UV damage signatures are commonly encountered and

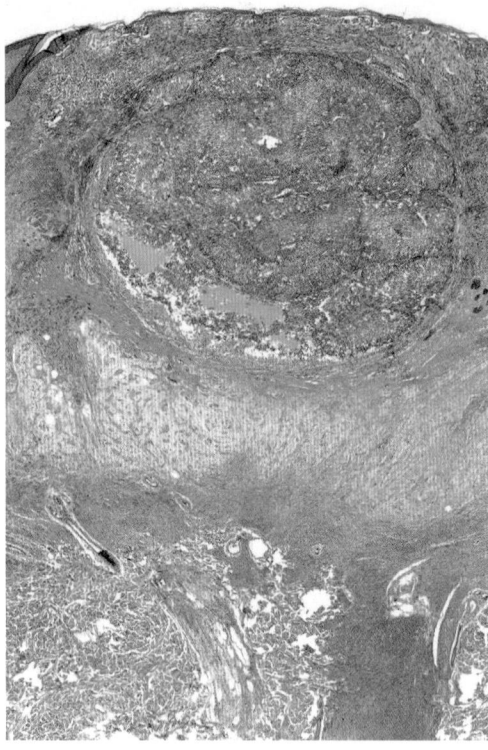

Fig. 26.116
Childhood melanoma: example of melanoma which has arisen in a giant congenital nevus.

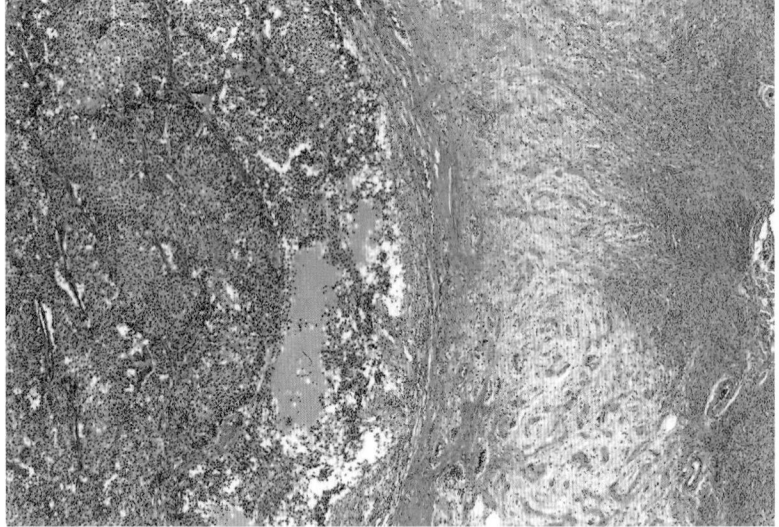

Fig. 26.117
Childhood melanoma: in this view, pleomorphic tumor cells are seen on the left; nevus is present on the right.

TERT promoter mutations are common, excepting the cases arising in congenital nevi.[49]

As with adult melanoma, the most important prognostic indicators are Breslow thickness and presence of ulceration. Melanoma in children should be reported in exactly the same way as adult melanoma.[51]

Differential diagnosis

Clinicopathological correlation is of great importance when considering a diagnosis of melanoma in a child, particularly in the first few years of life. Significant cytological atypia affecting junctional and dermal components accompanied by pagetoid spread and mitotic activity is not uncommon in congenital nevi, especially those affecting neonates.

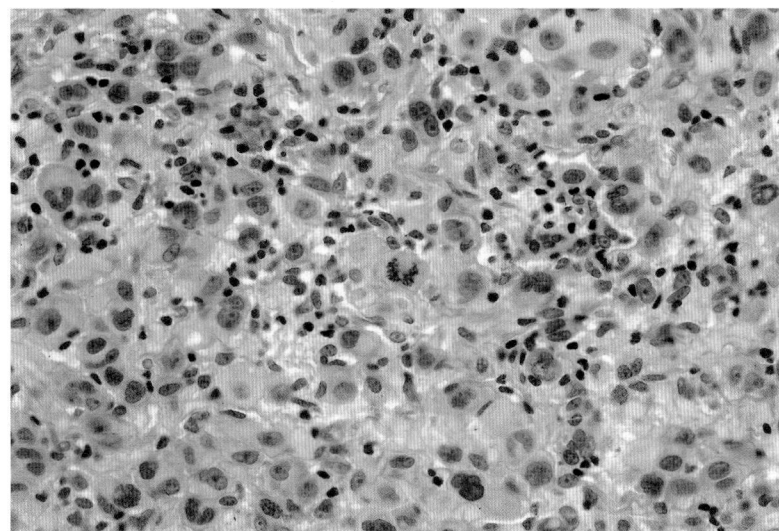

Fig. 26.118
Childhood melanoma: in the center of the field is an atypical mitotic figure.

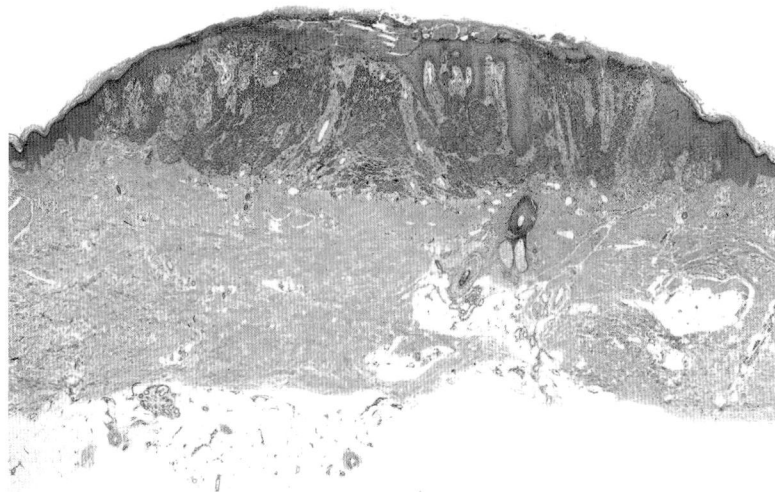

Fig. 26.119
Childhood melanoma: this tumor, which presented as a nodular lesion, arose in a girl aged 13 years. By courtesy of M. Little, MD, University College Hospital, Galway, Ireland.

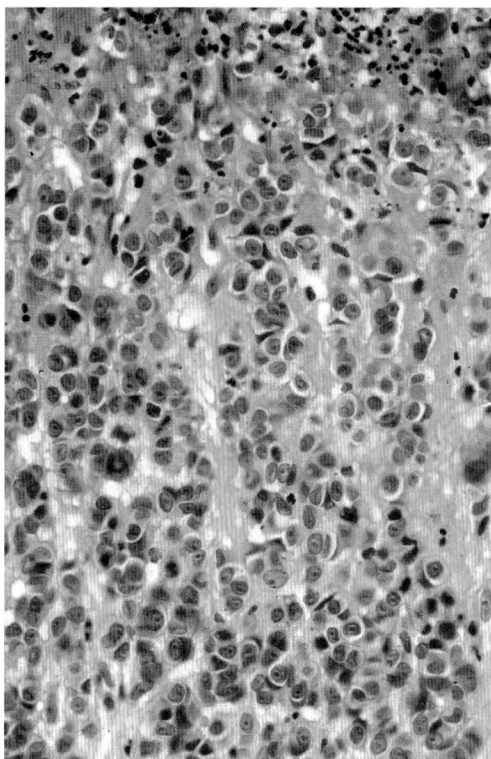

Fig. 26.120
Childhood melanoma: there is surface ulceration. By courtesy of M. Little, MD, University College Hospital, Galway, Ireland.

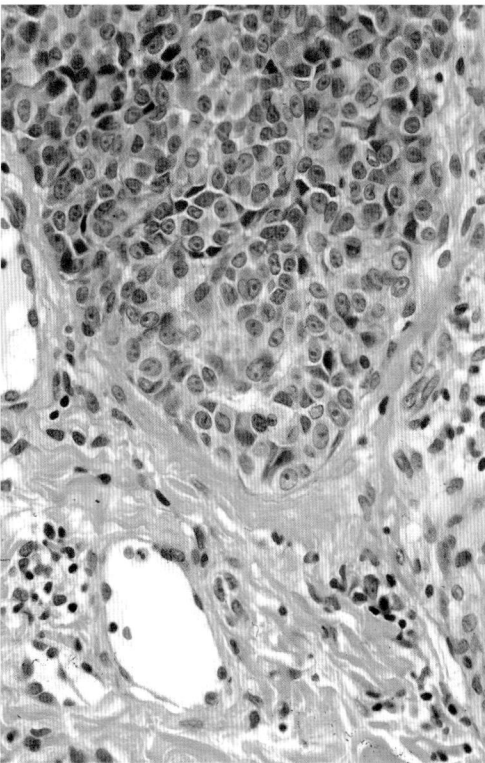

Fig. 26.121
Childhood melanoma: there is no maturation with depth. Note the sharply delineated lower border. By courtesy of M. Little, MD, University College Hospital, Galway, Ireland.

Dermal squamomelanocytic tumor

Clinical features

Reports of this tumor are exceedingly rare in the pathology literature.[1-6] Patients present with brown or purple-black facial nodules measuring up to 1.0 cm in diameter. The age range documented is 32–94 years and there have been less than 15 cases reported with equal sex distribution.[5] A precursor lentigo maligna has been documented in one case.[1] The relatively short follow-up information (mean 2.7 years) has shown no evidence of recurrence or metastasis.[2] A recently reported 'metastatic' case purportedly showing micrometastasis to a sentinel lymph node has an appearance much more characteristic of a capsular nevus.[6,7]

Histologic features

Although a precursor lesion or origin from the epidermis may be identifiable, the tumor may present as an upper dermal nodule independent of any epidermal connection (Fig. 26.124).[2] A case limited to the epidermis has also been described.[3] It consists of a sharply delineated, lobular tumor composed of intimately admixed malignant squamous epithelium and a usually less prominent population of malignant melanocytes (Figs 26.125 and

26.126).[2] Matrical differentiation has also been described.[5] The two populations are distinctive morphologically, but the distinction is highlighted by S100 protein or other melanocytic markers and cytokeratin immunohistochemistry (Fig. 26.127).[2]

Basomelanocytic tumor

Clinical features

Basomelanocytic tumor is a very rare biphasic neoplasm similar, or perhaps related, to the dermal squamomelanocytic tumor described above.[1]

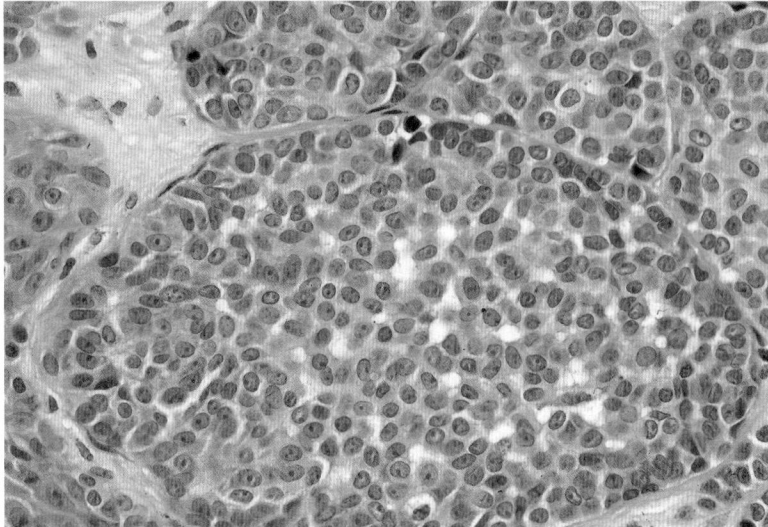

Fig. 26.122
Childhood melanoma: the presence of expansile nodules is an important diagnostic clue. By courtesy of M. Little, MD, University College Hospital, Galway, Ireland.

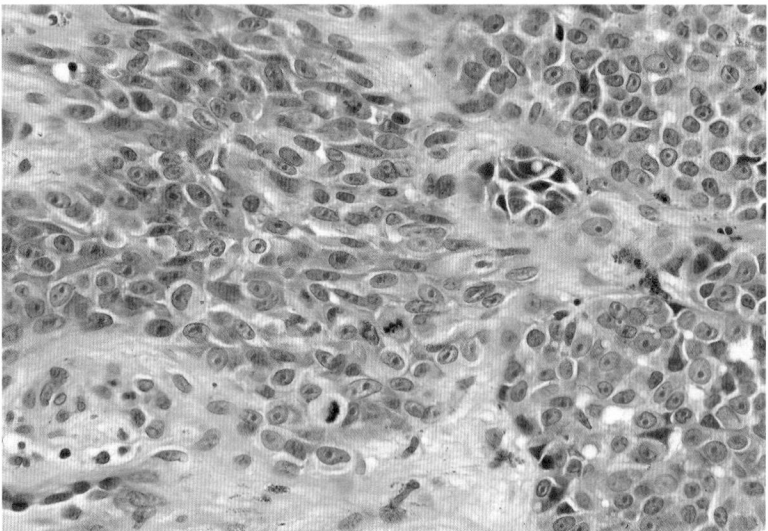

Fig. 26.123
Childhood melanoma: multiple dermal mitoses are present in this field. By courtesy of M. Little, MD, University College Hospital, Galway, Ireland.

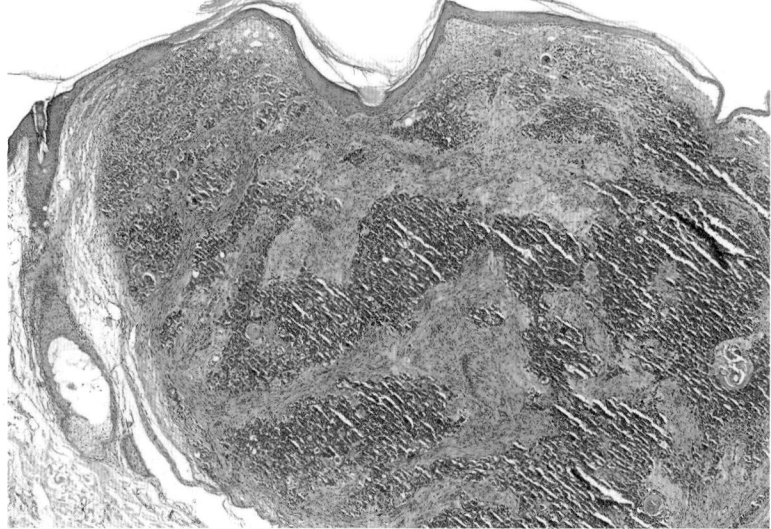

Fig. 26.124
Dermal squamomelanocytic tumor: low-power view of a facial tumor. By courtesy of S. Poole, MD, Beth Israel Deaconess Medical Center, Boston, USA.

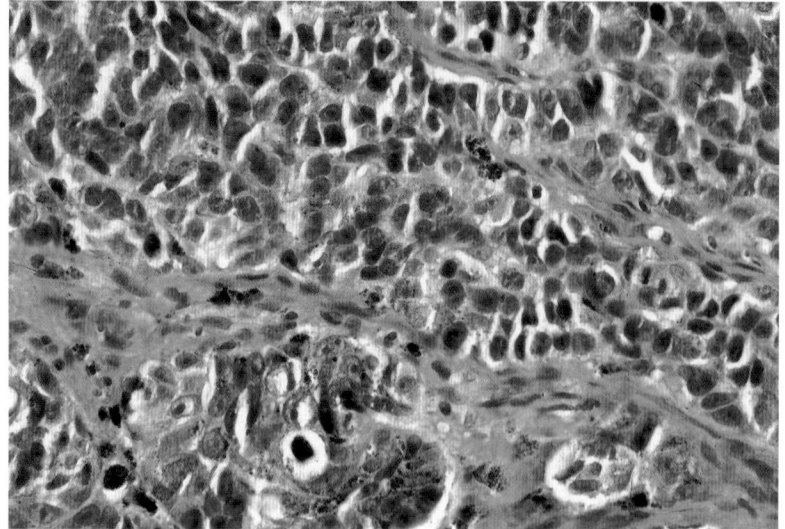

Fig. 26.125
Dermal squamoproliferative tumor: in this field, the tumor is composed of variably pigmented cells with irregular hyperchromatic nuclei. By courtesy of S. Poole, MD, Beth Israel Deaconess Medical Center, Boston, USA.

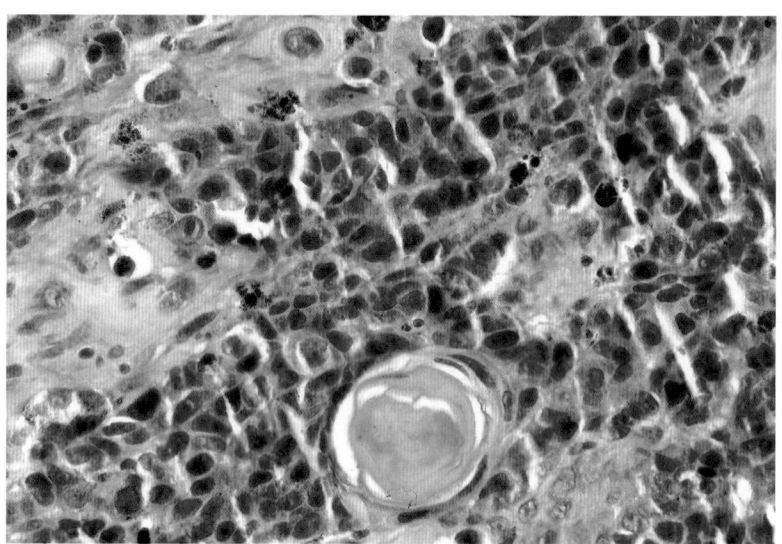

Fig. 26.126
Dermal squamoproliferative tumor: focal squamous differentiation is evident. By courtesy of S. Poole, MD, Beth Israel Deaconess Medical Center, Boston, USA.

However, basomelanocytic tumor is a combination of basaloid carcinoma and melanoma.[2-4] As would be expected, the melanocytic component of the tumor appears to be the more aggressive component and has been reported to metastasize with fatal outcome.[3]

Histologic features

In this combined tumor, the basaloid component in the few described cases can take the appearance of a basaloid squamous cell carcinoma or be more basal cell carcinoma-like (*Fig. 26.128*). Unlike so-called collision tumors, biphasic tumors show an intimate association of the epithelial and melanocytic components. An intraepidermal component is not always present. Cases of melanoma metastatic to a basal cell carcinoma or colonization by melanoma in situ have been described as mimics of basomelanocytic tumor.[5,6]

The melanoma component stains with traditional melanocytic markers such as S100 protein, MART-1, and HMB-45 (*Fig. 26.129*). Cytokeratins, including AE1/AE3, mark the basaloid component, and Ber-EP4 can also be positive (*Fig. 26.130*).[3,4] Characteristic copy number alterations can be seen in the melanoma component.[1]

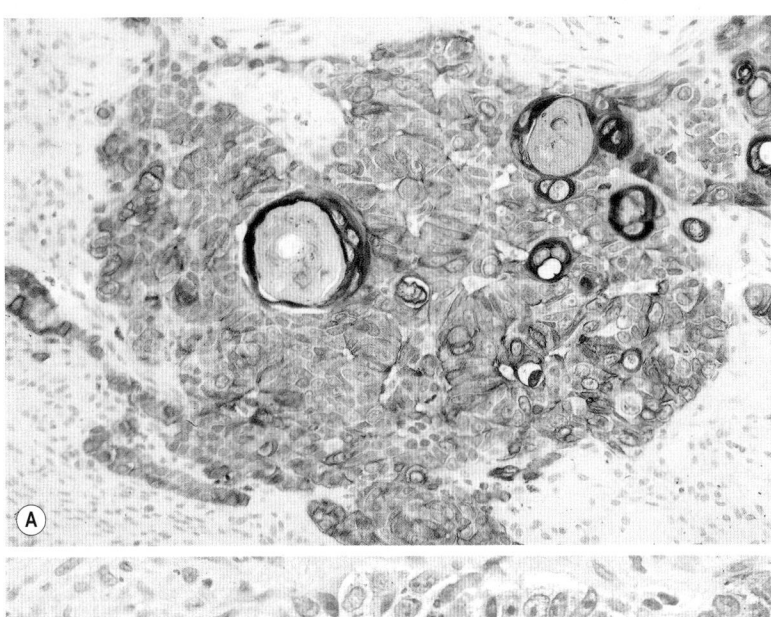

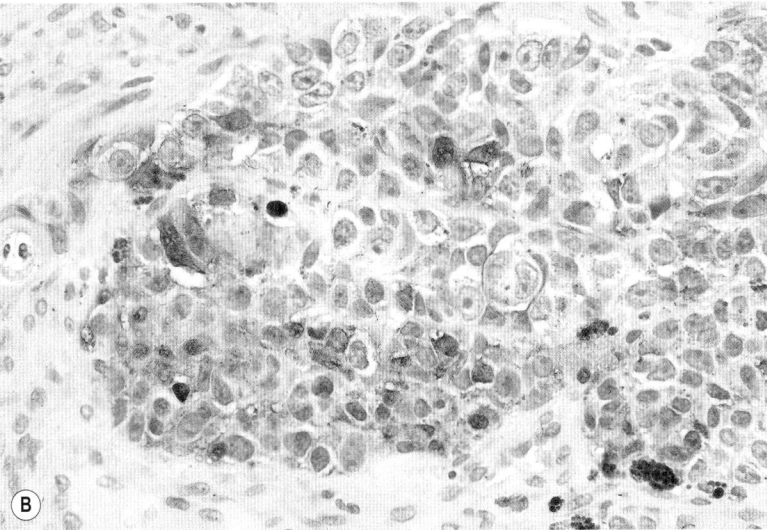

Fig. 26.127
Dermal squamoproliferative tumor: (**A**) the squamous component is highlighted with keratin immunohistochemistry; (**B**) S100 protein. By courtesy of S. Poole, MD, Beth Israel Deaconess Medical Center, Boston, USA.

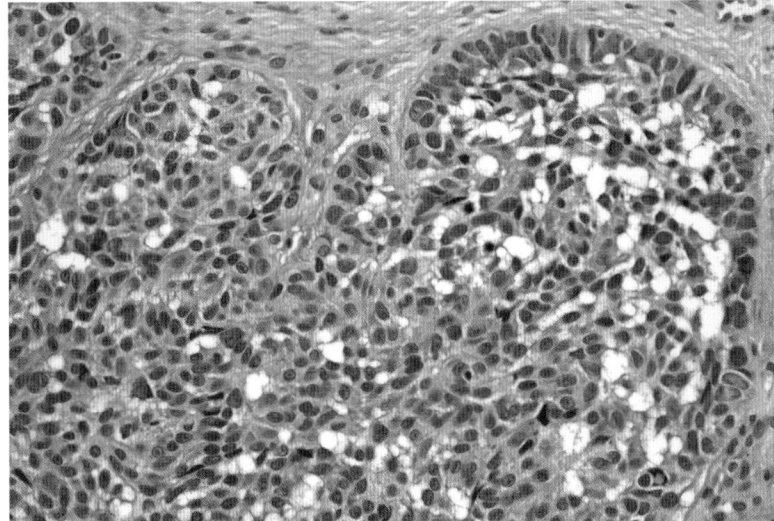

Fig. 26.128
Basomelanocytic tumor: surrounding undifferentiated tumor cells is a striking palisade of basophilic cells typical of basal cell carcinoma. By courtesy of L. Erickson, MD, Mayo Clinic, Rochester, Minnesota.

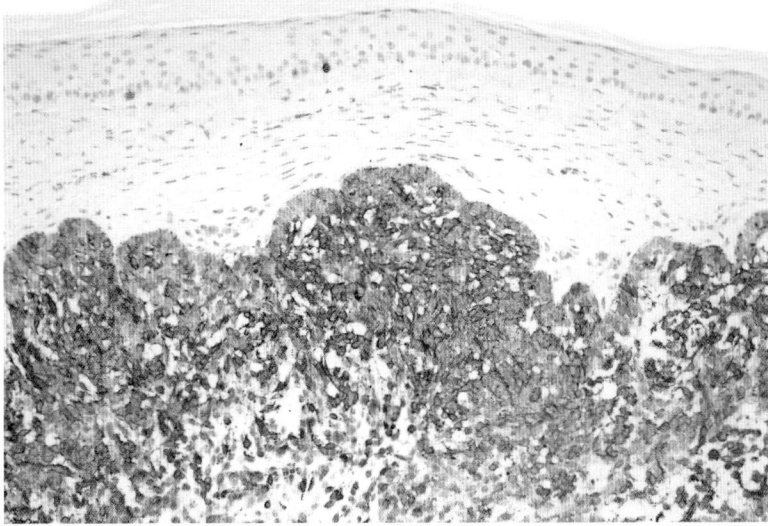

Fig. 26.129
Basomelanocytic tumor: the inner cells express HMB-45. Mart-1 was also positive. By courtesy of L. Erickson, MD, Mayo Clinic, Rochester, Minnesota.

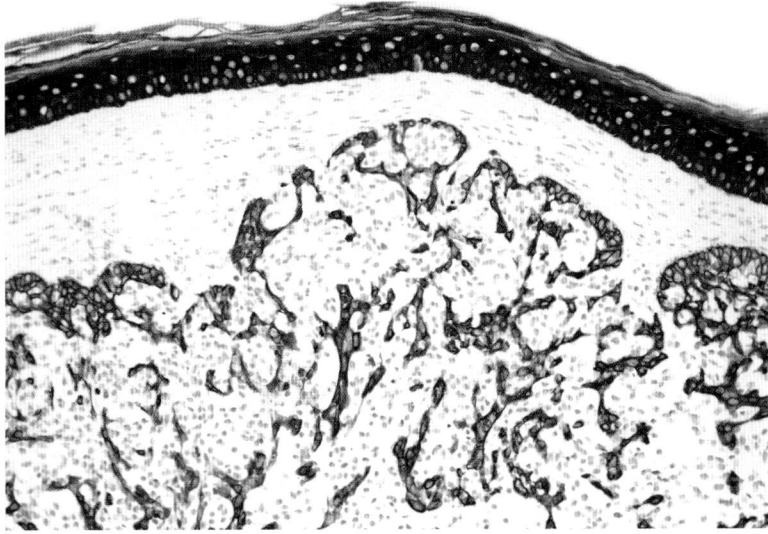

Fig. 26.130
Basomelanocytic tumor: the background population of basaloid cells expresses keratin. By courtesy of L. Erickson, MD, Mayo Clinic, Rochester, Minnesota.

Lentiginous melanoma

Clinical features

This type of melanoma should be distinguished from acral lentiginous melanoma. These tumors have a propensity for the shoulders and upper back in elderly patients while the lower legs, particularly in younger female patients, may also be affected.[1-6] Similar to lentigo maligna, this form of melanoma may be associated with an extended in situ phase of many years, and in an important number of cases there is a precursor lesion. The latter have been described as atypical lentiginous melanocytic nevus and dysplastic atypical nevus of the elderly with some questioning whether these lesions are truly malignant.[7-9] Additional study is required to further define and characterize this seemingly distinct lesion.

Histologic features

Lentiginous melanoma, as the name implies, consists of a primarily single cell array of melanocytes achieving confluence at least focally with limited associated junctional nests (*Figs 26.131–26.133*). Pagetoid intraepidermal ascent can be noted but it tends to be very focal when present. Epidermal atrophy is not present and there is preservation of normal rete architecture

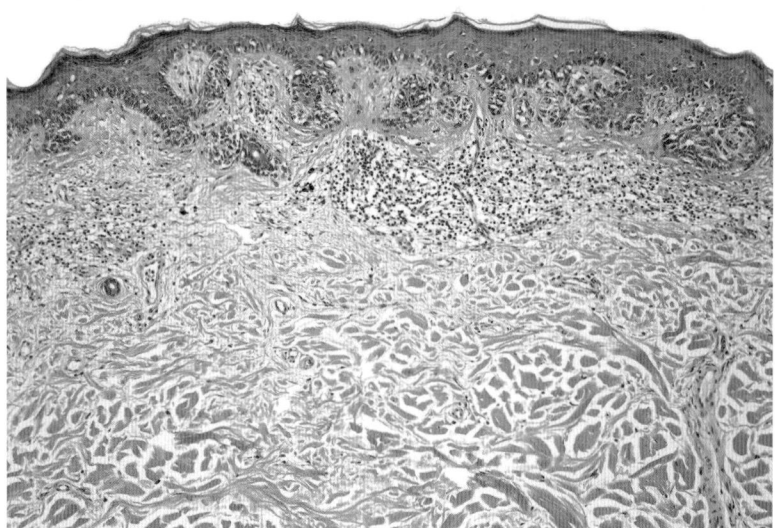

Fig. 26.131
Lentiginous melanoma: in this field, there is a lentiginous and focally nested atypical melanocytic proliferation. Note the upper dermal lymphocytic infiltrate.

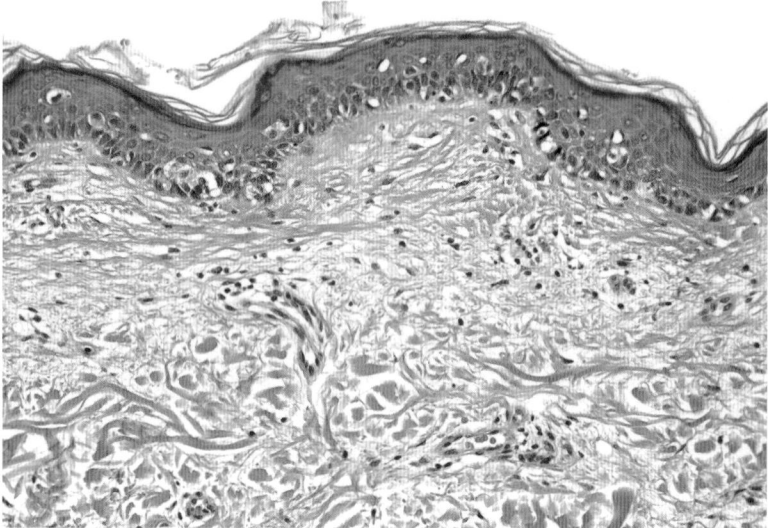

Fig. 26.132
Lentiginous melanoma: the tumor cells are predominantly basally located. There is no evidence of solar elastosis.

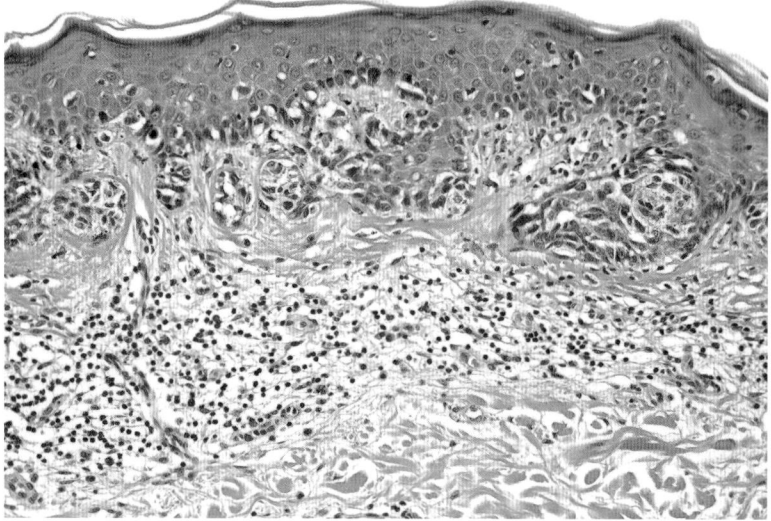

Fig. 26.133
Lentiginous melanoma: junctional nests showing moderate to severe cytological atypia are evident.

at the dermal–epidermal junction. Cytological atypia varies and may not be prominent, and solar elastosis is not a feature. These features help separate this entity from other forms of lentiginous melanoma. Melanocytic stains may be helpful to better visualize the increased density of atypical melanocytes. These lesions may be more readily recognized in larger excision specimens as the features may be difficult to discern in smaller biopsies.[2] As stated before, in many lesions there is evidence of a lentiginous nevus with variable atypia, suggesting a precursor lesion. This is the reason the diagnosis can be missed in small biopsies.

Primary dermal melanoma

Clinical features

The described cases of this apparently rare presentation of melanoma show a dermal nodule lacking an identifiable in situ component or association with a pre-existing nevus.[1-4] Published series indicate that this presentation of melanoma represents less than 1% of all melanomas.[5-7] A wide anatomic distribution is reported, but the head and neck region and extremities are the most common sites. In one study, in a cohort of 13 patients, the average Breslow depth was 9.6 mm with 92% survival at a mean of about 4 years.[8,9] Subsequent studies have documented a somewhat less impressive but still relatively favorable 88% 5-year survival in a cohort of nine cases with a median Breslow thickness of 3.4 mm.[6] A series of 49 cases with mean Breslow depth of 3.0 mm and mean mitotic rate of 4.3 per mm^2 is also reported.[7] A caveat of this latter series is that 14 cases showed association with a pre-existing intradermal nevus and average follow-up was only 26 months. Nineteen percent of patients developed locoregional recurrence and 6% showed distant metastases; only one patient died of disease. Traditional AJCC parameters did not correlate with outcome. These studies suggest that this tumor behaves much less aggressively than comparable traditional nodular melanoma. Others examining a larger series of 101 cases defined as a solitary dermal melanoma (as distinct from melanoma of unknown primary which usually presents as an isolated lymph node metastasis) within larger well-characterized cohort of 12,817 patients found no difference in outcome compared to stage-matched traditional melanomas.[5] Other studies show various results, but most include melanoma of unknown primary which could skew the results.[10-14] Indeed, in all of these papers, it is unclear whether the authors are describing the same tumor. Much more study is needed to refine our definitions and understanding of this possible entity and delineate its natural history. At the present time, this presentation is probably best assessed and reported as a standard melanoma with risk proportional to the assessed Breslow depth, though a note suggesting that such cases have been described to have more indolent behavior would certainly be appropriate.

Histologic features

The lesion is characterized by a nodular deposit of melanoma composed of epithelioid to spindled cells in the dermis and/or subcutis. Spitzoid and blue nevus-like features have been noted in some cases, but many have the appearance of traditional melanoma.[7] Some cases have conspicuous mitoses, but overall a Ki-67 index may be lower than that seen in comparable cases of nodular melanoma or metastatic melanoma.[8] It would be extremely important to distinguish these cases from metastatic melanoma or melanoma of unknown primary, both of which have vastly different staging implications.[15] This can be challenging and indeed such cases have now been described to have BRAF and NF1 mutations as well as P16/CDKN2A loss and other copy number aberrations similar to traditional cutaneous melanoma.[7,16] Explanations for this entity include an origin in association with follicular melanocytes and complete regression of a prior intraepidermal component. More recently, de la Fouchadiere and colleagues have described five cases of non-pigmented dermal melanoma each with a CRTC1-TRIM11 fusion that are dermal based and nodular in outline.[17] Cytology ranges from epithelioid to spindled sometimes with scattered multinucleate cells. In some ways the appearance is similar to that of clear cell sarcoma which can also sometimes be confined to the dermis.[18] Behavior is low grade. This lesion would appear to fall within the spectrum of primary dermal melanoma though where it falls in the end in the spectrum between melanoma and dermal clear cell sarcoma remains to be seen.

Molecular classification of melanoma

Over the last decade significant molecular data have shed new light on differences between melanoma subtypes. This continues to inform an emerging classification, which integrates epidemiology, clinical and histopathological features with patterns of somatic mutations and mutational mechanisms. This final portion of the melanoma chapter focuses on conceptual information regarding the molecular classification of melanoma and its correlation to UV damage, as well as the progression from melanoma in situ to invasive and metastatic melanoma. Molecular data continue to inform our traditional classification schemes, validating them in some instances and expanding them in others. While traditional classification categories of melanoma are still employed, the molecular characterization of melanocytic neoplasia continues to progress and will have to be continually integrated with the traditional features to establish a classification system that correctly describes distinctive phenotypes but is firmly based in the underlying mechanistic alterations that are in large part caused by genetic alterations.

Melanoma epidemiology

Melanomas are most common in Caucasians, where they typically arise on sun-exposed skin. In patients under the age of 50, the highest density is found on the trunk and extremities. In patients older than 50, the highest density of melanomas is found on the head and neck. The high frequency of melanoma and non-melanoma skin cancers in Caucasians is considered to be the result of light skin pigmentation with the consequence of increased UV-induced mutagenesis. Some aspects of skin color variation are likely due to selective advantage during human evolution that optimizes benefits from solar radiation (e.g., lighter skin pigmentation to enhance vitamin D synthesis) in less sunny climates. Association studies have revealed common polymorphisms in pigmentation genes are genetic factors controlling skin color, tanning ability, and freckling, with some variants increasing melanoma risk. These pigmentation genes include the melanocortin receptor one (MC1R), its antagonist the agouti signaling protein (ASIP), tyrosinase (TYR), tyrosinase-related protein (TYPR), the P-gene mutated in oculocutaneous albinism type II (OCA2), ion exchange proteins of the solute carrier family SLC24A5, SLC24A4, and SLC45A2 (MATP), and the interferon regulatory factor IRF4 or MUM1.[1]

Decreased pigmentation in Caucasian skin leads to decreased protection from UV radiation and results in increased somatic mutations in skin cells, including melanocytes. However, increased melanoma susceptibility in Caucasians may not be entirely attributed to differences in skin pigmentation, because albinos of African descent do not share the increased incidence of melanomas, while they do suffer more frequently from cutaneous squamous cell carcinoma.[2] Melanin, which is present in Caucasian skin and absent in albinos who lack functional tyrosinase, appears to have both protective and deleterious effects for DNA. Mutations from UV radiation continue to accumulate in the skin for hours after removal from UV light.[3] These 'dark' mutations do not occur in albino mice lacking melanin. In mice with intact melanin production, these mutations were twice as frequent in those with increased pheomelanin (due to MC1R mutation) versus those with high eumelanin, implicating melanin, particularly pheomelanin, as a critical factor in these 'dark' mutations. Further evidence is found in transgenic mouse models in which melanoma development after UVA radiation only occurs in black mice with intact melanin production and not in albino mice.[4]

Melanoma and UV radiation

The establishment of a causal link between UV radiation and melanoma formation requires several considerations. UV radiation causes a wide spectrum of mutations. Among these UV signature mutations, pyrimidine dimers resulting in C>T or CC>TT transitions are the most common and are due to a direct photochemical reaction with the DNA. However, mutations in common melanoma oncogenes such as BRAF and NRAS typically do not

indicate such a signature.[5,6] For example, the most common mutation at BRAF codon 600 is a T to A transition and thus does not match the classical UV signature.[7] The fact that these mutations lack a UV signature does not exclude a role for UV radiation in their formation, as they can form as the result of indirect consequences of UV radiation such as the formation of reactive oxygen species. Furthermore, activating an oncogene requires mutations to change very specific amino acid sequences in the protein, whereas abrogating a tumor suppressor protein's function can occur through numerous possible mutations (missense, nonsense, and frameshift mutations). Therefore, mutations that activate oncogenes tend to cluster in a few critical hotspots, whereas mutations in tumor suppressor genes are more widespread and enriched for damaging mutations that truncate or scramble the DNA sequence. The need for specific growth promoting mutations in oncogenes such as BRAF and NRAS therefore significantly skews the mutations observed in these genes. The causative role for UV radiation in mutagenesis of melanomas on sun-exposed skin is clearly demonstrated by the high burden of UV signature mutations in the tens to hundreds of thousand mutations found in the genomes of cutaneous melanomas and by the observation that mutations in critical genes such as the TERT promoter, CDKN2A, P53, and PTEN are indeed enriched for UV signature mutations.[8,9]

However, not all melanoma subtypes harbor genomic damage attributable to UV radiation. Melanomas arising on the palms and soles, nail beds, and mucosal sites, as well as uveal melanoma, typically lack the high mutation burden with a UV signature found in cutaneous melanomas. This indicates that while UV radiation plays a critical role in the pathogenesis of some melanoma subtypes, it does not in others. This could also explain why acral and mucosal melanomas affect all world populations independent of skin complexion.[10]

Melanoma is composed of distinct subtypes

There is considerable variation in the clinical and histopathological presentation of melanomas that partially depends on the anatomic site in which the tumor arises and how much ultraviolet radiation exposure has occurred. As outlined previously in this chapter, these differences formed the traditional 'histogenetic' classification of melanoma as initially proposed in the Sydney Classification.[11] There has been considerable controversy on the justification of this classification and opponents have long posited that melanoma is a single disease, with the variation in clinical and pathological features representing secondary phenomena. This belief stemmed both from the lack of difference with regards to prognosis of advanced disease and the inability in the past to predict a different response to therapy between subtypes.[12] In addition, there was significant overlap in the defining phenotypic features that hindered unequivocal classification of a considerable portion of primary tumors.[13]

Considerable progress has now been made in the identification of genetic alterations in melanoma and has provided strong support for the concept of biologically distinct melanoma types. This is consistent with work leading to the discovery and validation of clinically relevant genetic subtypes that have emerged in other malignancies such as lung and colon cancer. This is a decisive trend in oncology that is critical for the implementation of precision cancer medicine. Mutations in specific genes, mutational signatures, and other genetic alterations such as genome-wide chromosomal aberrations correlate with specific clinical and histopathological features of melanoma, providing genetic support for the original concept that melanomas fall into different categories of diseases. New genetic data offer an opportunity to integrate causal genetic alterations with clinical or histopathological disease attributes, as well as predisposing and environmental factors. The emerging melanoma subtypes that integrate clinicopathological features overlap considerably with the original 'histogenetic' melanoma types, but offer a more nuanced picture of the categories. This continuity is satisfying and underscores the enduring importance of thoughtful clinicopathological characterization as a basis for initial classification. The extent of UV radiation damage can serve as an initial branch point in the classification of melanoma: melanomas found in skin with high cumulative sun damage (high-CSD), low cumulative sun damage (low-CSD), and melanomas on sites with negligible (e.g., acral) or no sun exposure (e.g., mucosal).

Melanoma on sun-exposed skin

Epidemiological data alone suggest differences between melanomas from sun-exposed skin and melanomas on acral or mucosal sites, the latter of which do not show variation in incidence between races. Additionally, the anatomic site of origin and the cumulative dose of UV radiation are two intricately linked features that are strongly associated with distinctive clinical and histopathological presentations of melanoma. Melanomas on the head and neck tend to occur in older individuals with a peak incidence of about 72 years of age.[14] The skin surrounding these melanomas typically shows signs of chronic sun damage, as evidenced by pronounced solar elastosis and other signs of chronic sun-induced damage such as solar lentigines and actinic keratoses.[15] Total cumulative UV dose appears to represent a major risk factor for these melanomas. The traditional lentigo maligna variant of melanoma falls into the high-CSD category.

By contrast, melanomas involving the trunk arise earlier in life, with a peak incidence at around age 54, and signs of chronic sun damage (severe solar elastosis) are typically absent.[14] The drop in incidence of melanomas on the trunk after age 54 suggests that it is not the cumulative dose of UV radiation but timing of UV exposure that plays a decisive role in these melanomas, with a particular window of vulnerability present earlier in life. Epidemiological studies demonstrate that exposure to UV irradiation in childhood plays an important role in the pathogenesis of melanoma in general.[16] Patients with melanomas on the trunk, but not with melanomas on chronically sun-exposed sites such as the face, have more melanocytic nevi, suggesting a common pathogenesis between low-CSD melanomas and nevi.[17] This is supported by the fact that low-CSD melanomas more frequently have adjacent precursor nevi than CSD melanomas and that nevi and low-CSD melanomas share a high frequency of BRAF V600E mutations. A functional scale for assessing sun damage has been proposed to grade the degree of solar elastosis involving the dermis.[18,19] Recent studies have demonstrated how melanomas progress from such nevi through the acquisition of additional UV-associated mutations.[20] The fact that most nevi arise during childhood and adolescence furthers highlights the possibility of a window of vulnerability towards UV radiation early in life for these types of melanocytic neoplasms.[21] Genetic data also support the concept of distinct melanoma types based on sun-exposure as discussed below.[22]

Melanoma with low cumulative sun damage (low-CSD)

Low-CSD melanomas occur most frequently in patients under 50 on the trunk or extremities and show a low to moderate degree of solar elastosis histopathologically. $BRAF^{V600E}$ mutations are very common (approximately 70%) in low-CSD melanomas, representing the main driver mutation, followed by NRAS mutations (approximately 20%).[19,23] BRAF mutant melanomas frequently exhibit specific histomorphological features such as increased upward scatter of intraepidermal melanocytes (pagetoid scatter), a predominance of nests over single cells, thickening of the involved epidermis, a sharper demarcation toward the adjacent uninvolved epidermis, and constituent tumor cells that are larger, rounder, and more heavily pigmented (Fig. 26.134).[24] Simple combinations of these independently associated features predicted BRAF mutation status with 90% accuracy in one study.[24] These histomorphological criteria also performed better in predicting mutation status than the traditional WHO melanoma classification, indicating the potential for developing improved classification schemes that define more biologically homogeneous subsets. This is increasingly relevant with the increased use of targeted therapies to specific genetic alterations including BRAF inhibitors[25] and KIT inhibitors.[26-28]

The shared high incidence of $BRAF^{V600E}$ mutations in melanocytic nevi and low-CSD melanomas supports a common etiology with regard to UV radiation and timing of exposure. Approximately one-fourth to one-third of melanomas arise within histopathologically identifiable precursor nevi, with low-CSD melanomas representing the main melanoma type in which precursor nevi can be identified.[29] Frequently only melanoma in situ is present with the associated nevus, the latter of which remains identifiable in the underlying dermis. The melanoma in situ harbors the same initiating mutation as the precursor nevus (typically BRAF or NRAS), with additional genetic aberrations such as TERT promoter mutation or heterozygous CDKN2A

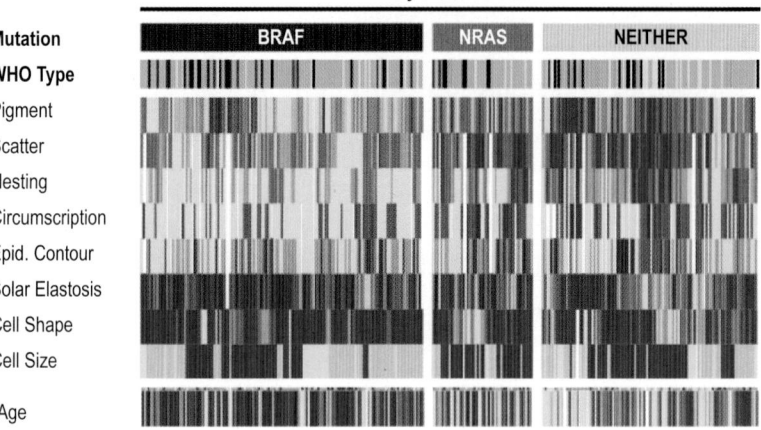

Fig. 26.134

Morphological and clinical features of 302 primary melanomas by mutation status: the heat map shows the features that are significantly associated with mutation status for three groups of melanomas: BRAF mutant, NRAS mutant, or neither mutation. The scores for the features in the following rows range from shades of blue (low score) to gray (intermediate scores) to yellow (high scores): pigmentation of neoplastic melanocytes, upward scatter of intraepidermal melanocytes, nesting of melanocytes, degree of solar elastosis, cell size, and patient age. For circumscription, yellow indicates an abrupt transition from involved to adjacent uninvolved skin, gray scores represent a continuous transition, and blue scores a discontinuous transition. Epidermal contour ranges from yellow (acanthotic) to blue (atrophic) of the epidermis involved by the melanoma. Cell shapes range from blue (round) to yellow (spindled). Samples are listed in columns and are ordered within each category using agglomerative hierarchical clustering. The color codes for WHO types are superficial spreading melanoma (SSM) green, lentigo maligna melanoma (LMM) yellow, nodular melanoma (NM) red, and acral lentiginous melanoma (ALM) orange. Unclassifiable samples are in black.

loss.[20] The latter mutations reflect the importance of replicative senescence and maintaining G1/S checkpoint control in preventing nevi from progressing to melanoma. UV signature mutation profiles implicate UV radiation as the driving factor in this transformation of nevi to melanoma.[20]

Progression from in situ to invasive melanoma involves additional genetic alterations required for unrestrained growth outside the confines of the epidermis. Ability to grow and survive in the dermis alone is not indicative of malignant transformation, as the cells of melanocytic nevi already have this property. Loss of cell cycle checkpoint regulation is critical in unleashing or increasing the proliferative capacity associated with invasive melanoma as evidenced by frequent homozygous loss of the CDKN2A gene encoding both p16 and p14ARF in the transition from in situ to invasive melanoma. Additional mutations in genes encoding critical tumor suppressor proteins such as TP53 and PTEN occur later in the progression to more advanced stage disease.[20] Additionally, invasive melanomas must evade antitumor immune surveillance through mechanisms such as induction of immune tolerance.

The vast majority of melanomas exhibit some degree of genomic instability in the form of chromosomal gains and losses. This instability seems to coincide with the transition from benign melanocytic nevi to melanoma in situ, as nevi tend to not have chromosomal copy number changes, whereas they can be detected in melanoma in situ.[20] The instability may be related to telomere shortening and end-to-end fusion of sister chromatids with eroded telomeres that result in dicentric chromosomes that can rupture during mitosis. The selective advantage of TERT promoter mutations early during melanoma progression suggests that replicative senescence becomes an early barrier to transformation. TERT promoter mutations only lead to marginal telomerase expression, which manages to preserve critically short telomeres but cannot fully suppress telomere fusions resulting in instability that generates DNA copy number changes.[30] This explains why the telomeres of melanomas with TERT promoter mutations remain short.[30,31]

While there are some similarities in the patterns of the chromosomal gains and losses across melanoma subtypes, significant differences exist with

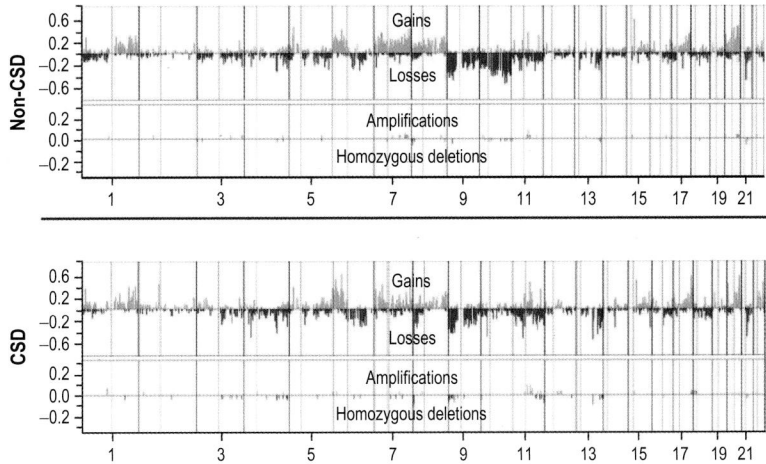

Fig. 26.135
Frequencies of DNA copy number changes in non-CSD and CSD melanomas: the upper histogram for each melanoma type shows the frequencies of gains (*green*) and losses (*red*), and the lower histogram shows amplifications (*green*) and homozygous deletions (*red*). The x axis represents the genomic position from chromosome 1 to 22. Vertical solid blue lines mark the boundaries between chromosomes, and the vertical dashed gray lines mark the position of the centromeres.

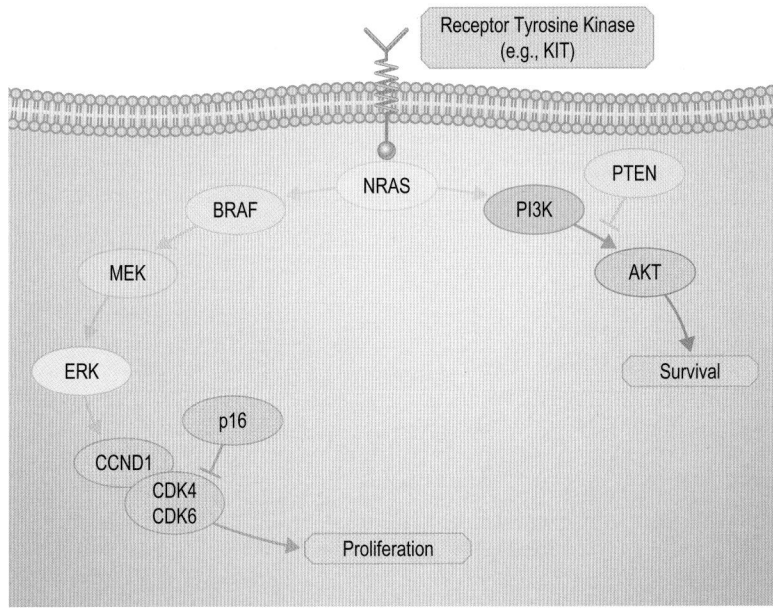

Fig. 26.136
Simplified schematic of pathways important in melanoma: downstream from certain receptor tyrosine kinases lies Ras which bifurcates to the BRAF/ERK and PI3K/AKT pathways leasing to proliferation and survival. It appears that activation of both of these pathways (and others) is required for melanoma development and these are grouped in a rational fashion. For instance, activating mutations in *KIT*, *NRAS*, and *BRAF* are mutually exclusive since they activate the same pathways and loss of PTEN is seen with *BRAF*, but not *NRAS* mutation, because *NRAS* activates the PI3K pathway while *BRAF* does not. These combinations will likely have therapeutic relevance as more specific inhibitors are developed.

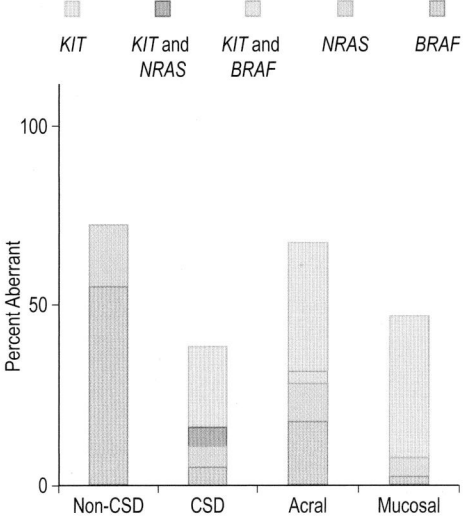

Fig. 26.137
Frequency distribution of genetic alterations in *BRAF*, *NRAS*, and *KIT* among four groups of melanoma: non-CSD, melanomas on skin without chronic sun-induced damage; CSD, melanomas on skin with chronic sun-induced as evidenced by the presence of marked solar elastosis; acral, melanomas on the soles, palms, or subungual sites; mucosal, melanomas on mucosal membranes. One CSD melanoma had a *KIT* and an *NRAS* mutation, and one acral melanoma had a *KIT* and a *BRAF* mutation.

By contrast, activating mutations in *NRAS* activate both the MAP kinase and the PI3 kinase pathway, therefore obviating the need for a loss of PTEN in tumors with *NRAS* mutations.[32] Point mutations in the catalytic subunit of PI3 kinase have also been found in a small minority of melanomas.[33]

Gains of chromosome 7 are more common in low-CSD melanomas.[19] *BRAF* resides at 7q34 and the copy number increase reflects duplication of the mutant *BRAF* allele, which provides a proliferative advantage.[34,35] Copy number increases of *CCND1* encoding cyclin D1 at chromosome 11q13 represent an additional distinguishing feature as they occur infrequently in low-CSD melanomas, while present in up to 50% of high-CSD melanoma.[19,36] These genetic changes demonstrate how both the major proliferative and survival pathways are activated during melanoma progression. This can be accomplished through different combinations of mutations and chromosomal aberrations such as activating mutations in upstream tyrosine kinase receptors such as *KIT* or *NRAS* which activate both the MAP kinase pathway and PI3K pathway, or through combinations of activating mutations in *BRAF* combined with loss of *PTEN* (*Fig. 26.136*).

Melanoma with high cumulative sun damage (high-CSD)

High-CSD melanomas typically occur in Caucasians over age 50 mostly on the head and neck and display marked solar elastosis histopathologically. In contrast to low-CSD melanomas, high-CSD melanomas typically have no associated precursor nevus, arising 'de novo' in the epidermis. These melanomas are often characterized by an extended in situ stage, in which the neoplasm can grow to the size of several centimeters over many years prior to becoming invasive. Genomic data on the in situ stage of high-CSD melanoma are limited. Approximately 20% of such in situ melanomas have *BRAF* mutations, although *BRAF^{non-V600E}* mutations (e.g., *BRAF^{V600K}*) are more frequent than *BRAF^{V600E}* mutations in this group.[37] In addition to the striking difference in *BRAF* mutations between high-CSD and low-CSD melanomas (15% vs 70%),[34,38] additional genetic differences have also been found. For instance, some studies report up to 30% of high-CSD melanomas harbor mutations or DNA copy number increases of *KIT*, whereas *KIT* mutations are rare in low-CSD melanomas (*Fig. 26.137*).[39] Differences in the mutation frequency of *NRAS* have been reported by some, but do not appear to be a consistent finding.[19,40]

Desmoplastic melanoma represents a specific variant of melanoma that occurs in chronically sun-damaged skin and has a high mutation burden that typically exceeds that of all other melanomas (median 62 mutations/Mb compared to approximately 15/Mb in low-CSD melanoma).[41] The mutational profile of desmoplastic melanoma has a strong UV radiation profile and is notable for the complete absence of *BRAF* and *NRAS* hotspot mutations and a high prevalence of inactivating *NF1* mutations, which can also be detected in the overlying in situ component.[41,42] In addition, there are recurrent mutations in the promoter of *NFKBIE*, which encodes an inhibitor of nuclear factor NF-κB signaling, and inactivating mutations in *TP53*, *CDKN2A*, *ARID1A*, *ARID2*, and *RB1*. *TERT* promoter mutations are also

respect to tumors based on the degree of UV exposure.[19] Gain of chromosome 6p and loss of 6q are common in both low-CSD and high-CSD melanomas, but chromosome 10 loss occurs in 40% of low-CSD melanomas and fewer than 10% of CSD melanomas (*Fig. 26.135*). The region commonly lost on chromosome 10 contains the tumor suppressor *PTEN*, which encodes a negative regulator of the PI3 kinase pathway and is considered to represent the major selective force for chromosome 10 loss. *BRAF* mutations only activate the MAP kinase pathway, which explains the advantage of concurrent *PTEN* loss to activate the PI3 kinase pathway (*Fig. 26.136*).[32]

Table 26.3
Genes implicated in melanoma development

Gene	Function	Associated with melanoma susceptibility
ACD/POT1/TERF2IP	Nuclear proteins that bind telomeres and prevent inappropriate recombination events	Yes
ARID1/ARID2	Chromatin remodeling	
BAP1	Deubiquitinase that binds to BRCA1 and is involved with chromatin dynamics	Yes
BRAF	Protein kinase in the MAP kinase pathway	
CDKN2A	Encodes p16, an inhibitor of cyclin-dependent kinases, and p14, an inhibitor of MDM2	Yes
CDK4	Cyclin-dependent kinase that phosphorylates Rb	Yes
CTNNB1	Encodes beta-catenin, an adherens junction protein that signals in the WNT pathway	
ERBB4	EGFR family of tyrosine kinase receptors involved in differentiation and proliferation	
GNAQ/GNA11	G-protein coupled receptor that activates phospholipase C-beta	
KIT	Tyrosine kinase receptor activating multiple pathways in cell survival and proliferation	
MC1R	Encodes the melanocortin 1 receptor that binds melanocyte stimulatory hormone	Yes
MGMT	DNA repair protein	Yes
MITF	Transcription factor in melanocyte development	Yes
NF1	Encodes neurofibromin that negatively regulates RAS signaling	
NRAS	Tyrosine kinase receptor that activates the MAP kinase and PI3K pathways	
POLE	DNA polymerase subunit involved in DNA repair	Yes
PTEN	Lipid phosphatase antagonist of PI3K pathway	Yes
RAC1	GTPase involved in cell growth	
SLC45A2	Transporter protein in melanin synthesis	Yes
TERT	Encodes telomerase which maintains telomere length; can be amplified or have promoter mutation	Yes
TP53	Encodes tumor suppressor p53	
XP genes	Xeroderma pigmentosum genes encode nucleotide excision repair proteins	Yes

common in desmoplastic melanomas.[41] Desmoplastic melanomas have fewer chromosomal copy number alterations than most other melanomas, though focal amplifications of oncogenes such as EGFR, CDK4, CCND1, MDM2, TERT, and MAP3K1 and focal deletions in tumor suppressor genes such as CDKN2A occur.[41]

Numerous other recurrent genetic alterations have been discovered in melanomas on sun-exposed skin including amplifications or mutation of MITF and activating mutations in CTNNB1, encoding β-catenin. MITF is a basic helix-loop-helix (hHLH)-leucine zipper protein that plays a role in the development of melanocytes.[43] β-catenin is a critical signaling component of the WNT pathway where it acts as an adherens junction protein that can also function as a transcription factor and is mutated in a small subset of melanomas.[44,45] It is also increasingly clear that telomere-related proteins are critical factors in melanoma development. Germline mutations in components of the telomere shelterin complex (e.g., POT1, ACD, TERF2IP), which is responsible for capping telomere ends and preventing recombination events, have been linked with familial melanoma.[46] Mutations in the promoter of TERT, a gene encoding the protein component of telomerase, have also been described in familial melanoma and in 35% to 70% of sporadic melanomas.[47,48] TERT promoter mutations are the most common mutations in melanoma and have a UV signature C>T pattern. The predisposing mutations in TERT and other telomere-related factors are thought to contribute to increasing melanoma risk by increasing telomere length and extending the replicative lifespan of neoplastic cells, thereby increasing the likelihood of acquiring the additional mutations required for transformation.[49] Numerous additional genes have been implicated in melanoma, many of which are listed in Table 26.3.

Melanomas on UV-protected sites
Acral and mucosal melanoma
The volar surfaces of the hands and feet are minimally exposed to UV radiation, and glabrous skin has a thicker epidermis with a very thick stratum corneum providing additional UV protection. The nail matrix is protected by the proximal nail fold and the nail plate. With the exception of the lips and the bulbar conjunctiva, mucosal sites in which melanoma arise are not exposed to sunlight. Genomic analyses with CGH and DNA sequencing in melanomas from these UV-protected sites show a high degree of genomic instability reflected by frequent chromosomal aberrations, with focused gene amplifications in particular and a low mutation burden (Fig. 26.138).[19,50–53] The mucosal example in Fig. 26.138 in particular shows copy number changes affecting virtually every chromosome. Although mucosal melanomas are typically detected with considerable latency and therefore tend to be thicker than the primaries of the other melanoma categories, this high degree of genomic instability can already be demonstrated in thinner lesions. In other cancers, gene amplifications usually arise late during progression and often are a sign of adverse prognosis.[54] By contrast, in acral melanoma these amplifications arise very early during progression and can already be detected at the in situ stage.[50]

Gene amplifications typically arise through repeated cycles of double-stranded DNA breaks and subsequent end-to-end fusions of chromatids and thus indicate a loss of control over genomic integrity. The cause of this loss of control and subsequent genetic instability is currently unclear since TP53 and other known instability-inducing mutations are uncommon in these melanomas. While it is evident that UV radiation does not play a significant role in these melanomas, it is currently unresolved whether or not there are specific carcinogens involved in the pathogenesis of acral and mucosal melanomas or whether they arise as a consequence of stochastic alterations without external influence. The marked differences in the degree of genomic instability and mutation burden between melanomas on sun-protected sites and those on sun-exposed skin indicates that the types of genetic insults are fundamentally different between these melanoma subtypes. In sun-exposed melanomas UV photoproducts and oxidative damage are the predominating drivers of tumorigenesis, whereas double-stranded DNA breaks as part of breakage-fusion-bridge cycles and/or other yet to be

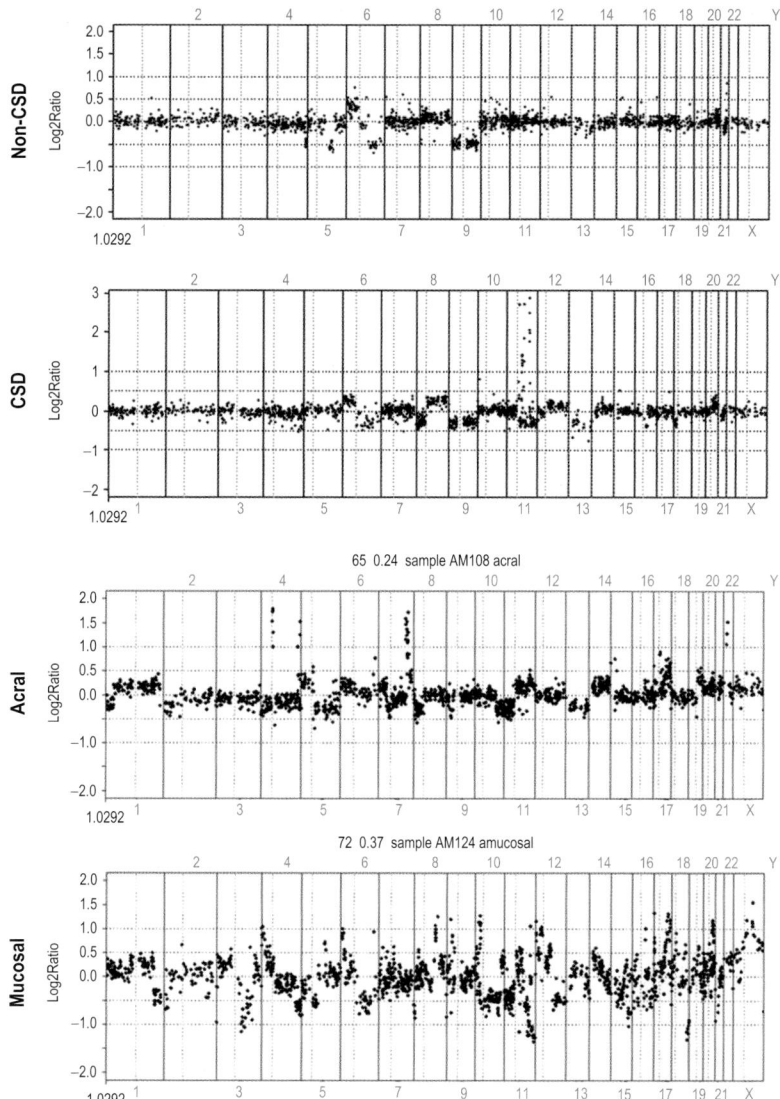

Fig. 26.138

Differences in the degree of genomic instability among melanoma types: representative examples of array CGH profiles of non-CSD, CSD, acral, and mucosal melanoma. The y axis represents the copy number for each array element (average value of a triplicate measurement) expressed as the $\log_2$ of the ratio of the tumor to reference fluorescence intensities. Values between +0.25 and −0.25 would be considered normal; values above that range are gains and below that range are losses. Values above 0.9 would be considered amplifications. In practice, a more complex assessment that takes into account the signal-to-noise ratio for each individual case is used.[33] The x axis represents the genomic position from chromosome 1p to 22.

discovered mechanism(s) appear critical for acral and mucosal melanoma formation.

This chromosomal instability in acral and mucosal melanoma occurs early in disease progression and has even been detected in histopathologically normal appearing melanocytes around acral melanoma in situ, so-called field cells or field effect (*Fig. 26.139*).[55] Field cells harbor some, but not all of the gene amplifications found in the adjacent melanoma, indicating that they are precursors of the histopathologically manifest form of melanoma in situ (*Fig. 26.140*). These cells represent clonal expansions of melanocytes with severe genetic alterations stemming from loss of control over maintenance of genomic integrity. Such genetic changes are qualitatively different from point mutations in oncogenes such as *BRAF*, as they indicate loss of protective factors that preserve genomic integrity. Field cells are therefore best interpreted as an early form or precursor of melanoma in situ. These fields of neoplastic melanocytes can be extensive, present up to >1 cm beyond the histopathologically detectable in situ portion, and the size of the field is completely independent of tumor thickness, further demonstrating

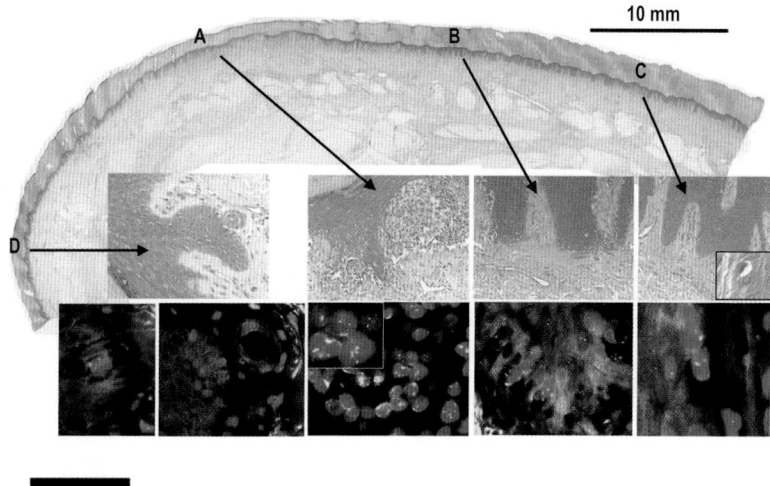

Cyclin D1
hTERT

Fig. 26.139

Field cells in acral melanoma: the top panel shows an acral melanoma with close-ups of four particular areas underneath. Area A shows superficially invasive melanoma that by FISH shows amplification of CCND1 (cyclin D1) and TERT telomerase reverse transcriptase (clusters of red and green signals in blue stained nuclei, respectively). Area B shows melanoma in situ with amplification of CCND1 and normal copy number of hTERT. Areas C and D show histopathologically uninvolved epidermis which by FISH harbors single basal melanocytes with amplification of CCND1 (clusters of red signals within blue stained nuclei). In the second FISH panel for area D a melanocyte with CCND1 amplification is situated in an eccrine duct.

that they reflect an early progression phase of disease.[55] Once their clinical relevance has been defined, the determination of field effect may offer a more objective guidance for the size of surgical margins for removal of primary melanomas than the current empirically derived recommendations.

Although acral and mucosal melanomas share a high incidence of chromosomal aberrations, including frequent gene amplifications, the genomic regions affected by these copy number alterations differ significantly between the two.[19] The most commonly amplified site in acral melanomas is the *CCND1* locus encoding cyclin D1 on chromosome 11q13. Another commonly amplified site includes the *TERT* telomerase locus on chromosome 5p15. However, while approximately 50% of acral melanomas amplify *CCND1*, mucosal melanomas typically do not. Instead, a subset of mucosal melanomas amplifies cyclin dependent kinase 4 (*CDK4*) on chromosome 12q14, encoding the binding partner of cyclin D1.[19] CDK4 is normally inhibited by p16 function, which functions as the gatekeeper of the G1/S transition point. In mucosal melanomas, the amplification of *CDK4* is mutually exclusive with deletions at the p16 locus, indicating that these genomic aberrations may be functionally equivalent. Mucosal melanomas also have recurrent mutations in *SF3B1*, a gene commonly mutated in uveal melanoma, which is typically not found in acral melanoma.[56]

In contrast to the high number of chromosomal copy number changes and amplifications in acral and mucosal melanomas, their mutational burden is much lower than sun exposed melanomas. Many of the mutations show a pattern of mutagenesis seen with aging in which there is spontaneous deamination of 5-methylcytosine at CpG dinucleotides.[31] UV signature mutations are absent for the most part. Most genetic studies of acral and mucosal melanoma focus on invasive melanoma, with very little published on the in situ stage. *BRAF*^{V600E} mutation in acral melanoma in situ has been reported,[57] but the incidence of *BRAF* mutation in acral melanoma (approximately 15–20%) is significantly lower than in low-CSD melanomas (approximately 70%) and even lower in mucosal melanoma (approximately 5%), suggesting *BRAF* mutation initiates a comparatively small percentage of these melanomas.[34,58–63] *NRAS* mutation and *KIT* mutation or amplification are more frequently found in acral and mucosal melanoma.[58,64,65] These two mutations activate the MAP kinase pathway and drive proliferation, so it is logical to assume they occur in the early proliferative phase of

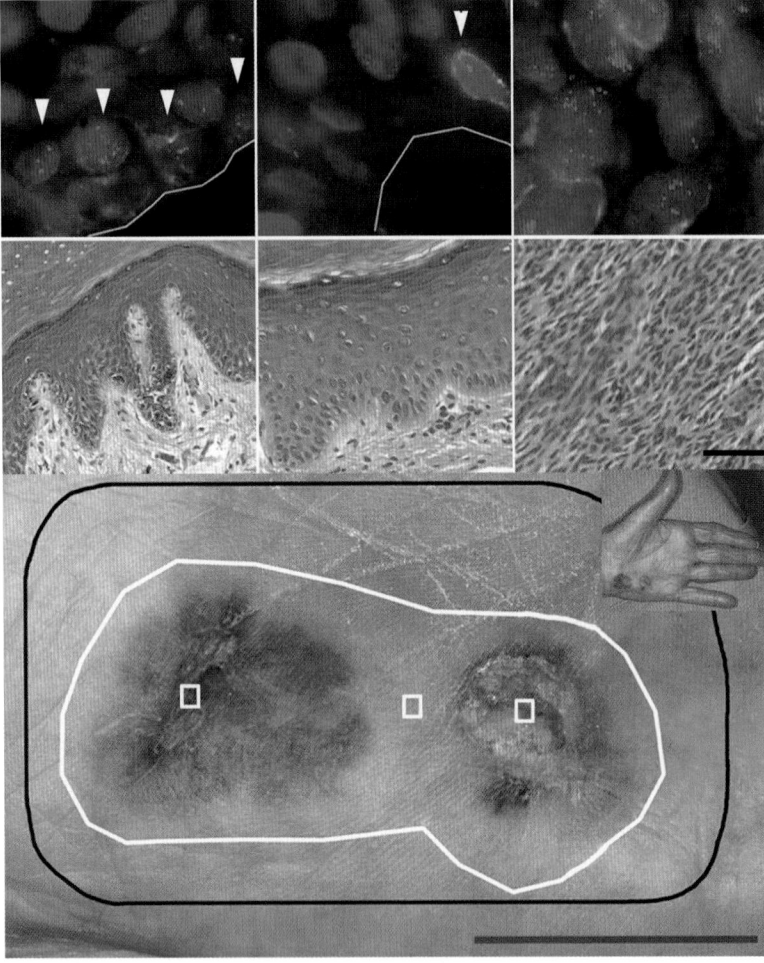

Fig. 26.140
Field cells in acral melanoma: bottom panel: clinical picture with (1) melanoma in situ; (2) clinically, dermoscopically, and microscopically normal skin; (3) invasive melanoma of 3.0-mm thickness. Black line, surgical margin; white line, field cell margin identified by amplification of 11q13. Middle and upper panels, respectively: H&E and FISH for areas 1–3. FISH images represent one focal plane, so not all signals are visible. A green immunofluorescent labeled Melan-A antibody was used to aid in identifying basal melanocytes. Cells with amplification of 11q13 are highlighted by arrowheads for areas 1 and 2 (upper panels).

melanoma in situ on acral and mucosal sites. Future studies are necessary to confirm this supposition. *TERT* promoter mutations are less common in acral melanoma (approximately 10%),[58] but *TERT* gene amplification is frequently seen and has been documented in acral melanoma in situ.[66]

While mutations in the receptor tyrosine kinase *KIT* often occur in acral and mucosal melanomas, similar to high-CSD melanomas, their incidence varies by anatomic site.[34,56,58,67–69] Anorectal and vulvovaginal have the highest number of *KIT* mutations (approximately 35%).[56,68–70] Anorectal melanomas also have frequent *NF1* and *SF3B1* mutations (20% each), the latter of which is often present in uveal melanomas.[56] Twenty percent of acral and penile melanomas have *KIT* mutations[58,68] while oral melanomas have approximately 10% *KIT* mutation prevalence.[62,63] While early clinical trials of unselected melanoma patients failed to show any efficacy with *KIT* inhibitors,[71] subsequent case reports and follow-up studies indicate that when melanoma patients with confirmed *KIT* mutations are selected for, dramatic responses to KIT inhibitors such as imatinib and other agents do occur.[26–28,72–74] Although the majority of melanomas with genetic alterations in *KIT* overexpressed the protein as determined by CD117 immunohistochemistry, increased immunoreactivity does not reliably predict responding patients.[39,75–77] Patients with *KIT* amplification without mutation do not appear to significantly benefit from the KIT inhibitor therapy.[72–74]

The melanoma categories in which genetic alterations of *KIT* are found frequently show a lentiginous growth pattern and poor circumscription

toward the uninvolved epidermis. These growth characteristics may be related to biological effects of *KIT* activation. *KIT* is essential for melanoblast migration from the neural crest into the skin and for homing into epithelial structures during development. If constitutively active *KIT* is introduced into human melanocytes in vitro, it induces a migratory phenotype resembling a lentiginous pattern.[78] Aberrant KIT signaling in melanoma may therefore help explain the field effect described for melanomas on acral skin (*Figs 26.139* and *26.140*).[50]

Melanocytic tumors arising without associations to epithelial structures

Most melanocytic neoplasms, benign melanocytic nevi as well as melanomas, originate from melanocytes situated within epithelial structures throughout the body and have mutations in genes such as *BRAF*, *NRAS*, *NF1*, and *KIT*. However, a subset of melanocytic neoplasms arises without an apparent connection to epithelial structures and does not show these mutations.[38,79] One category, uveal melanoma, arises from melanocytes within the choroidal plexus, the ciliary body, and the iris of the eye and is biologically distinct from cutaneous melanoma by a very strong propensity to metastasize to the liver.[80] It also differs in the presence of certain chromosomal aberrations such as frequent loss of chromosome 3, which serves as a negative prognostic indicator in uveal melanoma.[81] In the skin, intradermal melanocytic proliferations, which can be congenital or acquired, present in diverse ways ranging from discrete blue papules (blue nevi) to large blue-gray patches affecting the conjunctiva and periorbital skin (nevus of Ota), shoulders (nevus of Ito), and the lower back (Mongolian spot).[82] A potential connection between intradermal melanocytic neoplasms and uveal melanoma is suggested by the fact that nevus of Ota represents a risk factor for uveal melanoma in Caucasians. In addition, blue nevi can show cytological similarities to uveal melanoma.[80] Interestingly, while uveal melanomas strongly express KIT on immunohistochemistry, they lack mutations in the *KIT* gene.[79]

A forward genetic screen in mice identified germline mutations in the heterotrimeric G-protein subunits *GNAQ* and *GNA11* that cause skin hyperpigmentation by inducing a subtle intradermal proliferation of melanocytes.[83] *GNAQ* and *GNA11* are members of the q class of G-protein alpha subunits and are involved in mediating signals between G-protein coupled receptors (GPCRs) and downstream effectors.[84] Somatic mutations in *GNAQ* are found in 83% of blue nevi, 50% of blue nevus-like melanoma ('malignant blue nevi'), and 46% of uveal melanomas.[85] The mutations in human tumors differed from the genetic variants discovered in the mouse screen. In human melanocytic tumors, all mutations occurred exclusively at codon 209, which is homologous to codon 61 of *NRAS* family members and leads to constitutive activation. GNAQ activates protein kinase C (PKC) family members PKCδ and ε via the release of diacylglycerol (DAG) by phospholipase Cβ.[86] In vitro studies show that the *GNAQ*^{Q209L} mutation transforms melanocytes with efficiencies comparable to *NRAS* mutations and leads to activation of the MAP kinase pathway. This MAP kinase activation occurs specifically through recruitment of RasGRP3 to the cell membrane by DAG and its phosphorylation and activation by PKC δ and ε. RasGRP3 then activates RAS to initiate MAP kinase pathway signaling.[86] When introduced into murine melanocytes, mutant GNAQ induces heavily pigmented tumors that morphologically resemble the spectrum of human blue nevi and pigmented epithelioid melanocytomas, confirming its role in driving these tumor types.[85]

While GNAQ or GNA11 mutations are sufficient to initiate growth of these melanocytic neoplasms (*Fig. 26.141*), additional genomic aberrations are required for transformation into melanoma (e.g., uveal melanoma, blue nevus-like melanoma). Additional mutation or loss of the tumor suppressor *BRCA1-associated protein 1 (BAP1)* gene in uveal melanoma is associated with a poor prognosis and has also been found in the transformation of blue nevi to melanoma.[87,88] Recurrent *SF3B1* and *EIF1AX* mutations have also been found. They typically occur in mutually exclusive fashion from BAP1 loss and are associated with a more indolent disease course.[89,90] Array CGH profiling of cellular blue nevi, atypical cellular blue nevi, and blue nevus-like melanoma shows increasing genomic instability during progression through these stages, with most nevi having no chromosomal aberrations and a

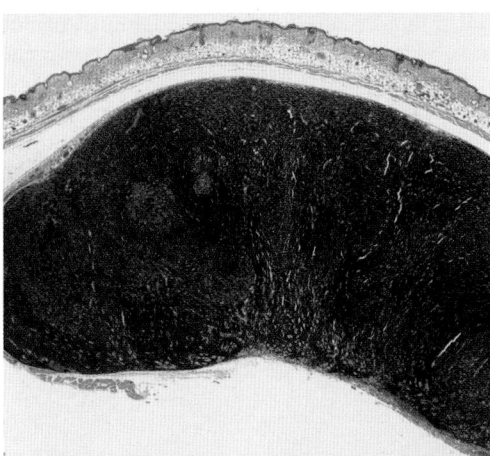
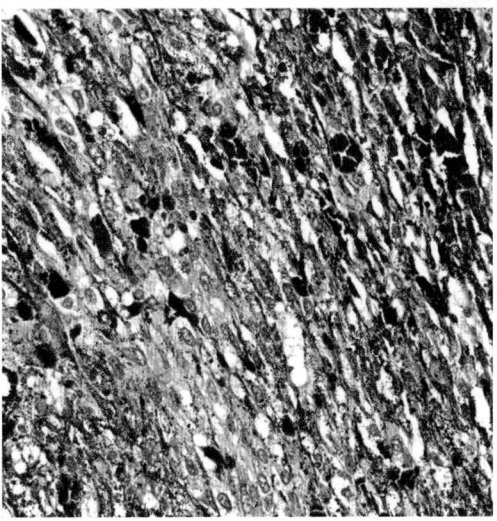

Fig. 26.141
An animal model of *GNAQ* mutant melanocytes: mouse melanocytes stably transduced with mutant *GNAQ*, but not with wild-type *GNAQ*, induce highly pigmented tumors of spindled and epithelioid melanocytes after 10 weeks

minority of atypical cellular blue nevi showing one to two chromosomal aberrations.[88,91] Blue nevus-like melanomas exhibit multiple chromosomal aberrations (typically ≥3) including recurrent deletions of chromosomes 1p, 3p, 4q, 6q, 8p, 9, 16, and 17q and recurrent gains of chromosomes 6p, 8q, 20, and 21q.[88,91]

Another signaling pathway implicated in the pathogenesis in tumors that share phenotypic features with blue nevi is the protein kinase A (PKA) pathway. Loss-of-function mutations in a regulatory subunit of PKA (encoded by *PRKAR1A*) are found in epithelioid blue nevi associated with Carney complex and result in hyperactivation of PKA with subsequent activation of the MITF transcription factor.[92] Such mutations have also been detected in a subset of tumors designated as pigmented epithelioid melanocytomas.[93]

Spitzoid melanoma

Spitzoid melanocytic neoplasms represent a class of neoplasia with a range of malignant potential from Spitz nevi at the benign end to spitzoid melanoma at the malignant end, and atypical Spitz tumors as a biologically intermediate category. Spitz nevi are defined by distinct histopathological features and an age distribution skewed towards children. They have a distinctive mutational landscape that distinguishes them from common nevi, which include activating mutations in *HRAS* and kinase fusions of *ROS1*, *NTRK1*, *NTRK3*, *ALK*, *BRAF*, *RET*, or *MET*.[94–97] Spitz nevi tend to have no chromosomal aberrations with the exception of lesions with isolated chromosome 11p gain, which is typically associated with an oncogenic *HRAS* mutation on the duplicated chromosomal arm.[94] Some Spitz nevi can also have isolated copy number increase of distal chromosome 7q, which indicates fusions of *BRAF* or *MET* mapping in this area.[96,97]

Atypical Spitz tumors have similar oncogenic alterations as Spitz nevi, but have some additional chromosomal aberrations, often with loss of chromosome 9. Spitzoid melanoma, when defined by solely by histologic

features, appears to be a heterogeneous category with the majority of cases representing *BRAF* and *NRAS* mutant melanoma[98] rather than melanomas that evolved from bona fide Spitz nevi or atypical Spitz tumors with *HRAS* mutations or various kinase fusions. The genetic features of bona fide Spitzoid melanomas, i.e., melanomas that originate from Spitz nevi or are closely related to them molecularly, are currently poorly characterized. Both homozygous loss of *CDKN2A*[99] and *TERT* promoter mutation[100] appear to occur in some lethal Spitzoid melanomas, though the small number of cases reported with these aberrations limits the generalizability of these findings.

Emerging concepts in metastatic melanoma

The traditional concept of melanoma progression to metastasis starting from primary invasive melanoma and spreading through lymphatics to regional lymph nodes, and then from regional lymph nodes to distant sites is inadequate in explaining the observed biological behavior of metastatic melanoma. Phylogenetic analysis of separate metastatic foci in melanoma patients shows genetically distinct populations within the same patient, indicating that parallel seeding of metastatic sites occurs from the primary tumor followed by subsequent separate genetic evolution at the sites of metastasis.[101–103] Metastatic 'reseeding', in which cells from a distant metastatic site travel to other sites of metastasis and proliferate,[104] may also occur and could explain the emergence of multifocal treatment resistance to targeted therapies in some patients.[105] Some evidence supporting WNT pathway activation in the progression to metastatic melanoma has been reported,[101,106] and *MITF* amplification has been found to be more prevalent in metastatic disease.[107] However, multiple genetic analyses of primary tumors and metastases have not identified a distinct set of genetic changes that reproducibly predict progression to metastasis.[108–110]

The Cancer Genome Atlas

The Cancer Genome Atlas (TCGA) is a National Institute of Health (NIH)-sponsored cooperative effort to comprehensively analyze various cancer types. The TCGA published results on a collaborative, multi-platform analysis of 333 melanomas with a high percentage of metastatic melanomas (80%, mostly regional lymph node metastases) representing the largest study of melanoma to date.[111] This study categorized melanoma by DNA mutations, copy number alterations, gene expression (RNA), non-coding RNA, methylation, protein expression, and histologic images linked to a database with clinical annotation and follow-up. In this analysis, melanomas were classified into four types: *BRAF*, *RAS*, *NF1*, and triple-wild type (WT). The first three types had >90% UV signature mutation profile with high-frequency *TERT* promoter mutations corresponding to the low-CSD and high-CSD melanoma classes. The triple WT melanoma mutation profile was only 30% UV signature with <10% *TERT* promoter mutation and had more copy number changes and fusion driver events, corresponding to the category of acral and mucosal melanomas. RNA expression analysis identified three clusters with significantly different survival rates, with the 'immune' signature subgroup having the most favorable survival rates and the 'keratin' signature subgroup showing an adverse prognosis.[111] This and additional studies demonstrating prognostic value from histologic documentation of lymphocytic infiltrates as well as expression profiling of the immune response in these tumors have been reported as well.[112] A separate TCGA study of primary uveal melanoma cases (n = approximately 80%) demonstrated the near universal detection of *GNAQ* and *GNA11* mutations as well as poor prognosis associated with chromosome 3 monosomy (loss of the tumor suppressor *BAP1*) on chromosome 3p.[90] In addition, *EIF1AX* and *SF3B1* mutations were associated with distinct copy number alteration and methylation patterns within the chromosome 3 disomy group that corresponded to better prognosis.

Summary

Genetic analyses have revealed that deregulation of a few key signaling pathways is critical in melanoma formation. Common key events include activating mutations in the MAP kinase (proliferation) and PI3 kinase (survival) pathways and inactivating mutations in the RB1 pathway (cell cycle control). Kinase activation can occur at the receptor level (*KIT* mutations and fusions of receptor tyrosine kinases such as *MET*, *RET*, *ALK*, *ROS1*,

NTRK1, NTRK3) often activating both the MAP kinase and PI3 kinase pathways or further downstream (*NRAS, PTEN, BRAF, PI3KCA*) activation of a pathway. The mutation patterns often correlate with the anatomic site of the primary tumor and clinical and histologic features. These driver mutations initiate proliferation in early stages of melanocytic neoplasia and are followed by loss of cell cycle checkpoint inhibition (e.g., p16, Rb), dysregulation of chromatin remodeling proteins (e.g., ARID1/2), and protection from replicative senescence through *TERT* gene amplification or *TERT* promoter mutation. Mutations in *GNAQ/GNA11* in uveal melanoma, blue nevi, and related tumors have highlighted additional signaling pathways of relevance in subsets of melanocytic neoplasia. The advent of high-throughput genomic tools has initiated the construction of sets of critical genetic alterations in melanoma which will in time complete the foundation for comprehensive classification of melanoma that will continue to integrate genomic alterations with established phenotypes and is expected to significantly improve prognostication and treatment stratification.

Access **ExpertConsult.com** for the complete list of references

See
www.expertconsult.com
for references and
additional material

Tumors of the conjunctiva

CHAPTER
27

Amy Y. Lin

Introduction

Anatomy and histology of the conjunctiva

The conjunctiva is a mucous membrane that covers the surface of the eyeball and posterior aspect of the eyelid that functions to protect the eye and allow the eyelids to move smoothly over the globe (*Fig. 27.1*).[1] It is divided into four main regions: limbus, bulbar, fornix, and palpebral (tarsal) conjunctiva.

The limbus (*Fig. 27.2*) is lined by nonkeratinizing stratified squamous epithelium, 8–10 cells thick, with stem cells in the basal layer. Melanocytes are present to protect stem cells from ultraviolet (UV) light damage. Darker-pigmented individuals are more heavily pigmented at the limbus compared with lighter-skinned individuals. The limbal basement membrane is wavy, with rete peg-like formations called the palisades of Vogt.[2] The limbus is a common site of squamous and melanocytic neoplasms.

The bulbar conjunctiva is lined by nonkeratinizing stratified squamous epithelium with scattered goblet cells, mostly in the inferior and nasal portions (*Fig. 27.3*).[1] The connective tissue stroma, called the substantia propria, is loose in the bulbar conjunctiva.

The fornix is lined by pseudostratified columnar epithelium with numerous goblet cells. The substantia propria is loose and contains lymphocytes and plasma cells that form the conjunctiva-associated lymphoid tissue (CALT) (*Fig. 27.4*).[2] Accessory lacrimal glands (glands of Krause) are also present.

The palpebral or tarsal conjunctiva lines the posterior surface of the eyelid (*Fig. 27.5*). It is lined by nonkeratinizing epithelium containing goblet cells. The substantial propria is very thin and tightly adherent to the tarsus. Accessory lacrimal glands (glands of Wolfring) are present at the superior aspect of the tarsus in the upper eyelid.[1]

The conjunctival substantia propria contains numerous lymphatic vessels. Therefore, malignant neoplasms of the conjunctiva tend to spread to regional lymph nodes.

The caruncle is the fleshy tissue present in the medial interpalpebral angle of the eye. It is a specialized area of conjunctiva lined by nonkeratinized stratified squamous epithelium with hair follicles, smooth muscle, sebaceous glands, adipose tissue, accessory lacrimal glands, and sweat glands in the stroma.[1] The plica semilunaris is another specialized portion of the conjunctiva just lateral to the caruncle with similar histologic features to other areas of the conjunctiva. Rarely, cartilage is present in the stroma.

Diagnostic approaches

Because the conjunctiva is readily visible, tumors and other lesions are usually recognized and diagnosed at a relatively early stage. An experienced ophthalmologist can often make an accurate diagnosis with careful external ocular examination and slit-lamp biomicroscopy. The bulbar, palpebral, and upper and lower forniceal conjunctiva, as well as the cornea, must be evaluated for tumor involvement, and lesions should be photographed to document the tumors and their margins. Corneal involvement by squamous or melanocytic neoplasia may be subtle, and appear as gray surface opacity.

Definitive diagnosis of conjunctival or corneal tumors requires histologic examination. Small (≤4 clock hours limbal tumor or ≤15 mm basal

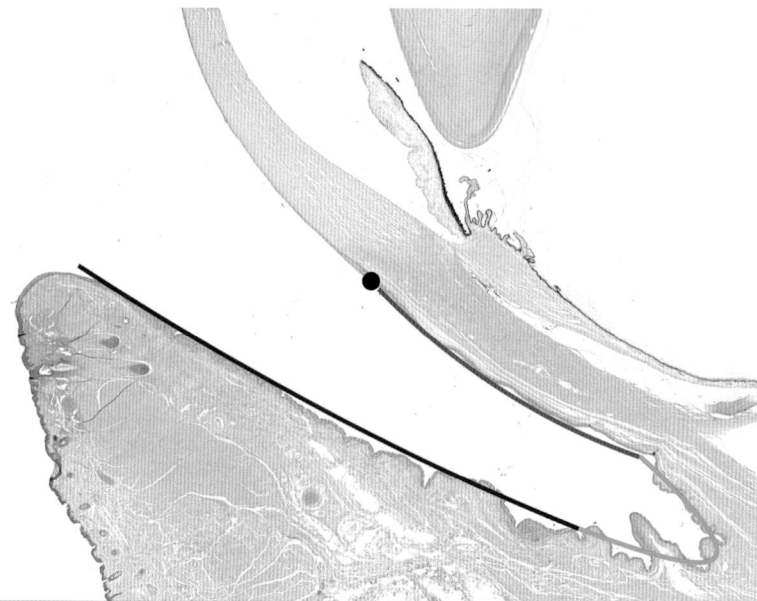

Fig. 27.1
Normal eye structure: a sagital section of an exanteration specimen illustrates the different regions of the conjunctiva – limbus in black, bulbar conjunctiva in pink, fornix in green and palpebral (tarsal) conjunctiva in dark blue.

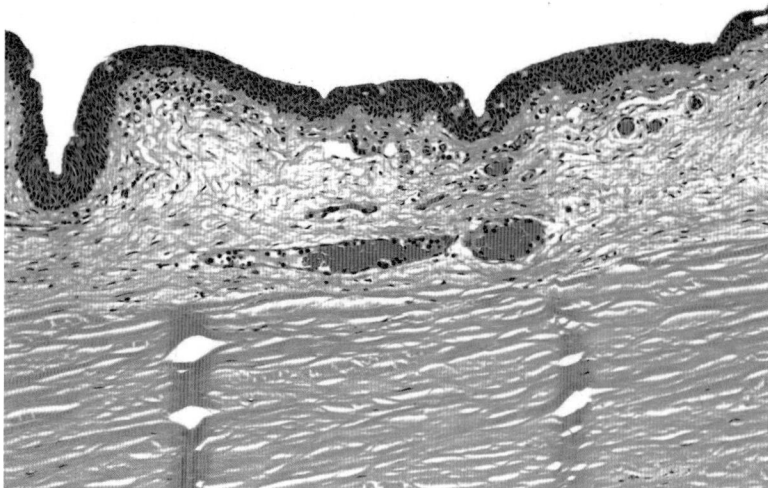

Fig. 27.3
Normal bulbar conjunctiva: histology shows squamous mucosa with scattered goblet cells and loose connective tissue in the substantia propria.

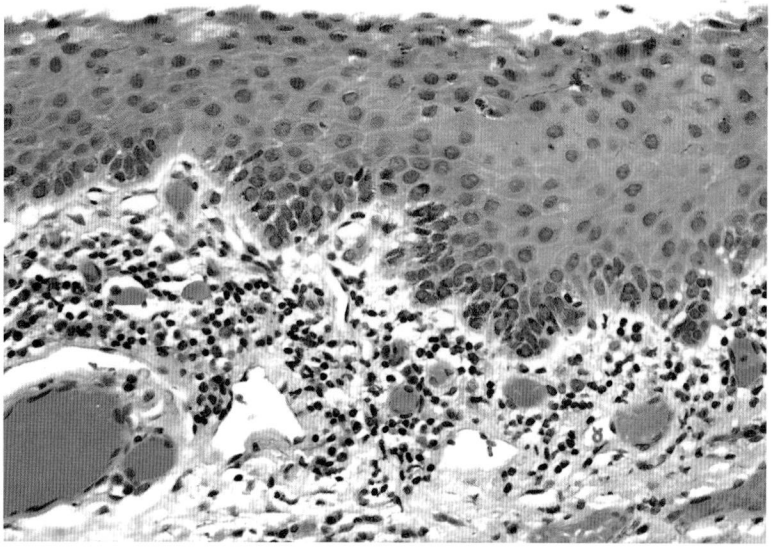

Fig. 27.2
Normal limbus: histology shows nonkeratinizing squamous epithelium and palisades of Vogt with melanin pigmentation of the basal epithelium and scattered intraepithelial dendritic melanocytes.

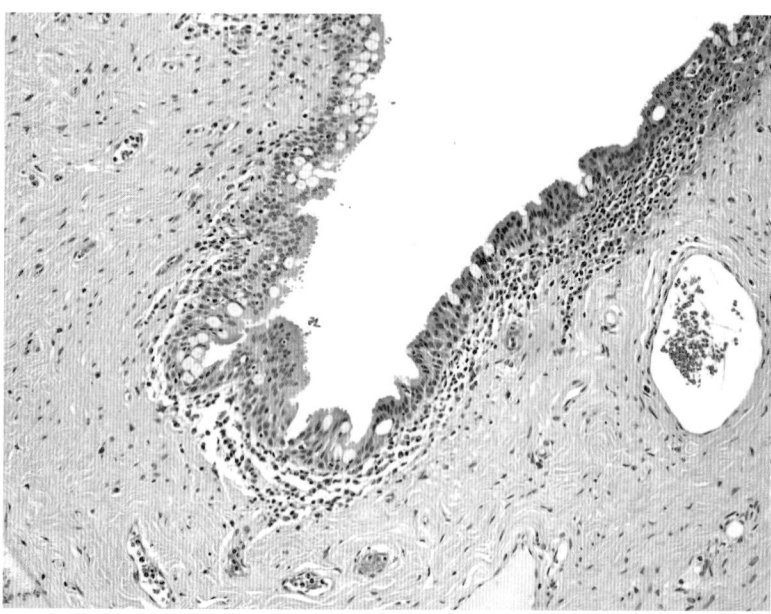

Fig. 27.4
Normal fornix: histology shows pseudostratified columnar epithelium with numerous goblet cells and lymphocytes and plasma cells in the substantia propria.

dimension), asymptomatic, benign appearing tumors are usually observed, and biopsied when there is evidence of growth or malignant change. For small tumors that are symptomatic or suspected to be malignant, complete removal (excisional biopsy) is recommended. For large lesions (>4 clock hour limbal tumor or >15 mm basal dimension), incisional biopsy is recommended because complete removal can severely compromise the ocular surface or may not be possible. Extensive conjunctival resection decreases the number of goblet cells, which interferes with corneal wetting. The resultant dry eye predisposes the patient to corneal ulceration and painful loss of vision.[3] Incisional biopsy is also appropriate for tumors that are treated with radiotherapy, chemotherapy, or local means such as cryotherapy or topical chemotherapy, such as lymphoid tumors, metastatic tumors, and some cases of squamous cell carcinoma and primary acquired melanosis (PAM). Exfoliative cytology can be a helpful adjunct in select cases, but only provides information about superficial layers of the lesion and not the degree of invasiveness.[4]

Classification

Tumors of the conjunctiva are generally classified by tissue or cell of origin, and whether the tumor is benign or malignant. Most conjunctival tumors are epithelial or melanocytic in origin.[5,6] Hematopoietic tumors, such as lymphomas and leukemias, can occur in the conjunctiva. Other conjunctival tumors are from various elements of the conjunctival stroma, including vascular, fibrous, neural, histiocytic, myogenic, myxoid, and lipomatous. Other groups of conjunctival tumors include hamartomas and choristomas, caruncular tumors, metastatic and secondary tumors, and tumorlike lesions.

The classification of conjunctival tumors in this chapter is based on the second edition of the World Health Organization (WHO) International Histological Classification of Tumors[6] with consultation of other major texts.[4,6–9] The tumors discussed in this chapter are listed in Table 27.1.

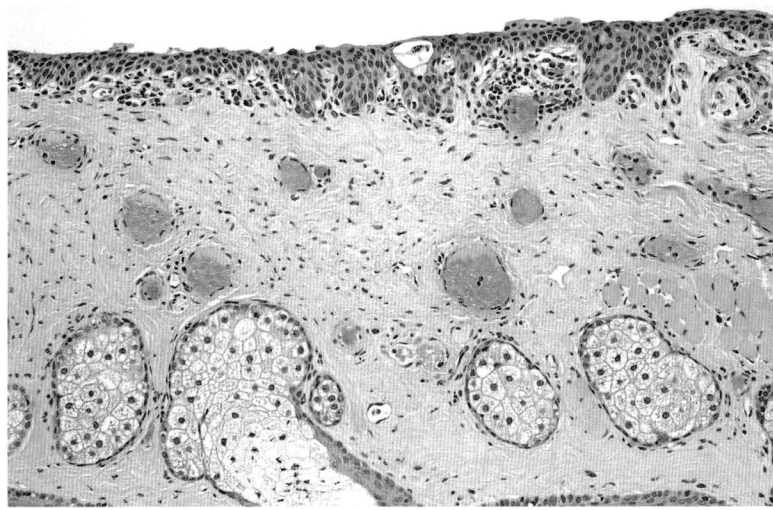

Fig. 27.5
Normal palpebral (tarsal) conjunctiva: histology shows squamous mucosa tightly adherent to the tarsus, which contains sebaceous glands, called Meibomian glands.

Congenital lesions

Congenital lesions are usually hamartomas or choristomas, and diagnosed in infancy and childhood.

Dermoid

Clinical features

Epibulbar dermoid (*Fig. 27.6*) is a congenital lesion that is most commonly located inferotemporally at the limbus. It is well circumscribed, tan-yellow, and may have fine hair protruding from the surface. The lesion may be isolated, or associated with Goldenhar syndrome (oculoauriculovertebral dysplasia).[1] Patients should be evaluated for preauricular skin append-ages, hearing loss, eyelid colobomas, mandibular hypoplasia, and vertebral abnormalities.[2] Dermoid can cause astigmatism and amblyopia.

Histologic features

Epibulbar dermoid is composed of dense fibrous tissue containing dermal appendages, such as hair follicles, sebaceous glands, sweat glands, and sometimes adipose tissue, lined by nonkeratinizing stratified squamous epi-thelium (*Fig. 27.7*).

Dermolipoma

Clinical features

Dermolipoma is a congenital lesion, most commonly located superotempo-rally in the fornix. Patients may be asymptomatic for years, and present in adulthood with a mass that appears soft and yellow with fine hairs on the surface. The lesion may extend into the orbit and onto the bulbar conjunctiva.[1]

Histologic features

Dermolipoma is composed of variable amounts of fibrous connective tissue and adipose tissue, lined by conjunctival epithelium. Pilosebaceous units and lacrimal gland tissue may be present. Dermolipoma may be associated with Goldenhar syndrome.

Osseous choristoma

Clinical features

Osseous choristoma is a rare congenital lesion that presents as an epibulbar mass superotemporally, usually in early infancy or childhood.[1,2] The lesion

may be adherent to the extraocular muscle sheath, overlying conjunctiva, or underlying sclera.[1]

Histologic features

Osseous choristoma is composed of mature cortical bone surrounded by fibrous connective tissue (*Fig. 27.8*).[1]

Lacrimal gland choristoma

Clinical features

Lacrimal gland choristoma is a congenital lesion that presents as an asymp-tomatic, pink stromal mass superotemporally or temporally in young chil-dren. It has also been described in the limbal area.[1] Rarely, the lesion may be cystic.[2]

Histologic features

Lacrimal gland tissue is present in the conjunctival stroma.

Complex choristoma

Clinical features

Complex choristoma contains tissue derived from two germ layers. The clin-ical appearance depends on the components of the lesion: for example, a tumor with lacrimal gland tissue may appear pink; one with dermal tissue may appear yellow-white, and one with cartilage, smooth and blue-gray.[1] Complex choristoma may be associated with nevus sebaceous of Jadassohn. Patients should be evaluated for nevus sebaceous of the face, as well as neurological features, such as seizures, mental retardation, arachnoid cyst, and cerebral atrophy.[1]

Histologic features

Complex choristomas may include a combination of ectopic tissues, includ-ing dermal tissue with adipose tissue and dermal appendages, lacrimal gland tissue, smooth muscle, cartilage, and bone (*Figs 27.9* and *27.10*).[2]

Epithelial tumors

Epithelial tumors are located on the surface of the conjunctiva. They gener-ally have irregular, granular, or papillary surfaces and may be leukoplakic or gelatinous in appearance. Epithelial tumors can be superficial and thin, or thick and fleshy. In this section, we will discuss a number of benign epithe-lial tumors, including more common entities (e.g., squamous papilloma and epithelial cyst) and rare entities (e.g., keratoacanthoma, hereditary benign intraepithelial dyskeratosis [HBID], dacryoadenoma, oncocytoma, kera-totic plaque, and actinic keratosis), as well as premalignant and malignant epithelial tumors (i.e., ocular surface squamous neoplasia [OSSN], which includes squamous cell carcinoma).

Squamous papilloma and inverted papilloma

Clinical features

Squamous papilloma is a common benign tumor, comprising 14.5% of epi-thelial lesions excised from the conjunctival sac and 13% to 32% of all tumors of the caruncle.[1] It is a pink to red fleshy lesion with finger-like pro-jections that may be pedunculated or sessile (*Fig. 27.11*). Those arising at the lid margin or caruncle tend to be pedunculated, whereas those arising at the limbus are usually sessile. The growth pattern may be exophytic, mixed exo- and endophytic, or rarely, endophytic (inverted). It is more common in males than females, and can occur in children and adults (mean age, 39.6 years; range, 17–84).[2] Lesions may be single or multiple, and most commonly arise medially and inferiorly.[2] Squamous papilloma is associ-ated with human papillomavirus (HPV), usually types 6 and 11.[3] Lesions may recur, and rarely progress to carcinoma. Inverted papilloma is rare, with 10 reported cases in the literature since it was described in 1979,

Table 27.1

Classification of conjunctival tumors

Hamartomas and choristomas Dermoid Dermolipoma Osseous choristoma Lacrimal gland choristoma Complex choristoma	Cavernous hemangioma Racemose hemangioma Varix Lymphangiectasia Lymphangioma Kaposi sarcoma Angiosarcoma

Epithelial tumors
Benign epithelial tumors
Squamous papilloma
Keratotic plaque
Keratoacanthoma
Reactive epithelial hyperplasia (pseudoepitheliomatous hyperplasia)
Inverted papilloma
Hereditary intraepithelial dyskeratosis
Oncocytoma
Dacryoadenoma
Cysts
	Fibrous tumors
	Fibroma
	Fibrous histiocytoma
	   Benign
	   Malignant
	Nodular fasciitis

	Neural tumors
	Neurofibroma
	   Localized
	   Diffuse
	Neurilemmoma (schwannoma)
	Granular cell tumor

Premalignant and malignant epithelial tumors
Actinic keratosis
Conjunctival intraepithelial neoplasia
Epithelial dysplasia
Carcinoma in situ
Squamous cell carcinoma
   Spindle cell carcinoma
   Mucoepidermoid carcinoma
   Adenoid squamous carcinoma
   Involvement in sebaceous gland carcinoma
   Xeroderma pigmentosum
	Histiocytic tumors
	Xanthoma
	Juvenile xanthogranuloma
	Reticulohistiocytoma

	Myxoid tumors Myxoma
	Myogenic tumors Rhabdomyosarcoma
Melanocytic tumors *Benign melanocytic tumors* Junctional nevus Compound nevus Subepithelial nevus Inflamed juvenile conjunctival nevus Spitz nevus Blue nevus Primary acquired melanosis (PAM) without atypia Congenital melanosis Complexion-associated melanosis (racial melanosis)	***Lipomatous tumors*** Lipoma Herniated orbital fat Liposarcoma
	Hematopoietic tumors Benign reactive lymphoid hyperplasia Lymphoma Leukemic infiltrates

Premalignant and malignant melanocytic lesions
PAM with atypia
Malignant melanoma
   arising in junctional nevi
   arising in PAM with atypia
   arising de novo
	Metastatic and secondary tumors
	Metastatic tumors from distant organs
	Extraocular extension of intraocular tumors
	Conjunctival involvement by eyelid tumors
	Conjunctival involvement by lacrimal gland and other orbital tumors

	Caruncular tumors Of conjunctival tissue origin Of epidermis and skin appendages origin
Benign and malignant stromal tumors *Vascular tumors* Lobular capillary hemangioma (pyogenic granuloma) Capillary hemangioma	**Lesions simulating conjunctival tumors** Pinguecula and pterygium Amyloidosis

and has more benign, less aggressive behavior compared with its sinonasal counterparts.[1]

Histologic features

Squamous papilloma has a frondlike growth pattern with fibrovascular cores (*Fig. 27.12*). Given the association with HPV, koilocytosis and occasionally, varying degrees of dysplasia, typically low-grade, may be seen. In one study, 40% of squamous papillomas had some degree of inflammation.[2]

Inverted papilloma is an epithelial proliferation surrounding fibrovascular cores with an endophytic growth pattern. Goblet cells or cysts are typically identified within the tumor; hence, Jakobiec and colleagues[4] suggested the term 'inverted mucoepidermoid papilloma' to reflect these features. Inverted papilloma may be misdiagnosed histologically as squamous cell carcinoma. Features distinguishing inverted papilloma from squamous cell carcinoma include: well-defined, circumscribed margins; blending of the lesion with surface epithelium that is not dysplastic; no sharp demarcation between proliferating epithelium and normal surface epithelium; no obvious cytological atypia or conspicuous mitotic figures; absence of prominent perilesional inflammatory infiltrate; presence of multiple cysts with goblet cells; and presence of eosinophilic globoid cytoplasmic inclusions that represent inspissated mucus. Additionally, HPV is usually negative in inverted papilloma, and p53 and Ki67 are usually low (10–20% compared with >50% in dysplasia and carcinoma for p53; <1% compared with >25% in dysplasia and carcinoma for Ki67) by immunohistochemistry.[1]

Reactive epithelial hyperplasia

Reactive epithelial hyperplasia (pseudoepitheliomatous hyperplasia, pseudocarcinomatous hyperplasia) occurs secondary to irritation caused

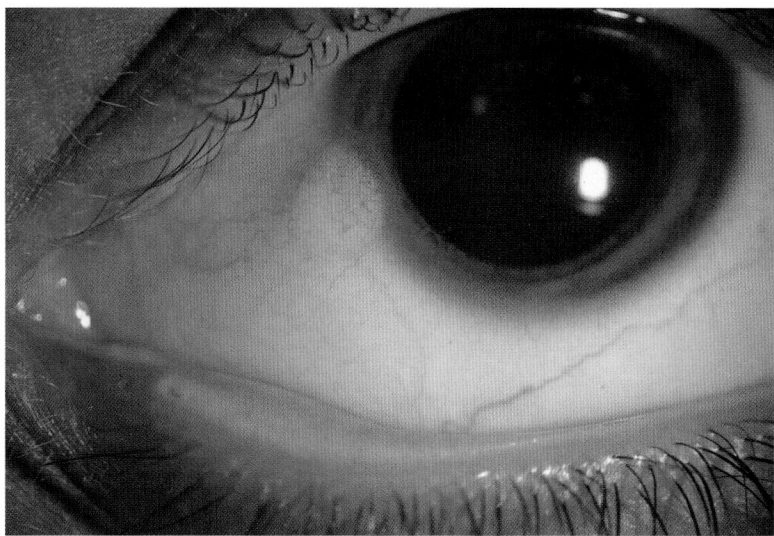

Fig. 27.6
Limbal dermoid: clinical photograph showing an elevated, yellow-white lesion at the limbus inferonasally.

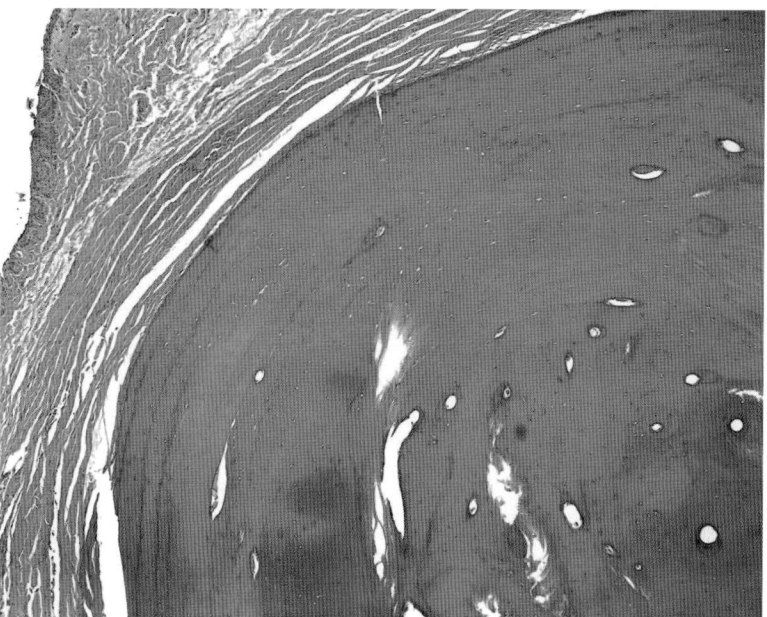

Fig. 27.8
Osseous choristoma: histology shows mature compact bone surrounded by connective tissue.

Keratoacanthoma

Clinical features

Keratoacanthoma is a rare lesion with fewer than 20 reported cases[1] that grows rapidly, over a period of 3 to 4 weeks. It most frequently occurs at the temporal limbus. The lesion is a white nodular mass with a hyperkeratotic area and surrounded by dilated blood vessels, and may be clinically indistinguishable from squamous cell carcinoma.

Histologic features

Keratoacanthoma of the conjunctiva shows similar features to that of the skin, with crateriform architecture filled with keratin. The surrounding epithelium is acanthotic and hyperkeratotic with focal parakeratosis and dyskeratosis. A chronic inflammatory infiltrate is often present at the base. Cytological atypia is usually mild,[1,2] but some cases may demonstrate marked atypia, causing difficulty in distinguishing from well-differentiated squamous cell carcinoma.

Hereditary benign intraepithelial dyskeratosis

Clinical features

HBID is a rare, autosomal dominant condition that presents at birth or early childhood, characterized by elevated plaques on the nasal or temporal bulbar conjunctiva and oral mucosa. The majority of patients trace their ancestry to the Haliwa-Saponi Native American tribe in North Carolina.[1-6] Some patients are Caucasian French. Lesions may involve the cornea and be associated with hyperemia and foreign body sensation. Using genetic linkage analysis, the gene for HBID in Native Americans was located to chromosome 4 (4q35).[3] In a group of Caucasian French patients, next-generation sequencing identified a novel missense mutation in the NLRP1 gene on chromosome 17 (17p13.2).[5]

Histologic features

Histopathology shows acanthotic epithelium with hyperkeratosis and dyskeratosis. Chronic inflammation is present at the base. There is no invasion of underlying tissue. Exfoliative cytology may be a useful alternative for patients who are suspected to have HBID, but are unable to undergo biopsy.[6] Cytological features include rounded squamous epithelial cells with dense homogenous orange cytoplasm and hyperchromatic oval or crenated nuclei, occasionally accompanied by small lymphocytes.[6]

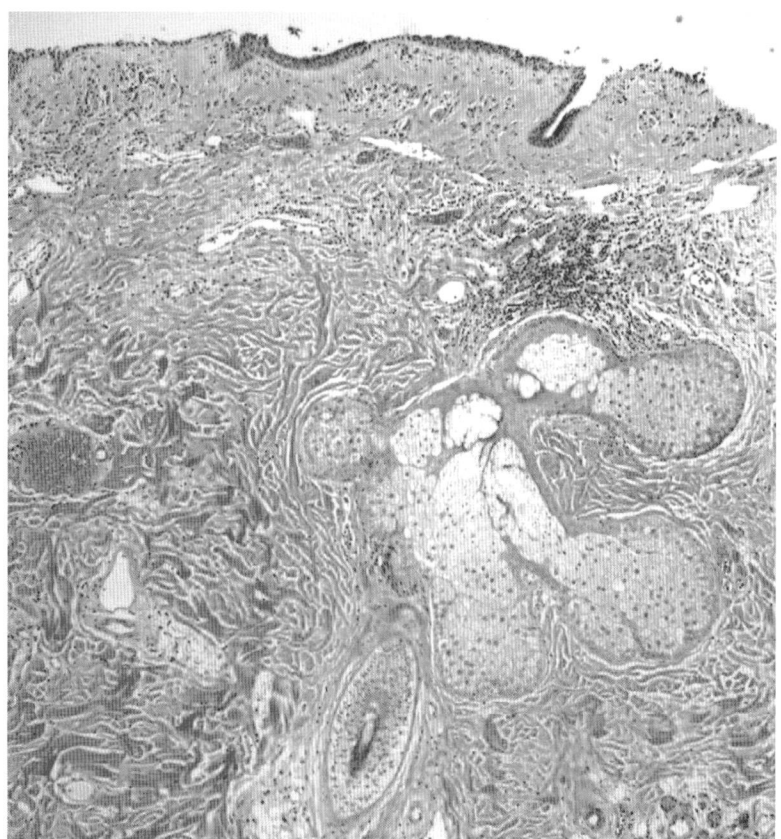

Fig. 27.7
Limbal dermoid: histology shows dermal type collagen and skin adnexal structures, including hair follicle and sebaceous gland.

by concurrent or pre-existing stromal inflammation.[1-3] It presents as an elevated, leukoplakic pink lesion that usually occurs in the limbic area. Histologically, it shows acanthosis, hyperkeratosis, or parakeratosis and subepithelial inflammation. Mitotic figures may be present, but cytological atypia is generally absent. Clinically and histologically, reactive epithelial hyperplasia may be difficult to differentiate from conjunctival squamous cell carcinoma. An infiltrative growth pattern, marked cytological atypia, and excessive mitotic activity (including atypical forms) obviously favor the latter diagnosis.

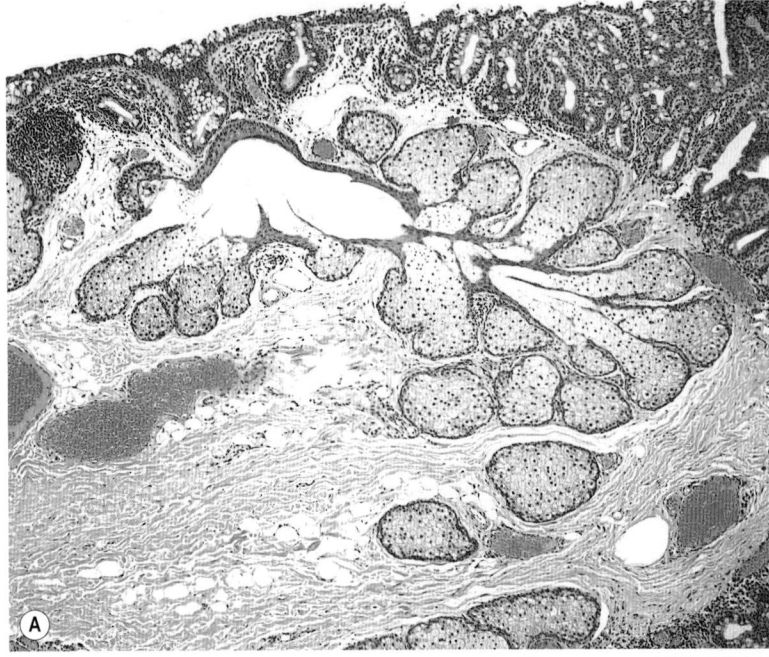

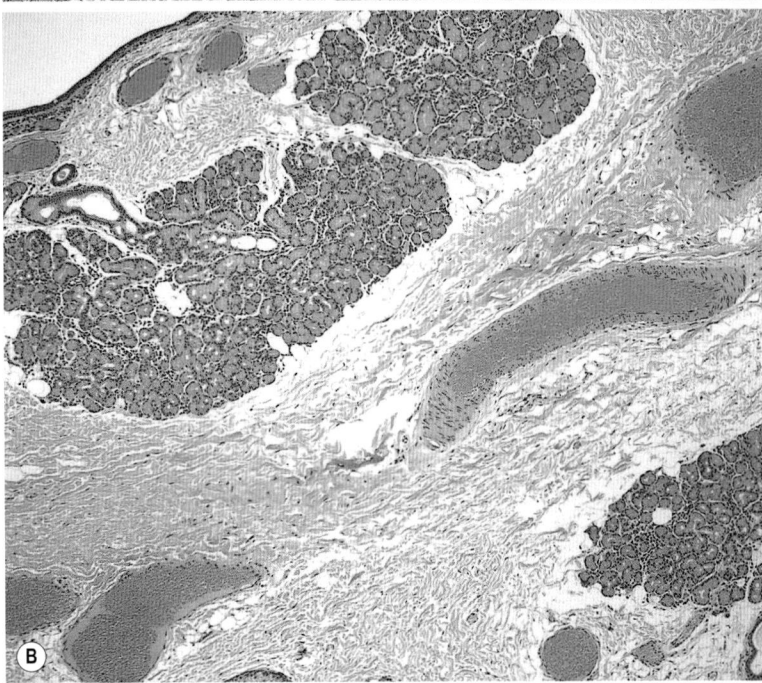

Fig. 27.9
Complex choristoma: (**A**) one area of the lesion contained dermal type collagen and adipose tissue with skin appendages (sebaceous glands). (**B**) In a different area of the lesion, lacrimal gland tissue was identified.

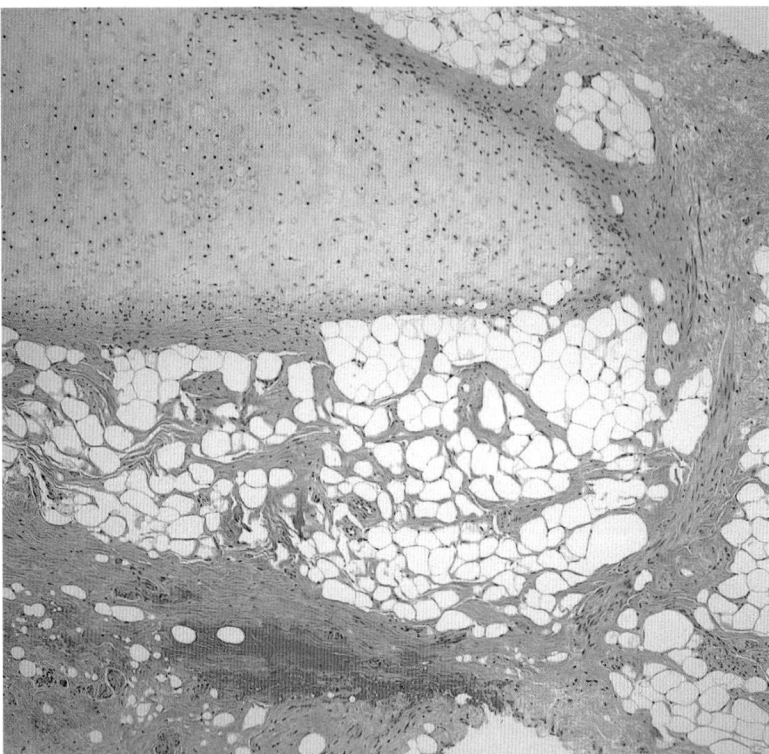

Fig. 27.10
Complex choristoma: histology shows a mixture of fibroadipose tissue, smooth muscle, and cartilage.

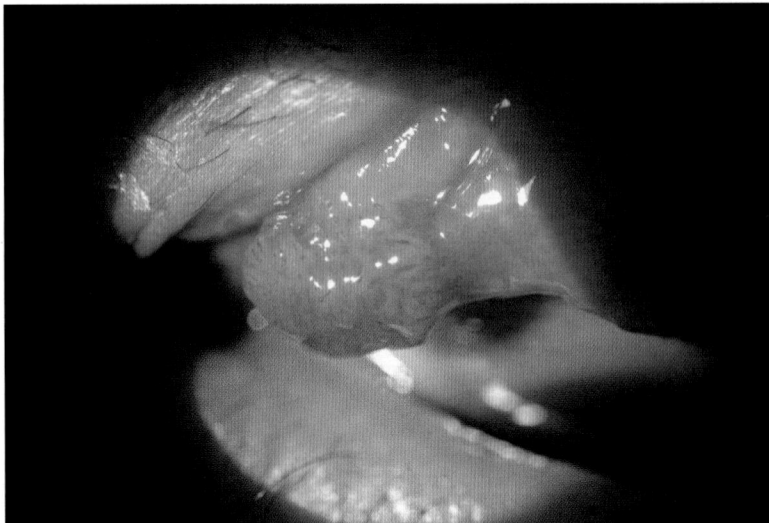

Fig. 27.11
Squamous papilloma: an exophytic tarsal lesion.

Dacryoadenoma

Dacryoadenoma is a rare, benign conjunctival tumor that appears as a pink mass.[1] Histologically, dacryoadenoma is a proliferation of metaplastic surface epithelium that forms tubular and glandular structures similar to the lacrimal gland. Myoepithelial cells are associated with the acinar-type epithelium, and goblet cells are also present.[2]

Oncocytoma

Clinical features

Oncocytoma is a benign tumor that usually arises in the caruncle of older, female patients (*Fig. 27.13*). Patients typically present with a fleshy, sub-epithelial, orange-red or dark blue mass, often with intralesional cysts.

Ultrasound biomicroscopy may show mixed solid and cystic components.[1] Oncocytoma may also arise from lacrimal sac, lacrimal gland, or eyelid.

Histologic features

Oncocytoma is a circumscribed nodule of epithelial cells with abundant, granular eosinophilic cytoplasm arranged in nests, cords, or sheets that may form glandular or ductal structures (*Fig. 27.14*). Carcinomatous transformation is very rare.[1]

Epithelial cysts

Clinical features

Conjunctival cysts are common lesions that may be congenital or most often, acquired. They may occur spontaneously, or after surgical or nonsurgical

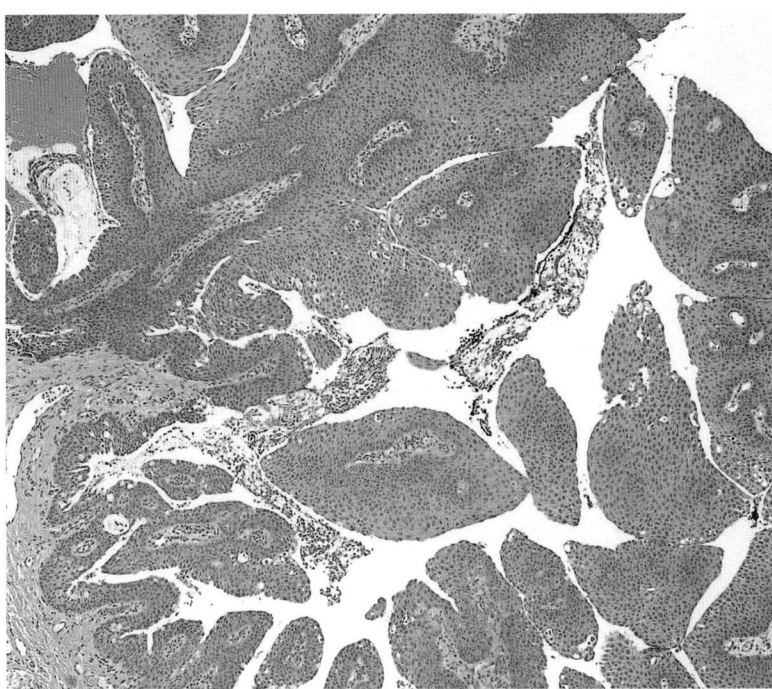

Fig. 27.12
Squamous papilloma: histology shows fronds of nonkeratinized squamous epithelium surrounding central fibrovascular cores.

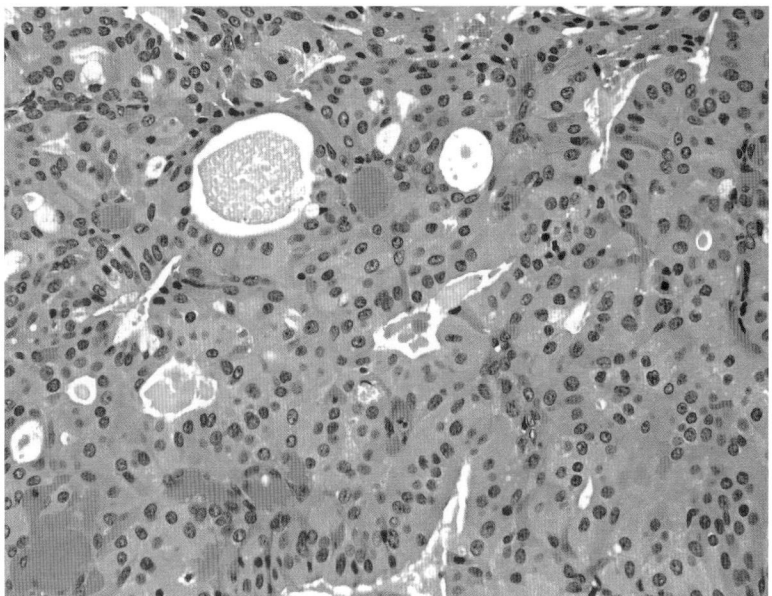

Fig. 27.14
Oncocytoma: histology of a lesion in the substantia propria of the caruncle shows large cells with eosinophilic cytoplasm arranged in glandular structures.

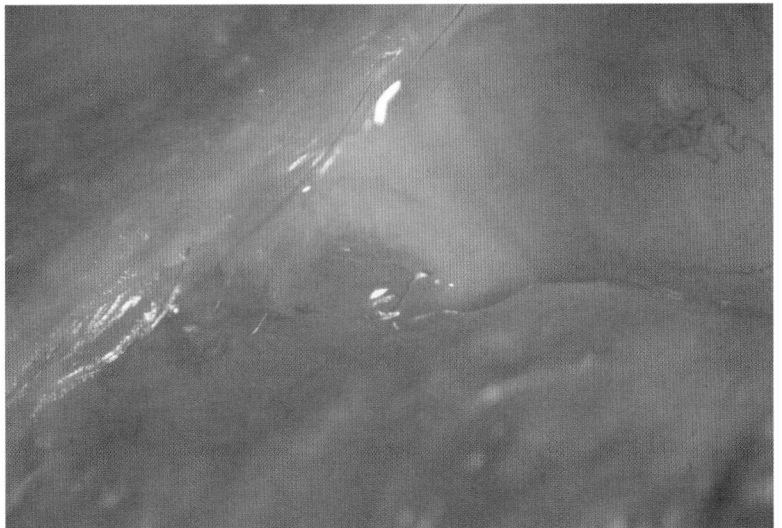

Fig. 27.13
Oncocytoma: subepithelial, fleshy orange-pink lesion in the caruncle.

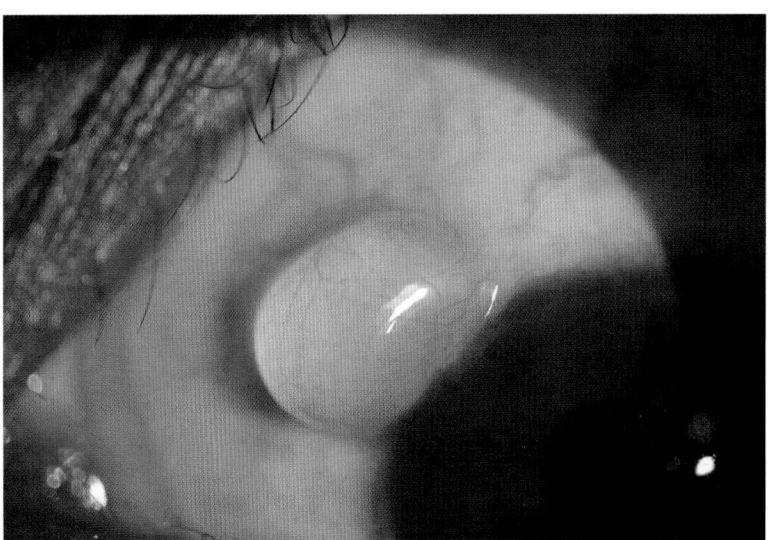

Fig. 27.15
Epithelial cyst: clinical appearance of a cyst adjacent to the limbus.

trauma.[1,2] Acquired cysts are mostly implantation (epithelial inclusion) cysts of surface epithelium. Ductal cysts, which arise from accessory lacrimal glands, are also common. Cysts appear smooth and translucent, and contain clear fluid (*Fig. 27.15*).

Histologic features

Epithelial inclusion cysts are lined by conjunctival epithelium and contain clear fluid. Ductal cysts are lined by a double layer and contain periodic acid-Schiff (PAS)-positive material (*Fig. 27.16*).

Keratotic plaque and actinic keratosis

Clinical features

Keratotic plaque and actinic keratosis are clinically indistinguishable and manifest as a flat, white plaque on the interpalpebral bulbar conjunctiva or limbus. Keratotic plaque has little to no malignant potential, whereas actinic keratosis is a precancerous lesion.[1-3]

Histologic features

Keratotic plaque is composed of acanthotic epithelium with keratinization and parakeratosis. Actinic keratosis is similar, and often occurs over a chronically inflamed pinguecula or pterygium.[1-3] There is variable cytological atypia that ranges from minimal to severe (*Fig. 27.17*).[1]

Premalignant and malignant epithelial tumors

OSSN encompasses a spectrum of conjunctival and corneal tumors ranging from low-grade dysplasia to carcinoma in situ and invasive squamous cell carcinoma.[1] Noninvasive squamous epithelial neoplasms (i.e., mild dysplasia, moderate dysplasia, severe dysplasia, and carcinoma in situ) are referred to as conjunctival intraepithelial neoplasia (CIN).

Clinical features

OSSN occurs worldwide. The incidence of squamous cell carcinoma varies based on geographic location with more than 12 cases per million per year in Uganda,[2] 1.4 per million per year in Western Australia,[2] 0.3 per million

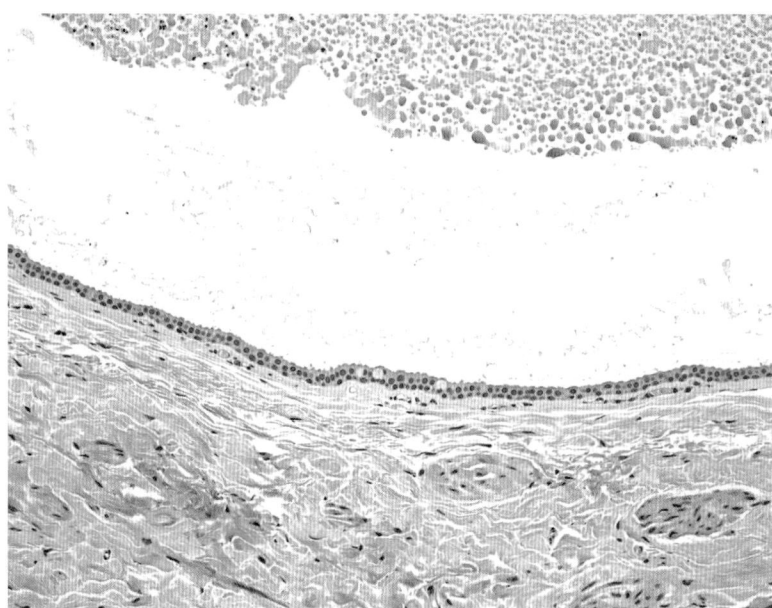

Fig. 27.16
Epithelial cyst: histology shows a cystic space filled with epithelial debris and lined by two layers of cuboidal epithelium with rare goblet cells.

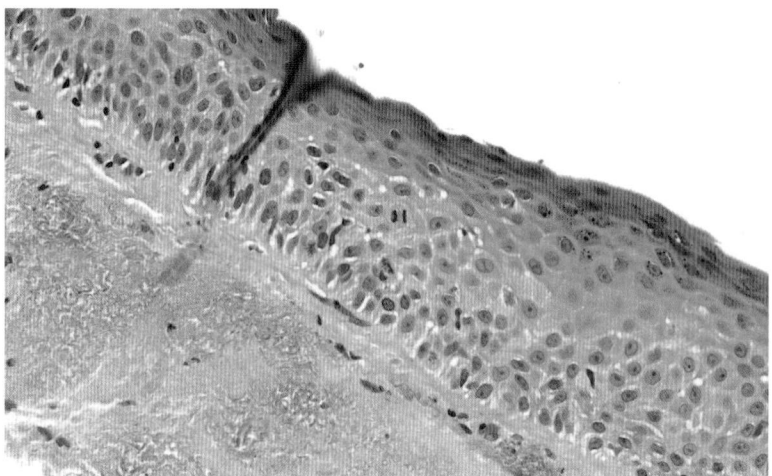

Fig. 27.17
Actinic keratosis: histology shows acanthotic epithelium with surface keratinization and mild cytological atypia with increased mitotic activity. Actinic elastotic degeneration is present in the substantia propria.

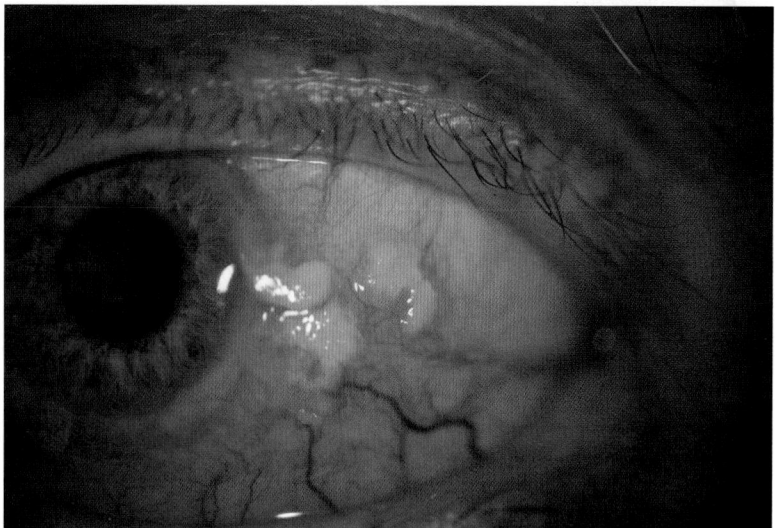

Fig. 27.18
Ocular surface squamous neoplasia (OSSN): there is a flat leukoplakic and slightly erythematous bulbar conjunctival lesion adjacent to the temporal (9 o'clock) limbus of a left eye. Dilated feeding vessels are seen.

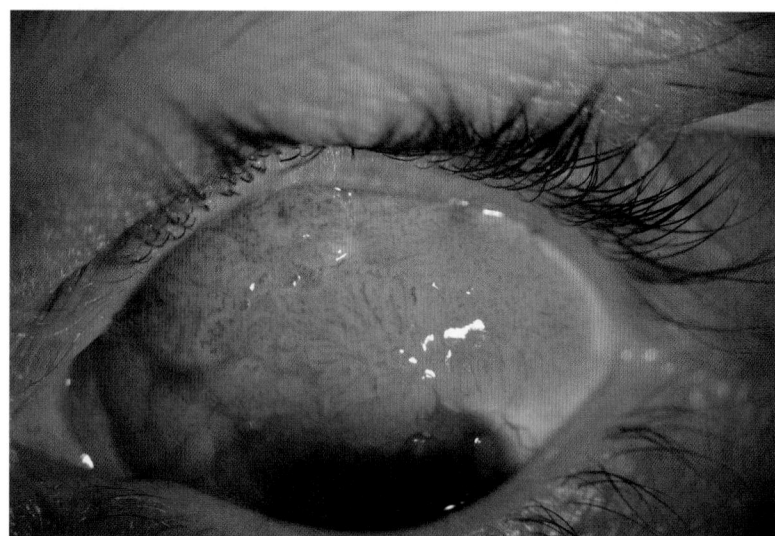

Fig. 27.19
Ocular surface squamous neoplasia (OSSN): a large, fleshy papillomatous lesion extends over the superior bulbar conjunctiva at the limbus and extends onto the cornea.

per year in the United States,[3] and less than 0.2 per million per year in the United Kingdom. Newton et al. found that the incidence of squamous cell carcinoma decreased by 49% for each 10° increase in latitude, which is related to the degree of UV sunlight exposure.[2]

OSSN usually occurs in older men in temperate climates, but both sexes are affected equally in Africa.[4] The difference is thought to be due to increased prevalence of human immunodeficiency virus (HIV) infection in the African population. In one study of 101 eyes from the United States, the median age was 71 years (range, 37–96 years) and 67% of patients were male.[5] In developed countries, it is thought that older men are at higher risk for OSSN because of greater cumulative UV light exposure.[6]

Solar UV light, particularly UVB rays, is a major risk factor.[2–4] Lesions are usually located within the interpalpebral fissure, arising from the limbus, particularly in the nasal quadrant. The nasal aspect of the limbus is particularly vulnerable because direct sunlight received at the temporal aspect of the limbus is focused nasally, where the limbal basal cells contain less melanin.[4] Other risk factors include human HPV and HIV infection. High-risk HPV types promote oncogenesis through inactivation of Rb and p53.[4] HPV-16 has been detected in conjunctival dysplasia and carcinoma.[7] However, one study showed no statistically significant association between the presence of

anti-HPV antibody and risk of conjunctival squamous neoplasia, suggesting that HPV alone may be insufficient to cause OSSN.[8] Patients affected by HIV have an 8-fold increased risk of developing OSSN. Possible mechanisms that HIV contributes to tumorigenesis include weakened tumor surveillance, potentiation of oncogenic viruses such as HPV, and inducing a state of persistent inflammation.[4] Not surprisingly, tumors that develop in HIV-positive patients are generally larger, higher grade, and more likely to recur.[9]

Clinically, CIN appears as a sharply demarcated, fleshy, sessile, or elevated lesion, most commonly at the limbus, where the stem cells are located, with conjunctival and/or corneal involvement (Figs 27.18–27.20). The lesion may appear gelatinous, leukoplakic, or papilliform.[5,6,9] Invasive squamous cell carcinoma (Fig. 27.21) is generally larger and more elevated than CIN, but it may be difficult to distinguish one from the other. It is gray-white and exophytic, usually surrounded by inflamed conjunctiva. Rarely, tumors may demonstrate a diffuse growth pattern that mimics chronic conjunctivitis.

OSSN is considered a low-grade malignancy. Lesions are usually confined to the ocular surface, but can recur and infrequently metastasize. Reported recurrence rates are 17% to 24% for dysplasia and 30% to 41% for squamous cell carcinoma.[5] Most recurrences are confined to the ocular surface,

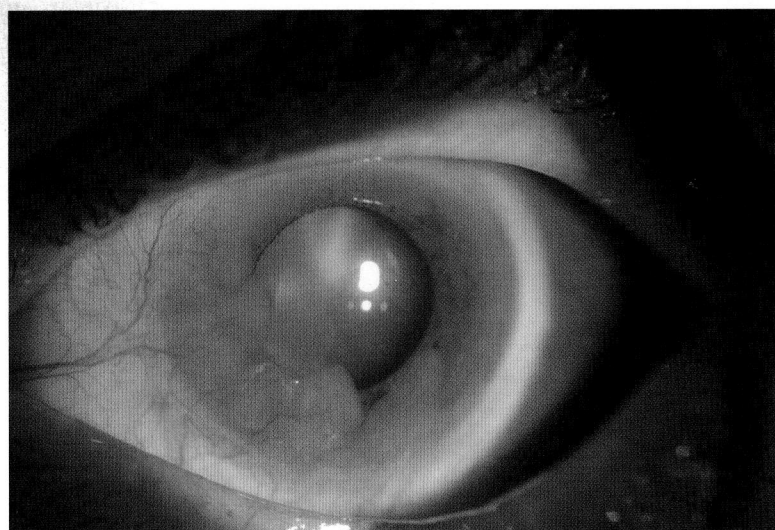

Fig. 27.20
Ocular surface squamous neoplasia (OSSN): an irregular, gray-white opacity of the corneal epithelium with prominent vascularization extends from 4 o'clock to 12 o'clock. The conjunctiva at the limbus inferiorly appears irregular and gelatinous. This patient had dysplasia and squamous cell carcinoma.

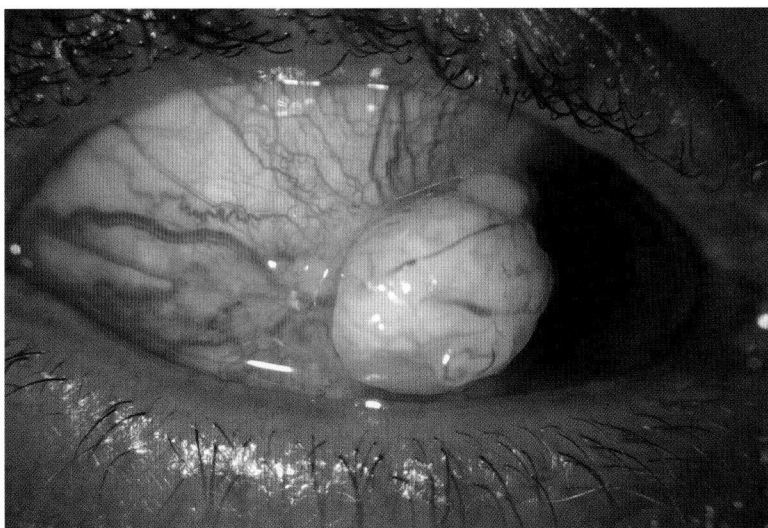

Fig. 27.21
Squamous cell carcinoma: a large, white exophytic mass with large feeder vessels is present at the temporal (3 o'clock) limbus of a right eye, surrounded by inflamed conjunctiva.

and can be treated locally or with excision. This is thought to be due to the difficulty in determining tumor edges and margins.[10] Factors associated with higher risk of recurrence in OSSN include a higher T category, particularly T3 (tumor invades adjacent structures, excluding orbit) and T4 (tumor invades orbit with or without further extension) using the American Joint Committee on Cancer – TNM (AJCC-TNM) staging system (*Table 27.2*). T category is also an important prognostic indicator of poor outcome.[5,10] Larger tumor size of at least 2 cm and diffuse growth pattern also increase the risk of recurrent disease.[10]

Intraocular invasion is rare, but can occur in older patients who had multiple excisions for one or more recurrences of squamous cell carcinoma near the limbus.[11] Tumors can also invade into the orbit. Metastatic conjunctival squamous cell carcinoma is extremely rare, occurring in advanced neglected cases.

Histologic features

Definitive diagnosis is based on histopathological examination of a biopsy. However, other approaches have been explored, such as vital staining,

Table 27.2

Carcinoma of the conjunctiva: definition of tumor, lymph node, metastasis (TNM) staging

Pathological and clinical staging	
Primary tumor (T)	
TX	Primary tumor cannot be assessed
T0	No evidence of primary tumor
Tis	Carcinoma in situ
T1	Tumor ≤5 mm greatest dimension
T2	Tumor >5 mm great dimension, without invasion of adjacent structures
T3	Tumor invades adjacent structures, excluding orbit
T4	Tumor invades orbit with or without further extension
T4a	Tumor invades orbital soft tissues without bone invasion
T4b	Tumor invades bone
T4c	Tumor invades adjacent paranasal sinuses
T4d	Tumor invades brain
Regional lymph nodes (N)	
NX	Regional lymph nodes cannot be assessed
N0	No regional lymph node metastasis
N1	Regional lymph node metastasis
Distant metastasis (M)	
MX	Distant metastasis cannot be assessed
M0	No distant metastasis
M1	Distant metastasis

Ref: AJCC-UICC Ophthalmic Oncology Task Force. Carcinoma of the conjunctiva. In: Edge S.E., Byrd D.R., Carducci M.A., Compton C.A., eds. AJCC Cancer Staging Manual. 7th ed. New York, NY: Springer; 2009:531–533.

exfoliative cytology, impression cytology, and high-frequency ultrasonography. In some studies, topical application of methylene blue and 1% toluidine blue had a high sensitivity for the detection of OSSN when performed with clinical examination.[6] Exfoliative cytology[12,13] and impression cytology[14] may be helpful adjuncts for diagnosis of OSSN, especially in patients who refuse biopsy. By impression cytology, cellular features of OSSN include keratinized dysplastic cells often accompanied by hyperkeratosis, syncytial-like groupings, and nonkeratinized dysplastic cells. Invasive squamous cell carcinomas may show significant keratinization and greater degree of inflammation, or little evidence of keratinization and presence of one or more macronucleoli. However, because considerable overlap exists between intraepithelial and invasive squamous lesions, cytological methods do not reliably distinguish intraepithelial disease from invasive lesions.[14] High-frequency ultrasonography may be helpful to assess the extent of OSSN for local invasion prior to surgery.[15]

Dysplastic lesions (CIN) are classified as mild, moderate, or severe dysplasia based on the extent of epithelial involvement. Dysplastic changes originate in the basal layers and extend toward the surface, with mild, moderate, and severe dysplasia involving the lower one-third, up to two-thirds, and greater than two-thirds of the epithelial thickness, respectively. Mitotic figures are frequent and may be atypical. The involved epithelium is thickened and sharply demarcated from the adjacent normal-appearing conjunctival epithelium. Some lesions may have fronds of proliferating blood vessels and connective tissues, mimicking sessile papilloma.

Carcinoma in situ shows total loss of normal cellular maturation with cytological atypia (*Figs 27.22* and *27.23*). Surface keratinization may be present, and mitotic figures can be seen in all layers of the epithelium. Invasive squamous cell carcinoma has similar cytological features to carcinoma in situ, but has invaded through the basement membrane into the conjunctival substantia propria. It is characterized by lobules, nests, and cords of atypical squamous cells with individual cell dyskeratosis and variable degrees of keratinization (*Figs 27.24* and *27.25*). Mitotic activity is

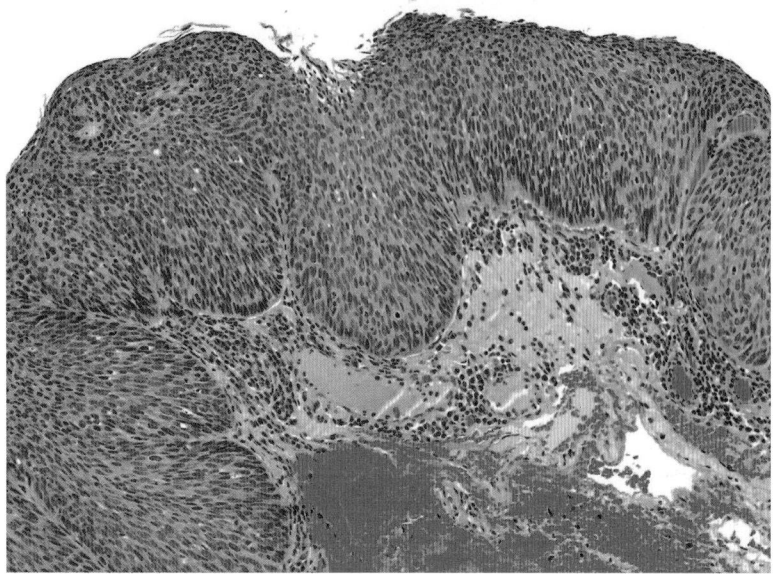

Fig. 27.22
Ocular surface squamous neoplasia (OSSN), carcinoma in situ: histology shows acanthosis with dysplasia affecting the full thickness of the epithelium. Chronic inflammation is present at the base of the lesion.

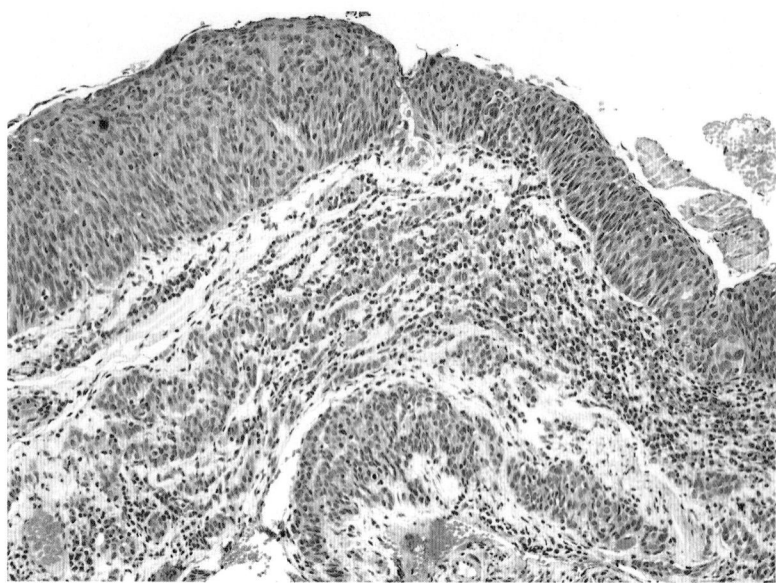

Fig. 27.24
Squamous cell carcinoma: histology shows invasion of the conjunctiva substantia propria by nests and cords of poorly differentiated tumor cells. No significant keratinization is seen.

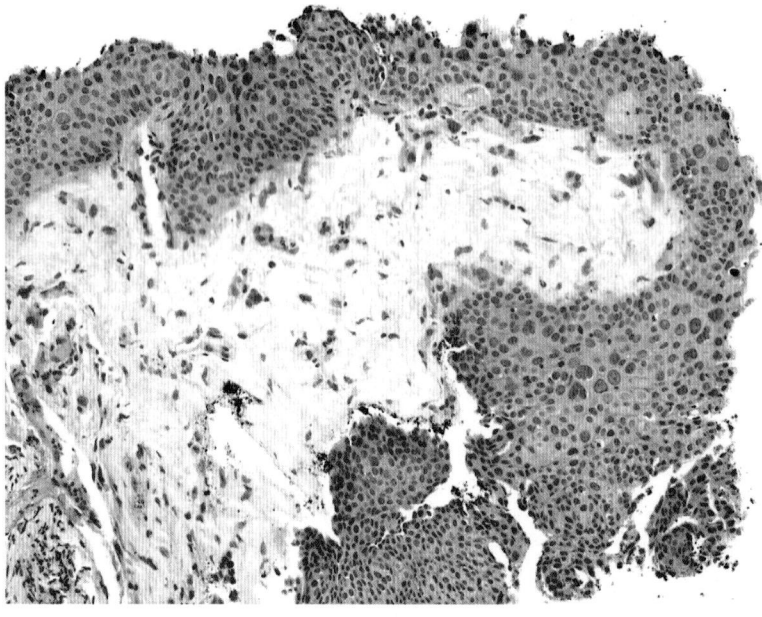

Fig. 27.23
Ocular surface squamous neoplasia (OSSN), carcinoma in situ: histology shows full-thickness dysplasia. There is marked cytological atypia with nuclear enlargement, pleomorphism, and hyperchromasia.

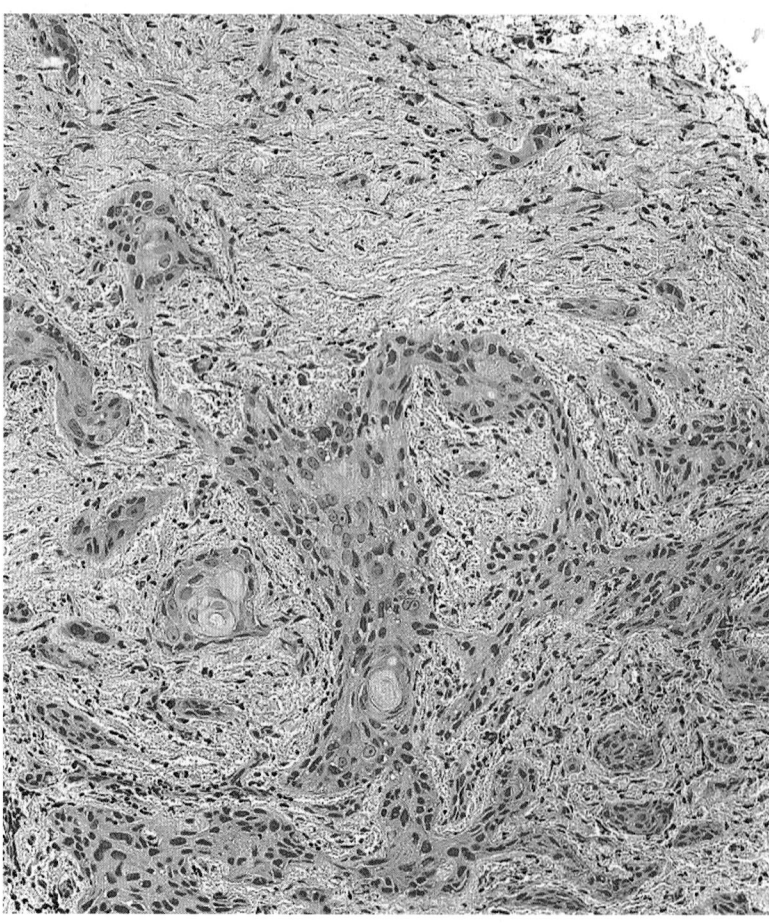

Fig. 27.25
Squamous cell carcinoma: medium power view of the invasive component shows marked solar elastosis of the substantia propria and keratinization of tumor cells.

usually low, and atypical mitotic figures may be seen. Ohara and colleagues, using immunohistochemistry for Ki-67 proliferation index, showed that dysplasia (CIN) and squamous cell carcinoma have significantly higher proliferation compared with normal. Additionally, sebaceous gland carcinoma, an important differential diagnosis, has a significantly higher proliferation index compared with squamous cell carcinoma.[16] Immunohistochemical stains for adipophilin and androgen receptor may also be helpful in differentiating sebaceous gland carcinoma from squamous cell carcinoma.[6] In darkly pigmented patients, OSSN may be pigmented because of abnormal proliferation of melanocytes, simulating melanoma. OSSN of the cornea typically occurs as extension of a limbal lesion; isolated corneal involvement is rare.[17]

Three variants of squamous cell carcinoma deserve special mention because of more aggressive biological behavior compared to conventional squamous cell carcinoma. These variants may invade the eyeball or orbital tissue or metastasize. Mucoepidermoid carcinoma is composed of an admixture of epidermoid cells, intermediate cells, and mucous-producing cells that stain positively with special stains for mucopolysaccharides. Spindle cell carcinoma is composed of infiltrating spindled cells with oval vesicular nuclei,

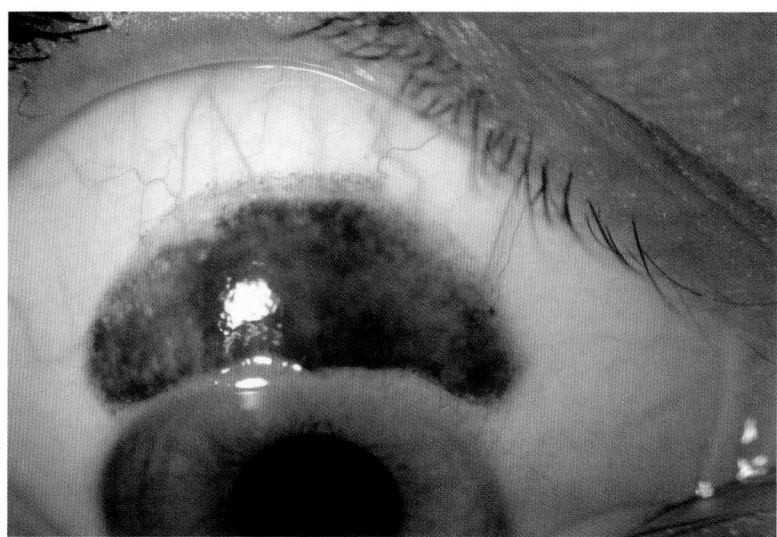

Fig. 27.26
Conjunctival nevus: there is a pigmented lesion on the superior bulbar conjunctiva. Note the cysts within the lesion.

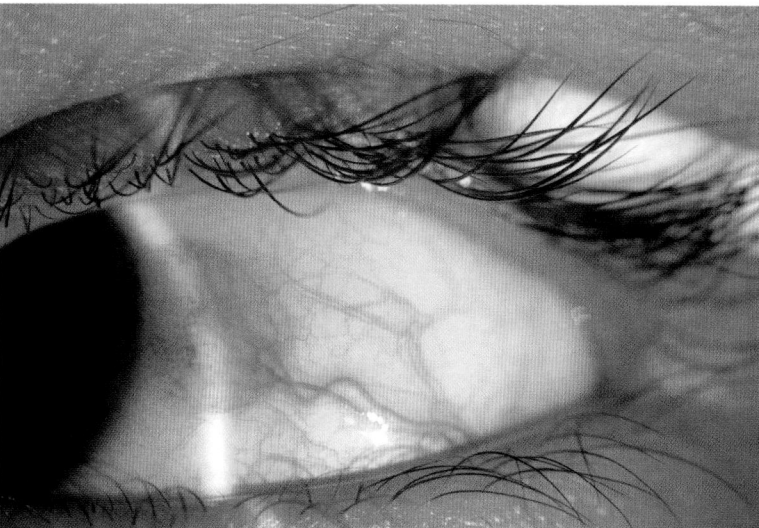

Fig. 27.27
Conjunctival nevus: a circumscribed tan lesion is on the temporal bulbar conjunctiva of a left eye. Prominent feeder vessels, as seen here, may be present in one-third of conjunctival nevi.

and large nucleoli. The overlying epithelium is acanthotic with variable degrees of dysplasia. By immunohistochemistry, spindle cells are immunoreactive to keratin. Adenoid squamous carcinoma has foci of pseudoglandular spaces due to acantholysis of neoplastic squamous cells. Extracellular hyaluronic acid is present, and intracellular mucin is absent.[18]

Melanocytic tumors

Most pigmented conjunctival lesions are derived from melanocytes. In this section, we will discuss conjunctival nevus, a common conjunctival tumor, as well as complexion-associated melanosis, PAM, a potential precursor of melanoma, and malignant melanoma. Other causes of conjunctival pigmentation should be considered in the differential diagnosis, including aggregation of melanophages in the substantia propria; some systemic diseases, such as Addison disease or ochronosis; use of certain medications, such as tetracycline or topic epinephrine; or deposition of metals, such as silver (argyrosis).

Conjunctival nevus

Clinical features

Conjunctival nevus is the most common melanocytic tumor of the conjunctiva, comprising 23% to 29% of conjunctival tumors in several large series.[1,2] Conjunctival nevi may be divided into congenital (appearing within the first 6 months of life) or acquired (appearing more than 6 months after birth) types.

In one large series of 410 conjunctival nevi,[2] the mean age is 32 years with a wide range of 2–93 years. The majority of patients are Caucasian, and there is equal sex predilection. Most lesions are located on the bulbar conjunctiva (72%) (Figs 27.26–27.28), caruncle (15%), or plica semilunaris (11%). Nevi are rarely found in the fornix, tarsal conjunctiva, or within the cornea; therefore, pigmented lesions in these areas should raise suspicion for PAM or melanoma. Conjunctival nevus most commonly develops near the limbus.[1,2] The most common clinical presentation is the appearance of a spot on the eye. Pain is very rare.

Clinically, the tumor is most commonly brown, and less often tan or nonpigmented. Intralesional cysts are present in the majority of lesions. Feeder vessels and intrinsic vessels, which may be prominent in conjunctival melanoma, can be seen in approximately one-third of cases.[2]

Histologic features

Histologically, conjunctival nevi are described as junctional, compound, or subepithelial, which may be considered as stages of evolution.[1] Junctional

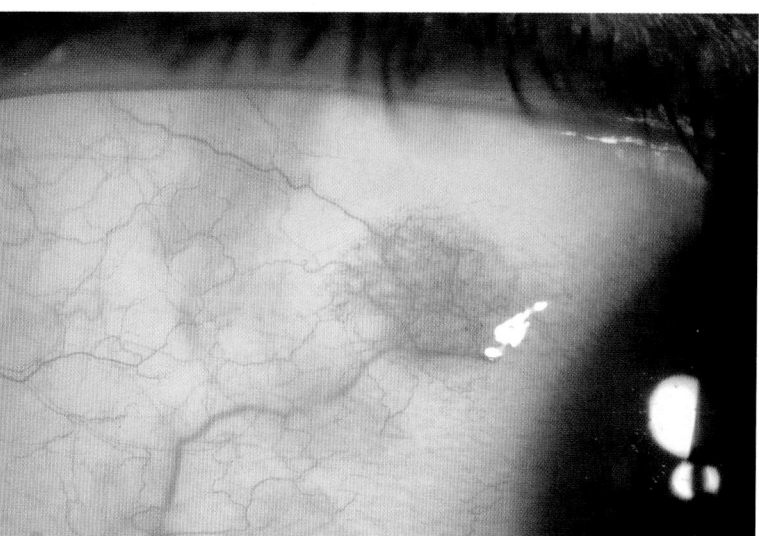

Fig. 27.28
Conjunctival nevus: a circumscribed, lightly pigmented lesion with intralesional cysts is on the bulbar conjunctiva.

nevi are found only early in life and have nests of nevus cells along the interface of the epithelium and substantia propria. Junctional nevus cells generally have abundant cytoplasm. As intraepithelial nevus cells begin dropping off into the substantia propria, dragging surface epithelium with them, nevus cells and intraepithelial inclusions expand the substantia propria. The nevus becomes thicker clinically. A nevus with cells in the epithelium and substantia propria is a compound nevus (Fig. 27.29). The intraepithelial component of a compound nevus should not extend much beyond the lateral edges of the subepithelial component. The presence of melanocytes individually or in nests far beyond the lateral margins of the subepithelial component should raise suspicion for intraepithelial atypical melanocytic hyperplasia, also known as PAM with atypia, which is a precursor lesion for melanoma. Over time, the nevus may become disconnected from the overlying epithelium and reside completely in the substantia propria. This type of nevus is designated as subepithelial nevus (Fig. 27.30) and is analogous to intradermal nevus of the skin. Compared with intraepithelial nevus cells, those in the substantia propria generally have less cytoplasm, especially toward the base, which reflects maturation. Some nevus cells may contain intranuclear cytoplasmic inclusions. Binucleated and multinucleated cells may be identified, and are

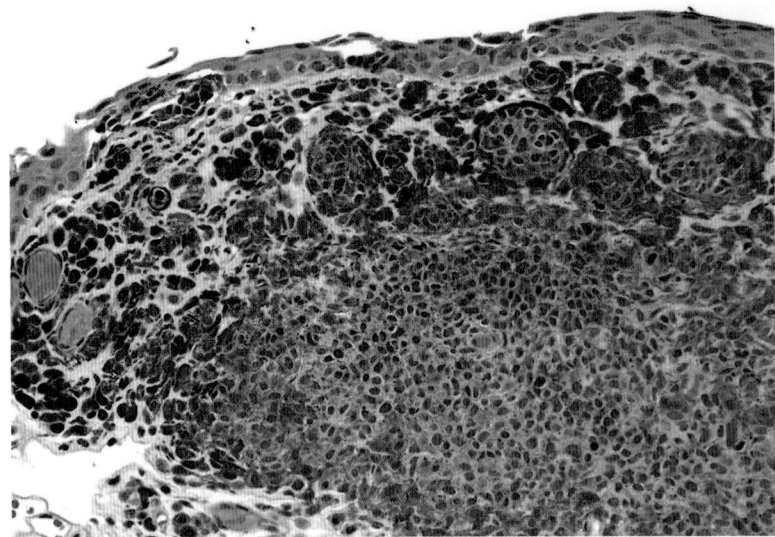

Fig. 27.29
Compound nevus: junctional nests and involvement of the substantia propria is evident.

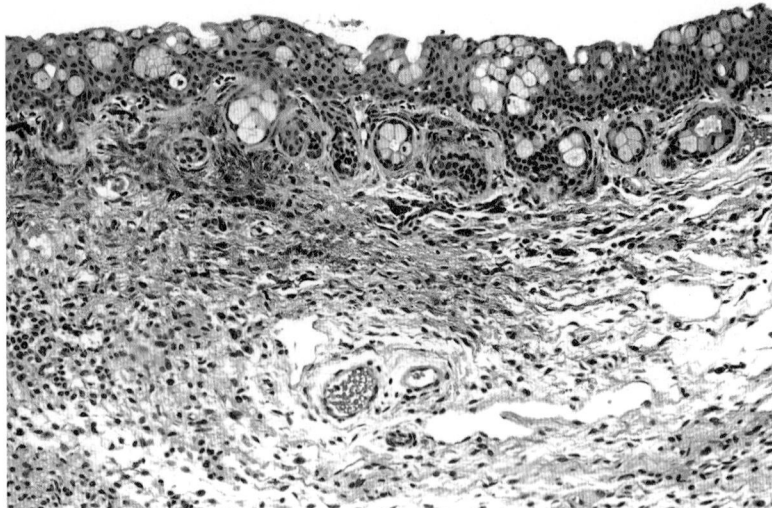

Fig. 27.31
Combined nevus: histology shows nests of common nevus cells and more pigmented spindle and dendritic cells.

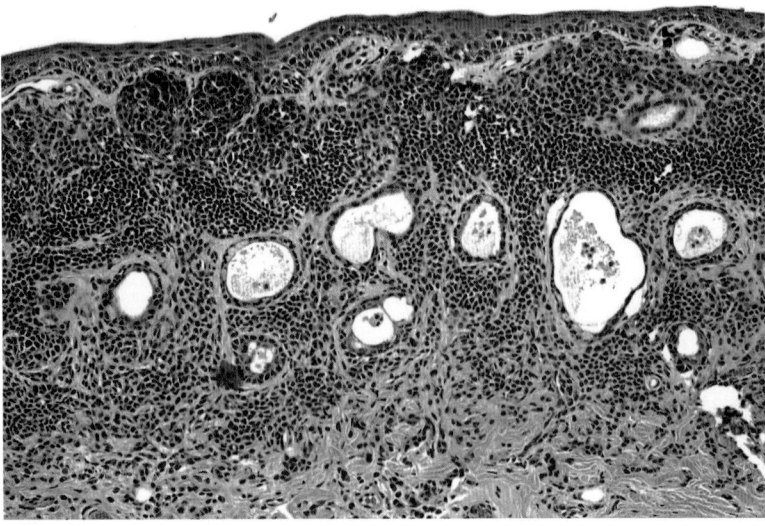

Fig. 27.30
Subepithelial nevus: nevus cells are present in the substantia propria without junctional nests. Epithelial cysts are present within the lesion. Note how there is increased melanin pigmentation of the superficial nevus cells compared to those toward the base.

not indicative of malignancy. Two distinct types of nevus cells, balloon cells and spindle cells, can be seen in otherwise typical conjunctival nevi. Balloon cell nevi have rarely been reported.[3] Occasionally, conjunctival combined nevi are encountered.[4]

Spitz nevus

Clinical features

Conjunctival Spitz nevus is a very rare melanocytic lesion that usually occurs in children and adolescents.[1,2] The lesion is nonpigmented and grows rapidly, raising suspicion for melanoma, although melanoma is extremely uncommon in children.

Histologic features

In contrast to typical conjunctival nevus, which may contain spindle cells within the epithelium that are oriented parallel to the surface, Spitz nevus

is composed of fascicles of spindle nevus cells that are usually oriented perpendicular to the surface and are uniformly and symmetrically arranged. Mitotic figures or brisk expression of MIB-1[2] in Spitz nevi reflect rapid clinical growth and do not indicate malignancy.

Blue nevus

Clinical features

Conjunctival blue and cellular blue nevi are rare lesions that arise from neural crest cells that do not reach the epithelial surface during embryonic migration. Clinically, the lesion is sharply demarcated and appears brown or black.[1] Lesions may be unifocal or multifocal and occur at any site of the conjunctiva.[2] There is only one reported case of malignant melanoma arising from blue nevus.[3]

Histologic features

Conjunctival blue nevus is composed of uniformly pigmented spindle-shaped cells in the substantia propria. Dendritic melanocytes are also present. Cellular blue nevus has lightly pigmented nodules of uniform spindle cells surrounded by heavily pigmented dendritic melanocytes.[3] When elements of blue nevus are present with a common acquired or congenital nevus of the conjunctiva, it is termed combined nevus (*Fig. 27.31*).[4]

Inflamed juvenile conjunctival nevus

Clinical features

Inflamed juvenile conjunctival nevus is a benign, usually amelanotic, juxtalimbal lesion in children and adolescents (*Fig. 27.32*). It may grow rapidly, raising concern for malignancy. Patients often have history of allergy, allergic conjunctivitis, or vernal conjunctivitis.[1] This association is supported by one study that showed increased expression of nerve growth factor, eosinophils, and mast cells in inflamed juvenile nevus and modulation of eosinophil properties by lesional fibroblasts, partly through nerve growth factor.[2] Intralesional cysts may be seen clinically.

Histologic features

Inflamed juvenile conjunctival nevi have intraepithelial and stromal melanocytic nests with solid and cystic inclusions, goblet cells, and chronic inflammatory infiltrates with eosinophils and plasma cells (*Fig. 27.33*).[1,3] Rapid growth of a clinically inflamed nevus indicates inflammatory infiltration and cystic enlargement rather than malignant transformation.

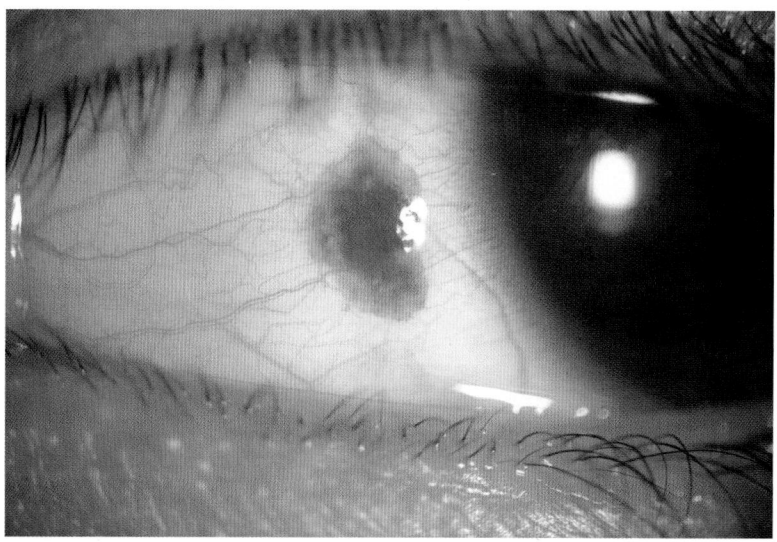

Fig. 27.32
Inflamed juvenile nevus: partially pigmented inflamed juvenile nevus on the bulbar conjunctiva at 9 o'clock. Intralesional cysts are seen.

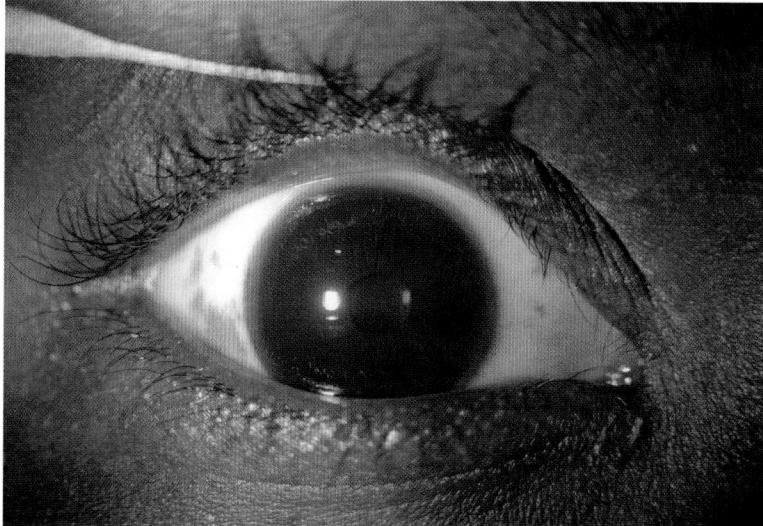

Fig. 27.34
Congenital melanosis oculi: clinical view of the right eye showing slate gray pigmentation of the sclera.

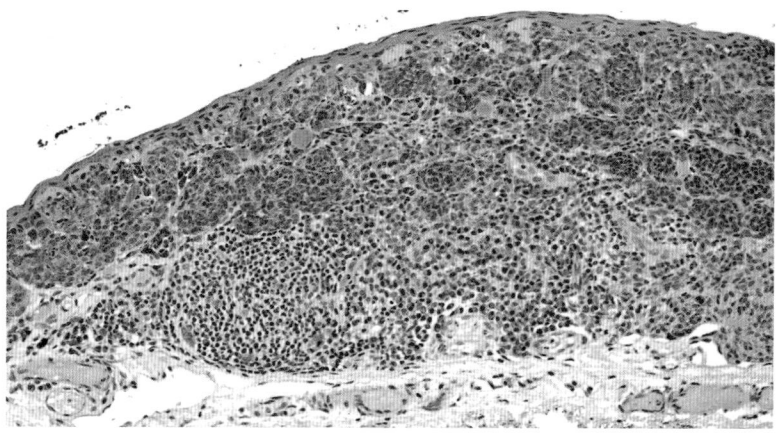

Fig. 27.33
Inflamed juvenile nevus: nests of nevus cells are admixed with lymphocytes and plasma cells.

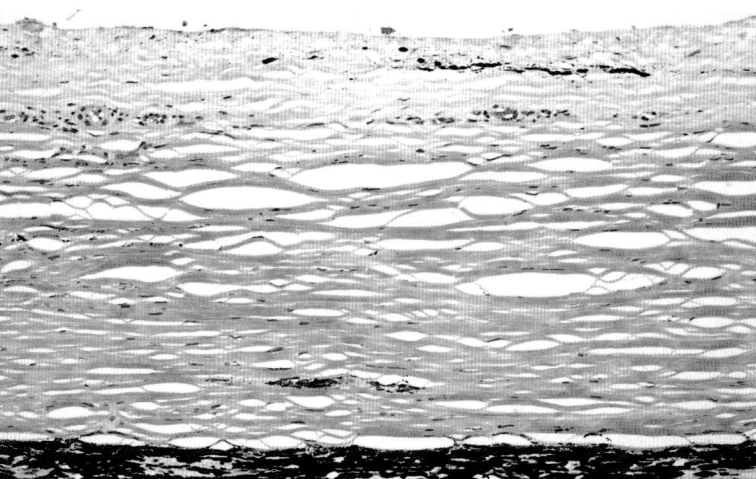

Fig. 27.35
Congenital melanosis oculi: pigmented dendritic melanocytes are present within episcleral and scleral tissues. The choroid is also heavily pigmented.

Congenital melanosis oculi (congenital ocular melanocytosis)

Clinical features

Congenital melanosis oculi or congenital ocular melanocytosis is characterized by flat, spiculated slate-gray pigmentation of the sclera sometimes surrounding episcleral lymphatics and blood vessels (*Fig. 27.34*). The periocular skin, orbit, meninges, and soft palate may be affected.[1] Although the conjunctiva is not involved, the lesion is included here because it is considered in the clinical differential diagnosis of conjunctival pigmented lesions. When periocular skin is involved, the condition is called nevus of Ota or oculodermal melanocytosis. Patients with congenital melanosis oculi have approximately 1 in 400 risk of developing uveal melanoma; however, conjunctival melanoma has not been described in these patients.[2]

Histologic features

Pigmented dendritic melanocytes are present in the episcleral and scleral tissues (*Fig. 27.35*). The conjunctiva is not involved.

Complexion-associated conjunctival pigmentation (racial melanosis)

Clinical features

Complexion-associated melanosis is a common, bilateral condition characterized by diffuse or patchy, flat pigmentation of the conjunctiva in patients with dark skin complexion, including African-Americans, Hispanics, Asians, and whites.[1] The pigmentation is concentrated around the limbus and may involve the cornea. It rarely involves the fornix or palpebral conjunctiva. The distribution of pigmentation may be asymmetric, but this should raise suspicion for PAM, a unilateral, potentially premalignant condition (see next section).

Histologic features

Histologically, there is hyperpigmentation of basal conjunctiva squamous epithelial cells without melanocytic hyperplasia or cytological atypia.[1]

Primary acquired melanosis

PAM is a clinical term used to describe localized or diffuse flat pigmentation of the conjunctiva.[1,2] Lesions are primary because they cannot be attributed to a known cause, such as Addison disease. Lesions are acquired rather than congenital, as they usually occur in middle-aged or older individuals rather than in children, and occur in the conjunctiva, not the episclera, sclera, or uveal tract as those seen in congenital ocular melanosis.[3,4]

Several terms have been previously used to describe what is now referred to PAM, including senile freckle or lentigo melanosis, precancerous melanosis, benign acquired melanosis, primary idiopathic acquired melanosis, and intraepithelial melanocytic hyperplasia.[5,6] The terminology has created

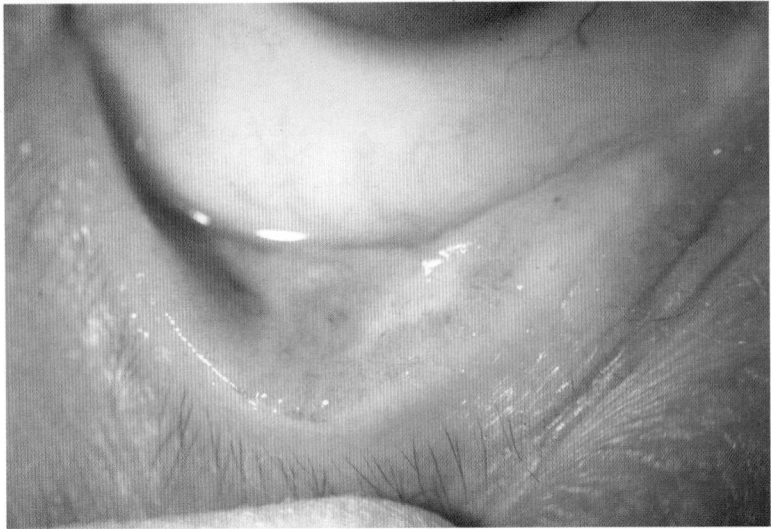

Fig. 27.36
Primary acquired melanosis (PAM): clinical view of PAM on the lower tarsal conjunctiva that appears like sprinkled cinnamon.

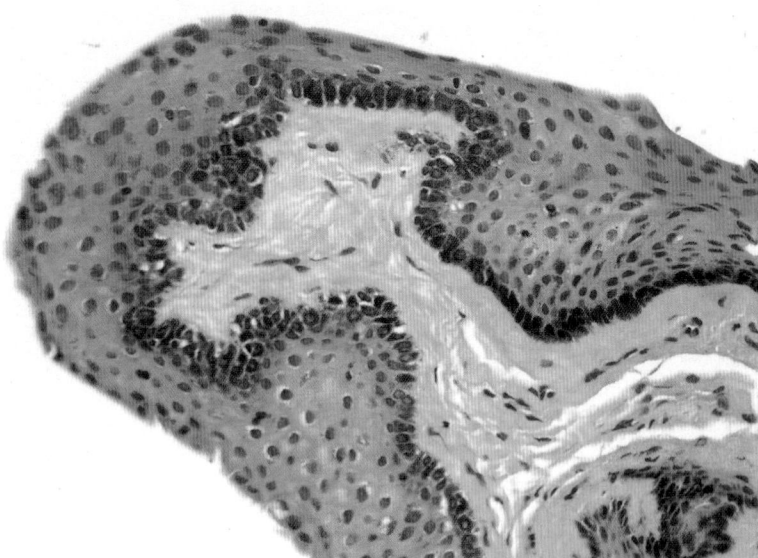

Fig. 27.37
Primary acquired melanosis (PAM) without atypia: there is uniform pigmentation of the basal layer of the epithelium without melanocyte atypia.

challenges because PAM comprises a set of lesions with variable clinical behavior. Most recently, Damato and Coupland[7] proposed the term 'conjunctival melanocytic intraepithelial neoplasia (C-MIN)' without and with atypia in place of PAM without and with atypia. This term has not gained widespread use. C-MIN without atypia, defined by intraepithelial melanocytic proliferation confined to the basal layer of the epithelium without cytological features of atypia, is problematic because it is unclear whether this truly represents neoplasia or melanocytic hyperplasia. As the WHO continues to use the term PAM as a histologic designation in the classification of conjunctival melanocytic proliferations,[2] and ophthalmologists are familiar with the clinical implications of PAM, we strongly recommend the continued use of the term PAM without or with atypia to describe these lesions.

Clinical features

PAM without atypia and PAM with atypia cannot be distinguished clinically.[5] PAM is unilateral flat, brown pigmentation of the conjunctiva in Caucasian patients (*Fig. 27.36*), typically middle-aged or elderly. It may occur in young adults, but not in children.[4] When observed over time, lesions wax and wane – they enlarge and regress; darken and lighten. Lesions diagnosed histologically as PAM without atypia do not progress to melanoma. In contrast, almost half of PAM with atypia lesions progress to melanoma. In one study, the median interval between biopsy diagnosis of PAM with atypia and biopsy diagnosis of melanoma was 2.5 years.[5] PAM may involve the cornea, and in such cases, should be scraped off the surface of Bowman layer to preserve the natural boundary against tumor penetration into the corneal stroma.[1]

Pathogenesis and histologic features

PAM without atypia is characterized by melanin pigmentation of the conjunctival epithelium with or without hyperplasia of cytologically benign melanocytes (*Fig. 27.37*).

Lesions that feature cytologically atypical melanocytes are designated PAM with atypia. When evaluating the histology of PAM with atypia, the pathologist must consider both cytological and architectural features. Cytologically, atypical melanocytes have different shapes and sizes, and tend to fall apart from one another and from adjacent epithelium. Cells may be small and round, spindled, or epithelioid. Small- to medium-size cells usually have high N/C ratio, and small to medium hyperchromatic nuclei without nucleoli. Epithelioid cells have large nuclei, discernible cytoplasm, and sometimes visible nucleoli or vesicular features. Architecturally, atypical melanocytes may be distributed along the epithelial basement membrane (basilar hyperplasia pattern), segregated into nests along the epithelial basement membrane, or dispersed as intraepithelial nests or individual cells upward into the epithelium (pagetoid spread) (*Fig. 27.38*). In some areas,

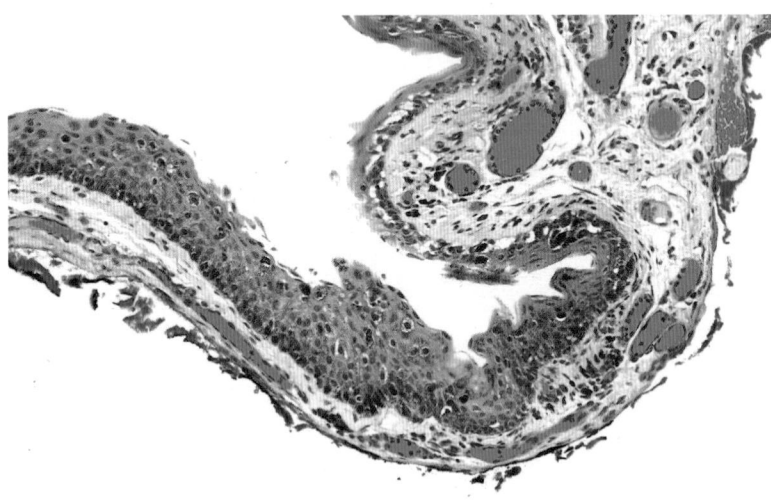

Fig. 27.38
Primary acquired melanosis (PAM) with atypia: large, hyperchromatic atypical melanocytes are confluent along the basal layer. In some areas upward migration of atypical melanocytes is seen (pagetoid spread).

atypical melanocytes may completely replace the epithelium (analogous to cutaneous melanoma in situ) (*Fig. 27.39*).[3,8]

PAM with atypia is heterogeneous with variable risk of recurrence or progression to invasive melanoma. For example, Folberg et al.[5] found that progression to melanoma was more frequent if basilar hyperplasia was not the dominant histologic pattern (90% progressed) or if epithelioid cells were present (75% progressed). Histologic scoring systems have been proposed that stratify PAM with atypia into groups with low or high risk of recurrence, invasion, and metastasis.[9,10] Lesions are scored based on architectural and cytological features without or with Ki-67 immunostaining. Sugiura et al.[3] showed that the features associated with low risk of invasion or metastasis were lesions with single cell lentiginous growth pattern, and composed of small- to medium-size cells with high nuclear-to-cytoplasmic ratio, and small to medium hyperchromatic nuclei without nucleoli. Lesions with high risk of invasion or metastasis were characterized by epithelioid tumor cells. The architectural pattern is variable, and at least focal single cell invasion of the substantia propria is frequently identified.

Potential diagnostic pitfalls include: interpretation of bulbous projection of intraepithelial nevus cells into the substantia propria, clusters of

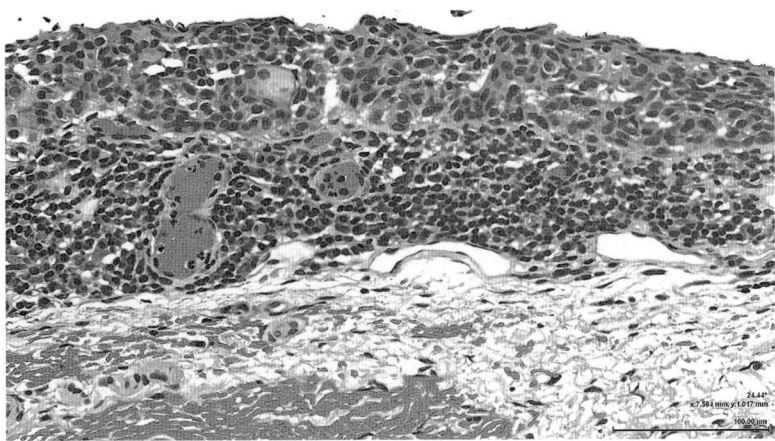

Fig. 27.39
Primary acquired melanosis (PAM) with atypia: atypical melanocytes almost completely replace the epithelium in this area. This degree of involvement could be considered by some pathologists as melanoma in situ. A bandlike chronic inflammatory infiltrate is present at the base.

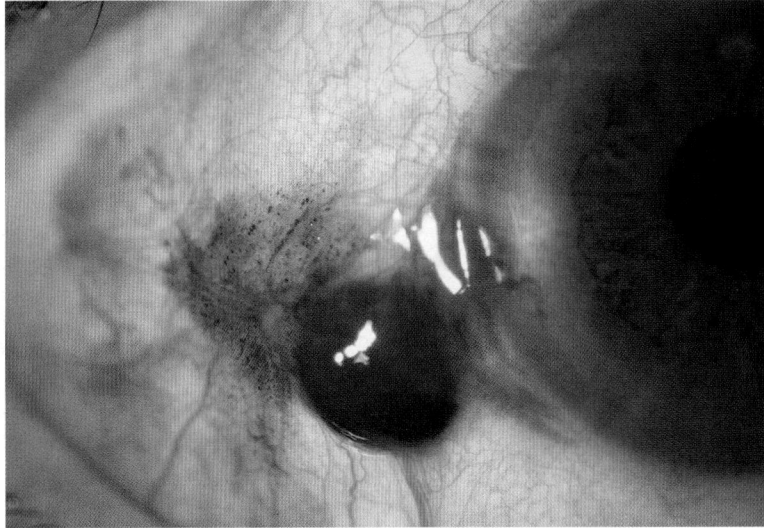

Fig. 27.40
Conjunctival melanoma: there is a melanoma of the perilimbal bulbar conjunctiva with feeder vessels entering the tumor. The large area of pigmentation of the bulbar conjunctiva surrounding the tumor likely represents PAM. Pigmentation also extends onto the corneal surface.

melanophages in the substantia propria, or involvement of pseudoglands of Henle by PAM as invasive melanoma; interpretation of tangential sections of basal hyperplasia or pigmentation of goblet cells as pagetoid spread; interpretation of pagetoid intraepithelial spread of sebaceous carcinoma as pagetoid spread of PAM.[1]

Chowers and coworkers, using immunohistochemistry for Ki-67 and proliferating cell nuclear antigen (PCNA), showed that PAM with atypia has significantly higher proliferative activity than PAM without atypia.[11] Maly et al. showed that >1% Ki-67 staining of PAM with atypia correlated with more aggressive behavior. Use of Ki-67 immunostaining may provide helpful information about the biological behavior of PAM with atypia.[9] Sharara and coworkers found significantly higher expression of HMB-45 in PAM with atypia than in PAM without atypia and also in conjunctival nevi.[12] Use of HMB-45 may be helpful for pathologists to distinguish between benign and malignant conjunctival melanocytic lesions.

Differential diagnosis

The main differential diagnoses include complexion-associated melanosis, ephelis, junctional nevus, ocular melanocytosis, and conjunctival melanoma. Complexion-associated melanosis may be distinguished clinically by its bilateral nature, and presence in darker complexioned individuals. Ephelis is a flat, unilateral pigmented lesion that occurs in the sun-exposed portions of the interpalpebral conjunctiva, and histologically identical to PAM without atypia. A flat, pigmented lesion on the tarsal conjunctiva or fornix could not be ephelis due to lack of sun exposure. The diagnosis of junctional nevus of the conjunctiva should only be made in childhood. Even so, histologic examples are exceedingly rare. Histologic features that may be helpful in distinguishing junctional nevus from PAM with atypia include the presence in the latter of pagetoid spread, pigmentation of adjacent squamous epithelial cells, and discohesiveness of melanocytes with one another and adjacent epithelium.

PAM lesions can be distinguished from ocular melanocytosis because PAM lesions are tan-brown and movable. In ocular melanocytosis, the lesion is blue-gray, immobile, and usually multifocal. Conjunctival melanoma is typically elevated or nodular, but may appear flat in its early stages, particularly when it arises from PAM with atypia.

Conjunctival melanoma

Conjunctival melanoma is a rare, unilateral tumor with a mortality rate of 23% to 30%.[1,2] It is often lumped together with uveal melanoma and referred to collectively as 'ocular melanoma'. However, these tumors have distinct clinical behaviors and histologic features, and should be approached as separate entities.

It may arise de novo or in the context of conjunctival nevus and/or PAM with atypia.

Clinical features

The reported incidence of conjunctival melanoma is 0.2 to 0.5 per million among white populations,[1,3] and it comprises 3% of ocular cancers registered by the United States Veterans Administration.[4] Similar to cutaneous melanoma, there is evidence of increased incidence of conjunctival melanoma in the United States from 1973 to 1999. This trend was seen in white men but not in white women.[3]

Population-based data have indicated that an equal number of men and women develop conjunctival melanoma,[5] but recent studies have shown a higher incidence among males.[3,6] It is more common in middle-aged and older persons, between the fourth and seventh decades of life,[5] and only a few cases have been reported in children.[7,8] Conjunctival melanoma is much less common among black and other non-white populations[3,5]; according to one study, the white-to-black ratio is 13.6 : 1.0.[9]

Ocular and oculodermal melanocytosis, cutaneous melanoma, and dysplastic nevus syndrome are not associated with conjunctival melanoma.[1]

Melanoma is typically a thickened brown, tan, or pink mass with feeder vessels and intrinsic vascularity.[10] Tumors can involve any part of the conjunctiva (Figs 27.40–27.43), as well as the caruncle, plica semilunaris, and cornea. Primary melanoma of the cornea is very rare. More commonly, corneal involvement is intraepithelial and associated with an adjacent limbal melanoma. Lesions confined to the corneal epithelium should be removed using absolute alcohol.[10] Spread of atypical melanocytes into the corneal stroma is usually due to prior excision of a limbal melanoma that used lamellar dissection of the involved cornea (lamellar keratectomy).[11]

In one study, the 10-year cumulative incidence of regional metastasis was 11% with a higher trend for tumors thicker than 2 mm.[12] Other risk factors for metastasis include involvement of the fornix, palpebral conjunctiva, or caruncle; local tumor recurrence[12]; and positive tumor margins[10].

Local recurrence is common and occurs in half of patients, usually within 5 years of treatment of the primary tumor.[1] The mean time to recurrence is 2.5 years.[1] Risk factors associated with recurrence include melanoma location (not touching the limbus) and positive resection margins on pathological examination.[10] Conjunctival melanoma may spread locally in the conjunctiva before metastasizing regionally and systemically. 'In-transit' metastases are small secondary tumor nodules thought to be caused by local lymphatic spread within the conjunctiva.[1] 'Local metastasis' due to melanoma cell dissemination during tumor excision has also been reported.[1]

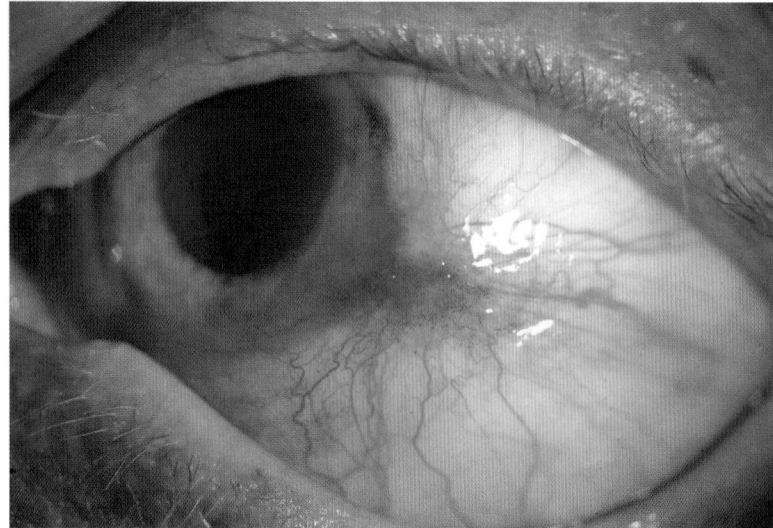

Fig. 27.41
Conjunctival melanoma: this tumor is more pink-brown with increased vascularity. The widespread pigmentation of the bulbar conjunctiva around the limbus and on the peripheral cornea likely represents PAM in this Caucasian patient.

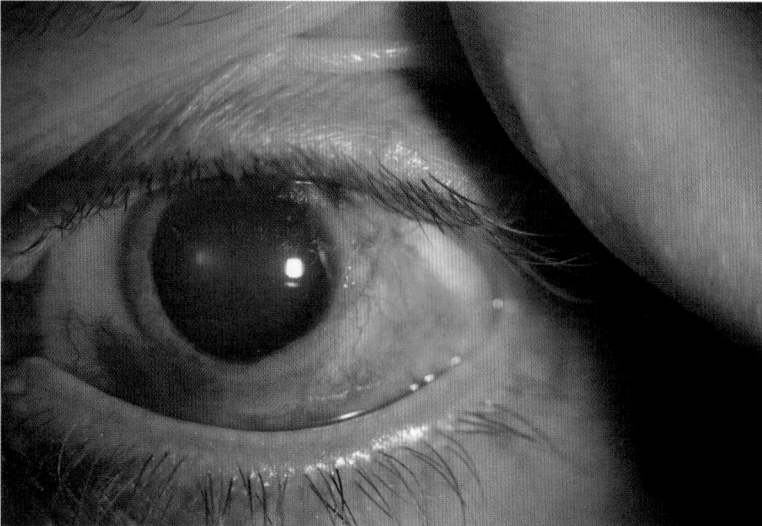

Fig. 27.42
Conjunctival melanoma: this tumor is more diffuse, surrounding the limbus for at least 180°. There is some nodularity at 3 o'clock. The tumor is relatively amelanotic with inflammation and prominent intrinsic vascularity.

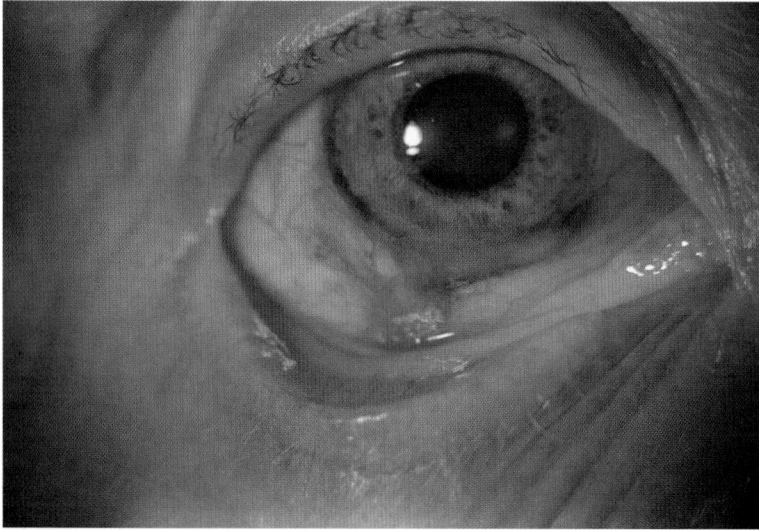

Fig. 27.43
Conjunctival melanoma: there is a melanoma involving the inferior bulbar conjunctiva, extending to the fornix.

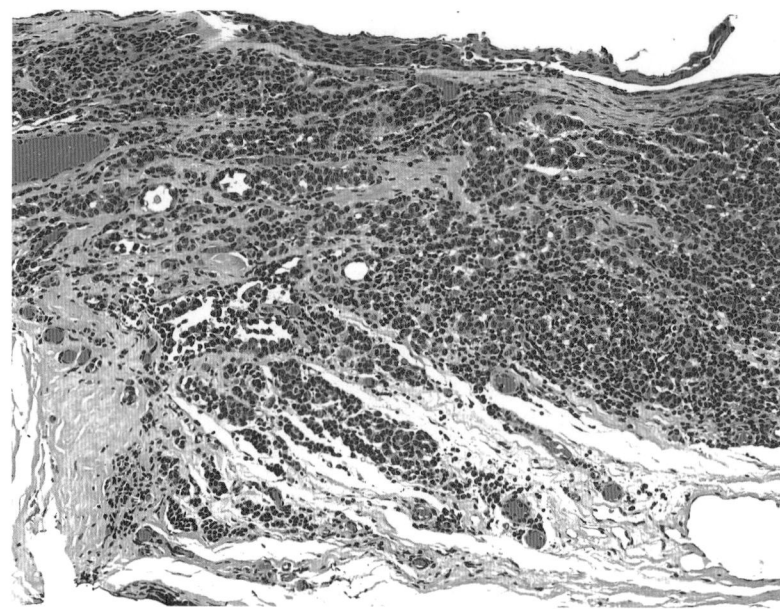

Fig. 27.44
Conjunctival melanoma: histology of *Figure 27.42*. The tumor arises in the context of primary acquired melanosis (PAM) with atypia, and shows nests of small, polyhedral, amelanotic melanoma cells invading the substantia propria. The tumor is quite vascular, and tumor nests intermingle with chronic inflammation.

Regional lymph node metastasis to parotid (preauricular) and submandibular regions occurs in 20% to 40% of patients.[1,10,13,14] Melanomas involving the nasal conjunctiva tend to metastasize to submandibular lymph nodes, whereas those involving the temporal conjunctiva tend to metastasize to the parotid (preauricular) lymph nodes.[15] Regional metastases occur at a median of 23 (range, 12–108) months after diagnosis of primary conjunctival melanoma.[15] Risk factors for regional metastasis include non-limbal location, tumor thickness >2 mm, large basal diameter, positive resection margins, orbital extension, and nodular tumor shape.[13] Sentinel lymph node biopsy has been suggested for patients with melanoma in a non-limbal location and thickness >2 mm[13]; however, its use is controversial because there is still debate over the overall survival benefit.[16] Systemic metastasis most commonly occurs in the brain, liver, and lung.

Pathogenesis and histologic features

Most tumors develop on the interpalpebral bulbar conjunctiva; however, there is no clear evidence that UV radiation causes conjunctival melanoma.

Definitive diagnosis depends on histologic examination. Most cases can be accurately diagnosed using light microscopy (*Figs 27.44–27.46*). Histologically, conjunctival melanoma may contain mixtures of four cell types: small, polyhedral; spindle; balloon; and round epithelioid cells with eosinophilic cytoplasm (*Fig. 27.47*).[1,4,17] Melanoma is often accompanied by intraepithelial PAM with atypia. Sometimes, melanomas may be associated with a conjunctival nevus. Occasionally, desmoplastic stroma may be seen.

Histologic features that predict adverse prognosis include tumor thickness[2] and size; positive surgical margins; tumor location[18]; presence of Pagetoid spread; histologic evidence of lymphatic spread[18]; and tumor cell proliferation as determined by immunohistochemistry for Ki-67. Various studies attempting to identify a critical tumor thickness that may serve as a prognostic factor for conjunctival melanoma have found values ranging from 0.8 to 4.0 mm.[1,2,10,18] Tumor thickness is measured using an ocular micrometer, calibrated to the working microscope, going from the surface of the conjunctival epithelium to the point of deepest invasion.[2] Larger tumors, greater than 10 mm, are also associated with worse prognosis.[1] Tumor location in the palpebral, conjunctiva, fornix, plica, caruncle, and lid margin are associated with higher mortality compared with bulbar melanoma.[1,18] Sex, age, and tumor origin (PAM, nevus, or de novo) are not useful prognostic indicators.[18] The pathologist's report should include information to guide the ophthalmic surgeon's treatment of the patient, particularly the adequacy of the lateral and deep margins, and tumor thickness.

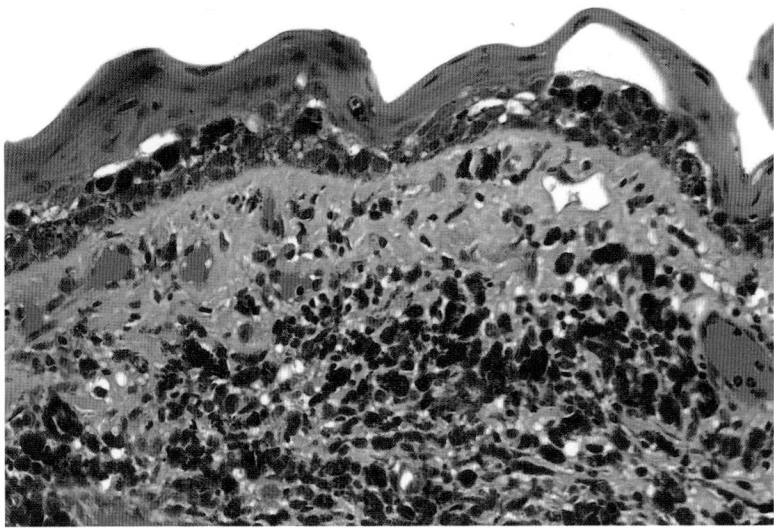

Fig. 27.45
Conjunctival melanoma: low-power view of a melanoma adjacent to the limbus (cornea is at the right of the image). Note how the intraepithelial component extends well beyond the subepithelial part of the tumor.

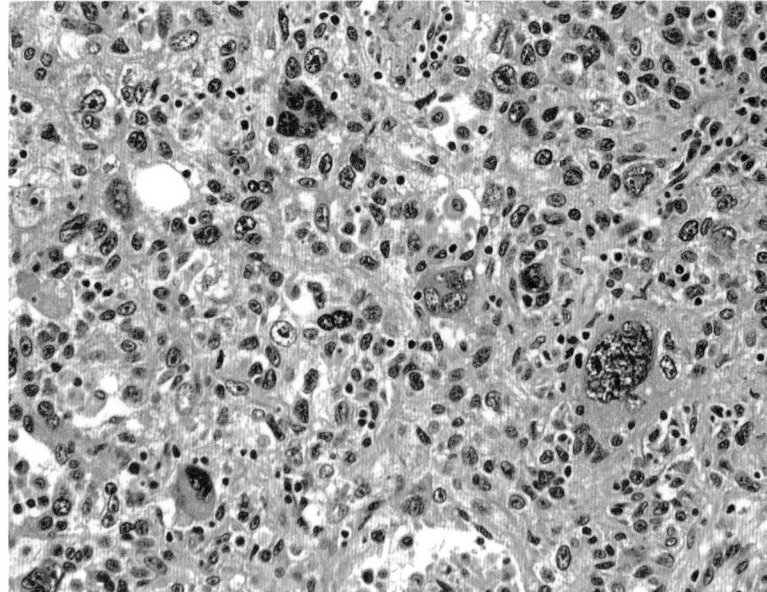

Fig. 27.47
Conjunctival melanoma: in this example, there are large, pleomorphic epithelioid cells and tumor giant cells with abundant eosinophilic cytoplasm and nuclei with prominent nucleoli.

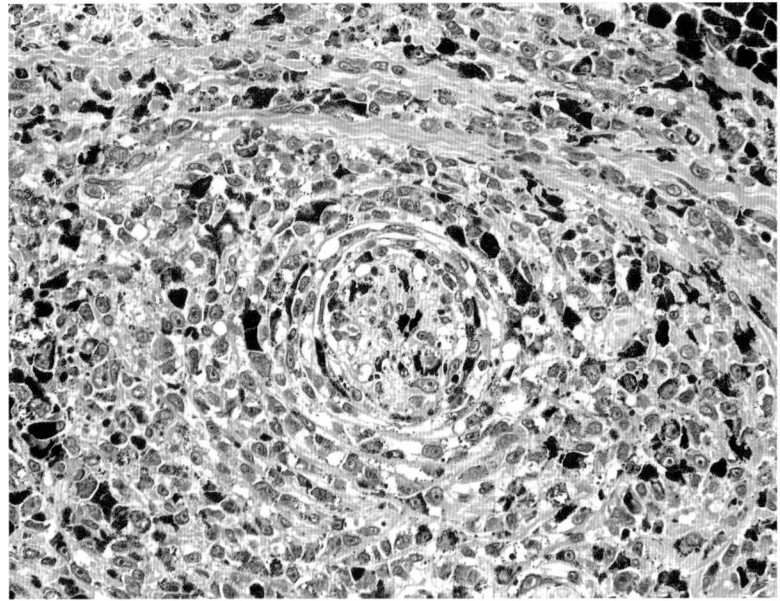

Fig. 27.46
Conjunctival melanoma: there is intraneural and perineural involvement.

BRAF mutation may be seen in 50% of primary and metastatic conjunctival melanomas. In one study, BRAF V600E mutation was detected in 82% of cases with BRAF mutation. The presence of BRAF mutation was more frequent in younger patients and in melanomas that arose from a nevus but was not associated with prognosis.[19] Targeted therapies with BRAF and MEK inhibitors can improve survival in patients with BRAF-mutated metastatic cutaneous melanoma. Routine testing of all conjunctival melanomas for BRAF V600E mutation by immunohistochemistry or molecular analysis may predict responsiveness to Vemurafenib if the patient develops metastatic disease.[20]

Differential diagnosis

Differential diagnosis includes conjunctival nevus, extraocular extension of intraocular uveal melanoma, metastases to the conjunctiva, epithelial lesions with acquired pigmentation (e.g., squamous papilloma, CIN, invasive squamous cell carcinoma), and others (e.g., staphyloma, subconjunctival hematoma, foreign bodies).[1]

Clinical features that favor melanoma over conjunctival nevus include (1) new development of a lesion in an adult patient; (2) location in the

palpebral conjunctiva or fornix; and (3) adherence to underlying sclera.[1] Histologic features that favor melanoma over conjunctival nevus include (1) intraepithelial, pagetoid growth; (2) intraepithelial proliferation that extends significantly lateral to the edge of the subepithelial component, which represents PAM with atypia; (3) inflammation at the base of the lesion; (4) mitoses; (5) absence of cellular maturation at the base of the lesion; and (6) presence of melanin within lesional cells toward the base (typically, nevus cells at the base tend to be amelanotic).[4]

Epibulbar extension of uveal melanoma or melanocytoma should also be considered (Fig. 27.48); in these cases, the trans-scleral nature of the lesion can be identified by high-frequency ocular ultrasonography.

Hematopoietic tumors

Lymphoproliferative disorders, including conjunctival lymphoma

Lymphoproliferative disorders of the conjunctiva encompass a spectrum that includes benign lymphoid hyperplasia, atypical lymphoid hyperplasia, and lymphoma.

Clinical features

A small percentage of patients with benign lymphoid hyperplasia and atypical lymphoid hyperplasia may develop systemic lymphoma.[1,2] Extent of disease at presentation is the most important prognostic factor for the development of lymphoma.[1] Conjunctival lymphoma primarily occurs in older patients (the median age was 63 years in one series),[2] but has been described in patients 33 months to 92 years old.[3] Extranodal marginal zone lymphoma (EMZL) and follicular lymphoma (FL) commonly present in patients in their late 60s, whereas diffuse large B-cell lymphoma (DLBCL) and mantle cell lymphoma (MCL) occur in patients in their 70s.[3] Overall, conjunctival lymphoma does not have gender predilection; however, certain subtypes occur more frequently in one gender. For example, conjunctival EMZL occurs more frequently in women, and DLBCL and MCL occur more frequently in men.[3]

Patients usually present with a salmon-colored, fleshy mass on the conjunctiva (Fig. 27.49). Less commonly, patients present with ptosis, epiphora, blurred vision, proptosis, or diplopia. The lesion is usually unilateral, but may be bilateral. Most lesions are located on the bulbar conjunctiva or fornix, in the superior and inferior quadrants, hidden underneath the eyelid. Although some tumors may occur in the caruncle or plica semilunaris,

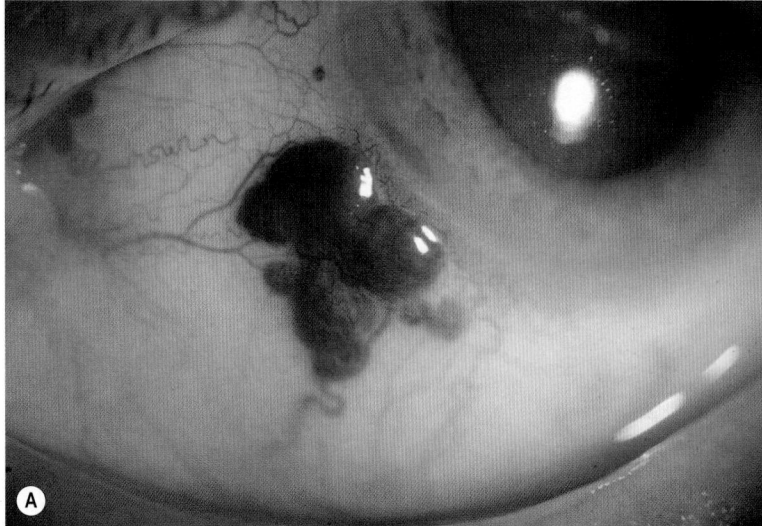

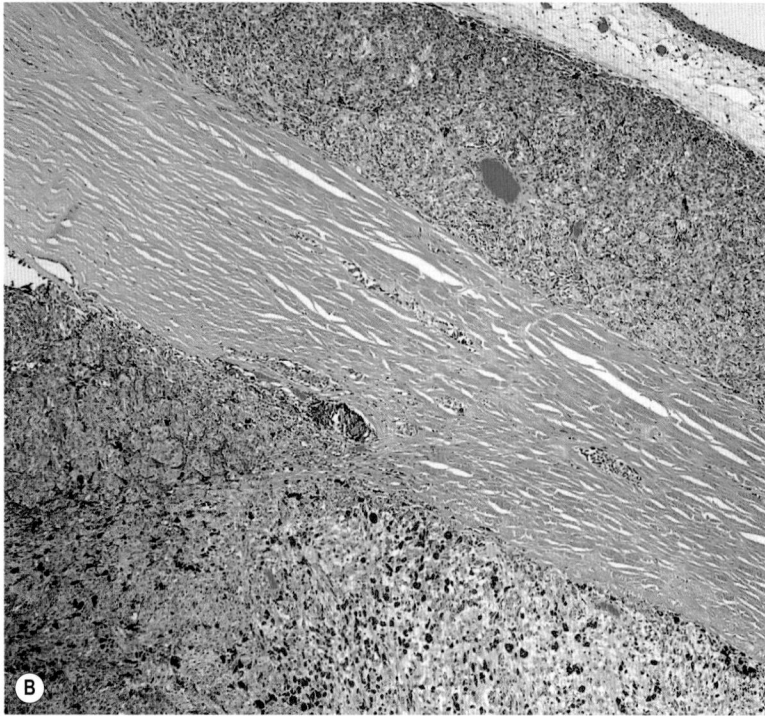

Fig. 27.48
Extraocular extension of a ciliary body melanoma. (**A**) A brown-black multilobulated tumor with large feeder vessels is adjacent to the limbus. A portion of the intraocular component peeks out from the anterior chamber angle. (**B**) Histology shows a ciliary body melanoma that invades through the sclera to the subconjunctival space.

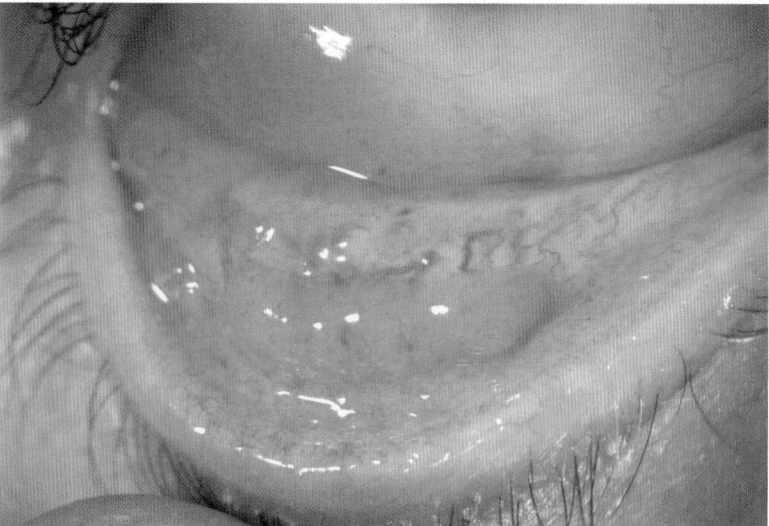

Fig. 27.49
Conjunctival lymphoma: two pink salmon patch lesions are seen – one along the inferior bulbar conjunctiva and the other in the fornix.

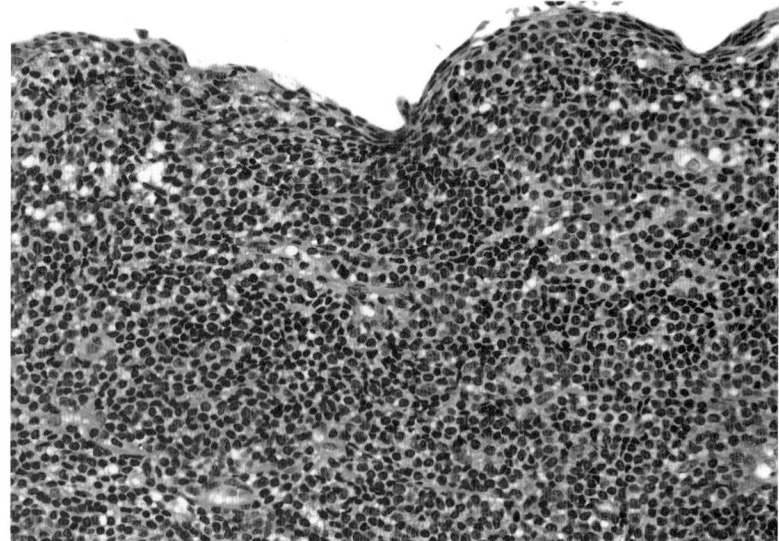

Fig. 27.50
Conjunctival lymphoma: the substantia propria is infiltrated by sheets of small monocytoid lymphocytes.

conjunctival lymphoproliferative lesions rarely occur on the palpebral conjunctiva.

Conjunctival lymphoid tumors may be associated with involvement of other ocular sites and systemic involvement. The most common other ocular sites of involvement include the orbit (15%), uvea (4%), eyelid (3%), and vitreous (1%).[2] The most common systemic sites of tumor include lymph nodes (53%), abdomen (19%), and bone marrow (8%). Approximately one-third of patients with conjunctival lymphoid tumors have systemic lymphoma. Patients with bilateral conjunctival involvement are more likely to have systemic lymphoma.

Conjunctival lymphoma generally has a good prognosis, with no progression or recurrence in 90% of patients during 1-year follow-up. Conjunctival MCL has a worse prognosis with approximately 15% of patients experiencing progression or recurrence in 1 year. Conjunctival T-cell lymphoma is even worse, with approximately 50% of patients experiencing progression or recurrence during the 1-year follow-up.[3]

Pathogenesis and histologic features

Differentiating between benign and malignant conjunctival lymphoid tumors by clinical examination is not possible. Biopsy is necessary to establish the diagnosis. Reactive lymphoid hyperplasia is characterized by dense infiltrates of a mixture of small T- and B-lymphocytes in the conjunctival substantia propria with lymphoid follicles and germinal center formation.[4]

The majority of lymphomas are B-cell non-Hodgkin lymphomas (*Fig. 27.50*).[2–4] The most frequent subtype is EMZL, identified in 81% of cases in one review of 1014 conjunctival lymphoid neoplasms,[3] followed by FL, comprising 8% of cases, and MCL and DLBCL, each comprising 3% of cases.

Chronic antigenic stimulation, autoimmune disorders, and genetic abnormalities may all contribute to the pathogenesis of conjunctival lymphoma.[5] Chronic antigenic stimulation is thought to be involved in the development of EMZL because the tumor is often preceded by benign, chronic inflammation. *Helicobacter pylori*, *Chlamydia psittaci*, and hepatitis C have been suggested as possible contributing agents. Regarding other types of lymphoma of the conjunctiva, investigators have shown associations between Epstein-Barr virus (EBV) and conjunctival NK/T-cell lymphoma and lymphomatoid granulomatosis; and human T-cell lymphotropic virus type 1 (HTLV-1) with adult T-cell lymphoma of the conjunctiva.[3] A number of autoimmune diseases are associated with increased risk of lymphoma; however, an association between autoimmune diseases and conjunctival lymphoma is not well established.

Several chromosomal abnormalities occur in ocular adnexal lymphomas, which include conjunctival lymphomas. For EMZL, the following translocations may be seen: t(11;18)(q21;q21) involving API2 and MALT1 is present in approximately 20% of conjunctival EMZLs and is related to oxidative damage; t(14;18)(q32;q21) translocation involving IGH and MALT1; t(3;14)(p14;q32) involving FOXP1 and IGH; and t(1;14)(p22;q32) involving Bcl-10 and IGH.[5] All of these translocations except for the one involving the *FOXP1* gene lead to the formation or upregulation of proteins that result in activation of nuclear factor κB (NFκB). Trisomy 18 is commonly present in conjunctival EMZL, found in up to 67% of patients.[3] In conjunctival FLs, the typical t(14;18)(q32;q21.3) translocation involving BCL2 and IGH may be seen, leading to overexpression of the anti-apoptotic protein BCL2.[3] In conjunctival MCL, the t(11;14)(q13;q32) translocation involving cyclin D-1 and IGH may be seen. The overexpression of the cyclin D-1 gene leads to cell cycle dysregulation and enhanced proliferation.[3]

Leukemic infiltrates

Clinical features

Leukemic infiltrates most commonly involve the retina and choroid, and may rarely involve the conjunctiva.[1] Fewer than 20 cases of biopsy-proven conjunctival leukemic infiltrates are reported in the English literature[2]; however, autopsy studies show that more patients have conjunctival involvement that may not be recognized premortem. Some patients may also have associated orbital involvement. Most cases are acute leukemias[3] or lymphocytic leukemias[4]. Conjunctival leukemic infiltrates may be the presenting sign of leukemia or indication of relapse. Conjunctival involvement is consistent with good visual acuity, with no reports of vision reduction associated with conjunctival infiltration; however, prognosis is poor, with a median survival of 3 months.[2] Clinically, the lesions occur on the bulbar or palpebral conjunctiva, are firm and nontender, and are usually associated with hemorrhage. Conjunctival leukemic infiltration responds well to systemic chemotherapy.[5]

Histologic features

Leukemia cells are present in the substantia propria, may be diffuse or patchy, and tend to localize around blood vessels.[2,5] It is thought that there may be higher concentrations of adhesion molecules present in the endothelial cells of arterioles and capillaries in the conjunctival stroma.

Conjunctival stromal tumors

The conjunctival stroma contains vascular, fibrous, neural, and other tissues. Benign and malignant tumors may originate from these tissues; however, conjunctival stromal tumors are rare, comprising 6.6% of conjunctival tumors in one large series of 1643 tumors.[1] Stromal tumors generally have smooth surfaces. Tumor color can be helpful for differential diagnosis. For example, vascular tumors are red, pink, or sometimes blue; fibrous tumors are usually white; and neural, histiocytic, and lipomatous tumors are yellow.

Vascular tumors

Lobular capillary hemangioma (pyogenic granuloma)

Clinical features

Lobular capillary hemangioma (LCH; pyogenic granuloma) is polypoid form of capillary hemangioma, characterized by a lobulated, purple-red appearance with smooth surface that may become ulcerated and bleed.[1] It arises in response to tissue injury from inflammation or surgical[2] or nonsurgical trauma. Rarely, lesions can involve the cornea.[3]

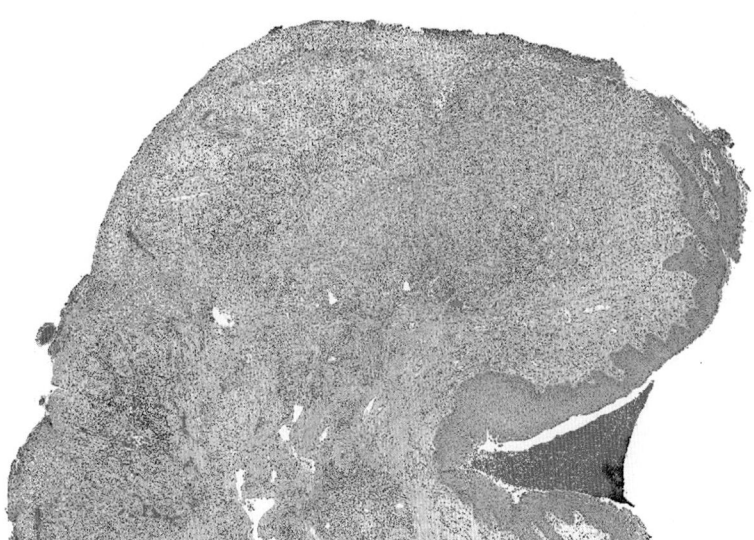

Fig. 27.51
Lobular capillary hemangioma (pyogenic granuloma): histology shows a polypoid mass with surface ulceration composed of numerous blood vessels accompanied by an inflammatory infiltrate.

Histologic features

LCH is a lobulated mass composed of numerous blood vessels with abundant small capillaries in an edematous, fibromyxoid matrix often with a diffuse inflammatory infiltrate composed of lymphocytes, plasma cells, and neutrophils (*Fig. 27.51*).[3]

Capillary hemangioma

Clinical features

Conjunctival capillary hemangioma is similar to its cutaneous counterpart. It presents in infancy as a red stromal mass, and may be associated with capillary hemangioma of the skin or orbit. The lesion may enlarge over several months and spontaneously involute. Patients are most often observed, but surgical resection or local or systemic prednisone can be used for treatment.[1]

Histologic features

Similar to capillary hemangiomas elsewhere, conjunctival capillary hemangioma shows numerous capillary channels and endothelial cell proliferation.

Cavernous hemangioma

Clinical features

Cavernous hemangioma is a rare tumor in the deep conjunctival stroma in young children that appears red or blue.[1] It may cause occasional bloody tears.[2] It is managed by local resection.

Histologic features

Cavernous hemangioma is composed of ectatic vascular channels lined by endothelial cells and separated by fibrous septa.

Varix and racemose hemangioma

Clinical features

Varix and racemose hemangioma are rare tumors of the conjunctiva. Varix may enlarge with Valsalva maneuver. Management should be conservative and include observation and symptomatic treatment because there is a risk of prolonged bleeding with surgery.

Racemose hemangioma is a raised, multilobular lesion that resembles a cluster of grapes[1] and may be associated with Wyburn-Mason syndrome.[2] The lesion can be managed conservatively with observation.

Histologic features

Histologically, varix is a fusiform saccular dilation of a pre-existing vein lacking an elastica. The lesion can undergo thrombosis with intravascular papillary endothelial hyperplasia and phlebolith formation.[1] Some consider it to be a lymphangioma.[2] Racemose hemangioma has irregularly sized vascular lumens with variably thickened muscular walls with fibrosis and lack of elastic lamina and intervening capillary bed.[2]

Kaposi sarcoma

Clinical features

Prior to the HIV/acquired immunodeficiency syndrome (AIDS) era, Kaposi sarcoma (KS) was a rare malignancy of the conjunctiva that mainly occurred in elderly, immunosuppressed patients. It is now encountered mostly in patients with AIDS, usually late in the course of the disease, although conjunctival KS may be the first sign of HIV/AIDS.[1] Rarely, KS may appear in HIV negative, non-immunosuppressed patients.[2–4]

Conjunctival KS may be single or multiple, and appear as a dark red to purple painless lesion that may be initially mistaken for a subconjunctival hemorrhage. As it grows it may become elevated and nodular, causing irritation and foreign body sensation. The patient may have KS lesions elsewhere on the body.

Histologic features

Similar to KS elsewhere, it is composed of spindle-shaped cells with elongated oval nuclei and slit-like vascular channels lined by bland endothelial cells. By immunohistochemistry, tumor cells are positive for vascular markers, such as CD31, Erg, and CD34, as well as human herpesvirus (HHV)-8.[3]

Lymphangiectasia

Clinical features

Lymphangiectasia is a rare condition where normal conjunctival lymphatics are dilated within the bulbar conjunctiva. Patients usually present with ocular irritation, and focal or diffuse chemosis.[1] Sometimes, conjunctival lymphatics may be filled with blood due to abnormal connections between the conjunctival lymphatic and vascular systems. This is referred to as 'lymphangiectasia haemorrhagica conjunctivae'.[2] The condition may be congenital, associated with primary lymphedema, but is most often secondary to disruption or obstruction of lymphatic pathways by inflammatory or neoplastic disease processes, surgery, or radiotherapy.[1]

Histologic features

Lymphangiectasia is characterized by dilated lymphatic channels lined by flattened endothelium with edema of the surrounding lamina propria. The lymphatic channels may contain proteinaceous fluid. Scattered inflammatory cells and fibroblastic proliferation or scarring may be seen in the surrounding lamina propria. The overlying epithelium may show squamous metaplasia and keratinization. Immunohistochemistry for D2-40 may be helpful to differentiate capillaries from lymphatic channels.[1]

Conjunctival lymphangioma

Clinical features

Lymphangioma may be an isolated conjunctival lesion or the superficial component of an orbital lymphangioma. It usually manifests in the first decade of life as a multiloculated mass with variably sized clear cystic channels and sometimes blood.[1,2] When hemorrhage occurs in the lesion, it is referred to as 'chocolate cyst'.

Histologic features

Lymphangioma is a nonencapsulated lesion composed of variably sized, thin-walled channels lined by D2-40-positive endothelium and scattered lymphoid aggregates around the walls.[3]

Fibrous tumors

Fibroma/solitary fibrous tumor

Clinical features

Fibroma and solitary fibrous tumor are rare in the conjunctiva.[1,2] Clinically, fibroma appears as a white stromal mass. In the periocular region, solitary fibrous tumor more commonly occurs in the orbit. In the one reported case of conjunctival solitary fibrous tumor, the lesion was a well-circumscribed, firm pink mass in the fornix.[2]

Histologic features

Microscopically, fibroma is composed of dense fibrous connective tissue with bland appearing mesenchymal cells compressed between parallel layers of collagen lamellae.[1] There is no significant vascularity or inflammation. The cells have fibroblast features by immunohistochemistry (vimentin positive; S100 protein, smooth muscle actin, CD34, and CD99 negative).[1]

Histologically, solitary fibrous tumor resembles those seen in the pleura, composed of spindle cells and thin, parallel collagen bands. The cells may be arranged in short, ill-defined fascicles or randomly in a 'patternless pattern'. Areas of hyalinization are usually present. By immunohistochemistry, solitary fibrous tumor is typically positive for CD34, Bcl2, CD99, and vimentin and negative for desmin, cytokeratin, S100 protein, and muscle-specific actin and smooth muscle actin.[2]

Benign and malignant fibrous histiocytoma

Clinical features

Fibrous histiocytoma (FH) is a mesenchymal tumor that can show benign or malignant features.[1] In the ocular region, FH more commonly occurs in the orbit, and rarely arises in the conjunctiva. Tumor location is mostly the limbus,[1] and less frequently, bulbar conjunctiva,[2] caruncle,[3] and tarsal conjunctiva.[4] Clinically, the lesion appears as a firm, tan, dome-shaped subconjunctival mass with vessels over the surface. The tumor is usually unilateral, but two cases of bilateral FH have been reported.[5,6] In Kim et al.'s[1] review of 23 previously reported cases of FH, the mean age was 39 years, and there was no gender predilection. Malignant FH, now referred to as pleomorphic undifferentiated sarcoma, can metastasize to regional lymph nodes and distant organs, resulting in death.[7] Both benign and malignant FH can recur; therefore, complete excision with careful examination of the margins is advised.

Histologic features

FH is composed of fibroblasts arranged in a focal storiform pattern and lipid-laden histiocytes. Features of malignancy include increased mitotic activity, cytological atypia, and pleomorphism with multinucleated tumor giant cells. Immunohistochemical stains may be used to rule out other spindle cell tumors, such as melanoma, spindle cell carcinoma, and schwannoma.

Nodular fasciitis

Clinical features

Nodular fasciitis is a benign proliferation of fibroblasts and myofibroblasts that rarely occurs in the ocular region, including orbit and eyelid. Eight cases of epibulbar nodular fasciitis have been reported in the literature.[1] Although it was thought to be a response to repeated trauma or inflammation, it is now thought to be a transient neoplasm associated with a MYH9-USP6 gene fusion.[2–4] The most common locations are at extraocular muscle insertions, and at the limbus with involvement of the cornea.[1,2] Epibulbar nodular fasciitis is thought to originate from Tenon capsule.[5]

Histologic features

Nodular fasciitis is a round or oval unencapsulated nodule composed of spindled to stellate fibroblasts and smooth muscle actin-positive myofibroblasts in a myxoid to fibrous background arranged haphazardly in a 'tissue culture' appearance. Extravasated red blood cells and scant inflammatory cells may be present. Numerous mitotic figures may lead to misdiagnosis as sarcoma.

Neural tumors

Neurofibroma

Clinical features

Neurofibroma is a peripheral nerve tumor that occurs rarely in the conjunctiva. It may be solitary, plexiform, or diffuse. Plexiform neurofibroma is associated with neurofibromatosis type 1. Solitary neurofibroma is usually not associated with systemic disease. It presents as a slow-growing, nodular, amelanotic epibulbar mass in adults.[1-3] Plexiform neurofibroma is diffuse.

Histologic features

Neurofibroma is composed of Schwann cells and fibroblasts in a fibromyxoid matrix. Solitary neurofibromas may be circumscribed, but not encapsulated. It consists of spindle cells with elongated, slender, sometimes wavy nuclei (*Fig. 27.52*). Scattered mast cells and nerve axons are present. By immunohistochemistry, S100 protein is generally positive throughout most of the tumor. CD34 highlights perineural fibroblasts, and neurofilament highlights axons within the lesion.

Schwannoma (neurilemmoma)

Clinical features

Schwannoma is a very rare tumor of the conjunctiva, with seven reported cases in the English literature.[1] The tumor typically presents as an amelanotic, well-circumscribed, subconjunctival mass.[2]

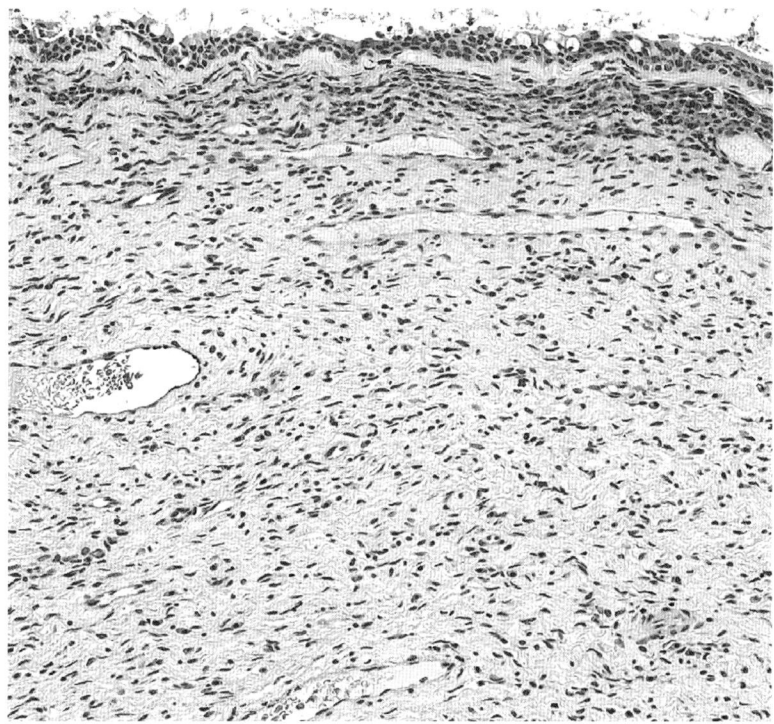

Fig. 27.52
Neurofibroma: the tumor is composed of cells with eosinophilic cytoplasm and wavy nuclei.

Histologic features

Schwannoma is composed of spindle-shaped cells with eosinophilic cytoplasm and fascicular or palisade arrangement. There is no cytological atypia or atypical mitoses. By immunohistochemistry, tumor cells are strongly positive for S100 protein.[1]

Granular cell tumor

Clinical features

Granular cell tumor is rare in the conjunctiva and caruncle.[1] It appears as a pink to red stromal mass that may be clinically indistinguishable from other well-circumscribed tumors.[2]

Histologic features

Granular cell tumor is composed of sheets of large polygonal cells with small, bland-appearing nuclei and abundant granular eosinophilic cytoplasm. The granular cytoplasm is PAS positive and diastase resistant. There may be overlying pseudoepitheliomatous hyperplasia. By immunohistochemistry, tumor cells are positive for S100 protein and neuron-specific enolase.

Histiocytic tumors

Xanthoma

Clinical features

Xanthoma is very rare in the conjunctiva. It appears as a yellow, subepithelial, smooth epibulbar nodule adherent to the underlying sclera. It may be bilateral in patients with xanthoma disseminatum, a nonhereditary condition in adults characterized by widespread xanthomas of skin and mucous membranes and normal serum lipoprotein studies.[1]

Histologic features

Xanthoma is composed of foamy histiocytes with scattered Touton giant cells. In xanthoma disseminatum, the lesion may be microscopically indistinguishable from xanthogranuloma.

Xanthogranuloma

Clinical features

Juvenile xanthogranuloma (JXG) is an uncommon non-Langerhans cell histiocytic skin disorder that primarily affects infants and young children. In and around the eye, the iris and eyelids are most frequently involved. The conjunctiva, ciliary body, optic nerve, and orbit are affected less frequently. Solitary JXG of the corneoscleral limbus is a rare form of ocular involvement seen in infants and children, and few adult cases have also been reported.[1,2] Clinically, the lesion is a yellow-pink to yellow-orange stromal mass (*Fig. 27.53*). Patients may or may not have systemic findings.

Histologic features

JXG is composed of numerous foamy histiocytes with scattered Touton giant cells, and scattered lymphocytes, plasma cells, eosinophils, and some neutrophils (*Fig. 27.54*).[2] By immunohistochemistry, lesional cells are positive for the macrophage markers CD68 and CD163 and often, but not always, negative for S100 protein. CD1a and Langerin are negative.

Reticulohistiocytoma

Clinical features

Reticulohistiocytoma is a rare benign conjunctival lesion that usually occurs as an isolated skin nodule or as part of multicentric reticulohistiocytosis, a systemic disorder. Reported cases of reticulohistiocytoma in the ocular

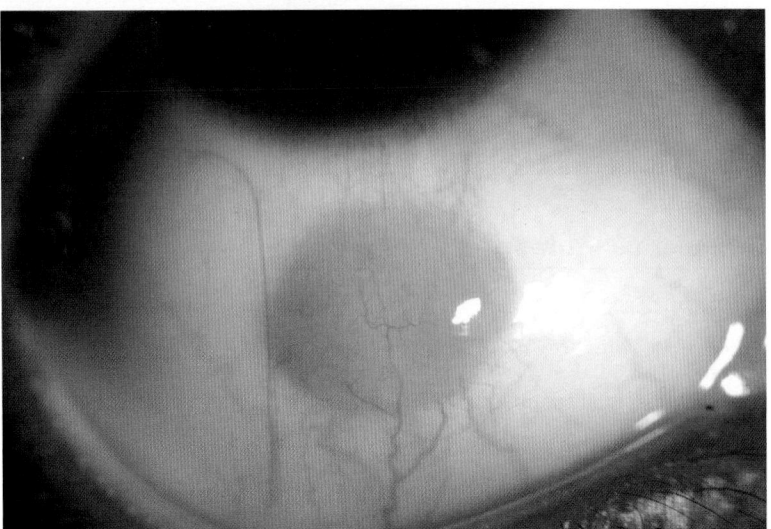

Fig. 27.53
Juvenile xanthogranuloma: a circumscribed yellow-orange lesion is on the inferior bulbar conjunctiva.

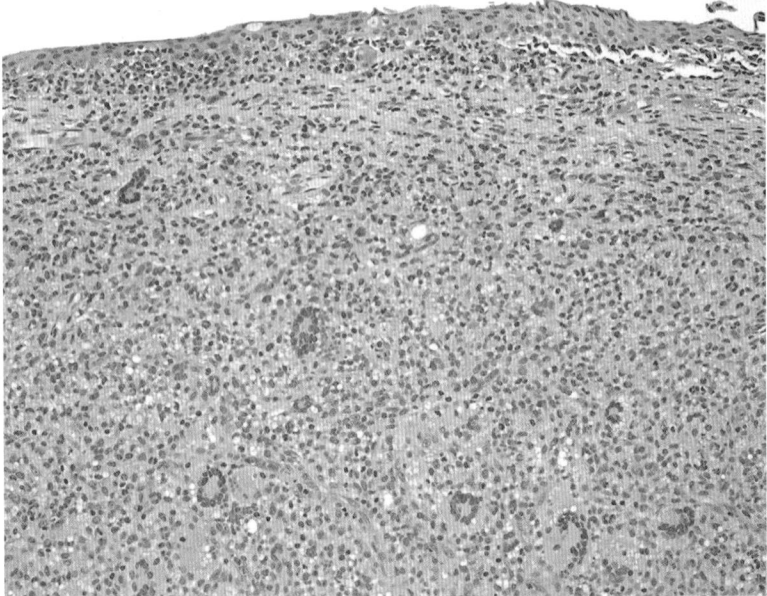

Fig. 27.54
Juvenile xanthogranuloma: histology shows histiocytes with scattered Touton giant cells.

surface have been solitary, painless masses localized to the cornea and limbus without systemic disease.[1]

Histologic features

Reticulohistiocytoma is composed predominantly of large mononuclear cells and scattered multinucleated cells with eosinophilic ground-glass cytoplasm and large nuclei with prominent nucleoli.

Conjunctival myxoma

Clinical features

Conjunctival myxoma is a rare, benign mesenchymal tumor with 41 cases reported in the literature since 1913.[1] It affects males and females equally, mostly adults, with mean age at presentation of 47.6 years (median age, 49 years; range, 11–80 years).[1] Lesions may be localized or associated with Carney complex, which includes cutaneous and cardiac myxomas, multiple

pigmented lesions, and endocrine overactivity.[2] The lesion is a slow-growing, painless, well-circumscribed, yellow-pink, fleshy, translucent-to-solid mass on the bulbar conjunctiva.[1,2]

Histologic features

Myxoma is a paucicellular tumor composed of spindle- and stellate-shaped cells within a loose mucoid, myxoid stroma.[1–3] Some tumor cells may have small intranuclear vacuoles, and some may have clear intracytoplasmic inclusions. The stroma is composed of Alcian-blue-positive, hyaluronidase-sensitive hyaluronic acid mucopolysaccharides and chondroitin sulfates with a network of reticulin fibers, small blood vessels, and collagen fibers. Few mast cells may be present in the stroma.[2,4] Histochemical stains for mucicarmine and colloidal iron are also positive in the tumor stroma, while PAS and oil red O stains are negative. By immunohistochemistry, tumor cells show strong immunoreactivity for vimentin and focal reactivity for a-smooth muscle actin, but negative for S100 protein, desmin, and myoglobin.[1,5] Ki-67 proliferation index is low (<5% of tumor cells).[4]

Myogenic tumors

Rhabdomyosarcoma

Clinical features

In the ocular region, rhabdomyosarcoma (RMS) most commonly occurs in the orbit. It is the most common primary orbital malignancy in children, comprising 5% of pediatric tumors.[1,2] Primary conjunctival RMS is rare.[1,2] In one series of 33 consecutive patients with primary ophthalmic involvement by RMS, the conjunctiva was the primary site in 4 patients (12%), and all of these patients had orbital involvement.[3] Similar to orbital RMS, the tumor is most commonly located superiorly.[3] Clinically, the lesion appears as a soft, gelatinous, fleshy pink mass with numerous grape-like vesicles.[2] Early in the clinical course, the lesion grows rapidly.[4] Differential diagnosis may include inflammatory lesions such as allergic conjunctivitis, or other tumors such as lymphoma, Langerhans cell histiocytosis, and lymphangioma.[1,3] Initial workup should include orbital imaging with CT or MRI to determine the extent of the lesion and location for surgical planning.[1,3]

Histologic features

RMS of the conjunctiva is typically botryoid type, which is considered a variant of embryonal RMS that occurs in mucosal sites.[2] The tumor consists of a bandlike layer of spindle cells just beneath the epithelium, termed the cambium layer, and spindled and round rhabdomyoblasts with eosinophilic cytoplasm and enlarged, hyperchromatic nuclei within a myxoid matrix.[4] Cross striations are seen in <10% of cases. By immunohistochemistry, tumor cells are positive for desmin, myogenin, and myoglobin.

Lipomatous tumors

Clinical features

True lipomatous tumors of the conjunctiva are very rare. However, herniated orbital fat located under the conjunctiva is not uncommon and may be mistaken for a lipomatous tumor.[1–4] This occurs predominantly in the middle-aged and elderly. There is a striking predilection for males.[5,6]

Histologic features

Histologically, the features of herniated fat were originally mistaken as representing pleomorphic lipoma.[1] Thus it is composed of adipocytes of various sizes with associated fibrous septa. Adipocytes containing intranuclear vacuoles and floret giant cells are present (Fig. 27.55), often accompanied by a mixed inflammatory cell infiltrate.[5] Mitotic activity is absent. The floret cells express CD34.[6]

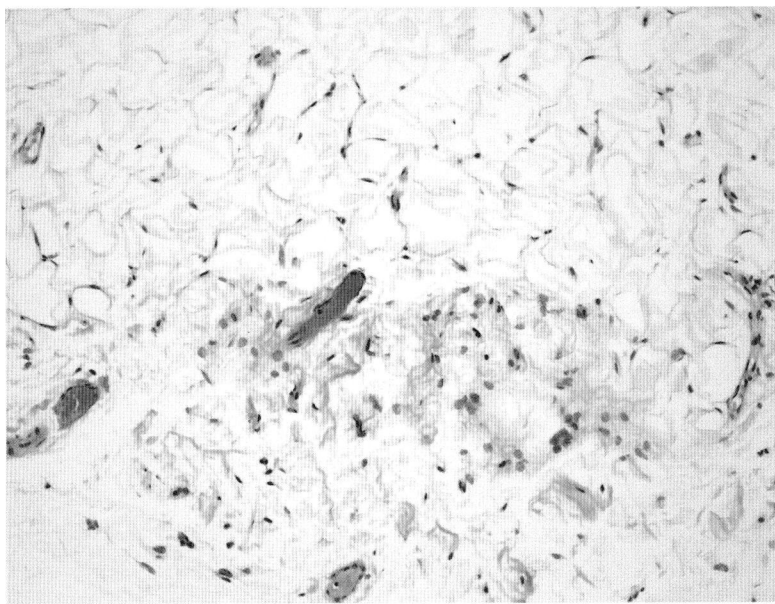

Fig. 27.55
Herniated orbital fat: histology shows mature adipose tissue with scattered floret giant cells.

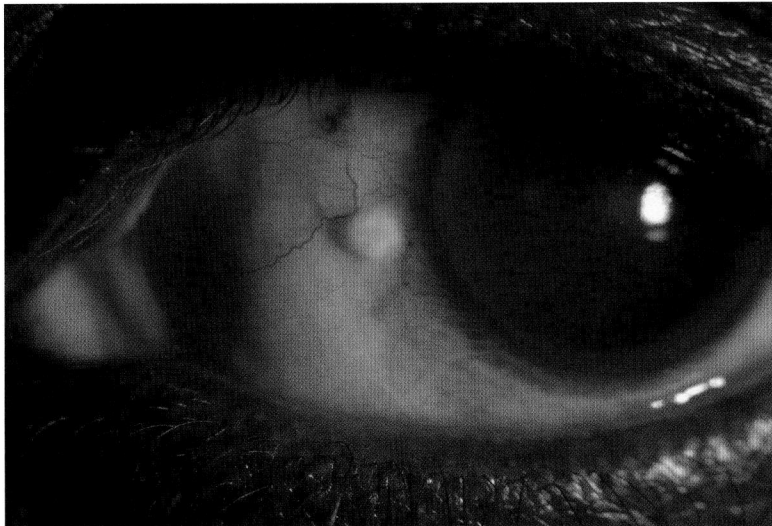

Fig. 27.56
Pinguecula: a yellow-white mass is seen on the nasal bulbar conjunctiva.

Other tumorlike lesions

Some non-neoplastic conditions, such as pinguecula and pterygium, foreign body, inflammation, and amyloidosis, can simulate neoplasms.[1]

Pinguecula and pterygium

Clinical features

Pinguecula is a localized yellow-white elevated mass, most commonly found in the nasal conjunctiva adjacent to the limbus (*Fig. 27.56*). Pterygium is a localized yellow-white elevated area found in the nasal or temporal conjunctiva that extends onto the cornea. Both are the result of UV light damage.[1]

Histologic features

Histologically, pinguecula and pterygium are characterized by actinic (basophilic) degeneration of the substantia propria. Pterygium also features dissolution of Bowman layer and fibrovascular proliferation.

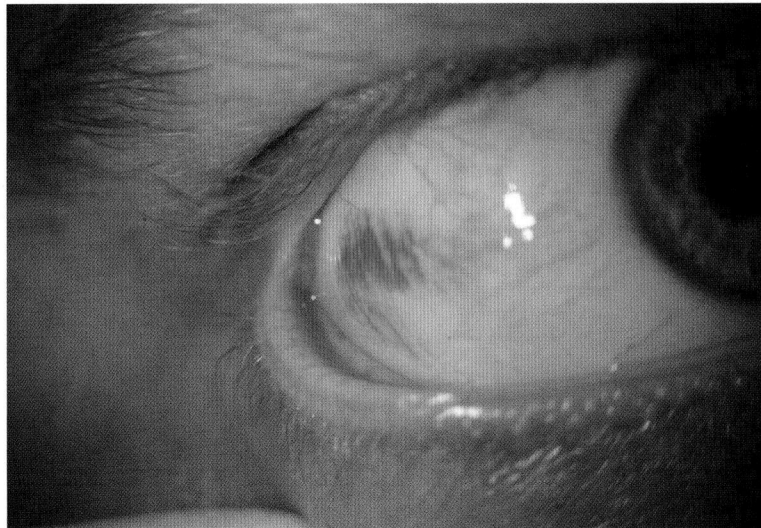

Fig. 27.57
Conjunctival amyloidosis: a yellow, waxy lesion with overlying subconjunctival hemorrhage is seen on the temporal bulbar conjunctiva.

Amyloidosis

Clinical features

Conjunctival amyloidosis is an uncommon condition that is usually localized and rarely associated with systemic involvement. It is usually seen in middle-aged adults. Patients present with confluent fusiform lesions or polypoid papules with a waxy or yellow color. Some patients may present with subconjunctival hemorrhage (*Fig. 27.57*) or blepharoptosis. Conjunctival amyloidosis usually affects the palpebral conjunctiva, but any part of the conjunctiva may be affected. Systemic evaluation for primary systemic amyloidosis and lymphoma is warranted.[2,3]

Histologic features

Conjunctival amyloidosis is characterized by homogeneous eosinophilic deposits in the conjunctival substantia propria that are Congo red and thioflavin T positive (*Fig. 27.58A and B*). With Congo red and polarized light, the deposits show apple-green birefringence and dichroism (*Fig. 27.58C*).

Metastatic and secondary tumors

Metastatic tumors

Metastatic tumors to the eye and ocular adnexa are usually found in intraocular structures, such as the iris and choroid, or the orbit. Rarely, metastases may be present in the optic nerve, eyelids, and conjunctiva. Conjunctival metastases usually appear when the systemic malignancy is advanced stage, and there is evidence of other ocular or organ metastases.[1] Tumors may appear anywhere on the conjunctiva, most commonly the bulbar conjunctiva. Lesions may be solitary or multiple. The most common primary tumors are breast carcinoma and cutaneous melanoma. Metastases from lung carcinoma, laryngeal carcinoma, gastric adenocarcinoma, bladder carcinoma, colon adenocarcinoma (*Fig. 27.59*), and seminoma have also been reported. Clinically, metastatic carcinomas are fleshy, stromal tumors that are yellow or pink, whereas metastatic cutaneous melanoma may be pigmented. Conjunctival metastases can be treated with excision, radiation therapy, or chemotherapy. Prognosis is poor, with a mean survival of 9 months between conjunctival metastasis and death.[1]

Secondary tumors

The conjunctiva can be secondarily involved by extension of tumors from the eyelid or orbit, or extraocular extension of an intraocular tumor.[2] Sebaceous gland carcinoma of the eyelid is particularly important because it often exhibits pagetoid invasion of the conjunctival epithelium (*Fig. 27.60*),

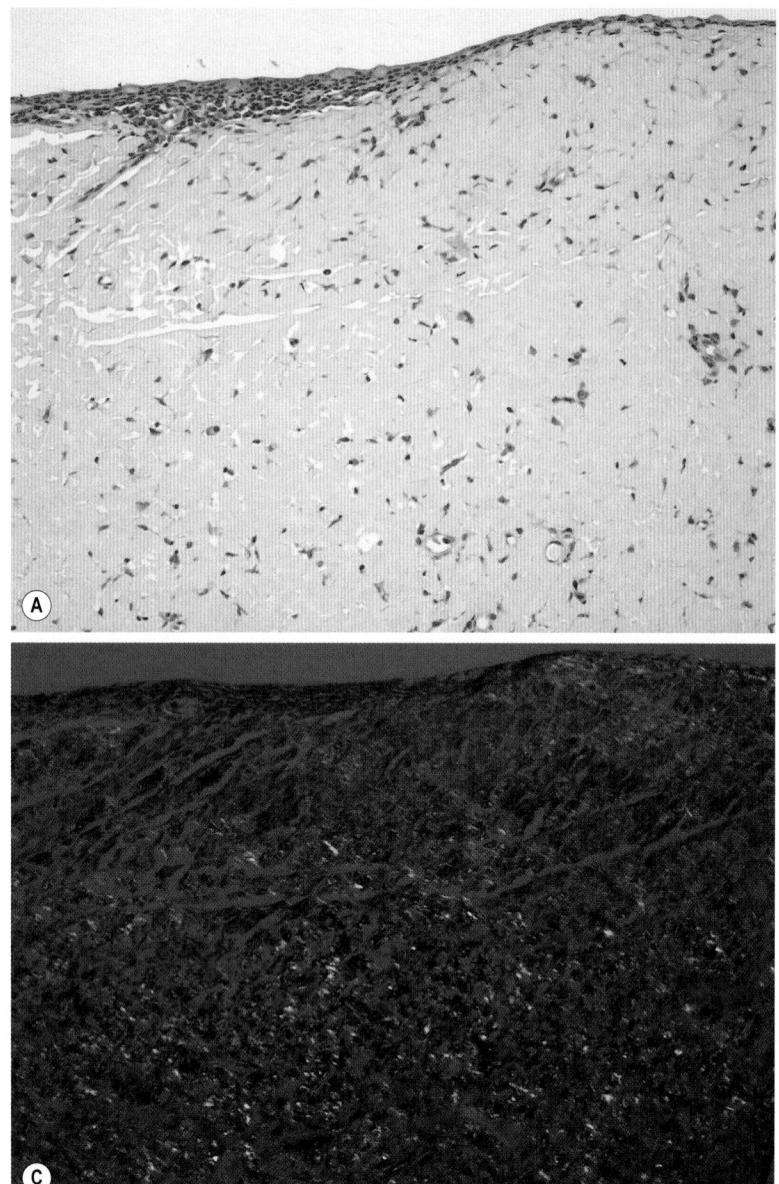

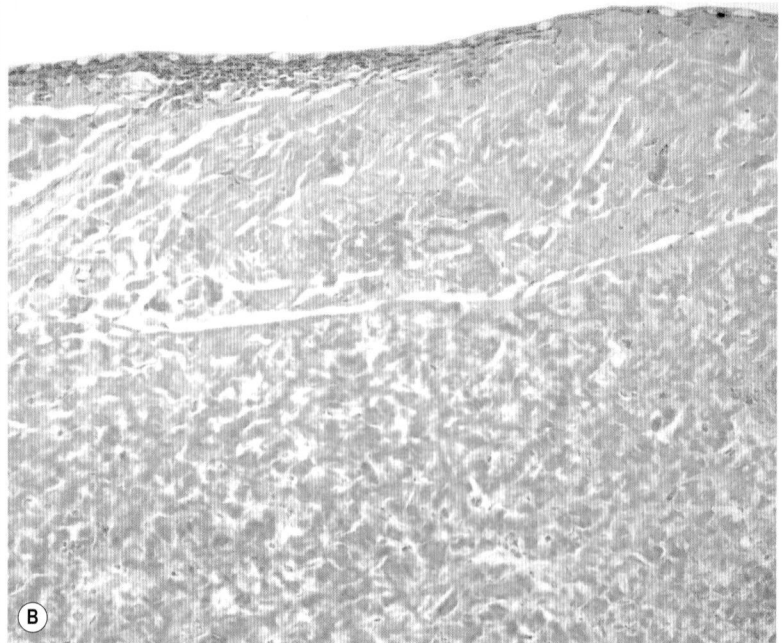

Fig. 27.58
Conjunctival amyloidosis: (**A**) histology shows amorphous eosinophilic deposits in the substantia propria embedded with scattered spindle to stellate shaped cells and blood vessels. (**B**) The deposits are positive for Congo red. (**C**) With polarized light, the deposits show apple-green birefringence.

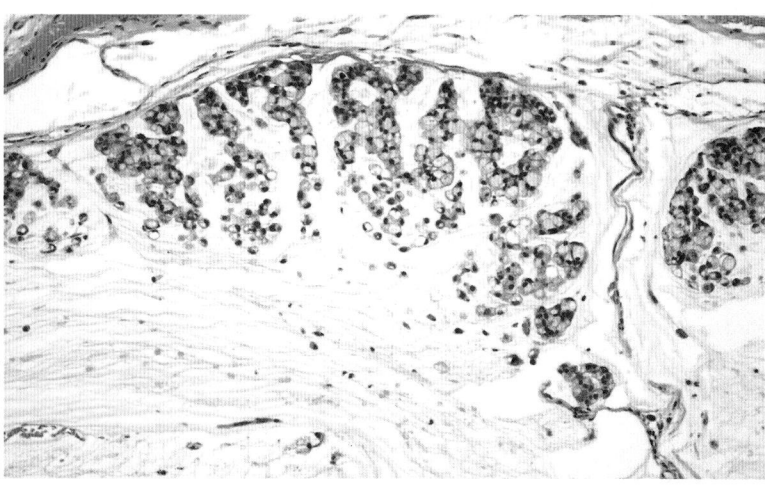

Fig. 27.59
Metastatic carcinoma: histology shows groups of signet ring cells floating in pools of mucin. Tumor cells were CK7-, CK20+, CDX2+ by immunohistochemistry, consistent with colorectal primary.

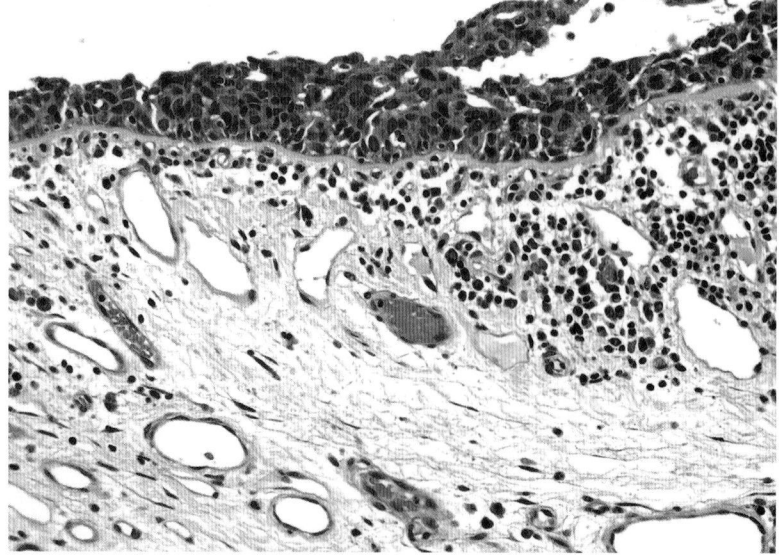

Fig. 27.60
Sebaceous gland carcinoma: the epithelium is completely replaced by sebaceous carcinoma. It is important to look carefully for cells with foamy cytoplasm.

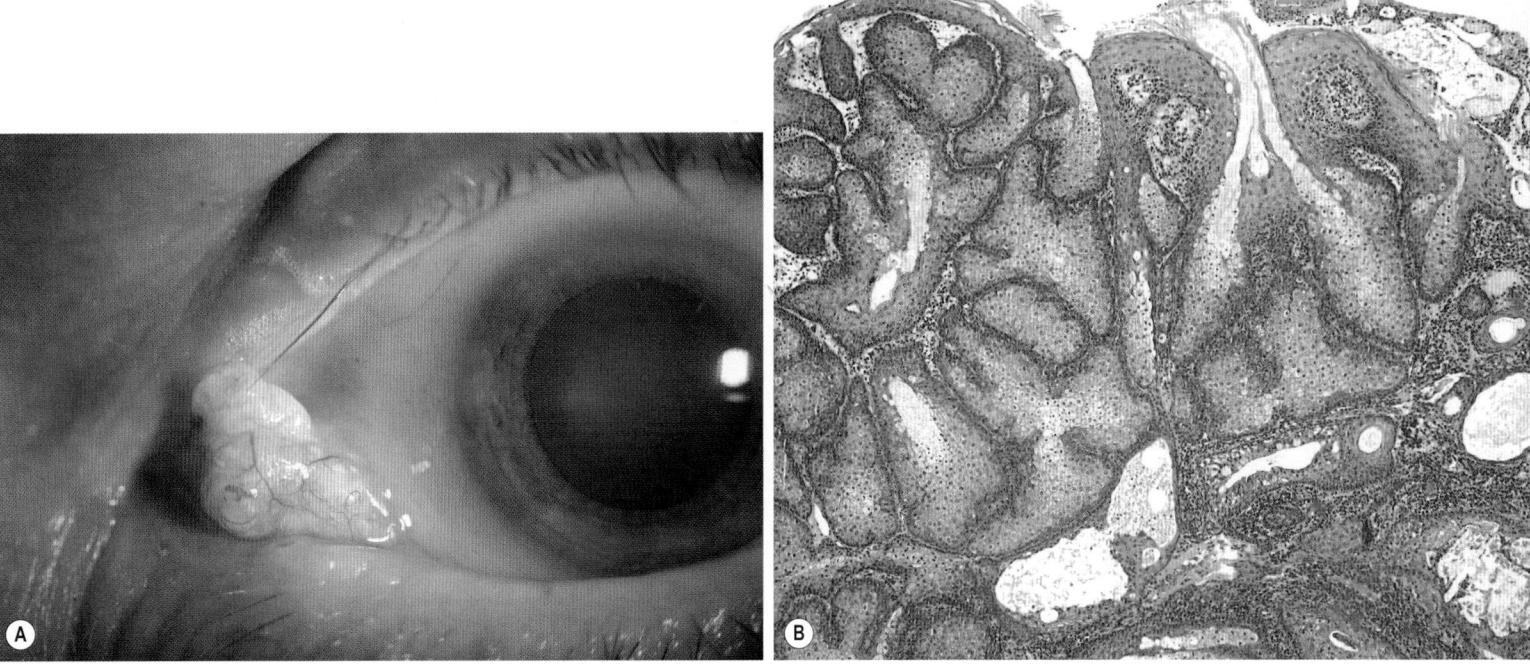

Fig. 27.61

Sebaceous adenoma, caruncle. (**A**) A polypoid yellow-pink lesion protrudes from the caruncle. (**B**) Histology shows lobules of sebaceous glands with a more prominent basal layer.

which may clinically mimic chronic unilateral blepharoconjunctivitis, or histologically mimic OSSN, and result in delayed diagnosis. Orbital tumors, such as RMS in children or lymphangioma, may first present in the conjunctiva. Ciliary body melanoma that extends through the sclera into the subconjunctival tissue may simulate conjunctival melanoma.

Tumors of the caruncle

Tumors of the caruncle are rare, comprising 1% or less of all surgical ophthalmic specimens submitted[1-3] and approximately 4% of conjunctival tumors[4]. A wide variety of lesions may be seen due to the underlying structures of the caruncle, including nonkeratinizing stratified squamous epithelium with goblet cells, hair follicles, sebaceous glands (*Fig. 27.61*), sweat glands, and accessory lacrimal tissue. Preoperative clinical diagnosis is reported to be correct in only about half of cases (range, 37–52%).[3] The vast majority of lesions, approximately 95%, are benign.[1-3,5] The most frequent tumors are nevus (range, 43–60%) and squamous papilloma (range, 7–23%). Although malignant lesions are rare, they may be fatal. Malignant melanoma, sebaceous gland carcinoma, basal cell carcinoma, and lymphoma have all been described. Due to the difficulty in clinical diagnosis, malignancy is clinically overestimated; thus, any suspected malignant lesion should be excised and examined by an experienced pathologist.

Access **ExpertConsult.com** for the complete list of references

Sentinel lymph node biopsies

Alistair J. Cochran

See
www.expertconsult.com
for references and
additional material

Introduction

This chapter is based on the author's previous publications on this topic.[1–4]

Management of patients with primary melanoma in vertical growth phase who have no evidence of regional nodal metastases on palpation or ultrasound has been controversial for many years.

Until recently, the treatment options were:

- observation with lymphadenectomy delayed until regional metastases became clinically evident (watch and wait),
- elective (prophylactic) regional lymph node dissection after microscopic identification of a primary melanoma (*Fig. 28.1*).

Neither option is ideal. While observation spares the approximately 80% of patients who never develop regional nodal metastases from morbid lymph node surgery:

- it delays lymphadenectomy beyond the optimum time for the 20% of patients who develop regional metastases,
- it allows melanoma metastases to spread to nonsentinel nodes (NSNs),
- it permits the evolving melanoma to achieve a higher AJCC stage.

To resolve this dilemma, Morton, Cochran, and colleagues at UCLA and The John Wayne Cancer Institute developed the techniques of lymphatic mapping (LM) and sentinel node biopsy (SNB).[5]

Studies of melanoma patients early in the evolution of regional nodal tumor spread showed that most had metastatic melanoma in a single node, the remaining lymph nodes in the regional basin being free of tumor.[6] From this observation, we hypothesized that if it were possible to identify the individual node that was susceptible to these earliest metastases for surgical excision and histologic scrutiny, it would be possible to accurately stage the regional basin on the basis of a relatively minor surgical procedure. Lymphoscintigraphy, in which a radioactive isotope, such as 99mTc antimony sulfide, is injected around the site of a primary tumor, reliably identifies the lymph node basin(s) that receive lymph from that specific site.[7] If the lymphoscintigram is read 'early', it is possible to identify the individual lymph node that first receives the isotope (*Fig. 28.2*).[8] The location of that node can then be marked on the overlying skin. Animal experiments had previously shown that marker dye injected in anatomically definable areas of the skin drained reliably to a specific lymph node (*Fig. 28.3*).[9] Combination of lymphoscintigraphy and intraoperative insertion of vital dye and isotope permitted the reliable identification of the first lymph node on the direct lymphatic drainage pathway from a primary melanoma, which, because it 'guards' the remaining lymph nodes of the group, we called the sentinel node (SN) (*Fig. 28.4*).[1] In a study of 223 melanoma patients who had an SNB followed by completion lymph node dissection (CLND) regardless of whether or not the SN contained melanoma, we showed that if the SN was tumor free there was a less than 1% chance that NSNs would contain metastases. If the SN contained tumor, there was a 16% chance that NSN would contain metastases.[1] These findings led to the development of an NIH-funded international randomized clinical trial (MSLT-I) in 2001. This compared (1) patients with intermediate-thickness primary melanoma (1 mm and thicker or Clark level IV of any thickness), without clinically detectable regional or disseminated metastatic melanoma, who had wide excision and SNB with immediate CLND if the SN contained tumor, followed by observation, with (2) CLND only if the patients developed clinically detectable nodal metastases during observation. Analysis of the results of MSLT-I has shown that SNB is a low-morbidity procedure and is the most accurate staging technique available for melanoma.[10] Patients treated by SNB with immediate CLND if the SN contained tumor had significantly longer disease-free survival relative to observed patients. Patients who had CLND delayed until nodal metastasic disease became clinically detectable, had significantly more tumor-positive nodes, were staged at a higher AJCC level, and had a significantly less favorable survival than patients with tumor in the SN who had an immediate CLND.[11]

LM and SNB, in addition to wide use in the management of patients with cutaneous melanoma, have been applied to nonmelanoma skin cancers, including Merkel cell carcinoma, squamous carcinoma, and appendageal carcinomas. The techniques are also used to manage patients with cancers of organs other than the skin. SN procedures have been widely performed for breast cancer. The approach is also used for patients with cancers of the upper and lower gastrointestinal tract, vulva and cervix, lung, and thyroid.

Accurate identification of the true SN and its precise histopathological assessment are essential for accurate staging, individualized prediction of the likelihood of metastases in NSNs, subsequent extranodal metastases,

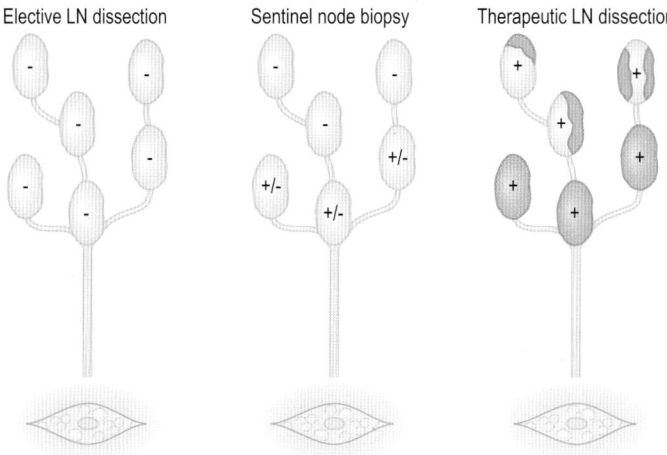

Elective LN dissection   Sentinel node biopsy   Therapeutic LN dissection

Fig. 28.1
Approaches to managing patients with intermediate-thickness primary melanoma without clinically detectable lymph node metastases:

- Elective (prophylactic) lymph node dissection (*left panel*). All lymph nodes in the draining lymph node group are excised immediately after microscopic identification of a primary melanoma (preferably removed by excision biopsy). By this approach, the 80% of patients who have no nodal metastases are subjected to a morbid operation that is unlikely to confer clinical benefit.
- Observation after wide excision of a primary melanoma with lymphadenectomy delayed until regional metastases are clinically evident (*right panel*). This spares the approximately 80% of patients who never develop regional node metastases morbid lymph node surgery, but delays, beyond the optimum time, lymphadenectomy for the 20% of patients who eventually develop nodal metastases, with highly negative clinical consequences.
- Lymph node mapping with sentinel node biopsy (*middle panel*). This low-morbidity technique selectively identifies the lymph node(s) most susceptible to early metastases. Only patients with tumor in the SN receive complete lymph node dissection.

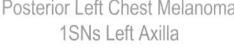
Posterior Left Chest Melanoma
1SNs Left Axilla

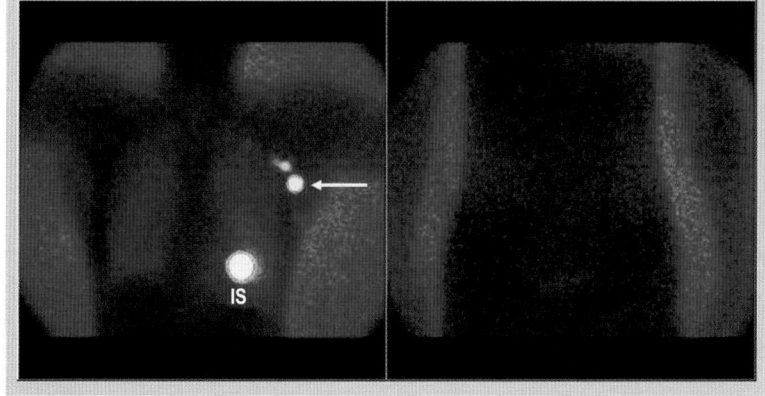

IS

Fig. 28.2
Identification of a left axillary sentinel node (SN) by lymphoscintigraphy in a patient with a primary melanoma on the left mid back: two 20 MBq, 0.1 mL injections of 99mTc antimony sulfide were made on either side of a small excision biopsy site (*IS*). On the left is an anterior view of the shoulders, axilla, and chest showing the prominent SN (*white arrow*) and limited spread of tracer to a second-tier node above the SN. On the right is an anterior view of the pelvis showing no evidence of drainage to groin nodes. By courtesy of R. Uren, MD, Sydney, Australia.

and death from melanoma. SN tumor status also assists in determination of the need for additional surgical and nonsurgical therapy. The responsibility for correct identification of the SN lies with the nuclear medicine physicians and surgeons. Correct determination of the presence or absence of tumor in the SN is the responsibility of the pathologist.

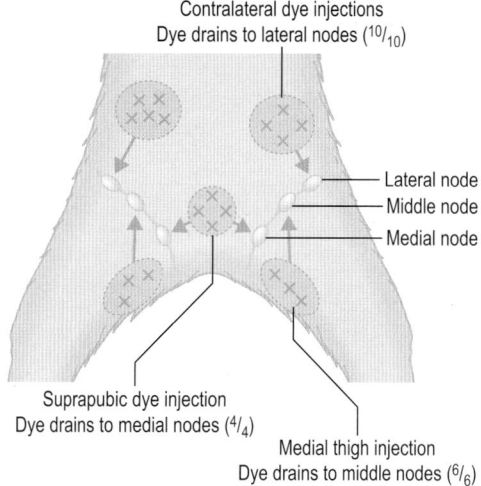

Contralateral dye injections
Dye drains to lateral nodes ($^{10}/_{10}$)

Lateral node
Middle node
Medial node

Suprapubic dye injection
Dye drains to medial nodes ($^4/_4$)

Medial thigh injection
Dye drains to middle nodes ($^6/_6$)

Fig. 28.3
Animal study: this demonstrates that dye injected in specific areas of the skin drains reliably to predictable lymph nodes. Dye injected in the lower lateral abdomen, the suprapubic area, and the upper medial thigh passed reliably to the lateral, medial, and middle lymph nodes, respectively. By courtesy of Wong etc.

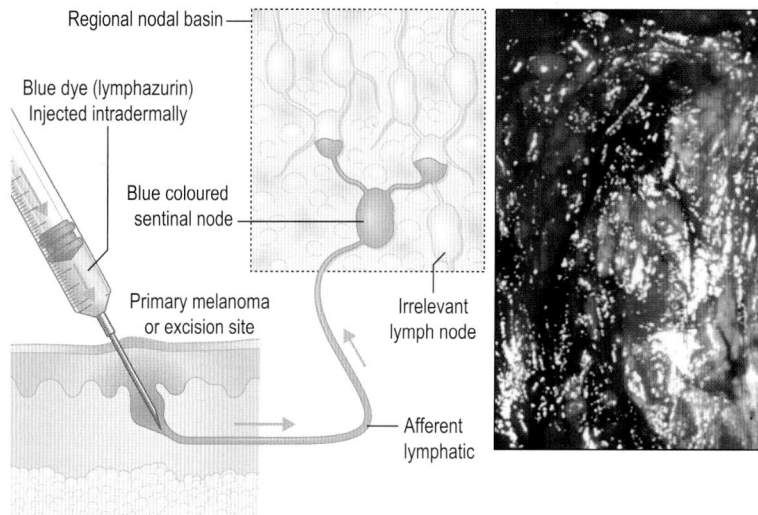

Regional nodal basin
Blue dye (lymphazurin) Injected intradermally
Blue coloured sentinal node
Primary melanoma or excision site
Irrelevant lymph node
Afferent lymphatic

Fig. 28.4
Diagram and photograph of the sentinel node (SN) technique as originally applied: blue dye (lymphazurin) is injected intradermally around the primary melanoma or biopsy site. The surgeon then explores the lymph node area identified by prior lymphoscintigraphy as the lymph drainage destination from the site of the primary tumor. Blue-colored afferent lymphatics (*lower two-thirds of the right panel*) are identified and followed to the blue-colored sentinel node (*upper mid area of the right panel*). Note that the SN is not necessarily the node that is anatomically closest to the primary site.

Laboratory management and gross evaluation of sentinel nodes

SNs arrive at the laboratory, fixed or fresh, as a single cleanly dissected lymph node, a single node in a mass of fat, or as multiple nodes embedded in fat. Surgeons may mark SN with clips or stitches to indicate where afferent lymphatics enter the node, to localize blue-stained segments of the node (evidence supporting SN status) and to highlight areas suspicious for tumor. Requisition forms usually refer to the nodes as SNs, less often as 'blue nodes', and occasionally simply imply SN status by appending the radioactive count detected intraoperatively.

Most patients have a single SN, but two and three nodes claimed to be SNs may be submitted. The number of nodes claimed as sentinel may reflect:
- the timing of isotope introduction at lymphoscintigraphy,
- whether additional isotope is injected at the beginning of surgery,

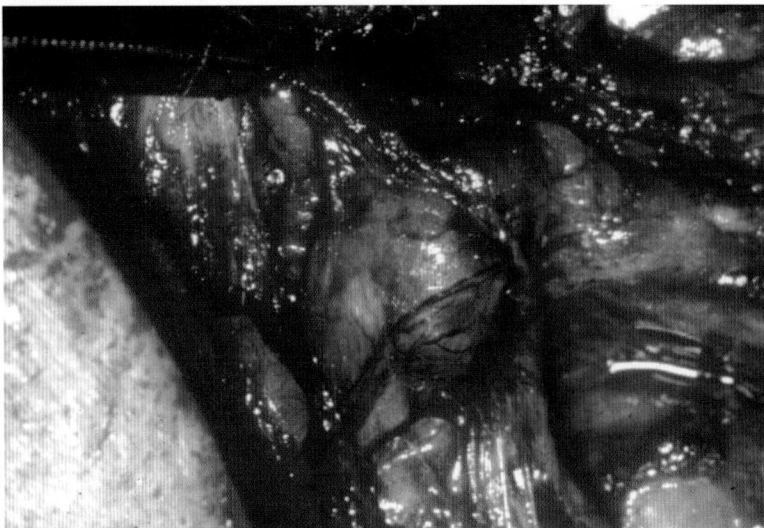

Fig. 28.5

Lymphazurin-stained blue sentinel node in situ. Persistence of visible dye is unusual when the specimen arrives in the pathology department.

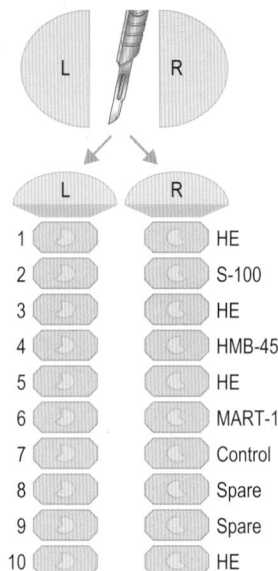

Fig. 28.6

Technique for sampling sentinel node (SN): the SN is bisected through the longest meridian. The nodal halves are placed cut face down in cassettes and fixed in formalin, ideally for 12–24 hours. Larger nodes may need to be cut more extensively, but additional slices should be cut parallel to the initial cut and parallel to the meridian (see text). Ten full-face serial sections are cut from both faces of the node and stained by H&E (sections 1, 3, 5, and 10), S100 (section 2), HMB-45 (section 4), and MART-1 (section 6). Sections 7–9 are reserved as spares. If tumor cells are not found in the initial 20 sections, cut from both halves of the SN of a patient with a thick primary melanoma (and thus significantly at risk for nodal metastases); additional sections may be prepared and examined, although the yield from this additional evaluation is likely to be low.

- the time taken by the surgeon to detect all lymph nodes that demonstrate increased radioactivity.

If many lymph nodes are submitted, the specimen is probably the product of a partial regional lymph node dissection rather than a true SNB. SNB, as originally described, provides a limited specimen that contains critical metastasis-susceptible nodal tissue, permitting a more detailed examination than is practicable for the multiple lymph nodes included in lymphadenectomy specimens.[1] Surgeons need to be aware that there are significant labor and expense issues when SN evaluation is required for specimens that contain multiple lymph nodes.

SN specimens are most informative if they are free of artifacts due to crush or cautery. SN may be partially dissected free of associated fat by the pathologist to facilitate processing, but it is good practice to leave a rim of fat so that entering lymphatics can be assessed for the presence of tumor. During dissection, the SN should be examined for blue coloration (*Fig. 28.5*) (although dye has usually dispersed by the time the specimen arrives at the laboratory). SN are measured (maximum length × width × thickness in millimeters) and exactly bisected through the longest meridian because melanoma cells first reach the subcapsular sinus via the afferent lymphatics, which mostly enter the node in the plane of the central meridian.[2] Cut surfaces are scrutinized for metastases, collections of melanin, or carbon pigment (from tattoos or deliberately introduced by the surgeon). This inspection is improved by use of a hand lens or dissecting microscope. Imprints can be prepared at this stage for cytological evaluation (see below). The SN halves are placed cut face down in cassettes and fixed in formalin (*Fig. 28.6*), ideally for 12–24 hours, although a lesser period may be acceptable if the specimen arrived at the laboratory in an appropriate volume of formalin. Larger nodes may need to be cut more extensively, but additional slices should be cut parallel to the initial cut and parallel to the meridian.

Confirmation of the sentinel status of submitted lymph nodes

Correct identification of the SN is primarily the responsibility of the nuclear medicine physicians and surgeons. Because of technical problems during nuclear medicine and surgical procedures, lymph nodes submitted as sentinel may not be true SN. Tumor within an SN can obstruct and divert lymph flow to another node, leading to incorrect designation of that node that contains blue dye and shows enhanced radioactivity as sentinel. Preoperative ultrasonography can identify nodal metastases larger than 5 mm (and some claim that smaller deposits are detectable by ultrasound).[1,2] If putative tumor deposits detected by ultrasound are confirmed as melanoma by fine needle aspiration, the patient may be considered for CLND instead of SNB.

The accuracy of currently used mapping agents is time dependent. The blue dye is not usually visible by the time that the SN is examined in the laboratory, and may have passed on to second-tier (nonsentinel) nodes. The radioactive isotope decays rapidly from the peak emission values measured in the operating room, and few laboratories have the equipment or expertise necessary to measure radioactivity. There is a need for a stable, inert marker that, after intradermal injection with the blue dye/isotope mixture, would selectively accumulate in SN and be readily visible on standard microscopic examination. Such a reagent would allow pathologists to confirm the actual status of nodes claimed to be sentinel.

Carbon particles injected intradermally with blue dye accumulate preferentially and usually exclusively in SN.[3] Particles accumulate in subcapsular sinuses and lymphoid tissues around the entry point of afferent lymphatics (*Fig. 28.7*). The location of these particles fortuitously indicates the area of the lymph node most likely to harbor metastatic tumor cells, since the carbon particles are delivered to the SN via the same lymphatics as tumor cells shed by the primary melanoma.[4] This approach cannot be used in patients with carbon-based permanent black tattoos of skin in the catchment area of the SN because tattoo pigment frequently tracks to regional lymph nodes. Drug regulations vary from country to country, and widespread use of this interesting and potentially valuable technique must await the clearance of substantial regulatory hurdles.

In Australia, antimony sulfur colloid is routinely used for lymphoscintigraphy prior to SNB.[5] Scolyer and coauthors report the use of inductively coupled plasma mass spectrometry of tissue sections to confirm SN status by detection of increased amounts of antimony: however, this approach is still in development and is not presently available for routine use.[6]

Can tissue from a sentinel node ethically be made available for research?

Accurate determination of the presence or absence of tumor in the SN is essential for correct staging of patients and to allow planning of optimal management. Identification of tumor status of an SN may be difficult as the amount of tumor present may be very small and occupy a limited area of the SN. Underassessment of the SN has serious consequences. Patients who develop ipsilateral regional nodal metastases after a reportedly tumor-free SN (false-negative SN) have an outcome that is at least as bad and possibly worse than that of patients who develop clinically detectable metastases in the regional nodes during observation after wide excision.[1] Not all false-negative SN can be attributed to pathologist error. Some are due to misidentification of an NSN as sentinel during lymphoscintigraphy or at surgery. Others reflect vagaries of the biology of melanoma spread. For example, while at the time of SNB there may be no tumor cells visible in the SN or at the excised primary site, clinically undetectable tumor cells present in the afferent lymphatics may arrive in the nodal basin after the SNB has been performed, seed in the remaining lymph nodes, and with time grow to clinically detectable size. Pathologists should therefore be extremely cautious in providing SN tissue to investigators until after the SN tumor status has been established.

That said, there is a legitimate need to determine whether novel techniques such as reverse transcriptase polymerase chain reaction (RT-PCR) (see below) can detect small amounts of clinically relevant tumor that are not readily identified by standard histopathological approaches. Equally, there is a need to investigate the biology of the SN to determine the molecular and cellular events that underlie SN susceptibility to metastases and to possibly develop therapies that will reverse such susceptibility. Research that can utilize formalin-fixed, paraffin-embedded tissue is not usually problematic: the provision of unfixed tissue is more difficult. Pathologists need to meet investigators to develop an understanding of the tissue requirements of the scientists and, in turn, to explain the professional and regulatory limitations that govern how and when tissue may be provided for research. Such meetings, conducted in good faith, will usually allow the development of a mutually acceptable approach. For example, we have on occasion been willing to provide interleaved sections with one section going for histology and the next for research. This has the great advantage of providing precise histologic and cytological control for the biological observations. Given the small amount and limited location of tumor in most SN, we are opposed to protocols where half of the SN is given away for scientific evaluation. Sampling and disposition of the SN must be controlled by the pathologist who is responsible for preparing the formal pathology report on the tumor status of the SN.

Intraoperative evaluation of sentinel nodes

Early in our development of LM/SNB, we evaluated the SN by intraoperative frozen sections and rapid immunohistochemistry to make possible immediate CLND if the SN contained tumor.[1] This had the advantage of sparing patients a second anesthetic and surgical procedure. However, experience has shown that evaluation of SN from melanoma patients on the basis of intraoperative frozen sections is relatively unreliable. Preparation of a full-face frozen section is necessary to allow complete evaluation of the subcapsular sinus where early tumor is often detected. To obtain a section that includes the entire subcapsular sinus from a frozen block often requires that many of the initial sections are discarded, leading to loss of substantial nodal tissue. Since SN metastases are frequently very small and selectively located in the area of the nodal meridian, limited diagnostic tissue may be entirely lost with these initial discarded sections. Additionally, identification of single melanoma cells or small clusters of melanoma cells or nevocytically differentiated melanoma cells is more difficult in frozen sections than in well-stained slides from fully fixed tissues. We and other authors strongly believe that melanoma-draining SNs should be evaluated using thin sections cut from well-fixed paraffin-embedded tissues.[2,3] If intraoperative assessment is requested, visual assessment of the cut face of the node for deposits of tumor is recommended, using a hand lens or dissecting microscope if necessary. Cell smears may be obtained by scraping the nodal cut surfaces, or tumor imprints prepared by pressing the cut surfaces of SN onto glass slides for cytological evaluation (*Fig. 28.8*). Interpretation of such preparations can be challenging if the melanoma cells are few in number or small and nevocytically differentiated, and the opinion of an experienced cytopathologist is likely to be necessary.

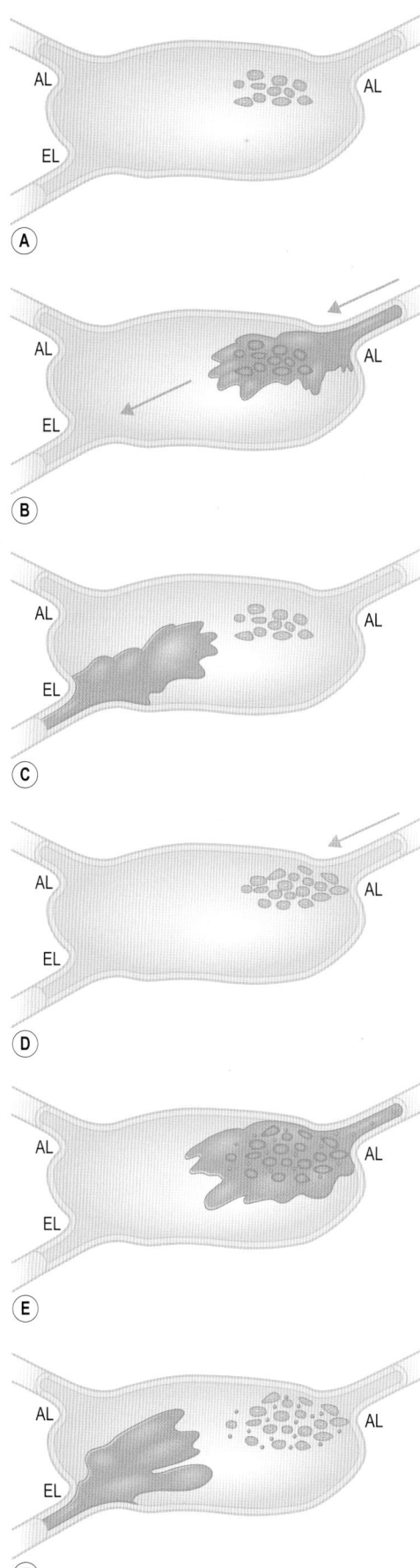

Fig. 28.7
Use of carbon particles to confirm the sentinel status of a lymph node and focus the search for tumor cells: (**A**) the upper three parts show the dynamics of passage of blue dye through an SN that contains a small focus of tumor cells. (**B** and **C**) The blue dye enters via the afferent lymphatic (AL) from the area of the primary tumor (via the same lymphatic that delivered the tumor cells) and rapidly passes through the lymph node to exit via the efferent lymphatic (EL). (**D**) The lower three parts show the identical sequence, but with carbon particles added to the blue dye. In contrast to the blue dye: (**E** and **F**) the carbon particles persist in the node, confirming its sentinel status and indicate the point of entry of the afferent lymphatic where tumor cells are most likely to be detected; (**B**) carbon particles free and within macrophages in a lymph node that received lymph from the site of a black tattoo.

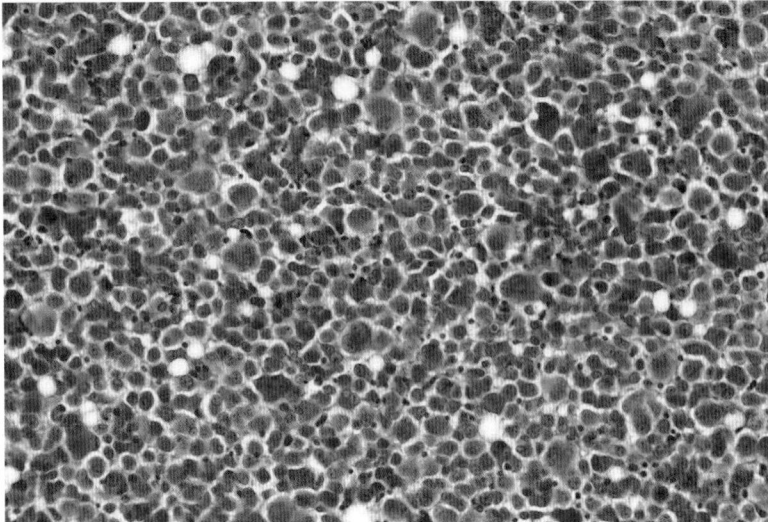

Fig. 28.8
Imprint of sentinel node showing melanoma cells: inguinal node from a patient with a vulvar primary melanoma. Most imprints are less obvious than this and show a minority of tumor cells admixed with abundant lymph node cells. Specialist cytopathological evaluation is often required.

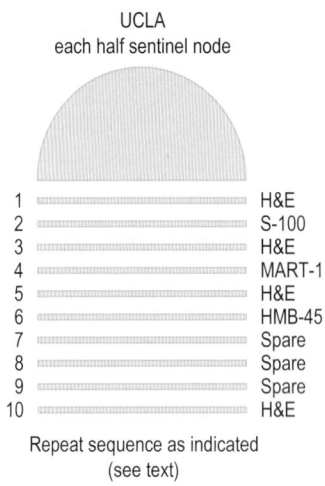

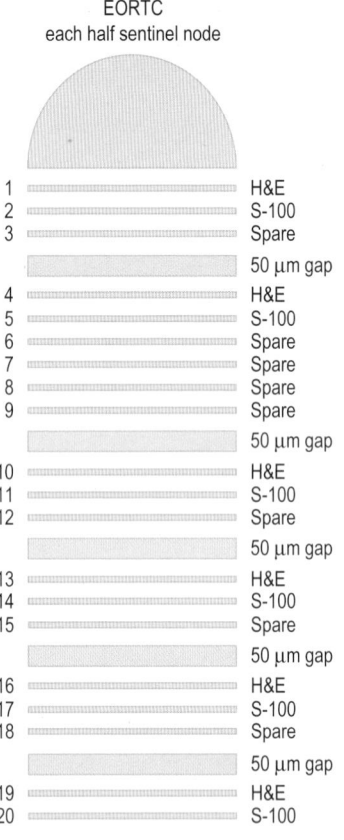

In large or round lymph nodes the 50 μm gap may be increased up to a maximum of 100 μm

Fig. 28.9
Guidelines (left panel, UCLA sampling; right panel, EORTC sampling): the left column depicts long-standing recommendations from UCLA that the two halves of the sentinel node are intensively sampled using H&E and immunohistochemistry on sequential full-face sections. This approach intensively samples the parameridional tissues, uses three separate immunomarkers of varying sensitivity and specificity, but does not evaluate the more peripheral parts of the node. This technique detects melanoma in 16% to 20% of sentinel nodes, a frequency identical to the ipsilateral failure rate of patients treated by wide excision alone. The right column depicts the node sampling technique adopted by the EORTC Melanoma Group. This uses H&E staining and S100 protein (spare sections may be used for additional immunomarkers). It samples more peripheral portions of the two halves of the sentinel node and is reported to detect melanoma in up to 33.8% of sentinel nodes. The clinical significance of the additional positive nodes detected in this way will become clear from extended follow-up studies that are in progress. This approach calls for some additional technical effort and a significant increment in pathologist work.

The need to evaluate multiple levels of the sentinel node

Sectioning

There is wide agreement on the general principles that govern acceptable histologic examination of SN from melanoma patients, but limited consensus on optimum sectioning and staining protocols. Multiple sections should be cut from each half of the SN and stained with hematoxylin and eosin (H&E) and immunohistochemically, using antibodies directed to melanoma-associated epitopes. The number of sections to be stained conventionally and by immunohistochemistry and the interval between sections for evaluation remain subject to debate.

In initial studies of nodal micrometastases, we observed that early melanoma metastases are usually located in a relatively narrow band of tissue adjacent to the longest nodal meridian.[1] Thus carefully sampling the tissues adjacent to the nodal meridian should detect the subgroup of melanoma patients with early nodal metastases. In this study, additional sampling of more peripheral areas of the node did not increase the proportion of melanoma-positive lymph nodes. This is in contrast to other tumors, such as breast cancer, where the tumor cells spread more widely across the nodal surface, and thus more extensive sampling progressively increases the proportion of tumor-positive lymph nodes. On the basis of these findings in lymph nodes from melanoma patients, we have consistently recommended examination of 10 full-face serial sections cut from both faces of the node and stained by H&E (sections 1, 3, 5, and 10), S100 (section 2), HMB-45 (section 4), MART-1 (section 6), and SOX-10 (section 7).[1] Sections 7–9 are retained as spares. If tumor cells are not found in the initial 20 sections cut from both halves of an SN of a patient with a primary melanoma thicker than 1.2 mm (and thus significantly at risk for nodal metastases), additional sections may be prepared and examined, although the yield from this additional evaluation is, in our experience, low. This approach detects melanoma in 16–20% of SNB specimens, a figure that varies according to the thickness of the primary melanomas included in the study group and that is closely similar to the rate of development of clinically detectable metastatic melanoma in the ipsilateral regional lymph nodes of patients observed for up to 10 years after wide excision of a primary melanoma.[2] It is arguable that this relatively simple focused sampling protocol detects most or all of the clinically significant melanoma deposits in SN.[3]

Recent studies, however, have reported that more extended sampling to allow evaluation of sections cut from deeper areas of SN identifies melanoma metastases in some patients where sections closer to the nodal meridian were tumor free.[4–8] The clinical significance of these additional melanoma cells detected by extended sampling remains unknown, and elucidation of their biology will require that patients be followed for up to 10 years.

Cook and coworkers have reported that examination of six pairs of sections cut at 50-μm intervals and stained respectively with H&E and S100 detects melanoma in up to 33.8% of SNs.[5] Spare sections are cut at each level and retained to permit additional immunohistochemistry in the event of ambiguous results from initial sections. These studies were undertaken because the authors had encountered practical difficulty in accurately cutting the SN through the true meridional plane and wished to reconcile reported differences in the rate of detection of tumor-positive SN by histopathology and molecular techniques (RT-PCR) (see below). A modification of this protocol has recently been adopted by the European Organisation for Research and Treatment of Cancer (EORTC) and is currently a requirement for evaluation of the SN of melanoma patients entering EORTC clinical trials (Fig. 28.9).

In choosing a protocol for sampling SNs, pathologists, in consultation with their surgical colleagues, should balance the need for accuracy with cost and workload considerations.[9]

The role of immunohistochemistry in detecting tumor in sentinel nodes

It may be extremely difficult to identify single melanoma cells or small clusters of melanoma cells (micrometastases) in H&E-stained sections. Without the assistance of immunohistochemistry, even experienced pathologists may overlook small amounts of tumor in up to 12% of SN specimens (*Fig. 28.10*). For this reason, and to minimize delays in reporting, immunohistochemical studies are best ordered at the time of initial processing. It is important to be selective in choosing the antibodies to be used in this evaluation.[1] Antibodies to S100 protein detect nuclear and cytoplasmic epitopes in virtually all melanomas, including desmoplastic melanomas (100% sensitive for melanoma), but are relatively non-specific, staining dendritic leukocytes in the nodal paracortex (*Figs 28.11* and *28.12*), some sinus histiocytes, fat cells within and outside lymph nodes, Schwann cells of node-associated nerves, and capsular/trabecular nevus cells (*Figs 28.13–28.15*). Some pathologists dislike antibodies to S100 because of this non-specificity, but with experience it is usually relatively easy to separate clusters of dendritic cells (DC) that tend to lie toward the periphery of paracortical nodules from melanoma cells, which are usually larger and nondendritic and are characteristically located in the subcapsular zone and deeper parenchymal tissues (*Figs 28.16* and *28.17*). Dendritic cells may be encountered in the subcapsular and other nodal sinuses, in which case they are regarded as immature DC (originally Langerhans cells) migrating from the skin to the nodal paracortex. Melanoma cells can be dendritic, but this morphology is usually observed in the radial growth phase of lentiginous melanomas and is exceedingly rare in vertical growth phase or metastatic melanoma. Paradoxically, nodal dendritic leukocytes in some SNs may be poorly dendritic or nondendritic. This is considered to indicate down-regulation of the paracortical dendritic cells as part of the tumor-induced immune suppression that affects SNs.[2] Nondendritic cells are recognized by their location in the nodal paracortex and characteristic immunophenotype: S100 positive, MART-1, SOX-10, and HMB-45 negative.

The epitopes detected by MART-1 and HMB-45 are located in the cytoplasm of melanoma and other melanocyte-derived cells. Such epitopes are more specific for cells of melanocytic lineage than S100, but are not expressed by the cells of up to 25% of melanomas, particularly metastatic melanomas.[1] Antityrosinase antibodies are also relatively specific, but of comparably limited sensitivity. There are reports of the use of combinations of antibodies (antibody cocktails), but these seem to be no more sensitive than S100 and do not allow the critical separation of melanoma cells from nevus cells on the basis of immunophenotype (see below).

Pathologist error accounts for some, but not all, cases of false-negative SNB, where – despite a reportedly negative SN – the patient later develops metastatic melanoma in the ipsilateral nodal basin (3–5% in most published series). Such cases may also reflect incorrect identification of the SN by nuclear medicine or at surgery, or a quirk of biology in which, at the time of SNB, the eventually metastatic tumor cells have departed the primary site, but have not yet arrived at the nodal basin. It is highly important to minimize the frequency of false-negative SN as patients in this category have an unfavorable prognosis, comparable to that of patients who develop nodal metastases during a period of observation after wide excision of a primary melanoma.[3]

False-positive assessment of an SN is relatively uncommon, but may lead to patients being subjected to immediate CLND, an operation that is associated with considerably more morbidity than SNB alone and that confers no benefit on patients without nodally metastatic melanoma.[3] False positivity is usually due to misinterpretation of benign cells in the lymph node as melanoma cells. Misidentification often involves macrophages (*Figs 28.18* and *28.19*), particularly melanin-containing macrophages and macrophages that have phagocytosed melanosomal fragments that express the epitopes of MART-1/Melan-A or HMB-45 released from disrupted melanoma cells, dendritic leukocytes, and capsular and trabecular nodal nevus cells. Confusion

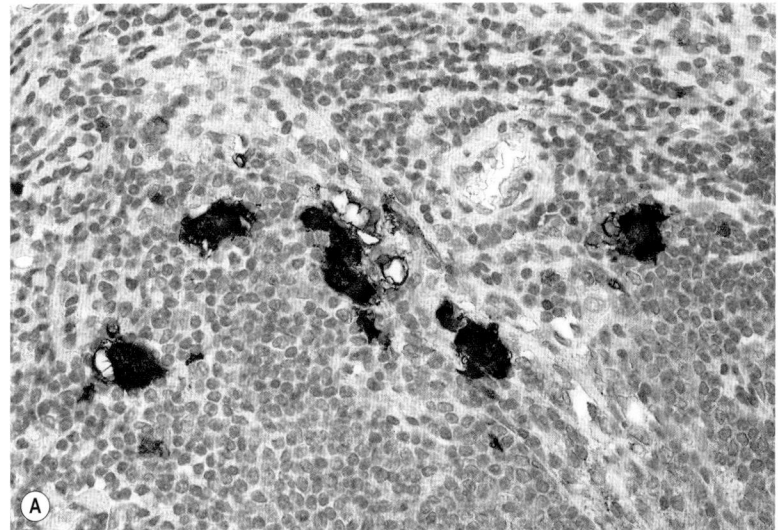
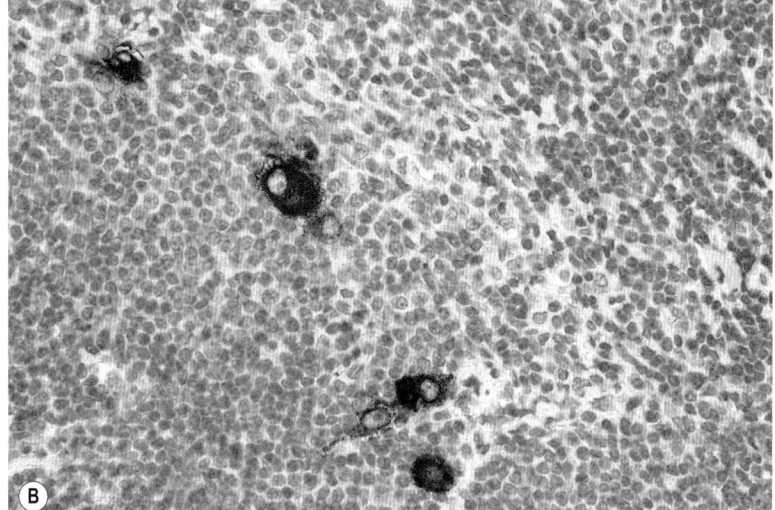
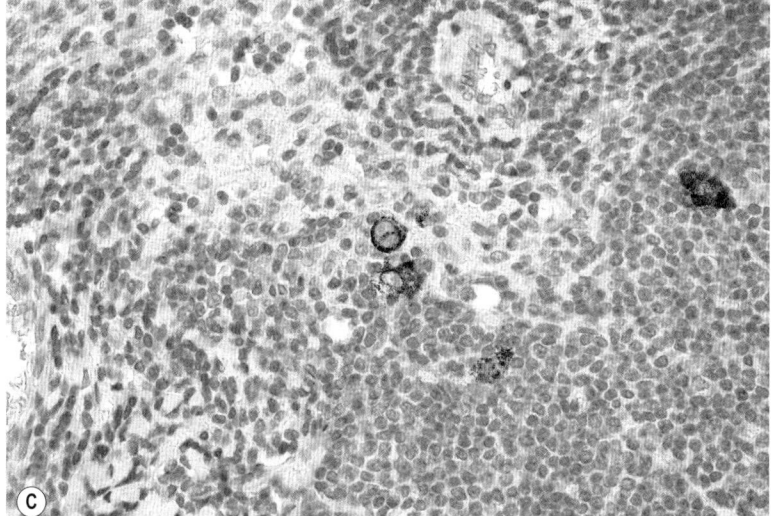

Fig. 28.10

Single melanoma cells immunohistochemistry: detected by their expression of (**A**) S100 protein; (**B**) MART-1/Melan-A; and (**C**) HMB-45. In the illustration of the HMB-45-stained section, there is a granular macrophage below and to the right of the central melanoma cells.

between melanin-containing macrophages and immunopositive melanoma cells may be reduced by using a colored chromogen, such as aminoethylcarbazole or alkaline phosphatase (followed by 'fast red'), in place of brown diaminobenzidine that may be misinterpreted as melanin (*Fig. 28.20*). However, since colored chromogens are less frequently used, pathologists may find such preparations more difficult to interpret. Other potential sources of false-positivity are S100-positive Schwann cells of intranodal and perinodal nerves (*Fig. 28.21*), ganglion cells, and mast cells. Distinction of these potential confounding cells is usually achieved by scrutiny of their cytology, their location in or adjacent to the lymph node, and immunophenotype. SNs, particularly inguinal SNs removed from older patients, may show extracellular HMB-45 reactivity associated with calcified foci in the collagen of the nodal trabeculae.

We have encountered an unusual potential cause of a false-positive interpretation of an SN in patients where a small piece of melanoma is included on the slide as a positive control. In rare instances, cells from the positive control tissue may detach and float over to settle on top of the nodal section under evaluation. The keys to identifying these 'internal floaters' are to recognize that the tumor cells are not in the plane of the section and then to confirm that the 'floater' tumor cells are morphologically and immunophenotypically identical to the cells of the positive control tissue.

Microscopic evaluation of sentinel nodes for metastatic melanoma

It is useful to examine the immunohistochemically stained sections first since MART-1/Melan-A, HMB-45, SOX-10, and S100 protein stains can detect truly small numbers of melanoma cells that are difficult to identify in H&E preparations. The entire slide is scanned at low power, and the

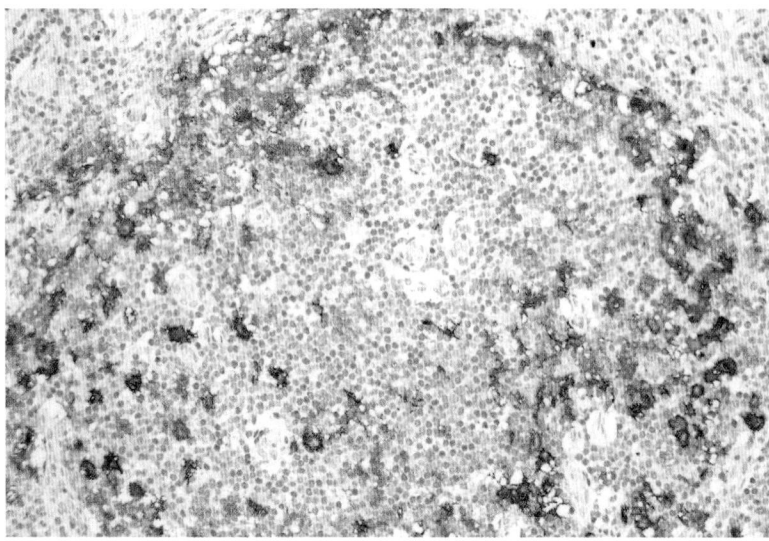

Fig. 28.11
Lymph node stained for S100 protein: the illustration shows a paracortical nodule with an abundant population of polydendritic dendritic cells (DCs) that tend to cluster in a ring around the periphery of the paracortical tissue. This classic distribution of DCs is best seen at moderate magnification. DC may also be encountered in the lymph node sinuses and less abundantly in B-cell areas. In addition to their distribution, the presence of multiple complex dendritic processes, relatively small size, and lack of a prominent S100 positive nucleus allows separation of these cells from melanoma cells. Additionally, DC do not express MART-1/Melan-A or HMB-45. In some SN, DC may lose their dendrites, and this may present more of a diagnostic challenge.

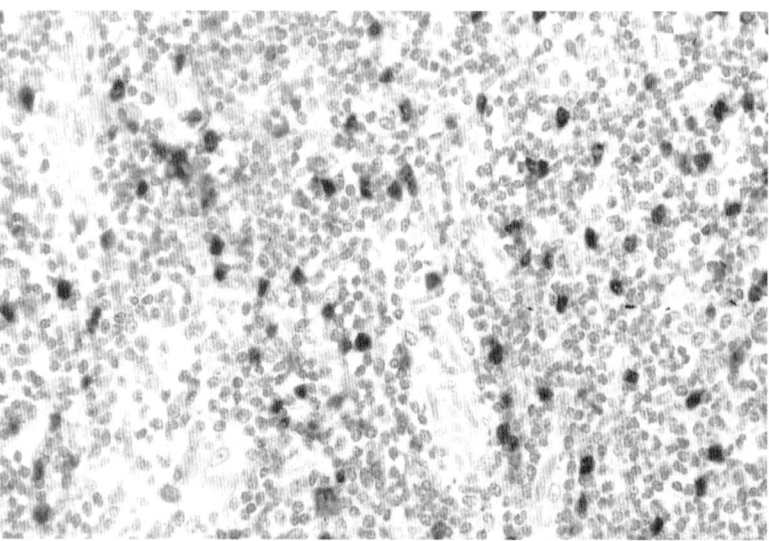

Fig. 28.12
Poorly dendritic and nondendritic DC in a sentinel node: reduced expression of dendrites by DC is viewed as evidence that they are down-regulated by tumor-induced immune suppression. Nondendritic DC are recognized by their scattered distribution in nodal paracortex and sinuses and their characteristic immunophenotype: S100 positive, MART-1 and HMB-45 negative.

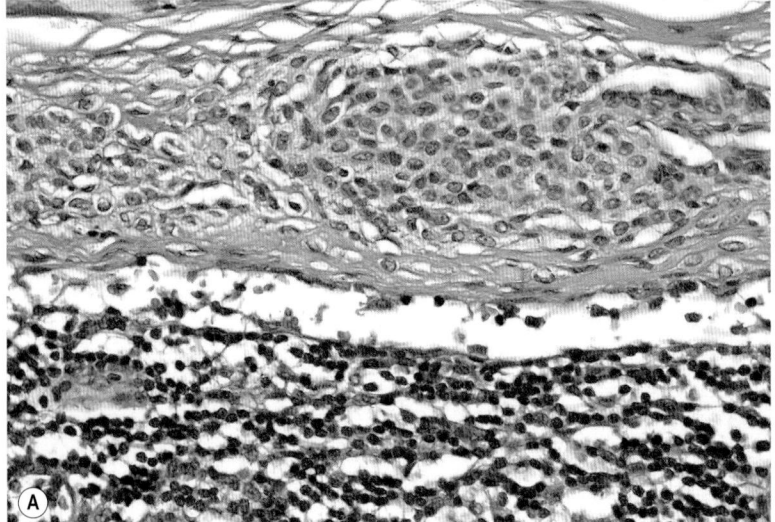
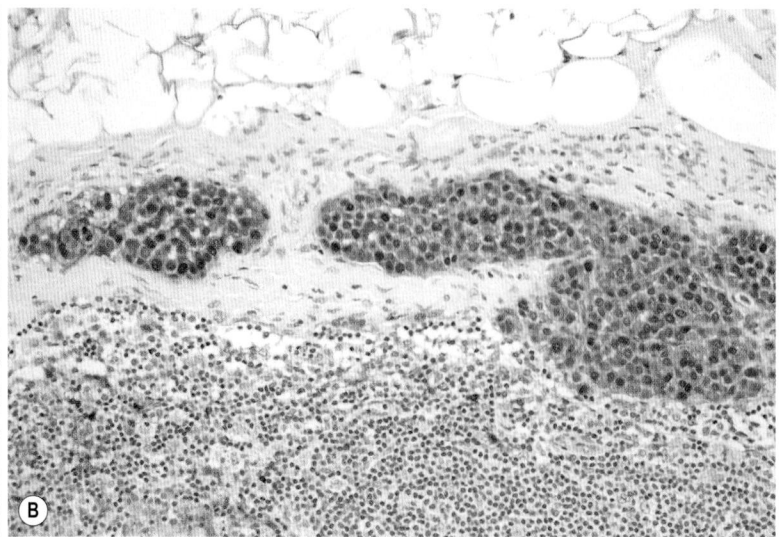

Fig. 28.13
Capsular nevus: (**A**) shows a nevus that is clearly confined to a slightly expanded nodal capsule (H&E). Nevus cells are smaller than most melanoma cells, have limited cytoplasm, usually show only traces of cytoplasmic melanin, and may resemble large lymphocytes. Their nuclei are bland and lack large nucleoli or mitoses. (**B**) A capsular nevus stained for S100 demonstrating epitope in nuclei and cytoplasm.

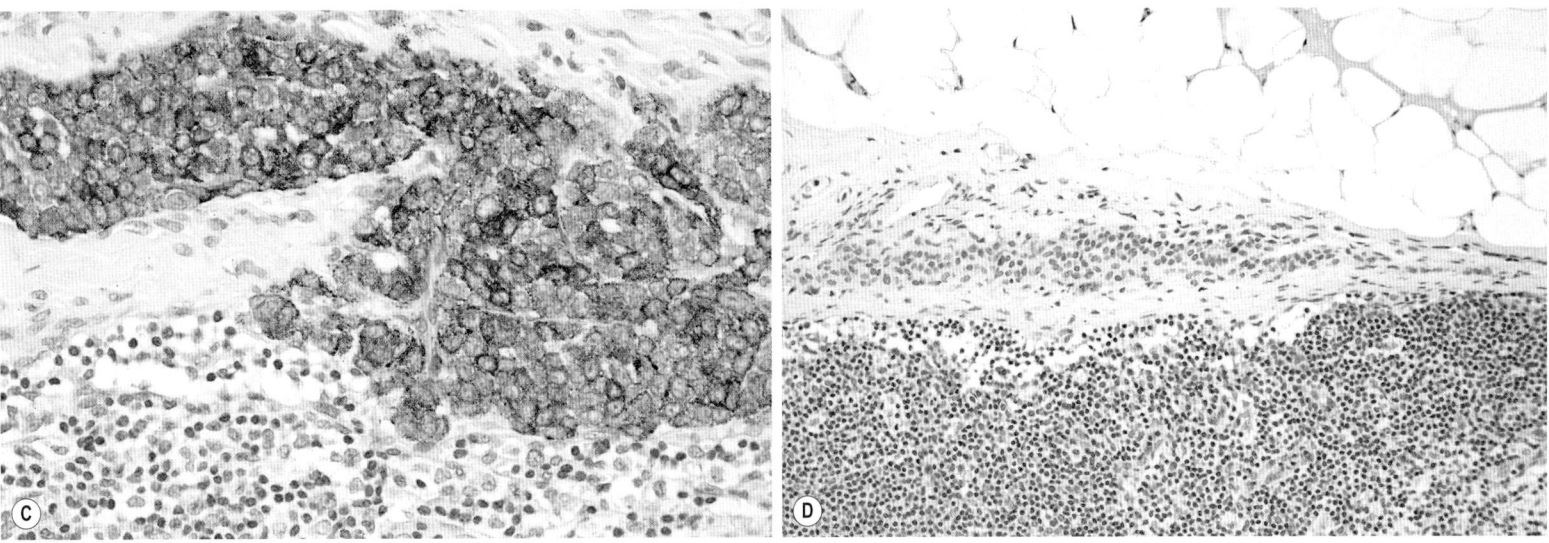

Fig. 28.13, cont'd
(**C**) A capsular nevus stained for MART-1/Melan-A demonstrating epitope confined to the cytoplasm. (**D**) A capsular nevus stained for HMB-45. The great majority of nevus cells do not express HMB-45, although occasional cells may show a trace of epitope in the cytoplasm.

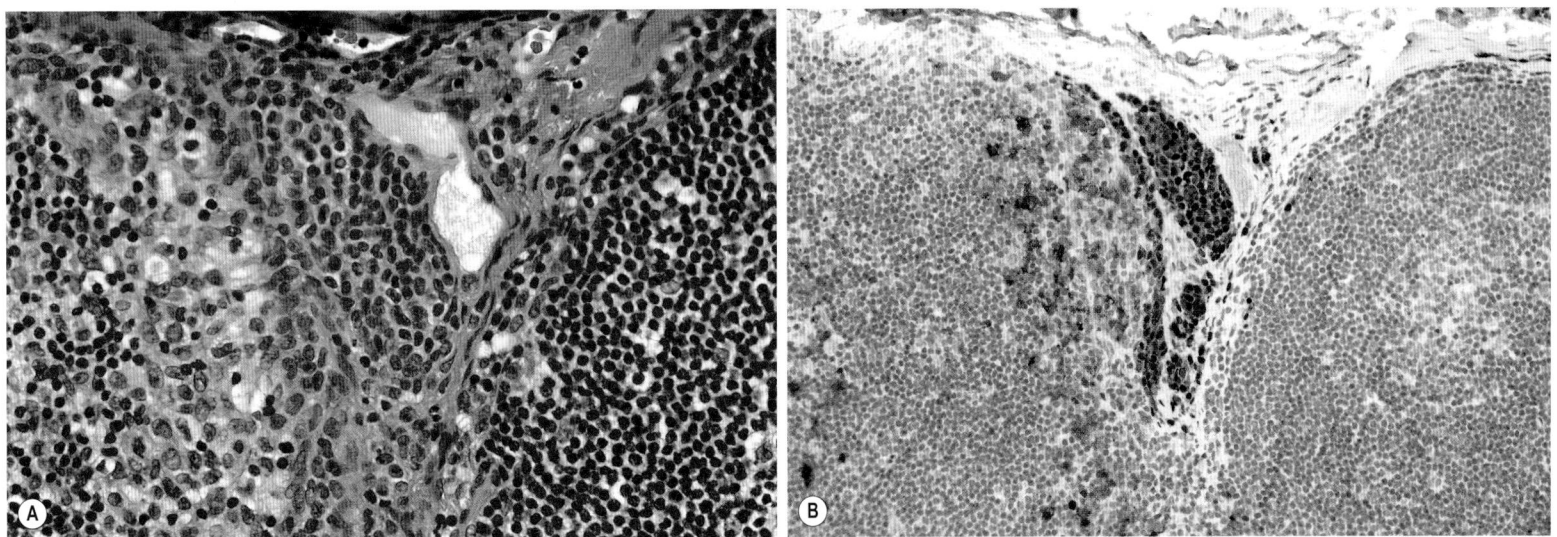

Fig. 28.14
Trabecular nevus cells: (**A**) shows a column of nevus cells located in a nodal trabeculum and flanked by a peritrabecular sinus and lymphoid parenchyma; (**B**) shows the same trabecular nevus stained for S100 and again flanked by a peritrabecular sinus and lymphoid parenchyma. The S100 positive cells in the peritrabecular sinus and parenchyma are dendritic cells.

different nodal compartments are assessed, starting with the subcapsular sinus, the commonest location of early metastases (*Fig. 28.22*). Tumor cells may occupy substantial areas of the node or be few, and singly dispersed or organized as microcolonies in subcapsular sinuses, lymphoid parenchyma, and deeper sinuses. The afferent lymphatics should be specifically evaluated for the presence of tumor. Tumor in afferent lymphatics, including intracapsular lymphatics, has the same clinical implications as intranodal tumor and is equivalent to a positive SN (*Fig. 28.23*). High-power (× 400) fields are examined to confirm the cytology and nature of single or clustered melanocyte-derived cells. Extracapsular extension (*Fig. 28.24*) is infrequent, especially when the tumor burden is small, but should be recorded if present.

Separation of nevus cells and metastatic melanoma in sentinel nodes

Benign nevus cells can be identified in the connective tissue architecture of up to 24% of lymph nodes, predominantly in the capsule and trabeculae.[1,2]

The great majority of nodal nevus cell collections derive from cutaneous nevi in the catchment area of the lymph node, the nevus cells apparently reaching the node via afferent lymphatics. Careful scrutiny will often show that benign nevi abut and deform adjacent dermal lymphatics. In rare instances, nodal nevi may be the result of aberrant migration of neural crest-derived melanocyte precursors (melanoblasts) during embryogenesis or even of melanocyte stem cells.[3] Accurate discrimination of nodally located benign nevi from melanoma cells is very important. This requires careful consideration of the location of the melanocyte-derived cells in the nodal architecture and detailed assessment of their cytology and immunophenotype. Melanoma cells are mostly larger than nevus cells (although the occasional nevoid melanoma may present a considerable diagnostic challenge) and are commonly located in the subcapsular sinus and deeper lymphoid tissues of the node. Unlike nevus cells, melanoma cells are seldom present in the nodal capsule other than within afferent lymphatics. Cytological features that may be used to distinguish melanoma from nevus cells include large cell size, high nuclear to cytoplasmic ratio, prominent nucleoli, and mitotic figures (especially atypical mitoses). Both melanoma and nevus cells

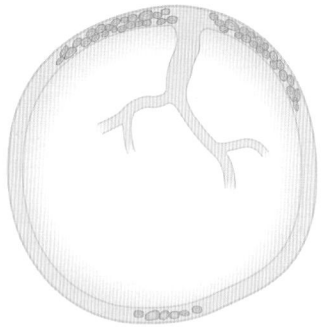

(A)   Nevocytes in lymph node capsule

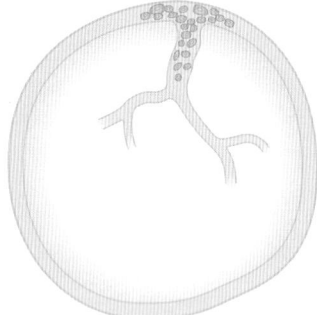

(B)   Nevocytes in trabeculum of lymph node

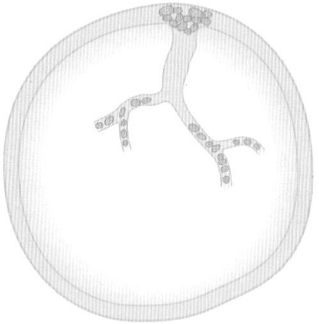

(C)   Nevocytes in arborized trabeculae of lymph node

may contain finely dispersed small melanin granules (single melanized melanosomes that are just visible under the microscope) that indicate melanin synthesis within the cell (*Fig. 28.25*). The amount of melanin in melanoma cells is widely variable, but in most instances (with the notable exception of the cells of heavily melanized cellular blue nevi) is greater than that encountered in the cells of melanocytic nevi. Coarse melanin granules (aggregates of melanosomes that are readily visible under the microscope) are characteristic of melanin-containing macrophages (melanophages), but may be seen, admixed with smaller melanin granules, in some melanoma cells. Melanoma cells are almost always S100 protein-positive (staining of nuclei and cytoplasm), SOX-10 (nuclear staining), most (up to 85%) stain positively for MART-1/Melan-A and HMB-45, and Ki67 reactive nuclei are present at relatively high frequency.

Conventional nodal nevus cells are smaller than most melanoma cells, have limited cytoplasm, usually show only traces of cytoplasmic melanin, and may resemble large lymphocytes. Their nuclei are bland and lack prominent nucleoli or mitoses. They stain positively for S100 protein, SOX-10, MART-1/Melan-A, and P16[4], but weakly or negatively for Ki67 and HMB-45.[5] Up to 25% of melanoma patients have capsular or trabecular nevus cells in one or more regional node(s). Location of nevi in connective tissue is usually obvious, although it may be necessary to use a connective tissue stain to rule out extension into the subcapsular parenchyma. Extension of nevi into perivascular stroma or ultrafine reticulations of the trabeculae can make interpretation difficult, because on initial appraisal the nevus cells may appear to be located in the nodal parenchyma,[6] a location that is more characteristic of melanoma metastases. Connective tissue stains such as Masson trichrome and reticulin may help by disclosing the complex arborizing pattern of nodal stroma.

Is there a role for SNB in the evaluation of melanocytic lesions of uncertain metastatic potential?

The morphology and immunophenotype of some primary cutaneous melanocytic lesions may be insufficiently typical to allow their certain assignment to the category of melanoma or nevus: lesions of uncertain malignant potential.[1-5] The majority of lesions falling into this category are atypical cellular blue nevi, atypical spitzoid lesions, and deep penetrating nevi. In such cases, the surgeon will usually excise the lesion with a margin of local clearance appropriate for a primary melanoma of similar thickness, and

Fig. 28.15
Diagram demonstrating the relationship of capsular and trabecular nevus cells to the lymph node: note that the nevus cells can also be present in fine arborizations of the nodal trabecular frame work (which may only become visible with special stains for collagen and reticulin). In the absence of special staining, it may be incorrectly assumed that such cells are free within the nodal parenchyma and they may be incorrectly interpreted as melanoma metastases.

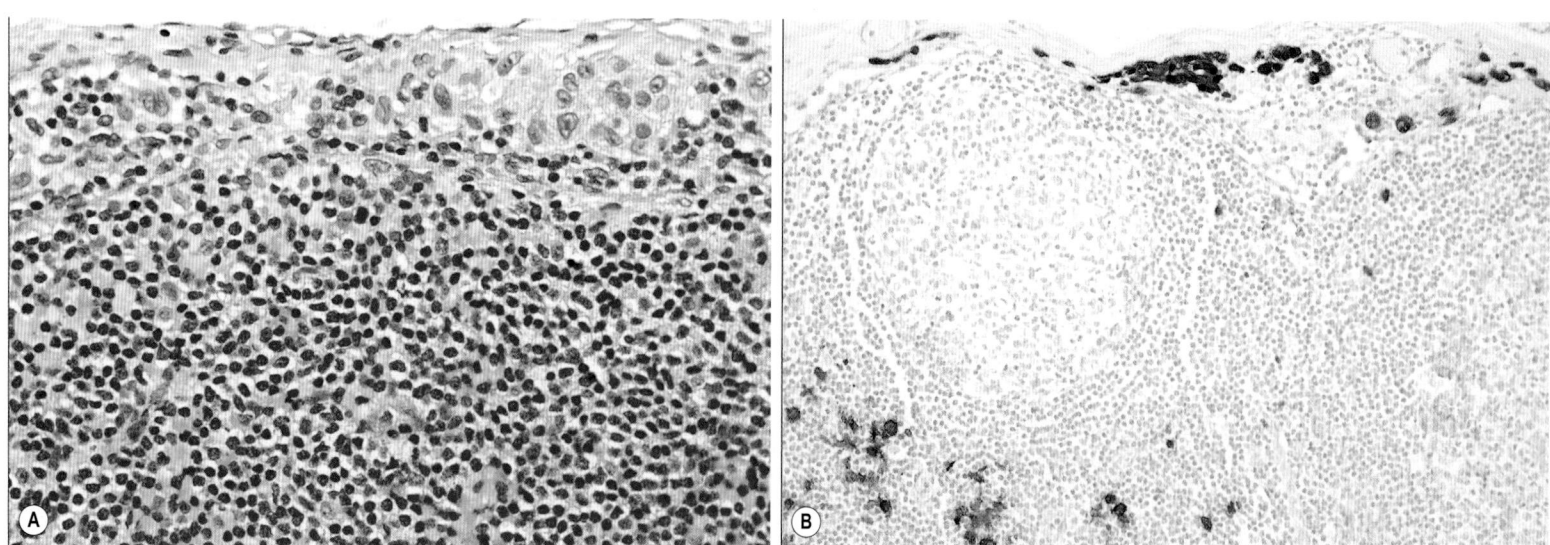

Fig. 28.16
Subcapsular sinus melanoma metastases: (**A**) this shows a ribbon of melanoma cells sandwiched between the nodal capsule and the nodal parenchyma (H&E). (**B**) There is a small collection of S100-positive melanoma cells immediately deep to the capsule. Note that deeper in the node there are S100 positive dendritic cells that lack the prominent nuclear staining by S100 that is seen in the melanoma cells. Most of these are poorly dendritic, but some have well-developed dendritic processes.

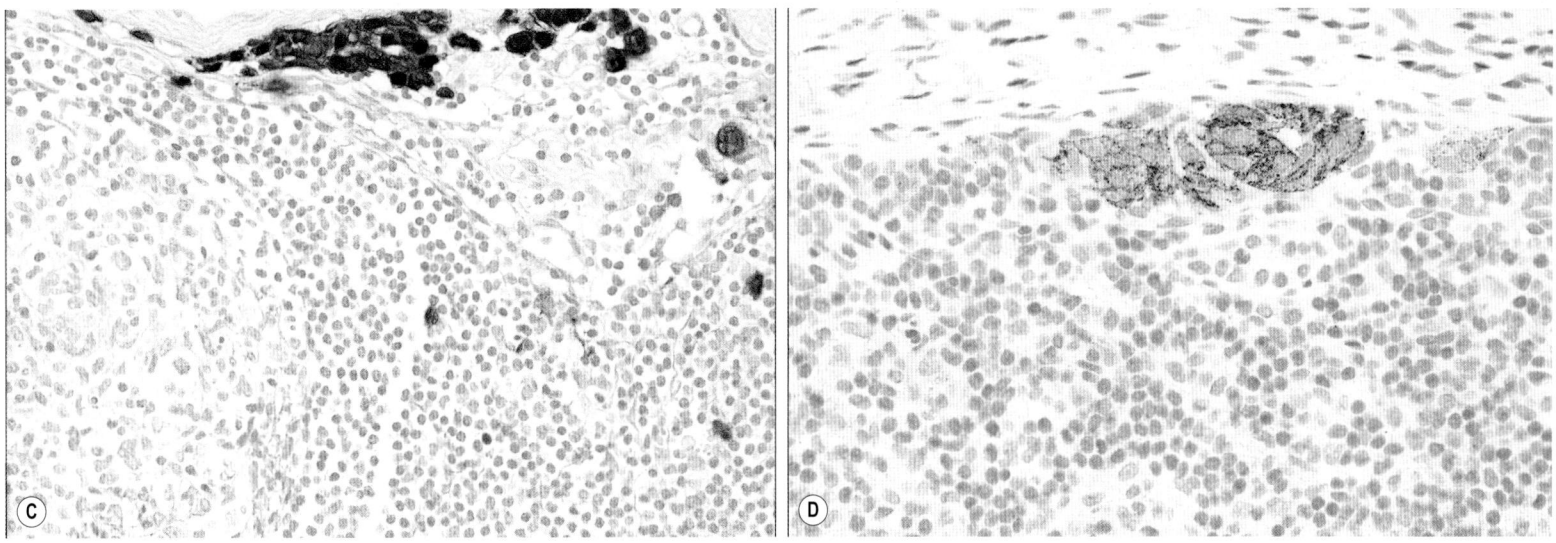

Fig. 28.16, cont'd
(C) Detail of the subcapsular melanoma in (B); (D) shows subcapsular melanoma expressing HMB-45. This lesion also expressed MART-1/Melan-A with a similar cytoplasmic pattern of staining (not shown).

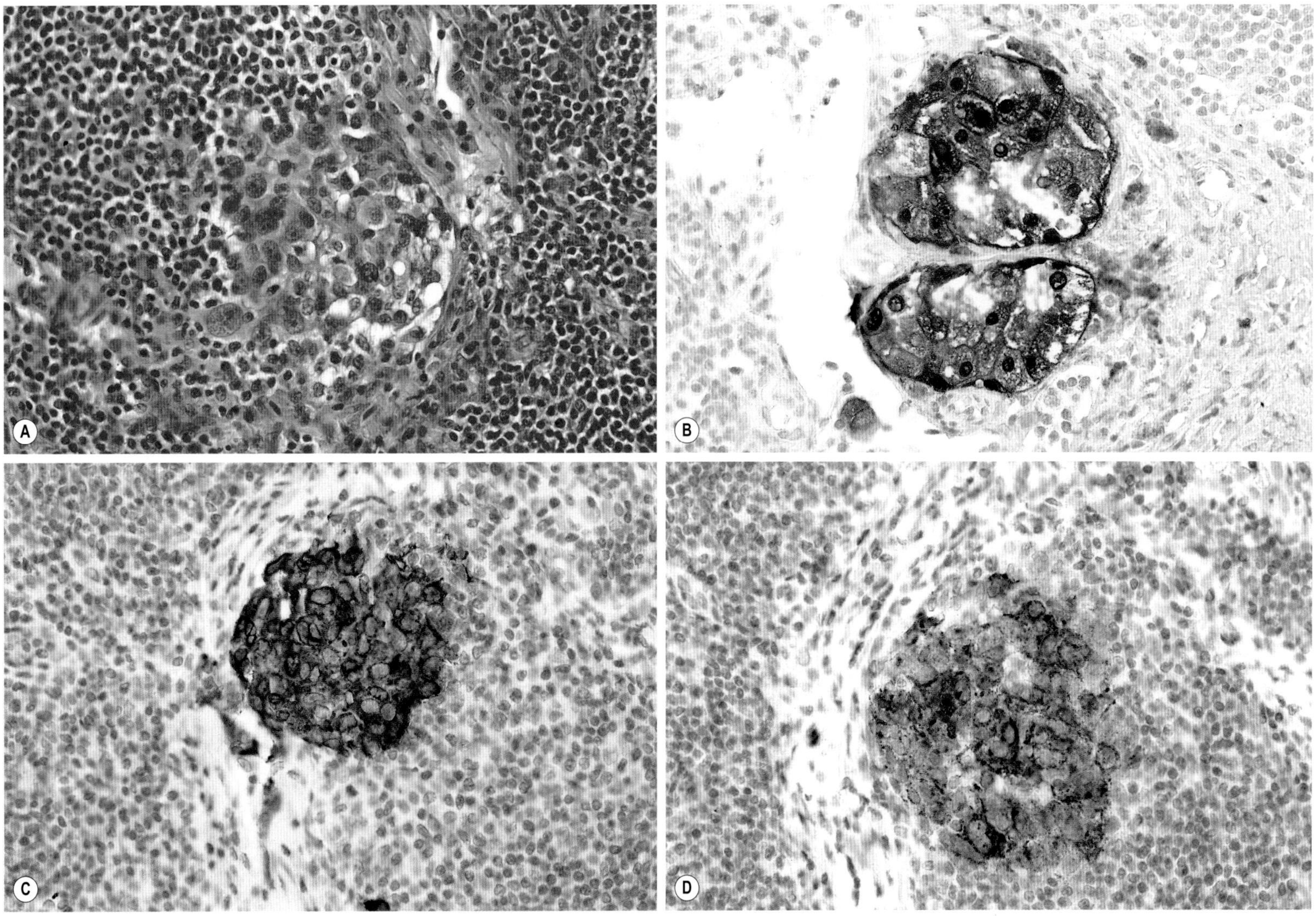

Fig. 28.17
Parenchymal melanoma metastases: these panels show a metastasis of melanoma located deep in the nodal parenchyma. (A) While visible in an H&E-stained section, the fact that (B) the amelanotic lesion expresses S100 protein, (C) MART-1/Melan-A, and (D) HMB-45 confirms that it is a melanoma.

review the pros and cons of SNB with the patient. If an SNB is performed and the SN shows no evidence of a melanocytic lesion, this may represent a nevus without capacity to extend to the nodes or a melanoma that has not (yet) metastasized to the regional nodes, but which may later develop clinically detectable metastases in distant sites. In such cases, CLND is not indicated. If a nodal melanocytic lesion is identified but is confined to the lymph node capsule or trabeculae, there is again no indication for immediate completion lymphadenectomy. If lesional cells are confined to the nodal capsule (other than the special case of melanoma cells in an afferent lymphatic) and

trabeculae, it is likely that they are collections of benign nevus cells (see above). If the node contains tumor that is truly located in the parenchyma, CLND and adjuvant therapy may be considered because a true parenchymal location strongly favors metastatic melanoma. The use of SNB in evaluation of melanocytic lesions of uncertain malignant potential is opposed by some, who argue that SNB is not appropriate for lesions with limited malignant potential that are not customarily treated by regional nodal surgery. The situation is further complicated by the fact that some patients with atypical spitzoid lesions atypical cellular blue nevi and pigmented epithelioid melanocytomas are found to have ostensibly parenchymal tumor deposits in the SN that closely resemble lymph node metastases and yet such lesions do not seem to extend to additional NSNs or to visceral sites. The biology and clinical management of these 'borderline' lesions is poorly understood and clearly needs more formal evaluation. Since the last edition of this book, the use of SNB in the management of melanocytic lesions of uncertain malignant potential has decreased. While a proportion of these patients may have lesional cells in the SN, the incidence of additional nodal tumor at CLND and the frequency of visceral metastases and melanoma death in these patients is essentially zero.

Molecular biology techniques in the assessment of sentinel nodes from melanoma patients

Since it is not possible histologically to examine the entire SN, it is possible that conventional microscopy may fail to detect some melanoma metastases in SNs of patients with limited tumor burden. This argues for more extensive nodal sampling[1] and/or the introduction of novel approaches such as the RT-PCR.[2] Molecular staging is currently standard in the management of hematological malignancies. The possibility that RT-PCR might identify melanoma cells in SNs in which extensive histologic and immunohistological evaluation reveals no evidence of tumor has attracted considerable interest. However, there is currently no compelling reason to abandon microscopy and analyze SN exclusively by RT-PCR. The techniques commonly used to extract mRNA for evaluation by RT-PCR destroy the tissue and prohibit identification of the specific cell from which the enhanced signal was derived. A molecular signal for a melanoma-associated marker, in addition to originating from a melanoma cell, might also derive from capsular and trabecular nevi, Schwann cells of intranodal nerves or macrophages that have ingested melanosomes or other organelles from melanoma cells. Concerns have been expressed that overinterpretation of RT-PCR results carries the

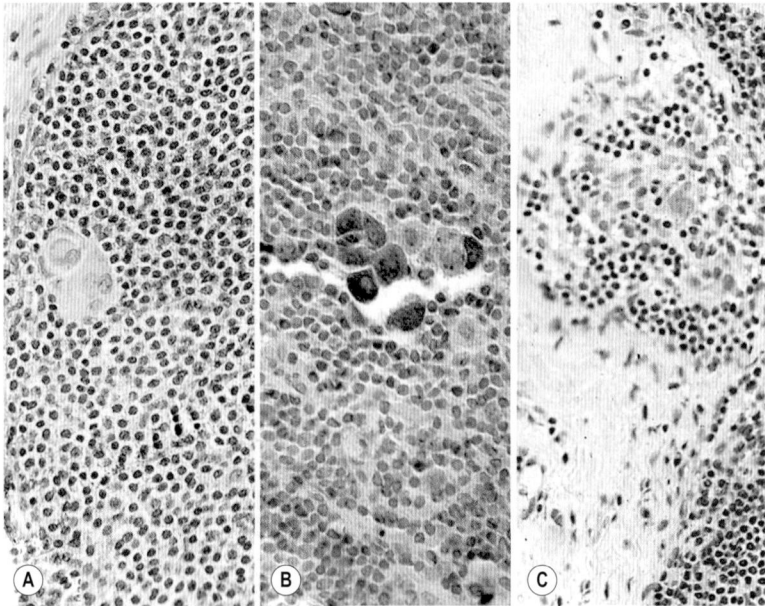

Fig. 28.18
Care must be taken to avoid the overinterpretation of nodal macrophages as melanoma cells. In panel (**A**), relatively large epithelioid macrophages are scattered among lymphocytes in a subcapsular position. These cells were negative for S100, MART-1/Melan-A, and HMB-45. Panel (**B**) shows a collection of relatively large macrophages containing abundant coarsely granular melanin (melanophages). These cells were negative for S100, MART-1/Melan-A, and HMB-45. Panel (**C**) shows a small granuloma-like collection of epithelioid macrophages. These cells were negative for S100.

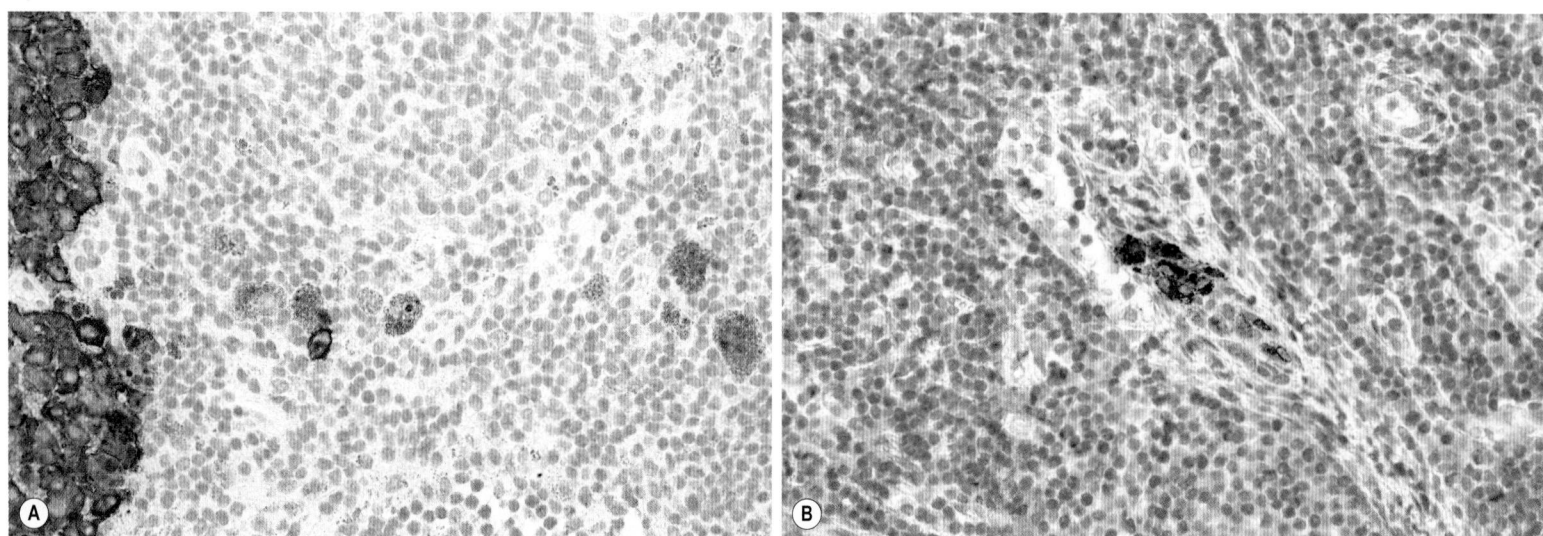

Fig. 28.19
Nodal macrophages: a further problem with nodal macrophages is that they may ingest fragments of melanosomes that express melanoma-associated epitopes from disrupted melanocytic cells and react positively in immunohistochemical studies: (**A**) shows a MART-1/Melan-A-stained section with metastatic melanoma at the left and toward the right scattered macrophages that contain MART-1/Melan-A positive granules; (**B**) shows a collection of macrophages that contain coarse HMB-45 positive granules.

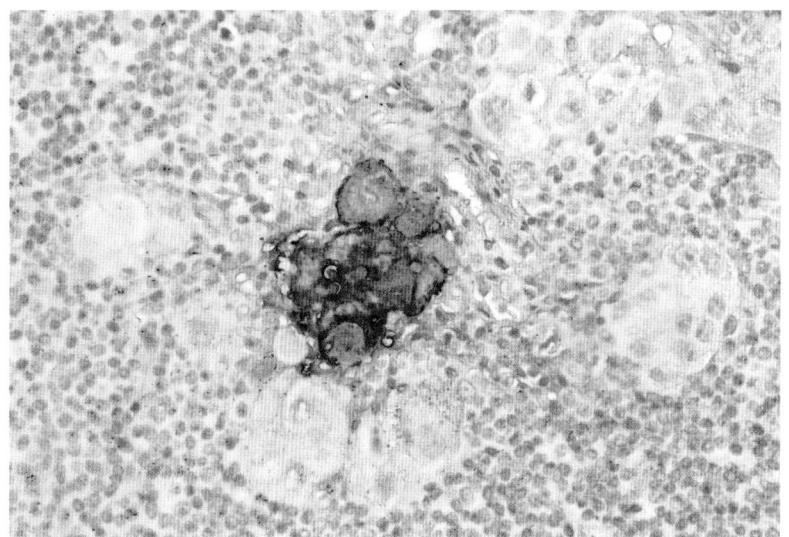

Fig. 28.20
Melanoma: this small collection of melanoma cells stains positively for HMB-45 and is highlighted by the red chromogen aminoethylcarbazole. Note the granuloma-like collections of melanin-containing macrophages that surround these cells. Traces of AEC-highlighted, HMB-45 positive material are present in some of the macrophages.

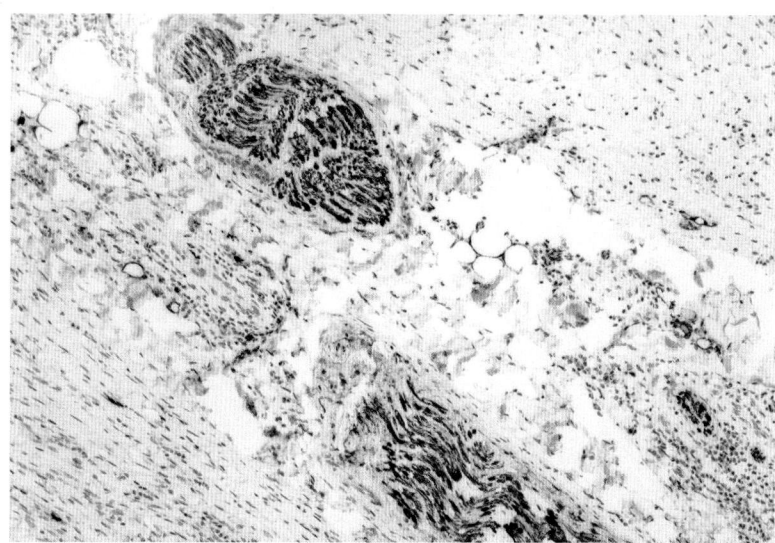

Fig. 28.21
Perinodal nerve: the Schwann cells are stained with an antibody to S100. While the neural nature of such structures is usually (as in this case) readily apparent, there may occasionally be a problem in distinguishing neural structures from melanoma cells in a lymphatic or free in the tissue. This type of problem is most likely to occur when the nerves are intranodal or if the tissue section is thick or from poorly fixed material. Nerves stain negatively with antibodies to MART-1/Melan-A and HMB-45.

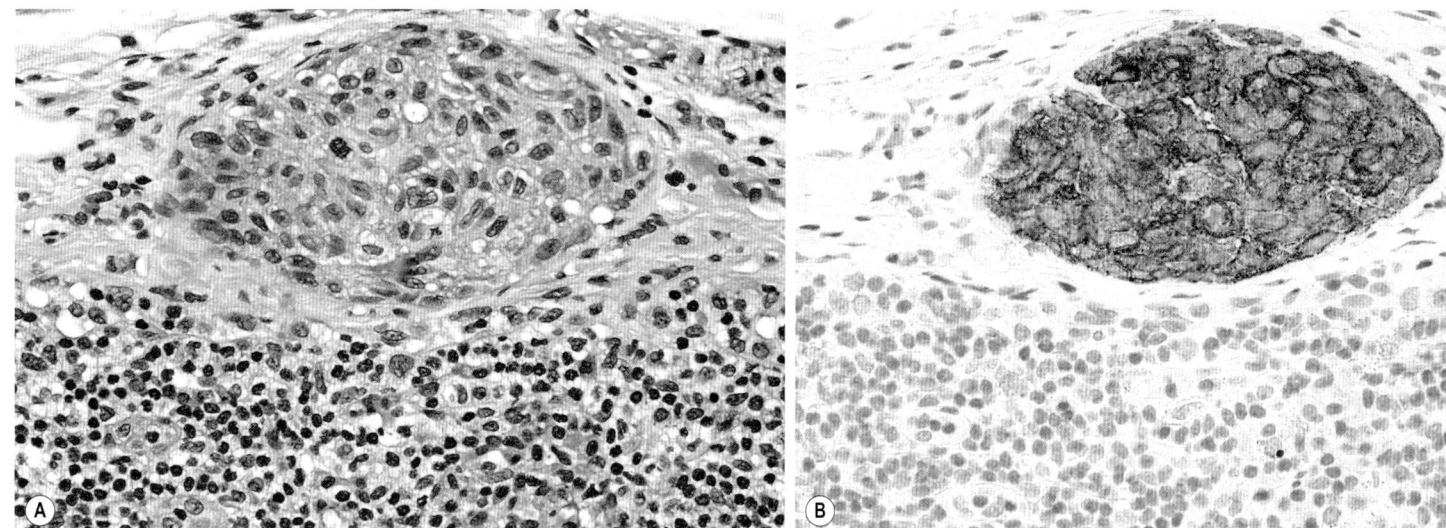

Fig. 28.22
Metastatic tumor in afferent lymphatics: (**A**) melanoma in the intracapsular segment of an afferent lymphatic of a sentinel lymph node (H&E); (**B**) MART-1/Melan-A. In the presence of these appearances, the sentinel node should be reported as positive.

risk of overtreatment.[3] Mocellin and coworkers, in a careful meta-analysis, have shown that a positive PCR reaction in the SNs of melanoma patients is significantly correlated with TNM stage, disease recurrence, and overall and disease-free survival.[4] These authors did, however, find extensive heterogeneity between the results obtained in the 22 sizeable studies that they analyzed. They conclude that 'the available evidence is somewhat conflicting and probably is not sufficient to conclude that PCR status is a prognostic indicator reliable enough to be implemented clinically in the therapeutic decision-making process'. However, they consider that their findings 'justify additional investigations of the prognostic power of PCR analysis of sentinel lymph node (SLN) in patients with cutaneous melanoma'. The efficacy and clinical relevance of molecular analysis of SN are being studied in the second Multicenter Selective Lymphadenectomy Trial (MSLT-II), sponsored by the National Cancer Institute in the United States.

Prediction of outcome based on the extent of nodal replacement by tumor and its distribution within the sentinel node

Clinical outcome and the likelihood of death from melanoma correlate with the number of lymph nodes that contain melanoma metastases,[1] but pathologists may further refine that assessment by measuring the size of nodal metastases and specifying their location within the SN. Building on earlier (pre-SN) studies[2] of the morphometric assessment of the area and micrometer-assessed diameter of nodal melanoma metastases (*Fig. 28.26*), Starz and coworkers[3] reported that the micrometer-measured depth of tumor penetration from the inner surface of the SN capsule correlated directly with the likelihood of metastases in NSNs in the same nodal drainage basin (*Fig. 28.27*). Wagner and coworkers[4] correlated SN tumor volume

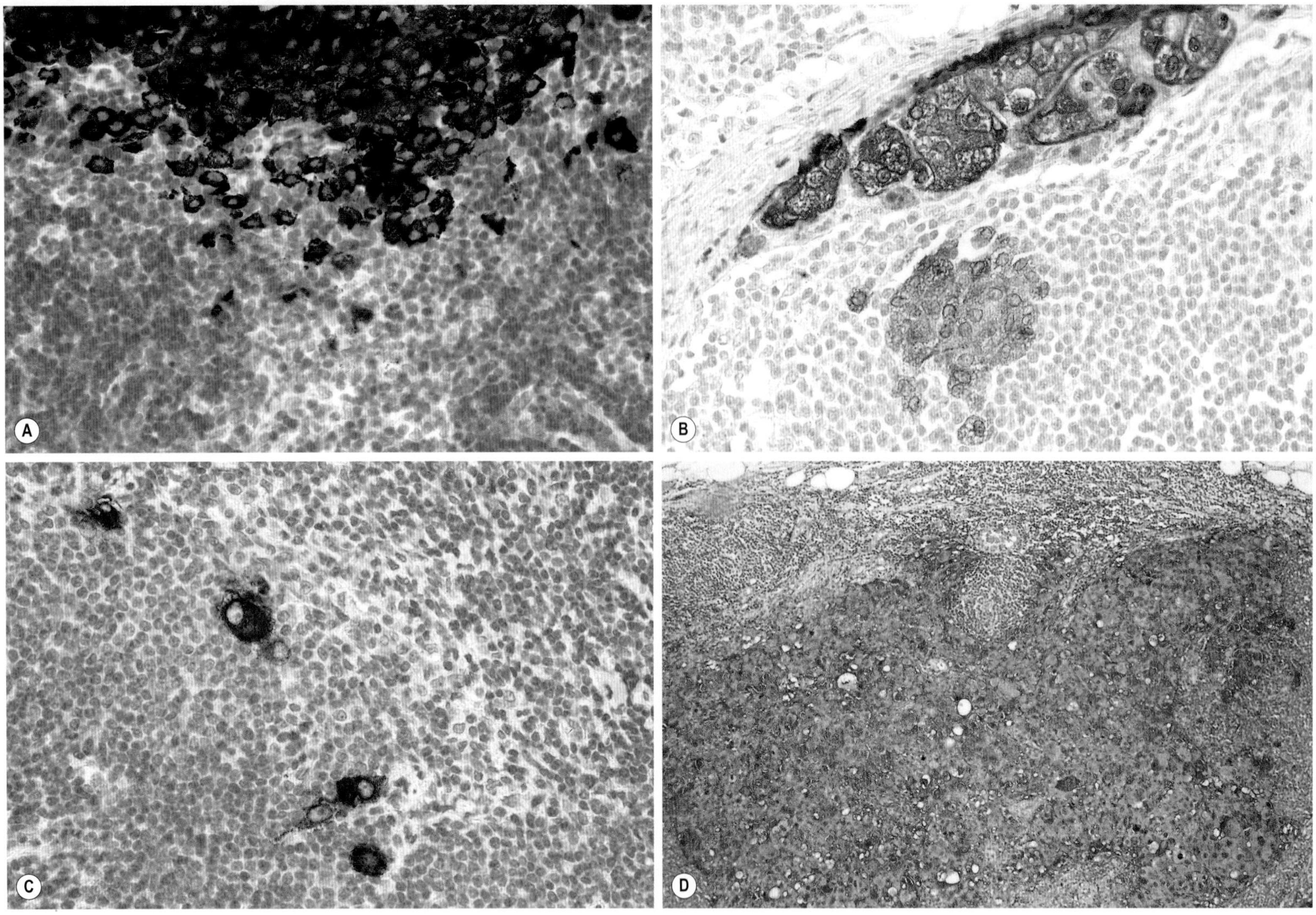

Fig. 28.23
Metastatic melanoma in the nodal parenchyma: (**A**) early extension of metastatic melanoma from the subcapsular sinus into the nodal parenchyma (HMB-45); (**B**) subcapsular metastatic melanoma with subjacent parenchymal melanoma metastases arranged as single tumor cells and a micrometastasis (MART-1/Melan-A); (**C**) single melanoma cells in the nodal parenchyma (MART-1/Melan-A); (**D**) macrometastasis in the nodal parenchyma (S100 protein-red chromogen-aminoethylcarbazole).

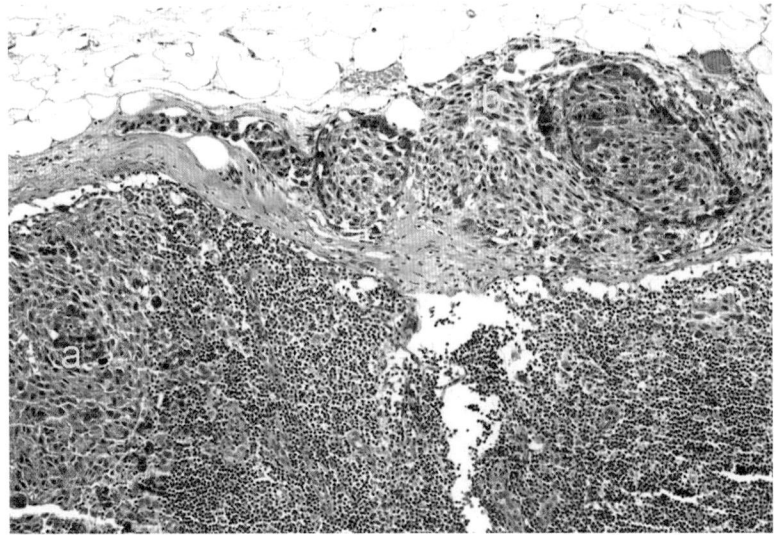

Fig. 28.24
Extracapsular extension of melanoma from a sentinel lymph node: tumor extends through the capsule and into the adjacent perinodal fat. By courtesy of R.R. Huang, MD, UCLA, California, USA.

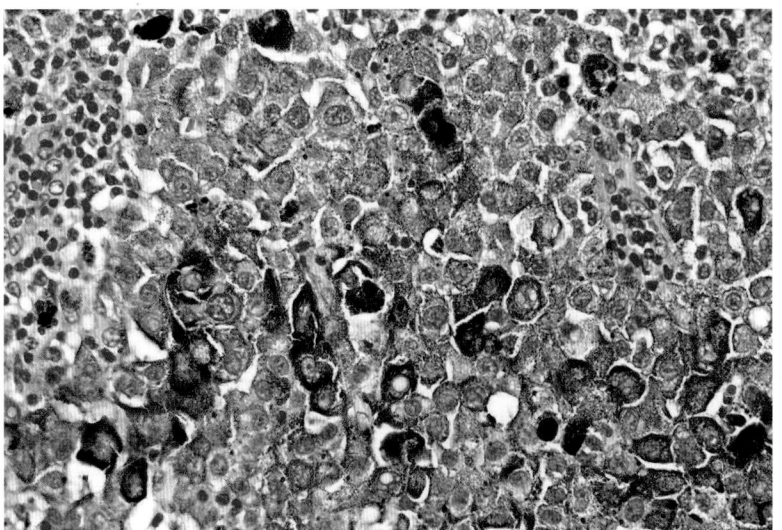

Fig. 28.25
Nodal metastatic melanoma: the great majority of cells in this illustration are melanoma cells, but a minority have coarse granules of melanin and are regarded as melanin-containing macrophages (melanophages).

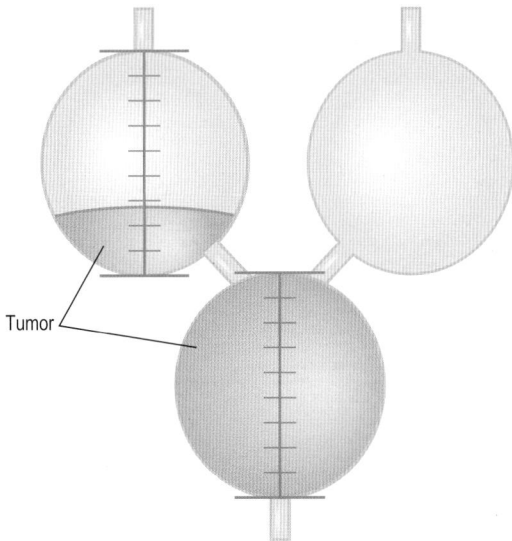

Fig. 28.26
Assessment of clinical outcome and the likelihood of death from melanoma correlate with the number of lymph nodes that contain melanoma metastases, but pathologists may further refine that assessment by measuring the size of nodal metastases. This can be recorded either as the proportional area of the lymph node occupied by tumor or using a micrometer to relate tumor maximum diameter to nodal maximum diameter.

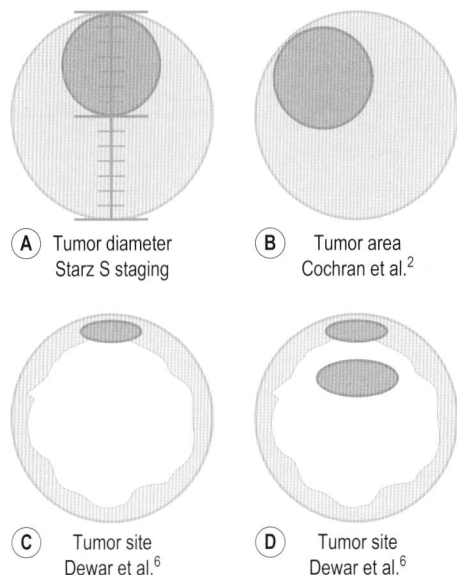

(A) Tumor diameter
Starz S staging

(B) Tumor area
Cochran et al.[2]

(C) Tumor site
Dewar et al.[6]

(D) Tumor site
Dewar et al.[6]

Fig. 28.27
Approaches to the prediction of clinical outcome based on tumor burden and distribution in the sentinel node: (A) shows the Starz approach[12], in which a micrometer measures the depth of penetration of the metastasis from the internal aspect of the nodal capsule to the deepest invasive tumor cell; (B) the measured area of the metastatic tumor is related to the area of the lymph node (proportional area); (C) A simpler approach is to record the diameter of the largest metastatic deposit; (D) the Dewar approach, in which it is determined whether the tumor is confined to the subcapsular sinus (relatively favorable) or also involves the parenchymal tissues (less favorable).

with outcome, and Cochran and coworkers,[5] using computer-linked morphometry, calculated the percentage area of the SN replaced by melanoma to predict the likelihood of NSN metastasis, recurrence, and death from melanoma. Dewar and coworkers[6] reported that the anatomical location of melanoma metastases in the SN strongly predicted NSN metastases. In their study, metastases confined to the subcapsular zone were not associated with additional metastases, whereas patients with metastases in the lymph node

parenchyma more often had additional nodes that contained metastases. Van Akooi and coworkers[7] confirmed that the maximum dimension of the largest nodal tumor deposit is related to prognosis. They found that metastases <0.1 mm in diameter were infrequently associated with metastases in NSNs or unfavorable clinical outcomes during short-term follow-up. Govindarajan and coworkers[8] also reported that tiny SN metastases (<0.2 mm in diameter in their study) were not associated with further disease, but Scheri and coworkers[9] have shown that even very small SN metastases can be associated with reduced survival. These important issues remain under extensive study and should yield clearly applicable and clinically relevant criteria by which nodal tumor burden can be assessed.

It is therefore likely that critical decisions regarding the need for CLND and deployment of adjuvant therapy will depend on the pathologist's assessment of tumor burden and location in the SN.[10,11] Currently, none of the available measures of tumor burden or disposition in the SN, individually or in combination, is sufficiently accurate that it can serve as the sole basis for treatment decisions. Such observations can effectively assist in the placement of patients in high- and low-risk categories for recurrence and death from melanoma. Pathologists may therefore wish to provide information on (for example) the Starz micrometer depth diameter of the largest metastasis and whether tumor is confined to the subcapsular zone or extends into the nodal parenchyma.[12]

Pathological evaluation of nonsentinel nodes

Metastases are identified in the NSNs of 17–25% of patients found to have metastatic melanoma at SNB. Such metastases are usually limited to a single NSN and usually replace less of that node than does the tumor identified in the SN. While SNs are studied in detail, using multiple sections and immunohistochemistry, most NSNs undergo a relatively superficial examination: bisection with both halves stained by H&E. There has been some interest in whether the routine use of immunohistology to evaluate NSNs would improve patient management, but data from Scolyer and coworkers[1] and Wen and coworkers[2] suggest that the return from such studies would be low. Immunohistochemical study of NSNs might be more appropriate in the relatively few patients where the amount of tumor in the SN is substantial, but this possibility requires further study.

The impact of complete lymph node dissection after positive sentinel lymph node biopsy in melanoma-specific survival

Since the last edition of this book, we completed the initial phase of the MSLT-II trial, an international, multicenter trial randomizing subjects with SLN metastases diagnosed by standard pathology or a multimarker molecular assay to immediate CLND or observation with nodal ultrasound.[1] The primary endpoint was melanoma-specific survival (MSS), and the secondary endpoints disease-free survival and cumulative rate of nonsentinel nodal metastases. Immediate CLND was not associated with improved MSS in the 1934 evaluable subjects (CLND 76% vs. observation 78%, at 5 years, median follow-up of 43 months, p = 0.42). Disease-free survival was better in the CLND group (61% vs. 57% at 5 years, p = 0.048) due to better control of regional nodal disease (89% vs. 74% at 5 years, p <0.001). In the CLND group, 11.5% had nonsentinel nodal metastases that were a strong independent negative prognostic factor. Cumulative nonsentinel nodal metastases affected 26% of the observed group at 5 years, versus 22.9% in CLND recipients (p = 0.005). Immediate CLND does not improve MSS in patients with SLN metastases, but does improve regional tumor control and provides significant prognostic information. Careful regional nodal observation is an acceptable alternative management approach in patients with SLN metastases. These findings are similar to the observations of Leiter et al.[2] As these findings are entirely new, oncologists will need to review current recommendations for the management of regional lymph nodes in melanoma to determine how to use this new information in treatment planning.[3–5] In the future, pathologists may be asked to review fewer CLNDs and patients will be spared the substantial side effects of extensive excision of regional lymph nodes.

Table 28.1

Standardized form for reporting characteristics of the SN. This template may be modified to fit local practices and requirements

Worksheet for evaluation of sentinel node pathology

Patient name: _____   Date of birth: _____

Hospital number: _____   Pathology number: _____

Anatomic site of sentinel node: _____

Specimen type: _____

Surgeon-dissected node(s):   Number of nodes: _____   Color: _____   Radioactivity*

Fatty nodule: _____   Number of nodes:* _____   Color: _____   Radioactivity**

	Node 1	Node 2	Node 3	Node 4	Node 5	Node 6
Node length (mm)						
Node width (mm)						
Bisected (yes/no)						
1 mm slices (number)						
Number of tumor foci						
Subcapsular tumor (yes/no)						
Parenchymal tumor (yes/no)						
Extracapsular spread (yes/no)						
Diameter largest deposit (mm)						
Depth of tumor (from capsule) (mm)						
Tumor as % nodal area						
Tumor immunophenotype						
S100 ±						
MART-1 ±						
HMB-45 ±						
Other ±						
Other ±						
Nevus: Capsule ± trabeculum						

*After dissection in Pathology.
**Radioactive count from requisition sheet.

Lymphatic mapping and sentinel node biopsy for nonmelanocytic neoplasms

The SN approach is widely used for nonmelanocytic tumors, and early attempts to develop the concept were based on studies of squamous cell carcinoma (SCC) of the penis.[1] Since then, there have been numerous reports of the use of these approaches for the management of patients with cutaneous SCC, particularly SCC of the male and female genitalia.[2-4] There are also several reports of the successful application of SNB in patients with Merkel cell carcinoma[5-9] and carcinomas of the skin appendages, and it has been proposed that this approach may also find use in managing patients with sebaceous carcinoma or extramammary Paget disease.[4] The techniques are applied to patients with nonmelanoma skin cancer in exactly the same way as for melanoma, although each class of tumor requires the use of antibodies specific to the class of tumor that is being evaluated.

Reporting the sentinel node

Pathologists may find it useful to develop a pro forma worksheet to facilitate the inclusion of all clinically relevant information obtainable from examination of SNs. *Table 28.1* shows an example of such a worksheet that could be modified to fit local practices.

Access **ExpertConsult.com** for the complete list of references

See
www.expertconsult.com
for references and
additional material

Cutaneous lymphoproliferative diseases and related disorders

CHAPTER
29

John Goodlad and Eduardo Calonje

Classification of lymphomas

The classification of lymphomas and hematopoietic neoplasms has undergone radical changes in philosophy and diagnostic criteria since the early days of Lukes and Collins, Rappaport, and the subsequent Updated Kiel classification and the Working Formulation. The majority of these earlier classifications relied mainly on morphology to differentiate between entities, and were designed to be applicable to nodal disease with little or no attention being paid to extranodal sites (including the skin) or other clinical considerations. More recently, the input of immunohistochemistry enabled recognition of B- and T-cell variants, rapidly followed by the establishment of more detailed and discriminatory criteria for the diagnosis of specific entities. The identification of consistent genetic abnormalities in association with distinct lymphoma subtypes (i.e., the t(14:18) translocation in follicular lymphoma and the t(2:5) translocation in anaplastic large cell lymphoma) has further strengthened precise classification. As a result, modern lymphoma classification schemes recognize entities on the basis of shared morphological, immunophenotypic, genetic, and clinical features, ensuring more relevant disease categories and greater diagnostic consistency.

This more systematic approach achieved general acceptance with the publication of the revised European and American lymphoma (REAL) classification in 1994.[1] However, although the REAL classification recognized certain cutaneous lymphoproliferative disorders as independent entities, it failed to address the fact that certain lymphomas arising primarily in the skin were biologically distinct from morphologically and phenotypically similar neoplasms occurring in lymph nodes. The European Organisation for Research and Treatment of Cancer (EORTC) classification, proposed by the Cutaneous Lymphoma Study Group of the EORTC, sought to address these deficiencies. This was designed for cutaneous lymphomas with a greater emphasis on the unique clinical features of some primary cutaneous lymphomas, but otherwise employed a similar philosophy to that used in the REAL classification.[2] It was originally based on the data derived from 626 patients in the records of the Dutch Registry for Cutaneous Lymphoma, and later validated in several large studies with follow-up data from >1300 patients.[2-5] This classification subdivided primary cutaneous lesions into indolent, aggressive, and provisional categories based on behavior as determined by clinical experience (Table 29.1). This was a major step forward because it provided a precise definition for a number of primary cutaneous lymphomas and recognized differences in biological behavior (and thus potential treatment requirements) between nodal and cutaneous primary disease. For example, CD30-positive (ALK-negative) large T-cell lymphomas arising in lymph nodes are high-grade tumors, with a mortality of up to 63%, whereas morphologically and immunophenotypically identical tumors arising primarily in the skin are clinically low grade, and have a mortality of less than 5%.[6,7]

Many of the advances made in the EORTC classification were not recognized in the update of the REAL classification published jointly with the World Health Organization (WHO) in 2001.[8] This generated considerable controversy, particularly with respect to B-cell neoplasms. Arguments used against the EORTC approach included complaints of too broad a definition

of primary cutaneous follicle center cell lymphoma and the appropriateness of designating large B-cell lymphoma of the leg as a separate entity.[9,10] Dissension also reigned over use of the term primary cutaneous 'immunocytoma' as opposed to marginal zone lymphoma, immunocytoma at that time being inclusive of lymphoplasmacytic lymphoma, an entity distinct from marginal zone lymphoma.

These differences were resolved following meetings of members of both classification systems in Lyon and Zurich in 2003 and 2004, respectively. This resulted in a consensus WHO-EORTC classification first published in 2005.[11,12] The entities delineated in this system were subsequently incorporated, with refinements of some diagnostic criteria and the addition of new entities, into the WHO classification of tumors of the hematopoietic and lymphoid tissue published in 2008, with further modifications in the 2016 revision.[13,14] The terminology and criteria used in this latest update will be used in this chapter. The main lymphoma subtypes that primarily affect the skin are listed along with their expectant clinical behavior in Table 29.2.

Table 29.1

EORTC classification of primary cutaneous lymphomas

Primary CTCL	Primary CBCL
Indolent	
Mycosis fungoides	Follicle center cell lymphoma
Mycosis fungoides + follicular mucinosis	Immunocytoma(marginal zone B-cell lymphoma)
CD30+ large cell CTCL Anaplastic Immunoblastic Pleomorphic	
Lymphomatoid papulosis	
Intermediate	
	Large B-cell lymphoma of the leg
Aggressive	
Sézary syndrome	
CD30– large cell CTCL Immunoblastic Pleomorphic	
Provisional	
Granulomatous slack skin	Intravascular large B-cell lymphoma
CTCL, pleomorphic small/ medium-sized	Plasmacytoma
Subcutaneous panniculitis-like T-cell lymphoma	

Abbreviations: *CTCL*, Cutaneous T-cell lymphoma; *CBCL*, cutaneous B-cell lymphoma; *EORTC*, European Organisation for Research and Treatment of Cancer. Modified from: Willemze, R., et al. (1997) *Blood*, 90, 354–371.

Table 29.2

Lymphoma subtypes and behavior as defined in WHO-EORTC classification of cutaneous lymphoma

WHO-EORTC subtype	Behavior
Cutaneous T-cell lymphoma	
Mycosis fungoides	Indolent
MF variants	
Folliculotropic MF	Indolent
Pagetoid reticulosis	Indolent
Granulomatous slack skin	Indolent
Sézary syndrome	Aggressive
Adult T-cell leukemia/lymphoma	Aggressive
Primary cutaneous CD30+ lymphoproliferative disorders	
Primary cutaneous anaplastic large cell lymphoma	Indolent
Lymphomatoid papulosis	Indolent
Subcutaneous panniculitis-like T-cell lymphoma	Indolent
Extranodal NK/T-cell lymphoma, nasal type	Aggressive
Primary cutaneous T-cell lymphoma, unspecified	
Primary cutaneous aggressive epidermotropic CD8+ T-cell lymphoma*	Aggressive
Hydroa vacciniforme-like lymphoma	Aggressive
Cutaneous γ/δ T-cell lymphoma	Aggressive
Primary cutaneous acral CD8+ T-cell lymphoma*	Indolent
Primary cutaneous CD4+ small/medium-sized pleomorphic T-cell lymphoproliferative disorder*	Indolent
Cutaneous B-cell lymphoma	
Primary cutaneous marginal zone lymphoma	Indolent
Primary cutaneous follicle center lymphoma	Indolent
Primary cutaneous large B-cell lymphoma, leg type	Intermediate
Primary cutaneous large B-cell lymphoma, other	Intermediate
Primary cutaneous intravascular large B-cell lymphoma	Intermediate

*Provisional entities.
Abbreviations: *MF*, Mycosis fungoides; *WHO-EORTC*, World Health Organization-European Organisation for Research and Treatment of Cancer.
Modified from: Swerdlow S.H., et al. (2016). *Blood*, 127, 2375–2390.

T-CELL LYMPHOMAS

Mycosis fungoides

Clinical features

Mycosis fungoides (MF) (Gr. *mykes*, fungus; L. fungus + Gr. *eidos*, form), although rare, represents the commonest form of primary cutaneous T-cell lymphoma.[1-7] Alibert named it, in 1806, after the mushroom-like tumors that develop in the terminal stages of the illness (*Fig. 29.1*). The annual incidence in the United States varies from 0.36 to 0.46 cases per 10^5 of the population,[8-10] with approximately 1000 new cases diagnosed per year.[1,11] The incidence in Europe is somewhat less.[12] There is predilection for males (2:1). It is more common in blacks (2:1) and less common in Asians and Hispanics.[2,8,11,13] Any age group may be involved, but there is a higher incidence in the fourth to sixth decades. MF in children is discussed separately (see below).

The course and outcome is unpredictable, ranging from a protracted, persistent, relatively benign illness through to a widespread malignancy with high morbidity and mortality.[3]

In addition to the classical (Alibert) form, patients may present with a poikilodermatous variant (poikiloderma atrophicans vasculare, large plaque parapsoriasis) or with erythroderma (Hallopeau-Besnier). The last should not be confused with Sézary syndrome, which represents an erythrodermic leukemic manifestation of T-cell lymphoma, and usually develops de novo.

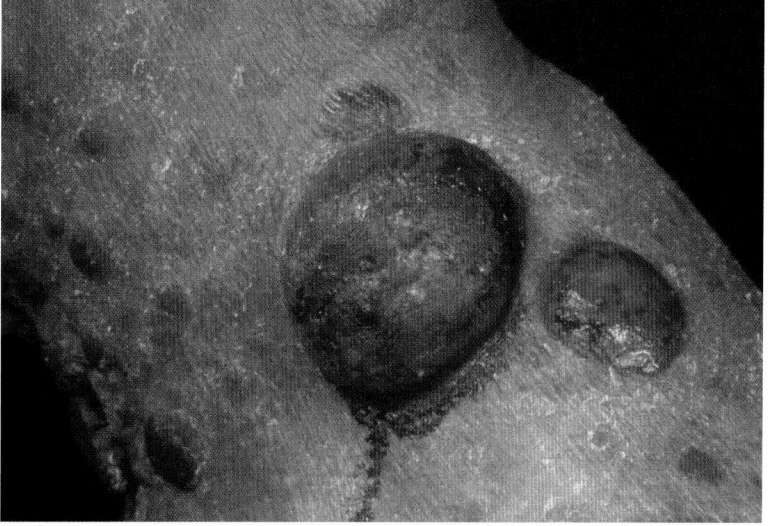

Fig. 29.1
Mycosis fungoides: this patient has advanced tumor-stage mycosis fungoides. Such massive ulcerated tumor nodules are a rare manifestation. By courtesy of the Institute of Dermatology London, UK.

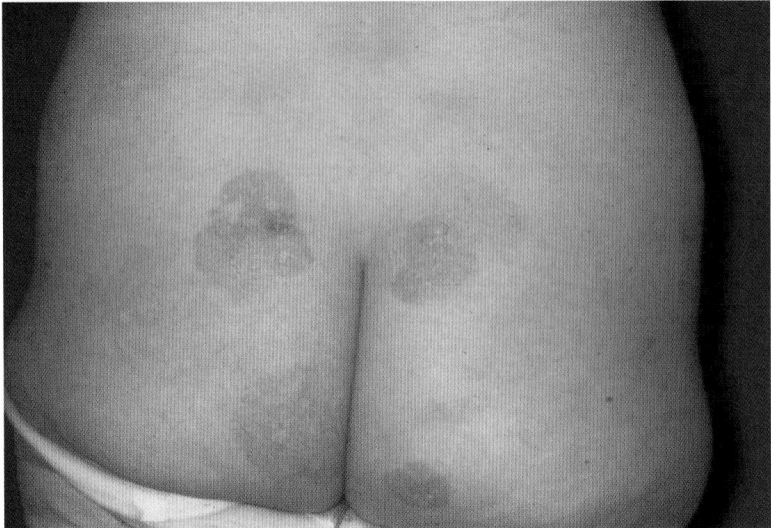

Fig. 29.2
Mycosis fungoides (patch stage): these irregular, erythematous, and scaling lesions are present in a typical distribution on the buttocks. By courtesy of R.A. Marsden, MD, St George's Hospital, London, UK.

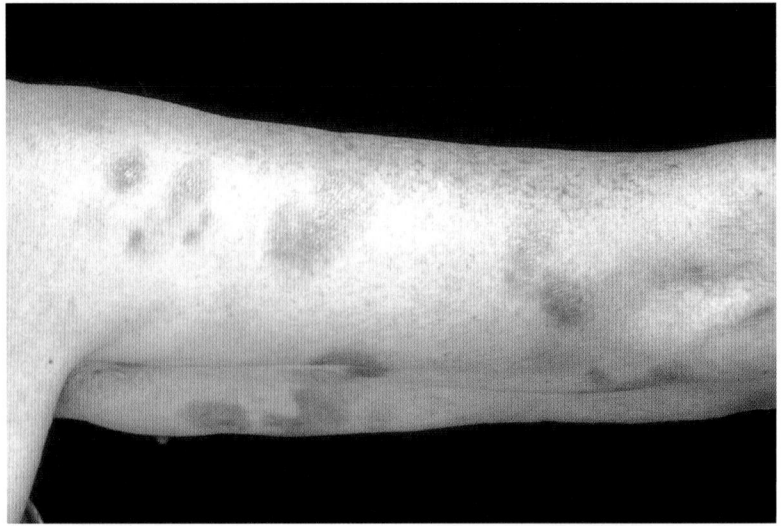

Fig. 29.3
Mycosis fungoides: multiple patches are present on this patient's arm. By courtesy of the Institute of Dermatology, London, UK.

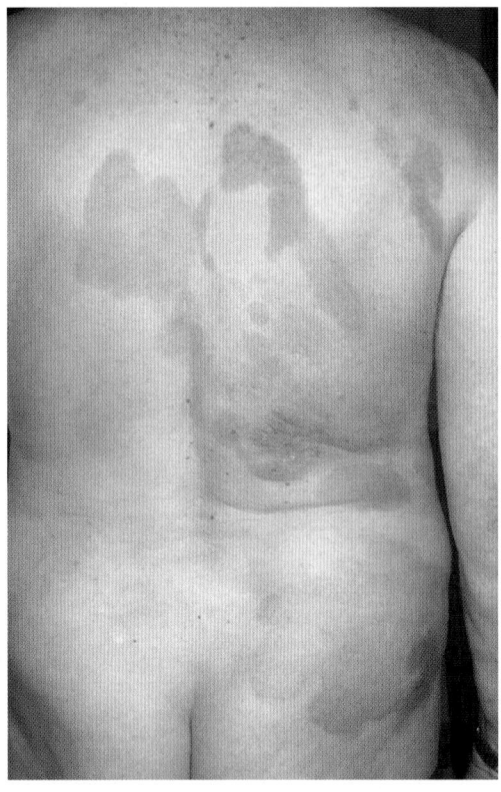

Fig. 29.4
Mycosis fungoides: lesions sometimes have a generalized distribution. By courtesy of the Institute of Dermatology, London, UK.

MF presenting with tumor nodules from the outset, so-called tumeur d'emblée mycosis fungoides (Vidal Brocq), is no longer recognized as an entity. Such cases are likely to represent other variants of T-cell lymphoma including cutaneous anaplastic large cell lymphoma or primary cutaneous T-cell lymphoma, unspecified (CD30-negative large cell lymphoma).

Rarer presentations include bullous, follicular, hypopigmented, verrucous/hyperkeratotic, pustular, lichenoid papular, palmoplantar psoriasiform, granulomatous, and acanthosis nigricans-like variants. These are clinically unusual cases that run a similar course to that of classic MF, and are not considered separate entities. In contrast, folliculotropic mycosis fungoides, pagetoid reticulosis, and granulomatous slack skin disease have distinct clinicopathological features and are recognized as biologically distinct variants of MF in the WHO classification.[14,15]

Classic MF is traditionally divided into patch, plaque, and tumor stages.[2] This is, however, a somewhat arbitrary classification because all stages may be present simultaneously in one individual while other patients never progress beyond the patch stage.[15,16] In addition, patch stage lesions obviously merge with plaques.

The early erythematous lesions are irregular, asymmetrical, slightly scaly, variably sized pink or red patches (Fig. 29.2). Many lesions show signs of atrophy, and in some lighting conditions they appear smooth and shiny. While lesions are more commonly present on the trunk, limb girdles, breasts, and flexures; they can also be more widespread (Figs 29.3 and 29.4).

The clinical differential diagnosis includes discoid, atopic or contact allergic dermatitis, psoriasis, and, in particular, chronic superficial scaly dermatitis (small plaque parapsoriasis).[17–22] Patients, usually middle aged, present with erythematous scaly persistent patches, showing predilection for the limbs and trunk, that are sometimes likened to cigarette paper.[20,23] While the lesions may be round or oval, they often have a finger-like appearance – hence, the alternative designation digitate dermatosis (Fig. 29.5). The patches tend to be uniform in size, shape, and color, contrasting vividly with the great variability of those of mycosis fungoides.

Adverse drug reactions may also mimic mycosis fungoides. Patients can present with multiple infiltrated plaques or erythroderma that are histologically indistinguishable from mycosis fungoides.[22] Drugs which have been particularly implicated are the anticonvulsants (including phenytoin, barbiturates, carbamazepine), cardiac drugs such as atenolol and angiotensin-converting enzyme (ACE) inhibitors, antihistamines, ciclosporin, and allopurinol.[22,24–26]

Patients sometimes develop foci of poikiloderma within a more typical background. In others, the entire eruption may be poikilodermatous – so-called poikiloderma atrophicans vasculare (Gr. poikilos, spotted, mottled, varied) (large plaque parapsoriasis).[17] They present with small numbers of large plaques showing a predilection for the breasts, buttocks, hips, abdomen, and major flexures (Fig. 29.6). Individual features of the plaques include atrophy, telangiectases, and variable hypo- and hyperpigmentation with erythema (Fig. 29.7). The appearances have been likened to those of chronic radiation damage. Further progression may be similar to that of classic mycosis fungoides, although it appears that fewer patients develop tumor-stage mycosis fungoides.[27]

Further progression of patch stage disease leads to the development of an increased number of indurated plaques (Figs 29.8 and 29.9). The lesions can be quite bizarre and, not uncommonly, due to central regression, they have an annular or serpiginous appearance (Fig. 29.10). Plaques are sometimes extremely hyperkeratotic, particularly on the palms and soles (see mycosis fungoides palmaris et plantaris, page 1421).

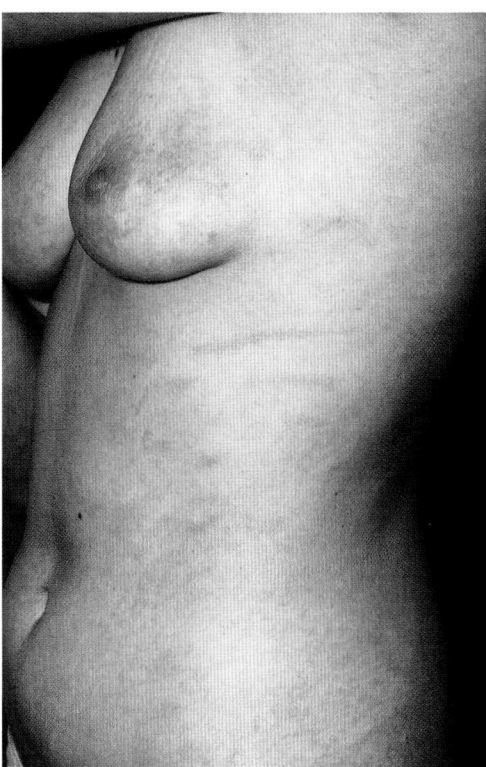

Fig. 29.5
Superficial scaly dermatitis: this patient shows digitate erythematous lesions in a characteristic distribution. By courtesy of R.A. Marsden, MD, St George's Hospital, London, UK.

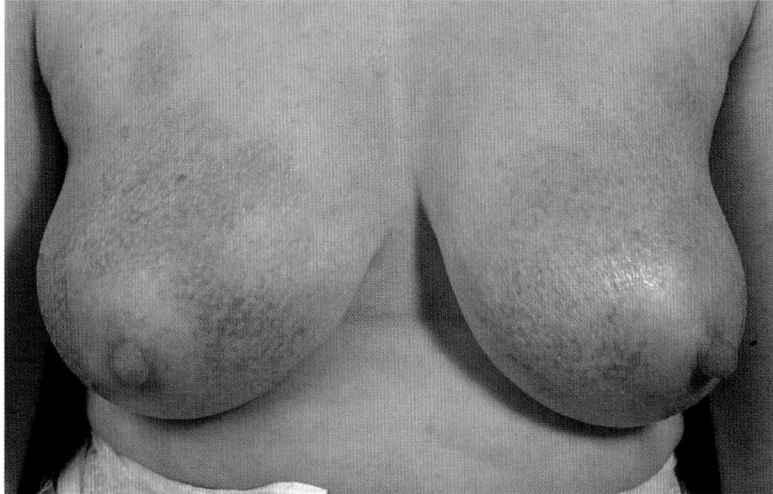

Fig. 29.6
Mycosis fungoides (poikiloderma atrophicans vasculare): early lesion showing slight scaling and dilated vasculature. By courtesy of the Institute of Dermatology, London, UK.

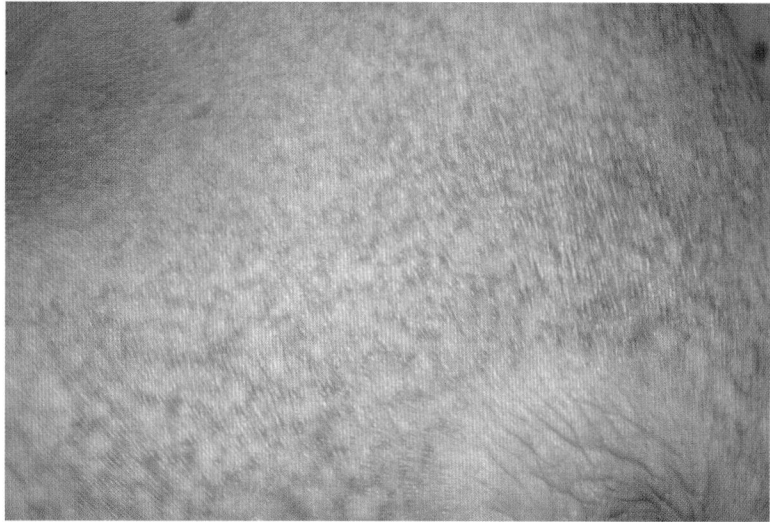

Fig. 29.7
Mycosis fungoides (poikiloderma atrophicans vasculare): this field shows the typical features of reticulate pigmentation, atrophy, scaling, and telangiectasia. By courtesy of the Radcliffe Infirmary, Oxford, UK.

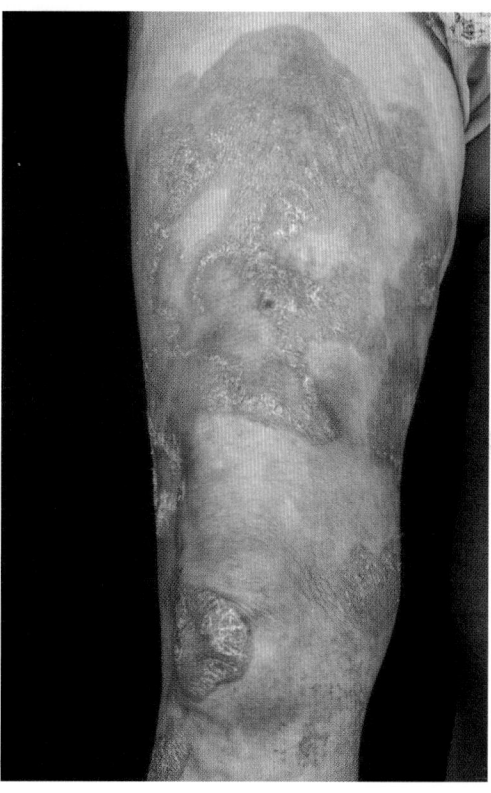

Fig. 29.8
Mycosis fungoides: large erythematous plaques with scaling. By courtesy of the Institute of Dermatology, London, UK.

A small proportion of patients develop tumors (*Figs 29.11–29.13*). Sometimes ulcerative lesions are seen (*Fig. 29.14*). The face, scalp, and intertriginous areas are particularly affected.[28]

Clinical staging relates to the extent of disease and the presence or absence of cutaneous tumor nodules and erythroderma. It is based on the system proposed by the International Society for Cutaneous Lymphomas (ISCL) and the EORTC.[29] This scheme takes account of advances in molecular biology, immunohistochemistry, and imaging, as well as new data on prognostic variables. It assesses the extent and nature of the skin lesions present, extent of nodal involvement, visceral involvement, and the presence and degree of any peripheral blood involvement (*Table 29.3*). Combinations of these parameters (stage) can be used to determine prognosis and

are essential for determining treatment.[30,31] Outcome in mycosis fungoides is varied. When only patches and plaques are present at presentation, and cover 10% of body surface area (T1), survival is no different from that of age-matched controls.[17,32–34] Patients with patches and plaques covering >10% body surface area (T2) have a median survival of 10–12 years and a 25% risk of progression, whilst the median survival for patients with tumors (T3) or erythroderma (T4) is only 4–5 years.[33,34] Visceral involvement carries a very poor prognosis, with median survivals of only 1–2 years.[31,34] Lymph node enlargement is common and does not necessarily indicate pathological involvement. Its impact on prognosis is often overshadowed by the extent of skin lesions. The presence of abnormal circulating cells and the tumor burden in the peripheral blood are also important parameters to assess as

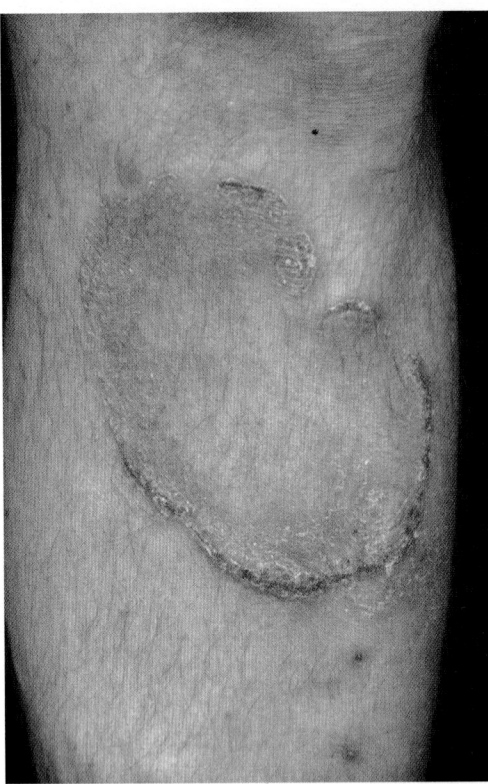

Fig. 29.9
Mycosis fungoides: high-power view. By courtesy of the Institute of Dermatology, London, UK.

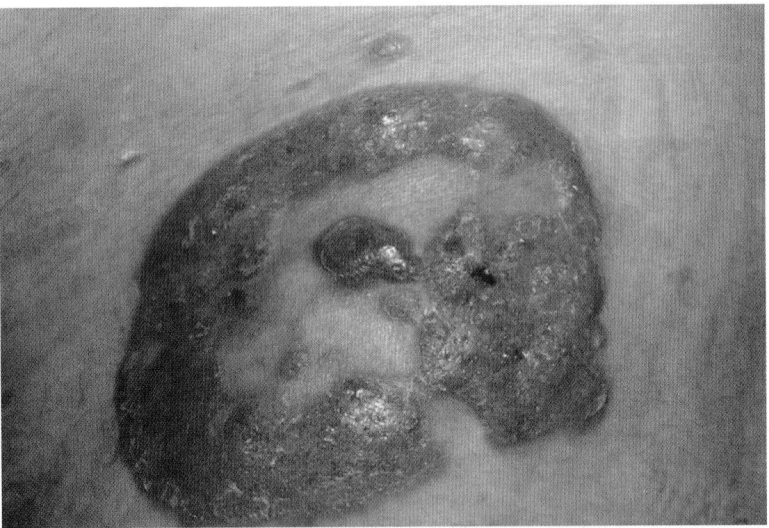

Fig. 29.10
Mycosis fungoides: close-up view of an annular lesion. By courtesy of the late N.P. Smith, MD, Institute of Dermatology, London, UK.

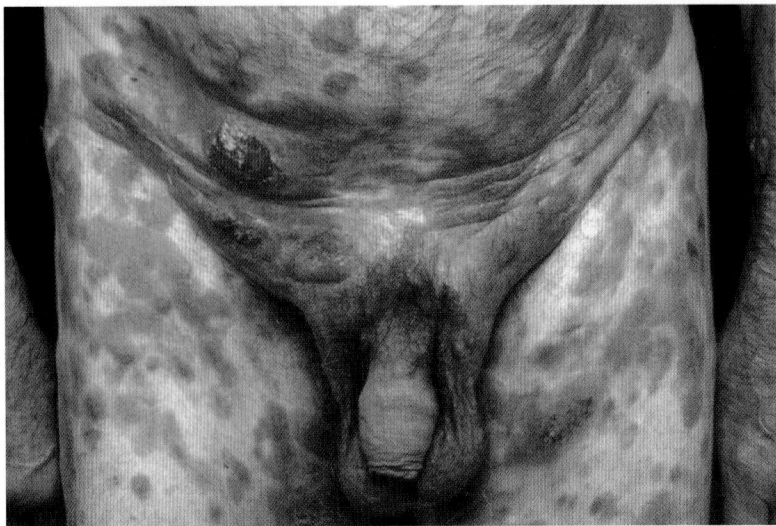

Fig. 29.11
Mycosis fungoides: multiple tumors have arisen against a background of plaque stage disease. By courtesy of the Institute of Dermatology, London, UK.

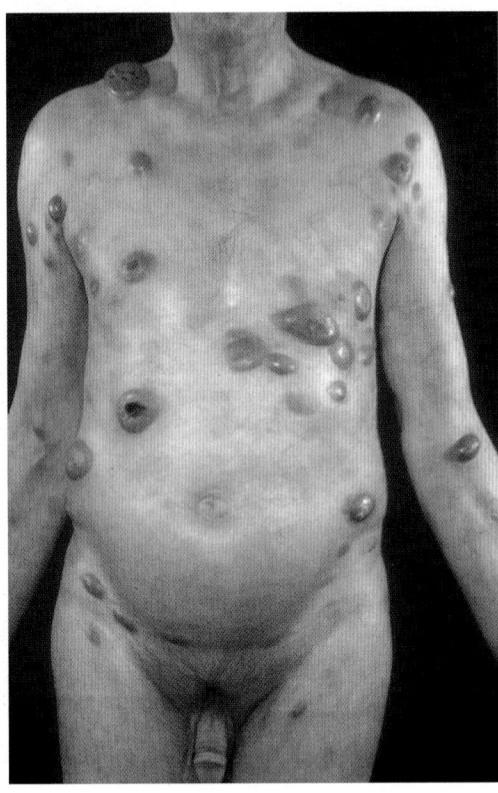

Fig. 29.12
Mycosis fungoides (tumor stage): there are multiple tumor nodules in a background of patches and plaques. By courtesy of the Institute of Dermatology, London, UK.

they are of independent prognostic significance.[33,35,36] The patient should therefore be thoroughly investigated to assess the extent of skin lesions and to determine whether there is nodal, visceral, or hematological spread.

Raised levels of lactate dehydrogenase (LDH), soluble interleukin (IL)-2 receptor, erythrocyte sedimentation rate (ESR), and raised blood eosinophil count are other markers of poor prognosis.[37–43] Transformation to large cell lymphoma also relates to adverse outcome.

Infection is the major cause of death, with *Staphylococcus aureus*, Enterobacteriaceae and *Pseudomonas aeruginosa* being the most frequent pathogens.[1,2,44–46] Beta-hemolytic streptococcus, herpes simplex, and varicella-zoster infections are also of importance.[45]

Patients with mycosis fungoides also have an increased risk of epithelial tumors, including carcinoma of the lung and colon, and B-cell non-Hodgkin lymphoma (NHL).[47–49]

Pathogenesis and histologic features

Mycosis fungoides is a neoplastic proliferation of monoclonal T cells from the outset.[50–54] While monoclonal lymphoid populations have been described in apparently non-neoplastic conditions, such as pityriasis lichenoides acuta, lichen aureus, lichen planus, pigmented purpuric dermatosis, allergic contact dermatitis, and drug reactions, the presence of a clonal TCR gene rearrangement is highly suggestive of a lymphomatous process, particularly when the same clone is found in more than one lesion or in one patient over time.[54–65] Furthermore, recurrent chromosomal abnormalities have been found in some cases including loss of chromosomes 1p, 17p, 10q/10, 13q, and 19, as well as gains of 4/4q, 17q/17, and 18.[66]

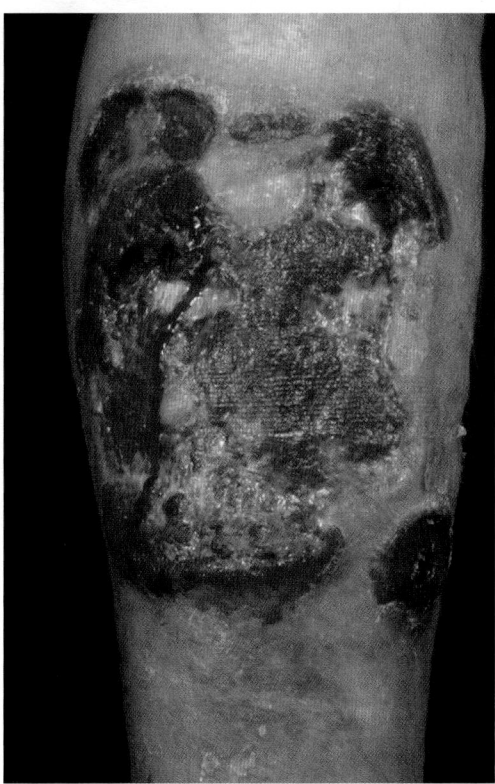

Fig. 29.13
Mycosis fungoides: this patient shows advanced disease with a fungating tumor on the knee. By courtesy of the Institute of Dermatology, London, UK.

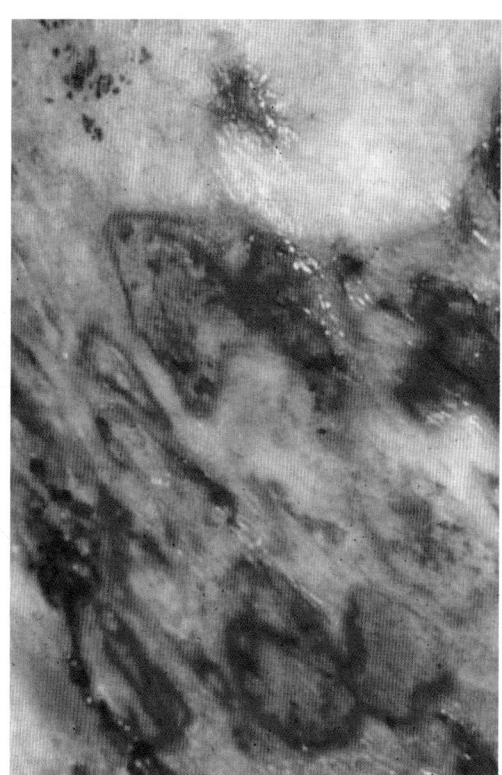

Fig. 29.14
Mycosis fungoides: ulcerative lesions, as seen in this patient, are a rare manifestation. By courtesy of A. du Vivier, MD, King's College Hospital, London, UK.

Table 29.3
ISCL/EORTC revision to clinical and pathological staging of mycosis fungoides

Stage	Description	TNMB
IA	Limited patches, papules and/or plaques covering <10% skin surface area (T1); no evidence of nodal (No), visceral (M0) or significant blood involvement (B0), or low blood tumor burden (B1)	$T_1N_0M_0B_{0,1}$
B	Generalized patches, papules and/or plaques covering ≥10% skin surface area (T2); no evidence of nodal (No), visceral (M0) or significant blood involvement (B0), or low blood tumor burden (B1)	$T_2N_0M_0B_{0,1}$
II	Any extent of patches, papules and/or plaques (T! 0r T2); clinically abnormal nodes showing DL (N1) or early involvement by MF (N2); no evidence of visceral (M0) or significant blood involvement (B0), or low blood tumor burden (B1)	$T_{1,2}N_{1,2}M_0B_{0,1}$
IIB	One or more tumors (≥1.5 cm diameter) (T3); up to early lymph node involvement (N2); no evidence of visceral (M0) or significant blood involvement (B0), or low blood tumor burden (B1)	$T_3N_{0-2}M_0B_{0,1}$
III	Erythema covering ≥80% skin surface area; up to early lymph node involvement (N2); no evidence of visceral (M0) or significant blood involvement (B0), or low blood tumor burden (B1)	$T_4N_{0-2}M_0B_{0,1}$
IIIA	Stage III with no significant blood involvement	$T_4N_{0-2}M_0B_0$
IIIB	Stage III with low blood tumor burden	$T_4N_{0-2}M_0B_1$
IVA1	Any degree of skin involvement; up to early lymph node involvement; no evidence of visceral spread; high blood tumor burden (B2: >1000 Sezary cells/ml with positive clone)	$T_{1-4}N_{0-2}M_0B_2$
IVA2	Any degree of skin involvement; partial or complete effacement of node by MF (N3); no visceral involvement; any degree of blood involvement	$T_{1-4}N_3M_0B_{0-2}$
IVB	Any degree of skin involvement with visceral involvement, irrespective of nodal or blood involvement	$T_{1-4}N_{0-3}M_1B_{0-2}$
Modified from Olsen, E., et al. (2007) *Blood*, 110, 1713–1722.		

As with many malignancies, the etiology and pathogenesis of mycosis fungoides is likely to be multifactorial. Specific causative agents and precise pathogenetics are unknown.[67]

There is little evidence of genetic predisposition to mycosis fungoides. Familial occurrence is exceptional.[68,69] However, a number of studies have inconsistently linked various human leukocyte antigen (HLA) types with mycosis fungoides. For example, HLA-B8 and HLA-AW19 have been found with increased frequency in mycosis fungoides patients from the United Kingdom, whereas an association with HLA-DR5 (DRB1*11) and DQB1*03 was demonstrated in North American Caucasians.[70–73] In studies from Israel, no association with HLA class I alleles was detected.[74]

It is thought that mycosis fungoides most probably develops as a consequence of chronic antigenic stimulation, either to long-term exposure to irritant substances or infective agents. Epidemiological studies have variously pointed toward occupational exposure to metals, plastics, cutting oils, solvents, glass, pottery, and ceramics, or working as a crop or vegetable farmer, painter, woodworker, or carpenter.[10,75–79] A pathogenetic role for infective agents has also long been postulated.[3,67,80] A wide range of potential agents, particularly viruses, have been investigated including human T-cell lympho-tropic virus-I (HTLV-I), HTLV-II, Epstein-Barr virus (EBV), cytomegalovirus (CMV), human herpes virus (HHV) 6, HHV7, and HHV8. However, the results of various studies looking for evidence of these agents in MF have produced conflicting or inconclusive results.[6,67,81–84] Other organisms that have also been considered include *S. aureus*, persistent chlamydia infection, and *Borrelia burgdorferi*.[76,85–88] However, there is no strong evidence in favor of these agents playing a direct role in MF pathogenesis.[67] Nevertheless, it remains possible that various infectious agents are important initiators of the chronic lymphoproliferation from which lymphoma eventually develops, and a recent study has suggested that persistence of multiple infectious agents may be more important than any single one in isolation.[89]

A variety of recurrent genetic abnormalities have been identified in mycosis fungoides, although none are specific for this entity. They include deletions of chromosomes 1p, 17p, 10q, and 19, as well as gains on 4q, 18, and 17q.[90,91] Alterations in a number of tumor suppressor and apoptosis-related genes have also been detected. Silencing of p15, p16, Nav3, PTEN, and p53 due to mutations, promoter hypermethylation, or allelic loss have all been implicated in the progression from plaque to tumor stage.[92–96] More recently, massive parallel sequencing approaches have uncovered recurrent mutations in a multiple genes involved in epigenetic regulation, T-cell receptor signaling and particularly the JAK-STAT and NF-κB pathways.[97–100] These alterations are reflected, to a certain extent, by the gene expression profile and phenotype of the tumor cells in mycosis fungoides which display features of at least partially activated skin resident effector memory cells, with a unique expression of chemokine receptors and adhesion molecules, and a bias toward a Th2-type phenotype. These exclusive properties help explain some of the characteristic features of MF, and provide insight into the evolution and progression of the disease.

The neoplastic cells express cytokine receptors CCR4 and CCR10.[101,102] CCL17 and CCL22 are ligands for CCR4 and are present in high levels in skin lesions of affected patients.[90,101] CCL17 is also increased in the serum of patients with the disease and Sézary syndrome, as is CCL27, the ligand for CCR10.[67] Interaction of CCR4 and CCR10 with their respective ligands not only influences T-cell migratory properties, but promotes their survival via downstream activation of antiapoptotic pathways such as phosphatidylinositol-3-kinase and Akt.[67] Such chemokine interactions are therefore likely to be important in initiation and perpetuation of the skin lesions and may explain the marked propensity for the malignant cells to localize in the epidermis.[90]

MF cells also express cell surface adhesion molecules such as CD45RO and IL-2R, and there is evidence of constitutive activation of several intra-cellular signaling proteins in the JAK-STAT family of molecules, similar to that witnessed following stimulation of normal T cells via the IL-2 receptor.[91,103–107] This is likely to affect regulation of various aspects of cell survival and proliferation. Other factors may also contribute toward defects in normal apoptotic pathways in MF cells. For example, mutations of the Fas gene or abnormal splice variants of its transcript have been documented in MF and may protect against Fas-mediated stimulation of apoptosis.[92,108] Also, gene expression profiling studies have generated a genetic signature specific for MF. This is characterized by multiple genes involved in the tumor necrosis factor (TNF) signaling pathway, including several inhibitors of apoptosis.[109] Abnormalities in Fas and TNF signaling pathways may also contribute toward the constitutive activation of the NF-kappa B pathway noted in MF, further supporting a role for resistance to apoptosis in its pathogenesis.[110]

Tumor cells in MF also seem equipped to evade the host immune system. Cytotoxic T cells can induce apoptosis via engagement of Fas, expressed on the surface of the target cell, by Fas ligand (FasL). The aforementioned defects in FasL signaling in MF cells are therefore likely to protect against tumor-specific cytotoxic T-cell-mediated immunity.[90,92,108] Furthermore, the malignant cells in MF may express FasL, giving them the potential to eliminate tumor-specific CD8-positive cytotoxic T cells.[111] They also show down-regulation of Th1-associated genes, and express cytokines such as IL-4, IL-5, and IL-18, most in keeping with Th2-type T cells.[112–114] This Th2 bias, together with production of other immunomodulatory cytokines such as IL-10, transforming growth factor (TGF)-β, and soluble IL-2R may also

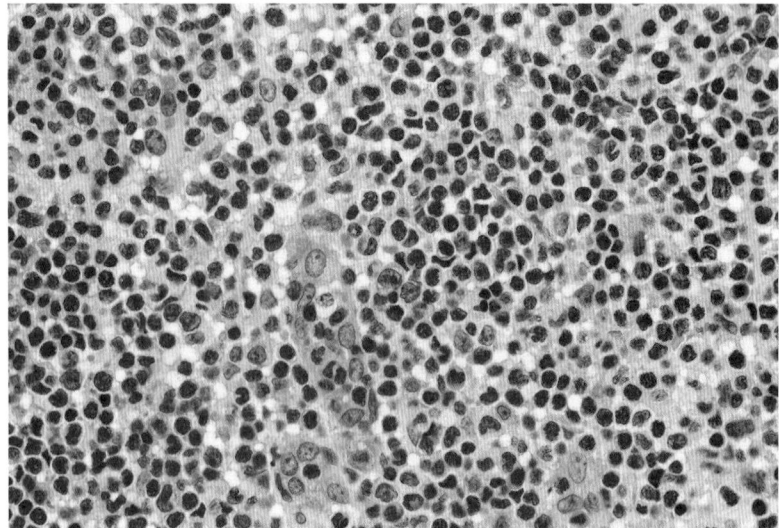

Fig. 29.15
Mycosis fungoides: the nuclei of the mycosis cells are hyperchromatic and highly irregular.

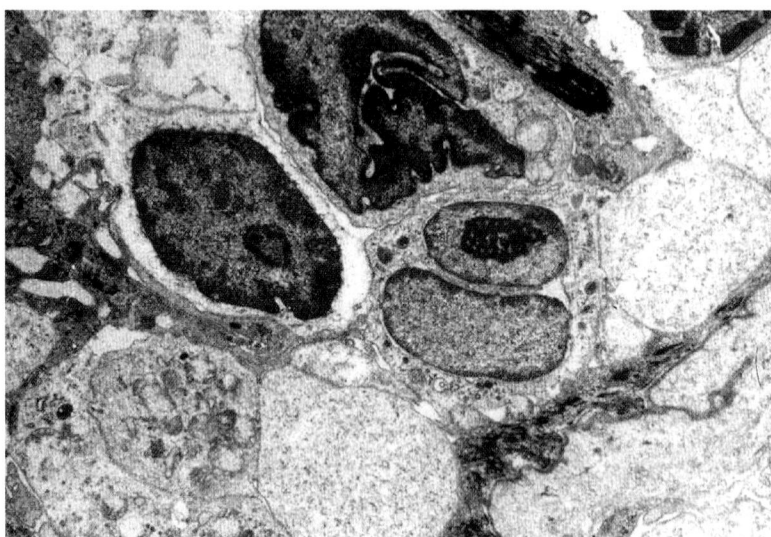

Fig. 29.16
Mycosis cells: note the highly convoluted (cerebriform nuclei).

contribute to suppressing the host antitumor immune response and partly account for the increased risk of infections and second malignancies.[115–118] Copy number gains and amplifications of JUNB, and JUNB overexpression have been documented in MF and may contribute to the Th2 bias, as JUNB promotes IL-4-mediated TH2 lymphocyte differentiation.[119,120]

The lymphocytes of MF are mature T cells that have transited through the lymph node and undergone antigenic stimulation. They show a particular tendency to colonize the epidermis (epidermotropism), although this is more evident in the patch and plaque forms than in tumor-stage disease where epidermotropism can be completely lost. To a lesser extent in early lesions, and more obviously in later stages, the infiltrate contains large cells with highly irregular, convoluted, or cerebriform nuclei, known as Sézary or mycosis cells (*Fig. 29.15*). Assessing their significance must be tempered with caution because identical cells (albeit in small numbers) are sometimes seen in the dermal infiltrate of a variety of dermatoses. Their presence must obviously be considered in the context of the accompanying histologic features and, in particular, in the light of the clinical information. Electron microscopically, mycosis/Sézary cells are characterized by a multilobed hyperconvoluted nucleus with conspicuous peripheral chromatin margination (*Fig. 29.16*).

Epidermotropism is, therefore, the histologic hallmark of MF.[121–130] It is related to the stage of the disease and the degree of differentiation of the

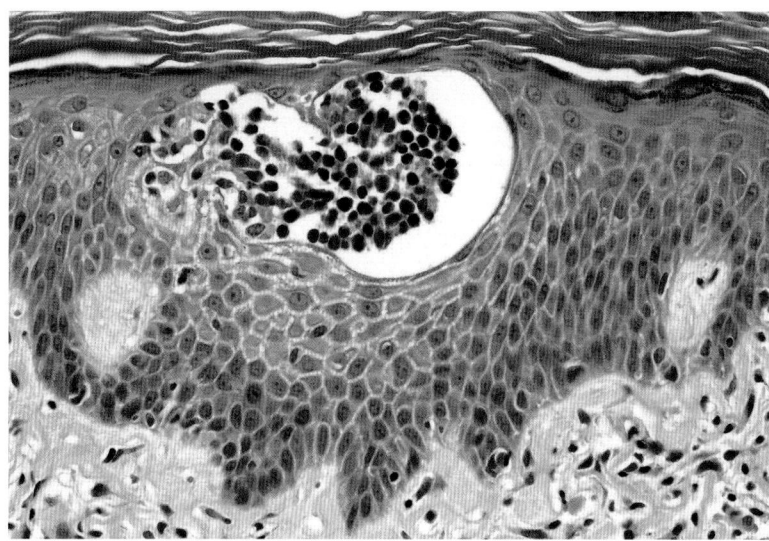

Fig. 29.17
Mycosis fungoides: a typical Pautrier microabscess composed of hyperchromatic atypical lymphocytes.

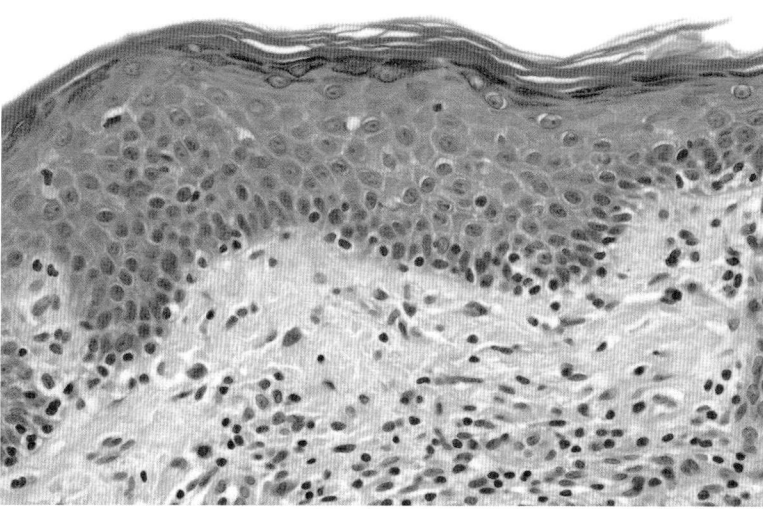

Fig. 29.19
Mycosis fungoides (patch stage): high-power view of atypical lymphocytes tagging the dermal–epidermal junction.

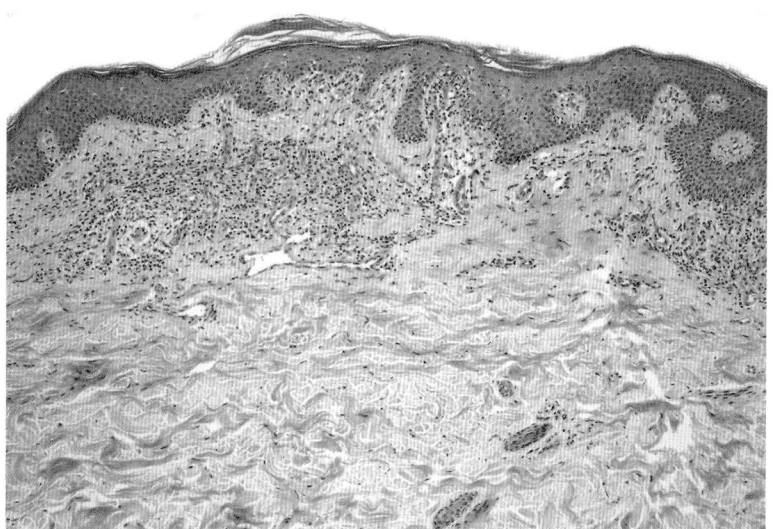

Fig. 29.18
Mycosis fungoides (patch stage): this biopsy of an early lesion shows focal parakeratosis, acanthosis, atypical lymphocytes 'tagging' the dermal–epidermal junction and a superficial perivascular lymphohistiocytic infiltrate.

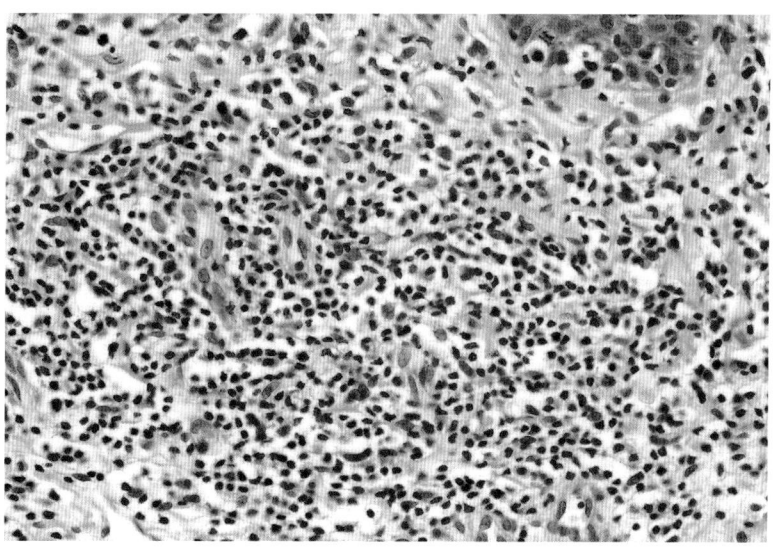

Fig. 29.20
Mycosis fungoides (patch stage): there is a superficial perivascular lymphohistiocytic infiltrate. Atypical cells are not seen.

lymphocytes. With the development of tumor stage MF, large transformed cells are conspicuous and epidermotropism is commonly lost. Epidermotropism as seen in cutaneous T-cell lymphoma differs from exocytosis of lymphocytes as seen in dermatitis/eczema in that there is usually no or only very mild spongiosis and vesiculation is not usually a feature. The presence of atypical lymphoid cells in an intraepidermal vesicle (the Pautrier microabscess) is typical, although not diagnostic, of mycosis fungoides (*Fig. 29.17*). Similar features may be seen, though less often, in Sézary syndrome, adult T-cell leukemia/lymphoma (ATLL), actinic reticuloid, and drug-induced T-cell pseudolymphomas.

Patch stage mycosis fungoides

The histopathological features of the early patch stage of MF are usually subtle and easily overlooked (*Fig. 29.18*). Multiple biopsies are commonly necessary to reach a diagnosis. The epidermis may be of normal thickness, slightly acanthotic, or less commonly atrophic, and often there is mild hyperkeratosis with focal parakeratosis. Basal cell hydropic degeneration is sometimes noted. Within the epidermis, there are characteristically small numbers of atypical irregular lymphoid cells, each surrounded by a clear halo, although in very early lesions they may sometimes be absent (*Fig.*

29.19). Occasionally, small numbers of larger typical cells may also be evident. Palisading of lymphocytes along the basal layer of the epidermis is a diagnostic pointer. Individual necrotic keratinocytes are seen in some cases. A lymphohistiocytic infiltrate surrounds the vessels of the superficial vascular plexus and extends into the papillary dermis (*Fig. 29.20*). Eosinophils and plasma cells are present in small numbers or absent.[128,131] Red cell extravasation is sometimes evident. Pigmentary incontinence is common. The connective tissue of the papillary dermis is occasionally increased with coarsening of the collagen bundles (although this is more typical of plaque stage disease).[128] In the more advanced patch stage, increasing numbers of atypical cells may make the diagnosis more obvious, although frank Pautrier microabscesses are uncommon (*Figs 29.21* and *29.22*).

Sometimes, prior treatment with steroids or PUVA before biopsy masks the features, making the diagnosis virtually impossible, emphasizing the necessity for careful clinicopathological correlation (*Figs 29.23–29.26*).

Plaque stage mycosis fungoides

In established plaque stage disease, there is usually little difficulty in establishing the correct diagnosis. There is compact hyperkeratosis, patchy parakeratosis, and the epidermis is commonly acanthotic, frequently adopting

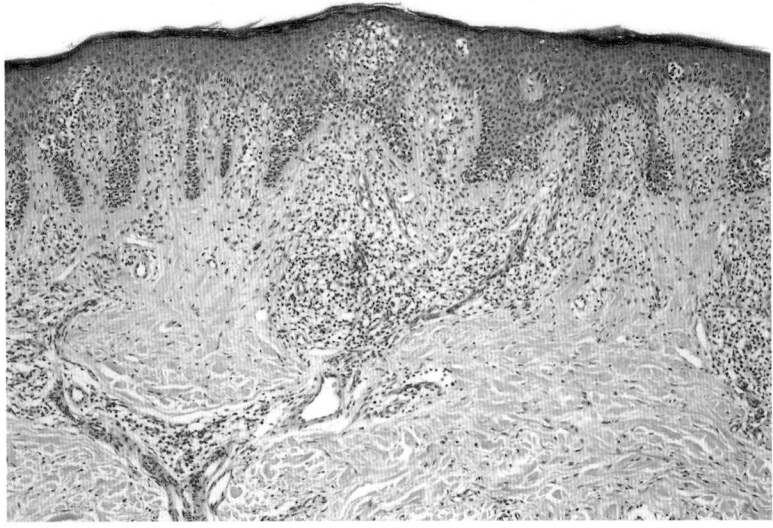

Fig. 29.21
Mycosis fungoides (patch stage): the epidermis shows psoriasiform hyperplasia in this more advanced example. Even at this magnification, epidermotropism is conspicuous.

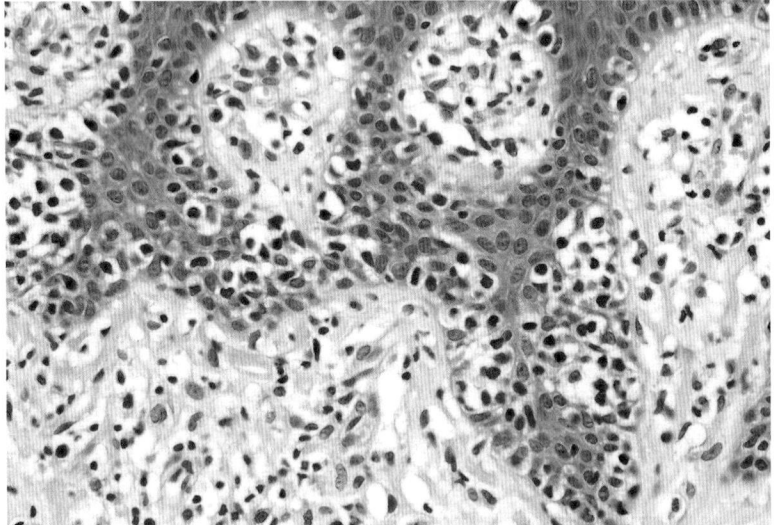

Fig. 29.22
Mycosis fungoides (patch stage): high-power view of atypical lymphocytes with well-developed halo.

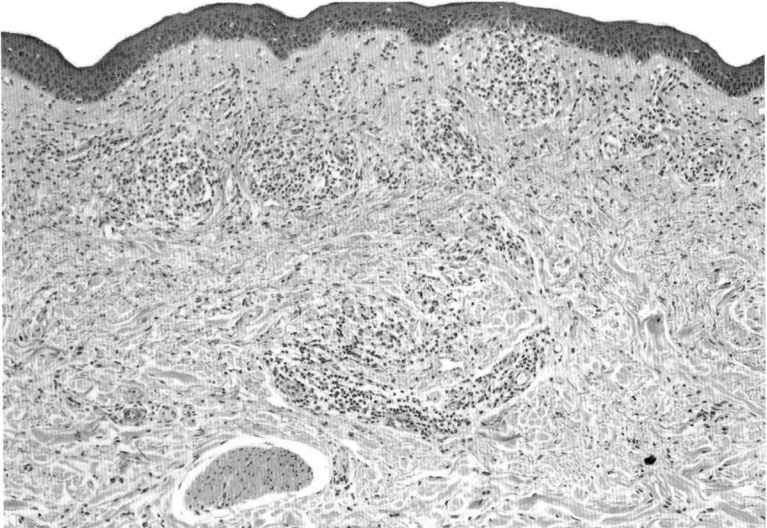

Fig. 29.23
Mycosis fungoides: the case illustrated here and in *Figs 29.24–29.26* demonstrates the effects of prior treatment with PUVA before biopsy. Note the dermal perivascular and interstitial lymphocytic infiltrate.

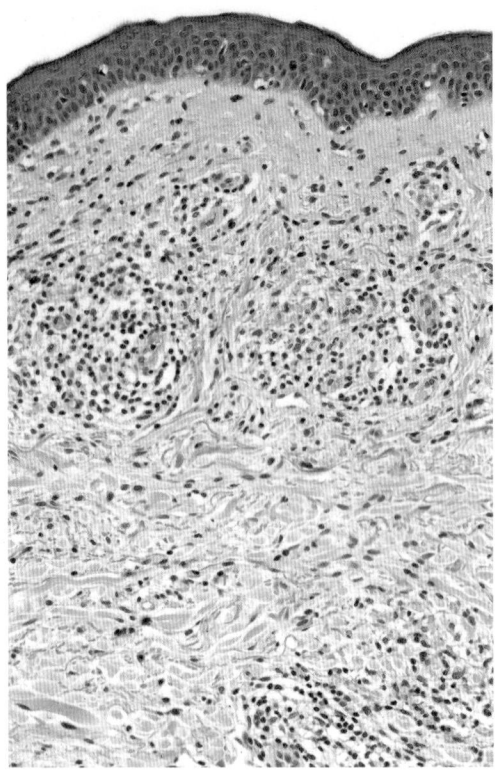

Fig. 29.24
Mycosis fungoides: higher-power view of *Fig. 29.23*.

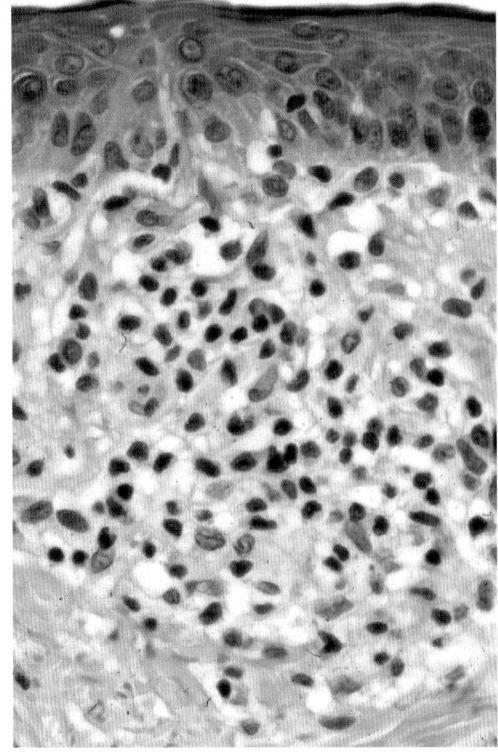

Fig. 29.25
Mycosis fungoides: mild cytological atypia is evident.

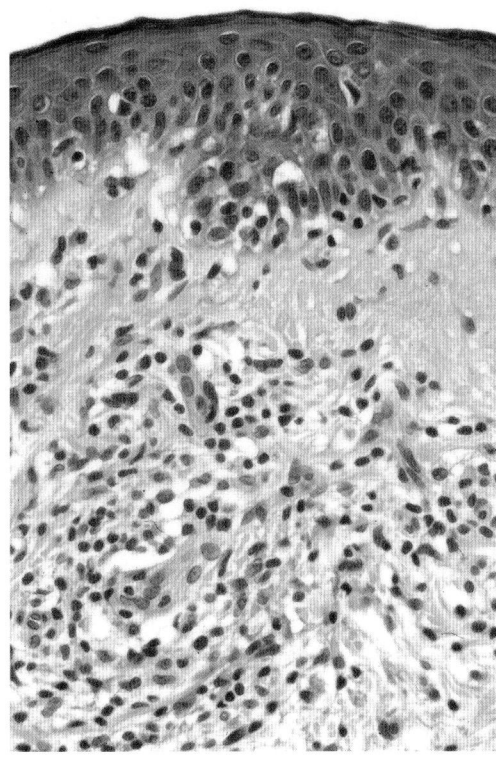

Fig. 29.26
Mycosis fungoides: there is just a hint of epidermotropism. This case illustrates the importance of clinicopathological correlation. A repeat biopsy following a period with no therapy showed typical features.

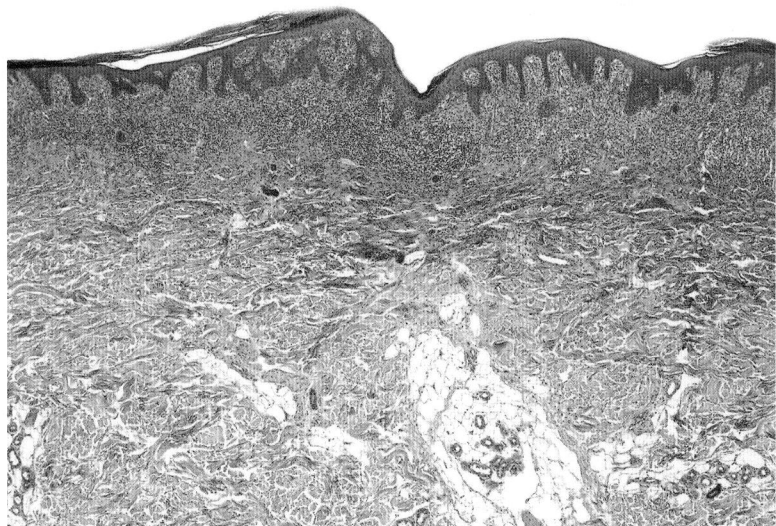

Fig. 29.27
Mycosis fungoides (plaque stage): there is focal parakeratosis and marked psoriasiform hyperplasia.

a psoriasiform appearance (*Fig. 29.27*). The infiltrate is much more intense than in the patch stage, and large numbers of atypical mononuclear cells are commonly present in the epidermis (*Figs 29.28* and *29.29*). Occasionally, however, epidermotropism is absent, particularly in patients who have been treated topically. In the dermis, the distribution is predominantly superficial and bandlike in character. Mycosis/Sézary cells may be present singly or in clusters or exceptionally replace almost the entire epidermis.

Pautrier microabscesses are not uncommon, being identified in 17–37.5% of cases.[127] The infiltrate may obscure the dermal–epidermal junction, and cytoid bodies are sometimes present. Occasionally, the additional histologic features of confluent hyperkeratosis, irregular acanthosis, extensive basal cell hydropic degeneration, and apoptosis mimic lichen planus.

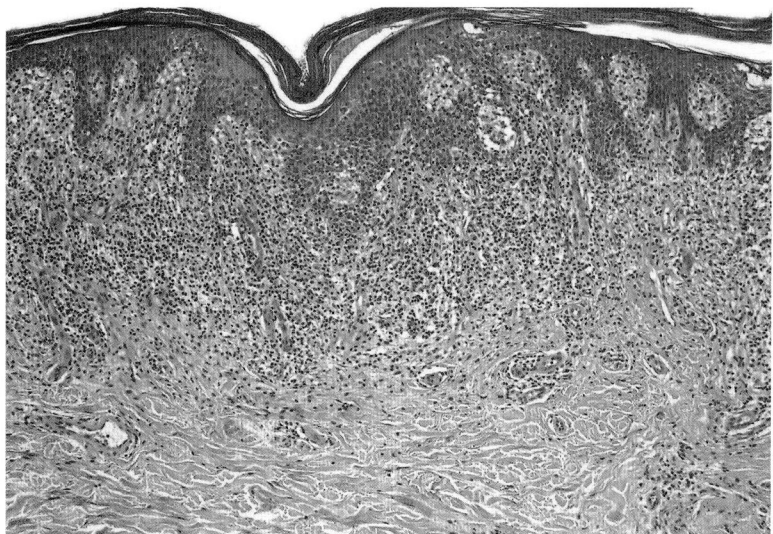

Fig. 29.28
Mycosis fungoides (plaque stage): there is a dense upper dermal bandlike infiltrate.

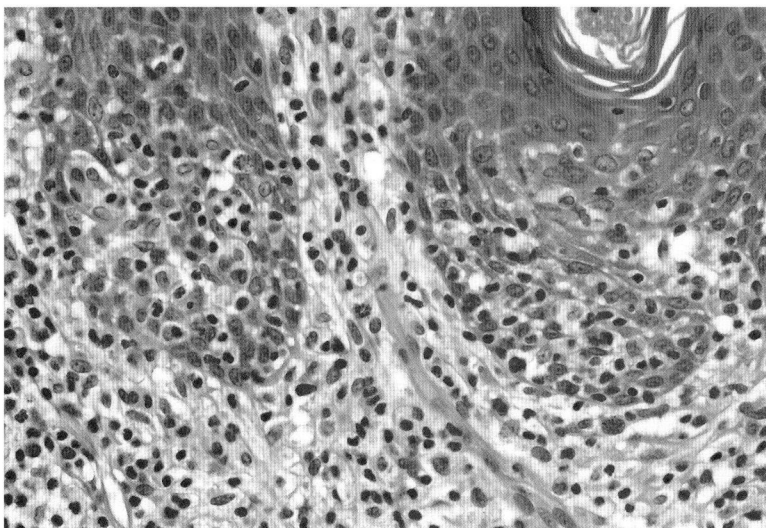

Fig. 29.29
Mycosis fungoides (plaque stage): there is a dense population of atypical lymphocytes with marked epidermotropism.

In addition to the epidermal changes, follicular epithelium may be involved, and sometimes follicular mucinosis is evident. There may also be infiltration of sweat duct epithelium by the malignant cells (syringotropism).

In poikilodermatous lesions, the epidermis is typically flattened, atrophic, and covered by a scale of hyperkeratosis or parakeratosis (*Fig. 29.30*). Hypergranulosis is not usually a feature. Necrotic keratinocytes are occasionally seen. There is often hydropic degeneration of the basal layer of the epidermis (*Fig. 29.31*). Epidermotropism is a constant feature and occasionally mycosis/Sézary cells may be noted. In the dermis, there is a bandlike or perivascular lymphohistiocytic infiltrate. Pigmentary incontinence is usually a feature, and often telangiectatic vessels are evident. The superficial dermis may be scarred.

Verrucous lesions which show pseudoepitheliomatous hyperplasia and crusting with associated hyperkeratosis and parakeratosis may be clinically confused with deep mycoses and even keratoacanthoma.

The dermal infiltrate often contains an admixture of reactive inflammatory cells, including eosinophils, plasma cells, and histiocytes, in addition to atypical lymphocytes.[127] Occasionally, multinucleate giant cells are evident and mitoses are sometimes seen. Coarse collagen bundles with or without increased numbers of fibroblasts are commonly present in the papillary dermis (*Figs 29.32* and *29.33*).

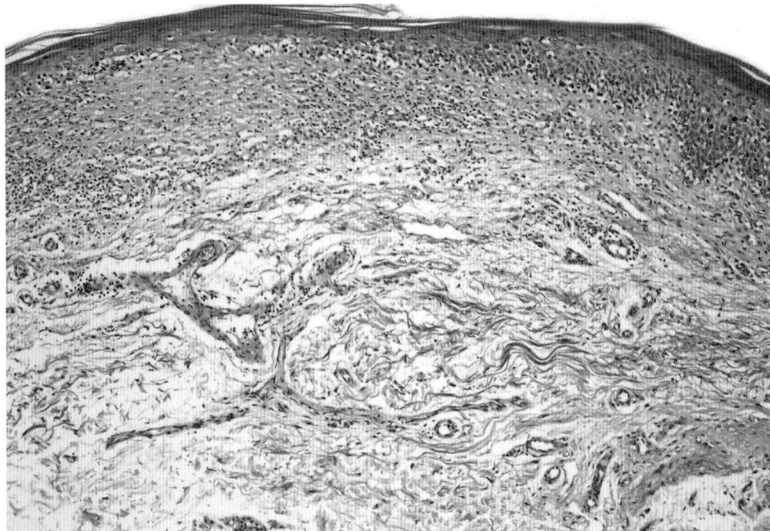

Fig. 29.30
Mycosis fungoides (poikiloderma atrophicans vasculare): there is hyperkeratosis, epidermal atrophy, marked basal cell hydropic degeneration, and fibrosis.

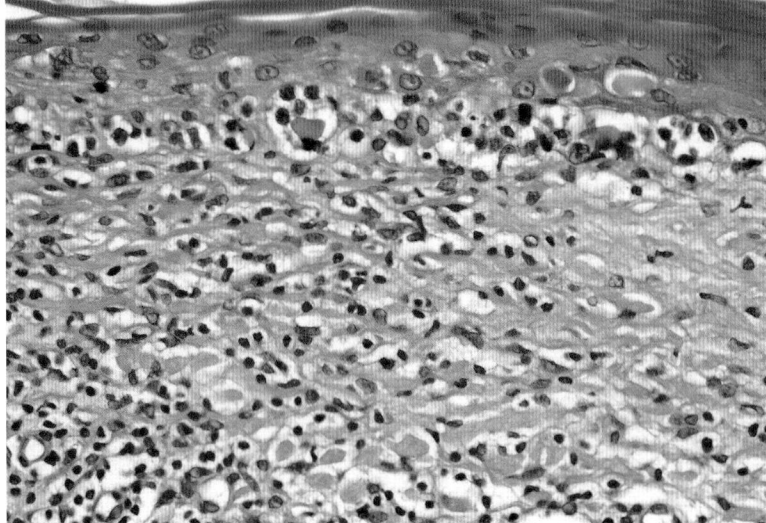

Fig. 29.31
Mycosis fungoides (poikiloderma atrophicans vasculare): there is liquefactive degeneration of the basal layer, and cytoid bodies are present. Note the scattered intraepidermal atypical lymphocytes.

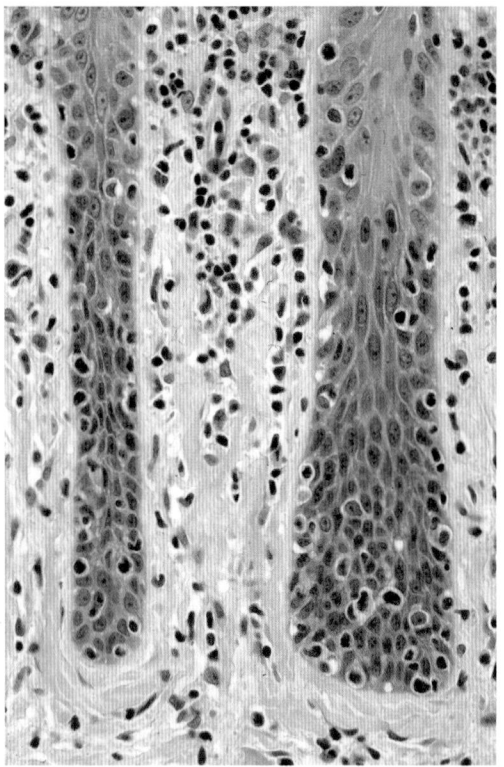

Fig. 29.32
Mycosis fungoides (plaque stage): note the vertically orientated fibrous tissue. This results from chronic scratching.

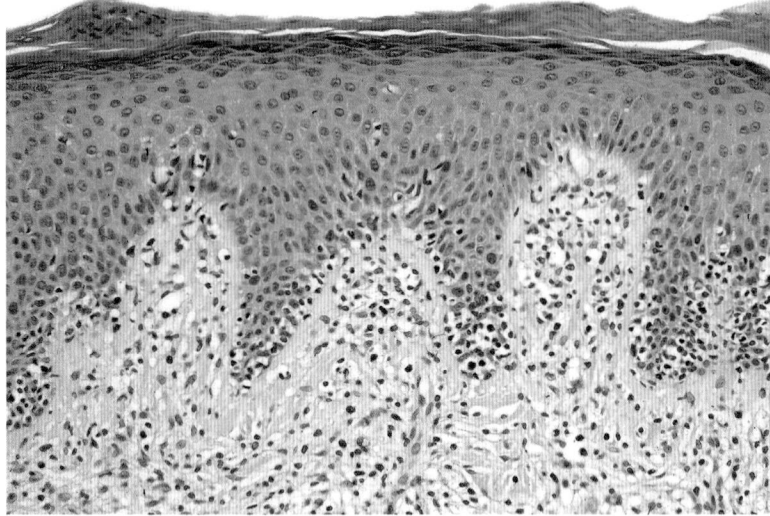

Fig. 29.33
Mycosis fungoides (plaque stage): in this example, the scarring is more marked.

Tumor stage mycosis fungoides

In tumor stage MF, a very dense infiltrate occupies the dermis, sometimes extending into the subcutaneous fat (*Figs 29.34–29.38*). A top-heavy configuration may be apparent. The lesions are often ulcerated, and epidermotropism is typically either slight or absent. The infiltrate, which may be diffuse or show an ill-defined nodular outline, in addition to containing mycosis/Sézary cells, often has large numbers of highly pleomorphic cells. Mitotic figures are conspicuous and frequently abnormal.

A broad spectrum of histologic changes has been described in biopsies of early stage MF, and many of these overlap with features seen in inflammatory dermatoses.[131,132] The following have been reported to be useful when trying to establish a definite diagnosis in such situations:[123,124,127,133]

- lymphocytes in linear array at the dermal–epidermal junction (linear epidermotropism),
- hyperconvoluted lymphocytes within the epidermis (epidermal cerebriform cells),
- disproportionate epidermotropism,
- Pautrier microabscesses,
- epidermal lymphocytes larger than dermal lymphocytes,

- wiry bundles of papillary dermal collagen associated with a lichenoid infiltrate,
- lymphocyte atypia, although characteristic, is often not apparent in early lesions,
- mitotic activity is of little value in early disease.

However, two multivariate analyzes produced conflicting results as to which of these features was the most helpful.[127,133] This emphasizes the need for good clinicopathological correlation, and is the reason why diagnostic algorithms incorporating clinical, pathological, and molecular findings have been proposed (see below). It is also important to be aware of a patient's current treatment when assessing a biopsy specimen, since local treatments may mask any tendency to epidermotropism.

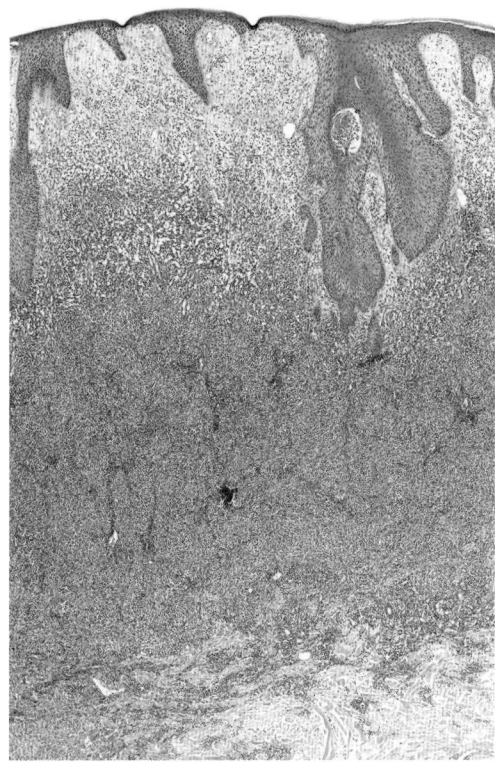

Fig. 29.34
Mycosis fungoides (tumor stage): an intense infiltrate is present in the dermis.

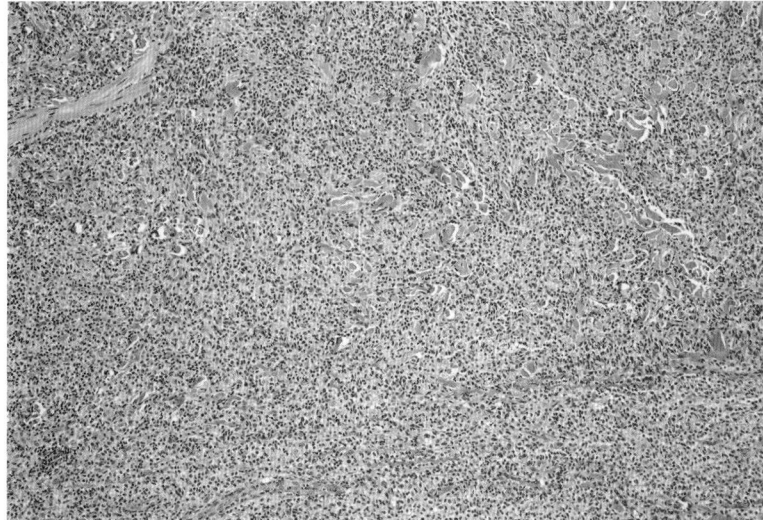

Fig. 29.35
Mycosis fungoides (tumor stage): note the dissection of collagen.

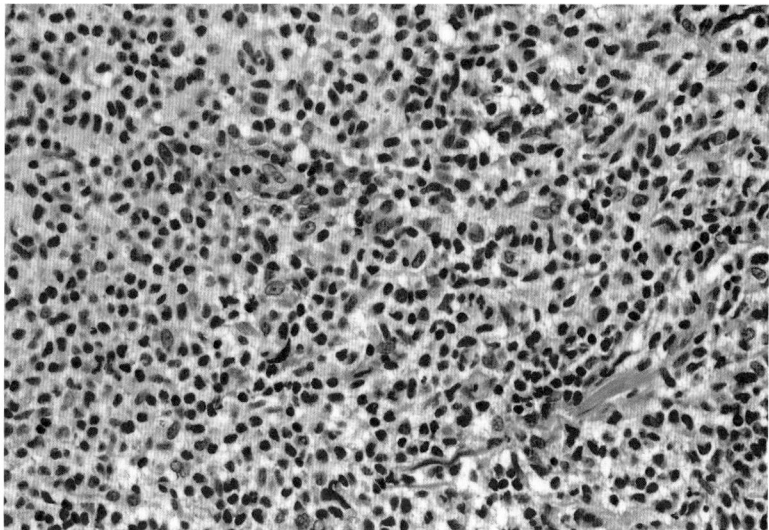

Fig. 29.36
Mycosis fungoides (tumor stage): there is a uniform population of mycosis cells.

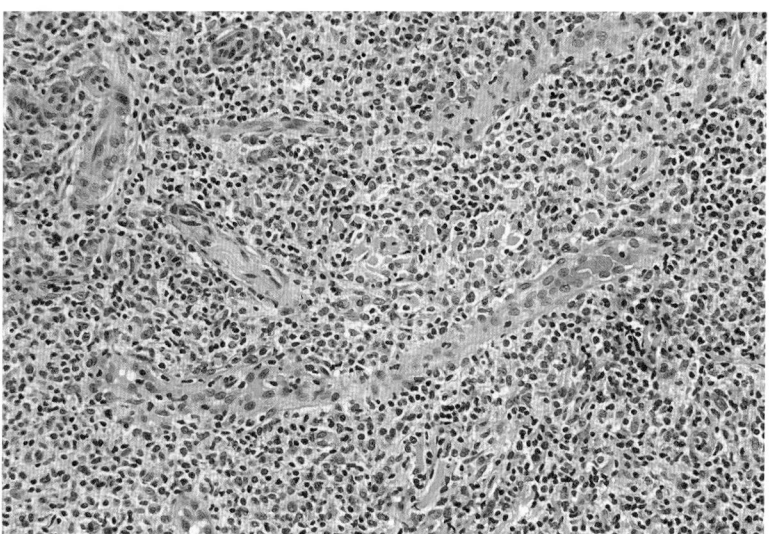

Fig. 29.37
Mycosis fungoides (tumor stage): this view demonstrates the conspicuous vasculature.

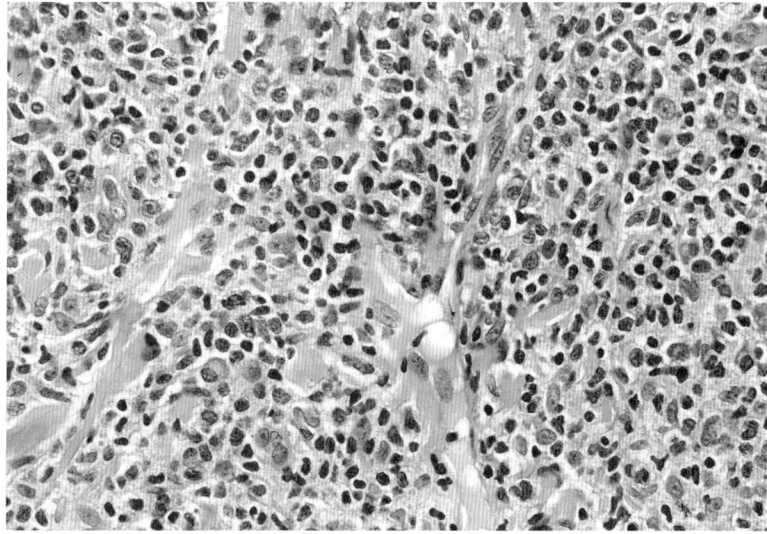

Fig. 29.38
Mycosis fungoides (tumor stage): high-power view.

MF is commonly characterized by accumulation and proliferation of CD4+, CD45RO-positive helper/memory T lymphocytes, although occasionally a CD8+ and even CD4/CD8-phenotypes may be seen (*Figs 29.39* and *29.40*). The latter has no bearing on prognosis. The lymphocytes usually also express the pan-T-cell antigens CD2, CD3, CD5, and CD7, as well as TCRαβ and cutaneous lymphocyte antigen (CLA).[96,111] CD7 is often focally lost very early, and it is not of diagnostic value as its expression is also often lost in reactive conditions (*Fig. 29.41*), as are less frequently CD2, CD3, or CD5.[24,134] CD25 (IL-2 receptor) is positive in up to 50% of cases, and the T-follicular helper cell marker, PD1, is also frequently expressed.[135,136] CD30 expression correlates with transformation but has no prognostic implications. Unlike some other cutaneous T-cell lymphomas, MUM1, as identified by the MUM1p antibody, is rarely expressed.[137] Aberrant expression of CD20 is occasionally seen, and this is not associated with expression of

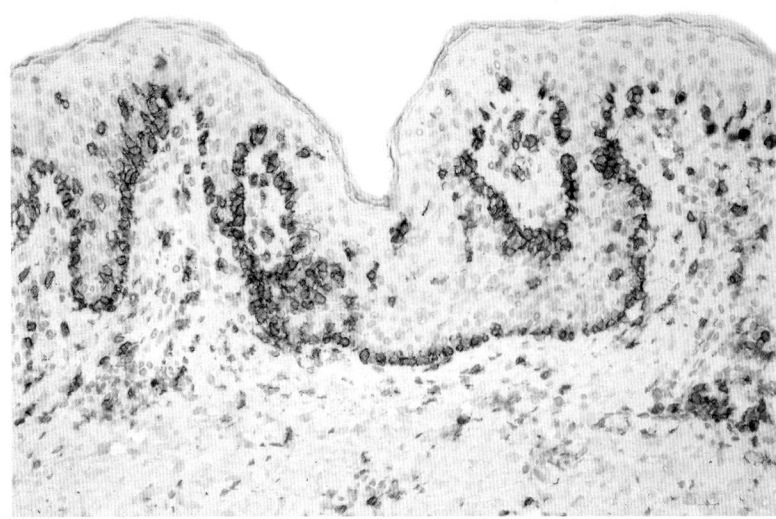

Fig. 29.39
Mycosis fungoides: intraepidermal lymphocytes are highlighted with CD3 immunohistochemistry. Note the conspicuous tagging.

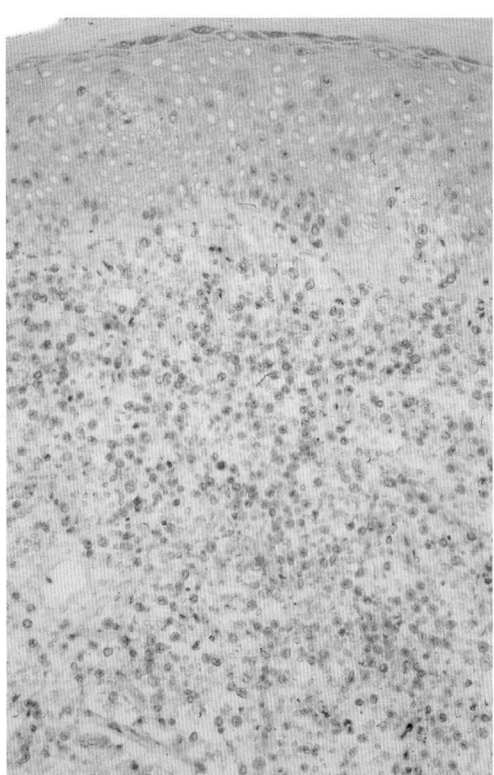

Fig. 29.41
Mycosis fungoides: CD7 is absent.

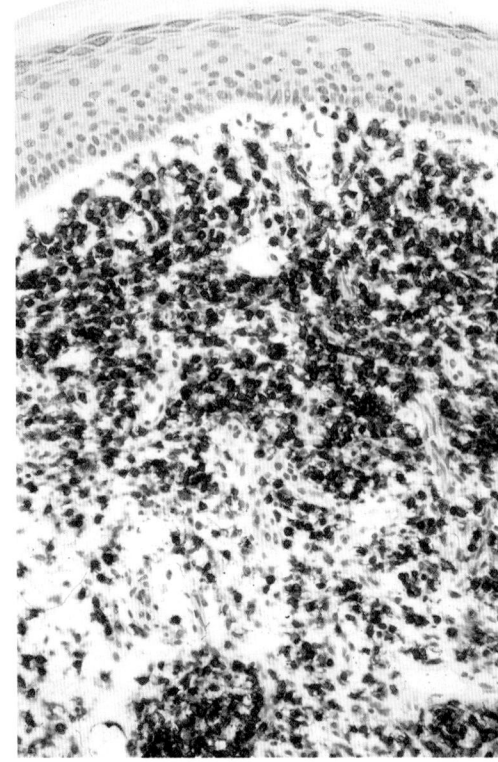

Fig. 29.40
Mycosis fungoides: the lymphocytes express CD4.

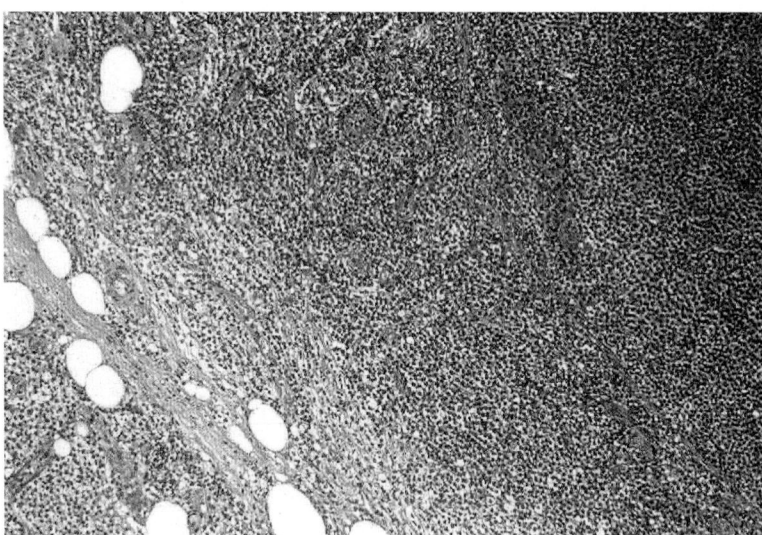

Fig. 29.42
Mycosis fungoides: this lymph node biopsy shows partial replacement by mycosis cells. Note the spillover into the pericapsular fat.

other B-cell markers.[138] Expression of TCRγδ is rarely found, and this has no bearing on behavior or prognosis in the context of classic cutaneous T-cell lymphoma (mycosis fungoides).[139]

Evidence of a clonal T-cell receptor gene rearrangement may be identified by Southern blot or polymerase chain reaction (PCR) in the majority of cases.[53–60] Overall, TCR gene rearrangements can be anticipated in up to 100% of cases of tumor stage, 50–100% of plaque stage, and 50–78% of patch stage MF.[43] The results should, however, be interpreted with caution since TCR gene rearrangements have been described in a number of inflammatory dermatoses including discoid lupus erythematosus, lichen planus, lichen sclerosus, and pityriasis lichenoides et varioliformis acuta (PLEVA).[58–64]

Dermatopathic lymphadenopathy with lymph node involvement

Lymphadenopathy is frequently present in MF but does not always correlate with histologic evidence of lymphomatous involvement. The features of dermatopathic lymphadenitis are characterized by a marked infiltration of the nodal paracortical region by large numbers of histiocytes, including interdigitating reticulum cells and Langerhans cells.[140–144] Occasional plasma cells and eosinophils may be present. The histiocytes often contain melanin. At this stage, there is no distortion of the lymph node architecture. With progression, careful study of the paracortex may reveal infiltration by mycosis/Sézary cells (*Fig. 29.42*). These are best identified around the postcapillary venules (*Figs 29.43* and *29.44*). At first, they may be present singly or in

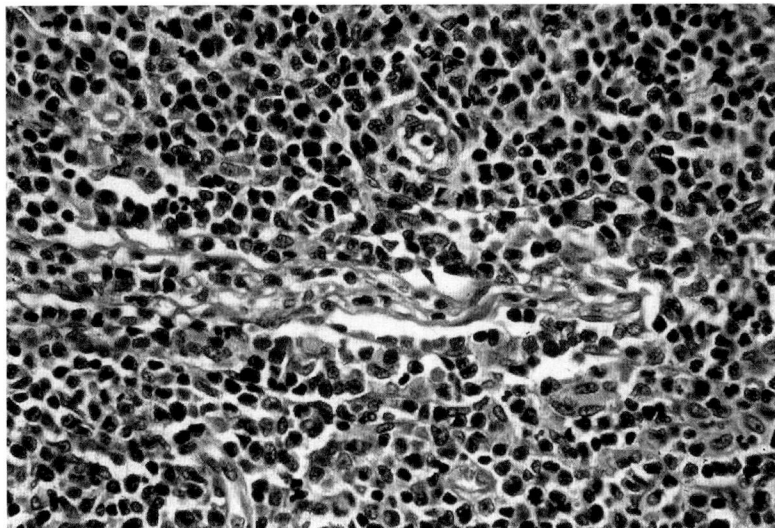

Fig. 29.43
Mycosis fungoides: higher power view shows a monomorphic infiltrate of Sézary cells.

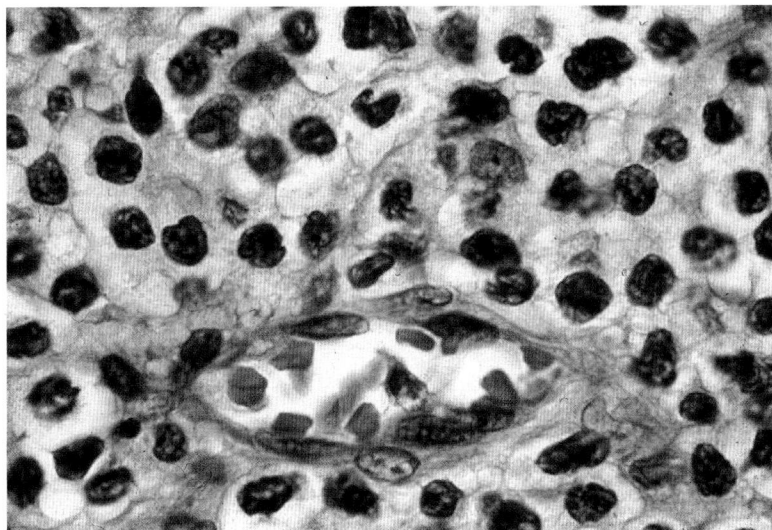

Fig. 29.44
Mycosis fungoides: mycosis cells surround a postcapillary venule.

small groups, but in advanced disease sheets of tumor cells are evident and the nodal architecture is effaced.

Historically, two histologic staging systems have been used to document the degree of lymph node involvement. Both record the number and distribution of 'abnormal' lymphocytes within the nodal parenchyma, but differ in their definition of what constitutes 'abnormal'. In the NVI/VA system, neoplastic cells are defined as lymphocytes with cerebriform, irregularly folded, hyperconvoluted nuclei irrespective of size.[145,146] The Dutch system only accepts cerebriform cells >7.5 microns in diameter as neoplastic.[144] Both of these approaches have been incorporated into a simplified version in the proposed ISCL/EORTC staging system.[30] In this, minor degrees of lymph node involvement are grouped with changes of dermatopathic lymphadenopathy, since the prognostic impact of the former is unclear.[30] Partial and complete effacement of lymph node architecture clearly impacts on survival and is worthy of separate consideration.[30] The results of clonality studies can also be included in lymph nodes showing possible early involvement. However, there is no clear evidence that the presence of a clone detected by PCR in an uninvolved or minimally involved lymph node has any added impact on outcome. The definitions of the various stages are summarized below, and a comparison of the various systems is shown in *Table 29.4*:

- N0N: clinically abnormal nodes therefore no biopsy required (abnormal node ≥1.5 cm),

Table 29.4

Pathological staging systems for lymph nodes in mycosis fungoides

Updated ISCL/EORTC classification	Dutch system	NCI-VA classification
N1	Grade 1: dermatopathic lymphadenopathy	LN0: no atypical lymphocytes seen LN1: scattered atypical lymphocytes, not in clusters LN2: many atypical lymphocytes arranged in clusters of 3–6 cells
N2	Grade 2: early involvement by mycosis fungoides	LN3: aggregates of atypical lymphocytes observed but lymph node architecture preserved
N3	Grade 3: lymph node architecture partially effaced by lymphoma Grade 4: complete effacement of lymph node architecture by lymphoma	LN4: partial or complete effacement of the lymph node architecture by lymphoma

Modified from Olsen, E., et al. (2007) *Blood*, 110, 1713–1722.

- N1: clinically abnormal nodes; dermatopathic lymphadenopathy; atypically lymphocytes may be present but only singly or in small clusters (3–6 cells),
  – N1aNo: evidence of monoclonal T-cell population by PCR,
  – N1b: clonal T-cell population detected by PCR,
- N2: clinically abnormal nodes; aggregates of atypical cells present but nodal architecture preserved,
  – N2aNo: evidence of monoclonal T-cell population by PCR,
  – N2b: clonal T-cell population detected by PCR,
- N3: clinically abnormal nodes; partial or complete effacement of nodal architecture,
- Nx: clinically abnormal nodes; no histologic confirmation.

Differential diagnosis

Skin biopsies from patients with MF often show features that are also seen in various benign dermatoses.[131,132] Patch stage mycosis fungoides must be distinguished in particular from chronic superficial dermatitis, which is typically a mild spongiotic process. Lymphocyte atypia and epidermotropism are not features. Lymphomatoid drug reactions may be histologically indistinguishable from MF. Differential diagnosis requires consideration of a constellation of clinical, histologic, immunohistochemical, and molecular features. This is recognized in the diagnostic algorithm recently proposed by the ISCL.[24] This system assigns weighted scores to multiple criteria, up to a maximum of six, a diagnosis of MF requiring a total of at least four. This is an eminently sensible approach, but as yet there are only limited reports of its usefulness.

MF showing marked epidermotropism should be distinguished from CD8+ primary cutaneous epidermotropic T-cell lymphoma. ATLL commonly presents with histologic features indistinguishable from mycosis fungoides.

Tumor stage MF may be confused with other lymphomatous infiltrates, particularly if the cells are very pleomorphic and especially if epidermotropism is absent. Often, only careful review of the clinical information, taken in conjunction with the histologic features of previous biopsies (if available) and immunohistochemistry, allows the correct diagnosis to be made.

Transformation of mycosis fungoides

Large cell transformation in MF occurs in 10–23% of cases in larger series in which all stages of mycosis fungoides are included as the denominator.[1–3]

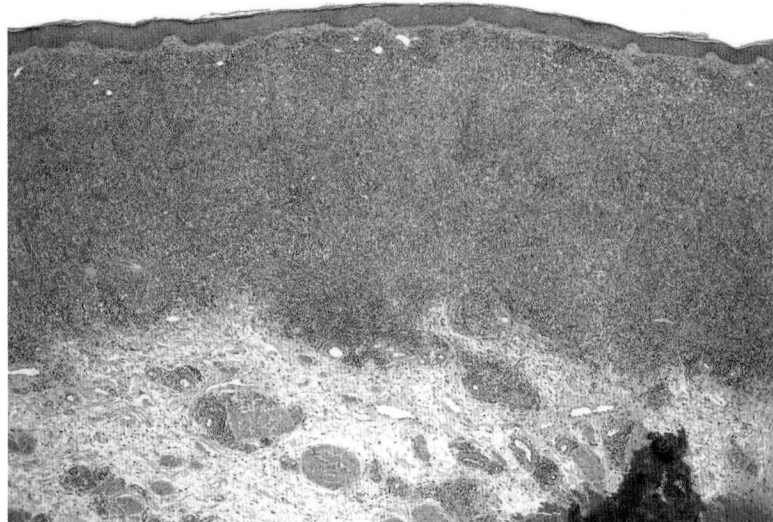

Fig. 29.45
Mycosis fungoides (transformation): there is an intense dermal infiltrate.

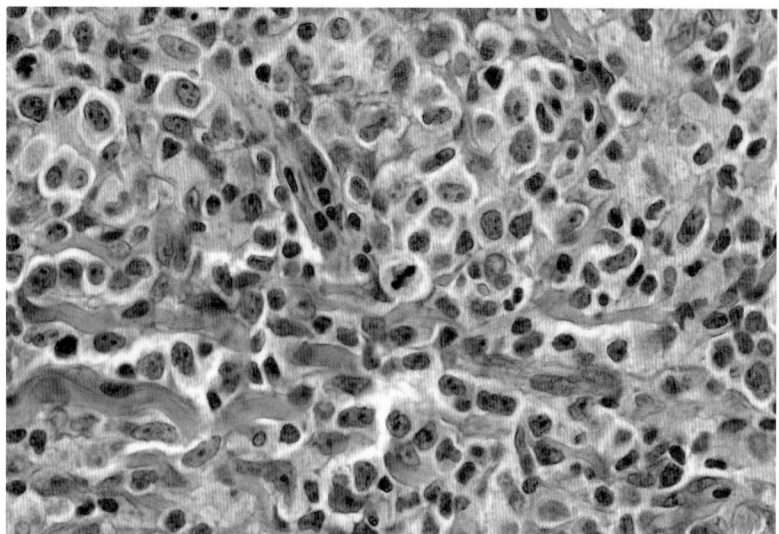

Fig. 29.47
Mycosis fungoides (transformation): note the central mitotic figure.

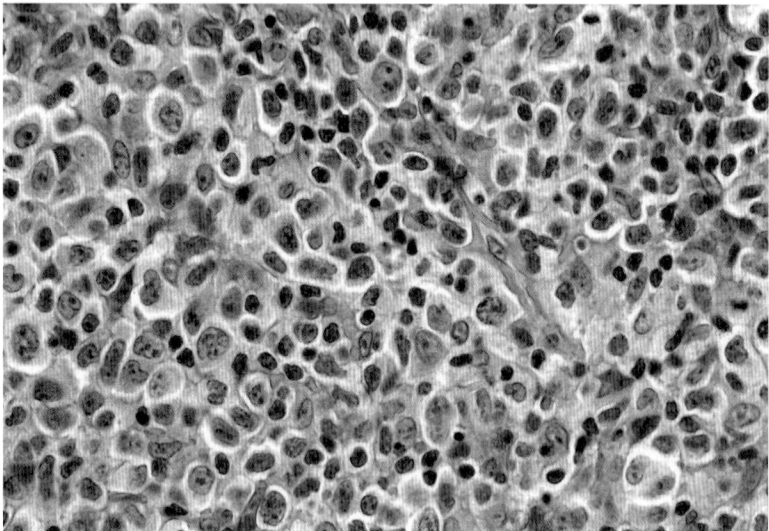

Fig. 29.46
Mycosis fungoides (transformation): the infiltrate is composed predominantly of blast cells with large vesicular nuclei and prominent nucleoli.

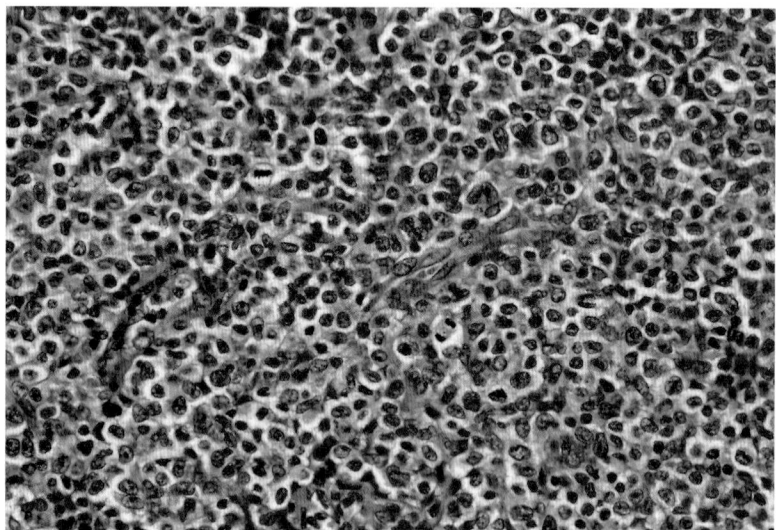

Fig. 29.48
Mycosis fungoides (transformation): multiple mitotic figures are present.

Transformation is associated with a very poor prognosis and predicts for inferior outcome even in patients with advance stage disease.[1-5] Median survival from transformation ranges from 11 to 36 months.[2-4]

The pathogenesis of large cell transformation in MF is unknown. p53 overexpression has been correlated with transformation, but this is not associated with a p53 gene mutation and is of uncertain significance.[6] More recently, loss of CDKN2A/CDKN2B as well as overexpression of micro-RNAs miR-93-5p, miR-181a, miR181b, miR-34a, and miR-326 have been documented at high frequency in transformed MF, but the role these abnormalities play in disease progress remains undetermined.[7,8]

Large cell transformation may be recognized when the infiltrate contains 25% or more large cells or if there is a discrete tumor cell nodule (Fig. 29.45).[1,4] Large cells are defined as being four or more times the size of a small lymphocyte.[1] They have prominent vesicular or hyperchromatic nuclei, often with conspicuous nucleoli and abundant cytoplasm (Fig. 29.46). Nuclear pleomorphism is common, and giant cells (including Reed-Sternberg-like variants) are sometimes present. Mitotic activity is usually marked and abnormal forms may be identified (Figs 29.47 and 29.48). Although in most instances the tumor is of the large cell phenotype, pleomorphic and immunoblastic variants have also been documented.[4,9,10] The immunophenotype is similar to prototypical mycosis fungoides, although there is more frequent loss of CD7, CD2, and CD5. The transformed tumor cell population is typically CD4+ although these may acquire a cytotoxic phenotype with expression of cytotoxic molecules such as TIA-1, perforin, and granzyme B. Exceptionally, CD8+ variants have been described. Some degree of CD30 expression is seen in 30–50% of cases, and in half of these, 75% of the infiltrate express this antigen. Expression of CD30 is not associated with prognosis. CD25 expression is also seen in many cases (Fig. 29.49).[2,3,11] In addition, although small and large B cells are often prominent in infiltrates of transformed MF, aberrant CD20 expression has also been confirmed on the surface of the neoplastic T cells.[3,12]

It is most important to distinguish CD30-positive large cell transformation from lymphomatoid papulosis or cutaneous anaplastic large cell lymphoma, which may also develop in patients with MF (especially lymphomatoid papulosis). Both conditions can be distinguished on clinical grounds, and clinical course is often the only distinguishing feature.[3]

Classic mycosis fungoides with unusual clinical manifestations

This section describes a group of mycosis fungoides cases with unusual clinical features that run a similar course of classic MF. They may display overlapping features, and can be seen in patients with otherwise typical lesions of MF.

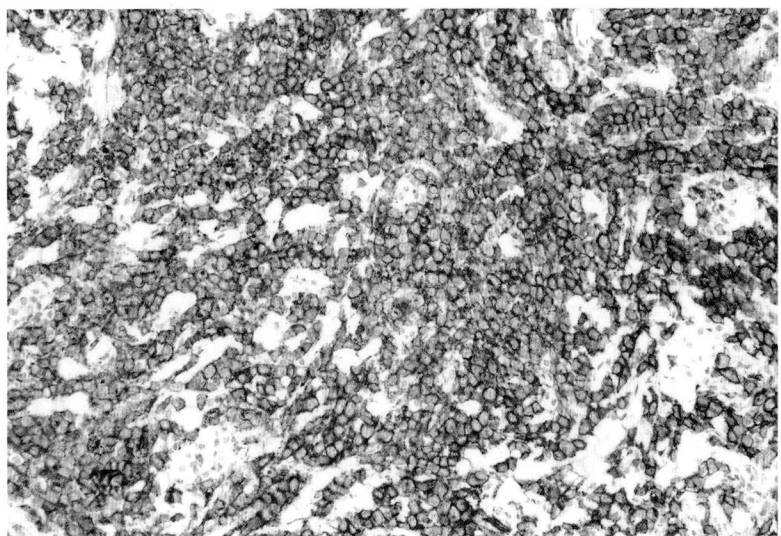

Fig. 29.49
Mycosis fungoides (transformation): the tumor cells express CD30.

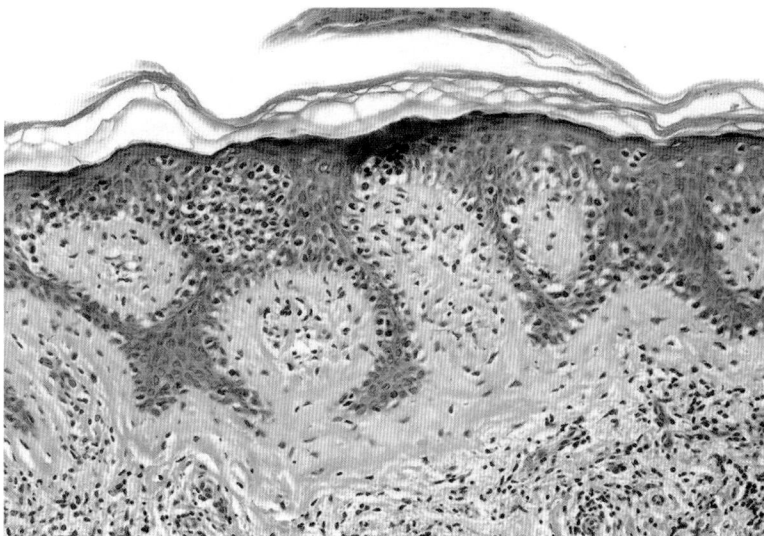

Fig. 29.51
Childhood mycosis fungoides: there is parakeratosis, psoriasiform hyperplasia, and an atypical lymphoid infiltrate.

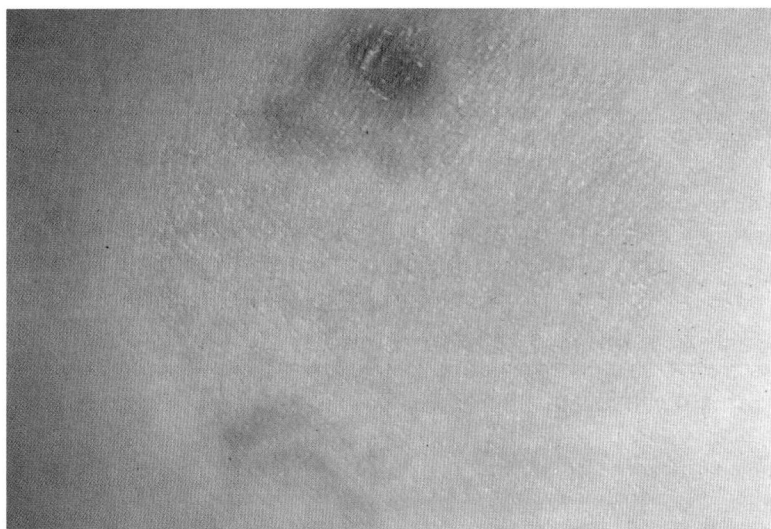

Fig. 29.50
Childhood mycosis fungoides: patch-stage lesion on the trunk of a child. By courtesy of J. Williams, MD, Harvard Medical School, Boston, USA.

Mycosis fungoides in children and adolescents

Clinical features

Mycosis fungoides in children and adolescents accounts for 0.5–2.7% of cases in the literature.[1–16] In one population-based registry, the incidence of MF in patients under 20 years of age was 0.05 per 100 000 persons. In addition, in young adults with MF, presentation may well have been much earlier although this has not necessarily been documented.[12] The youngest patient documented was 22 months at diagnosis.[11] As in adults, males are affected more often than females.

In most patients, presentation is as patch or plaque stage disease, and hypopigmented variants are particularly prevalent in childhood (Fig. 29.50).[17] Exceptionally, unilesional disease has been documented.[14,18] Although there are very rare cases in which children have developed fatal tumor stage disease, leading some authors to postulate that the prognosis in children is worse than in adults, these are very much in the minority. In general, prognosis is good and relates to the disease stage.[3,5,10,19] In fact, it has been shown that children fare slightly better than adults overall in terms of both 5- and 10-year survival (93% vs. 81% and 74% vs. 68%, respectively) although this does not reach statistical significance.[12]

Histologic features

HTLV-I serology has been positive in one documented patient with hypopigmented lesions.[13] The significance of this is uncertain.[20,21]

MF in childhood and adolescence is histologically indistinguishable from the disease in adults (Fig. 29.51).

The immunophenotype in most cases is CD2+, CD3+, CD4–, CD5+, CD7–, and CD8+. A CD8+ phenotype is also commonly encountered in hypopigmented variants (see below).[16,18,22]

Hypopigmented mycosis fungoides and hyperpigmented mycosis fungoides

Clinical features

Mycosis fungoides associated with hypopigmentation is a rare occurrence and may be clinically confused with vitiligo, pityriasis alba, tinea versicolor, annular lichenoid dermatosis, and postinflammatory hypopigmentation.[1,2] It is more often seen in children and adolescents.[3–15] The sex ratio is equal. Dark-skinned patients are particularly affected, although there is a small number of reports in Caucasians (Figs 29.52 and 29.53).[16–20] Patients present with asymptomatic or rarely pruritic, slightly scaly, hypopigmented patches, most often affecting the trunk and extremities. Very occasionally, a macular presentation is seen.[21,22] In general, this variant is indolent with a good prognosis. Exceptional cases of markedly hyperpigmented MF have been documented.[23,24]

Pathogenesis and histologic features

The pathogenesis of hypopigmentation is uncertain. Ultrastructural studies have been conflicting. Some authors have demonstrated melanocyte degenerative changes including dilatation of the rough endoplasmic reticulum, mitochondrial swelling, cytoplasmic vacuolation, and incompletely melanized melanosomes with keratinocytes containing normal numbers of melanosomes.[4,16] These changes are thought to represent a non-specific response to cellular injury with no evidence of a block of melanosome transfer to keratinocytes. Other authors, however, have documented impaired melanosome transfer in the absence of any evidence of melanocyte injury.[15]

Histologically, hypopigmented lesions are usually indistinguishable from classical mycosis fungoides except for the presence of very marked pigment incontinence. Some reports note striking epidermotropism mimicking pagetoid reticulosis.[1,3,4,16] The immunophenotype is also usually identical. There is a number of reports of cytotoxic suppressor CD8+ T cells predominating in the epidermal infiltrate, which probably reflects the disproportionate number of childhood and juvenile-onset cases in most series.[13–15,25]

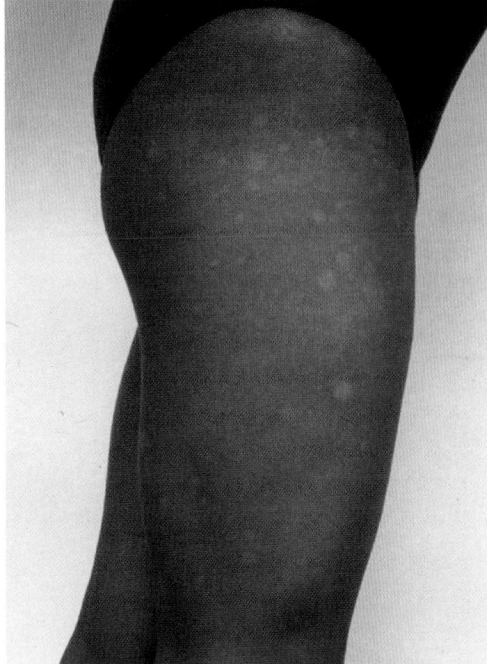

Fig. 29.52
Hypopigmented mycosis fungoides: this variant predominantly affects dark-skinned races. From the collection of the late N.P. Smith, MD, Institute of Dermatology, London, UK.

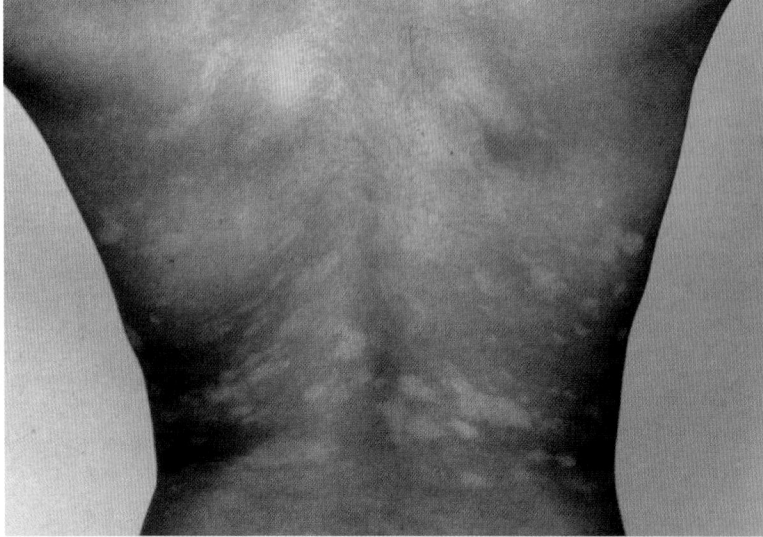

Fig. 29.53
Hypopigmented mycosis fungoides: patches of variable sizes, some of which appear infiltrated. From the collection of the late N.P. Smith, MD, Institute of Dermatology, London, UK.

Hyperpigmented lesions have been characterized by marked elongation of the rete ridges with increased pigmentation and conspicuous dermal melanophages superimposed upon the changes of MF.[23,26]

Mycosis fungoides and ichthyosis

Clinical features

There is only a small number of cases documenting presentation of MF as acquired ichthyosis.[1-6] In one study, they accounted for 3.5% of all patients with MF.[6] Patients have generally shown a fine scaly eruption resembling autosomal dominant ichthyosis vulgaris. The condition may be localized to the lower limbs or may be more widespread.[4,6] A more typical presentation

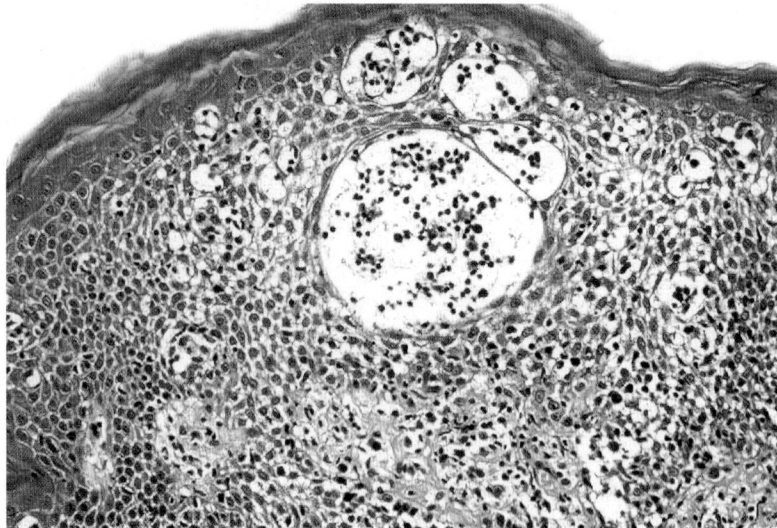

Fig. 29.54
Vesiculobullous mycosis fungoides: intraepidermal spongiotic vesiculation. This may reflect an allergic response to topical treatment. Atypical lymphocytes are present.

of MF may be seen.[6] Comedo-like lesions have also been described overlapping with folliculotropic MF.[3]

Histologic features

Histologically, the features of ichthyosis (hyperkeratosis, acanthosis with a thinned granular cell layer) are superimposed upon MF. The immunophenotype when reported has usually been CD2+, CD3+, and CD4+, with loss of CD7, apart from one CD8+ case.[4-6]

Vesiculobullous mycosis fungoides

Clinical features

Bullous MF is exceptional. Lesions, which may resemble bullous pemphigoid, pemphigus vulgaris, or pemphigus foliaceus, can be generalized, although in some reports there is a predilection for the palms and soles.[1-9] Superimposed allergic contact dermatitis following topical therapy may give rise to spongiotic vesiculation.

Histologic features

The blisters may be subcorneal, intraepidermal, or subepidermal, although the last are most common (Fig. 29.54).[6] They develop as a result of tumor cell infiltration with possible cytokine release rather than as a consequence of a coexistent autoimmune bullous dermatosis. Immunofluorescence is invariably negative.[2,4,5]

Differential diagnosis

Gram stain and periodic acid-Schiff (PAS) should be performed to exclude secondary infection. Vesiculobullous mycosis fungoides must be distinguished from bullous pemphigoid arising in patients with pre-existent mycosis fungoides and sometimes complicating PUVA, ultraviolet (UV) B therapy, or other treatments such as topical methchlorethamine and interferon (IFN)-alpha.[10-13]

Pustular mycosis fungoides

Clinical features

Pustular lesions are very rare in cutaneous T-cell lymphomas including MF and erythrodermic variants such that there can be confusion with pemphigus and subcorneal pustular dermatosis.[1,2] A palmoplantar pustulosis-like variant has also been documented. Similar lesions may be encountered in patients with psoriasis and MF.[3-5]

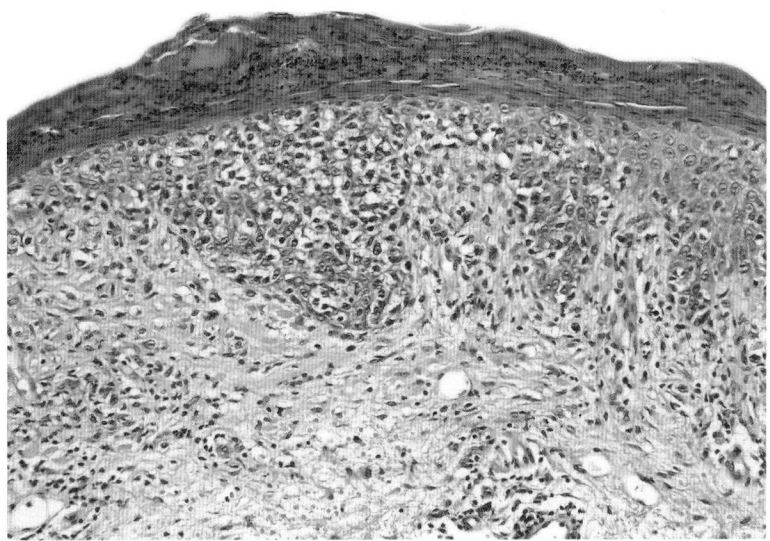

Fig. 29.55
Pustular mycosis fungoides: early pustule formation arising in a background of patch stage disease.

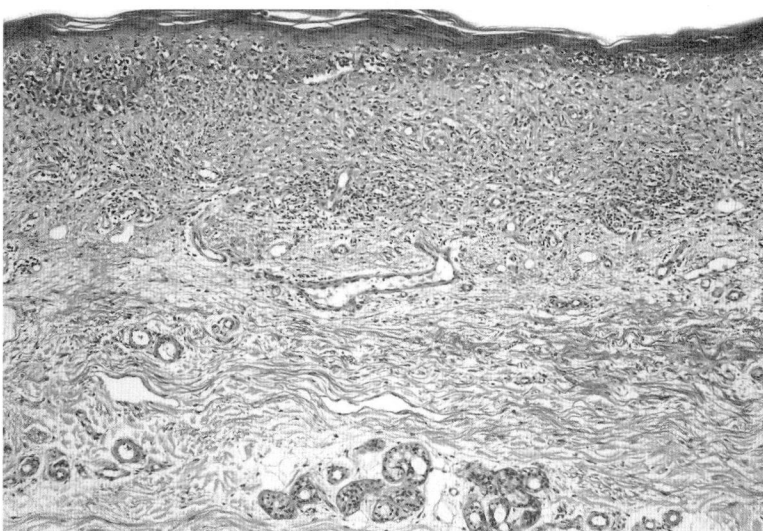

Fig. 29.56
Purpuric mycosis fungoides: this specimen comes from a patient with poikiloderma atrophicans vasculare.

Pathogenesis and histologic features

The cause of pustulation is unknown. Histologically, the pustular lesions may be related to subcorneal neutrophil abscesses (i.e., true pustules) or else reflect conspicuous Pautrier microabscesses (*Fig. 29.55*).[1,2]

Differential diagnosis

PAS and Gram stains should be performed to exclude a secondary infection. Pustular lesions have been described in a patient with MF as a result of demodex folliculitis.[6]

Pigmented purpura-like mycosis fungoides

Clinical features

Exceptionally, MF presents with purpuric lesions simulating a pigmented purpuric dermatosis.[1-9] However, in the latter, the eruption is generally restricted to the lower legs, whereas in MF the eruption is more often generalized and there is usually a background of more typical clinical lesions.[3]

Histologic features

Histologically, there can be considerable overlap with both conditions showing lymphocytes aligned along the epidermal side of the dermal–epidermal junction, red cell extravasation, and hemosiderin deposition (*Figs 29.56* and *29.57*). In purpuric mycosis fungoides, however, the epidermotropism is likely to be more marked and the dermal infiltrate tends to be deeper and denser. In addition, careful scrutiny is necessary for atypical lymphocytes present in mycosis fungoides and not in pigmented purpuric eruptions. Although theoretically a clonal T-cell population could be taken as supportive of a diagnosis of a lymphomatous process, clonal populations have been identified in a background of otherwise typical pigmented purpura.[3,10]

In the vast majority of cases, pigmented purpuric dermatosis tends to be self-limited, resolving in a few months or sometimes years, and does not progress to mycosis fungoides. There are, however, a sufficient number of cases where pigmented purpura appears to have progressed or been associated with lymphoma so that a prolonged and careful follow-up is warranted.[11,12]

Palmoplantar mycosis fungoides

Palmar and plantar involvement during the course of MF occurs in up to 11.5% of patients.[1] Purely palmar/plantar involvement is exceedingly

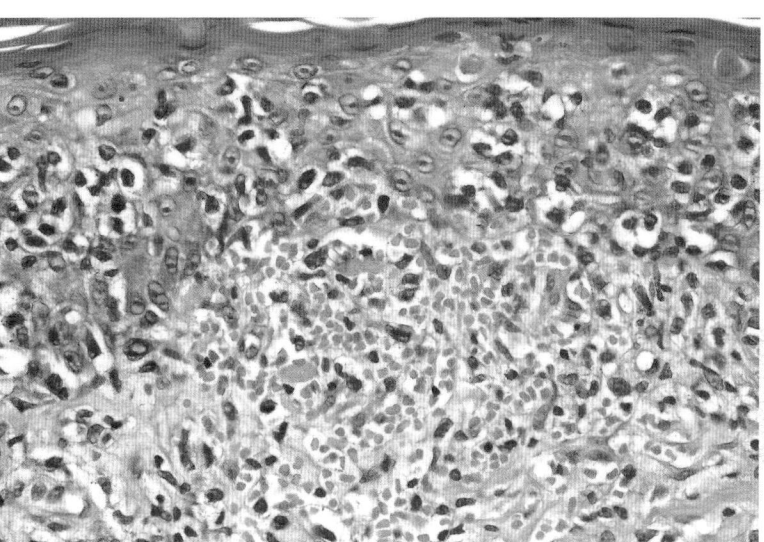

Fig. 29.57
Purpuric mycosis fungoides: high-power view showing red cell extravasation.

rare, accounting for only 0.6% of cases in a series of 722 patients with mycosis fungoides.[1] Patients present with erythematous, hyperkeratotic, scaly palmar, and/or plantar plaques that may be initially misdiagnosed as contact dermatitis, palmoplantar psoriasis, dermatophyte infection, or pompholyx.[1-8]

The literature concerning this condition is confusing. While some authors have used the term to describe a variant of MF, others have used it synonymously for pagetoid reticulosis. Although there are undoubtedly similarities, palmoplantar MF contrasts with pagetoid reticulosis by the invariable CD4+ T-helper nature of the infiltrate in contrast to pagetoid reticulosis where the immunophenotype is CD8+ or CD4–/CD8– as often as it is CD4+ and in which the infiltrate is almost entirely epidermotropic.[9,10]

Verrucous/hyperkeratotic mycosis fungoides

Very rarely, patients with MF present with large verrucous crusted lesions that may be clinically mistaken for a halogenoderma, or deep fungal or atypical mycobacterial infection.[1-5] Lesions are sometimes quite widespread. Occasionally, they are located acrally and might then be better classified as palmoplantar MF or pagetoid reticulosis.

Unilesional mycosis fungoides

Clinical features

Unilesional (solitary) MF is very rare. Patients usually develop a solitary, slowly growing patch or plaque, typically on the trunk or upper extremity.[1–9] Although most documented cases have been in adults, there are occasional instances of childhood presentation.[3,10] Folliculotropic and hypopigmented variants have been reported.[3,4] Although complete remission is generally achieved following treatment (e.g., with excision, localized electron beam therapy or topical nitrogen mustard), occasional recurrences have been noted and noncontiguous spread may occur after many years.[5,6] Systemic spread and death have not been described, reflecting the excellent prognosis of early-stage disease.

Histologic features

Histologically, unilesional MF is indistinguishable from the more usual multilesional variant. Clonal TCR gene rearrangements are present in up to 50% of cases.

'Invisible' mycosis fungoides

It has long been recognized that clinically normal skin may be affected histologically in MF.[1,2] Exceptionally, MF may present with intense pruritus and no clinically visible lesions but with evidence of histologic involvement – so-called invisible mycosis fungoides.[3]

Mycosis fungoides with unusual histologic features

A minority of cases of otherwise classic MF display unusual histologic features. These have perhaps been granted unwarranted significance in the literature through designation with specific names. Nevertheless, although not biologically distinct entities, these different histologic patterns merit recognition in order to heighten awareness of the spectrum of changes that can be seen in MF. Spongiosis is sometimes prominent, and in other cases a bandlike infiltrate closely mimicking lichen planus may be seen. In the former situation, the underlying changes are those of MF, and in the latter scenario there is often migration of lymphocytes above the basal cell layer of the epidermis, lymphocytes appear to extend into basal keratinocytes rather than stay in the junction as they do in lichen planus, and other features of MF are present.

Granulomatous mycosis fungoides

Clinical features

A granulomatous infiltrate is seen in up to 4% of cases of MF.[1–16] The clinical features are indistinguishable from those of typical MF; patients present with papules, plaques, and tumors, and may run a stepwise progression (*Fig. 29.58*).[13] Most reported cases have been described in adults, but exceptional cases occur in children.[7,17] It may rarely be seen in association with sarcoidosis or generalized granuloma annulare, and an ichthyosis-like presentation has been reported.[10,11,16,18–21] Granulomas are thought to represent an immunologically mediated reaction to the tumor, and was initially supposed to indicate a favorable prognosis.[22] However, there are examples of rapidly progressing forms of the disease, so other factors are likely to be more important in determining outcome.[8,14,18,23–26]

Granulomatous inflammation is also commonly encountered in folliculotropic MF and may be seen in up to one-quarter of cases.[26] In this situation, the granulomatous inflammation represents a reaction to ruptured hair follicles.

Histologic features

In all cases, there are underlying features of MF. The associated granulomas are usually sarcoid type, often accompanied by foreign body and Langhans giant cells (*Figs 29.59–29.61*).[13] While this may represent only a minor component of the infiltrate, in many cases it can constitute 25% or more with the

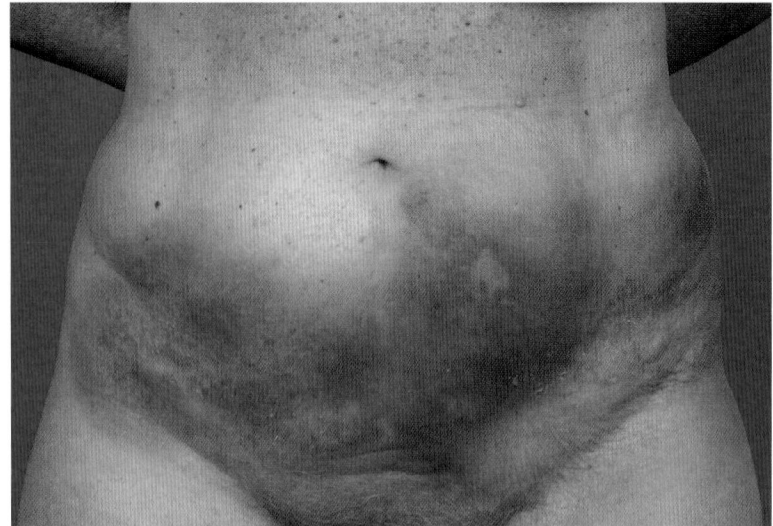

Fig. 29.58
Granulomatous mycosis fungoides: indurated coalescing plaques on lower abdomen. By courtesy of M. Duvic, MD, the MD Anderson Cancer Center, Houston, Texas, USA.

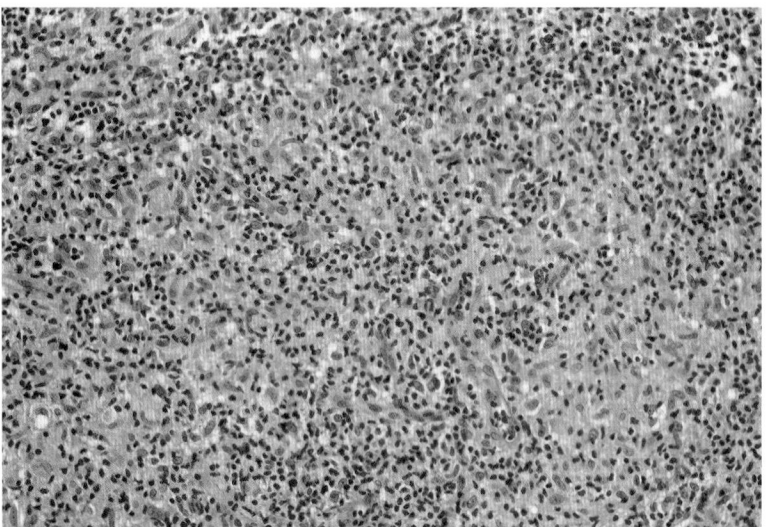

Fig. 29.59
Granulomatous mycosis fungoides: in this field there is a well-developed granulomatous inflammatory infiltrate with a background of atypical lymphocytes.

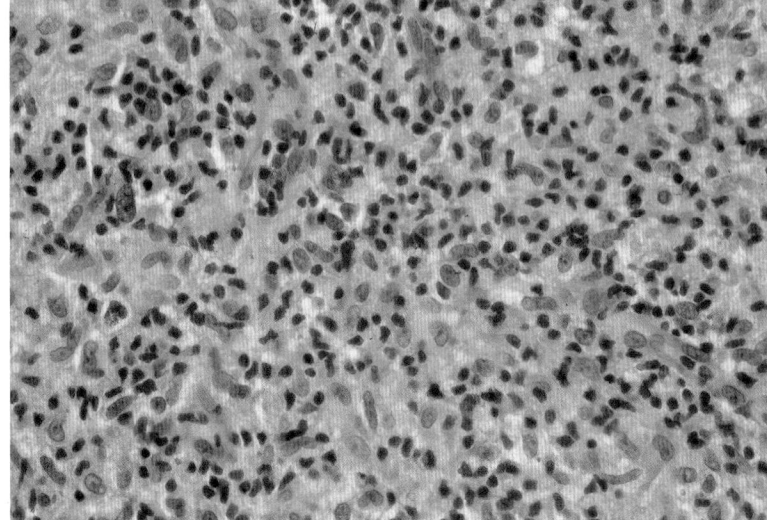

Fig. 29.60
Granulomatous mycosis fungoides: high-power view.

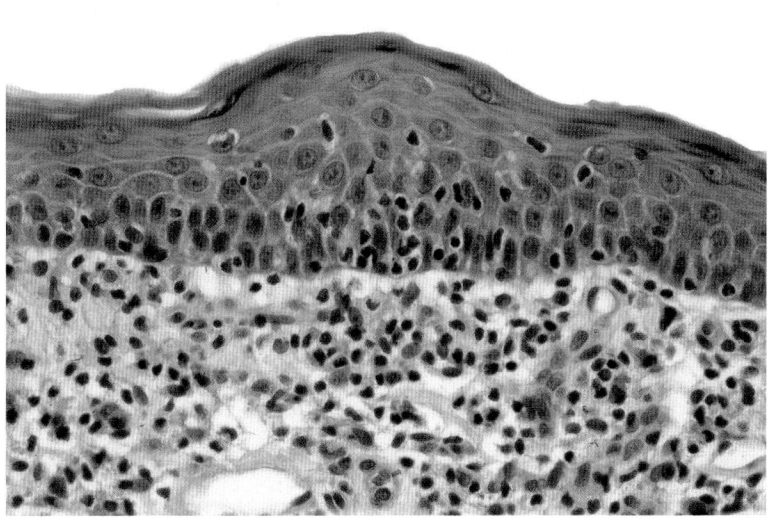

Fig. 29.61
Granulomatous mycosis fungoides: epidermotropism with lymphocyte tagging.

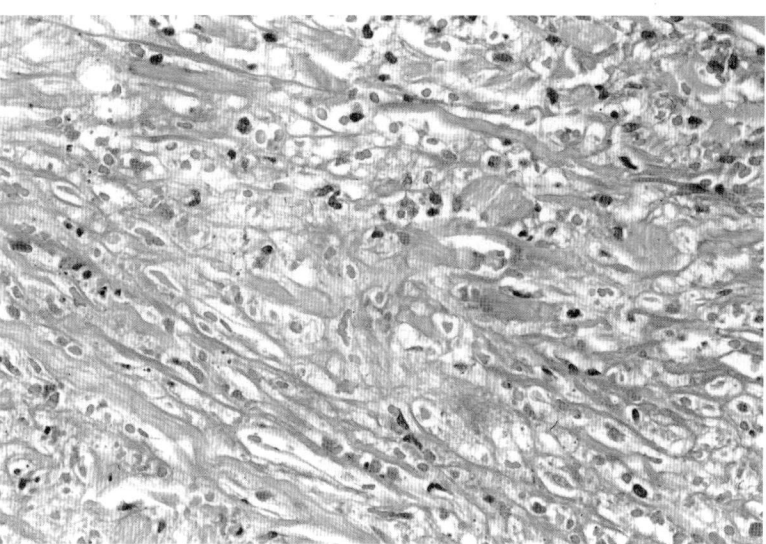

Fig. 29.63
Granulomatous mycosis fungoides: close-up view of necrobiosis.

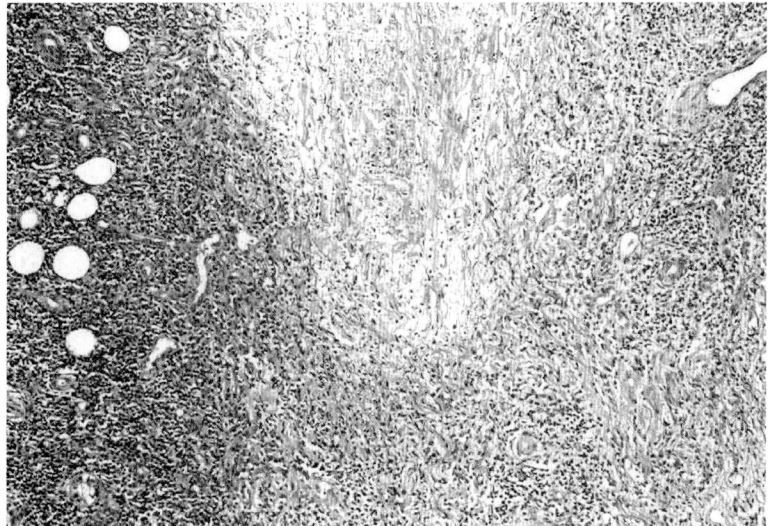

Fig. 29.62
Granulomatous mycosis fungoides: this case shows necrobiosis-like features. The collagen fibers are swollen and eosinophilic.

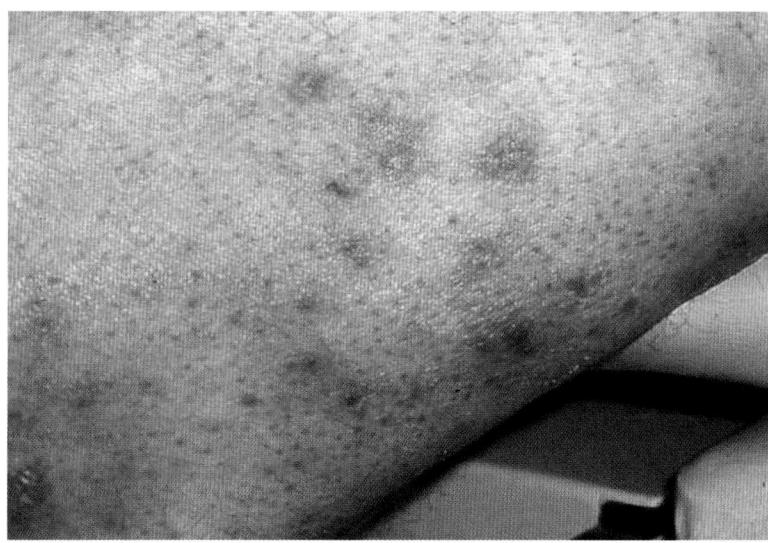

Fig. 29.64
Syringotropic mycosis fungoides: distinct papules are present on this patient's arm. By courtesy of H. Naeem, MD, Harvard Medical School, Boston, USA.

potential for misdiagnosis as an inflammatory or infective condition.[5,13,21,27] Lymphophagocytosis is sometimes present, and elastophagocytosis is common.[28] In some instances, palisading histiocytic granulomata reminiscent of granuloma annulare or necrobiosis lipoidica are noted (*Figs 29.62* and *29.63*), whilst in others the granulomata are tuberculoid.[2,3,29] Special stains for microorganisms should be performed to exclude an infection.

Differential diagnosis

Granulomatous MF can be distinguished from granulomatous slack skin in which the infiltrate is usually much denser and regularly involves the subcutis. The granulomata are generally less well formed, and there is more lymphophagocytosis in the latter. The loss of elastic tissue is typically focal in granulomatous MF, and very prominent in granulomatous slack skin. However, histologic overlap may be seen and reliable distinction relies on clinical correlation.[11,29]

Granulomatous inflammation has been described as a feature in a range of other cutaneous lymphomas, and these must also be considered in the differential diagnosis. These include subcutaneous panniculitic T-cell lymphoma, Sézary syndrome, small/medium pleomorphic T-cell lymphoproliferative disorder, primary cutaneous anaplastic (CD30+) large cell lymphoma, angioimmunoblastic T-cell lymphoma (AITL), peripheral T-cell lymphoma secondarily involving the skin, and primary cutaneous B-cell lymphoma (PCBCL).[27,30-32]

Syringotropic mycosis fungoides

Clinical features

Syringotropism in MF is a very rare occurrence, usually manifesting as small papules arising in a background of patch or plaque stage disease. Less often, it may present de novo.[1-12] It most frequently accompanies the folliculotropic variant of MF.[3,7,8,12,13]

The so-called syringolymphoid hyperplasia presenting with localized alopecia and anhidrosis is likely to represent a form of syringotropic T-cell lymphoma.[1,2] In rare cases, biopsies show subtle changes with no evidence of lymphoid atypia, and these patients should be monitored carefully with repeat biopsies for evidence of lymphoma.[8,9]

Syringotropism in MF is seen most frequently in males (12:5).[12] In general, lesions are localized, presenting as erythematous or brown patches and plaques with superimposed papules, often accompanied by localized hair loss (*Fig. 29.64*).[10,12] Ulceration and scarring are not uncommon. Hypoesthesia and anhidrosis may be seen.[1-3,5] Because of the deep-seated

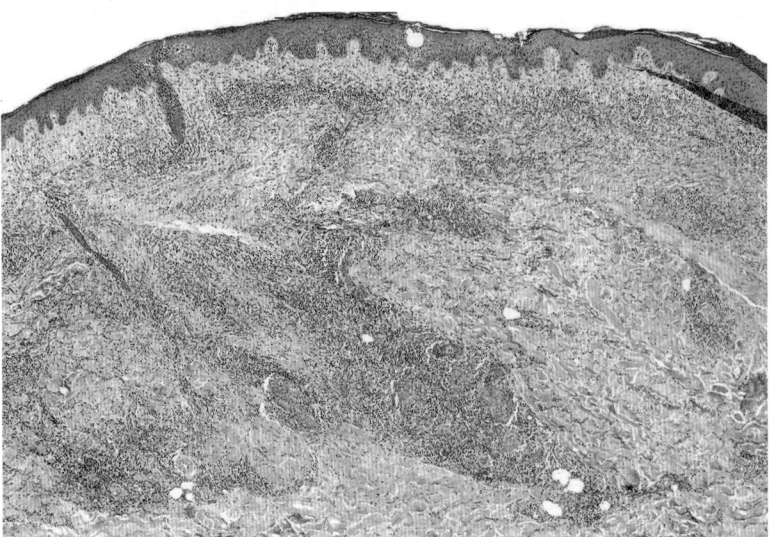

Fig. 29.65
Syringotropic mycosis fungoides: low-power view showing a distinctly nodular lymphoid infiltrate.

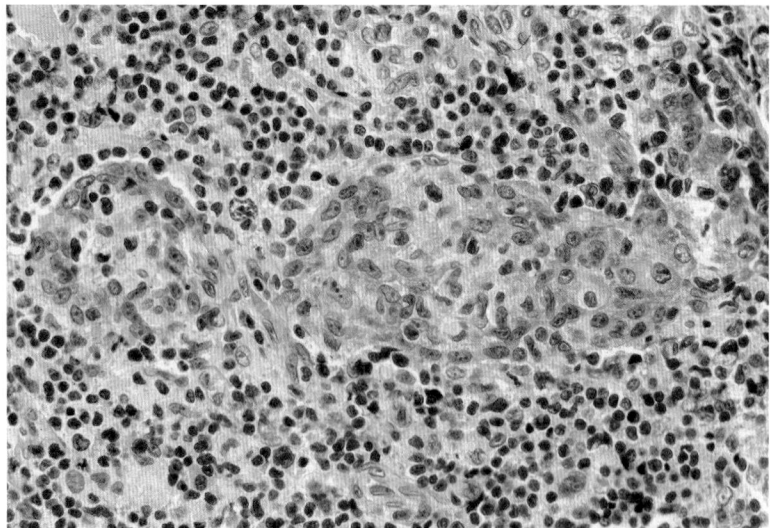

Fig. 29.67
Syringotropic mycosis fungoides: the lymphocytes have infiltrated the sweat gland epithelium.

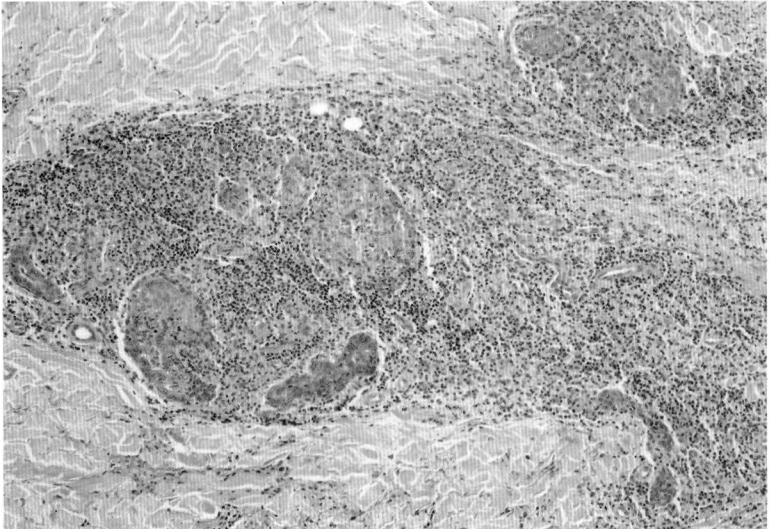

Fig. 29.66
Syringotropic mycosis fungoides: the infiltrate is centered on hyperplastic sweat glands.

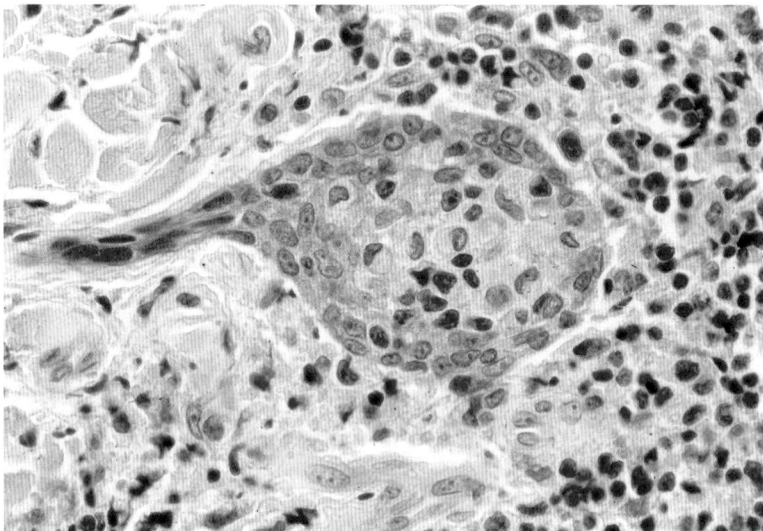

Fig. 29.68
Syringotropic mycosis fungoides: in this field, there is marked hyperplasia of the sweat gland epithelium.

nature of the infiltrate, response to skin directed therapies may be poor and localized radiotherapy required.[12]

Histologic features

Lesions are characterized by dense lymphoid infiltrates surrounding and infiltrating the sweat gland and ductal epithelium (*Figs 29.65–29.67*). In those patients in whom a diagnosis of lymphoma is apparent, there are conspicuous atypical lymphoid cells with enlarged, irregular, and hyperchromatic nuclei. The sweat gland epithelium may be hyperplastic, and frequently the lumen is obliterated (*Fig. 29.68*). Follicular mucinosis or folliculotropic MF is sometimes present and in those lesions arising in a background of typical MF, an atypical superficial dermal infiltrate with epidermotropism is seen.

The lymphocytes express CD2, CD3, CD4, and CD45RO.[4,6] Loss of CD7 has been documented.[5,10] Keratin immunohistochemistry can be of value in highlighting destroyed sweat gland epithelium. TCR gene rearrangements assists in making the diagnosis.[5,8,12]

Mycosis fungoides with dermal mucin

Very exceptionally, widespread dermal mucin deposition (unrelated to follicular mucinosis) has been described in MF.[1] In one case, mucin deposition

was accompanied by a storiform spindle cell proliferation.[2] Clinically, the latter lesions were reminiscent of scleromyxedema.[2] Whether this represents a genuine variant or coincident expression of two disorders is uncertain.

Distinct variants of mycosis fungoides

In contrast to the above, the following three entities have distinctive clinicopathological features that mark them out as biologically distinct variants of MF.[1]

Folliculotropic mycosis fungoides

Clinical features

Folliculotropic MF is a rare, biologically distinct variant of MF characterized by follicular infiltrates of cerebriform T cells, often with sparing of the epidermis. While a number of cases are associated with follicular mucinosis, this is not a prerequisite for making the diagnosis,[1–3] despite earlier reports suggesting that lymphomas with and without this feature should be regarded separately.[4–6] The disease has been described under different names including follicular MF,[5–10] pilotropic MF,[4,11] folliculotropic MF,[2] MF

Fig. 29.69
Folliculotropic mycosis fungoides: this patient shows a large abdominal scaly patch. By courtesy of H. Naeem, MD, Harvard Medical School, Boston, USA.

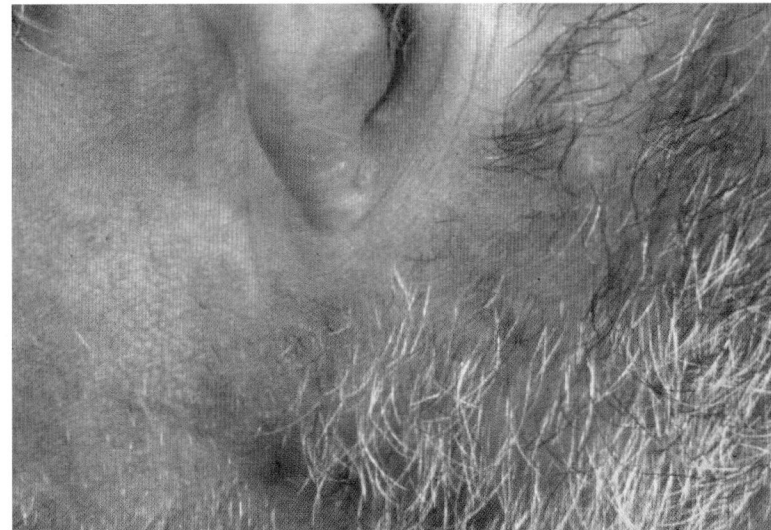

Fig. 29.71
Folliculotropic mycosis fungoides: erythematous lesions are present in the beard area and on the neck. The patient had associated mycosis fungoides. By courtesy of the Institute of Dermatology, London, UK.

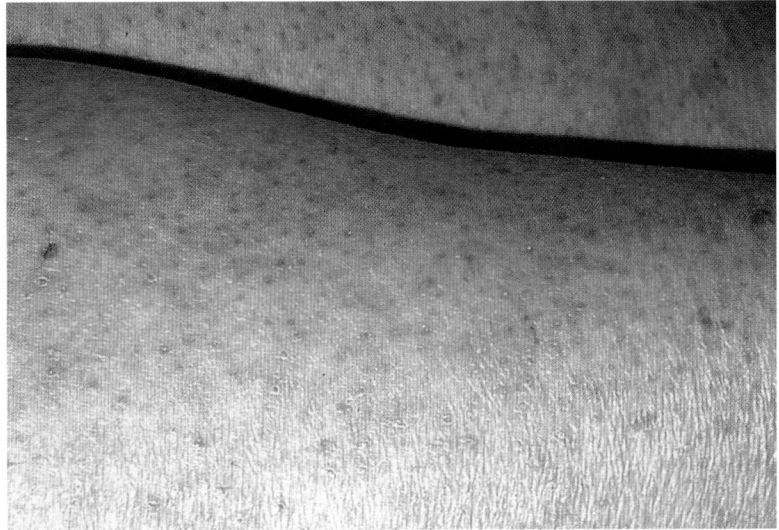

Fig. 29.70
Folliculotropic mycosis fungoides: follicular lesions are present on the legs. By courtesy of H. Naeem, MD, Harvard Medical School, Boston, USA. Reproduced from Liu V and McKee PH. Cutaneous T-cell Lymphoproliferative disorders: approach for the surgical pathologist and clarification of confused issues. Advances in Anatomic Pathology. 2002, 9:79–100, with permission from Lippincott Williams & Wilkins.

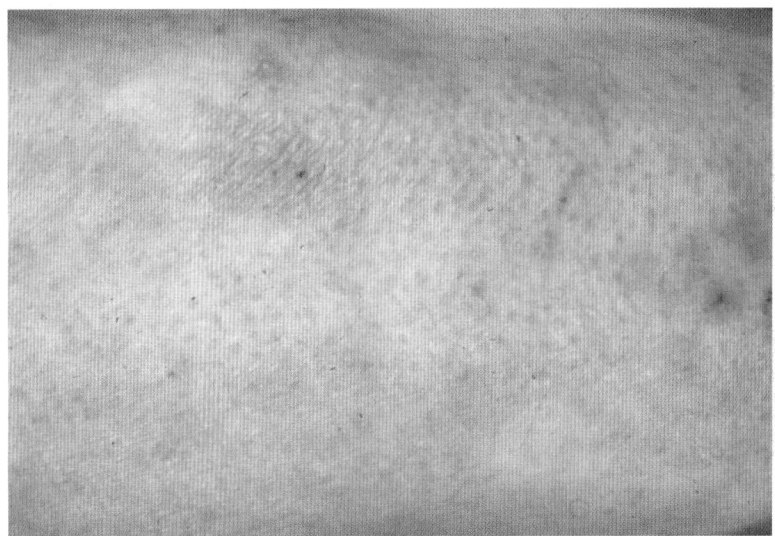

Fig. 29.72
Folliculotropic mycosis fungoides: grouped follicular papules are present. The patient had associated mycosis fungoides. By courtesy of the Institute of Dermatology, London, UK.

presenting with follicular mucinosis,[12] MF-associated follicular mucinosis,[13] and basaloid folliculolymphoid hyperplasia with alopecia.[14]

Follicular MF is more common in middle aged to elderly males.[1-3] It has predilection for the head and neck, particularly the face and scalp, although lesions are frequently seen on the trunk.[1-3] Involvement of the limbs may also be seen. Most patients present with patches, plaques, or grouped papules (Figs 29.69–29.73).[1-3] Tumor stage lesions may also be encountered.[2,3] Intense pruritus and alopecia are common. Less frequent are acneiform lesions such as comedone-like cysts, pustules, or milia.[1,3] Some patients present with spiky keratosis. In lesions associated with sweat gland involvement, hypohydrosis may also be a feature.[15] Mucinorrhea and erythroderma are rarely seen.[3]

The principal reason for distinguishing folliculotropic MF as a specific entity is because it is more difficult to treat than classic MF and has a higher incidence of disease progression with worse prognosis. Early-stage folliculotropic MF has a significantly poorer progression-free, disease-free, and overall survival than classic MF and displays outcomes more similar to those seen in tumor stage MF.[1-3,16,17] This may in part be due to the fact that folliculotropic MF is generally more refractory to treatment, with lower rates of complete remission. However, even when treated more aggressively at the outset, outcomes are poor,[1] and there may be intrinsic differences in tumor cell biology that contribute to outcome.[14,16]

Histologic features and pathogenesis

The pathogenesis of folliculotropic MF is unknown, although it has been speculated that folliculotropism is mediated through intracellular adhesion molecule 1 (ICAM-1) expression by follicular epithelium and lymphocyte function-associated antigen (LFA-1) expression by the lymphoid cells.[4] Gene expression profiling studies have also shown that folliculotropic MF cases tend to express genes associated with inflammation and pathways involved with epidermal proliferation, and to cluster with cases of typical MF of advanced stage with poor prognosis.[14]

The defining histologic feature of this variant is infiltration of hair follicle epithelium by medium to large cerebriform cells (Figs 29.74–29.81).[1,3] Collection of acid mucopolysaccharides within the involved follicles (follicular mucinosis) is present to varying degrees but is often absent.[1,3] Other histologic features include basaloid follicular hyperplasia, granulomatous inflammation, numerous eosinophils in and around hair follicles, and follicular

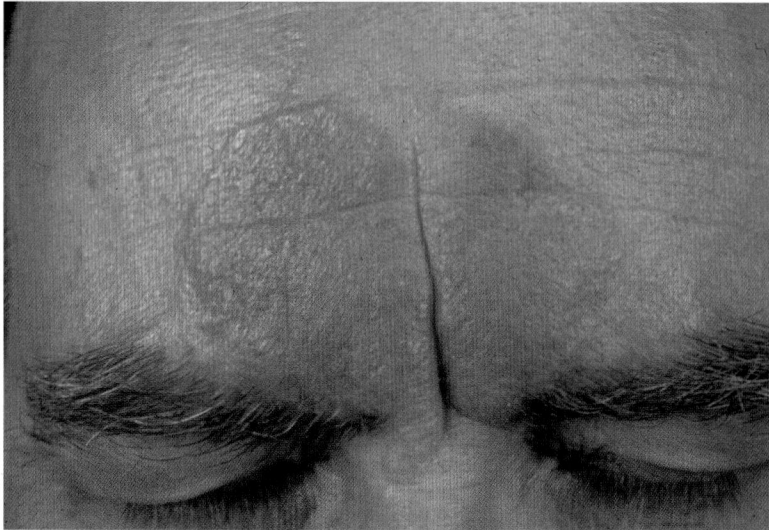

Fig. 29.73
Folliculotropic mycosis fungoides: mycosis fungoides-associated erythematous plaque. By courtesy of the Institute of Dermatology, London, UK.

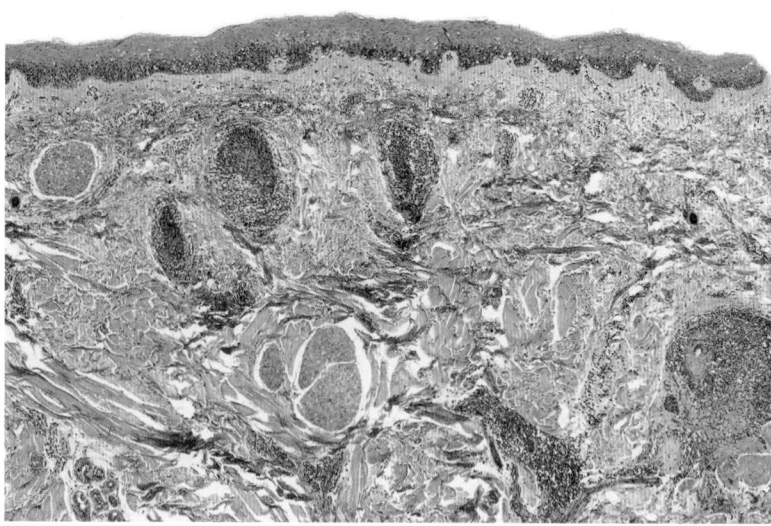

Fig. 29.76
Folliculotropic mycosis fungoides: this specimen comes from the leg. The follicles are ensheathed by an atypical lymphoid infiltrate.

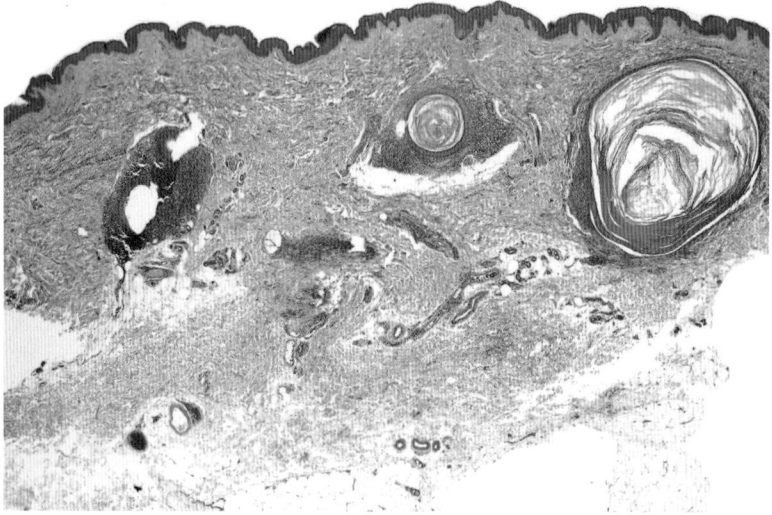

Fig. 29.74
Folliculotropic mycosis fungoides: scanning view showing a folliculocentric lymphoid infiltrate.

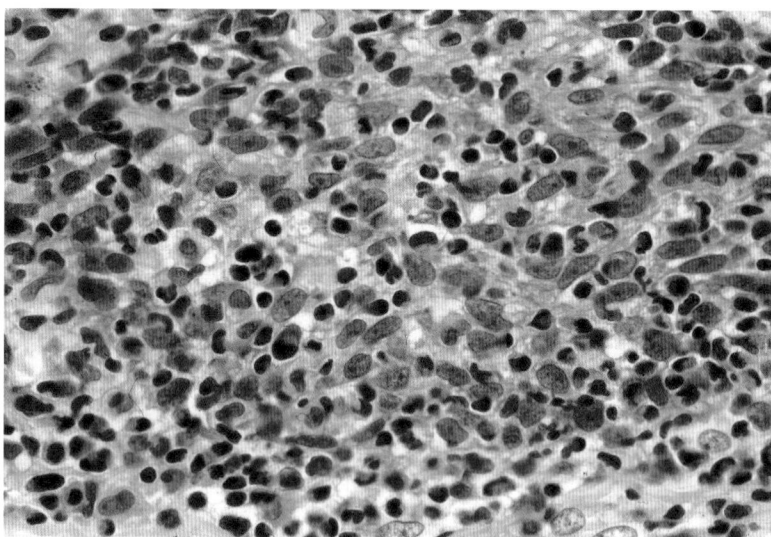

Fig. 29.77
Folliculotropic mycosis fungoides: the follicular epithelium is infiltrated by atypical lymphocytes.

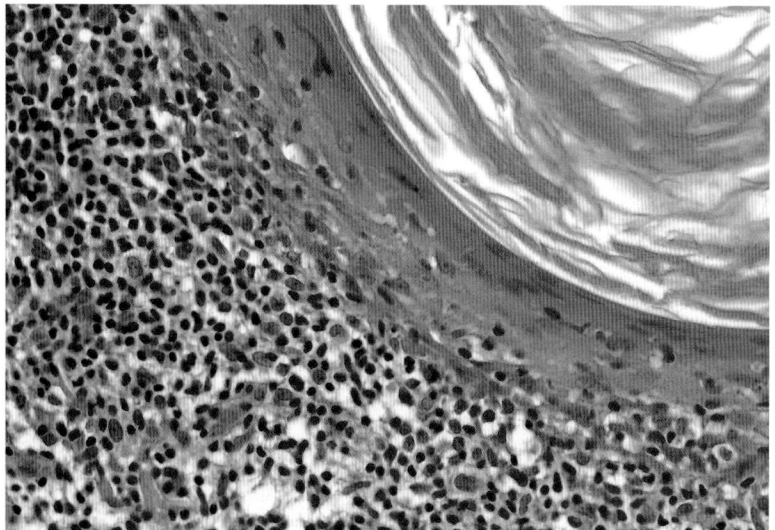

Fig. 29.75
Folliculotropic mycosis fungoides: note the atypical lymphocytes investing the follicle.

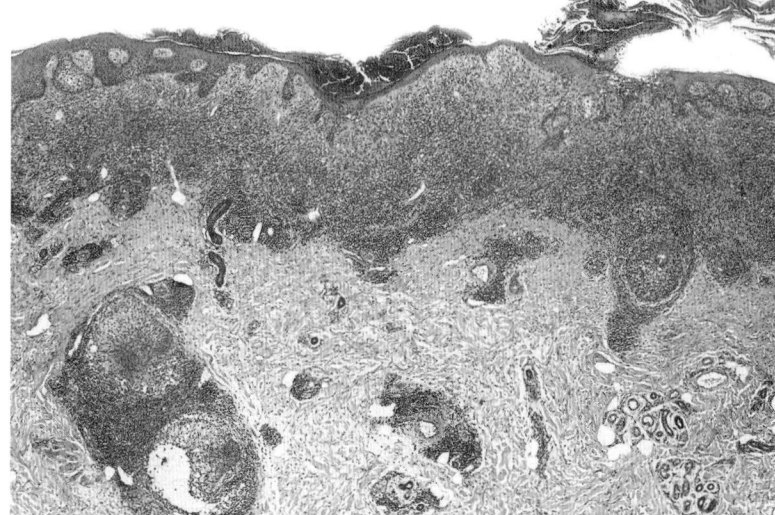

Fig. 29.78
Folliculotropic mycosis fungoides: in addition to a superficial bandlike infiltrate, there is follicular involvement.

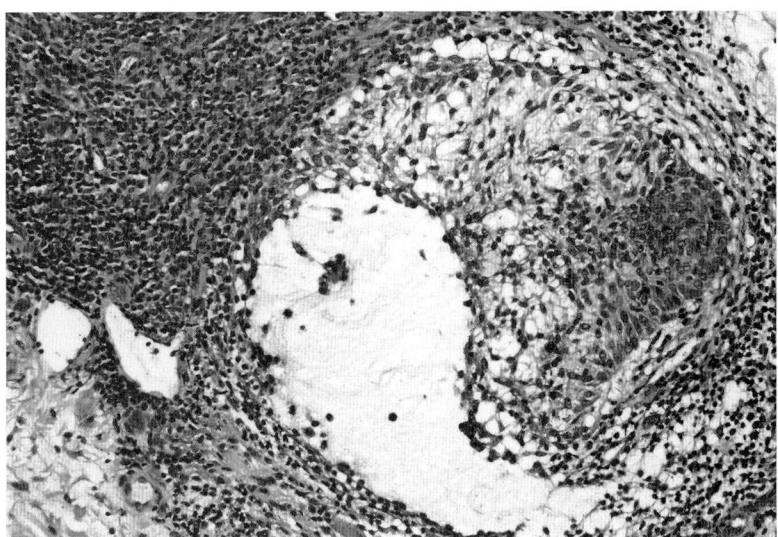

Fig. 29.79
Folliculotropic mycosis fungoides: there is striking follicular mucinosis.

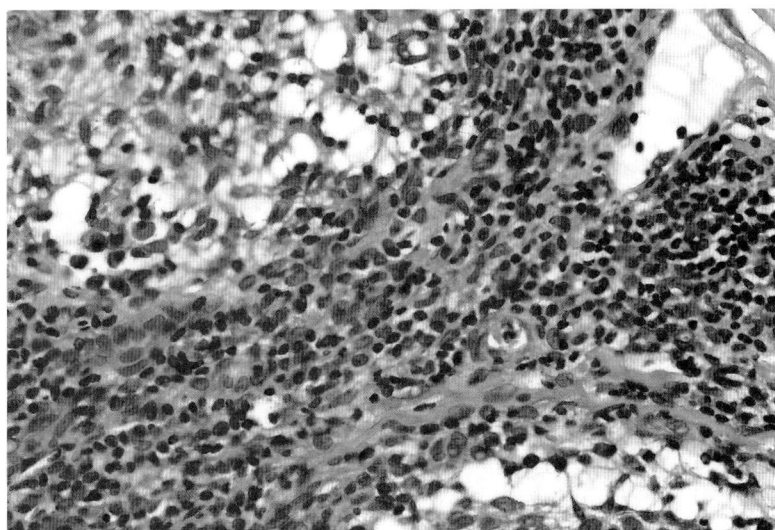

Fig. 29.80
Folliculotropic mycosis fungoides: high-power view.

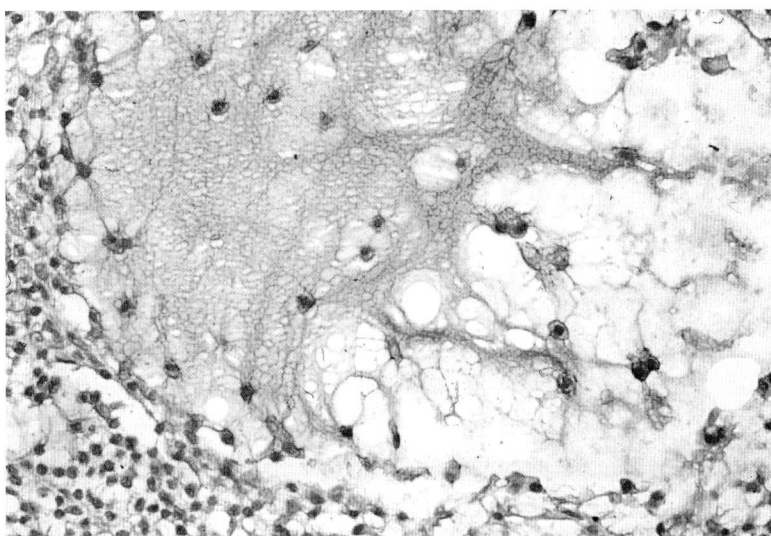

Fig. 29.81
Folliculotropic mycosis fungoides: the mucin stains positively with Alcian blue at pH 2.5.

cystic change even with formation of epidermoid cysts and comedone-like lesions.[1,16,17] Basaloid follicular hyperplasia refers to the proliferation of basaloid cells extending from follicles, or complete basaloid transformation of hair follicles with infiltrating atypical lymphocytes.[1,18] Granulomatous inflammation is usually secondary to ruptured hair follicles. Other non-specific changes may be seen including neutrophilic pustular lesions, syringotropism, prominent interface dermatitis of the follicular epithelium or epidermis, and epidermotropism involving nonfollicular epithelium.[16,17] Not infrequently, blast cells are numerous, and large cell transformation may be seen in some cases.[1,3]

The neoplastic lymphocytes in folliculotropic mycosis fungoides usually have a T-helper phenotype. Blast cells, when present, are often CD30 positive.[1,3]

Differential diagnosis

Folliculotropic MF must be distinguished from lichen planopilaris, pseudolymphomatous folliculitis, eosinophilic folliculitis, follicular lymphomatoid papulosis, and follicular mucinosis/alopecia mucinosa.[5]

In lichen planopilaris, there is a bandlike infiltrate, colloid bodies are conspicuous, and atypical folliculotropic lymphocytes are lacking. It may be difficult to distinguish folliculotropic MF from pseudolymphomatous folliculitis. In the latter, the hair follicles have an activated appearance, destruction of hair follicles is absent, and lesions tend to be solitary and resolve spontaneously.[19] Although PCR was originally said to show polyclonal patterns of gene rearrangement, examples of 'clonal pseudolymphomatous folliculitis' have been described.[20] Follicular mucinosis may be present incidentally or in conditions such as eosinophilic folliculitis of both Ofuji disease and HIV-associated cases, but atypical folliculotropic lymphocytes are not present.[21,22] Clinical features are more helpful in distinguishing follicular lymphomatoid papulosis from folliculotropic MF, in particular, the presence of crops of spontaneously regressing papules.[2]

Follicular mucinosis and alopecia mucinosa

The terms alopecia mucinosa and follicular mucinosis have often been used synonymously in the literature, creating much confusion.[1] Follicular mucinosis is a histologic reaction pattern that may be seen in a variety of conditions including Ofuji disease, HIV-associated eosinophilic folliculitis, angiolymphoid hyperplasia, *Pityrosporum* folliculitis, arthropod bite, melanocytic nevi, and lentigo maligna.[2–10] Alopecia mucinosa is the term historically given to the constellation of clinical features seen in cases of follicular mucinosis unattributable to other cutaneous or extracutaneous diseases (idiopathic alopecia mucinosa) or when follicular mucinosis occurs in association with MF or Sézary syndrome (secondary alopecia mucinosa) (*Figs 29.82–29.85*). Most of the latter probably represent examples of folliculotropic MF. Moreover, several studies have demonstrated that there are no repeatable, dependable clinical, histologic, or molecular findings that allow idiopathic alopecia mucinosa to be distinguished from follicular mucinosis associated with lymphoma.[1,11] This applies even to cases presenting as solitary lesions in young adults, running an indolent course. Over 50% of these cases show a monoclonal pattern of T-cell receptor gene rearrangement by PCR, even when no evidence of overt lymphoma is seen at presentation or during the course of follow-up.[11,12] It therefore seems likely that 'idiopathic' alopecia mucinosa is not a distinct entity, but a form of localized MF with good prognosis, and the term idiopathic alopecia mucinosa should be discontinued.[1,11] Of course, this interpretation raises questions as to the veracity of the association between folliculotropic MF and poor prognosis. It suggests that folliculotropic MF can show the same spectrum of behavior as classic MF, some cases remaining localized to the skin with the affected patients having a normal life expectancy.

Pagetoid reticulosis

Clinical features

Pagetoid reticulosis (PR) is rare and characterized by localized lesions and a prominent intraepidermal proliferation of neoplastic lymphocytes.[1]

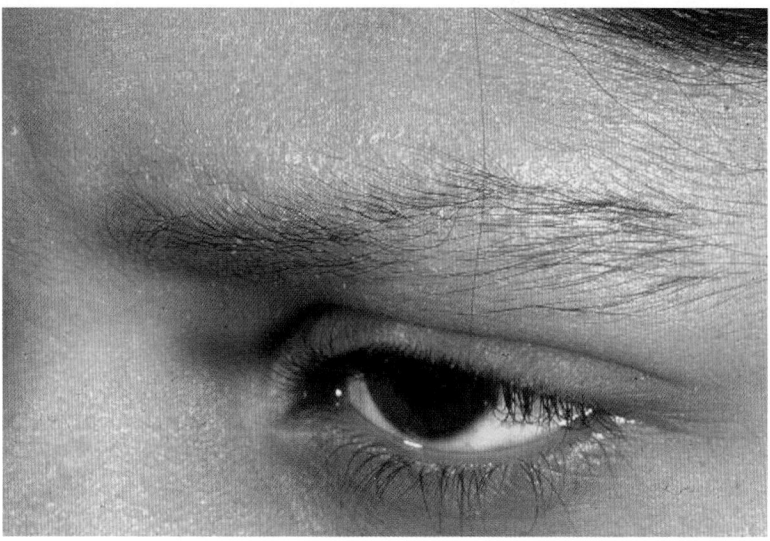

Fig. 29.82
Alopecia mucinosa: eyebrow involvement showing alopecia. By courtesy of the Institute of Dermatology, London, UK.

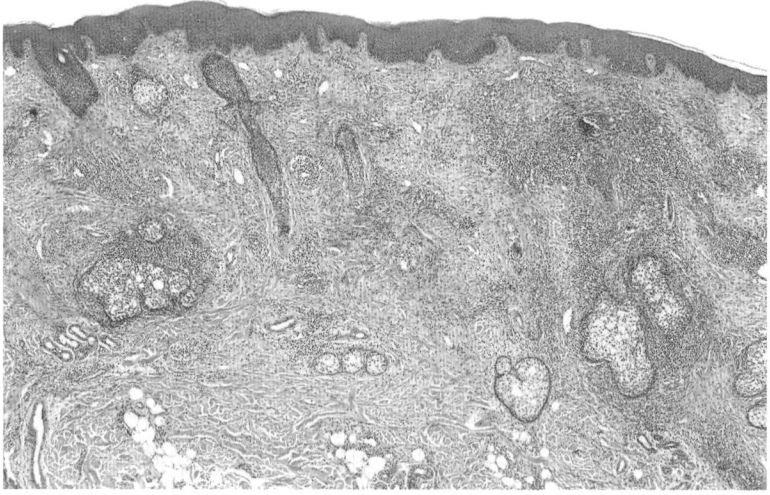

Fig. 29.83
Alopecia mucinosa: low-power view showing a striking perifollicular infiltrate. The patient did not have associated mycosis fungoides and the pathogenesis of this lesion is unknown.

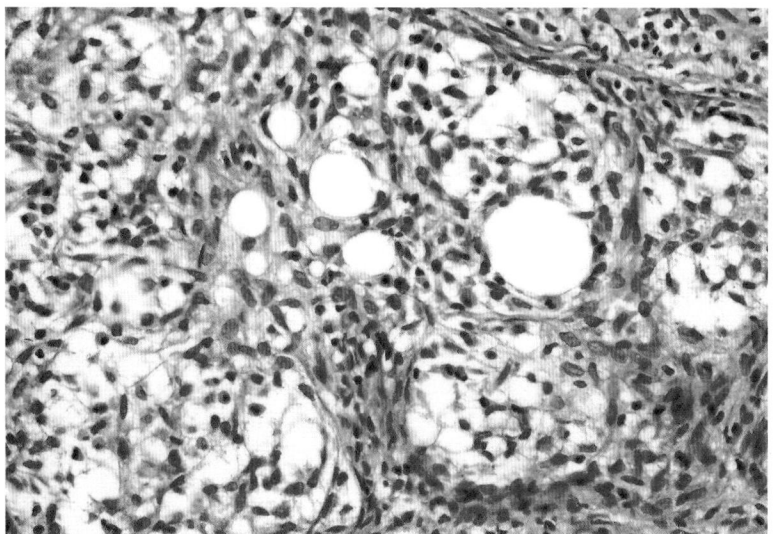

Fig. 29.84
Alopecia mucinosa: there is follicular mucinosis associated with a heavy eosinophil infiltrate.

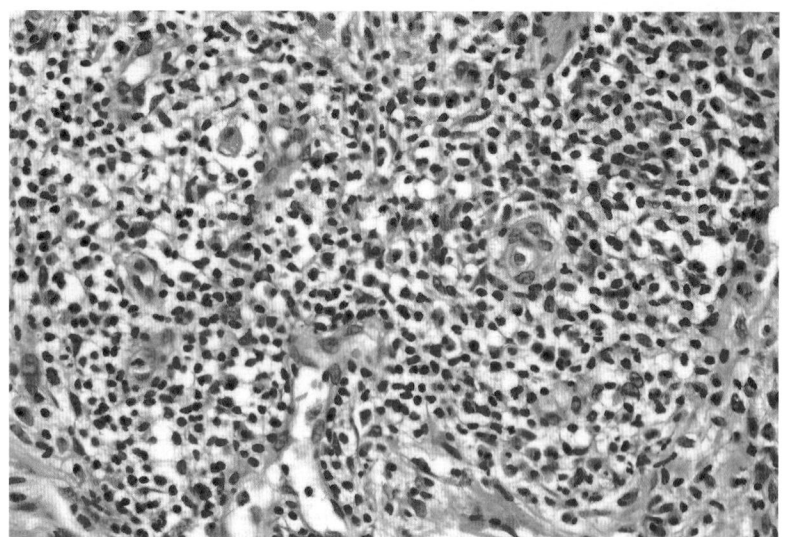

Fig. 29.85
Alopecia mucinosa: within the dermis is a dense lymphohistiocytic and eosinophil infiltrate. There are no atypical lymphocytes.

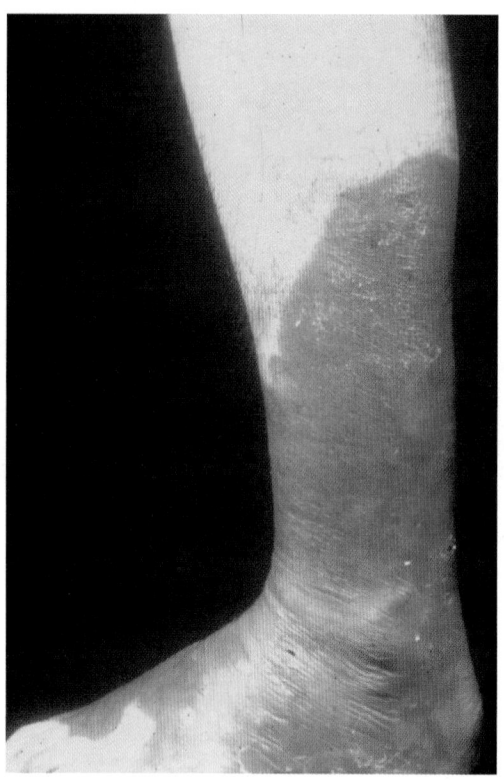

Fig. 29.86
Pagetoid reticulosis: this extensive erythematous lesion shows scaling and a sharply demarcated border. By courtesy of M.M. Black, MD, Institute of Dermatology, London, UK.

Historically, localized and disseminated forms of pagetoid reticulosis have been described under the names Woringer-Kolopp disease and Ketron-Goodman disease, respectively. However, most cases of disseminated pagetoid reticulosis are likely to represent examples of aggressive epidermotropic CD8-positive cutaneous T-cell lymphoma, cutaneous γ/δ T-cell lymphoma, or tumor stage mycosis fungoides, and the term pagetoid reticulosis should be reserved only for the localized form of the disease.[1,2]

Most cases present as a solitary, erythematous lesion which typically enlarges slowly to form a thick plaque or localized group of plaques, with evolution often taking many years. There is a marked predilection for the extremities. Plaques tend to be scaly and have sharply demarcated borders (*Fig. 29.86*). They can measure up to 30 cm in diameter.[3] Ulceration, verrucosity, and tumor formation are frequent complications. The lesions can

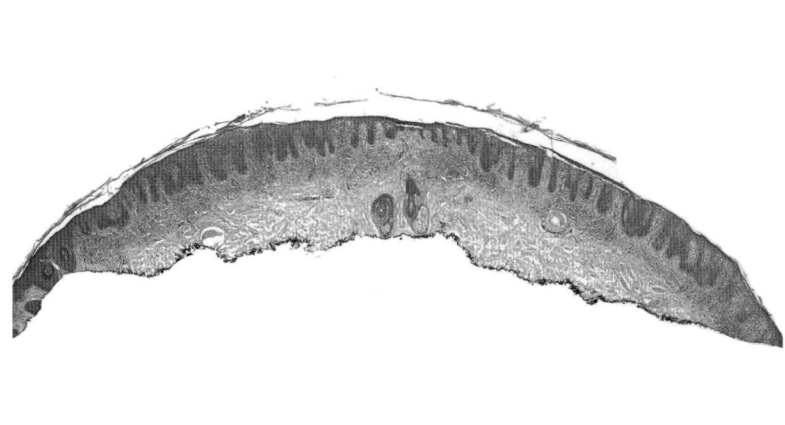

Fig. 29.87
Pagetoid reticulosis: scanning view showing characteristic psoriasiform hyperplasia.

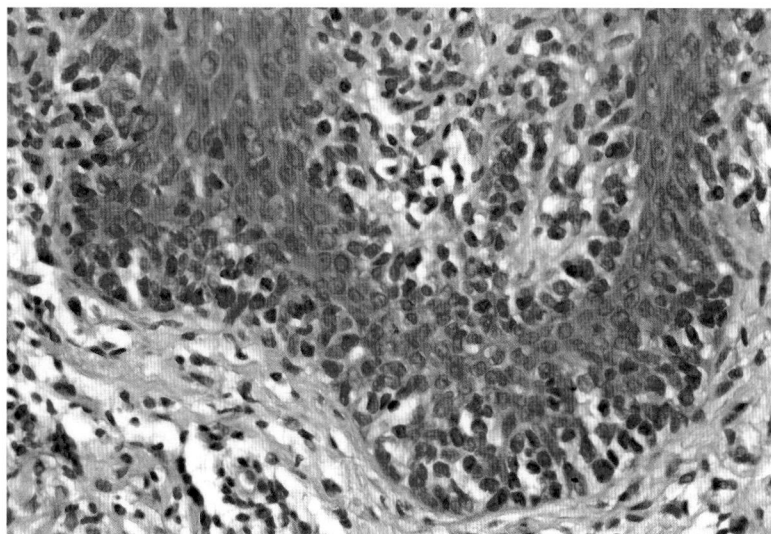

Fig. 29.89
Pagetoid reticulosis: high-power view of epidermotropism.

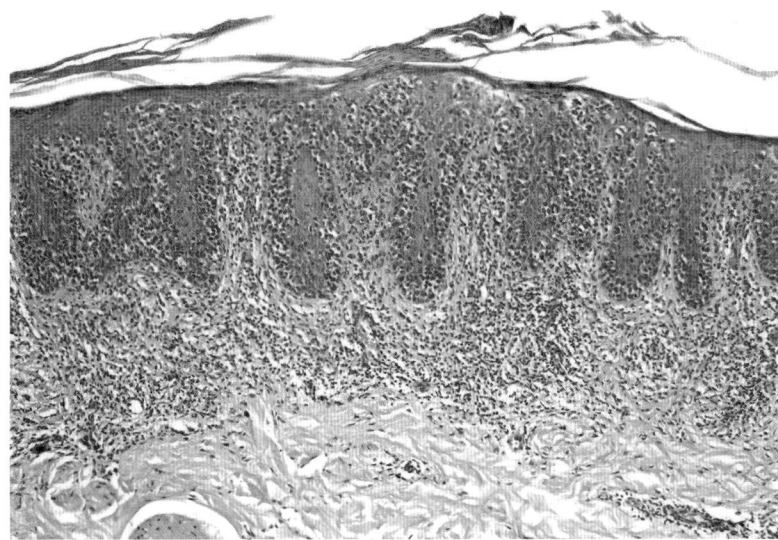

Fig. 29.88
Pagetoid reticulosis: atypical mononuclear cells are predominantly seen in the lower aspects of the elongated epidermal ridges.

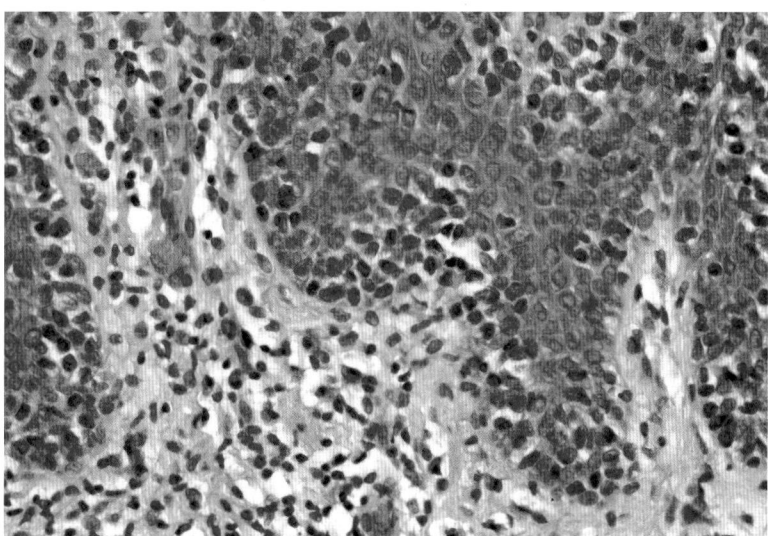

Fig. 29.90
Pagetoid reticulosis: note that the atypical lymphocytes are largely restricted to the epidermis.

easily be clinically misdiagnosed as a plaque of Bowen disease, superficial basal cell carcinoma, discoid eczema, psoriasis, or even extramammary Paget disease.[4] Regional lymph nodes may be enlarged, although histologically they show reactive changes only. The disorder usually has an indolent course and responds to excision or radiotherapy. However, recurrences either at the same or a distant site are not uncommon. Occasional cases are relatively resistant to therapy and behave in a more progressive fashion. Prolonged follow-up is therefore advisable.[3]

Pathogenesis and histologic features

Histologically, PR is characterized by an almost completely intraepidermal infiltrate of atypical mononuclear cells. Occasional reports documenting expression of CLA and $\alpha_E\beta_7$ (CD103; an adhesion molecule that binds to E-cadherin on epithelial cells) by the tumor cells suggest an important role for adhesion molecules in the extreme epidermotropism characteristic of this condition.[5,6]

The epidermis shows hyperkeratosis and/or parakeratosis in association with acanthosis, which often adopts a psoriasiform appearance. The epithelium is infiltrated (particularly in the lower reaches) by medium to large lymphocytes with large and irregular nuclei, and abundant vacuolated cytoplasm (*Figs 29.87–29.90*). A perinuclear halo is commonly present. The cells may adopt a single-cell diffuse distribution, show Pautrier microabscess-like configurations, or be present in large lacunae. Mitotic figures are sometimes conspicuous. Involvement of adnexal epithelium is often a feature. The superficial dermis contains a perivascular lymphohistiocytic infiltrate, but atypical cells are very sparse or absent.[3,7]

PR represents a proliferative lesion of CD45+ hematopoietic cells that are of T-cell derivation. They show expression of the pan-T-cell antigens CD2, CD3, and CD5, but CD7 is frequently lost or down-regulated (*Fig. 29.91*).[3,6,8,9] Both T-helper (CD4+) and T-suppressor/cytotoxic (CD8+) phenotypes have been reported.[6,8–11] Although CD4/CD8 double negative forms have also been described, such cases may represent examples of γ/δ T-cell lymphomas.[4,8,12–14] Loss of CD45RO (UCHL-1), a marker of memory T cells, has been documented by some authors.[3,8,14] High levels of expression of CD30 (>50%) and Ki-67 (50%) may be demonstrated.[3,8,9] The dermal infiltrate consists of immunophenotypically normal T cells (CD4+/CD8– and CD4–/CD8+) with an admixture of B cells and macrophages.[6] Keratinocyte HLA-DR expression has been noted.[7] Most cases tested show a monoclonal pattern of TCR gene rearrangement.[3,5,9,12]

Differential diagnosis

Pagetoid reticulosis should be distinguished from mycosis fungoides palmaris et plantaris. The latter is invariably of a CD4+ phenotype and is

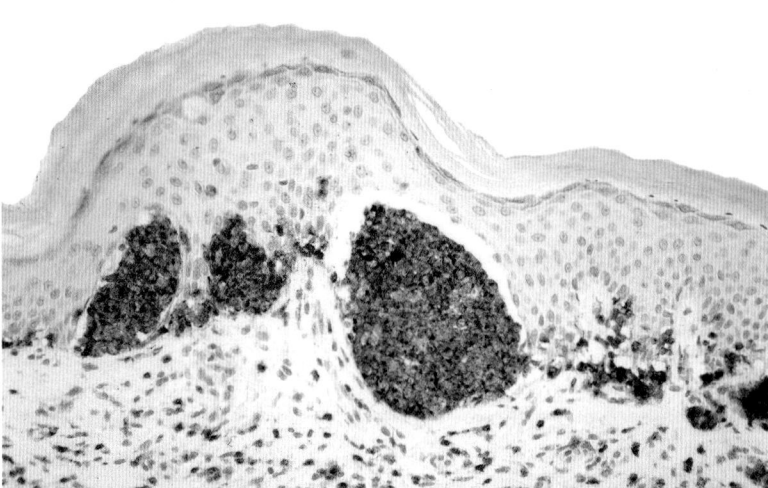

Fig. 29.91
Pagetoid reticulosis: the atypical lymphocytes can be highlighted with CD2 as shown in this example.

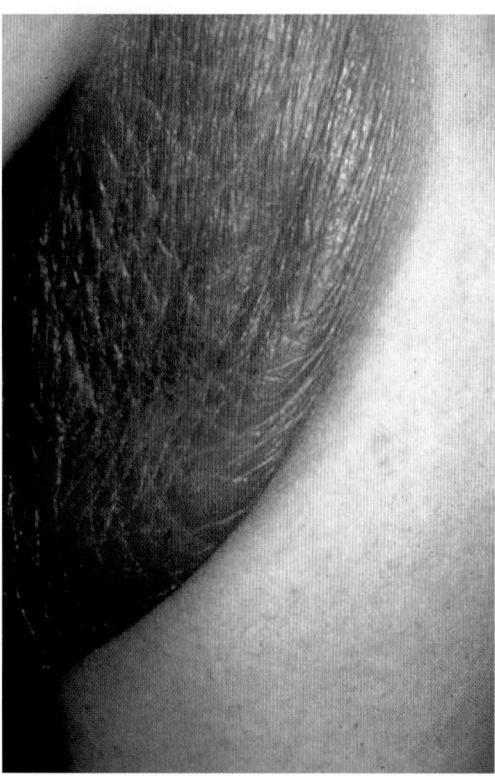

Fig. 29.92
Granulomatous slack skin: pendulous flexural folds of erythematous, indurated skin, as seen in this patient's axilla, are characteristic. By courtesy of P.E. LeBoit, MD, University of California, San Francisco, USA.

clinically characterized by thin plaques in contrast to the thickened and often verrucous lesions of PR. Histologic distinction is mainly based in the presence of prominent epidermotropism in the latter. The main differential diagnosis is with primary cutaneous CD8-positive aggressive epidermotropic cytotoxic T-cell lymphoma. The distinction is mainly clinical as in the latter the disease is aggressive with widespread cutaneous lesions and poor prognosis. Histologically, the appearances are identical, but a number of cases of pagetoid reticulosis have a CD4 phenotype. However, primary cutaneous CD8-positive aggressive epidermotropic cytotoxic T-cell lymphoma tends to display a more prominent dermal infiltrate.

Granulomatous slack skin disease

Clinical features

Unlike granulomatous mycosis fungoides, granulomatous slack skin is recognized as a distinct variant of MF in the WHO classification.[1,2] It is an exceedingly rare disease, with fewer than 50 cases documented to date.[3–33] It shows a predilection for Caucasians, with male predilection. Most patients are in the third to fifth decades of life.[19] Children are exceptionally affected.[19]

Presentation is initially as asymptomatic, erythematous, or red–purple papules and plaques. With progression, atrophy supervenes with loss of elastic tissue, and boggy pendulous folds of redundant skin reminiscent of cutis laxa develop. There is predilection for the inguinal and axillary regions (*Fig. 29.92*), although involvement may be more widespread. Lesions may develop de novo or less often present within a background of patch or plaque stage mycosis fungoides.[19] The affected areas are generally resistant to treatment and commonly recur following surgery. Progression is very slow over many years, and by itself does not appear to be life threatening. However, affected patients have high risk of developing a second lymphoma in up to 50% of cases. The latter may arise concurrently, precede, or follow the development of slack skin lesions.[15,20] In the majority of cases, patients develop Hodgkin lymphoma (HL) or other NHLs.[13,15,16,20,23] Leukemia and Langerhans cell histiocytosis (LCH) may also occur.[23–26]

Pathogenesis and histologic features

Monoclonal TCR gene rearrangements have been identified in almost all cases tested.[7–10,12,16,17,20,28,31] Trisomy 8 has been documented in two cases and a t(3;9)(q12;p24) in another.[12,17,29] The latter did not involve the JAK2 gene located on chromosome 9p.[25,29]

In its early stages, the histologic features are reminiscent of evolving mycosis fungoides with focal epidermotropism. Within the superficial dermis is a bandlike or perivascular lymphohistiocytic infiltrate accompanied by multinucleate giant cells. The lymphocytes are irregular and small- to

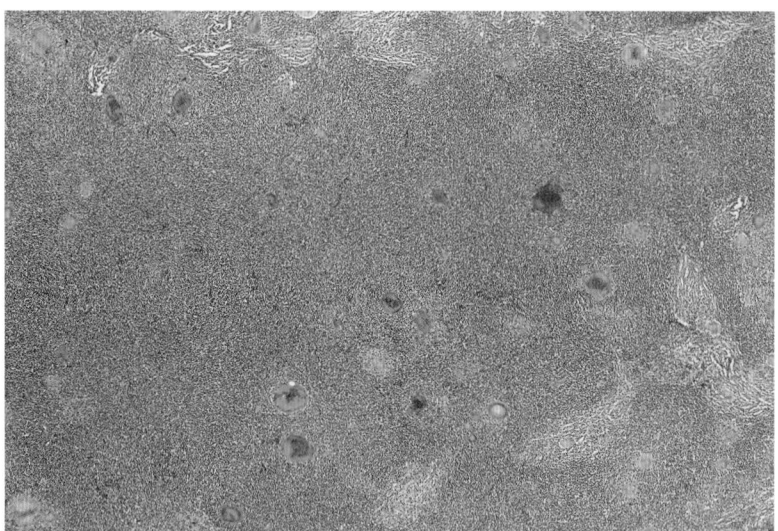

Fig. 29.93
Granulomatous slack skin: the dermis is extensively infiltrated by a dense lymphocytic infiltrate. Even at this magnification, multinucleate giant cells are conspicuous. By courtesy of P.E. LeBoit, MD, University of California, San Francisco, USA.

medium-sized with hyperchromatic nuclei. Typical mycosis fungoides/Sézary syndrome cells are sparse or absent.

In established lesions, the histologic features are both dramatic and diagnostic. There is a dense infiltrate of atypical, irregular, and convoluted lymphocytes often involving the dermis and even extending to the subcutis (*Figs 29.93–29.95*). Mycosis fungoides cells are sometimes conspicuous. Epidermotropism, folliculotropism, and Pautrier microabscesses may be seen but are not usually prominent.[12,17,18,34] Many histiocytes and individual scattered multinucleate giant cells are present in association with the dermal infiltrate and display prominent lymphophagocytosis and elastophagocytosis.

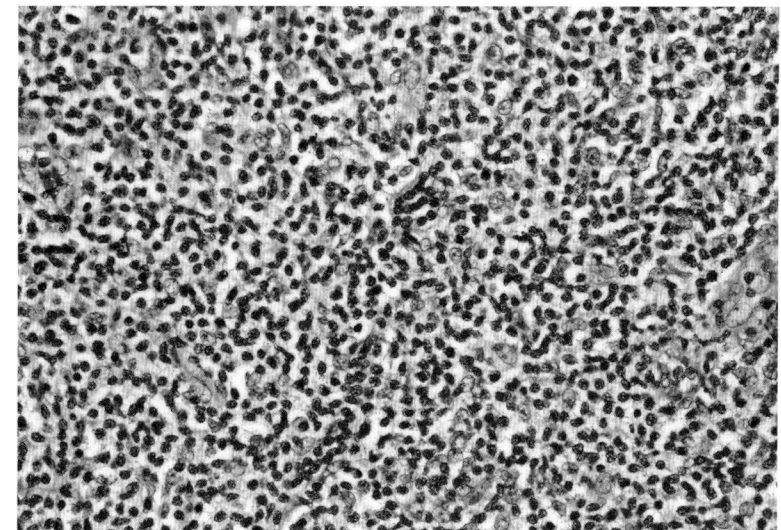

Fig. 29.94
Granulomatous slack skin: there is a background population of pleomorphic lymphocytes typical of mycosis fungoides. By courtesy of P.E. LeBoit, MD, University of California, San Francisco, USA.

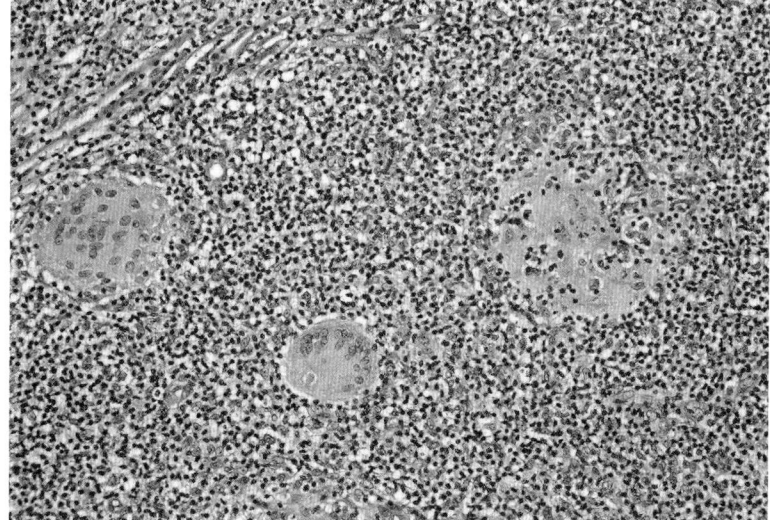

Fig. 29.95
Granulomatous slack skin: medium-power view showing lymphophagocytosis. By courtesy of P.E. LeBoit, MD, University of California, San Francisco, USA.

Discreet granulomas including noncaseating granulomata are sometimes a feature. The giant cells characteristically have numerous nuclei, and special stains show widespread loss of the dermal elastic tissue. A background population of small lymphocytes, plasma cells, and eosinophils may also be seen. Granulomatous vasculitis has been reported in one patient, and granulomas in the absence of overt lymphoma has been described in lymph nodes and spleen.[11,20] In addition, dissemination of the neoplastic clone and associated granulomatous inflammation to lymph nodes and bronchus has been reported.[11,28,30]

The lymphocytes are predominantly of the helper T-cell phenotype and express CD4 and CD45RO. They may show loss or diminished expression of CD3, CD5, and/or CD7.[17,20] Rare CD30-positive cells are identified. The giant cells express histiocytic markers. Many of the surrounding histiocytes can be labeled with CD1a, suggesting that they represent Langerhans cells or dermal dendritic cells.

Differential diagnosis

Granulomatous slack skin shows considerable histologic overlap with granulomatous mycosis fungoides, since elastophagocytosis may be a feature of both conditions. Although the distinction is best made clinically, in granulomatous mycosis fungoides elastic tissue loss is typically focal rather than

widespread, the giant cells usually contain fewer nuclei than in granulomatous slack skin, and lymphophagocytosis is distinctly uncommon. Other lymphomas that may be associated with prominent granulomatous inflammation should also be considered.[35,36]

Sézary syndrome

Clinical features

Sézary syndrome is a rare variant of cutaneous T-cell lymphoma, accounting for <5% of cases and characterized by erythroderma, blood involvement, and a poor prognosis.[1] Sézary syndrome belongs to the broader spectrum of erythrodermic cutaneous T-cell lymphomas. Also within this group are cases of erythroderma arising in patients with mycosis fungoides (erythrodermic mycosis fungoides), and cases of cutaneous T-cell lymphoma not conforming to mycosis fungoides or Sézary syndrome (erythrodermic cutaneous T-cell lymphoma, not otherwise specified). Cutaneous T-cell lymphoma with peripheral blood findings of Sézary syndrome but without erythroderma is not included, but diagnosed as 'mycosis fungoides with leukemic involvement'.

Erythroderma is defined as a disease state in which there is diffuse erythema involving >80% of the skin surface, with or without scaling.[2] It may be seen in cutaneous T-cell lymphoma as well as in a variety of other benign and malignant conditions. The latter include other lymphomas such as B-cell chronic lymphocytic leukemia, ATLL, and T-prolymphocytic leukemia.[3] Benign causes include psoriasis, atopic and contact dermatitis, drug rash, and pityriasis rubra pilaris. Idiopathic erythroderma refers to cases with no identifiable etiology.[2]

Diagnosis is usually at least in part dependent on peripheral blood findings, and the ISCL recommends adherence to a rigorous set of criteria designed to reflect the increased blood tumor burden and poor prognosis associated with Sézary syndrome.[2] These have largely been adopted in the WHO/EORTC classification of skin lymphomas[1] and include;

- an absolute Sézary cell count of 1000 cells/mm³ or more,
- a CD4/CD8 ratio of 10 or higher caused by an increase in CD3+ CD4+ cells by flow cytometry,
- aberrant expression of pan-T-cell markers (CD2, CD3, CD4, CD5) by flow cytometry; deficient CD7 expression on T cells (or expanded CD4+/CD7– cells = 40%) represents a tentative criterion of Sézary syndrome,
- increased lymphocyte counts with evidence of a T-cell clone in the blood by Southern blot or PCR technique,
- a chromosomally abnormal T-cell clone.

It should be noted that some peripheral blood findings may overlap with those of nonmalignant causes of erythroderma. For example, small numbers of Sézary cells may be seen in benign conditions and rarely even exceed the threshold of 1000/mm³.[3] The presence of very large (diameter >14 µm) Sézary cells is a more specific but less sensitive finding.[3] Some of the flow cytometric parameters are also relatively insensitive and are also occasionally seen in benign dermatoses.[3–5] It may, therefore, be prudent to look for other cytometric parameters that suggest the presence of a neoplastic clone in the peripheral blood.[6] These include the presence of expanded populations of CD4+CD27– T cells, CD4+CD26– T cells (with or without CD27), or an excess of T cells expressing a particular Vβ chain as part of their T-cell receptor.[3,7–16] Expression of CD158 in combination with other markers may also be useful in identifying the malignant population in the peripheral blood of patients with Sézary syndrome.[16–19] T-cell clones detectable by PCR or Southern blot are also rarely encountered in blood samples from patients with benign erythroderma, and can be seen as an incidental finding in the elderly.[20,21] A more clinically meaningful result is obtained when an identical clone can be demonstrated in other tissues, including lymph node or skin.[3,22,23]

Sézary syndrome shows a predilection for males (3:2) and occurs most commonly in the fifth to seventh decades.[24,25] Black populations are affected twice as often as white populations.[26] It is intensely pruritic and is characterized by infiltrative erythroderma (Fig. 29.96). In addition, patients often show edema of the skin and scaling, which may be particularly marked

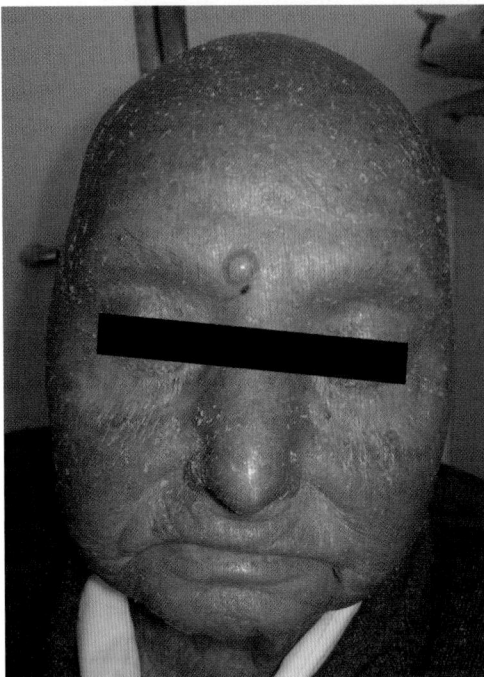

Fig. 29.96
Sézary syndrome: the facial skin is indurated and covered by a scale. Note the alopecia. By courtesy of M. Blanes, MD, Alicante, Spain.

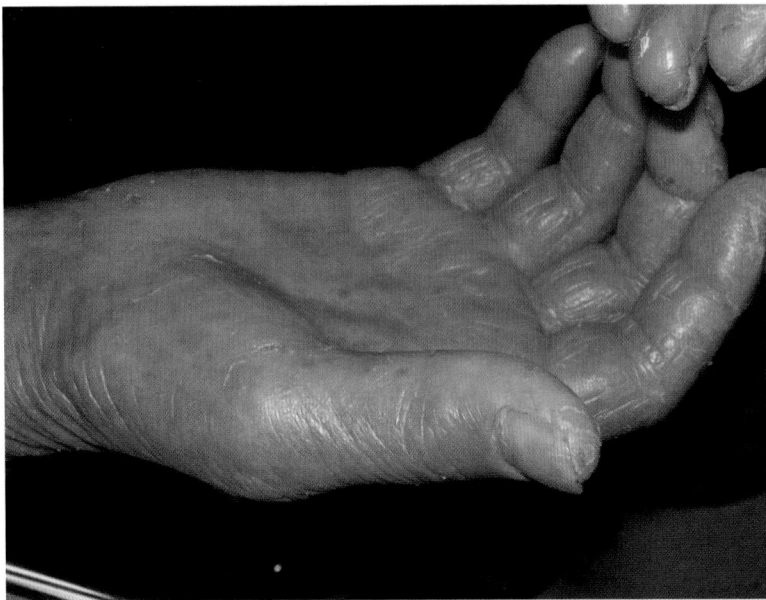

Fig. 29.97
Sézary syndrome: palmar keratoderma is often present. By courtesy of M. Blanes, MD, Alicante, Spain.

on the palms and soles (palmoplantar keratoderma) (Fig. 29.97). Hepatomegaly, alopecia, ectropion, and nail dystrophy are common manifestations, and lymphadenopathy is common.[24]

The outcome of the disease is variable but it is often associated with poor prognosis.[24,27–33] Median survival figures of 45–48 months are often quoted, and a recent study reported a 5-year survival of 51.4%.[30,32,33] Patients with visceral involvement fare particularly badly. Documented important prognostic indicators have included lymph node status, absolute Sézary cell count, fast evolution of the disease, large cell transformation and serum LDH and beta-2-microglobulin levels.[30,32,33,34] The cause of death may be the tumor itself or overwhelming secondary infection. Visceral spread is similar to that of advanced mycosis fungoides.

Erythrodermic cutaneous T-cell lymphoma should be classified as stage 4 disease.

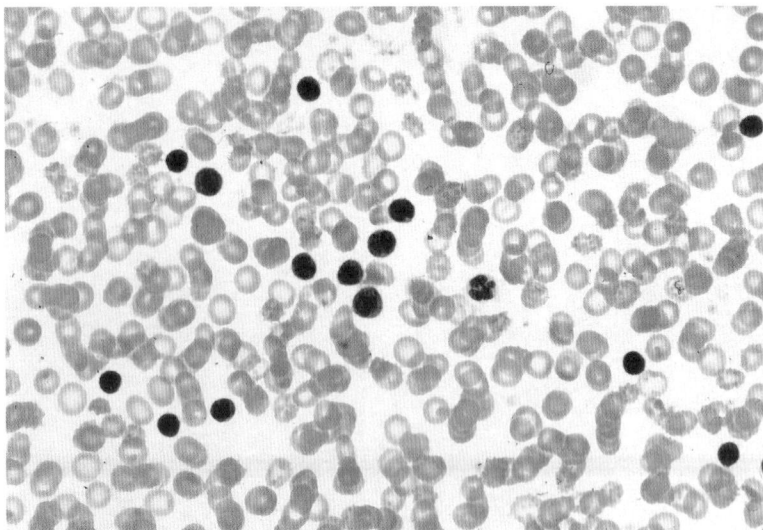

Fig. 29.98
Sézary syndrome: peripheral blood smear showing large numbers of Sézary cells. By courtesy of the Institute of Dermatology, London, UK.

Pathogenesis and histologic features

The etiology of Sézary syndrome remains unknown. No consistent viral, environmental, or occupational causative factor or hereditary mutation has been found.[35] Most cases show evidence of chromosomal instability with complex karyotypes and/or large numbers of chromosomal abnormalities.[36–39] This genetic complexity has been confirmed in more recent genomic analyzes. These studies also demonstrate consistent genomic alterations affecting genes involved in cell cycle and epigenetic regulation as well as the T-cell receptor and JAK/STAT signaling pathways.[40,41] Genomic differences between Sézary syndrome and mycosis fungoides have also been described, suggesting that these two entities may not be as closely related as previously thought.[42,43]

The term Sézary cell is synonymous with 'mycosis cell', 'Lutzner cell', and 'cerebriform lymphocyte'.[2] On electron microscopy, Sézary cells have characteristic hyperconvoluted (cerebriform) nuclei.[44–46] They may be classified into three subtypes in peripheral blood smear according to size (Fig. 29.98):[2]

- small Sézary cells (Lutzner cells): 8–11 μm,
- intermediate-sized Sézary cells: 11–14 μm,
- very large Sézary cells: >14 μm.

Very large Sézary cells tend only to be seen in association with lymphoma where they correlate with a worse prognosis, but it is important to remember that circulating Sézary cells of small and intermediate size may be found in a number of benign conditions including contact dermatitis, atopic dermatitis, erythrodermic psoriasis, erythrodermic eczema, actinic reticuloid, and pseudolymphomatous drug reactions.[2,47–49] They may even be found in the blood of healthy elderly people.[50,51]

Diagnostic biopsies contain significant numbers of atypical lymphocytes with cerebriform nuclei (Sézary cells), although they are often in the minority.[52,53] In 20–40% of cases these cells display epidermotropism, and the histologic features are similar to those seen in mycosis fungoides (Figs 29.99–29.101).[6,32,52] In the remainder of diagnostic cases, epidermotropism is absent and the lymphoid infiltrate assumes a perivascular or superficial dermal bandlike distribution.[6,32,52] Uniform small lymphocytes often predominate, but there are sufficient identifiable small, intermediate, and/or large Sézary cells to permit a diagnosis of Sézary syndrome, given the appropriate clinical setting. In a minority of nonepidermotropic cases, the dermal infiltrate consists entirely of large atypical lymphocytes and the histologic features are those of a large cell lymphoma.[6,33,52] In one series, adnexal involvement was frequently seen and included follicular mucinosis in rare cases.[33]

Biopsies of patients with Sézary syndrome are reported to show non-specific and/or nondiagnostic features in around 40% of cases. Earlier studies using less precise diagnostic criteria may have included examples of

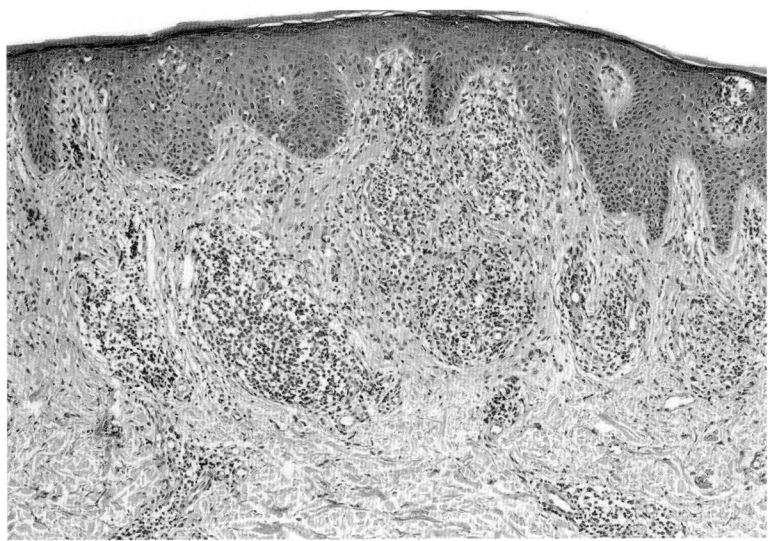

Fig. 29.99
Sézary syndrome: there is hyperkeratosis with acanthosis and a dense upper dermal lymphocytic infiltrate.

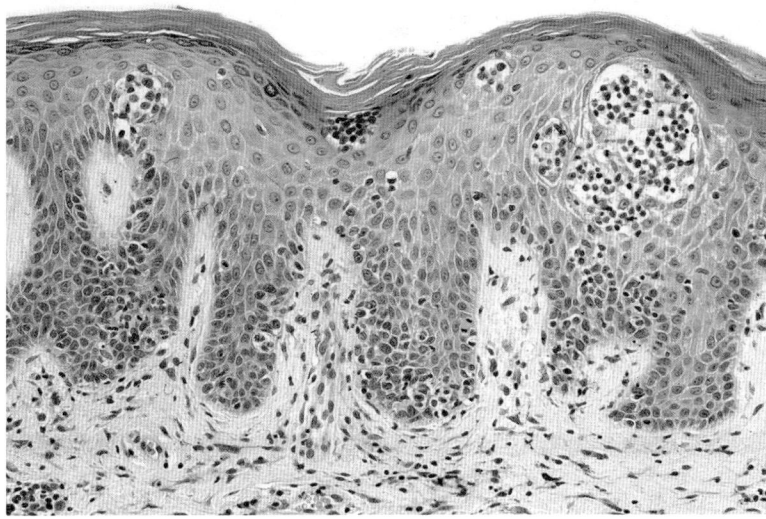

Fig. 29.101
Sézary syndrome: in this field, there are multiple Pautrier microabscesses.

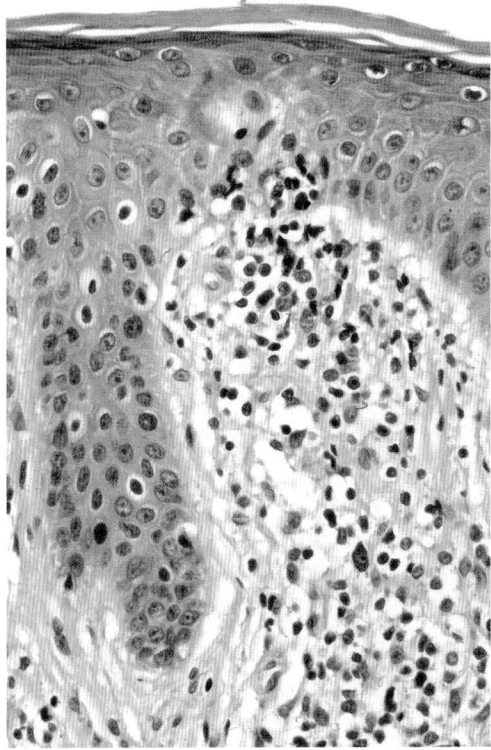

Fig. 29.100
Sézary syndrome: occasional atypical lymphocytes are present within both the epidermis and the dermis.

benign erythroderma, leading to an overestimate in the proportion of such cases. However, a significant proportion of cases lack diagnostic features even in more recent studies in which Sézary syndrome was more stringently defined.[4–6,32,52,53]

In some studies, >50% of biopsies show features that are not diagnostic of lymphoma. These include cases with a predominantly dermal infiltrate with few, if any, recognizable Sézary cells, as well as cases showing features consistent with chronic dermatitis.[19–21]

Occasional nondiscriminatory additional features in diagnostic and non-diagnostic biopsies include acanthosis, parakeratosis, spongiosis, basal layer damage, and dermal fibrosis. A mixture of inflammatory cells including histiocytes, eosinophils, neutrophils, and plasma cells is sometimes seen.[6,52,53]

The difficulty in arriving at a histologic diagnosis has in part been attributed to a loss of epidermotropism in Sézary cells. It is speculated that this is due to accumulation of Th2-polarized neoplastic lymphocytes in the skin, resulting in reduced production of IFN-γ, leading to decreased production of IFN-γ inducible protein-10 and ICAM-1 by keratinocytes.[3] Topical treatment prior to biopsy and inadequate sampling may also contribute to the frequent lack of diagnostic features. However, even when both these criteria are satisfied, the diagnosis may remain elusive.

Lymph nodes usually show features of dermatopathic lymphadenopathy but may show partial or complete effacement of the architecture by lymphoma. In contrast to mycosis fungoides, large transformed cells are not usually conspicuous.[54,55]

By immunohistochemistry, Sézary cells are typically CD2+, CD3+, CD4+, CD5+, CD8–, TCRαβ+, CLA+, and CD45RO+ T cells.[2,33,52] CD7 is commonly diminished or absent, and CD2, CD3, and CD5 are sometimes lost.[2,32] CD4–/CD8+ variants have been described, and occasionally a CD4+/CD8+ phenotype is encountered. PD1 is often positive. CD158 can be demonstrated on neoplastic cells if frozen tissue is available.[56]

Monoclonality may be demonstrated in skin biopsies of patients with Sézary syndrome. Such finding is best regarded as significant, particularly when an identical clone is demonstrated in peripheral blood.[3,22,23]

Primary cutaneous CD30-positive T-cell lymphoproliferative disorders

Primary cutaneous CD30-positive T-cell lymphoproliferative disorders are collectively the second most common group of cutaneous T-cell lymphomas, accounting for approximately 30% of cases.[1,2] This category comprises a spectrum of disease with overlapping histologic and immunophenotypic characteristics, and encompasses lymphomatoid papulosis at one end and primary cutaneous anaplastic lymphoma at the other.[3] Clinical appearances and disease course are critical for determining the diagnosis. 'Borderline' is the term applied to cases in which the distinction between lymphomatoid papulosis and primary cutaneous anaplastic large cell lymphoma cannot be readily made, usually because of a discrepancy between the clinical and pathological features.[2,3] Cases of CD30-positive transformed mycosis fungoides are excluded, as are other systemic CD30-positive large T- and B-cell lymphomas involving the skin.

Lymphomatoid papulosis

Clinical features

First described in 1968, lymphomatoid papulosis is a chronic, self-healing eruption.[1] It is now classified as an indolent lymphoproliferative disorder in the WHO classification.

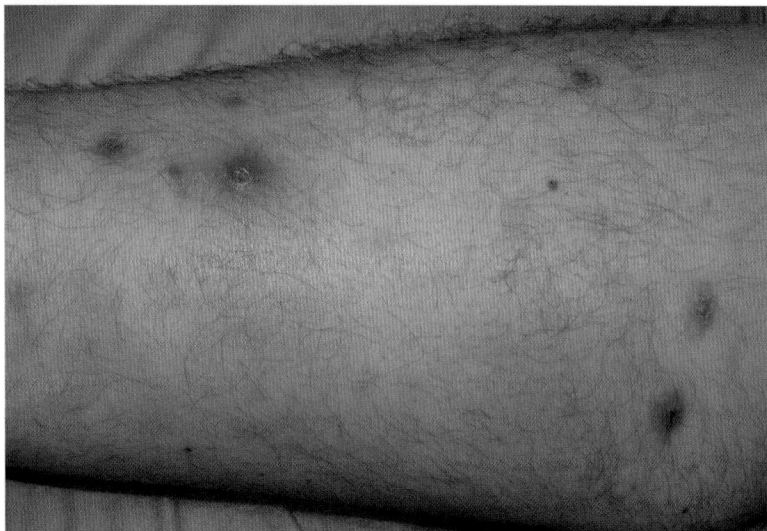

Fig. 29.102
Lymphomatoid papulosis: multiple variably sized papules on a limb. Courtesy of Dr Teresa Estrach Panella, Barcelona, Spain.

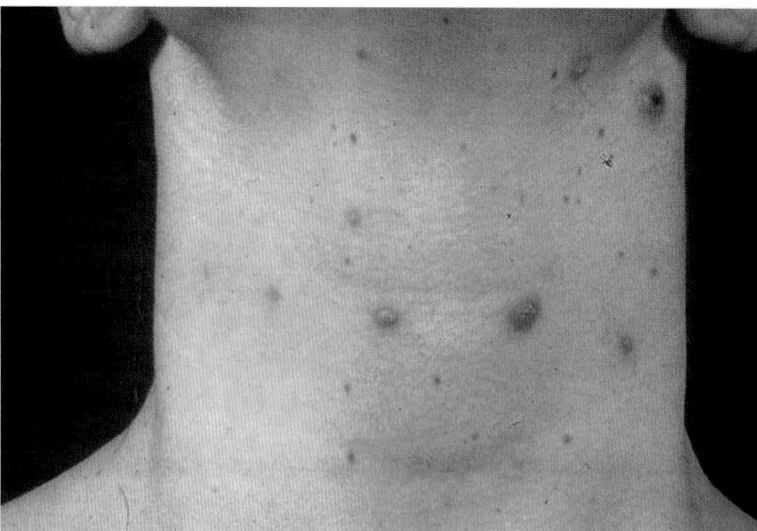

Fig. 29.104
Lymphomatoid papulosis: in this example, lesions are present on the neck. By courtesy of the Institute of Dermatology, London, UK.

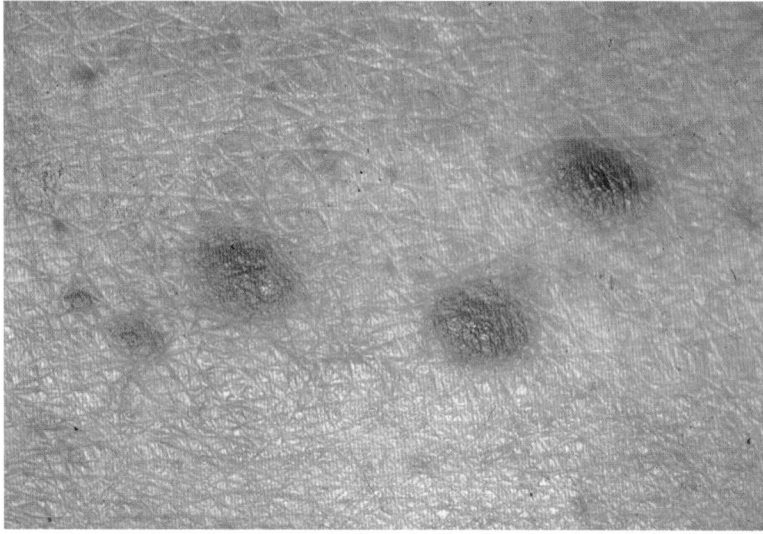

Fig. 29.103
Lymphomatoid papulosis: close-up view of erythematous papules. By courtesy of R.A. Johnson, MD, Massachusetts General Hospital, Harvard Medical School, Boston, USA.

Lymphomatoid papulosis occurs more frequently in males (2 : 1). Patients are usually in their fifth decade, although a wide age range, including children, may be affected.[2–8] The typical presentation is crops of erythematous papules, 0.5–1.0 cm across, which develop over the course of 3–4 weeks, become hemorrhagic and necrotic, and then heal, forming atrophic scars (*Figs 29.102–29.104*). The clinical features often overlap with those of pityriasis lichenoides acuta. Other lesions may be larger and nodular, and heal with deep varioliform scars. The condition commonly presents on the trunk and limbs, but occasionally other sites are involved. Numbers of lesions are variable, ranging from several to hundreds and take from a few weeks to several months to regress.[9]

Rare clinical variants have been described. In regional lymphomatoid papulosis, lesions are limited to one body region for years, and seem to be more common in children.[10–13] Mucosal involvement is exceptional.[14–17] Oral lesions present as recurring and spontaneously regressing painful ulcers, nodules, or erythematous indurated plaques.[15,17] Follicular and pustular variants have been described, as has a hydroa vacciniforme (HV)-like

presentation in Japan.[18–21] Pediatric and adolescent disease constitutes 6–10% of cases.[3,4] The clinical presentation may be alarming, with the rapid development of large ulcerating lesions in addition to the usual papular eruption. However, the disease is otherwise typical.[4,22–24]

Lymphomatoid papulosis may run a short self-limiting course, or a more protracted course of 5–10 years or longer. Whatever the scenario, the outcome is generally benign, with treatment only being required when lesions are particularly numerous and/or cosmetically disturbing.[4] However, between 9% and 19% of cases are associated with another lymphoma, such as mycosis fungoides, primary cutaneous anaplastic large cell lymphoma, or HL.[3,25–29] The lymphoma may precede, arise concurrently with, or succeed lymphomatoid papulosis. The occurrence of lymphomatoid papulosis lesions restricted to the site of mycosis fungoides lesions has been described as persistent agmination of lymphomatoid papulosis.[30,31]

Pathogenesis and histologic features

The pathogenesis remains undetermined. Most cases appear to represent clonal proliferations of T lymphocytes, more likely a T-regulatory cell subset.[3,28,32–35] Some studies have shown a high rate of apoptosis probably contributing to regression.[36,37] This may be mediated by death-receptor pathway signaling via cell surface Fas (CD95) signaling and/or due to increased levels of the proapoptotic protein bax.[3,38–41] An autocrine or paracrine growth control mechanism has been proposed, mediated by TGF-β secretion and signaling. Mutations of TGF-β signaling receptor genes results in disease progression.[34,42,43] More recently, a distinctive subset of lymphomatoid papulosis cases characterized by predominantly localized lesions presenting in elderly patients and associated with chromosomal rearrangements involving 6p25.3 has been described.[44]

In cases of lymphomatoid papulosis associated with another lymphoma, a common clonal identity can often be demonstrated, suggesting a common stem cell giving rise to both.[34,45–50] This theory, supported by cytogenetic findings, holds that different tumor cell phenotypes with distinct histopathologies and behaviors arise from accumulated genetic alterations in subclones of a common, occult stem cell.[34,45–50]

Patients with lymphomatoid papulosis exhibit a variety of pathologies. An awareness of this spectrum is important as many of the patterns encountered can be mistaken for more aggressive lymphomas. The different types described overlap and may be seen in different biopsies from the same patient. Traditionally, the different patterns of lymphomatoid papulosis have been designated subtypes with a letter of the alphabet appended for identification. This is a rather arbitrary subdivision but is adhered to herein to highlight the range of specific features that may be encountered.[51]

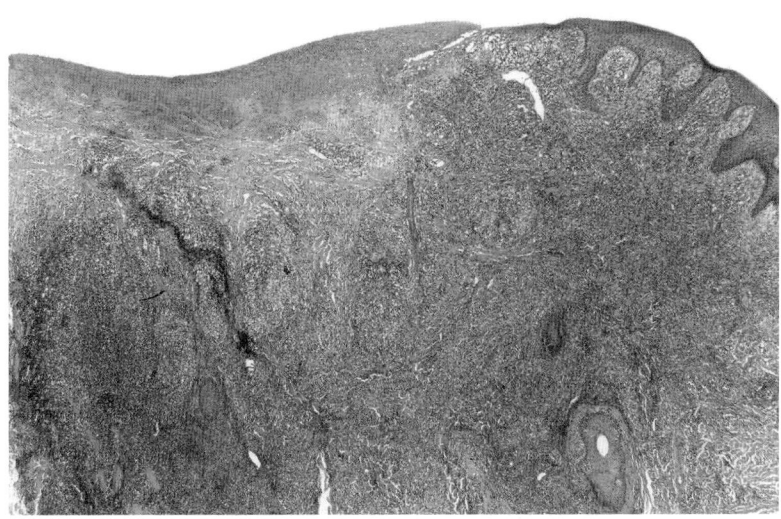

Fig. 29.105
Lymphomatoid papulosis: low-power view showing ulceration and a dense dermal infiltrate.

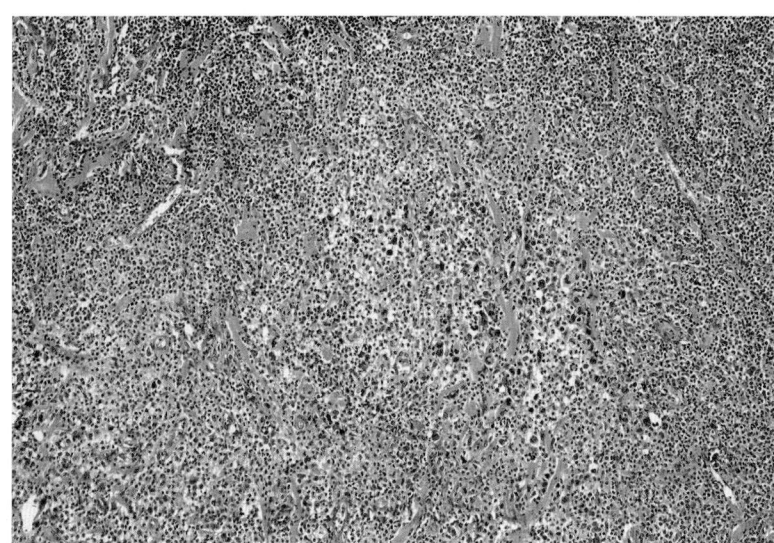

Fig. 29.107
Lymphomatoid papulosis: dense dermal infiltrate. Even at this magnification, the cytological atypia is obvious.

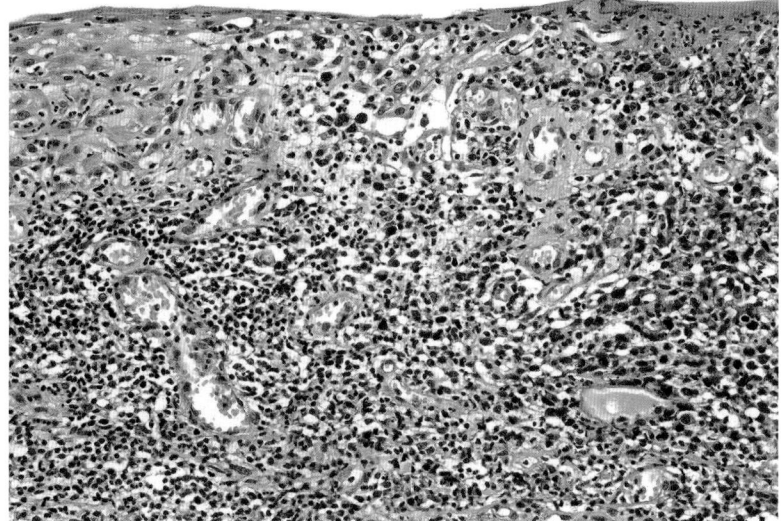

Fig. 29.106
Lymphomatoid papulosis: the epidermis is infiltrated by atypical pleomorphic lymphocytes.

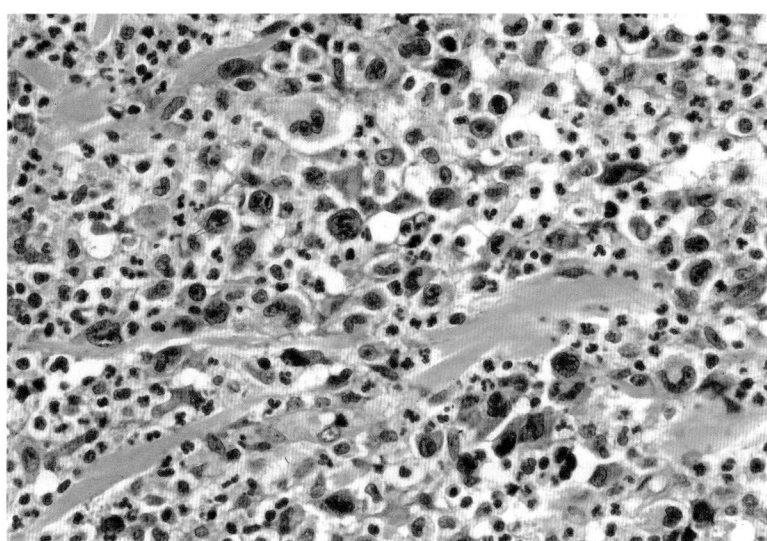

Fig. 29.108
Lymphomatoid papulosis: the lymphocytes have highly irregular hyperchromatic or vesicular nuclei. Note the background population of neutrophils.

- Type A pattern (75–80% of cases) consists of a mixed, wedge-shaped dermal and rarely focally subcutaneous infiltrate containing large anaplastic cells (15–30 μm in diameter) with pleomorphic vesicular nuclei containing prominent nucleoli and abundant cytoplasm (*Figs 29.105–29.109*). These may be multinucleate and can resemble Reed-Sternberg cells. Mitotic figures are frequent (*Fig. 29.110*). In established lesions, these cells are scattered or arranged in small clusters, and admixed with neutrophils, eosinophils, plasma cells, lymphocytes, and histiocytes. Epidermotropism of large atypical cells is rare.[3]
- Type B pattern (5–10% of cases) has a preponderance of small to medium-sized lymphocytes with pleomorphic irregular and enlarged nuclei (*Figs 29.111* and *29.112*). The infiltrate displays a bandlike distribution in the upper dermis. Epidermotropism is prominent, and it simulates plaque stage mycosis fungoides, although Pautrier microabscesses, halos, and basal lymphocytic palisades are usually absent.[9]
- In type C pattern (7–10% of cases), the infiltrate is nodular with large clusters or cohesive sheets of type A cells with relatively few inflammatory cells. The features may be identical to those seen in

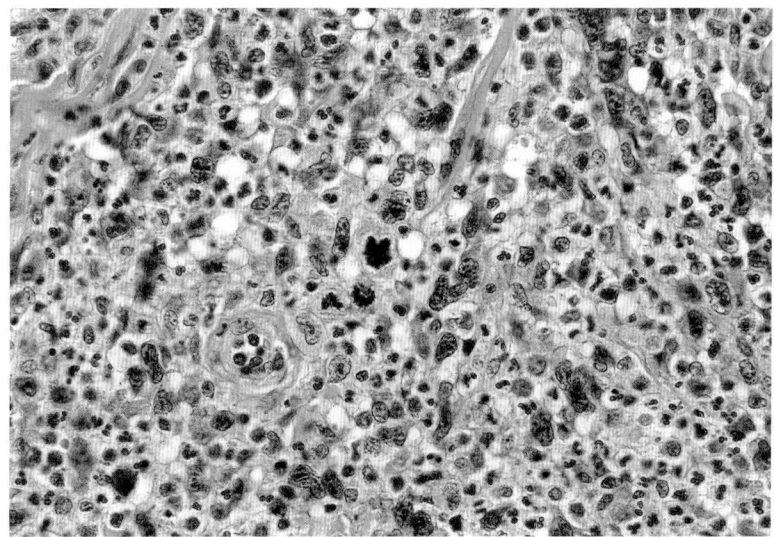

Fig. 29.109
Lymphomatoid papulosis: multiple mitotic figures are present.

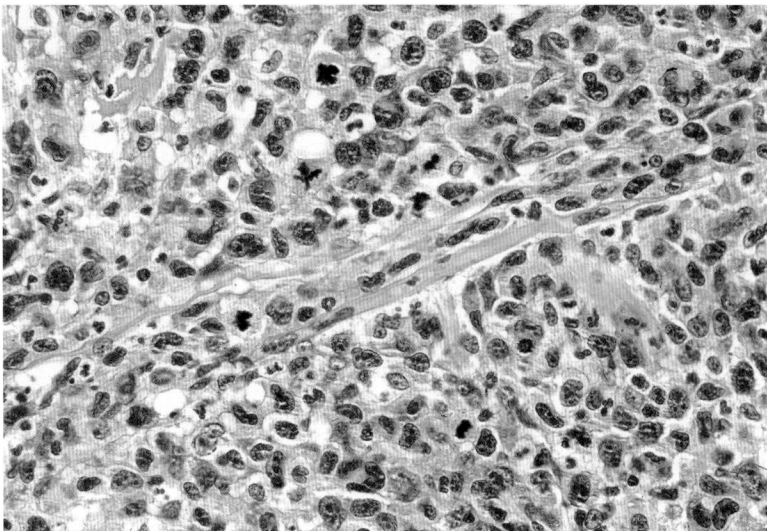

Fig. 29.110
Lymphomatoid papulosis: an atypical mitosis is seen just above the center of the field.

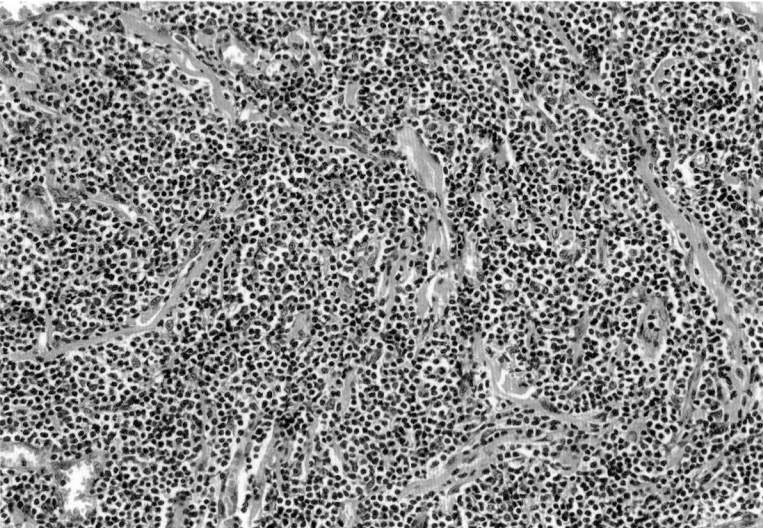

Fig. 29.111
Lymphomatoid papulosis: there is a dense infiltrate of type B cells.

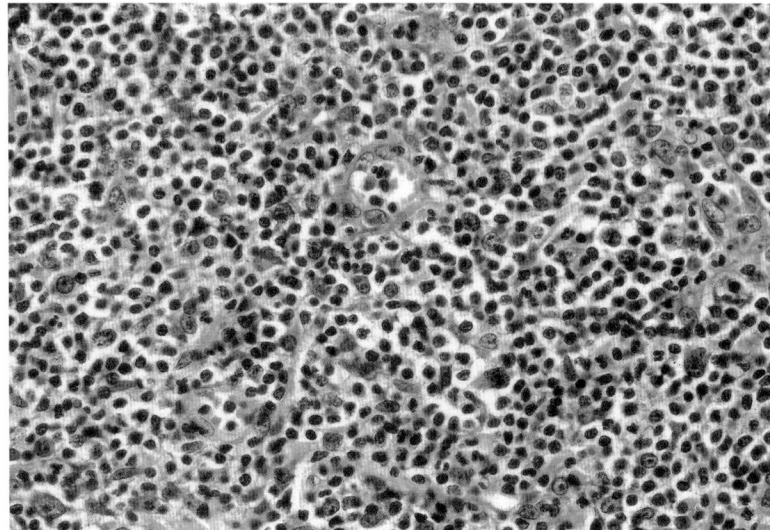

Fig. 29.112
Lymphomatoid papulosis: the type B cells have enlarged, irregular hyperchromatic nuclei and scanty cytoplasm reminiscent of mycosis cells.

primary cutaneous anaplastic large cell lymphoma, and the two processes are only distinguished on the basis of clinical features.[4]

- Type D lymphomatoid papulosis is associated with prominent epidermal hyperplasia and marked epidermotropism. The intraepidermal lymphocytes are usually larger than those seen in type B lesions and express CD8 rather than CD4. However, large anaplastic cells, as seen in types A and C lymphomatoid papulosis, are usually absent.[52]

- So-called type E lymphomatoid papulosis is characterized by an angioinvasive growth pattern with destruction of blood vessel walls. The infiltrating lymphocytes may be small, medium, or large and are admixed with eosinophils and neotrophils. There is often associated necrosis. Clinically, these patients are slightly different from those with classical lymphomatoid papulosis, presenting with relatively few papulonodules that evolve into large flat ulcerations (eschar-like) measuring up to 4 cm in diameter.[53]

- A type F lymphomatoid papulosis has also been proposed for cases exhibiting prominent folliculotropism, although this is not an uncommon feature seen in association with other patterns of infiltration.[3,54,55] Secondary changes, including follicular mucinosis, hyperplasia of hair follicle epithelium, folliculitis, and granulomatous inflammation, often ensue.[3,55]

- Recently, a specific subtype of lymphomatoid papulosis associated with a specific genetic abnormality has been described in a small number of patients.[56] All have translocations involving the DUSP22-IRF4 locus at 6p25.3. These patients present with one to several eruptive papulonodular lesions limited to a single body area. Biopsy shows a cohesive nodular dermal infiltrate of medium to large blast cells. The overlying epidermis shows extensive colonization by small to medium lymphocytes, often with cerebriform nuclear contours. Pautrier microabscess-like collections may be seen, and the epidermal changes often resemble those seen in pagetoid reticulosis.[56]

It should be noted that not all cases of lymphomatoid papulosis neatly subclassify into the variants described above. In up to 10% of cases, there are overlapping features of two or more subtypes within a single lesion, and lesions displaying different patterns may be present at different sites and/or times within a single patient.[3,57,58]

Other features are common to all of the subtypes. Dermal edema and hemorrhage are often conspicuous. Some vessels may show fibrin deposition and occlusion. Reactive epidermal changes are variable, depending on the stage of evolution of the papule. Early lesions show intercellular edema and occasional intraepidermal lymphocytes. Intermediate lesions are characterized by variable necrosis of keratinocytes, intercellular edema, and intraepidermal cells, many of which are atypical. Intraepidermal polymorphs and erythrocytes are commonly found. Late lesions are characterized by extensive epidermal necrosis, ulceration, and the formation of a scaly, parakeratotic crust. Occasionally, there is striking pseudoepitheliomatous hyperplasia such that misdiagnosis as a squamous cell carcinoma or keratoacanthoma may result.[59]

Rare histologic patterns described include a myxoid variant with a sarcoma-like appearance and a syringotropic example.[3,60,61]

In all histologic patterns, the atypical lymphoid cells express CLA and are usually CD4+ and CD8−, although occasionally CD4−/CD8+ (type D and type E in particular), CD4−/CD8− and CD4+/CD8+ variants are encountered.[3,52,53,62] Cytotoxic molecules, such as TIA-1, perforin, and granzyme B, are usually identifiable, irrespective of the CD4/CD8 status.[3,63] There is variable expression of the pan-T-cell antigens, CD2, CD3, CD5, and CD7.[4] The anaplastic cells in the types A and C variants express CD45 and CD30, but not CD15, or p80/ALK1 reactivity with CD25 may also be seen (*Fig. 29.113*).[45,64–69] Although epithelial membrane antigen (EMA) is usually negative, it may be focally positive in some cases. Conversely, in type B lesions, CD30 is often, although not always, negative.[3,33] Although earlier studies suggested an absence of CD56, more recently expression of this molecule has frequently been seen.[3,68,69] In general, tumors of natural killer (NK)/T-cell origin have been generally associated with a very poor prognosis, but this does not appear to be the case in lymphomatoid papulosis. Most cases (75–80%) of lymphomatoid papulosis are also positive for IRF4 (MUM1), but this protein is also expressed in most primary cutaneous

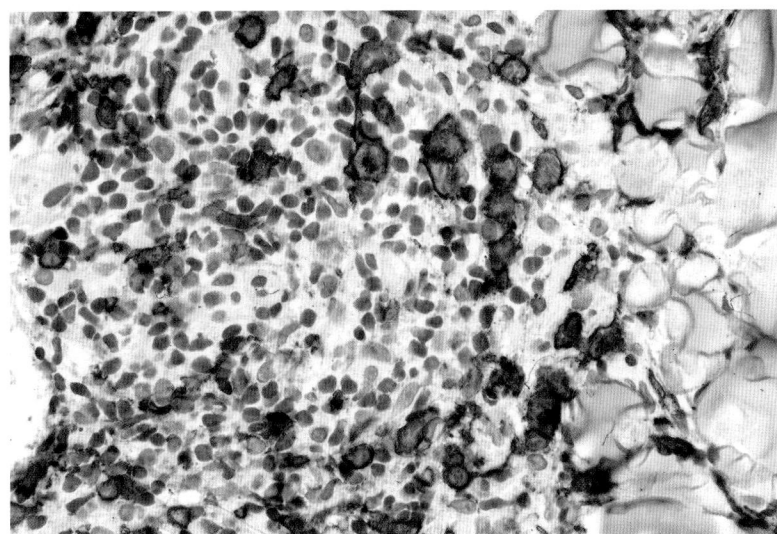

Fig. 29.113
Lymphomatoid papulosis: numerous CD30+ cells are present.

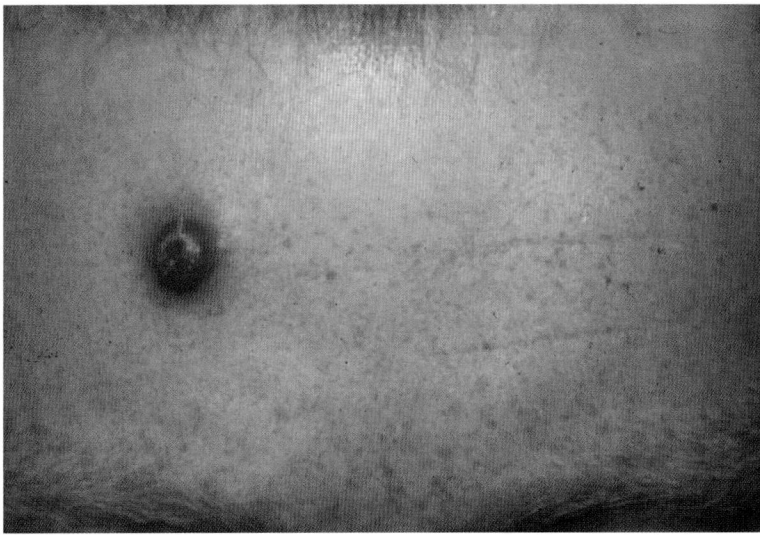

Fig. 29.114
Primary cutaneous anaplastic large cell lymphoma: erythematous, ulcerated tumor nodule on the forehead. By courtesy of the Institute of Dermatology, London, UK.

anaplastic large cell lymphomas and is not a useful marker for distinguishing between these two ends of a spectrum.[70,71] Some cases of lymphomatoid papulosis type D express TCR-γ.[72]

TCR gene rearrangements are detected in approximately 60% of cases.[3,26,32,33,44]

Differential diagnosis

Expression of CD30 is not a reliable discriminator for differentiating cutaneous CD30+ T-cell lymphoproliferative disorders from reactive inflammatory skin conditions or other types of lymphoma. An increasing number of infectious skin diseases have been shown to contain significant numbers of CD30+ cells and mimic lymphomatoid papulosis. These include cutaneous lesions in various viral infections, including herpes virus, molluscum contagiosum, parapox virus (milker's nodule), EBV, HTLV-1, and HIV.[67,70,73–78] Lesions of scabies, syphilis, and superficial fungal infections may also contain CD30+ cells.[66,79,80] Noninfectious cutaneous inflammatory processes, such as pityriais lichenoides et varioliformis acuta, atopic dermatitis, and drug reactions (particularly to anticonvulsants), may also harbor small numbers of CD30+ cells.[81–84] Cutaneous eruption of lymphocyte recovery may also contain CD30+ cells.[66,85]

In most of these disorders, the CD30+ cells lack the anaplastic features and are present in fewer numbers than in lymphomatoid papulosis. They also tend to be scattered, rather than in small clusters, but this is not always the case.[66] However, close clinicopathological correlation remains essential.

Type B and type D lymphomatoid papulosis displaying epidermotropism may be impossible to distinguish from other epidermotropic lymphomas such as mycosis fungoides (including pagetoid reticulosis) and primary cutaneous CD8-positive aggressive epidermotropic T-cell lymphoma on the basis of pathological features. In such situations, the diagnosis is dependent on the clinical features.

Primary cutaneous anaplastic large cell lymphoma

Primary cutaneous anaplastic large cell lymphoma is a tumor composed of at least 75% of CD30-positive T cells.[1,2] These latter may display anaplastic, pleomorphic, or immunoblastic morphology. The outcome is similar irrespective of histologic subtype.[1,3,4] The prognosis is excellent, particularly when compared to other CD30-positive large cell lymphomas involving the skin. The latter include transformed mycosis fungoides, as well as nodal/systemic ALK-positive and ALK-negative anaplastic large cell lymphoma with cutaneous dissemination. Primary cutaneous CD30-negative large cell lymphomas are also excluded from this category because of their much more aggressive behavior and poorer prognosis.[1,4,5]

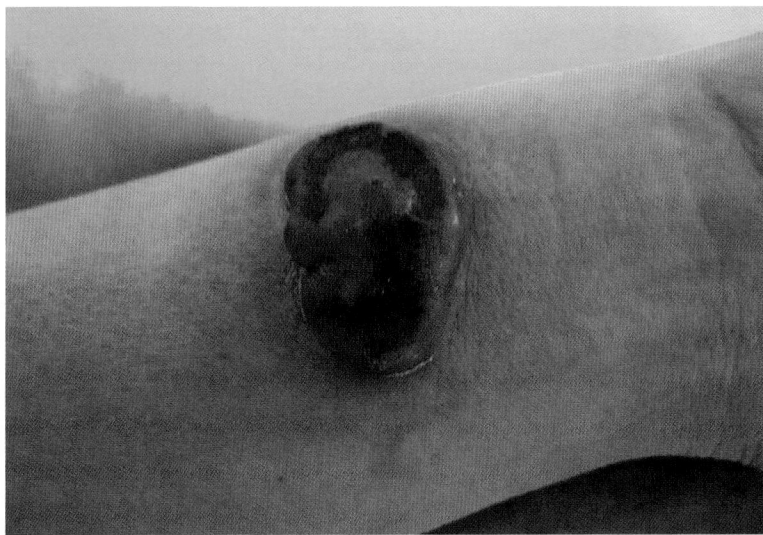

Fig. 29.115
Primary cutaneous anaplastic large cell lymphoma; large ulcerated nodule on the forearm. Courtesy of Dr Teresa Estrach Panella, Barcelona, Spain.

Clinical features

Primary cutaneous anaplastic large cell lymphoma occurs mainly in the seventh decade. Although a wide age range may be affected, childhood cases are rare and, unlike systemic anaplastic large cell lymphoma, there is no bimodal age distribution.[6–9] There is male predilection. Most cases (approximately 80%) present with a solitary erythematous or violaceous, often ulcerated nodule or group of nodules/papules restricted to a single region (Figs 29.114 and 29.115). The extremities are particularly involved. Multifocal disease, defined as two or more lesions at multiple anatomic sites, is seen in around 20% of cases (Fig. 29.116).[1–6]

Clinical behavior varies: 42% of lesions are associated with partial or complete regression; such variants were described as 'regressing atypical histiocytosis' in the older literature.[6,10–12] A further 42% are associated with one or more recurrences, but only 10–20% are associated with extracutaneous (generally nodal) spread.[6] There does not, however, appear to be any significant difference in behavior between those that are confined to the

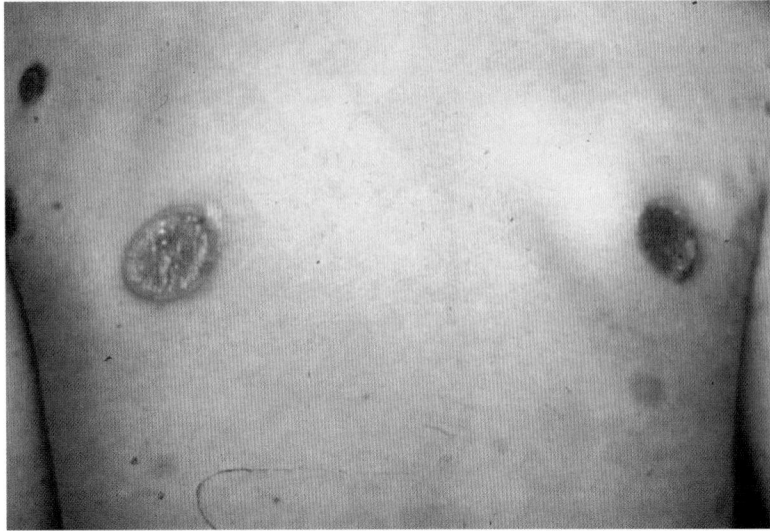

Fig. 29.116
Primary cutaneous anaplastic large cell lymphoma: multiple lesions affecting different regions are present in this patient. By courtesy of the late N.P. Smith, MD, Institute of Dermatology, London, UK.

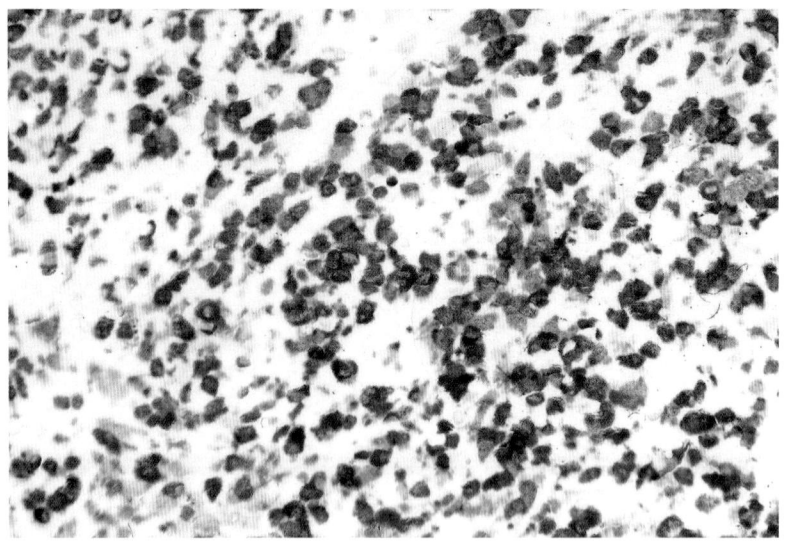

Fig. 29.117
Secondary cutaneous anaplastic large cell lymphoma: this example of metastatic disease is ALK positive.

skin and those that spread to one draining lymph node region.[6] The 5- and 10-year disease-related survival ranges from 91% to 96% for patients with primary disease (depending on whether or not there is concomitant lymph node involvement) compared with 24% for patients with secondary cutaneous involvement by nodal CD30-positive large T-cell lymphoma.[6] Risk factors for tumor progression are unknown.[6]

Pathogenesis and histologic features

Primary cutaneous anaplastic large cell lymphoma is a neoplasm of activated skin-homing T lymphocytes which appear to show a Th2-type bias of cytokine production.[13-15] They have clonally rearranged T-cell receptor genes but are deficient in T-cell receptor and T-cell receptor associated proximal signaling molecules.[16]

The pathogenesis is unknown.[17-22] Consistent cytogenetic abnormalities have been identified and a variety of oncogenes implicated, including JUNB, but specific mechanisms of tumor development have yet to be elucidated.[23-25] As with lymphomatoid papulosis, it is possible that expression of the proapoptotic protein bax and/or death-receptor (CD95) signaling may contribute to the spontaneous regression of some cases and the generally favorable outcome.[26,27]

Primary cutaneous anaplastic large cell lymphomas typically lack the t(2;5)(p23;q35) and resulting overexpression of the NPM-ALK fusion protein normally associated with this translocation.[28] Nevertheless, rare cases of ALK protein and ALK gene translocation positive lymphomas presenting primarily in the skin have recently been described and appear to be associated with a similarly favorable prognosis.[29] In addition, cases of primary cutaneous anaplastic large cell lymphoma displaying cytoplasmic ALK expression but lacking evidence of an underlying genetic abnormality are noted.[30,31] Thus, even if bona fide cases of ALK-positive primary cutaneous anaplastic large cell lymphoma do exist, they are currently best excluded from this category until there is sufficient information to better understand their biology and predict their behavior (Fig. 29.117). A further finding is the presence of translocations involving the DUSP22/IRF4 locus at 6p25.3 that have been documented in around 20% of cases, although this is not specific for primary cutaneous anaplastic large cell lymphoma, also being found in a similar percentage of systemic ALK-negative anaplastic large cell lymphomas and a small subset of lymphomatoid papulosis cases.[32-35]

In contrast to lymphomatoid papulosis where the infiltrate is largely restricted to the dermis, in primary cutaneous large cell lymphoma, the tumor (which is often ulcerated) commonly extends into the subcutaneous fat or deeper tissues. Rare cases confined to the subcutis have also been reported and occasionally an angiodestructive growth pattern is evident.[36-39]

Fig. 29.118
Primary cutaneous anaplastic large cell lymphoma: low-power view showing the superficial part of a large tumor nodule.

A number of histologic variants are recognized, with a similar spectrum of appearances to that seen in systemic ALK-positive anaplastic large cell lymphoma.[36,40-42] Most commonly, the tumor cells display an anaplastic morphology with abundant cytoplasm and pleomorphic vesicular nuclei with clumped heterochromatin and prominent nucleoli (Figs 29.118–29.121). Some cells may show cytoplasmic vacuolation and even assume a signet ring appearance.[36] Bizarre forms are common and include multinucleated giant cells resembling Reed-Sternberg cells, as well as cells with nuclei arranged in wreath configurations (Fig. 29.122). Lymphophagocytosis may be seen (Fig. 29.123). Mitoses including atypical forms are common (Fig. 29.124).

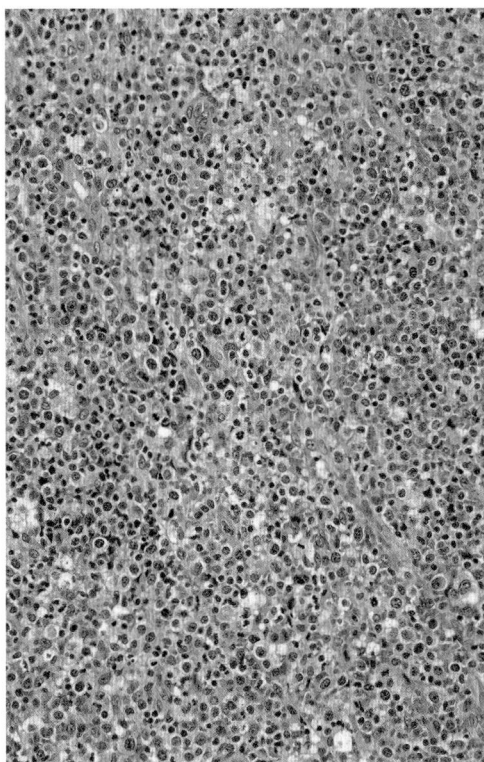

Fig. 29.119
Primary cutaneous anaplastic large cell lymphoma: the tumor is composed of anaplastic cells with vesicular nuclei containing prominent eosinophilic nucleoli.

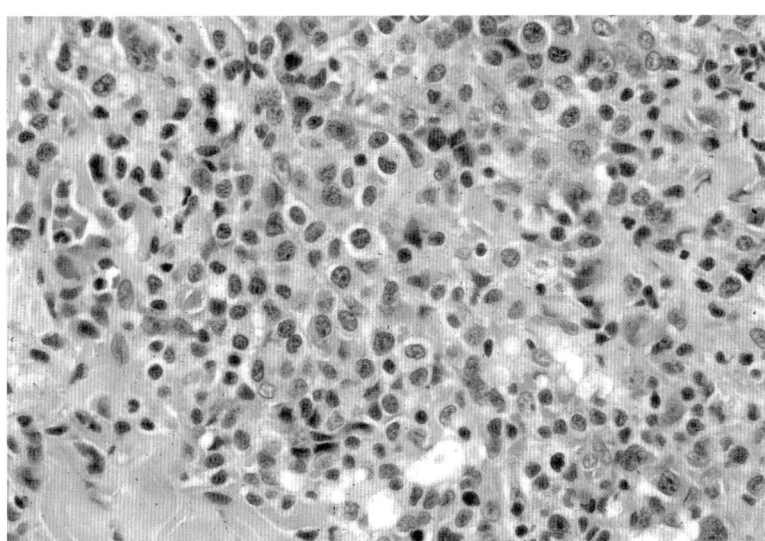

Fig. 29.120
Primary cutaneous anaplastic large cell lymphoma: the tumor cells have abundant ill-defined amphophilic cytoplasm and vesicular nuclei.

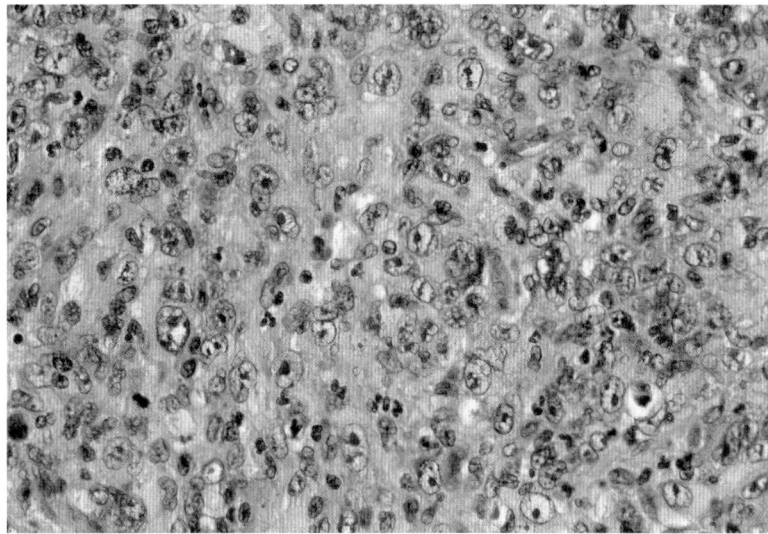

Fig. 29.121
Primary cutaneous anaplastic large cell lymphoma: in this example, single, central basophilic nucleoli are conspicuous.

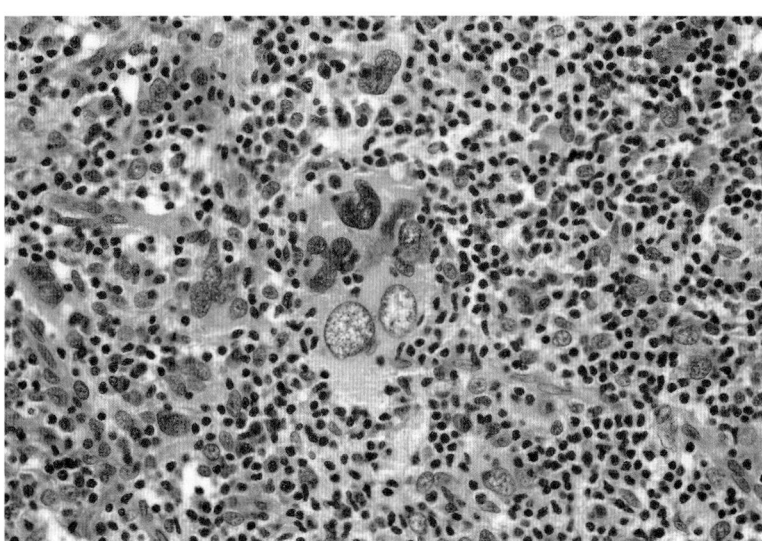

Fig. 29.122
Primary cutaneous anaplastic large cell lymphoma: note the anaplastic multinucleated tumor cells.

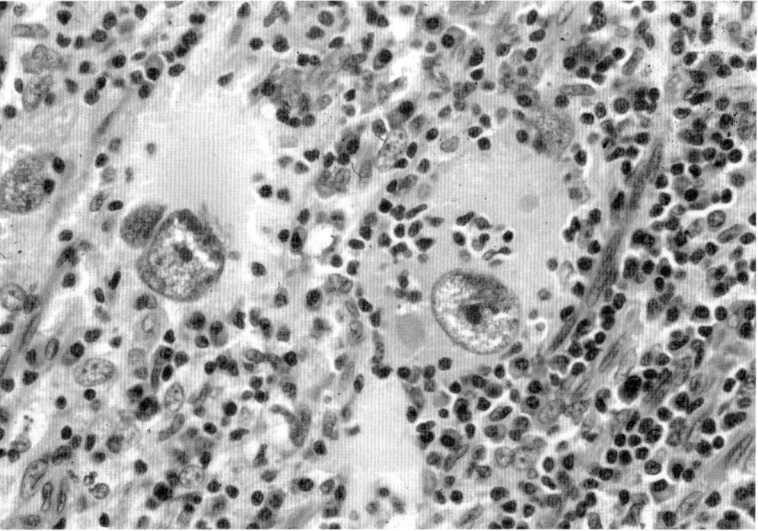

Fig. 29.123
Primary cutaneous anaplastic large cell lymphoma: the tumor giant cells show lymphophagocytosis.

Less often, tumor cells have a pleomorphic or immunoblastic appearance. Small cell (pleomorphic) variants may resemble tumor stage mycosis fungoides and are rare (Figs 29.125 and 29.126).[36] They are characterized by an infiltrate of atypical hyperchromatic and only weakly CD30+ cerebriform T lymphocytes with much smaller numbers of anaplastic large cells and inflammatory cells.[4,36,43,44] Rarely, the tumor cells may have a pleomorphic spindle cell morphology, myxoid stroma, or a storiform growth pattern, mimicking a sarcoma.[45–47]

The tumor cells grow in large nests or diffuse sheets (occasionally leading to a mistaken diagnosis of metastatic carcinoma or melanoma) commonly

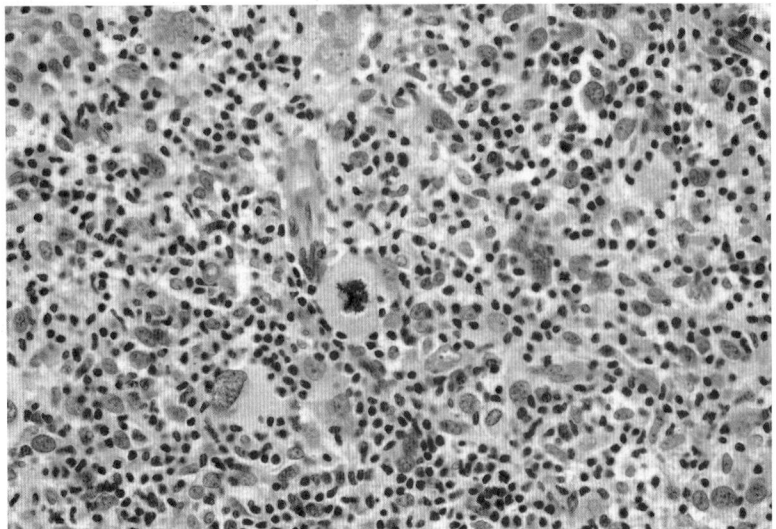

Fig. 29.124
Primary cutaneous anaplastic large cell lymphoma: abnormal mitoses are present.

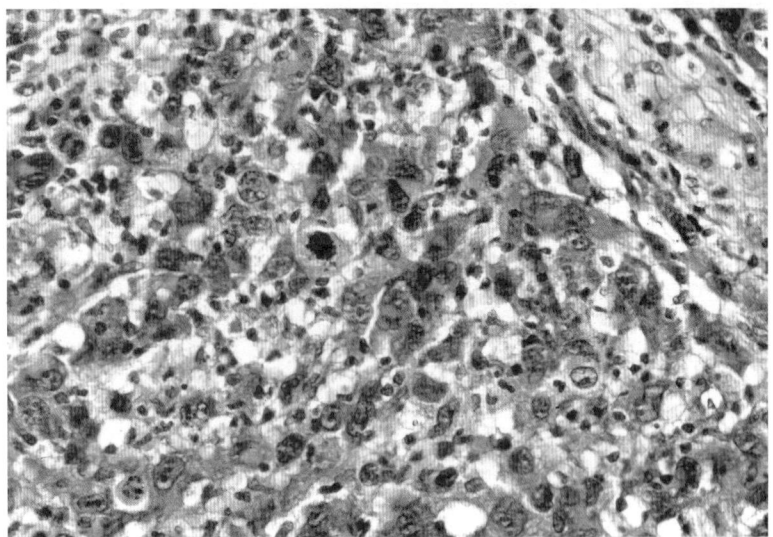

Fig. 29.127
Primary cutaneous anaplastic large cell lymphoma: in some lesions, the tumor cells grow in cohesive cords such that a carcinoma may first be suspected.

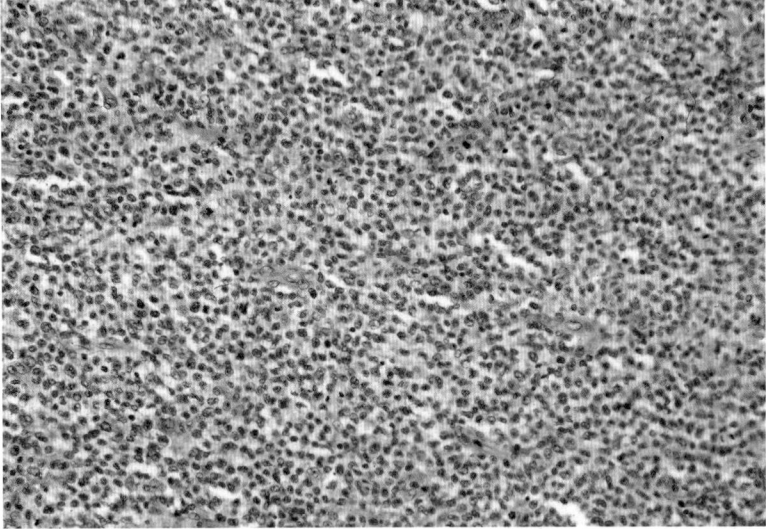

Fig. 29.125
Primary cutaneous anaplastic large cell lymphoma: small cell variant characterized by a uniform population of tumor cells with hyperchromatic nuclei.

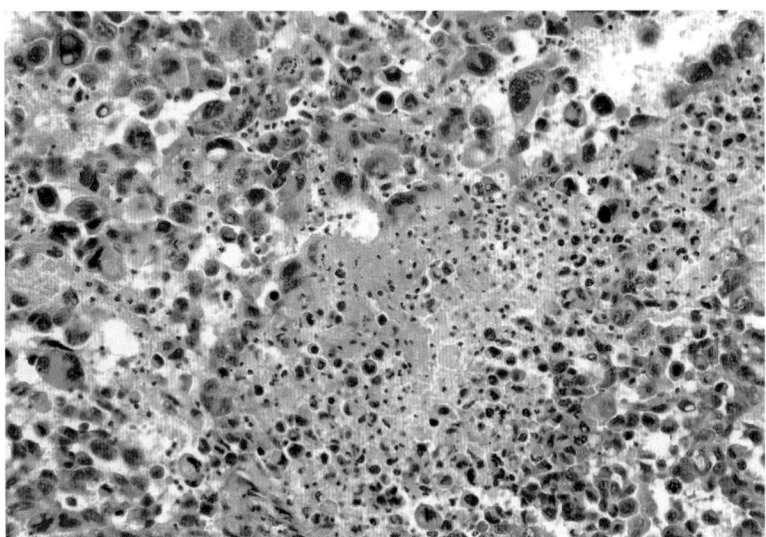

Fig. 29.128
Primary cutaneous anaplastic large cell lymphoma: widespread necrosis is present.

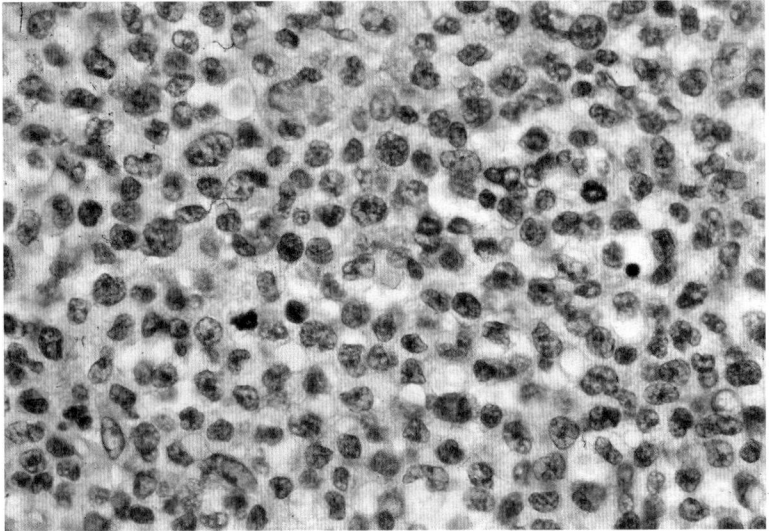

Fig. 29.126
Primary cutaneous anaplastic large cell lymphoma: small cell variant. The nuclei are darkly staining and cytoplasm is minimal.

showing areas of necrosis (*Figs 29.127* and *29.128*). Intralymphatic permeation is relatively common.[48,49] Epidermotropism may be seen in up to 40% of cases.[36] Pseudoepitheliomatous hyperplasia may be marked, closely mimicking malignancy, especially in small biopsies.[4,36,50]

Inflammatory cells including neutrophils, eosinophils, histiocytes, lymphocytes, and plasma cells are frequent (*Figs 29.129* and *29.130*). Rarely, neutrophils are so conspicuous that an inflammatory process such as a pustular/infective dermatosis may initially be suspected (neutrophil-rich variant, pyogenic lymphoma).[36,51,52] It has been suggested that the intense neutrophil infiltrates result from IL-8 production by the tumor cells.[53] In other cases, large numbers of eosinophils are present and may represent the disease described as eosinophilic histiocytosis.[36,54,55] A lymphohistiocytic variant characterized by the presence of numerous histiocytes, which may display hemophagocytosis, has also been described.[36,56] Some cases harboring translocations of the IRF4-DUSP22 locus may show distinctive features, similar to those seen in lymphomatoid papulosis associated with the same genetic abnormality. These cases exhibit a biphasic pattern characterized by nodular and diffuse dermal infiltrates of large cells with overlying pagetoid reticulosis-like changes, the intraepidermal lymphocytes generally being of small size.[57]

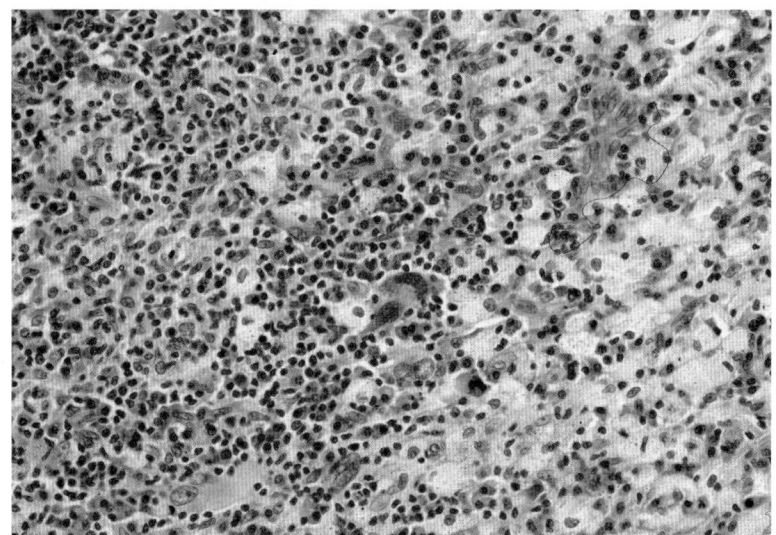

Fig. 29.129
Primary cutaneous anaplastic large cell lymphoma: abundant histiocytes as shown in this field account for misdiagnosis as inflammatory malignant fibrous histiocytoma.

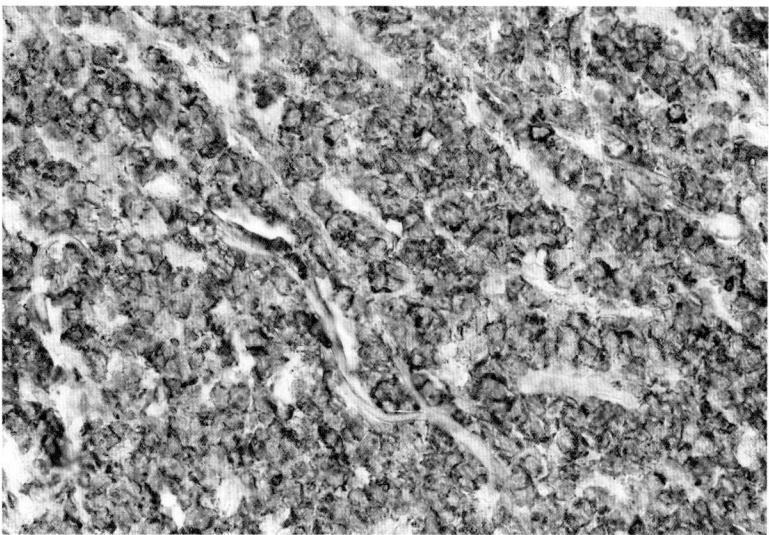

Fig. 29.131
Primary cutaneous anaplastic large cell lymphoma: the tumor cells are uniformly CD30 positive.

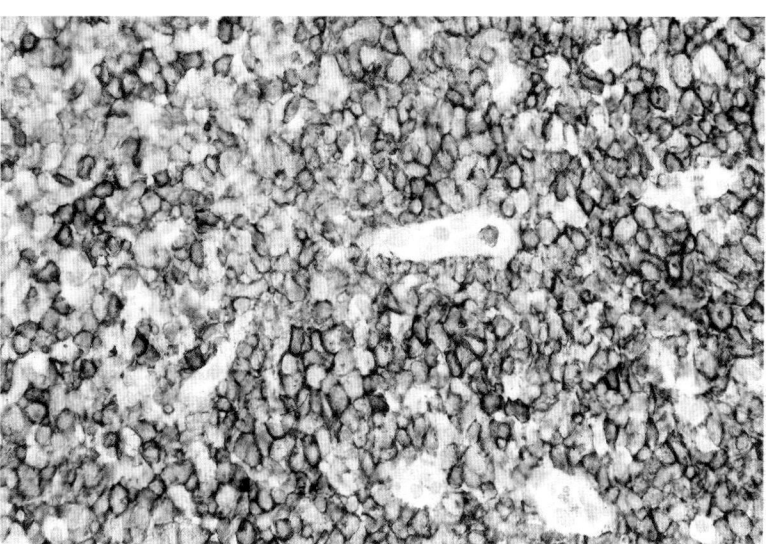

Fig. 29.132
Primary cutaneous anaplastic large cell lymphoma: the cells coexpress CD4 (same case as *Fig. 29.131*).

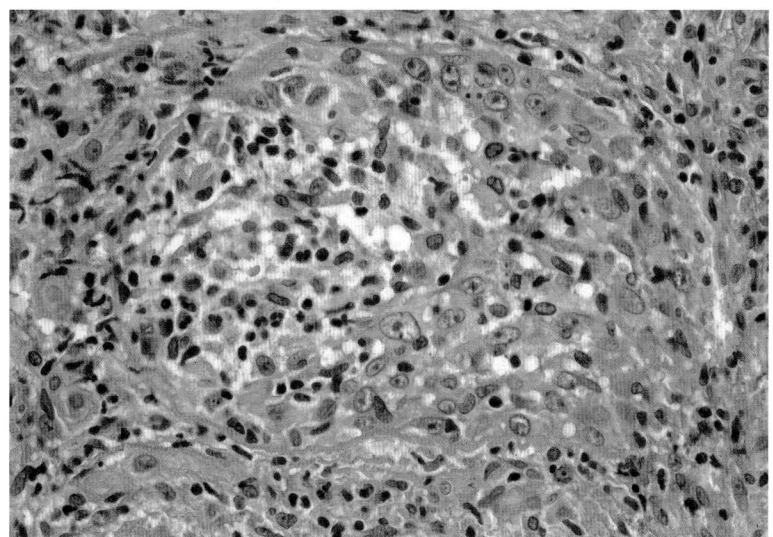

Fig. 29.130
Primary cutaneous anaplastic large cell lymphoma: numerous eosinophils are present in this example.

By definition, 75% or more of the tumor cells express membranous and Golgi CD30 (Ber-H2/Ki-1) (*Fig. 29.131*). Most cases display an activated CD4+ T-cell phenotype, although occasionally CD8+ or null cell variants are encountered (*Fig. 29.132*). There is variable loss of various pan-T-cell antigens. The majority of cells express cytotoxic molecules TIA-1, perforin, or granzyme B.[2,58,59] CD25, CD71, and HLA-DR are also usually present.[60] CD15 is typically absent. In contrast to primary nodal variants, EMA is almost invariably absent in primary cutaneous lesions although it may sometimes be evident in children (*Fig. 29.133*). Staining for ALK1 is also usually negative (see above).[7] Spindle cell variants may express smooth muscle actin.[46] Fascin is expressed in up to 64% of cases of CD30-positive anaplastic large cell lymphoma, compared with only 24% of cases of lymphomatoid papulosis.[61] Occasional CD56+ tumors have been documented, but this does not appear to be associated with prognosis.[62–64] IRF4 (MUM1) may also be expressed but has limited utility in distinguishing primary cutaneous anaplastic large cell lymphoma from lymphomatoid papulosis, transformed mycosis fungoides, and systemic T-cell lymphoma secondarily involving the skin.[32,65,66]

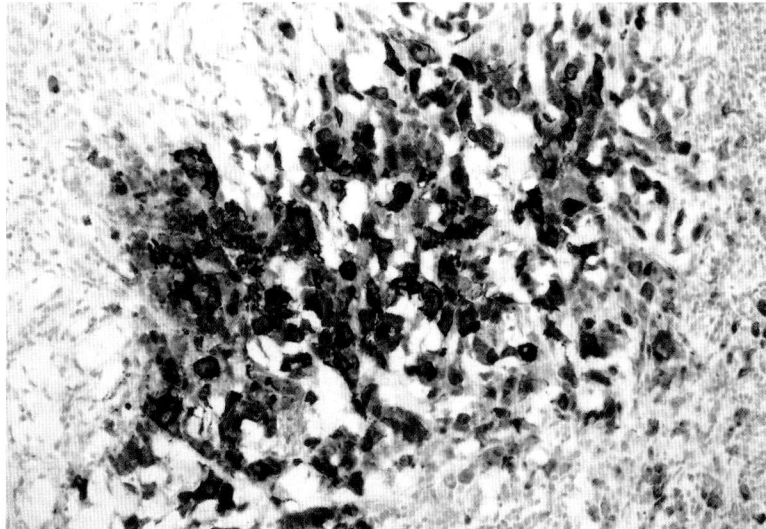

Fig. 29.133
Cutaneous anaplastic large cell lymphoma: in this example, the tumor cells express epithelial membrane antigen. This case proved to represent a metastasis from a nodal primary lesion.

Differential diagnosis

Clinical correlation is essential in differentiating primary cutaneous anaplastic large cell lymphoma from other CD30+ large cell lymphomas that may arise in, or disseminate to, the skin. The clinical appearance of lesions and course of disease are the only reliable discriminants of primary cutaneous anaplastic large cell lymphoma and lymphomatoid papulosis types A and C. Primary cutaneous anaplastic large cell lymphoma may also be indistinguishable from transformed CD30+ mycosis fungoides, and this possibility should always be excluded by careful clinicopathologic correlation. Staging, including CT of chest and abdomen and bone examination, is essential in excluding dissemination of nodal CD30+ large T-cell lymphomas, such as ALK+ and ALK– anaplastic large cell lymphoma and some examples of peripheral T-cell lymphoma, unspecified.[6]

Immunohistochemistry and genetic analysis may facilitate distinction from nodal ALK+ anaplastic large cell lymphoma, with the above caveats. Immunohistochemistry will also permit distinction from rare cases of CD30+ large B-cell lymphoma involving the skin, and will facilitate distinction of spindle cell variants from spindle cell carcinoma, spindle cell melanoma, dermal sarcomas, inflammatory pseudotumor (IPT), follicular dendritic cell (FDC) sarcoma, dendritic reticulum cell sarcoma, and spindle cell leukemic infiltrates.[46,67,68]

Inflammatory conditions containing CD30+ cells are more likely to be mistaken for lymphomatoid papulosis than cutaneous anaplastic large cell lymphoma.

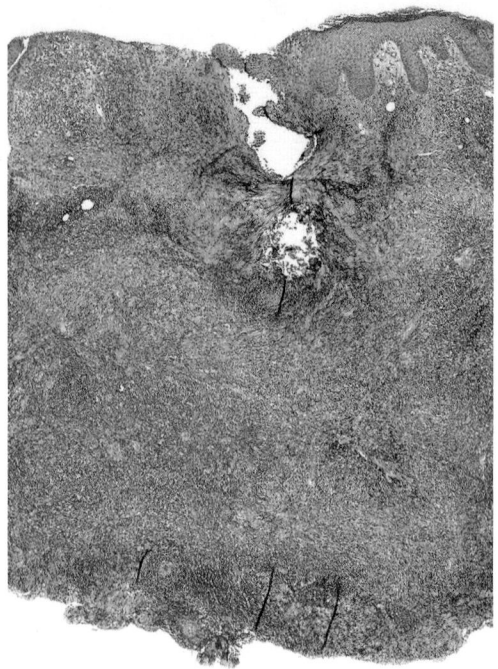

Fig. 29.134
Primary cutaneous CD4-positive small/medium T-cell lymphoproliferative disorder: this is a punch biopsy of a solitary cutaneous tumor nodule. There is a uniform infiltrate of pleomorphic lymphoid cells.

Primary cutaneous CD4-positive small/medium T-cell lymphoproliferative disorder

Clinical features

Primary cutaneous CD4-positive small/medium T-cell lymphoma was included as a provisional entity in the 2008 WHO classification.[1] It remains a provisional entity in the 2016 update although the nomenclature has been altered to primary cutaneous CD4-positive small/medium T-cell lymphoproliferative disorder to reflect the uncertain malignant potential associated with such lesions.[2] It has been suggested to represent a limited clonal response to an unknown stimulus, lacking sufficient criteria to designate a malignancy.[2] It is defined as a proliferation of small to medium-sized CD4-positive pleomorphic T cells in patients lacking patches or plaques typical for mycosis fungoides.[1] It is rare, accounting for approximately 2–3% of all primary cutaneous T-cell lymphomas.[1,3]

Females and males appear to be equally affected.[4] The age range is wide, and most patients are adults, with a median age at presentation in the sixth decade; pediatric cases may be encountered.[4–7] The majority of patients present with solitary or localized asymptomatic, erythematous to purple papulonodules or plaques, particularly on the head and neck and upper trunk.[3–10] A minority of patients present with large tumors or multiple lesions.[5,8,9] The prognosis is good. Early series quoted 5-year survivals of around 80%.[3] However, more recent reports in which the majority of patients presented with solitary or localized lesions, have a much more favorable outcome with survival approaching 100%.[10] Those with multiple lesions/large tumors run a more aggressive clinical course.[5,6,8,9]

Histologic features

Histologically, the tumor is composed of a fairly uniform population of small to medium-sized lymphocytes with pale scanty cytoplasm and hyperchromatic irregular noncerebriform nuclei in a perivascular, bandlike, nodular, or diffuse fashion, often involving the entire dermis and sometimes extending into the subcutis (Figs 29.134 and 29.135).[4,5,8–10] By definition, large cells make up less than 30% of the population.[1,6] Mitotic figures are rare and epidermotropism is absent, or focal (Fig. 29.136).[4–6,10] Lymphocytes, neutrophils, eosinophils, and plasma cells may sometimes be present, and rarely there is a granulomatous component.[4,7] Formation of germinal centers is not usually seen.

Tumor cells have a T-helper phenotype, and there may be loss of CD7 and rarely CD2 and/or CD5 (Fig. 29.137).[4,6,9,11] CD30, cytotoxic molecules,

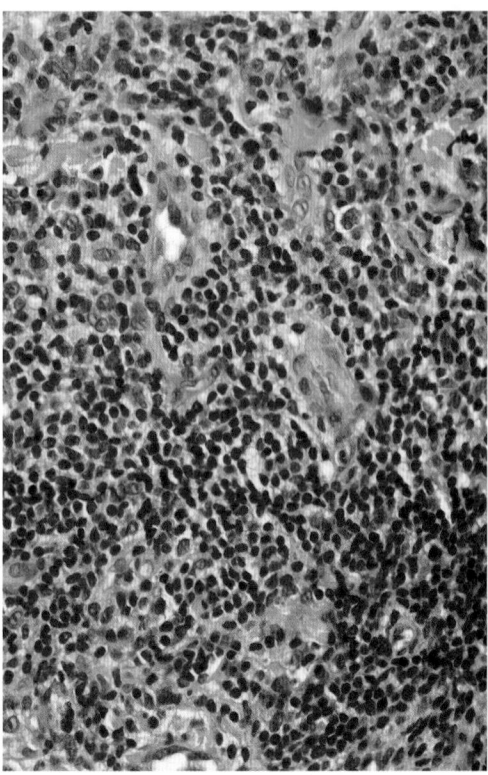

Fig. 29.135
Primary cutaneous CD4-positive small/medium T-cell lymphoproliferative disorder: the tumor cells have irregular hyperchromatic nuclei and minimal cytoplasm. Distinction from mycosis fungoides depends on clinicopathological correlation.

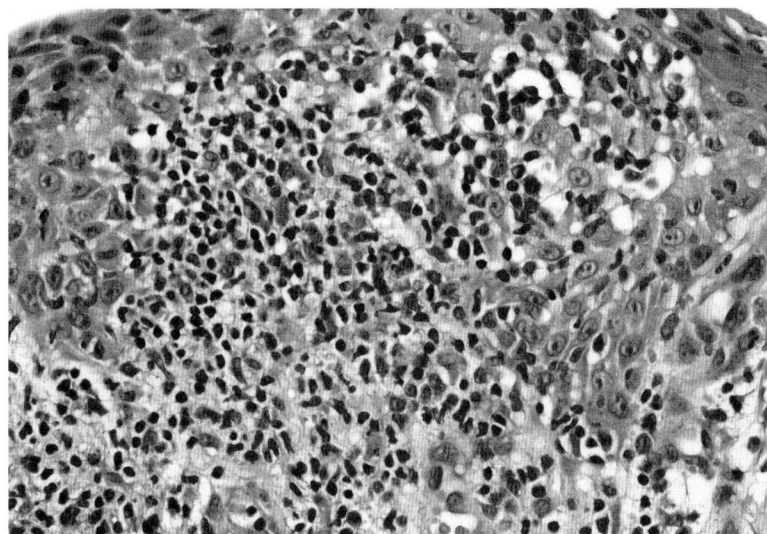

Fig. 29.136
Primary cutaneous CD4-positive small/medium T-cell lymphoproliferative
disorder: this example shows focal epidermotropism, heightening the histologic
resemblance to mycosis fungoides.

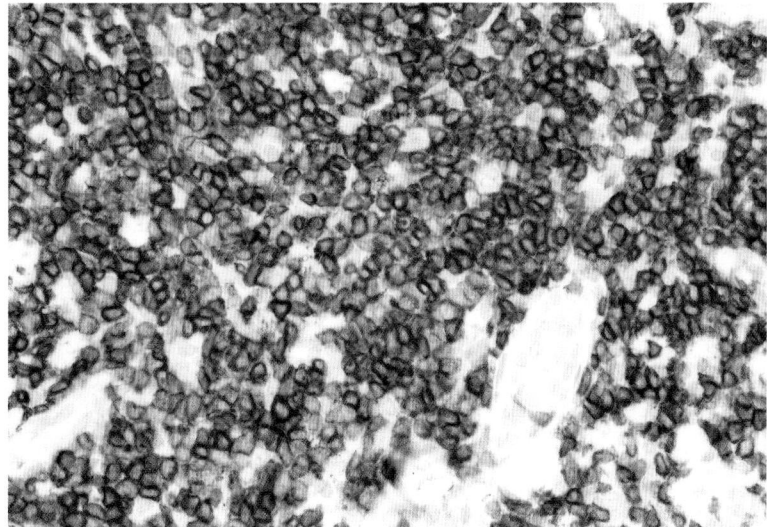

Fig. 29.137
Primary cutaneous CD4-positive small/medium T-cell lymphoproliferative disorder:
the tumor cells express CD4.

and EBV are negative.[5] The neoplastic lymphocytes also show reactivity with
antibodies to PD1 and BCL6, with lesser numbers also usually expressing
CXCL13 and ICOS, but they are usually CD10 negative.[5,11,12] PD1-positive
cells are often seen in clusters, but this is not specific. Based on the immunoprofile, it has been suggested that primary cutaneous CD4-positive small/
medium T-cell lymphoproliferative disorder is a lesion of T-follicular helper
cells, although the absence of CXCR5 in the clonal lymphocytes casts some
doubt on this hypothesis.[12] Antibodies to CD20 highlight B lymphocytes.
These are often numerous and include blast cells that may coexpress CD30,
and are often surrounded by the PD1-positive lymphocytes.[9,11,12]

Clonal rearrangements of the T-cell receptor genes are found in the
majority of cases.[4,7,9,11,12]

Differential diagnosis

Primary cutaneous small/medium-sized T-cell lymphoma should be distinguished from tumor stage mycosis fungoides, lymphomatoid papulosis, subcutaneous panniculitis-like T-cell lymphoma, and T-cell pseudolymphoma.[6]
The distinction depends as much on clinical information as on histologic
and immunophenotypic investigations. The distinction with T-cell pseudolymphoma is not clear-cut. T-cell pseudolymphomas often presents with a

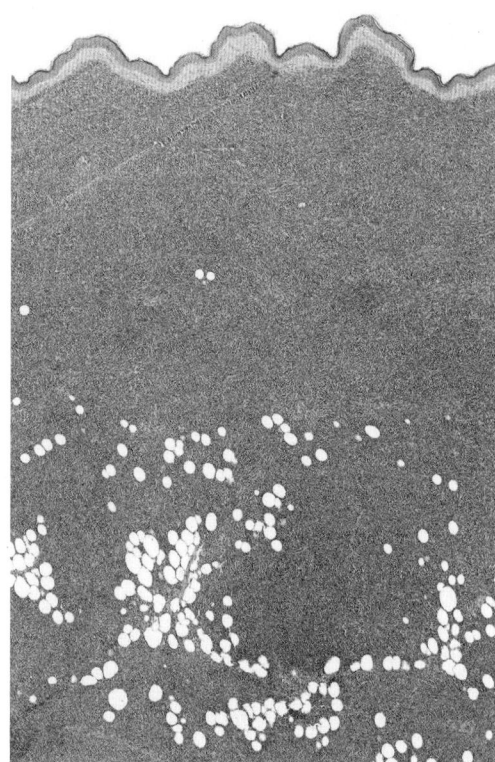

Fig. 29.138
Indolent CD8-positive lymphoid proliferation of the ear: low-power view of dense
dermal infiltrate extending into the subcutis. Note the grenz zone. Courtesy of Dr.
T. Petrella, MD, Dijon, France.

solitary plaque or nodule, and recent studies have shown considerable pathological overlap, including clonality and expression of T-follicular helper cell
markers.[13,14] This has led some to propose that most cases previously called
T-cell pseudolymphoma would now be classified as primary cutaneous
CD4-positive small/medium T-cell lymphoproliferative disorder.[13,14]

Primary cutaneous acral CD8+ T-cell lymphoma

Clinical features

Primary cutaneous acral CD8+ T-cell lymphoma appears for the first time
as a provisional entity in the 2016 update of the WHO classification.[1] It is
the name now proposed for a variant of cutaneous T-cell lymphoma first
described as 'indolent CD8-positive lymphoid proliferation of the ear' in a
very small series of cases in 2007.[2] Since this original publication, additional
cases have been reported, all with similar pathological and clinical features,
but with a broader distribution of lesions, including elsewhere on the face,
particularly the nose, and other acral sites.[3-10] Presentation is with asymptomatic, slow-growing, often solitary papules, nodules, or plaques on the
ear (helix or earlobe), elsewhere on the face, particularly the nose, or the
hands and feet.[2-10] The behavior seems to be indolent with no dissemination.

Pathogenesis and histologic features

The pathogenesis is unknown. Histologically, the epidermis appears unremarkable, and it is separated from a diffuse prominent dermal, and focally
subcutaneous infiltrate by a grenz zone (Fig. 29.138). Tumor cells are
medium-sized and fairly monotonous with a blast-like appearance, irregular
nuclei, and a small nucleolus (Fig. 29.139). The proliferative activity is low.
By immunohistochemistry, tumor cells stain for CD3, CD8, CD45RA, and
cytotoxic granules including granzyme B (Fig. 29.140). CD4 and CD30 are
negative, and there may be loss of other T-cell markers including CD2 and
CD5. A few reactive B cells are present in the background. A T-cell clone is
usually demonstrated.[2-10]

Despite these features of malignancy, and irrespective of the blast cell
morphology and cytotoxic T-cell phenotype, this is an indolent process.

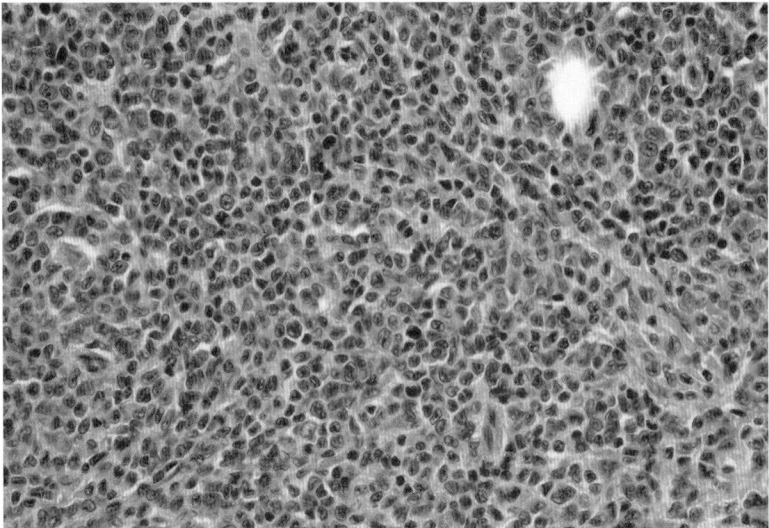

Fig. 29.139
Indolent CD8-positive lymphoid proliferation of the ear: the infiltrate is composed of a uniform population of blast cells. Courtesy of Dr. T. Petrella, MD, Dijon, France.

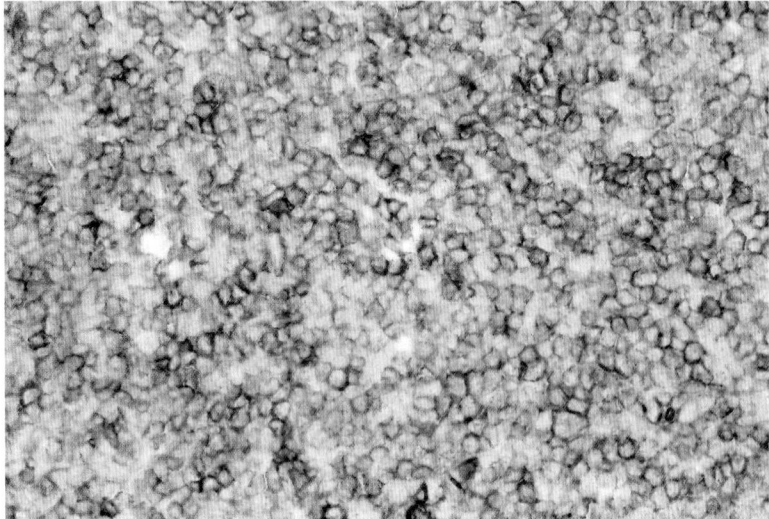

Fig. 29.140
Indolent CD8-positive lymphoid proliferation of the ear: the tumor cells are positive for CD3. Courtesy of Dr. T. Petrella, MD, Dijon, France.

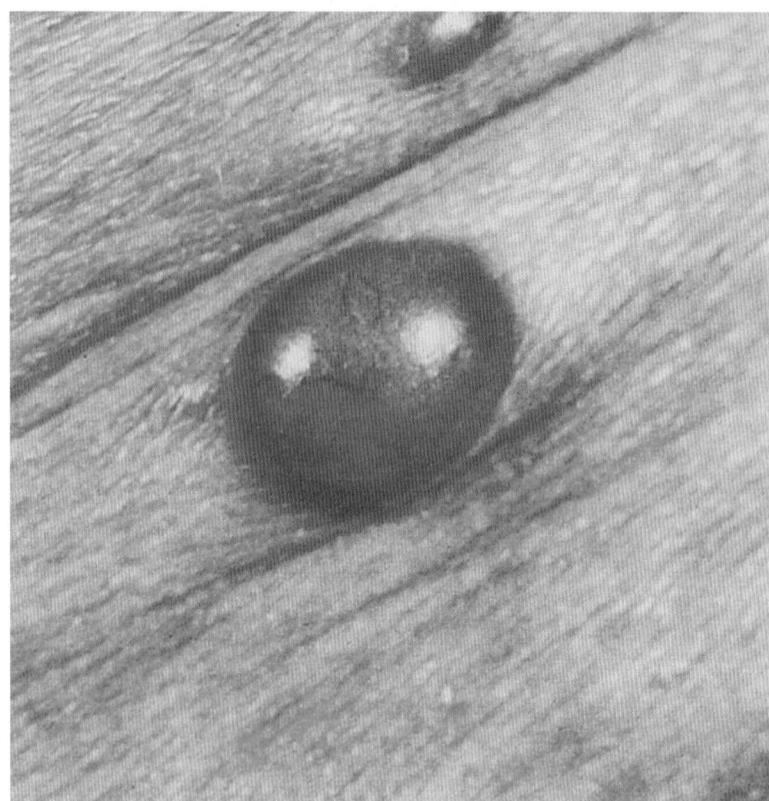

Fig. 29.141
Angioimmunoblastic T-cell lymphoma: an erythematous maculopapular eruption on the anterior chest wall and anterior axillary fold. By courtesy of M.G. Bernengo, MD, Clinica Dermatologica, Turin, Italy.

Cases treated with only locally directed therapy, including biopsy or excision alone, almost invariably go into complete remission and, although relapses may occur, no disease related deaths have yet been reported.[2–10]

The main challenge is therefore to differentiate these lesions from the other lymphomas with a cytotoxic phenotype that often exhibit a more aggressive behavior.[11] Clinicopathological correlation should help discriminate from other specific cutaneous lymphomas that occasionally express CD8 rather than CD4 such as mycosis fungoides, pagetoid reticulosis, primary cutaneous anaplastic large cell lymphoma, lymphomatoid papulosis, or others which are also characterized by a cytotoxic phenotype, including CD8 expression in some or all cases. The latter include subcutaneous panniculitis-like T-cell lymphoma, primary cutaneous CD8-positive aggressive epidermotropic cytotoxic T-cell lymphoma, primary cutaneous γ/δ T-cell lymphoma, and extranodal NK/T-cell lymphoma of nasal type. However, the distinction may not always be clear-cut, and localized nonepidermotropic cutaneous CD8-positive lymphoproliferations with a poor outcome have previously been described.[12] Expression of CD68 by the neoplastic lymphocytes may help as it has recently been reported to be specific for primary cutaneous acral CD8+ T-cell lymphoma, although the utility of this marker has yet to be tested in large series of cases.[13]

Angioimmunoblastic T-cell lymphoma

Clinical features

Angioimmunoblastic T-cell lymphoma (AITL) is a peripheral T-cell lymphoma characterized by systemic disease including generalized lymphadenopathy, hepatosplenomegaly, anemia, and hypergammaglobulinemia.[1] The reported male/female ratio is variable, but age of presentation is in the sixth or seventh decades.[1–6] The disease is usually in an advanced stage at presentation with generalized lymphadenopathy and frequent hepatosplenomegaly, bone marrow and skin involvement, and systemic symptoms.[1–6] Pleural effusions, ascites, arthritis and/or arthralgia, ear, nose, and throat involvement, and neurological manifestations may also be present.[1–6] Often, patients have hemolytic (Coombs positive) anemia, polyclonal hypergammaglobulinemia, raised LDH, leukocytosis, including eosinophilia, or lymphopenia and thrombocytopenia.[1–4,6] Additional autoimmune phenomena may be encountered including cold agglutinins, cryoglobulins, circulating immune complexes, smooth muscle antibody, rheumatoid factor, and antinuclear antibodies.[1,2,4,7]

Cutaneous lesions occur in up to 50% of patients at presentation and/or relapse.[6–9] Skin involvement manifests as a pruritic maculopapular eruption on the trunk and extremities; this may mimic a viral exanthem or drug hypersensitivity reaction, and in some cases skin lesions may follow drug administration (*Figs 29.141* and *29.142*).[8–12] Other reported manifestations include urticaria, erythroderma, erosions, petechiae, purpura, papulovesicular prurigo-like lesions, plaques, and tumor nodules.[8,13,14]

The outlook for patients with AITL is poor, and while the initial response to treatment is good, it tends to be short-lived.[1,3,5,6] The median survival is <36 months, and 5-year overall survival is between 30% and 35%.[1,3,5,6] Death is often due to infectious complications.[3,7,15]

Pathogenesis and histologic features

AITL is a malignancy of follicular helper T cells, as evidenced by the immunophenotype and gene expression profile.[2,3,16–20] Chromosomal

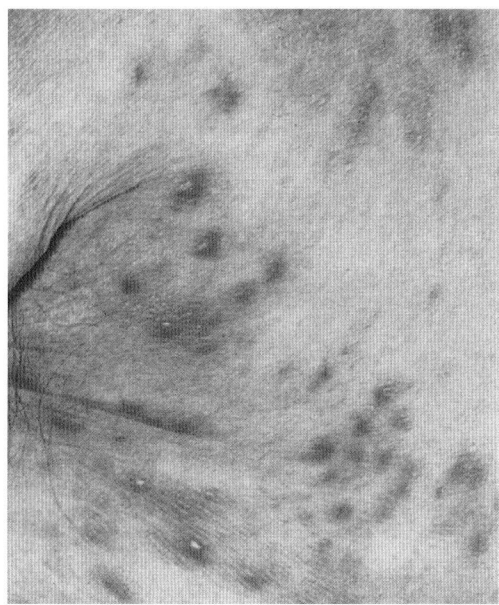

Fig. 29.142
Angioimmunoblastic T-cell lymphoma: a nodular deposit was also present. By courtesy of M.G. Bernengo, MD, Clinica Dermatologica, Turin, Italy.

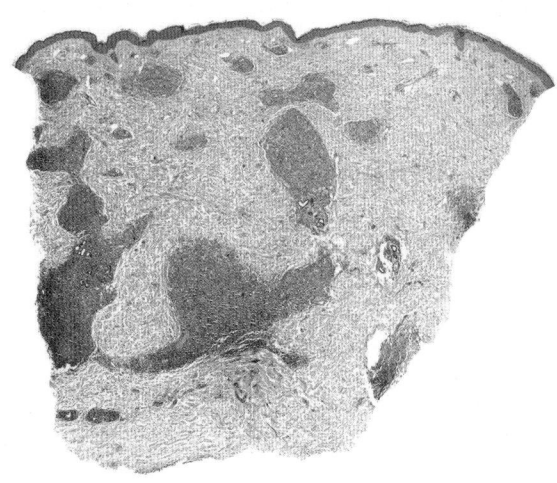

Fig. 29.143
Angioimmunoblastic T-cell lymphoma: this biopsy shows a striking granulomatous dermal infiltrate.

abnormalities have been detected in AITL, the most common being trisomies of chromosomes 3, 5, 18, and 19, gain of chromosome X, and deletion of chromosome 7.[2,4,21] Comparative genomic hybridization (CGH) has also documented gains of 11q13, 19, and 22p, and losses of 13q in a subset of cases.[22] More recent studies have shown that mutations of epigenetic regulators, such as RHOA, TET2, DNMT3, and IDH2, are common in AITL, although only IDH2 mutations appear to be relatively specific for this subtype of T-cell lymphoma.[23–28]

Lymph nodes involved by AITL typically show partial effacement of their architecture by a polymorphic infiltrate, mainly in paracortical areas. The sinuses are usually preserved, but perinodal connective tissues are often involved. In the early stages of the disease, there may be hyperplastic B-cell follicles, but frequently follicles are regressed or absent.[1–3,29] Paracortical areas show marked proliferation of high endothelial venules and a mixed population of lymphocytes, plasma cells, eosinophils, and histiocytes. The neoplastic lymphocytes are usually of intermediate size with abundant clear or pale cytoplasm.[1–3] They are typically found in small clusters around follicles and high endothelial venules. Small reactive lymphocytes are also present, as are scattered large B immunoblasts, some resembling Reed-Sternberg cells.

Biopsies of cutaneous lesions most often show superficial or superficial and deep perivascular or rarely periadnexal lymphocytic infiltrates that are suspicious or diagnostic of lymphoma. The infiltrates range from sparse to dense, contain pleomorphic atypical lymphocytes, and are associated with vascular hyperplasia with prominence of endothelial cells.[8,30,31] Less commonly, the changes are non-specific, comprising superficial perivascular infiltrates of small lymphocytes showing no atypia, eosinophils, and sometimes plasma cells.[8,30] Mild interface changes have been described in a number of cases in one series.[30] Biopsies showing leukocytoclastic vasculitis and granulomatous inflammation are seen in some cases (Figs 29.143 and 29.144).[8,32,33] Rarely, the associated and sometimes neoplastic B-cell expansion may dominate the histologic picture, masking the underlying T-cell lymphoma.[31,34] Most often, the B-cell proliferation resembles diffuse large B-cell lymphoma (DLBCL), but in others it may mimic lymphoplasmacytic or marginal zone lymphoma, or a plasma cell neoplasm.[29,34,34]

Tumor cells often best highlighted in lymph nodes are CD4 positive, and usually express CD2, CD3, and CD5, although significant numbers of reactive CD8-positive T cells may also be present. In common with follicular T-helper cells, at least a proportion express CD10, CXCL13, PD1, and sometimes bcl6.[1,2,16,17,19,20,35,36] CD20 highlights the B immunoblasts, and these are often positive for EBV by in situ hybridization. Irregular, expanded FDC meshworks, often in the vicinity of high endothelial venules,

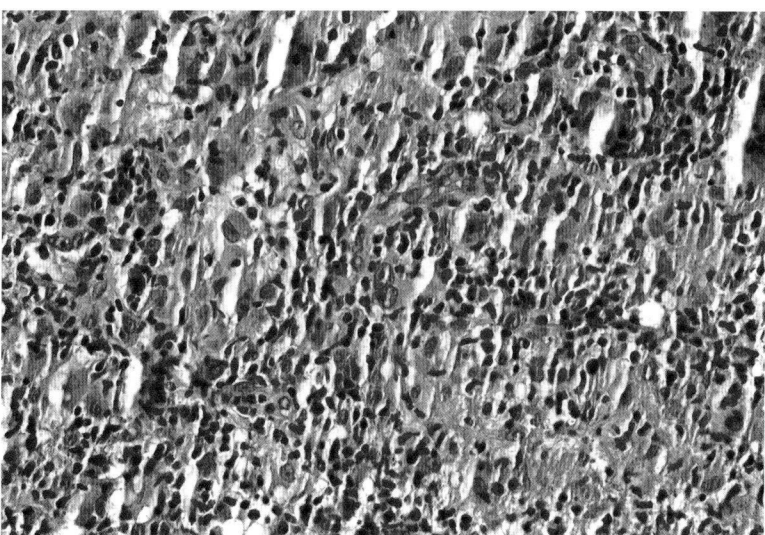

Fig. 29.144
Angioimmunoblastic T-cell lymphoma: note numerous histiocytes and scattered atypical cells.

are highlighted by CD21, CD23, CD35, and/or CNA42. In the skin, it is often harder to identify the neoplastic lymphocytes, but immunohistochemistry with antibodies to CXCL13 seems to be sensitive and specific.[30]

Clonal rearrangements of the TCR gene are identifiable in lymph nodes in most cases, and correlate well with the presence of CXCL13-positive tumor cells in the skin.[11,30,37,38] Clonal immunoglobulin gene rearrangements are seen in 20–30% of cases and correspond to expanded populations of EBV-positive B cells.[37,38]

Differentiating cutaneous involvement by AITL from reactive cutaneous infiltrates is best achieved by correlation with the lymph node pathology and clinical features. In certain situations, staining for CXCL13 and gene rearrangement studies may prove useful.[30]

Adult T-cell leukemia/lymphoma

Clinical features

Adult T-cell leukemia/lymphoma (ATLL) is a systemic disease induced by human T-cell leukemia virus type 1 (HTLV-1) with variable clinical manifestations, and frequent skin involvement. It was first described on the island of Kyushu in southwestern Japan.[1–3] It also occurs in the Caribbean,

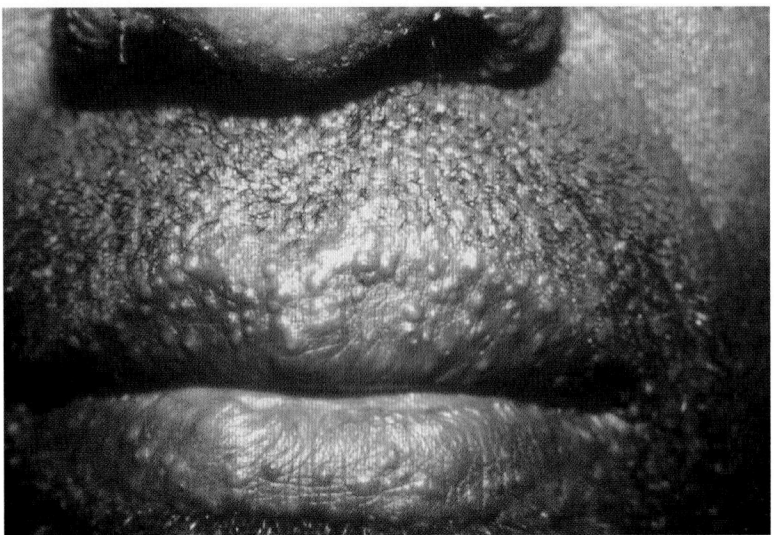

Fig. 29.145
Adult T-cell leukemia/lymphoma: in this case, multiple papules are seen on the lips. By courtesy of the Institute of Dermatology, London, UK.

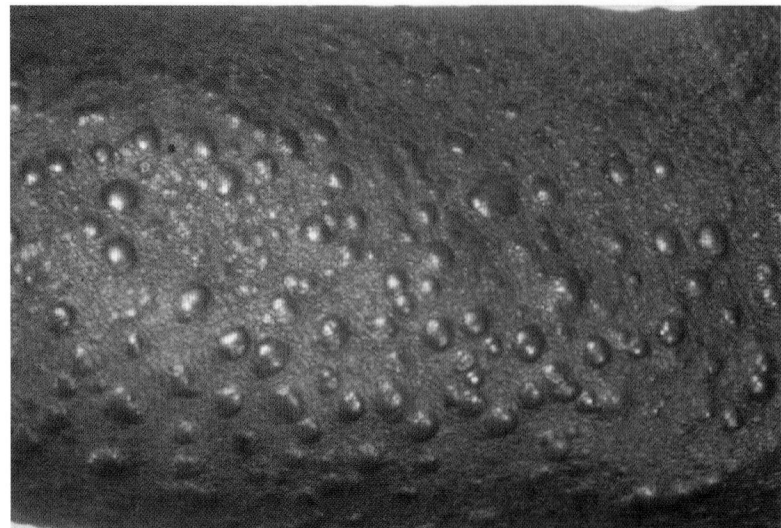

Fig. 29.146
Adult T-cell leukemia/lymphoma: innumerable papules and nodules are present on the arm. By courtesy of the Institute of Dermatology, London, UK.

northeastern South America, southeastern United States, Central Africa, and the Pacific basin.[4,5] Cases are occasionally diagnosed in the rest of the United States and Europe as a consequence of immigration.[6] The disease predominantly affects adults, pediatric cases being rare.[7]

There may be a prodromal phase, but once established, four variants are recognized: acute, chronic, smoldering. and lymphomatous:[1,2,8]

- Acute ATLL (55%): This is the most common subtype, usually presenting with an abrupt onset, and is characterized by a leukemic phase. Hypercalcemia, with or without lytic bone lesions, constitutional symptoms, and raised LDH are typical. A very high white cell count, numerous circulating neoplastic lymphocytes, neutrophilia, and eosinophilia are common. Skin lesions are present in about 50% of cases, and there may be lymphadenopathy and hepatosplenomegaly.
- Chronic ATLL (20%): A lymphocytosis may be present with few circulating atypical lymphoid cells. Hypercalcemia is absent and serum LDH is normal or only slightly raised (less than or equal to twice the upper limit of normal). Skin lesions, including an exfoliative rash, may occur and there may be mild lymphadenopathy and/or splenomegaly.
- Smoldering ATLL (5%): The lymphocyte count is normal but >5% of circulating lymphocytes are abnormal T cells. Hypercalcemia is absent. Skin and pulmonary involvement are frequent. Lymphadenopathy or hepatosplenomegaly are absent. Serum LDH is normal or only slightly raised (less than or equal to 1.5 times the upper limit of normal).
- Lymphomatous ATLL (20%): Peripheral blood involvement is seen in this variant, the disease being characterized by prominent lymphadenopathy, usually of advanced stage. Hypercalcemia is less frequent than in the acute form of the disease, but skin lesions are common.

Cutaneous lesions are reported in 43–72% of cases and may be seen in all forms of the disease, but are less common in the lymphomatous subtype (*Figs 29.145 and 29.146*).[2,9–13] Skin lesions are somewhat heterogeneous, presenting as papules, nodules, tumors, plaques, or erythema/erythroderma.[10,14,15] Rarely, pompholyx-, keloid-, and granuloma-like lesions and hyperpigmented, purpuric, vesicular, and bullous lesions are seen.[10,16,17] A cutaneous variant, in which monoclonal lymphocytes proliferate in skin only, has been proposed.[14,18–20] This is because such cases are associated with a poorer prognosis than smoldering ATLL (the category in which most would currently be grouped), but a much better outcome than the other variants.[14,21]

Many patients have a T-cell-associated immunodeficiency and are immunocompromised. Opportunistic infections, including *Pneumocystis jiroveci* pneumonia, candidiasis, cryptococcosis, CMV, and strongyloidiasis, are common. Prognosis is related to the clinical subtype, age, serum calcium, and LDH levels and, for cases with cutaneous involvement, the type of skin lesion, those with patches and plaques doing relatively well, whilst those with eryhtroderma have a particularly poor outcome.[1,2,22] The median survival for acute and lymphomatous variants ranges from around 2 weeks to 1 year while patients with chronic and smoldering forms can survive for up to 2 years or longer.[1,23] Death is usually due to infection, hypercalcemia, or tumor burden.

Pathogenesis and histologic features

ATLL develops only in HTLV-1 infection and the malignant cells contain integrated HTLV-1 provirus, providing strong support for a causative role.[24] HTLV-1 is transmitted via peripheral blood (intravenous drug abuse, sexual intercourse), blood products, or from mother to child transplacentally or via breast milk. However, a relatively low proportion of infected individuals go on to develop ATLL, the cumulative risk for males being 6.6% and for females 2.1%.[24,25] There is also a long latent period, most cases seeming to follow transmission by breastfeeding, with the average age of a Japanese patient being 60 years.[24,26] This implies that an as-yet unidentified cofactor is necessary for transformation.

HTLV-1 proviral DNA is randomly integrated into host cell DNA with transcription of viral genes. Expression of the transcriptional transactivator protein, Tax, and/or the HTLV-1 basic leucine zipper factor seems to be important for transformation. These may act via downstream effects on cell cycle progression and/or apoptosis following activation of the NF-κB pathway.[24,26,27]

Complex karyotypes are seen in ATLL together with a variety of clonal chromosomal abnormalities.[4,28–33] Mutations or loss of function of a number of tumor suppressor genes, including cyclin-dependent kinase inhibitors (p15, p16), p53, and Rb have also been identified, particularly in the lymphomatous and acute variants.[34,35] Overexpression of p21 may also occur.[36] Recurrent mutations involving the RHOA, TET2, and CCR4 genes have also been demonstrated in a significant percentage of cases.[36–39]

Circulating leukemic cells have characteristic morphology with hyperlobated pleomorphic nuclei that sometimes resemble a clover leaf, with condensed chromatin and inconspicuous nucleoli.[40] They contain acid phosphatase, β-glucuronidase, and acid-naphthyl acetate esterase.[41] Immunophenotypically, they are helper/inducer T lymphocytes.[42]

In tissues, a broad spectrum of cytological appearances may be seen including pleomorphic small, medium, and large cell, anaplastic large cell, Hodgkin-like and AITL-like (*Figs 29.147 and 29.148*).[43] Cutaneous lesions may show perivascular, nodular, or diffuse patterns of infiltration.[14] In erythematous lesions, tumor cells are located in the upper dermis and are small to medium-sized lymphocytes with mild nuclear irregularity and few mitotic figures. In papules and nodules, a pan-dermal and sometimes subcutaneous nodular or diffuse infiltrate is seen. The lymphocytes are usually of medium to large size with highly irregular nuclear outlines, coarsely

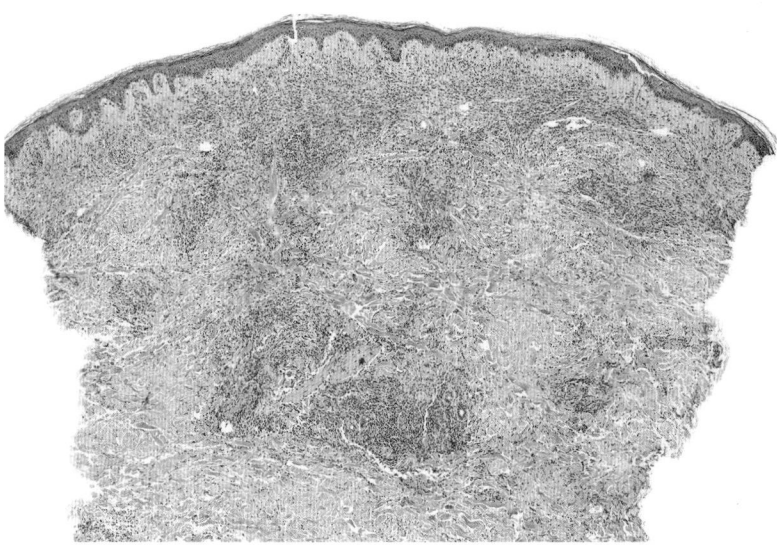

Fig. 29.147
Adult T-cell leukemia/lymphoma: there is a dense infiltrate within the dermis.

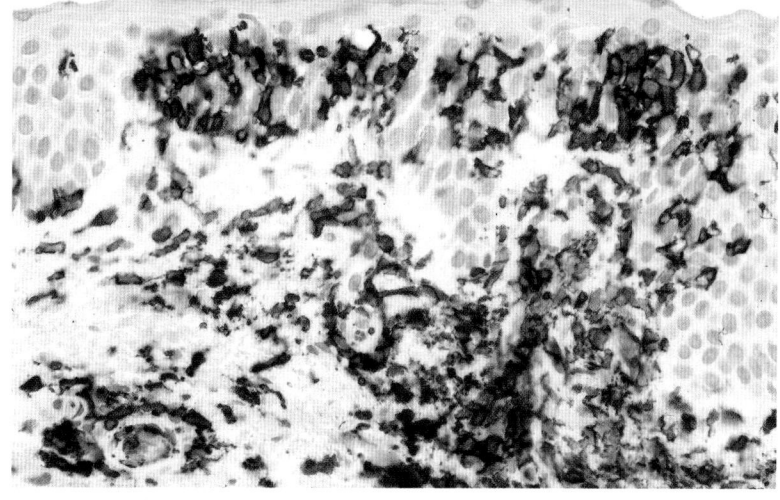

Fig. 29.149
Adult T-cell leukemia/lymphoma: the lymphocytes are CD4+ T-helper cells.

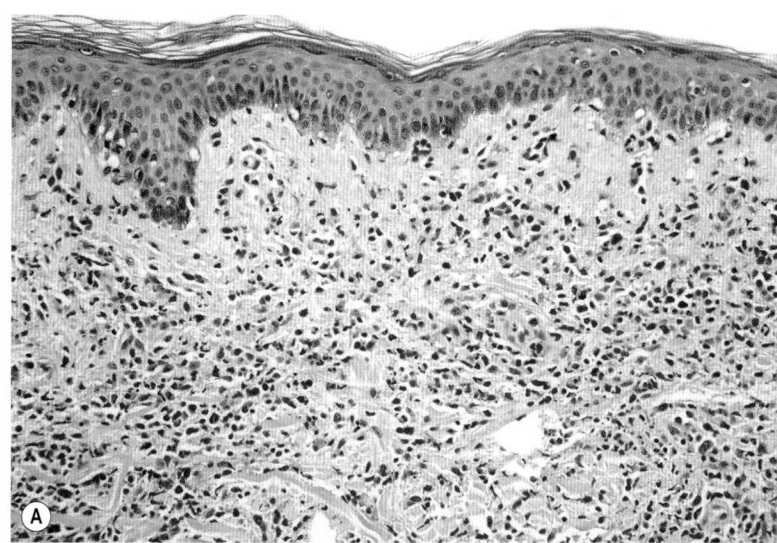

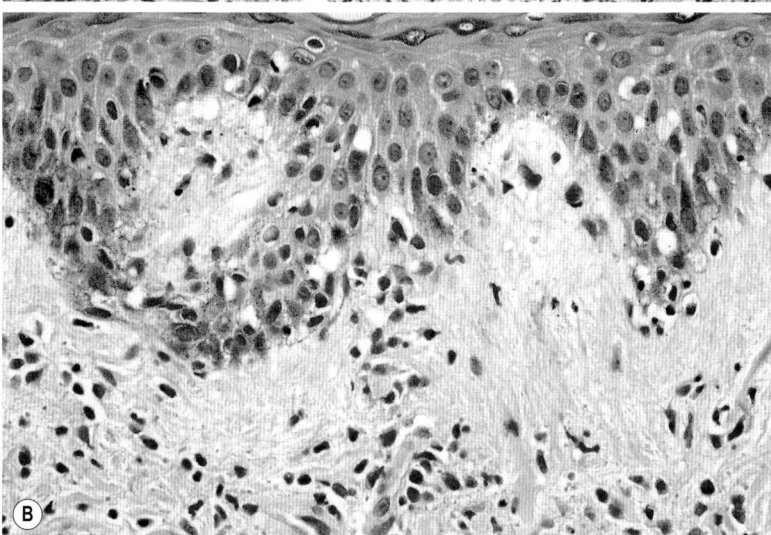

Fig. 29.148
(A, B) Adult T-cell leukemia/lymphoma: the infiltrate is composed of an admixture of small and large pleomorphic lymphocytes. Note the epidermotropism. Distinction from mycosis fungoides depends on clinicopathological correlation.

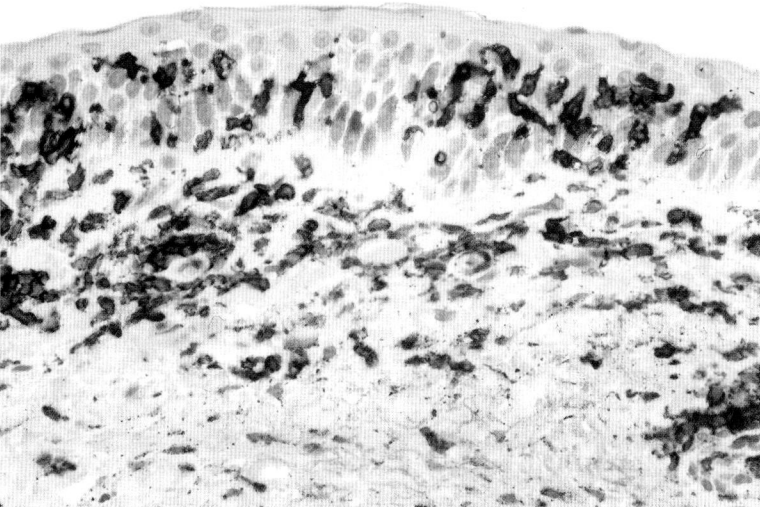

Fig. 29.150
Adult T-cell leukemia/lymphoma: there is uniform CD25 expression.

clumped chromatin, and sometimes prominent nucleoli. Blast-like cells, cerebriform giant cells, and Reed-Sternberg-like cells are present in some cases, and mitotic figures are frequent. Epidermotropism, with Pautrier microabscesses, may be seen, most frequently in association with perivascular infiltrates and lesions resemble mycosis fungoides or Sézary syndrome.[1,5,13,14,42–44] Histiocytes, plasma cells, and sometimes eosinophils are often evident.[42,44] Rare cases are associated with follicular mucinosis and granulomas are exceptional.[16,45–48]

In addition to bone marrow, skin, and lymph node involvement, widespread tumor infiltration is commonly present in the lung, liver, kidney, gastrointestinal tract, and central nervous system (CNS), in decreasing order of frequency.[16]

The cells are usually CD2+, CD3+, CD4+, CD5+, CD25+, and CD7– (Figs 29.149 and 29.150).[1,5] CD8+ variants have occasionally been documented, and rarely the tumor cells express both CD4 and CD8.[1,42] The large transformed cells may express CD30 but are negative for ALK1 and cytotoxic molecules. The tumor cells also frequently express the chemokine receptor CCR4 and FoxP3, suggesting a relationship to T-regulatory cells.[49]

Differential diagnosis

ATLL may show considerable overlap with mycosis fungoides and Sézary syndrome. The acute onset and typical lack of a patch stage are useful discriminants.[5] In cases of doubt, the diagnosis of ATLL may be firmly established serologically or by the identification of HTLV-I sequences in tumor DNA.

Subcutaneous panniculitis-like T-cell lymphoma

Clinical features

Subcutaneous panniculitis-like T-cell lymphoma (SPTCL), first described in 1991, is a rare tumor that may be associated with hemophagocytic syndrome.[1] Previously, many cases may have been variously reported as cytophagic histiocytic panniculitis, Weber-Christian disease, histiocytic lymphoma, malignant histiocytosis, or histiocytic medullary reticulosis.[2,3] SPTCL became recognized as a distinct entity in the 2001 WHO Classification.[4-6] However, since then, it has become increasingly evident that distinction should be made between cases of alpha-beta and gamma-delta T-cell lineage, on the basis that the former usually display a CD4–, CD8+, CD56– phenotype and a favorable prognosis, and the latter, which are most often aggressive tumors with a CD4–, CD8–, CD56+ phenotype.[7-15] The current EORTC/WHO classification, and its 2016 update, therefore reserves the term SPTCL for alpha-beta positive cases, while gamma-delta cases are regarded as a separate entity, 'gamma-delta cutaneous T-cell lymphoma'.[16,17]

There is predilection for females (2:1).[15] SPTCL is seen in a wide age range, including children and the elderly.[17-20] Up to 20% of patients are <20 years old at diagnosis with a median age of 36 years.[15] Presentation is with erythematous or violaceous nodules or deep-seated plaques measuring from <1 to >20 cm (Fig. 29.151).[1,15] Ulceration is uncommon.[15,17] In most cases, lesions are generalized at presentation and involve the limbs and trunk, followed rarely by the face, neck, axilla, groins, and buttocks (Fig. 29.152). Patients with solitary or localized lesions are relatively uncommon.[15] B symptoms are seen in 50% of patients, and anemia, cytopenias, raised ESR, and deranged liver function tests are common.[15] There is usually no lymphadenopathy, and while hepatosplenomegaly may be seen, this is not due to lymphomatous infiltration.[7,15,16] A hemophagocytic syndrome is seen in up to 20% of cases, characterized by hepatosplenomegaly, coagulopathy with widespread bleeding, weight loss, fever, and myalgia.[1,15]

Although earlier literature suggests that SPTCL is an aggressive disease with a high mortality, this is largely due to the inclusion of gamma-delta-positive cases.[7,12,15] If more stringent criteria are used to define the entity, then SPTCL has a favorable prognosis with 5-year overall and disease-specific survival rates of 80–90%.[15] Cases associated with a hemophagocytic syndrome have a poorer prognosis, with a 5-year overall survival of only 46%.[5,10] Although polychemotherapy may be required, particularly in patients with hemophagocytic syndrome, first-line treatment with immunomodulatory agents, such as steroids and ciclosporin A, may be effective in some patients.[21,22] SPTCL usually remains confined to the skin throughout its course, with death occurring due to hemophagocytic syndrome or complications of treatment.[1,7]

Histopathological features

The etiology of SPTCL is unknown. A significant percentage of cases are associated with autoimmune disease, particularly lupus erythematosus, and lupus erythematosus panniculitis (LEP) and SPTCL may exhibit overlapping clinical and pathological features.[15,23-27] Thus, it has been proposed that there is a spectrum of disease encompassing LEP and SPTCL at either end.[23-27] This is supported by recent gene expression profiling studies demonstrating up-regulation of genes in SPTCL that are also associated with autoimmune disorders, including lupus.[28] SPTCL also harbors chromosomal abnormalities that identify it as a specific subgroup among cutaneous T-cell lymphomas.[29]

The infiltrate typically involves fat lobules with limited septal involvement. There may be some extension into the deep reticular dermis, but the superficial dermis and epidermis are usually spared.[1,15] Angioinvasion and angiodestruction are uncommon.[15] Neoplastic lymphocytes vary in size and comprise small to intermediate-sized lymphocytes with only scattered large cells. Nuclei are hyperchromatic and cytoplasm is scanty (Figs 29.153–29.158).[15] Rimming of individual fat cells is typical, but may be focal and is not specific.[30] Karyorrhexis and fat necrosis are almost always present, usually in association with histiocytes, and occasionally granulomatous inflammation.[10,15,16] Histiocytes are frequently vacuolated, may contain phagocytosed nuclear debris, or display erythrophagocytosis. Reactive small lymphocytes may also be seen, while neutrophils and eosinophils are rare.[1,15,16,30] Plasma cells and lymphoid follicles are also sparse except in cases overlapping with LEP.[27]

Tumor cells display a cytotoxic phenotype and are CD3+, CD4–, CD8+ with expression of the cytotoxic molecules granzyme B, TIA-1, and perforin, although rarely CD4+, CD8–, and CD4–, CD8– cases may occur.[17,29] Loss of the pan-T-cell antigens CD2, CD5, and CD7 occurs in 10%, 50%, and 44% of cases, respectively.[15] CD30 is usually negative, and rarely few

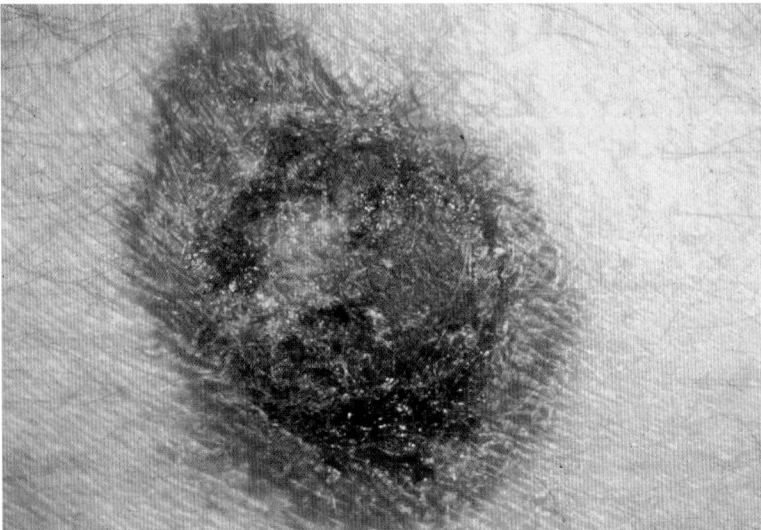

Fig. 29.151
Subcutaneous panniculitis-like T-cell lymphoma: this patient presented with multiple, ulcerated nodules on the legs. By courtesy of D. McGibbon, MD, Institute of Dermatology, London, UK.

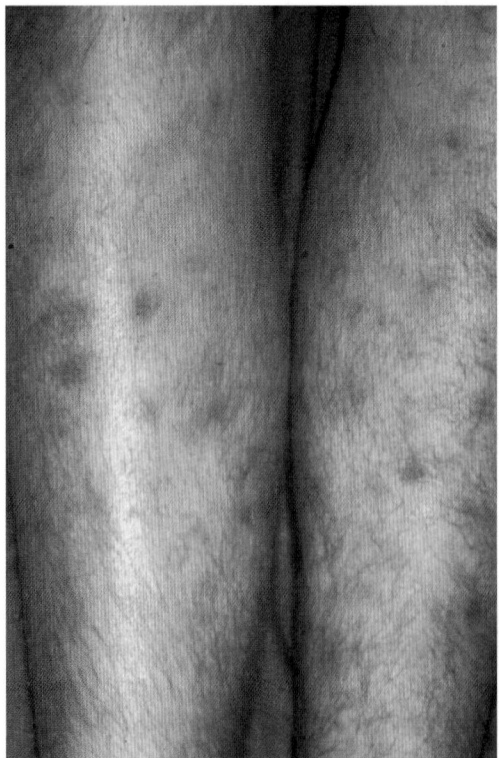

Fig. 29.152
Subcutaneous panniculitis-like T-cell lymphoma: in this picture, the lesions are reminiscent of erythema nodosum. By courtesy of D. McGibbon, MD, Institute of Dermatology, London, UK.

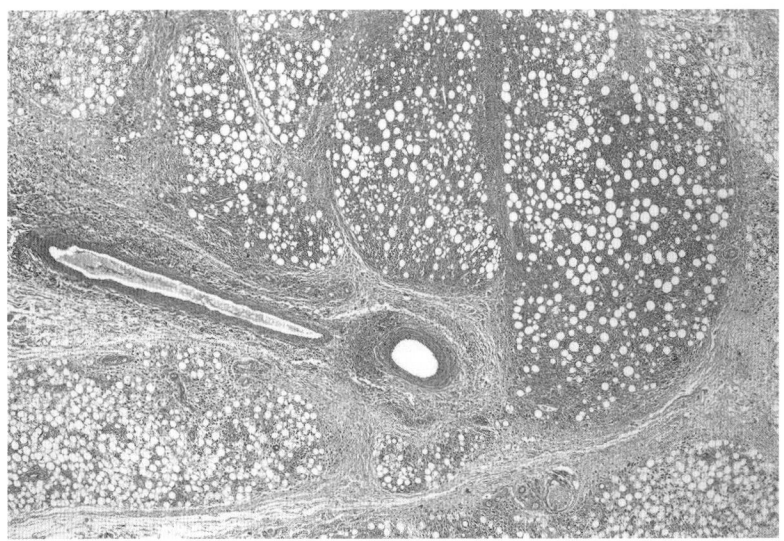

Fig. 29.153
Subcutaneous panniculitis-like T-cell lymphoma: there is a dense infiltrate in the subcutaneous fat, giving rise to a characteristic lacelike appearance.

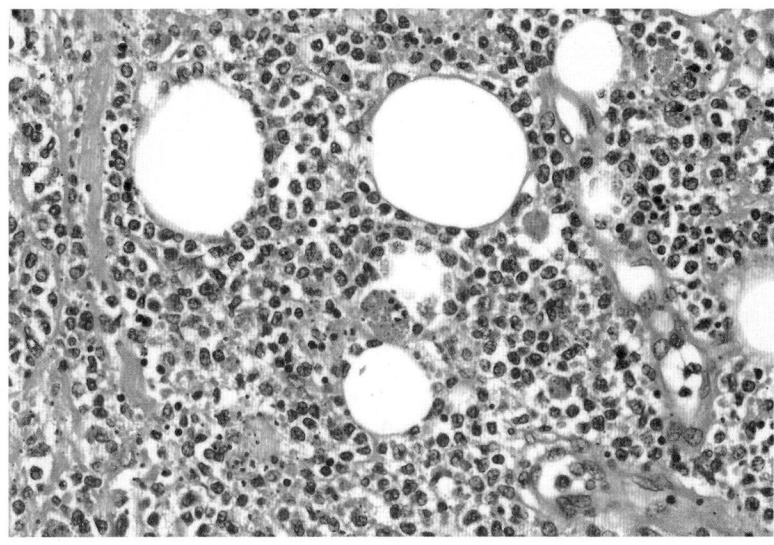

Fig. 29.156
Subcutaneous panniculitis-like T-cell lymphoma: this field shows conspicuous erythrophagocytosis.

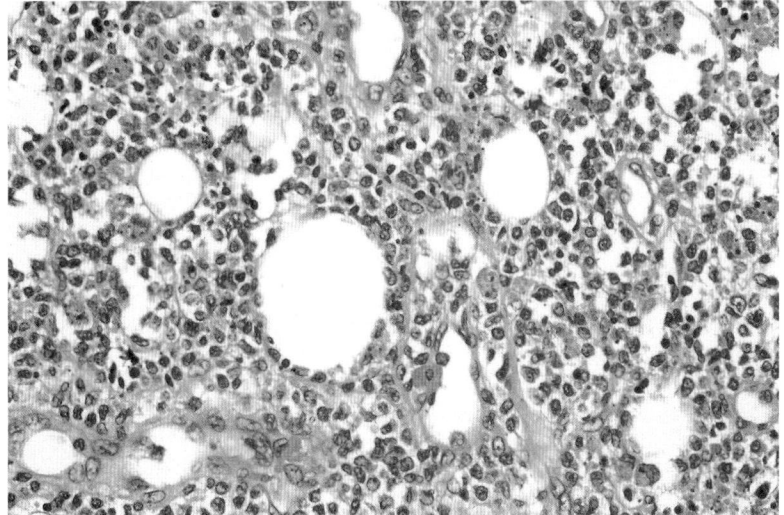

Fig. 29.154
Subcutaneous panniculitis-like T-cell lymphoma: the tumor cells have variably vesicular or hyperchromatic nuclei. Note the characteristic rimming of the adipocytes.

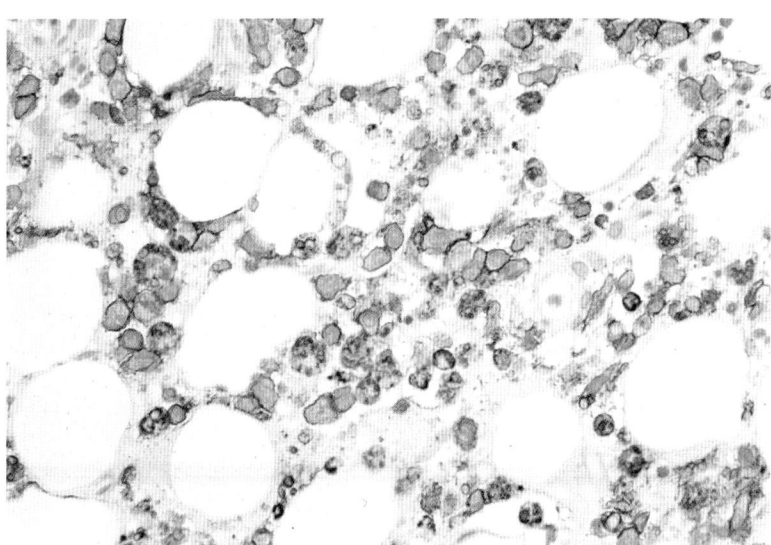

Fig. 29.157
Subcutaneous panniculitis-like T-cell lymphoma: the lymphocytes express CD3.

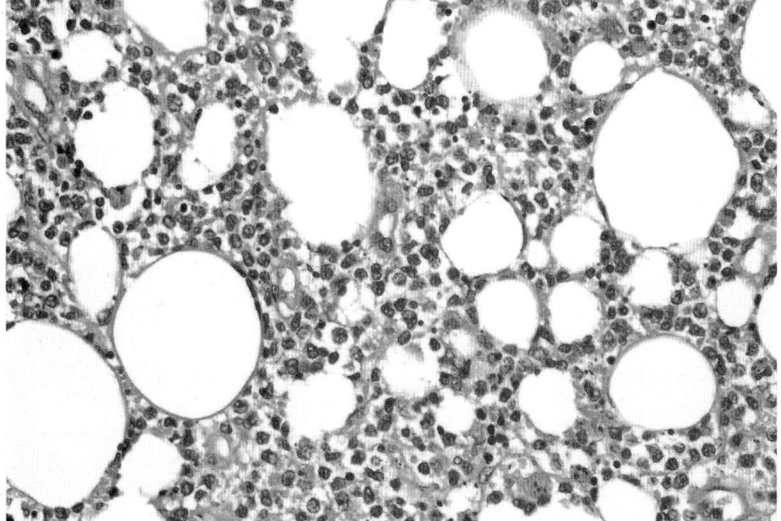

Fig. 29.155
Subcutaneous panniculitis-like T-cell lymphoma: there is an admixture of tumor cells and histiocytes.

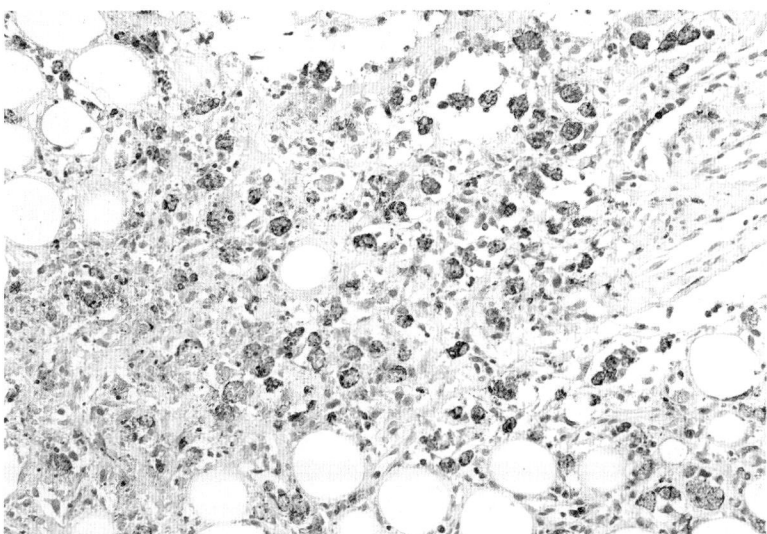

Fig. 29.158
Subcutaneous panniculitis-like T-cell lymphoma: the histiocytes are highlighted by CD68.

CD56+ cells are seen.[15,29] Beta F1 is usually identifiable, commensurate with an alpha-beta phenotype. EBV is absent, apart from exceptional cases from Asia.[15,30]

Clonal rearrangements of the T-cell receptor genes are generally identified.[15]

Differential diagnosis

The main differential diagnosis includes cutaneous gamma-delta T-cell lymphoma and extranodal T/NK-cell lymphoma, nasal type.[9–11,31–34] Immunohistochemistry should readily help distinguish between these entities. Cutaneous gamma-delta T-cell lymphomas are usually CD4–, CD8–, lack beta F1, and typically express CD56. Extranodal T/NK-cell lymphomas usually lack CD3 as well as CD4 and CD8, and express CD56. Moreover, staining for EBV is invariably positive.

LEP may be difficult to distinguish from SPTCL. It may be prudent to screen all cases of suspected SPTCL for lupus erythematosus.[15] In general, a diagnosis of LEP should be strongly considered when numerous plasma cells, areas of hyalinization, and reactive germinal centers are seen, with epidermal involvement. Aggregates of CD123 positive plasmocytoid dendritic cells may also be seen. A polyclonal pattern of gene rearrangement would also favor a diagnosis of lupus.

Extranodal NK/T-cell lymphoma, nasal type

Clinical features

Natural killer (NK) cells are members of the innate immune system that mediate major histocompatibility complex (MHC)-unrestricted target cell lysis without prior antigen exposure.[1] True NK cells are characterized by germline TCR genes, absence of a fully assembled TCR-CD3 complex on the cell surface, and expression of CD16 and CD56.[1] They typically possess cytotoxic granules.[1,2]

NK cells and cytotoxic T cells are closely related and share certain phenotypic features. Cytotoxic T cells often express NK-associated antigens such as CD56, and NK cells may react with antibodies to T-cell-associated antigens including CD2, CD7, and CD8.[1,3] The diagnostic category of NK/T-cell lymphoma reflects this blurred distinction, and while most cases belonging to this entity are genuine neoplasms of NK cells, inclusion of cases displaying some features of a cytotoxic T-cell phenotype is also permitted.[4]

Examples of NK/T-cell lymphoma have previously been described as lethal midline granuloma, polymorphic reticulosis, and angiocentric T-cell lymphoma. However, these diagnostic categories also contain a variety of other malignancies that share some clinical (e.g., involvement of upper respiratory tract or skin) and pathological (e.g., an angiocentric growth pattern, expression of CD56) features with NK/T-cell lymphoma. These entities have now been separated into their own categories, such as lymphomatoid granulomatosis (LG), γ/δ T-cell lymphoma, and subcutaneous panniculitis-like T-cell lymphoma. Most patients are adults with a median age at presentation of around 50 years and a slight male predominance. It is more common in East Asian countries such as China, Korea, and Japan, rare in Europeans, and relatively frequently encountered in Native Americans in Mexico and South and Central America.[4–13] As the name implies, most cases are extranodal in location with predilection for the upper aerodigestive tract, particularly the nasal cavity, nasopharynx, paranasal sinuses, and palate.[14] It is characterized by destructive midline lesions and involvement of the nasal cavity, nasopharynx, paranasal sinuses, and/or palate. Orbital swelling and edema may be prominent.[4,11,15] Other extranodal sites may also be involved including skin, soft tissue, gastrointestinal tract, and testis, and in some cases disease is present in the absence of nasal involvement (so-called 'extranasal type').[14,16–18] After the upper aerodigestive tract, skin is the most frequently involved site of presentation, and in rare cases the disease may be primary cutaneous in origin.[5,16,19–23] Cutaneous lesions consist of multiple nodules or plaque, sometimes ulcerated. Vasculitis, panniculitis-like, and cellulitis-like appearances may occur.[19,20,24,25] Lesions present at more than one anatomic site, with predilection for the trunk and/or limbs.[5,20] However, sometimes they are solitary, restricted to one anatomic site, and this seems to be more common in the skin.[19]

Systemic symptoms (fever, malaise, and weight loss) and the hemophagocytic syndrome may be present.[16,24–28] Lymph nodes are involved as part of disseminated disease and only rarely represent primary disease.[8,29,30] Bone marrow and peripheral blood involvement is uncommon and when present raises the possibility of aggressive NK-cell leukemia.[31]

The survival rates for extranodal NK/T-cell lymphoma have been very poor, with more than 60% of patients succumbing to disease, often within a matter of months. However, response and survival rates have improved with more aggressive treatments.[4,16] The most important prognostic factor is the presence or absence of nasal disease, those with nasal involvement having a significantly superior survival compared to 'extranasal' cases.[14] A particularly poor prognosis appears to be associated with extranodal NK/T-cell lymphoma presenting primarily as cutaneous disease compared to nasal or other extranodal sites.[16,19–21,23,32]

Pathogenesis and histologic features

Extranodal NK/T-cell lymphoma is strongly associated with EBV, and some cases arise in the context of immunosuppression.[29,33–36] Most Japanese patients are infected with type A EBV with a 30-base-pair deletion in the LMP1 gene, suggesting a pathogenetic role for the virus.[37,38] Various cytogenetic abnormalities have been described. By conventional cytogenetics, deletions of 6q are common, whilst CGH and loss-of-heterozygosity studies reveal frequent DNA gains and losses.[39–41] Mutations or partial deletions of various genes may also occur, including TP53, TP73, CDKN2A, CDKN2B, MDM2, FAS, KIT, RAS, ATR, and STAT3.[39,42–47] Inactivation of PDRM has also been implicated in disease pathogenesis.[48,49]

The poor response to treatment in NK/T-cell lymphoma has been attributed to overexpression of multidrug resistance proteins.[50,51] The extensive coagulative necrosis seen in many cases and attributed to vascular occlusion by lymphoma cells may also be due to release of cytokines and chemokines by tumor cells.[52]

Skin biopsies show a dense, nodular, or diffuse dermal infiltrate, which often extends into the subcutaneous fat (Fig. 29.159).[4,21,24,53–55] The infiltrate is typically angiocentric, often angiodestructive, and associated with extensive zonal necrosis (Figs 29.160 and 29.161). Epidermotropism is exceptional. Tumor cells are variable, ranging from small to medium or large with irregular, granular, or vesicular chromatin, inconspicuous or small nucleoli, and moderate amounts of pale or clear cytoplasm (Fig. 29.162).[4,53,55] Mitoses are abundant. Small lymphocytes, plasma cells, histiocytes, and eosinophils may be seen. Florid pseudoepitheliomatous hyperplasia is noted at mucosal sites.[4]

Cases with an NK-cell phenotype typically express CD2 and CD56, as well as cytoplasmic but not membranous CD3. Cytotoxic molecules (TIA-1,

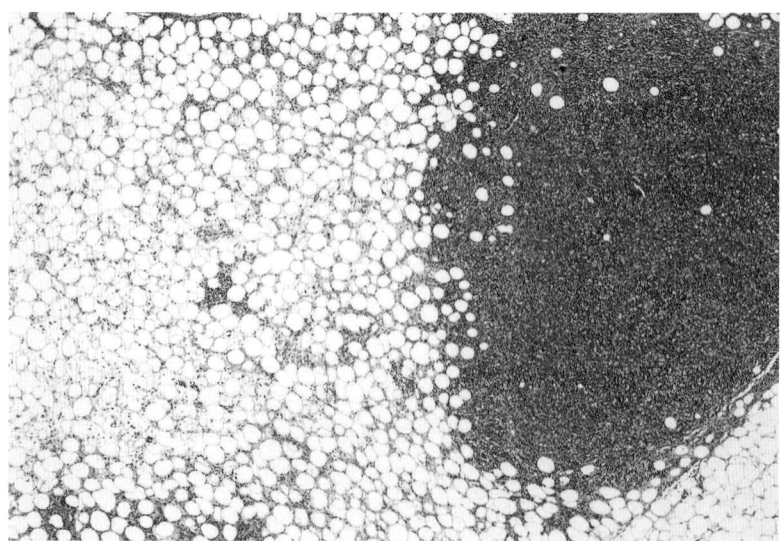

Fig. 29.159
Extranodal NK/T-cell lymphoma: this case presented with nodules in the subcutaneous fat clinically reminiscent of erythema nodosum. There is extensive infiltration of the dermis and subcutaneous fat by atypical lymphocytes.

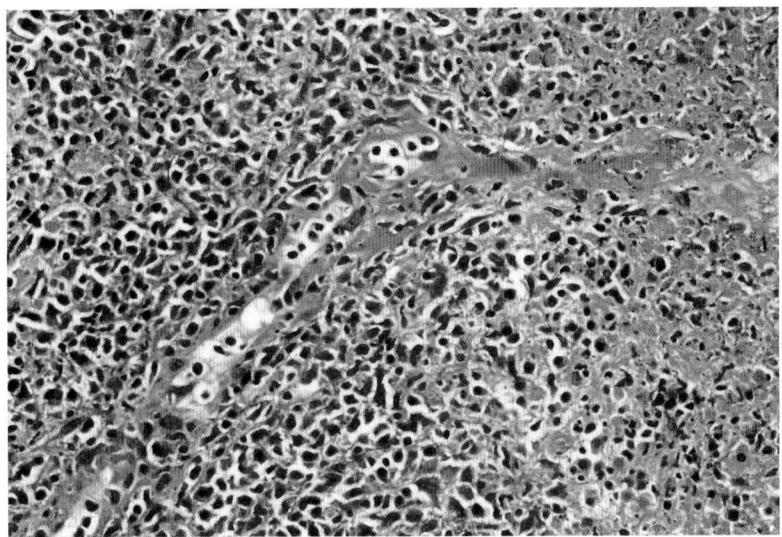

Fig. 29.160
Extranodal NK/T-cell lymphoma: in this example, there is fibrinoid necrosis affecting a large venule.

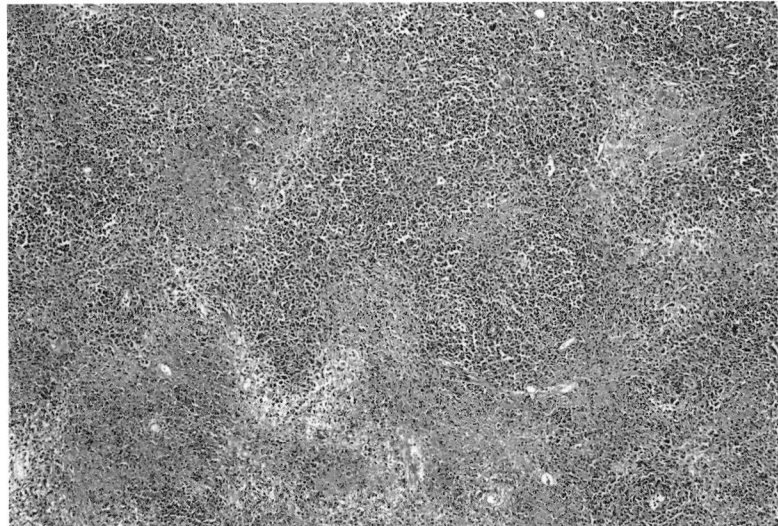

Fig. 29.161
Extranodal NK/T-cell lymphoma: massive geographic necrosis is a characteristic feature.

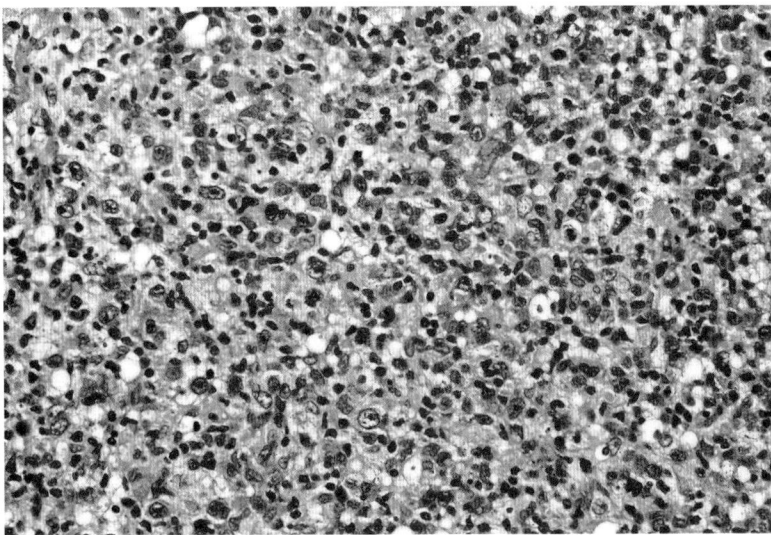

Fig. 29.162
Extranodal NK/T-cell lymphoma: the tumor cells have large vesicular nuclei with prominent nucleoli.

granzyme B, perforin) are present, but other T-cell-associated antigens, including CD3, CD4, CD5, CD7 and CD8, are usually lacking, as are the NK-cell antigens CD16 and CD57.[2,4,10,14] Extranodal NK/T-cell lymphoma of NK-cell origin also display a germline pattern of T-cell receptor gene rearrangement.[4,56,57] A T-cell lineage is documented in 10–40% of cases and is associated with expression of one or more of CD2, CD3, CD4, CD5, CD7, and CD8, together with cytotoxic molecules and/or a monoclonal T-cell receptor gene rearrangement.[16,21,58]

Differential diagnosis

Before the advent of immunophenotyping, NK/T-cell cutaneous lymphoma and lymphomatoid granulomatosis were readily confused. It now recognized that lymphomatoid granulomatosis represents an EBV-positive clonal B-cell proliferation associated with a brisk reactive T-cell infiltrate. Immunohisto-chemistry and in situ hybridization for EBV should also allow most cases to be readily distinguished from other lymphoma subtypes including subcutaneous panniculitis-like T-cell lymphoma, blastic plasmacytoid dendritic cell neoplasm (BPDCN), primary cutaneous CD8+ aggressive epidermotropic cytotoxic T-cell lymphoma, cutaneous γ/δT-cell lymphoma, and peripheral T-cell lymphoma, unspecified.[14] There may be considerable pathological overlap between extranodal NK/T-cell lymphoma and HV-like lymphopro-liferative disorder, separation often being largely dependent on clinical features. HV-like lymphoproliferative disorder typically presents in a younger age group and has a protracted, rather than a rapidly progressive, course.

Primary cutaneous CD8-positive aggressive epidermotropic cytotoxic T-cell lymphoma

The majority of cutaneous T-cell lymphomas (CTCLs) consist of lympho-cytes with the phenotype of resting or activated CD4-positive memory T cells. However, a proportion exhibit a CD8-positive cytotoxic phenotype. Expression of CD8 may be characteristic of a particular entity, as in subcu-taneous panniculitis-like T-cell lymphoma. CD8 expression may occasionally be seen in lymphoma subtypes that more commonly express CD4, including typical cases of mycosis fungoides, pagetoid reticulosis, lymphomatoid pap-ulosis, and cutaneous anaplastic large cell lymphoma.[1-8] In addition, there is a subset of CD8-positive lymphomas with a distinctive clinical presentation and aggressive clinical course, suggesting a specific entity, primary cutane-ous CD8-positive epidermotropic cytotoxic T-cell lymphoma.[2,9-16] This was a provisional entity in the 2008 WHO classification and remains so in the 2016 update.[17,18] Examples may previously have been described as general-ized pagetoid reticulosis (Ketron-Goodman disease) or mycosis fungoides d'emblee.[17]

Clinical features

Primary cutaneous CD8-positive aggressive epidermotropic cytotoxic T-cell lymphoma accounts for less than 1% of all CTCLs. Most patients are adults who present with a generalized, rapidly progressive eruption consisting of erythematous patches and plaques, verrucous hemorrhagic papules, nodules, and tumors with occasional oral involvement (*Fig. 29.163*).[1,11,14,16,19-22] Disease progression is relentless, with widespread vis-ceral metastases to uncommon sites including the testis, lungs, spleen, and CNS (without lymphadenopathy) and high mortality (mean survival time, 32 months).[1,9,11,14,16,20-22]

Histologic features

Histologically, lesions are characterized by a highly epidermotropic atypi-cal lymphoid infiltrate (*Figs 29.164* and *29.165*), usually with a pagetoid appearance and usually lacking Pautrier microabscesses.[21] Associated epi-dermal necrosis is common.[1,9,20,21] The tumor cells display varying cytology but are often of medium to large size with enlarged hyperchromatic nuclei. A dermal infiltrate is almost always present and often extends to the deep reticular dermis or subcutaneous fat.[20,21] Angiocentricity and angioinvasion are also frequently present.[11,15,20,21] Syringotropism and folliculotropism can be seen. Histiocytes, eosinophils, and plasma cells might also be noted.

The tumor cells are of alpha/beta phenotype, react with antibodies to beta F1, and express CD3 and CD8 (*Fig. 29.166*). They usually express

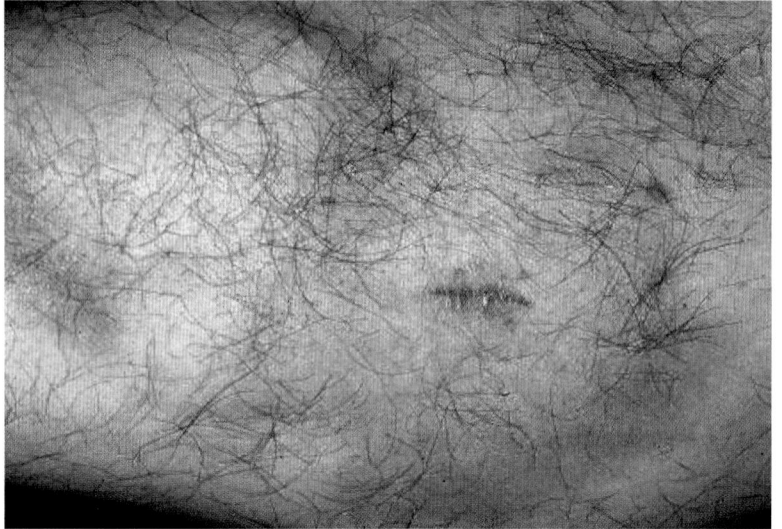

Fig. 29.163
Primary cutaneous CD8+ aggressive epidermotropic T-cell lymphoma: note the large erythematous plaque. By courtesy of R.A. Johnson, MD, Massachusetts General Hospital, Harvard Medical School, Boston, USA.

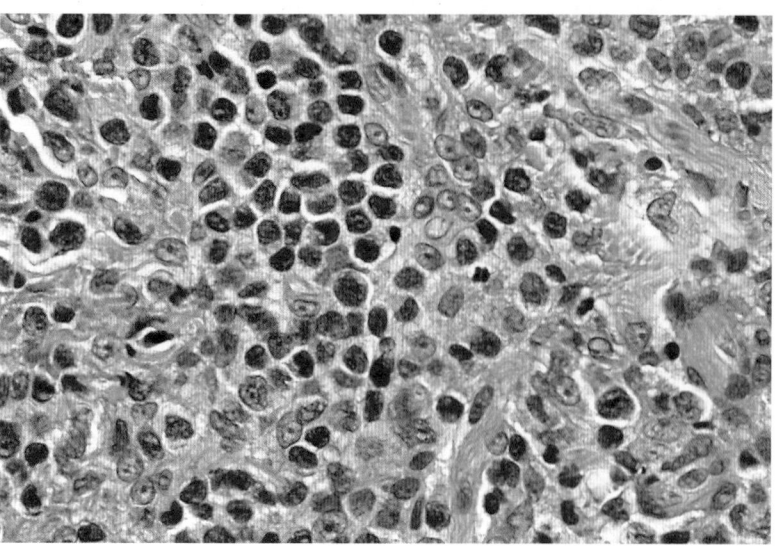

Fig. 29.165
Primary cutaneous CD8+ aggressive epidermotropic T-cell lymphoma: the lymphocytes have enlarged, irregular hyperchromatic nuclei.

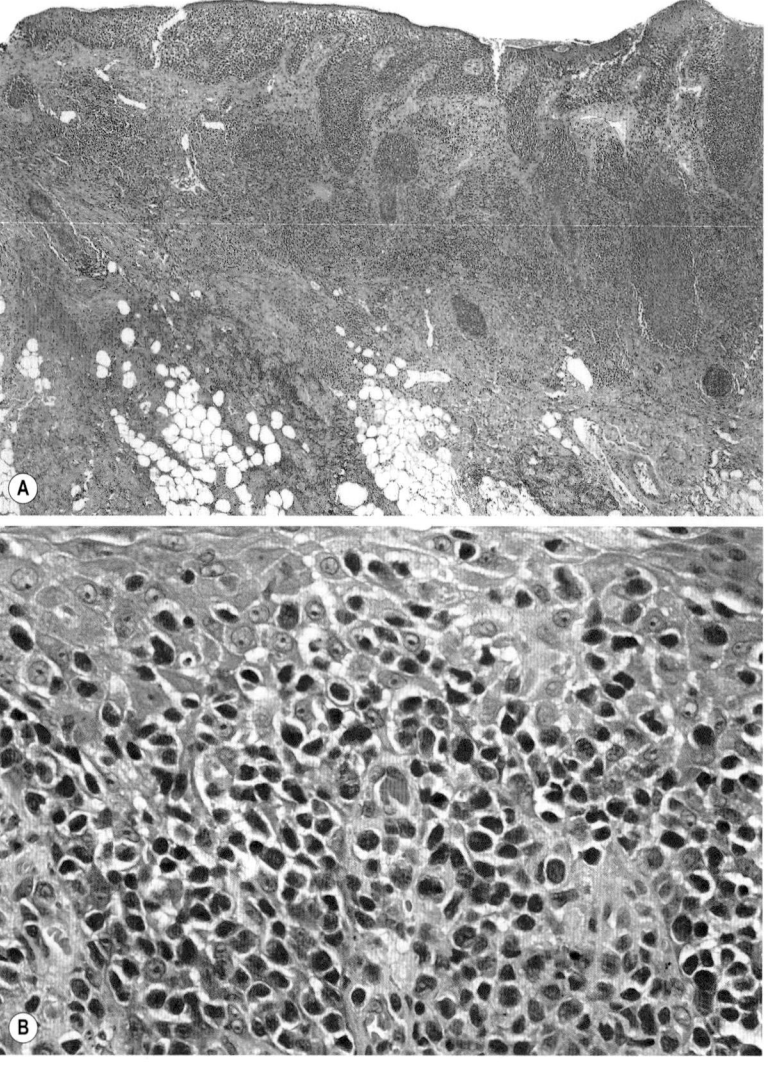

Fig. 29.164
(**A**, **B**) Primary cutaneous CD8+ aggressive epidermotropic T-cell lymphoma: there is a dense superficial perivascular and bandlike upper dermal infiltrate with marked epidermotropism.

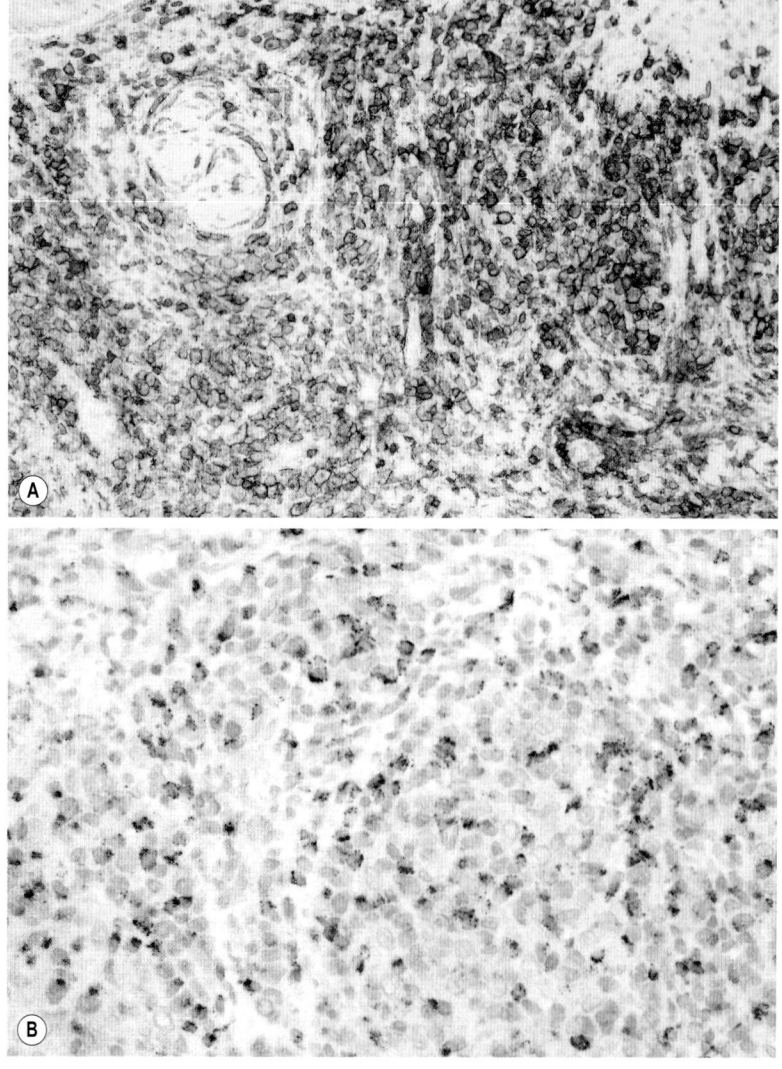

Fig. 29.166
(**A**, **B**) Primary cutaneous CD8+ aggressive epidermotropic T-cell lymphoma: (**A**) the lymphocytes express CD8; (**B**) TIA1 is positive.

CD7, while CD2 and CD5 are frequently lost, and CD4 is negative.[1,9,15,17,20,21] TIA1 is detectable, but perforin and granzyme B may be negative.[1] There is no association with EBV infection.[1,15,20,21] Flow cytometry results suggest that the tumor cells may express CD15, and that circulating CD8-positive tumor cells are detectable in peripheral blood, although the latter seems to be antibody dependent.[22–24]

Differential diagnosis

Clinical correlation is paramount in distinguishing primary cutaneous CD8-positive epidermotropic cytotoxic T-cell lymphoma from other CD8-positive lymphoproliferations that may also display marked epidermotropism. These include mycosis fungoides, pagetoid reticulosis, and some cases of lymphomatoid papulosis. In particular, short history and disseminated nature of lesions at presentation, together with the rapid clinical course, sets primary cutaneous CD8-positive epidermotropic cytotoxic T-cell lymphoma apart.[20] Distinction from primary cutaneous gamma-delta T-cell lymphoma, which is occasionally CD8-positive, can be achieved by determining the nature of the surface T-cell receptor by staining with antibodies to the BF1, γ, and/or δ subunits.

Hydroa vacciniforme-like lymphoma

Clinical features

HV was historically defined in Western countries as a photosensitivity disorder of childhood characterized by development of papules and vesicles on sun-exposed skin of the face and dorsum of hands. Lesions evolve to crusts that heal, leaving varicelliform scars.[1] In most cases, the onset is in childhood with resolution during early adult life. There are no associated systemic symptoms. Conversely, HV-like lymphoma was the name given to a clinical syndrome clinically very similar to HV but with a more aggressive clinical course. This was described predominantly in children from East Asia, Latin America, and Mexico. Patients with HV-like lymphoma present with marked facial edema and recurring vesiculopapular rashes with development of large ulcers and crusts. Healing of these lesions is associated with severe scarring and disfigurement. Unlike classical HV, the skin lesions develop on sun-exposed and non-sun-exposed skin. In addition, systemic symptoms are usually present in the form of fever, weight loss, hepatosplenomegaly, and lymphadenopathy. There is frequent association with severe mosquito bite hypersensitivity, and the prognosis is often poor with a fatal outcome.[2–9] Past names for this condition include edematous scarring vasculitic panniculitis, hydroa-like lymphoma, and angiocentric cutaneous T-cell lymphoma of childhood.[2,3] Cases referred to as severe HV-like eruption are probably part of the spectrum.[10,11] This entity was incorporated into the 2008 WHO classification and considered separate from classical HV.[12]

Further analysis of cases has shown considerable clinical and pathological overlap between patients originally designated classical HV and HV-like lymphoma, and there is a lack of reproducible morphological, immunophenotypic, and molecular findings to allow the distinction of these two putative entities.[9,13,14] It has therefore been proposed that there is a spectrum of EBV-associated T/NK-cell lymphoproliferations with HV-like cutaneous manifestations. Classic, self-resolving HV lies at one end of this spectrum and HV-like lymphoma with an aggressive clinical course at the other.[9,13,15,16] Consequently, the currently preferred approach is to include all such lesions under the heading of HV-like lymphoproliferative disorder (LPD), and this is the recommended nomenclature used in the 2016 update of the WHO classification.[17]

The clinical features of HV-like LPD are as described above. All cases run a waxing and waning course. Extensive and disfiguring skin lesions, involvement of non-sun-exposed sites, and a potentially fatal clinical course characterize the more severe form of the illness. Cases that behave aggressively typically have severe symptoms at presentation. Death results from progression to T- or NK-cell lymphoma or leukemia, hepatic failure, or the consequences of treatment.[13] There is no standard treatment. Multiagent chemotherapy and radiotherapy offer little benefit, and these modalities may also increase the chances of dying from sepsis or liver failure.[3,4,14,18,19] Immunomodulatory therapies, using agents such as prednisolone, IFN-α,

chloroquine, and thalidomide may offer a better alternative as frontline treatment and have been shown to provide temporary remission or improvement of symptoms.[2,3,14,19]

Pathogenesis and histologic features

It is presumed that EBV is involved in driving proliferation of latently infected lymphocytes. Deletions of the long arm of chromosome 6 are seen, as in other EBV-associated lymphomas.[20,21]

Histologically, HV-like LPD is characterized by a perivascular and periadnexal lymphoid infiltrate. This may be relatively sparse in some cases with only few reactive appearing lymphocytes, but in others the infiltrate is dense with obvious cytological atypia manifesting as large cells with irregular nuclei, prominent nucleoli, and abundant clear cytoplasm. There may be associated angiodestruction with extension into the subcutaneous fat. There is no epidermotropism, but spongiotic vesicles are often present and lesions are frequently ulcerated.[13]

By definition, the infiltrating cells are positive for EBV by in situ hybridization, although they only rarely express LMP1 and are negative for EBNA2.[13] They typically account for only a proportion of the infiltrate (10–40%), with the remaining cells being reactive.[9,13] The phenotype of the EBV-positive cells is variable. In some cases they display a T-cell phenotype (60–70%), whilst others are proliferations of NK cells (30–40%).[9,13,14,18] The majority of cases of T-lineage show clonal rearrangement of the T-cell receptor gene.[13] The presence of more extensive, deeper infiltrates, often with involvement of the subcutis, tends to correlate with more severe symptomatology. Cases with an NK phenotype more often suffer from severe hypersensitivity to mosquito bite, more often have a prominent eosinophil component to the infiltrate, and show a tendency toward panniculitic lesions.[13,22,23] However, there are no pathological features that reliably predict clinical course.

Differential diagnosis

Demonstration of EBV in the neoplastic cells is essential in differentiating HV-like LPD from other entities that may also display an angiocentric and angiodestructive growth pattern, including primary cutaneous aggressive epidermotropic CD8-positive T-cell lymphoma and primary cutaneous γδ T-cell lymphoma. There is considerable pathological overlap between HV-like LPD and extranodal NK/T-cell lymphoma, and separation may be largely dependent on clinical features. HV-like LPD presents in a younger age group and has a more protracted course dominated by recurring papules and vesicles, with or without systemic symptoms and organomegaly, rather than progressively destructive masses.[13,14,16,24,25]

Primary cutaneous gamma/delta T-cell lymphoma

Clinical features

Gamma/delta T cells are cytotoxic members of the innate immune system.[1,2] They represent about 5% of the mature lymphocyte population and preferentially localize to epithelial-rich tissues and mucosal surfaces (skin, intestine and reproductive tract, and the sinusoidal areas of the spleen).[1,2] Tumors of gamma/delta T cells mirror this physiological distribution.

Primary cutaneous gamma/delta T-cell lymphoma (PCGD-TCL) is now recognized as a distinct entity in the most recent (2016) WHO classification and includes cases previously referred to as subcutaneous panniculitis-like T-cell lymphoma with a gamma/delta phenotype, and examples of CD4/CD8 double-negative cutaneous T-cell lymphoma.[3–8] Mucosal gamma/delta T-cell lymphoma is a closely related entity, but hepatosplenic gamma/delta T-cell lymphoma is biologically distinct, being derived from functionally immature gamma/delta T cells, which seem to belong to a different Vδ subset than the lymphocytes of PCGD-TCL.[8–12]

PCGD-TCL comprises only about 1% of all cutaneous T-cell lymphomas.[4,8,13,14] Most cases arise in adults, mainly males, with a wide age range (13–84 years; median, 59 years).[4,8,13,14] Presentation is with plaques reminiscent of mycosis fungoides, nodules, and (in some patients) subcutaneous lesions (Fig. 29.167).[5,11,15–19] There may be ulceration.[4,6,8,10,13,20,21] Lesions are usually generalized at presentation, with preferential involvement of

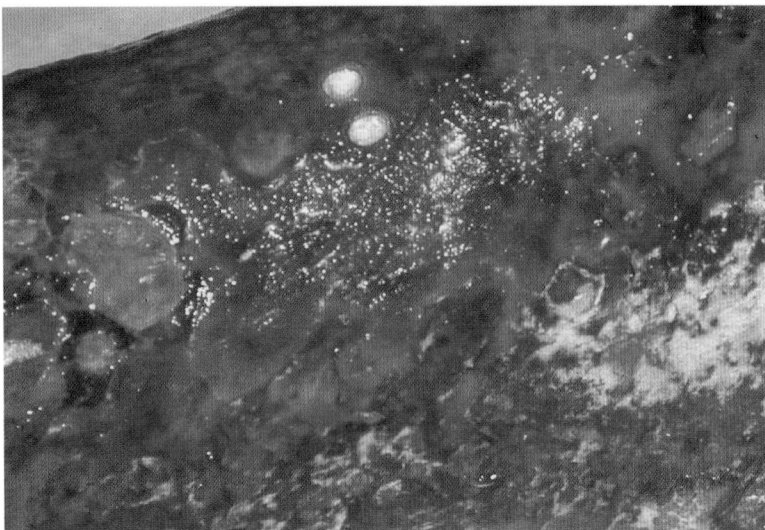

Fig. 29.167
Primary cutaneous gamma/delta T-cell lymphoma: this patient has extensively ulcerated lesions. By courtesy of M. Bosenberg, MD, University of Vermont, USA.

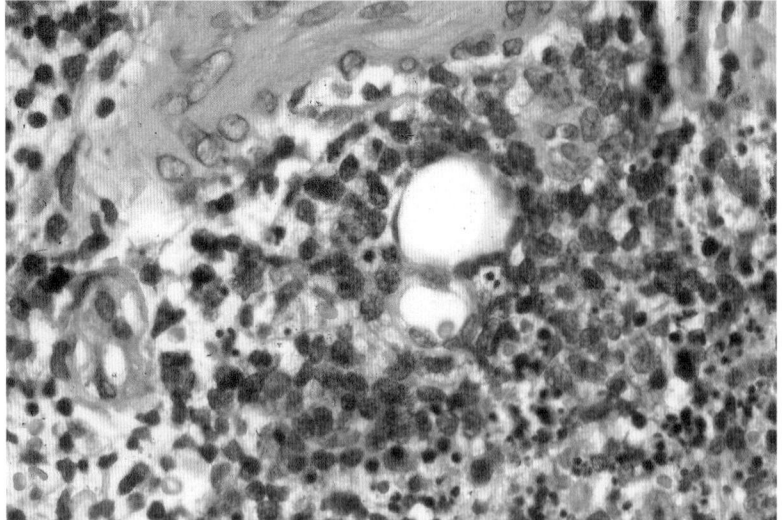

Fig. 29.169
Primary cutaneous gamma/delta T-cell lymphoma: the lymphocytes have irregular hyperchromatic nuclei. By courtesy of M. Bosenberg, MD, University of Vermont, USA.

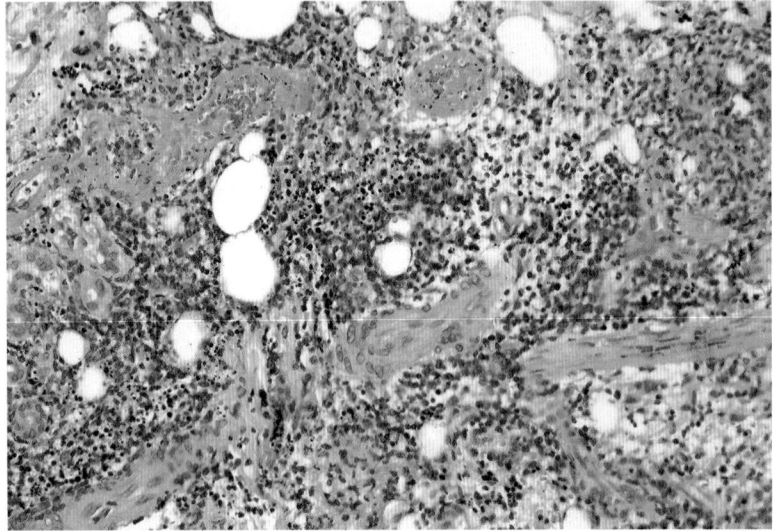

Fig. 29.168
Primary cutaneous gamma/delta T-cell lymphoma: the subcutaneous fat is infiltrated by markedly atypical lymphocytes. Note the vessel wall necrosis and thrombosis. By courtesy of M. Bosenberg, MD, University of Vermont, USA.

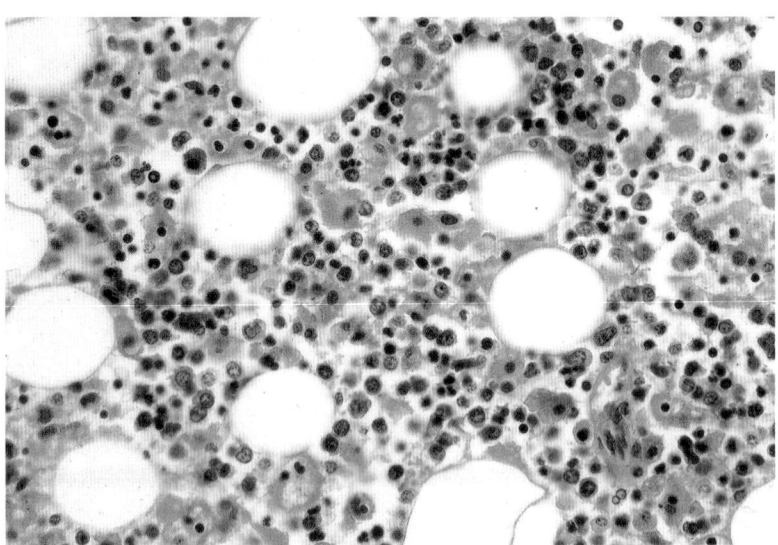

Fig. 29.170
Primary cutaneous gamma/delta T-cell lymphoma: this field shows marked erythrophagocytosis. By courtesy of M. Bosenberg, MD, University of Vermont, Vermont, USA.

the extremities and also the trunk.[4,13,15,16,22] Hemophagocytic syndrome occurs in up to 25% of patients, and the majority of patients have B symptoms.[4,8,13,16] The disease is resistant to treatment and the prognosis is poor, with a median survival of 15 months.[4,13] Cases with prominent subcutaneous involvement may carry a poorer prognosis than those with disease limited to the epidermis and dermis.[13,16] It has recently been suggested that a subgroup of gamma-delta cutaneous T-cell lymphomas in which epidermotropic cells represent more than 75% of the infiltrate, are distinctive and have better prognosis than those that are predominantly dermal and/or subcutaneous.[23]

Histologic features

Three major histologic patterns are recognized, but more than one pattern can be present in different biopsies from the same patient, or even within a single biopsy.[4,13,16,21,22] Plaques are characterized by epidermotropic infiltrates. The degree of epidermotropism may range from mild to pagetoid reticulosis-like.[11,15,16,21] Tumors may show predominantly dermal involvement, can be separated from the epidermis by a grenz zone, and extend into subcutaneous fat (Figs 29.168 and 29.169).[15] In subcutaneous lesions, the features closely resemble subcutaneous panniculitis-like T-cell lymphoma,

including rimming of fat cells, although dermal and epidermal involvement is usually also present (Fig. 20.170).[4,5,11–13,16,24] Tumor cells are medium to large with coarsely clumped chromatin. Blast cells are usually relatively infrequent. Necrosis and angioinvasion are common.[4,13,16]

By definition, the neoplastic lymphocytes in PCGD-TCL should express a gamma/delta heterodimer on the cell surface. This can now be demonstrated by antibodies to TCR-gamma in paraffin sections.[16,24] The tumor cells typically express CD2, CD3, and also CD7; CD5 is usually absent.[16,24] Most cases lack both CD4 and CD8, although occasional CD8-positive cases are reported, and there is strong expression of the cytotoxic molecules TIA-1, perforin, and granzyme B.[4,5,8,13,15,16,22] CD56 is often expressed, particularly in subcutaneous cases, but may be negative.[4,16,19,22,24] EBV is usually absent.[10,13,20,22]

TCR-gamma and TCR-delta genes are clonally rearranged.[16] The TCR-beta gene may be rearranged or deleted, but is not expressed.

Differential diagnosis

The differential diagnosis of PCGD-TCL includes subcutaneous panniculitis-like T-cell lymphoma and extranodal NK/T-cell lymphoma. The combination of clinical features and gamma/delta phenotype should allow a correct diagnosis to be established in most cases. Extranodal NK/T-cell lymphoma is almost invariably EBV positive.[8,13,22] In addition, rare cases of mycosis fungoides and lymphomatoid papulosis express a $\gamma\delta$ phenotype.[24] Clinical correlation is required to separate these from PCGD-TCL.

Peripheral T-cell lymphoma, not otherwise specified

Peripheral T-cell lymphoma, not otherwise specified, is a heterogeneous group of nodal and extranodal mature T-cell lymphomas that do not fit into one of the well-defined subtypes of T-cell lymphoma/leukemia.[1-5] They not uncommonly involve the skin as a primary or secondary manifestation of disease. When presenting in the skin, they display aggressive behavior with a similarly poor outcome, whether or not there is concomitant lymph node involvement.[4] Cases which do not fit well into any of the above described categories of cutaneous T-cell lymphoma should, therefore, be assigned to this group. Cutaneous involvement by systemic T-cell lymphoma is mainly seen in patients with mature T cell or T-cell/NK lymphoma (40% of cases) and less frequently with anaplastic large cell lymphoma (10%) and angio-immunoblastic lymphoma (5%).[6]

BENIGN CUTANEOUS INFILTRATES THAT CAN BE MISTAKEN FOR CUTANEOUS T-CELL LYMPHOMA (CUTANEOUS T-CELL PSEUDOLYMPHOMA)

Cutaneous pseudolymphoma does not constitute a distinct entity, but is a term used to describe lymphoid infiltrates that simulate malignancy histologically and sometimes also clinically.[1] Cases can be broadly divided into those mimicking T-cell lymphomas (cutaneous T-cell pseudolymphoma) and those masquerading as B-cell neoplasms (cutaneous B-cell pseudolymphoma). This rather arbitrary distinction is based on the histologic pattern and predominant cell type.[1] Many examples contain significant numbers of B cells, often arranged in follicles, and fall into the category of cutaneous B-cell pseudolymphoma. Cases mimicking T-cell lymphoma are less common.[2-5]

Cases of cutaneous T-cell pseudolymphoma (CTPL) may be idiopathic, but many can be classified as distinct clinicopathological entities, the main ones being lymphomatoid drug eruptions, lymphomatoid contact dermatitis, pseudolymphomatous angiokeratoma (APACHE), T-cell rich angiomatoid polypoid pseudolymphoma (TRAPP), pseudolymphomatous folliculitis, chronic actinic dermatitis (CAD), persistent arthropod bite reaction, lymphomatoid keratosis, and atypical cutaneous lymphoproliferative disorder of HIV infection.[1,6-14] Several of these specific entities are discussed below, or elsewhere in this or other chapters. Many idiopathic cases show considerable overlap with primary cutaneous CD4-positive small/medium pleomorphic T-cell lymphoproliferative disorder, and may well be part of the same spectrum of disease.[15,16]

Intravascular pseudo-T-cell lymphoma

Clinical features

Rarely, intralymphatic aggregates of CD30 positive or, less commonly, CD30 negative blastic cells are seen in skin biopsies performed in the setting of trauma or various inflammatory and neoplastic pathologies including lichen sclerosus, hidradenitis suppurativa, and hemangioma.[1-6] The behavior appears to be benign with no adverse effects in any of the cases reported so far.

Histologic features

A variable number of dermal lymphatics appear dilated by a proliferation of blastic cells that are frequently, but not always, CD30 positive (*Figs 29.171–29.173*). Other T-cell markers including CD3 and CD4 are usually expressed. B-cell markers are negative. The proliferating cells are usually polyclonal.

Differential diagnosis

The differential diagnosis includes intravascular T, NK/T, or B cell lymphoma and intravascular histiocytosis. Clinicopathological correlation, immunophenotyping, and clonality studies are crucial to establish the right diagnosis.

Pseudolymphomatous angiokeratoma

Clinical features

Pseudolymphomatous angiokeratoma (acral pseudolymphomatous angio-keratoma, APACHE) was originally described as a disorder presenting as unilateral, asymptomatic, red, angiomatous papules and nodules on acral sites of children with equal sex incidence and predilection for the hands and feet, particularly the digits.[1-3] However, similar cases have rarely been described in adults with a wider anatomic range including elsewhere on the limbs and the trunk. It is likely that the latter represent examples of T-cell rich angiomatoid polypoid pseudolymphoma (TRAPP, see below). Lesions tend to be persistent and are exceptionally linear.[4-8]

Pathogenesis and histologic features

The etiology is unknown and there is no relation with angiolymphoid hyperplasia (epithelioid hemangioma) as has been suggested.[9] The epidermis appears flattened, and there may be some degree of interface change. In the underlying dermis, there is a prominent, often diffuse infiltrate composed of lymphocytes and variable numbers of plasma cells. Cytological atypia is absent. In the background, there are numerous, small,[1] thin-walled vascular channels. T cells tend to predominate with both CD4+ and CD8+ T cells represented.[10,11] Rarely, B cells are prominent. Unlike other angiokeratomas,

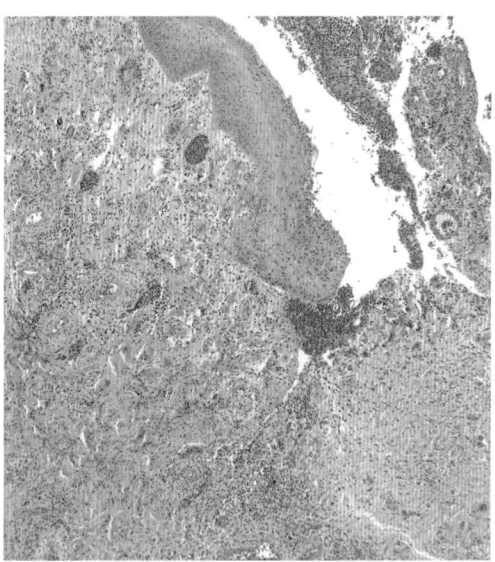

Fig. 29.171
Intravascular pseudo-T-cell lymphoma: numerous dilated lymphatic channels containing blastic lymphoid cells.

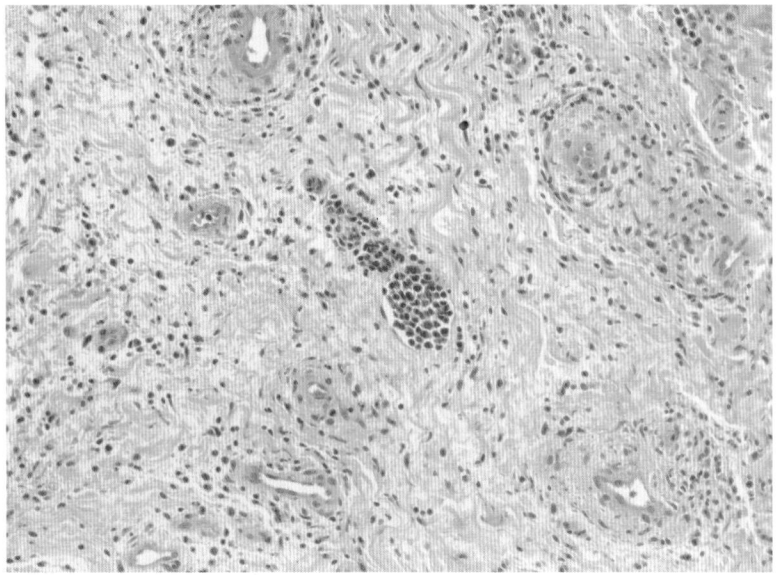

Fig. 29.172
Intravascular pseudo-T-cell lymphoma: closer view of a dilated lymphatic vessel containing blastic lymphoid cells.

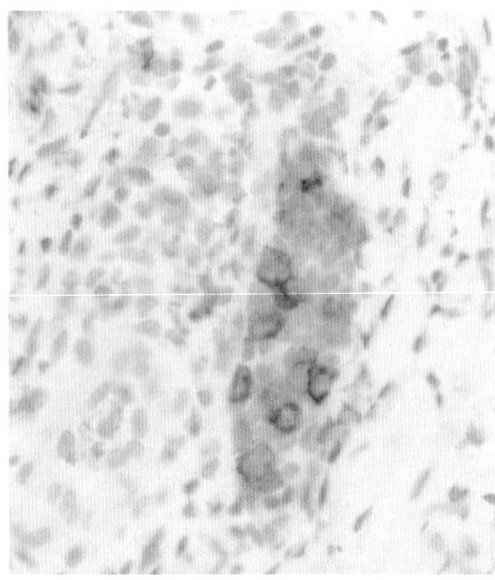

Fig. 29.173
Intravascular pseudo-T-cell lymphoma: many but not all of the blastic cells T cells are positive for CD30.

the endothelial cells in pseudolymphomatous angiokeratoma appear to express WT1.[12]

T-cell rich angiomatoid polypoid pseudolymphoma

Clinical features

T-cell rich angiomatoid polypoid pseudolymphoma (TRAPP) is a distinctive variant of cutaneous pseudolymphoma.[1] Lesions are solitary and present as a small (less than 1 cm) polypoid angiomatous papule with predilection for the head and trunk. It clinically resembles a nonulcerated pyogenic granuloma, and patients are predominantly young adults with some predilection for females. Regression is not usually seen. There is no tendency for local recurrence.

Pathogenesis and histopathological features

The pathogenesis of TRAPP is unknown. The typical histology consists of a polypoid, nonulcerated diffuse and well-circumscribed infiltrate often separated from a thinned epidermis by a grenz zone (Figs 29.173–29.175). In

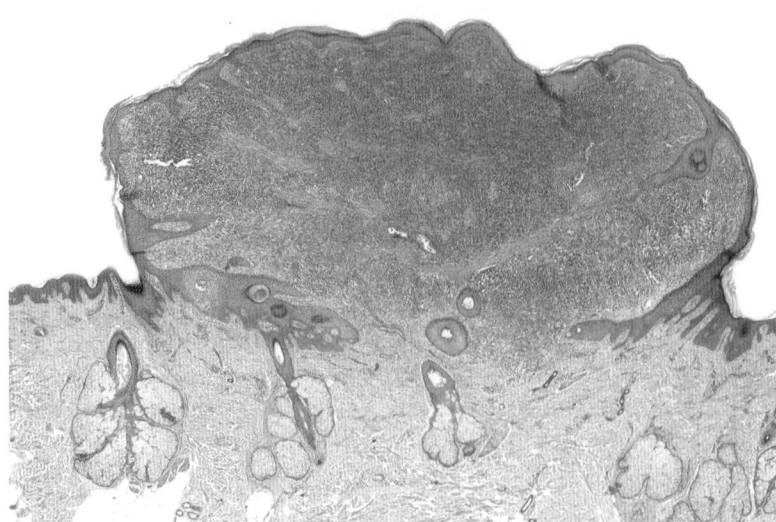

Fig. 29.174
T-cell rich angiomatoid polypoid pseudolymphoma (TRAPP): scanning view of polypoid nodule.

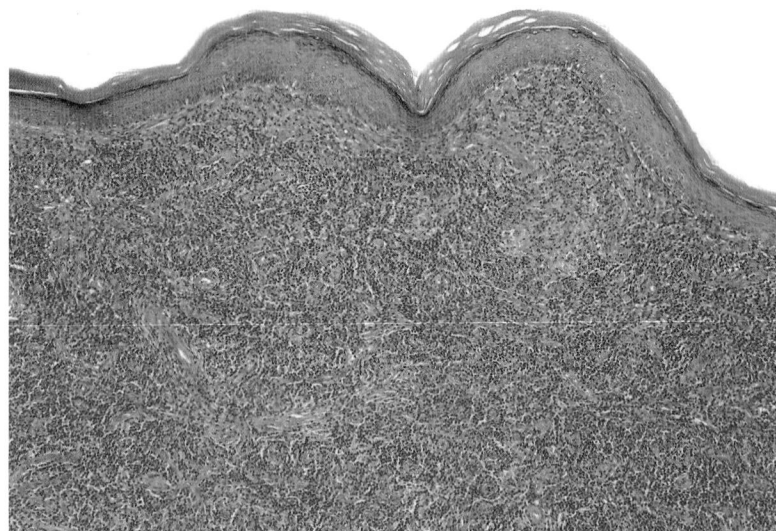

Fig. 29.175
T-cell rich angiomatoid polypoid pseudolymphoma (TRAPP): medium-power view showing lack of epidermal involvement.

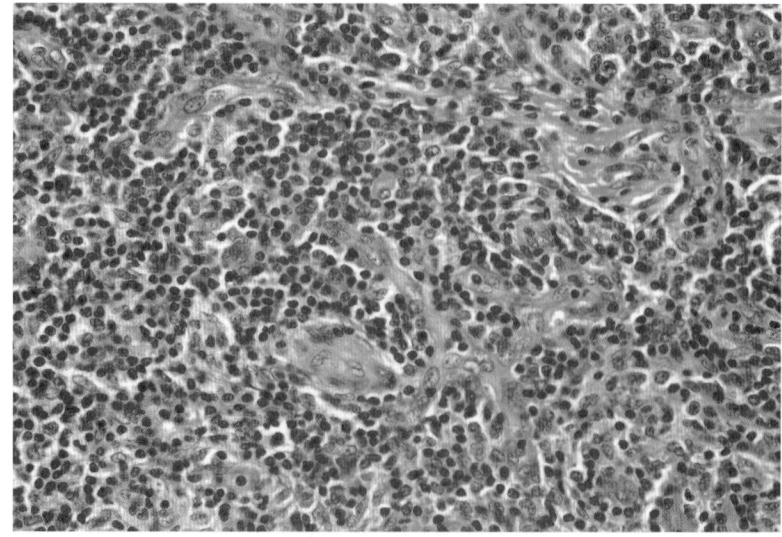

Fig. 29.176
T-cell rich angiomatoid polypoid pseudolymphoma (TRAPP): high-power view of blood vessels and small lymphocytes.

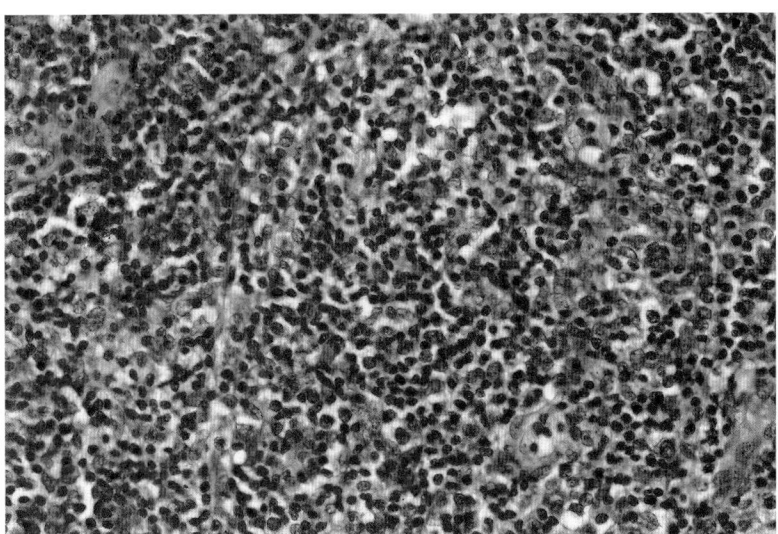

Fig. 29.177
T-cell rich angiomatoid polypoid pseudolymphoma (TRAPP): detailed view of infiltrate.

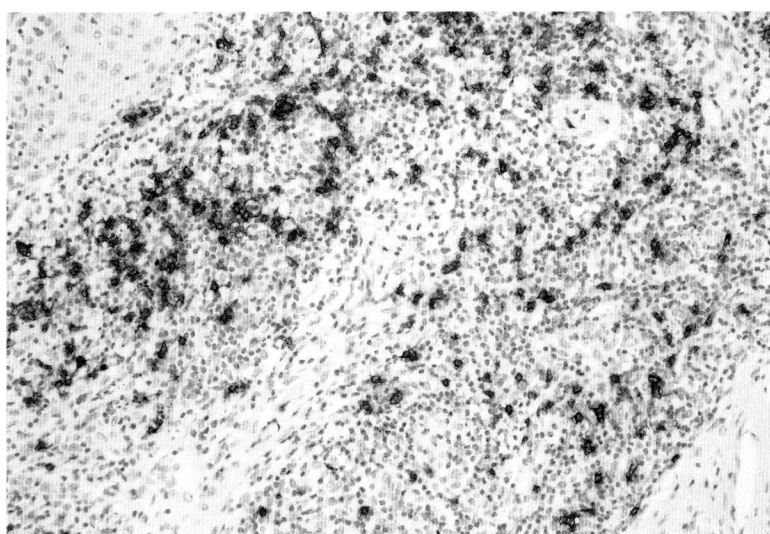

Fig. 29.179
T-cell rich angiomatoid polypoid pseudolymphoma (TRAPP): small numbers of CD20-positive lymphocytes are also seen.

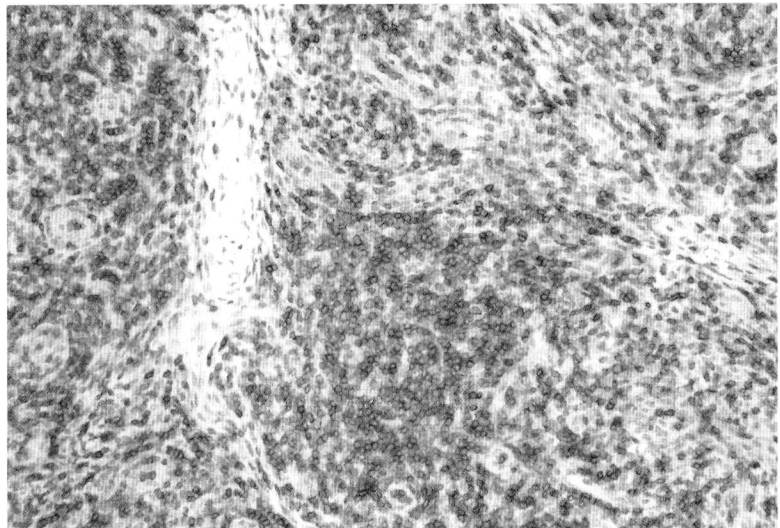

Fig. 29.178
T-cell rich angiomatoid polypoid pseudolymphoma (TRAPP): the lymphocytes express CD3.

the background, there are numerous small blood vessels lined by plump but not epithelioid endothelial cells. These vessels have features of high endothelial venules seen in lymph nodes (*Fig. 29.176*). The infiltrate consists mainly of CD3-positive lymphocytes, and both CD4+ and CD8+ cells are represented (*Figs 29.177–29.179*). B cells are sparse. Cytological atypia is not seen. Eosinophils and plasma cells may be seen. Old lesions display some degree of fibrosis.

Differential diagnosis

The main differential diagnosis is with pseudolymphomatous angiokeratoma (APACHE).[2-4] Similar lesions have also been described under different rubrics including papular angiolymphoid proliferation with epithelioid features in adults and children (PALEFACE) and angiolymphoid hyperplasia with high endothelial venules (APA-HEL).[5,6] There is undoubtedly some overlap with pseudolymphomatous angiokeratoma (APACHE). However, TRAPP occurs on the head and trunk, it presents as a solitary lesion, with adult predilection, and it is always polypoid with an epithelial collarette and lack of interface change.

Drug-induced pseudolymphoma

This is discussed in Chapter 14.

Pseudolymphomatous folliculitis

Clinical features

Pseudolymphomatous folliculitis is uncommon and presents in the head and neck region as solitary red or violaceous, nonulcerated, solitary nodules, measuring up to 3 cm in diameter.[1-6] The sexes are affected equally, and most patients are in their fourth or fifth decade.[2,4] Surgery seems to be adequate treatment since only one case of recurring lesions has been reported.[4] Even when not fully excised, lesions tend to spontaneously regress.[2,3]

Pathogenesis and histologic features

The etiology in the vast majority of cases is unknown. One case had a history of previous insect bite, in two a history of antecedent trauma, and in another, *B. burgdorferi* DNA was demonstrated.[1,2,4] The striking folliculocentricity and conspicuous dendritic cell population suggest that the condition most probably represents an exuberant hypersensitivity reaction to an as yet unidentified follicular antigen.

The salient diagnostic features are the presence of a dense nodular or diffuse folliculocentric infiltrate, together with hyperplasia and distortion of pilosebaceous units.[2,4,5] The infiltrate is usually separated from the epidermis by a grenz zone and may involve the subcutis.[2-4] It consists of lymphocytes with variable numbers of histiocytes, plasma cells, and, in some cases, eosinophils.[1,2,4] The lymphocytes are usually small, although in some cases medium to large lymphocytes are present, either with irregular hyperchromatic nuclei or an immunoblastic appearance.[2,4] Lymphoid follicles are rare.[4] The histiocytes generally have an epithelioid appearance and are often clustered around infiltrated hair follicles and sebaceous glands.[2] Small noncaseating granulomata can be seen.[4]

The infiltrate consists of a mixed population of T and B cells.[2,3] CD8+ T cells are sparse.[3] In most cases, T cells predominate, but in some B cells are present in equal or greater numbers.[4] The epithelioid histiocytes react with antibodies to CD68 whilst antibodies to S100 protein and CD1a highlight collections of perifollicular dendritic cells.[2-4] There is no evidence of immunoglobulin light chain restriction in the B-cell rich variants.[2-4]

Gene rearrangement studies were uniformly negative in a Japanese series, but a recent large study from Europe demonstrated clonal T-cell receptor rearrangements by PCR in about 50% of patients, and clonal immunoglobulin gene rearrangement in three out of 42 cases.[2,4] In one case, both the T-cell receptor and immunoglobulin heavy chain gene were clonally rearranged.[4] Clonal cases of pseudolymphomatous folliculitis show no clinical or pathological differences to nonclonal ones.[4] However, the median follow-up of 3 years in this study is too short to draw definite conclusions. If clonality is found, then close follow-up is advisable.[4]

It is questionable whether pseudolymphomatous folliculitis is truly distinct from other cutaneous lymphoid hyperplasias in which hair follicle hyperplasia is absent. However, it is important to distinguish pseudolymphomatous folliculitis from cases of lymphoma, especially as follicular hyperplasia has also been reported, albeit rarely, in a variety of primary and secondary cutaneous lymphomas of T- and B-cell type.[4] The presence of solitary lesions, absence of an aberrant phenotype, and demonstration of polyclonality by light chain immunohistochemistry all favor a benign diagnosis. However, as evidenced above, care must be taken interpreting the results of gene rearrangement studies, as not all molecularly clonal lesions are lymphomas.

Atypical cutaneous lymphoproliferative disorder of HIV infection

Clinical features

Also known as pseudo-Sézary syndrome, this rare condition presents with widespread, pruritic, and often erythematous patches, papules, and plaques.[1–7] Lesions are sometimes lichenified.[4,7] Hyperpigmentation is common and occasionally hypopigmentation is noted.[5,7,8] Erythroderma, palmoplantar keratoderma, and photosensitivity are also described.[2,5,6,8] Patients typically have advanced HIV disease with severe immunosuppression.[5,7] Lymphadenopathy is present in a minority of patients, and circulating Sézary-like cells may be detected.[2,8] The clinical course is chronic and may be modified by introduction of antiretroviral therapy.[9] Exceptionally, cutaneous T-cell lymphoma supervenes.[7]

Pathogenesis and histologic features

The etiology is unknown although the infiltrate has been shown to be HIV specific and directed toward a variety of antigens.[8] There is no evidence of a drug-related pathogenesis.[7] Photosensitivity may be an initiating event, at least in some patients.[2] HTLV-I proviral DNA has been identified in the skin and peripheral blood of two patients but is absent in others.[2,4]

Histologically, there is a superficial and deep perivascular and perifollicular polymorphous infiltrate composed of lymphocytes, eosinophils, plasma cells, and rare neutrophils accompanied by an atypical mitotically active lymphoid population with enlarged irregular nuclei containing prominent nucleoli.[2,7] Mycosis/Sézary cells may be present.[2,4,7] Epidermotropism is variably present, being reported in some cases but described as absent or minimal in others.[1,2–4,6–10]

The lymphoid cells are CLA+, CD2+, CD3+, CD5+, CD8+, and TCRβ+.[2,3,5–8] CD7 may be diminished.[3,7] CD4, CD15, and CD30 are negative.[7] B cells are absent. TCR gene rearrangement studies are negative.[2,3,6]

Chronic actinic dermatitis

Clinical features

Chronic actinic dermatitis (CAD) (actinic reticuloid, photosensitivity dermatitis) is a rare chronic photosensitivity reaction of unknown pathogenesis that is of particular importance because it may resemble a lymphoma.[1–5]

The disease occurs predominantly in middle aged or elderly males.[6,7] Young adults of either sex, however, may also be affected.[5,8–11] In addition to Caucasians and Asians, CAD sometimes presents in the black population.[11–13] The prevalence in Scotland has been estimated as 16 per 100 000.[14] A history of allergic contact dermatitis, chronic atopic dermatitis, seborrheic dermatitis, or polymorphous light eruption is not uncommon.[5,15] Indeed, a preliminary diagnosis of contact allergy is often documented before the significance of the photosensitive component is realized. Patients develop an intensely pruritic, scaly, erythematous eruption, which is initially limited to the sun-exposed areas, particularly the face, back of the neck, and the hands.[1,7] However, lesions also develop on covered sites. Involvement of the eyelids may point toward an allergic contact reaction.[5] With further progression, edematous, lichenified, thickened plaques and smooth-topped papules develop (*Figs 29.180* and *29.181*).[6] In severe cases, lesions may become confluent on exposed areas, giving rise to a leonine facies. Patients

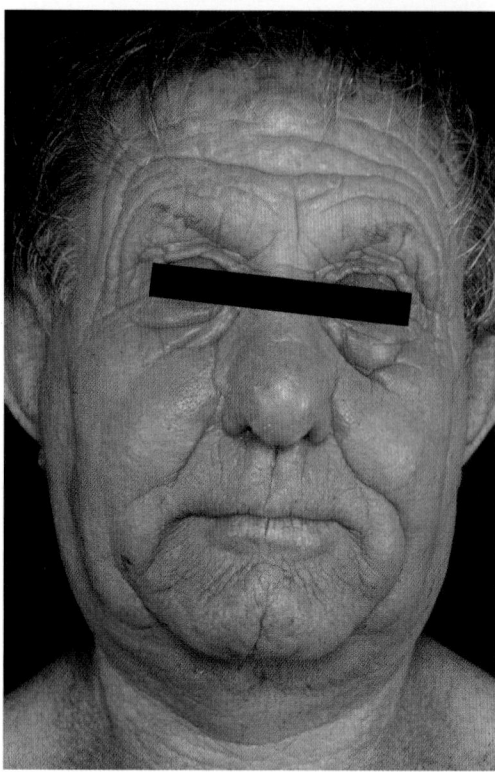

Fig. 29.180
Chronic actinic dermatitis: marked erythema, edema, and thickening of the skin. From the collection of the late N.P. Smith, MD, The Institute of Dermatology, London, UK.

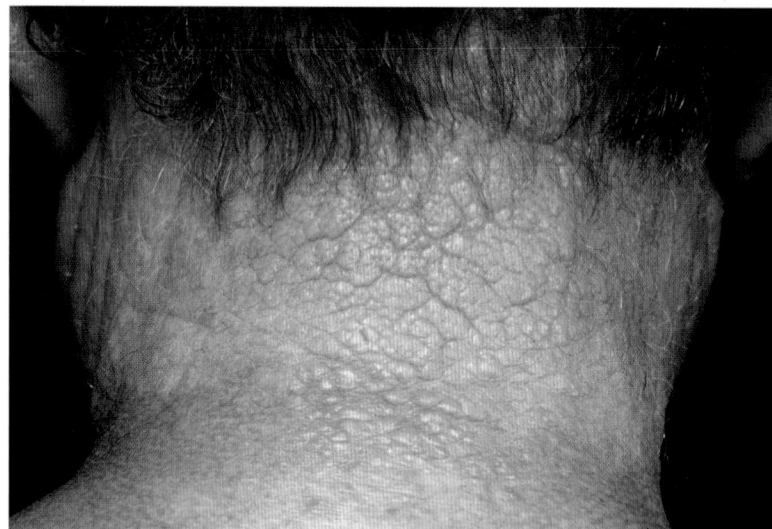

Fig. 29.181
Chronic actinic dermatitis: prominent lichenification. From the collection of the late N.P. Smith, MD, The Institute of Dermatology, London, UK.

with CAD are prone to episodes of erythroderma, which may resemble Sézary syndrome, and in some cases there is palmoplantar involvement.[15] Circulating Sézary cells are common and sometimes present in high numbers (2.5–18% of white cells), particularly in erythrodermic patients when a reversed helper/suppressor T-cell ratio is commonly found.[2,16–19] Lymphadenopathy is frequently present. Improvement of the photosensitivity may occur over time, and rarely there is also resolution of the contact allergy.[20] A case associated with adult T-cell leukemia has been reported.[21]

Pathogenesis and histologic features

CAD is associated with sensitivity to ultraviolet (UV) B (290–320 nm), UVA (320–400 nm), and parts of the visible spectrum (400–700 nm).[16] Patients

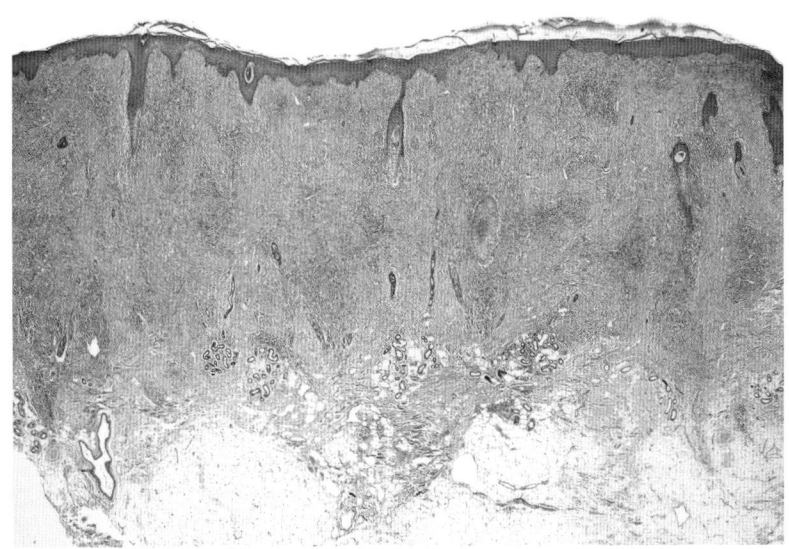

Fig. 29.182
Chronic actinic dermatitis: a dense infiltrate extends throughout the dermis and fibrosis is evident.

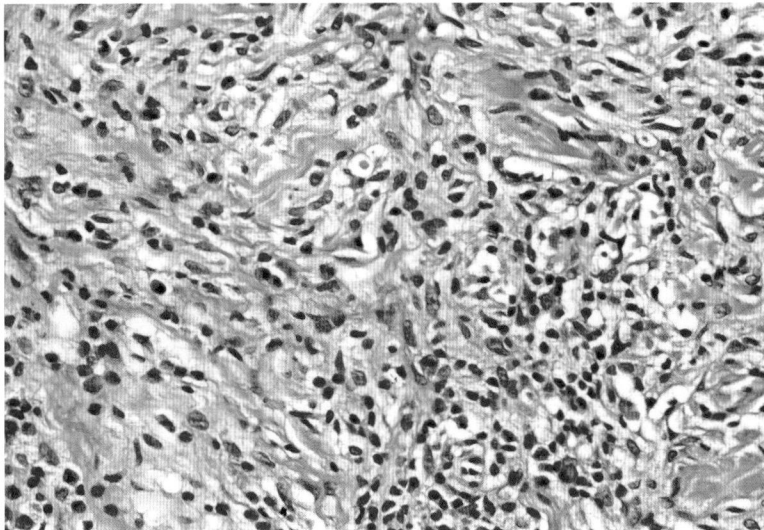

Fig. 29.183
Chronic actinic dermatitis: the infiltrate consists of lymphocytes, eosinophils, and histiocytes.

also commonly show evidence of contact allergy, and sesquiterpene lactone mix, composite oleoresins, rubber components, potassium dichromate, sunscreens components (benzophenone, butyl methoxydibenzoylmethane, and ethylhexyl benzophenone), fragrances including musk ambrette, and, most recently, p-phenylenediamine, parthenium, and xanthium have been incriminated.[6,22-24] Occasional patients are HIV positive.[7] It has been suggested that impaired antigen recognition and increased levels of antigen-specific suppressor T cells, which develop as a consequence of UV hypersensitivity, may result in a state of chronic low-grade antigen stimulation and the subsequent development of an atypical cellular immune reaction.[25]

The histologic features are variable. Biopsy specimens from less severely affected patients may show only the features of a chronic dermatitic process: parakeratosis, acanthosis, spongiosis, and a superficial perivascular chronic inflammatory cell infiltrate.[1,7,16] In patients with more extensive involvement, there is commonly a very dense cellular infiltrate involving the papillary and reticular dermis, sometimes extending into the subcutaneous fat (Fig. 29.182).[6,7] The infiltrate is composed of lymphocytes, histiocytes, and variable numbers of eosinophils and plasma cells (Figs 29.183 and 29.184). Multinucleate stellate myofibroblasts are common, and occasionally giant cells are a conspicuous feature.[7,16] The latter appear to be particularly related to foci of elastolysis.[6] Of importance is the occasional finding of large atypical and hyperchromatic cerebriform lymphoid cells and large transformed cell forms, which can raise the suspicion of a cutaneous lymphoma.[6] Mitoses can be conspicuous. The epidermis may show exocytosis, but Pautrier microabscess-like features are only rarely evident (Fig. 29.185). Fibrosis of the superficial dermis is a common manifestation.

Ultrastructural examination of specimens from patients with CAD have demonstrated large numbers of Sézary-type cells.[2,3,19]

The lymph nodes usually show the features of dermatopathic lymphadenopathy, but rarely Sézary cells are identified in the paracortical region and sinuses.[6]

The results of immunohistochemistry are variable. In general, CD4+ helper T cells are more common in the cellular infiltrate in early lesions but, with increasing severity, the CD8+ suppressor subset usually predominates.[6,7,16,26,27] IgE-positive dendritic cells are frequently present in the dermal infiltrate.[6,27]

Although a small number of cases with associated lymphoma have been documented, these may be coincidental.[6,28-30] DNA flow cytometry studies have given conflicting results, varying from complete absence of aneuploidy to presence in 63% of patients.[25,31] TCR gene rearrangement studies usually resolve this dilemma.[32,33] Although occasional cases demonstrate a clonal population, in a more recent study of 12 cases of CAD, no TCR gene rearrangements were identified.[33-36] In the largest series published to date, none of the 231 patients with CAD had an associated lymphoma.[37]

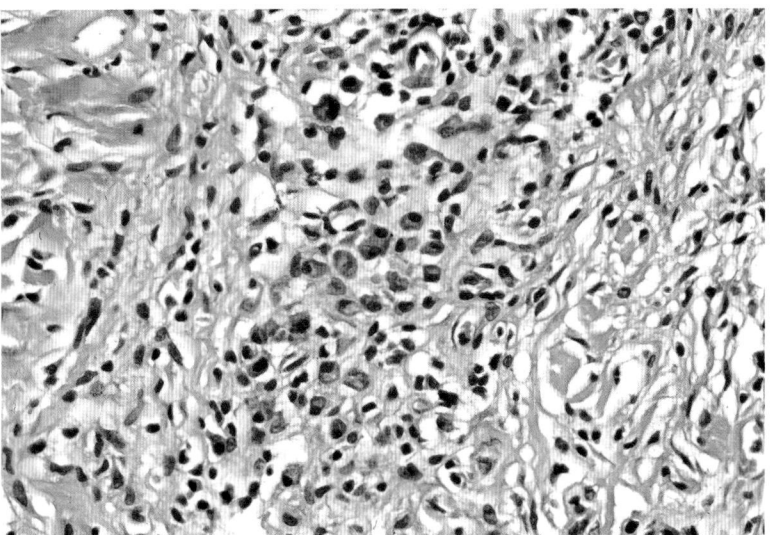

Fig. 29.184
Chronic actinic dermatitis: conspicuous plasma cells are present.

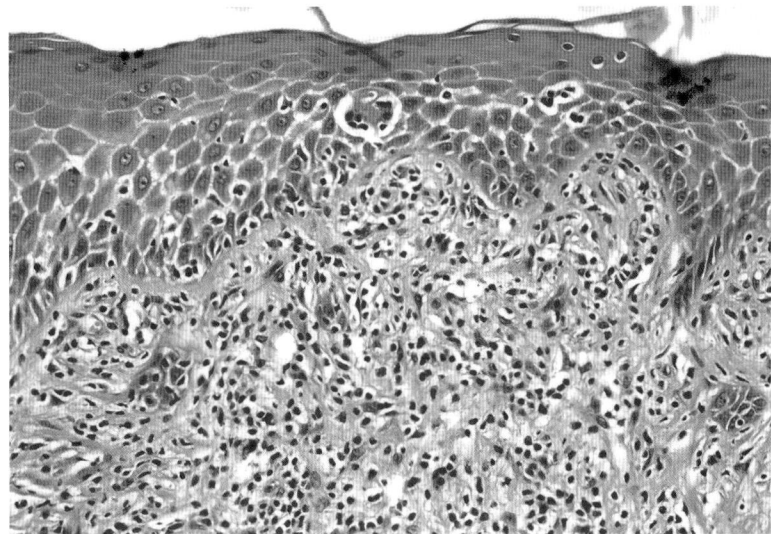

Fig. 29.185
Chronic actinic dermatitis: there is mild cytological atypia. Focal epidermotropism is evident.

Differential diagnosis

In the absence of an adequate clinical history, actinic reticuloid may be histologically confused with patch/plaque stage mycosis fungoides or Sézary syndrome. The matter is further complicated by the rare occurrence of erythrodermic cutaneous T-cell lymphomas with severe photosensitivity.[38] Histologic points of diagnostic help include the presence of multinucleate stellate myofibroblasts, eosinophils and plasma cells, and the absence of Pautrier microabscesses in CAD. The CD8+ phenotype of actinic reticuloid contrasts with the CD4+ proliferation characteristic of mycosis fungoides and Sézary syndrome.[15,33] Similarly, study of the peripheral blood may reveal a decreased or even reversed CD4:CD8 ratio.[32]

Lymphocytic infiltrate of the skin (Jessner)

This condition is discussed in Chapter 8.

B-CELL LYMPHOMAS

B-cell lymphomas, which are defined as arising primarily in the skin, include:
- extranodal marginal zone B-cell lymphoma of mucosa-associated lymphoid tissue (MALT lymphoma),
- cutaneous follicle center lymphoma,
- primary cutaneous diffuse large B-cell lymphoma, leg type (PCDLBCL-LT).

The skin may also be involved secondarily in a wide range of mature B-cell lymphomas including, in particular, mantle cell lymphoma (MCL), B-chronic lymphocytic leukemia/small lymphocytic lymphoma (CLL/SLL), intravascular large B-cell lymphoma (IVLBCL), lymphomatoid granulomatosis, plasmablastic lymphoma (PL), and post-transplant lymphoproliferative disorder (PTLD).

Since B-cell lymphomas presenting in the skin may be either primary or metastatic, staging is essential to distinguish between the two.

Primary cutaneous B-cell lymphoma

The diagnosis and differential diagnosis of cutaneous B-cell lymphocytic infiltrates is challenging. The topic has been confusing for a number of reasons including the belief that the presence of lymphoid follicles invariably implies a reactive process. This is now known to be completely false, reactive follicles being a characteristic feature of marginal zone lymphomas. In addition, the literature has been bedeviled by the use of time-honored – but now rather meaningless – descriptive nomenclature and eponyms (Spiegler-Fendt sarcoid, lymphocytoma cutis, large cell lymphocytoma, Crosti reticulohistiocytoma (RH) of the dorsum, and lymphadenoma benigna cutis) that were largely used before the advent of immunohistochemistry and molecular/genetic studies. Such terms should be abandoned.

In general, most PCBCLs are low grade with little tendency to nodal or systemic spread.

However, it is not always possible to confidently distinguish between a benign and a malignant infiltrate, particularly when the sample obtained is inadequate. In such instances, a guarded report should always be given, with a recommendation for repeat biopsy when relevant, combined with careful follow-up.

Primary cutaneous marginal zone B-cell lymphoma

Clinical features

Extranodal marginal zone lymphoma of mucosa associated lymphoid tissue (MALT lymphoma) is the third commonest form of NHL, and 11% of cases occur primarily in the skin, accounting for 2–7% of primary cutaneous lymphomas.[1-4] Most, if not all, tumors previously labeled primary cutaneous immunocytoma and cutaneous follicular lymphoid hyperplasia with monotypic plasma cells belong to this group.[5-9] By definition, primary cutaneous marginal zone lymphoma (PCMZL) is stage IE at presentation.

The literature contains conflicting results as to sex predominance.[10-19] The age range is wide, but most patients are older than 40 years (median, 50 years).[20-22] Presentation is with solitary lesions or clusters of asymptomatic, reddish/reddish brown to violaceous or purple papules, nodules, and plaques measuring from 1 to 10 cm in diameter.[11,12,18,19] The trunk (particularly the back) and arms are predominantly affected. Head and neck involvement is less common.[10,11,16,17,22] Lesions may be solitary or localized, affect multiple anatomical sites simultaneously, or rarely be generalized.[16,18,19] Exceptionally, a serum monoclonal immunoglobulin is encountered. B-symptoms are absent and serum LDH and beta-2 microglobulin levels are normal.[12,18] Anetoderma may rarely be seen in the skin overlying the lesions. Rare cases present following solid organ transplantation.[23]

Surgery or radiotherapy is used for localized or scattered multifocal lesions, and extensive disease is managed with chemotherapy or electron beam.[18,19,24] Most patients achieve complete remission, but cutaneous relapse is common in up to 50% of cases.[19]

Dissemination to lymph nodes, liver, spleen, parotid gland, orbit, breast, intestine, and bone marrow has been reported.[10,12,18,19] Prognosis is excellent, with 5-year survivals of 90–100%.[4,9,18] High-grade transformation is exceptional.[18]

Pathogenesis and histologic features

In contrast to the mucosae, the skin does not have an associated B-cell lymphocyte population. It has been suggested that skin associated lymphoid tissue (SALT) may develop following chronic antigen stimulation with eventual development of B-cell lymphoma analogous to the extranodal MALT-type lymphomas complicating chronic infection by *Helicobacter pylori* in the stomach, *Chlamydia psittaci* (ocular adnexal MALT lymphomas), *Campylobacter jejuni* (immunoproliferative small intestinal disease), or that have developed in association with autoimmune diseases (Hashimoto thyroiditis and Sjögren syndrome).[25-29] Immunoglobulin variable region gene analysis supports such a role for antigen in stimulating the growth of PCMZL.[30] A proportion of PCMZL may be related to infection by *B. burgdorferi* in certain geographic locations (e.g., Scotland, Austria, France), and there is anecdotal evidence that some cases resolve following antibiotic therapy.[11,31-37] However, there appears to be no link between PCMZL and *B. burgdorferi* in many other regions (e.g., United States, Italy, Asia), and not all *Borrelia*-related cases respond to antibiotics.[38-41] Rare cases have been reported with tattoos and vaccinations.[42,43]

Extranodal marginal zone lymphomas are derived from postgerminal center memory B cells, often showing plasmacytic differentiation and gene expression profile.[44] A variety of chromosomal translocations have been identified in MALT lymphomas as a group. These include t(11;18)(q21;q21), resulting in an apoptosis inhibitor 2 (API2)–MALT1 fusion gene, t(14;18)(q32;q21), juxtaposing the MALT1 gene with the immunoglobulin heavy chain (IGH) gene, t(1;14)(p14;q32), translocating the BCL10 gene to the IGH gene, and t(3;14)(p14.1;q32) involving IGH and FoxP1. The first three of these are relatively specific for MALT lymphoma and all target the NF-κB pathway, albeit in different ways.[28] The translocations have different incidences in MALT lymphomas from different sites. t(11;18)(q21;q21) and t(1;14)(p14;q32) predominate in MALT lymphomas of the stomach and lung, but the former is only very rarely seen in PCMZL and occurrence of the latter has yet to be documented.[28,45-51] t(14;18)(q32;q21) has been demonstrated in some cases of PCMZL in a few studies but has not been identified in others.[47-50,52] Rare cases of t(14;18)(q32;q21) with a BCL2/IGH translocation have also been reported in PCMZL, occasionally concurrent with an IGH/MALT translocation.[52] One study documented t(3;14)(p14.1;q32) in 2/20 PCMZL, but this translocation is not specific for extranodal marginal zone lymphoma.[53,54] Another non-specific finding is the

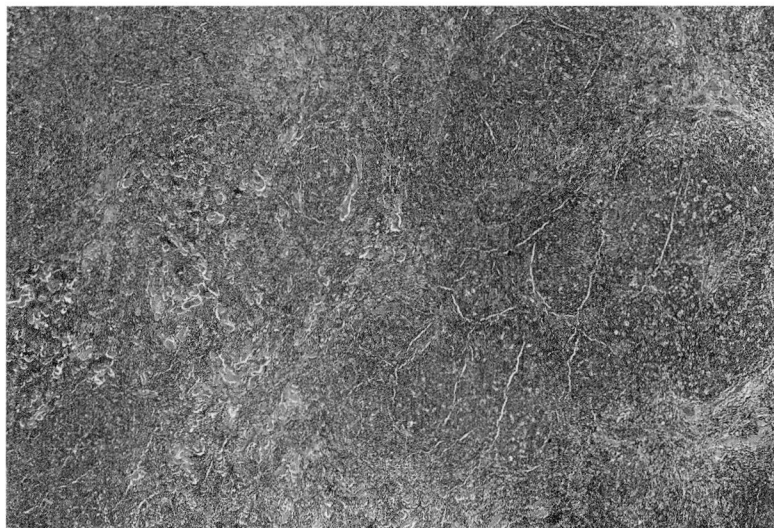

Fig. 29.186
Primary cutaneous marginal zone B-cell lymphoma: there is a dense deep dermal lymphoid infiltrate.

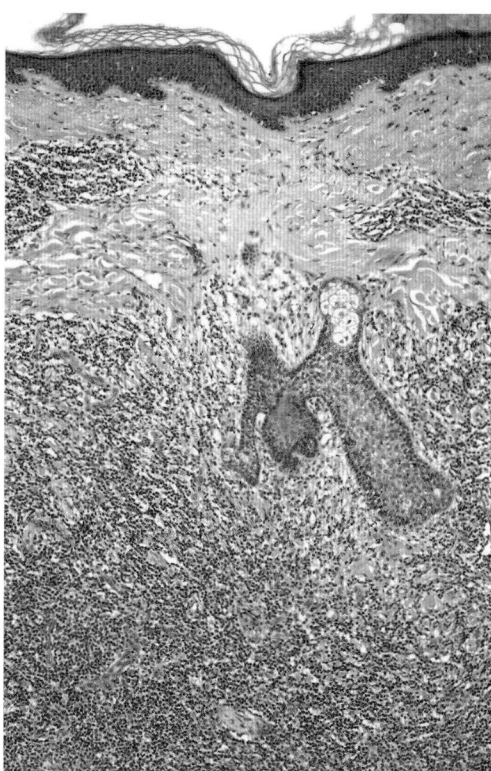

Fig. 29.188
Primary cutaneous marginal zone B-cell lymphoma: note the uninvolved grenz zone.

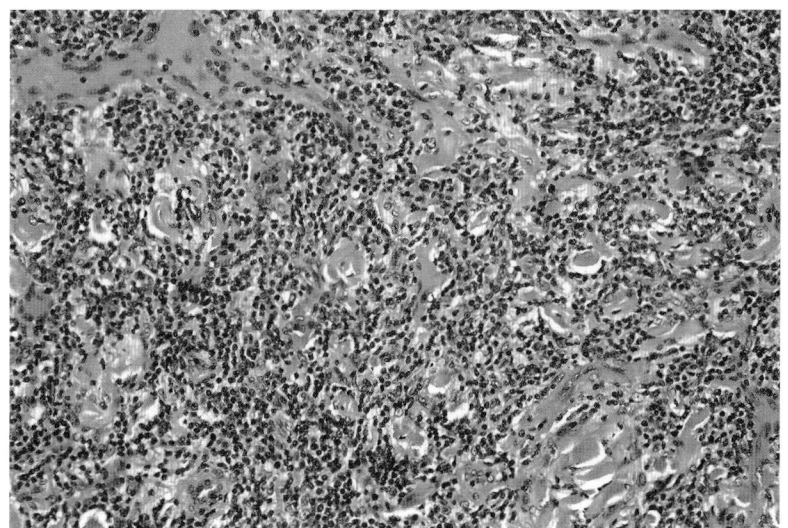

Fig. 29.187
Primary cutaneous marginal zone B-cell lymphoma: note the dissection of collagen.

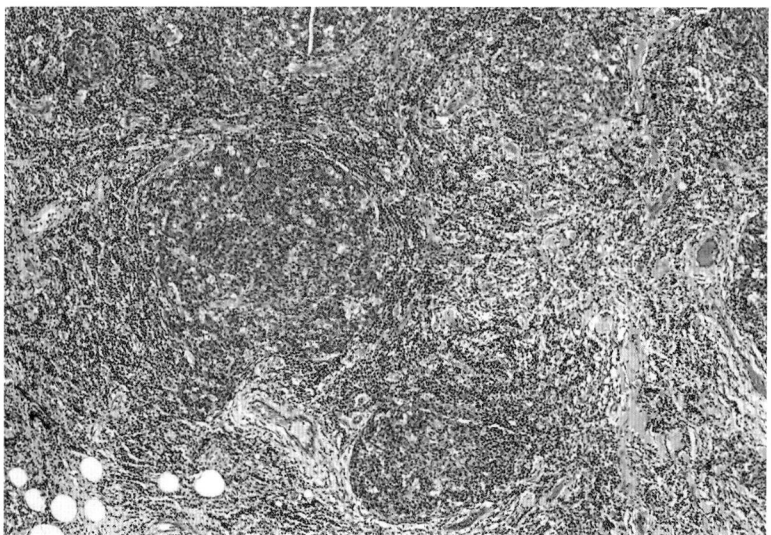

Fig. 29.189
Primary cutaneous marginal zone B-cell lymphoma: multiple lymphoid follicles with germinal centers are present.

presence of trisomies 3 or 18 in a few cases.[47,48] Mutations and/or deletions of TNFAIP3 are commonly encountered in MALT lymphoma of the ocular adnexa and salivary gland but, as yet, no detailed mutational analysis of PCMZL has been undertaken.[55–59] MYD88 mutations are not found.[60]

Biopsies of PCMZL show a nodular or (less frequently) diffuse infiltrate involving the reticular dermis, often extending into the subcutaneous fat (Figs 29.186 and 29.187).[11,16,18] A grenz zone is usually present and ulceration is exceptional (Fig. 29.188).[16] The infiltrate contains reactive lymphoid follicles, often with germinal centers and distinct mantle zones surrounded by a pale-staining infiltrate of marginal zone cells (Fig. 29.189).[10,11,14,16,18] These are often described as centrocyte-like with slightly irregular nuclei, dense chromatin, inconspicuous nucleoli, and modest amounts of pale or watery cytoplasm (Fig. 29.190). Extension into the germinal center (follicular colonization) is often evident, and cells with more abundant cytoplasm (i.e., monocytoid B cells) may be seen (Figs 29.191–29.193). Lymphoepithelial lesions are rare and when present may affect the hair follicles and the sweat glands (Fig. 29.194).[19] Mitoses are inconspicuous.[12] Lymphoplasmacytoid cells are typically present, and these are accompanied by mature plasma cells which are characteristically conspicuous and often comprise the majority of discernible neoplastic cells in PCMZL (Fig. 29.195). They tend to predominate at the edge of the infiltrate and under the epidermis.[11,18]

Dutcher bodies (eosinophilic intranuclear inclusions) are sometimes seen.[12] Variable numbers of centroblasts, immunoblasts, histiocytes, and eosinophils are present, and in some tumors multinucleate giant cells and granulomata are identified (Figs 29.196 and 29.197).[15] Exceptional cases displaying prominent epidermotropism have been described.[61,62]

The tumor cells are CD20+, PAX-5, and CD79a+, often with aberrant coexpression of CD43, but they are otherwise CD10–, CD23–, bcl-6–, and cyclin D1– (Fig. 29.198).[11,14,17,18] Staining for CD5 has rarely been reported in marginal zone lymphoma occurring in the skin and at other extranodal sites.[63,64] Bcl-2 is positive. Monotypic light chain expression is commonly identified and clonal IgH rearrangements are frequently detected (Figs 29.199 and 29.200).[11,18] Unlike most other MALT lymphoma, PCMZL are typically class-switched, expressing IgG rather than IgM, and this is often

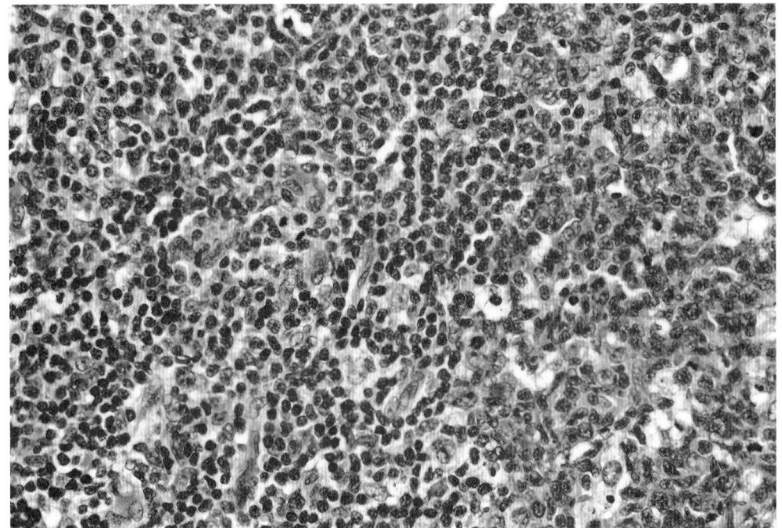

Fig. 29.190
Primary cutaneous marginal zone B-cell lymphoma: tumor cells are present on the left of the field with a germinal center on the right. Note the nuclear hyperchromatism.

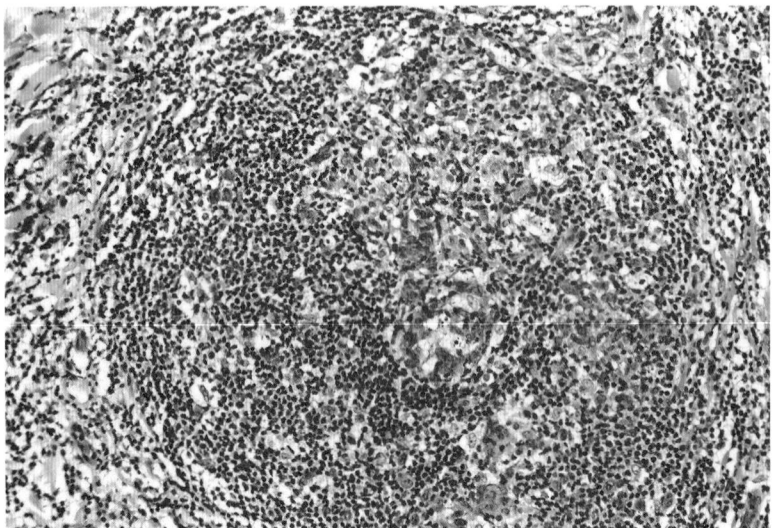

Fig. 29.191
Primary cutaneous marginal zone B-cell lymphoma: medium-power view of residual germinal center surrounded by tumor cells.

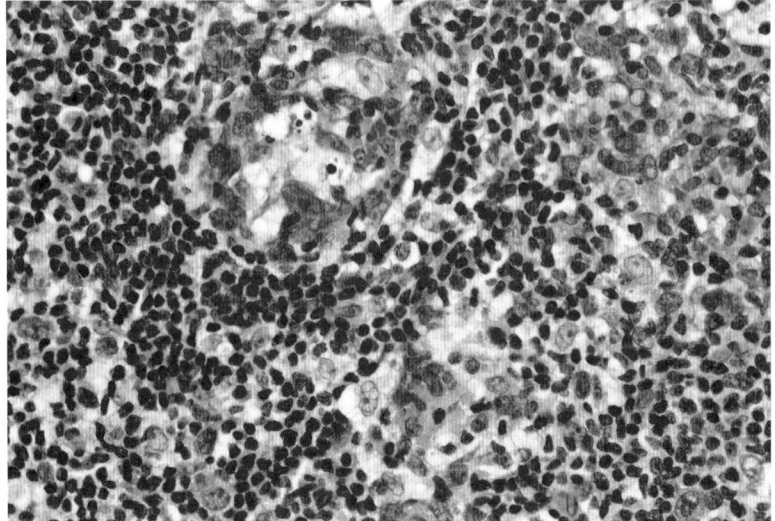

Fig. 29.192
Primary cutaneous marginal zone B-cell lymphoma: high-power view of *Fig. 29.191* showing follicular colonization.

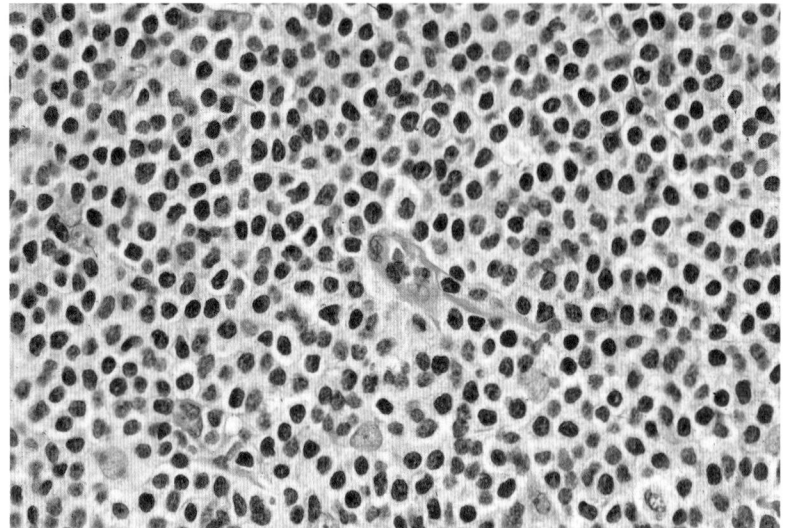

Fig. 29.193
Primary cutaneous marginal zone B-cell lymphoma: this field shows a uniform population of monocytoid B cells.

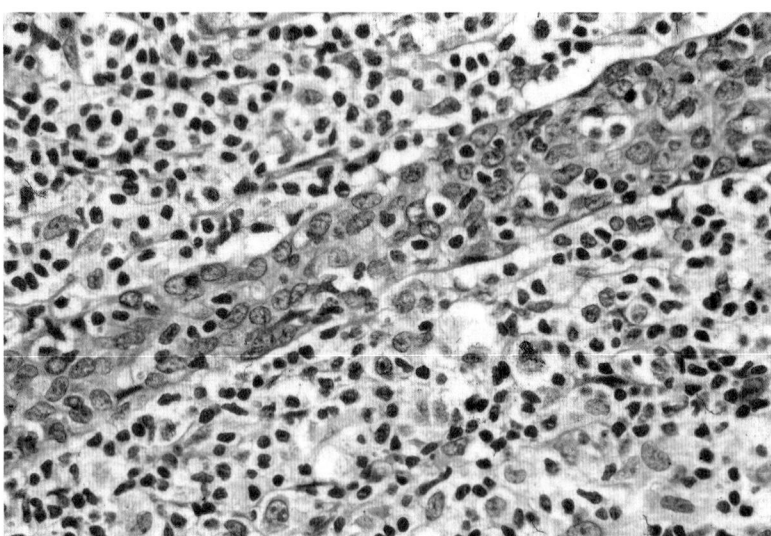

Fig. 29.194
Primary cutaneous marginal zone B-cell lymphoma: infiltration of sweat gland epithelium is present in this lymphoepithelial lesion. Note the nuclear irregularity and pale-staining cytoplasm.

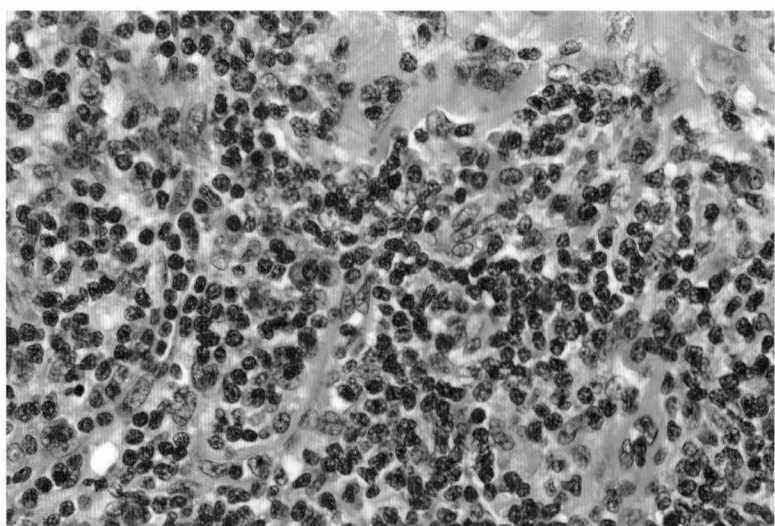

Fig. 29.195
Primary cutaneous marginal zone B-cell lymphoma: scattered plasma cells are present.

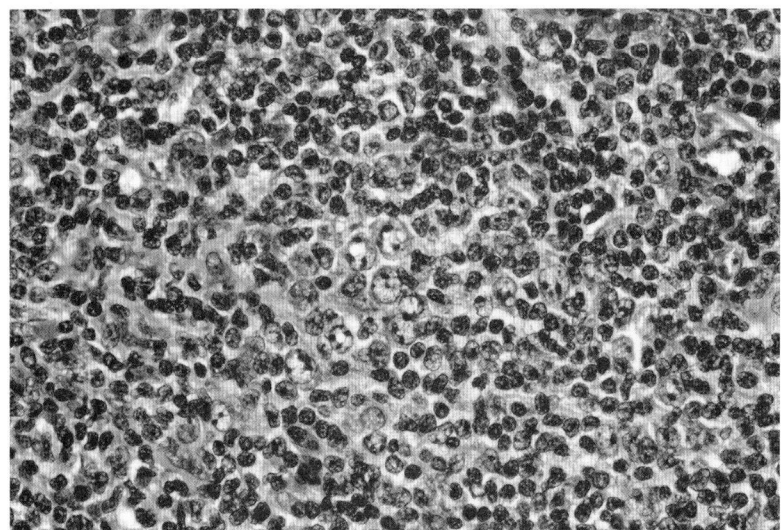

Fig. 29.196
Primary cutaneous marginal zone B-cell lymphoma: centroblasts with multiple nucleoli are present.

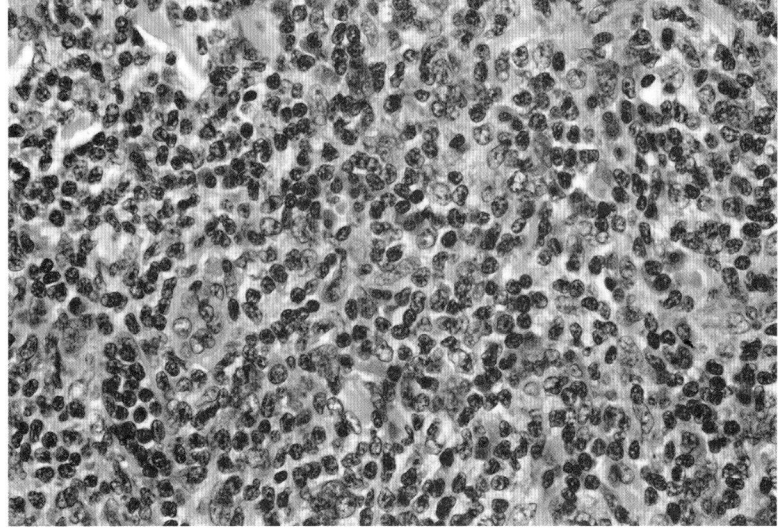

Fig. 29.197
Primary cutaneous marginal zone B-cell lymphoma: this field shows conspicuous eosinophils.

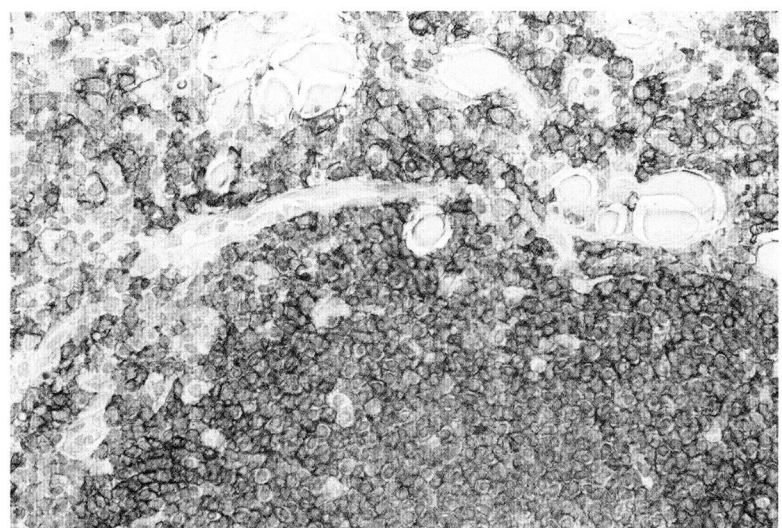

Fig. 29.198
Primary cutaneous marginal zone B-cell lymphoma: the tumor cells express CD20.

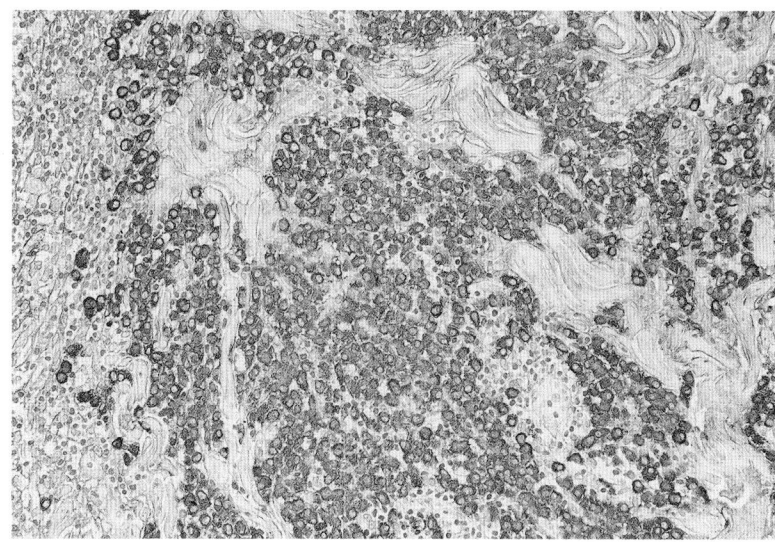

Fig. 29.199
Primary cutaneous marginal zone B-cell lymphoma: kappa light chain is strongly expressed.

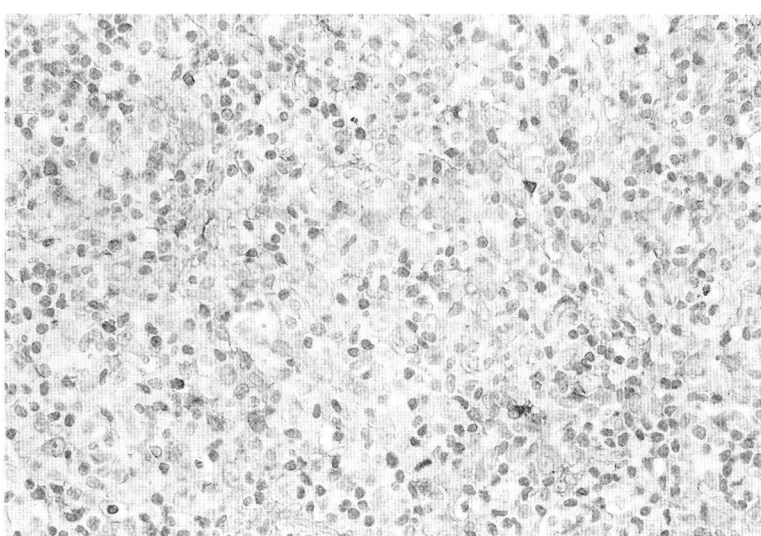

Fig. 29.200
Primary cutaneous marginal zone B-cell lymphoma: lambda light chain is negative.

of IgG4 subtype.[64–66] PCMZL arising in the post-transplant setting are positive for EBV.[23] Small numbers of CD30+ large transformed cells may be present.[18] The associated reactive follicles are CD10+ and bcl-6+, but bcl-2– and the presence of a follicular architecture can be highlighted by CD21, CD23, and/or CD35 expression, which identify FDCs (*Fig. 29.201*). There is a background population of unremarkable T cells.

Differential diagnosis

B-cutaneous lymphoid hyperplasia (B-CLH) and PCMZL are often difficult to distinguish from one another as they may share many histologic features, including a 'top-heavy' or 'bottom-heavy' distribution, reactive lymphoid follicles, a grenz zone, and a polymorphic interfollicular infiltrate.[13] However, close attention to detail should permit a proportion of cases to be reliably diagnosed as PCMZL, and others to be designated as B-CLH. Reactive follicles are said to be seen more frequently in PCMZL.[13] However, this should never be used as the sole criterion for a diagnosis of lymphoma; rather, it should stimulate a search for more definitive features in the interfollicular areas, as should the presence of partially colonized follicles. These include aggregates of marginal zone cells, confluent sheets of plasma cells, and Dutcher bodies.[13] Immunohistochemistry is required to confirm the B lineage of cells with a marginal zone appearance, since activated T cells

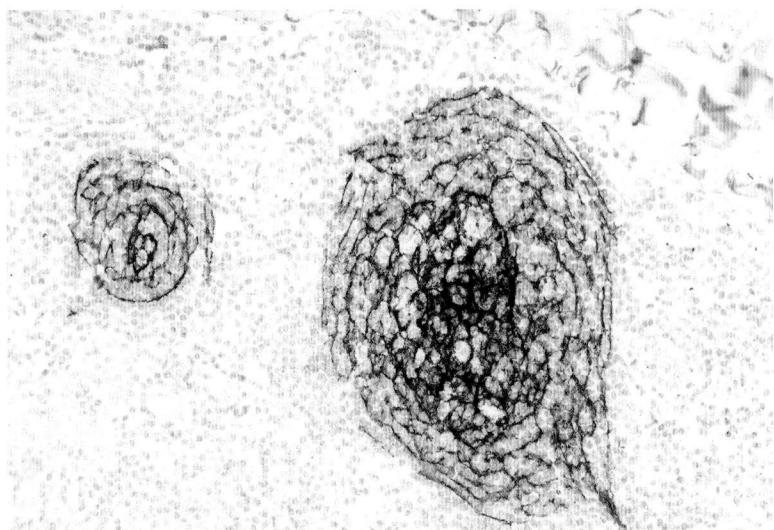

Fig. 29.201
Primary cutaneous marginal zone B-cell lymphoma: the germinal centers are highlighted with CD21 immunohistochemistry.

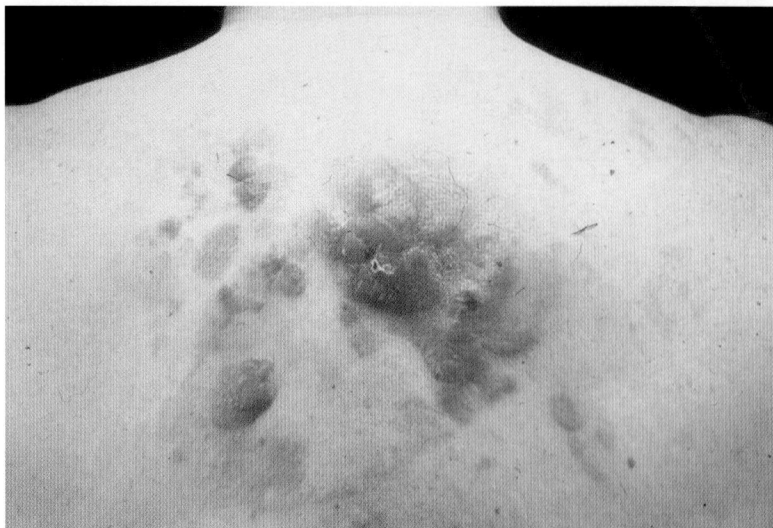

Fig. 29.202
Primary cutaneous follicle center lymphoma: presentation on the back was once known as reticulohistiocytoma of the dorsum (Crosti lymphoma). Note the aggregate of erythematous tumor nodules. By courtesy of the Institute of Dermatology, London, UK.

may also possess irregular nuclei and clear cytoplasm. Demonstration of a B-cell:T-cell ratio of >3:1 and aberrant expression of CD43 by B lymphocytes are the other features associated with a diagnosis of lymphoma.[13] It may be difficult to demonstrate expression of immunoglobulin light chains on the surface of B lymphocytes. However, assessment of cytoplasmic light chain expression by plasma cells is relatively straightforward, and the presence of monotypic plasmacytoid cells at the periphery of the infiltrate is a common finding in PCMZL.

Some authors consider demonstration of clonal immunoglobulin gene rearrangement as an important discriminator between B-CLH and cutaneous B-cell lymphoma.[67,68] However, clonality has also been demonstrated in some cases showing histologic features of B-CLH.[69,70] The significance of these findings is unclear. Several studies have shown no correlation between the presence of a B-cell clone and clinical presentation, development of further lesions, or progression to overt lymphoma.[69–72] Nevertheless, B-CLH may evolve into lymphoma, and it is possible that there is a continuous spectrum of B-lymphoproliferative disorders, with polyclonal B-CLH at one end and overt clonal cutaneous B-cell lymphoma at the other.[69–72] In between lie cases displaying histologic features of B-CLH but harboring occult oligo- or monoclonal populations of B lymphocytes which may occasionally evolve into full-blown lymphoma. For practical purposes, patients with 'clonal B-CLH' should probably be staged/investigated in the same way as those with definite cutaneous lymphoma, but managed along the lines of B-CLH.

PCMZL may also resemble primary cutaneous follicle center lymphoma (PCFCL), particularly when the latter has a follicular growth pattern. However, the follicles in PCFCL are neoplastic and tend to have a monotonous appearance with few tingible body macrophages, no differentiation into light and dark zones, an absence of mantles, and generally a lower proliferation index than reactive germinal centers. They may express bcl-2, unlike the reactive follicles in PCMZL, although this is not always the case, and follicular colonization by marginal zone cells can complicate the distinction. Staining for bcl-6 and/or CD10 may highlight interfollicular aggregates of neoplastic follicle center cells, allowing distinction form PCMZL, which is usually CD10 and bcl-6 negative.[17]

Distinction of PCMZL and cutaneous infiltration by CLL or MCL is usually straightforward on the basis of morphology and immunophenotype. The neoplastic lymphocytes of CLL usually express CD5 and CD23, whilst those of MCL are CD5 and cyclin D1 positive.

Primary cutaneous follicle center lymphoma

Much of the controversy surrounding this entity was resolved following the introduction of the new WHO-EORTC classification.[1] PCFCL consists of neoplastic lymphocytes that resemble the centrocytes and centroblasts of a normal germinal center. Unlike nodal follicular lymphoma, a follicular architecture is not a prerequisite for diagnosis, and often cases have a diffuse pattern of growth.[2] PCFCL largely equates with the entity primary cutaneous follicle center cell lymphoma, as defined in the original EORTC classification.[3] Cases previously described as primary cutaneous follicular lymphoma are included in this category, as are a proportion of cases included in series of primary cutaneous diffuse large B-cell lymphoma.[3–11] In addition, examples of this entity in the skin of the back have been referred to as RH of the dorsi or Crosti lymphoma (Fig. 29.202).[12]

Clinical features

PCFCL is the most common type of PCBCL, accounting for just less than 60% of cases in large series.[2,13] There is predilection for males, and the median age at presentation is >50 years.[7,12–14] Clinically, there are firm, erythematous to violaceous plaques, nodules, and/or tumors of variable but sometimes large size. The vast majority of cases (≈80%) present with solitary or localized lesions, multifocal lesions being rare.[1,2,8,13] There is predilection for the head and neck, particularly the scalp, and trunk; rare cases occur on the legs.[1,2,6,8,11,13–16] Disease should be limited to the skin at presentation in order to qualify as PCFCL.

Radiotherapy is the treatment of choice for solitary or localized lesions, and rituximab is used for more generalized disease.[17] Cutaneous relapses are frequent (≈30% of cases). The overall prognosis is excellent with a 5-year survival of >95%. Systemic combination chemotherapy is rarely required, when there is very extensive cutaneous disease, rare examples associated with systemic dissemination, and possibly also for cases arising on the leg, since the latter appear to have a less favorable prognosis.[2,6,8,15,17]

Pathogenesis and histopathological features

The neoplastic lymphocytes are of follicle center origin. Gene expression profiling studies show a pattern similar to that seen in DLBCL of germinal center type, and there is frequent amplification of c-REL.[17–20] Follicular lymphoma, which arises predominantly in lymph nodes, is another neoplasm of follicle center cells, and is characterized by a t(14;18)(q32;q21) juxtaposing the BCL2 gene with the immunoglobulin heavy chain.[21] This translocation is seen in around 90% of cases of nodal follicular lymphoma, but PCR-based assays identify it in only a relatively low proportion of PCFCL.[4–6,10,15,22–26] A higher incidence of t(14;18)(q32;q21) is seen in some series of PCFCL studied by fluorescence in situ hybridization (FISH) but not in others.[27–29] However, even the highest reported incidence (41–47%) is lower than that seen in nodal follicular lymphoma, and the fact that many FISH-positive cases are PCR negative suggests that different pathogenetic mechanisms are

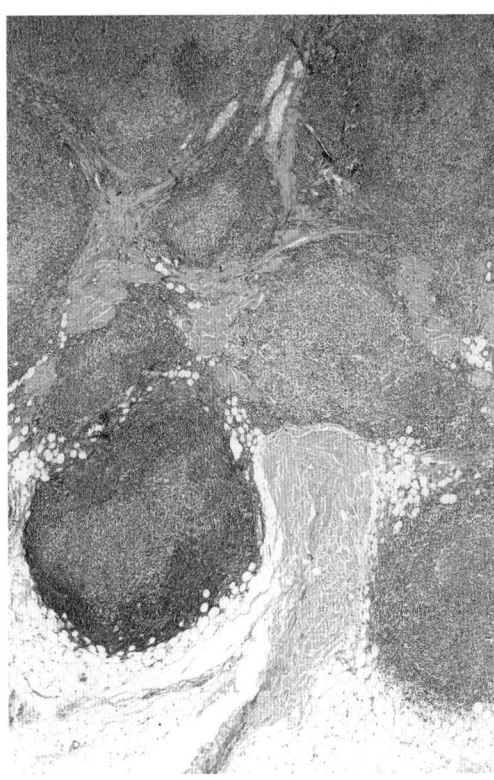

Fig. 29.203
Primary cutaneous follicle center lymphoma: there is a dense nodular infiltrate with a distinctive follicular pattern. By courtesy of G. Pinkus, MD, Brigham and Women's Hospital and Harvard Medical School, Boston, USA.

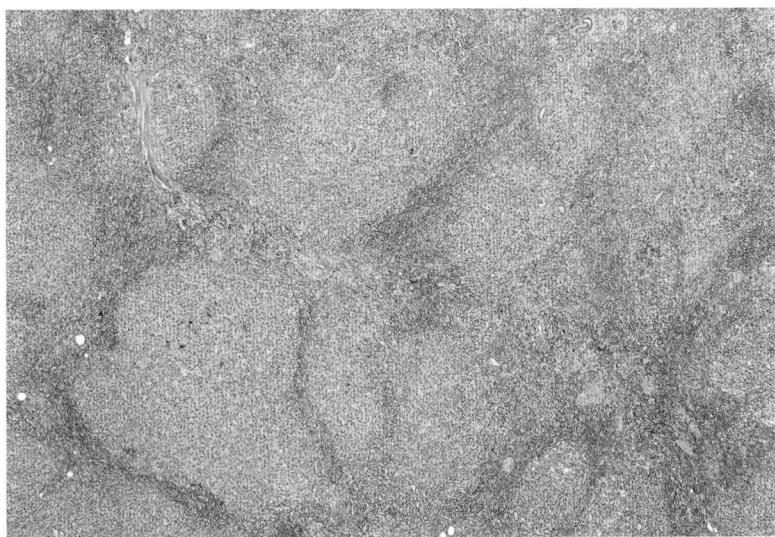

Fig. 29.204
Primary cutaneous follicle center lymphoma: note the conspicuous tumor follicles. By courtesy of G. Pinkus, MD, Brigham and Women's Hospital and Harvard Medical School, Boston, USA.

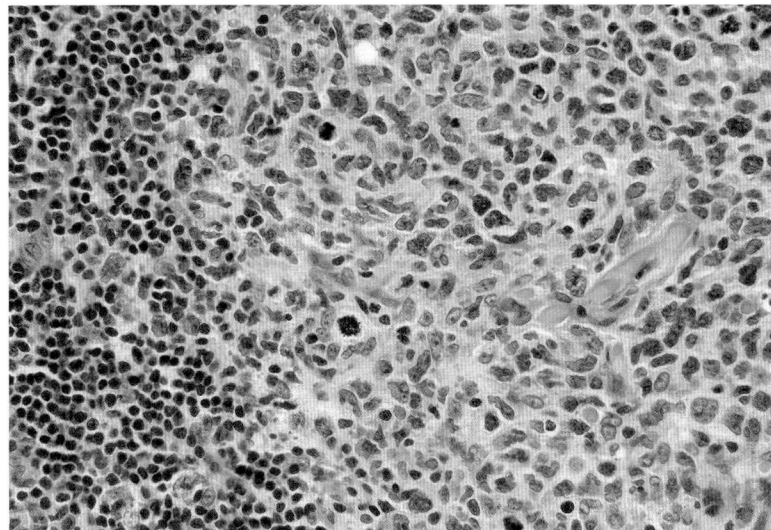

Fig. 29.205
Primary cutaneous follicle center lymphoma: the follicles are composed of a uniform population of tumor cells. Note the mitoses. By courtesy of G. Pinkus, MD, Brigham and Women's Hospital and Harvard Medical School, Boston, USA.

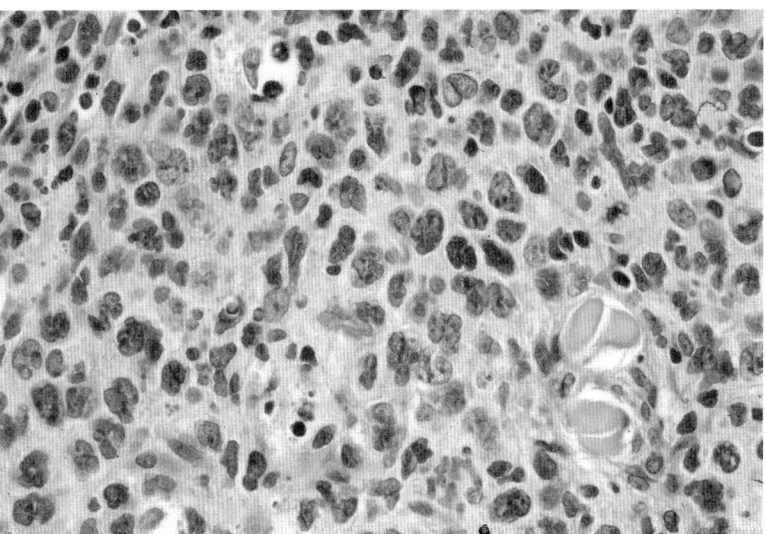

Fig. 29.206
Primary cutaneous follicle center lymphoma: the tumor consists of centrocytes with irregular, hyperchromatic nuclei. By courtesy of G. Pinkus, MD, Brigham and Women's Hospital and Harvard Medical School, Boston, USA.

at work in many PCFCLs.[27,28,30] A t(3;14)(q27;q32) has also been documented in a small number of cases and a del 1p36 in one.[27,28]

The infiltrate shows a perivascular and periadnexal distribution, but may diffusely fill the dermis. The majority of cases lack follicles (64%), but some show a follicular and diffuse pattern of growth or, less commonly, a purely follicular architecture.[1–3,14,31] The neoplastic lymphocytes are predominantly medium to large centrocytes, or centroblasts (*Figs 29.203–29.206*). Centrocytes have angulate, twisted, or cleaved nuclei with inconspicuous nucleoli and scant cytoplasm; centroblasts have round or oval nuclei with vesicular chromatin, with one to three nucleoli and a narrow rim of cytoplasm. Follicles have a monotonous appearance, generally have few tingible body macrophages, and show no differentiation into light and dark zones. Mantles are either absent or only poorly formed. Aggregates of neoplastic follicle center cells are present in the interfollicular areas.[4,6,14] Cases with a predominantly diffuse growth pattern contain a majority of large centrocytes with scattered polylobated cells and few centroblasts.[3,9,12,14,31] A spindle cell morphology is rarely encountered.[32–35] The neoplastic lymphocytes show consistent expression of CD20 and bcl-6 (*Figs 29.207* and *29.208*). CD10 expression varies. It is usually present when follicles are prominent, but negative in cases with a diffuse growth pattern (*Fig. 29.209*).[2,8,15,30,36,37] Early studies reported a virtual absence of bcl-2 protein expression, and although this protein is in fact probably expressed in the majority of cases, it is usually weak and often difficult to discern against a background of strongly positive T cells.[2,4,6,8,23,27,28,37–39] Strong positivity for both CD10 and bcl-2 should raise suspicion of secondary cutaneous involvement by nodal follicular lymphoma. Staining for CD5 and cyclin D1 is negative, and there is rare expression of CD23, CD30, MUM1, or FOXP1 (*Fig. 29.210*).[4,10,11,14,36,40] A unique case positive for EBV has also been described.[41] The proliferation rate of neoplastic germinal centers is lower than that seen in reactive germinal centers. The expanded follicular nodules can be highlighted with CD21, which can be negative in diffuse lesions (*Fig. 29.211*).[20,36]

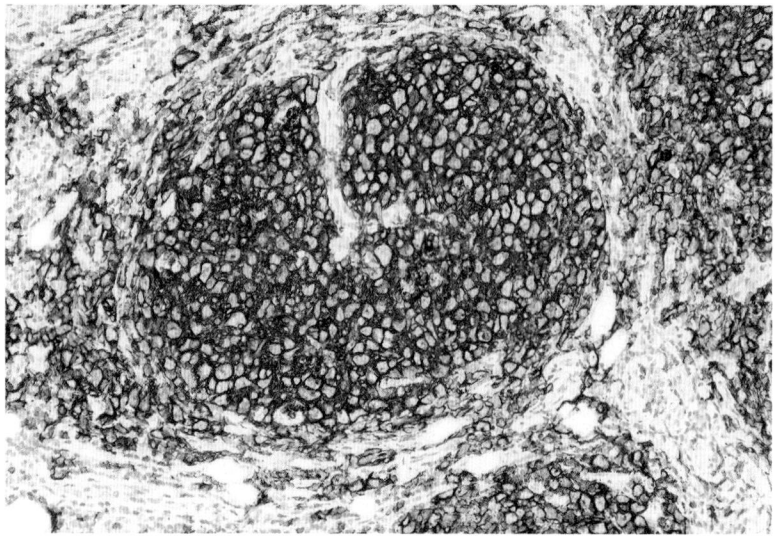

Fig. 29.207
Primary cutaneous follicle center lymphoma: the tumor cells express CD20. By courtesy of G. Pinkus, MD, Brigham and Women's Hospital and Harvard Medical School, Boston, USA.

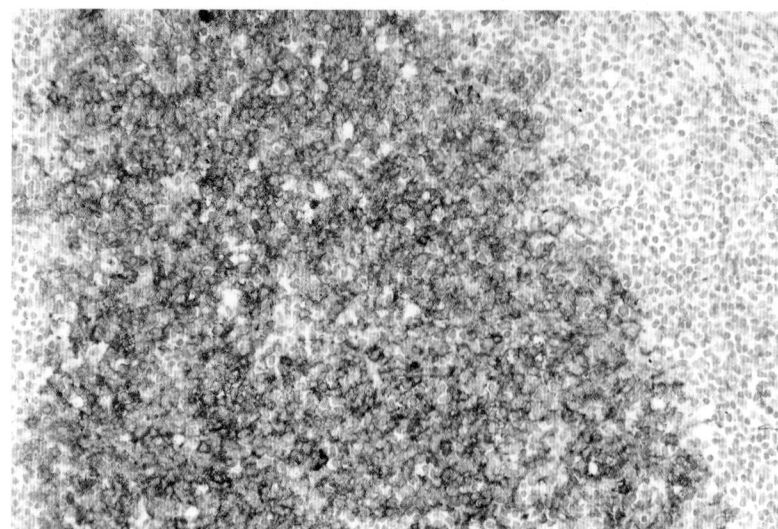

Fig. 29.209
Primary cutaneous follicle center lymphoma: in this example, CD10 is strongly expressed.

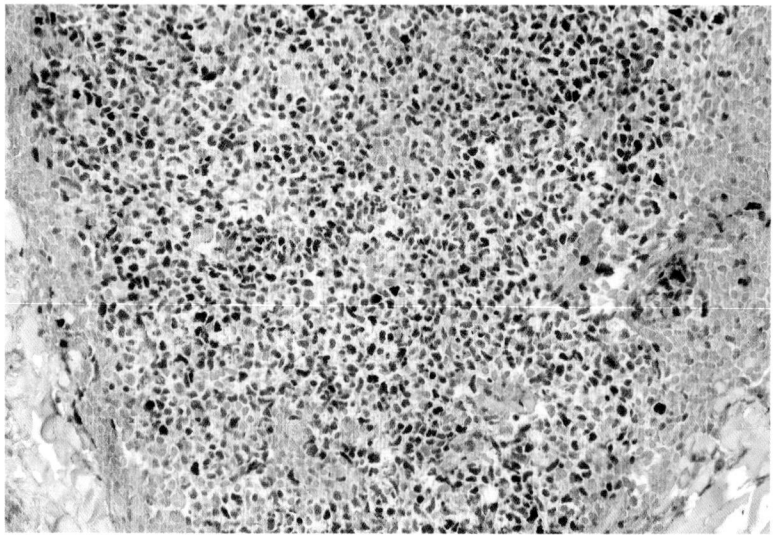

Fig. 29.208
Primary cutaneous follicle center lymphoma: the tumor cells are bcl-6 positive. By courtesy of G. Pinkus, MD, Brigham and Women's Hospital and Harvard Medical School, Boston, USA.

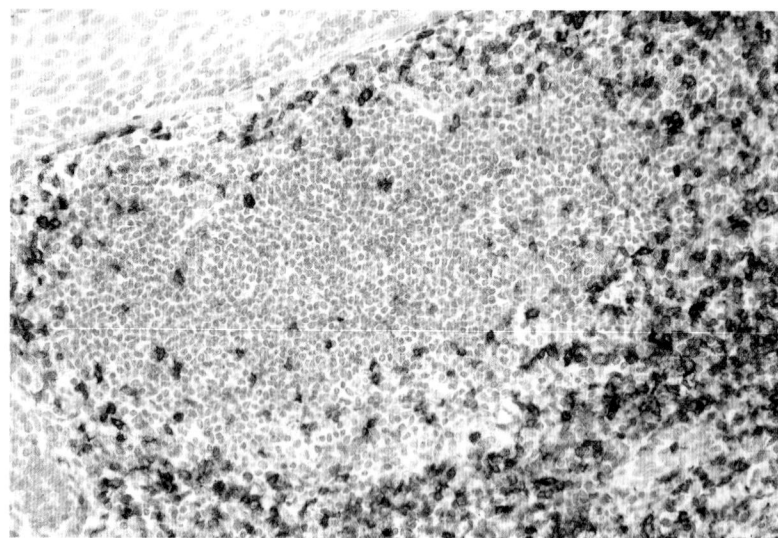

Fig. 29.210
Primary cutaneous follicle center lymphoma: CD5 is absent. By courtesy of G. Pinkus, MD, Brigham and Women's Hospital and Harvard Medical School, Boston, USA.

Clonality may be confirmed by light chain restriction (although this is often difficult due to low levels of surface immunoglobulin expression), IgH gene rearrangement, or, in some cases, by the presence of the t(14;18) translocation.[36]

Differential diagnosis

PCFCL with a diffuse growth pattern is usually composed of large cells and is not easily mistaken for reactive conditions. However, cases with a follicular growth pattern may be difficult to differentiate from B-CLH. It is not possible to reliably discriminate B-CLH from PCFCL on the basis of the architectural features at scanning magnification.[42]

Determining whether the lymphoid follicles are reactive or neoplastic is the main way of making this distinction. Neoplastic follicles typically have a monotonous appearance, lack well-formed mantles, show no differentiation into light and dark zones, and have relatively few tingible body macrophages. PCFCL are also composed predominantly of large centrocytes. By comparison, reactive follicles usually show differentiation into light and dark zones, tend to have higher numbers of mitotic figures and tingible body macrophages, and contain a higher proportion of centroblasts and immunoblasts.[42] However, in the skin, reactive follicles may lack mantles, especially

when associated with *B. burgdorferi* infection.[15,43] Immunohistochemical demonstration of bcl-2 in the follicle center cells confirms a diagnosis of lymphoma. Neoplastic follicles often have a low proliferation fraction compared with reactive follicles, and staining for Ki-67 may also highlight the presence of zonation in the latter. However, bcl-2 expression is often weak and may be negative in PCFCL, and cases composed predominantly of large cells may display a high proliferation fraction (*Fig. 29.212*). In such situations, a careful search for CD10 and/or bcl-6 positive interfollicular cells is necessary; extrafollicular CD10 B cells are only seen in lymphoma and are not a feature of reactive lymphoid tissue.

MCL can be distinguished from PCFCL by the expression of CD5 and cyclin D1 in the former.

Primary cutaneous diffuse large B-cell lymphoma, leg type

Clinical features

The once controversial entity of large B-cell lymphoma of the leg, proposed in the original EORTC classification, has gained general acceptance

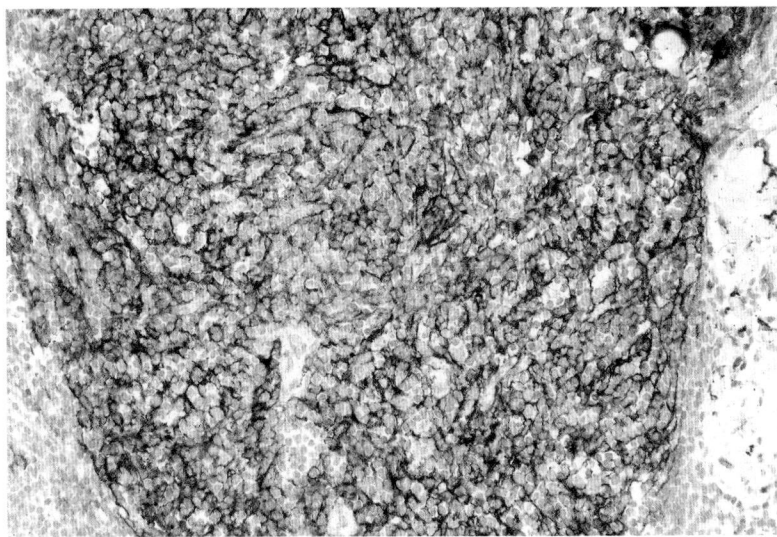

Fig. 29.211
Primary cutaneous follicle center lymphoma: the tumor follicles are highlighted with CD21 immunohistochemistry. By courtesy of G. Pinkus, MD, Brigham and Women's Hospital and Harvard Medical School, Boston, USA.

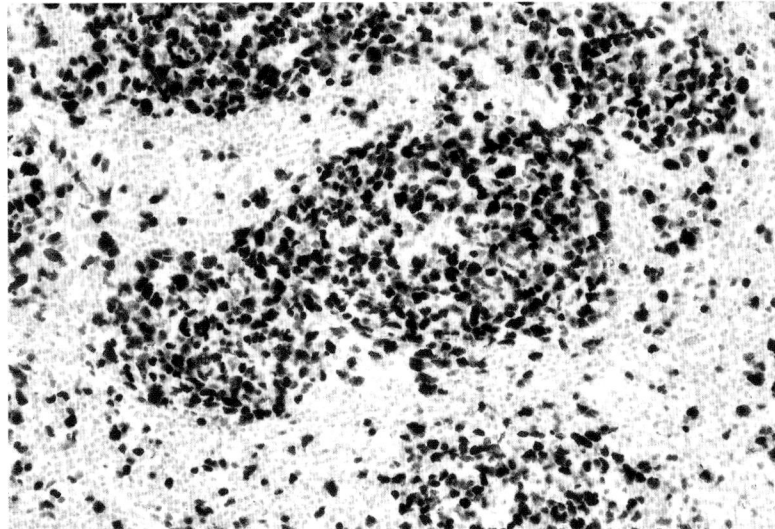

Fig. 29.212
Primary cutaneous follicle center lymphoma: this high-grade lesion shows very brisk proliferative activity with MIB-1. By courtesy of G. Pinkus, MD, Brigham and Women's Hospital and Harvard Medical School, Boston, USA.

following an increasing number of publications associating location in the lower limb with poor outcome in primary cutaneous lymphomas composed of large B cells.[1–5] However, lymphomas displaying similar clinicopathological features also occur above the waist, and this has led to the use of the less anatomically restricted term of primary cutaneous diffuse large B-cell lymphoma, leg type (PCDLBCL-LT).[6,7]

PCDLBCL-LT accounts for around 20% of all PCBCLs.[6,8] Most patients are elderly females (male/female ratio 1:3.4), with a median age at presentation >70 years.[7–11] Presentation is usually with multiple red or bluish-red nodules or tumors and, less commonly, patches, plaques, subcutaneous tumors, and ulcers.[2,4,5,7,9–12] Solitary lesions are relatively infrequent. About 10–15% of cases present at a site different from the leg (trunk, upper limbs, and head and neck).[7–11] Multifocal disease is seen in 5–20% of cases.[8,9,11] The recommended treatment is as for systemic diffuse large B-cell lymphoma (DLBCL).[13] Relapses and extracutaneous dissemination, to lymph nodes and/or viscera, are common (55–69% and 17–47% of patients, respectively), with relatively frequent CNS involvement.[8,9,11] Historically, the 5-year disease-specific survival was quoted at approximately 50%, but a more recent study suggests an improved outcome (74% overall 5-year

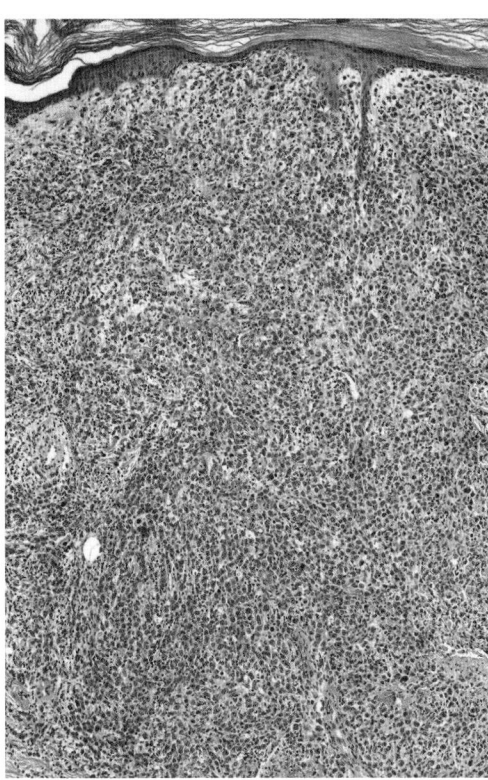

Fig. 29.213
Primary cutaneous diffuse large B-cell lymphoma, leg type: there is a dense dermal infiltrate which, in this case, abuts the overlying epithelium.

survival) following routine addition of Rituximab to CHOP-like chemotherapeutic regimens.[2,4,8,10,11,14]

Pathogenesis and histologic features

Primary cutaneous diffuse large B-cell lymphoma is a tumor of postgerminal center B cells that displays a gene expression profile similar to that seen in activated B-cell-like DLBCL, as well as one that suggests constitutive activation and inhibition of the intrinsic apoptosis pathway.[15–17] In common with activated B-cell-like DLBCL at other sites, there is a relatively high incidence of mutations involving NF-κB pathway genes, particularly MYD88.[18–21] Translocations involving MYC, BCL6, IGH, and, rarely, BCL2 may be found.[19,22,23] In addition, more than half of cases show amplifications of 18q21.31-q21.33, a region encompassing the BCL2 and MALT1 genes, providing an explanation for the high levels of bcl-2 expression seen in this neoplasm. Loss of 9p21.3, harboring the CDKN2A gene encoding p16 and p14ARF, or inactivation by promoter hypermethylation, is also common and may be a poor prognostic indicator.[19,24–27]

Biopsies show a diffuse dermal infiltrate composed of sheets of centroblasts and immunoblasts that effaces adnexal structures (*Figs 29.213–29.215*). A grenz zone is present and ulceration may be seen. Centroblasts have little cytoplasm and round to oval vesicular nuclei typically containing multiple small nucleoli dispersed adjacent to the nuclear membrane. Immunoblasts have more abundant basophilic cytoplasm and the nucleus contains a single large eosinophilic nucleolus. Mitotic figures are plentiful. A few reactive T cells are present.[2,4,6–8,11]

Tumor cells express CD20 and CD79A, and are almost always strongly positive for bcl-2, MUM1/IRF4, and FOXP1, although negative staining for bcl-2 and MUM1/IRF4 is reported in up to 10% of cases (*Fig. 29.216*).[5,8,10,14,28–30] Staining for bcl-6 is usually positive and CD10 is negative (*Fig. 29.217*).[5,8,30]

Differential diagnosis

Primary cutaneous diffuse large B-cell lymphoma must be differentiated from DLBCL secondarily involving this skin, which is done by staging, and PCFCL. PCFCL and PCDLBCL-LT are primarily distinguished on the basis of cell morphology, the former containing a predominance of cleaved cells

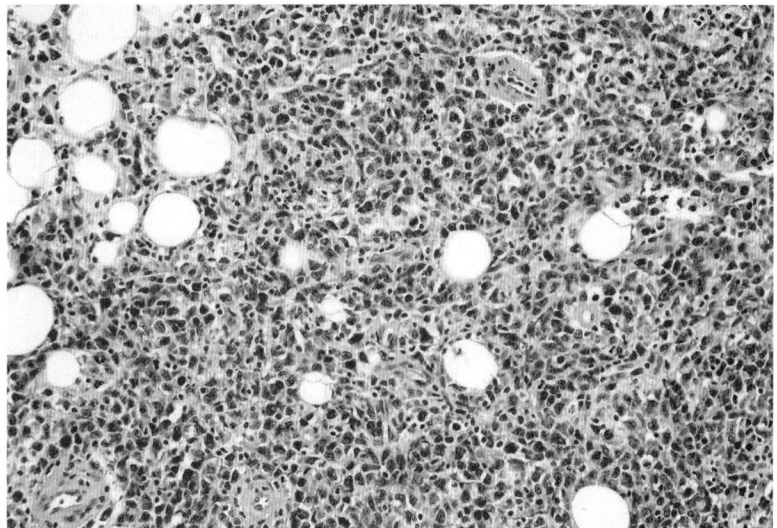

Fig. 29.214
Primary cutaneous diffuse large B-cell lymphoma, leg type: the tumor extends into subcutaneous fat.

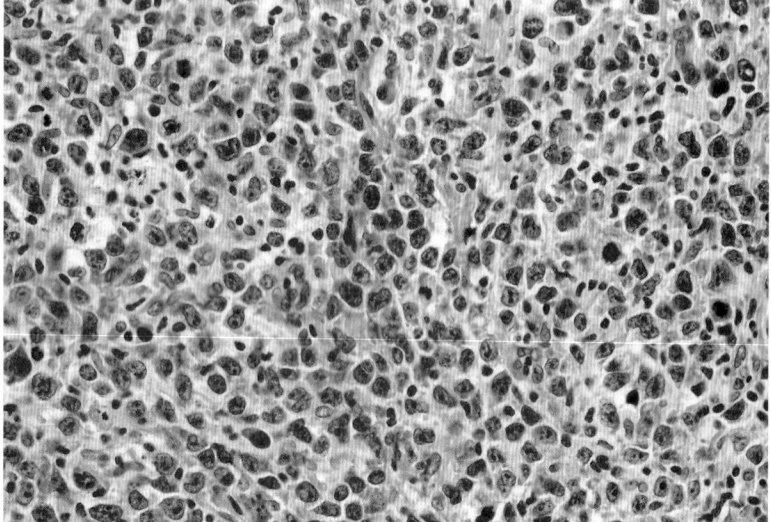

Fig. 29.215
Primary cutaneous diffuse large B-cell lymphoma, leg type: the tumor is composed of an admixture of centroblasts and immunoblasts. Note the mitotic activity.

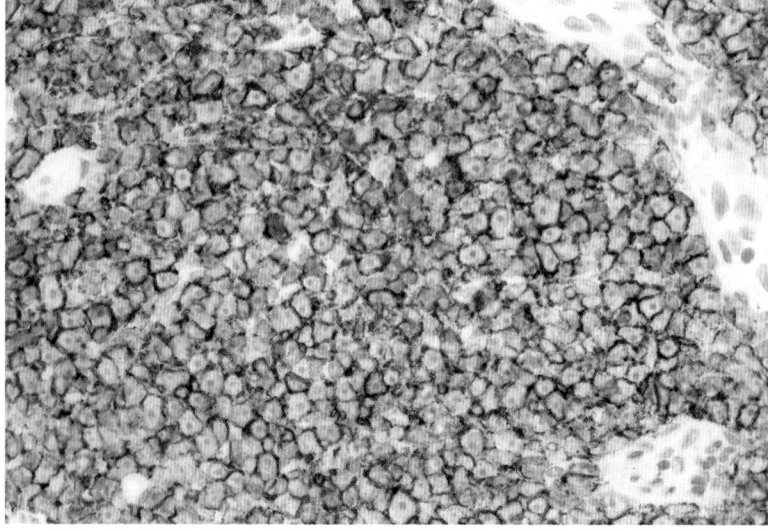

Fig. 29.216
Primary cutaneous diffuse large B-cell lymphoma, leg type: the tumor cells show uniform expression of CD20.

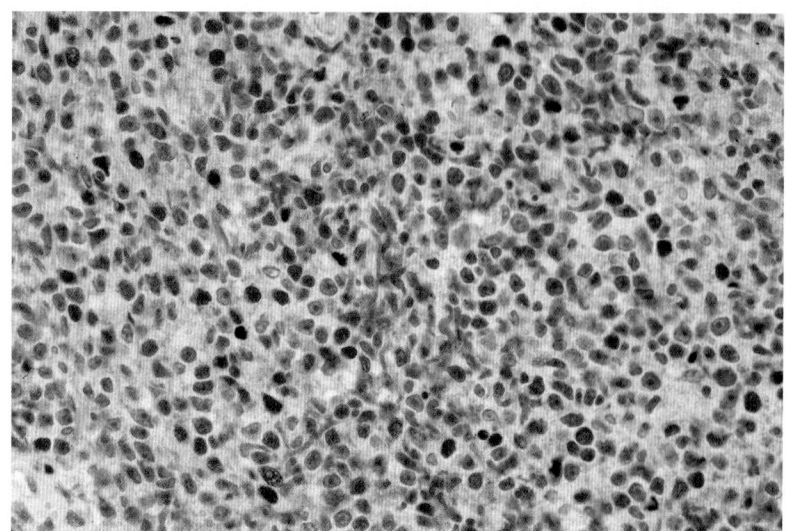

Fig. 29.217
Primary cutaneous diffuse large B-cell lymphoma, leg type: bcl-6 is strongly expressed.

and the latter diffuse sheets of round cells. However, distinction is difficult and is subject to interobserver variation.[2] Other factors that suggest a diagnosis of PCFCL are the presence of a significant admixture of T cells, a stromal reaction, and remnants of FDC networks, as demonstrated by antibodies to CD21, CD23 and/or CD35. Strong staining for bcl-2, MUM1, and FOXP1, and expression of IgM favor a diagnosis of PCDLBCL-LT.[8,31-33] MCL disseminating to skin can also bear close pathological resemblance to PCDLBCL-LT, but can be distinguished by cyclin D1 expression and demonstration of a CCND1 translocation.[33]

Primary cutaneous diffuse large B-cell lymphoma, other

Primary cutaneous diffuse large B-cell lymphoma, other (PCDLBCL-O) was a term introduced in the original EORTC–WHO classification.[1] It was used for rare cases of large B-cell lymphoma arising in the skin that could not be comfortably categorized as primary cutaneous diffuse large B-cell lymphoma, leg type (PCDLBCL-LT) or PCFCL. It was suggested that it would include variants of DLBCL that usually represent a skin manifestation of a systemic lymphoma, such as plasmablastic lymphoma or T-cell/histiocyte-rich large B-cell lymphoma. This approach was slightly modified in the WHO classification of skin tumors published in 2006. In this text, both T-cell/histiocyte-rich large B-cell lymphoma and plasmablastic lymphoma are considered separate from PCDLBCL-O.[2] PCDLBCL-O is largely restricted to lymphomas showing features typical of PDLBCL-LT but lacking bcl-2 expression.[2] However, more recent publications suggest no significant clinical differences between bcl-2-positive and bcl-2-negative PCDLBCL-LT, and several authors accept the latter as part of the spectrum of PCDLBCL-LT.[3,4]

Plasmablastic lymphoma is discussed below as an example of a systemic lymphoma that may present in the skin. T-cell/histiocyte-rich large B-cell lymphoma arising primarily in the skin is exceedingly rare and characterized by scattered large neoplastic B cells with a background of numerous (>90%) reactive T cells. Clinically, such cases show similarities with PCFCL and PCMZL and may merely represent an exaggerated T-cell infiltrate in association with other, specific forms of PCBCL. Cutaneous T-cell/histiocyte-rich large B-cell lymphoma does not appear to be related to the nodal form of the disease, which is much more aggressive.[5-8]

PCDLBCL-O is therefore not an entity, but a holding category into which large B-cell tumors can be placed until such time as the diagnosis becomes obvious, or future studies clarify gray areas in the current classification system. In view of its apparent poor prognosis, PCFCL arising on the leg might be viewed in such a light.

Secondary cutaneous involvement by B-cell lymphoma

The following lymphomas not infrequently involve the skin. Cutaneous lesions may be the presenting feature, and in some cases disease may remain confined to the skin for lengthy periods. However, such tumors are no different from morphologically identical neoplasms that disseminate to the skin during relapse and/or progression.

Mantle cell lymphoma

Clinical features

Mantle cell lymphoma(MCL) (mantle zone lymphoma, centrocytic lymphoma, lymphocytic lymphoma of intermediate grade) is a rare peripheral B-cell lymphoma thought to be derived from naive pregerminal center B cells of the inner mantle zone.[1] It accounts for approximately 3–10% of NHL subtypes.[2] It is more common in old adults (median, 60 years) with predilection for males (2:1–4:1).[1,3,4]

MCL is a nodal disease that frequently disseminates to extranodal sites. Most cases are advanced stage (stage III or IV) at diagnosis. Generalized lymphadenopathy is the most frequent presentation (87–90%). Infiltration of bone marrow (80%), spleen (47–60%), and liver (13%) is frequent. The gastrointestinal tract (18–20%) and Waldeyer ring (10–12%) are also often affected, and most cases of lymphomatous polyposis of the intestine are due to this lymphoma. Neoplastic lymphocytes are typically found in peripheral blood using flow cytometry, and rarely there may be a leukemic picture.[5–8] 'B' symptoms (clinical symptoms of pyrexia (sometimes periodic), weight loss, and night sweats) are present in 14% to 40% of patients.[3,4] Anemia, low serum albumin, raised LDH, and β_2-microglobulin levels are common.[3,4] Cutaneous involvement is exceptional, and although MCL may present in the skin, it is almost invariably associated with systemic disease.[9–13] Presentation is with erythematous nodules or tumors on the trunk or extremities, although indurated plaques, macules, and a maculopapular rash may occur.[9–12] It can also be associated with cutaneous paraneoplastic phenomena. Several cases of insect bite-like reactions, similar to those more commonly seen in CLL, have been described. These manifest as a polymorphous rash comprising multiple pruritic, erythematous papules, nodules, plaques, and/or vesicles, that usually precede, but may follow, the diagnosis of lymphoma.[14–18] Hypersensitivity reactions to mosquito bites, similar to those seen in association with NK/T-cell lymphomas, have also been described.[19,20]

The median survival is only of 3–5 years.[1,21] The most consistent prognostic indicators are a high mitotic or Ki-67 index and a blastoid or pleomorphic morphology.[1,7,8,22,23] An indolent non-nodal leukemic variant characterized by involvement of peripheral blood, bone marrow, and often spleen is now recognized. Unlike more usual MCL, the neoplastic lymphocytes possess mutated immunoglobulin heavy chain genes and are SOX11 negative.[24]

Pathogenesis and histopathological features

MCL is associated with a t(11;14)(q13;q32) translocation in most cases.[1,3,4,25–27] This results in dysregulation of the PRAD1/CCND1 gene with overexpression of cyclin D1, a protein that is critical to cell cycle regulation.[28,29] A variant translocation involving CCND1 and light chain genes may also occur.[30] Most cases also contain a high number of non-random secondary chromosomal aberrations, some of which correlate with more aggressive behavior.[31–33] A subset of MCLs lack t(11;14)(q13;q32) and do not overexpress cyclin D1. These cases show identical morphologic and clinical features as cyclin D1-positive cases and share the same gene expression profile, except that they express high levels of cyclin D2 or cyclin D3. Some have a t(2;12)(p12;p13) juxtaposing the cyclin D2 gene with the immunoglobulin lambda light chain gene.[34,35] Immunoglobulin light and heavy chain genes are rearranged in many cases, but the V regions are usually either unmutated or show only low levels of somatic hypermutation.[36,37]

Nodal tumors may show a nodular, diffuse, or mixed growth pattern.[1–3,5,38,39] In nodular variants, the nodules represent reactive follicles with a surrounding rim of tumor cells (mantle zone pattern) or are composed of a pure tumor cell population.[38,39] The infiltrate usually consists of a monomorphic population of small to medium-sized atypical lymphoid cells with irregular, hyperchromatic nuclei, inconspicuous nucleoli, and minimal cytoplasm.[1,3] Morphological variants include blastoid, pleomorphic, small cell, and marginal zone-like. In blastoid MCL, the cells are uniformly of intermediate to large size with a lymphoblast-like appearance. They have dispersed chromatin and a very high mitotic index (20–30/10 high-power fields [HPFs]). Pleomorphic MCL also comprises large cells, but these often have irregular nuclear outlines and prominent nucleoli. The neoplastic lymphocytes in the small cell variant resemble those seen in SLL, whilst the marginal zone-like cases have abundant pale cytoplasm.[1] Tumors may transform to a more aggressive variant with recurrence.[4] Hyalinized vessels, a background population of polyclonal plasma cells, and histiocytes are often seen.[1,3]

Cutaneous lesions vary from superficial perivascular to nodular or diffuse dermal/subcutaneous monomorphic infiltrates (Figs 29.218–29.220).[9–12] Small/intermediate and blastoid variants may be encountered.[11] Insect

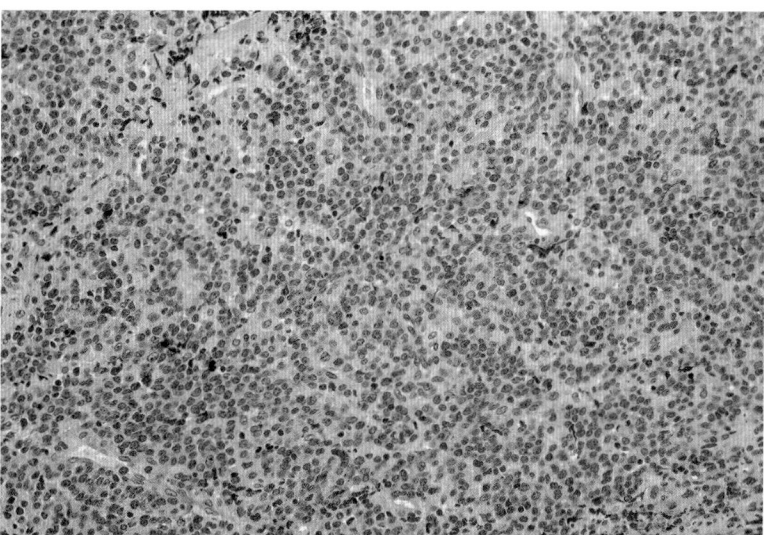

Fig. 29.218
Mantle cell lymphoma: this lesion presented in the subcutaneous fat. The tumor consists of a monomorphic population of lymphoid cells with hyperchromatic nuclei. By courtesy of G. Pinkus, MD, Brigham and Women's Hospital and Harvard Medical School, Boston, USA.

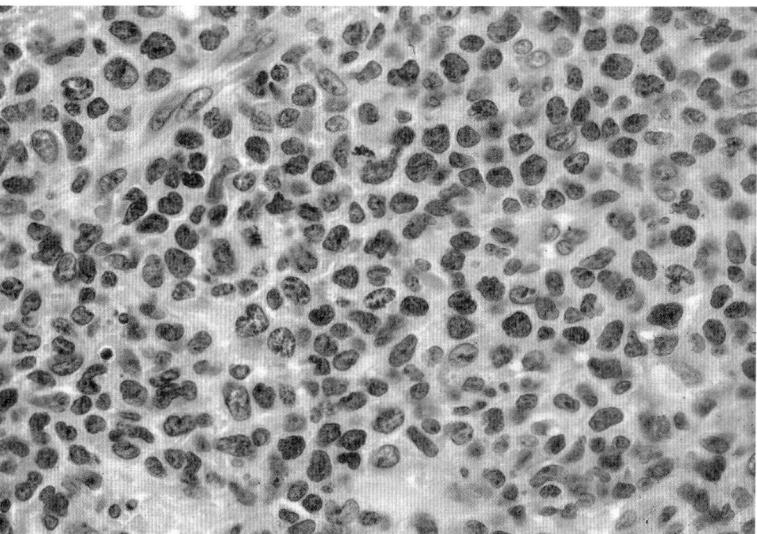

Fig. 29.219
Mantle cell lymphoma: nuclei are irregular. Note the mitosis. By courtesy of G. Pinkus, MD, Brigham and Women's Hospital and Harvard Medical School, Boston, USA.

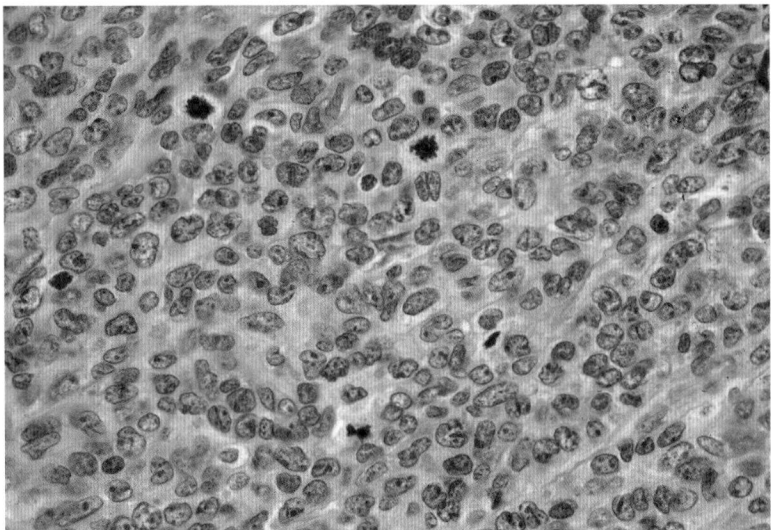

Fig. 29.220
Mantle cell lymphoma: in this field, nucleolated forms are present, and there are multiple mitoses. By courtesy of G. Pinkus, MD, Brigham and Women's Hospital and Harvard Medical School, Boston, USA.

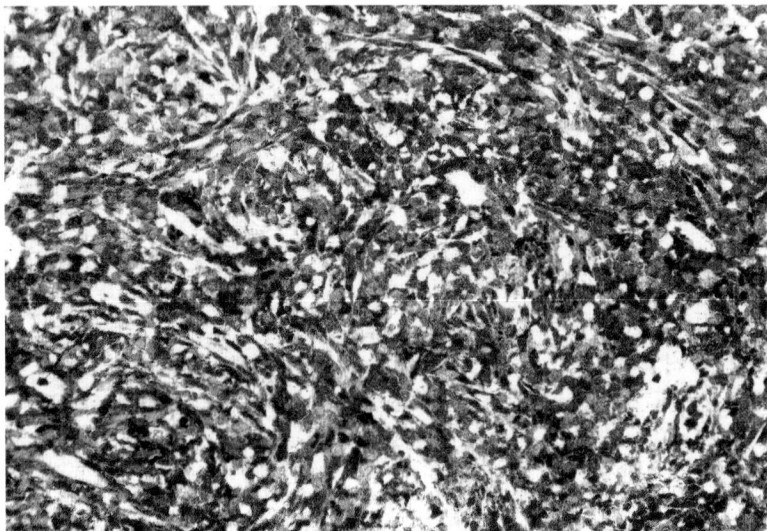

Fig. 29.221
Mantle cell lymphoma: the tumor cells uniformly express cyclin D1. By courtesy of G. Pinkus, MD, Brigham and Women's Hospital and Harvard Medical School, Boston, USA.

bite-like reactions seen in MCL show a superficial and deep perivascular and interstitial lymphocytic infiltrate with numerous eosinophils. Neutrophils are also usually plentiful and nuclear dust may be seen, but there is no fibrinoid necrosis of vessel walls. In biopsies of papules, nodules, and plaques, there is either no epidermal involvement or only mild spongiosis. Vesicular lesions show marked subepidermal edema and dermal–epidermal separation.[14]

Tumor cells are of B-cell origin (CD20+ and CD79a+) with coexpression of surface IgM and IgD, and more often show lambda than kappa light chain restriction.[1] They typically express CD5, CD43, cyclin D1, bcl-2, and SOX11, and are usually negative for bcl-6 and CD10 (*Fig. 29.221*).[1,40] Cases with aberrant CD5 negative or CD10 or bcl-6 positive phenotypes can occur.[1,41,42] CD23 is negative or weakly positive. Bcl-2 is positive, as is cyclin D1, in nearly all cases (i.e., those harboring a t(11;14)(q13;q32)). A high proliferation index is usually evident.

Cyclin D1 immunohistochemistry is valuable with paraffin-embedded material (91% sensitivity). However, in those cases that are negative or indeterminate, interphase FISH may be of particular value in demonstrating the t(11;14) translocation.[12,43,44] Amplification of the t(11;14) genomic

breakpoint by PCR suffers from scattering of the breakpoints, and it is much less sensitive.[43] The diagnosis may also be confirmed by reverse transcription PCR (RT-PCR) demonstration of cyclin D1 transcript overexpression.[43] It should also be remembered that rare cases lack t(11;14). Thus, when confronted with a CD5-positive, cyclin D1-negative lymphoma with the morphological features of MCL, consideration should be given to staining for SOX11, cyclin D2, and/or cyclin D3 to avoid a misdiagnosis.

Differential diagnosis

MCL must be distinguished from other small B-cell lymphomas that may disseminate to the skin, including follicular lymphoma and B-small lymphocytic lymphoma/chronic lymphocytic leukemia, cutaneous follicle center lymphoma, and PCMZL. Differentiation from primary cutaneous diffuse large B-cell lymphoma, leg type (PCDLBCL-LT) may also be problematic.[45] Follicular lymphoma and cutaneous follicle center lymphoma are typically CD5–/CD10+, marginal zone lymphoma, and PCDLBCL-LT are CD5–/CD10– and small cell lymphocytic lymphoma is CD5+CD23+/CD10–. All are cyclin D1 and SOX11 negative.[3,46,47]

B-chronic lymphocytic leukemia/small lymphocytic lymphoma

Clinical features

B-chronic lymphocytic leukemia/small lymphocytic lymphoma (CLL/SLL) is a neoplasm of small, antigen-experienced B lymphocytes.[1] CLL is defined on the basis of a persistent (≥3 months) lymphocytosis of $\geq 5 \times 10^9$/L.[1,2] SLL is the term applied to cases without a leukemic blood picture, in which there is tissue infiltration by cells displaying morphological and immunophenotypic features of CLL, lymphadenopathy, absence of cytopenias due to bone marrow infiltration, and a peripheral blood lymphocyte count of $<5 \times 10^9$/L.[2]

CLL is the commonest leukemia in Western populations and accounts for 6–7% of all NHL seen in tissue biopsies.[3,4] The mean age at presentation is 65 years with predilection for males.[1] Usually, there is involvement of peripheral blood and bone marrow and frequent infiltration of lymph nodes, liver, and spleen. Other extranodal sites may also be involved and specific infiltrates are seen in the skin in 1–2% of cases.[5,6]

There is predilection for the face, scalp, upper trunk, and extremities.[7,8] In general, however, the infiltrates appear to be fairly randomly distributed and are sometimes generalized.[7,9,10] Lesions consist of papules, nodules, tumors, or plaques. Occasionally, pruritic erythroderma or bullous lesions may be seen (*Fig. 29.222*).[6–9,11] Mucosal involvement is exceptional. Fingertip hypertrophy and macrocheilia are rare manifestations.[12,13] In some patients, the tumor cells localize to the site of previous viral (e.g., herpes simplex or zoster) or *Borrelia* infection.[5,11,14–17] They may also home into epithelial neoplasms, such as squamous cell carcinoma and basal cell carcinoma, as well as sites involved by other lymphoproliferative disorders.[18,19] The homing of CLL lymphocytes to skin affected by other pathologies has no bearing on prognosis.

Patients are at increased risk of second malignancies, including nonmelanoma skin cancer, and such tumors may have unusual clinical presentations and/or display atypical histologic features.[5,20,21] Cutaneous viral infections are more frequent, commonly severe in nature, and may, in part, be a consequence of therapy.[5,22] Exaggerated responses to mosquito bites and insect bite-like reactions have also been described.[23–27]

The disease is indolent with a relatively good medium- to long-term prognosis.[1] Infiltration of skin does not appear to specifically affect the prognosis, although overall stage of the disease does.[6,11,28,29] Biological markers are also important in predicting outcome. Cases with somatically mutated immunoglobulin genes and with del13q14.3 appear to do better. Poor prognosis is associated with nonmutated cases, cases expressing Zap70 and CD38, and those with deletions of 11q22-23, 17p, and 6q.[30–33] Additional adverse prognostic indicators include a rapid lymphocyte doubling time in peripheral blood and raised serum markers of increased cell turnover (thymidine kinase, sCD23, β_2-microglobulin).[34] Transformation to diffuse large B-cell lymphoma occurs in 2–8% of cases (Richter syndrome), and to classic

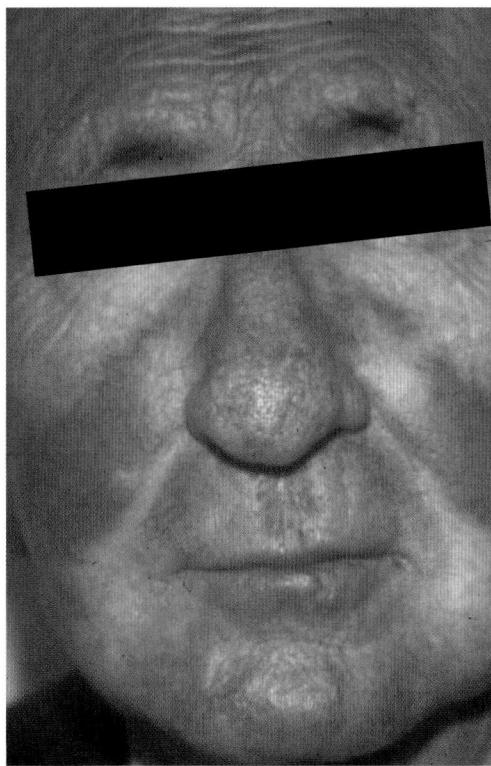

Fig. 29.222
Chronic lymphocytic leukemia. There is intense facial erythema. By courtesy of R.A. Marsden, MD, St George's Hospital, London, UK.

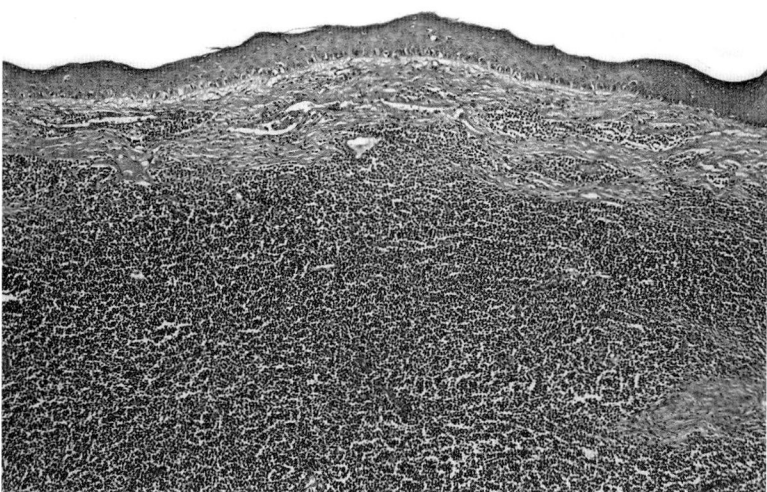

Fig. 29.223
Chronic lymphocytic leukemia: there is an intense lymphoid infiltrate in the dermis.

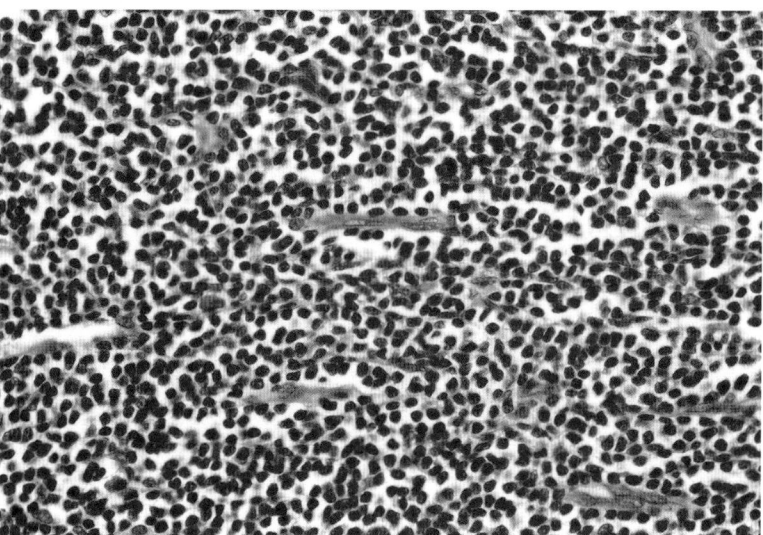

Fig. 29.224
Chronic lymphocytic leukemia: the infiltrate consists of a pure population of small lymphocytes.

HL in <1%. Such high-grade transformation is associated with a dismal prognosis (median survival of <1 year).[1]

Pathogenesis and histopathological features

Tumor cells show a very restricted use of immunoglobulin and light chain variable regions, suggesting that chronic stimulation by antigen or auto-antigen plays an important role in disease pathogenesis.[35] There is a very strong familial and geographic association (CLL is very rare in the Far East), implying a genetic predisposition.[1] The commonest genetic abnormalities are del13q14.3 (50%), trisomy 12 (≈20%), del11q22-23, del17p13, and del6q21.[33,36–38] 13q14.3 harbors two microRNA genes (miR-16-1 and miR-15a), 11q22-23 the ATM gene, and 17p13 the TP53 gene, implicating their products in the etiology and/or pathogenesis of CLL.[32,33,39]

The cutaneous deposits are variably perivascular, nodular, diffuse, or rarely bandlike in distribution with frequent involvement of the subcutis.[11] Although a grenz zone is often present, there may be focal and mild epidermotropism and rarely ulceration.[8,40] Adnexal infiltration is often a feature and, in some cases, the adnexae may be destroyed.[40] The infiltrate is composed predominantly of darkly staining small lymphocytes with round nuclei, clumped chromatin, and inconspicuous or small nucleoli. These are usually admixed with scattered small to medium-sized cells with more prominent nucleoli (prolymphocytes), and intermediate to large cells with vesicular nuclei and single central eosinophilic nucleoli (paraimmunoblasts; *Figs 29.223* and *29.224*).[1,8,10,40] In rare cases, ill-defined, pale-staining areas containing mainly prolymphocytes and paraimmunoblasts are seen, such 'proliferation centers' being much more common in lymph nodes infiltrated by CLL. Hodgkin and Reed-Sternberg-like cells are rarely seen.[41] Lymphocytic vasculitis is sometimes evident.[40] Granulomatous inflammation is also sometimes seen, particularly in those lesions which localize to sites of previous herpetic infection.[15] Cutaneous CLL associated with granuloma annulare-like changes also occurs.[42]

Occasionally, blister formation is a feature in leukemic deposits of CLL.[6,7,43] The blisters are predominantly subepidermal, with or without a multilocular intraepidermal component.[7] Epidermal necrosis accompanied by blood vessel wall necrosis is sometimes conspicuous and numerous eosinophils may be present.[43] Blood vessel wall granular IgG and C3 have occasionally been described.[7] Intra- and extravascular eosinophil basic protein has been identified in two cases.[43] Bulla may also be seen in biopsies of the exaggerated insect bite-like reactions, the typical features of which are superficial and deep perivascular infiltrates consisting of lymphocytes, eosinophils, and neutrophils.[25,44]

The presence of large numbers of blastic B cells should raise the possibility of the development of large cell lymphoma (Richter syndrome) with its attendant high mortality.[6]

Immunohistochemically, the tumor cells of CLL are CD5, CD20, CD23, CD43, and bcl-2 positive (*Figs 29.225* and *29.226*). They do not react with antibodies to CD10 or bcl-6. They are also negative for cyclin D1 apart from occasional positivity in cells within proliferation centers.[1,8,45]

Differential diagnosis

CLL must be differentiated from other small B-cell lymphomas that may infiltrate skin. Clinical features, particularly the presence of a significant lymphocytosis, will often provide a clue, and immunohistochemistry usually permits reliable subclassification.[46]

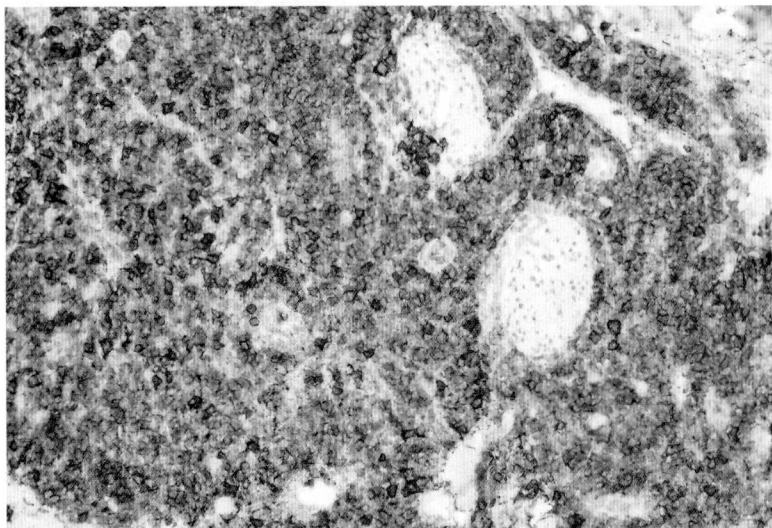

Fig. 29.225
Chronic lymphocytic leukemia: there is uniform expression of CD20.

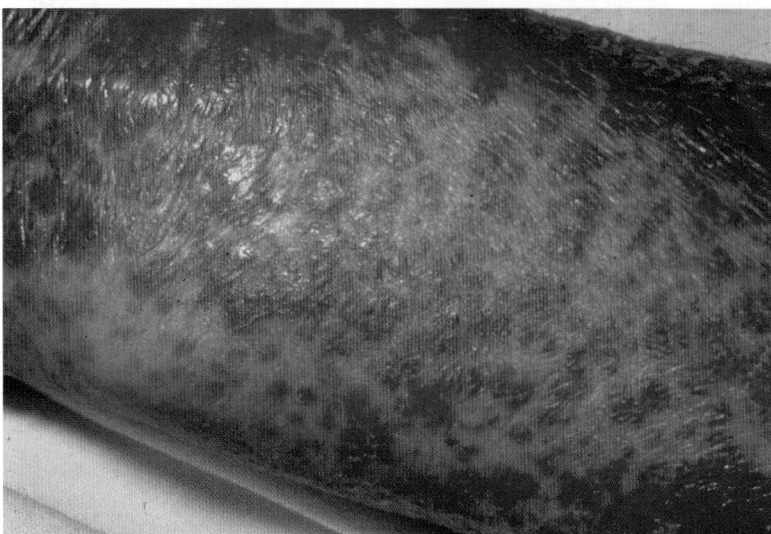

Fig. 29.227
Lymphomatoid granulomatosis: there are raised annular erythematous lesions on the arms, shoulders, and chest. By courtesy of J. Zifell, MD, Walter Reed Army Medical Center, Washington DC, USA.

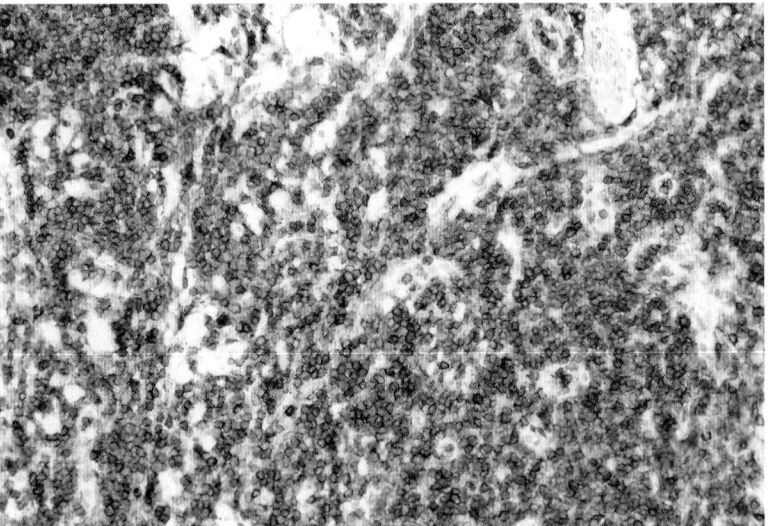

Fig. 29.226
Chronic lymphocytic leukemia: the tumor cells are strongly positive for CD5.

Lymphomatoid granulomatosis

Clinical features

Lymphomatoid granulomatosis (angiocentric lymphoma, angiocentric immunoproliferative lesion) (LG) is a rare extranodal B-cell proliferative disorder associated with a reactive T-cell infiltrate, EBV infection, immunosuppression, and an angiocentric, angioinvasive, and angiodestructive lymphoid infiltrate.[1-7] LG may present at virtually any age, from late childhood to old age, but most cases occur in the fourth to sixth decades with male predominance (2–3 : 1).[2-5,8-10]

LG is primarily a pulmonary disease, with lung involvement being present in >90% of patients at presentation. However, a number of other sites are commonly affected including the skin (25–50%), the brain (26%), kidneys (32%), and liver (29%). Involvement of the upper respiratory and gastrointestinal tracts, spleen, and lymph nodes is rare.[2-5,7] Patients usually present with chest pain, cough, and dyspnea in addition to pyrexia, malaise, and weight loss.[2-4] The chest radiograph commonly shows bilateral round nodular opacities or, less commonly, diffuse fluffy infiltration.[11] CNS involvement is associated with poor prognosis and may manifest as confusion, ataxia, epilepsy, upper motor neuron signs, cranial nerve palsies, and peripheral neuropathies.[7] Myalgia, arthralgia, and gastrointestinal symptoms are rare.

Dermatological manifestations of LG are varied. Lesions are usually multiple, and more than one type of lesion may be present in the same patient. The most frequent presentation is with dermal and/or subcutaneous nodules or papules, on the extremities and/or trunk.[6,12] Plaques, macular erythema, and maculopapular and folliculitis-like eruptions have also been described, and rare cases may present as vesicles, ichthyosis, anhidrosis, alopecia, and necrobiosis lipoidica-like lesions (Fig. 29.227).[3,6,12,13] Cutaneous lesions may be transient, even when left untreated, and may precede (10–15% of cases), coincide with, or follow pulmonary manifestations.[6,8,12,14] Cutaneous involvement does not appear to influence the outcome of the disease.

Although some patients follow a waxing and waning course with rare spontaneous remissions, LC is generally an aggressive disease. The median survival in a large series was <2 years.[3] Durable responses at least for grade 1 and 2 lesions have been achieved with IFN-α therapy.[15,16] Grade 3 lesions should be treated with multiagent chemotherapy similar to diffuse large B-cell lymphoma.[1,2,4,15,17]

Pathogenesis and histologic features

Lymphomatoid granulomatosis is an EBV-associated B-cell proliferative disorder in which the T-cell predominant population is reactive.[15] EBV has been identified by in situ hybridization, Southern blot analysis, and PCR and double labeling has identified the virus within B cells,[18-23] and clonal rearrangements of the Ig heavy chain are present.[12,23,24] Distinct clones of B cells may be found in different lesions within the same patient, indicating that clonal expansion of EBV-infected B cells takes place simultaneously at different sites.[12-15] In rare cases, clonal T-cell receptor gene rearrangements have been reported. This seems analogous to the occasional but well-documented finding of reactive clonal or oligoclonal T-cell proliferations in association with acute and chronic EBV infection.[10,12,25,26]

There is an association with underlying immunodeficiency.[24,27] The risk of LG is increased in allogeneic organ transplant recipients and in patients with Wiskott-Aldrich syndrome, HIV infection, and X-linked lymphoproliferative syndrome.[9,27-31] LG has also been described in association with CLL and angioimmunoblasic T-cell lymphoma, hematological malignancies well known to be associated with defects in T-cell function.[32] Moreover, laboratory analysis usually reveals evidence of reduced immune function in patients presenting with lymphomatoid granulomatosis in the absence of a history of predisposing immunodeficiency.[15,33] The vascular changes that are often present and lead to tissue necrosis are believed to result from EBV-related up-regulation of the chemokines IP-10 and Mig, which are known to damage vascular endothelial cells and to promote adhesion of T cells.[12,34]

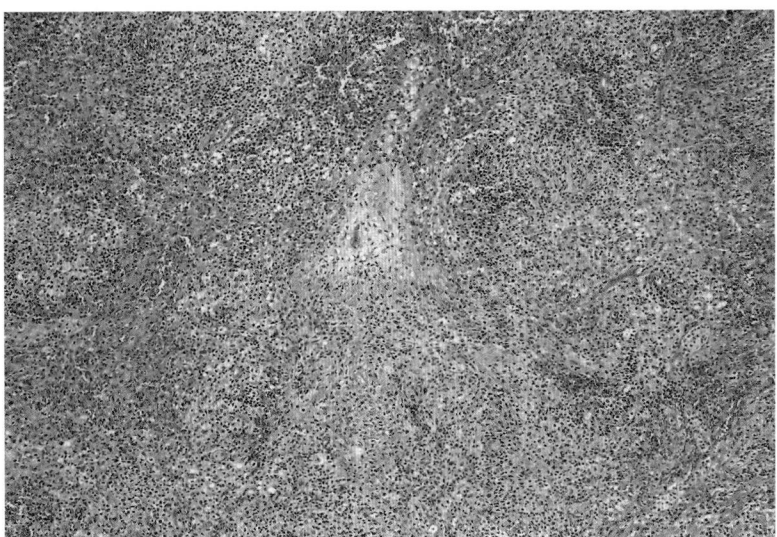

Fig. 29.228
Lymphomatoid granulomatosis: there is a multinodular tumor cell infiltrate.

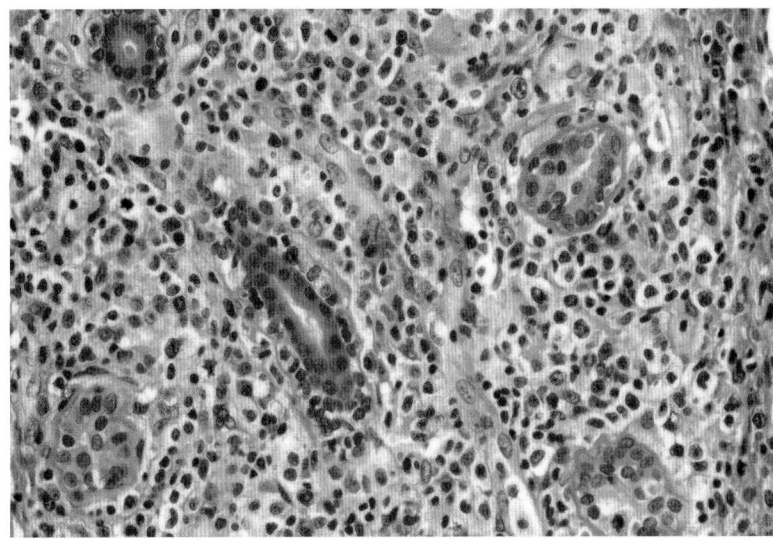

Fig. 29.230
Lymphomatoid granulomatosis: high-power view of dermis showing atypical lymphoid cells.

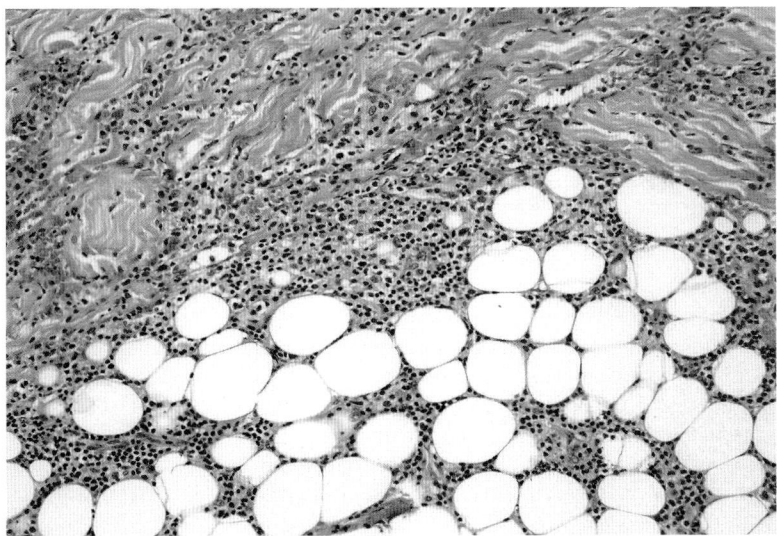

Fig. 29.229
Lymphomatoid granulomatosis: the infiltrate extends into the subcutaneous fat.

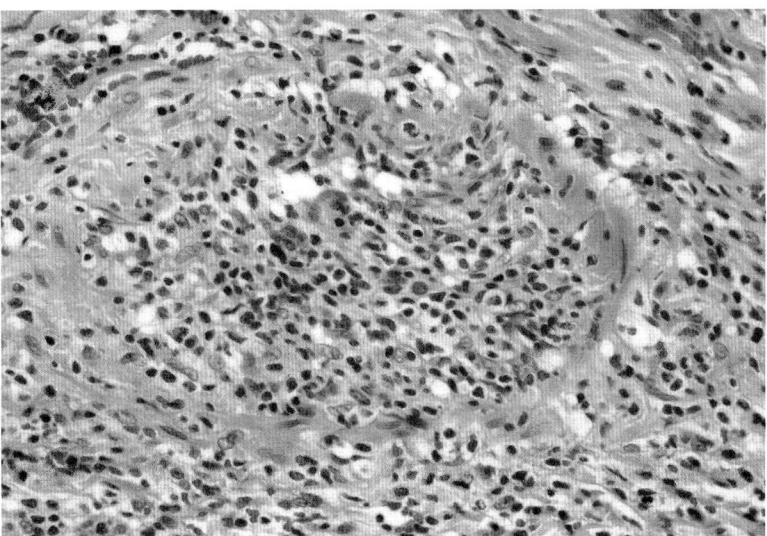

Fig. 29.231
Lymphomatoid granulomatosis: there is striking vascular involvement.

Biopsies of nodules and papules provide the most diagnostic histology when there is cutaneous involvement, as the changes in plaquelike lesions are often non-specific.[12] LG is characterized by a perivascular angiodestructive and periadnexal superficial and deep polymorphous lymphoid infiltrate that may extend into the subcutis with focal formation of granulomas due to fat necrosis (Figs 29.228–29.231).[1–4] Granulomas are not otherwise seen in the disease despite its name. Small lymphocytes predominate and are accompanied by plasma cells, histiocytes, and large transformed lymphoid cells. In some instances, the small lymphocytes have irregular or slightly enlarged nuclei, and this has been referred to as 'atypia' by some authors, although there is no nuclear hyperchromasia or cytological features of malignancy.[12] The large transformed cells often resemble immunoblasts, but some are large with abundant cytoplasm and pleomorphic vesicular nuclei and prominent nucleoli. Multinucleate forms may be seen and some resemble Hodgkin cells, although classic Reed-Sternberg cells should not be present.[1] Neutrophils and eosinophils are generally inconspicuous or absent.[1] Infiltration of blood vessel walls (both arteries and veins) is usually seen, and there may be fibrinoid necrosis with widespread coagulative necrosis of the surrounding parenchyma.[2–4]

By immunohistochemistry, the background population of lymphocytes is CD3+ T cells, predominantly of the CD4+ helper subtype. The large atypical transformed cells, however, are B cells with a CD20+/CD79a+ immunophenotype.[1,4] CD30 is often present but CD15, CD56, and CD57 are invariably negative.[4,15,23,24,35] A variable number shows evidence of EBV, and this is better demonstrated by in situ hybridization for EBV-encoded RNA (EBERs) than with immunohistochemistry for latent membrane protein 1 (LMP1). EBV is harder to demonstrate in cutaneous than in pulmonary lesions.[22] Light chain restriction is only rarely identified, and then in the cytoplasm of cells displaying plasmacytoid differentiation.[1] The angioinvasive component also commonly comprises reactive CD4+ T-helper cells.

Grading

The prognosis of LG is, to some extent, a reflection of the histologic grade. Tumors with a more overt lymphomatous appearance have a more aggressive behavior. Grade is related to the proportion of EBV-positive B cells relative to the reactive background.[1,2,4,15,24,36]

- Grade I lesions are highly polymorphous and show no lymphocytic nuclear atypia. Blast cells are inconspicuous and often only detected in immunohistochemically stained sections. Necrosis is absent or very focal. EBV+ cells are very sparse (<5 per HPF with in situ hybridization).
- Grade II lesions show lymphocytic cytological atypia, and large transformed cells are more numerous and may form small clusters. Necrosis is common. EBV+ cells number 5–20 per HPF.

- Grade III lesions are frankly lymphomatous, although a polymorphous inflammatory background infiltrate is seen. Large atypical transformed cells are readily identifiable and may form larger aggregates. EBV+ cells are very conspicuous (>50 per HPF) and may present as confluent sheets.

When a uniform population of EBV+ blasts is present with no inflammatory background then a diagnosis of LG is no longer tenable, and the lesion should be regarded as diffuse large B-cell lymphoma.

Differential diagnosis

Wegener granulomatosis differs clinically from LG by its upper respiratory tract involvement and by the presence of necrotizing vasculitis accompanied by granulomatous inflammation. Lymphoproliferative disorders which can be confused with LG usually also display a partial angiocentric/angiodestructive growth pattern and include extranodal NK/T-cell lymphoma, Epstein-Barr virus-positive mucocutaneous ulcer (EBV+ MCU) and EBV-positive diffuse large B-cell lymphoma. Pulmonary involvement is uncommon in extranodal NK/T-cell lymphoma, and although also associated with EBV infection, is characterized by a CD3–, CD20–, CD3ε+, CD56+ phenotype. EBV+ MCU and EBV-positive diffuse large B-cell lymphoma show considerable pathological overlaps with parts of the LG spectrum, and clinical features must be taken into account in order to arrive at the correct diagnosis. EBV+ MCU is always localized without formation of a mass lesion. Pathologically, it is a circumscribed lesion with a confining rim of small T cells at the base and sides of the infiltrate. Characteristic lung changes should be seen in order to make a diagnosis of LG and, unlike EBV-positive diffuse large B-cell lymphoma, lymph node involvement is typically absent.

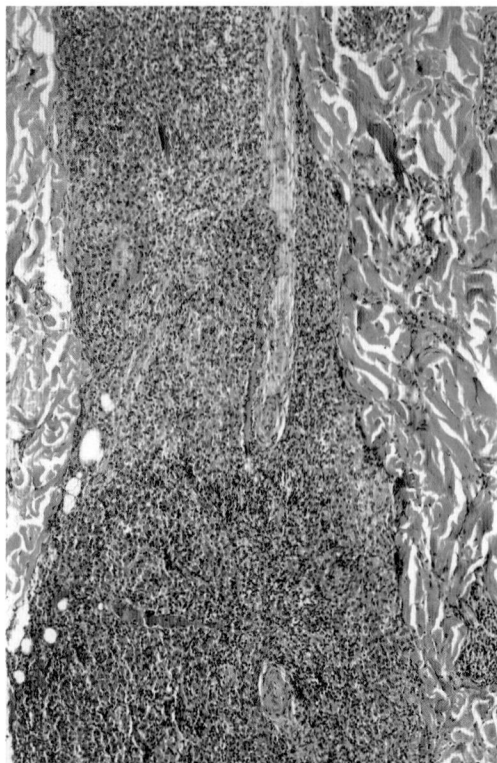

Fig. 29.232
Plasmacytoma: there is a dense dermal infiltrate. By courtesy of J. Cohen, MD, Dermatopathology Laboratory, Tucson, Arizona, USA.

Cutaneous manifestations of plasma cell myeloma and primary cutaneous plasmacytoma

Clinical features

A wide variety of skin conditions are associated with plasma cell neoplasms, apart from the manifestations of specific infiltration by tumor cells. Many are associated with deposition of monoclonal immunoglobulin or one of its fragments. These include amyloidosis and cryoglobulinemia. Others are specific diseases in their own right but show an association with plasma cell dyscrasias. These include neutrophilic dermatoses, leukocytoclastic vasculitis, scleromyxedema, scleroderma, subcorneal pustular dermatoses, necrobiotic xanthogranuloma, subcorneal pustular dermatosis, and POEMS syndrome.[1,2] In addition, there is a miscellaneous group of non-specific conditions that includes pruritus, infections, and drug reactions.[1,2] A more detailed account of these disorders can be found elsewhere in this book or in review articles.[1,2] This section deals with the consequences of cutaneous infiltration by the neoplastic process.

Skin involvement is relatively rare in plasma cell myeloma, occurring in 3–4% of cases at presentation and approximately in 5% of cases at relapse or disease progression.[3] Cutaneous involvement most often represents terminal expression of plasma cell myeloma or widespread extramedullary plasmacytoma, but occasionally it precedes other manifestations of the disease.[2–8] It may develop as a consequence of hematogenous spread or direct extension from an underlying bony deposit.[2–4,9] Extramedullary dissemination of myeloma, including to cutaneous sites, is usually associated with a very poor prognosis, with most patients dying within months of its occurrence.[3,4,10]

Myelomatous deposits present as 1–5 cm in diameter, solitary, or more often multiple flesh-colored, red or violaceous nodules which affect the trunk, extremities, and face in decreasing order of frequency.[1–3]

Primary cutaneous plasmacytomas belong to the group of extraosseus (extramedullary) plasmacytomas. These are defined as neoplasms of plasma cells arising in tissues other than bone, and constitute 3–5% of all plasma cell neoplasms.[11,12] Eighty percent of cases arise in the upper respiratory tract, but occurrence in the gastrointestinal tract, lymph nodes, bladder, brain, thyroid, testes, parotid, and skin is also documented.[1] Consequently, primary cutaneous plasmacytomas are exceptional, with few genuine cases documented in the English-language literature.[2,13] Lesions, which may be

solitary or more often multiple, present on the face, trunk, limbs, scalp, and finger in decreasing order of frequency.[8,14–20] In most reports, they have been described as red to purple nodules or plaques. The middle aged and elderly are predominantly affected (mean, 60 years; range, 22–88 years), and there is a predilection for males (4:1).[13] Rare cases occur in solid organ transplant recipients.[2,21,22] Patients with single tumors may sometimes have a better prognosis, but multiple lesions are commonly associated with nodal and visceral involvement or development of plasma cell myeloma and a high mortality.[13,15,23] The overall death rate is at least 40%.[17] Occasionally, however, long-term disease-free survival is seen.[13]

Histologic features

The histologic features of primary cutaneous plasmacytoma and metastatic myeloma are similar. The infiltrate may be nodular or diffuse and is usually extensive, frequently involving the subcutaneous fat (Figs 29.232 and 29.233).[4,10] A distinct grenz zone is commonly present. An interstitial pattern of growth has been described in cases of secondary cutaneous involvement. Although in some well-differentiated examples the plasma cell nature of the infiltrate is obvious, with characteristic clock-face nuclei, more often the tumor cells are atypical, having distinctly angulated and often molded cytoplasmic borders with pleomorphic nuclei containing conspicuous nucleoli and granular eosinophilic cytoplasm.[3] Binucleate and multinucleate forms are often present, and mitotic figures may be abundant in less well-differentiated lesions.[3] Intracytoplasmic inclusions (Russell bodies) and intranuclear inclusions (Dutcher bodies), although not usually prominent, may sometimes be present.[5,10,19] Exceptionally, eosinophilic rhomboidal or needle-shaped crystals may be identified in the cytoplasm of tumor-associated histiocytes (crystal-storing histiocytosis), this being more often associated with plasma cell myeloma (Fig. 29.234).[24–27] A case of secondary mucinosis has also been reported.[28]

By immunohistochemistry, the plasma cells express CD38, CD79a, and CD138 (Fig. 29.235). They are usually CD19 negative and often lack CD20 and common leukocyte antigen.[4,13] Monotypic cytoplasmic Ig light chain is present (Figs 29.236 and 29.237). CD56 and cyclin D1 may be expressed, and occasionally there is positivity for EMA, HMB-45, and cytokeratin.[2]

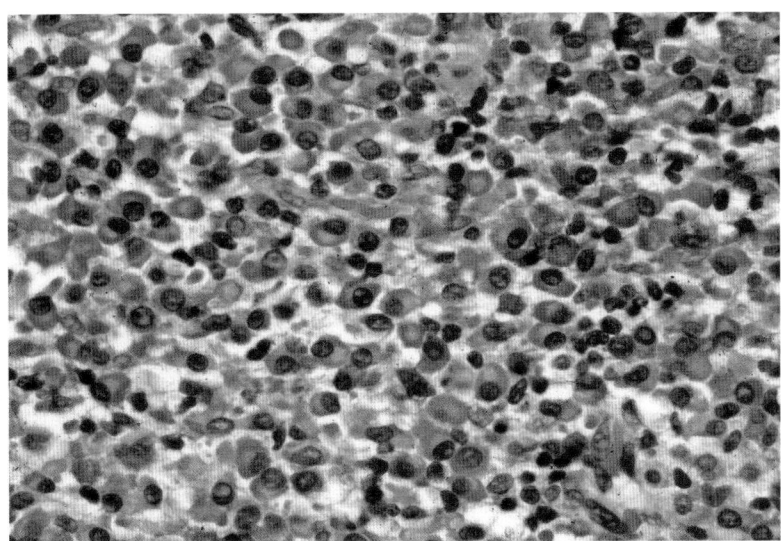

Fig. 29.233
Plasmacytoma: the infiltrate consists of an almost pure plasma cell population. By courtesy of J. Cohen, MD, Dermatopathology Laboratory, Tucson, Arizona, USA.

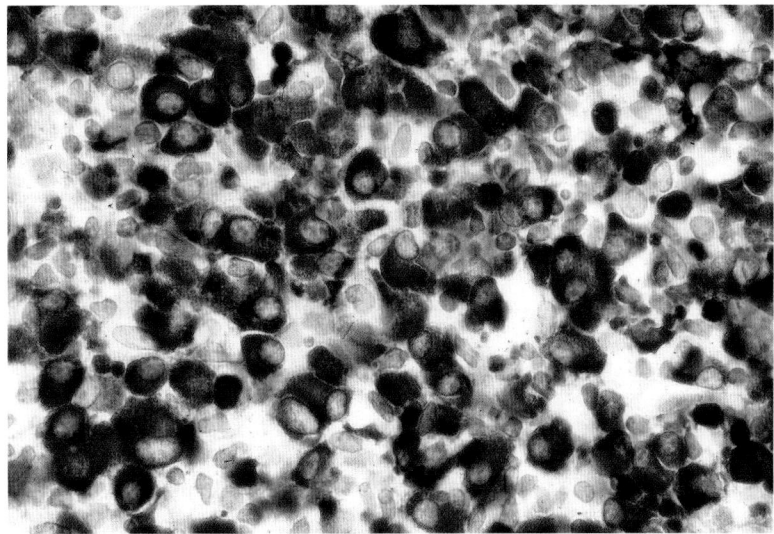

Fig. 29.236
Plasmacytoma: there is uniform kappa light chain expression. By courtesy of J. Cohen, MD, Dermatopathology Laboratory, Tucson, Arizona, USA.

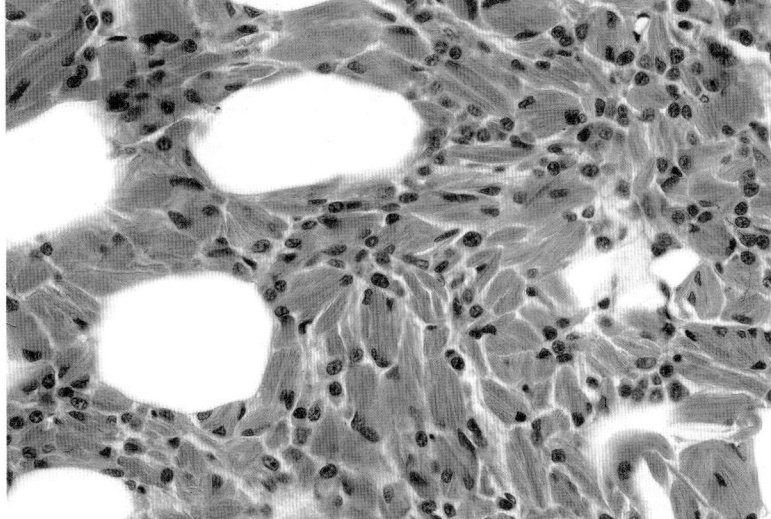

Fig. 29.234
Multiple myeloma: histiocytes containing needle-shaped crystals are evident – so-called crystal-storing histiocytosis. By courtesy of G. Pinkus, MD, Brigham and Women's Hospital and Harvard Medical School, Boston, USA.

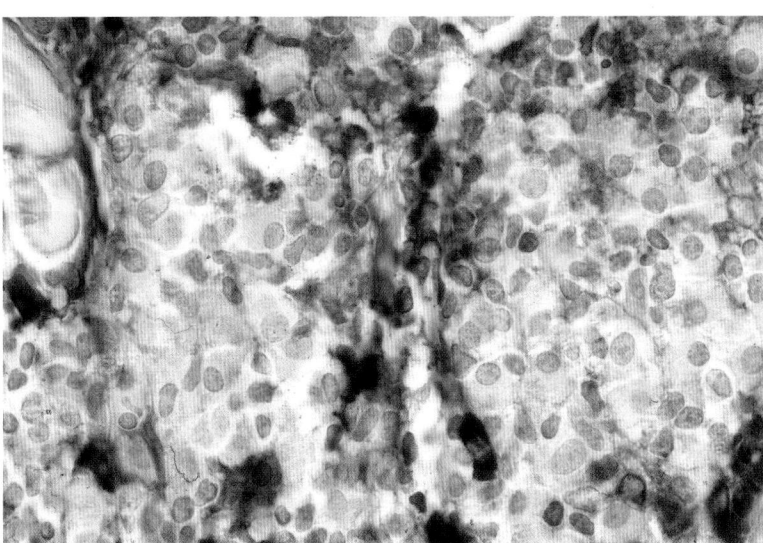

Fig. 29.237
Plasmacytoma: lambda light chain is absent. By courtesy of J. Cohen, MD, Dermatopathology Laboratory, Tucson, Arizona, USA.

Differential diagnosis

Differentiation of poorly differentiated forms of the disease from plasmablastic lymphoma is discussed in the section on plasmablastic lymphoma. Well-differentiated tumors are sometimes mistaken for plasma cell-rich conditions such as syphilis or *Borrelia* infection. If there is a significant background lymphocyte population, there may be confusion with primary cutaneous marginal zone B-cell lymphoma/immunocytoma or lymphoplasmacytic lymphoma. Distinction then rests on demonstrating a neoplastic component of lymphocytes, morphologically (marginal zone cells), with immunohistochemistry (CD20), or by flow cytometry. With poorly differentiated examples, the differential diagnosis can include high-grade lymphoma, carcinoma, or melanoma. In such instances, the immunohistochemistry panel of antibodies will require expansion.

Intravascular large B-cell lymphoma

Clinical features

Intravascular large B-cell lymphoma (IVLBCL) (angiotropic large cell lymphoma, intravascular lymphomatosis, intravascular malignant lymphomatosis, intravascular lymphoma) is a very rare type of lymphoma, frequently

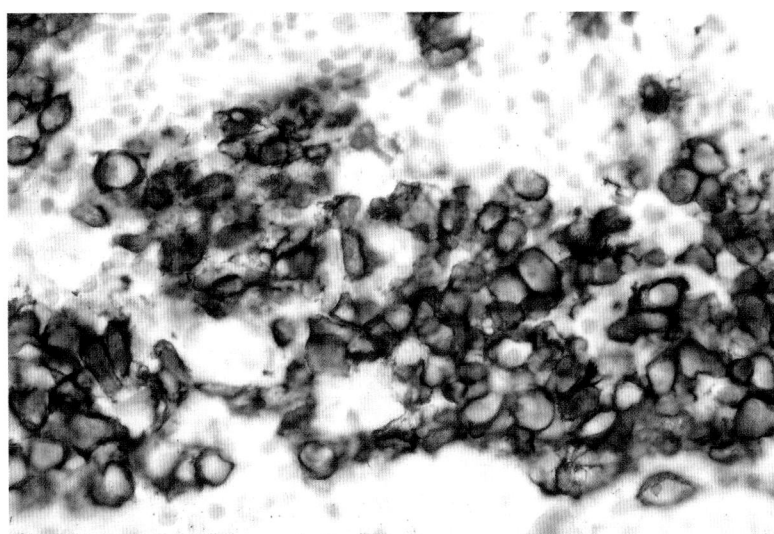

Fig. 29.235
Plasmacytoma: the tumor cells express CD138. By courtesy of J. Cohen, MD, Dermatopathology Laboratory, Tucson, Arizona, USA.

involving the skin and characterized by selective growth of neoplastic lymphocytes within blood vessels. It was formerly known as malignant angioendotheliomatosis because it was believed to be an endothelial malignancy.[1,2]

IVLBCL is mainly a neoplasm of elderly adults with roughly an equal sex incidence. Disease is usually widespread at presentation. As the symptoms are diverse and often non-specific, diagnosis may be delayed and is often made postmortem. The CNS and skin are the most common sites, but lung, kidney, gastrointestinal tract, genitourinary system, endocrine glands, liver, spleen, and bone marrow may also be involved. Lymph nodes are typically spared. B symptoms are common, and patients often have raised LDH, β_2-microglobulin, and ESR. Anemia is frequent and may be accompanied by leukopenia and thrombocytopenia. A monoclonal serum immunoglobulin is exceptional, and a hemophagocytic syndrome may be seen.[1,3–9]

Two major, often overlapping clinical patterns have been described. These occur predominantly in different geographic locations. In Western countries, symptoms are usually related to the organ involved, mainly skin and CNS.[5–7] In this subtype, a variant occurs that is limited to the skin. Patients tend to be younger (median age, 59 years), almost exclusively female, and usually have normal leukocyte and platelet counts, a lower incidence of B symptoms, and good performance scores.[5] The Asian variant, most frequent in Japan, often presents with multiorgan failure, liver and spleen involvement, pancytopenia, and typically a hemophagocytic syndrome. Bone marrow involvement is more common than in Western cases but skin involvement is less frequent.[6–10]

Skin lesions, whether restricted to the skin or occurring as part of more disseminated disease, vary in appearance, including erythematous or violaceous plaques and nodules particularly affecting the arms, thighs, trunk, and face. An inverted livedo reticularis-like pattern, gangrene, petechiae, purpura, ecchymoses, telangiectases, vasculitis, thrombophlebitis-like features, cellulitis, and 'peau d'orange'-like changes may also occur.[3,4,5,11–14] Erythema nodosum-like changes have been documented.[14] The condition may rarely present within the vascular channels of Kaposi sarcoma and in the lumina of a pre-existing cutaneous hemangioma.[15–18]

IVLBCL is an aggressive disease. Prognosis is similar in Western and Asian cases, except for patients with the cutaneous variant. The latter have a more favorable prognosis, particularly if there is only a solitary lesion. The 3-year overall survival for cutaneous cases is 56% compared with 22% for classical forms of the disease.[5]

Pathogenesis and histologic features

The etiology of IVLBCL is unknown although defects in expression of the homing receptors CD29 (β_1 integrin) and CD54 (ICAM-1) is postulated to account for the intravascular location of tumor cells.[19–21] Karyotypic abnormalities have been described in only one case.[21]

The neoplastic lymphocytes proliferate within vascular lumina, and there may be a minor, predominantly perivascular, extravascular component.[4,7,11] With the exception of large arteries and veins and lymphatics, any vessel may be involved including sinusoids in liver, spleen, and bone marrow.[1,7] The typical case consists of large lymphoid cells with scanty cytoplasm, vesicular nuclei, and prominent nucleoli (Figs 29.238 and 29.239). Mitoses are often conspicuous. Less commonly, the neoplastic lymphocytes may be of smaller size, or display an irregular nuclear outline with coarse chromatin.[7] Vascular occlusion is frequently evident, and pseudoglomeruloid structures may also be seen.[10] The lymphocytes are CD19, CD20, CD22, and CD79a positive (Fig. 29.240).[1] CD5 is positive in 38% of cases and CD10 in 13%, but as yet no clinical differences have been associated with expression of these antigens.[1,9,22,23] CD10-negative cases show strong expression of IRF4/MUM1. Cyclin D1 is negative.[22] Bcl-2 is usually positive, but the t(14;18) translocation is absent; bcl-6 expression is rare.[22] There is no association with EBV.[24]

Immunophenotypic and immunoglobulin gene rearrangement studies show clonality.[25,26]

Differential diagnosis

IVLBCL has to be distinguished from reactive angioendotheliomatosis. The latter is characterized histologically by numerous small blood vessels, lined by bland, sometimes plump, endothelial cells proliferating within

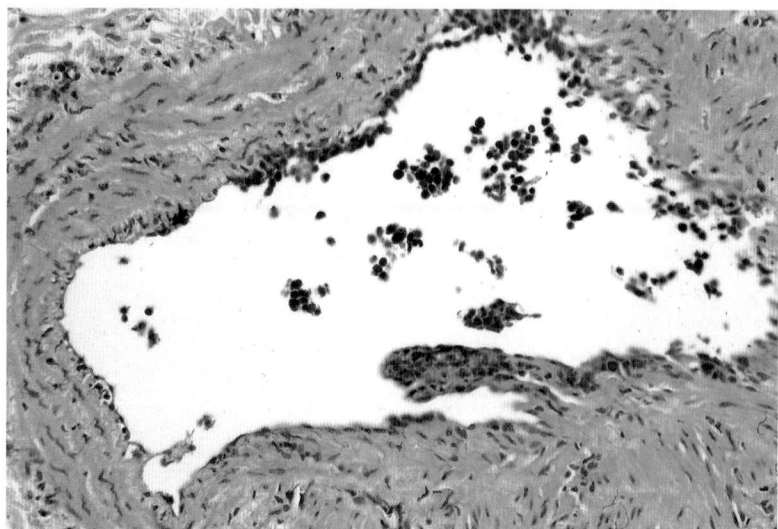

Fig. 29.238
Intravascular large B-cell lymphoma: the tumor cells have hyperchromatic irregular nuclei. In many places, they appear to be attached to the endothelium to give a hobnail appearance. By courtesy of J.-A. Vergilio, MD, Brigham and Women's Hospital and Harvard Medical School, Boston, USA.

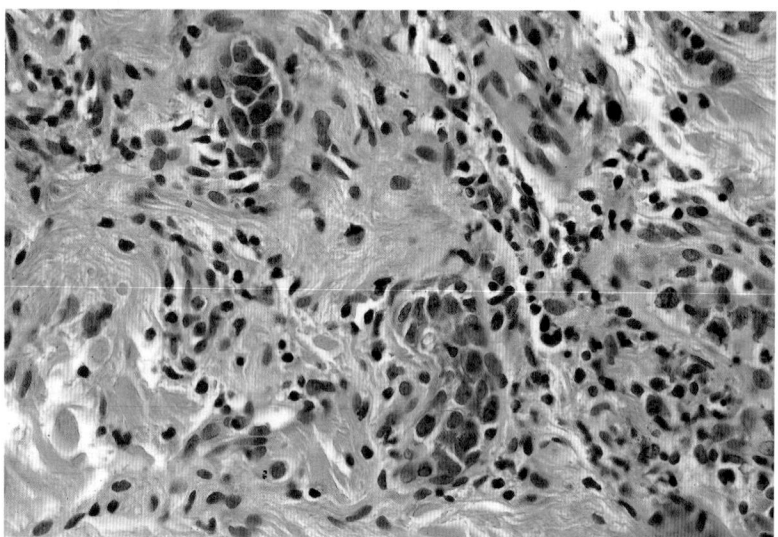

Fig. 29.239
Intravascular large B-cell lymphoma: aggregates of hyperchromatic and irregular lymphoid cells are present within small vessels. By courtesy of J.-A. Vergilio, Brigham and Women's Hospital and Harvard Medical School, Boston, USA.

pre-existing vascular channels.[11,27] Each vascular channel is surrounded by a layer of pericytes that may be highlighted by actin.[27] The endothelial cells are positive for endothelial cell markers and negative for LCA. Epithelioid angiosarcoma which may involve the skin primarily or secondarily with an exclusive intravascular location is characterized by large cells with abundant pink cytoplasm and a single prominent nucleolus that stain for endothelial cell markers including CD31 and ERG and are negative for lymphoid markers.

Other lymphomas may have an intravascular component, either in association with a predominant extravascular component (e.g., B-CLL, MCL, splenic marginal zone lymphoma) or occasionally as a predominant feature of the disease (e.g., splenic marginal zone lymphoma, hepatosplenic T-cell lymphoma). There are also rare, anecdotal reports of T-cell or NK-cell lymphomas and histiocytic neoplasms with intravascular growth.[7,10,28–35] The presence of extravascular disease in some cases, together with assessment of cytological features and immunophenotype, should allow reliable separation of most of these entities.[7] However, the relationship between rarely reported cases of IVLBCL associated with other types of NHL localized

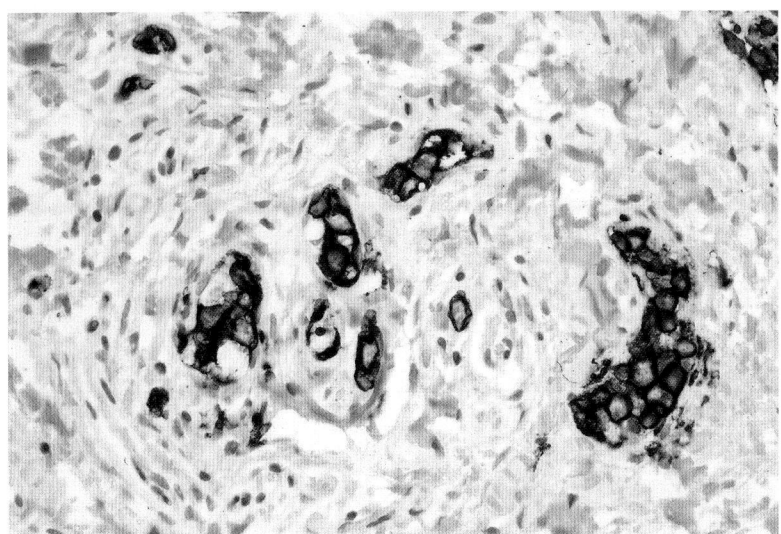

Fig. 29.240
Intravascular large B-cell lymphoma: the tumor cells express CD20. By courtesy of J.-A. Vergilio, Brigham and Women's Hospital and Harvard Medical School, Boston, USA.

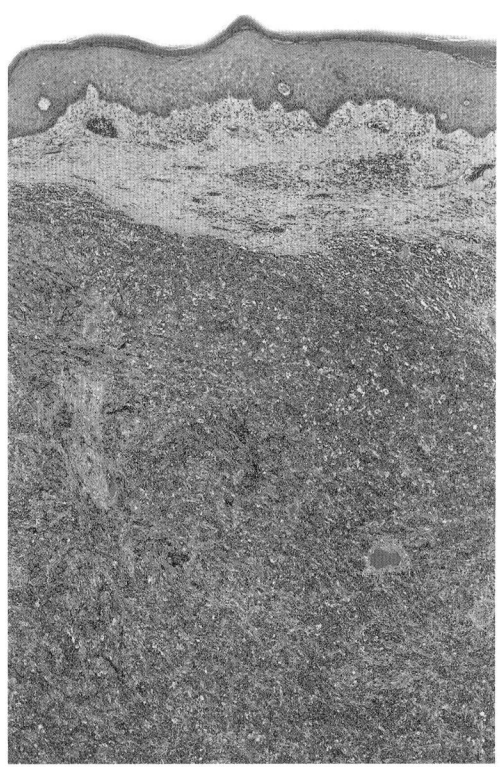

Fig. 29.241
Plasmablastic lymphoma: there is a dense dermal tumor cell infiltrate.

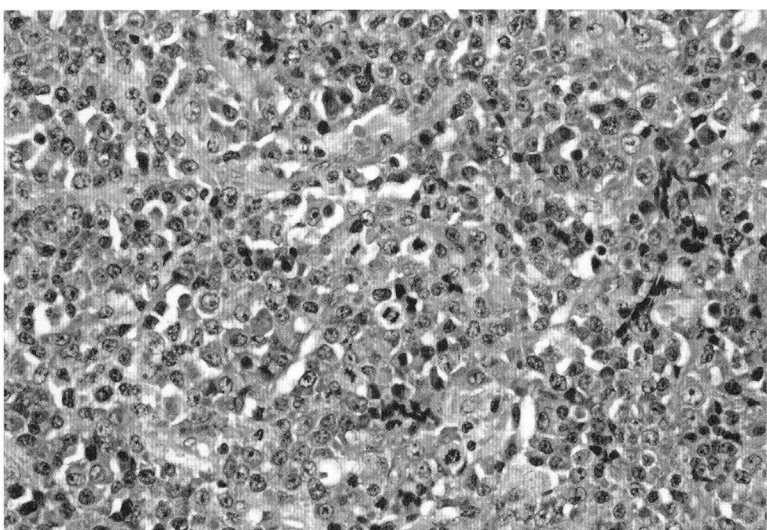

Fig. 29.242
Plasmablastic lymphoma: high-power view of plasmablasts with central nucleoli and occasional mature plasma cells.

in lymph nodes, including follicular lymphoma, marginal zone lymphoma, and diffuse large B-cell lymphoma, and 'pure' IVLCL remains to be determined.[4,7,22,31,36,37] Rare cases of intravascular lymphoma with a T- or NK-cell phenotype have also been reported. These are often associated with EBV, and their relationship to IVLBCL and extranodal NK/T-cell lymphoma, nasal type, remains to be determined.[38]

Lymphomas with an angiocentric and angiodestructive growth pattern (extranodal NK/T-cell lymphoma, lymphomatoid granulomatosis, cutaneous γ/δ T-cell lymphoma, and subcutaneous panniculitis-like T-cell lymphoma) should also be differentiated from IVLBCL. In these conditions, the neoplastic lymphocytes infiltrate vessel walls but are not intravascular as seen in IVLBCL. Immunohistochemistry is also discriminatory in intravascular aggregates of metastatic carcinoma and leukemia.[10]

Plasmablastic lymphoma

Clinical features

Plasmablastic lymphoma (PL) is a rare neoplasm of blastic cells displaying morphological and immunophenotypic features of terminal B-cell differentiation. Although originally described in the oral mucosa in HIV-positive individuals, and referred to as plasmablastic lymphoma of the oral mucosa in the 2001 WHO lymphoma classification, a broader spectrum of sites and clinical presentations is now appreciated.[1–3]

PL is seen most frequently in HIV-positive individuals, but is now also described following organ transplantation and in apparently immune competent individuals.[1,4–11] It has also been rarely documented in association with non-transplant-related iatrogenic immunosuppression.[12–14] A wide age range may be affected, including pediatric patients.[5] In the HIV-positive group the median age at presentation is 42 years, whilst HIV-negative and post-transplant patients tend to be older.[4,5] Males are more frequently affected than females in all groups. The vast majority of cases involve extranodal sites and are advanced stage (III/IV) at presentation.[4,5] The oral cavity is most frequently involved followed by the gastrointestinal tract and skin. Other sites include the anus, sinonasal cavities, orbit, bone, soft tissues, lung, and genitourinary system.[4–9,15,16] Lymph nodes are only rarely involved as the presenting site or as part of disease dissemination.[4–8]

Most patients present with masses.[1,3,7,8] Cutaneous involvement usually manifests as solitary or grouped, purple or erythematous nodules, or more rarely plaques on the extremities.[7,15,17–19] Most patients die within a year of diagnosis,[1,4,5] although the outlook may be less bleak in patients undergoing treatment with antiviral therapies.[10,20]

Pathogenesis and histologic features

Immunodeficiency predisposes to the development of plasmablastic lymphoma. As mentioned above, this may be due to HIV infection or a consequence of iatrogenic immunosuppression, usually in the post-transplant setting.[4,5] Patients with no obvious history of immunosuppression tend to be aged >50 years, and therefore may be intrinsically more prone to EBV-related lymphoproliferative disorders due to immunological deterioration or senescence.[4–6] EBV is present in neoplastic lymphocytes in the majority of cases and shows a type I latency, implying a significant role in the pathogenesis of at least some tumors.[1,4–8,21,22] Translocations involving the MYC gene are found in 50–67% of cases, suggesting a role for this oncogene in the majority of tumors.[4,5,12]

Histologically, plasmablastic lymphoma is characterized by sheets of blast cells with features of plasmablasts (*Figs 29.241* and *29.242*). These typically possess round, eccentrically placed nuclei with moderately clumped chromatin and a single central nucleolus, or several smaller peripherally placed nucleoli. There is moderate to abundant basophilic cytoplasm, often with a perinuclear hof. The mitotic index is high and apoptotic cells are frequent. In the oral cavity and nasal and paranasal areas, these blast cells predominate, giving a monomorphic appearance to the infiltrate.[1,3,4–8] However, at other extranodal sites and in lymph nodes, the cytological spectrum of tumor cells is broader and includes a larger proportion of cells showing greater degrees of plasmacytic differentiation.[1,4–8,21]

Immunohistochemically, tumor cells display a plasma cell phenotype with strong expression of plasma cell markers including CD138, CD79a, CD38, Vs38c, IRF4/MUM1, and BLIMP-1.[5,23] They should be negative for CD19, CD20, and pax5. CD45 may be expressed weakly, and CD10 and CD56 may also be positive, particularly in post-transplant patients.[4,5] Cytoplasmic immunoglobulins can be demonstrated in about 50% of cases (usually IgG and only very occasionally IgM or IgA) with either kappa or lambda light chain.[1,7,8,23] T-cell antigens such as CD2 and CD4 are occasionally aberrantly expressed.[5] The Ki-67 index is typically greater than 90%. EBV is detectable in up to 75% of cases using in situ hybridization for EBERs, but staining for LMP1 and EBNA2 is usually negative.[1,4,5,7,8,22,24] Despite one report to the contrary, HHV8 should not be present in the neoplastic lymphocytes.[1,4,5,8,23]

Immunoglobulin heavy chain genes are clonally rearranged, and somatic hypermutation is seen in a proportion of cases.[24]

Differential diagnosis

The differential diagnosis of PL includes other blastic lymphomas showing plasmablastic or plasmacytic differentiation. These include plasmablastic and anaplastic variants of plasma cell myeloma and plasmacytoma, diffuse large B-cell lymphoma with plasmacytic differentiation, Burkitt lymphoma with plasmacytic differentiation, ALK-positive large B-cell lymphoma, primary effusion lymphoma, and large B-cell lymphoma arising in HHV8-associated multicentric Castleman disease (CD).

Plasmablastic and anaplastic variants of myeloma/plasmacytoma share many morphological and immunophenotypic features with PL.[23] The presence of significant bone involvement, a monoclonal serum paraprotein, lower proliferation index, and negative staining for EBV favor a diagnosis of plasma cell myeloma. Diffuse large B-cell lymphoma with plasmacytic differentiation is usually strongly positive for CD20 and CD45, and these markers – together with coexpression of CD10 and bcl-6 – should also allow reliable discrimination of Burkitt lymphoma. ALK-positive large B-cell lymphoma is also morphologically similar to PL, may lack CD20 and CD45, and express plasma cell markers. However, such cases are always positive for ALK protein, with a granular cytoplasmic staining pattern, usually express cytoplasmic IgA, and often coexpress CD4 and CD57.[25]

The neoplastic lymphocytes in primary effusion lymphomas also lack B-cell markers, react with antibodies to plasma cell antigens including CD138 and Vs38c, and are frequently EBV positive. However, they tend to be larger and more pleomorphic than those seen in PL, and uniformly show nuclear positivity with antibodies to HHV8. In addition, location within body cavities strongly supports a diagnosis of primary effusion lymphoma, and while extracavitary examples of the tumor exist, they more frequently express B-cell antigens.[26] Large B-cell lymphomas arising in HHV8-associated multicentric CD were originally also referred to as PLs. However, they more frequently express CD20, are usually negative for EBV, and show cytoplasmic IgM lambda restriction. A background of plasma cell CD and stippled nuclear staining for the HHV8 also support this diagnosis over that of PL.

Other B-cell lymphomas secondarily involving the skin

Almost any other mature B-cell neoplasms may secondarily involve the skin. Those most likely to do so are follicular lymphoma, diffuse large B-cell lymphoma (DLBCL), and Burkitt lymphoma. Patients who develop cutaneous secondary lesions may present with either single or multiple tumor nodules (*Figs 29.243* and *29.244*).[1–3] Diffuse large B-cell lymphoma represents around 29% of systemic lymphomas involving the skin.[4] Staging,

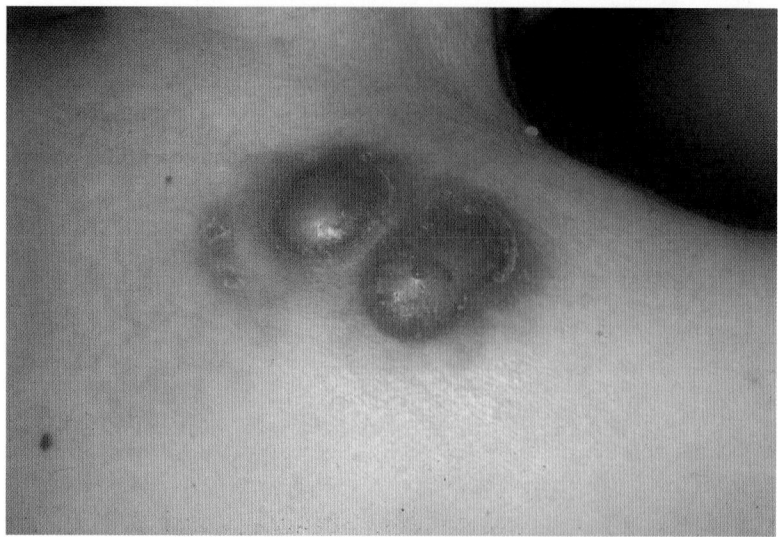

Fig. 29.243
Nodal B-cell lymphoma: skin involvement has presented with large tumor nodules showing surrounding erythema. By courtesy of R.A. Marsden, St George's Hospital, London, UK.

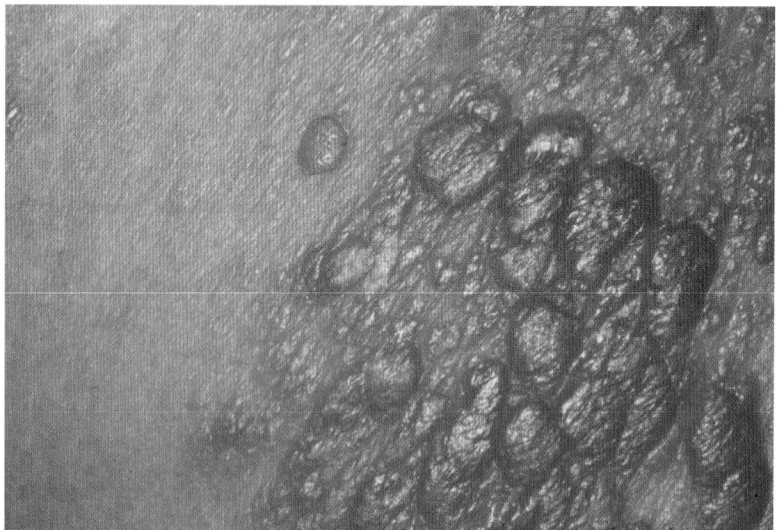

Fig. 29.244
Primary nodal B-cell lymphoma: there are numerous confluent erythematous papules. By courtesy of R.A. Marsden, St George's Hospital, London, UK

including full, thorough clinical examination, computerized tomography of trunk, and bone marrow examination, are mandatory for patients presenting with B-cell lymphoma presenting in the skin. The results of these studies should alert the pathologist to the possibility of underlying nodal disease, and may be the only reliable means of differentiating DLBCL from primary cutaneous diffuse large B-cell lymphoma, leg type, and large cell variants of PCFCL.

Pathological features favoring a diagnosis of nodal follicular lymphoma over cutaneous follicle center lymphoma include a prominent follicular architecture, strong staining of tumor cells with antibodies to CD10, bcl-6, and bcl-2, and the presence of t(14;18)(q32;q21); FISH is a more sensitive technique than PCR for demonstrating the latter.[5–9]

Burkitt lymphoma often presents as an extranodal mass, but cutaneous involvement is exceedingly rare and usually secondary.[10–12] It is characterized by a diffuse proliferation of medium-sized blasts with round nuclei, several small nucleoli, and a narrow rim of basophilic cytoplasm. There is a very high mitotic and apoptotic rate, and numerous tingible body macrophages. The phenotype is typically CD20+, CD10+, bcl-6+, and bcl-2–. A MYC translocation is always present, usually involving the immunoglobulin heavy chain, t(8;14)(q24;q32).

Cutaneous manifestations of Hodgkin lymphoma

Clinical features

Hodgkin lymphoma (HL) is a neoplasm of large atypical lymphoid cells, usually of B-cell origin, with an inflammatory background. Two distinct disease entities have been described under the banner of HL: nodular lymphocyte predominant HL and classical HL.[1] The latter can be subdivided into nodular sclerosis, mixed cellularity, lymphocyte rich, and lymphocyte depleted subtypes.[2] Cutaneous involvement in nodular lymphocyte predominant HL has not been reported, and this entity will not be discussed further. HL accounts for approximately 30% of all lymphomas in the United States and >95% are of the classical variety.[2,3] Classical HL is more common in males, and although it may develop at virtually any age, it shows two peaks: one in the second to fourth decades and the other in the elderly.[2] Virtually all cases present with nodal disease, with mediastinal involvement characterizing nodular sclerosing HL. Around 60% of patients have localized disease at presentation (stage I or II), and while splenic involvement is relatively common (20%), extranodal dissemination is rare.[2] B symptoms including pyrexia (sometimes periodic, known as Pel-Ebstein fever) are relatively frequent.

Cutaneous lesions are rare, being typically found in patients with advanced (stage IV) disease.[2,3] The incidence varies from 0.5% to 7.5%.[4,5,6] Involvement of the skin generally reflects direct extension from underlying nodal disease or retrograde lymphatic spread, hematogenous dissemination being exceptional.[7,8,9,10,11] It may be slightly more frequent in HIV-related cases.[12,13] More often, patients manifest paraneoplastic conditions including pruritus, prurigo-like papules, hyperpigmentation, xeroderma, ichthyosis, urticaria, erythroderma, eczematoid, and psoriasiform eruptions. Primary cutaneous HL is exceptionally rare.[14–16]

Patients with cutaneous involvement present with pink or reddish-brown papules, nodules, or plaquelike infiltrative, often ulcerated, lesions (Fig. 29.245).[4,5,6,17–19] The trunk is most commonly affected, often due to direct extension of mediastinal disease. In general, skin involvement is associated with a very poor prognosis, average survival being less than 1 year.[20] Cutaneous lesions are therefore graded as stage IV disease.

Pathogenesis and histopathological features

HL is now recognized as a tumor of B cells of germinal center derivation in the majority of cases.[2,21,22] Rare cases exhibit aberrant T-cell antigen expression.[2,23–25] The etiology is unknown although a number of abnormalities in cytokine and gene expression patterns have been documented, as well as

recurring chromosomal abnormalities.[2] There is also a significant association with EBV, particularly in cases of the mixed cellularity variant and in immunosuppressed patients.[13,15,20] It has also been speculated that cutaneous involvement is more frequent in HIV-positive patients and/or EBV-associated cases.[12,13,15] HL also sometimes develops in association with other lymphomas including mycosis fungoides, Sézary syndrome, lymphomatoid papulosis, anaplastic CD30+ large cell lymphoma, and primary cutaneous T-cell rich B-cell lymphoma.[26–30]

Cutaneous infiltrates of classical HL usually comprise a deep diffuse or nodular dermal infiltrate (Figs 29.246 and 29.247). As in lymph nodes, the diagnosis depends on identifying typical mononuclear, binucleate (or multinucleate) tumor cells, (designated Hodgkin cells and Reed-Sternberg cells, respectively, and Hodgkin-Reed-Sternberg (HRS) cells collectively) together with an appropriate inflammatory background (Fig. 29.248).[2,11] Classic Reed-Sternberg cells have abundant cytoplasm and have bilobed or multilobated nuclei (or are bi- or multinucleate). The nuclei are large and pale staining with a single prominent central nucleolus in each nucleus or lobe of nucleus. HRS cells account for the minority of cells in the infiltrate. The background inflammatory component comprises small lymphocytes (mainly

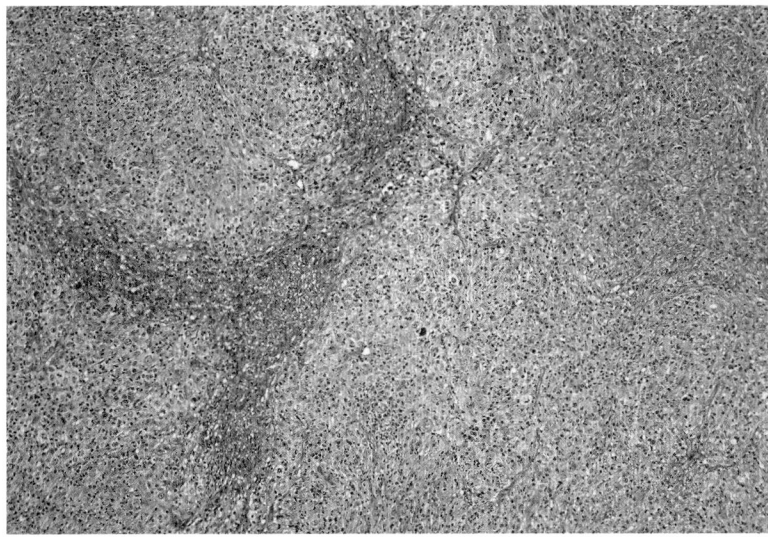

Fig. 29.246
Hodgkin lymphoma: subcutaneous deposit in a patient with known nodal disease. By courtesy of W. Grayson, MD, National Health Laboratory Service, Johannesburg, South Africa.

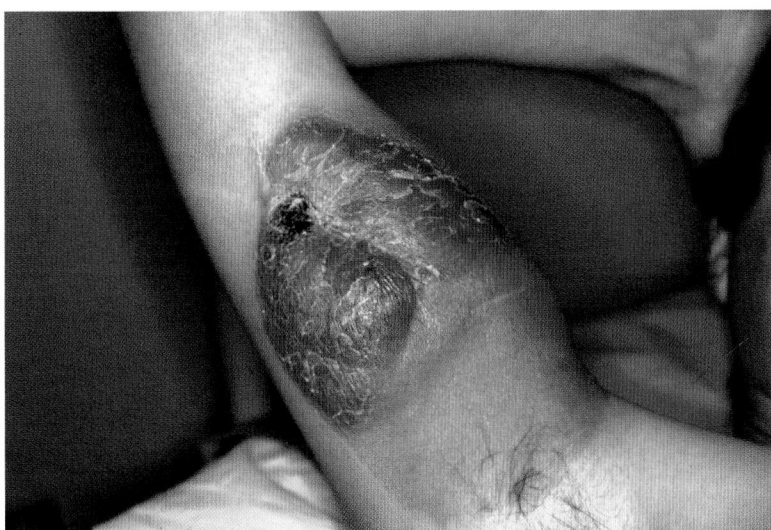

Fig. 29.245
Hodgkin lymphoma: this patient had stage IV disease. Cutaneous involvement presented as an ulcerated and encrusted plaque with tumor nodules on the arm of a middle-aged male. From the collection of the late N.P. Smith, MD, the Institute of Dermatology, London, UK.

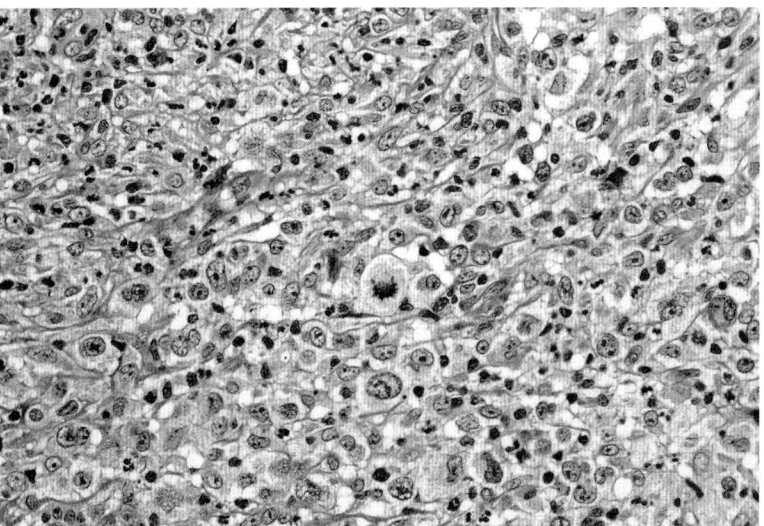

Fig. 29.247
Hodgkin lymphoma: high-power view of polymorphic infiltrate with central mitotic figure. By courtesy of W. Grayson, MD, National Health Laboratory Service, Johannesburg, South Africa.

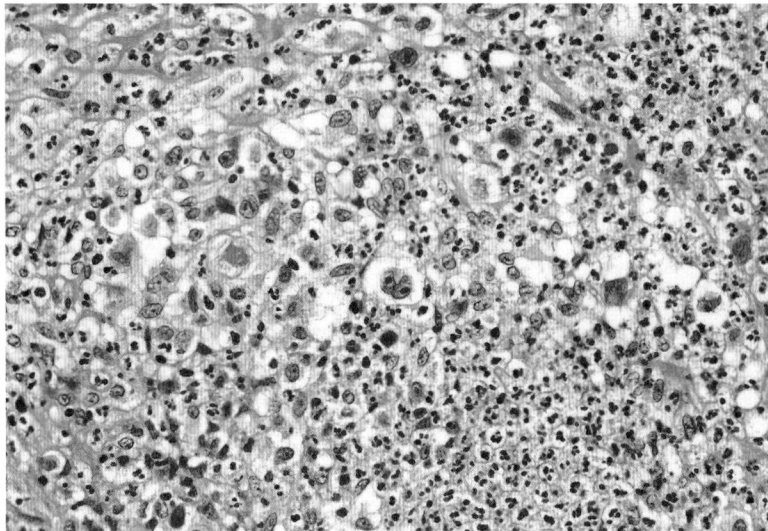

Fig. 29.248
Hodgkin lymphoma: a Reed-Sternberg cell is evident in the center of the field. By courtesy of W. Grayson, MD, National Health Laboratory Service, Johannesburg, South Africa.

T cells), together with variable numbers of histiocytes, plasma cells, eosinophils, and neutrophils.[2,11,31,32,33] Sclerosis may be evident in cutaneous lesions of classical nodular sclerosing HL.[31]

HRS cells are nearly always positive for CD30, and CD15 is demonstrable in 75–80% of cases, although it may be negative even when present in associated nodal lesions.[2,11,31-33] Staining for CD45, J-chain, CD75, and macrophage markers is negative. CD20 is often detectable but staining is weak, of variable intensity, and only present in a proportion of HRS cells.[2] Staining for pax5 and MUM1/IRF4 is positive, but one or both of OCT-2 and BOB.1 should be negative.[34] EMA and ALK1 are negative. EBV-positive cases react with antibodies to LMP1 and EBNA1, but not EBNA2, and EBERs are detectable using in situ hybridization (type II latency).[35] In a small number of cases, a minority of HRS cells show weak membranous or globular cytoplasmic staining for one or more T-cell antigens.[36] However, most such cases have clonal immunoglobulin gene rearrangements, suggesting that such reactivity is artifactual or represents aberrant expression.[25]

Differential diagnosis

The two most important differential diagnoses are lymphomatoid papulosis, cutaneous anaplastic large cell lymphoma and EBV+ MCU, since all of these conditions may contain Reed-Sternberg-like and Hodgkin-like cells that express CD30.

Lymphomatoid papulosis presents with a characteristic clinical history. The immunophenotype of the CD30+ cells includes CD45 (LCA)+, CD3+, and usually CD4+. CD15 is absent. A TCR gene rearrangement is present in many cases, which would also virtually exclude a diagnosis of HL.

Cutaneous anaplastic large cell lymphoma is localized to the skin and also expresses CD45, CD3, and most often CD4. Nodal tumors express EMA and ALK1 protein. A TCR gene rearrangement is present. The tumor cells do not express CD15.[37]

EBV+ MCU is a localized, circumscribed process typically contained by a peripheral rim of small T cells. It does not form a mass lesion.[38]

Methotrexate and other non-transplant iatrogenic-associated lymphoproliferative disorders

Clinical features

Methotrexate-associated lymphoproliferative disorder (MALD) was defined by the WHO in 2001 as a lymphoid proliferation or lymphoma in patients undergoing immunosuppressant treatment with methotrexate, mainly those with rheumatoid arthritis, psoriasis, and dermatomyositis, and often with associated EBV infection.[1] The lymphoid proliferation may mimic

a large B-cell lymphoma, an HL, or a polymorphous PTLD. In the most recently published WHO classification of hematological and lymphoid neoplasms, MALD has been put together under the rubric 'other iatrogenic immunodeficiency-associated lymphoproliferative disorders'.[2] The latter include similar lymphoproliferative disorders induced by antagonists of TNF-alpha including infliximab, adalimumab, and etanercept. TNF-alpha antagonists have only very rarely been associated with cutaneous lymphomas, and all cases so far have been T-cell lymphomas, mainly mycosis fungoides.[3-5] Other variants of T-cell lymphoma associated with this therapy include Sézary syndrome, CD30-positive anaplastic large cell lymphoma, subcutaneous panniculitis-like T-cell lymphoma, and cutaneous gamma/ delta T-cell lymphoma.[6-10] Cessation of the anti-TNF-alpha therapy may induce improvement or, more rarely, regression of the disease. The great majority of MALD occur in patients with rheumatoid arthritis and much less commonly in those with psoriasis or dermatomyositis.[1] About 40% of cases are extranodal, and the skin may rarely be involved primarily.[11-18] Most cases of MALD represent diffuse large B-cell lymphoma and HL. Less frequently, patients may present with follicular lymphoma, Burkitt lymphoma, peripheral T-cell lymphoma, and polymorphic lymphoplasmacyite infiltrates. Complete regression of the lesions may occur after cessation of methotrexate therapy, particularly in cases associated with EBV.

Pathogenesis and histopathological features

Immunosuppression is clearly associated with the development of these disorders, and in many cases, particularly Hodgkin disease and less commonly diffuse large cell lymphoma, there is an association with EBV. Immunosuppression related to old age only may induce similar processes.[19] The duration and intensity of immunosuppression are important factors as is the type of disease for which the patient is being treated. Patients with rheumatoid arthritis have an increased risk of developing lymphoma compared to the normal population. This may be due to chronic antigenic stimulation leading to immune dysregulation. In the setting of drug-induced immunosuppression, the risk of developing an immunoproliferative disorder appears increased.

The histologic appearances are identical to those seen in the specific type of lymphoma not associated with immunosuppression. Cases of MALD affecting the skin are often diffuse CD30+ large B-cell lymphomas and may be angiocentric.[16,17] Other cases have a more polymorphic appearance with variable numbers of blast cells, including Reed-Sternberg-like cells and often large numbers of T cells.[20] EBV can be demonstrated mainly by in situ hybridization in cases of HL, diffuse large B-cell lymphoma, and the more polymorphic proliferations. Clonality is often demonstrated, and in rare cases, both a T- and a B-cell clone may be demonstrated, which may indicate a composite lymphoma.[18]

Cutaneous post-transplant lymphoproliferative disorders

Clinical features

Post-transplant lymphoproliferative disorders (PTLDs) are defined by the WHO as lymphoid or plasmacytic proliferations secondary to immunosuppression in patients with solid organ, bone marrow, or stem cell allograft transplant.[1] The spectrum of PTLD is very wide and includes polyclonal and monoclonal B cell (usually, but not always, EBV driven) and T-cell proliferations. The incidence of PTLD is around 2%, and the prognosis is variable with survival of between 50% and 80%.[2] Presentation is usually early in lesions driven by EBV and late in those not driven by the virus. The incidence of PTLD is higher in children, in those that are seronegative for EBV at the time of transplantation, and in patients with heart–lung, lung, or gastrointestinal transplants.[1] Renal transplant patients have a lower incidence of PTLD. Extranodal involvement is common, particularly in the lungs, gastrointestinal tract, CNS, and even the transplanted organ. Cutaneous involvement by PTDL is very rare with no more than 30 cases reported in the literature.[2-20] It is usually restricted to the skin, and may affect children and adults, with no sex predilection. Presentation is with single or multiple papules, nodules, or plaques that may involve the limbs, trunk,

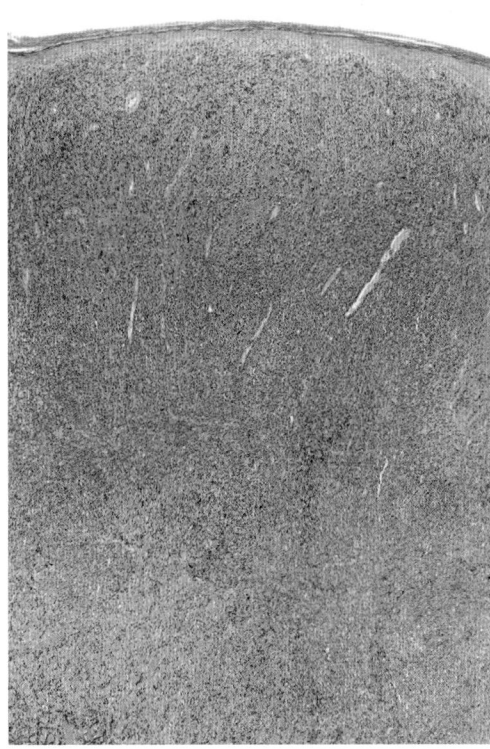

Fig. 29.249
Post-transplantation B-cell lymphoproliferative disorder: this patient developed a large perianal plaque following renal transplantation. The tumor regressed following reduction in immunosuppression.

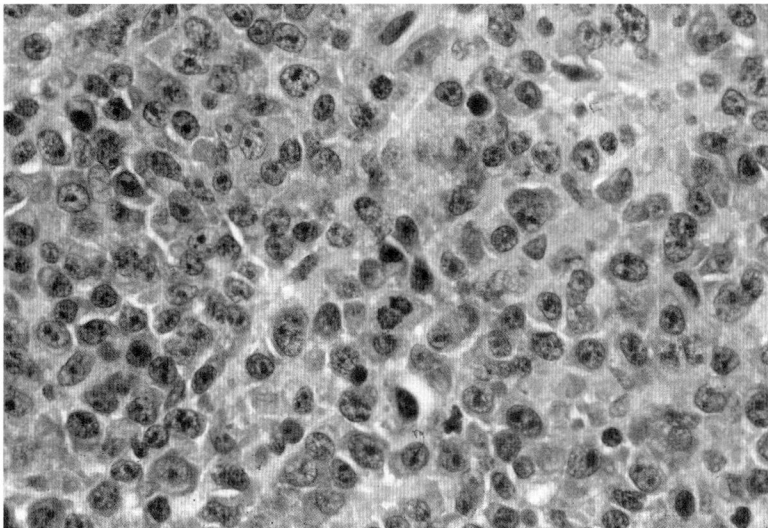

Fig. 29.250
Post-transplantation B-cell lymphoproliferative disorder: high-power view showing plasmacytoid differentiation.

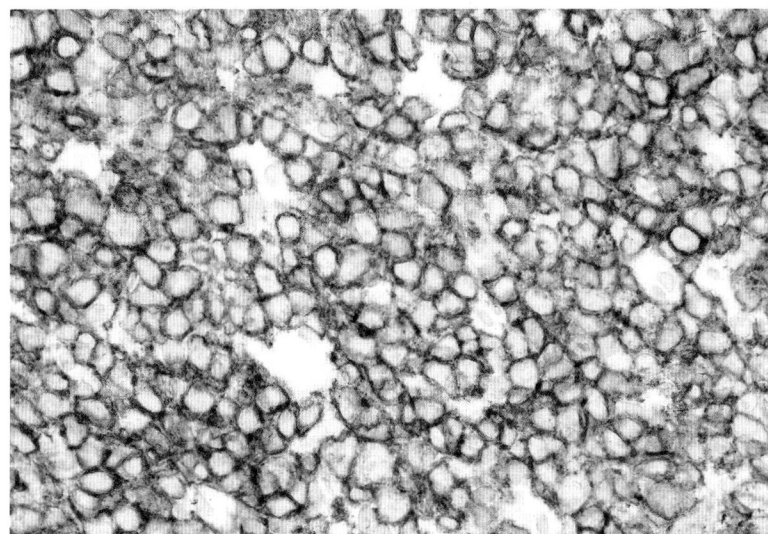

Fig. 29.251
Post-transplantation B-cell lymphoproliferative disorder: the tumor cells express CD138.

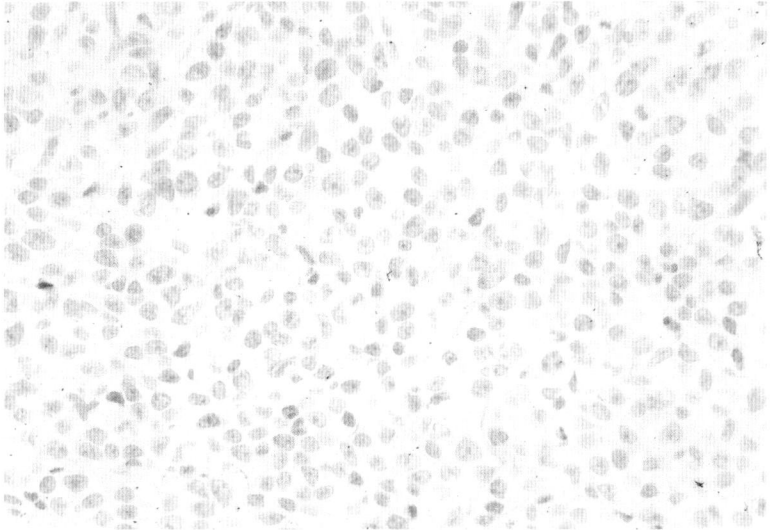

Fig. 29.252
Post-transplantation B-cell lymphoproliferative disorder: CD20 is negative.

or face. Patients with cutaneous disease tend to have good prognosis, and improvement or complete regression is seen with reduction or cessation of immunosuppression.

Pathogenesis and histopathological features

As mentioned above, most cases of B-cell proliferations are driven by EBV. The pathogenesis in cases negative for EBV is not clear but may be due to other viruses or chronic antigenic stimulation. Histologically, PTDL have been divided into early lesions (plasmacytic hyperplasia), polymorphic PTDL, and monomorphic PTDL.[1] Early lesions of PTDL consist of hyperplasia of plasma cells with mature lymphocytes and occasional immunoblasts. EBV is usually demonstrated and clonality is absent. In polymorphic PTDL, there is a prominent dermal and often subcutaneous infiltrate composed of mature plasma cells, immunoblasts, and small to medium-sized irregular lymphocytes (*Figs 29.249–29.253*). Some cells may resemble Hodgkin or Reed-Sternberg cells.[1,20] EBV and a B-cell clone are usually demonstrated. Monomorphic PTDL includes B and T/NK lymphomas that occur in an immunocompetent host, but most indolent B-cell lymphomas, with the exclusion of marginal zone lymphoma, are not included.[21,22] Monomorphic T-cell PTDLs are much less common than those of B-cell lineage. Any type of T-cell lymphoma may be seen, and in the skin, mainly anaplastic large T-cell lymphoma has been described.[11-16] A T-cell clone is usually demonstrated, but EBV is only exceptionally detected.[14]

Epstein-Barr virus-positive mucocutaneous ulcer

Clinical features

Epstein-Barr virus-positive mucocutaneous ulcer (EBV+ MCU) is a relatively recently described entity that arises in association with iatrogenic immunosuppression for autoimmune disease or post-organ transplant, as well as in apparently healthy elderly individuals, presumptively on a background of immune senescence.[1-5] In cases associated with autoimmune disease, the most commonly implicated drug is methotrexate.[1,3,4,6] It has

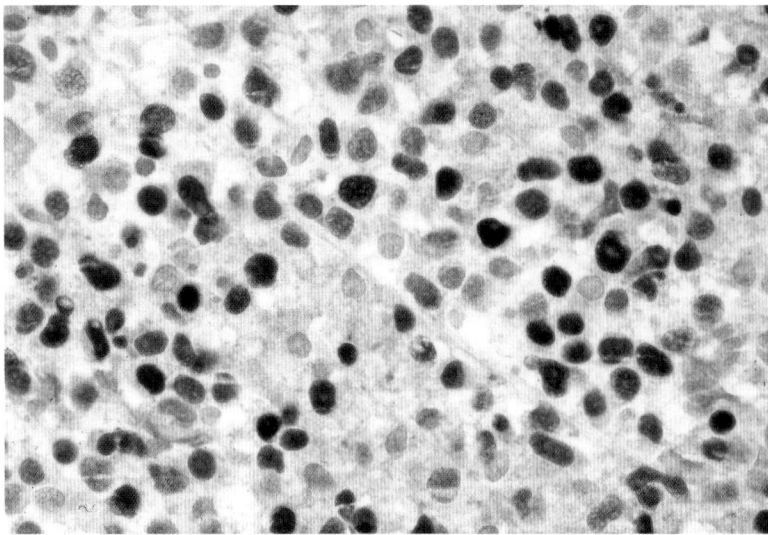

Fig. 29.253
Post-transplantation B-cell lymphoproliferative disorder: in situ hybridization for
Epstein-Barr virus is diffusely positive.

Pathogenesis and histologic features

It is hypothesized that, in patients developing EBV+ MCU, immune surveillance is reduced to a level that is only just sufficient to maintain EBV in a dormant state systemically. Localized factors are then thought to tip the balance toward an EBV-driven lymphoproliferation at a specific affected site. This often corresponds to locations where EBV-infected cells are prevalent, such as Waldeyer ring.[1]

The characteristic ulcer is circumscribed and shallow. A polymorphous infiltrate is present in the base of the ulcer, comprising variable numbers of immunoblasts and large atypical Reed-Sternberg-like cells. These are admixed with small lymphocytes, plasma cells, histiocytes, and eosinophils. In a significant proportion of cases, there is vascular invasion with thrombosis and sometimes necrosis. The deep aspect of the infiltrate is sharply defined by a rim of small lymphocytes. In squamous mucosa and skin there may be reactive epithelial atypia, and pseudoepitheliomatous hyperplasia may be encountered.[1,5] The immunoblasts and Reed-Sternberg-like cells are EBV-positive B cells that are uniformly CD30, and in some, CD15 positive. CD20 is often down-regulated, but there is typically expression of PAX5, MUM1, OCT2, and usually, BOB1.[1,5] Staining for EBV reveals a type II or type III latency pattern in most.[1,5,6] The background small lymphocytes are of T-lineage, and antibodies to CD3 are useful in highlighting the constraining rim of T lymphocytes at the base and sides of each lesion. Monoclonal immunoglobulin gene rearrangement can be identified in around 50% of cases. Clonal T-cell receptor rearrangements are often also detectable and are thought to be a consequence of a restricted but reactive T-cell repertoire.[1,3,5]

Differential diagnosis

The differential diagnosis of EBV+ MCU includes lymphomatoid granulomatosis, EBV-positive diffuse large B-cell lymphoma, and EBV-positive classical HL. There is considerable overlap in the cytological composition, and phenotype of these three entities and differentiation is often reliant on clinical features. The localized nature of EBV+ MCU and absence of a mass lesion are the most important features.[1,3–5,10] Peripheral blood EBV-DNA load may also be useful, and a putative diagnosis of EBV+ MCU should be questioned if elevated.[5] If the biopsy is adequate, pathological features may also be of help. EBV+ MCU is always sharply circumscribed with a band of small T cells at the base of the lesion, whereas more infiltrative patterns are seen with lymphomatoid granulomatosis and EBV-positive diffuse large B-cell lymphoma. EBV+ MCU may also resemble classical HL. However, the clinical criteria described above should also help in this situation. In addition, classical HL presenting as extranodal disease in the absence of nodal involvement is extremely rare, and the Reed-Sternberg-like cells in EBV+ MCU typically express CD45 and have an intact B-cell program.

been incorporated into the revised 2016 WHO Classification of lymphoid neoplasms as a provisional entity.[7]

Patients present with a solitary, well-circumscribed, often painful, ulcerating lesion at a mucosal or cutaneous site. Oropharyngeal mucosa is the most frequent site of presentation, and cutaneous involvement is often perioral, although other acral sites or trunk may be affected.[1,3,6] Examples have been described throughout the gastrointestinal tract, and patients occasionally present with a variety of abdominal symptoms, including abdominal emergencies.[5] Crucially, clinical examination and/or imaging fails to detect an underlying mass lesion. There is also no associated lymphadenopathy or splenomegaly.[5] EBV-DNA is typically undetectable in peripheral blood, in contrast to many other types of EBV-associated lymphoproliferative disorders.[5]

EBV+ MCU is an indolent disease. Spontaneous regression is frequent in apparently immunocompetent elderly individuals and reduction in immunosuppression is sufficient for most patients receiving therapeutic immunosuppression. Most patients do not suffer relapse, although a relapsing and remitting course without progression may occasionally be seen.[1–4,8,9]

BENIGN CUTANEOUS INFILTRATES THAT CAN BE MISTAKEN FOR CUTANEOUS B-CELL LYMPHOMA (SO-CALLED CUTANEOUS B-CELL PSEUDOLYMPHOMA)

Reactive cutaneous lymphoid infiltrates that can simulate B-cell neoplasms include B-CLH (so-called cutaneous B-cell pseudolymphoma), cutaneous (systemic) plasmacytosis, and IPT.

B-cutaneous lymphoid hyperplasia

Clinical features

B-cutaneous lymphoid hyperplasia (cutaneous B-cell pseudolymphoma) is a generic term employed to denote reactive lymphoid infiltrates with a significant B-cell component that simulate B-cell lymphoma. It encompasses a variety of different clinicopathological scenarios with a common histologic endpoint; it is best described as B-cutaneous lymphoid hyperplasia (B-CLH). The historical terminology for this group of disorders includes

sarcomatosis cutis, lymphocytoma cutis, lymphadenosis benigna cutis, and pseudolymphoma of Spiegler and Fendt.[1] In some instances, a precipitating cause can be identified. Examples include arthropod bites,[2,3] Borrelia infection,[4–7] trauma,[8] vaccinations,[9–11] injected drugs or antigens for hyposensitization,[12,13] acupuncture,[1] gold pierced earings,[14–16] tattoos,[17–19] and varicella-zoster infection scars.[20–22] However, in most cases, the cause remains unknown.

The clinical features depend to a certain extent on the situation in which the B-cell pseudolymphoma arises. Idiopathic cutaneous B-cell pseudolymphoma probably constitutes the largest group and is most frequent on the face (cheek, nose, earlobe) (70%), chest, and upper extremities. There is predilection for females (3:1), and white races are affected more often than black (9:1).[1] B. burgdorferi is probably the commonest cause in endemic regions in Europe, although cutaneous B-cell pseudolymphoma is a rare

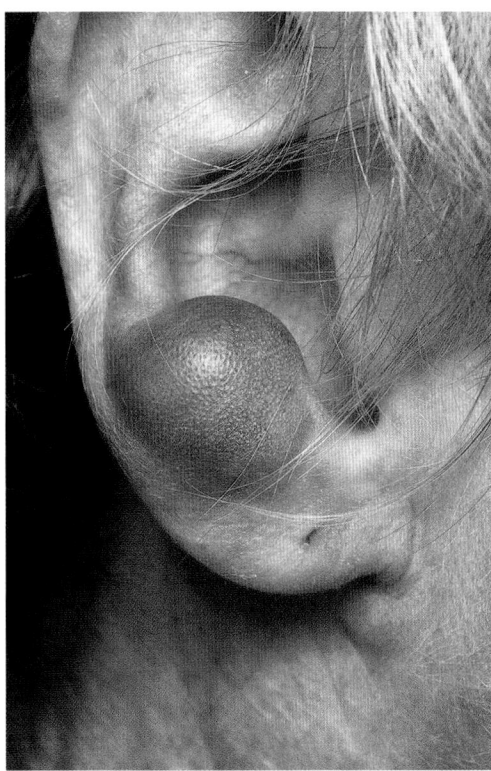

Fig. 29.254
B-cutaneous lymphoid hyperplasia: the earlobe is a commonly affected site. Lesions are usually solitary. By courtesy of the Institute of Dermatology, London, UK.

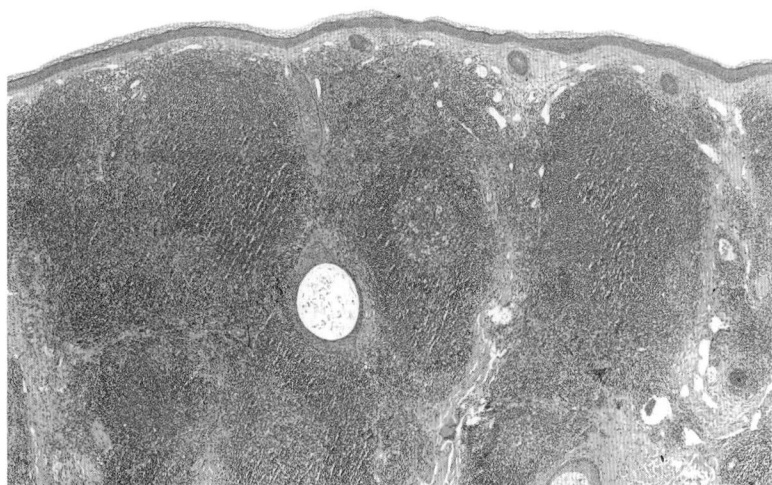

Fig. 29.255
B-cutaneous lymphoid hyperplasia: there is a dense dermal lymphoid infiltrate with conspicuous germinal centers.

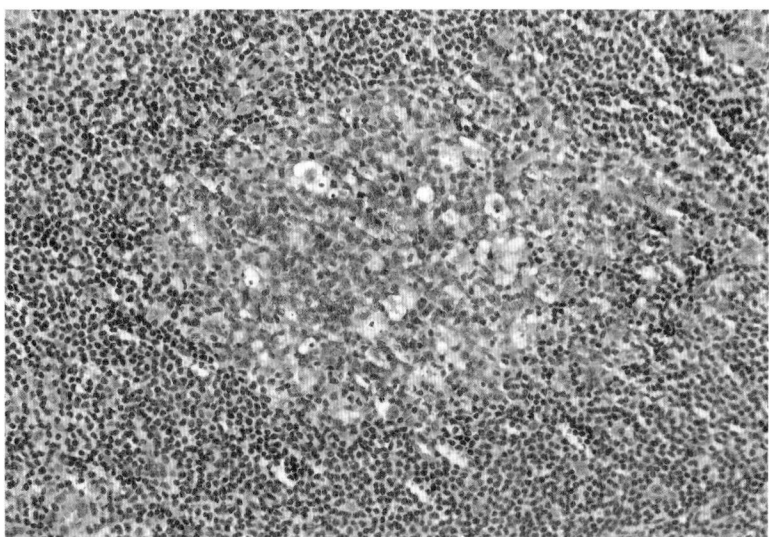

Fig. 29.256
B-cutaneous lymphoid hyperplasia: there are prominent tingible body macrophages within the germinal center.

manifestation of Lyme disease, showing a prevalence of only 0.6–1.3% in patients with serological and/or clinical evidence of infection.[5,23,24] Specific skin lesions usually develop within a few weeks to months of a tick bite, usually in the nipple region, genital region, or on the ear lobe (*Fig. 29.254*).[1,7,25] They may develop de novo or arise in a background of erythema chronicum migrans.[7]

Whatever the cause, most patients present with solitary, small, erythematous to plum-colored or bluish plaques and nodules. Ulceration is very rare and multiple lesions uncommon. Most cases run a benign clinical course, and many resolve following removal of the causative stimulus, although in some the process is chronic and recalcitrant to treatment.[1] Examples of B-CLH evolving into overt B-cell lymphoma are also well documented, and it is possible that a spectrum of disease exists.[6,26–29] Follow-up of all patients is therefore advisable.

Pathogenesis and histopathological features

Persistent antigenic stimulation is the presumed cause of B-CLH in cutaneous B-cell pseudolymphoma, particularly when a precipitating cause can be identified. For example, *B. burgdorferi*-specific DNA is present in many *Borrelia*-associated cases of cutaneous B-cell pseudolymphoma. Mouthparts have been identified in skin biopsies showing B-CLH developing in association with arthropod bites, and adjuvant (aluminum hydroxide) has been demonstrated at the site of vaccination-associated cutaneous B-cell pseudolymphoma.[2,7,17,30] Tattoo-induced B-CLH appears to occur principally in association with red tattoo pigment and only rarely with green or blue tattoos.[1,17–19] A case of B-CLH has also been documented in a patient with Sjögren syndrome, raising the possibility of autoantigenic stimulation in some cases.[31] In addition, certain dendritic cell subtypes are present in greater numbers in B-CLH than cutaneous B-cell lymphomas, further implicating persistent antigenic stimulation in the pathogenesis.[32–34]

Histologic features reported to be relatively specific for cutaneous B-cell pseudolymphoma in the historical literature including a 'top heavy' distribution, do not hold up to modern-day scrutiny, especially as many of the early series mistakenly included examples of cutaneous B-cell lymphoma in their cohorts of pseudolymphoma.[8,35] In fact, low-power examination often reveals a diffuse, vaguely nodular infiltrate that fills the dermis and sometimes involving the subcutis (*Fig. 29.255*). In less florid examples, the infiltrate tends to be nodular and perivascular and periadnexal in distribution, but may still extend to the deep reticular dermis and subcutis. A grenz zone is often present, but exocytosis and spongiosis may be seen, and other epidermal changes, such as atrophy, hyperplasia, and parakeratosis, are relatively frequent.[7,36,37]

The lymphoid tissue is similar to reactive lymphoid tissue at sites where it is more usually encountered (e.g., lymph nodes, tonsils). Lymphoid follicles are almost always present. These may be primary in nature, and composed of closely packed small lymphocytes, but in most cases reactive germinal centers are also prominent.[7,25,36,37] Germinal centers comprise an admixture of large centroblasts, small and large centrocytes, and tingible body macrophages. Whilst a compressed mantle of small lymphocytes is the norm in germinal centers at other sites, it is often lacking in B-CLH, particularly in cases associated with *Borrelia* infection.[7,25,38] Reactive germinal centers have a high proliferation rate and often appear 'zoned', with darkly staining areas full of proliferating centroblasts and lighter zones in which centrocytes predominate (*Figs 29.256* and *29.257*). The interfollicular areas are populated by a polymorphic infiltrate with predominant small lymphocytes, scattered blast cells, histiocytes, plasma cells, and sometimes eosinophils.[7,25,36,37]

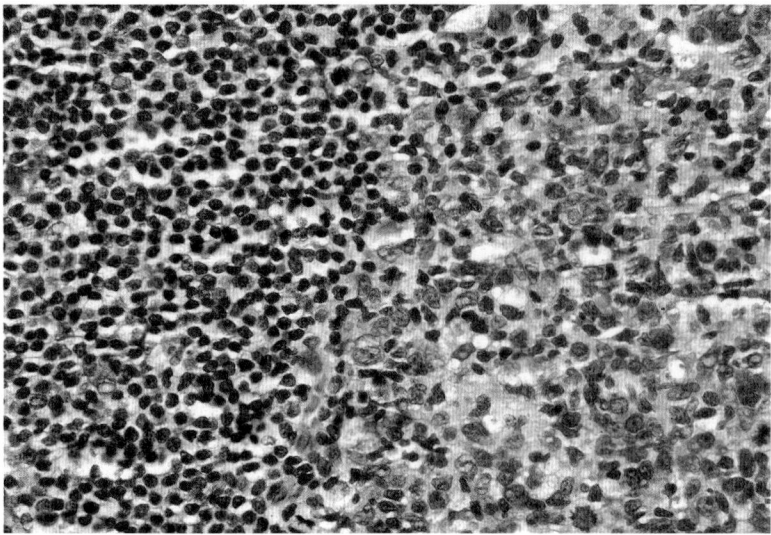

Fig. 29.257
B-cutaneous lymphoid hyperplasia: high-power view of edge of germinal center and adjacent population of mature small lymphocytes.

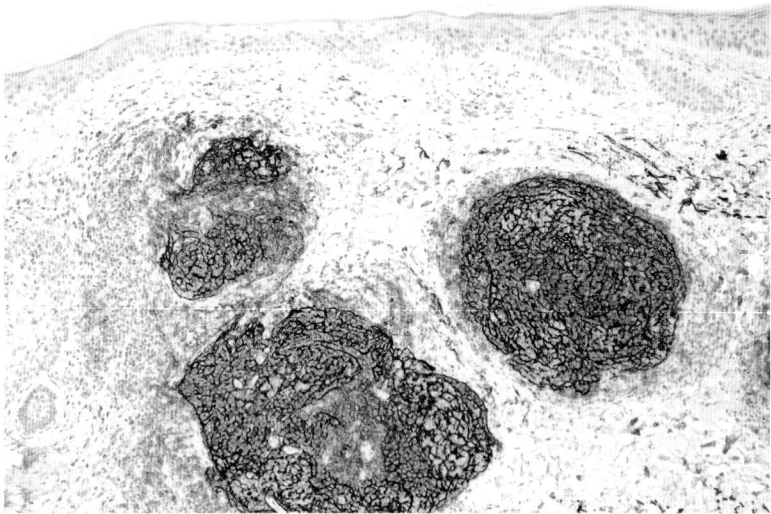

Fig. 29.258
B-cutaneous lymphoid hyperplasia: the follicular architecture is outlined by demonstration of the follicular dendritic cell population (CD21).

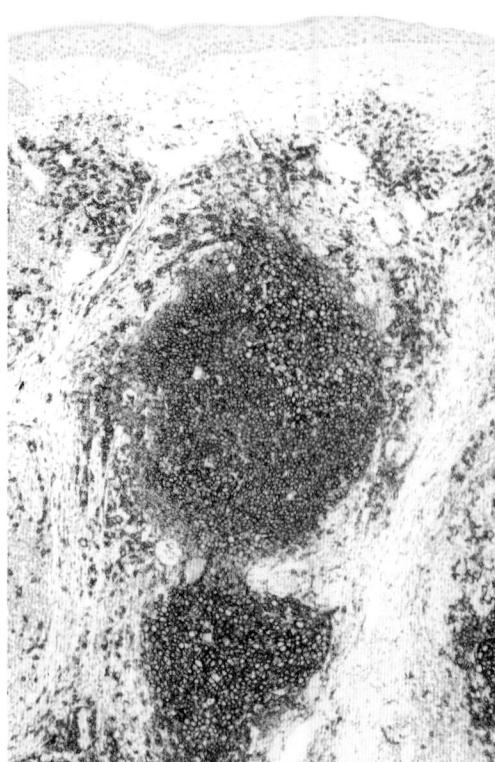

Fig. 29.259
B-cutaneous lymphoid hyperplasia: the B-cell component is outlined with CD20 immunohistochemistry.

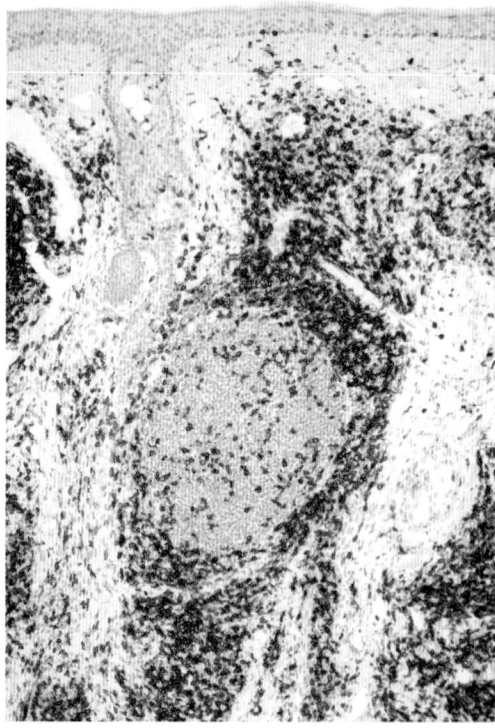

Fig. 29.260
B-cutaneous lymphoid hyperplasia: a layer of T cells (CD3) surrounds the B-cell nodules.

Lymphoid follicles can be identified immunohistochemically by antibodies marking the FDC networks (CD21, CD23, and CD35) (*Fig. 29.258*). Primary B-cell follicles contain a uniform population of small B lymphocytes (CD20 positive), many of which coexpress CD23 (*Fig. 29.259*). The germinal center B cells express CD10 and bcl-6, but lack bcl-2. T cells predominate in the interfollicular areas, although small numbers of B cells are also seen (*Fig. 29.260*), including a proportion of the scattered blasts (*Fig. 29.260*). These typically show no expression of CD10. Immunohistochemistry or in situ hybridization for light chains shows a polytypic pattern of staining for the B lymphocytes and plasma cells (*Figs 29.261* and *29.262*).[7,25,36,37,39]

PCR clonality assays most often show a polyclonal pattern of immunoglobulin gene rearrangement. However, clonality has been demonstrated in lesions otherwise typical for B-CLH.[40–42]

Differential diagnosis

The main differential diagnoses of B-CLH are primary cutaneous marginal zone lymphoma and cutaneous follicle center lymphoma, as discussed previously in the relevant sections on these entities. Briefly, in marginal zone lymphoma there are sheets of marginal zone cells, a predominance of interfollicular B lymphocytes, and aberrant B-cell expression of CD43.[36,43]

Neoplastic follicles in PCFCL, or follicular lymphoma secondarily involving the skin, typically have a monotonous appearance with no zonation, relatively few tingible body macrophages and mitotic figures, and a low proliferation fraction. In secondary follicular lymphoma, the neoplastic follicles are also usually bcl-2 positive, although this is less often the case for PCFCL.[37,39]

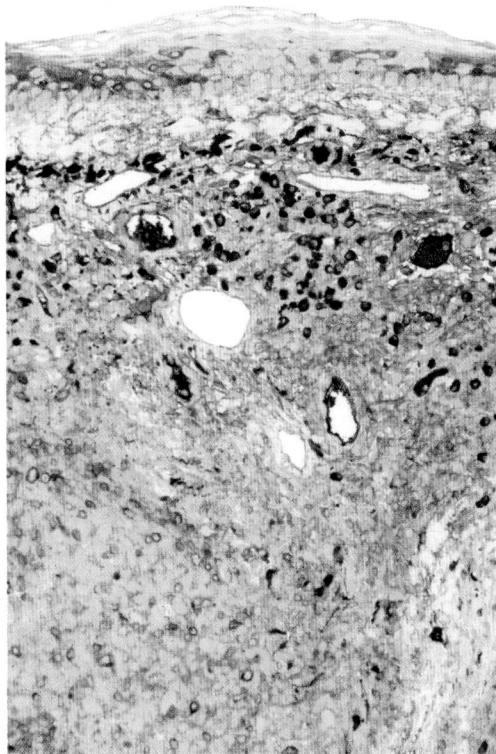

Fig. 29.261
B-cutaneous lymphoid hyperplasia: kappa plasma cells are scattered throughout the infiltrate.

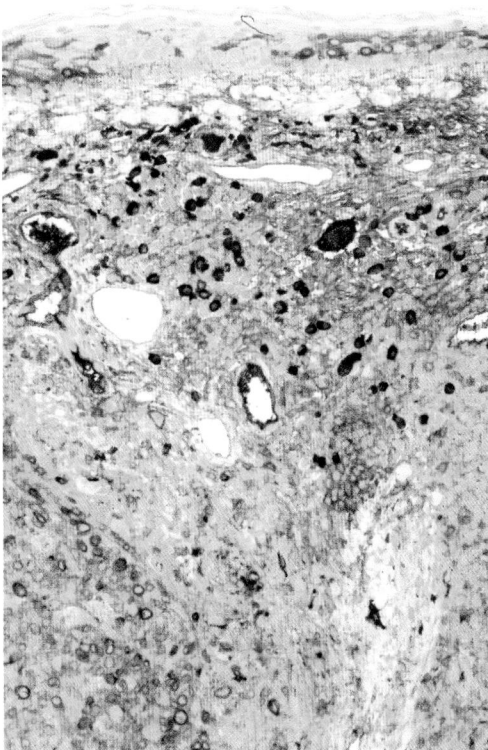

Fig. 29.262
B-cutaneous lymphoid hyperplasia: similar numbers of lambda plasma cells are present.

B-CLH associated with *Borrelia* infection may also mimic large B-cell lymphoma, since the follicles contain numerous centroblasts with a lack of zonation, often lack mantles and may coalesce to form large areas with predominance of blast cells. Moreover, in some cases, there are apparent interfollicular aggregates of CD10 and/or bcl-6-positive B cells. Such a

finding would normally be indicative of lymphoma, but in this situation the aggregates probably represent small cross sections of follicle centers that are devoid of mantles. A benign diagnosis is favored by the presence of numerous tingible body macrophages and an associated mixed reactive infiltrate of small lymphocytes, histiocytes, eosinophils, and plasma cells.[7,38]

Demonstration of monoclonality by in situ hybridization or light chain immunohistochemistry is strong evidence of lymphoma, but immunoglobulin gene rearrangement studies are less conclusive in view of the well-documented examples of clonal B-CLH.[28,29,40,41] Moreover, interpretation of molecular results is further hampered by the relatively high incidence of pseudoclonality encountered when performing PCR on skin biopsies.[44]

Cutaneous and systemic plasmacytosis

Clinical features

Cutaneous plasmacytosis is rare and has been mainly documented in Asians, particularly Japanese, and consists of a triad of cutaneous lesions, superficial lymphadenopathy, and polyclonal hypergammaglobulinemia.[1-7] Because of the relatively high frequency of plasmacytosis infiltrates at extracutaneous sites, the current preferred nomenclature is cutaneous and systemic plasmacytosis (CSP).[5-7] Cases in Caucasians are very rare.[8-11] There is male predilection (approximately 2.8:1), and the median age at presentation is 49 years (range, 15–75 years).[6] Rarely, it occurs in children.[12,13] The skin lesions comprise widespread, frequently pruritic, reddish-brown macules, papules, nodules, and plaques. The trunk is most often affected.[3,5-7] In patients with scalp involvement, alopecia can occur.[14] There may be systemic involvement (systemic plasmacytosis) with hepatosplenomegaly and constitutional symptoms.[2,6,15] Rare associations include lymphoid interstitial pneumonia, tuberculosis, and syphilis.[16-18] The ESR is usually raised, and in some patients antinuclear factor may be present. Investigations to exclude myeloma are invariably negative.

CSP generally has a favorable prognosis although occasional cases run a more aggressive clinical course with infiltration of viscera, and one case has been associated with development of T-cell lymphoma.[15]

Pathogenesis and histopathological features

The cause is not known, although IL-6, a cytokine involved in mediating differentiation of activated B cells to plasma cells, is implicated in its pathogenesis. Serum IL-6 levels are elevated, and this cytokine has been demonstrated in lesional cells.[19-22] In addition, cases of CSP successfully treated with steroids show reduced levels of IL-6 in serum and lesional tissues.[21,22]

Histologically, there is a dermal superficial to deep perivascular and periadnexal infiltrate of mature plasma cells that may extend into the subcutis (*Figs 29.263* and *29.264*).[1,3,5-7] By definition, cytological atypia and mitotic activity are absent. Lymphocytes and histiocytes may be present in small numbers, and lymphoid follicles are reported in some cases. By immunohistochemistry, the plasma cells are polyclonal.[1] Staining for HHV8 is negative.[15]

Bone marrow and lymph nodes are infiltrated by mature polyclonal nonatypical plasma cells.

Differential diagnosis

Disseminated plasma cell myeloma, cutaneous plasmacytoma, and cutaneous marginal zone lymphoma may all harbor significant numbers of plasma cells but these are monoclonal, and often atypical in the case of plasma cell neoplasm. A monoclonal serum immunoglobulin is absent in CSP.

CSP shows overlapping features with the plasma cell variant of multicentric CD. Multicentric CD may rarely involve the skin and some authors maintain that the two conditions are related.[6,23] That notwithstanding, multicentric CD is typically a more severe illness frequently associated with anemia, thrombocytopenia, and HIV infection, features not found in cutaneous plasmacytosis.[15,23] HHV8 is often present in multicentric CD.[24]

CSP lacks the prominent dermal sclerosis seen in IPT, a solitary lesion displaying plasma cell granuloma-like features, and should not fulfill the criteria required for a diagnosis of IgG4-related disease (IgG4-RD).[25] The condition must also be differentiated from the dermal plasma cell infiltrates

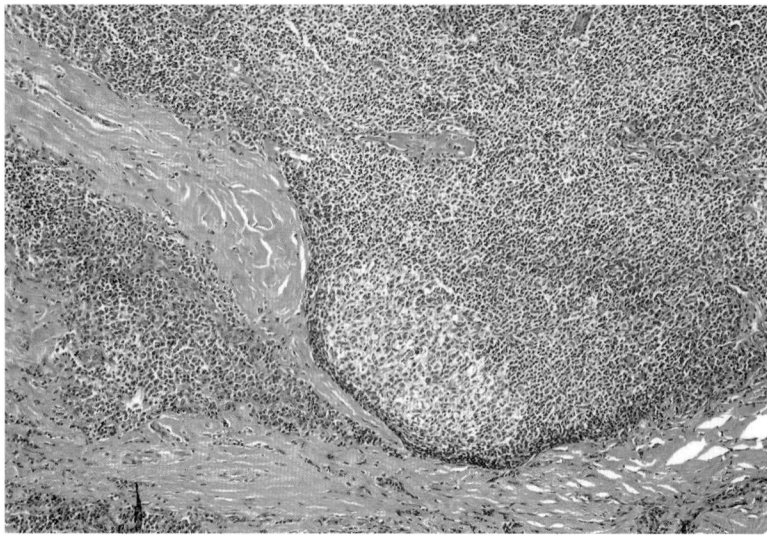

Fig. 29.263
Cutaneous plasmacytosis: there is a dense dermal infiltrate. A lymphoid follicle is present toward the center of the field. By courtesy of K. Busam, MD, Memorial Sloan-Kettering Cancer Center, New York, USA.

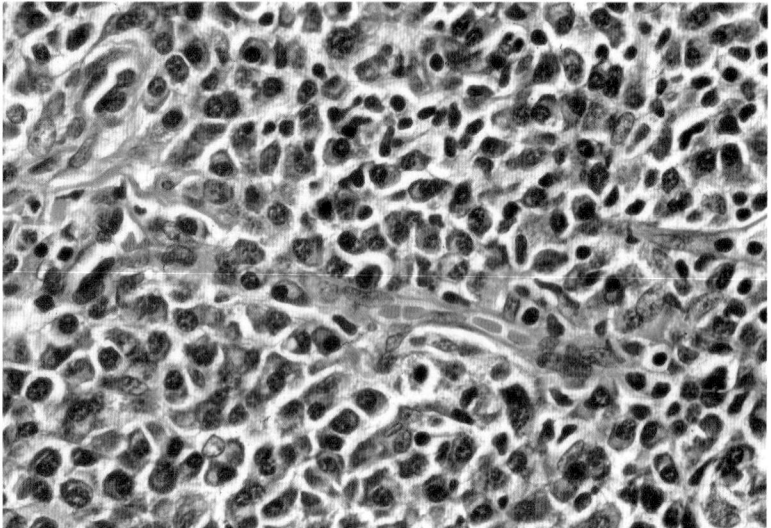

Fig. 29.264
Cutaneous plasmacytosis: the infiltrate consists of a monotonous population of mature plasma cells. By courtesy of K. Busam, MD, Memorial Sloan-Kettering Cancer Center, New York, USA.

associated with infections including syphilis and Lyme disease and also connective tissue diseases.[1,3,5,6] Infiltrates in these disorders tend to be more sparse, and clinical correlation is usually discriminatory.

IgG4-related disease

Clinical features

IgG4 is the least common of the four IgG subclasses of antibody. It has a low affinity for target antigen and does not activate compliment. It plays a role in parasitic infection and allergic conditions such as asthma, eczema, as well as certain bullous disorders.[1] IgG4-related disease (IgG4-RD) was first recognized following studies of autoimmune pancreatitis.[2,3] A similar disease process was subsequently documented at many other sites, and many previously recognized conditions are now acknowledged to lie within the spectrum of IgG4-RD.[4] The latter include salivary gland lesions such as Mikulicz syndrome and Kuttner tumor, Reidels thyroiditis, and eosinophilic angiocentric fibrosis of orbit and upper respiratory tract.[4] A recent

consensus conference has now produced recommendations for a unifying nomenclature, interpretation of pathological findings, and diagnostic criteria.[5–7]

A diagnosis of IgG4-RD requires the presence of a mass or swelling showing characteristic pathological features and a raised serum IgG4 ($\geq$135 mg/dl).[7] One or more organs may be involved. If all criteria are met, a diagnosis of IgG4-RD can be made. However, if only some are present then descriptive terminology should be used mentioning that increased numbers of IgG4-positive plasma cells are present and that IgG4-RD is a possibility. Follow-up may help clarify the diagnosis in ambiguous situations. Once a diagnosis is made, it is recommended that site-specific nomenclature be used, preceded by the common terminology, 'IgG4-related'. Most patents are middle aged or elderly males.[4,8] Presenting symptoms are often related to the mass lesion, and constitutional symptoms are usually lacking. Serum immunoglobulins, including IgG4, are usually, but not always, raised.[4,8]

The most common sites of presentation are pancreas (IgG4-related pancreatitis), biliary tree (IgG4-related sclerosing cholangitis), salivary glands (IgG4-related sialadenitis), and periorbital tissues and lacrimal gland (IgG4-related orbital inflammation and dacryoadenitis), but virtually any organ can be involved.[4,5,8] Skin involvement is rare and usually associated with extracutaneous disease; however, in rare instances skin may be the primary site of disease.[4,8–14] Lesions are typically erythematous itchy plaques or subcutaneous nodules which are often localized close to the main areas of underlying organ involvement.[9,10,14] Hence, they are frequently found in the head and neck region, particularly on or behind the ear or in the vicinity of the submandibular gland.[9,10,14] Other manifestations of cutaneous involvement that have been described include prurigo-like nodules, rosacea-like papules and pustules, scleroderma-like lesions, xanthogranuloma, and papules and nodules mimicking angiolymphoid hyperplasia with eosinophilia.[9,15–18]

IgG4-RD typically responds well to corticosteroids if diagnosed in its early stages. Problems usually arise as a consequence of established fibrosis which may require surgical intervention.[4,8]

Pathogenesis and histologic features

IgG4-RD appears to be an autoimmune disease.[19] Its key pathological features are the presence of a dense lymphoplasmacytic infiltrate, often with germinal centers and eosinophils, fibrosis which is focally storiform, and obliterative phlebitis.[6] The absolute plasma cell count varies depending on the age of the lesion biopsied and the site of involvement.[6] It has been proposed that >200 plasma cells/hpf are required before considering a diagnosis of IgG4-related skin disease.[6] However, this figure was derived from a relatively low number of cases and may be an overestimate.[6,14] The plasma cells are polytypic with increased numbers expressing IgG4; an IgG4/IgG ratio of >40% is considered a prerequisite for diagnosis. In the skin, the infiltrate tends to be nodular and involves the dermis and/or subcutaneous fat. Fibrosis is less commonly encountered than at some other sites.[14]

Differential diagnosis

The pathology of IgG4-related skin disease overlaps considerably with that of several other dermatoses and may mimic cutaneous plasmacytosis, angiolymphoid hyperplasia with eosinophilia, Kimura disease, Rosai-Dorfman disease, multicentric CD, and cutaneous B-cell pseudolymphoma.[12,15,18,20–23] It should be noted that many of these disorders also contain IgG4-positive plasma cells. Hence, close clinicopathological correlation with adherence to diagnostic guidelines is required in order not to under- or overdiagnose IgG4-RD. PCMZL may also contain IgG4-positive plasma cells, but these are monotypic and monoclonal.[24]

Cutaneous Castleman disease

Clinical features

Castleman disease (CD) (giant lymph node hyperplasia, angiofollicular lymph node hyperplasia) is a rare B-cell lymphoproliferative disorder mainly involving lymph nodes, with unicentric (usually no systemic symptoms) or multicentric (usually with systemic symptoms) involvement and associated in a percentage of cases with HIV/AIDS and HHV8 infection.[1] However, not all cases associated with HHV8 infection are HIV positive. Two main histologic variants occur, namely, the hyaline vascular type predominantly seen in unicentric disease and the plasma cell type mainly seen in multicentric disease and in cases associated with HIV infection. Cutaneous involvement in CD is exceptional, with only a handful of cases reported and mainly associated with the multicentric plasma cell variant of the disease. Cutaneous presentation is with papules, nodules, or plaques and involvement has been reported on trunk and limbs and rarely on the face.[2-9]

Pathogenesis and histologic features

CD appears to be due to secretion of IL-6 both in idiopathic cases and in those associated with HHV8.[1,10] In cutaneous lesions, there is a dermal and sometimes subcutaneous infiltrate composed mainly of polyclonal plasma cells with no cytological atypia.[2,3,5-7] Increased vascularity is usually present in the background. In rare cases, the appearance is more similar to that seen in the hyaline vascular type of disease, with bands of sclerosis surrounding an infiltrate with atrophic germinal centers and expanded mantle zones in an onion ring pattern.[4,8]

Inflammatory pseudotumor of the skin

Clinical features

Inflammatory pseudotumor (IPT) encompasses a heterogeneous group of disorders characterized histologically by varying proportions of inflammatory cells, hyalinized collagenous stroma, and myofibroblastic proliferations. Many historical cases would probably now be considered to lie within the spectrum of IgG4-RD. Some, corresponding to many cases referred to as plasma cell granuloma, are probably reactive and may be related to infectious processes, while others likely represent genuine neoplasms with clonal cytogenetic abnormalities, and include patients with a t(2;5) and overexpression of ALK1.[1-7] The latter are often referred to as inflammatory myofibroblastic tumors.

IPT has been reported in virtually every body site, including rare cutaneous cases.[8-16] A wide age range may be affected, and there is no obvious sex predilection.[1] IPT presents as a solitary slow-growing nodule that usually measures between 1 and 3 cm in diameter.[17] Cutaneous variants are invariably benign and do not usually recur following excision.

Pathogenesis and histologic features

The pathogenesis is unknown, particularly for those tumors displaying plasma cell granuloma-like features. It is most likely that such cases represent either an inflammatory reaction pattern to an as-yet unidentified stimulus or the end stage of a chronic vasculitis, possibly in response to a local persistent antigen.[8,18] Lesions with a prominent spindle cell component probably represent a true neoplasm, similar to inflammatory myofibroblastic tumor, but to date none has shown overexpression of ALK1.[8]

Histologically, two main patterns are seen.[8] 'Plasma cell granuloma-like' lesions present as nonencapsulated, sharply demarcated dermal and/or subcutaneous nodules with a prominent infiltrate composed of small lymphocytes, lymphoplasmacytoid cells, and numerous plasma cells (Figs 29.265–29.267). Reactive follicles, eosinophils, and neutrophils may be seen. There is background of thick hyalinized collagen bundles, often intersecting or forming an onionskin pattern with focal perivascular accentuation and prominent high endothelial venules. A marked spindle cell component is not seen.[8,9,16] A similar heavy inflammatory cell infiltrate is present in the other main pattern, but in these cases the nodules are poorly circumscribed, display a prominent dermal bland spindle cell proliferation mainly in fascicles, and bear a closer resemblance to inflammatory myofibroblastic tumor described at other sites. There are intervening bundles of thick hyalinized collagen.[8,10,12,13]

Immunohistochemistry highlights B-cell aggregates with intervening small T cells and polyclonal plasma cells. EBV and HHV8 are negative, and PCR shows a polyclonal pattern of immunoglobulin gene rearrangement. Spindled cells, when present, express smooth muscle actin and muscle-specific

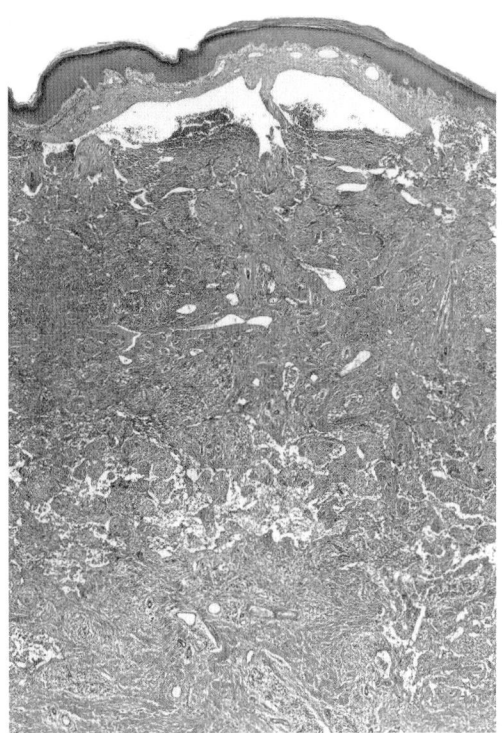

Fig. 29.265
Inflammatory pseudotumor of the skin: low-power view showing dermal infiltrate, hyalinized collagen bundles, and increased vascularity.

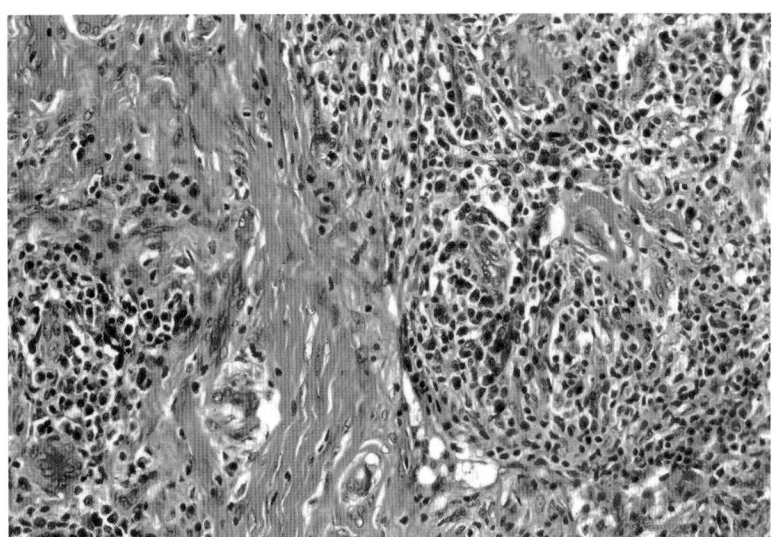

Fig. 29.266
Inflammatory pseudotumor of the skin: higher-power view of collagen and lymphoid infiltrate.

actin, consistent with myofibroblasts, but in the small number of cases tested are negative for ALK1, CD21, CD34, and S100.[8,17]

Differential diagnosis

Plasma cell granuloma-like lesions are most likely to be mistaken for a superficial lymph node or a cutaneous lymphomatous deposit, particularly cutaneous plasmacytoma, metastatic myeloma, or PCMZL. The first can be excluded by the absence of a subcapsular sinus and the polymorphous nature of the infiltrate. Lymphoma is excluded by the invariable polyclonal nature of the infiltrate.[8-10] Epithelioid hemangioma (angiolymphoid hyperplasia with eosinophilia) is differentiated on the basis of its vascular characteristics, particularly the presence of epithelioid endothelial cells, and often

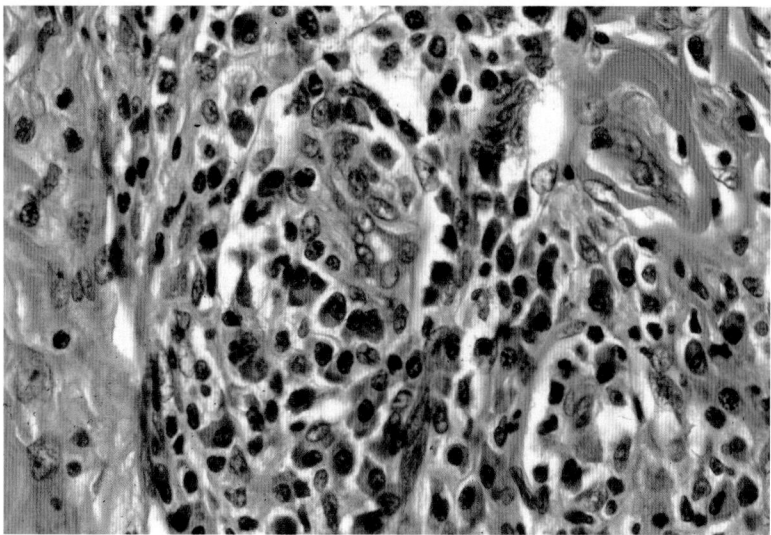

Fig. 29.267
Inflammatory pseudotumor of the skin: the infiltrate consists of lymphocytes and conspicuous plasma cells.

prominent eosinophils. Kimura disease is morphologically similar, but clinically most patients are Asian and there is peripheral blood eosinophilia and raised serum IgE.

Lesions with prominent spindle cells are more likely to be confused with other spindled cell tumors, with differential diagnosis including solitary fibrous tumor, FDC sarcoma, and nodular fasciitis.

Differentiation from IgG4-RD requires close clinicopathological correlation and application of agreed diagnostic criteria.[19]

Pretibial lymphoplasmacytic plaque

Clinical features

Pretibial lymphoplasmacytic plaque first described as isolated benign primary cutaneous plasmacytosis is a variant of pseudolymphoma that characteristically occurs in children and adolescents with marked predilection for the pretibial area.[1,2] Most cases described so far have been in Caucasians. Presentation is as a solitary, red-brown, long-standing (often years) scaly, erythematous plaque varying in size from less than 1 to 4 cm.[1-6] Papular lesions may also be seen. The behavior is benign, but treatment is difficult.

Pathogenesis and histologic features

The etiology of the process is unknown. The epidermis displays acanthosis and hyperkeratosis with focal parakeratosis. In the underlying superficial and deep dermis, there is a moderate to prominent perivascular and periadnexal mononuclear cell infiltrate composed of lymphocytes and numerous mature plasma cells.[1-6] In some cases, focal interface inflammation of the epidermis and sweat glands is seen. Occasional epithelioid cell granulomas are rarely identified.

Differential diagnosis

Primary cutaneous plasmacytosis is characterized clinically by multiple plaques with predilection for the trunk, occurs almost exclusively in Asians, and consists histologically of an infiltrate composed almost exclusively of mature polytypic plasma cells. Acral pseudolymphomatous angiokeratoma of children (APACHE) consists of warty papular lesions, usually on acral sites, and it is characterized histologically by more prominent epidermal changes and a dermal predominantly lymphocytic infiltrate with few plasma cells and a prominent proliferation of small vascular channels. T cell-rich angiomatous polypoid pseudolymphoma (TRAPP) presents as a single polypoid lesion, with predilection for adults and consists of a prominent dermal infiltrate composed of T lymphocytes with few plasma or no plasma cells and numerous small blood vessels.

HISTIOCYTIC DISORDERS

The histiocytoses are a group of heterogeneous reactive and neoplastic disorders in which cells of the dendritic or monocyte–macrophage lineage proliferate in various tissues, including the skin. They have been the source of considerable confusion due to their relative rarity, the use of imprecise terminology, and a lack of knowledge of the precise lineage of lesional cells.

The term 'histiocyte' denotes a group of tissue-based immune cells that includes both macrophages and dendritic cells. Macrophages display strong phagocytic capabilities and function predominantly as antigen presenting cells, whereas dendritic cells are primarily accessory cells with antigen presenting functions.[1,2] Distinction between these two groups is often not clear since both cell types display considerable plasticity, their characteristics changing according to their stage of development and/or the influence of the microenvironment in which they are present. This results in considerable functional, morphological, and immunophenotypic overlap.[1-3]

The majority of histiocytes originate from a CD34+ bone marrow progenitor, although some may derive from mesenchymal cells (e.g., FDCs) or even lymphocytes. A simplistic view of subsequent development holds that one of two pathways is followed with maturation into either CD14– or CD14+ cells. The former give rise to Langerhans cells while the latter are the source of dermal dendritic cells or monocyte/macrophages.[4]

The system used to define the various entities in this edition is based on the recent revised classification of histiocytoses and neoplasms of the macrophage-dendritic cell lineage recently proposed by the Histiocyte Society.[5] This classification takes cognisance of histologic, phenotypic, molecular, clinical, and imaging characteristics. It recognized five groups of diseases:

- cutaneous and mucocutaneous (non-Langerhans cell) histiocytoses,
- Rosai-Dorfman disease (RDD),
- malignant histiocytoses,
- hemophagocytic lymphohistiocytosis (HLH) and macrophage activation syndrome.

Historically, LCH has been separated from non-Langerhans cell histiocytoses.[1,6] However, the discovery of shared genetic abnormalities and clinical features between LCH and Erdheim-Chester disease (ECD) has led to both being grouped within the Langerhans cell-related group, together with indeterminate cell histiocytosis. Cutaneous and mucocutaneous histiocytoses encompass the xanthogranuloma family of diseases as well as multicentric reticulohistiocytosis (MRH). Cutaneous RDD is also included in this group, separated from classical sporadic RDD and RDD secondary to predisposing inherited conditions. Malignant histiocytosis includes cases previously diagnosed as histiocytic sarcoma (HS), interdigitating dendritic cell (IDC) sarcoma, Langerhans cell sarcoma (LCS), and indeterminate cell sarcoma. These may arise de novo or secondary to other malignancies. Lastly, there is a category of HLH and macrophage activation syndrome, which may be related to an inherited genetic disorder or secondary to other etiologies. These disorders are detailed in Table 29.5.

Two additional entities not listed in the table are discussed first, these are cutaneous Kikuchi-Fujimoto disease (KFD) and intralymphatic histiocytosis (IH).

Table 29.5
The histiocytoses

Langerhans cell family of histiocytoses
Langerhans cell histiocytosis
Congenital self-healing histiocytosis
Indeterminate dendritic cell tumor
Erdheim-Chester disease
Cutaneous and mucocutaneous histiocytoses (non-Langerhans cell)
Xanthogranuloma family
• Juvenile xanthogranuloma
• Benign cephalic histiocytosis
• Generalized eruptive histiocytosis
• Xanthoma disseminatum
• (scalloped cell granuloma)
• Papular xanthoma
• Progressive nodular histiocytosis
• (spindle cell xanthogranuloma)
(Cutaneous Rosai-Dorfman disease)
Multicentric reticulohistiocytosis
Malignant histiocytoses
Langerhans cell sarcoma
Follicular dendritic cell sarcoma
Interdigitating dendritic cell sarcoma
Histiocytic sarcoma
Hemophagocytic lymphohistiocytosis

Cutaneous Kikuchi-Fujimoto disease

Clinical features

Kikuchi-Fujimoto disease (KFD) (Kikuchi-Fujimoto disease, histiocytic necrotizing lymphadenitis) is a relatively rare self-limited reactive disorder that characteristically presents with cervical lymphadenopathy, systemic symptoms including fever, weight loss, and sweating, and tends to be more common in young females, particularly in the Far East. Children may also be affected. Cutaneous involvement in KFD has been described in up to 40% of patients.[1-14] Specific cutaneous lesions of KFD include macules and papules and more rarely nodules, plaques, pustules, or ulcerated lesions. Subcutaneous lesions are rare.[14] They can occur anywhere in the body with predilection for the face, trunk, and upper limbs. Non-specific cutaneous associations of the disease include leukocytoclastic vasculitis and erythema multiforme.[15-17] An association with lupus erythematosus has also been described.[18-21] However, the histologic features of the lymphadenitis seen in lupus erythematosus are identical to those seen in KFD, and therefore it is likely that the patients reported in the literature had lupus erythematosus from the outset. In a single case, cutaneous disease has been associated with Sjögren syndrome.[22]

Pathogenesis and histologic features

Although a possible relationship with a viral infection including EBV has been suggested, this has not been proven in most cases.[23] Histologic criteria for the diagnosis of KFD have recently been proposed based on a series of cases. The most consistent findings include hydropic degeneration of basal cells, necrotic keratinocytes, and a superficial and deep perivascular and focally interstitial infiltrate composed of lymphocytes and histiocytes with variable amounts of nuclear debris in the absence of neutrophils. A proportion of the histiocytic cells are plasmacytoid monocytes. Some histiocytes have a crescentic nucleus that is pressed against the cytoplasmic membrane.[14] Involvement of the subcutis is seen in up to 60% of cases.[14] Epidermal changes include acanthosis, hyperkeratosis, and parakeratosis, and there is often papillary dermal edema. Other inflammatory cells including plasma cells and eosinophils are rare. Interstitial mucin is sometimes identified. The histiocytes are positive for CD68 and CD163 and may be positive for myeloperoxidase.[24] The plasmacytoid monocytes are positive for CD123. The lymphocytes are T cells, and there seems to be a more prominent number of CD8-positive cells.

Differential diagnosis

The differential diagnosis includes pityriasis lichenoides, lupus erythematosus, and the adverse antibiotic-induced eruptions associated with EBV infection.[14,25] In pityriasis lichenoides, there are necrotic keratinocytes and hydropic degeneration of basal cells. However, the infiltrate is predominantly lymphocytic, and nuclear debris, if present, are very focal. Distinction from lupus erythematosus is extremely difficult, particularly as the lymph node changes may be identical. Distinction is based on clinicopathological correlation, immunofluorescence, and the scarcity of histiocytes and presence of plasma cells in cutaneous lesions of lupus erythematosus. The histologic features of the adverse antibiotic-induced eruptions associated with EBV infection are identical to those seen in KFD, and distinction is based on the clinical information.

Intralymphatic histiocytosis

Clinical features

Intralymphatic histiocytosis (IH) (intravascular lymphangitis, intravascular histiocytosis) is a rare disorder with relatively few cases described in the literature so far.[1-11] It is more common in middle aged to elderly females with predilection for the upper and lower limbs and less commonly the face. Almost half of the cases associated with rheumatoid arthritis present in the vicinity of joints affected by the disease.[2-4,6,11] The appearance varies from ill-defined plaques to a pattern mimicking livedo reticularis. In some patients there is association with another form of chronic inflammation, whilst in others there no apparent associated disease.[11] A role for chronic inflammation is supported by reports of IH arising in postoperative scars following insertion of metallic joint prosthesis and following mastectomy in breast cancer, as well as cases occurring in association with colonic cancer, tonsillitis, and vulval ulceration.[5-10] Response to therapy is poor, and persistence tends to be the rule.

Pathogenesis and histologic features

The pathogenesis of IH is unknown, and the disorder may represent a non-specific reaction pattern associated with various inflammatory conditions. Focal changes identical to those seen in IH can be identified in a number of inflammatory processes and even in association with tumors. Chronic inflammation associated with lymphedema and lymphangiectasia may be the trigger for the intravascular proliferation of histiocytes.[6] Histologically, dilated, irregular thin-walled vascular channels are seen in the reticular dermis and many contain aggregates of cells with a histiocytic appearance including pale cytoplasm and vesicular, reniform nuclei with an inconspicuous nucleolus (*Fig. 29.268*). These cells are positive for histiocytic markers including CD68 and can occasionally be positive for myeloperoxidase.[6] Cytological atypia is not a feature, and there are no mitotic figures. The histiocytes can be associated with lymphocytes and neutrophils, and a perivascular infiltrate composed of lymphocytes and plasma cells is often present. Endothelial cells may be slightly prominent and occasionally display focal proliferation. The lymphatic nature of the vascular channels is confirmed by positivity of the endothelial cells for podoplanin, LYVE-1, and Prox-1.[2,6]

Differential diagnosis

The differential diagnosis includes reactive angioendotheliomatosis and intravascular lymphoma. It has been suggested that reactive angioendotheliomatosis and IH are part of the same spectrum, but this is unlikely.[12,13] The former is a proliferation of endothelial cells that fill pre-existing blood vessels and frequently result in formation of new vascular channels. The proliferation involves blood vessels and not lymphatics as in IH. In intravascular lymphoma, an aggressive disease usually presenting with systemic dissemination, atypical and mitotically active lymphoid cells mostly with a B-cell phenotype fill dilated vascular channels. Morphology and immunohistochemistry should allow easy distinction between the two entities.

A further differential diagnosis is a recently described entity under the name intravascular histiocytosis with hemophagocytosis. Only three cases

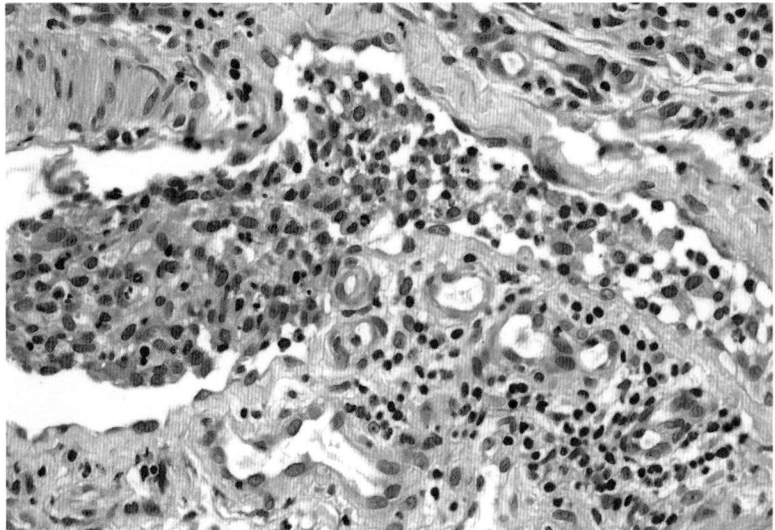

Fig. 29.268
Intralymphatic histiocytosis: innumerable histiocytes are present within the lumen of this dermal vessel.

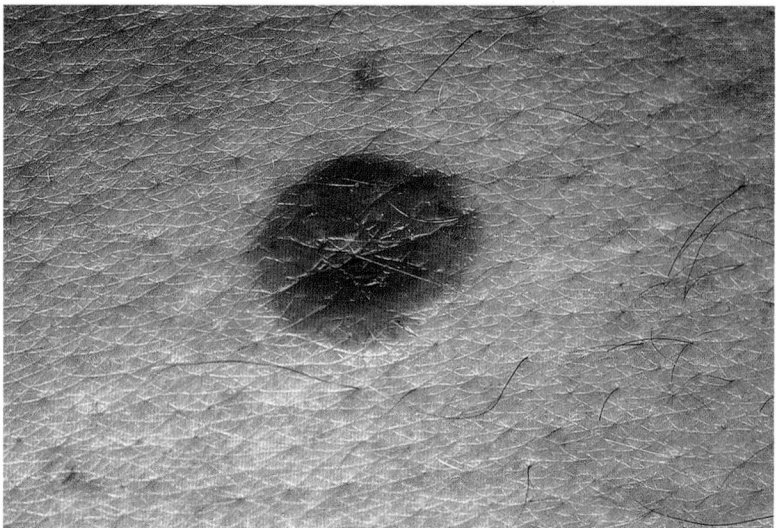

Fig. 29.269
Unifocal LCH (eosinophilic granuloma): this example is a raised erythematous plaque. By courtesy of the Institute of Dermatology, London, UK.

have been reported, and presentation is with a reticulated symmetrical erythema with predilection for the skin of the breasts.[14] The channels involved appear to be blood vessels, not lymphatics, and distinctively there is intravascular hemophagocytosis.

Langerhans (L) group of histiocytosis

The prototypical L group histiocytosis is, of course, LCH. LCH is grouped together with indeterminate cell histiocytosis, with which it shares many morphological and immunophenotypic features, and ECD, which display many similar genetic abnormalities.

Langerhans cell histiocytosis

Clinical features

Langerhans cell histiocytosis (LCH) (histiocytosis X, Langerhans cell granulomatosis) is a neoplastic clonal proliferation of Langerhans cells with variable clinical presentation. LCH can be localized to a single site, involve multiple sites within a single system (usually bone), or present as a disseminated multisystem disease.[1,2] Previously, and prior to the realization that they represented parts of a spectrum of a single disease process, different synonyms were appended to different clinical presentations. These included eosinophilic granuloma (solitary lesions), Hand-Schüller-Christian disease (multiple lesions), and Letterer-Siwe disease (disseminated disease and/or visceral involvement). Congenital self-healing reticulohistiocytosis (Hashimoto-Pritzker disease) is regarded by some as part of the spectrum of Langerhans cell histiocytoses, but is discussed separately.[3-5]

LCH is an extremely rare condition with an estimated incidence in children of 1–5 per million of the population per year.[6-8] Most cases occur in childhood, although the true incidence in adults is unknown. There is a male predilection.[6-9]

Patients with unifocal disease (eosinophilic granuloma) are usually older children or adults. Bone and adjacent soft tissue are the most frequently affected sites, particularly the skull, femur, vertebrae, pelvic bones, and ribs. Less commonly, localized disease occurs in lymph nodes, skin, lung, brain, or oral mucous membranes (*Fig. 29.269*).[7,10] Bone lesions are usually lytic with cortical erosions, while at other sites unifocal LCH presents as mass lesions or lymphadenopathy. Cutaneous lesions are deep dermal and/or subcutaneous nodules.[8,11,12]

Patients with unisystem, multifocal LCH (most examples of Hand-Schüller-Christian disease) are usually children in the first 5 years of life, but the age range is wide (*Figs 29.270* and *29.271*).[13-17] Bone and adjacent

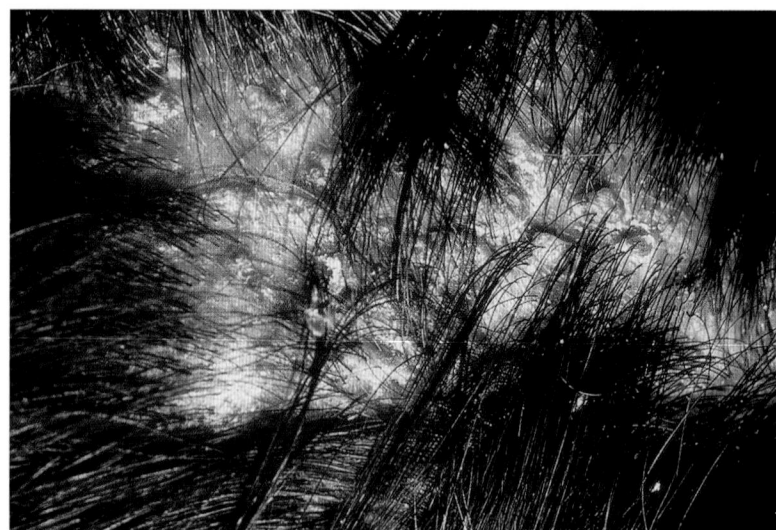

Fig. 29.270
Multifocal chronic LCH: scalp involvement with scale crust and hair loss. By courtesy of the Institute of Dermatology, London, UK.

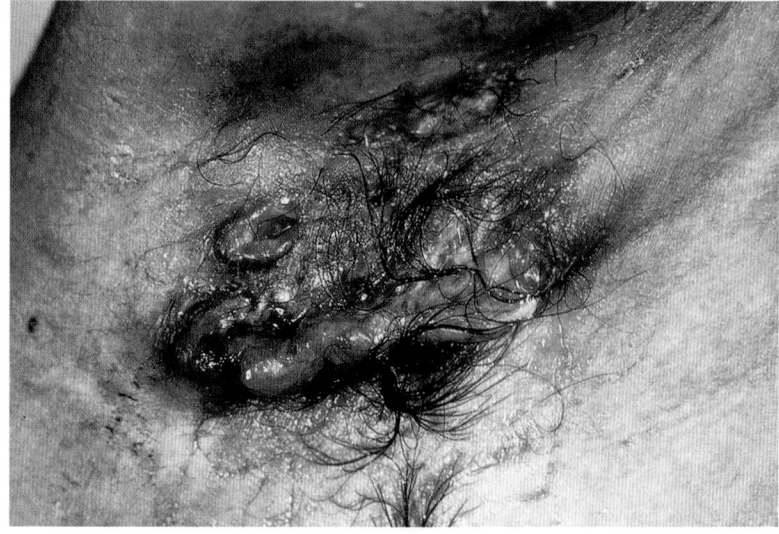

Fig. 29.271
Multifocal chronic LCH: note the vegetative lesions in the axilla. By courtesy of the Institute of Dermatology, London, UK.

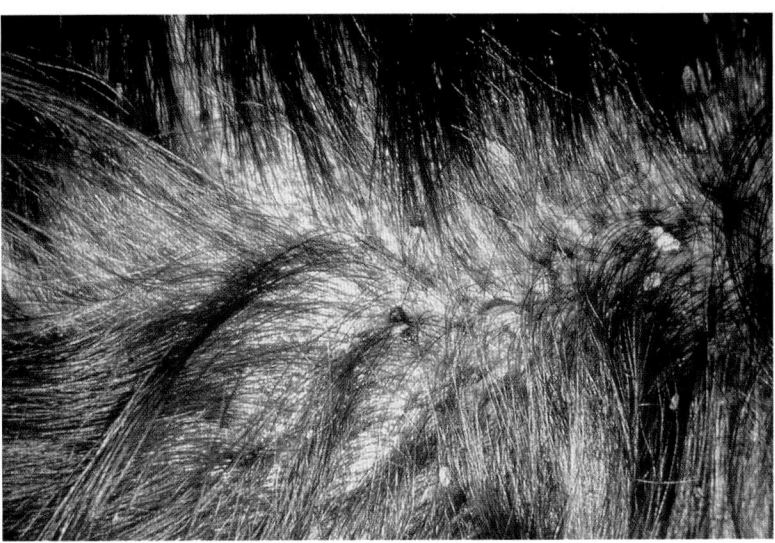

Fig. 29.272
Acute generalized LCH: this scalp shows a characteristic erythematous and scaly eruption. By courtesy of D. Burrows, MD, Royal Victoria Hospital, Belfast, UK.

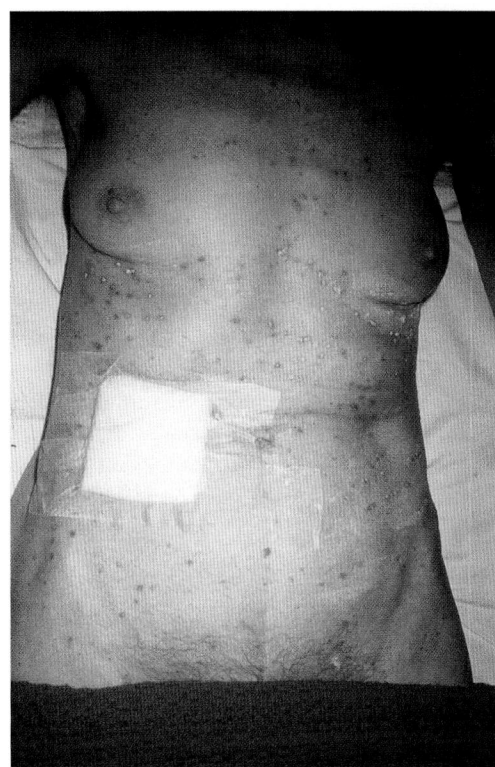

Fig. 29.274
Acute generalized LCH: there are scattered scaly papules over the thorax and abdomen. By courtesy of B. Monk, MD, Kings College Hospital, London, UK.

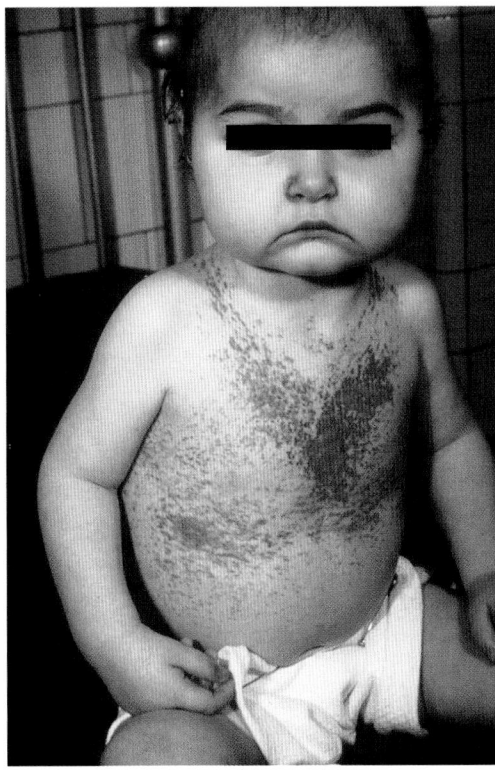

Fig. 29.273
Acute generalized LCH: erythematous eruption showing a characteristic seborrheic distribution. By courtesy of D. Burrows, MD, Royal Victoria Hospital, Belfast, UK.

soft tissue are most frequently involved, with patients presenting with multiple or sequential destructive bone lesions. The skull and mandible are characteristic sites, and secondary effects may produce the classic triad of osteolytic skull lesions, hypopituitarism-induced diabetes insipidus, and exophthalmos.[8,18] Chronic otitis externa is frequent due to involvement of the mastoid or petrous temporal bones.

Multisystem LCH (Letterer-Siwe disease and more extensive presentations of Hand-Schüller-Christian disease) usually presents in infants, and may be present at birth or develop in the neonatal period, although some of these cases may represent examples of congenital self-healing histiocytosis (CSH) (Figs 29.272 and 29.273).[7,8,13,19–22] Exceptionally, adults are affected (Fig. 29.274).[23–26] There is predilection for skin, bone, liver, spleen, bone

marrow, lymph nodes, and lung.[7,24] Cutaneous lesions are tiny widespread erythematous, or brownish-red, papules and patches with predilection for the scalp, chest, back, groins, and axillae.[27] Perineal and mucosal lesions are common. The rash is often described as eczematoid or seborrheic, although this refers more to distribution than morphology.[28] Less commonly, lesions are petichial, purpuric, vesicular, pustular, erosive, or even nodular.[8,24,28] In lesions with follicular prominence, the appearances may mimic Darier disease.[23,25] Symptoms include fever, weight loss, lymphadenopathy, hepatosplenomegaly, and pancytopenia.[8] Radiological studies frequently disclose bone involvement (radiolucent defects), particularly in the skull, ribs, and femur, and miliary or nodular infiltrates in the lungs where, less often, multiple cysts may be found. A hemophagocytic syndrome is a rarely seen in multifocal disease.[29] An increased incidence of associated malignancies including acute lymphoblastic leukemia, acute nonlymphoblastic leukemia, HL and NHL, retinoblastoma, medulloblastoma, osteosarcoma, and basal cell carcinoma has been noted, although some of these may be treatment related.[30–33]

Age is probably not as important as disease extent in determining the prognosis. Patients with unifocal LCH at presentation have a ≥99% survival.[1,2,13,14,34] Approximately 10% of patients with multifocal disease die from their illness, while 60% run a chronic course and only 30% achieve complete remission.[35,36] Involvement of bone marrow, liver, and lung are reported to be particularly high-risk factors.[1,2] Large therapeutic trial suggest that the initial response to chemotherapy is the best predictor of outcome.[37–41] Responders have an overall survival of 88–91% compared with 17–34% for nonresponders.[37–41] More recently, encouraging results have been obtained using BRAF inhibitors such as vemurafenib.[42] Occasionally, patients with unifocal disease subsequently develop multisystem involvement, and even those showing a good response to treatment may suffer from long-term sequelae, including hypothalamic–pituitary dysfunction, cognitive dysfunction, and cerebellar symptoms.[1,2,43,44] All patients therefore require long-term follow-up.

The precise nature of large clusters or sheets of Langerhans cells, seen occasionally in association with some neoplasms or tumorlike conditions, remains to be fully determined, and this includes most cases of isolated LCH of the lung in adults that seems to represent a polyclonal proliferation associated with cigarette smoking.[45–48] In some instances, proliferations of LCH may represent a transdifferentiation process. For example, cases of LCH associated with T-lymphoblastic leukemia have been shown to share the same clonal T-cell receptor gene rearrangement, indicative of origin from the same tumor stem cell.[49] However, in other instances, LCH-like proliferation associated with various lymphoproliferative disorders appear to represent a localized reactive phenomenon.[50]

Pathogenesis and histologic features

Langerhans cell histiocytosis appears to represent a unique combination of oncogenesis and immune dysregulation.[51] Investigations using X-chromosome linked DNA probes or human androgen receptor inactivation (HUMARA) assays have shown the lesional cells to be clonal.[44,46,50,52] They also display a less mature phenotype than normal activated Langerhans cells, and show overexpression of various cell cycle related products such as TGF-β receptors I and II, MDM2, p53, p21, p16, Rb, and bcl-2.[53–57] The heterogeneous pattern of expression of these factors suggests a degree of regulation, and may explain the slow growth and variable outcome of LCH lesions.[53]

The local microenvironment also appears to play a role in pathogenesis and the resultant sequelae, such as fever, fibrosis, bone resorption, and necrosis.[58,59] Serum cytokine levels, including IL-17A, fms-like tyrosine kinase ligand (FLT3-L), macrophage colony stimulating factor (M-CSF), and vascular endothelial growth factor (VEGF), are elevated in patients with LCH and, in some instances, correlate with extent and severity of disease.[60–62] Similarly, high levels of various cytokines have been demonstrated in Langerhans cells, T cells, macrophages, and eosinophils in lesions of LCH including interleukins 1α, 2, 4, 5, 7, 10, and 11, TNF-α, IFN-γ, GM-CSF, and leukemia inhibitory factor (LIF).[63] Expression of TNF, IL-11, and LIF has also been shown to correlate with disease severity.[63,64]

Recurrent *BRAF pV600E* mutations are present in around 50% of LCH, whilst *MAP2K1* mutations are found in a further 19%.[65–72] These mutations result in constitutive activation of the *MAPK* signaling pathway, as do less commonly found mutations in other *MPAK* pathway genes such as *ARAF* and *MAP3KI*.[72,73] Mutations affecting other signaling pathways, including *PIK3CA*, *PICK1*, and *PICK3R2* have also been implicated.[70,74]

Tumor cells have a rather uniform appearance. They are oval in shape and possess moderately abundant, lightly eosinophilic cytoplasm, and large infolded or reniform vesicular nuclei with thin nuclear membranes and inconspicuous nucleoli. Nuclei often have longitudinal nuclear grooves (coffee bean shape) (*Figs 29.275–29.277*). Mitotic figures are variable (*Fig. 29.278*). Neoplastic cells are admixed with variable numbers of eosinophils and, in some cases, with histiocytes (including foam cells and multinucleate forms), neutrophils (often sparse), small lymphocytes, and plasma cells

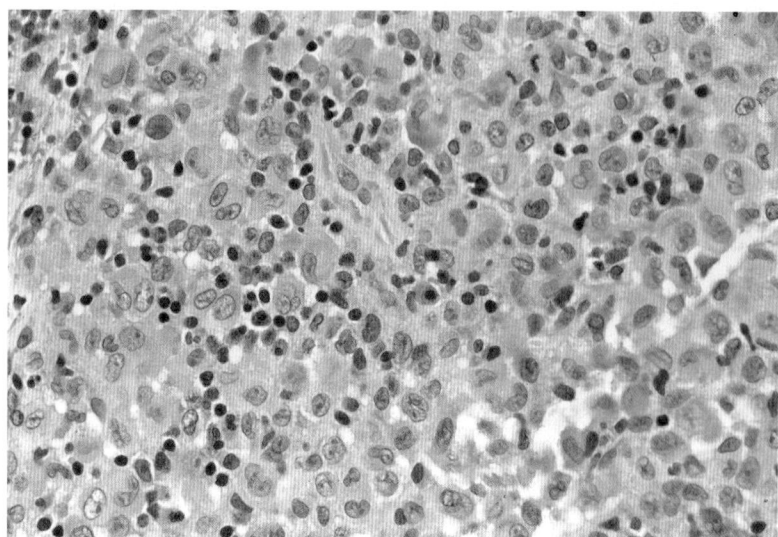

Fig. 29.276
Acute generalized LCH: the infiltrate consists of histiocytes with abundant eosinophilic cytoplasm. Note the lymphocytes and eosinophils.

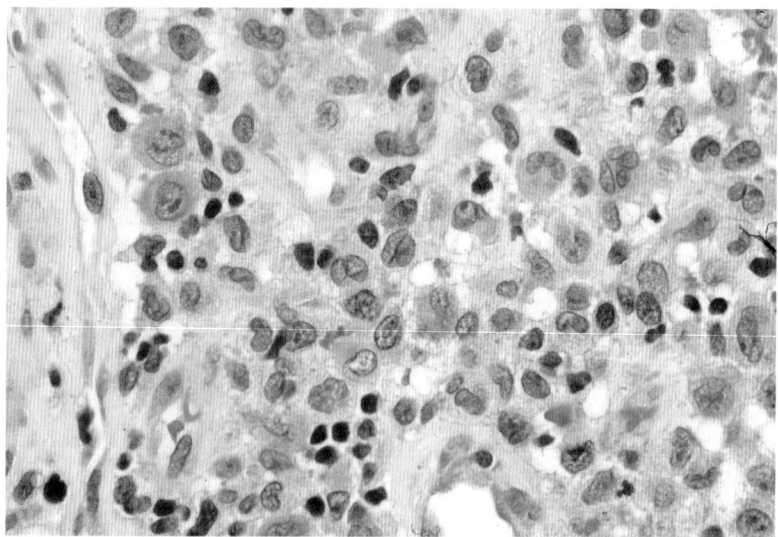

Fig. 29.277
Acute generalized LCH: this field shows typical coffee bean, vesicular nuclei; a nucleus with a longitudinal groove is present in the center of the field.

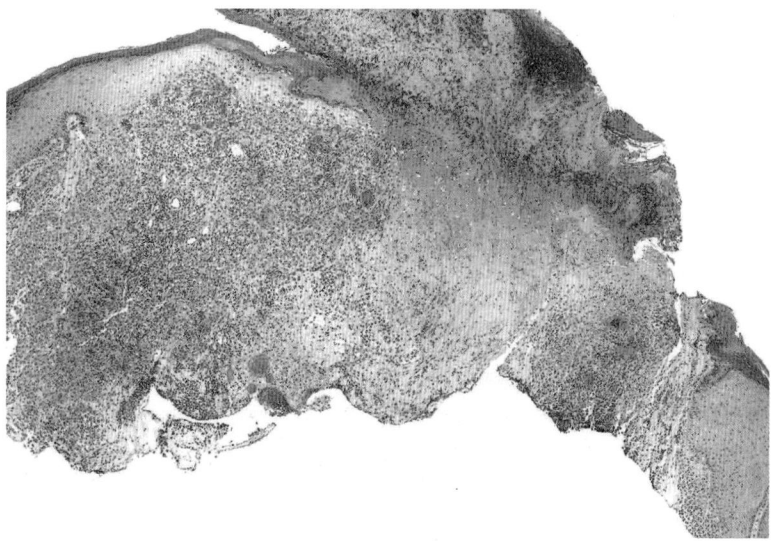

Fig. 29.275
Acute generalized LCH: scanning view of an ulcerated and crusted lesion showing a dense dermal infiltrate.

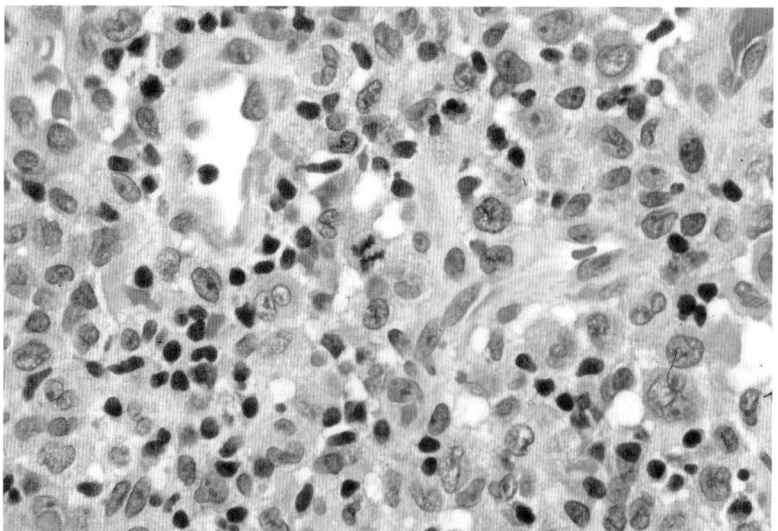

Fig. 29.278
Acute generalized LCH: note the mitotic figure.

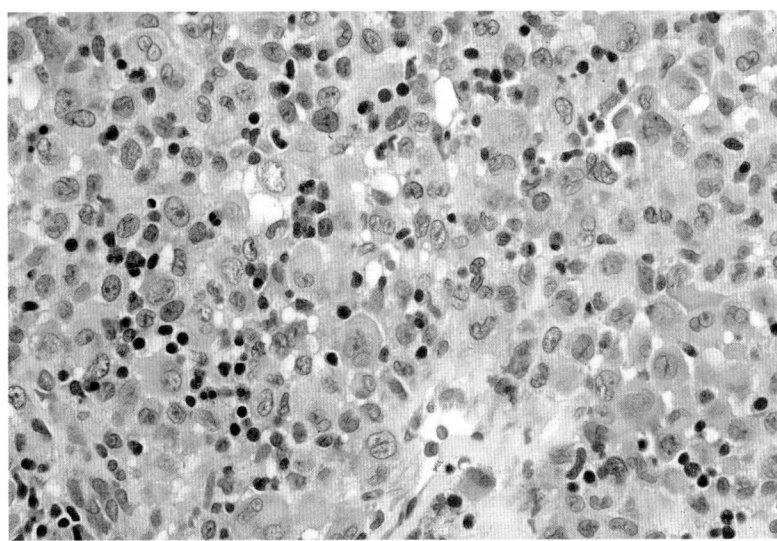

Fig. 29.279
Acute generalized LCH: the conspicuous eosinophils seen here are a variable finding.

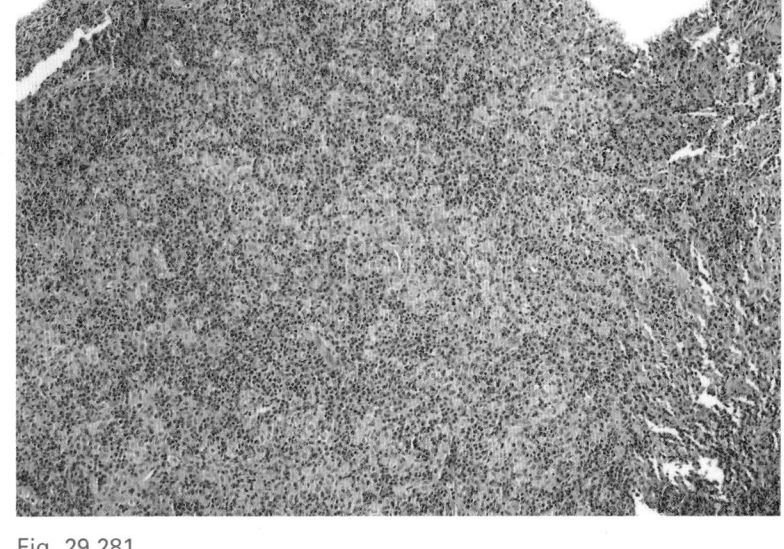

Fig. 29.281
Unifocal LCH (eosinophilic granuloma): low-power view of an oral lesion.

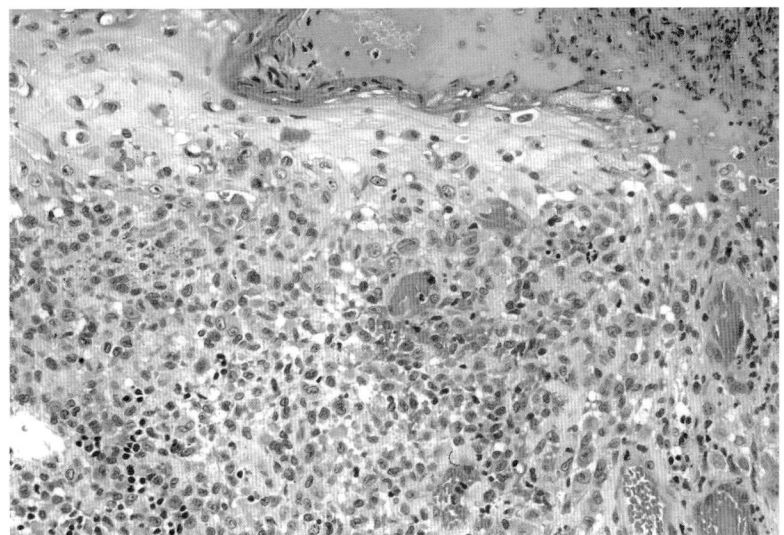

Fig. 29.280
Acute generalized LCH: high-power view showing infiltration of the overlying epidermis, a common feature.

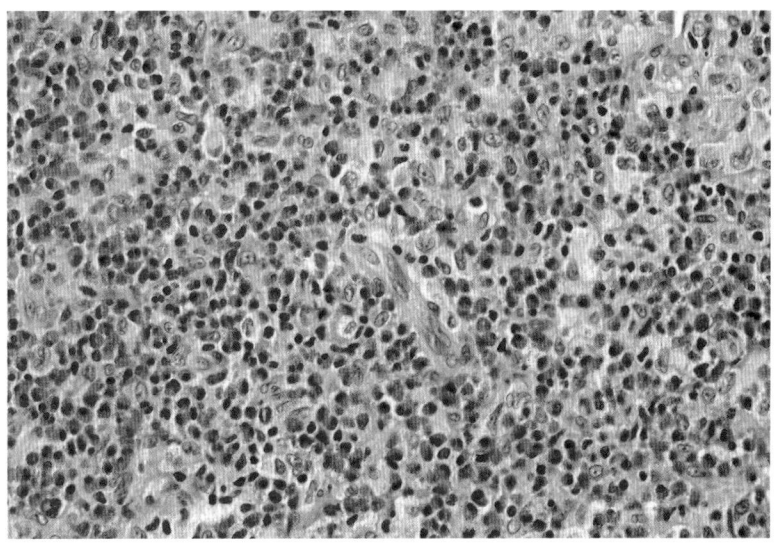

Fig. 29.282
Unifocal LCH (eosinophilic granuloma): note the numerous eosinophils.

(*Fig. 29.279*). Eosinophils are numerous in some lesions and may form abscesses with central necrosis rich in Charcot-Leyden crystals. In early lesions, Langerhans cells predominate along with eosinophils and neutrophils, but in later lesions there are increased foamy histiocytes and fibrosis.[7]

In fully developed cutaneous papules and plaques, the infiltrate is usually dense and bandlike, and may obscure the dermal–epidermal junction. Extravasated red blood cells and epidermotropism with formation of intraepidermal Langerhans cell microabscesses are frequent (*Fig. 29.280*).[8] In some cases, the infiltrate shows a periadnexal, particularly follicular, distribution.[25]

Lymph node involvement varies from sinusoidal lesions through to partial or complete architectural destruction by tumor cells.[7] Exceptionally, a sarcoid-like granulomatous infiltrate has been described.[75] In the liver, the infiltrate most often affects the portal tracts and may be associated with bile duct proliferation; a diffuse infiltrate is typically found in the spleen. Bone lesions show a widespread infiltrate, often coupled with fibrosis. Lung lesions comprise a diffuse infiltrate, involving alveoli and alveolar walls, and peribronchial and subpleural deposits. Fibrosis and cysts are common.

The histologic features of focal chronic lesions (eosinophilic granuloma) are similar to those seen in multifocal LCH except that the eosinophils are perhaps present in greater numbers (*Figs 29.281–29.283*).

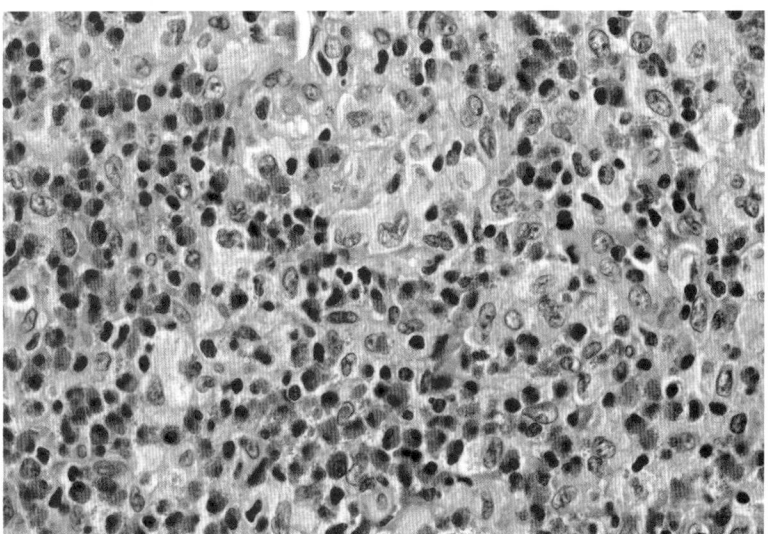

Fig. 29.283
Unifocal LCH (eosinophilic granuloma): high-power view showing typical Langerhans cells.

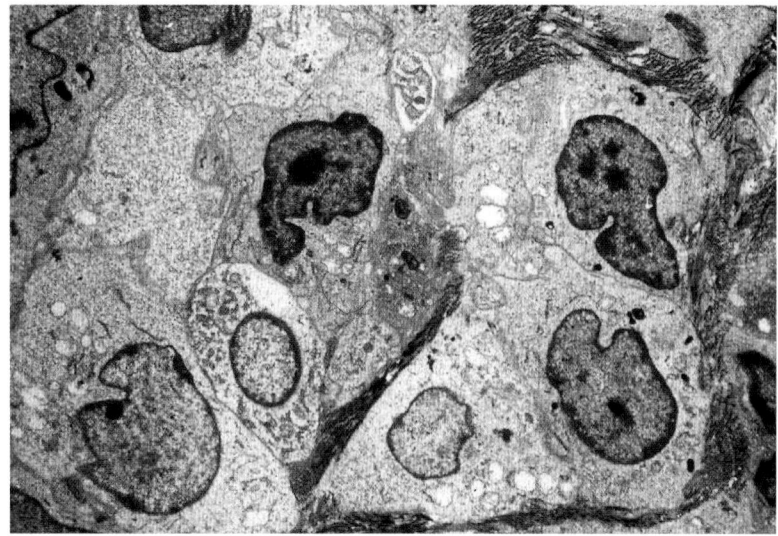

Fig. 29.284
Acute generalized LCH: the infiltrate is composed almost entirely of Langerhans cells. Note the horseshoe-shaped nuclei and abundant cytoplasm.

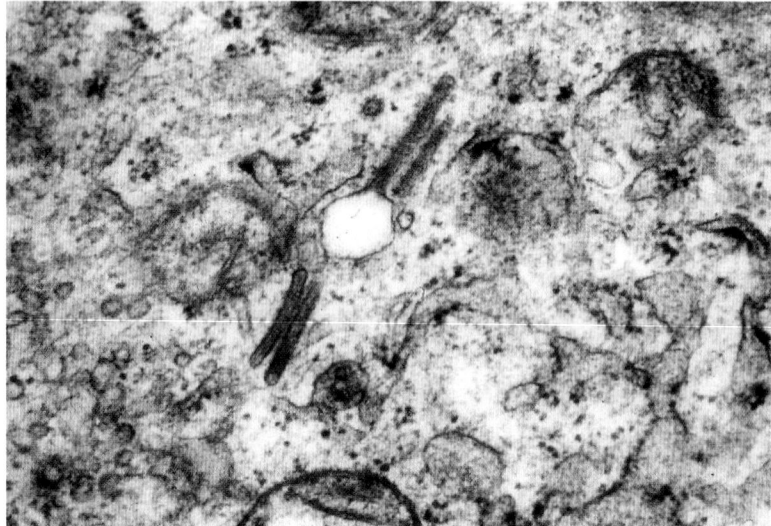

Fig. 29.285
Acute generalized LCH: numerous Birbeck granules are present.

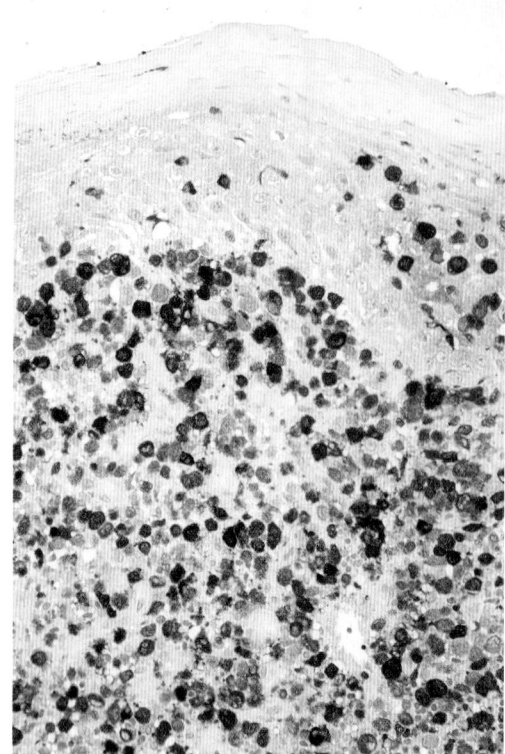

Fig. 29.286
Acute generalized LCH: the Langerhans cells show uniform expression of S100 protein.

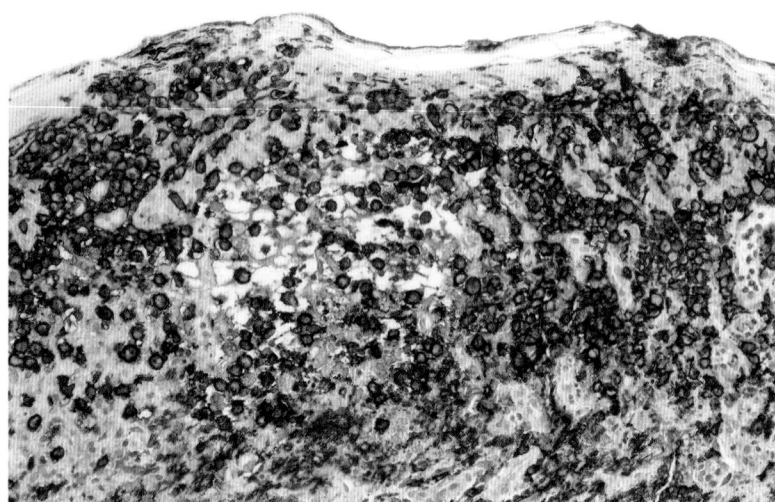

Fig. 29.287
Acute generalized LCH: CD1a is also strongly positive.

The hallmark of Langerhans cells is the presence of Birbeck granules, which form in the endosomal recycling area of the cell.[76] They are tennis racquet- or rod-shaped organelles measuring 200–400 nm (length) by 33 nm (width), with a zipper-like appearance along the 'handle' when viewed by electron microscopy (*Figs 29.284* and *29.285*). Although specific for Langerhans cells, immunohistochemistry has superseded electron microscopy in confirming the diagnosis of LCH.[9]

Langerin (CD207) is an antibody to a transmembrane C-type lectin that associates with Birbeck granules, and it is the most sensitive and specific marker for Langerhans cells.[53,77,78] Langerhans cells also typically express CD1a, CD4, and S100, and are also positive for vimentin, CD68, and HLA-DR (*Figs 29.286* and *29.287*).[7-9,79] Staining for other B- and T-cell markers, FDC markers (CD21, CD35), and CD30 is negative. The Ki-67 index is highly variable.[9]

Differential diagnosis

Langerhans cell histiocytosis must be distinguished from other histiocytic and dendritic cell neoplasms, including HS and tumors of follicular and IDCs, as well as deposits of acute leukemia. Most cases can be resolved by immunohistochemistry, particularly when antibodies to langerin are available.[9,53,59] LCS is differentiated on the basis of overt cytological atypia,

its generally very high mitotic index, and less prominent inflammatory background.[7]

Langerhans cell sarcoma

Clinical features

Langerhans cell sarcoma (LCS) (malignant histiocytosis X, malignant Langerhans cell tumor) is a very rare high-grade neoplasm with overtly malignant features.[1-4] Almost all reported cases are in adults, with a median age of 39 years (range, 10–72 years) and female predilection.[1-4] Skin and underlying soft tissue are most commonly involved. However, LCS is often high stage at presentation (44% stage III/IV), and there is frequent multiorgan involvement with spread to lymph nodes, lungs, liver, spleen, and bone.[1,3-8] Skin lesions may manifest as generalized papules and nodules at presentation, but more often acral sites (particularly the leg) are affected by a single tumor nodule. Twenty-two percent of cases are primarily nodal, and hepatosplenomegaly and pancytopenia may be seen in 22% and 11% of cases, respectively.[1] A leukemic phase has also been described in two cases, although the phenotype of the circulating cells in the most recent report was not that of Langerhans cells.[9,10] Prognosis is poor with >50% mortality, although occasional cases have a more favorable prognosis.[1,11]

Pathogenesis and histologic features

The pathogenesis of LCS is largely unknown. Cases may arise de novo but have also been described in patients with Langerhans cell histiocytosis as well as in association with other hematological malignancies, including B-lymphoblastic leukemia, follicular lymphoma, CLL, and hairy cell leukemia.[12–17] A clonal relationship has been demonstrated in such situations and BRAF mutation has also been identified in a sporadic case.[13,15,16,18]

Tumor cells are malignant with pleomorphic nuclei containing clumped chromatin and prominent nucleoli.[1,7,11] There is often little to suggest a Langerhans cell origin, although some cells may possess complex nuclear grooves similar to those seen in LCH cells. Mitotic figures are numerous (>50 per 10 HPFs).[4] Scattered eosinophils and occasional small lymphocytes may be present.[1,8,19]

Ultrastructural or phenotypic evidence of Langerhans cell differentiation must be confirmed. Electron microscopy may reveal Birbeck granules and the immunophenotype is usually identical to that seen in Langerhans cell histiocytosis, although staining for individual markers may be focal and patchy.[1,4] Immunoglobulin and T-cell receptor genes are Germline except in cases related to other lymphomas.[13,15,16,20]

Differential diagnosis

LCS must be differentiated from other sarcomas involving the skin, and this is usually achieved by immunohistochemistry. Cases are separated from LCH on the basis of their malignant cytological features and aggressive clinical course.

Congenital self-healing histiocytosis

Clinical features

Congenital self-healing histiocytosis (CSH) (congenital self-healing reticulohistiocytosis, Hashimoto-Pritzker disease) is a rare condition and is classified as a congenital self-healing variant of LCH.[1–9] The sexes are affected equally.

Lesions are present at birth or develop in the perinatal period. They usually consist of widespread erythematous, blue or brown, 2–15 mm diameter macules, papules, and nodules, with sparing of mucous membranes. A solitary red–brown asymptomatic nodule is seen in 30% of cases.[10–15] Central ulceration with necrosis and crusting is often present. Vesicular or bullous lesions can also occur.[16–20] Healing of the latter may leave anetoderma-like scarring.[16] There is predilection for scalp, face, trunk, and proximal extremities, and the palms and soles are sometimes involved.[1] A single retinal lesion has been described.[21] Very rarely, extracutaneous manifestations including hepatomegaly and mild hematological abnormalities including lymphocytosis occur.[5,16] In contrast to LCH, the lesions invariably regress, usually 3–4 months, leaving hypo- or hyperpigmented macules or patches.[8] Recurrences are not usually a feature, but patients with CSH require continued observation as there are a small number of patients who go on to develop LCH-like features with recurrent lesions, bone involvement, and diabetes insipidus.[22,23] Patients with vesiculobullous lesions may be at particular risk.[21]

Histologic features

There is an upper dermal infiltrate of epidermotropic large histiocytes with eosinophilic cytoplasm and notched or reniform vesicular nuclei.[8,14,24] Neutrophils, eosinophils, lymphocytes, and xanthoma cells are also often present. CSH is histologically indistinguishable from LCH, although it has been reported that a high content of eosinophils, necrosis, and ulceration are more frequently encountered in the former.[8] Occasionally, cells with glassy,

eosinophilic cytoplasm reminiscent of the 'ground glass' cells of RH are evident.[5] In contrast to LCH, abundant reticulin fibers are present in CSH, surrounding either individual cells or groups of cells, and PAS-positive cytoplasmic inclusions are frequently seen.[5,16,25] The latter may include punctate and ring forms representing glycogen or diffuse cytoplasmic staining indicating the presence of neutral glycosaminoglycans.[5]

Immunohistochemically, the infiltrate is indistinguishable from LCH, and tumor cells are positive for S100 protein, CD1a, CD4, and HLA-DR.[1]

Ultrastructurally, in addition to Birbeck granules (present in 10–25% of cells), tumor cells contain myelin-like dense bodies and, less often, phagolysosomes filled with laminated membranous debris and paracrystalline material.[1,2,5,6] The latter do not appear to have been described in LCH.

Differential diagnosis

In view of the histologic and immunohistochemical similarities, distinction of CSH from multisystem LCH depends on the absence of severe systemic involvement and regression of lesions in the former condition.

Indeterminate dendritic cell tumor

Clinical features

Indeterminate dendritic cell tumor (IDCT) (indeterminate cell histiocytosis) is very rare and composed of so-called indeterminate cells, an alleged cutaneous dendritic cell subset displaying histologic and some ultrastructural and immunophenotypic features of Langerhans cells, but lacking Birbeck granules. Most cases occur in adults, but examples in children and exceptional congenital lesions have been reported.[1–6] No sex predilection is seen.

Lesions may be solitary or multiple with wide anatomic distribution. Solitary lesions usually present as soft red nodules measuring up to 1 cm in diameter, and may be ulcerated.[2,6–8] Multiple lesions are usually red–brown papulonodules ranging from a few millimeters to 1 cm in diameter and tend to appear in successive crops.[1,2,7–15] Disease is almost always localized to the skin with no systemic symptoms. Rare cases with visceral involvement and a solitary ocular example have been described.[3–6,16] The prognosis is generally good. Most cases undergo complete or partial regression without recurrences, a more aggressive course being rare.[3,7]

Pathogenesis and histologic features

The origin of indeterminate cells is still debated. It has been proposed that they are immature Langerhans precursor cells that have yet to acquire Birbeck granules, or that they are derived from Langerhans cells and have lost Birbeck granules as they migrate toward lymph nodes or that they belong to an independent group of epidermal/dendritic cells.[8,9,13,17] Rare cases are association with leukemia or lymphoma, raising the possibility of a common precursor or so-called 'transdifferentiation' in some instances.[7,13,18,19]

Histologically, IDCT is characterized by a dermal infiltrate that may extend into the subcutis, composed of cells that resemble Langerhans cells (Figs 29.288–29.290).[4,5] Epidermal involvement is absent.[11,12] The constituent cells are usually ovoid or rarely have a more spindle cell morphology.[4,5] They possess abundant eosinophilic cytoplasm and oval-to-indented nuclei; nuclear grooves are sometimes seen.[4,5,12] Multinucleate giant cells may also be present, as may clusters of lymphocytes, but eosinophils are usually absent.[4,5]

Some reports of IDCT describe a predominance of histiocytes with a scalloped or vacuolated appearance and cases with Touton-type giant cells, xanthomatized cells, neutrophils, eosinophils, and plasma cells.[1,2,9,10,12,13,19] However, it is possible that this broader morphological spectrum results from inclusion of variants of other forms of non-Langerhans cell histiocytosis, particularly xanthogranuloma, in which there is aberrant S100 protein or CD1a expression.[20]

The neoplastic cells in IDCT are consistently S100 and CD1a positive but are negative for langerin (Figs 29.291–293).[17,19] They lack B- and T-cell markers and are negative for CD30 and FDC markers (CD21, CD23, CD35). Positivity for CD4, CD45, CD68, CD163, factor XIIIA, lysozyme, and HLA-DR is variable, as is the Ki-67 index.[3–6,9,13,15,19] One case was clonal with the HUMARA assay.[4]

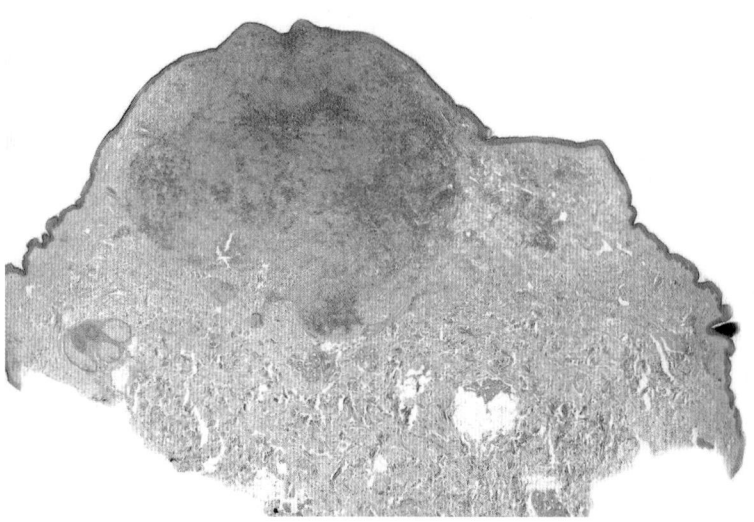

Fig. 29.288
Indeterminate dendritic cell tumor: scanning view of circumscribed dermal tumor nodule.

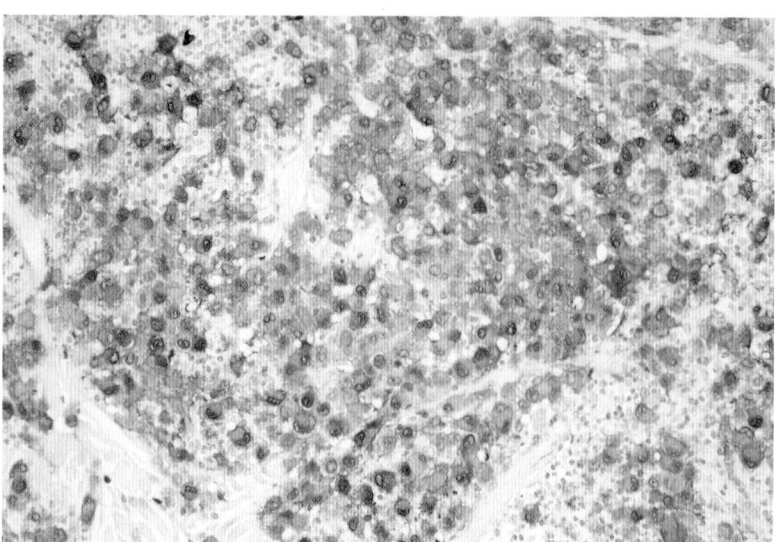

Fig. 29.291
Indeterminate dendritic cell tumor: the tumor cells are S100 positive.

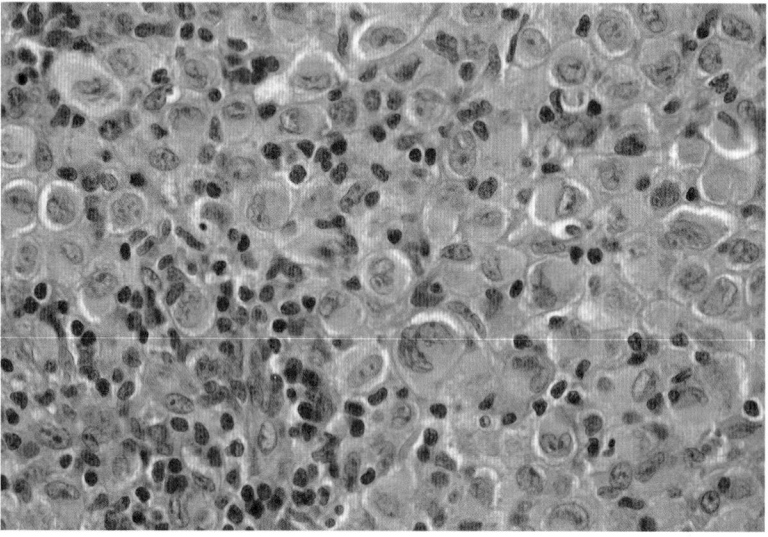

Fig. 29.289
Indeterminate dendritic cell tumor: the appearances are identical to those of Langerhans cell histiocytosis.

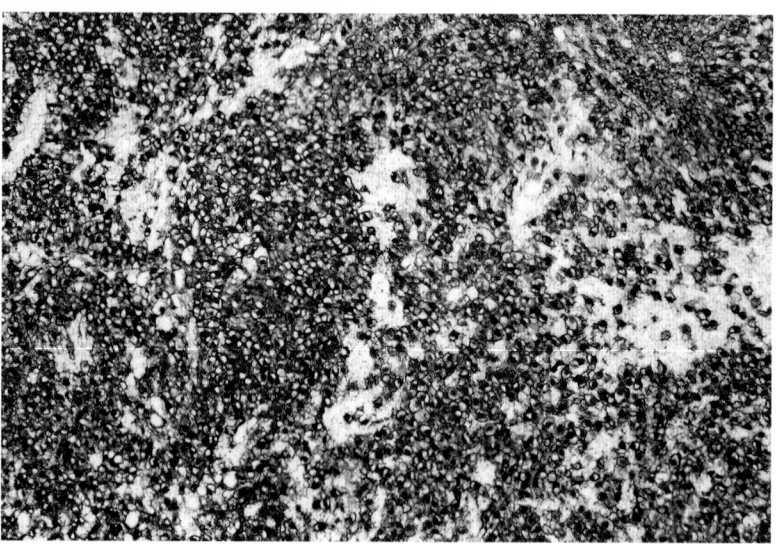

Fig. 29.292
Indeterminate dendritic cell tumor: there is strong expression of CD1a.

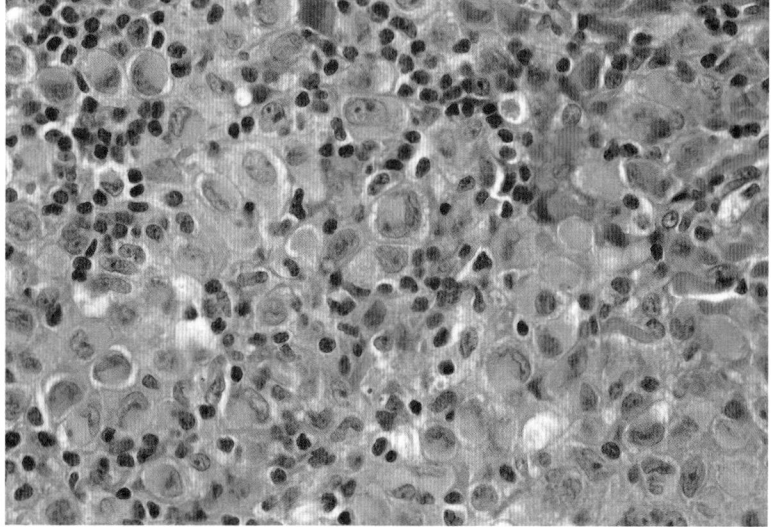

Fig. 29.290
Indeterminate dendritic cell tumor: note the presence of reniform nuclei and delicate nuclear grooves.

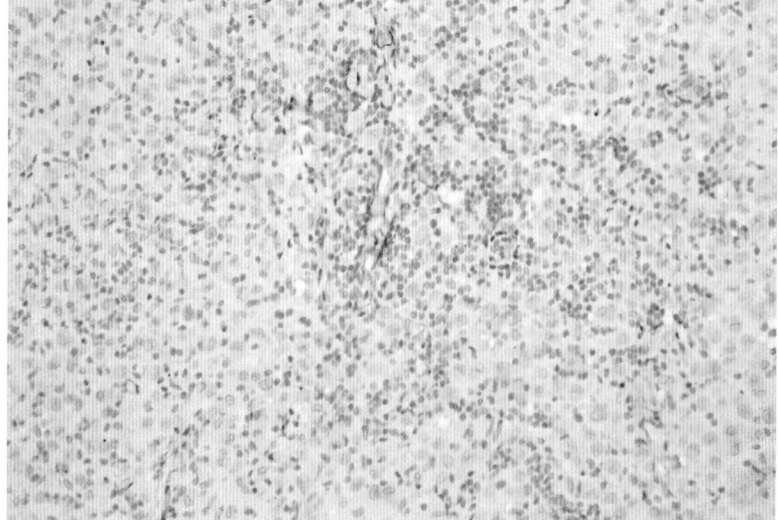

Fig. 29.293
Indeterminate dendritic cell tumor: langerin is negative.

By definition, no Birbeck granules are seen on electron microscopy, although there is abundant cytoplasm containing lysosomes, phagosomes, and well-developed endoplasmic reticulum.[2,7,14]

Differential diagnosis

IDCT must be distinguished from LCH. Points of distinction include lack of epidermotropism and absence of Birbeck granules. However, electron microscopy may not be available and distinction is not always possible. Differential expression of langerin (CD207) is therefore a useful surrogate for separating these entities.[17,19] Uniform expression of CD1a and S100 protein usually allows distinction of IDCT from other forms of non-Langerhans cell histiocytosis.

Erdheim-Chester disease

Clinical features

Erdheim-Chester disease (ECD) is a rare, but increasingly recognized, histiocytosis. Until recently, ECD was considered a non-Langerhans cell histiocytosis and classified as a subset of xanthogranulomatosis, but in the light of more recent molecular findings is now thought to be better grouped along with Langerhans cell histiocytosis.[1,2] Most cases are diagnosed between the ages of 40 and 70 years, and there is possibly a male predominance.[3,4] The diagnosis is made by identifying characteristic histologic and radiological findings in the appropriate clinical context. Bone scan or PET scan typically demonstrate symmetrical diaphyseal and metaphyseal osteosclerosis in the legs, particularly the distal ends of the femur and proximal tibia.[5]

Infiltration of nearly every organ system has been reported in ECD, but the most commonly affected tissues are bone, large vessels, heart, retroperitoneum, orbit, lung, CNS, and endocrine system.[4-11]

Skin is involved in 20-32% of cases.[4,12,13] The most frequent manifestation is the presence of xanthelasma, usually in the form of yellowish plaques in the periorbital area.[3,14-17] These may also occur on the trunk, extremities, scalp, and face.[18-22] Lesions may also appear as erythematous to brown patches and plaques on the leg, back and trunk.[3]

ECD has a varied clinical course. Some patients have few symptoms and an indolent course, whilst others have progressive, potentially lethal disease. CNS involvement is a poor prognostic sign.[2,5] There is no recognized treatment, although recent reports suggest that BRAF inhibitors may be very effective in patents harboring the appropriate mutation.[23]

Pathogenesis and histologic features

BRAF mutations are found in around 55% of cases, indicating that this is a truly neoplastic disease.[24,25] ECD histiocytes also express a characteristic proinflammatory cytokines and chemokines which are also present in the serum of affected patients, suggesting that the inflammatory milieu plays an important role in the pathogenesis of the clinical manifestations.[26,27]

Biopsy of lesional tissue reveals numerous lipid-laden foamy histiocytes in a variably fibrotic background. Multinucleate and Touton-type giant cells may also be present.[3] In the skin, this process tends to extend into the deeper reticular dermis, unlike classic xanthelasma, and fibrosis may be less marked.[3] The histiocytes express CD68, CD163, and, variably, FXIIIA, but are negative for CD1a, S100 and langerin.[3,5] In a proportion of cases, there may also be a component of Langerhans cell histiocytosis in the lesional tissue.[3,28]

Differential diagnosis

The pathological features are indistinguishable from those of juvenile xanthogranuloma (JXG)/xanthogranulomatous histiocytosis. Accurate diagnosis is therefore dependent on careful clinical pathological correlation and adherence to consensus guidelines, although demonstration of a BRAF mutation may also be helpful.[2] The histiocytes in ECD are morphologically and phenotypically different from those seen in Langerhans cell histiocytosis, the latter expression CD1a, S100 and langerin.

CUTANEOUS AND MUCOCUTANEOUS HISTIOCYTOSES

This group of histiocytoses are non-Langerhans cell histiocytoses that are localized to skin and/or mucosa, some of which may be associated with systemic involvement. It includes a wide variety of entities, most of which belong to the xanthogranuloma family. The revised classification of histiocytoses proposed by the Histiocyte Society also includes cutaneous RDD and MRH within this category.

Xanthogranuloma family

The JXG family of disorders is rare, but constitutes the most frequently encountered types of non-Langerhans cell histiocytosis. Common to all subtypes is a proliferation of histiocytes and Touton-type giant cells, with a characteristic phenotype, displaying features of both macrophage and dendritic cell differentiation. Thus, the histologic appearances of all subtypes of 'xanthogranuloma' are similar and, for practical purposes, indistinguishable. Nevertheless, they have a broad clinical spectrum of disease, with many parallels to that seen in LCH. Manifestations include patients with solitary or multiple skin lesions, presentation with large deeply situated masses, and widespread disease with systemic involvement. As in LCH, the majority of cases with disseminated and/or systemic disease occur in children, most within the first 10 years of life, and half before the age of 1 year. Solitary lesions may be seen at any age. Although biologically a benign disorder, a variety of clinical outcomes may be experienced. There is a high tendency for cutaneous lesions to undergo spontaneous resolution, but systemic lesions may persist for long periods of time and cause significant, site related, morbidity. Progression of disease is encountered in some rare instances.

Historically, patients suffering from disorders of this type have been grouped together on the basis of constellations of shared clinical features.

JXG constitutes the largest group. Most patients are children with solitary or multiple skin lesions, soft tissue or visceral tumors with rare mucous membrane involvement and systemic disease. Patients presenting with generalized disease are subdivided on the basis of age and distribution of lesions, into benign cephalic histiocytosis (children, localized to skin), generalized eruptive histiocytoma (young adults, localized to skin) and xanthoma disseminatum (XD) or ECD (adults with systemic disease). XD almost always has a cutaneous component. 'Xanthogranulomatous' disorders in middle-aged adults and the elderly usually manifest as progressive nodular histiocytosis. Other, even less frequently encountered, less well-defined, and rather more spurious entities are also best included within this family of diseases. These include solitary spindle cell xanthogranuloma, scalloped cell xanthogranuloma, and papular xanthoma (PX).

These putative entities show considerable clinical overlap and, in view of their relatively uniform pathological features, are probably best regarded as different manifestations of the same disease process. Nevertheless, the clinical details of each will be outlined separately below, in order that the reader can relate to the pleitropic nomenclature and somewhat confused literature that surrounds these disorders.

Juvenile xanthogranuloma

Juvenile xanthogranuloma (JXG) (xanthogranuloma, nevoxanthoendothelioma, xanthoma multiplex) arises in the first 5 years of life, usually in the first year, and may be present at birth.[1-4] However, up to 20% of cases develop in adolescents and young adults, and it also occurs in adults and elderly patients.[4-10] Sex incidence is equal, and most patients are Caucasian.[4,11,12]

JXG is usually limited to the skin, but may arise at extracutaneous sites, with or without concomitant cutaneous lesions. Approximately two-thirds

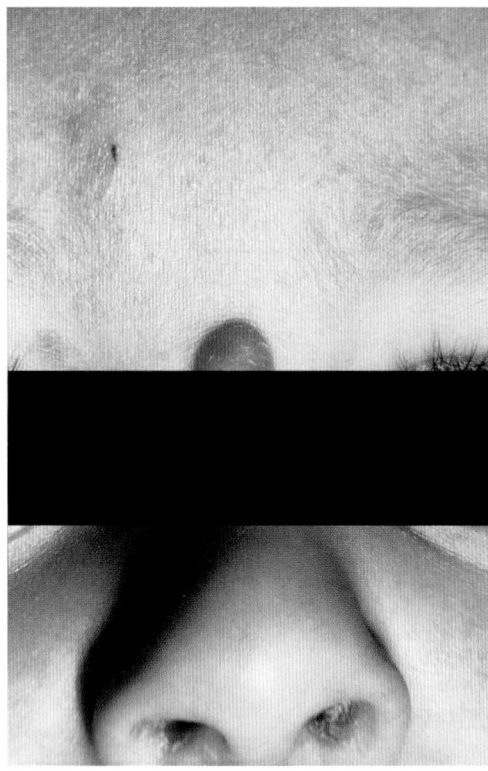

Fig. 29.294
Xanthogranuloma: there is a characteristic reddish-brown nodule on the bridge of the nose of this infant. By courtesy of R.A. Marsden, MD, St George's Hospital, London, UK.

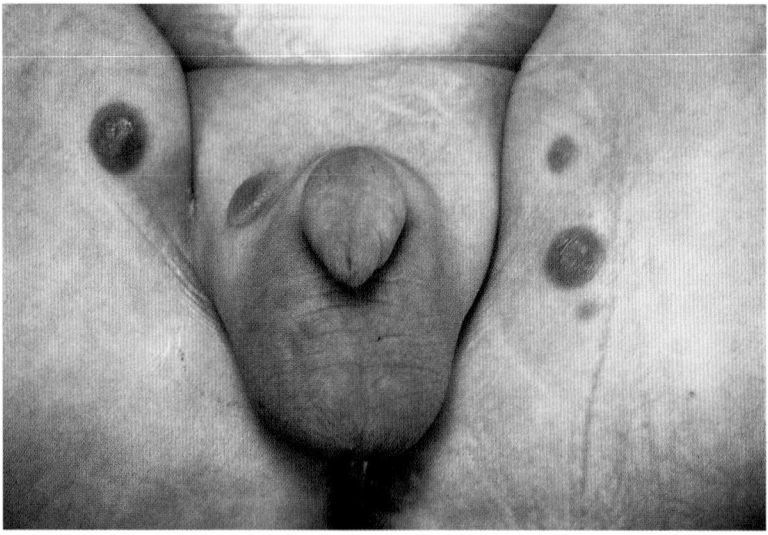

Fig. 29.295
Xanthogranuloma: this child has multiple lesions. By courtesy of the Institute of Dermatology, London, UK.

of cases present as a solitary cutaneous nodule, typically in the head and neck region, followed by the trunk or upper limbs (*Fig. 29.294*).[4,11,12] Multiple skin lesions are much less common (approximately 7% of cases) (*Fig. 29.295*).[4] Patients are usually young children (median age, 5 months) with head and neck involvement. In one series, nearly all cases were male.[4] Cutaneous lesions are usually described as yellowish, orange, red-brown, or flesh-colored papules or nodules and rarely plaques measuring a few millimeters to several centimeters in diameter. The appearances may mimic a Spitz nevus or mastocytoma.[11] Lesions are usually asymptomatic, although pruritus may be a feature and rarely they are painful.[12]

Rare presentations include giant, clustered (agminate), and lichenoid forms.[11] Giant lesions are >2.0 cm in diameter, and most commonly affect

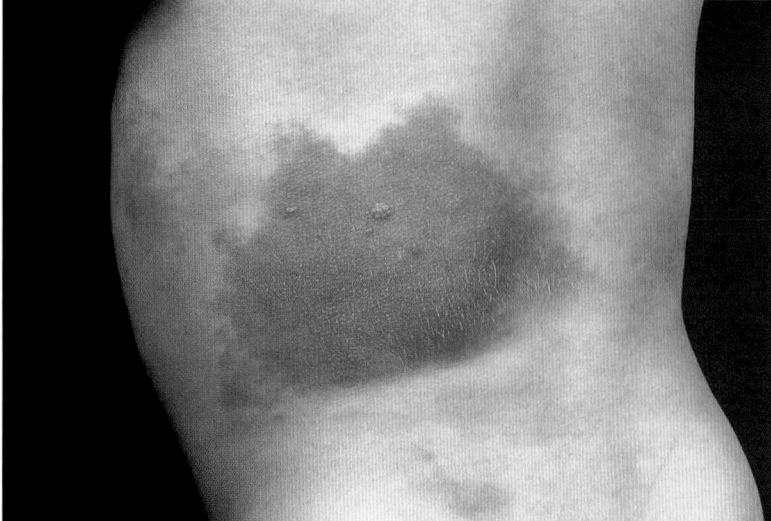

Fig. 29.296
Xanthogranuloma: this is a rare example of xanthogranulomata presenting in a child with neurofibromatosis type I. By courtesy of the Institute of Dermatology, London, UK.

the upper trunk and proximal limbs, predominantly in girls (5:1).[11,13–16] Congenital presentation is common and ulceration is often seen.[11] The agminate variant is exceptional, presenting as clustered papules, and may be associated with alopecia.[17,18] In contrast to the more usual sites, the arm and leg have been affected. One case of lichenoid JXG has been described.[19]

Extracutaneous involvement is seen in up to 25% of cases and may take the form of a solitary lesion without associated skin disease.[4,20] Solitary extracutaneous lesions usually present as a large subcutaneous (up to 3 cm in diameter) or soft tissue (usually >4 cm diameter) mass. The soft tissues of the head and neck are most frequently involved, and rarely lesions occur on the trunk and limbs, and in the abdomen–pelvis.[4,21–24] The orbit is another common site.[2,3,25,26] Patients with ocular involvement are under 2 years of age, and most present with a unilateral asymptomatic iris tumor, a red eye with signs of uveitis, unilateral glaucoma, and spontaneous hyphema.[12,25,26] Solitary lesions can also occur in bone, tongue, nasal cavity and paranasal sinuses, and lung.[4]

Visceral disease is usually multifocal and associated with multiple skin lesions.[4] Organs involved include liver, spleen, lungs, and CNS, and less commonly in the heart, oropharynx, muscle, kidney, bone, pancreas, peripheral nerve, ovaries, testes, and adrenal gland.

Skin lesions tend to flatten, disappearing over months to years, sometimes leaving atrophic or hypopigmented scars. Most systemic lesions also completely regress within 3 to 6 years.[1–3] Rare fatalities have occurred in patients with CNS or hepatic involvement.[4,27–29] There is a well-documented association between JXG and neurofibromatosis type I and/or juvenile myelomonocytic leukemia (*Fig. 29.296*).[9,30–32] In cases associated with leukemia, JXG usually precedes or presents concurrently.

Benign cephalic histiocytosis

Benign cephalic histiocytosis is exceptional and presents in early childhood.[33–41] The age at onset ranges from 3 to 34 months (mean, 13.5 months).[34] The sexes are equally affected. Early lesions are erythematous, round or oval maculopapules that enlarge to form 2–8 mm diameter, brownish-yellow papules distributed most often on the face, particularly the cheeks, eyebrows, and forehead (*Fig. 29.297*). Not infrequently, they later spread to affect the shoulders, proximal limbs, trunk, and pubic area.[34,35]

Numbers of lesions are variable, ranging from solitary to hundreds of papules.[34] The mucous membrane, palms, and soles are unaffected and there is generally no evidence of systemic involvement. An exceptional case with diabetes insipidus and a further case with insulin-dependent diabetes mellitus have been reported.[40,42] Spontaneous regression always occurs, leaving transitory hyperpigmented lesions, which subsequently disappear completely.

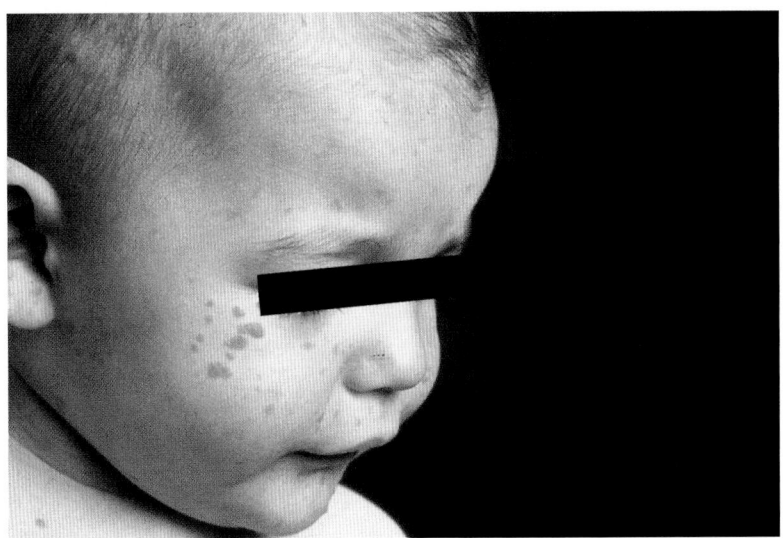

Fig. 29.297
Benign cephalic histiocytosis: numerous erythematous macules and papules are present on this infant's forehead and cheek. By courtesy of R. Gianotti, MD, Universitá di Milano, Milan, Italy.

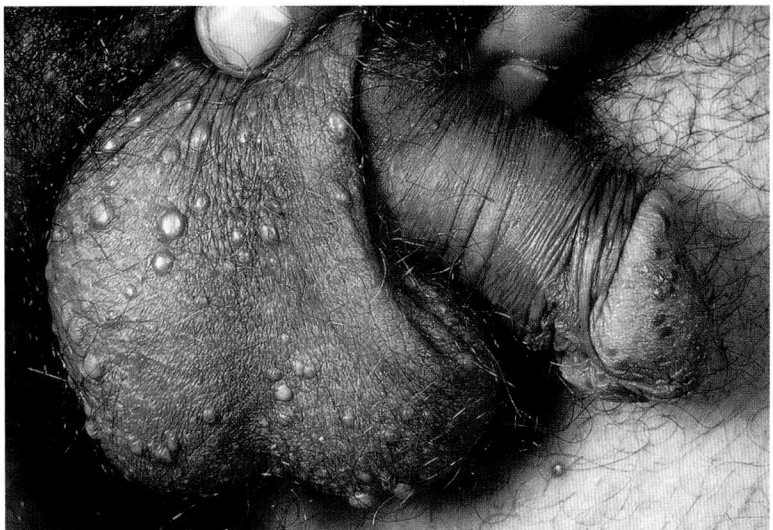

Fig. 29.299
Xanthoma disseminatum: typical papules on the scrotum. By courtesy of the Institute of Dermatology, London, UK.

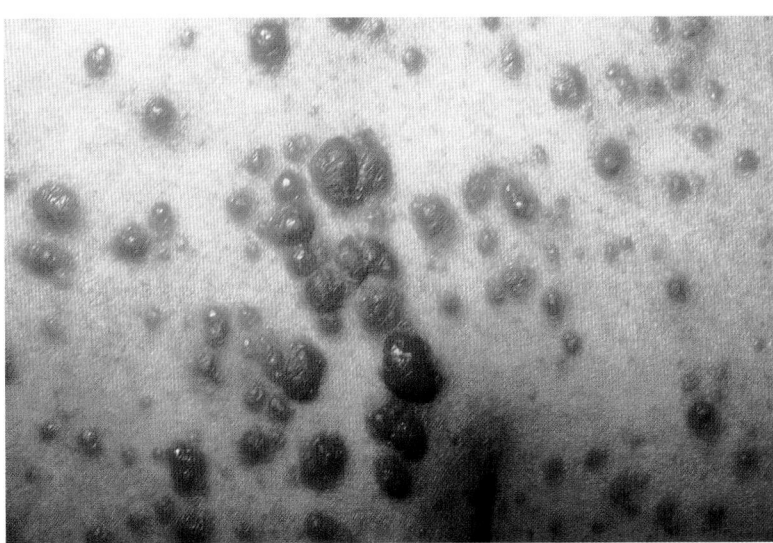

Fig. 29.298
Generalized eruptive histiocytoma: this middle-aged patient developed hundreds of asymptomatic papules on the trunk and limbs. By courtesy of R.M. Mackie, MD, Western Infirmary, Glasgow, UK.

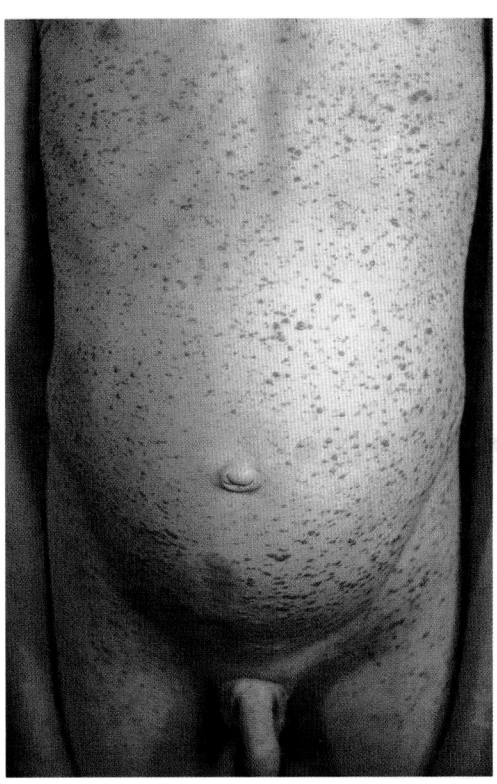

Fig. 29.300
Xanthoma disseminatum: in this patient, lesions are generalized. By courtesy of the Institute of Dermatology, London, UK.

Generalized eruptive histiocytosis

Generalized eruptive histiocytosis (generalized eruptive histiocytoma) is a rare condition characterized by recurrent, asymptomatic, symmetrical crops of small (1–10 mm) tan, erythematous or blue-red, firm, discrete papules or rarely nodules on the face, trunk, and arms, and occasionally the legs (Fig. 29.298).[43–50] Warty lesions and lesions in a seborrheic distribution are exceptional.[44,48,51,52] Mucous membranes, palms, and soles are generally spared.[2,6,8,9] Visceral involvement is not a feature and lipids are normal.[49] Lesions may last from months to years.[6] Spontaneous resolution to leave hyperpigmented atrophic anetoderma-like macules is common, with complete resolution of all lesions.[48,49] Adults are most often affected, with rare cases in children.[51–60] Umbilicated lesions in children mimic molluscum contagiosum.[55,56,60] Two patients have been described in which an early presentation as generalized eruptive histiocytoma evolved into typical XD, emphasizing the considerable overlap in the non-X group of histiocytosis.[55,56]

Xanthoma disseminatum and scalloped cell xanthogranuloma

Xanthoma disseminatum (XD) usually develops in young adults (<25 years), with rare cases in children and in the elderly.[61–68] There is a male predilection.[61,62]

Early lesions are red-yellow papules, nodules, and plaques, with predilection for the flexures (Fig. 29.299). Occasionally, lesions may be generalized (Fig. 29.300).[69,70] They tend to be progressive, sometimes confluent, and as maturation ensues lesions become brown (Figs 29.301 and 29.302).[71] Mucous membranes are involved in 30–50% of cases with lesions in the larynx, pharynx, mouth, trachea, epiglottis, tongue, and lower gastrointestinal tract.[72] These may be associated with significant morbidity,

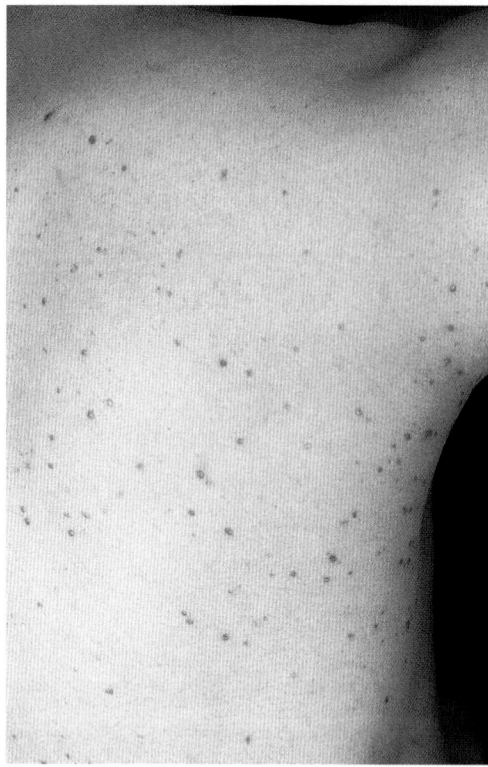

Fig. 29.301
Xanthoma disseminatum: note the widespread erythematous papules. By courtesy of the Institute of Dermatology, London, UK.

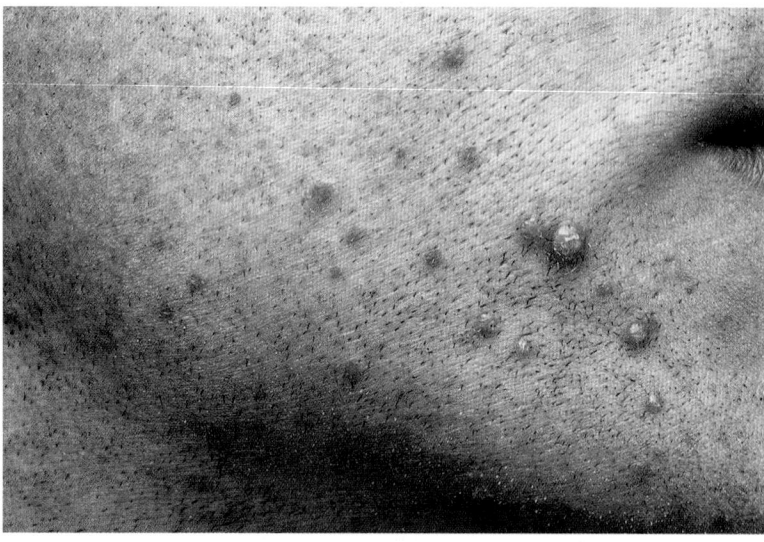

Fig. 29.302
Xanthoma disseminatum: multiple lesions are present on the cheek. By courtesy of the Institute of Dermatology, London, UK.

including hoarseness, respiratory embarrassment, and problems with closure of the mouth or with defecation.[71,73,74] Lower respiratory tract involvement resulting in respiratory failure has also been rarely reported.[12,65,68]

Systemic disease is frequently encountered, the most common manifestation being diabetes insipidus, which occurs in about 40% of cases and is due involvement of the hypothalamus–pituitary region.[74,75] The diabetes insipidus is usually both mild and transient. Meningeal lesions are rare and give rise to epilepsy. Ocular involvement affecting the cornea and conjunctiva occurs in approximately 20% of patients.[62] Rarely, bone disease is a feature with progressive and osteolytic lesions.[63,71,76,77] Hepatic involvement is very rare.[64]

A rare association with multiple myeloma and Waldenström macroglobulinemia has been reported.[78,79]

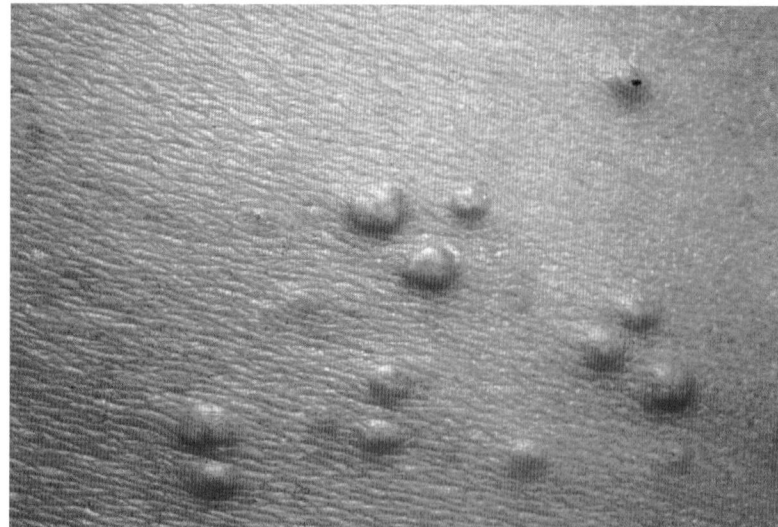

Fig. 29.303
Papular xanthoma: typical bright yellow papules. By courtesy of the Institute of Dermatology, London, UK.

The clinical course is usually benign. However, although there is usually spontaneous resolution of lesions, this commonly takes a few years and up to 40 years in some cases.[80,81] Exceptional fatalities may occur due to respiratory failure, or involvement of the lower respiratory tract or of the CNS.[67,68,82–84]

Scalloped cell xanthogranuloma has been described in one series in which it was proposed that it represents the solitary counterpart of XD.[85,86] Tumors present on the back, head, and neck of young adults (particularly males) as 5–10 mm diameter yellow or red papules and nodules.[86]

Papular xanthoma

Papular xanthoma (PX) is exceptional, presenting most often as disseminated, asymptomatic 2–15 mm diameter, round, yellow to orange discrete papules and nodules with predilection for the head, trunk, and upper limbs, and rarely mucous membranes (*Fig. 29.303*).[61,87–95] The flexures are typically spared.[88] Rarely, the distribution is more limited.[96] There is a slight female predilection. Only two cases presented with systemic involvement. One of these involved the larynx, and the other involved the conjunctiva, gums, ears, and upper airways.[97,98] Lesions were congenital in a single case.[99] Most patients are normolipemic, although there is one case associated with primary dysbetalipoproteinemia.[89] In adults, the lesions appear to be persistent, whereas in childhood, lesions appear to be self-healing.[90] In one case, resolution followed oral doxycycline.[98] A variant – so-called progressive PX in which disfiguring chronic lesions may be accompanied by mucosal involvement – has been described and shows considerable overlap with progressive nodular histiocytosis.[95]

Solitary lesions may be seen mainly on the trunk, followed by the extremities and the head and neck, in children or middle-aged adults, with marked predilection for males (4:1).[94]

Progressive nodular histiocytosis and spindle cell xanthogranuloma

Progressive nodular histiocytosis is very rare.[100–108] Presentation is usually with small yellowish papules or large nodules measuring up to 5.0 cm in diameter with predilection for the trunk.[104] Rarely, a leonine facies is a feature.[105,106] Mucosal lesions are exceptional.[107] Spontaneous regression is not usual. The sex distribution is equal, with predilection for the fifth and sixth decades.[104] Serum lipids are generally normal. Rare associations include hypercholesterolemia, chronic myeloid leukemia, and hypothalamic involvement with precocious puberty and growth failure.[106,108]

Solitary spindle cell xanthogranuloma predominantly affects younger adults (20–40 years) with equal sex incidence. Anatomic distribution is wide including the head, neck, upper trunk, and extremities, in decreasing order of frequency. Lesions are slightly elevated to dome-shaped yellow-brown papules or nodules.[104]

Pathogenesis and histologic features

The pathogenesis of this group of disorders is unknown, as is the precise cell of origin. Derivation from a dermal/interstitial dendritic cell is currently favored, in view of the phenotype shared by the dominant histiocytes in all cases, particularly expression of factor XIIIA, fascin, and macrophage markers.[20,109–111] Monocytes/macrophages, indeterminate cells, and plasmacytoid monocytes (plasmacytoid dendritic cells) have also been suggested as likely sources of the main cell type.[4,11,23,112,113] Although foam cells are a prominent feature, serum lipids are normal. This had led some to propose that lipid accumulates in histiocytes as a result of enhanced uptake and intracellular biosynthesis.[114] It has also been suggested that viruses, such as CMV and varicella, or physical factors, may act as triggering stimuli, but this remains speculative.[30,115–118] Clonality has been demonstrated in one case.[119] BRAF mutations are not typically seen.[120]

The diseases referred to in this section overlap clinically and histologically, suggesting that they represent a continuous spectrum of disease, the manifestations of which are determined by the state of maturation of the constituent cells.[110] Thus, disorders of histiocytes at the most immature end of the spectrum tend to arise in early life, run a short clinical course, and undergo spontaneous resolution, i.e., JXG and benign cephalic histiocytosis. Generalized eruptive histiocytosis and XD are proposed to be proliferations of more mature histiocytes, occurring in young adults. Although spontaneous resolution is the norm, the clinical course is longer, from months to many years. Progressive nodular histiocytosis lies at the most mature end of the spectrum. Middle-aged adults and the elderly are most commonly affected; the histiocytes display a fully matured spindled morphology, and the disease is progressive, resistant to treatment, and shows no tendency to spontaneous resolution. This approach is useful, not least in that it acts as a useful aide memoire for the various clinical manifestation of this group of diseases.[3,85,110] It has also been proposed that the morphology of the constituent histiocytes within a lesion can be used to predict maturational status, and hence permit pathological discrimination between entities. Vacuolated or lightly eosinophilic histiocytes predominate in immature lesions, scalloped and/or xanthomatized histiocytes in more mature cases, and spindled histiocytes in the most mature. Although there is some evidence to support this, histologic differentiation of entities is often irreproducible in practice.[3,85]

Lesions in the JXG family are typically well-circumscribed dermal nodules comprising a dense cellular infiltrate. The epidermis is normal, although attenuation over the lesion may be seen (*Figs 29.304* and *29.305*). Mononuclear and multinucleate histiocytes make up the majority (95%) of cells.[85] Mononuclear histiocytes are most frequently small, round, or oval cells with ill-defined lightly eosinophilic, often vacuolated cytoplasm. The nuclei are round to oval with euchromatin and sometimes prominent, albeit small, nucleoli.[4,7,103,121–124] Mitotic figures may be seen (*Fig. 29.306*). Variations on this theme include: larger xanthomatized cells with finely vacuolated, foamy, cytoplasm; 'scalloped' histiocytes with angulated, scalloped, or jagged borders; and spindle-shaped histiocytes, sometimes with mildly vacuolated cytoplasm and occasionally showing a storiform pattern.[85] The multinucleate cells are typically Touton-type and are present in 85% of lesions but are not a prerequisite for diagnosis. They are very large cells with wreath-like nuclei encircling a central eosinophilic core with a peripheral rim of xanthomatized, foamy cytoplasm (*Fig. 29.307*). Multinucleate foreign body-like giant cells are rare. Other inflammatory cells are usually present to varying degrees, particularly small lymphocytes, but also eosinophils, neutrophils, and even plasma cells can be present (*Fig. 29.308*).

Lesions of JXG typically contain histiocytes with a variety of appearances, those with lightly eosinophilic and/or vacuolated cytoplasm predominating (*Figs 29.309–29.311*). Xanthomatized histiocytes predominate in PX, and scalloped histiocytes in XD and scalloped cell xanthogranuloma. Progressive nodular histiocytosis and spindle cell xanthogranuloma are characterized by a predominance of spindled histiocytes (*Figs 29.312* and *29.313*). Early lesions are characterized by an abundance of cells with

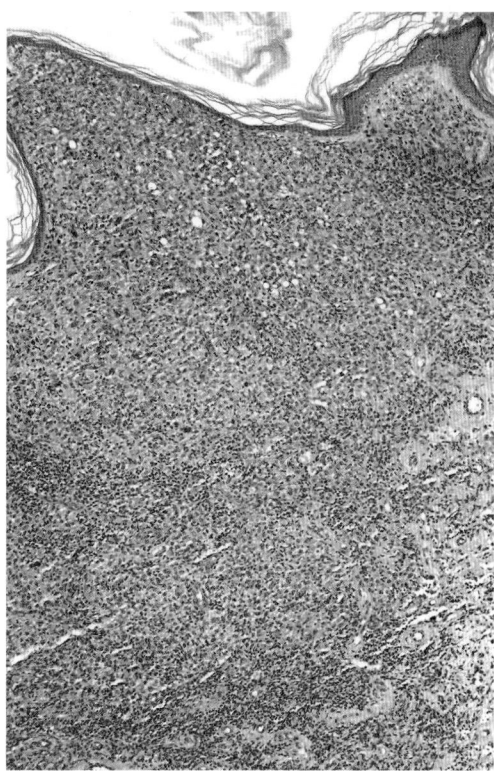

Fig. 29.304
Xanthogranuloma (generalized eruptive histiocytoma): there is a dense infiltrate occupying the papillary and reticular dermis.

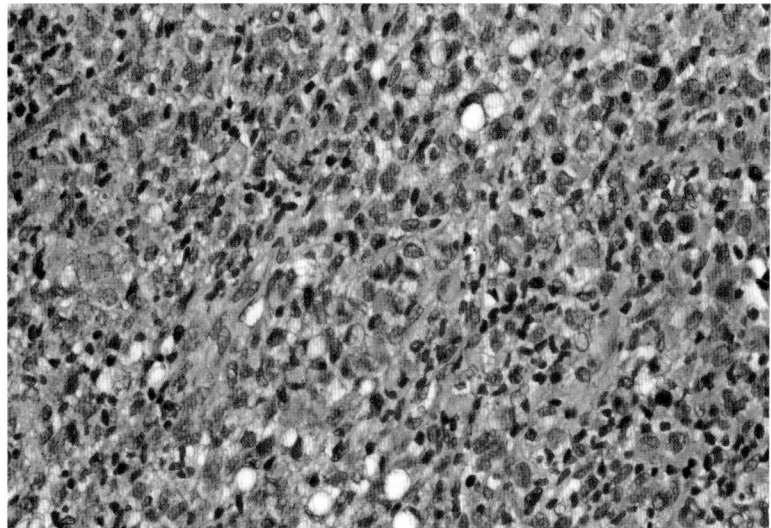

Fig. 29.305
Xanthogranuloma (generalized eruptive histiocytoma): there is a uniform population of nonxanthomatized histiocytes.

lightly vacuolated cytoplasm, which become progressively lipidized (xanthomatized) with age. Spindled cells represent the most aged end of this spectrum. Systemic lesions more frequently lack Touton-type giant cells, and spindled cells are often present and may predominate.[1,4,21,85,109,113,125]

The immunophenotype of the main histiocytic component is the same in all variants of the JXG family. There is positive staining for the macrophage markers CD14, CD68 (both coarse granular cytoplasmic pattern), and CD163 (surface and cytoplasmic) (*Fig. 29.314*). Dendritic cell markers are also expressed, fascin always, and factor XIIIA frequently. Staining for S100 may be positive in up to 25% of cases. CD1a and langerin are negatvie.[113]

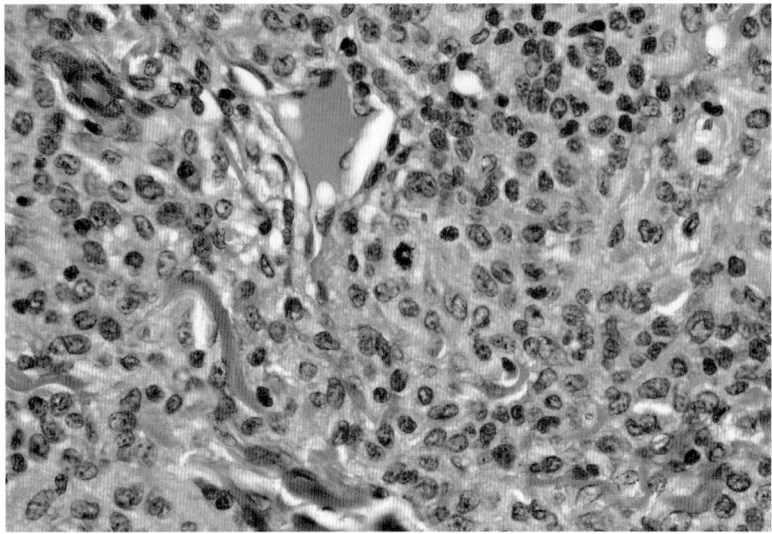

Fig. 29.306
Xanthogranuloma: note the mitotic figure.

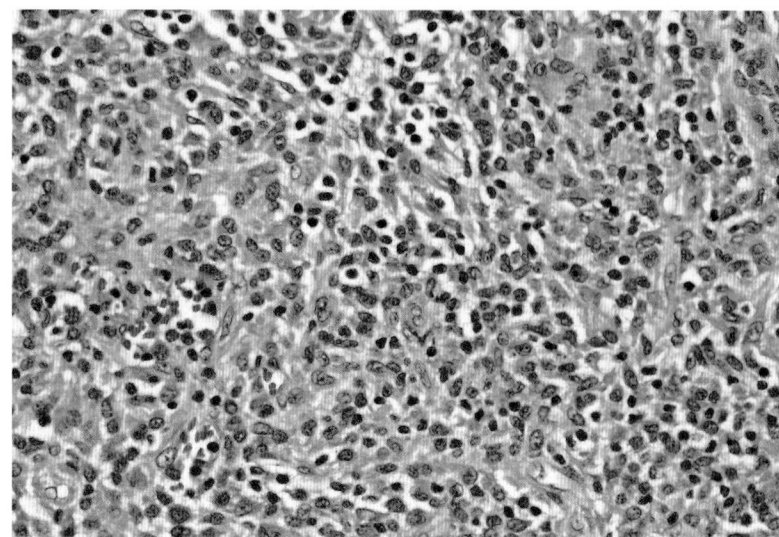

Fig. 29.308
Xanthogranuloma: note the background population of lymphocytes.

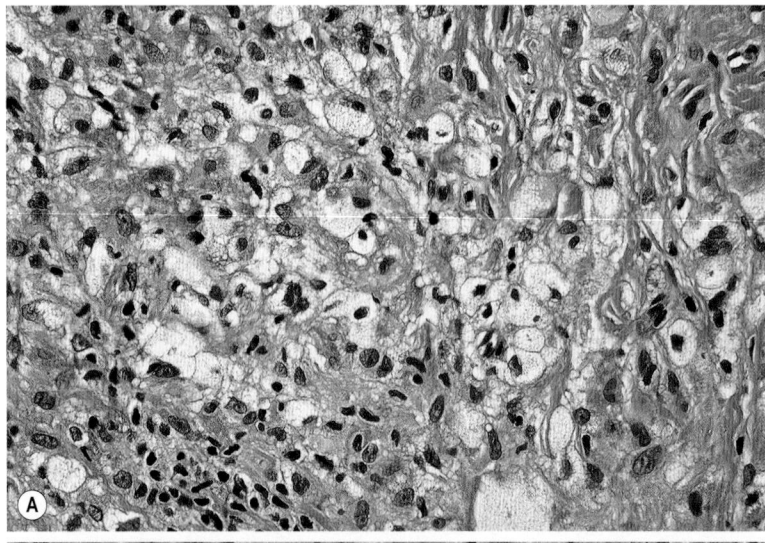

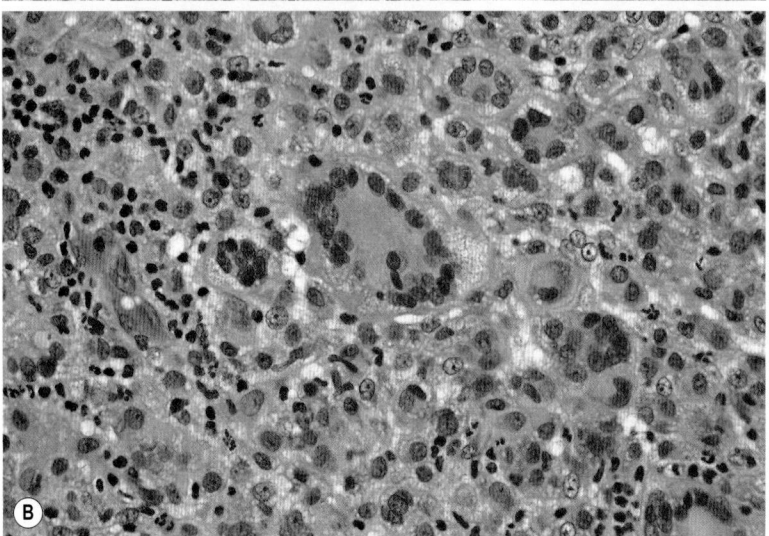

Fig. 29.307
(A, B) Xanthogranuloma: (A) high-power view showing xanthomatized cells;
(B) high-power view of a typical Touton giant cell.

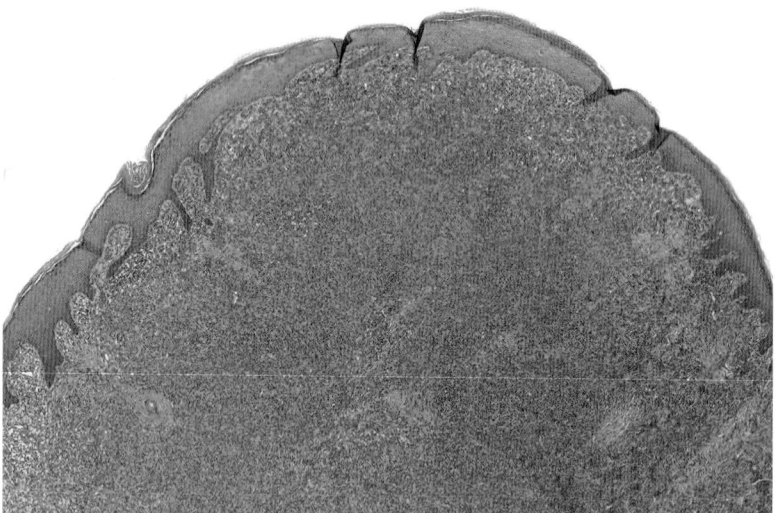

Fig. 29.309
Xanthogranuloma: the dermis is expanded by a dense cellular infiltrate.

Differential diagnosis

Although there may be histologic variation between the different members of the JXG family, it is not possible to reliably distinguish them on pathological grounds alone. This is done primarily on the basis of clinical features. All types of xanthogranuloma are distinguished from cutaneous xanthomas by the lack of an inflammatory component and/or multinucleate cells in the latter and normal levels of serum lipids in the former. Langerhans cell histiocytosis is differentiated on immunophenotypic grounds, being uniformly positive for S100 and also expressing CD1a and langerin. RH is usually composed of larger histiocytes with typical eosinophilic ground-glass cytoplasm, and lacks Touton-type giant cells. In Rosai-Dorfman disease, the histiocytes are larger and usually paler staining, show emperipolesis, and are positive for S100. Xanthogranulomas with a prominent spindle cell component may resemble dermatofibroma. However, the distinctive phenotype of xanthogranulomas, and often the clinical features, should allow these two entities to be easily separated.

Rosai-Dorfman disease

Clinical features

Rosai-Dorfman disease (RDD) (sinus histiocytosis with massive lymphadenopathy) is a rare, benign, self-limiting illness characterized by a reactive

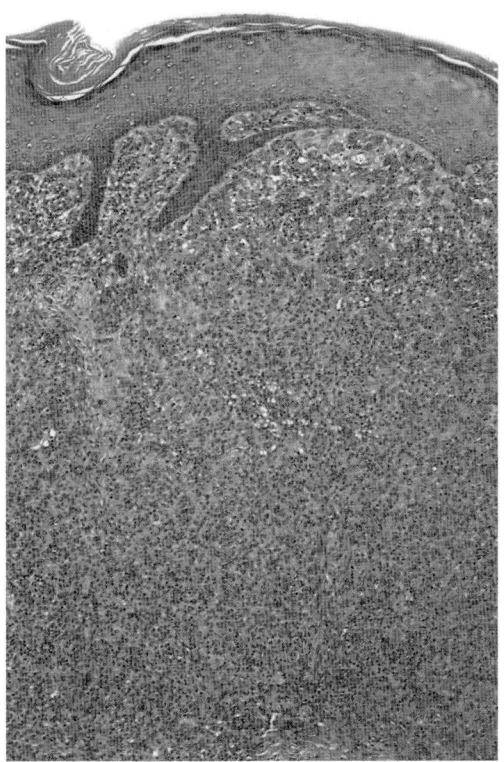

Fig. 29.310
Xanthogranuloma: medium-power view of *Fig. 29.309*.

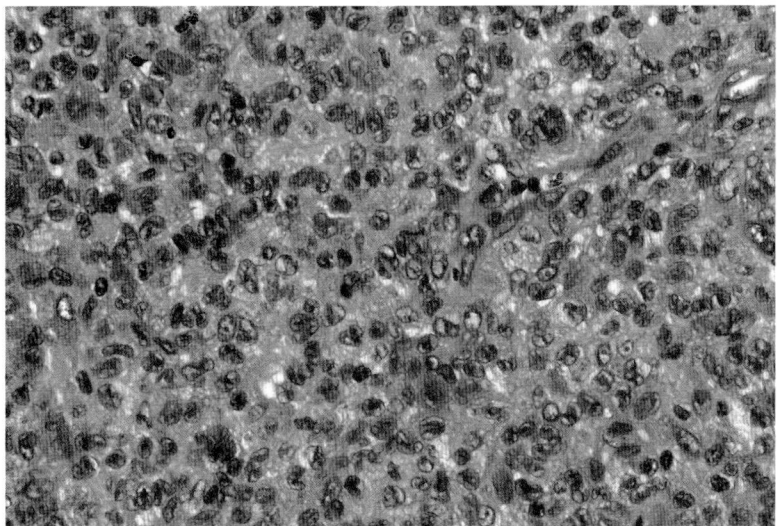

Fig. 29.311
Xanthogranuloma: in early lesions xanthomatized forms are often absent.

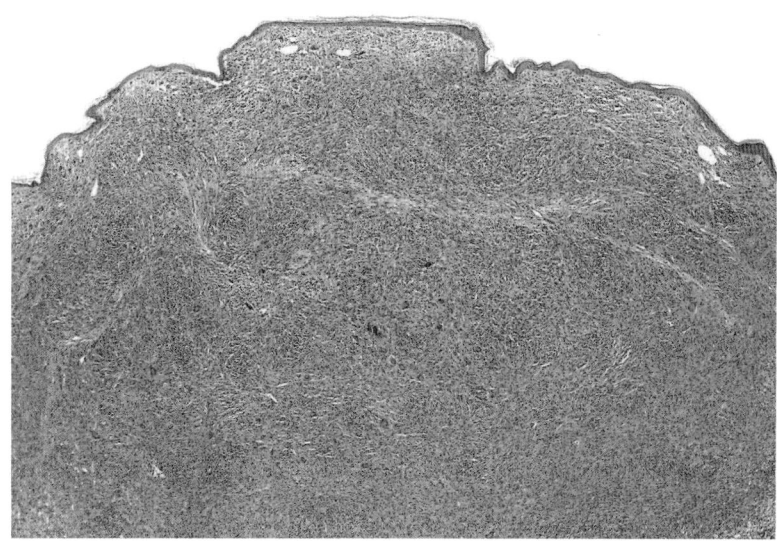

Fig. 29.312
Xanthogranuloma: scanning view of a dermal nodule.

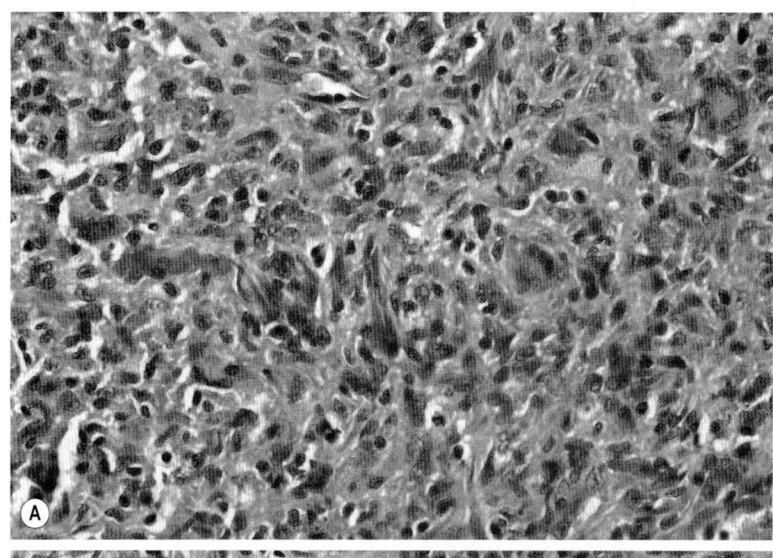

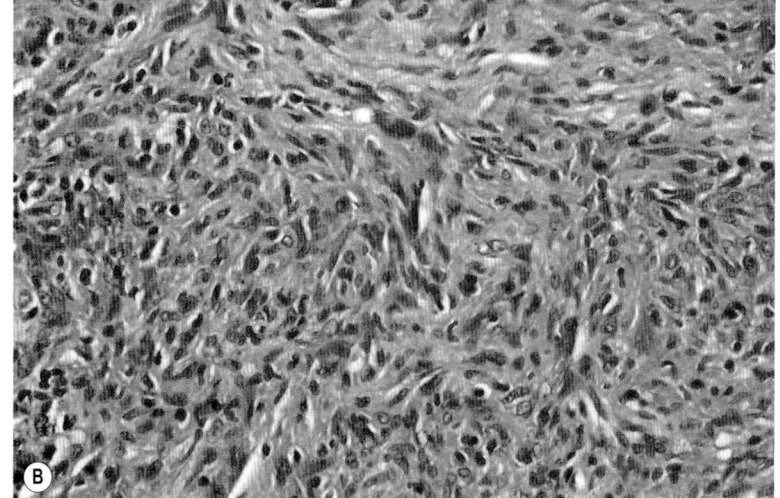

Fig. 29.313
(**A**, **B**) Xanthogranuloma: spindle cells predominate in old lesions such that dermatofibroma is often considered in the differential diagnosis.

proliferation of histiocytes that phenotypically appear to be macrophage–dendritic cell hybrids.[1–3] Age range is wide with predilection for the first and second decades of life and a slight male predominance.[1–3] Blacks and whites are most often affected, while it is rare in Asians.[4] Clinically, it is characterized by massive, painless, frequently bilateral, cervical lymphadenopathy associated with pyrexia, night sweats, leukocytosis with neutrophilia, raised ESR, and a polyclonal hyperglobulinemia.[1–5] Occasionally, other groups of lymph nodes may be involved. Extranodal deposits are common (43% of cases) and are most frequently encountered in skin and subcutis, orbit, bone, and CNS coverings, although virtually any organ can be affected.[2,4–10]

Skin lesions are present in 9% of cases and are not uncommonly seen in the absence of lymph node and other extracutaneous disease, or systemic abnormalities.[5–8,11–17] The latter situation, referred to as cutaneous RDD, seems to occur in a somewhat older age group (fifth decade of life; range,

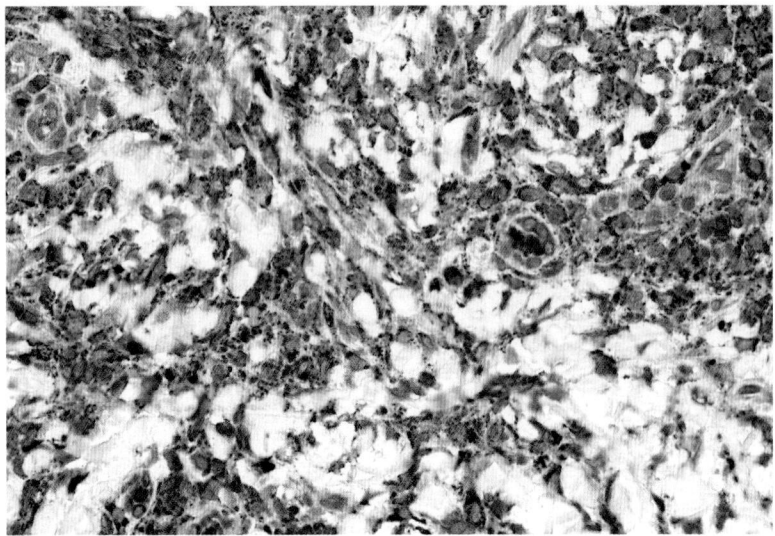

Fig. 29.314
Xanthogranuloma: the histiocytes show strong expression of CD68.

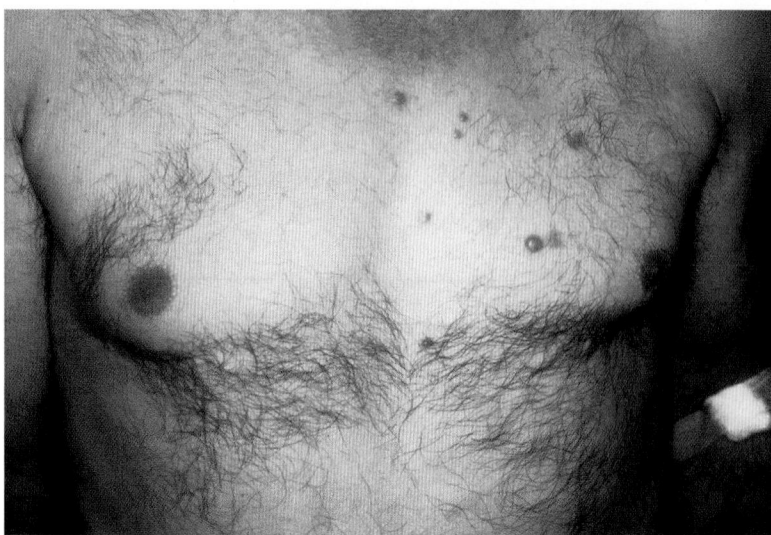

Fig. 29.316
Rosai-Dorfman disease: there are scattered erythematous papules on the left chest. By courtesy of J. Rosai, MD, National Cancer Institute, Milan, Italy.

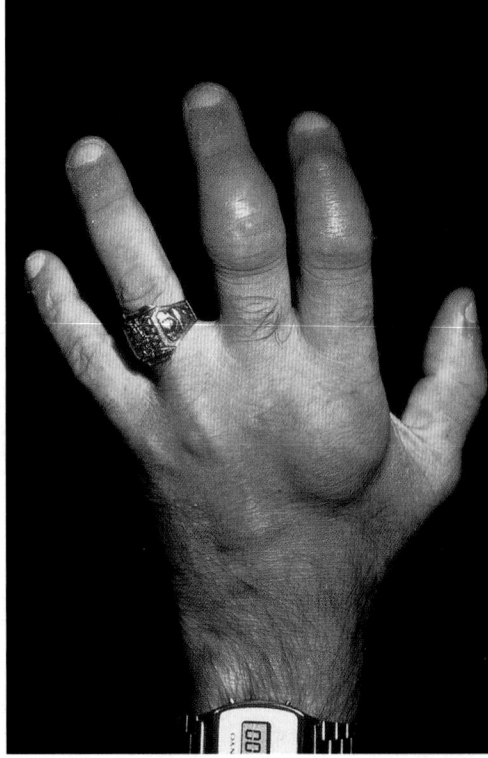

Fig. 29.315
Rosai-Dorfman disease: there is diffuse swelling involving the hand, index, and second fingers. By courtesy of N.S. Pennys, MD, University of Miami School of Medicine, Miami, USA.

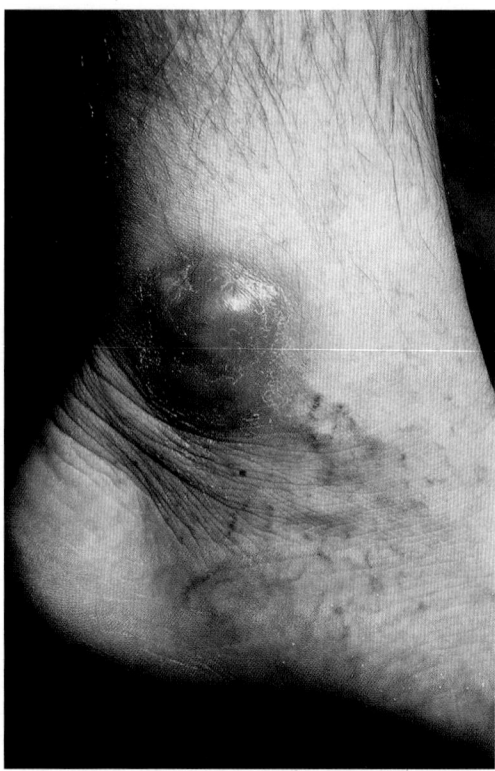

Fig. 29.317
Rosai-Dorfman disease: a brownish-red nodule with scaling overlies the medial malleolus. By courtesy of N.S. Pennys, MD, University of Miami School of Medicine, Miami, USA.

15–77 years), is more frequent in females, and has a higher prevalence in Asians compared to classic nodal disease.[11,13,16–18]

Cutaneous disease presents as xanthomatous, erythematous, or red-brown papules, nodules, or plaques, that may be single, clustered, or widespread (*Figs 29.315–29.318*). The trunk and limbs are most frequently involved.[7,13–17] Acne rosacea-like, giant granuloma annulare-like, acneiform, and pustular lesions, and a vasculitis-like appearance have rarely been described.[12,14,19,20] Subcutaneous lesions also occur.[21]

Most patients with RDD run a benign clinical course with partial or complete spontaneous remission, although this may take a number of years, and episodes of relapse are possible.[2,4,9] Residual atrophic brown macules may persist after resolution.[3] Fatalities are encountered in approximately

5% of patients, as a result of related immunological abnormalities or malignancies (including HL, NHL, leukemia, or solid tumors), or due to the secondary effects of disease at vulnerable sites such as the CNS or upper respiratory tract.[3,9,22,23]

Pathogenesis and histologic features

The etiology is unknown. The proliferating histiocytes are polyclonal, and it has been postulated that RDD may represent a disorder of cell-mediated immunity due to cytokine dysregulation and/or an exuberant response to an infective (possibly viral) agent.[14,19,24,25] There is no convincing evidence for an EBV infection.[26] The role of human herpesvirus (HHV) is uncertain. Current evidence suggests that neither HHV6 nor HHV8 is implicated in the

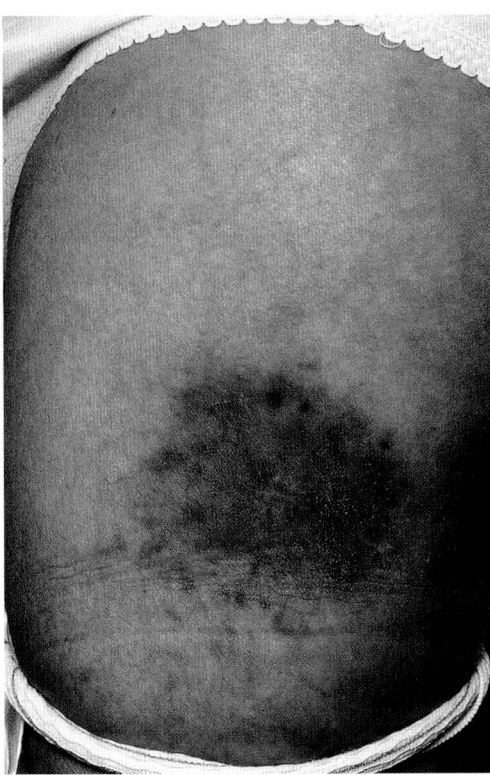

Fig. 29.318
Primary cutaneous Rosai-Dorfman disease: this patient presented with a hyperpigmented indurated plaque. Reproduced with permission from Brenn, T. et al. (2002) American Journal of Dermatopathology, 24, 385–391.

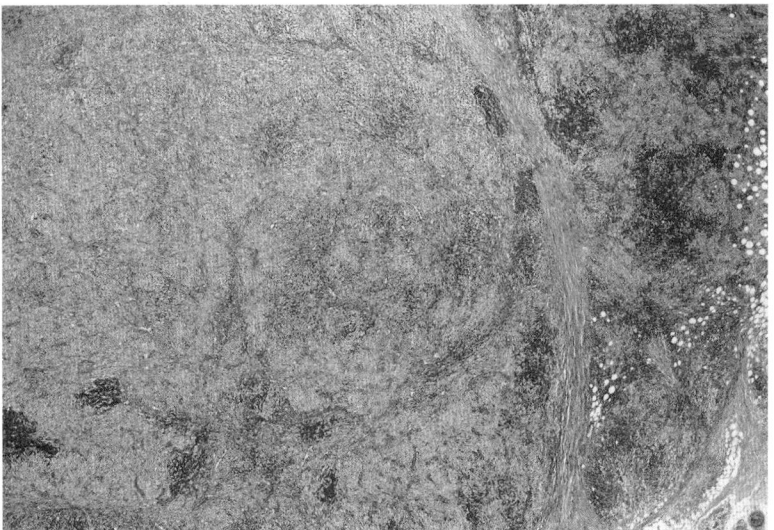

Fig. 29.319
Rosai-Dorfman disease: scanning view showing a dense multinodular cellular infiltrate. Note the lymphoid follicles which are often seen in this condition.

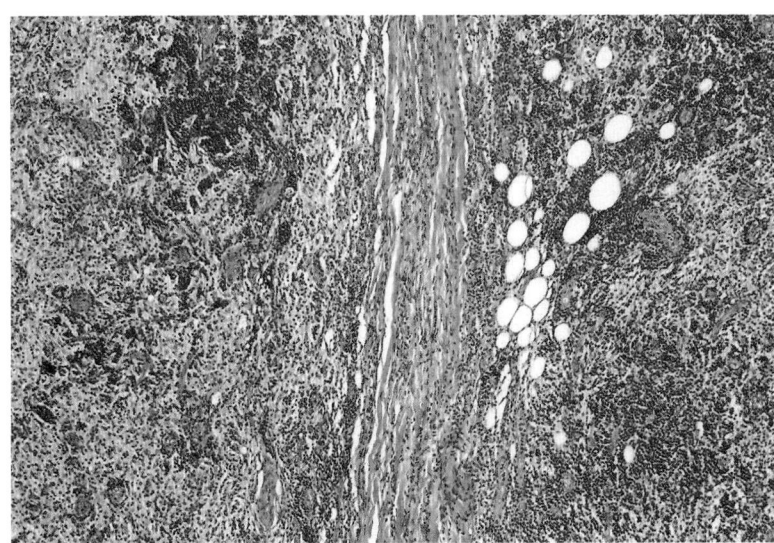

Fig. 29.320
Rosai-Dorfman disease: medium-power view showing two large nodules.

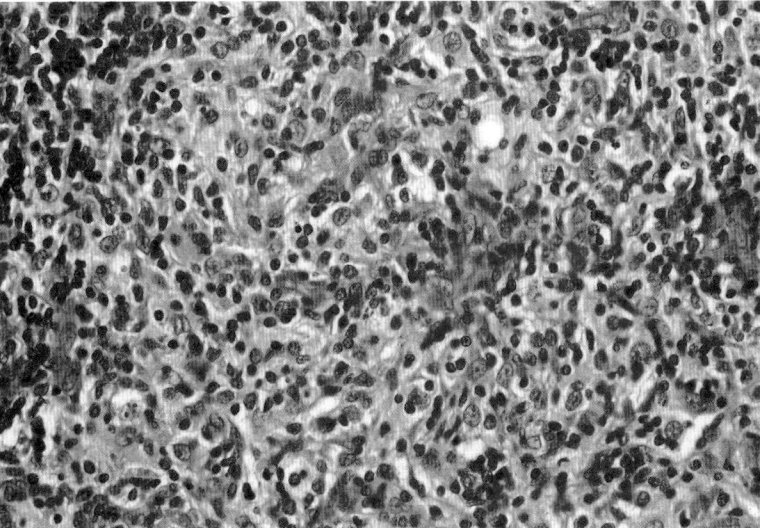

Fig. 29.321
Rosai-Dorfman disease: the infiltrate consists of large histiocytes with abundant eosinophilic cytoplasm admixed with lymphocytes and occasional plasma cells.

majority of cases.[27] Rosai-Dorfman-like changes are seen in association with other conditions. These include autoimmune hemolytic anemia, systemic lupus erythematosus, and juvenile idiopathic arthritis.[28] Rosai-Dorfman-like changes are also seen in 41% of patients with autoimmune lympho-proliferative syndrome type 1a who have mutations in *TNFRSF6* affecting the *FAS* gene, as well as in patients in Faisalabad Histiocytosis and 'H' syndrome.[29–31] Because of these varied associations, it may be that RDD represents a reaction pattern rather than a single distinct entity. *BRAF* mutations are not found.[32,33]

The lymph node findings are characteristic.[2] The node sinuses are dilated and contain very large numbers of histiocytes, characterized by abundant, pale-staining eosinophilic cytoplasm with irregular (feathery) borders, large, centrally placed vesicular nuclei with a single distinct nucleolus.[1,2,4] Mitotic figures are rare. Characteristically, the cytoplasm of the histiocytes appears to contain lymphocytes, red blood cells, and/or granulocytes, a feature known as emperipolesis. Some cells have foamy cytoplasm and some may be multinucleate. Plasma cells are common.

The skin lesions are characterized by a dense cellular infiltrate involving the dermis and sometimes the subcutis (*Fig. 29.319*).[7,11,13,16,17] There may be associated acanthosis or, rarely, collarette formation. Ulceration is uncommon. The infiltrate typically has a nodular appearance, and occasionally a lobular pattern is seen (*Fig. 29.320*). It is composed of sheets of histiocytes similar to those described in the lymph node, although emperipolesis may be less conspicuous (*Figs 29.321* and *29.322*). Cytological atypia is absent and xanthomatized cells are rare. There is often an admixture of lymphocytes, plasma cells, neutrophils, and eosinophils (*Fig. 29.323*). An increase in vascularity is sometimes a feature, and in certain cases stromal fibrosis with a storiform pattern is seen.[13,18] Rarely, lymphoid follicles with germinal centers are apparent.[14,16] Intravascular involvement has been described.[27]

In rare cases, localized proliferations of Langerhans cells resembling microscopic foci of Langerhans cell histiocytosis are noted.[16,34] It is not clear whether this represents transdifferentiation, coincidence of two separate pathologies, or a reactive Langerhans cell proliferation.

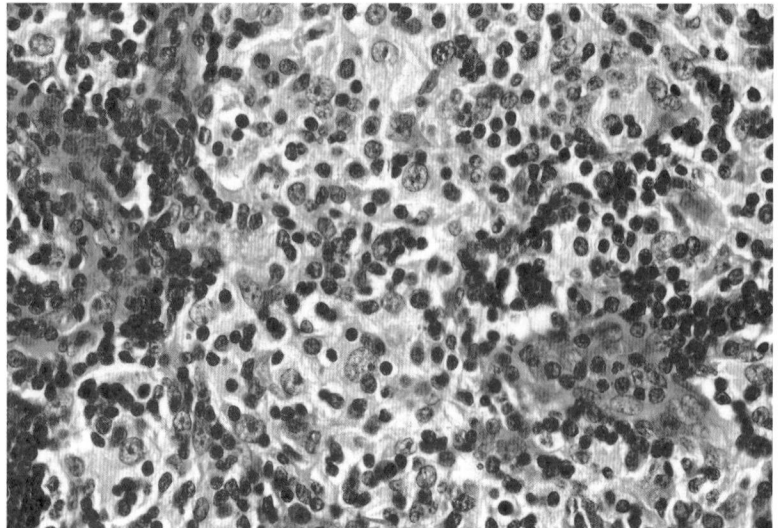

Fig. 29.322
Rosai-Dorfman disease: high-power view showing emperipolesis.

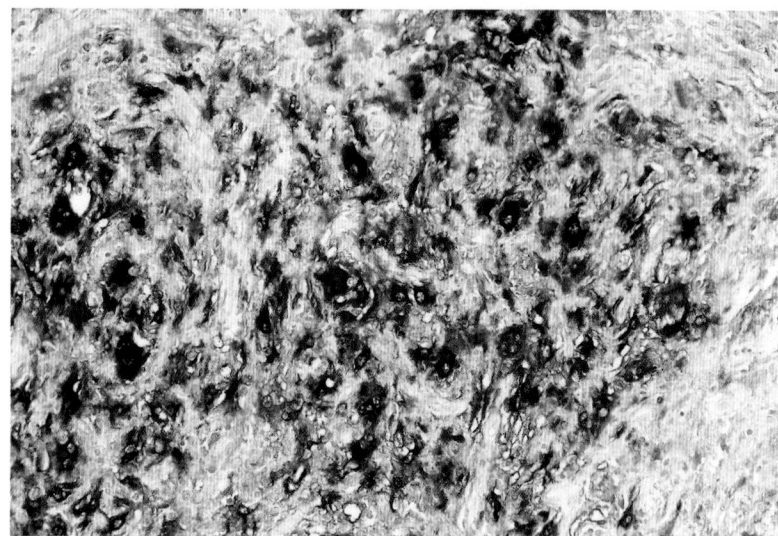

Fig. 29.324
Rosai-Dorfman disease: the histiocytes are S100-protein positive.

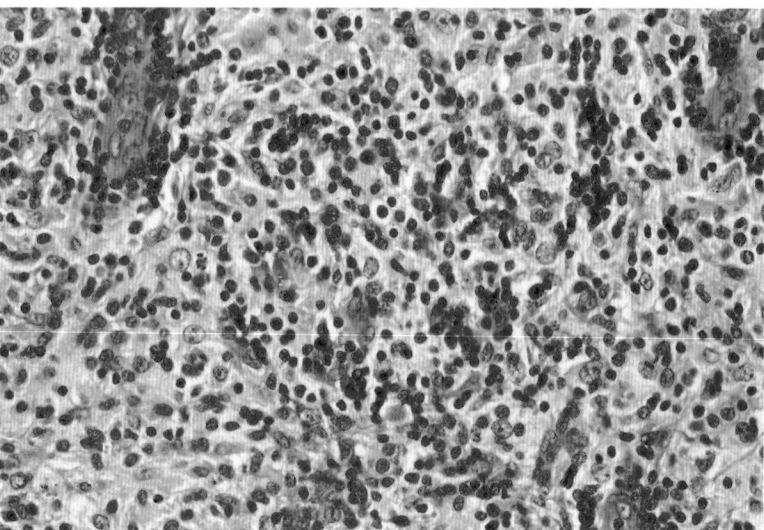

Fig. 29.323
Rosai-Dorfman disease: in this high-power view, there are admixed lymphocytes and plasma cells.

The histiocytes express S100 protein, the macrophage markers CD68, CD14, and CD163 (both strong surface staining) (*Fig. 29.324*). Factor XIIIa, CD1a, and langerin are negative.

Ultrastructurally, the histiocytes have undulating villous cytoplasmic processes.[1]

Differential diagnosis

Skin deposits in RDD may be confused histologically with eruptive xanthomata. However, histiocytes in xanthomata are usually S100 negative and lack emperipolesis. Langerhans cell histiocytosis can be differentiated by the smaller size of the histiocytes, the typical folded reniform nucleus, epidermotropism, and positive staining for CD1a and langerin.[7] In reticulohistiocytosis, the histiocytes have prominent eosinophilic ground-glass cytoplasm and are usually negative for S100. In the JXG family of disorders, the histiocytes are often factor XIIIa positive, and negative or focally positive for S100. Some of the plasma cells in RDD disease may express IgG4, and some authors proposed that there is some overlap between RDD and IgG4-RD.[35,36] Separation of these two entities should be based on recently published criteria that take into account pathological and clinical features as well as the serum IgG4 level.

Multicentric reticulohistiocytosis and reticulohistiocytoma

Clinical features

Multicentric reticulohistiocytosis (MRH) (lipoid dermatoarthritis, giant cell reticulohistiocytosis) is a rare non-Langerhans cell histiocytosis characterized by a cutaneous eruption, usually associated with a severe arthropathy, frequent mucous membrane involvement, and occasional visceral symptoms.[1–3] Most patients are adults aged >40 years (mean age at presentation, 43 years; range, 6–71 years).[3–7] There is female predilection (3:1).[2–5] Two-thirds of patients present with arthropathy and invariably develop skin lesions within months to a few years. Cutaneous lesions represent the primary complaint in 20% of patients, and while many go on to develop joint symptoms, in some the disease remains in the skin (referred as generalized cutaneous reticulohistiocytosis).[1,2] Cutaneous lesions present on the face (predominantly ears, nose, and paranasal areas), the hands (dorsum and lateral aspects of the fingers, nail folds), neck, and trunk. Multiple reddish-brown to yellow papules and nodules measuring from a few millimeters to 2 cm in diameter are seen.[2–4,8–11] Sometimes they coalesce to form plaques with a cobblestone appearance. Nail fold changes present a characteristic 'coral band' pattern.[5] The interphalangeal joints of the hand are the most frequently affected joints, and there may be shortening of the fingers with an 'opera glass' deformity when both proximal and distal interphalangeal joints are involved – so-called 'main en lorgnette'.[5,8] Less often, there is involvement of the knees, wrists, shoulders, hips, ankles, feet, and elbows, in decreasing order of frequency.[2]

Mucous membrane lesions are present in 50% of patients, and affect the oral cavity, pharynx, and nose. Involvement of other sites is rare and include the lungs, heart, liver, breast, stomach, thyroid, submandibular gland, skeletal muscle, and bone.[2,12–22] Hyperlipidemia is reported in 30–50% of cases, and patients often have xanthelasmata.[23] An internal malignancy is found in 30–50% of patients, including carcinoma of the breast and stomach and, more rarely, carcinoma of the cervix, colon, lung, and ovary, lymphoma, leukemia, sarcoma, and melanoma.[23–32] An association with autoimmune disease is described in 15–27% of cases, including polymyositis, Sjögren syndrome, hypothyroidism, primary biliary cirrhosis, vitiligo, Hashimoto thyroiditis, and lupus erythematosus.[1,3,5,33–35] Concomitant vasculitis is rarely seen.[8] Some cases have been linked to infection.[3] Non-specific symptoms including weight loss, fever, and weakness are rare.

The outcome of the disease is unpredictable. Cutaneous lesions may resolve spontaneously or persist. In around 50% of patients, joint symptoms remain stable or diminish over many years. However, in the remainder, disease is progressive with disabling and destructive arthropathy.[4,8]

RH (solitary epithelioid histiocytoma) refers to solitary cutaneous lesions, histologically identical to those in MRH.[36–38] Patients are usually young adults (mean and median age at presentation, 35 years), although age range is wide. There is no sex predilection. Clinically, a papule or nodule measuring up to 1 cm in diameter on the skin or mucous membranes is seen. Trunk, head and neck, or extremities may be the presenting site but, unlike MRH, fingers are not involved.[36]

Pathogenesis and histologic features

The pathogenesis of MRH and RH is unknown. An abnormal macrophage response to different stimuli has been proposed. An immunological basis for the histiocytic reaction in MRH is possible in view of the relationship with infection, autoimmune disease, and internal malignancy.[9] There may be a more localized trigger in RH, but this has not been proven.[39]

Cutaneous lesions in MRH and RH are identical and consist of a well-defined collection of uniform pink histiocytes and multinucleated giant cells, with somewhat eosinophilic, finely granular, ground-glass cytoplasm. The infiltrate is mainly dermal, but rarely erodes the basal epidermis or extends into superficial subcutis (Figs 29.325–29.328). Scattered inflammatory cells, including lymphocytes, granulocytes, and plasma cells, may also be present.

The histiocytes and multinucleate giant cells are consistently positive for CD68, CD163, and Ki-M1p and react variably with antibodies to Ham56

and factor XIIIa. They are negative for CD1a and S100.[1,2,36] The giant cells are diastase-PAS positive (Fig. 29.329).

Synovial lesions show similar histology.[6]

Differential diagnosis

In cases with systemic features, the clinical history is paramount. Solitary RH may be distinguished from JXG by the absence of lipidized cells and Touton giant cells and the typical eosinophilic cells with ground-glass cytoplasm. However, JXG may have scattered cells similar to the latter. Distinction from a melanocytic lesion is made by negative staining for melanocytic markers.

Hemophagocytic lymphohistiocytosis

Clinical features

Hemophagocytic lymphohistiocytosis (HLH) (hemophagocytosis syndrome) represents a complex group of disorders that share a final common pathway culminating in hemophagocytosis and associated signs and symptoms. They are divided into primary and secondary HLH. Primary HLH equates with familial forms of the disease and is usually associated with an inherited genetic disorder, although a family history may be negative, and HLH in these patients may be triggered by infections.[1,2] Secondary variants include

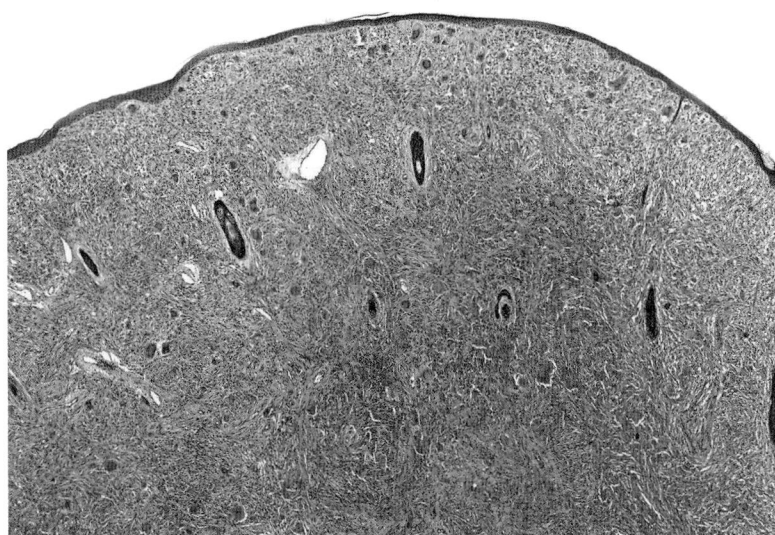

Fig. 29.325
Reticulohistiocytoma: the dermis is expanded by a dome-shaped nodule composed of large histiocytes.

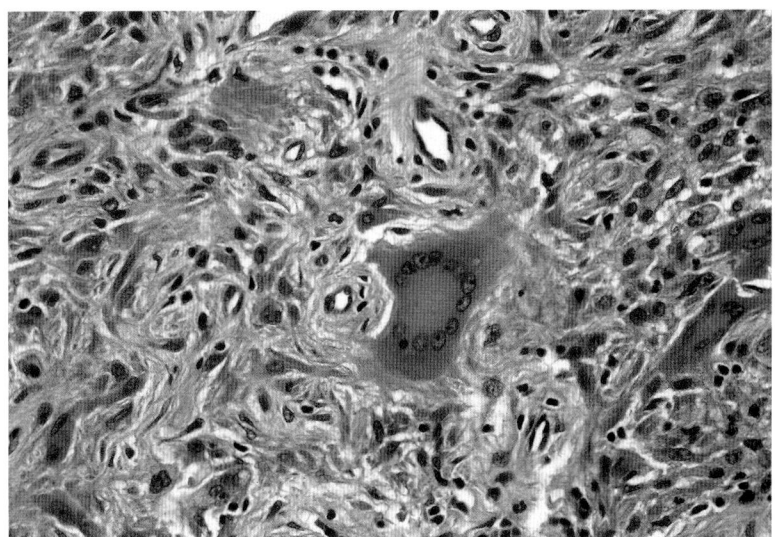

Fig. 29.327
Reticulohistiocytoma: characteristic multinucleate giant cell with ground-glass cytoplasm.

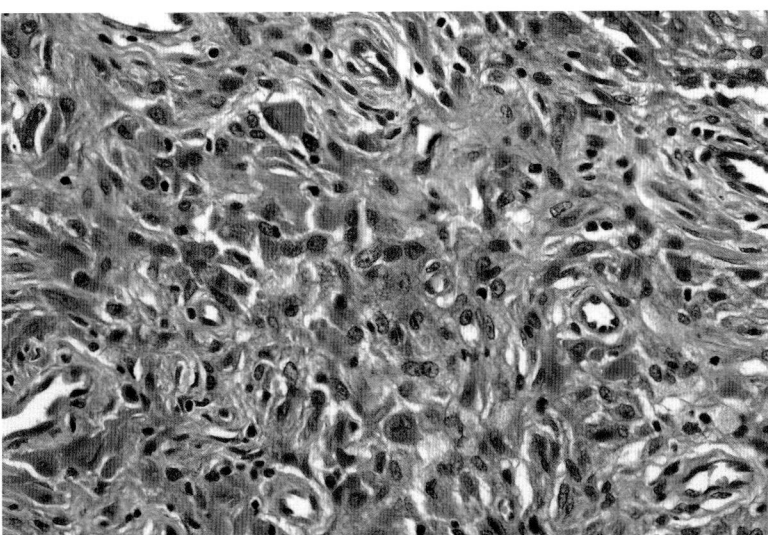

Fig. 29.326
Reticulohistiocytoma: the histiocytes have copious eosinophilic cytoplasm.

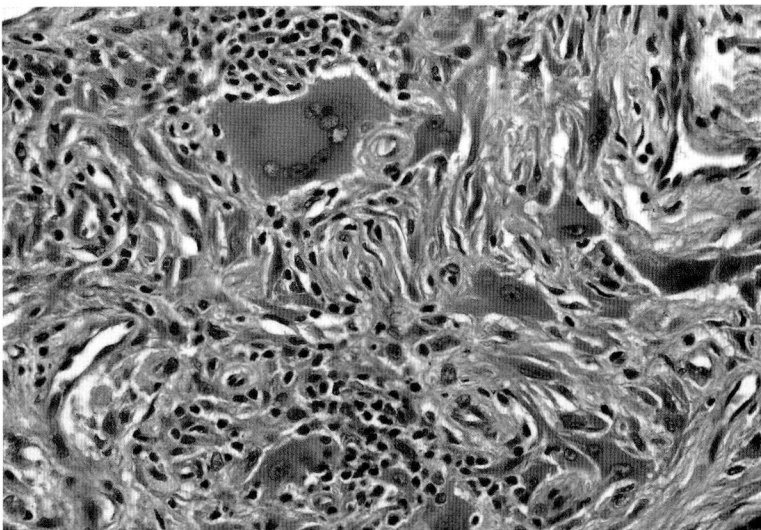

Fig. 29.328
Reticulohistiocytoma: lymphocytes are also present.

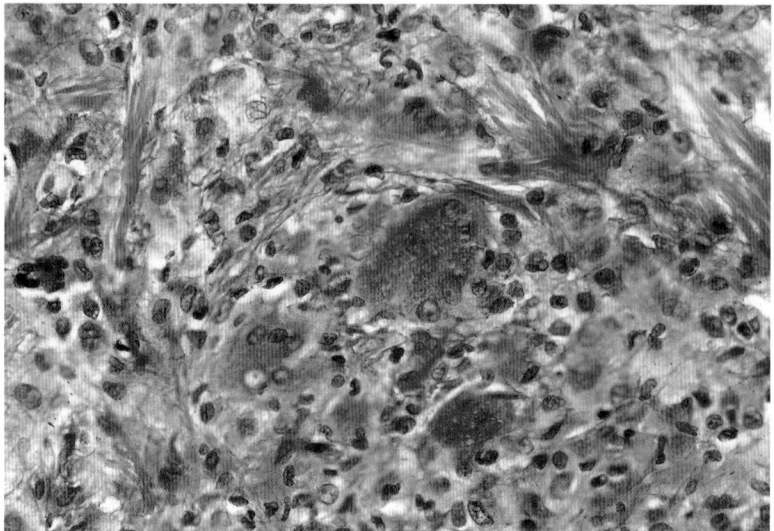

Fig. 29.329
Reticulohistiocytoma: the giant cells are PAS positive, diastase resistant.

HLH associated with inherited immune deficiencies (e.g., Chédiak-Higashi syndrome, X-linked lymphoproliferative syndrome, and Griscelli syndrome), and acquired HLH in patients with immune system defects. In the latter, HLH is triggered by severe infection with viruses (especially EBV and CMV), other infectious agents (e.g., leishmaniasis) or malignancy (particularly various lymphomas). HLH may also complicate autoimmune disease, including macrophage activation syndrome in systemic juvenile arthritis, adult-onset Still disease, and lupus erythematosus.[3]

Familial HLH occurs in around 1 in 50 000 live-born children and usually presents at <1 year of age, and exceptionally in older children and adults.[4–6] Acquired HLH tends to occur in older age groups.

The diagnostic criteria for HLH have been revised and are based on the signs and symptoms typically seen in hemophagocytic syndromes.[1] To establish the diagnosis, five of the following criteria should be present:
- fever,
- splenomegaly,
- cytopenias affecting more than two lineages,
- hypertriglyceridemia and/or hypofibrinogenemia,
- hemophagocytosis in bone marrow, spleen or lymph nodes,
- no evidence of malignancy,
- low or absent NK-cell activity,
- raised ferritin; and raised soluble CD25.

Alternatively, primary forms of the disease may be diagnosed if a specific genetic mutation consistent with familial HLH can be identified.[1]

Other clinical and laboratory findings often seen in HLH include cerebromeningeal symptoms, lymphadenopathy, jaundice, edema, skin rashes, abnormal liver function tests, hypoproteinemia, hyponatremia, raised very low density lipoprotein (VLDL), and reduced high density lipoprotein (HDL).[1] Skin manifestations are seen in up to 65% of patients and include a transient purpuric or hemorrhagic maculopapular eruption, erythroderma, and morbilliform erythema.[7]

Despite recent advances in treatment, only about 50% of patients are cured.[1,3,8]

Pathogenesis and histologic features

Natural killer (NK) cells play an important role in regulating the macrophage response following activation by various infectious agents. In all types of HLH, there appears to be a defect in NK target cell killing leading to uncontrolled activation of macrophages.[1,3,9,10] Familial HLH is characterized by defects in genes critical to cytotoxic granule formation, movement, or exocytosis. About 15–50% of cases have mutations in the perforin gene, 15–30% defects in the UNC13D gene, and other mutations in the STX11 gene.[3,11–19] Inherited disorders that predispose to the development of HLH also typically harbor defects in genes involved in cytotoxic granule formation and/or function, or key regulatory signaling effects of lymphocytes,

e.g., mutations in LYST in Chediak-Higashi syndrome or SH2D1a, or SAP in X-linked lymphoproliferative syndrome.[3,20–22] Molecular defects predisposing patients to other secondary HLH disorders have yet to be delineated.

The levels of many cytokines are raised in HLH, mostly as a consequence of this loss in regulatory processes, and they may account for some of the typical signs and symptoms. For example, raised interleukin-1 may be a cause of fever, and increased levels of TNF-α and IFN-γ may account for fatigue, wasting, and pancytopenia. TNF-α has also been implicated in down-regulation of lipoprotein lipase, explaining the raised serum triglycerides.[3]

Histologically, the infiltrate consists of mature lymphocytes (including activated forms) and macrophages showing phagocytosis of any or all hemopoietic elements, and particularly affecting the spleen, lymph nodes, bone marrow, liver, and CSF.[23] Cutaneous involvement occurs in less than 10% of cases, and the features are usually non-specific, consisting of a perivascular lymphohistiocytic infiltrate. Hemophagocytosis is rarely a feature.[7,23] The histiocytes are CD68 positive.

Crystal-storing histiocytosis

Clinical features

Crystal-storing histiocytosis is an extremely rare condition characterized by deposition of crystalline material in the cytoplasm of histiocytes.[1–3] About 90% of the cases have been described in patients with lymphoplasmacytic neoplasms, including lymphoplasmacytic lymphoma (immunocytoma), monoclonal gammopathy of uncertain significance, multiple myeloma, extramedullary plasmacytoma, MALT lymphoma, and large cell B-cell lymphoma.[1,4–8] Much more infrequently (in up to 10% of the cases), crystal-storing histiocytosis has been associated with non-neoplastic disorders, including various inflammatory diseases (e.g., rheumatoid arthritis, pulmonary infections, and Crohn disease), metabolic states (cystinosis), and drugs (clofazimine).[1] Localized variant, defined as a single deposit involving only one organ or site, and generalized variant of the disease, involving two or more distant organs or sites, have been recognized.[1]

Primary cutaneous involvement is exceptional, and the literature on this aspect is limited to six cases only, all associated with lymphoplasmacytic neoplasms.[3,9–11] These patients presented with either swelling, indurated plaques, pruritic rash, or erythematous asymptomatic subcutaneous nodules and tumors (Fig. 29.330) with no particular site of predilection. Cutaneous crystal-storing histiocytosis can develop early in the course of neoplastic disease and is not necessarily associated with an aggressive clinical course.[3]

Histologic features

The condition is characterized by the presence of histiocytes containing eosinophilic crystals which have been likened to Gaucher cells (pseudo-Gaucher cells) admixed with lymphoma cells (Fig. 29.331).[6] The crystals are variably polygonal to rhomboid or needle-shaped and stain positively with PAS and phosphotungstic acid hematoxylin (Fig. 29.332).[9,10] The crystals are usually composed of kappa light chain with no consistent association with any particular heavy chain.[3] Erythrophagocytosis may also be evident.[6]

The histiocytes express CD68, and sometimes immunoglobulin heavy and light chains may be stained weakly.[6]

Ultrastructurally, the crystals are sometimes membrane bound (of lysosomal derivation) and display platelike, rectangular, trapezoid, and rhomboid shapes with a distinct hexagonal lattice structure.[6,9,10] The tumor cells may also contain intracytoplasmic crystals.[6]

Follicular dendritic cell sarcoma and interdigitating dendritic cell sarcoma

Clinical features

Follicular dendritic cell (FDC) sarcoma and interdigitating dendritic cell (IDC) sarcoma are exceptional neoplasms of antigen-presenting dendritic cells. FDCs are of mesenchymal origin, reside in the primary and secondary lymphoid follicles, and play a major role in the induction and maintenance

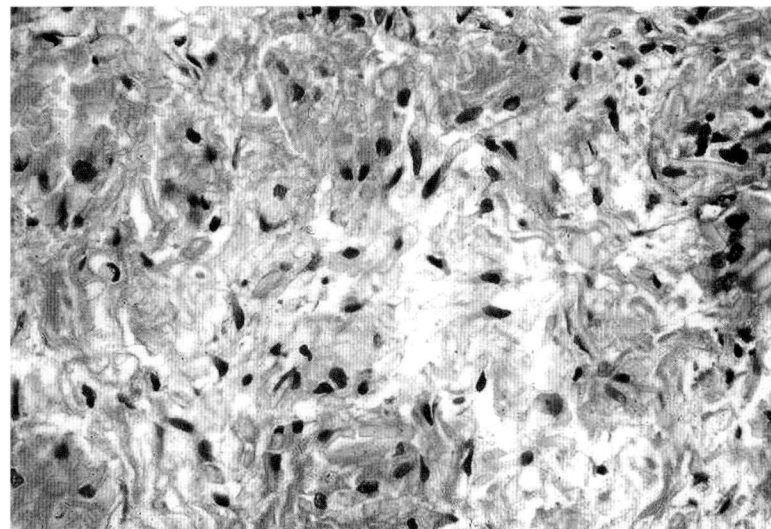

Fig. 29.332
Crystal-storing histiocytosis: the cytoplasm contains large eosinophilic crystals.

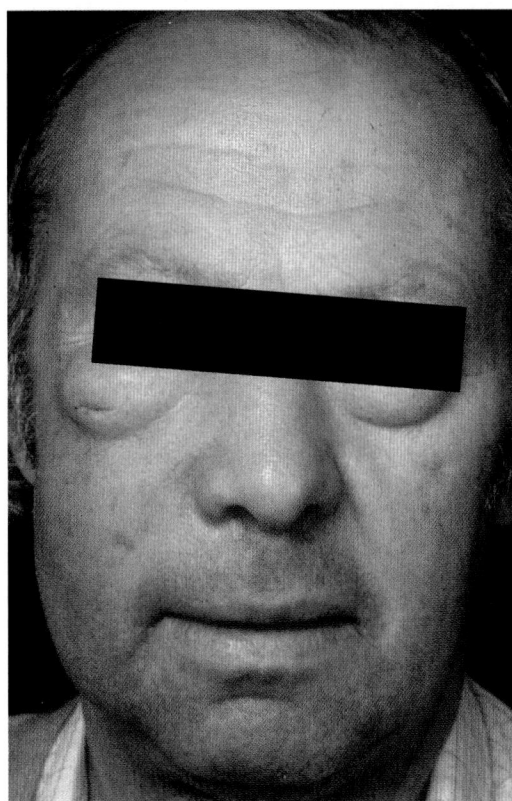

Fig. 29.330
Crystal-storing histiocytosis: this patient presented with marked swelling of the face and the eyelids.

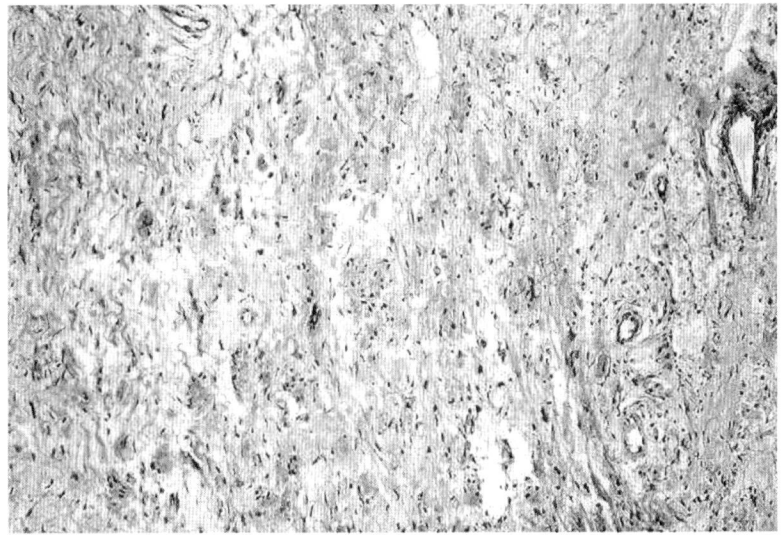

Fig. 29.331
Crystal-storing histiocytosis: within the dermis are large histiocytes with abundant eosinophilic cytoplasm.

of the humoral immune response.[1,2,3] IDCs are bone marrow-derived cells, typically found in the T-cell areas of peripheral lymphoid organs, and they stimulate resting T cells during a primary immune response.[2,4,5]

FDC and IDC sarcomas occur in a wide age range, including children, but most patients are adults, mainly in the fifth decade.[3,6–12] Sex distribution is about equal, apart from IPT-like FDC sarcomas, in which there is a marked female predominance.[3,6,7–9,11] Both tumor types arise most commonly in lymph nodes, particularly cervical lymph nodes for FDC sarcoma. Up to one-third of cases present at extranodal sites.[3,6,7–9] Extranodal FDC sarcoma has been most frequently reported in the upper aerodigestive tract (oral cavity and tonsil), soft tissues, liver, and gastrointestinal tract, whilst IDC sarcoma has been documented in the mediastinum, nasopharynx,

intestine, mesentery, spleen, and testes, among other sites.[3,6,11,12] Skin involvement in both types of tumor is very rare, and is often part of disseminated disease.[3,6,13–20]

Disease is localized at presentation in the majority of cases (77%), more frequently in FDC (85%) than IDC sarcoma (60%).[8] Clinical behavior is more that of a low-grade soft tissue sarcoma than lymphoma, with an intermediate risk of local recurrence and distant metastasis (≈30%).[3,6,21,22] Intra-abdominal location and large tumor size have also been associated with a poorer prognosis.[21,23]

Pathogenesis and histologic features

An association between FDC sarcoma and hyaline vascular CD has been reported, and it has been proposed that FDC proliferation in CD predisposes to dysplastic change, with evolution into FDC sarcoma.[3,17,21,24–26] EBV-encoded RNA is present in almost all tumor cells in a subset of IPT-like FDC sarcomas arising in the liver and spleen. The virus has been shown to be present in monoclonal and episomal forms.[27–31] BRAF mutations have been identified in FDC sarcoma, as have loss of function alterations in tumor suppressor genes involved in negative regulation of NF-κB activation and cell cycle progression.[32,33] In addition, some FDC sarcomas harbor copy number gains of 9p24, implicating PD-1L and PD-2L and immune evasion in disease pathogenesis.[34] A proportion of IDC sarcoma are also associated with hematological malignancies including CLL, follicular lymphoma, T-lymphoblastic leukemia, diffuse large B-cell lymphoma, and mycosis fungoides.[6]

The neoplastic cells in FDC sarcoma are spindled to oval in shape with eosinophilic cytoplasm and indistinct cell borders. Nuclei are oval or elongated with vesicular or finely granular chromatin, and generally small but distinct nucleoli. (Figs 29.333–29.335).[3,19,21] Nuclear pseudoinclusions are common and binucleate and multinucleate cells may be seen. Most cases appear cytologically bland, but significant atypia may be seen in some cases. The growth pattern is fascicular, storiform, sheetlike, or nodular. The mitotic count is variable (0–50/10 HPF) but usually relatively low (0–10/10 HPF). Areas of necrosis may be seen. Small lymphocytes, scattered between the tumor cells and forming perivascular aggregates, are common.[3,7,8,11]

IDC sarcoma shows a similar fascicular, storiform, and/or whorled growth pattern, and involves the T-cell areas in nodal forms. The tumor cells are large fusiform spindle-shaped cells with abundant eosinophilic cytoplasm and indistinct cell borders. Nuclei are spindled to ovoid with finely dispersed chromatin and distinct nucleoli of small to large size. Occasional multinucleate cells may be seen and the degree of cytological atypia is variable. The mitotic count is usually low (<5/10 HPF) and necrosis is rare. Lymphocytes, and less commonly plasma cells, are usually present. The morphology is very similar to, and often indistinguishable from, FDC sarcoma.[6,7,9]

Fig. 29.333
Follicular dendritic cell tumor: there is a heavy dermal infiltrate consisting of pale-staining follicular dendritic cells associated with a background population of lymphocytes. By courtesy of N.L. Harris, MD, Massachusetts General Hospital and Harvard Medical School, Boston, USA.

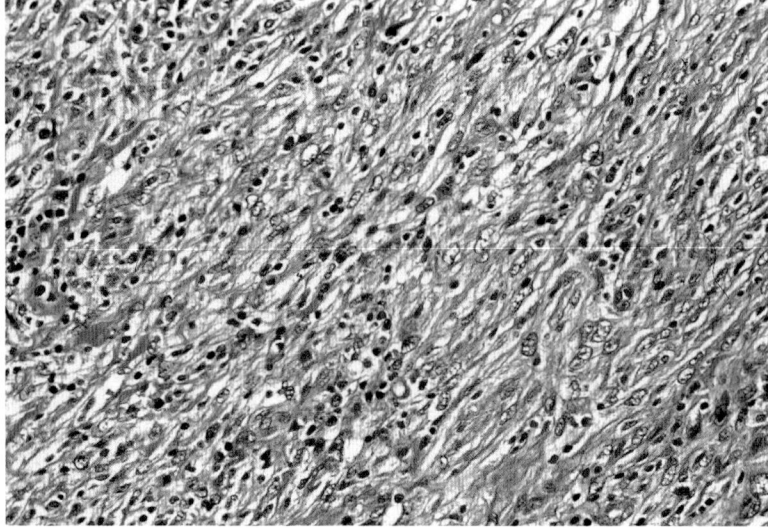

Fig. 29.334
Follicular dendritic cell tumor: the tumor cells are arranged in loose fascicles. By courtesy of N.L. Harris, MD, Massachusetts General Hospital and Harvard Medical School, Boston, USA.

Tumor cells in FDC sarcoma react positively with one or more FDC makers, including CD21, CD23, CD35, KiMP4, and CAN.42.[3,7,8,19] CXCL13 and clusterin have been proposed as useful markers for FDC sarcoma, particularly with respect to other dendritic cell tumors.[34–36] Staining for vimentin, fascin, epidermal growth factor receptor, HLA-DR, and desmoplakin is often positive. CD68, S100, and EMA are variably expressed.[7,19,37,38] Cytokeratin is very rare and when present is seen in <10% of neoplastic cells.[11] Rarely, tumor cells express CD20 and/or CD45.[19] Staining for CD1a, lysosyme, myeloperoxidase, CD34, CD3, CD79A, CD30, and HMB-45 is negative. The admixed small lymphocytes may be predominantly B or T cells or a mixture of both.[19,21]

In IDC sarcoma, tumor cells are consistently S100 and vimentin positive, and CD1a and langerin negative. Variable, often weak, reactivity is seen with antibodies to CD68, lysosyme, and CD45. FDC markers (CD21, CD23, CD35, CAN.42), myeloperoxidase, CD34, markers of B- and T-cell lineage, CD30, EMA, and cytokeratins are negative. The background small lymphocytes are almost always T cells.[6,7,9,19]

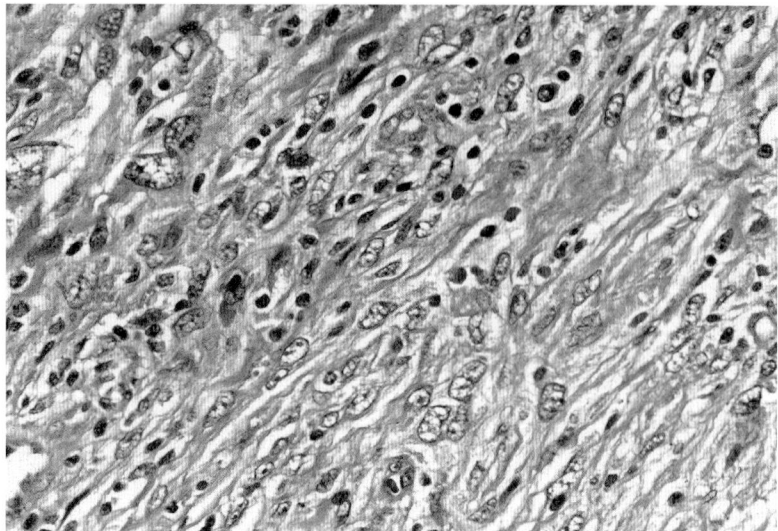

Fig. 29.335
Follicular dendritic cell tumor: the spindle cells have eosinophilic cytoplasm and elongated vesicular nuclei. By courtesy of N.L. Harris, MD, Massachusetts General Hospital and Harvard Medical School, Boston, USA.

Ultrastructurally, cells in FDC sarcoma are characterized by villous processes united by desmosomal attachments.[21] Birbeck granules and lysosomes are absent. IDC sarcoma possesses complex interdigitating cell junctions lacking well-formed desmosomes. Scattered lysosomes may be present but there are no Birbeck granules.[19]

Differential diagnosis

FDC and IDC sarcomas are underrecognized, particularly at extranodal sites, and up to one-third of cases are misdiagnosed at initial evaluation.[11,19,39] Once FDC and IDC sarcoma enter the differential diagnosis, appropriate immunohistochemistry should permit reliable distinction from each other, and from other neoplasms, such as Langerhans cell histiocytosis and LCS, HS, melanoma, and spindle cell carcinoma.

Histiocytic sarcoma

Histiocytic sarcoma (HS) (histiocytic lymphoma, malignant histiocytosis) is a very rare malignant proliferation of cells displaying morphological and immunophenotypic features of mature histiocytes.[1,2] Many cases diagnosed before the era of immunohistochemistry and molecular techniques are now recognized to be examples of diffuse large B-cell lymphoma, anaplastic large cell lymphoma, or other NHLs.[3–8] The historical literature is therefore difficult to interpret. However, there are a few well-documented, bona fide reports of HS including a few larger cohorts.[2,8–23]

Most patients are adults in the fourth or fifth decade of life but the age range is wide.[2,8,19,23] A male predominance is reported in some series.[8,19,23] The majority of lesions appear to arise at extranodal sites, particularly the intestinal tract, skin, and soft tissues.[1,2,8,9,15,16,18–23] Involvement of the spleen, CNS, and other extranodal sites is rare.[10–13,17,21,23,24] Cutaneous lesions are most often described as red or violaceous nodules. Rare cases present with systemic disease and multiple sites of involvement ('malignant histiocytosis').[7,23,25] Some patients present with fever, weight loss, hepatosplenomegaly, and pancytopenia.[8,19,23]

The majority of patients (70%) present with advanced-stage disease (stage III or IV), which is associated with a 60–80% mortality.[1,2,8,23] However, more localized disease may be seen, in which case the outcome appears more favorable.[19,23]

Pathogenesis and histologic features

The etiology and pathogenesis of HS are unknown. Few cases are associated with mediastinal germ cell tumors, mostly malignant teratoma plus or minus yolk sac tumor. This raises the possibility that HS derives from the same progenitor cell as the germ cell tumor.[26,27] Other cases occur in

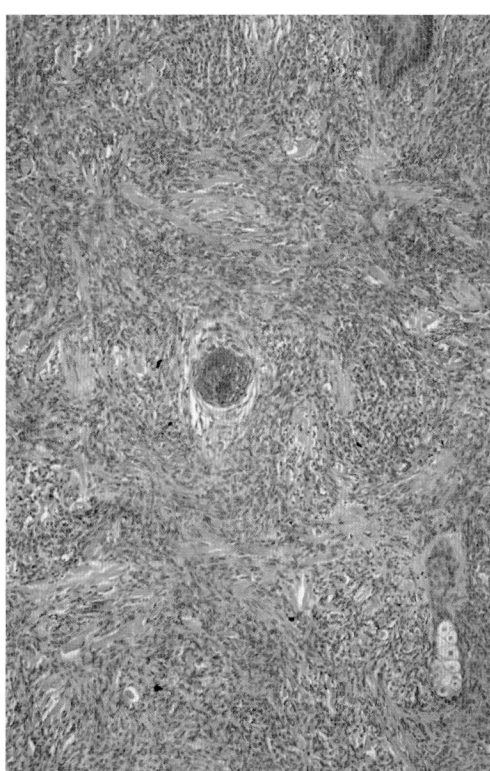

Fig. 29.336
Histiocytic sarcoma: there is a dense cellular infiltrate extending from the dermis into subcutaneous fat. By courtesy of C.D.M. Fletcher, MD, Brigham and Women's Hospital and Harvard Medical School, Boston, USA.

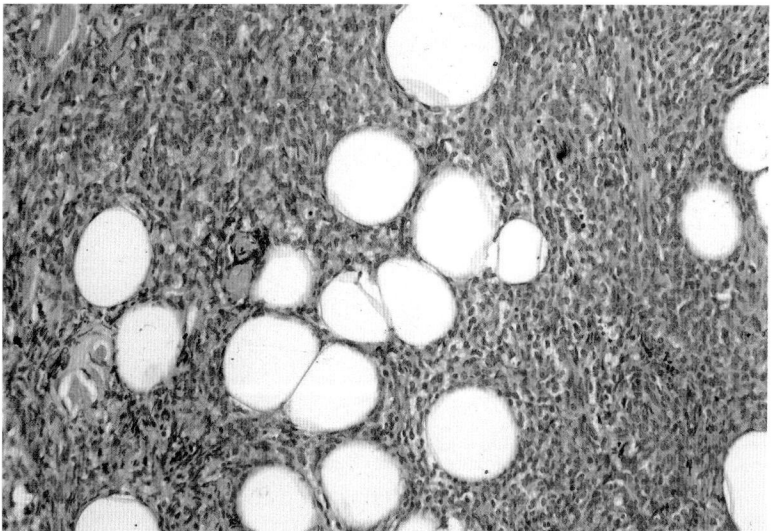

Fig. 29.337
Histiocytic sarcoma: the infiltrate extends into the subcutaneous fat. By courtesy of C.D.M. Fletcher, MD, Brigham and Women's Hospital and Harvard Medical School, Boston, USA.

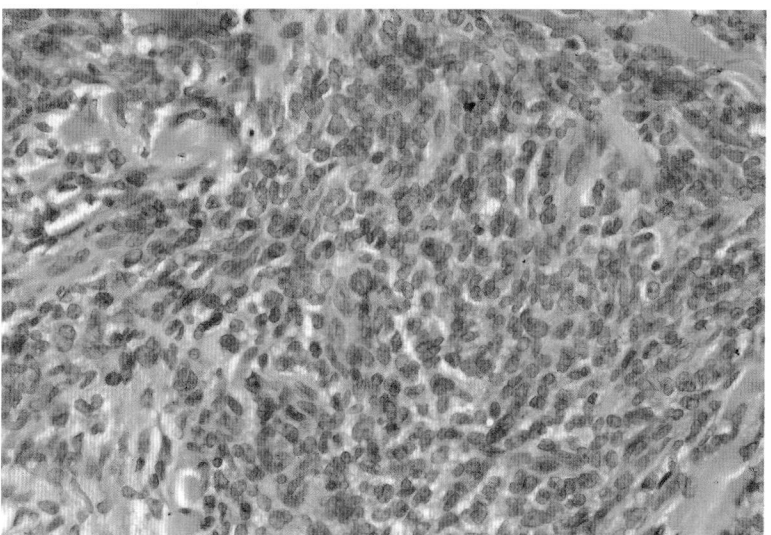

Fig. 29.338
Histiocytic sarcoma: the histiocytes have eosinophilic cytoplasm and vesicular nuclei. By courtesy of C.D.M. Fletcher, MD, Brigham and Women's Hospital and Harvard Medical School, Boston, USA.

association with other hematological malignancies, including NHL, myelodysplasia, and leukemia.[2,8,19,23,28] In a small cohort of tumors, the same BCL2 translocation and/or immunoglobulin gene rearrangement as the follicular lymphoma with which they were associated was demonstrated.[29] Thus, some neoplasms may arise as a consequence of transdifferentiation, alterations in transcription factor expression resulting in malignant lymphoid cells being diverted to a histiocytic pathway of differentiation.[29] Mutations of the *BRAF* gene have been identified in a relatively high proportion of cases in one study.[30]

Histologically, there is a diffuse, often 'bottom heavy', extension from the reticular dermis into the subcutis (*Figs 29.336* and *29.337*). Epidermotropism is not a feature and a grenz zone is frequently evident.[23] Tumor cells are large with moderate to abundant eosinophilic cytoplasm and often with fine vacuoles (*Fig. 29.338*). Nuclei tend to be eccentrically placed. They range from round to oval vesicular to multilobed, twisted, and sometimes bizarre variants occasionally mimicking Hodgkin or Reed-Sternberg cells.[3,14,20] Nucleoli are prominent and frequently multiple. Mitotic activity is variable; mitoses are generally conspicuous and often abnormal.[8,19,23] Spindle cell sarcoma-like features with a storiform growth pattern and xanthomatous forms may occur.[19,20,23] Erythrophagocytosis is infrequent.[23] Lymphophagocytosis may be a feature.[19,20,23] Areas of necrosis may be seen, but are not usually extensive, and vascular invasion is rare.[8,19,22] A prominent inflammatory cell infiltrate consisting of lymphocytes, neutrophils, and occasionally eosinophils and plasma cells is sometimes seen.[1,19,23]

Immunohistochemistry shows positivity for CD163, CD68, and/or lysozyme, the latter often showing accentuation in the Golgi region (*Figs 29.339* and *29.340*).[1,8,19,23,31] There is often weak positive staining for CD45, CD45RO, and CD4, and occasionally weak expression of CD15.[1,19,21–23] Staining for S100, usually weak and focal, is sometimes seen, suggesting a degree of dendritic cell differentiation.[8,19,23] CD1a, and even langerin staining, is exceptional but only in a very small minority of cells.[19,32] In such instances, it may be difficult or impossible to distinguish HS from LCS. Markers of other specific lines of differentiation, including FDC (CD21, CD35), lymphocyte (CD3, CD5, CD20, CD79a, pax5), myeloid (CD33,

myeloperoxidase), melanocytic (HMB-45, Melan A), and epithelial (cytokeratins) are absent.[1,8,19,23]

Ultrastructurally, the tumor cells have conspicuous lysosomes. Birbeck granules, desmosomal attachments, and interdigitating junctions are absent.[8,14,23]

In most cases, the antigen receptor genes are in a germline configuration. However, clonal immunoglobulin and T-cell receptor gene rearrangements have been rarely documented.[3,28] The explanation for this may be transdifferentiation from pre-existing NHLs, or the so-called 'lineage promiscuity' due to the primitive nature of the neoplastic cells.[2,8,29]

Differential diagnosis

Diagnosis of HS is dependent on demonstrating a histiocytic lineage in the tumor cells, while excluding other lines of differentiation, and is often a diagnosis of exclusion. Undifferentiated diffuse large B-cell lymphoma, anaplastic large cell lymphoma, and other NHLs can usually be recognized or reliably excluded if a broad immunohistochemical panel is employed. Melanocytic neoplasms usually express HMB-45 and/or melan A, and undifferentiated carcinomas one of the many keratins. Acute myeloid leukemia (AML) should react with CD33 and sometimes myeloperoxidase.

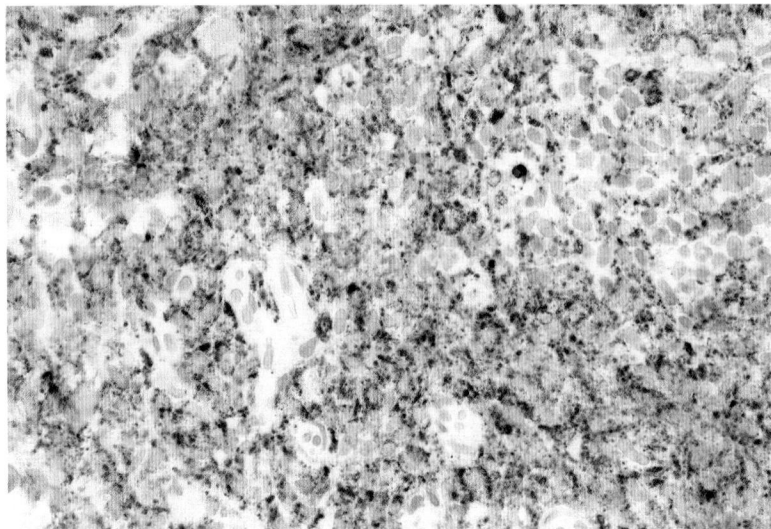

Fig. 29.339
Histiocytic sarcoma: the tumor cells express CD68. By courtesy of C.D.M.
Fletcher, Brigham and Women's Hospital and Harvard Medical School, Boston,
USA.

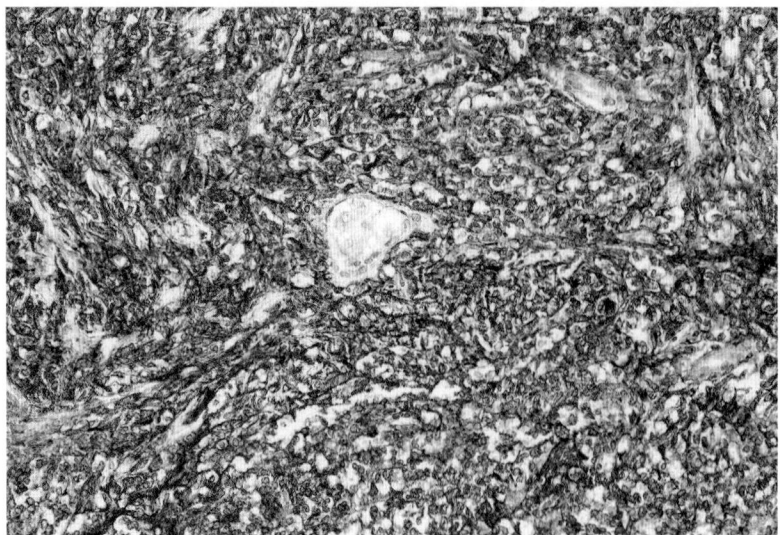

Fig. 29.340
Histiocytic sarcoma: note the diffuse lysozyme expression. By courtesy of C.D.M.
Fletcher, Brigham and Women's Hospital and Harvard Medical School, Boston,
USA.

CUTANEOUS LEUKEMIC INFILTRATES AND PRECURSOR CELL NEOPLASMS

Introduction

Leukemias are neoplastic proliferations of leukocytes and their precursors in the bone marrow and peripheral blood. The subtypes can be broadly categorized into those of myeloid and lymphoid cells, as well as into tumors of mature leukocytes ('chronic leukemias') or their blast-cell precursors ('acute leukemias). Not surprisingly, in view of high levels of circulating tumor cells, leukemic infiltrates often involve other tissues. The manifestations of several of the chronic leukemias (e.g., CLL, adult T-cell lymphoma/leukemia) are discussed elsewhere in this chapter, as are several lymphomas and myeloproliferative neoplasms that may present in skin and have a leukemic phase (e.g., MCL, mastocytosis). Chronic myeloid and myelomonocytic leukemias may also involve the skin, but only rarely.[1-3] This section deals primarily with malignant neoplasms of hematopoietic precursor cells that may present with cutaneous disease, i.e., AML, blastic plasmacytoid dendritic cell neoplasm, and precursor lymphoblastic leukemia/lymphoma (LLL).

A detailed account of precursor cell neoplasms is beyond the scope of this textbook, and the following is only a very general overview. Historically, the French–American–British (FAB) system was used to classify cases of AML. This was morphologically based on and related to the type and degree of differentiation of the constituent blast cells. However, over recent years it has become increasingly apparent that a number of specific genetic alterations are found in AML, and these predict for clinical behavior and outcome. These were incorporated into the 2001 WHO classification, and used to define a category of 'AML with recurrent genetic abnormalities'. Other categories recognized at this time included AML with multilineage dysplasia, therapy-related AML, and AML, not otherwise categorized. The latter group was subdivided on morphological grounds using a modified FAB approach, and included cases of myeloid sarcoma (MS).[4-9]

The updated WHO classification published in 2008 further refined this classification. Two changes are of particular relevance to the skin. First, MS was recognized as a specific subtype for the first time. In addition, the entity previously known as 'blastic NK cell lymphoma' was renamed 'blastic plasmacytoid dendritic cell neoplasm', and moved from the general category of neoplasms of mature T cells and NK cells into the category of variants of AML.[10,11] Although the principles of classification remain the same, the 2016 update of the WHO classification further refine the diagnostic criteria and categories to accommodate advances in knowledge, particularly with respect to recent discoveries in gene mutations.[12] Importantly, blastic

plasmacytoid dendritic cell neoplasm and MS remain as distinct entities, the latter as a unique presentation of AML of any subtype.[12]

Tumors of lymphoid precursors are referred to as lymphoblastic leukemias and/or lymphomas. They are subdivided into those of T-cell type and those derived from B cells. B-LLL is further subclassified according to the presence of specific genetic abnormalities that correlate with distinctive clinical or phenotypic properties with prognostic implications.[13-15] As with AML, diagnostic criteria have been refined and new provisional entities added to both T- and B-cell categories.[12]

The dermatological manifestations of leukemia include a wide variety of non-specific lesions such as purpura and ecchymoses, adverse drug reactions, opportunistic infections, acute or chronic graft-versus-host disease, leukocytoclastic vasculitis, pyoderma gangrenosum, Sweet disease, and a rare intraepidermal vesicular eruption mimicking transient acantholytic dermatosis (Grover disease) and Hailey-Hailey disease.[16-18] Leukemic vasculitis may also be encountered.[19] Non-specific cutaneous lesions may also be seen in patients with myelodysplastic syndromes, hematological disorders that are characterized by chronic refractory cytopenias, infections, and hemorrhage.[2,3,20,21] These include cutaneous vasculitis, photosensitivity, prurigo nodularis, Sweet disease, pyoderma gangrenosum, erythema elevatum diutinum, subcorneal pustular dermatosis, and relapsing polychondritis.[22-28]

Myeloid sarcoma

Clinical features

Myeloid sarcoma (MS) is defined as a tumor or mass of myeloblasts, with or without maturation, occurring at a site other than the bone marrow. The term leukemia cutis is often used to denote cases with skin involvement. MS occurs in the absence of other evidence of acute myeloid leukemia (ML) in about 25% of cases. A diagnosis of MS equates with one of AML, and the patient should be investigated, classified, and treated accordingly.[1-6] In 35% of cases, MS is diagnosed simultaneously with another hematological malignancy, most frequently AML, but sometimes a myeloproliferative neoplasm or a myelodysplastic syndrome.[1-3,7-10] In the remaining cases (approximately 40%), there is a previous history of hematological malignancy or myelodysplasia.[1-3,11-13] Thus, MS may be the first sign of relapse in a patient with AML previously in complete remission, or indicate transformation to acute leukemia in patients with myeloproliferative disorders or

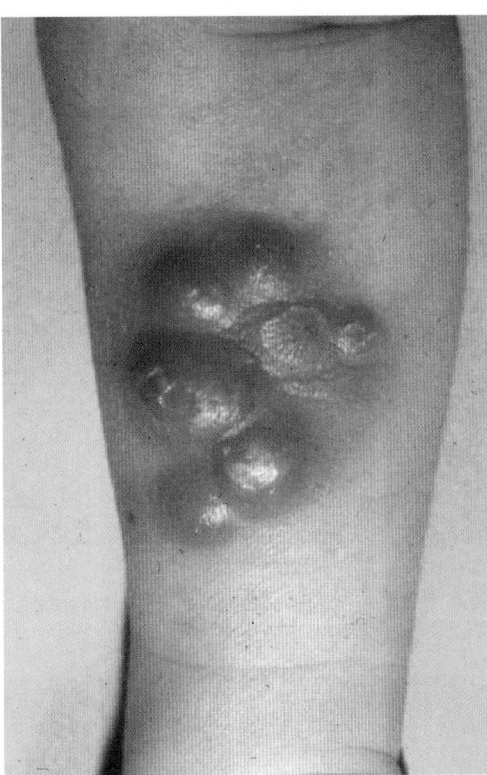

Fig. 29.341
Myeloid sarcoma: there are erythematous nodules on the medial aspect of the lower leg of this young child.

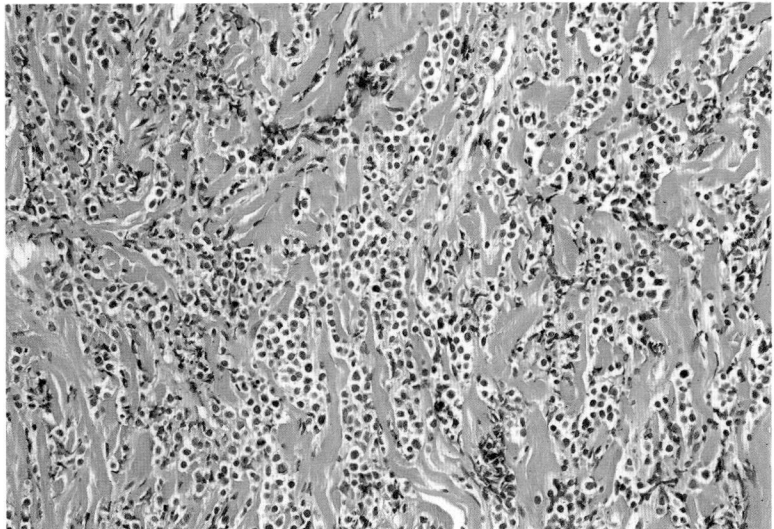

Fig. 29.342
Myeloid sarcoma: there is a heavy dermal infiltrate with prominent dissection of collagen.

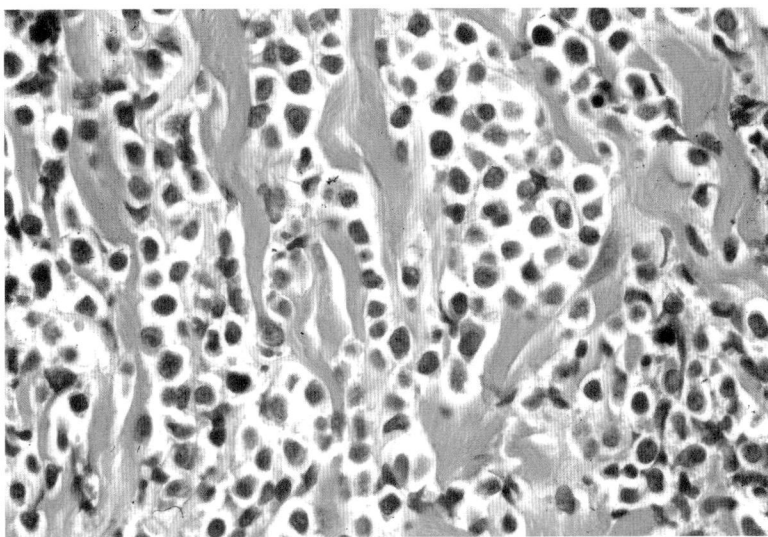

Fig. 29.343
Myeloid sarcoma: the blast cells have darkly staining nuclei and minimal cytoplasm.

myelodysplastic syndromes. The commonest sites of presentation are in the skin (28.2%), lymph nodes (16.35%), testes (6.5%), intestine (6.5%), bone (3.25%), and CNS (3.25%), although virtually any tissue may be affected.[2,3]

Cutaneous MS is relatively uncommon and reported in between 2% and 30% of AML patients.[14–19] There is an equal sex incidence, and it is seen in a wide range of ages.[11,14,20,21] There is no clear site predilection, and the clinical appearances are varied and often non-specific. Erythematous or violaceous papules and nodules (which may be purpuric) are the most frequent clinical findings, but infiltrative plaques and, less commonly, macules, ulcers, and rarely blisters, are also sometimes seen (*Fig. 29.341*).[20–23] Oral manifestations are not uncommon and include papules, nodules, and ulcers. Gingival hypertrophy may be found in patients with acute monocytic and myelomonocytic leukemia.[22–27]

Previously, it was suggested that skin involvement by AML was a poor prognostic indicator.[15,28,29] However, a large study of MS showed that clinical behavior and response to therapy was not influenced by age, sex, anatomic location, de novo presentation, clinical history related to other myeloid neoplasms, histologic features, immunophenotype, or cytogenetic findings.[2] Patients treated with intensive chemotherapy and bone marrow transplantation have the best chance of survival.[2,30]

Pathogenesis and histologic features

The pathogenesis of MS is theoretically the same as for AML. In the few cytogenetic studies performed, an increased incidence of MLL rearrangements, monosomy 7, and trisomy 8 have been noted.[2,18,31] Mutations of nucleophosmin-1 are also frequent, as they are in AML as a whole.[3] A high incidence of t(8;21)(q22;q22) has also been reported, and appears to be associated with pediatric and/or orbital tumors.[2,32–35]

Cutaneous lesions consist of a moderate to dense dermal infiltrate, displaying a nodular or diffuse growth pattern, and sometimes involving the subcutis. Perivascular or periadnexal accentuation is frequent. The epidermis is typically spared.[11,14,21,36,37] The tumor cell cytology is variable and dependent on the direction and degree of differentiation. Most cases comprise medium to large blasts, which often infiltrate in rows between collagen bundles, and frequently display a monoblastic or myelomonocytic

appearance.[2,11,15,36,37] Varying degrees of granulocytic differentiation may be seen, and immature eosinophils are common (*Figs 29.342 and 29.343*).[21,29]

The immunophenotype varies depending on the degree and type of maturation present. In cutaneous MS, this is often monocytic or monoblastic in nature. There may be expression of myeloid markers, such as myeloperoxidase, CD33, and CD117, but often at lower frequency compared to AML confined to bone marrow. Conversely, expression of CD4, CD14, CD68, and CD163 is more frequent. CD56 may also be expressed, but CD123 and CD303 are only present in a small minority, and CD34 is often also negative.[11,20,36,37]

Differential diagnosis

The main differential diagnoses include blastic plasmacytoid dendritic cell neoplasm, LLL, large B-cell lymphomas, and small round blue cell tumors of childhood. Immunohistochemistry and clinical information should make the diagnosis relatively easy, although a broad range of antibodies may be required. The greatest overlap is with blastic plasmacytoid dendritic cell neoplasm, and this is most reliably distinguished by demonstrating evidence of plasmacytoid dendritic cell differentiation (e.g., CD123, BDCA-2) and absence of myeloid markers other than CD33 (e.g., myeloperoxidase).

Blastic plasmacytoid dendritic cell neoplasm

The cell of origin of blastic plasmacytoid dendritic cell neoplasm (BPDCN) has proven elusive, resulting in a variety of terms including:

- blastic NK-cell lymphoma,
- agranular CD4+ NK-cell leukemia,
- blastic NK-cell leukemia/lymphoma,
- agranular CD4+CD56+ hematodermic neoplasm/tumor.[1–6]

However, BPDCN has been demonstrated to derive from precursors of plasmacytoid dendritic cells, hence the new name and its grouping together with variants of AML in the most recent WHO classification.[7–10]

BPDCN accounts for <1% of all acute leukemia cases and 0.7% of cutaneous lymphomas.[8,11,12] There is no known racial or ethnic predilection. The male/female ratio is ≥3:1.[8,10] The age range is wide (<1–103 years), but most patients are elderly.[8,13–15] Almost all cases have cutaneous lesions at presentation, and there is frequent involvement of bone marrow and peripheral blood (60–90%) and lymph nodes (40–50%), although virtually any organ can be affected.[5,13–16]

Lesions may be solitary or often multiple, affecting the trunk, head, and extremities.[13–17] They are typically erythematous or red-brown nodules, tumors, or plaques, or bruise-like lesions.[8,10,13–17] Rare cases remain localized to the skin for lengthy periods (i.e., >6 months). More commonly, the clinical course is aggressive with involvement of bone marrow, peripheral blood, and other sites, and the development of cytopenia.[2,8,10,17,18] Initial responses to treatment are relatively common, but most patients relapse within a short space of time. Median survival is only 12–14 months.[8,10,18] Exceptional patients have a better prognosis with long-term remissions; mostly young patients, those treated with allogeneic stem cell transplants, and possibly those with a more immature plasmacytoid dendritic cell phenotype.[5,16–21] Patients receiving ALL/lymphoma-type induction therapy seem to fare slightly better than those receiving AML-type therapy.[18]

In 10–20% of cases, BPDCN are associated with, or develop into, a myelodysplastic syndrome, myelomonocytic leukemia, or AML.[5,13–17,22–24]

Pathogenesis and histology

A derivation from precursors of plasmacytoid dendritic cells is now well established on the basis of antigen and chemokine receptor expression, in vitro functional assays, gene expression profiling, and studies on a tumor-derived cell line.[8,9,16,20] Cytogenetic analysis has mostly revealed complex karyotypes with no specific abnormalities, but consistent changes including recurring anomalies affecting 5q21 or 5q34, 12:12p13, or chromosome 13, loss of 6q or del 6q23-qtr, monosomy 15p, and monosomy 9.[23] A CGH array study has identified recurrent alterations in chromosome 4, chromosome 9, and chromosome 13, at sites containing tumor suppressor genes, but again none is specific for BPDCN.[9] There is no association with EBV.[11,17]

Histologically, there is a monotonous dermal infiltrate that may extend into the subcutis, but typically spares the epidermis (Fig. 29.344).[8,10,15,17] Angioinvasion and coagulative necrosis are not usually seen. The infiltrate consists of medium-sized blasts possessing irregular nuclei with finely dispersed chromatin and one to several small nucleoli (Fig. 29.345). Cytoplasm is moderate or scanty, agranular, and usually slightly basophilic ('gray-blue').

The blast cells characteristically express CD4, CD43, and CD56, although both CD56- and CD4-negative variants have been described.[13] Markers of plasmacytoid dendritic cells, such as CD123 (interleukin-3α-chain receptor), BDCA2 (CD303), and TCL1, are also found.[13] CD68 reactivity is seen in more than half of cases, and CD7, CD33, and TdT may also be expressed.[8,13,19] One study suggests that there may be a spectrum of differentiation within BPDCN, the most primitive examples expressing TdT but not BDCA2 or CD7, whilst the more mature lesions are TdT negative but positive for BDCA2 and CD7; the latter have a worse prognosis.[19] Staining for other T cell, B cell, and myeloid markers is usually negative.[10,13,17]

In most instances, the B-cell and T-cell receptor genes are in a germline configuration. Clonal T-cell receptor rearrangement is rarely seen.[5,16,17,24]

Differential diagnosis

Blastic plasmacytoid dendritic cell neoplasm must be differentiated from other blastic malignancies expressing CD56. Extranodal NK/T-cell lymphoma lacks CD4 and is consistently positive for EBV. In the 10–20% of

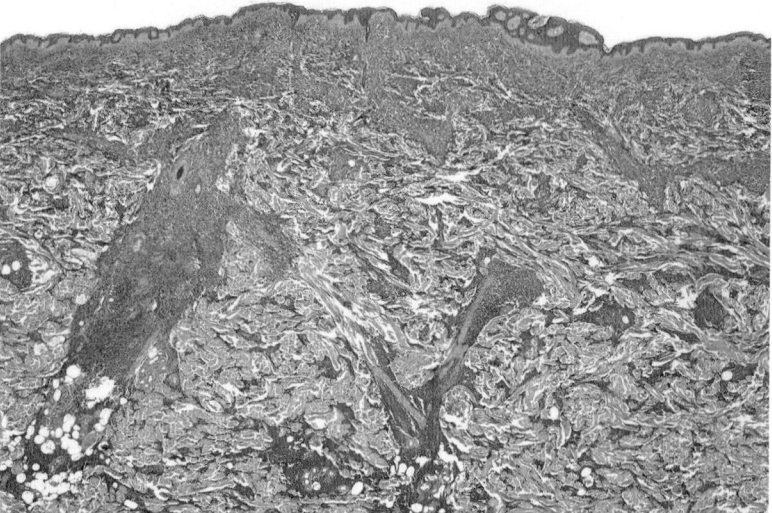

Fig. 29.344
Blastic plasmacytoid dendritic cell neoplasm: there is a dense perivascular, perifollicular, and interstitial cellular infiltrate.

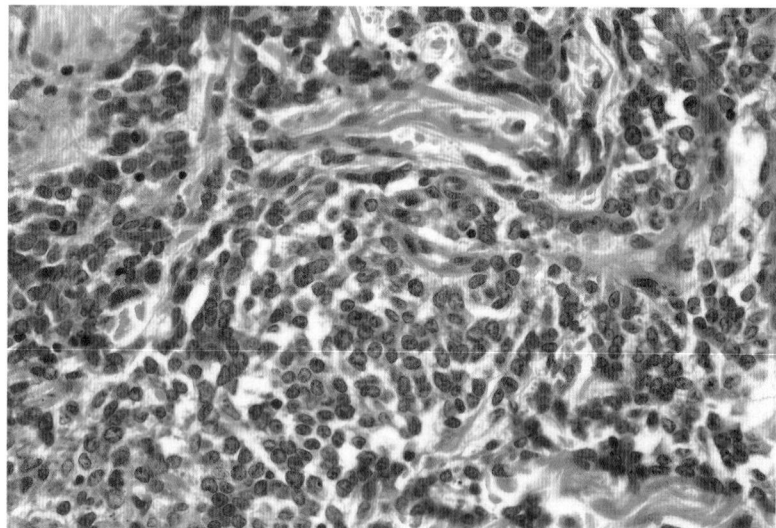

Fig. 29.345
Blastic plasmacytoid dendritic cell neoplasm: the infiltrate consists of a uniform population of cells with basophilic cytoplasm, round to oval nuclei, and small nucleoli.

AML cases that are CD4 and/or CD56 positive, distinction is more difficult. Expression of myeloid markers other than CD33 favors a diagnosis of AML, while detection of plasmacytoid dendritic cell markers such as CD123 or BDCA2 points toward BPDCN. Mature T-cell lymphomas involving the skin may also express CD56, with or without CD4, but these generally show features typical for other specific entities such as anaplastic large cell lymphoma, lymphomatoid papulosis, and mycosis fungoides. Care must be taken to distinguish BPDCN from the massive accumulation of plasmacytoid dendritic cells that is occasionally seen at nodal or extranodal sites in patients with myeloid neoplasia, particularly chronic myelomonocytic leukemia. The latter are morphologically mature and CD56 negative.[25]

Precursor lymphoblastic leukemia/lymphoma

Lymphoblastic leukemia/lymphomas (LLLs) are neoplasms of lymphoid precursor cells (lymphoblasts) of T or B lineage. Conventionally, the term lymphoma is used when the disease is a mass with no or minimal peripheral blood or bone marrow involvement; leukemia is reserved for cases with extensive blood and bone marrow involvement.[1,2] The majority of lymphoblastic leukemias are of B-cell type, whilst ≈90% of lymphoblastic lymphomas are of T lineage.[2,3] However, T-lymphoblastic lymphoma typically presents with disease in the mediastinum and lymph nodes, whereas

B-lymphoblastic lymphoma displays a predilection for skin, soft tissue, bone, and lymph nodes.[2,4,5,6] Thus, infiltrates of B lymphoblasts are the most frequently encountered form of precursor lymphoid neoplasm in the skin.[7–12]

Cutaneous LLL of all types account for <10% of cutaneous lymphoid malignancies.[13–15] Most patients are children or young adults. The typical presentation is with an erythematous or violaceous nodule or tumor, cases of B-lymphoblastic lymphoma showing a predilection for the head and neck region.[4,8,16,17] Cutaneous disease may occur in isolation (so-called 'primary cutaneous lymphoblastic lymphoma') or be associated with other extranodal deposits and/or a leukemic component.[4,10,18–20] However, even in solitary skin disease, patients should always be regarded as having systemic disease.

LLL is an aggressive neoplasm but is often responsive to treatment. The prognosis is more favorable in children, and better for B-LLL than T-LLL, at least in younger patients. Cure rates in children with B-LLL are ≈80%.[1,2,21] Cutaneous involvement does not appear to be a poor prognostic indicator.[7]

Pathogenesis and histologic features

LLLs is associated with a complex series of genetic abnormalities, some of which correlate with pathogenesis and clinical outcome.[1,2,21,22]

Histologically, there is a monotonous diffuse dermal infiltrate consisting of medium-sized blasts with scanty basophilic cytoplasm, finely dispersed chromatin, and inconspicuous or small but distinct nucleoli. The nuclear contours may be smooth or irregular but do not correlate with lineage. Mitotic figures are frequent. Tumor cells are often seen dissecting between collagen bundles, and crush artifact is frequent.[4,5,13,16,17]

There is consistent expression of TdT, CD43, and CD99.[8,10,16,17,23] Tumor cells are often also CD10 positive, particularly in B-cell neoplasms, but may be negative for CD45.[4,16,17] Neoplasms of T lineage are usually CD7 positive, showing variable expression of other T-cell markers such as CD1a, CD2, CD3, CD4, CD5, and CD8.[17,24] Cases of B-LLL express one or more B-cell-associated antigens, most frequently pax5, CD19, and CD79a, and less often CD20.[4,13,16,17] Both T-LLL and B-LLL may occasionally express myeloid markers such as CD33, but myeloperoxidase is always negative.[1,2,21]

Clonal immunoglobulin heavy chain and T-cell receptor gene rearrangements are usually seen in B-LLL and T-LLL, respectively. Light chain gene rearrangements are less frequently found, as they occur later in B-cell ontogeny. Lineage infidelity is frequent, i.e., T-cell receptor gene rearrangements in B-lineage neoplasms or immunoglobulin gene rearrangements in T-cell neoplasms.[4,25,26]

Differential diagnosis

The main differential diagnosis is with other blast cell neoplasms, including AML, blastic plasmacytoid dendritic cell neoplasm, and blastic forms of lymphoma (e.g., large B-cell lymphomas, extranodal T/NK-cell lymphoma), and small round blue cell tumors. A broad panel of antibodies is required to facilitate distinction of AML and blastic plasmacytoid dendritic cell neoplasm (see above), while the presence of TdT will exclude cases of lymphomas of mature/peripheral lymphocytes with blast cell morphology. Other small cell tumors of childhood lack TdT, as well as specific T-cell or B-cell antigens such as CD7 and CD79a.[18]

Cutaneous extramedullary hematopoiesis

Clinical features

Extramedullary hematopoiesis (EMH) (myeloid metaplasia) describes the development of hematopoietic tissue outside the bone marrow. Most frequently, EMH is associated with an underlying myeloproliferative neoplasm or myelodysplastic syndrome, usually chronic idiopathic myelofibrosis.[1–9] Rarely, it is seen following marrow replacement by lymphoma or metastatic carcinoma, in storage disorders, and in patients with severe anemia from many causes, including hereditary spherocytosis, sickle cell anemia, Rhesus incompatibility, and twin-to-twin transfusion.[5,7] It has also been described following severe intrauterine infection and in patients receiving myeloid growth factors.[5,7,10,11]

EMH is mainly seen in the liver and spleen. EMH elsewhere is rare.[10,12–14] The clinical presentation in skin is variable, lesions being described as solitary or multiple, skin colored or red-purple papules, nodules, and plaques. Ulcers and blisters are rare.[5,7,12,13] EMH may rarely present as an incidental finding in pilomatricoma, spindle cell lipoma, pachydermoperiostosis, and pyogenic granuloma.[10,15–20]

Pathogenesis and histologic features

The pathogenesis of EMH is unknown and possibly multifactorial. EMH associated with myeloid disorders probably results from displacement of abnormal hematopoietic stem cells.[21,22] It may also represent a compensatory phenomenon following marrow replacement by fibrosis or by neoplastic cells. Another hypothesis is that locally or systemically produced myelostimulatory factors induce extramedullary differentiation of adult stem cells into cells of hematopoietic lineage. This last theory may explain the incidental localized occurrence of EMH in cutaneous lesions in the absence of underlying bone marrow abnormalities.[10,15]

Histologically, EMH consists of varying proportions of erythroid (nucleated) precursors, immature granulocytes, and megakaryocytes. The last may secrete fibrogenic cytokines with resultant fibrosis and the development of a so-called sclerosing extramedullary hematopoietic tumor.[8] In some examples, one or more of the three main cell lines is inconspicuous and the appearances of the hematopoietic precursors may provide a clue to the nature of the underlying abnormality. For example, large atypical megakaryocytes are sometimes seen in cases associated with idiopathic myelofibrosis, prominent granulopoiesis in patients with chronic myeloid leukemia, and erythropoiesis in polycythemia vera or hemolytic anemias.[10,13,21,22]

In cases associated with spindle cell lipoma and pilomatrixoma, EMH is seen in the marrow spaces between bony trabeculae, and is present in the stroma of the pyogenic granuloma-associated cases.[15–20]

Immunohistochemistry may be helpful in confirming the lineage of hematopoietic precursor cells. Antibodies to glycophorin A identify red blood cell precursors, antimyeloperoxidase and antineutrophil elastase stain myeloid precursors, and CD42b and CD61 stain megakaryocytes.

Differential diagnosis

EMH can generally be distinguished from leukemia cutis by the presence of precursor elements, usually belonging to more than one cell line and displaying maturation.

Mastocytosis

Mastocytosis was regarded as a myeloproliferative disorder in the 2008 WHO Classification of myeloid malignancies.[1] However, major advances in the understanding of the disease has led to it now being categorized as a separate disease entity in the 2016 update of the WHO classification.[2] It is a heterogeneous disorder, characterized by clonal proliferation and accumulation of mast cells in one or more organ systems. The clinical course ranges from asymptomatic, sometimes spontaneously regressing disease with a normal life expectancy, to highly aggressive forms associated with multiorgan failure and short survival.[1,3–5] Mastocytosis is subdivided into different categories on the basis of extent and distribution of organ involvement, degree of impairment of organ function, and other clinical and laboratory findings.[1–9] The two main subtypes are systemic mastocytosis (20% of cases), and a more common, skin-limited form of the disease referred to as cutaneous mastocytosis (80% of cases). Systemic mastocytosis is characterized by involvement of bone marrow and/or other extracutaneous organs, although skin may also be involved in up to 50% of cases. Diagnosis of systemic mastocytosis requires fulfillment of at least one major and one minor, or three minor criteria (Table 29.6).

The majority of systemic mastocytosis cases belong to an indolent group, but rare aggressive variants also exist, and are defined according to further clinical and laboratory parameters. The following subtypes of mastocytosis that will be recognized in the 2016 update of the WHO classification are:[2]

- cutaneous mastocytosis,
- systemic mastocytosis,
  - indolent systemic mastocytosis,
  - smoldering systemic mastocytosis,
  - systemic mastocytosis with an associated hematological neoplasm,
  - aggressive systemic mastocytosis,

Table 29.6
Criteria for diagnosing mastocytosis

Cutaneous mastocytosis

Typical clinical findings of urticaria pigmentosa/maculopapular cutaneous mastocytosis or solitary mastocytoma with appropriate histologic mast cell infiltrates in skin biopsy. Absence of criteria for systemic mastocytosis.

Systemic mastocytosis

Requires presence of major criterion and one minor criterion, or at least three minor criteria.

Major criterion:

Multifocal infiltrates of mast cells in bone marrow and/or other extracutaneous organ(s); must be ≥15 mast cells/aggregate

Minor criteria:

1. >25% spindle shaped or otherwise atypical mast cells in biopsy sample
2. Activating point mutation at codon 816 of *KIT*
3. Aberrant expression of CD2 and/or CD25 by mast cells
4. Serum tryptase >20 ng/mL in absence of associated clonal myeloid disorder

Modified from Horny, H.P., et al. (2008) WHO classification of tumors of haematopoietic and lymphoid tissues. Swerdlow, S.H., Campo, E., Harris, N.L., et al (eds). Lyons: IARC Press, pp 54–63.

- mast cell leukemia,
- mast cell sarcoma.

A full discussion of the intricacies of this subclassification is beyond the scope of this text (see references 1–3 and 5), and although general clinical features of systemic mastocytosis are summarized below, detailed discussion is limited to cutaneous disease.

Clinical features

Patients may be affected at any age. Cutaneous mastocytosis is most common in children, may be present at birth, and up to half of cases manifest in the first 6 months of life. It is much less frequent in adults, most cases of skin involvement in this age group being associated with systemic mastocytosis.[5,10–12] Systemic mastocytosis generally arises after the second decade. There is no clear sex or ethnic predilection.[13,14] Skin lesions are common in mastocytosis, overall being present in 80% of patients, including 50% of cases of systemic mastocytosis. Bone marrow is almost always involved in systemic mastocytosis, and there may rarely be a leukemic blood picture with significant numbers of circulating mast cells.[15–20] Virtually any other tissue may be involved, but the most frequently reported are spleen, lymph node, liver, and gastrointestinal tract.[7,8,15,18,21–23]

Symptoms are often related to release of a wide range of mast cell mediators, as well as to the direct effects of organ infiltration. These include histamine, eicosonoids, proteases, and heparin. They may induce localized or more generalized reactions such as anaphylaxis, flushing, headache, urticarial rhinitis, palpitations, and hypotension with syncope.[4,24,25] Gastrointestinal symptoms include vomiting, colicky abdominal pain, peptic ulceration, and diarrhea.[4,7] In the skin, mast cell degranulation also accounts for the common presence of pruritus, a positive Darier sign, and dermographism (*Fig. 29.346*). Darier sign refers to localized swelling or urticaria induced by stroking of a lesion; this may reach bullous proportions.

Constitutional symptoms of fatigue, weight loss, fever, and musculoskeletal complaints including bone pain, osteopenia, osteoporosis, fractures, arthralgias, and myalgias may be seen. Minimal splenomegaly is sometimes seen, and rarely there may be lymphadenopathy and hepatomegaly.[4,8,18,21,22,26] Peripheral blood eosinophilia is the most commonly reported hematological abnormality, but others include anemia, leukocytosis, neutropenia, and thrombocytopenia.[15,17,27–30] Serum tryptase is usually elevated in systemic mastocytosis, and a persistently raised level constitutes one of the minor diagnostic criteria. It is normal or only minimally elevated in cutaneous mastocytosis.[1,4,31] The presence of circulating mast cells is rarely observed and is a diagnostic criterion for mast cell leukemia.[4] In addition, an association with myeloid or lymphatic malignancy has been documented in up

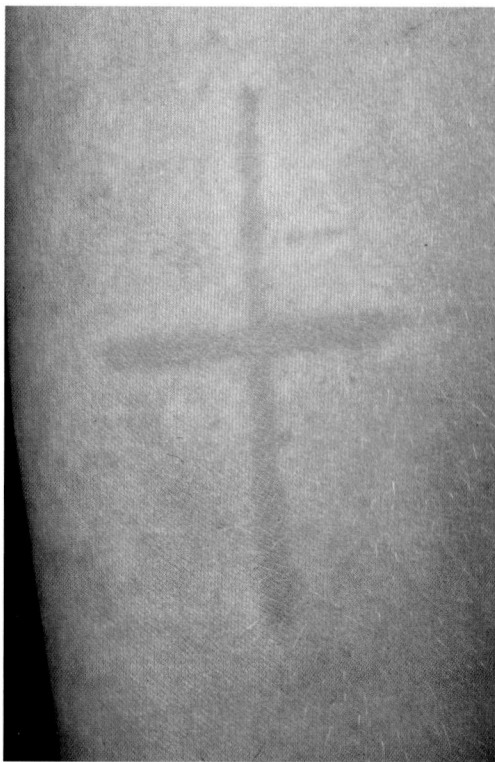

Fig. 29.346
Mastocytosis: a classic example of dermographism.

to 30% of patients with systemic mastocytosis, either preceding, concurrent with, or succeeding the mast cell disease. This is usually chronic myelomonocytic leukemia, but may be myelodysplasia, AML, lymphoma, or any other recognized hematological malignancy.[4,5,17,32–37] Such cases fall into the systemic mastocytosis category of 'systemic mastocytosis with an associated hematological neoplasm'.[2]

Cutaneous involvement in the absence of criteria for systemic mastocytosis is subdivided into one of three clinicopathological variants:
- solitary mastocytoma,
- maculopapular mastocytosis/urticaria pigmentosa,
- diffuse mastocytosis.

Skin is also frequently involved in indolent forms of systemic mastocytosis, but much less often not in aggressive variants. It may also be a presenting site for very rare cases of mast cell sarcoma.

Solitary cutaneous mastocytoma

This is a solitary lesion that occurs almost exclusively in children with no obvious site predilection, although a study suggested an affinity for the extremities (*Fig. 29.347*). It accounts for 10–20% of cases of mastocytosis.[24,38–41] Lesions are nodular with a reddish or yellow color, and usually do not exceed 1 cm in diameter.[4,24,38–40] They may be associated with flushing attacks.[13,39] Most cases resolve spontaneously, whilst the few cases that persist are cured by excision.[4,11,35,38]

Maculopapular cutaneous mastocytosis/urticaria pigmentosa

Maculopapular cutaneous mastocytosis is the commonest manifestation of mastocytosis, accounting for 80% of cutaneous cases, and with an approximate incidence of 1:1000–1:8000 live births.[4,39,40] It presents most frequently in children, with no sex predilection.[35] Lesions may present at birth or during the first year of life. They are pruritic, erythematous, or red-brown, round to oval macules, papules, and plaques, often measuring up to 2–3 cm in diameter (*Figs 29.348* and *29.349*).[4,13] They occur predominantly on the trunk, although any region (including the mucous membranes) may be affected.[24,40] Darier sign is characteristically positive and patients may show

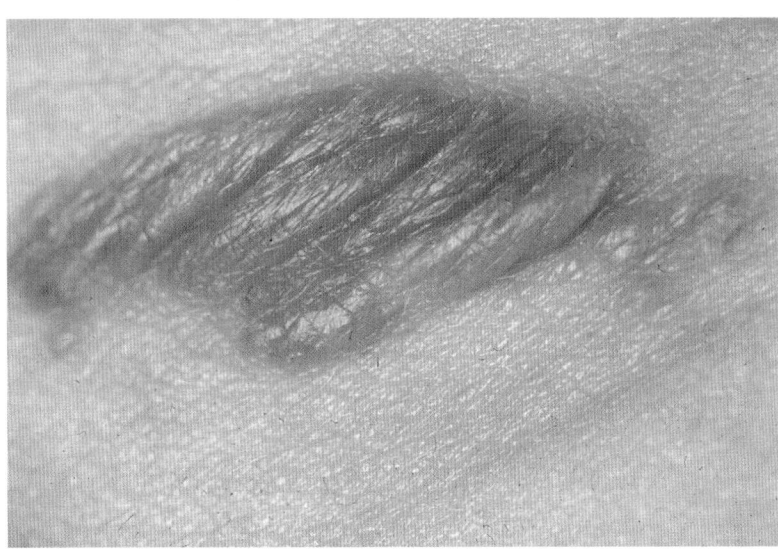

Fig. 29.347
Mastocytoma: edematous, erythematous plaque in a child. From the collection of the late N.P. Smith, MD, the Institute of Dermatology, London, UK.

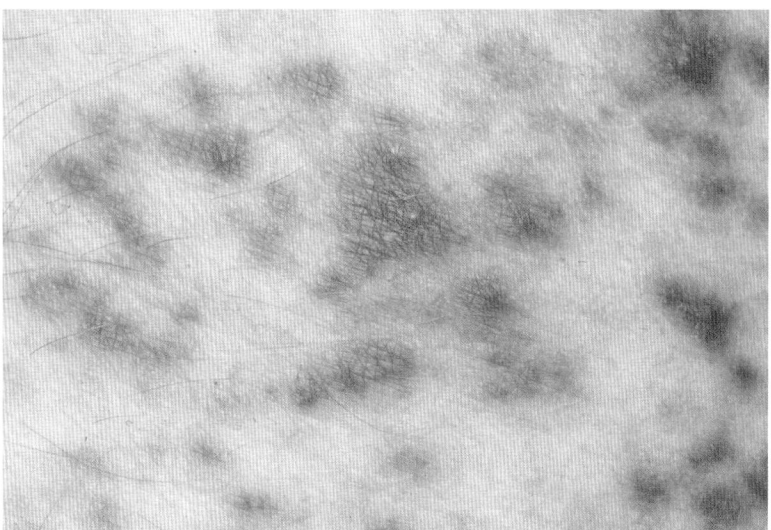

Fig. 29.349
Urticaria pigmentosa: in this example, the macules and papules are erythematous. From the collection of the late N.P. Smith, MD, the Institute of Dermatology, London, UK.

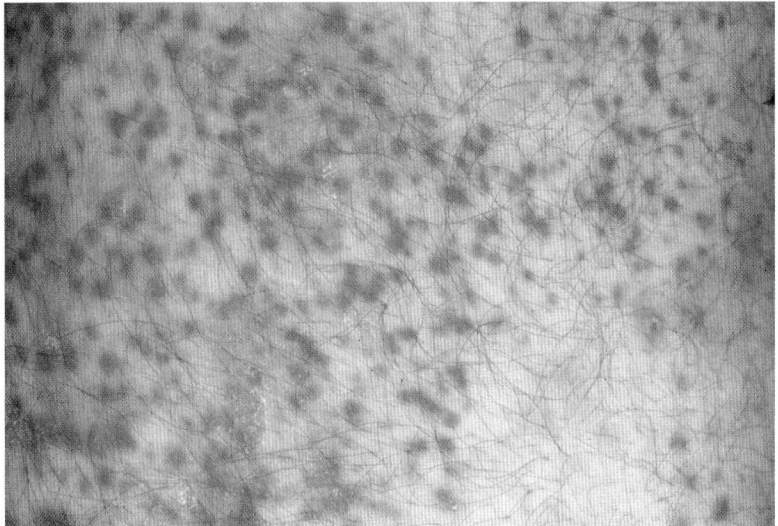

Fig. 29.348
Urticaria pigmentosa: numerous brown macules and papules are present. From the collection of the late N.P. Smith, MD, the Institute of Dermatology, London, UK.

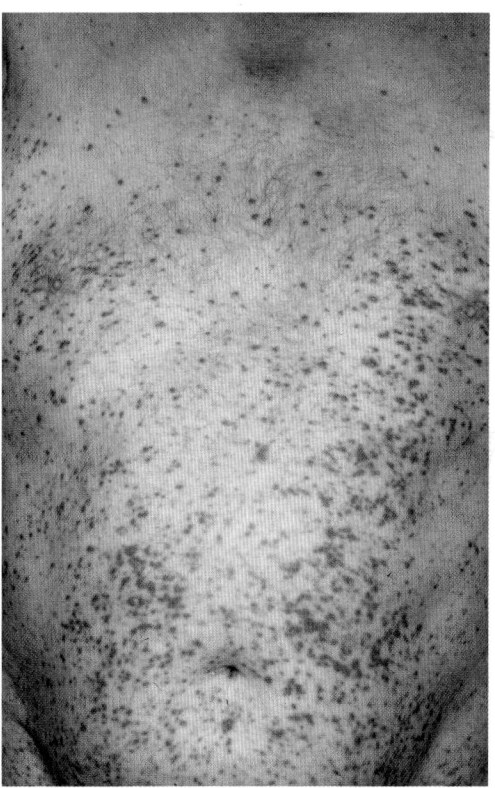

Fig. 29.350
Urticaria pigmentosa: note the generalized distribution of the lesions. From the collection of the late N.P. Smith, MD, the Institute of Dermatology, London, UK.

generalized dermographism. Blisters develop occasionally; rarely, these may be generalized and mimic a primary or acquired bullous dermatosis.[42] In adults, lesions are more often disseminated, more heavily pigmented, and tend to be macular (*Fig. 29.350*).[11] Telangiectasia may be present, hence the name, telangiectasia macularis eruptiva perstans.[13,38,43,44]

Most childhood cases resolve spontaneously before or during puberty. Adult cases tend to persist, and systemic mastocytosis should always be ruled out.[1,11,12,38,45] Even when systemic mastocytosis is present, the course tends to be indolent and has no effect in survival.[12]

Diffuse cutaneous mastocytosis

This is very rare and affects mainly children and only rarely adults.[13,46–48] The skin is erythrodermic, often itchy, and, due to the widespread infiltrate of mast cells, has a thick doughy or boggy consistency, with accentuation of surface markings. Occasionally, the skin may have a red, yellow-brown, 'peau d'orange', or grain leather ('peau chagrine') appearance.[38] Lichenification is sometimes evident. Urtication and blister formation following mild trauma are usual.[38,46] Generalized blistering may occur, sometimes mimicking staphylococcal scalded skin syndrome or bullous erythema multiforme.[49–51] Diffuse cutaneous mastocytosis commonly resolves by the

third to fifth years.[11] Systemic symptoms include flushing, hypotension, shock, and diarrhea.[11]

Cutaneous involvement in systemic mastocytosis

This is almost invariably of the urticaria pigmentosa type and is regularly seen in indolent systemic mastocytosis.[52] It is rare in aggressive mastocytosis and exceptional in mast cell leukemia.[11]

Mast cell sarcoma

Mast cell sarcoma is extremely rare, and although it presents initially as a solitary lesion, there is invariably rapid dissemination and a terminal phase

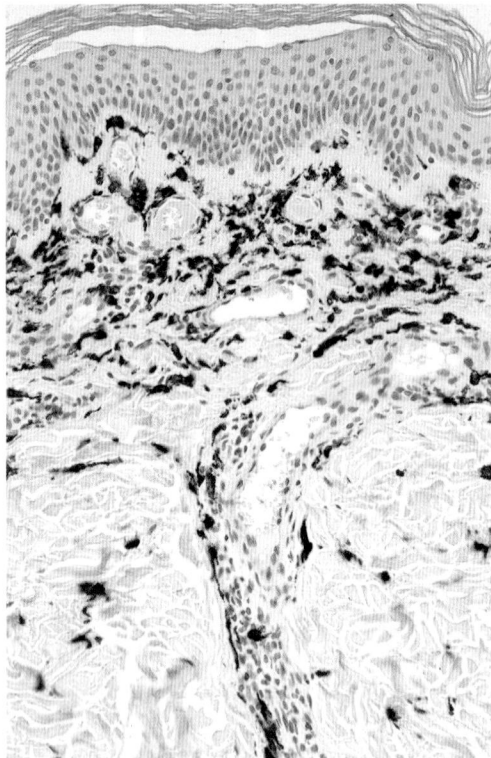

Fig. 29.351
Urticaria pigmentosa: the mast cells are positive for tryptase.

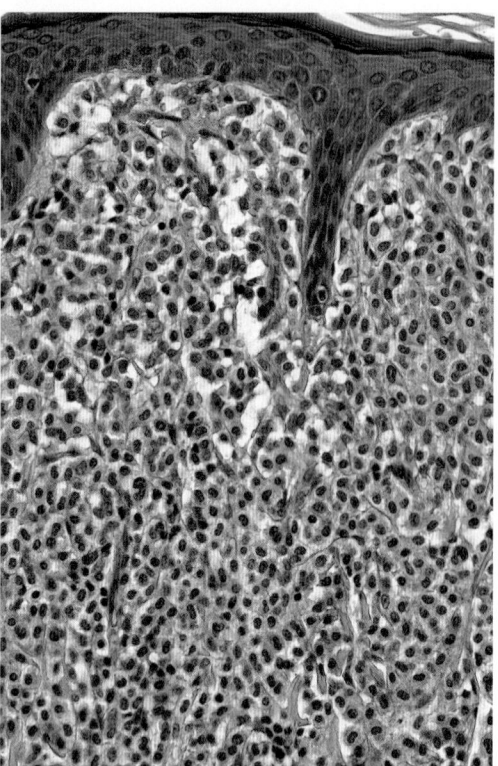

Fig. 29.352
Urticaria pigmentosa: there is a dense dermal cellular infiltrate.

resembling mast cell leukemia. It has been documented in the larynx, large bowel, meninges, bone, and skin.[1,52–55]

Pathogenesis and histologic features

Somatic activating point mutations within the KIT gene on chromosome 4q12 are common in mastocytosis.[5,56–58] The majority of these affect codon 816 in the tyrosine kinase domain, and involve substitution of Val for Asp (D816V).[56–63] This is seen in ≥95% of adult patients with systemic mastocytosis, but only in about one-third of patients with cutaneous mastocytosis.[58,61–63] The frequency of point mutations other than D816V is significantly higher in cutaneous than in systemic mastocytosis.[5,38,58,62–64] These mutations result in constitutive activation of KIT with subsequent oncogenic effects on downstream pathways that influence cell survival and function, and some render the tumor resistant to treatment with tyrosine kinase inhibitors such as imatinib.[56,65] Increased expression of antiapoptotic proteins has also been documented in mast cells in the skin and bone marrow of patients with mastocytosis.[13,66]

Normal mast cells are usually oval to polygonally shaped cells with moderately abundant, eosinophilic or amphophilic cytoplasm containing numerous small, faintly visible granules. Mast cells are metachromatic when stained with Giemsa or toluidine blue and contain cytoplasmic tryptase (Fig. 29.351). Nuclei are round to oval in shape with clumped chromatin and indistinct nucleoli. They are occasionally binucleate or multinucleate. When nuclei are centrally placed, a 'fried egg' appearance is present. A spindled morphology is frequent.[14,18] In normal skin, mast cells are seen perivascularly and scattered throughout the dermis, but do not form clusters.

In mastocytosis, the neoplastic mast cells are histologically indistinguishable from normal, and diagnosis depends on assessing their number, distribution, and immunoprofile. In particular, aggregates of mast cells must be present for an unequivocal diagnosis. Within the macules and papules, the mast cells are usually seen predominantly in the papillary dermis and they have normal appearance (Figs 29.352 and 29.353). There may be edema of the papillary dermis and if the lesion has been traumatized before biopsy, subepidermal vesiculation is sometimes evident mainly in solitary mastocytoma.[39]

As a rule, there are generally fewer mast cells in adult than childhood cutaneous mastocytosis. Changes may be quite subtle and consist only of a mild increase in perivascular mast cells in the papillary dermis, particularly in biopsies from patients showing clinical features of telangiectasia macularis eruptive perstans (Figs 29.354 and 29.355).

In the larger nodular lesions and in solitary mastocytomas, tumorlike deposits fill the entire dermis and often extend into the subcutis (Figs 29.356 and 29.357).

Basal cell hyperpigmentation of the overlying epidermis is a common feature in urticaria pigmentosa. It is found particularly in older lesions in the maculopapular lesions and less so in nodules.[67] Superficial lymphocytes and histiocytes may be evident, especially in the adult-onset variant.[67] Eosinophils are often seen, particularly if the lesion has been rubbed before biopsy.

Immunohistochemistry

Mast cells express CD33, CD5, CD68, CD117, tryptase, and chymase. CD117 is perhaps the most sensitive but not a specific marker for mast cells (Fig. 29.358). Chymase is highly specific but its detection is less sensitive. Myelomonocytic markers such as CD14, CD15, and CD16 are absent, as are most T- and B-cell markers.[4,68–71] Neoplastic mast cells differ from their normal counterparts in that they express CD2 and/or CD25. Moreover, expression of CD25 in skin lesions is a predictor for underlying systemic disease.[72]

Differential diagnosis

Increased numbers of mast cells may be seen in many inflammatory disorders. Such reactive mast cell infiltrates may be difficult to differentiate from cases of cutaneous mastocytosis in which the neoplastic infiltrate is relatively sparse. Clinical information may be helpful, but to be certain of a diagnosis, clusters of mast cells should be seen. This may take more than one biopsy to demonstrate. In addition, immunohistochemistry may be helpful, with expression of CD2 and/or CD25 facilitating differentiation of neoplastic mast cells from reactive ones.[1]

Access **ExpertConsult.com** for the complete list of references

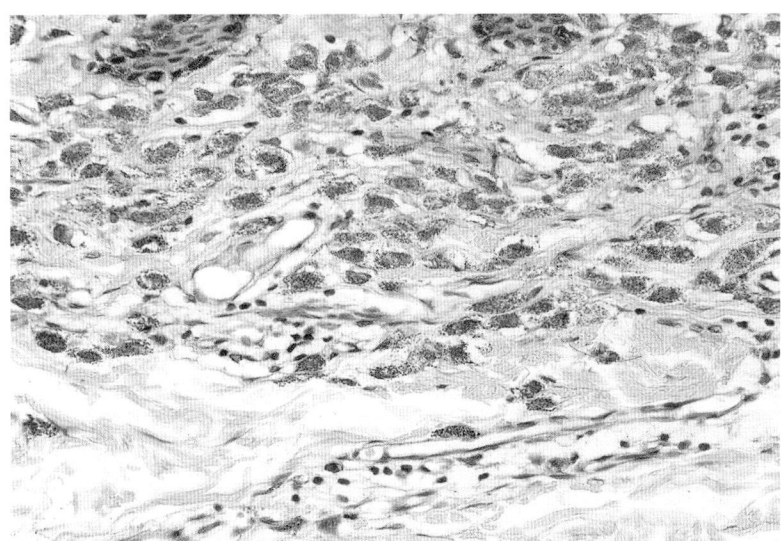

Fig. 29.353
Urticaria pigmentosa: the mast cells stain for chloracetate esterase.

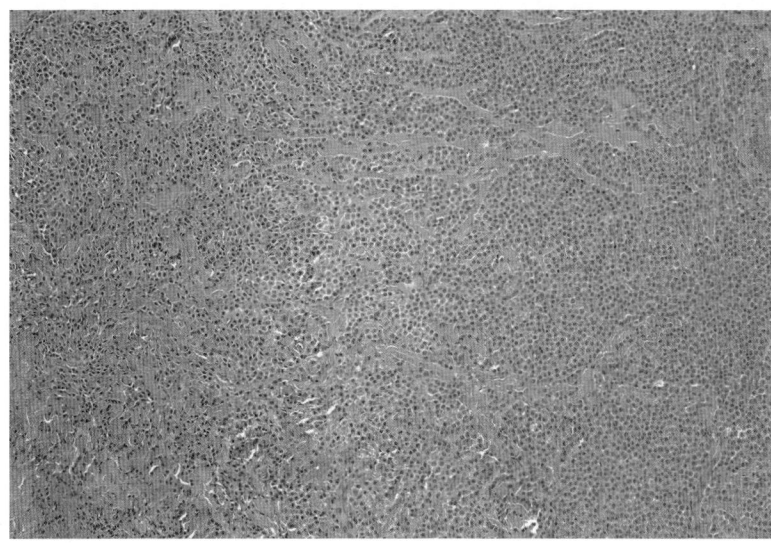

Fig. 29.356
Mastocytoma: the tumor cells have abundant eosinophilic cytoplasm and uniform darkly staining nuclei.

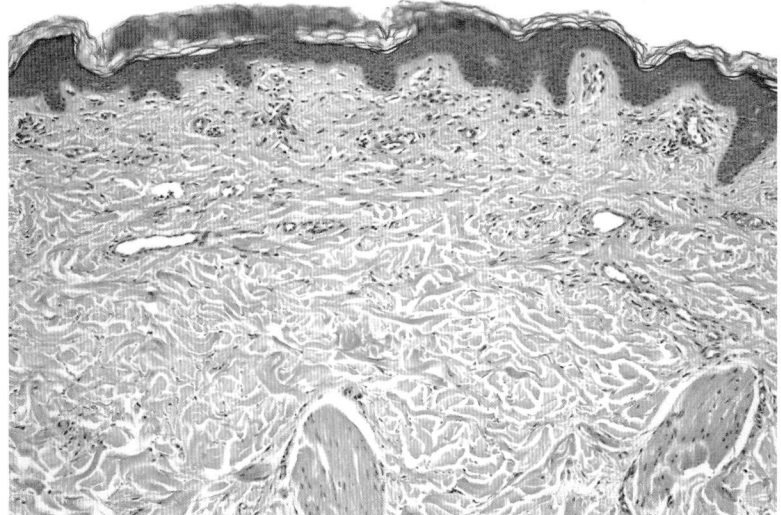

Fig. 29.354
Telangiectasia macularis eruptiva perstans: the features are often very subtle and easily missed. There is telangiectasia and a very slight perivascular infiltrate.

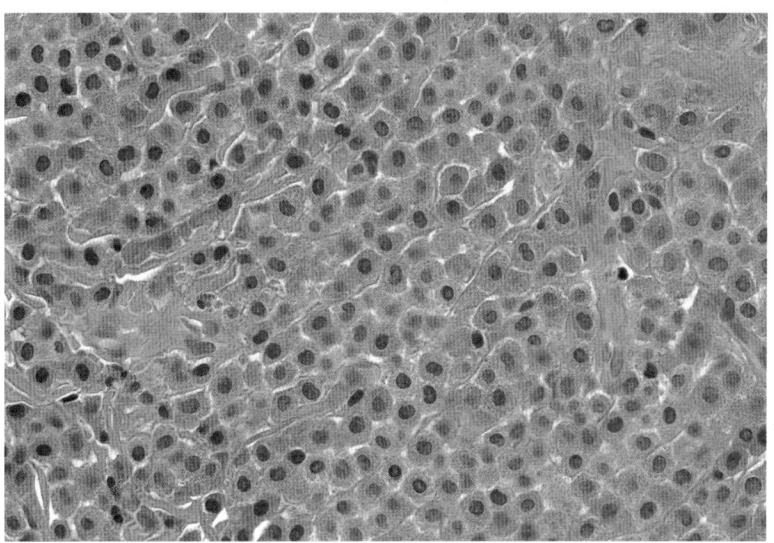

Fig. 29.357
Mastocytoma: high-power view.

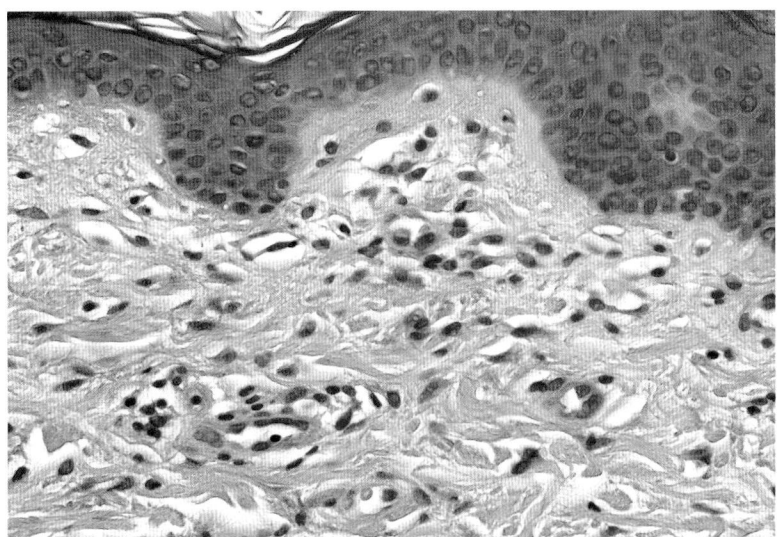

Fig. 29.355
Telangiectasia macularis eruptiva perstans: in this variant, the mast cells often adopt a spindled morphology.

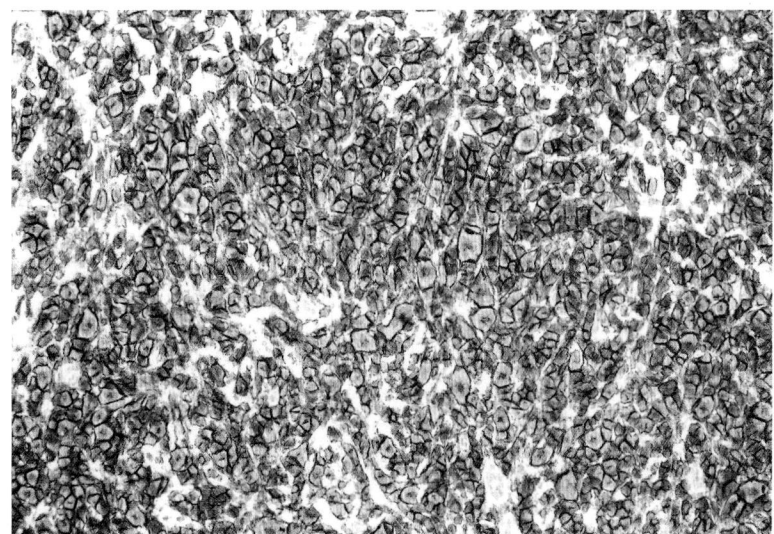

Fig. 29.358
Mastocytoma: CD117 is strikingly positive.

Cutaneous metastases and Paget disease of the skin

See
www.expertconsult.com
for references and
additional material

CUTANEOUS METASTASES

Secondary involvement of the integument by a malignant tumor may represent a metastatic phenomenon (such as following vascular or lymphatic emboli) or occur as a direct consequence of contiguous spread through tissue spaces or lymphatic and vascular channels (*Figs 30.1* and *30.2*).[1,2] In addition, tumor deposits may be accidentally implanted during surgical procedures.[3,4] Rarely, cutaneous metastasis may be the presenting feature of a visceral malignancy.[5-7]

On histologic grounds alone, the differential diagnosis between metastatic tumors in the skin and primary cutaneous tumors can be challenging. This discrimination is of a paramount importance due to the profound implications for prognosis and subsequent therapy. Detection of cutaneous metastases usually indicates disseminated disease and a poor prognosis.

Determining the origin of the tumor is often very difficult and sometimes impossible, although careful use of ancillary techniques – particularly immunohistochemistry and, very rarely, electron microscopy – can give the pathologist some useful pointers in the right direction.

When unusual intradermal tumors are encountered, particularly in elderly patients, a high index of suspicion is always necessary, since the unwary can easily mistake a small deposit of metastatic breast duct carcinoma for an adnexal tumor. Care with tissue specimens, by both the clinician and the pathologist, is always mandatory. Poorly fixed lymphomatous infiltrates, for example, may be misdiagnosed morphologically as cutaneous neuroendocrine carcinoma, while artifactual crushing may result in confusion with metastatic small cell carcinoma. Ancillary studies such as immunohistochemistry should be engaged when histologic detail is compromised.

Clinical features
Incidence, primary sites and chronology of presentation

The more frequent sites for secondary tumor deposits are lymph nodes, liver, lungs, adrenals, brain, bone, ovaries, and kidneys with some variation based on primary tumor type. The skin is a relatively uncommon site for presentation of metastasis; recorded frequencies have varied from 0.7% to 9% of all cases of metastatic malignant disease.[2,7-9] A meta-analysis including over 20000 patients with carcinoma, and excluding melanoma, found the incidence of cutaneous metastases to be 5.3%.[10] Considering the fact that the skin is the largest organ in the body, it is unclear why this relatively low incidence of metastasis from internal malignancy is observed. As initially described in 1889 by Stephen Paget in his 'seed and soil' hypothesis, the tumors preferentially metastasize to those organs with an intrinsically favorable environment.[11,12] It is therefore possible that the skin may provide the proper environment for colonization and survival of only a few types of

tumors.[13] The role of the unique microenvironments composed of various immune and stromal cells present at different body sites in the metastatic process is the topic of much research.[14]

Cutaneous metastases present most commonly a few months or years after the primary tumor has been diagnosed.[15] There are rare reports of metastatic tumors arising decades after the diagnosis of the primary neoplasm.[16] Cutaneous metastases develop most commonly at the same time as internal metastases.[17] Less frequently, a metastasis is diagnosed concurrent with the primary tumor or represents the initial manifestation of the disease.[8] In a study by Brownstein and Helwig, skin metastases were the presenting sign of the disease in 37% of men and in 6% of women.[8] This discrepancy may reflect the fact that although metastatic breast carcinoma represents the most common skin metastasis in women, currently breast cancer is usually diagnosed fairly early in the course of the disease as opposed to many other internal malignancies. Cutaneous metastases from some primary sites appear more likely to be the first sign of the disease. These include lung cancer (60% of cases), renal cancer (53% of cases), and ovarian cancer (40% of cases), but the incidence of skin metastasis as the initial presenting symptom is likely falling dramatically from these historical levels with earlier clinical detection of internal disease in contemporary medicine. A more contemporary study suggests that where cutaneous metastases do occur, they can be the initial sign of metastases beyond the regional lymph nodes.[9] Although cutaneous metastases may present at any age, the greatest incidence is in the fifth to seventh decades.

The relative frequencies of the underlying primary neoplasms largely reflect the incidence of the various tumors that occur in humans.[9] In Western communities, the most common sources of cutaneous metastases in males include the lungs (24%), large intestine (19%), melanoma (13%), squamous carcinoma of the oral cavity (12%), kidney (6%), stomach (6%), and esophagus (3%) (*Fig. 30.3*).[8,18] In females, the primary tumor site is most often the breast (69%), while other important sources include the large intestine (9%), melanoma (5%), ovaries (4%), and uterine cervix (2%) (*Fig. 30.4*).[8,18] With the increased incidence of cigarette smoking in females, carcinoma of the bronchus is of growing importance. Much less common primary sites have been reported including thyroid, adrenal, endometrium, urinary bladder, and pancreas.[9,19] Prostate carcinoma, despite its high incidence in men, is among the least common primary site to result in cutaneous metastases, perhaps a practical demonstration of the seed and soil hypothesis discussed above.

In a study by Lookingbill, melanoma was the most common source of metastatic disease in the skin in men and the second most common source

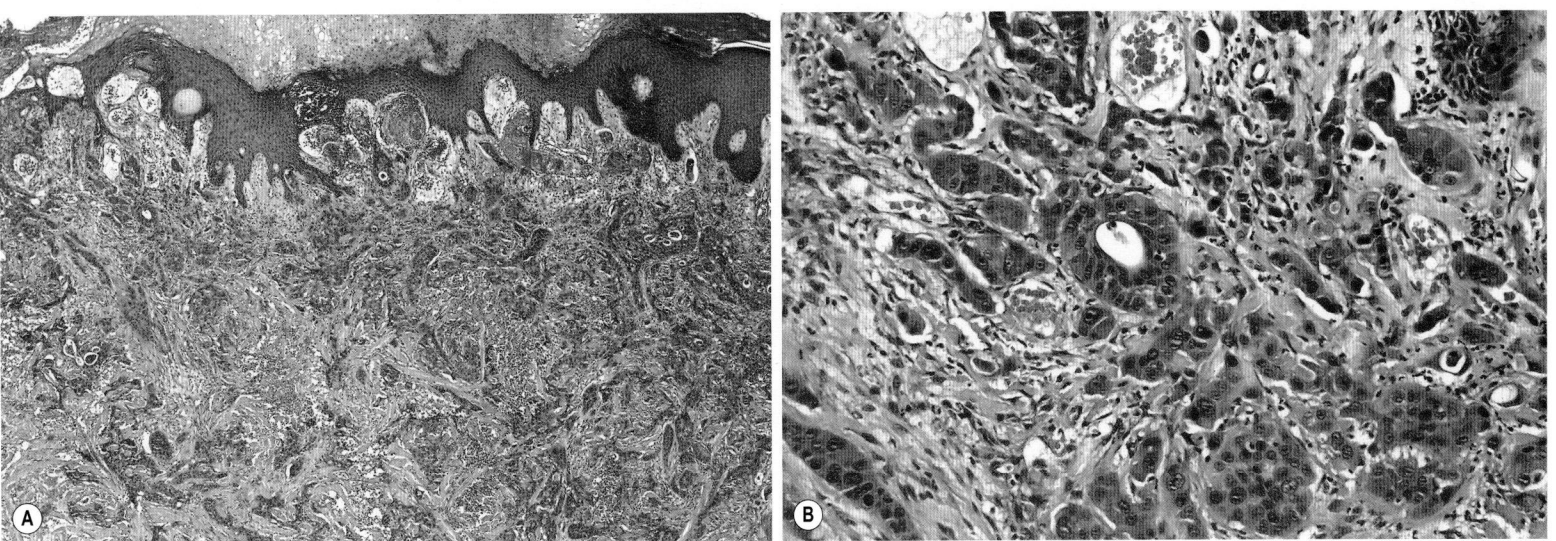

Fig. 30.1
Metastatic breast carcinoma: (**A**) this field shows metastatic poorly differentiated breast ductal carcinoma; (**B**) high-power view showing focal ductal differentiation.

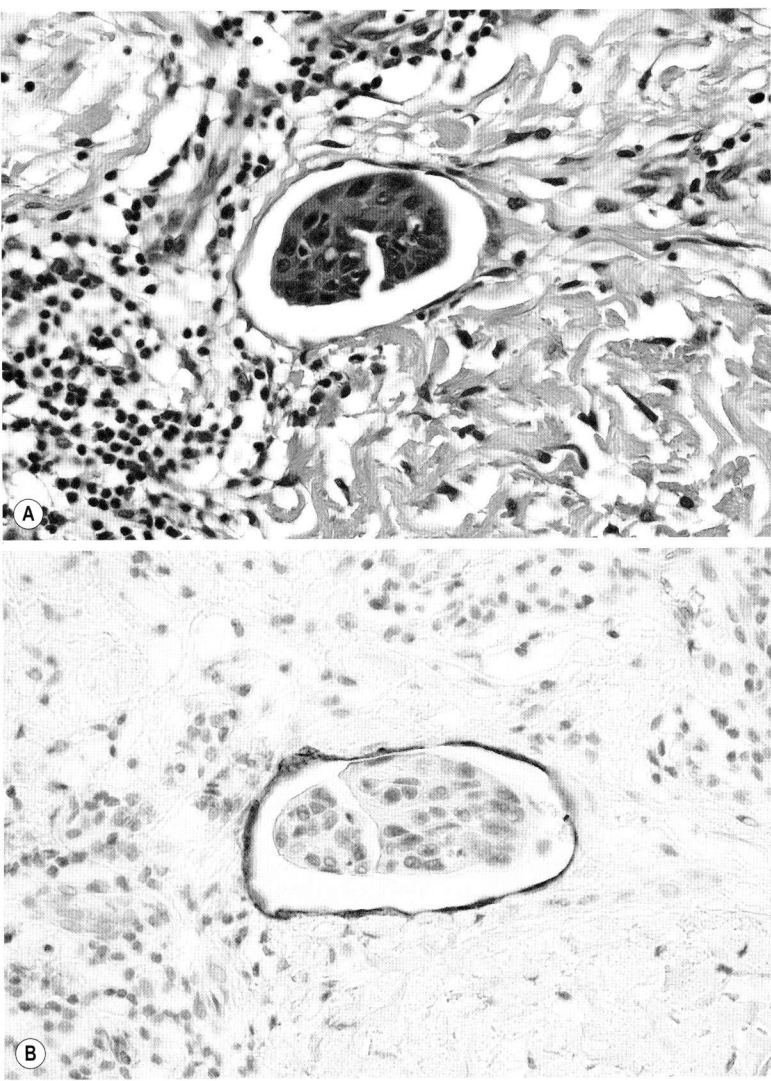

Fig. 30.2
Metastatic breast carcinoma: (**A**) lymphovascular invasion is present; (**B**) the vessel endothelium shows strong D2-40 expression.

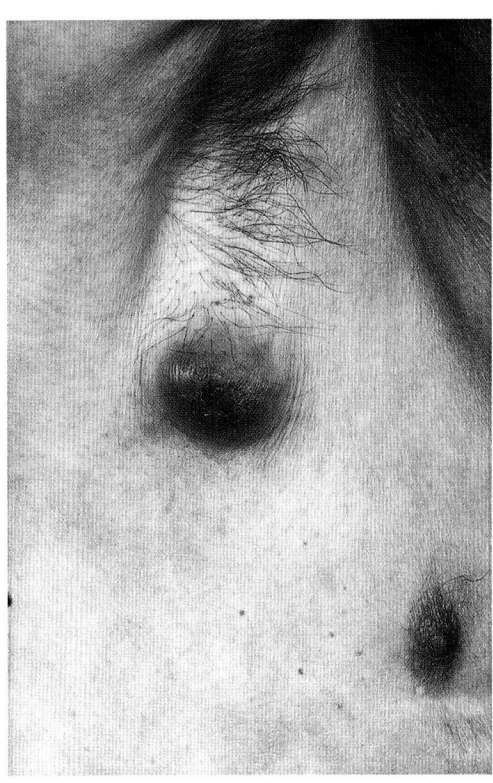

Fig. 30.3
Metastatic bronchial carcinoma: the lung is the commonest source for cutaneous metastases in males. By courtesy of R.A. Marsden, MD, St George's Hospital, London, UK.

for women (*Fig. 30.5*).[9] A study from India has shown that the most common primary sites of cutaneous metastasis are the lung and esophagus in men and the breast and ovaries in females.[20]

With the exceptions of leukemia and lymphoma, cutaneous metastases from underlying malignancies in children are very rare. However, around 50% of malignant cutaneous tumors in children represent metastatic disease.[21] Interestingly, and in contrast to adults, cutaneous metastases represent the first manifestation of the disease in up to 84% of cases.

The most common childhood tumors metastasizing to the skin are rhabdomyosarcoma and neuroblastoma, reflecting the incidence of these tumors in this age group (*Fig. 30.6*).[22] Neuroblastoma is most often seen in neonates. In this age group, neuroblastoma presents with skin metastases in up to 32% of cases.[23]

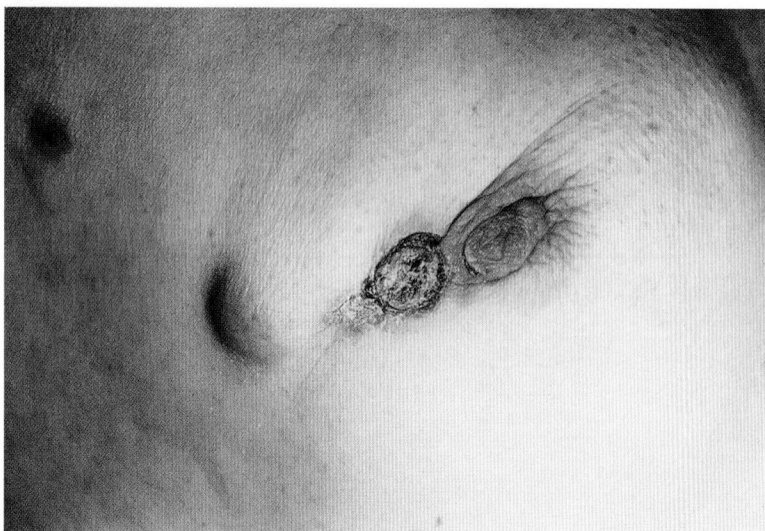

Fig. 30.4
Carcinoma of the breast: there is a small ulcerated tumor to the left of the nipple, as well as two pale nodular cutaneous metastases. By courtesy of R.A. Marsden, MD, St George's Hospital, London, UK.

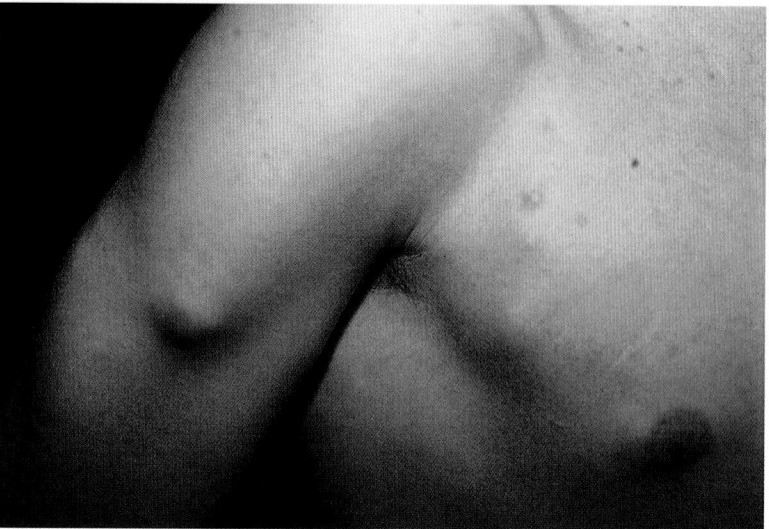

Fig. 30.6
Metastatic neuroblastoma: there are multiple metastases on the chest wall and arm. By courtesy of Drs José María Ricart and Amparo Marquina Vila, Hospital Peset, Valencia, Spain.

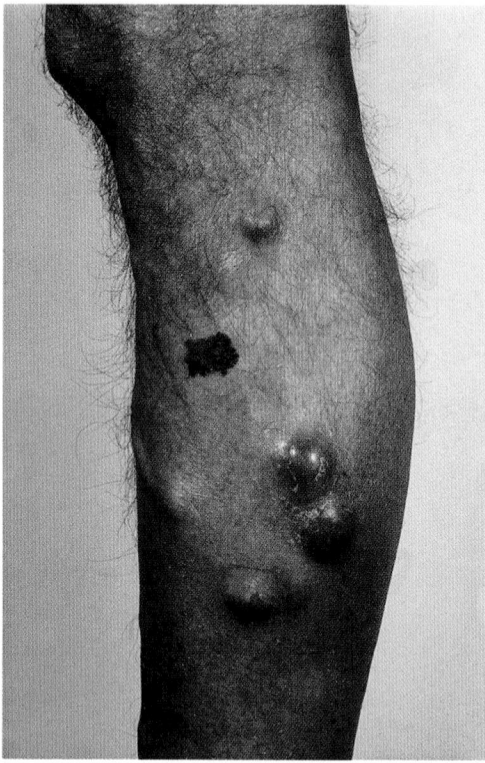

Fig. 30.5
Malignant melanoma: pink nodules of metastatic tumor are present on the lateral aspect of the lower leg of a male. By courtesy of A. du Vivier, MD, King's College Hospital, London, UK.

Rare tumors metastasizing to skin in children include osteosarcoma, choriocarcinoma, Ewing sarcoma, malignant rhabdoid tumor, melanoma, paraganglioma, and nasopharyngeal carcinoma. Choriocarcinoma presenting as a metastatic tumor in a neonate is associated with a primary placental tumor, which can also spread to the mother.[24] As with adults, central nervous system tumors only exceptionally spread to the skin in children.[25] In the vast majority of children with metastatic carcinoma in the skin, the source of the primary tumor is almost invariably determined after thorough and comprehensive investigation.[26] An unknown primary is truly exceptional.

Cutaneous metastases in young adults are rare, reflecting the general low incidence of cancer in this age group.

Although not always the rule, the location of a cutaneous metastasis often reflects the site of the underlying tumor.[27] The anterior chest, abdomen, head, and neck regions are the most common sites for metastatic tumors. Multiple sites of cutaneous metastases (involving two or more anatomic regions) have also been reported. Metastases to the skin of the face and neck are most often associated with a squamous carcinoma of the oral cavity, although lung, kidney, and breast may also represent rare sources of such metastases. Carcinoma of the breast most frequently spreads to the anterior chest wall, while bronchial and lung tumors tend to metastasize to the chest wall and upper extremities (*Fig. 30.7*). Gastrointestinal tumors usually involve the anterior abdominal wall but may present in other areas such as the face and scalp[28]; pelvic neoplasms show a predilection for the perineal region. Primary tumors of the prostate, bladder, and colon can spread to the penis or scrotum.[29–34] Intra-abdominal tumors, including those of the stomach, colon, ovary, endometrium, urinary bladder, fallopian tube, prostate, cervix, and pancreas, sometimes metastasize to the skin of the umbilicus to form the so-called Sister Mary Joseph nodule (*Fig. 30.8*).[35–48] Rarely, a metastatic breast carcinoma or mesothelioma can present as a Sister Mary Joseph nodule. Umbilical metastases represent the first manifestation of disease in about 14% of cases.[44]

Metastases to the limbs are uncommon, most often resulting from spread of primary cutaneous melanoma. Sometimes, these present in a subungual location. Subungual metastases can also complicate carcinoma of the stomach, lung, esophagus, kidney, colon, and breast.[49–53] Subungual metastases from a choriocarcinoma have also been reported.[54]

Melanoma and neoplasms associated with vascular invasion (e.g., renal cell carcinoma, thyroid follicular carcinoma, and choriocarcinoma) lack such a tendency towards regional localization (*Figs 30.9 and 30.10*).

Some tumors are characterized by a predilection to metastasize to certain sites.[55] For example, ocular melanoma selectively spreads to the liver. In addition to skin, lung, bowel, and brain are also common sites for melanoma metastasis.[55]

Involvement of the scalp is not uncommon, accounting for up to 5% of all metastases.[56–58] Sometimes, it may represent a primary manifestation of the underlying malignancy.[1,8,59–61] In a large series of malignant tumors of the scalp from Taiwan, metastatic disease accounted for 12.8% of cases.[62] The most common primary site in both men and women in this series was the lung. Tumors most likely to spread to the scalp include those of the breast, lung, colon, stomach, and kidney (*Figs 30.11 and 30.12*). Scalp metastases are particularly common in renal cell carcinoma. A plaque of alopecia is the usual manifestation, but occasional cases of metastatic breast carcinoma without alopecia have also been described.[59,62] Amongst sarcomas, leiomyosarcoma shows a particular propensity for scalp metastases.[63]

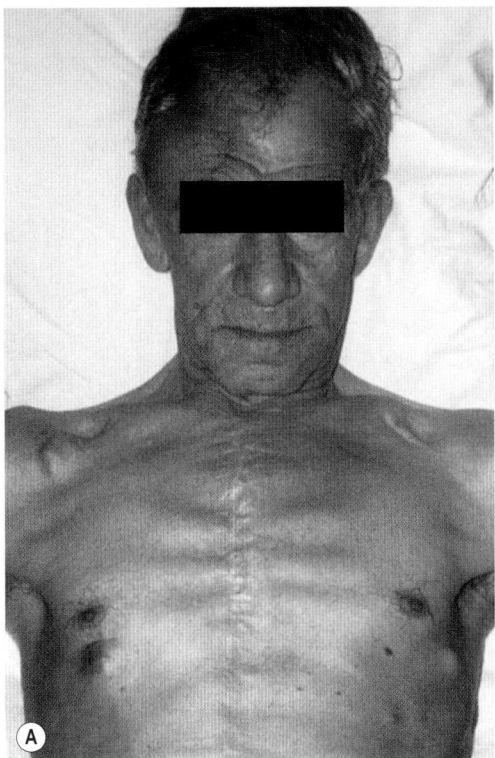
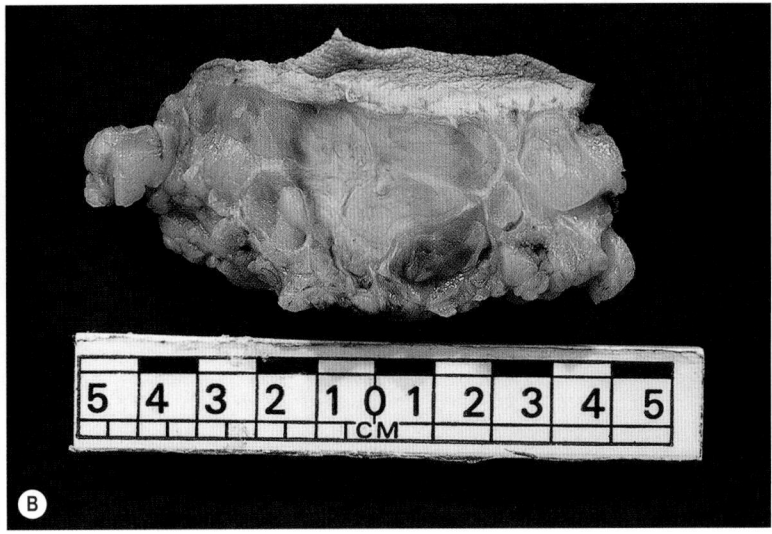

Fig. 30.7
Metastatic carcinoma of bronchus: (**A**) there are disseminated nodular cutaneous lesions involving the anterior chest wall, right shoulder, and forehead; (**B**) note the sharply circumscribed tumor nodule with focal necrosis. (**A**) By courtesy of R.A. Marsden, MD, St George's Hospital, London, UK.

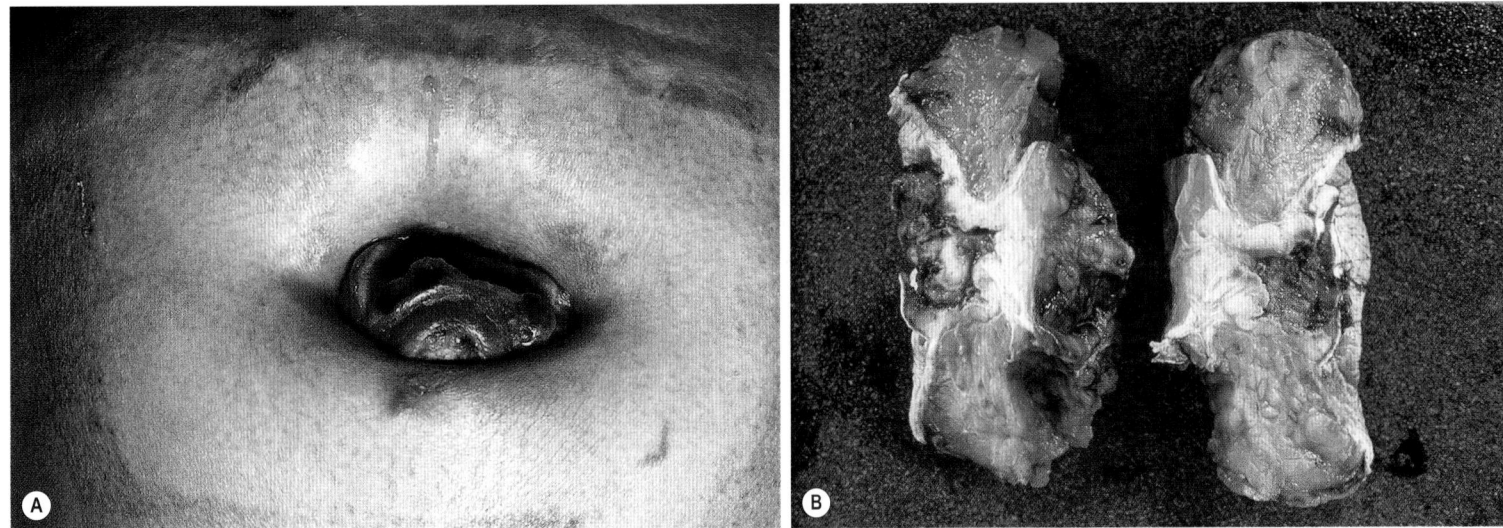

Fig. 30.8
Sister Mary Joseph nodule: (**A**) umbilical metastasis from a large bowel carcinoma; (**B**) bisected surgical specimen consisting of umbilical tissue containing an ulcerated deposit of pale tumor. The primary lesion was a poorly differentiated colonic adenocarcinoma. (**A**) By courtesy of the Institute of Dermatology, London, UK.

Of the various patterns of cutaneous metastasis, the most common is development of a nodule or group of nodules (frequently in a surgical scar), typically painless, rapidly growing, freely mobile, and often flesh colored (*Figs 30.13–30.16*).[8] Most lesions are less than 3 cm in greatest diameter. Unless traumatized, they rarely ulcerate. Other patterns of cutaneous metastases include micropapules, plaques, and lesions simulating scars. Scar-like lesions can be seen in metastases from the breast, stomach, lung, and kidney.[64]

The clinical appearance of some metastases mimics a number of benign dermatological conditions such as erythema annulare centrifugum, contact dermatitis, cellulitis, kerion, chancre, follicular cyst, condyloma, and even a cutaneous horn.[65–70] Other clinical presentations include zosteriform and elephantiasiform lesions, facial lymphedema (*Fig. 30.17*), and hemorrhagic blisters.[71–78] Zosteriform metastases have occurred with many malignancies including melanoma, squamous cell carcinoma, porocarcinoma, angiosarcoma, and carcinomas of the breast, ovary, colon, bronchus, tonsil, prostate, and bladder, and transitional carcinoma of the renal pelvis.[73,79–81]

Cutaneous metastasis can also mimic primary cutaneous tumors such as pyogenic granuloma, cylindroma, keratoacanthoma, blue nevus, Kaposi sarcoma, angiosarcoma, and melanoma.[82–90]

Hemorrhagic cutaneous metastatic nodules usually imply a primary renal cell carcinoma, thyroid follicular carcinoma, or choriocarcinoma. Pigmented

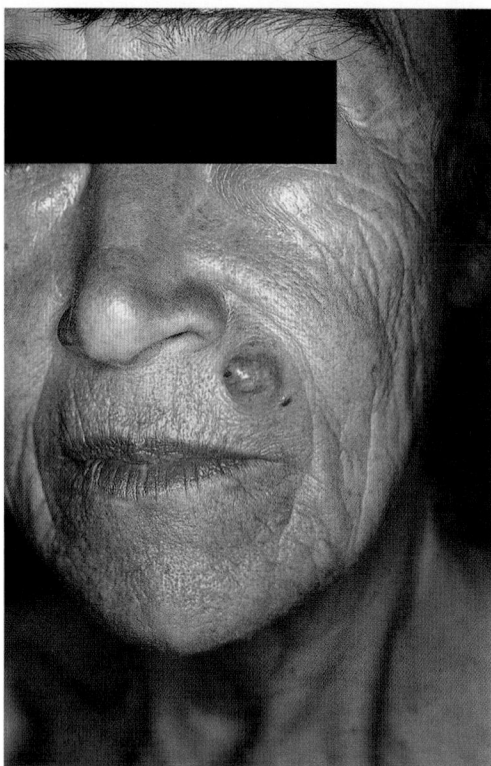

Fig. 30.9
Metastatic thyroid carcinoma: tumors, which spread primarily by vascular invasion, do not show regional localization. By courtesy of Dr. Orlando Duenàs, Bogota, Columbia.

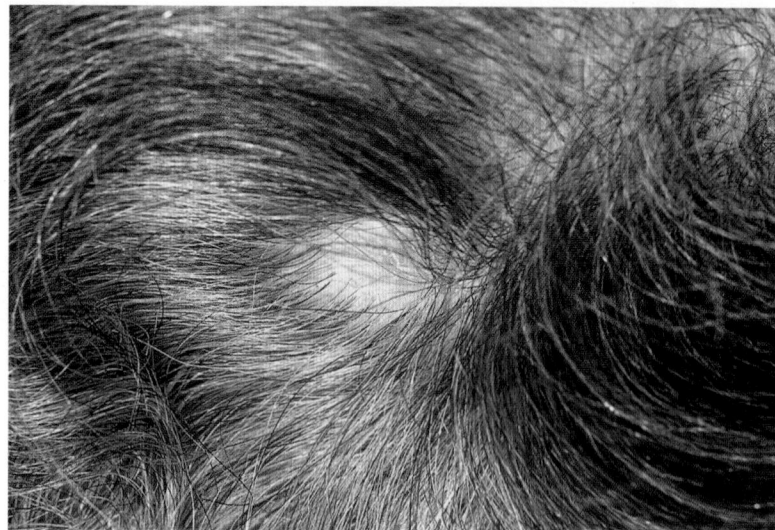

Fig. 30.11
Metastatic carcinoma of breast: scalp lesion associated with focal alopecia. By courtesy of M. Shaw, MD, St Thomas' Hospital, London, UK.

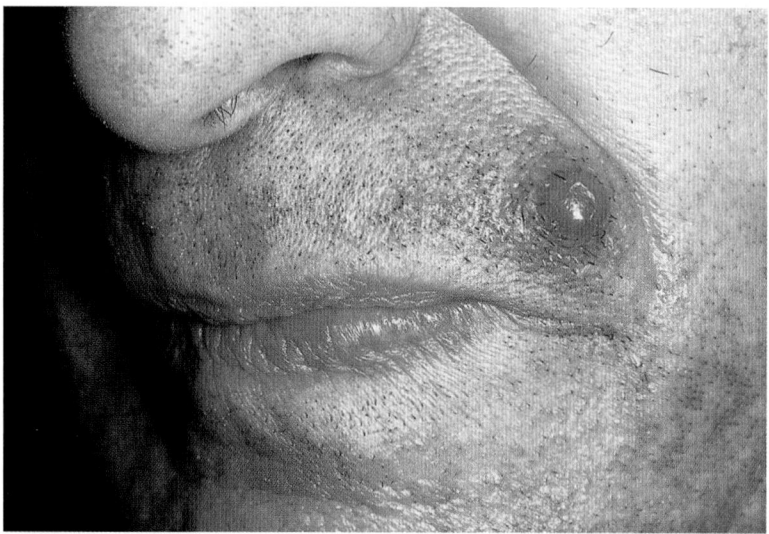

Fig. 30.10
Metastatic renal cell carcinoma: cutaneous metastases are typically erythematous and vascular, and may be misdiagnosed as pyogenic granuloma. By courtesy of R.A. Marsden, MD, St George's Hospital, London, UK.

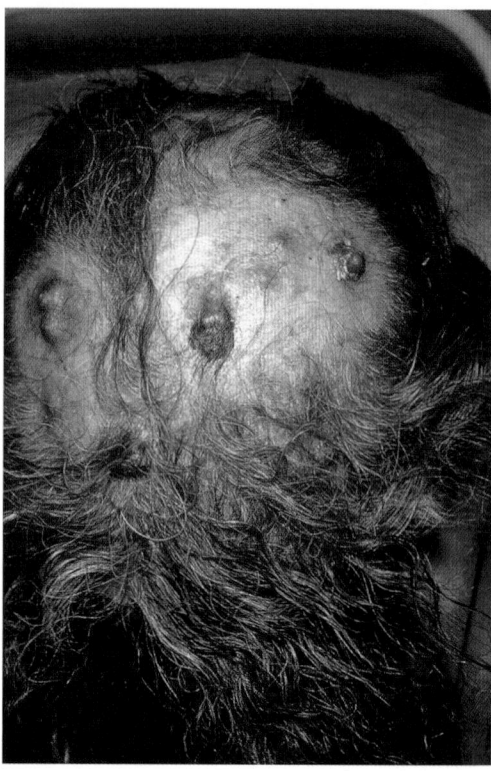

Fig. 30.12
Metastatic carcinoma of kidney: scalp lesions associated with numerous nodules and alopecia. By courtesy of R.A. Marsden, MD, St George's Hospital, London, UK.

metastases can mimic a melanoma.[91,92] The pigmented nature of the tumor is most likely due to epidermotropic metastasis that causes damage to the epidermis and subsequent pigmentary incontinence.

Exceptionally, metastases to benign cutaneous lesions such as nevi have been documented.[93,94] Unusual presentation of metastases includes spread to skin with radiation changes and to sites of surgical procedures.[95] The latter include scars following removal of abdominal organs or mastectomy sites, percutaneous biopsies or fine needle aspirates, pericardiocentesis, thoracocentesis, and sites of implantation of biliary catheters.[64,96–101]

There are other modes of presentation of cutaneous metastases which are particularly, but not exclusively, related to breast cancer. Inflammatory

cutaneous metastasis (carcinoma erysipelatoides) is fairly rare and results from massive lymphatic obstruction by tumor with associated edema.[102–105] It presents as a tender, erythematous, warm plaque (Fig. 30.18) located in most cases on the anterior chest wall (particularly in females with pendulous breasts). Clinically, it may be misdiagnosed as cellulitis or erysipelas, but theoretically, at least, it may be distinguished by the absence of fever and leukocytosis. Inflammatory cutaneous metastases have also been described with carcinoma of the prostate, lung, large bowel, pancreas, stomach, kidney, ovary, tonsil, parotid, uterus, esophagus, melanoma, and bladder.[106–114] Also associated with a poor prognosis are breast metastases presenting on the anterior chest wall as violaceous telangiectatic papules,

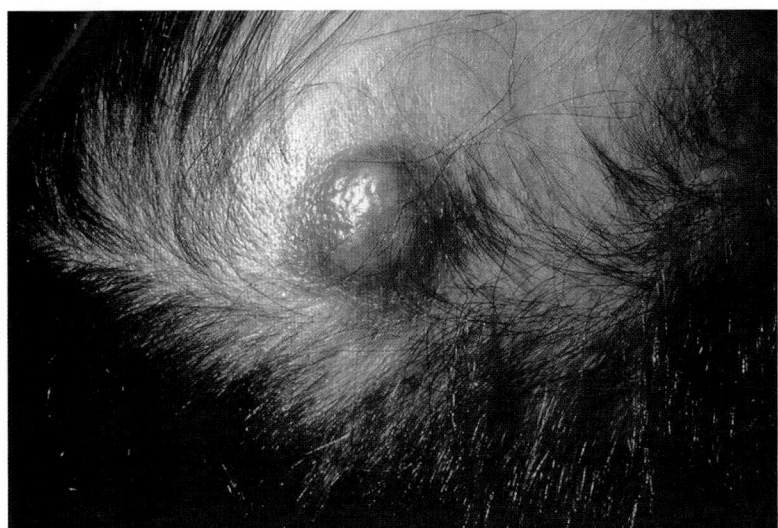

Fig. 30.13
Metastatic carcinoma: most metastases present as a flesh-colored or erythematous nodule. By courtesy of Drs José María Ricart and Amparo Marquina Vila, Hospital Peset, Valencia, Spain.

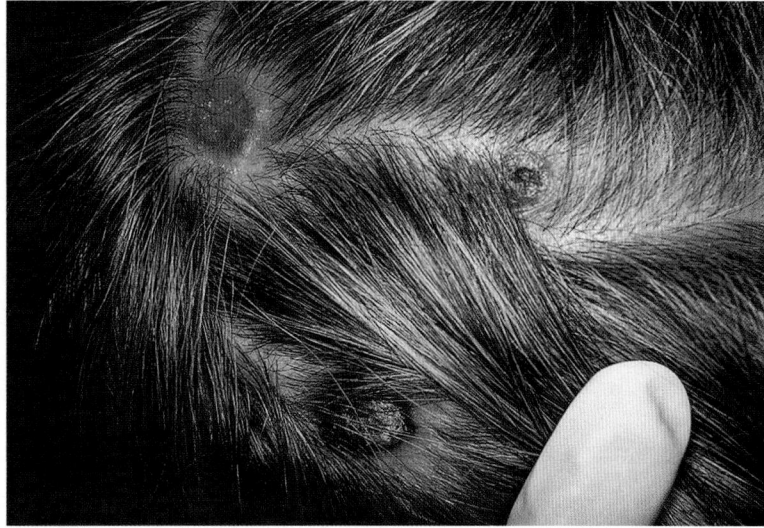

Fig. 30.15
Metastatic breast carcinoma: multiple tumor deposits are present on this patient's scalp – a common site of presentation following vascular invasion. By courtesy of Drs José María Ricart and Amparo Marquina Vila, Hospital Peset, Valencia, Spain.

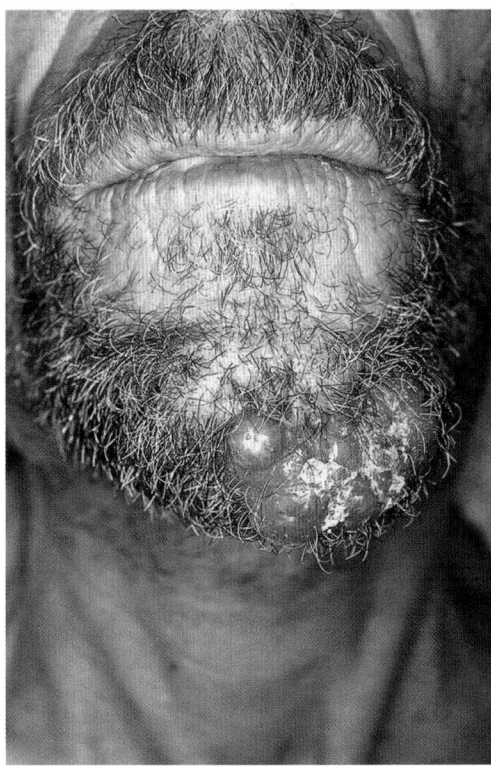

Fig. 30.14
Metastatic carcinoma: there are matted tumor nodules on the chin. The patient had a gastric carcinoma. By courtesy of Drs José María Ricart and Amparo Marquina Vila, Hospital Peset, Valencia, Spain.

A clinical variant that sometimes causes diagnostic confusion is the sclerodermatous (eburneous) metastasis usually associated with tumors having a dense fibrous stroma, such as carcinoma of the breast and pancreas.[120] The lesion is usually nontender and nonpruritic, and is most often located on the scalp with associated alopecia, so-called alopecia neoplastica. The latter may be confused with lichen planopilaris, pseudopélade, lupus erythematosus, alopecia areata, keloid, and morpheaform basal cell carcinoma.[8,124] Alopecia neoplastica has also been described in association with metastatic colonic carcinoma to the scalp.[125]

Neonates with metastatic neuroblastoma often present with multiple firm, blue-gray nodules in a typical appearance described as the 'blueberry muffin' syndrome. This presentation, however, is not specific and can also be seen in lymphoma, leukemia, vascular tumors, and congenital infections.[22]

Rare cutaneous metastases

Some tumors have only very exceptionally been reported with skin metastases. Many of these primary tumors are themselves quite uncommon. These include glioblastoma, glioma, eccrine porocarcinoma or hidradenocarcinoma, pheochromocytoma, ameloblastoma, parotid adenocarcinoma (including malignant pleomorphic adenoma), chordoma, malignant thymoma, seminoma, Leydig cell tumor, papillary serous carcinoma of the uterus and of the ovary, ovarian malignant Brenner tumor, gallbladder adenocarcinoma, adrenocortical carcinoma (including a case presenting with cutaneous metastasis 30 years after the primary), transitional bladder carcinoma, hepatocellular carcinoma, carcinoid tumor, neuroendocrine tumors, mesothelioma, anaplastic carcinoma of the thyroid, medullary thyroid carcinoma, Sertoli cell tumor, salivary adenoid cystic carcinoma, cholangiocarcinoma, paraganglioma, and pancreatic mucoepidermoid carcinoma.[9,39,58,84,126–154] Other cases include metastases of myoepithelial carcinoma including one case in a child, well-differentiated fetal adenocarcinoma, adenocarcinoma of rete testis, malignant sacrococcygeal teratoma, prostatic small cell carcinoma, mucinous sweat duct carcinoma, adenocarcinoma arising in a longstanding nevus sebaceus of Jadassohn, small-cell neuroendocrine carcinoma of the uterine cervix, squamous cell carcinoma of the ureter, an exceptional case of acinic cell carcinoma of salivary gland presenting with cutaneous metastases 20 years after the primary, and a malignant blue nevus of the scalp with distant metastasis to the back.[155–166]

Sarcomas mainly involve the skin as a result of direct extension from the underlying subcutis or deeper soft tissues. Cutaneous metastatic sarcoma, which represents less than 3% of all cutaneous metastases, has been described in association with leiomyosarcoma arising in different organs including the uterus and small intestine, epithelioid sarcoma, chondrosarcoma, osteosarcoma including a postirradiation lesion, undifferentiated

vesicles, or nodules resembling lymphangioma circumscriptum.[115–117] This is known as carcinoma telangiectaticum, and it may also be seen rarely with lung carcinoma. The lesions are sometimes purpuric and hemorrhagic and resemble a vasculitic process.[118] Other manifestations of breast cancer are *peau d'orange*, representing dermal edema due to obstruction of superficial cutaneous lymphatic vessels and carcinoma *en cuirasse*, an intensely sclerotic plaque of tumor (*Fig. 30.19*).[1,102–105,119,120]

Metastatic breast carcinoma infrequently presents in the inframammary crease in a characteristic pattern mimicking dermatitis or resembling a primary epithelial tumor including basal cell and squamous cell carcinoma.[121–123]

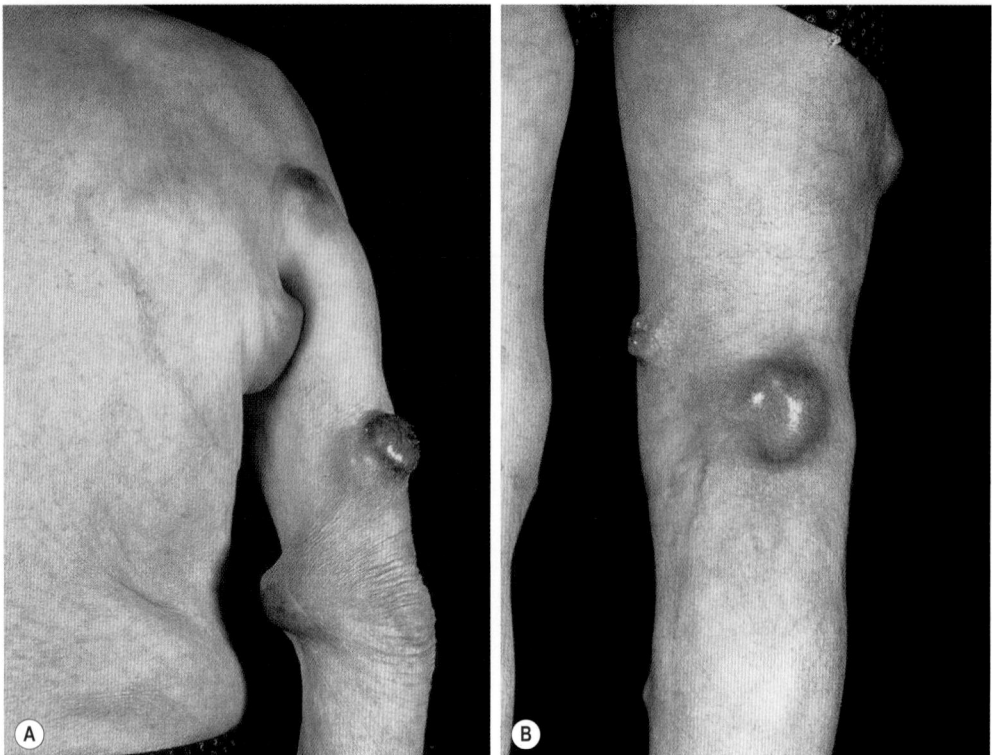

Fig. 30.16
Metastatic melanoma: tumor deposits are present on (**A**) the arm and (**B**) the leg. By courtesy of the Institute of Dermatology, London, UK.

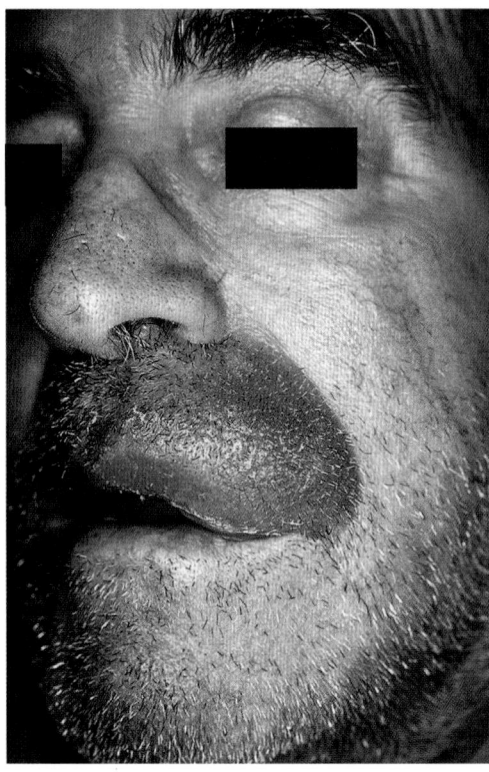

Fig. 30.17
Metastatic bronchial carcinoma: in this patient, the tumor deposit has resulted in a lymphedematous lesion. By courtesy of Drs José María Ricart and Amparo Marquina Vila, Hospital Peset, Valencia, Spain.

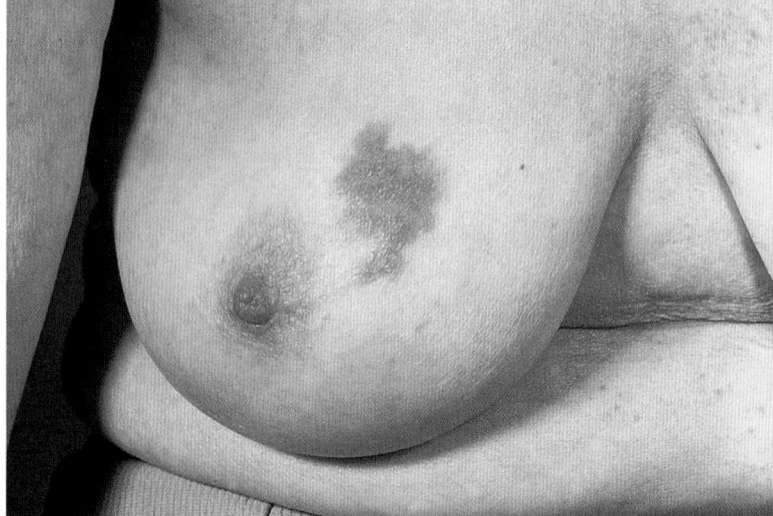

Fig. 30.18
Metastatic carcinoma of breast: an inflammatory cutaneous metastasis usually presents as a tender, warm, erythematous plaque. By courtesy of R.A. Marsden, MD, St George's Hospital, London, UK.

derived from the chondrosarcomatous component of a metaplastic (sarcomatoid) breast carcinoma has also been described.[185] A case of cutaneous metastasis from osteosarcoma has been reported as the first manifestation of disease.[186] Atrial myxoma may embolize to the skin, particularly in the context of Carney complex.[187–189]

Prognosis

The presence of cutaneous metastases is usually (although not invariably) an ominous sign. The average survival is about 6 months after diagnosis.[7,34,190] However, some patients may have long survival. This reflects both improvement in cancer therapy and the biological behavior of the individual tumor.[18] For example, neuroblastoma in children can mature or undergo complete regression, and patients with renal cell carcinoma can have a long

pleomorphic sarcoma, giant cell tumor of bone, fibrosarcoma, rhabdomyosarcoma, gastrointestinal stromal tumor, synovial sarcoma, alveolar soft part sarcoma, Ewing sarcoma, myxofibrosarcoma, angiosarcoma, PEComa, and pleomorphic liposarcoma.[60,63,167–184] In the authors' experience, metastatic leiomyosarcoma is most commonly encountered. A cutaneous metastasis

Fig. 30.19
Peau d'orange: this typical clinical appearance is not due to tumor infiltration, but represents severe cutaneous lymphedema caused by lymphatic blockage at a distant site.

survival following removal of the primary tumor and the metastases. In general, patients with cutaneous metastases from the upper digestive tract, upper respiratory tract, lung, and ovary have very poor survival.[18] In a study involving 200 patients with cutaneous metastases, Schoenlaub and coauthors reported median survival times of 13.8 months for breast cancer, 2.9 months for lung cancer, and 6.5 months for all other cancers.[190]

Histologic features

Histologic interpretation of a cutaneous metastasis depends upon a complete knowledge of the patient's clinical history (past and present), coupled with adequate experience of the wide range of histologic features of tumors.

The most challenging differential diagnosis of cutaneous metastases is with primary cutaneous tumors, especially with those of adnexal origin. On histologic grounds alone, several features are traditionally used to distinguish between these entities. One of the features in favor of a primary cutaneous tumor is continuity with the epidermis or growth into skin appendages (i.e., an in situ component). However, it is important to remember that tumors such as hidradenocarcinoma are strictly intradermal and do not connect with overlying epidermis, and also that epidermotropic metastases are not infrequent. Another useful clue for a primary cutaneous tumor is identification of the benign counterpart within the lesion (such as areas of benign spiradenoma within a spiradenocarcinoma). One finding that is seldom noted in the literature is the more frequent presence of entrapped, 'passenger' melanocytes within primary cutaneous lesions in contrast to metastatic tumors where they are rarely seen. The most useful histologic features in favor of a cutaneous metastasis include location in the deep dermis or subcutaneous tissue, multifocality, and more frequent presence of lymphovascular invasion. It is important to be aware that while these histologic findings may be useful in the diagnosis of cutaneous metastases they are not completely reliable. They should be used in combination with the clinical history and, in the majority of cases, immunohistochemical studies that may help in identification of the tumor origin. On some occasions, however, the finding of poorly differentiated adenocarcinoma or squamous carcinoma will permit only a list of the more likely sites of the primary lesion.

Immunohistochemistry, electron microscopy and fine needle aspiration cytology

Immunohistochemistry is of particular value in distinguishing between various carcinomas, melanomas, lymphomas, and pleomorphic sarcomas (Figs 30.20–30.24). With respect to metastatic adenocarcinoma, however, it is more difficult to accurately predict the likely site of the primary neoplasm.[1,2] With a few specific exceptions, including thyroid (thyroglobulin), prostatic carcinoma (prostate specific antigen, prostatic acid phosphatase),

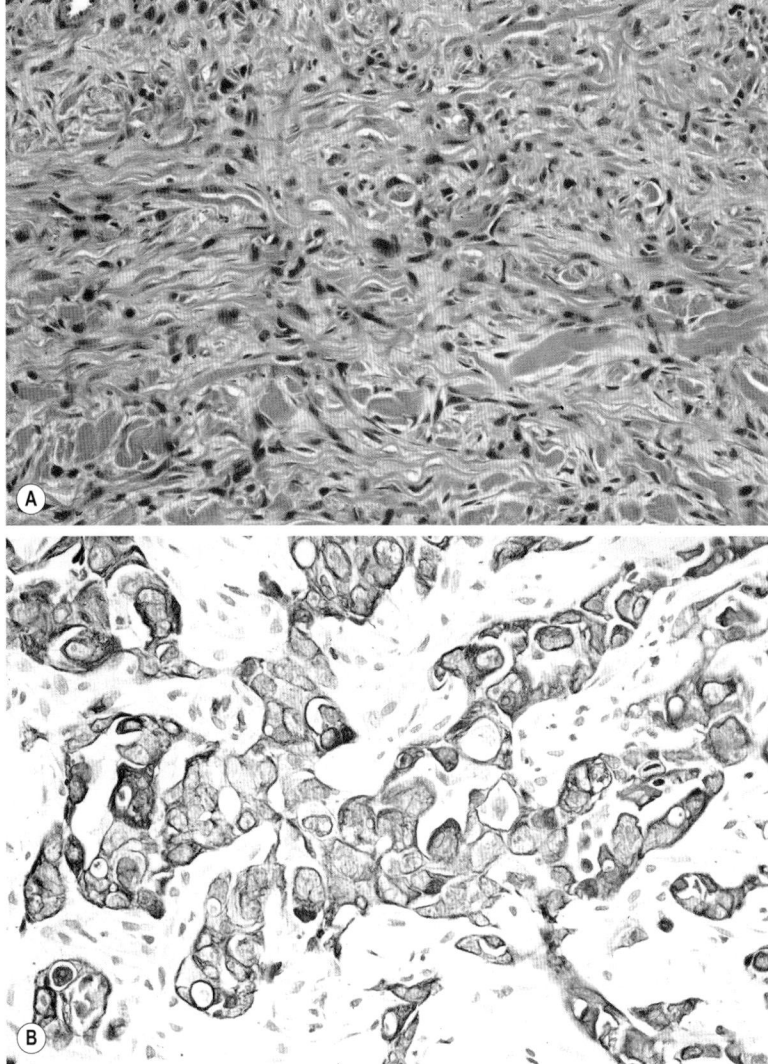

Fig. 30.20
Metastatic carcinoma: (A) this field shows a deposit of metastatic, poorly differentiated bronchial adenocarcinoma; (B) the tumor cells show intense keratin expression, thereby confirming their epithelial nature.

and hepatocellular carcinoma (hepatocyte paraffin 1 and α-fetoprotein),[3] if the precise diagnosis is not apparent after careful scrutiny of hematoxylin and eosin stained sections then it is less than likely that immunohistochemistry will be of definite help in resolving the problem.[1,4]

Immunohistochemistry can sometimes play an important role in the assessment of metastasis associated with an occult primary tumor. An enormous range of antibodies is now available, and a large proportion is suitable for use with routine, formalin-fixed, paraffin-embedded tissues. Difficulties, however, are often experienced due to lack of specificity or poor sensitivity. It is essential that the practitioner be aware of the often wide range of cell types that may express any particular antigen and that the use of panels of immunohistochemical studies is more helpful than single stains. Virtually, all new markers initially heralded as highly specific in an initial publication follow a natural history of decreasing specificity in subsequent reports.

Distinction between primary cutaneous and metastatic neuroendocrine carcinoma is usually made by the presence of positive dotlike perinuclear staining for low molecular weight cytokeratin (CK) 20 and neurofilament protein expression in the former and absence of staining in the latter.[5,6] Apart from the skin, CK20 is only expressed consistently in neuroendocrine carcinomas of salivary gland origin.[5] In contrast, bronchial neuroendocrine carcinoma expresses CK7. Although these findings are useful in the differential diagnosis in most cases, caution is recommended before basing a diagnosis on a single immunohistochemical result. Some cases of lung small cell carcinoma express CK20, and there are also reported

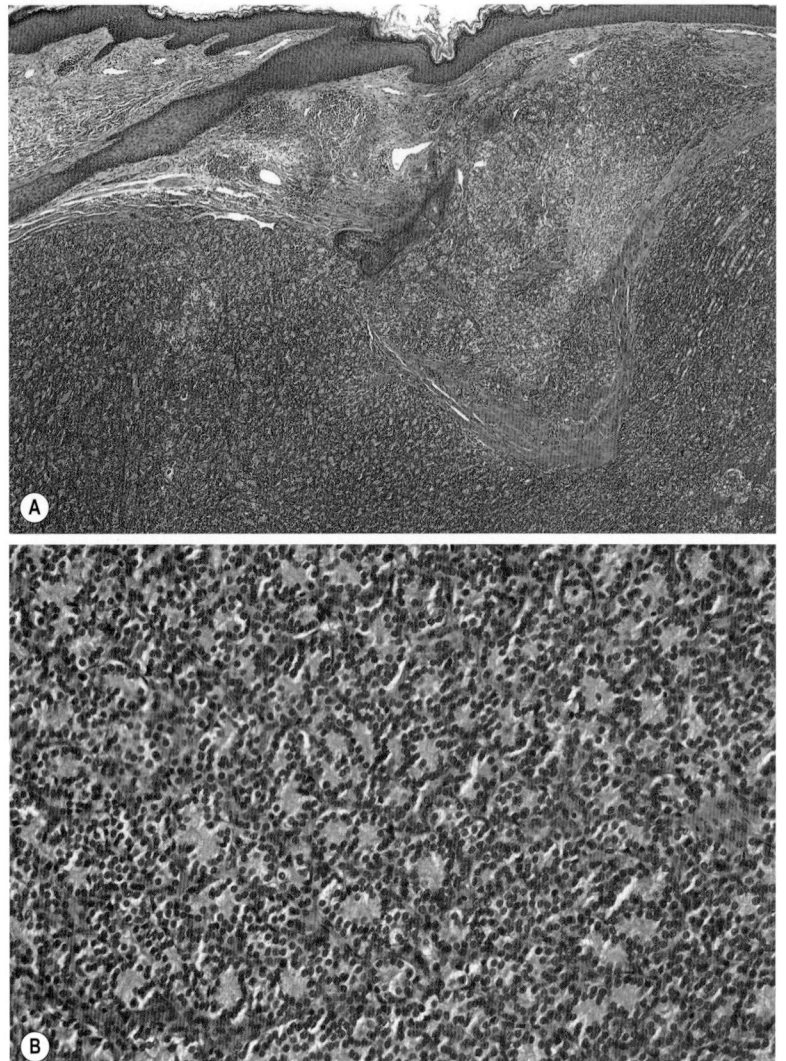

Fig. 30.21
Metastatic thyroid follicular carcinoma: (**A**) low-power view; (**B**) typical follicles are evident.

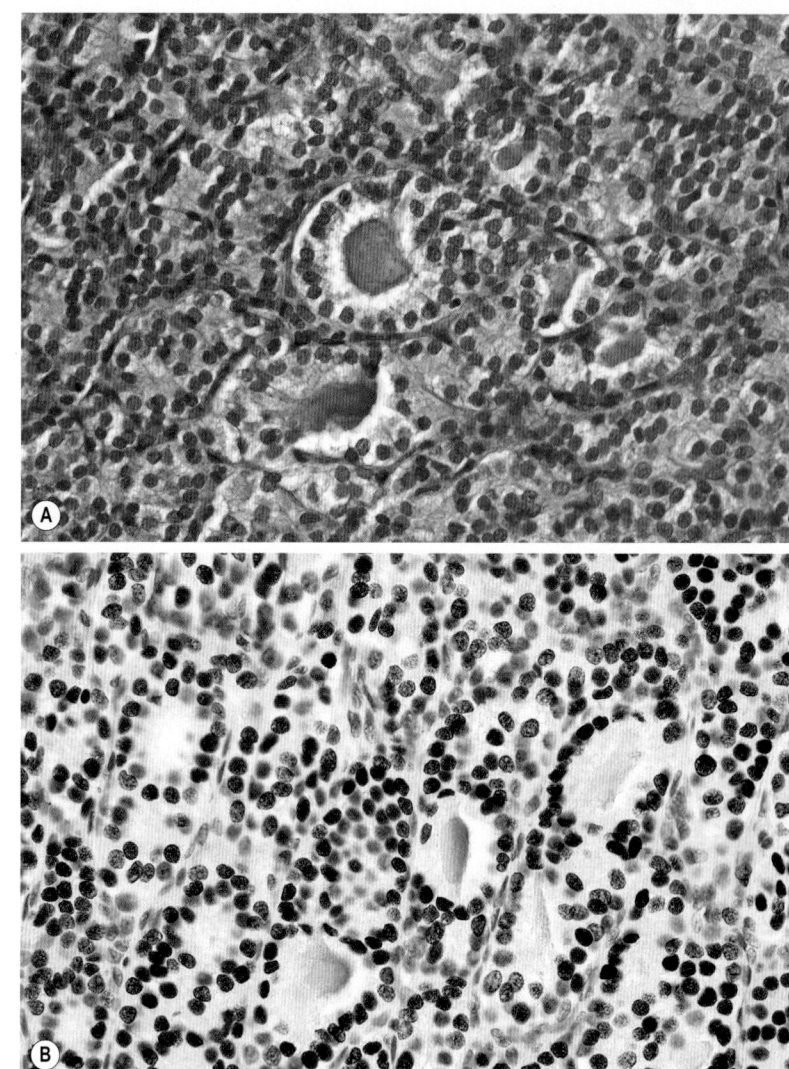

Fig. 30.22
Metastatic thyroid follicular carcinoma: (**A**) focal colloid production is seen; (**B**) the nuclei show strong nuclear staining for TFF-1.

cases of cutaneous neuroendocrine carcinoma (Merkel cell carcinoma) that are CK20-negative.[7–10] The use of thyroid transcription factor 1 (TTF-1) can also be of help in the distinction between a primary cutaneous and a metastatic bronchial neuroendocrine carcinoma: TTF-1 is negative in the former but present in the latter.[11,12] However, occasional cases of Merkel cell carcinoma have been shown to be positive for TTF-1.[13,14] Although CK20 is most commonly used, other cytokeratins, such as CAM 5.2, also label the tumor cells of primary cutaneous neuroendocrine carcinoma. A further marker has been described as useful in the distinction between pulmonary small cell carcinoma and Merkel cell carcinoma.[13] MASH-1 (raised against Achaete-scute complex-like 1) is an important protein in the development not only of the brain but also of the neuroendocrine system. MASH-1 tends to be positive in pulmonary small cell carcinoma in up to 83% of cases but appears to be uniformly negative in Merkel cell carcinoma.[13]

Historically, gross cystic disease fluid protein 15 (GCDFP-15), estrogen receptor (ER), and progesterone receptor (PR) have been used as markers for breast differentiation. However, it is important to note that GCDFP-15, ER, PR, and Her2/neu have all been shown to be also expressed in cutaneous adnexal neoplasms, reflecting the close relationship between the sweat gland and the breast.[15–19] For this reason, these markers should be used with caution if utilized in an attempt to distinguish primary cutaneous lesions from metastatic breast tumors.

Staining for other low molecular weight keratins such as CK7 is of limited value in the differential diagnosis of metastatic carcinoma. Although this marker is absent from many carcinomas – including those originating in prostate, colon, kidney, and thymus – it is present in the majority of carcinomas arising in other organs, and therefore its specificity is very limited.[20] CK7 has been shown to be expressed in both primary cutaneous adnexal neoplasms and cutaneous metastases, mainly from the lung and breast.[21] However, the pattern of CK7 labeling is distinctly different between the two categories: only focal in primary adnexal neoplasms, present in the inner luminal cells lining tubules and cysts, whereas there is strong and diffuse staining in metastatic adenocarcinomas.[21] However, using CK7 and CK20 in combination with GCDFP-15 can be useful in determining whether a case of extramammary Paget disease is primary or metastatic.[22–24] Primary perianal and extramammary Paget disease tends to be positive for CK7 and GCDFP-15 and negative for CK20, while metastatic rectal adenocarcinoma is usually negative for the former two markers and positive for the latter.[22–24] The transcription factor GATA3 is seen in over 80% of both breast and urothelial carcinomas.[25]

Gastrointestinal metastasis to the skin can often be suspected by the presence of 'dirty' necrosis (intraluminal necrotic debris), commonly seen in primary and metastatic intestinal adenocarcinoma. The pattern of strong CK20 expression and lack of CK7 expression favors a metastasis from an intestinal primary tumor. Carcinoma originating in the hepatobiliary or upper gastrointestinal tract may be also CK7-positive and/or CK20-negative. CDX2, a homeobox gene encoding an intestinal epithelial transcription factor, initially considered a specific marker for gastrointestinal tract origin, has also been reported in other tumors, including ovarian mucinous tumors of the intestinal type, pulmonary mucinous adenocarcinoma, bladder adenocarcinoma, and endometrial carcinoma, and rare tumors of the lung (non-mucinous), bladder (urothelial), and head and neck.[26–28] Villin is an

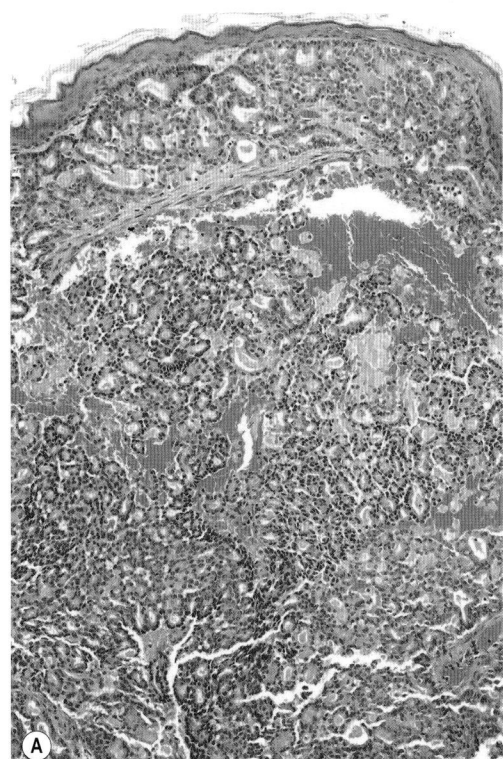

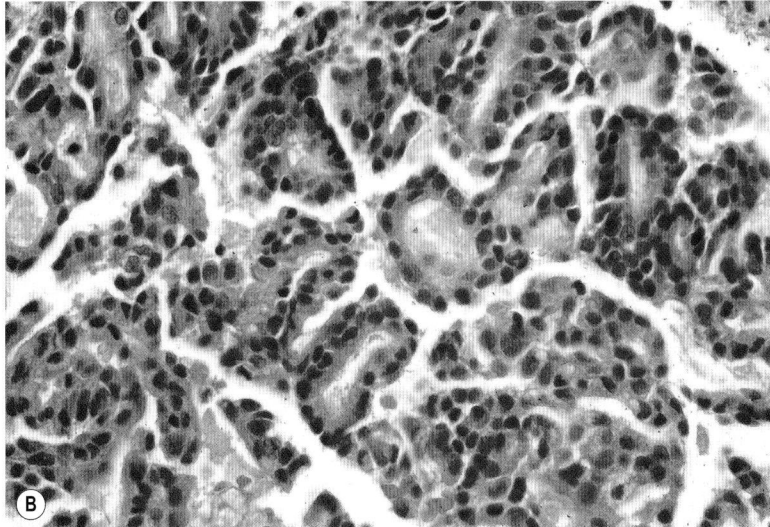

Fig. 30.23
Metastatic pancreatic carcinoma: (**A**) low-power view; (**B**) the tumor shows a well-developed glandular structure.

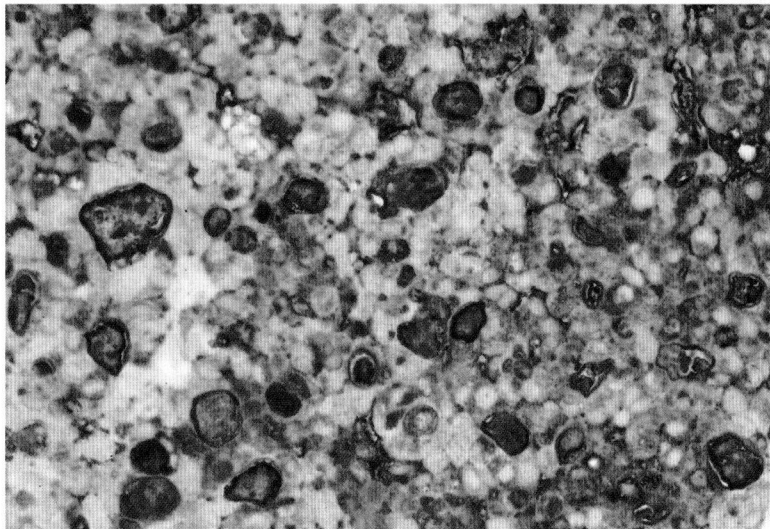

Fig. 30.24
Metastatic pancreatic carcinoma: the tumor cells are strongly CA 19-9 positive.

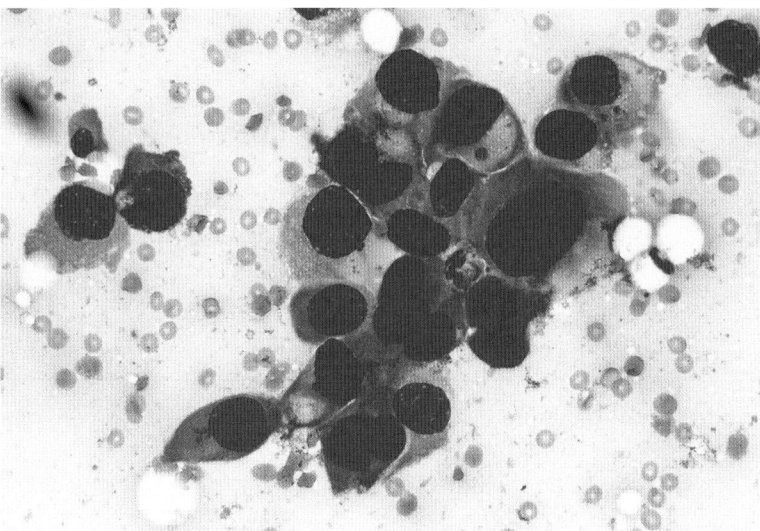

Fig. 30.25
Fine needle aspirate: this specimen from a cutaneous nodule shows large pleomorphic adenocarcinoma cells. By courtesy of G.T. McKee, MD, Massachusetts General Hospital, Boston, USA.

additional marker that may help to distinguish between colorectal (positive) and ovarian metastatic deposits (negative).[29]

Cutaneous metastases from the lung often express CK7 and lack CK20. Additionally, approximately 75% to 85% of primary pulmonary adenocarcinomas express TTF-1, but is also seen in thyroid carcinomas.[30,31] Napsin A is expressed in up to 80% of pulmonary adenocarcinomas as well as ovarian clear cell and renal cell and papillary carcinomas.[32]

The great majority of adrenocortical neoplasms will coexpress Melan A/MART1, inhibin, and calretinin. Prostatic carcinoma will usually express PSA, PAP, androgen receptor (AR), and the transcription factor NKX3-1.[28] The transcription factor PAX8 is a sensitive marker for carcinomas of the ovary, thyroid, and kidney.[28,33]

Formalin-fixed, paraffin-embedded tissue may be reprocessed for electron microscopy, and ultrastructural investigation of such material may throw light on the likely source of the primary neoplasm. Traditionally, if possible, a small portion of fresh tissue was processed for electron microscopy. Identification of cellular markers, such as desmosomes, intracytoplasmic mucin, melanosomes, and membrane-bound neurosecretory granules, may

be helpful in pointing to the correct diagnosis. Use of this technique to identify tumors of uncertain differentiation has become exceedingly rare with the wide availability of numerous immunohistochemical markers.

Over the past few decades, the enthusiasm for fine needle aspiration cytology has grown. The technique in many circumstances has proven to be a highly satisfactory alternative to more conventional excisional, punch, or tru-cut biopsy specimens. In the dermatopathology setting, it can be of particular value in assessing potential metastatic tumors, especially if the patient is unfit or unwilling to undergo further operative procedures (*Figs 30.25* and *30.26*).[34] Fine needle aspiration cytology is a fast, inexpensive, and effective method of confirming the diagnosis in the majority of cases. Where appropriate, the technique also permits the application of immunohistochemical investigations, fluorescent in situ hybridization (FISH), and polymerase chain reaction (PCR)-based techniques.

Individual tumors

Squamous carcinoma

Metastatic squamous carcinoma reflects a wide variety of primary sites including the bronchus (30% of metastatic lung tumors), esophagus (less

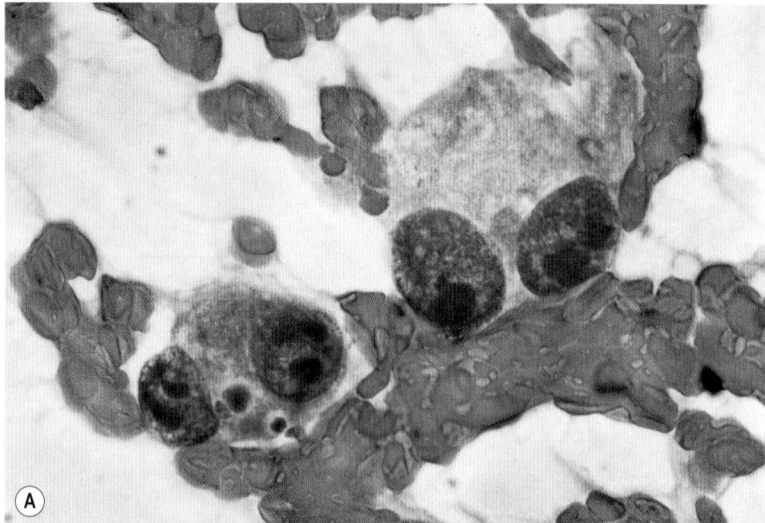

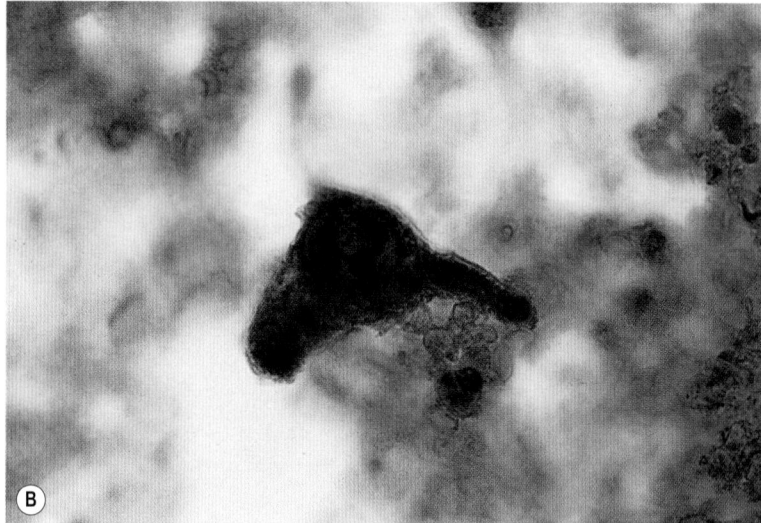

Fig. 30.26
Fine needle aspirate: this is an example of metastatic malignant melanoma. Note (**A**) the large nucleoli and (**B**) the intracytoplasmic pigment. By courtesy of G.T. McKee, MD, Massachusetts General Hospital, Boston, USA.

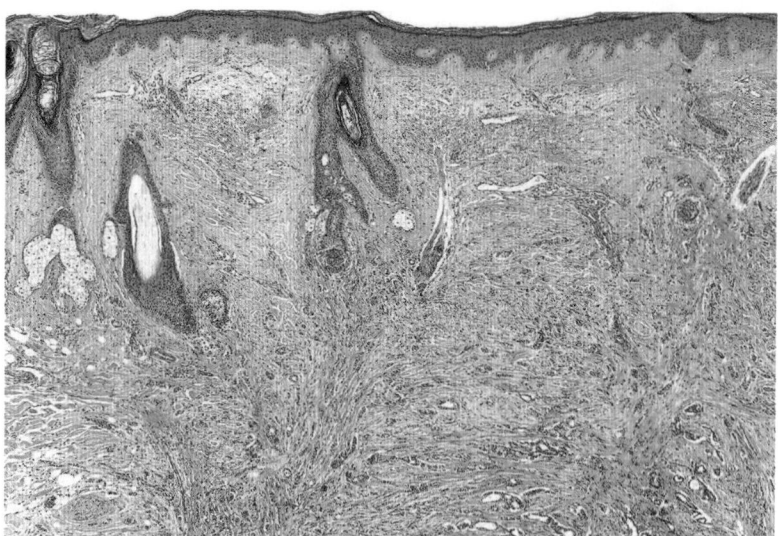

Fig. 30.27
Metastatic carcinoma of breast (alopecia neoplastica): scalp biopsy from a middle-aged female shows extensive infiltration of the dermis by tumor, resulting in loss of pilosebaceous structures.

carcinoma is frequently positive for this marker, while adenocarcinoma is negative except in areas of metaplastic squamous differentiation.[28,50] Adenocarcinomas are also often positive for low molecular weight keratins such as CAM 5.2.

Anaplastic and spindle cell variants may be mistaken for lymphoma, melanoma, atypical fibroxanthoma/dermal pleomorphic sarcoma, and even sarcoma. In such lesions, immunocytochemistry is usually essential. It is important to use antibodies reactive against a broad spectrum of keratins or a cocktail of antibodies because restricted antibodies such as CAM 5.2 are usually negative.

Adenocarcinoma

Adenocarcinomatous deposits are by far the most common cutaneous metastasis, with the breast being the most frequent source (up to 23% of cutaneous metastases, the vast majority of which occur in women).[35,38,51] Lung and large intestine are also important sources of metastatic adenocarcinoma.[52,53] Other primary sites include the stomach, prostate, pancreas, endometrium, thyroid gland, ovaries, and endocervix.[4,35,38,54–61] Antibodies against lineage restricted transcription factors are available for many cancer types and will be discussed further below.

Metastases from carcinoma of the breast have a variety of appearances, depending to some extent on the nature of the primary tumor (*Figs 30.27–30.31*).[62] Nodular deposits and carcinoma *en cuirasse* consist of a diffuse infiltrate of undifferentiated cells with hyperchromatic nuclei and minimal cytoplasm. Metastatic breast carcinoma to the eyelid is seen with some frequency, and at that site the tumor cells sometimes have a prominent histiocytoid appearance.[63] Rarely, metastatic adenocarcinoma of the breast, prostate, and colon can present with epidermotropism, and confusion with primary cutaneous carcinoma or superficial spreading melanoma may ensue.[43,64] Exceptionally, metastatic breast carcinoma mimics a granular cell tumor or contains melanin pigment resembling a melanoma.[65–67]

Typical of a breast metastasis, especially the lobular type, is the presence of linear dissection of tumor cells between adjacent collagen bundles (stacked-penny or 'single-file' appearance) (*Fig. 30.32*). Similar appearances may be seen with a number of other tumors including those of the prostate, stomach, and pancreas, and small cell carcinoma. Lymphoma, sclerosing epithelioid fibrosarcoma, and primary cutaneous neuroendocrine tumor may occasionally adopt an identical pattern. There may be obvious glandular differentiation, but it is unusual for this to predominate (*Fig. 30.33*). Inflammatory carcinoma is characterized by a widespread infiltration of the subepidermal and deeper lymphatic channels, and, in the telangiectatic variant, vascular involvement may also be apparent[68] (*Figs 30.34*

than 2% of esophageal cancers disseminate to the skin), oral cavity, larynx, and cervix.[35–41] It may less frequently arise from a squamous carcinoma elsewhere on the integument, anus, vulva, penis, vagina, and tonsil.[42] Poorly differentiated metastases often cause difficulties, and multiple sections may have to be scrutinized carefully before foci of squamous differentiation (keratinization or intercellular bridges) are detected. An important point is that it is not possible to distinguish metastatic poorly differentiated squamous cell from transitional cell tumors in the absence of keratinization. In addition, the site of origin of squamous cell carcinomas is generally not distinguished by morphological or immunohistochemical markers.

Usually, the metastatic tumor does not connect with the overlying epidermis. Exceptionally, however, a metastatic squamous cell carcinoma can present as an epidermotropic and/or folliculotropic metastasis, making distinction from a primary tumor very difficult. This phenomenon has been described in a metastatic laryngeal carcinoma, in a carcinoma from the lip, and in metastases from a primary cutaneous squamous cell carcinoma.[43,44] High molecular weight keratins such as CK 5/6 can also be used for the diagnosis of squamous cell carcinoma, particularly in poorly differentiated tumors, but this does not allow a distinction between primary and metastatic neoplasms.[28,45,46] Both p63 and p40 can also be used as markers that suggest squamous origin if characteristic morphological features are lacking.[47–49]

The use of CK14 has been advocated as being helpful in distinguishing between a squamous cell carcinoma and an adenocarcinoma. Squamous cell

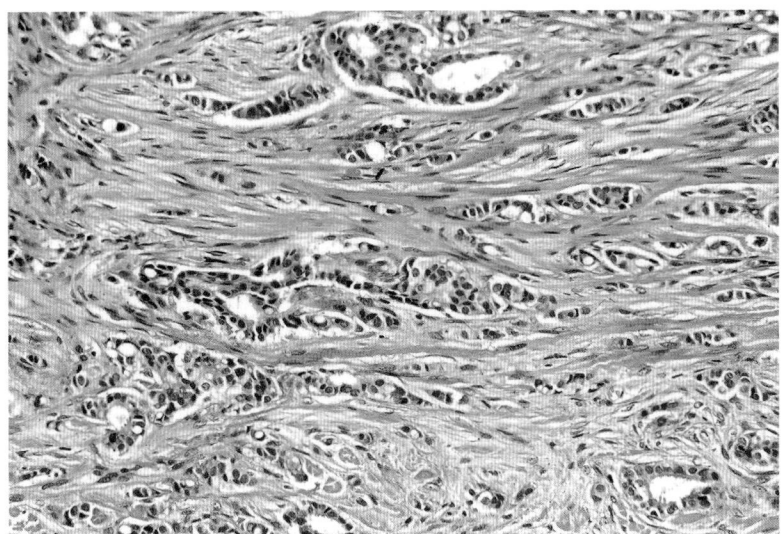

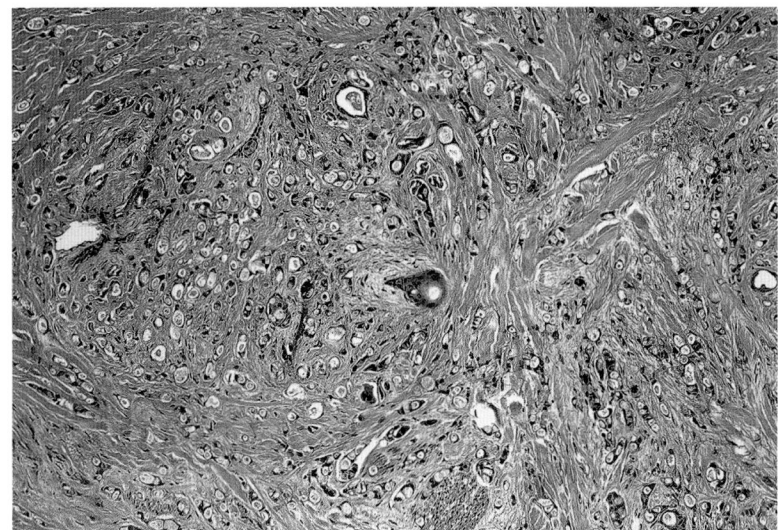

Fig. 30.28
Metastatic carcinoma of breast (alopecia neoplastica): the tumor infiltrate is composed of cords of tumor cells dispersed in a dense fibrous stroma. Note the glandular differentiation.

Fig. 30.30
Sclerodermatous metastatic carcinoma of breast: the cells are dispersed in a very dense fibrous stroma.

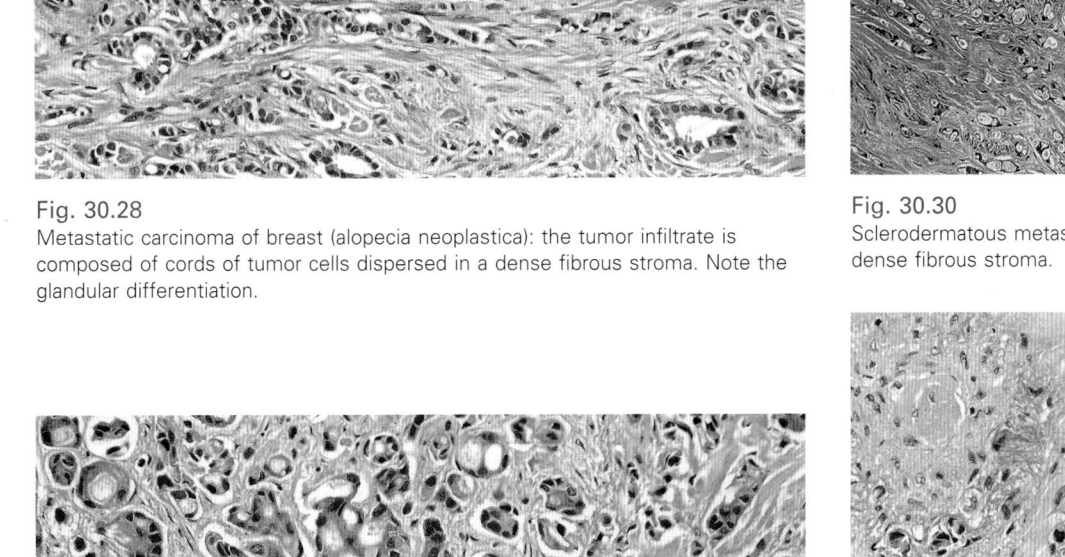

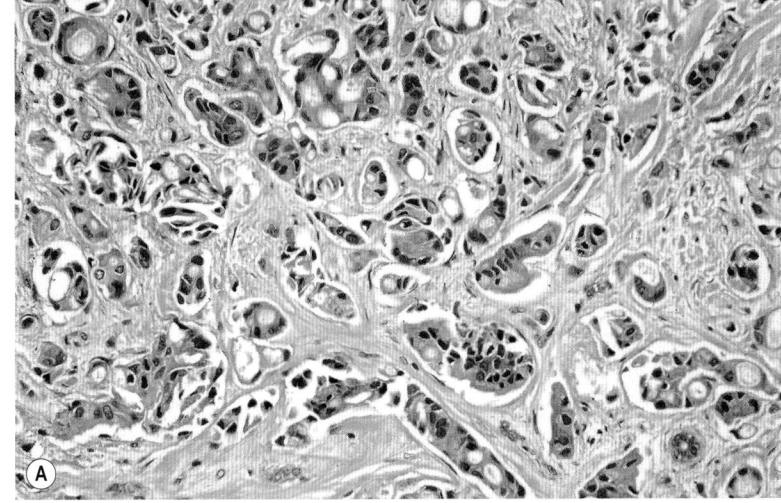

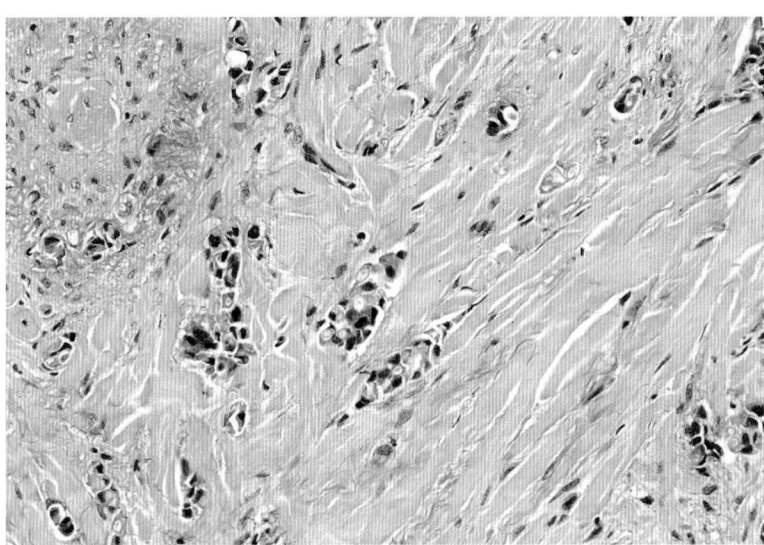

Fig. 30.31
Sclerodermatous metastatic carcinoma of the breast: higher-power view.

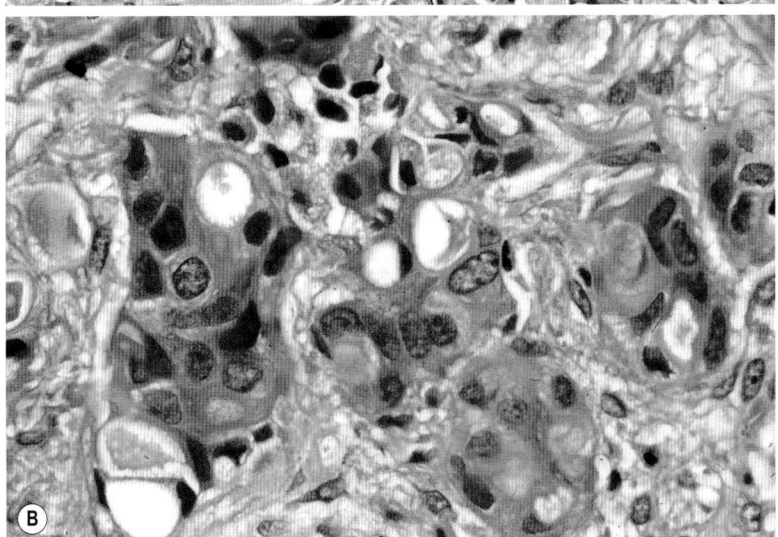

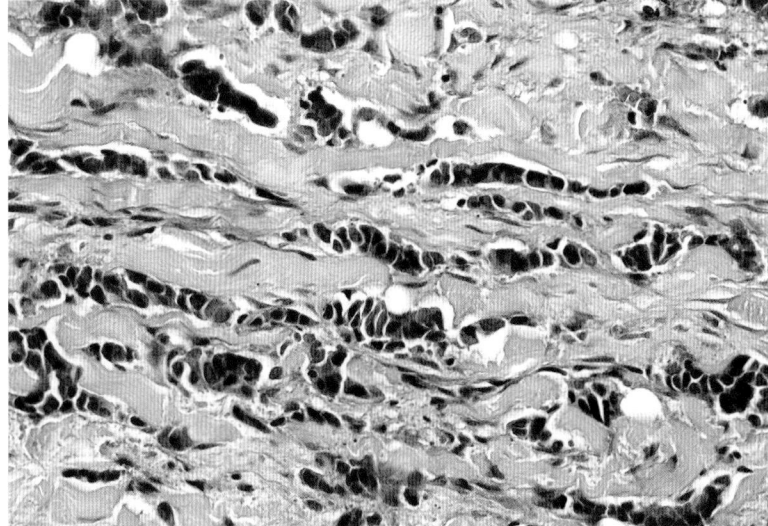

Fig. 30.29
Metastatic carcinoma of the breast (alopecia neoplastica): (A) this example is much more high grade. Note the pleomorphism; (B) intracytoplasmic lumina are present.

Fig. 30.32
Metastatic carcinoma of breast: the characteristic stacked-penny appearance is well demonstrated in this field. By courtesy of J. Cohen, MD, Dermatopathology Laboratory, Tucson, USA.

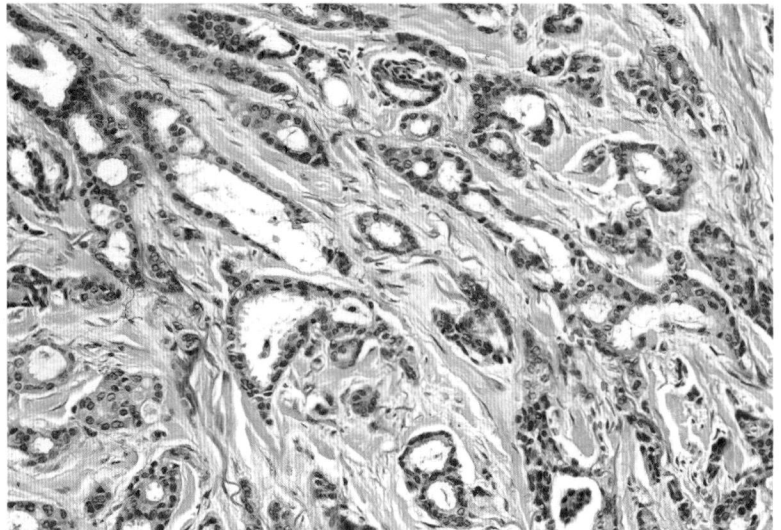

Fig. 30.33
Metastatic carcinoma of breast: in this example, there are well-developed ducts.

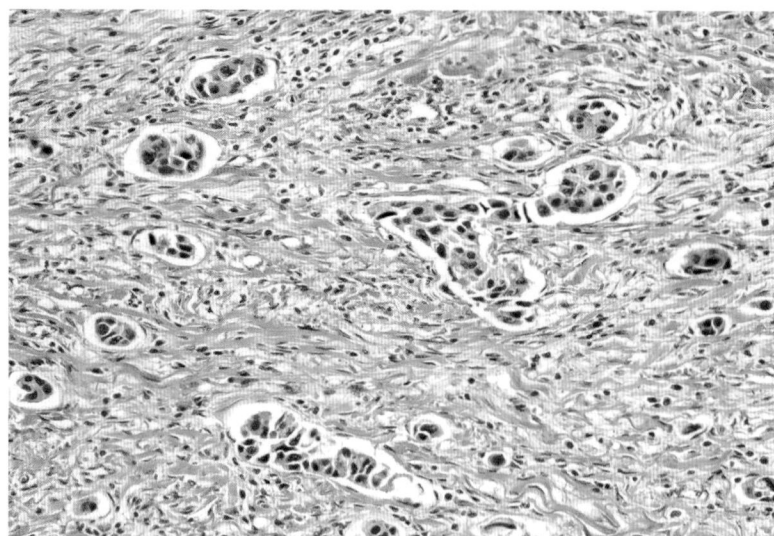

Fig. 30.35
Inflammatory carcinoma: in this example, innumerable vessels were affected.

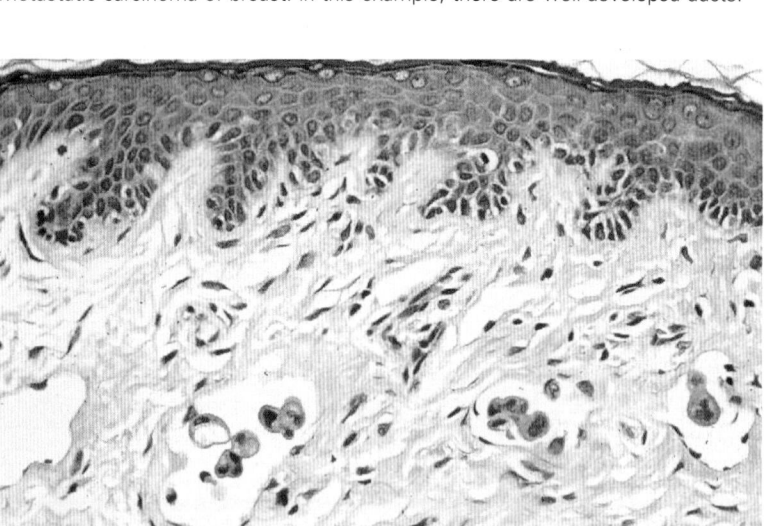

Fig. 30.34
Inflammatory carcinoma: there is involvement of the superficial dermal lymphatics.

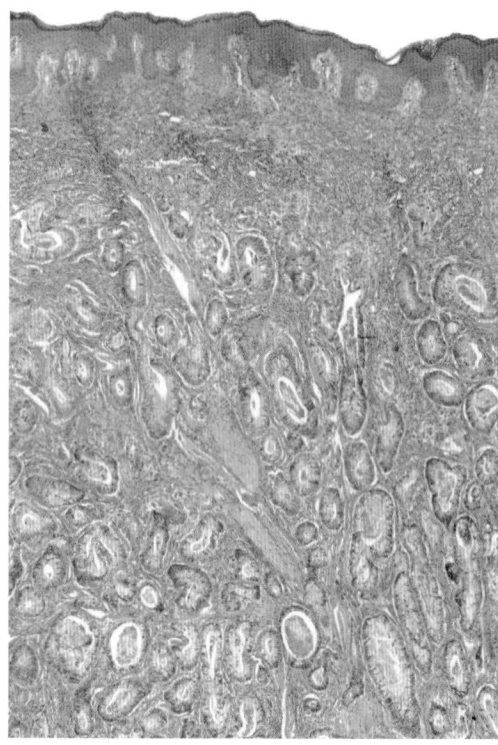

Fig. 30.36
Metastatic colonic adenocarcinoma: there is widespread infiltration of the dermis. Note the well-formed ductal structures.

and *30.35*). A well-differentiated glandular architecture, with focal necrosis, is more typical of a primary tumor in the large intestine or rectum (*Figs 30.36–30.39*). In anaplastic variants, the features of the tumor cells may be indistinguishable from those of a high-grade lymphoma. Immunohistochemical techniques are often necessary to establish the correct diagnosis. Some CD30-positive anaplastic large cell lymphomas fail to express leukocyte common antigen (CD45). It is important to include a range of antibodies to both B- and T-cell antigens before excluding the diagnosis of disseminated lymphoma. It must also be remembered that nodal CD30-positive anaplastic large cell lymphoma not uncommonly expresses epithelial membrane antigen (EMA), which may therefore be a diagnostic pitfall for the unwary.

Metastatic tumors with a papillary growth pattern may reflect a number of different sites, including the colon, ovary, thyroid gland, stomach, and even the lung (*Figs 30.40* and *30.41*).[58–60] Certain distinguishing features sometimes permit differentiation between various papillary metastases. Concentrically laminated calcified psammomatous bodies may be conspicuous in both serous (ovarian) carcinoma and thyroid papillary carcinoma. The latter, however, may be further identified by colloid production, nuclear grooving, and characteristic 'Orphan Annie' nuclei.[35] Intranuclear cytoplasmic pseudoinclusions are also sometimes a feature. The immunohistochemical demonstration of thyroglobulin production is confirmatory. Cutaneous metastasis of papillary thyroid carcinoma with prominent clear cell change

may mimic a primary adnexal tumor such as a clear cell hidradenocarcinoma. A percentage of cases of metastatic papillary thyroid carcinoma show BRAF (V600E) mutations detectable by immunohistochemistry using the VE1 antibody or other molecular methods, a feature that is absent in follicular carcinoma of the thyroid and in hidradenocarcinoma, allowing distinction in difficult cases.[69,70]

Perhaps one of the most challenging differential diagnoses lies between metastatic adenocarcinoma and a primary cutaneous adnexal carcinoma showing well-developed ductal differentiation. Eccrine carcinomas, including microcystic adnexal carcinoma and hidradenocarcinoma in particular, can commonly mimic adenocarcinoma metastatic to the skin from a variety of primary sites, most commonly breast, lung, gastrointestinal tract, or ovary. Eccrine adenoma can also enter the differential diagnosis in such cases because of the duct formation, but the absence of an infiltrative growth

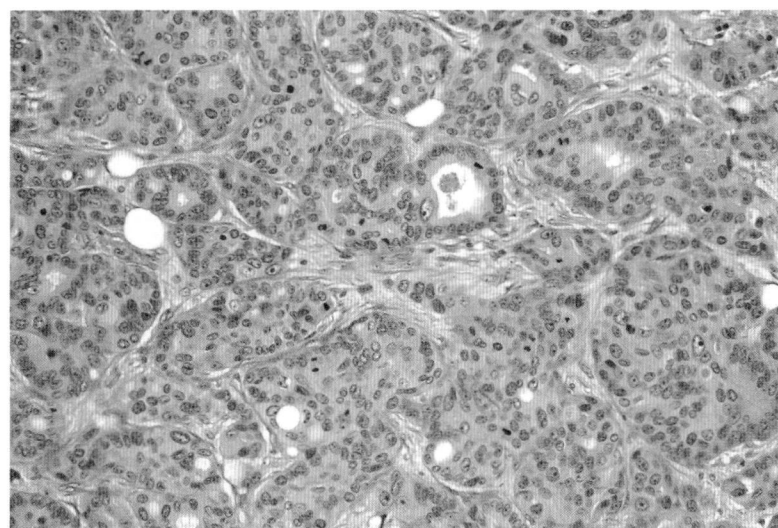

Fig. 30.37
Metastatic colonic adenocarcinoma: high-power view.

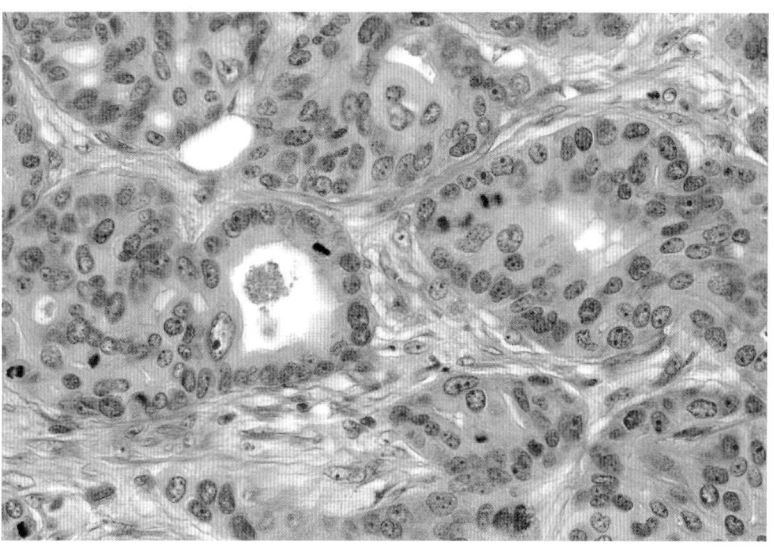

Fig. 30.38
Metastatic colonic adenocarcinoma: there is conspicuous mitotic activity.

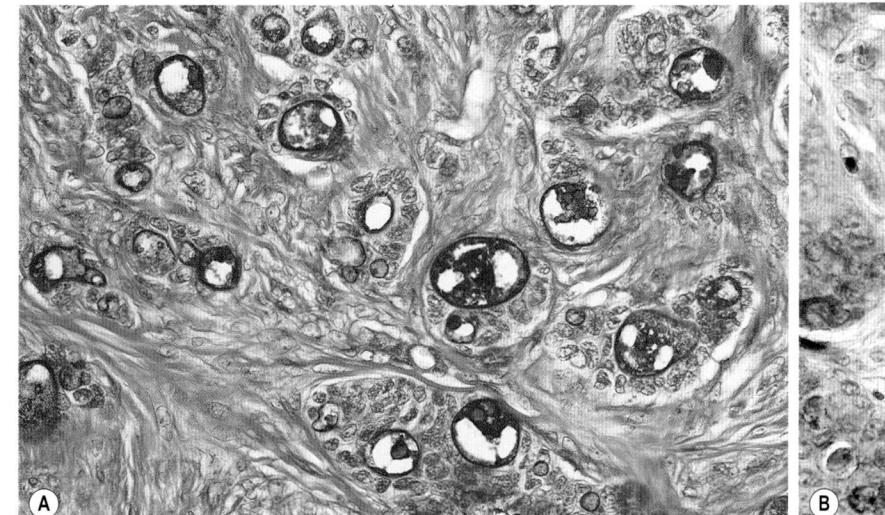
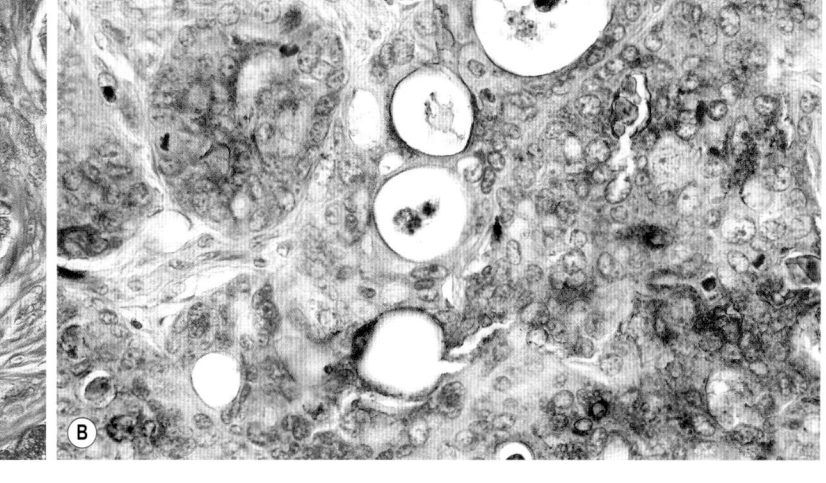

Fig. 30.39
Metastatic colonic adenocarcinoma: (A) the tumor is strongly PAS positive, diastase resistant; (B) the epithelial lining is outlined by carcinoembryonic antigen.

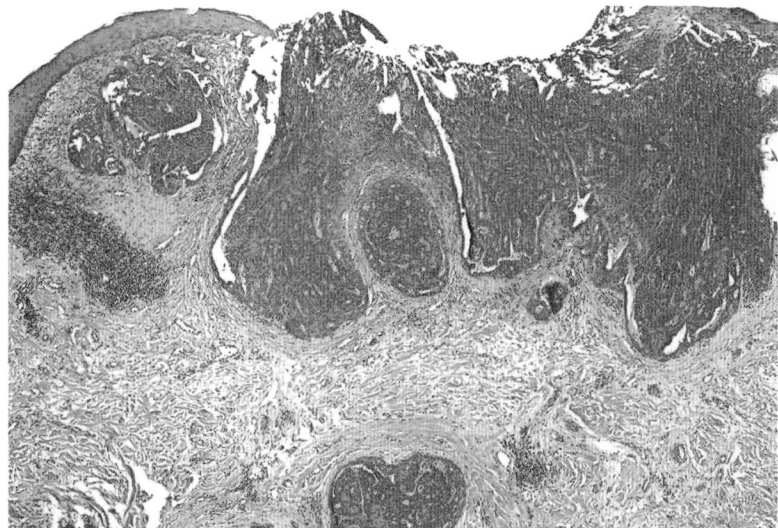

Fig. 30.40
Metastatic thyroid papillary carcinoma: an ulcerated, multifocal carcinoma with a papillary configuration is present in the superficial and deep dermis.

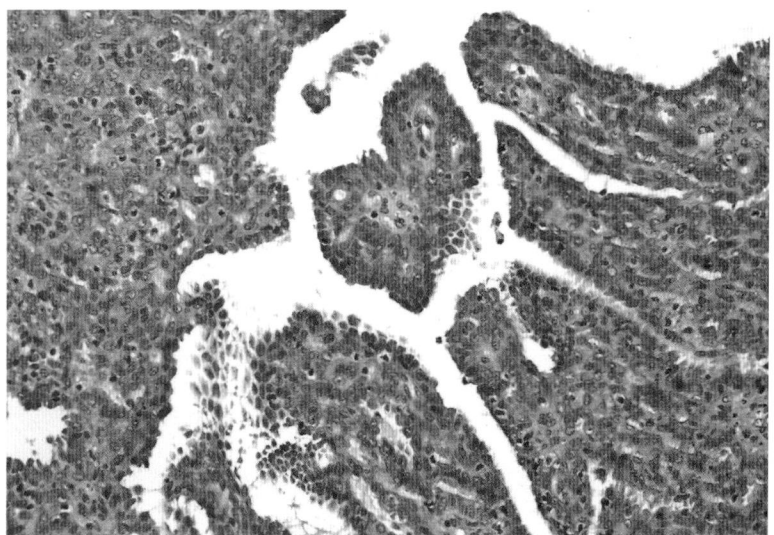

Fig. 30.41
Metastatic thyroid papillary carcinoma: the papillae are covered with tall columnar epithelial cells.

pattern and cytological atypia will generally distinguish this entity from a cutaneous adenocarcinomatous visceral metastasis. Distinction between these entities, particularly eccrine ductal carcinoma, can be very difficult based on histology alone; immunohistochemistry is sometimes very useful.

It has been suggested that p63 can be used as a marker to distinguish primary adnexal tumors from metastatic adenocarcinoma in the skin: p63 is generally expressed in cutaneous adnexal tumors and is lacking in metastatic adenocarcinomas (breast, gastrointestinal tract, lung).[21,71] It is important to note, however, that p63 immunohistochemical staining cannot be used to distinguish between primary and metastatic squamous cell carcinomas (whether of lung or head and neck origin) or metastatic urothelial carcinomas since it can be routinely identified in the normal basal cells of skin and other stratified epithelia, as well as in prostatic and respiratory epithelium.[72,73] p63 is also a marker for myoepithelial cells of the breast.[67] Recently, p40 has been suggested as having better specificity for distinguishing primary skin adnexal tumors from cutaneous metastases, but has similar caveats and drawbacks to those discussed above for p63.[74]

These observations have also been supported by other studies. Qureshi and coworkers studied 15 metastatic carcinomas to the skin including 14 adenocarcinomas and 1 urothelial carcinoma.[21] Only one of the adenocarcinomas displayed partial p63 expression, and this was a poorly differentiated esophageal carcinoma. Sariya and coworkers found that when used as a single marker, a positive p63 stain had the highest sensitivity (96%) for primary adnexal tumors and a negative p63 stain had the highest positive predictive value for a metastasis.[75] Kanitakis and coworkers also reported that the large majority (88.5%) of primary skin tumors express p63 while 89% of the metastatic tumors to skin are p63-negative.[76] Ivan and coworkers have also demonstrated that strong p63 expression is retained in those rare cases of metastatic sweat gland carcinoma to other skin sites and lymph nodes.[77] The use of p63 in a panel of immunohistochemical studies may therefore be of value in the differential diagnosis of metastatic adenocarcinoma to skin from primary cutaneous tumors showing ductal differentiation. Although additional studies are needed, p40 may show superior specificity over p63 in distinguishing primary and metastatic tumors.[74]

Another immunohistochemical marker that has been reported as useful in the differential diagnosis of cutaneous metastases from primary cutaneous adnexal neoplasms is CK5/6, which is expressed in the majority of primary cutaneous adnexal neoplasms, but only rarely in cutaneous metastases of internal adenocarcinoma.[46] A further marker, podoplanin (D2-40), has also been reported as positive in primary adnexal tumors and not in metastatic tumors of various origin (lung, breast, gastrointestinal, or genitourinary tracts).[78] A subsequent study suggests pairing p63 with D2-40 (podoplanin) to increase the specificity in this setting.[79] Calretinin, a calcium-binding protein expressed in mesothelial, epithelial, and stromal cells, has been found to be positive in metastatic tumors but also in some cases of primary cutaneous neoplasms.[75]

Appropriate assessment of the histologic features in combination with a complete clinical history and utilization of a carefully selected immunohistochemical panel should help resolve the majority of diagnostic problems. However, it must be emphasized that a diagnosis should never be based solely on immunohistochemical findings.

Mucinous carcinoma

Mucinous carcinoma is characterized by compartments created by fibrous strands, which contain pools of mucin and floating nests of tumor cells. These usually have ample cytoplasm, centrally placed vesicular nuclei, and only mild cytological atypia. Although mucinous carcinoma may sometimes arise as a primary tumor in the skin (most commonly as a slow-growing nodule on the head or neck of older men), on occasions it represents metastatic spread from sites such as the breast, stomach, colon, rectum, and pancreas (*Fig. 30.42*).[80–82]

Distinction between a primary and a metastatic tumor is usually not possible on histologic grounds alone, although in a large case series, Kazakov and coworkers reported that the presence of an in situ component is particularly helpful in the diagnosis of primary cutaneous neoplasms. However, the absence of such a component does not exclude the diagnosis.[81,83] Dirty necrosis has been reported as a constant histologic finding in metastatic

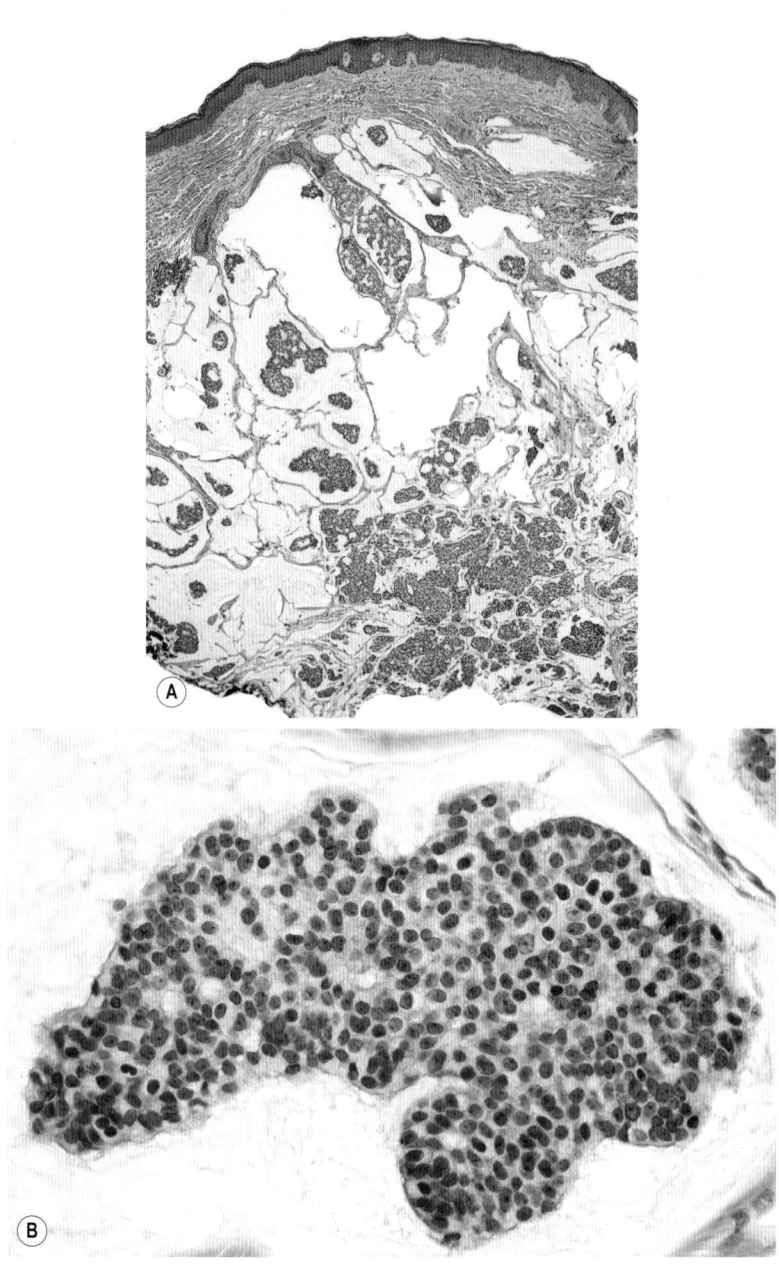

Fig. 30.42
Metastatic mucinous carcinoma: (**A**) low-power view of a deposit of metastatic mucinous carcinoma; (**B**) high-power view. Primary and metastatic diseases are histologically indistinguishable unless an in situ component is identified in the former.

adenocarcinoma of intestinal origin.[81] Mucinous carcinoma found in the skin of the trunk usually represents metastatic disease from internal primary tumors.[81]

'Signet ring' metastases, in which intracellular mucin accumulation results in compression of the nucleus to the cell periphery, may be seen with gastric, large intestinal, and pancreatic primary tumors (*Fig. 30.43*). Rarely, they may also arise in the endocervix and gallbladder. Signet ring cell change may be seen in a number of cutaneous tumors including sweat gland carcinoma, melanoma, squamous cell carcinoma, and basal cell carcinoma.

Of historical interest, the type of mucin can help distinguish between primary cutaneous mucinous carcinoma and cutaneous metastases of a gastrointestinal primary. In primary cutaneous mucinous carcinoma, the mucin contains abundant sialomucin, and is therefore Alcian blue positive at pH 2.5, but not at pH 1.0 or 0.4.[84] The mucin seen in gastrointestinal mucinous carcinomas that metastasize to the skin contains sulfamucins, which

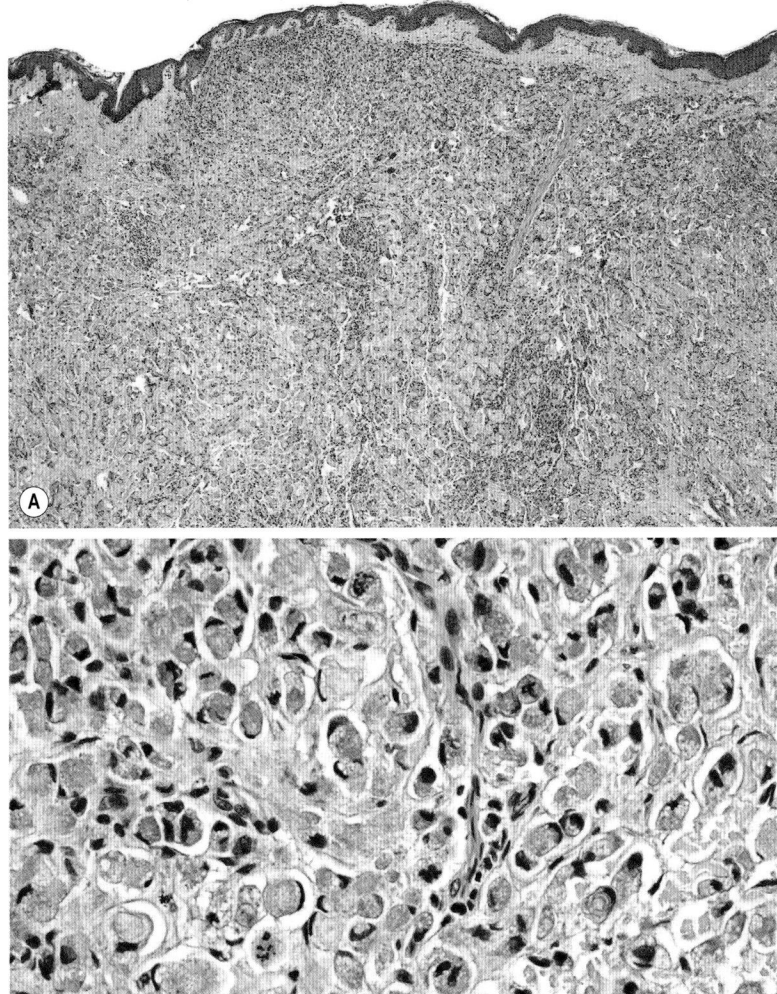

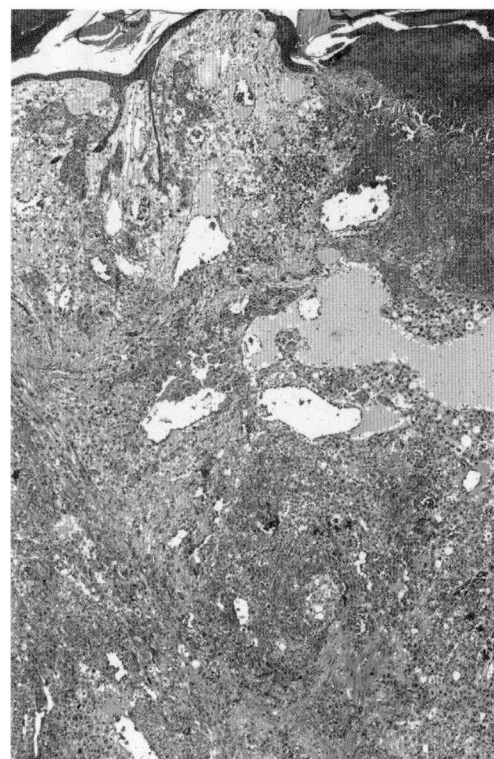

Fig. 30.44

Metastatic testicular choriocarcinoma: low-power view showing a hemorrhagic tumor filling the dermis. By courtesy of D. Lowe, MD, St Bartholomew's Hospital, London, UK.

Fig. 30.43

Metastatic signet-ring cell carcinoma: (**A**, **B**) the dermis is completely replaced by a pure population of signet ring cells.

are Alcian blue positive at a pH of 1.0 and 0.4.[85] However, these stains are not commonly performed at variable pH levels in most laboratories.

Gastrointestinal mucinous tumors metastatic to the skin generally retain CK20 expression, which is not seen in primary cutaneous mucinous sweat gland carcinoma.[81,86,87] Strong CDX2 expression has been well documented in gastrointestinal metastases to other visceral organs, and has been observed in isolated cases of mucinous cutaneous metastases of intestinal origin.[88,89] SATB2 has similar sensitivity (80–90%) for metastatic tumors of gastrointestinal origin and may have increased or complementary specificity with CDX2.[90,91] GATA3 has been reported in primary cutaneous mucinous carcinoma and thus cannot be used to favor breast origin.[92] If an in situ component of cutaneous mucinous adenocarcinoma is identified, the surrounding myoepithelial cells may label for p63, CK5/6, calponin, or smooth muscle actine (SMA).[76,77,81,83] Metastatic mucinous carcinomas are usually negative for p63.[77]

Adenoid cystic carcinoma

Primary cutaneous adenoid cystic carcinoma is rare and therefore must be distinguished from metastatic disease. Sources of a systemic primary tumor include salivary gland, lacrimal gland, cervix, bronchus, or breast.[93,94] In clinical practice, however, these visceral tumors are usually slowly-growing lesions in which cutaneous presentation would be most unlikely, although isolated cases of such have been described.[95,96] The majority of adenoid cystic carcinomas in the skin therefore represent primary neoplasms. Metastatic lesions most often arise from the salivary gland.[97,98] A subset of primary cutaneous adenoid cystic carcinomas can harbor MYB rearrangements as

seen with the t(6;9)(q22~23;p23~24) resulting in MYB-NFIB fusions present in salivary adenoid cystic carcinomas.[99]

Choriocarcinoma

Choriocarcinoma, although usually a gestational tumor, may also be derived from the testis and, more rarely, the mediastinum, ovary, and, exceptionally, a placental site trophoblastic tumor.[100] Associated with a marked propensity for vascular invasion, cutaneous metastases are not uncommon.[100–105] The tumor is characteristically hemorrhagic and necrotic; frequently, viable tissue is only recognizable at the periphery.

Choriocarcinoma is a tumor of trophoblastic tissue: the cytotrophoblast, the proliferative component, and the syncytiotrophoblast, the hormonally active element. The lesion is composed of a variable admixture of these two cell types, and no chorionic villi are found (Figs 30.44 and 30.45). The cytotrophoblast consists of regular polyhedral cells, arranged in sheets and cords, each with pale cytoplasm and a fairly large vesicular nucleus, often with a prominent nucleolus. Mitotic figures may be conspicuous and are frequently abnormal. In contrast, the syncytiotrophoblast is composed of very large pleomorphic cells with abundant, somewhat basophilic, cytoplasm. They are frequently multinucleate and are often seen in intimate association with the neighboring cytotrophoblast (Fig. 30.46). Immunohistochemical demonstration of gonadotrophin is a useful diagnostic aid (Fig. 30.47). Choriocarcinoma components from testicular mixed tumors as well as postpartum cases can metastasize to skin.[106–109]

Clear cell carcinoma

Metastatic clear cell carcinoma is typically derived from the kidney, but other sources include the lungs, liver, and the mesonephric clear cell carcinomas of the ovaries, endometrium, cervix, and vagina.[110–112] The tumor is composed of cords, alveoli, and, occasionally, tubular structures consisting of uniform clear cells containing both lipid and glycogen (Figs 30.48–30.51). The stroma is usually delicate and highly vascular, often resulting in conspicuous areas of hemorrhage and therefore accounting for the characteristic clinical appearance of such a metastasis. It must be histologically differentiated from clear cell squamous carcinoma, clear cell hidradenocarcinoma, clear

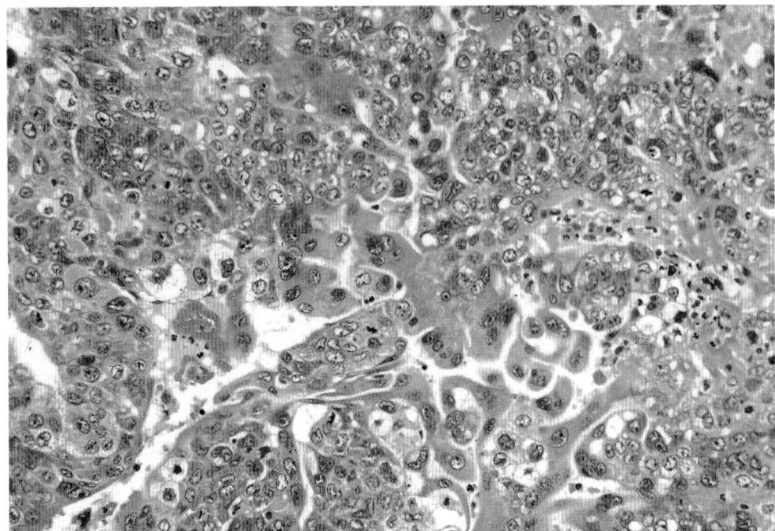

Fig. 30.45
Metastatic testicular choriocarcinoma: the cytotrophoblast is ensheathed by the syncytiotrophoblast, characterized by irregular pleomorphic vesicular nuclei with prominent eosinophilic nucleoli, dispersed in an abundance of slightly basophilic cytoplasm. By courtesy of D. Lowe, MD, St Bartholomew's Hospital, London, UK.

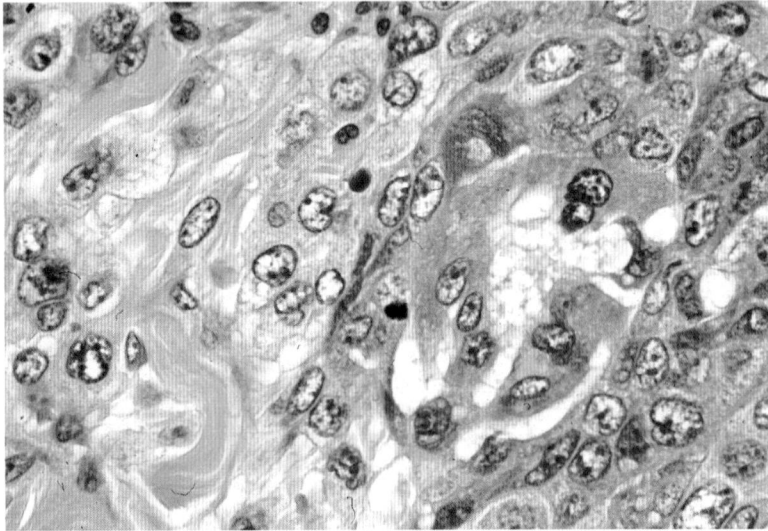

Fig. 30.46
Metastatic testicular choriocarcinoma: high-power view. By courtesy of D. Lowe, MD, St Bartholomew's Hospital, London, UK.

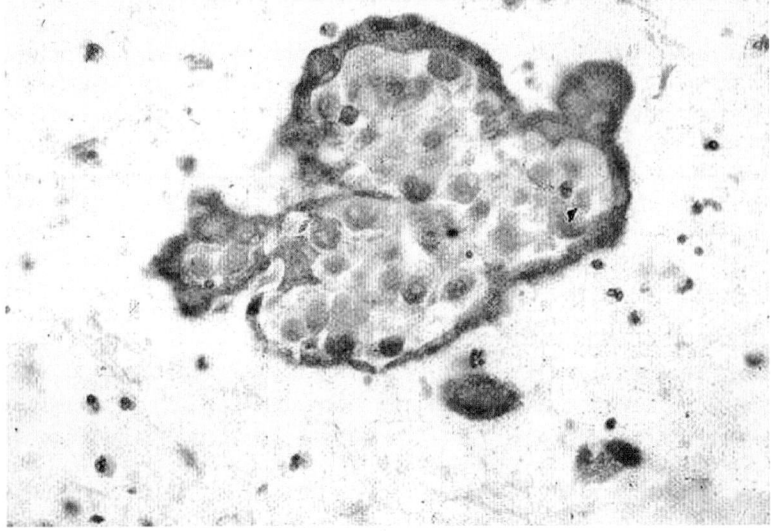

Fig. 30.47
Metastatic testicular choriocarcinoma: there is strong labeling for human chorionic gonadotrophin (fine needle aspiration).

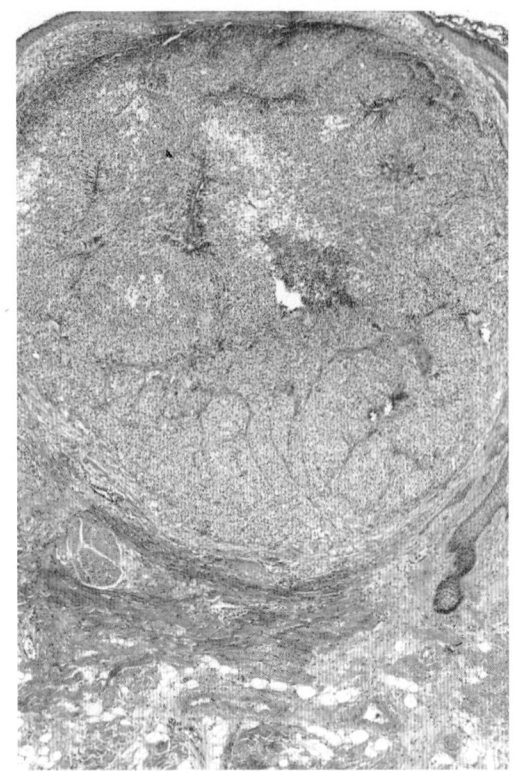

Fig. 30.48
Metastatic renal (clear cell) carcinoma: there is a well-circumscribed tumor nodule in the dermis.

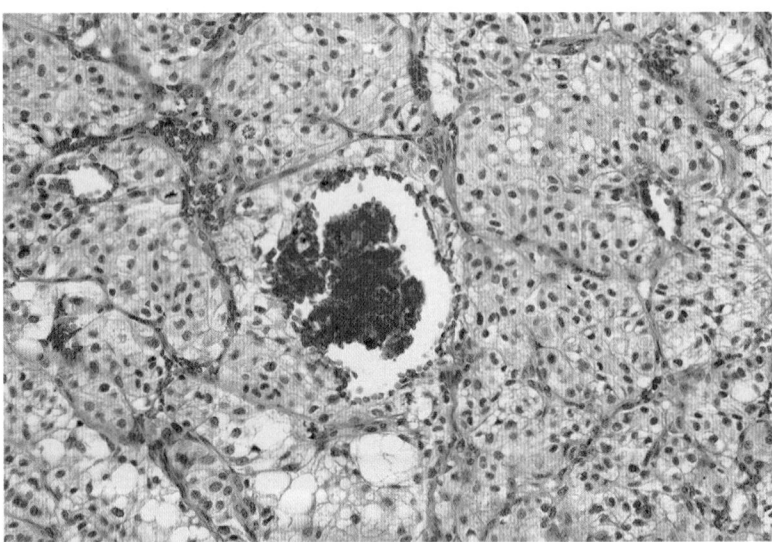

Fig. 30.49
Metastatic renal (clear cell) carcinoma: note the clear cells and characteristic hemorrhage.

cell porocarcinoma, trichilemmal carcinoma, sebaceous carcinoma, amelanotic clear cell melanoma, PEComa, and clear cell sarcoma (melanoma of soft parts).

Immunohistochemical studies can be used as an adjuvant in the differential diagnosis, but they are not very specific. Primary renal cell carcinoma has been shown to express CD10 (common acute lymphoblastic leukemia antigen [CALLA]) and also in cutaneous metastatic disease.[113–116] The renal cell carcinoma marker (RCC-Ma) has a high specificity and moderate sensitivity for cutaneous metastases of renal cell carcinoma.[117] As such, a positive result with RCC-Ma is highly suggestive of a diagnosis of metastatic renal cell carcinoma; however, a negative result does not exclude the diagnosis.[118] PAX8 is a lineage-specific transcription factor that is positive in kidney tumors, but also in ovary and thyroid, so use in panels with careful consideration of the differential diagnosis is needed.[28,119,120]

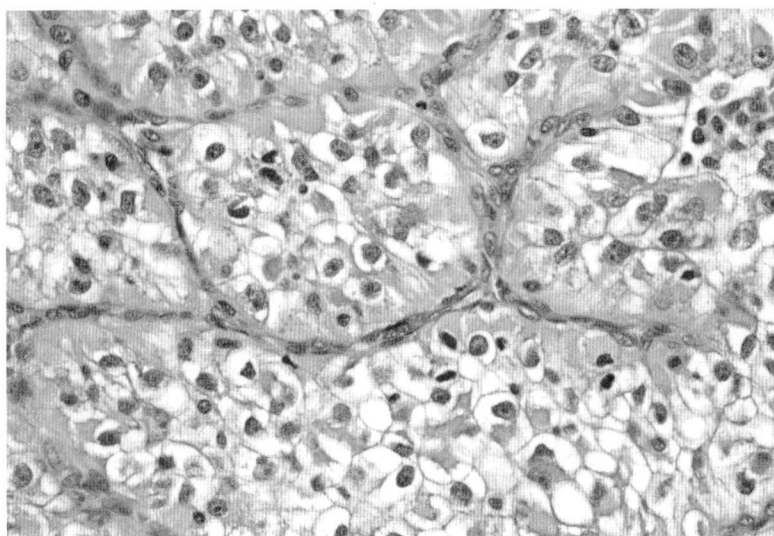

Fig. 30.50
Metastatic renal (clear cell) carcinoma: the clear cell appearance is due to the accumulation of glycogen and lipid.

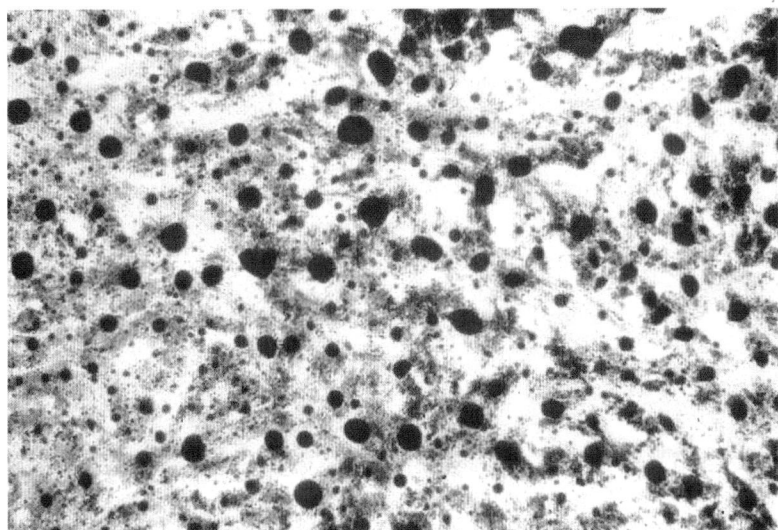

Fig. 30.51
Metastatic renal (clear cell) carcinoma: oil red O staining for lipid is strongly positive.

Neuroendocrine carcinoma (small cell carcinoma)

Metastatic neuroendocrine carcinoma is recognized by its distinctive features of small, hyperchromatic, and round to oval nuclei with barely perceptible cytoplasm (Fig. 30.52). Typical of the tumor is the presence of abundant basophilic nuclear debris around its vasculature.

Tumors from which bronchial neuroendocrine carcinoma must be differentiated include neuroendocrine tumors arising elsewhere (e.g., from skin, gastrointestinal tract, and uterus), medullary carcinoma of the thyroid, small cell melanoma, and poorly fixed specimens of lymphoma.[121,122] Immunohistochemically, these tumors express a range of antigens including low molecular weight keratin (CAM 5.2), EMA, neuron-specific enolase, chromogranin, synaptophysin, CD56, PGP 9.5, and bombesin. Medullary carcinoma of the thyroid expresses calcitonin. Neuroendocrine carcinoma of the salivary gland and cutaneous tumors consistently show perinuclear dotlike positivity for CK20, and this is useful in their differential diagnosis from other metastatic neuroendocrine carcinomas.[5,6] Both Merkel cell carcinoma and non-Merkel cell primary cutaneous neuroendocrine carcinomas should also receive diagnostic consideration.[123–127] Some recent data suggest that determining the site of origin of neuroendocrine carcinomas could be of utmost importance.[128] Although for many metastases clinical correlation

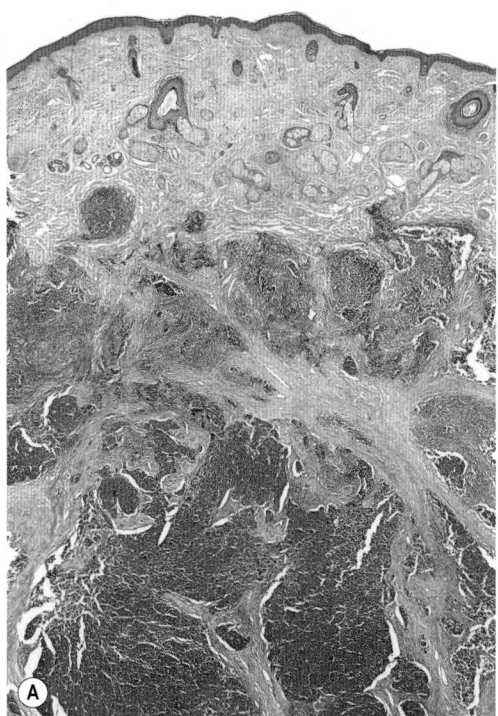

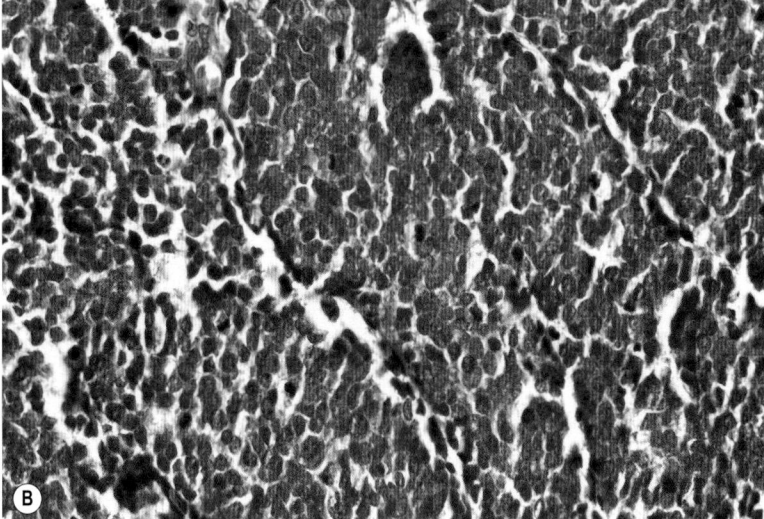

Fig. 30.52
Metastatic small cell carcinoma: (A, B) in the absence of clinical history or immunohistochemistry, it would not be possible to distinguish this metastasis from a primary cutaneous neuroendocrine carcinoma.

often provides the answer, immunohistochemistry is often an important aid in reaching a diagnosis. More recently with advances in molecular diagnostics, it has been suggested that the use of a 92-gene cancer classifier is also a very useful way to predict the site of origin of neuroendocrine tumors.[129]

Mesothelioma

Metastatic cutaneous mesothelioma is exceptional.[130,131] Most cases of cutaneous involvement by mesothelioma result from direct extension or are a consequence of implantation from surgical procedures. The most common sites of metastases are the trunk, face, and scalp. Rare cases of metastatic disease to the umbilicus and penis have been described.[132,133]

Histologically, mesothelioma can present with an epithelioid, sarcomatoid, or mixed morphology. Most mesotheliomas are predominantly epithelioid and, in this setting, distinction from a metastatic adenocarcinoma can be very difficult (Fig. 30.53).[134] An exceptional case with pagetoid metastatic

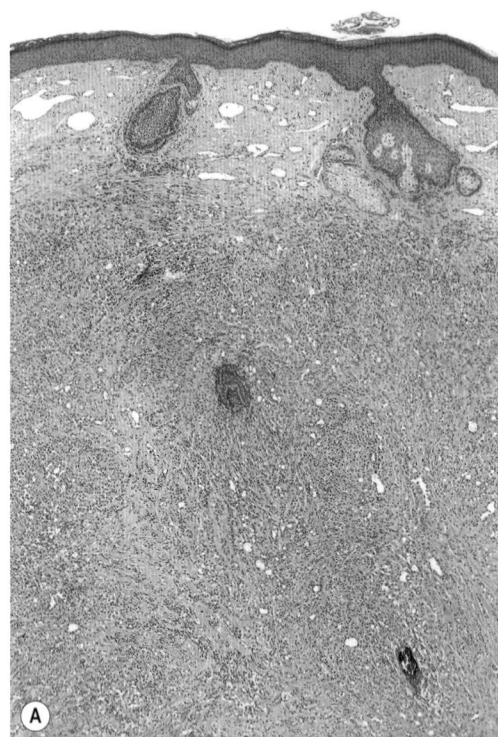

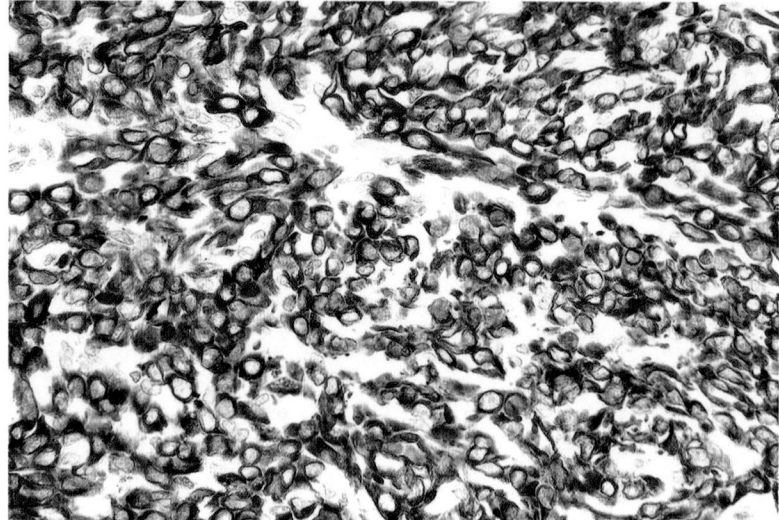

Fig. 30.54
Metastatic mesothelioma: the tumor cells are strongly positive for calretinin.

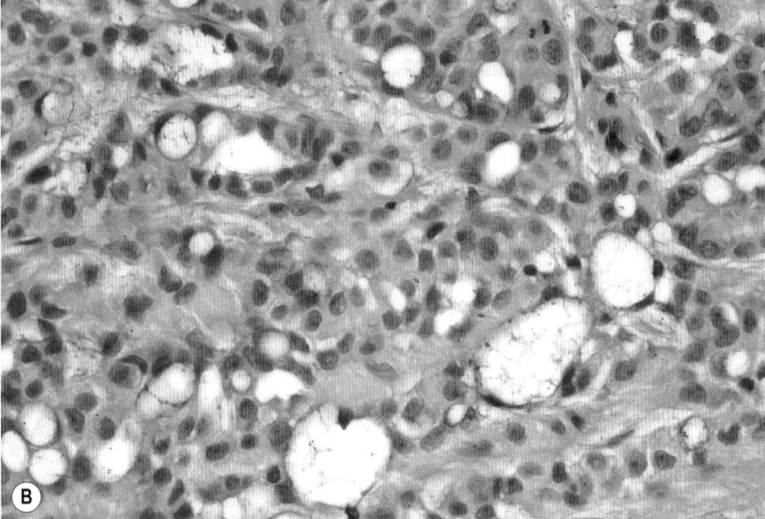

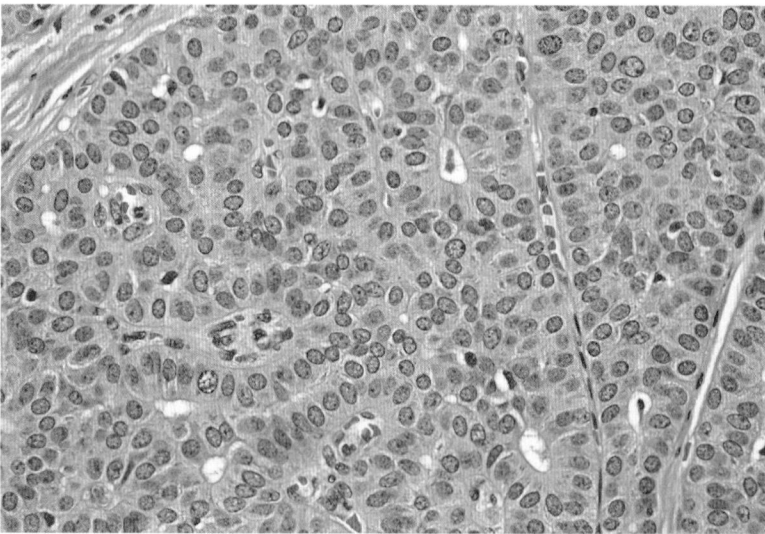

Fig. 30.55
Metastatic carcinoid tumor: note the uniform nuclear morphology, eosinophilic cytoplasm and acini.

Fig. 30.53
Metastatic mesothelioma: (**A**, **B**) the features are indistinguishable from poorly differentiated carcinoma.

spread has been described.[133] There are no antibodies that are entirely specific for mesothelioma. Immunohistochemical markers including keratin, carcinoembryonic antigen (CEA), B72.3, Leu-M1, WT1, and Ber-EP4 are used routinely to try to establish a diagnosis.[28,135,136] Mesotheliomas tend to be negative for all these markers except for keratin, which is consistently positive, and Ber-EP4. Staining for CK5/6 can also be helpful, as mesotheliomas are positive for this marker and metastatic adenocarcinomas tend to be negative.[137] Calretinin may be positive in mesotheliomas, but is not specific (*Fig. 30.54*).[74]

Ultrastructurally, mesothelioma cells contain numerous characteristic elongated surface microvilli.

Carcinoid tumor

Carcinoid tumor is uncommon, shows a predilection for females, and presents most often in the seventh decade. Although primary cutaneous lesions do occur very exceptionally, it is most probable that a cutaneous lesion represents metastatic disease.[138–142] The majority of carcinoid tumors arise in the terminal ileum and appendix; those at the latter site are almost invariably benign. The rest develop in the colon, stomach, bronchus, and, very rarely, in the gallbladder and in ovarian teratoma. The bronchus appears to be the most common primary site in the setting of cutaneous metastasis.[143] Rarely, patients can present with symptoms of the carcinoid syndrome.

There is usually, although far from invariably, a positive argentaffin reaction; some tumors require the presence of an additional reducing agent – the argyrophil reaction. Occasional tumors, however, show neither of these reactions.

Histologically, the tumor has a characteristic appearance of variably sized nodules of strikingly uniform cells (*Fig. 30.55*). The cells have regular, round to oval, vesicular nuclei and show a tendency towards peripheral palisading. The cytoplasm is eosinophilic, and granules may be especially evident at the periphery of the nodules. Mitotic activity is usually low. Diagnosis can be confirmed by a variety of techniques including the diazo reaction, the Masson-Fontana technique, and Pearse lead-hematoxylin reaction. In addition, the tumor cells express chromogranin, synaptophysin, PGP 9.5, CD56, and neuron-specific enolase (*Figs 30.56* and *30.57*). Carcinoid tumors are usually negative for CK5/6 and p63, and this may be useful in the distinction from benign cutaneous adnexal tumors as the latter tend to be positive for these markers.[144]

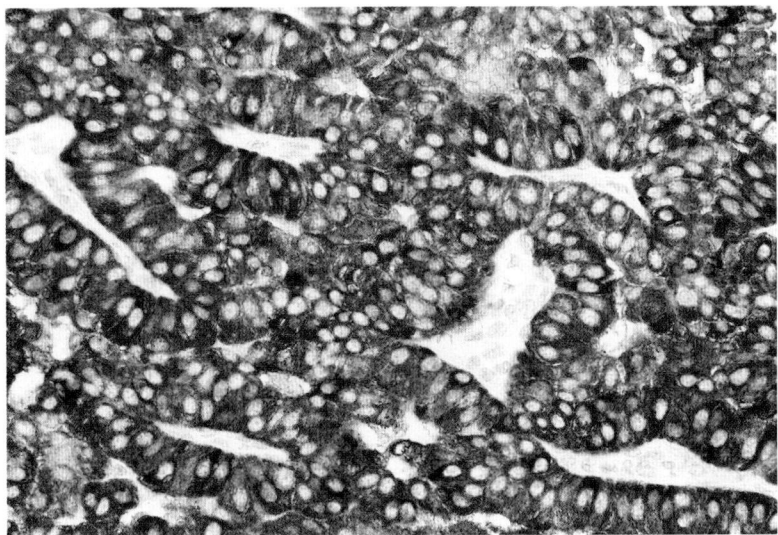

Fig. 30.56
Metastatic carcinoid tumor: the tumor cells are strongly positive for synaptophysin.

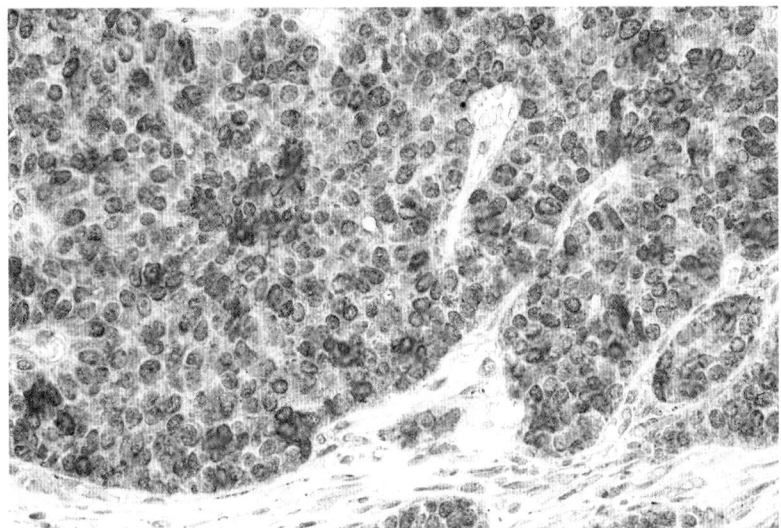

Fig. 30.57
Metastatic carcinoid tumor: neuron-specific enolase (NSE) is also expressed.

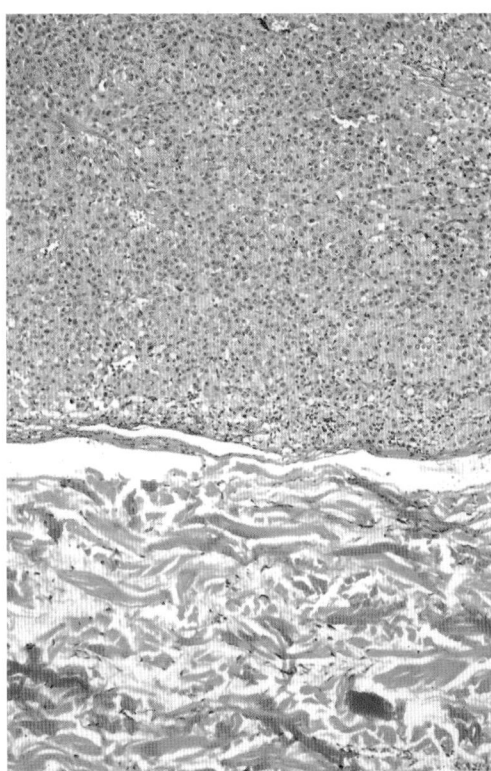

Fig. 30.58
Metastatic melanoma: the circumscribed, nodular growth pattern is very suggestive of a metastasis. Although amelanotic, the tumor cells expressed S100 protein and HMB-45.

Metastatic melanoma

Melanoma is the third most common source of cutaneous metastases (*Fig. 30.58*).[35] Metastatic melanoma usually poses little diagnostic difficulty. In up to 5% of patients, a metastatic melanoma to skin is the first manifestation of the disease; if amelanotic, the histologic differential diagnosis can be extremely challenging.[145] Amelanotic spindle cell deposits may be confused with spindle cell squamous carcinoma, atypical fibroxanthoma, or metastatic spindle cell sarcomas, particularly leiomyosarcoma. In these instances, the use of the Masson-Fontana reaction may reveal melanin pigment in quantities insufficient for easy detection using conventional hematoxylin and eosin staining. The diagnosis may also be facilitated by the use of S100 protein, Melan-A, MITF-1 (microphthalmia transcription factor 1), SOX10, and HMB-45 immunohistochemistry. Malignant smooth muscle tumors are distinguished by immunohistochemical evidence of actin, desmin, and h-caldesmon expression. Although most cases of metastatic melanoma lack an epidermal component, metastatic melanoma may occasionally be associated with prominent epidermotropism.[146–149] In this setting, distinction from a primary melanoma is far from easy. When amelanotic, immunohistochemistry may be necessary to exclude the diagnosis of extramammary Paget disease. On histologic grounds alone, amelanotic melanoma with balloon cell change or the exceptional signet ring change can be very difficult to distinguish from primary adnexal or metastatic tumors.[150]

MAMMARY AND EXTRAMAMMARY PAGET DISEASE

Clinical features

Paget disease of the nipple and areola is an uncommon disease, almost always associated with an underlying in situ or invasive mammary duct carcinoma that may or may not be clinically detectable at the time of diagnosis.[1,2] In exceptional cases, an underlying tumor cannot be found.[3–5] Very rare cases present outside the nipple and the areola elsewhere in the breast, and one case presented on the thoracic wall at the site of a mastectomy.[6,7] It is predominantly a disease of females in their fifth or sixth decade, although rarely it affects males.[1,4] The condition is usually unilateral but can be bilateral in exceptional cases.[8] It presents as pink or red, weeping, erosive, often scaly plaques that may be mistaken for eczema or psoriasis (*Figs 30.59* and *30.60*). Occasionally, particularly in males, Paget disease may present as a pigmented lesion mimicking melanoma, and the clinical and histologic differential diagnosis can be difficult.[9,10] Presentation as multiple pigmented macules has also been described.[11] In the light of histologic confirmation of the diagnosis of mammary Paget disease, further investigations to locate the associated neoplasm is mandatory. Very rare cases have been reported in association with ectopic breast tissue including a supernumerary nipple.[12,13] The prognosis of mammary Paget disease depends on the size and characteristics of the underlying breast carcinoma.[14] Patients with mammary Paget disease but undetectable breast mass have a better prognosis.

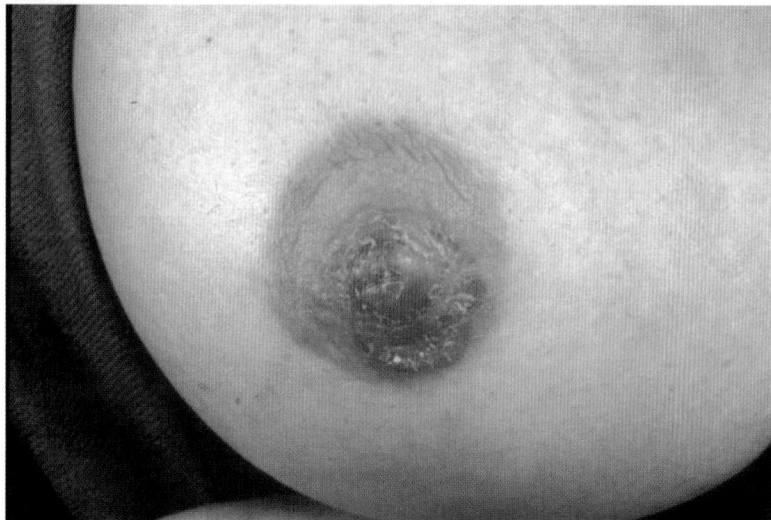

Fig. 30.59
Mammary Paget disease: the nipple shows erythema and erosion. From the collection of the late N.P. Smith, MD, the Institute of Dermatology, London, UK.

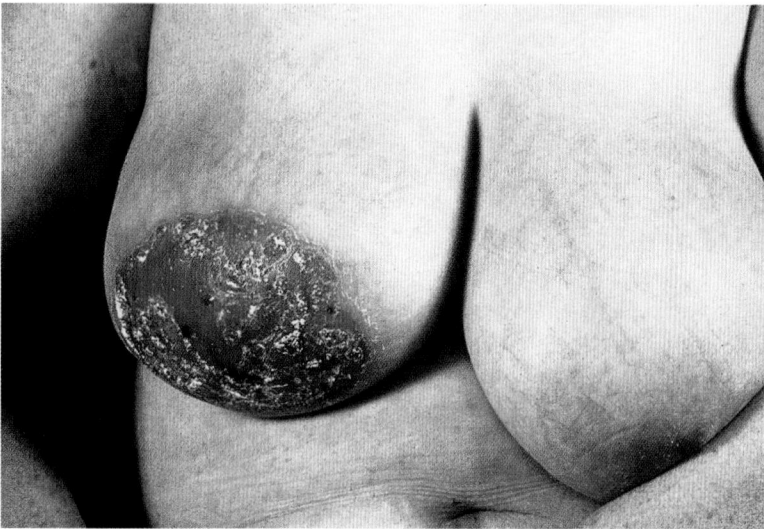

Fig. 30.60
Mammary Paget disease: this patient showed very extensive involvement with crusting of the nipple and areola. By courtesy of the Institute of Dermatology, London, UK.

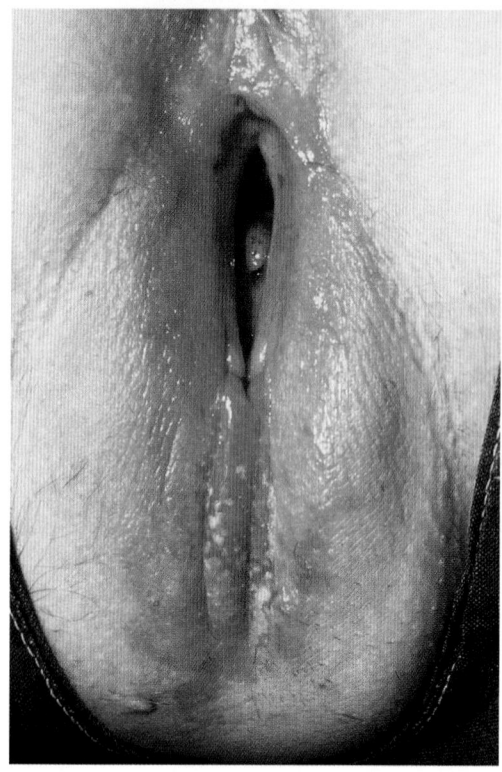

Fig. 30.61
Extramammary Paget disease: there is extensive involvement of the vulva and perineum. By courtesy of the late M. Ridley, MD, Whittington Hospital, London, UK.

Extramammary Paget disease presents in areas rich in apocrine sweat glands. It is a rare condition that usually occurs in the sixth to eighth decades with a female predominance.[2,15,16] In Asians the disease is more common in males. Caucasians are more frequently affected. Vulva is the most common site of extramammary Paget disease, accounting for approximately 65% of cases, followed by the perianal region.[2,16–20] Perianal extramammary Paget disease has an equal incidence in men and women. In males, the scrotum is the most common site of involvement.[21] Less commonly, it may arise on the penis, axilla, umbilicus, eyelid, and external auditory meatus.[22–25] Presentation at other sites is vanishingly rare but includes the face, scalp, knee, abdomen, anterior chest away from the breast, esophagus, and oral cavity.[26–33] Rarely, multifocal lesions and concomitant presentation in the genitalia and axilla have been documented.[18,34] An exceptional occurrence in the same patient of vulval and breast Paget disease with underlying cancer at both sites has been reported.[35] Multiple lesions of Paget disease involving the areola, axilla, and genital skin in the same patient and without underlying breast or genital skin carcinoma has also been described.[36] Interestingly, the mucin core protein expression suggested that the lesions more likely represented multifocal extramammary Paget disease than synchronous extramammary and mammary disease.

The onset of disease is insidious. Pruritus is often a major symptom and may precede the appearance of clinically detectable lesions.[19,21,37] The lesions are sometimes painful and present as single or multicentric erythematous, well-demarcated plaques that may become ulcerated, erosive, scaly, or eczematous (Fig. 30.61). In the later stages, tumor nodules may be evident. It has been suggested that patients who present with an 'underpants' pattern of erythema usually have an ominous prognosis.[38] This clinical appearance is due to lymphatic invasion and is often associated with regional lymph node involvement and distant metastases. Rarely, extramammary Paget disease presents with hypopigmented macules or can clinically mimic lichen sclerosus.[39–41] Epidermal papillomatous hyperplasia has been described in extramammary Paget disease and may resemble condyloma acuminatum.[42]

Extramammary Paget disease has been described in a familial context including the occurrence in two siblings.[16,43] An exceptional case of a basal cell carcinoma arising within a plaque of extramammary Paget has been documented.[44] Coexistence with hidradenoma papilliferum is also exceptional.[45]

Local recurrences are frequent in extramammary Paget disease. In vulval disease, a local recurrence rate ranging from 34% to 40% has been reported in retrospective series.[15,19,46] The recurrence rate reaches 50% in vulval extramammary Paget disease with underlying adenocarcinoma.[19] In perianal disease the reported local recurrence rate is 37%, and in peno-scrotal disease it is 22%.[47–49] The risk of local recurrence is reduced by wide local excision but the recurrence rate is high, varying from 33% to 60%.[16] With Mohs micrographic surgery, the risk of local recurrence is 12.2%.[50] A small recently published study has proposed a novel method of evaluating subclinical extension of disease with three-dimensional images using a tissue-cleaning method with CK7 immunostaining and two-photon microscopy.[51]

Poor prognosis is associated with invasive disease, an underlying dermal adenocarcinoma, association with an internal carcinoma, lymphovascular invasion, and lymph node metastasis.[5,52,53] Invasive disease is more common in females, Caucasians, in the eighth decade of life, and with predilection for the vulva in females and the scrotum in males.[54] Up to 80.4% of patients present with localized disease, 17.1% present with locoregional spread, and 2.5% present with distant metastases.[54] It has been shown that patients with invasive extramammary Paget have an increased risk of non-synchronous secondary malignancies, mainly involving the colon, rectum, and anus, and the initial site of disease usually predicts the site of secondary malignancies.[54] It has been suggested that disease involving the clitoris has a more aggressive behavior.[55] Extramammary Paget disease of the vulva may rarely extend to involve the vagina, cervix, or urethra.[56,57] Spontaneous regression has been exceptionally documented after incomplete excision.[58]

High expression of chemokine receptors CXCR4 and/or CXCR7 by tumor cells in extramammary Paget correlates with regional lymph node metastasis and lymphovascular invasion and is also associated with shorter progression free-survival and cancer-specific survival.[59]

The role of sentinel lymph biopsy in extramammary Paget disease has been evaluated in a small number of studies, most of which analyzed a limited number of cases with short follow-up.[60–62] The largest retrospective study of 151 patients found that patients with clinical lymphoadenopathy had worse prognosis than those without lymphadenopathy and also than those without clinical lymphanodenopathy but positive sentinel lymph node biopsy. Sentinel lymph node positivity was associated with lymphovascular invasion and dermal invasion. Survival, however, was not influenced by sentinel lymph node status.[63] It is not clear whether survival advantage was influenced by lymph node dissection in patients with positive lymph node biopsy. The second retrospective study of 45 patients with microinvasive disease involving the papillary dermis or with deeper invasion into the reticular dermis found an incidence of sentinel lymph node positivity in patients with microinvasion of 4.1% and for those with reticular dermal invasion of 42.8%.[64] The 5-year survival for patients with positive sentinel lymph node was 24%. Involvement of the reticular dermis and subcutaneous tissue was shown to be an independent prognostic factor predicting sentinel lymph node positivity. Sentinel lymph node status, however, in contrast to the previous study, was an important predictor of survival in patients with invasive disease.

Pathogenesis and histologic features

Mammary Paget disease is almost always associated with carcinoma of the breast. It has been hypothesized that Paget disease originates from the underlying mammary carcinoma, migrating via the lactiferous ducts to the surface epithelium of the nipple and areola.[1,2] Mammary Paget disease is most commonly associated with in situ or invasive ductal carcinoma of breast, but it has been rarely described in association with invasive papillary carcinoma and mucinous breast carcinoma.[65,66]

In very rare cases of mammary Paget disease, no underlying breast carcinoma is identified by palpation or imaging studies.[3–5] It has been postulated that in such cases the disease might be derived from Toker cells.[67,68] These represent mammary gland-related cells and are normally found in approximately 10% of the histologically normal epidermis of the nipple.

The pathogenesis of extramammary Paget disease remains controversial.[69–73] In the majority of cases, it represents an intraepidermal adenocarcinoma most likely derived from the intraepidermal sweat duct. In a minority of cases, it represents an epidermotropic metastasis or spread from an associated sweat gland carcinoma. Usually, the tumor is of apocrine derivation, although occasionally eccrine-derived lesions may be encountered. It is particularly important to note that extramammary Paget disease may also represent an epidermotropic metastasis from a distant malignant neoplasm, such as carcinoma of the rectum, bladder, urethra, prostate, endocervix, or stomach.[70,73–77] This is particularly true for perianal lesions in which an associated rectal adenocarcinoma is present in as many as one-third of cases.[18,73] The overall incidence of association with an internal carcinoma is about 15%. Paget disease of the vulva is associated with an underlying vulval adenocarcinoma in 4% of cases, and purely intraepithelial disease may become invasive in 12% of cases.[19,55] Coexistence of vulval Paget disease with ovarian teratoma has been noted.[78] Paget disease of the eyelid is associated with carcinoma of Moll glands, while involvement of the external auditory meatus is associated with ceruminous gland carcinoma. Patients with extramammary Paget disease, therefore, must also be screened for an underlying malignancy.

The precursor cell of origin in extramammary Paget disease not associated with an underlying carcinoma is still speculative. Pluripotential germinative cells in the epidermis and/or adnexae have been hypothesized as precursors of the disease. Toker cells have been identified in vulval epidermis, more precisely within the mammary-like glands of the vulva present in the interlabial sulcus between labia majora and labia minora.[79] Mammary-like glands of vulva have histologic characteristics resembling both the female breast and sweat glands.[80–82]

It has also been suggested that extramammary Paget disease could be a result of proliferation of adnexal stem cells residing in the infundibulo-sebaceous unit of hair follicles and adnexal structures, since Paget cells label for CK15 and CK19, which are considered markers of follicular stem cells located in the hair follicle bulge region.[83]

PIK3CA mutations associated with low levels of hypermethylated DCL1 in patients with advanced age have been demonstrated in extramammary Paget disease, suggesting a pathogenetic role.[84]

The finding of germline mutations in mismatch repair genes in cases of extramammary Paget disease raises the possibility that these mutations may play a role in the pathogenesis of the disease.[85]

Histologically, in both mammary and extramammary Paget disease, the epidermis is often acanthotic with hyperkeratosis, parakeratosis, or ulceration. There is infiltration by variable numbers of large cells with abundant, clear, or sometimes eosinophilic cytoplasm, containing prominent vesicular nuclei (*Figs 30.62–30.65*). Mitotic figures may occasionally be identified.

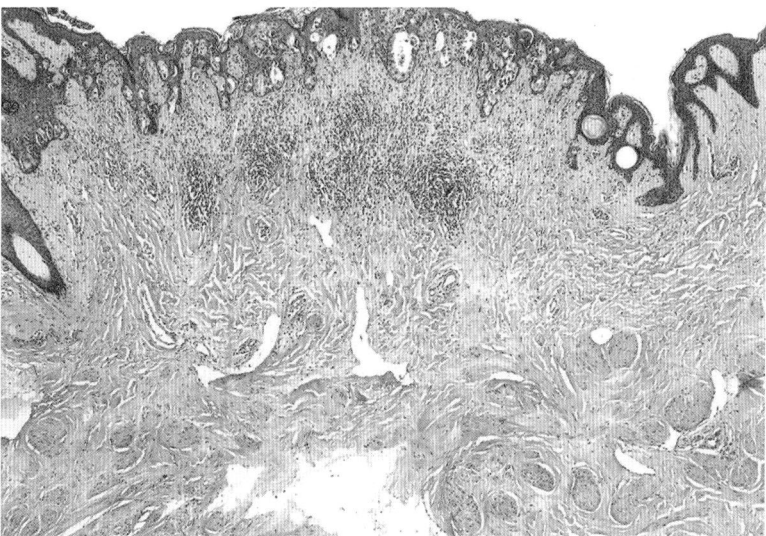

Fig. 30.62
Mammary Paget disease: low-power view showing extensive tumor infiltration of the epidermis. Intraepithelial glands can also be seen.

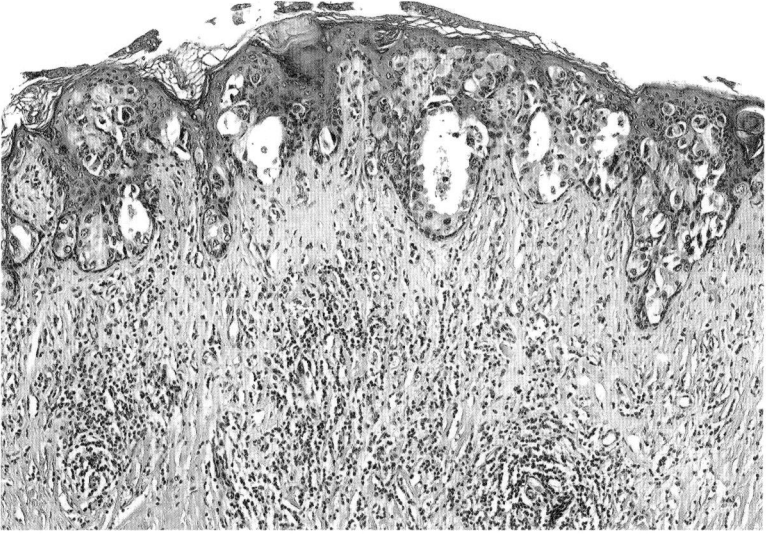

Fig. 30.63
Mammary Paget disease: higher-power view.

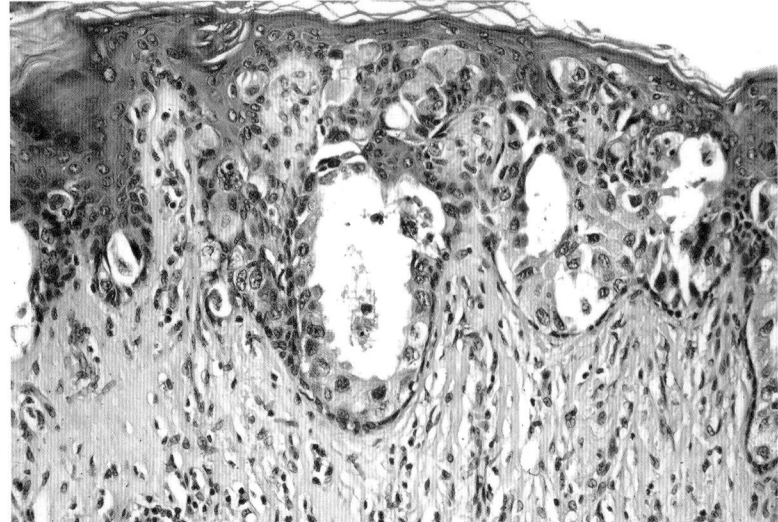

Fig. 30.64
Mammary Paget disease: in this field, there is glandular differentiation.

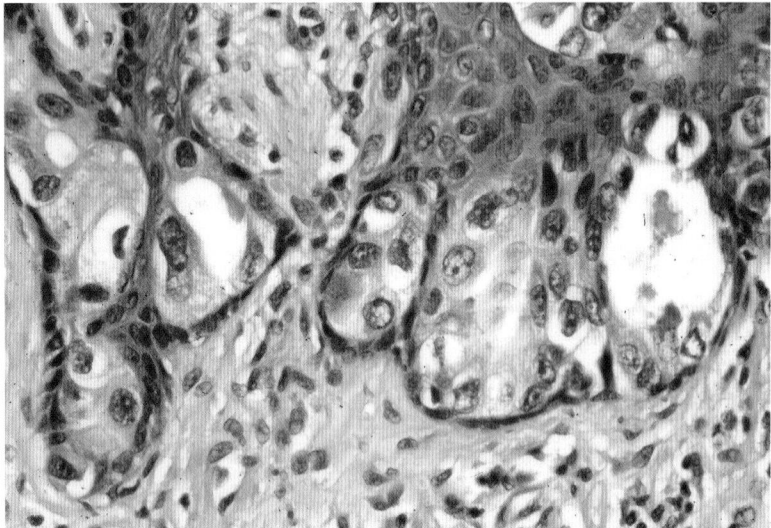

Fig. 30.65
Mammary Paget disease: the tumor cells have abundant eosinophilic cytoplasm and large vesicular nuclei with prominent nucleoli.

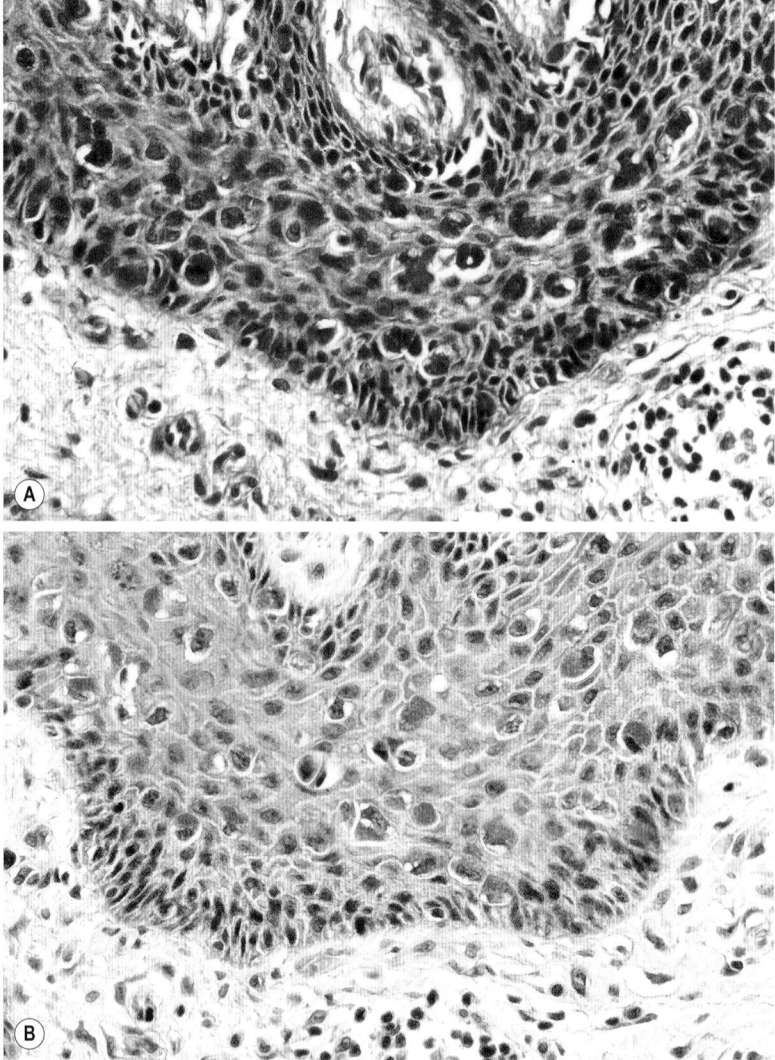

Fig. 30.66
Extramammary Paget disease: (**A**, **B**) the tumor cells are PAS positive, diastase resistant; the mucin is positive with the mucicarmine stain.

The cells are present singly or in clusters and are usually scattered throughout all layers of the epidermis. Involvement of skin adnexae is noted and can be prominent.[86] Occasionally, glandular or acinar differentiation is seen, and signet ring cells with intracytoplasmic mucin may be identified.[64] In rare cases, tumor cells can show marked cytological atypia in what has been described as the anaplastic variant of Paget disease.[87] In this instance, distinction from Bowen disease can be very difficult without the use of special stains and immunohistochemistry (see below). It must be remembered, however, that Bowen disease of the nipple is exceptional.[88] Pigmentation may be seen in both types of Paget disease and can lead to confusion with a melanoma. Tumor cells may be pigmented or there can be colonization of the involved epidermis by non-neoplastic dendritic melanocytes.[89]

Biopsies from patients with anogenital Paget disease frequently show associated epidermal lesions, which have been divided into three types: squamous hyperplasia, papillomatous hyperplasia, and fibroepithelioma of Pinkus-like hyperplasia.[90,91] The last of these is more commonly seen in perianal Paget disease and, if found in a biopsy, it should prompt a search for evidence of Paget disease.[91] Syringocystadenocarcinoma papilliferum in situ-like changes and exceptionally eccrine syringofibroadenoma-like changes may be seen.[92] Syringoma-like structures both in the dermis involved by the process and beyond have also been described.[93] Any of these patterns of hyperplasia may obscure the histologic features of Paget disease. Squamoid

metaplasia of Paget cells can be also seen and may hinder the correct diagnosis.[94] Coexistent changes of carcinoma in situ and invasive squamous cell carcinoma are rarely present. This finding is likely to be coincidental, as demonstrated in a study in which human papillomavirus (HPV) was found in the squamous element but not in the coexistent Paget disease.[42]

Frequently, though not invariably, the cells stain positively with the diastase–periodic acid-Schiff (PAS) reaction, mucicarmine, and zirconyl hematoxylin, indicating the presence of neutral mucopolysaccharides (*Fig. 30.66*).[95] Much less often, acid mucopolysaccharides may be identified by the Alcian blue reaction. Immunohistochemistry, however, is a more reliable method to confirm the diagnosis (*Figs 30.67–30.69*).

Immunohistochemically, Paget cells are usually positive for low molecular weight cytokeratins such as CK7, CAM 5.2, AE1/AE3, and EMA. There is variable expression for polyclonal CEA. GCDFP-15 has been reported in approximately 50% of cases and is typically positive in primary extramammary Paget disease and negative in secondary disease.[96–102] GATA3 has also been reported as a sensitive marker of Paget disease.[103]

Initial reports considered CK7 staining as fairly specific for extramammary Paget disease, but further publications have demonstrated its relative lack of specificity.[99,104,105] Both Toker and Merkel cells in the epidermis are positive for CK7.[95] This is particularly evident in cases where there is Toker cell hyperplasia. Pagetoid Bowen disease and actinic keratosis can also be positive for CK7.[105–109] Tumor cells in secondary extramammary Paget disease, especially associated with underlying colonic carcinoma, are usually positive for both CK7 and CK20. This observation is of value, since tumor

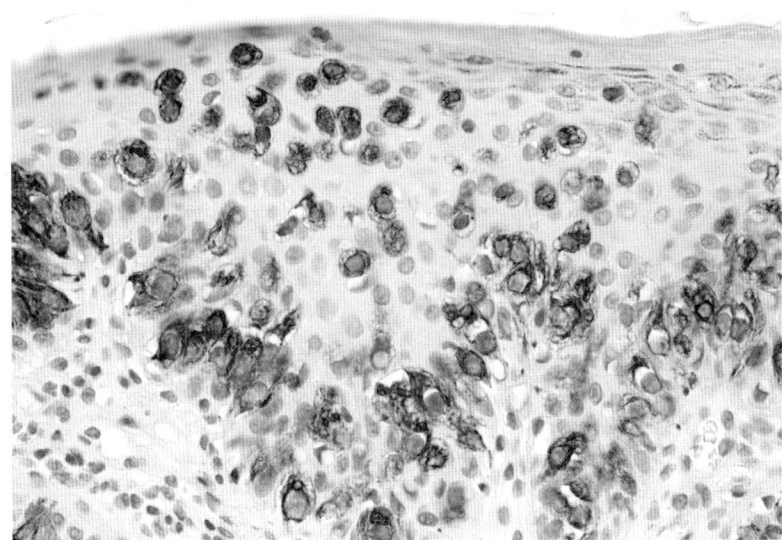

Fig. 30.67
Extramammary Paget disease: the tumor cells express cytokeratin.

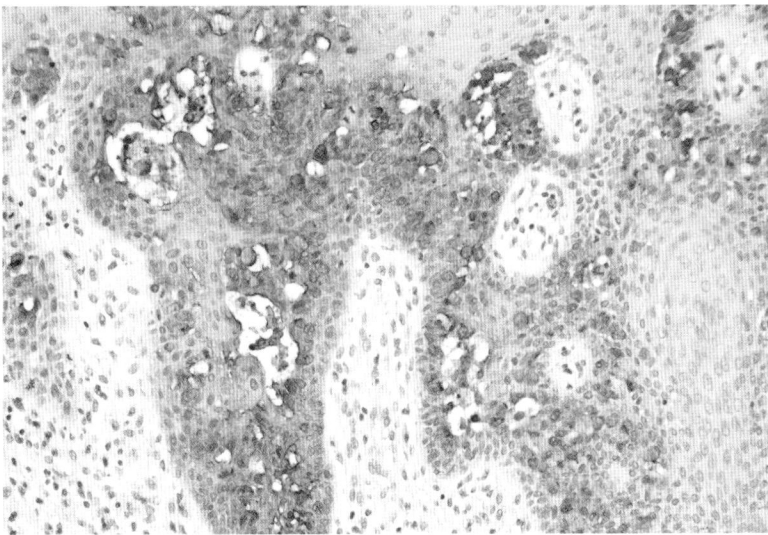

Fig. 30.68
Extramammary Paget disease: EMA is also positive.

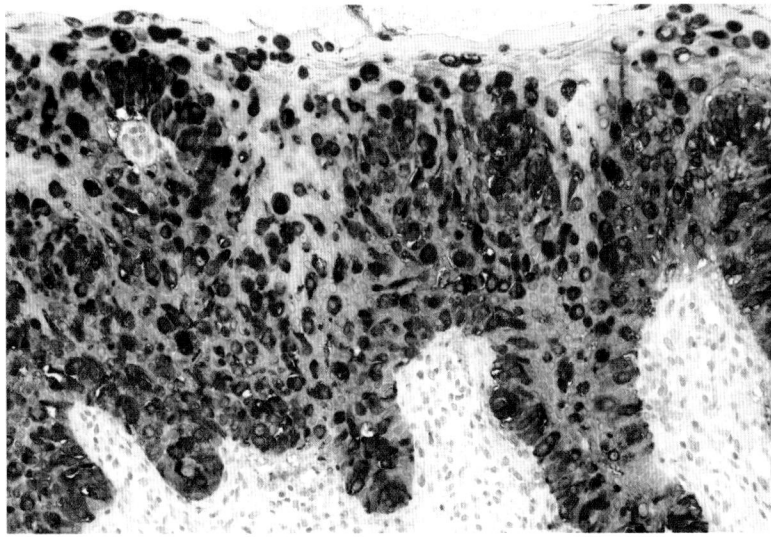

Fig. 30.69
Extramammary Paget disease: there is strong CEA expression

cells in primary extramammary Paget disease tend to be positive for CK7 but negative for CK20.[104,110,111] However, staining for CK20 is not entirely specific.

Expression of mucin core proteins may be useful in the diagnosis of both mammary and extramammary Paget disease.[112–114] MUC1 is consistently positive in tumor cells in mammary and extramammary Paget disease.[109–112] MUC1, however, is also expressed by normal Toker cells.[111] MUC5AC is frequently positive in tumor cells of primary extramammary Paget disease and less commonly in tumor cells of secondary extramammary Paget disease. When primary intraepithelial disease becomes invasive, expression of MUC5AC decreases or is lost.[115] Tumor cells do not usually express MUC2 in primary extramammary Paget disease, but it may be expressed in cases associated with rectal adenocarcinoma.[112]

S100 protein, HMB-45, SOX10, and MART-1 are usually negative in Paget disease. Cases of pigmented Paget disease, in which increased melanin pigment in the surrounding keratinocytes or melanocytic hyperplasia is seen, require careful morphological analysis in order to correctly interpret the immunohistochemically labeled dendritic processes of the intraepidermal melanocytes, rather than labeling of the malignant (Paget) cells.[116]

The majority of cases of mammary and extramammary Paget disease are negative for PR and have a low expression of ER.[117] In contrast, AR, Her-2/neu, and COX-2 are commonly expressed in mammary and extramammary Paget disease.[118–121] However, a study has found that although Her-2/neu is consistently expressed in mammary Paget disease, this is not the case in extramammary Paget disease of the vulva.[122] Variable positivity for AR is seen particularly in cases unassociated with internal malignancy and when there is negative staining for estrogen and PRs.[117,119,123] Expression of AR by tumor cells has led to suggestions that treatment may be based on hormonal therapy such as that given in prostatic cancer.[123] Similarly, reports of overexpression of Her-2 protein and Her-2/neu amplification by fluorescence in situ hybridization in cases of Paget disease also suggest the possibility of clinical use of molecular targeted therapy against the Her-2 pathway.[124,125] Her-1 (epidermal growth factor receptor [EGFR]), Her-3, and Her-4 are usually negative in both variants of Paget disease.[115]

RCAS1 (receptor-binding cancer antigen expressed on SiSo cells) has been reported as a highly sensitive marker in extramammary Paget disease.[126,127] Uroplakin III is positive in extramammary Paget disease secondary to urothelial carcinoma but negative in other cases of Paget disease.[128,129] Prostate-specific antigen is expressed in those cases associated with prostatic adenocarcinoma.[76]

CD23, a marker of lymphoid cells, is strongly expressed in the cells of the eccrine and apocrine secretory coils and was positive in all cases of mammary and extramammary Paget disease published. This marker was negative in cases of melanoma in situ, pagetoid Bowen disease, and sebaceous carcinoma, suggesting that it may be a useful marker in the histologic differential diagnosis of these entities.[130] Claudins 3 and 4 consistently stain cells in Paget disease of the nipple, and claudin 5 identifies cells in 50% of cases.[131] These markers are negative in melanocytic lesions and actinic keratoses and may of some help in differential diagnosis.

Overexpression of nuclear p53 has been found to correlate with stromal invasion in vulval disease.[132] The combined high expression of Ki-67 and cyclin D1 is also strongly associated with invasive lesions of extramammary Paget disease.[133] The presence of lymphatic invasion highlighted by D2-40 in an immunohistochemical study has been shown to be a strong predictor of nodal metastasis in extramammary Paget disease.[134]

Although immunohistochemistry is useful in the diagnosis of both mammary and extramammary Paget disease, a diagnosis should be based on close correlation of the histologic features, a panel of immunohistochemical studies, and the relevant clinical history. Immunohistochemistry may also be important for evaluation of surgical margins, which are important to reduce the risk of recurrence.[135]

Differential diagnosis

In most cases, the diagnosis of cutaneous Paget disease poses little difficulty. Occasionally, however, it may be confused with superficial spreading melanoma (especially pigmented cases) or with carcinoma in situ (actinic keratosis and Bowen disease), particularly examples with pagetoid morphology.[102]

Table 30.1
The differential diagnosis of extramammary Paget disease

	Extramammary Paget disease (primary)	Extramammary Paget disease (secondary)	Bowen disease	Superficial spreading melanoma
Diastase–periodic acid-Schiff	+	+	–	–
Mucicarmine	+	+	–	–
Alcian blue (pH 2.5)	+	+	–	–
Colloidal iron	+	+	–	–
Zirconyl hematoxylin	+	+	–	–
Masson-Fontana	–	–	–	+
Pankeratin	+	+	+	–
CAM 5.2	+	+	–	–
Cytokeratin 7	+	+	±	–
Cytokeratin 20	Usually –	Usually +	–	–
Epithelial membrane antigen	+	+	–	–
Carcinoembryonic antigen	+	+	–	–
GCDFP-15	+	–	–	–
S100 protein	–	–	–	+
Melan-A	–	–	–	+
P63	–	–	+	–
CEA	+	+	–	–

None of these techniques in isolation provides an absolute mechanism of establishing the correct diagnosis: a battery of tests is usually required.
GCDFP-15, Gross cystic disease fluid protein 15.

Histologic criteria are often enough to establish a diagnosis.[136] However, in rare challenging cases, immunohistochemistry is a valuable aid to reach the correct diagnosis. Melanocytic markers including S100 protein, SOX10, HMB-45, and Melan-A are negative in Paget cells.[111] Tumor cells in Bowen disease/actinic keratosis are usually negative for CAM 5.2, GCDFP-15, c-erbB-2, and for diastase-PAS, Alcian blue, and zirconyl hematoxylin (*Table 30.1*). It has been suggested that p63 constitutes a useful marker for differentiation from pagetoid Bowen disease which labels for p63 while Paget disease does not.[137–139] Mammary Toker cells are negative for p63.[140] Although CK7 expression is valuable in confirming a diagnosis of Paget disease, it is important to remember that both Bowen disease and pagetoid actinic keratosis may also be positive for this marker. It has been suggested that expression of RANKL, but not of PD1, is helpful in distinguishing Paget from Pagetoid Bowen as tumor cells are positive in the former but negative in the later.[141]

An exceptional case of a chemotherapy reaction to ixabepilone, an antimitotic agent, mimicking Paget disease as a result of epidermal mitotic arrest has been reported.[142]

Adult Langerhans cell histiocytosis may mimic Paget disease of the nipple, but the epidermotropic lesional cells are strongly positive for CD1a, langerin, and S100 and negative for Paget-specific immunomarkers.[143]

Pagetoid dyskeratosis is a distinctive histologic change, usually representing an incidental finding in biopsies taken from diverse sites including the cervix, lips, and hemorrhoids.[144–146] It is thought to develop as an abnormal keratinocyte proliferative response to friction. Cytological atypia is usually absent, and the cells are located higher in the epidermis (*Fig. 30.70*). They are negative for mucin stains and also for CEA.

Clear cell papulosis presents as multiple hypopigmented macules and papules and is considered to represent Toker cell hyperplasia, without cytological atypia. The immunohistochemical profile is similar to Paget disease, but stains for mucin are usually negative.[147,148]

Access **ExpertConsult.com** for the complete list of references

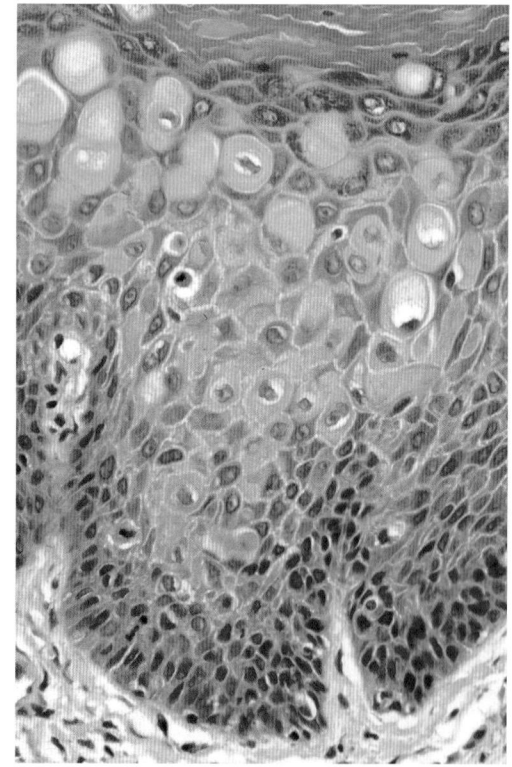

Fig. 30.70
Pagetoid dyskeratosis: the keratinocytes in the upper epidermis have abundant eosinophilic pale cytoplasm. They are diastase–PAS negative.

See
www.expertconsult.com
for references and
additional material

Tumors of the hair follicle

CHAPTER

31

Hair nevi

Clinical features

Localized variations of hair growth or hair follicle numbers are more easily appreciated clinically than histologically.[1-3] Increased growth of terminal hairs may be seen over a spina bifida defect and also occurs in hairy congenital melanocytic nevus and Becker nevus.

Hair follicle nevus

Clinical features

Hair follicle nevus (congenital vellus hamartoma) is an extremely rare hamartomatous lesion, which is usually evident at birth or develops in childhood as a small (less than 1 cm in diameter) solitary papule on the face, the preauricular area, and the ear.[1-13] Extrafacial occurrence is uncommon, and occasional cases presenting in adults have also been described.[2,6,14,15] Rarely, hair follicle nevi are multiple and may then be arranged in a linear distribution following the lines of Blaschko or they can be associated with epidermal nevus-like lesions.[16,17] An association with ipsilateral alopecia, leptomeningeal angiomatosis, and frontonasal dysplasia has been documented.[11,18]

Histologic features

Histologically, hair follicle nevus is characterized by a proliferation of mature vellus hair follicles, some of which are associated with small sebaceous glands. The follicles appear to be at the same stage of differentiation and are located abnormally high within the dermis. The perifollicular fibrous sheath is thickened and the follicles are embedded in fibrous tissue. Smooth as well as striated muscle may rarely be present, and the lesion is occasionally associated with a calcified nodule.[8,10]

Differential diagnosis

Hair follicle nevus is distinguished from fibrofolliculoma by the absence of a central cystic space.[4,7] The presence of cartilage and adipose tissue favors a diagnosis of accessory tragus.[19]

Woolly hair nevus

Clinical features

Woolly hair nevus is an exceedingly rare, nonhereditary condition characterized clinically by a well-defined area of tightly curled hair on the scalp (Fig. 31.1).[1-16] The hair is frequently thinner and lighter in color compared to the surrounding normal hair, and combing is difficult. There is no gender predilection.

Three distinct groups of patients are identified:
- those in whom the nevus is present at birth or develops within the first 2 years of life and there are no associated findings,
- those in whom the nevus is associated with an ipsilateral epidermal nevus; this occurs in about 50% of affected patients,[1,3,6,7,10,11,13,15]
- those in whom the nevus presents in early adulthood (acquired progressive kinking of hair).[17-26] This variant is very rare.

The term 'acquired progressive kinking of hair' has, however, been applied to a number of presentations. Most commonly, it refers to progressive kinking of hair in androgen-dependent locations with the subsequent development of androgenic alopecia.[18,23-25]

Woolly hair nevus has also been associated with systemized linear epidermal nevus, precocious puberty, incontinentia pigmenti, and ocular abnormalities such as persistent papillary membrane.[1,4,8,14,27]

Histologic features

No consistent abnormalities in hair morphology have been reported.[5,8,9] On histologic sectioning, there is curving of the lower third of the follicle.[12] Whole exome sequencing has revealed a recurrent somatic HRAS mutation in two patients.[28]

Comedo nevus

Clinical features

Comedo nevus (comedone nevus, nevus comedonicus) represents an uncommon abnormality of pilosebaceous development and presents as an usually

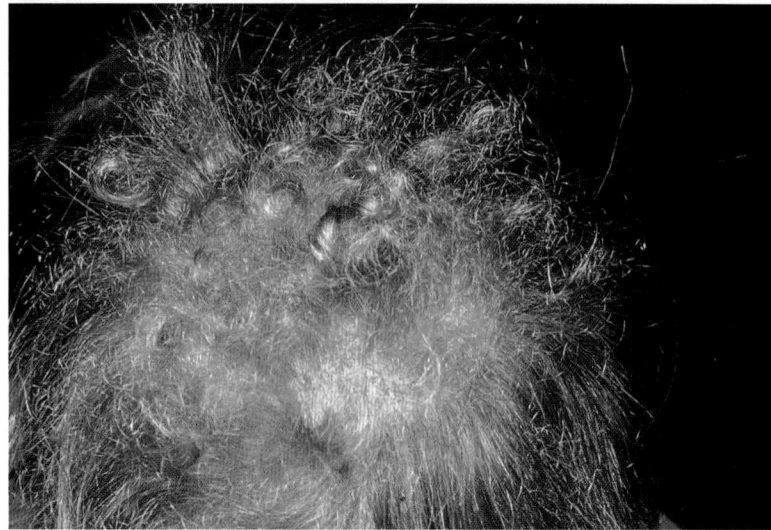

Fig. 31.1
Woolly hair nevus: the extremely curled hair on the top of the head contrasts with the normal straight hair on the side. By courtesy of the Institute of Dermatology, London, UK.

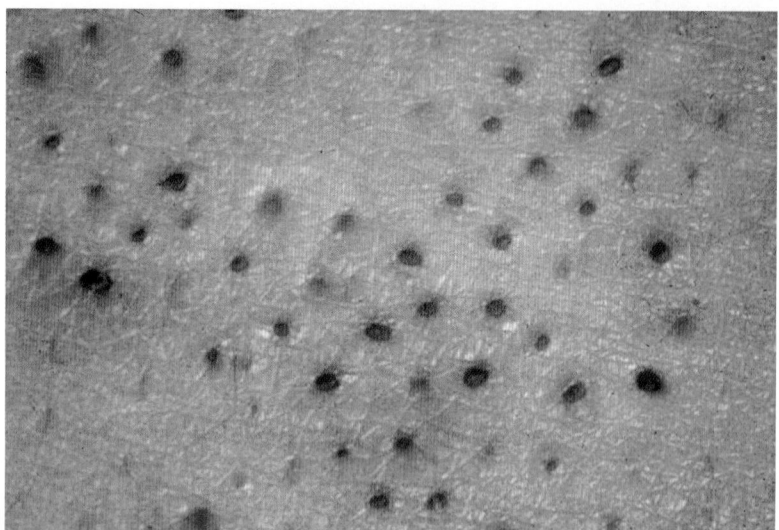

Fig. 31.3
Comedone nevus: close-up view. By courtesy of R.A. Marsden, MD, St George's Hospital, London, UK.

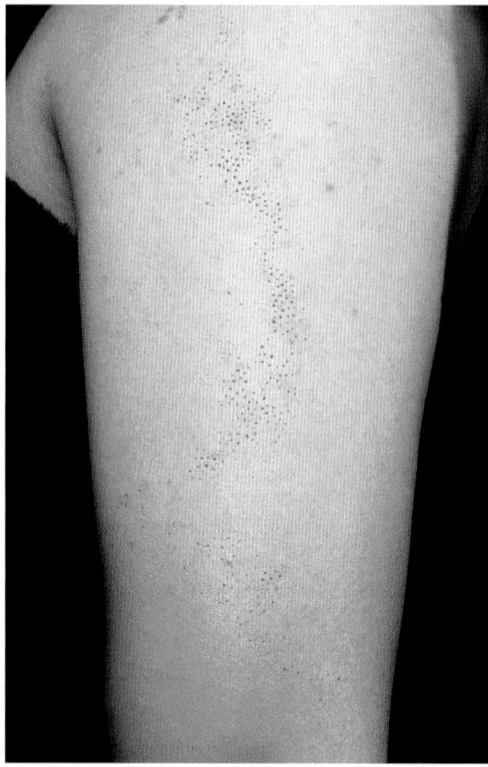

Fig. 31.2
Comedone nevus: there is a linear band of comedones. By courtesy of R.A. Marsden, MD, St George's Hospital, London, UK.

asymptomatic group of comedones, which may be localized or arranged in a linear, sometimes zosteriform, pattern, frequently following the lines of Blaschko.[1–3] The lesions are typically unilateral, but rare cases with bilateral involvement have been reported.[4–6] The face, neck, or upper trunk is most commonly affected (Figs 31.2 and 31.3).[1,2] Rarely, involved regions include the genital area in addition to the palm and wrist.[7–9] Very occasionally, the condition is much more extensive and widely distributed about the body.[1,10–12] Lesions are usually present at birth or develop within the first two decades of life.[13] There is an equal sex incidence.[2,14] The nevus sometimes shows inflammatory changes and sinuses; fistulae and severe scarring may be evident.[2,12,15]

Clinically, plugged sweat pores in a linear distribution may mimic comedones. Nevus comedonicus is sometimes associated with other cutaneous

disorders such as ichthyosis, linear morphea, lichen striatus, trichilemmal cysts, accessory breast tissue, hidradenoma papilliferum, and syringocystadenoma papilliferum in addition to follicular tumors including trichofolliculoma, dilated pore of Winer, and pilar sheath acanthoma, keratoacanthoma, as well as basal cell and squamous cell carcinoma.[16–24] An occasional association with systemic manifestations (nevus comedonicus syndrome) has been documented, including scoliosis, fused vertebrae or hemivertebrae, spina bifida occulta, finger deformity, clinodactyly, polydactyly, and syndactyly of fingers and toes, rudimentary toe, cataracts, microcephaly, seizures, EEG abnormalities, and transverse myelitis.[11,20,25–32]

Pathogenesis and histologic features

A mutation in the fibroblast growth factor receptor 2 (FGFR2) gene identical to that documented in Apert syndrome has been identified in a nevus comedonicus but not in unaffected skin from the same patient.[33] This finding suggests that nevus comedonicus syndrome may potentially represent a mosaic presentation of Apert syndrome, which shares at least some of the skeletal manifestations observed in patients with nevus comedonicus syndrome.[33] Whole exome sequencing has identified a NEK9 mutation in three patients with nevus comedonicus. NEK9 is speculated to disrupt normal follicular development.[34]

The epidermis is hyperkeratotic and variably acanthotic or atrophic. Occasionally, it shows irregular proliferation into the adjacent dermis.[2] Arising from it are large numbers of atrophic cystically dilated hair follicles containing abundant keratinous debris (Fig. 31.4). Sebaceous glands are usually normal, but sometimes they are diminished in number or size.[1,2,10] Infection or leakage of cyst contents can result in a focal acute or granulomatous inflammatory response. Epidermolytic hyperkeratosis may be an additional feature and the presence of follicular cysts resembling dilated pores of Winer has been described.[35–40]

Basaloid follicular hamartoma

Clinical features

Basaloid follicular hamartoma is a rare condition with varied clinical expression.[1] Solitary, localized, linear nevoid, generalized, and inherited variants are recognized.[2–4]

- Solitary: this presents in the elderly and show a slight female predominance. It affects the face, scalp and, less frequently, the shoulder, trunk, and extremities, presenting as a flesh-colored papule 1–2 mm in diameter.[1,5] Clinical misdiagnosis as basal cell carcinoma is common.

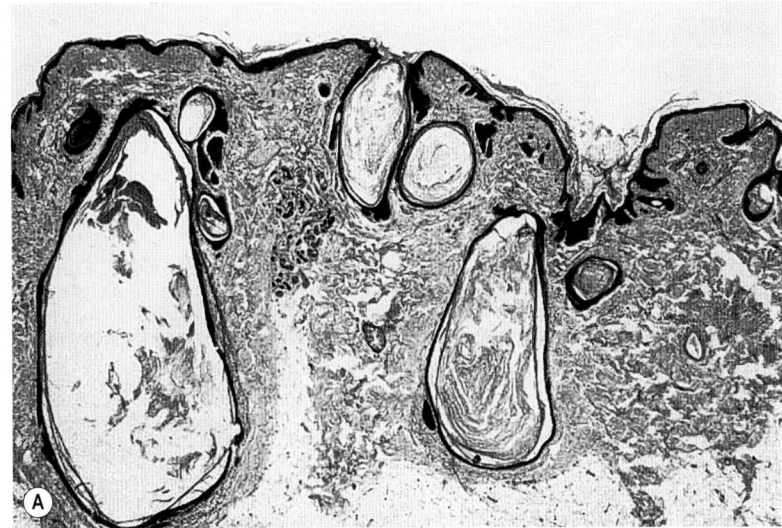

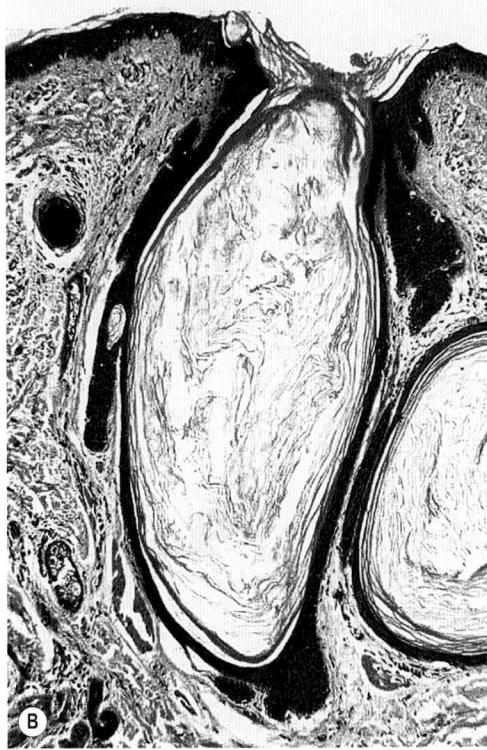

Fig. 31.4
Comedone nevus: (**A**) the lesion is characterized by both open and closed comedones; (**B**) shown in higher power.

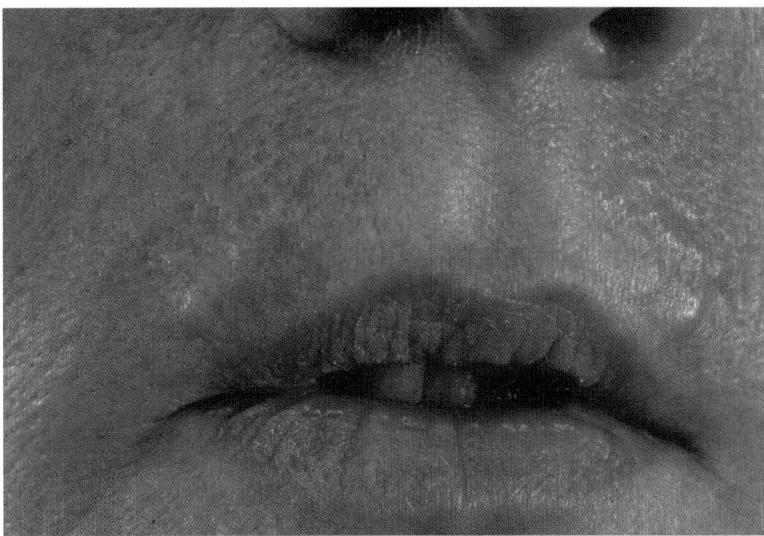

Fig. 31.5
Basaloid follicular hamartoma: note the pale infiltrated plaques involving the upper lip. By courtesy of the late N.P. Smith, MD, Institute of Dermatology, London, UK.

- Localized: the localized form which affects the head, particularly the scalp, presents in the third or fourth decade as an erythematous or slightly hyperpigmented plaque, sometimes associated with milia and alopecia.[3,6–10] Congenital lesions have also been described.[8,9]
- Linear nevoid: the congenital linear nevoid variant (linear unilateral basal cell nevus with comedones) may cover a large area, such as a dermatome, a quadrant, or even half of the body surface. Plaques are pale brown and covered with follicular papules (*Fig. 31.5*).[3,4,11–15] Alopecia, basal cell carcinoma, epidermal cysts, and comedones may also be present.
- Segmentally arranged: this recently reported variant is characterized by the presence of segmentally arranged basaloid follicular hamartomas associated with osseous and dental malformations and cerebral defects.[16–19]
- Generalized: the generalized form presents with infiltrated plaques on the face, alopecia totalis, and systemic manifestations including myasthenia gravis, cystic fibrosis, thyroid disorders, hyperhidrosis, and systemic lupus erythematosus (*Fig. 31.6*).[2,4,20–26] Systemic manifestations

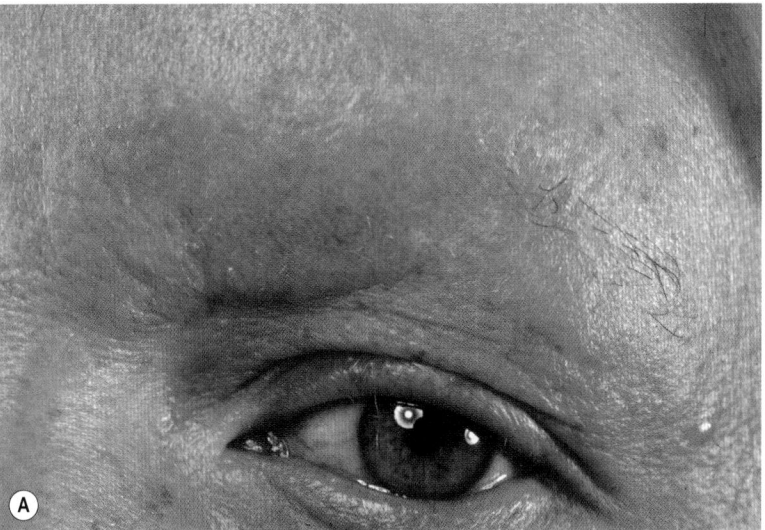

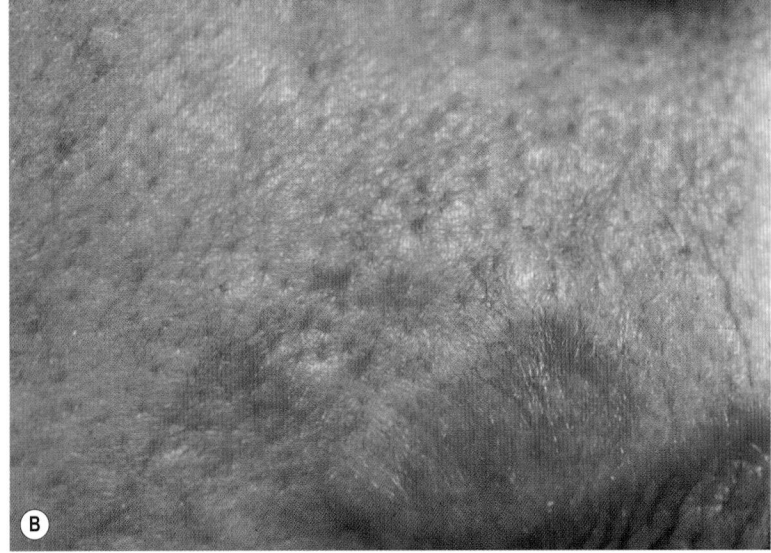

Fig. 31.6
Basaloid follicular hamartoma: (**A**) note loss of hair in the eyebrow and (**B**) a cobblestone appearance. From the collection of the late N.P. Smith, MD, Institute of Dermatology, London, UK.

are not invariably present, and a generalized presentation has also been reported in association with acrochorda and seborrheic keratoses in a patient with chondrosarcoma.[15,26,27]

- Inherited: the inherited familial variant typically is transmitted as an autosomal dominant trait.[1,15,28–30] Patients present in adulthood with innumerable small flesh-colored or pigmented papules on the head, neck, trunk, and anogenital region. It may be associated with systemic manifestations including partial alopecia and cystic fibrosis. An autosomal dominant basaloid follicular hamartoma syndrome has been reported; this presents at birth or in early childhood with innumerable milia, comedone-like lesions, and skin-colored to hyperpigmented papules on the face, trunk, and extremities, associated with hypertrichosis and pits of the palms and soles.[31,32]

Pathogenesis and histologic features

Molecular studies have demonstrated the importance of the sonic hedge-hog (Shh) signaling pathway in the development of basal cell carcinoma. Published data have implicated alterations in this pathway in the molecular pathogenesis of basaloid follicular hamartoma.[33]

Within the spectrum of this condition, two types of lesion may be seen. The epidermis is often structurally normal, although dilated follicles containing keratin debris are sometimes present.

- Most commonly, the hamartomatous proliferation appears as thin anastomosing strands and branching cords of small basaloid cells admixed with squamous cells embedded in a loose fibrous stroma affecting the majority or all of the pilosebaceous units (*Fig. 31.7*).[1–4] In some examples, an origin from the overlying epidermis has also been documented.[6,11] The epithelial islands are commonly orientated with their vertical axes perpendicular to the skin surface. Peripheral palisading of tumor cells reminiscent of basal cell carcinoma can be conspicuous (*Fig. 31.8*). The hamartomas show no evidence of pleomorphism and mitotic activity is not a feature. Occasionally, there are small foci of keratinization and horn cyst formation.[1,11] Melanin pigmentation within the epithelium is sometimes evident, and stromal amyloid deposition may be a feature.[1]
- On other occasions, the features are indistinguishable from those of trichoepithelioma, the lesion consisting of anastomosing trabeculae and lobules of basaloid cells embedded in a densely cellular fibrous stroma (*Fig. 31.9*).[20,21,34] Abortive hair germs, foci of keratinization, and peripheral palisading are additional features.[24] Occasionally, nodular basal cell carcinoma is present within an otherwise typical hamartomatous lesion.[6,11,35]

By immunohistochemistry, basaloid follicular hamartoma shows scarce expression of bcl-2 and Ki-67.[13,36] The surrounding stroma contains conspicuous CD34+ cells.[36] Intralesional CK20-positive cells are also present.[37]

Differential diagnosis

Basaloid follicular hamartoma can be distinguished from basal cell carcinoma by the absence of a retraction artifact separating the tumor strands from the adjacent dermis, inconspicuous mitotic activity, and apoptosis. Immunohistochemically, basal cell carcinoma shows strong expression of bcl-2 and marked proliferative activity with MIB-1.[13,38,39] A CD34+ spindle cell population does not surround the tumor nodules or strands of basal cell carcinoma.[13]

Dilated pore

Clinical features

Dilated pore (Winer) is a common, usually solitary, lesion which presents as a large comedone on the face or neck, typically in an adult.[1] There is a slight male predilection (2:1).[2] Development of basal cell carcinoma within a dilated pore has rarely been reported.[3]

Histologic features

The dilated pore consists of a keratin-plugged, cystically dilated hair follicle, which is usually superficially located, although occasionally it extends

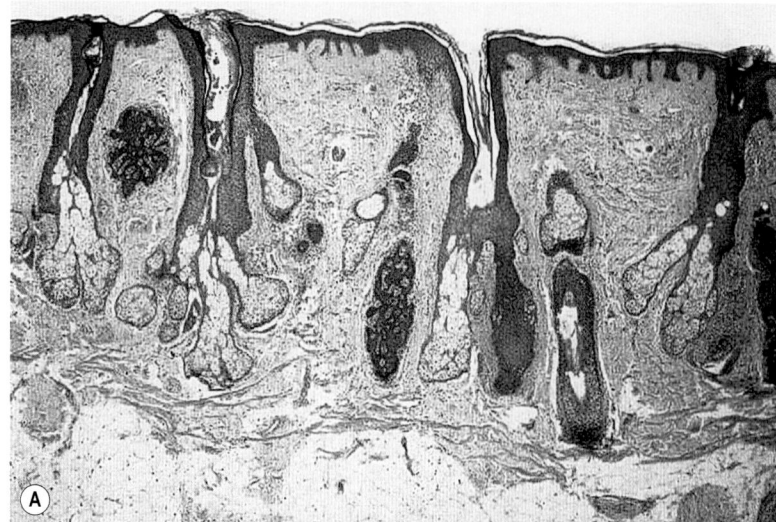
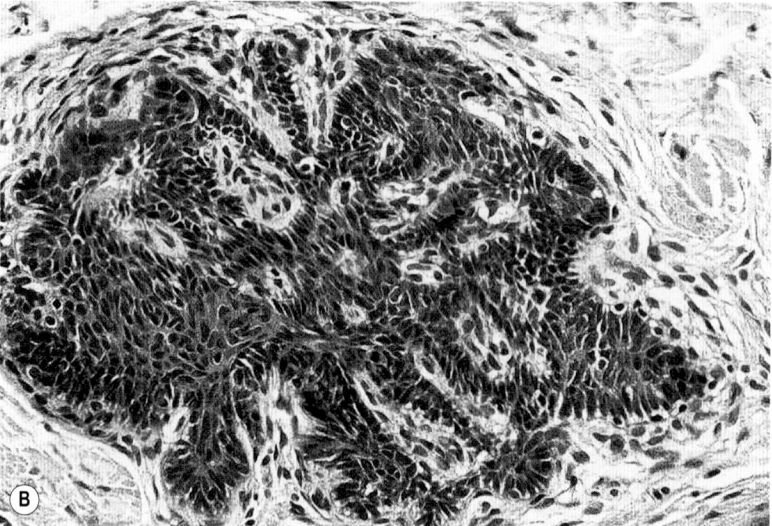

Fig. 31.7
Basaloid follicular hamartoma: (**A**) adjacent to each pilosebaceous unit is a hamartomatous lesion; (**B**) note the anastomosing strands of small basophilic cells and the spindle cell connective tissue stroma. By courtesy of the late N.P. Smith, MD, Institute of Dermatology, London, UK.

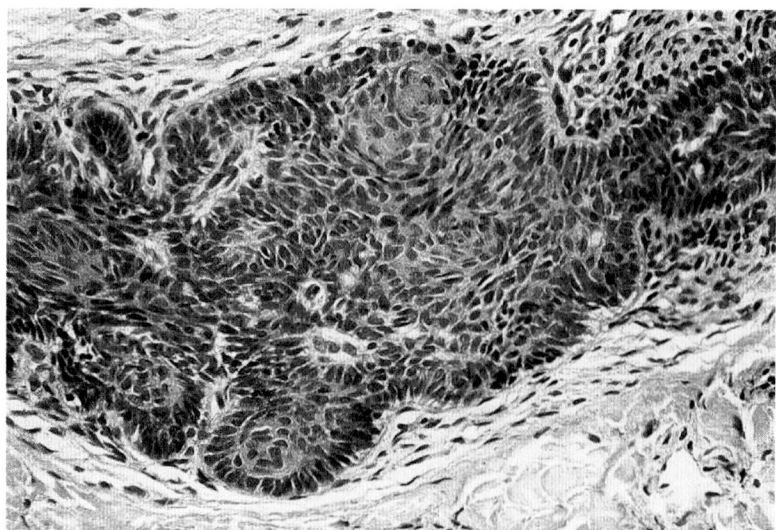

Fig. 31.8
Basaloid follicular hamartoma: note the peripheral nuclear palisading. By courtesy of the late N.P. Smith, MD, Institute of Dermatology, London, UK.

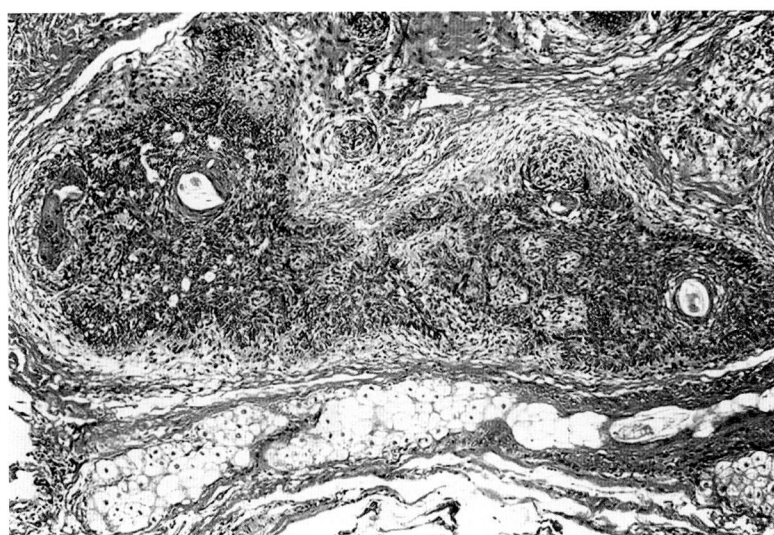

Fig. 31.9
Basaloid follicular hamartoma: in this example, the features are indistinguishable from those of a trichoepithelioma. Note the lacelike epithelial islands and the conspicuous stroma. By courtesy of the late N.P. Smith, MD, Institute of Dermatology, London, UK.

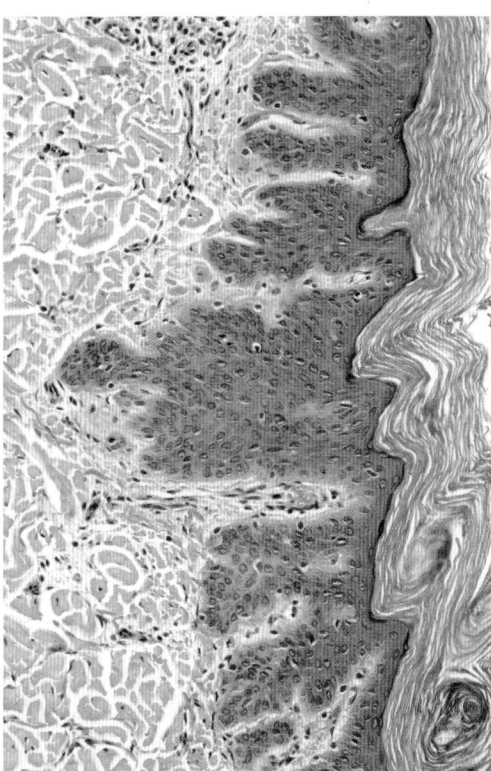

Fig. 31.11
Dilated pore: the epithelium on the lateral aspect of the pore shows irregular budding, a characteristic feature.

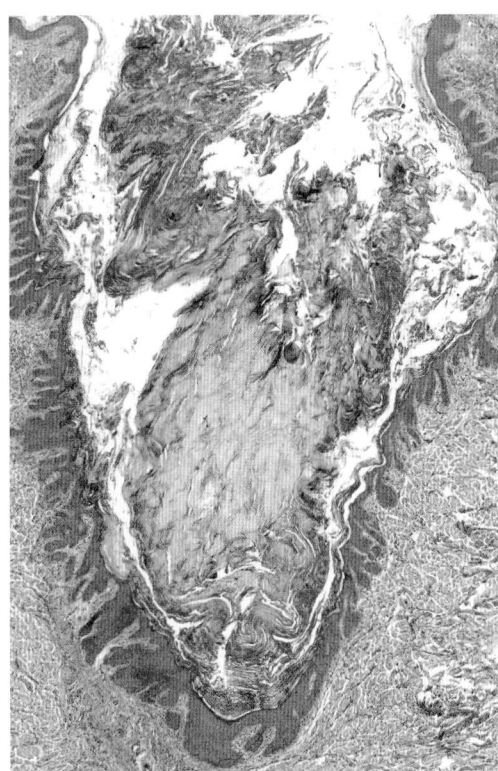

Fig. 31.10
Dilated pore: note the follicular dilatation and keratin plugging.

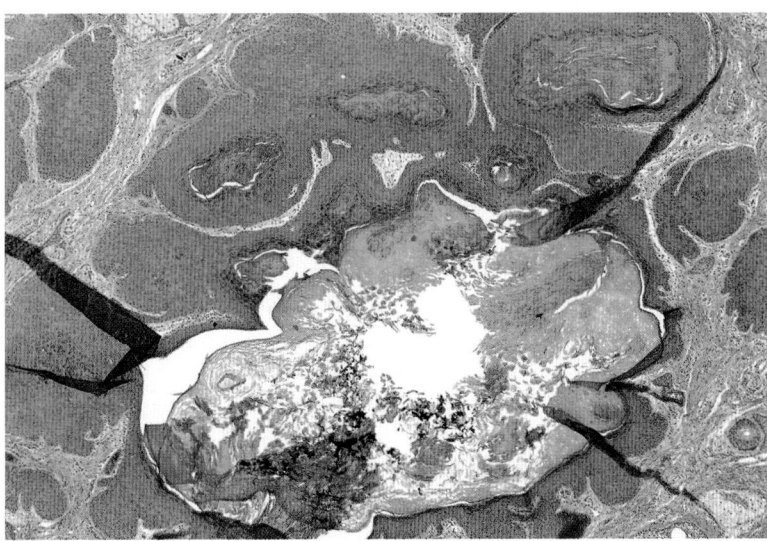

Fig. 31.12
Pilar sheath acanthoma: arising from the epidermis is a cystic invagination. Note the marked lobular epithelial proliferation.

into the subcutaneous fat (*Fig. 31.10*).[2,4,5] It is lined by stratified squamous epithelium, which is typically acanthotic, particularly in the deeper aspect of the comedone. Characteristically, the epithelium proliferates as irregular strands into the adjacent dermis (*Fig. 31.11*). Vellus hairs and sebaceous glands are sometimes present within the cyst wall.

Pilar sheath acanthoma

Clinical features

Pilar sheath acanthoma, which is usually located on the upper lip, consists of a solitary asymptomatic, small (0.5–1 cm) skin-colored nodule with a central pore containing keratinous debris.[1-5] It occurs equally in men and women.

Histologic features

Arising from the epidermis is a multilobulated cystic invagination from which numerous tumor lobules extend into the surrounding dermis and sometimes involve the subcutaneous fat or skeletal muscle (*Fig. 31.12*).[1] The cyst wall is composed of keratinizing stratified squamous epithelium with a granular cell layer. The lobules are of pilar epithelium which, due to the presence of glycogen, may be vacuolated (*Fig. 31.13*).[2,3] Peripheral palisading of nuclei can be a feature, and occasionally a diastase-resistant, periodic acid-Schiff (PAS)-positive hyaline sheath encircles the lobules (*Fig. 31.14*). Keratinization is usually infundibular and accompanied by keratin

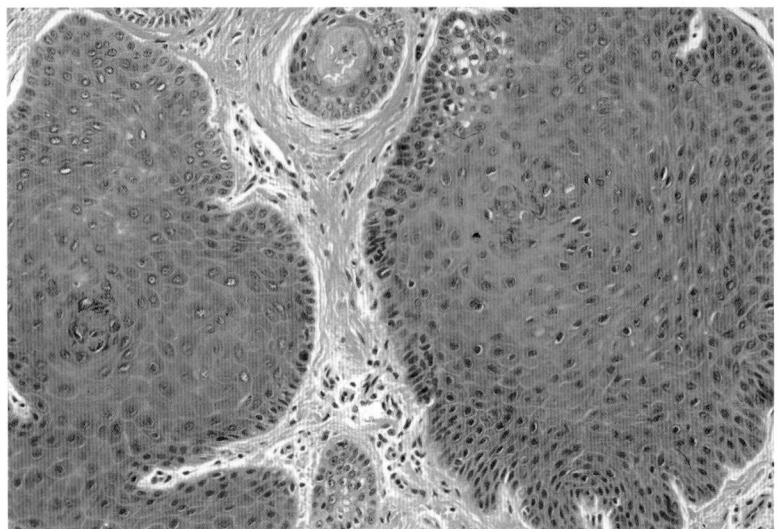

Fig. 31.13
Pilar sheath acanthoma: the tumor lobules are composed of outer root sheath squamous epithelium. There is no cytological atypia.

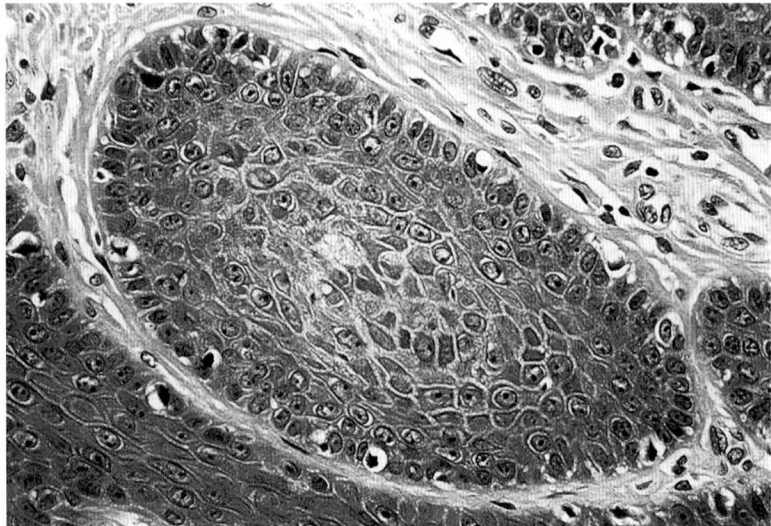

Fig. 31.14
Pilar sheath acanthoma: the epithelial lobules are surrounded by an eosinophilic hyaline basement membrane. By courtesy of N.A. Wright, MD, Royal Postgraduate Medical School, London, UK.

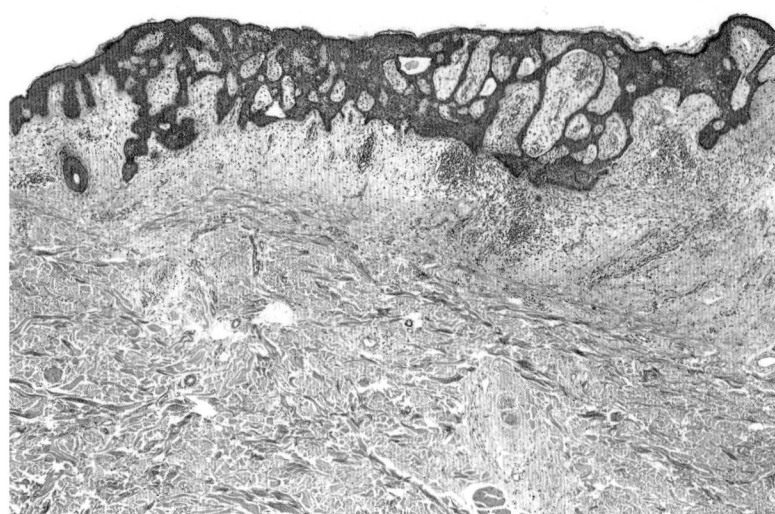

Fig. 31.15
Follicular infundibulum tumor: the tumor consists of anastomosing islands of basophilic cells showing multiple points of attachment to the overlying epithelium. The tumor is oriented parallel to the surface.

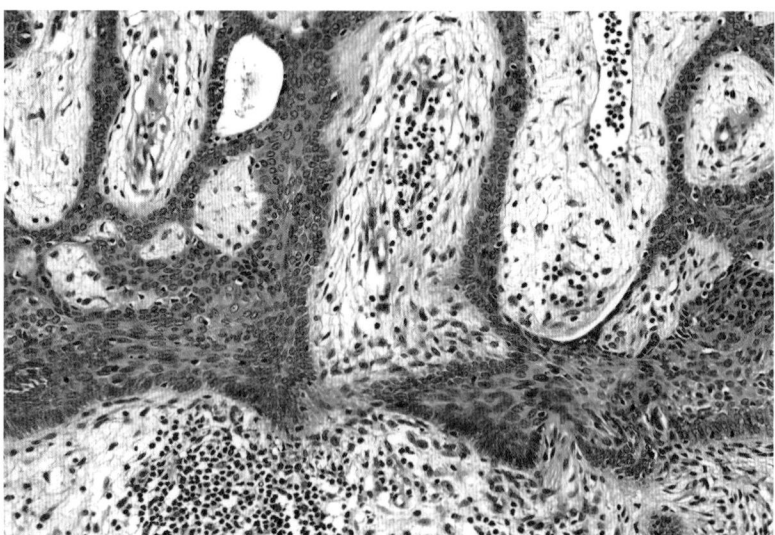

Fig. 31.16
Follicular infundibulum tumor: note the striking palisading.

cyst formation. Occasionally, however, the latter shows a trichilemmal epithelial lining.[3] A tumor stroma is usually inconspicuous.

Follicular infundibulum tumor (infundibuloma)

Clinical features

Follicular infundibulum tumor is a rare lesion that occurs most frequently on the head and neck. It presents as an asymptomatic, solitary, scaly nodule up to 1.5 cm in diameter often misdiagnosed clinically as basal cell carcinoma.[1–8] It is more common in females and affects the middle aged and elderly.[5,8] Rarely, it presents with multiple lesions, and an eruptive variant has been documented.[8–14] Tumor of follicular infundibulum may arise within an organoid nevus, and occasionally it is associated with Cowden disease.[7,11,15]

Histologic features

The lesion is characterized by a fenestrated epithelial plate connected to the epidermis at multiple points and showing a point of attachment to the follicular external root sheath of adjacent vellus hairs (Fig. 31.15).[2,5] The

tumor cells are pale staining due to glycogen and show peripheral palisading (Fig. 31.16).[2] An eosinophilic basement membrane is usually evident.[2] A characteristic feature is marked condensation of elastic fibers outlining the base of the lesion.[2] Eccrine and sebaceous differentiation have rarely been reported, and one example has been described in association with a trichilemmal tumor.[16–18]

By immunohistochemistry, the tumor cells are Ber-EP4 negative and intratumoral CK20-positive cells are present.[8]

Trichoadenoma

Clinical features

Trichoadenoma is a rare tumor that most commonly presents on the face and to a lesser extent the buttocks of adults, occurring equally in men and in women.[1–7] Very occasionally, the neck, upper arm, and thigh may be affected. Congenital and childhood presentation is unusual.[4,8,9] The solitary asymptomatic lesions are soft or firm nodules 3–50 mm in diameter and variably yellowish or erythematous in color. They rarely present as linear and verrucous plaques.[3,9] Development of a trichoadenoma within a dermal nevus is likely to be coincidental.[10] Trichoadenoma is completely benign.

Histologic features

Trichoadenoma is believed to be midway between trichoepithelioma and trichofolliculoma in terms of morphological differentiation and probably reflects differentiation toward the infundibular portion of the pilosebaceous canal.[1,5,11]

The epidermis is normal. Within the dermis is a well-defined fibroepithelial tumor composed of keratinous cysts and a conspicuous fibrovascular stroma (*Fig. 31.17*). The cyst wall is composed of squamous epithelium, which manifests epidermoid keratinization (with a granular cell layer) (*Fig. 31.18*). Solid epithelial islands may also sometimes be evident. There is generally no evidence of hair follicle formation, although in the verrucous variant (verrucous trichoadenoma), the cysts regularly contain vellus hairs.[3,8]

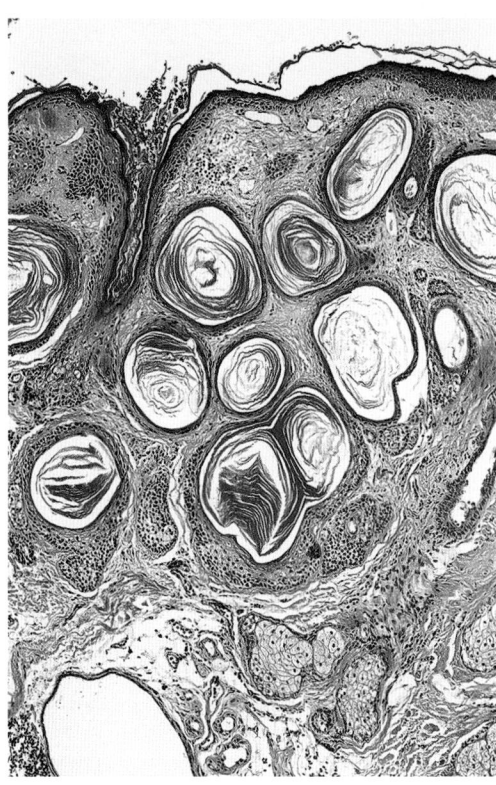

Fig. 31.17
Trichoadenoma: note the numerous keratocysts, many with a thick epithelial lining.

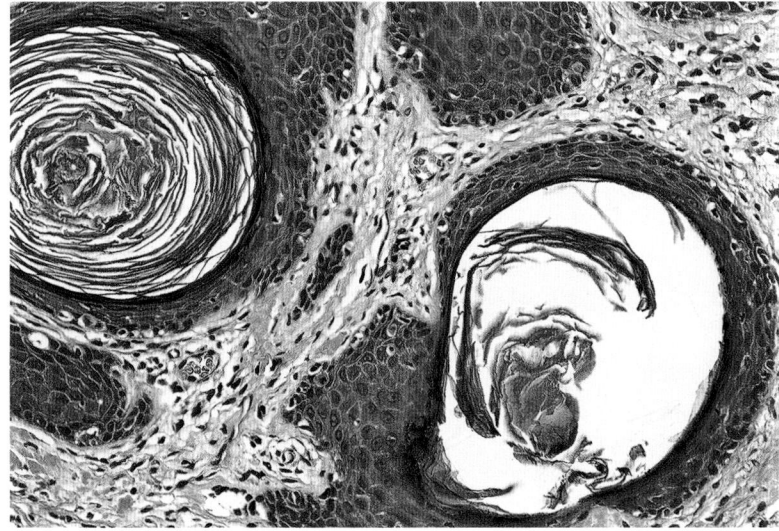

Fig. 31.18
Trichoadenoma: the cysts are lined by stratified squamous epithelium. Keratinization is epidermoid in type.

Immunohistochemistry reveals retained CK20-positive intratumoral Merkel cells. Tumor cells are negative for Ber-EP4 and androgen receptor.[12]

Trichilemmoma and Cowden disease

Clinical features

Trichilemmoma may be solitary or multiple.[1-4] The solitary variant occasionally develops within a pre-existent nevus sebaceus, but most often it presents as a single, small, warty or smooth, skin-colored papule on the face of older adults.[2-8]

The presence of multiple trichilemmomas is diagnostic of Cowden (multiple hamartoma) disease.[9-11] This disorder is characterized by multiple hamartomas and a high risk of breast and thyroid carcinoma with variable expression and age-related penetrance. The incidence of this autosomal dominant condition is estimated at approximately 1:200 000, and there appears to be a female predominance of 3:1.[11]

The facial lesions are skin colored and often very numerous, occurring predominantly around the mouth, nose, and ears. Patients may also develop trichilemmomas on the neck. Dermal fibromas are common and acrochorda are often present.[12] Also seen in Cowden disease are skin-colored or brownish scaly acral keratoses with a predilection for the dorsal and ventral aspects of the hands and feet (*Fig. 31.19*). Punctate keratoses of the palms and soles may also be evident (*Fig. 31.20*). Other cutaneous manifestations include vitiligo, lipomas, hemangiomas, neurofibromas, schwannomas, and xanthomas.

Oral lesions are common and include papules and polyps of the tongue, palate, lips, and buccal mucous membranes (*Fig. 31.21*). A cobblestone appearance is characteristic, due to gingival oral fibromas (*Fig. 31.22*).

Cowden disease is also associated with a wide variety of systemic manifestations. Most importantly, these include carcinomas of the breast, thyroid, and endometrium as well as macrocephaly and L'hermitte-Duclos disease (dysplastic cerebellar gangliocytoma).[13-18] Other manifestations are thyroid adenomas and goiter, fibrocystic disease of the breast, renal cell carcinoma, ovarian cysts and dysgerminoma, uterine fibroids, and colonic polyps.[13-17,19] The clinical diagnosis of Cowden disease is currently based on the constellation of major and minor criteria established by the International Cowden Consortium (*Box 31.1*).[13] Over 90% of patients are believed to manifest a phenotype by age 20. The risk of breast cancer is estimated at 25% to 50% and the risk of thyroid cancer is approximately 10%.[20]

Pathogenesis and histologic features

The susceptibility gene for Cowden disease has been mapped to 10q22-23 and identified as the tumor suppressor gene PTEN.[21,22] Germline mutations in

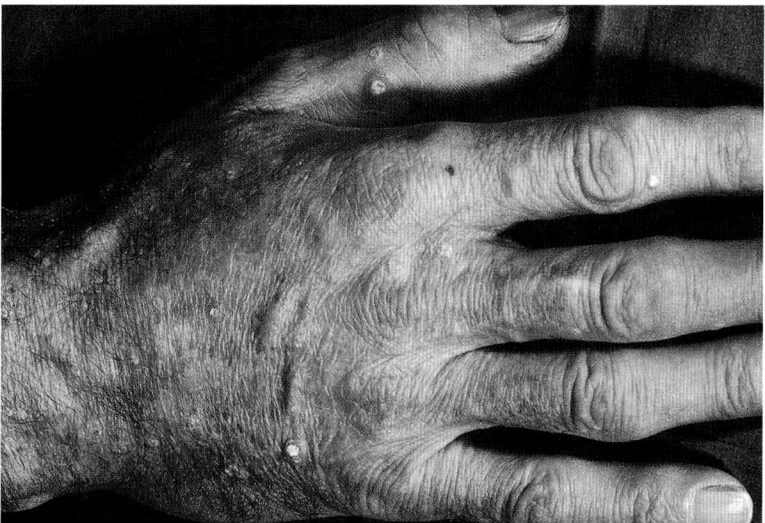

Fig. 31.19
Cowden disease: there are numerous keratoses on the back of this male patient's hand. By courtesy of R. Graham, MD, and R. Emmerson, MD, Royal Berkshire Hospital, Reading, UK.

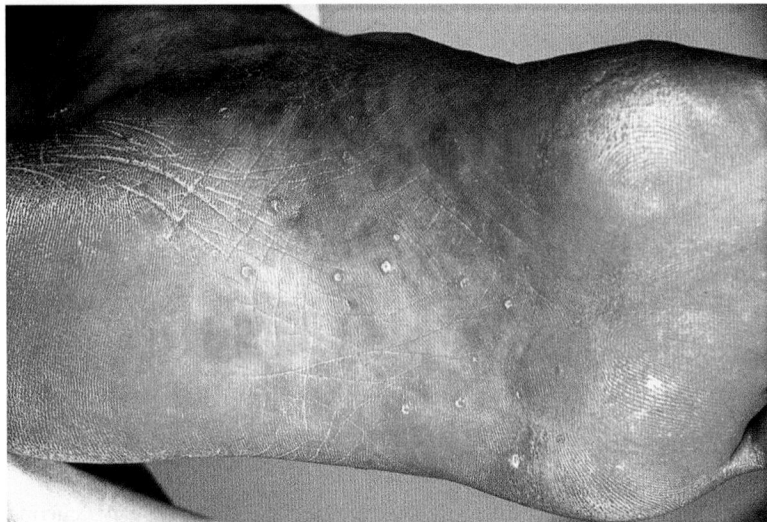

Fig. 31.20
Cowden disease: note the presence of multiple plantar keratoses. By courtesy of R. Graham, MD, and R. Emmerson, MD, Royal Berkshire Hospital, Reading, UK.

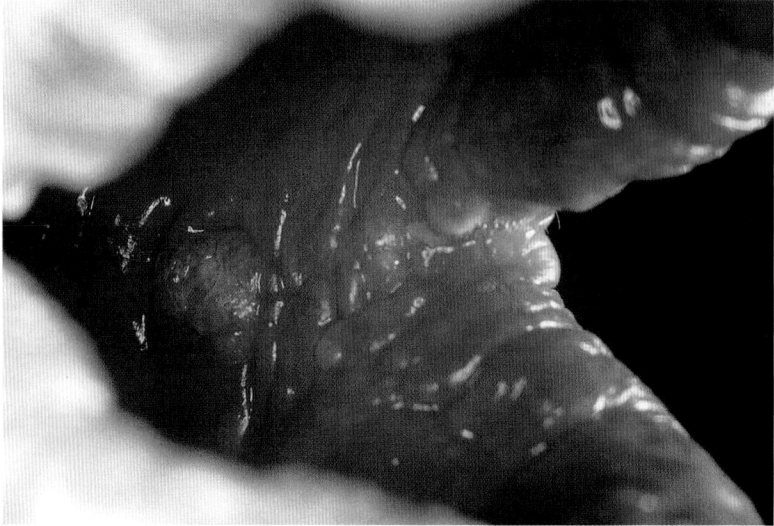

Fig. 31.22
Cowden disease: this patient shows the typical cobblestone appearance of the buccal mucosa. By courtesy of R. Graham, MD, and R. Emmerson, MD, Royal Berkshire Hospital, Reading, UK.

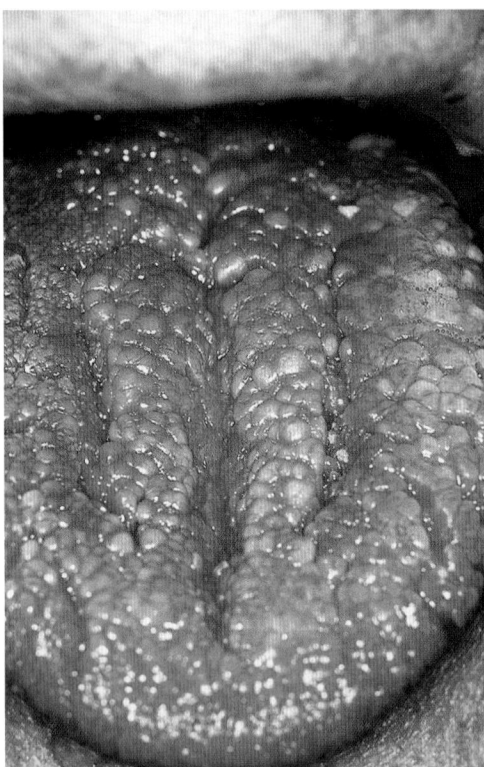

Fig. 31.21
Cowden disease: the innumerable shiny papules on this patient's tongue are characteristic. By courtesy of R. Graham, MD, and R. Emmerson, MD, Royal Berkshire Hospital, Reading, UK.

Box 31.1

International Cowden Consortium revised operational criteria for the diagnosis of Cowden disease (2000)

Pathognomonic criteria
- Mucocutaneous lesions
  - facial trichilemmomas
  - acral keratoses
  - papillomatous papules
  - mucosal lesions

Major criteria
- Breast carcinoma
- Thyroid carcinoma (nonmedullary), especially follicular thyroid carcinoma
- Macrocephaly (megalencephaly) (say, ≥95th centile)
- L'hermitte-Duclos disease (LDD)
- Endometrial carcinoma

Minor criteria
- Other thyroid lesions (e.g., adenoma or multinodular goiter)
- Mental retardation (say, IQ ≤75)
- Gastrointestinal hamartomas
- Fibrocystic disease of the breast
- Lipomas
- Fibromas
- Genitourinary tumors (e.g., renal cell carcinoma, uterine fibroids) or malformation

Operational diagnosis in a person
- Mucocutaneous lesions alone if:
  (a) there are six or more facial papules, of which three or more must be trichilemmoma, or
  (b) cutaneous facial papules and oral mucosal papillomatosis, or
  (c) oral mucosal papillomatosis and acral keratoses, or
  (d) palmoplantar keratoses, six or more.
- Two major criteria, one of which must be macrocephaly or LDD
- One major and three minor criteria
- Four minor criteria

Operational diagnosis in a family where one person is diagnostic for Cowden disease
- The pathognomonic criterion/criteria
- Any one major criterion with or without minor criteria
- Two minor criteria

Journal of the Medical Genetics, 2000; 37, 828–30, reproduced with permission from the BMJ Publishing Group.

PTEN are present in approximately 80% of patients with this syndrome.[23,24] The PTEN tumor suppressor gene is a lipid phosphatase mediating cell cycle arrest and apoptosis. Germline mutations in this gene have also been observed in other syndromes including the Bannayan-Riley-Ruvalcaba syndrome, characterized by macrocephaly, lipomatosis, hemangiomatosis, and speckled penis, in addition to Proteus syndrome.[25–30]

Solitary trichilemmoma, which represents proliferation of the follicular outer root sheath, appears as a small solid lobule or a group of close-set lobules connecting with the epidermis (*Figs 31.23* and *31.24*).[1,31,32] If early lesions are examined, the tumor may often be seen to arise in relation to the follicular external root sheath. The lobules characteristically show peripheral nuclear palisading and are composed of uniform small cells with round

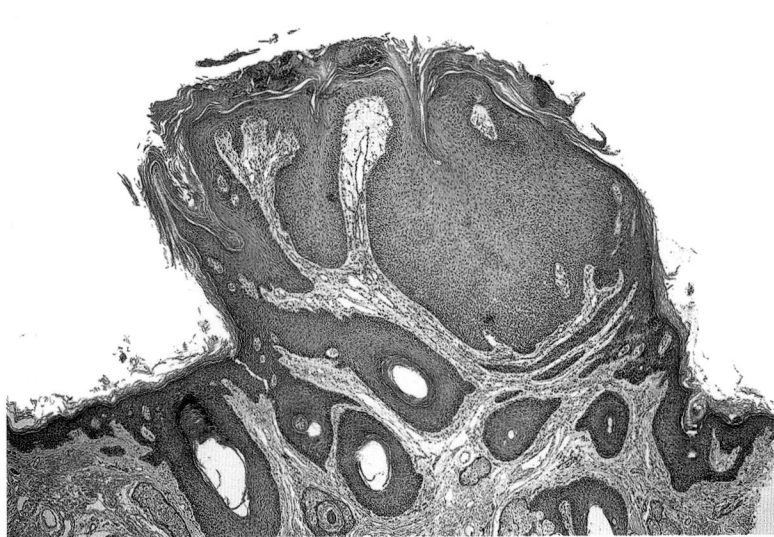

Fig. 31.23
Trichilemmoma: this facial lesion presented clinically as a small warty papule.

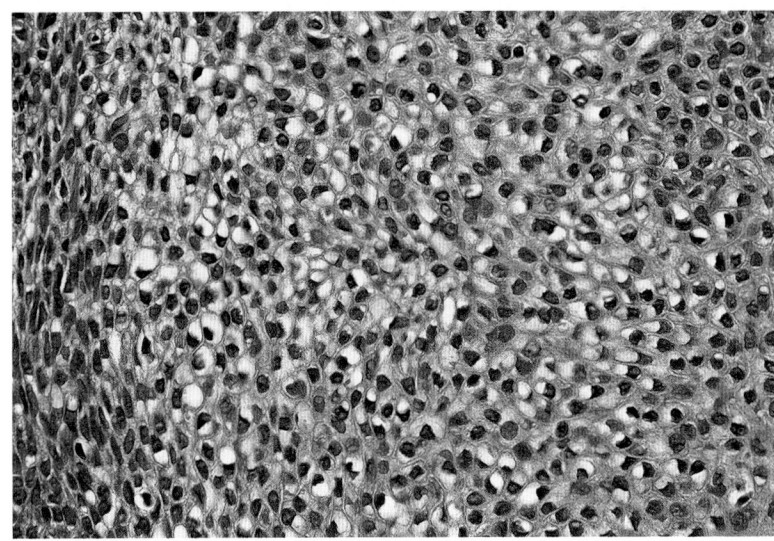

Fig. 31.25
Trichilemmoma: close-up view showing cytoplasmic vacuolation.

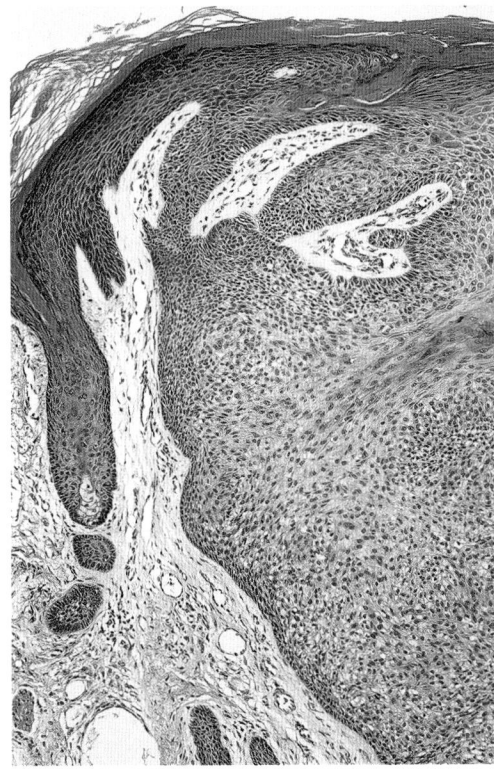

Fig. 31.24
Trichilemmoma: the tumor is composed of small, uniform cells showing cytoplasmic vacuolation.

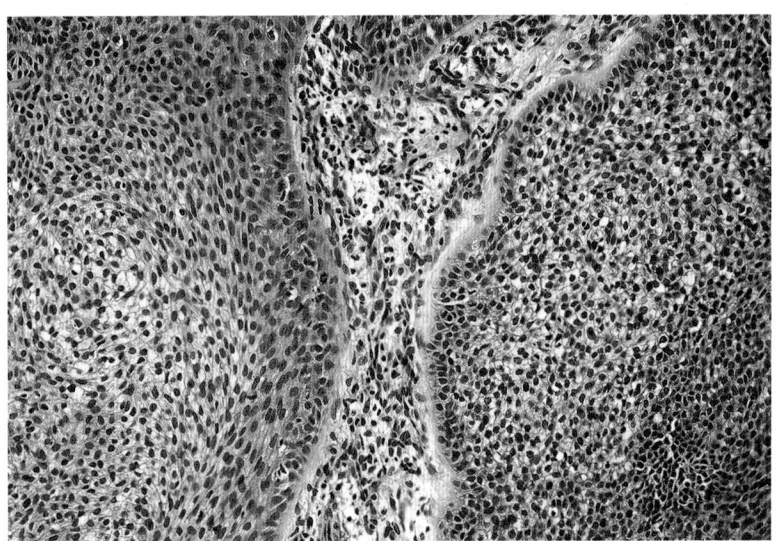

Fig. 31.26
Trichilemmoma: note the nuclear palisading.

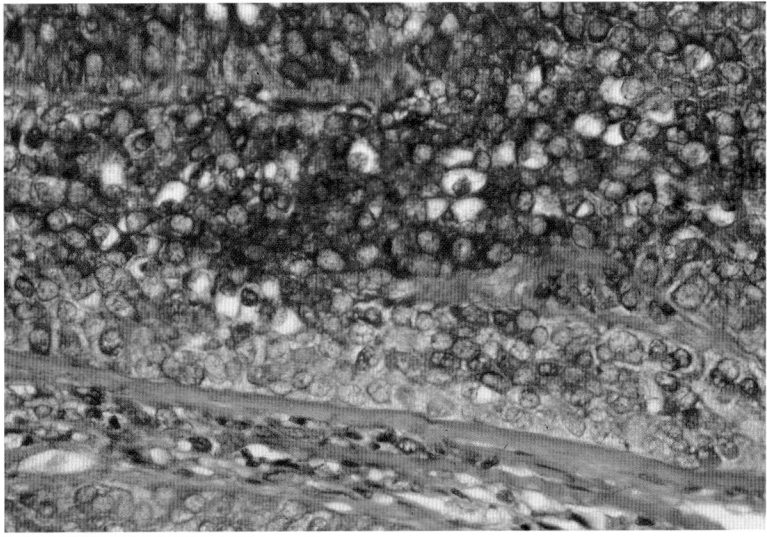

Fig. 31.27
Trichilemmoma: the PAS stain is strikingly positive.

or oval vesicular nuclei (*Figs 31.25* and *31.26*). Pleomorphism is not a feature, and mitoses are usually absent. A heavy glycogen content results in many of the tumor lobules having a conspicuous clear cell component (*Fig. 31.27*). A dense eosinophilic, diastase-resistant, PAS-positive hyaline mantle surrounding individual lobules is a typical feature (*Fig. 31.28*). CD34 is positive in tumor cells.[33] Keratinization is usually minimal, superficial, and trichilemmal. Occasionally, however, there may be marked keratinization in association with follicular dilatation and squamous eddy formation, resulting in histologic resemblance to an irritated seborrheic wart – so-called keratinizing trichilemmoma.[12,34] It can also be argued that the latter represents an overlap between a trichilemmoma and an inverted follicular keratosis. The surface epithelium is hyperkeratotic or parakeratotic, and sometimes a cutaneous horn is present (*Fig. 31.29*).[1]

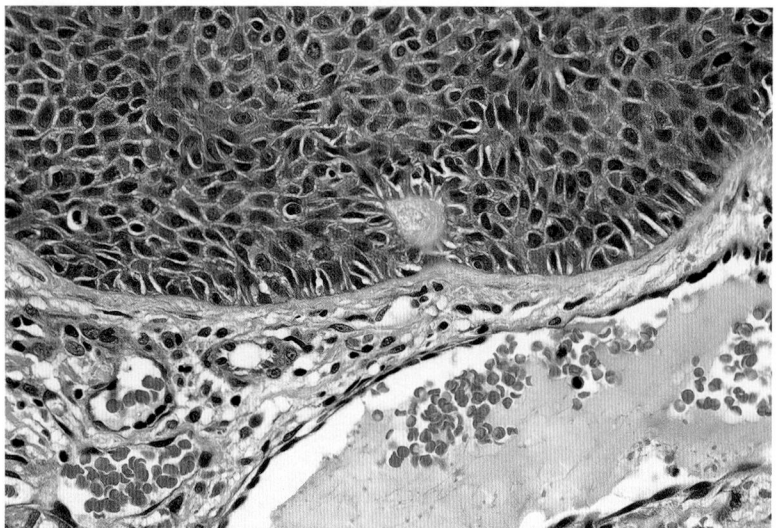

Fig. 31.28
Trichilemmoma: an intensively eosinophilic hyaline mantle surrounds the tumor lobules.

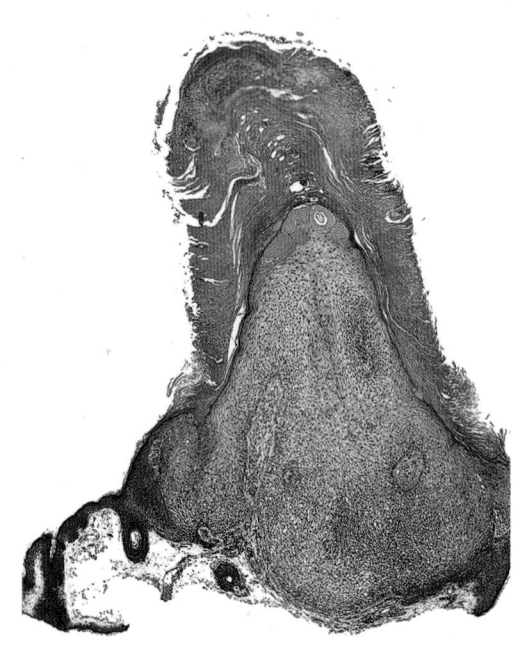

Fig. 31.29
Trichilemmoma: this lesion presented with a cutaneous horn.

In Cowden disease, about 50% of the facial lesions show features typical of trichilemmomas; most of the others show non-specific appearances of benign verrucous acanthomas. Occasional tumors show features intermediate between trichilemmoma and follicular infundibulum tumor or irritated seborrheic keratosis.[35] Filiform wartlike lesions may also be present.[35] The nonfacial keratoses show a grossly thickened keratin horn in association with a prominent granular cell layer and epidermal hyperplasia, sometimes reminiscent of acrokeratosis verruciformis or verruca vulgaris.[36]

The dermal fibromas often show a distinctive appearance, consisting of dense hyalinized bundles of collagen arranged in a whorled pattern reminiscent of storiform collagenoma.[12,37] There is typically abundant mucin and these lesions are therefore often strongly PAS-positive.

The oral lesions are all fibrous hamartomas and are composed of hyperplastic squamous epithelium overlying a fibrovascular core (fibroepithelial polyp).

By immunohistochemistry, complete loss of PTEN expression in trichilemmomas is highly indicative of an underlying Cowden syndrome. While reduced PTEN staining may be observed, complete loss of expression is rare in sporadic trichilemmomas.[38,39]

Differential diagnosis

Trichilemmoma is most easily confused with hidroacanthoma simplex and eccrine poroma. The presence of a distinct peripheral palisade and hyaline eosinophilic mantle, CD34 positivity, and absence of ductal differentiation and/or intracytoplasmic lumina are helpful diagnostic discriminants. Epithelial membrane antigen (EMA) and carcinoembryonic antigen (CEA) immunohistochemistry may be of value to identify the last.

Desmoplastic trichilemmoma

Clinical features

This rare variant of trichilemmoma, which appears to be more common in males, presents as a solitary, slowly growing, skin-colored or erythematous, dome-shaped papule.[1-7] Lesions, which are usually less than 1 cm in diameter, are found predominantly on the face, although the scalp, neck, chest, and vulva may sometimes be affected.[3] Occasionally, it arises within a pre-existent nevus sebaceous, and coexistence with basal cell carcinoma has been described.[8-10] There is no association with Cowden disease.

Histologic features

Desmoplastic trichilemmoma shows a characteristic biphasic tumor cell population. At the periphery, typical lobules of conventional trichilemmoma are present (Fig. 31.30). Toward the center, however, these merge with narrow irregular cords of smaller epithelial cells distributed in a dense, often pale eosinophilic hypocellular stroma containing diastase-resistant, PAS-positive, and Alcian blue-positive material (Fig. 31.31).[2,3] A chronic inflammatory cell infiltrate composed of lymphocytes and plasma cells may be evident in the adjacent dermis.[2] The tumor may rarely be colonized by pigmented dendritic melanocytes.[11]

The desmoplastic variant is of particular importance because its central sclerotic zone sometimes results in overdiagnosis as trichilemmal carcinoma or confusion with squamous cell and morpheaform basal cell carcinoma, particularly in small samples.

Trichilemmoma expresses keratin in addition to CD34, but not EMA or CEA.[2,12,13]

Differential diagnosis

Distinction from squamous cell carcinoma may be difficult in small samples containing only the pseudoinfiltrative squamoid component. However, tumor cells are negative for CD34 in the former and positive in desmoplastic trichilemmoma.

Trichilemmal carcinoma

Clinical features

Trichilemmal carcinoma is a rare tumor located predominantly on sun-exposed skin of the elderly.[1] Sites of predilection therefore include the face, scalp, neck, and dorsum of the hand.[2-4] The eyelid and the thigh have also rarely been involved.[5,6] The age range is wide, but the tumor usually presents in patients in the seventh to ninth decades, with a mean age of 71 years.[1-4] Lesions are variably described as single papules, nodules, and plaques, which are frequently ulcerated and sometimes crusted. They are usually erythematous or flesh colored and measure 0.5-2.0 cm in diameter. Development of a cutaneous horn is an unusual manifestation.[7] Presentation with multiple tumors and occurrence in colored races are extremely rare. Trichilemmal carcinoma has been described in association with localized pretibial pemphigoid and has arisen within burn scars, seborrheic in addition to solar keratoses, and Bowen disease.[8-14] It may also arise in the setting of immunosuppression following solid organ transplantation.[15-17]

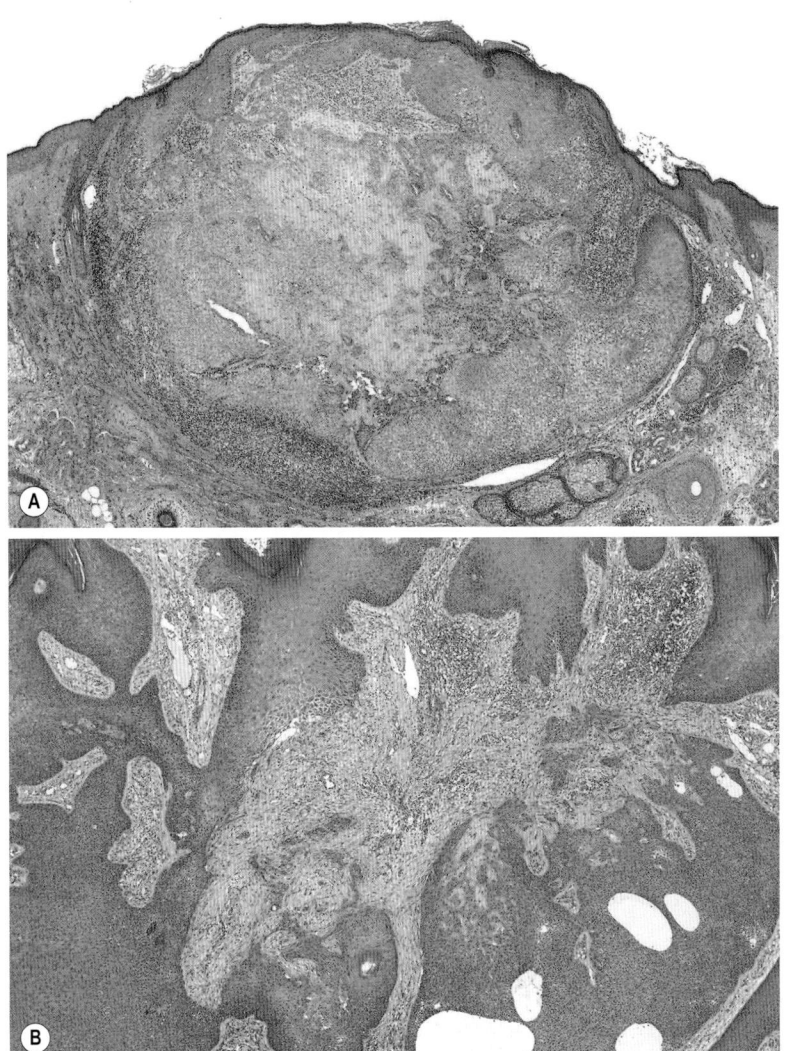

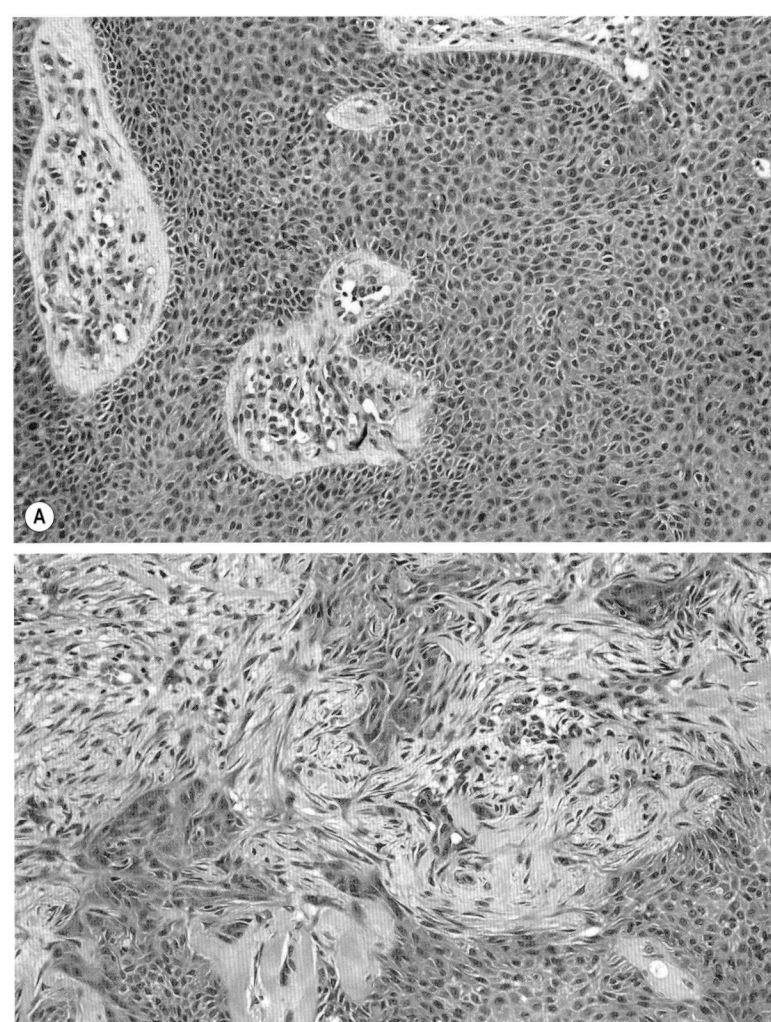

Fig. 31.30
Desmoplastic trichilemmoma: (**A**) note the epidermal origin. In the center of the lesion there is marked sclerosis; (**B**) the periphery of the tumor shows the typical features of trichilemmoma.

Fig. 31.31
Desmoplastic trichilemmoma: (**A**) high-power view; (**B**) note the admixture of epithelial strands and dense hyalinized collagen. This appearance is easy to mistake for a malignant tumor.

Despite histologic features suggestive of likely aggressive behavior, this tumor appears to have an indolent course. Recurrence and perineural infiltration are exceedingly rare, and metastatic spread is very rare.[18,19]

Histologic features

Although the tumor can be purely intraepidermal (trichilemmal keratosis), more commonly it is associated with an invasive component, which may extend to the deep dermis or even into the subcutaneous fat.[1,2,4] The intraepidermal variant is often centered on, and sometimes partially replaces, the pilosebaceous follicles with frequent involvement of the interfollicular epithelium.[2]

Invasive tumor commonly displays continuity with both the epidermis and hair follicles. It shows a variety of features including diffuse, lobular, and trabecular growth patterns (*Fig. 31.32*).[4] A pushing rather than infiltrating lower border is generally present. The neoplastic epithelium consists of large cells with diastase-sensitive, PAS-positive clear cytoplasm (see *Fig. 31.34*). There is a striking tendency to trichilemmal keratinization (i.e., in the absence of a granular cell layer) (*Fig. 31.33*). Nuclear pleomorphism is variable, ranging from mild in well-differentiated examples through to marked in high-grade tumors. Mitotic activity is often conspicuous and abnormal forms may be found (*Fig. 31.35*). Large tumors commonly show foci of hemorrhage and/or necrosis.[3] The periphery of the tumor lobules is characterized by nuclear palisading and subnuclear vacuolation, and sometimes a hyalin mantle is evident. Some tumors are characterized by

an infiltrative growth pattern such that distinction from squamous cell carcinoma depends on identification of pilar keratinization (*Figs 31.36* and *31.37*). Occasional features include acantholysis, intracytoplasmic eosinophilic inclusions, and focal pagetoid spread.[1,2,4] A lymphocytic/plasma cell infiltrate is often present. Neuroendocrine differentiation with expression of chromogranin, synaptophysin, and CD56 in tumor cells is exceptional.[20]

Immunohistochemistry reveals high molecular weight keratin expression.[1] The tumor is usually CEA and EMA negative, although expression of the latter has occasionally been documented.[3]

Differential diagnosis

Trichilemmal carcinoma must be distinguished from other malignant clear cell tumors, including clear cell squamous carcinoma, clear cell porocarcinoma, and clear cell hidradenocarcinoma. Clear cell squamous carcinoma has an infiltrative growth pattern in contrast to the pushing border of trichilemmal carcinoma and typically lacks the peripheral palisading and hyalin mantle. Squamous carcinoma is often EMA positive. Porocarcinoma and hidradenocarcinoma, by definition, show evidence of ductal differentiation and/or intracytoplasmic lumen formation, which can often be accentuated by the diastase–PAS reaction or immunohistochemically by EMA or CEA expression. Rarely, malignant melanoma may show a clear cell pattern. In cases of doubt, the identification of melanin pigment by the Masson-Fontana reaction or the use of S100 protein or HMB-45 immunocytochemistry should readily establish the correct diagnosis.

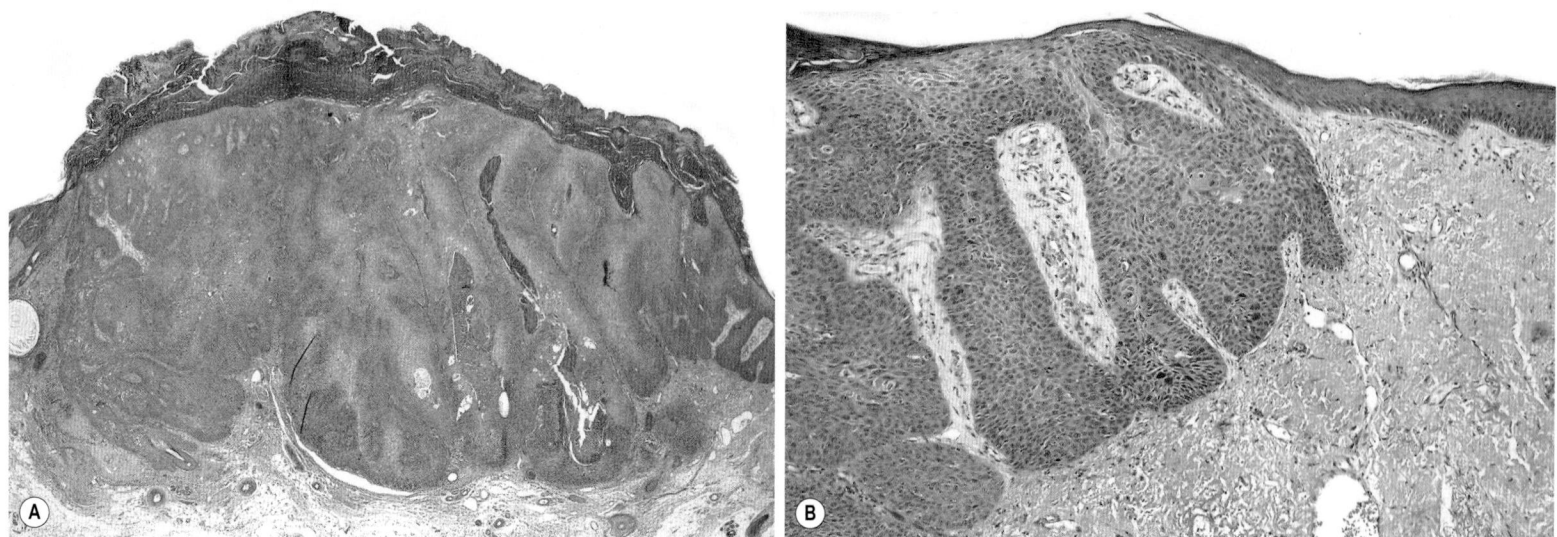

Fig. 31.32
Trichilemmal carcinoma: (**A**) this scanning view shows a well-defined tumor composed of lobules of epithelium, with a sharply defined lower border; (**B**) higher-power view of the tumor surface.

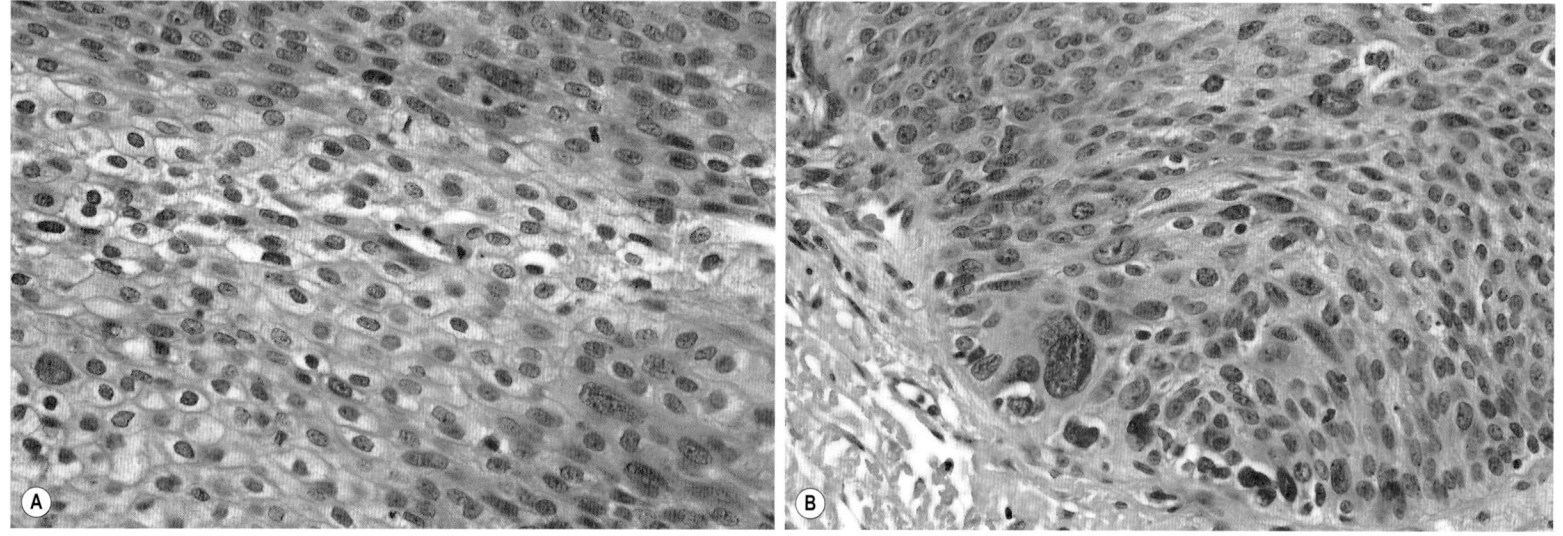

Fig. 31.33
Trichilemmal carcinoma: (**A**) there is clear cell change; (**B**) there is marked nuclear pleomorphism.

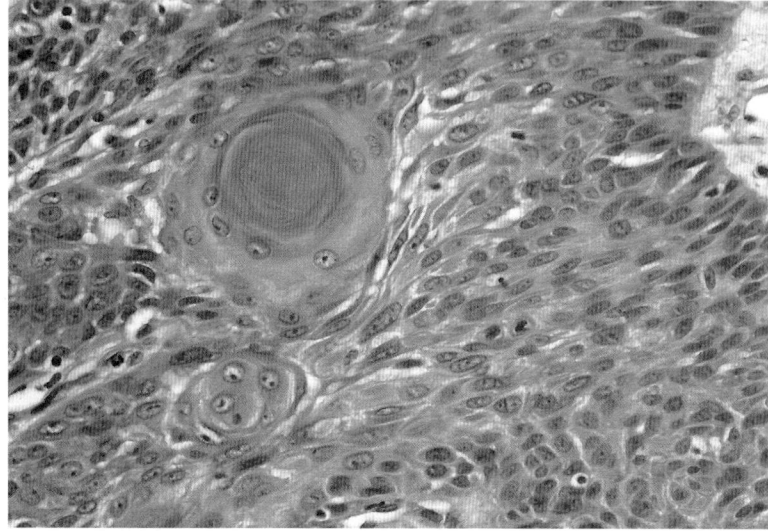

Fig. 31.34
Trichilemmal carcinoma: this view shows pilar keratinization.

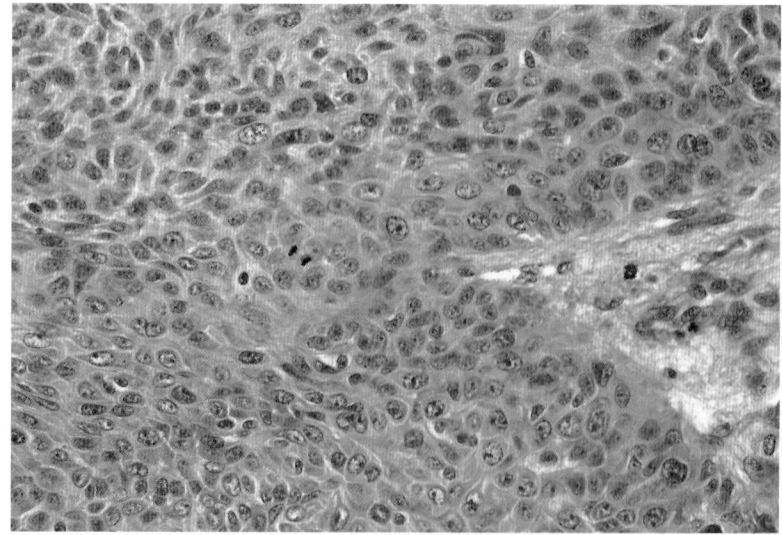

Fig. 31.35
Trichilemmal carcinoma: note the mitotic activity.

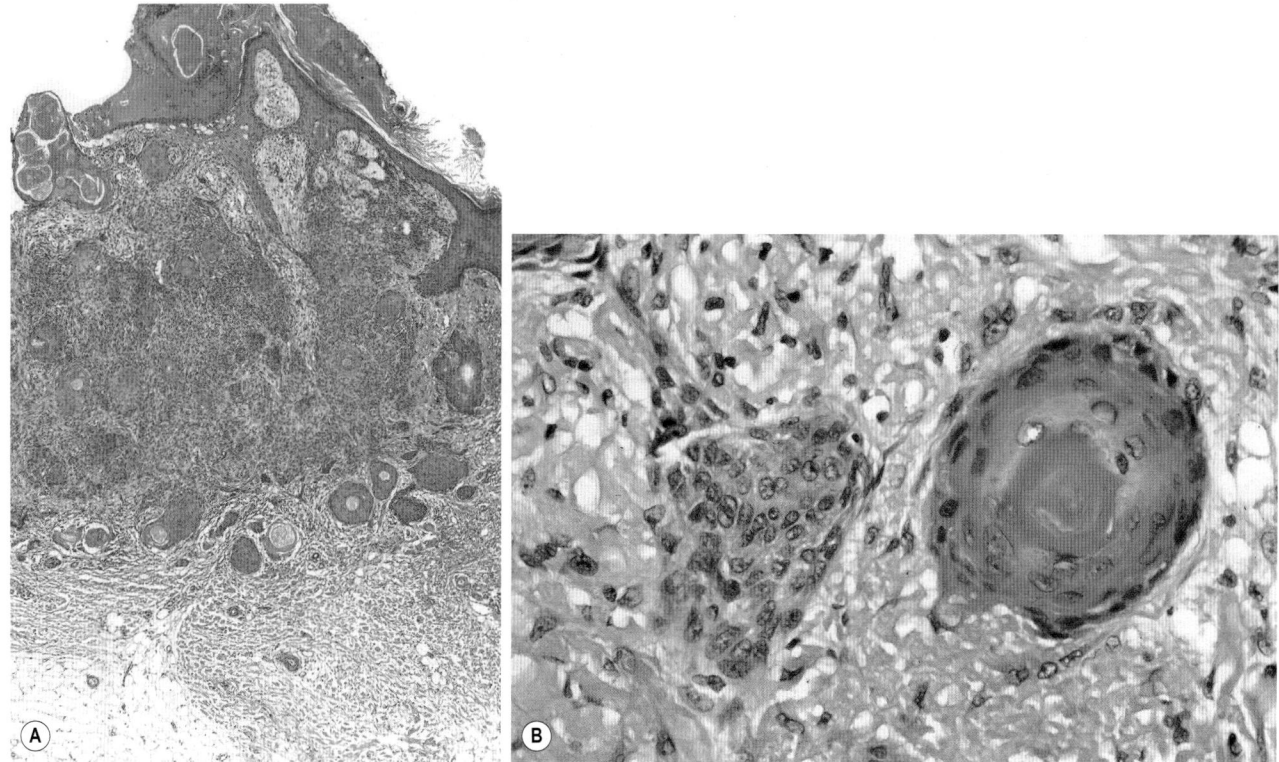

Fig. 31.36
(**A, B**) Trichilemmal carcinoma: this example shows an infiltrative growth pattern reminiscent of squamous cell carcinoma. There is widespread pilar-type keratinization.

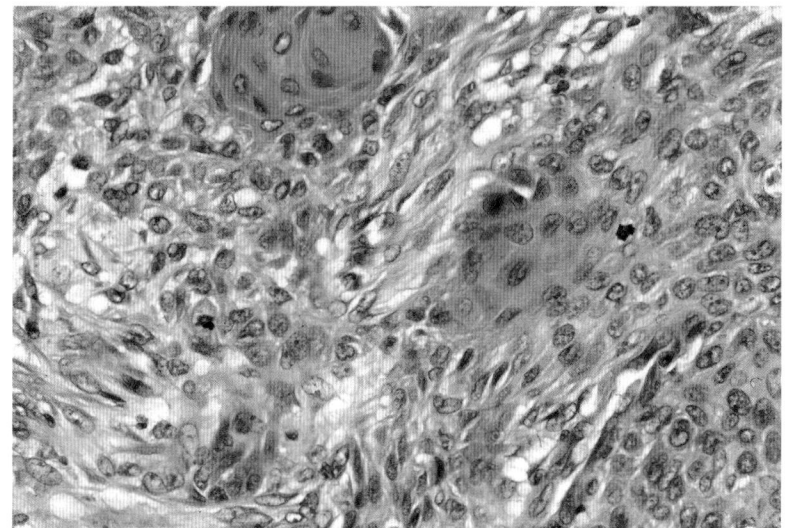

Fig. 31.37
Trichilemmal carcinoma: high-power view showing multiple mitoses.

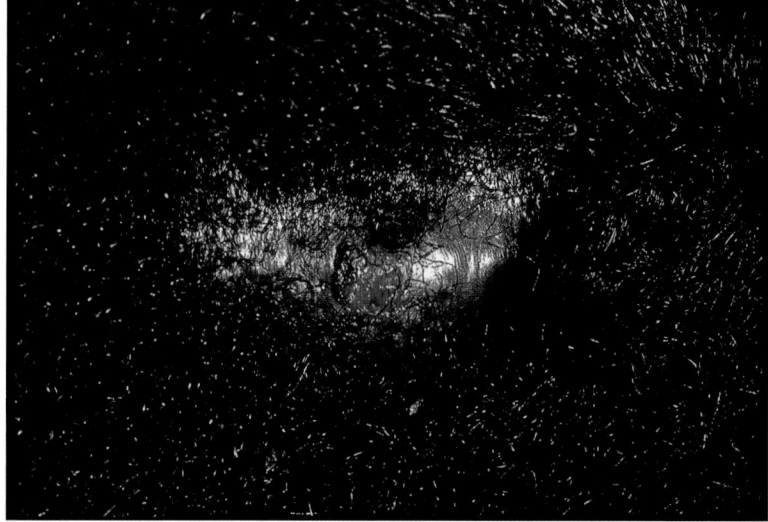

Fig. 31.38
Pilar tumor: an ulcerated lesion is present on the scalp, a characteristic site. By courtesy of R.A. Marsden, MD, St George's Hospital, London, UK.

Proliferating trichilemmal (pilar) cyst

Clinical features

The proliferating trichilemmal cyst (pilar tumor of the scalp) is a rare, usually benign, tumor of external root sheath derivation and, in most instances, appears to develop within the wall of a pre-existent pilar cyst.[1-3] A wide range of anatomic sites including the trunk, and rarely the extremities, nose, eyelid, and vulva may be affected, but the majority (90%) occur on the scalp (*Fig. 31.38*).[4-16] Rarely, it arises in the background of an epidermal nevus or nevus sebaceous.[17-19] There is a marked female predominance of 6:1. Lesions present as usually solitary, slowly growing, often multinodular, soft tumors in the deep dermis, often extending into the subcutaneous fat.[7,20,21] They are commonly large, measuring up to 6 cm or more in diameter (*Fig. 31.39*).[14,22] Occasional patients have multiple tumors, and not infrequently there is a background of one or more simple pilar (trichilemmal) cysts.[23-25]

Pilar tumors occasionally involve the deeper soft tissue or even extend to bone, but recurrences following inadequate excision are uncommon.[7,26] Locally destructive behavior and metastases to regional lymph nodes are rare.[23,27-33] Tumors regarded as 'malignant proliferating pilar tumors' have potential for local recurrence, distant metastasis, and disease-related mortality.[34,35]

Pathogenesis and histologic features

The proliferating trichilemmal cyst is thought to develop initially as a focus of epithelial proliferation in a trichilemmal cyst, perhaps as a consequence of trauma or chronic inflammation.[2,3]

It consists of a lobulated intradermal mass of squamous epithelium, which may simulate a squamous cell carcinoma, but has individual lobules with a characteristically sharply defined and regular noninfiltrative border (*Fig. 31.40*). Peripheral palisading is often present, and lobules may be

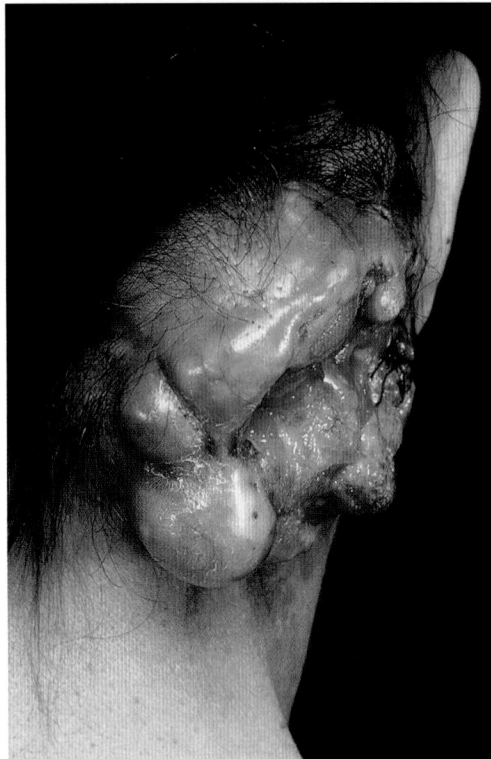

Fig. 31.39
Pilar tumor: this is a more severe example in which multiple tumors are evident. By courtesy of the Institute of Dermatology, London, UK.

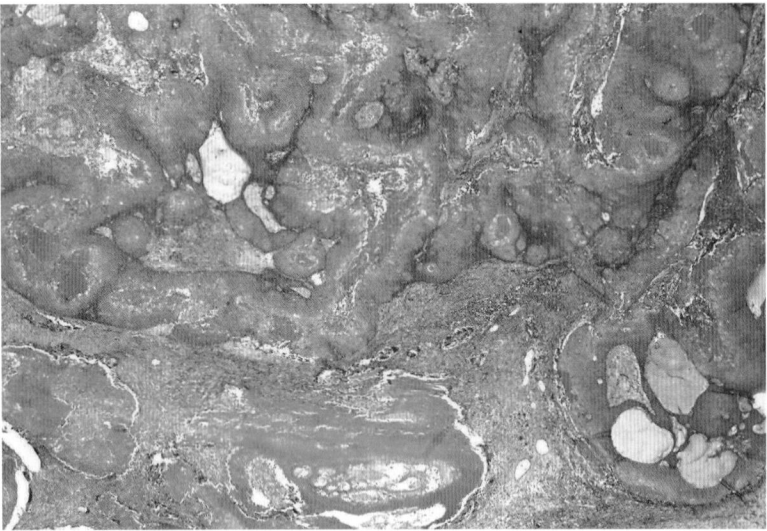

Fig. 31.40
Pilar tumor: low-power view showing multiple lobules composed of squamous epithelium. Note the characteristic pushing margin contrasting with the usual infiltrative growth pattern of squamous cell carcinoma.

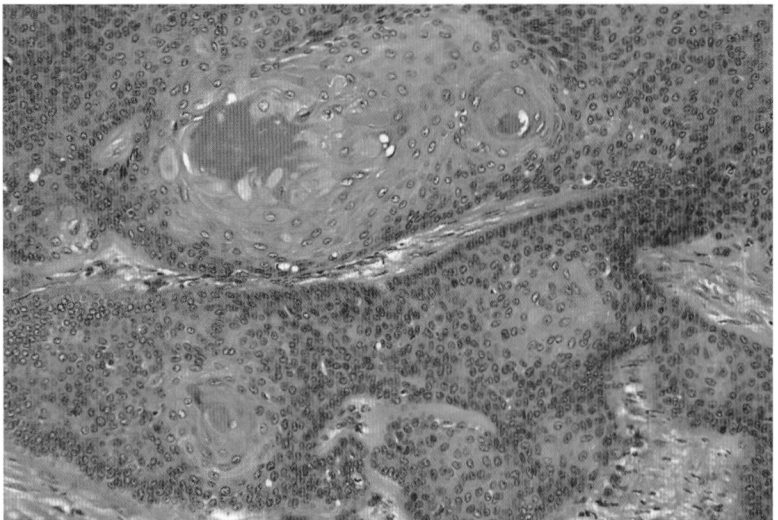

Fig. 31.41
Pilar tumor: peripheral nuclear palisading is present.

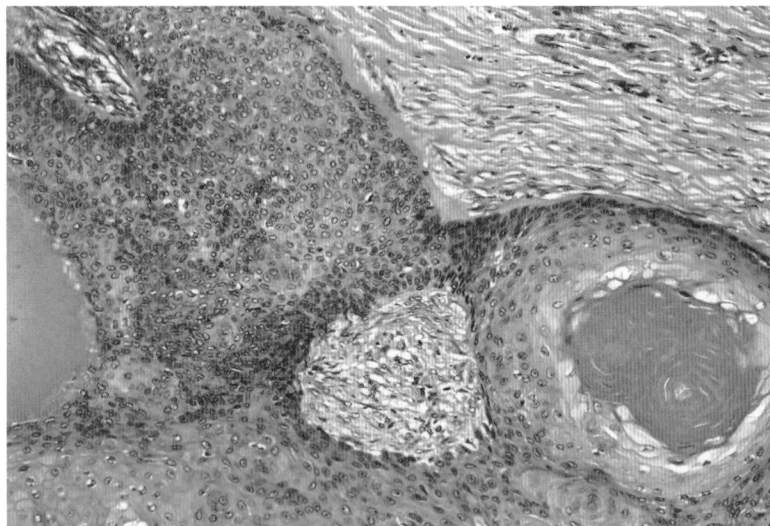

Fig. 31.42
Pilar tumor: at the edges of the lobules, there is an intensely eosinophilic, thickened basement membrane.

surrounded by a thickened refractile basement membrane (*Figs 31.41* and *31.42*). Cyst formation is not usually a prominent feature. Widespread trichilemmal keratinization associated with necrosis is characteristic (*Figs 31.43* and *31.44*). A granular cell layer is therefore usually absent, although occasionally a few parakeratotic cells may be seen at the edge of the keratinous necrotic centers. Frequently, the keratinous debris is associated with a foreign body giant cell reaction and calcification may be present (*Fig. 31.45*).[36] Sometimes, due to glycogen accumulation, the tumor may contain large numbers of clear cells (*Fig. 31.46*). Some areas of the tumor may manifest epidermoid keratinization or outer root sheath maturation, and therefore individual cell keratinization and squamous eddy formation may be features (*Fig. 31.47*). Occasionally, mild cellular atypia is seen, but mitotic figures are in general limited to the basal epithelium and are rarely abnormal (*Fig. 31.48*).

Malignant proliferating pilar tumors show a spectrum of histologic features ranging from in situ foci of increasing nuclear and cytoplasmic pleomorphism accompanied by numerous and often atypical mitotic figures through to frankly invasive lesions that are often accompanied by a destructive growth pattern (*Figs 31.49–31.51*).[4,7,21,23,26–34,37–42] Spindle cell sarcomatous features have also been documented.[28,37,43] Experience is limited to a small number of case reports, but features of ominous significance include clinical findings such as rapid increase in size, tumor size >5 cm, nonscalp location, and/or foci of necrosis or ulceration in addition to histologic findings of infiltrative growth, abundant mitotic figures (including atypical forms), and marked cytological atypia.[31,43] In a more comprehensive attempt to correlate histologic features with outcome, three distinct groups have emerged in an analysis of 76 tumors. Tumors showing circumscribed silhouettes and pushing borders, mild nuclear atypia and lack of necrosis, atypical mitoses, and perineural or lymphovascular invasion are characterized by benign behavior with no increased risk for local recurrence or distant metastasis. In contrast, tumors showing irregular outlines and infiltrative growth with involvement of deep dermis and subcutis may have potential for locally destructive growth, while metastatic potential was observed in tumors with an invasive growth pattern in addition to marked nuclear atypia, atypical

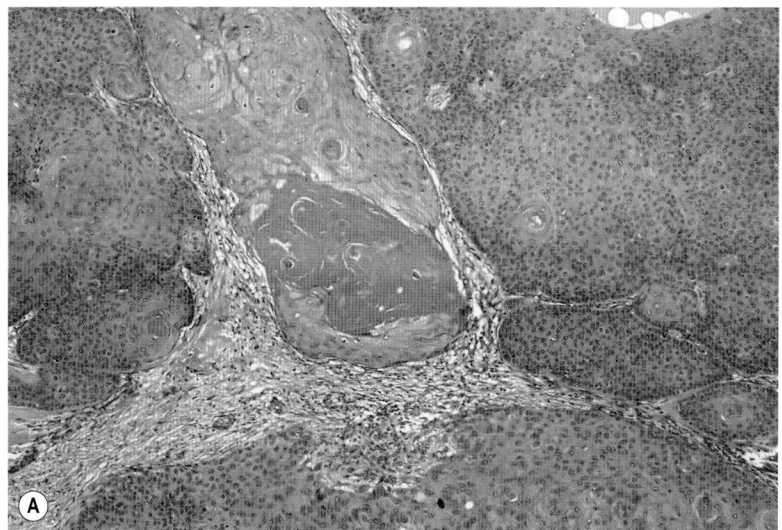

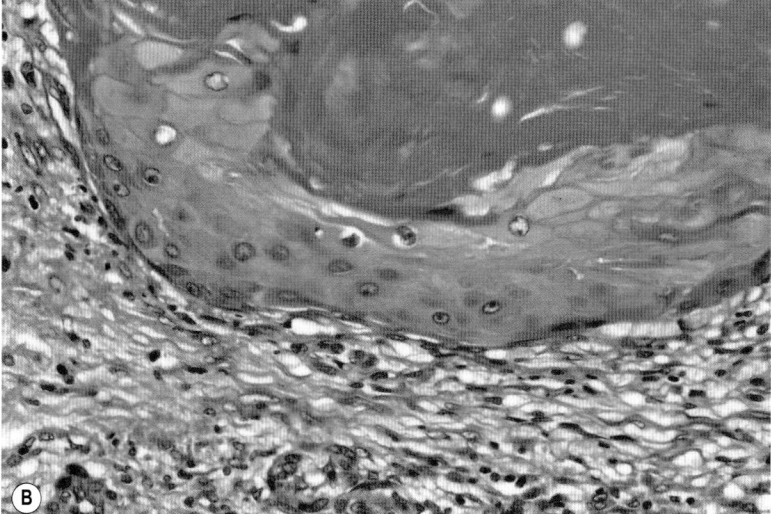

Fig. 31.43
(**A**, **B**) Pilar tumor: the epithelium shows pilar keratinization, i.e., in the absence of a granular cell.

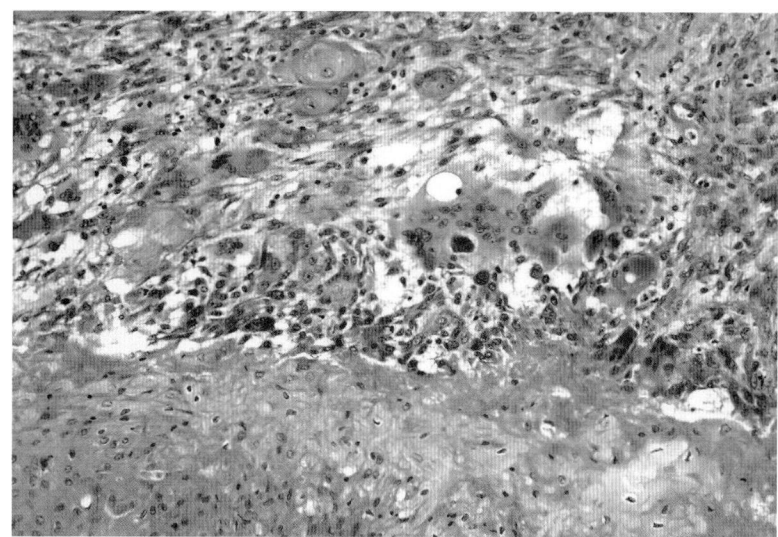

Fig. 31.45
Pilar tumor: the presence of free keratin within the dermis commonly evokes a foreign body giant cell reaction.

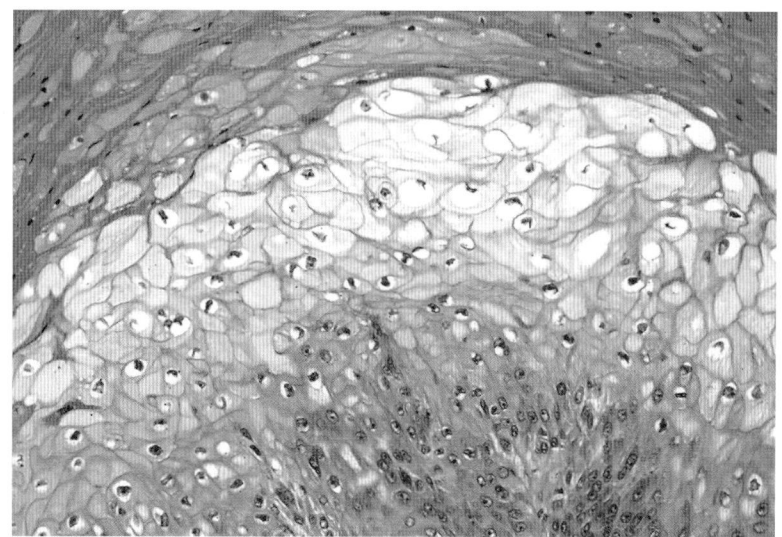

Fig. 31.46
Pilar tumor: note the clear cells, which result from glycogen accumulation.

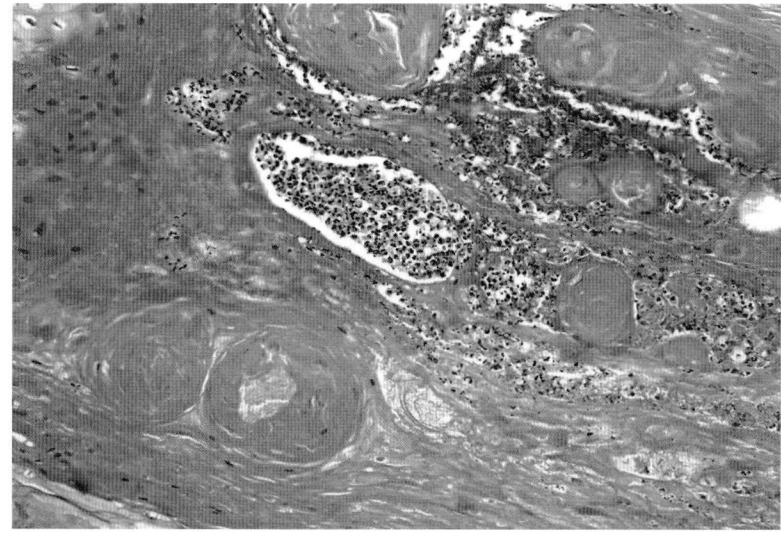

Fig. 31.44
Pilar tumor: foci of necrosis are commonly present.

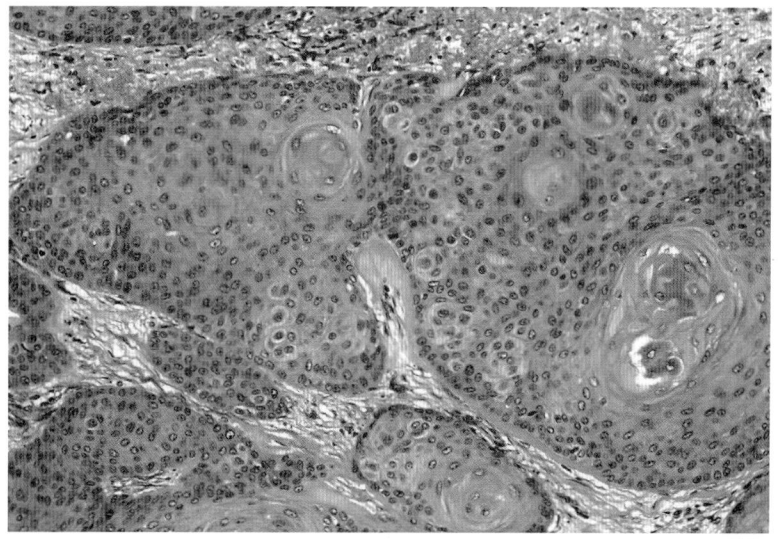

Fig. 31.47
Pilar tumor: this field shows conspicuous squamous eddies.

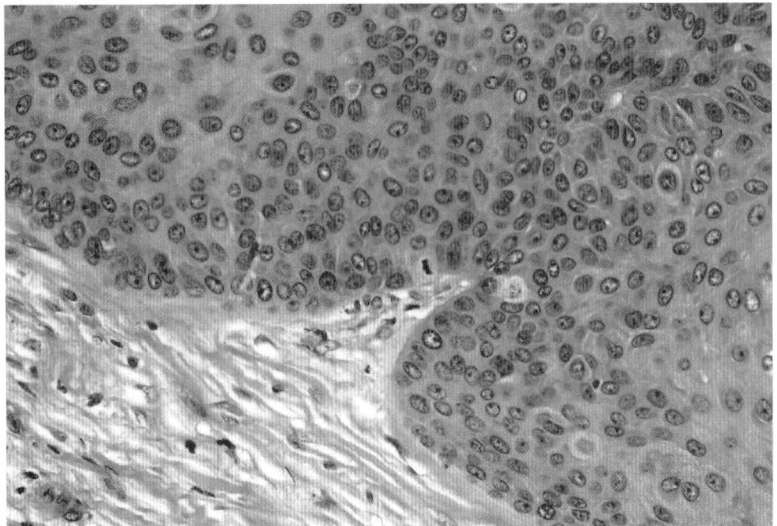

Fig. 31.48
Pilar tumor: mitotic figures, as shown in this field, are generally inconspicuous.

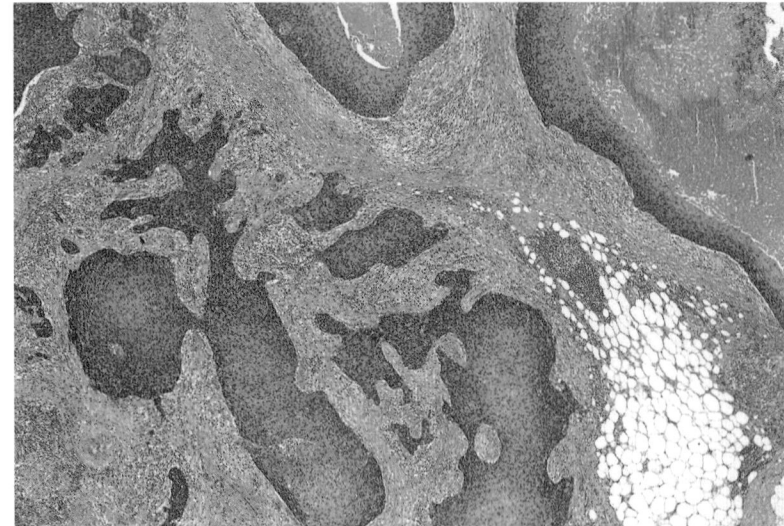

Fig. 31.50
Malignant pilar tumor: medium-power view of the carcinomatous component.

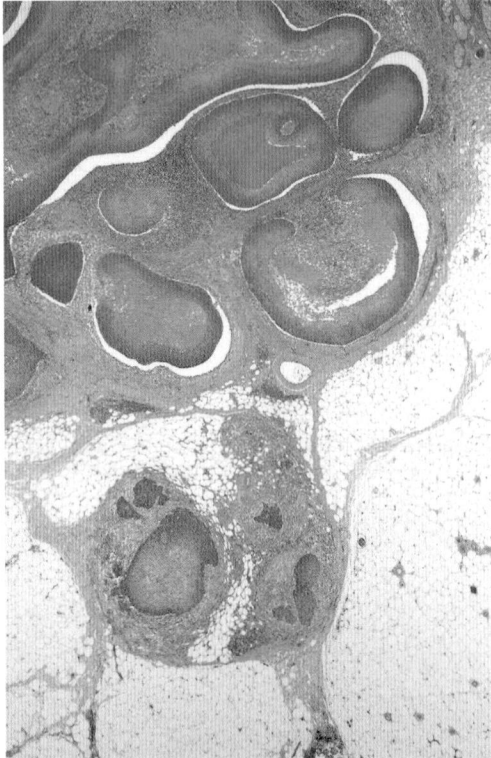

Fig. 31.49
Malignant pilar tumor: low-power view showing a typical pilar tumor associated with a carcinomatous infiltrating component.

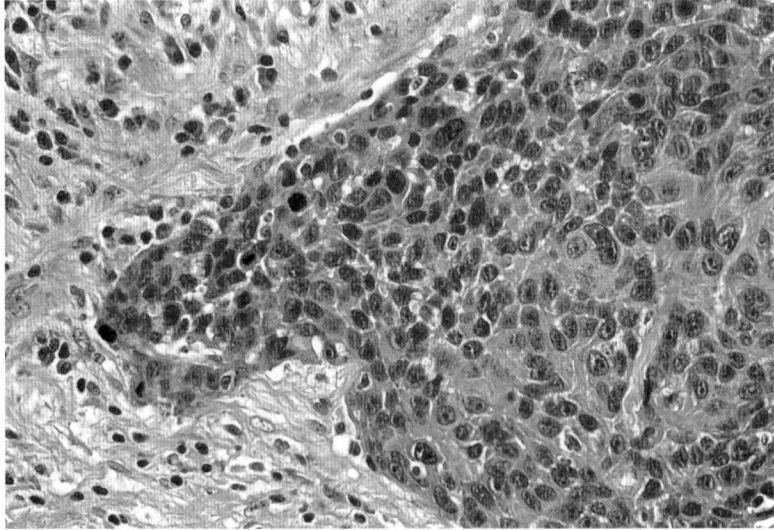

Fig. 31.51
Malignant pilar tumor: the nuclei are hyperchromatic and irregular, and multiple mitoses are present.

Pilomatrixoma

Clinical features

Pilomatrixoma (pilomatricoma, calcifying epithelioma of Malherbe) usually represents a solitary lesion, but occasionally multiple tumors are evident as part of an autosomal dominant disorder.[1–6,7] Rarely, it may represent a dermatological marker of systemic disease (e.g., myotonic dystrophy, Gardner syndrome, or MYH-associated polyposis [MAP]).[8–21] Multiple pilomatrixomas have also been reported in patients with Turner syndrome, trisomy 9, Rubinstein-Taybi syndrome, Sotos syndrome, and spina bifida.[22–28] Synchronous appearance of multiple tumors is exceptional.[29]

It presents as a slowly growing, firm-to-hard nodule of around 0.5–3 cm on the head, upper limbs, neck, trunk, and lower limbs, in decreasing order of frequency (*Fig. 31.52*).[2,20,30–32] The cheek is the most commonly affected site.[33,34] Unusual locations include the spermatic cord and paratesticular region.[35,36] Large chalky deposits are sometimes evident, and calcification may be revealed by radiology. Tumors are rarely extremely large, measuring up to 12 cm in diameter (giant pilomatrixoma).[37–43] The overlying skin can be bluish, and show dilated vessels, bullous, anetodermic, or perforating changes.[44–68]

mitoses, and geographic necrosis with or without perineural or lymphovascular invasion.[35] Malignant proliferating pilar tumors may display aneuploidy, an increased proliferative index, and loss of staining for CD34 and wild-type p53 protein.[44–46] Malignant proliferating pilar tumor has been reported to occur in patients with keratosis-ichthyosis-deafness (KID) syndrome and shows risk for distant metastasis and associated mortality.[31,47]

Differential diagnosis

Usually, proliferating trichilemmal cysts can be distinguished from squamous cell carcinoma by the presence of multiple circumscribed nodules showing a noninfiltrative palisaded border, sometimes accompanied by a hyaline basement membrane and showing abundant trichilemmal rather than epidermoid keratinization.

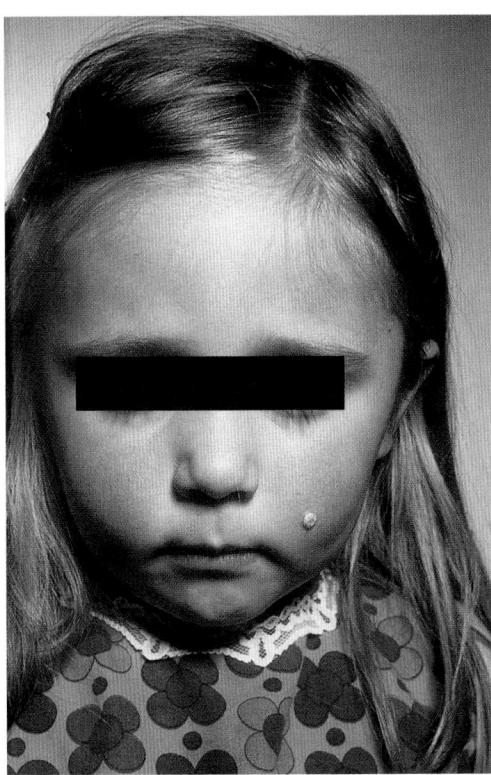

Fig. 31.52
Pilomatrixoma: note the small chalky nodule on the cheek of this young girl, a characteristic site. By courtesy of R.A. Marsden, MD, St George's Hospital, London, UK.

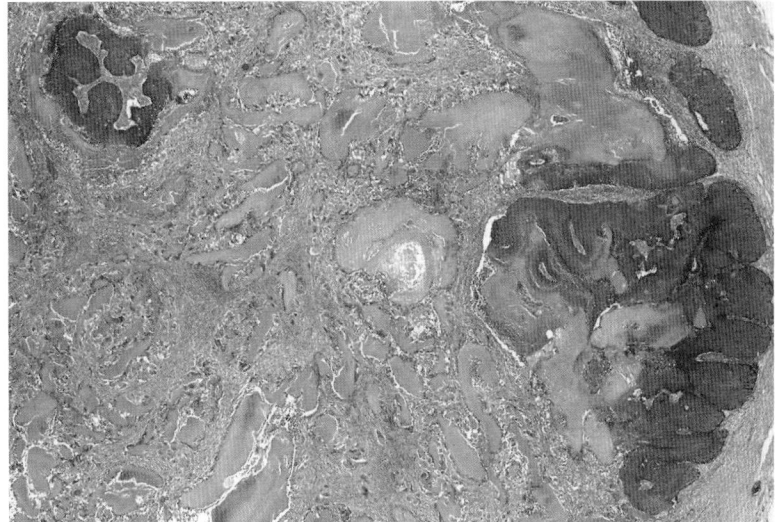

Fig. 31.53
Pilomatrixoma: this low-power view shows the typical biphasic population.

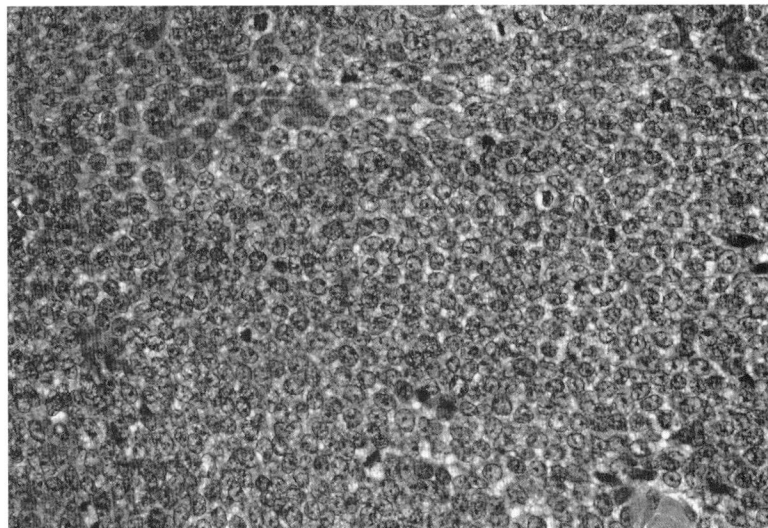

Fig. 31.54
Pilomatrixoma: early lesions are composed predominantly of sheets of germinative basaloid cells with uniform nuclei and small nucleoli.

Young people are mainly affected, with some 60% of cases being excised before 20 years of age and most before 10 years.[3,69] There is a female predominance.[2,30,33,34,69–72] More recent studies, however, have documented a somewhat wider age distribution with a second peak among those in their sixth and seventh decades of life.[4,9,73–75] Surgical excision is curative although there is local recurrence in 2% to 3% of cases.[1,33,34,71,76]

Pathogenesis and histologic features

Recently, insights have been gained into the molecular pathogenesis of pilomatrixoma implicating β-catenin as a key molecule. β-Catenin is an important intracellular protein with a dual role. It has a structural function and is involved in cell-cell junction formation by binding to cadherins as well as α-catenin, thereby providing a link between adherens junctions and the actin cytoskeleton.[77–79] It is also part of the Wnt/wingless signal transduction pathway and mediating transcriptional activation of target genes such as c-myc and cyclin D1.[80–82] Cytosolic β-catenin is phosphorylated at its N terminus and is subsequently subject to ubiquitin-mediated degradation involving the APC gene.[83,84] Wnt signaling prevents phosphorylation of β-catenin leading to its cytosolic accumulation. Cytosolic β-catenin then interacts with lymphoid enhancer factor-1/T-cell factor (Lef-1/Tcf) to form a nuclear transcription factor complex.[85,86] β-Catenin stabilization caused by truncating mutations in its N terminus (which prevents phosphorylation) has been shown to result in the formation of pilomatrixoma in a mouse model.[87] These observations have led to the identification of mutations in the N-terminal portion of β-catenin in human pilomatrixoma predominantly affecting direct sites of phosphorylation.[88–95] By immunohistochemistry, pilomatrixoma expresses cyclins D1, D2, and D3 and β-catenin nuclear staining within the basaloid/matrix cells while only cytoplasmic and membranous staining is observed in areas of maturation/transitional area. Staining is absent in ghost cells.[96–101] Analogous to the findings in anagen hair follicles, the sequential expression of hair keratins is preserved in the transitional layer of pilomatrixoma, and there is subsequent loss of expression in the ghost cell layer.[102,103] While cortical differentiation of matrix cells in anagen hair follicles is accompanied by LEF-1/α-catenin induced expression of the hair keratin hHa1, nuclear coexpression of LEF-1 and α-catenin is

not observed in the outer transitional layer of pilomatrixoma, arguing that cortical differentiation in pilomatrixoma is not under the control of the Wnt signaling pathway.[104,105]

Mutations in the β-catenin gene have also been identified in other tumors showing morphological overlap with pilomatrixoma including basal cell carcinoma with ghost cell differentiation, cribriform trichoblastoma, and craniopharyngioma.[95]

Differentiation of pilomatrixoma toward the hair matrix is supported by a number of studies on keratin, S100, and gene expression involved in the α-catenin pathway, and apoptosis represents the main mechanism leading to ghost cells.[88,98,106–113]

Pilomatrixoma is a tumor that expresses differentiation toward the hair matrix; hair shaft formation is therefore not a feature. The epidermis is usually normal, although rarely transepidermal elimination of tumor in addition to anetoderma-like changes and blister formation have been documented.[3,48–55] Situated within the dermis and sometimes extending into the subcutaneous fat is a multilobulated tumor, which may on occasion be surrounded by a fibrous pseudocapsule of compressed adjacent connective tissue elements (Fig. 31.53). Individual tumor lobules are composed of a variable admixture of basaloid and ghost cells; the former predominate in evolving lesions and the latter in mature lesions.[114] Basaloid cells are small and uniform with round vesicular nuclei and prominent nucleoli (Fig. 31.54). Early lesions may show very brisk mitotic activity, but this is never abnormal and is indicative of a rapid growth phase rather than malignant potential (*Fig. 31.55*). With tumor maturation, the basaloid cells transform into ghost cells, acquiring abundant eosinophilic cytoplasm and developing small hyperchromatic nuclei (*Fig. 31.56*). Eventually, the nuclei are lost, leaving sheets of intensely eosinophilic keratinous debris in which the ghost outlines of tumor cells are faintly visible, and giant cells are often present (*Fig. 31.57*). Keratinization in pilomatrixoma is therefore predominantly pilar, although occasionally small foci of epidermoid keratinization may be found. An additional feature in some tumors is melanin pigment within both basaloid cells and tumor histiocytes.[3,115] Calcification is seen in 80% of lesions, more commonly in those that have achieved maturity.[73] Basophilic stippling of ghost cells is the most common expression (*Fig. 31.58*). Rarely, large calcific concretions are present, and in 20% of cases ossification takes place (*Figs 31.59* and *31.60*).[73] Bone morphogenetic protein-2 (BMP-2), an important molecule involved in bone and cartilage formation, has been demonstrated in shadow cells by immunohistochemistry and may play a role in bone formation in pilomatrixoma.[116] Stromal amyloid deposition and focal clear cell change are occasionally seen (*Fig. 31.61*), and differentiation toward other aspects of the hair follicle including the follicular infundibulum and the inner root sheath as well as follicular germinal cells is a rare finding.[117]

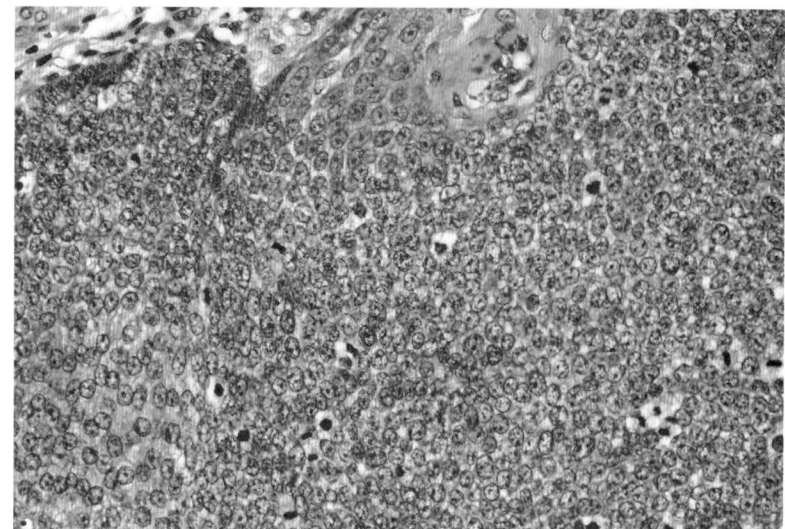

Fig. 31.55
Pilomatrixoma: note the presence of conspicuous mitotic figures. These are often numerous in early lesions and are not a cause for alarm.

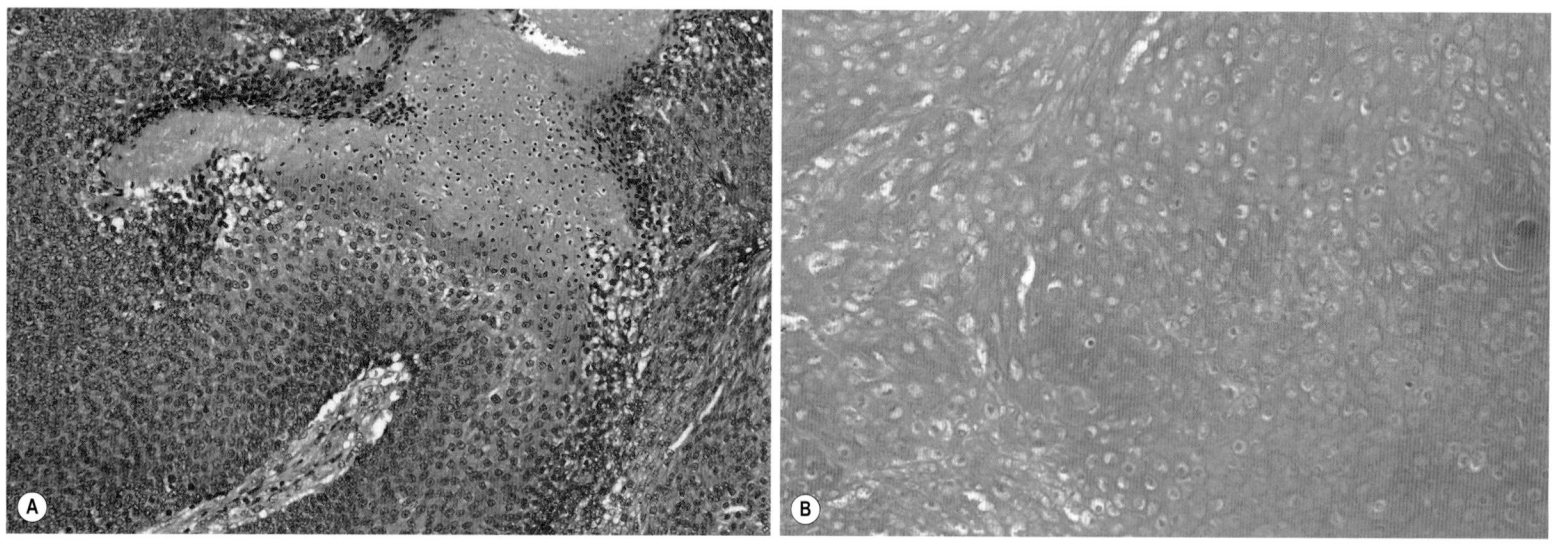

Fig. 31.56
(**A, B**) Pilomatrixoma: with maturation, the cells become larger, acquire abundant eosinophilic cytoplasm, and show nuclear pyknosis.

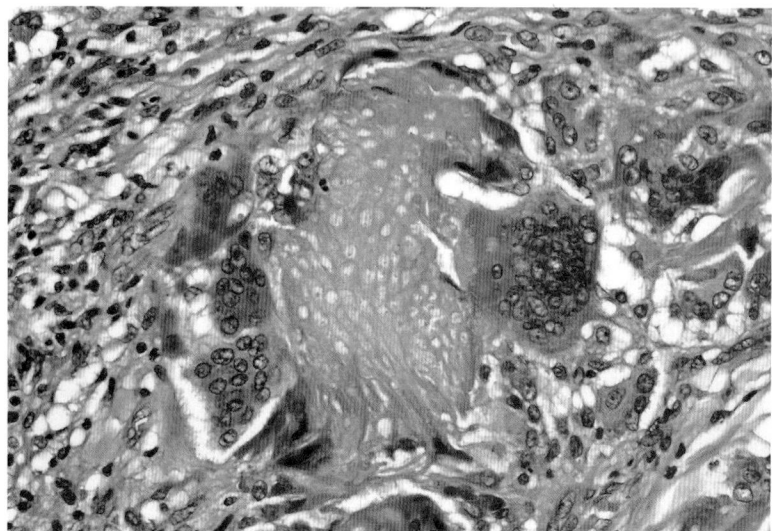

Fig. 31.57
Pilomatrixoma: a foreign body giant cell reaction is commonly present.

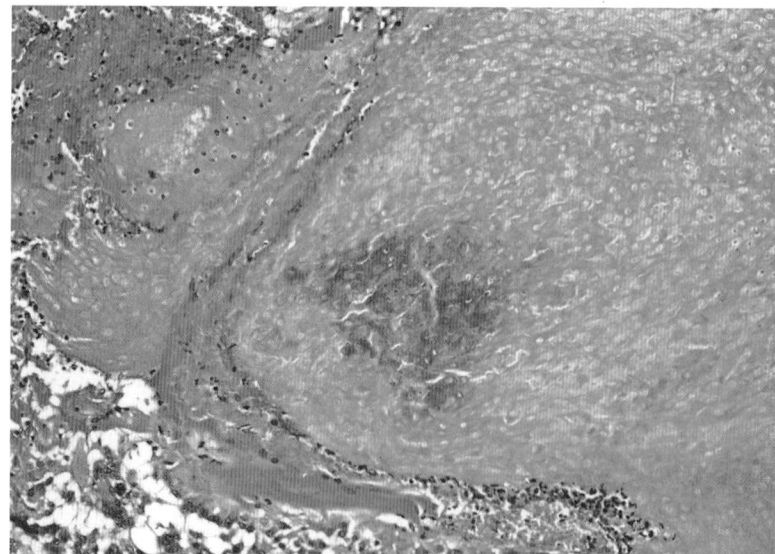

Fig. 31.58
Pilomatrixoma: note the fine basophilic calcification.

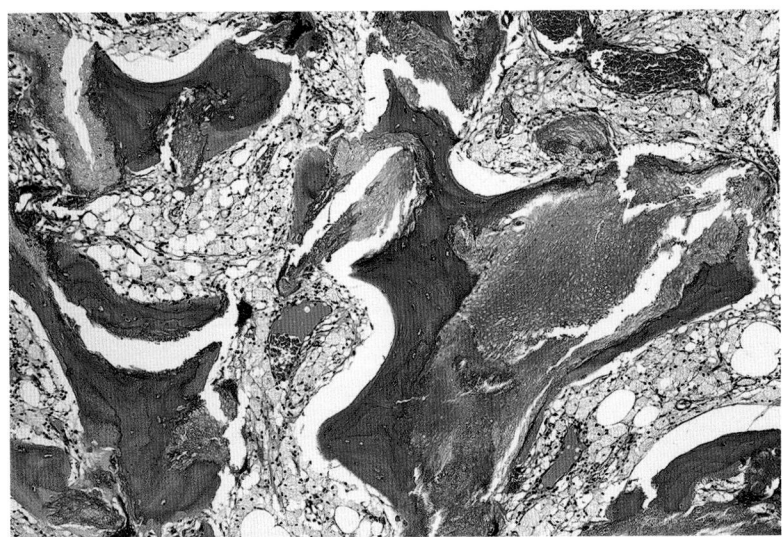

Fig. 31.59
Pilomatrixoma: this tumor shows widespread osseous metaplasia including the formation of marrow spaces.

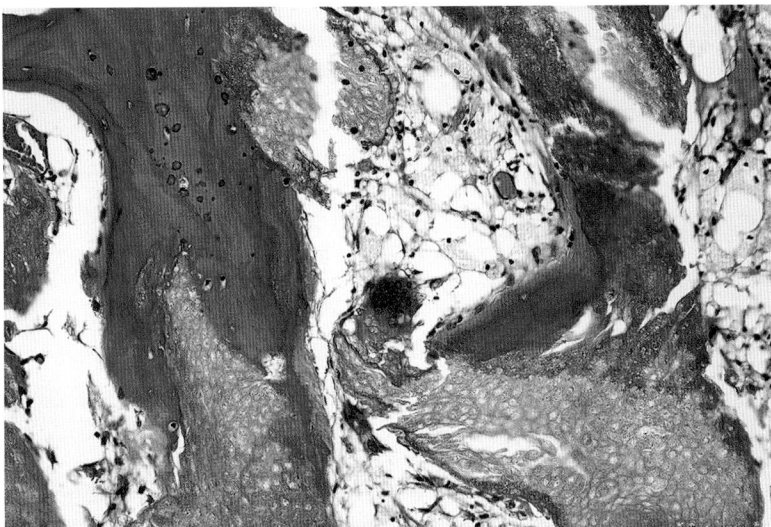

Fig. 31.60
Pilomatrixoma: high-power examination shows foci of ghost cells contrasting with the more eosinophilic osteoid.

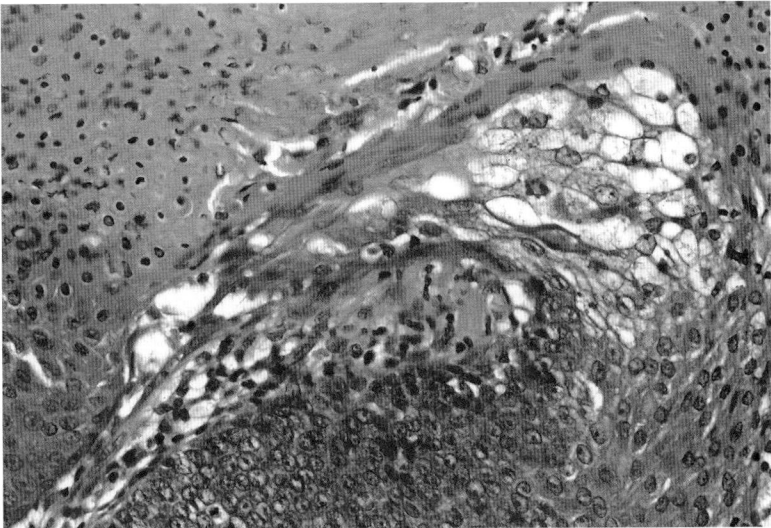

Fig. 31.61
Pilomatrixoma: high-power view showing focal clear cell change.

Pilomatrixomas in the elderly generally show features similar to those of the childhood variant. Occasionally, however, atypical features include basaloid cell pleomorphism, loss of polarity, nuclear hyperchromatism, and marked mitotic activity including atypical forms.[73,118] This variant has also been referred to as proliferating pilomatrixoma.[118–120] Lymphatic and perineural spread are not features. These atypical variants do not appear to behave in any way differently from more conventional lesions. Nevertheless, their complete removal with careful follow-up is advised.

An unusual tumor showing features of pilomatrixoma in an intraepidermal location with cutaneous horn formation has been described as pilomatricomal horn.[121] This tumor is characterized by papillomatous and thickened epidermis composed of well-defined lobules of matrical cells budding into papillary dermis. Tumor cells mature to produce ghost cells, and there is an overlying keratinaceous horn.

Differential diagnosis

Although ghost cells are characteristic of pilomatrixoma, they can also be seen in a variety of other follicular neoplasms including infundibular cysts, trichoepithelioma, and its desmoplastic variant.[122,123] Matrical differentiation may also sometimes be seen in basal cell carcinoma and combined cysts.

Pilomatrix carcinoma

Clinical features

Pilomatrix carcinoma (malignant pilomatrixoma, matrical carcinoma) is rare, approximately 130 cases having been documented in the English literature.[1–41] The tumor, which shows a predilection for males (4:1), most frequently presents in adults as a mass ranging in size from 0.5 to 20 cm (mean 4 cm) on the posterior neck, back, scalp, and retroauricular region and may rarely be pigmented.[1,9,30,39–43] Other locations include the extremities, shoulder, breast, axilla, hip, and groin.[9,10,15,16,25,35–38] Pilomatrix carcinoma exceptionally occurs in children.[36,37] It has arisen, albeit rarely, in a background of multiple benign pilomatrixomas and also at the site of treatment of a pilomatrixoma.[18,35]

Recurrences are common, but metastases are limited to a handful of cases that particularly affect drainage lymph nodes and the lung and rarely other sites including bone.[1–8,10–14,19–21,38,44–46] In general, therefore, pilomatrix carcinoma appears to be a low-grade neoplasm, with wide excision being the treatment of choice.[1,9] Local recurrence increases the risk for the development of metastatic disease.[41] Careful review of the literature suggests that at least some examples of malignant pilomatrixoma (particularly earlier reports) may represent misdiagnoses resulting from overinterpretation of the often brisk mitotic activity seen in evolving lesions. The biological behavior of these tumors therefore requires further study.

Pathogenesis and histologic features

Analogous to pilomatrixoma (see above), the Wnt signaling pathway and β-catenin have been shown to be involved in the molecular pathogenesis of pilomatrix carcinoma. Cytoplasmic and nuclear staining for β-catenin in addition to nuclear staining for cyclin D1 is present in the basaloid cell population, and there are mutations in the N terminus of β-catenin.[38,47] Interestingly, the spectrum of mutations is similar to that reported in benign pilomatrixoma.[38,48] This indicates that further molecular alterations in addition to a disturbance of the Wnt signaling pathway must be necessary for a pilomatrixoma to undergo malignant change.[49]

Features that raise the possibility of malignant potential include large size (4 cm or more in diameter), an infiltrating border with involvement of fascia or skeletal muscle, basaloid cell predominance, nuclear pleomorphism, conspicuous eosinophilic nucleoli, abnormal mitotic figures, areas of confluent tumor necrosis, stromal desmoplasia, and vascular, lymphatic or perineural invasion (Figs 31.62–31.67). It should be noted that brisk mitotic activity is a common feature in early benign lesions, and on its own should not necessarily be a cause for alarm. Many of the documented cases of pilomatrix carcinoma have contained 30 or more mitoses per 10 high-power fields.[1] This, however, should not be used as the sole criterion for a diagnosis of malignancy. Pigmentation of pilomatrix carcinoma may occasionally

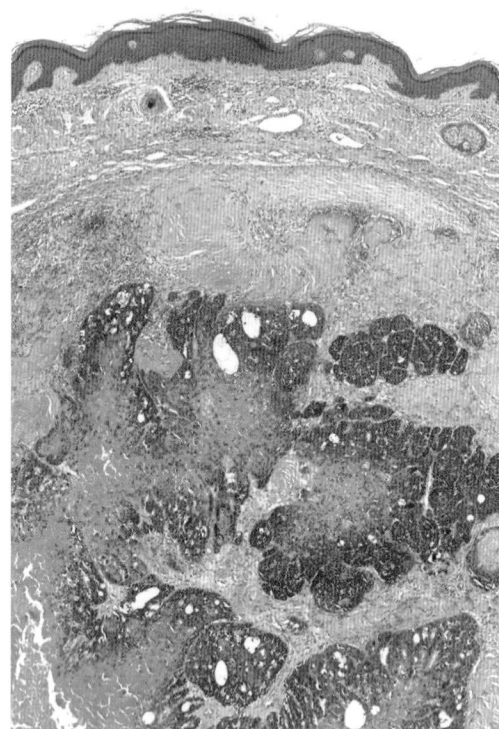

Fig. 31.62
Pilomatrix carcinoma: low-power view of irregular tumor lobules.

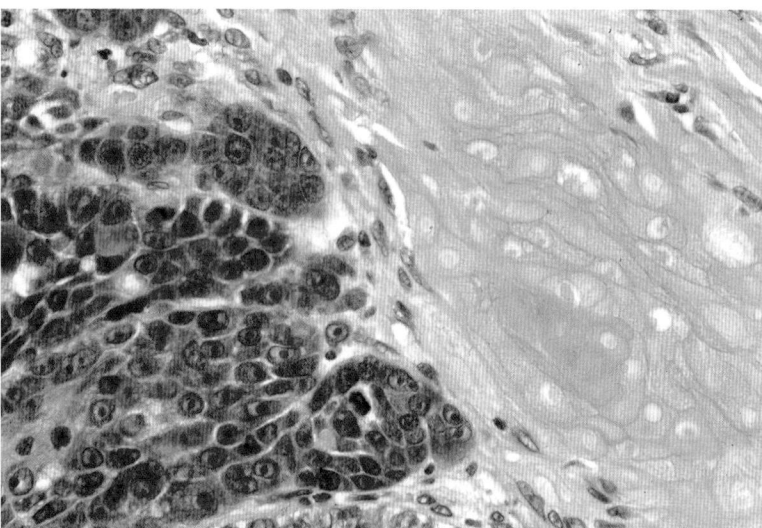

Fig. 31.63
Pilomatrix carcinoma: the tumor is composed of basophilic cells. Note the ghost cells.

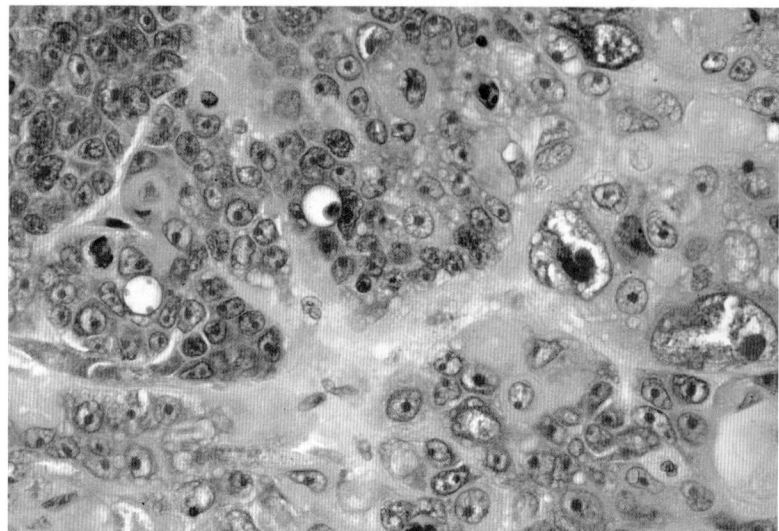

Fig. 31.64
Pilomatrix carcinoma: there is marked nuclear pleomorphism with prominent nucleoli.

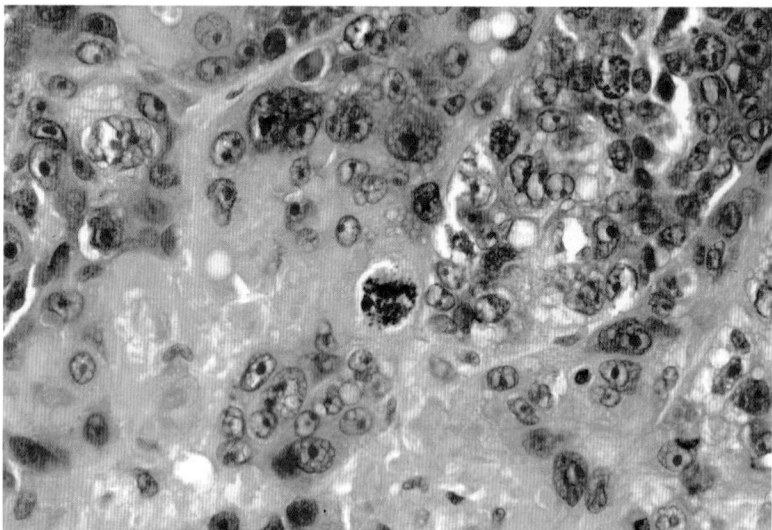

Fig. 31.65
Pilomatrix carcinoma: an abnormal mitotic figure is present.

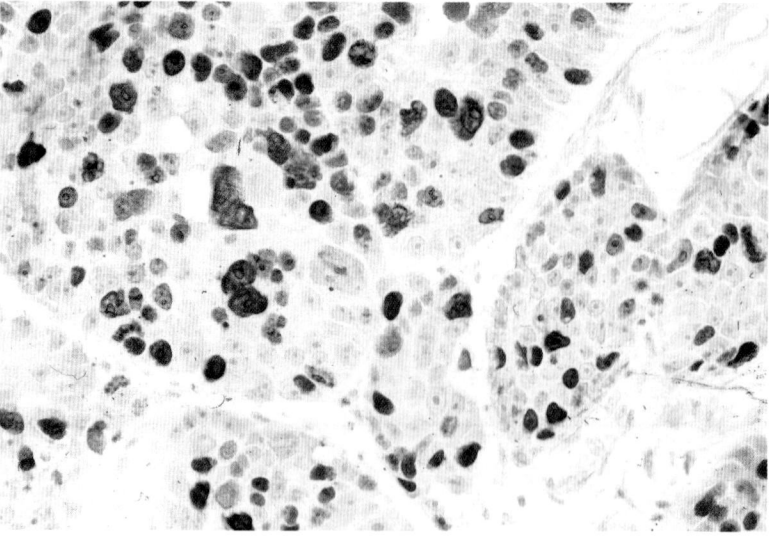

Fig. 31.66
Pilomatrix carcinoma: there is striking Ki-67 expression.

be observed due to increased accumulation of melanin pigment within tumor cells or colonization of the tumor by pigmented dendritic melanocytes.[9,30,39,50] Exceptionally, malignant pilomatrixoma has been described in association with MFH-like stromal features.[14]

Melanocytic matricoma

Clinical features

Melanocytic matricoma is a recently described entity, with less than 20 cases having been reported to date.[1–4] It presents clinically as a small (less than 1 cm) well-circumscribed purple to black papule on sun-damaged skin in the elderly (sixth to seventh decade).[1–3,5,6] Affected sites have included the nose, preauricular area, chest, back, hand, and forearm.[1–3,6] An agminated

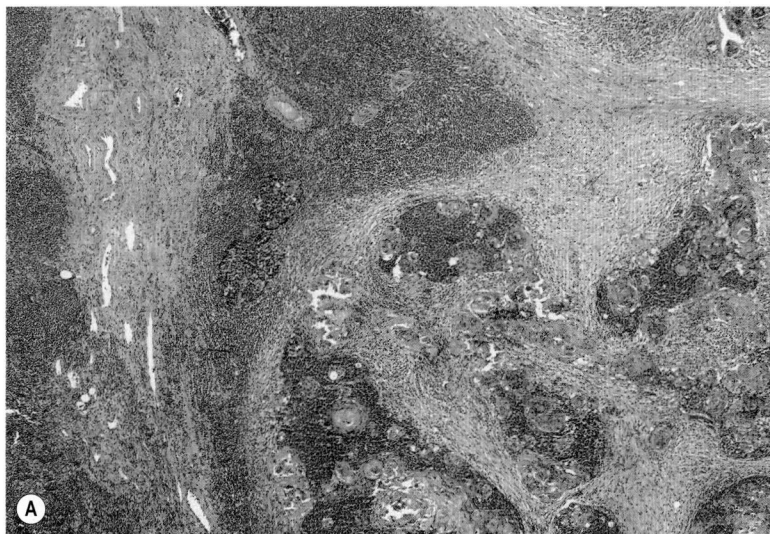

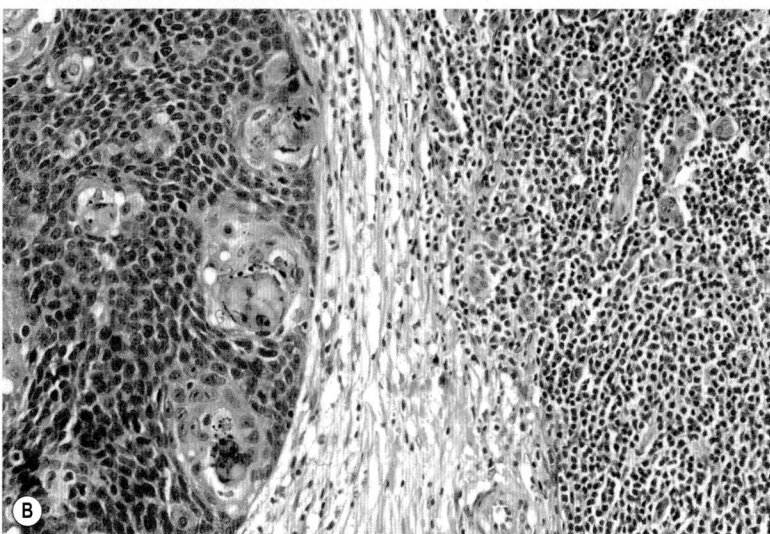

Fig. 31.67
(**A**, **B**) Pilomatrix carcinoma: lymph node metastasis.

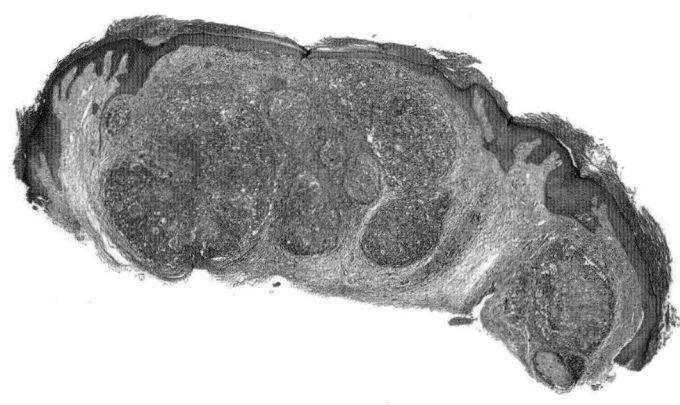

Fig. 31.68
Melanocytic matricoma: there is a multinodular dermal tumor.

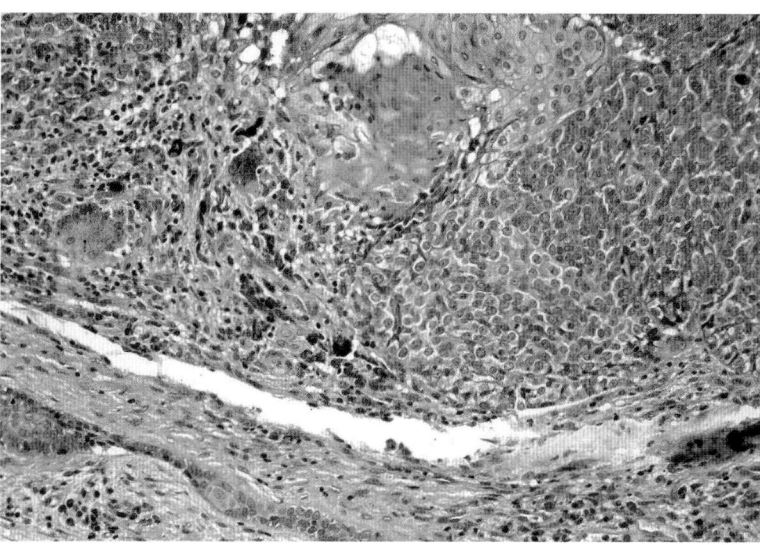

Fig. 31.69
Melanocytic matricoma: focal ghost cell change is present. Note the dendritic melanocytes.

presentation has also been documented.[7] The clinical differential diagnosis includes pigmented basal cell carcinoma, hemangioma, and melanoma. After complete excision, none of the lesions has recurred or harmed the patient (longest follow-up period is 2 years).[1–3] Further studies, however, will be necessary to determine this lesion's true biological potential.

Pathogenesis and histologic features

Melanocytic matricoma presents histologically as a well-circumscribed dermal tumor showing asymmetrical pigmentation (*Figs 31.68* and *31.69*).[1–3] It is arranged in solid nests and lobules composed of basaloid cells with scant amounts of cytoplasm and prominent nucleoli reminiscent of matrical and supramatrical cells (*Figs 31.70–31.72*). Cytological atypia as well as mitotic figures may be present. Dispersed singly and in small aggregates are ghost cells within the tumor, and pigmented dendritic melanocytes are admixed. Surrounding the tumor is a sclerotic stromal response containing melanophages. The dermis and overlying epidermis reveal changes of significant sun damage including elastosis, epidermal atrophy, and actinic keratoses.[1–3] Colonization by atypical epithelioid melanocytes has been reported recently.[8,9] The biological significance of this finding is uncertain as there was no adverse outcome after complete excision. Rare cases have been reported as 'malignant melanocytic matricoma' because of an infiltrative or pushing tumor growth, marked nuclear pleomorphism, and the presence of brisk and atypical mitotic figures.[10–12] Clinical follow-up of these cases is limited, and it is uncertain at this point whether these histologic features are truly signs of malignancy or whether they may be part of a histologic spectrum of melanocytic matricoma.

By immunohistochemistry, the basaloid cells show membranous staining for both P- and E-cadherin as well as nuclear and cytoplasmic staining for β-catenin reminiscent of the hair bulb of anagen hair and also implicating β-catenin in its pathogenesis.[8,13]

Differential diagnosis

The main histologic differential diagnoses include pilomatrixoma, pilomatrix carcinoma, and basal cell carcinoma with matrical differentiation.

Melanocytic matricoma shows overlapping features with both pigmented pilomatricoma and pilomatrix carcinoma, and reliable distinction may not always be possible.

Despite the presence of cytological atypia and abundant mitotic figures, the tumors are small, well circumscribed, and lack atypical mitoses, necrosis, lymphovascular invasion, and may thereby be distinguished from pilomatrix carcinoma in many instances. Nevertheless, tumors displaying such features should be viewed with caution, and complete excision would be prudent.

Basal cell carcinoma with matrical differentiation is characterized by foci of typical basal cell carcinoma composed of basaloid nests showing peripheral palisading and stromal retraction artifact.

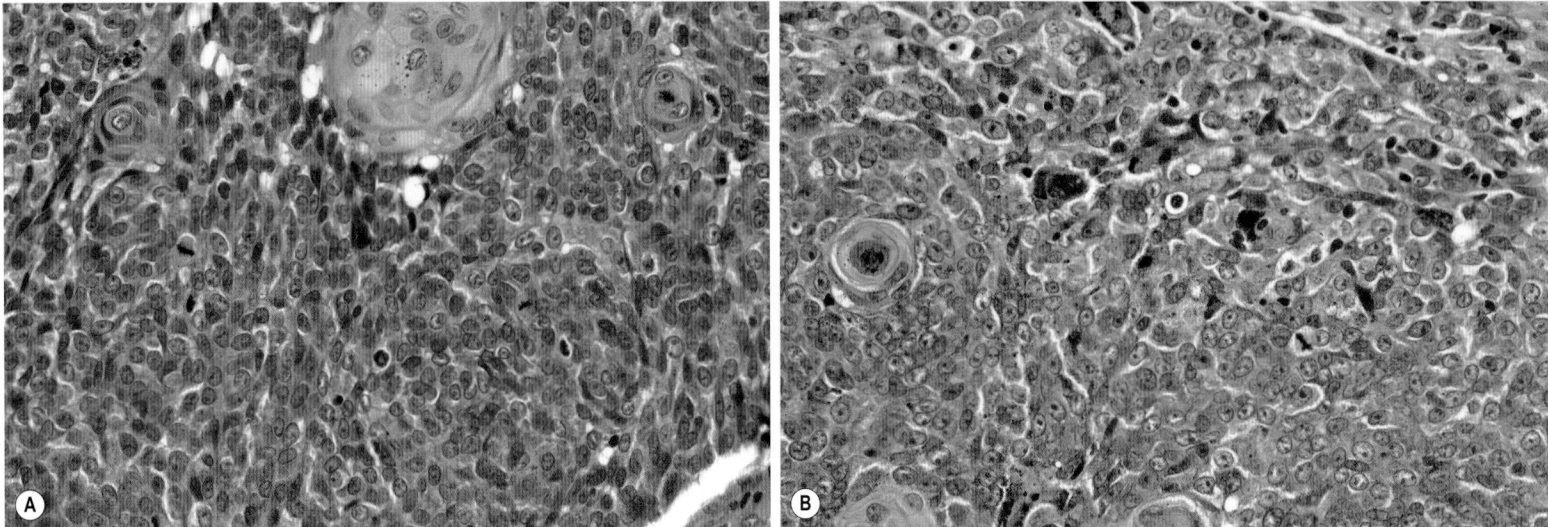

Fig. 31.70
Melanocytic matricoma: (**A**) the tumor is composed of basophilic cells with mild nuclear pleomorphism and conspicuous mitotic activity; (**B**) high-power view showing melanocytes.

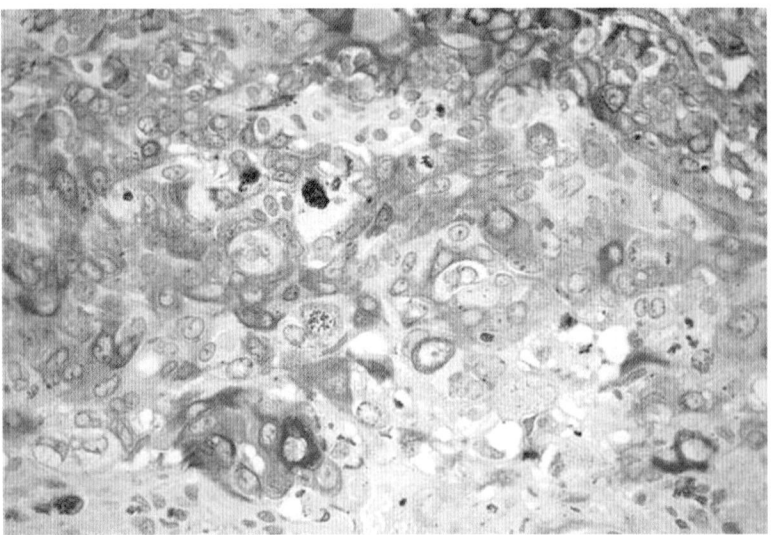

Fig. 31.71
Melanocytic matricoma: the matrical cells express keratin.

Trichofolliculoma

Clinical features

Trichofolliculoma is a not uncommon hamartoma that usually arises on the face and presents as a single, dome-shaped, 0.5- to 1.0-cm-diameter papule with a central pore.[1–7] It is occasionally found on the scalp or neck and has been rarely described on the vulva.[7–9] A wide age range is affected, although lesions are very rare in children or infants.[8,10,11] Characteristic, although not diagnostic, is the presence of one or more silky, white, thread-like hairs (trichoids) growing out of the central opening (*Fig. 31.73*).[8] Rarely, trichofolliculoma may coexist with a basal cell carcinoma.[12]

Pathogenesis and histologic features

It consists of a cystic cavity (dilated hair follicle) lined by stratified squamous epithelium (including a granular cell layer), which can usually be shown to arise from the surface epithelium (*Fig. 31.74*).[1,2] The cavity contains keratinous debris and hair shaft fragments.[8] Arising from its wall are numerous hair follicles, each surrounded by a clearly defined perifollicular sheath (*Figs 31.75* and *31.76*). Secondary budding with further abortive

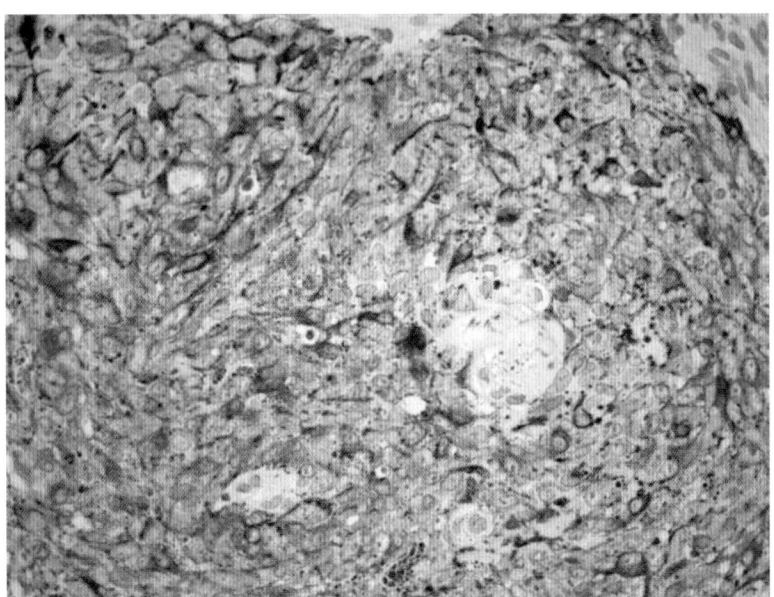

Fig. 31.72
Melanocytic matricoma: the dendritic melanocytes are highlighted with HMB-45.

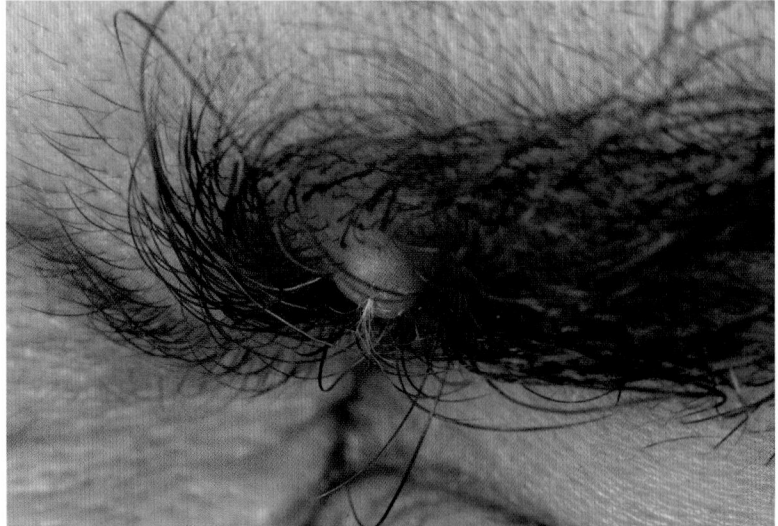

Fig. 31.73
Trichofolliculoma: characteristic dome-shaped nodule with protruding trichoids. From the collection of the late N.P. Smith, MD, the Institute of Dermatology, London, UK.

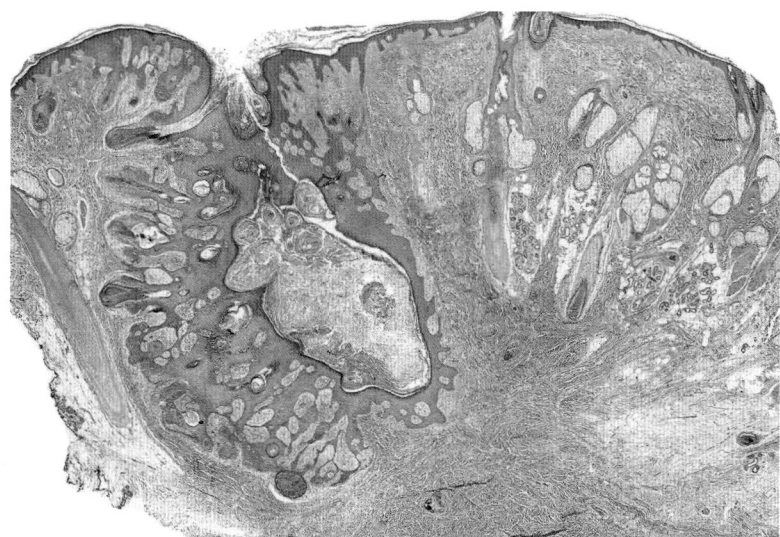

Fig. 31.74
Trichofolliculoma: scanning view showing a cystically dilated follicle communicating with the epidermis. Note the secondary follicles arising from the lateral wall.

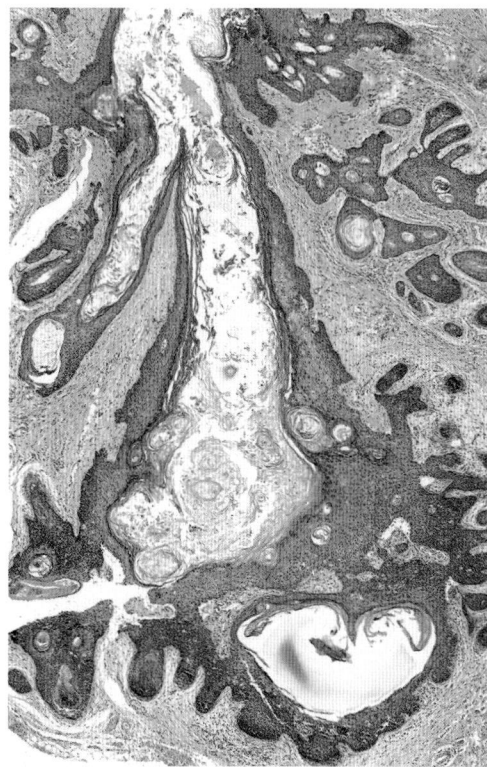

Fig. 31.75
Trichofolliculoma: this example emphasizes the numerous secondary follicles.

pilar differentiation may be seen. Small primitive sebaceous acini and keratocysts are occasionally present.

Stromal granulomatous inflammation surrounding hair shaft fragments and focal calcification are sometimes present, and focal acantholytic dyskeratosis may be an incidental finding.[8,13]

An analysis of the histologic features demonstrates that trichofolliculoma shows a morphological spectrum corresponding to the hair follicle cycle, and it has been postulated that the very late stage of trichofolliculoma is identical to folliculosebaceous cystic hamartoma (see below).[14,15] The early-stage trichofolliculoma is characterized by several curved vellus hair follicles leading into an infundibulum without cystic dilatation, whereas the late stage shows changes of catagen and telogen hair follicles and more prominent sebaceous differentiation.[14]

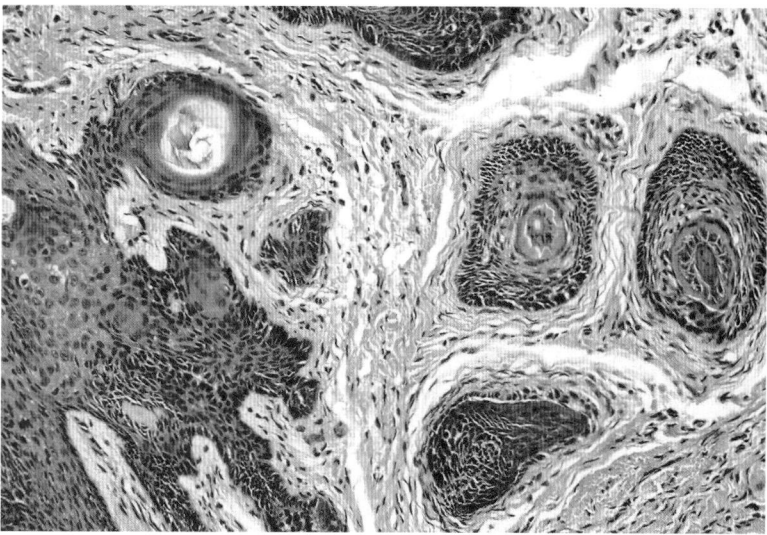

Fig. 31.76
Trichofolliculoma: high-power view of secondary follicles.

Folliculosebaceous cystic hamartoma

Clinical features

Folliculosebaceous cystic hamartoma is a rare hamartomatous lesion with follicular, sebaceous, and mesenchymal elements.[1–13] It typically presents as a small (around 1 cm in diameter) solitary symmetrical papule or nodule with a predilection for the central face, especially the nose.[1,2,14–18] Genital location as well as a giant variant have been described to involve extrafacial sites.[3,4,19–22] Patients typically present in young adulthood, but the age distribution is wide and lesions present at birth have been described.[1,2,5,6,13–15,18,22] A example has been reported in association with a port-wine stain, and multiple tumors have been documented in the setting of a giant nevus lipomatosus superficialis.[23–25] There is no association with Torre-Muir syndrome.

Pathogenesis and histologic features

Folliculosebaceous cystic hamartoma is a dermal-based lesion composed of an infundibular cystic cavity similar to trichofolliculoma (*Fig. 31.77*). Within the cavity, keratinaceous debris and sebaceous secretions are found.[1,2,5,7] Hair shafts may occasionally be identified but are absent in the majority of cases.[15,26] Although initially thought to be uncommon, epidermal communication may be present.[1,14] Numerous small sebaceous lobules are connected to the cavity via sebaceous ducts (*Fig. 31.78*). Hair follicles at various stages in the follicular cycle are occasionally observed, and sometimes these are malformed (*Fig. 31.79*).[13] Small cystic apocrine glands may also be present.[13] The epithelial component is surrounded by a dense laminated collagenous fibroplasia, and the fibroepithelial unit is separated from the adjacent mesenchymal proliferation by cleftlike spaces (*Fig. 31.80*).[1,2,5,7]

Mesenchymal elements including collagen, elastic fibers, adipose, and vascular tissue represent an integral component of this tumor, and indeed in some examples they may predominate.[1,8] The folliculosebaceous elements are embedded in a distinctive, variably collagenous stroma composed of spindled cells with eosinophilic cytoplasm and tapered hyperchromatic nuclei (*Fig. 31.81*). Abundant mature adipocytes are often present and there is a conspicuous vascular component, often showing perivascular fibroplasia (*Fig. 31.82*).[13] In some tumors, mucin deposition has been noted, and this may show striking perivascular accentuation (*Fig. 31.83*). A background of an acquired intradermal nevus is occasionally noted.[18] A neural component has also been described.[9,12] Studies on keratin and filaggrin expression demonstrate differentiation toward the follicular infundibulum, the sebaceous duct, and sebaceous cells.[27]

Differential diagnosis

Although, at first sight, this lesion bears a similarity to trichofolliculoma, particularly the sebaceous variant, the more usual lack of communication

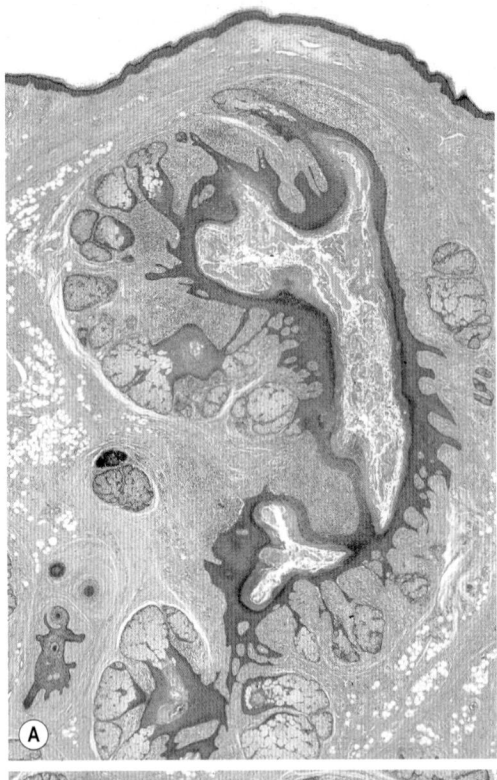

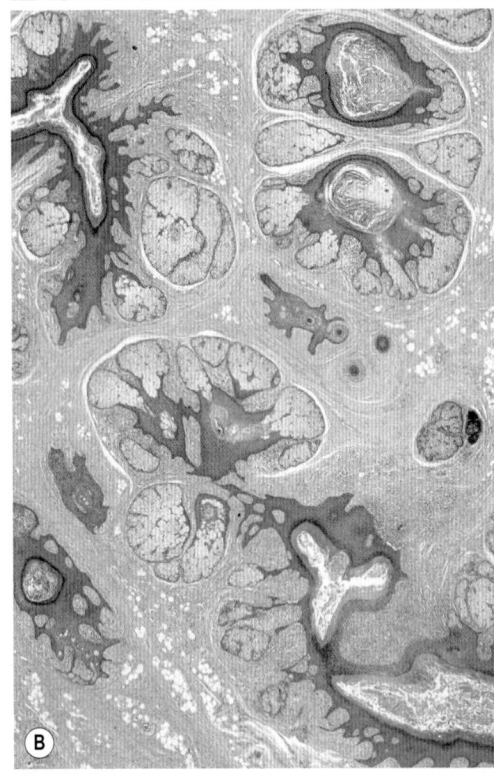

Fig. 31.77
Folliculosebaceous cystic hamartoma: (A) scanning view showing cystic cavity with conspicuous sebaceous glands embedded in a dense stroma; (B) oblique section of cyst emphasizing the sebaceous glands. By courtesy of C. Steffan, MD, Palm Springs, California, USA.

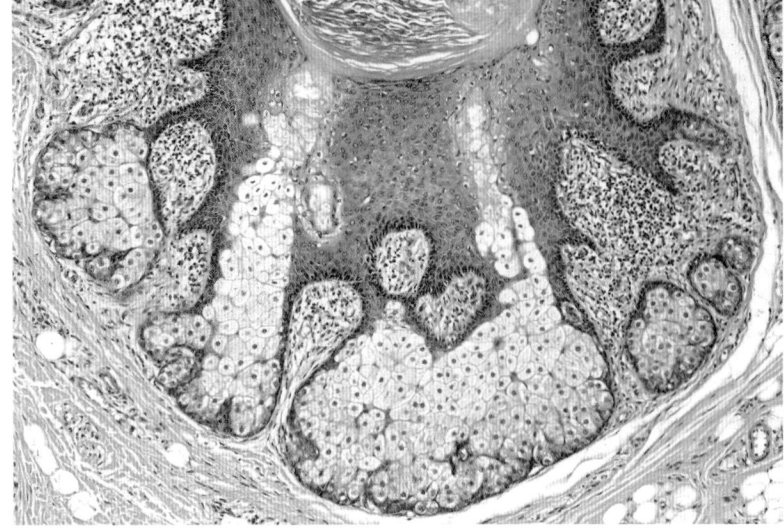

Fig. 31.78
Folliculosebaceous cystic hamartoma: the sebaceous glands communicate with the cyst through small ductules. By courtesy of C. Steffan, MD, Palm Springs, California, USA.

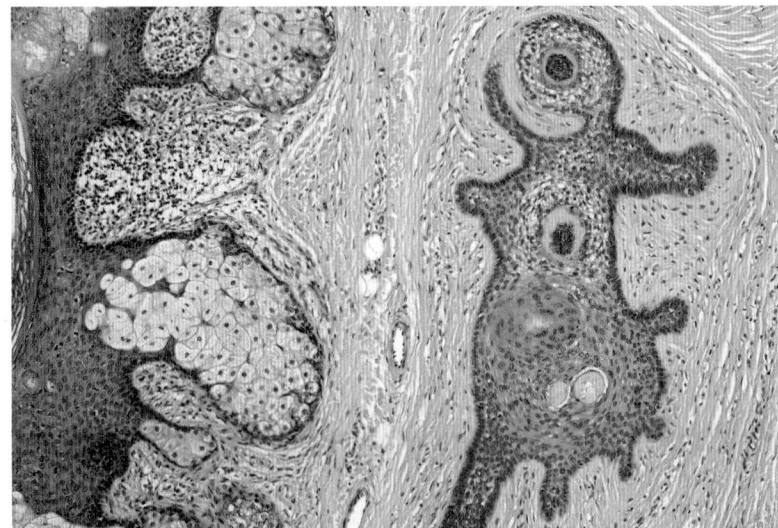

Fig. 31.79
Folliculosebaceous cystic hamartoma: malformed hairs as shown in this field are sometimes present. By courtesy of C. Steffan, MD, Palm Springs, California, USA.

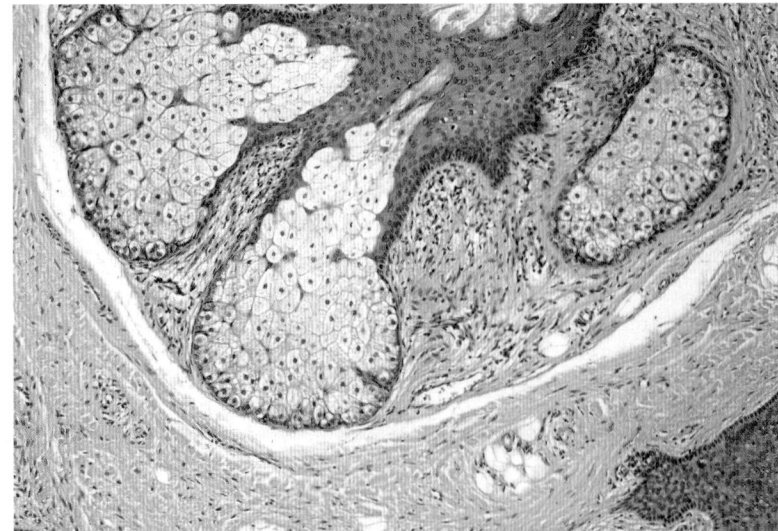

Fig. 31.80
Folliculosebaceous cystic hamartoma: note the cleftlike space, a characteristic feature. By courtesy of C. Steffan, MD, Palm Springs, California, USA.

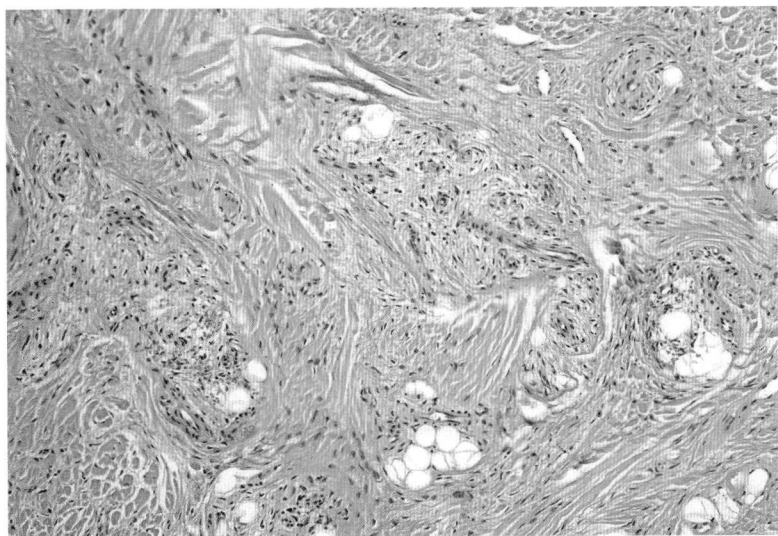

Fig. 31.81
Folliculosebaceous cystic hamartoma: a dense spindle cell stroma is an integral component of the tumor. By courtesy of C. Steffan, MD, Palm Springs, California, USA.

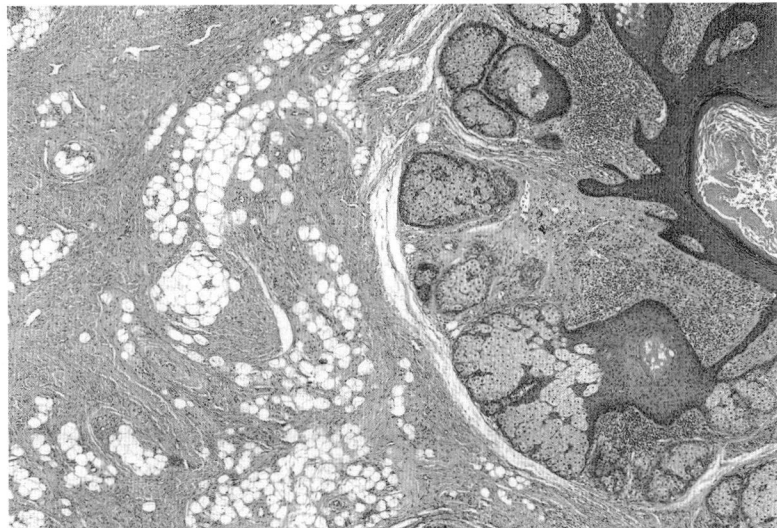

Fig. 31.82
Folliculosebaceous cystic hamartoma: mature adipocytes are regularly present in this tumor. By courtesy of C. Steffan, MD, Palm Springs, California, USA.

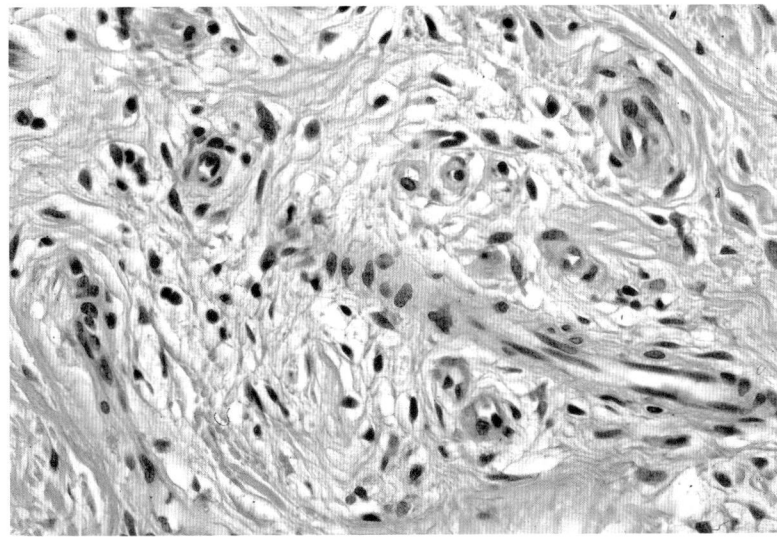

Fig. 31.83
Folliculosebaceous cystic hamartoma: high-power view showing perivascular mucin deposition. By courtesy of C. Steffan, MD, Palm Springs, California, USA.

with the surface epithelium, combined with the conspicuous stromal components present in this hamartomatous lesion, serves as helpful histologic discriminants.

Sebaceous trichofolliculoma

Clinical features

Sebaceous trichofolliculoma is a rare hamartomatous condition and represents a variant of trichofolliculoma. It presents as a depressed lesion up to 1 cm across, usually on the nose and only rarely on the scrotum and penis (*Fig. 31.84*).[1-3] It is associated with one or more fistulous openings from which protrude terminal hairs, vellus hairs, and trichoids. Typically, lateral pressure does not express any debris. The lesion neither communicates with the paranasal sinuses nor causes any bony destruction.

Histologic features

It consists of a multilocular crateriform cavity lined by epidermoid stratified squamous epithelium (*Fig. 31.85*).[1] Additional small laterally orientated sinuses may drain into the central cavity, which contains hairs of varying size as well as keratinous debris. Arising from the wall of the cyst are numerous sebaceous lobules associated with terminal hairs, vellus hairs, and trichoids.

Differential diagnosis

Sebaceous trichofolliculoma may be distinguished from sebaceous hyperplasia, the latter merely representing a grossly enlarged solitary sebaceous gland not associated with hair follicle formation.

Sebaceous trichofolliculoma must be differentiated from dermoid cyst and median nasal dermoid fistula.

- *Dermoid cysts* do not communicate with the surface epithelium, smooth muscle is often present in proximity to the cyst wall, and eccrine and apocrine glands are sometimes evident.
- *Median nasal dermoid fistula* is a rare developmental abnormality in which nasal fusion is associated with the sequestration of fetal

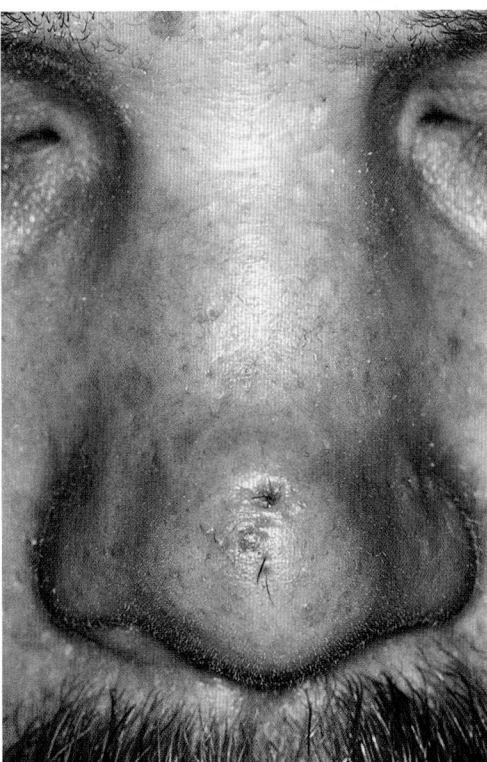

Fig. 31.84
Sebaceous trichofolliculoma: there is a characteristic pit-shaped depression on the tip of the nose. Note the protruding hairs. By courtesy of G. Plewig, MD, Düsseldorf, Germany.

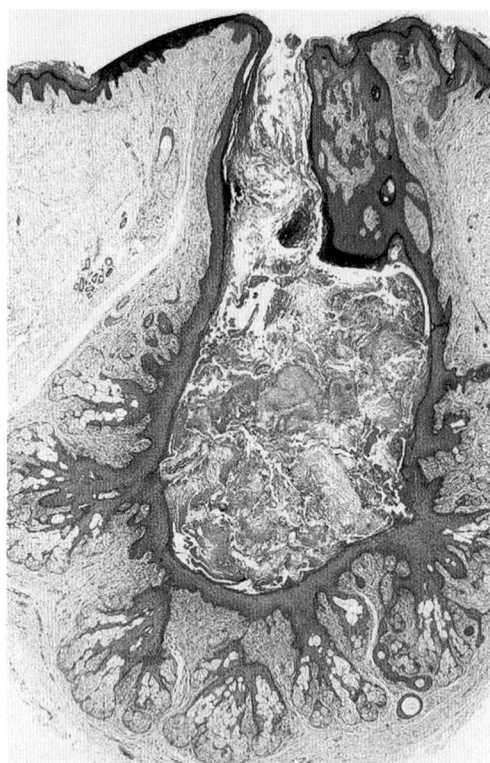

Fig. 31.85
Sebaceous trichofolliculoma: this cystically dilated follicle is lined by squamous epithelium showing infundibular keratinization. Numerous sebaceous lobules are present.

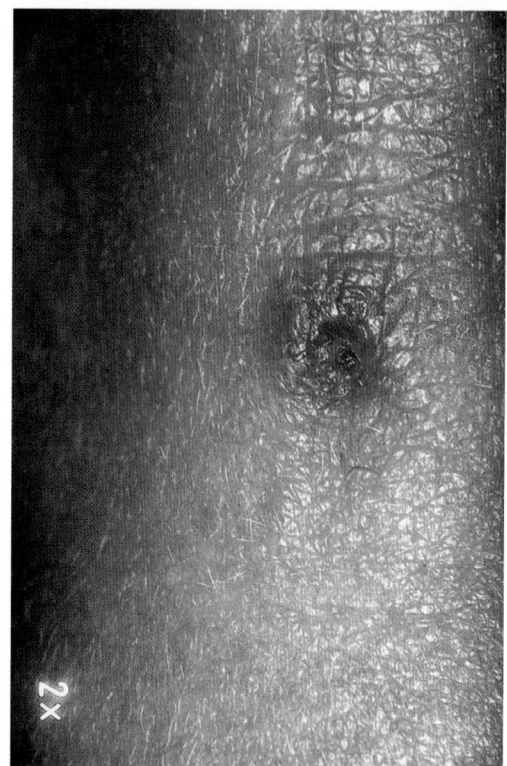

Fig. 31.86
Median nasal dermoid fistula: on the dorsum of the nose is an erythematous crateriform depression. By courtesy of D. Shuttleworth, MD, University of Wales, Cardiff, UK.

ectoderm, the proliferation of which results in the development of the fistula.[4,5] Patients present with an erythematous pit in the midline or dorsum of the nose (Figs 31.86 and 31.87). Typically, small hairs protrude from the opening of the fistula. Histologically, the fistula is lined by keratinizing stratified squamous epithelium. Numerous hair follicles are associated with the fistula wall, but sebaceous, apocrine, and eccrine glands are not present (Fig. 31.88). The importance of the median nasal dermoid fistula is that it may communicate with an anterior meningoencephalocele.

Trichoepithelioma

Clinical features

Trichoepithelioma is a hamartomatous condition that shows less follicular differentiation than a trichofolliculoma. The lesion may be multiple and familial or solitary.

Multiple familial trichoepithelioma

Multiple familial trichoepithelioma (epithelioma adenoides cysticum [Brooke]) is inherited in an autosomal dominant fashion with diminished expression in males and onset during puberty.[1] Patients present with multiple, small, skin-colored papules in a roughly symmetrical distribution located predominantly on the face (Figs 31.89 and 31.90).[2] The nasolabial folds, eyebrows, eyelids, and cheeks are most commonly involved.[2,3] Other sites including the scalp, neck, extremities, buttocks, and genital area may also be affected.[2,4-9] The lesions are usually asymptomatic and commence as translucent skin-colored papules, which sometimes show slight surface telangiectasia. They slowly enlarge to reach a maximum diameter of about 0.5 cm. Rarely, ulceration occurs, usually at a very late stage. Lesions are occasionally pigmented. A linear and dermatomal distribution has also been reported.[5]

Patients with epithelioma adenoides cysticum rarely develop any significant systemic manifestations. An association with renal and pulmonary cysts and with malignant lymphoepithelial lesion of the parotid gland has,

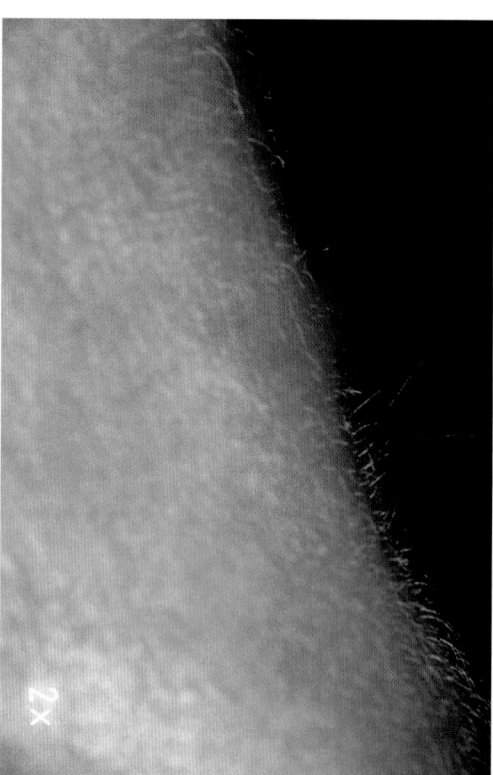

Fig. 31.87
Median nasal dermoid fistula: the presence of protruding white hairs is characteristic. By courtesy of D. Shuttleworth, MD, University of Wales, Cardiff, UK.

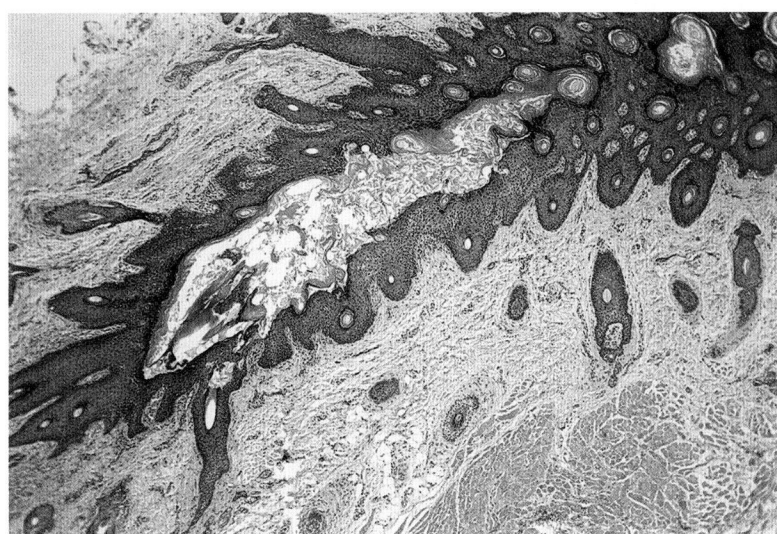

Fig. 31.88
Median nasal dermoid fistula: the fistula, which communicates with the surface epidermis, is lined by hair-bearing epithelium. By courtesy of D. Shuttleworth, MD, University of Wales, Cardiff, UK.

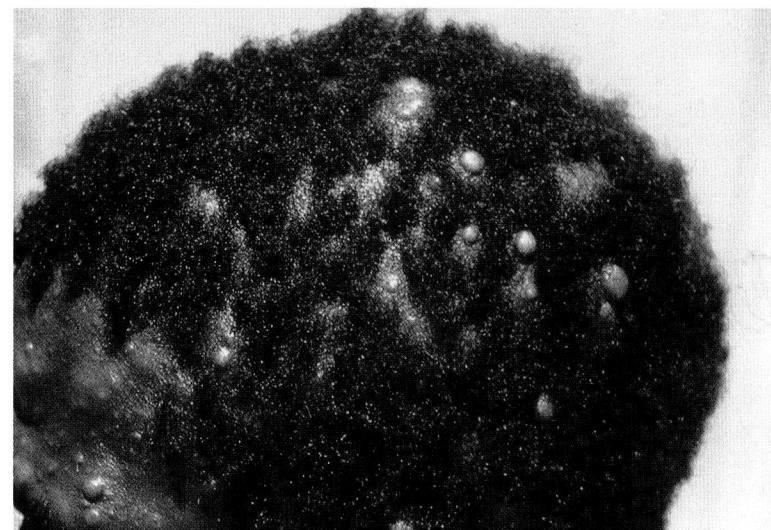

Fig. 31.90
Trichoepitheliomas: note the numerous skin-colored papules and nodules on this girl's scalp and forehead. By courtesy of R.A. Marsden, MD, St George's Hospital, London, UK.

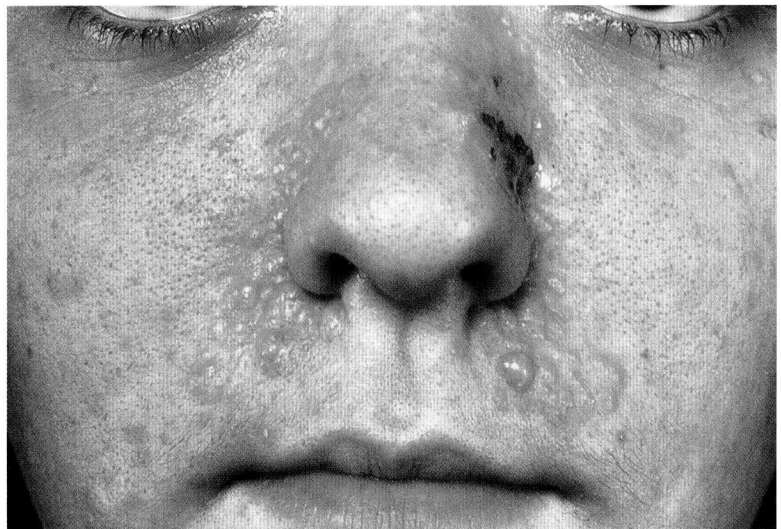

Fig. 31.89
Trichoepithelioma: this patient has familial multiple trichoepitheliomas. Note the presence of multiple skin-colored papules about the nasolabial folds. By courtesy of the Institute of Dermatology, London, UK.

however, been documented.[10,11] Very rarely, a coexistent basal cell carcinoma may be found.[12–16]

Although initial genetic linkage analysis mapped the disease to a region on chromosome 9p21, subsequent studies have failed to confirm this observation. Instead, mutations in the CYLD gene on chromosome 16q12-q13 have been consistently identified in multiple families, analogous to Brooke-Spiegler syndrome.[17–28] These data emphasize that multiple familial trichoepithelioma may indeed represent part of a disease spectrum that also includes familial cylindromatosis and Brooke-Spiegler syndrome.

Brooke-Spiegler syndrome

The autosomal dominant Brooke-Spiegler syndrome (familial cylindromatosis or turban tumor syndrome) is characterized by multiple cylindromas in addition to spiradenomas, multiple trichoepitheliomas, and milia.[29–54] While penetrance is high, there is great variability in presentation among patients. Within the same family some patients may present with either multiple cylindromas or trichoepitheliomas only, or a combination of both. Patients present with skin lesions in early adulthood, and there is a female predilection. While cylindromas typically present on the scalp and may grow to

large size and confluence (turban tumor), the multiple trichoepitheliomas are largely located centrofacially.[2] Tumors frequently show hybrid features such as spiradenocylindromas, and sebaceous differentiation may be a feature.[55] Patients also develop other hair follicle tumors such as trichoblastoma and cutaneous lymphadenoma.[55] Additional syringomas are rare and may be an incidental association.[56] Parotid gland tumors such as membranous-type basal cell adenoma, a histologic mimic of cylindroma, may rarely develop as well as cylindroma of the breast parenchyma.[57–64] Both the salivary gland tumor as well as the cylindromas infrequently undergo malignant change.[31,58,65–67] Malignant transformation in trichoepithelioma (high-grade trichoblastic carcinoma) and development of a carcinosarcoma have also been documented in patients with Brooke-Spiegler syndrome and multiple familial trichoepithelioma.[68–70]

Rombo syndrome

Rombo syndrome comprises multiple trichoepitheliomas, milia, vermiculate atrophy, basal cell carcinoma, vellus hair cysts, peripheral vasodilatation, and cyanosis.[71] It is an exceedingly rare condition, with a possible autosomal dominant mode of inheritance.[72] Skin lesions present in childhood and basal cell carcinomas develop in early adulthood.[72]

A further familial form has been associated with nail dystrophy, alopecia, and myasthenia gravis.[73–76]

Solitary trichoepithelioma

Solitary trichoepithelioma usually presents as a 0.5-cm-diameter, asymptomatic, flesh-colored nodule on the face of an adult. It is occasionally seen at other sites, including the scalp, neck, back, vulva, mons pubis, and proximal extremities.[2,77,78]

Trichoepithelioma is occasionally associated with melanocytic (banal or blue) and epidermal nevi.[79–82]

Pathogenesis and histologic features

The Brooke-Spiegler syndrome has recently been mapped to chromosome locus 16q12-13, and the candidate gene identified as the tumor suppressor gene CYLD.[47–52] Mutations resulting in inactivation of the CYLD gene have been reported, with tumors showing loss of heterozygosity for the wild-type copy, a characteristic finding for tumor suppressor genes.[32,33,35,47] CYLD mutations have now also been identified in families with multiple familial trichoepithelioma and familial cylindromatosis, suggesting phenotypic variation of the same underlying disease.[18,19,21–28,30,83] However, no genotype–phenotype correlation has emerged thus far.

More recently, insights into the molecular function of CYLD have been gained. CYLD is a deubiquinating protein that interferes with the tumor necrosis factor alpha (TNF-α)/NF-κb pathway by targeting multiple important signaling molecules such as TRAF2 (tumor necrosis factor receptor-associated factor 2), NEMO as well as bcl-3, among others. CYLD is therefore involved in the regulation of various important functions including inflammation, cell survival, proliferation, and tumorigenesis.[84–86] Lack of CYLD results in constitutive NF-κb pathway activation as well as decreased apoptosis.[87–91] The precise mechanism detailing how NF-κb pathway activation is involved in tumorigenesis is, however, not fully understood.

Keratin expression profiles in trichoepithelioma demonstrate differentiation toward the outer root sheath.[92] In contrast to data on multiple familial trichoepithelioma and the Brooke-Spiegler syndrome, the Shh signaling pathway appears to be involved in the pathogenesis of solitary trichoepithelioma. Analogous to basal cell carcinoma, somatic mutations and loss of heterozygosity of the patched gene (PTCH) have been detected in a subset of trichoepitheliomas.[93,94] Transgenic mice overexpressing GLI-1, a protein involved in the Shh signaling pathway, develop basal cell carcinoma as well as adnexal tumors reminiscent of trichoepithelioma and cylindroma, and high GLI-1 transcript levels have been detected in both basal cell carcinomas as well as trichoepitheliomas.[95,96]

The tumor sometimes shows continuity with the epidermis, which may appear normal or slightly hyperkeratotic and thinned with loss of the rete ridge pattern. Ulceration, however, is exceedingly rare. Typical trichoepithelioma is characterized by numerous horn cysts free within the dermis and within lobules of basaloid cells (Figs 31.91 and 31.92).[2] Admixed with the horn cysts are lobules of tumor cells indistinguishable from those of basal cell carcinoma, being basophilic with minimal cytoplasm and showing peripheral palisading (Fig. 31.93). In trichoepithelioma, however, the perilobular connective tissue sheath is more conspicuous and is frequently associated with the formation of juxtaepithelial round or oval fibroblastic aggregates – papillary mesenchymal bodies (Fig. 31.94).[97] These are believed to represent primitive papillary mesenchyme. Sometimes they indent the lobules to produce a hair bulblike appearance. The lobules of basaloid cells are frequently associated with thin epithelioid strands resulting in a frondlike appearance (Fig. 31.95). Trichoepitheliomas not uncommonly show a foreign body giant cell reaction to free keratin, and occasionally foci of calcification are evident. Amyloid deposits are uncommon.[98–100]

Some trichoepitheliomas, however, may show little keratin cyst formation.[2] Instead, the tumor is composed of a rather circumscribed lesion in which discrete lobules of basaloid cells are widely dispersed throughout an abundant connective tissue stroma (Figs 31.96 and 31.97). Tumors with this particular pattern are likely to have arisen at extrafacial sites. Rarely, epithelial giant cells and multinucleated forms have been observed in tumor lobules.[101]

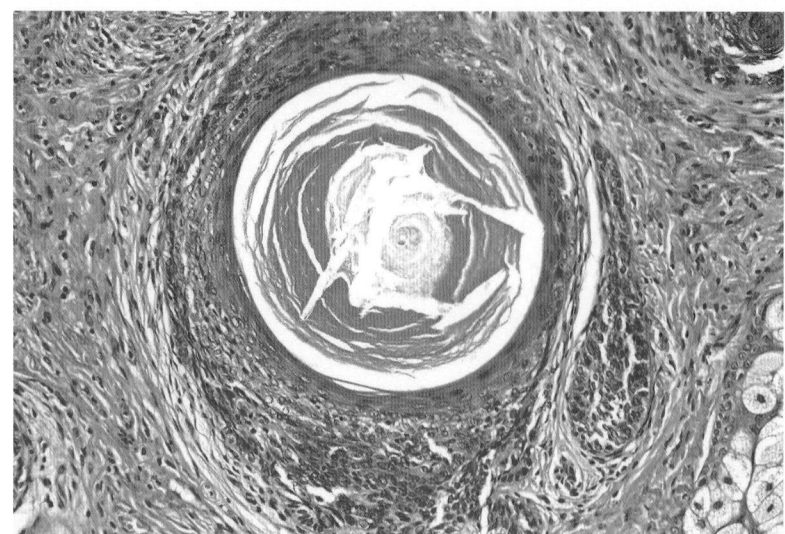

Fig. 31.92
Trichoepithelioma: the keratocysts show infundibular keratinization.

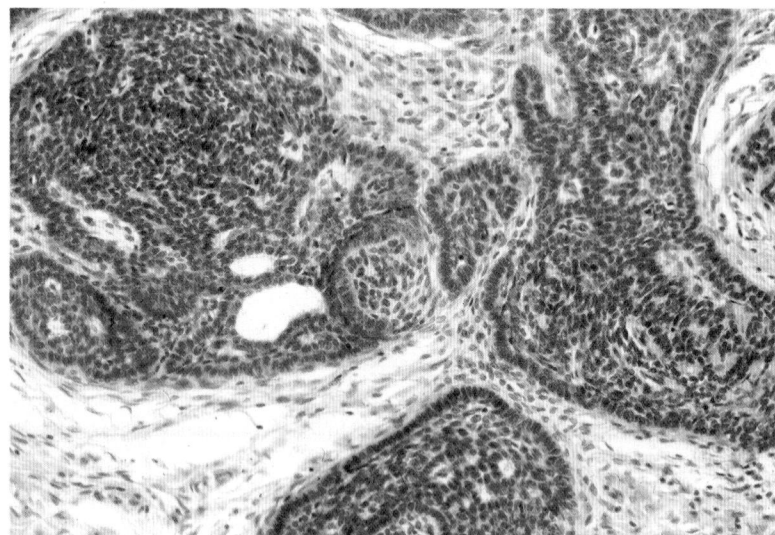

Fig. 31.93
Trichoepithelioma: in this area, the tumor lobules show conspicuous peripheral palisading and are enveloped in a dense connective tissue sheath. A papillary mesenchymal body is evident in the center of the field.

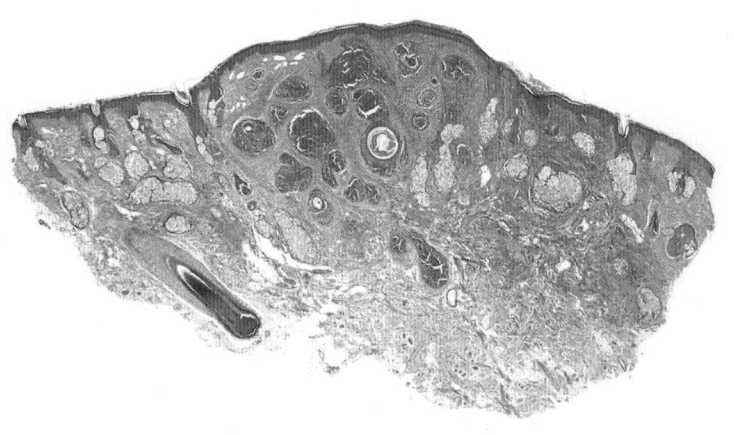

Fig. 31.91
Trichoepithelioma: this scanning view shows the typical appearances of lobules of basaloid cells and keratocysts.

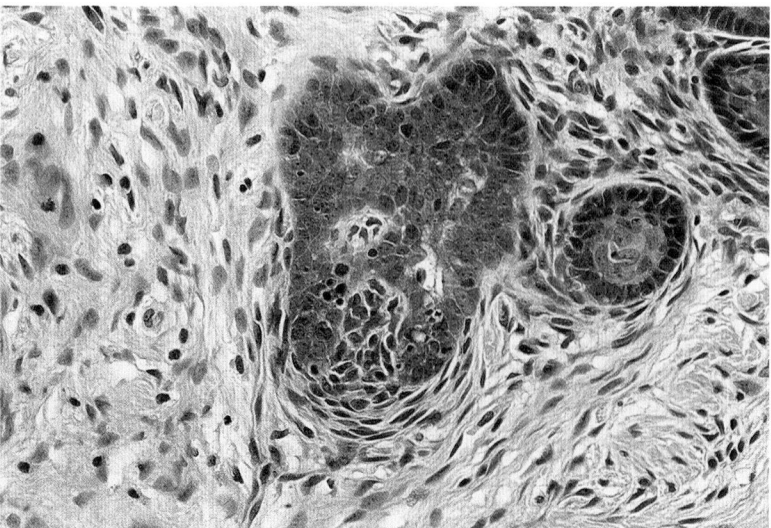

Fig. 31.94
Trichoepithelioma: high-power view of a papillary mesenchymal body.

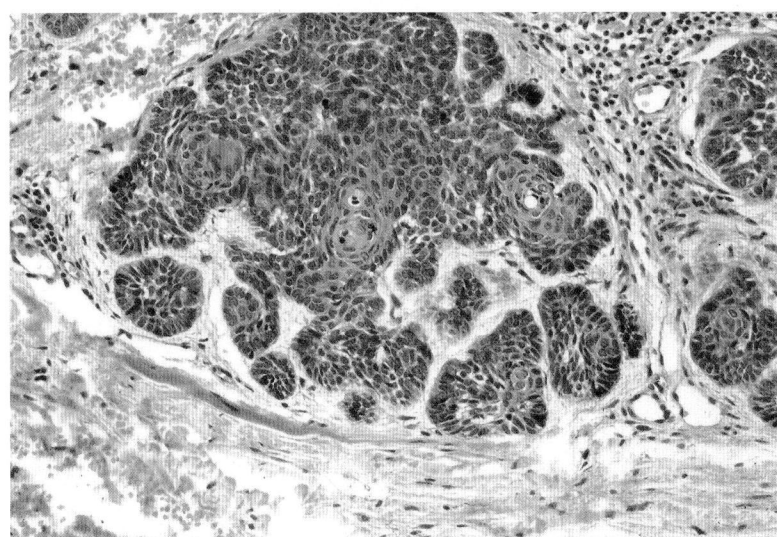

Fig. 31.95
Trichoepithelioma: in this view, the tumor has a delicate frondlike pattern.

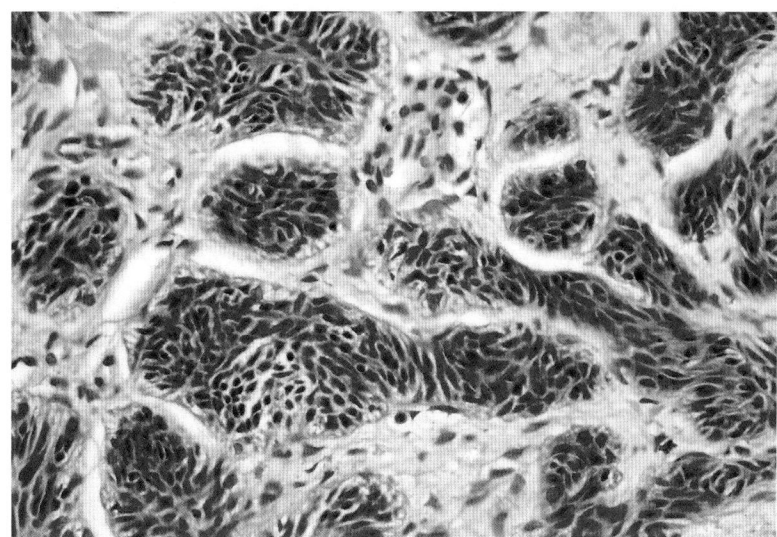

Fig. 31.97
Trichoepithelioma: the tumor is composed of small cells with uniform darkly staining nuclei.

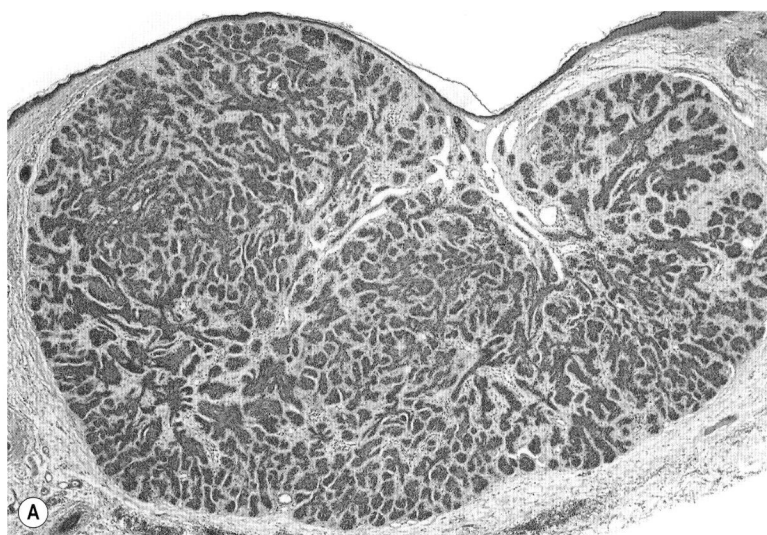

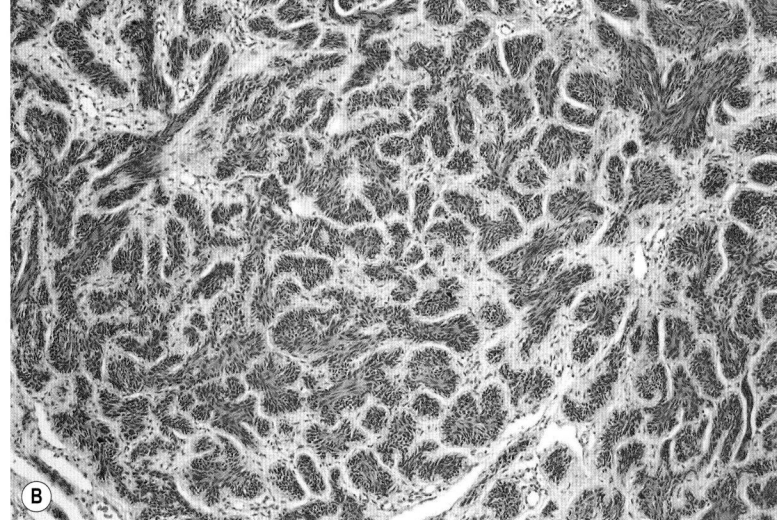

Fig. 31.96
(**A**, **B**) Trichoepithelioma: in this example, the tumor is composed of small basophilic lobules surrounded by a dense fibrous stroma. Keratocysts are not present.

Table 31.1

Immunohistochemical profile of basal cell carcinoma (BCC), trichoblastoma (TB), and trichoepithelioma (TE)

	BCC	TB	TE
bcl-2 (epithelium)	+ (diffuse)	± (peripheral)	± (70%; peripheral)
CD10 (epithelium)	+ (86%)	±	± (15%)
CD10 (stroma)	–	+	+ (92%)
CD34 (stroma)	±	±	+
Androgen receptor (epithelium)	+ (78%)	–	–
Intratumoral CK20-positive Merkel cells	–	+ (70%)	n/a

Differential diagnosis

Sometimes the histologic appearances of trichoepithelioma are difficult to distinguish from those of keratotic basal cell carcinoma. The presence of ulceration and/or a marked tumor–stroma retraction artifact with mucin deposits argue in favor of the latter, whereas marked epithelial frond formation, and more particularly, papillary mesenchymal body with hair bulb formation, are indicative of the former.[98] Mitotic figures and apoptotic cells may be present in both conditions.[98] Immunohistochemistry may play a useful role in the differential diagnosis although the cytokeratin (CK) expression pattern is largely similar.[97,102] Only CK15, which is expressed in most trichoepitheliomas but not in basal cell carcinoma, appears to be of some value.[103,104] Expression of bcl-2 is consistently found to be diffuse in basal cell carcinoma while it is predominantly peripheral in trichoepithelioma.[102,105] PHLDA1 is expressed in the majority of trichoepitheliomas while it is frequently lost in basal cell carcinoma.[106] The MIB-1 proliferative index and p53 nuclear staining are increased in basal cell carcinoma compared to trichoepithelioma, and androgen receptor expression is observed in the majority of basal cell carcinomas while it is absent in trichoepitheliomas.[107,108] In addition, the stroma surrounding trichoepithelioma contains CD34+ cells, whereas these are largely absent in basal cell carcinoma.[109] CD10 staining in trichoepithelioma is predominantly located in the stromal rather than the epithelial component while the opposite is true for basal cell carcinoma (*Table 31.1*).[110] However, none of the above-mentioned immunohistochemical stains can be used with complete confidence in the differential diagnosis and should not be relied on.[111] A clinical history of numerous small facial papules is highly suggestive of epithelioma adenoides cysticum. If the lesion is solitary and the diagnosis is in doubt, it is probably in the patient's safest interest to treat it as a keratotic basal cell carcinoma.

Trichoepithelioma shows considerable histologic overlap with trichoblastoma, and indeed some authors might classify it as such.

Desmoplastic trichoepithelioma (sclerosing epithelial hamartoma)

Desmoplastic trichoepithelioma was originally thought to represent a syringoid variant of trichoepithelioma. It was subsequently described simultaneously as desmoplastic trichoepithelioma and sclerosing epithelial hamartoma.

Clinical features

Desmoplastic trichoepithelioma is an asymptomatic, slowly growing lesion that usually presents on the face or neck of young adults, with favored sites being the cheek, chin, and forehead (*Figs 31.98* and *31.99*).[1-13] Congenital presentation is rare.[14] Lesions are usually solitary, although patients with multiple tumors have occasionally been documented.[15,16] It shows a predilection for females (4:1).[2,13] The tumor is 3–8 mm in diameter, hard and annular, white or yellow, with a depressed or atrophic center and an elevated border.[2,17] Typically, the lesion does not ulcerate. Occasionally, milia

are also present. Desmoplastic trichoepithelioma is not seen in patients with the multiple trichoepithelioma syndromes, and familial occurrence is exceptional.[18,19]

Histologic features

Desmoplastic trichoepithelioma is quite different from conventional trichoepithelioma. It consists of a triad of narrow epithelial strands, keratinous cysts, and a desmoplastic stroma (*Figs 31.100* and *31.101*).[1,3,4]

The epidermis may be normal, atrophic, or mildly acanthotic. Marked pseudoepitheliomatous hyperplasia is a rare finding.[20,21] Occasionally, a central depression is evident. Situated within the upper and mid-dermis is a variable admixture of linear and branched epithelial strands and keratinizing cysts embedded in a dense fibrous and often collagenous stroma (*Figs 31.102* and *31.103*). The cysts consist of a peripheral border of small cuboidal basal cells with prominent nuclei and scanty cytoplasm. These mature to form squamous epithelium, which in turn undergoes epidermoid keratinization. Epithelial strands sometimes bud from the cyst walls.[1] A foreign body giant cell reaction due to released keratin is very common. Calcification is also frequently seen, and occasionally bone formation occurs (*Fig. 31.104*).[22]

The epithelial strands (which sometimes unite with the epidermis) are composed of small cuboidal basaloid cells in a layer 1–3 cells thick. Mitotic activity is very rare and pleomorphism is never a feature. Peripheral

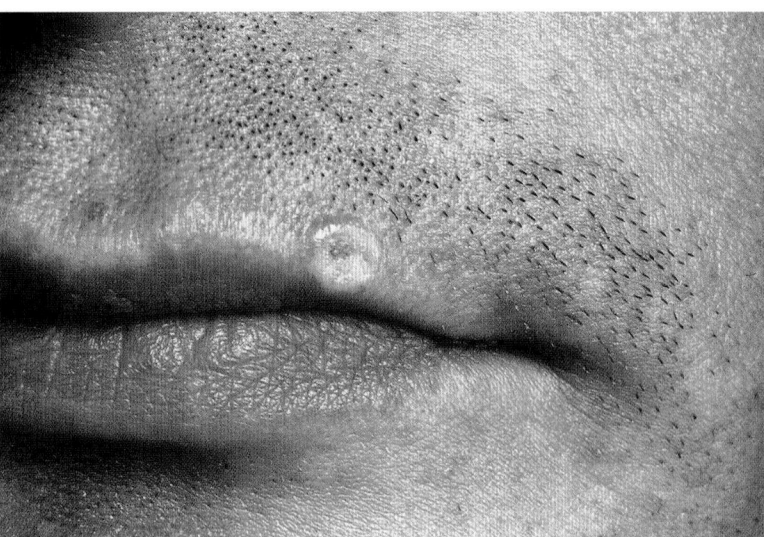

Fig. 31.98
Desmoplastic trichoepithelioma: there is a white annular lesion with a rolled upper border reminiscent of basal cell carcinoma. By courtesy of the Institute of Dermatology, London, UK.

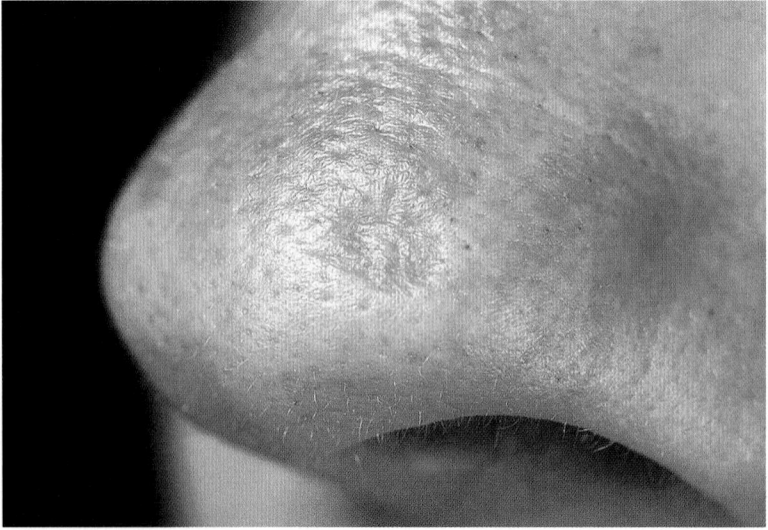

Fig. 31.99
Desmoplastic trichoepithelioma: this example on the nose presented as a depressed area of scarring. By courtesy of the Institute of Dermatology, London, UK.

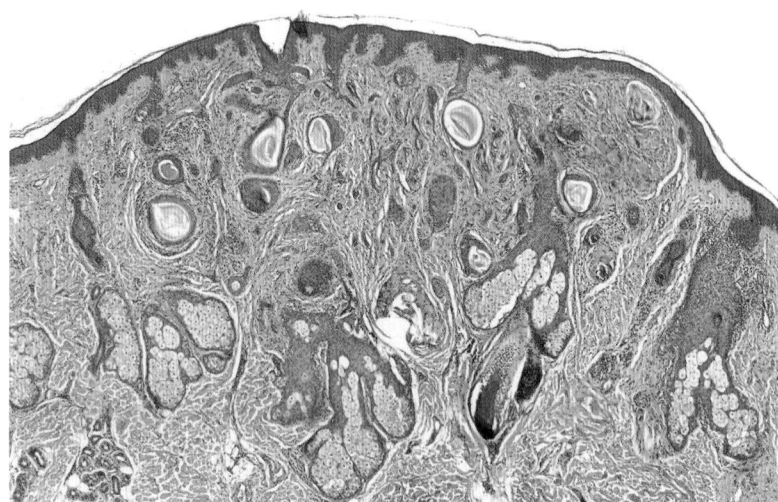

Fig. 31.100
Desmoplastic trichoepithelioma: low-power view showing the typical features. Note the keratocysts and epithelial strands embedded in a dense fibrous stroma.

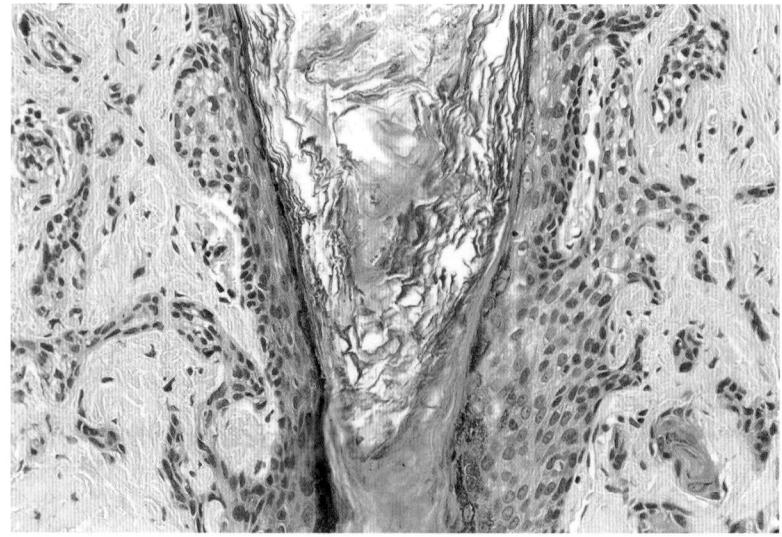

Fig. 31.101
Desmoplastic trichoepithelioma: in this example, a follicular origin is evident.

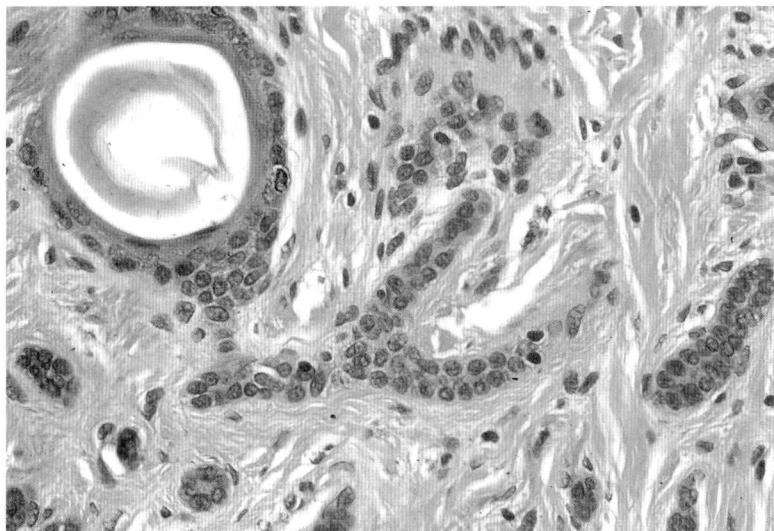

Fig. 31.102
Desmoplastic trichoepithelioma: note the narrow strands of small basophilic cells embedded in a dense collagenous stroma.

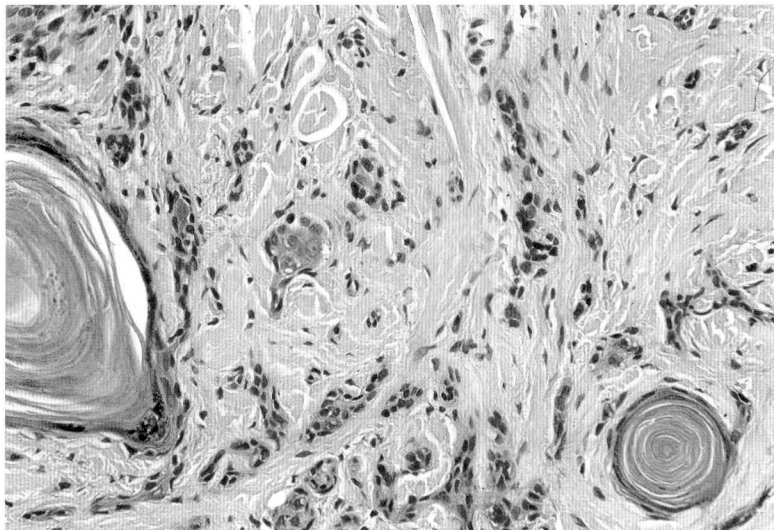

Fig. 31.103
Desmoplastic trichoepithelioma: the cysts show epidermoid keratinization.

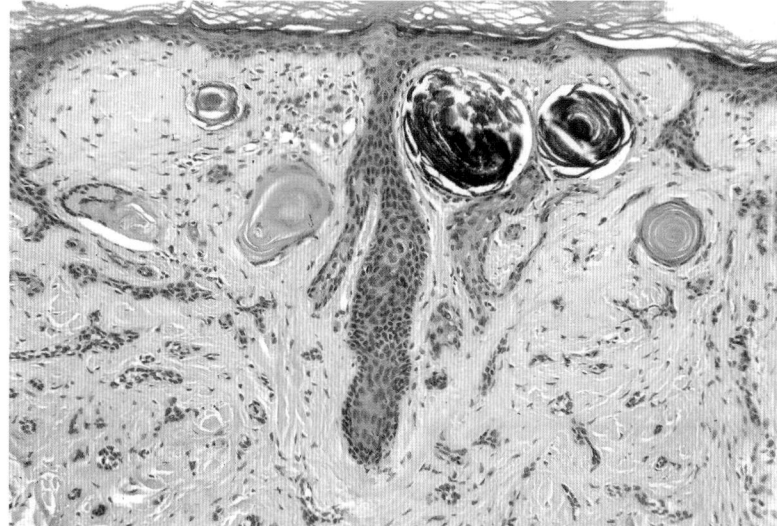

Fig. 31.104
Desmoplastic trichoepithelioma: focal calcification as shown in this field is a very common feature.

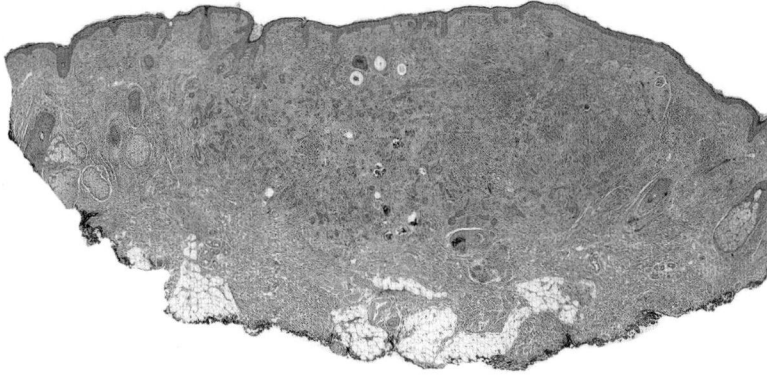

Fig. 31.105
Desmoplastic epithelioma: this example shows a coexistent dermal nevus.

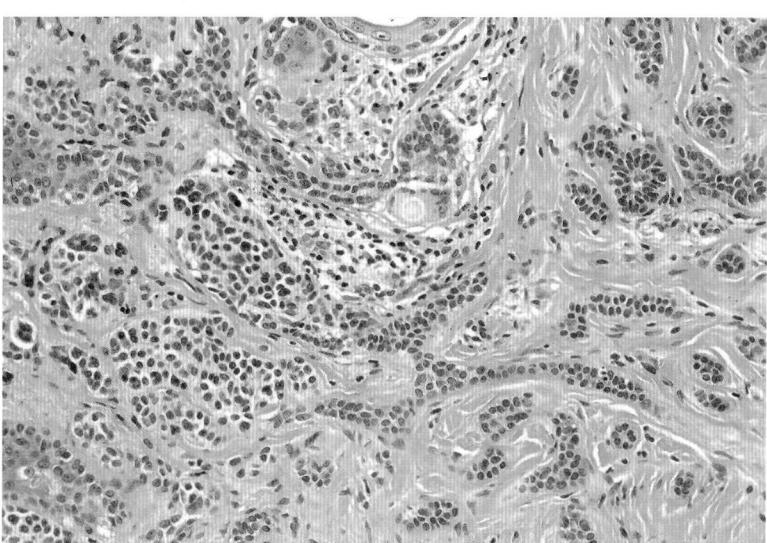

Fig. 31.106
Desmoplastic trichoepithelioma: high-power view.

palisading is absent. Occasionally, aggregates of ghost cells are evident.[23] The tumor cells are PAS-negative. The tumor stroma is dense and often appears hyalinized. Merkel cells are seen and represent an integral component of the tumor.[24,25]

Perineural infiltration is rarely seen in desmoplastic trichoepithelioma.[26]

P53 and bcl-2 are not expressed, and the MIB-1 proliferation index is extremely low.[27] In contrast to morpheaform basal cell carcinoma, there is no expression of the matrix metalloproteinase stromelysin-3 in perilesional fibroblasts and the surrounding stroma contains CD34+ cells.[28–30]

Occasionally, desmoplastic trichoepithelioma coexists with an intradermal nevus including blue nevus (*Figs 31.105* and *31.106*).[22,31–35] Whether this is fortuitous or represents melanocyte-induced epithelial hyperplasia, as has been suggested, is uncertain.[32,36] It does, however, occur sufficiently frequently to suggest that the association is not random. Desmoplastic trichoepithelioma has also been described in a varicella scar.[37]

Differential diagnosis

Desmoplastic trichoepithelioma is most likely to be confused with morpheaform basal cell carcinoma.[3,4,23] It differs by its symmetry, and absence of peripheral palisading, necrosis, retraction artifact, and mitotic activity. Desmoplastic trichoepithelioma rarely ulcerates. Morpheic basal cell carcinoma is not usually associated with horn cyst formation. By immunohistochemistry, CK20-positive Merkel cells are identified in most desmoplastic trichoepitheliomas but only in a small subset of basal cell carcinomas.[38] P75 neurotrophin receptor and PHLDA1 are expressed in desmoplastic trichoepithelioma but less frequently in infiltrative or morpheic basal cell carcinoma.[39–42] In contrast, fibroblast activation protein is expressed by

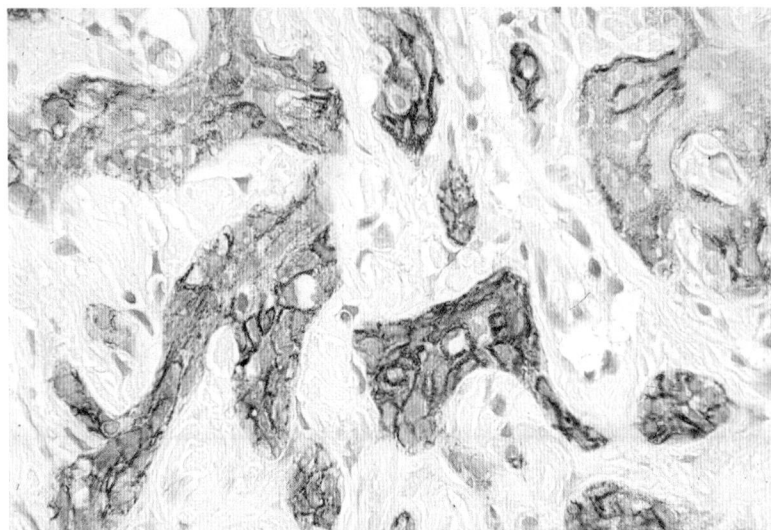

Fig. 31.107
Desmoplastic trichoepithelioma: the tumor cells express EMA, but there is no evidence of ductal differentiation.

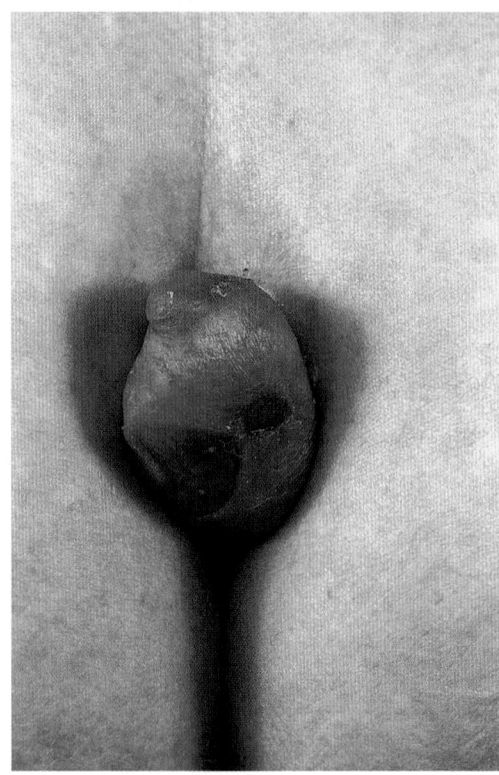

Fig. 31.108
Trichoblastoma: this ulcerated, polypoid lesion is present between the buttocks, one of the characteristic sites. By courtesy of E. Wilson Jones, MD, Institute of Dermatology, London, UK.

the peritumoral stromal cells of infiltrative and morpheic basal cell carcinoma but not desmoplastic trichoepithelioma.[43] Most cases of desmoplastic trichoepithelioma are negative for androgen receptor.[38,44] Similar to basal cell carcinoma, desmoplastic trichoepithelioma stains positively for Ber-EP4 and this marker is not useful in the distinction from basal cell carcinoma.[45]

Occasionally, particularly when only small biopsies are available for study, desmoplastic trichoepithelioma may be mistaken for syringoma, microcystic adnexal carcinoma, or eccrine epithelioma (eccrine syringoid carcinoma). The presence of duct formation or intracytoplasmic lumina, as determined with the use of diastase–PAS staining or by assessing EMA and CEA immunohistochemistry, excludes a tumor of follicular differentiation (Fig. 31.107).[46,47] Furthermore, mitoses are more common and CK19 expression is more common in microcystic adnexal carcinoma, and CD23 expression is not identified in desmoplastic trichoepithelioma.[48,49]

Trichoblastoma

Trichogenic tumors are neoplasms recapitulating the germinative hair bulb and its associated mesenchyme.[1] Their nomenclature is, however, exceedingly confusing. Analogous to odontogenic neoplasms, Headington classified these tumors according to the relative amounts of epithelial and mesenchymal components and the presence of stromal inductive change.[2] Purely epithelial tumors were labeled trichoblastoma while mixed epithelial and mesenchymal tumors were referred to as trichoblastic fibroma or trichogenic trichoblastoma in the presence of hair follicle differentiation.[2,3] Individual neoplasms are, however, capable of showing varying degrees of differentiation, and the originally proposed classification is too strict and limited.[4] In addition, subsequent reports of trichogenic neoplasms have used a variety of designations, confusing classification of these tumors even further. For example, tumors resembling trichoblastic fibroma have been referred to as giant solitary trichoepithelioma, subcutaneous trichoepithelioma, or immature trichoepithelioma. More recently, entities such as trichogerminoma, rippled-pattern trichoblastoma, rippled-pattern trichomatricoma, and melanotrichoblastoma have also been described. These tumors display some unique histologic features but also share features of the traditional trichogenic tumors. While it is important to recognize distinct histologic patterns within a neoplasm, it is equally important that classification is comprehensible and meaningful. Since the clinical presentation and behavior of the aforementioned entities are similar and a variety of histologic patterns may be seen in any one tumor, trichogenic tumors in this text are unified under the single heading trichoblastoma.

Cutaneous lymphadenoma has been shown to represent a variant of trichoblastoma and is likely synonymous with trichoblastoma with adamantinoid features. Due to its distinctive morphological features, it is discussed separately.

Clinical features

Trichoblastoma presents clinically as a slowly growing, solitary, well-circumscribed nodule located predominantly in the head and neck area with predilection for the scalp, but other anatomic sites including trunk, proximal extremities, perianal, and genital region may also be affected (Fig. 31.108).[1,4–38] Lesions rarely present as infiltrative plaques and these are almost invariably located on the face, especially the cheeks, where they have been referred to as 'plaque-variant' of trichoblastic fibroma.[5,6] Trichoblastomas are frequently present for multiple years before initial biopsy, and they usually grow to a large size – 3 cm or more in diameter; some examples have reached 8–10 cm across.[7–10] Any age group (except young children) may be affected, but most commonly patients are in their fifth to seventh decades.[1,4–38] The tumor occurs equally in men and women except for the plaquelike facial lesion where there is a striking female predominance of 9:1.5. There is no relationship with familial multiple trichoepitheliomas, but trichoblastoma has been described in a patient with Birt-Hogg-Dubé syndrome and in one patient with Curry-Jones syndrome, characterized by multiple malformations involving brain and skull abnormalities, polysyndactyly, as well as defects of eyes, skin, and gastrointestinal tract.[39,40] Lesions are typically skin colored, although a pigmented variant has also been documented.[11,12] They are rarely related to a dilated pore.[41] Development of trichoblastoma as well as basal cell carcinoma has been reported as a complication of radiation treatment for ringworm infection of the scalp.[42]

Trichoblastoma typically behaves in a benign fashion. Malignant change has, however, been rarely described (see below).[13,43–54]

Histologic features

Trichoblastoma is a well-circumscribed but unencapsulated nodular tumor spanning the entire dermis, characteristically extending into subcutaneous tissue (Fig. 31.109). A purely subcutaneous location may rarely be seen.[1,3,15–18,55,56] It is devoid of epidermal or follicular derivation and characterized by variably sized epithelial nests closely resembling basal cell

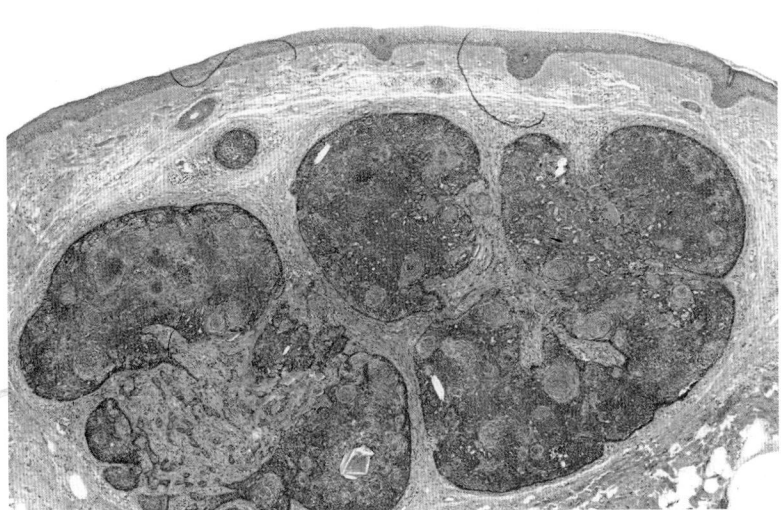

Fig. 31.109
Trichoblastoma: low-power view of a pseudoencapsulated multinodular basaloid cell population. Note the absence of a retraction artifact. The stromal component is best seen in the center of the field.

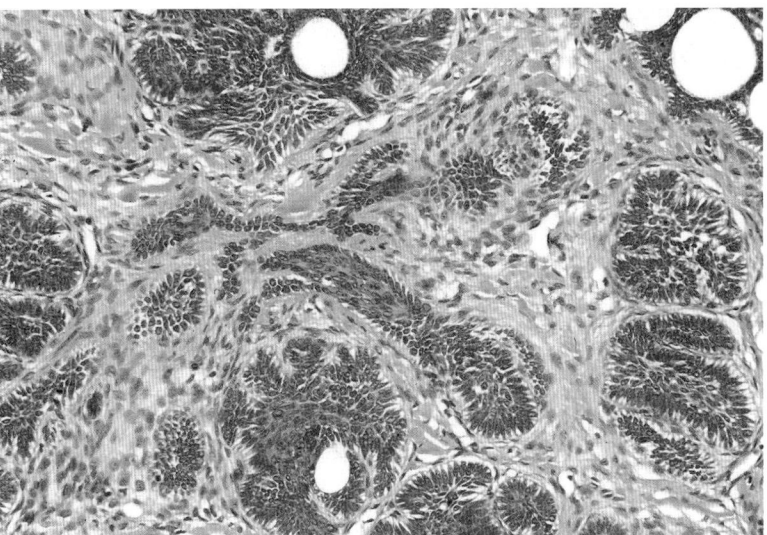

Fig. 31.111
Trichoblastoma: high-power view showing epithelial strands and stroma.

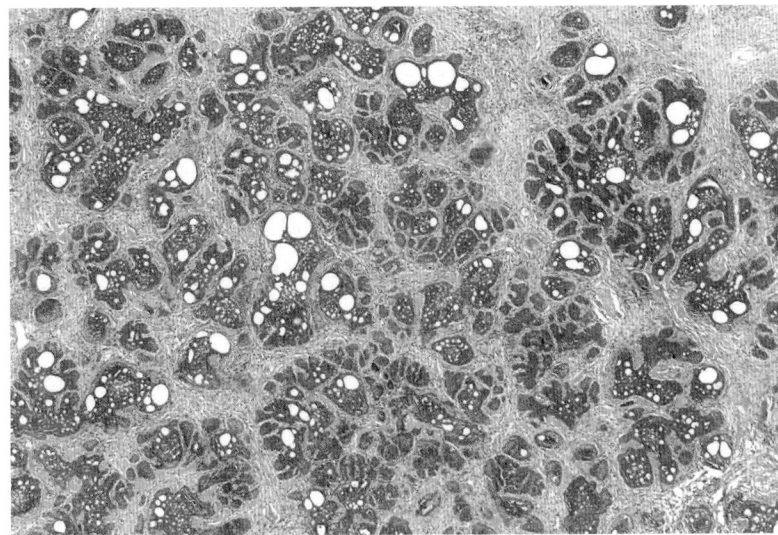

Fig. 31.110
Trichoblastoma: scanning view of a trichoepithelioma-like variant (trichoblastic fibroma) showing an admixture of basophilic tumor lobules and foci of adenoid change. Note the abundant densely cellular stroma.

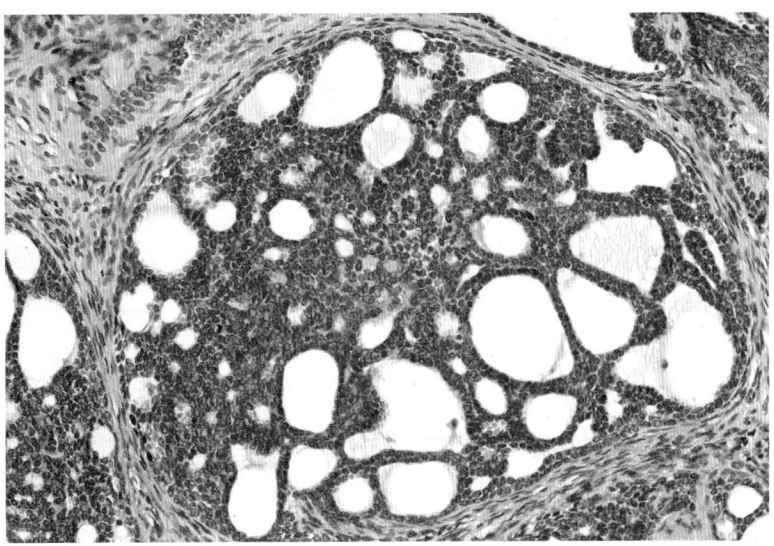

Fig. 31.112
Trichoblastoma: stromal mucin deposition results in adenoid foci as shown in this field. This feature may cause confusion with adenoid basal cell carcinoma.

carcinoma. Peripheral palisading is conspicuous but there is stromal condensation around tumor lobules, and cleft artifact is not a prominent feature. The amount of surrounding stroma as well as 'stromal induction' is variable between different tumors as well as within the same lesion.

The tumor described as trichoblastic fibroma is characteristically biphasic, being composed of lobules of basaloid cells intimately associated with a conspicuous fibromyxoid stroma (*Fig. 31.110*).[1,5,19] Larger lobules and their stroma are often arranged in a mosaic pattern, while the smaller islands of tumor cells are set in close clusters with little intervening stroma. Tumor cells are small and basophilic with minimal cytoplasm. They often show peripheral palisading. Pleomorphism is not a feature, but mitotic activity is frequently brisk and apoptotic bodies may be evident. Some of the lobules have associated narrow epithelial strands, giving rise to 'antler-like' patterns (*Fig. 31.111*).[15,17] Occasionally, a cribriform appearance is evident (*Fig. 31.112*).[1] Sometimes the large lobules are associated with keratin cyst formation although much less frequently than seen in trichoepithelioma. Keratinization is usually epidermoid in nature, but pilar type may also be represented. The small tumor lobules sometimes form whorls or squamous

eddies around a central space or keratinized core, and occasionally focal glycogen-rich clear cell change is evident.[1]

The fibromyxoid stroma is an important, integral component of the tumor (*Fig. 31.113*). It comprises both stellate and spindled cell fibroblasts and characteristically is associated with primitive hair papilla formation – so-called papillary mesenchymal bodies, which often indent the adjacent epithelium (*Fig. 31.114*).[1]

At the opposite end of the spectrum, some tumors are predominantly composed of large basaloid epithelial lobules showing peripheral palisading and only scant sclerotic intervening stroma with no or only little evidence of stromal induction (*Figs 31.115* and *31.116*).[9,11,12,18,21–25] Within the tumor lobules, cells may take on a spindle appearance and align to form nuclear palisading reminiscent of Verocay body formation. This pattern can be focal or extensive, and tumors such as this have been referred to as rippled-pattern trichoblastoma (rippled-pattern trichomatricoma) (*Figs 31.117* and *31.118*).[9,21–25] Sebaceous differentiation is sometimes observed in this variant.

Tumors described as trichogerminoma show additional distinctive histologic features.[13,14,57] They are composed of small basaloid epithelial lobules and nests separated by thin fibrous strands. The lobules are composed of

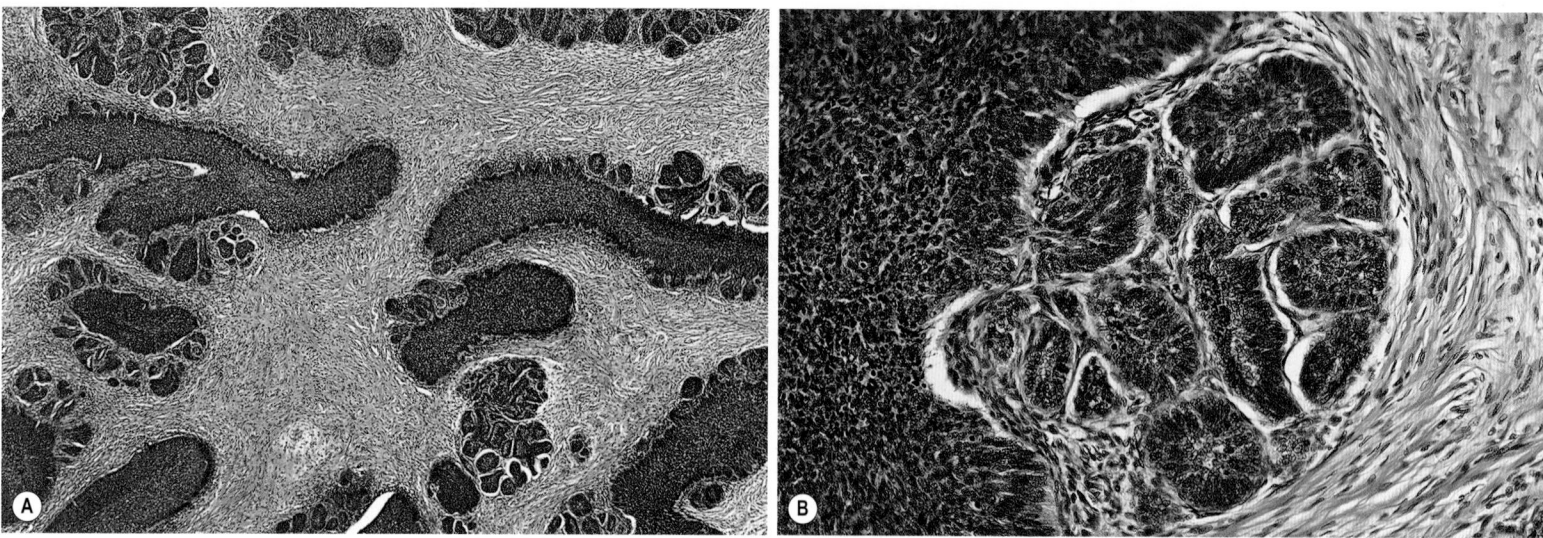

Fig. 31.113
(**A**, **B**) Trichoblastoma: in this example, there is a conspicuous stromal component. Note the peripheral palisading.

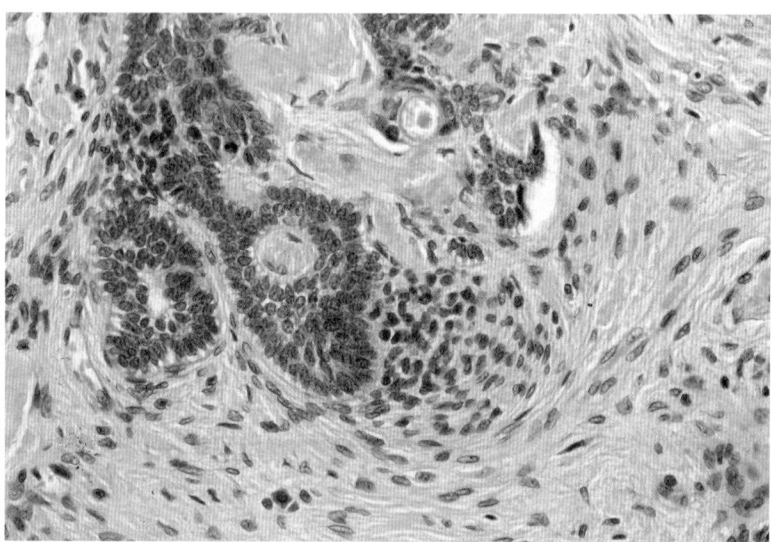

Fig. 31.114
Trichoblastoma: condensation of the stroma has resulted in primitive hair papilla formation (papillary mesenchymal body).

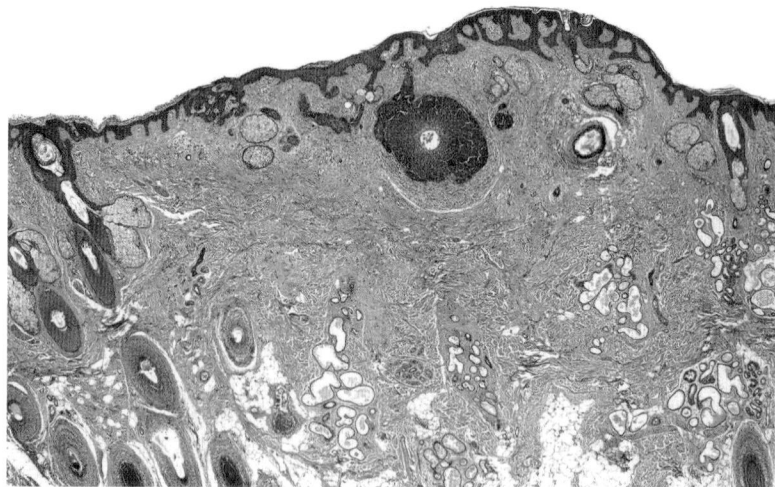

Fig. 31.115
Trichoblastoma: this example, which arose in a nevus sebaceous, consists solely of an epithelial component. There is little stromal induction. In the past, such lesions were regarded as basal cell carcinoma.

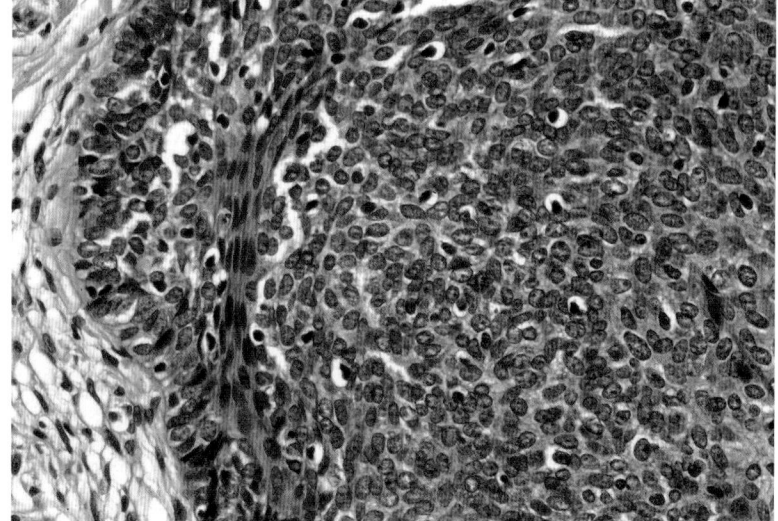

Fig. 31.116
Trichoblastoma: high-power view.

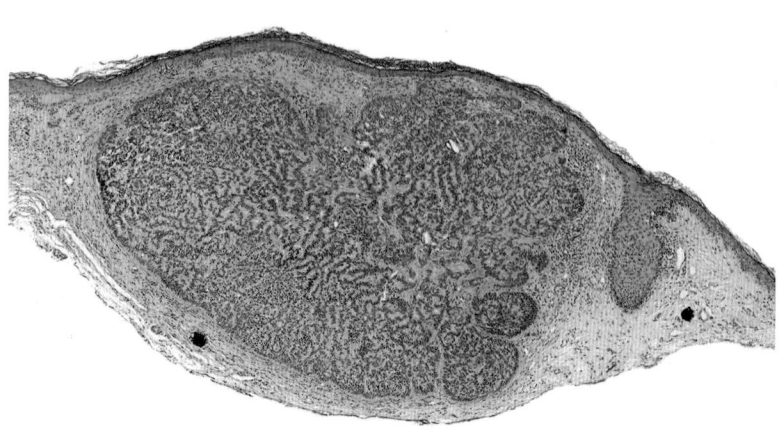

Fig. 31.117
Trichoblastoma: rippled-pattern variant showing prominent palisading.

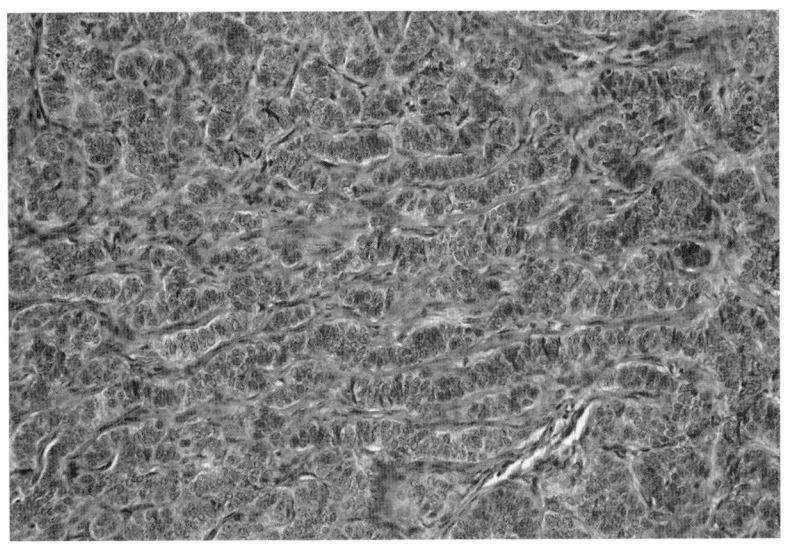

Fig. 31.118
Trichoblastoma: high-power view.

densely packed basaloid cells reminiscent of 'Zellballen' and closely resemble the hair bulb (*Fig. 31.119*). A peripheral palisade surrounds them.

Trichoblastoma is rarely heavily pigmented and contains abundant intralesional dendritic melanocytes (*Figs 31.120–31.122*). This variant has been referred to as pigmented trichoblastoma or melanotrichoblastoma.[11,12,58]

Occasionally, abundant clear cell change (clear cell trichoblastoma) may be evident, and ductal as well as sebaceous differentiation has been described.[13,24,25,59–65]

Nodular trichoblastoma with adamantinoid features is a distinctive variant thought to be synonymous with cutaneous lymphadenoma.[37]

Panfolliculoma is an exceedingly rare and unusual tumor.[36,66] It falls into the spectrum of trichoblastoma but shows unique histologic features with differentiation toward all elements of the hair follicle. It is well demarcated and symmetrical, and both solid and cystic with a wide range of differentiation toward germinal hair bulb and papilla as well as follicular matrix and inner and outer root sheath.[67,68] Focal sebaceous differentiation has also been reported.[69] Rarely, the tumors are intraepidermal.[70,71]

A rare subset of tumors is characterized by an infundibular cyst with additional germinative and matrical follicular differentiation. These tumors have been referred to as trichoblastic infundibular cysts or cystic trichoblastoma.[72,73]

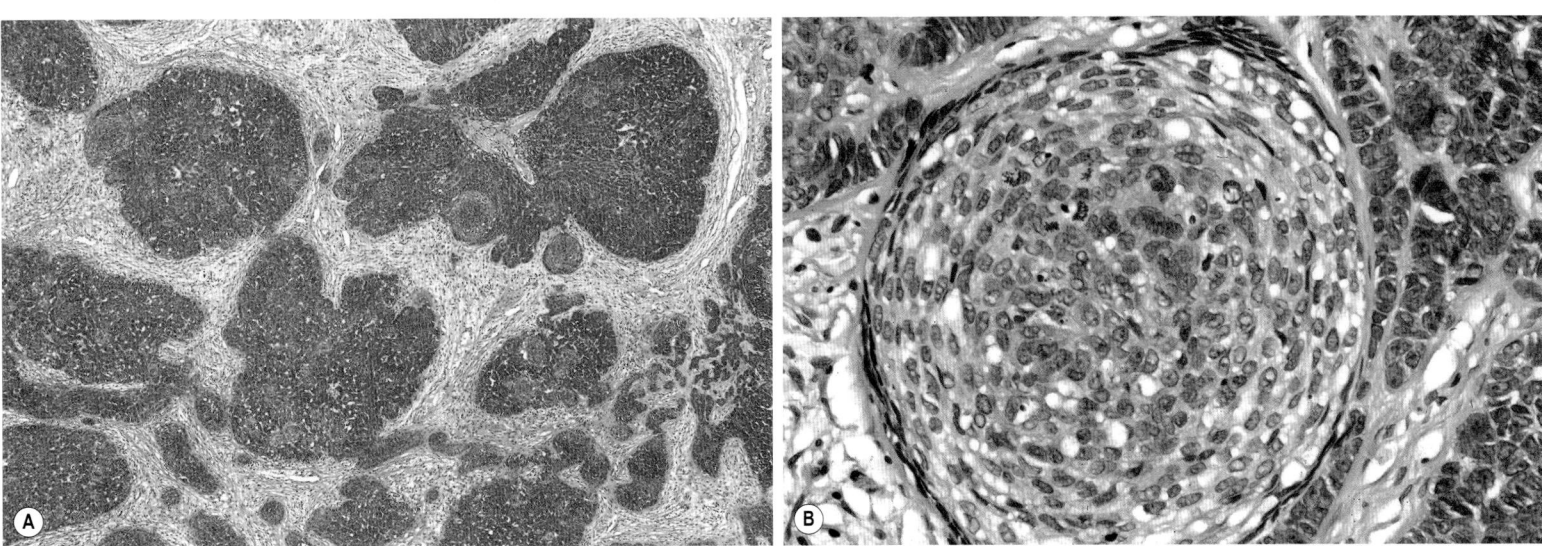

Fig. 31.119
(**A**, **B**) Trichoblastoma (trichogerminoma): this example consists predominantly of a germinative component comprising basaloid cells admixed with distinct pale micronodules (Zellballen).

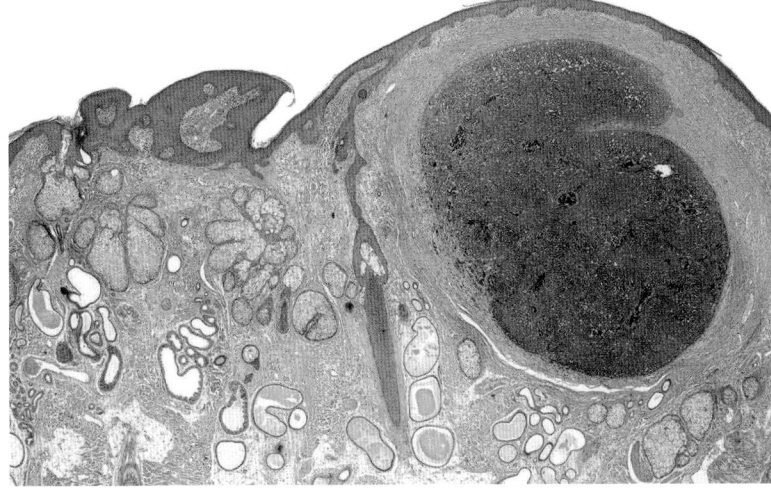

Fig. 31.120
Pigmented trichoblastoma: this lesion developed in a background of nevus sebaceous. There is heavy melanin pigmentation.

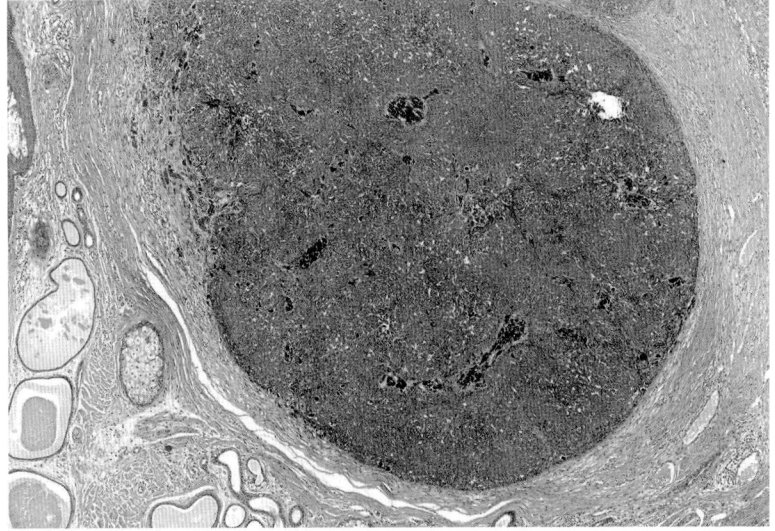

Fig. 31.121
Pigmented trichoblastoma: medium-power view. There is abundant pigment.

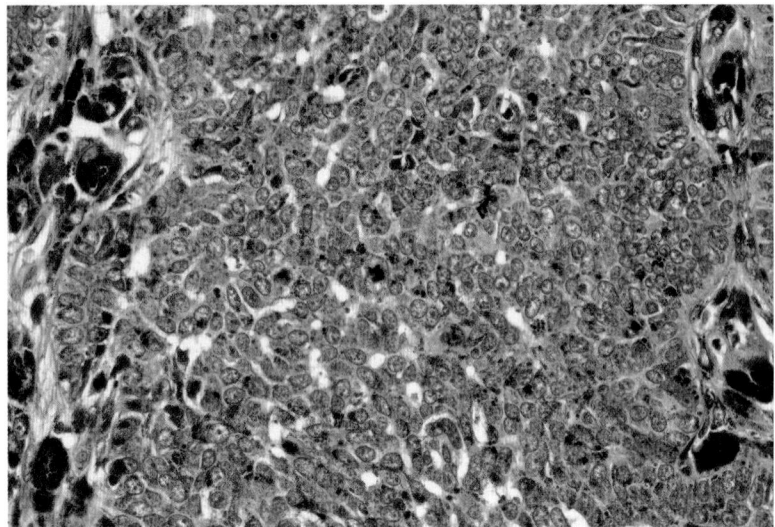

Fig. 31.122
Pigmented trichoblastoma: melanin pigment is present within tumor cells, dendritic cells, and macrophages.

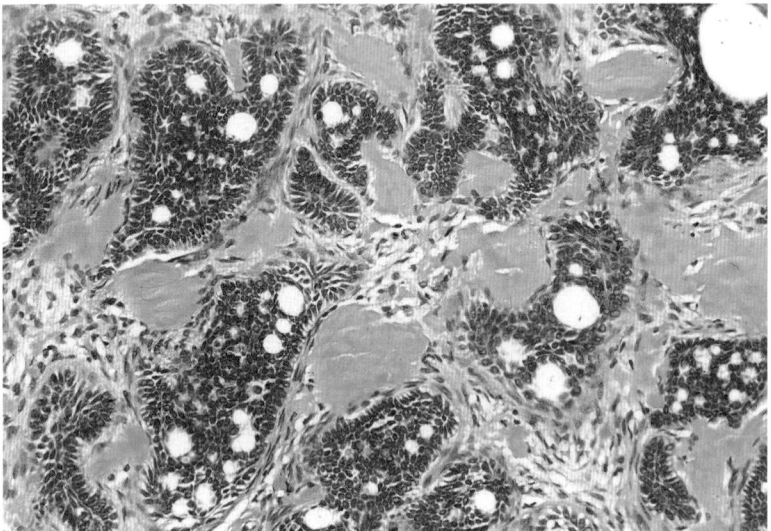

Fig. 31.123
Trichoblastoma: in this example, there are conspicuous amyloid deposits.

A mild chronic inflammatory cell infiltrate is sometimes present, and mast cells are often conspicuous. Amyloid deposits are commonly found within the stroma, and focal calcification is sometimes evident (*Figs 31.123 and 31.124*).[11,33] Merkel cells frequently populate trichoblastoma.[74,75]

Trichoblastoma may arise within a nevus sebaceous and rarely occurs in a poroma (see *Fig. 31.115*).[58,61,76–87]

Occasionally, areas morphologically reminiscent of basal cell carcinoma may arise within an otherwise typical trichoblastoma, raising concern for malignant change.[88]

Immunohistochemical studies of CK expression have revealed the presence of CKs 6, 8, 14, 17, and 19, and absence of hair keratins in trichoblastoma, trichoepithelioma, and basal cell carcinoma, thereby demonstrating differentiation toward the follicular outer root sheath.[89–93] Lack of CK7 expression in trichoepithelioma compared with both trichoblastoma and basal cell carcinoma has been documented.[90] Analogous to basal cell carcinoma and pilomatricoma, CD10 is expressed in most trichoblastomas.[65,94] In contrast to basal cell carcinoma, however, trichoblastoma does not express androgen receptor and is often colonized by CK20-positive Merkel cells (see *Table 31.1*).[88,95] Merkel cells, however, are more frequently seen in superficial trichoblastomas.

By molecular analysis, a mutation in β-catenin (CTNNB1) has been identified in 1 of 15 trichoblastomas studied and HRAS mutations were seen in 11% of sporadic trichoblastomas.[96,97] In contrast, no mutations in the PTCH, KRAS, or BRAF gene have been detected.[97,98]

Differential diagnosis

Trichoblastoma is most commonly mistaken for conventional trichoepithelioma and nodular basal cell carcinoma.

It is much larger than conventional trichoepithelioma and is situated within deep dermis and subcutaneous tissue, while 'conventional' trichoepithelioma is centered in mid-dermis. Trichoblastoma shows less keratinization and is devoid of epidermal or follicular origin.

Lack of epidermal origin, more conspicuous stroma with prominent papillary mesenchymal bodies, and absence of retraction artifact are useful diagnostic features in excluding basal cell carcinoma. It is, however, often extremely difficult to make this distinction with confidence, especially on a small biopsy specimen. Complete excision is therefore the treatment of choice.

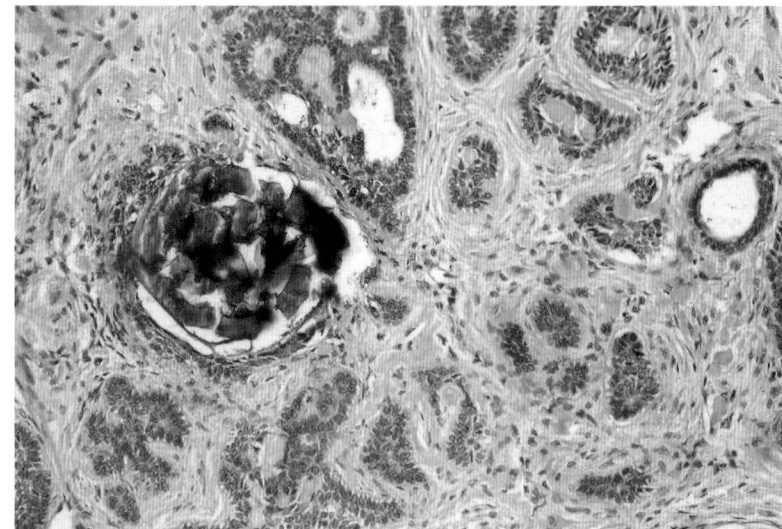

Fig. 31.124
Trichoblastoma: focal calcification is a not uncommon feature.

Malignant trichoblastoma

Trichoblastoma is a biphasic tumor characterized by an epithelial as well as an intimately associated stromal component in varying proportions. The malignant change in trichoblastoma may be related to its epithelial component (trichoblastic carcinoma), its stromal component (trichoblastic sarcoma), or both (trichoblastic carcinosarcoma).

Clinical features

Malignant trichoblastoma is a tumor of the elderly, presenting in the fifth to the eighth decade of life.[1–17] There is no gender predilection and a wide range of anatomic sites is affected. Malignant trichoblastoma has also been documented in the setting of Brooke-Spiegler syndrome and familial multiple trichoepithelioma.[12,13,18] Tumors in this setting may present at an earlier age.[12]

Trichoblastic carcinoma: two distinct forms, low- and high-grade variants, have been reported in the literature.[1–14]

- *Low-grade trichoblastic carcinoma*: these are characterized by morphological features of trichoblastoma but have an infiltrative growth pattern with involvement of deeper tissues such as skeletal muscle.[1–8] They have also been referred to as 'plaque variant of trichoblastic fibroma' and 'aggressive trichoblastoma'.[1–3,6,7] Clinical presentation is of a large plaque measuring multiple centimeters with a strong predilection for the face.[1–8] There are only few documented examples in the literature, and clinical follow-up is limited. Although no adverse outcome such as local recurrence or metastasis has been documented, we have seen a number of cases with local recurrence. Complete removal and follow-up is advisable.

- *High-grade trichoblastic carcinoma*: the characteristic feature of this tumor is the presence of a high-grade, undifferentiated carcinoma arising in the background of a trichoblastoma or trichoepithelioma. Only eight cases of this rare tumor have been reported to date.[9–14,19] A wide range of anatomical sites is affected, with predilection for the trunk and extremities. The head and neck area appears to be involved less often. The clinical presentation is that of a frequently ulcerated tumor measuring multiple centimeters. A deeply pigmented tumor has been reported as malignant melanocytic trichoblastoma.[14] Typically, there is a history of a longstanding lesion over many years, which has shown recent and rapid growth.[9–12] An additional history of a systemic malignancy has been elucidated in some patients, and one tumor arose in a patient with Brooke-Spiegler syndrome and another in the setting of familial multiple trichoepithelioma. High-grade trichoblastic carcinoma has potential for aggressive clinical behavior, and distant metastasis and death from disease have been documented in two patients.[9,10]

Only one case of *trichoblastic sarcoma* and four cases of *trichoblastic carcinosarcoma* have been documented in the literature so far. All tumors have affected the elderly. The documented trichoblastic carcinosarcomas have presented as ulcerated tumors affecting the ear, cheek, neck, and sacral area.[11,16–18] The trichoblastic sarcoma presented on the neck as a 4-cm mass.[15] A history of a longstanding tumor with recent change and rapid growth similar to high-grade trichoblastic carcinoma may be elucidated. A carcinosarcoma has also developed on the back in a patient with Brooke-Spiegler syndrome.[18] Follow-up is limited but no adverse outcome has been reported thus far.

Histologic features

Low-grade trichoblastic carcinoma: this neoplasm is characterized by an asymmetrical dermal-based tumor with infiltrative margin and extension into deeper structures including skeletal muscle. It is composed of basaloid epithelial nests and strands with intimately associated stroma and papillary mesenchymal body formation.[1–8] Cytological atypia is mild but mitotic activity can be present. Keratinization and keratocyst formation may be focal findings (*Figs 31.125–31.128*).

High-grade trichoblastic carcinoma: the characteristic histologic feature of this rare neoplasm is the presence of an undifferentiated, morphologically high-grade carcinoma arising in the background of a trichoblastoma, cutaneous lymphadenoma, or trichoepithelioma.[9–13,19] Tumors involve dermis and subcutis without epidermal connection. The malignant component

shows a solid and expansile growth with pushing or infiltrative borders. It is composed of atypical basaloid cells showing varying degrees of nuclear pleomorphism arranged in nests and ribbons. Spindle cell differentiation as well as focal peripheral palisades, squamoid features, and external root sheath differentiation may be additional findings. Mitotic figures are numerous, including atypical forms. Frank necrosis is frequently present. Melanin deposits may rarely be present, leading to the clinical impression of a pigmented tumor.[14] Diagnosis rests on recognition of a pre-existing trichoblastoma or trichoepithelioma (*Figs 31.129–31.131*).

Trichoblastic sarcoma: this circumscribed biphasic tumor involves dermis and subcutis and is characterized by pushing rather than diffusely infiltrative borders.[15] It is composed of tumor lobules containing a central benign-appearing epithelial element associated with a bland stromal component reminiscent of trichoblastoma/trichoepithelioma. Focal sebaceous differentiation may also be present. The highly cellular sarcomatous component is located peripherally as a nodular and expansile area sharply demarcated

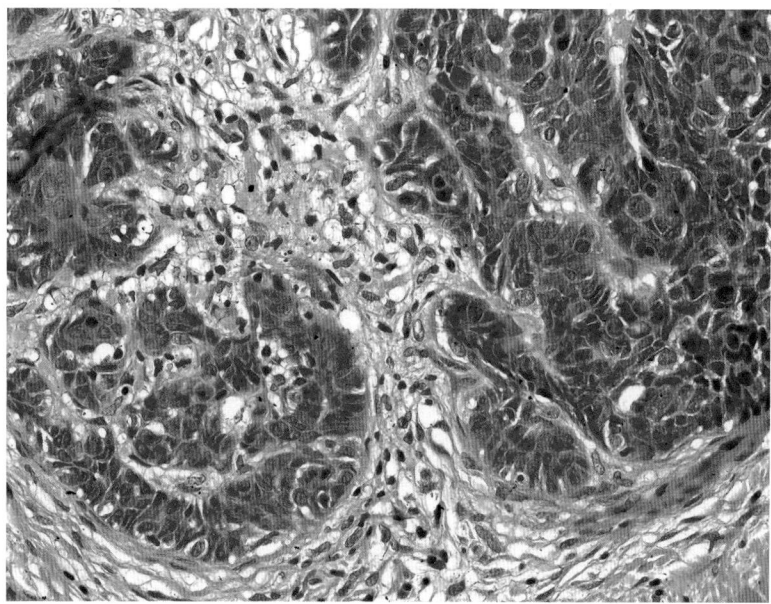

Fig. 31.126
Malignant trichoblastoma: high-power view showing nuclear atypia and increased mitotic activity. Courtesy of D. Kazakov, MD, Charles University Medical Faculty Hospital, Pilsen, Czech Republic.

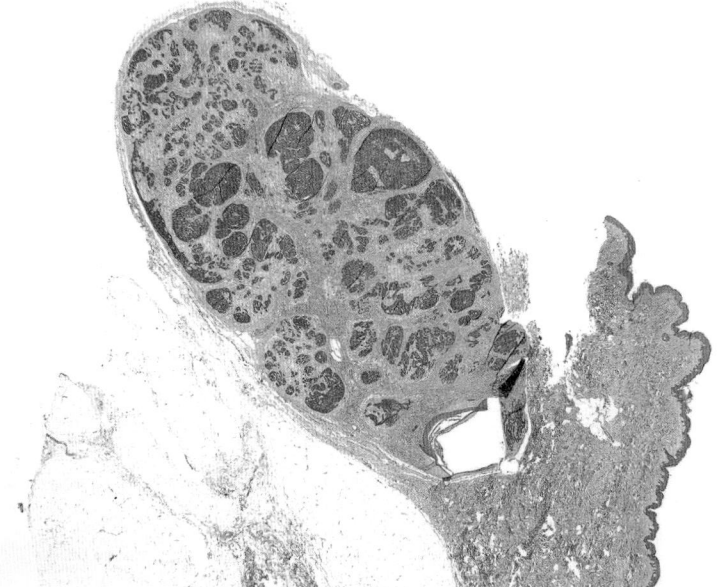

Fig. 31.125
Malignant trichoblastoma: scanning view showing a pseudoencapsulated tumor composed of variably sized nests of basaloid cells. Courtesy of D. Kazakov, MD, Charles University Medical Faculty Hospital, Pilsen, Czech Republic.

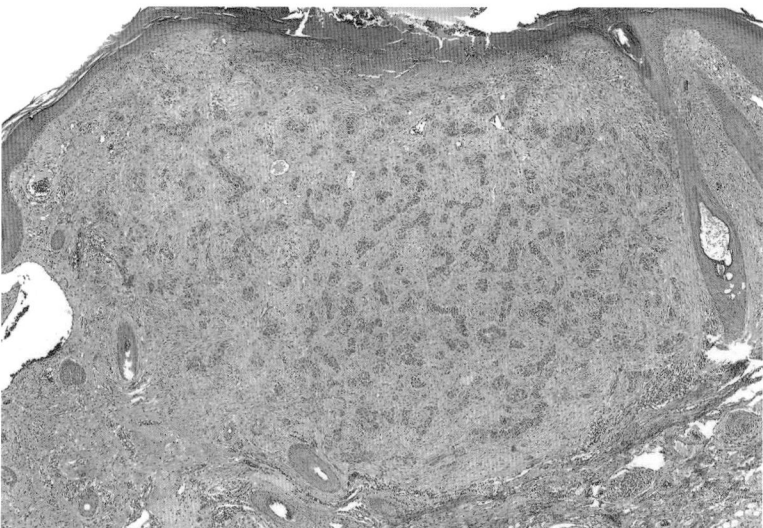

Fig. 31.127
Malignant trichoblastoma: ulcerated tumor. Note the epithelial strands and associated stroma. Courtesy of D. Kazakov, MD, Charles University Medical Faculty Hospital, Pilsen, Czech Republic.

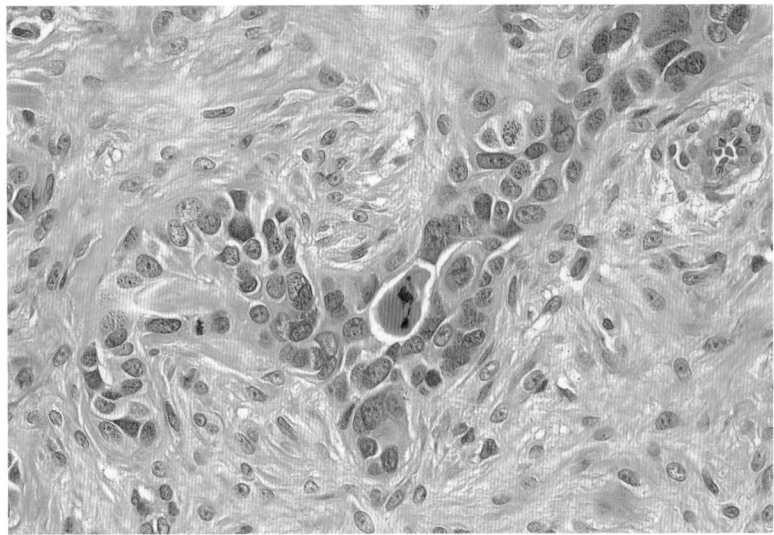

Fig. 31.128
Malignant trichoblastoma: high-power view showing marked nuclear pleomorphism and mitotic activity. Courtesy of D. Kazakov, MD, Charles University Medical Faculty Hospital, Pilsen, Czech Republic.

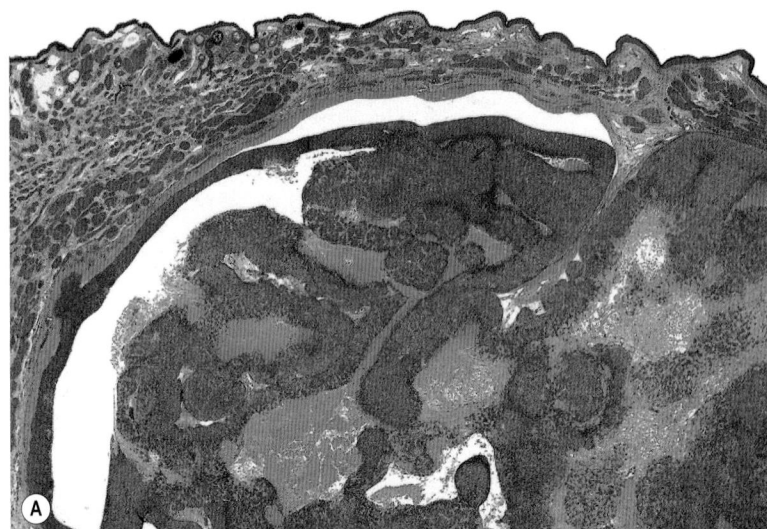

Fig. 31.129
Malignant trichoblastoma: (A) low-power view of a biphasic tumor. Benign trichoepithelioma is seen in the left upper quadrant; elsewhere, there is a cystic and necrotic carcinomatous nodule; (B) high-power view of benign component.

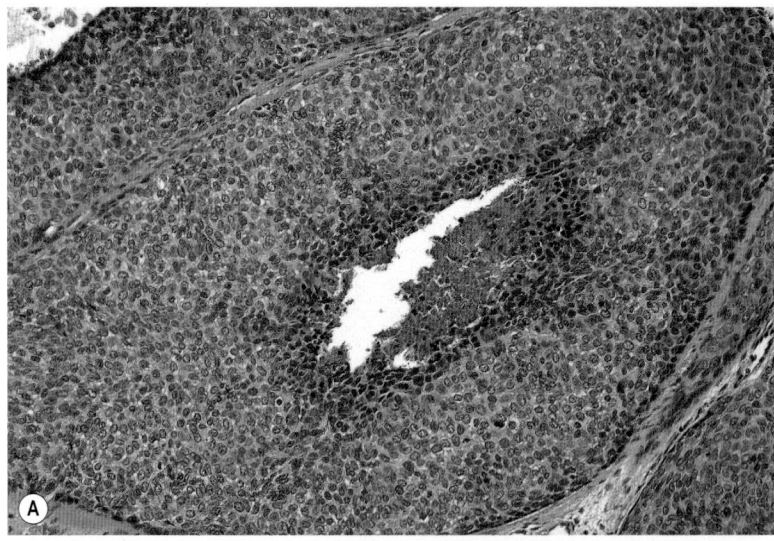

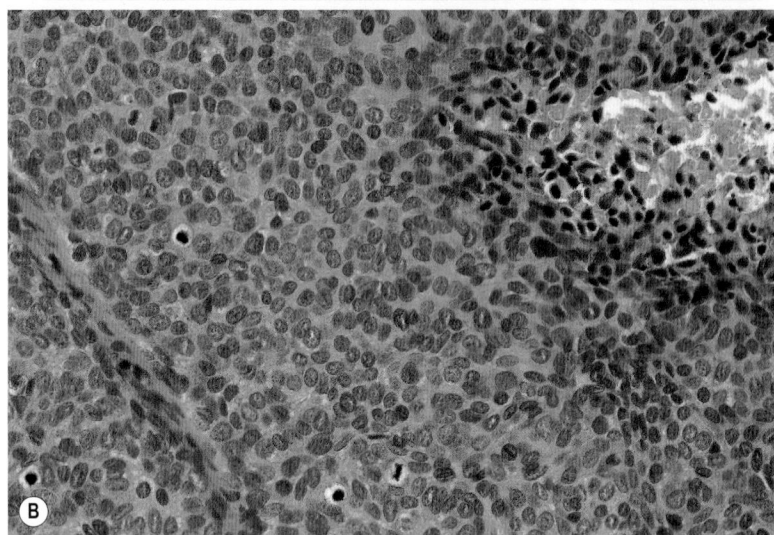

Fig. 31.130
(A, B) Malignant trichoblastoma: the tumor is composed of multiple nodules of basaloid cells showing central necrosis.

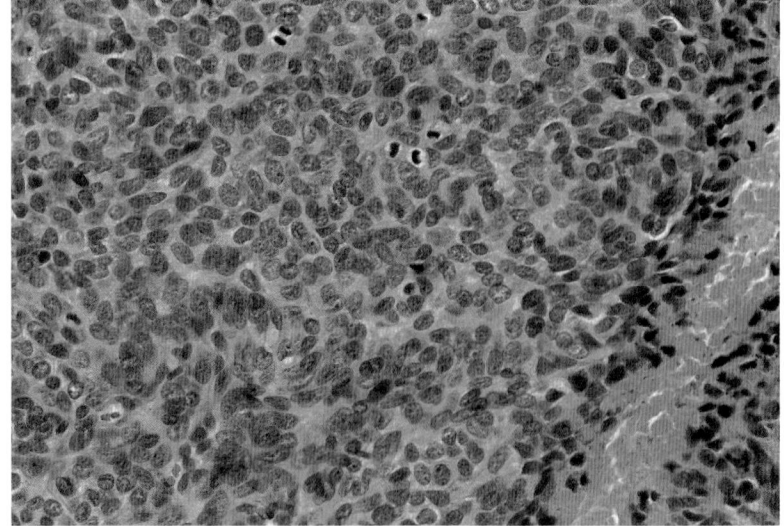

Fig. 31.131
Malignant trichoblastoma: there is nuclear pleomorphism and multiple mitoses are evident.

from the rest of the tumor. It lacks epithelial elements and is composed of large pleomorphic and bizarre-appearing cells which frequently are multinucleated. Mitotic activity is brisk and includes atypical forms. In areas, the sarcomatous elements infiltrate into the benign epithelial elements of the tumor.

By immunohistochemistry, the sarcomatous component focally expresses smooth muscle actin but is negative for CKs, desmin, and S100.

Trichoblastic carcinosarcoma: this tumor is characterized by the presence of a malignant epithelial component showing trichoblastic differentiation associated with malignant mesenchyme.[11,16–18] These asymmetric and expansile tumors may show exo- and endophytic growth with ulceration of the overlying epidermis. The epithelial component forms tumor nodules of varying size in areas showing a cribriform or fenestrated architecture. Tumor lobules consist of basaloid cells with scant cytoplasm and significant cytological atypia and nuclear pleomorphism. There is nuclear crowding, increased mitotic as well as apoptotic activity, and a peripheral palisade may be evident.[16,17] Surrounding the epithelial tumor lobule is a multilayered rim of medium-sized stromal cells with scant cytoplasm and pale, vesicular nuclei. These cells form concentric layers around the epithelial lobules and, in areas, they are arranged to form so-called continuous papillae.[16,17] In other areas, they show diffuse and patternless growth within a slightly myxoid matrix. Nuclear pleomorphism and crowding is prominent, and increased and atypical mitotic activity is evident. In a case reported as 'high-grade' trichoblastic carcinosarcoma, an additional pleomorphic spindle cell component was present.[17]

By immunohistochemistry, the stromal component is negative for CK and EMA as well as actin, desmin, CD31, and CD34. The MIB-1 proliferative index is high, and p53 expression is observed in both stromal and epithelial components.[16]

Differential diagnosis

The main differential diagnosis of 'low-grade' trichoblastic carcinoma is with trichoblastoma and basal cell carcinoma as they show morphological features of trichoblastoma but infiltrative growth more reminiscent of basal cell carcinoma. As discussed above, complete excision may be the treatment of choice until further data regarding clinical behavior become available.

'High-grade' trichoblastic carcinoma has a wide differential diagnosis including Merkel cell carcinoma and sebaceous carcinoma as well as cutaneous metastasis from visceral primary carcinomas. The diagnosis is based entirely on identification and recognition of a pre-existing trichoblastoma or trichoepithelioma.

Trichoblastic carcinoma differs from carcinosarcoma by the presence of a benign, rather than malignant, mesenchymal component. The differential diagnosis of carcinosarcoma further includes primary or secondary sarcomas to the skin and, analogous to 'high-grade' trichoblastic carcinoma, the diagnosis rests on recognition of the trichoblastic nature of the epithelial component.

Trichoblastic carcinosarcoma shows overlapping features with other cutaneous carcinosarcomas and especially sarcomatoid (metaplastic) basal cell carcinoma. Trichoblastic carcinosarcoma appears to be morphologically distinct, based largely on its epithelial–mesenchymal interaction with formation of follicular germlike structures.

Cutaneous lymphadenoma (lymphoepithelial tumor of the skin)

Cutaneous lymphadenoma is a rare neoplasm of disputed histogenesis. Differentiation toward the pilosebaceous unit has been postulated, and some authors have included it within the category of trichoblastoma (trichoblastoma with adamantinoid features).

Clinical features

It presents as a usually slowly growing, skin-colored, sometimes indurated, papule, nodule, or plaque, up to 1 cm in diameter and clinically mistaken for dermatofibroma, sebaceous hyperplasia, and basal cell carcinoma.[1–23] It shows a predilection for the head, particularly the face, and only rarely are the legs affected (*Fig. 31.132*).[2,3,13] The sex incidence is equal. Although the

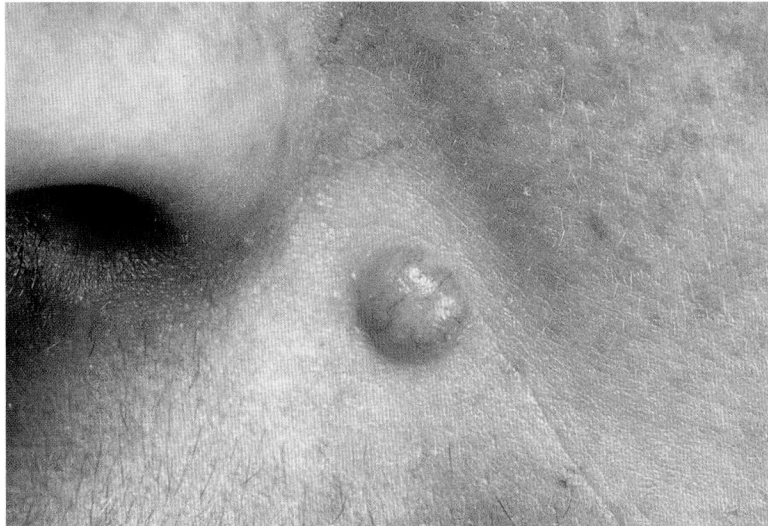

Fig. 31.132
Cutaneous lymphadenoma: this lesion presented as a dome-shaped nodule on the cheek, a commonly affected site. By courtesy of the Institute of Dermatology, London, UK.

age range is wide (newborn to 75 years), most patients are in the fourth or fifth decade.[2,4,16,22,23]

Recurrence and metastasis have not yet been documented and local excision appears curative.[5] A case showing transformation to carcinoma (malignant trichoblastoma) has recently been reported.[24]

Pathogenesis and histologic features

Cutaneous lymphadenoma was originally thought to differentiate toward the pilosebaceous unit.[2,3] Arguments in favor of this hypothesis included the presence of occasional sebaceous cells within the tumor lobules and connection with follicular structures.[2,3] This view has been challenged by reports proposing sweat gland differentiation due to the presence of ductlike structures.[8,9,11,22] It is, however, not clear at this point whether their presence represents true ductal differentiation or entrapment of pre-existing structures, as was originally suggested.[2] More recent data, including immunohistochemical profiling, postulate pilar differentiation; these data advocate classification as a variant of trichoblastoma (adamantinoid trichoblastoma.)[13,14,25]

Cutaneous lymphadenoma is primarily located in the dermis, although sometimes the superficial subcutaneous tissue is affected and is characterized by irregularly shaped lobules and trabeculae of epithelial cells enmeshed in a dense fibrous stroma, rarely containing Alcian blue (pH 5.0)-positive mucin (*Fig. 31.133*).[2,7] The tumor is well delineated but unencapsulated; occasionally, connection with the epidermis or a hair follicle is evident.[2,3,5,6] Lobules are composed of a peripheral rim of one or more layers of small basaloid cells, sometimes showing palisading, surrounding a core of large glycogen-rich cells with vesicular nuclei and often containing large nucleoli (*Fig. 31.134*).[2,5] Mitotic activity is not usually a feature.

An integral component is the presence of large numbers of small lymphocytes admixed with the epithelial cells; germinal center formation can be seen in the adjacent stroma (*Fig. 31.135*).[4] Occasionally, foci of central keratinization are present and rare isolated sebaceous cells may be identified.[2,5] Small ductlike structures are sometimes observed within the lobules.[2,8,9,12,22] Their epithelial lining may show decapitation secretion and their luminal surfaces stain positively with antibodies against EMA. Cutaneous lymphadenoma has been described adjacent to an osteoma, and synchronous presentation with syringoid eccrine carcinoma has been reported.[6,12]

Immunohistochemically, the epithelial cells express keratin and sometimes EMA, but they are consistently CEA negative (*Fig. 31.136*).[2,4,5] The infiltrate is composed of a mixture of B and T lymphocytes with a predominance of the latter.[2,7] CK20+ Merkel cells may be present, and S100 protein-positive dendritic cells are often conspicuous (*Fig. 31.137*).[4,14,26] These coexpress CD1a and likely represent Langerhans cells.[14] The peripheral layer in cutaneous lymphadenoma stains positively for bcl-2 and CK17.[14,26] Scattered

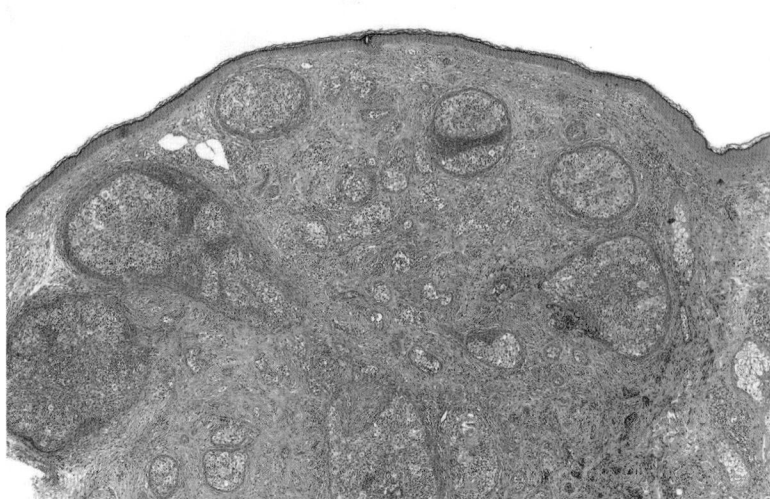

Fig. 31.133
Cutaneous lymphadenoma: scanning view showing multiple epithelial nodules embedded within a dense fibrous stroma.

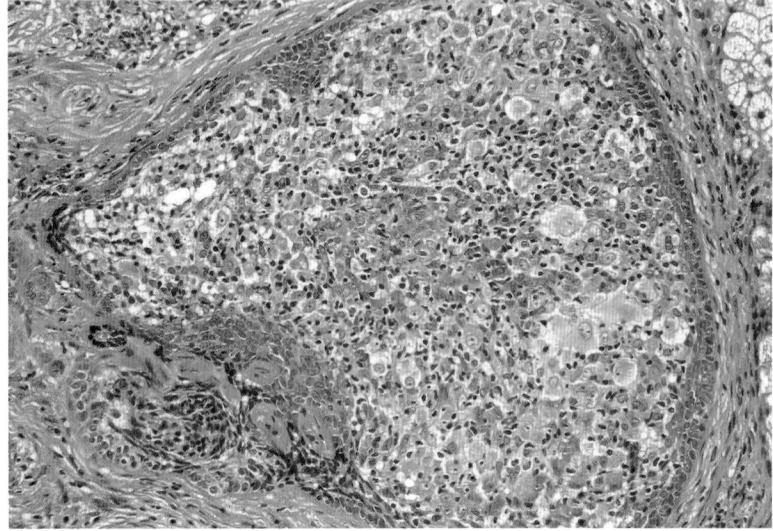

Fig. 31.134
Cutaneous lymphadenoma: the epithelial component consists of a rim of basaloid cells surrounding a clear or pale-stained cell population.

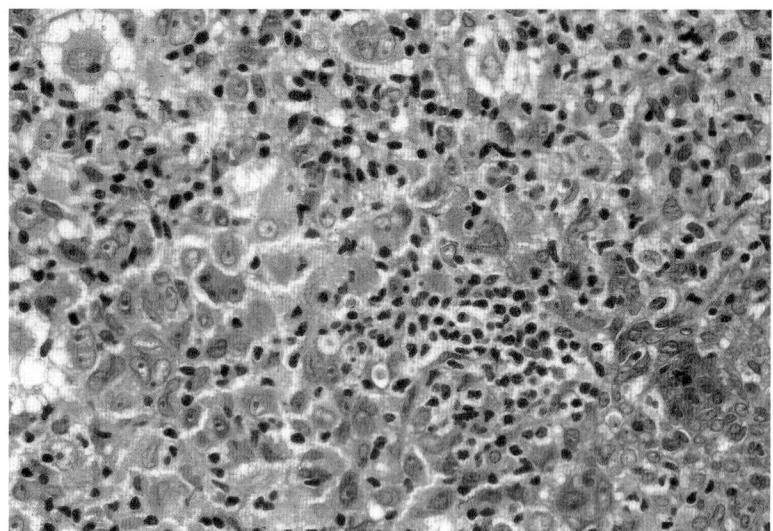

Fig. 31.135
Cutaneous lymphadenoma: the tumor cells have abundant cytoplasm and large vesicular nuclei with prominent nucleoli. Note the conspicuous lymphocytes.

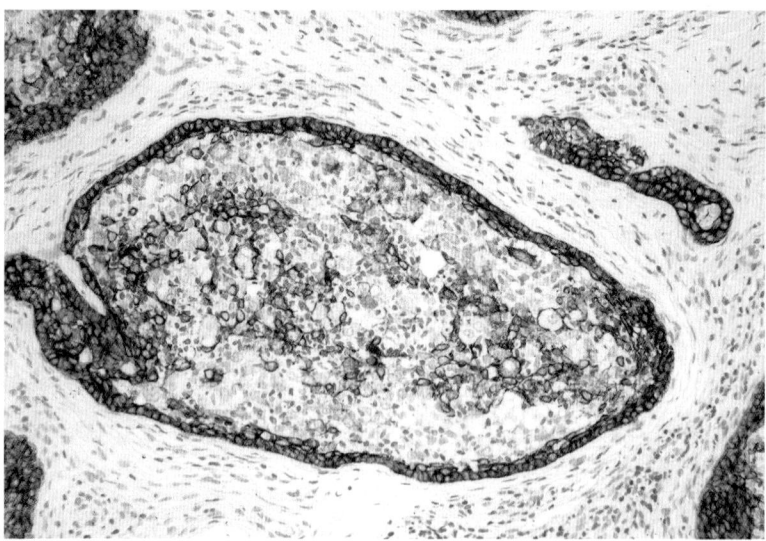

Fig. 31.136
Cutaneous lymphadenoma: the tumor cells express keratin (MNF-118).

within the center of the lobules are CD30+ cells, which have been variably interpreted as representing activated lymphocytes and histiocytes.[10,14]

Differential diagnosis

Cutaneous lymphadenoma should not be confused with lymphoepithelial-like carcinoma of the skin.[2] The latter represents a poorly differentiated tumor with a very heavy admixture of lymphocytes, reminiscent of nasopharyngeal lymphoepithelioma.[27]

Perifollicular fibroma

Clinical features

Perifollicular fibroma is a very rare nevoid lesion of the perifollicular sheath. It may be single (congenital or acquired) or multiple (late onset) and presents as a 1- to 5-mm-diameter, asymptomatic, flesh-colored, or erythematous papulonodule most commonly located on the face or neck.[1–5] Occasionally, the trunk is affected.[6] Perifollicular fibromas have been documented in association with colonic polyps and may be inherited as an autosomal dominant trait (Hornstein-Knickenberg syndrome) and with the Birt-Hogg-Dubé syndrome.[4,7–11] The two conditions are closely related if not identical.[9,10]

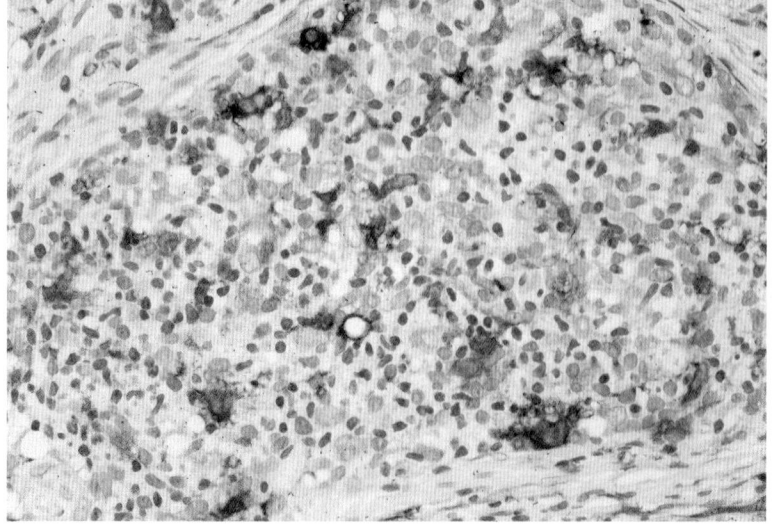

Fig. 31.137
Cutaneous lymphadenoma: note the S100 protein-positive dendritic cells.

Pathogenesis and histologic features

The lesion consists of concentric layers of cellular fibrous tissue producing an 'onion skin' effect around a normal hair follicle (*Figs 31.138* and *31.139*).[1,12] An artifactual cleft often separates the fibroma from the adjacent connective tissue. Occasionally, a chronic inflammatory cell infiltrate is present within the lesion and around the blood vessels in the superficial dermis.

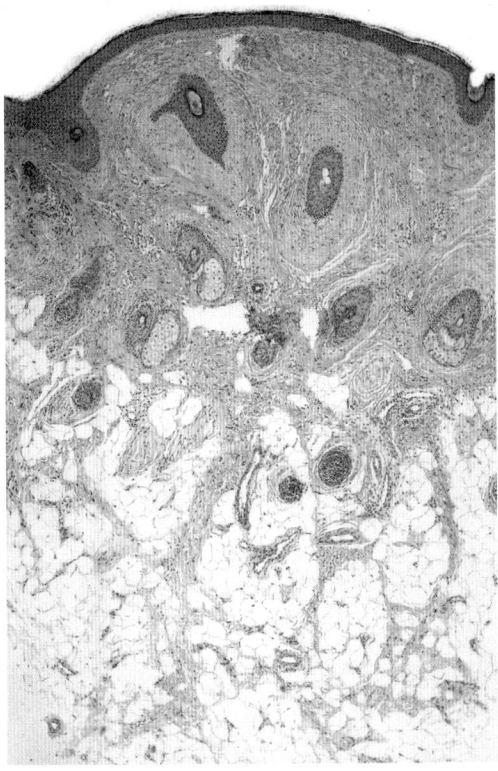

Fig. 31.138
Perifollicular fibroma: the hair follicles are surrounded by a dense connective tissue sheath. Note the retraction artifact.

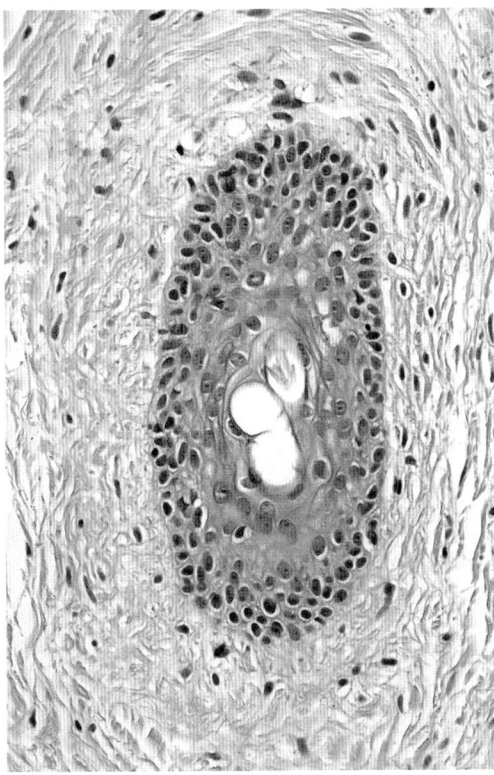

Fig. 31.139
Perifollicular fibroma: in addition to fibrous tissue, there are excessive glycosaminoglycans.

Fibrofolliculoma

Clinical features

Fibrofolliculoma very rarely presents as a solitary facial papule.[1,2] More often, multiple lesions are seen, which represent either an isolated condition or an autosomal dominant syndrome.[1,3,4] In one instance, a series of patients with multiple fibrofolliculomas had familial thyroid medullary carcinoma.[5] The presence of multiple fibrofolliculomas has also been described in association with a connective tissue nevus.[6] Fibrofolliculoma has been reported in association with nevus lipomatosis and in a patient with tuberous sclerosis.[7,8] Patients with multiple fibrofolliculomas may have multiple trichodiscomas and acrochorda (Birt-Hogg-Dubé syndrome).[9–12]

Fibrofolliculomas present as dome-shaped, pale yellow or white papules, 2–4 mm in diameter, with a predilection for the scalp, forehead, face, and neck (*Fig. 31.140*). Lesions may also be found on the chest and back, and antecubital and popliteal fossae.[3] Some papules are umbilicated with a keratinous plug, while others contain hairs. Presentation is most common in the third decade of life.[3,6,9]

Histologic features

Fibrofolliculoma is a benign hamartomatous condition combining proliferation of the perifollicular fibrous and external root sheaths.[1,13] It has a unique and very distinctive histologic appearance, which is centered on the infundibulum. A section through the middle of a papule reveals a well-formed hair follicle, which is often cystically dilated and contains keratinous debris or a hair shaft (*Fig. 31.141*). Surrounding the infundibulum is a circumscribed proliferation of loose connective tissue containing fine collagen and excess hyaluronic acid. Rarely, this may contain bizarre-appearing multinucleated stromal cells, giving rise to an ancient-type or pseudosarcomatous appearance.[14] Elastic fibers are absent.[3,6] Epithelial strands, 2–4 cells thick, arise from the infundibulum, anastomose and rejoin the infundibulum or unite with the stratum germinativum of the sebaceous gland, to give an

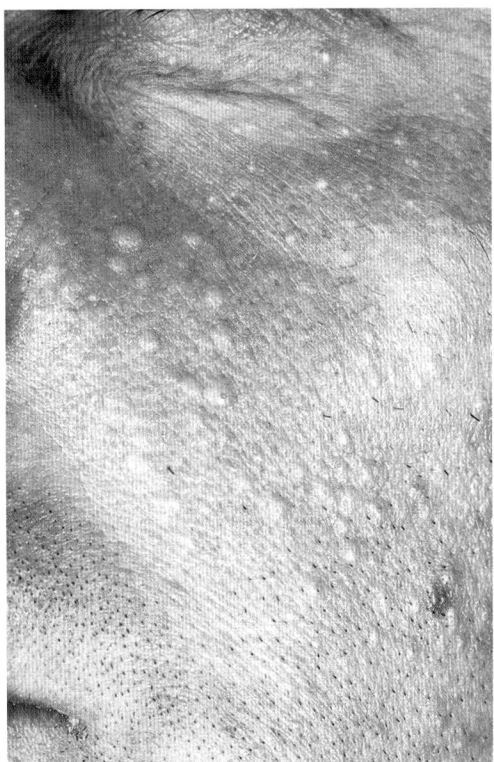

Fig. 31.140
Fibrofolliculoma: note the numerous pale facial papules. By courtesy of R.A. Marsden, MD, St George's Hospital, London, UK.

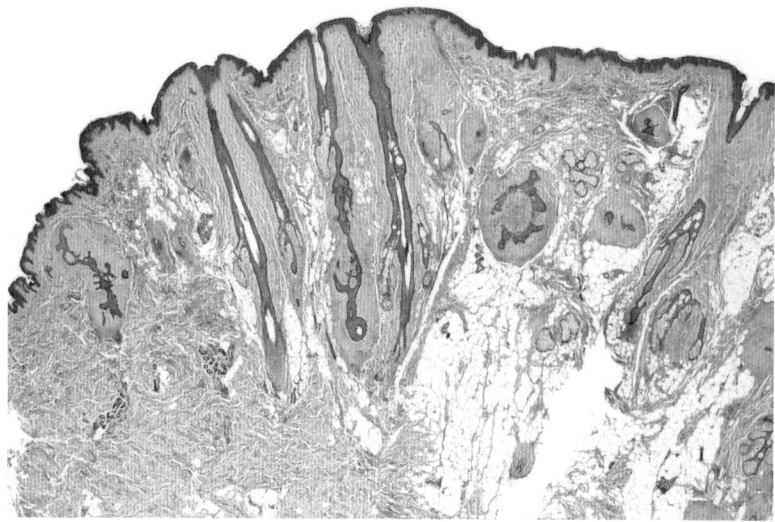

Fig. 31.141
Fibrofolliculoma: this combination of outer root sheath and perifollicular fibrous sheath proliferation is pathognomonic.

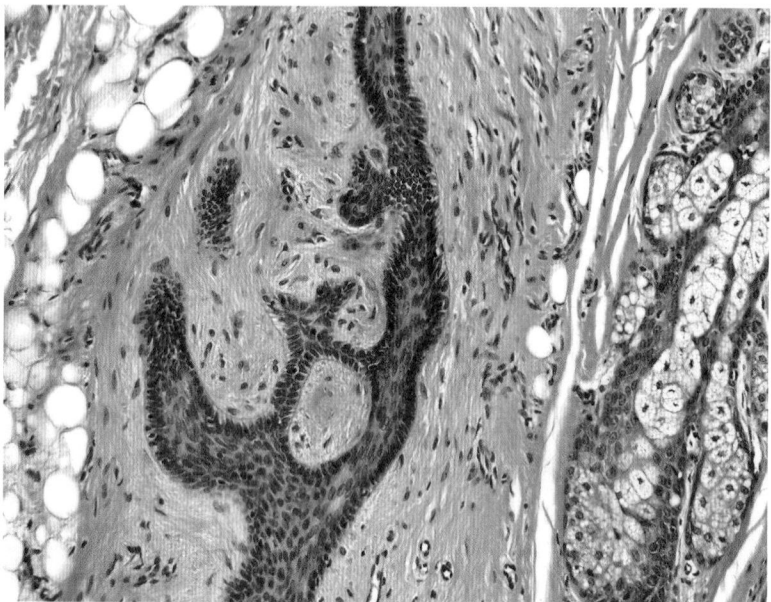

Fig. 31.142
Fibrofolliculoma: high-power view.

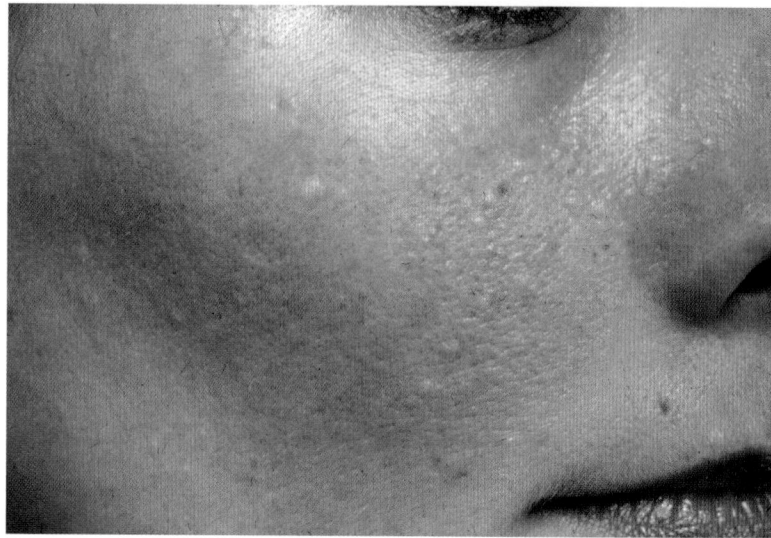

Fig. 31.143
Birt-Hogg-Dubé syndrome: note multiple facial papules. From the collection of the late N.P. Smith, MD, the Institute of Dermatology, London, UK.

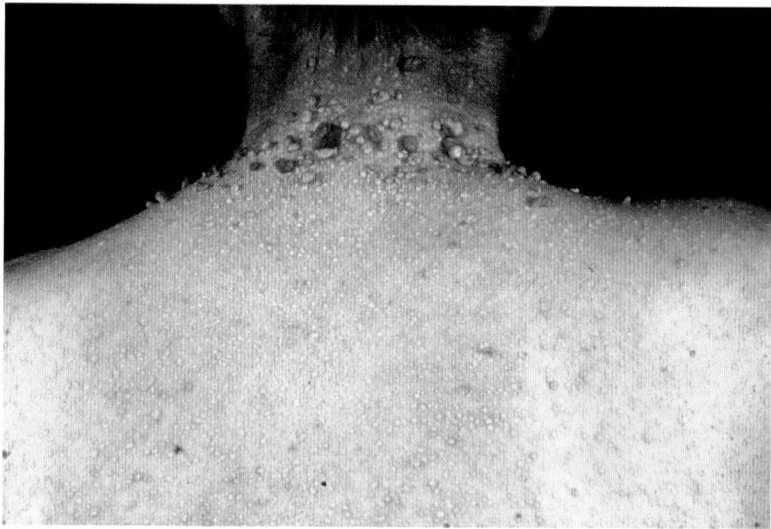

Fig. 31.144
Birt-Hogg-Dubé syndrome: neurosis papules are seen some with features of acrochorda. From the collection of the late N.P. Smith, MD, the Institute of Dermatology, London, UK.

appearance reminiscent of scaffolding (*Fig. 31.142*). Residual sebaceous glands are often incorporated into the nevus. Some papules show histologic features combining fibrofolliculoma with trichodiscoma. The acrochorda may show features of a fibroepithelial polyp or focal fibrofolliculomatous change.

Trichodiscoma, Birt-Hogg-Dubé, and Hornstein-Knickenberg syndromes

Clinical features

Trichodiscoma is a hamartomatous proliferation of the mesodermal component of the hair disc (haarscheibe), which represents a slowly adapting mechanoreceptor.[1] Patients present with hundreds of small (1–5 mm) asymptomatic, round, sharply circumscribed, firm, dome-shaped or flat, flesh-colored papules, which are widely distributed about the body.[1,2] Lesions are sometimes associated with vellus hairs. There are no associated systemic abnormalities.

In some patients, the condition is inherited as an autosomal dominant.[3] The association of multiple trichodiscomas with fibrofolliculomas and

acrochorda was originally described in 1977 and is now referred to as the Birt-Hogg-Dubé syndrome.[4,5] This autosomal dominant genodermatosis is clinically characterized by multiple firm papules on the face, neck, and trunk; pedunculated lesions resembling acrochorda may also be present (*Figs 31.143–31.145*). Importantly, there is an association with internal disease, especially renal tumors and lung disease including recurrent spontaneous pneumothorax, lung cysts, and bullous emphysema.[6–13] Renal tumors are frequently bilateral and cosegregate in a dominant fashion. Histologically, their spectrum encompasses oncocytoma and chromophobe in addition to papillary renal cell carcinoma.[7–9,14–16] An association with intestinal polyps and intestinal malignancy has been proposed, but to date it is uncertain whether this truly represents part of the syndrome since no unequivocal evidence has been documented.[7,17–20] A number of other systemic manifestations have been reported including medullary thyroid carcinoma, follicular adenoma of the thyroid, multinodular goiter of the thyroid, oncocytoma of the parotid gland, chorioretinal scars, multiple lipomata and angiolipomata, neural tumors, parathyroid adenoma, connective tissue nevus, and multiple facial angiofibromas.[4,6,8,17–27] The significance of these associations is unclear.

Hornstein-Knickenberg syndrome is reminiscent of Birt-Hogg-Dubé syndrome. It is characterized by the presence of multiple perifollicular fibromas presenting as numerous papules on the face, neck, and trunk in association

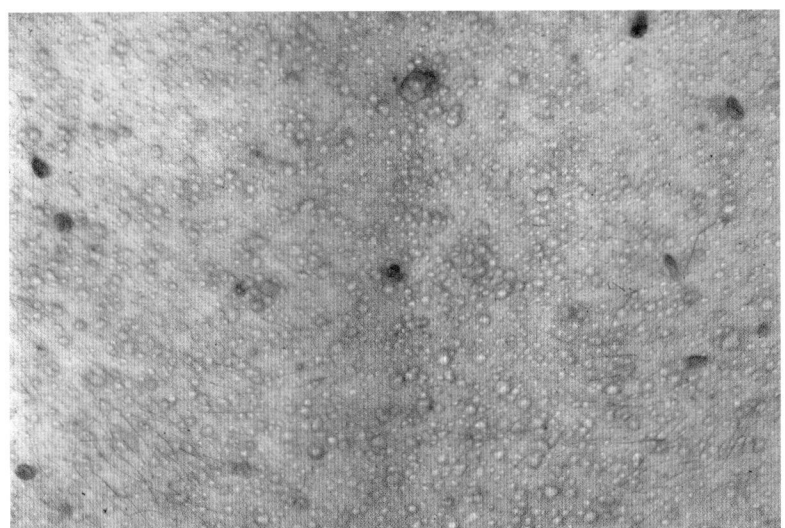

Fig. 31.145
Birt-Hogg-Dubé syndrome: papular lesions can be numerous and confluent. From the collection of the late N.P. Smith, MD, the Institute of Dermatology, London, UK.

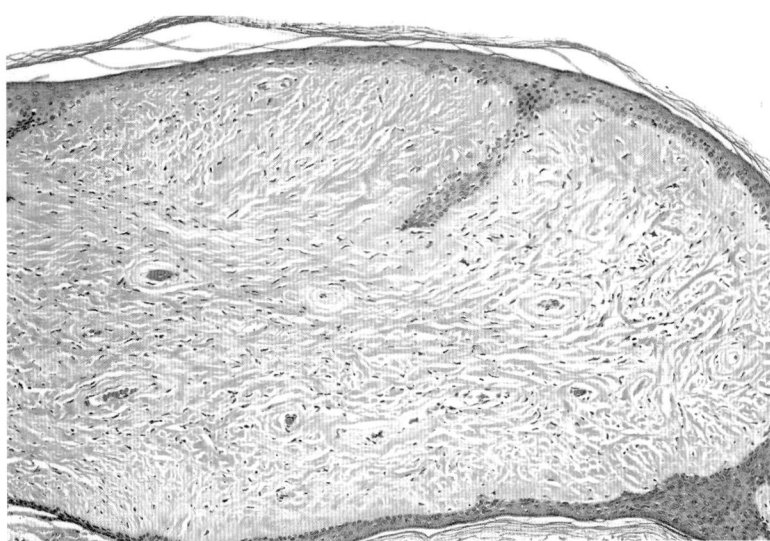

Fig. 31.147
Trichodiscoma: the core of the lesion consists of edematous connective tissue. By courtesy of V. Liu, MD, Harvard Medical School, Boston, and E. Page, MD, Lahey Clinic, Burlington, USA.

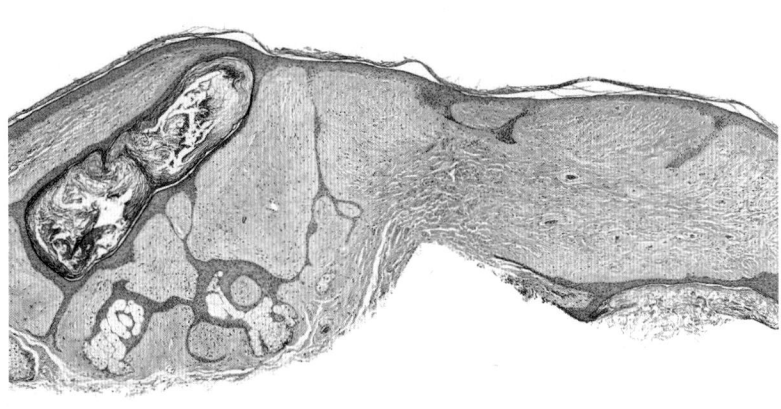

Fig. 31.146
Trichodiscoma: scanning view showing the raised papule with lateral collarette. By courtesy of V. Liu, MD, Harvard Medical School, Boston, and E. Page, MD, Lahey Clinic, Burlington, USA.

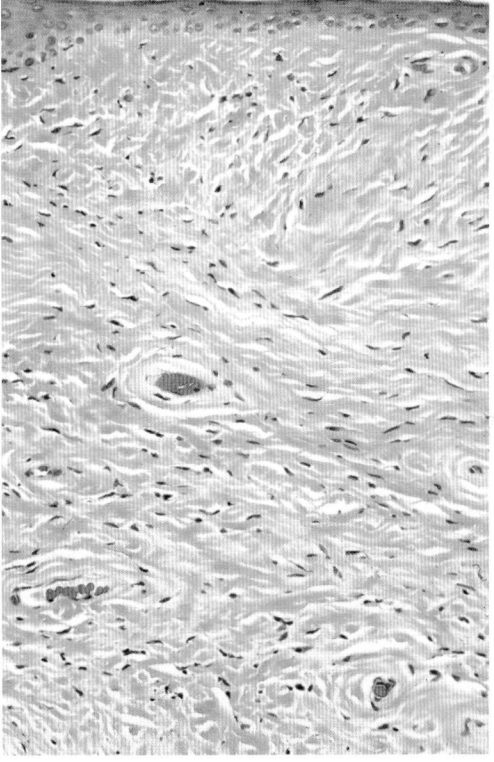

Fig. 31.148
Trichodiscoma: the tumor characteristically contains admixed thin- and thick-walled blood vessels. By courtesy of V. Liu, MD, Harvard Medical School, Boston, and E. Page, MD, Lahey Clinic, Burlington, USA.

with adenomatous polyps and adenocarcinoma of the colon.[28–30] More recent data suggest that perifollicular fibroma and fibrofolliculoma/trichodiscoma likely represent a morphological spectrum and that Hornstein-Knickenberg syndrome and Birt-Hogg-Dubé syndrome are manifestations of the same condition.[20,31–33]

Pathogenesis and histologic features

Recent studies have excluded a number of candidate genes for Birt-Hogg-Dubé syndrome, and the susceptibility locus has been mapped to chromosome 17p11.2.[34–37] The candidate gene (BHD) has recently been identified, and this encodes for a novel protein, folliculin.[37] Although its precise function and mechanism of action remain unknown, folliculin is likely a tumor suppressor gene and involved in the mammalian target of rapamycin (mTOR) pathway similar to other hamartoma syndromes.[38–40] Multiple mutations in the folliculin gene have been identified in patients with Birt-Hogg-Dubé syndrome including insertions, deletions, frame shift, and splice site mutations as well as missense and nonsense mutations.[41–49]

Trichodiscoma is always topographically related to a hair follicle, although multiple sections may be necessary to confirm this.[1] The overlying epidermis is flattened, but laterally there is a collarette (Fig. 31.146).

It is composed of an unencapsulated, elliptical, loosely woven admixture of collagen, reticulin, and thin elastic fibers with abundant acid mucopolysaccharides and containing bland-appearing spindle cells (Fig. 31.147).[1–3] Occasionally, the stromal compartment may show lipomatous metaplasia, and it may contain atypical stromal cells.[50] Focal hyalinization may sometimes be evident.[3] A regular feature is the presence of multiple thin-walled blood vessels with PAS-positive basement membranes within the substance of the tumor (Fig. 31.148).[2] A thick-walled vessel with a narrow lumen and conspicuous endothelial cells often enters the tumor, usually approaching from the vicinity of a hair follicle. Melanin pigment within small fusiform and stellate cells (presumably Schwann cells) is characteristic. Occasionally, multinucleate cells are evident.[3] Examination of serial sections sometimes reveals a peripheral nerve entering the lesion. In contrast to the hair disc, Merkel cells are not present in trichodiscoma.

By immunohistochemistry, spindle cells may react with CD34 antibodies but are negative for S100, SMA, EMA, and desmin.[51,52]

Neurofollicular hamartoma (spindle cell predominant trichodiscoma)

Clinical features

Neurofollicular hamartoma is a rare benign tumor that lies within the spectrum of trichodiscoma and fibrofolliculoma. Despite its name, true neural differentiation is not a feature, and more recently the term 'spindle cell predominant trichodiscoma' has been proposed to reflect this.[1] The tumor is now thought to represent the cellular end of a morphological spectrum with trichodiscoma.[1] It presents clinically as a small, skin-colored, dome-shaped, firm papule, less than 1 cm in diameter.[2-5] Lesions are almost invariably located on the face, with a strong predilection for the nose or nasolabial fold.[2-5] Adults are affected predominantly in the fourth or fifth decade, and there is no gender predilection. The clinical differential diagnosis typically includes fibrous papule, basal cell carcinoma, and dermal nevus.

Histologic features

Neurofollicular hamartoma is a well-circumscribed, dermal-based tumor composed of epithelial and mesenchymal components.[2-5] The epithelial component consists of distorted and hyperplastic pilosebaceous units with prominent sebaceous glands accompanied by a proliferation of basaloid and ductal epithelium. Surrounding and embedding this epithelial component is a somewhat myxoid and fibrillary stroma containing elongate and wavy spindle cells arranged in loosely formed fascicles. Focal palisading may be present, and atypia of the stromal cells, so-called ancient-type or pseudo-sarcomatous change, may be noted.[6,7] Small nerve twigs are interspersed and mast cells are sometimes prominent.[2-5] The stromal and epithelial components appear intimately associated. The features of neurofollicular hamartoma are reminiscent of trichodiscoma and fibrofolliculoma, and these entities possibly represent a morphological spectrum.[3]

Variable expression of S100 protein is identified within these tumors.[2-5] However, S100 positivity is likely present within intralesional S100-positive dendritic cells rather than the lesional spindle cells.[1,3] Furthermore, there is no significant expression of NSE, synaptophysin, GFAP, NFP, EMA, or Leu-7, arguing against true neural differentiation.[1-5] Spindle cells express CD13 and CD34 as well as CD10 and are negative for actin, desmin, Melan-A, and factor XIIIa.[1,8]

Access **ExpertConsult.com** for the complete list of references

See
www.expertconsult.com
for references and
additional material

Tumors and related lesions of the sebaceous glands

CHAPTER

32

Ectopic sebaceous glands

Clinical features

Sebaceous glands are normally found in association with a hair follicle. However, at several mucosal sites, they may develop independently, presenting as small 1- to 3-mm yellow to white papules (Fordyce spots), which can be accentuated when the mucosa is stretched.[1] Lesions of the oral cavity commonly present on the vermilion border of the lip and the buccal mucosa.[1,2] On the vulva, Fordyce spots affect the medial aspect of the labia majora while in males the glans penis is involved.[3] Prevalence varies, but some large studies place the incidence of oral lesions at greater than 25%.[1,2,4] Incidence increases with age since Fordyce spots are not commonly seen in infants.[1,2] They are of little consequence and likely represent a normal physiological variant since such a large proportion of the adult population is affected.[5] Rarely, lesions on the lip become a cosmetic nuisance.[6]

Similar tiny papules are sometimes seen on the areola of the female breast where they are known as Montgomery tubercles.[7-10] These may be associated with vellus hairs or lactiferous ducts, and occasionally in adolescence they are complicated by the development of a small breast lump, which discharges thin secretions.[11] Such lesions tend to resolve spontaneously. Sebaceous hyperplasia of the areola has been reported in both women and men (see below), but its relationship to Montgomery tubercles (if any) is unclear.[12]

Occasionally, ectopic sebaceous glands have been identified in the esophagus, gastroesophageal junction, uterine cervix, vagina, sole of the foot, thymus, and tongue.[13-25] Rarely, these lesions have been described as extensively involving the esophagus.[23]

Histologic features

These lesions are all characterized by the presence of well-formed lobules or small clusters of sebocytes located high in the lamina propria and opening directly onto the epithelial surface.

Sebaceous hyperplasia

Clinical features

Sebaceous hyperplasia is a common condition that is frequently clinically misdiagnosed as basal cell carcinoma. It most often presents on the face of older adults, particularly males (Fig. 32.1).[1] Lesions are, however, occasionally encountered in children.[2-4] The forehead and cheeks are predominantly affected, and occasionally diffuse facial involvement occurs (Fig. 32.2).[1,4,5] Other less common sites include the chest, ocular caruncle, penis, scrotum, and vulva.[6-12] A linear variant presenting has been described on the penis, head and neck region, and chest.[13-16]

Lesions – which may occur individually, in groups, or as a sheet of papules – present as yellowish, dome-shaped asymptomatic papules 1–2 mm in diameter.[1,17] Larger variants measuring 1.0 cm or more in diameter are occasionally seen (giant solitary/senile sebaceous hyperplasia).[18-21] The papule is umbilicated, and individual lobules emanating out from the center can often be identified with a hand lens. Distinctive dermatoscopic features including cumulus sign, crown vessels, and milia-like cysts have been described.[22,23]

Rarely, postpubertal sebaceous hyperplasia occurs, either as an isolated phenomenon or more rarely in association with anhidrotic ectodermal dysplasia.[24,25] Familial cases, sometimes with early onset, have also been described.[26-28] One variant is termed presenile diffuse familial sebaceous hyperplasia.[29] Sebaceous hyperplasia is significantly increased in transplant patients, particularly in males following renal transplantation, and this is likely to be related to therapy with ciclosporine A.[30-36] Eruptive cases in this setting are rarely described.[37,38] A case in an immunosuppressed patient with Senear-Usher syndrome (pemphigus erythematosus) has been reported.[39]

Ectopic sebaceous glands with associated hyperplasia have been described in the oral mucosa and on the areola where lesions may be bilateral (areolar sebaceous hyperplasia).[40-49]

Pathogenesis and histologic features

Although sebaceous development is profoundly affected by androgens, their mode of action in sebaceous hyperplasia may be limited.[50,51] Since these lesions do not regress, it is unclear that they truly represent hyperplasia, which is a reversible phenomenon. Nonetheless, the name sebaceous hyperplasia is certainly indicative of a well-defined clinicopathological entity.

Studies have indicated that overexpression of the mEDA-A1 splice variant of *EDA* which encodes ectodysplasin, a member of the tumor necrosis factor (TNF) ligand family, induces sebaceous hyperplasia in transgenic mice.[52] This transcription factor is involved in skin adnexal development, acting through the nuclear factor-kappaB (NF-κB) and JNK pathways.[52,53] Hemizygous *EDA* pathogenic variant males (X-linked) or biallelic pathogenic variants in *EDAR*, *EDARADD*, or *WNT10A* pathogenic variants in males or females cause hypohidrotic ectodermal dysplasia (HED).[54,55] The relevance

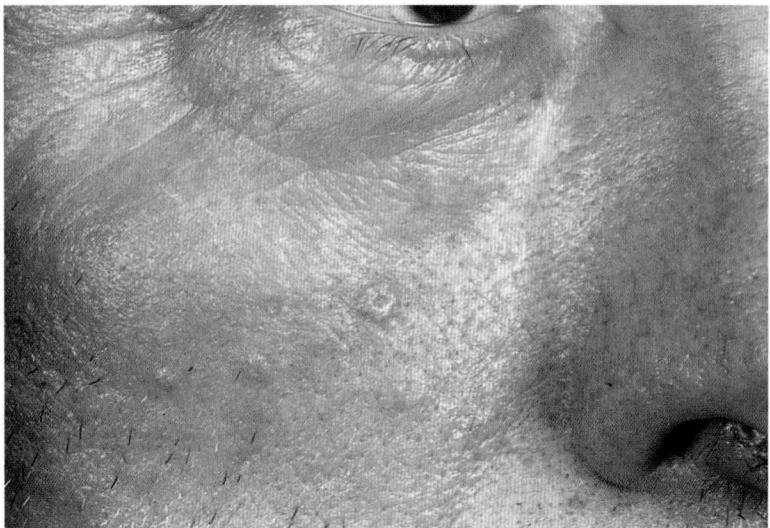

Fig. 32.1
Sebaceous hyperplasia: multiple lesions are present on the cheek. Note the central umbilication. By courtesy of the Institute of Dermatology, London, UK.

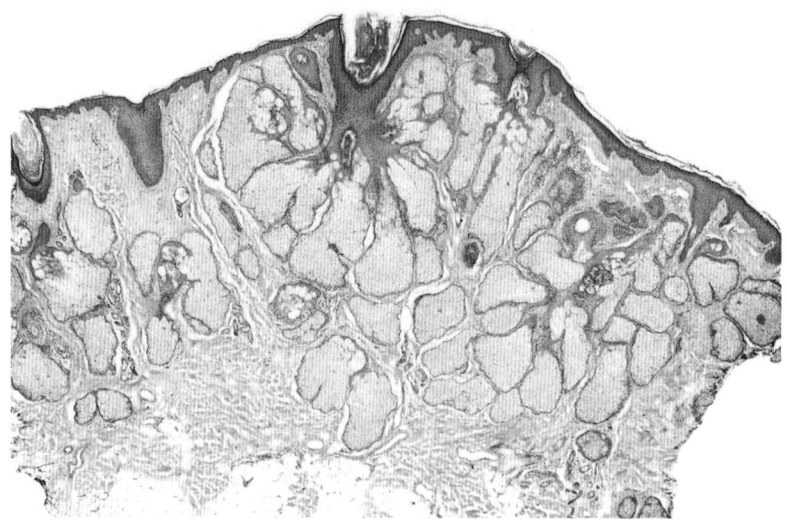

Fig. 32.3
Sebaceous hyperplasia: scanning view showing sebaceous glands grouped around a cystic infundibulum.

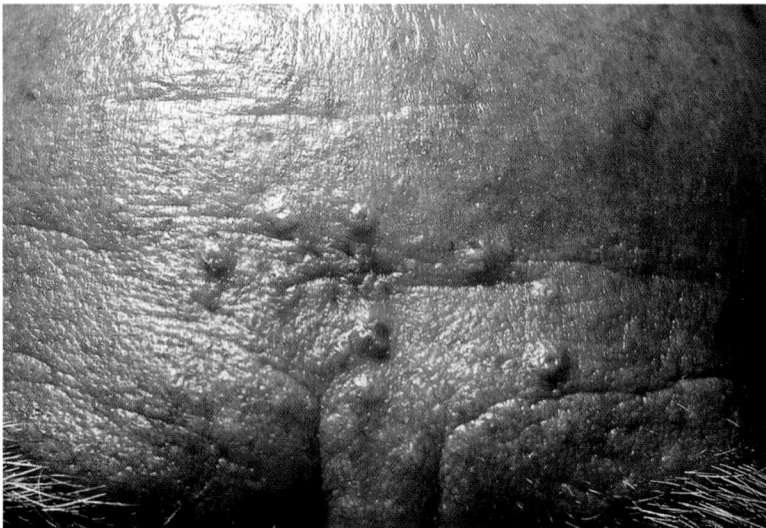

Fig. 32.2
Sebaceous hyperplasia: in this example, a group of papules is present on the forehead, a characteristic site. By courtesy of R.A. Marsden, MD, St George's Hospital, London, UK.

Nevus sebaceous

Clinical features

Nevus sebaceous (Jadassohn, organoid nevus) is not uncommon and often presents at birth although it usually does not cause the patient to seek medical attention until the second to fourth decades.[1–3] Lesions have been described in up to 0.3% of neonates.[4] The sex distribution is equal.

Nevus sebaceous is single, round or oval, well circumscribed, and usually measures 1–6 cm in greatest dimension. It commonly affects the head and neck, particularly the scalp where it presents as a yellowish, flat, or mamillated patch of alopecia (Fig. 32.6). Other sites of predilection include the forehead, temples, around the central face, and behind the ears.[1–3] Rarely, lesions have been documented at other sites including the trunk, breast, limbs, oral cavity, external auditory canal, and perianal region.[3–8] It becomes rather warty during childhood and in adolescence shows marked enlargement with development of a waxy surface under the influence of pubescent hormonal stimulation.[3] In adulthood, any further change is likely to be due to the development of a range of usually benign but sometimes malignant tumors of variable differentiation (Fig. 32.7).[1–3] Less frequently, nevus sebaceous presents as a linear lesion, often behind the ear.[2] Sometimes the lesion is very extensive, and a zosteriform variant has been noted.[9] A few cases of familial nevus sebaceous showing paradominant transmission have been described.[10–16]

Very rarely, congenital nevus sebaceous is associated with other abnormalities, particularly neurological symptoms.[17] Involvement tends to be linear and frequently parasagittal with a wide distribution on the head and scalp, and sometimes it extends to the neck and shoulder.[18,19] Most such cases are classified as linear nevus sebaceous syndrome, which presents with a triad of nevus sebaceous, seizures, and mental retardation.[9,18,19] In practice, however, seizures and mental retardation are not regularly present. Ocular abnormalities are common and other organ systems may also be affected.[19] The seizures are sometimes intractable to medical treatment and may require surgical intervention.[20] Reported complications include unilateral megaencephaly, a hamartomatous intracranial mass, hemimegaencephaly, cerebral arteriovenous malformation, a desmoplastic neuroepithelial tumor, hemifacial asymmetry, complex conjunctival colobomas or choristomas, corneal dermoid, macular and optic nerve hypoplasia, optic glioma, nonparalytic strabismus, partial oculomotor palsy, microphthalmia, retinal detachment, sensorineural deafness, inner ear malformation with hearing loss, rickets, uvula bifida, premature tooth eruption, cleft secondary palate, and diffuse pulmonary angiomatosis.[21–40] Extensive surgical resection with reconstruction may sometimes be required.[41] This condition forms part of the Schimmelpenning syndrome (Schimmelpenning-Feuerstein-Mims syndrome,

of this finding to human sebaceous hyperplasia remains to be determined, although interestingly and perhaps incongruously, sebaceous hyperplasia as mentioned above has been reported in the setting of HED.[24,25,56]

Very recently, activating mutations in *HRAS*, *KRAS*, and *EGFR* have been documented in a subset of sebaceous hyperplasia, suggesting that despite the term hyperplasia, these lesions might be best considered as neoplasia.[57]

In solitary papules, the individual gland is hyperplastic and situated higher in the dermis than normal (Fig. 32.3).[58] Individual lobules are increased in number but are not appreciably different in size compared with normal sebaceous glands. The individual lobules drain into a central duct, which is often associated with a hair follicle, through single or multiple follicular infundibula (Figs 32.4 and 32.5).[59] In confluent lesions, multiple sebaceous glands are similarly affected. In both variants the dermis is normal, except for a variable degree of elastosis.

Mucosal sebaceous hyperplasia is not associated with a hair follicle, and the lobules empty into a single duct that opens directly onto the surface.[41,48]

Sebaceous hyperplasia overlying a benign fibrous histiocytoma (dermatofibroma) has been documented, including its dermatoscopic features.[60–63]

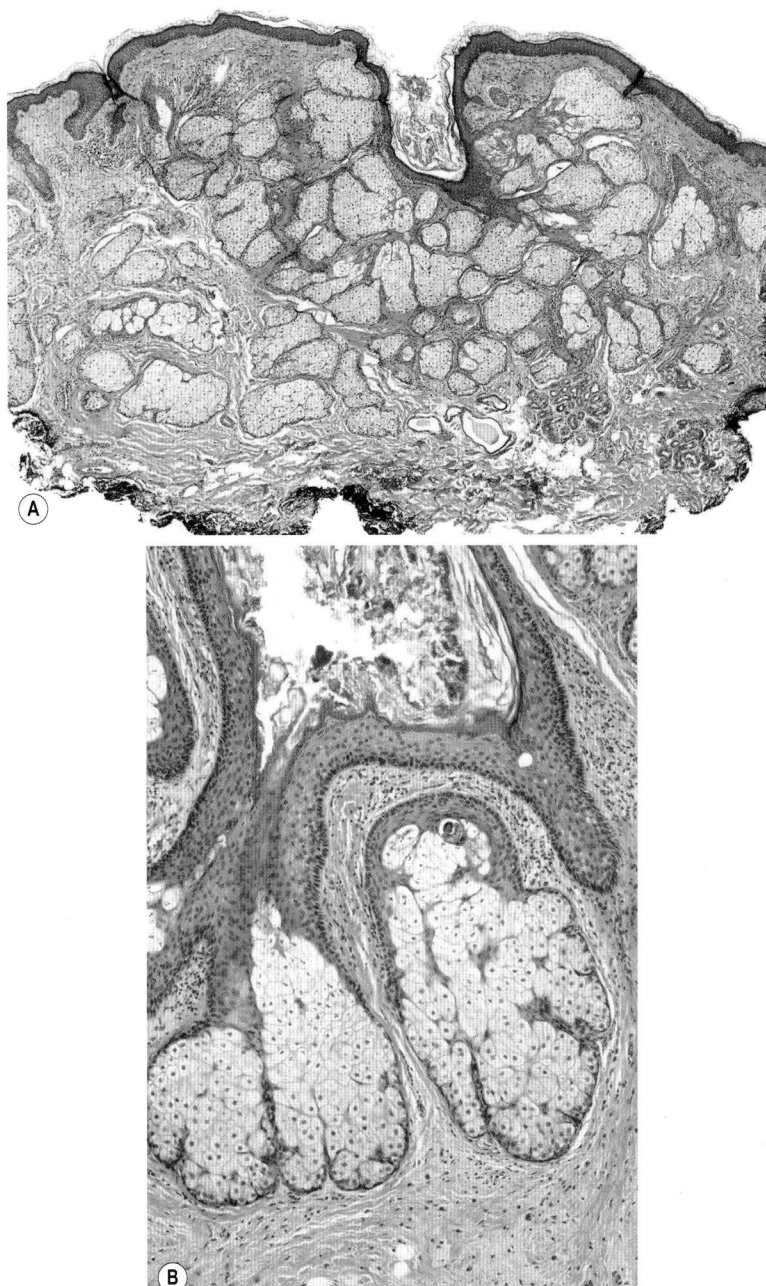

Fig. 32.4
(**A**, **B**) Sebaceous hyperplasia: the sebaceous lobules drain through short ductules into the central duct.

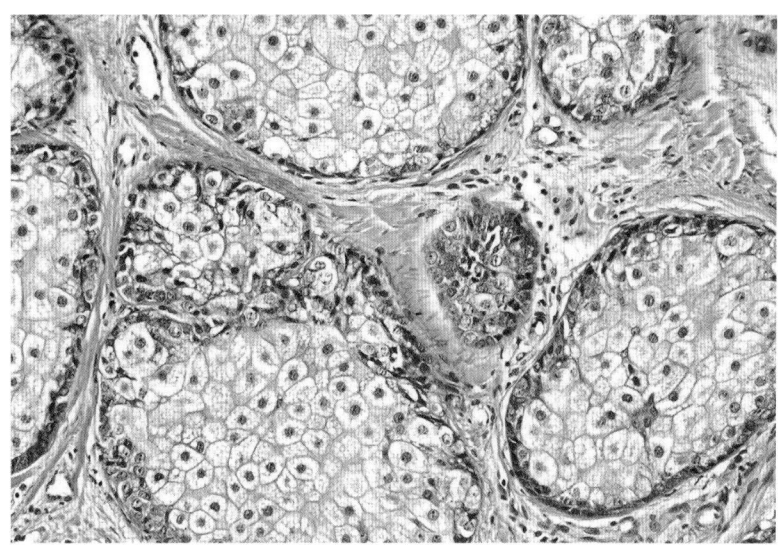

Fig. 32.5
Sebaceous hyperplasia: the hyperplastic sebaceous lobules mirror the normal sebaceous gland and consist of an outer layer of basaloid cells surrounding mature sebaceous cells with eosinophilic bubbly cytoplasm.

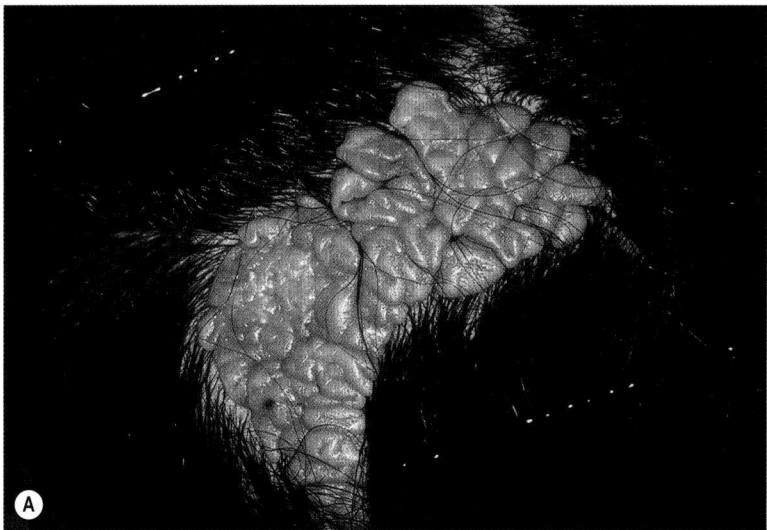

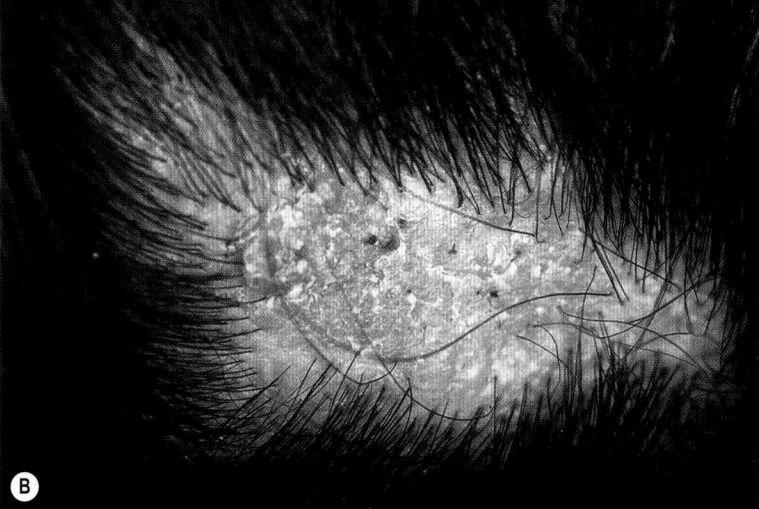

Fig. 32.6
Nevus sebaceous: (**A**) lesions most commonly affect the scalp; (**B**) this example shows the characteristic yellow cerebriform appearance. By courtesy of R.A. Marsden, MD, St George's Hospital, London, UK.

organoid nevus phakomatosis), which represents a distinct clinicopathological subset of the epidermal nevus syndrome.[42–44] SCALP syndrome has been described as consisting of the combination of nevus sebaceous, central nervous system malformations, aplasia cutis congenita, limbal dermoid, and pigmented nevus.[45]

Nomenclature and classification schemes for the epidermal nevus syndrome are complex, with overlapping entities and variable associated defects.[46] Nevus sebaceous can coexist with other epidermal nevi, including verrucous epidermal nevus, possibly representing a continuum of manifestations.[47]

Other rare associations, not clearly syndromic and perhaps incidental, include melorheostosis, mediastinal lipomatosis, and familial retinoblastoma.[48–50] Nevus sebaceous has also been reported in a child with nevoid basal cell carcinoma syndrome.[51] A nevus sebaceous has been reported as a paired phacomatosis pigmentokeratotica with speckled lentiginous nevus of the abdominal wall in which an embryonal rhabdomyosarcoma arose in one exceptional case.[16]

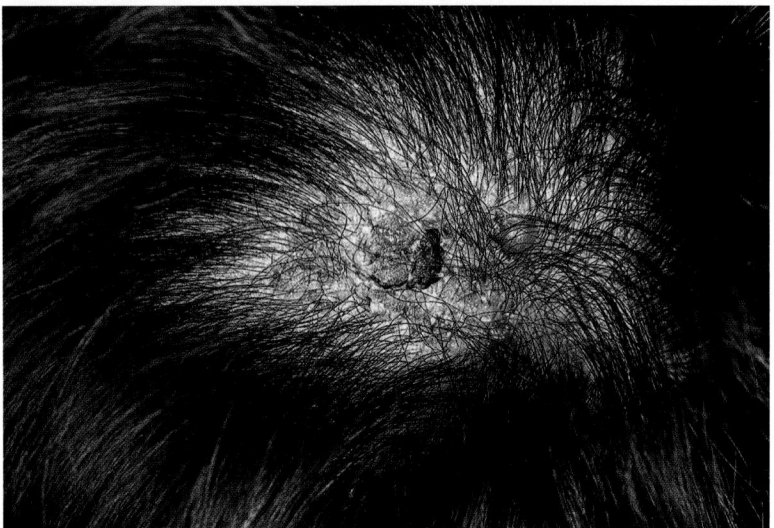

Fig. 32.7
Nevus sebaceous: in this example, basal cell carcinoma has developed in a nevus sebaceous. Courtesy of J.C. Pascual, MD, Alicante, Spain.

Pathogenesis and histologic features

Deletion of the *PTCH* gene has been reported in nevus sebaceous.[52] The *PTCH* pathway is involved in cutaneous patterning and development.[53-56] This finding has some relevance, particularly in the context of the disordered epithelium and appendageal structures characteristic of this lesion. However, such *PTCH* deletions have not been confirmed by others and additional research is necessary.[57] More recently, nevus sebaceous has been recognized to be associated with RAS family mutations – primarily in *HRAS* (in particular, c.37G>C; p.Gly13Arg) and much less frequently *KRAS*.[58,59] The condition is now conceptualized as a mosaic RASopathy produced from a section of skin with a RAS mutation.[60,61] When not limited to the skin, these mosaic mutations can produce the more severe effects seen in some of the nevus sebaceous associated disorders. The diverse family of epidermal nevus syndromes appear to have similar genetic origins, though the characteristic mutations vary.[46] A mouse skin graft model with nevus sebaceous-like lesions which appear to have been induced by aberrantly transplanted dermal fibroblasts has been described, demonstrating that stromal epithelial interactions may also be of importance.[62]

Nevus sebaceous is a complex lesion comprising abnormalities of the epidermis, hair follicle, and sebaceous and sweat glands. The epidermis may be acanthotic or papillomatous and foci of abortive hair papillae-like proliferations are commonly seen (*Figs 32.8* and *32.9*). The epithelium in older lesions sometimes contains foci of pale-staining glycogen-rich cells, suggesting outer root sheath differentiation reminiscent of trichilemmoma.

Sebaceous glands are variably hyperplastic and excessive, diminished in number, or even absent (*Fig. 32.10*). In early infancy, the sebaceous glands often show a transient enlargement under the lingering influence of maternal hormones, but they then diminish in size until adolescence when they undergo marked proliferation. This is followed by a tendency to involution with increasing age. Virtually all lesions show irregularities of morphology and distribution of sebaceous glands. Commonly, they are located at an abnormally high level within the dermis, sometimes communicating directly with the surface of the epidermis (*Fig. 32.11*). Often, they appear unrelated to a hair follicle. A punched-out defect at the periphery of a lobule is occasionally seen, presumably representing coalescence of several mature lipid-laden sebaceous epithelial cells.

A very common finding is an absence or great reduction in the number of mature hair follicles. This is invariable in scalp lesions. In many cases, ectopic apocrine glands are present within the lower dermis.

Nevus sebaceous is frequently complicated by development of a variety of other benign cutaneous neoplasms including syringocystadenoma papilliferum, trichoblastoma-like lesions, trichilemmoma, sebaceous neoplasms, keratoacanthoma-like lesions, viral wart, seborrheic keratosis,

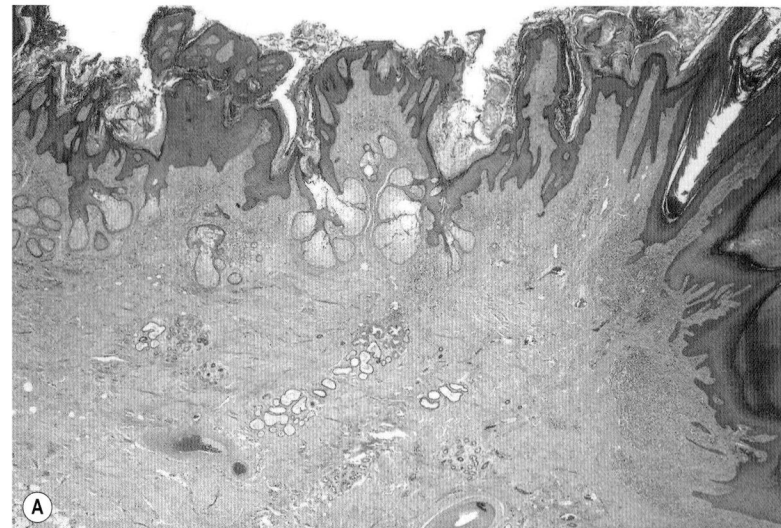

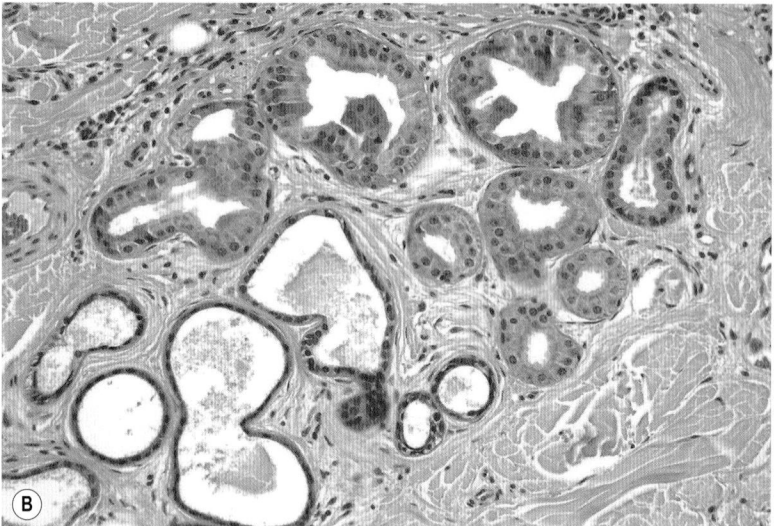

Fig. 32.8
Nevus sebaceous: (**A**) there is marked papillomatosis with hyperkeratosis. Note the almost complete absence of hair follicles. Apocrine glands are present in the center of the field; (**B**) high-power view showing apocrine glands.

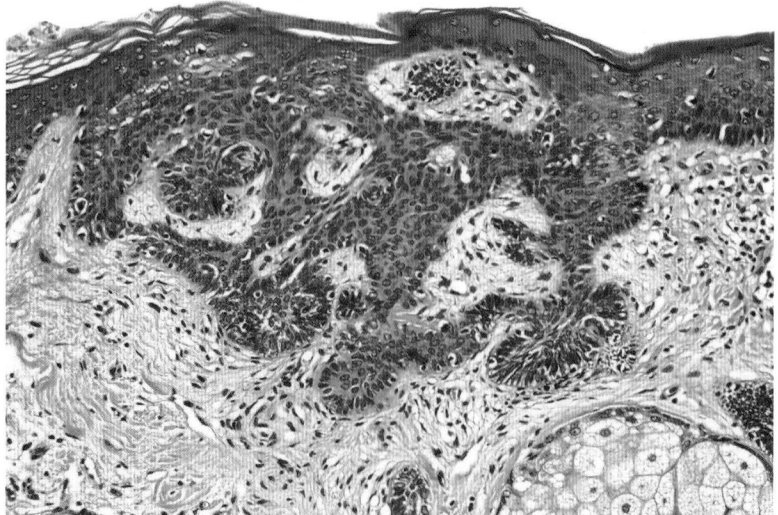

Fig. 32.9
Nevus sebaceous: several primitive hair germlike proliferations arising from the epidermis are seen in this field. Note the peripheral palisading.

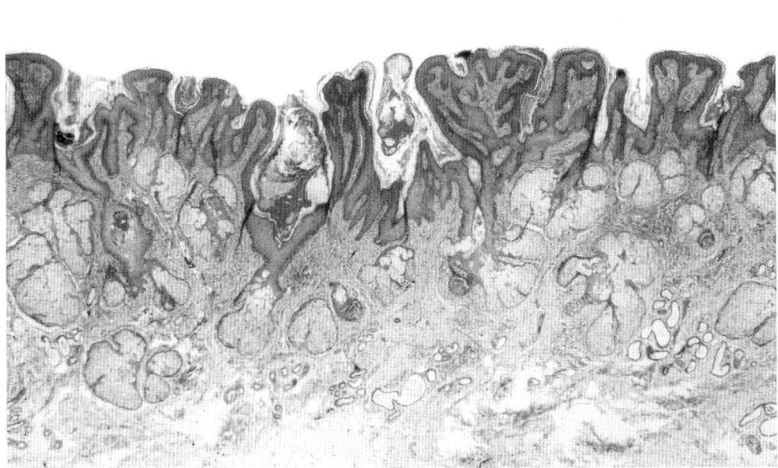

Fig. 32.10
Nevus sebaceous: in this example, there are excessive numbers of sebaceous glands. Note the absence of hair follicles.

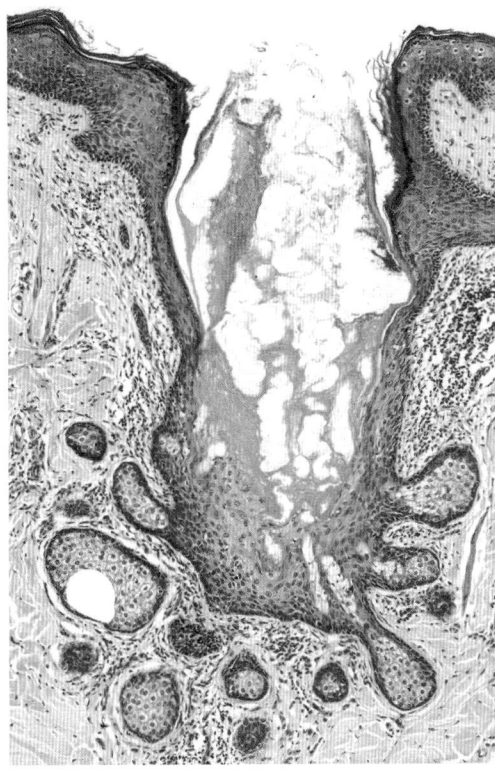

Fig. 32.11
Nevus sebaceous: in this field, the sebaceous gland communicates directly with the epidermis.

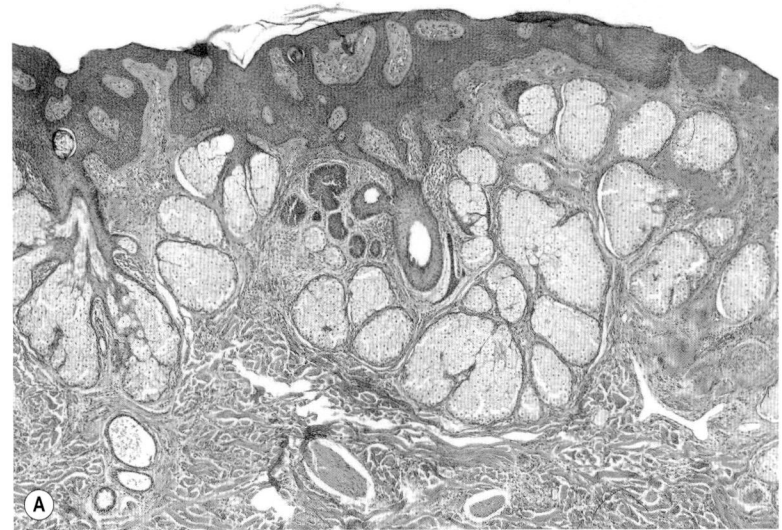

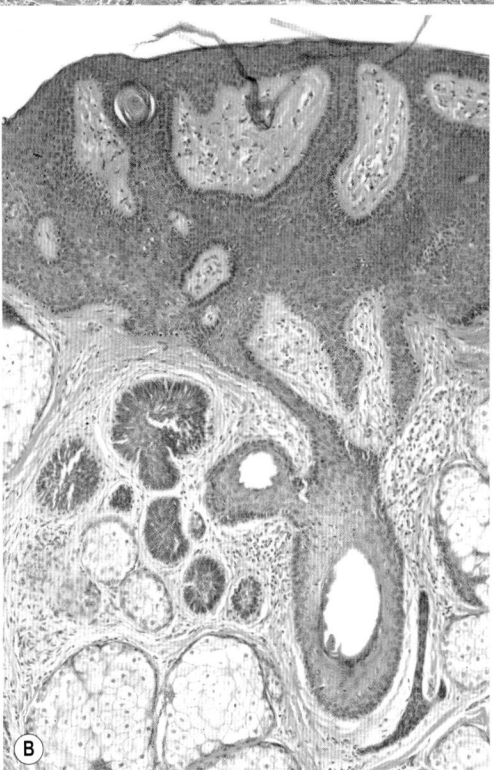

Fig. 32.12
Nevus sebaceous: (**A**) a small evolving trichoblastoma is present in the center of the field; (**B**) these lesions were previously regarded as basal cell carcinoma.

giant cutaneous horn, spiradenoma, pilar leiomyoma, nodular hidradenoma, dermal lipoma, banal melanocytic nevus, combined blue and speckled lentiginous nevus, infundibuloma, apocrine cystadenoma, tubular apocrine adenoma, syringoma, and extramedullary hematopoiesis.[1,63-72] Large studies indicate that syringocystadenoma papilliferum (2–5%) and trichoblastoma-like proliferations (2–7%) are the most commonly encountered lesions while trichilemmoma and sebaceoma are present in 2% to 3% of cases, with other lesions being less frequent (*Figs 32.12–32.16*).[72-75] The benign secondary lesions show associations with the site of the lesion and age of the patient.[74] These benign secondary lesions show the same *HRAS* and *KRAS* mutations as seen in the nevus sebaceous; additional mutations have not been demonstrated.[58-61] Many of the secondary tumors seen in nevus sebaceous are also associated with RAS family mutations when

encountered outside of this context and thus are sufficient as a cause.[76,77] Why secondary tumors are only seen in a subset of lesions is unclear. This process could be sporadic or perhaps be due to the mosaic nature of nevus sebaceous and thus which cell types and lineages harbor the mutations. Malignant tumors are much less often seen and include basal cell carcinoma, squamous cell carcinoma, melanoma, sebaceous carcinoma, eccrine porocarcinoma, dermal leiomyosarcoma, apocrine carcinoma, microcystic adnexal carcinoma, and trichilemmal carcinoma.[1,73,74,78-87] These malignant secondary tumors have not been well studied for additional mutations. Historically, basal cell carcinoma was thought to represent the most common malignant neoplasm arising in association with nevus sebaceous with incidences reported as high as 20%.[1-3] Other more recent studies, however, have much lower prevalences and indicate that the majority of cases of basal cell carcinoma arising in nevus sebaceous are more accurately classified as benign trichoblastoma-like lesions, although authentic basal cell carcinoma is occasionally seen, primarily in older patients (postpuberty).[72,73,88-90] Both benign and malignant secondary lesions are more commonly encountered in adults, although children may also rarely be affected with malignancy

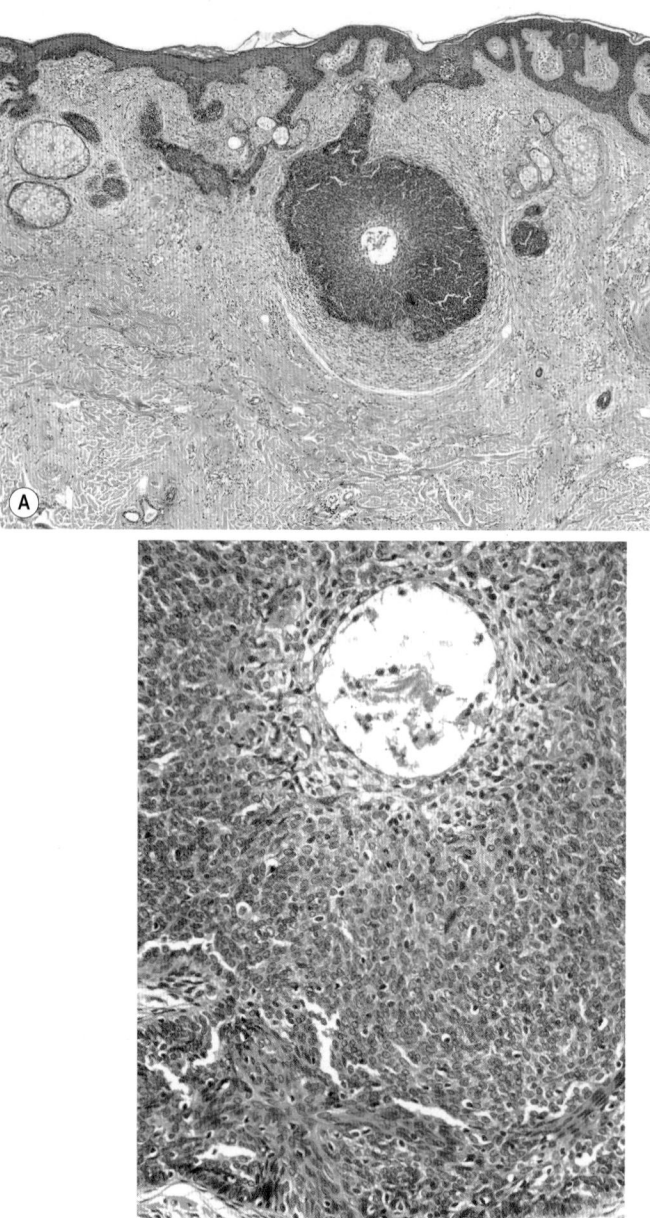

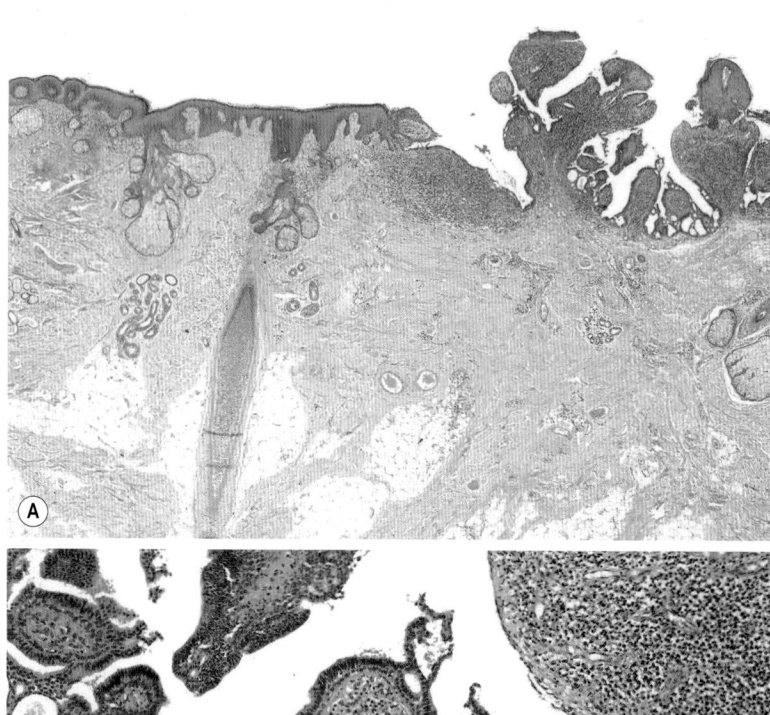

Fig. 32.14
(**A**, **B**) Nevus sebaceous: this example shows a syringocystadenoma papilliferum. Note the villous processes covered by a double layer of epithelium.

Fig. 32.13
Nevus sebaceous: (**A**) multinodular trichoblastoma; (**B**) the tumor cells have very regular, small, round-to-oval nuclei. Note the absence of mitoses or apoptosis.

being exceedingly rare.[73,78,88–91] Nonetheless, the currently perceived scarcity of malignancy in childhood nevus sebaceous has called into question the necessity of early prophylactic excision.[92,93] Nevus sebaceous not uncommonly shows multiple tumorlike proliferations.[89,91] Sometimes, these defy precise classification.[89]

Steatocystoma and sebocystomatosis

Clinical features

Steatocystoma multiplex, characterized by autosomal dominant inheritance, usually presents in adolescence.[1,2] Some cases lack a family history and are considered to be sporadic.[3] Although the sternal region is commonly affected tumors males, and the axillae and groins en females, lesions (which are invariably multiple) may involve most of the upper trunk and face. More localized variants presenting on the face, scalp, nose, acral sites, vulva, and scrotum have been described.[4–16] Scrotal cases can show calcification.[17,18] A linear form is very infrequently encountered.[10,19,20]

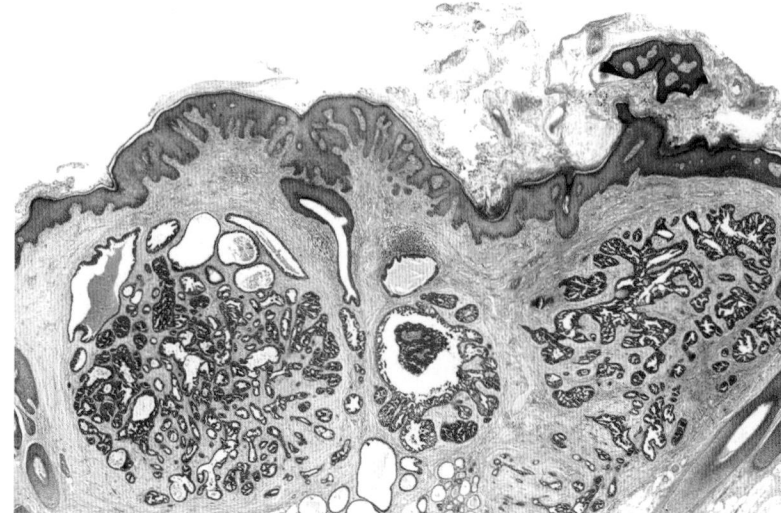

Fig. 32.15
Nevus sebaceous: this apocrine papillary adenoma arose in a background of nevus sebaceous.

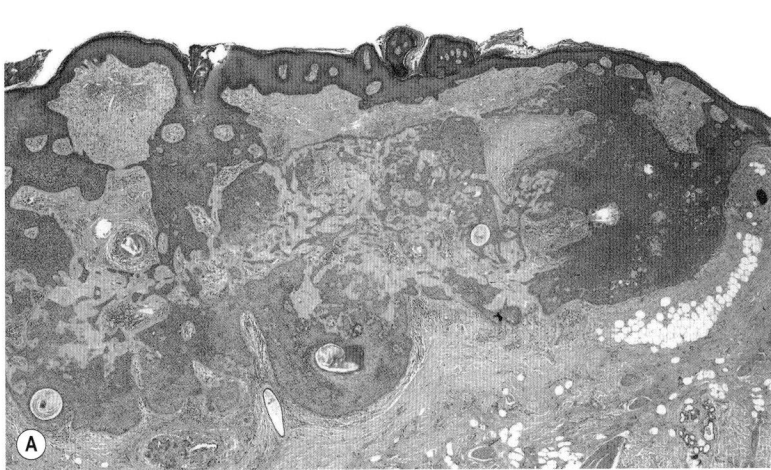

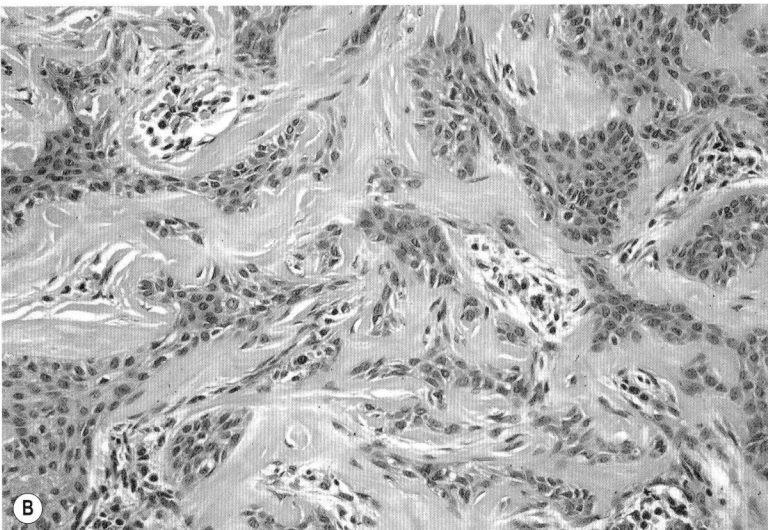

Fig. 32.16
(**A**, **B**) Nevus sebaceous: desmoplastic trichilemmoma arising in a background of nevus sebaceous.

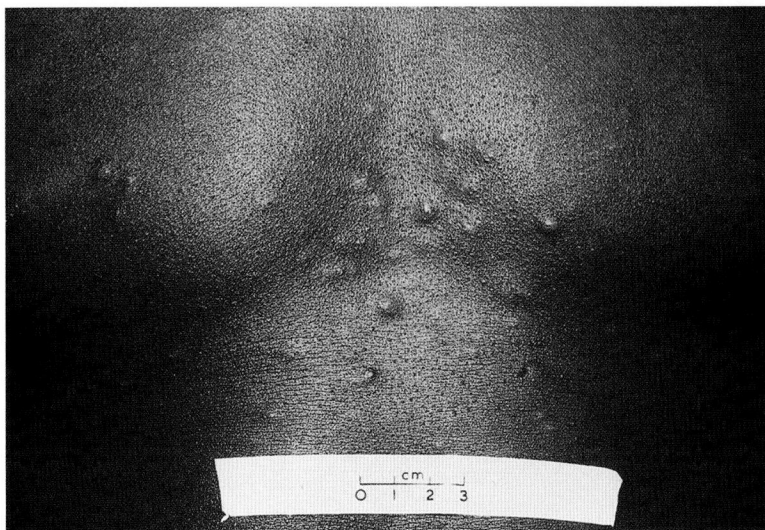

Fig. 32.17
Steatocystoma multiplex: numerous small yellowish papules are present on the chest. By courtesy of R.A. Marsden, MD, St George's Hospital, London, UK.

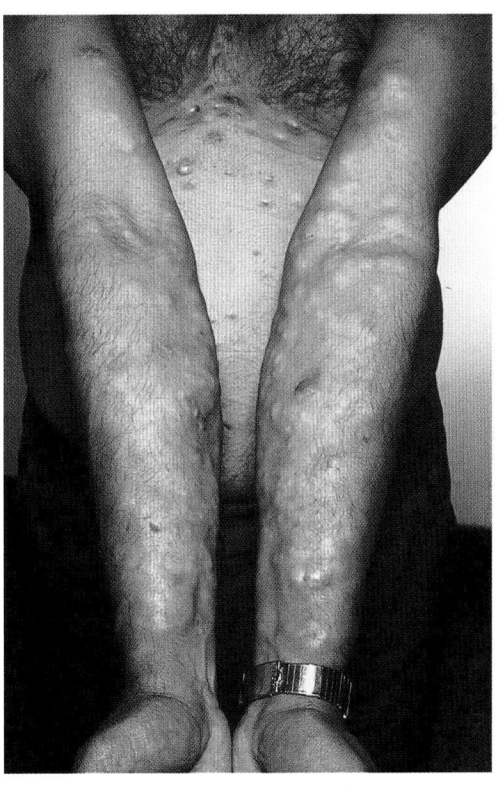

Fig. 32.18
Steatocystoma multiplex: a rather more extensive case showing involvement of the arms in addition to the chest and abdomen. By courtesy of R.A. Marsden, MD, St George's Hospital, London, UK.

Early small dome-shaped lesions are rather translucent, changing to a yellowish color with age (*Figs 32.17* and *32.18*). Puncta are not obvious, but comedones are often associated features.[21] Spontaneous rupture of the cysts sometimes results in steatocystoma multiplex suppurativum characterized by inflammation and scarring reminiscent of acne conglobata.[22–25]

Rarely reported associations include natal teeth, hidradenitis suppurativa, bilateral preauricular sinuses, multiple trichoblastomas, familial hypobetalipoproteinemia, cerebellar ataxia, intracranial dermoid, LEOPARD syndrome (lentigines, electrocardiographic conduction defects, ocular hypertelorism, pulmonary stenosis, abnormalities of the genitalia, retarded growth with short stature, deafness), familial syringoma, polycystic kidney disease 1 (Alagille syndrome), and Lowe (oculocerebrorenal) syndrome.[26–35] Spherulocystic disease (myospherulosis) has also been described.[36]

Steatocystoma simplex, in which patients present with a solitary lesion, shows an equal sex incidence and usually affects adults.[37] The cysts are asymptomatic and well circumscribed. They are particularly found on the face or neck, chest, axillae, and arms.[38] Involvement of the oral cavity and ocular caruncle has been described, albeit uncommonly.[39–41]

On occasion, steatocystoma multiplex and eruptive vellus hair cysts have been described in the same patient, suggesting a possible pathogenic relationship.[3,42–49]

Pathogenesis and histologic features

Mutations in *KRT17* (encoding keratin 17), which is expressed in the nail matrix, hair follicles, and sebaceous glands, have been documented in families with steatocystoma multiplex.[50–53] Similar mutations have also been described in the autosomal dominant disease pachyonychia congenita 1 (formerly known as Jadassohn-Lewandowsky type) caused by *KRT16* mutations and pachyonychia congenita 2 (formerly known as Jackson-Lawler type) caused by *KRT17* mutations; mutations in *KRT6A* and *KRT6B* underlie the other forms of this disease.[54–56] The cysts in pachyonychia type 1 are sometimes described more as pilosebaceous cysts than true steatocysts.[57] Cysts are more common in the *KRT17* cases than in the other types.[57] These shared mutations offer a pathogenetic basis for occasional cases of these two conditions occurring in the same individual.[58–61] The presence of a mutation in *KRT17* within a single family cohort can lead to affected

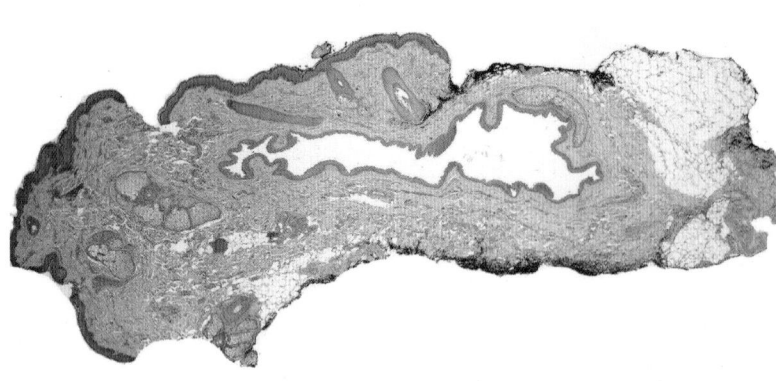

Fig. 32.19
Steatocystoma multiplex: this low-power view shows a collapsed empty cyst lined by squamous epithelium.

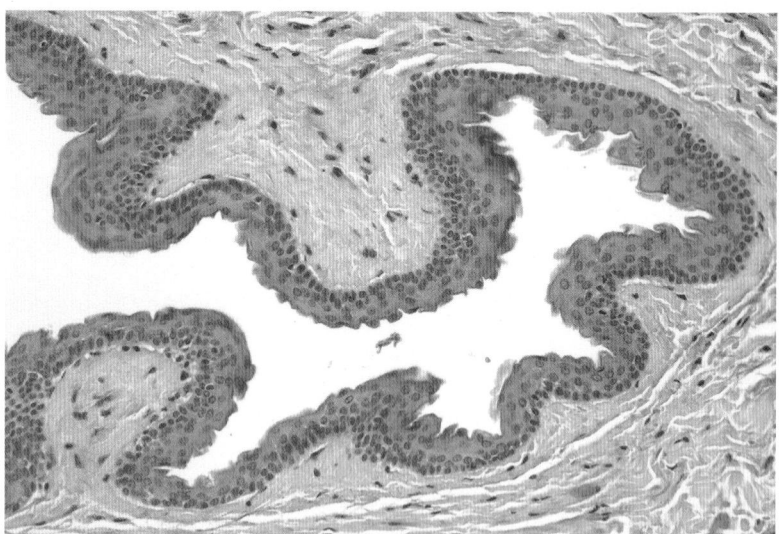

Fig. 32.21
Steatocystoma multiplex: a thick, wavy refractile hyaline cuticle covers the surface of the epithelium.

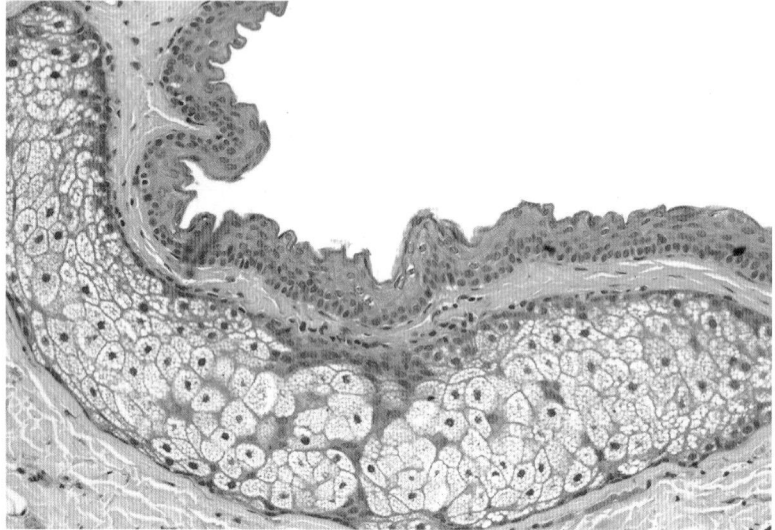

Fig. 32.20
Steatocystoma multiplex: the presence of sebaceous glands within the cyst wall is a characteristic feature.

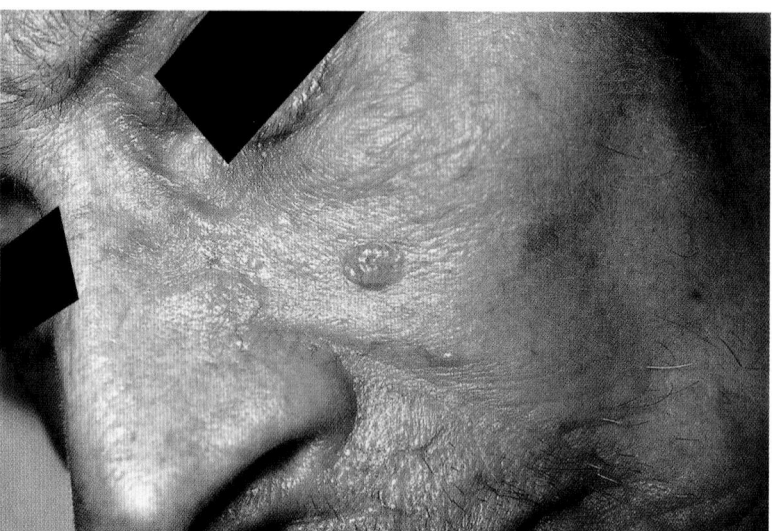

Fig. 32.22
Sebaceous adenoma: note the yellow papule on the cheek of this elderly patient. By courtesy of R.A. Marsden, MD, St George's Hospital, London, UK.

members with only pachyonychia congenita type II or only steatocystoma multiplex.[54] Mutations in *KRT17* have not been described in steatocystoma simplex.

It is of some relevance that eruptive vellus hair cysts have also been described in association with pachyonychia congenita since a number of authors believe that there is significant morphological overlap between eruptive vellus hair cyst and steatocystoma.[3,43,44,47,49,62–65] Although eruptive vellus hair cysts express keratin 17, steatocystoma also expresses keratin 10 and thus other authorities believe that the two conditions can be clearly distinguished.[54,66] Mutations in KRT17 have not been described (or carefully explored) in the familial or sporadic forms of eruptive vellus hairs cysts, and thus the exact pathogenic relationship between these two lesions remains to be determined.[48]

Steatocystoma probably represents a true sebaceous cyst since its lining mirrors the point where the sebaceous duct enters the hair follicle.[67] The thin-walled dermal cyst is usually collapsed and folded, appearing empty except for sebaceous debris and rarely a hair fragment (*Figs 32.19* and *32.20*).[37] The lining typically comprises a few cells forming stratified squamous epithelium and maturing into a homogeneous, undulating eosinophilic cuticle without the formation of a granular layer (*Fig. 32.21*).[38] Sebaceous

glands are an almost invariable feature, either within the squamous lining itself or adjacent to it.

The lesions of steatocystoma multiplex and simplex are histologically indistinguishable.

Sebaceous adenoma

Clinical features

Sebaceous adenoma is rare and frequently misdiagnosed clinically as a basal cell carcinoma. It presents most often in older people (mean age, 60 years) as a tan, pink-to-red, or yellow papulonodule measuring approximately 0.5 cm in greatest dimension.[1–3] Occasionally, it has a polypoid appearance.[2] The face (particularly the nose and cheek) and scalp are most often affected (*Figs 32.22* and *32.23*).[2] Less commonly affected sites include the ear and medial canthus, and occasionally lesions have been described on the trunk, leg, arm, and penis.[2,4,5]

Sebaceous adenoma forms part of the spectrum of the Muir-Torre syndrome, particularly those that arise outside the head and neck region.[6–9] Occasional reports have documented its presence in patients with the

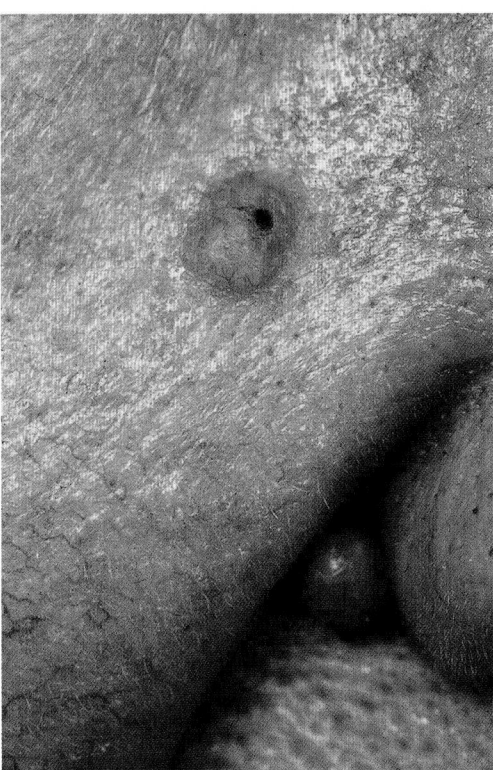

Fig. 32.23
Sebaceous adenoma: this example is dome-shaped and has a slightly scaly surface. By courtesy of R.A. Marsden, MD, St George's Hospital, London, UK.

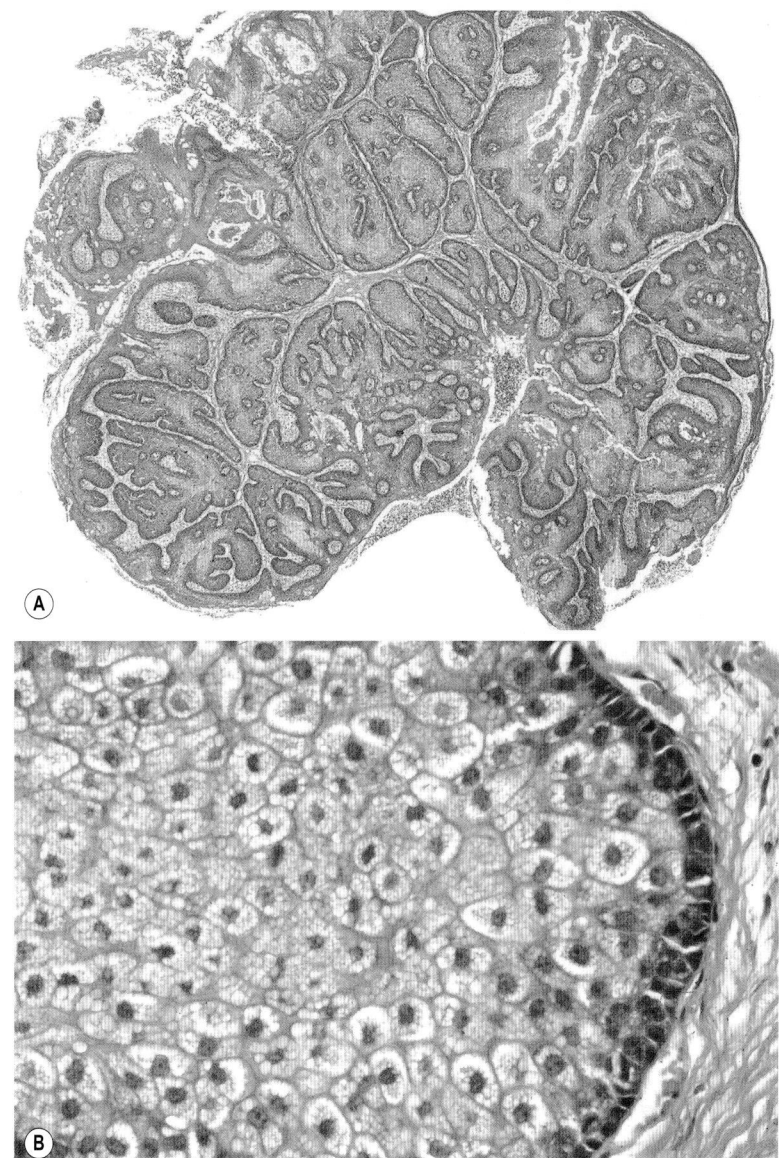

Fig. 32.24
Sebaceous adenoma: (**A**) this example has been shelled out. Note the circumscribed border; (**B**) there is a peripheral layer of basophilic germinative cells and inner sebaceous cells with bubbly cytoplasm and crenated nuclei.

acquired immunodeficiency syndrome (AIDS).[10,11] Rarely, it may develop intraorally, possibly in association with Fordyce papules.[3,12-18] Sebaceous adenoma has rarely been described in the submandibular and parotid glands.[19-22]

Pathogenesis and histologic features

Inactivating mutations in *LEF1*, the gene encoding a transcription factor in the Wnt/β-catenin pathway, have been documented in a subset of sebaceous adenomas.[23] This pathway is involved in fate selection of follicular stem cells to adopt sebaceous differentiation and may also directly promote tumorigenesis.[24,25] The hedgehog and c-Myc pathways may also be involved in tumorigenesis.[24,26] Broader sequencing methods have revealed mutations in *CDKN2A*, *EGFR*, *CTNNB1*, *KRAS*, and *TP53*.[27]

The tumor is multilobulated and sometimes appears to replace the surface epithelium (*Fig. 32.24*).[1,2] Individual lobules, often surrounded by a collagenous pseudocapsule, mirror the structure of a normal sebaceous gland. At the periphery are a variable number of layers of small germinative cells with round or oval vesicular nuclei and scanty cytoplasm.[2,3] This increased number of basaloid or germinative cells allows separation from sebaceous hyperplasia, which has at most two layers of basal cells.[28] The basaloid cells blend with the usually more centrally located mature sebaceous cells, which are much larger and have pale-staining foamy cytoplasm and central crenated hyperchromatic nuclei.[28,29] Occasionally, peripheral palisading is a feature.[2] Some lobules show cystic degeneration and others appear to communicate directly with the surface epithelium. By convention, more than half of the lobule in sebaceous adenoma is composed of mature sebaceous cells.[28]

Sometimes, giant sebaceous adenomas are encountered which may show increased mitotic activity in the basaloid cell component (*Figs 32.25* and *32.26*). This should not be interpreted as implying malignant potential.

The intervening dermis may contain a chronic inflammatory cell infiltrate including lymphocytes, histiocytes, and plasma cells.[30] An overlying cutaneous horn has been described.[31]

A large study has shown substantial interobserver variation in the diagnosis of circumscribed sebaceous neoplasms within the categories of sebaceous adenoma, sebaceoma, and sebaceous carcinoma.[32]

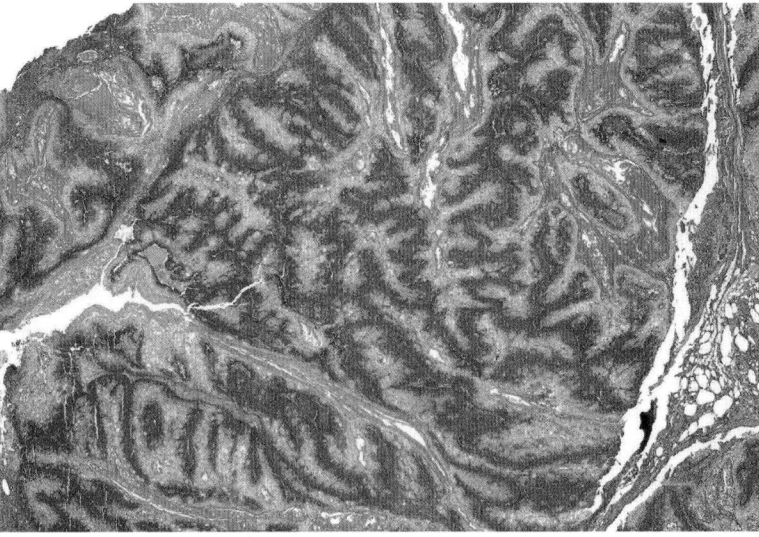

Fig. 32.25
Sebaceous adenoma: part of an ulcerated giant variant.

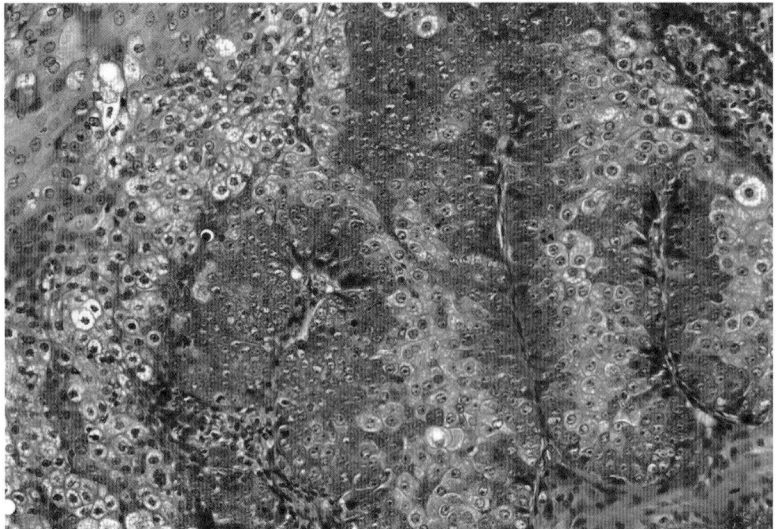

Fig. 32.26
Sebaceous adenoma: higher-power view showing retention of the architecture with peripheral basaloid cells and inner sebocytes. Note the mitotic figures.

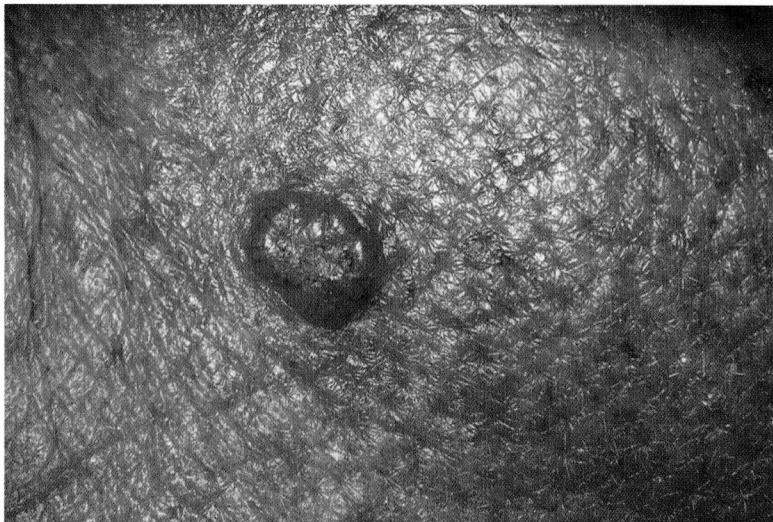

Fig. 32.27
Sebaceoma: yellowish nodule on the forehead of an elderly patient. By courtesy of the Institute of Dermatology, London, UK.

Sebaceous epithelioma

Few terms have caused as much confusion in dermatopathology as sebaceous epithelioma. This tumor has been variably recognized as a distinct lesion, as a variant of sebaceous adenoma, as an intermediate stage between sebaceous adenoma and basal cell carcinoma, and as a synonym for basal cell carcinoma with sebaceous differentiation. Troy and Ackerman introduced the term sebaceoma to help clarify this morass and proposed that the term sebaceous epithelioma be abandoned.[1] Sebaceoma is clearly defined and distinguishable from sebaceous hyperplasia, sebaceous adenoma, and sebaceous carcinoma. Over time, use of sebaceous epithelioma as a diagnostic term has declined; most recent papers use this terminology primarily in the canine setting or historically in reviews.[2-5] The publications that have documented tumors described as sebaceous epithelioma have illustrations that are clearly not those of basal cell carcinoma with sebaceous differentiation and are indistinguishable from the description of sebaceoma.[6-9] While we have sympathy with the view of Dinneen and Mehregan that 'the term sebaceous epithelioma has merit for historical reasons and because the tumor can be locally destructive', we believe that its continued use will only perpetuate the confusion in the literature.[9] Sebaceoma appears to be established as the diagnostic terminology of choice for this tumor and, as in the third and fourth editions, we have adopted the term sebaceoma and no longer recognize sebaceous epithelioma as an entity. The alternative term sebomatricoma, which includes sebaceous adenoma and sebaceoma as opposite ends of a spectrum of benign sebaceous tumors, has not received significant support in the literature.[10,11]

Sebaceoma

Clinical features

Sebaceoma presents as a yellow-to-orange or flesh-colored papule, nodule, or tumor measuring approximately 1–3 cm in diameter (Fig. 32.27).[1-7] A giant variant measuring up to 6.0 cm in greatest dimension has also been described.[2,8] The tumor presents more often in females (4:1) though one large recent series should support a more equal distribution and, while a wide age range may be affected (29–87 years), the majority of patients are in the sixth to ninth decades.[9] Lesions predominantly affect the face and scalp, although a single report has described a case developing on the chest.[4] Sebaceoma arising in continuity with a seborrheic keratosis has been documented and some examples have arisen within nevus sebaceous[2,3,10-13] Importantly, sebaceoma may reflect associated Muir-Torre syndrome.[4,5,9,14,15]

Recurrences or metastasis has not been reported.

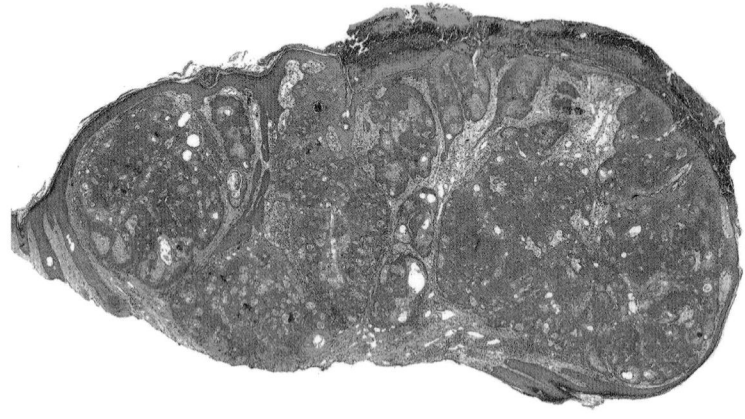

Fig. 32.28
Sebaceoma: there is a multinodular dermal tumor showing multiple points of origin/contact with the epidermis.

Histologic features

Sebaceoma is centered in the dermis and only rarely affects the subcutaneous fat (Figs 32.28 and 32.29).[1] Epidermal involvement is often present. It consists of multiple variably sized, discrete nodules, symmetrically distributed and separated by dense eosinophilic connective tissue (Fig. 32.30).[1-4] The nodules are composed of an admixture of basaloid cells and mature sebocytes lacking an organized lobular architecture.[1] Peripheral nuclear palisading and cleftlike spaces separating the tumor nodules from the adjacent stroma are absent.[1]

The basaloid cells are small and uniform with minimal indistinct cytoplasm and round to oval nuclei, sometimes containing small nucleoli (Fig. 32.31). There is no nuclear pleomorphism and mitotic activity is generally sparse, although as with other basaloid cutaneous neoplasms (e.g., pilomatrixoma) it can sometimes be prominent. The sebaceous cells appear mature with eosinophilic bubbly cytoplasm and scalloped nuclei, but this process is usually distributed in multiple pockets throughout the proliferation rather than being centralized, as seen in sebaceous adenoma. Duct formation is frequently present and cysts containing sebaceous debris lined by an eosinophilic cuticle are often present within the nodule or at its edges (Figs 32.32 and 32.33). Focal glandular differentiation with apocrine features has been

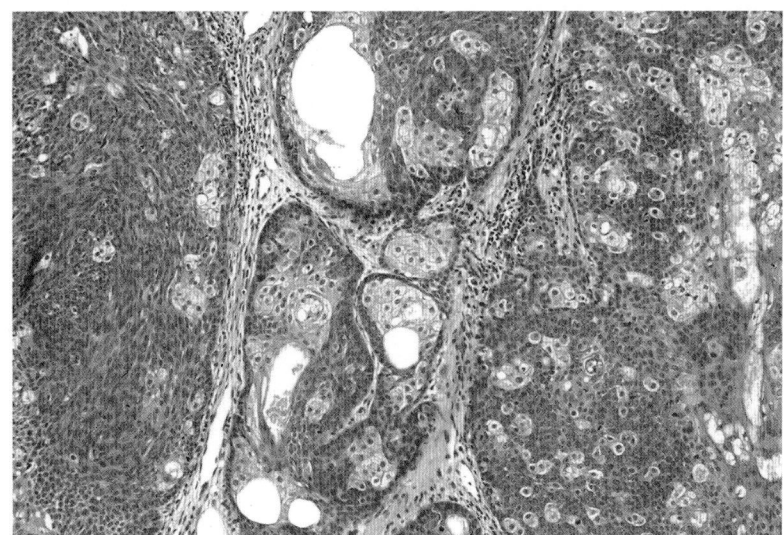

Fig. 32.29
Sebaceoma: the tumor is composed of multiple lobules separated by connective tissue septa.

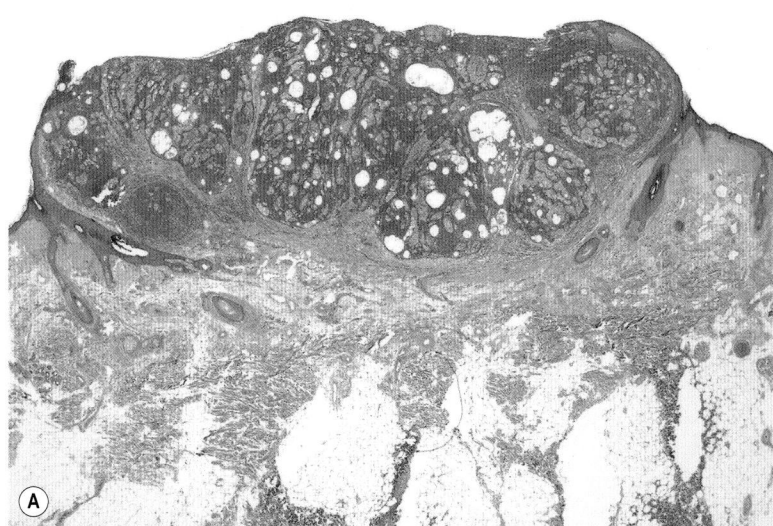

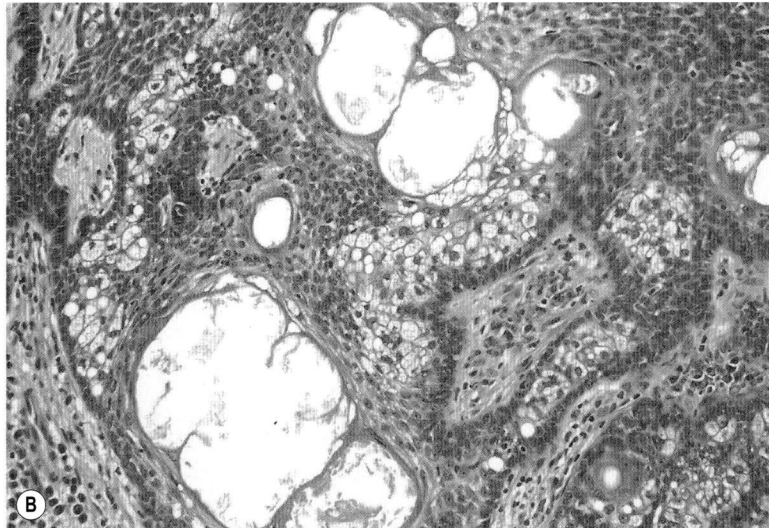

Fig. 32.30
Sebaceoma: (A) scanning view showing conspicuous cyst formation; (B) high-power view of cysts.

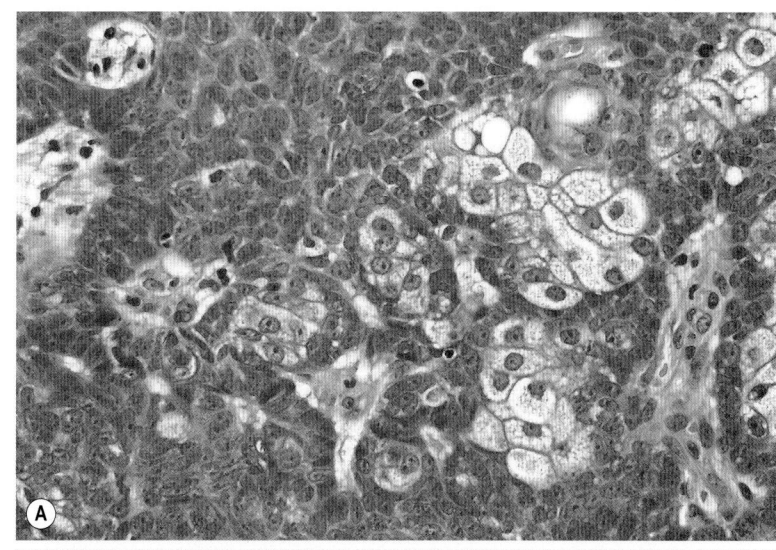

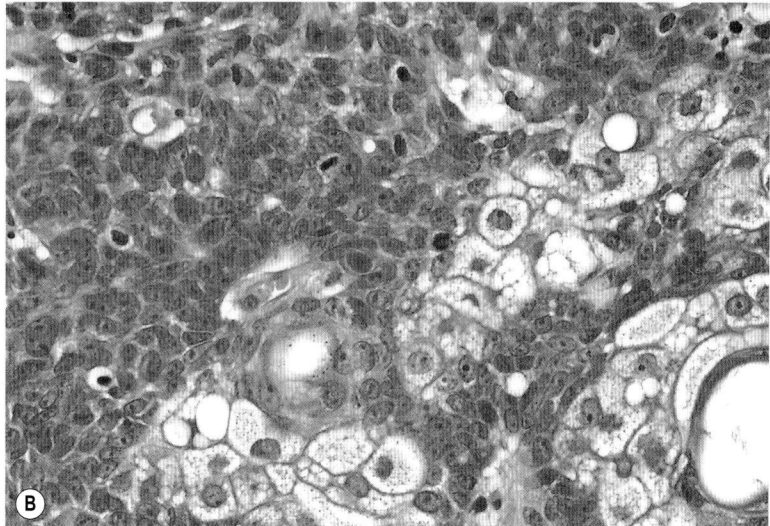

Fig. 32.31
Sebaceoma: (A) the tumor consists of a random admixture of basaloid cells and mature sebocytes; (B) in this field, there are two mitoses. There is no significant atypia.

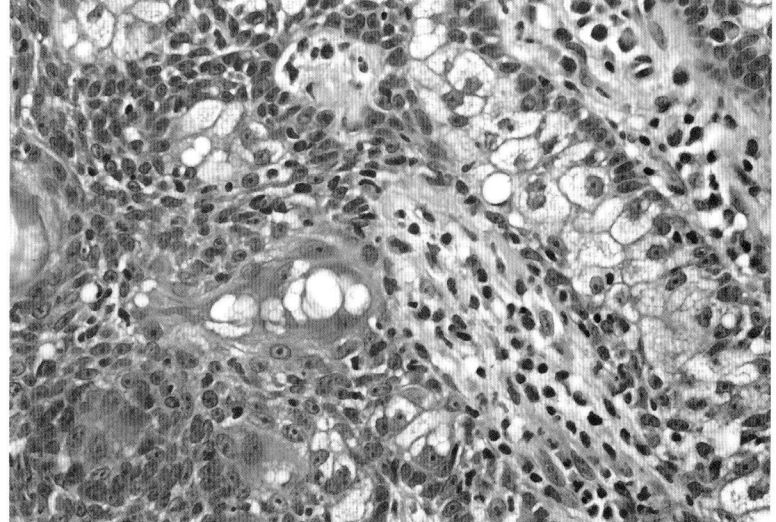

Fig. 32.32
Sebaceoma: ductal differentiation is commonly present.

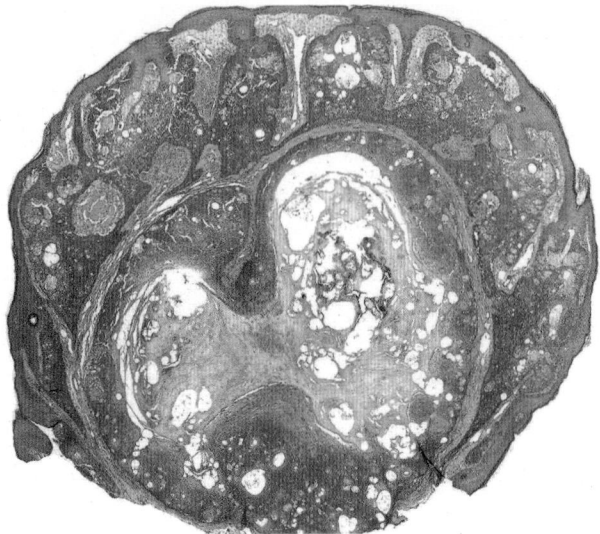

Fig. 32.33
Sebaceoma: this is a scanning view of a rare cystic variant showing central degenerative features.

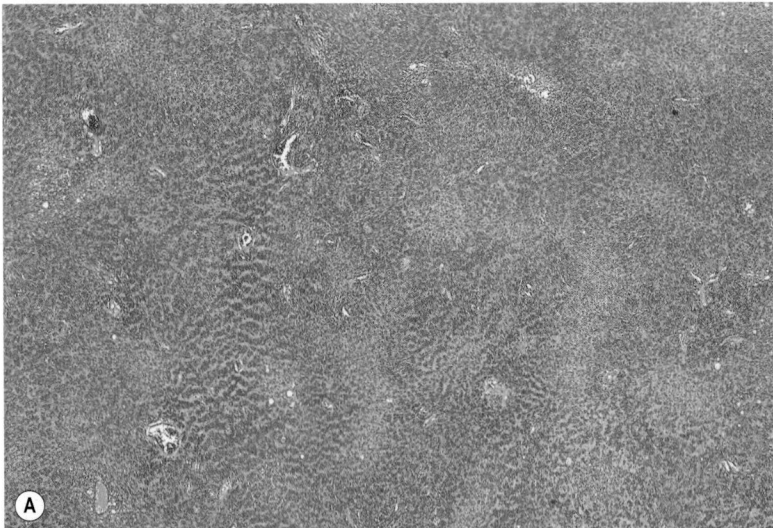

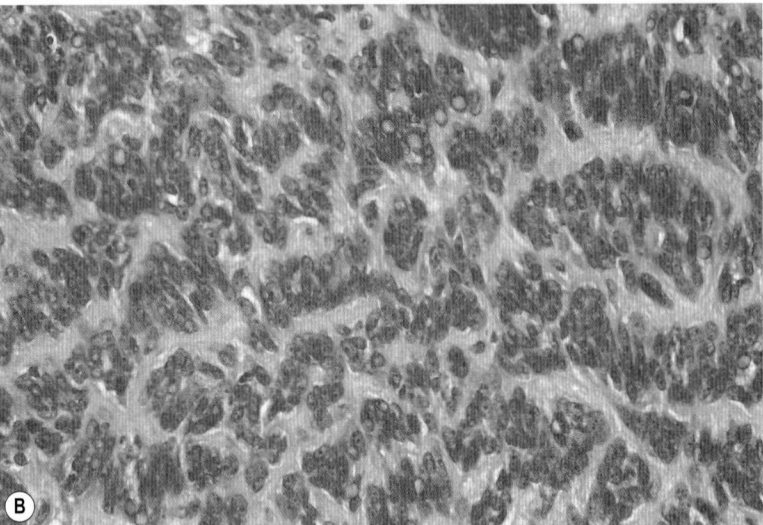

Fig. 32.34
Sebaceoma: (**A**) palisaded variant, which shows considerable histologic overlap with rippled-pattern trichoblastoma; (**B**) stromal hyalinization has resulted in this trabecular pattern (high-power view).

noted on rare occasion.[16–18] While holocrine secretion is regularly present, tumor necrosis in the basaloid component is not a feature.

Occasional tumors may show superficial elements reminiscent of seborrheic keratosis or verruca vulgaris.[2] Sebaceomas with carcinoid-like, reticulated, cribriform, and rippled or Verocay body-like features have also been described (*Fig. 32.34*).[6,7,16,19–21] Infundibulocytic structures and prominent squamous metaplasia have recently been noted as rare features.[22]

Differential diagnosis

Sebaceoma can be distinguished from sebaceous adenoma in which a lobular architecture with distinct and regular maturation (mimicking the normal sebaceous gland) is typically present. Sebaceous adenoma generally presents as a solitary nodular lesion in the superficial dermis, frequently replacing the overlying epidermis in whole or in part. It should be noted, however, that focal sebaceous adenoma-like features may sometimes be seen in a background of more typical sebaceoma.[2] In such instances, the final diagnosis of sebaceous adenoma or sebaceoma may well be arbitrary. Of more importance is distinction from well-differentiated sebaceous carcinoma and recognition that the lesion could represent a cutaneous marker of Muir-Torre syndrome.

Sebaceoma should not be confused with basal cell carcinoma showing sebaceous differentiation which first and foremost is clearly a basal cell carcinoma showing peripheral palisading and cleft formation and in which the sebaceous differentiation is merely an incidental finding. Immunohistochemistry using epithelial membrane antigen (EMA) and D2-40, which are expressed by sebaceoma, and Ber-EP4, which labels basal cell carcinoma, may be helpful in limited biopsies, but the distinction can usually be made morphologically in intact specimens.[23,24]

Sebaceous carcinoma is characterized by significant nuclear pleomorphism, nucleolar prominence, and conspicuous mitotic activity. Although in well-differentiated variants the tumor may have a distinct lobular architecture with smooth regular margins, thereby resulting in diagnostic confusion, less well-differentiated examples typically display an infiltrating growth pattern.

Sebaceoma should also be differentiated from trichoblastoma with sebaceous differentiation.[4] This latter tumor invariably shows focal hair germ differentiation, and papillary mesenchymal bodies are often evident. Peripheral nuclear palisading and stromal induction are also generally present.

When sebaceoma was originally defined, the authors intended it to replace the confusing term sebaceous epithelioma and to clearly define a novel entity distinct from both sebaceous adenoma and basal cell carcinoma with sebaceous differentiation.[1] Others have proposed an alternative term, sebomatricoma, to include lesions previously designated sebaceoma, sebaceous epithelioma, superficial epithelioma with sebaceous differentiation,

the sebaceous neoplasms associated with Muir-Torre syndrome, and those arising in nevus sebaceus.[25] This alternative designation has not received support in the subsequent literature. Sebaceoma has become a widely adopted and useful diagnostic category. We agree that the term of sebaceous epithelioma is confusing and should no longer be used. Of utmost importance is recognition that a variety of benign sebaceous lesions with variable architecture and proportion of basaloid cells form the benign end of the Muir-Torre spectrum. Sebaceoma represents a more cellular and less architecturally organized variant (*Fig. 32.35*). Recognition of this cellularity is important to avoid confusion with sebaceous carcinoma. The term sebaceoma clearly recognizes this increased cellularity as benign.

Superficial epithelioma with sebaceous differentiation

Clinical features

Superficial epithelioma with sebaceous differentiation is a rare tumor, with less than 25 cases having been documented.[1–14] Multiple names have been used, including reticulated acanthoma with sebaceous differentiation.[15] Most often, it presents on the face.[1–3] Two cases, however, have been described on the back, and a single patient with multiple lesions involving the face, axilla, trunk, and thigh has been reported.[4–6] Lesions are usually 1 cm or less in diameter, but cases of up to 2 cm have been encountered.[4] They present as flesh-colored or yellow-to-brownish papules, nodules, or plaques. The age

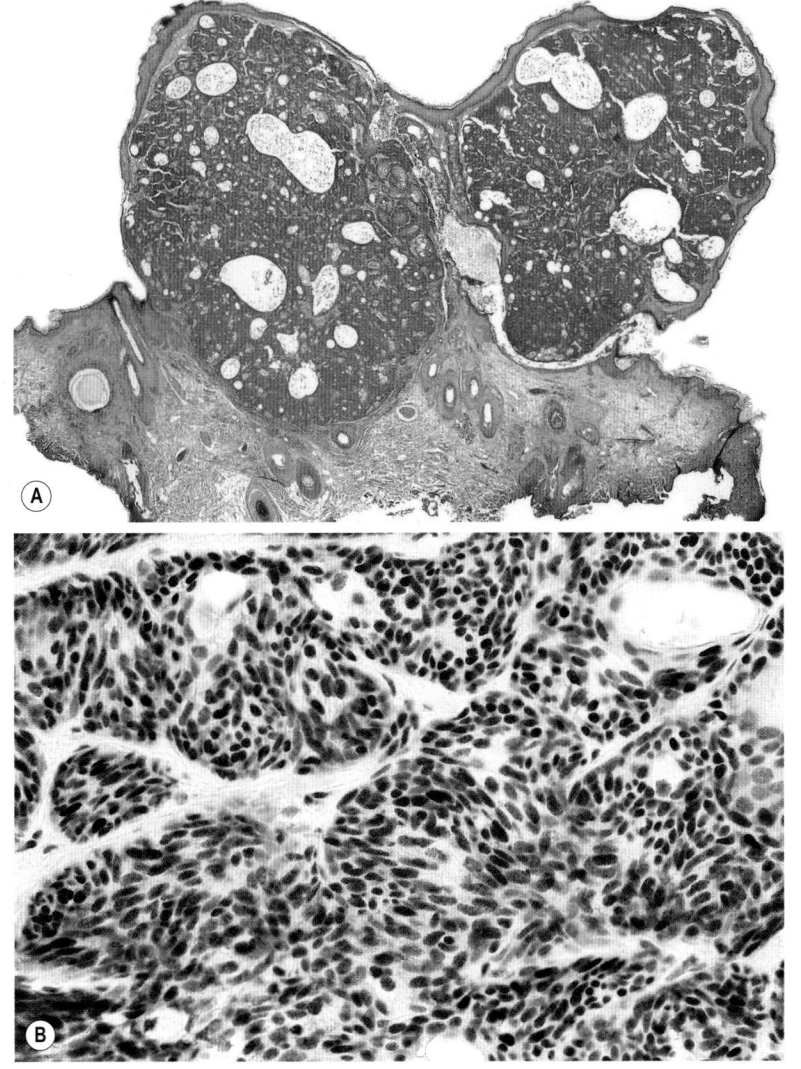

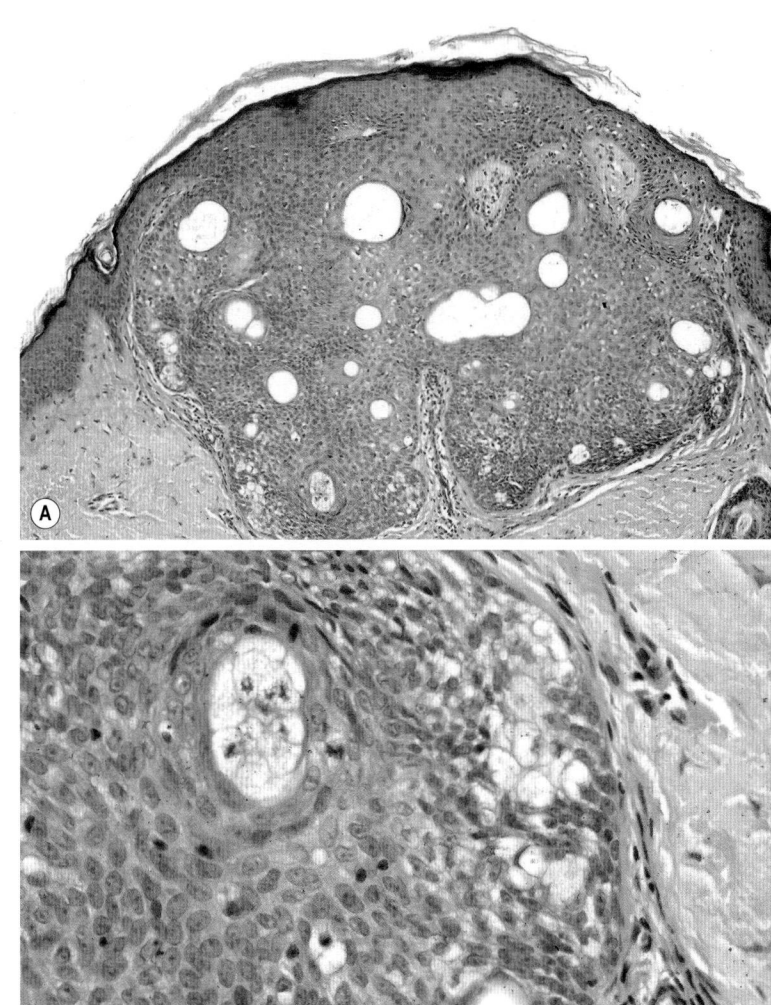

Fig. 32.35
Sebaceoma: (**A**) this example was not associated with Muir-Torre syndrome; (**B**) MSH-2.

Fig. 32.36
Superficial epithelioma with sebaceous differentiation: (**A**) there is a circumscribed focus of epidermal thickening with duct formation; (**B**) foci of sebaceous differentiation are evident. Courtesy of E. Farmer, MD, Virginia Commonwealth University, Virginia, USA.

distribution is wide (38–79 years) but the mean age is 60 years.[4] There is no clear gender predilection.[7]

The relationship of this tumor to Muir-Torre syndrome is unknown, although one patient has had a family and personal history of esophageal and colon carcinoma.[1,15,16] A case is reported to have arisen in the context of nevus sebaceous.[12] Recurrences following local excision have not been described.[4]

Histologic features

The tumor is characterized by a sharply defined and well-circumscribed, platelike epidermal growth with elongated, thickened rete ridges that anastomose in a reticular pattern (*Fig. 32.36*).[1] Merging with the more superficial keratinocytes is a cytologically bland basaloid cell population in which are admixed mature sebocytes, singly and in clusters.[1] Mitotic activity may be evident and is sometimes brisk, but cytological atypia is not a feature.[1] Ductal differentiation and keratin-filled cystic spaces are also present, and occasionally squamous eddies are a feature.[1,4] Melanin pigmentation has been described.[1] Peripheral palisading is not a feature, and cleftlike spaces separating the tumor from the adjacent dermal connective tissue are absent.

Differential diagnosis

Superficial epithelioma with sebaceous differentiation should be distinguished from follicular infundibulum tumor. The latter is also characterized by a platelike epithelial proliferation suspended from the epidermis. However, the tumor trabeculae are characteristically thin, vacuolated, and often surrounded by a thickened eosinophilic basement membrane. In addition, follicular infundibulum tumor does not contain keratin-filled cysts or generally show sebaceous differentiation, although a single published case showed features of both tumors.[17]

Seborrheic keratosis with sebaceous differentiation also enters the differential diagnosis.[8] This lesion, however, shows the features of an acanthotic variant of seborrheic keratosis with only small numbers of mature sebaceous cells scattered randomly throughout the epithelium.

A single case has been reported with the squamous portion descending from the surface epithelium and showing a reticulated pattern.[18]

Sebomatricoma

The term sebaceous epithelioma has been the source of considerable confusion, largely because different authors have taken it to mean different things while others have used it indiscriminately without precise definition. Thus, sebaceous epithelioma has been used as a synonym for basal cell carcinoma with sebaceous differentiation or else to represent a variant of sebaceous adenoma.

To overcome this problem, Troy and Ackerman introduced the term sebaceoma, which clearly described a tumor distinguishable from sebaceous hyperplasia, sebaceous adenoma, sebaceous carcinoma, and basal cell carcinoma with sebaceous differentiation.[1] They recommended that the term sebaceous epithelioma be abandoned. In a similar vein, Sánchez Yus's group proposed the term sebomatricoma to describe a spectrum of tumors ranging from sebaceous adenoma to sebaceoma.[2-4] Although this has some merit, since sebaceous adenoma and sebaceoma do show an element of overlap and may both be associated with Muir-Torre syndrome, the term sebomatricoma has not received great support in the subsequent literature.[5] In addition, the unusual benign sebaceous neoplasms associated with Muir-Torre syndrome were also included in this definition. The issue was a little clouded, however, since the authors also recommended inclusion of superficial epithelioma with sebaceous differentiation and sebaceous neoplasms arising within nevus sebaceus.[4] In addition, this term would group sebaceous neoplasms clearly associated with the Muir-Torre syndrome and lesions such as follicular infundibulum tumor that can rarely show sebaceous differentiation but probably have no connection with the Muir-Torre syndrome. As a spectrum, while perhaps intriguing from a developmental standpoint, this grouping may not have clinical utility.[6]

Basal cell carcinoma with sebaceous differentiation

Clinical features

Basal cell carcinoma with sebaceous differentiation is exceedingly rare, few cases having been published with even fewer photomicrographs.[1-4] Despite this fact, the entity is commonly cited in reviews.[5-7] It arises in the distribution expected for basal cell carcinoma, with the most common site being the face. Lesions are sometimes multiple.[2,3] Its behavior appears no differently than other basal cell carcinomas.

Pathogenesis and histologic features

It is not clear whether basal cell carcinoma with sebaceous differentiation forms part of the spectrum of the Muir-Torre syndrome. Some authors have reported an association with internal malignancy, but diagnostic criteria within this family of neoplasms have evolved significantly since that report.[3] In addition, since traditional basal cell carcinomas are associated with mutations in patched (*PTCH1*), *p53*, and *BAX* (bcl-2 associated X-protein) and not the genetic defects in DNA mismatch repair (MMR) seen in the Muir-Torre syndrome, a true relationship may not be present.[8-12] Basal cell carcinomas are increasingly conceptualized as adnexal in origin, and thus it is not surprising that numerous adnexal elements are reported within this tumor.

Basal cell carcinoma with sebaceous differentiation shows features of basal cell carcinoma with proliferation of palisading basaloid cells, usually in a nodular form, retraction artifact, and loose stroma rich in mucin. Within these nodules are foci of variable numbers of mature sebocytes, sometimes with formation of cysts due to holocrine secretion.

Sebaceous carcinoma

Clinical features

Sebaceous carcinoma is rare and has traditionally been divided into two groups: an aggressive periocular variant comprising about 75% of cases and an extraocular form considered by some to be less aggressive.[1-5] More recent observations, however, indicate that this distinction is inappropriate, since a significant number of extraocular tumors are associated with metastases and appreciable mortality.[6-10] Indeed, a recent retrospective review of 1349 sebaceous carcinoma cases followed over a 31-year period from the Surveillance, Epidemiology, and End Results (SEER) database of the National Cancer Institute indicated no difference in overall survival between groups with periocular and nonocular sebaceous carcinoma.[11,12]

Periocular sebaceous carcinoma

The periocular variant is more common than the cutaneous or extraocular form and presents in the mid-1960s.[13] It arises in association with the ocular sebaceous glands. At least five types of sebaceous adnexae are recognized in the eye. The meibomian glands (tarsal glands) are modified sebaceous glands that are associated with the tarsal plates of both the upper and lower eyelids.[14] They are relatively large structures that are not associated with

hair follicles and which discharge through squamous epithelium-lined ductules into a larger central duct that ultimately empties at the margin of the eyelid. These glands contribute to the lipid content of tears.[14] The glands of Zeis are associated with the eyelashes at the lid margin. Also recognized are the sebaceous glands of the caruncle, eyebrows, and those of the tiny vellus hairs on the surface of the eyelid.[9]

Sebaceous carcinoma is the second or third most common malignant tumor of the eyelid after basal cell carcinoma (and probably squamous cell carcinoma), accounting for 1.5% to more than 25% of tumors in several large series from referral centers.[9,15-20] It is a significantly more common diagnosis in series from Asia, but it is not clear that Asian populations in the United States have a higher incidence. The difference may well be due to a relatively low incidence of other malignant tumors such as basal cell carcinoma and squamous cell carcinoma in this population.[9,11,21] Most series from other regions place the incidence at approximately 1% to 5% of malignancies of the eyelid.[9,13]

Tumors generally arise in association with the meibomian gland, and present as a steadily enlarging, nonulcerated mass that usually involves the upper eyelid.[22] Occasionally, tumors develop from the glands of Zeis and from the sebaceous glands of the eyelid, caruncle, and eyebrow.[1] Sometimes they are multicentric or diffuse.[23-25] Occasionally, they present in younger patients.[24] There was believed to be a slight female preponderance, but this is not clearly demonstrated in the other largest studies to date.[11,22,26]

The tumor is very rarely diagnosed clinically, as presentation is notoriously varied. Many lesions are mistaken for basal cell carcinoma, squamous cell carcinoma, and even as a chalazion or chronic blepharoconjunctivitis.[22,27] The metastatic rate with subsequent mortality is high, approaching 25%.[11,22] Aggressive local behavior with intracranial extension may also occur.[28] Prognosis is particularly poor when both the upper and lower eyelids are involved.[22] Other poor prognostic features are multicentric presentation, duration of symptoms greater than 6 months, distinctly infiltrative architecture, pagetoid involvement of the skin epithelial surface of the eyelid, and lymphovascular or orbital invasion.[22] These features have not be formatted into an established three-tiered grading system.[29] The metastatic and mortality rate can be significantly lowered (to 18%) with early detection and treatment.[30-32] The organs most often affected include the regional nodes with subsequent involvement of lung, liver, brain, and bone.[9] Metastatic disease is a poor prognostic sign with a 50% 5-year mortality in one study.[22] Sentinel lymph node biopsy may be helpful for disease staging.[33-35] American Joint Committee on Cancer (AJCC) staging of the primary tumor by clinical and pathological features as well as regional lymph node and distant metastasis show prognostic influence, though the largest tumor dimension alone is not a helpful feature.[36]

Sebaceous carcinoma has been documented in retinoblastoma patients treated with radiotherapy, although it has also been reported in these patients in the absence of such treatment and occurring in a considerably younger age range.[37-39] Tumors associated with human immunodeficiency virus (HIV) infection have also been reported.[40] Periocular sebaceous carcinoma is generally believed to be less frequently associated with DNA MMR deficiency and the Muir-Torre syndrome than is the extraocular form, though the literature varies on this point.[26,41-43]

Extraocular sebaceous carcinoma

Extraocular sebaceous carcinoma accounts for approximately one-quarter of all cases.[6,7,9,11] It commonly presents on the head and neck where sebaceous glands are more concentrated (*Fig. 32.37*). Approximately one-quarter of the extraocular tumors arise at other regions including the trunk and thigh and, rarely, the genitalia.[1,7,11,44-46] Other exceptionally affected sites include the nasal vestibule, breast, nipple, finger, foot, and external auditory canal.[47-51]

Traditionally, males are thought to be affected more often than females in a ratio of up to 2:1, but this has varied among authors and is less pronounced in the more recent comprehensive reviews and large series.[7-9,11,52,53] The majority of patients are in their seventh decade.[7,8] Exceedingly rare cases in children have been described.[54] The tumor presents as a sometimes ulcerated pink to yellow-red nodulocystic lesion measuring up to 8 cm in diameter.[1] It has usually been present for at least 6 months, and often much longer,

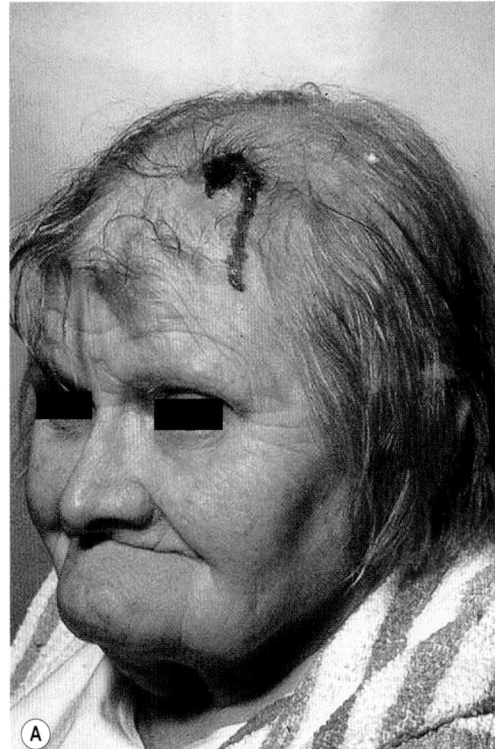

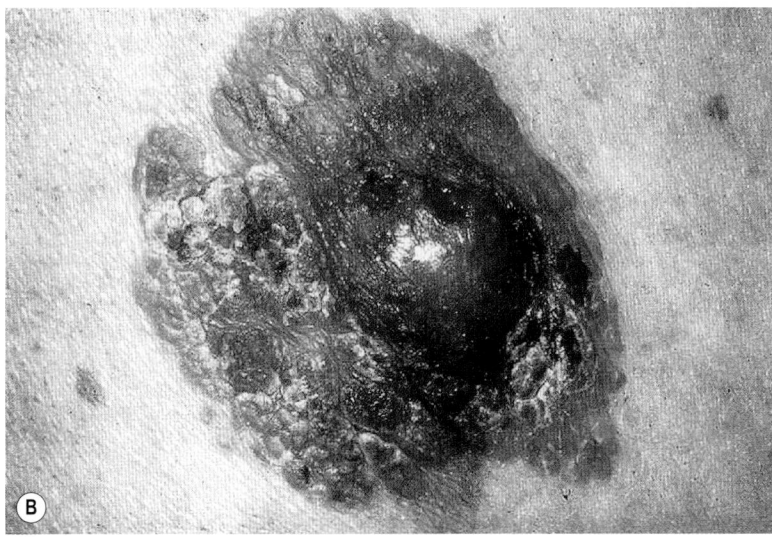

Fig. 32.37
Sebaceous carcinoma: (**A**) an encrusted tumor on the scalp of an elderly patient; (**B**) a more extensive lesion showing a central, erythematous, dome-shaped nodule. By courtesy of D.H. McGibbon, St Thomas' Hospital, London, UK.

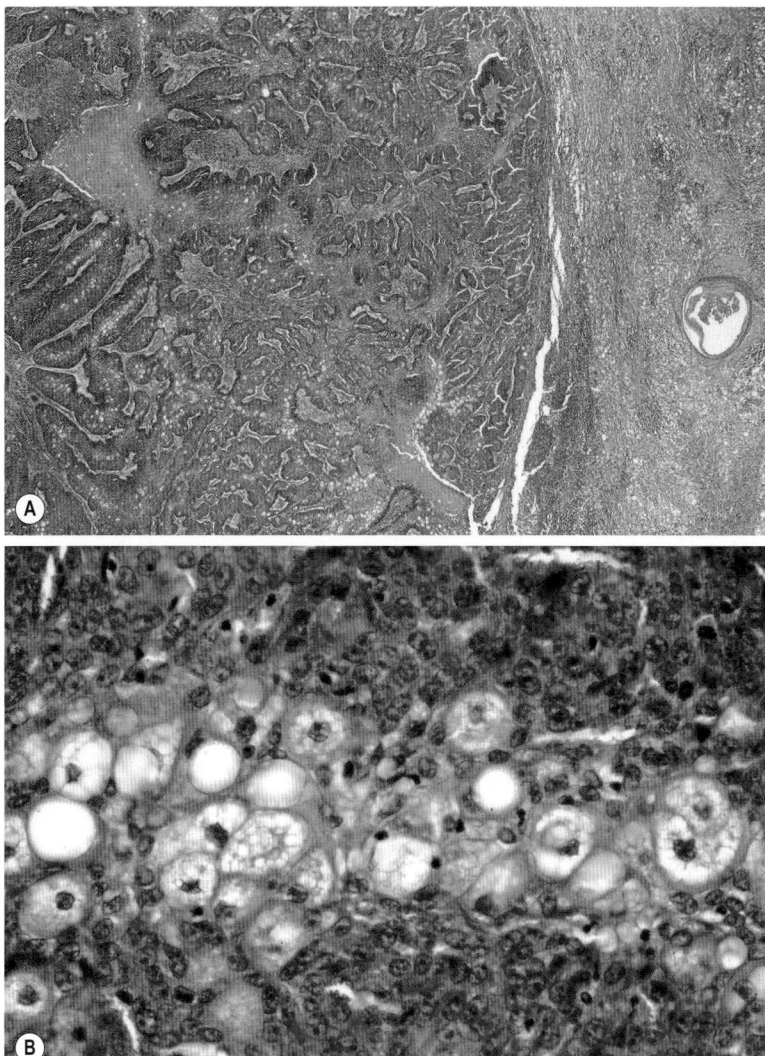

Fig. 32.38
Sebaceous carcinoma: (**A**) the tumor consists of irregular lobules and trabeculae composed of an admixture of dark-staining germinative cells and small numbers of differentiated sebaceous cells; (**B**) high-power view.

before diagnosis. Metastasis and mortality are believed by many authors to approximate to that of periocular tumors, and the pattern of metastasis is similar.[6–11] Sebaceous carcinoma has been reported in association with xeroderma pigmentosum and Bowen disease of the vulva.[55,56] A series has been described in immunosuppressed organ transplant patients, but such cases are exceptional.[57,58] It can also complicate nevus sebaceous.[59–62]

Sebaceous carcinoma may also very rarely arise at noncutaneous sites. Documented cases have been described in the oral and buccal mucosa, tongue, hypopharynx, pulmonary bronchus, lung, parotid and submandibular glands, uterine cervix, and in dermoid cysts or benign cystic teratomas of the ovary.[63–73] These could arise in association with ectopic sebaceous glands. The parotid gland is the most common of the noncutaneous sites, and other benign sebaceous neoplasms have also been described at this location.[8,9,68,74,75] Sebaceous lymphadenoma and the exceedingly rare sebaceous lymphadenocarcinoma are also seen in the parotid, but have not been reported in skin.[75,76]

Both periocular and extraocular carcinoma represent the malignant end of the spectrum of sebaceous lesions seen in Muir-Torre syndrome; cases from such patients tend to appear at a somewhat younger age.[77] Association of periocular sebaceous carcinoma with the Muir-Torre syndrome appears to be less prominent than the extraocular types.[26] In particular, sebaceous carcinomas from outside of the head and neck region may be most indicative of the Muir-Torre syndrome, though more than one such tumor and younger age are also important factors.[77]

Pathogenesis and histologic features

In general, the etiology of sebaceous carcinoma is unknown although ultraviolet radiation is probably of importance, and occasional tumors have followed therapeutic cutaneous irradiation.[7,22,78,79] Periocular cases from Asia show a frequent association with human papillomavirus (HPV) infection, but this has not been replicated in series from other regions.[80,81] Mutation and nuclear accumulation of TP53 and increased expression of the c-erB-2 oncogene have also been noted.[81,82] Nuclear accumulation of p53 and c-erB-2 expression may correlate with a poor outcome.[83] Dysregulation of the cell cycle as assessed by loss of appropriate compartmentalization of p21 (WAF1) has been described.[84] Pathogenesis may differ based on association with the Muir-Torre syndrome.[85]

Histologically, extraocular tumors are characterized by a variety of irregular lobular patterns or, less frequently, diffuse growth in the upper dermis, usually showing foci of continuity with the overlying epidermis (*Figs 32.38* and *32.39*). Infiltration of subcutaneous fat or skeletal muscle may

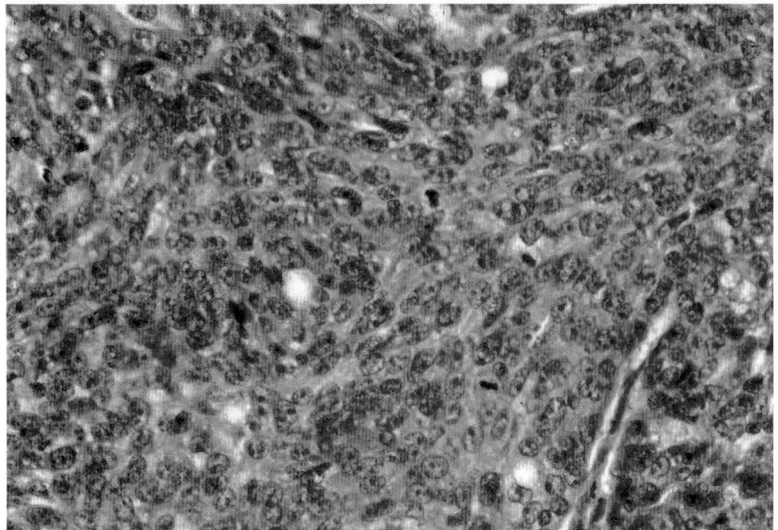

Fig. 32.39
Sebaceous carcinoma: in this high-power view showing an almost pure basaloid cell population, there are conspicuous mitoses.

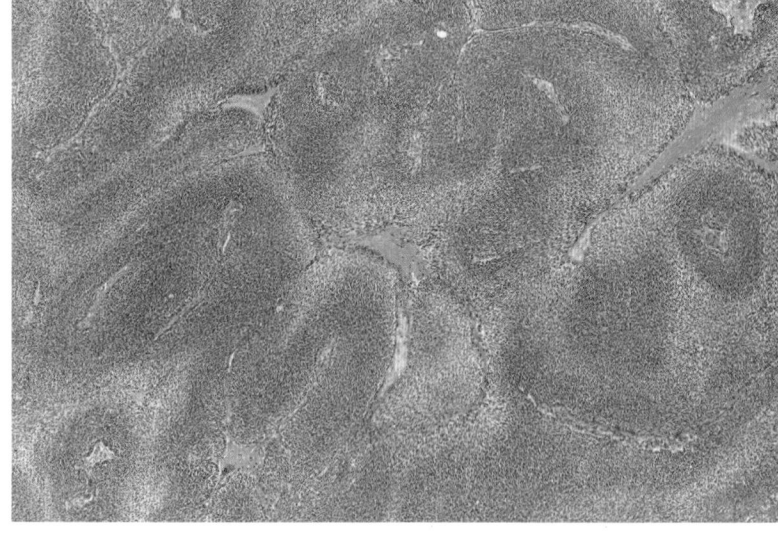

Fig. 32.41
Sebaceous carcinoma: poorly differentiated variant composed almost entirely of undifferentiated cells.

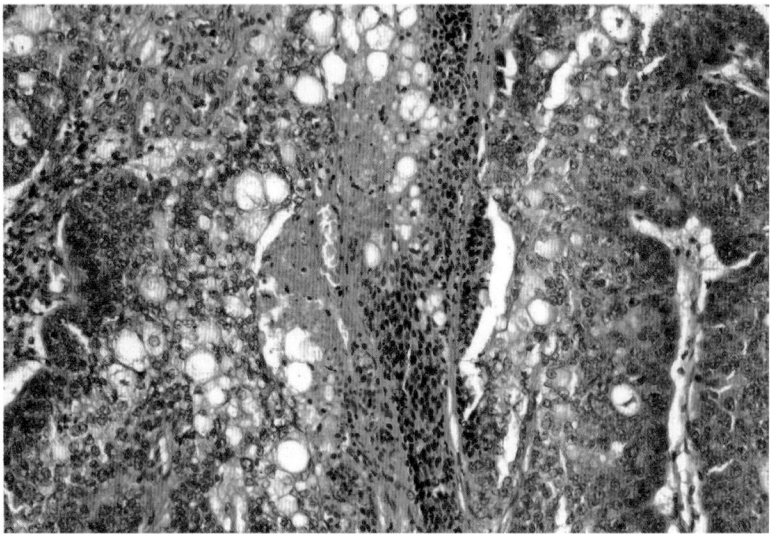

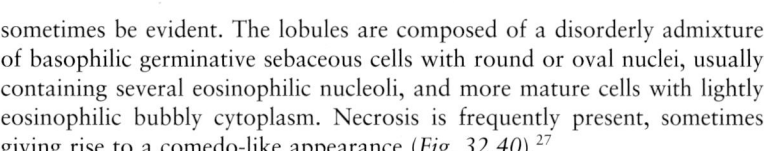

Fig. 32.40
Sebaceous carcinoma: high-power view showing admixture of basaloid and differentiated cells. Note the tumor necrosis.

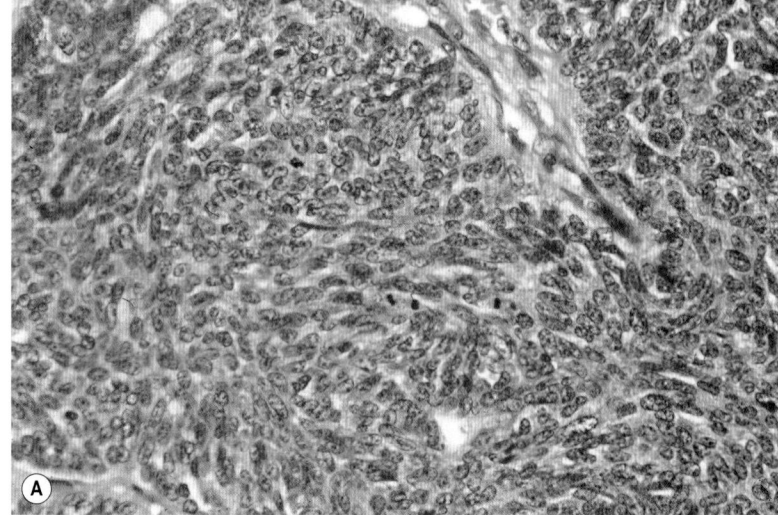

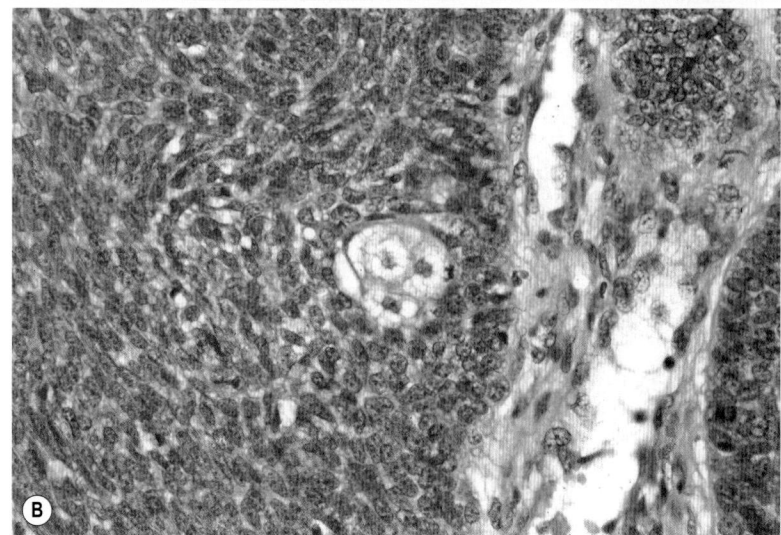

Fig. 32.42
Sebaceous carcinoma: (A) the tumor shows marked mitotic activity; (B) only a very tiny focus of sebaceous differentiation is evident.

sometimes be evident. The lobules are composed of a disorderly admixture of basophilic germinative sebaceous cells with round or oval nuclei, usually containing several eosinophilic nucleoli, and more mature cells with lightly eosinophilic bubbly cytoplasm. Necrosis is frequently present, sometimes giving rise to a comedo-like appearance (Fig. 32.40).[27]

In poorly differentiated examples, the tumor cells are more hyperchromatic and may contain minimal lipid (Figs 32.41 and 32.42). Peripheral palisading is occasionally seen, but is never marked. Keratinization resulting in diagnostic confusion with squamous cell carcinoma is sometimes a feature, and there may be an associated foreign body giant cell reaction. The tumor cells in poorly differentiated lesions usually show marked nuclear and cytoplasmic pleomorphism and frequent, often abnormal, mitoses. Infiltration of the perineural space and lymphatic or vascular invasion are variable features. More recently, intraepidermal or pagetoid spread has been recognized in a few cases of extraocular lesions, and an in situ form of the disease has been described.[86–90] A rippled or carcinoid-like pattern similar to that described for sebaceoma has also been reported.[91,92] Very rarely, apocrine differentiation has been reported.[93–95]

Special staining for lipid is usually positive (Fig. 32.43). If the diagnosis is in doubt, ultrastructural examination typically reveals nonmembrane-bound intracytoplasmic lipid inclusions (Fig. 32.44).[27]

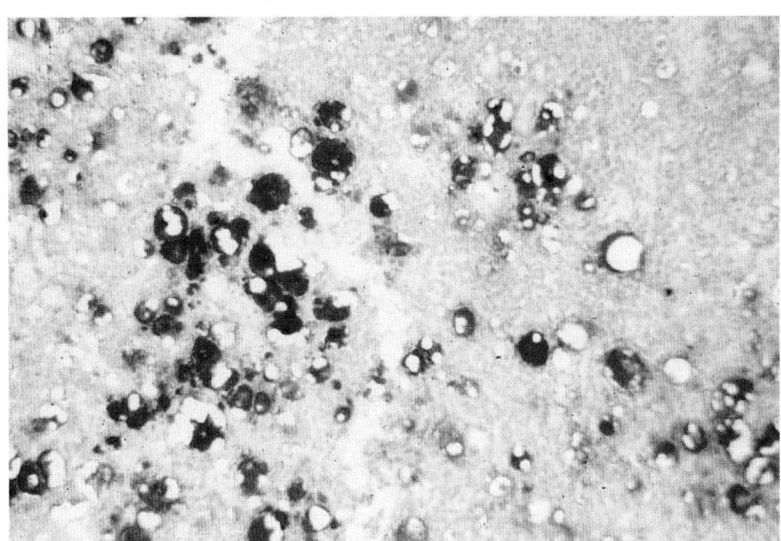

Fig. 32.43
Sebaceous carcinoma: a positive lipid stain aids in the differential diagnosis.

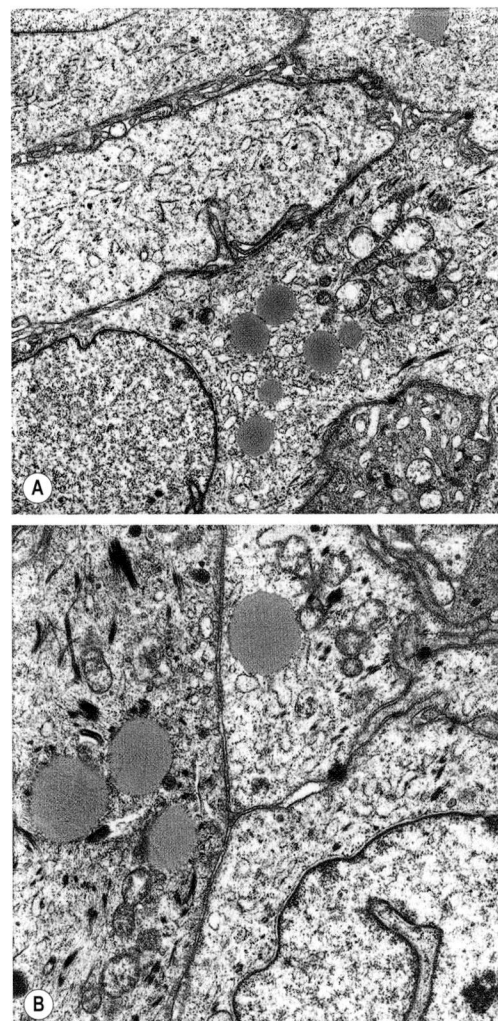

Fig. 32.44
Sebaceous carcinoma: (**A**) ultrastructural examination shows prominent nonmembrane-bound lipid vacuoles; (**B**) shown in high power. Note the tonofilaments and desmosome.

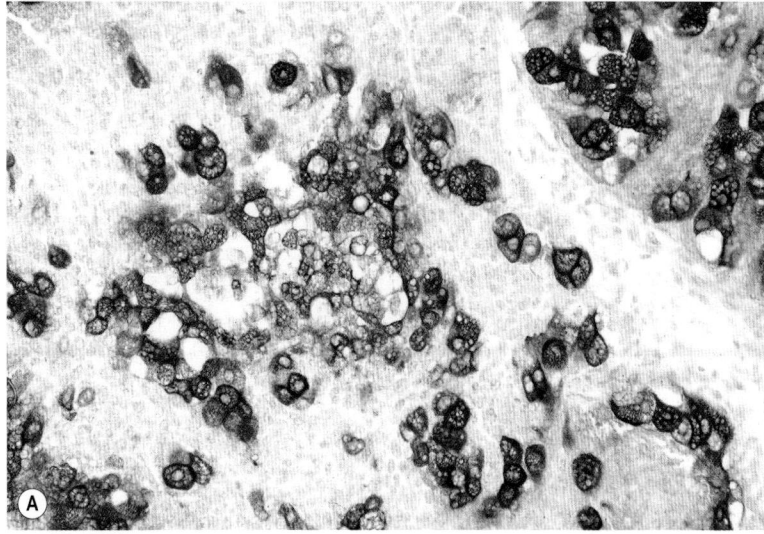

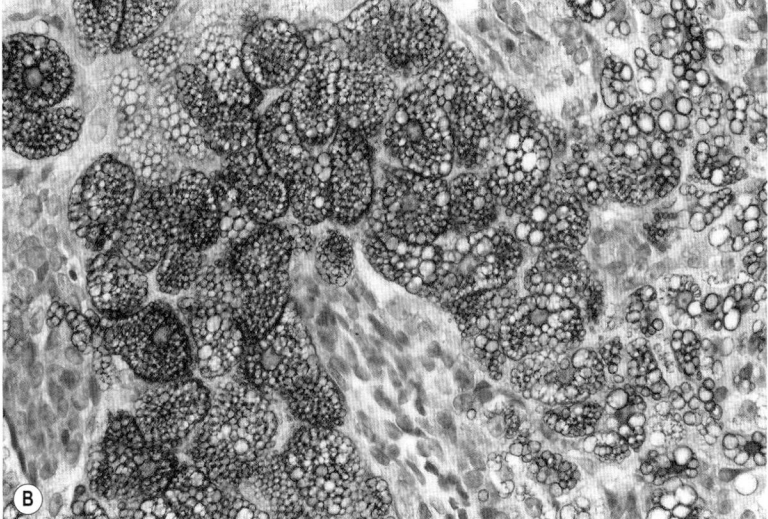

Fig. 32.45
Sebaceous carcinoma: (**A**) the tumor cells show strong epithelial membrane antigen expression; (**B**) adipophilin is positive.

With immunohistochemistry, sebaceous carcinoma is characterized by strong EMA and adipophilin (see under differential diagnosis) expression, but is carcinoembryonic antigen (CEA) negative (*Fig. 32.45*). Cytokeratin 7, androgen receptor (AR), progesterone receptor membrane component 1 (PGRMC1), squalene synthetase, and alpha/beta hydrolase domain-containing protein 5 (ABHD5), and GATA3 can also be expressed to varying degree and prevalence.[96,97] Nuclear expression of AR is common and recent reports also identify the unusual pattern of nuclear factor XIIIa as common in cells showing sebaceous differentiation, though this experience is not universal and could be related to antigen retrieval or antibody/clone selection.[96–100]

The periocular variety has similar histologic features, but is further characterized by a striking tendency to show pagetoid spread and/or bowenoid carcinoma in situ in the overlying conjunctival epithelium or epidermis (*Figs 32.46–32.49*).[22,27,89,101] Initial histopathological misdiagnosis is common despite the presence of sebaceous differentiation.[12] Grading systems have been devised stressing classification by either tumor cytological differentiation or architectural growth pattern,[22,27,29] These systems are not uniformly applied and their prognostic significance is not well established.

Poor prognostic indicators include multicentricity, size greater than 1 cm in diameter, poor differentiation, extensive tissue infiltration, and vascular or lymphatic involvement.[22]

Differential diagnosis

Sebaceous carcinoma is distinguished from benign sebaceous neoplasms with conspicuous germinative basaloid cells by its more irregular architecture, pleomorphism, nucleolar prominence, mitotic activity, and abnormal mitotic figures. Sometimes, some, but not all, of these features make for a diagnostic challenge.[102,103]

Occasionally, however, well-differentiated variants merge into a histologic continuum with other sebaceous tumors. In cases of doubt, particularly

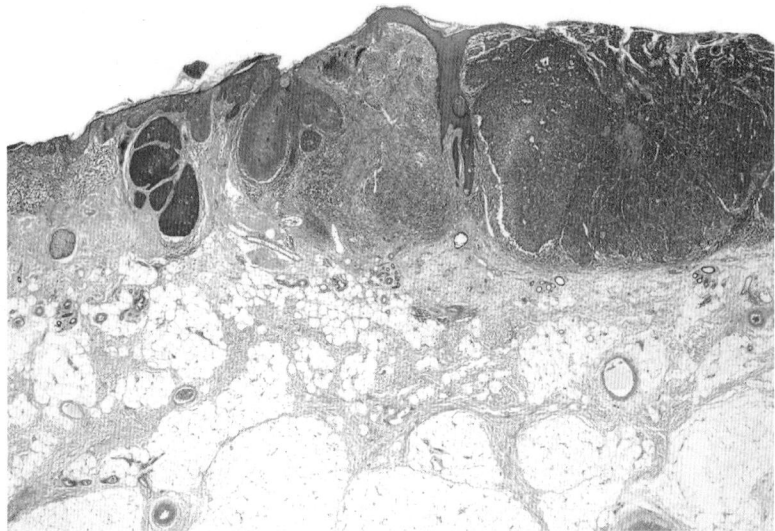

Fig. 32.46
Sebaceous carcinoma: this is a periocular variant.

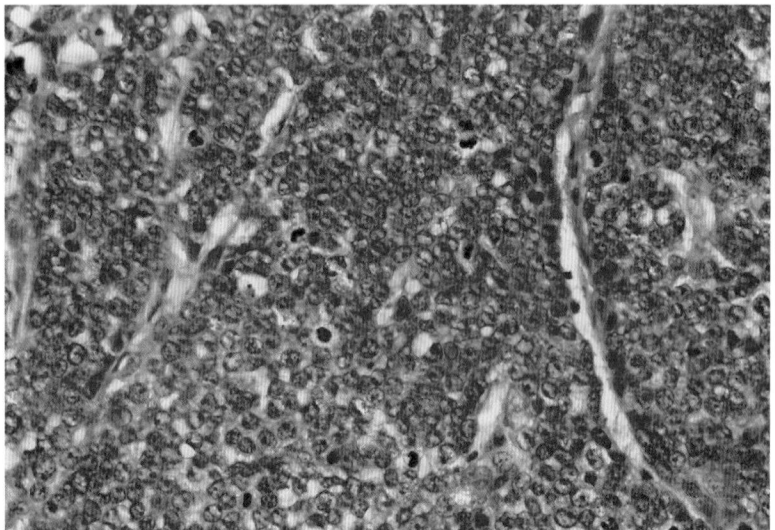

Fig. 32.47
Sebaceous carcinoma: the tumor is poorly differentiated. Note the conspicuous mitotic activity.

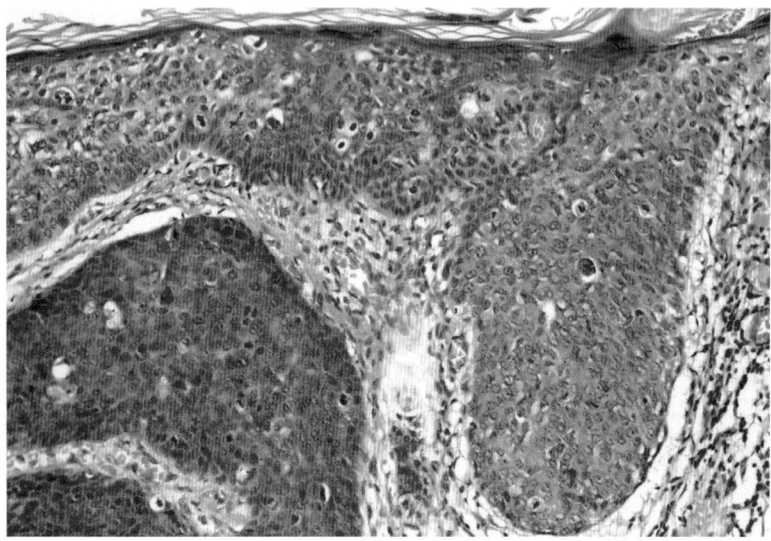

Fig. 32.48
Sebaceous carcinoma: the surface epithelium shows striking bowenoid features.

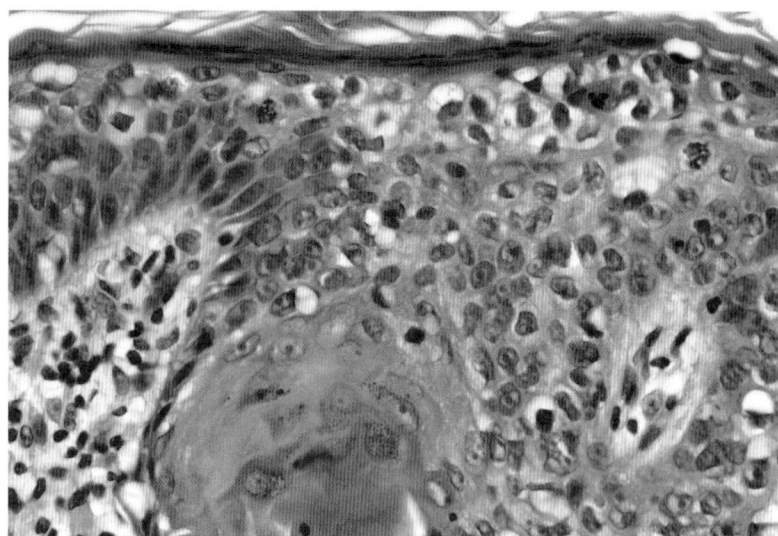

Fig. 32.49
Sebaceous carcinoma: high-power view superficially showing focal sebaceous differentiation.

with periocular lesions, it is probably in the patient's best interests to regard the tumor as a sebaceous carcinoma. It should be noted that unlike the extraocular sites, malignant cases greatly outnumber benign cases in the periocular region. Much literature is devoted to differentiating periocular sebaceous carcinoma from other periocular neoplasms such as the much more common basal cell and squamous cell carcinomas as biopsies from this region are often minute.

It may be differentiated from clear cell squamous carcinoma and clear cell hidradenocarcinoma by positive staining for lipid and negative periodic acid-Schiff, Alcian blue, or mucicarmine staining for glycogen and mucin. Others have stressed that a dimorphic staining pattern of basal cells and mature sebocytes with cytokeratin, EMA, and Ber-EP4 may be of assistance in demonstrating sebaceous differentiation, particularly in small biopsies.[98,104–106] Fat stains can be useful in the rare situation where fresh tissue is available and detection of sebaceous differentiation with immunohistochemistry for subclasses of the human milk fat globules has been reported.[107] An immunohistochemical marker applicable to fixed tissue is adipophilin, and the related perilipin, which mark proteins associated with intracellular vesicles that contain lipids (see Fig. 32.45B).[21,57,108] Adipophylin appears to be more sensitive than perilipin and is thus more widely adopted.[108] A definite intracellular vesicular staining pattern is needed to confirm specificity with this stain against clear cell and other neoplasms in this differential diagnosis.[109,110] An additional important differential diagnosis is balloon cell melanoma, which may be identified by positive S100 protein, HMB-45, or MART-1 (melanoma antigen recognized by T cells 1) reactions.

Muir-Torre syndrome

In 1967, Torre and Muir each reported an individual patient with multiple cutaneous tumors and gastrointestinal malignancies.[1–3] Where this association has been seen to be familial (autosomal dominant, 59%), the title 'family cancer syndrome' has been applied.[4,5] There appears to be a high degree of penetrance, but expression of the syndrome is variable.[6] More than 300 patients with Muir-Torre syndrome have now been reported. Sebaceous adenoma, sebaceoma, both ocular and extraocular sebaceous carcinoma, and keratoacanthoma have all figured in the cutaneous findings (Fig. 32.50).[4,6–9] Professor Torre defines the syndrome as having at least one cutaneous sebaceous neoplasm and at least one visceral cancer – no family history is required.[8] Association with keratoacanthoma is much less frequently documented especially in the more recent literature, but scattered reports remain.[10,11]

Traditionally, sebaceous adenoma is the most specific marker for the syndrome, but sebaceoma may have a similar degree of association, and multiple lesions increase the specificity.[8,12] One series indicates that up to 40%

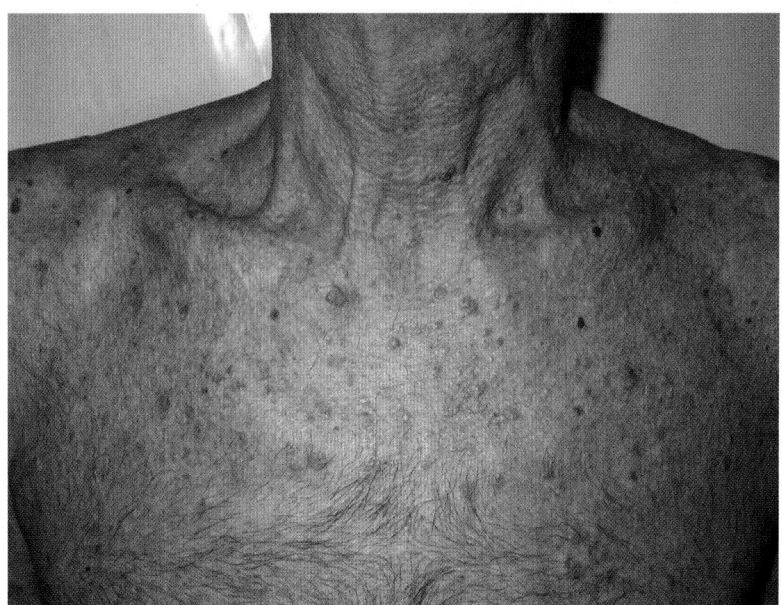

Fig. 32.50
Muir-Torre syndrome: this patient has innumerable small tumors on the anterior chest wall and neck. Courtesy of J.C. Pascual, MD, Alicante, Spain.

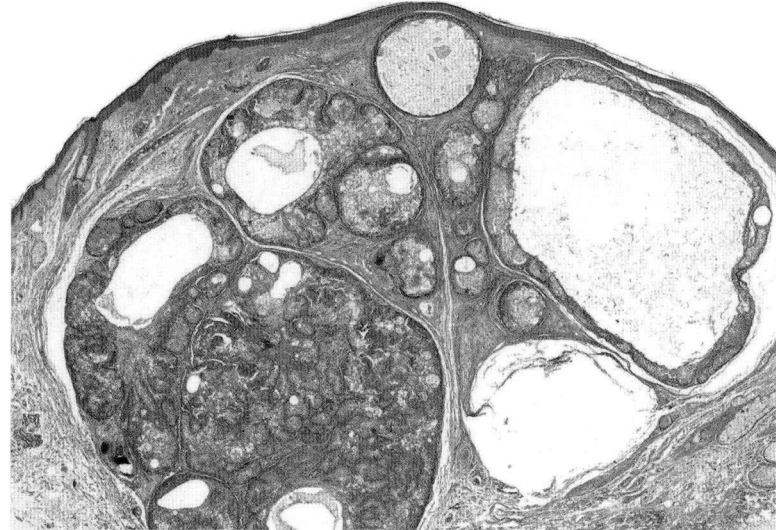

Fig. 32.51
Muir-Torre syndrome: sebaceous tumors showing cystic change as seen in this example are suggestive but far from diagnostic of Muir-Torre syndrome.

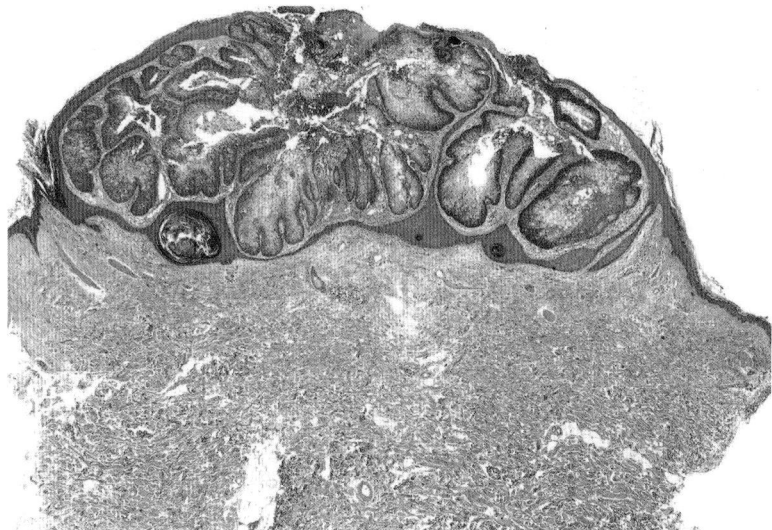

Fig. 32.52
Muir-Torre syndrome: sebaceous tumors showing a keratoacanthoma-like architecture sometimes indicate Muir-Torre syndrome. Note the epidermal collarette.

of adenomas are associated with internal malignancy, but referral bias likely affects the prevalence in various series; the association with sebaceous carcinoma appears to be lower.[6,8,13,14] Indeed, a study of 664 cutaneous sebaceous carcinomas using the SEER database of the National Cancer Institute over a three-decade period indicated that the risk of internal malignancy in those patients was greatly elevated over that seen in a cohort of patients with periocular sebaceous carcinoma.[15] The skin tumors may antedate the presentation of the internal malignancies by several years, although more often they are a subsequent or simultaneous development.[6,16] Some series show a slight male predominance and presentation ranges from the third to the ninth decade, but is most common in the fifth and sixth decades.[6,7] AIDS and other immune suppressive states may induce expression of the syndrome.[17–24]

The internal neoplasms in the Muir-Torre syndrome, which can be multiple, generally behave less aggressively and overall survival is improved.[6,7,20,25,26] Current emphasis on screening and early detection will likely further improve prognosis. Common associations include gastrointestinal ($\approx$53%), bladder and renal pelvis ($\approx$11%), endometrium ($\approx$10%), breast ($\approx$5%), and hematological malignancies ($\approx$5%).[4,25,27,28] Less common associations include mycosis fungoides, adrenal cortical carcinoma, prostate carcinoma, malignant astrocytoma, and various sarcomas.[13,29–32] Intestinal polyps are present in at least a quarter of cases (although not to the degree seen in familial adenosis polyposis coli syndrome) and correlates strongly with the presence or development of colorectal carcinoma.[16,25,33,34] The colonic carcinomas tend to be proximal in distribution (60%) and up to 50% of patients will have more than one primary tumor.[16] It is important to note that on occasion a single sebaceous tumor, including an ocular lesion, has been found to be associated with a visceral carcinoma.[35–38] Since sebaceous tumors (excluding simple hyperplasia) are uncommon, it is prudent to draw the attention of the physician to the possibility of an underlying systemic neoplasm when such a lesion is diagnosed. Clinical screening with formal risk assessment are also extremely helpful in this context.[12]

The sebaceous lesions of Muir-Torre syndrome sometimes have unique histopathological features, and some authors consider that many tumors cannot be classified using existing categories.[39–43] In particular, cystic sebaceous lesions devoid of a connection with the overlying epidermis and sebaceous tumors with keratoacanthoma-like architecture have been described (Figs 32.51 and 32.52), but their specificity for the Muir-Torre syndrome in an unselected series is unclear.[41,42,44–46] The cystic lesions may show significant proliferative activity in their basaloid rims.[42] Cytological atypia has been noted, and it has been proposed that these lesions represent low-grade malignancies, although confirmation of an aggressive biological behavior is lacking.[43] The sensitivity and specificity of these findings for the Muir-Torre syndrome is unknown. Sebaceous tumors that are readily classifiable also represent markers for this syndrome.

A cancer syndrome known as Lynch syndrome or hereditary non-polyposis colorectal carcinoma (HNPCC) is the most common form of inherited colorectal carcinoma and represents up to 1% to 3% of all colorectal malignancies.[47,48] Despite the previous name of HNPCC, Lynch syndrome is also associated with endometrial, urological, ovarian, hepatobiliary, and other internal malignancies.[49] This syndrome is associated with an inherited defect in one allele or copy of a DNA MMR gene.[50] Subsequent loss of the other wild-type allele leads to genetic instability during replication at repetitive sequences of DNA known as microsatellites.[51] This phenomenon is known as microsatellite instability (MSI) and is characteristic of tumors associated with this syndrome.[50] MSI is present in the tumors of approximately 70% of patients with Lynch syndrome; the underlying defect in the remainder is unknown.[52] Malignancies associated with MSI are generally less aggressive than their same-stage counterparts.[53] The two major MMR proteins involved are MLH1 and MSH2, though isolated loss of either MSH6 or PMS2 alone has been rarely reported as well.[50,53–60] In cases of MSH2 loss, MSH6 nuclear protein expression is usually also lost due to protein instability or

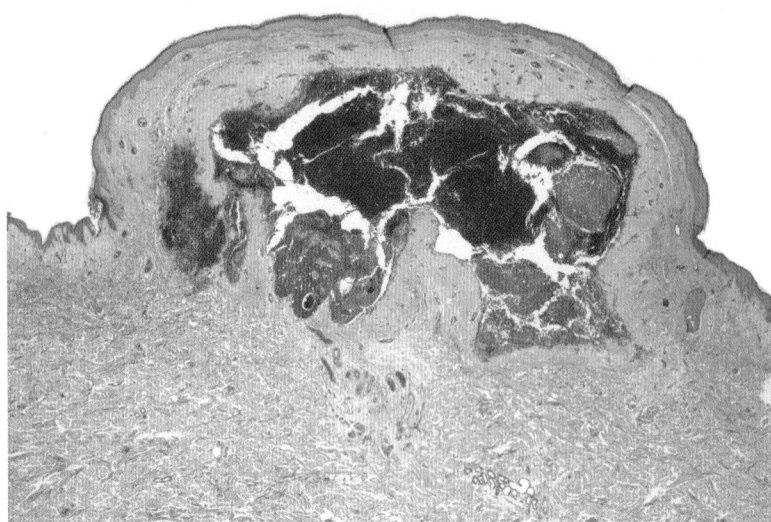

Fig. 32.53
Muir-Torre syndrome: this tumor arose in a patient with known Muir-Torre syndrome.

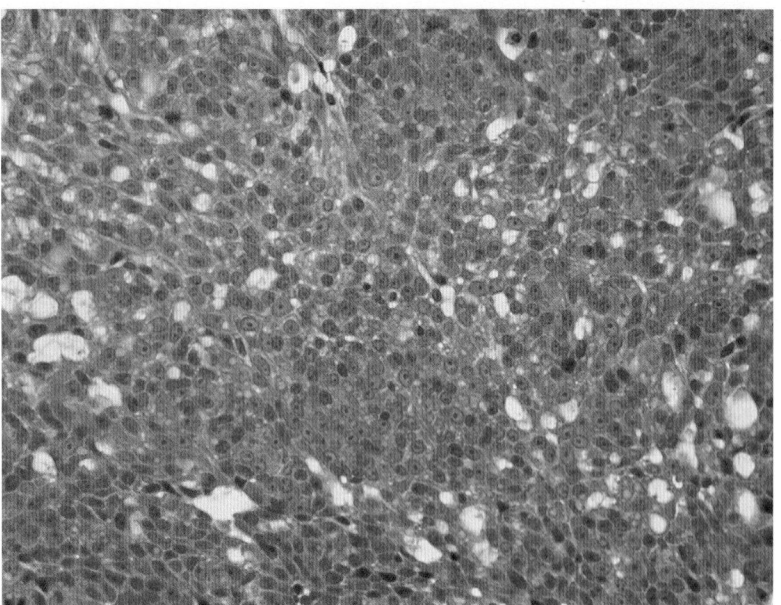

Fig. 32.54
Muir-Torre syndrome: high-power view showing focal sebaceous differentiation.

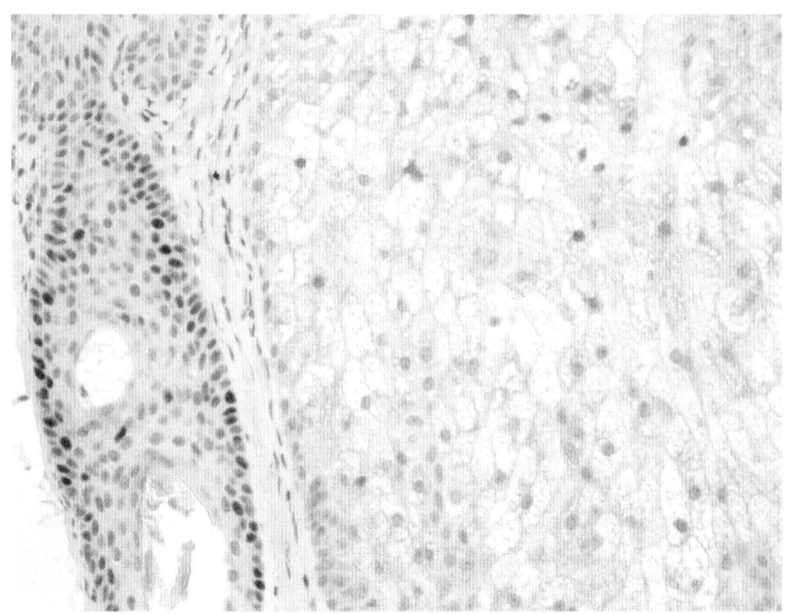

Fig. 32.55
Muir-Torre syndrome: there is complete absence of MSH2 expression.

downregulation.[45] Loss of nuclear PMS2 expression and sometimes MSH6 loss are encountered in the context of primary MLH1 loss. Loss of MSH6 alone can occur in isolation on rare occasion in Muir-Torre syndrome.[59] Isolated PMS2 deficiency has not been formally reported in Muir-Torre syndrome, though with increased screening for *PMS2* associated Lynch syndrome cases, this may eventually be encountered. The Muir-Torre syndrome represents a subset of Lynch syndrome, and at least 70% of tumors from these patients show MSI as well.[52,61-64] Genetic alterations other than those in MMR genes, including fragile histidine triad (*FHIT*), have been suggested, but further confirmation is required.[65-68] In one study, the malignancies in patients with Muir-Torre syndrome associated with MSI presented at a significantly younger age (40 vs. 70 years).[61] The precise role of MSI in neoplastic transformation is unclear, but loss of tumor suppressor genes may be involved.[69-71] Recent work speculates that the cutaneous sebaceous tumors in Muir-Torre syndrome with MSI may be related to dysregulation of the β-catenin and PTCH signaling pathways.[72] Similar pathways may also be involved in spontaneous sebaceous neoplasms. Autosomal recessive loss of function mutations in the *MUTYH* gene causes MYH-associated polyposis (familial adenomatous polyposis 2). Rarely, cutaneous sebaceous tumors can be seen in this setting and would thus technically meet clinical criteria and constitute Muir-Torre syndrome.[73-77]

MSI can be assessed using a polymerase chain reaction (PCR)-based technique from formalin-fixed, paraffin-embedded tissue and is commonly identified in the sebaceous lesions and keratoacanthomas of Muir-Torre patients.[78-80] Immunohistochemistry to demonstrate loss of MMR proteins MLH1 and MSH2 is also available with excellent sensitivity and specificity (*Figs 32.35, 32.53–32.55*).[45,81-86] While germline disruption of MLH1 or MSH2 is evenly distributed in HNPCC, disruption of MSH2 is seen in the majority of Muir-Torre patients (>90%).[50,87-89] The cause of over-representation of the Muir-Torre syndrome among patients with MSH2 deficiency is not understood, but the precise location and type of mutation in the *MSH2* gene may result in a predisposition for sebaceous tumorigenesis.[64] Indeed, the great majority of patients with Lynch syndrome and MSH2-deficient internal tumors do not develop cutaneous tumors characteristic of the Muir-Torre syndrome.[47,49,50,52,88,89] Features of the Muir-Torre syndrome are recapitulated in a *Msh2*-deficient transgenic mouse model.[90]

Other internal malignancies can show MSI as a result of somatic loss of MLH1, usually by methylation suppression, a finding present in 10% to 15% of sporadic colonic and endometrial carcinomas as well as many other cancers at lower rates.[53,71] There is increased effort to identify such cases as new immuno-oncological treatments (checkpoint inhibitor therapy) show efficacy in such patients. The occurrence of sporadic cancers with somatic suppression of MMR genes is much more common than Lynch-associated

malignancies and does not imply heritability.[53] Loss of MLH1 is uncommon in sebaceous neoplasms, and somatic methylation suppression of MMR genes does not appear to be an important factor in their development.[91] Tumors occurring outside the head and neck region overwhelmingly show loss of MMR protein, particularly MSH2.[45] The finding of MSI and/or loss of MMR proteins in both the sebaceous cutaneous and internal tumors of a patient is strongly suggestive of the Muir-Torre syndrome.[61,63,82-84,87,88]

This issue of evaluating a single sebaceous tumor for DNA MMR protein loss, particularly in the absence of an internal malignancy, for evidence of Muir-Torre syndrome is complex. Until very recently, somatic loss of MSH2 or even MLH1 was not thought to be common in sebaceous neoplasia; thus, demonstration of loss in a sebaceous tumor by immunohistochemistry was considered as strongly suggestive of a germline deficit and thus the Muir-Torre syndrome. Many recent papers have been published showing high rates of DNA MMR protein loss in isolated sebaceous tumors and algorithms for work-up of such cases proposed.[12,45,92-97] In general, immunohistochemistry demonstrating DNA MMR protein loss is more common in adenomas than carcinomas, particularly the periocular carcinomas. Location outside of the head and neck region is more likely to be associated with DNA MMR protein loss in both adenomas and carcinomas. Recently, it has become apparent that the prevalence of MSI and DNA MMR protein loss is much higher in isolated sebaceous tumor cases than are the germline deficits in MHS2, MLH1, and MSH6 that underlie the majority of the Muir-Torre syndrome. This calls into question the positive predictive value of universal immunohistochemical screening of isolated cutaneous sebaceous tumors.[12,98,99] Somewhat surprisingly, there appears to be a high degree of somatic (non-germline) mutations in these genes in MSH2 (and less frequently MLH1 and MSH6) in sebaceous neoplasia; such cases would not be Muir-Torre syndrome patients as a heritable germline predisposition is required.[100,101] Thus, there is currently some reasoned reassessment of the value of universal testing of sebaceous tumor with DNA MMR immunohistochemistry or molecular MSI testing as a screen for Muir-Torre syndrome. There is now increased focus on clinical criteria such as family history of Lynch-associated cancers, age of the patient, and multiple sebaceous tumors. Recommendations will continue to evolve in this area over the next few years. Further confirmatory germline genetic testing is now more reliably and widely available with advances in DNA sequencing approaches. The critical component of involving formal genetic counseling professionals in this process should be recognized.

It is important to keep in mind that the absence of MSI and intact DNA MMR protein expression does not exclude the Muir-Torre syndrome.[61,82–85] Also, very rarely, cutaneous lesions other than sebaceous tumors or keratoacanthomas found in Muir-Torre patients may show MSI.[102,103] The immunohistochemical and molecular MSI testing of relevant cutaneous sebaceous neoplasms can certainly play a role in the work-up of these lesions, but the nuances above should be considered in whatever approach is adopted.[91–94,97,104–108]

Mantleoma

Clinical features

An intriguing entity showing possible differentiation toward the follicular mantle has been described only in a handful of cases.[1–3] It occurs solely on the face and often represents an incidental finding.[1] The tumor is benign. This lesion has not been associated with the Muir-Torre syndrome, though experience is limited.[2]

Pathogenesis and histologic features

First described by Felix Pinkus, the mantle is situated at the follicular infundibulum and in three dimensions appears like an inverted cup.[1] It is formed from thin strands of basaloid cells with variable sebaceous differentiation. Its exact nature is debated, but it may be related to sensory function or the formation of the sebaceous glands.[4] The term mantleoma has also been used to describe the trichodiscoma to fibrofolliculoma spectrum of tumors seen in Birt-Hogg-Dubé syndrome.[5,6] This relationship is uncertain and this use of the term mantleoma in this context is not widespread.

Although there may be considerable histologic variation, in essence mantleoma consist of folliculocentric cords and strands of basaloid cells containing variable numbers of sebocytes, and sometimes forming reticulated structures (Figs 32.56–32.58).[1] The associated connective tissue stroma may show mucin deposition and is separated from the adjacent dermis by cleftlike spaces. While not extensively documented in the literature, we have periodically noted this entity as an incidental finding.

Differential diagnosis

There is considerable morphological overlap with a similar benign adnexal tumor termed folliculocentric basaloid proliferation, but the relationship between these two lesions is unclear.[4] Some authors consider fibrofolliculomas and trichodiscomas, which can be markers for the Birt-Hogg-Dubé syndrome, to also show differentiation toward the mantle.[7]

Mantleoma displays histologic overlap with basaloid follicular hamartoma.[1,8,9] The latter condition, however, presents with multiple lesions and shows no evidence of sebaceous differentiation.

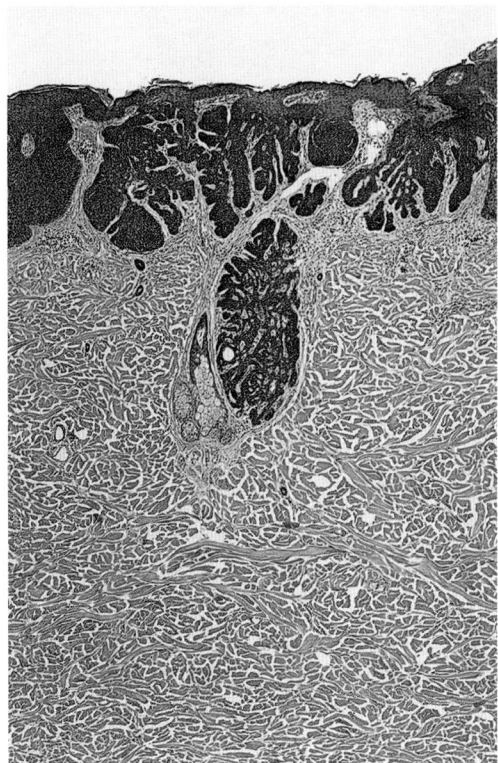

Fig. 32.56
Mantleoma: low-power view showing a lacelike proliferation of basaloid cells. By courtesy of C. Steffan, MD, Palm Springs, California, USA.

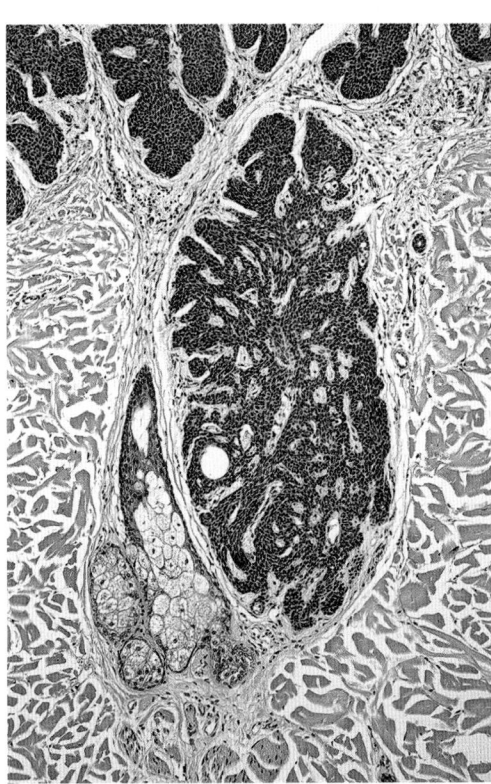

Fig. 32.57
Mantleoma: note the cleftlike space separating the tumor from the adjacent dermis and indented sebaceous gland. By courtesy of C. Steffan, MD, Palm Springs, California, USA.

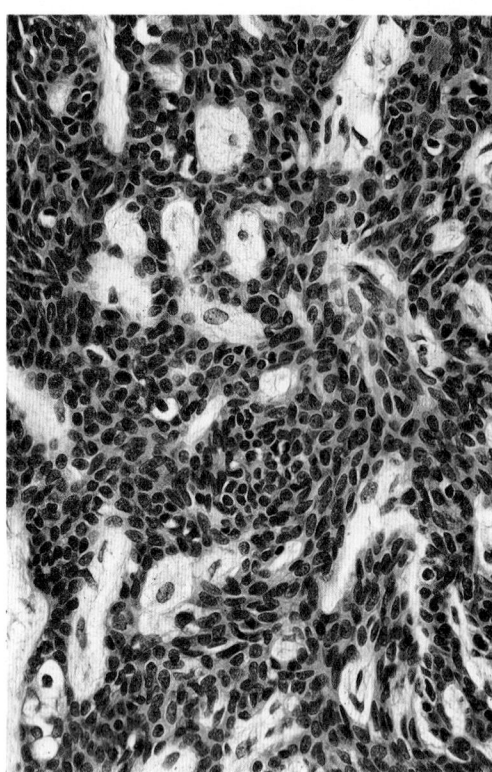

Fig. 32.58
Mantleoma: the tumor consists of a uniform population of small basaloid cells admixed with sebocytes. By courtesy of C. Steffan, MD, Palm Springs, California, USA.

Other cutaneous tumors showing sebaceous differentiation

A number of cutaneous epithelial or adnexal tumors can show a sebaceous component or differentiation.[1] This is not surprising since the skin adnexal structures arise from pluripotent stem cells.[2,3] Sebaceous differentiation in tumors of follicular derivation is not entirely unexpected given the intimate association of the pilar and sebaceous units.

Cutaneous tumors which may show sebaceous elements include cutaneous mixed tumor, microcystic adnexal carcinoma, syringocystadenoma papilliferum, tubular adenoma, poroma, porocarcinoma, proliferating trichilemmal cyst, panfolliculoma, fibrofolliculoma, trichofolliculoma, trichoblastoma, tumor of the follicular infundibulum, and pilar sheath acanthoma.[4–17]

The entity described as sebocrine adenoma is an alternative name for apocrine poroma and is characterized by sebaceous differentiation.[18,19]

A variety of unclassifiable mixed adnexal neoplasms with sebaceous differentiation have also been reported.[1,20–24]

Access **ExpertConsult.com** for the complete list of references

Tumors of the sweat glands

CHAPTER

33

See
www.expertconsult.com
for references and
additional material

Apocrine nevus

Clinical features

Apocrine nevus as defined by an excess of normal apocrine glands (apocrine hamartoma, hamartomatous apocrine gland hyperplasia) is a very rare and clinically heterogeneous condition. Most often it presents with a fleshy axillary swelling.[1–5] Erythematous or brown nodules on the neck, chest, and inguinal region, a plaque on the cheek, and multiple papules on the chest have also been documented.[6–11] Lesions are present at birth or develop in adulthood. Hyperhidrosis is not usually a feature. There is generally no underlying systemic disease, although one patient with a background of focal dermal hypoplasia (Goltz syndrome) and another with axillary apocrine carcinoma have been documented.[4,6,12] In addition, the development of syringocystadenoma papilliferum has been described within apocrine nevi.[13,14]

Histologic features

The lesion is characterized by excess mature apocrine glands in the reticular dermis, sometimes extending into the subcutaneous fat. Glands and ducts are represented.

Apocrine hidrocystoma and apocrine cystadenoma

Clinical features

Apocrine hidrocystoma is an uncommon cystic lesion and is most often solitary.[1–3] Despite its apocrine differentiation, it is rare at sites rich in normal apocrine glands.[3] It is usually found on the head and neck, commonly affecting the cheek (Fig. 33.1).[2,3] Multiple lesions have also been documented.[4–8] Those on the face are sometimes known as the Robinson variant, and these present most often in middle-aged females.[4,5,9] Multiple apocrine hidrocystomas are a feature of ectodermal dysplasia (Schöpf-Schulz-Passarge syndrome) and focal dermal hypoplasia (Goltz syndrome).[10–13] Similar lesions on the eyelids are also known as Moll gland cysts.[6,7] Rarely, it may present on the chest, shoulder, axilla, umbilicus, prepuce, vulva, penis, and the finger.[14–23] The diagnosis of an apocrine hidrocystoma or cystadenoma should be made with great caution on distal extremities as most represent digital papillary adenocarcinoma.[24] Penile variants are now thought at least in part to represent median raphe rather than true apocrine cysts. The cyst shows an equal sex incidence and arises most often in the middle aged.[15] Exceptionally, it has been described in childhood.[25]

It presents as an intradermal, moderately firm, dome-shaped, translucent, blue, bluish-black or purple cystic nodule measuring up to about 1 cm across. Giant variants measuring up to 7.0 cm in diameter are exceptionally encountered.[26–28] Apocrine hidrocystoma is not associated with a familial incidence. Although solitary apocrine hidrocystoma is said not to show seasonal variation, multiple lesions in some patients worsen in summer or with excessive heat and decrease during the winter months.[4,5] Apocrine hidrocystoma is an occasional feature of nevus sebaceous.[29]

Histologic features

Apocrine hidrocystoma consists of a large unilocular or multilocular cystic space situated within the dermis (Fig. 33.2).[3] A fibrous pseudocapsule is often present. Typically, the cystic spaces are lined by a double layer of epithelial cells: an outer layer of flattened vacuolated myoepithelial cells

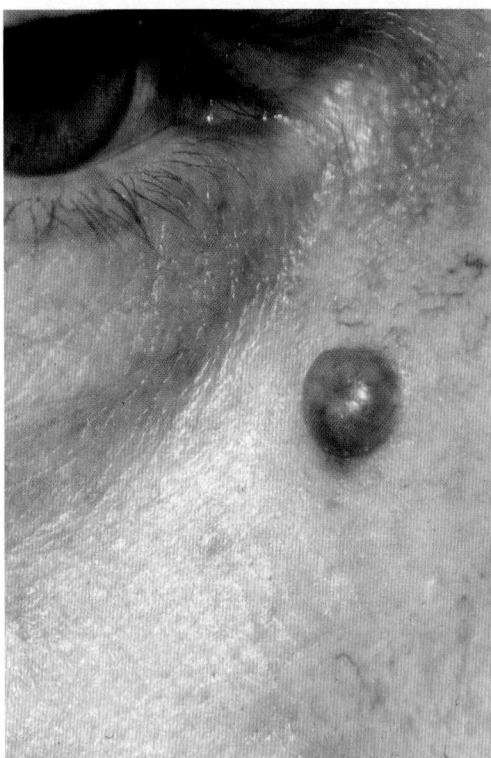

Fig. 33.1
Apocrine hidrocystoma: this shows a characteristic bluish translucent swelling on the cheek of a middle-aged male patient. From the collection of the late N.P. Smith, MD, the Institute of Dermatology, London, UK.

and an inner layer of tall columnar cells with eosinophilic cytoplasm and basally located, round or oval vesicular nuclei. Ultrastructural observations have confirmed the presence of myoepithelial in addition to secretory cells.[30] Decapitation secretion is usually present (*Fig. 33.3*). In lesions with prominent cystic change, the lining cells appear flattened. Diastase-resistant periodic acid-Schiff (PAS)-positive granules may be evident in the cytoplasm of the inner lining cells, and occasionally iron or melanin is also demonstrable.[3,15–17,31] In about 50% of lesions, numerous papillary projections are seen growing into the central cavity. Occasionally, the cyst cavity is partially replaced by a papillary or adenomatous proliferation (apocrine cystadenoma) (*Fig. 33.4*).[32]

Moll gland cyst is lined in part by apocrine-type epithelium and elsewhere by keratinizing squamous epithelium.[33]

The myoepithelial layer can be highlighted with smooth muscle actin (SMA), calponin and p63 immunohistochemistry (*Fig. 33.5*).[34] Staining with S100 protein is variable.

Differential diagnosis

There is often difficulty in distinguishing between apocrine hidrocystoma and eccrine hidrocystoma. This results largely from atrophy of the epithelial lining of the apocrine hidrocystoma due to cyst distension by excessive secretions. Eccrine hidrocystoma is thought to derive from cystic dilatation of a sweat duct.[35] Whether such a cyst is of eccrine or apocrine derivation is a moot point, since the two ductal systems are generally thought to be identical.[4,5] Some authors have proposed the alternative term ductal hidrocystoma to reflect this possible dual histogenesis.[5] Apocrine ducts, however, have been reported as expressing human milk fat globulin 1 (HMFG-1) whereas eccrine ducts are negative for this protein.[35] This may help separate true apocrine duct hidrocystoma from that of eccrine derivation. In any event, in hidrocystomas where decapitation secretion is unapparent, S100 protein Tumd α-SMA immunohistochemistry will readily resolve the problem since eccrine hidrocystoma is negative for both antibodies.[35–37] In addition, the luminal epithelial layer in apocrine hidrocystoma expresses keratins K7, K8, and K18, whereas in eccrine hidrocystoma the luminal layer expresses K1, K5, K10, and K14.[35,37]

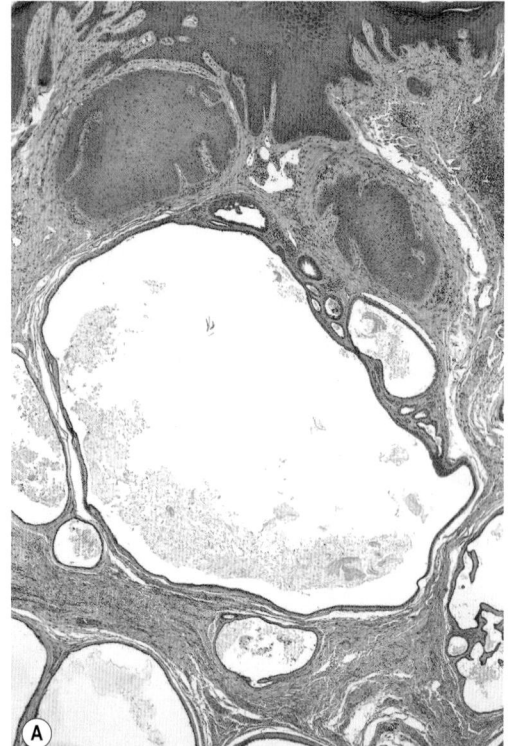

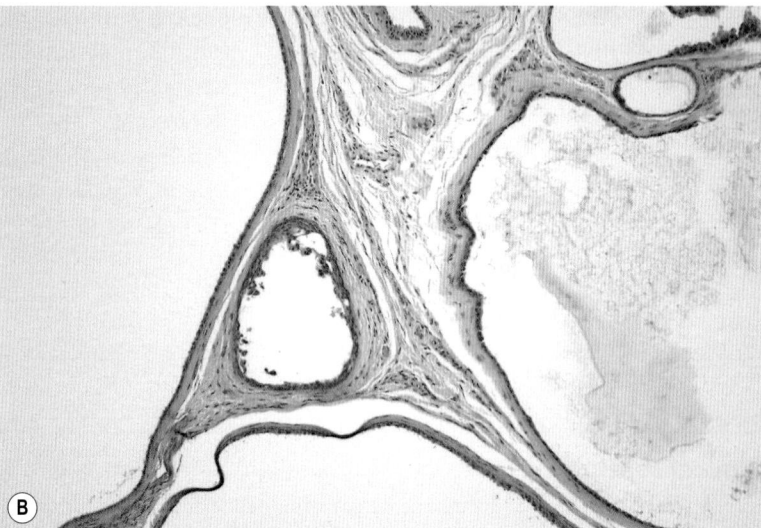

Fig. 33.2
(**A, B**) Apocrine hidrocystoma: this example consists of a multilocular cyst.

Hybrid epidermoid and apocrine cyst

Clinical features

This rarely documented entity presents as a usually less than 1.0 cm bluish or flesh-colored cystic papule or nodule. Lesions have been described on the nipple, eyelid, and lip.[1]

Histologic features

The cyst (which contains keratin debris) is lined in part by apocrine epithelium with decapitation secretion admixed with squamous epithelium showing a well-developed granular cell layer.

Syringocystadenoma papilliferum

Clinical features

Syringocystadenoma papilliferum is usually a solitary lesion, which may be present at birth or develop in childhood, and most commonly occurs on the

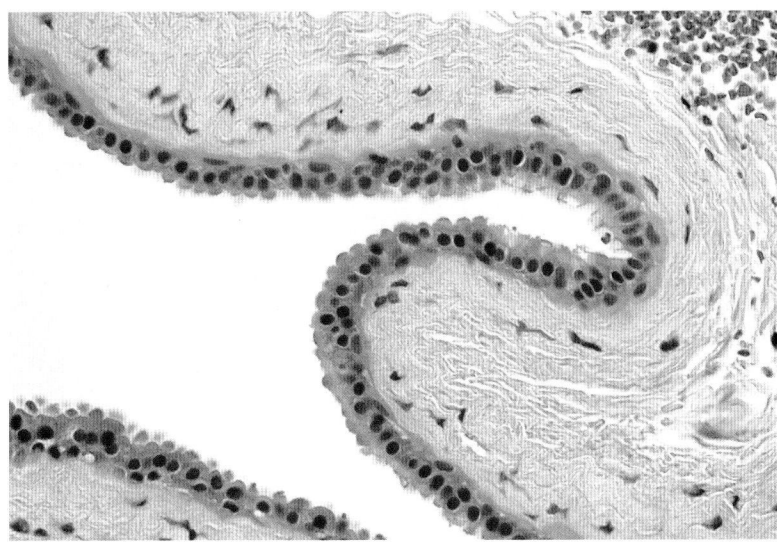

Fig. 33.3
Apocrine hidrocystoma: high-power view of lining epithelium showing decapitation secretion.

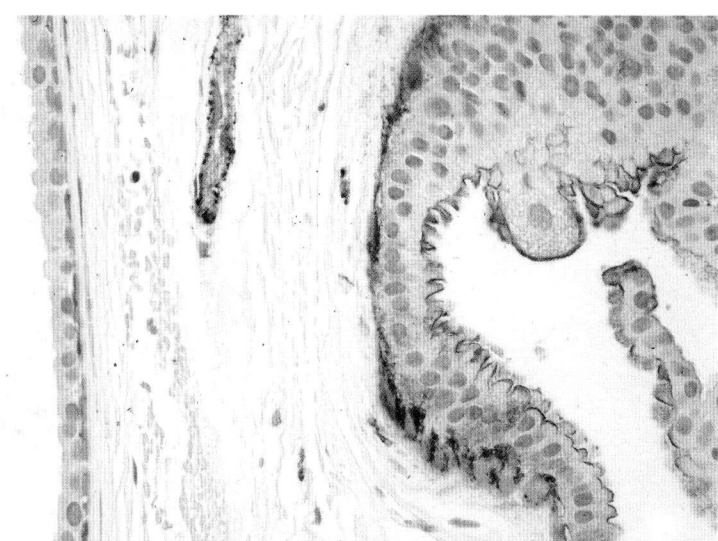

Fig. 33.5
Apocrine hidrocystoma: the outer myoepithelial cells express smooth muscle actin.

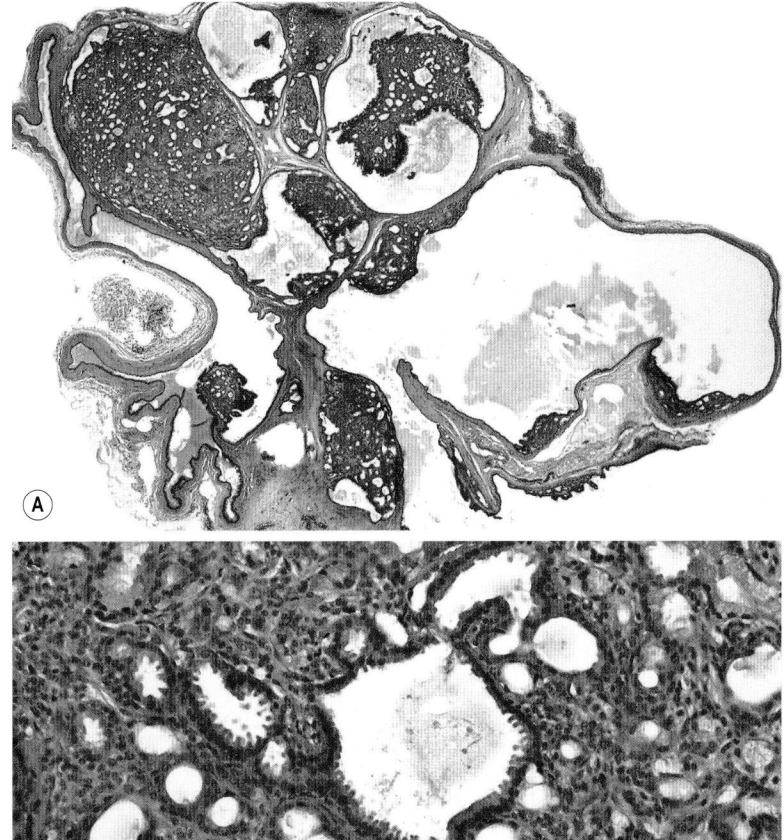

(A)

(B)

Fig. 33.4
(A, B) Apocrine papillary cystadenoma: this tumor (which presented on the skin of the neck) was cystic but contained both adenomatous and papillary components.

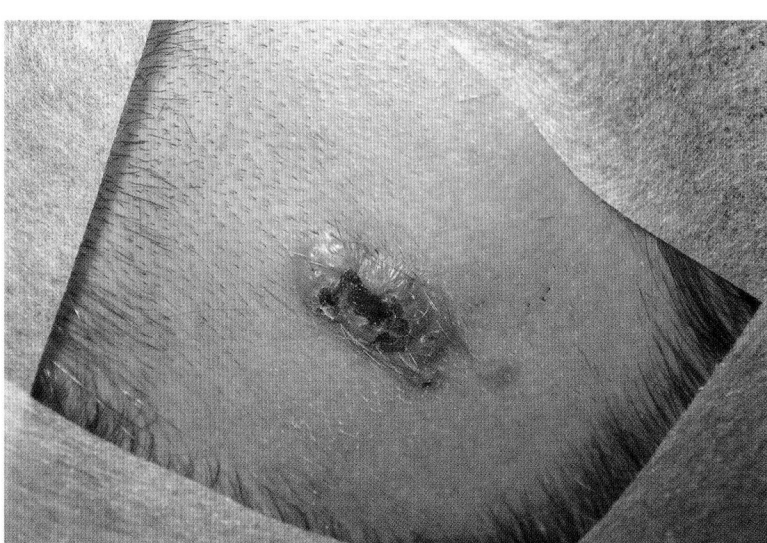

Fig. 33.6
Syringocystadenoma papilliferum: ulcerated, scaly plaque just prior to surgery. By courtesy of J.C. Pascual, MD, Alicante, Spain.

scalp.[1-5] It can also be found on the face, neck, trunk, and rarely the lower limbs (Fig. 33.6).[3] Surprisingly, it is not often present in the axilla, a site where apocrine glands are abundant. Rarely, lesions have been described on the eyelid, breast, arm, thigh, popliteal fossa, vulva, and scrotum.[6-16] Scalp involvement is commonly associated with nevus sebaceous (Fig. 33.7).[17-19] Syringocystadenoma papilliferum is thus found in between 5% and 19% of cases of nevus sebaceous, sometimes in association with trichilemmoma.[20,21] It has also been described in association with nevus comedonicus and in a patient with focal dermal hypoplasia (Goltz syndrome).[22,23]

Syringocystadenoma papilliferum most often presents as a gray or dark-brown papillary or rather warty, sometimes crusted, excrescence with a moist appearance. Less commonly, multiple small papules, occasionally in a linear or segmental distribution sometimes following Blaschko lines are seen.[3,24-29] Lesions may be excoriated due to pruritus, and those that develop on the scalp sometimes bleed due to the trauma of hair brushing or combing. Occasionally, there is central umbilication with drainage of sero-sanguineous secretions.[6] Multifocal disease is exceptional.[30]

Occasionally, syringocystadenoma papilliferum has been described in association with apocrine hidrocystoma, apocrine cystadenoma,

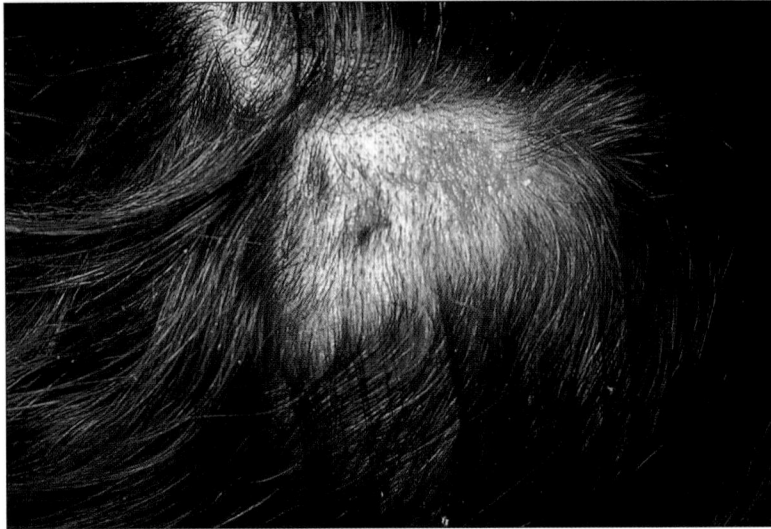

Fig. 33.7
Syringocystadenoma papilliferum: scalp tumor, which has arisen within a nevus sebaceous. By courtesy of the Institute of Dermatology, UMDS, London, UK.

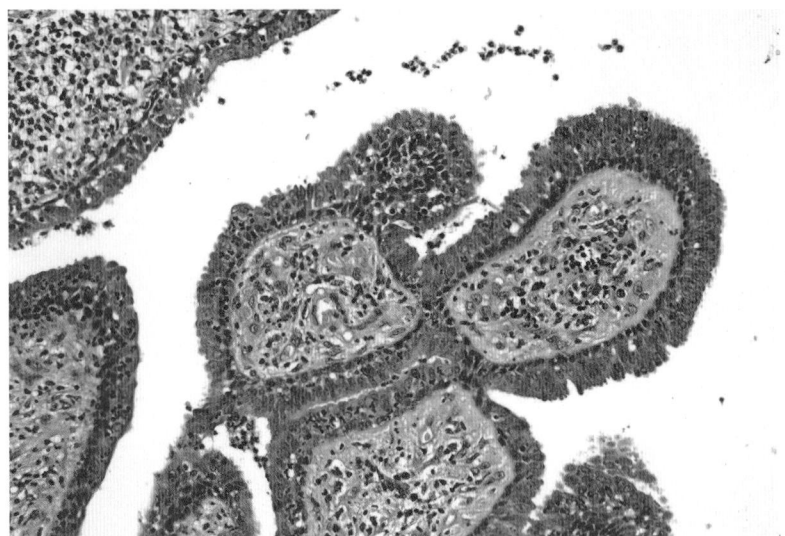

Fig. 33.9
Syringocystadenoma papilliferum: the papillae are covered by an outer layer of tall columnar cells with eosinophilic cytoplasm and an inner layer of small cuboidal myoepithelial cells with hyperchromatic nuclei.

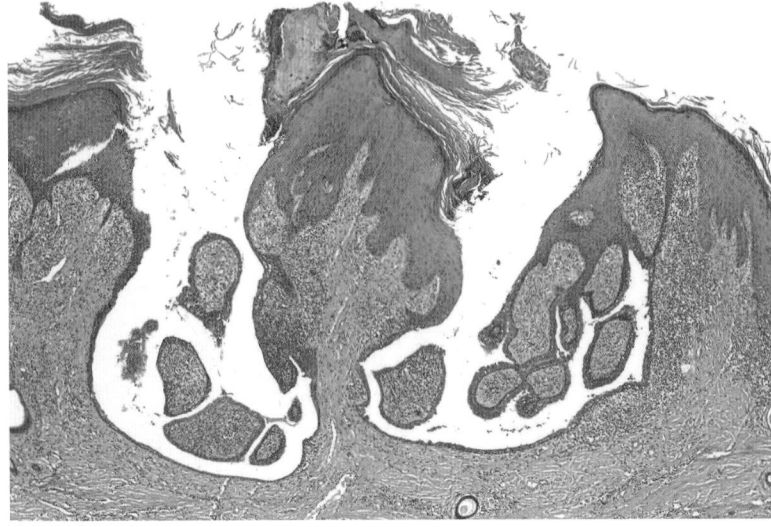

Fig. 33.8
Syringocystadenoma papilliferum: this exophytic lesion developed within a nevus sebaceous. Note that the surface is covered with squamous epithelium.

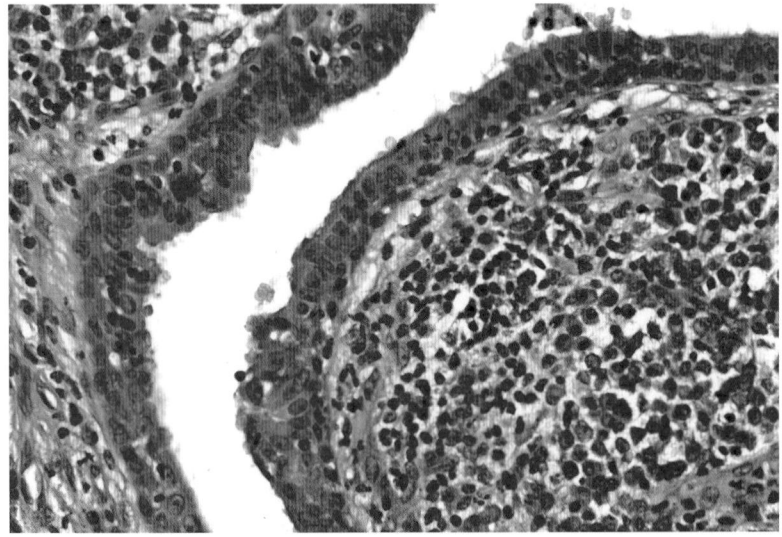

Fig. 33.10
Syringocystadenoma papilliferum: the stroma contains numerous plasma cells.

hidradenoma papilliferum, tubular apocrine adenoma, apocrine poroma, mixed tubulopapillary hidradenoma, as well as apocrine nevus.[18,31–36] It may also present with condyloma accuminatum, apocrine acrosyringeal keratosis, papillary eccrine hidradenoma, cutaneous horn, verrucous carcinoma, verrucous cyst, giant comedone, and poroma folliculare.[37–45]

Pathogenesis and histologic features

Although syringocystadenoma papilliferum is generally classified within the apocrine group, the results of electron microscopy, enzyme histochemistry, and immunocytochemistry are conflicting, variably offering support for both eccrine and apocrine derivation/differentiation.[3]

Genetically, deletion at 9q22 (PTCH) and at 9p21 (p16) have been identified in a subset of cases of syringocystadenoma papilliferum.[46] Sequencing analysis revealed frequent BRAF and HRAS mutations.[47,48]

Syringocystadenoma papilliferum has a characteristic and readily recognizable appearance. On low-power examination, it appears as an invagination from the overlying epidermis or else has an exophytic configuration (Fig. 33.8). Central to the diagnosis are superficially located epithelium-covered papillae, which communicate with ductlike structures in the deeper aspect of the lesion. At the surface, residual squamous epithelium is often hyperplastic and may show hyperkeratosis and parakeratosis. Superficially, the

villi can be covered by stratified squamous epithelium, but this soon gives way to a typical double-layered epithelium consisting of an inner zone of small cells with scant cytoplasm and oval hyperchromatic nuclei, and an outer zone of tall columnar cells with abundant eosinophilic cytoplasm and fairly large vesicular nuclei (Fig. 33.9). Decapitation secretion is often a feature. The glandular spaces are also lined by a double layer of epithelium. The papillary processes are supported by a fibrovascular core, which typically contains large numbers of plasma cells (Fig. 33.10). Although the histologic features of syringocystadenoma papilliferum are quite classic and characteristic, the morphological spectrum appears to be broad, and there may be at least some morphological overlap with tubular apocrine adenoma.[49] Syringocystadenoma papilliferum can show areas reminiscent of classic tubular apocrine adenoma as well as apocrine hidrocystoma and clear cell syringoma, and a tumor with focal sebaceous differentiation has also been reported to arise within a nevus sebaceous.[32–34,49–52]

Syringocystadenoma papilliferum expresses AE1/AE3, CAM 5.2, epithelial membrane antigen (EMA), and carcinoembryonic antigen (CEA).[12,33,53,54] The inner layer is positive for SMA.[12] The results of markers of apocrine differentiation are variable. Some authors have found gross cystic disease fluid protein 15 (GCDFP-15) and HMFG-1 negative.[10,39] Others have found GCDFP-15 and/or HMFG-2 present.[12,53]

Syringocystadenocarcinoma papilliferum

Clinical features

Only very rare cases of syringocystadenocarcinoma have been described.[1–24] These have included three in situ variants.[1,5,6–8,20–26] There are insufficient cases to allow for meaningful clinical data other than documenting that they have been described particularly on the scalp, but the forehead, temple, neck, chest, breast, back, and perianal region have also been affected. The sex incidence is equal and patients have been middle aged or elderly (range 46–81 years). Patients presented with verrucous nodules or large plaques, usually of many years' duration. When documented, an episode of sudden rapid growth and tumor fixation to the underlying tissues has been evidence of malignant transformation. Occasionally, an association with nevus sebaceous has been documented.[26–28]

Thus far, these tumors appear to be low grade, with only one case having metastasized to regional lymph nodes.[3]

Histologic features

The majority of carcinomas have arisen in clearly recognizable benign precursor lesions. The malignant component may be recognized by nuclear atypia, multilayering, increased mitotic activity including abnormal forms, and dermal involvement in those cases associated with an invasive component. Intraepidermal pagetoid spread may be observed, and the invasive component may show additional differentiation toward squamous cell carcinoma.

Rarely, the development of mucinous adenocarcinoma or apocrine ductal carcinoma presenting in a syringocystadenoma papilliferum which had arisen in a nevus sebaceous has been documented.[27,28]

The tumor epithelial cells express AE1/AE3, EMA, and CEA.[6] HMFG-2 and GCDFP-15 are variably positive.[5,6]

Hidradenoma papilliferum

Clinical features

Hidradenoma papilliferum (papillary hidradenoma) in the vast majority of cases has been described in females.[1–9] Almost all cases have been reported in white women.[5] Patients are generally young or middle-aged adults (range 20–89 years).[6,7] There are only very rare documented cases reported in males, and some authors would regard such lesions as representing apocrine papillary cystadenomas.[7,10,11] The same might also be said for at least some examples of so-called ectopic hidradenoma papilliferum which have been described on the eyelid, nose, cheek, axilla, upper and lower limbs, chest, back, and external auditory canal.[12–17] The examples arising on the eyelid and external auditory meatus are likely derived from the gland of Moll and ceruminous gland, respectively.

The tumor presents as a small (1–2 cm in diameter), solitary, usually asymptomatic papule or nodule in a vulval, perineal, or perianal location.[4] Very occasionally, pain, tenderness, pruritus, burning, discharge, or bleeding may be encountered.[6] The tumor typically arises at sites of the anogenital mammary-like glands. Most often it affects the labium majus, but on occasion it has been described as involving the lateral aspect of the labium minus, the interlabial sulcus, the clitoris, posterior fourchette, and mons pubis (*Fig. 33.11*).[6,18] Lesions are round, solid, or cystic and sometimes umbilicated or ulcerated.[5]

Pathogenesis and histologic features

Hidradenoma papilliferum arises from apocrine glands or possibly the anogenital mammary-like glands, and it may represent the genital equivalent to intraductal papilloma of the breast with which it shares many morphological similarities.[19,20]

The epidermis may be normal, acanthotic, or ulcerated. The tumor forms a fairly well-demarcated nodule in the dermis or lamina propria and may sometimes show foci of continuity with the overlying epithelium (*Fig. 33.12*).[4,21] The lesion consists primarily of epithelium-covered papillary processes that project into cystic spaces. The epithelial lining is typically

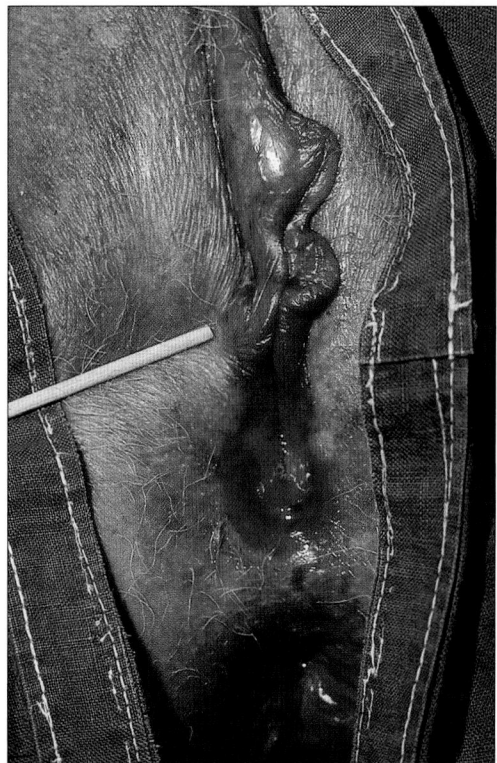

Fig. 33.11
Hidradenoma papilliferum: this example has caused erythema and ulceration below the right labium minus and around the introitus. By courtesy of the late M. Ridley, MD, Whittington Hospital, London, UK.

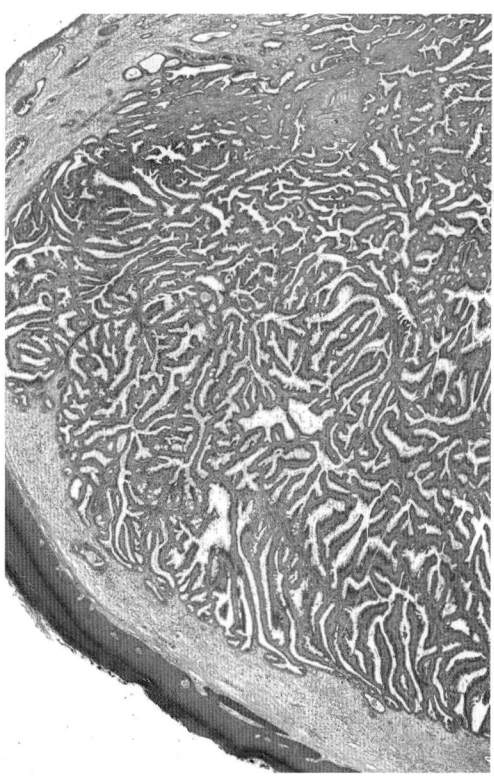

Fig. 33.12
Hidradenoma papilliferum: low-power view of an exophytic ulcerated nodule. The epidermal collarette is seen in the lower left of the field.

double layered, comprising inner small myoepithelial cells with oval hyperchromatic nuclei and outer tall columnar cells with eosinophilic cytoplasm, sometimes manifesting decapitation secretion (*Fig. 33.13*). Prominent oxyphilic metaplasia of the epithelial cells, in areas showing mild nuclear pleomorphism, may be a focal feature.[8,9] Occasionally, the lining is only one cell

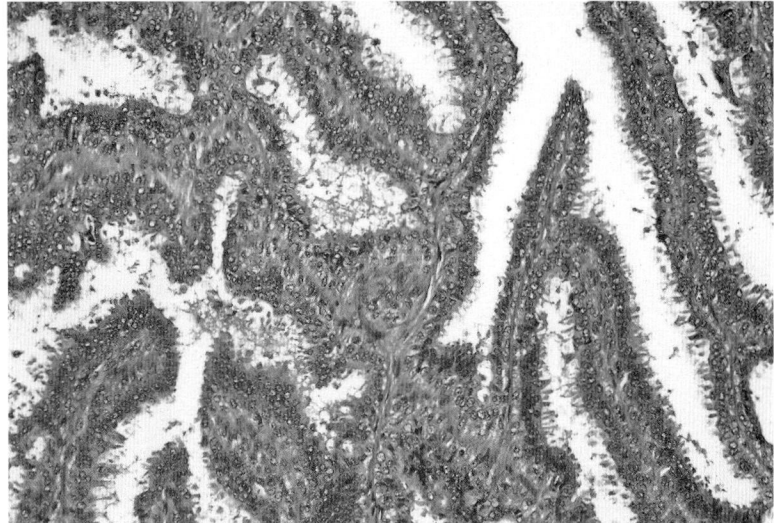

Fig. 33.13
Hidradenoma papilliferum: a double layer of epithelium covers the epithelial fronds. Decapitation secretion is conspicuous.

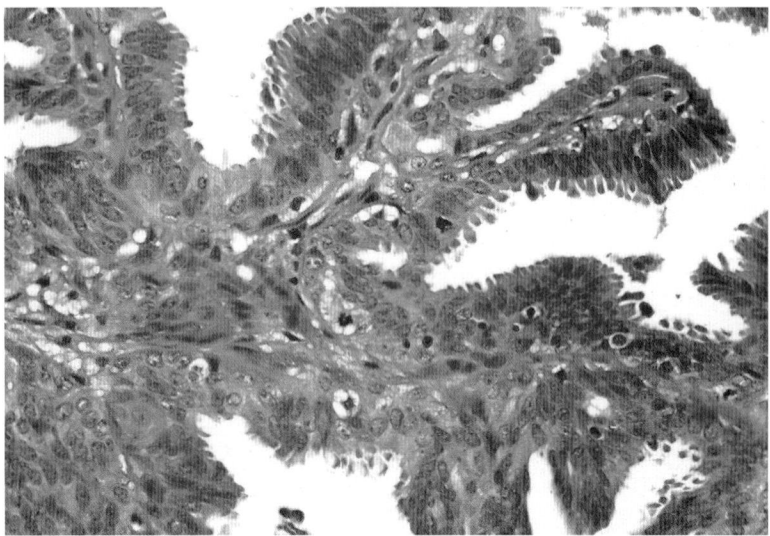

Fig. 33.14
Hidradenoma papilliferum: in the center of the field are two mitotic figures.

thick (columnar). Diastase-resistant, PAS-positive intracytoplasmic granules are usually present. The presence of normal mitotic activity has no sinister implication (*Fig. 33.14*).[22] The larger villi have a fibrous core in which occasional ductular structures may be identified, sometimes forming a cribriform pattern. Often, the fibrous tissue surrounding the tumor is compressed to form a pseudocapsule. An inflammatory cell component is not a significant feature although aggregates of lymphocytes and plasma cells have been described in the stroma of ectopic lesions.[14] The tumors may show overlapping histologic features with syringocystadenoma papilliferum.[23] Rare observations include a focally solid growth pattern composed of small monomorphous cells with lumen formation, a spindle cell population as well as areas resembling sclerosing adenosis, usual and atypical ductal hyperplasia in the breast.[8,24] Uncommonly, focal sebaceous differentiation may be a feature.[4,17]

Exceptionally rarely, a malignant variant may be encountered including intraductal carcinoma.[25–29] In the single example encountered by the authors, focal areas showing an extensive infiltrative growth pattern accompanied by marked nuclear pleomorphism and conspicuous, sometimes abnormal, mitotic activity were identified against a background of typical benign morphology. The outcome in this case is unfortunately not known. Coincidental hidradenoma papilliferum in a patient with vulval Paget disease has been described.[7,30]

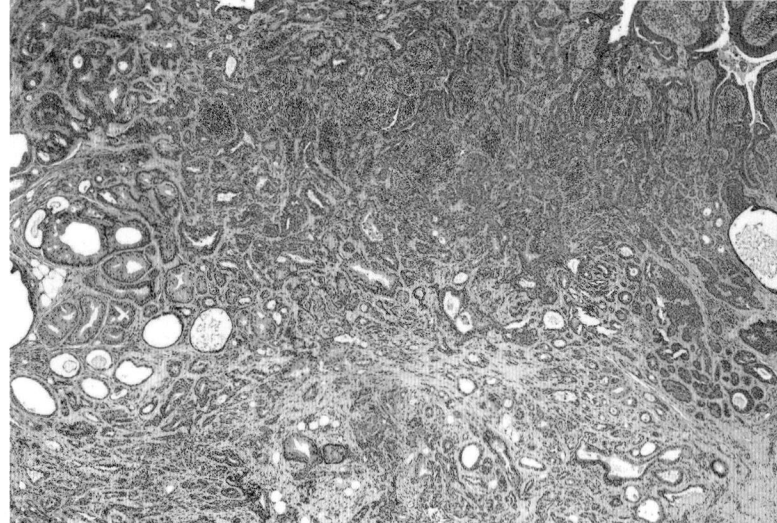

Fig. 33.15
Apocrine tubular adenoma: this example from the face consists of variably sized tubules, many showing cystic dilatation.

Ultrastructurally, hidradenoma papilliferum shows features of apocrine differentiation.[31]

Immunohistochemically, the epithelial cells express low molecular weight keratin, EMA, CEA, HMFG, and GCDFP-15.[7,32] Estrogen and, to a lesser extent, progesterone receptors are positive, and androgen receptor is expressed in up to 20% of tumors.[32–34] The myoepithelial cells express S100 protein and SMA.[32]

Genetically, the tumors may show mutations in the PIK3Ca and AKT1 genes, similar to intraductal papilloma of the breast.[20–36]

Human papillomavirus (HPV) types 16, 31, 33, 53, and 56 have been detected in a subset of anogenital lesions, but no definite causal role in the pathogenesis of this tumor has been established as yet and the significance of this finding is unclear.[8,37]

Tubular apocrine adenoma

Clinical features

Tubular apocrine adenoma (apocrine adenoma, tubulopapillary hidradenoma, papillary tubular adenoma) is a rare benign tumor which shows a female predominance (2:1) and a wide age distribution (18–78 years).[1–12] The scalp is most commonly affected although lesions have been described at a variety of other sites including the face, eyelid, axilla, leg, and genitalia.[3,5,8–11,13,14] The last, however, may represent an adenoma of the anogenital mammary-like glands.[10] Those that present on the scalp often arise in a background of nevus sebaceous and are sometimes associated with syringocystadenoma papilliferum.[12,15–19] The tumor generally presents as a dermal nodule 1–2 cm in diameter or pedunculated lesion, frequently of many years' duration, particularly those developing within a nevus sebaceous. The lesion is benign, and recurrence following excision is uncommon.

Histologic features

Histologically, tubular apocrine adenoma presents most often as a circumscribed intradermal nodule although in some cases the subcutaneous fat is involved. Sometimes the tumor communicates with the epidermis through ductlike structures or dilated follicular infundibula (*Fig. 33.15*). As mentioned above, there may be continuity with a syringocystadenoma papilliferum or an organoid nevus. It is composed of variably sized, well-formed tubules lined by a double- or multilayered epithelial cell layer comprising cuboidal or columnar forms with abundant eosinophilic cytoplasm and uniform round to oval nuclei (*Fig. 33.16*). There is no pleomorphism and mitoses are scanty. In those tubules showing glandular differentiation, the inner lining cells often show decapitation secretion while the outer layer is composed of flattened myoepithelial cells. Cystic change is common, and

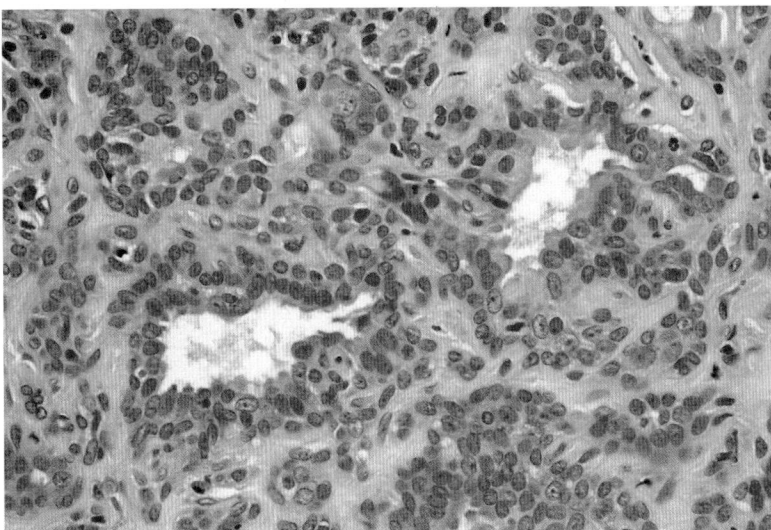

Fig. 33.16
Apocrine tubular adenoma: the tubules are lined by cuboidal to columnar epithelial cells with copious eosinophilic cytoplasm and focally showing decapitation secretion.

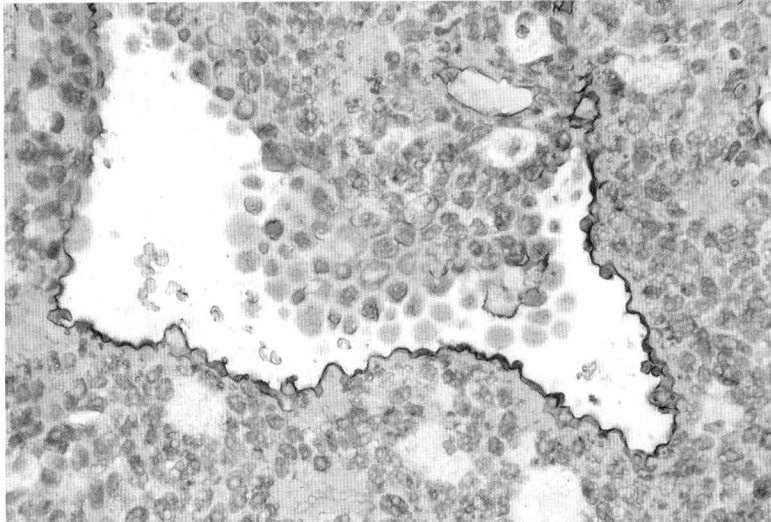

Fig. 33.17
Apocrine tubular adenoma: the luminal aspect of the tubules shows striking EMA positivity.

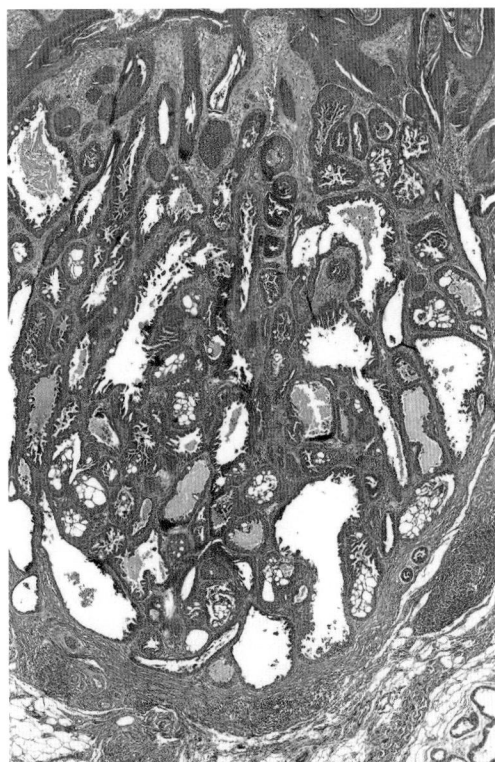

Fig. 33.18
Tubulopapillary hidradenoma: this example, which arose in a background of nevus sebaceous, shows a prominent papillary component.

in many tumors intraluminal papillae are present although usually these are devoid of a fibrovascular core. True papillae are, however, sometimes seen although these are generally evident in lesions associated with a syringocystadenoma papilliferum. The tumor has a well-developed connective tissue stroma in which only small numbers of chronic inflammatory cells are present. Areas of follicular and/or sebaceous differentiation may rarely be encountered.[20]

The luminal surface of the tubular lining epithelial cells shows strong expression of EMA and CEA (*Fig. 33.17*).[7,11,12,17] The cytoplasm is also sometimes weakly EMA positive.[12] HMFG-1 and GCDFP-15 may be present.[11] The myoepithelial cells can be highlighted with SMA or S100 protein immunohistochemistry.[11,12,17]

Ultrastructurally, the tubules are lined by cuboidal to columnar epithelial cells with conspicuous luminal microvilli and sometimes showing apical pinching or frank decapitation secretion. The cytoplasm contains prominent Golgi, conspicuous mitochondria, and lipid-rich secretory vacuoles. The outer layer shows features of myoepithelial cells.[12]

Differential diagnosis

Tubular apocrine adenoma must be distinguished from syringocystadenoma papilliferum, papillary eccrine adenoma, and papillary apocrine carcinoma.

Some tumors, particularly those arising in a background of an organoid nevus, develop in association with a syringocystadenoma papilliferum. Those that are wholly intradermal differ from syringocystadenoma papilliferum by the absence of true papillae with fibrovascular cores and by the absence of a plasma cell-rich inflammatory cell infiltrate. There may, however, be a morphological continuum between the two entities, and reliable separation is not always possible.[21]

Tubular apocrine adenoma can be distinguished from papillary eccrine adenoma in many cases by the presence of apocrine decapitation secretion and the common location on the scalp, especially when developing in association with syringocystadenoma papilliferum or organoid nevus. In some cases, however, the distinction is difficult or impossible (*Figs 33.18* and *33.19*). Occasional tumors show features of both lesions.[11] This has led some authors to suggest the alternative terms tubulopapillary hidradenoma and papillary tubular adenoma.[11,12,22]

Tubular apocrine adenoma differs from papillary apocrine carcinoma by the absence of an infiltrative growth pattern and cytological atypia. Mitoses are generally sparse and abnormal forms are absent.

Adenoma and adenocarcinoma of the anogenital mammary-like glands

The anogenital mammary-like glands combine the features of eccrine, apocrine, and mammary glands.[1–3] They are present in greatest concentration in the vulval interlabial sulcus. A range of tumors reminiscent of their mammary counterparts including epithelial hyperplasia, adenoma, fibroadenoma, phyllodes tumor, and in situ as well as invasive ductal carcinoma have been documented.[4–26] Pseudoangiomatous stromal hyperplasia (PASH) has also been documented.[26–28]

HPV has been detected in a single case of invasive ductal carcinoma.[29]

Nipple adenoma

Clinical features

Nipple adenoma (erosive adenomatosis, florid papillomatosis, superficial papillary adenomatosis) is a benign tumor which most often presents in

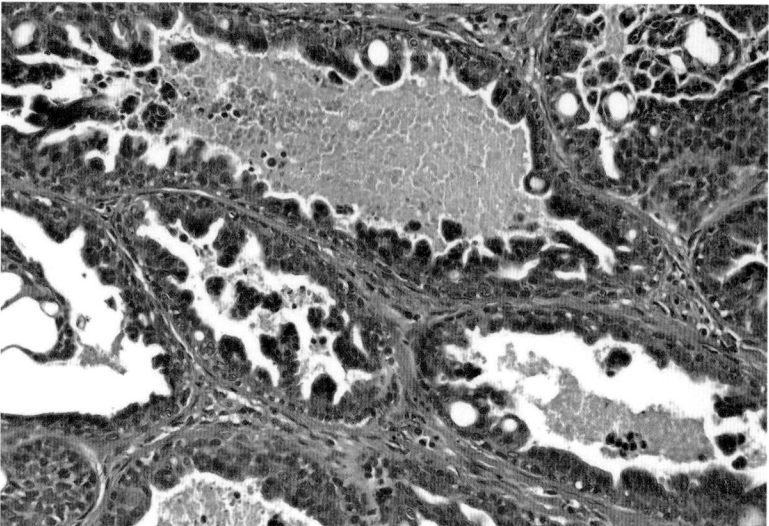

Fig. 33.19
Tubulopapillary hidradenoma: the tubules are lined by double-layered epithelium. The papillae are devoid of a fibrovascular core. It is often impossible to determine whether this tumor is of apocrine or eccrine differentiation.

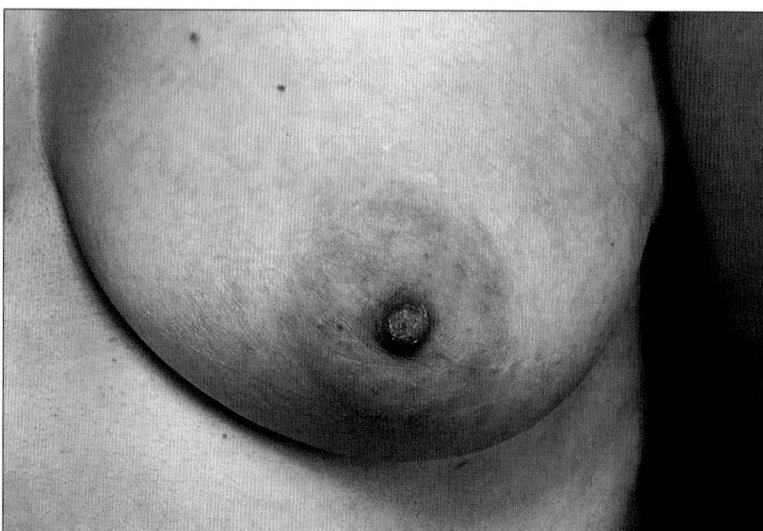

Fig. 33.20
Nipple adenoma: the nipple shows an ulcerated crusted lesion. By courtesy of the Institute of Dermatology, UMDS, London, UK.

middle-aged females with a peak incidence in the fifth decade.[1-8] Rarely, however, girls may be affected, and there are exceptional reports of the condition in males.[9-13] Patients present with erythematous, scaly or crusted, and sometimes eroded lesions clinically mistaken for eczematous dermatitis or Paget disease (*Fig. 33.20*).[1,6,14] Pruritus, irritation, pain, and burning are variable complaints.[9] A 0.5- to 1.5-cm tumor nodule and/or an increase in size of the nipple are sometimes present.[4,8] Some patients complain of nipple discharge or bleeding.

Histologic features

The tumor is unencapsulated and consists of adenomatous and papillary areas in varying proportion.[1] It usually communicates with the surface epithelium where cysts lined by an admixture of squamous and columnar epithelium are sometimes evident.[1] The glandular spaces are lined by tall columnar eosinophilic cells which invariably show decapitation secretion. A myoepithelial cell layer is present. Intraluminal papillomatosis is generally evident, and giant cells are sometimes seen.[1,9] Normal mitoses may be present. The papillae are devoid of a fibrovascular core and cytological atypia is absent. The stroma can be fibrotic or hyalinized, and in some

tumors this compresses the epithelium to give rise to a pseudoinfiltrative growth pattern.[1] A plasma cell-rich inflammatory cell infiltrate is sometimes evident in the surrounding connective tissue.

Genetically, the tumors show mutations in the PIK3CA gene in approximately 50% of cases.[15]

Syringomatous adenoma of the nipple

Clinical features

Syringomatous adenoma of the nipple is a rare tumor presenting as a firm unilateral mass of few centimeters on the breast predominantly affecting the nipple and subareolar area.[1-9] Bilateral presentation is rare, and the development within a supernumerary breast has also been reported.[10,11] It is a tumor of adulthood with a peak incidence in the fourth decade and a strong female predilection.[1-10] Presentation in males is exceptional.[9] Syringomatous adenoma of the nipple is a locally aggressive tumor with potential for recurrence if inadequately excised.[8,9] However, no distant metastasis or disease-related mortality has been documented, and complete excision with negative margins appears to be curative.[8,9]

Histologic features

The histologic features are reminiscent of microcystic adnexal carcinoma to which it may be closely related. The tumor shows an infiltrative growth pattern within dermis, along nipple ducts, and extending into breast parenchyma.[9,10] Infiltration of smooth muscle is a frequent feature and perineural infiltration may rarely be observed. The tumor is composed of small, well-formed ducts and basaloid epithelial strands within a fibrous stroma showing only little or no cytological atypia.[9,10] Tubular and squamous differentiation may be seen and keratocysts as well as dystrophic calcification are common.

By immunohistochemistry, the syringomatous adenoma of the nipple is composed of p63, CK5, and CK14 positive tumor cells and CK8 and CK18 positive glandular cells similar to low-grade adenosquamous carcinoma. It has recently been proposed that these may be closely related entities.[12]

Apocrine poroma

Clinical features

Apocrine poroma (poroma with divergent differentiation, complex poroma-like adnexal adenoma, sebocrine adenoma, sebaceous and apocrine adenoma, and poroma with sebaceous differentiation) is an uncommon tumor, which presents as an often slowly growing flesh-colored, erythematous papule, nodule, or plaque.[1-10] There is no site predilection, lesions having been described on the lip, cheek, eyelid, nose, abdomen, back, and limbs.[3,11,12] No cases presenting on the palms and soles have been documented to date. A wide age range may be involved (19–76 years). The sexes are affected equally.

The tumor is benign and recurrences are rare.[2]

Histologic features

Apocrine poroma in essence is defined as a poroma showing sebaceous differentiation with the occasional presence of follicular differentiation and foci of apocrine-like features. In terms of nomenclature, although sebaceous differentiation is the common link, the literature has focused on the apocrine element – hence the designation apocrine poroma. The presence of sebaceous, follicular, and apocrine features reflects the common embryological ancestry of the three units (the folliculosebaceous-apocrine unit).

Apocrine poroma – in common with its eccrine counterpart – is composed of anastomosing trabeculae, displaying multiple points of origin from the epidermis and located largely in the papillary and upper reticular dermis.[3] The individual cells are small and uniform with scanty cytoplasm and round to oval nuclei united by inconspicuous intercellular bridges. Foci of ductal differentiation with a well-developed eosinophilic cuticle are present. An example showing follicular infundibular origin in a patient with nevoid basal cell carcinoma has been reported.[4]

An infrequent feature is the presence of sebaceous cells, singly and in clusters with bubbly cytoplasm and crenated nuclei. Sebaceous ductlike tubular or cystic structures lined by squamous epithelium with an eosinophilic, scalloped cuticle and containing eosinophilic debris with pyknotic nuclei may also be present.[3] In some examples, hair germlike structures manifest as small collections of basaloid cells with peripheral palisading, and perifollicular sheathlike connective tissue are seen.[3,7,9] Occasional reports have described tubules lined by cells with intensely eosinophilic cytoplasm reminiscent of apocrine epithelium.[3,7] Although frank decapitation has generally been absent, it is well illustrated in the series of Yamamoto and coworkers.[6]

Wholly intraepidermal hidroacanthoma simplex-like and largely intradermal variants have been documented.[5,9] In addition, there is a report of an example associated with trichoblastoma.[10]

A case presenting on the areola has also been documented.[13] In it, however, there was no evidence of sebaceous, follicular, or apocrine differentiation. Although close proximity to the follicular infundibula was demonstrated, it is unclear whether the tumor might not have been better regarded as eccrine poroma.[13]

A metaplastic or sarcomatoid carcinoma has been shown to arise within an apocrine poroma (sarcomatoid apocrine porocarcinoma).[11]

Differential diagnosis

Diagnosis of apocrine poroma depends on exclusion of entrapped normal adnexae.

Intraepidermal variants may be differentiated from seborrheic keratoses with sebaceous differentiation by the presence of ducts, which may be highlighted with diastase–PAS staining or EMA/CEA immunohistochemistry.

Cutaneous oncocytoma

Clinical features

Oncocytomas rarely affect the skin. They are more commonly seen in the kidney, thyroid, parathyroid, and salivary glands. In the skin, they show a predilection for the lacrimal areas and they typically occur on the canthus, the eyelid, and rarely on the cheek as a small nodule.[1–4] The patients are elderly adults without significant gender predilection.[1–4] The clinical behavior is benign.

Histologic features

Cutaneous oncocytomas are well-circumscribed tumors within the dermis occasionally showing a connection with the overlying epidermis (Fig. 33.21).[1–4] Their growth pattern is solid and cystic with additional papillary and tubular areas. They are composed of large polygonal cells with abundant finely granular eosinophilic cytoplasm containing uniform nuclei with eosinophilic nucleoli (Fig. 33.22).[1–4] Nuclear pleomorphism and mitotic activity are not a feature.

By immunohistochemistry, tumor cells express pancytokeratin AE1/AE3 but they are negative for S100 and CD68. Luminal staining is noted for EMA and CEA.

Apocrine carcinoma

Clinical features

Apocrine adenocarcinoma is rare, and most documented cases have affected the axilla.[1–18] Occasionally, the tumor may present at a variety of other sites including the scalp, eyelid (Moll gland carcinoma), ear (ceruminous gland adenocarcinoma), anogenital region, chest, lip, and wrist, in descending order of frequency.[2,14,18–30] Tumors have also been described on the cheek, nipple, and fingertip.[11,31,32] Clinical data are limited in the majority of published cases, but most tumors present as single or multiple, sometimes ulcerated, often slowly growing nodules or plaques covered by erythematous or purple skin. A presentation as carcinoma erysipeloides has also been documented.[1–3,33] In some instances, tumors have been present for 30 years before diagnosis.[12] Occasional tumors have arisen within a nevus sebaceous, and invasive as well as in situ carcinoma has been documented

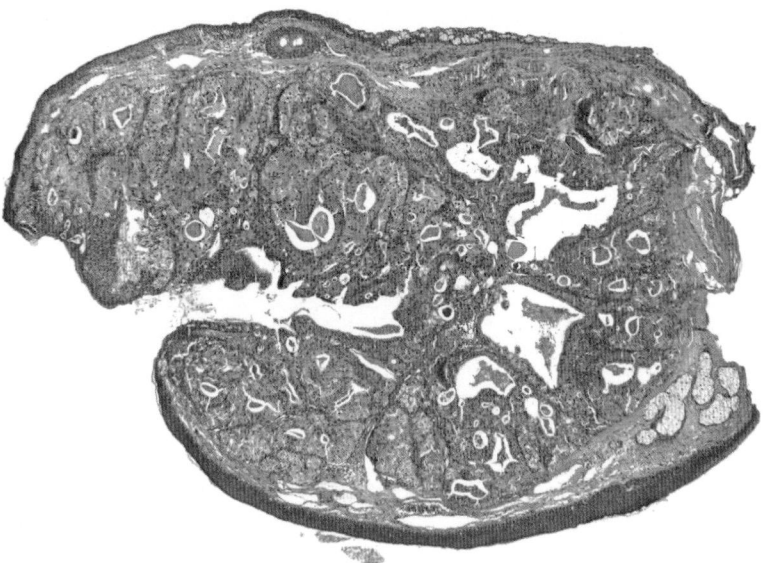

Fig. 33.21
Cutaneous oncocytoma: this well-circumscribed, nodular tumor is located at the mucosal–cutaneous junction of the eyelid and shows connection with the overlying epithelium. By courtesy of Katharina Flux, MD, Labor für Dermatohistologie und Oralpathologie, Munich, Germany.

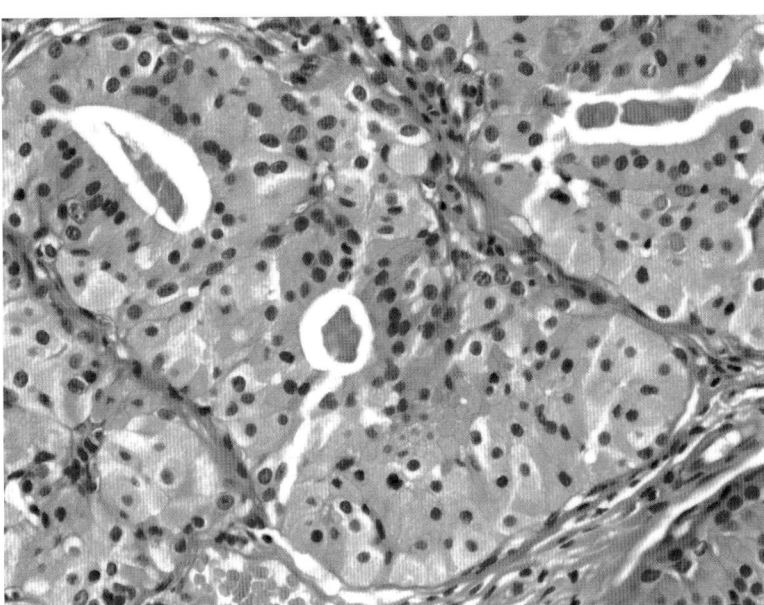

Fig. 33.22
Cutaneous oncocytoma: it is composed of large polygonal cells with abundant brightly eosinophilic and finely granular cytoplasm. Tubular differentiation is evident. By courtesy of Katharina Flux, MD, Labor für Dermatohistologie und Oralpathologie, Munich, Germany.

to arise in association with apocrine adenoma in the perianal area.[18,28,34–38] Patients with bilateral axillary apocrine carcinomas and associated apocrine hyperplasia have been reported in the Japanese literature.[16,39] Telangiectatic and inflammatory cutaneous metastatic disease similar to that described with breast carcinoma has been described.[24] Age at presentation is variable (18–91 years, mean 60 years) and the sex incidence is approximately equal.[1,2,18,40] There is no racial predilection.[2]

Apocrine carcinoma is often characterized by a prolonged course and, although recurrences (28%) and nodal metastases (50%) are common, the overall mortality is low. Bone and lung secondary deposits or more disseminated disease and tumor-related deaths have, however, been described.[1,2,5,11,12,18,22,24,41–44] Disease-related mortality was 24% in one study.[18] The median survival is 51.5 months, and positive lymph node status and metastatic disease are associated with poor overall survival.[40] In some patients,

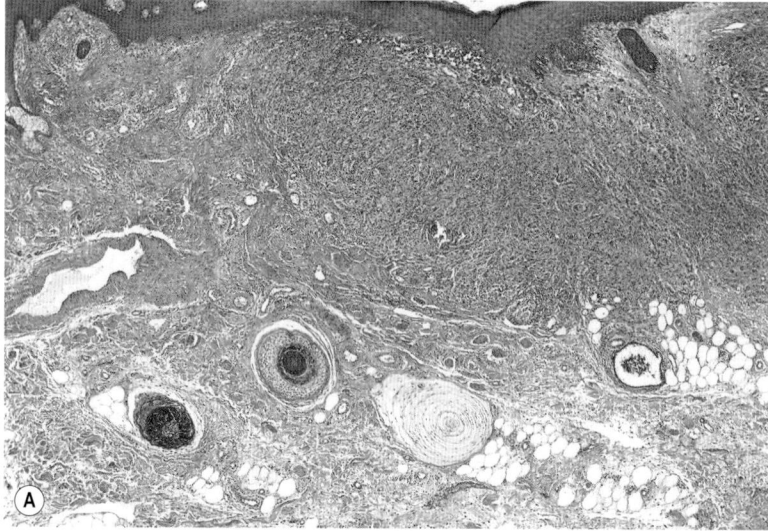

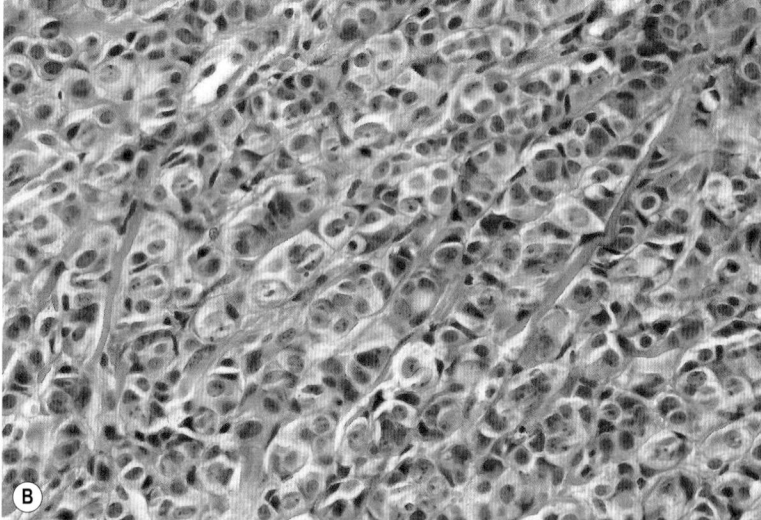

Fig. 33.23

(**A, B**) Apocrine carcinoma: this specimen comes from the vulva and shows diffuse infiltration by poorly differentiated adenocarcinoma. Note the nuclear pleomorphism and prominent nucleoli.

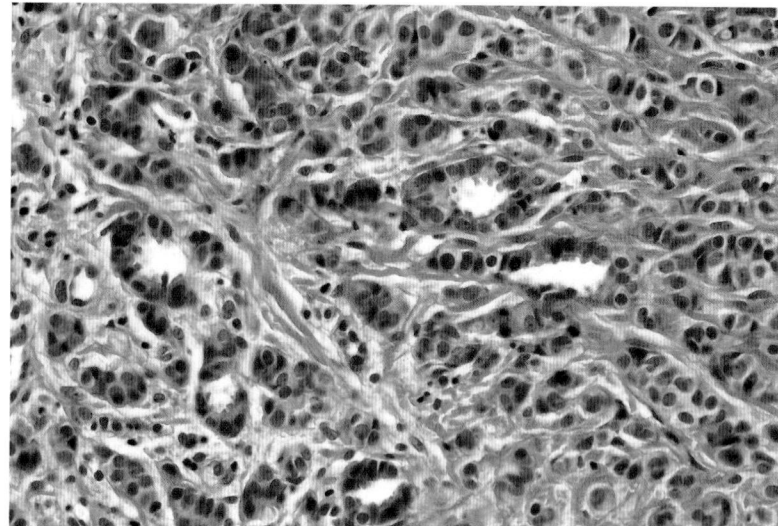

Fig. 33.24

Apocrine carcinoma: focal glandular differentiation and decapitation secretion is evident.

metastases are a very late development and therefore a very careful, prolonged follow-up is indicated.

Histologic features

Apocrine carcinoma is characterized by a variable glandular, tubular, papillary, tubulopapillary, or diffuse or solid growth pattern centered on the deeper dermis and frequently involving the subcutaneous fat (*Figs 33.23–33.26*).[1–3,18,45] Occasional tumors are cystic, and foci of necrosis are sometimes evident.[2] In contrast to apocrine adenoma, the tumor is usually poorly circumscribed, and typically an infiltrating border is present. Epidermotropism is sometimes a feature, and in some tumors frank Paget disease is present (*Fig. 33.27*).[2,11,13,18,23,24,46–48]

The epithelial cells have abundant eosinophilic cytoplasm, and decapitation secretion (albeit often focal) is invariably present (*Fig. 33.28*).[2,6] Nuclei are round or oval and vesicular and commonly contain a solitary prominent nucleolus (*Figs 33.29–33.31*). Focal squamous differentiation may occasionally be seen.[2] Exceptionally, sebaceous differentiation has been described.[26] Pleomorphism and mitotic activity are variable features, but become more prominent in poorly differentiated variants. The tumor is commonly accompanied by a dense hyaline stroma. A single filing growth pattern may be encountered in poorly differentiated tumors.[8–10,18,24] Apocrine carcinoma is characterized by intracytoplasmic diastase-resistant, PAS-positive granules, and intracytoplasmic iron is sometimes demonstrable.[2,16,22] Alcian blue (pH 2.5) and mucicarmine may also be positive but glycogen is uniformly absent.[9,13]

Normal apocrine glands are often found in close proximity to the tumor, and occasionally longstanding preexistent benign apocrine lesions (including hyperplasia, cystadenoma, cylindroma, syringocystadenoma papilliferum, and tubular adenoma) may be evident, raising the possibility of malignant transformation.[2,3,6,14,20,49] The apocrine glands sometimes show tumor infiltration/in situ carcinoma.[1,2,13,26] Perineural infiltration and lymphovascular invasion is occasionally seen.[18,22,26]

A small number of apocrine carcinomas showing signet ring cells reminiscent of invasive lobular carcinoma of breast have been reported.[18,50,51] These show a striking predilection for elderly males (10:1).[10] Although these have most frequently been described on the eyelids, they may also present in the axilla.[8–10] Apocrine carcinoma with focal mucinous carcinoma-like features has been documented.[23] An unusual tumor characterized by more circumscribed borders, epidermal connection, and atypical basaloid cells with duct formation and decapitation secretion has been reported.[52]

It has been proposed that tumors should be graded histologically according to the modified Bloom-Richardson method used in breast cancer as grade III lesions are associated with worse survival than those classified as grade I or II.[18]

Immunocytochemically, the tumor shows cytokeratin CAM 5.2, AE1/AE3, CK5/6, EMA, CEA, GATA3, and GCDFP-15 expression.[2,3,11,19,53] Lysozyme, α_1-antitrypsin, α_1-antichymotrypsin, and in some tumors S100 protein, are also present.[2,10] Myoepithelial cells as demonstrated by SMA or p63 are usually lost.[13,26,53] Androgen receptor is typically expressed and expression of estrogen receptor and progesterone receptor is seen in a significant subset of tumors.[18,53] In contrast, no HER2/neu expression is seen.[53] If fresh tissue is available, assessment of apocrine enzymes, including acid phosphatase and non-specific esterase, may be of diagnostic value.[6]

Electron microscopic findings, including luminal microvilli, conspicuous mitochondria, and large electron dense granules, have supported apocrine differentiation.[11,23]

Differential diagnosis

Primary cutaneous apocrine carcinoma is indistinguishable from metastatic mammary ductal apocrine carcinoma. With the exception of those rare lesions arising in a nevus sebaceous or showing focal continuity with an associated apocrine adenoma, careful breast assessment should be advised before accepting the diagnosis of primary cutaneous apocrine carcinoma, particularly for those lesions that present at an atypical location. By immunohistochemistry, primary cutaneous tumors are commonly adipophilin and HER2/neu negative and estrogen receptor (ER) and progesterone receptor (PR) positive. In contrast, mammary tumors are more likely to express adipophilin and HER2/neu with negative staining for ER and PR. Androgen receptor expression is nondiscriminatory.[53]

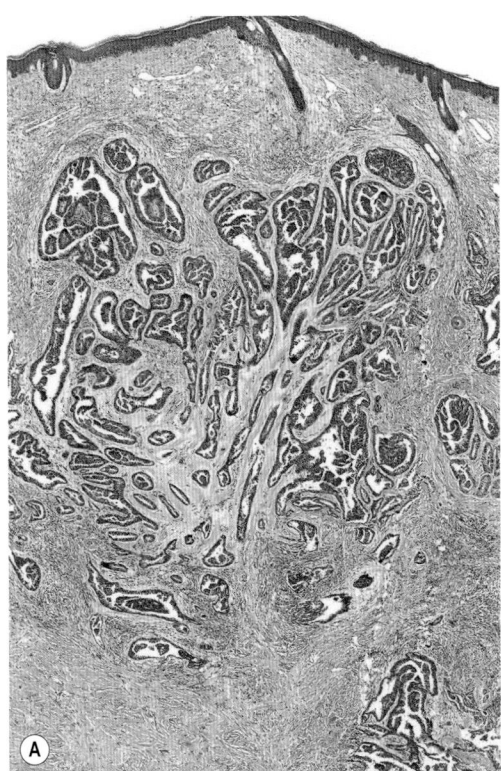

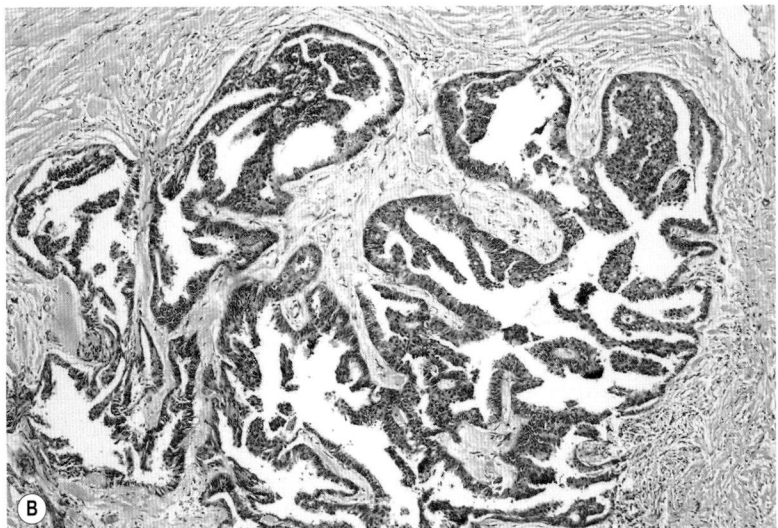

Fig. 33.25
(**A**, **B**) Apocrine carcinoma: this example from the face shows a striking papillary growth pattern.

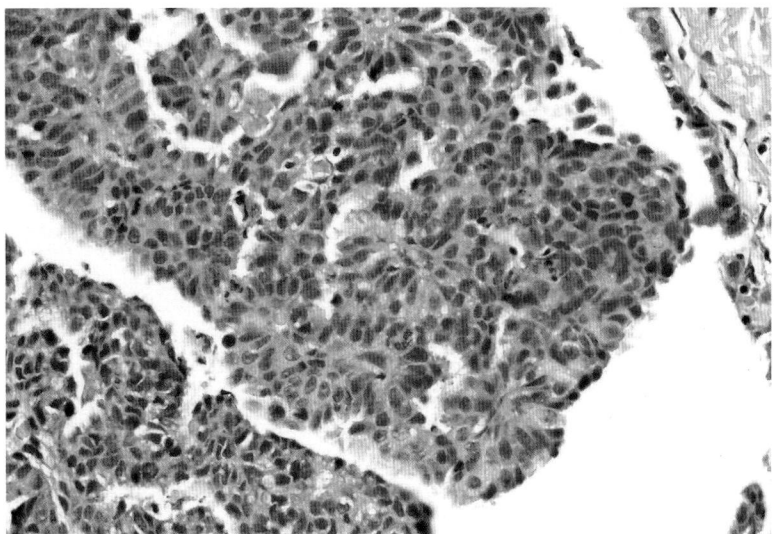

Fig. 33.26
Apocrine carcinoma: higher-power view showing multilayering, nuclear hyperchromatism, and pleomorphism.

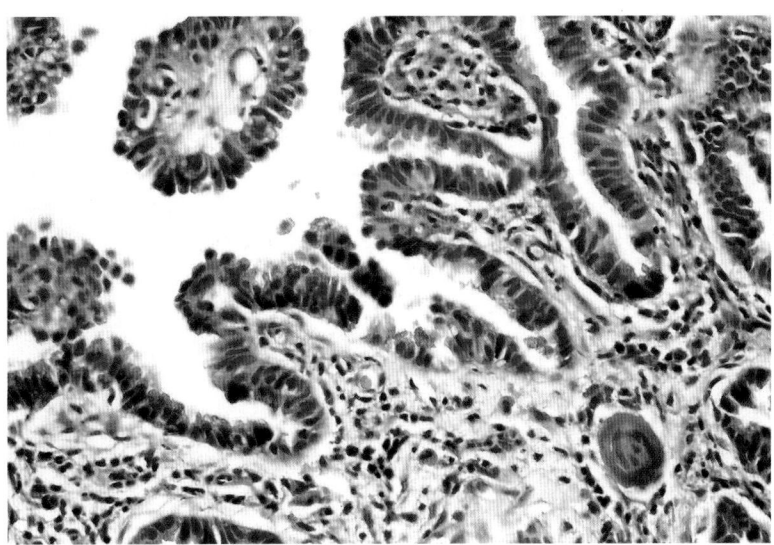

Fig. 33.27
Apocrine carcinoma: there is focal decapitation secretion.

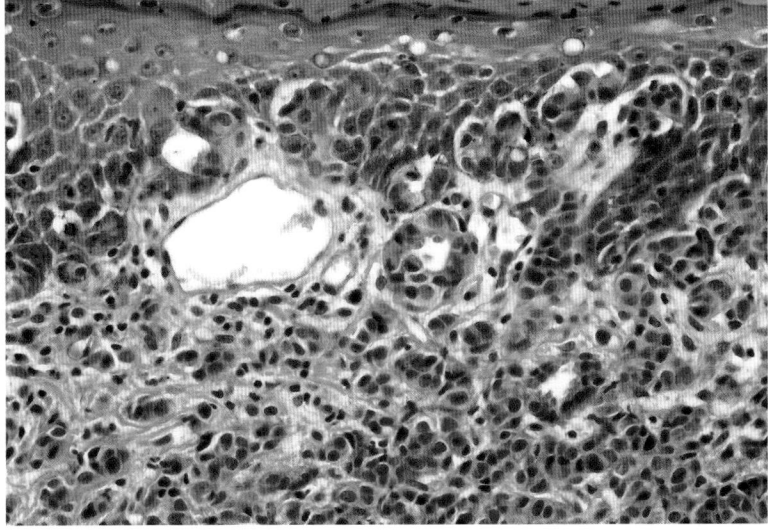

Fig. 33.28
Apocrine carcinoma: focal epidermotropism is evident (same case as *Figs 33.23* and *33.24*).

Primary cutaneous cribriform apocrine carcinoma

Clinical features

Primary cutaneous cribriform apocrine carcinoma is a rare and poorly documented but distinctive neoplasm currently regarded as a morphological variant of apocrine carcinoma.[1-4] It is, however, unclear whether this tumor has potential for malignant behavior and if it should be regarded as a carcinoma. As yet no recurrences, metastases or disease-related deaths have been reported. The tumor presents as firm 1- to 3-cm large nodules with a strong predilection for the limbs of middle-aged adults with a female predominance. The trunk and head and neck region are rarely involved.[3,4]

Histologic features

The tumors are circumscribed and symmetrical dermal based nodules, which may also extend into superficial subcutis (*Fig. 33.32*). They are composed of interconnecting nests and islands of basaloid cells with prominent duct formation giving rise to a cribriform architecture (*Fig. 33.33*). The tumor cells

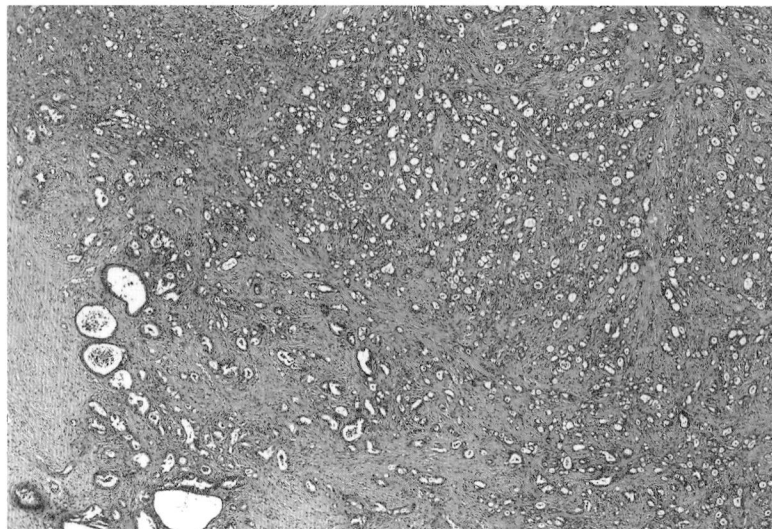

Fig. 33.29
Apocrine carcinoma: low-power view.

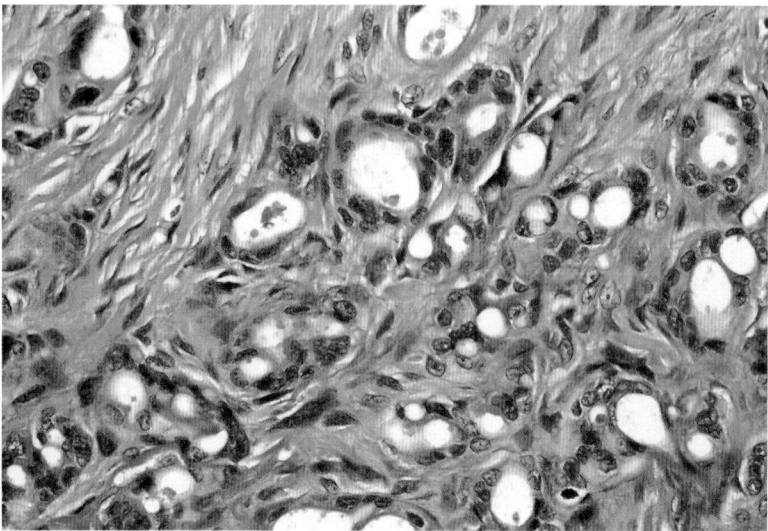

Fig. 33.30
Apocrine carcinoma: the tumor cells have abundant eosinophilic cytoplasm and large vesicular nuclei. Note the nuclear pleomorphism.

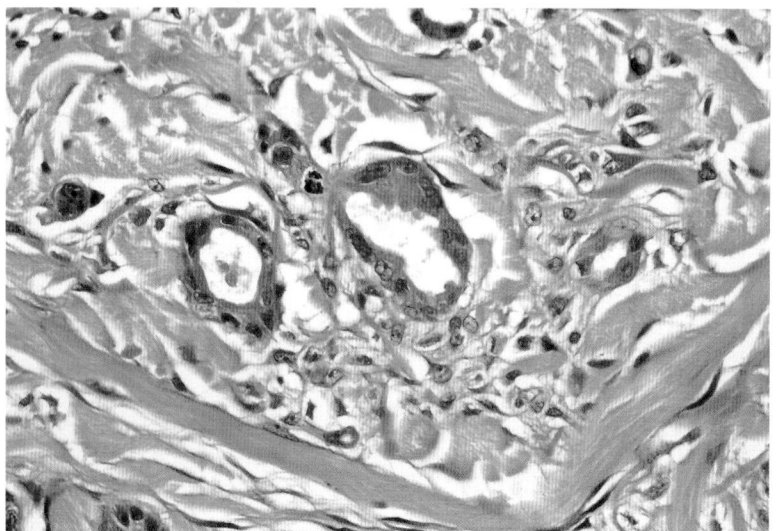

Fig. 33.31
Apocrine carcinoma: there is focal decapitation secretion.

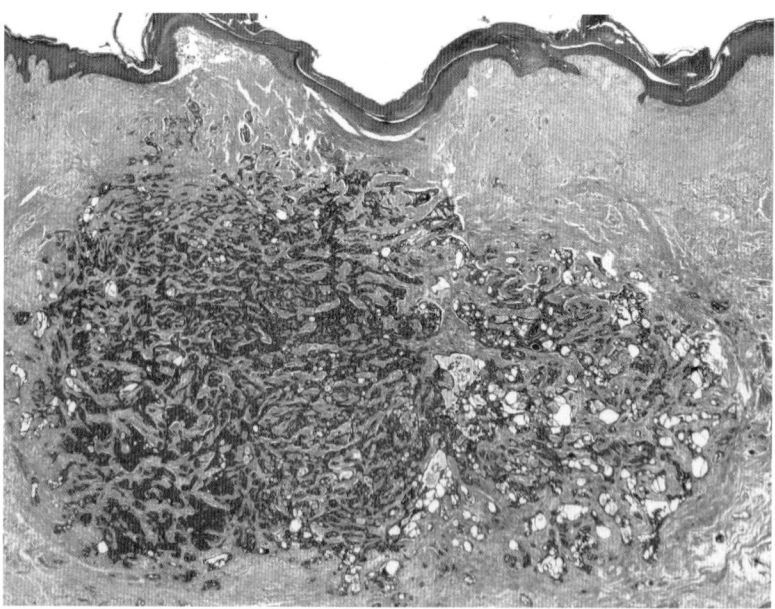

Fig. 33.32
Primary cutaneous cribriform apocrine carcinoma: this nodular tumor is based within dermis. It appears relatively circumscribed but unencapsulated. By courtesy of Fritjof Eckert, MD, Labor für Dermatohistologie und Oralpathologie, Munich, Germany.

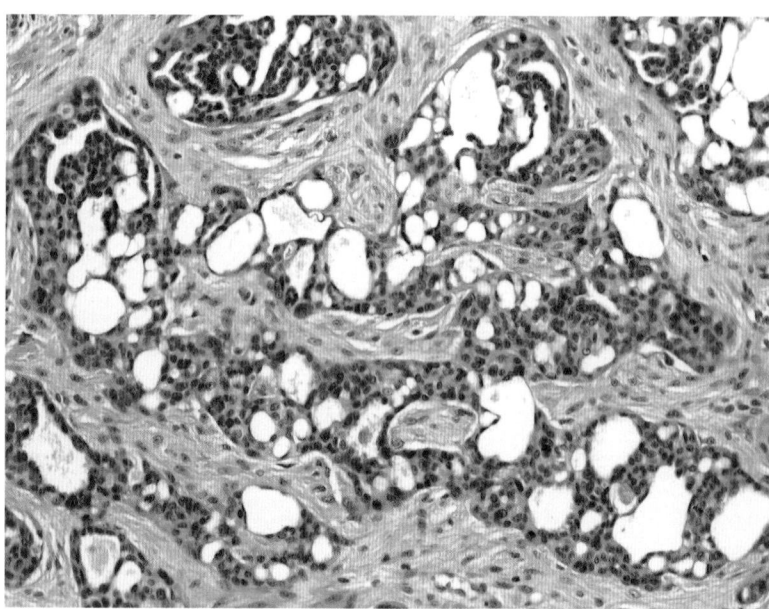

Fig. 33.33
Primary cutaneous cribriform apocrine carcinoma: it is composed of small epithelioid cells without nuclear pleomorphism. Prominent duct formation gives rise to the cribriform appearances. By courtesy of Fritjof Eckert, MD, Labor für Dermatohistologie und Oralpathologie, Munich, Germany.

show hyperchromatic nuclei but nuclear pleomorphism is limited. Mitoses are sparse and necrosis is rare. Focal decapitation secretion is noted as evidence of the apocrine differentiation. The tumor nests are separated by a fibrous stroma.

By immunohistochemistry, the tumor cells express cytokeratins AE1/AE3, MNF116, CAM 5.2 and CK7. CEA and EMA are expressed in the luminal cells. Patchy S100 staining has also been reported in tumor cells.[4] No staining is seen for CK20 and GCDFP-15 and no surrounding myoepithelial cell layer can be identified by p63, SMA, and calponin staining.[3]

Differential diagnosis

Nodular basal cell carcinoma may show a prominent cribriform pattern. It can be separated by the absence of duct differentiation and the presence of a peripheral palisade and stromal cleft artifact. Similarly, adenoid cystic carcinoma is characterized by a cribriform pattern and it shows additional duct differentiation. It shows however a more plaquelike architecture with a diffusely infiltrative growth pattern and almost invariable perineural invasion. In addition, the cribriform areas are composed of mucin filled pseudocysts rather than the florid ductal differentiation seen in primary cutaneous cribriform apocrine carcinoma. Papillary eccrine adenoma may show many low power similarities. It is however composed of well-formed tubules with a retained myoepithelial layer. In addition, cystic elements and papillary projections are also found. Finally, metastatic cribriform carcinoma of visceral origins, especially from the prostate and breast, needs to be considered. Definitive separation is possible only on clinical grounds.

Ceruminous gland tumors

Clinical features

Ceruminous gland tumors (ceruminoma) are rare and present as an often pedunculated nodule or cystic lesion in the external auditory canal, often associated with deafness and less commonly with tinnitus or otorrhea.[1-8] Pain is sometimes a feature as a result of otitis externa, ulceration, or malignancy.[7] Facial nerve palsy has occasionally been documented.[2,9] The age distribution is wide but tumors are most commonly seen in adulthood.[8] The sex incidence is equal.[5,8]

In the earlier literature, the term ceruminoma was often applied to all glandular tumors arising in the external auditory meatus. This resulted in considerable confusion since it lumped together both benign and malignant variants, the latter being the more common. Currently, ceruminous gland tumors are classified as benign, including apocrine adenoma and mixed tumor (pleomorphic adenoma), and malignant – ceruminous gland adenocarcinoma and adenoid cystic carcinoma.[1,2,6,10] In addition, cylindroma, syringocystadenoma papilliferum, and mucoepidermoid carcinoma have exceptionally been documented.[2,11]

Histologic features

The ceruminous glands are apocrine glands found predominantly within the dermis of the cartilaginous part of the external auditory canal.

Ceruminous apocrine adenoma presents as a circumscribed nodule composed of glands lined by a double layer of epithelium (Fig. 33.34).[4,8] The inner are cuboidal to columnar with eosinophilic cytoplasm often showing decapitation secretion. The outer are myoepithelial cells. Cystic change is sometimes present. Solid, acinar, and trabecular variants have been described.[5,8] Pleomorphism is absent and mitoses are scarce. Abnormal forms, by definition, are not a feature.

Ceruminous gland adenocarcinoma is characterized by an infiltrating growth pattern. Pure glandular and papillary variants are recognized. The cytology varies from deceptive, well-differentiated forms to high-grade tumors with marked pleomorphism and conspicuous mitotic activity (Fig. 33.35). Perineural infiltration is sometimes a feature and rarely extramammary Paget disease is seen.[12]

Differential diagnosis

Well-differentiated ceruminous gland adenocarcinoma may be difficult to distinguish from adenoma if the infiltrative border is not visible, as may be the case in small biopsy specimens. If there is any doubt, it is recommended that tumors be reported as having uncertain malignant potential with the final diagnosis deferred until the full excision specimen is available for study.[5]

Mixed tumor of the skin

Clinical features

Mixed tumor of the skin (chondroid syringoma) is not uncommon and presents as a slowly growing, firm, circumscribed, lobulated nodule within the dermis or subcutaneous fat. It is usually solitary and asymptomatic and most often affects the head and neck, particularly the nose, cheek, upper

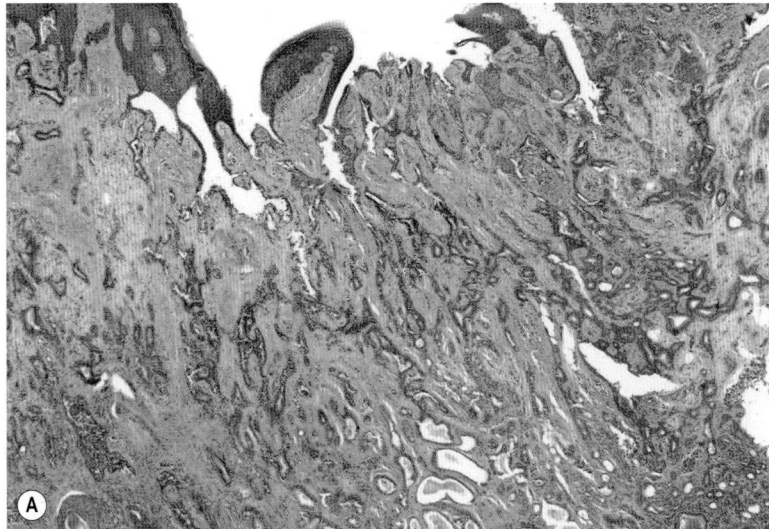
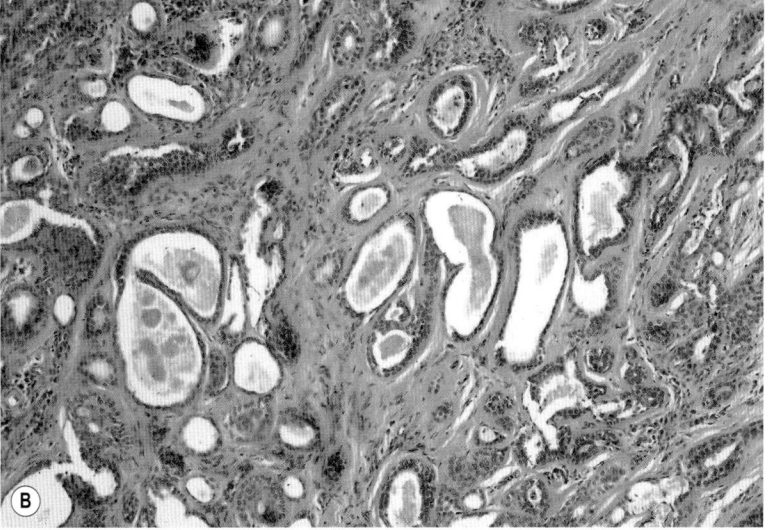

Fig. 33.34
(**A**, **B**) Ceruminous gland adenoma: this example shows continuity with the epidermis. The tumor shows tubule formation and multiple small cysts are apparent. The tubules are lined by a double layer of epithelium. The inner layer has abundant eosinophilic cytoplasm; the cells of the outer layer are cuboidal and represent myoepithelial cells. By courtesy of M. Bosenberg, MD, University of Vermont, Vermont, USA.

lip, scalp, forehead, chin, eyelids, and ear including the external auditory meatus, in descending order of frequency, although on occasions it may involve the axillae, trunk, or extremities (Figs 33.36 and 33.37).[1-9] Scrotal involvement has rarely been described.[10,11] Exceptional giant variants affecting the cheek and axilla have been documented.[8,12-15] Males are more commonly affected than females and the tumor typically presents in the middle aged.[9] Recurrences are rare.

Histologic features

Although the earlier literature argued variably for an eccrine or apocrine derivation, variants differentiating toward both (including follicular differentiation) are recognized.[16,17]

Most tumors are currently classified as apocrine type (apocrine chondroid syringoma). This is usually multilobulated and situated within the deep dermis and/or subcutaneous fat (Fig. 33.38). It forms a well-circumscribed mass in which a dominant component has a chondroid appearance (Figs 33.39 and 33.40). The lobules are separated by fibrous septa. The epithelial component is composed of nests and cords of cuboidal or polygonal cells with copious eosinophilic cytoplasm and basophilic nuclei.[1-3,12,17] They are distributed singly, in cords and nests or as irregular tubuloalveolar and ductal structures.

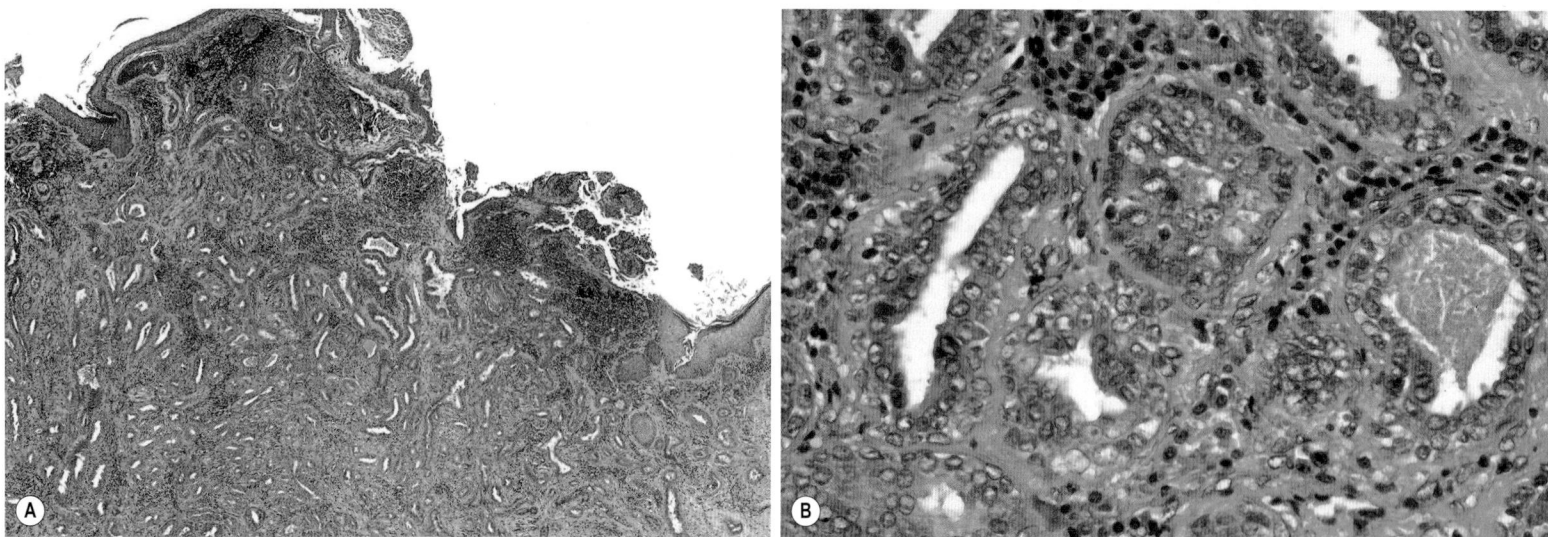

Fig. 33.35
Ceruminous gland adenocarcinoma: (**A**) low-power view of part of an ulcerated mass; (**B**) there is multilayering and nuclear pleomorphism.

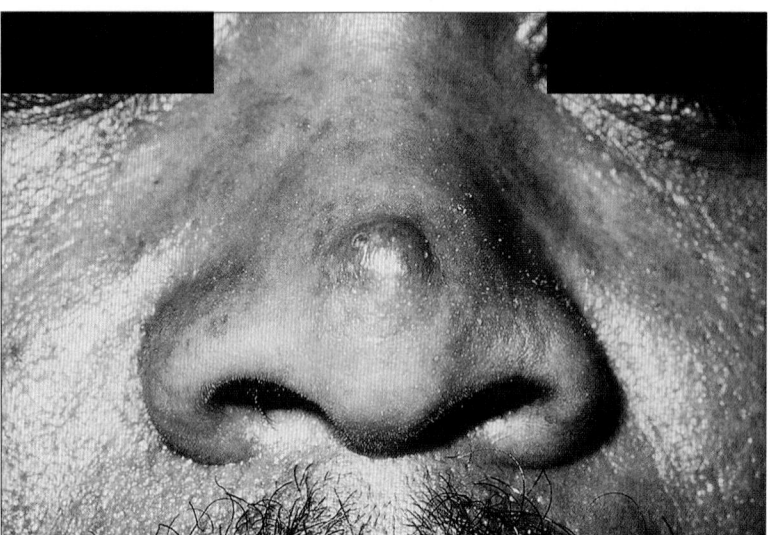

Fig. 33.36
Mixed tumor: this erythematous nodule is present at a characteristic site. By courtesy of R.A. Marsden, MD, St George's Hospital, London, UK.

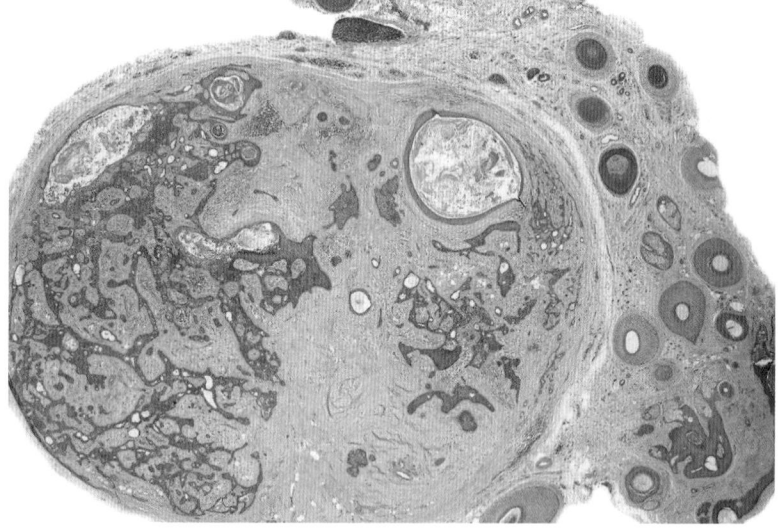

Fig. 33.38
Mixed tumor: at scanning magnification, the tumor is circumscribed and compresses the adjacent dermal connective tissue.

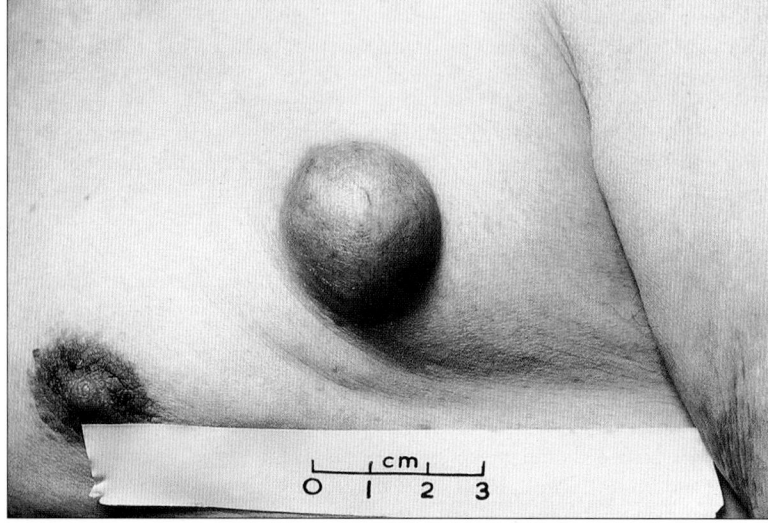

Fig. 33.37
Mixed tumor: lesions are more common in males and occasionally affect the thorax. By courtesy of R.A. Marsden, MD, St George's Hospital, London, UK.

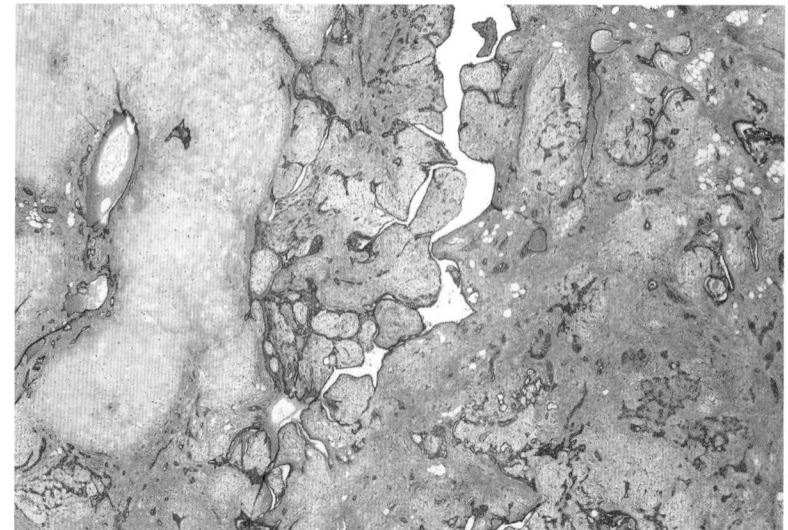

Fig. 33.39
Mixed tumor: this example has a well-developed chondroid stroma. There is conspicuous ductal differentiation and multiple cysts are present.

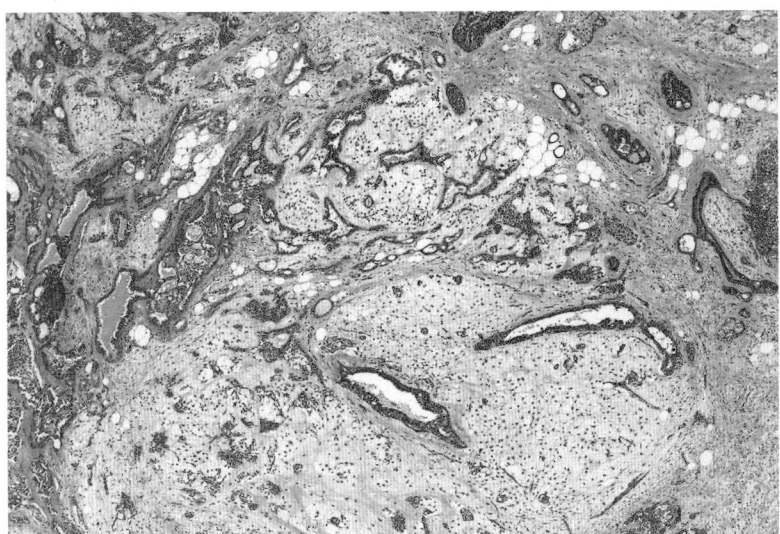

Fig. 33.40
Mixed tumor: higher-power view of chondroid component.

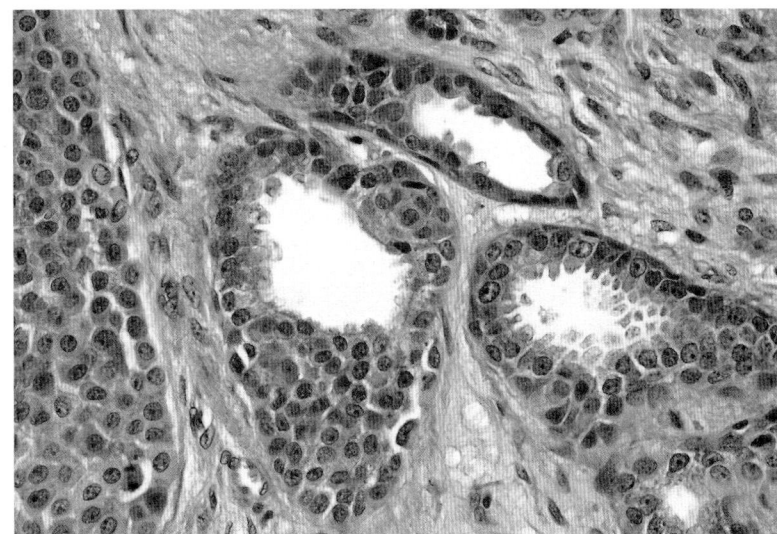

Fig. 33.42
Mixed tumor: this example shows well-developed decapitation secretion.

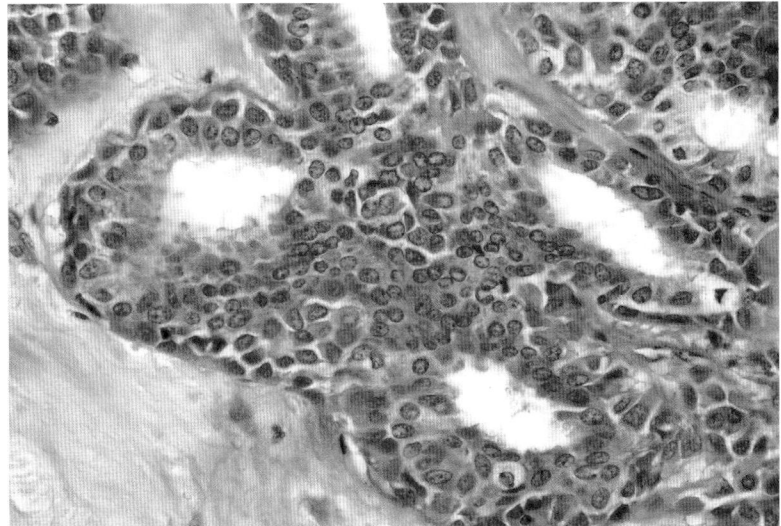

Fig. 33.41
Mixed tumor: the inner lining cells have abundant cytoplasm and vesicular nuclei; the outer myoepithelial cells have hyperchromatic spindled nuclei.

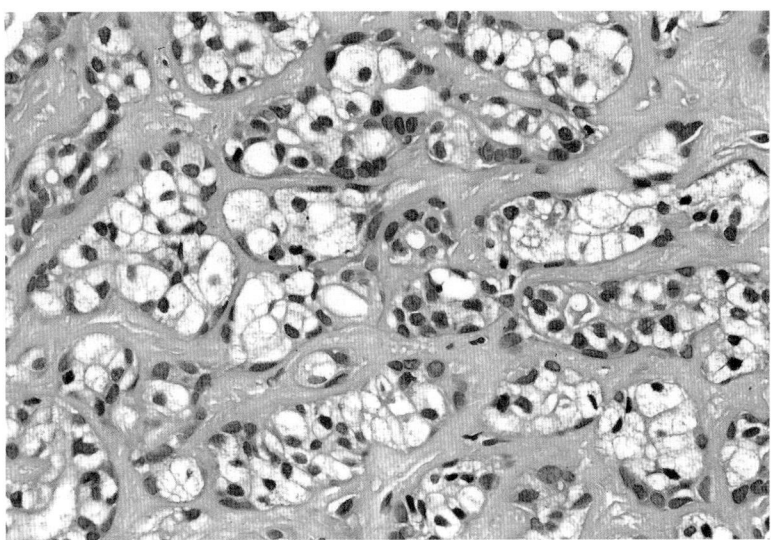

Fig. 33.43
Mixed tumor: clear cell change due to cytoplasmic glycogen is sometimes present.

The tubuloalveolar foci, which are believed to represent differentiation toward the secretory coil, are lined by two or more rows of epithelial cells, the outer layer being somewhat flattened and of myoepithelial derivation (Fig. 33.41). Apocrine decapitation secretion is sometimes evident and occasionally the epithelium has a lacelike pattern (Fig. 33.42). PAS-positive, diastase sensitive, glycogen-rich clear cells may be present (Fig. 33.43).[17] One or occasionally two layers of cells line the ducts, which represent differentiation toward the dermal sweat gland duct (Fig. 33.44). Cystic dilatation is common (Fig. 33.45). Occasionally, keratinous cysts and foci of squamous differentiation are present (Fig. 33.46).[1,17] In addition, clear cell change as well as mucinous, columnar, oxyphilic, and hobnail metaplasia of the epithelial component may be evident.[9] There is, however, no pleomorphism, mitoses are sparse, and necrosis is absent.

Not uncommonly, mixed tumor shows additional foci of follicular and sebaceous differentiation.[1,6,17–21] The former is characterized by the presence of infundibulocystic, isthmic as well as tricholemmal differentiation, hair bulbs and papillary mesenchyme in addition to foci of ghost cells reminiscent of pilomatrixoma.[6,9,20,21] Some tumors may be almost exclusively follicular. Sebaceous differentiation is present as foci of cells showing granular or bubbly cytoplasm and scalloped nuclei or as sebaceous ductlike structures with an eosinophilic, wavy, laminated, keratinized lining.[6,9,18] Rarely, pigmented dendritic melanocytes are a feature.

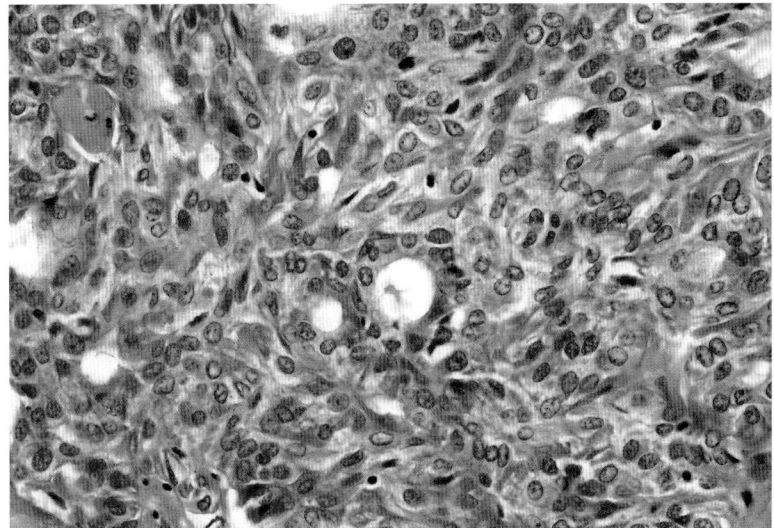

Fig. 33.44
Mixed tumor: the ducts are lined by cuboidal epithelium and show a well-developed cuticle.

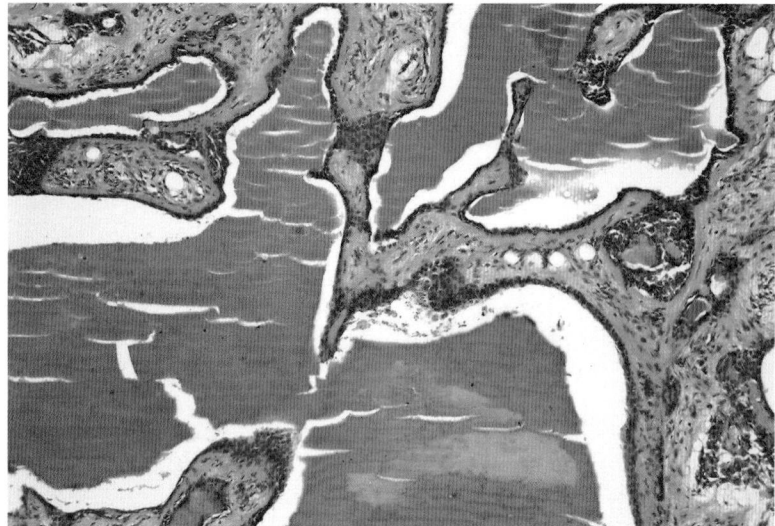

Fig. 33.45
Mixed tumor: this example shows marked cystic change.

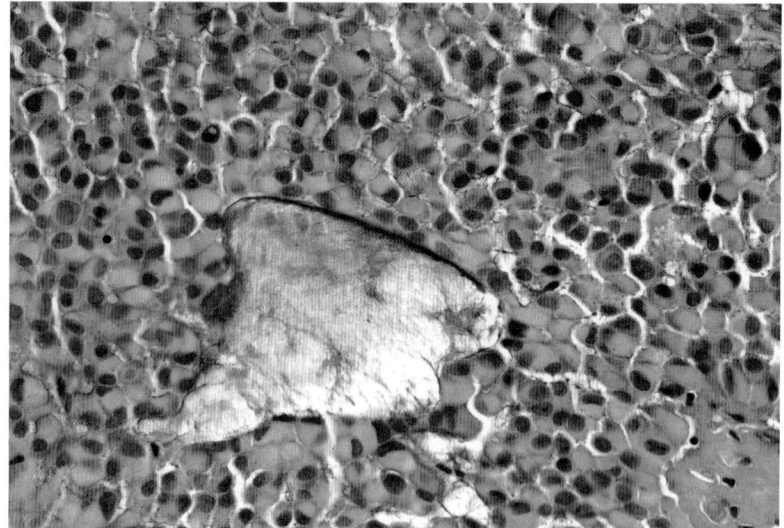

Fig. 33.47
Mixed tumor: this example shows conspicuous hyaline/plasmacytoid cells.

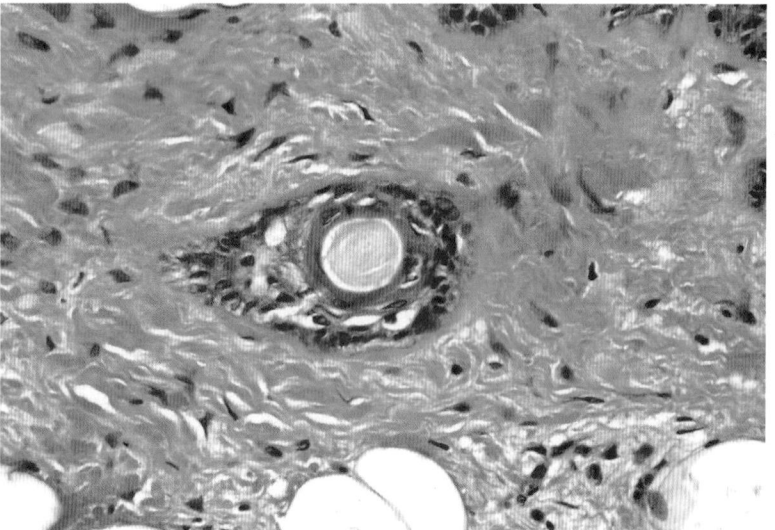

Fig. 33.46
Mixed tumor: keratocysts, as shown in this field, are sometimes present.

The myoepithelial component may show hyaline (plasmacytoid), spindled cell, or clear cell differentiation.[9,22–26] The hyaline (plasmacytoid) cells are characterized by abundant ground-glass eosinophilic cytoplasm and an eccentric nucleus. They are present singly within the stroma or as distinct noncohesive aggregates (Fig. 33.47).[17,22–27,28] Spindled cell myoepithelial cells are also present within the chondroid matrix and are responsible for its production.[29–31] Clear cell change of the myoepithelial component may be an additional finding. Transition between polyhedral cells and spindled cells or foci of squamous differentiation may be seen.[27] The stroma is of variable appearance. Characteristically, it is composed of homogeneous bluish chondroid (Fig. 33.48). In other areas it is myxoid or densely collagenous, eosinophilic, and hyalinized (Fig. 33.49). Positive Alcian blue or green staining at pH 2.5 indicates the presence of acid mucopolysaccharides (Fig. 33.50).[17] Sometimes, abundant mature fat is present ('lipomatous mixed tumor') (Fig. 33.51).[8,9,32–36] Some tumors may show foci of calcification, and on rare occasions osteoid with marrow spaces has been described.[6,16,18,37–42]

Less often, the tumor is composed of small glandular and tubular structures lined by a single layer of cuboidal epithelium dispersed in a mucinous and/or chondroid stroma (Figs 33.52 and 33.53).[16,17] This is sometimes referred to as the eccrine variant (eccrine chondroid syringoma).[4,16] Occasionally, these tumors may show a cribriform architecture and clear or hyaline cell change of the epithelial component and cartilaginous or sclerotic stromal change with ossification, lipomatous metaplasia and ossification.[43]

Exceptionally, hidrocystoma-like features have been described.[44]

Cutaneous mixed tumors with atypical histologic features but benign clinical behavior have been described.[45] Atypical architectural features include lesional asymmetry and slightly infiltrative tumor edges without capsular invasion.[45] More often, the atypical findings relate to the cytological features. Mild cytological atypia of epithelial cells in ductular structures may be present but the most frequent finding is the presence of scattered multinucleated pleomorphic and bizarre-appearing cells within the myoepithelial component of the tumor. By immunohistochemistry, these cells are characterized by a myoepithelial phenotype.[45]

There are occasional reports of diagnosis of mixed tumor by fine needle aspiration cytology.[46–48] In view of the difficulty sometimes encountered in distinguishing between benign and malignant variants, a complete excision with histologic study should always be performed.

Immunocytochemically, the inner epithelial cell layer is characterized by high and low molecular weight keratin (AE1/AE3), EMA, CEA, and GCDFP-15 expression (Fig. 33.54).[17,49–52] The outer cells express vimentin, S100 protein, SOX10, and sometimes SMA and muscle-specific actin (MSA) (Fig. 33.55).[39,40,51–55] Stromal cells are vimentin and S100 protein positive.[39,40]

A more detailed immunohistochemical study of stromal cells in mixed tumor has shed some light on their likely nature.[27] The authors classified them into the following three subtypes:

- Hyaline cells express CAM 5.2, but not cytokeratin 10 (CK10), CK14, SMA, or MSA, indicative of simple epithelium. A rim of CK14+ cells possibly representing ductal basal cell or myoepithelial differentiation may surround them. The additional presence of S100 and focal GFAP expression, however, argues for myoepithelial differentiation.[56]
- Polyhedral cells express CK14, but not CK10, SMA, or MSA, and may represent myoepithelial cells or sweat duct basal cells.
- Spindled cells express CK14, SMA, and MSA, but not CAM 5.2 or CK10, and are therefore thought to be of myoepithelial derivation.[27]

A number of in-depth investigations of keratin expression in mixed tumor have been published.[56–58] The results suggest that all elements of the sweat gland are represented although whether the tumor arises in or differentiates toward the apocrine or eccrine sweat gland apparatus remains uncertain.

Genetically, most cutaneous mixed tumors show rearrangement of the PLAG1 gene and immunohistochemical expression of PLAG1 analogous to pleomorphic adenomas of the salivary gland.[59–61] A small subset of tumors show EWSR1 gene rearrangement as seen in myoepitheliomas of the skin.[62]

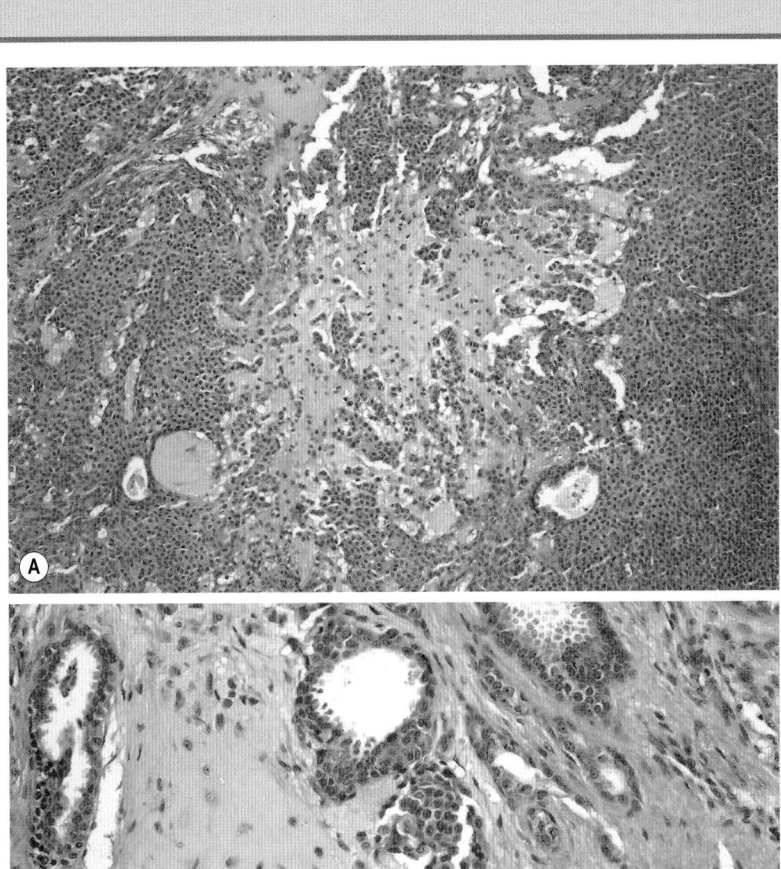

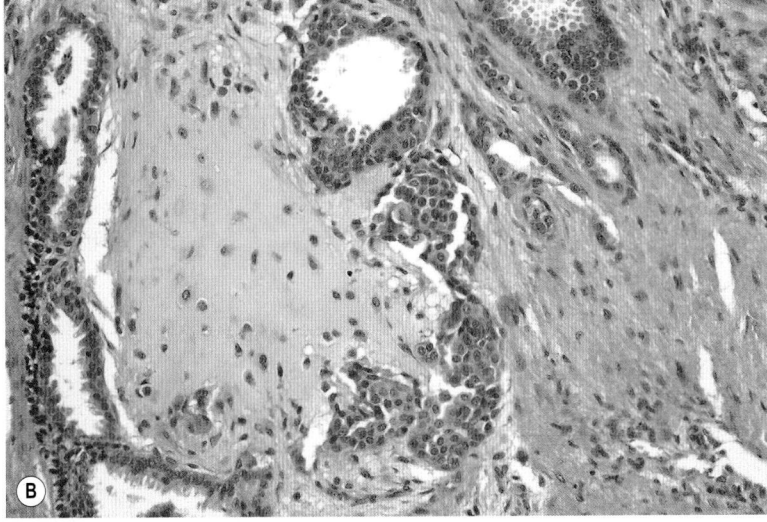

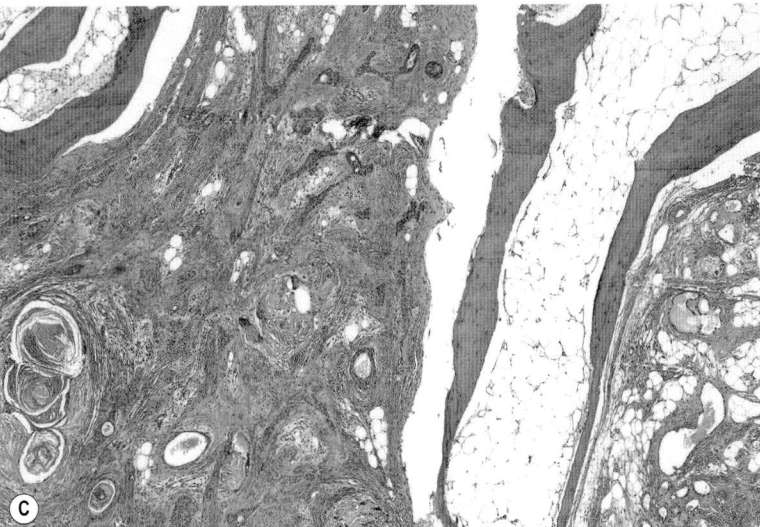

Fig. 33.48
Mixed tumor: (**A**, **B**) in this field, the stroma has a chondroid appearance; (**C**) this example shows well-developed bone with marrow cavities.

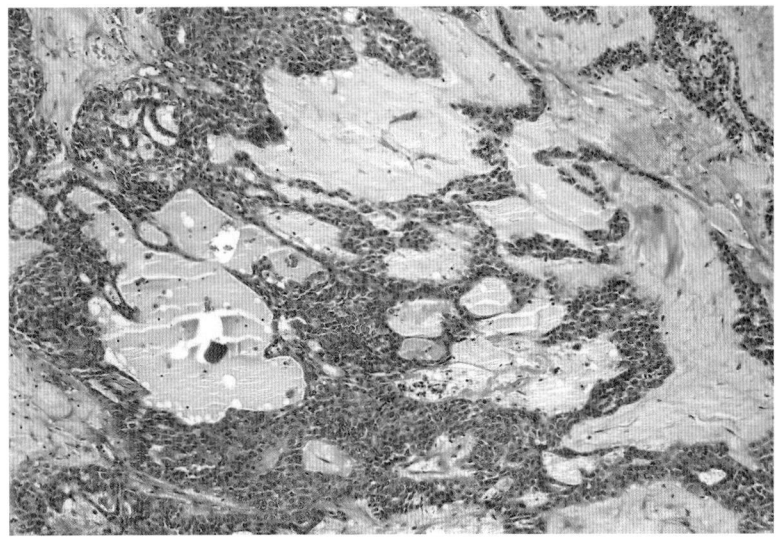

Fig. 33.49
Mixed tumor: myxoid change due to abundant mucopolysaccharide is commonly present.

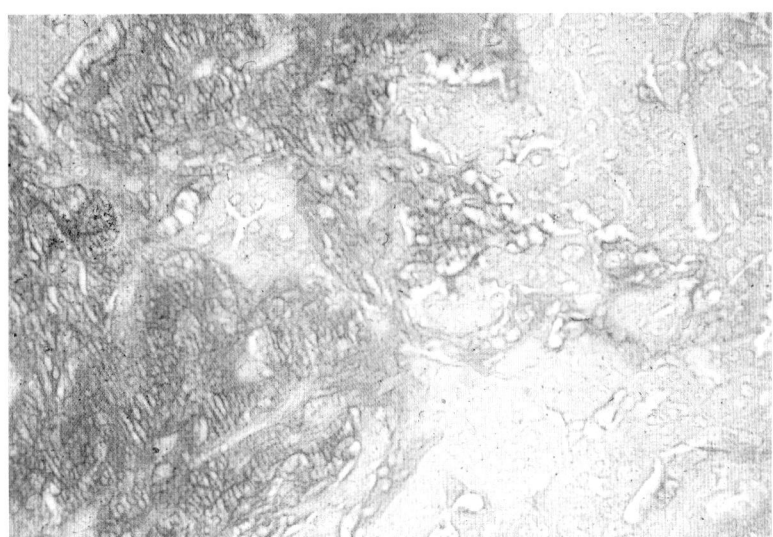

Fig. 33.50
Mixed tumor: the stroma stains strongly with Alcian green.

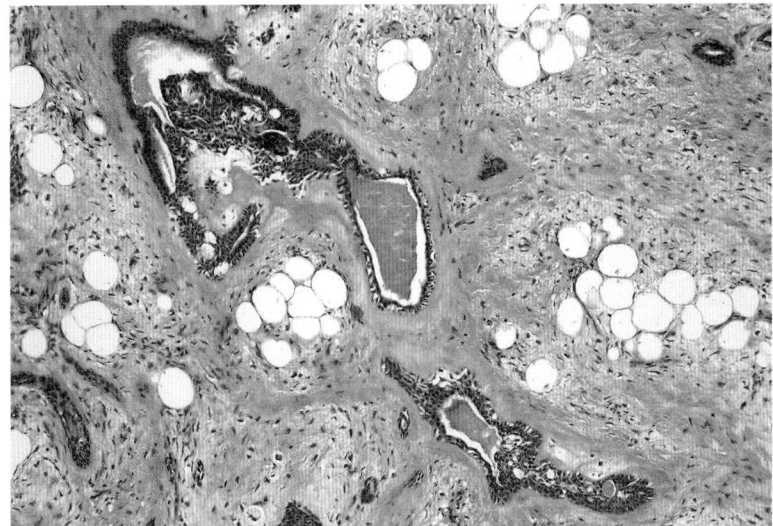

Fig. 33.51
Mixed tumor: foci of mature adipocytes are often an integral component of the tumor.

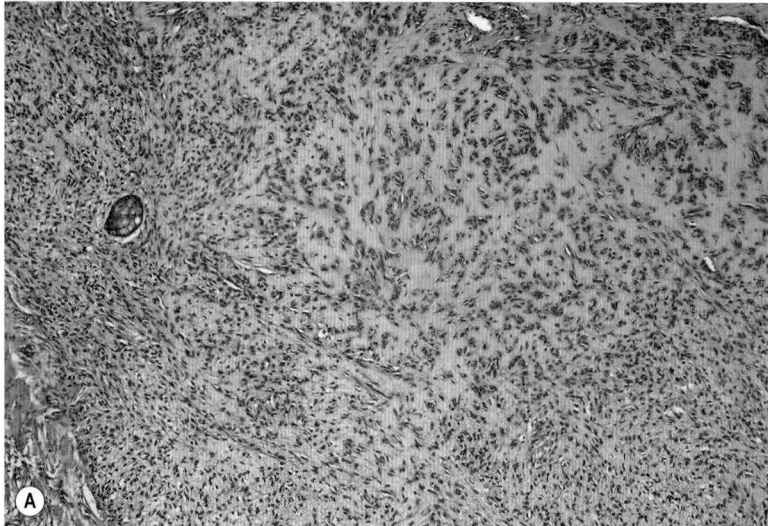

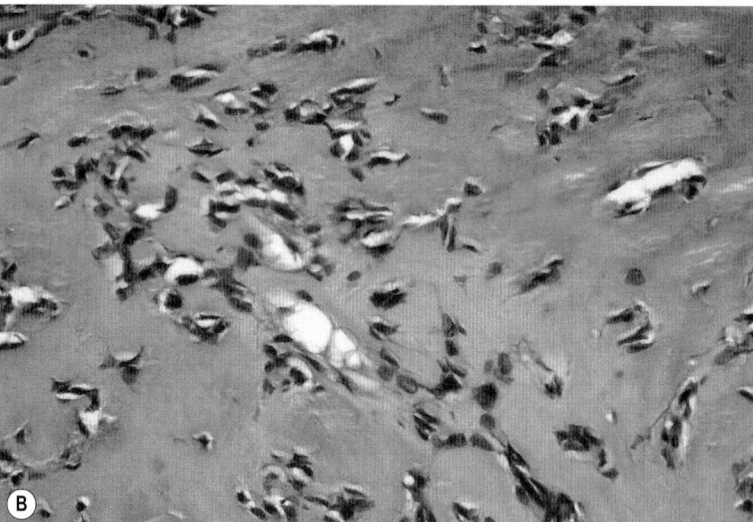

Fig. 33.52
(**A**, **B**) Mixed tumor: eccrine variant showing small, ductlike structures dispersed in a hyalinized stroma.

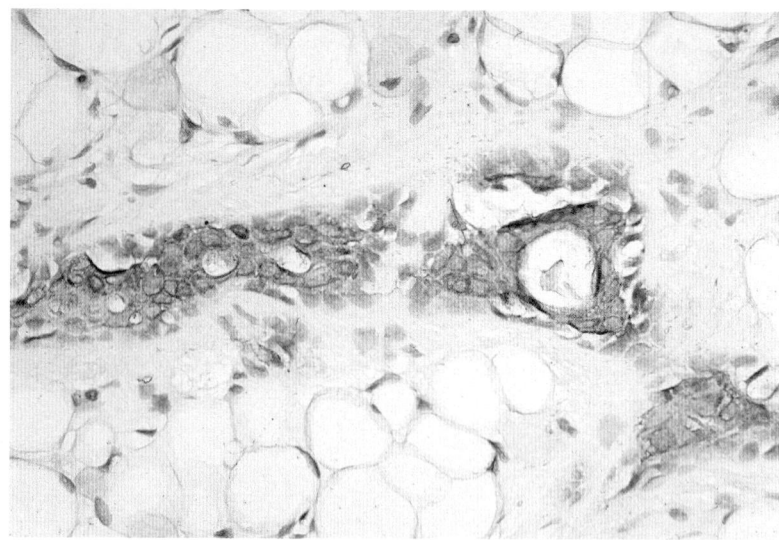

Fig. 33.54
Mixed tumor: the inner layer of epithelial cells shows strong EMA expression.

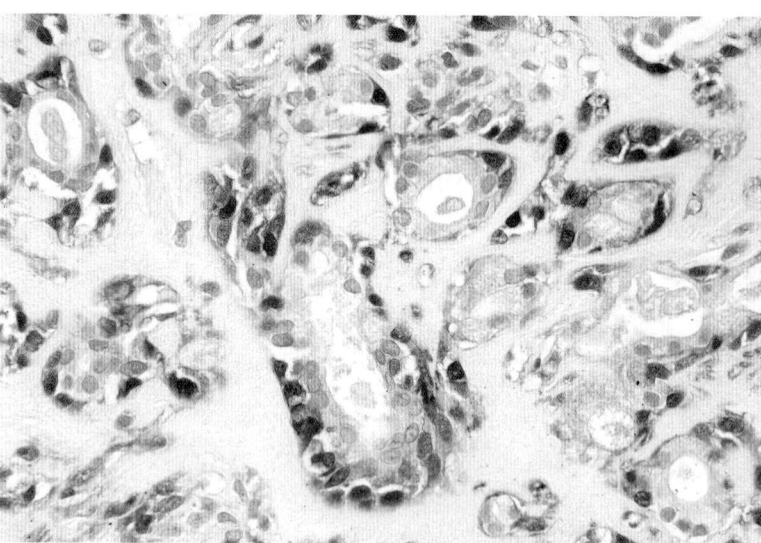

Fig. 33.55
Mixed tumor: in this example, the myoepithelial cells are highlighted with S100 protein immunohistochemistry.

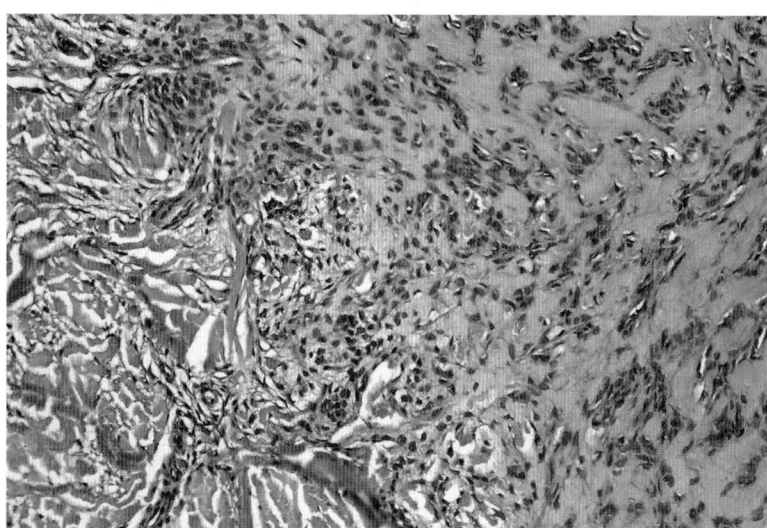

Fig. 33.53
Mixed tumor: focal clear cell change is seen in this example.

Malignant mixed tumor

Clinical features

Malignant mixed tumor (malignant chondroid syringoma) is an extremely rare tumor.[1–19] Approximately 50 cases have been described to date. Although the majority of tumors have developed de novo, there are some documented examples which appear to have arisen within a preexistent benign mixed tumor.[4,6,8,14] The tumor predominantly affects the distal extremities (the foot being the common site), shows a predilection for females (2:1), and most often arises in the sixth decade although there is a wide age range (18–89 years).[15] Clinically, the tumor is not distinctive and presents as a flesh-colored or erythematous nodule.

Malignant mixed tumor is an extremely high-grade neoplasm with a metastasis rate of approximately 60% and a mortality of roughly 25%.[9] The lymph nodes, lungs, and bone are predominantly affected.[4,10–14,17,20]

Histologic features

Ideally, the diagnosis of malignant mixed tumor should depend upon the identification of a benign precursor lesion (*Figs 33.56–33.60*). This, however, has only rarely been histologically documented.[4,6,14] In the majority of cases, diagnosis depends upon identification of foci of mucoid stroma

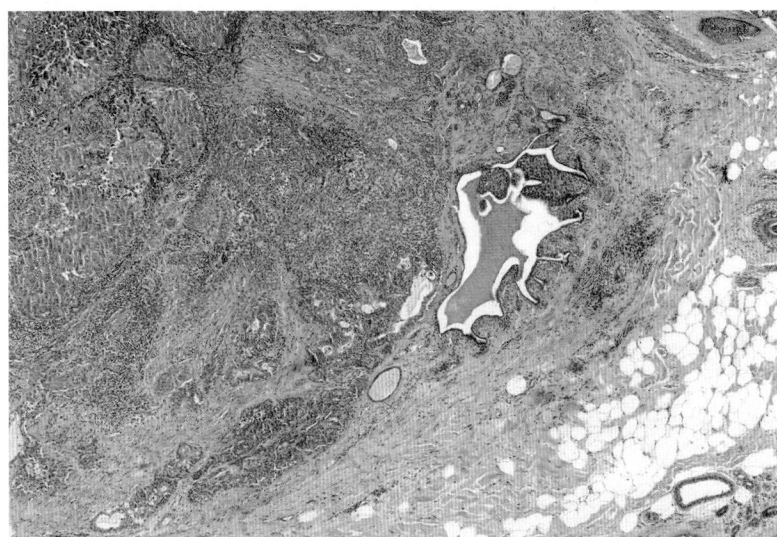

Fig. 33.56
Malignant mixed tumor: this specimen comes from a longstanding lesion. Residual benign precursor is seen to the right of center.

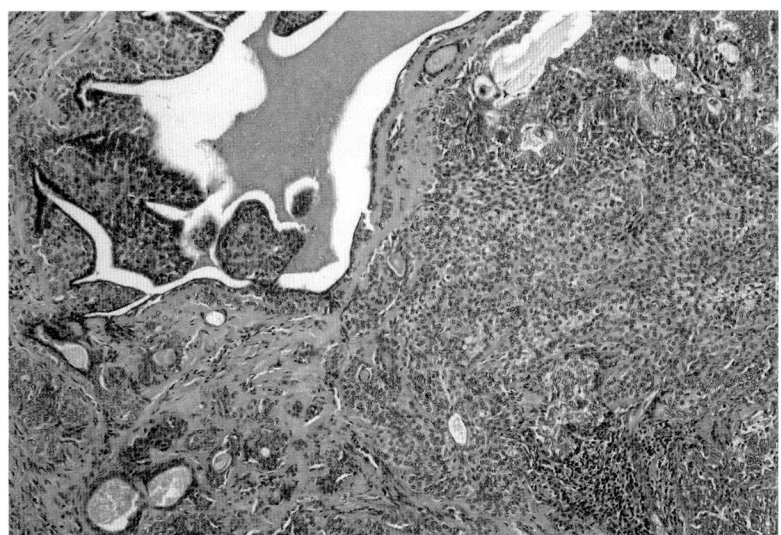

Fig. 33.57
Malignant mixed tumor: benign tumor on the left merges with carcinoma on the right.

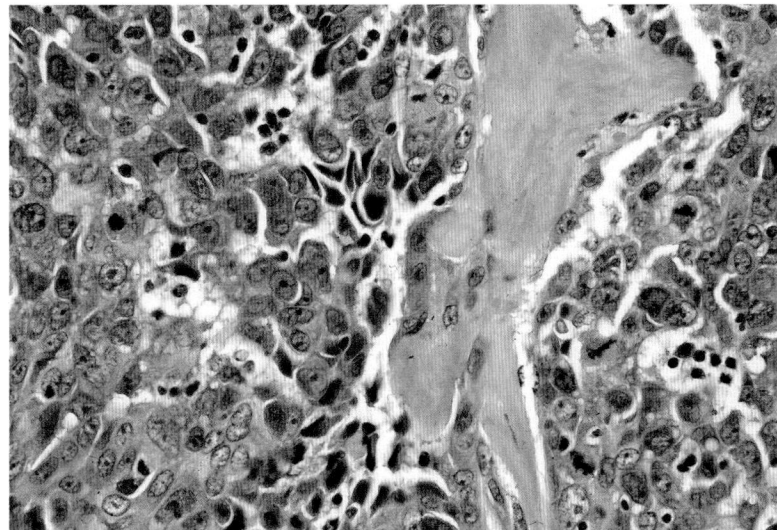

Fig. 33.58
Malignant mixed tumor: the carcinoma cells have large vesicular nuclei with prominent eosinophilic nucleoli. Multiple mitoses are present.

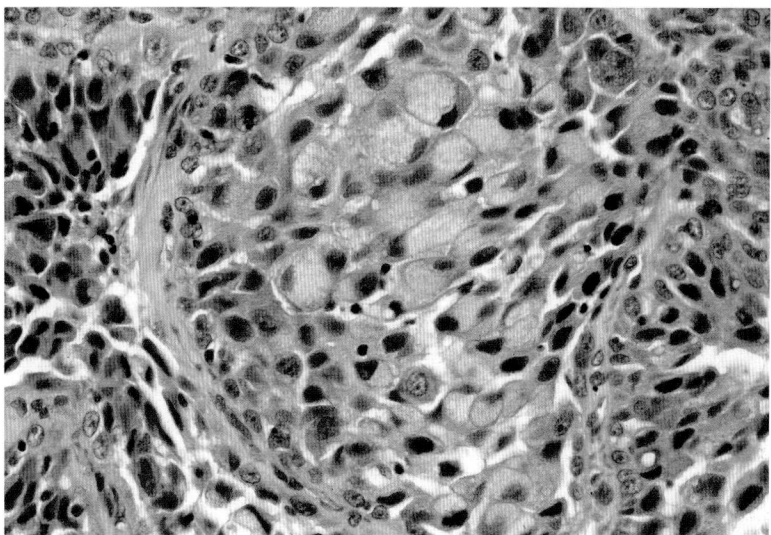

Fig. 33.59
Malignant mixed tumor: focally, the tumor cells show signet ring cell change.

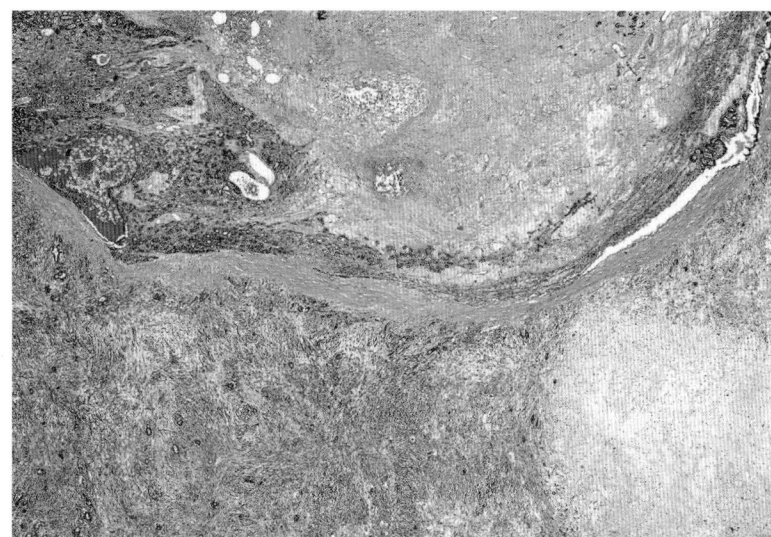

Fig. 33.60
Malignant mixed tumor: this example is a recurrent lesion on the foot. Residual benign tumor is present in the upper-left quadrant. Chondroid stroma is evident in the lower-right field.

and chondroid differentiation as with its benign counterpart. Criteria suggestive of malignant potential include an infiltrative growth pattern, epithelial nuclear and cytoplasmic pleomorphism, excessive or abnormal mitotic activity, and tumor necrosis (*Figs 33.61–33.63*). Vascular and lymphatic invasion or metastases obviously confirm the diagnosis. Impaired tubular differentiation, excessive mucoid matrix, and abundant, poorly developed chondroid elements may also point toward a diagnosis of malignancy, and frank chondrosarcomatous or osteosarcomatous differentiation may be present.[3,9,17] Some tumors which have metastasized have been deceptively bland. An infiltrative growth pattern or evidence of satellite lesions in such tumors should be viewed with concern and the tumor widely excised, with careful follow-up recommended.[16]

The tumor often shows multiple satellite lesions in the adjacent dermis or subcutaneous tissue, which may result in incomplete excision and account for the high risk of recurrence.[15]

There is one instance of malignant mixed tumor recognized by fine needle aspiration cytology.[12]

Immunohistochemically, the epithelial cells express pankeratin, AE1/AE3, CAM 5.2, EMA, CEA, and variably S100 protein.[5,6,8–11] Intracytoplasmic lumina may be outlined with CEA.[9] The stromal cells are S100 protein positive [9,10] and variably express keratin.[9] SMA has been variably reported as present or absent.[10,11]

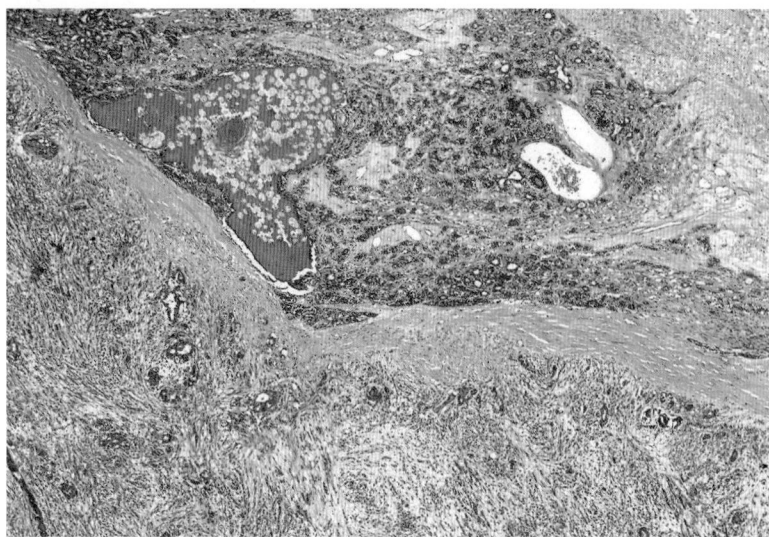

Fig. 33.61
Malignant mixed tumor: residual benign tumor showing cysts and ducts lined by a double-layered epithelium. Carcinoma is present in the lower field.

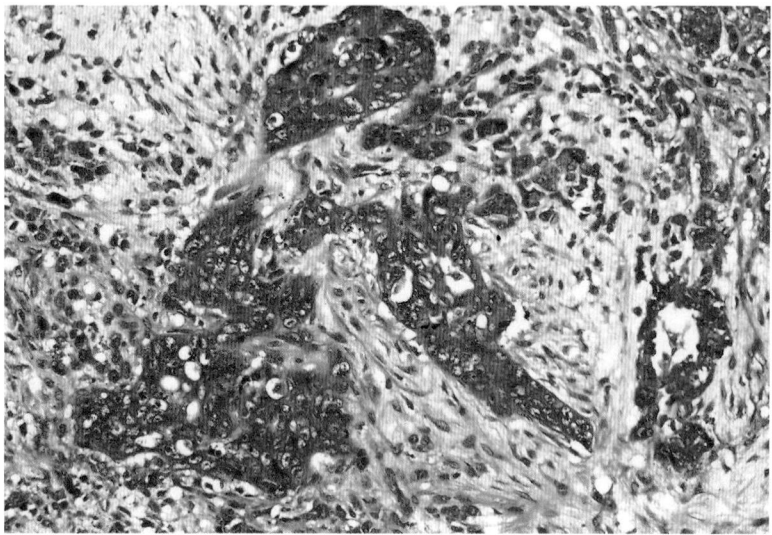

Fig. 33.62
Malignant mixed tumor: the malignant component shows focal glandular differentiation.

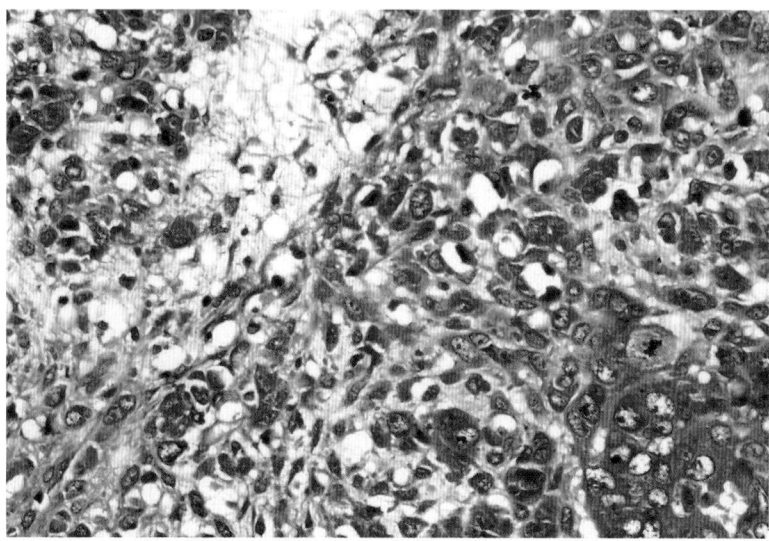

Fig. 33.63
Malignant mixed tumor: note the nuclear pleomorphism and mitotic activity.

Differential diagnosis

Malignancy in mixed tumor relates solely to the epithelial proliferation. If nuclear pleomorphism and mitotic activity affect the chondroid component, a diagnosis of metaplastic carcinoma (carcinosarcoma) is more appropriate. Other tumors in which a mucinous or chondroid matrix is evident, including mucinous carcinoma, extraskeletal myxoid chondrosarcoma, and metastatic skeletal chondrosarcoma, may occasionally have to be excluded.

Myoepithelioma and malignant myoepithelioma

Clinical features

Myoepithelioma is a rare tumor which arises in the dermis, subcutaneous fat or soft tissues.[1-19] Analogous to salivary gland tumors, cutaneous myoepitheliomas are composed of the myoepithelial and stromal components of mixed tumors but lack the ductal epithelial component.[7,8] The age range at presentation is wide (newborn–93 years) but there is a predilection for adolescents and young adults.[1-3,5-8,18] Males appear more frequently affected than females. Cutaneous tumors present as firm or hard, well-circumscribed, flesh-colored, gray, or violaceous nodules ranging in size from 0.5 to 2.5 cm (mean 1.1 cm).[7] Tumors located within soft tissue may present as larger masses measuring up to 12 cm (mean 3.8 cm) while malignant myoepithelioma may reach up to 20 cm.[8] There is a predilection for the extremities and limb girdles but the head, neck, and trunk are also affected.[2-4,6-8,18] Local recurrence may be a complication, but distant metastasis and disease-related death are rare.[3,7,8,15] While few data are available regarding morphologically malignant tumors of skin, those presenting in soft tissue show an increased risk of local recurrence (40–50%), high metastatic potential of 30% to 50%, and high disease-associated mortality.[8,18,10]

Histologic features

Myoepithelioma is composed of an unencapsulated, often dome-shaped, circumscribed nodule consisting of a pure population of myoepithelial cells with no evidence of glandular or ductal differentiation as is seen in the more commonly encountered mixed tumor (Figs 33.64 and 33.65).[5-7] The overlying epidermis may be hyperplastic and sometimes a well-developed collarette is present.[1] A variety of cell types are encountered, including epithelioid, spindled, histiocytoid, and plasmacytoid (hyaline) cells; occasionally clear cells are a feature.[3] These may show a solid sheetlike, reticular, or whorled and occasionally fascicular arrangement.[2,6,7] Some tumors are characterized by a multinodular growth pattern. There is generally no significant nuclear pleomorphism, nucleoli are inconspicuous, and mitoses usually

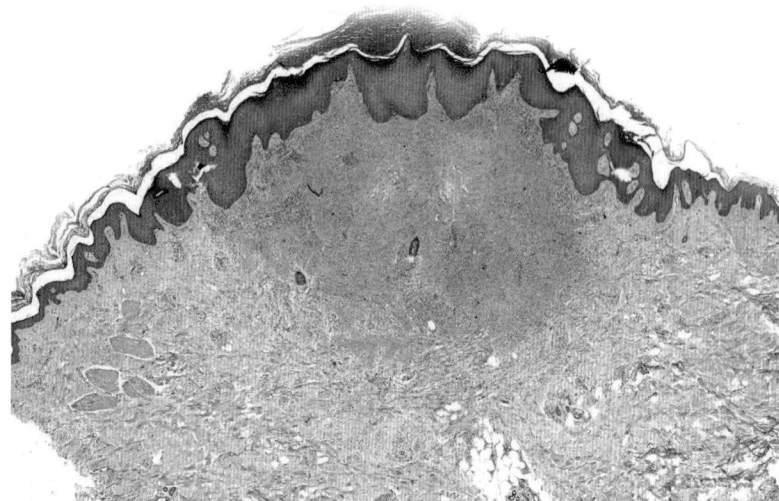

Fig. 33.64
Myoepithelioma: scanning view showing a circumscribed upper dermal tumor nodule. By courtesy of L. Cohen, MD, Cohen Dermatopathology, Massachusetts, USA.

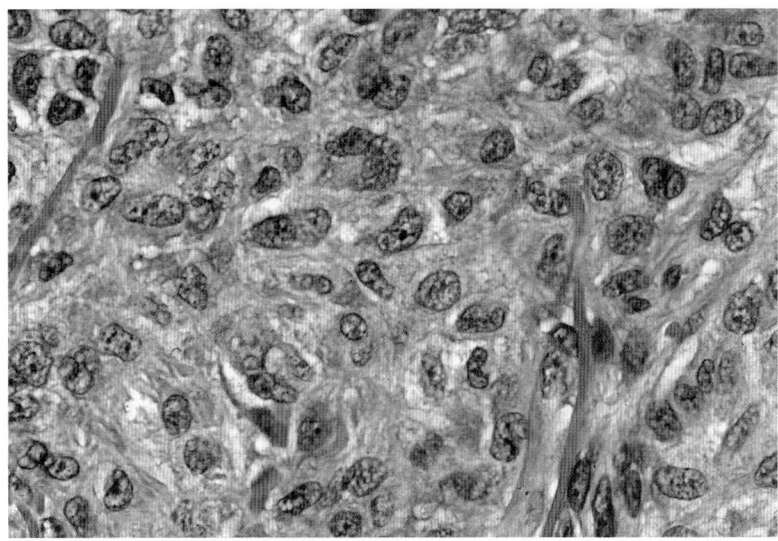

Fig. 33.65
Myoepithelioma: the tumor cells have eosinophilic cytoplasm and round to oval or spindled vesicular nuclei with prominent nucleoli. By courtesy of L. Cohen, MD, Cohen Dermatopathology, Massachusetts, USA.

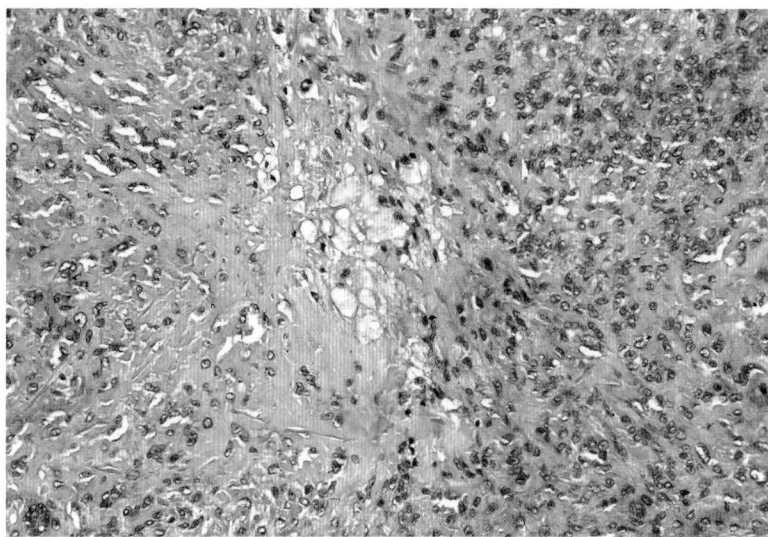

Fig. 33.67
Myoepithelioma: in this field, there is marked stromal hyalinization. By courtesy of L. Cohen, MD, Cohen Dermatopathology, Massachusetts, USA.

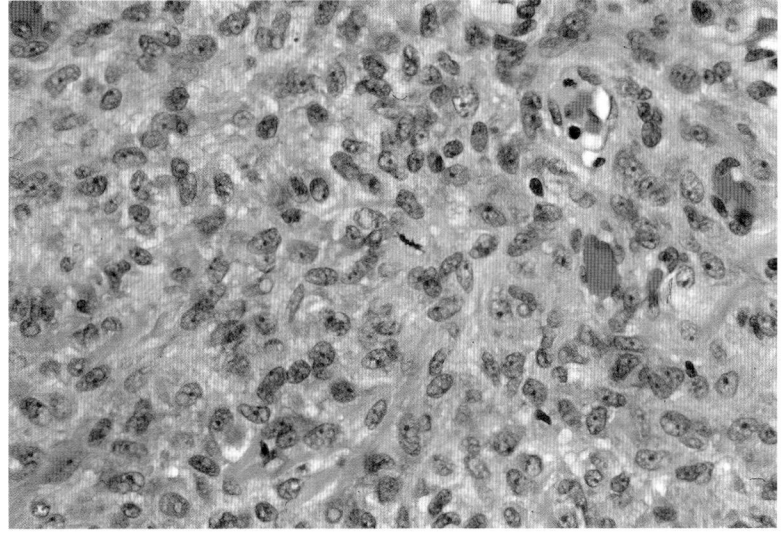

Fig. 33.66
Myoepithelioma: a mitosis is present in the center of the field. By courtesy of L. Cohen, MD, Cohen Dermatopathology, Massachusetts, USA.

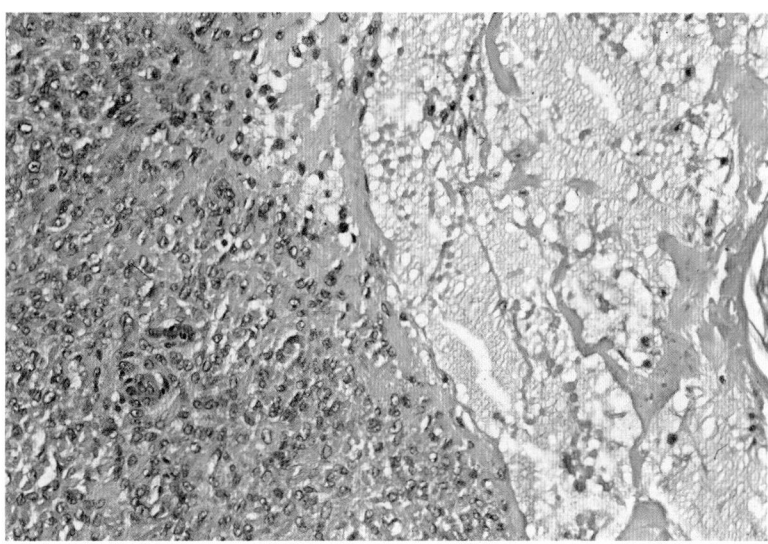

Fig. 33.68
Myoepithelioma: myxoid change, as shown in this field, is sometimes present. By courtesy of L. Cohen, MD, Cohen Dermatopathology, Massachusetts, USA.

scanty (*Fig. 33.66*).[1] Intranuclear cytoplasmic pseudoinclusions are sometimes present. The stroma is typically myxoid or hyaline (*Figs 33.67* and *33.68*).[3,6–8] Cartilagenous differentiation or osseous metaplasia is only rarely present.[8,18] In some tumors conspicuous mature adipocytes are present.[1,4,7] Occasionally, radially orientated collagenous crystalloid inclusions are a feature.[3] These are composed predominantly of type I collagen with type III collagen at their periphery.[3] Rarely, colonization by dendritic melanocytes may be a feature.[17] A subset of tumors is known as cutaneous syncytial myoepithelioma. The tumors present in dermis and are less well circumscribed. They are characterized by a sheetlike growth of ovoid to spindle cells with palely eosinophilic cytoplasm, syncytial cell borders, and vesicular nuclei with small nucleoli (*Figs 33.69* and *33.70*). Occasional mitoses are present, but there is no significant cytological atypia. Adipocytic metaplasia is frequently noted in this subtype of myoepithelioma.[7,20]

Malignant myoepithelioma is characterized by marked nuclear pleomorphism, conspicuous nucleoli, a high mitotic rate, and necrosis.[6–8,18] Lymphovascular invasion or perineural infiltration may also be present.[18] The behavior of cutaneous and soft tissue myoepitheliomas is, however, unpredictable and local recurrence and even distant metastasis as well as disease-related mortality have been documented in tumors lacking cytological features of malignancy. Reliable criteria for malignancy are therefore difficult to establish.

Ultrastructurally, intermediate filaments with focal densities are prominent and the tumor cells are surrounded by a well-developed basal lamina.[2] Desmosomes may be present.[1]

By immunohistochemistry, expression of cytokeratin and/or EMA together with S100, SOX10, and/or GFAP in tumor cells is required to document their myoepithelial phenotype.[21,22] The cutaneous syncytial variant is typically cytokeratin negative and EMA positive.[7,20] In addition, expression of calponin and SMA may be seen (*Fig. 33.71*).[6–8] Nuclear staining for p63 may be seen but desmin is only rarely expressed.[6,7] INI1 expression is lost in a subset of tumors.[23,24] Malignant variants show an identical profile.[6]

Cytogenetic studies on one case of malignant myoepithelioma have revealed complex findings with deletion of 3p, gain of 16q, and monosomy of chromosomes 13 and 15.[14] EWSR1 gene rearrangements are present in around 45% of soft tissue myoepitheliomas and myoepithelial carcinomas and in 80% of cutaneous syncytial myoepitheliomas. As yet identified translocation partners include POU5F1, ATF1, PBX1, PBX3, and ZNF444.[25–32] PLAG1 gene rearrangements are rare in myoepithelial tumors without duct differentiation.[33–35]

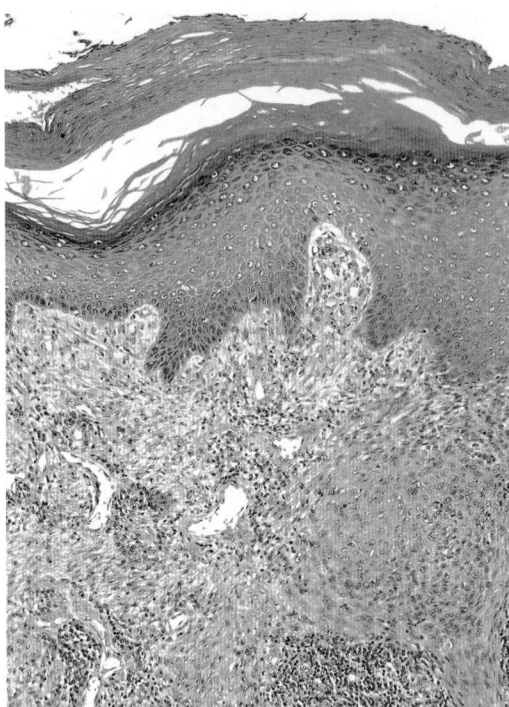

Fig. 33.69
Syncytial myoepithelioma: dermal tumor composed of sheets of pale eosinophilic cells. There is inflammation in the background.

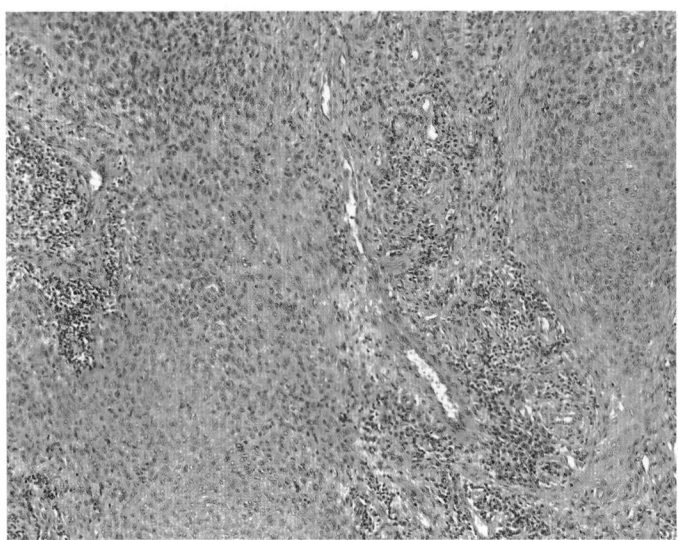

Fig. 33.70
Syncytial myoepithelioma: ovoid or slightly elongated cells with syncytial pale eosinophilic cytoplasm and vesicular nuclei with a small nucleolus.

Eccrine nevus

Clinical features

Eccrine nevus (nevus sudoriferous, sudoriferous hamartoma) is a rare hamartoma of the eccrine unit which typically presents in childhood or adolescence.[1-15] Clinical manifestations are variable and include localized areas of hyperhidrosis (localized unilateral hyperhidrosis). The condition may also develop in association with cutaneous lesions including solitary papules, nodules, patches, or plaques frequently showing brownish discoloration.[1-4,6-14] These cutaneous findings may also present in the absence of hyperhidrosis. There is a predilection for the upper extremities. Lesions may be grouped in a linear arrangement but are rarely multiple, and congenital presentation is infrequent.[3,6,7,12]

Pathogenesis and histologic features

Histologically, eccrine nevi are characterized by increased sized or number of eccrine coils. Infrequently, abundant mucin or an angiomyxoid stroma surrounds the coils, when the term mucinous eccrine nevus is applied.[15-20,21]

Adnexal polyp of neonatal skin

Clinical features

Adnexal polyp of neonatal skin presents as a small congenital polypoid and typically solitary cutaneous lesion. It is skin colored and regresses within a few days of birth.[1,2] The incidence reported in a large Japanese study is estimated at 4%.[2,3] It almost exclusively affects the areola of the breast, but other sites such as the eyelid, cheek, periauricular and scapular regions, axilla, arm, hypochondrium, scrotum, and labium majus may also be involved.[1-3]

Pathogenesis and histologic features

Histologically, the polyp consists of centrally located adnexal structures including hair follicles, sebaceous glands, and well-formed eccrine units. Arrector pili muscle and apocrine structures are absent. Keratinous cysts are sometimes present.[2]

Eccrine syringofibroadenoma

Clinical features

Eccrine syringofibroadenoma (acrosyringeal nevus) is uncommon. It may show a variable presentation, ranging from solitary lesions to multiple papules and nodules arranged in a symmetrical or linear nevoid pattern.[1,2] Distribution is wide and includes the face, back, abdomen, buttock, extremities, and rarely the nail.[2-4] The age of onset ranges from 16 to 80 years; most patients, however, were in their seventh or eighth decade.[1] A stratification according to five clinically distinct subgroups has been proposed[5,6]:

- *Solitary eccrine syringofibroadenoma*: this variant presents as a single, often verrucous-like lesion in the middle aged or elderly.[2,5,7-19] The anatomical distribution is wide with a predilection for the lower extremity.[5]
- *Multiple eccrine syringofibroadenoma associated with ectodermal dysplasia*: patients in this subgroup typically present with multiple erythematous papules predominantly affecting the limbs and especially the palms and soles.[5,20-26] Presentation is in adolescence and is associated with ectodermal dysplasia. The accompanying cutaneous manifestations frequently include eyelid hidrocystoma, hypotrichosis, hypodontia, and nail hypoplasia, a constellation also referred to as the Schöpf-Schulz-Passarge syndrome.[27]
- *Multiple eccrine syringofibroadenoma without associated cutaneous findings*: the lesions typically occur on the palms and soles of the elderly without associated cutaneous anomalies.[1,5,28,29]
- *Nonfamilial unilateral linear eccrine syringofibroadenoma*: this extremely infrequent presentation is nonfamilial and lesions are present unilaterally as multiple papules and plaques in a linear arrangement.[2,30-32] A wide age range is affected but patients typically present in adolescence or early adulthood and there is a predilection for the extremities.
- *Reactive eccrine syringofibroadenoma*: eccrine syringofibroadenoma may also be present as an unusual reactive epithelial change complicating other cutaneous disease including inflammatory dermatoses in addition to neoplasia. It has been associated with longstanding venous stasis, nail trauma, chronic ulceration of the foot, burn scar ulcer, leprosy, nevus sebaceous, enterostomy site, bullous pemphigoid, epidermolysis bullosa, erosive palmoplantar lichen planus, epithelioid hemangioendothelioma, and squamous cell carcinoma.[3,23,33-48]

Recurrences are not a feature, but malignant transformation within a longstanding eccrine syringofibroadenoma has been postulated.[37,49]

Pathogenesis and histologic features

Whether presenting as a solitary tumor or in a nevoid distribution, the histologic features are remarkably similar.[1,2,5,7,8,30] Arising from the epidermis at multiple points are thin anastomosing strands of uniform, small epithelial cells enclosing a fibrovascular stroma, which is often rich in acid mucopolysaccharides and sometimes contains a prominent lymphocytic and plasma

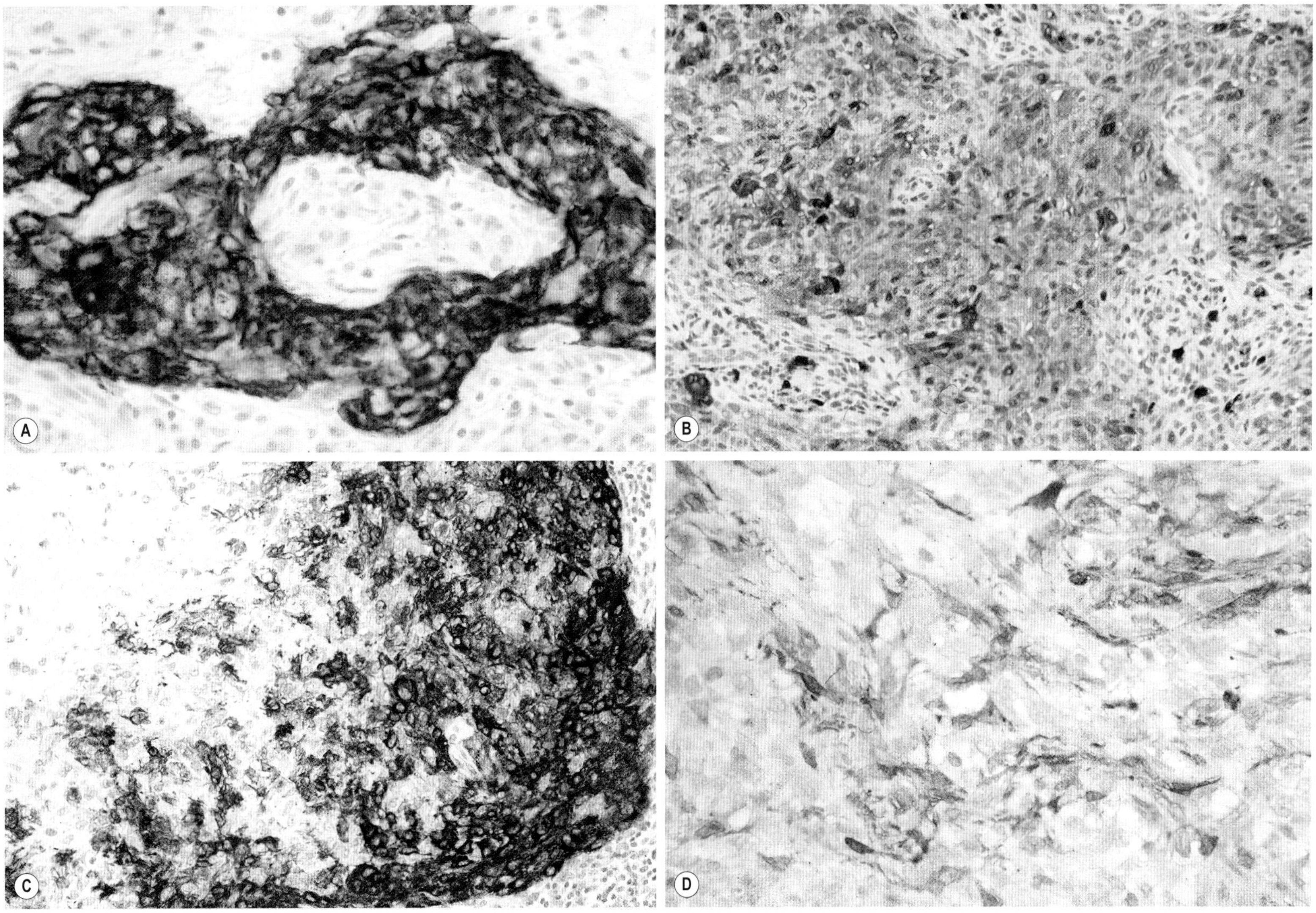

Fig. 33.71
Myoepithelioma: immunohistochemistry showing (**A**) EMA, (**B**) S100 protein, (**C**) smooth muscle actin, and (**D**) GFAP expression.

cell infiltrate (*Fig. 33.72*). The epithelial strands characteristically show ductal differentiation, often associated with a well-formed cuticle (*Figs 33.73* and *33.74*). Aggregates of clear cells may rarely be noted.[14,50] The epithelial cells are PAS positive and, in keeping with their eccrine derivation, contain oxidative enzymes, including succinic dehydrogenase, phosphorylase, and leucine aminopeptidase.[1]

Eccrine angiomatous hamartoma

Clinical features

Eccrine angiomatous hamartoma (eccrine angiomatous nevus) is a rare benign malformation characterized by both eccrine and vascular components. The clinical presentation is of a slowly enlarging nodule, plaque or papule with blue–purple discoloration and a predilection for the extremities, especially the legs.[1-27] Less frequently involved sites include the trunk and the head and neck area.[6,7,11,14,15,28] A wide age range, from 2 months to 73 years, may be affected, but presentation is usually in children (median 10 years).[1,29-32] In more than 50% of patients, the lesions are of congenital onset and there is no sex predilection.[1,26] Eccrine angiomatous hamartoma may present as single or multiple lesions ranging from very small (3 mm) to large lesions (up to 11 cm in size).[1,13,20,33,34] Rarely, patients have multiple, symmetrical lesions.[19,26] The cutaneous findings are frequently associated with pain, tenderness, hyperhidrosis, and (less frequently) hypertrichosis.[1,4] Eccrine angiomatous hamartoma has also developed in a patient with Cowden syndrome.[35]

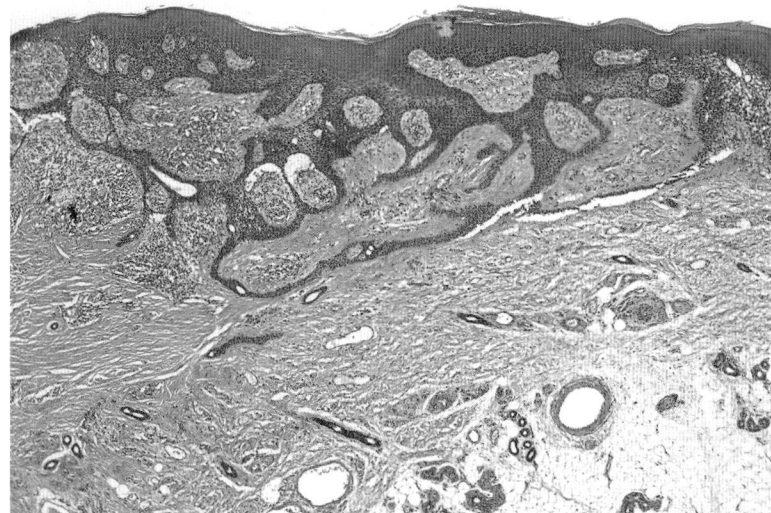

Fig. 33.72
Eccrine syringofibroadenoma: this lesion presented as a solitary tumor. Arising from the epidermis are numerous anastomosing strands of epithelium surrounded by a cellular fibrous stroma.

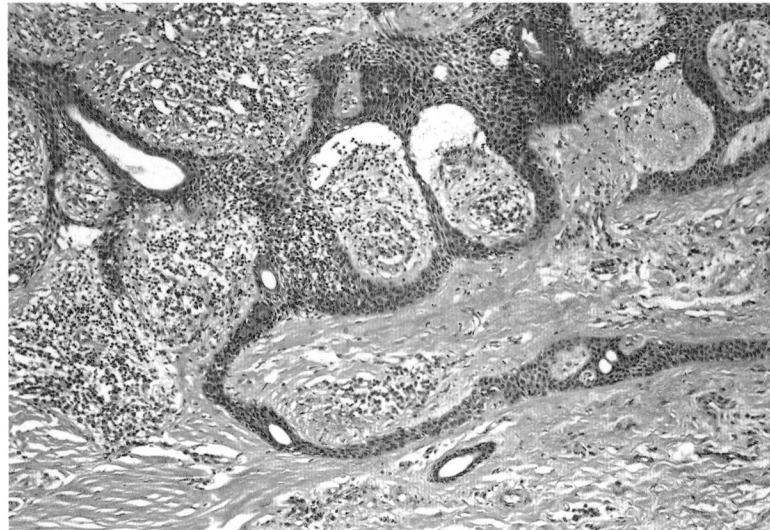

Fig. 33.73
Eccrine syringofibroadenoma: the epithelium is composed of uniform small cells with eosinophilic cytoplasm and small hyperchromatic nuclei. Ductal differentiation is present.

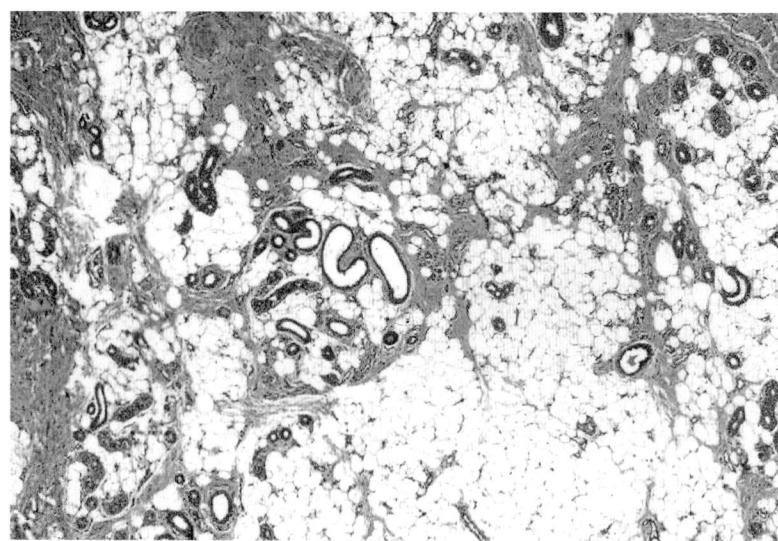

Fig. 33.75
Eccrine angiomatous hamartoma: this example involves the subcutaneous fat. There are widespread eccrine sweat gland units intimately associated with small vascular channels.

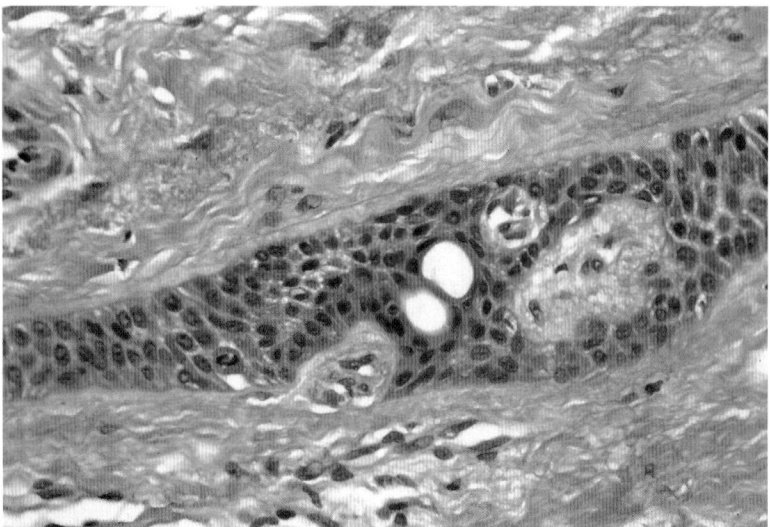

Fig. 33.74
Eccrine syringofibroadenoma: high-power view.

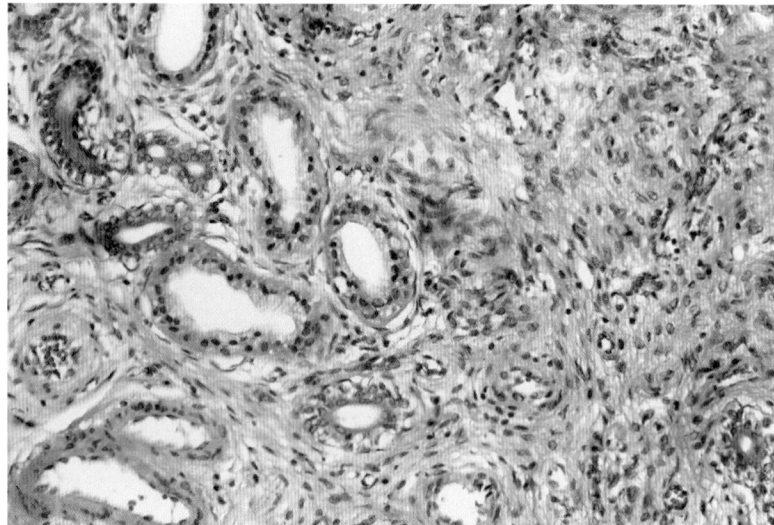

Fig. 33.76
Eccrine angiomatous hamartoma: higher-power view of the sweat glands and blood vessels.

Histologic features

Histologically, eccrine angiomatous hamartoma appears as a relatively circumscribed but unencapsulated lesion located within the mid to deep dermis and composed of increased numbers of occasionally dilated but mature-appearing eccrine glands (Figs 33.75 and 33.76).[1,4,19] Clear cell change may be a focal feature.[14,17] Eccrine duct formation is present, and intimately associated with the eccrine structures is a benign vascular proliferation (Fig. 33.77). This latter component is composed of small capillaries showing variable dilatation. It appears lobular but may rarely be ill defined.[1] Secondary changes such as thrombosis with evidence of recanalization or associated hemorrhage is sometimes a feature.[19] Other unusual findings include a lipomatous component, mucinous change, or pilar structures (Fig. 33.78).[10,11,15–17,19,36,37] The overlying epidermis is frequently unremarkable but occasionally verrucous features are present.[18] In addition, eccrine angiomatous hamartoma rarely may show features reminiscent of verrucous hemangioma or arteriovenous malformation.[38,39] It has also been documented adjacent to a spindle cell hemangioma.[37]

By immunohistochemistry, the vascular component is characterized by positive staining with endothelial markers.[5,7,15] Eccrine glands are positive for S100 protein, CEA, EMA, and cytokeratin as well as GCDFP-15.[5,15,19,21,40]

Porokeratotic eccrine ostial and dermal duct nevus

Clinical features

Porokeratotic eccrine ostial and dermal duct nevus is a rare hamartomatous lesion that was first described as 'comedo nevus of the palm' in 1979.[1]

Clinically, it presents at birth or in early childhood as multiple punctuate pits and papules, frequently showing comedo-like plugging (Figs 33.79 and 33.80).[1–32] The lesions may appear verrucous and are distributed in a linear arrangement. The palms and soles are almost exclusively affected, but rarely a generalized, widespread, and occasionally unilateral or dermatomal distribution is observed.[12,14,22–24,28–30,33] Late onset in adulthood is uncommon and there appears to be no gender predilection.[23,25] The concurrent occurrence of linear psoriasis and keratitis-ichthyosis-deafness (KID) syndrome has been reported, but no other associated anomalies are found.[8,19,27,34] Rarely, the lesions are complicated by the development of squamous cell carcinoma.[31,32]

Histologic features

The histologic features are distinctive and consist of a small epidermal invagination with an overlying prominent parakeratotic cornoid lamella-like tier (Fig. 33.81). This is frequently found in association with, and overlying, an

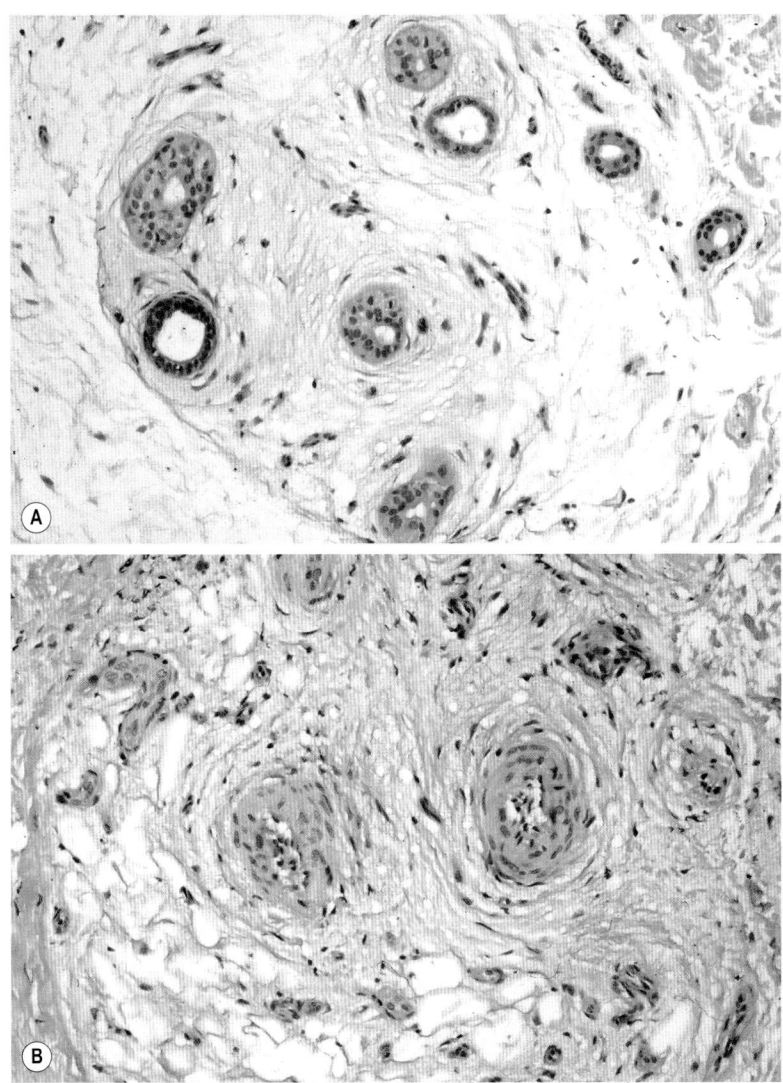

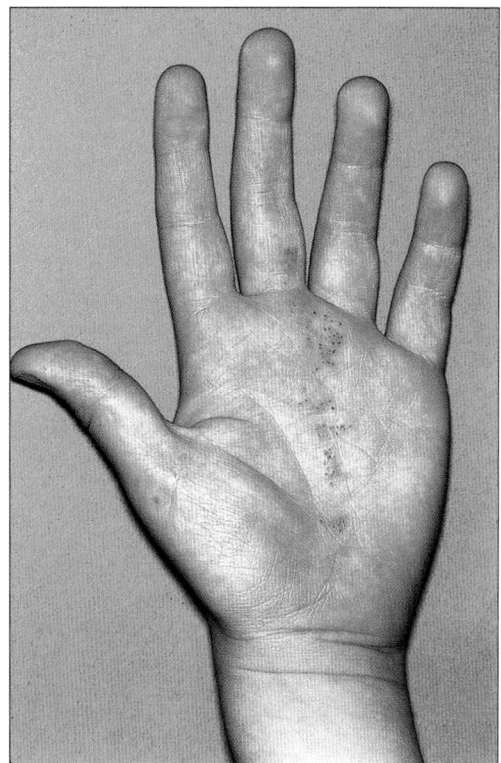

Fig. 33.79
Porokeratotic eccrine osteal and dermal duct nevus: note the linear distribution on the palm of the hand. By courtesy of R.A. Marsden, MD, St George's Hospital, London, UK.

Fig. 33.77
Eccrine angiomatous hamartoma: high-power views of (**A**) sweat glands and (**B**) the vascular component.

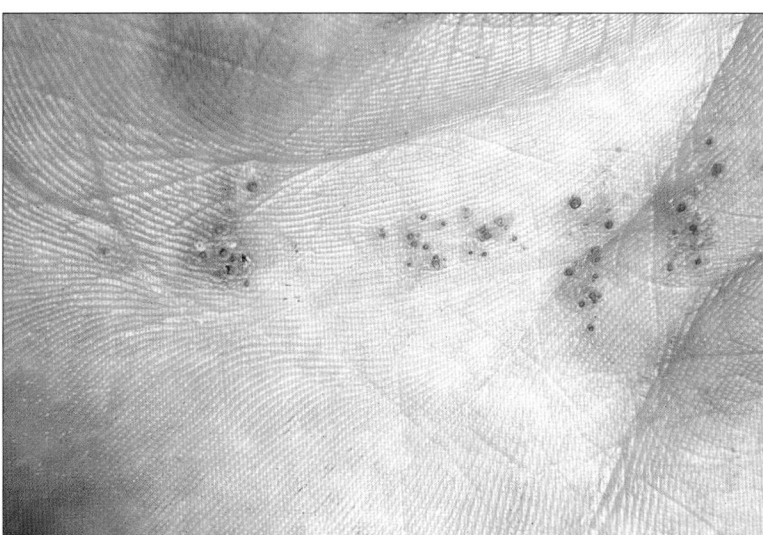

Fig. 33.80
Porokeratotic eccrine osteal and dermal duct nevus: each lesion consists of a dilated sweat pore containing keratinous debris. By courtesy of R.A. Marsden, MD, St George's Hospital, London, UK.

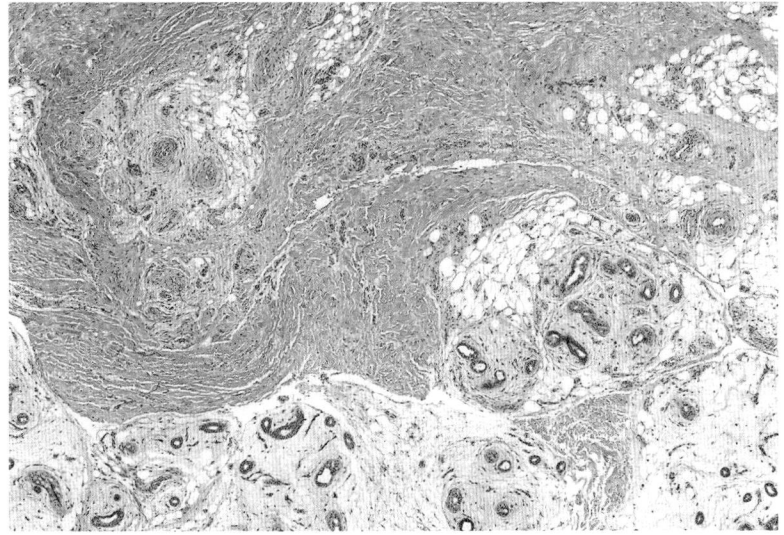

Fig. 33.78
Eccrine angiomatous hamartoma: this example shows a conspicuous mucinous component.

eccrine duct; sometimes it contains the tortuous acrosyringeal duct. Loss of the granular cell layer is seen at the base of the epidermal invagination and keratinocytes often appear vacuolated. Dyskeratotic cells may be evident.[1]

Genetically, the tumors show mutations in the GJB2 gene encoding the gap junction protein connexin 26.[35,36]

Eccrine hidrocystoma

Clinical features

Eccrine hidrocystomas are common and affect adults at any age.[1–3] Individual lesions vary in size from pinhead to pea-sized and appear as tense

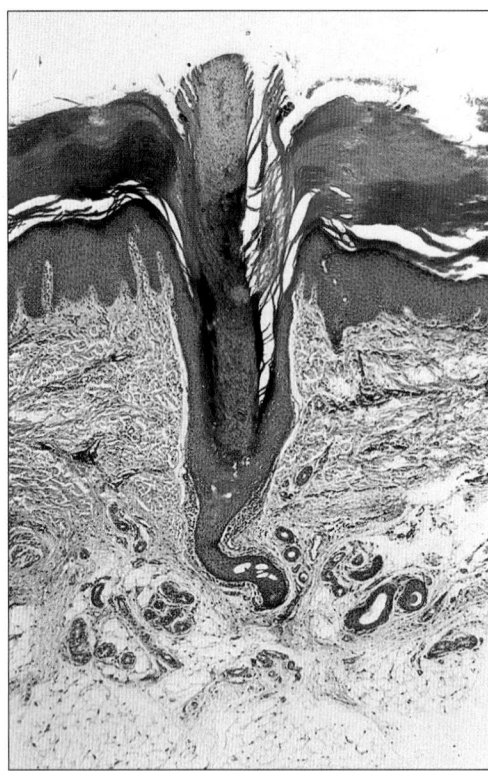

Fig. 33.81
Porokeratotic eccrine osteal and dermal duct nevus: there is gross hyperkeratosis with parakeratosis associated with marked dilatation of the acrosyringium and dermal duct. By courtesy of R.A. Marsden, MD, St George's Hospital, London, UK.

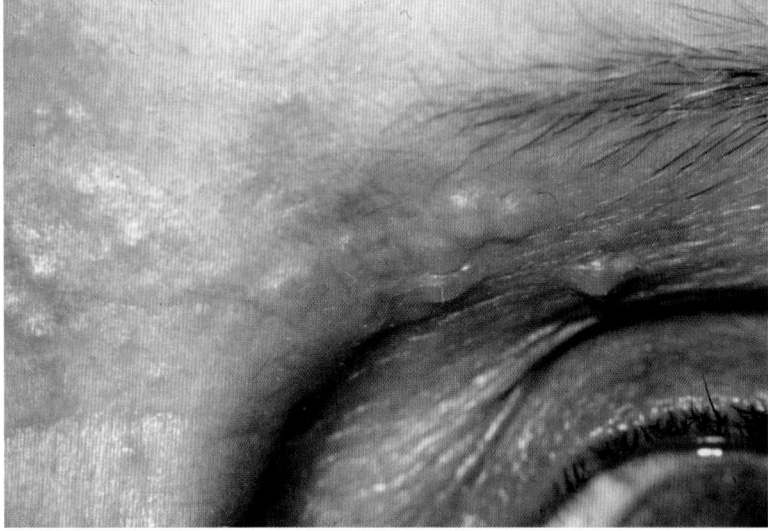

Fig. 33.82
Eccrine hidrocystoma: note the tense swellings adjacent to and below the eyebrow. From the collection of the late N.P. Smith, MD, Institute of Dermatology, London, UK.

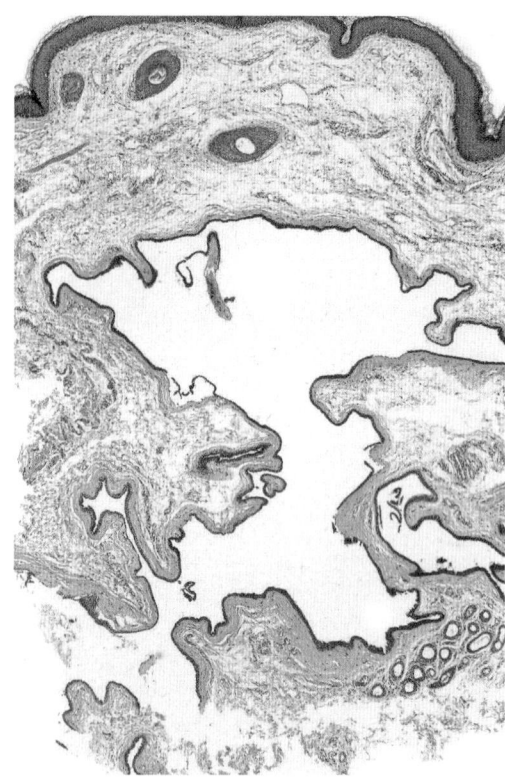

Fig. 33.83
Eccrine hidrocystoma: this tangential section from the eyelid shows a unilocular cyst.

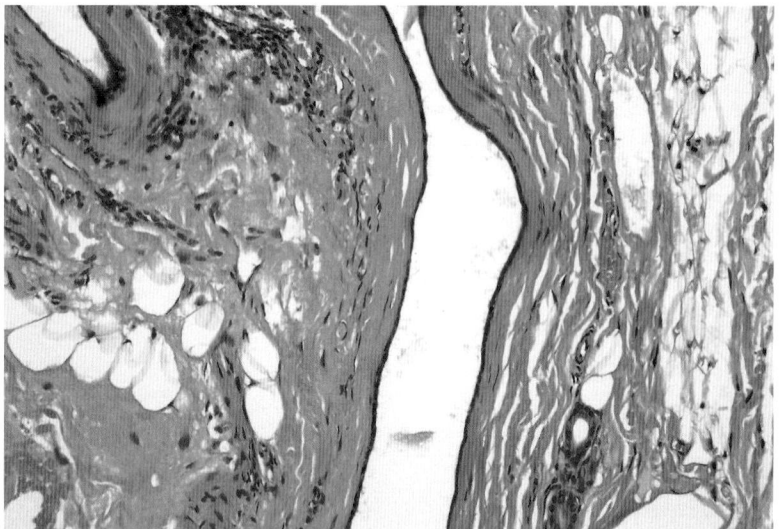

Fig. 33.84
Eccrine hidrocystoma: the cyst is lined by cuboidal epithelial cells. In contrast to apocrine hidrocystoma, there are no myoepithelial cells.

Pathogenesis and histologic features

Because of the clinical features and the fact that eccrine sweat ducts may empty into and drain from the cysts, it is thought that the lesion merely represents a massively dilated duct. The cause of the blockage is unknown, but it is not mechanical. The application of topical atropine or botulinum toxin resolves the lesion, lending support to a functional pathogenesis.[3,11,16]

Histologically, the hidrocystoma consists of one or several partially collapsed, unilocular cysts in the dermis, which are often situated adjacent to normal eccrine glands (Fig. 33.83). Serial sectioning sometimes shows continuity between the cyst epithelium and the lining of the proximal sweat duct.[3] The cyst wall is composed of a double layer of cuboidal epithelium with eosinophilic cytoplasm (Fig. 33.84).[3] Papillary projections are not usually evident.[1] Myoepithelial cells and decapitation secretion are not

vesicles located predominantly on the face, particularly periorbitally, but the trunk, popliteal fossae, external ear, and vulva may rarely be affected (Fig. 33.82).[1,4–7] Larger lesions sometimes have a bluish hue. Exceptionally, the cysts may be very large, reaching up to 8 cm.[8,9] Typically, the lesions wax and wane with circumstances that provoke sweat production; they are therefore exacerbated in summer, but may disappear clinically in the winter months.[3] There are two modes of presentation:

- More often, patients (with a slight female predilection, 3:2) have a solitary lesion.
- More rarely, patients (almost all female) develop numerous hidrocystomas, sometimes in the hundreds.[1,3,10–15]

present. A PAS-positive, diastase-resistant basement membrane is present, and the epithelial cells may contain glycogen. On occasions, compression of the adjacent dermal connective tissue results in a pseudocapsule.

In keeping with eccrine derivation, the cyst wall epithelium contains succinic dehydrogenase and phosphorylase.[2] The cytokeratin expression pattern in these lesions resembles that of the dermal eccrine ducts.[17,18]

Hidroacanthoma simplex

Clinical features

Hidroacanthoma simplex is a rare tumor and is usually clinically misdiagnosed as a seborrheic keratosis, basal cell carcinoma, or in situ squamous cell carcinoma (Bowen disease).[1] It presents most often on the distal extremities, although the chest, arm, and face may be affected (*Fig. 33.85*).[2] Lesions are generally hyperkeratotic erythematous or brown plaques.[3,4] The condition occurs equally in males and females, predominantly in the elderly.

Pathogenesis and histologic features

Hidroacanthoma simplex is a benign intraepidermal neoplasm derived from the acrosyringium. At low-power examination, the tumor appears as discrete circumscribed populations of cells within an irregularly acanthotic epidermis (*Fig. 33.86*).[2] Hidroacanthoma simplex therefore represents one cause of the intraepidermal epithelioma of Jadassohn (Borst-Jadassohn

phenomenon). Individual tumor cells resemble those of a poroma, being cuboidal or oval, with a vesicular nucleus containing a small nucleolus (*Fig. 33.87*). Intracytoplasmic glycogen can usually be demonstrated, and in some tumors this is so marked that a clear cell variant results.[5] Pigmented lesions associated with melanocyte colonization represent another unusual subtype.[6] On occasions, the tumor cells have a spindled appearance (*Fig. 33.88*).[2] Rudimentary duct formation and/or intracytoplasmic lumina are present, although multiple levels often have to be examined before they are identified.[7,8] By definition, the dermis is unaffected.

The tumor cells sometimes express EMA, but not CEA, although ductal differentiation/intracytoplasmic lumina may sometimes be highlighted with both antibodies.[9,10]

Occasional tumors showing nuclear and cytoplasmic pleomorphism with mitotic activity are encountered (*Figs 33.89 and 33.90*). These are best classified as in situ variants of eccrine porocarcinoma (malignant hidroacanthoma simplex).[11–19] Invasive tumor may result.

Differential diagnosis

Hidroacanthoma simplex must be distinguished from a seborrheic keratosis exhibiting a Jadassohn effect in which basaloid and squamous cells in the malpighian layer may show nesting or squamous eddy formation. Bowen disease may also rarely manifest an intraepidermal nesting appearance; the

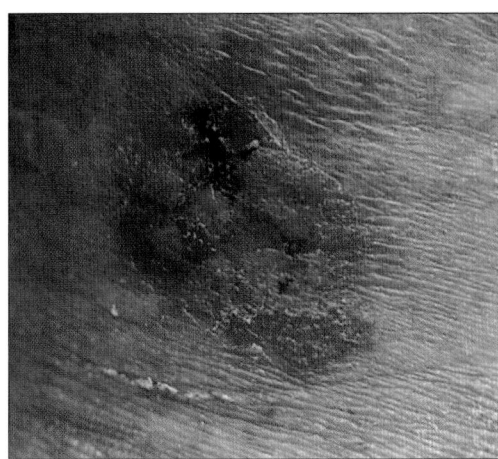

Fig. 33.85
Hidroacanthoma simplex: typical erythematous scaly lesion on the ankle. By courtesy of H. Woolfson, MD, Brook Hospital, London, UK.

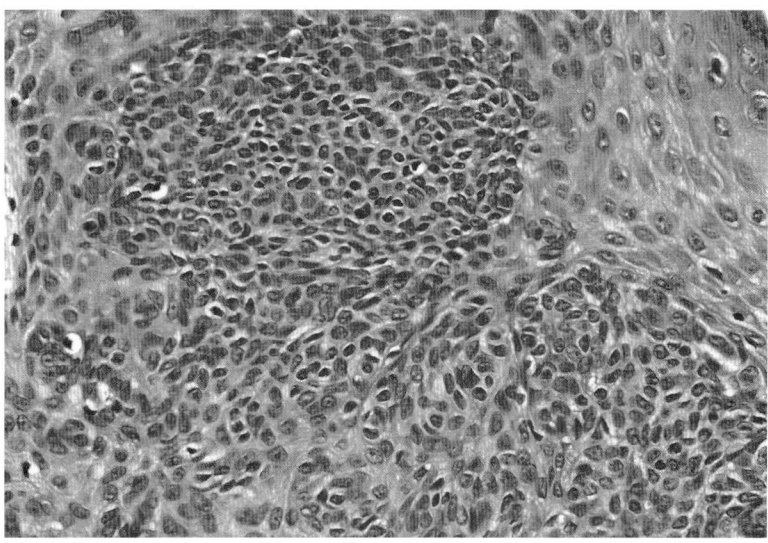

Fig. 33.87
Hidroacanthoma simplex: the tumor cells are smaller than the adjacent keratinocytes. They are very uniform and form intercellular bridges.

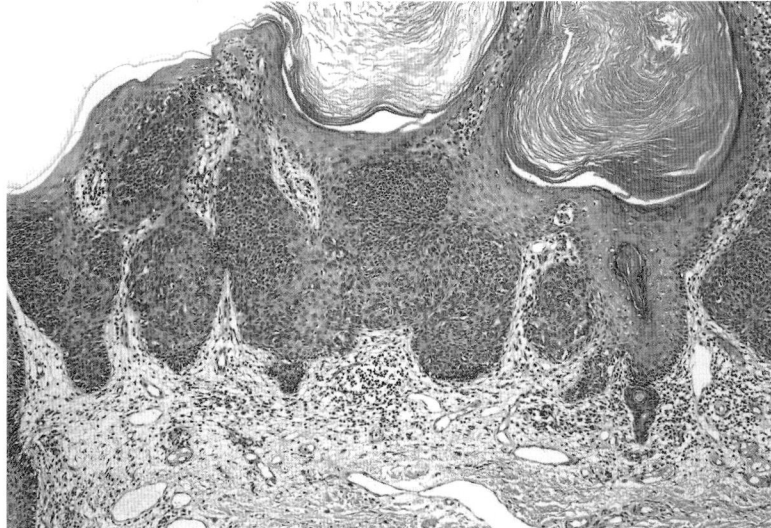

Fig. 33.86
Hidroacanthoma simplex: there is hyperkeratosis. Within the acanthotic epidermis are multiple discrete collections of tumor cells.

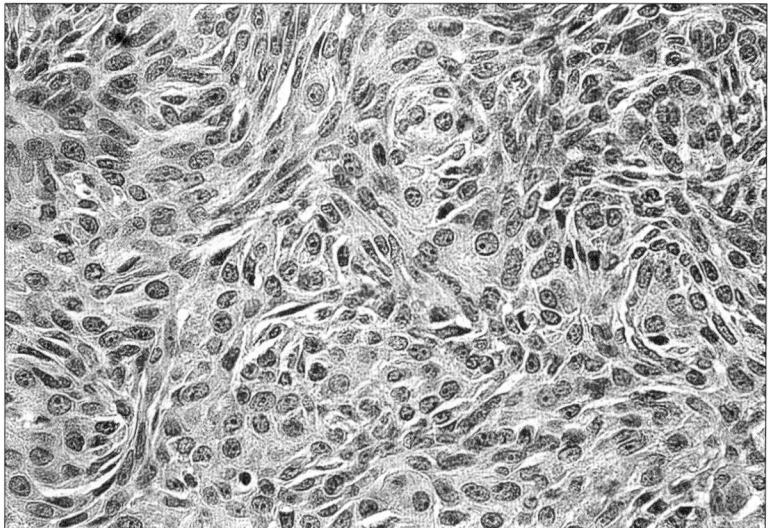

Fig. 33.88
Hidroacanthoma simplex: in this field, there is focal spindled cell morphology.

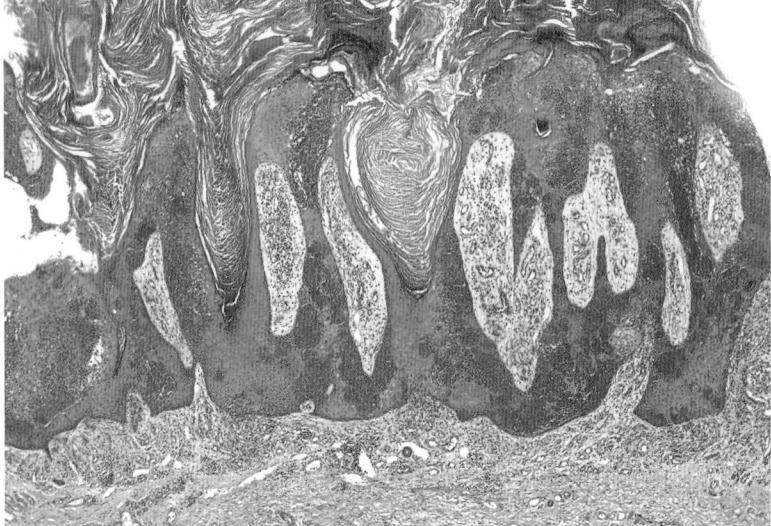

Fig. 33.89
Malignant hidroacanthoma simplex: this tumor arose on the shin. The epidermis appears verrucous and there is a distinct, nested basaloid cell population.

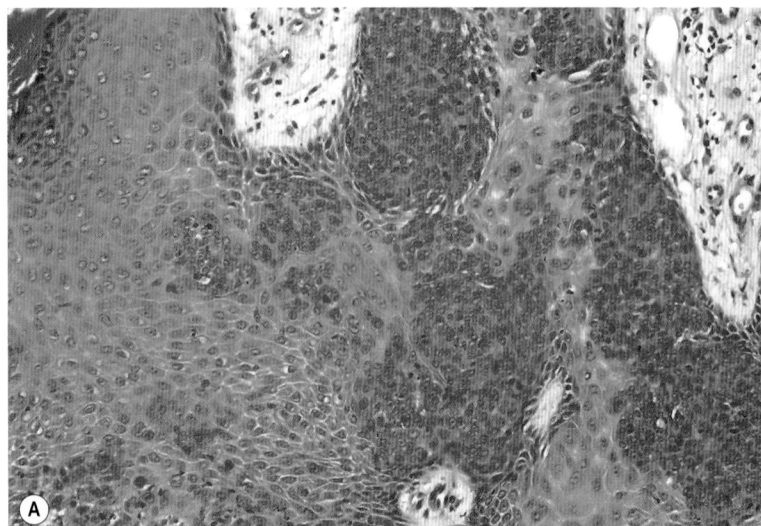

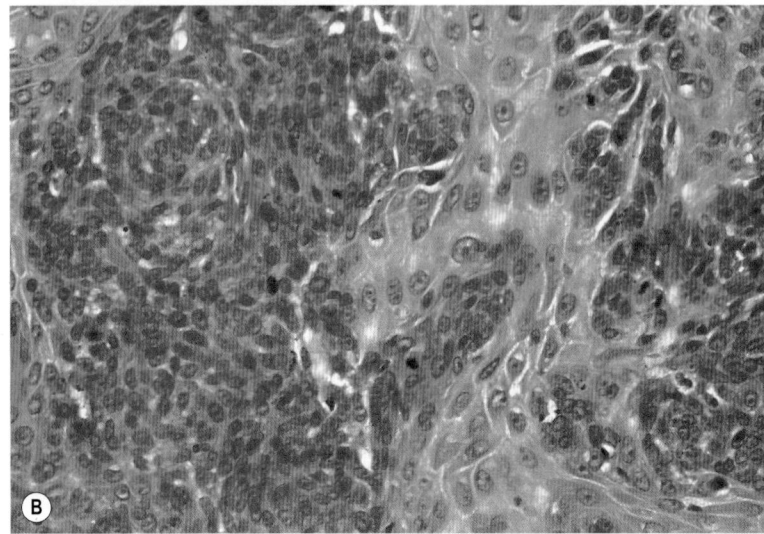

Fig. 33.90
(A, B) Malignant hidroacanthoma simplex: the basaloid cells have darkly staining nuclei. Nucleoli are prominent and mitoses conspicuous.

dysplasia and dyskeratosis should, however, make the diagnosis obvious, and in addition there is no evidence of ductal differentiation.

Eccrine poroma

Clinical features

Classically, this benign tumor, which presents as a solitary, sessile, skin colored to red, slightly scaly nodule, has been described most often on the sole or sides of the foot (*Fig. 33.91*).[1-3] This view has been challenged and a much wider distribution documented.[4] It may therefore also occur on the head, neck, scalp, chest, abdomen, proximal extremities, and hand (*Fig. 33.92*).[5-7] The external auditory canal has also been affected.[8] Lesions, which measure up to 3 cm in diameter, are usually asymptomatic, although bleeding after mild trauma is not uncommon. It is a tumor of adults and affects both sexes equally.[3] Presentation in childhood and congenital onset are unusual.[9,10] Multiple (poromatosis) and linear nevoid variants have been described, and tumors may occur in the setting of chronic scarring.[11-15]

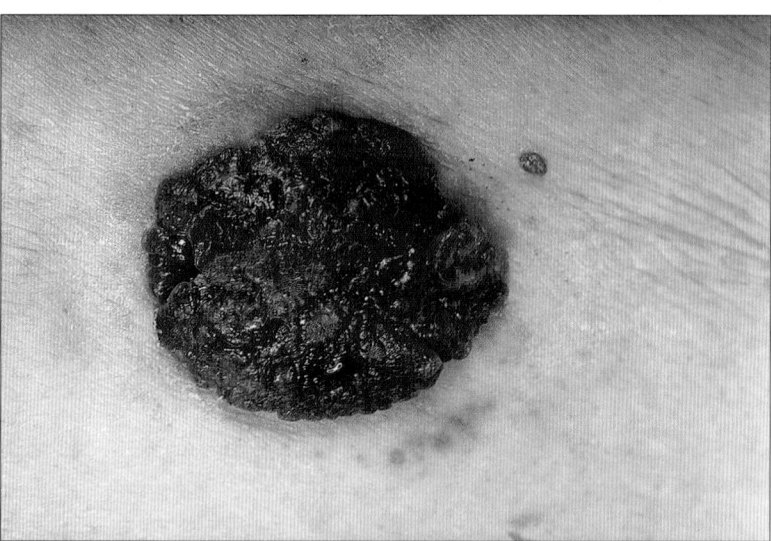

Fig. 33.91
Eccrine poroma: a dark-red nodule is present on the side of the foot, which is a characteristic site. By courtesy of R.A. Marsden, MD, St George's Hospital, London, UK.

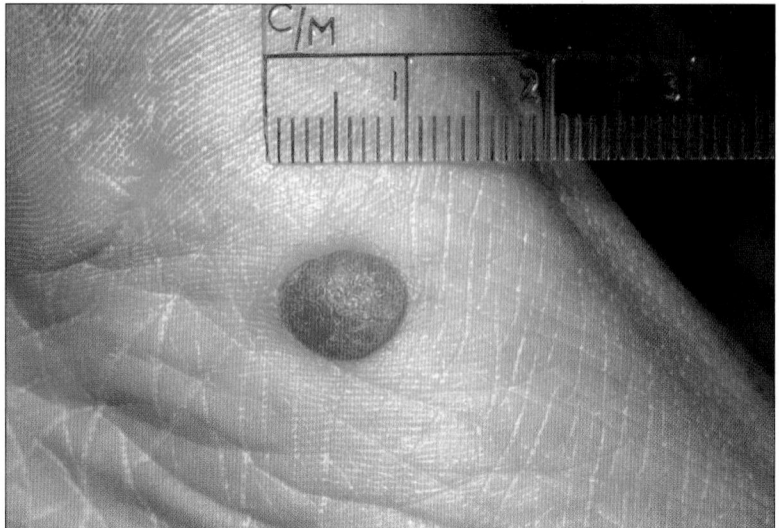

Fig. 33.92
Eccrine poroma: this example is present on the palm of the hand. By courtesy of the Institute of Dermatology, London, UK.

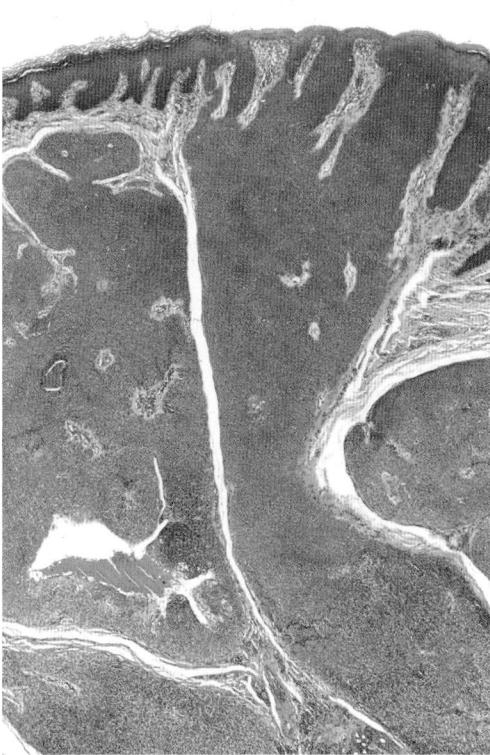

Fig. 33.93
Eccrine poroma: this scanning view shows interconnected epithelial downgrowths with multiple foci of attachment to the epidermis.

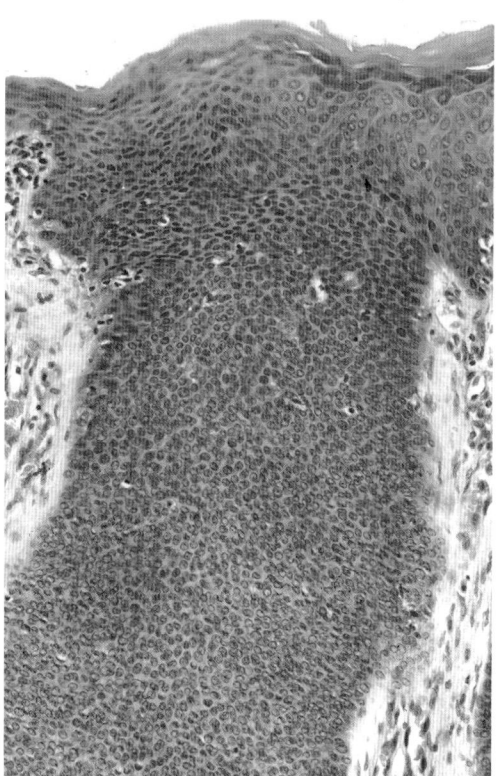

Fig. 33.94
Eccrine poroma: the tumor cells are much smaller than the adjacent keratinocytes.

Pathogenesis and histologic features

In general, the pathogenesis is unknown. There are, however, very occasional case reports documenting the development of multiple lesions in the site of previous electron beam and X-ray therapy.[16,17] One patient developed poromatosis in a background of hidrotic ectodermal dysplasia.[13]

Eccrine poroma is derived from cells of the outer layer of the acrosyringium and upper dermal eccrine duct. The tumor replaces the epidermis and grows down into the dermis in broad anastomosing bands (Fig. 33.93).[3] There is a sharp demarcation between the keratinocytes of the adjacent epidermis and the monomorphic, slightly smaller cuboidal poroma cells (Fig. 33.94). The tumor cells are united by conspicuous intercellular bridges (Fig. 33.95).[2] Peripheral nuclear palisading is not a feature. Confirmation of the diagnosis is provided by features of maturation, either into ductal lumina with a single row of luminal cells covered by an eosinophilic lining or, more frequently, into cystic spaces devoid of any formal lining. Intracytoplasmic lumina with refractile cuticular borders may also be seen (Fig. 33.96). The latter may be highlighted by diastase–PAS staining or EMA and CEA immunohistochemistry.[18,19] The tumor is supported by a delicate fibrovascular stroma. Eccrine poroma cells usually contain glycogen, although the staining is often patchy. Occasionally, pigmented variants with associated dendritic melanocytes and tumor cell melanin deposition are encountered.[10,20–27] These are of particular importance as they may be clinically mistaken for melanoma. Dystrophic calcification and transepidermal elimination of tumor nests are exceptional findings.[28,29]

Eccrine poroma shows marked phosphorylase and succinic dehydrogenase activity (Fig. 33.97).[2]

Comment

Benign eccrine ductal tumors – including hidroacanthoma simplex, eccrine poroma, dermal duct tumor, and eccrine hidradenoma – are in most instances readily recognizable as distinct histologic entities. Not surprisingly, however, considering their similar ancestry, overlap tumors are occasionally seen, and sometimes two or more subtypes may coexist in a particular lesion (overlap eccrine ductal tumors).[30]

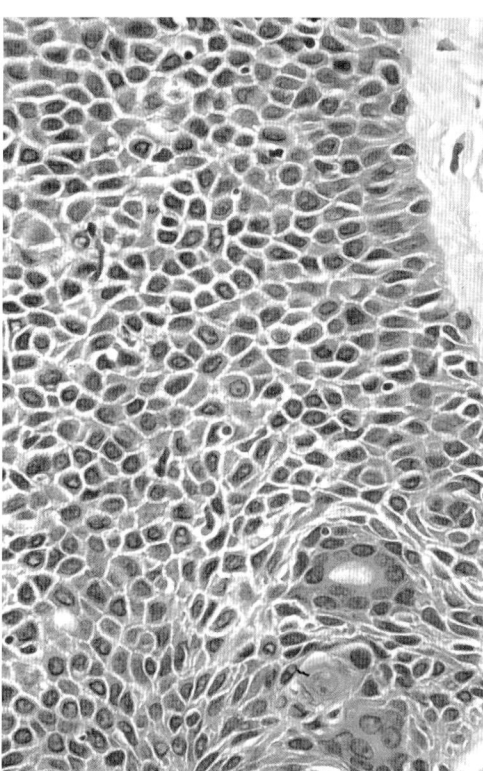

Fig. 33.95
Eccrine poroma: note the sharp boundary between the keratinocytes and tumor cells. Intercellular bridges are conspicuous.

Dermal duct tumor

Clinical features

Dermal duct tumor is a very rare benign tumor that usually occurs on the head and neck or limbs and presents as a nondescript, generally asymptomatic, flesh-colored or erythematous, firm nodule or papule measuring up

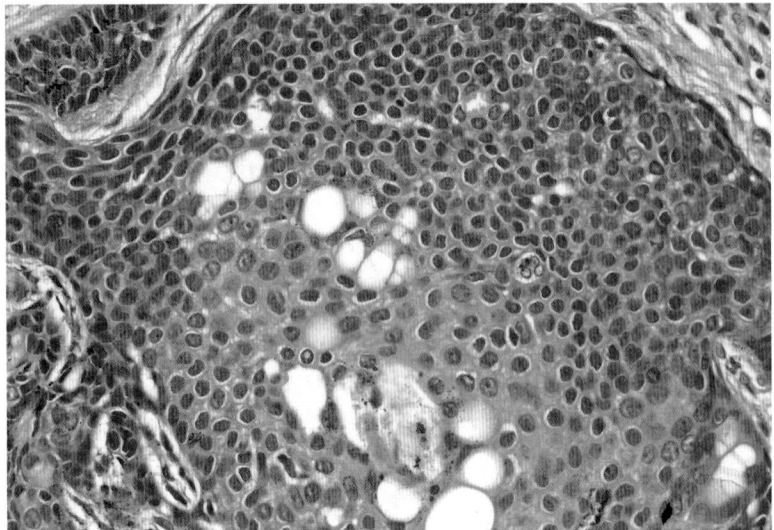

Fig. 33.96
Eccrine poroma: note the well-formed duct and there are conspicuous intracytoplasmic lumina.

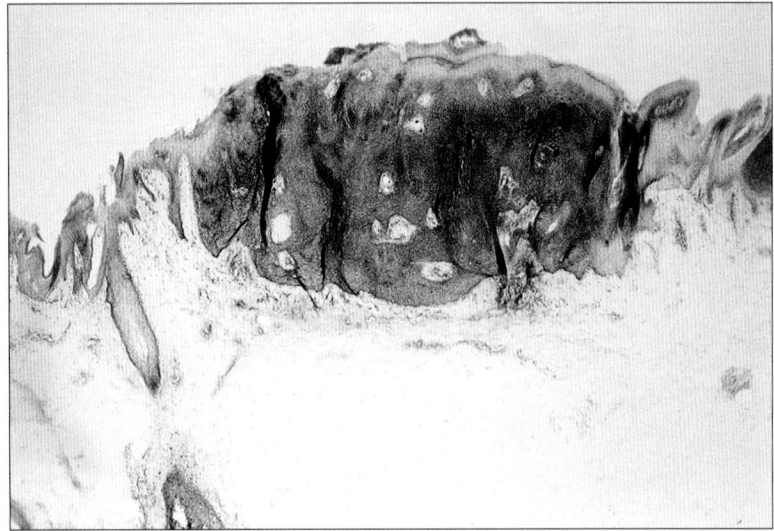

Fig. 33.97
Eccrine poroma: eccrine tumors can be identified by the presence of oxidative enzymes such as succinic dehydrogenase, as shown in this lesion. By courtesy of N. Ramnarain, FIMLS, Institute of Dermatology, London, UK.

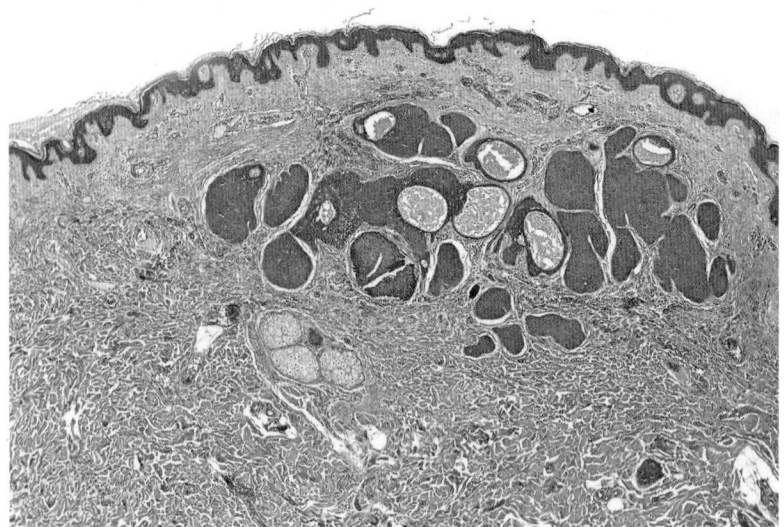

Fig. 33.98
Dermal duct tumor: this lesion is entirely intradermal. Note the circumscribed tumor nodules and scattered cysts.

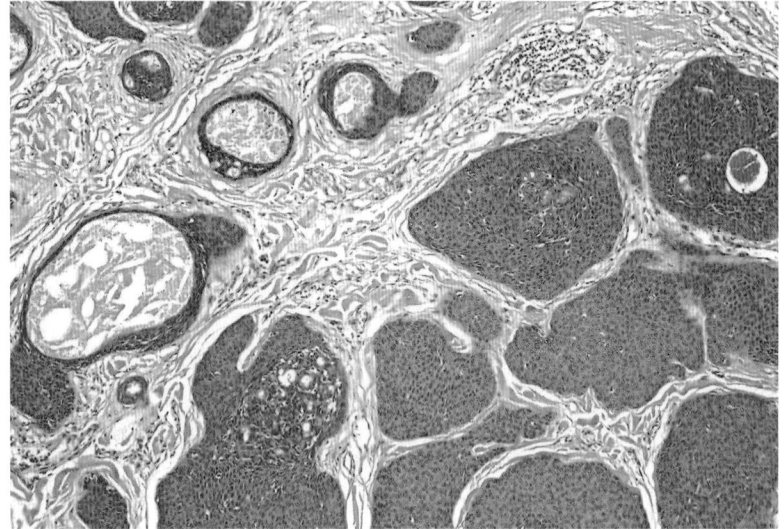

Fig. 33.99
Dermal duct tumor: there are multiple cysts and focal ductal differentiation is seen.

to 2 cm in diameter.[1–3] It is associated with a female preponderance (6:1) and tends to affect the elderly.

Pathogenesis and histologic features

The dermal duct tumor arises from the intradermal segment of the eccrine duct.[1] It is composed of large lobules of tumor in the mid and lower dermis; the epidermis is unaffected (Figs 33.98 and 33.99). The tumor consists of small uniform cuboidal cells showing maturation toward ductal lumina. The latter may be accentuated by the diastase–PAS reaction. Sometimes intracytoplasmic lumina are a feature, and occasionally cystic spaces are present (Fig. 33.100). Peripheral palisading is not usually a feature, the cells at the edges of the lobules tending to be rather flattened. Mitotic figures are not present. The tumor cells contain variable amounts of glycogen and, as further evidence of eccrine differentiation, both phosphorylase and succinic dehydrogenase activities may be demonstrated.[4] Occasionally, focal continuity with an intradermal eccrine duct has been demonstrated.[2]

Differential diagnosis

Dermal duct tumor is very rarely diagnosed since most apparent examples can be shown on deeper levels to demonstrate at least focal continuity with

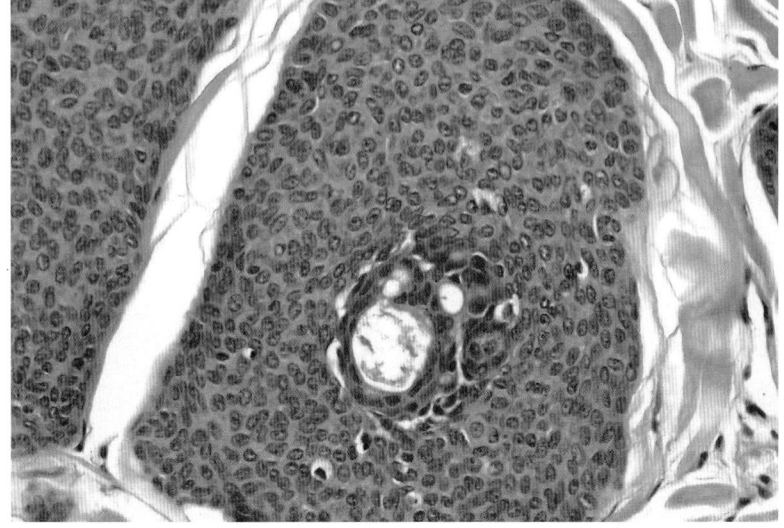

Fig. 33.100
Dermal duct tumor: high-power view.

the epidermis, when a diagnosis of poroma is then rendered.[5] Their distinction, in any event, is of little significance.

Eccrine porocarcinoma

Clinical features

Eccrine porocarcinoma (malignant eccrine poroma), in our experience, is the most frequently encountered malignant sweat gland tumor. It shows a slight predilection for females (1.3:1) and displays a propensity to affect the elderly, with a mean age at presentation of 73 years (range 12–91 years).[1-7] Very exceptionally, children are affected.[8] Lesions are not usually clinically distinctive, being described as verrucous plaques or polypoid growths measuring 0.4–20.0 cm in diameter (mean: 2.0 cm), often clinically misdiagnosed as squamous cell carcinoma, Bowen disease, seborrheic keratosis, or lobular capillary hemangioma (pyogenic granuloma) (Figs 33.101 and 33.102).[1,6] It presents most often on the lower limb, trunk, head, and upper limb in descending order of frequency.[6] However, virtually any site may be affected including the genitalia and nail bed.[9-12] Often, the tumor has been present for a long time, sometimes as much as 50 years, suggesting malignant transformation in a previous benign eccrine poroma.[2,4,6] Tumors are often ulcerated and many bleed on trauma. Eccrine porocarcinoma has also been reported in the setting of chronic arsenism.[13]

Eccrine porocarcinoma is prone to local recurrence (17%), is sometimes multiple, and is occasionally associated with nodal metastases (19%).[6] Some tumors are characterized by very aggressive local spread, and occasionally epidermotropic cutaneous metastases are encountered.[14-17] In some of the latter cases, identification of the primary may be very difficult or impossible. This is because some lesions appear purely intraepidermal and others display an invasive component. Systemic spread is rare (11%).[6,18] Although there are many case reports documenting mortality, we believe that this is an uncommon outcome.[19-24] In the substantial series published with sufficient follow-up information, the death rate amounts to only 7% to 11%.[1,3,6] Particularly aggressive behavior has, however, been reported from Japan with high rates of lymph node metastasis (50%) and associated mortality (33%).[25]

Pathogenesis and histologic features

In general, the pathogenesis of this tumor is unknown although occasional tumors have followed prior radiotherapy and one or two cases have arisen within a pre-existent organoid nevus.[6,26,27] Coexistent benign eccrine poroma is encountered in up to 11% of cases.[2,6,28] Rarely, a coexistent pigmented hidroacanthoma simplex or seborrheic keratosis is present.[29-31] p16 protein has been shown to be overexpressed in eight out of nine cases of eccrine porocarcinoma with absence of retinoblastoma (RB) protein expression.[32] No p16 gene mutation was discovered in the single tumor examined. A recent study detected Merkel cell polyomavirus in 68% of cases of porocarcinoma.[33]

The tumor may remain completely intraepidermal (in situ porocarcinoma) but is more often associated with an invasive intradermal component.[34]

The in situ variant is recognized by the presence of obvious poroma cells, with typical ductal lumina, associated with cytological features of malignancy including nuclear and cytoplasmic pleomorphism, nuclear hyperchromatism, and mitotic activity (frequently abnormal).[1]

Invasive malignant eccrine poroma invariably shows continuity with the surface epithelium and may be associated with a broad pushing deep margin or a more obviously infiltrative lower border (Figs 33.103 and 33.104). The former is a particular catch for the unwary unless the cytology of the lesion is carefully scrutinized. The tumor is most typically characterized by downgrowths of broad anastomosing bands of epithelium, composed of small cells united by small intercellular bridges and devoid of any tendency toward peripheral palisading (Fig. 33.105).[15,35,36] Occasionally, involvement of the surface epithelium manifests as a Borst-Jadassohn effect. Although some tumors appear deceptively bland and are only recognized as being malignant on the basis of their infiltrative growth pattern, the majority of tumors show nuclear pleomorphism and conspicuous, sometimes abnormal, mitotic activity (Figs 33.106 and 33.107).

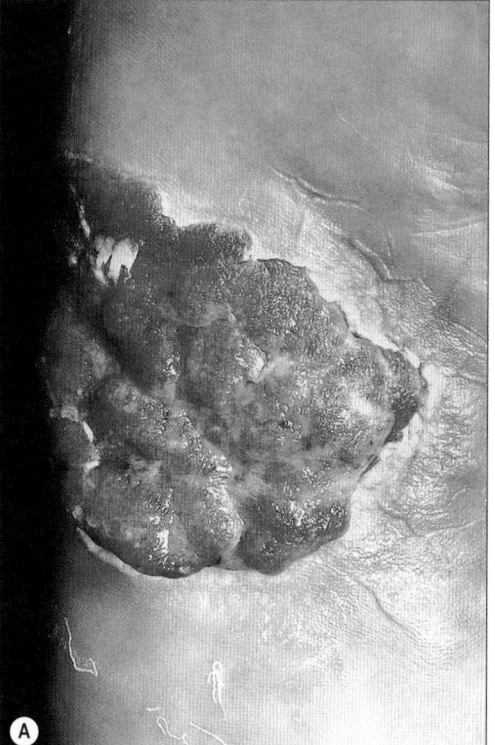

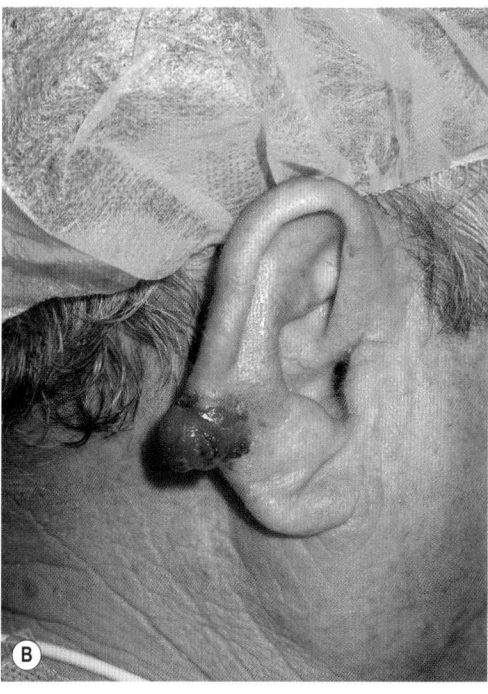

Fig. 33.101
Eccrine porocarcinoma: (**A**) this erythematous and ulcerated tumor plaque is present on the sole of the foot. By courtesy of R.A. Marsden, MD, St George's Hospital, London, UK. (**B**) The ear is a very unusual site. By courtesy of J.C. Pascual, Alicante, Spain.

Ductal differentiation and/or intracytoplasmic lumen formation is invariably evident and is often rendered more obvious by the use of the diastase–PAS reaction or the immunocytochemical demonstration of EMA or CEA expression (Figs 33.108 and 33.109). It is important not to misinterpret entrapped normal sweat ducts in which the epithelium is devoid of atypia as representing tumor ductal differentiation. Similarly, degenerative cytoplasmic vacuolation may initially suggest ductal differentiation, but it can be distinguished by the absence of a cuticle and negative EMA/CEA immunohistochemistry.

Lymphovascular invasion or spread along the perineural space is sometimes seen and tumor necrosis may be evident (Figs 33.110–112).[6,36]

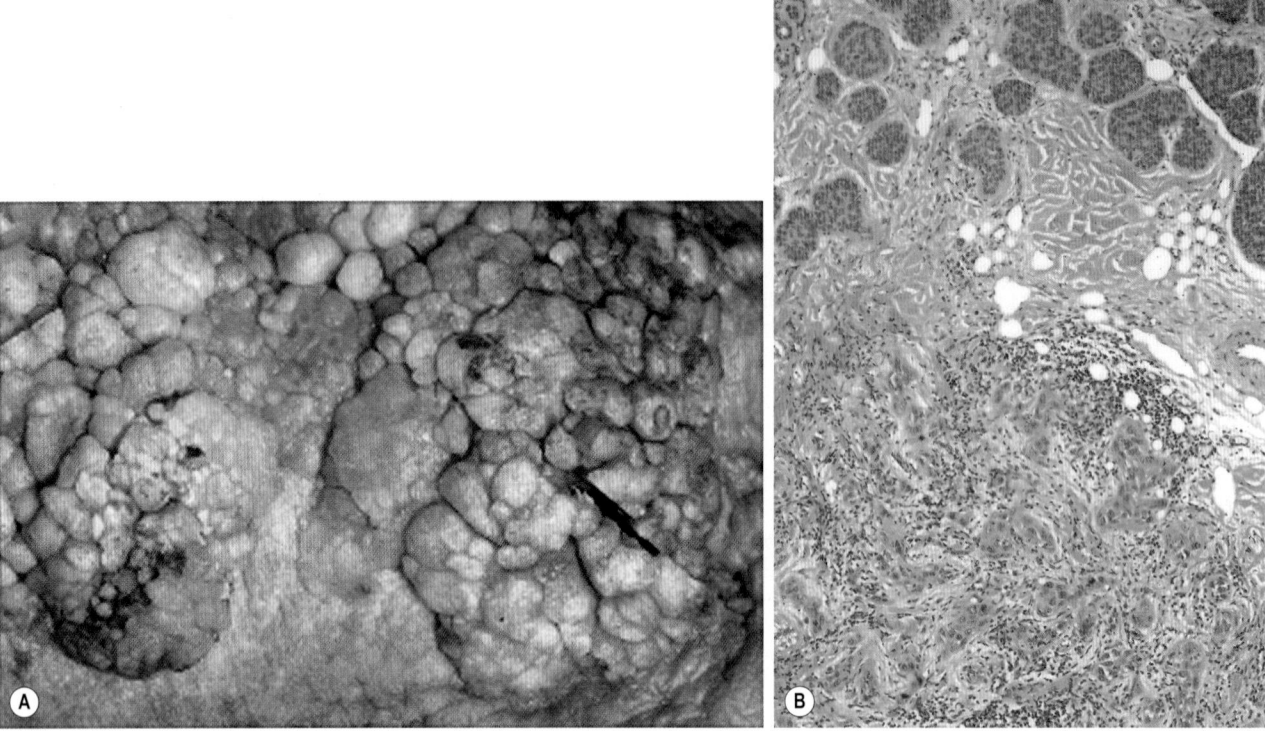

Fig. 33.102
Eccrine porocarcinoma: (**A**) the tumor is composed of numerous warty excrescences; (**B**) this example has arisen in a pre-existent benign poroma. Note the poroma above and invasive tumor below.

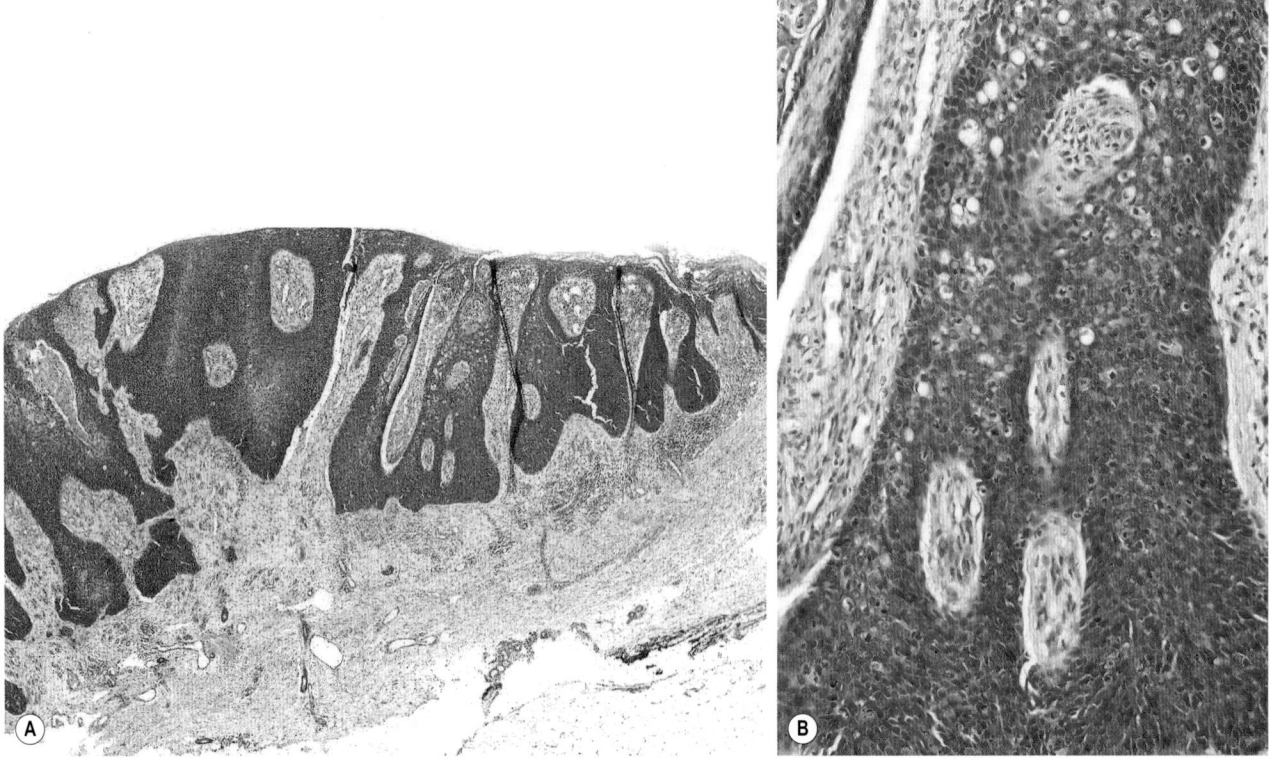

Fig. 33.103
Eccrine porocarcinoma: (**A**) in this example, the tumor has a broad pushing lower border; (**B**) the borders are sharply delineated and intracytoplasmic lumina are evident.

The tumor cells frequently contain glycogen, which may be sufficient to produce foci of clear cell change. Rarely, the latter feature predominates – the clear cell variant (*Figs 33.113* and *33.114*).[6,37,38] Squamous metaplasia is sometimes present and, uncommonly, the tumor may show foci of frankly bowenoid features with dyskeratosis or more obvious keratinization, usually affecting the more superficial aspect of the tumor (bowenoid porocarcinoma) (*Figs 33.115* and *33.116*).[2,6,39] Rarely, squamous features are extensive and these tumors resemble invasive squamous cell carcinoma on cursory examination (squamous variant of eccrine porocarcinoma).[40] However, areas of more obviously poromatous differentiation are invariably present.

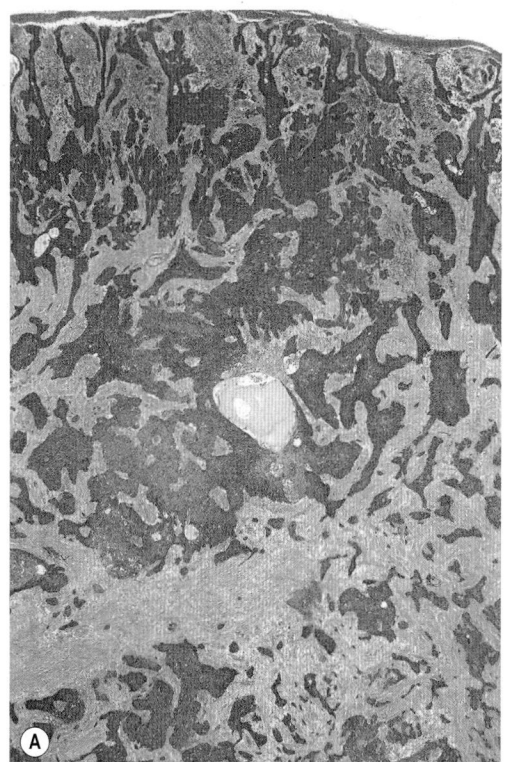

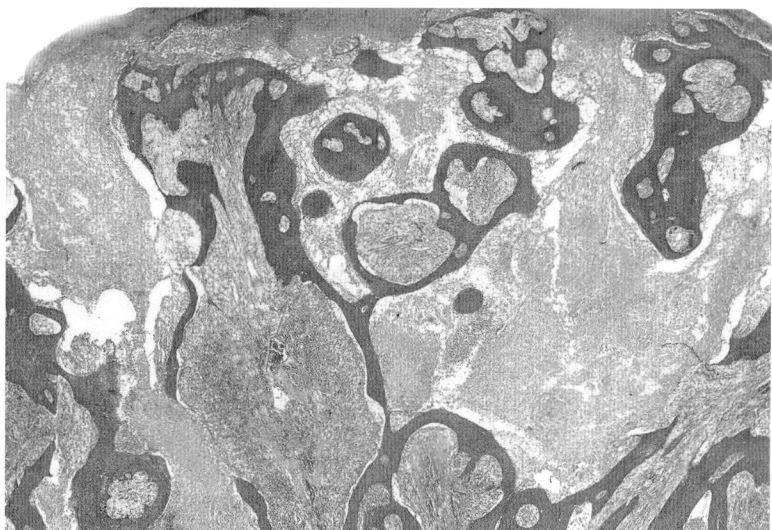

Fig. 33.105
Eccrine porocarcinoma: in this ulcerated example, the broad anastomosing trabeculae are well demonstrated. Note the necrosis.

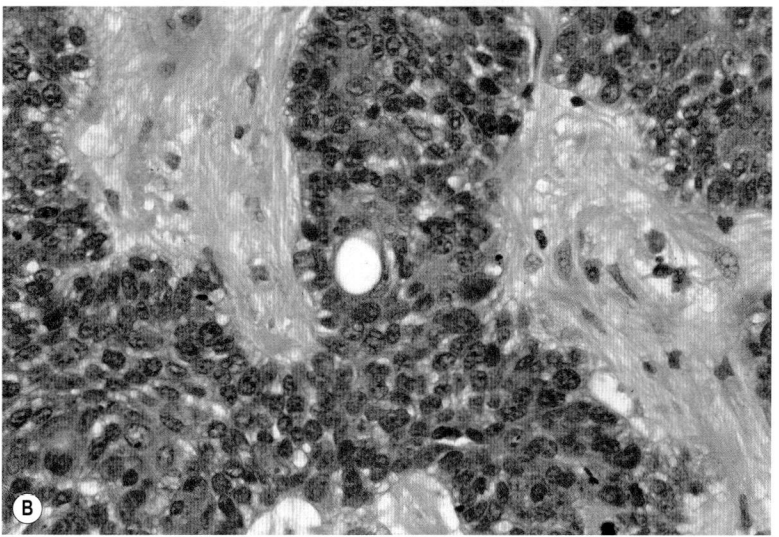

Fig. 33.104
Eccrine porocarcinoma (**A**, **B**): there is a very striking infiltrative growth pattern.

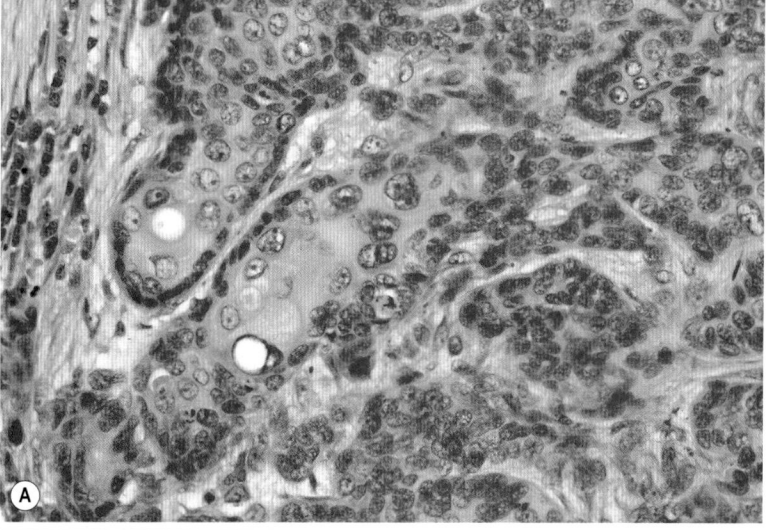

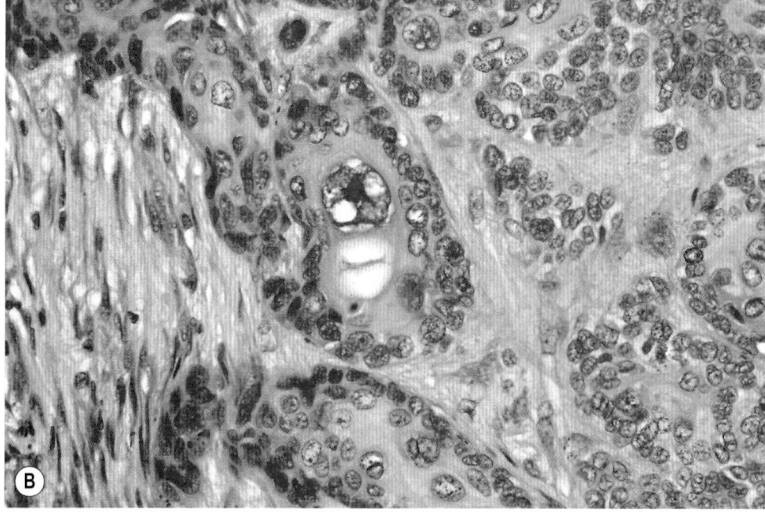

Fig. 33.106
(**A**, **B**) Eccrine porocarcinoma: the tumor cells have pleomorphic, vesicular nuclei. Note the intracytoplasmic lumina.

Colonization by melanocytes and pigmentation of tumor cell cytoplasm is sometimes a feature, particularly in the heavily pigmented races (pigmented porocarcinoma) (*Fig. 33.117*).[6,8,41,42] Other very rare variants, including giant cell, spindled cell, mucus cell, and metaplastic, porocarcinoma with Merkel cell carcinoma or sarcomatoid porocarcinoma, may be encountered (*Fig. 33.118*).[6,43–46] Exceptionally, porocarcinoma has been associated with syringoid eccrine carcinoma-like features, eccrine syringofibroadenoma-like foci, as well as areas resembling dermal ductular carcinoma.[6,43,47,48]

Cutaneous metastases show a propensity for epidermal, pagetoid involvement – epidermotropic eccrine carcinoma.[15,16]

The tumor cells express CK7, CK19, CAM 5.2, CD117, EMA, and CEA.[49,50] p53 protein has been shown to be overexpressed, but as this is also a feature of benign poromas, it would appear to be of no great significance.[22,51,52]

Prognostic indicators for eccrine porocarcinoma include mitotic activity, lymphovascular invasion, and tumor thickness.[6] Tumors with an infiltrating rather than pushing lower border are associated with a greater risk of recurrence.[6]

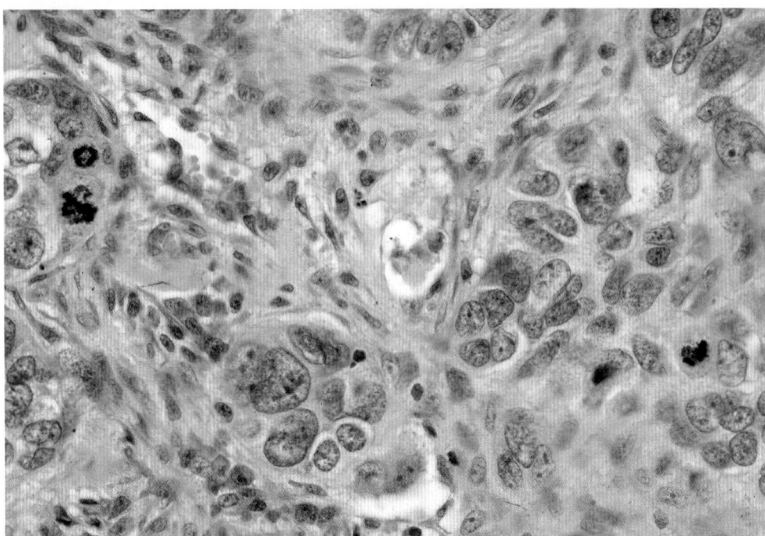

Fig. 33.107
Eccrine porocarcinoma: conspicuous mitoses are present.

Differential diagnosis

Malignant eccrine poroma may be distinguished from an infiltrating basal cell carcinoma by the presence of intercellular bridges and the absence of peripheral palisading. Ductal differentiation, intracytoplasmic lumina, and the small size of the tumor cells differentiate it from invasive squamous cell carcinoma with which it is frequently confused.

Syringoma

Clinical features

Syringomas are common tumors and present most often as multiple, symmetrically distributed, usually asymptomatic, small papules (1–3 mm) on the lower eyelids and upper cheeks (Fig. 33.119).[1,2] They appear at puberty or in early adult life and show a marked female predominance. Individual papules are firm and skin colored or slightly yellow (Fig. 33.120). Syringomas may, however, manifest a wide variety of clinical presentations. They may occur singly or in multiples on the scalp, forehead, neck, axillae, chest, abdomen, buttocks, extremities, or genitalia (male and female), periorally, or rarely, in a linear nevoid unilateral, segmental, or plaquelike pattern.[1,3,4–26]

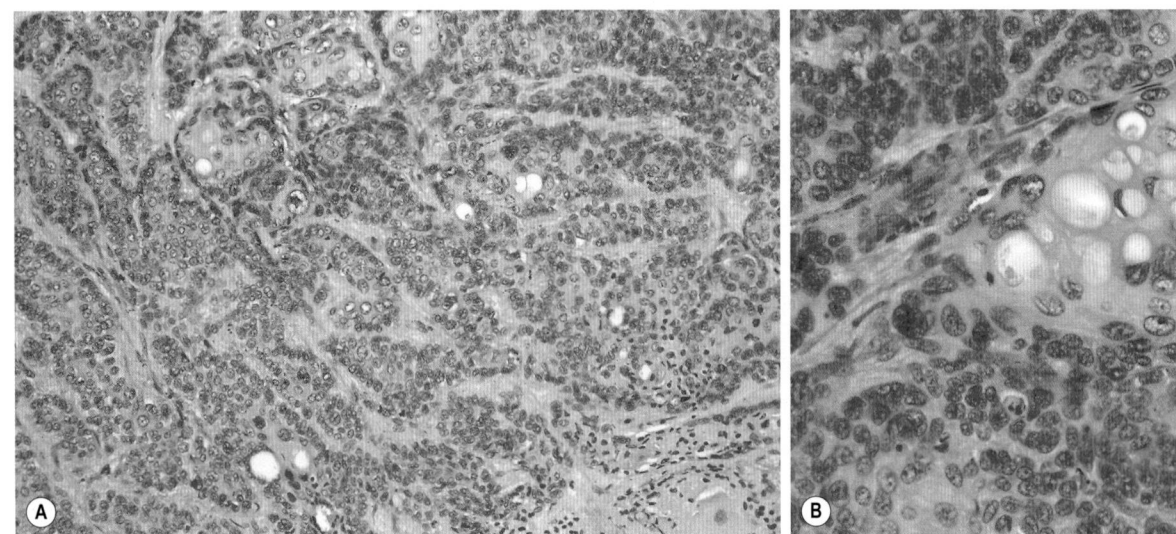

Fig. 33.108
(A, B) Eccrine porocarcinoma: ductal differentiation is an essential diagnostic feature.

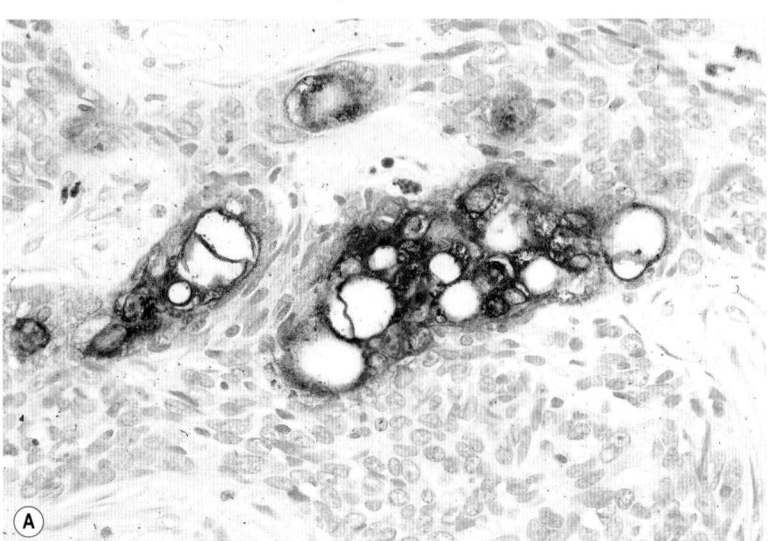

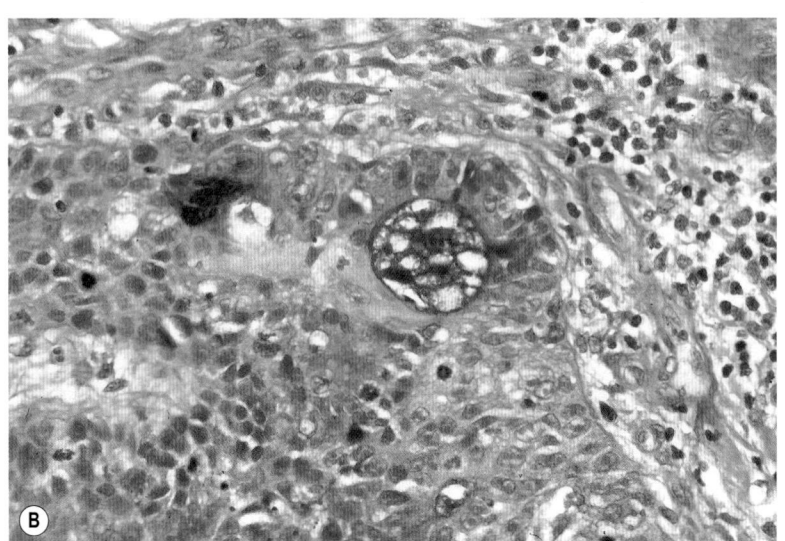

Fig. 33.109
Eccrine porocarcinoma: (A) ductal differentiation and intracytoplasmic lumina can be highlighted with EMA or CEA immunohistochemistry (EMA); (B) the luminal border of the duct is diastase resistant, PAS positive.

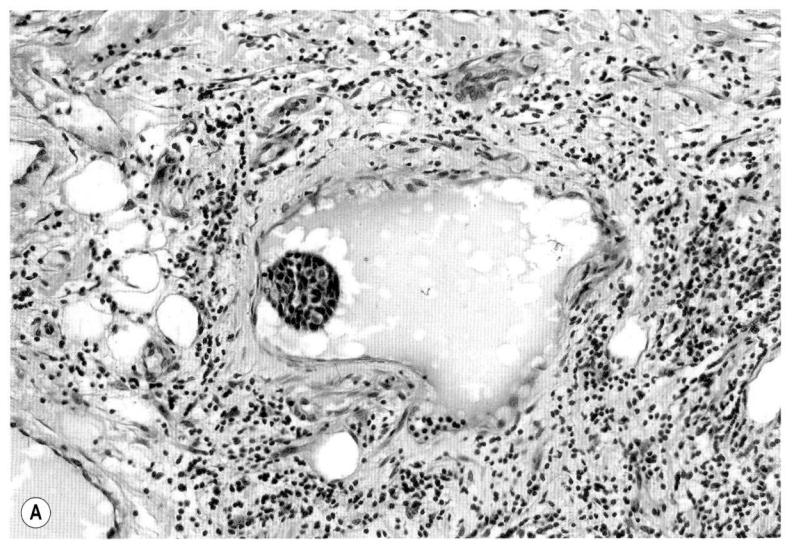

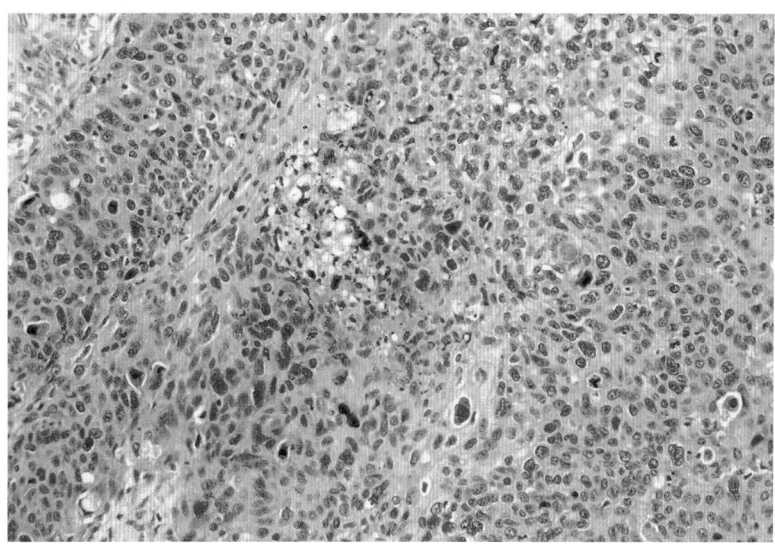

Fig. 33.112
Eccrine porocarcinoma: high-grade tumors commonly show areas of necrosis.

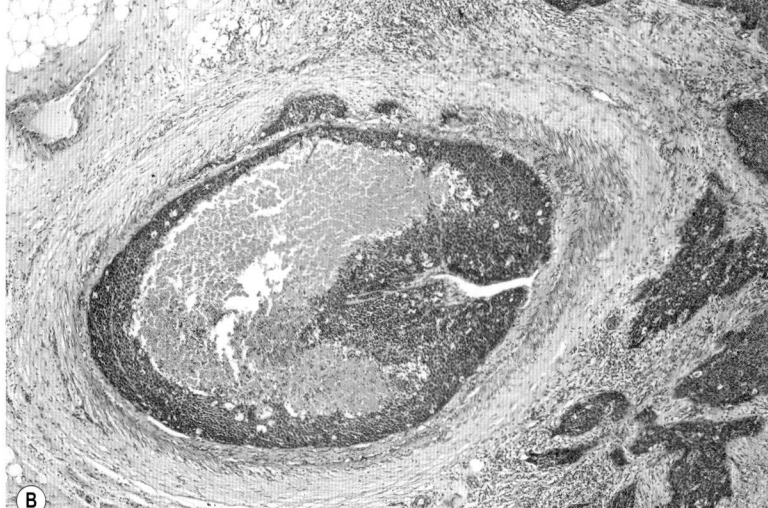

Fig. 33.110
(A, B) Eccrine porocarcinoma: lymphovascular invasion.

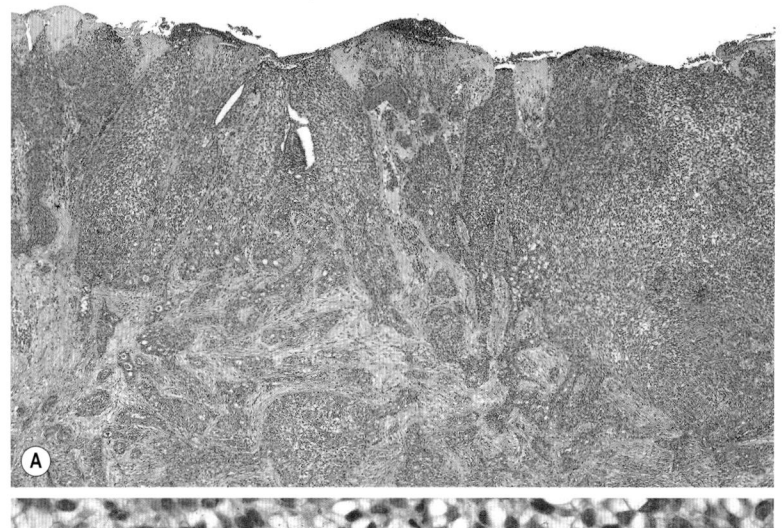

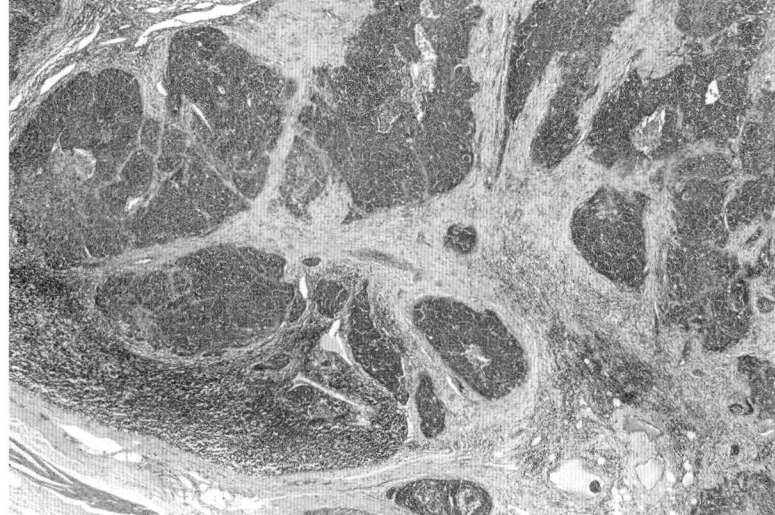

Fig. 33.111
Eccrine porocarcinoma: lymph node metastasis from the same patient as shown in Fig. 33.108B.

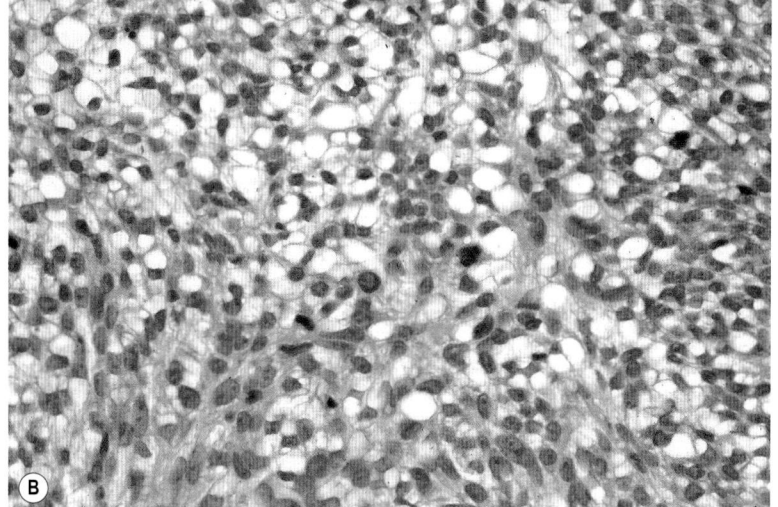

Fig. 33.113
Clear cell eccrine porocarcinoma: (A) there is striking cytoplasmic vacuolation; (B) high-power view.

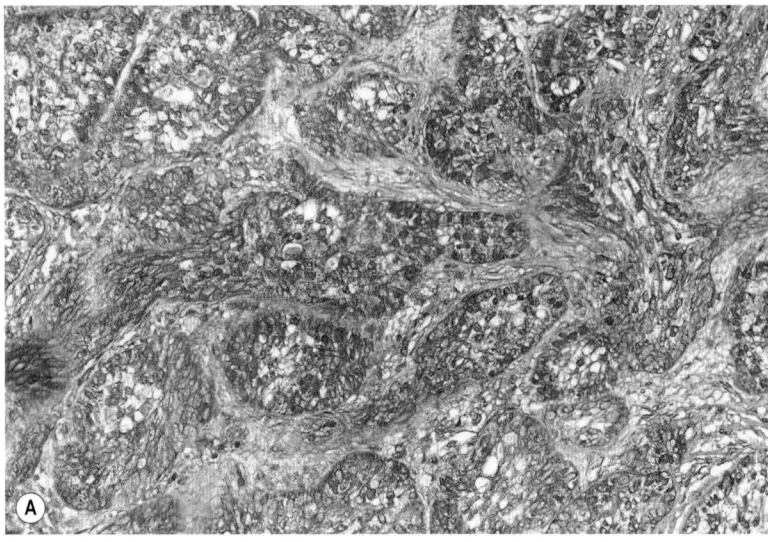

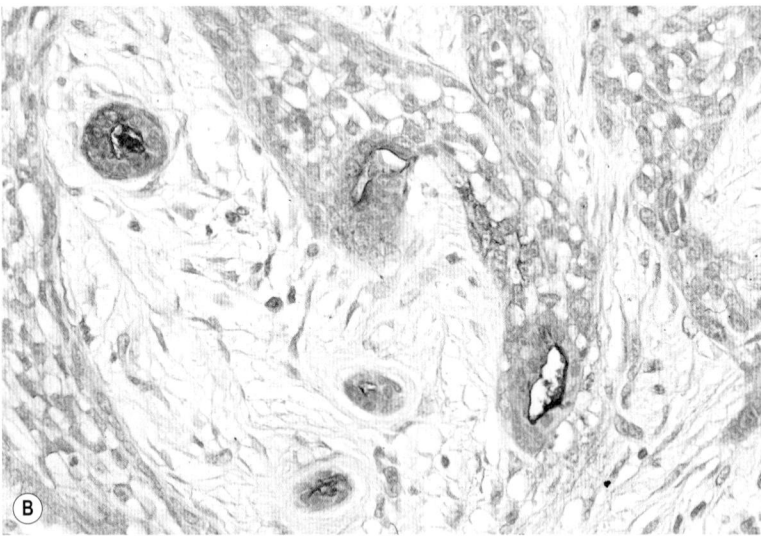

Fig. 33.114
Clear cell eccrine porocarcinoma: (**A**) the tumor cells are PAS positive; (**B**) EMA.

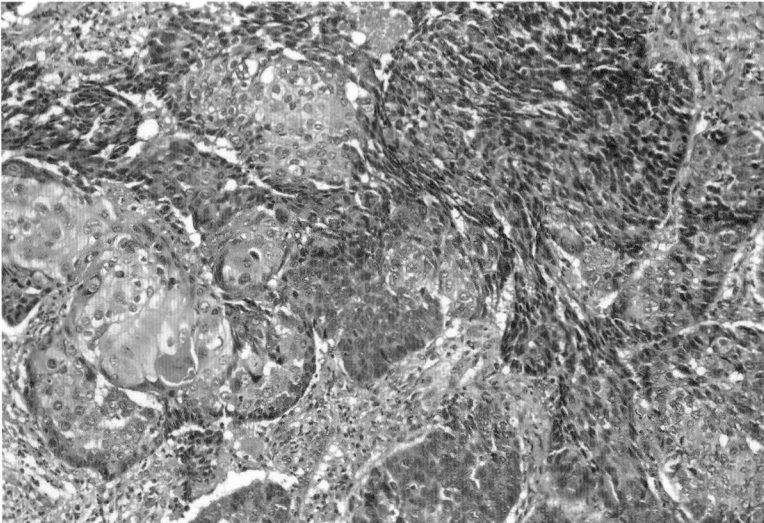

Fig. 33.115
Eccrine porocarcinoma: this example shows striking squamous differentiation with focal dyskeratosis.

A giant variant measuring up to 1 cm has also been described, and presentation as milia is an unusual finding.[27–31] Patients with vulval syringomas often have coexisting eyelid lesions, and vulval pruritus is a frequent presenting symptom.[12]

An eruptive variant has been described in which successive crops of papules appear on the anterior surfaces of young people.[32,33] Characteristic sites of involvement include the neck, chest, axillae, antecubital fossae, upper extremities, lower abdomen, and groins.[32,34] Occasional familial examples have been recorded.[34–39] Eruptive syringomas are more common in Orientals and are present in 18% of mature patients with Down syndrome.[40–43] They may rarely be associated with milium cysts and vermiculate atrophoderma (Nicolau and Balus syndrome).[44]

Pathogenesis and histologic features

Histochemical and electron microscopic studies have shown that the syringoma represents an adenoma of the acrosyringium, the intraepidermal eccrine sweat duct.[45,46] Immunohistochemical studies further confirm differentiation of this tumor toward the acrosyringium or dermal eccrine duct.[47–51] The epithelium of a syringoma therefore contains succinic dehydrogenase, phosphorylase, and leucine aminopeptidase.

The tumor is composed of interconnecting epithelial strands and ducts dispersed in a fibrous stroma within the upper dermis (*Fig. 33.121*). The ducts are lined by two layers of flattened cuboidal cells. There may be a cuticle lining the lumina, which frequently contains eosinophilic granular debris. Sometimes the ducts are associated with an epithelial strand, giving rise to the characteristic tadpole configuration (*Figs 33.122* and *33.123*). Occasionally, single glycogen-rich ductal cells are seen, and rarely all of the ductal cells contain glycogen, giving rise to the clear cell variant of syringoma. This appears to be particularly associated with diabetes mellitus.[52,53]

The milium-like variant of syringoma is characterized histologically by large epithelial-lined cysts containing keratinaceous material and located within superficial dermis.[28] The features are otherwise characteristic of syringoma, and the keratin-filled cysts are immunoreactive against CEA.

Differential diagnosis

Syringoma must be distinguished from desmoplastic trichoepithelioma, which typically features numerous keratocysts. Although there is obvious histologic overlap with eccrine epithelioma, the clinical features are quite different.[2] Eccrine epithelioma, which is a much more extensive tumor that may involve the subcutaneous fat, is associated with a markedly desmoplastic stroma. Syringoma-like features are not usually extensive and infiltration of the perineural space is often observed. Mitoses are not a feature of syringoma. Distinction from microcystic adnexal carcinoma may be impossible in small biopsies, and clinicopathological correlation is therefore crucial.

Papillary eccrine adenoma

Clinical features

Papillary eccrine adenoma is a rare tumor that predominantly involves the extremities.[1–12] It particularly affects blacks and shows a marked predilection for females (4:1).[1,6] The age at presentation is wide and children are occasionally affected.[1] The tumor presents as an erythematous, yellow or brown nodule measuring 0.5–4.0 cm in diameter.[1,6] Rarely, presentation as a cutaneous horn has been reported.[13] Most tumors are slow growing and are usually asymptomatic. The lesion is entirely benign, recurrences being extremely rare.[1]

Pathogenesis and histologic features

The tumor, which is most often situated in the mid and lower dermis, is well circumscribed although unencapsulated, and is composed of dilated branching ducts and cysts, which are usually dispersed in a dense, sometimes hyalinized, concentrically orientated stroma (*Fig. 33.124*).[8] The epithelial lining consists of two or more layers of small eosinophilic cells with regular, round, or oval nuclei containing small nucleoli (*Fig. 33.125*).[1] Papillary projections are frequent, and occasionally a delicate cribriform pattern is evident. Foci

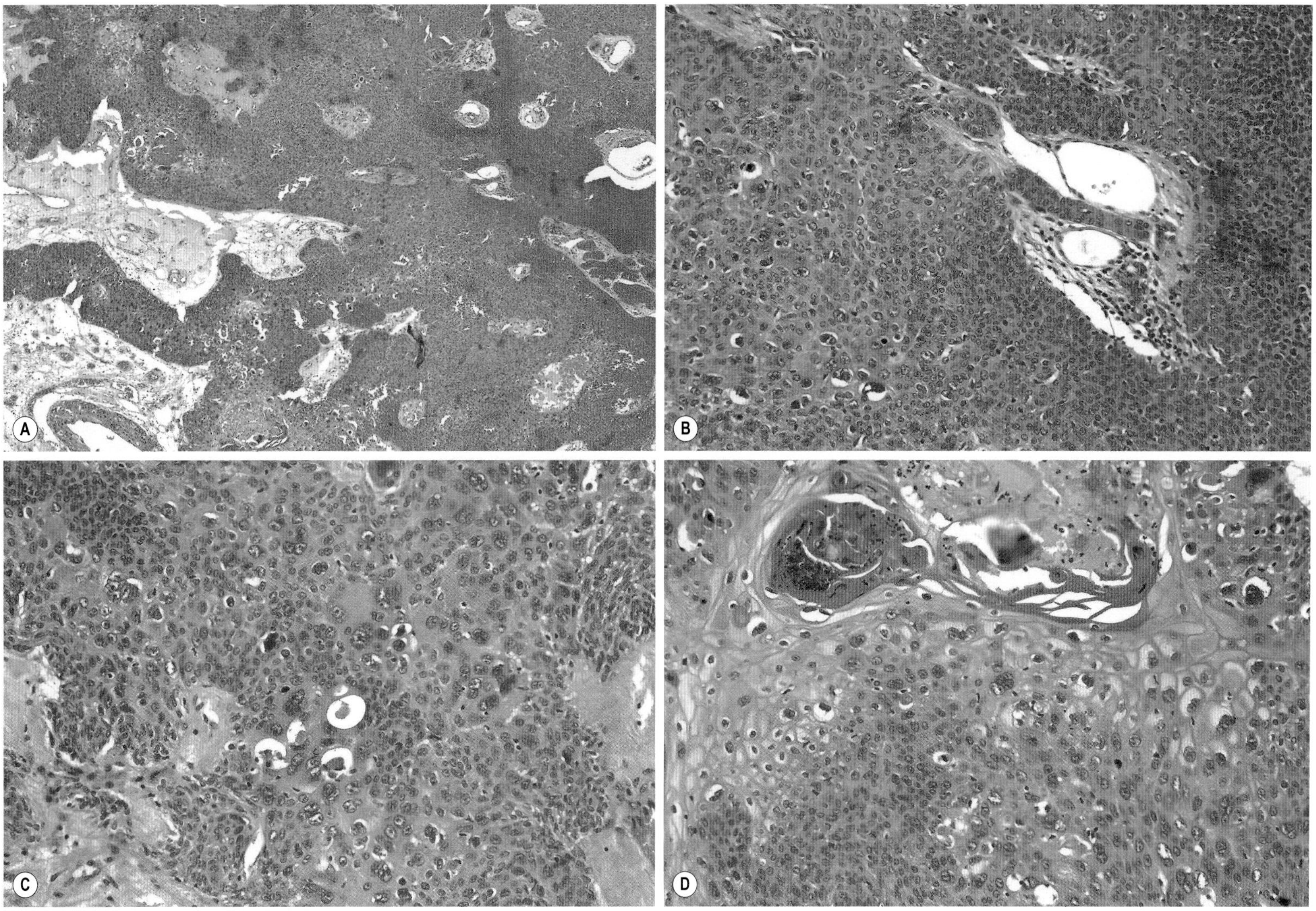

Fig. 33.116
Bowenoid porocarcinoma: (**A**) low-power view showing obvious poromatous features; (**B**) junction between the bowenoid and poromatous areas; (**C**) this field comes from near to the surface and there is squamous differentiation; (**D**) high-power view near to surface showing marked keratinization. It is very easy to misdiagnose this variant as squamous cell carcinoma.

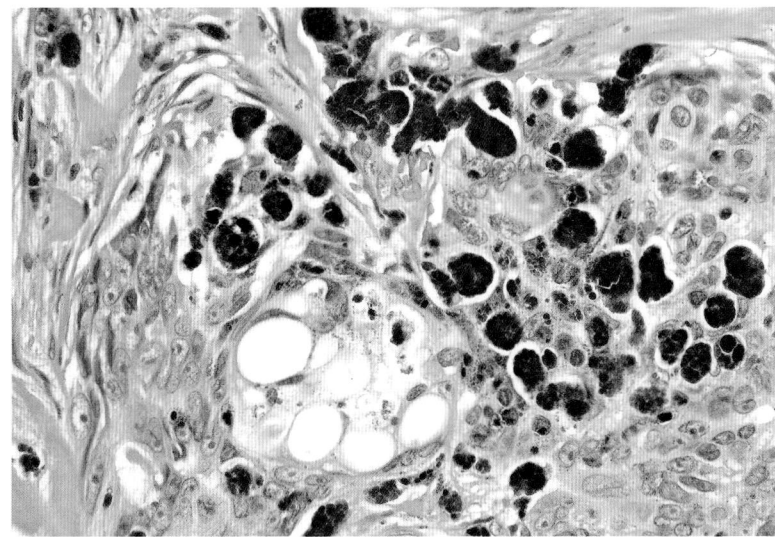

Fig. 33.117
Eccrine porocarcinoma: pigmented variants due to melanocyte colonization are common in colored races. By courtesy of W. Grayson, MD, University of Witwatersrand, University of Johannesburg, South Africa.

of clear cell change due to cytoplasmic glycogen are sometimes present.[8] The lumen contains diastase-resistant, PAS- and Alcian blue-positive material. Decapitation secretion, by definition, is absent. Nuclear pleomorphism is not a feature and mitoses are either absent or scanty (*Fig. 33.126*). Abnormal forms are not seen. Necrosis and perineural infiltration are not present. The tumor may be associated with a lymphocyte and plasma cell infiltrate, sometimes accompanied by lymphoid follicles.[1,8]

Immunohistochemically, the epithelium displays keratin (CK8 and CK14), EMA, and CEA expression.[5–7,12,14–18] S100 protein and SMA are also sometimes present.[5,6,12,14,16,18] Expression of IKH-4, a marker of eccrine glandular differentiation, is also found.[19] Histochemical studies have confirmed the presence of amylophosphorylase, and ultrastructural studies also suggest ductal differentiation.[9,10]

Differential diagnosis

Papillary eccrine adenoma must be distinguished from aggressive digital papillary adenocarcinoma.[20] The latter typically has a more infiltrative growth pattern and shows nuclear and cytoplasmic pleomorphism with conspicuous mitotic figures. Distinction from tubular apocrine adenoma is based on the presence of decapitation secretion and absence of papillary projections in the latter. However, both tumors overlap and it is likely that they are part of a spectrum.

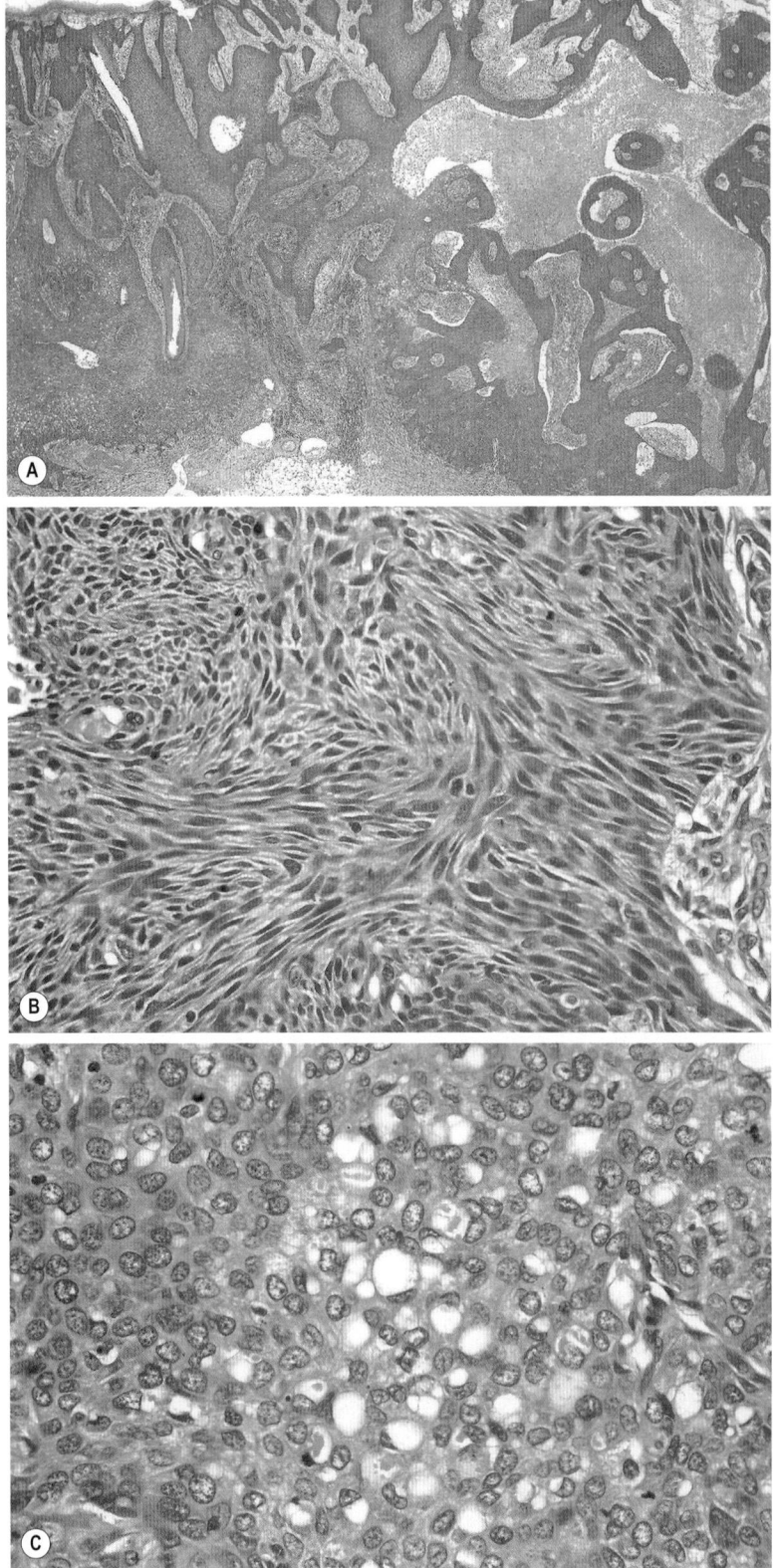

Fig. 33.118
Eccrine porocarcinoma: (**A**) low-power view of a spindle cell variant. There is extensive tumor necrosis. (**B**) High-power view of spindled cells; (**C**) the tumor shows striking ductal differentiation on the right side of the field.

Digital papillary adenocarcinoma

Clinical features

Digital papillary adenocarcinoma, formerly known as 'aggressive digital papillary adenocarcinoma', is a rare neoplasm with a wide morphological spectrum. The tumors were originally divided into adenoma and

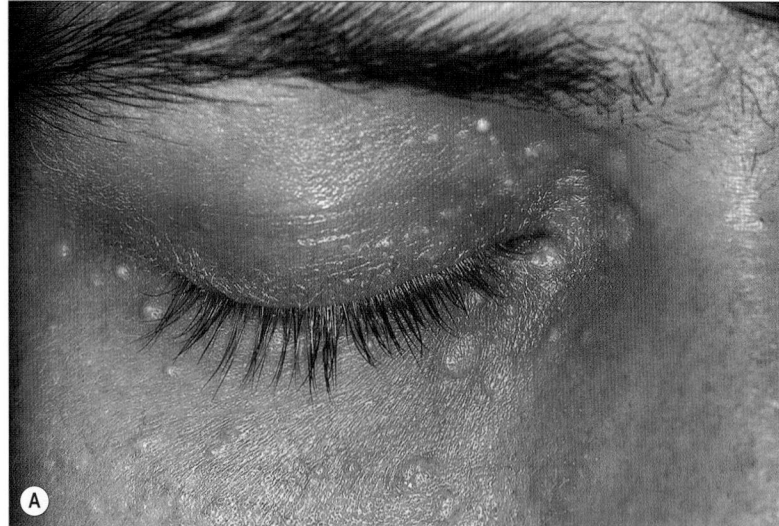

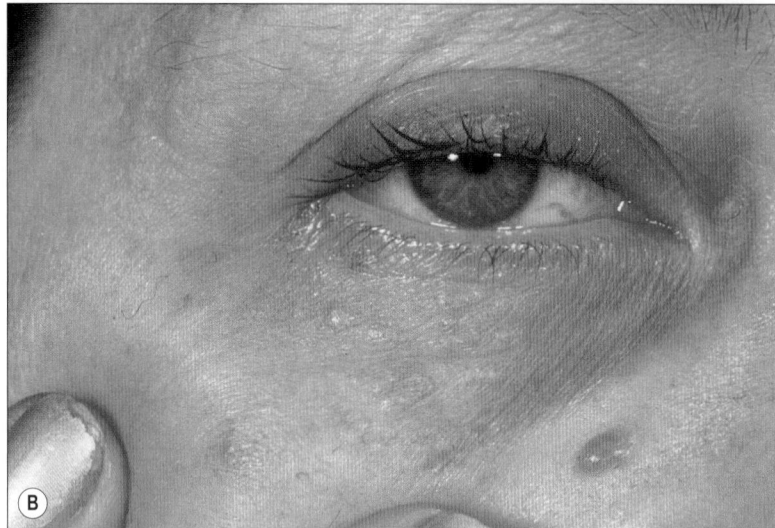

Fig. 33.119
(**A**, **B**) Syringoma: note the typical periorbital distribution of these small papules. (**A**) By courtesy of R.A. Marsden, MD, St George's Hospital, London, UK; (**B**) by courtesy of the Institute of Dermatology, London, UK.

adenocarcinoma.[1,2] It has now become apparent that the histologic features are not predictive of outcome and all tumors are regarded as potentially malignant.[3–5] The currently preferred terminology is cutaneous digital papillary adenocarcinoma.[5–7] The tumors affect the distal extremities, particularly the fingers and toes and adjacent skin of palms and soles.[1,3–6,8–22] The single most common site is the volar aspect of the digit tip between the nail bed and distal interphalangeal joint.[1,3] Lesions present in the adult (median 52 years) as solitary, usually asymptomatic nodules, measuring from less than 1 cm to multiple cm in diameter with a median of 2 cm. Adolescents may also be affected.[5,18] There is a strong male predominance with a male/female ratio of 7:1.[1,5] The presenting symptom is a mass frequently accompanied by pain.[3] The overall local recurrence rate is roughly 30% but is significantly lower (5%) after adequate surgical treatment with re-excision or amputation.[3] Irrespective of treatment or the presence of local recurrence, the rate of distant metastasis is approximately 14% to 25%.[3,5] Metastatic disease most commonly affects the lung and lymph nodes. The disease course is often protracted with potential for distant metastasis to develop years after the initial presentation.[5] Death from disease has been documented, but the overall mortality rate is low.[1,3,5,7,23,24] Sentinel lymph node biopsy, in addition to local treatment, has been performed in rare instances, but its value has not been assessed in larger prospective trials as yet.[25,26]

Pathogenesis and histologic features

Digital papillary adenocarcinoma is of particular importance because it may be mistaken for apocrine hidrocystoma/cystadenoma or a metastasis of

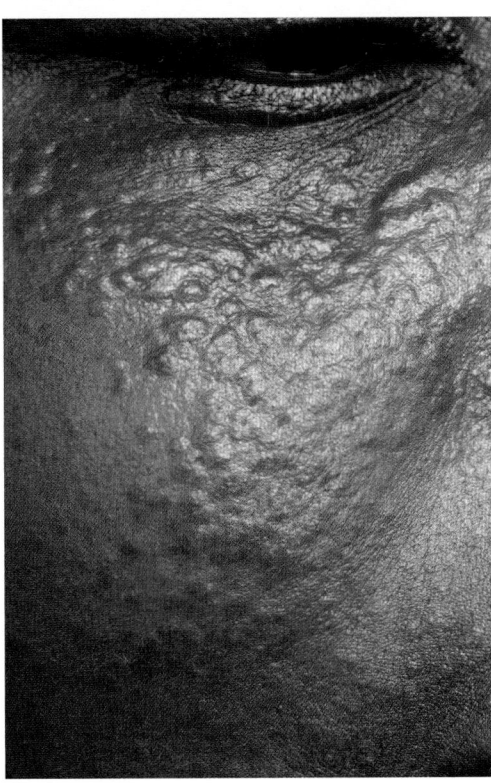

Fig. 33.120
Syringoma: there is extensive involvement of the cheek. From the collection of the late N.P. Smith, MD, Institute of Dermatology, London, UK.

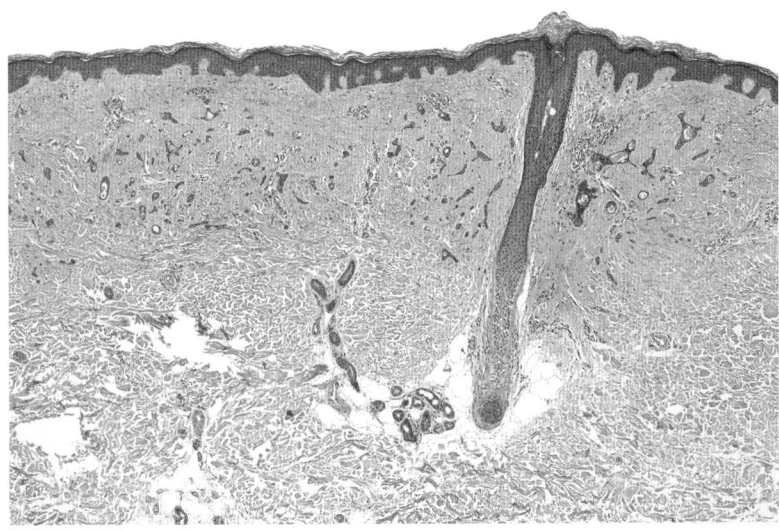

Fig. 33.121
Syringoma: characteristic epithelial strands and small cysts are present in the dermis. There is a dense, sclerotic fibrous stroma.

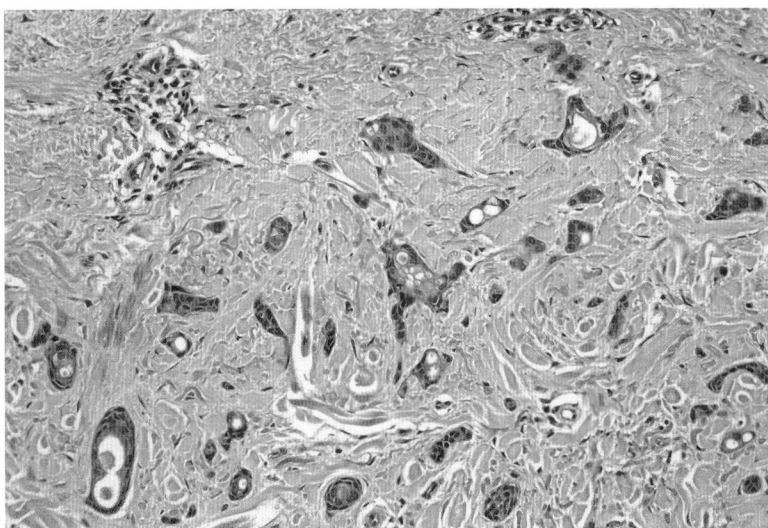

Fig. 33.122
Syringoma: note the epithelial strands and ductal differentiation.

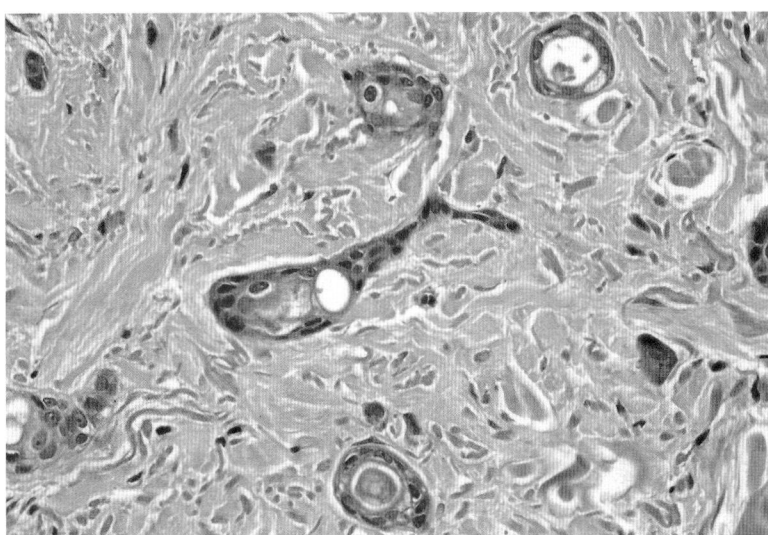

Fig. 33.123
Syringoma: this field shows the characteristic tadpole appearance.

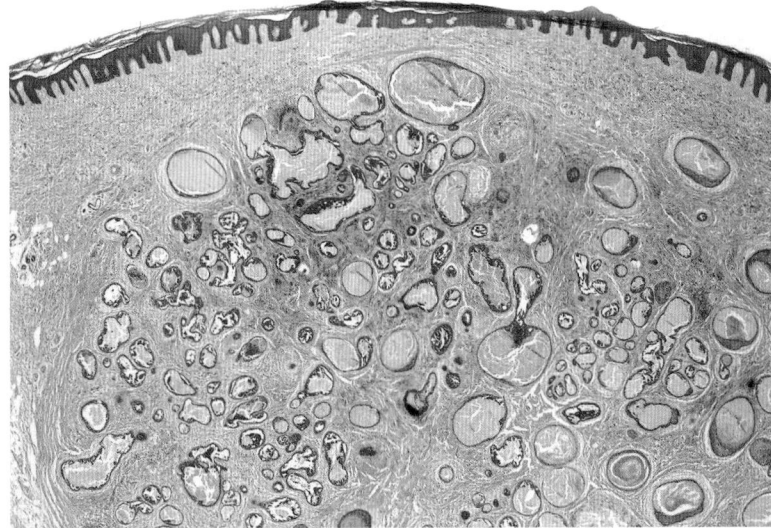

Fig. 33.124
Papillary eccrine adenoma: the lesion is composed of dilated ducts and cysts dispersed in a fibrous stroma.

papillary adenocarcinoma of mammary, thyroid, or colonic origin.[22] Knowledge of the entity combined with careful evaluation of histologic features and, when necessary, immunohistochemistry should, however, resolve the great majority of diagnostic dilemmas.

The tumor, which is located in the deeper dermis, often involves the subcutaneous fat and may infiltrate skeletal muscle, tendon, or bone. It is composed of multiple cystic epithelial nodules showing both glandular and papillary morphology separated by fairly dense fibrocollagenous stroma (*Figs 33.127* and *33.128*).[1,5] Tumors occasionally communicate with the overlying epidermis and may be predominantly solid.[3] The glands are lined by one or two layers of cuboidal or columnar epithelium with eosinophilic cytoplasm and round or oval vesicular nuclei. The papillary component is variable and ranges from simple epithelial strands through to

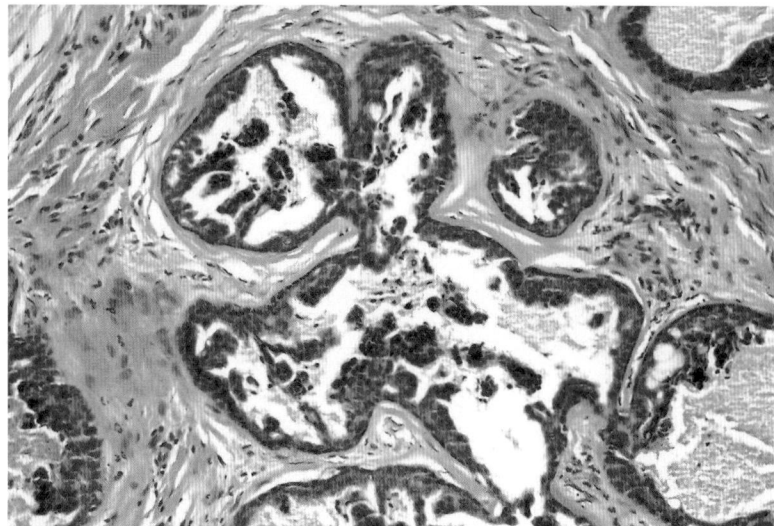

Fig. 33.125
Papillary eccrine adenoma: the cysts are lined by a double layer of uniform cuboidal cells. Tiny papillary processes are present.

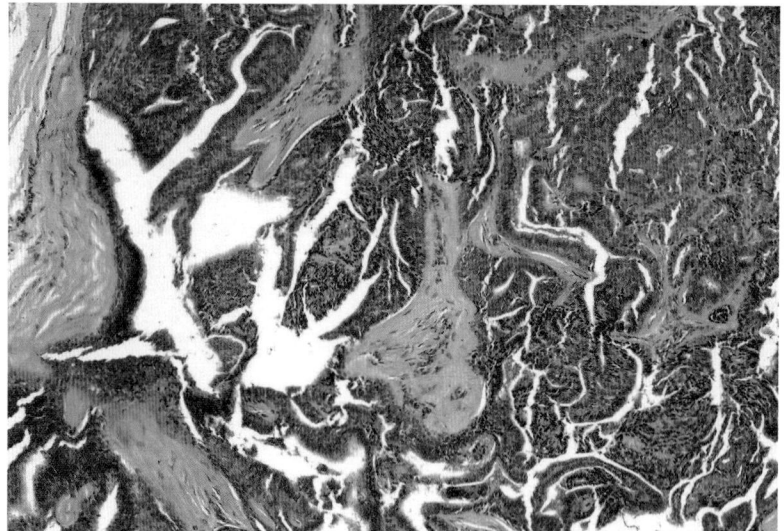

Fig. 33.128
Digital papillary adenocarcinoma: the papillae have a fibrovascular core.

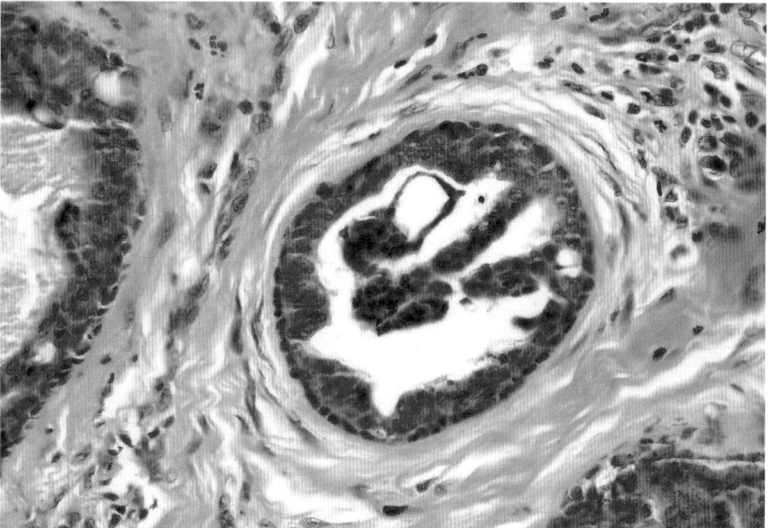

Fig. 33.126
Papillary eccrine adenoma: high-power view. There is no pleomorphism.

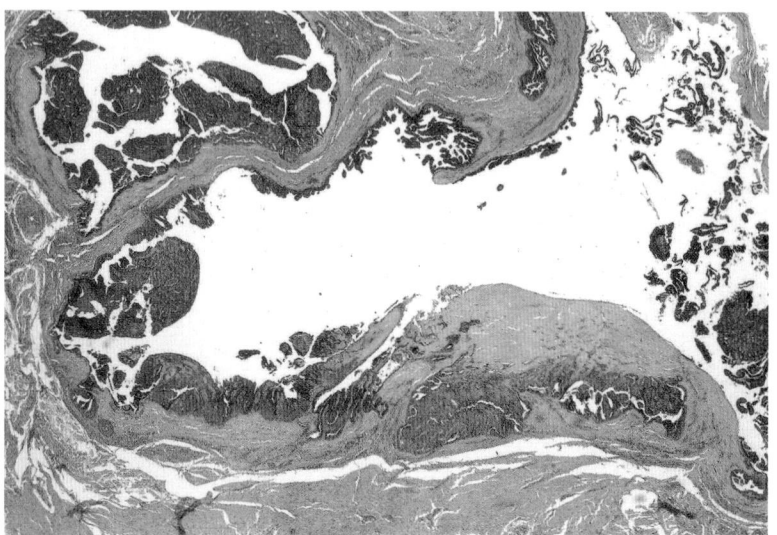

Fig. 33.127
Digital papillary adenocarcinoma: this example is partially cystic. Note the papillary processes covered by multiple layers of basophilic epithelium.

more structured elements composed of a connective tissue core covered by one or more layers of epithelium (Fig. 33.129). Squamous metaplasia, clear cell change, and spindled cell foci are commonly present.[1,3,5] Decapitation (apocrine-type) secretion is sometimes a feature.[3] Differentiation is variable, with some tumors showing more obvious nuclear pleomorphism, hyperchromatism, mitotic activity, and necrosis. Other findings include extensive and deep infiltration, and lymphovascular involvement.

Immunohistochemically, the epithelium shows strong keratin staining, and luminal differentiation is highlighted by CEA and EMA staining. A second myoepithelial component is demonstrated by S100 protein, SMA, calponin, and p63 immunohistochemistry.[5] Demonstration of a myoepithelial cell layer is particularly helpful in the exclusion of a metastatic papillary carcinoma from a visceral primary site. The differentiation from apocrine cystadenoma is difficult on morphology as there may be significant histologic and immunohistochemical overlap. It is important to remember that apocrine cystadenoma is distinctly rare on the digits and that most reported cases represent innocuous appearing examples of cutaneous digital papillary adenocarcinoma.[22]

Only little is known of the underlying genetics of these tumors. A recent screen for oncogenic mutations in 50 genes revealed a BRAF-V600E mutation in one of nine tumors only.[27]

Hidradenoma

Clinical features

Hidradenoma (clear cell hidradenoma, solid–cystic hidradenoma, clear cell myoepithelioma, eccrine acrospiroma), which generally occurs on the head and neck or limbs (although any site may be affected), usually presents as a solitary, slowly growing, solid, or cystic nodule (Fig. 33.130).[1–6] The overlying skin may be flesh colored, erythematous, or blue.[1] Lesions typically measure about 1–2 cm in diameter and present most often in middle-aged adults or the elderly (range 3–93 years), with a slight predominance in females.[6] Giant variants measuring up to 12.0 cm in diameter have been documented.[7,8] Exceptionally, children are affected.[9–11] The tumors are sometimes symptomatic, with spontaneous oozing, hemorrhage, tenderness, pruritus, and burning.[1] Recurrences are uncommon.[3]

Pathogenesis and histologic features

The histogenesis of this tumor is uncertain. In keeping with an eccrine derivation, the tumor has been shown to contain large quantities of succinic dehydrogenase, amylophosphorylase, and leucine aminopeptidase.[2] Additionally, earlier reports showed that clear cell hidradenoma did not express markers of apocrine differentiation including GCDPF-15 and GCDFP-24.[12,13]

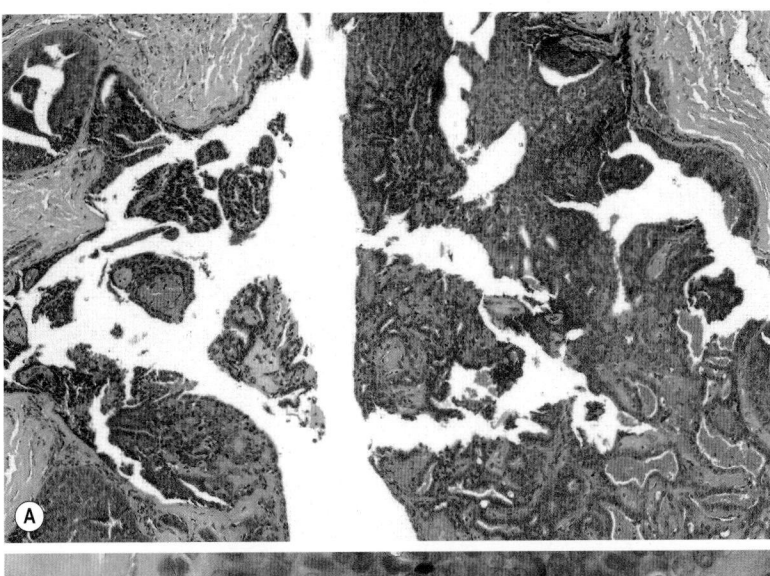

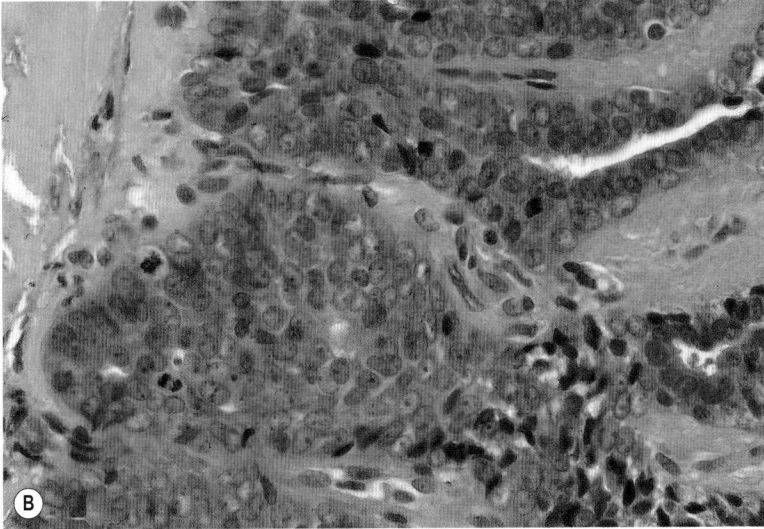

Fig. 33.129
Digital papillary adenocarcinoma: (**A**) medium-power view showing papillary processes; (**B**) there are prominent nucleoli and multiple mitoses are present.

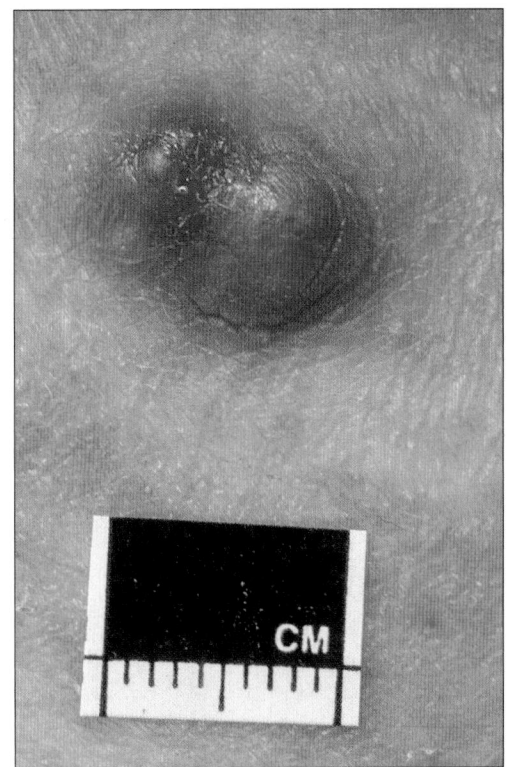

Fig. 33.130
Eccrine hidradenoma: this lesion presents as a solitary nodule most often on the head and neck or limbs. By courtesy of the Institute of Dermatology, London, UK.

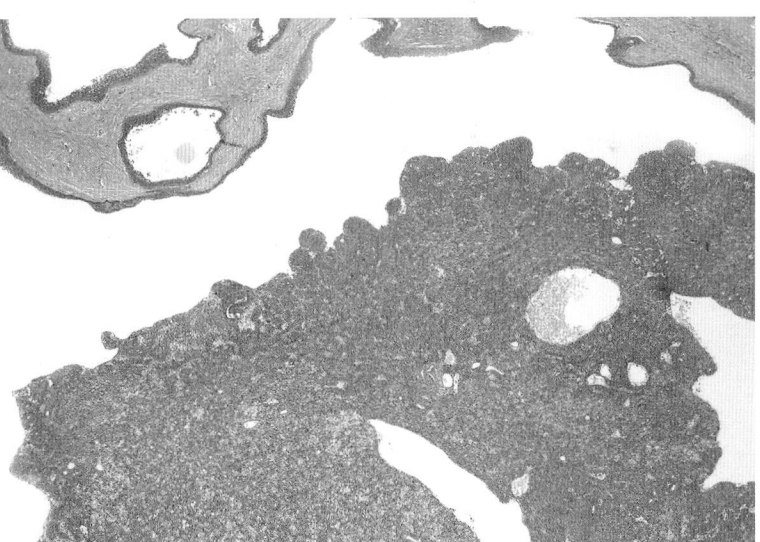

Fig. 33.131
Eccrine hidradenoma: this example shows multiple, variably sized cysts in addition to a solid component (solid-cystic hidradenoma).

However, this has been contested and a small series of cases was published in which GCDPF-15 was expressed.[14] On the basis of follicular continuity, decapitation secretion, mucin production, and the latter immunohistochemical finding, it has been proposed that clear cell variants are of apocrine derivation whereas only a minority of tumors composed of poroid and cuticular cells are of true eccrine derivation/differentiation (poroid hidradenoma).[5,14] A reproducible chromosomal translocation t(11;19)(q21;p13) involving the CRTC1 and the MAML2 genes has been reported in salivary gland tumors such as mucoepidermoid carcinoma and Warthin tumor and has also been detected in approximately 50% of hidradenomas.[15–18] This fusion appears to be particularly prevalent in tumors with clear cell features.[18,19] At least a subset of the remaining tumors has been found to harbor the chromosomal translocation t(6;22) involving the EWS and the POU5F1 genes.[20]

The tumor is circumscribed, but unencapsulated, and is composed of lobulated, sometimes cystic masses of cells in the upper or mid-dermis (*Figs 33.131* and *33.132*). Some tumors are associated with follicular structures whereas others display connection to or even replace the overlying epidermis, reminiscent of eccrine poroma. On occasions, the tumor may extend into the subcutaneous fat. The tumor has a biphasic cellular population: in some areas, it is composed of round, fusiform, or polygonal cells with eosinophilic cytoplasm and a round or oval vesicular nucleus showing nuclear grooves and conspicuous nucleolus, sometimes arranged in whorls; elsewhere, it consists of cells with clear cytoplasm containing a small, dark, often eccentrically located nucleus (clear cell hidradenoma) (*Figs 33.133* and *33.134*).[1,2,4,21,22] Transition between the two cell types is common. The

proportions and overlap of the two cell types vary within an individual tumor. Glycogen may be demonstrated in most of the tumor cells, but is in greater abundance in the clear cell areas (*Fig. 33.135*). The tumors are usually mitotically inactive. Tumor lobules may be intimately associated with dermal sweat glands or ducts, and occasionally the latter may be seen to be continuous with islands of tumor cells.[1] As mentioned above, focal apocrine decapitation secretion can be seen. Some tumors may show squamous differentiation, squamous eddy formation, or keratinization.[22,23] Mucin-rich goblet cells are an occasional finding, and rarely mucinous change is extensive (mucinous hidradenoma) (*Fig. 33.136*).[24] Sebaceous differentiation may also be a feature.[14,25–27] Exceptionally, hidradenoma has been demonstrated in continuity with mucinous syringometaplasia.[28]

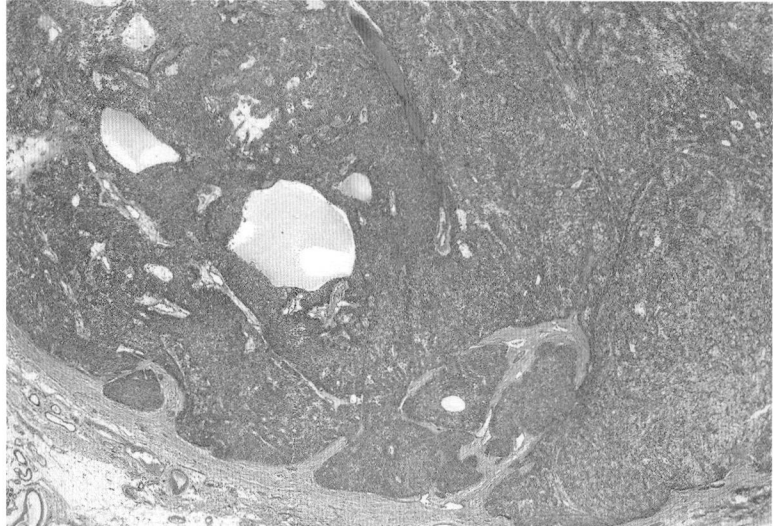

Fig. 33.132
Eccrine hidradenoma: low-power view of a circumscribed dermal tumor nodule.

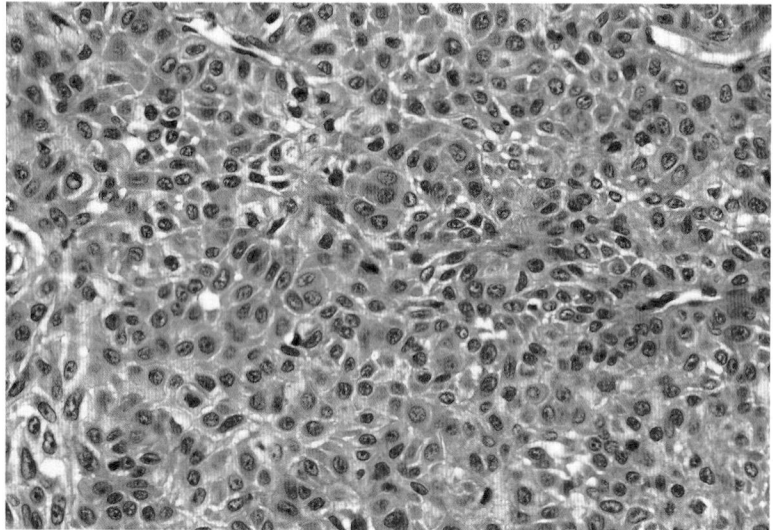

Fig. 33.133
Eccrine hidradenoma: high-power view showing uniform cells with eosinophilic cytoplasm.

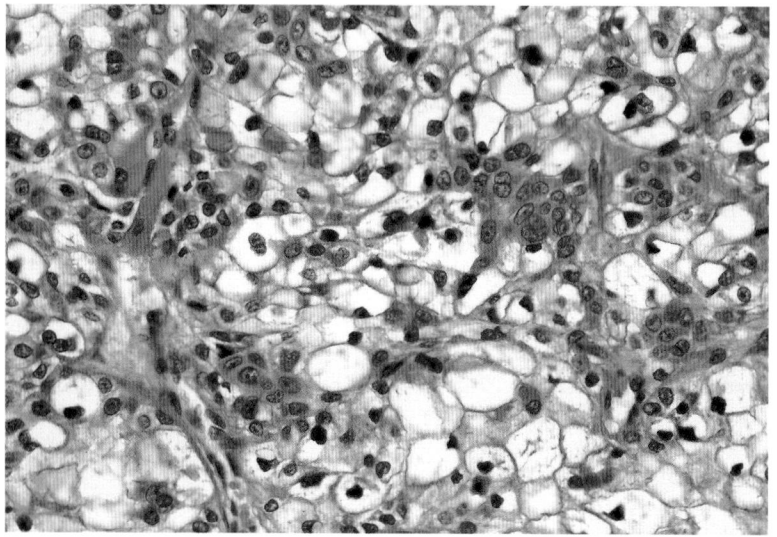

Fig. 33.134
Eccrine hidradenoma: in this field, the tumor consists of an admixture of cells with eosinophilic cytoplasm and glycogen-rich clear cell forms.

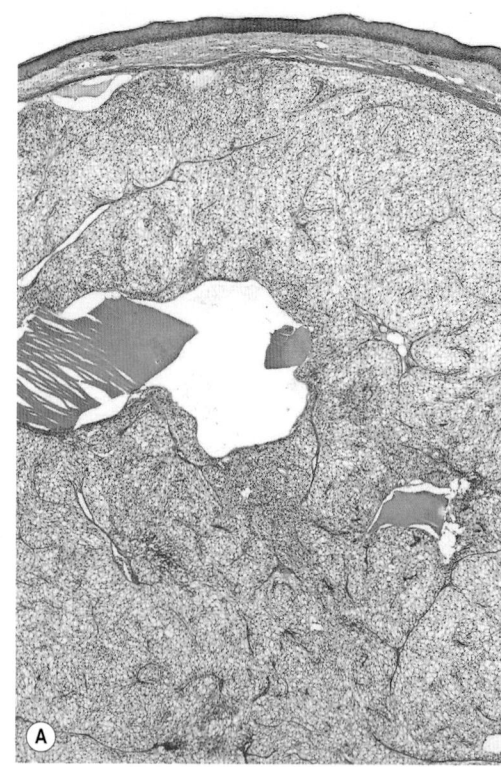

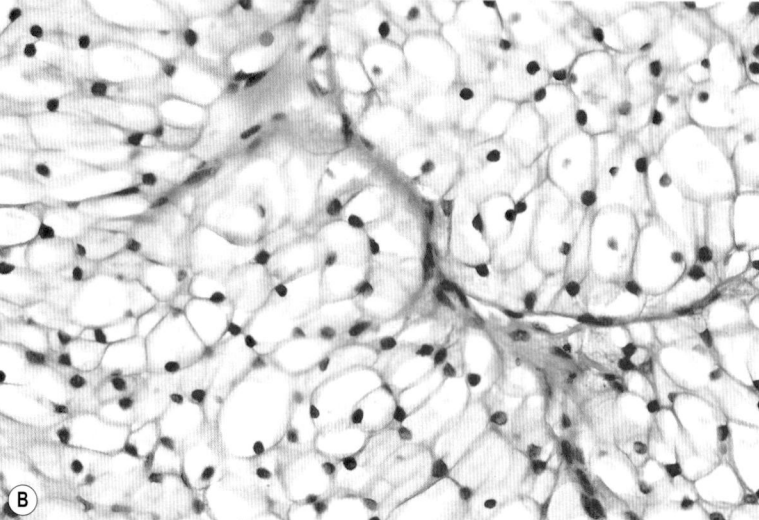

Fig. 33.135
(A, B) Eccrine hidradenoma: clear cell variant. The cells have clear cytoplasm and small hyperchromatic nuclei. The cytoplasm is PAS positive, diastase sensitive.

Ductlike structures are present in most tumors. These may appear as differentiated structures lined by a layer of cuboidal cells (Fig. 33.137). On other occasions, the tumor contains variably sized cystic cavities, sometimes comprising the vast bulk of the lesion (solid–cystic hidradenoma). Such cysts are lined by flattened cells and probably represent cystic degeneration. Ductal differentiation is also seen as foci of squamous cells surrounding irregular lumina complete with a diastase-resistant, PAS-positive cuticle resembling the acrosyringium (Fig. 33.138). The tumor lobules are surrounded by a definite stroma, which may be fibrovascular, collagenous, or even hyalinized (Fig. 33.139). Some tumors appear highly vascular, resulting in perivascular pseudorosettes and, occasionally, hemangiopericytoma-like areas. Occasionally, tumors may appear pigmented due to increased melanin pigment and colonization by pigmented dendritic cells.[29,30] Exceptional prominent intraneural growth has been reported in a case.[31] The tumor cells express AE1/AE3, EMA, and CEA.[12,15] The last two are of particular value in highlighting ductal differentiation.

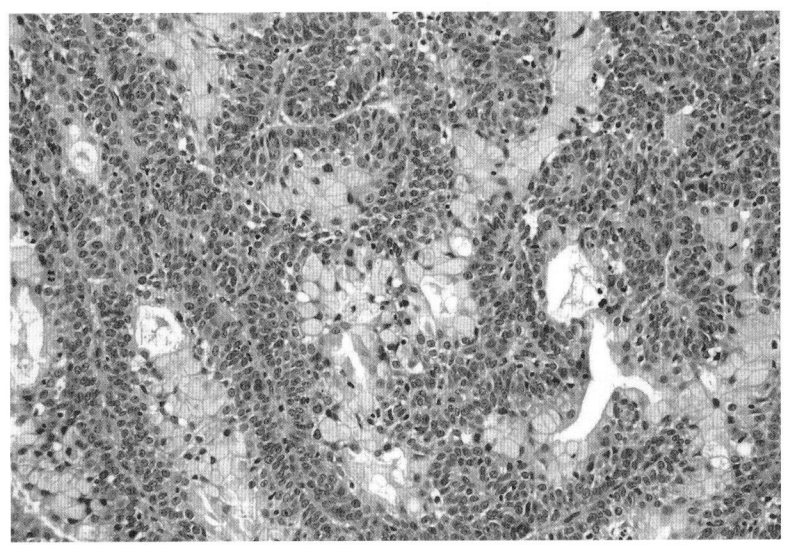

Fig. 33.136
Eccrine hidradenoma: in this field, there is mucinous metaplasia, which is an uncommon feature.

Comment

Occasionally, benign-appearing tumors show focal atypical features including nuclear pleomorphism and hyperchromatism, macronucleoli, giant cell forms, and prominent mitotic activity (two or more mitoses per 10 high-power fields) (*Figs 33.140* and *33.141*).[32] These appearances correlate with an increased risk of recurrence and possible malignant biological potential (atypical hidradenoma).[33] Wide re-excision and careful follow-up are therefore advisable for these worrisome lesions. In addition, high MIB-1 proliferative index (>11%) and phosphorylated histone H3 of >0.7% have been proposed to be associated with malignant rather than atypical hidradenoma.[34] Conversely, lymphovascular invasion and tumor deposits in locoregional lymph nodes have recently been reported in otherwise benign-appearing hidradenomas. With long-term follow-up, no adverse outcome was observed in these patients, and the findings likely represent the so-called benign metastasis. In practice, these findings should, however, be treated with caution and the tumors be regarded as atypical hidradenomas or as hidradenomas of uncertain malignant potential.[35,36]

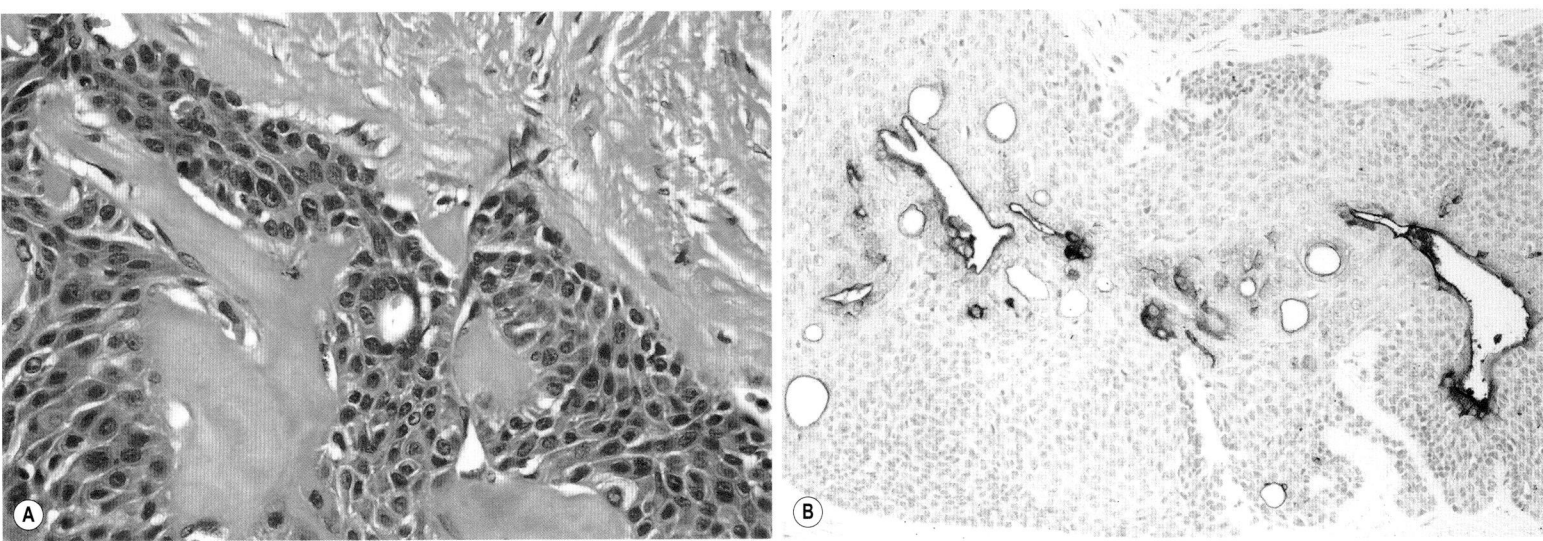

Fig. 33.137
Eccrine hidradenoma: (**A**) ductal differentiation as shown in this field is usually evident; (**B**) the ducts can be highlighted with EMA or CEA immunohistochemistry (EMA).

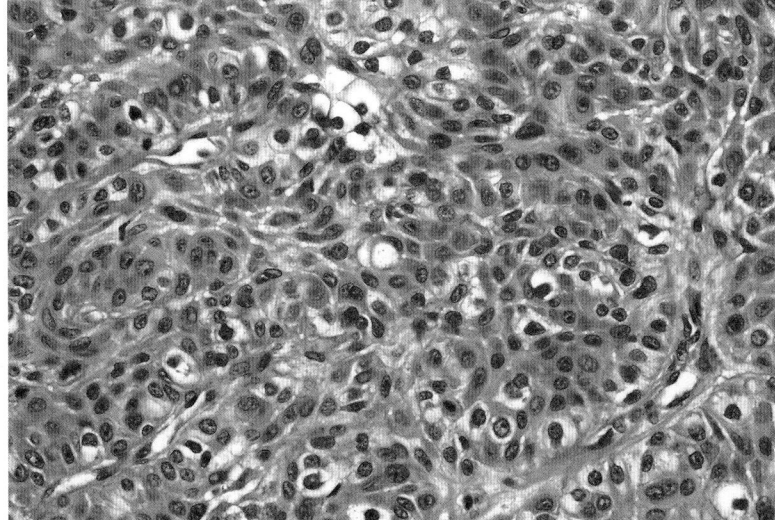

Fig. 33.138
Eccrine hidradenoma: note the intracytoplasmic lumen with eosinophilic cuticle.

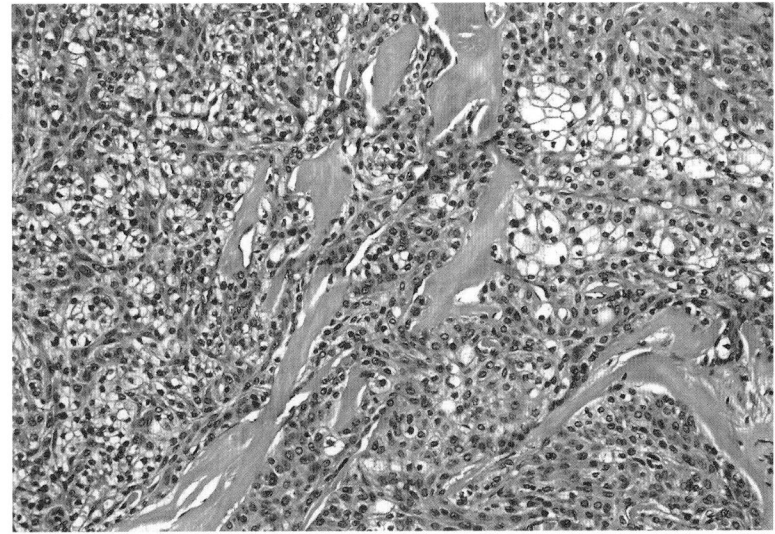

Fig. 33.139
Eccrine hidradenoma: in this field, the stroma is markedly hyalinized.

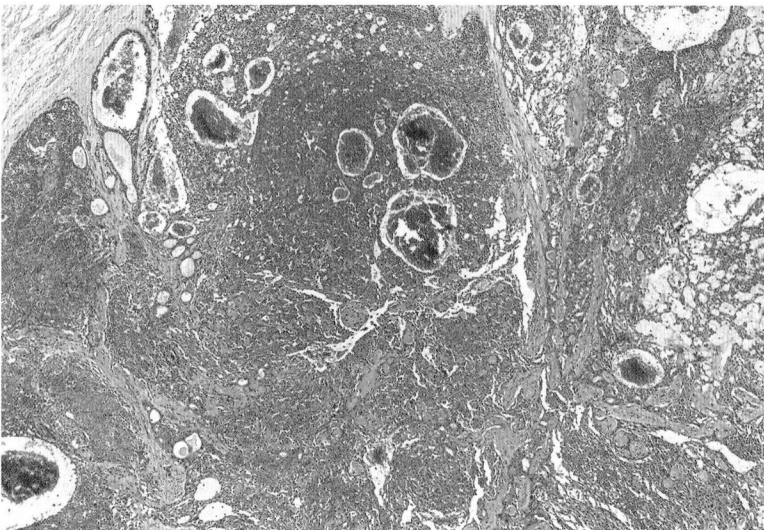

Fig. 33.140
Atypical eccrine hidradenoma: low-power view showing hemorrhage.

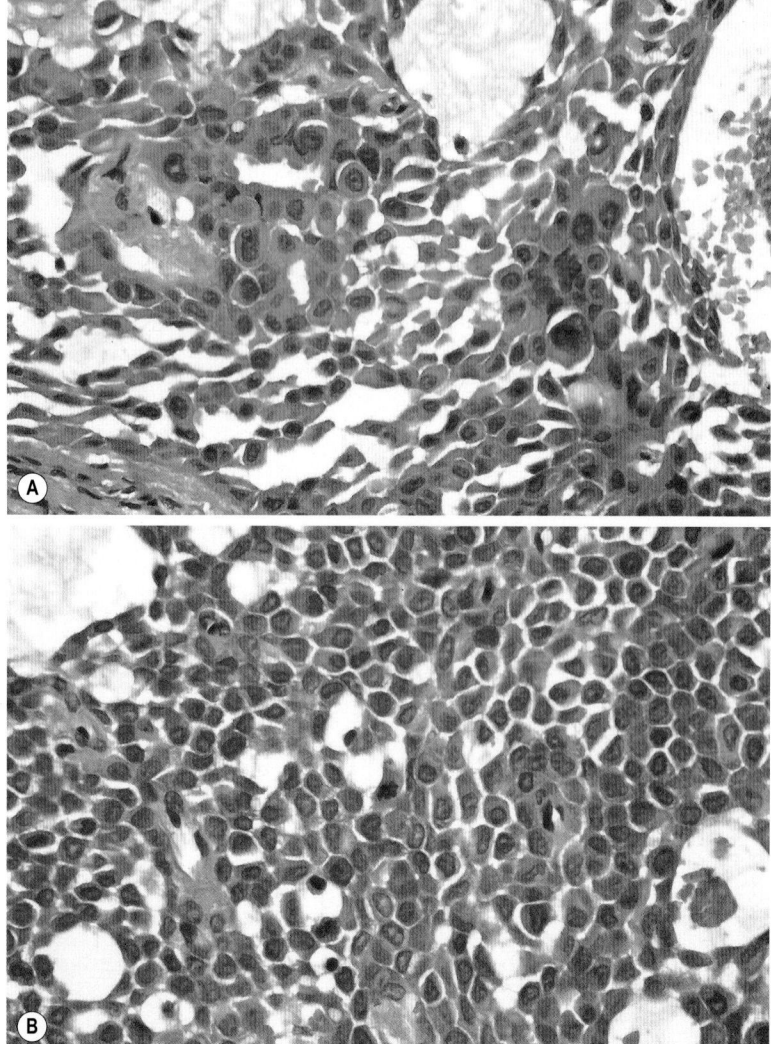

Fig. 33.141
Atypical eccrine hidradenoma. (**A**) Focal nuclear pleomorphism is present. There is hyperchromatism and nucleoli are prominent. (**B**) Mitotic figures are easily found. A complete excision with careful follow-up is advisable for patients with this borderline variant.

Clear cell hidradenocarcinoma

Clinical features

Clear cell hidradenocarcinoma (malignant acrospiroma, malignant nodular hidradenoma, malignant clear cell hidradenoma) is a rare neoplasm, with fewer than 100 cases documented in the literature. These have mainly represented single case reports, although there are a few small series.[1-30] Little clinical information is available other than that they present as intradermal nodular tumors said to have a predilection for the face and extremities.[2] The anatomic distribution is wide, and this tumor has been described at a very diverse range of sites including the scalp, lip, neck, chest wall, breast, back, leg, toe, and vulva. There is no gender predilection and the age range is wide, extending from childhood through to the elderly, with a predilection for middle aged to elderly adults.[30] Presentation at birth has also been documented.[4,19] These tumors appear to be generally aggressive with a high recurrence rate (50–75%). It is difficult to determine precise figures from the more recent literature, but in the few larger series both metastatic and mortality rates appear to be high.[12,28] The lymph nodes, lungs, and bones are the sites most commonly affected, and there may be a role for sentinel lymph node biopsy in addition to wide excision at time of diagnosis.[1,4,25,31]

Pathogenesis and histologic features

A pre-existing benign hidradenoma may be identified in a subset of tumors and, analogous to hidradenoma, the chromosomal translocation t(11;19) involving the CRTC1- and the MAML2 genes has also been found in hidradenocarcinoma, albeit less frequently (*Fig. 33.142*).[30] No data regarding the prevalence of the t(6;22) involving the EWS and the POU5F1 genes are available in hidradenocarcinoma as yet. Nuclear staining for p53 may be identified in a subset of tumors although a p53 mutation is only rarely detected in these tumors.[30]

Clear cell hidradenocarcinoma can be distinguished from eccrine porocarcinoma (in particular the clear cell variant) by an absence of epidermal origin or involvement. The tumor is composed most often of lobules of epithelium, although occasionally a diffuse growth pattern may be observed. A cystic variant may also be infrequently encountered (*Figs 33.143* and *33.144*). The epithelial cells, which show varying degrees of mitotic activity and nuclear pleomorphism, have characteristically vacuolated cytoplasm due to the presence of abundant glycogen (*Figs 33.145–33.147*). In some areas, cells with eosinophilic cytoplasm may also be evident. Occasionally, the tumor is composed predominantly of basaloid cells with little or no vacuolation and basal cell carcinoma may therefore enter the differential diagnosis. Nuclear peripheral palisading and retraction artifact, however, are not features of this neoplasm. Spindled cell differentiation, mucin-rich goblet cells, or signet ring cells are infrequently encountered.[32] Necrosis is variable but in some tumors it can be extensive or else it may present with comedo carcinoma-like features (*Figs 33.148* and *33.149*). It has been argued that at least some, if not all, of the cases reported as 'adnexal clear cell carcinoma with comedonecrosis' represent hidradenocarcinomas with extensive clear cell change and necrosis.[30,33] A case showing sarcomatoid/metaplastic features composed of pleomorphic spindled cells has also been reported.[30] Exceptionally, in situ carcinoma affecting adjacent sweat glands and pagetoid spread within the overlying epidermis have been described.[6,34]

A characteristic finding is the presence of intracytoplasmic ductal differentiation, sometimes showing a well-formed cuticular border; occasionally, well-formed ducts are also evident (*Fig. 33.150*). In case of doubt, the use of the diastase–PAS reaction and EMA or CEA immunohistochemistry are of value in highlighting these structures (*Fig. 33.151*).

Her-2/neu amplification as demonstrated by fluorescent in situ hybridization (FISH) is rare despite its relatively frequent expression immunohistochemically.[26,29,30]

Differential diagnosis

Clear cell hidradenocarcinoma can sometimes appear deceptively benign and yet be associated with metastatic disease. Clear cell hidradenoma may occasionally show mild focal cytological atypia and increased mitotic

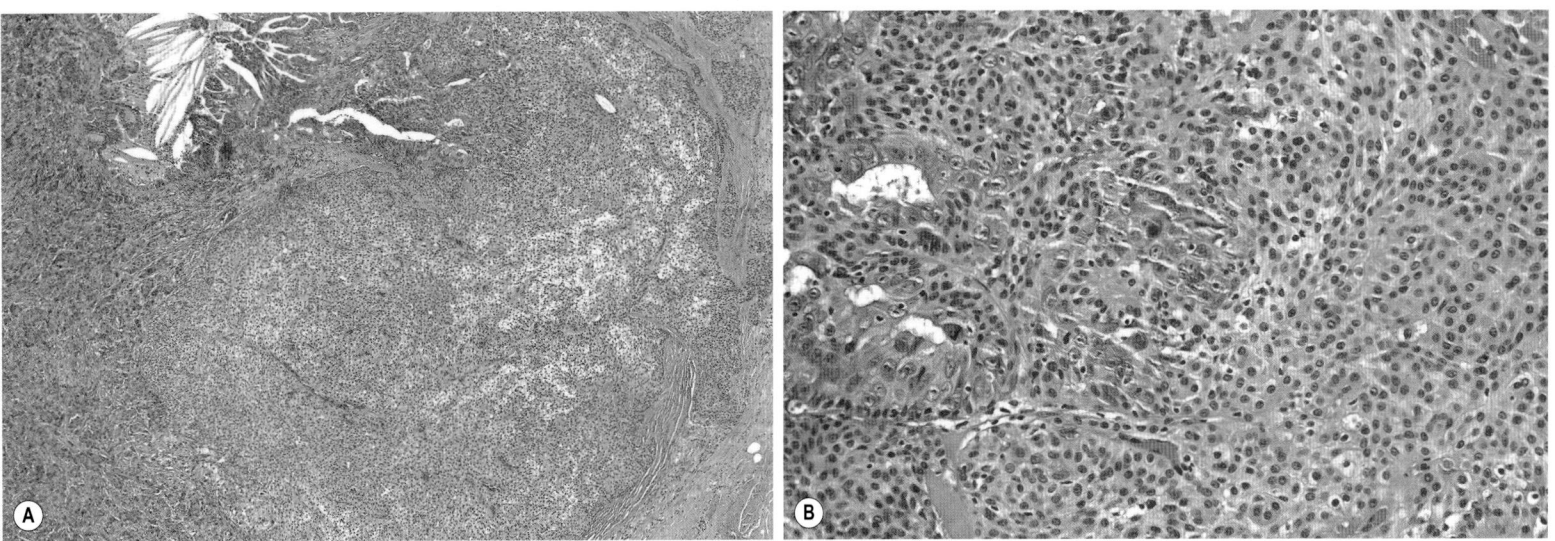

Fig. 33.142
Hidradenocarcinoma: (**A**) low-power view showing hidradenoma flanked on one side by poorly differentiated carcinoma; (**B**) high-power view.

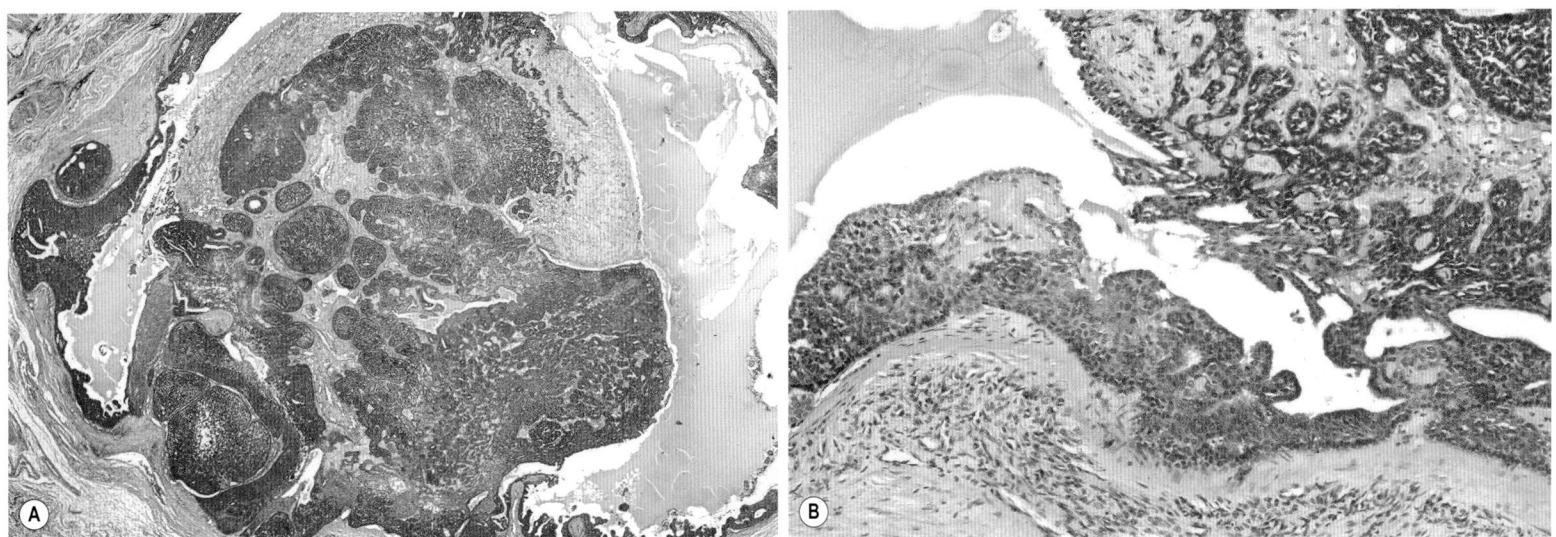

Fig. 33.143
(**A**, **B**) Hidradenocarcinoma: this is a cystic variant which presented on the forearm. It recurred four times despite apparently negative margins.

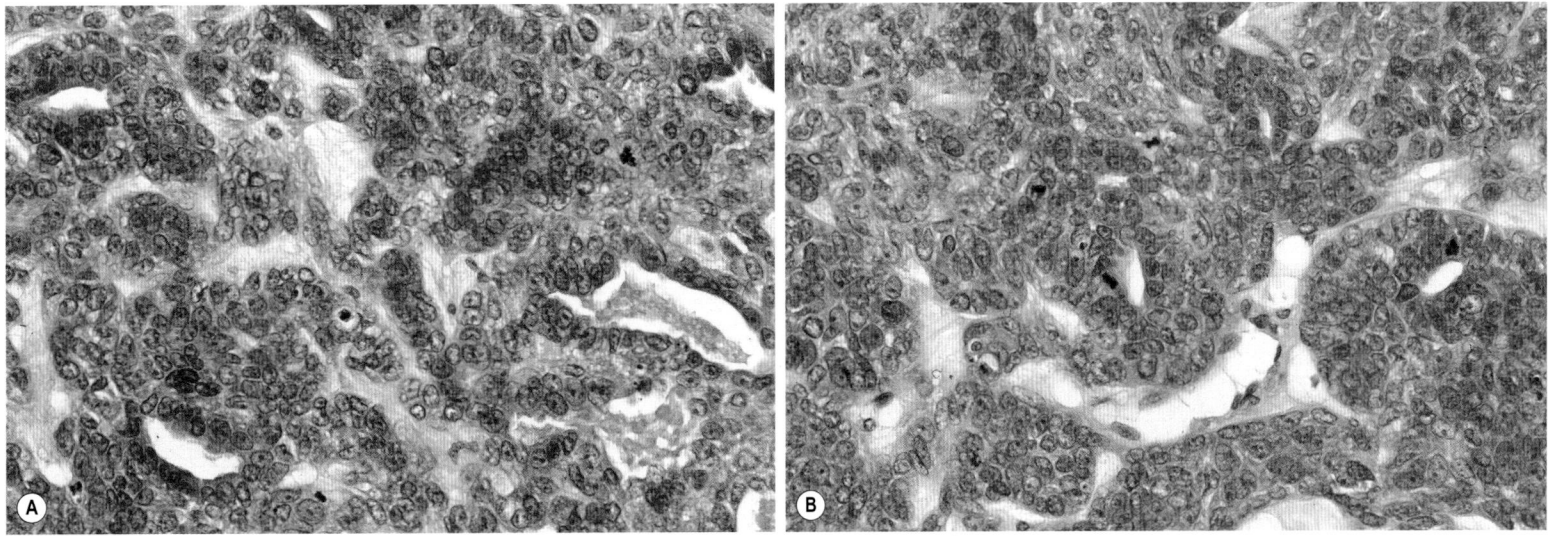

Fig. 33.144
(**A**, **B**) Hidradenocarcinoma: the tumor shows well-developed ducts. Mitoses are very conspicuous.

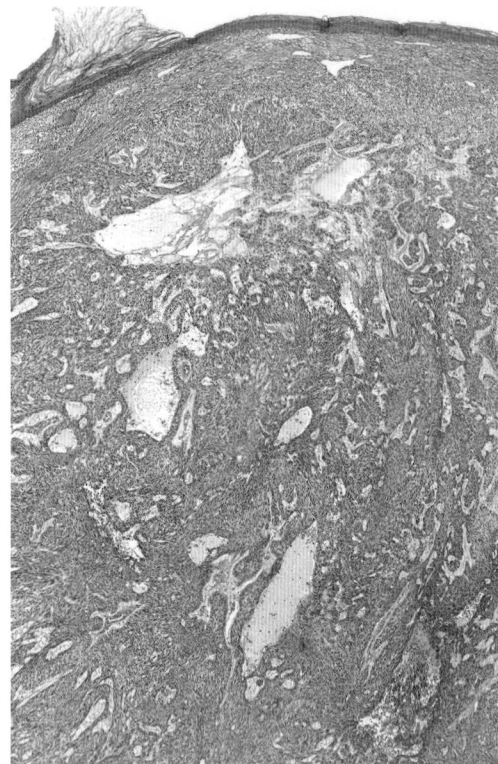

Fig. 33.145
Clear cell hidradenocarcinoma: in this example the tumor is composed of broad trabeculae.

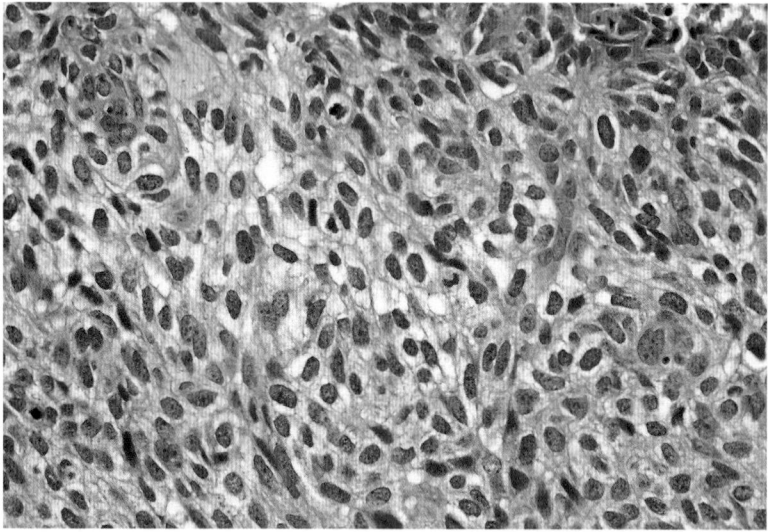

Fig. 33.146
Clear cell hidradenocarcinoma: the tumor cells have large vesicular nuclei and pale-staining or clear cytoplasm.

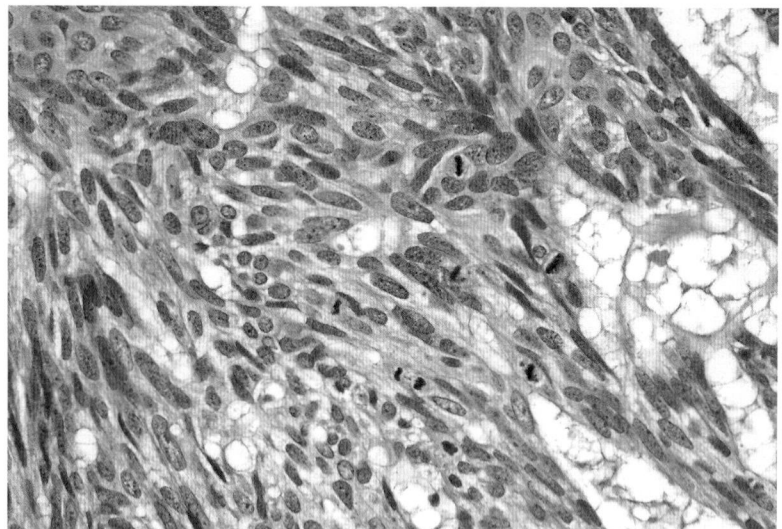

Fig. 33.147
Clear cell hidradenocarcinoma: numerous mitoses are present.

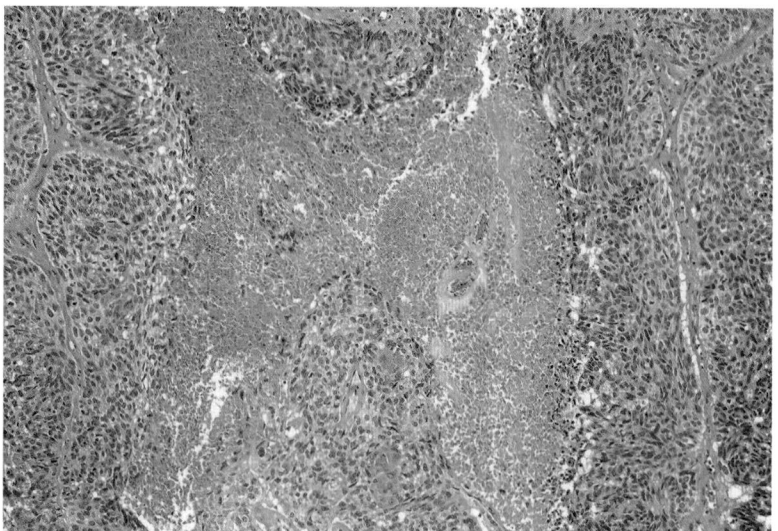

Fig. 33.148
Clear cell hidradenocarcinoma: the tumor shows extensive necrosis.

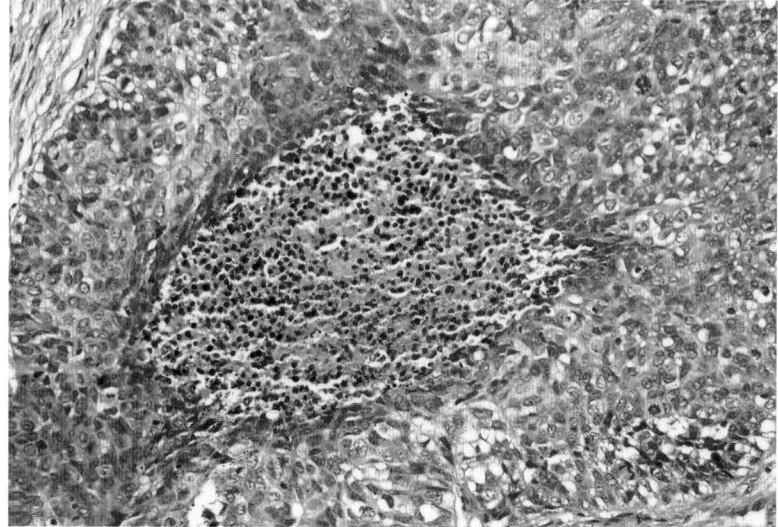

Fig. 33.149
Clear cell hidradenocarcinoma: in this example, central necrosis has resulted in a comedo carcinoma-like appearance.

activity (atypical hidradenoma). However, any tumor that shows brisk mitotic activity (particularly abnormal forms), cytological atypia, or an infiltrating growth pattern should be viewed with great caution. If it involves or is close to a margin, a wide excision is recommended.

It must also be distinguished from other tumors showing conspicuous cytoplasmic vacuolation including clear cell squamous carcinoma, trichilemmal carcinoma, and metastatic clear cell carcinoma from the kidney, bronchus, liver, and female genital tract. Rarely, clear cell melanoma may enter the differential diagnosis. Although on some occasions the diagnosis is not problematic, sometimes extensive clinical investigation and comprehensive immunohistochemistry are necessary before a diagnosis of a primary cutaneous tumor can be established.

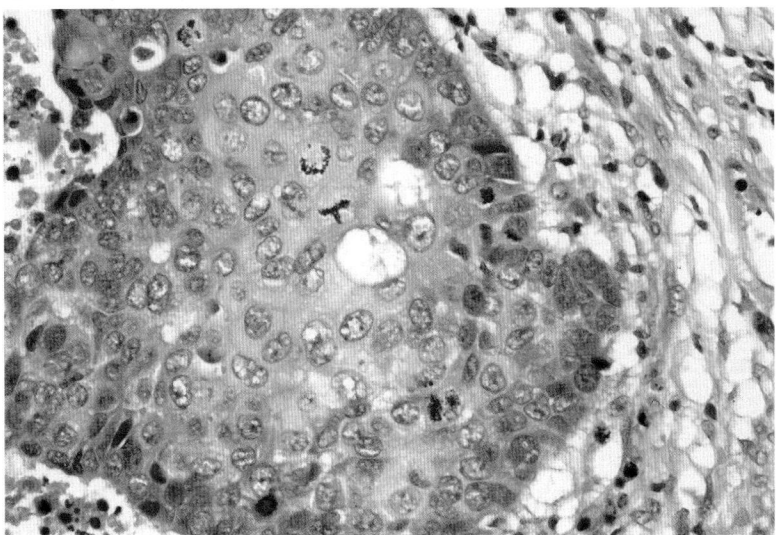

Fig. 33.150
Clear cell hidradenocarcinoma: well-developed glandular differentiation is evident.

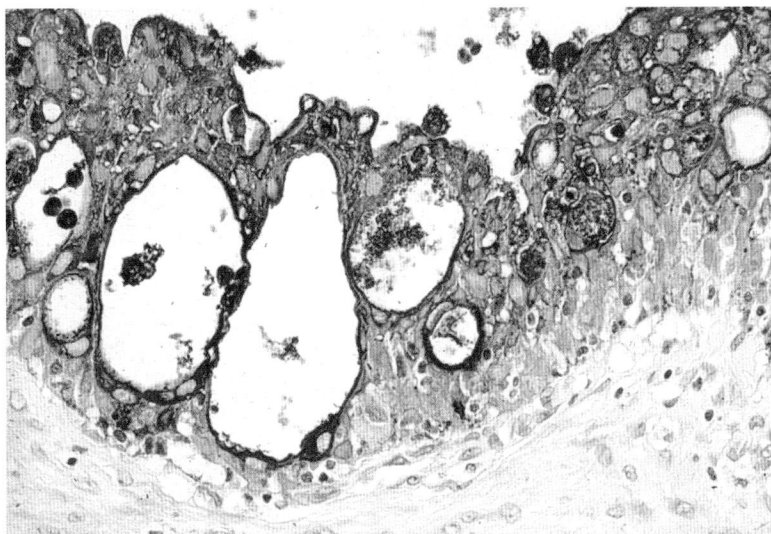

Fig. 33.151
Clear cell hidradenocarcinoma: numerous intracytoplasmic lumina are evident (EMA).

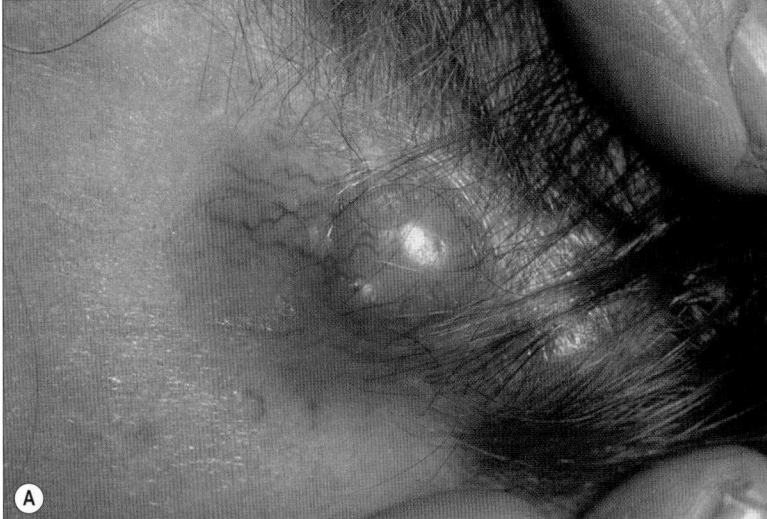

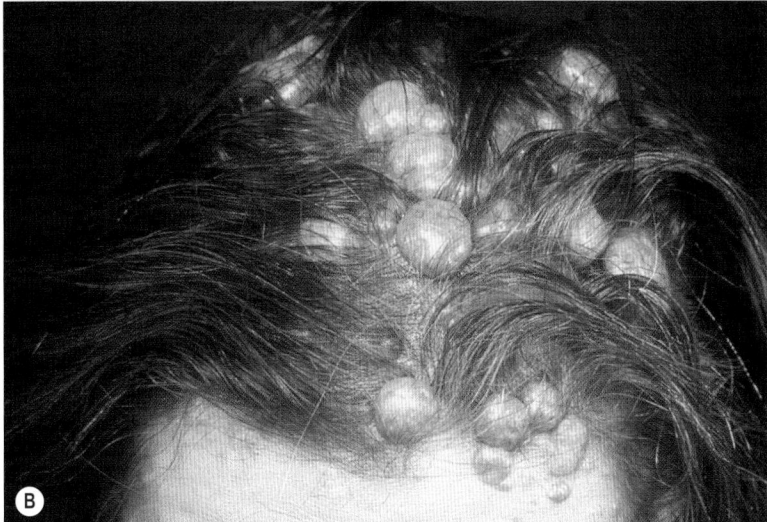

Fig. 33.152
Dermal cylindroma: (**A**) two dome-shaped nodules with associated telangiectasia are evident; (**B**) multiple lesions are present – turban tumor. By courtesy of the Institute of Dermatology, London, UK.

Dermal cylindroma

Clinical features

Dermal cylindroma is one of the more common benign adnexal tumors.[1] The vast majority (90%) occur on the head, neck, and scalp (60%) as slowly growing, sometimes painful, solitary pink or red dermal nodules averaging about 1 cm in diameter (*Fig. 33.152*).[1] Involvement of orbit, ear canal, abdomen, and breast is unusual.[2–8] There is a marked female preponderance (9:1).

Familial cases have been described and are typically associated with multiple tumors. Multiple cylindromas may be associated with facial trichoepitheliomas and also eccrine spiradenomas and milia, a constellation known as the autosomal dominant Brooke-Spiegler syndrome (familial cylindromatosis or turban tumor syndrome).[6–37] Penetrance in affected families is high but the clinical presentation is very variable, and within the same family individual members may present with multiple dermal cylindromas or multiple trichoepitheliomas or a combination of both in addition to eccrine spiradenomas and milia. Tumors may also show hybrid features of cylindroma and spiradenoma, and additional trichoepitheliomatous, trichoblastic, as well as sebaceous differentiation can be present.[37,38] Furthermore, patients sometimes develop other benign skin adnexal tumors including trichoblastoma,

cutaneous lymphadenoma, and syringoma.[38,39] Onset of the skin lesions is usually in early adulthood, and there is a predilection for females. Dermal cylindromas affect predominantly the scalp, but on occasions lesions may also be seen on the trunk and the extremities. A linear arrangement has been documented.[40] Scalp lesions can grow to a large size, and coalescence of numerous lesions is known as a 'turban tumor'. Trichoepitheliomas show a predilection for the centrofacial area.

Unusual presentations of this syndrome include the development of membranous-type basal cell adenoma of the parotid, a salivary gland tumor morphologically and pathogenetically related to dermal cylindroma, as well as malignant transformation within both dermal cylindromas and the salivary gland tumors.[12,41–50]

Pathogenesis and histologic features

Insights into the molecular pathways involved in these tumors have been gained through genetic analysis of patients with the Brooke-Spiegler syndrome. Using linkage analysis, this syndrome has been mapped to chromosome 16q12-q13, and a novel gene (CYLD) has been identified and subsequently cloned. CYLD represents a tumor suppressor gene. There is loss of heterozygosity of the wild-type copy in tumors. Germline mutations have been reported in patients with the Brooke-Spiegler syndrome, and somatic mutations are present in both solitary and familial tumors, resulting in inactivation of the CYLD gene.[13,14,16,28–33,51] The function of CYLD is only partially understood at this time. It belongs to the family of deubiquinating

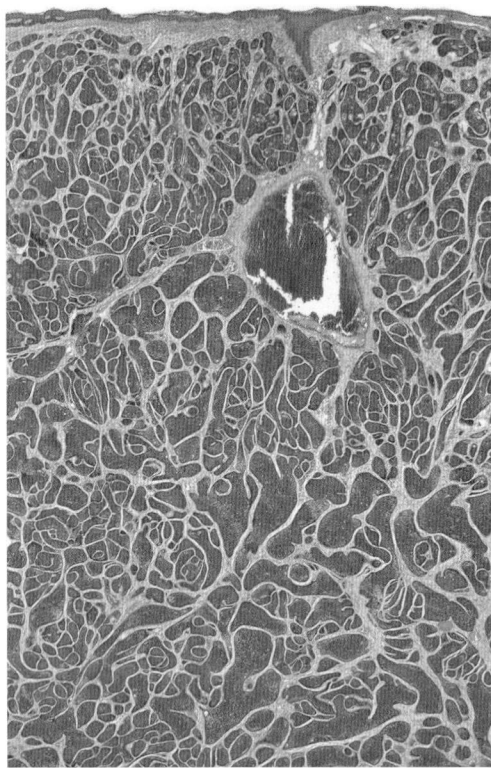

Fig. 33.153
Dermal cylindroma: this scanning view shows the complex interrelationship of the tumor lobules.

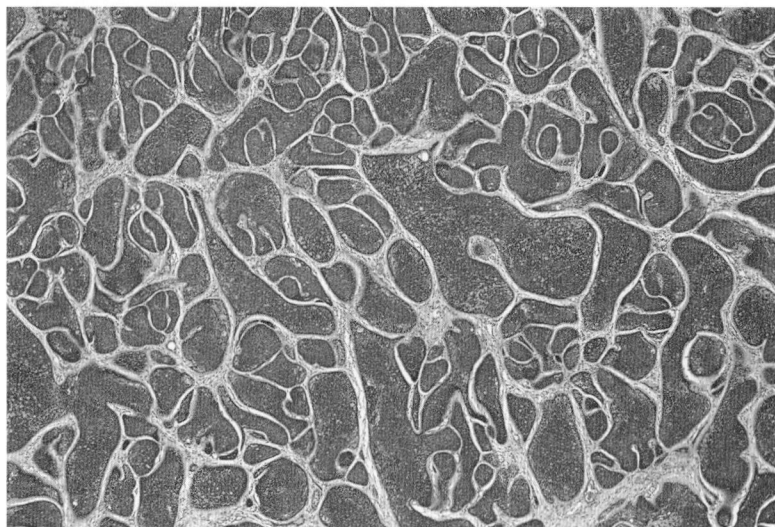

Fig. 33.154
Dermal cylindroma: the arrangement of the irregular lobules is reminiscent of pieces of a jigsaw.

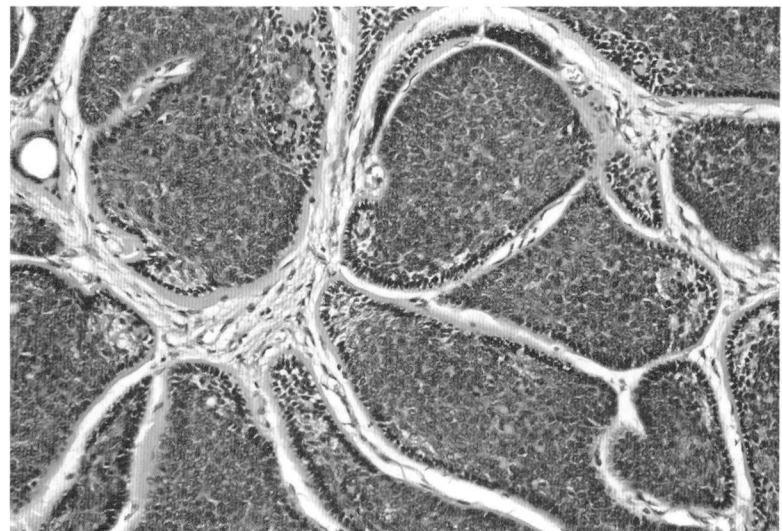

Fig. 33.155
Dermal cylindroma: each lobule consists of an outer layer of cells with small hyperchromatic nuclei and an inner zone of cells with oval vesicular nuclei. Each lobule is surrounded by a hyaline mantle.

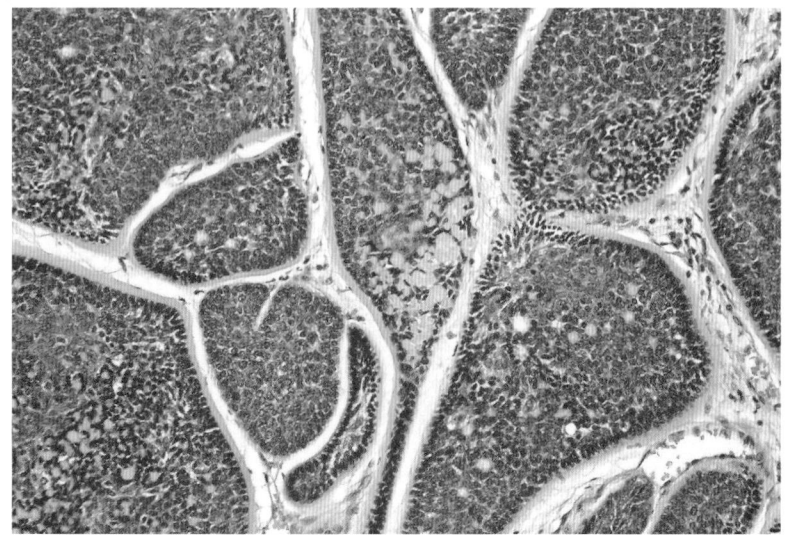

Fig. 33.156
Dermal cylindroma: the lobules contain deposits of hyaline material.

proteins and interferes with the tumor necrosis factor alpha (TNF-α)/NF-κb pathway, typically involved in mediating inflammation. Lack of CYLD results in NF-κb pathway activation in addition to decreased apoptosis.[52–55] How this NF-κb pathway activation is involved in tumorigenesis is currently unclear. An additional genetic event in cylindorma is the presence of the t(6;9)(q22-23;p23-24) translocation. Analogous to adenoid cystic carcinoma, it results in the MYB-NFIB fusion gene, one pathway leading to MYB overexpression, which can be detected by immunohistochemistry.[56] In the inherited, CYLD-defective tumors, the t(6;9) translocation is absent and MYB activation and overexpression occurs through other, as yet unidentified pathways.[57]

It has recently been proposed that cylindromas and spiradenomas are derived from hair follicle bulge and not from sweat glands. This is based on immunostaining for consistent staining of these tumors for the follicular stem marker CD200.[58]

Dermal cylindromas are remarkable for a prominent basement membrane-like structure surrounding tumor lobules. This is composed of proteins found at the normal dermal–epidermal junction including collagen types IV and VII, integrin $\alpha_4\beta_6$, and laminin 5.[59–62] Recent biochemical studies implicate improperly processed laminin[5] and low expression of integrin $\alpha_4\beta_6$ within the tumor, resulting in reduced numbers of hemidesmosomes and alterations in basement membrane structure.[63]

Dermal cylindroma, which is not encapsulated, is located in the upper dermis (*Fig. 33.153*). There is no connection with the overlying epidermis. Characteristically, the lesion is composed of multiple lobules arranged in a jigsaw or mosaic pattern (*Fig. 33.154*). Each lobule has an outer hyaline diastase-resistant, PAS-positive basement membrane (*Fig. 33.155*).[59–62] Hyaline droplets are typically seen in the center of the lobules and sometimes almost replace entire lobules (*Fig. 33.156*). Two cell types may be identified. Usually, although not invariably, situated at the periphery of the lobule are small cells with scanty cytoplasm containing a hyperchromatic nucleus. These surround larger cells with pale cytoplasm and an oval vesicular nucleus. Ductal lumina are usually present (*Fig. 33.157*). Often, there is morphological overlap between cylindroma and spiradenoma.[9,64,65] Such cases have been referred to as spiradenocylindroma.[64] Additional

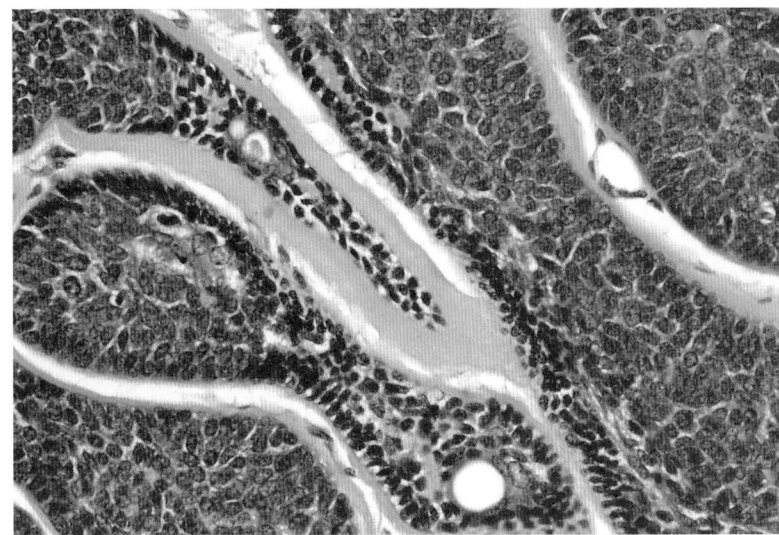

Fig. 33.157
Dermal cylindroma: ductal differentiation which is present at the edge of the field is an invariable feature.

trichoepitheliomatous, trichoblastic, and sebaceous differentiation has also been observed.[37,38]

Immunohistochemically, the ductal epithelium shows marked luminal CEA expression, but is HMFG negative.[66] The epithelial cells express CK6 and CK19 as well as CK7 and EMA.[67,68] Positive staining for SMA and S100 protein is evidence of myoepithelial differentiation, and staining with IKH-4 supports the eccrine nature of this neoplasm.[67-70]

Malignant cylindroma

Clinical features

Malignant cylindroma or cylindrocarcinoma forms a spectrum with spiradenocarcinoma, and tumors with overlapping features exist, so-called spiradenocylindrocarcinoma.[1,2] Cylindrocarcinoma is extremely rare with only approximately 50 histologically confirmed documented cases.[1,3-18] Diagnosis is dependent on the recognition of pre-existent benign tumor. Lesions may arise within solitary cylindromas or complicate the autosomal dominant multiple tumor variant, but the latter is more common.[12,13,18] Most malignant cylindromas have presented on the scalp, although the trunk, face, and extremities as well as the external auditory canal have occasionally been affected. There is a slight female predominance, and most patients are in their seventh to ninth decades. Clinical features suggestive of malignant transformation include ulceration, rapid growth, and bleeding.[9] This is a high-grade tumor with a recurrence rate of 36% and a metastasis rate of 46%, with the lymph nodes, liver, and vertebral column being particularly affected.[9,12]

Pathogenesis and histologic features

The etiology of malignant cylindroma in most instances is unknown. Several tumors, however, have developed following previous therapeutic radiation.[5,11]

Features suggesting possible malignant potential include an infiltrating growth pattern and loss of mosaic appearance, hyalin sheaths, and biphasic cellular distribution (Figs 33.158–33.161).[9] Nuclear and cytoplasmic pleomorphism, prominent nucleoli, and frequent or abnormal mitoses are also worrying features. Lymphatic and vascular invasion or infiltration of the perineural sheath also signifies an aggressive biological potential. Although most malignant cylindromas have represented variably differentiated adenocarcinomas, occasional tumors have displayed squamous or spindled cell features, and metaplastic/sarcomatous differentiation has been documented.[3,18]

Immunohistochemically, the tumor cells express CAM 5.2, EMA, and CEA.[3,6,9,12] S100 protein and GCDFP-15 expression are variable.[3,12] The tumors often express p53 immunohistochemically but they lack mutations

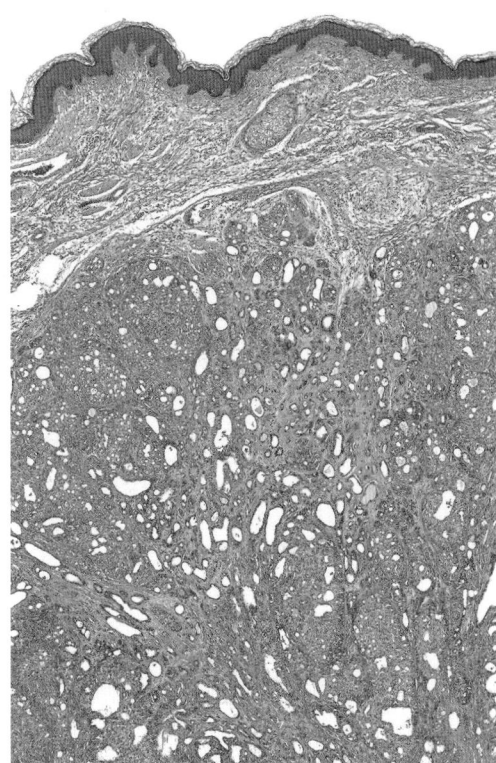

Fig. 33.158
Malignant cylindroma: low-power view showing tumor nodules with obvious ductal differentiation and cysts.

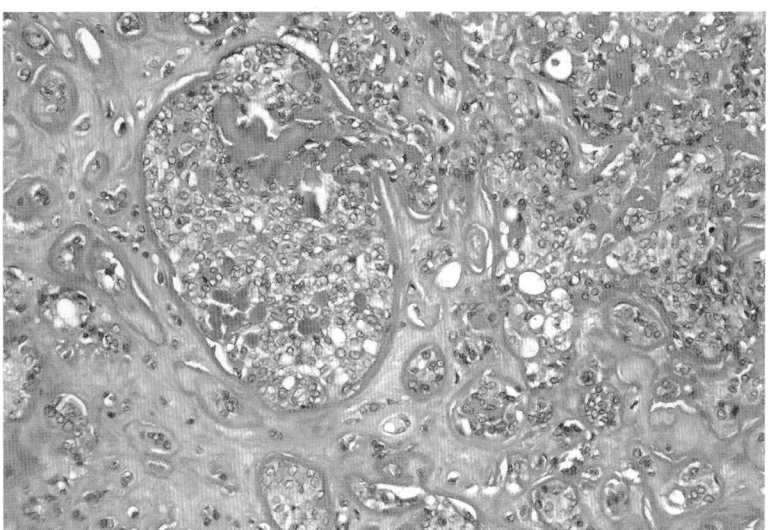

Fig. 33.159
Malignant cylindroma: scattered throughout the tumor are residual cylindromatous foci. Note the hyaline mantle.

in the TP53 gene. The p53 expression pattern is heterogeneous, and it is of limited use diagnostically to separate benign from malignant cylindroma.[19]

Eccrine spiradenoma

Clinical features

Eccrine spiradenoma is clinically rather distinct, as most examples are either tender or painful.[1,2] It presents as a usually solitary, intradermal, circumscribed, round or oval, firm lesion (Fig. 33.162). Often, the overlying skin is blue. Most tumors measure 0.3–5.0 cm in diameter, but occasionally giant variants are encountered.[3-6] Approximately 80% are present on the ventral aspect of the skin, most often affecting the upper half of the body.[1,2]

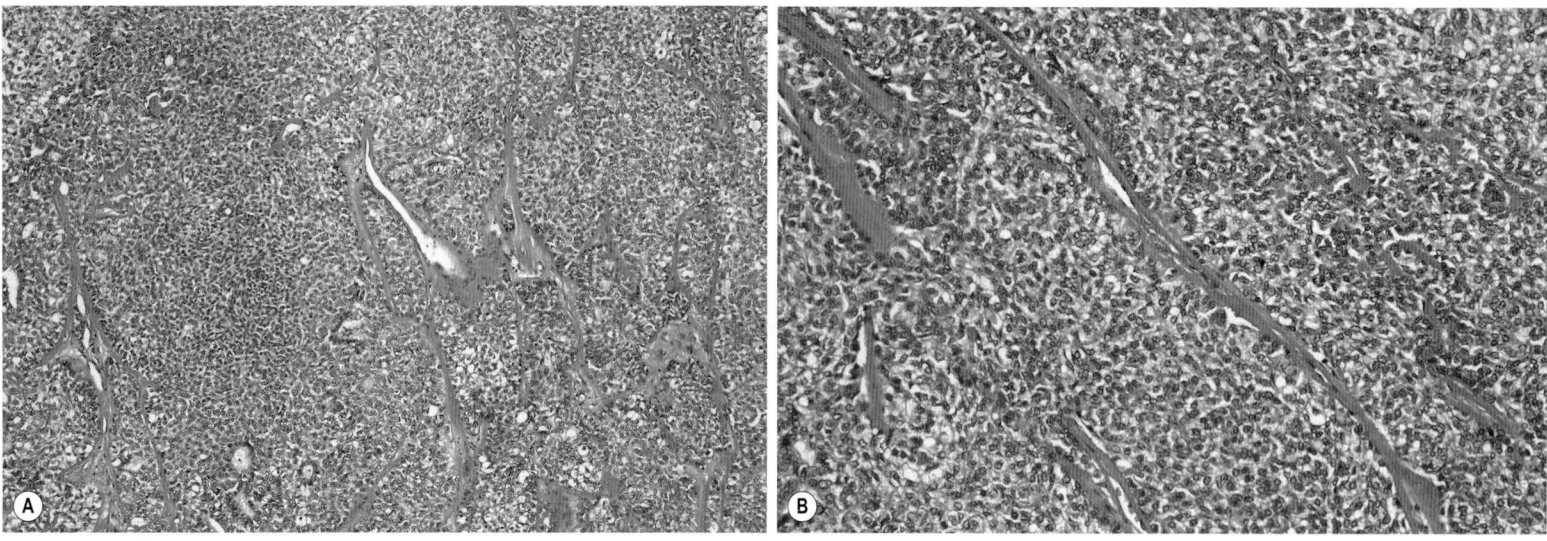

Fig. 33.160
Malignant cylindroma: (**A**) the dual cell population is lost and the tumor cells form expansile nodules and a sheetlike growth pattern; (**B**) higher-power view. Note the fibrous trabeculae.

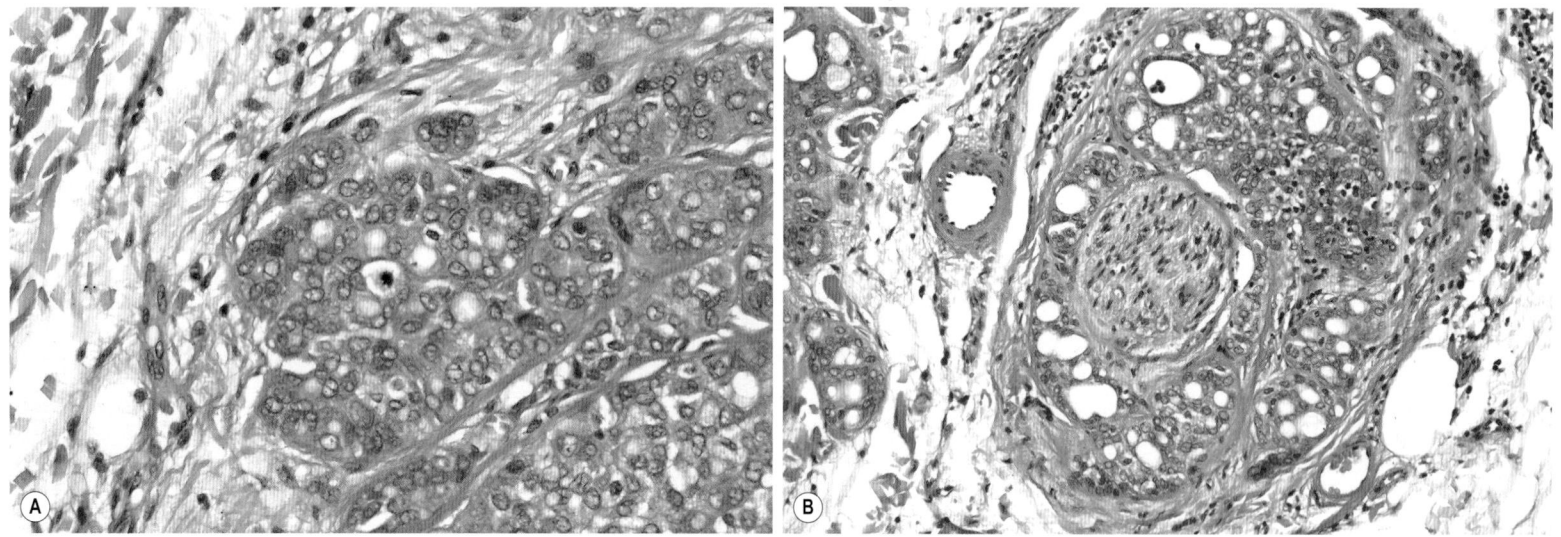

Fig. 33.161
Malignant cylindroma: (**A**) there is a centrally located mitotic figure. (**B**) This tumor showed perineural infiltration.

Unusual anatomic sites include the ear and postauricular area, eyelid, lip, and hand.[7-13] Although any age may be affected, most patients are in their second to fourth decades. Congenital onset or presentation in early infancy is unusual.[14,15] Multiple lesions occasionally occur and a linear or zosteriform variant has been described.[16-29] Multiple eccrine spiradenomas can be familial and are then inherited in an autosomal dominant pattern.[21] They may be associated with multiple trichoepitheliomas and cylindromas as well as, less frequently, trichoblastoma and cutaneous lymphadenoma (adamantinoid trichoblastoma) as part of the morphological spectrum of the Brooke-Spiegler syndrome.[19,22,28-33]

Pathogenesis and histologic features

Based on the positivity of tumor cells both in spiradenoma and cylindroma for the hair follicle bulge stem cell marker CD200, it has been proposed that the lineage of these tumors is follicular rather than sweat gland.[34]

Eccrine spiradenoma is characterized by the presence of one or more tumor lobules located in the dermis and sometimes extending into the subcutaneous fat (*Fig. 33.163*).[1,2] The overlying epidermis is normal. Due to nuclear crowding, the lobules are intensely basophilic. The tumor is usually encapsulated and is typically sharply circumscribed. Sometimes, a retraction artifact separates the capsule from the surrounding tissues, and not infrequently a nerve trunk may be identified in close proximity to the tumor

lobules. Exceptionally, extensive intraneural growth is seen. Tumor lobules contain two cell types. At the periphery of the lobule the cells are small with round hyperchromatic nuclei, whereas centrally they are larger with oval vesicular nuclei, often containing a small eosinophilic nucleolus, and have pale-staining or eosinophilic cytoplasm (*Figs 33.164–33.166*). Ductal differentiation is usually present (*Fig. 33.167*). An unusual and rare finding is the focal presence of small closely packed glandular structures with round lumina and composed of palely eosinophilic staining cuboidal to columnar cells. Luminal cells are typically surrounded by an additional myoepithelial layer. This pattern has been referred to as 'spiradenoma with an adenomatous component'.[35] With limited follow-up, these tumors showed benign behavior.[35] However, as this finding has also been found in association with severe cytological atypia and spiradenocarcinoma, its biological significance and potential are best regarded as uncertain at this time. A further rare morphological variant consists of adenoid cystic-like areas in spiradenomas with the formation of cribriform pseudocystic spaces filled with mucin or homogeneous eosinophilic material.[36]

Typically, eccrine spiradenoma does not contain glycogen. Mitoses are exceedingly rare. Some tumors may contain cystic cavities filled with diastase-resistant, PAS-positive finely granular eosinophilic material. The tumor lobules are supported by a delicate reticulin network, which demonstrates an alveolar pattern. Marked lymphedema may be present within the

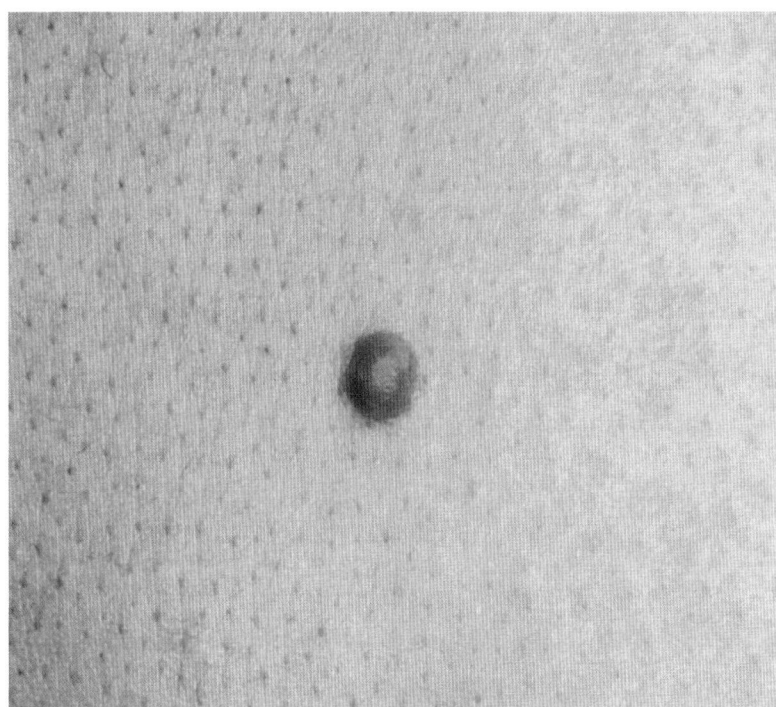

Fig. 33.162
Eccrine spiradenoma: this small nodule is typically tender or painful. By courtesy of D. McGibbon, MD, Institute of Dermatology, London, UK.

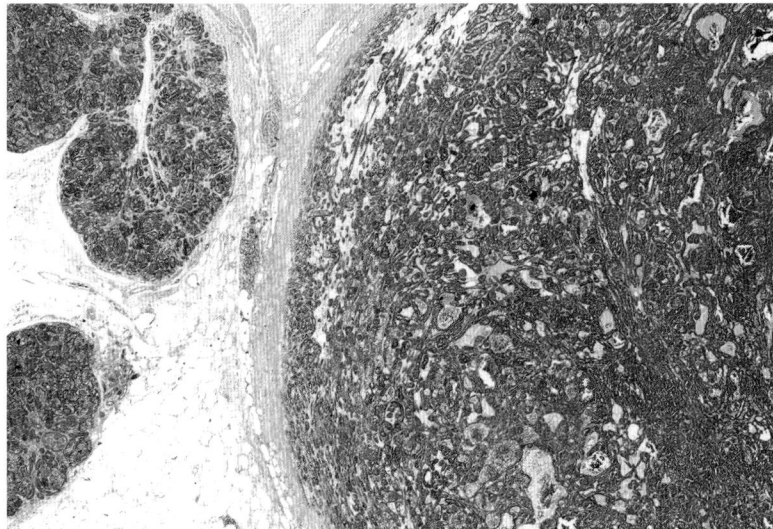

Fig. 33.163
Eccrine spiradenoma: in this example, there are three discrete tumor lobules. The largest appears encapsulated.

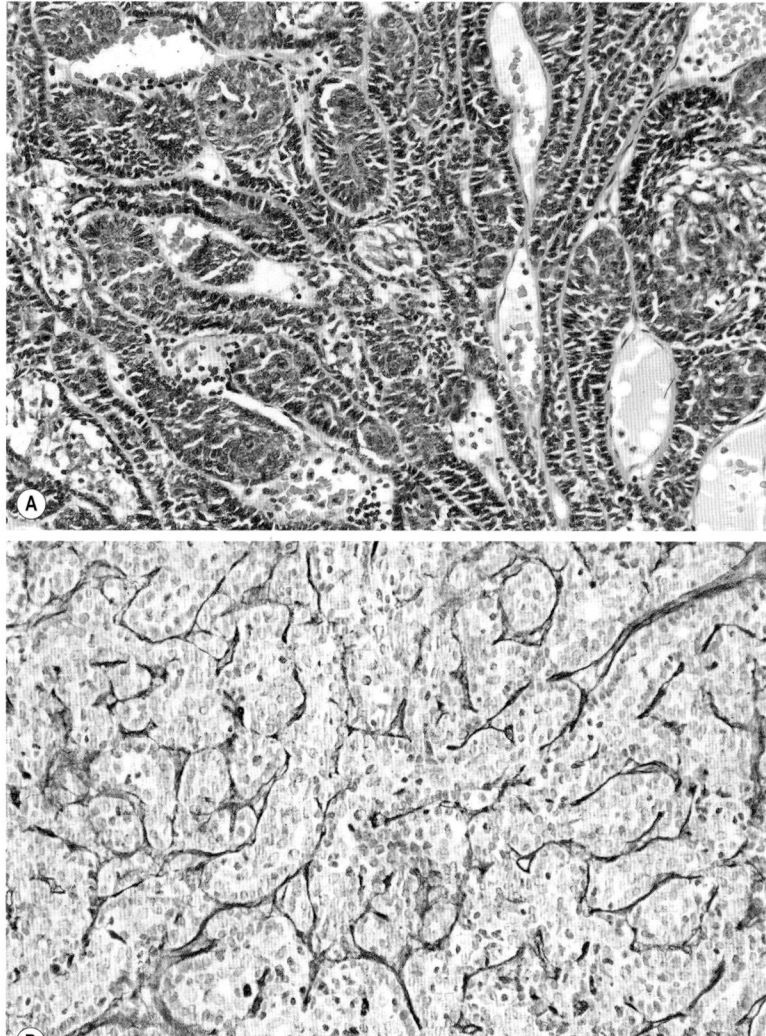

Fig. 33.164
(**A**, **B**) Eccrine spiradenoma: in this field, the biphasic cell population is evident. The outer layer cells have small hyperchromatic nuclei and minimal cytoplasm. These surround larger cells with round or oval vesicular nuclei and more conspicuous eosinophilic cytoplasm; the lobules are surrounded by a well-developed reticulin sheath.

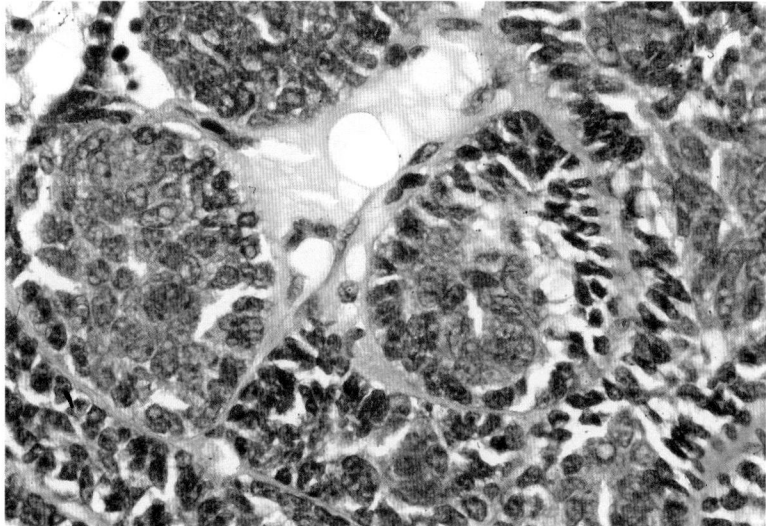

Fig. 33.165
Eccrine spiradenoma: close-up view of biphasic population.

tumor lobules and also in the surrounding connective tissue sheath (*Fig. 33.168*).[2] In a single case, extensive intraneural growth with no deleterious consequences was described.[37] Eccrine spiradenoma is richly vascular and on occasions conspicuous, widely dilated vascular channels may result in a superficial resemblance to an angioma, hemangiopericytoma, or glomus tumor (*Fig. 33.169*).[4] Prominent infarction can be seen in some cases with very little viable tumor left making diagnosis difficult. Variably sized perivascular spaces around one or more centrally located blood vessels are frequently present and are demarcated peripherally by palisading tumor cells and basement membrane material.[38] Rarely, hyaline droplets are present within the paler central component of the lobules. Occasionally, spiradenomas also show cylindromatous features (spiradenocylindroma), and less frequently trichoepitheliomatous as well as trichoblastomatous and sebaceous differentiation may be observed.[29,39–42]

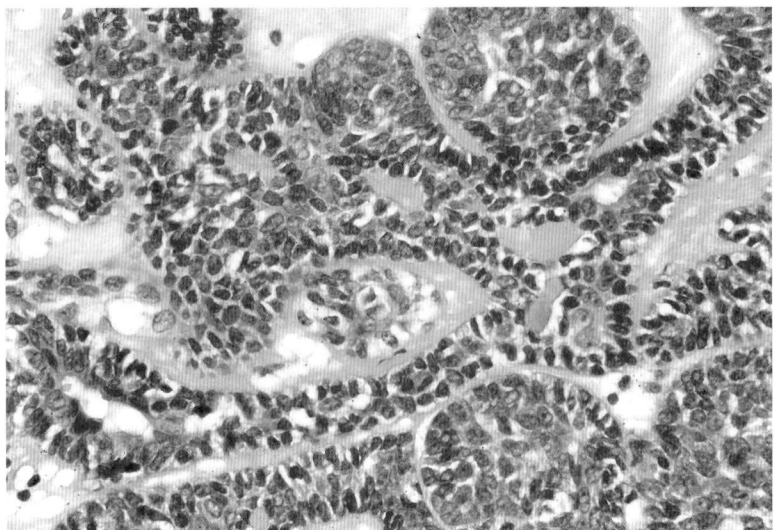

Fig. 33.166
Eccrine spiradenoma: in this field, the tumor lobules are surrounded by a thick hyaline mantle composed of basement membrane material.

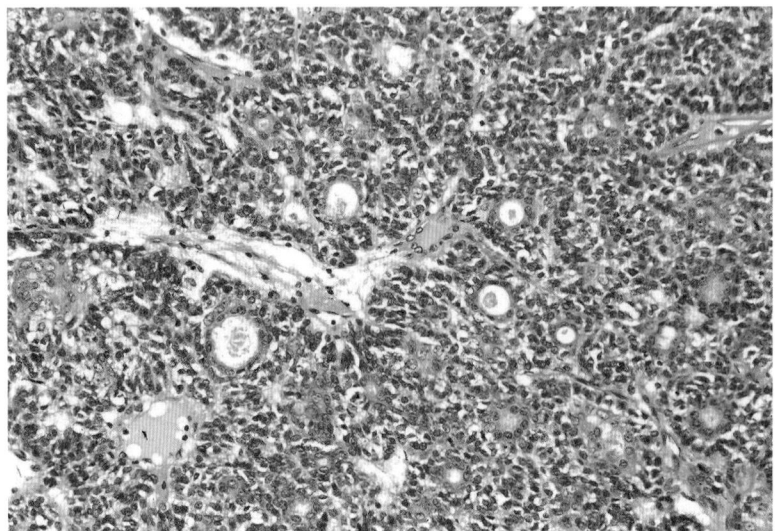

Fig. 33.167
Eccrine spiradenoma: in this field, there is extensive ductal differentiation.

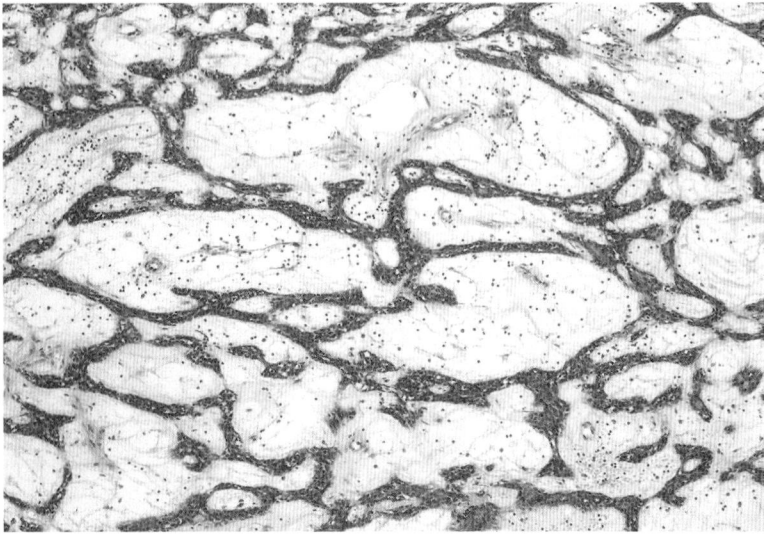

Fig. 33.168
Eccrine spiradenoma: very marked edema has resulted in this 'lymphangiectatic' variant.

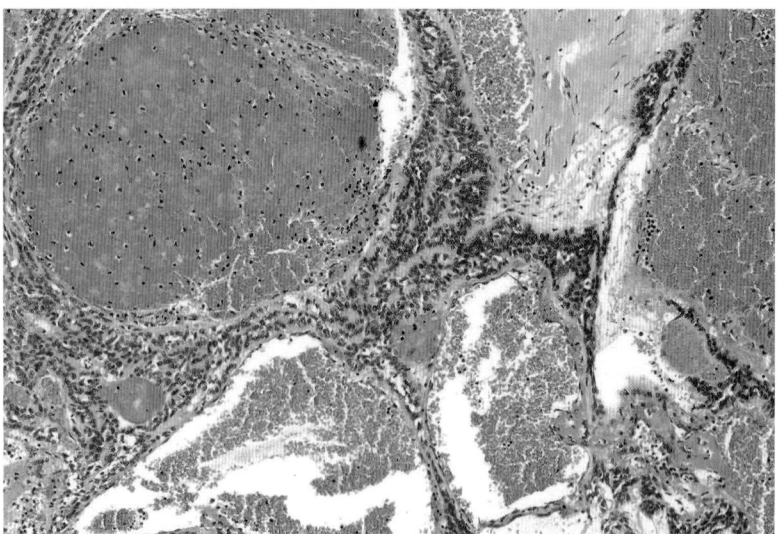

Fig. 33.169
Eccrine spiradenoma: note the widely dilated and congested vascular channels. This tumor is sometimes mistaken for a hemangioma or glomangioma.

By immunohistochemistry, eccrine spiradenoma expresses IKH-4 in keeping with its eccrine differentiation.[43] Tumor cells furthermore express CK7, CK8, and CK18 as well as EMA and CEA.[44,45] Myoepithelial differentiation is documented by positive staining for SMA and S100 protein.[45-49] The immunohistochemical findings are similar to those of dermal cylindroma and MYB overexpression as a surrogate marker for the t(6;9) translocation leading to the NFIB-MYB fusion gene is also noted.[50]

Differential diagnosis

Eccrine spiradenoma usually poses few diagnostic problems. Occasionally, however, particularly with small lesions in which ductal differentiation may not be obvious, the tumor may be mistaken for a lymphoid aggregate. The immunocytochemical demonstration of duct formation by EMA or CEA expression should rapidly resolve any diagnostic difficulty.

Eccrine spiradenocarcinoma

Clinical features

Eccrine spiradenocarcinoma (malignant eccrine spiradenoma) is an extremely rare neoplasm, with fewer than 100 examples having been documented in the English literature.[1-45] The clinical appearance is not distinctive, diagnosis being dependent on the recognition of a pre-existent benign counterpart.[2,44] It is characterized by a long history, often in decades, and in one case amounting to 70 years.[3,20,27,45] There is an equal sex incidence.[20] Elderly adults with a median age around 60 years are predominantly affected, but age at presentation is variable, ranging from 12 to 92 years.[6,19,20,27] A wide range of anatomical sites may be affected including the extremities, the trunk, and (less frequently) the head and neck.[20,27] Unusual locations are the external auditory canal and breast.[10,29,40] Presenting features have included a change in character including size, color, bleeding, and ulceration (*Fig. 33.170*).[4,20] Tumors are typically sporadic and solitary, but less frequently they may also present in the setting of Brooke-Spiegler syndrome.[44]

It is said to be a high-grade tumor with a reported recurrence rate of approximately 30%, a metastasis rate of 30% to 40%, and a mortality of 20%.[2,23,27,31,44] Preferred metastatic sites have been locoregional lymph nodes and lung followed by other visceral sites including brain, bone, liver, and kidney.[6-8,11,18,26,27,36,37] Accurate prognostic data are, however, difficult to obtain in such a rare entity (particularly as many documented examples are single case reports). The overall rates of recurrence and metastasis, as well as mortality, may indeed be lower.[20] More recent studies have shown that this is particularly true for the morphologically low-grade tumors.[44,46,47] Although these tumors have a documented 20% recurrence rate, the risk of

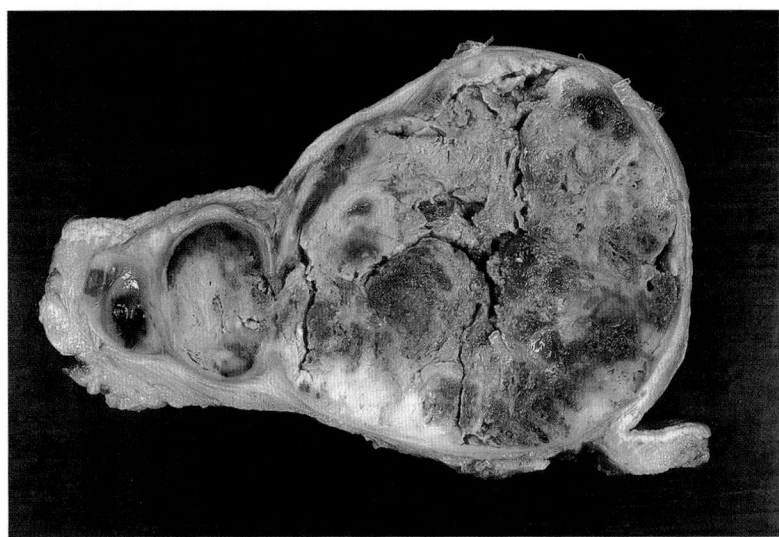

Fig. 33.170
Eccrine spiradenocarcinoma: this tumor had been present for many years. Note the necrosis and cystic degeneration. By courtesy of A.J. Blackshaw, MD, Bedford Hospital, Bedford, UK.

metastasis and mortality is negligible.[47] Distant metastasis and death from disease appears to occur only in morphologically high-grade tumors.

Treatment consists of wide excision. The benefit of sentinel lymph node biopsy and additional chemotherapy is not established at this point, and hormonal treatment such as tamoxifen could become a therapeutical option in estrogen receptor-positive tumors.[15]

Pathogenesis and histologic features

The diagnosis of malignant eccrine spiradenoma requires the recognition of an at least focal component of benign spiradenoma, which may be present to varying degrees (Figs 33.171–33.174).[2,4–6,20,44] The malignant features are not specific and include an infiltrating border, tumor necrosis, hemorrhage, lymphovascular invasion, and infiltration of the perineural sheath.[20] Cytological changes include loss of the dual cell population, nuclear pleomorphism, prominent nucleoli, and marked mitotic activity, including atypical forms (Figs 33.172–33.176). Malignant transformation change in spiradenoma can show two morphologically distinct patterns:[20]

- One pattern is that of an abrupt transition from a benign-appearing spiradenoma to frankly carcinomatous or sarcomatous areas (Figs 33.174–33.176). Carcinomatous change may be noted in the form of adenocarcinoma but squamous differentiation may also be seen.[20,25,44] Depending on the degree of differentiation of the carcinomatous

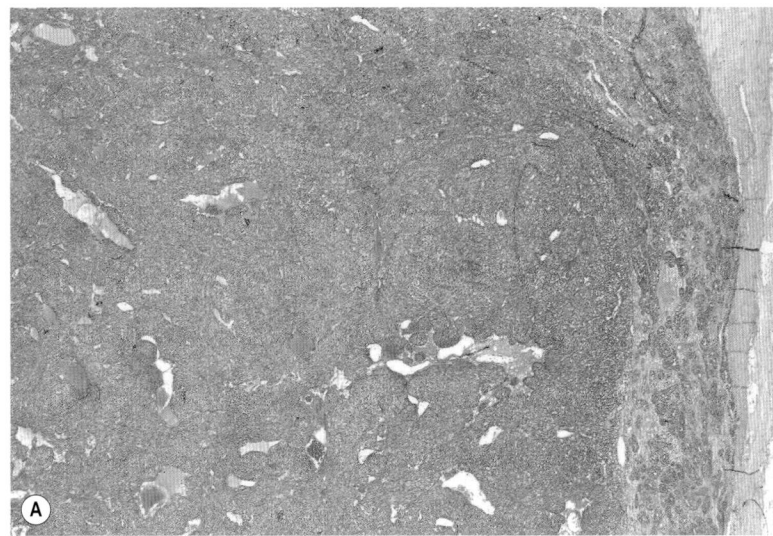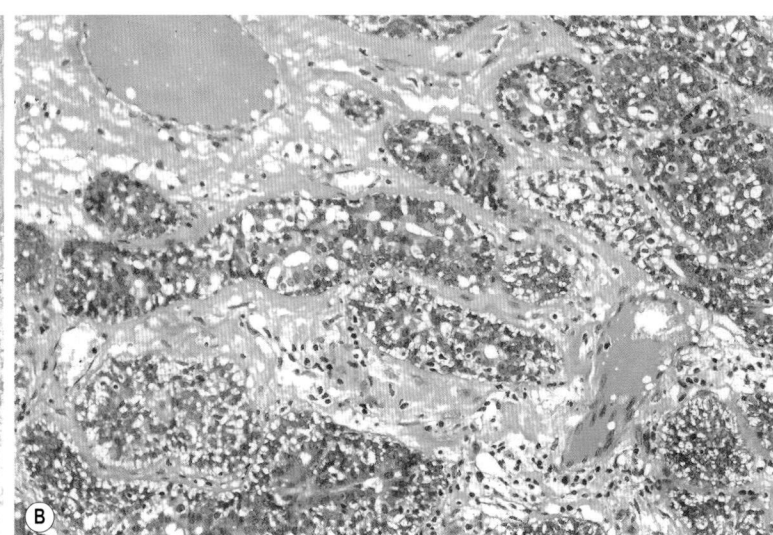

Fig. 33.171
Eccrine spiradenocarcinoma, morphologically low grade: (A) scanning view showing expansile nodular growth of the malignant component with adjacent benign eccrine spiradenoma; (B) high-power view of preexisting spiradenoma.

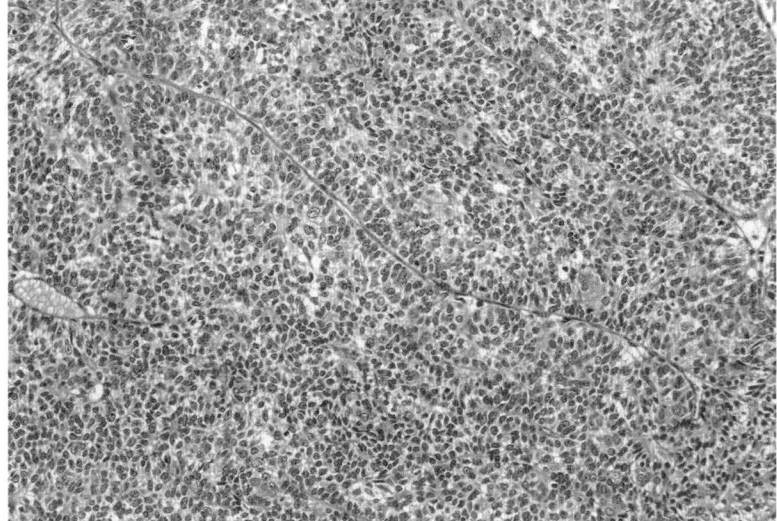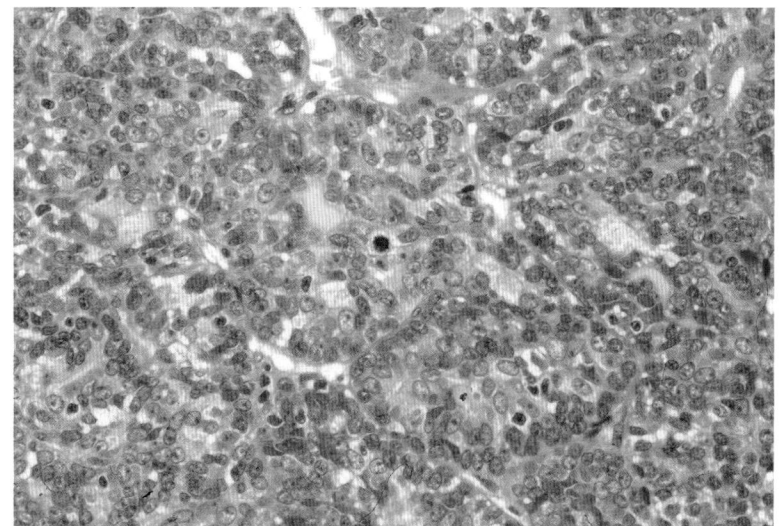

Fig. 33.172
Eccrine spiradenocarcinoma morphologically low grade: the tumor is composed of broad trabeculae. Note the loss of the dual cell population.

Fig. 33.173
Eccrine spiradenocarcinoma morphologically low grade: high-power view showing only mild cytological atypia but multiple mitoses.

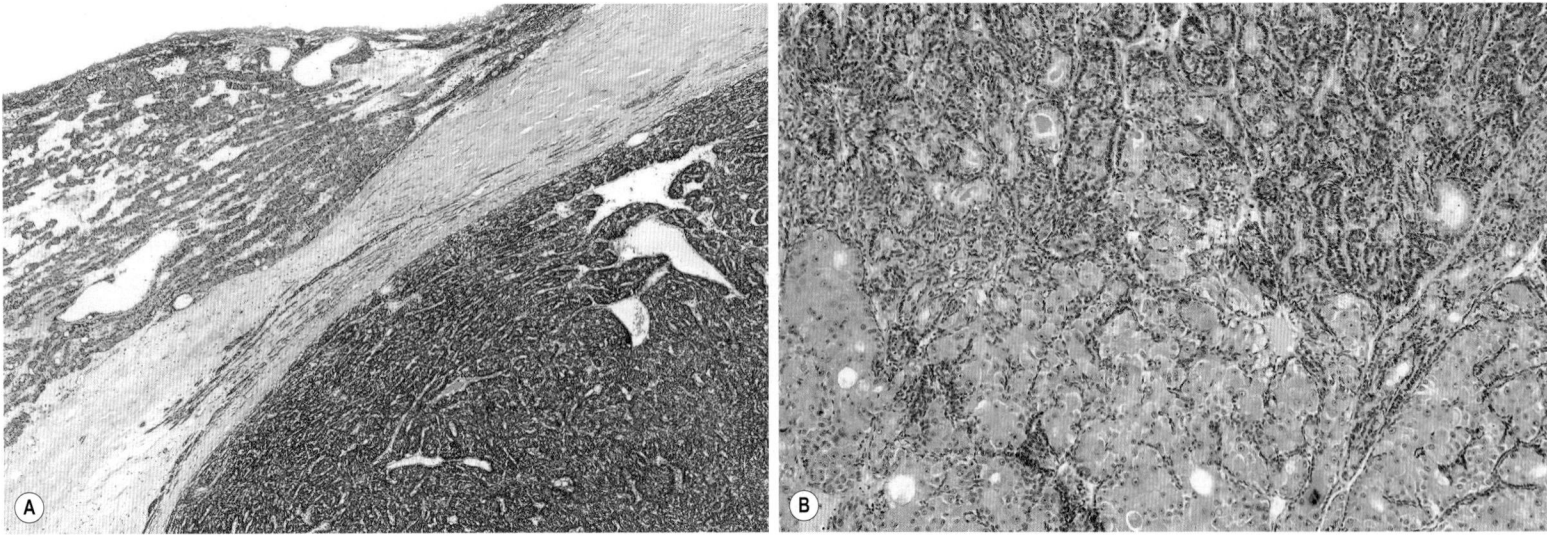

Fig. 33.174
Eccrine spiradenocarcinoma morphologically high grade: (A) precursor lesion; (B) note the biphasic population.

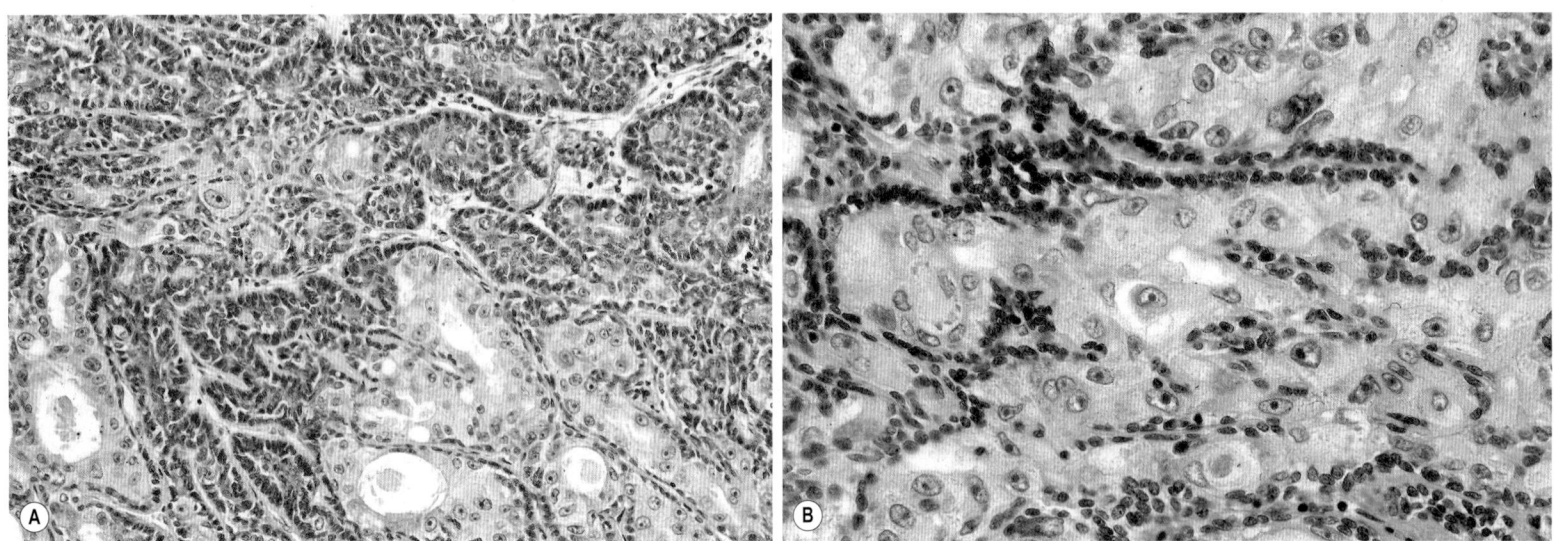

Fig. 33.175
(A, B) Eccrine spiradenocarcinoma morphologically high grade: these fields come from the junction of the benign and malignant components. There is nuclear pleomorphism and nucleoli are prominent.

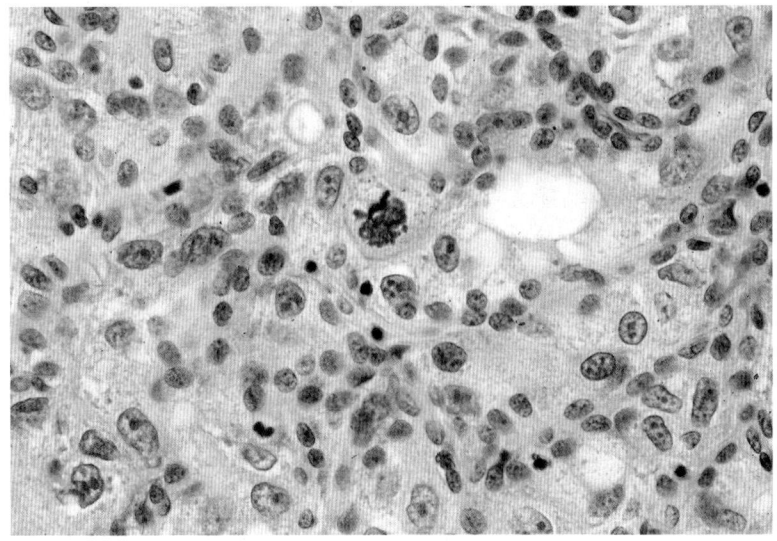

Fig. 33.176
Eccrine spiradenocarcinoma morphologically high grade: note the abnormal mitotic figure.

component, these tumors have recently been classified into 'salivary gland-type basal cell adenocarcinoma-like, high grade' and 'infiltrative adenocarcinoma, NOS'. Sarcomatous differentiation (carcinosarcoma) may be present in the form of a spindled cell, leiomyosarcomatous, osteosarcomatous, chondrosarcomatous, osteocartilagenous, or rhabdomyoblastic component.[7–9,15,18,19,26,28,29,33,44] Without identification of a benign component, these tumors would be difficult to classify.

- A second morphological type of malignant spiradenoma is characterized by a histologically low-grade tumor in which the lobular architecture of spiradenoma is retained (Fig. 33.171). Due to their close resemblance to salivary tumors, they have been termed 'salivary gland-type basal cell adenocarcinoma-like, low-grade'. These tumors are difficult to recognize at scanning magnification, but are characterized by loss of the dual cell population and are composed of a single component of only mildly to moderately atypical basaloid cells showing increased mitotic activity upon closer inspection (Figs 33.172 and 33.173).[11,20,47] A further clue is the absence of admixed intratumoral lymphocytes.

Additional morphological findings include squamous metaplasia and clear cell change as well as mucinous metaplasia.[44] An adenomatous component of small and densely packed, well-developed glands may also be present.[44]

Malignant change has also been documented in association with a pre-existing benign tumor showing morphological overlap between dermal cylindroma and eccrine spiradenoma (spiradenocylindrocarcinoma) and malignant cylindroma, spiradenocarcinoma, and spiradenocylindrocarcinoma likely represent the morphological spectrum of the same disease.[41,44,46]

Immunohistochemistry may be of help in highlighting ductal differentiation, the latter expressing EMA and CEA. The background population of cells expresses S100 protein and CAM 5.2 in addition to EMA.[1] The tumor cells may express estrogen receptor.[15,25] Overexpression of p53 may be seen in the malignant component, but mutations in the TP53 gene are rare.[48–50] Immunohistochemical use of p53 staining has not proven helpful to differentiate spiradenocarcinoma from a benign spiradenoma.[47,50] Similarly, the MIB1 proliferative index is elevated in malignant tumors. The changes are, however, not significant to be used for diagnostic purposes. In contrast, MYB staining has recently been shown to be lost at least in the morphologically low-grade tumors. This is diagnostically helpful to distinguish them from benign spradenomas.[47]

Syringoid eccrine carcinoma

Syringoid eccrine carcinoma, microcystic adnexal carcinoma, and adenoid cystic carcinoma show overlap and are probably variations on a single theme. However, in keeping with the current literature, they are classified as separate lesions in this chapter.

Clinical features

Syringoid eccrine carcinoma (eccrine epithelioma, basal cell tumor with eccrine differentiation) is rare and most commonly presents on the scalp, although tumors have also arisen on the face, neck, trunk, leg, forearm, dorsum of hand, and palm.[1–13] Clinical features are variable, ranging from a sometimes painful infiltrated plaque associated with alopecia through to a nonhealing ulcer reminiscent of basal cell carcinoma.[10] Lesions generally measure from 0.5 to 7.0 cm in greatest dimension. The tumor is characterized by a female preponderance (3:1) and most often affects the middle aged (range 42–74 years, mean 55 years).[10] It is frequently slowly growing and has often been present for many years, sometimes decades, before diagnosis. Syringoid eccrine carcinoma is therefore characterized by a protracted course, multiple recurrences, and aggressive behavior. Rarely, lymph node and pulmonary metastases have been documented, and one patient died from systemic spread.[6,13–15]

Pathogenesis and histologic features

The tumor is characterized by an infiltrate of basaloid cells showing ductular differentiation and set in a dense, often hyalinized, fibrous stroma (Figs 33.177 and 33.178). It is usually centered in the mid-dermis, and contact with or origin from the epidermis is uncommon. The tumor is typically deeply invasive and often extends to the subcutaneous fat, fascia or skeletal muscle. In some examples, the infiltrate is intimately associated with eccrine sweat glands and ducts.

The epithelial cells are small with oval hyperchromatic nuclei, ill-defined pale cytoplasm, and indistinct cell membranes. They are arranged in narrow cords and, in addition to duct formation, are sometimes associated with the development of cysts (Figs 33.179 and 33.180). Pleomorphism is not usually marked and mitotic activity is low. Intracytoplasmic glycogen is occasionally present. The lumen sometimes contains diastase-resistant, PAS-positive material. Rarely, the tumor epithelium may show striking vacuolation due to glycogen accumulation reminiscent of clear cell syringoma (Fig. 33.181).[4,7,10,16] Tadpole-like forms are sometimes evident, but squamous differentiation and cribriform patterns are generally not present (Fig. 33.182). In addition, keratocysts and features of follicular differentiation are absent. Infiltration of the perineural sheath is a common feature and undoubtedly contributes to the tumor's tendency to recurrence (Fig. 33.183).

Histochemically, syringoid eccrine carcinoma shows abundant phosphorylase, acid phosphatase, and succinic dehydrogenase activity.[2] Immunohistochemically, the tumor cells express high and low molecular weight keratin, EMA, CEA, and occasionally S100 protein (Fig. 33.184).[9,10,14,16–18] The ducts can be highlighted by EMA and/or CEA immunohistochemistry. In our experience, both of these antibodies should be included in the panel, as the staining characteristics of these tumors are quite variable.

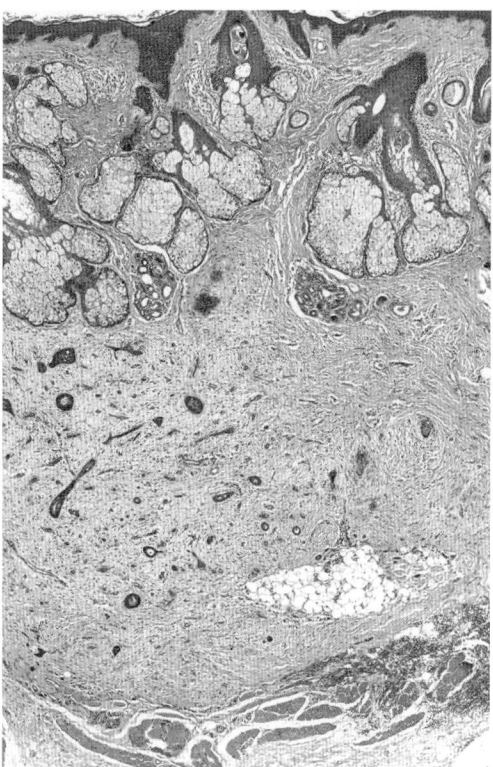

Fig. 33.177
Syringoid eccrine carcinoma: this is a tumor on the face. Note the darkly stained epithelium epithelial strands and cysts within the fibrosed dermis. The tumor extends to the skeletal muscle.

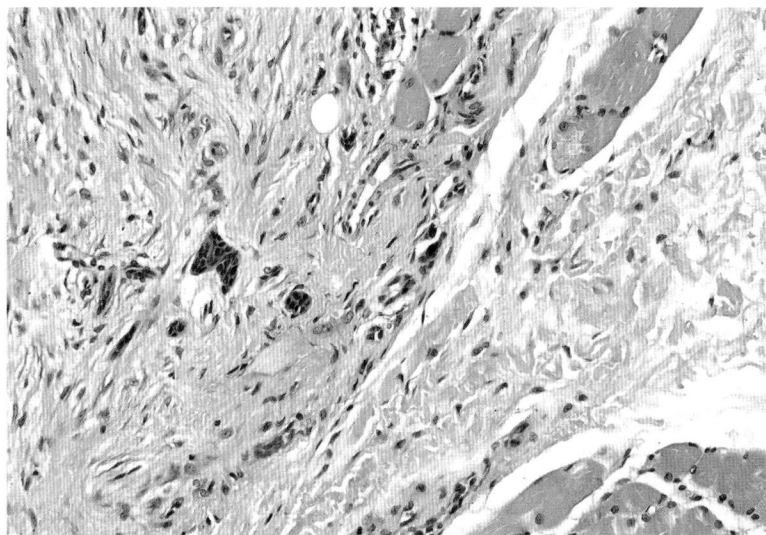

Fig. 33.178
Syringoid eccrine carcinoma: there is superficial involvement of the muscle.

Differential diagnosis

Syringoid eccrine carcinoma can be distinguished from microcystic adnexal carcinoma and adenoid cystic carcinoma by the absence of keratocysts, follicular differentiation, and cribriform morphology. It should, however, be noted that distinction is not always clear-cut and that on occasions typical sclerosing eccrine carcinoma may recur with focal cribriform features reminiscent of adenoid cystic carcinoma. It differs from basal cell carcinoma by the lack of retraction artifact and peripheral palisading and by the presence of EMA and CEA positivity. Basal cell carcinoma may rarely show ductal differentiation, but in our experience this finding is limited to nodular variants where there is no diagnostic difficulty. In those tumors unassociated with evidence of origin, the possibility of metastasis may have to

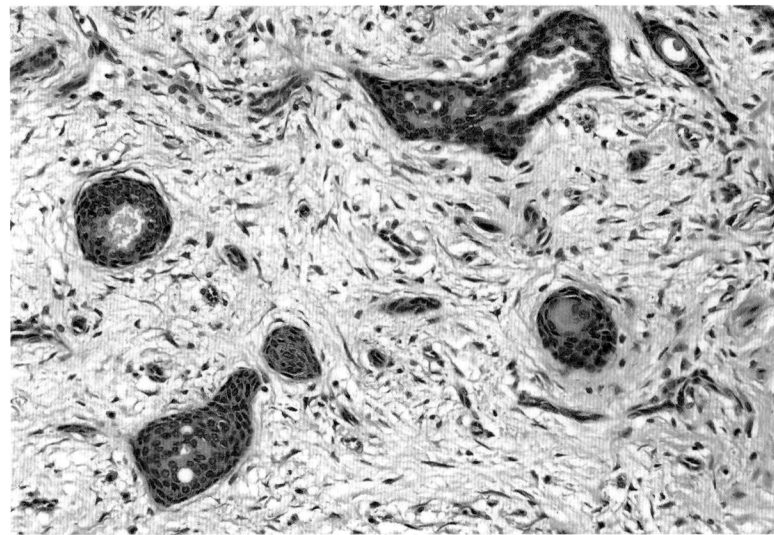

Fig. 33.179
Syringoid eccrine carcinoma: ductal differentiation, as shown in this field, is invariably present.

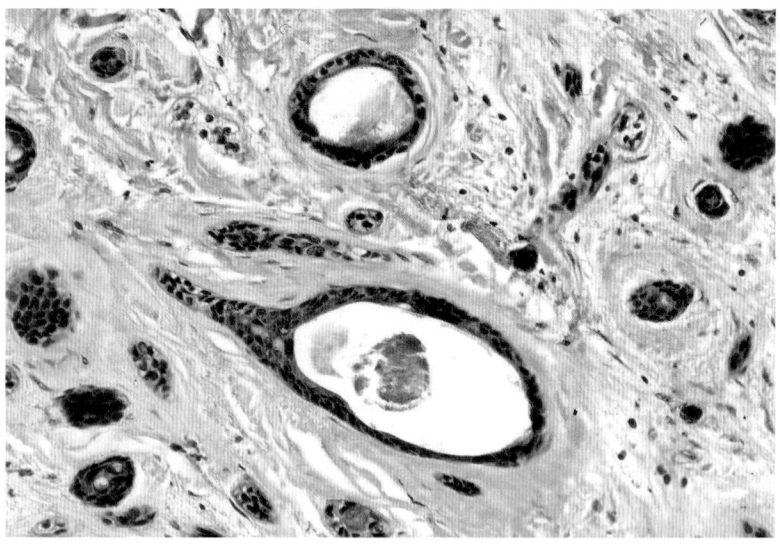

Fig. 33.182
Syringoid eccrine carcinoma: a 'tadpole' morphology reminiscent of syringoma is often seen.

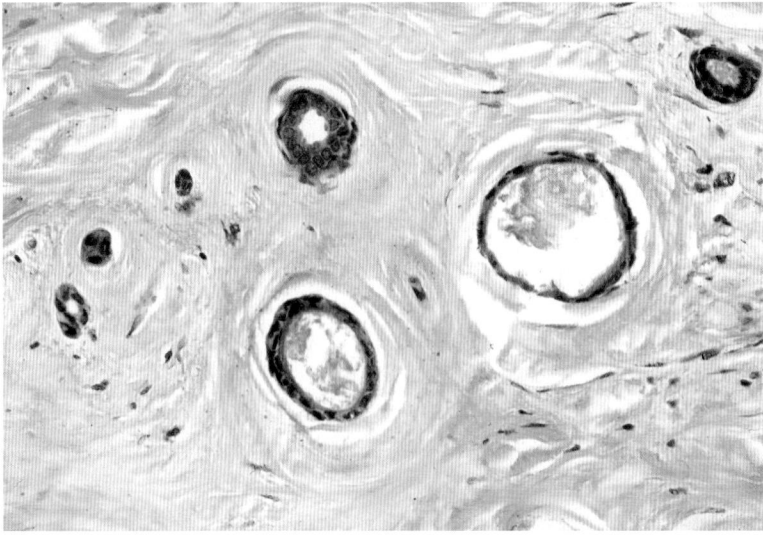

Fig. 33.180
Syringoid eccrine carcinoma: cysts are commonly seen.

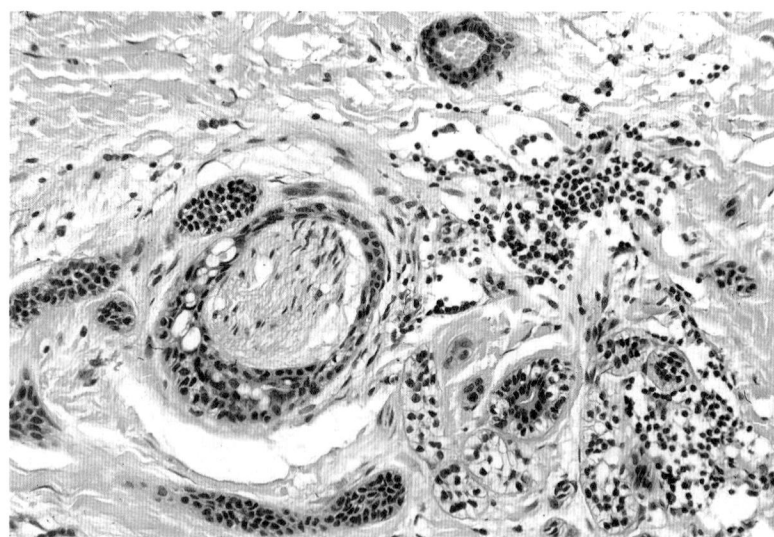

Fig. 33.183
Syringoid eccrine carcinoma: perineural infiltration is a common feature and in part accounts for the high recurrence rate.

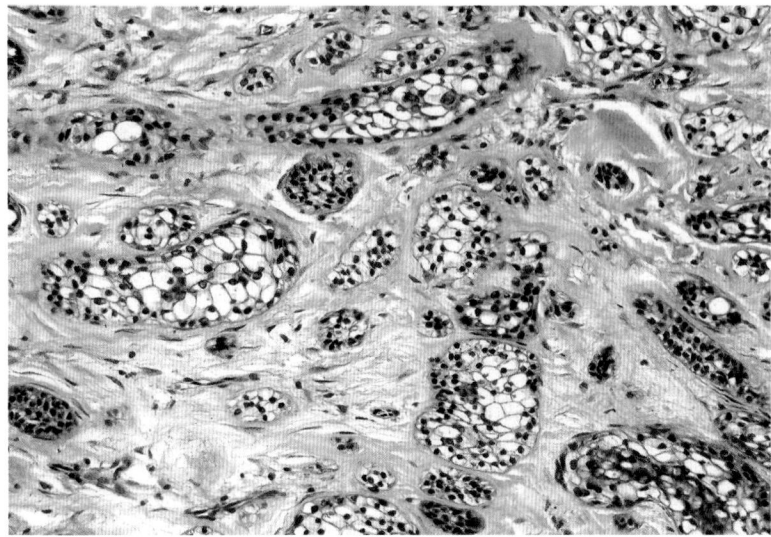

Fig. 33.181
Syringoid eccrine carcinoma: occasionally abundant intracytoplasmic glycogen results in this clear cell variant.

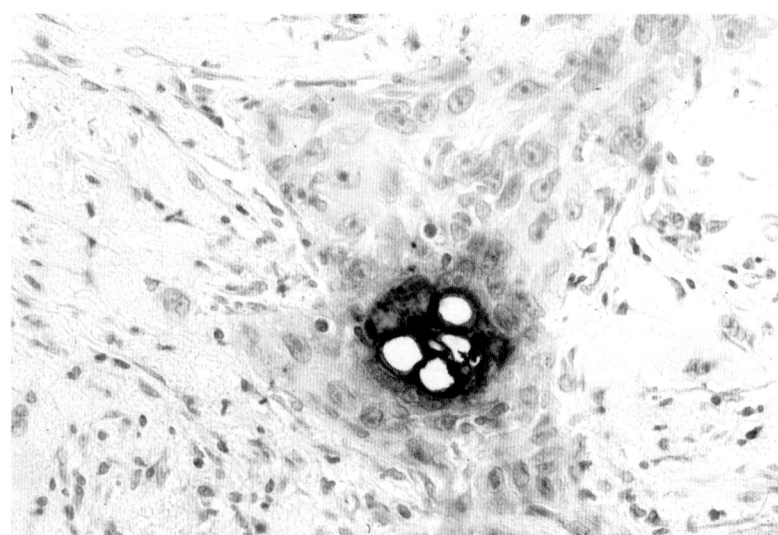

Fig. 33.184
Syringoid eccrine carcinoma: in this example, the ductal epithelium shows CEA expression.

be excluded by clinical investigation. The lack of expression of CK20 and GCDFP-15 may be of diagnostic help.[17,18]

Microcystic adnexal carcinoma

Clinical features

Microcystic adnexal carcinoma (sclerosing sweat duct (syringomatous) carcinoma, malignant syringoma, sweat gland carcinoma with syringomatous features, locally aggressive adnexal carcinoma, combined adnexal tumor) is a locally aggressive malignant adnexal tumor displaying sweat duct and follicular differentiation.[1-7] It is rare and, due to a combination of lack of familiarity and inadequate small punch or shave biopsies, it is frequently initially misdiagnosed, with potential serious consequences for the patient. The tumor is characteristically very indolent, with some examples having been present for decades before diagnosis.[6]

While there is a female preponderance in some series, overall the sexes are affected equally. The tumor presents in a wide age range (6–90 years) although the majority of patients are in their fifties or sixties.[8-10] There are very occasional reports of lesions arising in children.[11,12] The head (particularly the nasolabial and periorbital regions) is involved most often (*Figs 33.185* and *33.186*).[3,8,13-15] Lesions on the neck and scalp are uncommon, and the trunk, axilla, and breast are only rarely affected.[6,16-18] The left side of the face has been noted to be predominantly affected in two series, but this has not been confirmed in other reports.[6,19] Tumors have also been rarely described on the buttock, palm, toe, and vulva.[7,20] An orbital variant and an example arising in the tongue have recently been reported.[21-23]

The tumor presents as a slow-growing, flesh-colored, yellow or erythematous, firm or hard plaque or nodule, which may be associated with hyperkeratosis. Sometimes a central dell is evident. The margins are typically difficult to delineate. Indeed, the findings at surgery almost invariably disclose that the tumor extends several centimeters beyond the clinically visible lesion. Ulceration is unusual. Most tumors measure between 0.5 and 2.0 cm in diameter, but occasionally very large examples are encountered, measuring up to 12 cm in greatest dimension.[6,12] Although lesions are often asymptomatic, patients sometimes have pain, burning, or paresthesia due to perineural infiltration.[9,24] While the tumor has been predominantly reported in Caucasians, there is a small number of case reports documenting presentation in blacks, and a large series of Japanese patients has been reported.[7,25-27]

Microcystic adnexal carcinoma is an aggressive neoplasm often associated with considerable tissue destruction. With inadequate excision, recurrences are common, occurring in 30% to 40% of cases.[8,13] More recent series (particularly in patients following Mohs' surgery) have described low or even zero recurrence rates.[12,28,29] There is a small number of cases with associated local lymph node metastases.[14,30-34] Systemic spread and tumor-associated mortality is very exceptional.[35,36]

Pathogenesis and histologic features

In most cases, the etiology is unknown, but a small number of tumors have followed therapeutic cutaneous irradiation.[6,9,12,37-40] Other factors of possible importance include ultraviolet light and immunodeficiency.[31,41] There is one report documenting familial incidence in two sisters.[6] One or two tumors appear to have arisen within a pre-existent organoid nevus.[42,43] While the majority of tumors arise on sun-exposed skin, unlike squamous cell carcinoma, there is little evidence to suggest that p53 mutation is of any pathogenetic importance.[8,44]

The histogenesis of microcystic adnexal carcinoma remains uncertain. Although some authors believe that it shows only eccrine differentiation, others – on the basis of keratin immunohistochemistry and morphological features (see below) – postulate dual follicular and sweat gland differentiation.[1,8,45,46] The occasional finding of decapitation secretion and sebaceous differentiation has led some authors to propose derivation from the folliculosebaceous-apocrine unit.[46]

The tumor is poorly circumscribed, usually deeply infiltrating, and uncommonly shows an epidermal origin or connection with hair follicles. It expresses a constellation of features including numerous small to medium-sized keratocysts, usually superficially located and merging into

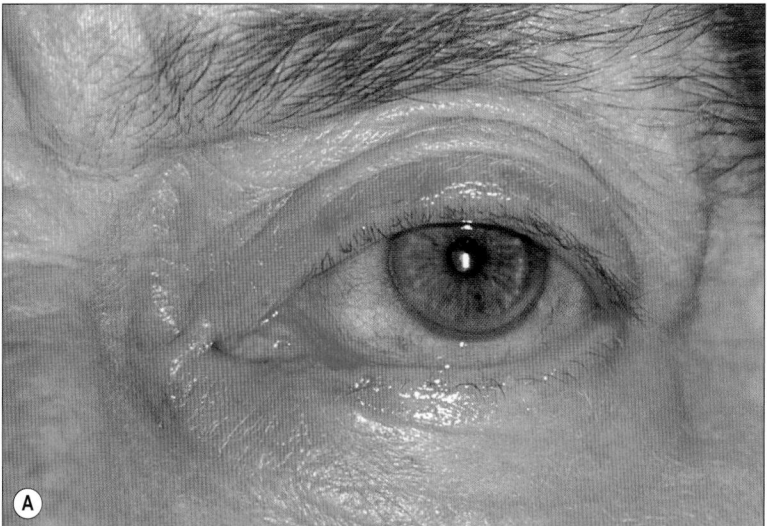

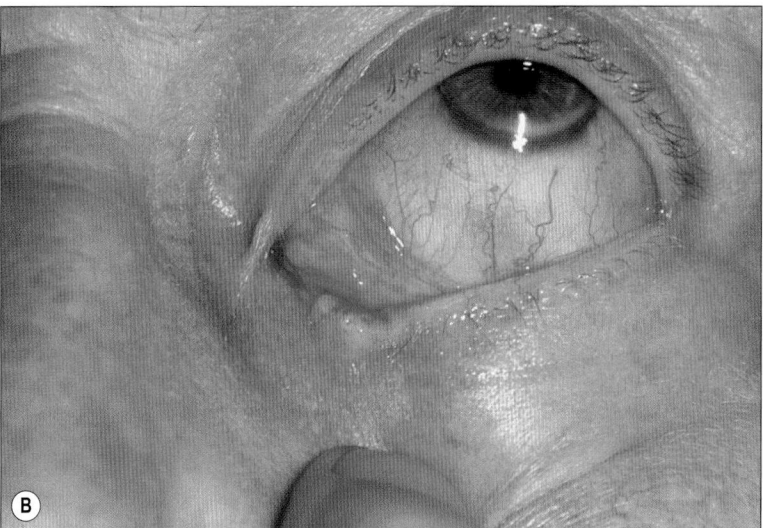

Fig. 33.186
(**A, B**) Microcystic adnexal carcinoma: there is a yellow ulcerated tumor on the lower eyelid near the inner canthus. By courtesy of J.M. Oliver, MD, Western Eye Hospital, London, UK.

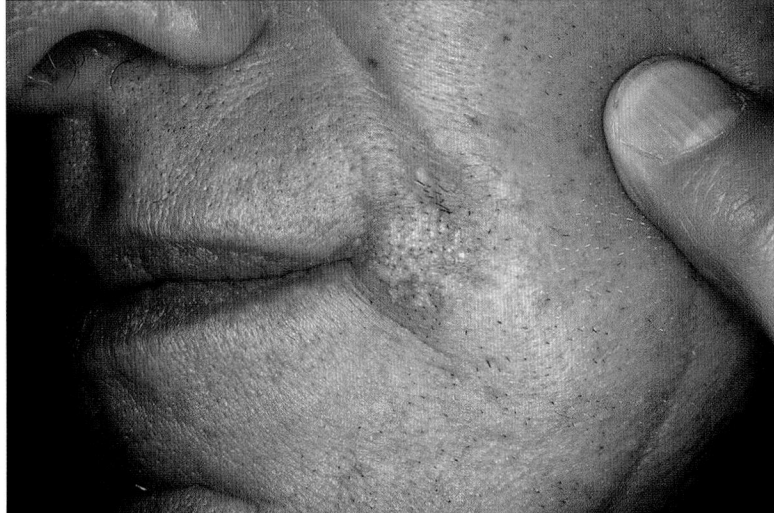

Fig. 33.185
Microcystic adnexal carcinoma: a scaly, erythematous swelling is present at the angle of the mouth. By courtesy of D. McGibbon, MD, Institute of Dermatology, London, UK.

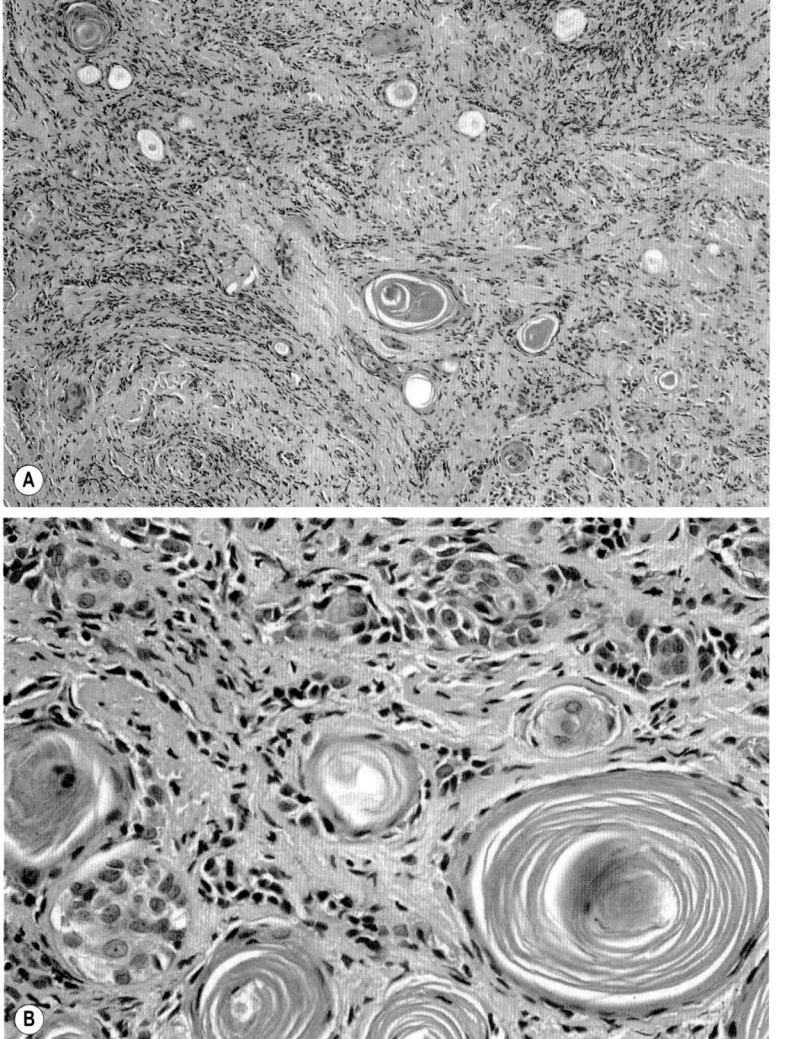

Fig. 33.187
Microcystic adnexal carcinoma: (**A**) the dermis is widely infiltrated by a tumor characterized superficially by the presence of keratocysts; (**B**) the latter typically show epidermoid keratinization.

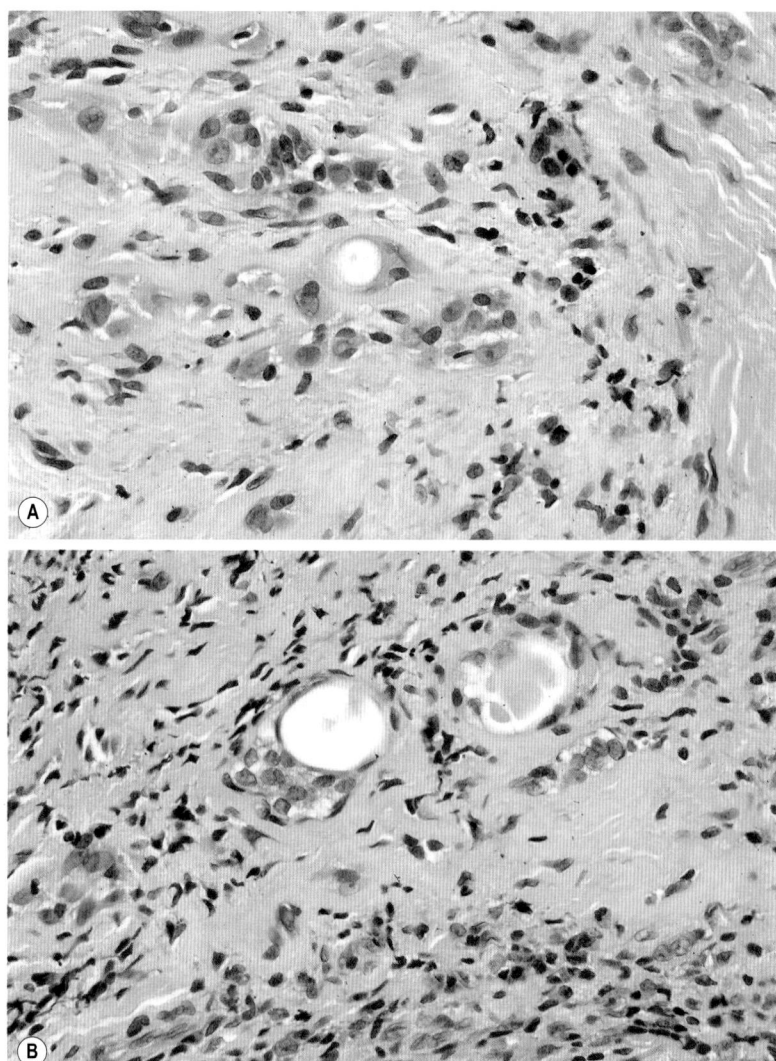

Fig. 33.188
(**A**, **B**) Microcystic adnexal carcinoma: the deeper component consists of narrow epithelial strands and small ductules.

smaller cysts, and solid strands of cells, many showing ductular lumina (*Fig. 33.187*).[1,3,24] In some examples, a tadpole-like morphology as seen in syringoma is a feature.[43] Very occasionally, the cyst contents are calcified. The deeper component consists of small solid strands with a highly infiltrative growth pattern (*Fig. 33.188*). Intracytoplasmic lumina are typically present and are a major diagnostic feature. A dense fibrous stroma surrounds all components and becomes more sclerotic in the infiltrative areas (*Fig. 33.189*). The subcutaneous fat and skeletal muscle are commonly affected. Invasion of bone has been documented in 13% of cases.[9,47–49] Perineural invasion is frequently observed (*Fig. 33.190*). Cytological atypia is rare and mitoses are uncommon. Glycogen-rich clear cells suggestive of external root sheath differentiation may be a feature, and occasionally large basaloid nodules with variable peripheral palisading reminiscent of trichoblastoma are present (*Figs 33.191–33.193*).[1,3,16,43,50,51] Shadow cells have also been described.[8] Sebaceous gland and duct (cuticular) differentiation has rarely been documented.[8,50] Apocrine-type decapitation secretion has been occasionally reported.[43]

Ultrastructural studies confirm the presence of ductal differentiation.[52]

With immunohistochemistry, the tumor cells express AE1/AE3 and EMA.[43,45] The latter is valuable for highlighting ductal differentiation or intracytoplasmic lumen formation as is CEA (*Fig. 33.194*).[38,43,45–47,52] In our experience, both of these antibodies should always be included in the panel, as the staining pattern is very variable. In addition, diastase–PAS may also

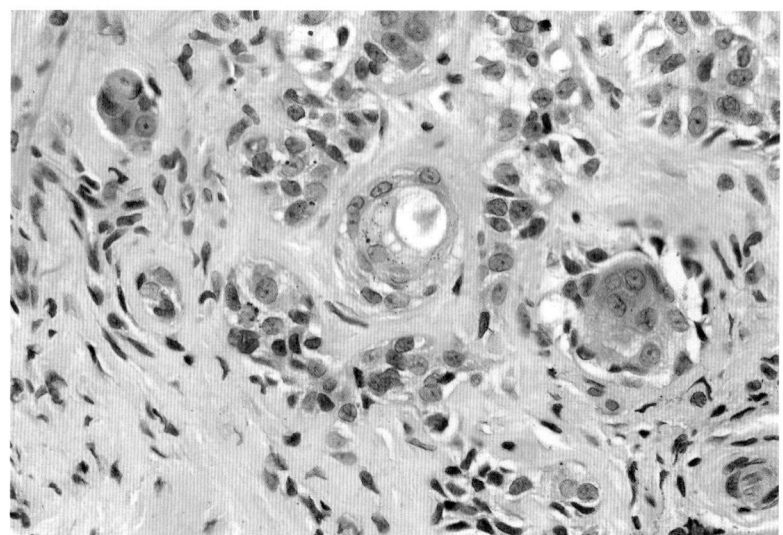

Fig. 33.189
Microcystic adnexal carcinoma: in this field, the stroma is hyalinized and has compressed the epithelial component. Note the ductal differentiation. This aspect of the tumor histology overlaps with eccrine epithelioma.

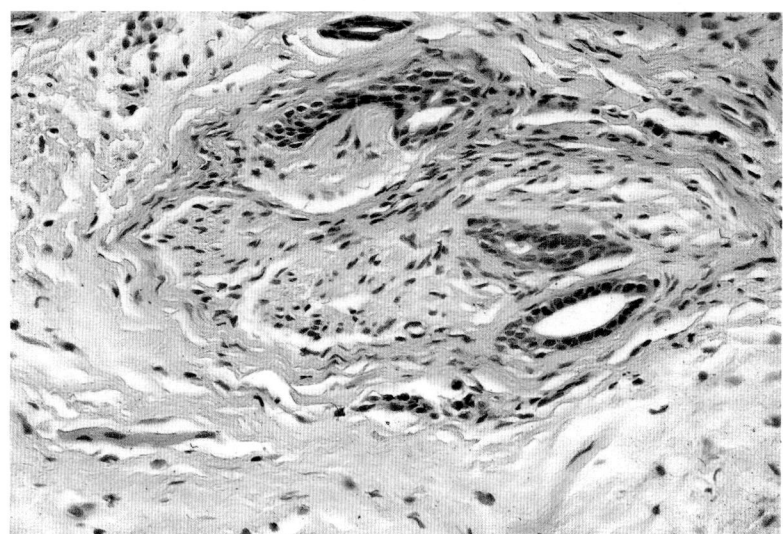

Fig. 33.190
Microcystic adnexal carcinoma: the tumor has infiltrated a nerve fiber.

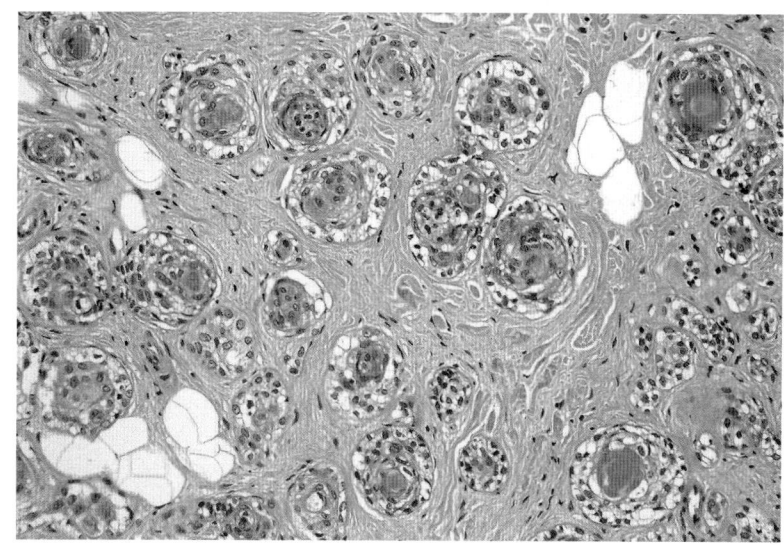

Fig. 33.191
Microcystic adnexal carcinoma: there is marked cytoplasmic vacuolation due to glycogen accumulation. Pilar keratinization is evident.

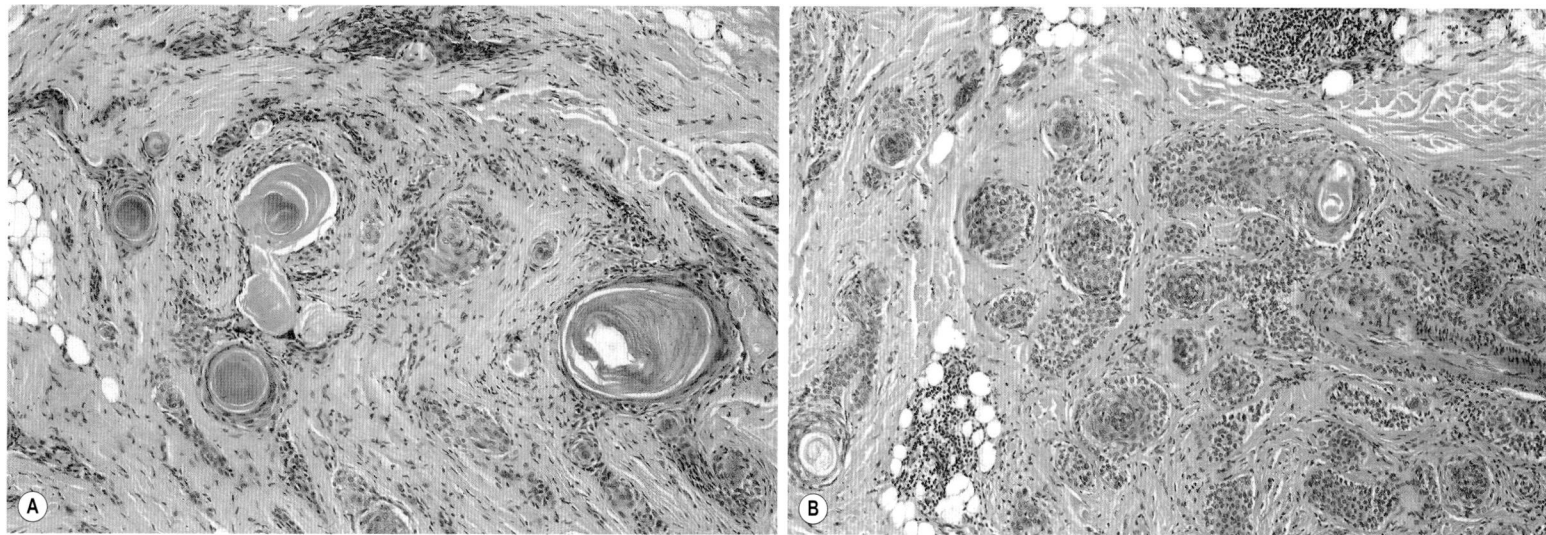

Fig. 33.192
Microcystic adnexal carcinoma: (A) in this field, the tumor shows typical features with conspicuous keratocysts; (B) elsewhere, there are discrete nodules of basaloid cells with peripheral palisading reminiscent of trichoblastoma.

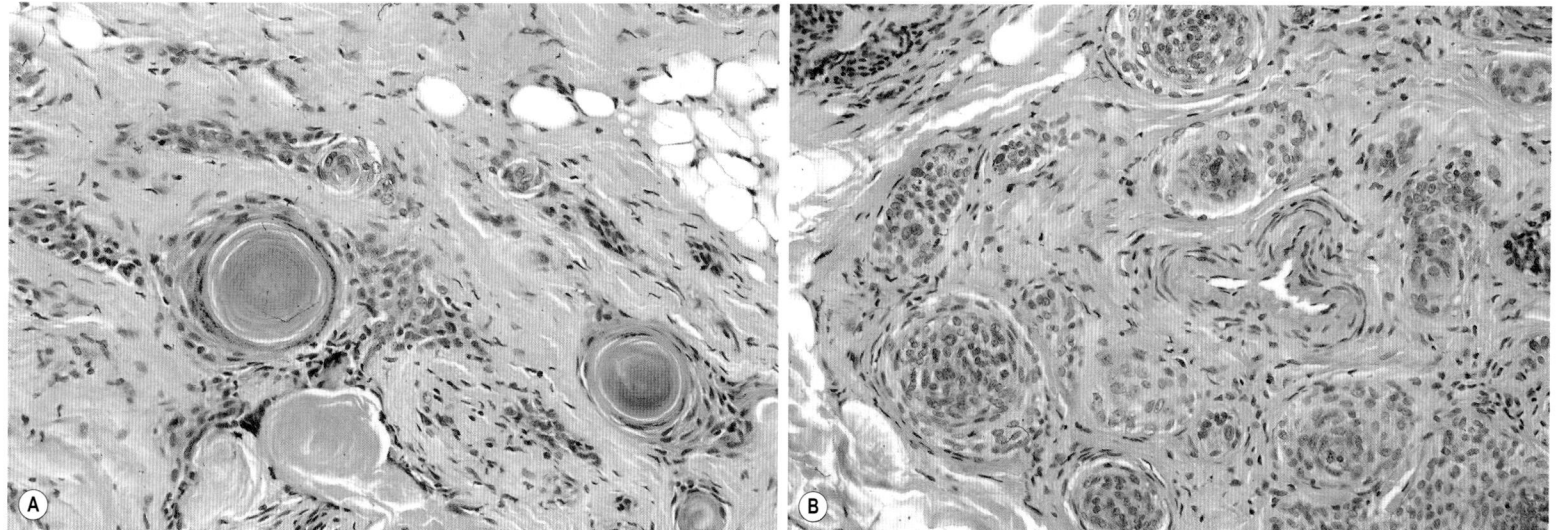

Fig. 33.193
(A, B) Microcystic adnexal carcinoma: high-power views of Fig. 29.186.

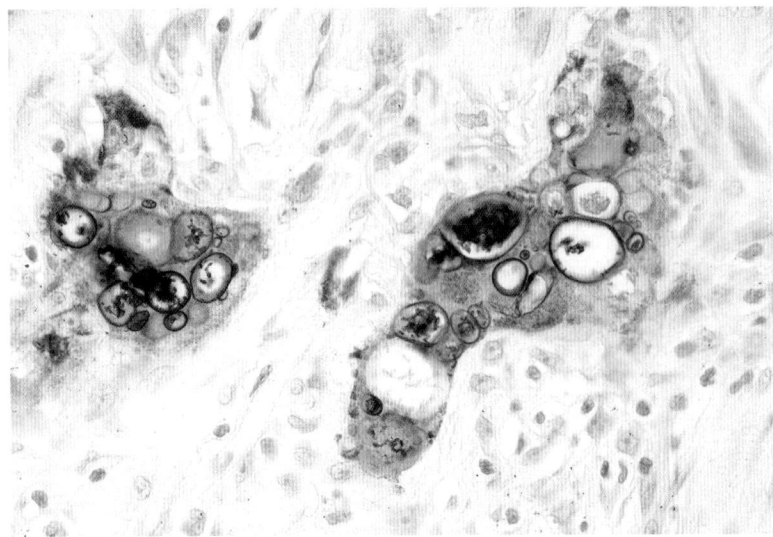

Fig. 33.194
Microcystic adnexal carcinoma: the ducts and intracytoplasmic lumina can be outlined by EMA and CEA immunohistochemistry (EMA).

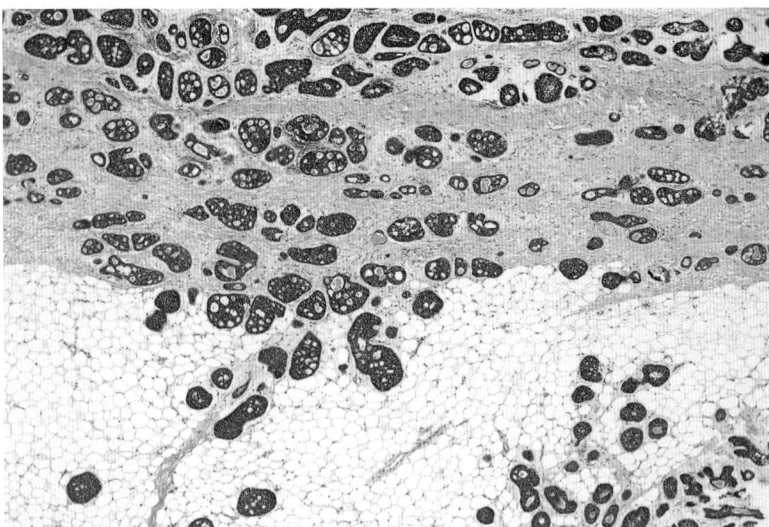

Fig. 33.195
Primary cutaneous adenoid cystic carcinoma: the tumor is composed of basophilic epithelium forming cords and ductular structures.

be of value in this context. S100 protein is negative. In support of follicular differentiation, the tumor expresses hard keratin (AE13 and AE14).[8,45] LeuM1 is also positive, and CK15 as well as Ber-EP4 expression may be observed.[39,53,54] Microcystic adnexal carcinoma shows a low proliferation rate as determined by MIB-1 immunohistochemistry.[8]

Differential diagnosis

Microcystic adnexal carcinoma must be distinguished from desmoplastic trichoepithelioma, trichoadenoma, syringoma, morpheaform basal cell carcinoma, and desmoplastic squamous cell carcinoma.[55]

- Microcystic adnexal carcinoma differs from desmoplastic trichoepithelioma by its deep and infiltrative growth pattern, perineural infiltration, and presence of ductal differentiation. These same features exclude trichoadenoma.
- Superficial biopsies may be difficult to distinguish from syringoma. The presence of keratocysts, mild nuclear atypia, and mitoses argues strongly against this diagnosis.
- Morpheaform basal cell carcinoma and desmoplastic squamous cell carcinoma are excluded on the basis of ductal differentiation and intracytoplasmic lumen formation. Although basal cell carcinoma may rarely show evidence of ductal differentiation, in our experience this occurs in nodular variants, when the correct diagnosis should be obvious.

Primary cutaneous adenoid cystic carcinoma

Clinical features

Primary cutaneous adenoid cystic carcinoma is a rare primary tumor of skin, with only around 100 cases having been described in the English literature.[1–15] Much more commonly, it is a tumor of the salivary glands and bronchus and may also arise within the breast, esophagus, cervix, prostate, vulva, and lacrimal and ceruminous glands.[2] The tumor shows a roughly equal gender distribution, affecting middle age or older (mean age 58 years), and it presents as a slowly growing, 0.5–8.0 cm in diameter crusted plaque or nodule, often of long duration.[6,14] Although a wide variety of sites may be affected, at least 40% have arisen on the scalp.[2] The breasts, back, and abdomen are also more often affected.[6] Perineal involvement is unusual.[11]

Primary adenoid cystic carcinoma of the skin is a much less aggressive tumor than its systemic counterpart. This is reflected by the fact that most cutaneous lesions are grade I. Although recurrence of the tumor is likely (57–70%), metastases to lymph nodes and the lung are relatively uncommon.[6,14–25] This contrasts with the approximately 50% metastasis rate of the salivary gland variant.[18] The high recurrence rate is a reflection

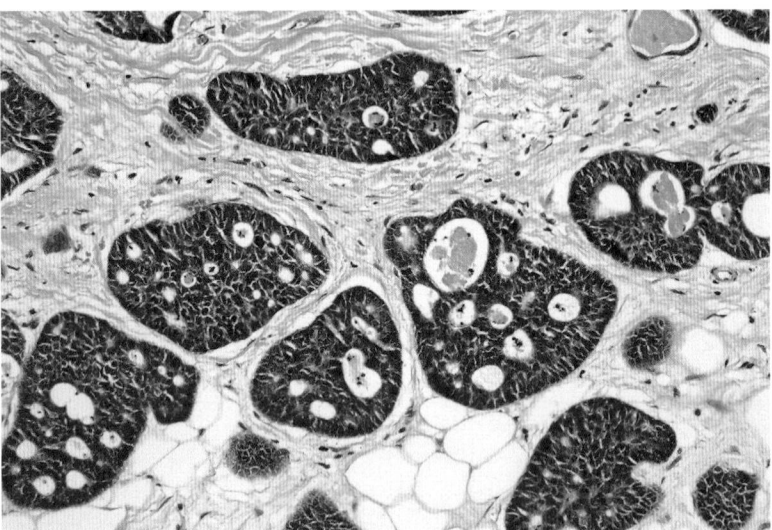

Fig. 33.196
Primary cutaneous adenoid cystic carcinoma: in this field, there is ductal differentiation and a focal cribriform pattern.

of the frequent presence of infiltration of the perineural space. Long-term follow-up is essential as presentation of recurrent tumor may be delayed for many years or even decades.

Cutaneous adenoid cystic carcinoma may also represent direct extension from an underlying salivary gland primary neoplasm.[26] Metastasis from a more distant site has been documented exceptionally rarely.[27–30]

Pathogenesis and histologic features

The histogenesis of this tumor is uncertain, and while some authors have argued apocrine derivation, citing the example of ceruminous gland variants (the ceruminous gland is a modified apocrine gland), others (on the basis of enzyme histochemistry) have favored an eccrine derivation.[17,20] Thus, adenoid cystic carcinoma is positive for succinic dehydrogenase and phosphorylase and negative for acid phosphatase and β-glucuronidase.[31]

The tumor has a characteristic basophilic low-power appearance due to nuclear hyperchromatism and crowding. It typically occupies the mid- and deep dermis and often extends into the subcutaneous fat (Fig. 33.195). There is no evidence of an epidermal origin. Adenoid cystic carcinoma is composed of variably sized islands of tumor cells dispersed in a loose fibrous and sometimes mucinous stroma (Fig. 33.196). The epithelium consists of fairly uniform cells with darkly staining nuclei, which sometimes contain

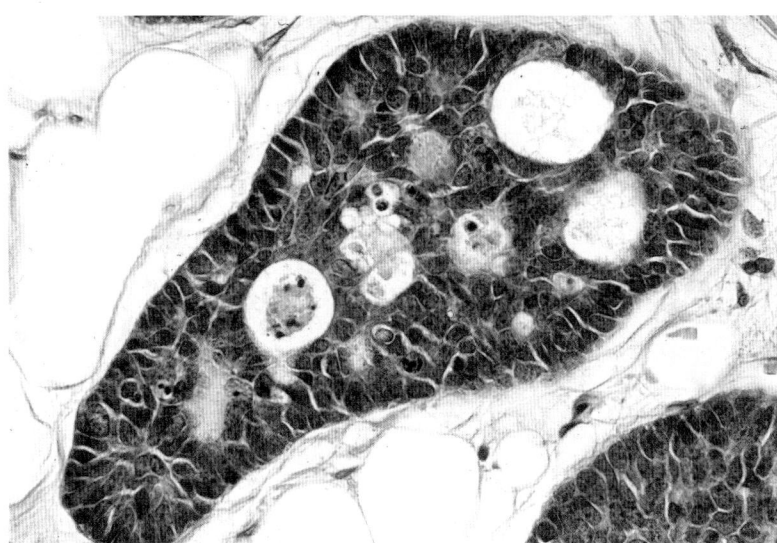

Fig. 33.197
Primary cutaneous adenoid cystic carcinoma: high-power view.

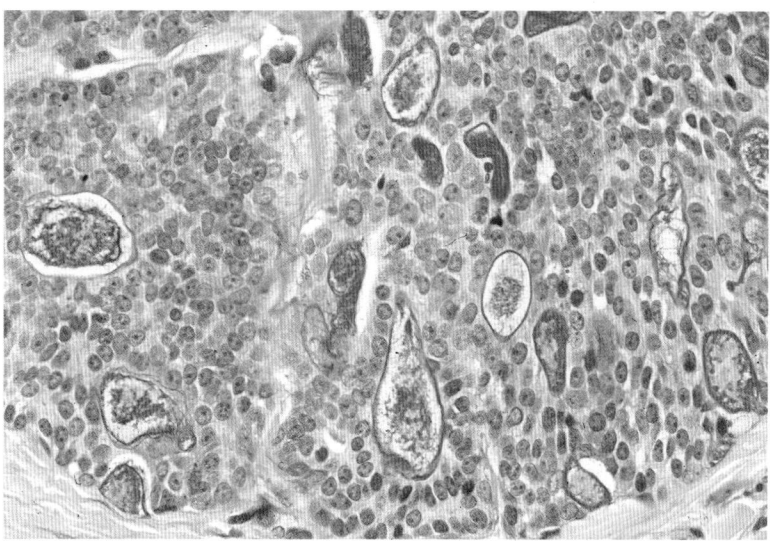

Fig. 33.199
Primary cutaneous adenoid cystic carcinoma: the hyaline membranes are strongly PAS positive (diastase resistant).

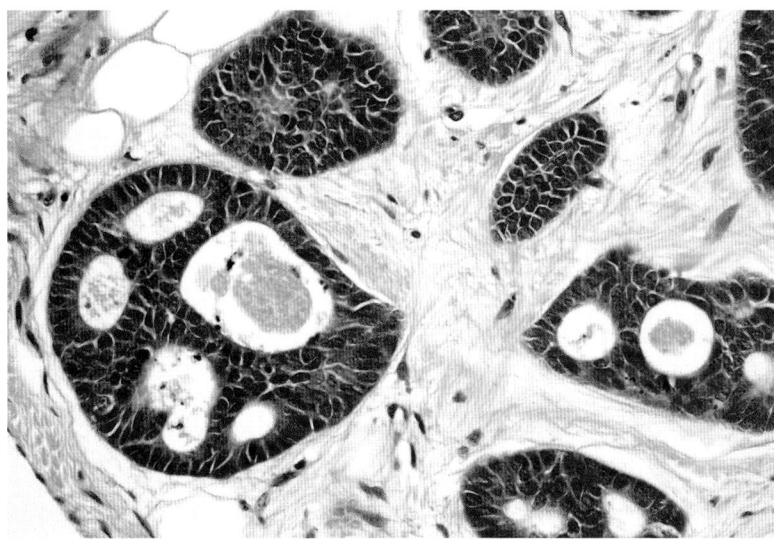

Fig. 33.198
Primary cutaneous adenoid cystic carcinoma: the pseudolumina are lined by thickened hyaline membranes formed from basement membrane constituents, notably type IV collagen and laminin.

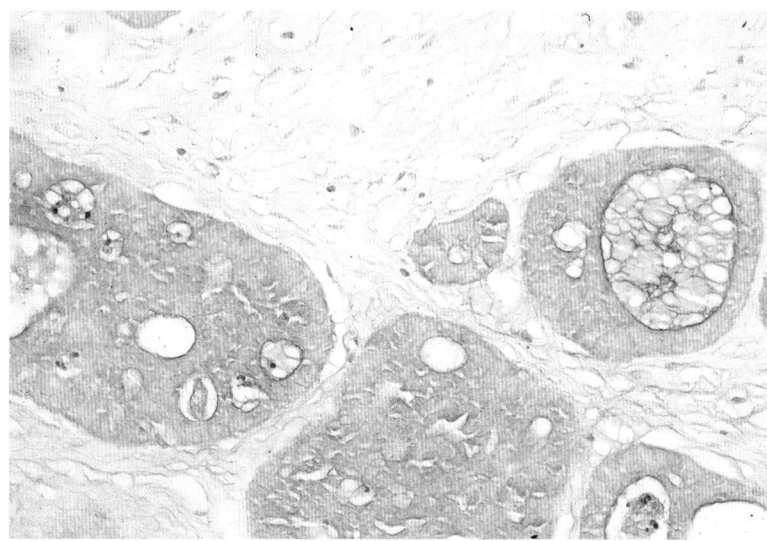

Fig. 33.200
Primary cutaneous adenoid cystic carcinoma: the luminal contents are strongly Alcian blue (pH 2.5) positive.

conspicuous, small, solitary nucleoli. Cytoplasm is minimal. Nuclear palisading is not a feature. Mitotic activity is usually sparse (*Fig. 33.197*).

A typical feature is the presence of excessive diastase-resistant, PAS-positive eosinophilic hyaline basement membrane-like material both between tumor cells and also surrounding individual lobules (*Figs 33.198* and *33.199*). Occasionally, it lines the luminal surface of cystic spaces (pseudolumina). The latter, which contain Alcian blue (pH 2.5)-positive hyaluronic acid and sulfated acid mucin, are a common feature, giving rise to the pathognomonic cribriform appearance (*Fig. 33.200*). Less frequently, tubular and diffuse patterns are encountered.[32] True ductal differentiation associated with mucin secretion is sometimes present. Adenoid cystic carcinoma typically shows an infiltrative border, and perineural spread is common (*Fig. 33.201*).

Immunohistochemically, the tumor cells express low and high molecular weight keratin, S100 protein (80% of cases), SOX10, and SMA, and variably CEA.[6,11,26,27,33] CD117 staining is observed in the majority of cases.[14,33] The presence of ductal differentiation can be confirmed with EMA and CEA (*Fig. 33.202*).[34,35] Ber-EP4 is focally positive and usually restricted to the areas with true ductal differentiation. The basement membrane material is composed of an admixture of collagens IV and V and laminin (*Fig. 33.203*).[31] Similar to adenoid cystic carcinoma of visceral sites, the

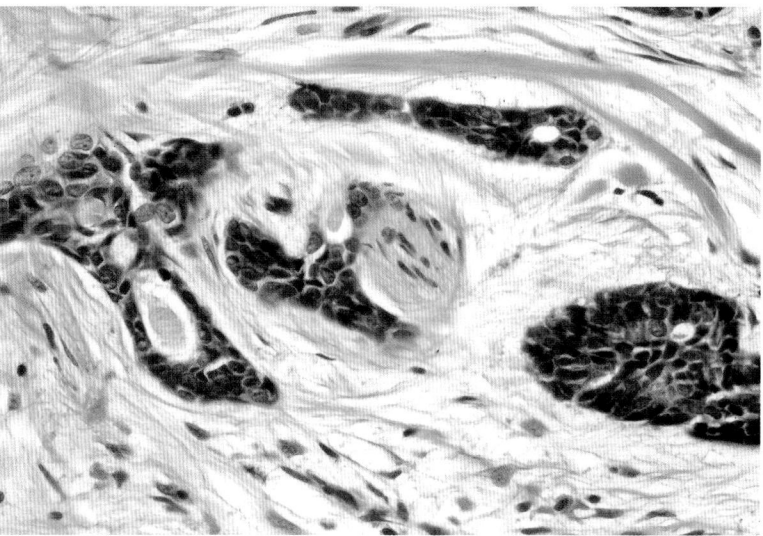

Fig. 33.201
Primary cutaneous adenoid cystic carcinoma: infiltration of the perineural space is a common manifestation.

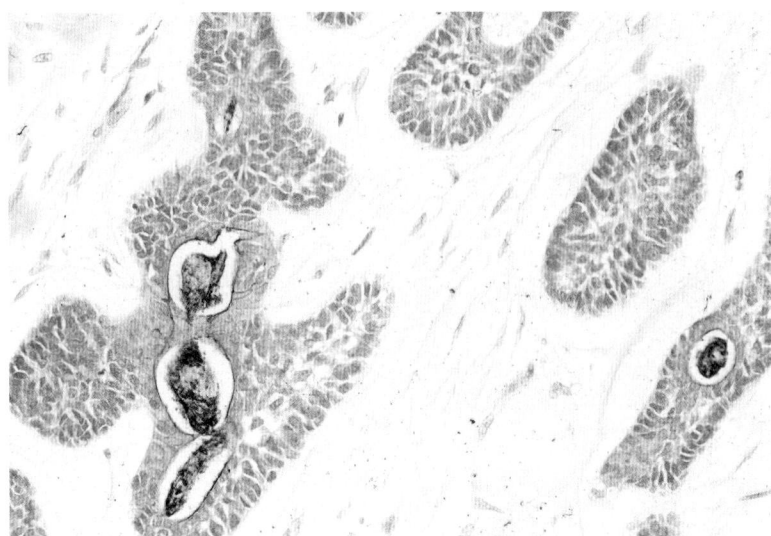

Fig. 33.202
Primary cutaneous adenoid cystic carcinoma: there is striking EMA expression along the luminal border.

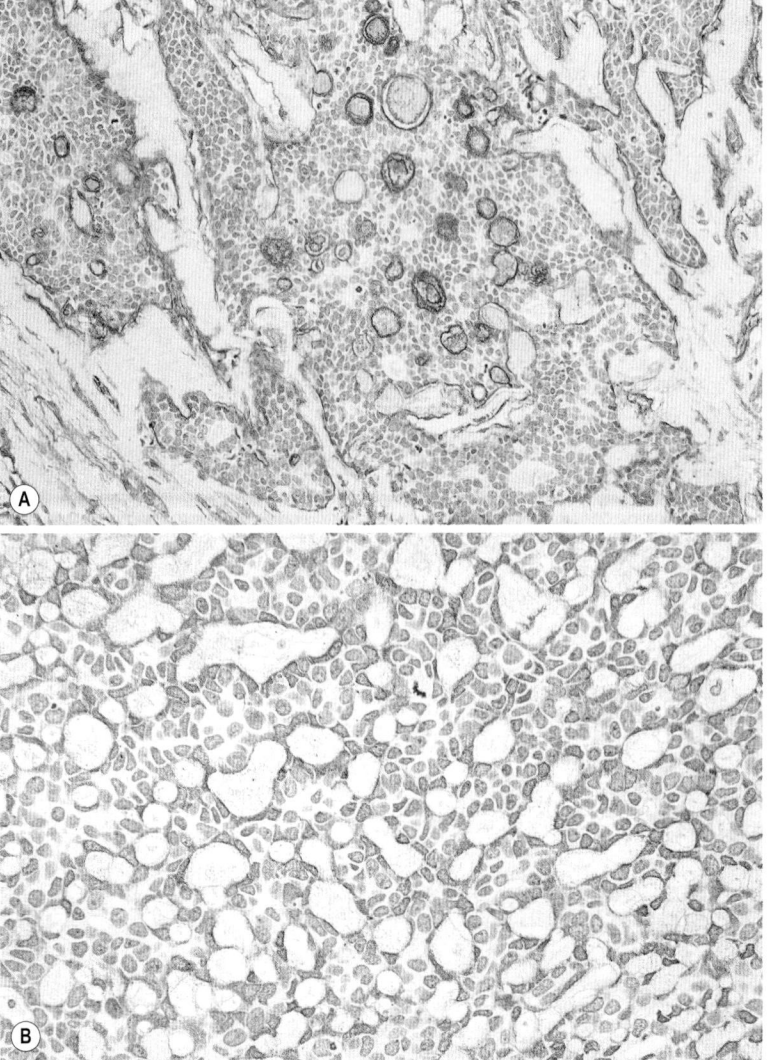

Fig. 33.203
Primary cutaneous adenoid cystic carcinoma: the hyaline membrane lining the pseudolumina is composed of (**A**) type IV collagen and (**B**) laminin.

cutaneous tumors show the characteristic t(6;9) translocation, resulting in the MYB-NFIB fusion gene with MYB activation and overexpression, which can be demonstrated immunohistochemically.[33,36]

Differential diagnosis

Cutaneous adenoid cystic carcinoma may be confused with adenoid basal cell carcinoma, particularly as both produce hyaluronic acid. However, an origin from the epidermis and stromal retraction are not seen in the former, while the latter is typically EMA, CAM 5.2, S100 protein, and CEA negative.[18]

As mentioned above, it must be stressed that direct extension from an underlying salivary gland tumor or metastasis should be excluded before accepting that a cutaneous lesion represents a primary tumor.

Primary cutaneous mucinous carcinoma

Clinical features

Primary mucinous carcinoma (cutaneous adenocystic carcinoma) is a rare neoplasm showing a predilection for the head and neck, particularly the eyelids, but on occasions affecting other sites including the scalp, face, ear, axillae, thorax, abdomen, groin, foot, hand, and vulva.[1-14] It presents as a slowly growing, flesh-colored, erythematous, or blue nodule.[1,5] Size at presentation is very variable, ranging from 0.5 to 8.0 cm in greatest dimension.[14,15] A wide range of ages may be affected (8–89 years), but the tumor particularly develops in the elderly (median age 62 years).[4,14] Primary cutaneous mucinous carcinoma usually follows a rather indolent course. Although it is locally aggressive and commonly recurs (26%), distant metastases are rare and usually only involve the regional lymph nodes.[3,6,7,12–14]

Pathogenesis and histologic features

The tumor is situated in the dermis and often involves the subcutaneous fat. It is compartmentalized by delicate fibrous septa, which enclose a lake of pale-staining mucin, in which are suspended islands of tumor cells (*Figs 33.204* and *33.205*). The latter are cuboidal with pink-staining, sometimes vacuolated cytoplasm, and centrally located round or oval vesicular nuclei (*Fig. 33.206*). Light- and dark-cell forms are occasionally distinguishable.[3] The tumor cells are cohesive. Signet ring forms are rarely a feature and mitoses are usually inconspicuous (*Fig. 33.207*), but decapitation secretion is a not infrequent finding. Rarely, a focal solid pattern is evident. Glandular differentiation is often present and sometimes a cribriform pattern is a feature.[14] An in situ component reminiscent of ductal carcinoma in situ of the breast with cribriform, solid, or micropapillary growth patterns may often be identified.[14] A subset of tumors is characterized by the additional presence of an invasive adenocarcinoma showing a solid or cribriform architecture, and comedo necrosis may be present.[14] Microcalcifications and psammoma body formation may be further features.[14] Foci of hemorrhage are commonly evident, but necrosis is not usually seen.

The mucin is diastase-resistant/PAS positive, hyaluronidase resistant/ Alcian blue positive (pH 2.5) and also stains with mucicarmine and colloidal iron (*Fig. 33.208*).[4] It is sensitive to sialidase, indicating the presence of nonsulfated sialomucin.[4] It is negative with Alcian blue at pH 1 and 0.4.[16]

The tumor cells express AE1/AE3, EMA, and CEA (*Fig. 33.209*).[8,9,16,17] In keeping with a derivation from the secretory lobule, CAM 5.2 is also often present, and tumor cells are CK7 positive but CK20 negative (*Fig. 33.210*).[18,19] S100 protein expression is variable.[8] p53 and c-erbB-2 are not expressed.[16] The tumor shows a low proliferation index with Ki-67.[16] Estrogen and progesterone receptors are positive (*Fig. 33.211*).[16,18,20,21] A rim of myoepithelial cells may be a focal finding which can be confirmed by immunohistochemistry for p63, CK5/6, calponin, and SMA.[14,18,19] Myoepithelial cells are preserved in areas of in situ carcinoma, and the presence of basement membrane material can be highlighted by collage type IV staining.[14] The identification of a myoepithelial component is useful in confirming the cutaneous origin of the tumor.

Neuroendocrine differentiation demonstrated by a positive Grimelius reaction and neuron-specific enolase (NSE), chromogranin, and synaptophysin immunohistochemistry has been described in a small number of cases

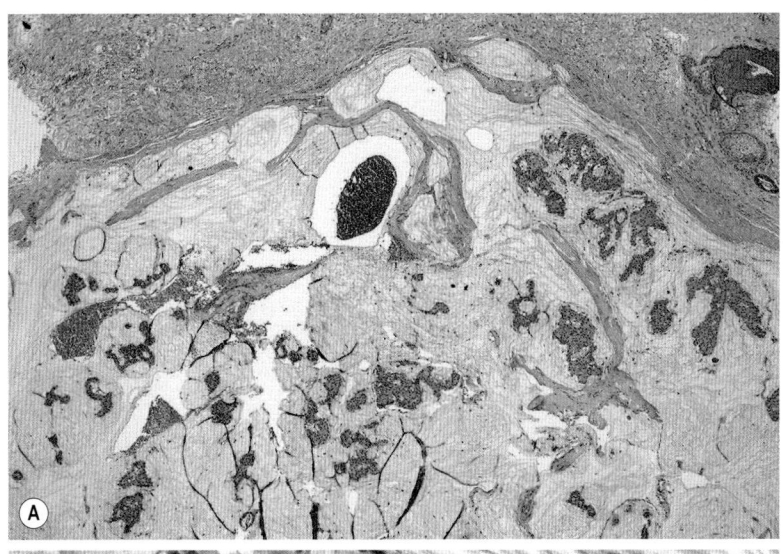

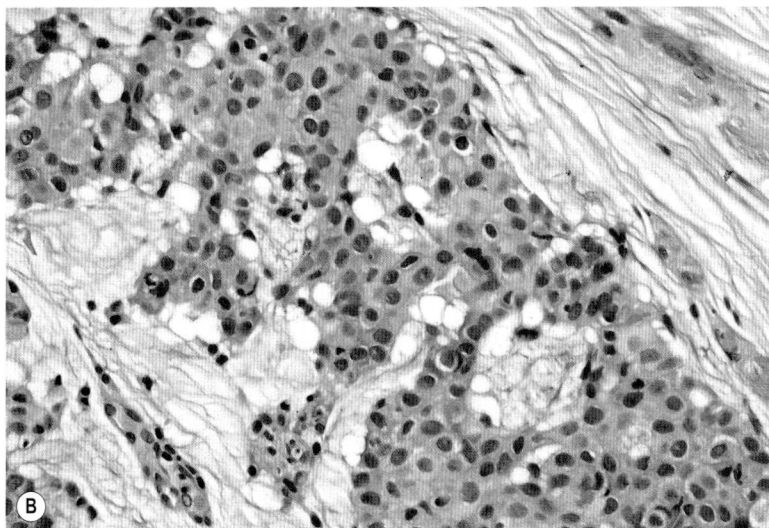

Fig. 33.204
(A, B) Primary cutaneous mucinous carcinoma: the epithelial component is widely dispersed in lakes of mucin.

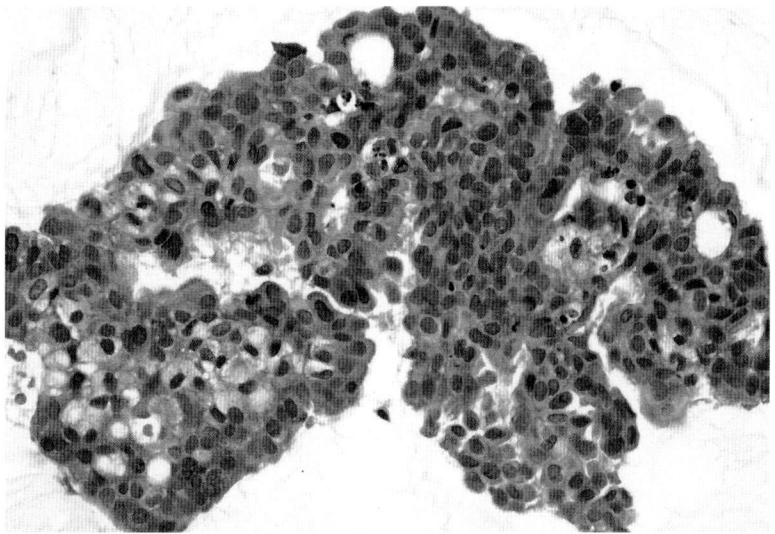

Fig. 33.206
Primary cutaneous mucinous carcinoma: the tumor cells are regular and have eosinophilic cytoplasm and small vesicular nuclei.

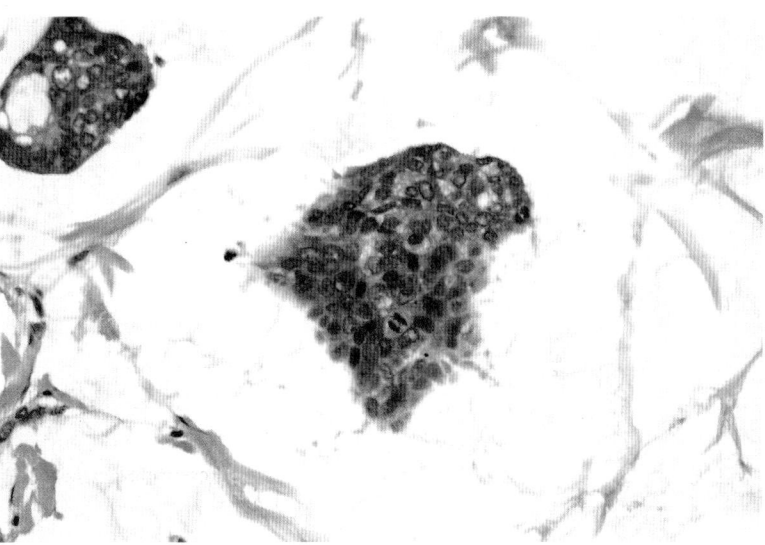

Fig. 33.207
Primary cutaneous mucinous carcinoma: mitotic figures, as seen in the center of the field, are typically sparse.

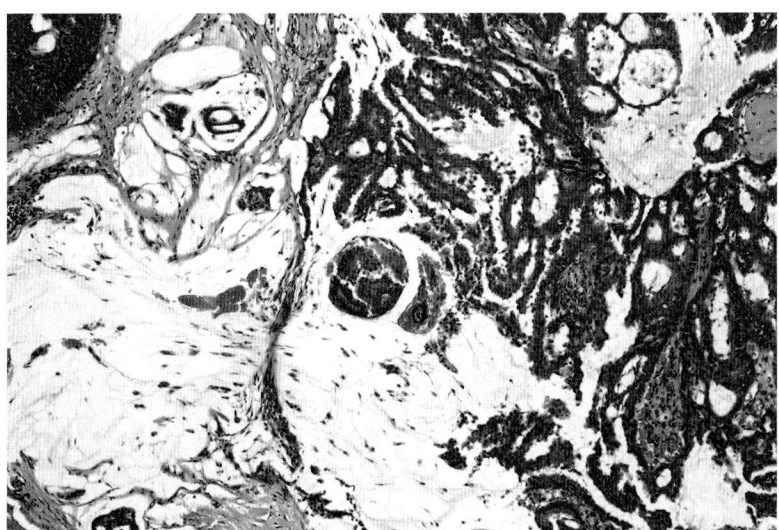

Fig. 33.205
Primary cutaneous mucinous carcinoma: less often the tumor adopts a papillary configuration.

(Figs 33.212 and 33.213).[16,17,20,22] Ultrastructural studies have confirmed the presence of membrane-bound granules.[17,22]

Ultrastructurally, the tumor is composed of an admixture of pale and dark cells, the latter containing mucin droplets.[2,5] Histochemistry supports an eccrine derivation, the tumor cells containing the oxidative enzymes succinic dehydrogenase, lactic dehydrogenase, and isocitric dehydrogenase.[2] Immunohistochemistry in a small number of cases has demonstrated expression of HMFG, GCDFP-15, GCDFP-24, and lysozyme in addition to focal decapitation secretion, suggesting that a subset may be derived from or differentiate toward the apocrine gland.[15,23]

Differential diagnosis

Cutaneous mucinous carcinoma may be histologically indistinguishable from metastatic lesions, particularly of mammary derivation.[24,25] Tumors from the gastrointestinal tract and ovary may also enter the differential diagnosis.[26] The clinical information in most instances will resolve any diagnostic problem. A breast carcinoma is most unlikely to present as a cutaneous metastasis. On the basis of statistics, therefore, a mucinous carcinoma arising on the face (particularly the eyelid) is almost certainly a primary lesion. On the other hand, a tumor presenting on the trunk is more likely to be secondary. Identification of an in situ component which usually requires

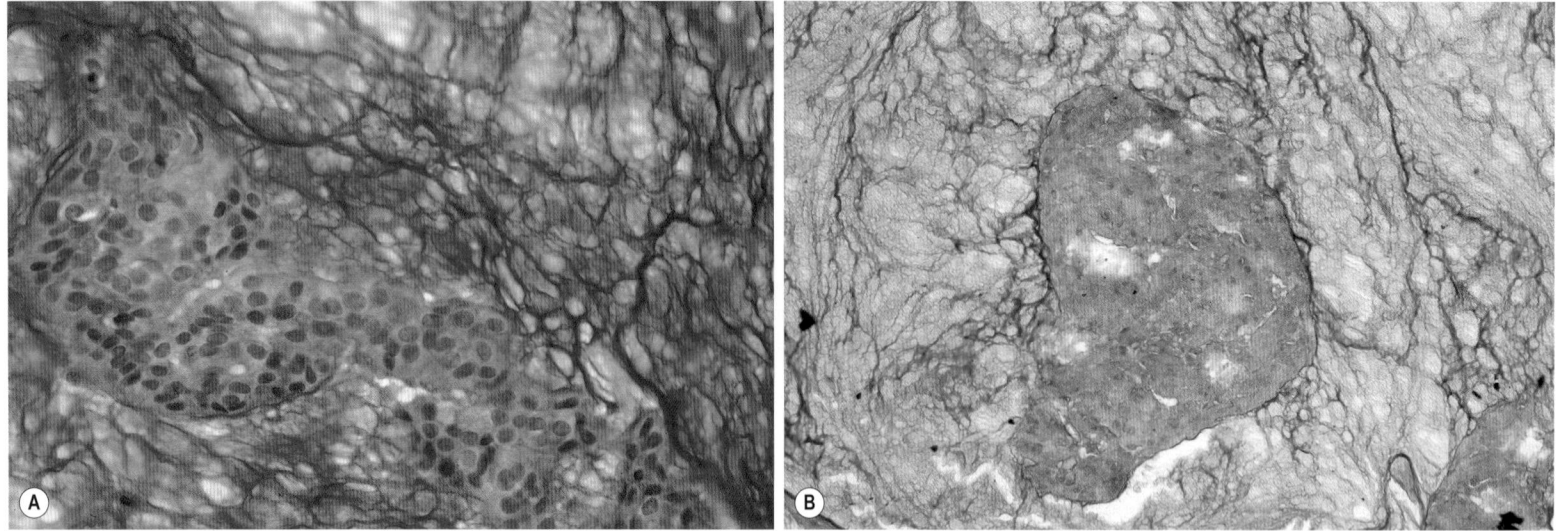

Fig. 33.208
Primary cutaneous mucinous carcinoma: (A) the mucin is PAS positive; (B) it stains with Alcian blue at pH 2.5.

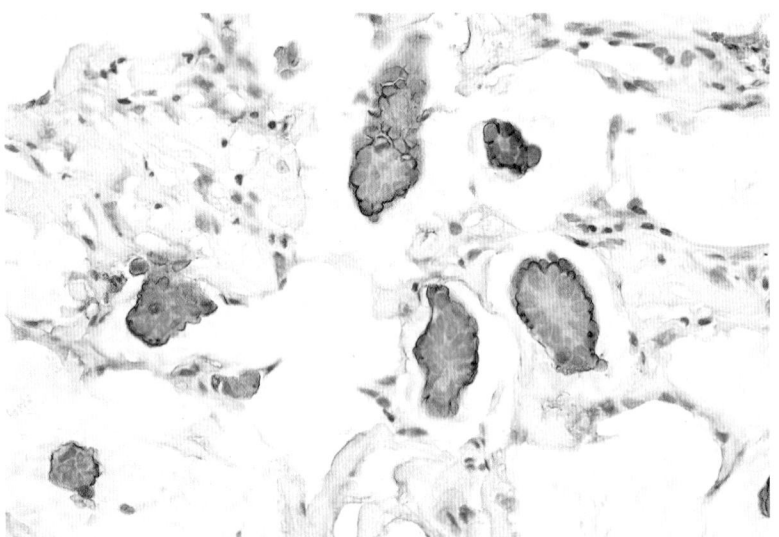

Fig. 33.209
Primary cutaneous mucinous carcinoma: there is prominent membranous labeling with EMA.

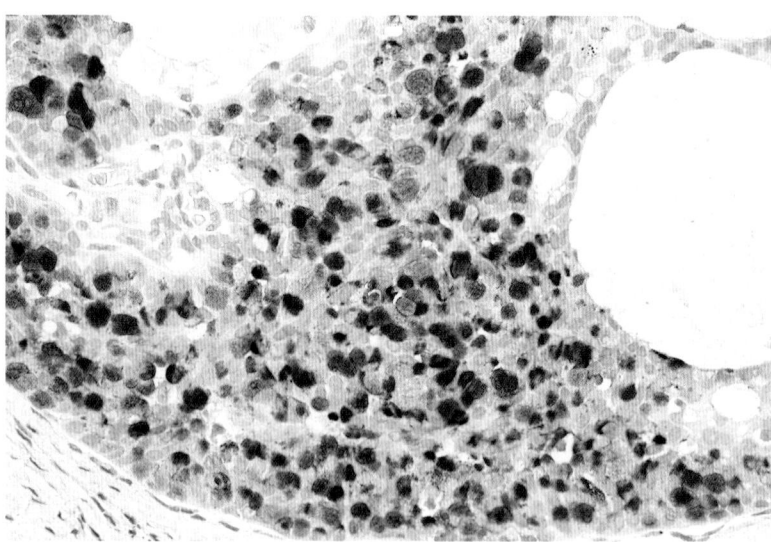

Fig. 33.210
Primary cutaneous mucinous carcinoma: the tumor cells express CAM 5.2.

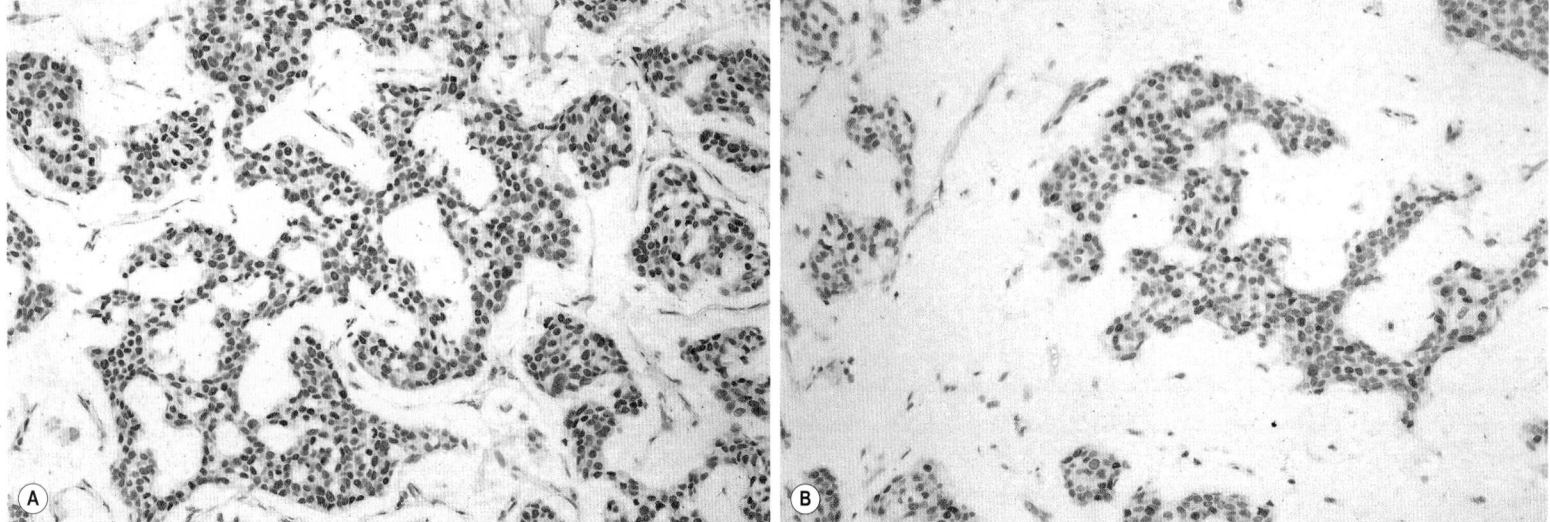

Fig. 33.211
Primary cutaneous mucinous carcinoma: the nuclei are positive for (A) estrogen and (B) progesterone receptors.

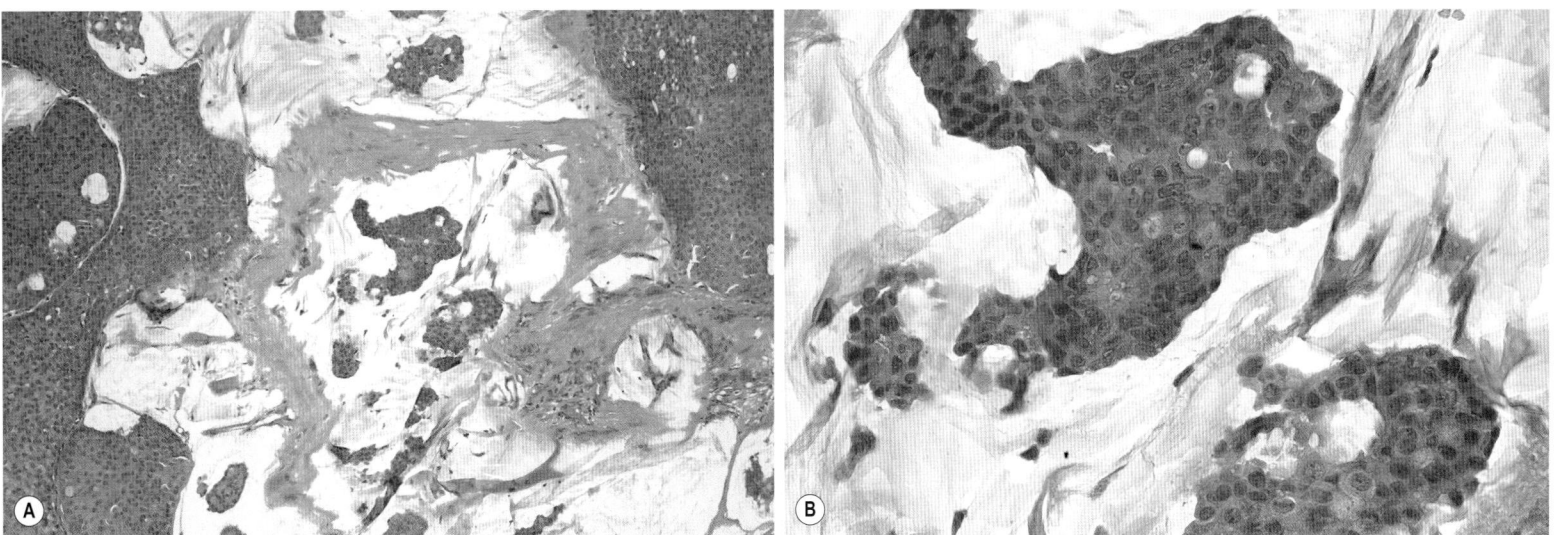

Fig. 33.212
(**A**, **B**) Primary cutaneous mucinous carcinoma: in this example, there is a predominant solid component.

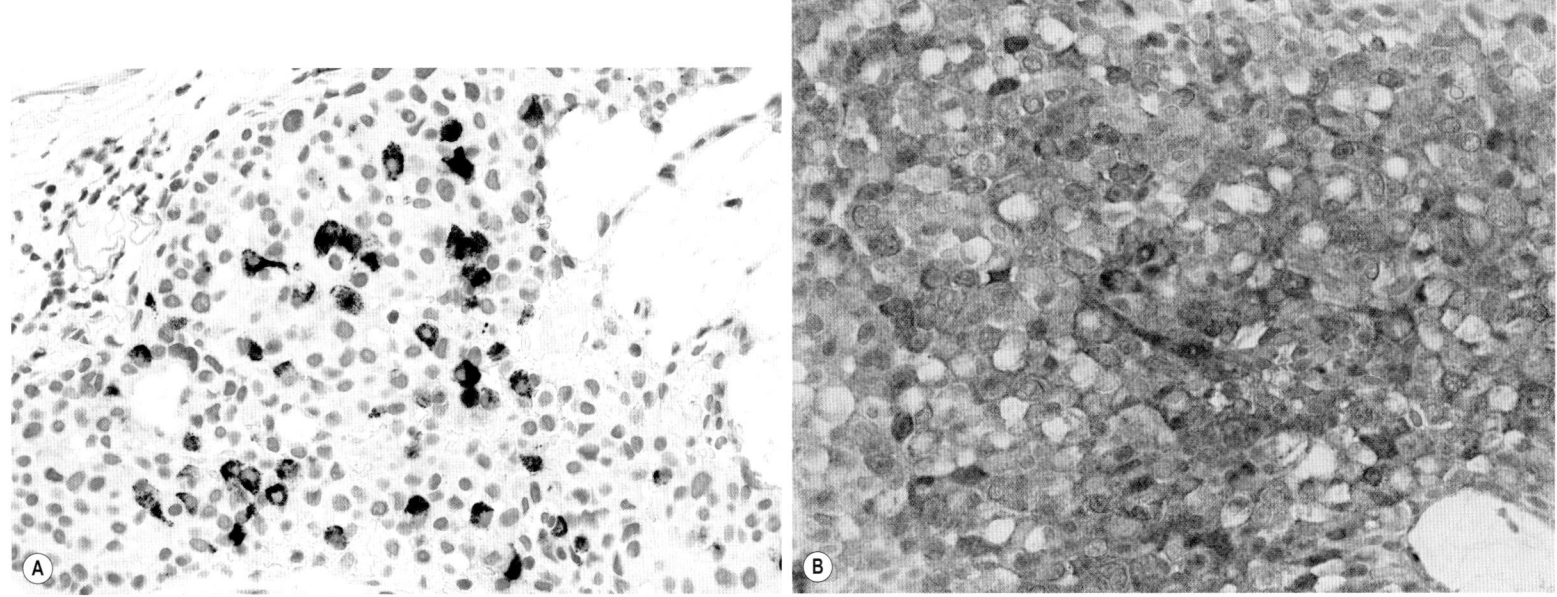

Fig. 33.213
Primary cutaneous mucinous carcinoma: the solid component expressed (**A**) chromogranin and (**B**) NSE.

extensive sampling is very useful as it allows confirmation of the primary nature of a given neoplasm.

Cutaneous mucinous carcinoma can be distinguished from gastrointestinal tumors on the basis of mucin histochemistry. In primary cutaneous tumors, the mucin contains abundant sialomucin (Alcian blue positive at pH 2.5) in contrast to gastrointestinal tumors, which produce sulfamucins (Alcian blue positive at pH 1.0 and 0.4).[3,4] In addition, primary cutaneous variants are CK20 negative in contrast to gastrointestinal lesions which characteristically express this keratin.[18] A further helpful clue is the identification of a myoepithelial layer in primary cutaneous mucinous carcinoma by immunohistochemistry for p63.[18,27]

Endocrine mucin-producing sweat gland carcinoma

Clinical features

Endocrine mucin-producing sweat gland carcinoma is a rare tumor with approximately 40 reported cases in the literature.[1–8] It is closely related to mucinous carcinoma and likely represents part of a morphological continuum or even a precursor. There is strong predilection for the eyelid, and

in particular the lower eyelid.[1–8] The cheek may also be affected.[2] It is a tumor of the elderly, with an average age at presentation of 70 years (range 48–84 years).[1–8] Females are more frequently affected than males.[2,8] Endocrine mucin-producing sweat gland carcinoma is regarded as a low-grade carcinoma with only rare recurrence but no reported metastasis as yet.[2,4,8]

Histologic features

Endocrine mucin-producing sweat gland carcinoma presents as a well-circumscribed uni- to multinodular tumor (*Fig. 33.214*). Tumor lobules are solid and cystic with papillary areas composed of uniform, medium-sized, round to oval cells with abundant cytoplasm and stippled chromatin pattern (*Fig. 33.215*).[1,2] Decapitation secretion may be a focal finding, and moderate cytological atypia as well as mitotic activity may be present. Intracellular mucin is seen within a subset of tumor cells as highlighted by mucicarmine staining. Small amounts of extracellular mucin may also be identified (*Fig. 33.216*). Areas of in situ carcinoma are recognizable in some tumors, and approximately 50% of cases are associated with small foci of conventional mucinous carcinoma.[2]

By immunohistochemistry, tumor cells express neuroendocrine markers such as chromogranin, synaptophysin, NSE, and CD57. They are cytokeratin

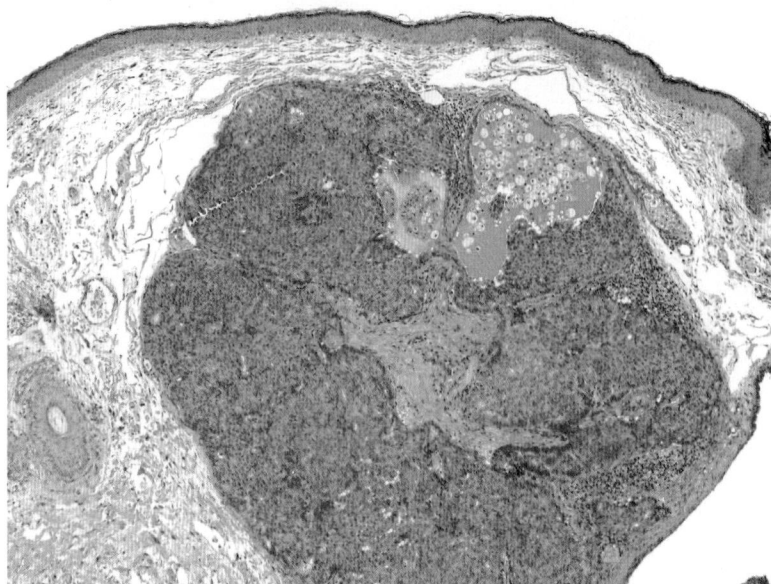

Fig. 33.214
Endocrine mucin producing sweat gland carcinoma: solid and partially cystic differentiation is observed in this nodular dermal based tumor.

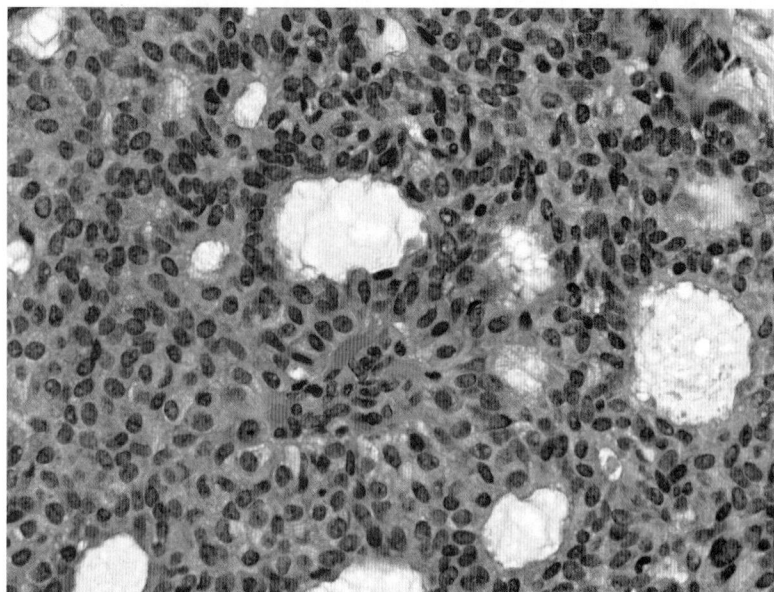

Fig. 33.216
Endocrine mucin producing sweat gland carcinoma: mucin-filled pseudocysts are seen within this tumor. There is no significant cytological atypia and the nuclei show a finely dispersed chromatin pattern.

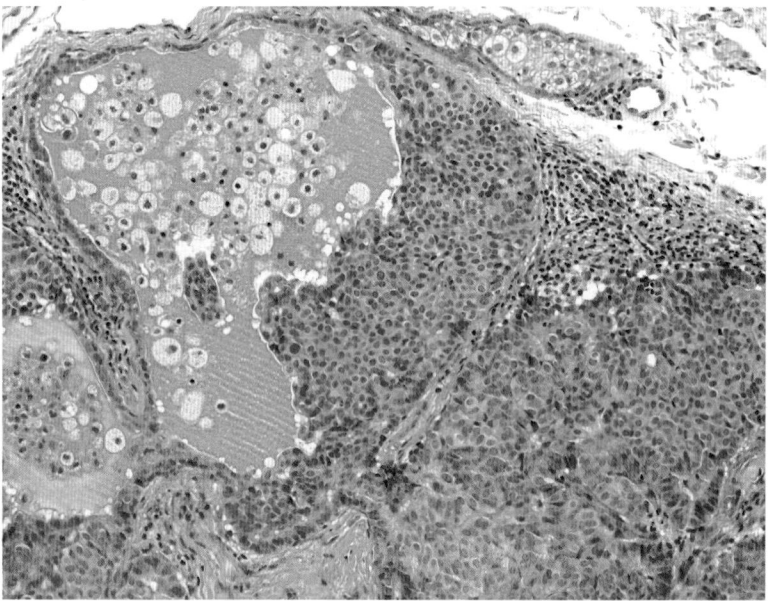

Fig. 33.215
Endocrine mucin producing sweat gland carcinoma: tumor cells are arranged in sheets with centrally placed round to ovoid nuclei and moderate amounts of cytoplasm. Focal cystic change is present.

and EMA positive and express CK7 but not CK20. All tumors tested also express estrogen and progesterone receptors. A myoepithelial cell layer, as highlighted with calponin, p63, and SMA, is preserved only in areas of in situ carcinoma.[2]

Mammary-type secretory carcinoma of the skin

Clinical features

Secretory carcinoma of the breast is a morphologically distinctive tumor, characterized by the t(12;15)(p13;q25) translocation leading to the ETV6-NTRK3 fusion gene.[1] These tumors have recently also been shown to arise in the salivary gland and the skin.[2–9] Primary cutaneous tumors present as small nodules with a mean size of 1.1 cm with a strong predilection for the axilla.[7] Rarely, the neck, flank, arm, and cheek have been

affected.[5–7,9] The patients are middle-aged adults, but the age range is wide (13–71 years). There is a female predilection. The behavior is benign with no recurrence or metastases reported after complete excision.

Histologic features

Secretory carcinoma of the skin are well circumscribed but unencapsulated tumors within the dermis (Fig. 33.217). They are composed of bland and uniform epithelioid cells with eosinophilic cytoplasm, vesicular nuclei, and small eosinophilic nucleoli. Prominent microcyst formation is present with intraluminal colloid-like secretions (Fig. 33.218).[3–9] Occasional mitotic figures may be encountered.

By immunohistochemistry, the tumor cells express cytokeratins AE1/3, Cam5.2, CK7, and S100 as well as STAT5 and mammaglobin. CEA and Ber-EP4 staining is negative. Like secretory carcinoma of the breast, the cutaneous tumors show the characteristic t(12;15)(p13;q25) resulting in the ETV6-NTRK3 fusion gene. The fusion gene can be detected by PCR. The ETV6 gene rearrangement can also be demonstrated by FISH.

Eccrine ductal carcinoma

Clinical features

Eccrine ductal carcinoma is a rare malignancy of major importance because it shows striking similarities to infiltrating ductal carcinoma of the breast and can therefore readily be mistaken for a metastasis. It shows a predilection for the head, neck, and extremities, and presents most often in the middle aged and elderly as a hard, usually nonulcerated, cutaneous nodule.[1–5] Unusual presentations include location on the vulva and the nipple and mimicking Paget disease.[3,6] The prognosis is poor, the tumor being associated with a high recurrence (70%) and metastasis rate (57%), with an overall mortality of 70%.[1]

Pathogenesis and histologic features

The tumor is situated in the lower dermis and often extends into the subcutaneous fat (Fig. 33.219). There is no evidence of epidermal origin and pagetoid spread is not a feature. Eccrine ductal carcinoma is characterized by nests and cords of cuboidal epithelium showing marked ductal differentiation (Figs 33.220 and 33.221).[1–3,6,7] Intracytoplasmic lumina are sometimes evident. Pleomorphism and mitotic activity are variable features, but are usually not marked. The tumor is associated with a dense, sometimes

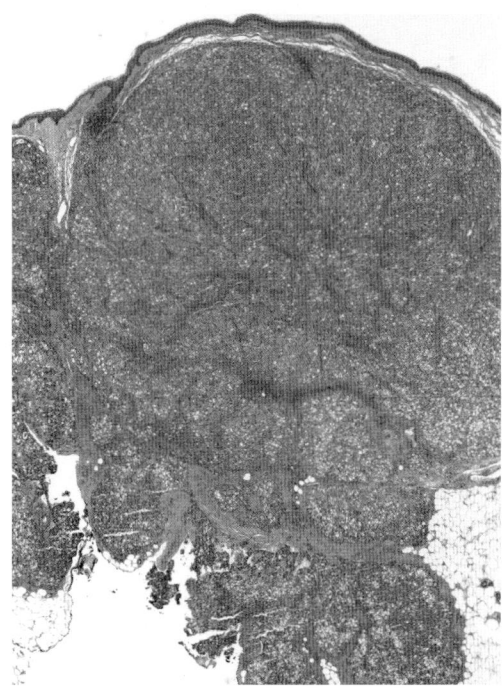

Fig. 33.217
Mammary-type secretory carcinoma of the skin: this multinodular tumor is based within dermis and also involves superficial subcutis. By courtesy of Bostjan Luzar, MD, PhD, Institute of Pathology, Ljubljana, Slovenia.

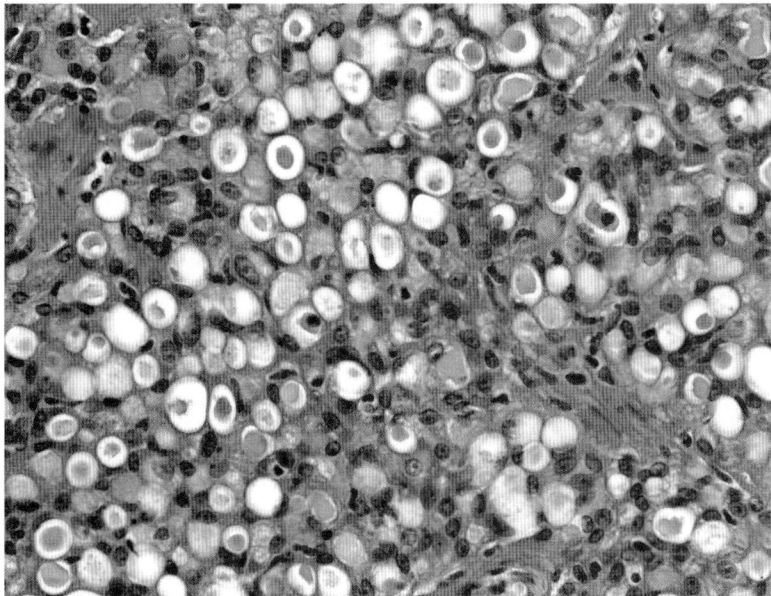

Fig. 33.218
Mammary-type secretory carcinoma of the skin: the uniform epithelioid tumor cells show prominent duct differentiation with a microcystic appearance. Also note the intraluminal eosinophilic colloidal material. By courtesy of Bostjan Luzar, MD, PhD, Institute of Pathology, Ljubljana, Slovenia.

sclerotic, fibrous stroma. Perineural infiltration and lymphatic and/or vascular invasion are commonly present.

By immunohistochemistry, the tumor cells are cytokeratin and CEA positive. They may also express estrogen and progesterone receptors, c-erbB-2, S100, and GCDFP-15 to varying degrees.[3,6,8,9]

Differential diagnosis

The histologic features are indistinguishable from those of invasive ductal breast carcinoma, and immunohistochemistry is of little value.[5,8] Before accepting such a tumor as being of primary sweat gland derivation, a careful clinical and radiological examination of the breasts is mandatory.[1] Rarely, metastatic large bowel carcinoma may result in an identical appearance.

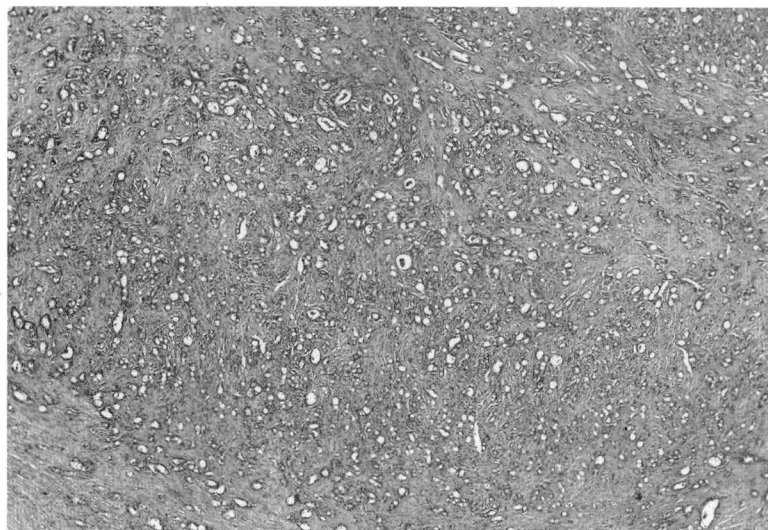

Fig. 33.219
Eccrine ductal carcinoma: the reticular dermis is extensively infiltrated by moderately differentiated adenocarcinoma, which is histologically indistinguishable from a metastasis. Note the dense fibrous stroma.

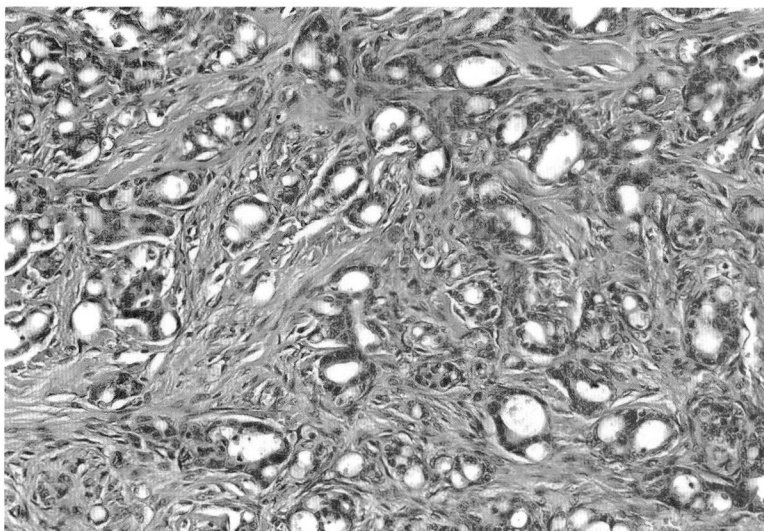

Fig. 33.220
Eccrine ductal carcinoma: there is widespread ductal differentiation.

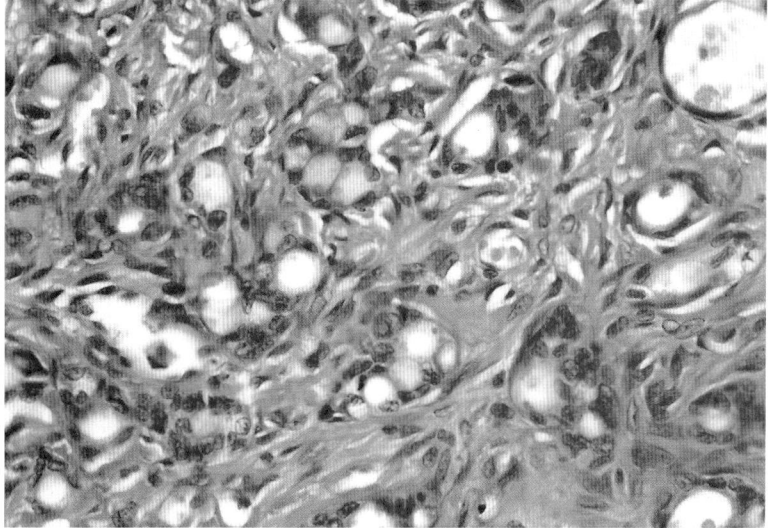

Fig. 33.221
Eccrine ductal carcinoma: intracytoplasmic lumina are evident in the center of the field. The diagnosis of this very rare tumor is one of exclusion. A metastasis must always be excluded.

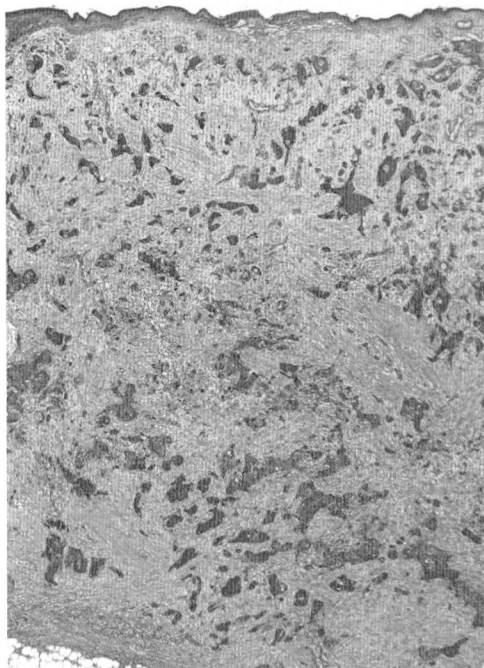

Fig. 33.222
Squamoid eccrine ductal carcinoma: the tumor shows a diffusely infiltrative growth pattern within dermis.

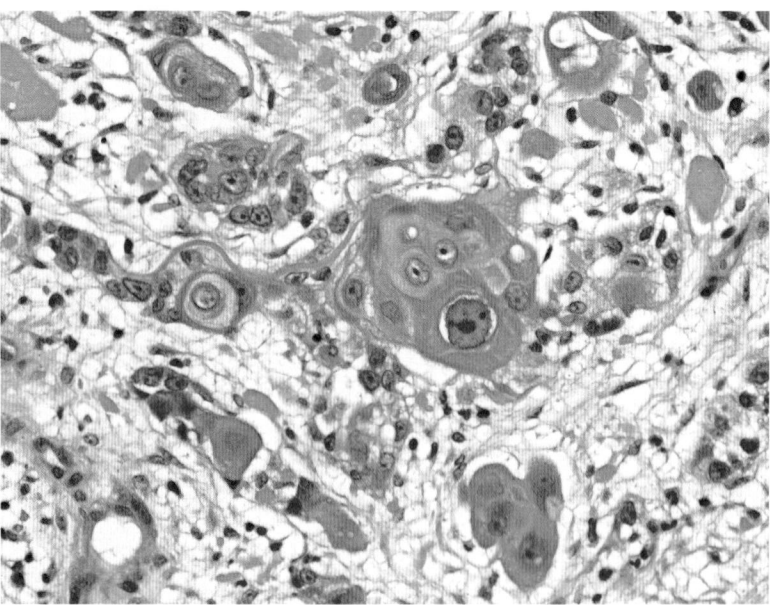

Fig. 33.223
Squamoid eccrine ductal carcinoma: in the superficial aspects, it shows features indistinguishable from squamous cell carcinoma.

Squamoid eccrine ductal carcinoma

Clinical features

Squamoid eccrine ductal carcinoma is a rare but likely underrecognized tumor.[1] It occurs in elderly adults with a male predominance as a solitary nodule on the head and neck area or extremities.[1–6] Tumor size measures up to 2 cm. The tumors have a high (25%) local recurrence rate. Metasases are mainly to locoregional lymph nodes. Distant metastasis and mortality are rare.[1]

Histologic features

Histologically, this tumor presents as a poorly demarcated and infiltrative neoplasm extending into deep dermis and subcutaneous tissue (*Fig. 33.222*).[1–4,7,8] Connection with the overlying epidermis or follicular structures may be evident, and ulceration is sometimes a feature.[1,2] An association with carcinoma in situ is often seen. The superficial aspect of the tumor shows prominent squamoid differentiation resembling squamous cell carcinoma (*Fig. 33.223*) and frequently connects with eccrine ducts at different levels.[2,3] Squamous eddies, horn cysts, and epithelial structures reminiscent of syringoma may also be present.[2] In the deeper reaches the tumor appears more infiltrative, and ductal differentiation in the form of a cuticle-like luminal structure is identified in addition to intracytoplasmic vacuoles (*Fig. 33.224*).[1–3] Marked cytologic atypia may be present in both ductal and squamoid elements and mitotic figures are present. Perineural infiltration is common but lymphovascular invasion has only rarely been reported.[1,2,7,8]

Ductal differentiation is confirmed with immunohistochemical staining for CEA and EMA. No reactivity is seen against S100 protein.[2,3]

Differential diagnosis

Squamous cell carcinoma can be excluded by the presence of ductal differentiation and connection with eccrine ducts. Immunohistochemistry for CEA and EMA will provide additional support. Squamous differentiation can also be observed in other adnexal tumors such as eccrine porocarcinoma. It is then more focal than and not as prominent as in squamoid eccrine ductal carcinoma.

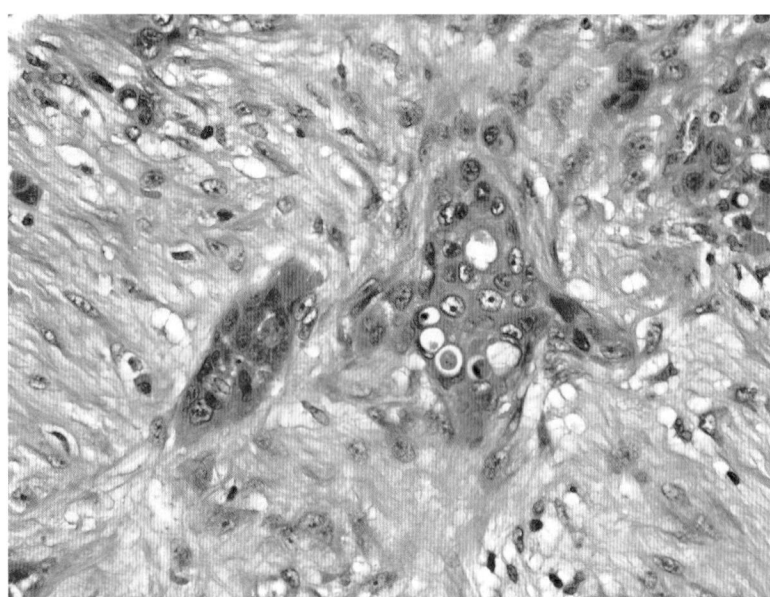

Fig. 33.224
Squamoid eccrine ductal carcinoma: in the deeper reaches, the tumor is composed of pleomorphic cuboidal cells arranged in strands in a desmoplastic stroma. Duct differentiation is present.

Polymorphous sweat gland carcinoma

Clinical features

This distinctive low-grade sweat gland carcinoma is not uncommonly mistaken for a cutaneous metastasis.[1–4] Only a small number of cases have been documented. Patients present with a slowly growing, smooth dermal nodule with a predilection for the limbs.[1,3] Many tumors have been present for 5 or even 10 years before presentation. Local recurrences are common, but lymph node metastases occur in fewer than 10% of cases.[1,3] There have been no tumor-associated deaths.

Histologic features

Histologically, polymorphous sweat gland carcinoma presents as a pseudoencapsulated deep dermal nodular growth associated with a wide range of histologic patterns including solid, trabecular, tubular, pseudopapillary, and cylindroma-like patterns.[1] Ductal differentiation is regularly present, and PAS- and mucicarmine-positive mucin may be evident.[1] The tumor cells are uniform with little cytoplasm and round to oval vesicular nuclei with prominent nucleoli. Mitoses are often conspicuous but abnormal forms are not a feature.[3] Perineural infiltration may rarely be seen but there is no tumor necrosis.[1] The stroma is often hyalinized and hemorrhage is common.

The tumor cells express keratin, CEA, and to a lesser extent EMA.

Primary cutaneous signet ring cell carcinoma

Clinical features

Signet ring cell carcinoma (histiocytoid carcinoma) is a rarely reported primary tumor presenting almost exclusively in the eyelid.[1] Bilateral eyelid involvement is uncommon.[2] The axilla may rarely be affected.[3–7] In the small number of cases published in the literature, it shows a striking predilection for males (5:1) and arises most often in the sixth decade (range 47–87 years, mean 63 years).[1,3,8–17] It is often slowly growing and presents as a non-specific thickening of the eyelid or as a mass.

The tumor is associated with an aggressive growth pattern commonly involving the orbit and with frequent recurrences. Lymph node spread has been described in 30% of cases.[11,13,14] Distant metastases are exceptional.

Histologic features

The tumor presents with a diffuse or widely infiltrating growth pattern typically associated with a single cell, 'stack of pennies' appearance. The tumor cells are variably described as histiocytoid with abundant eosinophilic cytoplasm containing small vacuoles and signet ring with a large intracytoplasmic vacuole compressing the nucleus to the periphery of the cell.[11,14] Nuclei may be hyperchromatic or vesicular and contain prominent nucleoli with variable mitotic activity. Mucin stains including D-PAS and Alcian blue are positive.[11]

With immunohistochemistry, the tumor cells express cytokeratins AE1/3, MNF116, CAM 5.2, CK7, EMA, CEA, p63 and variably estrogen receptor, progesterone receptor, lysozyme, GCDFP-15, and HMFG.[1,11,12,14]

Ultrastructural studies have confirmed the presence of intracytoplasmic lumina with microvilli and intracytoplasmic mucin.[14]

Differential diagnosis

Although a signet ring cell carcinoma of the eyelid is likely to represent a primary tumor, the diagnosis should never be made until the patient has been thoroughly investigated to exclude a metastasis from an underlying visceral primary tumor, particularly arising in the breast or gastrointestinal tract.

Access **ExpertConsult**.com for the complete list of references

CHAPTER

34

Cutaneous cysts

See
www.expertconsult.com
for references and
additional material

Although a wide variety of cysts may present in the skin, usually these turn out to be epidermoid (infundibular), trichilemmal, or glandular in nature (*Table 34.1*). It can sometimes be difficult to determine whether a structure is a true cyst, a sinus, a comedone, or an obliquely sectioned dilated hair follicle. Usually, the clinical information or further sections provide the answer, but the alternatives should always be borne in mind. The majority of cutaneous cysts are recognized as such clinically. However, a significant proportion of misdiagnoses do occur; therefore, it is advisable that all lesions are submitted for histologic confirmation.[1,2]

Follicular cysts

Most cutaneous cysts are derived from the pilosebaceous unit. Thus, epidermoid, pigmented follicular, and vellus hair cysts, and milia are each derived from the follicular infundibulum.[1] Pilar (trichilemmal cysts) are believed to originate in the follicular isthmus of anagen hairs. Steatocystoma is a cyst of the sebaceous duct. Cystic pilomatrixoma is derived from hair matrix cells, and hybrid cysts can originate from any of the above.[1]

Epidermoid cyst

Clinical features

Epidermoid (epidermal, infundibular) cysts, which occur particularly on the face, neck, and upper trunk, are believed to result from damage to the pilosebaceous units.[1] The vulval labia majora and scrotum are also sites of predilection. Rare lesions develop in non-hair-bearing areas like the soles (see below).[2] Young and middle-aged adults are most often affected, and the sexes are involved equally. Epidermoid cysts present as smooth dome-shaped swellings a few millimeters to a few centimeters across (*Fig. 34.1*). A punctum is usually present (*Fig. 34.2*).

The presence of multiple lesions may suggest the possibility of Gardner syndrome, which includes polyposis coli, jaw osteomas, and intestinal fibromatoses in addition to cutaneous cysts.[3,4] Less frequently, patients may manifest lipomas, pilomatrixomas (including epidermoid cysts with pilomatrical lining), and leiomyomas. Multiple lesions also occur in Gorlin-Goltz syndrome (see Chapter 24) and may be the first manifestation of the disease.[5] Subconjunctival epidermoid cysts appear to occur exclusively in patients with this syndrome.[6]

Multiple and often large epidermoid cysts are sometimes seen as a complication of ciclosporin therapy in transplantation recipients.[7,8] Multiple epidermoid cysts have also been described in association with imiquimod and vemurafenib therapy.[9,10]

Epidermoid inclusion cysts may also complicate penetrating trauma to the skin, such as by a sewing needle, with resultant implantation of squamous epithelium into the dermis (*Fig. 34.3*).[11,12] Lesions may rarely develop after genital mutilation,[13] after vaccination (BCG),[14] and after cosmetic surgical procedures including penile girth enhancement therapy[15] and abdominoplasty.[16]

It has been argued that since there is good agreement between the clinical and histologic diagnosis of epidermoid cysts, there is no need to submit these lesions for routine histologic examination. A study found a rate of concordance of about 80% between the clinical and histologic diagnosis, leading the authors to suggest that if the cyst is opened by the surgeon after excision and malodorous cheesy material is obtained, then the lesion can be discarded.[17] This is debatable as malignant changes may exceptionally develop within epidermoid cysts (see below). The incidence of malignancy, mainly squamous cell carcinoma developing in epidermoid cysts, was reported as 0.3% in a retrospective study.[18] However, most cysts developing malignancy become symptomatic, and it has therefore been proposed that excision should be performed only for symptomatic lesions.[19]

Pathogenesis and histologic features

Lesions develop as a result of obstruction of the upper part of the hair follicle or secondary to trauma (inclusion cysts).

Epidermoid cysts are unilocular, spherical, and are lined by an epidermis-like epithelium including a granular cell layer (*Figs 34.4–34.6*).[1] Exceptional multilocular lesions may occur.[20] The cyst contents of laminated keratin are believed to represent follicular infundibular derivation (the nonimplantation variant). In older lesions, the lining is often somewhat attenuated. Lichenoid inflammation of the wall indistinguishable from lichen planus may be seen. Acute inflammation may result in the subsequent disruption of the cyst wall, with the development of an intense foreign body giant cell reaction (*Fig. 34.7*). Sometimes this may be so marked that it completely destroys the cyst, and only focal dermal collections of keratin fragments remain (*Fig. 34.8*). It is not clear whether bacteria play an important role in the development of inflammation in epidermoid cysts. A study from Japan found an increased incidence of anaerobes in inflamed lesions as opposed to those without inflammation.[21] It remains to be established, however, whether this is the result of colonization or a true infection. Occasionally, the cyst lining may show epidermoid and focal trichilemmal keratinization. In the rare hybrid cyst, there is epidermoid keratinization in the

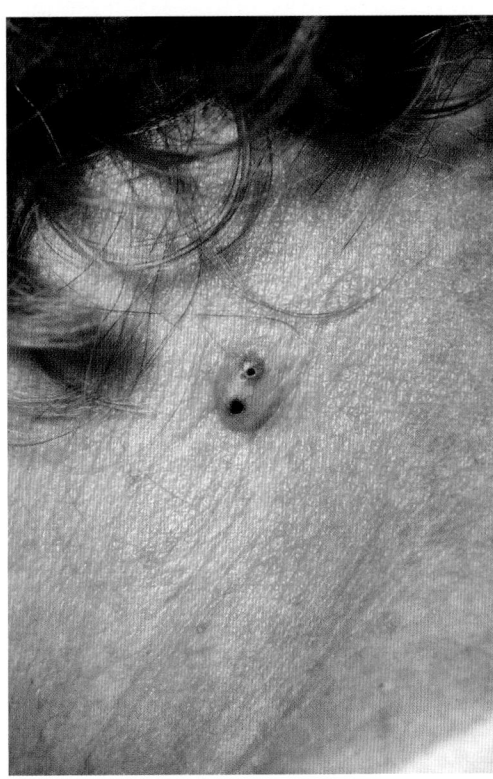

Fig. 34.1
Epidermoid cyst: a typical dome-shaped swelling with two puncta. By courtesy of R.A. Marsden, MD, St George's Hospital, London, UK.

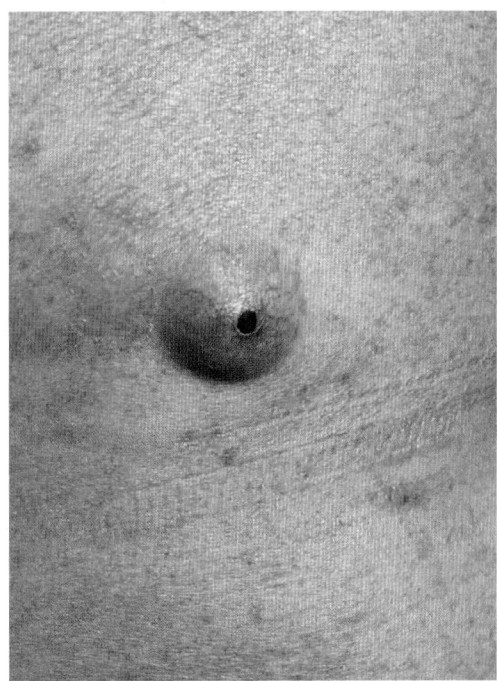

Fig. 34.2
Epidermoid cyst: close-up view of a punctum. By courtesy of the Institute of Dermatology, London, UK.

Table 34.1
Classification of cutaneous cysts

Keratinizing	Glandular
Epidermoid	Bronchogenic
Proliferating epidermoid	Thyroglossal duct
Hybrid cyst	Branchial
Verrucous	Cervical thymic
Epidermoid cyst of the sole	Ciliated
Comedonal	Median raphe
Milia	
Trichilemmal	
Vellus hair	
Steatocystoma	
Dermoid	

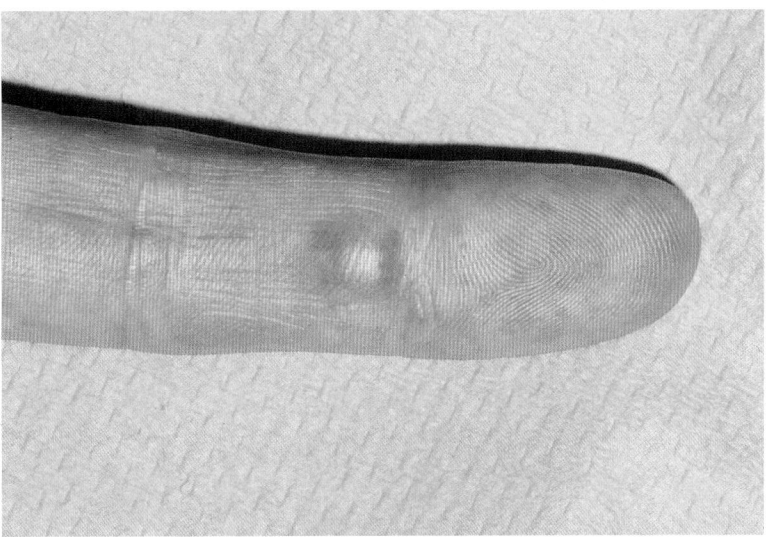

Fig. 34.3
Epidermoid cyst: this implantation variant is at a characteristic site. By courtesy of R.A. Marsden, MD, St George's Hospital, London, UK.

superficial half of the cyst and trichilemmal in the lower.[22] Exceptionally, a pigmented variant containing multiple terminal hair shaft fragments may be encountered (pigmented follicular cyst).[23,24] A case with numerous keratin spherules has been reported.[25]

In patients with Gardner syndrome, the cyst lining occasionally shows focal basaloid cell proliferation with ghost cell change, as seen in pilomatrixoma (*Fig. 34.9*).[26,27] Lesions outside this context may occur, including a case in a background of nevus sebaceous.[28,29] Thus, while highly suggestive, these cannot be considered pathognomonic.

The cysts in Gorlin-Goltz syndrome are usually hybrid with features of epidermoid cyst and steatocystoma.[30]

A case of multiple epidermoid cysts with lesions of angiofibroma in tuberous sclerosis patients associated with obstruction/trauma has been reported.[31]

Epidermoid cysts not uncommonly coexist with melanocytic nevi. This is of particular importance, as the resulting increase in size of the cyst may raise clinical suspicion of melanoma.[32,33] Most nevi are banal and dermal,

but cysts associated with compound nevi, congenital nevi, dysplastic nevi, blue nevi, and spindle cell nevi of Reed have also been documented.[33]

Malignant tumors may rarely develop within the wall of an epidermoid cyst including basal cell carcinoma, squamous cell carcinoma, and squamous cell carcinoma in situ (*Fig. 34.10*).[34–41] There are also rare case reports describing an epidermoid cyst in association with Paget disease and cutaneous neuroendocrine carcinoma (Merkel cell carcinoma).[42–44] There have been a reported case of melanoma arising in a lesion, an in situ melanoma associated with an adjacent cutaneous melanoma colonizing an epidermoid cyst, and there is a single further report of a melanoma in situ arising in a noncutaneous cerebellopontine angle epidermoid cyst.[45–47] Pilomatrixoma (in the absence of Gardner syndrome) in conjunction with an epidermoid cyst has also been documented.[48,49] Because epidermoid cysts with malignant change cannot be clinically reliably distinguished from their extremely common benign counterparts, histologic examination of all such cysts is recommended.[50]

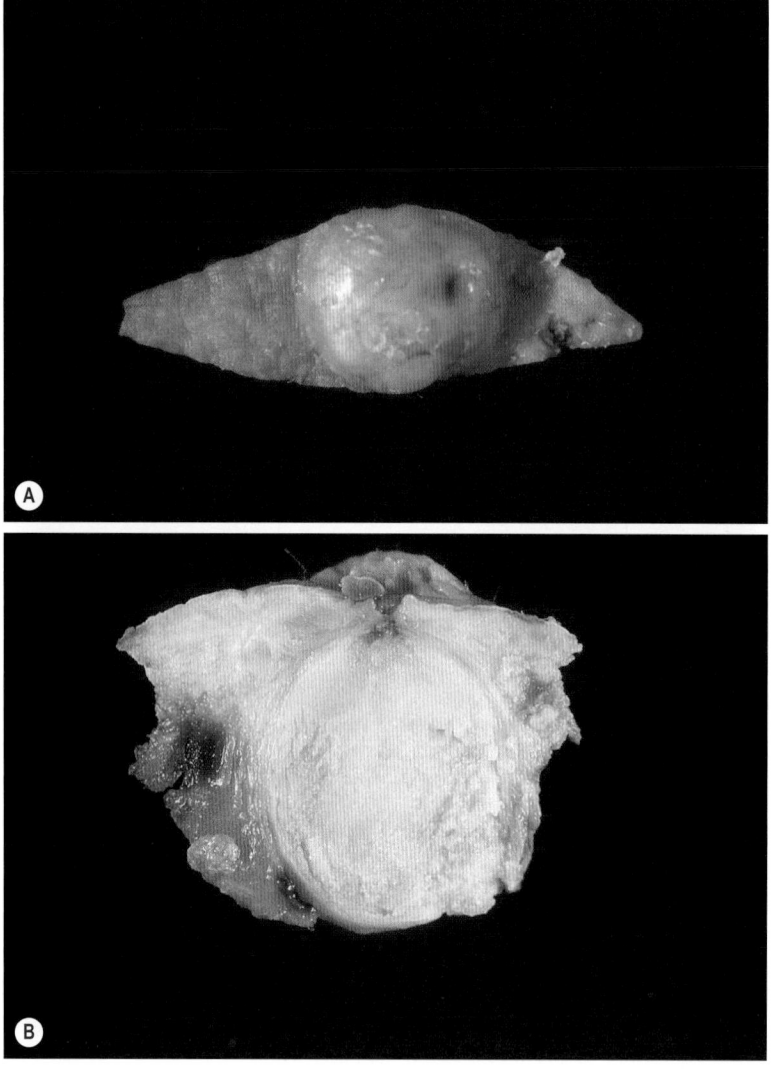

Fig. 34.4
(A, B) Epidermoid cyst: in this excision specimen, the punctum is clearly visible.

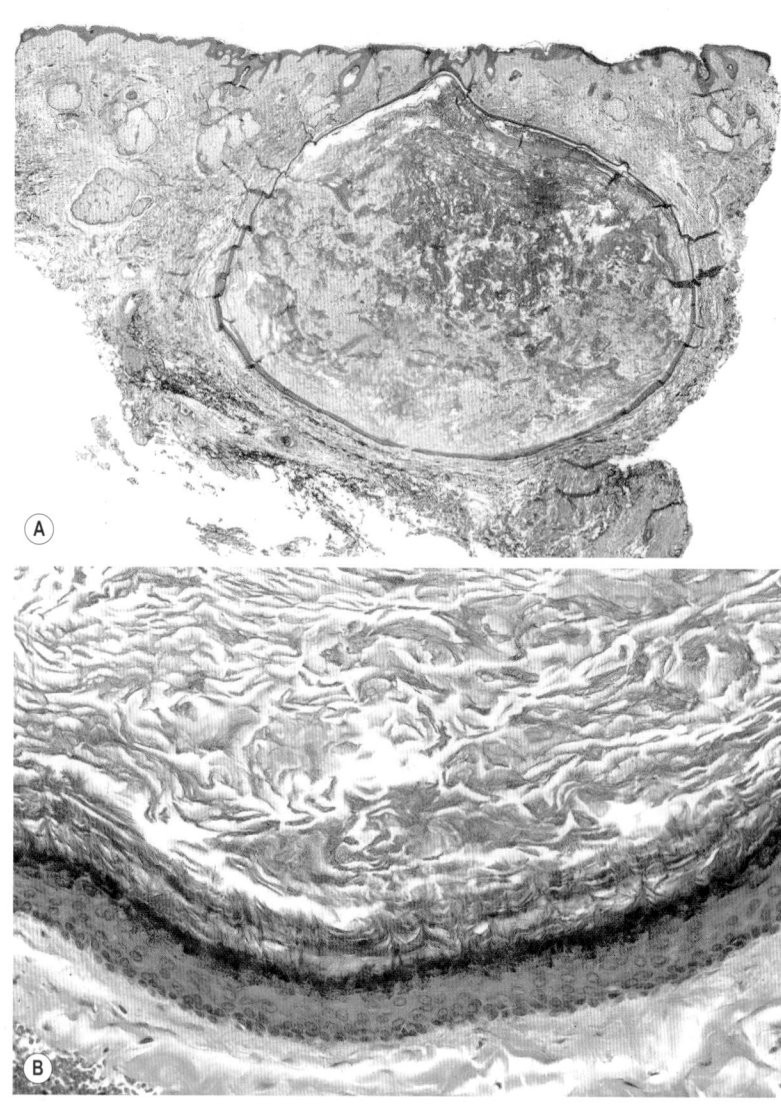

Fig. 34.6
Epidermoid cyst: (A) in this example, the punctum is present; (B) the cyst wall is composed of squamous epithelium and includes a granular cell layer. Note the laminated keratin.

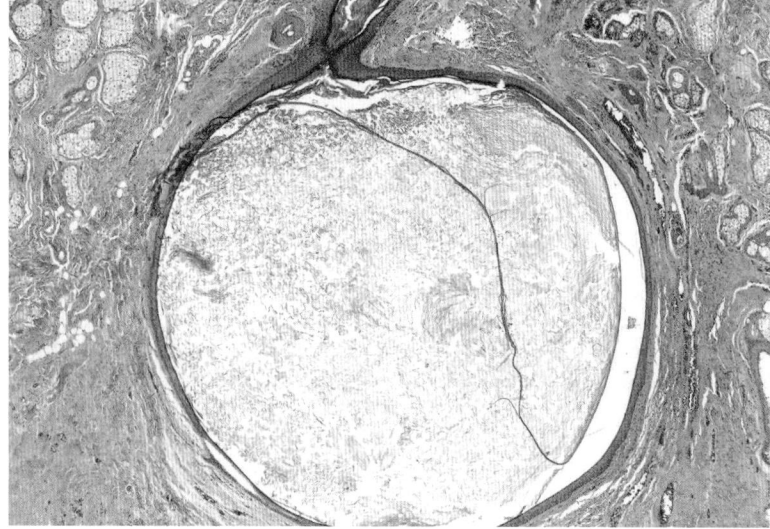

Fig. 34.5
Epidermoid cyst: a solitary lesion is present in the dermis.

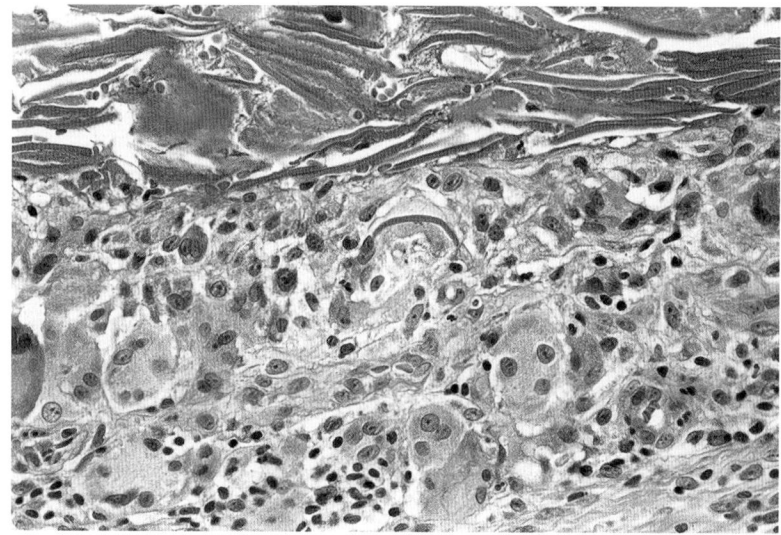

Fig. 34.7
Epidermoid cyst: rupture is associated with a foreign body granulomatous response. In the center of the field, a giant cell contains a keratin fragment.

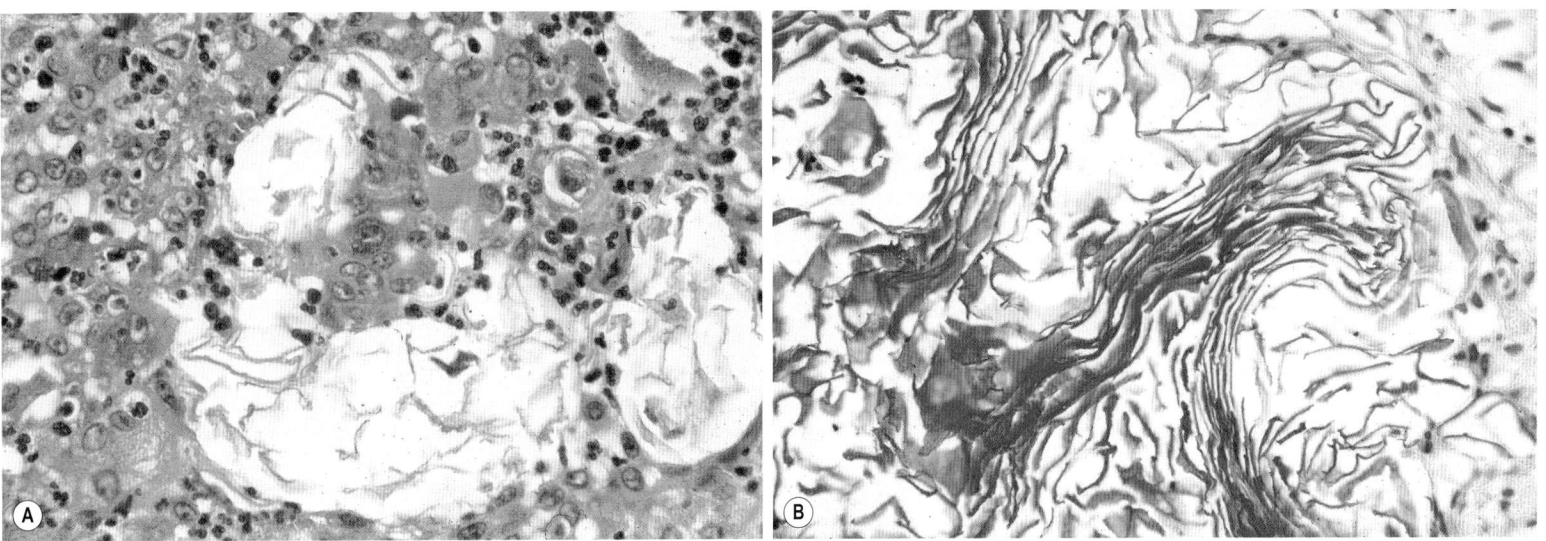

Fig. 34.8
Epidermoid cyst: (**A**) in this almost healed lesion, residual keratin lamellae, as seen in the center of the field, are all that is left of the ruptured cyst; (**B**) these may be highlighted by the Lendrum phloxine tartrazine reaction.

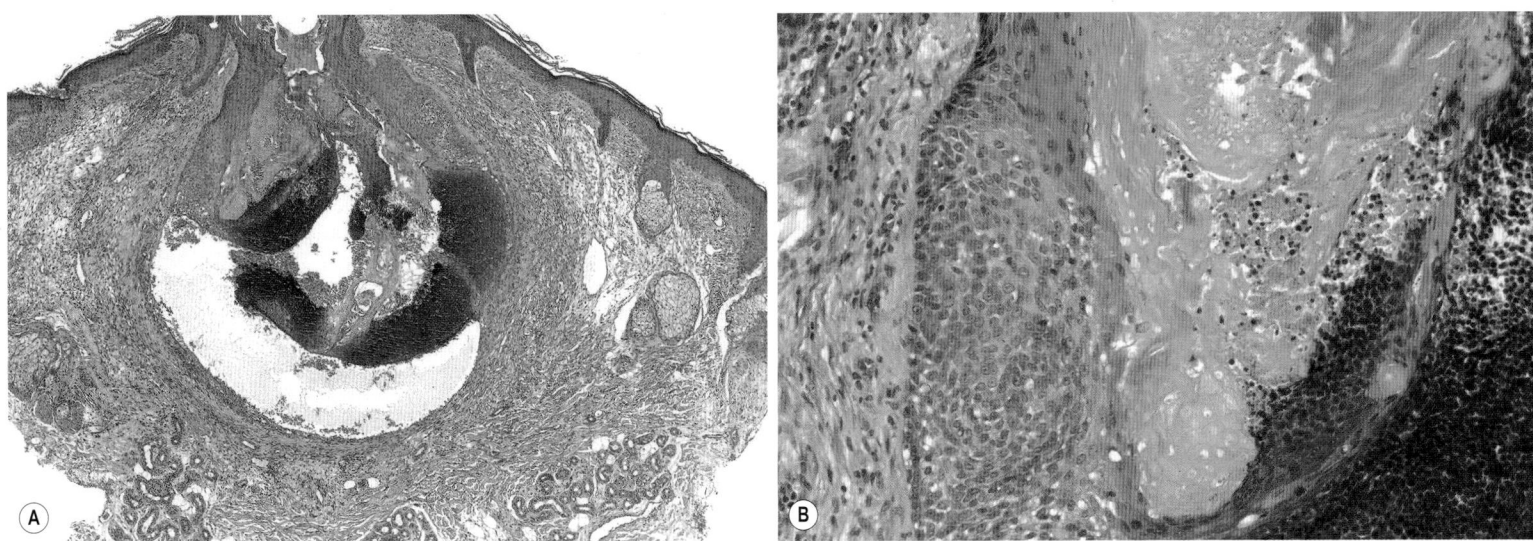

Fig. 34.9
(**A**, **B**) Epidermoid cyst: the lower half of the cyst wall shows matrical differentiation.

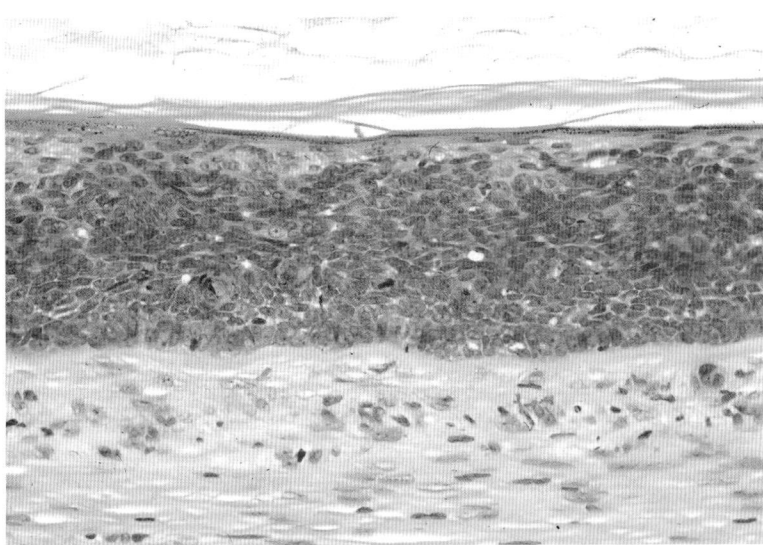

Fig. 34.10
Epidermoid cyst: in this example, the epithelial wall shows the features of carcinoma in situ.

Epidermoid cysts showing features of a range of cutaneous dermatoses have been described.[51] These include pemphigus, psoriasis, lichen planus, and Darier disease.[52–54] Changes of epidermolytic hyperkeratosis and involvement by molluscum contagiosum have also been described.[55,56] Human papillomavirus (HPV) associations are described below (see verrucous cyst and epidermoid cyst of the sole).

Proliferating epidermoid cyst

Clinical features

Proliferating epidermoid cyst is rare and poorly documented, with the majority of cases, in fact, describing the pilar/trichilemmal variant.[1,2] There are, however, very occasional reports of this entity, of which the comprehensive review from the Armed Forces Institute of Pathology is the most informative.[3,4]

The tumor shows a predilection for males (1.8:1) and, although a wide variety of sites may be affected, the majority appear to present on the pelvic area, scalp, and trunk in descending order of frequency.[4] Most patients are middle aged or elderly (range 21–88 years, mean 54 years). Occasional patients document the presence of a lesion for several decades, giving support to the concept that the resulting tumor has developed within a preexistent benign epidermoid cyst.[4] In this series, proliferating epidermoid cyst was associated with a 20% recurrence rate but metastases were not encountered.[4]

Histologic features

By definition, focal cyst wall lined by stratified squamous epithelium and showing a granular cell layer with epidermoid/infundibular keratinization must be evident. The proliferating component is variable and ranges from well-differentiated squamous epithelium with conspicuous squamous eddies reminiscent of inverted follicular keratosis through to multicystic, keratotic, and verrucous lesions.[4] Rarely, frank invasive carcinoma is encountered.

Hybrid cyst

The term hybrid cyst was originally introduced to describe a cyst in which the upper half showed features of an epidermoid cyst whereas the lower portion comprised a trichilemmal cyst.[1] There was a sharp distinction between the two linings. The spectrum was subsequently expanded to include cysts with a variety of dual linings including epidermoid cyst and pilomatrixoma, trichilemmal cyst and pilomatrixoma, epidermoid with both trichilemmal and pilomatrical features, and eruptive vellus hair cyst with trichilemmal cyst.[2-5] Cystic lesions with follicular germinative differentiation usually represent cystic trichoblastomas, cystic panfolliculomas, or even cystic follicular hamartomas.[6]

There are also a number of reports of cysts combining the features of eruptive vellus hair cyst and steatocystoma.[2,7-10] These are intriguing, given the potentially shared molecular pathogenic features of these processes likely involving keratin 17. Epidermoid cyst with apocrine hidrocystoma and pilomatrixoma with cystic trichilemmoma have also been described.[11,12] A lesion combining isthmic-catagen, pilomatrical, and syringocystadenoma papilliferum components has been described.[13] Hybrid cysts with follicular and apocrine differentiation seem to be more common on the eyelid.[14] Since all of these cysts are derived from various components of the hair follicle, their combination is not surprising. The characteristic cyst of Gardner syndrome, in which epidermoid features merge with pilomatrixoma, can also be regarded as a type of hybrid cyst.[15] The hybrid cysts associated with Gorlin-Goltz syndrome have been described under epidermoid cyst.

Verrucous cyst

Clinical features

The verrucous cyst is a variant of epidermoid cyst associated with HPV infection.[1-5] Adults are affected, and lesions may present at a wide variety of sites although the face, back, and (to a lesser extent) the arms and chest are most often involved.[5] The sexes are affected equally. The cysts show no particular distinguishing clinical features.[4]

Pathogenesis and histologic features

Verrucous cysts are associated with HPV infection as determined by polymerase chain reaction.[3,4] Thus far, HPV antigens have not been identified with immunohistochemistry. The subtype is unknown in most cases, but a single lesion with the HPV type 59 has been described.[6] HPV16 was demonstrated in a case of invasive squamous cell carcinoma arising from a verrucous cyst.[7] An unusual case of multiple verrucous cysts associated with epidermodysplasia verruciformis-associated HPVs (20, 24, alb-7, and 80) and epidermodysplasia verruciformis-like epidermal lesions in the setting of idiopathic CD4 lymphopenia (immunosuppression) has been described.[8]

Histologically, verrucous cyst shows focal features of a typical epidermoid cyst and rarely features of a trichilemmal cyst.[9] The greater part of the cyst wall, however, is lined by papillomatous, acanthotic squamous epithelium with hyperkeratosis, parakeratosis, and conspicuous hypergranulosis. Keratohyaline granules are enlarged and irregular, and occasionally koilocytes are seen.[2,3,5] In some lesions, the epithelium consists of an admixture of basaloid and squamous cells, and squamous eddies are prominent.[3] A lymphohistiocytic infiltrate is sometimes present in the surrounding dermis.

A lesion displaying melanocytic and sebaceous differentiation has been described.[10]

Differential diagnosis

Verrucous cyst differs from HPV-associated epidermoid cysts of the sole, which predominantly affect the Japanese and in which the morphology of the wall of the cyst is that of a typical epidermoid cyst.[11,12]

Epidermoid cyst of the sole

Clinical features

Epidermoid cyst of the sole has been described mainly in the Japanese.[1-5] A single case report documents the lesion in a non-Japanese.[6] Involvement of the palm has also been reported.[4] The cyst likely represents an implantation variant.[7] It is of particular interest as it has been shown to be associated with HPV infection in some cases (see below).[5] An exceptional giant lesion extending from the sole into the dorsum of the foot through the interosseous muscles has been described.[8]

Histologic features

Histologically, it is characterized by the presence of eosinophilic intracytoplasmic inclusions in the wall of the cyst and vacuolated cells in the keratin layer.[2,5] Parakeratosis with absence of the granular cell layer is sometimes noted in the more superficial portion of the cyst.[9] The cyst is filled with orthokeratotic keratin. Immunoperoxidase confirms the presence of viral antigen, and inclusions have been identified ultrastructurally.[2,5] HPV 57 and 60 have been demonstrated.[10,11]

Comedonal cyst

Clinical features

Acne, including chloracne (a condition characterized by the development of acneiform lesions in patients following exposure to the halogenated hydrocarbons), is the most common cause of comedone formation. Comedones are follicular retention cysts.[1] When they open directly onto the surface, a blackhead is visible clinically (*Fig. 34.11*). If the ostial canal is blocked, pigmented keratin is not visible and the medium-sized whitish papule is classified as a closed comedone or whitehead (*Fig. 34.12*).

Pathogenesis and histologic features

Follicular dilatation and hyperkeratosis (follicular plugging) are common features of facial skin. The development of an acne microcomedone is a further extension of that process. The fully developed blackhead contains abundant laminated keratin and cellular debris (*Fig. 34.13*). A large sebaceous gland with a small hair may be attached to the widely distended but patent follicle. If the lesion persists, the sebaceous gland and hair commonly atrophy (*Fig. 34.14*). A histologic section through a closed comedone will often miss the blocked connection with the epidermis, and sometimes a blackhead may appear as an intradermal cyst.

Differential diagnosis

Solar comedones (Favre-Racouchot disease) occur as a clinical triad of cysts, comedones, and elastosis around the orbit and malar areas of elderly patients, and are due to prolonged exposure to sunlight (*Fig. 34.15*) or very rarely secondary to radiotherapy.[2,3] Rarely, a plaquelike lesion may be seen.[4] Squamous cell carcinoma may rarely develop within a lesion.[5] Large thin-walled open and closed comedones are present in the upper dermis, accompanied by marked solar elastosis.[6] A small series of cases of what is regarded as a variant of Favre-Racouchot disease and including epidermoid cysts with vellus hairs and solar elastosis and presenting on the ears has been described.[7]

Open and closed comedones are also a feature of the congenital conditions familial comedones and familial dyskeratotic comedones. Both of these have an autosomal dominant mode of inheritance; the former is characterized by a greater number of lesions and an absence of dyskeratosis.[8-10]

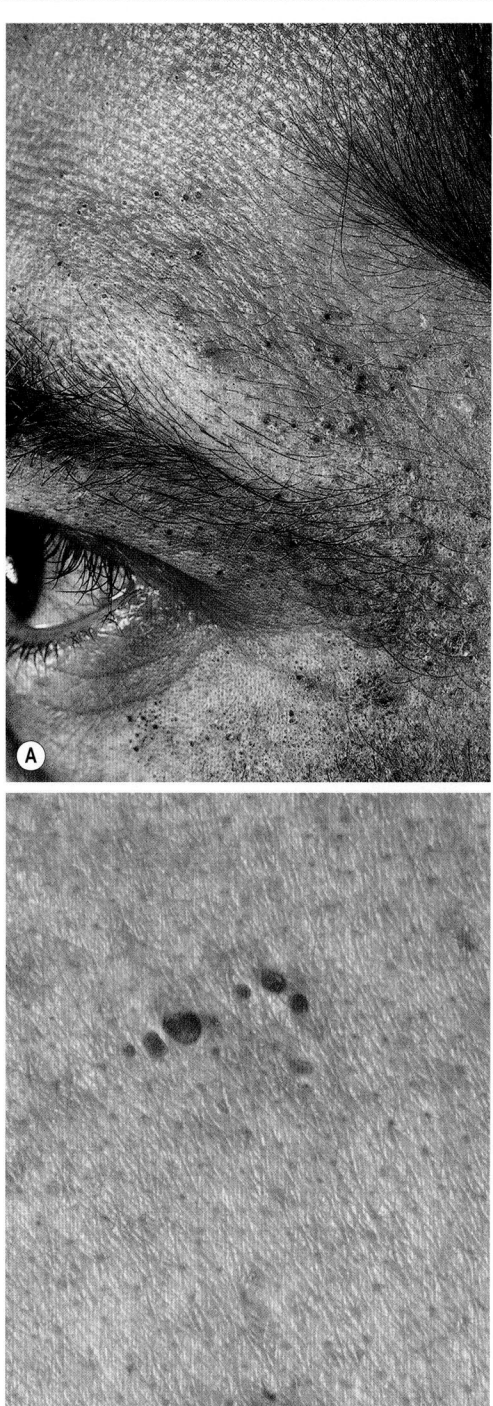

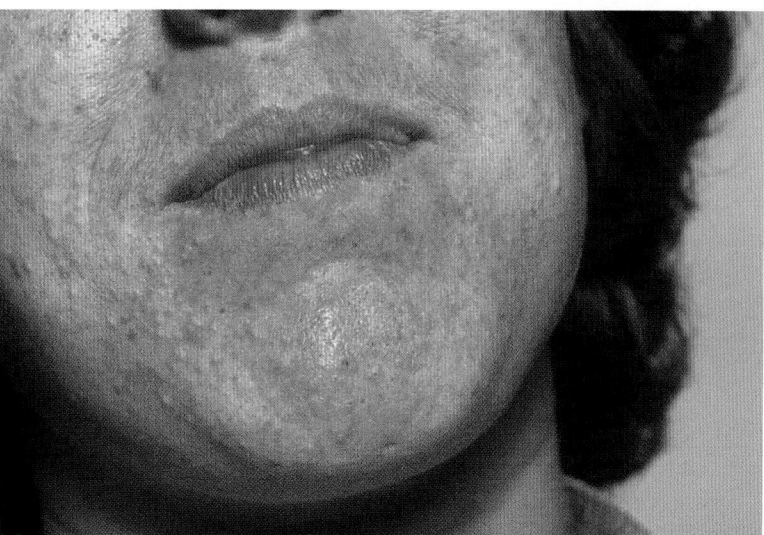

Fig. 34.12
Acne: numerous closed comedones (whiteheads) are present on this patient's cheek and chin. By courtesy of R.A. Marsden, MD, St George's Hospital, London, UK.

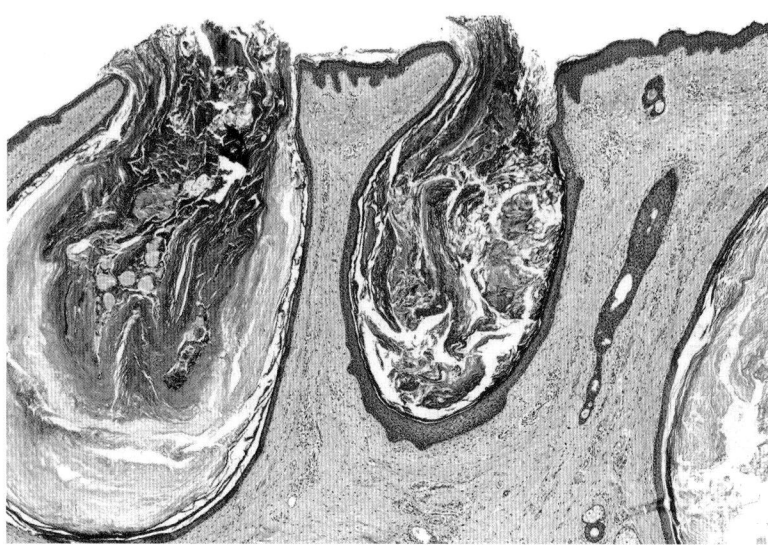

Fig. 34.13
Open comedone: the lesion consists of a cystically dilated hair follicle containing abundant keratin.

Fig. 34.11
Acne vulgaris: (**A**) typical open comedones (blackheads); (**B**) close-up view. (**A**) By courtesy of R.A. Marsden, St George's Hospital, London, UK; (**B**) by courtesy of the Institute of Dermatology, London, UK.

Rarely, late-stage follicular mucinosis and discoid lupus erythematosus may feature large thin-walled comedones as the dominant histologic component.

Milia

Clinical features

Milia are common superficial keratinous cysts that present as white or yellow dome-shaped nodules measuring 1–3 mm in diameter.[1,2] They may represent primary lesions when no cause can be identified or secondary variants usually following skin trauma or other injury.

Primary milia are seen in up to 50% of newborns and present on the face, upper trunk, and extremities.[3] These typically regress spontaneously. Children and adults can also be affected, when lesions are most often apparent on the face (forehead, eyelids, and cheeks) and the external genitalia (*Fig. 34.16*).[3] Possible association of persistent infantile milia with steatocystoma multiplex and eruptive vellus hair cysts has also been suggested.[4]

Secondary milia may complicate a wide range of conditions including follicular mucinosis, folliculotropic mycosis fungoides, lichen sclerosus, radiotherapy, herpes zoster infection, leishmaniasis, severe burns, dermabrasion, chemical peeling, cutaneous local steroid therapy, adverse drug reactions (e.g., benoxaprofen), contact dermatitis, tattoos, and in a case of generalized granuloma annulare with a photosensitive distribution.[3,5–17] Rarely, an association with bullae in systemic AL amyloidosis has been reported.[18] Multiple follicular cysts and milia resulting in cutis verticis gyrate have been described after brain radiotherapy during vemurafenib therapy for melanoma.[19] Lesions have also been described on the face and trunk during treatment with vemurafenib.[20] Milia are also a feature of a number of subepidermal blistering disorders including dystrophic

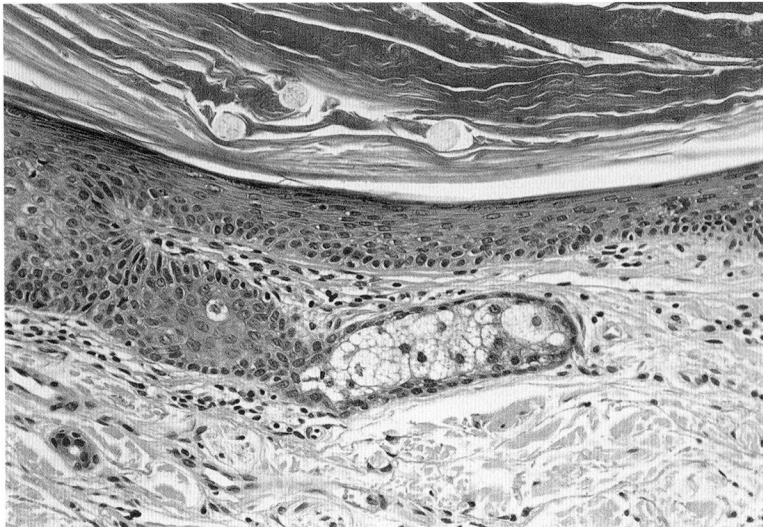

Fig. 34.14
Open comedone: the wall is composed of squamous epithelium. In addition to keratin, there are three pale-staining vellus hairs. Note the atrophic sebaceous gland.

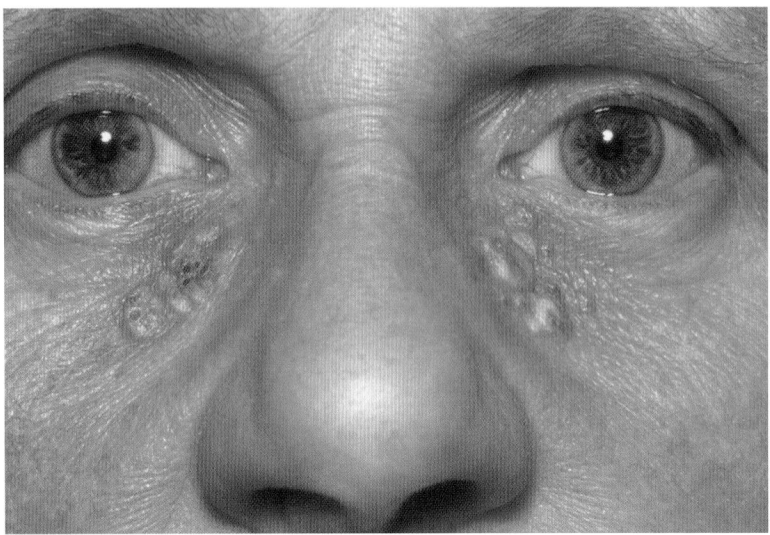

Fig. 34.15
Solar comedones: note the presence of blackheads and multiple yellow cysts.

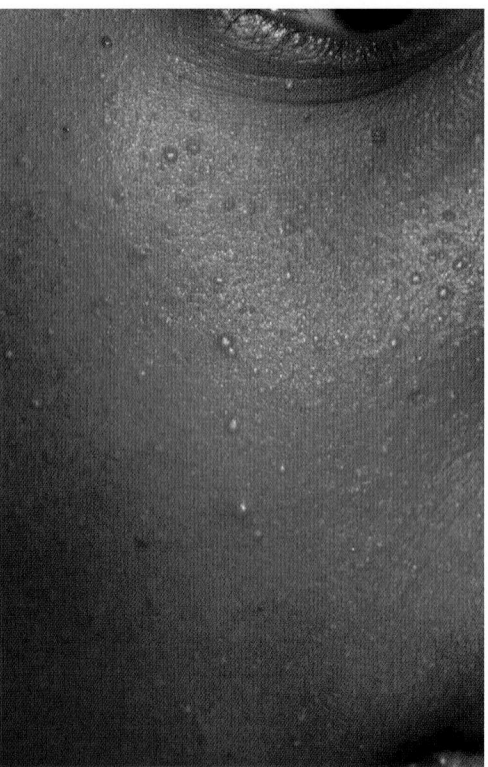

Fig. 34.16
Milia: numerous typical pale small spherical lesions are present. The cheek is a characteristic site. By courtesy of R.A. Marsden, MD, St George's Hospital, London, UK.

epidermolysis bullosa, epidermolysis bullosa acquisita, porphyria cutanea tarda, pseudoporphyria, and bullous pemphigoid.[21] Milia may exceptionally occur in dominant dystrophic epidermolysis bullosa at sites of intact skin and not in association with scarring, suggesting that it may represent a primary manifestation of the disease.[22] They may also be a feature of a variety of familial dermatoses including Rombo syndrome (facial anetoderma vermiculatum, telangiectasia, milia, hypotrichosis, acral erythema, cyanosis, and tendency to develop trichoepitheliomas and basal cell carcinomata), Bazex-Dupré-Christol syndrome (follicular atrophoderma, congenital hypotrichosis, basal cell carcinomas), familial multiple cylindromas, trichoepitheliomas, milia and spiradenomas (Brooke-Spiegler syndrome), Basan syndrome (diffuse congenital milia, transient neonatal acral bullae, and absence of dermatoglyphics), oral-facial-digital syndrome type 1, atrichia with papular lesions, hereditary vitamin D-dependent rickets type II, basal cell nevus syndrome, generalized basaloid follicular hamartoma syndrome, Nicolas-Balus syndrome (eruptive syringomas, milia, and atrophoderma vermiculata), KID syndrome, and hypotrichosis with light-colored hair and facial milia, and pachyonychia congenita type II.[23–26] Generalized congenital milia cysts have also been described in an infant with trisomy 13 syndrome.[27] Congenital familial milia with no other associations may also be rarely seen.[28]

Transverse nasal crease is a rare embryologic anomaly that presents at the junction of the middle and lower third of the nose.[29] The clinical presentation varies from a subtle erythematous line to a hypopigmented indentation. It has been suggested that what has been described as transverse nasal milia represents a clinical variant of transverse nasal crease.[29]

Rarely, milia present as a localized plaque variant (milia en plaque).[3,30–36] Such lesions are most often described around the ears. A small number of cases involving the eyelids have been documented, and there is one supraclavicular example.[31] One case that developed in a background of pseudoxanthoma elasticum has been described.[32] A further example in association with lupus erythematosus and another one in association with cryotherapy have also been reported.[37,38] In the small number of documented cases, the sex incidence is equal, and a wide age range has been affected (12–62 years). A congenital case has been described.[39] Bilateral lesions are exceptional.[40,41] There is no racial predilection.[33] Patients present with an edematous, erythematous plaque studded with numerous milia. Based on a single case with trichoepithelioma-like changes in the background, it has been suggested that this entity represents a variant of follicular hamartoma.[42]

Very occasional examples of eruptive milia have been described including rare cases in children.[4,43–45] Recently, these have been classified into spontaneous and autosomal dominant familial variants.[46] They may also represent a component of a genodermatosis.[4]

Pathogenesis and histologic features

Milia consist of miniature epidermoid cysts located in the superficial dermis just underneath the epithelium (Fig. 34.17). Attachment to a vellus hair follicle is often seen in the newborn variant. Secondary lesions may be related to hair follicles or eccrine sweat ducts. The latter are typically seen in milia associated with scarring blistering diseases. Primary lesions may also be associated with the eccrine duct.[47] Milia cysts occurring on palms and soles are likely derived from eccrine sweat ducts.[48]

The etiology of milia en plaque is unknown, although spectacles, earrings, and perfume have been suggested as possible causes.[33–35] In this variant, a background dense T-cell lymphocytic infiltrate is typically present.[33,34]

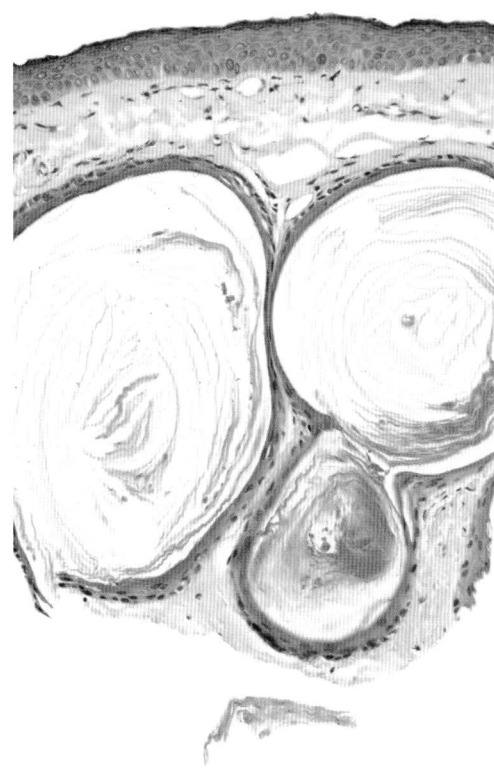

Fig. 34.17
Milia: the cysts are lined by keratinizing stratified squamous epithelium. A granular cell layer is present.

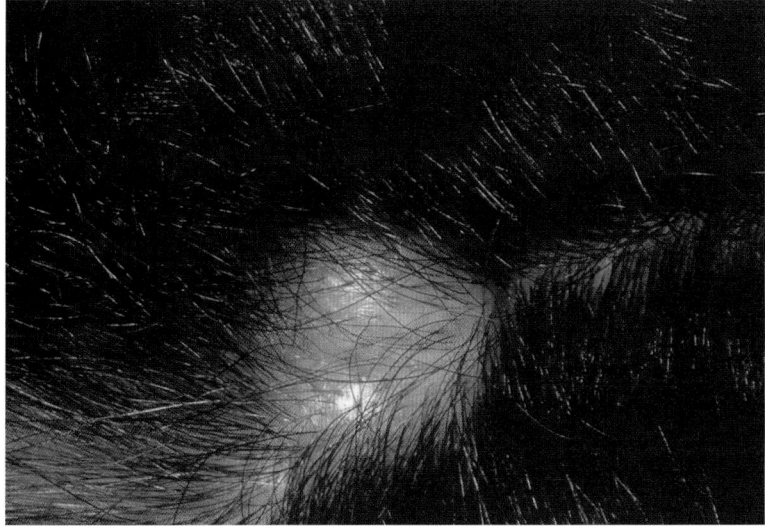

Fig. 34.18
Trichilemmal cyst: note the characteristic dome-shaped swelling on the scalp, a typical site. By courtesy of A. du Vivier, MD, King's College Hospital, London, UK.

Trichilemmal cyst

The outer root sheath of the hair follicle at the level of the follicular isthmus is recapitulated in the wall of trichilemmal (pilar) cysts.[1-3] It has been suggested that these cysts should be renamed as isthmic-catagen cysts. Their origin is unknown, but it has been suggested that they are produced by budding off from the external root sheath as a genetically determined structural aberration. Familial occurrence is seen in 75% of patients, in a pattern suggesting autosomal dominant inheritance.[4]

Clinical features

Trichilemmal cysts are found on the scalp in 90% of cases; they are solitary in 30% and multiple in 70% (Fig. 34.18).[4] Unusual sites such as the pulp of

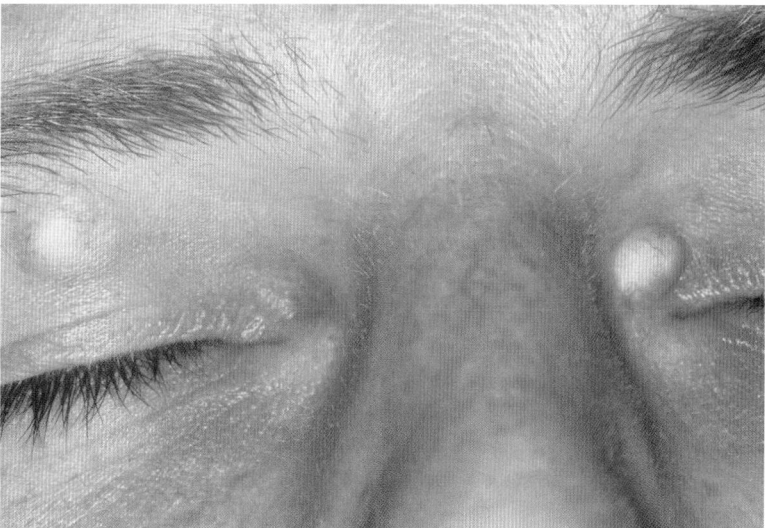

Fig. 34.19
Trichilemmal cyst: there are yellowish circumscribed nodules on the upper eyelids. By courtesy of R.A. Marsden, MD, St George's Hospital, London, UK.

a finger have been reported.[5] Proposed criteria for the diagnosis of hereditary trichilemmal cysts include: (1) lesions in at least two first-degree relatives or on three first- or second-degree relatives in two consecutive generations. (2) At least one of the affected persons diagnosed before the age of 45. (3) The presence of multiple or giant (>5 cm) or unusual histologic features including proliferating cysts or ossification.[6] A case of two female siblings presenting with multiple calcified trichilemmal cysts and alopecia universalis has been described.[7] They present as smooth, yellowish, dome-shaped intradermal swellings and are more common in females (Fig. 34.19). In contrast to epidermoid cysts, they are characteristically devoid of a punctum. It should be noted that the term 'sebaceous cyst' favored by many clinicians is a misnomer because such lesions represent either epidermoid or trichilemmal cysts. Typically, the cyst is encapsulated and uncomplicated lesions readily 'shell out' at surgery.[4] Acute inflammation is uncommon, and when it does occur it is usually of nonbacterial origin; its presence makes excision more difficult, with an increased likelihood of rupture. Exceptional cases of a lesion presenting with filiform hyperkeratosis, comedo-like lesions, and multiple trichilemmal cysts following Blaschko lines, have been described as trichilemmal cyst nevus (nevus trichilemmocysticus) and regarded as a complex organoid epidermal nevus.[8,9] A case of multiple giant trichilemmal cysts, one of which displayed transformation to a squamous cell carcinoma, has been reported.[10] Some lesions may be associated with the development of proliferating trichilemmal tumors (see Chapter 31).[11]

Histologic features

The cyst is surrounded by a fibrous capsule against which rests a layer(s) of small dark-staining basal cells. These merge with characteristic squamous epithelium composed of pale keratinocytes, which increase in height as they mature and transform abruptly into solid eosinophilic-staining keratin without forming a granular cell layer (Figs 34.20–34.22). Occasionally, small foci of epidermal keratinization (i.e., with a granular cell layer) may also be identified. Calcification occurs in 25% of lesions, regardless of the age or size of the cyst, and cholesterol clefts occur in up to 90% (Figs 34.23 and 34.24).[1,4] Osseous metaplasia may occur and exceptionally, extramedullary hematopoiesis has been described.[12,13] Secondary inflammation is manifest as an influx of inflammatory cells into the lumen of the cyst, in contrast to the granulomatous response that may surround an epidermoid cyst. In a small percentage of cases, there is budding of tiny daughter cysts from the parent.[14] Very rarely, sebaceous and apocrine differentiation are found in the cyst wall.[15] Exceptional cases of other neoplasms such as Merkel cell carcinoma colonizing or arising in a trichilemmal cyst have been reported.[16,17] Carcinoma in situ and squamous cell carcinoma may also rarely develop within trichilemmal cysts.[10,18]

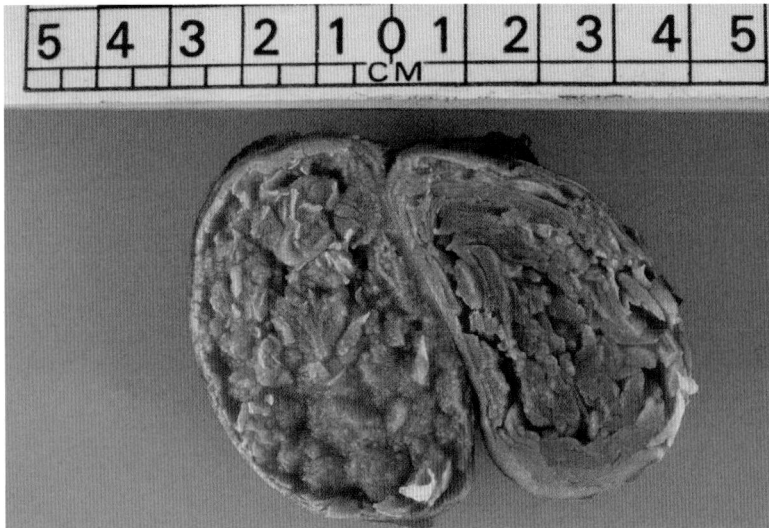

Fig. 34.20
Trichilemmal cyst: this shows the typical macroscopic appearance of cheesy lamellated contents.

Vellus hair cysts

Clinical features

Vellus hair cysts were originally reported in children and young adults of both sexes.[1-4] The sex distribution is equal and there is no racial predilection. Patients present with numerous asymptomatic, discrete, soft, flesh-colored or reddish-brown papules, 1–5 mm across, particularly over the parasternal area, although the distribution may be quite widespread.[4] A generalized distribution has been documented.[5] An exceptional case mimicking a nevus of Ota has been described.[6] Lesions may rarely be unilateral.[7] Occasional lesions are umbilicated, and squeezing may express white caseous material. Further cases have expanded the condition to include an inherited (autosomal dominant) variant, which may or may not be manifest at birth and is more likely to occur over the extensor aspects of the limbs.[3,8,9] Occurrence in twins has been reported.[10] A facial form, a patient presenting with a periorbital distribution, and a further patient with a single orbital lesion have been described.[11-14] Spontaneous involution is not uncommon.[2,15]

Vellus hair cysts have occasionally been associated with renal failure and a number of genodermatoses including pachyonychia congenita, anhidrotic ectodermal dysplasia, hidrotic ectodermal dysplasia, and rarely, Lowe syndrome (oculocerebrorenal syndrome characterized by Fanconi-type renal failure, mental retardation, and ocular abnormalities).[16-20] Occasionally, solitary lesions are encountered and may be large.[21]

Pathogenesis and histologic features

Eruptive vellus hair cysts most probably develop as a consequence of occlusion of the infundibulum of vellus hairs with resultant cystic dilatation and retention of keratinous debris and vellus hairs.[2] The primary cause of the obstruction is unknown. It has also been proposed that they represent follicular hamartomas.[8] Studies indicate that both eruptive vellus hair cysts and steatocystomas express keratin 17, with the latter also expressing keratin 10.[22,23] This overlap in keratin expression may help explain the underlying similarities and perhaps overlapping features of these two lesions; however, this opinion is not universal, and their exact relationship remains to be elucidated.[24-26]

The characteristic histology is that of a mid-dermal cyst containing laminated keratin and many vellus hairs (Figs 34.25 and 34.26).[2,4,15] The epithelial lining consists of several layers of squamous epithelium, often with a granular cell layer. Sometimes the cyst is in continuity with the epidermis, an atrophic follicle, or a pilomotor muscle.[3,4,15] Vellus hair cysts are more likely to open onto the surface in the congenital variant. Occasionally the cyst ruptures, and there is an associated foreign body giant cell reaction that may be associated with formation of cholesterol clefts.[27]

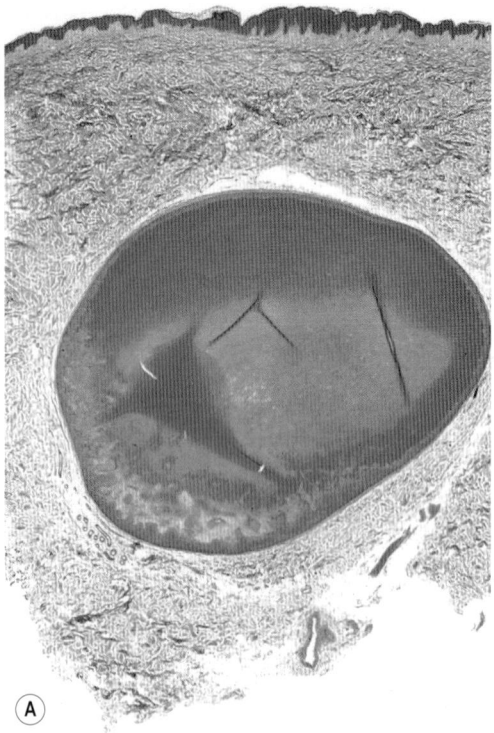

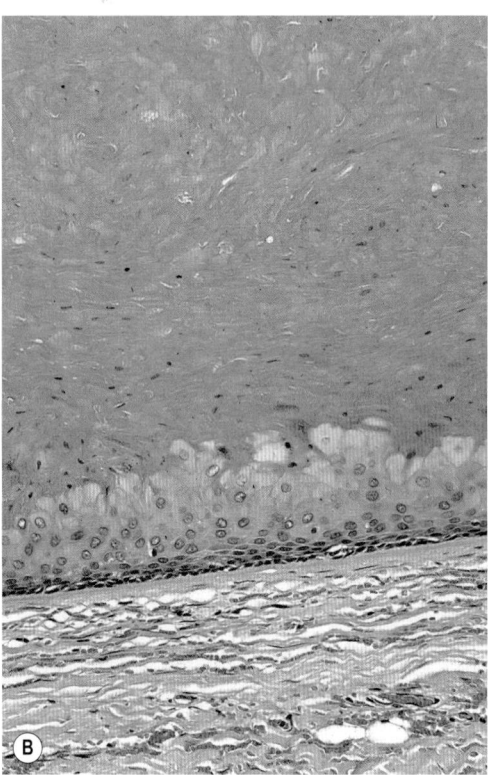

Fig. 34.21
(A, B) Trichilemmal cyst: these views show the homogeneous eosinophilic contents. Note the distinct basal cell layer.

Differential diagnosis

Eruptive vellus hair cysts show very marked clinical overlap with steatocystoma multiplex and can only be distinguished by histologic analysis.[28] Steatocystoma is characterized by an epidermoid lining without a granular cell layer. The innermost aspect of the cyst wall is covered by an undulating eosinophilic cuticle. Sebaceous glands are present in the wall of the cyst or in the immediate vicinity.

Sometimes, however, patients have both types of cyst simultaneously, and occasionally there are overlapping histologic features sometimes constituting a hybrid cyst.[28-30]

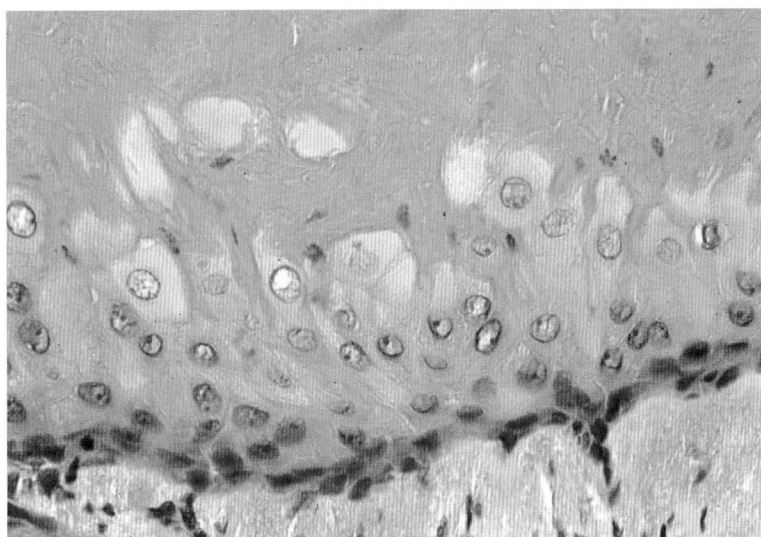

Fig. 34.22
Trichilemmal cyst: the cyst wall is composed of squamous epithelium and a granular cell layer is not present. The most superficial cells are larger, vertically orientated, and have abundant cytoplasm. Keratinization is abrupt.

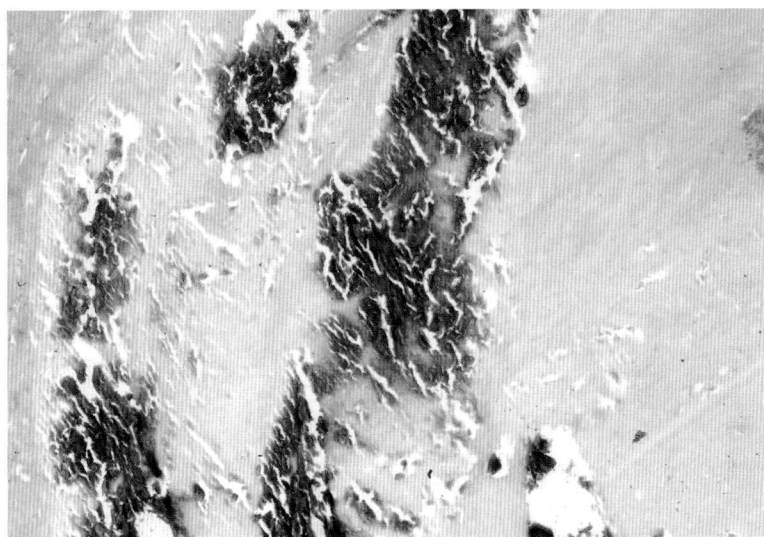

Fig. 34.23
Trichilemmal cyst: basophilic granular calcification is a frequent histologic finding.

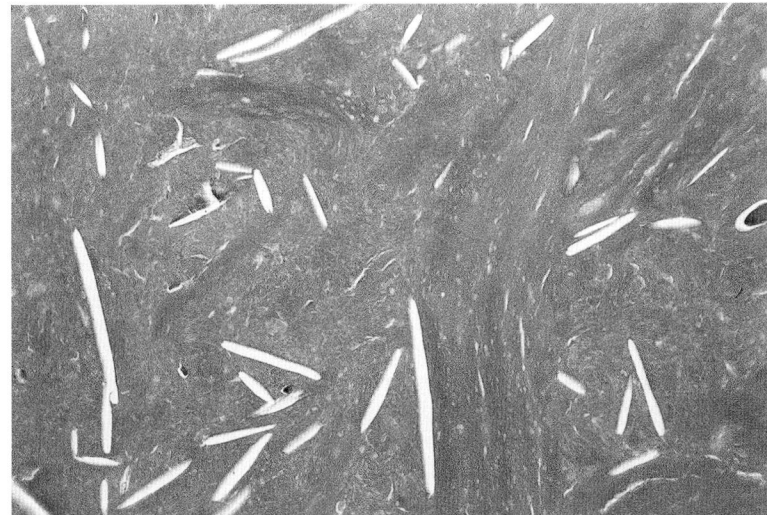

Fig. 34.24
Trichilemmal cyst: the empty spaces (cholesterol clefts) are a common feature of this lesion.

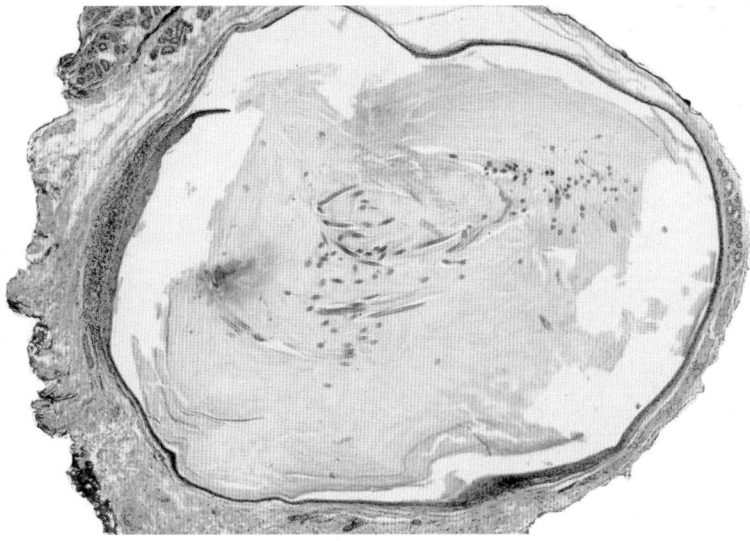

Fig. 34.25
Vellus hair cyst: this thin-walled cyst is present in the mid-dermis.

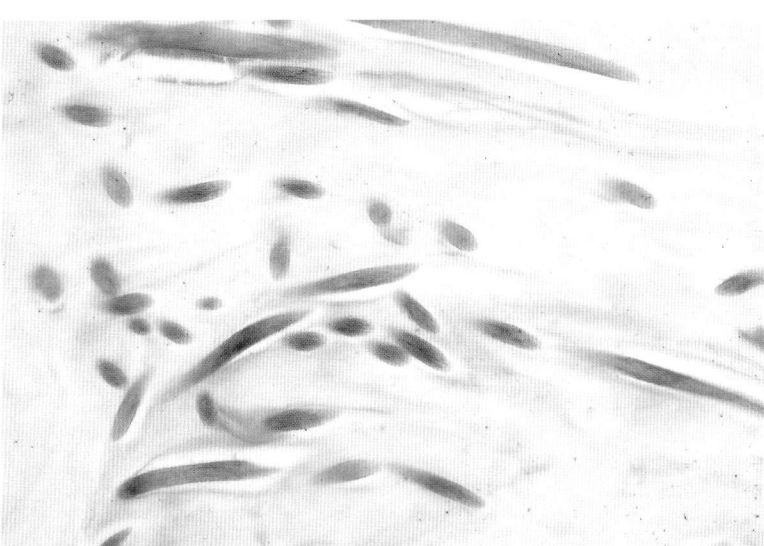

Fig. 34.26
Vellus hair cyst: on high power, the lumen contains numerous vellus hairs.

As noted above, differential keratin expression has been shown to distinguish the two cysts. Thus vellus hair cyst expresses K17 but not K10, whereas steatocystoma expresses K17 and K10.[31] Interestingly, mutations in the *KRT17* gene can cause both pachyonychia congenital type 2 and also a condition very similar or identical to steatocystoma multiplex.[32,33] The relevance of these findings to steatocystoma simplex and vellus hair cysts, if any, remains to be determined.

Dermoid cyst

Clinical features

Dermoid cysts result from the sequestration of cutaneous tissues along embryonal lines of closure.[1–5] The most common clinical appearance is that of a single nontender small subcutaneous nodule at birth on the lateral aspect of the upper eyelid (*Fig. 34.27*). Although slow enlargement is the rule, sometimes a sudden increase in size may occur, bringing the lesion to attention at a later age. Other potential sites of dermoid cysts include the midline of the neck, nasal root, nose, forehead, the mastoid area, anterior chest, and scalp.[3,6–8] The last is a particularly important site as the lesion may very occasionally show intracranial extension (dumbbell dermoid).[3,4] Midline occipital lesions are most often affected.[3] Dermoid cysts may also

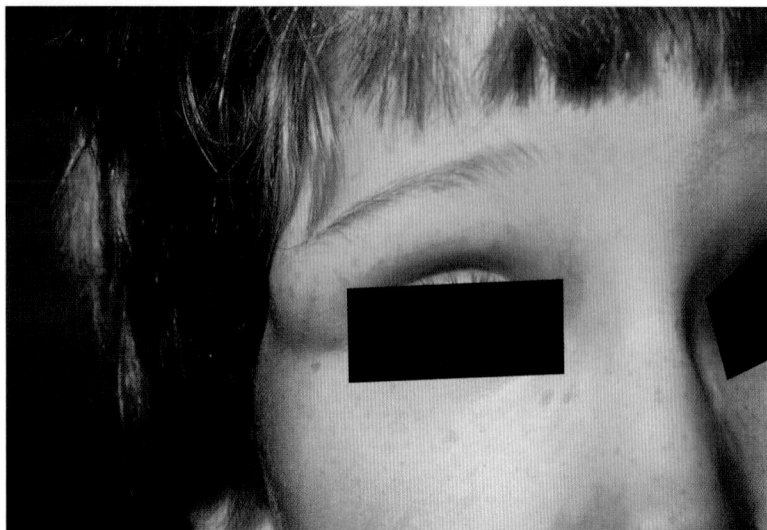

Fig. 34.27
Dermoid cyst: note the swelling adjacent to the upper eyelid – the external angular dermoid cyst. By courtesy of R.A. Marsden, MD, St George's Hospital, London, UK.

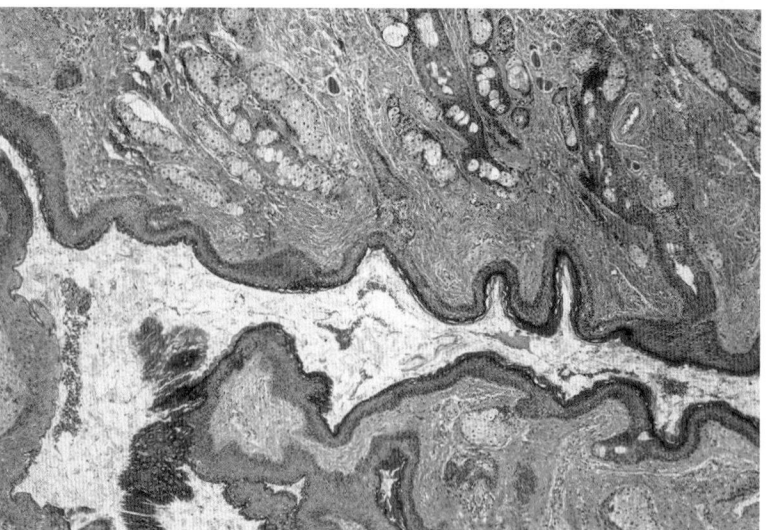

Fig. 34.28
Dermoid cyst: the cyst is lined by stratified squamous epithelium. Note the numerous sebaceous glands.

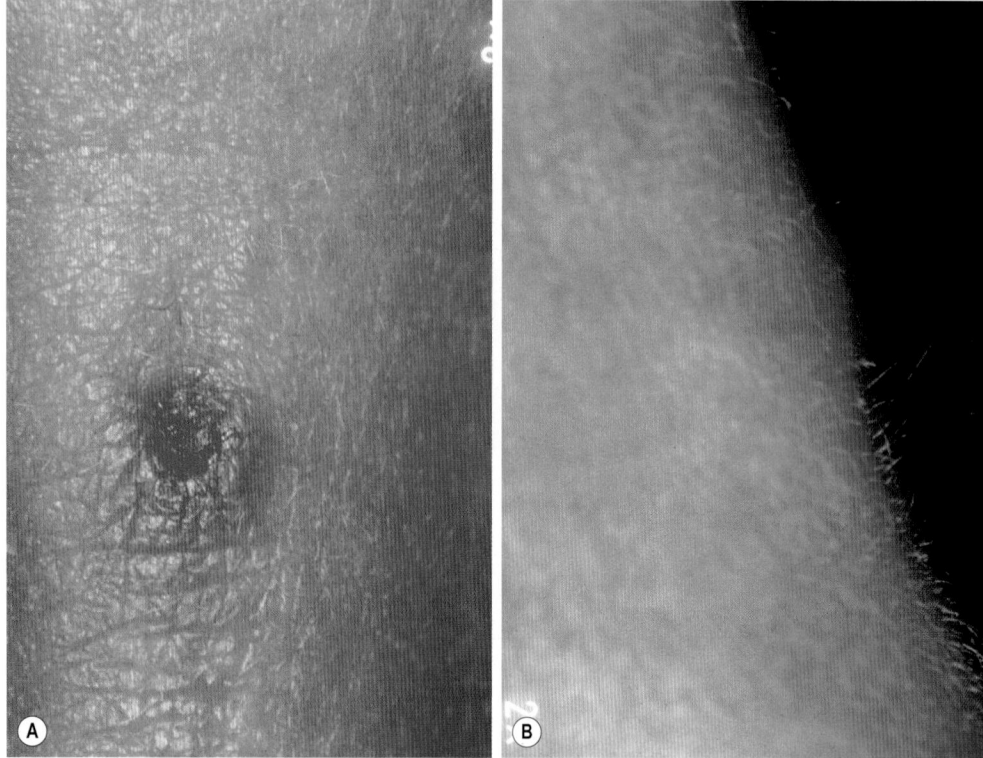

Fig. 34.29
Median nasal dermoid fistula: (**A**) on the dorsum of the nose is an erythematous crateriform depression; (**B**) the presence of protruding white hairs is characteristic. By courtesy of D. Shuttleworth, MD, Chichester, UK.

present on mid chest, sacrum, perineum, scrotum, penis, and ear.[5,9] Dermoid cysts are also encountered in the oral cavity and deeper noncutaneous sites.

Infection of a cranial dermoid cyst is a serious development as it may be complicated by central nervous system involvement.[3] Squamous cell carcinoma very rarely develops in the wall of the cyst.[10,11] Exceptionally, the development of carcinosarcoma has been described.[12] There are occasional reports of familial dermoid cysts, including one family associated with midline cleft lip.[13–15]

Pathogenesis and histologic features

The unilocular cysts are usually subcutaneous and may be attached to the periosteum. They are lined by stratified squamous epithelium with associated hair follicles and sebaceous glands (*Fig. 34.28*). Trichilemmal differentiation is exceptionally seen in the lining of the cyst.[16] Eccrine sweat glands are present in 35% of cases and apocrine glands in 15%. Smooth muscle can be present but – in contrast to benign cystic teratoma – cartilage and bone are not described. Some authors propose an embryological origin for these cysts, particularly in the nasal form.[17]

Antenatal diagnosis has been reported.[13]

Differential diagnosis

Dermoid cyst should be distinguished from congenital dermoid fistula, which presents at birth as a superficial fistula tract (*Figs 34.29 and 34.30*).[18–20]

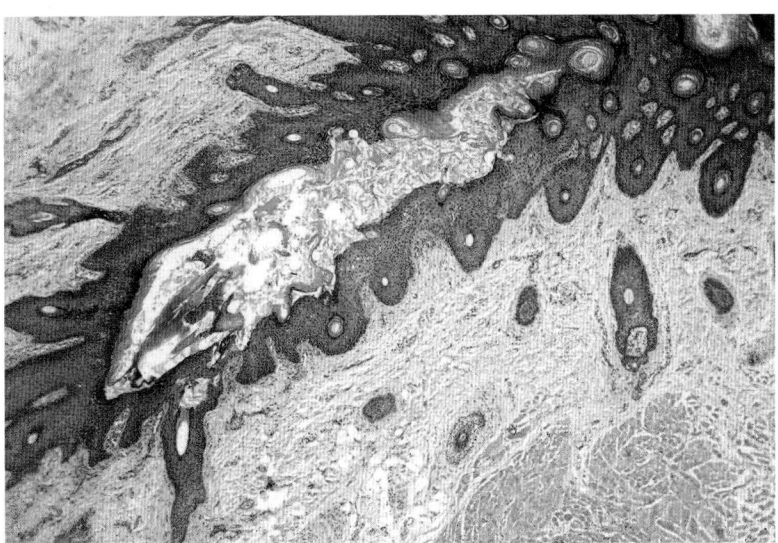

Fig. 34.30
Median nasal dermoid fistula: the fistula, which communicates with the surface epidermis, is lined by hair-bearing epithelium. By courtesy of D. Shuttleworth, MD, Chichester, UK.

Cutaneous mature cystic teratoma

Cutaneous mature cystic teratomas are exceptionally rare, but lesions presenting on the face, neck, and back have been documented.[1–3] To establish the diagnosis, representative elements from ectoderm, endoderm, and mesoderm should be identifiable.

Glandular cysts

Bronchogenic cyst

Clinical features

Bronchogenic cysts presenting in the skin are very rare, with fewer than 70 cases reported.[1–14] There is a marked predilection for males (4:1).[13] Most are situated on the precordium or overlying the suprasternal notch and are usually present at birth.[1–3] Occasionally, they are located about the shoulder, back, scapula, neck, abdomen, chin, and perianal area or present at a later age.[4,15,16] Clinical presentation is variable and includes cutaneous cystic nodules, sinuses, and even a papillomatous growth.[4,5] Occasionally, the cysts drain a mucinous fluid.[1,8] Most are asymptomatic, but some are tender or painful. Exceptionally, multiple lesions may be seen.[17]

Pathogenesis and histologic features

Bronchogenic cysts are believed to form from buds or diverticula that separate from the foregut during the development of the tracheobronchial tree; they may be intrapulmonary or peripheral. Cutaneous bronchogenic cysts may result from subsequent sequestration outside the chest cavity following fusion of the mesenchymal bars of the sternum or else from active migration prior to fusion.[13,14] Lesions overlying the scapula likely arose before the scapula developed, at the sixth week of gestation.[6]

The cutaneous bronchogenic cyst is situated within the dermis or subcutaneous tissue, and usually its lining is thrown into small folds. The epithelium is invariably pseudostratified cuboidal or columnar and ciliated, with mucus-secreting goblet cells in about 50% of cases.[2,13] Nonciliated cuboidal, columnar, and stratified squamous epithelium may also be identified. Smooth muscle supports the mucosa in 8% of cases.[1,12,13] Lymphoid follicles are found in only 25% of cases and then appear to be part of a secondary inflammatory response.[1] Seromucinous glands are also sometimes present.[2,5,12] Cartilage is evident in a minority of cases.[4,6,10,13] Not all of these features are necessarily present in any one particular cyst, and the diagnosis may then be in part dependent on clinicopathological correlation.[8,9]

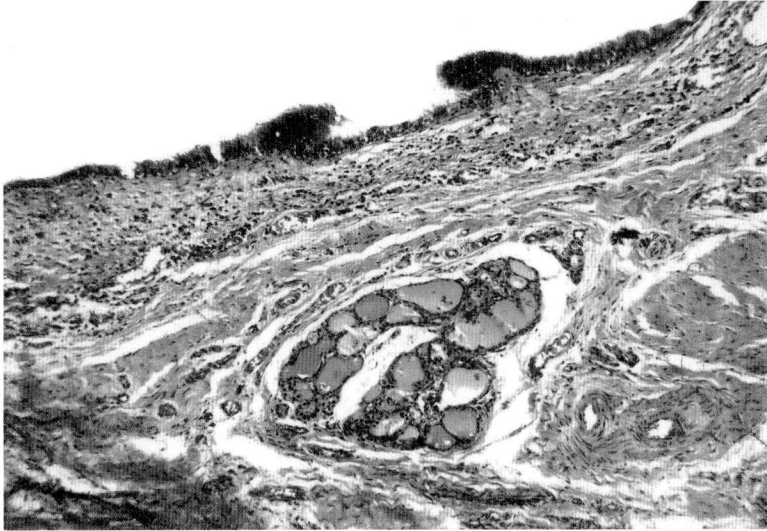

Fig. 34.31
Thyroglossal duct cyst: the cyst is lined by tall columnar epithelium. Note the colloid-containing thyroid follicles.

Cutaneous lung tissue heterotopia in which fully developed bronchioles and alveoli are present can be regarded as a variant.[18,19]

Immunohistochemistry has been only rarely documented. The lining epithelial cells express cytokeratin (AE1/AE3) but not carcinoembryonic antigen (CEA).[13]

Thyroglossal duct cyst

Clinical features

The thyroglossal duct cyst, which is a congenital anomaly representing a vestigial remnant of the tubular thyroid gland precursor, may present at any age including adulthood (predominantly in the fifth decade of life), but children in the first decade of life are most often affected.[1–10] Lesions are more common in males in children and in females in adults.[10] It is commonly found in the midline of the neck in the region below the hyoid bone as a fluctuant swelling up to 3 cm in diameter. It characteristically moves with swallowing.[11] The development of an associated sinus is a not uncommon complication more frequently seen in children.[10,12] An exceptional case of a recurrent lesion presenting with cutaneous blisters has been reported.[13]

Very occasional familial variants have been reported.[14] Most of these have displayed an autosomal dominant mode of inheritance although recessive forms are also recognized.[15–17] Although the number of documented families is small, there appears to be a predilection for females.[14]

Recurrence following surgery is low, varying from 2% to 6% of cases.[14,18]

Pathogenesis and histologic features

Thyroglossal duct cysts, which are variably lined by cuboidal, columnar, or stratified squamous epithelium, are frequently accompanied by an epithelial-lined tract.[1] Ciliated epithelium is also often present. The epithelial lining may be exclusively respiratory, squamous, or more often, in about half of the cases, a mixture of both.[10] In around 1% of cases, no epithelial lining is seen.[10] The adjacent tissues may show mucous glands, thyroid follicles (in 71% of cases), and a heavy lymphocytic infiltrate (Fig. 34.31). Occasionally, skin appendages (including hair follicles and sebaceous and sweat glands) are additionally found, resulting in histologic overlap with a dermoid cyst – the so-called mixed or hybrid cyst.[2,6] Smooth muscle is not present but skeletal muscle and adipose tissue are commonly seen.[10] In most cases, the hyoid bone is identified.[10]

Occasionally, histologic examination may reveal ectopic thyroid gland, thyroid adenoma, and in approximately 1% to 3% of cases, carcinoma.[10,19–26] The last are most often papillary adenocarcinoma, but follicular and squamous variants have also been described.[10,11] They sometimes represent an incidental finding following excision.

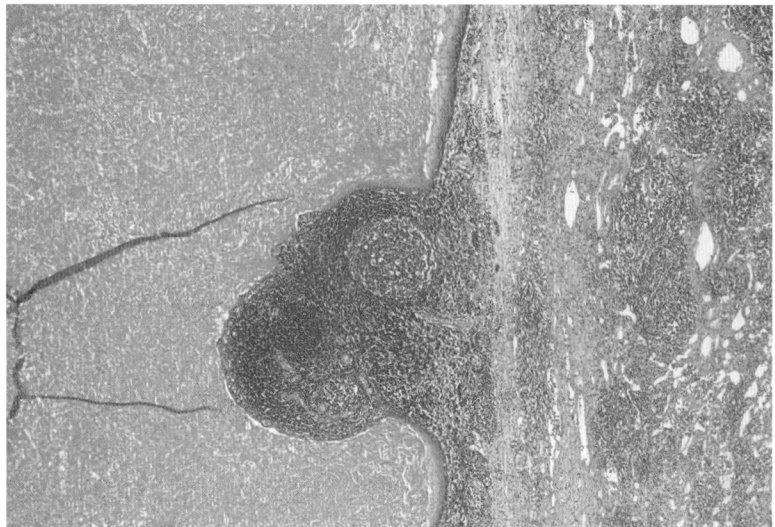

Fig. 34.32
Branchial cyst: the wall is composed of stratified squamous epithelium. Note the intense lymphocytic infiltrate.

Branchial cyst

Clinical features

The branchial (lymphoepithelial) cyst presents as a swelling near the angle of the jaw anterior to the sternomastoid muscle, most often at the junction of its upper one-third and lower two-thirds.[1–4] Lesions also present in deeper tissues. The cyst is asymptomatic and does not move on swallowing.[3] Patients are most commonly in their second or third decade. The sexes are affected equally.[3] Rare lesions are associated with a fistule. A single case was associated with a duplicated facial nerve.[5] Occasionally, bilateral cysts are present and then a familial tendency is sometimes in play.[6]

Pathogenesis and histologic features

The origin of the cyst is uncertain although it is generally considered to represent a developmental anomaly of the branchial arches. Possibilities include incomplete obliteration of branchial mucosa, remnants of the precervical sinus, or an origin from the thymopharyngeal duct.[3,7] Cystic degeneration of cervical lymph nodes has also been suggested.[7]

It is lined by stratified squamous or pseudostratified ciliated columnar epithelium (*Fig. 34.32*). Its wall typically contains lymphoid tissue in which germinal centers are usually conspicuous.[3] Occasionally, seromucinous glands may also be evident.[2] A case of nasopharyngeal branchial cleft cyst harboring a lymphoma and rare cases with a squamous cell carcinoma and papillary thyroid carcinoma (probably arising from ectopic thyroid tissue) have been reported.[8–14] In such cases, it is important to rule out a cystic lymph node metastasis from a primary elsewhere. It is important not to confuse a branchyal cyst with a rare cystic metastasis of a well-differentiated ciliated HPV-related carcinoma.[15]

Cervical thymic cyst

Clinical features

Cervical thymic cysts mostly affect children and present in the anterior triangle along a line from the angle of the mandible to the manubrium sternae.[1–6] Presentation in deeper tissues may also be seen. Lesions account for 0.3% to 1% of congenital neck masses.[7] Lesions only exceptionally present in adults.[8] The left side of the neck is affected in 68% of cases, the right side in 25% of cases, and the midline in 7% of cases.[3] Extension into the mediastinum is common.[5] The cyst may enlarge on Valsalva maneuver.

Pathogenesis and histologic features

The cyst develops from remnants of the thymopharyngeal duct which persist as the thymic precursor descends into the mediastinum.[3,4]

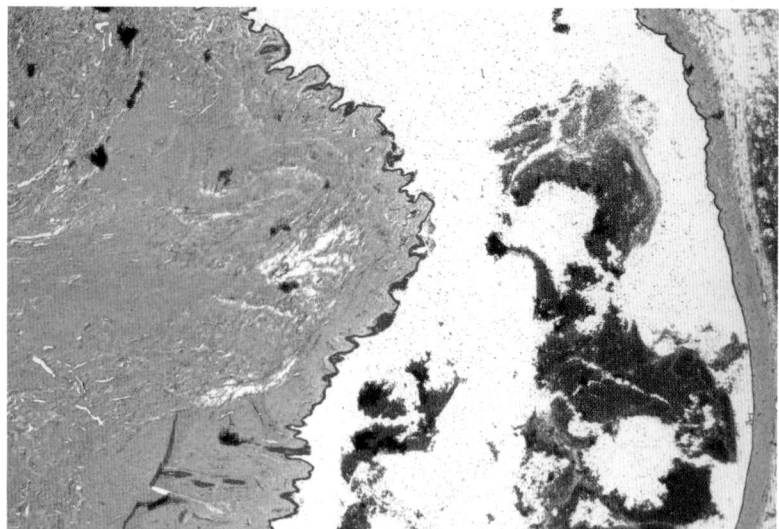

Fig. 34.33
Cutaneous ciliated cyst: note the papillary projections in the lower left of the field.

Cysts are unilocular or multilocular and contain clear, brown, red, or gelatinous material.[4,5,9] The lining epithelium is variably stratified squamous, cuboidal, columnar, pseudostratified, or ciliated.[1,3] Thymic remnants including Hassall corpuscles and cholesterol granulomata are also present.[1,3,10] The adjacent fibrous capsule often contains lymphocytic aggregates.[2] A lesion containing parathyroid tissue has been described.[11]

Cutaneous ciliated cyst

Clinical features

The term cutaneous ciliated cyst (cutaneous Müllerian cyst) most often refers to a solitary lesion which presents shortly after the menarche on the limb (including the digits) of young females (12–42 years).[1–13] The thigh, buttock, calf, and foot are affected, in decreasing order of frequency. The cysts are located in the deep dermis and/or subcutaneous tissue and are usually asymptomatic.[4] Occasionally, they become inflamed and painful and sometimes they rupture. Identical lesions have been described on the abdominal wall.[14,15]

Lesions have occasionally been described in males and at atypical sites including the back, shoulder, scalp, cheek, and scrotum.[16–24] These might better be classified as separate, distinct entities.

Pathogenesis and histologic features

Two theories have been proposed to explain the development of ciliated cysts. Those lesions which present on the limbs of young females are generally thought to be of Müllerian (paramesonephric) derivation, their presence representing a migration abnormality of fetal development (heterotopia).[2,3] In support of this hypothesis, authors have cited the close proximity of the paramesonephric duct to the developing limb bud, the striking predilection for females, the histologic similarity between the lining epithelium and that of the fallopian cord, and the absence of sweat glands in the near vicinity of the cyst wall.[13] Cysts arising at other sites and in males may represent metaplasia of the lining of a preexistent simple cyst of sweat duct derivation or else an entirely different histogenesis (see differential diagnosis).[5]

The cyst is unilocular or multilocular and has intraluminal papillary projections (*Fig. 34.33*). The lining, which is similar to that of normal fallopian tube, consists of cuboidal to columnar ciliated epithelium with frequent pseudostratified foci (*Fig. 34.34*).[6] Intercalated dark cells are also occasionally evident.[4] Squamous metaplasia is often a feature. Mucin-secreting cells have very exceptionally been described, and there are one or two reports of apocrine-like features.[2,8,11] Deep to the epithelium lie well-vascularized parallel bundles of collagen, but smooth muscle is not a feature.[1]

Ultrastructurally, the cilia have characteristic morphology with a central pair of microtubules, nine radially orientated pairs of microtubules,

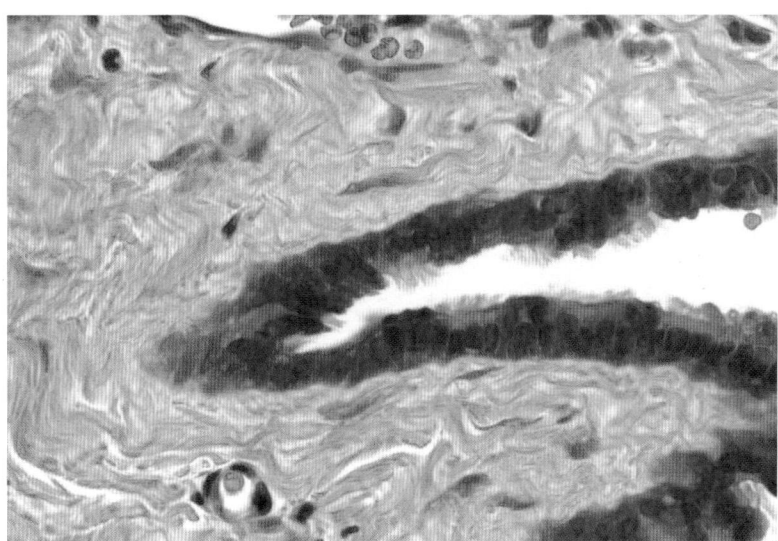

Fig. 34.34
Cutaneous ciliated cyst: the wall is lined by tall columnar cells. Cilia are evident in the center of the field.

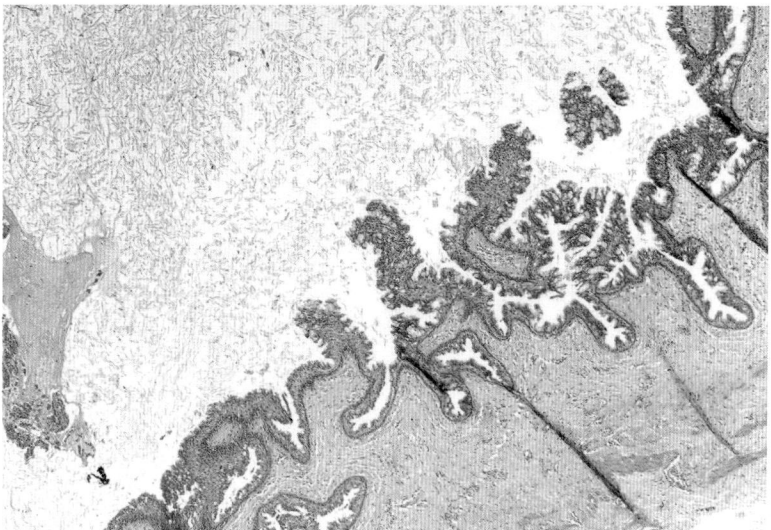

Fig. 34.35
Median raphe cyst: low-power view showing papillary processes covered by columnar epithelium.

basal bodies, and cross-striated rootlets.[7,8,13] Microvilli are sometimes evident.[8,14]

The lining cells express keratin and epithelial membrane antigen (EMA) but not CEA or desmin and smooth muscle actin (SMA).[8-10,14,15] One case, which presented on the cheek of a male and demonstrated an S100 protein and SMA positive myoepithelial layer, would be better classified as a sweat gland hidrocystoma with cilia metaplasia.[21] Desmin expression restricted to the apical aspect of the ciliated cells has been documented in one case.[8] Estrogen and progesterone receptors may be positive and S100 protein is occasionally present.[8,12,14] Positivity for PAX8 and WT-1 has also been reported in lesions arising in females supporting Müllerian differentiation in these lesions. [25-27] Single case reports also document expression of amylase and dynein.[3,10]

Differential diagnosis

Ciliated epithelial cells are also seen in bronchogenic, thyroglossal duct, branchial, and thymic cysts. They may also be present in mature cystic teratoma.

Median raphe cyst

Clinical features

Median raphe cysts (genitoperineal raphe cyst, parameatal cyst) are usually up to 1 cm across, contain clear fluid, and are most often noticed in the first three decades of life as an asymptomatic nodule, sometimes translucent, on the ventral aspect of the penis.[1-10] Rare lesions present as a cord-like or canal-like induration.[11] The glans is the most commonly affected site.[5] Lesions may also be seen along the ventral surface of the scrotum and on the perineum.[12-17] Perianal lesions are exceptional.[18] The cyst does not communicate with the urethra. Recurrences are uncommon.[1] Rarely, cysts develop in association with split median raphe.[19]

Pathogenesis and histologic features

The cyst is generally believed to result from anomalous fusion of the genitourethral folds and urethral plate, with resultant misplaced nests of urethral epithelium in the ventral midline.[11] Alternatively, some examples may result from misplaced periurethral glands (mucoid cyst) or aberrant urethral buds.[2,5] Similar malfusion of the labial–scrotal folds results in scrotal and perineal variants.[12]

Histologically, the cyst lining is variable. In most reports it consists of pseudostratified columnar epithelium, 1–4 cells thick (*Fig. 34.35*).[1,2,5] Uncommonly, diastase-resistant, periodic acid-Schiff (PAS)-positive mucinous, and stratified squamous epithelia are present (*Fig. 34.36*).[1,8,13] Glandular

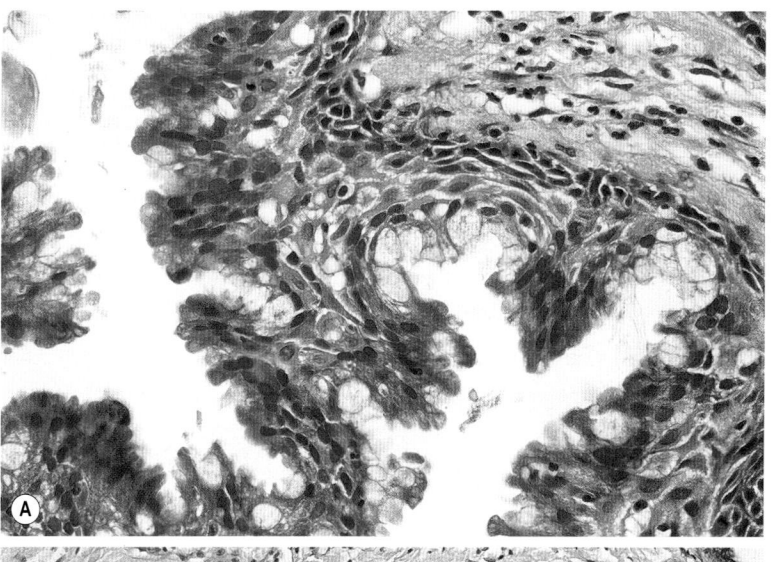

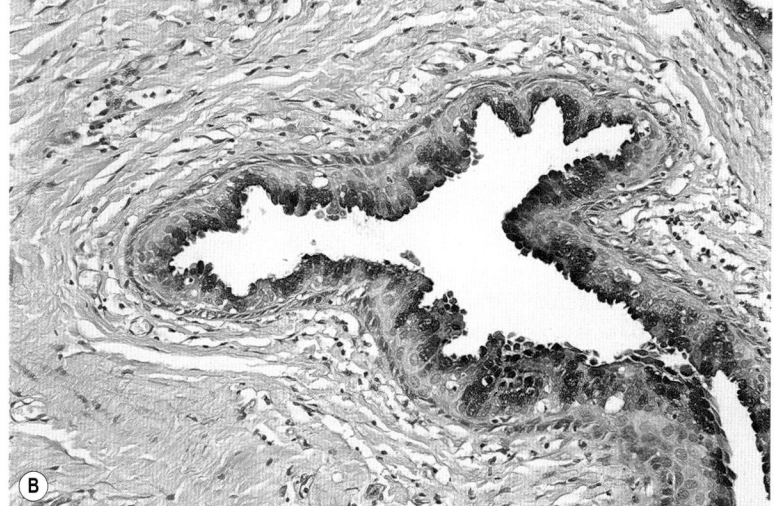

Fig. 34.36
Median raphe cyst: (**A**) the cyst is focally lined by mucus-containing epithelium; (**B**) the latter is PAS positive (diastase resistant).

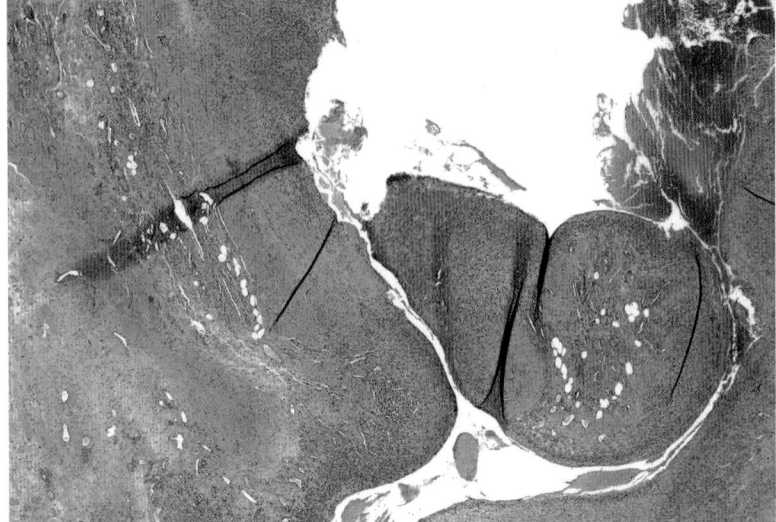

Fig. 34.37
Metaplastic synovial cyst: this example presented as a fistulous tract following abdominal surgery. Villous processes are evident.

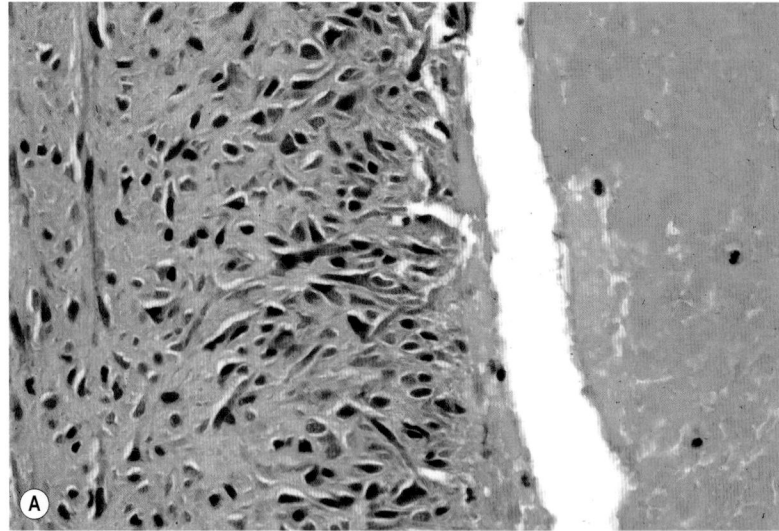

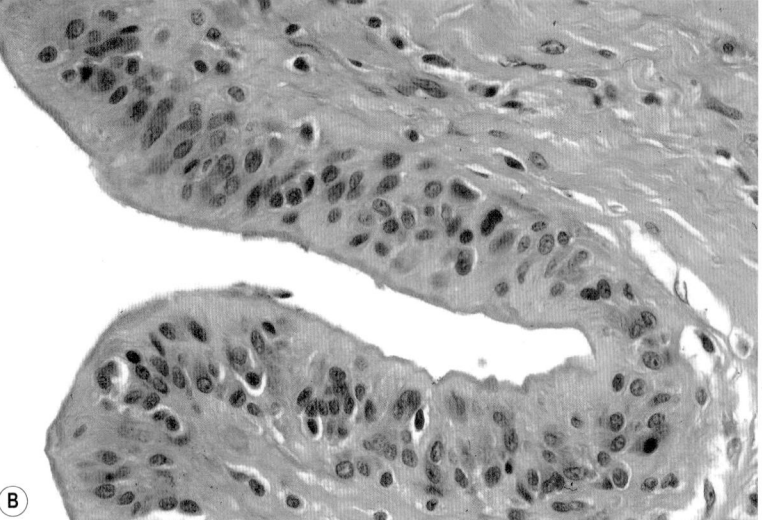

Fig. 34.38
(A, B) Metaplastic synovial cyst: the villi are covered by a layer of fibrin and vertically orientated spindle cells.

formation is very rare.[20] Metaplastic ciliated variants and admixed goblet cells are very occasionally seen.[9,10,13] Exceptionally, pigmented variants associated with intraepithelial dendritic melanocytes may be encountered.[6,21] One publication described linear small epidermoid cysts extending along the median raphe of the scrotum to the anal verge of a male infant. These may have resulted from entrapped squamous epithelial rests during the development of the raphe scroti.[12]

The epithelial cells are CK7 and CEA positive, and CK20 negative.[7,8] Focal neuroendocrine differentiation characterized by chromogranin and synaptophysin expression has been documented in two cases.[8]

Differential diagnosis

The midline site, the predominant pseudostratification, and the lack of both decapitation secretion and a myoepithelial layer distinguish median raphe cyst from apocrine cystadenoma. In addition, median raphe cysts do not express human milk fat globulin 1 (HMFG-1).[7]

Cutaneous metaplastic synovial cyst

Clinical features

First described by González and coworkers in 1987, cutaneous metaplastic synovial cyst is an uncommonly reported lesion which usually follows surgical or other trauma.[1–12] Patients present with an often tender dermal nodule adjacent to a scar and clinically diagnosed as a suture granuloma.[1] Lesions draining serosanguinous fluid sometimes communicate with the surface epithelium. Exceptionally, multiple lesions may be encountered.[7] Occasional examples have arisen without a history of trauma, most often in patients with severe rheumatoid arthritis.[7,9] Two cases have presented in patients with Ehlers-Danlos syndrome.[6,13] Lesions can occur at any site, and there is no sex or age predilection.[7] Local recurrence is very rare.[14]

Pathogenesis and histologic features

Seyle originally showed that a synovium-like membrane could develop in the connective tissue of rats following its disruption by the subcutaneous injection of air.[15] The experiment was later repeated, and similar observations have been reported following implantation of various prosthetic devices.[16–20]

Cutaneous metaplastic synovial cyst is not a true cyst since it lacks an epithelial lining. It is located in the dermis underneath a sometimes thickened epidermis with which it occasionally communicates through a fistulous tract (Fig. 34.37).[1] It contains multiple villous processes of two types: some are composed of hyalinized connective tissue covered by fibrin, whereas others are highly cellular and are lined by multilayered epithelioid cells

(Fig. 34.38).[1,4] The core of the second type is composed of admixed spindled and epithelioid cells and a mixed inflammatory cell infiltrate in which multinucleate giant cells are sometimes conspicuous. The lining cells are devoid of atypia, but multiple (normal) mitoses are sometimes present. The cyst is surrounded by chronically inflamed granulation and scar tissue.[3] Synovial metaplasia-like changes with papillary projections have rarely been described in association with oral mucoceles.[21]

The epithelioid cells regularly express vimentin and occasionally CD68, lysozyme, and α_1-antichymotrypsin.[1,2,9] They are consistently negative for keratins, CEA, EMA, S100 protein, SMA, and desmin.[2,4,6,9]

Pilonidal sinus

Clinical features

Pilonidal sinus (jeep disease) is a fairly common condition which shows a predilection for males (3–4:1) and presents most often in the second two decades.[1–4] Caucasians are predominantly affected.[3] The disease is very uncommon in blacks and exceptionally rare in Asians.[3] Although patients may very rarely be asymptomatic, the typical history is of a chronic painful draining sinus or multiple sinuses affecting the base of the spine or the intergluteal cleft.[2] Similar lesions have been described on the ear, scalp, chest, umbilicus, penis, vulva, anal canal, and axilla.[5–12] Similar interdigital variants may be encountered in barbers, hairdressers, sheep shearers, cow milkers, and dog groomers as a reaction to hair embedded in the dermis.[13–19] A subungual form has also been documented.[20]

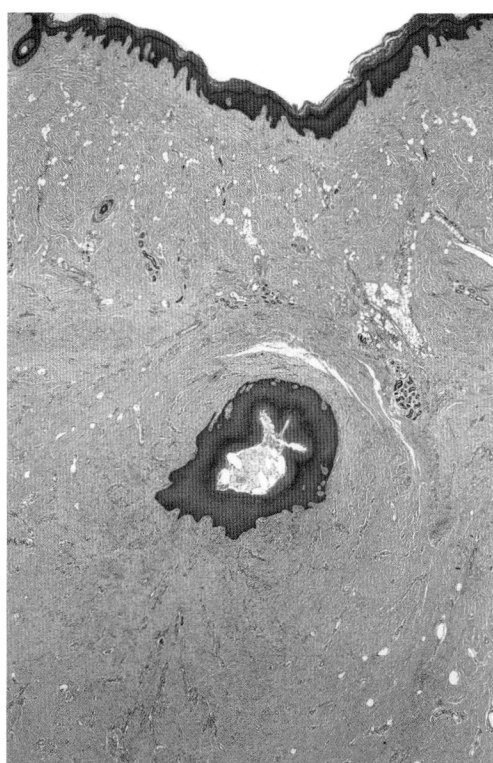

Fig. 34.39
Pilonidal sinus: the sinus is lined by stratified squamous epithelium. Note the surrounding scar tissue, chronic inflammation, and hemosiderin deposition.

There are a small number of reports of malignancy supervening in chronic sacrococcygeal pilonidal sinus with an estimated incidence of around 0.1%.[21-24]

Pathogenesis and histologic features

The sacrococcygeal variant appears to develop as a consequence of the patient's own hair penetrating the skin directly or via dilated follicular ostia.[2-4] Free hair in the gluteal cleft rubs against the adjacent skin and the friction from movement of the buttocks propels the shaft through the epithelium into the dermis where a foreign body granulomatous reaction results. It also results in a nidus for secondary infection and abscess formation.[3] Epstein-Barr virus-infected lymphocytes predominantly with a B phenotype have been found in more than half of the cases of pilonidal sinus in a study.[25] This is not thought to be related to the pathogenesis of the disease.

Superficially, the sinus is often lined by stratified squamous epithelium but toward the deeper reaches the wall consists of granulation and scar tissue surrounding intensely inflamed dermis containing one or more hair shaft fragments (Figs 34.39 and 34.40). Abscesses are commonly present, and foreign body multinucleate giant cells are usually conspicuous. Secondary infection with bacteria including Actinomyces may be seen.[26]

The rare malignancies are generally well-differentiated squamous cell carcinomas.[27] Morbidity and mortality are significant with local recurrence and metastasis in around a third of cases.[21] Immunosuppression can augment or complicate malignant degeneration.[22] Verrucous carcinoma has also been noted.[23] Very occasionally, basal cell carcinoma has been described and there is one example of adenocarcinoma.[28,29]

Dental sinus

Clinical features

Dental sinus tracts (odontogenic sinus) develop as a result of a periapical root infection or abscess.[1-7] Clinically, they present as papules, nodules, cysts, abscess, ulcers, or frank sinuses, usually associated with scarring.[4] In some patients, the dental abnormality is silent, which can result in delay in

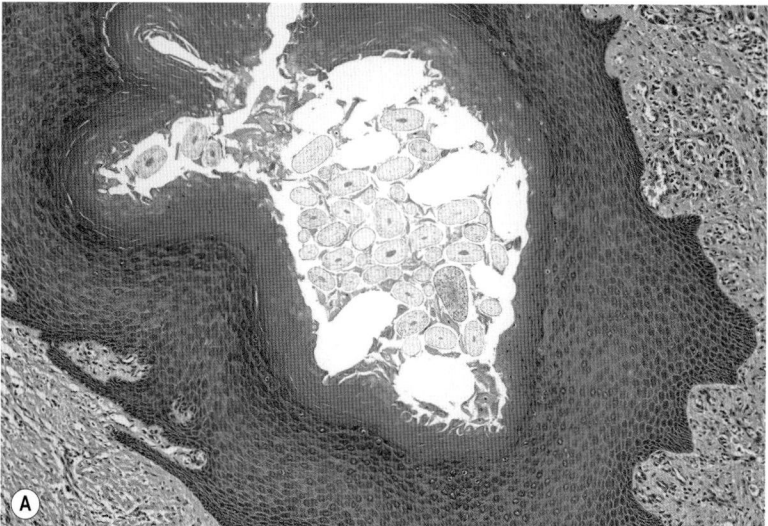
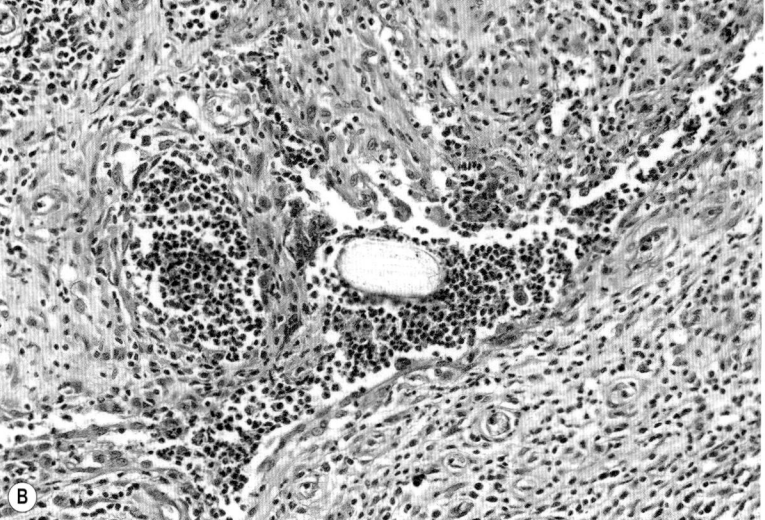

Fig. 34.40
(A, B) Pilonidal cyst: multiple hair shaft fragments are evident.

diagnosis or misdiagnosis.[8] Lesions may appear at a variety of sites on the head and neck, but the chin, submental region, and the cheek are most often affected (Fig. 34.41).[1] The lesion typically heals when the dental infection is cured.

Histologic features

Biopsy findings are non-specific and include a mixed inflammatory cell infiltrate with abscess formation and scarring, sometimes associated with a foreign body granulomatous component.

Mucinous syringometaplasia

Clinical features

Mucinous syringometaplasia (acral mucinous syringometaplasia, mucinous metaplasia, muciparous epidermal tumor) is a rare condition which most commonly presents on the soles of the feet or palmar aspect of the fingers as a 0.5- to 1.5-cm verrucous nodule, often diagnosed clinically as a viral wart.[1-8] Sometimes a central dell or sinus is present and occasionally a history of drainage of clear fluid is given.[7] Lesions occur less often at a variety of other sites including the neck, chin, chest, buttock, knee, and penis, when the appearance varies from a small plaque to a nodule.[6-8] Males are affected more often than females. The age at presentation is very variable, ranging from 15 to 66 years.[6] Duration of the lesion ranges from months to decades. The lesion is almost certainly reactive and does not recur following complete excision.[5-7]

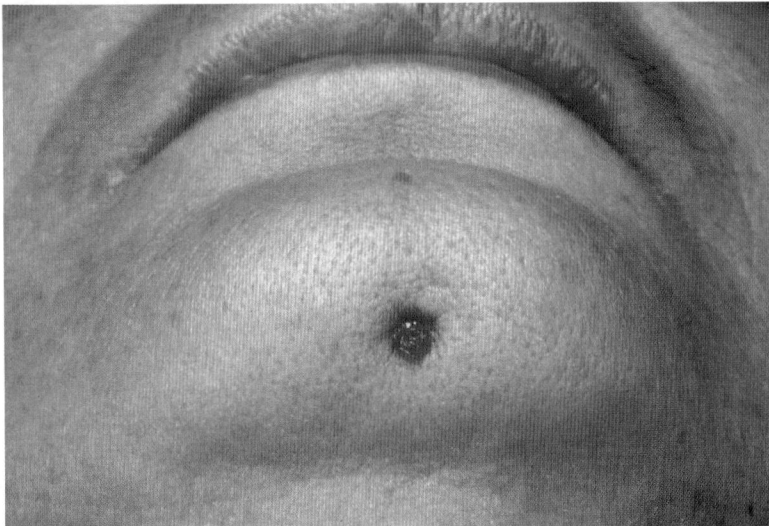

Fig. 34.41
Dental sinus: the chin is a commonly affected site. By courtesy of the Institute of Dermatology, London, UK.

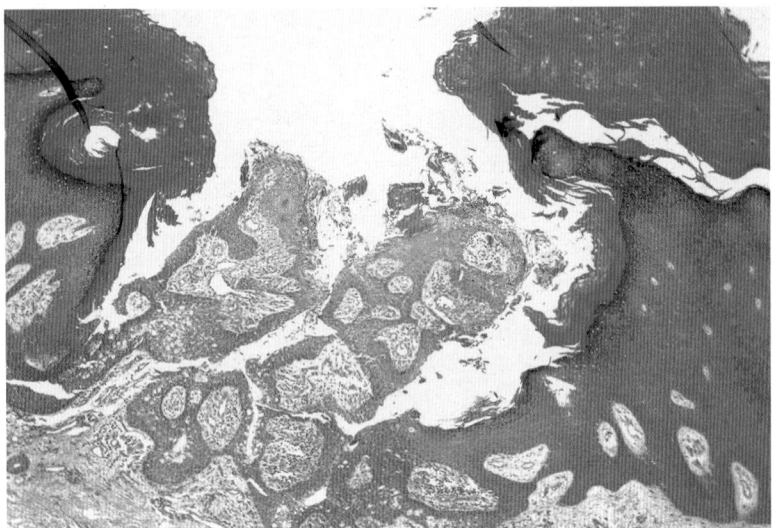

Fig. 34.42
Mucinous syringometaplasia: this lesion comes from the palm of the hand. Within the center of the defect are two epithelial-lined papillae. By courtesy of J. Grant, MD, Worthing Hospital, Worthing, UK.

Pathogenesis and histologic features

When first described, mucinous syringometaplasia was thought to represent a benign tumor – muciparous epidermal tumor.[1] Currently, however, it is generally believed to represent a metaplastic phenomenon principally affecting the superficial eccrine ducts and very rarely the apocrine duct.[9] The etiology is unknown although chronic trauma, pressure, and inflammation have been suggested as possible causes.[6,7]

Histologically, it is usually characterized by an epidermal invagination which is continuous at its base with eccrine ducts lined by nonkeratinizing squamous and mucin-containing epithelium (*Figs 34.42* and *34.43*).[5-7] These latter are sometimes seen in the epidermis, and goblet cells are often evident.[6] There is no significant pleomorphism and mitoses are sparse or absent.[6,8] The adjacent epidermis is hyperkeratotic, focally parakeratotic, and markedly acanthotic.[7] The underlying dermis commonly contains a heavy chronic inflammatory cell infiltrate with conspicuous plasma cells; fibrosis is often present.[6] In some cases, the ducts are continuous with the underlying dermal eccrine sweat ducts.[5] In one case, the changes extended to the eccrine secretory coil.[3] In other cases, no such continuity is demonstrable.[1,7,8]

The mucin-containing cells are positive for diastase–PAS, mucicarmine, colloidal iron (with and without hyaluronidase), and Alcian blue at pH 1 and 2.5.[5,7]

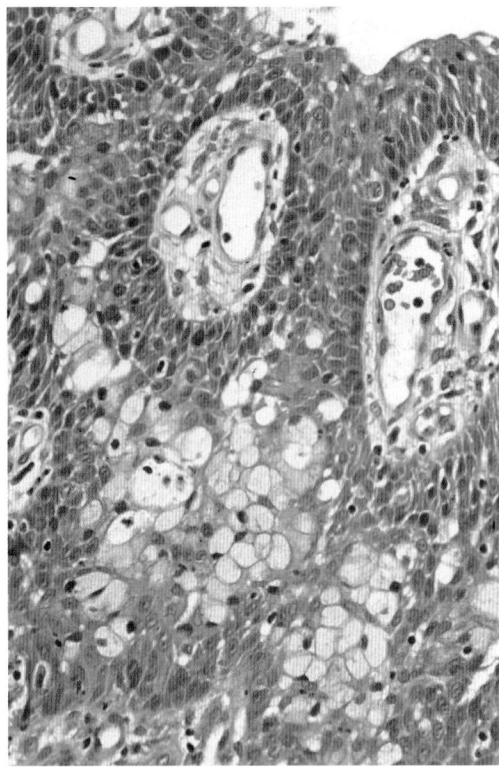

Fig. 34.43
Mucinous syringometaplasia: the epithelial lining contains numerous mucin-secreting cells. By courtesy of J. Grant, MD, Worthing Hospital, Worthing, UK.

Immunohistochemically, the mucin-containing cells express pankeratin, CAM 5.2, CEA, and EMA.[6-8] They are GCDPF-15 and S100 protein negative.[6,7]

Umbilical polyp and granuloma

The congenital umbilical polyp represents persistence of the distal-most segment of the vitelline (omphalomesenteric) duct, which connects the small intestine of the early fetus to the yolk sac. It usually disappears by about the seventh week of gestation. The most common manifestation of persistence is Meckel diverticulum, and the most serious consequence is an intestinal–umbilical fistula.[1] Cutaneous manifestations include polyps, sinuses, and cysts.[2-5,6] Less often, an umbilical polyp may arise from urachal remnants (urachal sinus or cyst).[7]

Clinical features

The lesions are usually noticed at birth, but presentation of sinuses and cysts may be delayed for days or years. Exceptionally, the lesion may not appear until late adulthood.[8] There is a marked predilection for males (6:1). The patient commonly presents with a bright red, 1- to 4-cm diameter pyogenic granuloma-like polyp on the umbilicus; secretions sometimes cause it to feel rather sticky or mucinous, and there may be damage to the surrounding skin, caused by acid or enzymes.[2,3]

The umbilical granuloma represents a granulation tissue polyp which sometimes develops in the umbilicus soon after separation of the cord. It is likely to be related to infection and presents as a 1.0-cm diameter or greater red polypoid lesion.

Histologic features

The polyp is associated with abrupt transition from stratified squamous to glandular epithelium of gastric, small intestinal, or colonic type (*Figs 34.44* and *34.45*).[9] Smooth muscle components of the bowel wall are sometimes present. Pancreas has also been identified.[8] Urachal lesions are composed of transitional cell epithelium.

The granuloma is composed of inflamed vascular granulation tissue.

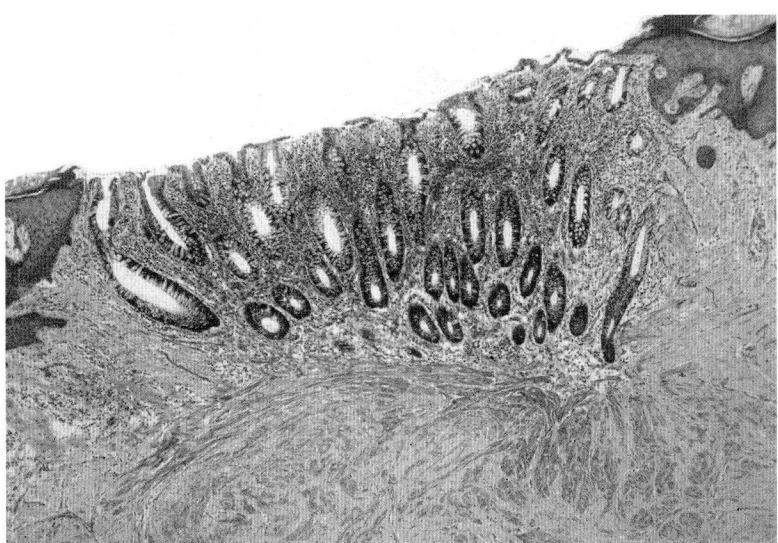

Fig. 34.44
Congenital umbilical polyp: in this example, the surface of the polyp is covered by large intestinal mucosa. Note the tubular glands. The fascicles of smooth muscle deep to the epithelium represent muscularis mucosae.

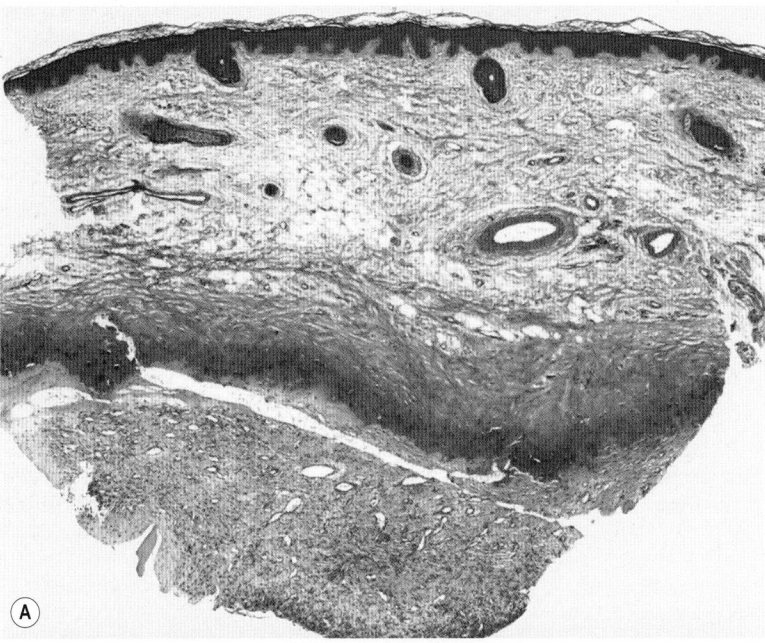

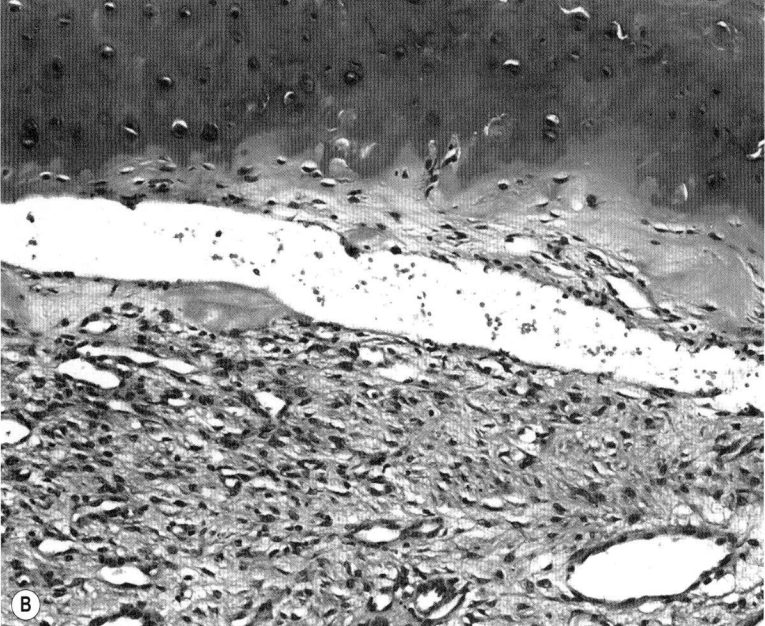

Fig. 34.46
Pseudocyst of the auricle: (A) cystic space within the cartilage; (B) the cavity is occupied by granulation tissue.

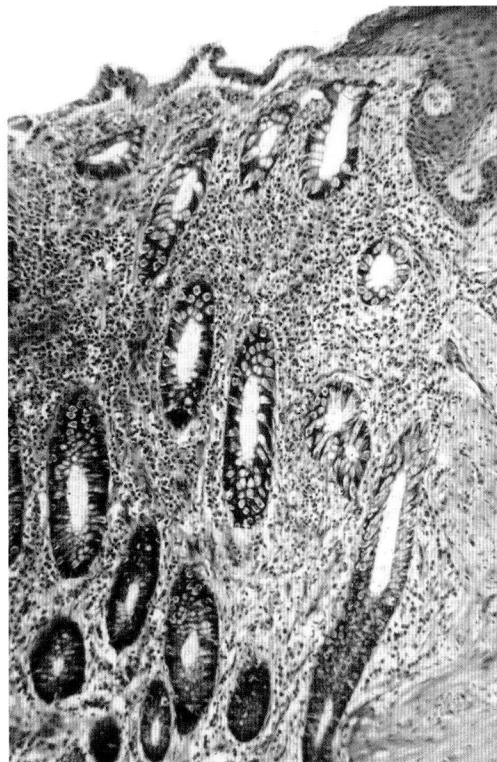

Fig. 34.45
Congenital umbilical polyp: note the continuity between the columnar and squamous epithelium.

Pseudocyst of the auricle

Clinical features

Pseudocyst of the auricle (endochondral pseudocyst) is uncommon and shows a predilection for males.[1-6] It presents as an asymptomatic, unilateral 1- to 5-cm swelling of the pinna.[5] The scaphoid or triangular fossa of the antihelix is predominantly affected.[7] Very occasionally, bilateral involvement may occur, and exceptionally the disease involves children.[8-10] Although there is a predilection for the Chinese, other Asian races and Caucasians can be affected.[11,12] If untreated, it may result in severe deformity of the ear.

Pathogenesis and histologic features

The etiology is unknown. Low-grade trauma, ischemia, embryological defect of cartilage development, and autoimmunity have been suggested as possible causes.[6,13] Repeated trauma in patients with ataxia has been associated with the condition.[14] A recurrent case has been described in the setting of atopic dermatitis.[15]

Grossly, the pseudocyst may contain 1–2 cc of serous fluid, rich in lactate dehydrogenase-4 and -5.[3,16] It is suggested that the presence of high lactate dehydrogenase levels results from trauma to the cartilage.[6] Histologically, the lesion presents as an intracartilaginous cystic space lacking an epithelial lining (Fig. 34.46). Degeneration of the adjacent cartilage is often evident. There are no significant inflammatory changes.

Access **ExpertConsult.com** for the complete list of references

CHAPTER 35

Connective tissue tumors

Eduardo Calonje, Vasileia Damaskou, Alexander J. Lazar

See
www.expertconsult.com
for references and
additional material

Introduction

Connective tissue tumors presenting primarily in the skin are relatively common. Because the majority of such lesions are benign and clinically nondistinctive they are sometimes neglected by clinicians. However, histologically they constitute a complex group of tumors showing various lines of differentiation and it can be difficult to classify a lesion as benign or malignant. Also, cutaneous or subcutaneous sarcomas, as well as various neoplasms of intermediate malignancy, are seen sufficiently frequently that some knowledge of their behavior and pathological appearances is mandatory for dermatologists and dermatopathologists alike.

Many benign soft tissue lesions – lipoma and fibrous histiocytoma being the most common – are often slow growing and asymptomatic. As a result, they frequently remain untreated unless they are a cosmetic nuisance, and so an accurate estimation of their incidence (which is probably relatively high) is impossible. However, sarcomas are relatively rare at any site, including the skin, accounting for less than 1% of all malignant neoplasms.

In this chapter, emphasis is placed upon those lesions that commonly present in the skin; various nondermatologic conditions are included for the sake of completeness and because they may be seen, albeit very occasionally, in dermatopathological practice.

When dealing with any soft tissue neoplasm, the single most important dictum to be strictly followed is that adequate tissue sampling, surgically and pathologically, is essential for accurate diagnosis. The range of diagnostic and non-specific histologic appearances seen in these tumors is very wide, reflecting the multipotentiality of mesenchyme; only by obtaining an overall view of a given neoplasm can a reliable diagnosis be made. In this regard, punch and shave biopsies can be exceedingly challenging or sometimes impossible to definitively diagnosis.

A number of cutaneous mesenchymal tumors have genetic features that can be helpful diagnostically. In general, malignant soft tissue tumors fall into the class of complex karyotype sarcomas (e.g., angiosarcoma and leiomyosarcoma) or simple genetic profile (e.g., clear cell sarcoma or dermatofibrosarcoma) often associated with a chromosomal translocation or, less often, with mutation or loss of a specific gene. An exhaustive discussion of the molecular diagnostics of soft tissue tumors is beyond the scope of this chapter, but see Chapter 2 for additional discussion of relevant techniques. Most of the molecular features discussed in this chapter can be used diagnostically when required, although some of the tests are available only in specialized centers.

ADIPOCYTIC TUMORS

Benign adipocytic tumors and tumorlike lesions

Lipoma

Clinical features

Lipomas are the most common connective tissue tumors.[1–3] They appear to occur more frequently in the obese, usually in middle and late adult life, may be multiple, especially in young adults, and are purportedly more common in females.[3] This, however, may only be a reflection of the greater tendency of women to request cosmetic attention for otherwise innocuous lesions. Lipomas are very uncommon in children and when present should raise the possibility of Bannayan-Riley-Ruvalcaba syndrome.[4] Congenital lipomas are very rare.[5] Multiple lesions may occur in a familial setting.[6] A case of multiple lipomas after total body electron beam therapy for mycosis fungoides has been reported.[7] Multiple lipomas have also been described in association with rosiglitazone, a peroxisome proliferator-activator receptor (PPAR) gamma agonist, in association with systemic chemotherapy for Hodgkin lymphoma and in Cowden disease.[8–10]

The lesions are found most often on the trunk, abdomen or neck, followed by the proximal extremities, and rarely on the face (particularly the forehead), scalp, hands or feet. Palmar lipomas are exceptional and may present with lesions simulating piezogenic pedal papules.[11] Periungual and subungual lesions are exceptional.[12,13] Trauma has been associated with induction of lipomas although it is not clear whether all of these lesions may represent pseudolipomas.[14,15] The latter sometimes includes an intravascular lesion.[16] Villous lipomatous proliferation of synovial membrane (lipoma arborescens) represents an infiltration of sub synovial connective tissue by adipose tissue.[17] Typically, lipomas originate subcutaneously, are slow growing, mobile and painless; sometimes they are multiple. Size varies and some lesions are very large. Dermal examples are often clinically confused with fibroepithelial polyps. Although the lesions are usually well circumscribed, the less common deep variants, which may arise in muscle or in association with a tendon sheath or nerve, are generally ill defined and infiltrative.

Subcutaneous lipomas are entirely benign and local excision is nearly always curative; recurrence is infrequent (less than 5%) and progression to liposarcoma virtually never occurs.

Pathogenesis and histologic features

Lipomas at all locations show clonal karyotypic abnormalities in up to 75% of cases.[18–25] The most common rearrangement involves the 12q13~15 region affecting the HMGA2 gene. The deregulation of HMGA2 appears to play a role in the genesis of the tumor. The most common translocation is t(3;12)(q27~28;q13~15) leading to a fusion gene HMGA2-LPP.[24,25] Many other translocations involving different chromosomes may be seen including 1p36, 1p32~34, 2p22~24, 2q35~37, 5q33, 9p21~22, 12p11~13, 13q12~14, and 4q27~28.[24,25] Other less common chromosomal aberrations include 6p21~23 (sometimes involving the HMGA1B), 13q11~12 and 12q22~24. The only translocation associated with 6p21~23 is t(3;6)(q27-28;p21~23).

The tumors are usually encapsulated, lobulated, and largely composed of univacuolated mature adipocytes, the nucleus and cytoplasm of which are compressed centrifugally (Fig. 35.1). The lobules are divided by delicate fibrous septa containing thin-walled vessels. Degenerative changes, often characterized by fibrosis, focal fat necrosis, or myxoid change, are not uncommon, particularly in long-standing or frequently traumatized cases (Figs 35.2–35.7). Prominent myxoid change and high vascularity are sometime present.[26] However, the majority of lipomas with prominent myxoid change (myxolipomas) are now considered to be part of the spectrum of spindle cell lipomas.[27] Foci of other fully differentiated mesenchymal elements, including bone or cartilage, can also be seen.

Although nuclear pleomorphism, hyperchromasia, and mitotic activity do not occur in lipomas, in any benign fatty lesion (or even in normal adipose tissue) occasional vacuolated nuclei known as lochkern may be seen (Fig. 35.8). These must not be confused with lipoblasts, the most important diagnostic feature of liposarcoma, which are characterized by multiple intracytoplasmic lipid vacuoles associated with scalloping of peripherally located hyperchromatic or bizarre nuclei. In some lesions there are septa of collagen between adipose tissue lobules and they are referred to as fibrolipomas or sclerotic lipomas. A variant of lipoma with predilection for acral sites (fingers, wrists, toes) and characterized by prominent collagenous or myxocollagenous stroma, bland stellate or spindle-shaped cells and scattered adipocytes has been described as sclerotic (fibroma-like) lipoma.[28] A further variant, known as fibrohistiocytic lipoma, has been reported.[29] Typically, it presents in the subcutis of the trunk and shows predilection for young men. Most lesions are small and asymptomatic. Tumors are well circumscribed and consist of lobules of mature adipocytes containing focal areas with plump spindle-shaped cells arranged in a fascicular or focal storiform pattern.[29] Rare lipomas may contain metaplastic bone.[30] Those containing sweat glands do not represent an adenolipoma but rather entrapment of normal glands by the tumor.[31–33] Lesions containing smooth muscle are rare, regarded as a distinct entity under the term myolipoma and tend to be deep seated.[27,34] Secondary changes including focal areas of fat necrosis with foamy histiocytes are often seen and some cases show membranous fat necrosis.[35]

Dermal lipomas are less well circumscribed and consist of scattered groups of mature adipocytes between collagen bundles (Figs 35.9 and 35.10). Nevus lipomatosus superficialis is histologically indistinguishable from dermal lipoma. The former term should therefore only be used, as a diagnostic term, in a specific clinical context (see below).

Differential diagnosis

The diagnosis of a lipoma is usually straightforward. Distinction from an atypical lipomatous tumor (adipocytic /lipoma-like variant) is mainly based on the presence of adipocytes varying in size and shape and with hyperchromatic nuclei in the latter. In addition, atypical stromal cells are usually present in the latter. The absence of lipoblasts is not a helpful finding as they are not always present in atypical lipomatous tumor. In particularly difficult cases, immunohistochemistry with MDM2 and CDK4 may be helpful (see under atypical lipomatous tumor). Dermal lipomas can be confused with pseudolipomatosis cutis. The latter is an artifactual incidental finding distinguished from a dermal lipoma by the presence of empty, round spaces simulating adipocytes but lacking nuclei and of variable size.[36]

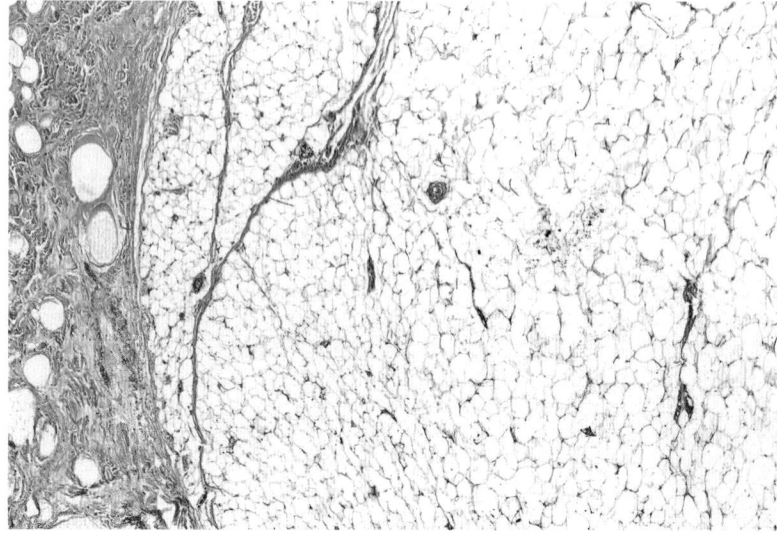

Fig. 35.1
Lipoma: low-power view showing a circumscribed encapsulated tumor composed of mature adipocytes.

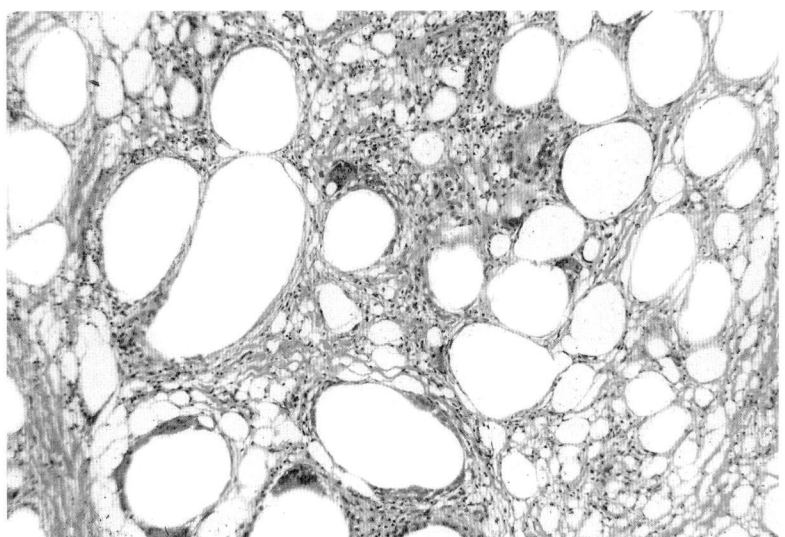

Fig. 35.2
Lipoma: post-traumatic fat necrosis.

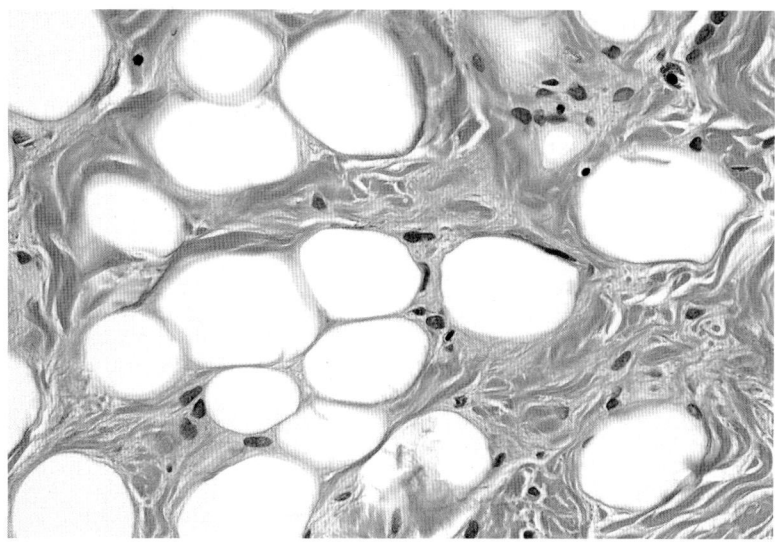

Fig. 35.5
Fibrolipoma: high-power view of Figure 35.4.

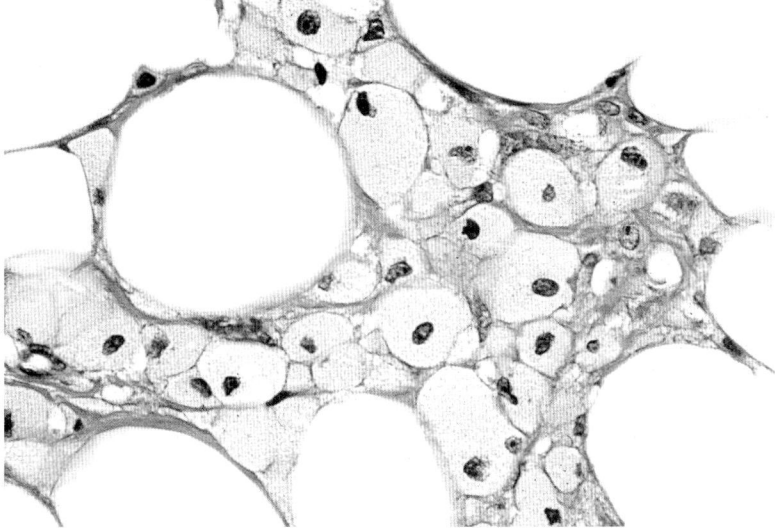

Fig. 35.3
Lipoma: note the lipid-laden xanthoma cells.

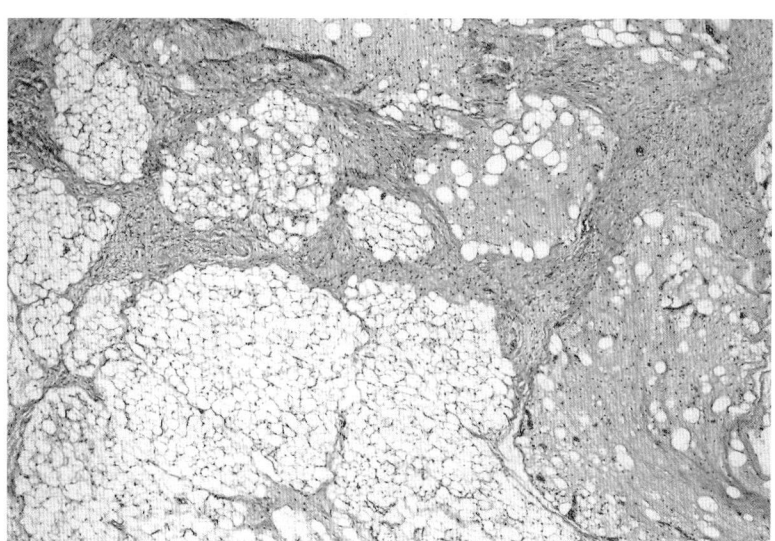

Fig. 35.6
Myxofibrolipoma: this variant of lipoma is characterized by fibrosis and foci of myxoid change. It is of no clinical significance.

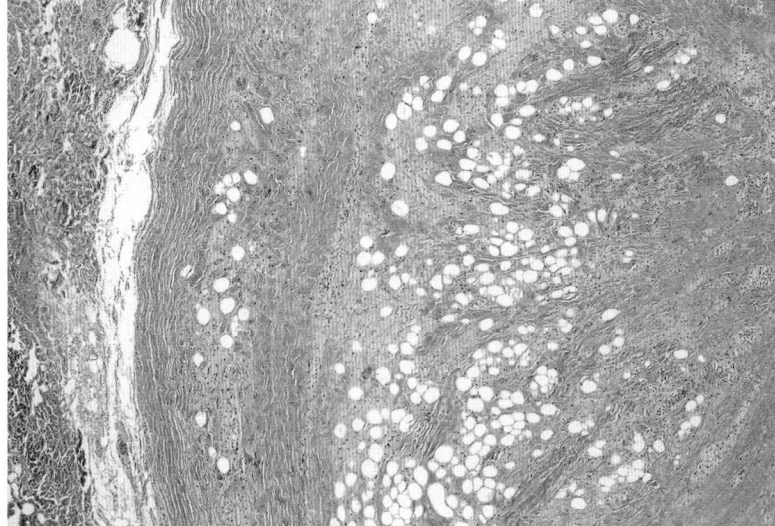

Fig. 35.4
Fibrolipoma: this term is sometimes applied to a lipoma with a prominent fibrous component.

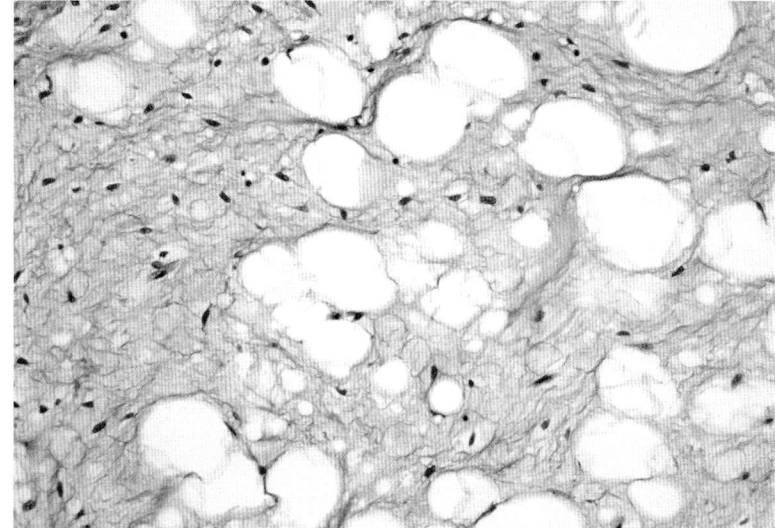

Fig. 35.7
Myxofibrolipoma: note the abundant mucinous matrix and spindled cells admixed with adipocytes.

Fig. 35.8
Lipoma: intranuclear lipid 'inclusions' (lochkern) should not be mistaken for lipoblasts.

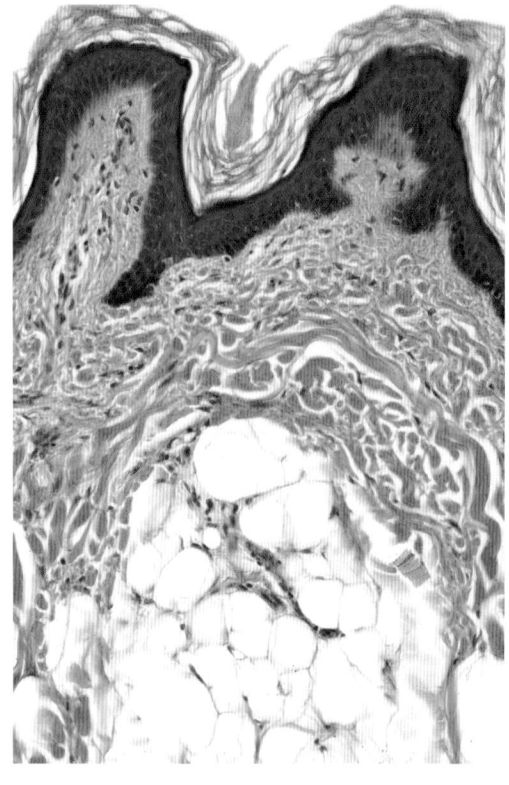

Fig. 35.10
Dermal lipoma: it is often separated from the epidermis by a grenz zone.

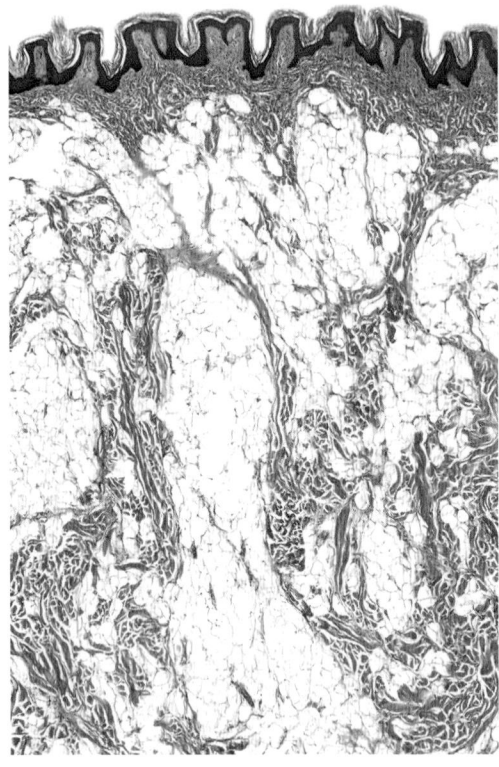

Fig. 35.9
Dermal lipoma: the dermal variant is often less well circumscribed and tends to dissect between the collagen fibers.

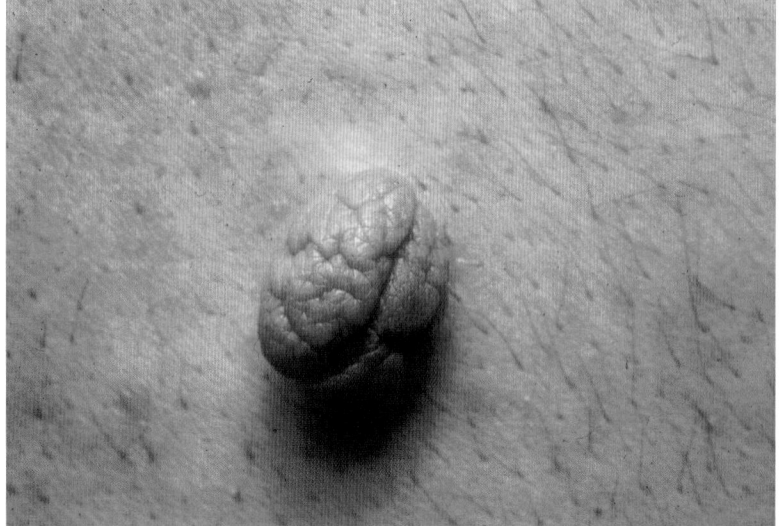

Fig. 35.11
Nevus lipomatosus superficialis: solitary lesions are often polypoid and have a soft consistency. By courtesy of the Institute of Dermatology, London, UK.

Nevus lipomatosus superficialis (Hoffman and Zurhelle)

Clinical features

Nevus lipomatosus superficialis is an uncommon form of connective tissue nevus, manifest principally by the deposition of fatty tissue in the dermis.[1-4] In its classical form, it is characterized by multiple papular, polypoid or plaque-like lesions, up to 2 cm in diameter, which almost always arise unilaterally on the posterior surfaces of the buttocks, upper thighs or lower back. More extensive and diffuse involvement may occur and patients present with prominent folds in what has been described as the Michelin tire appearance.[5-7] Typically, the lesions present in early childhood or adolescence. Unusual associations include co-occurrence with lipedematous scalp, folliculosebaceous cystic hamartoma, dermoid cysts, angiokeratoma of Fordyce, perifollicular fibromas, and trichofolliculoma.[8-13] A case associated with intramuscular lipomatosis has been reported.[14] A solitary form, usually seen in adults, shows a predilection for the same sites or occurs elsewhere and is more likely to represent a variant of fibroepithelial polyp or skin tag (*Figs 35.11* and *35.12*). Such lesions have been described as pedunculated lipofibroma.[15] In all types of nevus lipomatosus the sex incidence is equal. The papules or plaques, varying from skin-colored to yellow, are characteristically broad based and may show superficial comedone formation.

Pathogenesis and histologic features

The pathogenesis is unknown. In a single case, a 2p24 deletion has been described.[16]

Although alterations are seen in all the connective tissue elements in the dermis, the predominant feature is deposition of lobules of mature fat in variable quantities in the superficial dermis (*Fig. 35.13*).[3,17] These fatty lobules are located particularly around small blood vessels, the numbers of which are also increased. Areas of loose fibrous tissue, diminished elastic

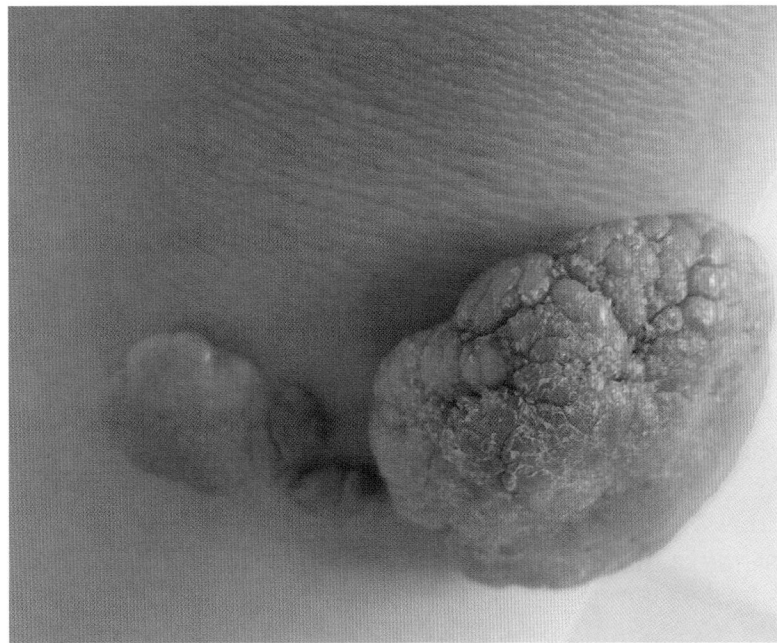

Fig. 35.12
Nevus lipomatosus superficialis: in this patient there are multiple papules and nodules. Courtesy of Dr Yi-Guo Feng, Xi'an Jiatong University, second affiliated hospital, China.

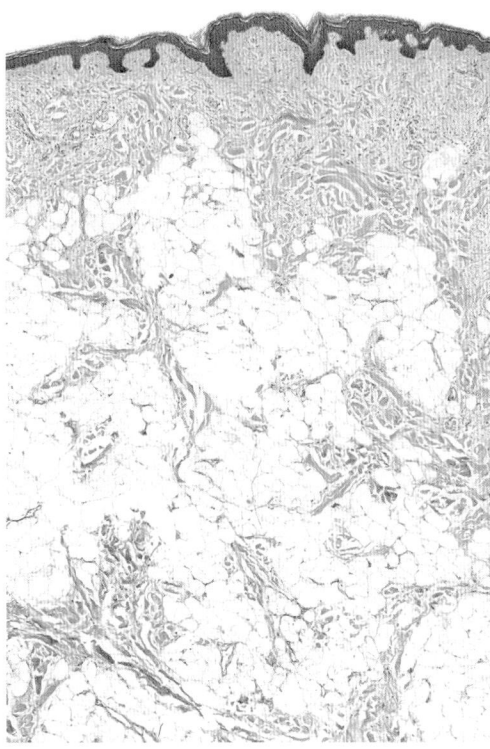

Fig. 35.13
Nevus lipomatosus superficialis: this specimen came from the lower back of a teenage male. There is widespread infiltration of the dermis by mature adipocytes.

fibers and reduced numbers of epidermal appendages may also be a feature. Entrapped hair follicles may appear cystically dilated.

A case with focal pagetoid spread of adipocytes and dystrophic calcification has been described.[18]

As mentioned previously, it has been argued that the solitary form represents a pedunculated, fat-containing skin tag or a lipofibroma. Although the distribution of fat in the superficial dermis makes this suggestion unlikely, the argument is semantic and of no practical value. Nevus lipomatosus superficialis is also histologically indistinguishable from the cutaneous nodules of focal dermal hypoplasia.

Lipomatosis

Clinical features

Lipomatosis is extremely rare and may present in several forms. Idiopathic forms include symmetric, diffuse and pelvic lipomatosis; the latter does not affect the superficial subcutaneous tissue.[1–17]

Two variants of lipomatosis affect the superficial subcutaneous tissue:
- Multiple symmetric lipomatosis (Launois-Bensaude) represents the commonest form and can be diffuse or localized.[1–3,5] In the diffuse variant, there is usually symmetrical involvement of the trunk or proximal limbs, head and neck, pelvis, and occasionally the tongue, abdominal cavity and the intestinal tract;[4,18] it is seen most often in children (particularly males), although adults may be affected. Single reports of associations with familial hyperlipidemia and tuberous sclerosis have been documented.[16,17] Some cases show an autosomal dominant inheritance, others are associated with myoclonic epilepsy with ragged red fibers (MERRF), and a number may be associated with diabetes mellitus.[6–9] The localized variant (multiple symmetric lipomatosis) is characteristically seen in the cervical region, back, shoulders and upper trunk, usually presents in middle-aged Mediterranean males with high alcohol intake, and is known as Madelung disease. Involvement of the mediastinum can be seen. Associated inspiratory dyspnea or obstructive sleep apnea may exceptionally occur.[10,11] The axillae and groins can also be affected. There is strong association with alcohol abuse and liver disease.[12] A variant of localized symmetrical lipomatosis restricted to the hands or the feet has been reported.[13,14]
- Asymmetric lipomatosis can present at any site and usually has no association with other diseases.[15] Single reports of associations with familial hyperlipidemia and tuberous sclerosis have been documented.[16,17]

A localized form of lipomatosis of the scalp has been reported as encephalocraniocutaneous lipomatosis (Haberland disease) and is associated with alopecia, aplasia cutis, nevus psiloliparus, skin tags and ocular and cranial abnormalities.[19–21] It is not associated with Proteus syndrome. A relationship with oculoectodermal syndrome has been proposed.[21] Congenital facial infiltrating lipomatosis refers to a disorder associated with hypertrophy of bones and soft tissues, macrodontia and premature dental eruption.[22,23]

In addition, cases associated with exogenous or endogenous production of steroids (steroid lipomatosis) with predilection for the face, central chest, upper mid-back and spinal epidural, retro-orbital and mediastinal tissue may occur.[24,25] An association with antiretroviral therapy (HIV lipodystrophy) has also been documented.[26,27]

In both idiopathic forms of lipomatosis, only radical surgery can prevent local recurrence. The disadvantages of recommending such treatment must be weighed against the possible functional impairment that the condition may induce.

Histologic features

Mitochondrial DNA damage has been suggested as a possible etiology of symmetric lipomatosis and in lipodystrophy induced by HIV therapy.[27,28] The localization of the lesions in multiple symmetric lipomatosis suggests an origin from brown fat.[29] The demonstration that cells cultured from lesions synthetize mitochondrial inner membrane protein, a marker of brown fat, gives further support to this theory.[29] Histologically, all forms are characterized by unencapsulated overgrowth of mature adipose tissue.

Adiposis dolorosa

Clinical features

Adiposis dolorosa (Dercum disease) is a rare disease characterized by painful, circumscribed areas with increased fat in a plaque-like distribution.[1–3] Usually, multiple body sites are involved but there is predilection for the buttocks, lower limbs and abdomen, particularly in juxta-articular areas.

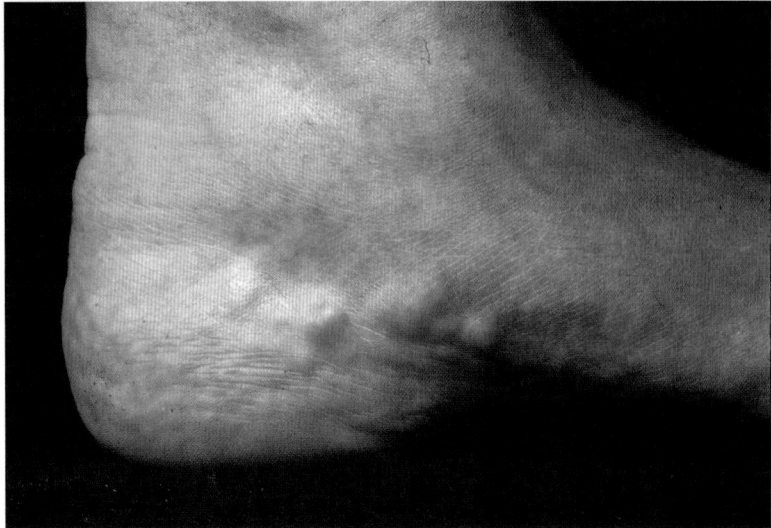

Fig. 35.14
Piezogenic pedal papules: note the multiple flesh-colored papules on the heel and lateral border of the foot. From the collection of the late N.P. Smith, MD, The Institute of Dermatology, London, UK.

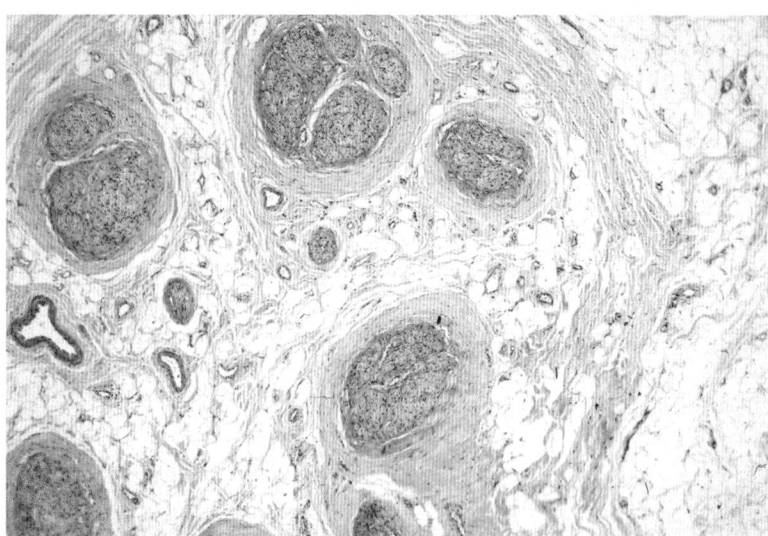

Fig. 35.15
Lipomatosis of nerve: note the extensive epineural fat deposition.

Localized disease is very rare and the breasts may be involved.[4,5] The condition is much more common in females, between the fourth and sixth decades of live, especially after the menopause, and patients often have associated obesity and psychological problems.[1-3] Occasional cases are inherited in an autosomal dominant manner.[6,7] A case associated with the use of corticosteroids, a further patient with hypercholesterolemia and severe atherosclerosis and one with lipomatous hypertrophy of the interatrial septum have been documented.[8-10] Pain occurs mainly as the result of palpation but may also occur spontaneously or as a result of movement.

A new classification of the disease has been proposed: (1) generalized diffuse without lipomas; (2) generalizsed diffuse associated with lipomas; (3) localized nodular; and (4) juxtaarticular.[11]

Pathogenesis and histologic features

The pathogenesis of adiposis dolorosa is unknown. Abnormal flow of lymph through the lymphatics within involved tissue has been suggested as an etiological factor.[12] Biopsy reveals mature adipose tissue with focal areas of fat necrosis and, exceptionally, granulomatous inflammation.

Piezogenic pedal papules

Clinical features

Piezogenic pedal papules characteristically present as multiple skin-colored papules on the heels (*Fig. 35.14*).[1-3] They show predilection for the internal aspect of the heels and are usually asymptomatic although pain may be elicited when the patient is standing. Lesions become more noticeable when the patient stands up as a result of pressure. Piezogenic pedal papules are common in patients with Ehlers-Danlos syndrome.[4,5] They have been described in athletes, including a marathon runner, ice-hockey players, skaters and in association with Prader-Willi syndrome.[6-9] Rare familial cases have been described.[10] An association with mitral valve prolapse and mitral valve insufficiency has been reported.[11-13]

Pathogenesis and histologic features

It is likely that trauma plays a role in the pathogenesis of the lesions.[6,7] A biopsy from a papule shows normal adipose tissue herniating into the dermis. This may mimic an intradermal lipoma but the clinical setting allows a diagnosis to be made. Rarely, prominent myxoid change and vascular proliferation can be seen.[14]

Lipomatosis of nerve

Clinical features

Lipomatosis of nerve (fibrolipomatous hamartoma of nerve, perineural fibrolipoma, perineural lipoma, intraneural lipoma) is a very rare hamartomatous condition usually occurring in children or young adults of either sex, around the wrists and hands, particularly along the distribution of the median nerve followed by the ulnar nerve and (less frequently) others including the brachial plexus and cranial nerves.[1-6] Presentation at birth is sometimes seen. It can be associated with macrodactyly of the fingers innervated by the involved nerve in up to one-third of cases.[1,7] Patients typically present with a slowly growing mass, which is either asymptomatic or associated with neurological symptoms including pain, paresthesia, loss of sensation or motor deficit. Carpal tunnel syndrome may develop when the median nerve is involved.[8,9] Although the lesion is benign, treatment is difficult, as surgical excision often results in permanent neurological deficit.[10]

Histologic features

The lesion is characterized by proliferation of mature fatty and fibrous tissue within the epineurium of a major nerve accompanied by prominent concentric perineural fibrosis (*Fig. 35.15*). In a handful of cases involving cervical and thoracic spinal nerves, the pathology was restricted to circumferential growth of fat around the epineurium.[11] Rarely, bone formation has been described.[12]

Lipoblastoma/lipoblastomatosis

Clinical features

Lipoblastoma is the circumscribed subcutaneous counterpart of lipoma seen in infancy and childhood.[1-6] Its diffuse form (lipoblastomatosis) is infiltrative and typically involves deeper structures, including muscle.

In either form, this condition most often presents in the first 9 years of life (exceptionally at birth, and 10% between the ages of 10 and 16), affects males more often than females, and is typified by a slowly growing, usually subcutaneous mass with size ranging from 1 to 15 cm.[1-7] Occasional cases may clinically mimic a hemangioma.[8] Most tumors involve the trunk and extremities, followed by the head and neck.[7,9] Presentation in the retroperitoneum, mediastinum, and a number of internal organs including the kidney, lung, and heart occurs rarely.[10-15] Intrascrotal tumors and

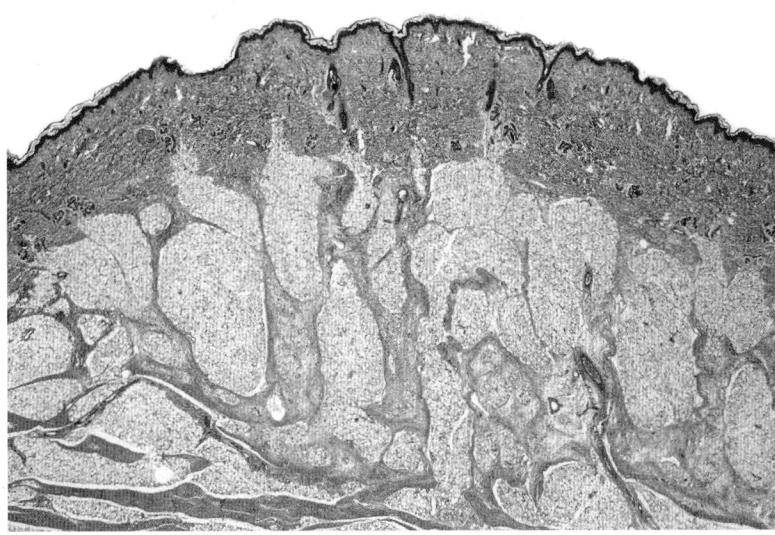

Fig. 35.16
Lipoblastoma: at low power, the tumor is lobulated and composed of mature fat cells and numerous multivacuolated lipoblasts.

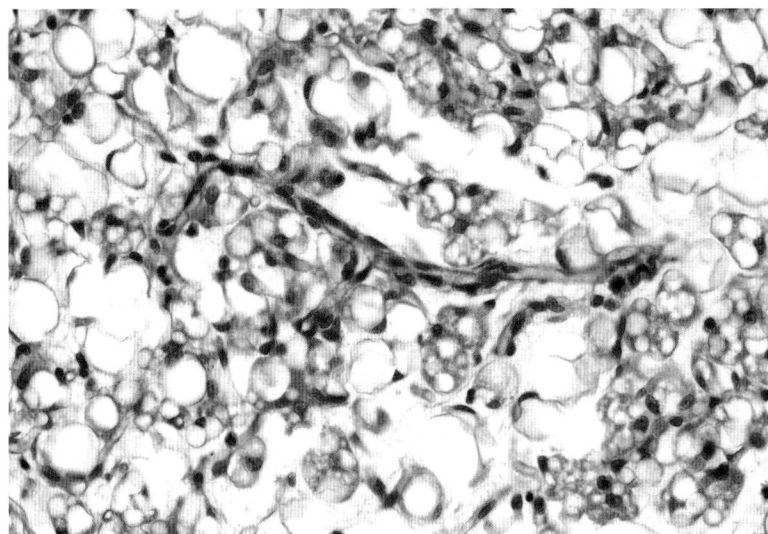

Fig. 35.18
Lipoblastoma: the adipocytes are of varying size. In the center of the field is a thin-walled, branched 'crow's foot' type of blood vessel.

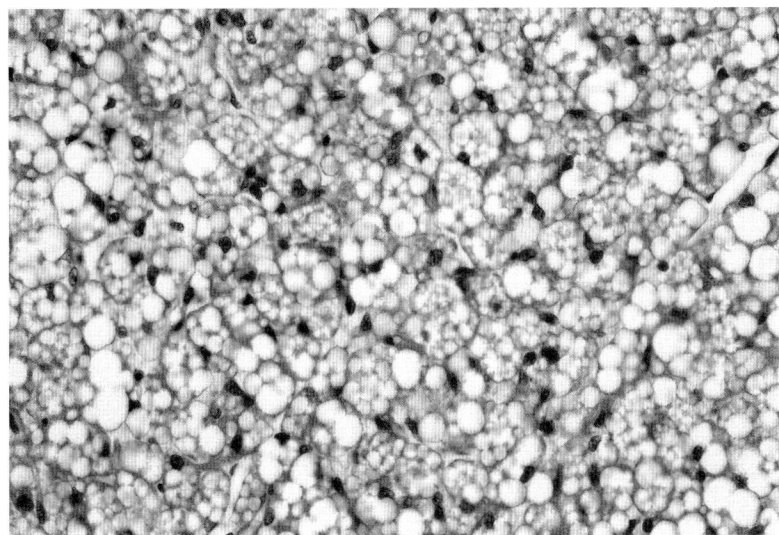

Fig. 35.17
Lipoblastoma: this field shows an admixture of adipocytes and multivacuolated lipoblasts.

association with accessory scrota have also been documented.[16–19] In the infiltrative type, local recurrence can occur following incomplete excision in up to 19% of cases.[3] Familial cases are noted.[7] In about 17% of patients central nervous system anomalies are noted including macrocephaly, developmental delay, autism, Sturge-Weber syndrome, and seizures.[7] Unusual associations include a patient with glomovenous malformations, epidermal nevus, temporal alopecia and heterochromia in addition to a lipoblastoma.[20] A further rare association with cleft palate has been described.[21]

One or more recurrences can occur in up to 46% of cases.[7]

Pathogenesis and histologic features

It has been shown that lipoblastoma has a consistent rearrangement of 8q11~q13, resulting in overexpression of the *PLAG1* oncogene.[22–33] Gene partners described as donating promoters include *HAS2*, *COL1A2*, *COL3A1*, *RAD51L1* and *RAB2A*.[34,35] Rarely additional chromosomal numerical abnormalities, mainly excess copies of chromosome 8, can be found.[7,18,29,30,33]

Lipoblastoma recapitulates developing fat and therefore contains varying proportions of mature adipocytes, lipoblasts and prelipoblasts arranged in a lobulated pattern and separated by loose fibrous connective tissue septa (*Figs 35.16* and *35.17*). The stroma is often myxoid with numerous small

capillaries giving a 'crow's feet' appearance (*Fig. 35.18*) and may contain very primitive stellate or spindled tumor cells. Hibernoma-like tumors can be seen.[32] Mitotic figures are uncommon; some cases show areas of extramedullary hematopoiesis.[2]

Positivity for S100 protein, CD34 and PLAG1 is seen.[7] In addition desmin may be positive in the spindle cells.[36] The degree of adipocytic differentiation does not predict risk of recurrence.[7] p16 is positive in rare tumors.[37]

Ultrastructural studies show adipocytes in different stages of development.[38]

Differential diagnosis

Distinction from myxoid liposarcoma, which is extremely rare in children, is made possible by the presence of prominent lobulation and the absence of nuclear hyperchromasia in lipoblastoma. Cytogenetics is very useful in allowing distinction between these tumors, as myxoid liposarcoma lacks rearrangement of 8q11~q13 and instead shows a consistent t(12;16)(q13;p11) involving the *DDIT3* and *FUS* genes. Cytogenetics is also very useful in tumors mimicking ordinary lipoma and hibernoma.[37,39] Human insulin injection may induce lipoatrophy with focal lipoblastoma-like changes.[40]

Lipoblastoma-like tumor of the vulva

A few cases of adipose tumors closely resembling lipoblastoma and presenting in the vulva of young to middle-aged patients have been described as lipoblastoma-like tumor of the vulva.[1–3] Lesions present as a nondescript mass, several centimeters in diameter, sometimes associated with pain. Local recurrence is exceptional. Lesions are lobulated with prominent myxoid change and a rich branching vascular network. Tumor cells vary in proportion and consist of adipocytes, bland spindle-shaped cells, and uni- or multi-vacuolated lipoblasts. Mitotic activity is minimal. Focal positivity for CD34 may rarely be seen. There is usually negative staining for HMGA2 and PLAG1 (as opposed to lipoblastoma) and also for S100 protein, MDM2 and CDK4. Based on the usual loss of RB1 expression, it has been suggested that these tumors are more likely related to spindle cell lipoma rather than lipoblastoma.[3]

Angiolipoma

Clinical features

Angiolipomas are benign lesions which, in contrast to simple lipomas, are seen most often in young adults and have a predilection for the subcutis of the upper limbs, particularly the forearm and less commonly the trunk.[1–3] Oral,

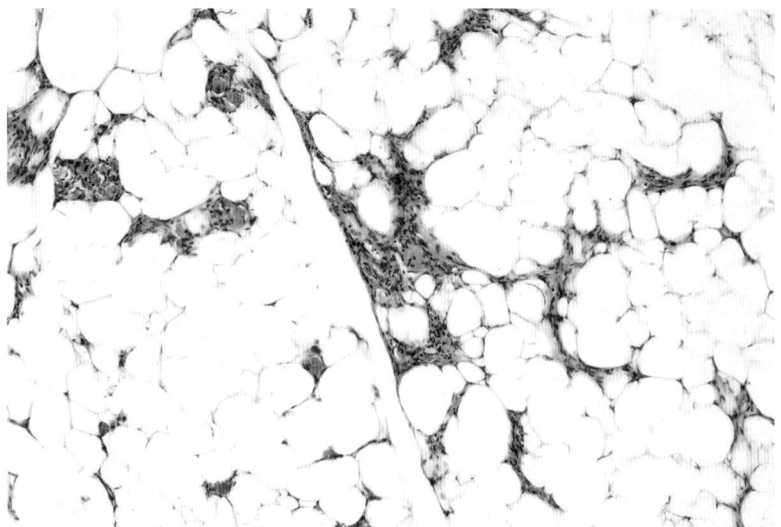

Fig. 35.19
Angiolipoma: admixed with the adipocytes are aggregates of small vessels.

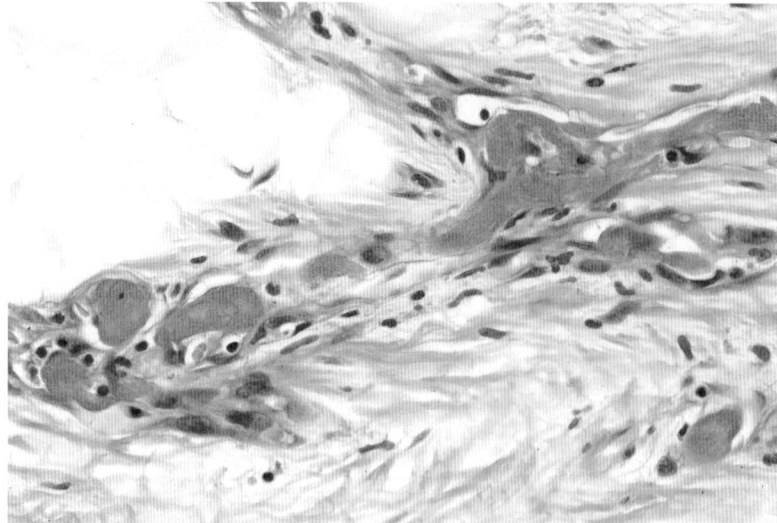

Fig. 35.20
Angiolipoma: vascular thromboses are an invariable feature. They are often found at the periphery of the tumor.

intra-articular, extradural, breast, and bronchial lesions are exceptional.[4–8] Familial cases are rarely seen.[9] Parenchymal, CNS and infiltrating intramuscular lesions are best regarded as variants of hemangiomas.[10]

The lesions are typically tender or painful, less than 2 cm in diameter, and may impart a reddish or bluish discoloration to the overlying skin. They are more often multiple than solitary and treatment can be problematic. Multiple lesions have exceptionally been documented in association with diabetes mellitus and as a complication of antiretroviral therapy (particularly with indinavir and saquinavir) in acquired immunodeficiency syndrome (AIDS).[11–14] A case of intravascular lymphomatosis as well as that of a B-cell lymphoma presenting in an angiolipoma have been documented.[15,16] Metastatic melanoma within an angiolipoma has also been described.[17] Giant angiolipomas are very rare.[18]

Pathogenesis and histologic features

Most cytogenetic studies in angiolipoma have consistently shown a normal karyotype.[19] In only a few tumors cytogenetic abnormalities have been demonstrated including a one with 46,Y,t(X;2)(p22;p12), one with complete loss of a chromosome 13 and two with structural aberrations of chromosome 13 involving the q12~q14 bands.[20,21] Interestingly, more recently, low-level mutations of protein kinase D2 was demonstrated in 80% of angiolipomas.[22] Aberrant expression of HMGA2 has been documented.[23]

The tumor, almost always encapsulated, is composed of mature adipocytes and varying proportions of irregular, anastomosing small blood vessels without endothelial atypia (Fig. 35.19). Luminal microthrombi are invariably present (Fig. 35.20). Although the blood vessels are usually seen in the periphery of the tumor, they may constitute most of the lesion. Such examples are known as cellular angiolipomas (Figs 35.21 and 35.22).[24–26]

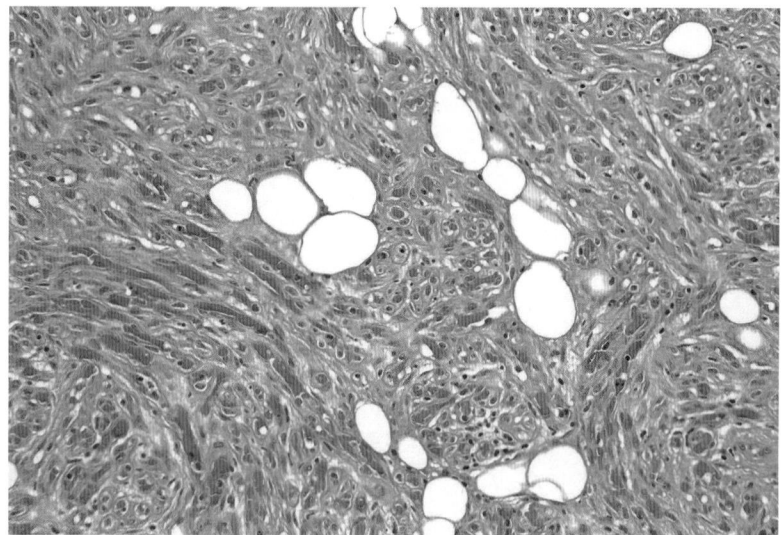

Fig. 35.21
Cellular angiolipoma: in this variant, bland spindled cells (possibly pericytes) predominate. The presence of adipocytes and capillary microthrombi confirms the diagnosis.

Differential diagnosis

Cellular angiolipoma can be confused with a vascular tumor, especially immature capillary hemangioma and kaposiform hemangioendothelioma.[17] The presence of mature adipocytes and capillaries with microthrombi allows distinction from immature capillary hemangioma. Kaposiform hemangioendothelioma may have capillaries with microthrombi in the periphery of tumor lobules, but mature adipocytes are absent.

Myolipoma

Clinical features

Myolipoma, (extrauterine lipoleiomyoma) is a benign adipocytic neoplasm predominantly seen in adult women.[1,2] Usually, it presents as an incidental, large (median size 10 cm), deep-seated mass in the retroperitoneum or abdomen and rarely in the pelvis or groin. Rarely, it may be seen as a

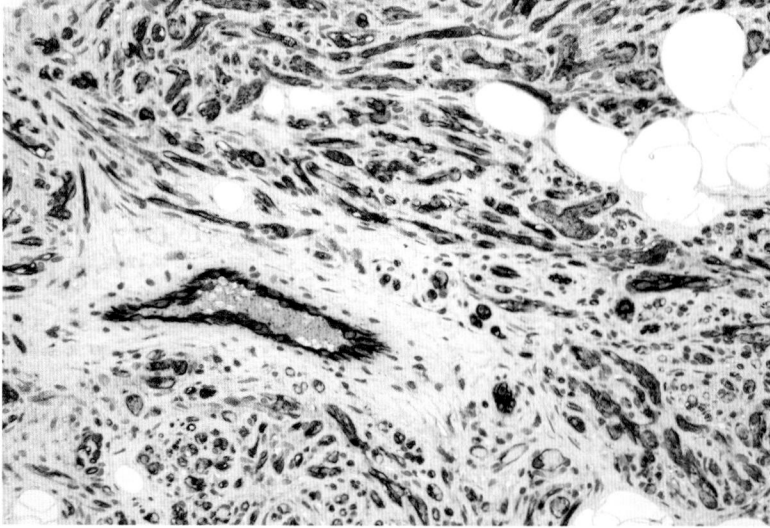

Fig. 35.22
Cellular angiolipoma: the vessels can be outlined with CD31.

smaller palpable subcutaneous lesion in the trunk and extremities. Complete surgical removal is curative.

Pathogenesis and histologic features

Fusion of the *HMGA2* and *C9orf92* genes with t(9;12)(p22;q14) has been reported in one case.[3] Myolipoma is well circumscribed with biphasic morphology; variable amounts of mature adipose tissue and well-differentiated smooth muscle fibers arranged in fascicles. Cytologic atypia is not seen. Necrosis is not observed. Unusual features include hypercellular fascicles, degenerative atypia, presence of hemosiderin or eosinophils, metaplastic bone or cartilage, and a round cell component.[2] By immunohistochemistry the smooth muscle nature of tumor cells is confirmed by positivity for SMA and desmin. Nuclear positivity of HGMA2 is seen in 2/3rd of cases.

Expression of estrogen and progesterone receptors has been reported.[2,4]

Differential diagnosis

Myolipoma must be differentiated from atypical lipomatous tumor/well-differentiated liposarcoma with smooth muscle differentiation based on the presence of cytologic atypia in the latter.[5,6] Moreover, myolipoma is usually negative for MDM2 and CDK4.[2] Angiomyolipoma is distinguished by the variable presence of thick-walled vessels and the expression of melanocytic markers, such as HMB45 and Melan-A.[6]

Chondroid lipoma

Clinical features

Chondroid lipoma is a distinctive tumor that presents predominantly in adult females, with a predilection for the proximal extremities and limb girdles.[1,2] Tumors in children are very rare.[3] Lesions are usually small and arise mainly in deeper soft tissues and (less commonly) in the subcutis. Rare examples present in the oral cavity, nasopharynx, and pelvis.[4–6] A case presenting within the peroneal nerve has been described.[7] Clinical features are not distinctive. Tumors are benign and there is no tendency for recurrence after simple excision.

Pathogenesis and histologic features

This tumor is characterized by t(11;16)(q13;p13) fusing *C11orf95* and *MLK2*.[8–11]

The lesion is well circumscribed, lobular and often encapsulated. It consists of an admixture of mature adipocytes, uni- or multivacuolated lipoblasts and hibernoma-like cells with granular eosinophilic cytoplasm in a myxoid and chondroid matrix, which can show hyalinization (*Figs 35.23*

and *35.24*). Fibrosis and hemorrhage are often seen. The matrix is composed of chondroitin sulfate.[12] Some tumor cells contain glycogen in the cytoplasm. Ossification is exceptional as is the presence of osteoclast-like giant cells.[13,14]

By immunohistochemistry, mature adipocytes are strongly positive for S100 protein; lipoblasts are only weakly positive for this marker. Chondroid lipomas show strong positivity for Cyclin D1.[11] Cytokeratin is very rarely focally positive.[2,11,12]

Electron microscopy confirms the presence of lipoblasts and mature fat cells. There is no evidence of true cartilaginous differentiation.[15]

Differential diagnosis

Myxoid liposarcoma usually lacks the presence of a 'chondroid-like' matrix and has a characteristic vascular pattern.

In myxoid chondrosarcoma there are no mature adipocytes, although some cells occasionally focally resemble lipoblasts.

Spindle cell lipoma/pleomorphic lipoma

Clinical features

Spindle cell lipoma is a comparatively uncommon variant and can be a source of histologic concern to the unwary.[1–3] Pleomorphic lipoma represents a variant of spindle cell lipoma, from which it is clinically and cytogenetically indistinguishable; it is entirely benign.[4–9]

Found predominantly in males, they arise mainly in the posterior portion of the neck, shoulder or upper back, and are characteristically seen in the sixth or seventh decade. Multiple lesions are rare and some are familial.[10,11] Rare cases can occur at other locations including the foot, hand, buttock, flank, oral cavity (including the tongue), larynx, orbit, soft tissues of the perianal area, perineum, groin, aortic valve, mediastinum and breast.[12–22] The last may represent an example of mammary-type myofibroblastoma of soft tissue, a lesion closely related to spindle cell lipoma.[23] Interestingly, lesions in women commonly occur in atypical locations.[24] They are more common on the extremities and face, are not infrequently dermal, and tend to occur at a younger age. They usually occur as a well-circumscribed, slowly growing, solitary, subcutaneous or (rarely, in up to 13% of cases) dermal lesion, less than 5 cm in diameter.[25–27] Intramuscular presentation is very rare.[28–31] A case has been reported at the site of an infantile fibrosarcoma treated with chemotherapy.[32] Spindle cell lipoma is an entirely benign,

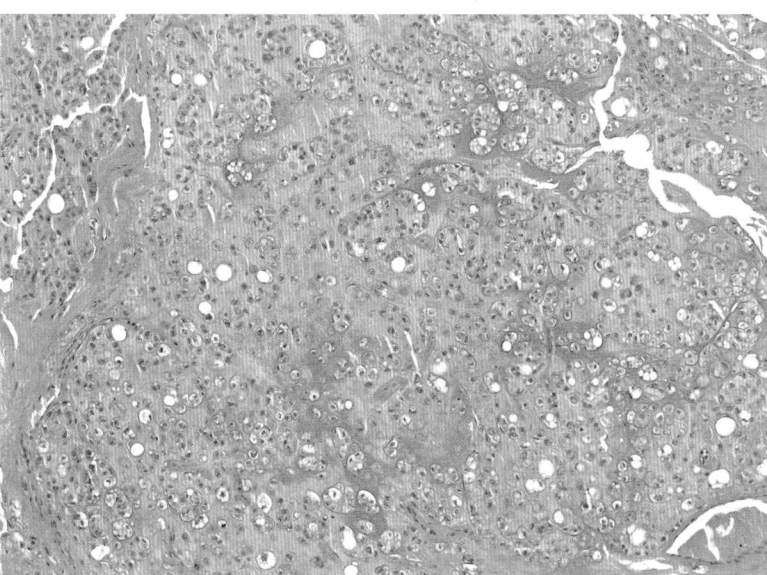

Fig. 35.23
Chondroid lipoma: myxoid and hyalinised stroma associated with variably vacuolated cells.

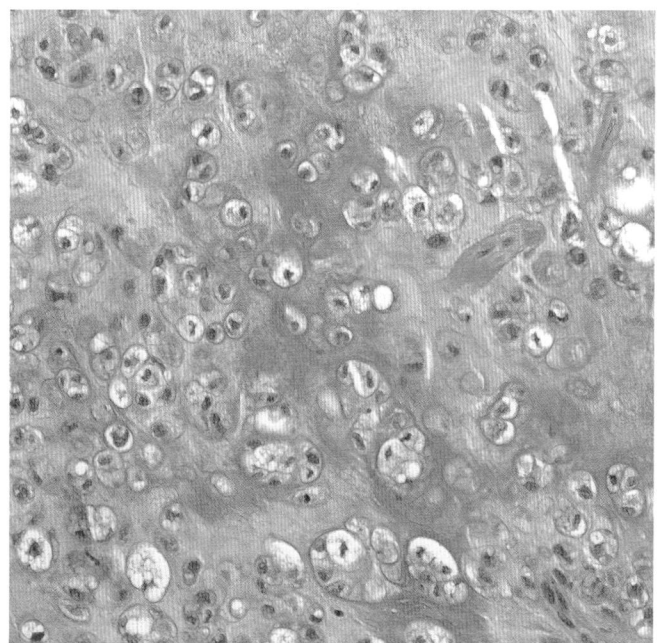

Fig. 35.24
Chondroid lipoma: high-power view highlighting wide range of lipoblastic differentiation.

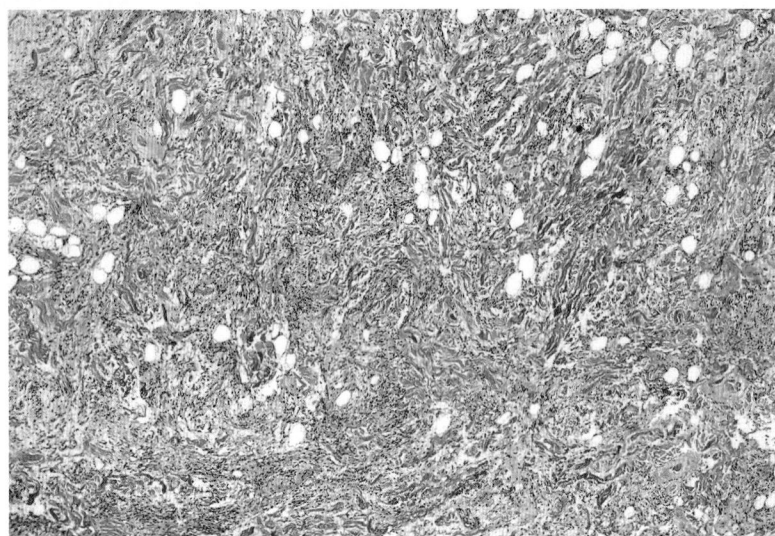

Fig. 35.25
Spindle cell lipoma: the tumor consists of an admixture of mature adipocytes and delicate spindle cells, often associated with broad bundles of hyalinized collagen.

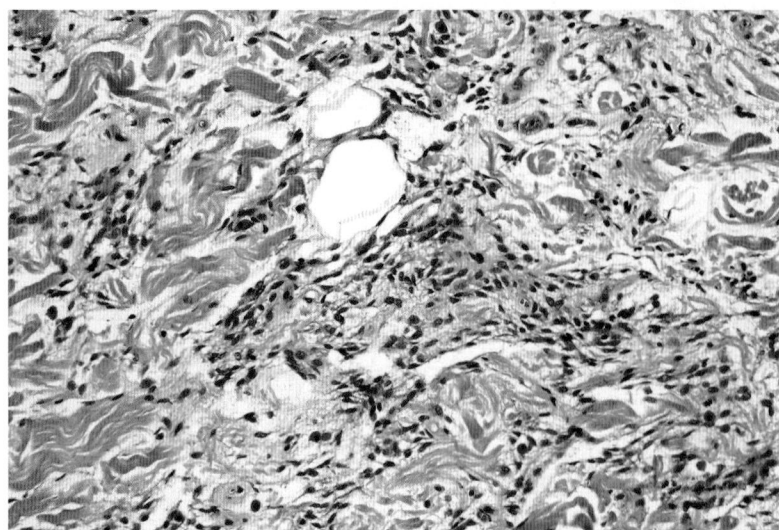

Fig. 35.26
Spindle cell lipoma: high-power view. Note the conspicuous mast cells.

nonrecurring lesion. Atypical spindle cell lipoma is a term proposed to refer to low-grade malignant adipose tumors with variable cellularity consisting of spindle cells with low to moderate cytologic atypia, adipocytes, lipoblasts, and myxoid stroma in varying proportions and with low potential for local recurrence (see below).[33–35]

Pathogenesis and histologic features

A number of chromosomal abnormalities have been found in spindle cell lipoma, identical to those found in pleomorphic lipoma. Monosomy or partial loss of chromosomes 13 and 16 are the most common alterations also seen in pleomorphic lipoma, strongly suggesting that these two lesions exist as a morphological continuum.[36–39] Interestingly, similar loss of 13q has been found in mammary-type myofibroblastoma and cellular angiofibroma, suggesting a close link between these tumors.[25,40–42] The 13q deletion seems to be involved in the activation of p38 mitogen-activated protein kinase induced by oxidative stress.[43]

Subcutaneous lesions tend to be well circumscribed while dermal tumors are ill defined.[27] Lesions located on the face usually display infiltration of skeletal muscle.[44] In addition to mature univacuolated adipocytes, irregular collections of slender spindled cells are seen with pale eosinophilic cytoplasm, uniform nuclei and rare mitoses (Fig. 35.25). Hyaline bundles of collagen and occasional giant cells may also be present, but lipoblasts are rarely identified. Mast cells are often numerous (Fig. 35.26). The relative proportions of adipose tissue to spindled cells vary between individual cases (Fig. 35.27). Some cases contain few or, rarely, no adipocytes at all.[45] Vascularity also varies and focal hemangiopericytoma-like areas are sometimes seen. Extensive myxoid change can lead to striking degenerative features with a pseudovascular pattern in which papillary structures project into empty spaces (Fig. 35.28). However, it has been shown that at least in some examples showing this change, the spaces are truly lined by endothelial cells, and these should be named angiomatous spindle cell lipoma.[46,47] Prominent myxoid change is more common in lesions presenting in the oral cavity. In addition to the histologic features of spindle cell lipoma, pleomorphic lipoma is characterized by numerous hyperchromatic and irregular multinucleated giant cells, with nuclei often arranged in a concentric floret pattern (floret giant cells) (Figs 35.29–35.31). Floret-like cells can also be seen in prolapsed orbital fat as a result of a degenerative process.[48] Mitotic figures may rarely be evident and occasional multivacuolated lipoblasts are sometimes present (Fig. 35.32). Lesions that show few or no adipocytes may pose a diagnostic challenge and this can be a feature of tumors with features of pleomorphic lipoma.[49,50]

The spindled cells are positive for CD34 but usually negative for S100 protein. However, positivity in the spindle cells for the later has been

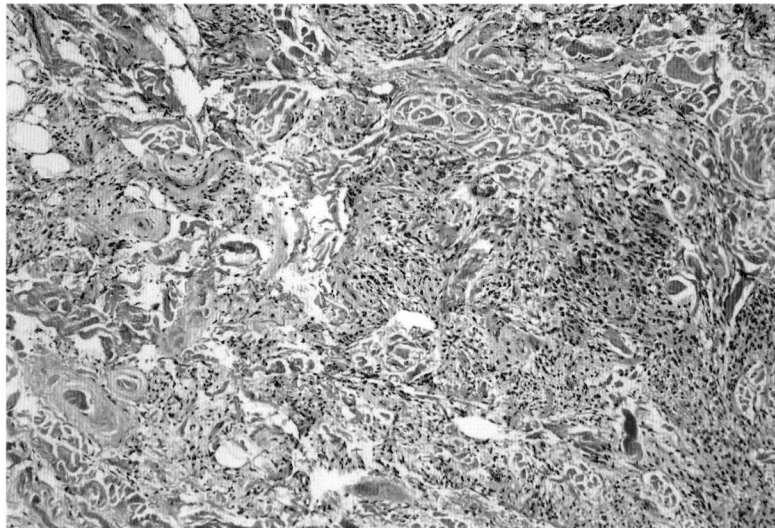

Fig. 35.27
Spindle cell lipoma: in some examples, the spindled cells predominate such that the lesion is easily mistaken for another connective tissue tumor.

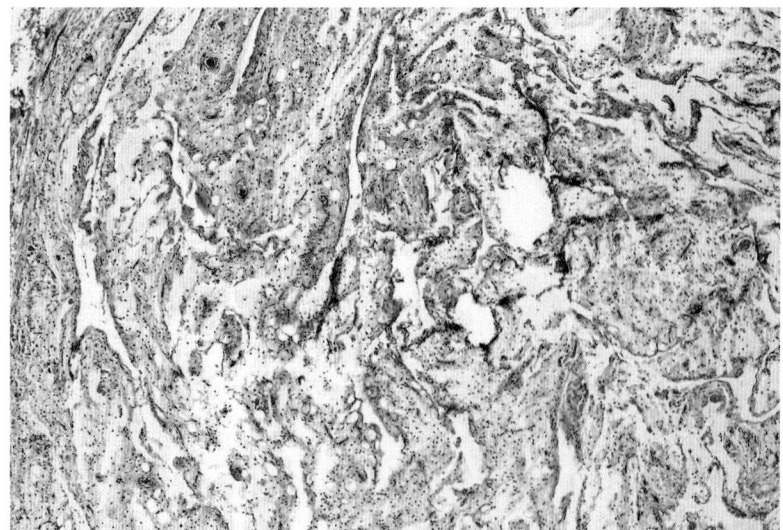

Fig. 35.28
Spindle cell lipoma: rarely, massive myxoid degeneration results in the formation of pseudovascular spaces (the so-called lymphangiomatous variant).

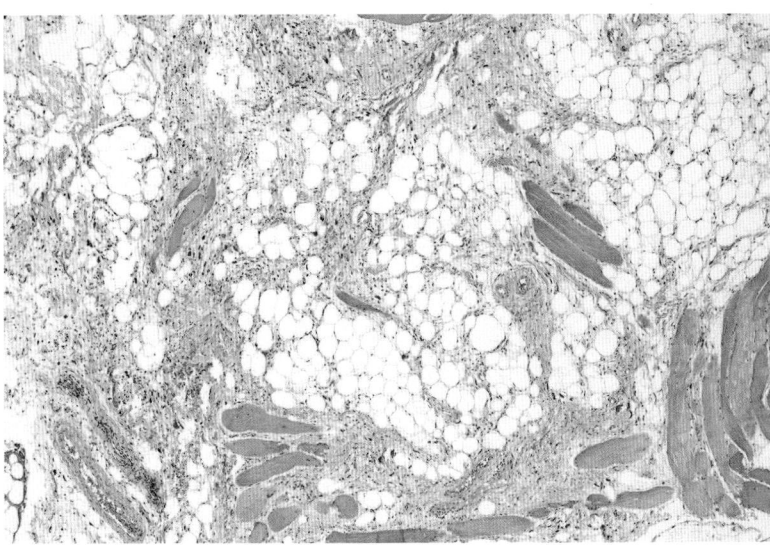

Fig. 35.29
Pleomorphic lipoma: this view shows adipocytes, thick collagen bundles, and spindled cells.

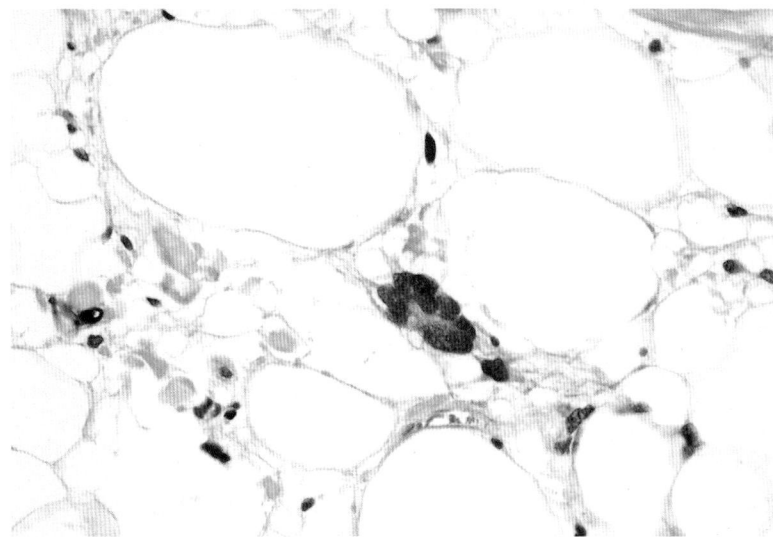

Fig. 35.32
Pleomorphic lipoma: high-power view.

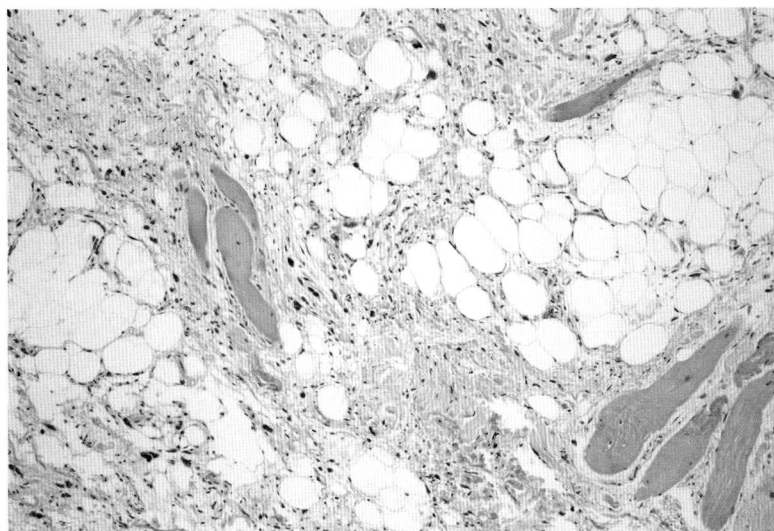

Fig. 35.30
Pleomorphic lipoma: multiple hyperchromatic giant cells are seen.

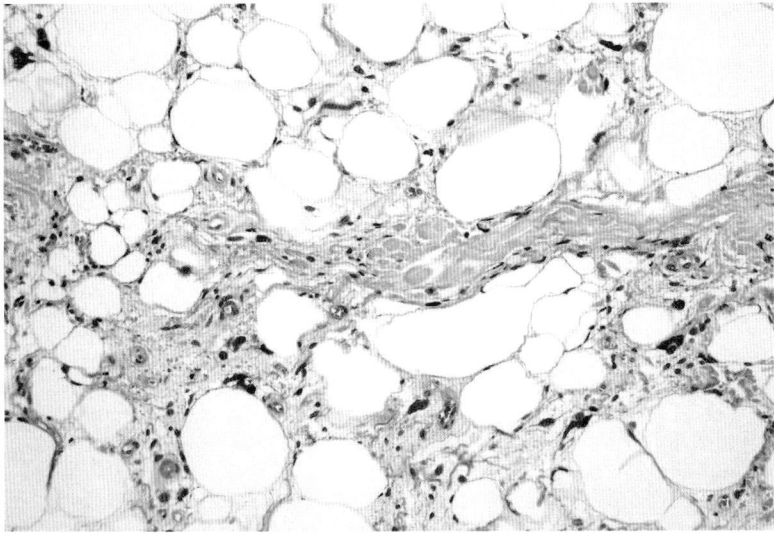

Fig. 35.31
Pleomorphic lipoma: conspicuous floret giant cells are present.

reported in some cases.[51] Estrogen receptor may be focally positive in some cases. Mature adipocytes are positive for S100. RB1 (retinoblastoma protein) is negative.

Ultrastructural studies show cells with features of mature adipocytes and spindled cells representing undifferentiated mesenchymal cells.[46]

Differential diagnosis

Although the clinical history may be sufficiently characteristic to aid the diagnosis, distinction from liposarcoma is made by the absence of either adipocytic atypia or variation in adipocyte size. Histologically comparable lesions involving deeper soft tissue should be classified as atypical spindle cell lipomatous tumor (previously termed spindle cell liposarcoma), reflecting their much greater tendency to recur.

Hibernoma

Clinical features

Hibernoma is a rare, invariably benign tumor resembling normal brown fat, which typically occurs in young adults with a slight female predominance. The tumor most often presents in the interscapular region and thigh followed by the axillae, chest wall and head and neck.[1–5] It is a slowly growing, highly vascular lesion that may attain a considerable size and is typified macroscopically by tannish-brown fatty tissue. The large majority of tumors are subcutaneous but about 10% of cases are intramuscular.[1] Lesions are benign and there is no tendency for local recurrence.

Pathogenesis and histologic features

In cytogenetic studies, hibernomas have shown consistent rearrangement at 11q13.[1,6,7] Additionally, MEN1 and/or AIP loss have been described.[8,9]

Hibernomas are classified histologically into four categories: typical (82% of cases), lipoma-like (7%), myxoid (9%), and spindled cell (2%).[1,3,10,11] Typical hibernoma is characterized by an admixture of multivacuolated large adipocytes with central nuclei, large cells with granular eosinophilic cytoplasm and mature univacuolated adipocytes (Fig. 35.33). They are usually encapsulated and lobulated, being subdivided by fine fibrous septa containing numerous small capillaries. Some cases have focal myxoid stroma and very few resemble spindle cell lipoma.[1,9] In a subset of lesions large lipoblast-like cells mimicking atypical lipomatous tumors may be conspicuous.[12]

Tumor cells show variable staining for S100 protein; in the spindle cell variant, the spindled cells are CD34 positive.[1] UCP1 positivity has been reported.[13]

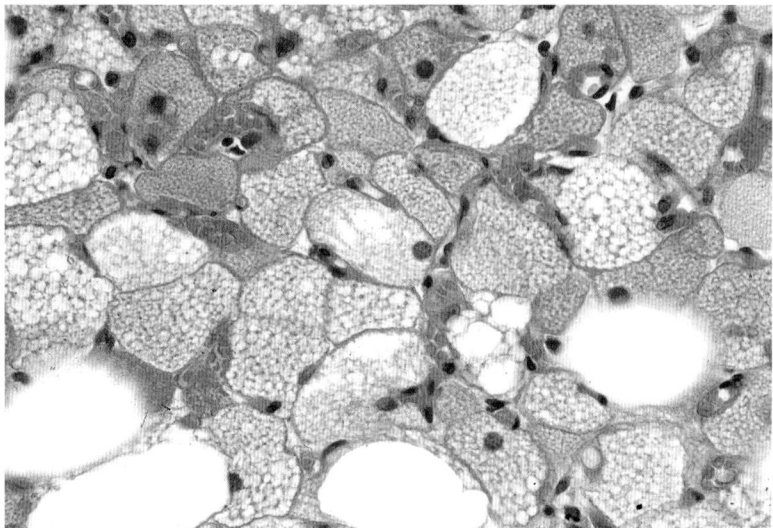

Fig. 35.33
Hibernoma: the admixture of mature adipocytes and large cells with eosinophilic granular cytoplasm is characteristic.

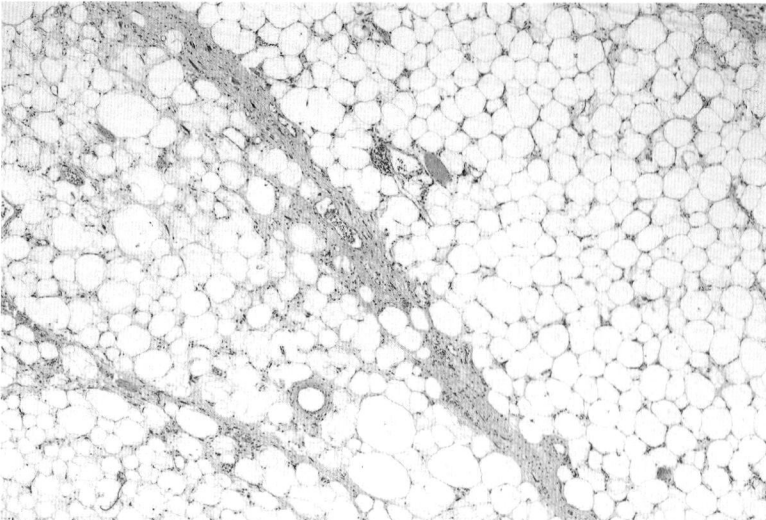

Fig. 35.34
Atypical lipomatous tumor: note the characteristic variation in adipocyte size and the scattered hyperchromatic cells.

Differential diagnosis

Distinction from a granular cell tumor is easy, as in the latter the cells are not vacuolated and there are no mature adipocytes. Lesions with lipoblast-like cells have areas that are otherwise typical of hibernoma and tumor cells are negative for *MDM2/CDK4*.

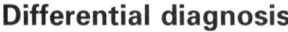

Adipocytic tumors of intermediate malignancy (locally aggressive)

Atypical lipomatous tumor

Clinical features

Atypical lipomatous tumors are usually deep seated and may occur in the subcutaneous tissue, within skeletal muscle, the retroperitoneum, the mediastinum, and the spermatic cord.[1–6] Visceral tumors are very rare. Subcutaneous tumors have a predilection for the legs (particularly the thighs) and the trunk.[2–6] Patients are more often male and usually present in their sixth and seventh decades, complaining of a slowly growing, painless mass measuring several centimeters. Deep-seated tumors, particularly those arising in the retroperitoneum, are usually very large by the time they are discovered.[7,8]

Most authors argue that the term 'well differentiated liposarcoma' should be reserved for deep seated tumors for which a complete surgical resection cannot usually be achieved: mediastinal, retroperitoneal and spermatic cord. These tumors frequently recur, as a result of incomplete excision, and can eventually undergo dedifferentiation.

Prognosis in atypical lipomatous tumors, as mentioned above, is closely related to site. Peripheral tumors are prognostically more favorable than their retroperitoneal counterparts: the smaller the tumor, the better the outlook. Subcutaneous tumors have a tendency for local recurrence due to incomplete excision but behavior is not aggressive and they do not metastasize unless they become dedifferentiated (see below). Dedifferentiation is exceptional in subcutaneous lesions.[9,10] Adjuvant radiotherapy following resection of tumors located in the extremities and trunk was associated with a reduction of local relapse risk in a large study.[11]

Pathogenesis and histologic features

From the cytogenetic point of view, ring or giant marker chromosomes with integration of variable portions of the 12q13~15 interval characterize ALT.[11–13] *MDM2* at 12q15 is virtually universally amplified.[14,15] *CDK4* is also usually amplified. Other frequently co-amplified genes include *HMGA2*,

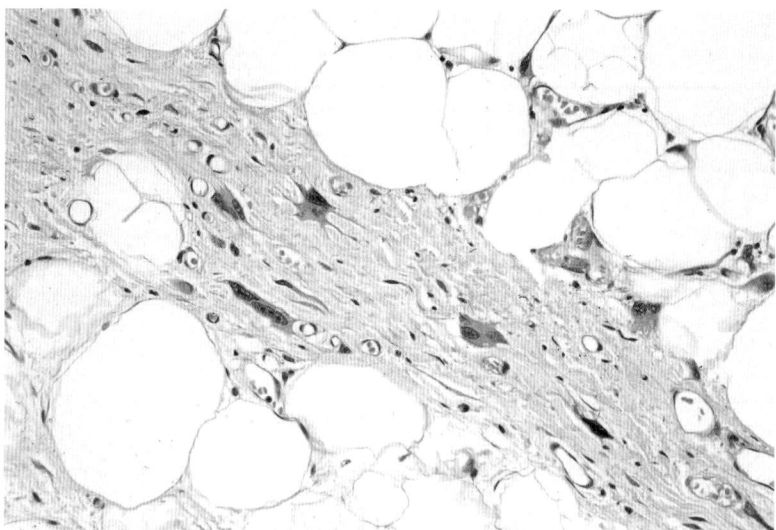

Fig. 35.35
Atypical lipomatous tumor: irregular hyperchromatic stromal cells are typically present, often in proximity to the septa.

YEATS4, *CPM* and *FRS2*. *ATF6* and *DUSP12* amplification has been found in some cases with 1q21~25 amplicon.[16]

Atypical lipomatous tumor has been traditionally subdivided into four variants: adipocytic, sclerosing, inflammatory and spindle cell.[2–6,17,18] In the latest WHO classification (2013) however, the well-differentiated variant of spindle cell liposarcoma is no longer considered as a morphological variant of atypical lipomatous tumor. Strictly defined, the latter is likely to represent part of the spectrum of a distinctive variant of low-grade adipocytic neoplasm termed atypical spindle cell lipomatous tumor (see below).[19,20]

- Microscopically, the adipocytic lipoma-like type is characterized by an appearance very similar to mature adipose tissue, but with scattered moderate nuclear pleomorphism, which is most prominent in the fibrous stroma, along with variation in adipocyte size and a few lipoblasts (*Figs 35.34–35.36*). Purely dermal lesions are rare.[1,21]
- The sclerosing type is always deep seated and consists of variably fibrillary or sclerotic collagenous tissue containing bizarre, often multinucleated cells and rare lipoblasts (*Fig. 35.37*). Both types show minimal, if any, mitotic activity. Atypical hyperchromatic cells are frequently seen in a perivascular location. Rare cases display a prominent mononuclear inflammatory cell infiltrate, often in a patchy distribution.

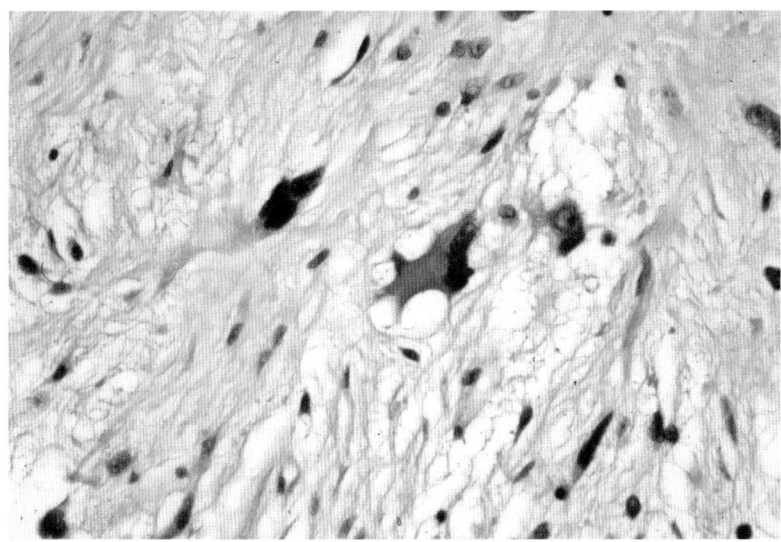

Fig. 35.36
Atypical lipomatous tumor: a multivacuolated lipoblast shown under high power.

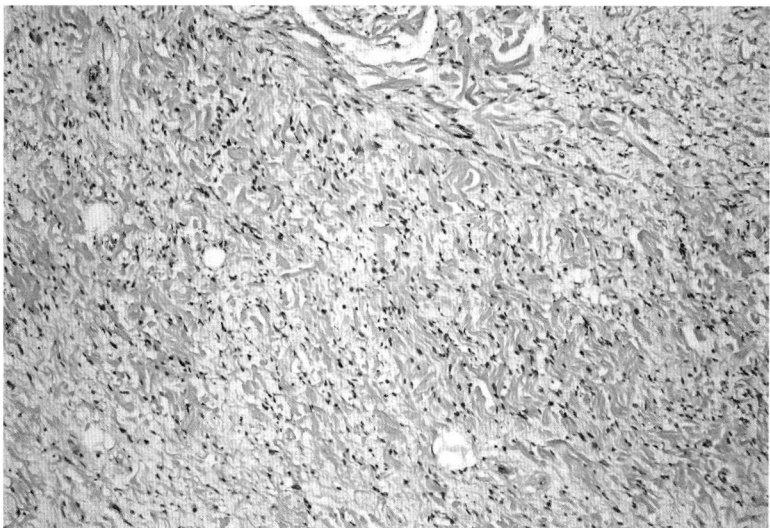

Fig. 35.38
Atypical spindle cell lipomatous tumor: in this example, the tumor consists predominantly of spindled cells with hyperchromatic nuclei. Only one or two adipocytes are present.

Differential diagnosis

Atypical lipomatous tumor (ALT) is distinguished from a lipoma by the variation in the size of the adipocytes and the presence of cells with hyperchromatic nuclei in the former condition. The changes seen in massive localized lymphedema associated with morbid obesity can mimic an atypical lipomatous tumor but the former lacks adipocytes with atypia and consists of large lobules of mature adipocytes with edema, thick septa and vascular proliferation within the septa.[34,35] Subconjunctival herniated orbital fat may be confused with an ALT, as the former often contains multinucleate floret-like giant cells (a mimic of pleomorphic lipoma), fibrous tracts and Lockhern cells. However, atypical cells within fibrous septae are absent in subconjuctival herniated fat.[36]

Atypical spindle cell lipomatous tumor

Atypical spindle cell lipomatous tumor is a distinct variant of lipomatous tumor of intermediate malignancy previously described under terms such as atypical spindle cell lipoma, spindle cell liposarcoma, well-differentiated spindle cell liposarcoma, and fibrosarcoma-like lipomatous neoplasm.[1-4] Tumors present as an asymptomatic or rarely painful subcutaneous or deep-seated mass, several centimeters in diameter, mainly in middle-aged males and with predilection for the limbs (hands and feet) and limb girdles.[1] Local recurrence is seen in about 12% of cases but there is no metastatic potential.

Only up to 50% of lesions are associated with heterozygous deletions of *RB1* correlating with loss of RB1 expression on immunohistochemistry. The histologic spectrum is wide and varies from hypocellular lesions with spindle cells displaying mild cytologic atypia, few mature adipocytes and prominent myxoid stroma to more cellular lesions, with spindle cells displaying mild to moderate cytologic atypia, lipoblasts, and less prominent stroma (*Figs 35.38–35.41*).[1] A subset of tumors mimicking pleomorphic lipoma and referred to as atypical pleomorphic lipomatous tumor is probably part of the same spectrum.[5] Our understanding of this tumor group and its morphological spectrum as well as molecular pathogenesis continue to evolve.

By immunohistochemistry, the spindle cells frequently express CD34 in up to two-thirds of cases, they are positive for S100 protein in about 40% of cases and for desmin in about one-fifth of cases.[1] MDM2 and CDK4 are rarely focally and weakly positive in tumor cells but are not co-expressed in the same tumor and not amplified genetically.[1]

Often this lesion is misdiagnosed as a low-grade malignant peripheral nerve sheath tumor, dermatofibrosarcoma protuberans, spindle cell lipoma,

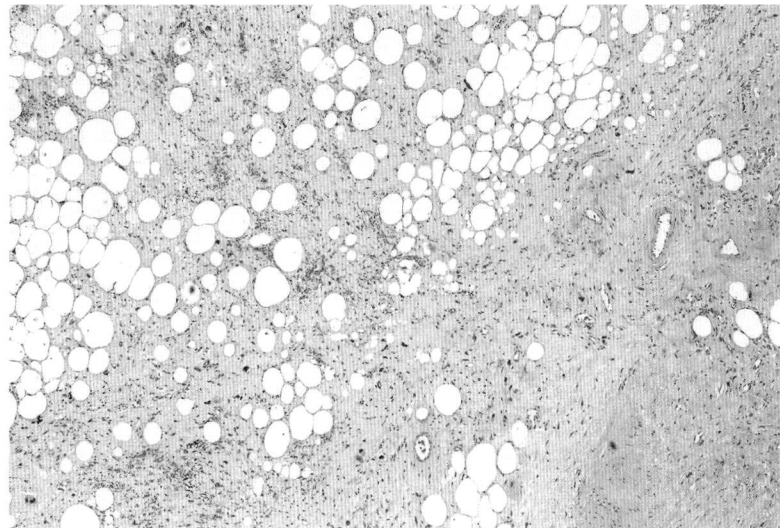

Fig. 35.37
Atypical lipomatous tumor: this field shows sclerotic collagenous tissue, adipocytes, and hyperchromatic cells.

- The inflammatory type, usually found in the retroperitoneum, displays a prominent mononuclear inflammatory cell infiltrate that can be so prominent as to obscure the real nature of the neoplasm.[22]

A mixture of morphological variants can be seen in the same tumor, especially in the deep-seated ones. The presence of lipoblasts is not required nor establishes the diagnosis. Metaplastic elements including cartilage, bone, and smooth muscle are sometimes a feature and should not be confused with dedifferentiation.[23]

Immunohistochemistry for MDM2 and CDK4 has been proposed as useful in the distinction of atypical lipomatous tumor/well-differentiated liposarcoma (ALT/WDLPS) from other benign lipomatous tumors. MDM2 and CDK4 tend to be positive in the former and negative in most of the latter.[24] However, a recent study found that immunohistochemistry for both markers has a sensitivity below 50%.[25] FISH and real-time PCR for amplification of *MDM2* is a more reliable method.[26-29] CISH or MLPA represent alternative sensitive methods.[30,31] p16 has also been advocated as useful in the distinction between ALT-WDLPS and lipoma as the latter do not express this marker.[32,33] However, the specificity is low and false positives may occur especially in small biopsies.[33] S100 protein is positive in adipocytes and some lipoblasts.

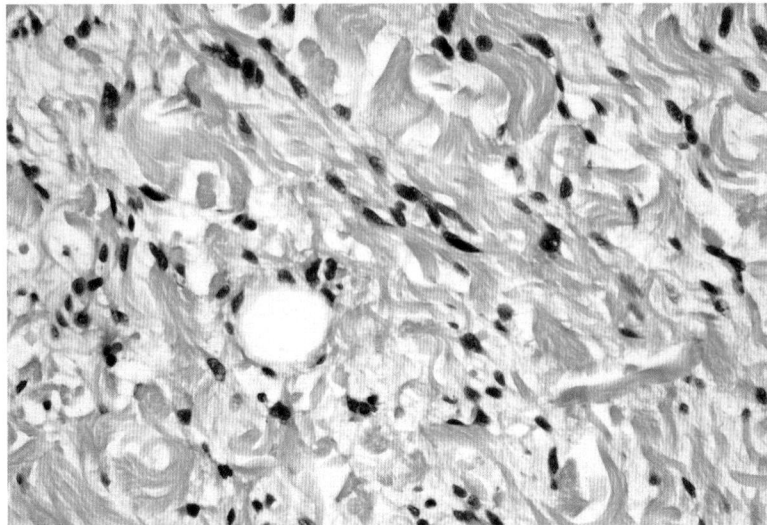

Fig. 35.39
Atypical spindle cell lipomatous tumor: high-power view of atypical spindle cells with hyperchromatic nuclei.

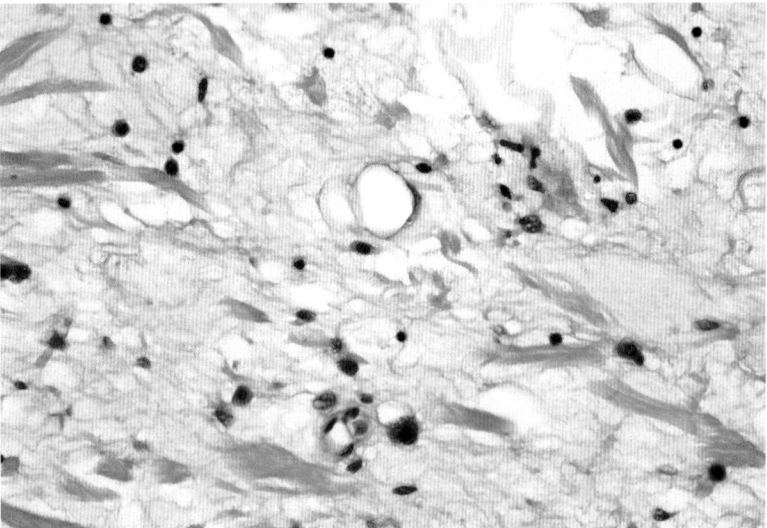

Fig. 35.40
Atypical spindle cell lipomatous tumor: high-power view showing signet-ring cell lipoblasts.

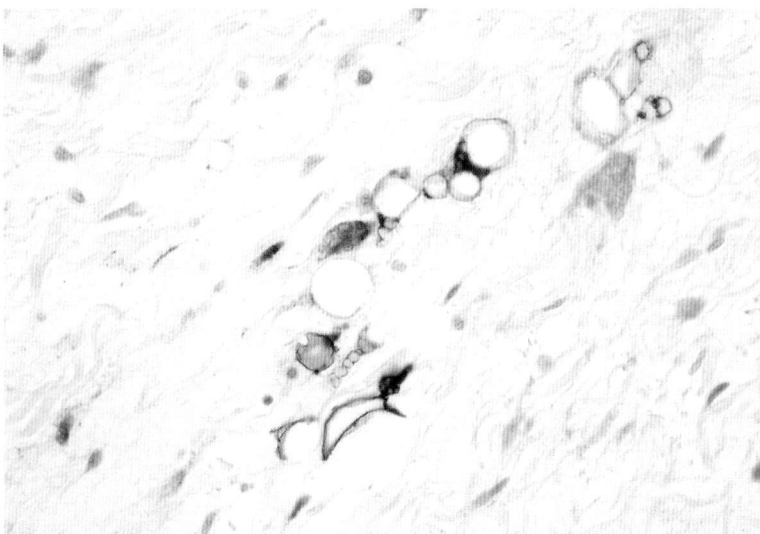

Fig. 35.41
Atypical spindle cell lipomatous tumor: the lipoblasts can be highlighted with S100 protein immunohistochemistry.

mammary-type myofibroblastoma, and fat-forming solitary fibrous tumor. Distinction from what some term low-grade dedifferentiated liposarcoma is important because of the difference in behavior.[6] In the latter, there is usually abrupt transition between a hypocellular and hypercellular tumor, there is more pleomorphism, and tumor cells display prominent diffuse positivity for MDM2 and CDK4.

Malignant adipocytic tumors

Liposarcoma

Clinical features

Despite being one of the most common soft tissue sarcomas, liposarcoma presents infrequently as a primary subcutaneous lesion and only exceptionally as a primary dermal tumor.[1]

Liposarcoma is traditionally divided into three subtypes:
- well-differentiated / dedifferentiated [2–7]
- myxoid, which includes the cellular (previously termed round cell) variant,[2–5,8,9]
- pleomorphic.[2–5,8–10]

Dedifferentiated liposarcoma

Dedifferentiation refers to a biphasic tumor containing an atypical lipomatous tumor and a sarcomatous undifferentiated component of variable grade. Dedifferentiation occurs mainly in deep-seated tumors (particularly those occurring in the retroperitoneum) and is exceptional in subcutaneous lesions.[11,12]

Myxoid liposarcoma

Myxoid liposarcoma occurs in adults, with a peak incidence between the fourth and fifth decades of life, and has no sex predilection.[9,13,14] Although rare in children and adolescents, it is the most common type of liposarcoma in this age group.[15] The majority of tumors arise in deep soft tissues, subcutaneous tumors being very rare.[16] The most common site is the lower limb, particularly the thigh. All tumors, without exception, tend to local recurrence, and metastases occur in approximately one-third of cases depending on the grade.[13,14,17] The presence of a cellular (previously termed round cell) component, necrosis and p53 overexpression has been found to be associated with poor prognosis.[17] The terminology of round cell liposarcoma is no longer favored under the WHO classification as round cell is not the only morphology adopted by the cellular (higher grade) variant of myxoid liposarcoma.

Pleomorphic liposarcoma

Pleomorphic liposarcoma is the least common variant of liposarcoma. There is no sex predilection, patients are elderly and tumors are deep seated, presenting mainly on the limbs.[18,19] Only exceptional tumors occur in the dermis or subcutis.[1,10,18,19] Tumors grow rapidly and there is a high tendency for local recurrence and metastasis.[18,19] While being by a wide margin the least common liposarcoma in deep soft tissue, it may be the most common liposarcoma to occur as a cutaneous primary.[10]

Pathogenesis and histologic features

Dedifferentiated liposarcoma shares the same cytogenetic alterations with atypical lipomatous tumor (well-differentiated liposarcoma), namely a ring or giant marker chromosome associated with amplification and overexpression of the 12q13~15 region containing *MDM2*. In addition, *JUN* (1p32), *ASK1* (6q23) and *TAB2* (6q25) amplification can be seen..[20–24]

Myxoid/round cell liposarcomas show a specific t(12;16)(q13;p11) fusing *DDIT3* and *FUS*. In a small subset of cases a t(12;22)(q13;q12) has been found where *EWSR1* substitutes for *FUS*. These translocations are seen in virtually all cases.[20–22,24–28]

No consistent cytogenetic abnormality has been demonstrated in pleomorphic liposarcoma, which often shows complex cytogenetic abnormalities with *TP53* mutations.[23,24,27]

Dedifferentiated liposarcoma is defined as a well-differentiated liposarcoma showing abrupt transition to a higher grade nonlipogenic sarcoma.[29]

Fig. 35.42
Myxoid liposarcoma: low-power view showing spindled cells in a myxoid stroma and conspicuous delicate vessels.

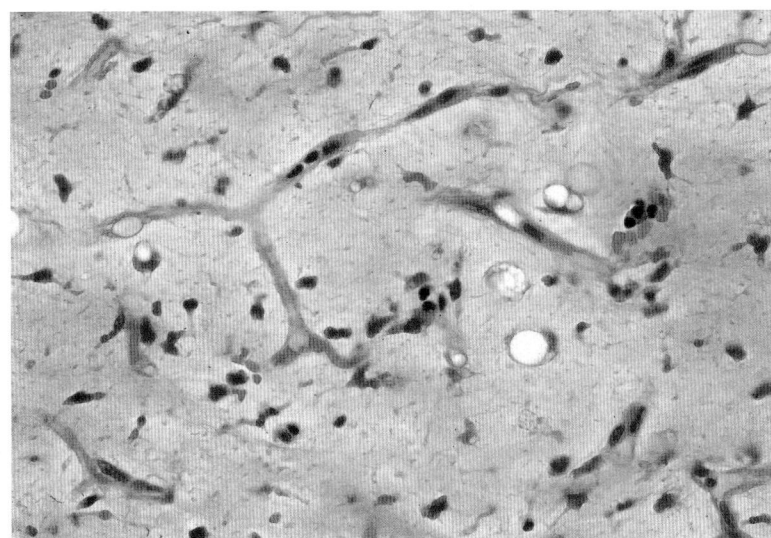

Fig. 35.44
Myxoid liposarcoma: this field shows a typical 'crow's-foot' type of blood vessel.

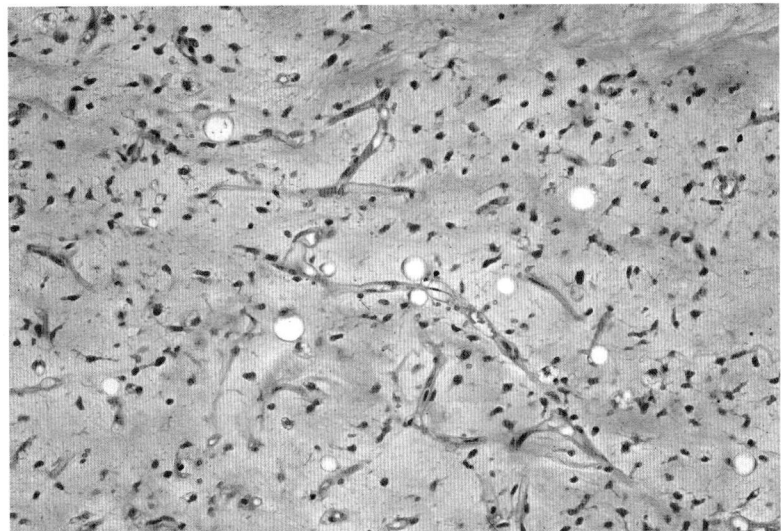

Fig. 35.43
Myxoid liposarcoma: medium-power view showing multiple signet-ring cell lipoblasts and conspicuous capillaries.

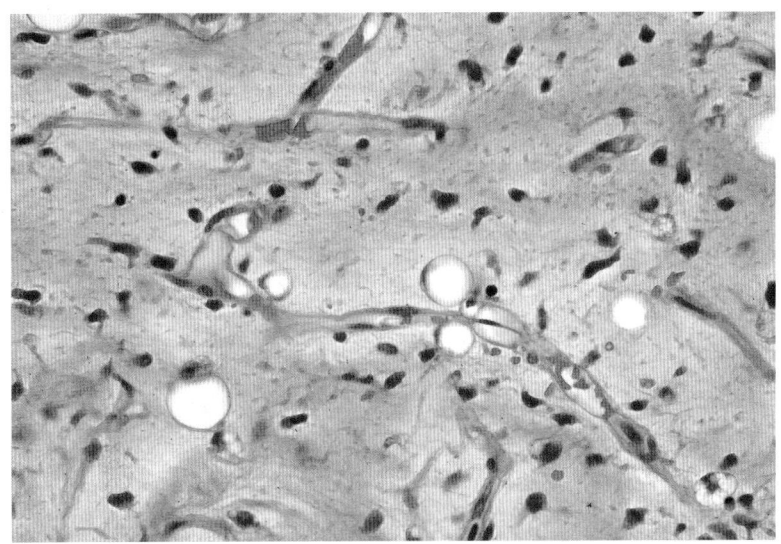

Fig. 35.45
Myxoid liposarcoma: multiple lipoblasts are present.

Less frequently the transition may be to a non-lipogenic low-grade sarcoma, but this terminology and the behavioral features are debated. In some cases, a well-differentiated area cannot be identified. Focal lipoblastic differentiation may be seen within the dedifferentiated areas.[30] This change can occur in a primary tumor and less often in a recurrence. Although in most cases the dedifferentiated component is pleomorphic, there are often focal less atypical areas that may mimic other tumors such as dermatofibrosarcoma protuberans. Moreover, local recurrences of dedifferentiated liposarcoma may be well-differentiated. Meningothelial-like whorls have also been documented.[31,32] Heterologous differentiation including osteosarcomatous, chondrosarcomatous, myogenic, and angiosarcomatous components is rarely seen.[33] Positive diffuse staining of MDM2 and/or CDK4 is a constant finding.

Myxoid liposarcoma is composed of fairly uniform stellate or spindled cells with small vacuoles set in a myxoid matrix composed of acid mucopolysaccharide (*Figs 35.42–35.45*).[3,5,13,14] Mucin pooling, producing a lymphangioma-like pattern, is common. Emphasis should be placed on the presence of a complex plexiform network of small thin-walled capillaries in a pattern resembling chicken-wire or 'crow's feet.' Mitoses are sparse. Lipoblasts are most easily identified at the periphery of the tumor. Occasionally,

extramedullary hematopoiesis may be seen. The presence of more cellular areas composed of uniform oval-to-round larger cells with hyperchromatic nuclei and inconspicuous cytoplasm indicates round cell change. This is associated with more aggressive behavior and such lesions are known either as combined myxoid and round cell liposarcoma or as high-grade myxoid liposarcoma (*Figs 35.46* and *35.47*).[5,6,29] The round cell component may predominate. Pure round cell liposarcomas are extremely rare in the subcutis, but mixed tumors are occasionally seen. Dedifferentiation in myxoid liposarcoma is exceptional.[34] S100 is positive in lipoblasts and variably positive in the round cell component. Immunohistochemistry for the cancer testis antigen NY-ESO-1 has been reported to be consistently positive in this group of tumors but not in other lesions that may be confused with them.[35]

Pleomorphic liposarcoma consists of highly pleomorphic spindle cells, lipoblasts, and numerous multinucleated multivacuolated giant cells (*Fig. 35.48*).[18,19,36] Identification of lipoblasts is vital in distinguishing this variant from other pleomorphic sarcomas.

Lipoblasts are variable present within all of these lesions and can be absent or very difficult to find in myxoid and well-differentiated liposarcoma. By definition, they are absent in the dedifferentiated liposarcoma component which is nonadipocytic. In exceptional cases, the dedifferentiated portion

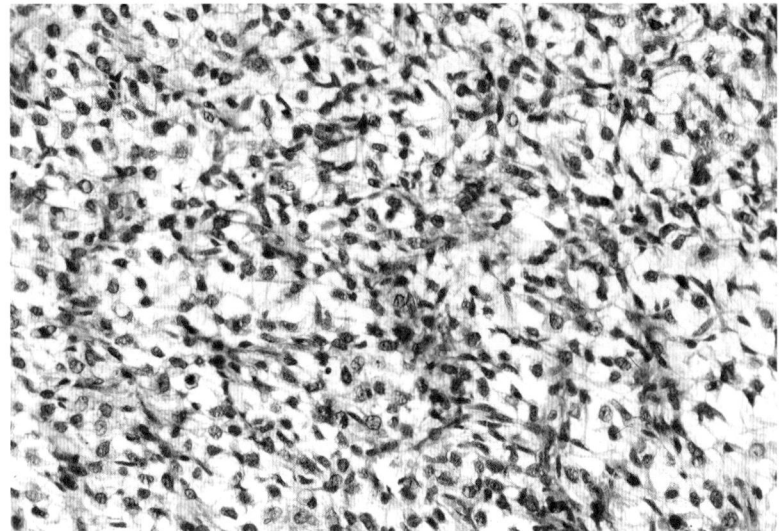

Fig. 35.46
Myxoid liposarcoma: round cell component. In this field, the tumor is much more cellular. The background vasculature is still visible.

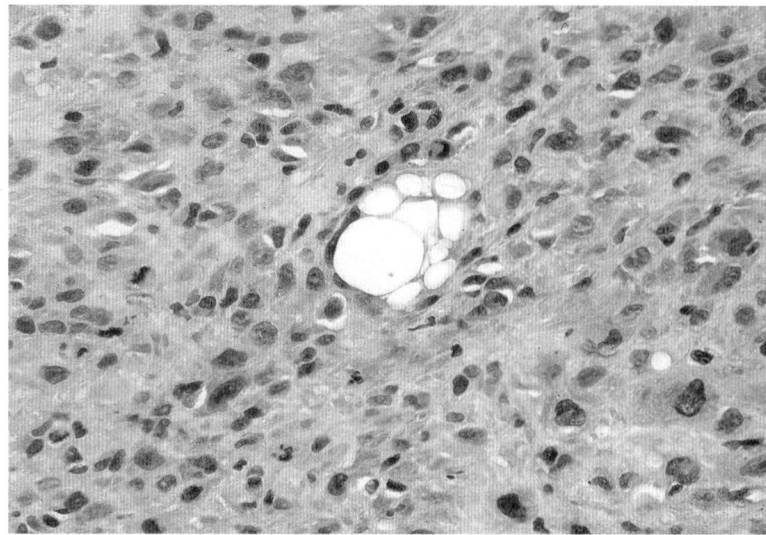

Fig. 35.48
Pleomorphic liposarcoma: recognition of this variant is dependent upon identification of lipoblasts among the highly pleomorphic cellular background.

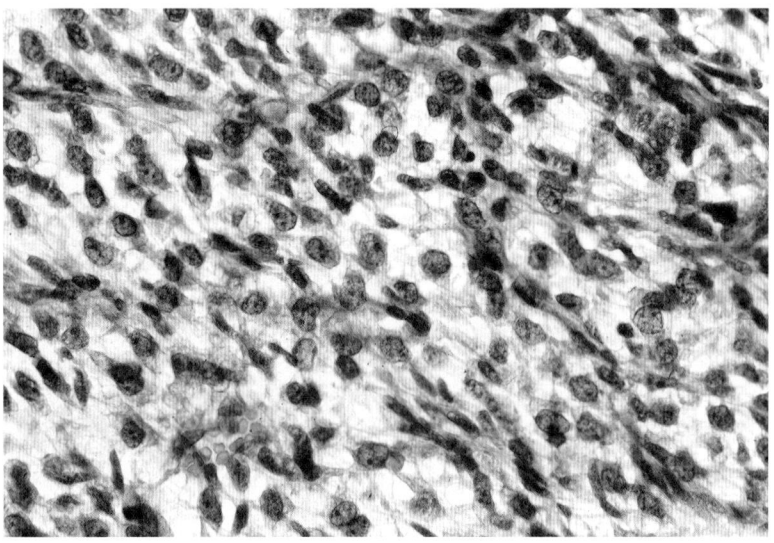

Fig. 35.47
Myxoid liposarcoma: round cell component. The nuclei are hyperchromatic and pleomorphic.

of liposarcoma can have a pleomorphic liposarcoma-like component, but 12q15 amplification and MDM2 and CDK4 expression are maintained. In pleomorphic liposarcoma proper, lipoblasts can range from diffusely present to very rare and focal. Typically, lipoblasts are highly variable in size, contain more than one well-defined or punched-out lipid vacuole, and have irregular, hyperchromatic (and sometimes multiple) nuclei, the margins of which are scalloped by the fat droplets.

Differential diagnosis

Nuclear positivity for MDM2 and or CDK4 will help establish the diagnosis of dedifferentiated liposarcoma in most cases (see also atypical lipomatous tumor).[37,38] Myxoid liposarcoma is distinguished from other sarcomas by its distinctive vessel morphology. In difficult cases molecular confirmation may be necessary.[16] Myxofibrosarcoma (myxoid malignant fibrous histiocytoma) is recognized by the lack of lipoblasts and the presence of more variable pleomorphism than present in myxoid liposarcoma. Distinction from lipoblastoma may be very difficult or impossible. However, liposarcoma is very rare in children and, in difficult cases, cytogenetic studies may be helpful (see lipoblastoma). The diagnosis of pleomorphic liposarcoma is based on the identification of lipoblasts in the background of a pleomorphic sarcoma and a lack of MDM2 and/or CDK4 nuclear positivity.

TUMORS OF FIBROUS, FIBROBLASTIC AND MYOFIBROBLASTIC TISSUE

Benign fibrous and myofibroblastic tumors and tumorlike lesions

Hypertrophic scar

Clinical features

Hypertrophic scars occur most frequently on the head and neck, chest, knees and shoulders and show no racial predilection.[1-3] Clinically, they may be distinguished from keloids by being less raised and not extending beyond the boundaries of the initiating injury. Unlike keloids, hypertrophic scars are far less prone to recur after treatment, but, in fact, precise distinction between these two lesions is not always possible and they represent a continuous spectrum.[4]

Pathogenesis and histologic features

Hypertrophic scar appears to be induced by over-activation of dermal wound healing pathways, in some ways similar to that of keloids below.[5-9] Transforming growth factor beta 1 has been associated with the induction of both hypertrophic scars and keloids by inducing production of collagen by fibroblasts particularly in early stages.[10] It has been proposed that abnormal blood vessel regulation may predispose to keloid and hypertrophic scar formation.[11] The Wnt pathway is activated as well, particularly in the proliferative phase.[12]

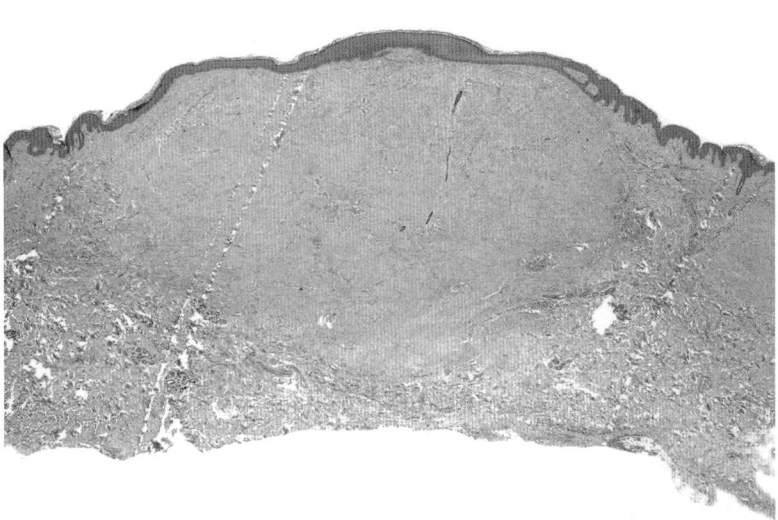

Fig. 35.49
Hypertrophic scar: within the dermis is a nodular fibrous lesion.

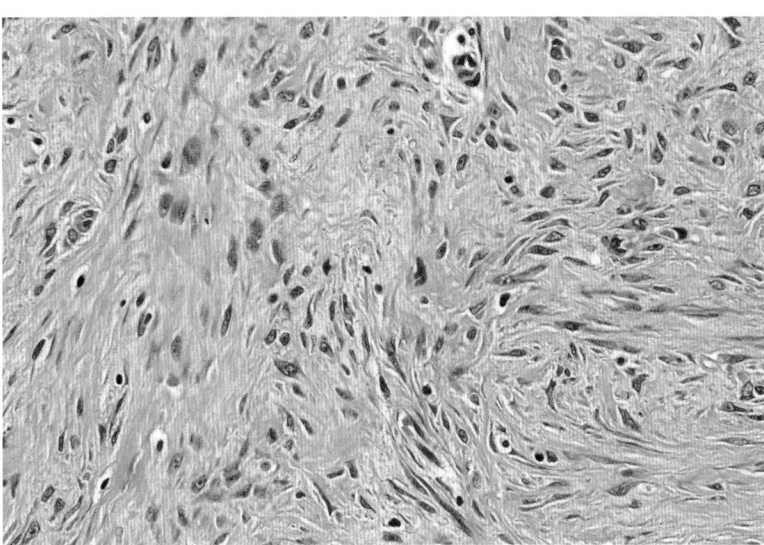

Fig. 35.51
Hypertrophic scar: note the spindled cells and collagenous stroma.

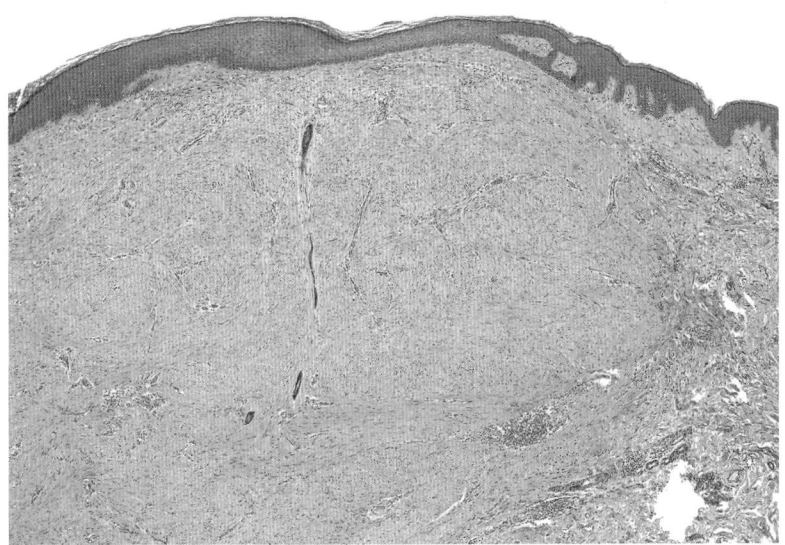

Fig. 35.50
Hypertrophic scar: the lesion is composed of banal fibroblasts with a variably collagenous stroma.

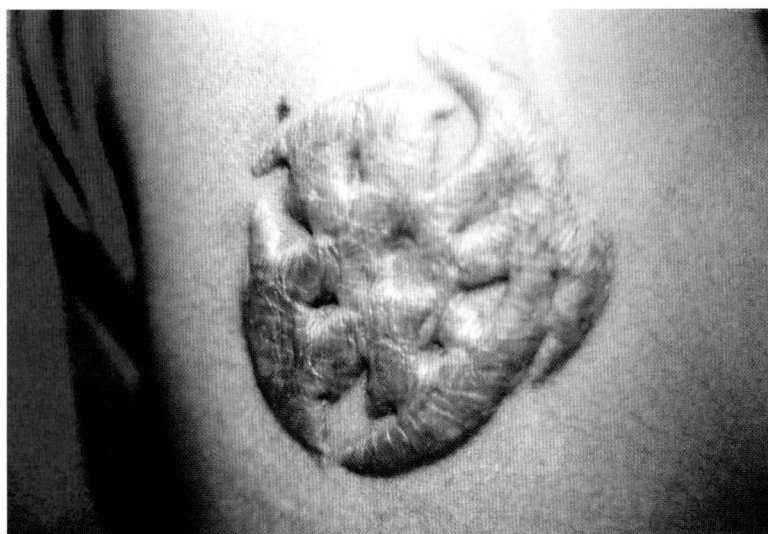

Fig. 35.52
Prominent keloid developing at the side of a tattoo. By courtesy of Dr J. Dayrit, Manila, The Philippines.

The appearances are typified by a somewhat non-specific dermal fibroblastic proliferation, which is often associated with epidermal atrophy (*Figs 35.49–35.51*). They tend to be more cellular than keloids, and hyalinized collagen fibers are far less prominent. Mitoses are sometimes noted. A nodular growth pattern is common. Evidence of a foreign body granulomatous reaction may sometimes be present.

Keloid

Clinical features

A keloid is a common reactive lesion that represents exuberant scar formation. It typically extends beyond the site of original injury.[1-5] Although keloids occasionally appear to arise spontaneously, it is believed that most develop as a direct result of local trauma, even if minor or unnoticed (*Figs 35.52–35.54*).[1-5] Keloids also develop as a result of inflammation in conditions such as acne vulgaris. The use of isotretinoin has also been linked to the development of keloids.[6] Eruptive keloids associated with aromatase inhibitor therapy, after chickenpox and as a paraneoplastic phenomenon, have been reported.[7-10] Although these lesions may arise at any age, they are most common in adolescents and young adults; they occur at least four times more frequently in patients of African descent and show a slight predilection for females. A positive family history is not uncommon and probably reflects a genetic predisposition to keloid formation.

Keloids usually occur on the head and neck (especially the ear), upper chest and arms, but may be seen at almost any cutaneous site although areas such as the hands and feet and the genitalia are very rarely affected.[11] Characteristically, they present as raised, well-circumscribed, rather smooth lesions, becoming progressively more indurated as time passes. They are occasionally itchy or tender and may be multiple, again reflecting individual susceptibility to their development. Irrespective of the treatment used, local recurrence is very common.

Pathogenesis and histologic features

The pathogenesis of keloids is not clear but seems to be multifactorial (see also under hypertrophic scar).[12] Genetic predisposition and local tissue

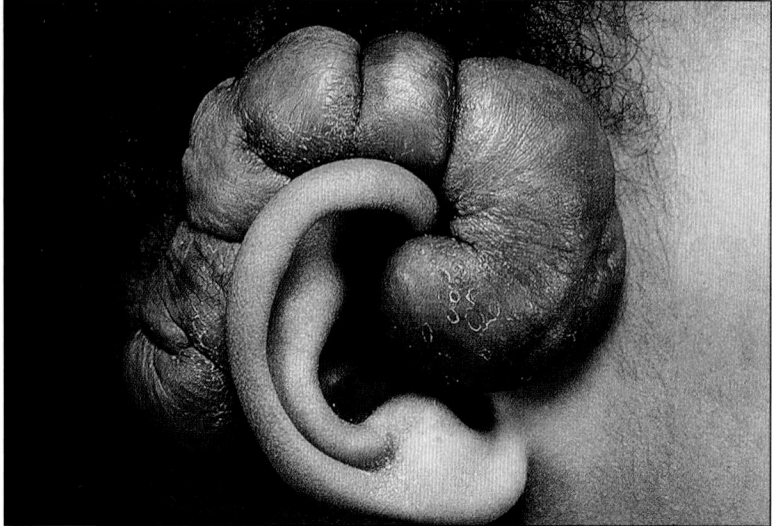

Fig. 35.53
Keloid: lesions commonly follow trauma and are a frequent complication of piercing. By courtesy of the Institute of Dermatology, London, UK.

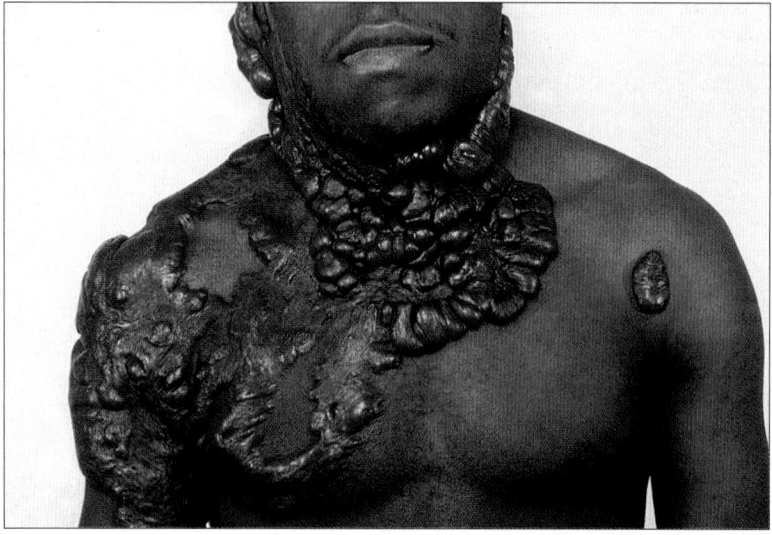

Fig. 35.54
Keloid: extensive keloid formation can be very disfiguring. By courtesy of the Institute of Dermatology, London, UK.

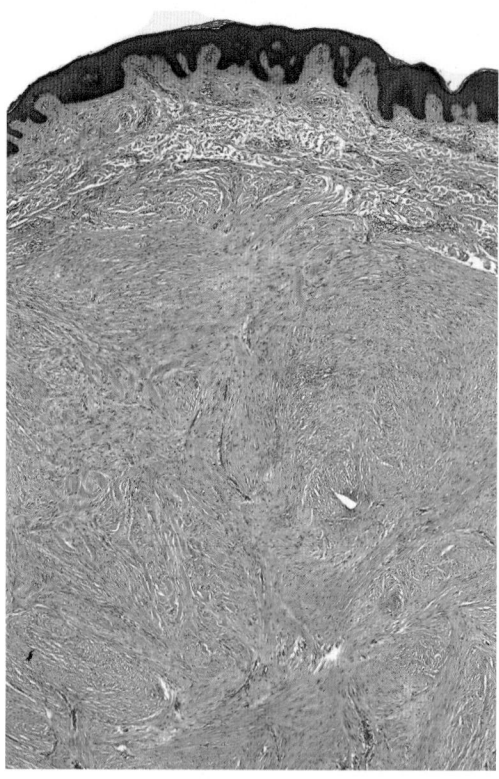

Fig. 35.55
Keloid: this lesion is distinguished from a hypertrophic scar by the presence of broad bundles of eosinophilic, hyalinized collagen.

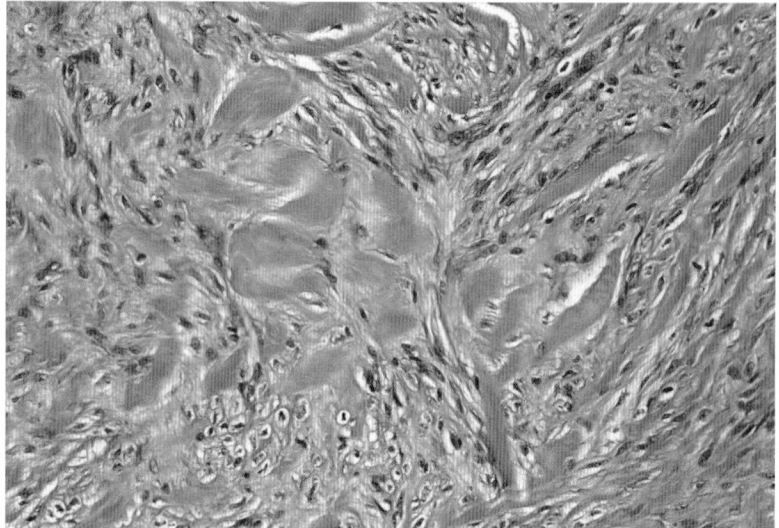

Fig. 35.56
Keloid: high-power view: note the swollen hyalinized collagen bundles admixed with bland spindled cells.

tension play an important role. Collagen synthesis is increased in keloids and the quality of the collagen produced is also different from that in normal skin. Apoptosis is reduced in fibroblasts in keloids.[13] There is an increased production of collagen I and III as demonstrated by an increase in levels of mRNA.[14] Transforming growth factor beta (TGF-β) seems to play an important role in wound healing and its increased production has been linked to the pathogenesis of keloids by activating the synthesis of collagen by fibroblasts.[15,16] The Wnt/β-catenin pathway associated with fibrosis and normal wound healing is strongly up-regulated and epigenetic changes affecting multiple profibrotic pathways are noted.[17–19]

The interaction between keratinocytes and fibroblasts appears to play an important role in the formation of keloids.[20] It has been demonstrated that when keloid fibroblasts are co-cultured with keloid keratinocytes there is increased production of soluble and insoluble collagen and procollagen III mRNA up-regulation.[21]

The histologic appearances are typified by a nodular fibroblastic proliferation and the presence of hypocellular, 'glassy', eosinophilic, thick hyalinized collagen fibers in the dermis (*Figs 35.55* and *35.56*). Early lesions may show a slight vascularity and foci of myxoid ground substance. Normal mitoses may occasionally be seen.

Nodular fasciitis

Clinical features

Nodular fasciitis is uncommon and represents a florid proliferative reactive process of unknown etiology.[1–8] It is most often seen in young or middle-aged adults of either sex, particularly on the limbs (especially the forearms) or trunk. Cases in children including newborns are rare and tend to favor the head and neck area (including the external auditory canal and oral cavity).[8–12] The lesion presents as a rapidly growing, subcutaneous nodule rarely exceeding 4–5 cm in diameter, and is typically painful or tender. Purely intramuscular lesions may rarely occur. The tumor develops with such speed that most patients present within 3 months of first becoming aware of a mass. Local recurrence may be a feature, but is sufficiently infrequent that its occurrence should raise the possibility of misdiagnosis. Recurrence seems to be more common in lesions of the head and neck mainly in

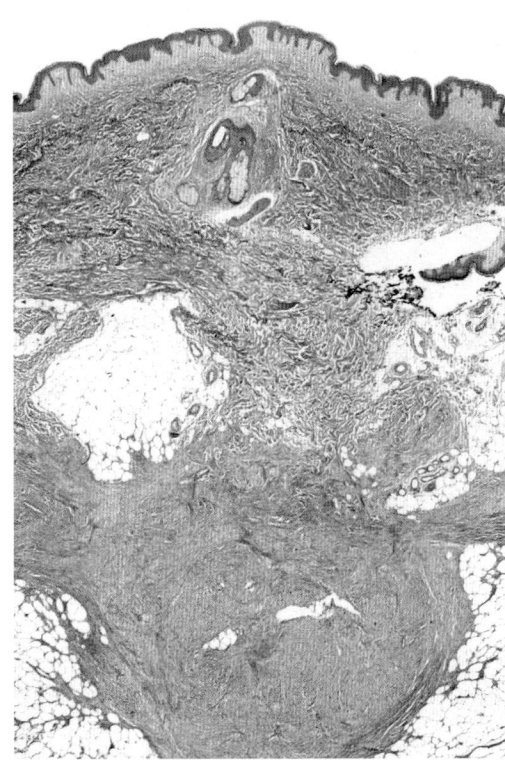

Fig. 35.57
Nodular fasciitis: low-power view showing a well-circumscribed example.

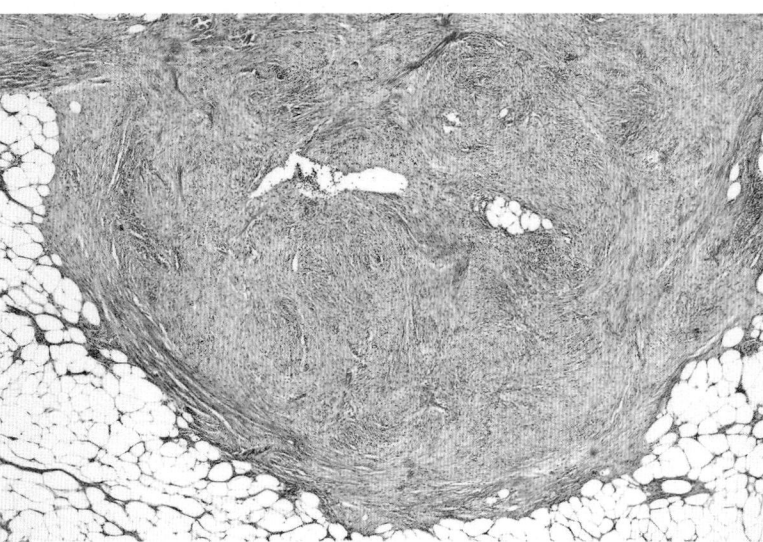

Fig. 35.58
Nodular fasciitis: this view highlights the circumscription.

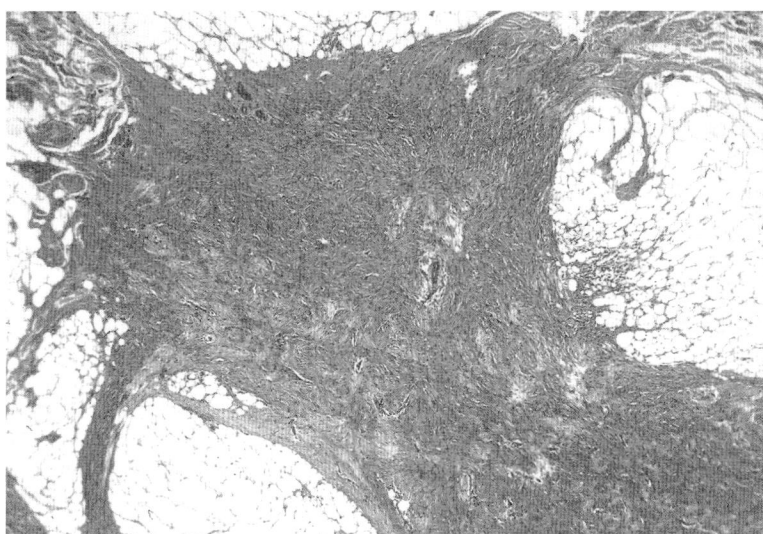

Fig. 35.59
Nodular fasciitis: in this lesion, there is a much more irregular border.

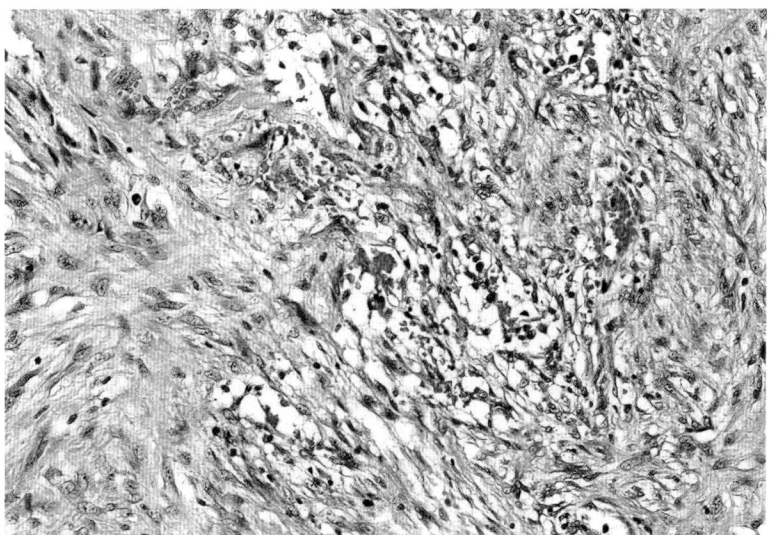

Fig. 35.60
Nodular fasciitis: the stroma is characteristically myxoid, which results in this feathery appearance.

children and in lesions presenting in the auricle.[13] Spontaneous regression may occur.[14] Intraneural and intra-articular lesions are very rare.[15–17] A case of nodular fasciitis developing at the margin of a second stage Mohs excision of a dermatofibrosarcoma protuberans has been described.[18] A case associated with etanercept therapy for psoriasis is probably coincidental.[19]

An exceptional case of nodular fasciitis with malignant behavior including multiple recurrences and metastatic spread and associated with PPP6R3-USP6 amplification has been described.[20]

Pathogenesis and histologic features

Initial studies of nodular fasciitis showed evidence of clonality, suggesting that the lesion is neoplastic.[21,22] Identification of an *MYH9-USP6* gene fusion has firmly established its neoplastic nature, and the tumor has been regarded as an example of transient neoplasm.[23–25] That is, the tumor has self-limiting growth followed by regression. Several additional novel fusion partners have been identified that use the promoters of genes other than *MYH9* to drive *USP6* overexpression.[24]

Nodular fasciitis is typified by a relatively well-circumscribed but unencapsulated mass composed of plump spindled cells set in a loose myxoid and collagenous stroma with a typically feathery, microcystic appearance (*Figs 35.57–35.60*). Numerous thin-walled blood vessels, often lined by rather prominent endothelial cells, ramify through the lesion, usually in a radial arrangement. Foci of hemorrhage and a sparse chronic inflammatory infiltrate composed largely of lymphocytes are usually present, and occasional cases contain foamy histiocytes and multinucleate osteoclast-type giant cells. The plump spindled cells (*Figs 35.61–35.63*) are mitotically active, but the mitoses are never atypical. The degree of cellularity and relative amounts of collagenous tissue and loose edematous stroma vary between lesions, probably reflecting the duration of the process. Extension into skeletal muscle is rare and mainly seen in lesions of the head and neck.[11]

Immunohistochemistry shows diffuse and strong positivity for smooth muscle actin and usually also calponin, but desmin and h-caldesmon are usually negative, in keeping with myofibroblastic differentiation (*Fig. 35.64*).[26]

Ultrastructurally, the tumor cells have abundant rough endoplasmic reticulum and contain aggregates of filaments with dense bodies deep to the plasma membrane (*Fig. 35.65*).

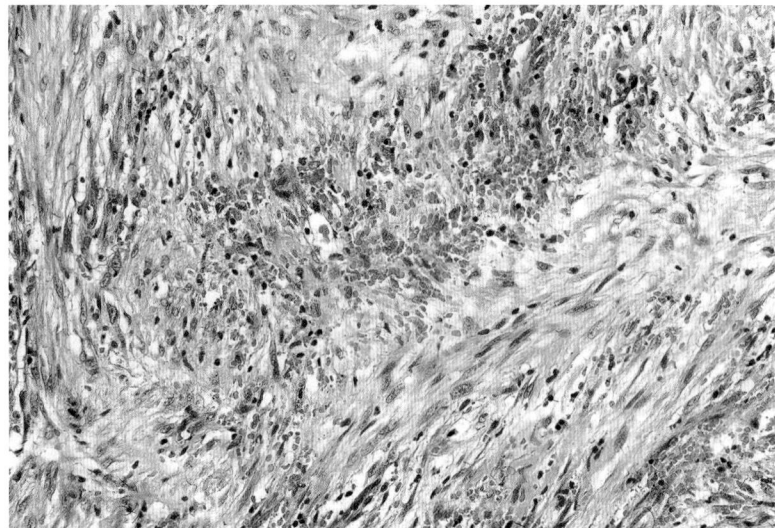

Fig. 35.61
Nodular fasciitis: foci of hemorrhage are commonly present.

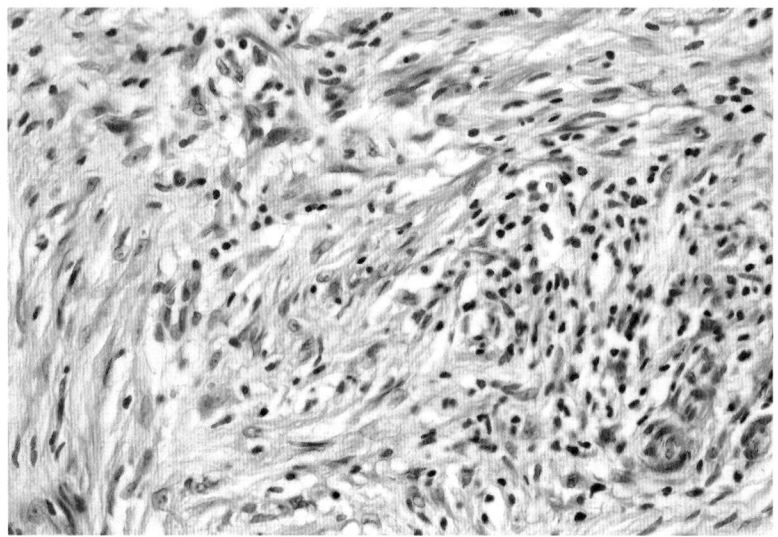

Fig. 35.62
Nodular fasciitis: small numbers of lymphocytes are usually evident.

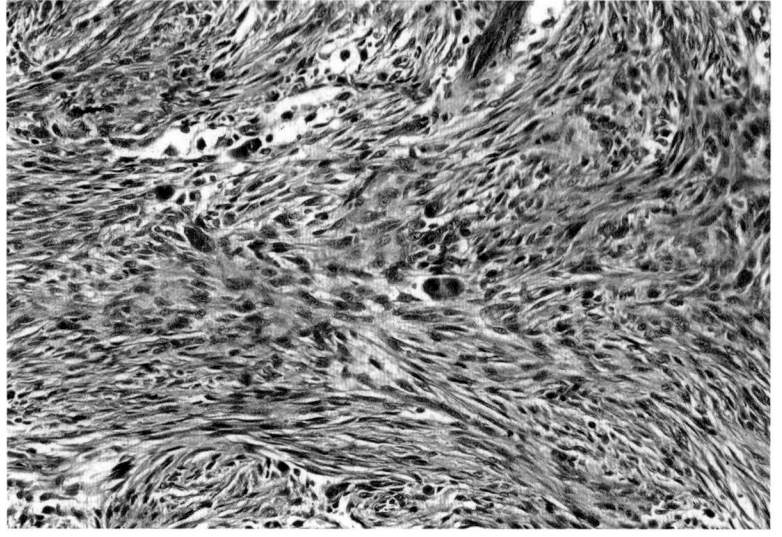

Fig. 35.63
Nodular fasciitis: in this example multiple giant cells are seen.

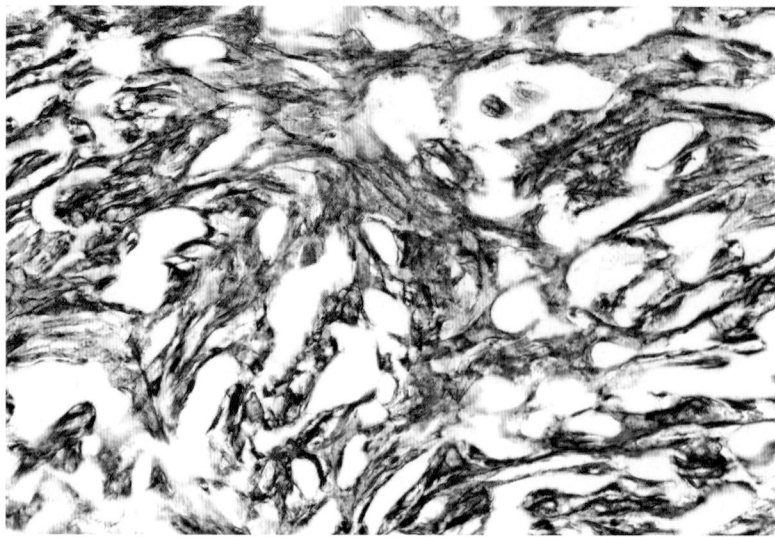

Fig. 35.64
Nodular fasciitis: the spindled cells show strong SMA expression.

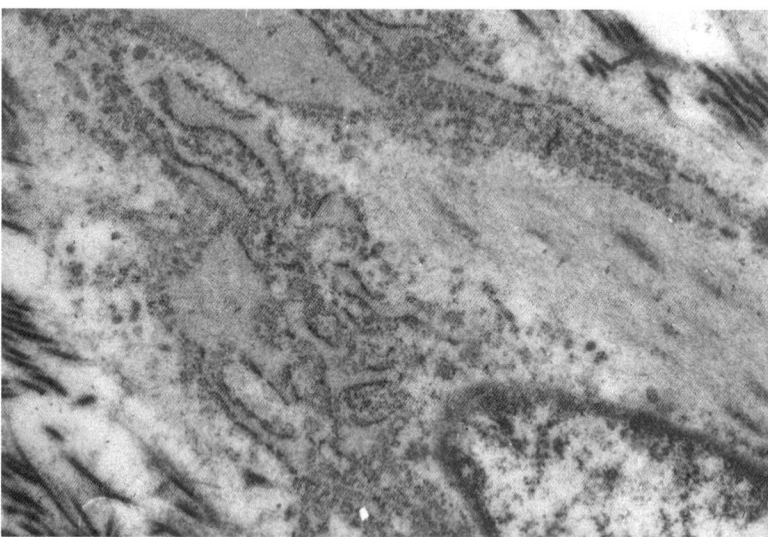

Fig. 35.65
Nodular fasciitis: ultrastructurally, the spindled cells show features of
myofibroblasts. Note the conspicuous rough endoplasmic reticulum and filaments
with dense bodies.

Variants

- Intradermal fasciitis refers to a very rare variant of fasciitis that
  primarily arises in the dermis with only focal extension into the
  subcutaneous tissue.[27–32] A polypoid architecture is exceptional.[33]
  Lesions on the ear may rarely extend into the underlying cartilage.[25]
  Histologic features are identical to those of the classic variant (*Figs
  35.66–35.68*) and tumors display the same molecular abnormality as
  that seen in the soft tissue counterparts.[24,25,32]
- Fasciitis ossificans describes the small proportion of cases of nodular
  fasciitis that show metaplastic formation of osteoid, mature bone or
  even cartilage.[5,34] A zoning pattern of maturation, as seen in myositis
  ossificans, is usually absent. In some cases, osteoid formation is only
  focal and calcification may be absent. Fibro-osseous pseudotumor of the
  digits is described below.
- Periosteal fasciitis arises from the periosteum and most often presents
  on the head of children (usually under the age of 2 years and with
  predilection for males). It is then known as cranial fasciitis when there
  is significant erosion of bone.[35,36] While histologically related to nodular
  fasciitis, it is not clear that this entity harbors the same fusion gene in
  the authors' experience.
- Proliferative fasciitis is described below.

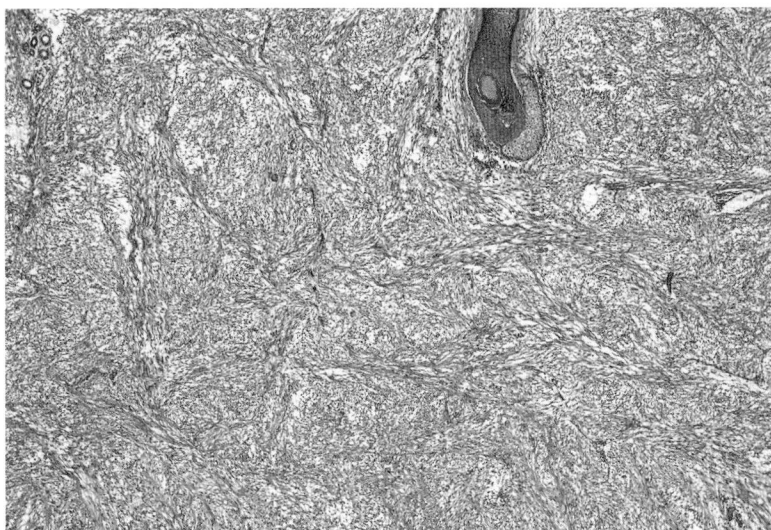

Fig. 35.66
Dermal fasciitis: low-power view showing a myxoid dermal spindled cell proliferation.

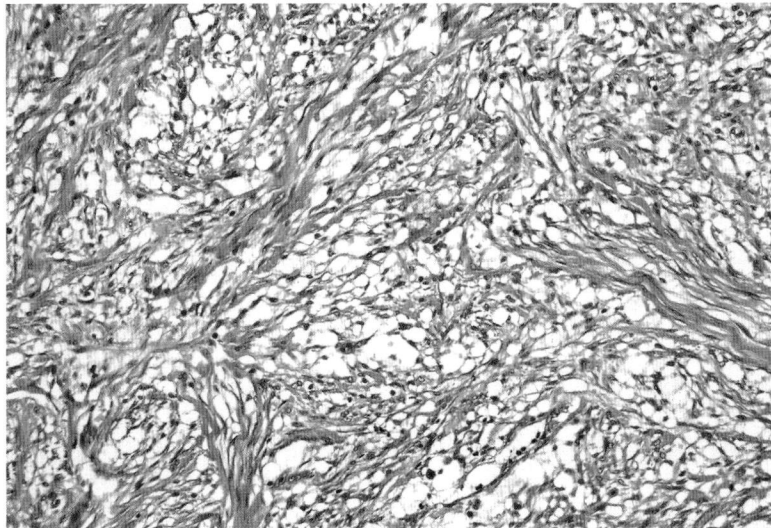

Fig. 35.67
Dermal fasciitis: the spindled cells have uniform vesicular nuclei with small nucleoli.

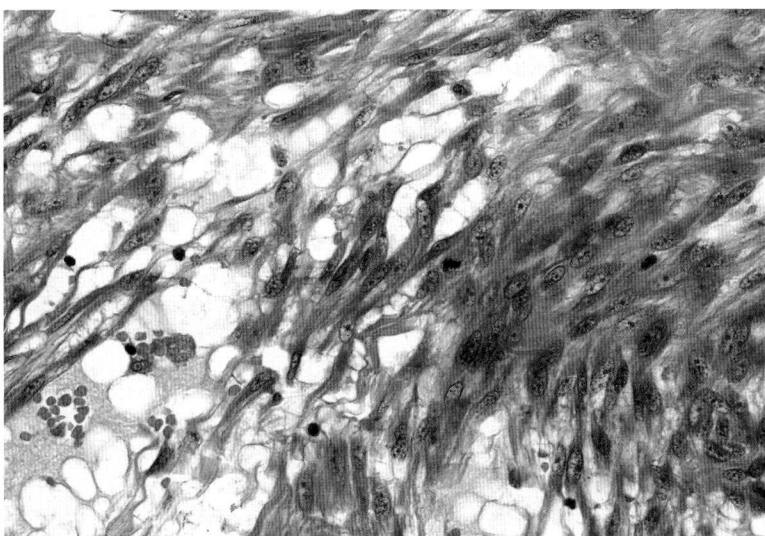

Fig. 35.68
Dermal fasciitis: normal mitoses are often present.

- Intravascular fasciitis is a very rare lesion seen most often in young adults. Intraoral cases have been described.[37] Although histologically very similar to typical nodular fasciitis, it involves the full thickness and lumen of a peripheral blood vessel (usually a vein), and therefore simulates vascular invasion.[7,37–39] To avoid a diagnosis of malignancy, careful attention should be paid to the bland histologic features.

Ultrastructural studies show cells with features of fibroblasts and myofibroblasts.

Differential diagnosis

Features that should raise the possibility of malignancy in diagnostically difficult lesions include abnormal mitotic figures, nuclear hyperchromasia or pleomorphism and necrosis. The dermal variant of nodular fasciitis can be distinguished from benign fibrous histiocytoma because the latter is more polymorphic and actin tends to be only focally positive or negative.

Proliferative fasciitis and proliferative myositis

Clinical features

Proliferative fasciitis tends to occur in older adults and quite often affects the subcutaneous tissue of lower limbs, but is otherwise clinically similar to typical nodular fasciitis.[1–3] Regression, sometimes rapid, may occur.[4] Intradermal lesions are exceptional.[5,6] Intravascular lesions have been reported.[7] Proliferative myositis is closely allied to proliferative fasciitis. It is a deep intramuscular lesion, which represents the deep counterpart of proliferative fasciitis; it is therefore rarely encountered in dermatology.[2,8,9] It usually occurs in the fifth and sixth decades, and most often affects the trunk or proximal upper limbs. Presentation in children is rare.[2,10] Both are regarded as a reactive conditions of rapid onset and are entirely benign. Most tumors are only a few centimeters in diameter. Simple excision is curative.[11]

Pathogenesis and histologic features

Cytogenetic studies have been reported in three cases of proliferative myositis. In two of them the presence of trisomy 2 was demonstrated and, in one, a t(6;14)(q23;q32) was identified.[12,13] It is not clear that proliferative fasciitis or myositis harbor the *MYH9-USP6* fusion characteristic of nodular fasciitis. Histologically, proliferative fasciitis is characterized by the presence of numerous basophilic ganglion-like giant cells, which are often multinucleated and may be mitotically active (*Figs 35.69* and *35.70*). Distinction from pleomorphic rhabdomyoblasts is afforded by the cytoplasmic basophilia, short history, and usually superficial nature of proliferative fasciitis.

Histologically, proliferative myositis is characterized by proliferating spindle cells and large basophilic ganglion-like cells distributed within the

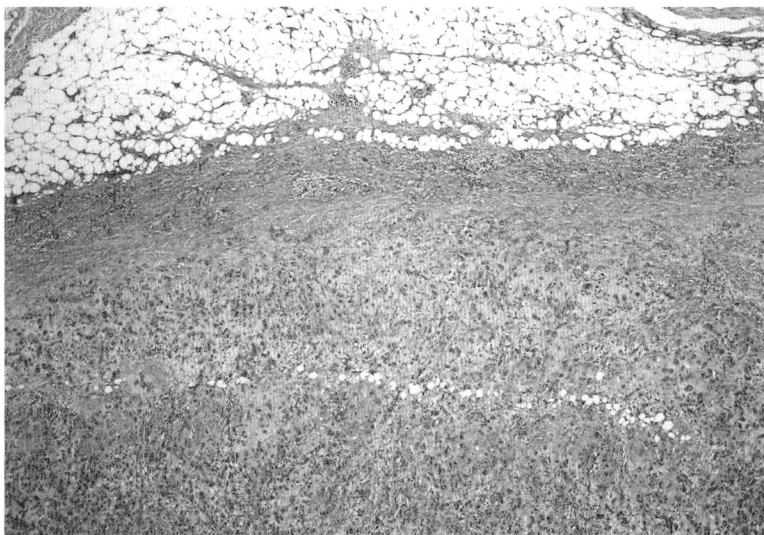

Fig. 35.69
Proliferative fasciitis: the fascia is thickened, edematous, and infiltrated by large numbers of ganglion-like giant cells.

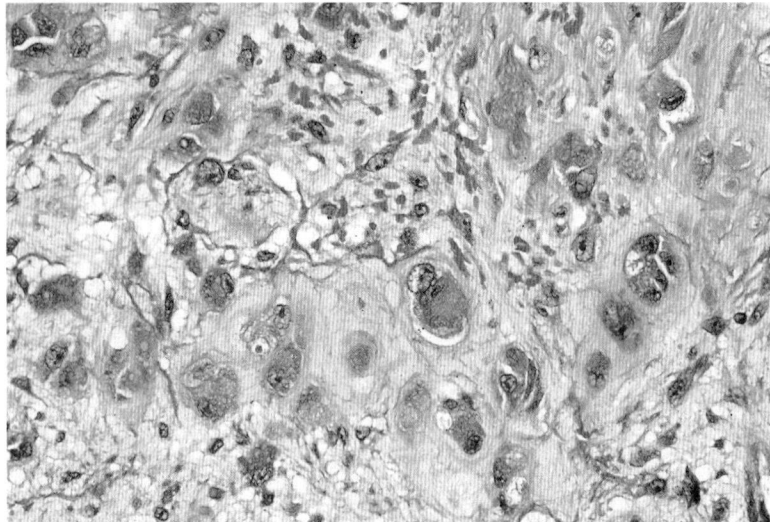

Fig. 35.70
Proliferative fasciitis: the ganglion-like cells have abundant eosinophilic cytoplasm and large vesicular nuclei containing prominent nucleoli.

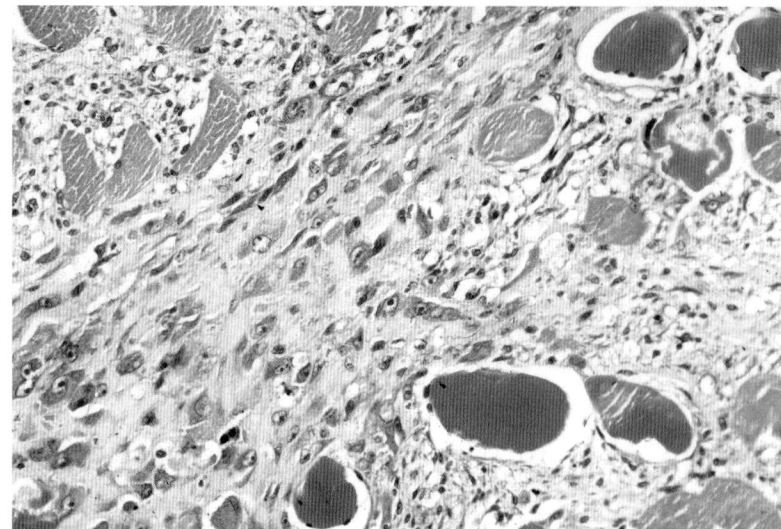

Fig. 35.72
Proliferative myositis: the giant cells have abundant cytoplasm and contain large vesicular nuclei with prominent intensely eosinophilic nucleoli.

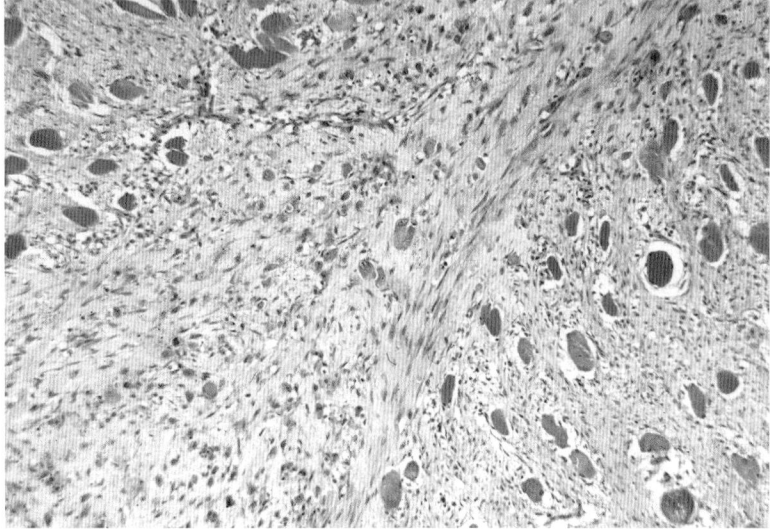

Fig. 35.71
Proliferative myositis: the muscle fibers are separated by a cellular infiltrate, giving a 'checkerboard' appearance.

fibrous tissue septa surrounding and dividing striated muscle fibers. These fibers are displaced rather than destroyed by the tumor and lesional cells alternating with skeletal muscle fibers produce a typical 'checkerboard' pattern (*Figs 35.71* and *35.72*). Normal mitotic figures are commonly found. Bone and cartilage may occasionally be seen.[14] Lesions in children tend to be more circumscribed, are more cellular and may show necrosis.[2]

The spindle-shaped proliferating cells are positive for actins (SMA and MSA) but negative for desmin, whereas the ganglion-like cells may be negative for actins and are negative for neural and epithelial markers.

Electron microscopy studies indicate that these cells have features of fibroblasts.[15,16] The flow cytometry profile of these lesions is diploid.[17]

Differential diagnosis

Distinction from a sarcoma may be difficult in small lesions, especially if close clinicopathological correlation is lacking. Most sarcomas have a larger size and although a 'checkerboard' appearance may be present in sarcomas or metastatic carcinomas, this is usually only focal and there is more tendency towards destruction of the surrounding muscle. A desmoid tumor lacks ganglion-like cells and usually replaces the muscle completely.

Fibro-osseous pseudotumor of the digits

Clinical features

This is a reactive myofibroblastic proliferation with bone formation, which occurs almost exclusively on the digits (*Fig. 35.73*).[1–4] It presents predominantly in young to middle-aged adults, with predilection for females. Cases in adolescents are rare. The fingers, particularly the proximal phalanx of the index finger are by far much more commonly affected than the toes. A single identical lesion occurred on the forehead.[3] The lesion grows rapidly (within a period between 2 to 6 weeks) and it is not attached to bone.[4] There is no tendency for local recurrence.

Pathogenesis and histologic features

The condition is more common in individuals exposed to repetitive manual labor.[4] It likely represents a superficial counterpart of myositis ossificans.

The tumor is ill-defined and similar to nodular fasciitis, except for the fact that there is formation of osteoid and mature bone (*Figs 35.74–35.76*). Edematous stroma, vascular proliferation and bundles of spindle-shaped myofibroblast-like cells are seen intermixed with osteoid and mature bone. Mitotic figures are present and their number depends on the age of the lesion. Proliferating cells are positive for smooth muscle actin and calponin.

Ischemic fasciitis

Clinical features

Ischemic fasciitis (also known as atypical decubital fibroplasia) is a relatively rare pseudosarcomatous fibroblastic/myofibroblastic condition that occurs over bony prominences.[1–3] The great majority of patients are elderly (between the sixth and ninth decades of life) and immobilized. However, cases in ambulatory and even in young patients have been described.[4–7] Lesions consist of an asymptomatic, subcutaneous, ill-defined mass only occasionally associated with ulceration. The majority of lesions arise in the deep subcutaneous tissue but involvement of the dermis and deeper soft tissues including skeletal muscle and tendons may also be seen.[4] Exclusive involvement of skeletal muscle is very rare.[4] Most tumors are less than 4 cm in diameter but larger lesions also occur. The usual sites are the shoulders, thighs, buttocks, sacral area and chest wall. Local excision is generally curative and recurrences are only seen in patients where the predisposing factor persists. A case of ischemic fasciitis associated with bizarre parosteal osteochondromatous proliferation has been documented.[8]

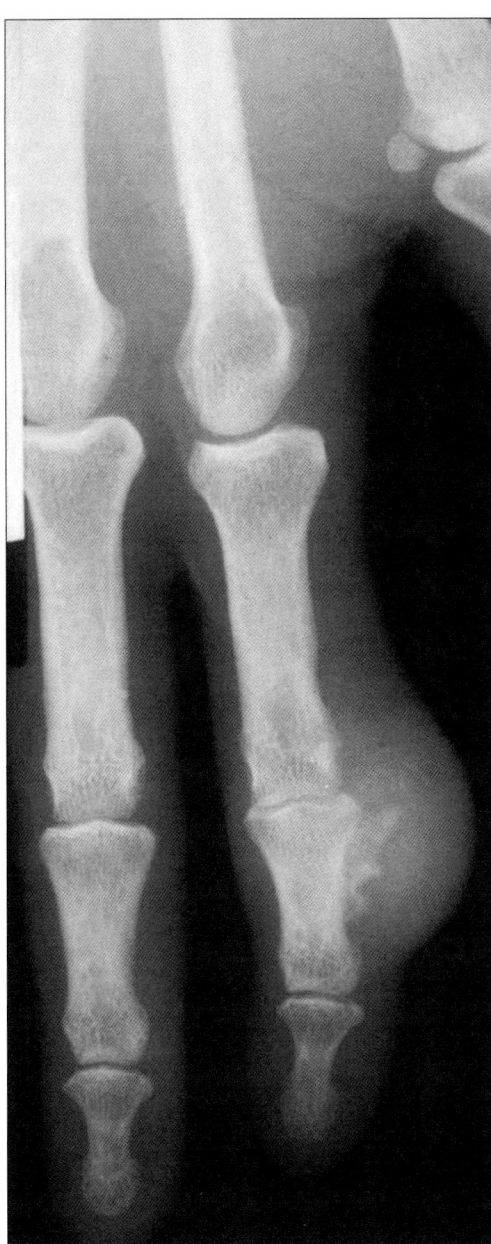

Fig. 35.73
Fibro-osseous
pseudotumor of the
digits: this lesion
presented as a rapidly
growing nodule. Note the
prominent calcification. By
courtesy of the Institute
of Dermatology, London,
UK.

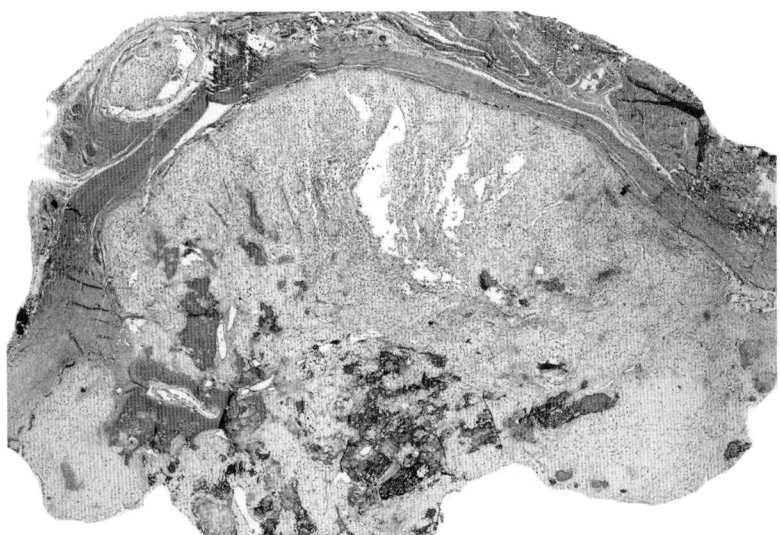

Fig. 35.74
Fibro-osseous pseudotumor of the digits: scanning view showing osteoid, foci of
calcification and a myxoid spindle cell tumor.

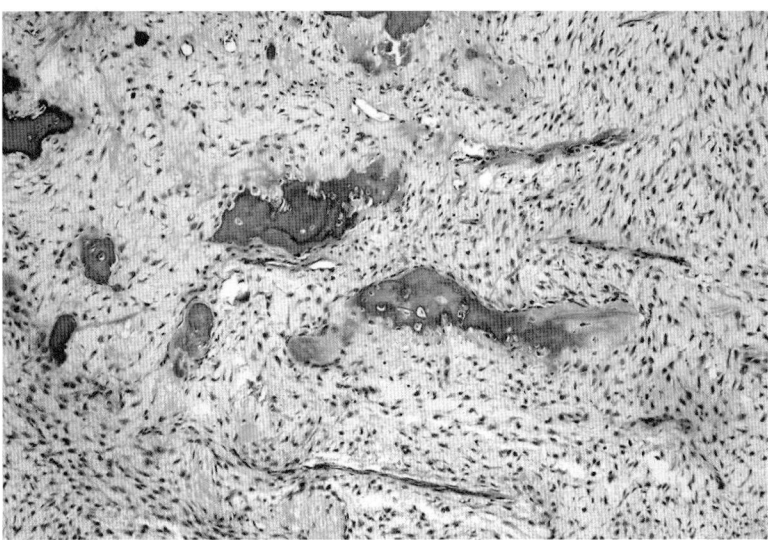

Fig. 35.75
Fibro-osseous pseudotumor of the digits: medium-power view showing calcified
osteoid and spindled cells within a myxoid matrix.

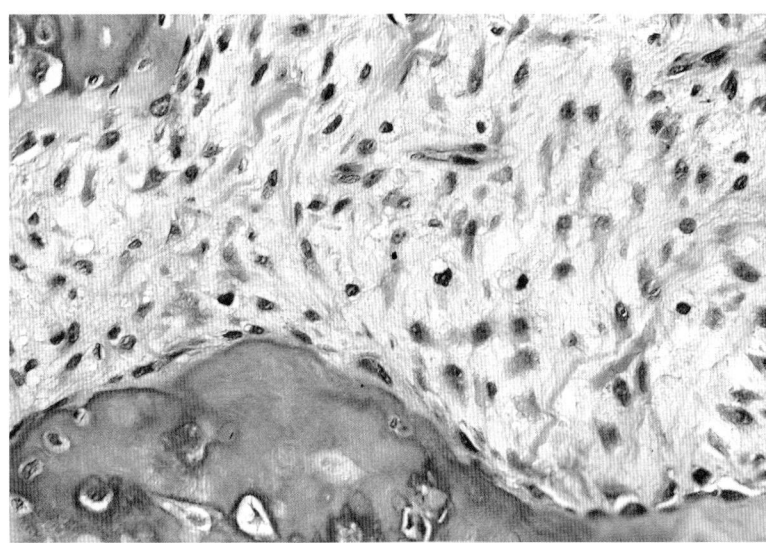

Fig. 35.76
Fibro-osseous pseudotumor of the digits: high-power view of tumor
myofibroblasts.

Pathogenesis and histologic features

The proliferation is thought to be due to ischemia induced by pressure
resulting from prolonged immobilization. However, a recent study has not
consistently found immobility or debilitation.[4] Some cases are triggered by
trauma.[4]

Histologically, lesions are multilobular and characterized by replacement
of the subcutaneous tissue by areas of fibrinoid necrosis and granulation
tissue (*Figs 35.77* and *35.78*). Myxoid change, hemorrhage and edema are
usually prominent. In the areas of necrosis there is marked fibrinoid change
and ghosts of necrotic adipocytes are seen. At the periphery there is vascular proliferation accompanied by variable numbers of spindle-shaped and
more round cells with irregular hyperchromatic nuclei and a single prominent basophilic nucleolus. Ganglion-like cells similar to those present in
proliferative fasciitis are also found and in these the nuclei contain smudged
chromatin (*Fig. 35.79*). Mitotic figures may be found but atypical forms are
generally not seen. Thrombosis of blood vessels is also a feature.

Immunohistochemistry shows that the cells in the proliferation are variably positive for smooth muscle actin (SMA), calponin and desmin.[4] In rare
cases positivity for MDM2, CDK4 and p16 can be seen.[5]

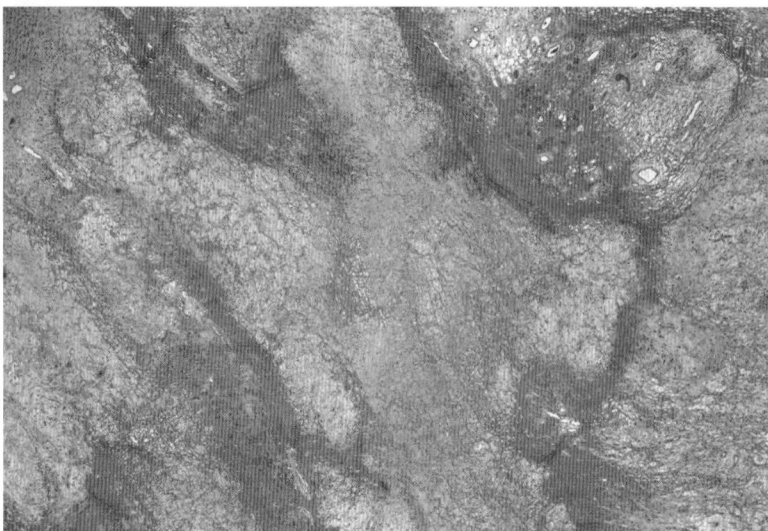

Fig. 35.77
Ischemic fasciitis: scanning view showing massive fibrin deposition with adjacent granulation tissue.

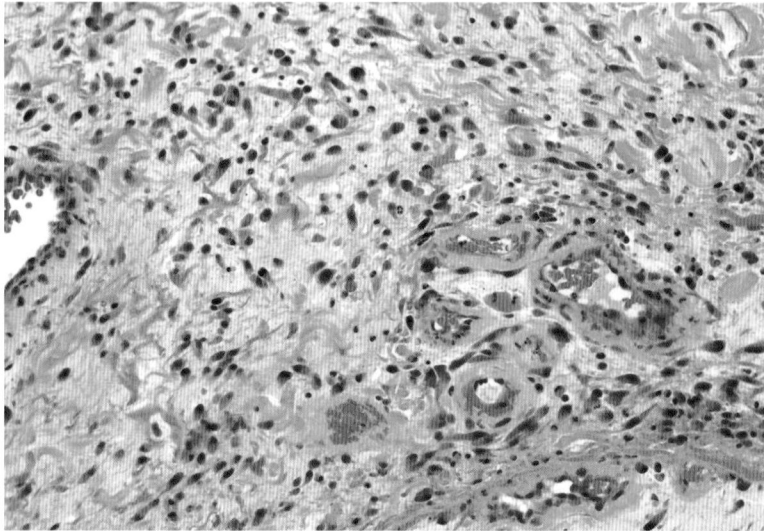

Fig. 35.78
Ischemic fasciitis: this field shows an atypical cellular population.

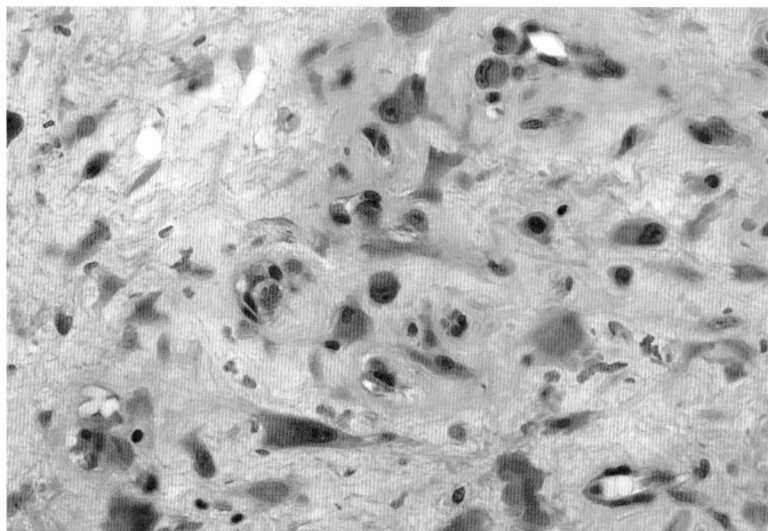

Fig. 35.79
Ischemic fasciitis: there are atypical spindled cells and histiocyte-like cells, some with a ganglion-like appearance.

Differential diagnosis

As already discussed, this lesion closely resembles proliferative fasciitis and many regard it as a variant of nodular fasciitis. However, the *MYH9-USP6* fusion characteristic of nodular fasciitis has not been documented in this condition. Distinction between ischemic fasciitis and a sarcoma is based on the relatively low mitotic count, the absence of atypical mitotic figures, and the low cellularity in the former lesion.

Elastofibroma

Clinical features

Elastofibroma is an uncommon, deep-seated pseudotumor that is thought to represent a degenerative and reactive change in elastic fibrous tissue.[1–5] It almost always arises in the infrascapular region, most often in the elderly, and is usually unilateral. There is only one report of a lesion developing in early life.[6] Rare cases have been reported in the hip, hand, olecranon, upper arm, eye and oral cavity.[7–9] Elastofibromatous changes are present in a number of samples obtained from patients operated for spinal canal compression.[10] Infrequently, lesions are bilateral and multiple;[11–13] Often, the second lesion is subclinical and can only be detected radiologically.[14] A visceral location is very rare but includes the trachea and gastrointestinal tract.[15] Females are predominantly affected and, although tumor size varies, fixation to the periosteum of the underlying ribs is invariable. Familial presentation has been described in up to 30% of cases.[5,16] Tumors are usually asymptomatic and may reach a large size. Simple excision is the treatment of choice but asymptomatic lesions do not necessarily need to be removed.[17,18] Recurrence is extremely uncommon.

Pathogenesis and histologic features

It is a commonly held belief that elastofibroma arises as a consequence of chronic frictional trauma between the scapula and underlying connective tissues, but a relationship with heavy manual labor is unsubstantiated. The theory that the process is a result of degeneration is given support by the finding of changes similar to those of elastofibroma in tissue taken in autopsies of elderly patients with no discernible mass.[19,20]

Cytogenetic studies have shown clonal and nonclonal structural changes, particularly aberrations of the short arm of chromosome 1.[21–24]

Elastofibroma is typically an ill-defined unencapsulated mass merging with adjacent connective tissue and composed of fairly acellular collagenous and adipose tissue containing numerous elastic fibers (*Figs 35.80* and *35.81*). These fibers, ideally demonstrated by an appropriate histochemical

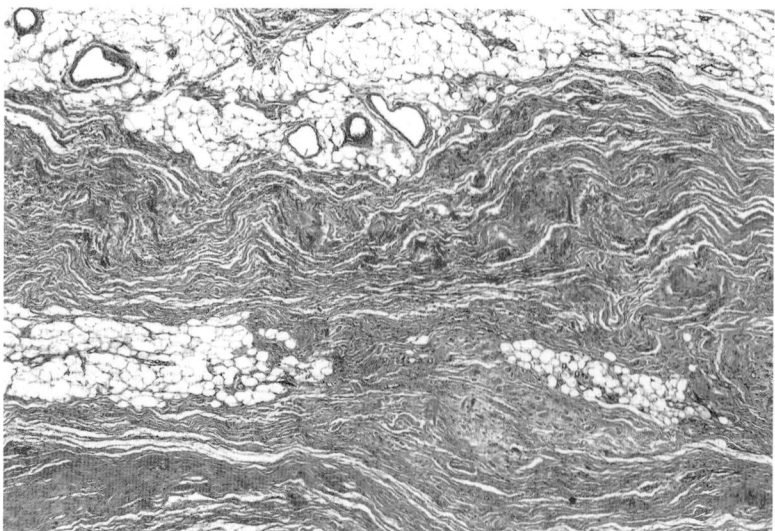

Fig. 35.80
Elastofibroma: there is an admixture of collagen bundles and thickened, irregular, eosinophilic elastic fibers.

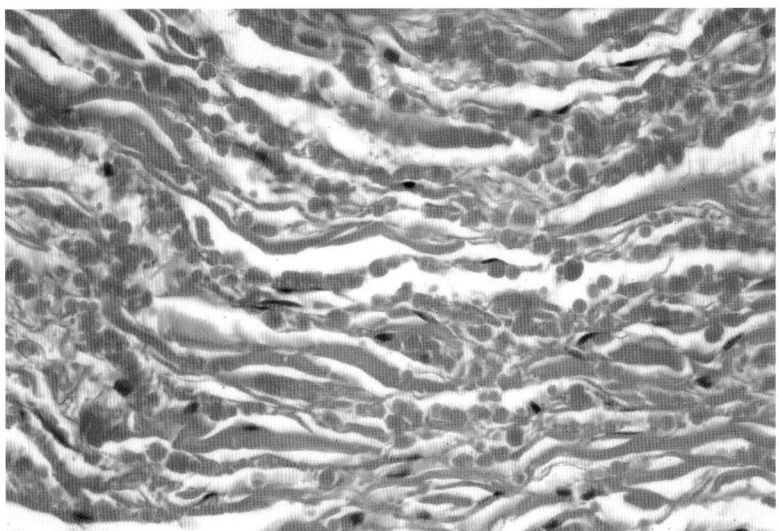

Fig. 35.81
Elastofibroma: the elastic fibers are fragmented and appear beaded.

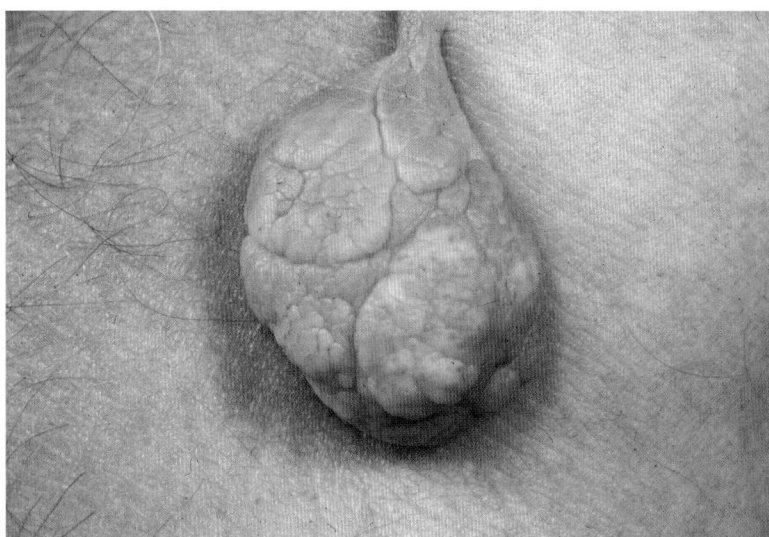

Fig. 35.83
Acrochordon: also known as a skin tag or fibroepithelial polyp, this soft polyp is exceedingly common. By courtesy of the Institute of Dermatology, London, UK.

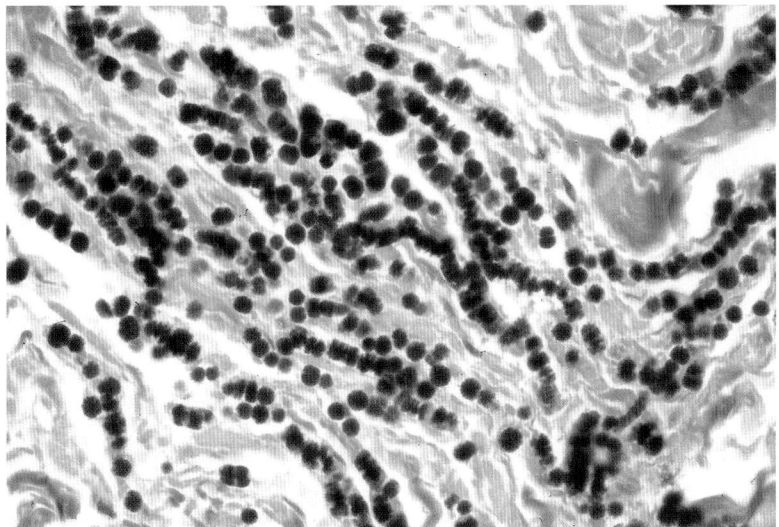

Fig. 35.82
Elastofibroma: the serrated edge so characteristic of this condition is seen in this elastic–van Gieson stained section.

stain, tend to be coarse, thick or globular, and are sometimes distributed as irregular masses (*Fig. 35.82*). It has been shown that the fibers represent true elastin and not elastotic collagen.[25,26] Amyloid deposition has been reported in one case.[27] The cells in the background tend to be positive for CD34 but negative for myofibroblastic markers.[28]

Differential diagnosis

Identification of the distinctive changes in the elastic fibers allows for easy recognition of the condition. Nuchal fibroma is distinguished from elastofibroma by the absence of altered elastic fibers and the presence of fairly thick collagen bundles in the former condition.

Fibroepithelial polyp (including pleomorphic fibroma)

Clinical features

Fibroepithelial polyps (acrochordon, skin tag, soft fibroma) are very common lesions that typically present in adults, especially obese females, with a predilection for the neck, axillae and groin.[1,2] Perianal lesions are also frequently encountered. Rare lesions have been documented in the umbilicus.[3]

These polyps are often multiple and can be associated with pregnancy. Contrary to what was proposed in the past, they do not appear to be a marker for colonic polyps.[4,5] An association with diabetes mellitus has been suggested.[6,7] Lesions are usually less than 1 cm in diameter and can be papular, filiform or pedunculated (*Fig. 35.83*). Rarely, tumors such as squamous cell carcinoma, keratoacanthoma and basal cell carcinoma may develop within a fibroepithelial polyp.[8–11] Lymphedematous fibroepithelial polyps have been documented in the glans penis and prepuce as a result of chronic condom and catheter use.[12] It has been suggested that fibroepithelial polyps should not be submitted for histologic examination since malignant tumors only very exceptionally show similar clinical features.[13] This is, however, controversial and, in our view, all should be carefully evaluated. Melanoma, for example, may very rarely grossly mimic a fibroepithelial polyp. Fibroepithelial polyps in children are very rare and their occurrence has been reported as a presenting sign of the nevoid basal cell carcinoma syndrome.[14] Lesions identical to fibroepithelial polyps have been described in the tongue of immunosuppressed patients and may also occur in the skin.[15,16] In these patients, the polypoid lesions show features of basal cell carcinoma. Fibroepithelial polyps can be associated with the rare Birt-Hogg-Dubé syndrome.

Histologic features

Fibroepithelial polyps show a normal or hyperplastic epidermis surrounding a core of fibrovascular tissue with loose or dense collagen fibers (*Figs 35.84 and 35.85*). Fat cells can be present and, if abundant, the lesion shows overlap with nevus lipomatosus superficialis. Focal pagetoid dyskeratosis may be an incidental finding in keratinocytes.[17]

Pleomorphic fibroma refers to a small proportion of cases of acrochordons that show cells with bizarre hyperchromatic and pleomorphic nuclei (*Figs 35.86 and 35.87*).[18] Multinucleation is also a feature, but mitotic figures are very few and never atypical. These cells are actin positive and the changes are likely to be the result of degeneration, as seen in other tumors such as pleomorphic lipoma and ancient schwannoma. Similar lesions have been described under the name cutaneous pseudosarcomatous polyp.[19,20] Changes similar to pleomorphic fibroma may also be seen in 'regressed' or hyalinized examples of solitary myofibroma or dermatomyofibroma.

By immunohistochemistry, cells may be positive for CD34.[21]

Differential diagnosis

Pleomorphic fibroma can be distinguished from a dermal atypical lipomatous tumor by the absence of an adipocytic component including lipoblasts in the former. MDM2 immunohistochemistry and *MDM2* gene amplification is not seen in pleomorphic fibroma.[22] In a single case report however,

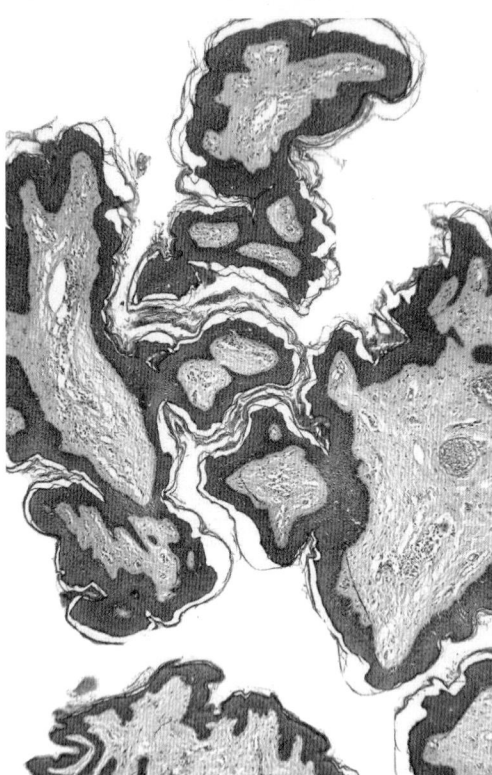

Fig. 35.84
Acrochordon: histologically, it consists of connective tissue covered by squamous epithelium.

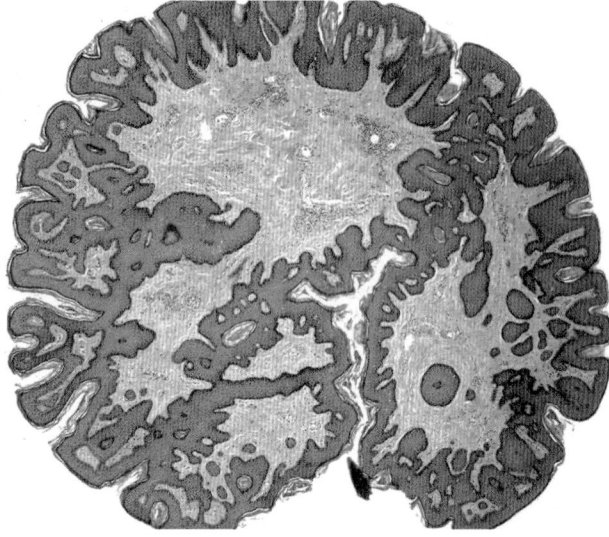

Fig. 35.85
Acrochordon: this unusually sectioned example shows the features to advantage.

MDM2 immunohistochemistry was positive in a pleomorphic fibroma but this was not associated with *MDM2* gene amplification.[23] Recently, uniform genetic loss of *RB1* (13q) has been documented in pleomorphic fibroma as well as recurrent losses in 10q, 16q, and 17p.[24] Loss of nuclear RB1 can also be demonstrated by immunohistochemistry.[24] This strongly suggests a genetic relationship to spindle cell and pleomorphic lipomas as well as cellular angiofibromas and mammary-type myofibroblastomas—all of which are known to harbor *RB1* loss.

Dermatomyofibroma

Clinical features

Dermatomyofibroma is a rare tumor that presents as a solitary, slowly growing, asymptomatic, skin-colored or hypopigmented plaque.[1–6] It usually presents on the upper trunk or neck of young adults, with a predilection for

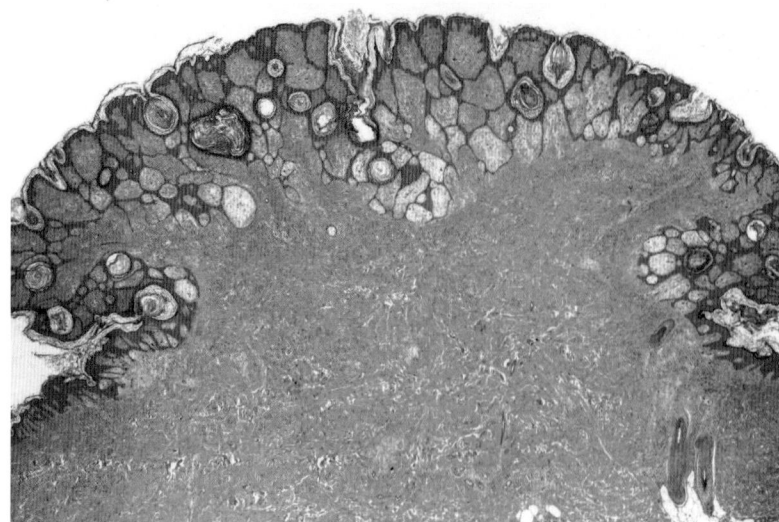

Fig. 35.86
Pleomorphic fibroma: this lesion is characterized by the presence of scattered mononuclear and multinucleated giant cells.

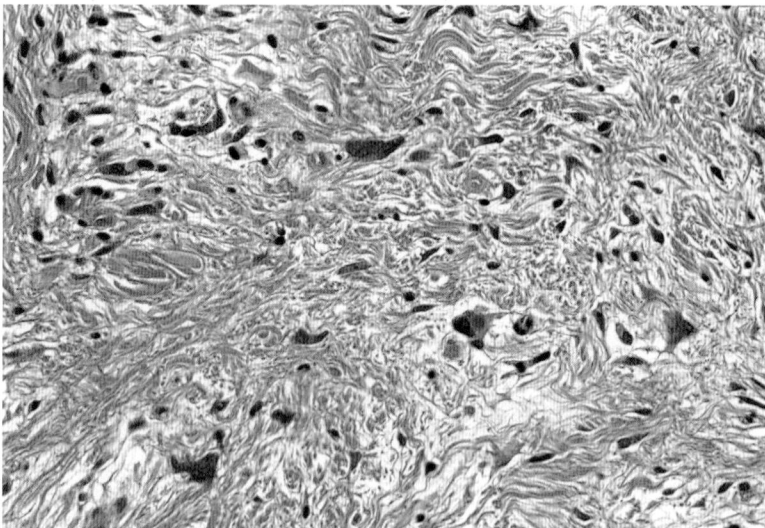

Fig. 35.87
Pleomorphic fibroma: note the fusiform and stellate cells with hyperchromatic irregular nuclei.

females. Most lesions are less than 4 cm in diameter. Tumors may resemble a plaque lesion of dermatofibrosarcoma protuberans or a keloid. An exceptional case presenting in a linear distribution, one with an annular configuration have been documented.[7,8] Rare cases occur in children and have predilection for the neck.[9–14] Multiple tumors are very rare.[15] Local recurrence is exceptional.

Histologic features

Histology is distinctive and shows a plaque-like proliferation of fascicles of bland spindled cells with pale eosinophilic cytoplasm and elongated vesicular nuclei with one or two nucleoli (*Figs 35.88–35.90*). These fascicles tend to be parallel to the epidermis. The papillary dermis is usually spared and there is entrapment, but no destruction of adnexal structures by the tumor. Focal extension into the subcutaneous tissue is sometimes seen and occurs mainly along the septa in a perpendicular fashion. Rare cases display prominent hemorrhage.[16] Myofibroblastic differentiation is suggested immunocytochemically by actin and calponin expression (*Fig. 35.91*). However, expression of actin and calponin is variable and may be focal or negative.[6] CD34 may be focally positive.[6] H-caldesmon and desmin are negative.

Electron microscopy shows cells with features of fibroblasts and myofibroblasts.[17]

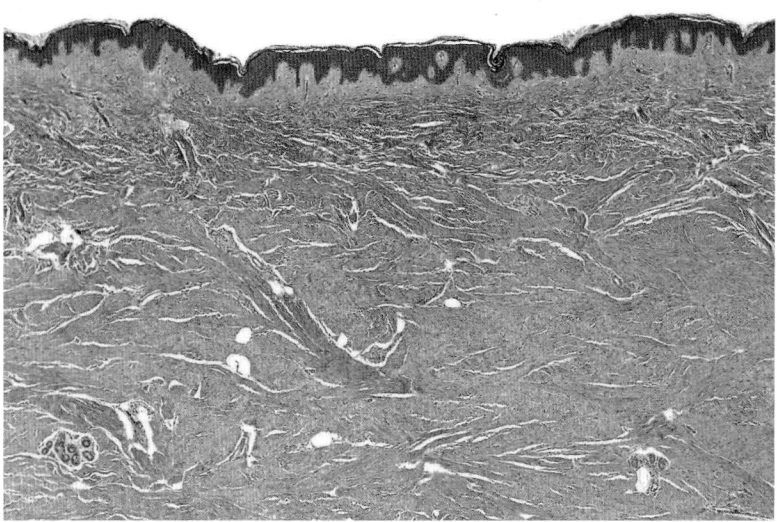

Fig. 35.88
Dermatomyofibroma: low-power view showing fascicles of spindled cells orientated parallel to the surface epithelium.

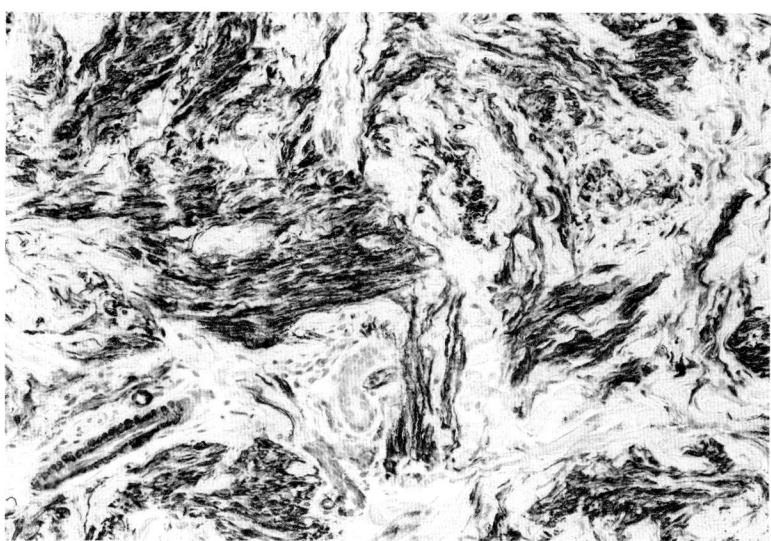

Fig. 35.91
Dermatomyofibroma: the tumor cells express smooth muscle actin.

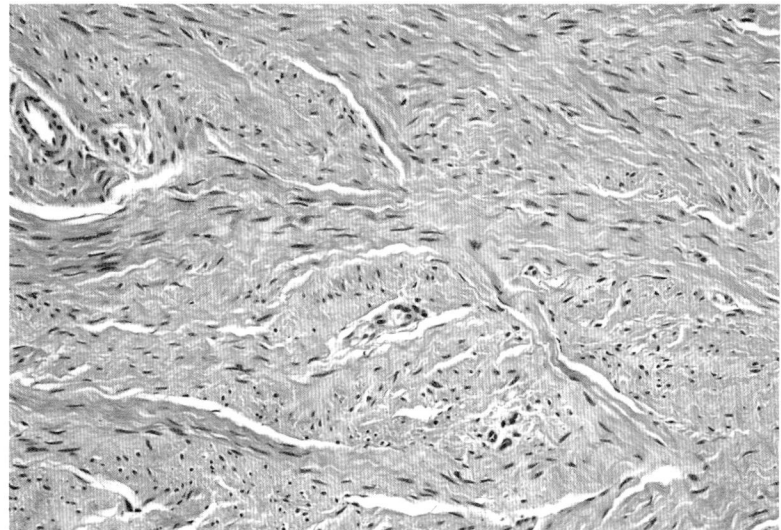

Fig. 35.89
Dermatomyofibroma: the fascicles grow between the dermal collagen bundles.

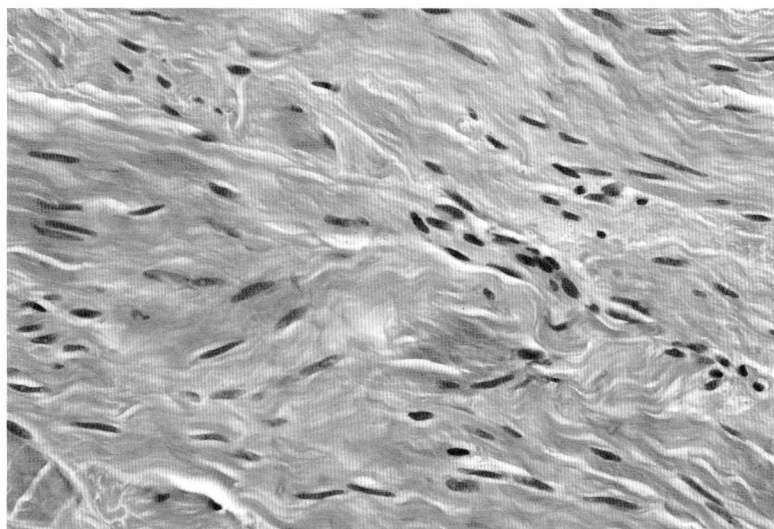

Fig. 35.90
Dermatomyofibroma: the tumor cells have eosinophilic cytoplasm and regular elongated nuclei.

Differential diagnosis

Dermatomyofibroma should be distinguished from plaque-stage dermatofibrosarcoma protuberans, in which the tumor cells are more basophilic and infiltrative. In addition, tumor cells in dermatofibrosarcoma protuberans are actin negative, and are usually diffusely positive for CD34. Dermatomyofibroma may also be confused with diffuse neurofibroma. The latter, however, is paler, lacks parallel orientation of tumor cells to the epidermis, and is S100 protein and CD34 positive. Rare hemorrhagic cases may be confused with nodular stage Kaposi sarcoma. However, in the latter condition, tumor cells are arranged in nodules, and are accompanied by numerous cleft-like spaces containing red blood cells. Inflammatory cells including plasma cells are always present, eosinophilic globules are prominent and all cases show nuclear reactivity with immunohistochemistry for human herpesvirus.[16]

Storiform collagenoma

Clinical features

Storiform collagenoma (also known as circumscribed storiform collagenoma and sclerotic fibroma) is a solitary skin-colored nodule, usually less than 1 cm in diameter.[1,2] It presents in adults of either sex and has a wide anatomical distribution. Simple excision is curative. Multiple lesions with identical histologic features are seen in Cowden disease (multiple hamartoma and neoplasia syndrome) and it has been suggested that they represent a marker for this condition.[3–6] In this setting, and also sporadically, such lesions have also been described in the oral cavity.[7–9] An exceptional case has been documented in the nail and a case associated with Rubinstein-Taybi syndrome in a young adolescent has been reported.[10,11]

Histologic features

Microscopically, storiform collagenoma is a well-circumscribed dermal nodule composed of hypocellular hyalinized collagen bundles separated by clefts and arranged in a storiform pattern (*Figs 35.92–94*). Rare spindle-shaped cells are occasionally seen. Occasional lesions display more cellularity and scattered pleomorphic cells as seen in pleomorphic fibroma; hence, a link has been suggested between both entities.[12,13] Tumor cells are positive for CD34 and CD99.[13] Giant cell collagenoma appears to be a variant of storiform collagenoma with scattered multinucleate giant cells, some of which have a bizarre appearance.[14,15]

On electron microscopy the lesional cells are seen to be separated from blood vessels by laminated concentric collagen resulting in a plywood-like pattern.[16]

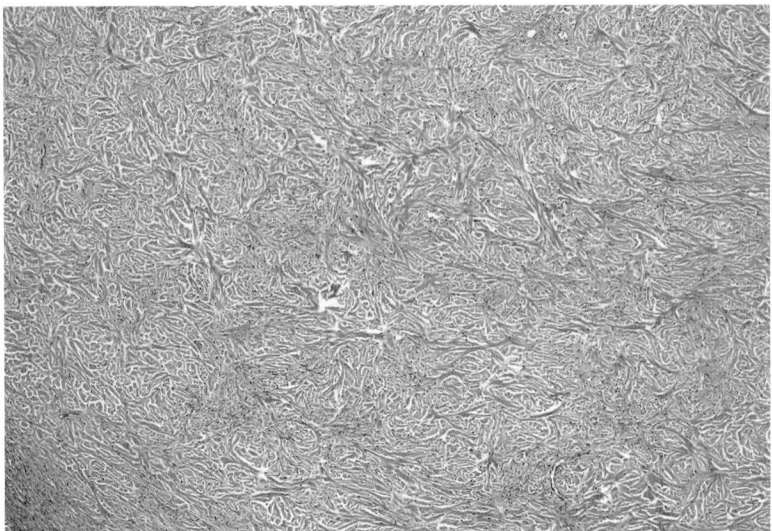

Fig. 35.92
Storiform collagenoma: the storiform arrangement of these eosinophilic collagen bundles is characteristic.

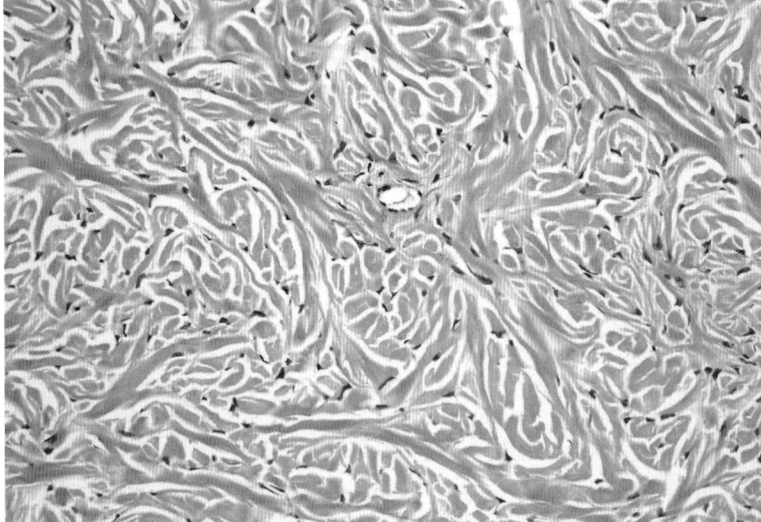

Fig. 35.93
Storiform collagenoma: high-power view.

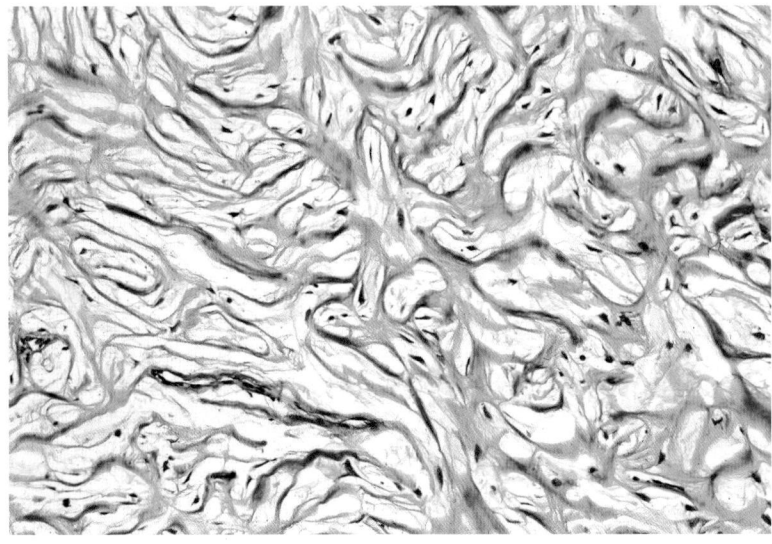

Fig. 35.94
Storiform collagenoma: the features are highlighted with Masson's trichrome stain.

Differential diagnosis

Areas simulating storiform collagenoma are sometimes seen in a variety of tumors, including fibroma of tendon sheath (which is never dermal), sclerotic fibrous histiocytomas, neurofibroma, fibroadenoma of axillary accessory breast tissue and even solitary myofibromas.[17-19] However, the distinctive histologic features of these latter conditions are usually apparent in neighboring fields. Dermal lipomas with prominent sclerosis may simulate a storiform collagenoma but mature adipocytes are always demonstrated in the former lesion.[20] Sometimes it may focally simulate sclerosing perineurioma but EMA is invariably negative. Focal changes simulating sclerotic fibroma may also be seen in inflammatory conditions such as erythema elevatum diutinum and folliculitis.[21]

Nuchal and nuchal-type fibroma

Clinical features

Nuchal fibroma (also known as collagenosis nuchae) is a distinctive dermal and subcutaneous tumor that tends to present mainly in the posterior neck of men between the third and fifth decades of life.[1-5] Despite the name, up to one-third of lesions can occur in other locations including the shoulder, back, and even the face and limbs (including a lesion on an ankle).[2-7] It has been proposed that lesions occurring in extranuchal sites should be described as nuchal-type fibroma. An association with diabetes has been documented.[5,8] Identical tumors – when multiple and presenting in children – are usually seen in Gardner syndrome (see below).[9,10] Only exceptionally are multiple lesions not associated with the later.[11] Tumors are asymptomatic and measure less than 3 cm in diameter. Local recurrence occurs in a small number of cases but this is not destructive. A case associated with dermatofibrosarcoma protuberans has been documented.[12] A tumor developing concomitantly with an inflammatory myofibroblastic tumor of the pleura was documented.[13]

Histologic features

Tumors are poorly circumscribed and composed of thick collagen bundles with a lobular architecture and few scattered fibroblasts (Figs 35.95 and 35.96). Entrapped fat and traumatic neuroma-like changes are often seen. Occasionally, there is focal infiltration of skeletal muscle. Mononuclear inflammatory cells are rare.

By immunohistochemistry, tumor cells are positive for CD34 and CD99 but negative for β-catenin, desmin and actin.[14]

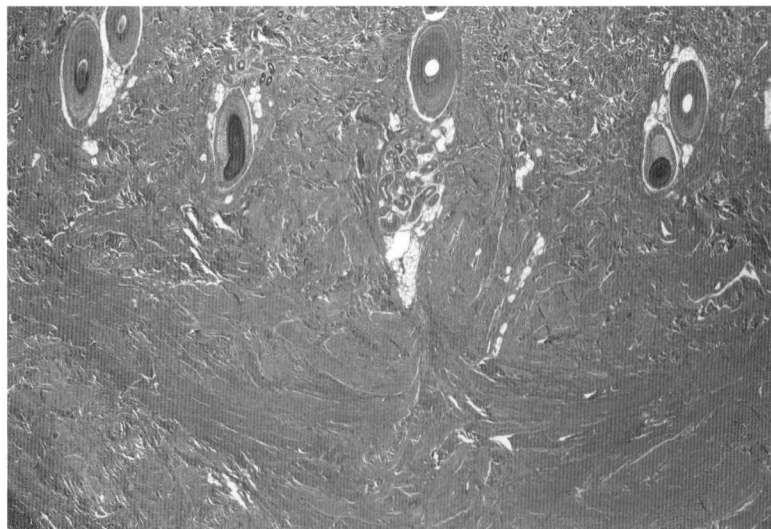

Fig. 35.95
Nuchal fibroma: the tumor consists of hypocellular collagen with a keloid-like appearance.

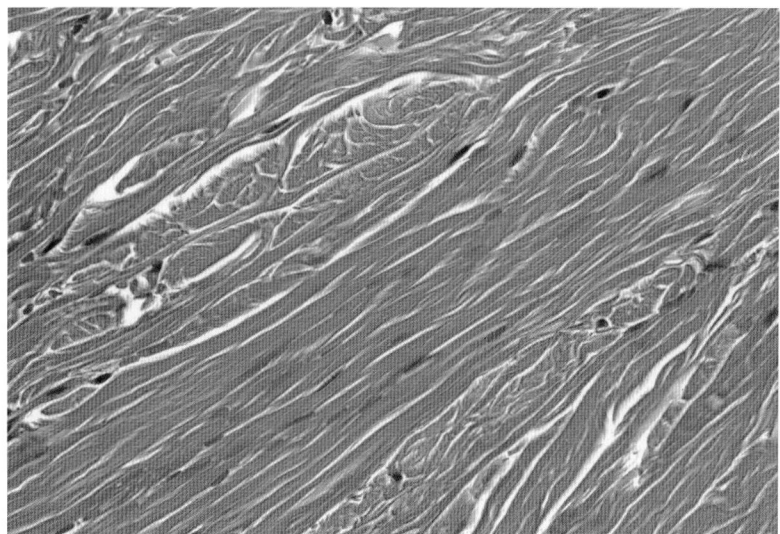

Fig. 35.96
Nuchal fibroma: high-power view.

Differential diagnosis

Distinction from Gardner fibroma may be very difficult. Nuclear accumulation of β-catenin is seen in Gardner fibroma but any lesion with morphological features of nuchal-type fibroma should be considered Gardner-associated until clinical work-up proves otherwise. Desmoid fibromatosis may show focal areas resembling a nuchal fibroma but, in most areas, tumors are more cellular and show prominent infiltration of surrounding tissues.[15]

Gardner fibroma

Clinical features

Gardner fibroma is a benign soft tissue tumor identical to nuchal fibroma, presenting in patients with Gardner syndrome (colonic adenomatous polyposis, epidermoid cysts), a familial adenosis poliposis (FAP) variant also associated with germline inactivating mutations in *APC*.[1] The tumor may be the first manifestation of the disease and lesions tend to be multiple, arising in children and at different sites including the neck, head, trunk and extremities.[2–4] Desmoid fibromatosis may develop at the sites of Gardner fibromas and the relationship of these two lesions is unclear. Lesions are poorly circumscribed, slow growing and range in size from 2 to 10 cm. Local recurrence is possible.

Pathogenesis and histologic features

These tumors are driven by overaction of the Wnt/β-catenin pathway secondary to inactivation of the *APC* gene.[1,5,6] Tumors are identical to nuchal fibroma (see above) but some lesions are more cellular and lack a lobular growth pattern.[7] A case associated with elastosis, traumatic neuroma and a *MUTYH* polymorphism has been described.[8] Immunohistochemistry to examine for nuclear accumulation of β-catenin can be helpful, but is not entirely specific.[9,10]

Nuchal fibrocartilaginous pseudotumor

Clinical features

Nuchal fibrocartilaginous pseudotumor is a rare distinctive proliferation described in adults and rarely in children.[1–4] Patients usually (but not always) have a previous history of neck injury and present with an asymptomatic mass on the posterior aspect of the neck at the junction of the nuchal ligament and the deep cervical fascia.[1,3] Tumors are only a few centimeters in diameter.

Histologic features

Histology shows a poorly circumscribed tumor consisting of moderately cellular fibrocartilaginous tissue within the nuchal ligament. Mitotic figures are rare and cytologic atypia is absent.

Tumor cells are positive for vimentin and CD34 and scattered chondroid cells stain for S100 protein.[5] Actin, desmin and keratin are negative.

Ultrastructural studies show cells with features of fibroblasts and chondroblasts. No myofibroblasts are identified.[5]

Fibromatosis colli

Clinical features

Fibromatosis colli is a rare condition seen only in infants and children. Most of the cases present within the first few weeks of life, with no sex predilection.[1–3] Typically, a mass involving the distal sternocleidomastoid muscle and measuring less than 3 cm in diameter is seen. The mass results in rotation of the head and torticollis. Lytic clavicular lesions have been reported.[4] A rare case associated with overlying hypertrichosis has been described.[5] Surgical treatment is required only in a small number of patients. The treatment of choice is physiotherapy. The majority of cases show spontaneous resolution.[3,6]

Pathogenesis and histologic features

Fibromatosis colli appears to be related to trauma, as often there is a history of intrauterine positional abnormalities or complicated deliveries.[1–3] Other musculoskeletal abnormalities can also be seen. An association with Wiedemann-Steiner syndrome has been reported.[7]

Histology shows partial replacement of skeletal muscle by collagenous tissue with poor cellularity. Degenerate muscle fibers are commonly seen.

By immunohistochemistry, tumor cells are positive SMA but negative for beta-catenin.

Differential diagnosis

Distinction from other types of fibromatosis is based on the typical clinical presentation and the presence of a predominantly collagenous hypocellular mass in fibromatosis colli. In addition, aberrant nuclear positivity for β-catenin is seen in most cases of fibromatosis, excepting superficial fibromatoses.

Calcifying fibrous tumor

Clinical features

Calcifying fibrous tumor (calcifying fibrous pseudotumor, childhood fibrous tumor with psammoma bodies) is rare and presents mainly in children and young adults with slight female predilection.[1–3] Most tumors occur in the gastrointestinal tract particularly the stomach, pleura, subcutaneous and deeper soft tissues, pleura, mesentery and retroperitoneum.[4–8] Exceptional oral, heart, lung and gallbladder examples have been documented.[9–12] Multiple lesions are very rare and appear to be mainly pleural.[13] Familial cases are uncommon.[14] Soft tissue lesions favor the extremities and trunk. Associations with Castleman disease, inflammatory myofibroblastic tumor and IgG4-related disease have been reported.[15–17] Size varies from 1 to 15 cm. Local recurrences may occur in up to 10% of cases.[18]

Pathogenesis and histologic features

The pathogenesis is unknown. Although a close relationship with inflammatory myofibroblastic tumor was proposed in the past, it is still considered a distinctive entity.[3]

Histology shows a well-circumscribed mass consisting of sclerotic hypocellular collagen with scattered mononuclear inflammatory cells consisting of lymphocytes and plasma cells (*Figs 35.97* and *35.98*). The latter may form focal aggregates. A striking feature is the presence of focal calcification with formation of psammoma bodies.[1,2]

Tumor cells are diffusely positive for CD34 and rare cells may be positive for actin and desmin.[3] ALK is negative.[3]

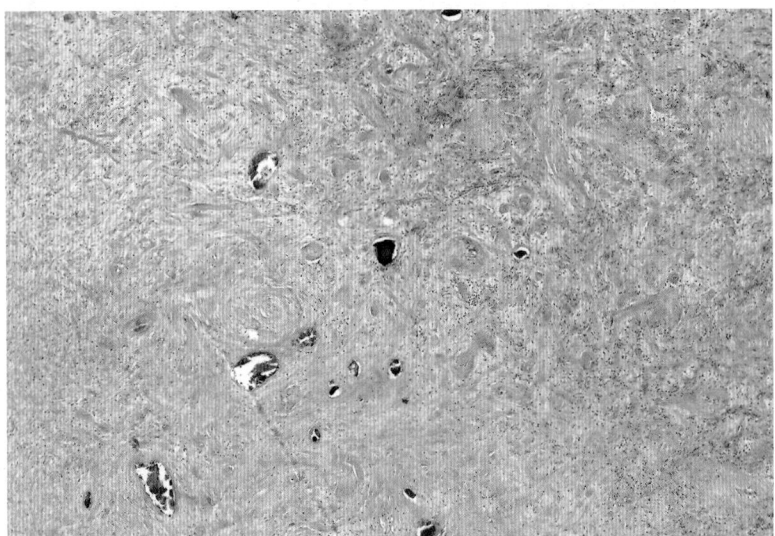

Fig. 35.97
Calcifying fibrous tumor: this example shows a relatively hypocellular tumor. Note the focal calcification.

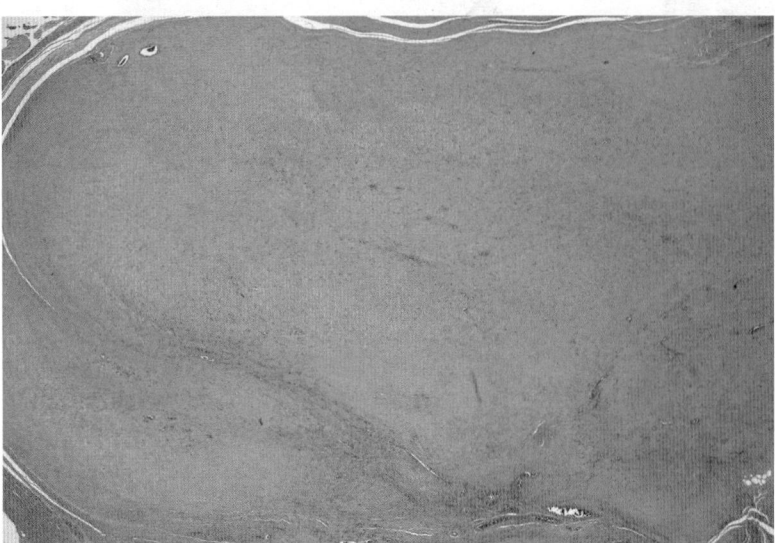

Fig. 35.99
Fibroma of tendon sheath: scanning view of a densely hyalinized nodule.

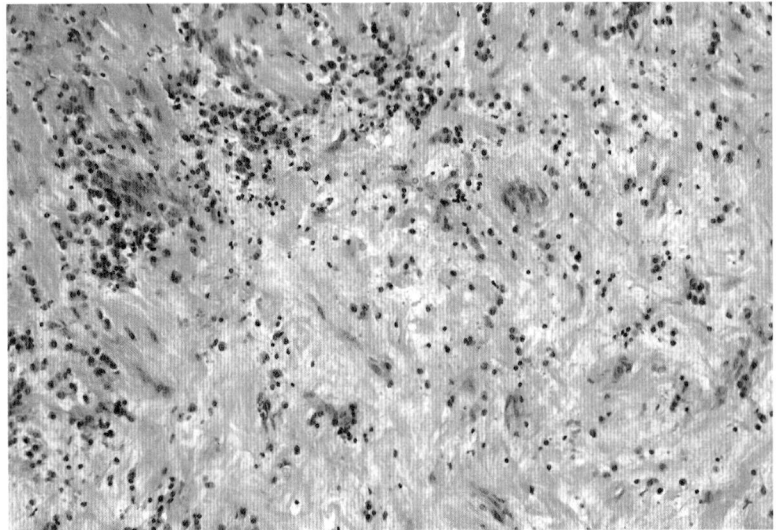

Fig. 35.98
Calcifying fibrous tumor: note the inflammatory cell infiltrate, which is often a feature of this tumor.

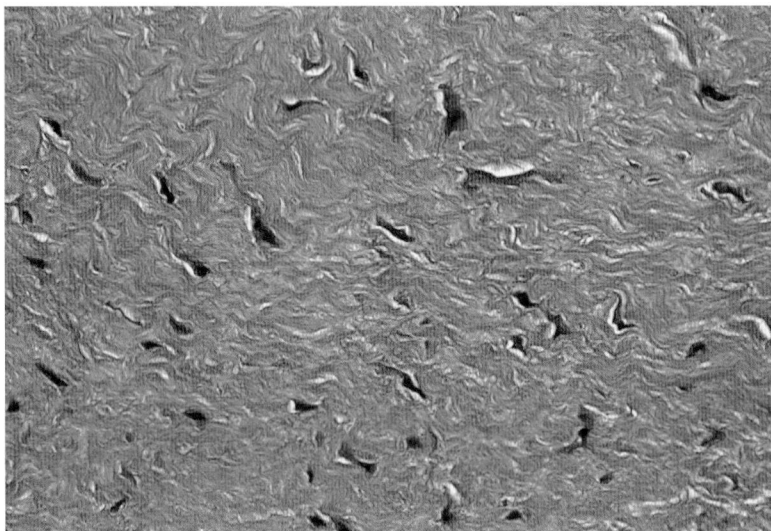

Fig. 35.100
Fibroma of tendon sheath: high-power view showing scattered myofibroblasts.

Differential diagnosis

The presence of a tumor combining sclerotic collagen, inflammation and calcification is distinctive and allows differential diagnosis from other tumors such as desmoplastic fibroblastoma.

Fibroma of tendon sheath

Clinical features

Fibroma of tendon sheath is a relatively common tumor and is usually seen in the third to fifth decades. It predominates in males (3:1) and is virtually confined to the extremities, especially the fingers (mainly the thumb and index), hands, wrists and more rarely the knees.[1-9] The lesion presents as a solitary, usually painless, subcutaneous nodule attached to a tendon or tendon sheath, particularly on the flexor aspect. It rarely exceeds 2 cm in diameter and is of variable duration. Exceptionally, bone erosion has been documented.[10] It may occur in an intra-articular location.[11-13] An association with carpal tunnel syndrome, trigger wrist and Guyon canal syndrome is occasionally seen.[9,14,15] Local recurrence may be seen in up to 24% of cases, almost always as a result of marginal or incomplete excision.[2]

Pathogenesis and histologic features

Cytogenetic studies in a case have found a t(2;11)(q31-32;q12).[16] The same cytogenetic abnormality has been found in collagenous fibroma (desmoplastic fibroblastoma) suggesting a genetic link between both entities.[17] However, a recent study, based on immunohistochemical positivity for FOSL1 in the latter but not in fibroma of tendon sheath, suggests that they represent distinct entities.[18] Furthermore, USP6 genetic rearrangements have been found in a subset of cellular, but not classic, fibromas of tendon sheath suggesting that they might represent underrecognized examples of tenosynovial nodular fasciitis.[19] A single case with a t(9;11)(p24;q13-14) translocation has also been reported.[20]

Fibroma of tendon sheath is a well-circumscribed encapsulated tumor with a lobulated appearance. It shows marked variation in cellularity and is composed of an admixture of dense, relatively acellular, fibrous tissue containing scattered uniform spindled cells and foci of myxoid change. Collagenous hyalinization and areas of increased cellularity, sometimes resembling nodular fasciitis, are commonly present (Figs 35.99 and 35.100). In uniformly cellular lesions the spindled cells are more often arranged in fascicles. These are composed of closely packed fibroblasts showing infrequent normal mitotic figures. A cardinal feature of this lesion, irrespective of the

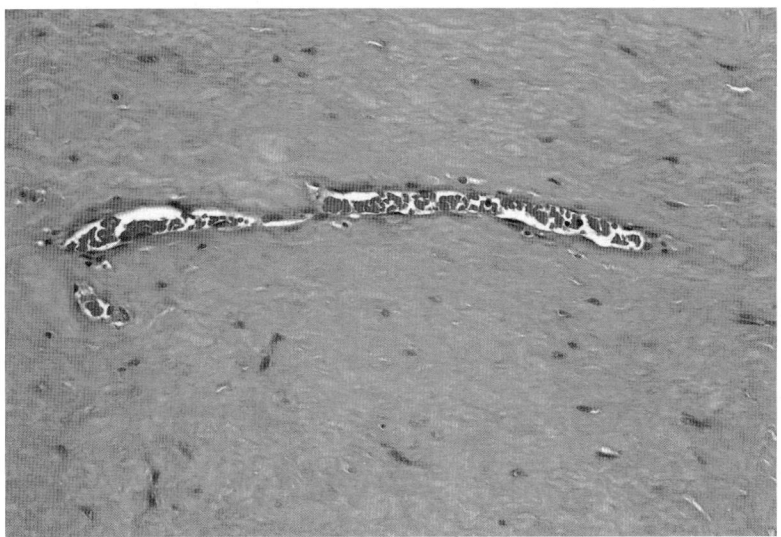

Fig. 35.101
Fibroma of tendon sheath: bland fibroblasts are evident in this field. Note the slit-like vessel.

Fig. 35.102
Desmoplastic fibroblastoma: a low-power view showing a paucicellular tumor with abundant collagen.

degree of collagenization, is the presence of numerous, usually slit-like, vascular spaces lined by normal endothelium (*Fig. 35.101*). A scattered chronic inflammatory infiltrate is not uncommon and some cases show rare, osteoclast-like giant cells and foamy macrophages focally mimicking a giant cell tumor of tendon sheath.

Differential diagnosis

The encapsulation and presence of a distinctive vascular pattern separate fibroma of tendon sheath from nodular fasciitis and fibromatosis. Dermal lesions composed of hypocellular eosinophilic concentric collagen, and considered in the past to be examples of fibroma of tendon sheath, probably represent examples of storiform collagenoma.

Desmoplastic fibroblastoma

Clinical features

Desmoplastic fibroblastoma (collagenous fibroma) is a distinctive, benign soft tissue tumor that mainly presents in a subcutaneous, fascial or intramuscular location.[1-4] Presentation in the dermis is very rare and in one of the reported cases, the patient had a long-standing history of pemphigus.[5-9] Lesions are asymptomatic and present as a slowly growing mass, most commonly located on the arm, shoulder, thigh, forearm, back and hands and feet.[4] Size varies from 1 to 20 cm but the majority of tumors measure less than 4 cm.

Unusual tumors presenting on the neck mimicking a goiter, on the face mimicking a parotid tumor, in the oral cavity (including the tongue), in a lacrimal gland and within a joint have been documented.[10-16] Most patients are middle-aged to elderly males but cases in younger patients and in children may rarely occur.[4,17] A case with bone involvement has been described.[18] The clinical behavior is entirely benign with no local recurrences reported in the literature to date.

Pathogenesis and histologic features

Cytogenetic studies in multiple cases have shown clonal abnormalities involving 11q12 which seems to be associated with deregulated expression of FOSL1.[19-24] This locus is identical to that found in a single case of fibroma of tendon sheath.[25] However, based on other studies, it is not likely that the entities are related (see fibroma of tendon sheath). One case with trisomy 8 has been reported.[26]

Tumors are fairly well circumscribed, round or oval and sometimes appear lobulated (*Figs 35.102* and *35.103*). Low-power examination reveals a lesion with very focal infiltration of surrounding tissues, poor cellularity

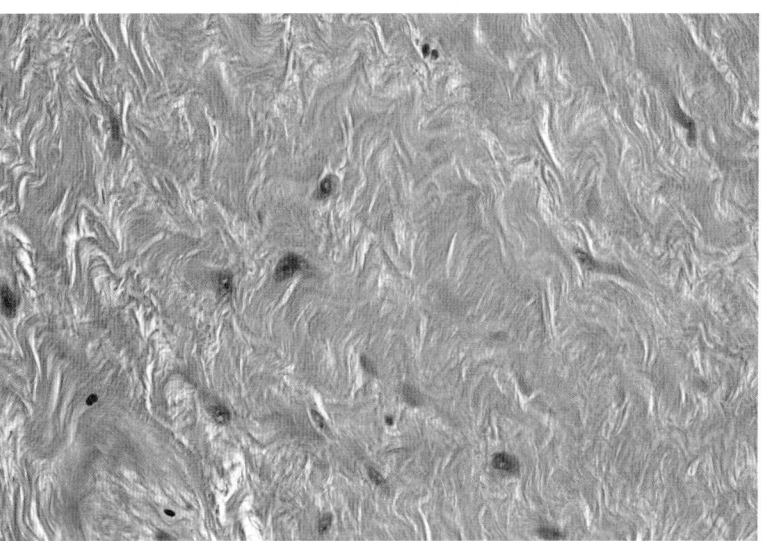

Fig. 35.103
Desmoplastic fibroblastoma: the tumor cells are fusiform or stellate. Mitotic figures are absent.

and a prominent collagenous stroma.[1-4] Tumor cells are elongated or stellate, with vesicular nuclei, a small nucleolus and pale cytoplasm. Mitotic figures are not seen. In some cases, there is focal myxoid change. Vascularity is not prominent and consists of small blood vessels with thin walls.

Immunohistochemistry shows diffuse positivity for vimentin, focal positivity for α-SMA and occasional positivity for keratin.[4] In addition tumor cells are uniformly positive for FOSL1.[27] There is negative staining for other markers including S100 protein, CD34 and desmin.

Ultrastructural studies suggest that the cells in the lesion are fibroblasts or myofibroblasts.[7,28]

Differential diagnosis

The main differential diagnosis is fibromatosis. The latter tumor has an infiltrative growth pattern, is cellular, tumor cells have an elongated appearance and there is a prominent vascular network. An old lesion of nodular fasciitis is usually more hyalinized, with focal inflammation and degenerative changes. Fibroma of tendon sheath almost always occurs in acral sites and has a prominent lobular architecture with a conspicuous vascularity. Also, tumor cells are negative for FOSL1.[27]

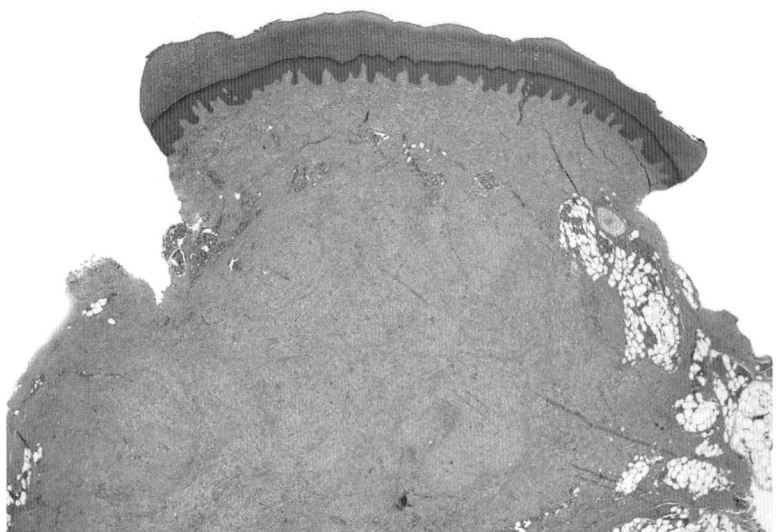

Fig. 35.104
Inclusion body fibromatosis: the tumor is composed of bland spindled cells with a collagenous stroma.

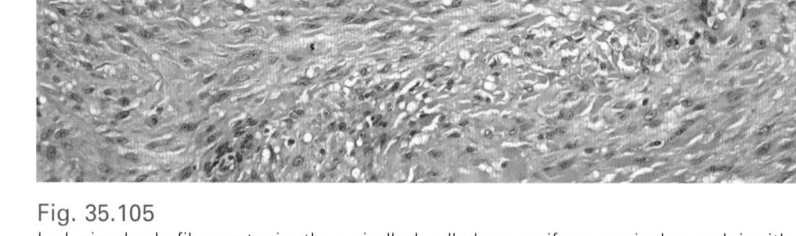

Fig. 35.105
Inclusion body fibromatosis: the spindled cells have uniform vesicular nuclei with small nucleoli.

Inclusion body fibromatosis

Clinical features

Inclusion body fibromatosis is a rare benign neoplasm initially described as infantile digital fibromatosis. The latter term derives from the fact that almost all cases arise on the fingers or toes of infants less than 3 years of age, and one-third of the cases are congenital.[1-7] However, rare cases have been reported in older children and in adults and at other sites, and a more accurate designation is that of inclusion body fibromatosis.[8-12] Typically, it presents as a small (usually less than 1 cm diameter), rapidly growing, dermal or subcutaneous nodule on the dorsal or lateral aspect of one of the digits; multiple lesions arising synchronously or separately on more than one digit (fingers and toes) are not uncommon. Lesions may also be seen elsewhere on the hands and feet.[7] Inclusion digital fibromatosis shows a marked tendency towards local recurrence after excision (up to 50%), but has no capacity to metastasize. Spontaneous regression is usually seen in most cases and therefore treatment should only be symptomatic.

Histologic features

The lesion is composed predominantly of an irregular mass of proliferating myofibroblasts, showing occasional normal mitoses, but no atypia, embedded in a dense collagenous stroma, which extends deeply from the dermis and may be attached to underlying osteoarticular structures (Fig. 35.104). The diagnostic sine qua non and characteristic feature is the presence of brightly eosinophilic intracytoplasmic inclusions in a variable number of the myofibroblasts (Figs 35.105 and 35.106) which can be seen as red inclusions with a Masson trichrome stain. A focal lymphocytic inflammatory cell infiltrate can be seen and it has been reported to be more common in areas with numerous inclusion bodies.[13] Tumor cells are usually positive for alpha smooth-muscle actin, calponin, and desmin.[7] Occasionally, they may be positive for h-caldesmon and beta-catenin (nuclear staining).[7] These inclusions are actin positive, especially in alcohol-fixed tissue, and the presence of these filaments has been demonstrated by immunoelectron microscopy.[14,15] The inclusions can also be highlighted with anti-calponin 1.[16] Positivity for actin may also be demonstrated if sections are pretreated with KOH.[17] The inclusions are composed of intermediate filaments measuring 5–7 nm. It is not clear why these inclusions are formed. It is very likely that they are the result of a defect in actin metabolism.[18] Other myofibroblastic lesions (including myofibrosarcoma), the stromal cells of phyllodes tumor, fibroadenoma, and some leiomyomas can rarely show similar actin-positive intracytoplasmic inclusions.[19-24]

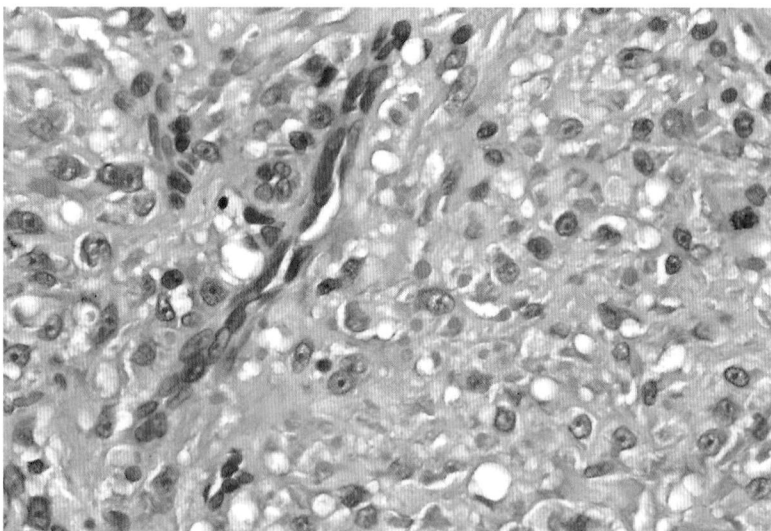

Fig. 35.106
Inclusion body fibromatosis: in this example, there are numerous inclusions.

Differential diagnosis

The presence of eosinophilic inclusions and the clinical history allow no differential diagnosis. Identical lesions may occur in the digits of patients with a syndrome consisting of terminal osseous dysplasia and pigmentary defects.[25,26] However, in these patients, inclusions are not seen.

Calcifying aponeurotic fibroma

Clinical features

Calcifying aponeurotic fibroma (also known as juvenile aponeurotic fibroma) is a very rare lesion seen predominantly in the first two decades of life, with a predilection for males.[1-3] It presents as a single small nodular or infiltrative mass, most often on the feet or hands, especially the palms. Involvement of other sites such as the head and neck, back, abdominal wall, legs and arms is very rare.[4,5] Multiple lesions are exceptional.[6] Bone involvement is extremely rare.[7] Local recurrence, particularly in younger patients, is common and occurs in up to 50% of cases.

Histologic features

An FN1-EGF gene fusion, not detected so far in any other neoplasm, has been reported as the main driver mutation in this tumor.[8]

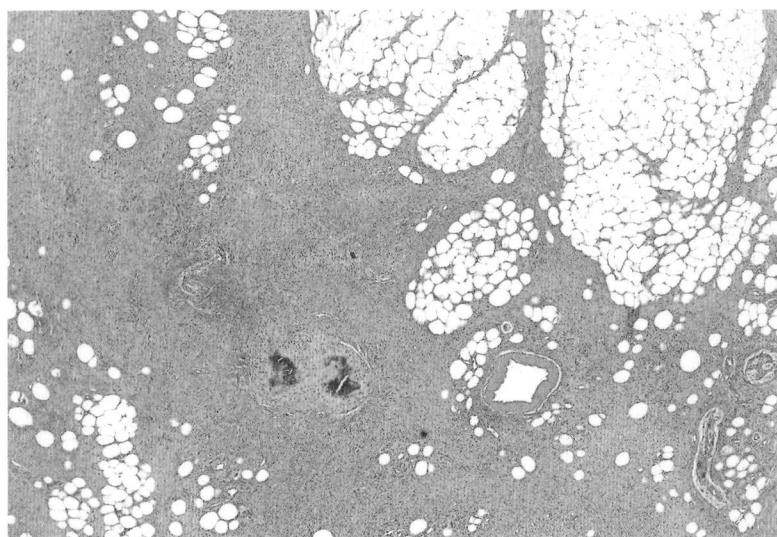

Fig. 35.107
Calcifying aponeurotic fibroma: an irregular infiltrative mass of fibroblastic tissue is present in the subcutaneous fat.

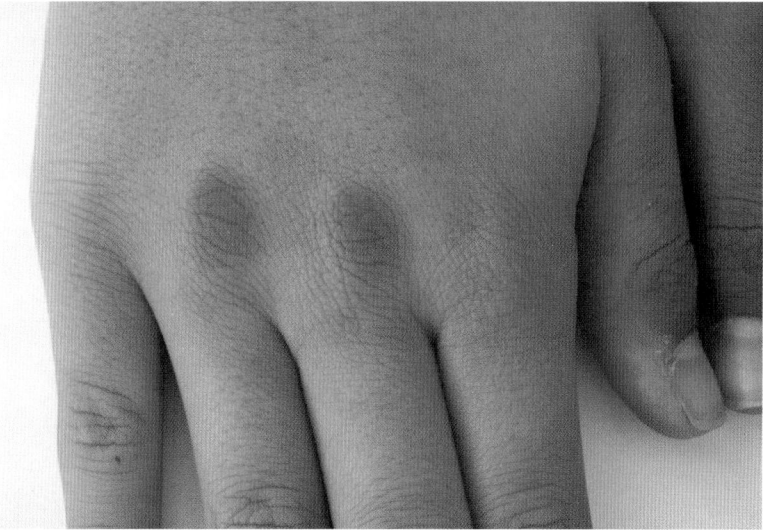

Fig. 35.109
Knuckle pad: typical thickened plaques are present over the interphalangeal joints and second metacarpophalangeal joint. By courtesy of M.M. Black, MD, Institute of Dermatology, London, UK.

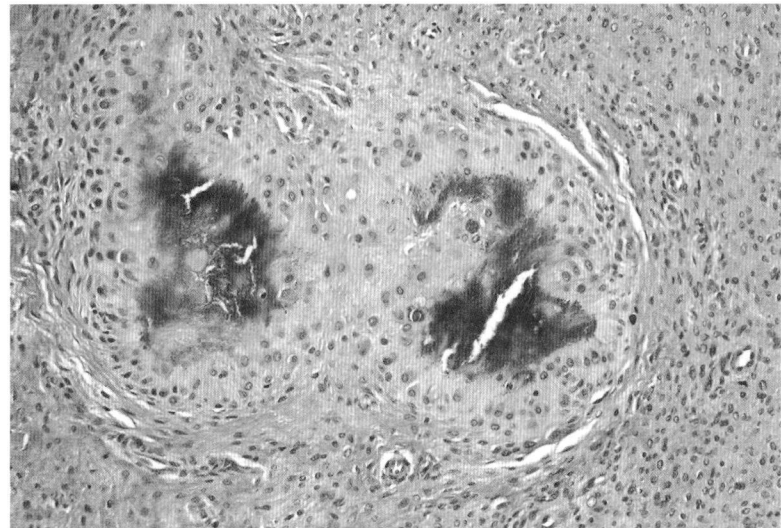

Fig. 35.108
Calcifying aponeurotic fibroma: in this section, there is chondroid metaplasia and there is focal basophilic calcification.

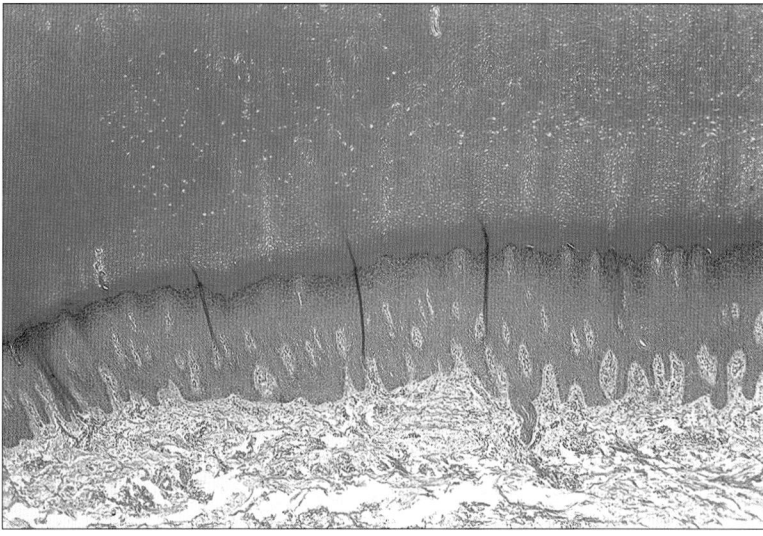

Fig. 35.110
Knuckle pad: in this section there is massive hyperkeratosis and acanthosis. The appearances are non-specific.

Calcifying aponeurotic fibroma characteristically forms an irregular mass of dense, fairly cellular, fibrous tissue invading subcutaneous and muscular structures widely (*Fig. 35.107*). Myofibroblasts tend to be plump with prominent nuclei. Usually, these cells have a linear or palisaded arrangement and comprise the bulk of the tumor. As the lesion matures, the calcified areas undergo chondroid metaplasia (*Fig. 35.108*). Extramedullary hematopoiesis may occasionally be seen.[9]

Differential diagnosis

The differential diagnosis includes palmar fibromatosis, which is rare in young people and tends to be fairly circumscribed, and soft tissue chondroma, which lacks the dense myofibroblastic component and is composed solely of cartilaginous tissue, which is often rather cellular.

Knuckle pad

Clinical features

Knuckle pads, which are regarded as a superficial variant of palmar fibromatosis, are not uncommon, rather banal lesions that rarely come to the attention of either clinicians or pathologists.[1-3] They present as fairly ill-defined foci of fibrous thickening over the metacarpophalangeal or proximal interphalangeal joints, most often in the middle aged (*Fig. 35.109*).[4-6] They may be familial, associated with Dupuytren contracture or plantar fibromatosis, secondary to repeated trauma or idiopathic. They are almost always asymptomatic. Knuckle pad-like lesions occur in epidermolytic palmoplantar keratoderma associated with mutations on keratin 9.[7-9] A case of knuckle pads with leukonychia and deafness has been documented.[10] An exceptional association with pseudoxanthoma elasticum is probably coincidental.[11]

Pathogenesis and histologic features

The etiology of knuckle pads is unknown but it has been suggested that they may be induced by knuckle cracking.[11] A case induced by trauma from playing video games has been reported.[12]

A knuckle pad is manifest as an area of non-specific fibrous proliferation in the dermis, often associated with overlying hyperkeratosis (*Fig. 35.110*).

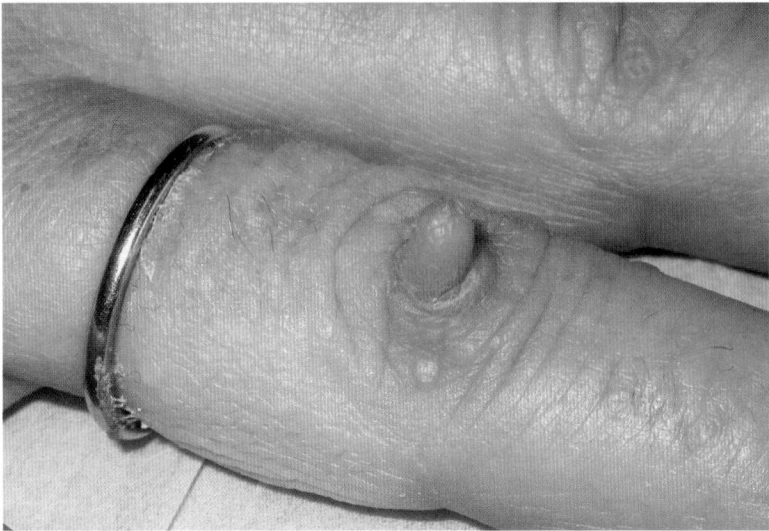

Fig. 35.111
Acquired digital fibrokeratoma: the resemblance to a supernumerary digit is striking. By courtesy of J.C. Pascual, MD, Alicante, Spain.

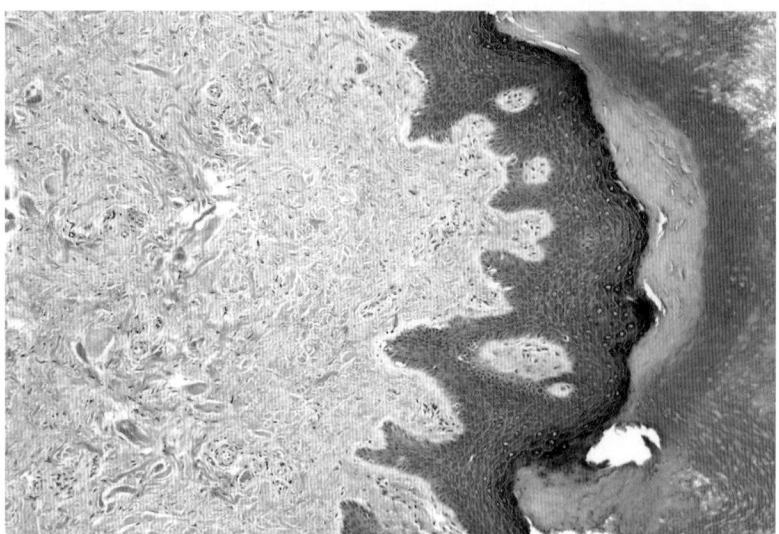

Fig. 35.113
Acquired digital fibrokeratoma: the core of the lesion consists of mature collagen bundles, fibroblasts, and small blood vessels.

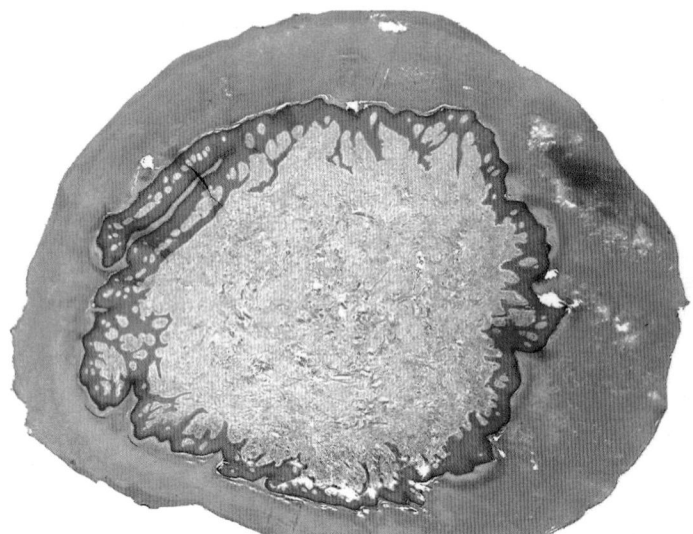

Fig. 35.112
Acquired digital fibrokeratoma: low-power view showing the hyperkeratotic acanthotic surface epithelium.

Acquired digital fibrokeratoma

Clinical features

Acquired digital fibrokeratoma is of no clinical significance and arises most often in adult life, affecting males more often than females.[1–3] It presents as a slowly growing firm nodule or excrescence, usually less than 1 cm in size, on the fingers or toes; as such, it may clinically resemble a supernumerary digit (*Fig. 35.111*). Periungual lesions are known as acquired periungual fibrokeratomas. A case with multiple lesions has been reported.[4] A similar lesion has been documented on the heel.[5,6] Some regard these lesions as traumatic, although with little supporting evidence. A case associated with ciclosporine treatment has been documented.[7] Acquired digital fibrokeratoma may be similar to the periungual fibroma that occurs in tuberous sclerosis but the latter tends to be multiple and has minimal or no epidermal component.[8]

Histologic features

Microscopically, fibrokeratomas are pedunculated lesions covered by variably acanthotic and hyperkeratotic skin (*Figs 35.112* and *35.113*). The core is composed of an admixture of dense collagen fibers containing a variable number of mature fibroblasts, small blood vessels and elastic tissue, all merging with the adjacent normal dermis. Within fibrokeratomas, small peripheral nerves or tactile corpuscles are inconspicuous in contrast to their prominence in accessory digits.

The clinical history allows their distinction from an accessory digit, periungual fibroma or knuckle pad. Local excision is curative.

Plaque-like CD34-positive dermal fibroma

Clinical features

This distinctive lesion was originally described as medallion-like dermal dendrocyte hamartoma to highlight the typical clinical appearance and also to suggest a possible line of differentiation towards dermal dendrocytes.[1] Since then, isolated case reports have been described and a small series was recently published challenging the theory regarding the line of differentiation and proposing the term plaque-like CD34-positive dermal fibroma.[2–5] Lesions usually present in young children, may be congenital, are rarely seen in adults and have predilection for the proximal limbs, neck, and upper trunk. Females are more often affected than males. Tumors usually measure several centimeters, are red or brown in color, and have a medallion-like appearance.[2–8]

Histologic features

Tumors are characterized by a band-like proliferation of fibroblast-like bland cells usually occupying the upper part of the dermis. Extension into the subcutaneous tissue is rare. Scattered small dilated vascular channels are present and tumor cells are interspersed with collagen bundles with decrease in elastic fibers. Superficial tumor cells have a vertical orientation to the epidermis and deeper cells usually have a horizontal orientation with regards to the epidermis. CD34 is positive in tumor cells and there is minimal focal staining for smooth-muscle actin and few factor XIIIa-positive cells.

Differential diagnosis

The main differential diagnosis is with early plaque-stage dermatofibrosarcoma protuberans. This is discussed under the latter condition.

Fibrous hamartoma of infancy

Clinical features

Fibrous hamartoma of infancy is a rare benign tumor of childhood, which although occasionally manifest at birth, usually presents in the first 2 years of life as a solitary, dermal and subcutaneous mass. Congenital lesions

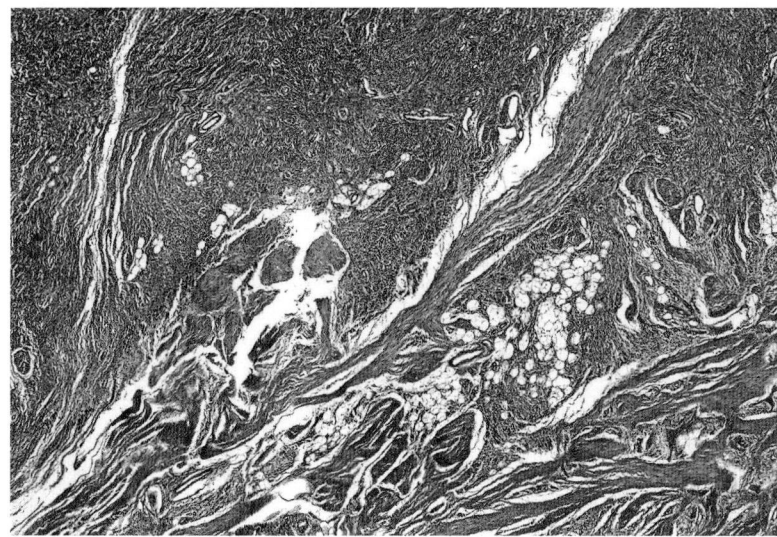

Fig. 35.114
Fibrous hamartoma of infancy: the tumor comprises mature fat, fibrous tissue, myofibroblastic elements, and circumscribed aggregates of undifferentiated mesenchymal cells.

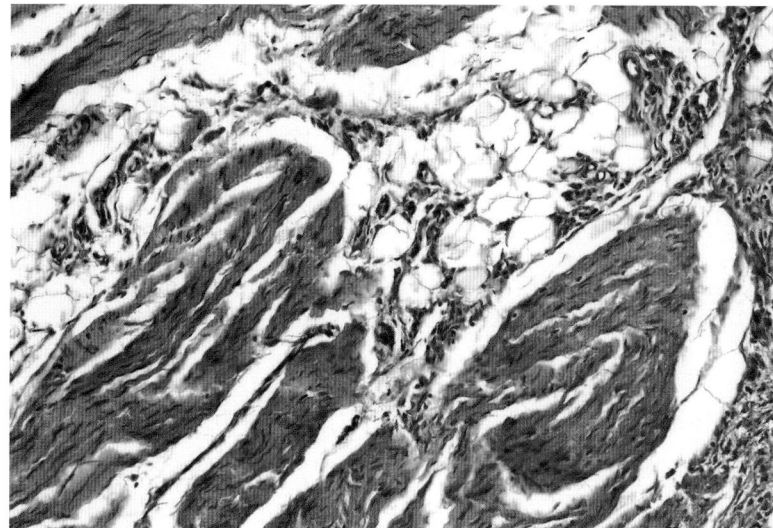

Fig. 35.115
Fibrous hamartoma of infancy: note the fascicles of myofibroblasts.

represent around 20% of cases. Tumors in older children are rare. Males are predominantly affected.[1-10] It occurs most often in the axilla, shoulder region, proximal upper limb, groin, back or forearm. Tumors rarely occur on the hands, feet, scrotum and scalp.[11-13] It typically presents as an asymptomatic, firm but mobile lesion up to 10 cm in diameter. Multicentric tumors are rare.[14,15] There is no family history. A likely coincidental association has been reported in a case of Williams syndrome and in a case of tuberous sclerosis.[16,17] Overlying hypertrichosis has been reported in one case.[18] Rarely, there may be local recurrence after inadequate excision. Sarcomatous features have been reported in two cases, one lost to follow-up and a further case with no aggressive behavior after 4 years of follow-up.[10]

Pathogenesis and histologic features

Cytogenetics in a single case revealed t(2;3)(q31;q21).[19] Two further cases have shown complex chromosomal translocations.[20,21] In a recent study, two tumors with sarcomatous features showed a hyperdiploid/near tetraploid karyotype suggesting that the lesion is likely to be neoplastic rather than hamartomatous.[10]

Fibrous hamartoma of infancy is an ill-defined lesion that merges with adjacent normal tissue and involves predominantly the deep dermis and subcutaneous fat. It is characterized by varying proportions of four components:[1-4]
- disorderly fibrous tissue (coarse bundles of collagenous fibrous tissue with blood vessels and inflammatory cells),
- orderly fascicles of eosinophilic myofibroblasts with wavy nuclei, which are actin positive (*Figs 35.114* and *35.115*),
- mature adipose tissue,
- primitive myxoid foci containing plump, undifferentiated mesenchymal cells arranged in whorls (*Fig. 35.116*).

The combination of these components produces an organoid pattern. A focal pseudoangiomatous may be observed in up to 50% of cases.[9] Areas of hyalinization with cleft lined tumor cells and mimicking giant cell fibroblastoma are commonly seen.[10] Occasional normal mitotic figures may be seen. Numerous thin-walled capillaries are also present. This distinctive appearance makes this tumor readily distinguishable from any other. Tumors with sarcomatous change display hypercellularity, cytologic atypia and increased mitotic activity.[10]

The myofibroblasts in the lesion stain positively for SMA and calponin. S100 and desmin are usually negative.[5,22-24] The more primitive cells stain variably for CD34. The latter is also positive in the pseudoangiomatous and giant cell fibroblastoma-like areas.

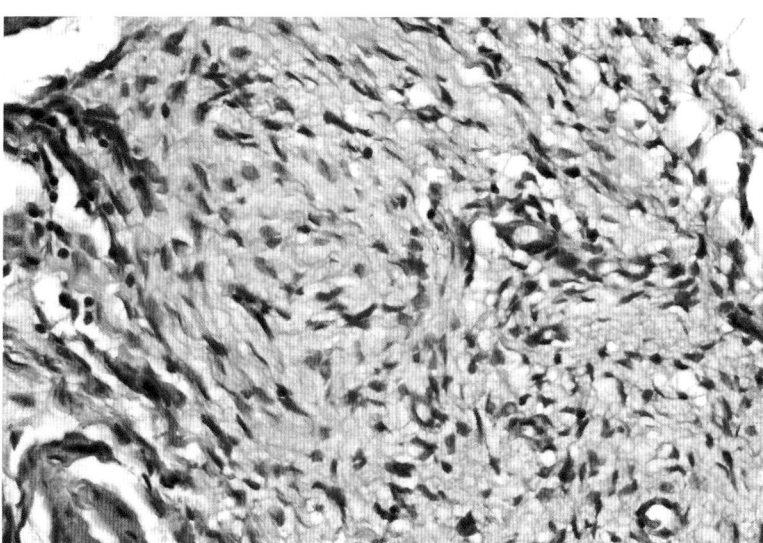

Fig. 35.116
Fibrous hamartoma of infancy: the primitive foci are composed of myxoid tissue containing small cells with round or oval vesicular nuclei.

Changes in the overlying eccrine glands have been described including hyperplasia with papillary projections, dilatation and squamous syringometaplasia.[24]

Ultrastructurally, cells within the more mature areas show features of fibroblasts and myofibroblasts. The cells in more undifferentiated myxoid areas show no specific features except for slender cytoplasmic processes.[5,22-25]

Differential diagnosis

The clinical presentation and histologic features usually allow a diagnosis to be made. In small biopsies, the spindle-shaped component in a myxoid stroma may be confused with a neurofibroma but this is only a focal change and cells are negative for S100 protein. Distinction from a myofibroma is based on the presence of a distinctive biphasic pattern in the latter tumor.

Fibroblastic connective tissue nevus

Clinical features

Fibroblastic connective tissue nevus is a rare newly described variant of connective tissue nevus which is described herein because of its resemblance to fibrous hamartoma of infancy.[1-3] It has been suggested that it might

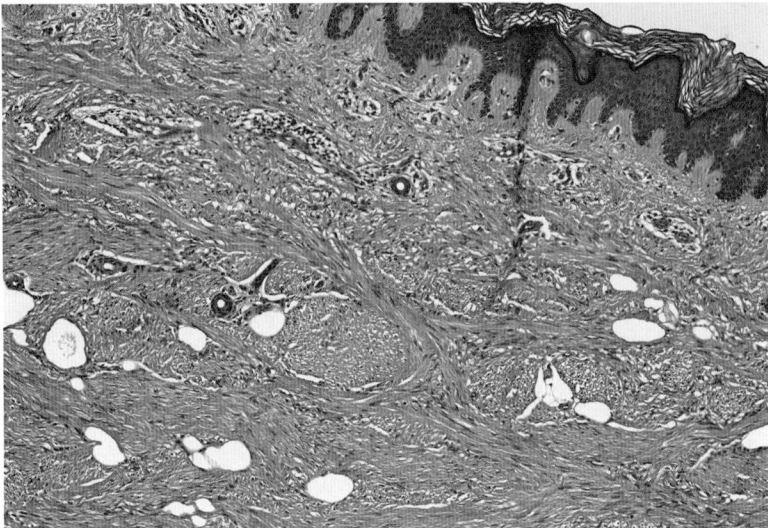

Fig. 35.117
Fibroblastic connective tissue nevus: there is a dermal and subcutaneous ill-defined hypocellular lesion with fibroblasts, collagen, and mature adipose tissue.

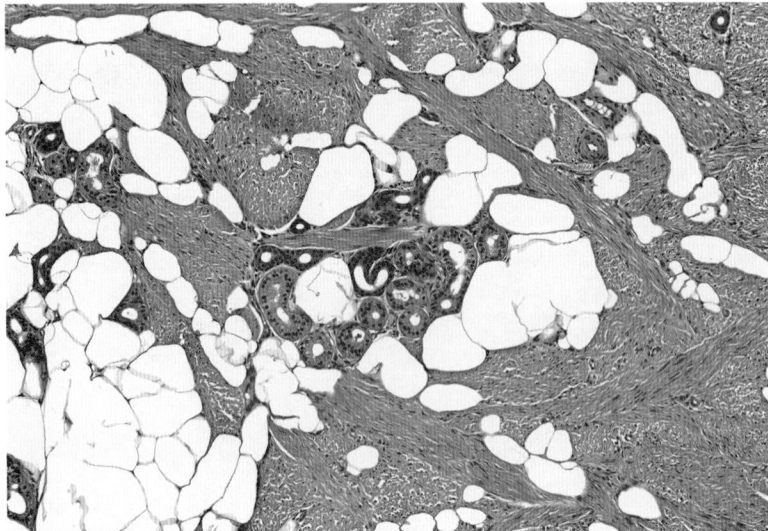

Fig. 35.118
Fibroblastic connective tissue nevus: somewhat hyalinized collagen, bundles of bland fibroblasts, and mature adipocytes.

represent a monophasic variant of fibrous hamartoma of infancy and it is considered a developmental abnormality.[1,3] It occurs more commonly in children, with predilection for females. Presentation in adults is uncommon. The lesion most commonly arises in the trunk, head and neck, and limbs as a single papule or nodule. A case presenting with agminated lesions has been described.[4] No recurrences have been reported, even after incomplete excision.[1-3]

Histologic features

Fibroblastic connective tissue nevus is a poorly circumscribed lesion arising in the deep reticular dermis sometimes involving the superficial subcutaneous fat (*Fig. 35.117*). The overlying epidermis is frequently papillomatous. The lesion is composed of fibroblastic or myofibroblastic cells, with pale eosinophilic cytoplasm, and an adipocytic component is often seen in the dermis (*Figs 35.118* and *35.119*). Entrapped adnexal structures are commonly observed. Elastic fibers are usually decreased or fragmented. CD34 is positive and SMA may be focally and weekly positive.[1,3]

Differential diagnosis

Distinction from the other CD34 positive fibroblastic lesions is usually straightforward.

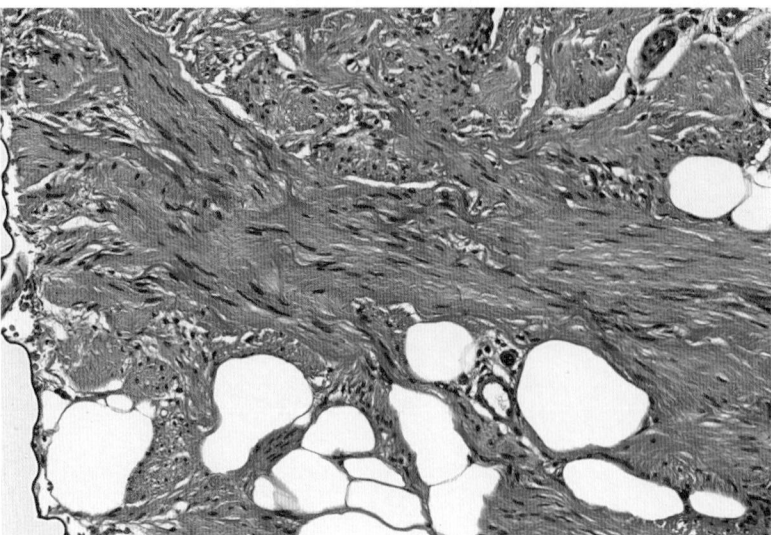

Fig. 35.119
Fibroblastic connective tissue nevus: high-power view highlighting fibroblasts and adipocytes.

Angiofibroma of soft tissue

Clinical features

Angiofibroma of soft tissues is a recently described subcutaneous or deep-seated tumor of likely fibroblastic nature which most often occurs adjacent to joints or fibrotendinous structures of extremities, usually the lower limbs. Unusual locations include trunk and pelvis. The age range is wide and there is female predilection. Lesions present as a fairly circumscribed painless mass of long duration. In some cases, however, an infiltrative growth may be seen, raising concerns for malignancy on imaging. From the limited data available, the tumor has an indolent course. Local recurrence is rare.[1-3]

Pathogenesis and histologic features

Angiofibroma of soft tissues is characterized by a recurrent t(5;8)(p15;q12) translocation resulting in *AHRR* and *NCOA2* gene fusions.[1,4-8] A *GTF21-NCOA2* fusion is rarely found.[5] In a single case in a child, a *GAB1-ABL1* fusion has been described.[3]

Histologically, the tumor is well circumscribed but unencapsulated. A focally infiltrative growth pattern may be seen. Lesions are characterized by a vascular and a fibroblastic bland spindle cell component of variable cellularity and low mitotic activity, embedded in a collagenous to myxoid stroma (*Figs 35.120* and *35.121*). The vascular component is variable: small sized branching vessels are prominent whereas larger vessels with ectatic lumina may be seen, usually at the periphery of the tumor. Sometimes the latter may be slitlike or with a staghorn appearance. Secondary degenerative changes such as vascular hyalinization, fibrinoid or ischemic necrosis, edema, and hemosiderin deposition are not uncommon. Mitotic activity is low. Typically, a perivascular inflammatory infiltrate is noted.[1,2] Tumor cells express CD163, ER, and nuclear NCOA2.[2,3,6] Other positive markers include EMA, CD68, PR, and CD34. Smooth muscle actin and desmin may also be focally positive. Cells are negative for S100, CK, MDM2, CDK4, and STAT6.

Mammary-type myofibroblastoma of soft tissue

Clinical features

This is a rare tumor identical to myofibroblastoma that occurs in the breast.[1] As with the latter tumor, it is most common in adult males and presents as an asymptomatic slowly growing subcutaneous mass with predilection for the groin/inguinal area. Cases in children are exceptional. Size varies but tends to be less than 2 cm. Lesions can also rarely occur on the trunk, breast, axilla, vaginal wall, paratesticular area, vulva, perianal area,

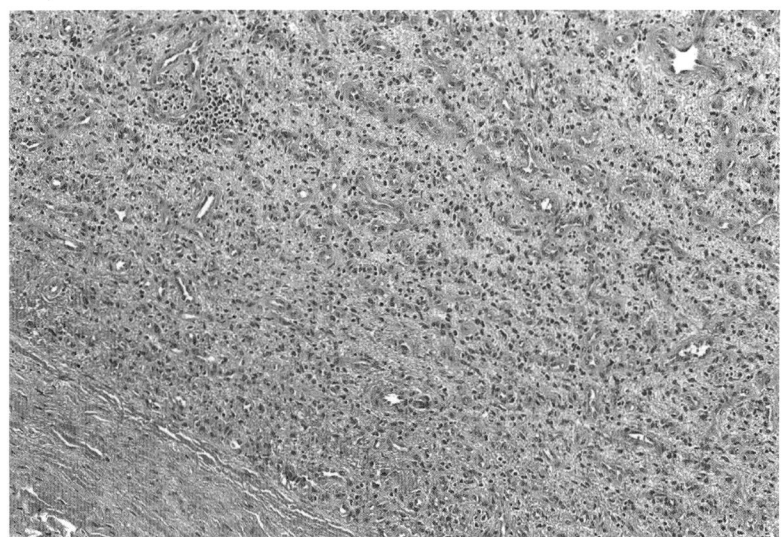

Fig. 35.120
Angiofibroma of soft tissue: a combination of short spindle-shaped cells and small vascular channels. By courtesy of C.D.M. Fletcher, MD, Brigham and Women's Hospital and Harvard Medical School, Boston, USA.

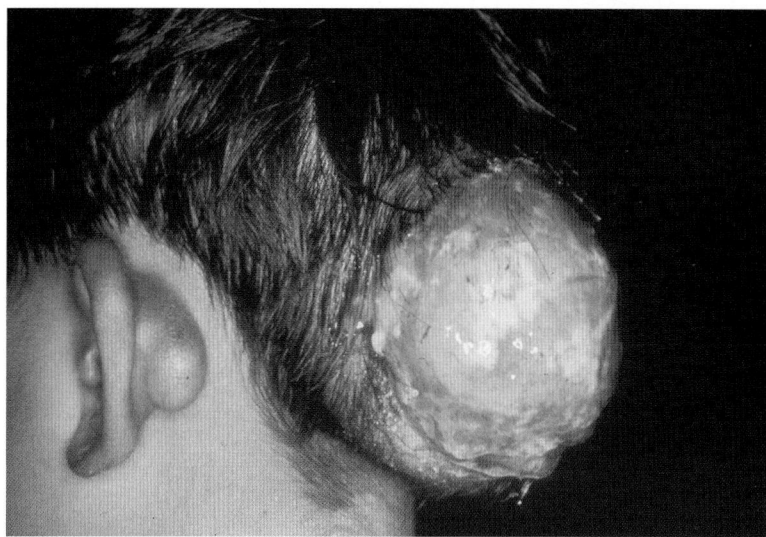

Fig. 35.122
Juvenile hyaline fibromatosis: there is a large circumscribed ulcerating mass. A smaller lesion is also present behind the left ear. By courtesy of Y. Kitano, MD, Osaka University School of Medicine, Japan.

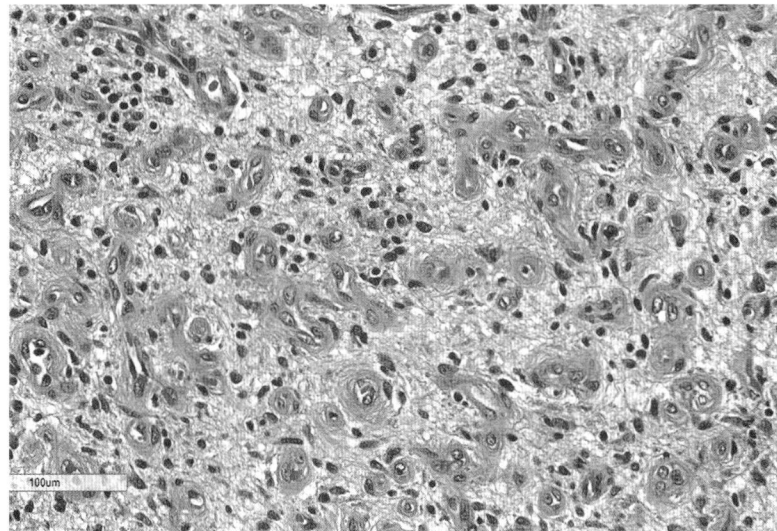

Fig. 35.121
Angiofibroma of soft tissue: abundant myxoid stroma. By courtesy of C.D.M. Fletcher, MD, Brigham and Women's Hospital and Harvard Medical School, Boston, USA.

and lower limb.[1-6] About 10% of cases occur in an intra-abdominal/retroperitoneal location.[2] There seems to be a predilection for tumors to occur along the milk line. Simple excision is the treatment of choice and there is no tendency for local recurrence.[2]

Pathogenesis and histologic features

Cytogenetic analysis has shown deletion or rearrangement of 13q14 that translates into loss of RB1 expression. Mammary-type myofibroblastoma appears to be part of a morphological spectrum that includes cellular angiofibroma and spindle cell lipoma (as well as pleomorphic lipoma and pleomorphic fibroma). These former tumors not only share morphological features but also the same cytogenetic abnormality.[2,7,8] There does not seem to be a relationship between solitary fibrous tumor and mammary-type myofibroblastoma.[9]

Tumors are well-circumscribed and composed of a mixture of bland spindled cells and variable, sometimes prominent, amounts of mature adipose tissue.[1] The spindled cells are arranged in fascicles and display a myofibroblast-like appearance with tapering nuclei and amphophilic cytoplasm with an indistinct cytoplasmic membrane. Nuclear palisading as seen

in schwannoma is sometimes seen.[2] Cytologic atypia is rare and mitotic figures are exceptional. Epithelioid cells may rarely be seen and sometimes scattered multinucleate cells can be identified. Blood vessels are small and tend to be inconspicuous. The stroma is often myxoid, mast cells are common, and hyalinized collagen bundles are intermixed with tumor cells.

Immunohistochemistry shows positivity for CD34 and desmin and loss of RB1 expression. Rare cases negative for CD34 and desmin may be seen.[2] Focal positivity for actin and calponin in a number of cases.[1]

Juvenile hyaline fibromatosis

Clinical features

Juvenile hyaline fibromatosis is an exceedingly rare autosomal recessive disfiguring condition of younger children and usually presents as cutaneous papules and nodules, multiple soft tissue masses of variable size that particularly affect the head and neck, and gingival hyperplasia (*Fig. 35.122*).[1-7] The back and flexures of the lower limbs may also be involved, resulting in flexion contractures. Often, joint contractures and gingival hypertrophy precede the cutaneous manifestations of the disease.[8] Other associations include mental retardation and osteolytic bone lesions, hyperpigmentation, osteosclerosis, scoliosis, atrial thrombus, and pericardial effusion.[9-12] A more localized and limited form of the disease has been documented.[13,14] In a single case, a squamous cell carcinoma developed in association with oral lesions.[15]

The only treatment is surgical excision of each lesion, but new tumors may continue to develop into adult life. Targeted therapy with proteasome inhibitors has been suggested as a therapeutic option.[16]

Infantile systemic hyalinosis is considered to be an allelic disorder with similar but more severe involvement, hyaline deposits in many organs, recurrent infections and death early in life, usually within the first 2 years.[17-21]

Pathogenesis and histologic features

Juvenile hyaline fibromatosis, thought to be due to a genetic abnormality of collagen production, may be seen in siblings, particularly of consanguineous parents.[2,22-24] Ultrastructural studies and skin fibroblasts from cultures have suggested defective synthesis of collagen within fibroblasts.[25-27] The disease results from an abnormal assembly of basement membrane material and collagen deposition is also abnormal.[19,20,28] The gene for the disease has been mapped to chromosome 4q21.[29] Multiple different mutations have been identified in this gene, which encodes capillary morphogenesis protein 2 (*CMG2*), also termed anthrax toxin receptor 2 (*ANTXR2*).[30-35] *ANTXR2* is a transmembrane protein induced during capillary morphogenesis.[19,20] The

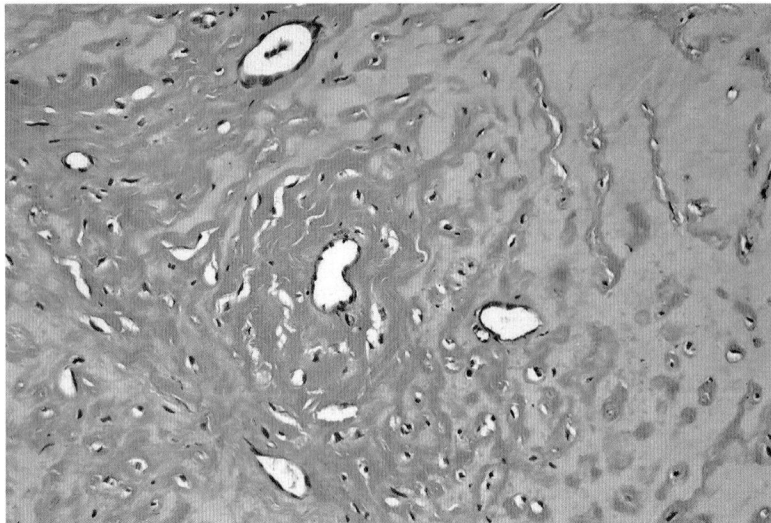

Fig. 35.123
Juvenile hyaline fibromatosis: this field is largely acellular and composed of intensely eosinophilic, hyalinized material. By courtesy of J. Sciubba, DDS, Baltimore, USA.

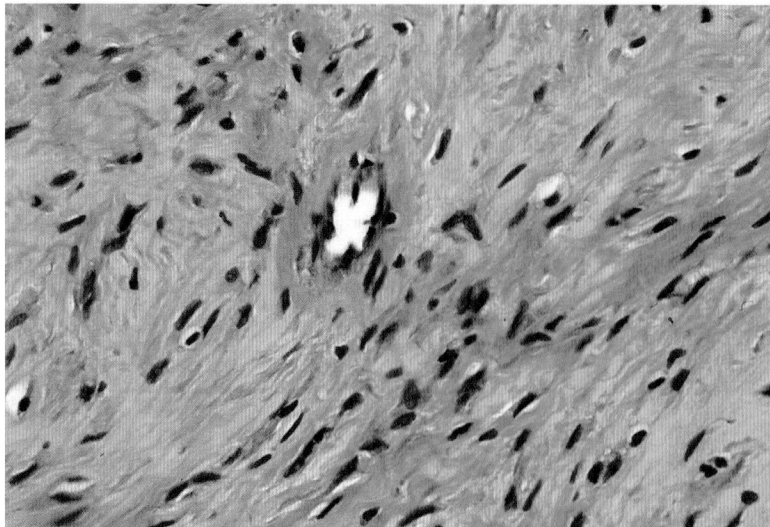

Fig. 35.125
Juvenile hyaline fibromatosis: the spindle cells are bland with hyperchromatic nuclei. By courtesy of J. Sciubba, DDS, Baltimore, USA.

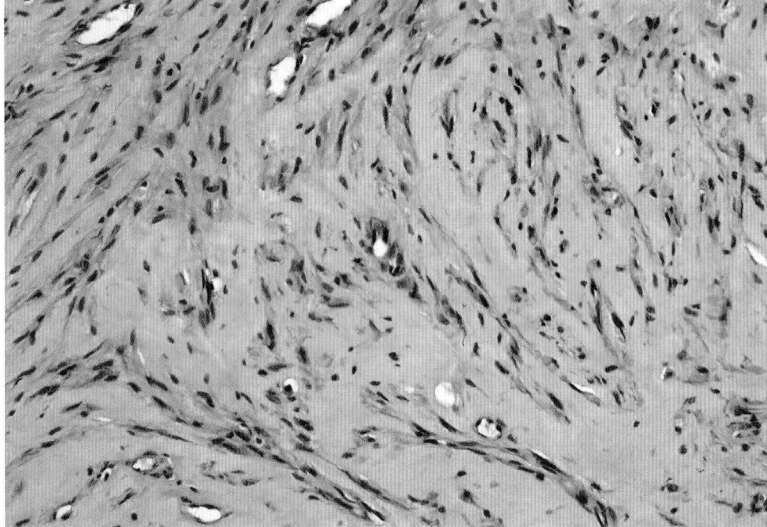

Fig. 35.124
Juvenile hyaline fibromatosis: other areas may be more cellular. By courtesy of J. Sciubba, DDS, Baltimore, USA.

protein binds laminin and collagen type IV and alterations in the protein result in abnormalities in the assembly of basement membrane material with the typical manifestations of the disease. Interestingly, ANTXR2 also serves as a receptor for anthrax toxin.[36] Infantile systemic hyalinosis has similar disease manifestations and *ANTXR2* mutations and it likely represents a disease spectrum with juvenile hyaline fibromatosis. The name of hyaline fibromatosis syndrome has been proposed to include both entitites.[37–43]

The tumors are largely composed of irregular poorly circumscribed masses of deeply eosinophilic, hyalinized, collagen-like material within which are embedded a variable (though usually small) number of fairly plump spindled cells (*Figs 35.123–35.125*). Hyalinization is rarely not prominent.[44] Scattered macrophages and multinucleated giant cells may also be seen.[25] Basophilic calcospherules have been documented.[44]

Electron microscopy shows mesenchymal cells with dilated rough endoplasmic reticulum, prominent Golgi complexes and vesicles with abundant fibrillogranular material.[45]

Differential diagnosis

The presence of multiple lesions arising in childhood and the characteristic histologic features narrow down the differential diagnosis. Infantile

myofibromatosis presents with multiple lesions but the histologic features are quite different from those of juvenile hyaline fibromatosis. Nuchal fibroma presents as a single lesion and is characterized by abundant collagen lacking masses of amorphous eosinophilic material.

Intermediate (locally aggressive) fibroblastic and myofibroblastic tumors

Locally aggressive fibrous lesions are defined as infiltrative neoplasms that are prone to local recurrence. They may be destructive, but never metastasize.

Palmar fibromatosis

Clinical features

Palmar fibromatosis (Dupuytren contracture) is a common condition that is largely confined to adults; its incidence increases with age.[1–6] Presentation in children is rare and occasional congenital cases may occur.[7,8] Males are affected more often than females and up to 4% of the adult male population, particularly the elderly, are thought to develop this lesion.[9] People of northern European descent are predominantly affected and women usually develop the disease much later in life than men.[10,11] The disease is much less common in Oriental Jews.[12] In contrast to keloid, Dupuytren contracture is comparatively uncommon in the dark-skinned races, but the incidence is increased in patients with plantar fibromatosis and knuckle pads. An association with diabetes and with Peyronie disease has also been documented.[13,14] Traditionally, the disease has been associated with alcoholism and epilepsy but this has not been substantiated in recent studies.[13,15] Bilateral involvement is common, but is usually asynchronous. There is an increased familial incidence, but no evidence of any relationship to either occupation or trauma.[16]

Typically, palmar fibromatosis begins as firm nodules in the distal palmar aponeurosis and culminates in disabling flexion at the metacarpophalangeal joints, especially in the ring finger, giving rise to a claw-like deformity and puckering of the palmar skin. Involvement of the wrist and of the interphalangeal joints is very rare.[17,18] Local recurrence is very common unless radical excision of the palmar fascia is performed.[9]

Pathogenesis and histologic features

The etiology is unknown. Although trauma has been suggested as an important factor, this has not been substantiated in a large study.[19] Array comparative genomic hybridization has shown no gene copy number changes.[20] Indinavir treatment in human immunodeficiency virus (HIV)-positive patients has been linked to the development of Dupuytren contracture.[21]

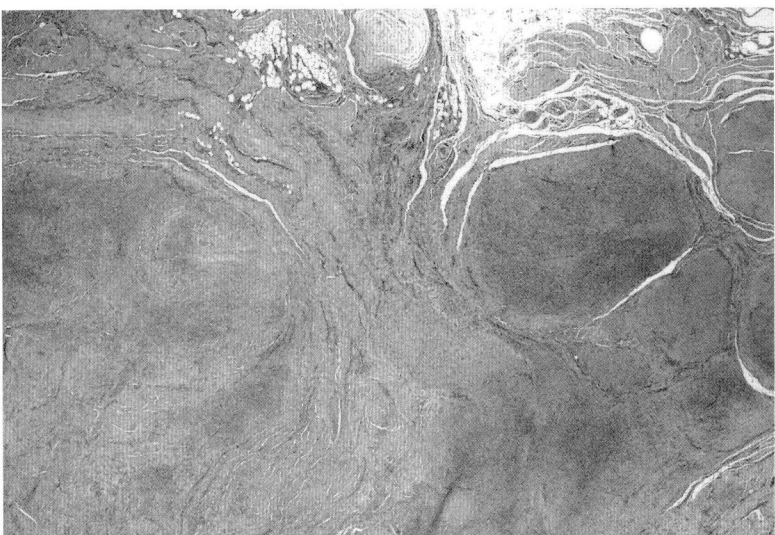

Fig. 35.126
Palmar fibromatosis: scanning view showing multiple nodules of hypercellular tissue with admixed hyalinized collagen.

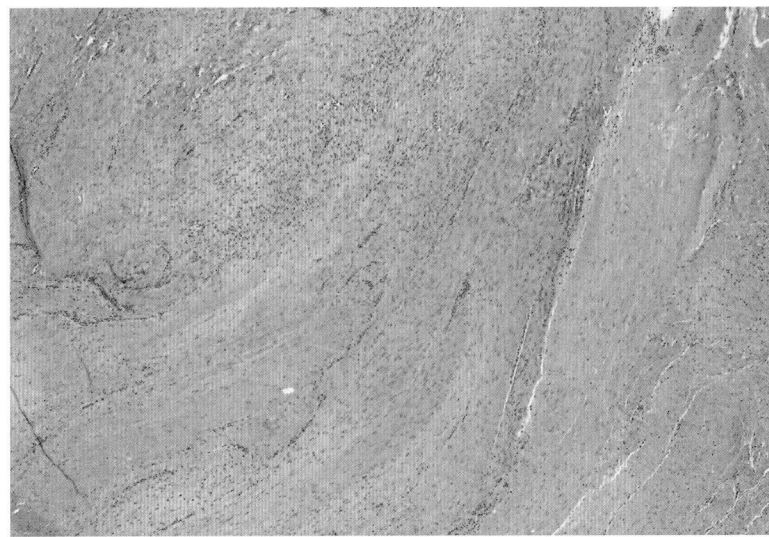

Fig. 35.128
Palmar fibromatosis: older lesions are characteristically hypocellular and consist largely of broad bundles of hyalinized collagen.

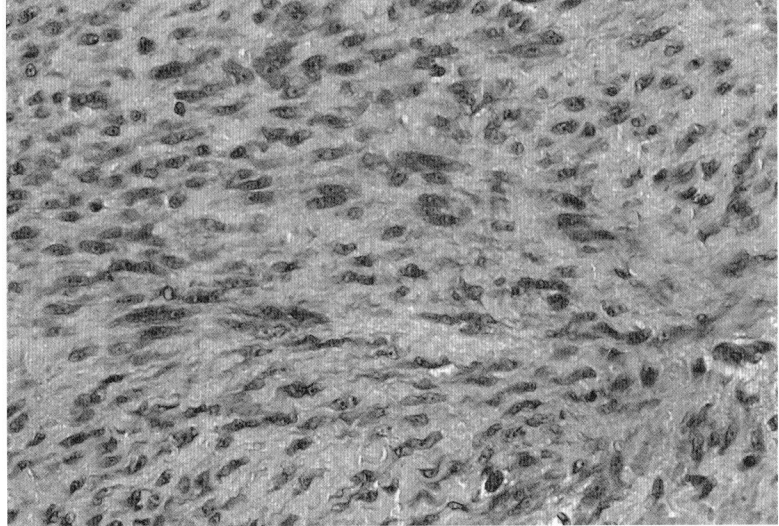

Fig. 35.127
Palmar fibromatosis: the lesion is composed of spindled cells with elongated vesicular nuclei containing small central nucleoli. Occasional normal mitotic figures are typical in early lesions.

TGF-β1, a multifunctional cytokine that plays a central role in wound healing, fibrosis and collagen deposition, is implicated in the pathogenesis of the disease.[22] While β-catenin is overexpressed, mutations in the encoding gene *CTNNB1* which are common in desmoid fibromatosis are not seen in palmar fibromatosis.[23–29] Overexpression of β-catenin does not seem to be related to risk of recurrence.[30] Periostin, an extracellular matrix protein, may have a role in the pathogenesis of the disease by inducing proliferation, contraction and apoptosis of fibroblasts.[31]

A heterozygous missense variant in the Asteroid Homolog 1 (*ASTE1*) has been described in a family with LMNA-related cardiomyopathy and palmar and plantar fibromatosis.[32]

The microscopic appearances of palmar fibromatosis depend, to some extent, upon the duration of the lesion. In the early stages, cellular nodules composed of uniformly plump, proliferating myofibroblasts develop in the palmar aponeurosis, and may show mitotic activity but without atypia (*Figs 35.126* and *35.127*). This proliferative process, which has very little collagenous stroma, gradually extends as an infiltrative mass into adjacent subcutaneous tissues.

With the passage of time, maturation of the fibrous tissue leads to late lesions characterized by large amounts of hypocellular, hyalinized collagen (*Fig. 35.128*). Scattered chronic inflammatory cells may be present at the periphery of the tumor, but there is no evidence of an active inflammatory process. Hemosiderin is uniformly absent, militating against a traumatic etiology. By immunohistochemistry, variable positivity for smooth muscle actin is seen, as expected in a myofibroblastic lesion. Desmin may be focally positive. Lesional cells are negative for CD34 and h-caldesmon. Nuclear β-catenin positivity is usually absent in superficial fibromatoses. However, occasional focal positivity may be seen. P16 is usually positive and estrogen receptor is expressed in many cases.

The degree of cellularity appears to correlate with the risk of local recurrence.[33]

Differential diagnosis

The only lesion that requires exclusion in the differential diagnosis is desmoid fibromatosis, which rarely occurs in the hand, is more uniformly cellular and tends to be deeper. Moreover, diffuse nuclear β-catenin positivity, although not specific for desmoid fibromatosis, is usually seen in the latter and not in palmar fibromatosis.

Plantar fibromatosis

Clinical features

Plantar fibromatosis (Ledderhose disease) is essentially the equivalent of palmar fibromatosis affecting the foot (although flexion deformity only rarely develops). The condition may be bilateral, usually arising asynchronously.[1,2] Although the overall age and sex distribution is similar to palmar fibromatosis, a significant proportion of cases occur in children or adolescents.[3] Familial cases including occurrence in twins are rare.[4,5] It is much less common than Dupuytren contracture and may be associated with it and with diabetes.[6] Characteristically, it presents as single or multiple nodules on the medial aspect of the sole, usually just distal to the pedal arch. A variant of plantar fibromatosis presenting in children and characterized by nodules on the anteromedial aspect of the sole has been documented.[7] Involvement of the plantar aspect of the heel in children is also seen.[8]

Although most cases are asymptomatic, patients may complain of discomfort or a burning sensation, particularly after walking. Neurological symptoms due to entrapment of nerves are exceptionally encountered.[9] Contracture of the toes is extremely rare.[10] Local recurrence is very common.[3,11] Plantar hyperkeratosis is a rare association.[12]

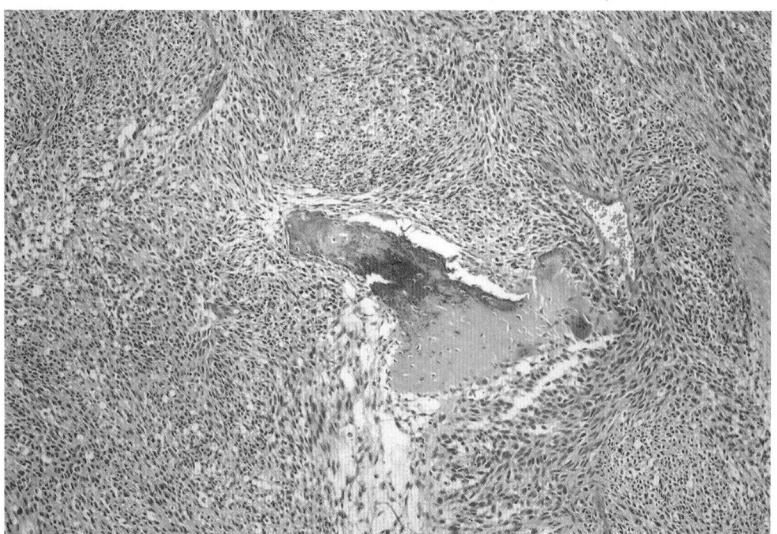

Fig. 35.129
Plantar fibromatosis: this example is strikingly cellular and shows focal osseous metaplasia.

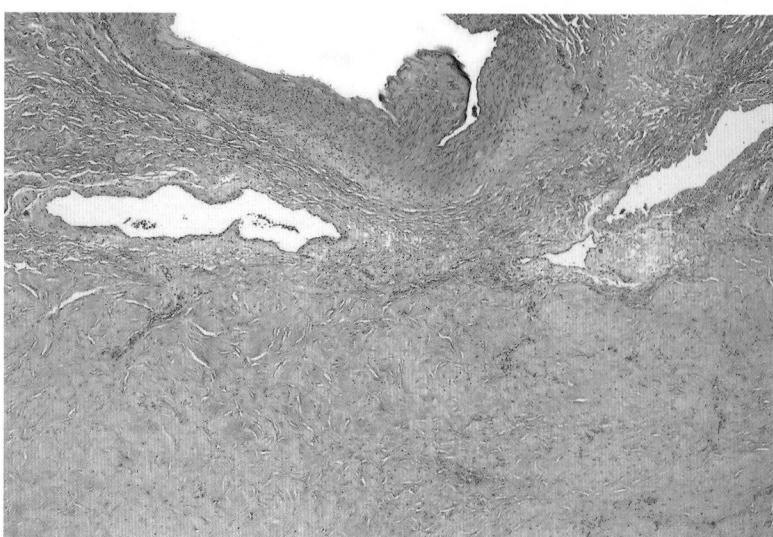

Fig. 35.130
Penile fibromatosis: biopsy from end-stage disease showing dense collagen without any significant inflammation. Despite its name, the condition most probably represents a reactive process.

Pathogenesis and histologic features

Cytogenetic studies have revealed trisomy 8 and trisomy 14.[13] Superficial fibromatoses are genetically distinct from deep fibromatoses in their lack of mutations in CTNNB1, the gene encoding β-catenin.[14–16]

The histologic and features are very similar to those of palmar fibromatosis; however, evidence of chronic inflammation or previous hemorrhage (both of which are probably secondary in nature) is more frequently present in plantar fibromatosis. Lesions also tend to be more consistently cellular and show much less tendency to hyalinize with time (Fig. 35.129). Scattered multinucleated giant cells may be seen.[17] Osseous metaplasia is exceptional.[18]

Penile fibromatosis

Clinical features

Penile fibromatosis (Peyronie disease) is an uncommon fibromatous lesion of the penis that results in pain or curvature on erection.[1–3] The etiology is entirely unknown and although it has traditionally been considered to be a form of fibromatosis it appears more likely to represent an unusual fibrotic reaction developing in response to chronic inflammation, veno-occlusive dysfunction, or trauma, maybe in combination with genetic factors.[4–7] Veno-occlusive dysfunction has been demonstrated by Doppler studies.[4] The prevalence of the disease is higher in diabetic patients and in those with low testosterone levels.[4,8] Hypertension and serum lipid abnormalities appear to have an impact in the severity of the symptoms and outcome.[9] A case was reported in association with methotrexate therapy.[10]

Peyronie disease usually presents as either solitary or multiple fibrous plaques adjacent to the corpora cavernosa, most often on the dorsal surface of the shaft. The peak incidence is in the fifth and sixth decades and there is no predilection for any particular racial group. The plaques rarely exceed 2 cm in diameter. The alleged rapidity of onset in many patients probably reflects the severe psychological problems that frequently develop. Spontaneous resolution is rare.

Histologic features

The microscopic appearances vary according to the duration of the condition. Early lesions are typified by a vasculitic and chronic inflammatory process in the loose connective tissue between the corpora cavernosa and penile fascia. This leads to an irregular reparative fibrotic process, culminating in the development of dense masses of hyalinized collagen with occasional foci of chronic inflammation (Fig. 35.130). Occasionally, metaplastic ossification may occur. There is no differential diagnosis.

Desmoid fibromatosis

Clinical features

Desmoid fibromatosis represents a group of deep-seated fibrous neoplasms which can present in a variety of clinical settings.[1–5] Although most cases are sporadic and solitary, some can be familial or associated with familial adenomatous polyposis (FAP, Gardner syndrome) and rare examples can be multicentric.[6,7] A further subgroup presents in children.[8] According to their anatomical distribution, desmoid tumors are classified into:
- extra-abdominal (around 60% of cases),
- abdominal (20–25%),
- intra-abdominal (15%).

All of these anatomical subsets typically occur between the second and fourth decades of life with a predilection for females. Extra-abdominal fibromatoses are often sporadic and solitary.[1,2] Most patients are young adults presenting with a slowly growing mass that may occasionally be painful. Tumors arise most often around the shoulder girdle or on the proximal lower limbs and rarely in the head and neck area, the latter group being commonest in children.[8] Subcutaneous involvement is an occasional feature. A small proportion of tumors arise in association with a previous scar or post radiotherapy. Desmoid tumors arising in the anterior abdominal wall are particularly common in females, especially during or after pregnancy.[3,5] Often, those arising after pregnancy appear at the site of the scar from a cesarean section. Many cases associated with FAP are intra-abdominal. Local recurrence is common even when excision is believed complete.[9,10]

Desmoid fibromatosis occurring in children less than 10 years of age is referred to as infantile fibromatosis.[11] Most patients with this form of fibromatosis present before the age of 5 and there is predilection for the head and neck, shoulder girdle or thigh.[8,12–14] Infiltration of neighboring tissues may be prominent.

A nonrandom association with gastrointestinal stromal tumor has been reported.[15] In addition, an association between desmoid fibromatosis and papillary thyroid carcinomas has been reported.[16]

Pathogenesis and histologic features

Familial adenomatous polyposis patients have germline inactivation of the adenosis polyposis coli gene (APC) which helps mediate the destruction of β-catenin.[17–19] The location and type of mutation in FAP appear to affect likelihood of desmoid development.[20,21] The tumors develop with loss of heterozygosity at the wild-type allele. Mutations in CTNNB1, the gene encoding β-catenin, are seen in approximately 85 % of sporadic desmoids.[22–25] Somatic mutations in APC can also be seen in sporadic cases.[26–28] All of these genetic deficits allow unregulated accumulation of β-catenin in the

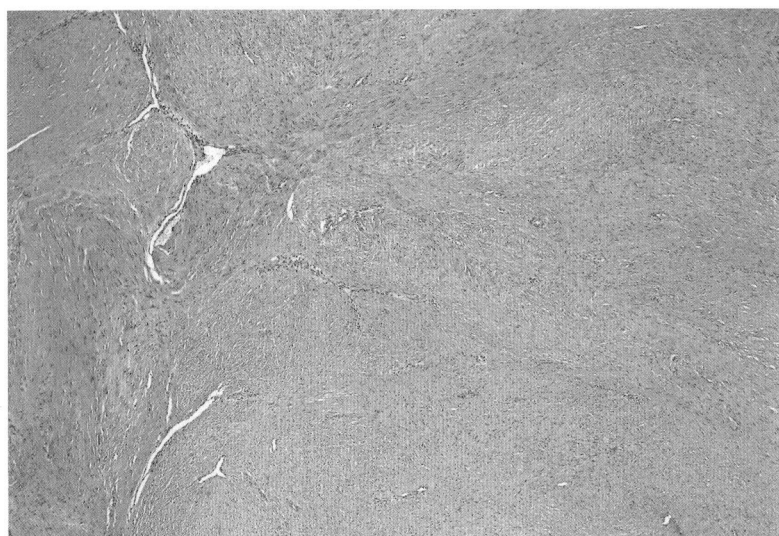

Fig. 35.131
Desmoid fibromatosis: low-power view showing cellular bundles with focal collagen deposition.

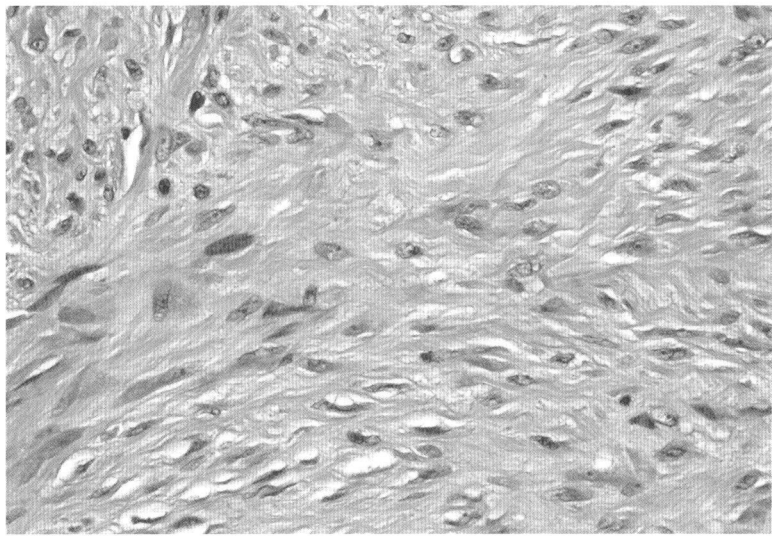

Fig. 35.133
Desmoid fibromatosis: the spindled cells have vesicular nuclei with small nucleoli. Mitoses are commonly present.

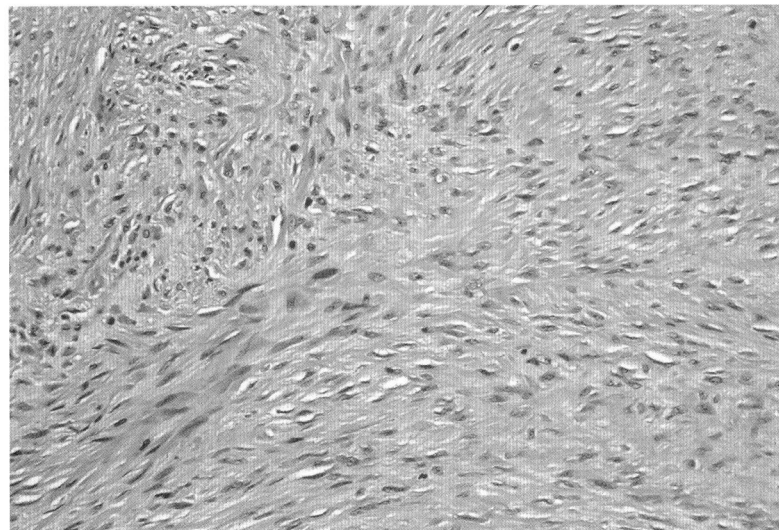

Fig. 35.132
Desmoid fibromatosis: the tumor is composed of spindled cells with a variable admixture of collagen.

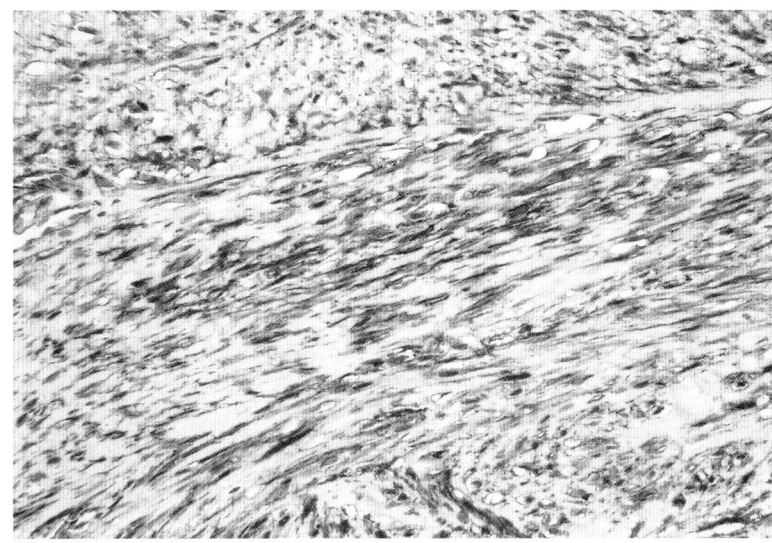

Fig. 35.134
Desmoid fibromatosis: the spindled cells are beta-catenin positive.

nucleus. Cytogenetic anomalies include trisomies of chromosomes 8 and/or 20 and loss of Y and 5q where *APC* is located.[29–32] Overactivation of the Wnt/APC/β-catenin pathway contributes to desmoid development by constitutive activation of pathways in common with fibrosis and scarring.[24,33,34] In addition to β-catenin, VEGF overexpression may play a role in progression of sporadic desmoid tumors.[35] Although etiologically there is clear evidence to suggest a genetic predisposition, this is probably secondarily influenced by trauma or sex hormones.[36] It has been shown that high levels of estrogens can promote, but do not initiate, growth of desmoid tumors. Moreover, it has been suggested that macrophages and microangiogenesis may play a role in the biological behavior.[37] *AKT1* and *BRAF* mutations have been found in pediatric cases.[38]

Histologic features are very similar in all subsets of desmoid tumor. Typical cases show a variegated appearance characterized by an admixture of plump spindled cells with rounded or tapering nuclei showing occasional mitotic figures embedded in a variably hyalinized or myxoid collagenous stroma (*Figs 35.131–35.133*). At the periphery of the lesion, skeletal muscle fibers, subcutaneous fat and fascia are irregularly infiltrated, resulting in bizarre atrophic, degenerative or reactive muscle cell forms. Peripheral collections of chronic inflammatory cells, particularly lymphocytes, are common.

In children, tumors may show a pattern typical of extra-abdominal fibromatosis or else may show a pattern consisting of more immature round cells in a myxoid background.

Immunohistochemical studies show variable positivity of tumor cells for actin and only rarely and focally for desmin. Demonstration of nuclear accumulation of β-catenin can be helpful, but is not entirely specific (*Fig. 35.134*).[23,39–41]

Occasional positivity for keratins and calretinin may lead to diagnostic pitfalls.[42] Cytoplasmic, but not nuclear, positivity for WT1 has been described in young type fibromatosis.[43] FAP-related lesions are also positive for COX2 and may be positive for cyclin D1 and TP53.[44]

Ultrastructural studies show cells with features of myofibroblasts and fibroblasts.

Differential diagnosis

The differential diagnosis is broad.[45,46] The most important differential diagnosis is fibrosarcoma, which shows greater cellularity, nuclear atypia, prominent abnormal mitotic activity, a much lower collagen content and, typically, a herring-bone pattern. Scarring or reactive fibrosis can show virtually identical findings and here history is helpful. Distinction from myofibroblastic tumors including myofibroma is based on the fact that desmoid tumor is deep seated and infiltrative and shows β-catenin nuclear staining. Myofibroblastic tumors tend to be negative for the latter marker. *CTNNB1* sequencing may be of help in challenging cases.[22,23,39,45,46] *CTNNB1* and *APC* genotyping can also aid screening for FAP when desmoid fibromatosis is diagnosed in children.[47]

Lipofibromatosis

Clinical features

Lipofibromatosis is a neoplasm that presents in children as a subcutaneous mass measuring from 1 to 7 cm and involving mainly the upper and lower limbs, with predilection for the hand.[1-4] Rare cases may present in the head and neck and back.[5-7] Cardiac and orbit lesions have been reported.[8,9] The rate of local recurrence or persistence is reported as being 72%.[1-4]

Pathogenesis and histologic features

In a single case a three-way translocation t(4;9;6) has been described.[10]

Histology reveals large amounts of mature adipose tissue combined with a focal spindled fibroblastic element that tends to be localized mainly in the septa of the fat or within the neighboring skeletal muscle.[1-3] Cytological atypia and mitotic figures are rare and univacuolated cells may be seen in the interface between the mature adipose tissue and the fibroblastic fascicles. Rarely, pigmented cells that are positive for melanocytic markers are seen.[6] Congenital infantile fibrosarcoma with lipofibromatosis-like areas may occasionally be seen.[11] Beta-catenin expression is not seen.[12]

Giant cell fibroblastoma

Clinical features

Giant cell fibroblastoma is a rare dermal or subcutaneous tumor that presents as a slowly growing mass up to 6 cm in diameter.[1-7] It commonly affects children under 10 years of age (almost two-thirds of cases), especially males, but lesions may also occur in young, middle-aged and elderly adults.[7] Exceptionally, a tumor may be congenital.[8] It has a wide anatomical distribution with predilection for the trunk (back, chest and abdomen) and (less commonly) the proximal extremities.[1-4] A tumor in the vulva and one in the penis have been reported.[9,10] Local recurrence is seen in up to 50% of cases after incomplete excision.[1-4] Some cases recur as dermatofibrosarcoma protuberans (see below) and this tumor is considered a pediatric form of this disease.

Pathogenesis and histologic features

Giant cell fibroblastoma shares the same chromosomal abnormalities as those of dermatofibrosarcoma protuberans (see below). There is a t(17;22) (q22;q13) resulting in fusion of the platelet-derived growth factor B-chain (*PDGFB*) and the collagen gene *COL1A1*. Ring chromosomes resulting from the t(17;22) are also seen.[11-14] Microscopically, giant cell fibroblastoma is a poorly circumscribed dermal and superficial subcutaneous lesion composed of bland to moderately pleomorphic spindle and multinucleated giant cells (frequently floret-like) in a conspicuous loose myxoid stroma, which is sometimes focally hyalinized and typically contains irregular gaping sinusoidal spaces simulating vascular lumina (*Figs 35.135* and *35.136*). The latter, however, are only lined discontinuously by hyperchromatic mononuclear or multinucleated giant cells, which do not stain for vascular markers (*Fig. 35.137*). Mitotic figures are only rarely seen. Focal hemorrhage and perivascular lymphocytes in an onion-skin pattern are common.[7] Exceptional tumors are purely dermal and rarely there is focal involvement of skeletal muscle.[7] Tumor cells are positive for CD34 and also for CD99.[15]

Ultrastructurally, and by immunohistochemistry, the tumor cells display fibroblastic features.

Giant cell fibroblastoma is closely related histogenetically to dermatofibrosarcoma protuberans, as demonstrated by the fact that some cases present combined histologic features, tumor cells in both lesions are CD34 positive and, more importantly, both tumors share the same cytogenetic abnormalities (see below) (*Figs 35.138* and *35.139*).[11-13,16,17] Cases of giant

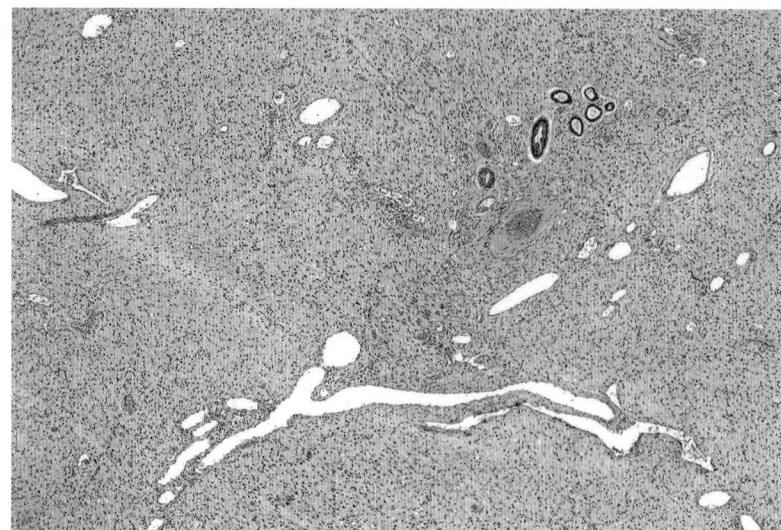

Fig. 35.135
Giant cell fibroblastoma: the admixture of dilated vessel-like spaces and mixed spindled and giant cells in a myxoid stroma is characteristic.

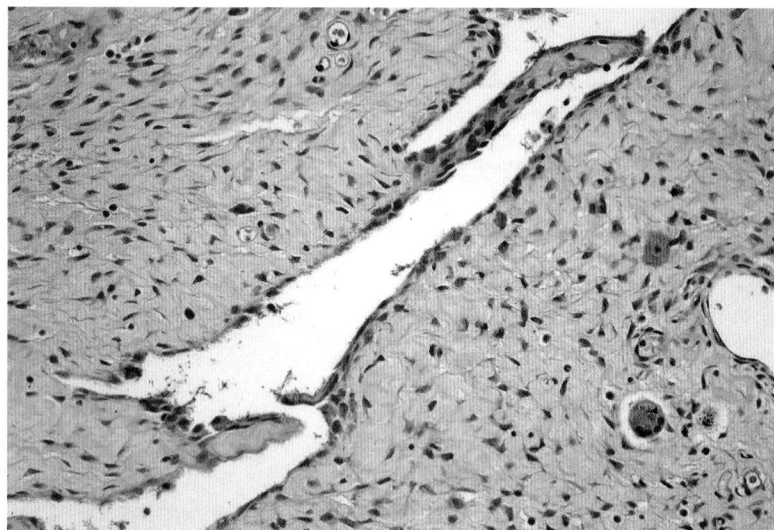

Fig. 35.136
Giant cell fibroblastoma: medium-power view showing blood-vessel–like space lined by tumor cells.

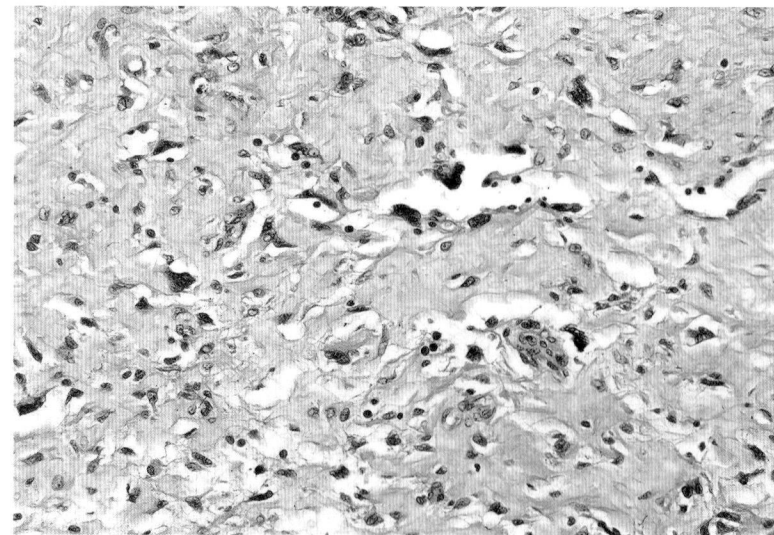

Fig. 35.137
Giant cell fibroblastoma: the sinusoid-like spaces are lined by multinucleate giant cells.

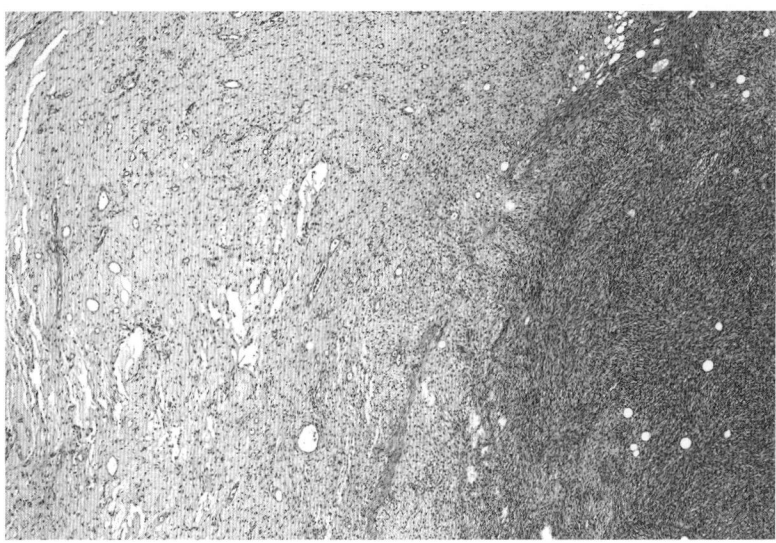

Fig. 35.138
Giant cell fibroblastoma: this lesion merges imperceptibly with typical dermatofibrosarcoma protuberans on the right side of the field.

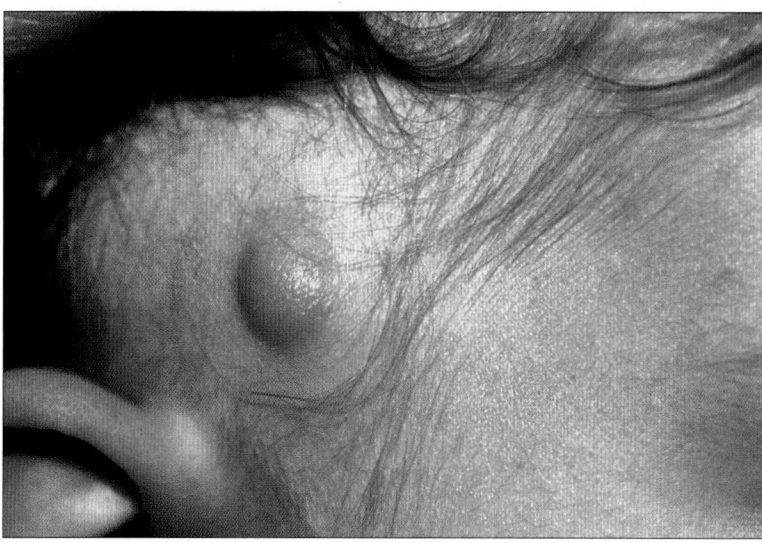

Fig. 35.140
Dermatofibrosarcoma protuberans: congenital lesions as shown here are exceedingly rare. By courtesy of the Institute of Dermatology, London, UK.

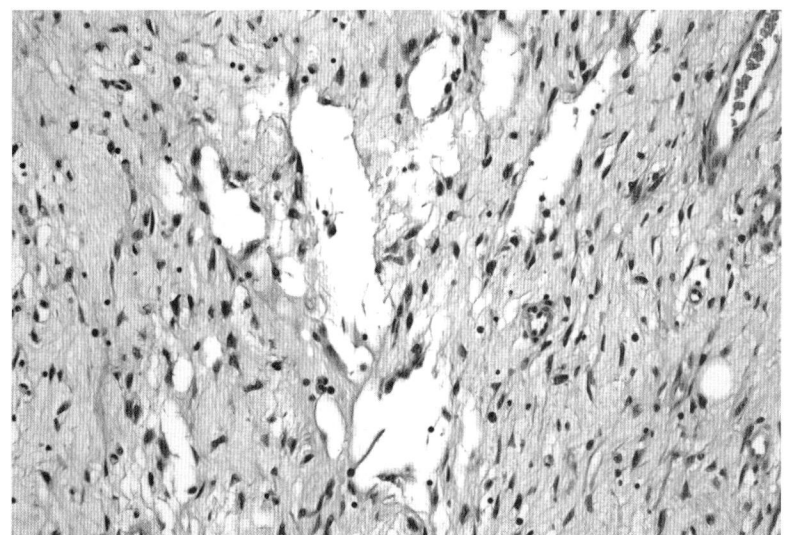

Fig. 35.139
Giant cell fibroblastoma: higher-power view of the left side of the field showing typical features.

cell fibroblastoma may recur as dermatofibrosarcoma protuberans and vice versa.[18,19] Bednár tumor (pigmented dermatofibrosarcoma protuberans) may also present primarily or recur with areas of giant cell fibroblastoma.[20,21] Mixed tumors may have fibrosarcomatous areas and myoid nodules.[7]

Differential diagnosis

Distinction from other myxoid tumors is readily made based on the biphasic appearance of solid and angiectoid areas with giant cells. Fibrous hamartoma of infancy may rarely show areas resembling giant cell fibroblastoma and in these areas tumor cells are also positive for CD34.[22] The diagnosis is usually established by the presence of the distinctive components seen in fibrous hamartoma of infancy.

Intermediate (rarely metastasizing) fibroblastic and myofibroblastic tumors

Low-grade malignant lesions are defined as neoplasms with a high recurrence rate and very low metastatic potential.

Dermatofibrosarcoma protuberans

Clinical features

Dermatofibrosarcoma protuberans typically presents in the third and fourth decades, shows a slight male predominance and is uncommon in the elderly.[1–5] However, many patients have a long preoperative history (often 10–20 years), probably corresponding to the plaque phase. In these patients a patch develops and may have features resembling morphea, atrophoderma, or an angioma.[6] Lesions can occur in children and some of these are congenital (*Fig. 35.140*).[1,4,7–17] Clinical diagnosis in this age group is difficult, as tumors often resemble a vascular birthmark.[6] Occurrence at sites of previous trauma (including scars, vaccination, an arteriovenous fistula, a decorative tattoo and leishmaniasis) and even post-radiation tumors have been documented.[18–25] Familial cases are exceptional and an association with HIV infection is probably coincidental.[26,27] Accelerated growth during pregnancy has been reported in a case.[27] Rare (probably coincidental) associations include multiple spindle cell lipomas and a nuchal fibroma.[28,29]

The tumor usually develops as a multinodular cutaneous mass, several centimeters in diameter that is slowly growing and appears to evolve from a dermal fibrous plaque stage. The overlying skin frequently shows a reddish-blue discoloration (*Figs 35.141–35.143*). Presentation as an atrophic plaque is seen in some cases (*Fig. 35.144*).[30,31] Polypoid tumors are exceptionally seen.[32] There is a marked predilection for the trunk (especially the abdominal wall and chest) and lower limbs (particularly the thighs). Involvement of distal extremities is very uncommon with most tumors developing on the foot (mainly the toes) and ankle and hardly any on the hands.[33–36] Rare tumors occur in the vulva and exceptional cases have been reported in the oral cavity, penis, and male breast.[37–45] Simultaneous occurrence of two tumors at different sites has been documented. Multicentric dermatofibrosarcoma protuberans in patients with adenosine deaminase-deficient severe combined immune deficiency has been documented.[46,47]

Purely subcutaneous tumors rarely occur and seem to have a predilection for head and neck.[48,49]

Local recurrence is frequent and varies in different series from 20% to 50% of cases.[1,5,50–56] However, in cases treated by wide excision or in those treated by Mohs micrographic surgery the rate of local recurrence is lower.[57–62] A frequent subject of debate is how wide the excision has to be to reduce the rate of local recurrence. Although the tendency in the past was to advocate several excisions with margins of several centimeters, more recent studies suggest that smaller excision margins of 2 cm achieve good local control in many cases.[63] Treatment with Mohs micrographic surgery using paraffin sections appears to be an excellent choice of treatment, allowing tissue conservation.[64] Other therapeutic options include excision

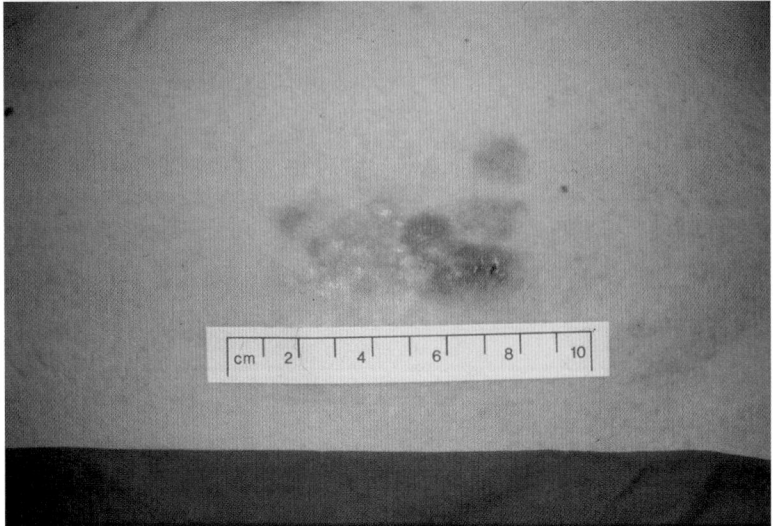

Fig. 35.141
Dermatofibrosarcoma protuberans: a typical multinodular reddish-blue plaque is present on the lower abdomen of a middle-aged female. By courtesy of M.H.A. Rustin, MD, Royal Free Hospital, London, UK.

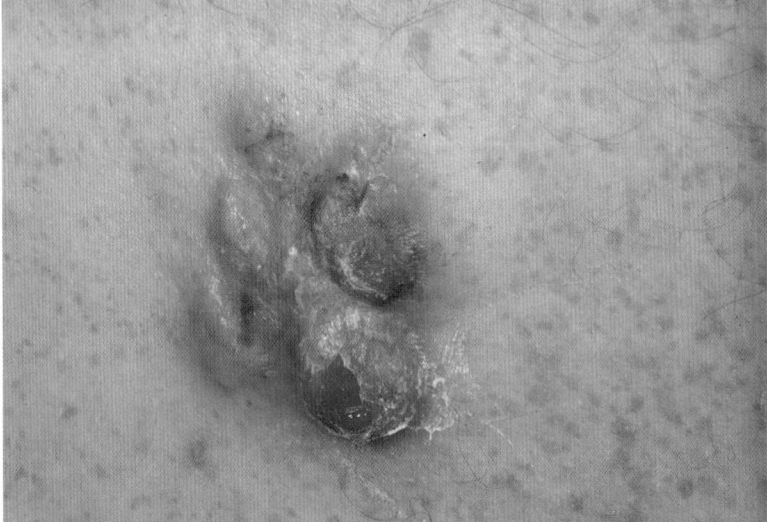

Fig. 35.142
Dermatofibrosarcoma protuberans: close-up view. By courtesy of M.H.A. Rustin, MD, Royal Free Hospital, London, UK.

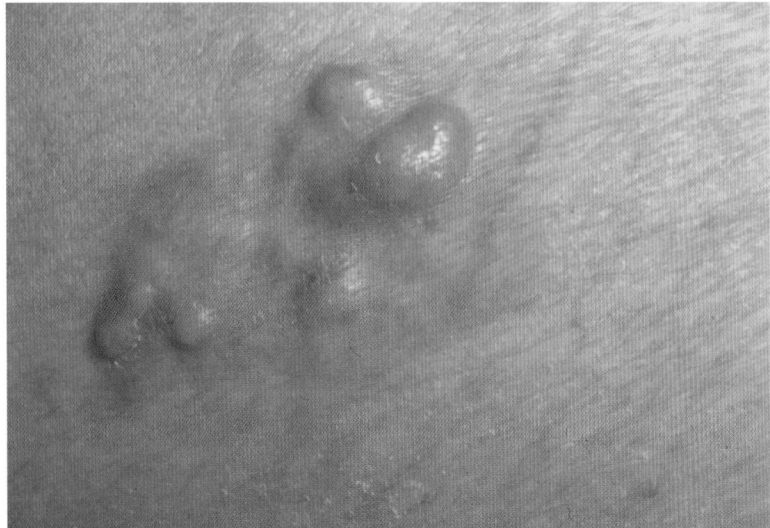

Fig. 35.143
Dermatofibrosarcoma protuberans: this example shows a combination of a plaque and nodules. By courtesy of the Institute of Dermatology, London, UK.

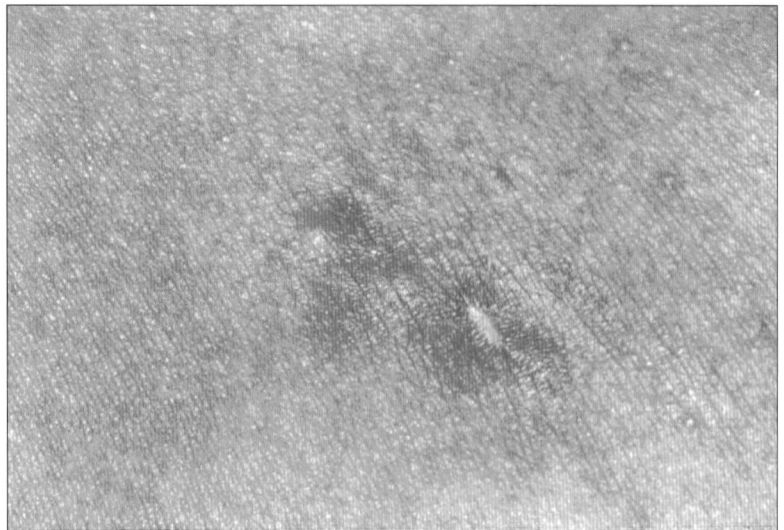

Fig. 35.144
Dermatofibrosarcoma protuberans: presentation as an atrophic plaque is rare. By courtesy of the Institute of Dermatology, London, UK.

with wide margins with or without radiotherapy, depending on the margin status. For recurrent or metastatic tumors, targeted therapy may be of help (see below). A multidisciplinary approach is the best option when dealing with challenging cases.[63–76] Intracranial invasion may occur in scalp lesions mainly after multiple recurrences.[77] Metastasis is exceedingly rare, less than 0.3% in our experience; many of the cases reported to have metastasized are supported by inadequate or even incorrect histologic evidence. Metastasis usually occurs after repeated recurrences, often with fibrosarcomatous transformation.[1–3,78–82] Fibrosarcomatous dermatofibrosarcoma protuberans recurs locally in 75% and the rate of metastasis is up to 23% of cases in some series.[78,79,83–85] However, in a more recent series, the rate of local recurrence (20%) and metastatic rate (10%) is much less than that reported in the past.[83] Aggressive behavior appears is suggested to be related to mitotic activity, pleomorphism and necrosis.[57,78,79,87]

Pathogenesis and histologic features

The genetic abnormalities found in dermatofibrosarcoma protuberans and giant cell fibroblastoma are identical, further indicating that they represent a spectrum.[88–90] As expected, other histologic variants of dermatofibrosarcoma protuberans – including Bednár tumor, dermatofibrosarcoma protuberans with granular cell change and fibrosarcomatous dermatofibrosarcoma protuberans – show the same cytogenetic abnormalities.[91–99] Ring chromosomes derived from chromosome 22 containing low-level amplified sequences from 17q22-qter and 22q10-q13.1 or t(17;22) are the most frequent finding.[90] In both the rings and linear der(22) a specific fusion of *COL1A1* and *PDGFB* is found. Ring chromosomes are mainly observed in adults, whereas translocations are present in all pediatric cases.[90] The breakpoint localization in *PDGFB* is remarkably constant, placing exon 2 under control of the *COL1A1* promoter. In contrast, the *COL1A1* breakpoint is variably located within the exons of the α-helical coding region (exons 6–49).[90,95–97]

Evidence of the *COL1A1-PDGFB* fusion by multiplex reverse transcription polymerase chain reaction or fluorescence in situ hybridization assays is present in almost all cases.[90,95–97,100]

A recent study of ordinary DFSP and tumors with fibrosarcomatous transformation suggested an association between the activation of the Akt-mTOR pathway proteins and PDGFR with progression from ordinary DFSP to fibrosarcomatous DFSP.[101] A case of fibrosarcomatous DFSP expressing programmed death-ligand 1 (PD-L1) in the metastasis but not in the primary tumor has been reported.[102]

Clonal evolution consisting of different somatic mutations and novel focal amplifications, has been found in metastatic samples but no in those obtained before metastasis is a single patient.[103] In a further study, no significant copy number alterations, insertion, or deletions was observed during imatinib treatment response.[104] However, emergence of 8 new

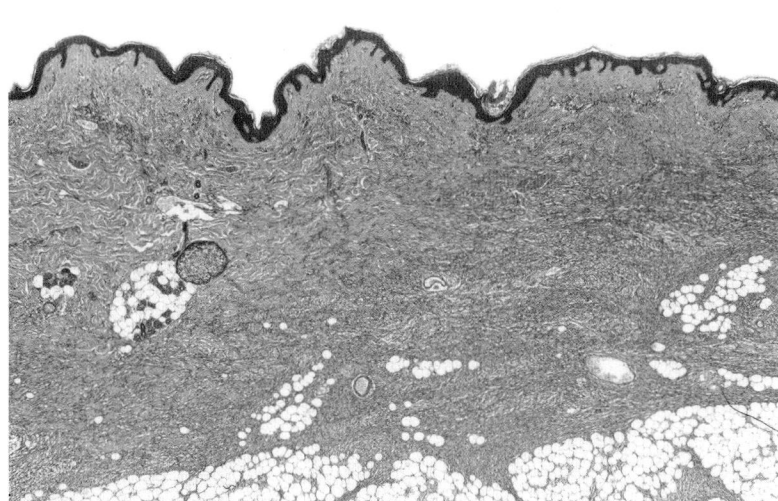

Fig. 35.145
Dermatofibrosarcoma protuberans: the lower dermis is replaced by a dense cellular infiltrate. In contrast to fibrous histiocytoma, the epidermis appears normal.

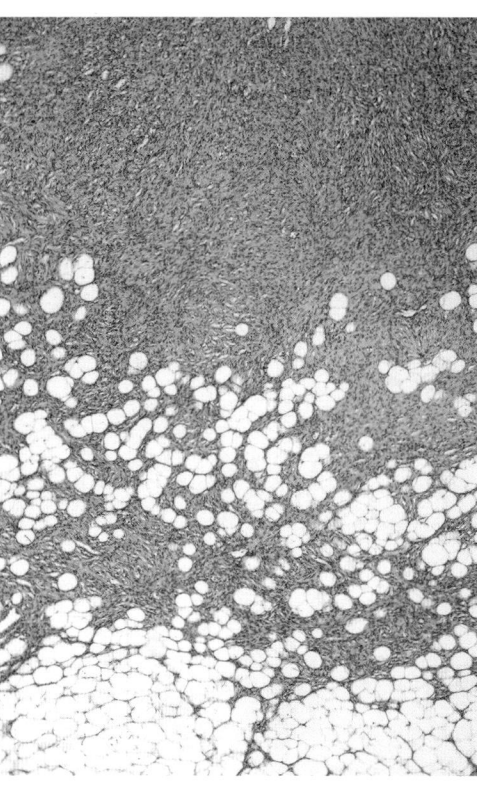

Fig. 35.146
Dermatofibrosarcoma protuberans: involvement of the subcutaneous fat is usual and typically results in a lace-like appearance.

non-synonymous somatic gene mutations in imatinib-resistant tumor tissue was identified.

PDGFB appears to act as a mitogen in tumor cells of dermatofibrosarcoma protuberans by autocrine stimulation of the *PDGF* receptor. Interestingly, imatinib mesylate (an antagonist of the *PDGF* receptor α tyrosine kinase) has been found to have an inhibitory effect in vivo and has been used with variable success in multiple cases of dermatofibrosarcoma protuberans (mainly in patients with unresectable or recurrent tumors and those with metastatic disease).[90,105-109] The rate of response has been estimated to be up to 50%.[110]

A single case of dermatofibrosarcoma protuberans-like tumor with COL1A1 copy number gain without t(17;22) has been described. In this case, tumor cells were positive for CD3 and H-caldesmon and very focally positive for EMA and SMA.[111]

The microscopic appearances vary little from case to case. The tumor is located in the dermis, but invariably shows diffuse irregular infiltration of the subcutaneous fat in a typical lace-like pattern or bundles of cells which ramify parallel to the epidermis (*Figs 35.145* and *35.146*). Rare cases may be mainly or exclusively subcutaneous.[48,49,112] Epidermal hyperplasia is very rare but does occur and the degree of hyperplasia seems to be inversely related to the distance of the tumor from the epidermis.[113]

The lesion is composed almost entirely of fairly uniform spindled cells with elongated nuclei showing little or no pleomorphism and scanty pale cytoplasm. The cells are characteristically arranged in a storiform or 'rush mat' pattern typified by numerous whorls of cells, sometimes centered around small blood vessels (*Figs 35.147–35.149*).

Mitotic activity, rarely abnormal in appearance, is scanty, not usually exceeding five mitoses per 10 high-power fields. Peripheral collections of chronic inflammatory cells are sometimes present, as are foci of myxoid degeneration, but necrosis is rarely a feature and is always minimal (*Fig. 35.150*). Cytological polymorphism is not a feature except in those infrequent cases showing overlap with giant cell fibroblastoma. However, in some cases, occasional nonpleomorphic giant cells are present. Focal histologic variation may be seen and includes areas of sclerosis, palisading, formation of Verocay-like bodies, granular cell change, meningothelial-like whorls and pseudocystic spaces.[114-120] In a case treated with imatinib mesylate prominent hyalinized collagen was seen.[121]

Immunohistochemically, tumor cells are usually diffusely positive for CD34 and negative for other markers including factor XIIIa, S100 protein, desmin, actin and, with rare exceptions, CD117 (*Fig. 35.151*).[122-124] Staining for EMA has been reported and, based on this finding, a perineural line of differentiation has been suggested although this marker is not specific.[125]

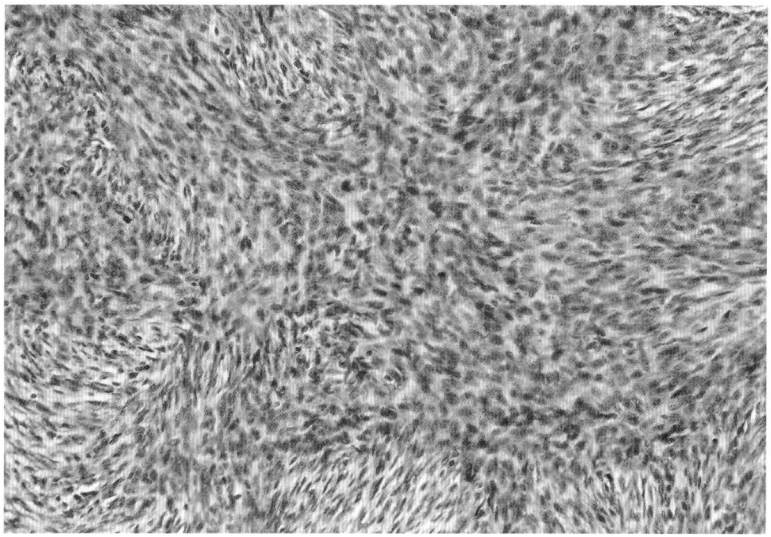

Fig. 35.147
Dermatofibrosarcoma protuberans: this field shows the characteristic storiform (*L. storia*, a rush mat) pattern.

CD99 is also positive in a number of cases.[126] Stromelysin, cathepsin K and D2–40 have been reported as useful markers in the differential diagnosis between dermatofibroma and dermatofibrosarcoma protuberans, as they tend to be positive in the former and negative in the latter.[127-129] Cthrc1 (collagen triple helix repeat containing-1) and Apo D, on the other hand, tend to be positive in dermatofibrosarcoma protuberans and negative in dermatofibroma.[130,131] Other markers that have been reported as useful in dermatofibrosarcoma protuberans include low-affinity nerve growth factor receptor (p75) and tenascin.[132] Tumor cells in dermatofibroma and dermatofibrosarcoma protuberans show positive staining with tenascin but staining of the dermal–epidermal junction overlying the tumor is only seen in dermatofibroma.[133]

Although the line of differentiation in dermatofibrosarcoma protuberans has been controversial for many years, it is increasingly being accepted as a fibroblastic tumor (*Figs 35.152* and *35.153*).[134,135]

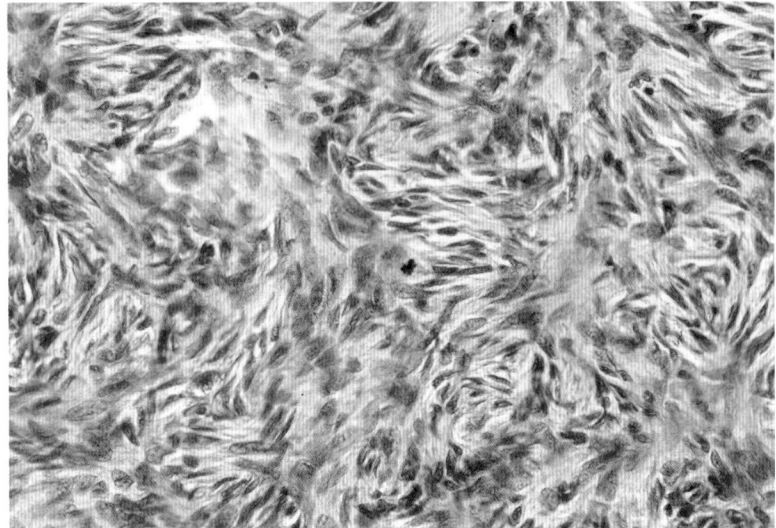

Fig. 35.148
Dermatofibrosarcoma protuberans: the storiform pattern comprises a central, almost syncytial, arrangement of cells with vesicular nuclei from which radiate the more delicate spindle cells with elongated darkly staining nuclei. Taken in context, this appearance is pathognomonic. Note the mitotic figure.

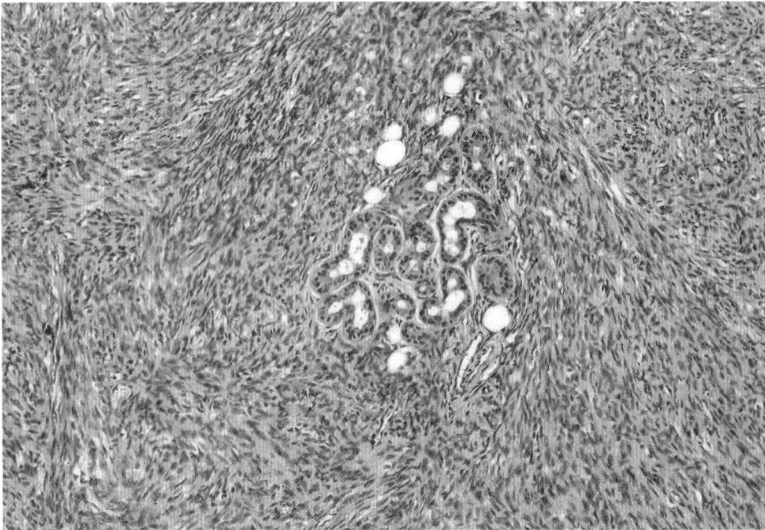

Fig. 35.149
Dermatofibrosarcoma protuberans: adnexal sparing is typically seen.

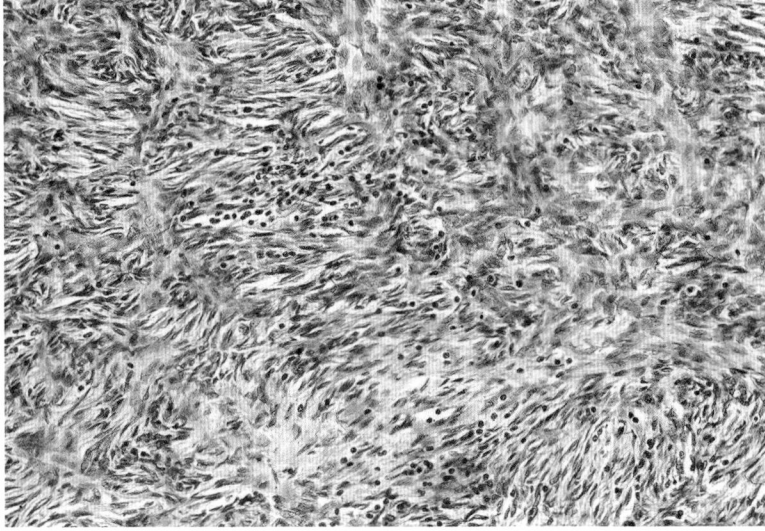

Fig. 35.150
Dermatofibrosarcoma protuberans: a diffuse lymphocytic infiltrate is present in this field.

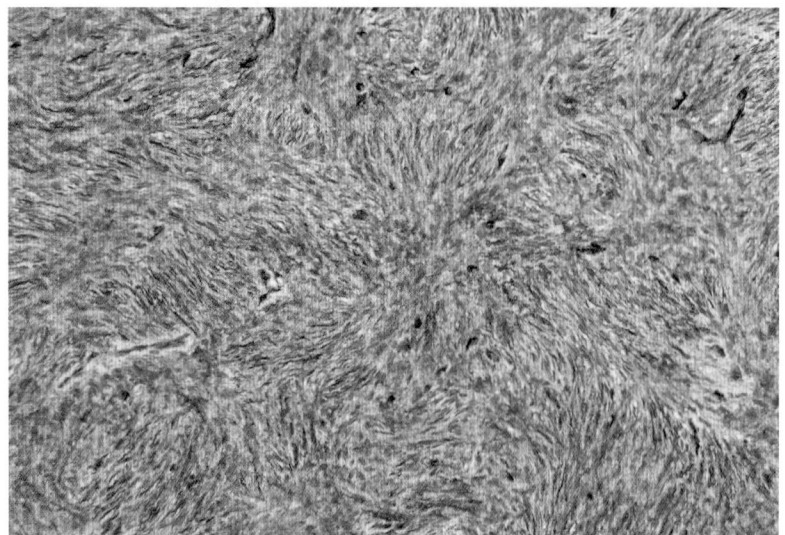

Fig. 35.151
Dermatofibrosarcoma protuberans: the tumor cells characteristically express CD34.

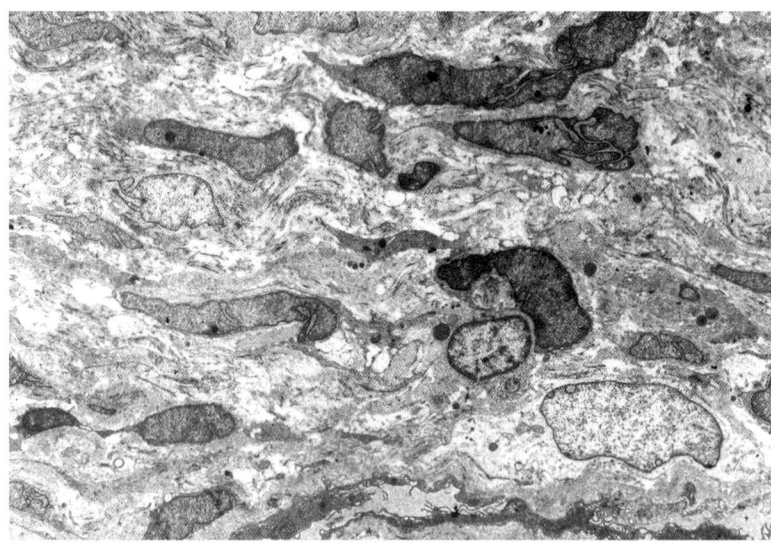

Fig. 35.152
Dermatofibrosarcoma protuberans: the tumor consists of a uniform population of fibroblasts typified by elongated nuclei and abundant rough endoplasmic reticulum.

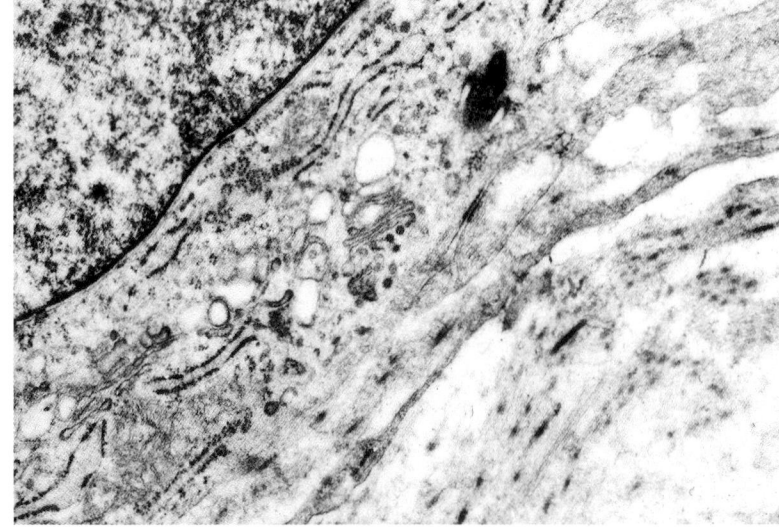

Fig. 35.153
Dermatofibrosarcoma protuberans: myofibroblastic differentiation is not a feature of this tumor.

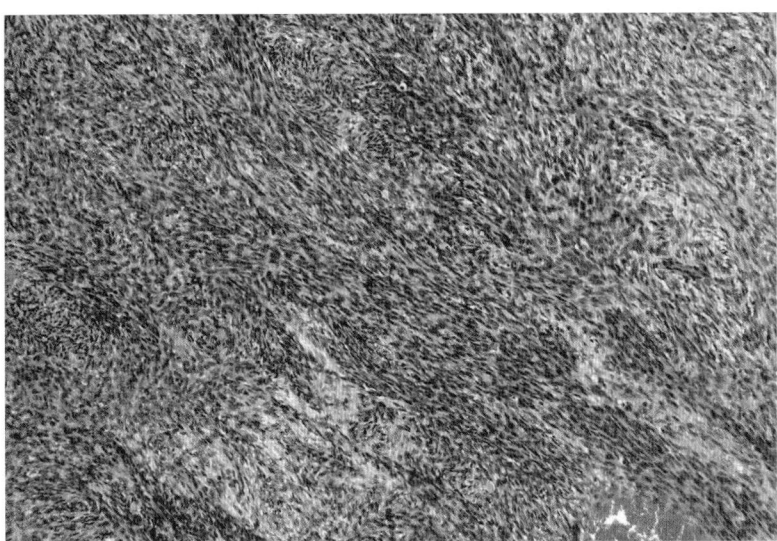

Fig. 35.154
Dermatofibrosarcoma protuberans: this is an example of fibrosarcomatous change. Note the characteristic herringbone pattern.

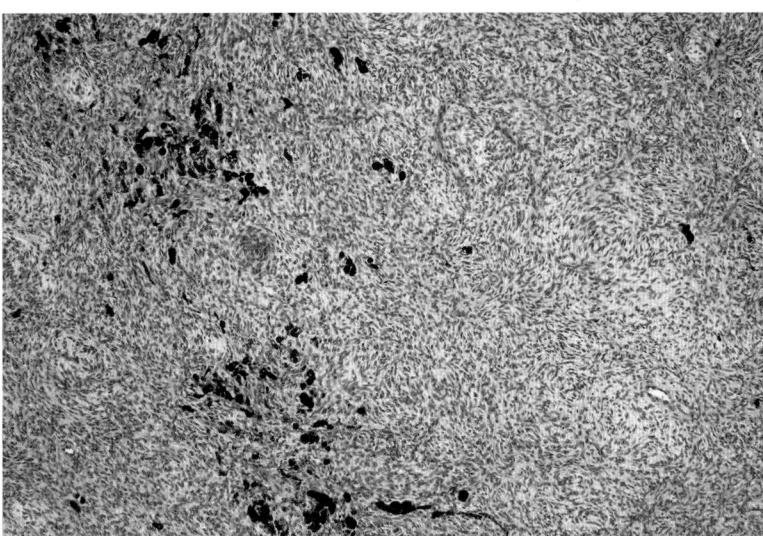

Fig. 35.156
Bednár tumor: except for the foci of pigmented cells, the appearances are identical to those of dermatofibrosarcoma protuberans.

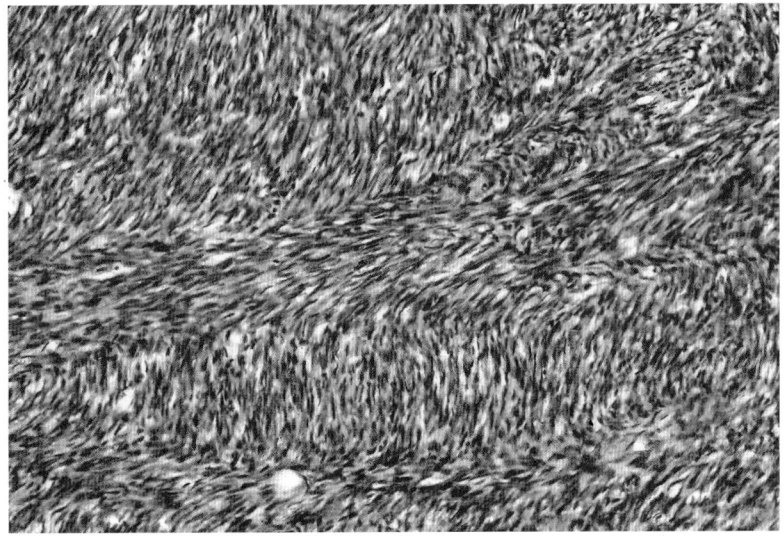

Fig. 35.155
Dermatofibrosarcoma protuberans: high-power view.

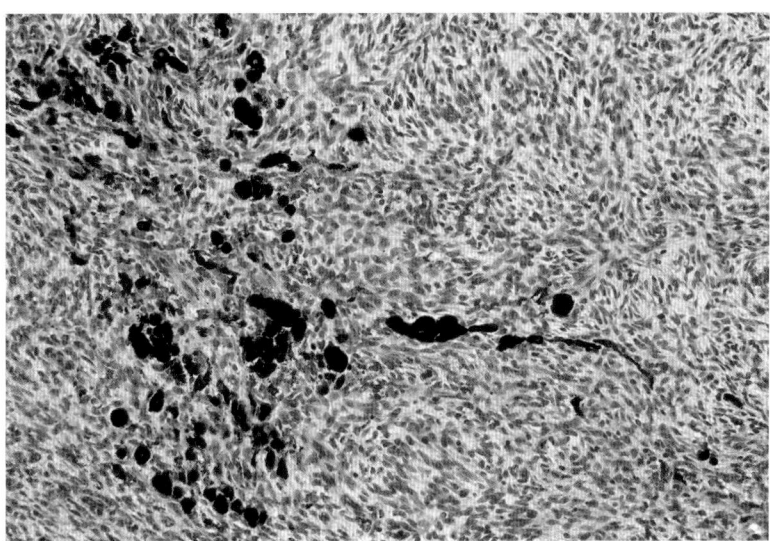

Fig. 35.157
Bednár tumor: the melanin pigment is contained within dendritic cells.

Fibrosarcomatous dermatofibrosarcoma

Fibrosarcomatous dermatofibrosarcoma is a variant in which a focal fascicular or 'herring-bone' pattern is present.[62–64,80] Fibrosarcomatous transformation may occur either de novo or in the recurrence of a typical dermatofibrosarcoma protuberans. These areas are more cellular, show more nuclear atypia and the mean mitotic count is higher than in typical dermatofibrosarcoma (*Figs 35.154* and *35.155*). Focal loss or less intense staining with CD34 is seen in the fibrosarcomatous areas.[86] Fibrosarcomatous dermatofibrosarcoma combined with Bednár may occur.[136] A case with formation of giant rosettes and one with a plexiform growth pattern have been reported.[137,138]

Progression in dermatofibrosarcoma protuberans to the fibrosarcomatous variant appears to be related to microsatellite instability and mutations in *TP53* as early and late events respectively.[139]

In rare cases, areas of a high-grade sarcoma may be found within an otherwise ordinary dermatofibrosarcoma protuberans.[140–144] These areas can mimic a myxofibrosarcoma or a pleomorphic malignant fibrous histiocytoma. It is not clear what the prognosis of these tumors is, as the occurrence of this phenomenon is very rare. Interestingly COL1A1-PDGFB fusion transcripts is also detected in sarcomatous areas of the tumor.[144]

Pigmented dermatofibrosarcoma

Pigmented dermatofibrosarcoma (also known as the Bednár tumor or formerly as pigmented storiform neurofibroma) contains dendritic melanocytes and small deposits of melanin pigment within an otherwise typical tumor (*Figs 35.156* and *35.157*).[145–147] The presence of melanocytes within the tumor is puzzling and is probably secondary to colonization. An alternative view proposes neuroectodermal multidirectional differentiation to explain this phenomenon.[148]

Myxoid dermatofibrosarcoma

Myxoid dermatofibrosarcoma is a term used to describe rare cases in which the more typical features may be only focally identifiable because of extensive myxoid degeneration (*Figs 35.158–35.160*).[149–151] Macroscopically, tumors are gelatinous. Thin-walled blood vessels are prominent. Myxoid change may occur in association with any variant of the tumor.[152]

Dermatofibrosarcoma with areas of giant cell fibroblastoma

Dermatofibrosarcoma with areas of giant cell fibroblastoma has already been discussed.

Fig. 35.158
Myxoid dermatofibrosarcoma protuberans: myxoid areas, as seen here, are nondiagnostic and therefore may cause confusion. A careful search should be made for more typical foci.

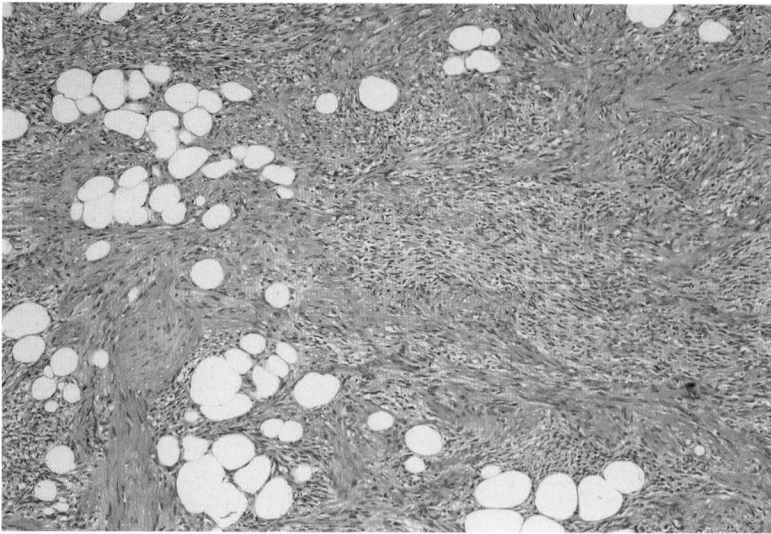

Fig. 35.161
Dermatofibrosarcoma protuberans: some tumors, particularly the fibrosarcomatous variant, contain nodules and bundles of myofibroblasts (the myoid variant).

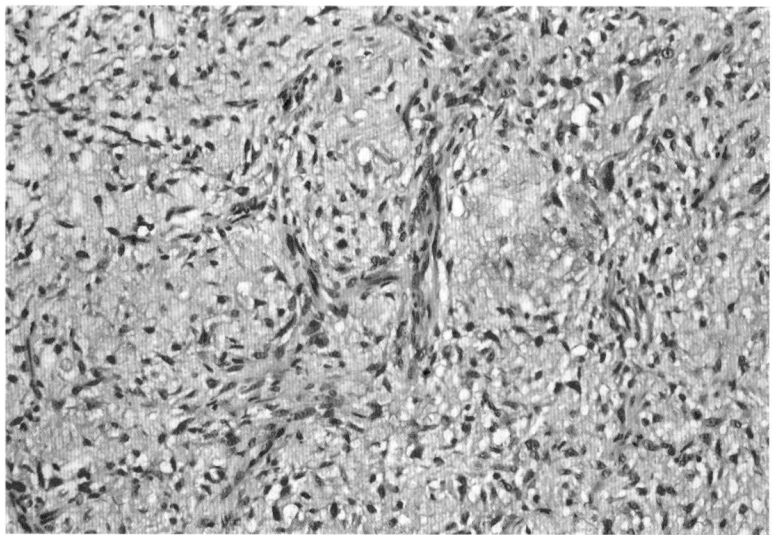

Fig. 35.159
Myxoid dermatofibrosarcoma protuberans: high-power view.

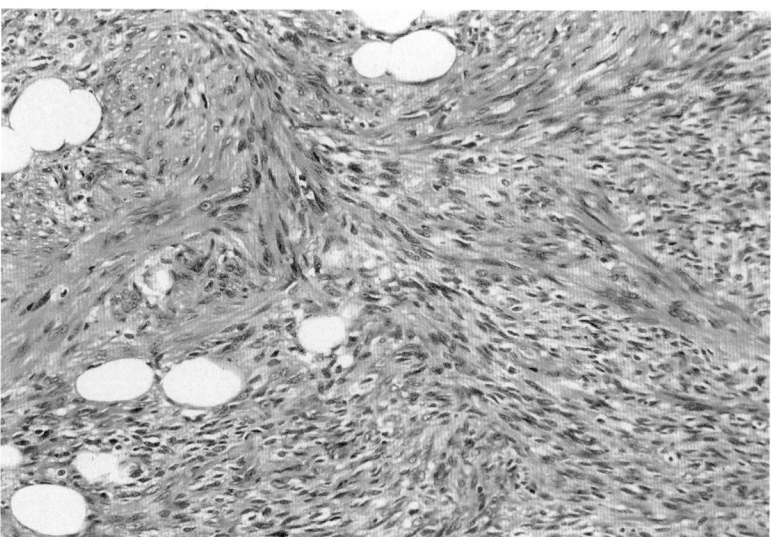

Fig. 35.162
Dermatofibrosarcoma protuberans: high-power view of Figure 35.170.

Dermatofibrosarcoma with myoid nodules

Dermatofibrosarcoma with myoid nodules refers to cases showing areas composed of bundles of eosinophilic SMA-positive spindle, desmin-negative cells indicating myofibroblastic differentiation (Figs 35.161 and 35.162).[153,154] Most cases of dermatofibrosarcoma protuberans with myoid nodules have fibrosarcomatous areas.[153,154] Small biopsies can cause confusion with myofibroblastic lesions, such as adult myofibroma, but other typical features of dermatofibrosarcoma are usually evident. It has been suggested that the myoid nodules do not represent true myofibroblastic differentiation but rather residual smooth muscle originating from blood vessels destroyed by the tumor.[155] However, the bundles of myoid cells are usually positive for actin and negative for desmin and H-caldesmon, suggesting myofibroblastic rather than smooth muscle origin/differentiation.

Flow cytometry studies in dermatofibrosarcoma protuberans often show aneuploidy.[156]

Differential diagnosis

The differential diagnosis includes fibrous histiocytoma, especially its cellular variant, dermatomyofibroma, perineurioma, plaque-like CD34-positive dermal fibroma (medallion-like dermal dendrocyte hamartoma) and neurofibroma (mainly in the superficial part of the tumor). Fibrous histiocytoma tends to be CD34 negative, shows cytological polymorphism, only a

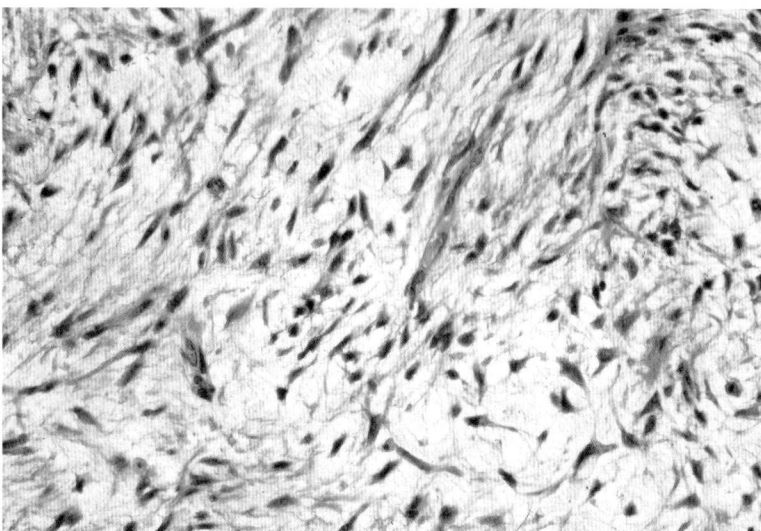

Fig. 35.160
Myxoid dermatofibrosarcoma protuberans: high-power view from a different case showing complete loss of the storiform growth pattern.

focal storiform pattern and limited superficial infiltration of the subcutis, usually in a radial pattern.[157] Epidermal changes (especially hyperplasia) are much more commonly associated with fibrous histiocytoma than with dermatofibrosarcoma protuberans. Cellular fibrous histiocytoma may show positivity for CD34 but this is often in the periphery of the tumor and associated with focal staining for SMA. Plaque-like CD34-positive dermal fibroma (medallion-like dermal dendrocyte hamartoma) has to be distinguished from the plaque stage of dermatofibrosarcoma protuberans.[158,159] The former occurs predominantly but not exclusively in children, is a neoplasm of the reticular dermis that tends not to extend to the subcutaneous tissue and consists of CD34-positive fibroblast-like cells with superficial cells oriented perpendicular to the epidermis and deep cells oriented parallel to the epidermis. The superficial part of a dermatofibrosarcoma protuberans may mimic neurofibroma, as the storiform pattern is usually lacking, and this is a particular problem in superficial samples.[160] Immunohistochemistry for CD34 and S100 is crucial as the latter is positive for both markers and the former positive for CD34. It has been suggested that there is a small subgroup of indeterminate fibrohistiocytic tumors of the skin in which it is not possible to distinguish accurately between dermatofibrosarcoma protuberans and fibrous histiocytoma because of histologic and immunohistochemical overlap; however, these tumors lack the *COL1A1-PDGFB* fusion transcript.[161,162] Distinction between neurofibroma and the myxoid variant of dermatofibrosarcoma is based on the storiform growth pattern, CD34 expression and S100 protein negative cells in the latter condition.

Myxoinflammatory fibroblastic sarcoma

Clinical features

Myxoinflammatory fibroblastic sarcoma (acral myxoinflammatory fibroblastic sarcoma, inflammatory myxohyaline tumor, inflammatory myxoid tumor of the soft parts with bizarre giant cells) is a distinctive, rare, low-grade tumor with marked predilection for the hands (around 80% of tumors mainly affecting fingers) and to a much lesser extent, the feet.[1–5] The ankles and wrists may also be involved and, rarely, tumors have been described on the forearm, upper arm, thigh, chest wall, face and nose.[6–10] Most tumors present in middle-aged adults, with exceptional lesions occurring in children and adolescents.[7] Tumors present as a slowly growing, ill-defined, dermal and subcutaneous (usually asymptomatic) mass measuring between 1 and 6 cm, and there is no sex predilection.[1,5,7] Larger tumors may also be seen.[4] An intramuscular location has rarely been reported.[5,11,12] Pain is an occasional symptom. The clinical diagnosis is usually an inflammatory process, a ganglion cyst or a giant cell tumor of tendon sheath. A case occurred in a renal transplant patient.[13] Local recurrences are seen in 22% to 67% of cases and may occur many years after the primary tumor has been excised. Regional lymph node metastasis has been reported in rare cases and distant metastases are exceptional, with only one patient dying of disease.[14–16]

Pathogenesis and histologic features

Cytogenetic studies have shown a t(1;10) with rearrangements of *TGFBR3* and/or *MGEA5* in about 18% of cases.[17,18] No functional fusion transcript is formed from the translocation, but upregulation of both *FGF8* and *NMP3*, two genes in the vicinity of *MGEA5*, does occur. Loss of material from chromosome 3 has also been reported and in rare individual cases further abnormalities include a t(2;6)(q31;p21) translocation, a complex karyotype one with supernumerary ring chromosomes composed of chromosome 3 material and one with duplication of chromosomes X and 19.[19–21] Based on morphological similarities and some cytogenetic studies it has been suggested that there is a relationship between myxoinflammatory fibroblastic sarcoma, hemosiderotic fibrolipomatous tumor and pleomorphic hyalinizing angiectatic tumor.[22–28] This view however, is not universally accepted.[18] Although it seems clear that hemosiderotic fibrolipomatous tumor and pleomorphic hyalinizing angiectatic tumor are related, it is not clear whether the latter two neoplasms are related to myxoinflammatory fibroblastic sarcoma. Furthermore, recurrent *BRAF* gene rearrangements have been recently found in myxoinflammatory fibroblastic sarcomas, but not in hemosiderotic fibrolipomatous tumors.[29]

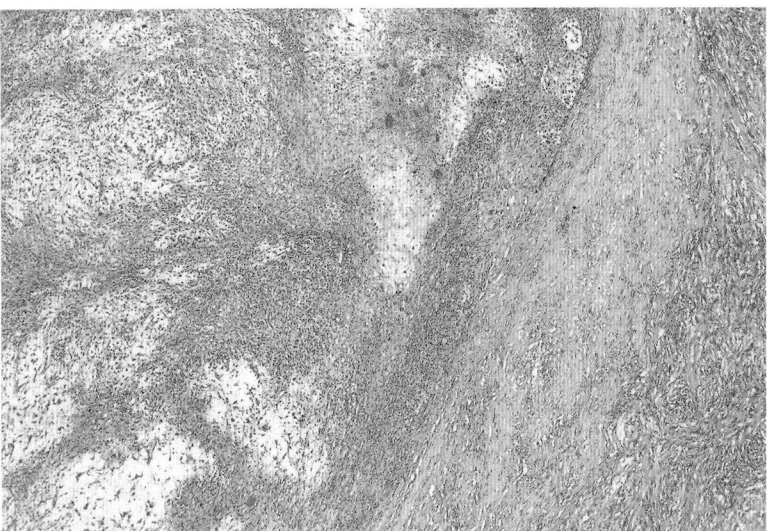

Fig. 35.163
Acral myxoinflammatory fibroblastic sarcoma: within the dermis is a multinodular tumor with striking myxoid change.

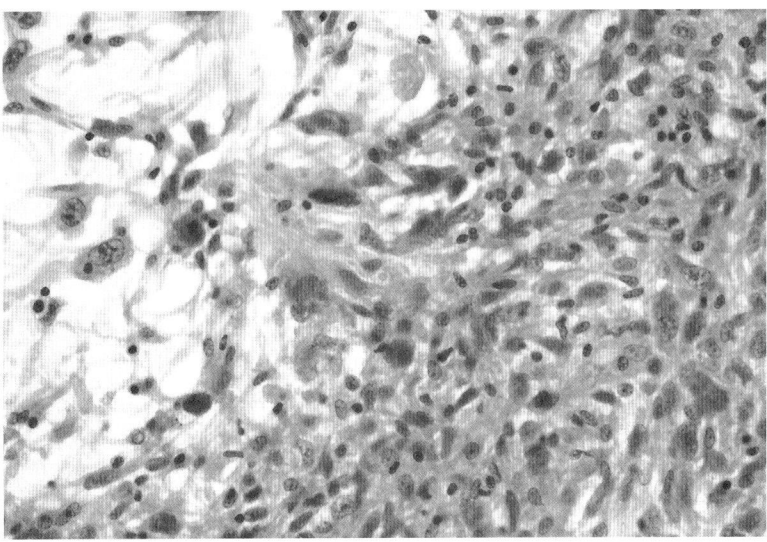

Fig. 35.164
Acral myxoinflammatory fibroblastic sarcoma: this lesion consists of stellate and histiocyte-like cells with scattered mononuclear inflammatory cells dispersed within the myxoid stroma.

Histology shows a multinodular and poorly circumscribed tumor with prominent myxoid change and focal areas of hyalinization (*Figs 35.163–35.165*). In the background, there are neutrophils, eosinophils, lymphocytes, plasma cells and variable numbers of pleomorphic mono- or multinucleated large cells with vesicular or hyperchromatic nuclei. These cells often have a prominent inclusion-like nucleolus. They may mimic ganglion cells, Reed-Sternberg cells or lipoblasts, and are sometimes masked by the intense inflammatory cell infiltrate. Hemosiderin deposition can be prominent. Mitotic figures, although present, are not conspicuous.

Tumor cells are positive for SMA, CD68, CD163, D240 and CD34. They may be focally positive for EMA and keratins; positivity for EGFR, D2-40 and S100 has also been reported.[4,5]

Differential diagnosis

Acral myxoinflammatory fibroblastic sarcoma is most likely to be mistaken for an inflammatory condition but the presence of bizarre tumor cells should alert the pathologist to the correct diagnosis. Distinction from myxofibrosarcoma is based on the absence of prominent inflammation in the latter condition and also the knowledge that myxofibrosarcoma is very rare on

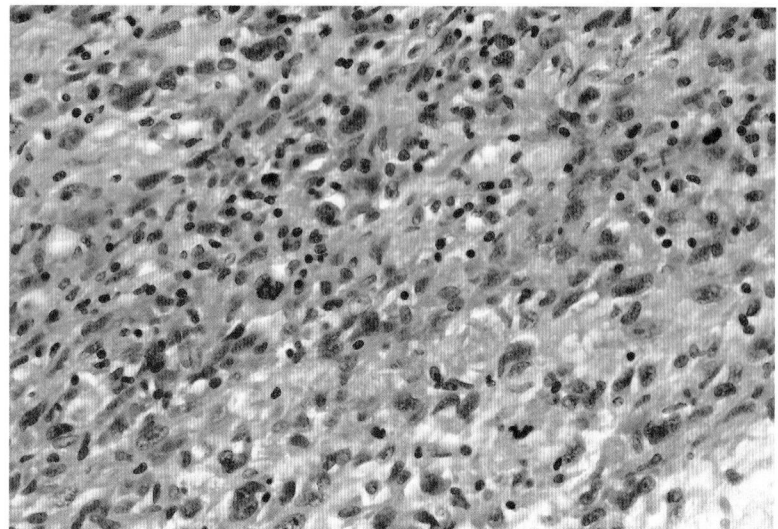

Fig. 35.165
Acral myxoinflammatory fibroblastic sarcoma: high-power view showing tumor cells with admixed lymphocytes and conspicuous eosinophils.

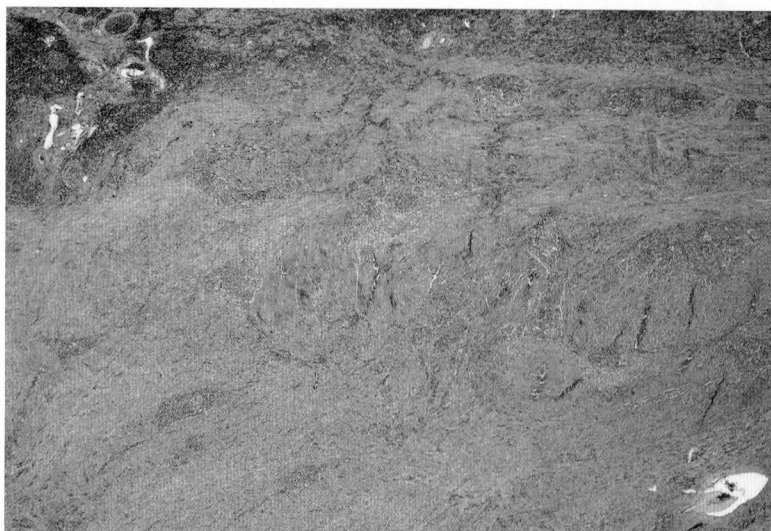

Fig. 35.166
Inflammatory myofibroblastic tumor: low-power view showing tumor, a heavy lymphocytic infiltrate, and background scar tissue.

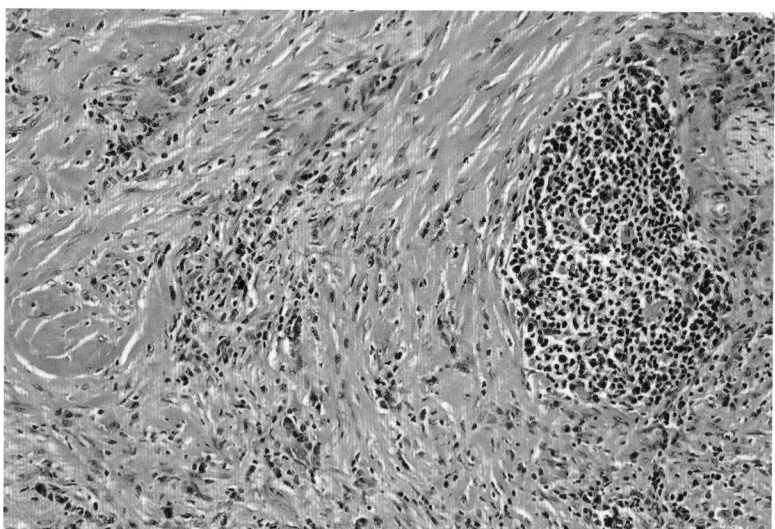

Fig. 35.167
Inflammatory myofibroblastic tumor: medium-power view with conspicuous myofibroblasts.

the hands and feet. Epithelioid sarcoma may enter the differential diagnosis. It often has areas of necrosis, tumor cells are epithelioid or short and spindled, and keratin is consistently positive.

Inflammatory myofibroblastic tumor

Clinical features

Inflammatory myofibroblastic tumor (inflammatory fibrosarcoma, inflammatory pseudotumor) is a term that includes a heterogeneous group of lesions characterized by proliferation of fibroblasts and myofibroblasts in a background of numerous inflammatory cells.[1-3] Most cases occur in children, usually in visceral organs (particularly the lung but also in the liver, heart, gastrointestinal tract, pancreas and urinary bladder), mesentery, omentum and (less commonly) the soft tissues (limbs and head and neck).[1-5] Oral, laryngeal, bone and lymph node lesions may also occur.[6-9] The tumor presents less frequently in young adults but is exceptional after the age of 30. Comparable examples in the skin have only exceptionally been reported.[4,10,11] Systemic symptoms including high erythrocyte sedimentation rate (ESR), anemia, fever and weight loss occur in up to 30% of cases. Rare associations include obliterative phlebitis and dermatomyositis.[12,13] Intestinal obstruction may be the cause of presentation in intra-abdominal tumors. Rare tumors have been described at the site of a tooth extraction and at the location of a pace maker.[14,15] The prognosis is good in most cases but local recurrences and exceptional metastasis occur.[16]

Excision is the most effective treatment. Targeted therapies seem promising.[17-19]

Epithelioid inflammatory myofibroblastic sarcoma is an aggressive variant of inflammatory myofibroblastic tumor with the ALK fused to *RANBP2* leading to a nuclear membrane or perinuclear distribution of ALK on immunohistochemistry.[20-24] It occurs in young adults, usually intra-abdominally and shows male predilection.[20]

Pathogenesis and histologic features

Rearrangement of the anaplastic lymphoma kinase (ALK) gene has been detected in more than half of inflammatory myofibroblastic tumors.[25-28] Immunohistochemical reactivity for the ALK protein is demonstrated in these tumors. In a subset of ALK negative tumors gene rearrangements and fusions in *ROS1*, *PDGFRB*, *ETV6*, *NTRK3* have also been documented.[29-32] Immunohistochemical expression of ROS1 correlates with *ROS1* gene rearrangements.[33]

Histologically the tumors are well circumscribed and those presenting in the skin are located in the deep dermis or subcutis. The proportion of fibroblasts/myofibroblasts varies among tumors. Lesions have prominent or moderate cellularity with a myxoid background or appear fairly hypocellular with areas of sclerosis and hyalinization often simulating a scar (*Fig. 35.166*). Focally, tumor cells have a histiocyte-like or Reed-Sternberg appearance and may resemble ganglion cells. In most tumors there is a variable mixed inflammatory cell infiltrate composed of numerous plasma cells, lymphocytes, histiocytes, neutrophils, eosinophils and occasional giant cells (*Figs 35.167* and *35.168*). Rare lesions do not display prominent inflammation. Germinal centers and proliferation of high endothelial venules may be a feature and, on low-power examination, lesions sometimes vaguely resemble a lymph node.

Tumor cells are usually positive for smooth muscle actin, muscle specific actin and calponin.[34] Focal desmin and cytokeratin positivity has also been reported and in up to 50% of cases there is cytoplasmic and less often nuclear positivity for anaplastic lymphoma kinase (ALK-1) which correlates with rearrangements at chromosome 2p23 with a variety of partners that change the cellular compartment localization of the constitutively active fusion kinase.[34-38] Recently, a new antibody (D5F3) for ALK, has been reported to show superior results.[39]

Some of these translocations are also seen in anaplastic large cell lymphoma.[40]

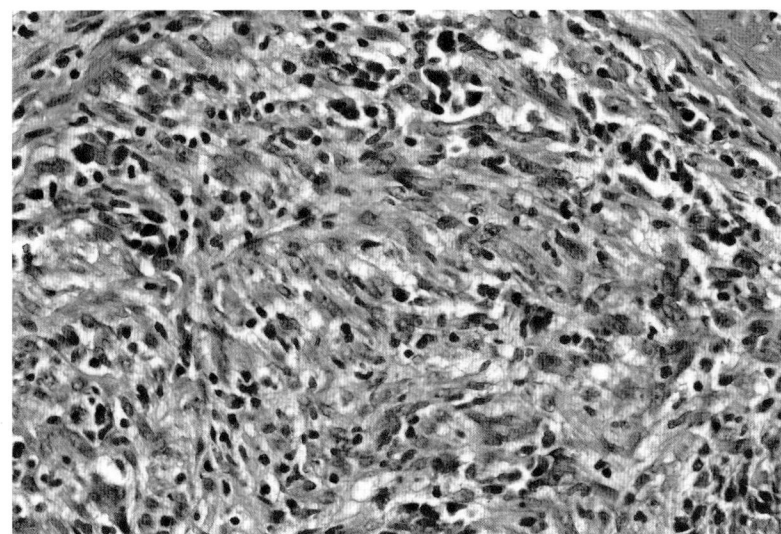

Fig. 35.168
Inflammatory myofibroblastic tumor: the tumor cells are admixed with lymphocytes, eosinophils, and plasma cells.

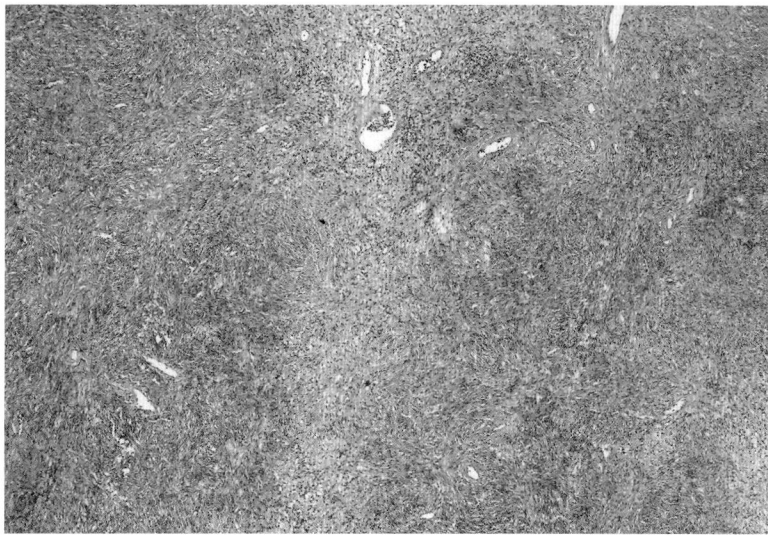

Fig. 35.169
Solitary fibrous tumor: low-power view of a spindle cell tumor with focal hyalinization. Note the prominent blood vessels.

Epithelioid inflammatory myofibroblastic sarcoma is composed of epithelioid cells and a minor spindle cell element in a myxoid stroma. Typically, an inflammatory cell infiltrate consisting mainly of neutrophils and lymphocytes is seen. Immunoreactivity for ALK, nuclear membrane or perinuclear, is distinctive. Tumor cells may also express SMA, desmin and CD30.[20–24]

Differential diagnosis

The main differential diagnosis is with other myofibroblastic tumors, mainly low-grade myofibroblastic sarcoma. The latter usually lacks inflammation, is more monomorphic and infiltrative and is not associated with positivity for ALK-1 or cytokeratin.[11]

Inflammatory processes, Epstein–Barr virus (EBV)-associated myofibroblastic proliferations, IgG4 sclerosing disease and dendritic reticulum cell sarcoma must be distinguished from inflammatory myofibroblastic tumor.[41–45] IgG4 positive cells can be seen in inflammatory myofibroblastic tumor suggesting a possible pathogenetic link.[46]

Solitary fibrous tumor

Clinical features

Solitary fibrous tumor is a distinctive neoplasm that presents mainly in the pleura but has increasingly been reported at numerous sites including solid organs, soft tissues (mainly limbs and head and neck) and (more rarely) the skin where a small number of cases have been documented.[1–10] Lesions also occur in the oral cavity and orbit. Almost any site can be affected.[11–13] Multiple tumors are very rare.[14] Most tumors present as a fairly circumscribed, slowly growing, asymptomatic mass in middle-aged to elderly patients, with no sex predilection. Rare cases, mainly in the pleura, are associated with hypoglycemia (Doege-Potter syndrome) and finger clubbing (Pierre-Marie-Bamberg syndrome).[15–19] Hypoglycemia can be due to the secretion of insulin-like growth factor 2 by tumor cells.[15–19] The majority of cases behave in a benign fashion, but a small percentage may recur locally or even metastasize to internal organs.[1–8] Aggressive behavior does not strictly correlate with morphology, as a number of tumors with no apparent histologic features suggestive of malignancy have metastasized. Several histologic parameters have been studied to predict clinical behavior. The most consistent reported parameter seems to be mitotic activity.[20–25] Positive resection margins correlate with recurrence and metastatic potential is higher in large (>10 cm) tumors.[21] A risk assessment model depending on patient age, tumor size, mitotic activity and necrosis has been proposed in which patients older than 55 with large tumors (> or = to 15 cm), necrosis and mitotic activity > or equal to 4 per 10 high power fields are more likely to have adverse outcome.[23,24] Extrathoracic tumors metastasize more

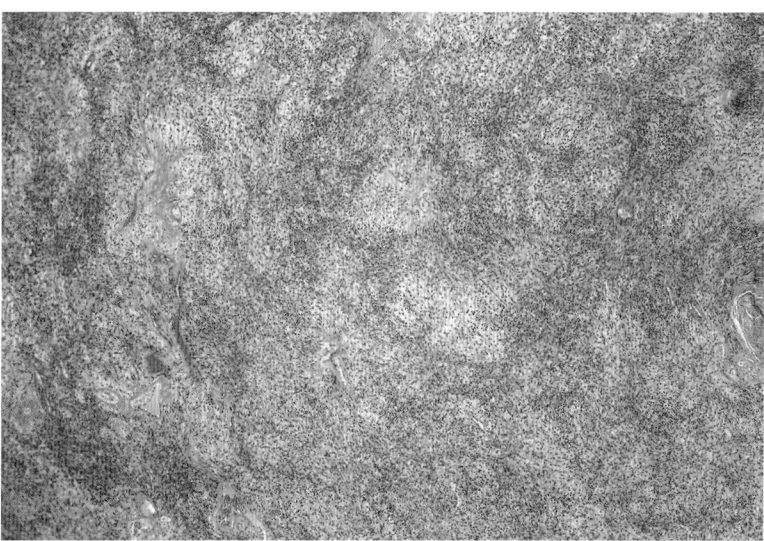

Fig. 35.170
Solitary fibrous tumor: medium-power view displaying alternating hyper- and hypocellular foci.

frequently than those occurring in the thorax.[22] Some studies suggest a correlation between behavior and fusion gene variants and also with overexpression of growth factors.[26–28]

Surgical excision is the treatment of choice. For aggressive or unresectable tumors radiotherapy and or systemic therapy may be considered.[29–33] Although cutaneous lesions may rarely recur, a more aggressive behavior has not been reported so far in these tumors.

Pathogenesis and histologic features

Inv12(q13q13)-derived *NAB2-STAT6* gene fusions have been consistently identified in solitary fibrous tumors.[27,28,34–41]

The features are those of a usually well-circumscribed tumor, typically described as having a patternless architecture (*Figs 35.169–35.171*). Hypo- and hypercellular areas alternate throughout the lesion and in the background there is prominent hyalinized collagen with a focal keloidal appearance and a prominent vascular network with a hemangiopericytomatous pattern and perivascular hyalinization (*Figs 35.172* and *35.173*). Tumor cells are round to short and spindled, with vesicular nuclei and little or no cytologic atypia. Mitotic activity is usually low. Myxoid change may be prominent and has been highlighted in a cutaneous tumor.[42,43] Accumulation of collagen may form amianthoid-like bodies. Mature adipocytes are sometimes a feature

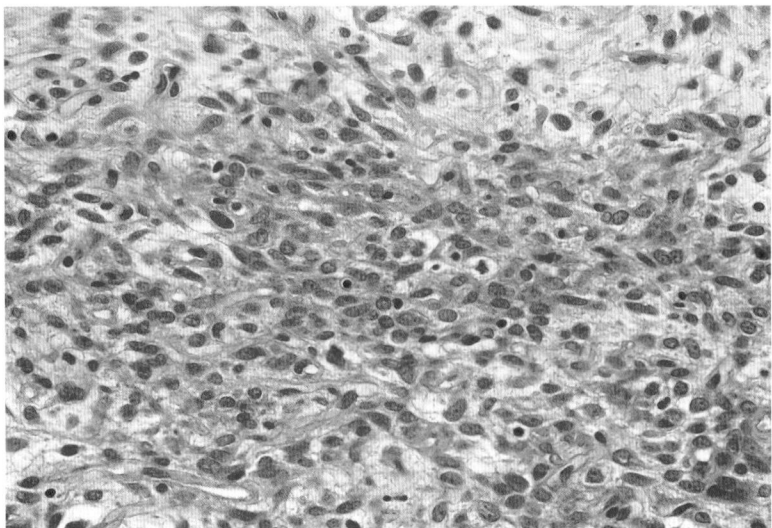

Fig. 35.171
Solitary fibrous tumor: tumor cells have eosinophilic or clear cytoplasm and oval to spindled basophilic nuclei.

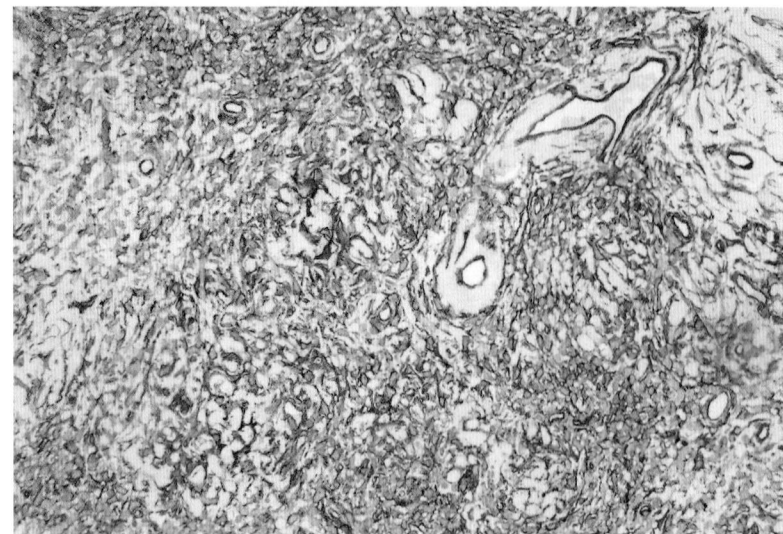

Fig. 35.174
Solitary fibrous tumor: the tumor cells show strong CD34 expression.

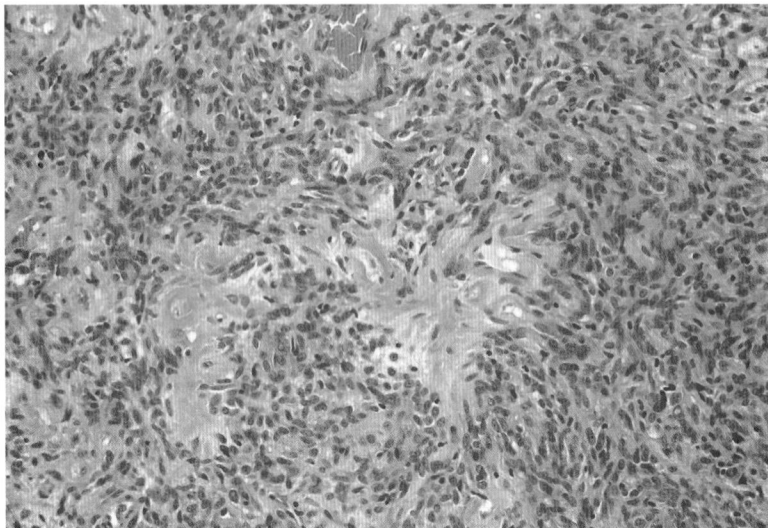

Fig. 35.172
Solitary fibrous tumor: foci of keloid formation are a characteristic feature.

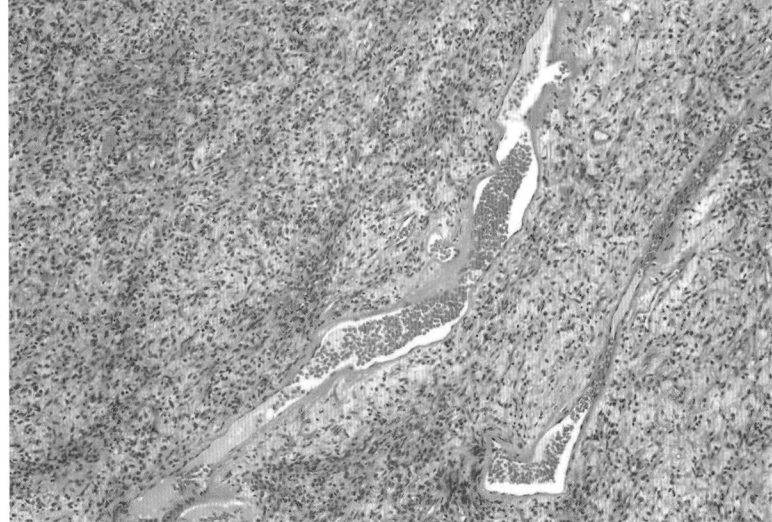

Fig. 35.173
Solitary fibrous tumor: hemangiopericytomatous vessels are often seen.

and can be prominent Such tumors were initially described as lipomatous hemangiopericytoma, are part of the spectrum of solitary fibrous tumor, and have been designated as fat forming solitary fibrous tumor.[44,45] Rare lesions may show histologic features of malignancy including cytologic atypia, increased mitotic activity, high cellularity and necrosis.[3] Giant cell angiofibroma is a variant of solitary fibrous tumor (giant cell rich solitary fibrous tumor) and is described below. Exceptional cases display abrupt transition to a high-grade sarcoma with loss of CD34 expression and strong reactivity of TP53 and P16.[45–51] This feature has been regarded as dedifferentiation and is associated with aggressive behavior and mortality. Heterologous elements (osteosarcomatous and rhabdomyosarcomatous) are exceptional.[47] Although some cases displaying dedifferentiation have been reported in soft tissues, this feature has not been reported in the skin.

By immunohistochemistry, tumor cells are almost invariably, diffusely positive for CD34 and for CD99 (*Fig. 35.174*), and in a smaller percentage of cases for SMA, EMA and bcl2.[52,53] S100 protein, desmin and cytokeratin may be positive focally. Nuclear immunoreactivity for STAT6 is consistent but not specific for solitary fibrous tumor as is GRIA2.[53–58] Nuclear β-catenin, PAX2 and PAX8 have been reported as positive in a subset of tumors.[41,59] Insulin-like growth factor 2 is highly expressed in tumor cells.[60]

Differential diagnosis

Distinction from a fibrous histiocytoma is based on the relative lack of circumscription, the polymorphism and the negative or only very focal positive staining for CD34 in the latter condition. Dermatofibrosarcoma protuberans is diffusely positive for CD34 and GRIA2 but is widely infiltrative and consists of monotonous cells arranged in a storiform pattern. Fat -forming variants should be differentiated from liposarcoma. Sometimes, depending on the predominant features, solitary fibrous tumor may resemble hemangioma, desmoid fibromatosis, sarcomas (mainly synovial sarcoma), atypical spindle cell lipomatous tumor, spindle cell carcinoma and spindle cell melanoma.[57,61,62]

Giant cell angiofibroma

Clinical features

Giant cell angiofibroma is a distinctive form of a giant cell-rich variant of solitary fibrous tumor occurring mainly in the orbit but also presenting elsewhere in the head and neck (including the oral cavity and pharynx), trunk, groin, vulva and perianal area.[1–9] An exceptional case in the mediastinum has also been described.[8] Patients are usually middle-aged adults and although orbital lesions have predilection for males, extraorbital lesions affect mainly females.[1–5]

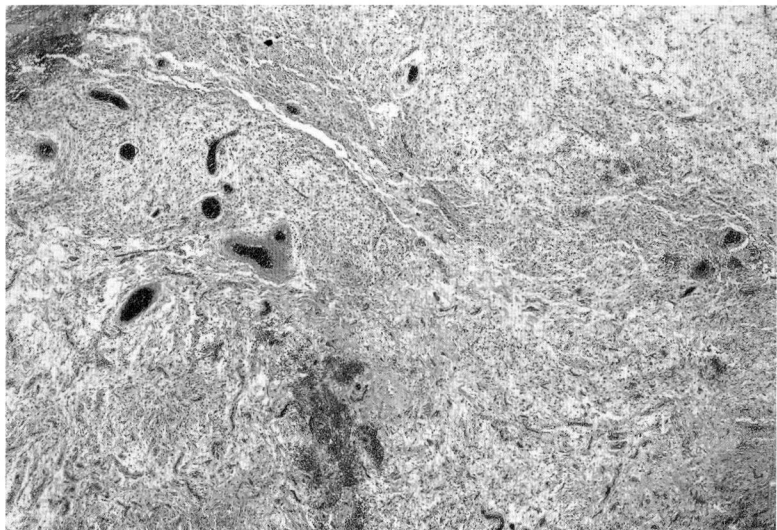

Fig. 35.175
Giant cell angiofibroma: low-power view showing prominent blood vessels and tumor cells dispersed in a myxoid stroma.

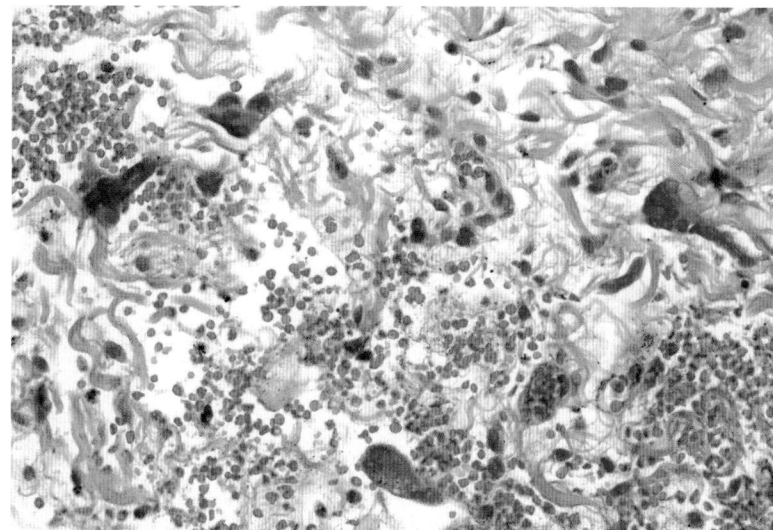

Fig. 35.177
Giant cell angiofibroma: note the tumor giant cells.

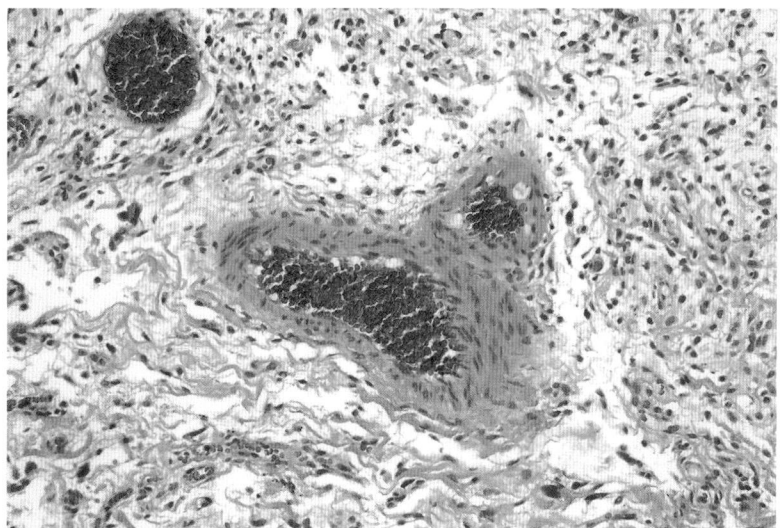

Fig. 35.176
Giant cell angiofibroma: high-power view.

Tumors are asymptomatic, subcutaneous, slowly growing and measure only a few centimeters in diameter. Local recurrence is rare. Aggressive behavior, however, has not been documented in any cases.

Pathogenesis and histologic features

Cytogenetic studies in a one case showed abnormalities of chromosome 6q, while another showed t(12;17)(q15;q23).[10,11] NAB2-STAT6 fusion transcripts have been identified in some cases of solitary fibrous tumor with giant cell angiofibroma-like features.[12]

Histology shows a well-circumscribed mass with variable cellularity composed of small or medium-sized vascular channels with thick walls, pseudovascular spaces, a combination of round and short spindle-shaped cells and a variable number of multinucleated giant cells (*Figs 35.175–35.177*). The latter often seem to be lining the pseudovascular spaces. Mitotic figures are rare. The stroma is myxoid or sclerotic.

Low-grade myofibroblastic sarcoma

Clinical features

Low-grade myofibroblastic sarcoma is a rare distinctive tumor that presents as a deep-seated mass in the limbs and head and neck of adults, with a

slight male predilection.[1–4] Tumors may rarely occur in bone, the oral cavity, heart, abdomen, stomach, breast, vulva, thoracic spine and larynx.[1–3,5–25] A single cutaneous tumor has been described.[12] A case in association with a desmoplastic melanoma has been reported.[26] Multicentricity is exceptional.[27] Local recurrence is common and metastatic disease is rare.[1,23,24]

Histologic features

Histology shows an infiltrative tumor composed of fascicles of cells with indistinct cytoplasmic margins, pale pink cytoplasm and elongated, vesicular nuclei. In some lesions there is variable cellularity. Cytologic atypia is not prominent but is always present. Mitotic activity tends to be low. In a single case intracytoplasmic hyaline inclusions have been reported.[28] It has been suggested that in tumors of the head and neck, aggressive behavior is associated with higher mitotic activity and necrosis.[29]

Tumor cells are positive for smooth muscle actin, muscle specific actin and calponin.[30,31] There may be focal positivity for desmin but h-caldesmon is negative.[30] ALK-1 and keratin are also negative a feature that allows distinction from inflammatory myofibroblastic tumor.[30] Beta-catenin shows no nuclear staining, a feature that allows distinction from desmoid fibromatosis.

Ultrastructural examination reveals subplasmalemmal bundles of myofilaments and fibronexus.[32]

Fibrosarcoma: infantile variant

Clinical features

Infantile fibrosarcoma presents before the age of 10 years. The great majority of patients are less than 2 years of age and tumors are often congenital with a predilection for males.[1–5] It frequently presents as a subcutaneous tumor with predilection for the limbs, but not uncommonly arises on the head and neck. Unusual locations include penis, scalp, lung, retroperitoneum, infratemporal area and heart.[6–9] Some tumors can be very large. The clinical course is much less aggressive than that of its adult counterpart and the 5-year survival is higher than 80%.[1–5] Local recurrence is seen in up to 25% of cases. Metastases are rare but may occur even before birth.[10,11] Cases associated hypercalcemia, a case associated with coagulopathy, one with fetal anemia and a further with urticaria pigmentosa have been described.[12–16] Clinically it may mimic vascular lesions or a sacrococcygeal teratoma.[17–19]

Pathogenesis and histologic features

Cytogenetic studies of infantile fibrosarcoma have shown a t(12;15)(p13;q26) resulting in activation of the *NTRK3* receptor tyrosine kinase gene, leading to a recurrent *ETV6-NTRK3* gene fusion.[20–22] This same translocation can

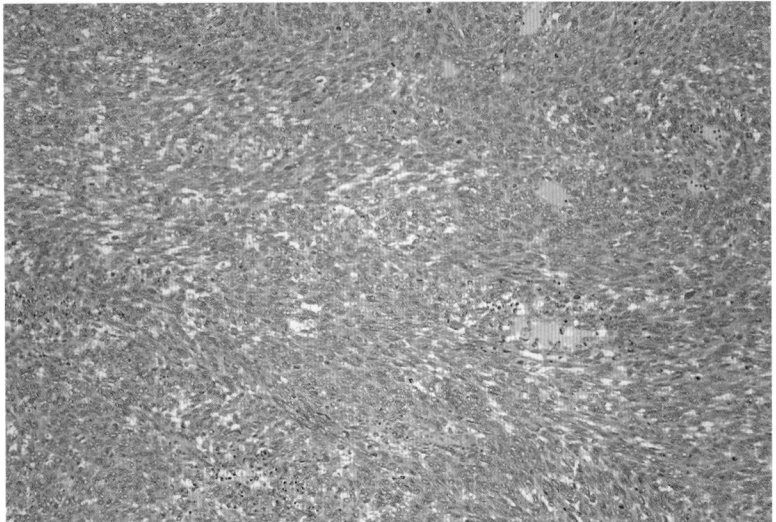

Fig. 35.178
Infantile fibrosarcoma: the tumor is densely cellular and an ill-defined herring-bone pattern is evident.

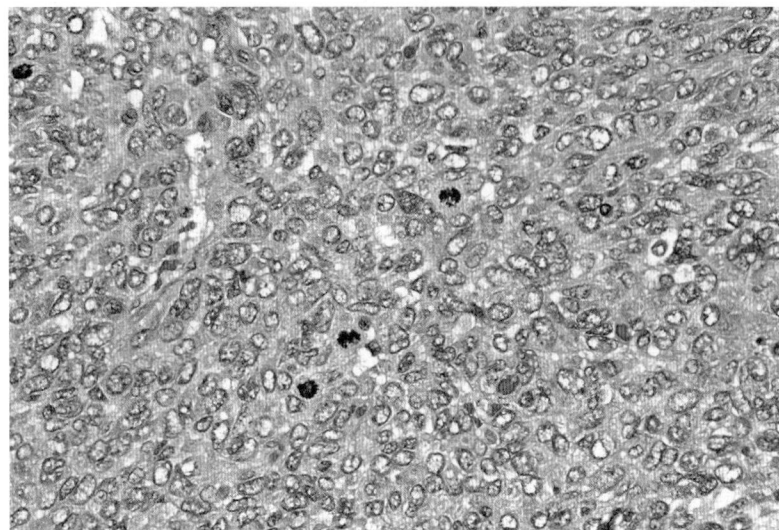

Fig. 35.180
Infantile fibrosarcoma: in this field the tumor cells are more epithelioid and show striking mitotic activity.

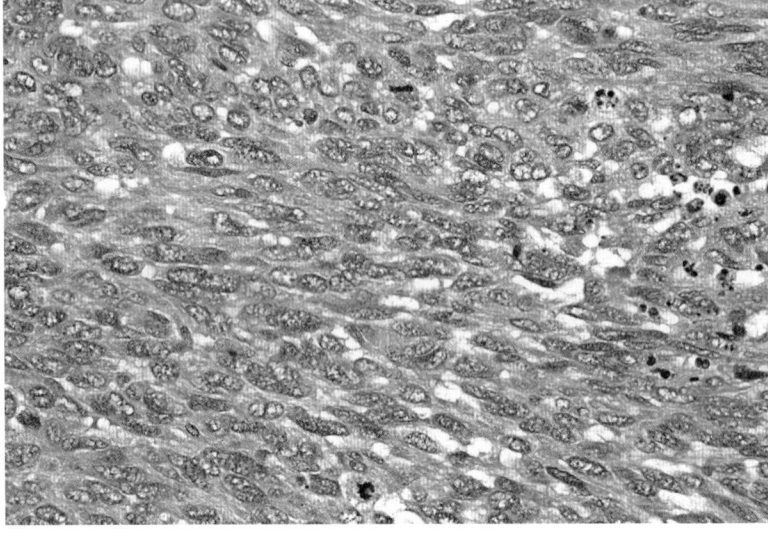

Fig. 35.179
Infantile fibrosarcoma: the tumor cells are basophilic and have regular elongated nuclei.

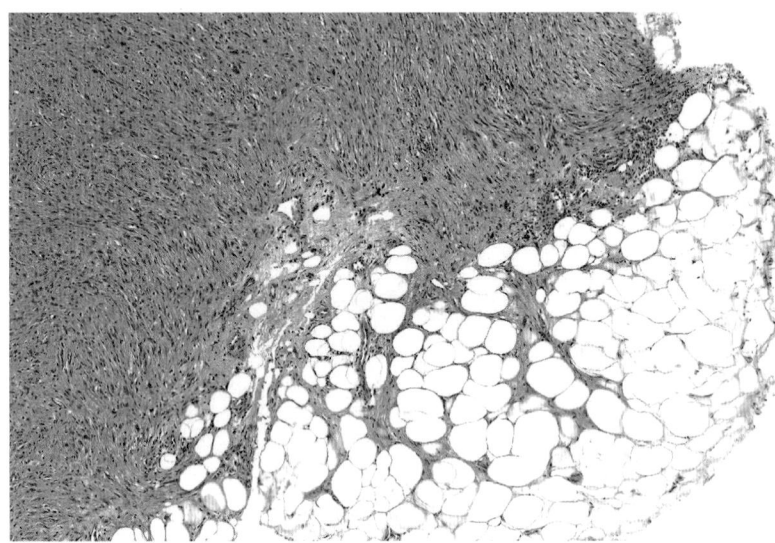

Fig. 35.181
Superficial CD34-positive fibroblastic tumor: pleomorphic spindle-shaped cells with nuclear enlargement and hyperchromatism.

also be associated with cellular congenital mesoblastic nephroma, which is considered its renal counterpart. This fusion has also been reported in other neoplasms such as acute myeloid leukemia, mammary type secretory carcinoma of the skin and salivary glands and secretory breast carcinoma.[20,23–25] EML4-NTRK3 fusion transcripts are also rarely found.[26] A small subgroup of cases displaying overlapping histologic features with infantile fibrosarcoma, occurring in older children and adolescents and with predilection for axial sites, display BRAF gene fusions.[27] In a further case with similar features a TPM3-NTRK1 fusion transcript was identified.[27]

Microscopic appearances are very similar to those of the adult variant (Figs 35.178–35.180). However, some cases show more primitive rounded cells and/or a hemangiopericytoma-like pattern mimicking myofibroma. A case with a lipofibromatosis-like component has been described.[28] Tumor cells are positive for vimentin and sometimes focally positive for actin.[29]

Ultrastructural studies show cells with features of fibroblasts.[29]

Differential diagnosis

Infantile myofibroma may contain focal areas resembling infantile fibrosarcoma.[30] Careful attention should be paid in such cases to identify areas typical of myofibromatosis. Cytogenetic analysis may also be of help.

Superficial CD34-positive fibroblastic tumor

Clinical features

Superficial CD34-positive fibroblastic tumor is a rare neoplasm of intermediate malignancy (locally aggressive) described in 2014 in a series of 18 cases.[1] Since then, another series of 11 cases and isolated cases reports have been published.[2–7] It presents in adults with a slight predilection for males. A suprafacial long-standing mass, usually in the lower limb, is the typical clinical presentation.[1,7] Local recurrence has not been reported, but in one case there was metastatic spread to a regional lymph node.[1] Complete surgical excision is the treatment of choice. Cases successfully treated with Mohs micrographic surgery have been reported.[8,9]

Pathogenesis and histologic features

Rearrangements of the TGFBR3 and MGEA5 genes have not been found.[1]

Histologically, tumors are fairly circumscribed, cellular, and composed of pleomorphic spindle to epithelioid cells arranged in fascicles and sheets (Figs 35.181 and 35.182). In contrast to the degree of pleomorphism, mitotic activity is low. Tumor cells may be large with abundant granular,

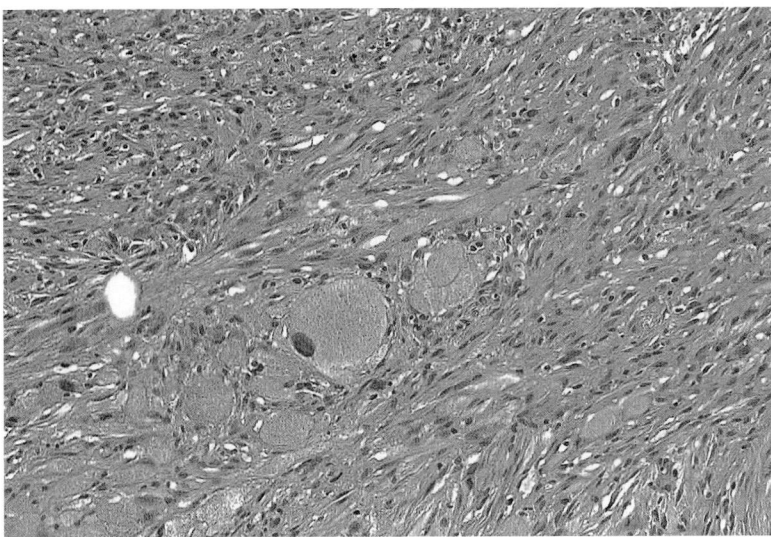

Fig. 35.182
Superficial CD34-positive fibroblastic tumor: focal granular cell change is frequent.

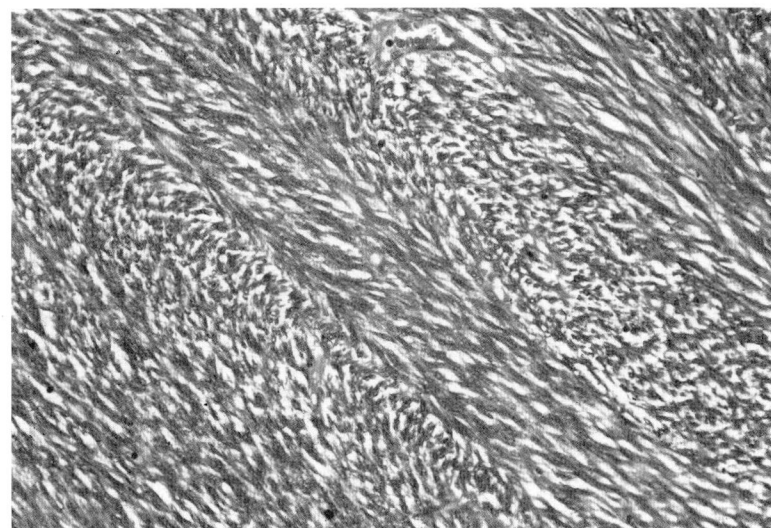

Fig. 35.184
Fibrosarcoma: marked basophilia and a herring-bone pattern of spindle cells are typical features of this lesion.

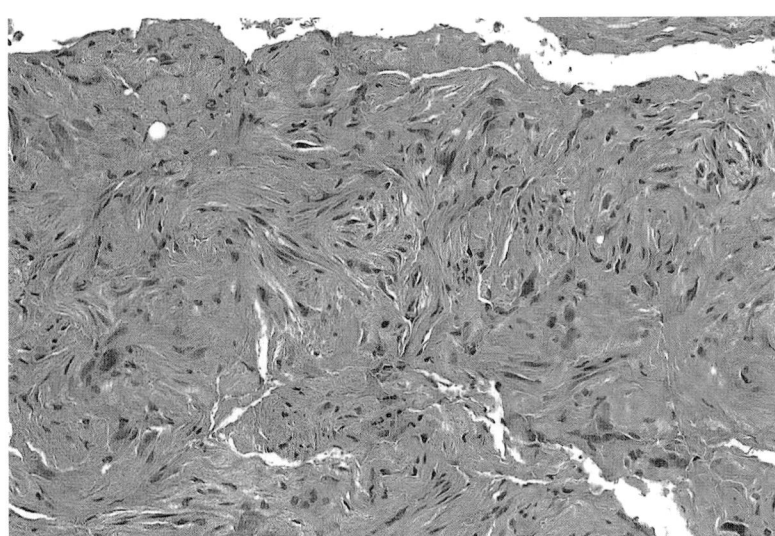

Fig. 35.183
Superficial CD34-positive fibroblastic tumor: extensive replacement of the subcutaneous tissue by a predominantly spindle cell tumor.

fibrillary xanthomatous or glassy cytoplasm; intranuclear and cytoplasmic inclusions are sometimes found. Focal granular cell change is frequent (*Fig. 35.183*). Arborizing vessels and a mixed inflammatory infiltrate are common features.[1,2]

Immunohistochemically, tumor cells are diffusely positive for CD34; focal staining for cytokeratin is seen in most cases.[1,2] FLI-1, ERG, S100 protein, desmin, and smooth muscle actin are negative. There is no overexpression of TP53 and SMARCB1 is retained.

Differential diagnosis

The combination of pleomorphic histology with very low mitotic index and diffuse CD43 expression in a superficial location is fairly distinctive. The main differential diagnosis is with myxoinflammatory fibroblastic sarcoma. In myxoinflammatory fibroblastic sarcoma, inflammatory cells are prominent, a number of cells display virocyte-like nuclear inclusions, and expression of CD34 is more focal. Cytogenetics studies may be of help in difficult cases (see also myxoinflammatory fibroblastic sarcoma).

Malignant fibroblastic tumors

Fibrosarcoma: adult variant

Clinical features

Contrary to age-old teaching, adult fibrosarcoma is now regarded as distinctly uncommon. With the aid of improved diagnostic techniques, many previous cases of fibrosarcoma would now be reclassified, most often as monophasic synovial sarcoma, solitary fibrous tumor or malignant peripheral nerve sheath tumor. True fibrosarcoma accounted for less than 1% of sarcomas among 100 000 adult sarcoma patients studied.[1]

Adult fibrosarcoma usually arises in the fifth and sixth decades, and shows a slight male predominance. It occurs most often in the lower limbs, followed by the upper limbs and trunk.[1–4] Tumors presenting in children are classified separately (see below). Fibrosarcoma is most often deep seated and asymptomatic. Only very occasional tumors are subcutaneous. There is a tendency for local recurrence and metastasis, with a 5-year survival of about 50%.

Pathogenesis and histologic features

A small proportion of adult tumors have been reported to be radiation induced but it is not clear whether all of these tumors represent true fibrosarcomas.[5]

Cytogenetic studies in a small number of fibrosarcomas have shown complex chromosomal abnormalities.[6,7] In two cases, tri- or tetrasomy of 2q has been described.[6]

Adult fibrosarcoma tends to be well circumscribed and is composed of relatively uniform spindled cells with little cytoplasm, typically arranged in a herring-bone pattern (*Figs 35.184* and *35.185*). There is usually minimal collagen production, mild pleomorphism can be present and the mitotic count varies. It is important to remember that tumors such as dermatofibrosarcoma protuberans and dedifferentiated liposarcoma may have areas identical to fibrosarcoma.

Immunohistochemistry shows that tumor cells are positive for vimentin and are occasionally focally positive for actin. Other markers including CD34, S100 protein, EMA and desmin are negative.

Ultrastructural studies show cells with features of fibroblasts and myofibroblasts.[8]

Differential diagnosis

All cases should be assessed for S100 protein, pankeratin and EMA expression to exclude malignant schwannoma and monophasic synovial sarcoma since the diagnosis of fibrosarcoma is one of exclusion. Leiomyosarcoma is composed of plumper spindle-shaped cells with abundant eosinophilic cytoplasm

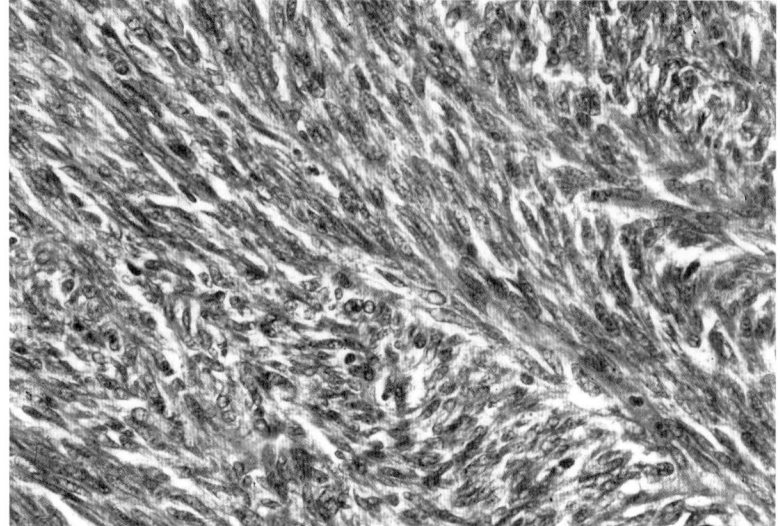

Fig. 35.185
Fibrosarcoma: the spindle cell borders are indistinct and their nuclei are elongated with thin tapered ends, unlike those in leiomyosarcoma and neurofibrosarcoma.

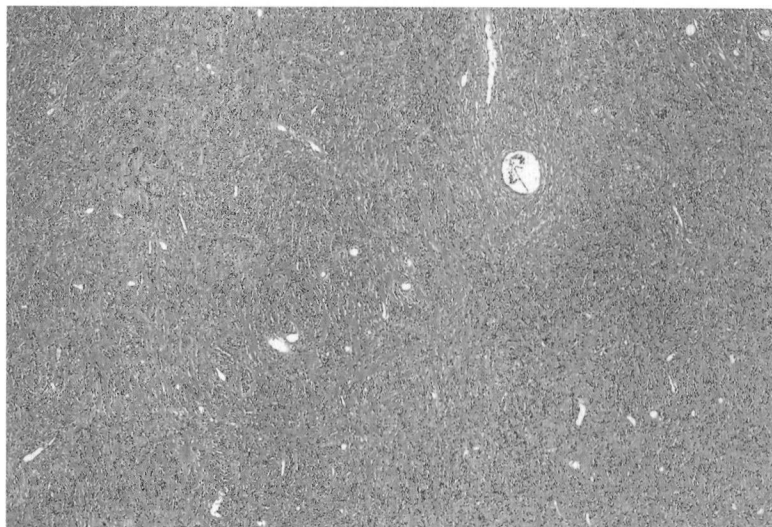

Fig. 35.186
Sclerosing epithelioid fibrosarcoma: low-power view showing a paucicellular infiltrate within a densely hyalinized stroma.

and cigar-shaped nuclei. Tumor cells are usually positive for desmin and staining for actin is more widespread than that seen in fibrosarcoma.

Sclerosing epithelioid fibrosarcoma

Clinical features

Sclerosing epithelioid fibrosarcoma is a very rare distinctive variant of fibrosarcoma. It involves deep soft tissues of the lower limbs/limb girdles followed by the trunk and upper limbs and rarely the head and neck (including the salivary gland and mouth) and bone.[1–6] Rare tumors can occur in the liver, colon, kidney, intra-abdominal soft tissues, pituitary gland, and skull.[7–15] One tumor developed after radiotherapy.[7] Patients are middle-aged adults and present with a variably painful mass. There is no sex predilection. There is a high recurrence rate of up to 50% and metastatic disease occurs in up to 40% of cases.[1–6]

Pathogenesis and histologic features

Recently, this tumor has been described in combination with low-grade fibromyxoid sarcoma (see below) with demonstration of the characteristic t(7;16)(q33;p11) in these mixed cases.[16,17] However, FUS rearrangements are uncommon in pure epithelioid fibrosarcoma, casting some doubt on the pathogenetic relationship between these two tumors in their pure, unmixed forms.[18] Recent reports suggest that EWSR1-CREB3L1 rearrangements are predominant over FUS and CREB3L2 rearrangements in pure sclerosing epithelioid fibrosarcoma.[19] In contrast, hybrid lesions recapitulate the genotype of low grade fibromyxoid sarcoma (most commonly, FUS-CREB3L2 fusion).[19,20]

The tumor is characterized by prominent hyalinization and relatively uniform, small, round or ovoid epithelioid cells with sparse and often clear cytoplasm arranged in cords and nests (Figs 35.186 and 35.187). Areas of typical fibrosarcoma may be seen. Focal calcification and bone formation are features that are sometimes present.

Tumor cells are generally positive for vimentin and beta-catenin. MUC4 is positive in the majority of cases; MUC4-positive cases are reported to be associated with a FUS gene rearrangement.[21] Some show focal positivity for EMA, S100 protein and more infrequently for neuron-specific enolase (NSE).[1,3] Rare tumors focally express keratin.[1]

Low-grade fibromyxoid sarcoma

Clinical features

Low-grade fibromyxoid sarcoma is a rare distinctive tumor which belongs within the spectrum of hyalinizing spindle cell tumor with giant rosettes.[1–20]

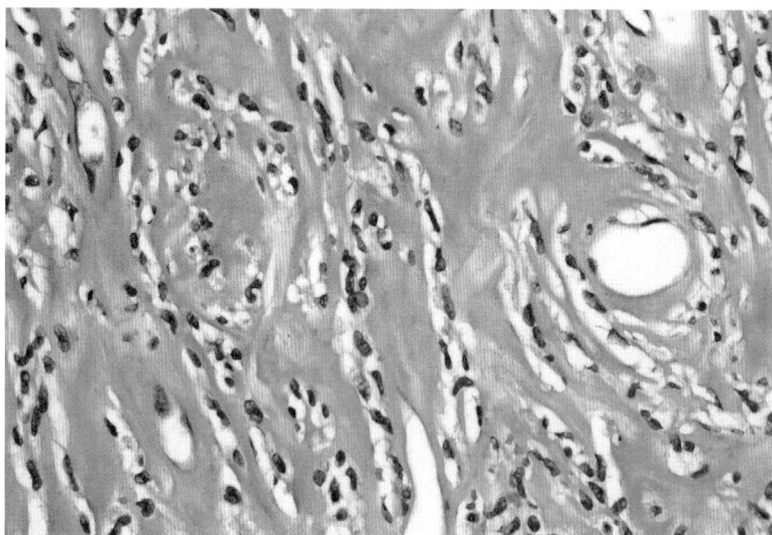

Fig. 35.187
Sclerosing epithelioid fibrosarcoma: the tumor cells characteristically show a single-file distribution.

It presents mainly in young adults or less commonly younger patients, including children as a slowly growing, asymptomatic large mass with a predilection for the limbs.[1–7,20,21] Most lesions are deep seated, may be intramuscular and some tumors are subcutaneous. Superficial lesions tend to be more common in children.[10] Unusual sites include intracranial, intrathoracic, mesenteric, omental, the ovary, the lung, the colon, the external anal sphincter and the falciform ligament.[11,22–24] Although the rates of local recurrence, metastasis and death were high in the first published series, a subsequent large series reported the rates of local recurrence, metastasis and death as 9%, 6%, and 2%, respectively.[3,4,6] Local recurrence and metastases may occur many years after excision of the primary tumor.[1,3,6,19–21] Cases associated with radiotherapy have been reported.[25,26]

Pathogenesis and histologic features

The vast majority of cases are associated with t(7;16)(q33;p11) fusing CREB3L2 and FUS; the former can be substituted by t(11;16)(p11;p11) with FUS-CREB3L1 fusion. CREB3L1 (11p11) is seen in a small subset of cases.[5,27–37] In some examples the fusion results in a supernumerary ring and these tumors appear to recur more frequently.[27]

Histology shows an infiltrative tumor with characteristic alternating myxoid and collagenous areas (Figs 35.188 and 35.189). Cellularity is

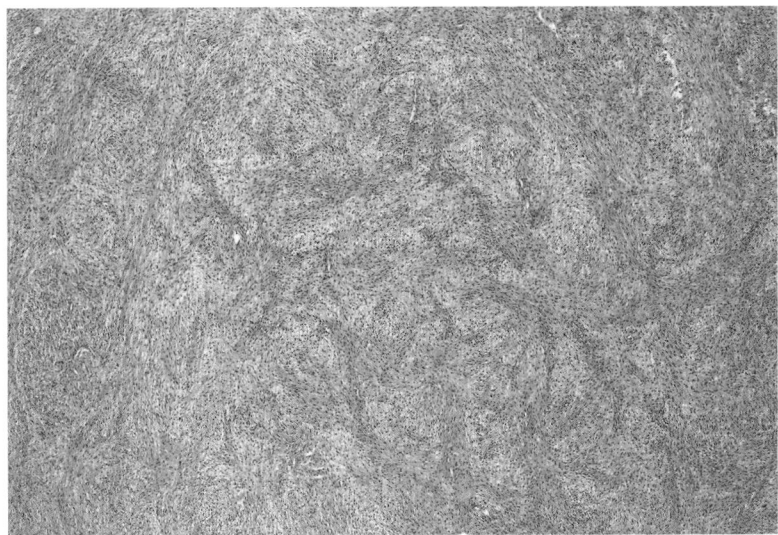

Fig. 35.188
Low-grade fibromyxoid sarcoma: this field shows cellular foci and adjacent myxoid regions.

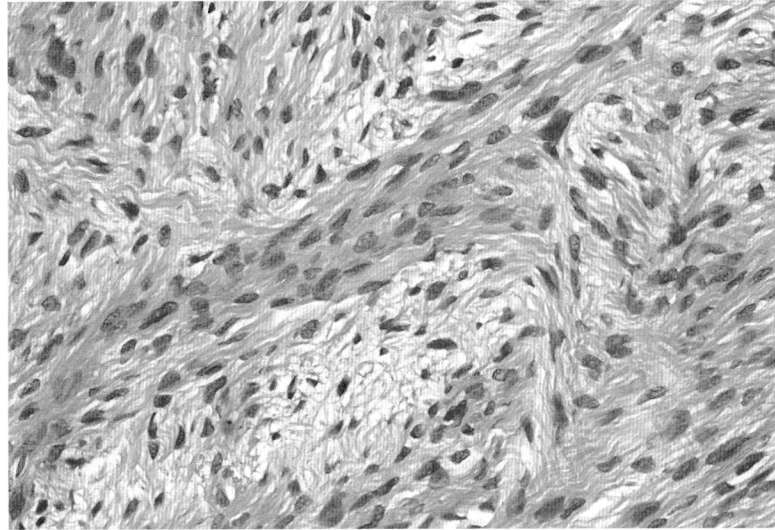

Fig. 35.189
Low-grade fibromyxoid sarcoma: high-power view.

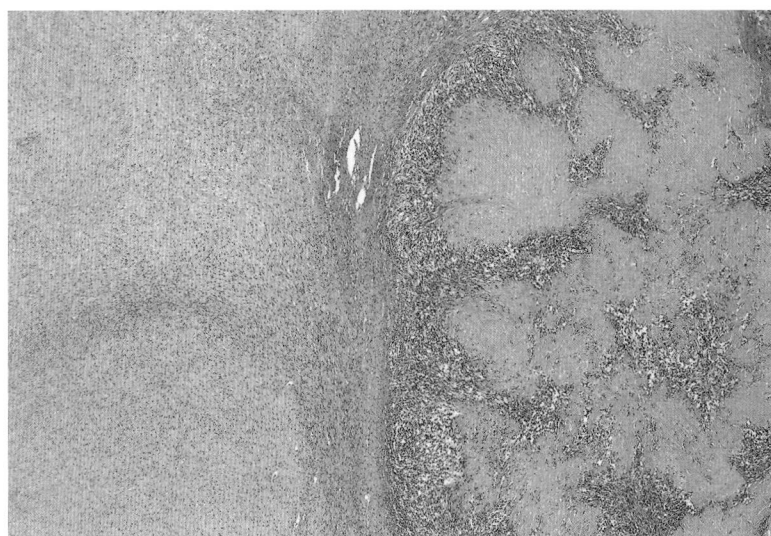

Fig. 35.190
Hyalinizing spindle cell tumor with giant rosettes: note the presence of giant rosettes containing abundant hyalinized collagen in the center.

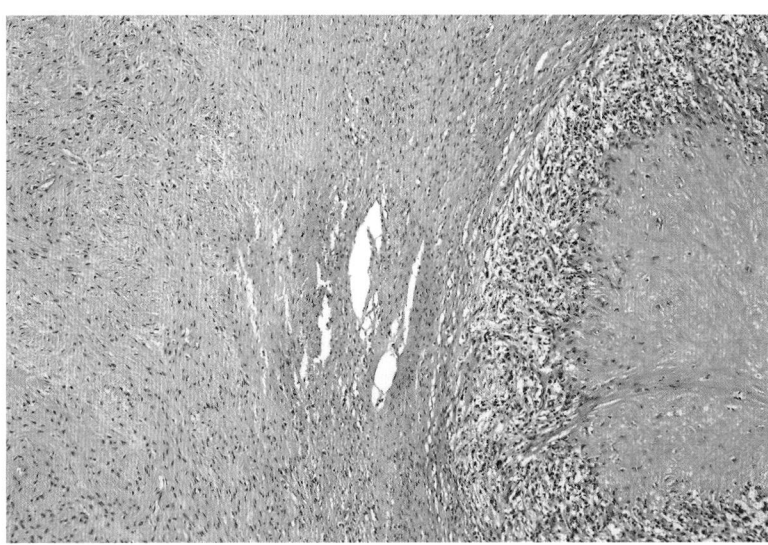

Fig. 35.191
Hyalinizing spindle cell tumor with giant rosettes: transition between bundles of bland elongated spindled cells and a giant rosette.

not prominent and tumor cells tend to predominate in the myxoid areas. Bundles of bland, elongated spindle-shaped cells with focal whorling are seen. Small blood vessels with surrounding fibrosis are often present and tumor cells may concentrate around vascular channels. Cytologic atypia is minimal and mitotic figures are very rare. In some cases, there is transition to areas with tumor cells that are focally epithelioid surrounding prominently hyalinized collagen with formation of giant rosettes (*Figs 35.190* and *35.191*). The latter neoplasm was previously considered a distinct entity termed hyalinizing spindle cell tumor with giant rosettes.[8,9,36] Rare cases contain focal areas resembling an ordinary fibrosarcoma or sclerosing epithelioid fibrosarcoma; it is still debated if the latter is related to low-grade fibromyxoid sarcoma (see also above).[4–6,34,35,37] Recurrences may exhibit nuclear pleomorphism.[21] A pediatric case mimicking ossifying fibromyxoid tumor has been documented.[38]

Immunohistochemistry shows staining for vimentin and very focal positivity for SMA and EMA. Claudin 1 is also often positive and this, coupled with positivity for EMA, may lead to a misdiagnosis of perineurioma.[39] However, Glut-1 tends to be positive in perineurioma and negative in low-grade fibromyxoid sarcoma.[40] MUC4 is a highly sensitive and specific marker of low-grade fibromyxoid sarcoma.[41] Ultrastructural studies show cells with features of fibroblasts.

Differential diagnosis

Distinction from myxofibrosarcoma is based on the presence of curvilinear blood vessels and at least focal prominent cytologic atypia with mitotic activity in the latter tumor.[42] Tumor cells in neurofibroma are wavier and myxoid, and collagenous areas do not alternate, but focal collagen deposition is seen between tumor cells. Furthermore, tumor cells in neurofibroma are S100 protein positive. In addition, none of the benign or malignant mimickers, with the exception of sclerosing epithelioid fibrosarcoma, is positive for MUC4.

Myxofibrosarcoma

Clinical features

Myxofibrosarcoma, formerly known as myxoid malignant fibrous histiocytoma is currently defined as a malignant fibroblastic tumor with pleomorphism, myxoid stroma and a distinctive curvilinear vascular pattern.[1] The tumor commonly presents in the limbs of the elderly and shows a slight predilection for males.[2–4] Up to 60% of cases arise in the subcutis and secondary involvement of the skin is common (*Fig. 35.192*).[5–7] Prognosis

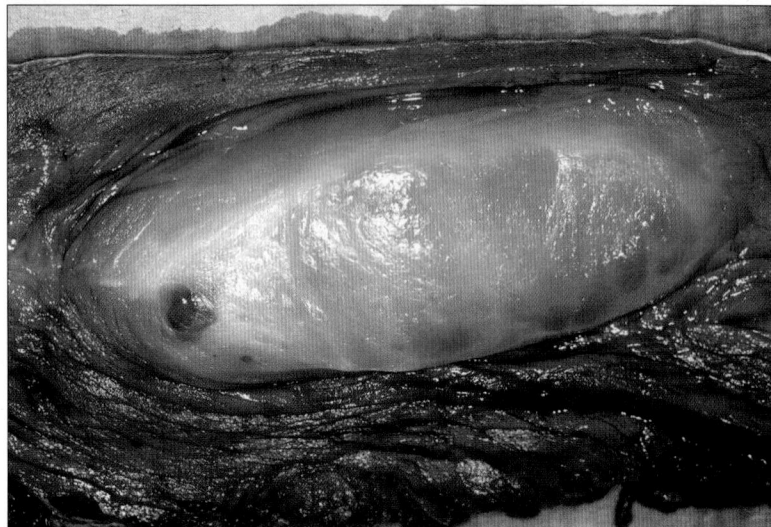

Fig. 35.192
Low-grade myxofibrosarcoma: note the multilobularity and prominent myxoid change. By courtesy of C.D.M. Fletcher, MD, Brigham and Women's Hospital and Harvard Medical School, Boston, USA.

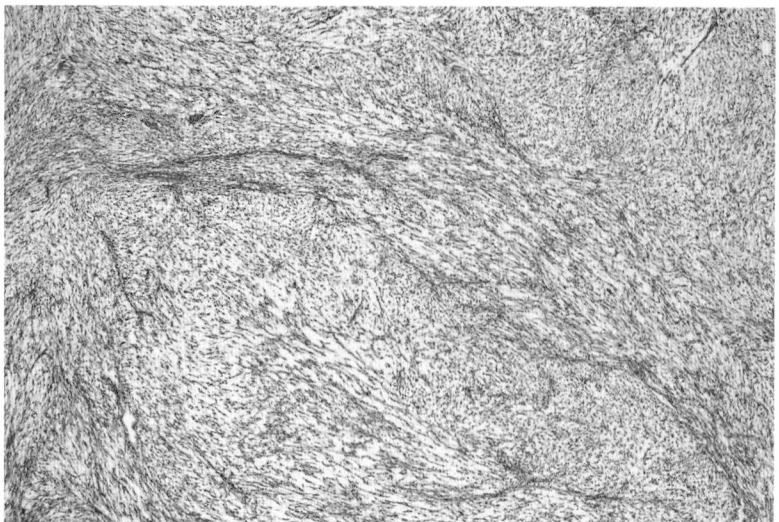

Fig. 35.193
Myxofibrosarcoma: low-grade lesions are relatively hypocellular and contain distinctive curvilinear vessels.

is related to histologic grading, but behavior tends to be indolent with a high tendency for local recurrence, occasional metastasis to regional lymph nodes and a 5-year survival of up to 70%.[4] Metastases are seen more commonly in deep-seated lesions and those with a high histologic grade.[4] Local recurrences appear to be associated with higher histologic grade and more complex cytogenetic abnormalities, surgical margins (close or involved) and old age.[8–12] Mortality is associated with tumor necrosis, large size and decrease in myxoid areas.[13]

Pathogenesis and histologic features

Karyotypes are highly complex and no recurrent genetic changes have been established. In addition, correlation of molecular events with malignant potential has been studied in some series. Gains at chromosome 7 have been described, and more recently, overexpression of MET (chromosome 7q31) have been reported in myxofibrosarcoma and this feature is associated with deeper, higher-grade tumors in more advanced stages.[14,15] A recent studies demonstrated mutations in *TP53*, *ATRX*, *PTEN*, *FGFR3*, *CDKN2A*, and *RB1*.[16,17] MET is a transmembrane receptor tyrosine kinase representing the only high-affinity receptor of hepatocyte growth factor (HGF). Ezrin, as protein associated with cell adhesion-mediated signaling, is over-expressed in myxofibrosarcoma and the expression correlates with poor prognostic factors including necrosis, high mitotic activity, high histologic grade and advanced stage.[18] Association of aggressiveness with down-regulation of p12CDK2AP1 has been reported.[19] Of interest, chondroitin sulfate synthase 1 expression has been reported as associated with malignant potential in soft tissue sarcomas with myxoid substance.[20] Domain-containing protein 2 (DCBLD2) is highly expressed in infiltrative myxofibrosarcoma.[21]

Histologically, appearances vary from low-grade, markedly myxoid, hypocellular lesions, to highly cellular, pleomorphic tumors with focal myxoid change. Tumor cells range from stellate to spindle shaped with variable pleomorphism. All tumors share a multinodular growth pattern, curvilinear thin-walled blood vessels, and a minimum of 10–20% of myxoid stroma with hyperchromatic stellate or spindle-shaped cells (*Figs 35.193–35.198*). Epithelioid cell change can be prominent, particularly in high-grade tumors.[22]

Tumor cells have ultrastructural features of fibroblasts and myofibroblasts and are only rarely focally for actin.[4,23,24]

Differential diagnosis

Distinction from superficial angiomyxoma is easy because the latter lacks cytologic atypia, is less cellular, is predominantly dermal and commonly has

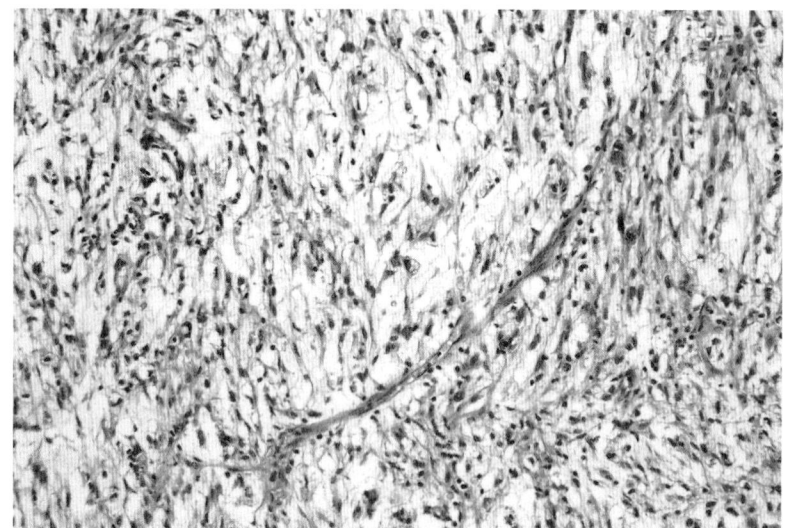

Fig. 35.194
Myxofibrosarcoma: the curvilinear vessels are characteristic.

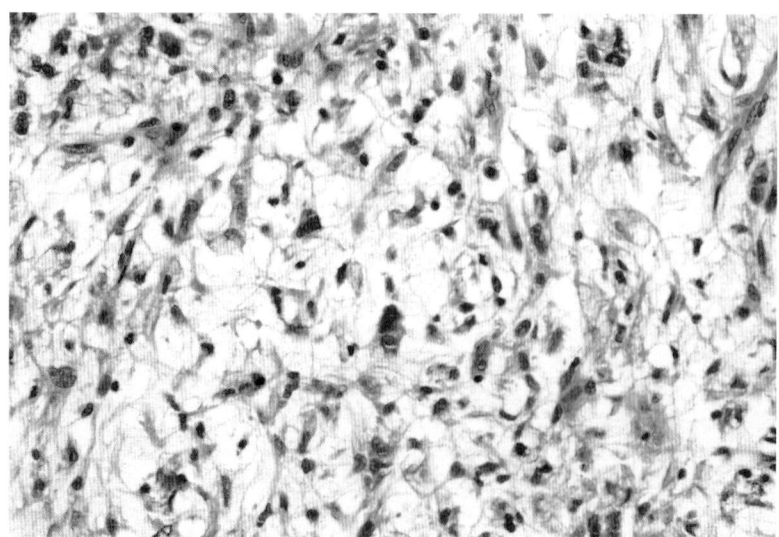

Fig. 35.195
Myxofibrosarcoma: note the pleomorphic tumor cells scattered in the myxoid matrix.

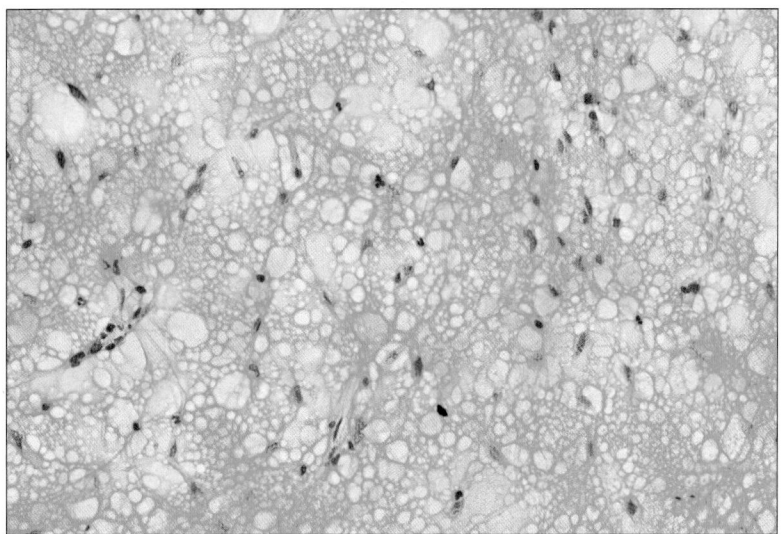

Fig. 35.196
Myxofibrosarcoma: the tumor stains strongly with Alcian blue at pH 2.5, indicating the presence of hyaluronic acid.

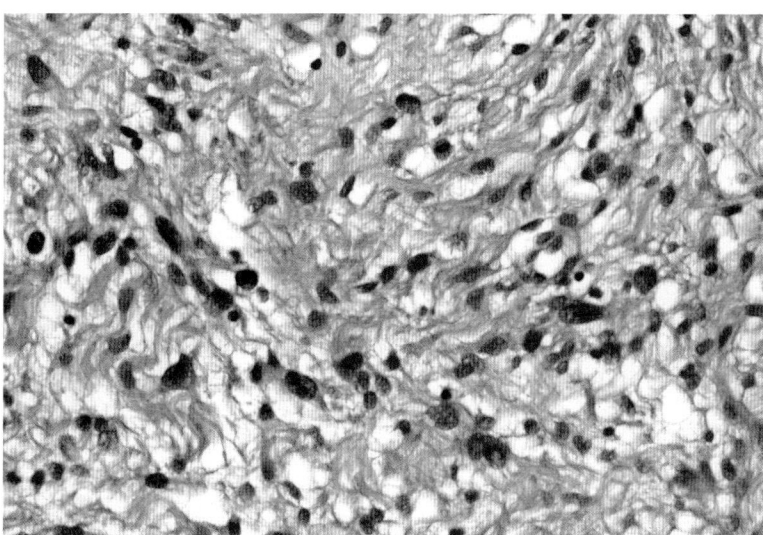

Fig. 35.198
Myxofibrosarcoma: there is marked nuclear pleomorphism.

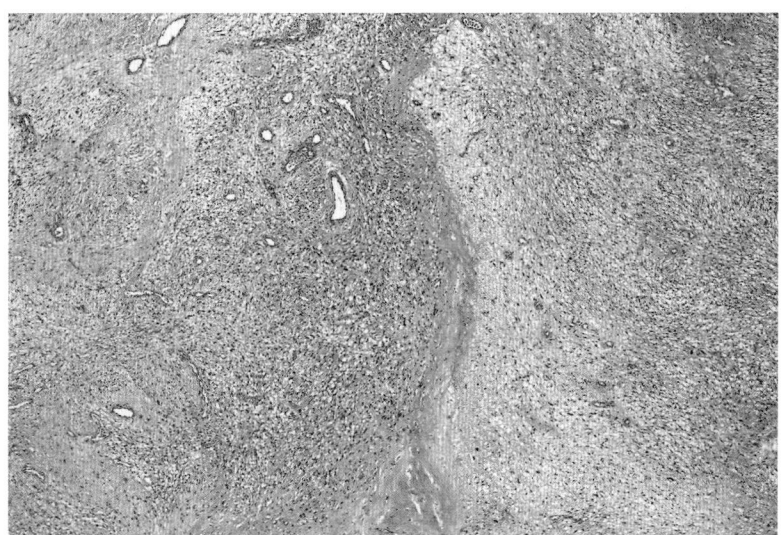

Fig. 35.197
Myxofibrosarcoma: in this field, the multinodularity is emphasized.

an epithelial component. Rare tumors can show focal changes mimicking a pleomorphic hyalinizing angiectatic tumor and sampling is very important to avoid a misdiagnosis.[25] In low-grade fibromyxoid sarcoma, there is no pleomorphism, mitotic figures are rare and curvilinear blood vessels are usually absent.[26] Immunohistochemical markers that have been reported to be of value in differential diagnosis from other myxoid soft tissue tumors include Claudin 6 and NY-ESO-1.[27,28] The former is expressed in myxofibrosarcoma and the latter is expressed in myxoid/round cell liposarcoma but not in myxofibrosarcoma.

FIBROHISTIOCYTIC TUMORS

A group of heterogeneous soft tissue tumors, many of which probably have little in common, is traditionally included under this heading. The term 'fibrohistiocytic' is essentially descriptive and refers to a light microscopic morphological resemblance of tumor cells to fibroblasts and histiocytes; it does not appear to have any relationship to line of differentiation or histogenesis. However, the term is retained in this chapter due to its widespread general use and because most tumors in this category are of uncertain histogenesis.

Benign fibrohistiocytic tumors and tumorlike lesions

Fibrous papule

Clinical features

Fibrous papule is a very common lesion that presents on the face of middle-aged adults, with predilection for the nose.[1–3] It is usually

skin-colored, asymptomatic and measures a few millimeters. Lesions with similar features occur in the tongue and are referred to as solitary oral fibromas.[4] A basal cell carcinoma arising within a fibrous papule of granular cell type has been reported.[5]

Pathogenesis and histologic features

Although in the past it was suggested that fibrous papule represents an old fibrosed nevus, several studies have demonstrated that this is not the case.[6–7] Mast cells may have a role in the development of fibrous papule.[8] A recent study showed activation of the Mammalian Target of Rapamycin Pathway, similar to tuberous sclerosis complex-associated angiofibroma.[9]

Histologically, the lesion is slightly raised, well circumscribed and located in the superficial dermis. It is composed of a collagenous stroma with increased vascular channels and scattered cells varying from spindle shaped to multinucleated (Figs 35.199 and 35.200). A case with multinucleated ganglion-like cells has been reported.[10] Mitotic figures are exceptional and some of the cells may show hyperchromatism. Variants with granular cell

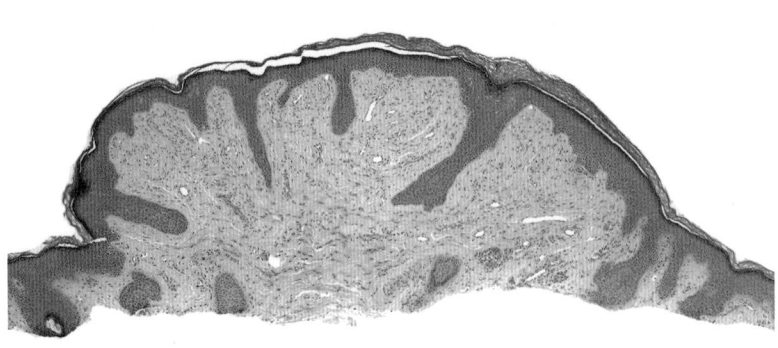

Fig. 35.199
Fibrous papule: shave biopsy from a lesion on the bridge of the nose. The dermis shows dense collagenous tissue.

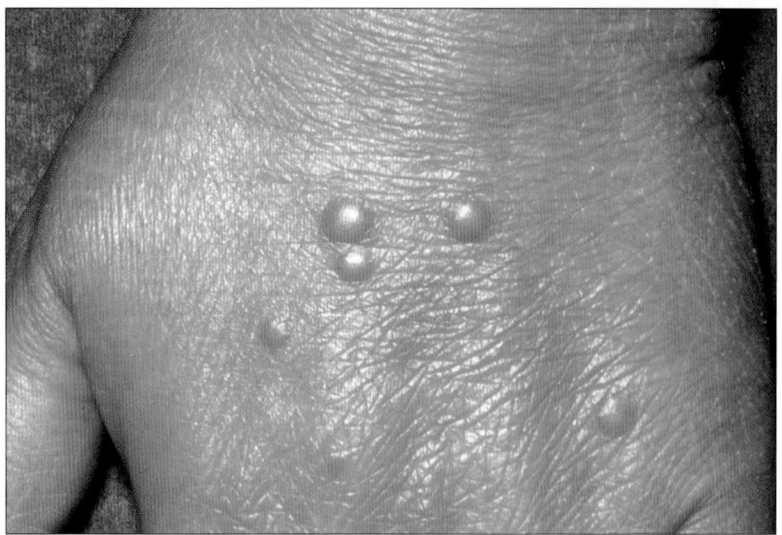

Fig. 35.201
Multinucleate cell angiohistiocytoma: multiple papules are present.

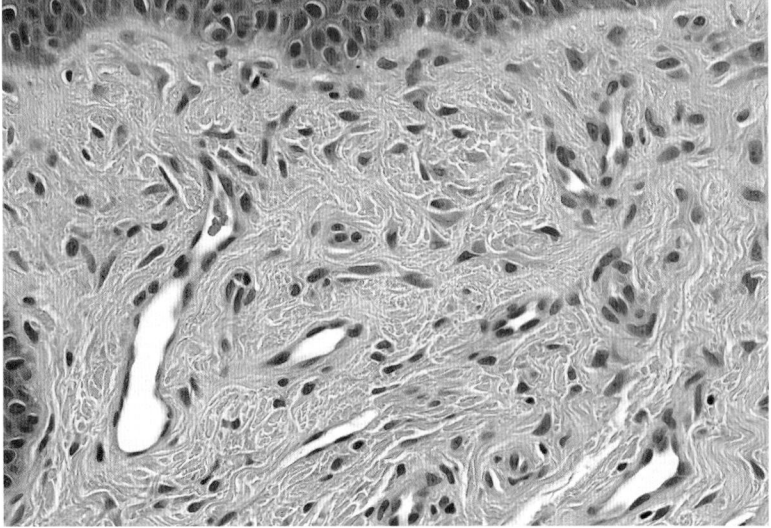

Fig. 35.200
Fibrous papule: high-power view of scattered dendritic cells.

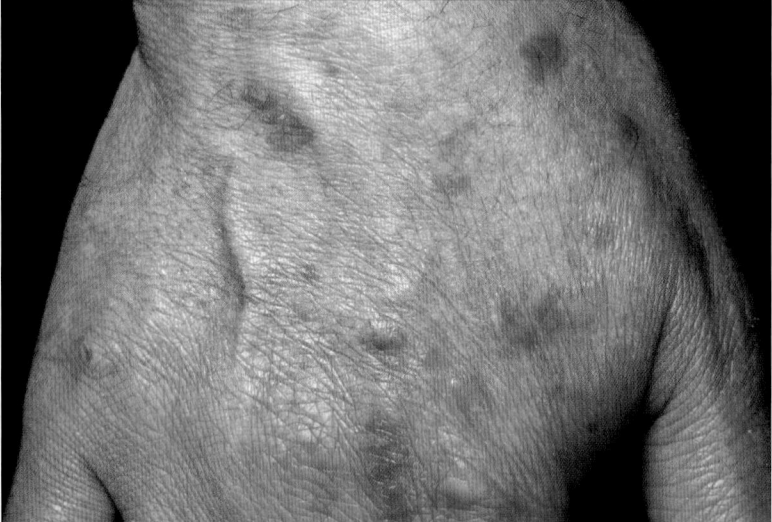

Fig. 35.202
Multinucleate cell angiohistiocytoma: the hand is a characteristic site. By courtesy of the Institute of Dermatology, London, UK.

change, clear cell change and epithelioid cells have been described.[11-16] Focal pigmentation and inflammation may be seen. Lesions with scattered pleomorphic cells overlap with pleomorphic fibroma. The overlying epidermis appears normal or slightly flattened.

By immunohistochemistry, the cells in the lesion are positive for factor XIIIa and may also be positive for CD34.[17-20] S100 protein is negative. Lesions with clear cells are positive for NKI/C3.[21]

Ultrastructurally, the cells have features of fibroblasts.[22,23]

Multinucleate cell angiohistiocytoma

Clinical features

Multinucleate cell angiohistiocytoma is a distinctive condition characterized by multiple, localized, angiomatous papules with predilection for the upper and lower limbs of middle-aged women (*Figs 35.201–35.203*).[1-6] The thigh and dorsum of the hands are frequent sites of involvement followed by face.[7] Generalized lesions are very rare.[8-11] A case developing during pregnancy has been reported.[12]

The lesions are asymptomatic and do not tend to regress spontaneously.[13] A case has been reported in the oral cavity another in vagina and a further lesion occurred in association with an iatrogenic arteriovenous fistula.[14-16] Dermoscopic features may be reminiscent of dermatofibroma.[17,18]

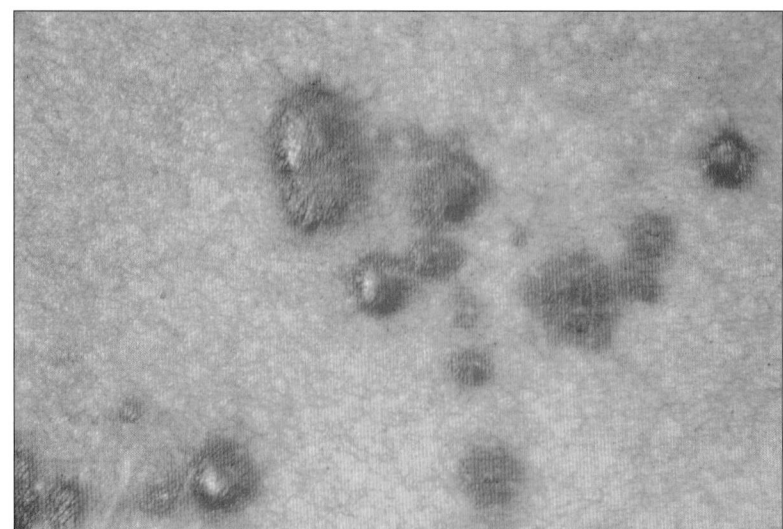

Fig. 35.203
Multinucleate cell angiohistiocytoma: in this example, the papules appear hemorrhagic. By courtesy of the Institute of Dermatology, London, UK.

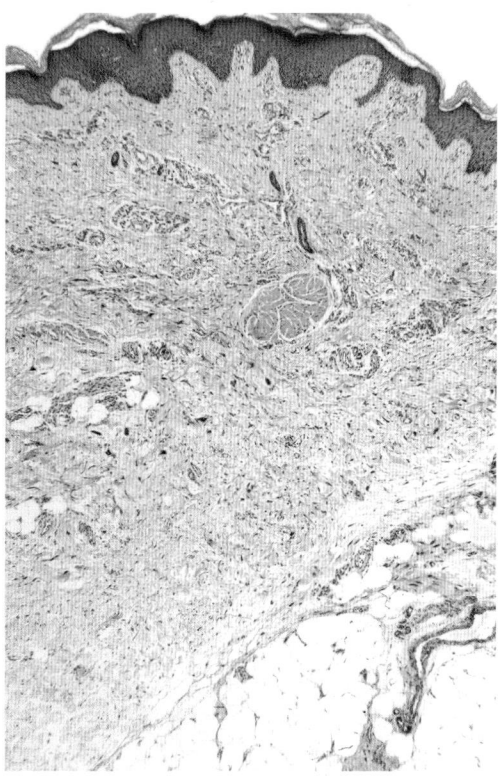

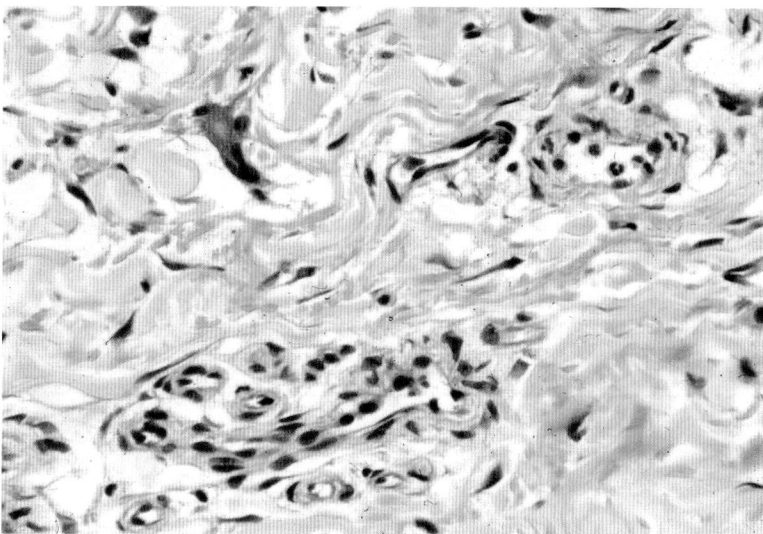

Fig. 35.204
Multinucleate cell angiohistiocytoma: within the dermis is a vascular and collagenous proliferative lesion with conspicuous multinucleate giant cells.

Fig. 35.206
Multinucleate cell angiohistiocytoma: high-power view of giant cell.

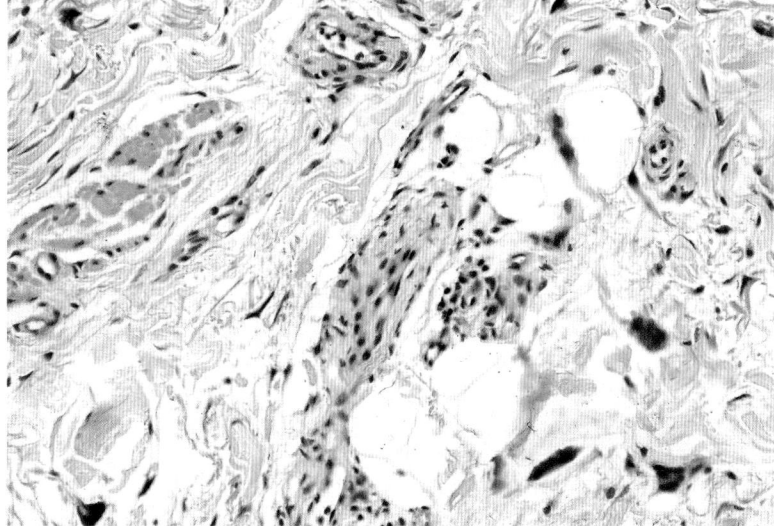

Fig. 35.205
Multinucleate cell angiohistiocytoma: medium-power view showing vessels with giant cells and pericytes.

Pathogenesis and histologic features

The pathogenesis is unknown but the lesions are much more common in females and the tumor cells express estrogen receptor alpha, suggesting a possible hormonal etiological role.[19] It is not clear whether it is a reactive or neoplastic condition.[17,20]

The epidermis appears unremarkable. In the superficial and mid dermis there is a proliferation of small, thin-walled vascular channels, each of which is surrounded by a layer of pericytes (*Fig. 35.204*). The surrounding dermis contains scattered multinucleate cells with angulated cytoplasm and a background of somewhat hyalinized collagen bundles (*Figs 35.205* and *35.206*). Occasional lymphocytes are also seen. An exceptional case with enlarged dermal nerves has been identified.[21] Hemosiderin deposition may be present.

The multinucleate cells are positive for CD68 and lysozyme while the interstitial cells may be positive for factor XIIIa.[7,21]

Differential diagnosis

An atrophic dermatofibroma can look remarkably similar to multinucleate angiohistiocytoma; however, the former presents as a single lesion. Distinction from Kaposi sarcoma is based on the presence of irregular, jagged, thin-walled vascular channels, absence of multinucleate giant cells and presence of plasma cells. Multinucleate angiohistiocytoma lacks HHV8 on immunohistochemistry.[22]

Fibrous histiocytoma (dermatofibroma)

Fibrous histiocytoma (dermatofibroma, sclerosing hemangioma, histiocytoma cutis, nodular subepidermal fibrosis) represents one of the most common benign cutaneous soft tissue tumors.[1–5] Over the years a number of variants have been described, and although they essentially highlight specific histologic features that can cause diagnostic confusion, some of them also correlate with characteristic clinical findings and behavior[6,7] (see below). However, it must be emphasized that the histologic features of several variants can coexist in the same lesion.[8]

Clinical features

Fibrous histiocytoma occurs most often in the middle aged and shows a slight female predominance. The majority of lesions are located on the limbs or (to a lesser degree) the trunk, and present as small, raised, hyperkeratotic cutaneous nodules usually less than 1 cm in diameter with a reddish-brown surface (*Figs 35.207* and *35.208*). Giant variants including a plaque-like variant are very rare.[9–12.]

A significant proportion of cases are said to be associated with previous minor local trauma, especially insect bites. They are slow growing and painless, and may sometimes be multiple. Eruptive lesions have been documented in the context of immunosuppression, HIV infection and highly active antiretroviral therapy (HAART).[13–19]

Simple excision is usually curative and local recurrence is exceptional except for some of the variants (see below) and in lesions occurring on the face, where the reported rate of local recurrence is 20%.[20] In some variants (e.g., atypical, aneurysmal, and cellular fibrous histiocytoma) and exceptional classic tumors, rare metastases have been reported.[21–28]

A small subgroup of these lesions originates in subcutaneous fat or in deeper structures (deep benign fibrous histiocytoma).[29,30]

Most fibrous histiocytomas show a typical dermoscopy pattern (peripheral delicate pigment network and a central white scar-like patch) but atypical patterns may mimic melanoma, vascular tumors, basal cell carcinoma, a collision tumor and even psoriasis.[31]

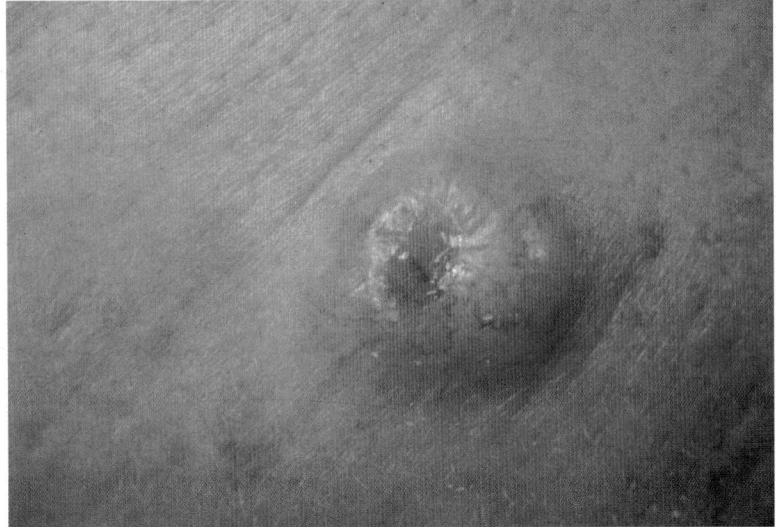

Fig. 35.207
Fibrous histiocytoma (dermatofibroma): this tumor most often presents as an erythematous raised lesion. Surface scaling is not uncommon. From the collection of the late N.P. Smith, MD, The Institute of Dermatology, London, UK.

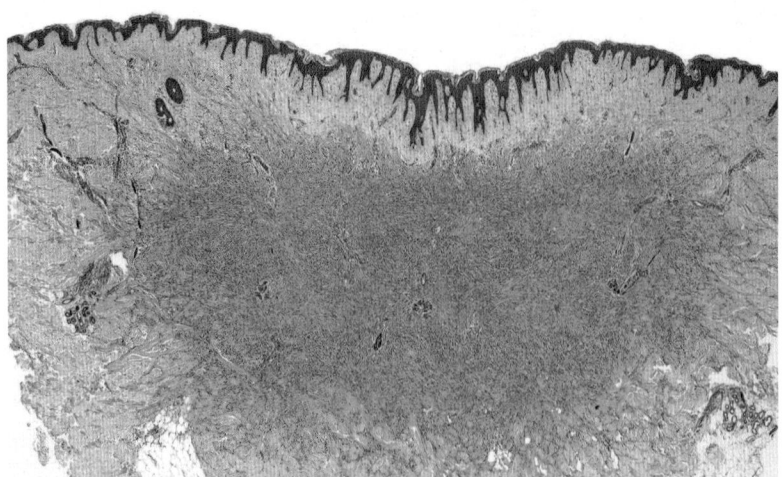

Fig. 35.209
Fibrous histiocytoma (dermatofibroma): scanning section showing the characteristic architecture. The lateral borders of the lesion interdigitate with the adjacent dermis. There is hyperkeratosis and acanthosis of the overlying epidermis.

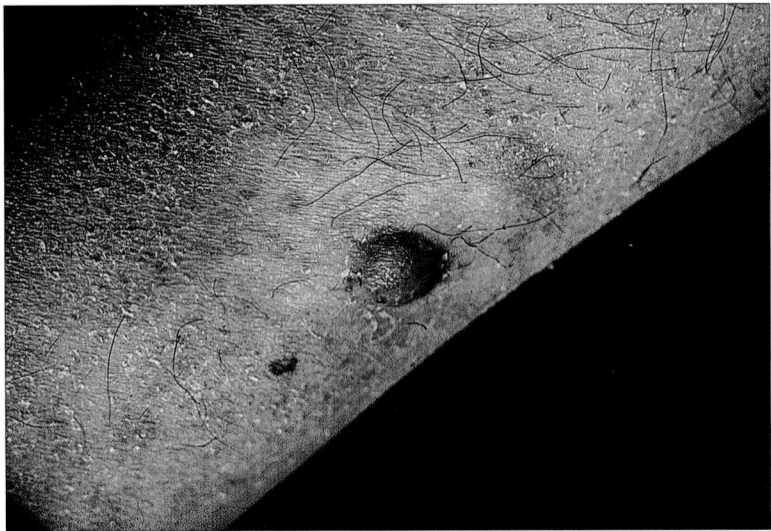

Fig. 35.208
Fibrous histiocytoma (dermatofibroma): dark brown (due to hemosiderin deposition) lesions are sometimes mistaken for melanocytic tumors, including melanoma. By courtesy of R.A. Marsden, MD, St George's Hospital, London, UK.

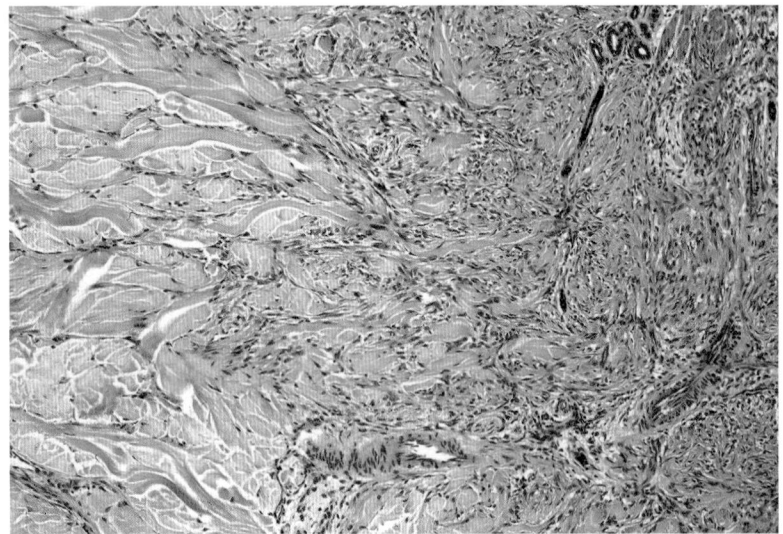

Fig. 35.210
Fibrous histiocytoma (dermatofibroma): the tumor extends into the adjacent normal dermis.

Pathogenesis and histologic features

For years, it was suggested that dermatofibroma represents a reactive process. Possible etiological associations included insect bites and even trauma such as body-piercing.[32] In later years it has become clear that the lesion represents a neoplastic process. Clinical evidence supporting the latter includes the following: tumors do not tend to regress spontaneously, in some variants there is variable potential for local recurrence, and a small number of cases have metastasized.[21–28,33] Cytogenetic analysis has provided further support to this theory. Clonality has been demonstrated in some examples of cellular fibrous histiocytoma.[34,35] More recently, further studies have demonstrated genetic aberrations by FISH analysis and RNA sequencing in rare examples of subsets of cutaneous fibrous histiocytoma (cellular and aneurysmal) and very exceptionally in regular lesions and deep fibrous histiocytoma.[36,37] Rearrangements of the protein kinase C genes (*PRKCB* and *PRKCD*) are seen in regular, epithelioid, cellular, and aneurysmal fibrous histiocytoma, and ALK rearrangements are only seen in the epithelioid variant.[37] Rearrangements of PRKC and ALK are mutually exclusive events; overexpression of these genes drives promoter swapping with a considerable variety of other gene fusion partners including *LAMTOR1*, *PDPN* and *CD63*. In another study,

DNA copy number changes by comparative genomic hybridization were detected in metastatic tumors and rare cases of nonmetastatic atypical and cellular variants.[27,38] The chromosomal aberrations were higher in metastatic cases resulting in death. With regards to aneurysmal fibrous histiocytoma, a translocation t(12;19)(p12;q13) was described and a pathogenetic role for *LAMTOR1-PRKCD* and *NUMA1-SFMBT1* has been suggested.[39,40]

The common variant is an ill-defined dermal lesion that may extend into superficial subcutaneous fat (*Figs 35.209–35.213*). It is largely composed of interlacing fascicles of slender spindled cells, sometimes in a focal storiform arrangement, set within a loose collagenous or (less often) myxoid stroma. Scattered between the spindled cells are foamy histiocytes, multinucleated giant cells and thin-walled blood vessels (*Figs 35.214–35.217*). Foci of chronic inflammatory cells, including lymphocytes and plasma cells, and hemosiderin deposition are frequently seen. A typical feature is the presence of individual hyaline collagen bundles surrounded by tumor cells in the periphery of the lesions.

Long-standing lesions show progressive hyalinization and decreased cellularity and are usually referred to as sclerosing or atrophic dermatofibroma.

All of these tumors, including the variants, may be associated with acanthosis or even pseudoepitheliomatous hyperplasia of the overlying epidermis

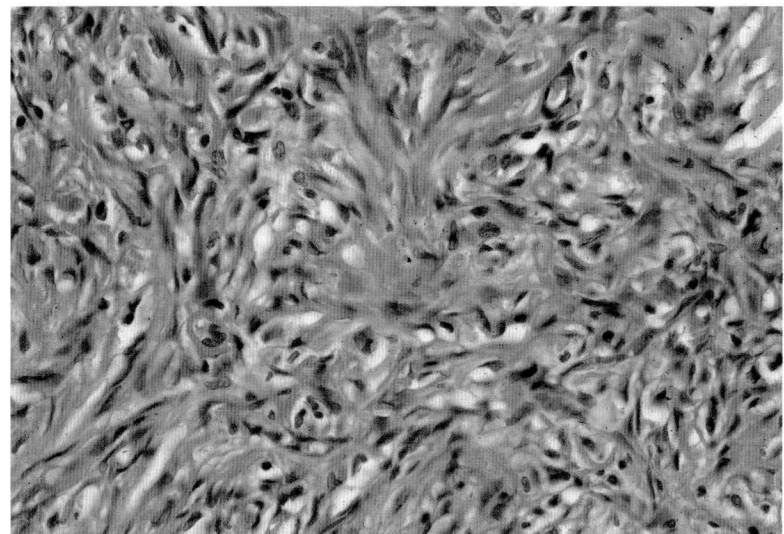

Fig. 35.211
Fibrous histiocytoma (dermatofibroma): high-power view showing storiform growth pattern.

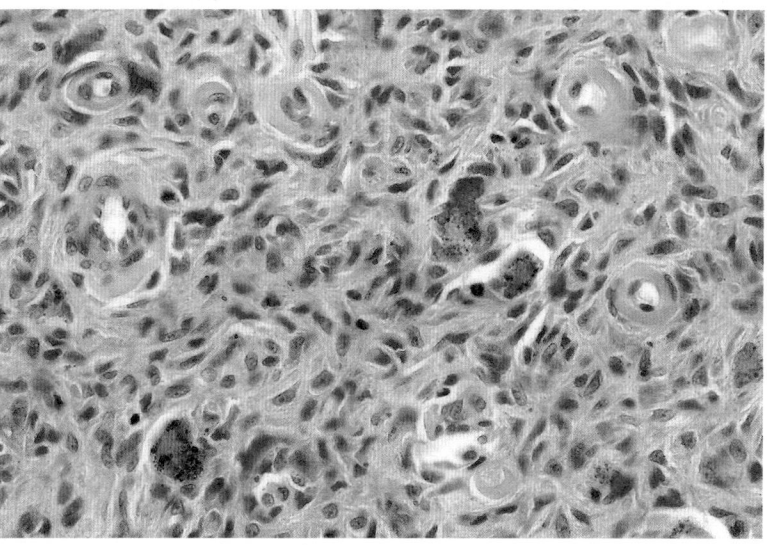

Fig. 35.214
Fibrous histiocytoma (dermatofibroma): scattered multinucleated giant cells are a not infrequent feature of this lesion. Note the hemosiderin pigment.

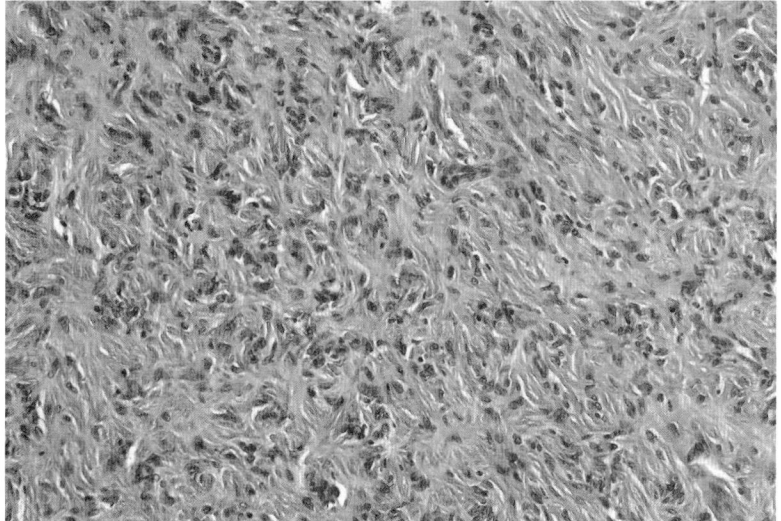

Fig. 35.212
Fibrous histiocytoma (dermatofibroma): the tumor is composed of uniform, interlacing spindle cells in a vaguely curlicue pattern embedded in a hyaline collagenous stroma.

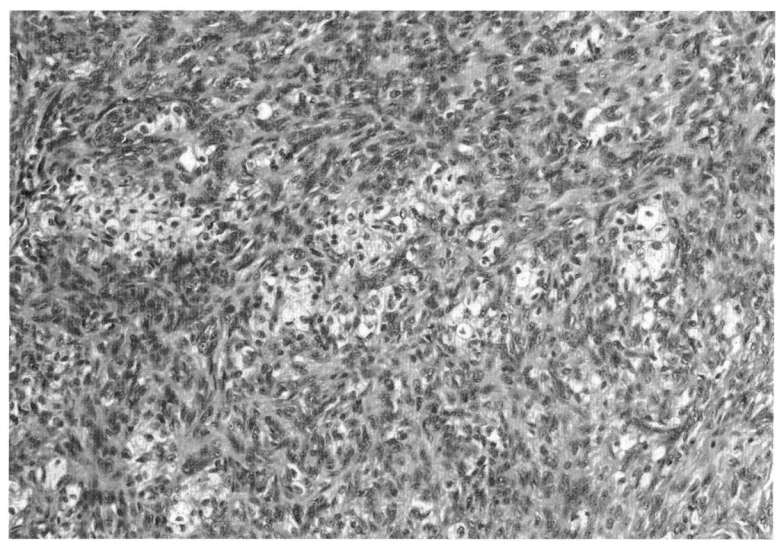

Fig. 35.215
Fibrous histiocytoma (dermatofibroma): lipid-laden histiocytes are commonly present.

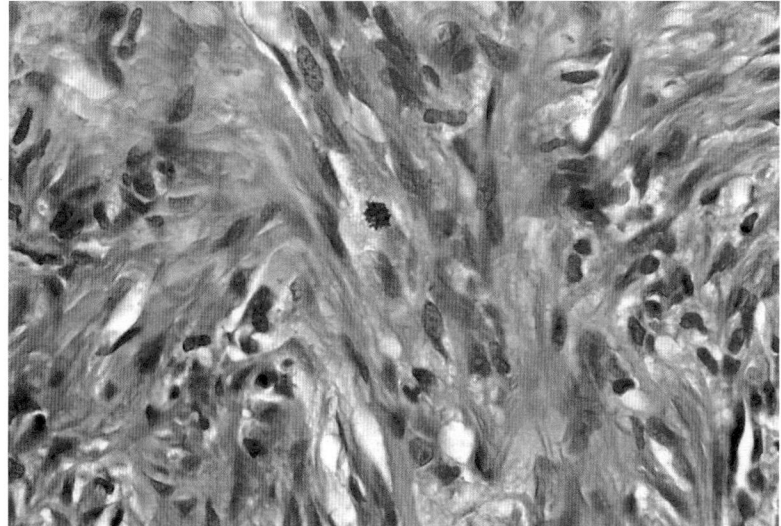

Fig. 35.213
Fibrous histiocytoma (dermatofibroma): occasional normal mitotic figures may be seen.

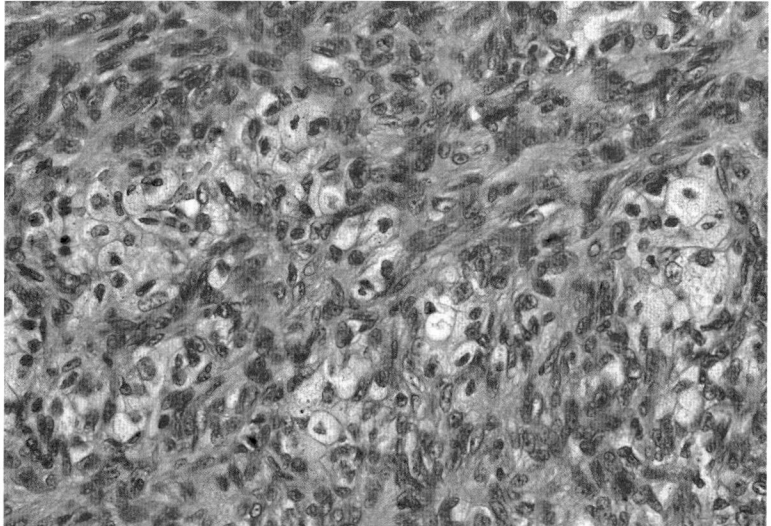

Fig. 35.216
Fibrous histiocytoma (dermatofibroma): high-power view.

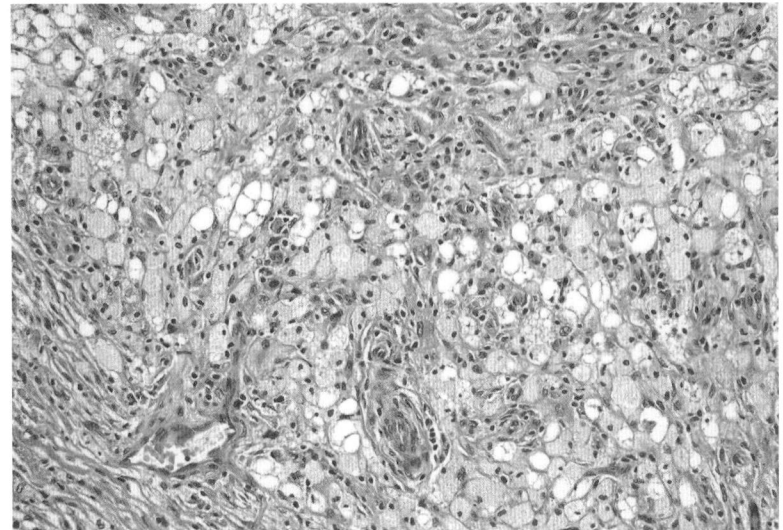

Fig. 35.217
Fibrous histiocytoma (dermatofibroma): when the lipid-laden histiocytes are numerous, this lesion is sometimes called histiocytoma cutis.

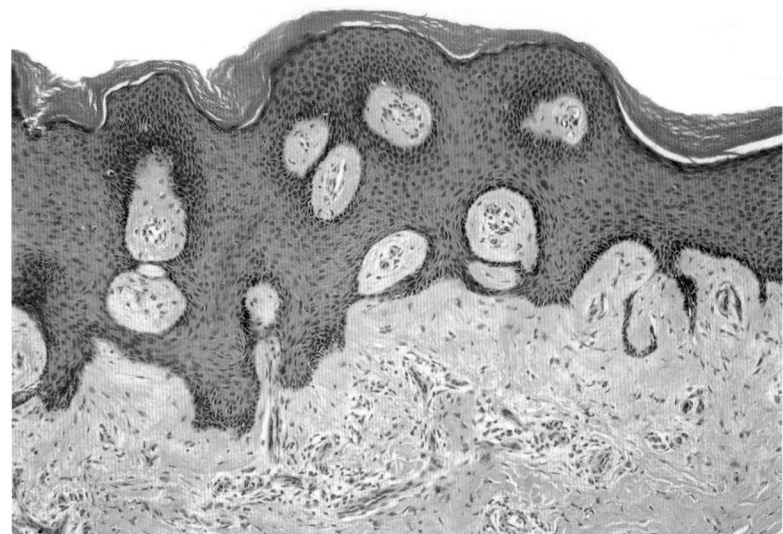

Fig. 35.219
Fibrous histiocytoma (dermatofibroma): the tumor is often separated from the epidermis by a grenz zone.

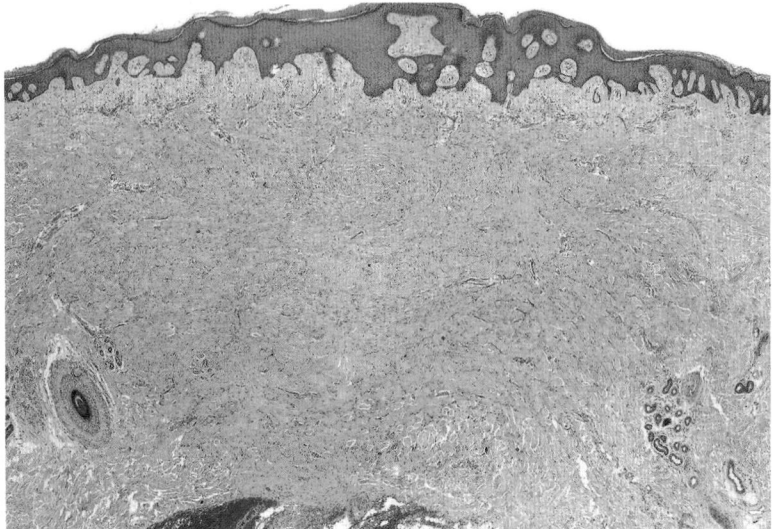

Fig. 35.218
Fibrous histiocytoma (dermatofibroma): the epithelium overlying the tumor is often acanthotic.

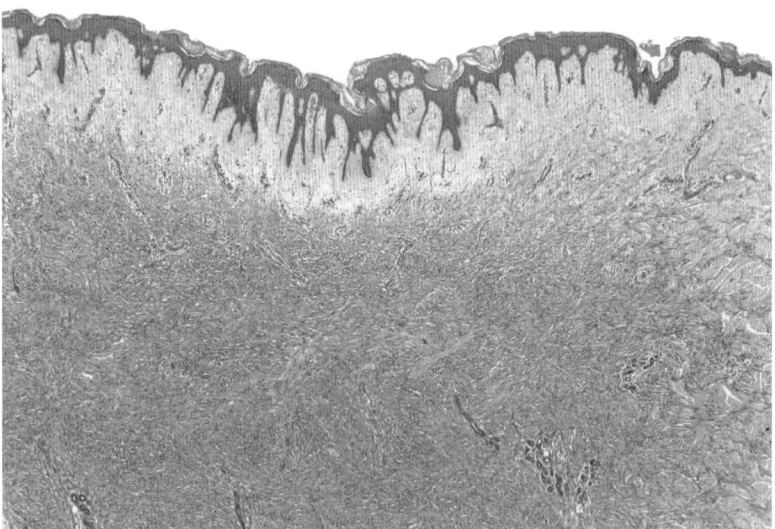

Fig. 35.220
Fibrous histiocytoma (dermatofibroma): in this example, there is an extensive grenz zone.

and hyperpigmentation of the basal cell layer (*Figs 35.218* and *35.219*). It has been suggested that epidermal growth factor may play a role in the pathogenesis of the epidermal hyperplasia.[41] A grenz zone of papillary dermal sparing is usually present (*Fig. 35.220*). Changes simulating seborrheic keratosis are common, followed by proliferation of clear cells mimicking a clear cell acanthoma, and proliferation of immature hair follicle-like structures closely resembling a trichoblastoma, and induction of sebaceous glands sometimes in a reticulate pattern (*Fig. 35.221*) [42,43] Mature hair follicles are rarely induced and more unusual epidermal changes including, epidermolytic hyperkeratosis, focal acantholysis and even Bowen disease, have also been described.[44,45] Most cases reported as basal cell carcinoma overlying dermatofibroma actually represent reactive induction of immature follicular structures rather than collision tumors.

A proportion of tumors, especially the cellular variant, stain focally for α-SMA and calponin, suggesting myofibroblastic differentiation (*Fig. 35.222*). It has been proposed that this lesion arises from a fixed dermal connective tissue cell, the dermal dendrocyte, which stains positively for factor XIIIa.[46] Although a number of cells within fibrous histiocytomas react with this marker, especially towards the edges of the lesion, these appear to be reactive cells and not true tumor cells. In contrast to dermatofibrosarcoma, CD34 expression is not usually a feature except in the cellular variant

of fibrous histiocytoma where focal positivity for this marker may be seen (see below). D2–40 is diffusely positive in dermatofibromas and only very focally positive or negative in dermatofibrosarcoma protuberans.[47]

Common dermatofibroma is usually easy to diagnose and problems with differential diagnosis generally only arise with its variants.[48]

Variants of dermatofibroma include:

- cellular fibrous histiocytoma,
- aneurysmal fibrous histiocytoma,
- epithelioid fibrous histiocytoma,
- atypical (pseudosarcomatous) fibrous histiocytoma,
- lipidized ('ankle-type') fibrous histiocytoma,
- clear cell fibrous histiocytoma,
- palisading cutaneous fibrous histiocytoma,
- atrophic dermatofibroma.

It is important to note that all variants of dermatofibroma except the epithelioid variant may overlap histologically.

Cellular fibrous histiocytoma

Cellular benign fibrous histiocytoma accounts for almost 5% of cutaneous fibrous histiocytomas.[48–50] It is most common in young adults, especially males, and has a predilection for the limbs and head and neck area (*Figs*

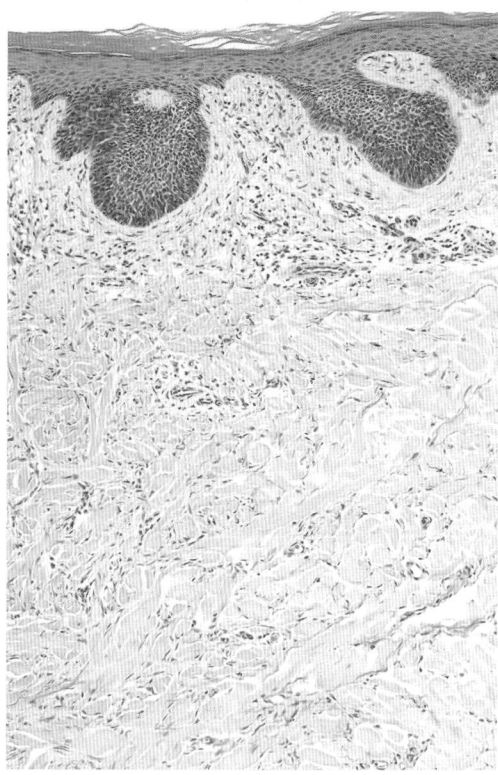

Fig. 35.221
Fibrous histiocytoma (dermatofibroma): proliferation of basaloid cells reminiscent of trichoblastoma.

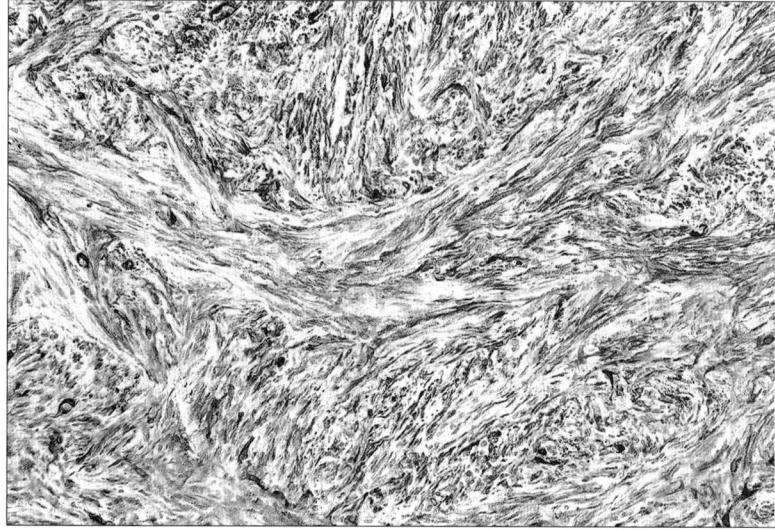

Fig. 35.222
Fibrous histiocytoma (dermatofibroma): this example shows strong smooth muscle actin expression.

35.223 and 35.224). These lesions are larger than common fibrous histiocytoma and have a high recurrence rate of up to 26%. Metastasis to regional lymph nodes, soft tissues and lungs has been reported in a small number of cases.[22–28] Development of satellite nodules has also been described.[26] In a further case, erosion of the phalanx occurred.[51] Histologic features do not allow prediction of those cases that ultimately metastasize.[26] Cases that may be more likely to metastasize appear to be those that recur early and on multiple occasions.

Histologically, lesions are highly cellular with a more prominent fascicular growth pattern (Figs 35.225–35.228). Frequently there is involvement of the superficial subcutis. Tumor cells tend to have more abundant eosinophilic cytoplasm, and normal mitotic figures are common (Fig. 35.229). Central necrosis is seen in some cases (about 10%). A pleomorphic sarcoma component has been described in a case of primary cellular fibrous histiocytoma and in a recurrent tumor.[27]

Immunohistochemistry shows variable (usually focal) staining for SMA (in most cases) and calponin and negative or only focal staining for CD34

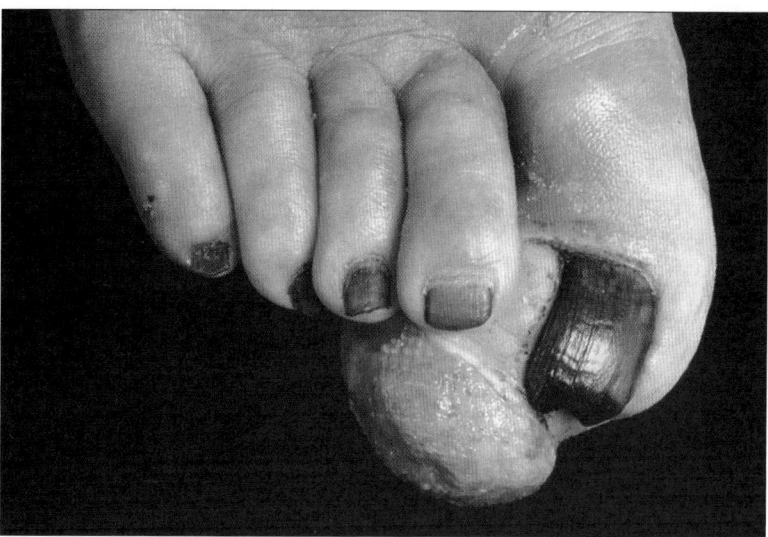

Fig. 35.223
Cellular fibrous histiocytoma: tumors may be large and sometimes present at unusual sites, as in this example. By courtesy of the Institute of Dermatology, London, UK.

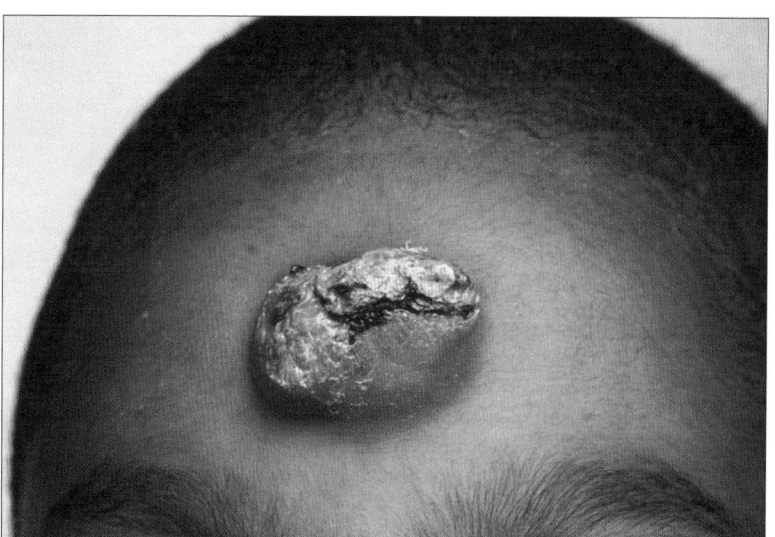

Fig. 35.224
Cellular fibrous histiocytoma: children may rarely be affected. Ulceration is sometimes a feature. By courtesy of the Institute of Dermatology, London, UK.

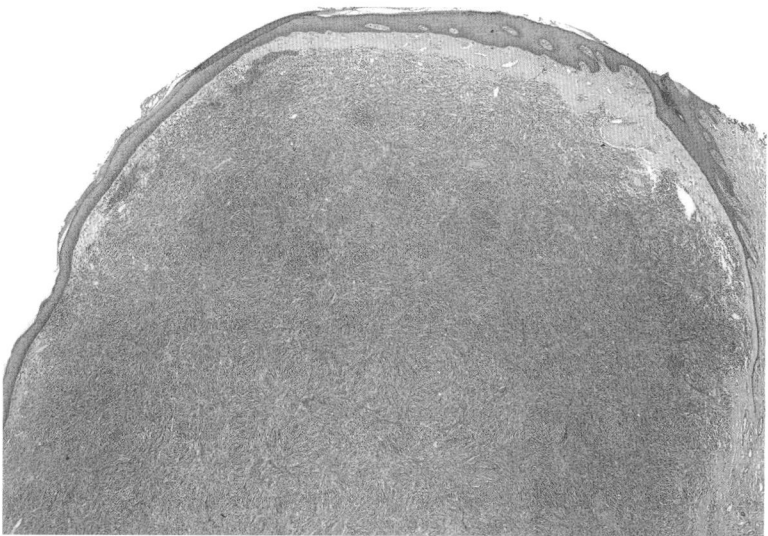

Fig. 35.225
Cellular fibrous histiocytoma: this variant of dermatofibroma is often a source of diagnostic confusion. It is larger than the conventional form and appears more cellular and mitotically active.

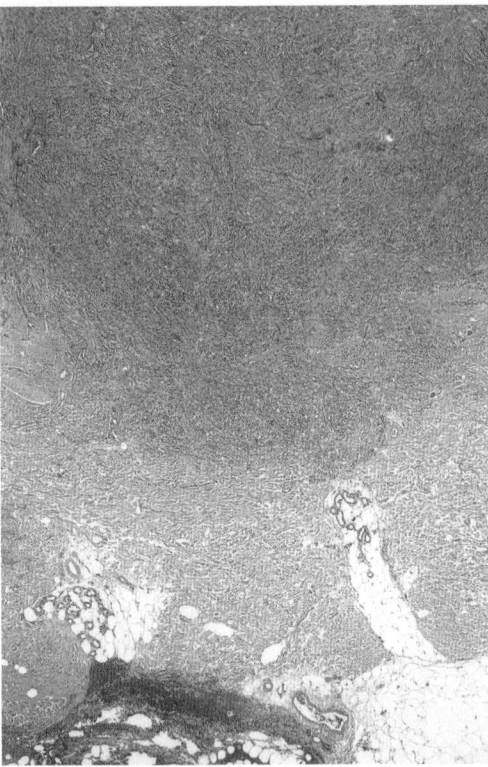

Fig. 35.226
Cellular fibrous histiocytoma: scanning view showing extension into the deep reticular dermis.

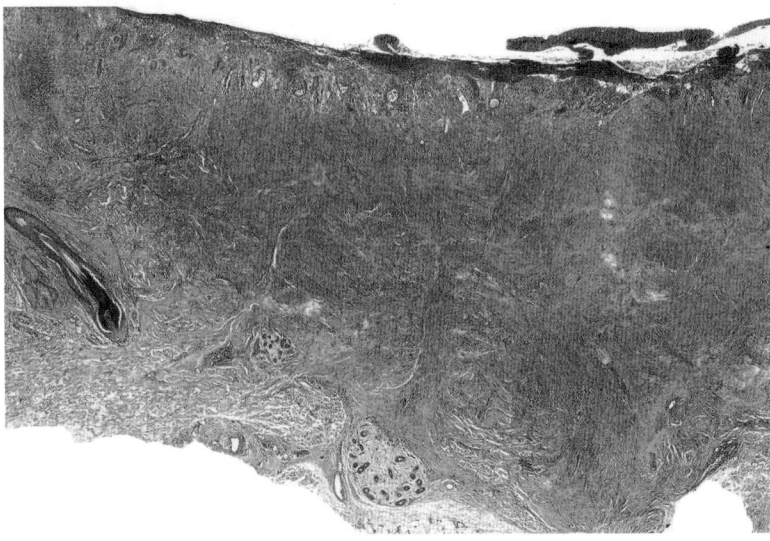

Fig. 35.227
Cellular fibrous histiocytoma: this example shows striking cellularity.

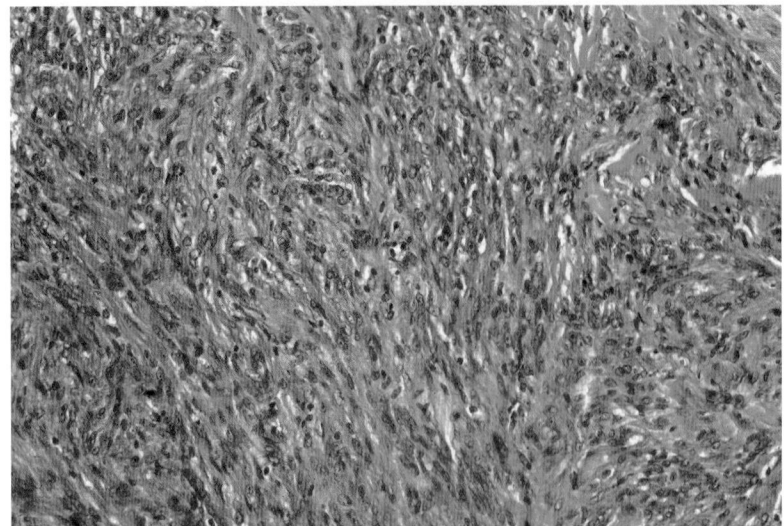

Fig. 35.228
Cellular fibrous histiocytoma: high-power view of Figure 35.226

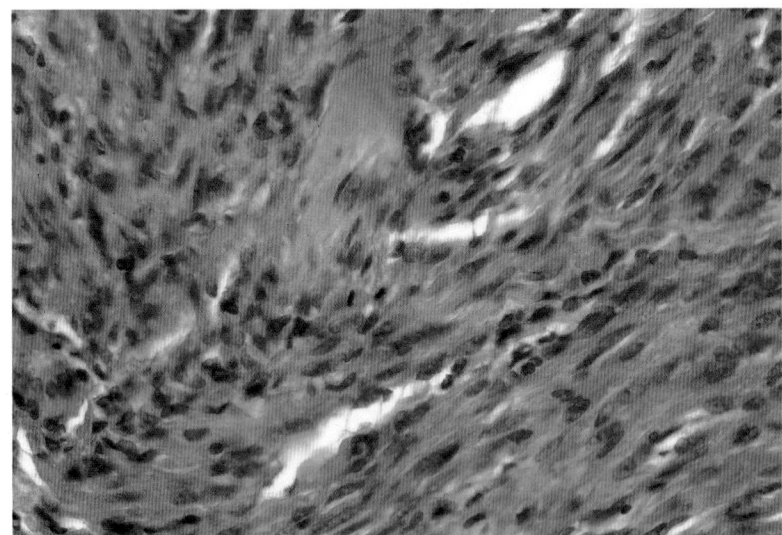

Fig. 35.229
Cellular fibrous histiocytoma: note the mitotic activity.

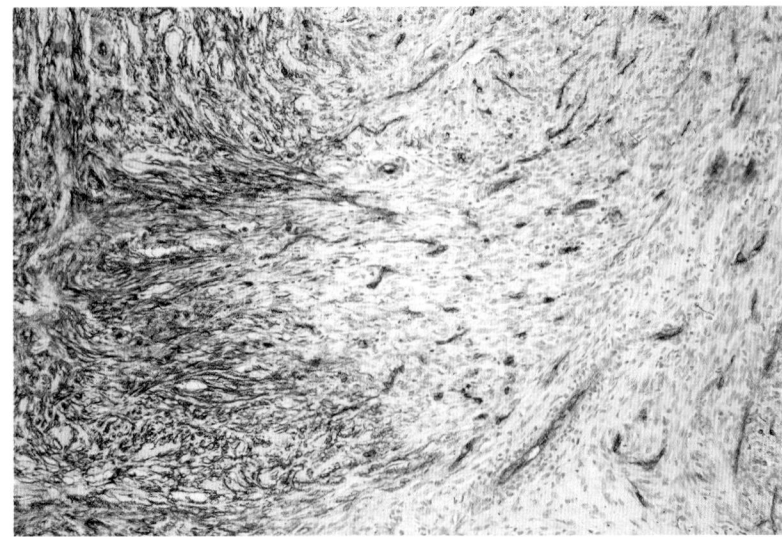

Fig. 35.230
Cellular fibrous histiocytoma: the tumor cells at the edge of the lesion often express CD34.

(*Fig. 35.230*). When the last is present, expression is limited to peripheral parts of the tumor. Focal desmin positivity may be seen in around a third of cases.[52]

Distinction from leiomyosarcoma is possible by the presence in the latter of cells with cigar-shaped nuclei, at least focal cytologic atypia, a uniform fascicular growth pattern, diffuse positivity for SMA, desmin and H-caldesmon and frequent focal positivity for keratin. Dermatofibrosarcoma protuberans has a monotonous, storiform growth pattern, monomorphous cells and diffuse positivity for CD34.

Aneurysmal fibrous histiocytoma

Aneurysmal benign fibrous histiocytoma represents less than 2% of fibrous histiocytomas and presents as a blue–brown nodule on the limbs of middle-aged adults, especially females (*Fig. 35.231*).[53–56] Rapid growth can be seen due to extensive hemorrhage, and clinical confusion with a melanocytic or vascular tumor is common. The rate of recurrence is around 19%.[54] Rare cases present with regional lymph node involvement.[26,27,54]

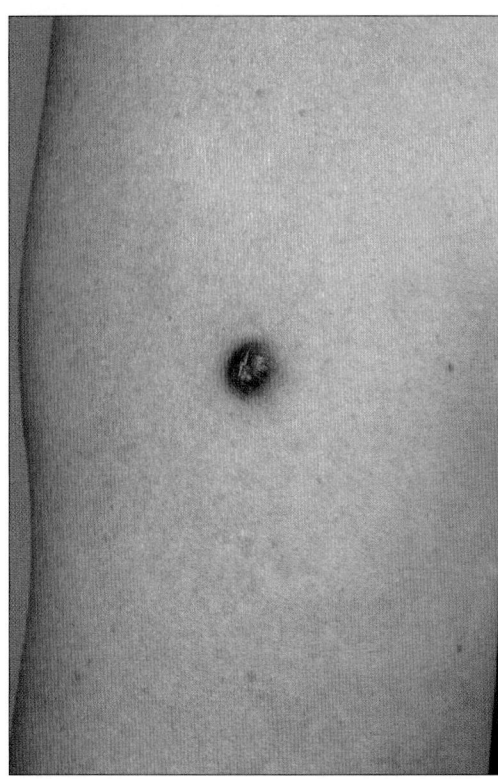

Fig. 35.231
Aneurysmal fibrous histiocytoma: this lesion presents as a hemorrhagic nodule. By courtesy of the Institute of Dermatology, London, UK.

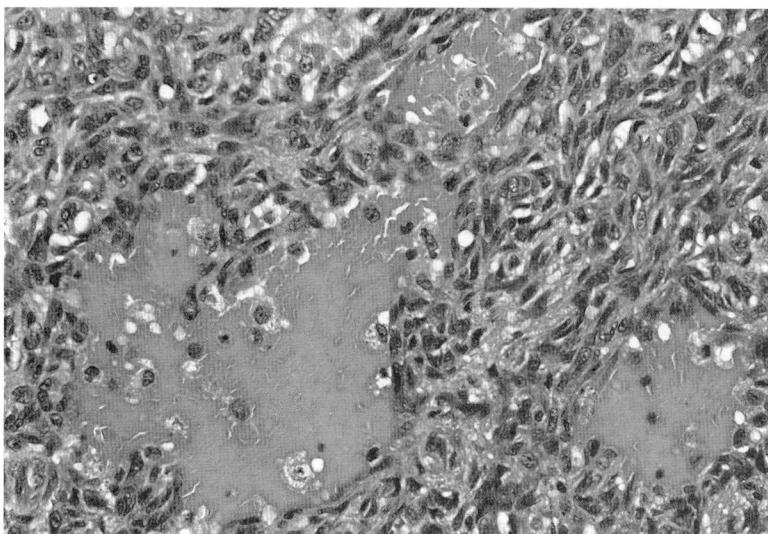

Fig. 35.233
Aneurysmal fibrous histiocytoma: the hemorrhagic spaces are devoid of an endothelial lining.

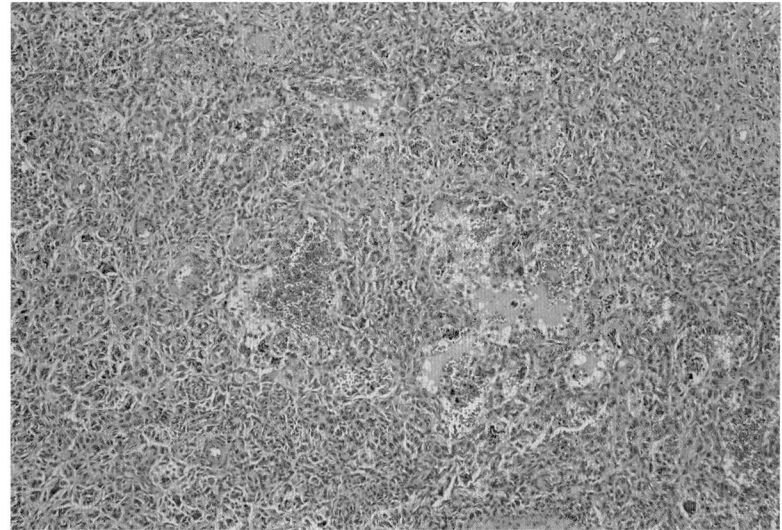

Fig. 35.232
Aneurysmal fibrous histiocytoma: a densely cellular infiltrate is present in the deeper dermis. Blood-filled cystic spaces are evident.

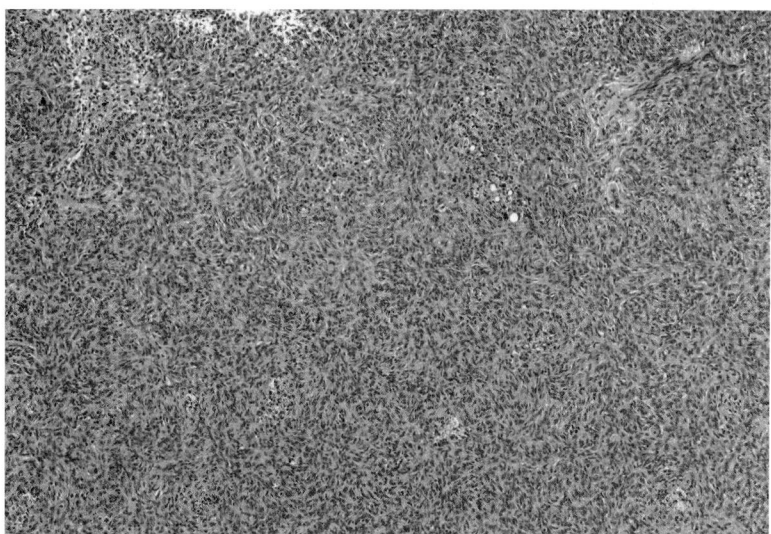

Fig. 35.234
Hemosiderotic fibrous histiocytoma: the marked vascularity and heavy hemosiderin content sometimes seen in this lesion gives a dark bluish-brown coloration, which clinically may cause confusion with melanoma.

Histologically, the most striking feature is the presence (especially towards the center of the lesion) of hemorrhagic irregular cleft-like and cystic spaces mimicking cavernous vascular channels, but without endothelial lining (*Figs 35.232* and *35.233*). Adjacent solid areas show the usual features of benign fibrous histiocytoma, but are often very cellular. Multifocal interstitial hemorrhage and intra- and extracellular hemosiderin deposition are prominent and normal mitotic figures are common (*Figs 35.234–35.236*). Due to the extensive secondary changes this lesion is frequently diagnosed as a vascular tumor, but typical features of fibrous histiocytoma are always present and endothelial markers are only positive in normal blood vessels.

Aneurysmal fibrous histiocytoma should not be confused with angiomatoid fibrous histiocytoma, the latter being an unrelated neoplasm with *EWSR1-CREB1* gene fusion. The latter is usually subcutaneous and is composed of monomorphic spindle-to-ovoid eosinophilic cells, which are usually desmin positive. A prominent lymphoplasmacytic infiltrate is commonly present. Some patients with the latter condition have striking systemic symptoms.

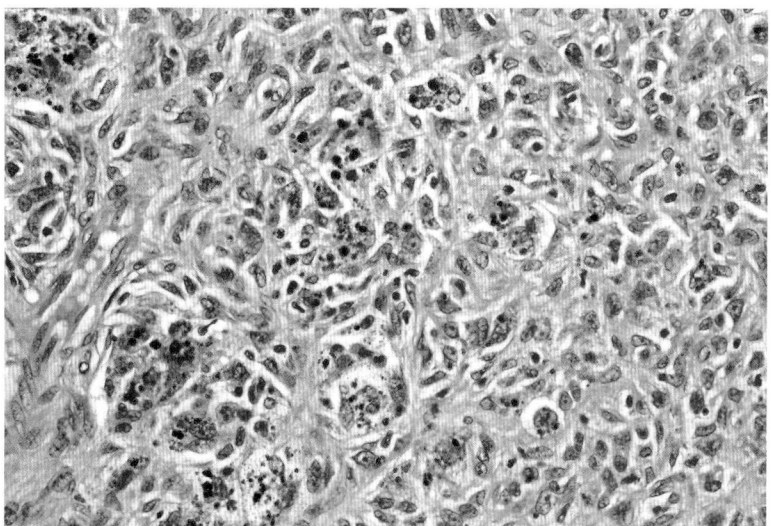

Fig. 35.235
Hemosiderotic fibrous histiocytoma: this variant is also sometimes known as sclerosing hemangioma.

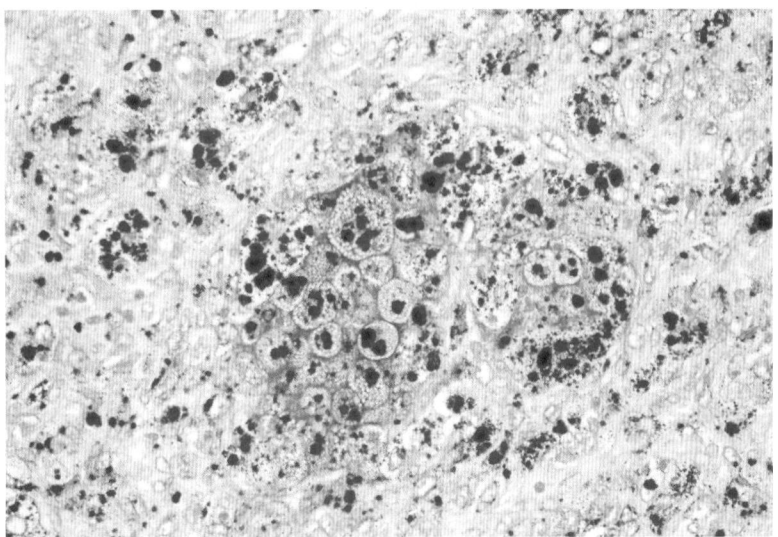

Fig. 35.236
Hemosiderotic fibrous histiocytoma: a Perl stain highlights the hemosiderin.

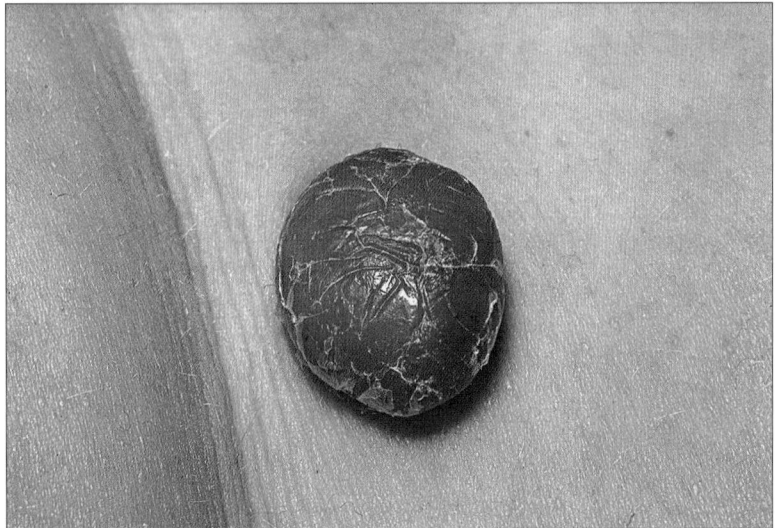

Fig. 35.237
Epithelioid benign fibrous histiocytoma: this variant typically presents as an erythematous polypoid lesion. By courtesy of the Institute of Dermatology, London, UK.

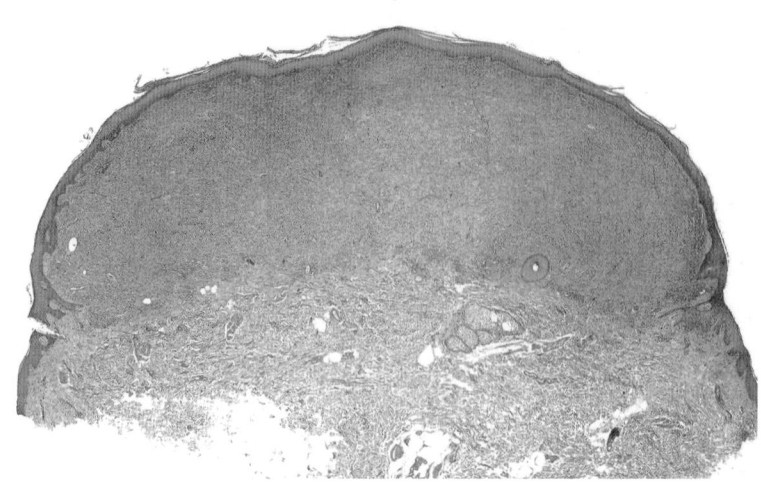

Fig. 35.238
Epithelioid benign fibrous histiocytoma: this low-power view shows a superficial tumor nodule with an associated epidermal collarette.

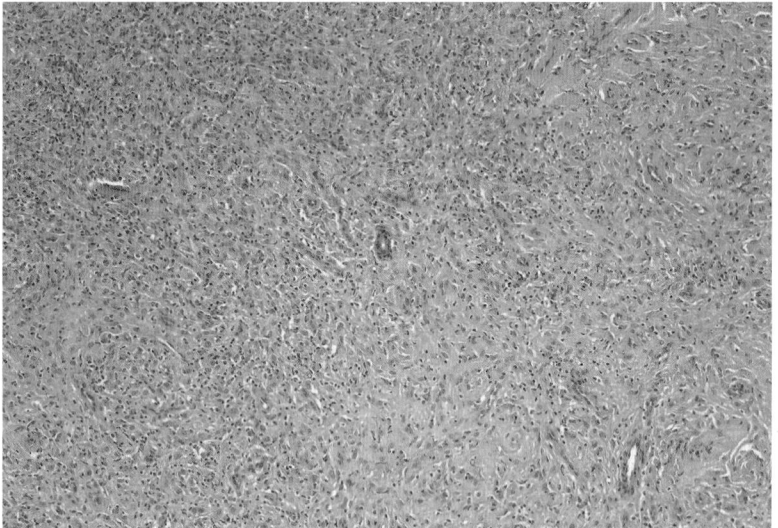

Fig. 35.239
Epithelioid benign fibrous histiocytoma: the tumor is composed of large cells with abundant eosinophilic cytoplasm. The infiltrate is uniform, in contrast to the more typical variant. Often, conventional features are identifiable elsewhere in the specimen.

Hemosiderotic fibrous histiocytoma probably represents a stage in the development of aneurysmal fibrous histiocytoma.

Epithelioid fibrous histiocytoma

Epithelioid fibrous histiocytoma is rare, has a wide age and anatomical distribution (with predilection for the proximal lower limb), and often presents as a polypoid red nodule, which is usually confused with a lobular capillary hemangioma (pyogenic granuloma) (*Fig. 35.237*).[57-60] Multiple lesions are exceptional and a lesion has been reported in the tongue.[61,62] A case with metastatic spread has been described.[26] Histologically, most tumors are superficial, but rare examples extend into the superficial subcutis. An epidermal collarette is often present and tumor cells are rounded with abundant eosinophilic cytoplasm and a vesicular nucleus with small eosinophilic nucleoli (*Figs 35.238–35.241*). Binucleate or multinucleate cells are common. Rarely, cells may have granular cell change.[63] Occasional normal mitotic figures may be evident. Some lesions are more myxoid and vascular. A rare variant of the tumor has been reported as chondroblastoma-like and consisting of pericellular calcification.[64] Immunohistochemistry reveals a population of CD34 positive cells and a population of factor XIIIa-positive dendritic cells.[65] Distinction from Spitz nevus is facilitated by the absence of a junctional component or nesting of tumor cells and negativity for S100

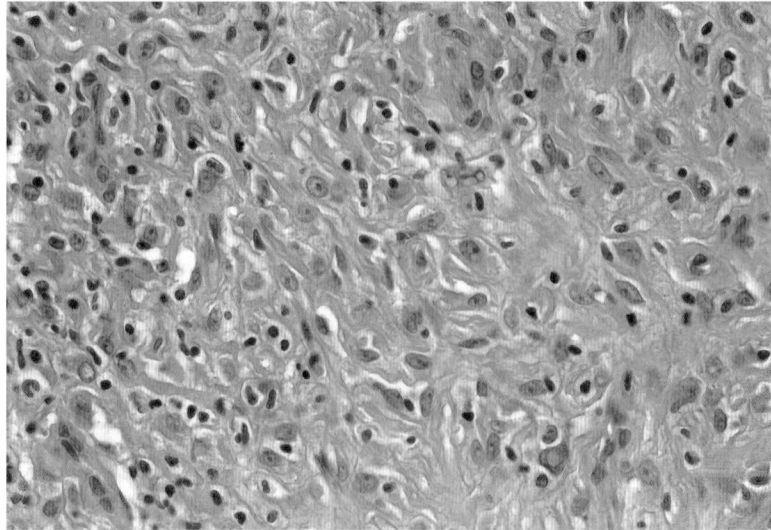

Fig. 35.240
Epithelioid benign fibrous histiocytoma: high-power view.

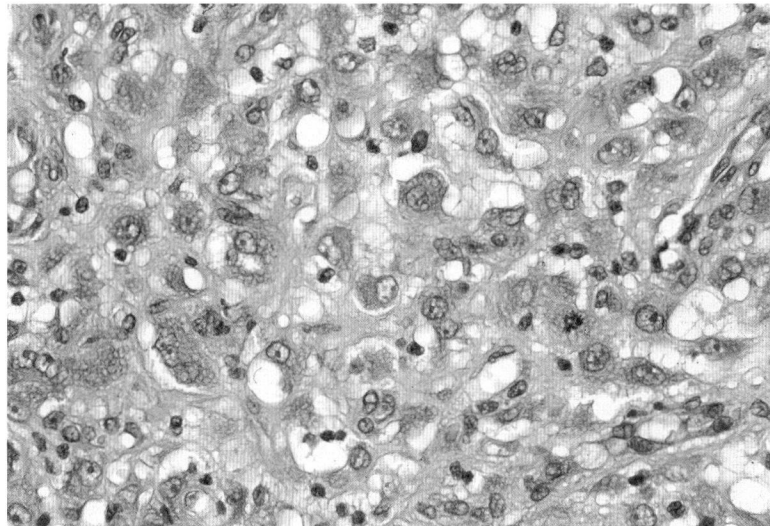

Fig. 35.241
Epithelioid benign fibrous histiocytoma: occasional normal mitotic figures may be present.

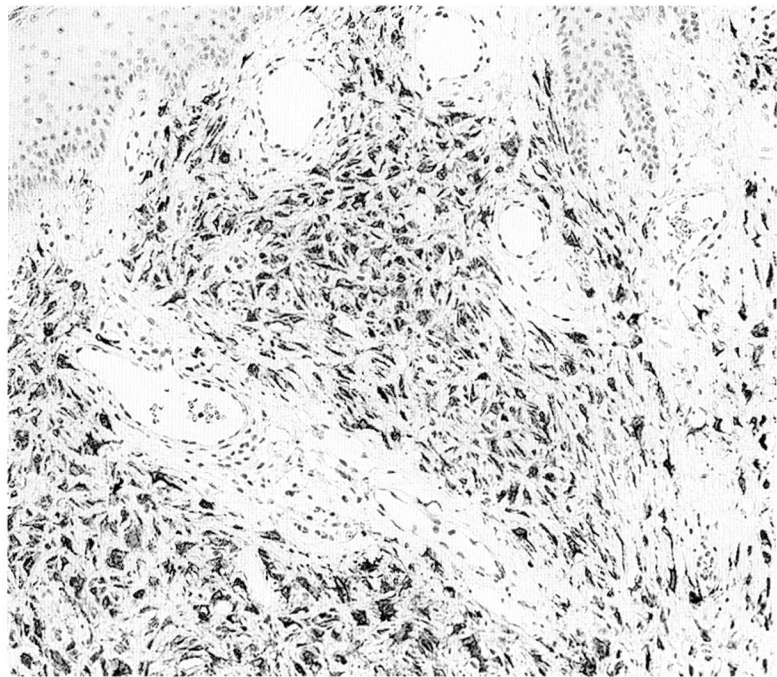

Fig. 35.242
Epithelioid benign fibrous histiocytoma: the tumor cells are often positive for ALK1.

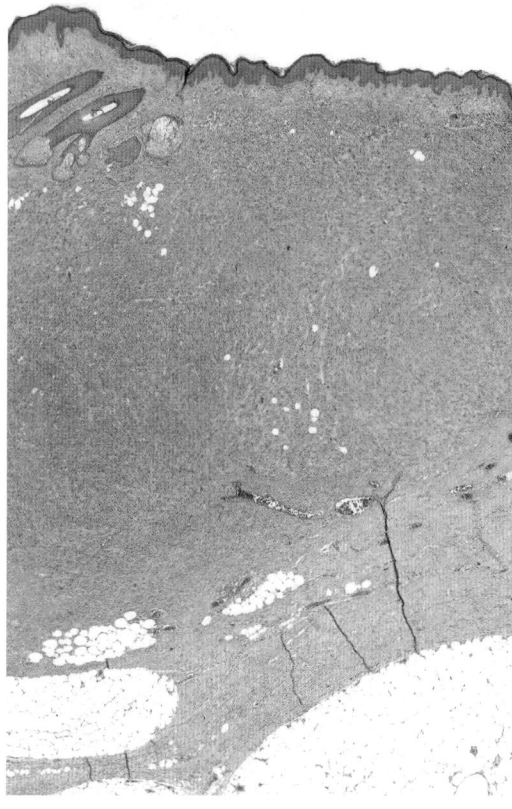

Fig. 35.243
Atypical benign fibrous histiocytoma: this cellular lesion extends into the subcutaneous fat.

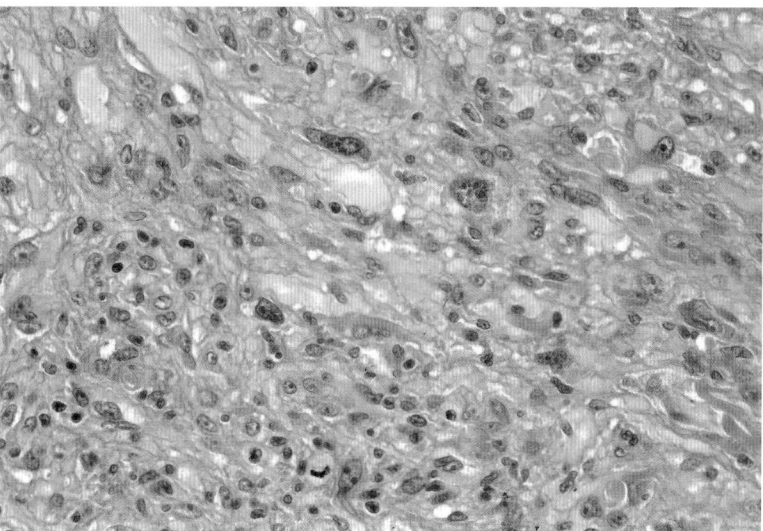

Fig. 35.244
Atypical benign fibrous histiocytoma: there is striking nuclear pleomorphism. Note the mitotic figure.

protein. Distinction from a cutaneous perineurioma with epithelioid cell change is made by the presence of diffuse EMA and claudin-1 positivity in the latter tumor. However, focal membranous EMA positivity is a frequent finding in epithelioid fibrous histiocytoma.[66] ALK expression is typically seen (in roughly 90% of cases) and is correlated with ALK rearrangements with a variety of partner genes including *SQSTM1, VCL, TMP3, EML4, PRKAR2A*, and others (*Fig. 35.242*).[67–69]

Atypical (pseudosarcomatous) fibrous histiocytoma

Atypical (pseudosarcomatous) fibrous histiocytoma is also known as dermatofibroma with monster cells.[21,70–73] Clinically, it has a predilection for the limbs with some tumors occurring on the trunk and head and neck. Lesions are usually papular or nodular but may be polypoid, and rare tumors measure up to several centimeters.[21] There is local recurrence in a minority of cases, and metastasis rarely occur with one patient dying as a result of systemic spread.[21,26,27]

Histologically, the lesion is mainly dermal but extends into the superficial subcutis in one-third of cases. In some areas, the tumor shows the features of a more typical fibrous histiocytoma (*Fig. 35.243*). However, a variable proportion of cells in the tumor have irregular, large and pleomorphic nuclei with prominent nucleoli (*Fig. 35.244*). Pleomorphism may be marked. The mitotic rate varies and may be high in some cases. Atypical mitotic figures are sometimes seen. An unusual feature is that of focal necrosis.[20] Histologic features do not allow prediction of the exceptional tumors that metastasize.[26]

Atypical fibrous histiocytoma should not be confused with atypical fibroxanthoma. The latter occurs in a completely different clinical setting (see below) and shows diffuse pleomorphism, cytologic atypia and numerous mitoses throughout.

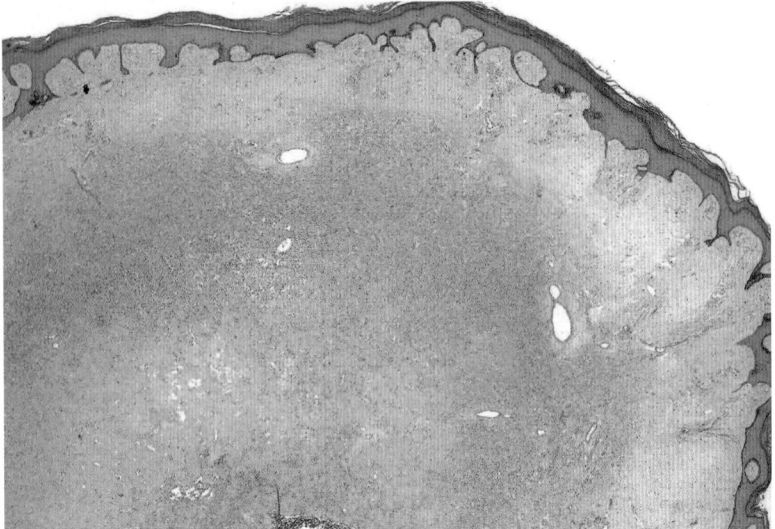

Fig. 35.245
Lipidized ('ankle-type') fibrous histiocytoma: this is a distinctive morphological subset characterized by a predominance of xanthoma cells associated with marked stromal hyalinization. By courtesy of R. Carr MD, Warwick Hospital, UK.

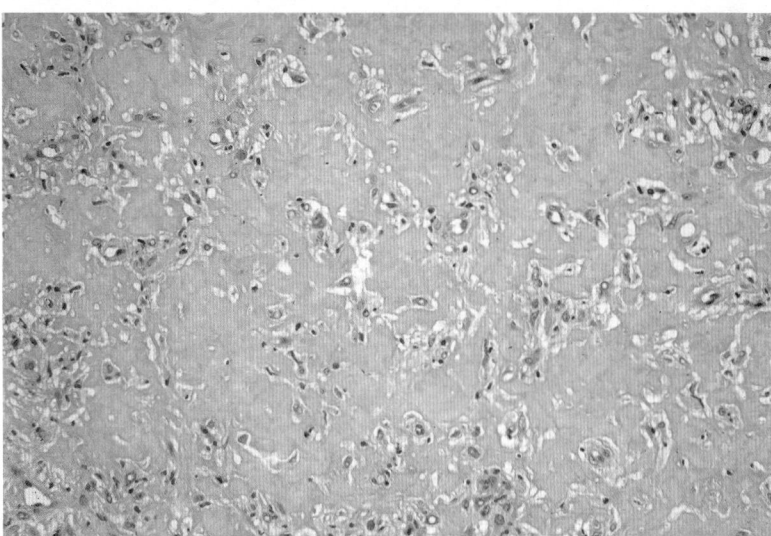

Fig. 35.247
Lipidized ('ankle-type') fibrous histiocytoma: this field shows densely hyalinized collagen reminiscent of amyloid. By courtesy of R. Carr MD, Warwick Hospital, UK.

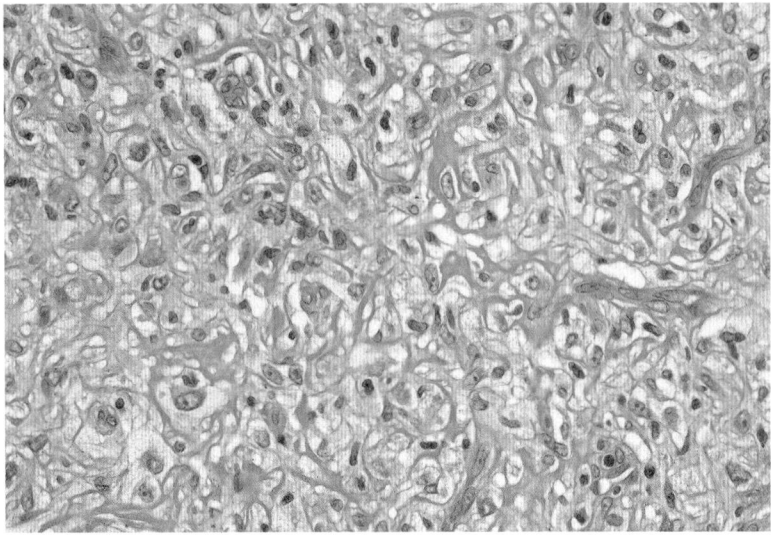

Fig. 35.246
Lipidized ('ankle-type') fibrous histiocytoma: high-power view of foamy histiocytes. By courtesy of R. Carr MD, Warwick Hospital, UK.

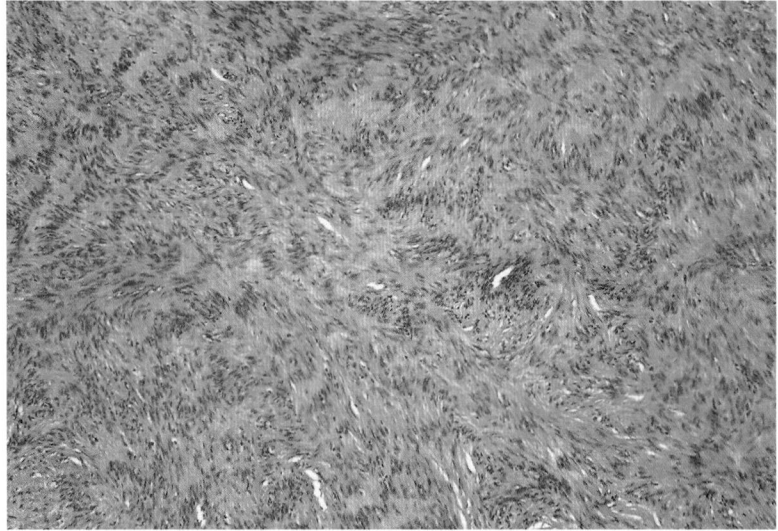

Fig. 35.248
Palisading fibrous histiocytoma: occasionally, palisading mimicking Verocay bodies may be a feature.

Lipidized ('ankle-type') fibrous histiocytoma

Lipidized ('ankle-type') fibrous histiocytoma presents as a polypoid yellow lesion on the lower leg.[74] Histologically, there is a predominance of foamy histiocytes surrounded by abundant, almost keloidal, hyalinized collagen bundles (*Figs 35.245–35.247*).

Clear cell fibrous histiocytoma

This is a very rare variant with no distinctive clinical features and with massive clear cell change throughout the lesion.[75–77] The overall architecture and morphological features are not usually typical of a fibrous histiocytoma and thus may represent an altogether unrelated tumor. It is likely that tumors previously described as clear cell fibrous histiocytoma represent the entity reported as dermal clear cell mesenchymal neoplasm.[78,79] Only a handful of cases of the latter entity have been described in adults with predilection for the lower limbs. Tumors consist of sheets of clear cells with vesicular nuclei that occupy the reticular dermis and may extend into the subcutaneous tissue. Cytologic atypia and mitotic figures are rare. Tumor cells are negative for most markers except vimentin, NKI/C3 and sometimes CD68. Behavior appears to be benign.

Palisading cutaneous fibrous histiocytoma

Palisading cutaneous fibrous histiocytoma refers to lesions that histologically show prominent nuclear palisading (*Figs 35.248* and *35.249*).[80,81] They appear to present most often on acral sites. Focally, there is a resemblance to schwannoma as the palisading mimics Verocay bodies. However, lesions are not encapsulated and tumor cells are S100 negative.

Atrophic dermatofibroma

Atrophic dermatofibroma probably represents the end stage of many dermatofibromas and is characterized clinically by an area of depression or retraction, often resembling a scar or even anetoderma.[82–84] Histologically, lesions are hypocellular and show prominent hyalinization of collagen (*Figs 35.250* and *35.251*). The changes may resemble those seen in multinucleate angiohistiocytoma but the latter usually presents with multiple clinical lesions.

Rare variants

Very occasionally, tumors can show prominent osteoclast-like giant cells (occasionally with ossification), granular cell change, cholesterol deposition, focal smooth muscle proliferation, marked myxoid change, keloidal change,

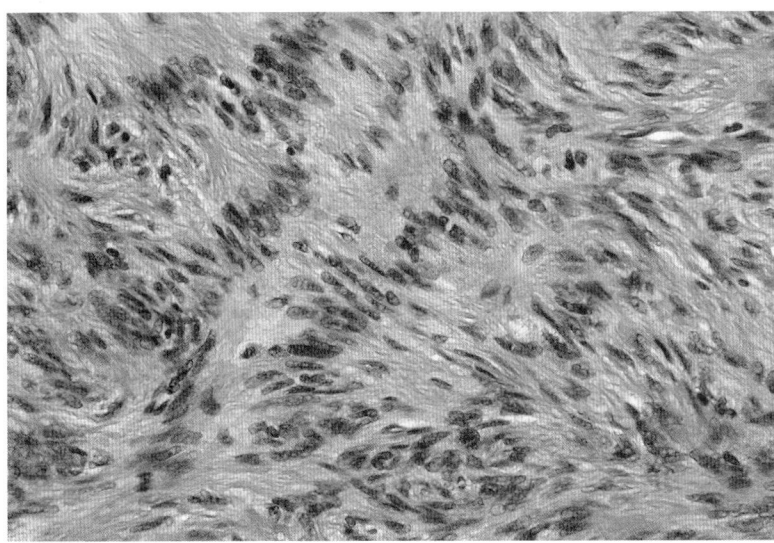

Fig. 35.249
Palisading fibrous histiocytoma: high-power view.

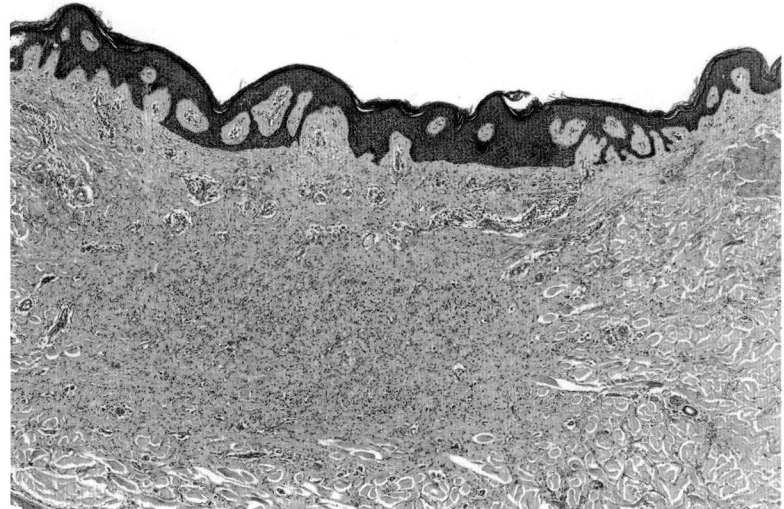

Fig. 35.250
Atrophic fibrous histiocytoma: this variant appears hypocellular and orientated parallel to the surface epithelium.

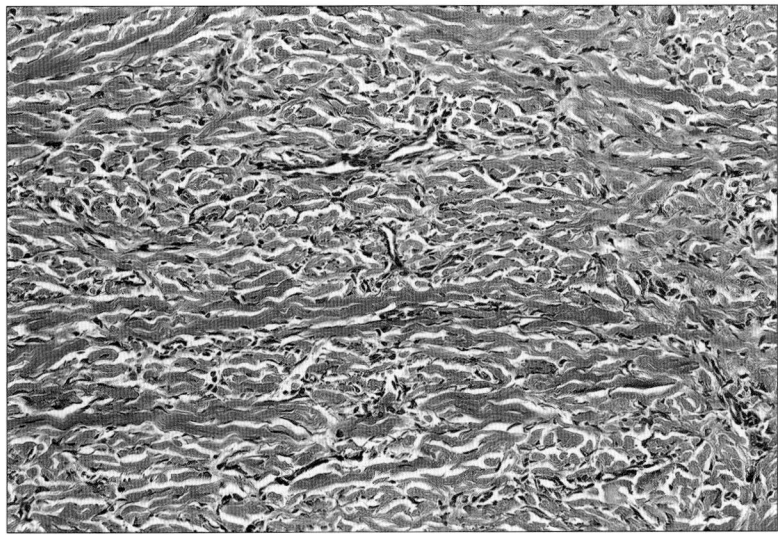

Fig. 35.251
Atrophic fibrous histiocytoma: the tumor cells are compressed by the collagenous component.

balloon cell change and signet-ring change.[85–102] Tumors may also present with a lichenoid pattern and in a single case intracytoplasmic eosinophilic globules were described.[103,104] Two cases of a tumor with scattered pigmented melanocytes, with CD34 positivity and overlapping histologic features between Bednar tumor and dermatofibroma have been reported.[105] Unfortunately, no cytogenetic studies were performed in these cases. A further case of a melanoma overlying a dermatofibroma has been reported.[106] Although inflammatory cells are a feature of most fibrous histiocytomas, formation of germinal centers is rare.[107] Cases with an angiokeloidal pattern have also been described.[108]

Cellular neurothekeoma

Clinical features

Cellular neurothekeoma usually presents on the head, neck and upper limbs followed by the trunk of children and young adults and shows predilection for females.[1–8] Tumors in elderly patients are rare.[9] Unusual sites of presentation include the maxilla, the bulbar conjunctiva, the oral cavity, the lip, the eyelid, hypopharynx, the ear and the vulva.[10–20] Lesions are long-standing skin-colored papules, which usually measure less than 1 cm and in most cases less than 2 cm in diameter. Multiple lesions and eruptive cases are exceptional.[8,21,22] A case in a patient with Guillain-Barre has been reported.[23] Local recurrence is rare and the figure of around 7% reported in large series likely reflects a referral bias.[7,8,24] Recurrent tumors are more common on the face.[7,24] Some cases present with atypical features (see below), raising the possibility of malignancy.[25–29] However, the behavior of these tumors is benign.

Hybrid tumors of perineurioma and cellular 'neurothekeoma' have been recently described (see below); the vast majority occur as a solitary papule on the lip.[30–33]

Pathogenesis and histologic features

Cellular neurothekeoma is no longer considered a tumor of neural lineage. Its origin remains obscure and although an association with plexiform fibrohistiocytic tumor has been proposed, this is not likely.[34]

Lesions are poorly circumscribed and located in the reticular dermis with frequent focal extension into the subcutis. Atypical variants (see below) extend deeper into the subcutaneous tissue and an exceptional example with purely subcutaneous presentation has been documented.[35] Facial tumors can focally involve the skeletal muscle. The tumor has a lobular growth pattern and consists of small nests and fascicles of epithelioid and short spindled cells with pale eosinophilic cytoplasm, vesicular nuclei and mild or no cytologic atypia (*Figs 35.252 and 35.253*). More prominent cytologic

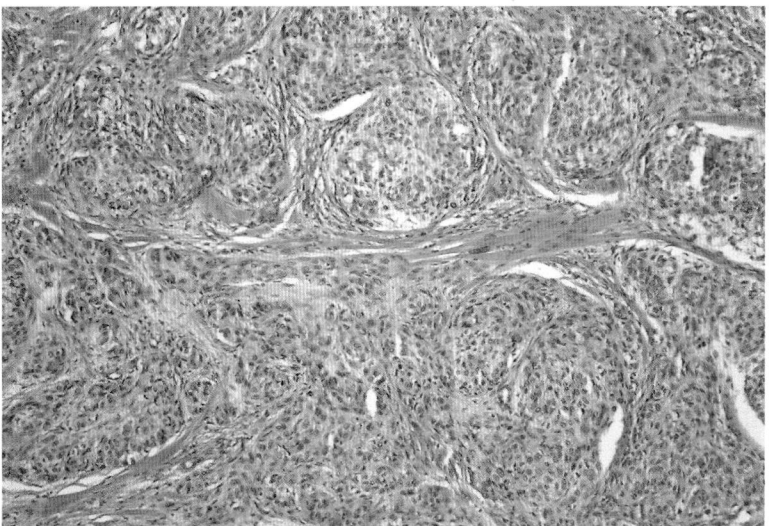

Fig. 35.252
Cellular neurothekeoma: the tumor consists of nests and fascicles of eosinophilic cells.

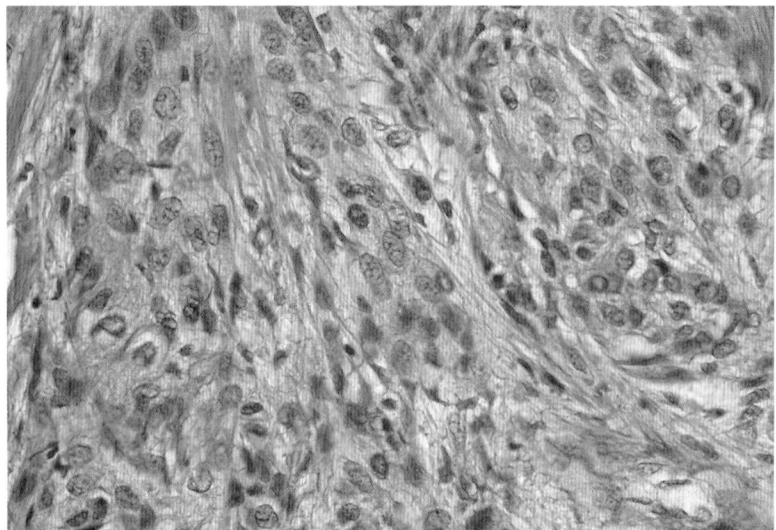

Fig. 35.253
Cellular neurothekeoma: the cells have abundant cytoplasm and vesicular nuclei.

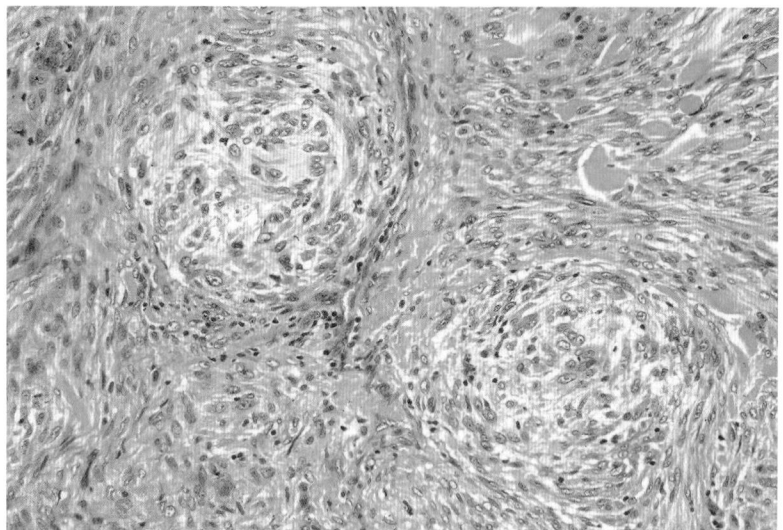

Fig. 35.255
Atypical cellular neurothekeoma: tumor cells show variation in size and there is cytologic atypia.

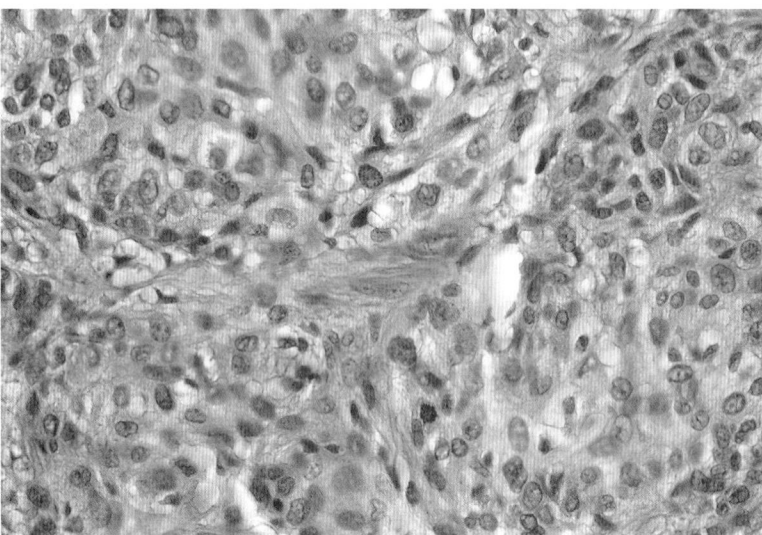

Fig. 35.254
Cellular neurothekeoma: mitoses are sometimes present.

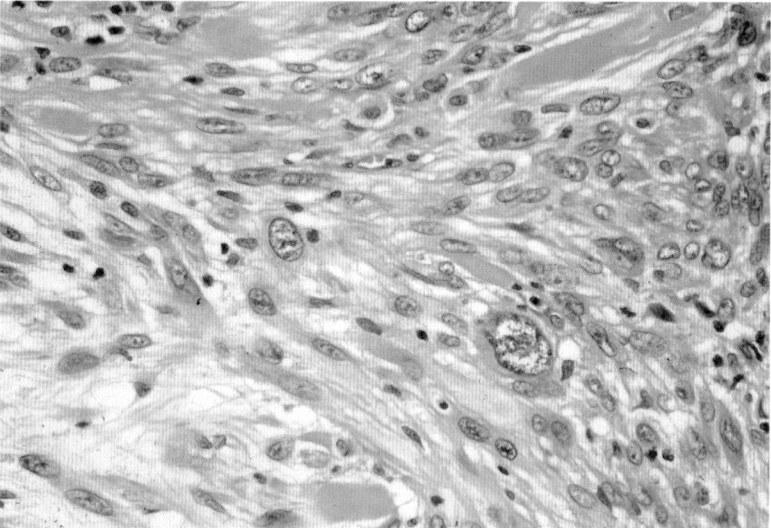

Fig. 35.256
Atypical cellular neurothekeoma: at higher power, note the marked nuclear pleomorphism.

atypia can be seen in up to 25% of cases.[7] Normal mitotic figures are fairly common and in some cases are prominent, and in exceptional instances atypical mitotic figures are found (Fig. 35.254).[8] Multinucleated giant cells including osteoclast-like giant cells can be seen. The collagen around the tumor cells sometimes appears somewhat sclerotic. In some cases, the latter change is prominent and these lesions are regarded as desmoplastic.[36–38] A predominantly plexiform pattern is very rare and in occasional cases larger lobules are identified.[7,39] A fascicular and a sheet-like pattern is exceptional.[28,40] Myxoid change is frequently observed and tends to be focal or more rarely predominant.[7,29,41,42] Two rare tumors containing melanin have been documented.[43]

Atypical cellular neurothekeoma is characterized by larger size, deep involvement, infiltrative growth pattern, vascular invasion, perineural invasion, high mitotic rate and marked cytologic atypia (Figs 35.255 and 35.256).[7,25,28,44] Lymphocytic cuffing, xanthomatoid areas, a pseudonevoid appearance and chondroid stroma may be seen.28 A case with neuroendocrine differentiation has also been reported.[45]

The histogenesis of this tumor remains enigmatic.[2–5] It has been suggested that the line of differentiation is fibroblastic/myofibroblastic and that it may represent part of the spectrum of plexiform fibrous histiocytoma.[7,46,47] Immunohistochemistry is quite distinctive, as cases are consistently S100 protein and SOX10 negative and NSE, NKI/C3 (described originally as a melanoma marker and a very non-specific marker) and CD10 positive

(Fig. 35.257).[7,8,48] Although it has been reported that NKI/C3 tends to be negative in tumors in which spindle cells predominate this is not our personal experience.[49] Although S100 protein is negative, S100A6 is positive in all reported cases.[50] A proportion of cases are focally positive for SMA.[2] PGP 9.5, microphthalmia transcription factor 1 (MITF-1) and podoplanin (D2–40) have also been reported as useful markers of cellular neurothekeoma.[49,51,52] A single case was positive for desmin.[7]

Hybrid tumors with features of perineurioma and cellular neurothekeoma are well-circumscribed, unencapsulated plexiform lesions composed of nests/nodules of tumor cells in a focally myxoid stroma.[30] Individual tumor cells are arranged in whorls or in a lamellar pattern. By immunohistochemistry most cells are strongly immunoreactive for S100A6, MITF1, NKI/C3, PGP9.5, EMA, and NSE. In some cases, there is weaker and focal positivity for CD34, claudin-1, and Glut-1. A biphasic non-plexiform hybrid tumor has also been reported.[32]

Differential diagnosis

Although the overall growth pattern with nesting somewhat resembles a melanocytic lesion, there is no epidermal component and lesions are S100 protein, HMB-45 and Melan-A negative. Nerve sheath myxoma is a predominantly acral tumor lacking cellular areas and composed of myxoid

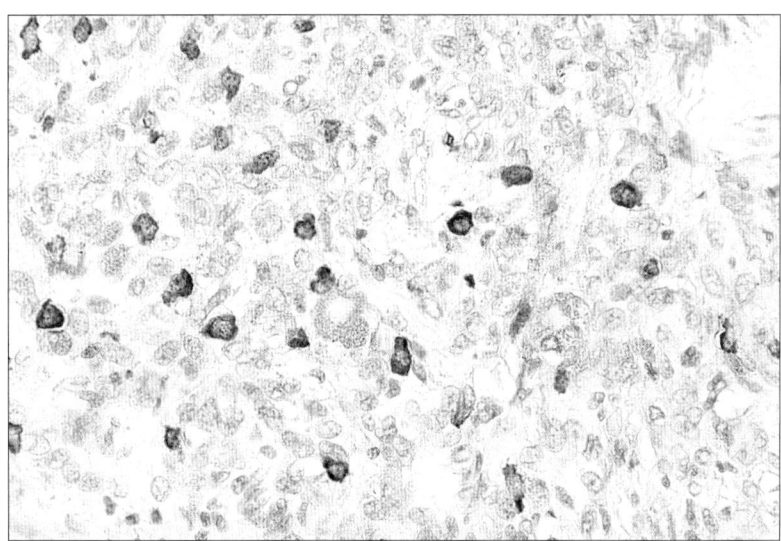

Fig. 35.257
Cellular neurothekeoma: the tumor cells express NKI-C3 but are S100 protein negative.

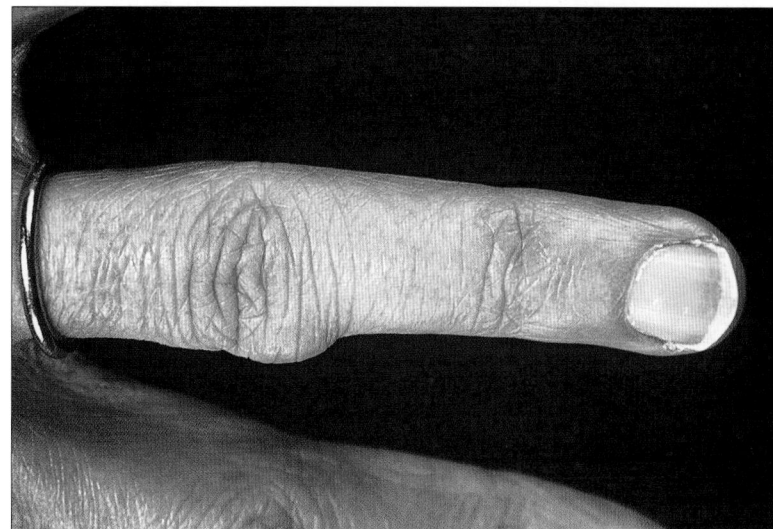

Fig. 35.258
Giant cell tumor of tendon sheath: this lesion presents as a firm nodule that most often affects the finger. By courtesy of H. du P. Menagé, MD, Institute of Dermatology, London, UK.

lobules of stellate cells which are positive for S100 protein and negative for NKI/C3.[53] MITF1 positivity may be of help when a plexiform fibrohistiocytic tumor is considered in the differential diagnosis.[54] PG9.5 is not a helpful marker as it has very low specificity.[55]

Deep benign fibrous histiocytoma

Clinical features

Deep benign fibrous histiocytoma is a rare tumor that presents most often between the fourth and fifth decades of life in the subcutis or deep soft tissues, with a predilection for males. It occurs mainly on the limbs followed by the head and neck and trunk.[1-4] Rare cases present in the mediastinum, retroperitoneum and pelvis.[1-3] Tumors are usually a few centimeters in diameter but larger tumors also occur. There is local recurrence in up to 22% of cases and two cases of metastatic lesions that resulted in death have been recorded.[2] These tumors did not look histologically different from nonmetastasizing lesions.[5]

Pathogenesis and histologic features

The pathogenesis is unknown but these tumors are the deep counterpart of dermal fibrous histiocytoma (dermatofibroma). Cytogenetic studies of a single case demonstrated a t(16;17)(p13.3;q21.3).[6] However, this change appears to be very rare as it was not demonstrated in a further six cases studied. Gene fusions involving protein kinase C (PRKC) genes have been described.[7]

Histologically, tumors are very similar to those occurring in the dermis. They are well-circumscribed and polymorphic (although less so than cutaneous counterparts), with a mixture of histiocyte-like cells, spindle-shaped cells and rare multinucleated giant cells and foamy cells. A sprinkling of lymphocytes is common. Areas of hemorrhage and cystic change are frequent. More monomorphic tumors very similar to cellular fibrous histiocytoma are common. Atypical variants of the tumor are rarely seen and are also identical to more superficial tumors.[8] Deep tumors have a more prominent storiform appearance. Mitotic activity may be seen and is usually no more than 5 per 10 HPFs. Up to 42% of cases display a hemangiopericytoma-like pattern and stromal hyalinization is present in 39% of cases.[2] A palisading pattern is exceptional.[9] Necrosis and lymphovascular invasion are very rarely seen.[4]

Immunohistochemically, tumor cells are often positive for CD34 and smooth muscle actin in about two-thirds of cases and very rarely for desmin.[2]

Differential diagnosis

The main differential diagnosis is with solitary fibrous tumor and dermatofibrosarcoma protuberans. The former is less monomorphic and displays hypo- and hypercellular areas lacking a storiform pattern and the latter is infiltrative with replacement of the subcutaneous tissue with a lace-like pattern. CD34 is of limited help as is tends to be positive in deep benign fibrous histiocytoma and in the latter tumors.

Giant cell tumor of tendon sheath

Clinical features

Giant cell tumor of tendon sheath (tenosynovial giant cell tumor: localized variant) is a frequently encountered tumor that occurs most often in the third to fifth decades and has a slight predilection for females.[1-6] Lesions in children are rare.[7-11] It occurs almost exclusively on the hands and feet, especially the fingers and less commonly the toes (Fig. 35.258).[1-6,12,13]

It presents as a slowly growing, usually painless nodule and is most often less than 2 cm in diameter. Multiple or bilateral lesions are uncommon.[14-19] This lesion has no malignant potential, but may recur locally in up to 30% of cases, usually as a consequence of incomplete excision.[1-7,20,21] It appears that there is increased risk of local recurrence in lesions involving the flexor and extensor tendons and the joint capsules.[22] Invasion of the underlying bone has been reported in up to 11% of cases.[23] Nerve-adherent tumors have been reported.[24]

The diffuse tenosynovial giant cell tumor is a rare variant which tends to involve the distal limbs, the larger joints of the limb girdles (especially the hip) and more rarely the vertebral column.[25-28] It is locally aggressive and there is quite often infiltration of extra-articular soft tissues and occasionally bone. Recurrence in up to a third of cases is common following incomplete surgical excision.[28] Exceptional tumors with benign histology may metastasize to regional lymph nodes, and tumors with sarcomatous change may develop distant metastases.[28,29]

Pathogenesis and histologic features

The reactive or neoplastic nature of giant cell tumor of tendon sheath has debated for years, and it has finally been confirmed as a neoplastic process.[30,31] The most common cytogenetic abnormality is t(1;2)(p13;q37) placing the colony-stimulating factor (CSF) under the COL6A3 promoter.[30-33] Substitution of COL6A3 by other promoters is also possible.[30] These cytogenetic abnormalities result in overexpression of CSF-1, but only in a small subset of cells.[34,35] The majority of apparently nonclonal cells, particularly macrophages, express CSF-1 receptor, a situation described as 'tumor landscaping effect'.[36] This may explain why some studies fail to demonstrate clonality.[37]

The tumors are usually lobulated and well defined, often with a fibrous pseudocapsule (Fig. 35.259). They are composed of mononuclear cells

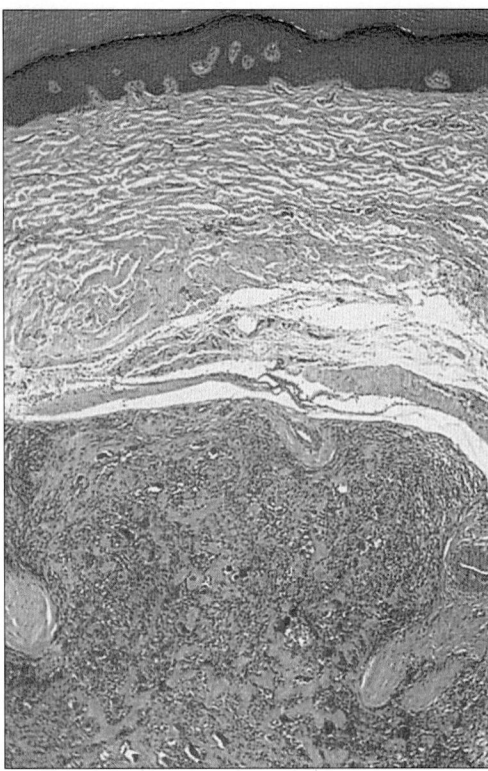

Fig. 35.259
Giant cell tumor of tendon sheath: low-power view showing a sharply circumscribed pseudo-encapsulated tumor.

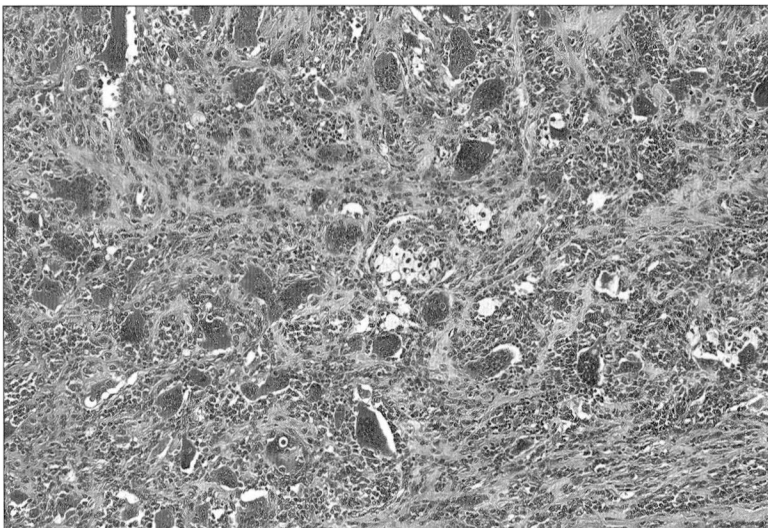

Fig. 35.260
Giant cell tumor of tendon sheath: higher-power view showing xanthoma cells and giant cells.

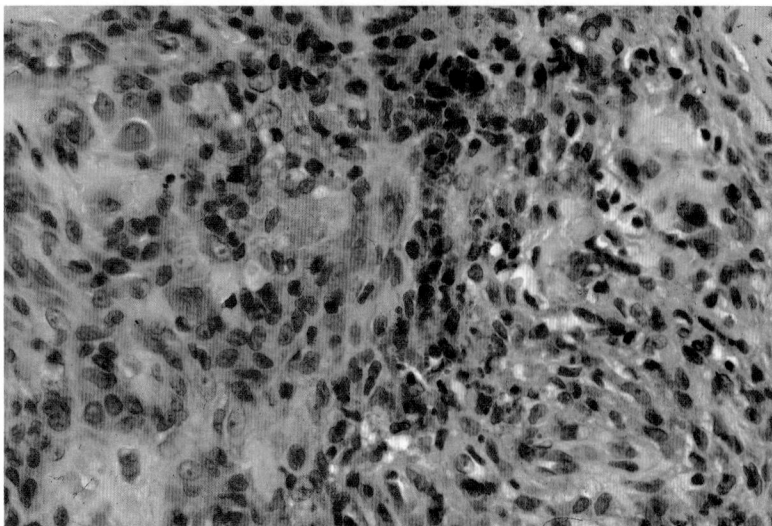

Fig. 35.261
Giant cell tumor of tendon sheath: there is conspicuous hemosiderin deposition.

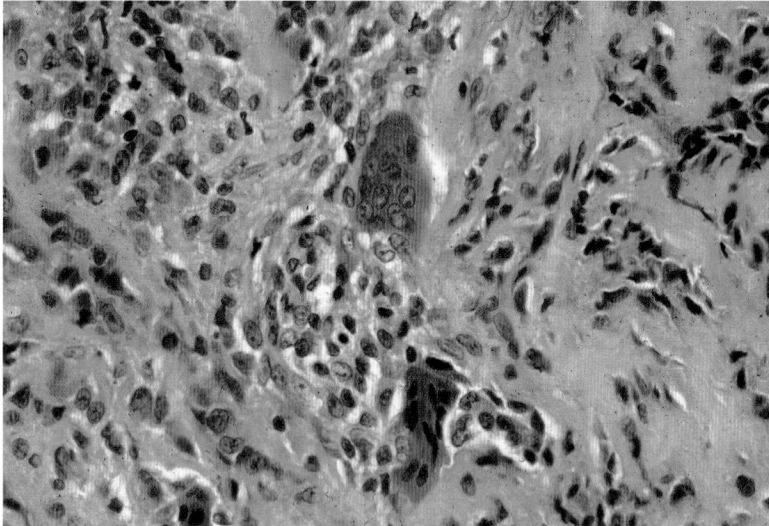

Fig. 35.262
Giant cell tumor of tendon sheath: osteoclast-like multinucleate giant cells are present.

with eosinophilic cytoplasm and vesicular nuclei, xanthomatous cells, siderophages, osteoclast-like multinucleated giant cells and mononuclear inflammatory cells (*Figs 35.260–35.262*).[38] The cells are typically set in a variably prominent collagenous stroma within which cholesterol clefts or evidence of previous hemorrhage in the form of stromal hemosiderin may be apparent. Normal mitotic figures are commonly seen and may be numerous. Old lesions can show prominent hyalinization. Tumors lacking giant cells and some with hepatoid cells have been reported.[39,40]

Immunohistochemically, some of the mononuclear cells and most of the osteoclastic giant cells are CD68, CD163 and CD45 positive. Actin may be focally positive in the mononuclear cells. Large mononuclear cells may express D2-40. Other markers are generally uninformative.

Histologic appearances of diffuse giant cell tumor are similar to those of the localized variant, except that cellularity is often higher, osteoclastic cells tend to be fewer and intralesional cleft-like spaces are common. An additional feature seen in most cases is the presence of a subpopulation of large, desmin-positive, dendritic histiocyte-like cells.[28] These have abundant

eosinophilic cytoplasm, large vesicular nuclei, paranuclear eosinophilic inclusions and rare intranuclear inclusions.[28]

Differential diagnosis

Fibroma of tendon sheath may be distinguished by its more uniform spindled cell appearance, its greater tendency for stromal hyalinization and the presence of characteristic slit-like vascular spaces. However, as mentioned under fibroma of tendon sheath, some cases show overlapping features.[41] Granulomatous inflammatory lesions are not usually circumscribed, show greater infiltration by chronic inflammatory cells and usually contain well-developed epithelioid granulomata. Diffuse-type lesions can be distinguished from synovial sarcoma by the absence of an epithelial lining in the clefts and negativity for epithelial markers.

Low-grade malignant fibrohistiocytic lesions

Giant cell tumor of soft tissues (and skin)

Clinical features

Giant cell tumor of soft tissues (also known as soft tissue giant cell tumor of low malignant potential) is regarded as the soft tissue counterpart of

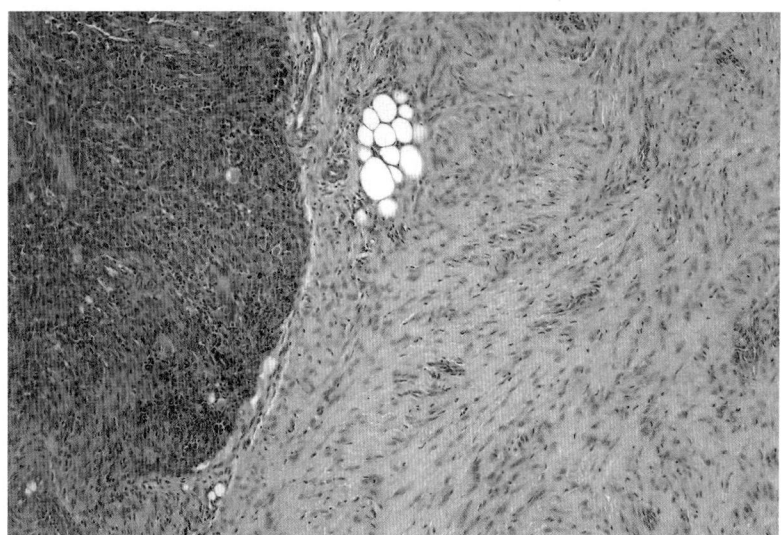

Fig. 35.263
Giant cell tumor of soft tissue: low-power view of the edge of a lesion.

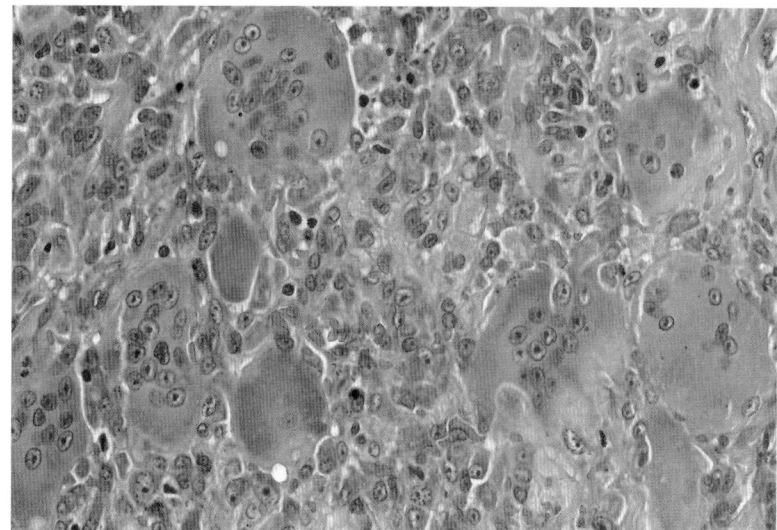

Fig. 35.264
Giant cell tumor of soft tissue: high-power view of osteoclast-like giant cells.

giant cell tumor of bone, although it seems to be genetically distinct (see below).[1–9] It is rare and presents mainly in adults, with no sex predilection. The great majority of lesions occur in the limbs followed by the trunk and only exceptionally in the head and neck.[10] Most tumors are well circumscribed and subcutaneous but dermal (exceptionally polypoid) and deeper lesions may occur.[6,11,12] The size ranges from less than 1 cm to up to 10 cm. In a single documented case, the tumor had been present for 46 years.[13] Local recurrence is seen in up to 10% of cases and metastases are exceptional and include one from a case arising in the skin.[1–3,14]

Pathogenesis and histologic features

The pathogenesis is unknown but rare associations with trauma, surgical scars and Paget disease of bone have been reported.[2,15,16] Although tumors are morphologically very similar to those presenting in bone, recent studies showed not only immunophenotypical differences between both lesions, but also failed to identify point mutations of the *H3F3A* gene often found in bone tumors in lesions presenting in soft tissues.[8,9]

Histology shows a well-defined tumor that is often multinodular and has focal areas of hemorrhage (*Fig. 35.263*). A peripheral shell of bone is seen in some cases. Focal areas of bone formation can also be present elsewhere in the tumor. Hemorrhage, aneurysmal bone cyst-like areas and sclerotic changes are additional features. Vascular invasion is found in up to one-third of the cases.[2,3] Tumor cells consist of a mixture of osteoclast-like giant cells and mononuclear cells (*Fig. 35.264*). The osteoclast-like giant cells often form nodular aggregates.

Both the osteoclast-like giant cells and the mononuclear cells are positive for CD68. Positive staining for actin may be focally present in mononuclear cells but not in the giant cells.[3] Exceptional focal positivity for keratin and S100 protein can be seen.[2]

Angiomatoid fibrous histiocytoma

Clinical features

Angiomatoid fibrous histiocytoma (previously known as angiomatoid malignant fibrous histiocytoma) is a rare tumor. It usually arises in the subcutaneous tissues and only exceptionally in the dermis of the extremities or trunk in children or young adults of either sex.[1–7] Presentation in the head and neck is exceptional.[8] Unusual sites include the lung, brain, mediastinum, vulva, retroperitoneum and ovary.[9–14] Lesions arising in deeper soft tissues are less common. A congenital example has been documented.[15] A case arising in the background of chronic radiodermatitis, a tumor developing in an HIV-positive child and one in a child with neuroblastoma have also been reported.[16–18] Most tumors are slow growing and less than 2 cm in diameter. Patients sometimes present with systemic symptoms including fever, weight

loss, anemia and paraproteinemia. Systemic symptoms usually disappear after removal of the tumor and might be caused by *EWSR1-CREB1* induced excess of interleukin-6 (IL-6).[19] There is local recurrence in 2–12% of cases.[2] Recurrences appear to be associated with deep-seated lesions, those with an infiltrative margin and lesions located in the head and neck.[2,20,21] Metastases to local lymph nodes occur in up to 1% of cases but behavior is usually benign with only very exceptional cases presenting with distant metastases and death.[22,23] No histologic features allow prediction of which tumors will recur or metastasize.

Pathogenesis and histologic features

The most common chromosomal translocation is t(2;22) resulting in *EWSR1-CREB1* in the large majority of cases. An *EWSR1-ATF1* or *FUS-ATF1* fusion is found in a small subset of cases.[17,18,20–30] *CREB1*, *ATF1* and *CREM* are closely related members of the cAMP response element binding protein (CREB) family. The same EWSR1-CREB1 and/or EWSR1-ATF1 fusion is also seen in clear cell sarcoma, clear cell sarcoma-like tumor of the gastrointestinal tract, primary pulmonary myxoid sarcoma, hyalinizing clear cell carcinoma of the salivary gland, clear cell odontogenic carcinoma, and most recently, a 'novel mesenchymal tumor with predilection for intracranial location.'[31–38] These fusions are thus among the most promiscuous in biology indicating that *EWSR1* fused to CREB family members can result in neoplastic, and usually malignant, transformation in a variety of cellular contexts – both mesenchymal and epithelial. The type of fusion found is not associated with prognosis. A recent study emphasizes the importance of performing RT-PCR in conjunction with FISH to increase the diagnostic yield.[39]

Angiomatoid fibrous histiocytoma is characterized by well-circumscribed nodules composed of relatively uniform, pale, round or short spindle-shaped eosinophilic cells with ovoid vesicular nuclei, interspersed with blood-filled pseudovascular spaces and foci of hemorrhage (*Figs 35.265–35.267*). Mitotic figures are usually not prominent. Typically, there is a dense lymphoplasmacytic mantle around and within the tumor, which thereby often simulates a lymph node. Cytologic atypia (which may be prominent) and mitotic activity may sometimes be more prominent but this does not correlate with behavior.[2,40] Scattered giant cells are seen. Other unusual histologic findings include a solid growth pattern lacking pseudoangiomatoid spaces, perivascular hyalinization, nuclear palisading, myxoid stroma with reticular arrangement reminiscent of myoepithelioma, sclerosis with a perineurioma-like pattern, and atypical mitotic figures.[41,42] Late-stage lesions may present with marked fibrosis.[43] A case of a 'pure' spindle cell tumor arising in the forearm musculature of a 19-year-old female has been reported.[44]

Immunohistochemically, tumor cells are positive in about 50% of cases for desmin and for muscle actin (HHF-35), but not for smooth muscle actin (*see Fig. 35.203*).[4] Positivity for EMA, CD68 and CD99 is usually seen in

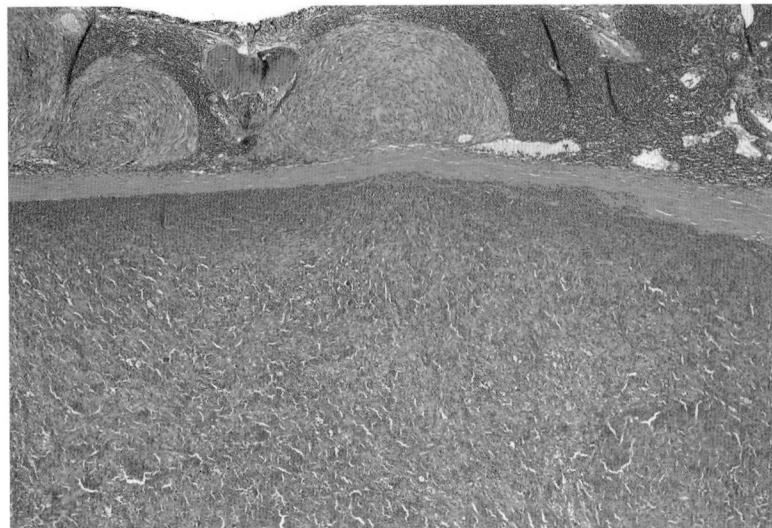

Fig. 35.265
Angiomatoid fibrous histiocytoma: viewed at low power, this condition sometimes resembles a lymph node. Note the multiple tumor nodules and foci of hemorrhage.

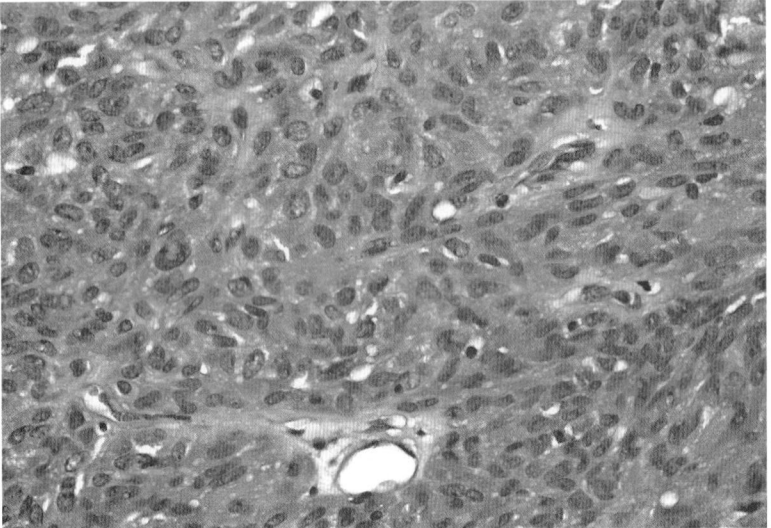

Fig. 35.266
Angiomatoid fibrous histiocytoma: the tumor cells are fairly uniform and have round or oval vesicular nuclei.

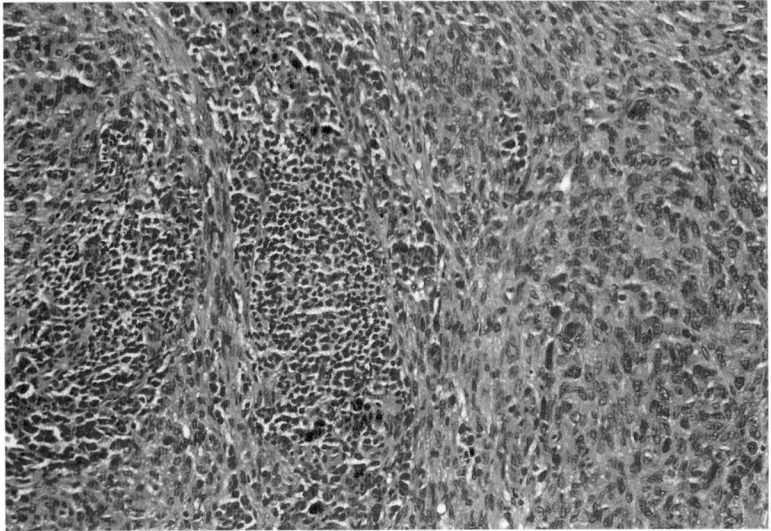

Fig. 35.267
Angiomatoid fibrous histiocytoma: medium-power view highlighting the lymphocytic infiltrate and hemosiderin deposition.

up to 50% of cases.[5,6] Tumor cells are negative for S100 protein, keratins and vascular markers. It is possible, combining morphology with immunophenotype, that these lesions show myoid (probably myofibroblastic) differentiation, although the combination of EMA and desmin is unusual.[4]

Ultrastructural studies show a variety of cells including fibroblastic, myofibroblastic, histiocyte-like or undifferentiated forms.[3,15,25]

Differential diagnosis

Distinction from aneurysmal fibrous histiocytoma is discussed under the latter entity.

Plexiform fibrohistiocytic tumor

Clinical features

Plexiform fibrohistiocytic tumor is a rare but distinctive neoplasm that most commonly presents on the limbs of children and young adults (more than 50% of patients are younger than 20 years) and has a slight predilection for females.[1-9] A single congenital case has been documented.[10] About 60% of the cases occur on the upper limbs (particularly the forearms, hands and wrists) followed by the lower limbs (about one-third of cases). Involvement of the trunk and face and neck is very rare.[1-3,11] Lesions present as an ill-defined nodule or plaque that predominantly involves the subcutaneous tissue but may extend into the dermis. Dermal variants of the tumor may occur.[7,12] There is a tendency for local recurrence varying from 12% to 37.5% of cases. Local lymph node metastasis has been reported in three cases and in one of these spread to the lungs was also seen.[1,2,13,14] Presentation in bone and multiple tumors are very rare.[15,16]

Pathogenesis and histologic features

Cytogenetic studies have been performed in some cases with differing clonal chromosomal abnormalities.[17-19] It has been suggested that plexiform fibrohistiocytic tumor and cellular neurothekeoma are part of the same spectrum, based on morphological and phenotypic similarities.[7,20] This is however, not a view that has been generally accepted.

Tumors are infiltrative and most are located mainly at the junction between the dermis and subcutaneous tissue, and occasionally there is involvement of underlying skeletal muscle (*Figs 35.268–35.271*). About one-third of cases are predominantly dermal.[7] Microscopic appearances vary according to the proportion of two main components, one of which may predominate:[1-3]
- fascicles of fibroblast/myofibroblast-like cells, which usually predominate (fibroblastic),
- nodules of histiocyte-like cells (histiocytic).

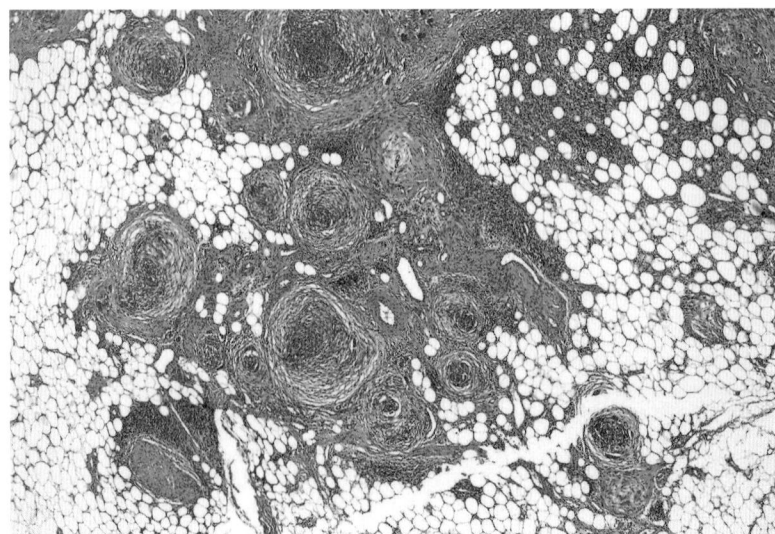

Fig. 35.268
Plexiform fibrous histiocytoma: the prototypical case consists of fibroblastic spindle cell areas in which there are nodules of histiocyte-like cells.

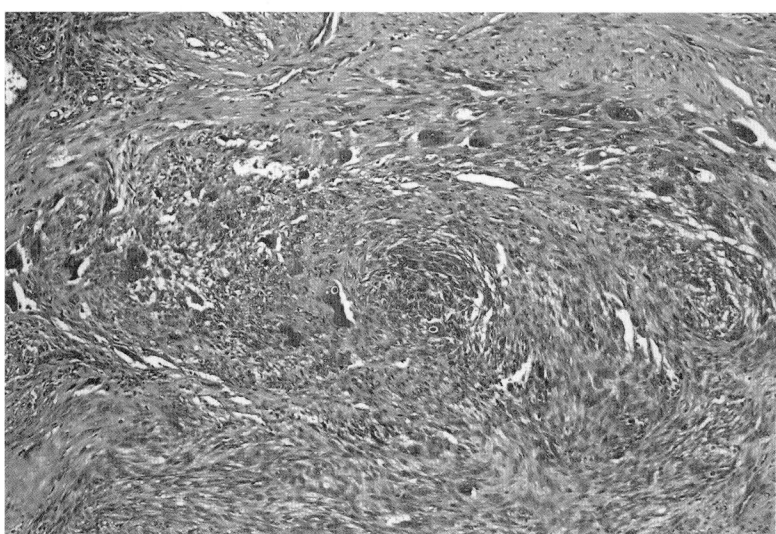

Fig. 35.269
Plexiform fibrous histiocytoma: there are prominent osteoclast-like giant cells.

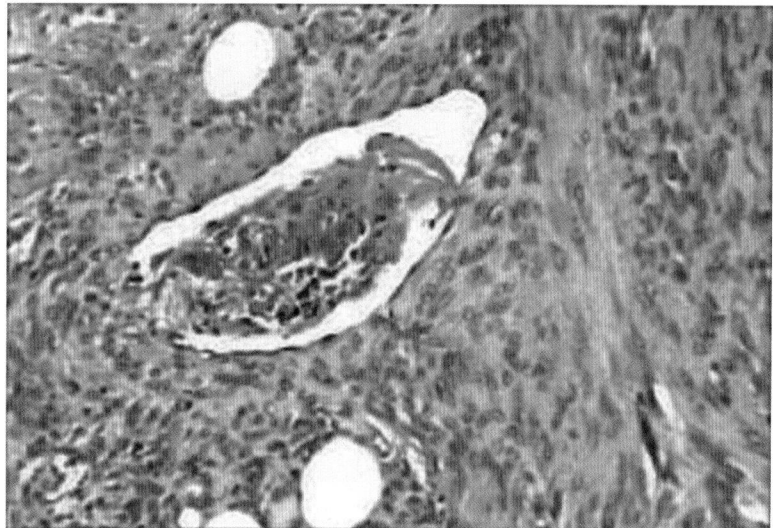

Fig. 35.272
Plexiform fibrous histiocytoma: vascular invasion as seen in this field is an occasional feature. It does not appear to be of prognostic significance.

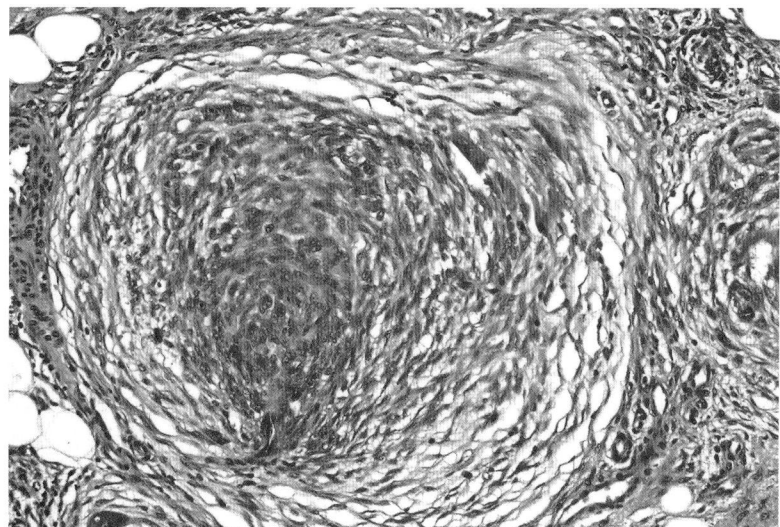

Fig. 35.270
Plexiform fibrous histiocytoma: high-power view of a histiocytic nodule.

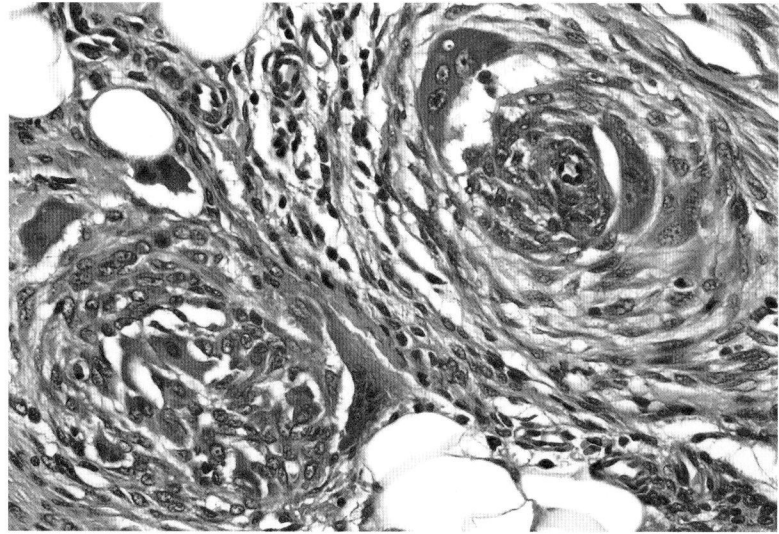

Fig. 35.271
Plexiform fibrous histiocytoma: the histiocyte-like nodules also contain multinucleate (usually osteoclast-like) cells and tend to show stromal hemorrhage.

Varying numbers of osteoclast-like giant cells are also present, mainly in the histiocytic variant. Areas of hemorrhage with hemosiderin deposition can be seen in and around the nodules, which may also show peripheral hyalinization. Often, the fibroblastic fascicles appear to radiate from a more solid central area. Entrapment of fat with the presence of microfat cells and myxoid change is occasionally observed. A focal lymphocytic inflammatory cell infiltrate is seen in most cases and it tends to be more prominent in the fibroblastic variant.[7] Perineural and peripacinian extension is rarely seen and in a few cases there is cytologic atypia and increased mitotic activity.[7,21] Occasionally, vascular invasion is present (*Fig. 35.272*). Bone formation has also exceptionally been documented. Dermal tumors spare adnexal structures. A variant of plexiform fibrohistiocytic tumor with prominent granular cell change has been described.[22] A myxoid stroma is an unusual finding.[23]

There are no histologic findings that allow prediction of tumors that will recur or metastasize.

By immunohistochemistry, most of the giant cells and some of the mononuclear cells within the nodules express CD68, while the spindle-shaped cells outside the nodules label for SMA and calponin.[2,3,6] Some of the mononuclear cells within the nodules are focally positive for SMA.[2,3] Myofibroblastic differentiation of the latter cells is also suggested by ultrastructural studies.[3,24]

Differential diagnosis

Cases with a prominent fibroblastic component may be confused with dermatomyofibroma and fibromatosis (*Fig. 35.273*). The former, however, is mainly dermal and the latter is deep seated. Both lack a plexiform growth pattern. Fibrous hamartoma of infancy has a typical organoid growth pattern and lacks histiocytic nodules with osteoclast-like giant cells. Dermal and deep benign fibrous histiocytomas usually have a more cohesive growth pattern and polymorphism is seen throughout the lesion. Other entities with a plexiform pattern (e.g, cellular neurothekeoma, dermal nerve sheath myxoma, plexiform schwannoma, and plexiform neurofibroma) can be differentiated with the use of immunohistochemical stains especially in small biopsies.[25,26] MITF may be of help in distinguishing, plexiform fibrohistiocytic tumor rich in histiocyte-like cells from cellular neurothekeoma especially in small samples, as in the former, tumor cells are negative for this marker, while in the latter they are very commonly diffusely positive.[27]

Atypical fibroxanthoma and pleomorphic dermal sarcoma

Clinical features

Atypical fibroxanthoma and pleomorphic dermal sarcoma are described together as they are likely to represent part of the spectrum of the same

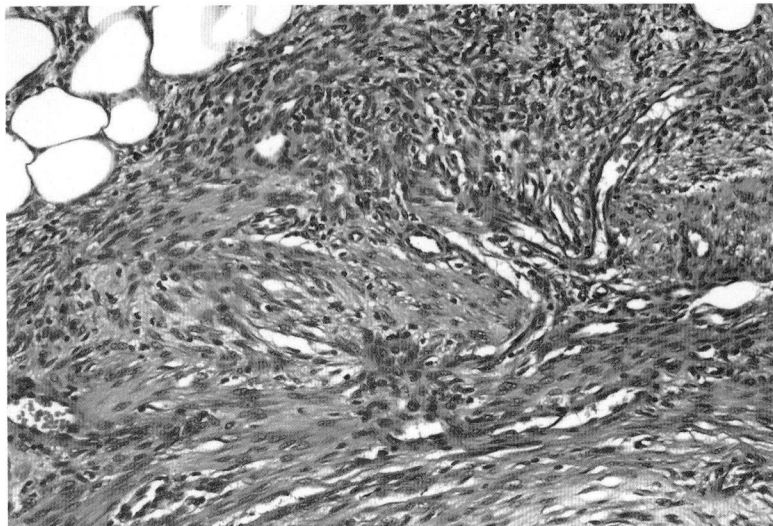

Fig. 35.273
Plexiform fibrous histiocytoma: note the fascicles of myofibroblasts infiltrating the subcutaneous tissue.

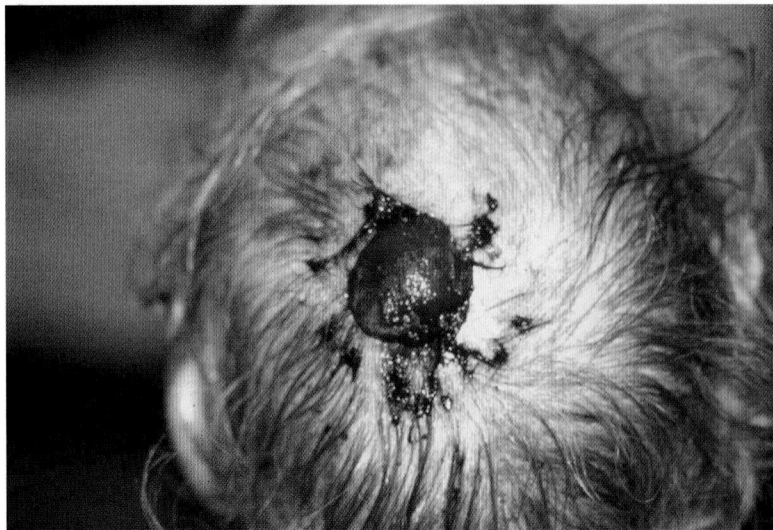

Fig. 35.275
Atypical fibroxanthoma: the scalp is another common site. This example is extensively ulcerated. By courtesy of R. Barlow, MD, Institute of Dermatology, London, UK.

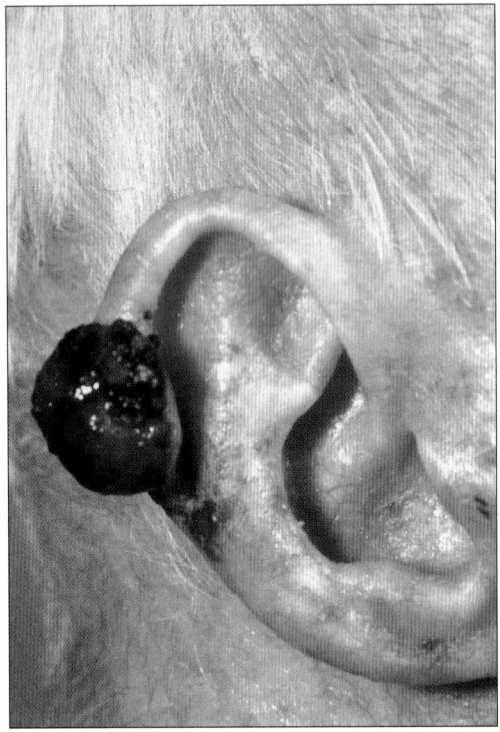

Fig. 35.274
Atypical fibroxanthoma: the tumor presents as an exophytic nodule, usually on sun-damaged skin of the elderly. The ear is a characteristic site. By courtesy of E. Wilson Jones, MD, Institute of Dermatology, London, UK.

neoplasm as suggested by clinical, histologic, immunophenotypic, and molecular features (see below).[1–9] Distinction between both is important because of the more aggressive behavior of the latter and it is based on histologic features as described below.

Tumors almost always present on the sun-exposed actinically damaged areas of the head and neck of individuals in the seventh or eighth decade of life.[1–6] An atypical fibroxanthoma in a 115 -year-old man has been reported.[10] Incidence figures depend on local climate and skin pigmentation. The lesion presents as a firm solitary cutaneous nodule, which is often ulcerated, rarely exceeds 3 cm in diameter and has typically been present for less than 1 year (Figs 35.274 and 35.275). Tumors may arise in the setting of xeroderma pigmentosum and solid organ transplantation.[11–16] Although the latter patients generally do not seem to be at increased risk of developing the tumor, multiple lesions developed in a heart transplant patient.[17] A case in an African-American woman, one following hair transplantation, another in the palpebral conjunctiva, one arising in the background of a nevus sebaceous, one at the site of a thermal burn and one on a pacemaker pocket have been reported.[18–23] However, as the pathogenesis of these tumors is

related to sun exposure, such a diagnosis should only be accepted in the setting of sun-damaged skin.

Complete excision is the treatment of choice. The overall rate of local recurrence is about 5% of patients and metastatic spread is very rare.[6,8,24–28] Most of the cases with metastasis reported in the older literature before immunohistochemistry was available are likely to represent examples of other pleomorphic malignancies and therefore most probably represent misdiagnoses. The great majority of tumors that metastasize are those classified as pleomorphic dermal sarcoma. In this group, a local recurrence rate of 28% and a metastatic rate of 10% has been reported.[7] A more recent study of a small series of cases has suggested a more aggressive course for dermal pleomorphic sarcoma with a metastatic rate of 20%.[29] Exceptional cases of atypical fibroxanthoma which do not fulfill the criteria for the diagnosis of pleomorphic dermal sarcoma may develop metastatic disease.[30] Metastatic lesions have been reported to lymph nodes, lungs and peritoneum.[24–28] An exceptional case with recurrence, satellite nodules and lymph node metastasis has been reported.[31]

The rate of local recurrence appears to be less in patients treated with Mohs micrographic surgery although this has not been confirmed in a recent study.[32–34]

Pathogenesis and histologic features

Etiologically, almost all cases are associated with solar or therapeutic irradiation damage. Support for the pathogenetic role of ultraviolet light in the genesis of this tumor is given by the recent demonstration of classical p53 UV-induced mutations (C–T and C–G transitions).[35] Further support comes from the demonstration of immunoexpression of UV photoproducts of cyclobutane pyrimidine dimers in atypical fibroxanthoma.[36] In a small percentage of cases, Merkel cell polyomavirus DNA has been detected but the significance of this finding is not clear.[37] Both atypical fibroxanthomas and pleomorphic dermal sarcoma have been found to have high number of similar recurrent mutations in multiple genes including FAT1, NOTCH1/2, CDKN2A, and TP53 as well as the TERT promoter. This strongly supports the contention that these two neoplasms are part of the same spectrum.[38,39]

Atypical fibroxanthomas are characteristically reasonably well-defined, predominantly dermal lesions, which may show extremely superficial invasion of subcutaneous fat in a small proportion of cases; they usually abut on the basal layer of the epidermis and ulceration is common (Figs 35.276–35.278). Most lesions are polypoid and often have an epidermal collarette. The deep margin is generally pushing.

The appearances comprise an admixture of spindle-shaped cells, histiocyte-like cells, xanthomatous cells and multinucleated giant cells, any or all of which may show marked pleomorphism, hyperchromasia and prominent mitotic activity (Figs 35.279–35.282). Abnormal forms are also

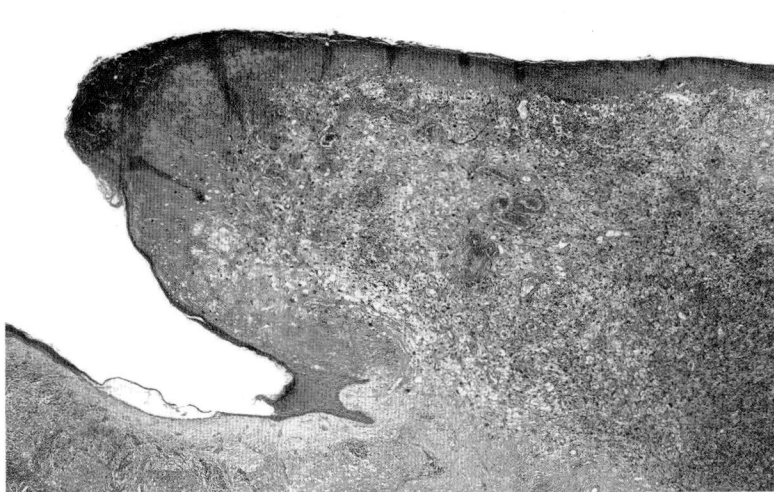

Fig. 35.276
Atypical fibroxanthoma: this low magnification shows an obviously pleomorphic intradermal spindle cell tumor which has eroded the epidermis. Note the lateral collarette.

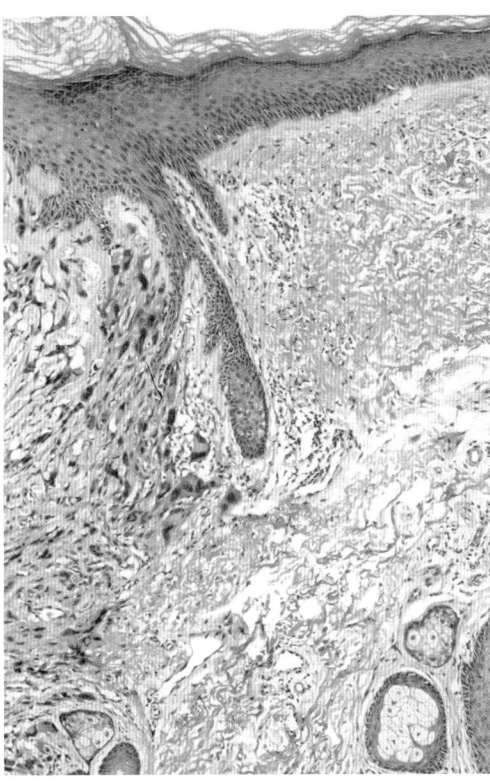

Fig. 35.278
Atypical fibroxanthoma: the adjacent dermis shows gross solar elastosis. There is no epidermal involvement.

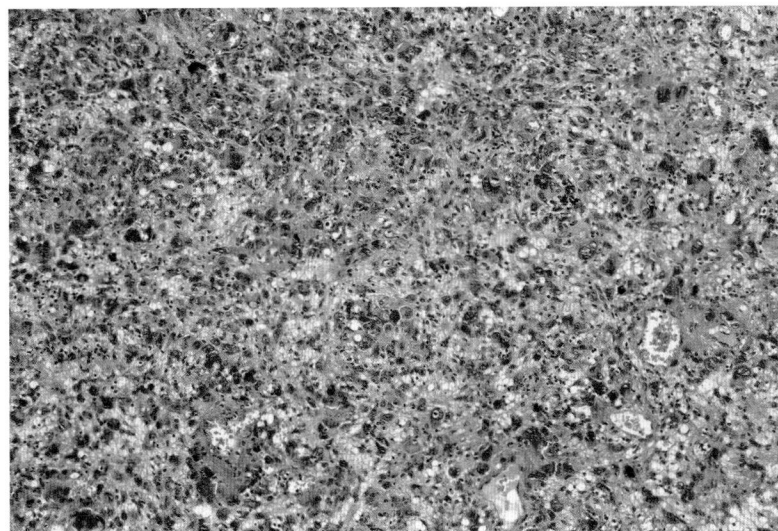

Fig. 35.277
Atypical fibroxanthoma: medium-power view showing a highly cellular and pleomorphic tumor cell infiltrate.

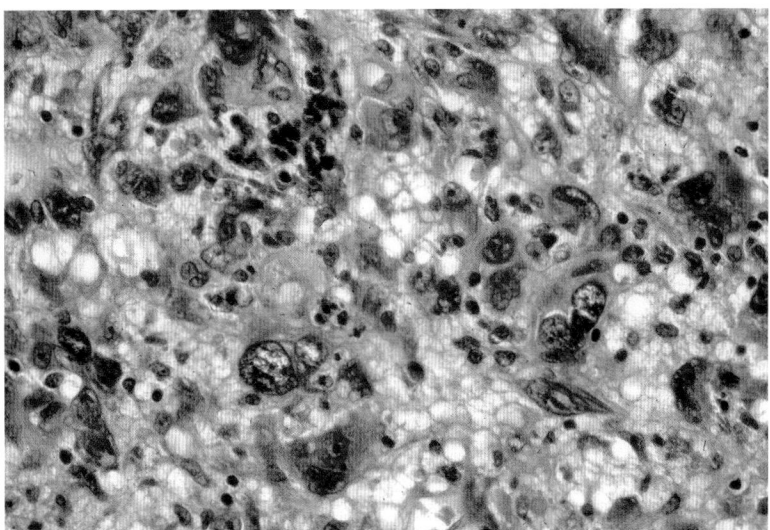

Fig. 35.279
Atypical fibroxanthoma: the tumor is composed of pleomorphic spindled and epithelioid cells with bizarre nuclei.

common. In some tumors, epithelioid cells may be prominent.[40] From a purely cytological point of view, therefore, atypical fibroxanthoma appears malignant. A chronic inflammatory infiltrate may be seen, particularly at the periphery of the tumor. The adjacent dermis shows marked solar elastosis.

Histologic variants of atypical fibroxanthoma include tumors with pigment, clear cell change, granular cell change, with osteoclast-like giant cells, myxoid change, and with keloidal change in the collagen.[40–58] Hemorrhage may be prominent and tumors may mimic a vascular lesion (Figs 35.283 and 35.284). Occasional cases display prominent sclerosis and even regression (focal or extensive).[59,60] An osteosarcomatous or chondrosarcomatous component, a lymphomatoid CD30-positive reaction and amyloid are exceptional.[61–64]

Spindle cell atypical fibroxanthoma is a relatively monomorphic variant which is composed predominantly of spindle-shaped cells with mild to moderate pleomorphism (Figs 35.285–35.287).[65]

Pleomorphic dermal sarcoma shows the same histologic spectrum described before but in addition the displays; invasion of the subcutaneous tissue, necrosis, lymphovascular invasion or perineural invasion (Figs 35.288–35.291).[7] Immunohistochemistry as described below is essential to confirm this diagnosis of exclusion as neoplasms like melanoma and sarcomatoid squamous cell carcinoma may display the latter findings.

By immunohistochemistry (Figs 35.292 and 35.293), the spindle cells are focally positive for SMA and calponin and the mononuclear and multinucleated cells are variably positive for CD68.[66–70] Focal positivity for EMA and p63 may also be seen. Other markers that are positive in tumor cells include CD99 and procollagen I.[71,72] CD163 is focally positive in some cases.[73] CD10 has been regarded as a useful marker, as most tumors show strong diffuse positivity for this marker.[74,75] However, any tumor with spindle cell morphology may show positivity for CD10, including sarcomas such as myxofibrosarcoma.[76] CD31 may be focally positive, albeit in a granular pattern analogous to the one observed in histiocytic markers. FLI1 may also be positive and this may lead to an erroneous diagnosis of angiosarcoma, especially in cases associated with hemorrhage.[77] In one case, focal positivity was reported for HMB-45 and MART-1 but only in the neoplastic giant cells.[78] In a further tumor with clear cell change, HMB-45 was expressed.[79] Tumor cells are negative for S100 protein, but may be positive for MITF.[80] Keratins, desmin, h-caldesmon and CD117 are negative.[69,81,82] An important pitfall is that a number of tumors contain a prominent number of reactive,

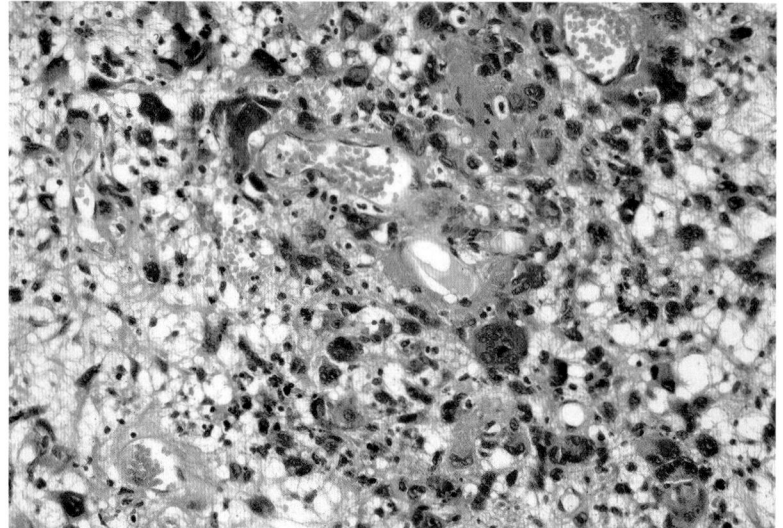

Fig. 35.280
Atypical fibroxanthoma: occasional osteoclast-like giant cells are present.

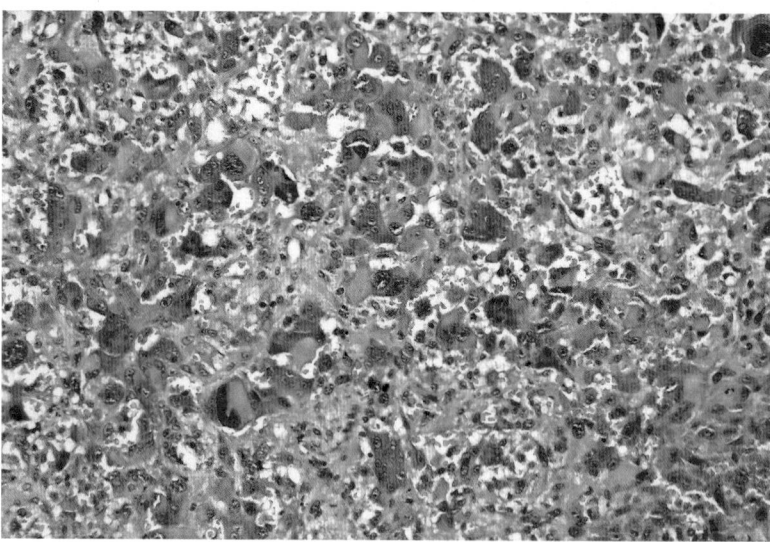

Fig. 35.283
Atypical fibroxanthoma: this is an example of an osteoclast-rich variant.

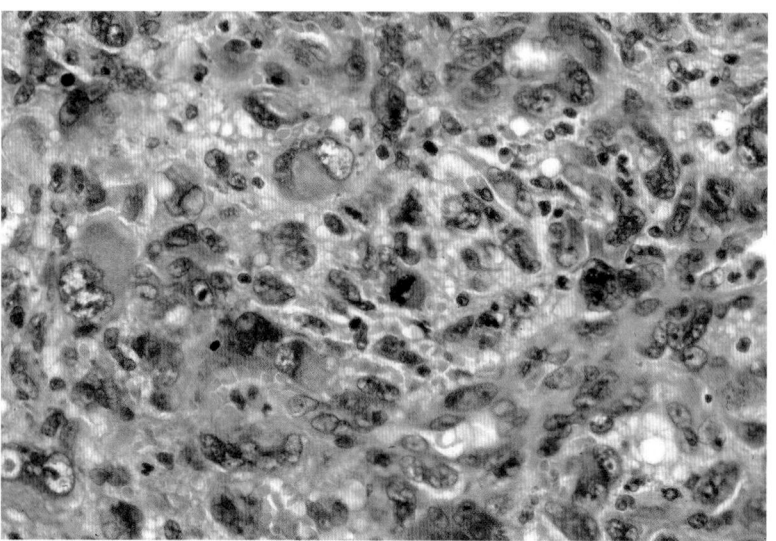

Fig. 35.281
Atypical fibroxanthoma: mitotic figures, often abnormal, are frequently present.

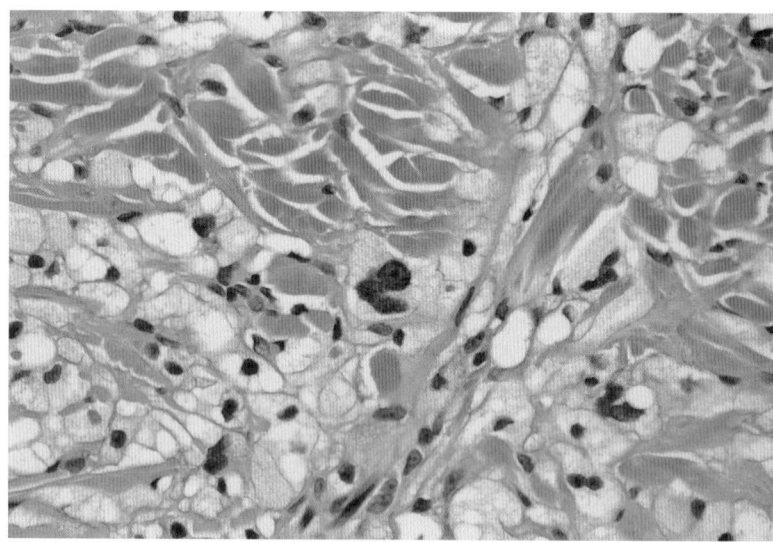

Fig. 35.284
Atypical fibroxanthoma: high-power view of a clear cell variant.

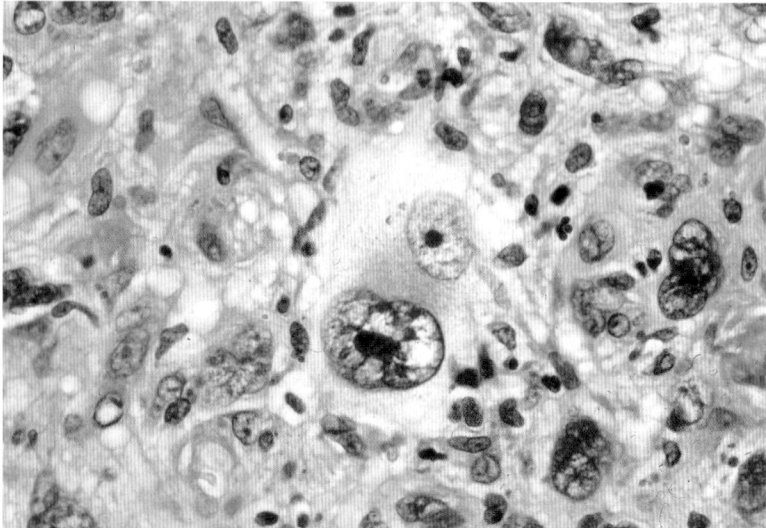

Fig. 35.282
Atypical fibroxanthoma: xanthomatized cells are commonly present. Note the conspicuous eosinophilic nucleoli.

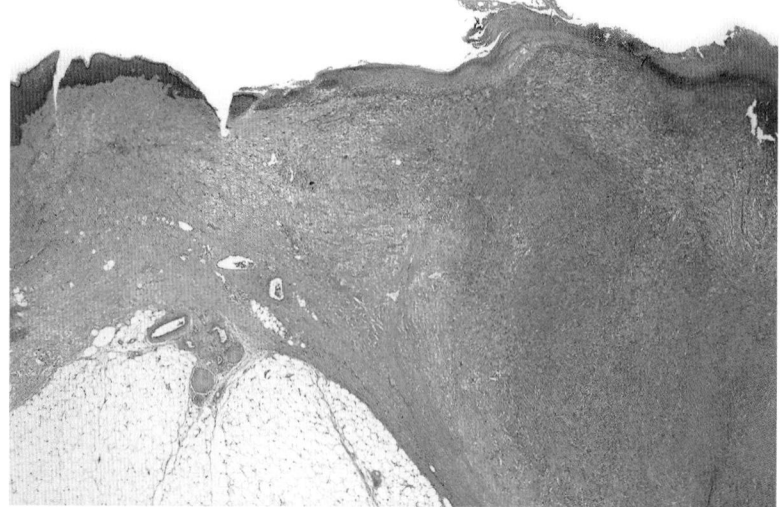

Fig. 35.285
Spindle cell atypical fibroxanthoma: the monomorphic appearance of the spindle cell variant differs considerably from conventional atypical fibroxanthoma.

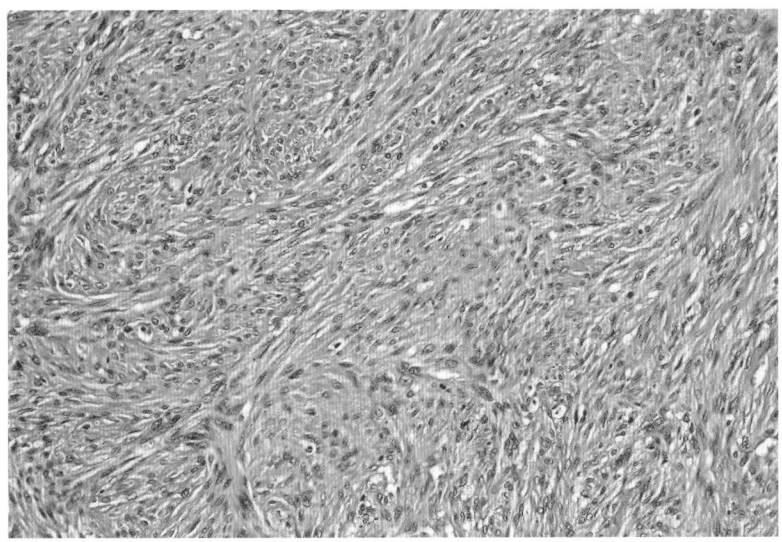

Fig. 35.286
Spindle cell atypical fibroxanthoma: cytologically, this lesion is easily confused with spindle cell melanoma or leiomyosarcoma.

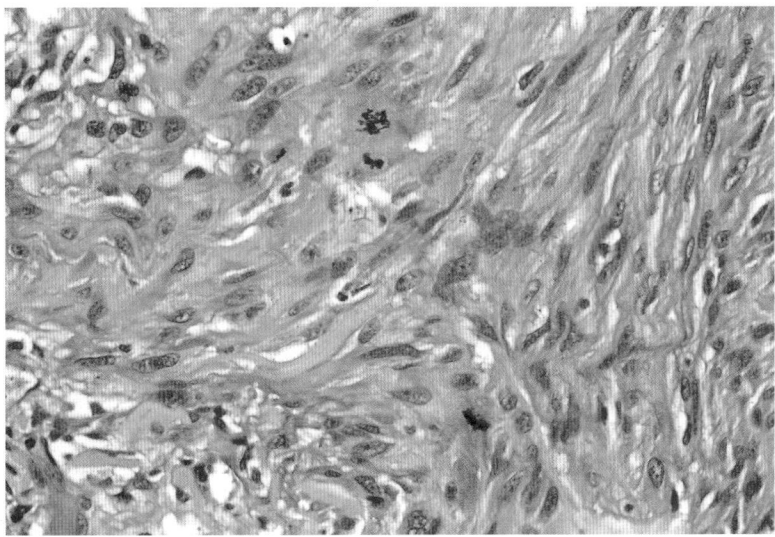

Fig. 35.287
Spindle cell atypical fibroxanthoma: there is brisk mitotic activity.

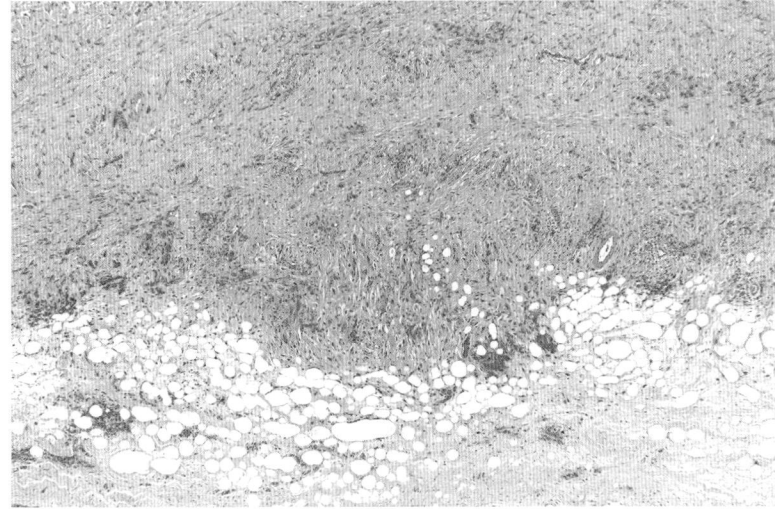

Fig. 35.288
Dermal pleomorphic sarcoma: prominent replacement of the subcutaneous tissue by a pleomorphic tumor.

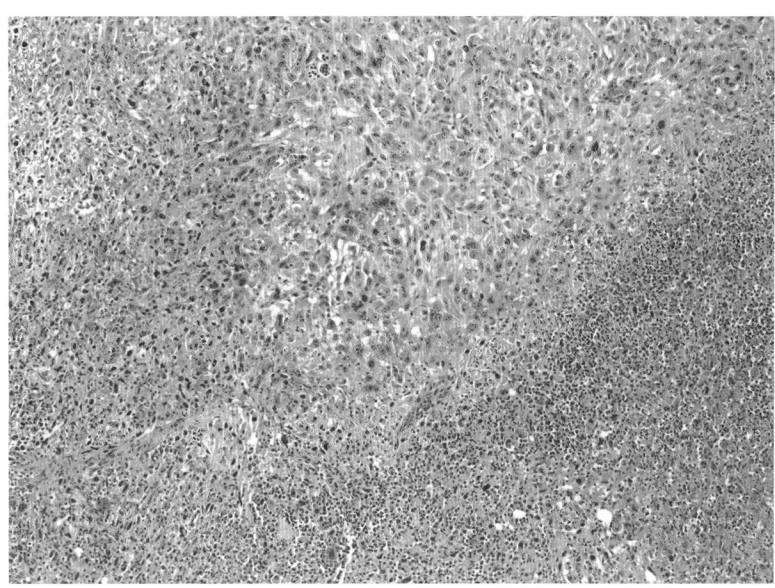

Fig. 35.289
Dermal pleomorphic sarcoma: prominent focal necrosis.

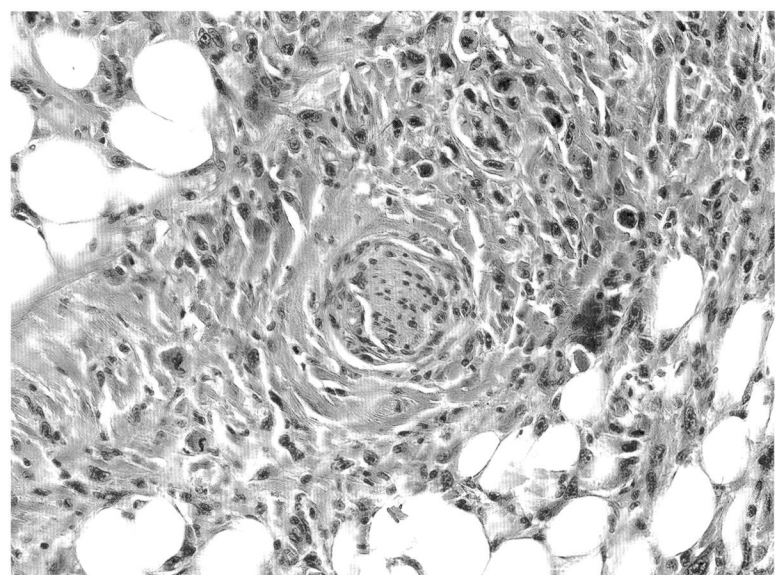

Fig. 35.290
Dermal pleomorphic sarcoma: perineural invasion.

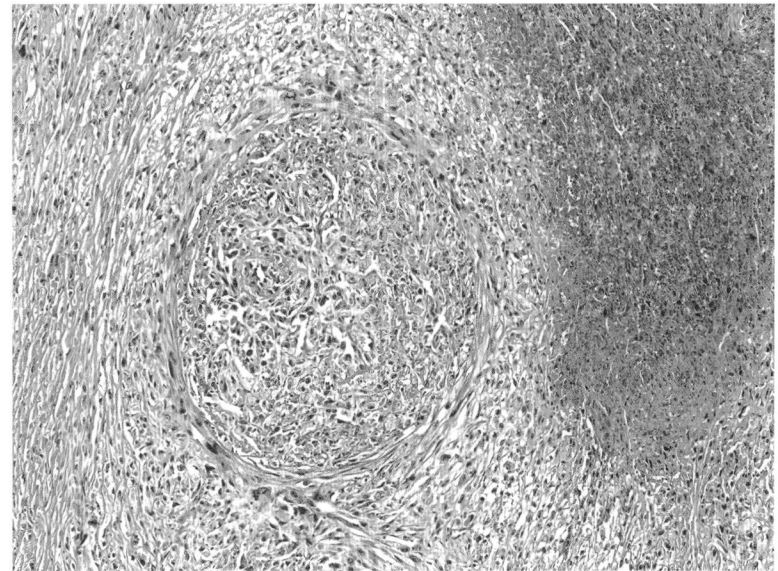

Fig. 35.291
Dermal pleomorphic sarcoma: necrosis and vascular invasion.

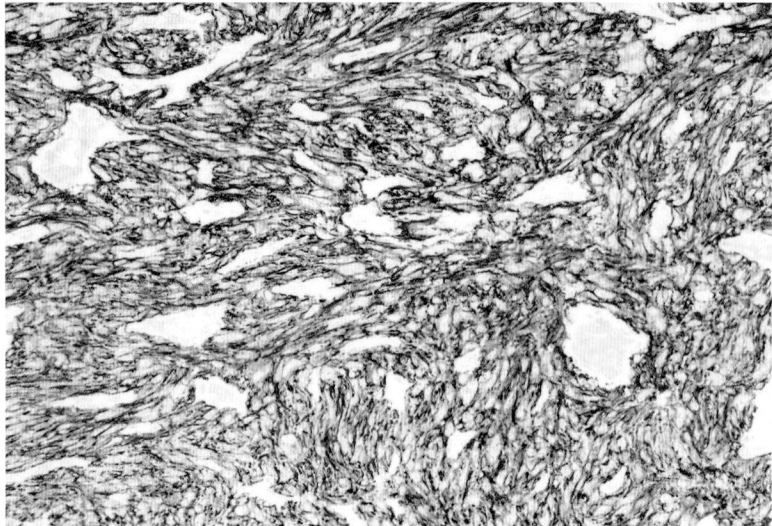

Fig. 35.292
Spindle cell atypical fibroxanthoma: the tumor cells express CD10.

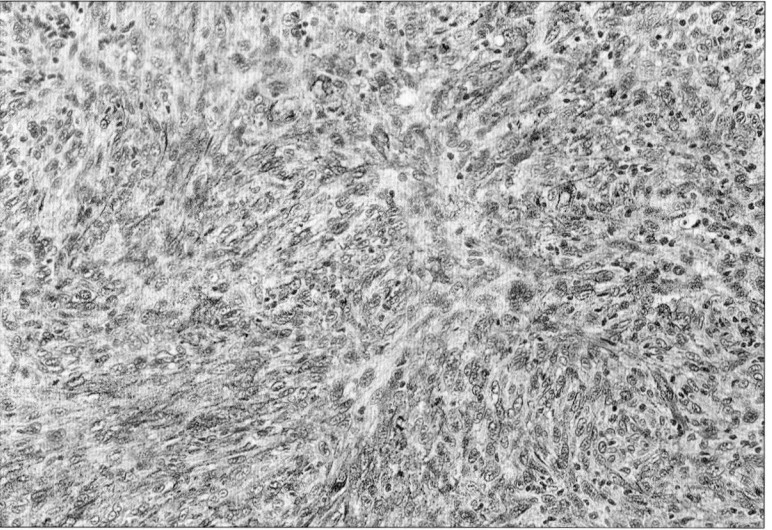

Fig. 35.293
Spindle cell atypical fibroxanthoma: note the diffuse expression of smooth muscle actin.

dendritic S100 protein-positive cells in the background, and this may be interpreted as positivity of tumor cells.

Differential diagnosis

Atypical fibroxanthoma and pleomorphic dermal sarcoma are diagnoses of exclusion.[83,84] Distinction from spindle cell variants of squamous carcinoma or melanoma is helped by adequate tissue sampling to detect an epithelial origin, a junctional component or more obviously differentiated areas, but this is not often found. Immunocytochemical stains for S100 protein, keratin and desmin expression should always be undertaken to exclude melanoma, spindle cell squamous cell carcinoma, an unusual metastasis or a leiomyosarcoma. P63 is a useful marker as it is diffusely positive in sarcomatoid squamous cell carcinoma and usually negative or minimally positive in atypical fibroxanthoma/pleomorphic dermal sarcoma.[85] It is important to highlight that sarcomatoid squamous cell carcinomas of the skin are often negative for CAM 5.2.

Merkel cell carcinoma, which recurred with features mimicking atypical fibroxanthoma, has been described as has a 'collision tumor' of these two types.[86,87] A collision with basal cell carcinoma and one with invasive melanoma have also been documented and this may represent a source of error in small samples.[88,89]

Tumors reported in the past as atypical fibroxanthoma occurring in non–sun-exposed skin of young patients represent examples of atypical fibrous histiocytoma.

Undifferentiated pleomorphic sarcoma (malignant fibrous histiocytoma)

Traditionally, undifferentiated pleomorphic sarcoma (malignant fibrous histiocytoma) has been regarded as the most common soft tissue sarcoma and five distinctive variants were originally described including pleomorphic, myxoid, angiomatoid, giant cell and inflammatory.[1–3] Over the years, however, it has become apparent that not only there is no true histiocytic differentiation in these tumors, but also that some of these variants have very little in common. The angiomatoid variant has been reclassified as angiomatoid fibrous histiocytoma. Moreover, the existence of a pleomorphic subtype (by far the most common tumor in the group) as an independent entity has been challenged.[4] In the current WHO classification (2013) the term 'malignant fibrous histiocytoma' is omitted. Under the heading 'tumors of unknown origin,' the term undifferentiated/unclassified sarcoma is used with the following subdivisions: spindle cell, pleomorphic, round cell, epithelioid, and NOS. Some of the round cell variants described as 'Ewing-like' are associated with specific translocations. Likely these will become distinctive entities outside of the undifferentiated sarcoma category in next WHO classification. These entities are briefly described in the Ewing sarcoma section (see page 1810).

Pleomorphic malignant fibrous histiocytoma as classically described is characterized histologically by prominent cytological pleomorphism, bizarre multinucleated giant cells, often a storiform pattern, and a mononuclear inflammatory cell infiltrate with foamy macrophages.[1–3] However, these features are non-specific and pleomorphic malignant fibrous histiocytoma as mentioned before, represents a waste basket for pleomorphic neoplasms, which, if studied by appropriate techniques such as immunohistochemistry and molecular methods, demonstrate a specific line of differentiation in the vast majority of cases.[4,5] Although most prove to be sarcomas (pleomorphic variants of leiomyosarcoma, rhabdomyosarcoma, liposarcoma), a small proportion represent melanomas or epithelial or even lymphoid neoplasms, and around 10% defy further classification.[4,6]

Excluding the spectrum of atypical fibroxanthoma/pleomorphic dermal sarcoma, other pleomorphic sarcomas are very rare in the skin and it is important to remember that the majority of 'sarcomatoid' cutaneous lesions are not true sarcomas but spindle cell variants of melanoma and carcinoma. Most true pleomorphic sarcomas in the skin represent extension from tumors arising in deeper soft tissues.

The groups described as giant cell malignant fibrous histiocytoma and inflammatory malignant fibrous histiocytoma, are no longer accepted as discreet entities. They are briefly discussed here for the sake of completeness to highlight that many of these lesions can be further subclassified into a distinctive group of neoplasms with the use of ancillary techniques.

Giant cell malignant fibrous histiocytoma represents a heterogeneous group of tumors, which have in common a multinodular growth pattern and the presence of multiple osteoclast-like multinucleated giant cells.[6] It was originally described in older individuals and show a predilection for the limbs. More than 50% of cases show neoplastic osteoid or bone formation and they are better classified as soft tissue osteosarcomas. A smaller proportion of tumors represent leiomyosarcomas rich in osteoclast-like giant cells and a further group of lesions is indistinguishable from giant cell tumor of bone.[7,8] The last has a benign histology and behavior is generally benign; as such it has been reclassified as giant cell tumor of soft tissue or soft tissue giant cell tumor of low-grade malignant potential (see page 1772).[9–11] It should be remembered that a variety of other lesions with a different phenotype, including atypical fibroxanthoma can be rich in osteoclast-like giant cells and that immunohistochemistry is an important aid in differential diagnosis.

Inflammatory malignant fibrous histiocytoma was originally described as a variant of so-called malignant fibrous histiocytoma presenting mainly in the retroperitoneum and other visceral soft tissues.[12,13] Since its original description, it has been proven, by the use of ancillary techniques, that in the majority of cases it represents a pattern of dedifferentiation in a dedifferentiated liposarcoma.

Undifferentiated pleomorphic sarcomas located superficially in the skin and subcutis, often display a highly infiltrative growth pattern.[14] Local recurrence is therefore common. These tumors display a complex karyotype and only TP53, RB1 and ATRX are noted to be significantly mutated.[15]

NERVE SHEATH AND NEUROECTODERMAL TUMORS AND TUMORLIKE LESIONS

Reactive lesions

Traumatic neuroma

Clinical features

Traumatic neuroma is not a true neoplasm but instead represents a proliferative hyperplastic response to peripheral nerve injury.[1,2] It may occur at any age or site, including subungual, oral cavity, penis, and rectum but is most often seen in young people, after severe accidental trauma or in older individuals following limb amputation (usually undertaken because of peripheral vascular disease), or other surgical procedures.[3-13] A case after hair transplantation has been reported.[14] However, trauma is not always severe and, in rare cases, a history of trauma cannot be elicited.[15-17] Associations with an arteriovenous aneurysm, a human bite and multiple lesions after deep burns have been documented.[18-20] Genital lesions, sometimes multiple, may be seen and are not always associated with known trauma.[21] Clinically, it presents as a small firm mass, which is often painful, but is sometimes associated with local anesthesia. Multiple recurrences of cutaneous carcinoma as a result of local tumor spread along the nerves of a traumatic neuroma have been reported.[22]

Histologic features

A traumatic neuroma is characterized by a variably well-defined, but unencapsulated, mass of numerous axons and Schwann cells embedded in scar tissue adjacent to the cut end of a damaged nerve (Figs 35.294 and 35.295). The newly formed neural tissue, failing to achieve continuity with the distal portion of the affected nerve, is arranged completely haphazardly. Nuclear pleomorphism and mitotic activity are not present. Dystrophic calcification is exceptionally seen.[23] Granular cell change can rarely occur in traumatic neuroma.[24,25] A rare oral lesion associated with intraepithelial proliferation of axons has been documented.[26]

Accessory digits often show the features of a traumatic neuroma and this may be the result of partial intrauterine amputation.[27]

Differential diagnosis

The clinical history, together with the typical histologic appearances, is usually sufficient to make a diagnosis. The presence of numerous axons as well as Schwann cells and fibroblasts allows ready distinction from a neurofibroma.

Digital pacinian neuroma

Clinical features

Digital pacinian neuroma (pacinian corpuscle hyperplasia) is a rare but distinctive type of neuroma that usually presents as a result of trauma to the fingers of adults.[1-4] Lesions are small and very painful.[5,6] A case has been associated with a Morton metatarsalgia.[6] Erosive bone changes have been documented in one patient.[7] Multiple lesions have been reported.[8]

Histologic features

Histologically, there are numerous pacinian corpuscles intermixed with small nerve fibers and surrounded by fibrous tissue (Figs 35.296 and 35.297).

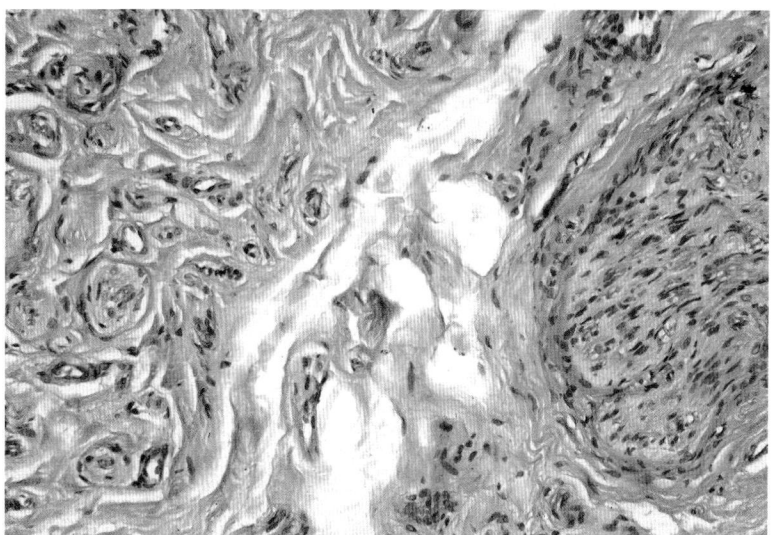

Fig. 35.295
Traumatic neuroma: high-power view.

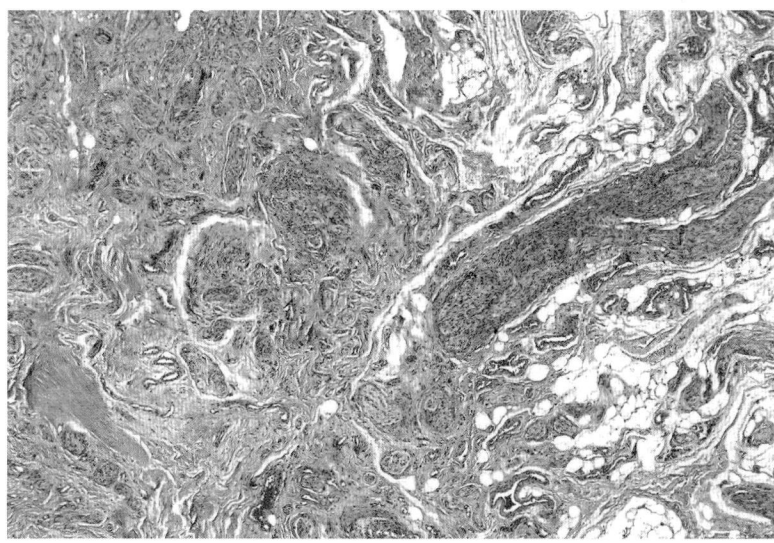

Fig. 35.294
Traumatic neuroma: arising from the cut end of this peripheral nerve is a proliferative spindle cell lesion.

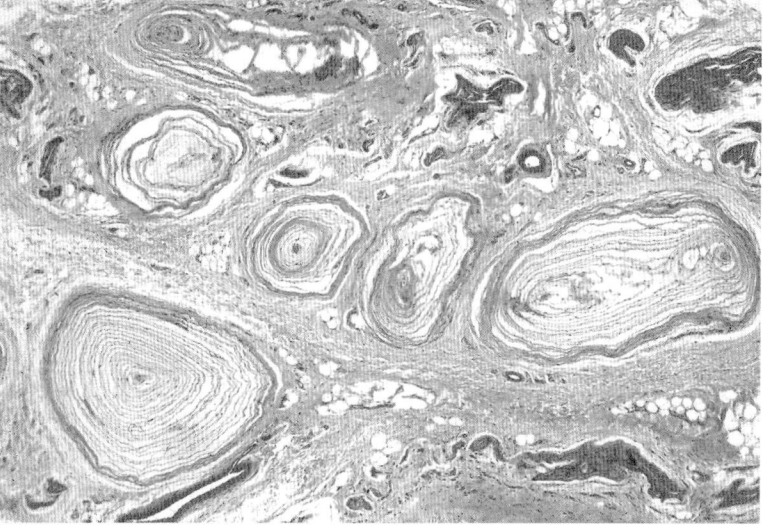

Fig. 35.296
Pacinian neuroma: this field shows an admixture of pacinian corpuscles, fibrous tissue and conspicuous nerve fibers.

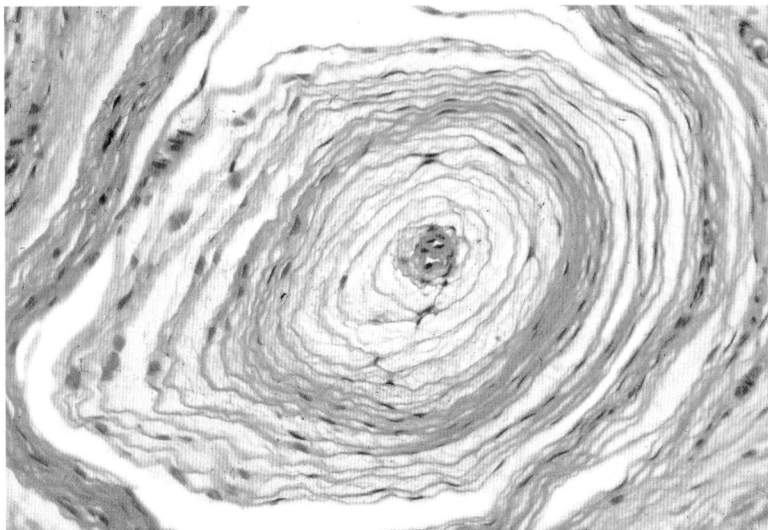

Fig. 35.297
Pacinian neuroma: high-power view showing the characteristic lamellated structure.

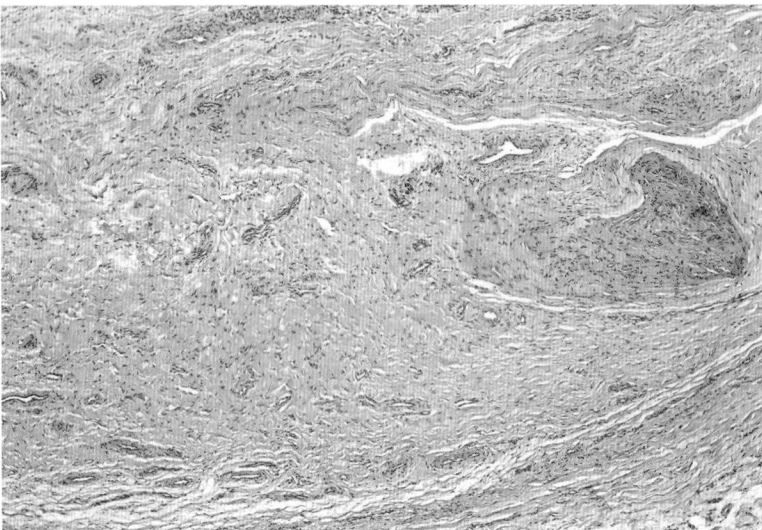

Fig. 35.298
Morton neuroma: the nerve trunk is markedly distorted by intense concentric fibrosis.

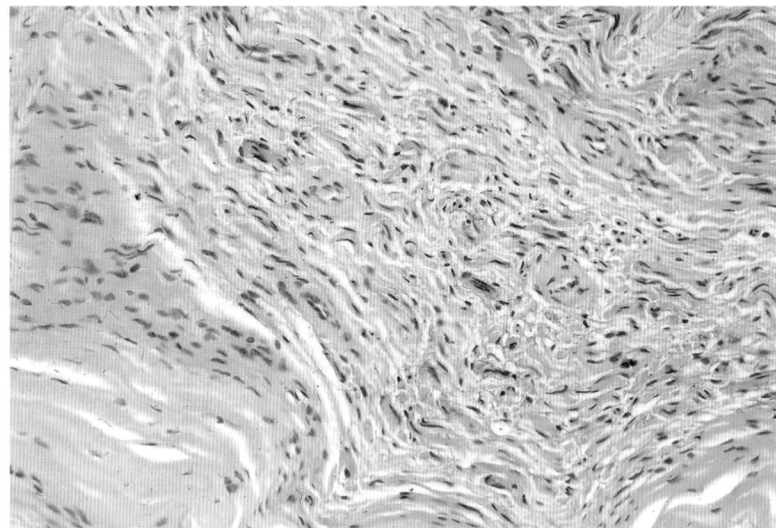

Fig. 35.299
Morton neuroma: high-power view showing numerous fibroblasts.

Morton neuroma

Clinical features

Morton neuroma (metatarsalgia) is also not a true neoplasm, but represents a degenerative response to chronic low-grade tissue damage.[1,2] It most often presents in adults, who complain of pain in the distal sole of the foot, usually when walking. Females are affected more often than males. Close examination reveals that the pain is often localized between (or over) the metatarsal heads, but a nodule or mass is not usually palpable. Bilateral involvement is rare.[3] If excision is undertaken, a localized, rather fusiform, expansion of one of the plantar digital nerves is seen. Excision is usually undertaken for symptomatic lesions but in a percentage of patients, pain resists or even gets worse.[4–8] A relationship between the width of the forefoot and the Greek foot has been suggested.[9,10]

Histologic features

Traditionally, histology has been described as revealing marked fibrosis of the endo-, epi- and perineurium associated with edematous change, marked degeneration and loss of nerve fibers (*Figs 35.298* and *35.299*). Fibrotic changes are often seen in the adjacent subcutaneous tissues and around blood vessels. However, a recent study comparing the histology of nerves excised from patients with Morton metatarsalgia with that of nerves from the same area excised from autopsy patients found no differences between both groups except for slightly thicker nerves in patients with the disease.[11] The authors concluded that histology has no role in confirming the diagnosis, a finding that has been supported by other studies.[12,13]

Dermal hyperneury

Clinical features

Dermal hyperneury is a well-recognized phenomenon which can be localized or multifocal.[1–7] When localized, it is usually associated with a trauma (including chronic scratching). It may be seen as an incidental finding in association with other cutaneous lesions or rarely in biopsies from notalgia paresthetica.[1–3] The multifocal form is generally considered syndromic; association with multiple endocrine neoplasia type IIB/MEN2B (RET at 10q11.21), Cowden syndrome (PTEN at 10q23.31), and neurofibromatosis type 2 (NF2 at 22q12.2) have been documented (see also mucosal neuromas), and it is very rare.[4–6] However, a subset of multifocal lesions are idiopathic and not associated with syndromes.

Histologic features

Histologically, in dermal hyperneury, hyperplastic and hypertrophic myelinated nerve bundles are seen scattered throughout the dermis.[7] When associated with an inflammatory infiltrate, it must be distinguished from an infectious process.[8]

Neural hamartomas

Mucosal neuroma

Clinical features

Mucosal neuromas are always multiple and have predilection for the mouth.[1–3] They may present as part of the multiple endocrine neoplasia syndrome type IIB (MEN 2B, Sipple; *RET* at 10q11.21), an autosomal dominant disease characterized by a marfanoid body habitus, dysmorphic facies, medullary carcinoma of thyroid and pheochromocytoma.[1–6] Laryngeal lesions may rarely also present in MEN2B.[7–9] Rare examples may present in the mouth and even the larynx in patients without MEN 2B.[10–12]

Pathogenesis and histologic features

SOS1 frameshift mutations cause pure mucosal neuroma syndrome unassociated with MEN 2B.[13]

Histologically, lesions are poorly circumscribed and consist of hyperplastic nerves in a haphazard and disorganized arrangement. An incomplete capsule surrounded by a layer of EMA-positive perineural cells is sometimes present.

Benign triton tumor

Clinical features

Benign triton tumor (neuromuscular hamartoma or choristoma, nerve rhabdomyoma) is very rare and usually presents with progressive pain or as a peripheral neuropathy in infants and children with no sex predilection.[1-12] Exceptional cases have been reported in adults.[13] Sciatic nerve and branchial plexus are the most common sites of occurrence but other sites such as spinal and head and neck including oral and orbit have been reported.[1-13] Intracranial cases are exceptional.[14] A case arising on the tongue and associated with embryonal rhabdomyosarcoma and ganglioneuroma (ectomesenchymoma) has been documented.[15]

Histologic features

Histologically an intimate admixture of neural and mature skeletal fibers is seen.[1,2,5]

Other hamartomas and choristomas

These include a group of miscellaneous acquired or congenital lesions with very few or only single case reports in the literature.

- Cutaneous ganglion cell choristoma or cutaneous ganglioneuroma presents as a solitary papule, usually on the trunk of adults.[1-7] A congenital case and one with multiple facial lesions have been documented.[8,9] Histologically, there is a dermal proliferation of mature ganglion cells admixed with Schwann cells and nonmyelinated axons. Ganglion cells are positive for glial fibrillary acid protein and Schwann cells are positive for S100 protein. Adipocytic metaplasia is exceptional.[10] Unusual examples include a case associated with a seborrheic keratosis, a lesion with a desmoplastic stroma and two with prominent overlying hyperkeratosis and acanthosis.[11-15]
- Congenital neurovascular hamartoma (NVH) of the skin is characterized by a proliferation of capillaries in a background of spindle cells that stain with NSE.[16] The two patients described with this lesion subsequently developed rhabdoid tumors and congenital neurovascular hamartoma has been proposed as a marker for this tumor.[17]
- In other lesions – variably called congenital neural hamartoma, cutaneous nerve hamartoma and linear cutaneous neuroma – there is a proliferation of Schwann cells or nerves.[18-20] A congenital cutaneous solitary hamartoma with mixed eccrine, neural, and lipomatous components has been described.[21]
- Congenital lesions containing hyperplastic pacinian corpuscles in the lower back with spina bifida occulta have been termed sacrococcygeal paciniomas while similar lesions on the buttock without underlying neural tube defects are described as multiple hairy pacinian neurofibromas.[22,23]
- A single case of an intraneural benign lesion displaying dual neural and melanocytic differentiation has been described under the rubric melanocytoneuroma.[24]

Benign neural tumors

It is controversial whether some of the lesions included under this heading are true neoplasms or, rather, represent hamartomas. However, they are included in this section because they have traditionally been considered neoplastic.

Solitary circumscribed neuroma

Clinical features

Solitary circumscribed neuroma (palisaded encapsulated neuroma) is a common but often unrecognized tumor that presents as a solitary, asymptomatic, skin-colored papule on the face (especially nose, nasolabial folds and cheeks) of middle-aged to elderly adults.[1-4] Lesions also seem to be relatively common in the oral cavity, particularly in the masticatory mucosa.[5] Rarely, acral lesions exceptionally multiple and bilateral may occur.[6] There is no sex predilection and most lesions are less than 1 cm in diameter. Other rare sites include the eyelid and penis.[7,9] Occasional cases present at other sites including the oral mucosa, nose and penis, and rarely multiple lesions have been described.[10-15] There is no known association with neurofibromatosis, although a relationship between solitary circumscribed neuroma and the mucocutaneous neuromas seen in multiple endocrine neoplasia (MEN2B) syndrome has been noted.[16] Multiple circumscribed neuromas in siblings have been reported.[17]

Histologic features

Typically, low-power examination reveals a well-circumscribed dermal nodule (Figs 35.300–35.303). However, the growth pattern in some lesions is multinodular or even plexiform.[5,11] Encapsulation is incomplete and the superficial part of the tumor often appears to merge with the surrounding dermis. Tumor cells are arranged in short fascicles separated by artifactual clefting and have wavy hyperchromatic nuclei and ill-defined pale eosinophilic cytoplasm. Palisading of nuclei is not as common as its original name might suggest. Occasional cases show degenerative nuclear changes or focal epithelioid morphology.[18] The epidermis is usually normal, but mild to prominent hyperplasia is sometimes a feature.[19] Commonly, a normal nerve

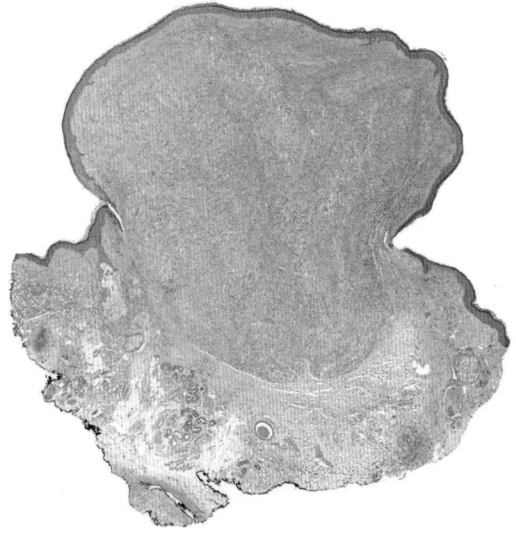

Fig. 35.300
Solitary circumscribed neuroma: the lesion is a well-circumscribed intradermal nodule.

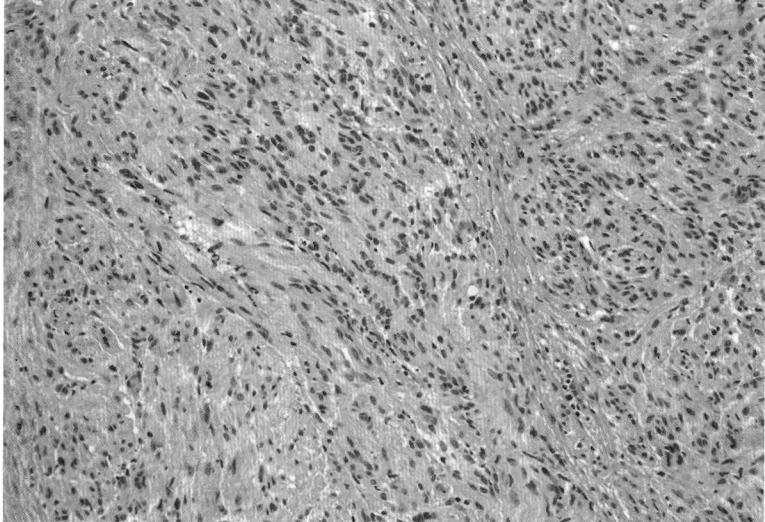

Fig. 35.301
Solitary circumscribed neuroma: medium-power view showing multinodularity.

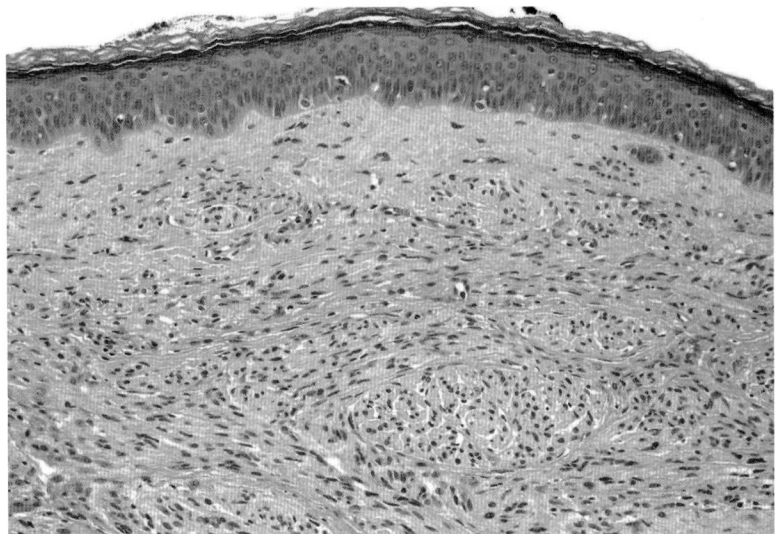

Fig. 35.302
Solitary circumscribed neuroma: note that the tumor merges imperceptibly into the papillary dermis.

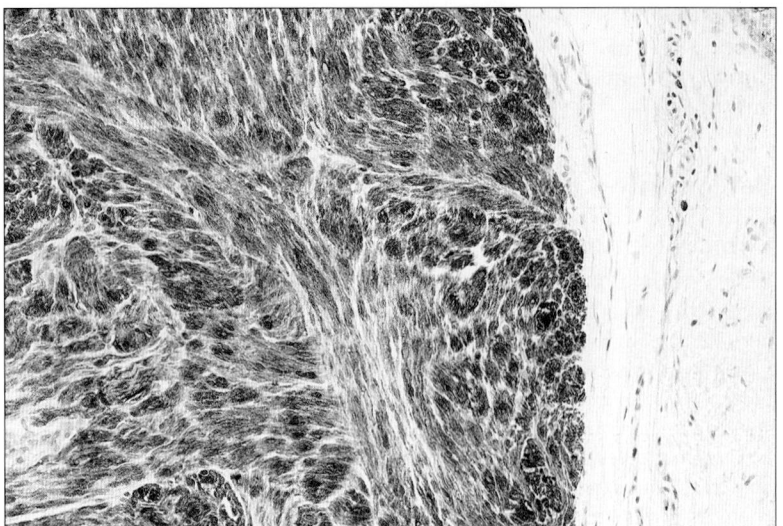

Fig. 35.304
Solitary circumscribed neuroma: the tumor cells express S100 protein.

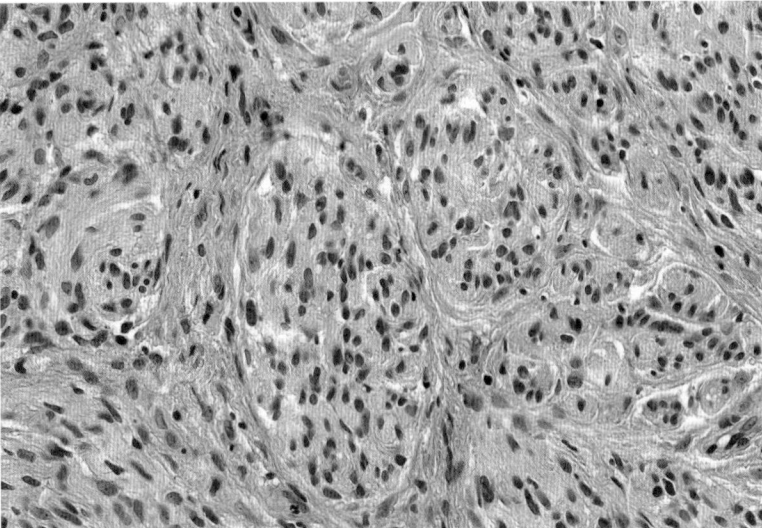

Fig. 35.303
Solitary circumscribed neuroma: the tumor is composed of pale-staining spindled cells with uniform elongated darkly staining nuclei.

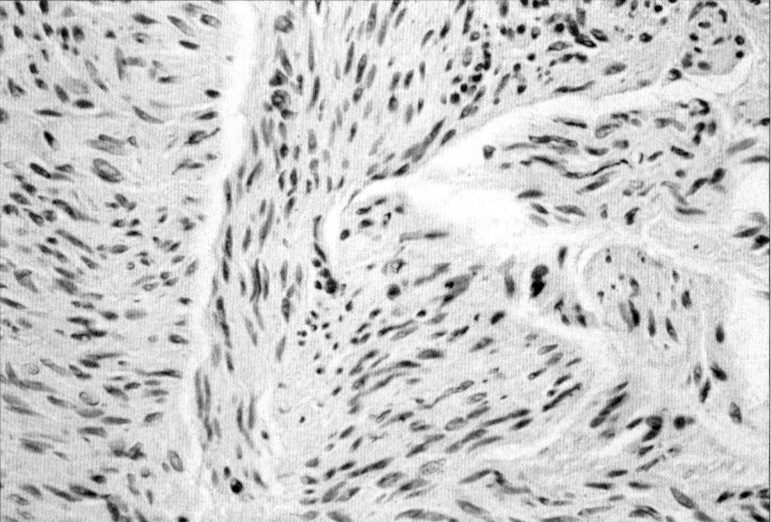

Fig. 35.305
Solitary circumscribed neuroma: the tumor contains numerous nerve fibers (neurofilament immunocytochemistry).

is identified near the base of the lesion, often entering (or fusing with) the lesional capsule. Prominent vascularity is occasionally present.[20]

By immunohistochemistry, most of the cells are S100 protein positive, in keeping with Schwann cells (*Fig. 35.304*). GFAP is negative.[5] Numerous axons can be identified with neurofilament protein and the cells in the capsule stain for EMA, as expected in normal perineurial cells (*Fig. 35.305*).[21,22] As the capsule tends to be partial and EMA can be weak, additional stains that help identifying the perineural cells include claudin 1 and Glut-1.[5]

Differential diagnosis

Distinction from neurofibroma and schwannoma is easy if attention is paid to the characteristic architecture and the presence of numerous intralesional axons.

Epithelial sheath neuroma

Clinical features

Epithelial sheath neuroma is a very rare distinctive lesion combining nerves and squamous epithelium.[1-3] The handful of cases reported so far have presented in adults as asymptomatic solitary lesions mainly on the back.

Pathogenesis and histologic features

The pathogenesis is unknown and there is no consensus as to whether the lesion is reactive or neoplastic.[1-5] In a case associated with trauma, a hyperplastic phenomenon mediated by IL-6 was suggested.[6]

Histology characteristically shows fairly prominent nerves in the superficial dermis encased by cytologically bland squamous epithelium (*Figs 35.306* and *35.307*). There is no evidence of a connection to the overlying epidermis or neighboring adnexal structures. A loose myxoid stroma, a lymphocytic infiltrate and prominent infundibular cysts may be seen.[4] Similar appearances may be seen in keratoacanthoma but in the latter there is evidence of inflammation and fibrosis accompanying the overlying tumor. In addition, the perineural invasion is usually deeply seated.

Schwannoma

Clinical features

Schwannomas (neurilemmomas) are common benign lesions, occurring most often in the fourth and fifth decades with an equal sex incidence and arising most frequently on the limbs (mainly the upper limbs) followed by the head and neck (including the oral cavity, orbit and salivary glands) (*Fig. 35.308*).[1-5]

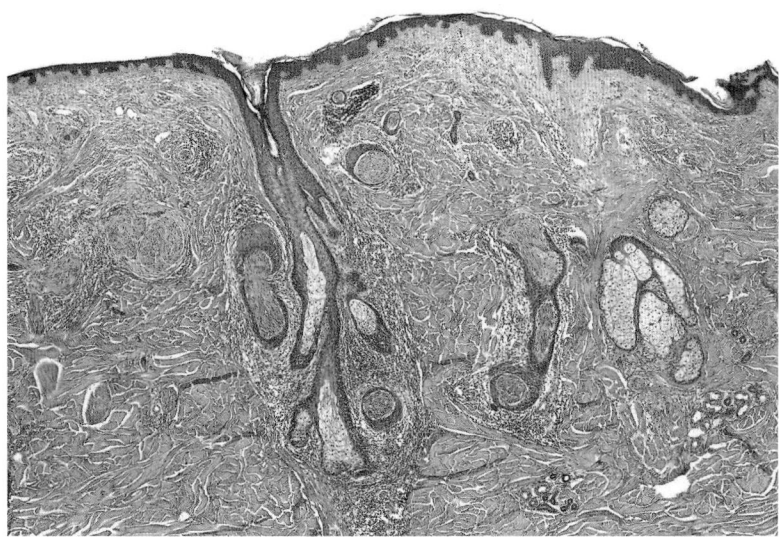

Fig. 35.306
Epithelial sheath neuroma: prominent nerves are present in the superficial reticular dermis encased by nests of bland squamous epithelium. By courtesy of L. Requena, MD, Madrid, Spain.

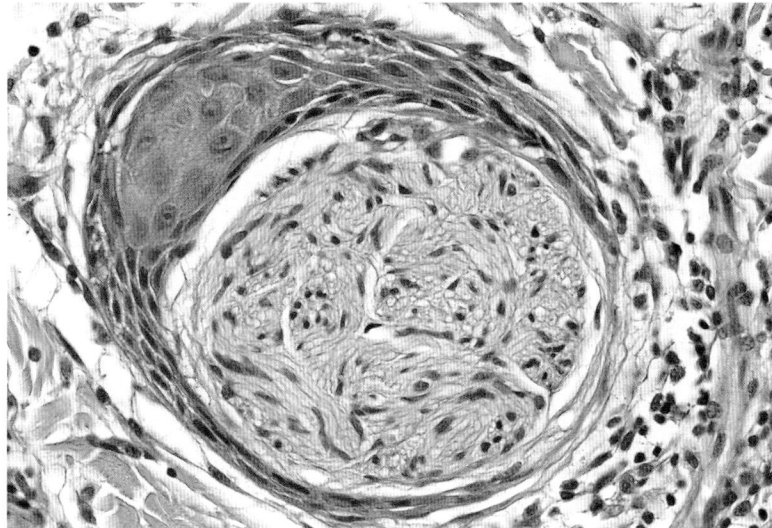

Fig. 35.307
Epithelial sheath neuroma: high-power view. By courtesy of L. Requena, MD, Madrid, Spain.

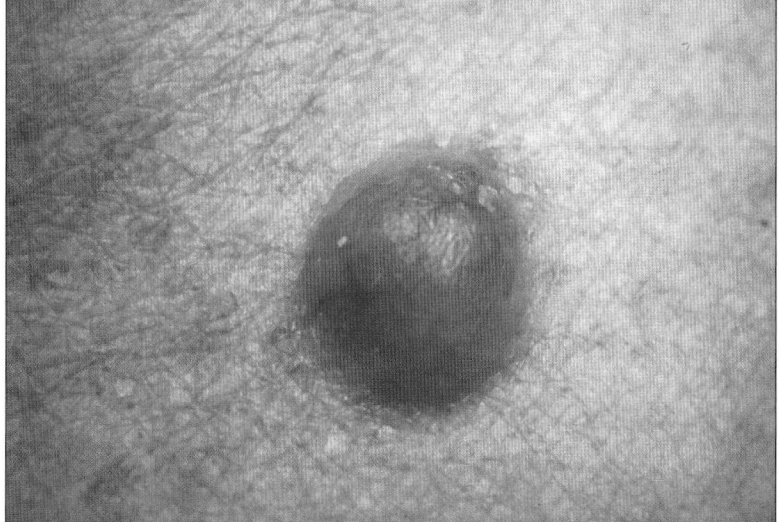

Fig. 35.308
Schwannoma: this tumor presents as a non-specific dermal nodule. By courtesy of the Institute of Dermatology, London, UK.

Lesions in children are very rare and exceptionally congenital.[6,7] They present most often as a solitary painless subcutaneous mass of variable size (exceptionally very large), but very occasionally they may be multiple and in this context are rarely associated with von Recklinghausen neurofibromatosis.[8,9] Prominent cystic change is occasionally seen. Purely dermal tumors are rare.[10,11] Cutaneous lesions exceptionally have an agminate pattern and one was associated with overlying anetoderma.[12,13] Tumors in the penis and vulva are exceedingly rare.[14,15] Some tumors occur in other locations including bone, gastrointestinal tract, pancreas, liver, retroperitoneum, mediastinum, trachea, nasopharynx, larynx, thyroid, adrenal gland and lymph node.[16-26] Neurological symptoms including pain and paresthesias are uncommon except in large deep-seated lesions; malignant change is exceedingly rare (see neurofibroma).[5,27,28] Exceptional cases include a cutaneous example that may have been associated with foreign material.[29] Recurrence after simple excision is very infrequent.[30]

Neurofibromatosis type II (NF2 gene at 22q12.2 encodin merlin protein) is characterized by acoustic schwannomas, cutaneous tumors and other central nervous system lesions including meningioma, cataract and retinal hamartoma.[31,32] About 59% of patients have skin tumors, the majority of which represent schwannomas.[32] Only rarely do patients develop neurofibromas or hybrid lesions. Café-au-lait spots may be present in up to 33% of patients but these tend to be fewer than in patients with neurofibromatosis type I.[32] The development of neurofibromas in neurofibromatosis type II may be due to interaction between neurofibromin and merlin, the NF2 gene product, in regulating the RAS proto-oncogene.[33,34] Cutaneous schwannomas are only rarely associated with neurofibromatosis type II.[35]

The National Institute of Health (NIH) diagnostic criteria for NFII are as follows:
- Bilateral vestibular schwannomas that do not require any additional features for diagnosis of the disease,
- First-degree relative with NF2 and either occurrence of unilateral vestibular schwannoma in patients younger than 30 or occurrence of two other associated lesions (e.g., glioma, meningioma, schwannoma, juvenile cortical cataract),
- Unilateral vestibular schwannoma and any two other associated lesions including glioma, meningioma, schwannoma, neurofibroma, or juvenile cortical cataract,
- Multiple meningiomas with any of the above lesions.[23]

The presence of multiple cutaneous schwannomas with or without similar lesions in spinal and other nerves has been termed schwannomatosis. Although it was initially doubted whether it represents a discreet entity or merely a variant of neurofibromatosis type II, it is now regarded as distinct.[32,36-45] Most cases appear to be sporadic but in a few an autosomal dominant pattern of inheritance has been described. Cases associated with multiple meningiomas and a family with predisposition to malignant rhabdoid tumors have been described.[46-50] Germline aberrations in INI1 / SMARCB1 (22q11) may be involved.

A new hereditary syndrome consisting of multiple schwannomas, multiple nevi and multiple vaginal leiomyomas has been described.[51] The nevi are congenital but the schwannomas and vaginal leiomyomas develop in adult life.

In a recent study it was found that children or young adults that develop solitary schwannoma or meningioma usually have genetic predisposition.[52]

Pathogenesis and histologic features

Cytogenetic studies in schwannomas have shown either loss of 22q material or monosomy 22, probably corresponding to the NF2 gene (22q12.2) encoding the neurofibromin 2 or merlin protein.[34,35,53,54]

Schwannomas are usually rounded and invariably encapsulated, and are typically found in the subcutaneous or deeper tissues; primary intradermal origin is unusual. Purely intraneural tumors are exceptional.[55] Microscopically, they are characterized by a classical biphasic pattern of cellular Antoni A and hypocellular Antoni B areas.
- Antoni A areas form the more cellular component of the lesion and are composed of fairly closely packed spindled cells with tapering, elongated, rather wavy nuclei; nuclear palisading is a prominent feature, producing the distinctive Verocay bodies (Figs 35.309–35.311). These

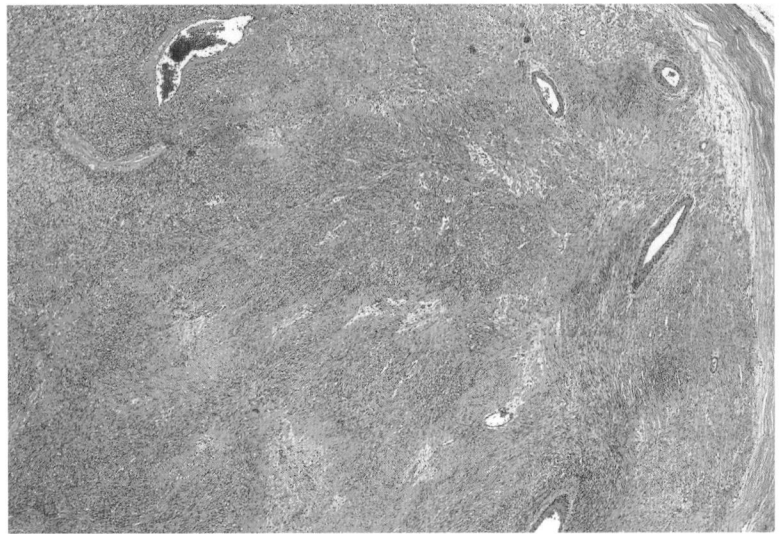

Fig. 35.309
Schwannoma: scanning view of spindle cell tumor with prominent blood vessels.
A capsule is seen on the right side.

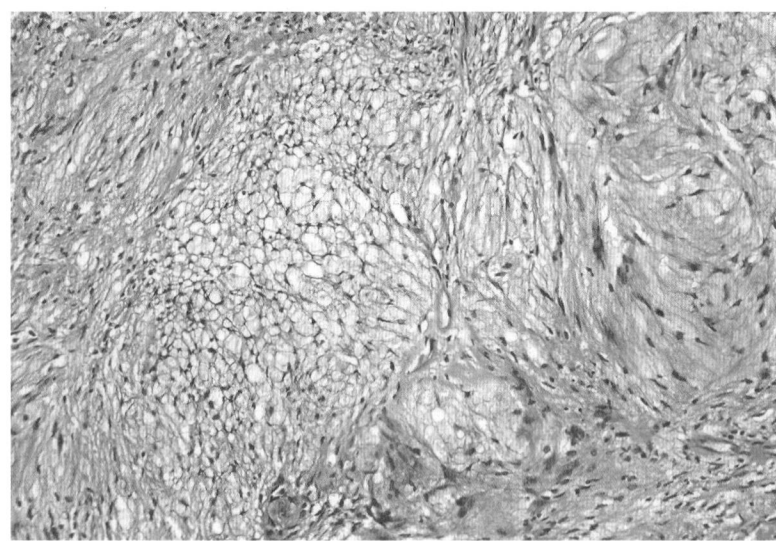

Fig. 35.312
Schwannoma: myxoid degeneration gives rise to Antoni B areas.

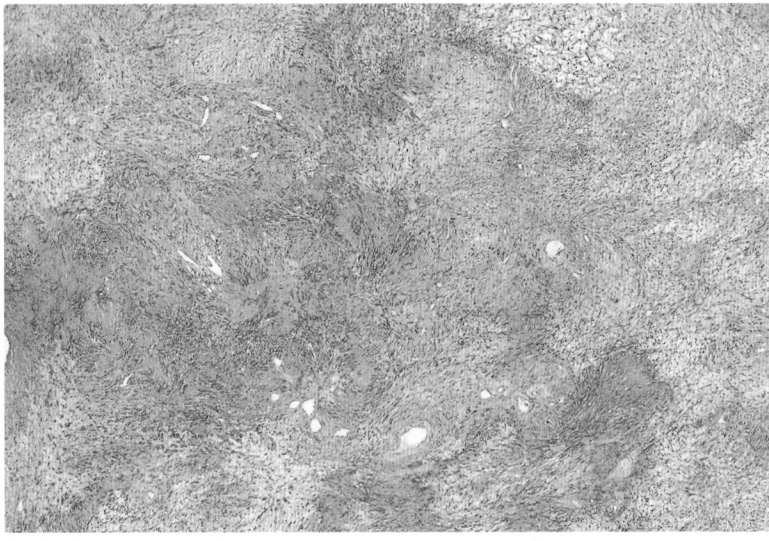

Fig. 35.310
Schwannoma: palisading is a characteristic feature.

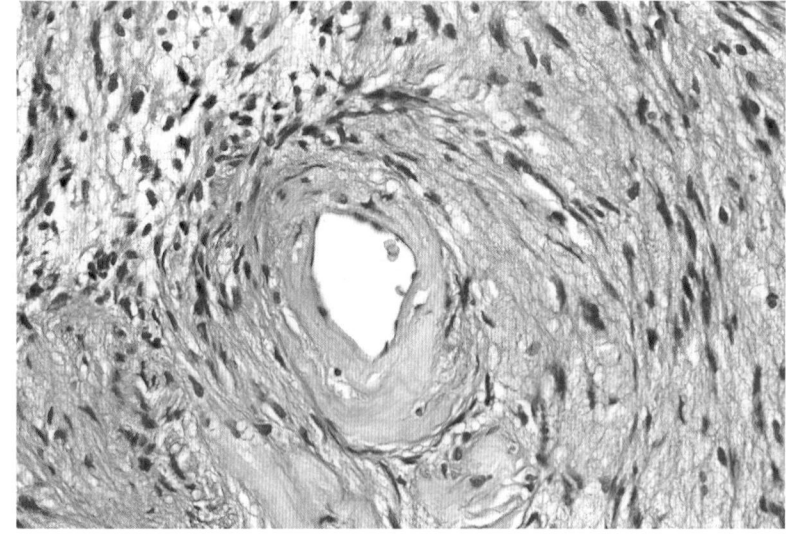

Fig. 35.313
Schwannoma: there is marked hyalinization of the blood vessel walls in Antoni B.

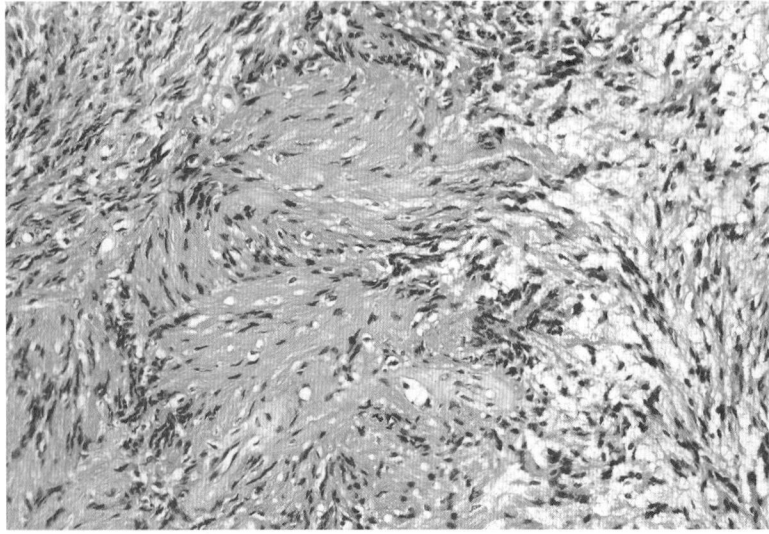

Fig. 35.311
Schwannoma: the Verocay body, typical of the Antoni A areas, is characterized by
two parallel rows of nuclei separated by Schwann cell processes.

are sometimes the predominant feature.[56] Verocay-like bodies may
be seen in a number of other tumors including dermatofibroma and
leiomyoma.[57] Degenerative nuclear pleomorphism and mitotic activity
are occasionally seen, but tend to be spatially unrelated. Hyalinization
of stromal collagen and focal dystrophic calcification are sometimes
present.

• Antoni B areas are typified by irregularly scattered spindled or stellate
cells set in an abundant loose myxoid stroma (*Fig. 35.312*). Within
these areas, scattered chronic inflammatory cells and small blood
vessels, often with hyalinized walls, are a prominent feature (*Fig.
35.313*). Focal degenerative changes, including microcystic change and
hemosiderin deposition, are not uncommon.

A schwannoma with collagenous spherulosis has been documented and in
one case meningothelial-like whorls were present.[58,59] An intravascular presentation is exceptional.[60]

The very rare finding of apparent glandular differentiation in benign
schwannomas represents proliferation of entrapped normal adnexal
structures.[61–64]

Though relatively rare, tumors exhibiting a hybrid appearance of
schwannoma and neurofibroma are increasingly recognized.[65–72] These can
be seen in patients with neurofibromatosis and often the neurofibroma is of

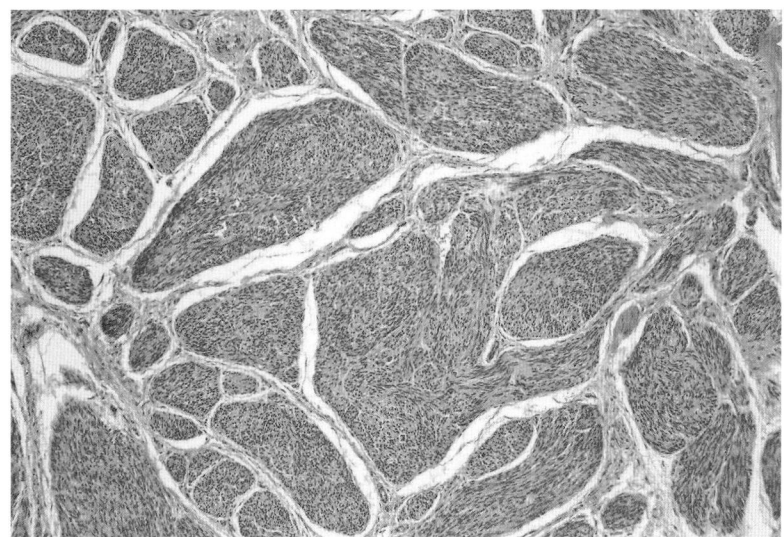

Fig. 35.314
Plexiform schwannoma: this small tumor is composed of multiple discrete nodules of schwannomatous tissue. Nuclear palisading and Verocay bodies are evident.

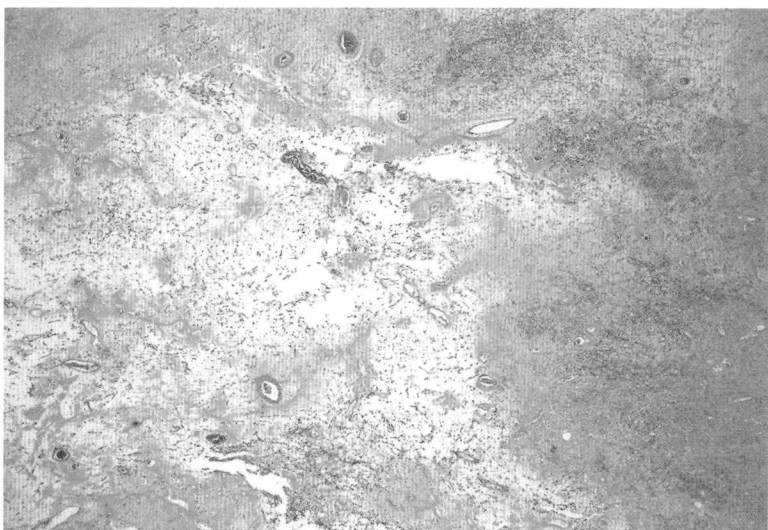

Fig. 35.315
Ancient schwannoma: degenerative changes have resulted in marked myxoid features with fibrosis and conspicuous vascularity.

the plexiform variant.[73] They appear to be overrepresented amongst patients with schwannomatosis and neurofibromatosis.[74] One hybrid case showed monosomy 22 (loss of *NF2* locus) as well as loss of function mutations in the *CTNNA3* gene (10q21.3).

The schwannomas seen in neurofibromatosis type II have been shown to contain axons.[76]

Malignant transformation often shows pleomorphic epithelioid cells and rarely there is divergent differentiation such as the presence of epithelioid angiosarcoma.[77–79]

Ultrastructurally, schwannomas are composed predominantly of Schwann cells and this is reflected immunohistochemically by S100 protein positivity in the majority of tumor cells. The capsule contains a layer of EMA-positive perineurial fibroblasts. GFAP and CKAE1/AE3 positivity may be seen mainly in deep seated tumors. SOX10, podoplanin and calretinin are positive in the majority of cases whereas positivity for CD34 is more focal.[80–85] Tumor cells express PDGFR-alpha, PDGFR-beta ligands and their cognate receptors as well as KIT, and it has been shown that imatinib mesylate inhibits a schwannoma cell line.[86,87]

Variants[88]

- Plexiform schwannoma is an uncommon tumor only very rarely associated with neurofibromatosis (mainly NF2) and tending to arise mainly on the head and neck or trunk of children or young adults.[89–98] These lesions represent about 4.3% of all schwannomas and around 15% of cutaneous schwannoma. It is usually a small intradermal or subcutaneous lesion characterized by multiple encapsulated nodules composed predominantly of Antoni A tissue (*Fig. 35.314*). Any histologic type of schwannoma may be represented in plexiform tumors, particularly the cellular variant. Cellular plexiform schwannoma occurs in infants and recurrence of trisomy 17 has been reported.[98] It shows lack of circumscription or an infiltrative growth pattern, increased cellularity and relatively high mitotic activity. These features may lead to a diagnosis of malignancy especially in small biopsies. There is no metastatic potential but local recurrence is not unusual.[89,98]
- A subgroup of plexiform and multinodular schwannomas affects major peripheral nerves. Deep-seated tumors also occur. Nuclear pleomorphism (mild to moderate), limited mitotic activity and focal necrosis (the latter in deep-seated examples) may be present, but recurrence is not a feature and there is no malignant potential. Distinction from plexiform neurofibroma is vital to avoid an inappropriate clinical diagnosis of von Recklinghausen disease (neurofibromatosis type 1). Rarely, tumors are associated with neurofibromatosis type 2 and schwannomatosis.

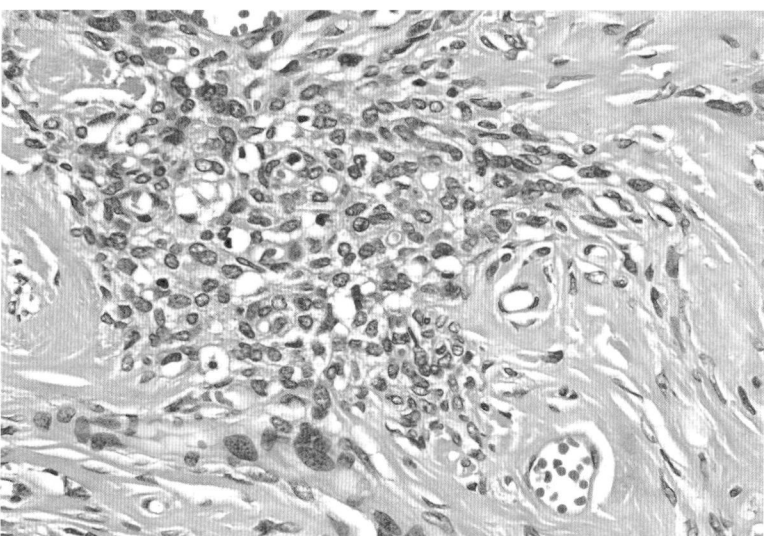

Fig. 35.316
Ancient schwannoma: focal nuclear pleomorphism should not be taken as having sinister implication. Mitotic activity is not present in these tumors.

- Ancient schwannoma, which is usually a more deeply located, long-standing lesion, is characterized by pronounced degenerative changes manifest as nuclear pleomorphism associated with extensive cyst formation, calcification, hyalinization or hemorrhage (*Figs 35.315* and *35.316*).[99] Mitoses, however, are rare.
- Cellular schwannoma only rarely presents subcutaneously as a large and encapsulated mass.[100–102] Microscopically, there is a marked increase in cellularity which, combined with a mainly fascicular architecture, may simulate a smooth muscle tumor (*Figs 35.317* and *35.318*). Verocay bodies are generally not seen. Xanthomatous cells and a lymphocytic infiltrate may be prominent (*Fig. 35.319*). Normal mitoses may number up to 10 per 10 high-power fields, but neither necrosis nor significant nuclear pleomorphism is a feature. Distinction from smooth muscle tumors is readily afforded by S100 positivity (*Fig. 35.320*).
- Malignant melanotic schwannian tumor (previously known as melanotic schwannoma, psammomatous melanotic schwannoma) is a rare lesion which, in addition to the features of a neural tumor, contains pigmented cells and usually displays psammoma bodies (*Fig. 35.321*).[103,104] Based on the observation that tumors recur and may metastasize, it has recently been proposed that all lesions should be

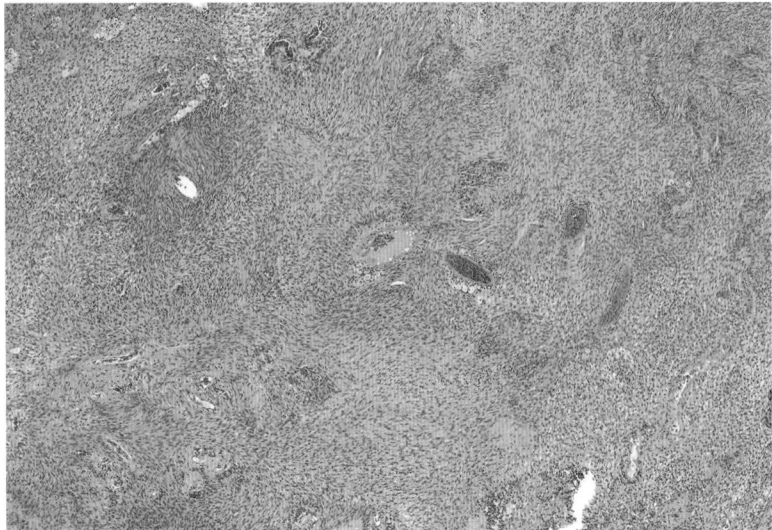

Fig. 35.317
Cellular schwannoma: typically, lesions are highly cellular, superficially resembling leiomyosarcoma.

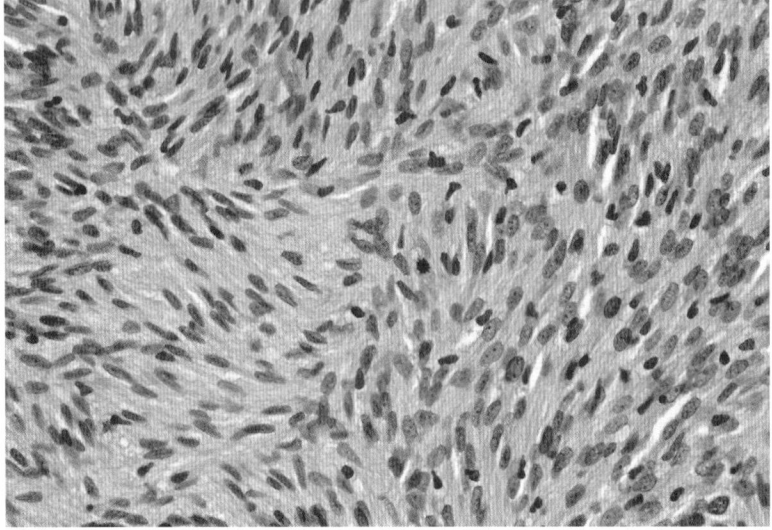

Fig. 35.318
Cellular schwannoma: scattered mitoses are commonly present.

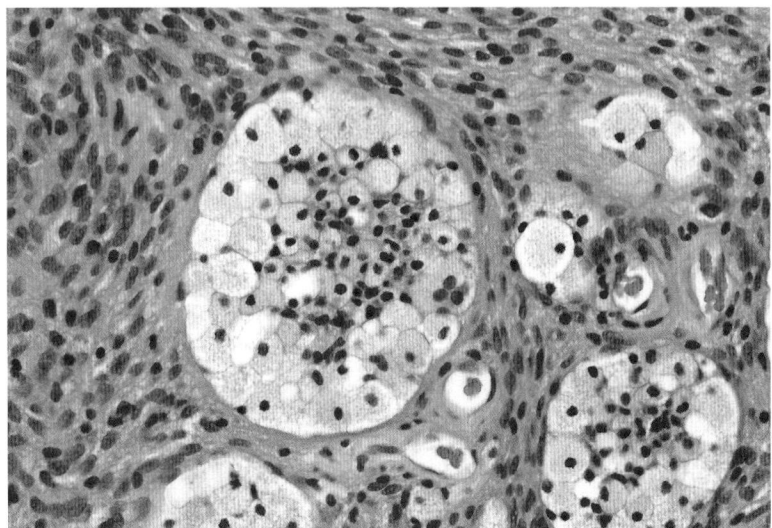

Fig. 35.319
Cellular schwannoma: although xanthomatous histiocytes may be seen in any type of schwannoma, they are particularly common in this variant.

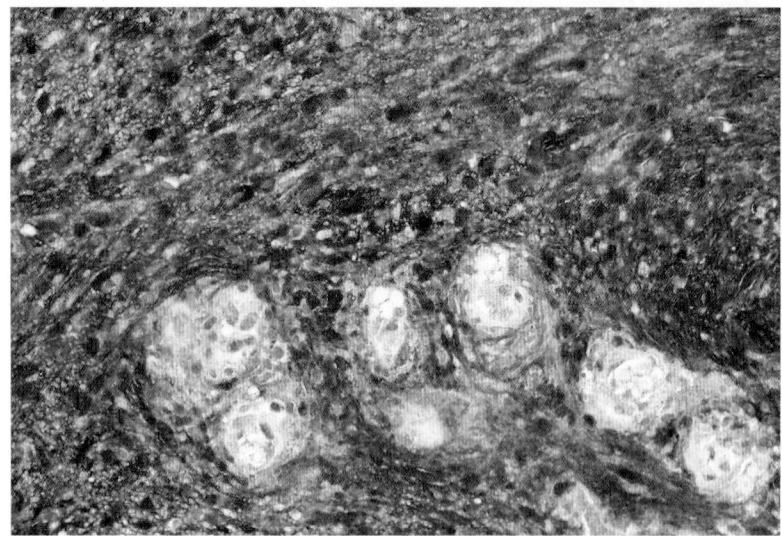

Fig. 35.320
Cellular schwannoma: the spindled cells are S100 positive.

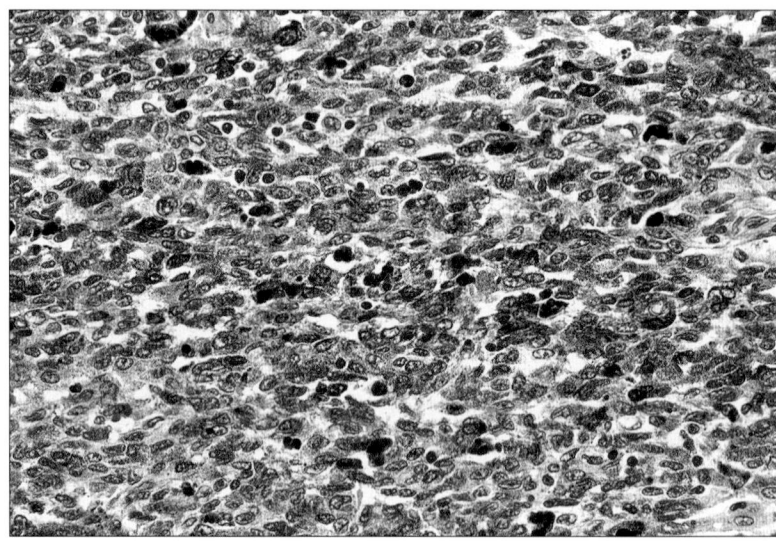

Fig. 35.321
Malignant melanotic schwannian tumor: this is usually a deep-seated lesion showing extensive melanin pigmentation. The nuclei are often grooved, resembling coffee beans.

labelled as malignant melanotic schwannian tumor. It arises most frequently around the spinal nerve roots and cutaneous presentation is very rare, with only 20 cases reported so far arising in the dermis or subcutaneous tissue, two of which have developed metastasis, and one patient died of disseminated disease.[105,106] Two cases arising in association with nevus of Ota have been documented.[107] The tumor is usually seen in association with Carney complex (myxomas, spotty pigmentation, and endocrine overactivity; autosomal dominant with mutation of *PRKAR1A*) (*Fig. 35.322*).[108,109] Lesions associated with the latter may also present with metastatic disease.[110] Tumor cells stain for S100 protein, SOX10 and other melanocytic markers. CD34 may also be positive.[111] Exceptionally a tumor may display a plexiform pattern.[112] Histologic features do not allow prediction of behavior, except for a mitotic rate of greater than 2 per 10 HPF, which correlates with metastases.[103,113]

- Pacinian schwannoma is a very rare tumor that presents as a solitary nodule, most often in the distal extremities. It is characterized histologically by an encapsulated mass composed of round or ovoid concentrically lamellated corpuscles (somewhat resembling pacinian corpuscles) set in a collagenous spindled cell stroma.[114,115] Although

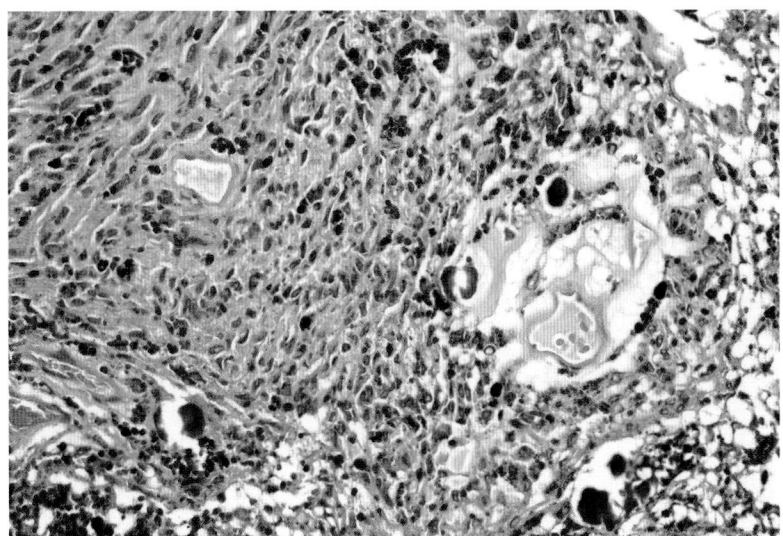

Fig. 35.322
Malignant melanotic schwannian tumor: psammoma bodies are a useful clue but are not always seen in this tumor.

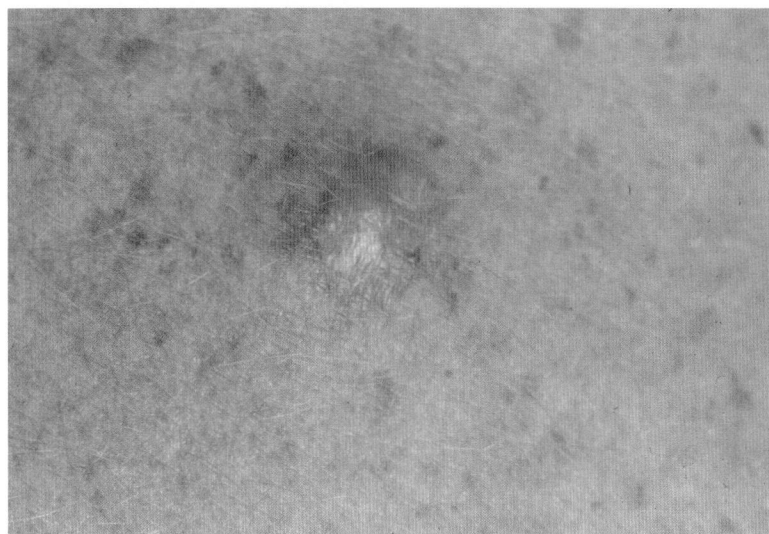

Fig. 35.323
Neurofibroma: erythematous nodule with surrounding simple lentigines. From the collection of the late N.P. Smith, MD, Institute of Dermatology, London, UK.

regarded in the past as pacinian neurofibroma, the histologic features are more in keeping with a schwannoma.

- Epithelioid schwannoma and neuroblastoma-like schwannoma are rare variants of schwannoma presenting mainly in the subcutis or dermis of adults with no sex predilection, and show overlapping features.[116–120] Deep-seated lesions, mainly intramuscular or gastrointestinal, are very rare.[116,117] An association with schwannomatosis 1 is exceptional.[116] Most lesions are small and only rarely very large tumors are observed.[116] There is predilection for the limbs followed by the trunk.[116,117] Histologically, tumors are well-circumscribed and composed of focal nests of epithelioid cells with amphophilic cytoplasmic arranged in cords and nests associated with a hyalinized or myxoid stroma. Areas with features of classic schwannoma are sometimes seen. Mitotic activity is usually low. Cases labelled as atypical are defined by high mitotic activity (equal or more than 3 mitoses per 10 HPFs) and variation in nuclear size. Tumor cells are positive for S100 And SOX10 and collagen type IV decorates cells in individual units or nests.[116,117] GFAP is variably positive. Melan-A and keratin are exceptionally positive.[116] The capsule contains EMA-positive cells. Around 42% of tumors show loss of SMARCB1/INI1 by immunohistochemistry.[117] In neuroblastoma-like schwannoma the epithelioid areas may mimic neuroblastoma and contain rosette-like structures with fibrillary collagenous centers.[121] Other areas of the tumor, however, are typical of a schwannoma. Lesions may rarely be plexiform.[122] A case with prominent collagen deposition and a hybrid tumor with perineurioma features have been documented.[123,124] The behavior is benign with hardly any risk of local recurrence even in cases labelled as atypical.[116,117] Tumors displaying transition to malignant epithelioid schwannoma are very rare.[117]
- Microcystic/reticular schwannoma usually presents in the gastrointestinal tract but a subset of cases occur in the skin as a multilobular proliferation with a microcystic, reticular, lace-like, or pseudoglandular pattern with prominent myxoid and/or mucinous material in the background.[125,126] Tumor cells show diffuse positivity for S100 protein, variable positivity for GFAP, and a discontinuous EMA-positive perineurium may be seen at the periphery of tumor lobules.

Schwannoma–perineurioma hybrid

Clinical features

Hybrid Schwannoma–perineurioma usually presents as an asymptomatic small subcutaneous, dermal or rarely deeper nodule, with an equal sex

incidence.[1,2] Lesions most commonly involve the lower limb followed by the upper limbs, with rare tumors occurring in the head and neck and trunk. Rare reported sites include pleural and internal auditory canal.[3,4] A possible association with radiation has been reported in one case.[5] It is not associated with neurofibromatosis. It is benign with little tendency for local recurrence.[6,7] Malignant transformation is exceptional. Simple excision is the treatment of choice.

Histologic features

Tumors are well circumscribed but lack a capsule and are composed of bland spindled cells with ill-defined pale cytoplasm and elongated nuclei with tapering ends. The distribution pattern of tumor cells is storiform, lamellar or whorled. Myxoid change can be present as can focal cytologic atypia that appears to be degenerative in nature. Antoni A and Antoni B areas are not a feature. Mitotic figures are rare. An infiltrative growth pattern and plexiform architecture are exceptional; cases with an epithelioid schwannoma component have been reported.[8,9] In one case a tumor was identified in a congenital melanocytic nevus.[10] By double staining, it has been demonstrated that tumor cells are either Schwann cells or perineural cells, with predominance of the former and no antigen coexpression.[1,2] Schwann cells are positive for S100 protein and SOX10 whereas perineural cells express EMA and CD34; tumor cells are usually positive for CD34, GFAP and claudin 1. Axons are rarely highlighted by neurofilament.[1,2,7,11–13]

Neurofibroma

Clinical features

Neurofibroma is perhaps the commonest tumor of nerve sheath origin.[1–3] In the majority of cases it is solitary and unassociated with any other systemic features; however, multiple lesions are not rare and form a cardinal feature of neurofibromatosis type I (von Recklinghausen disease). In its sporadic form, this tumor presents in a somewhat younger age group than schwannoma, as a polypoid or nodular soft lesion; in contrast to the latter it is frequently cutaneous and may arise anywhere in the integument (Figs 35.323 and 35.324). Cases of multiple lesions induced by radiotherapy have been reported.[4,5] Isolated cutaneous tumors tend to be sporadic. Deeper and larger lesions are much more concerning for syndromic association, especially when they display plexiform features.

It is essential that any patient found to have a neurofibroma, even if seemingly in isolation, should be carefully examined for other stigmata of neurofibromatosis. Neurofibromas, particularly the plexiform variant in neurofibromatosis type I, have an undoubted, albeit uncommon, tendency to undergo malignant change, but such transformation is exceedingly rare

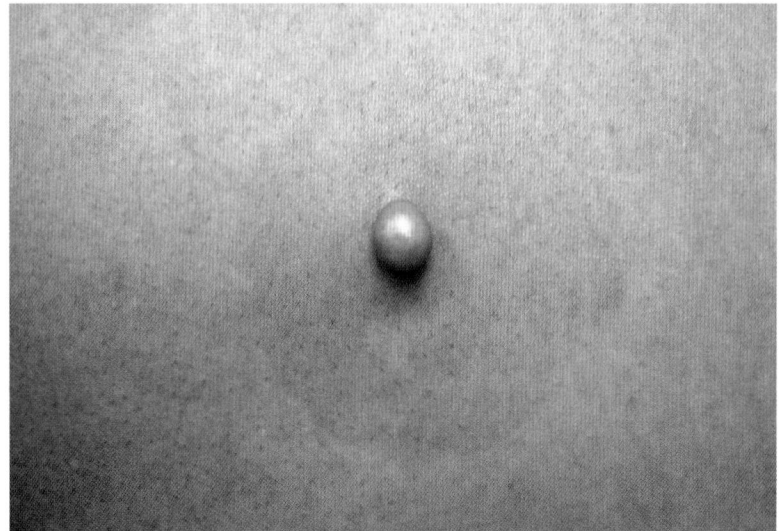

Fig. 35.324
Neurofibroma: this example presented as a circumscribed firm exophytic nodule. By courtesy of J. Dayrit, MD, Manila, The Philippines.

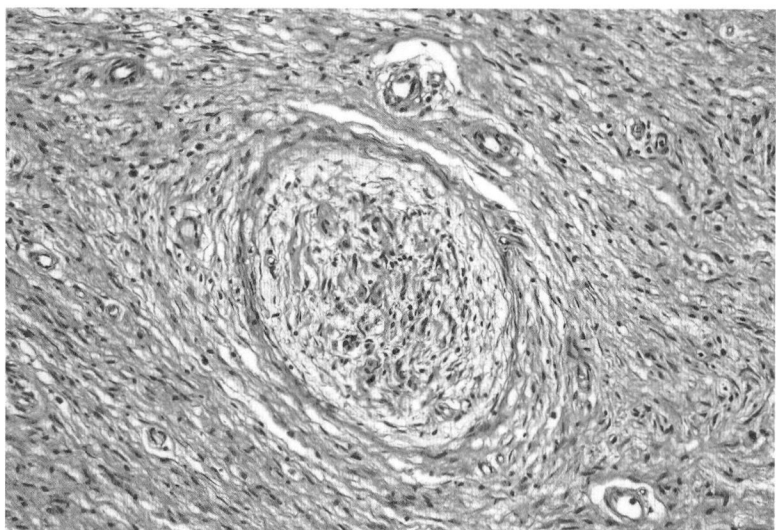

Fig. 35.326
Neurofibroma: a large nerve trunk is present in the center of the field.

Fig. 35.325
Neurofibroma: the tumor is composed of small spindled cells with indistinct cell borders.

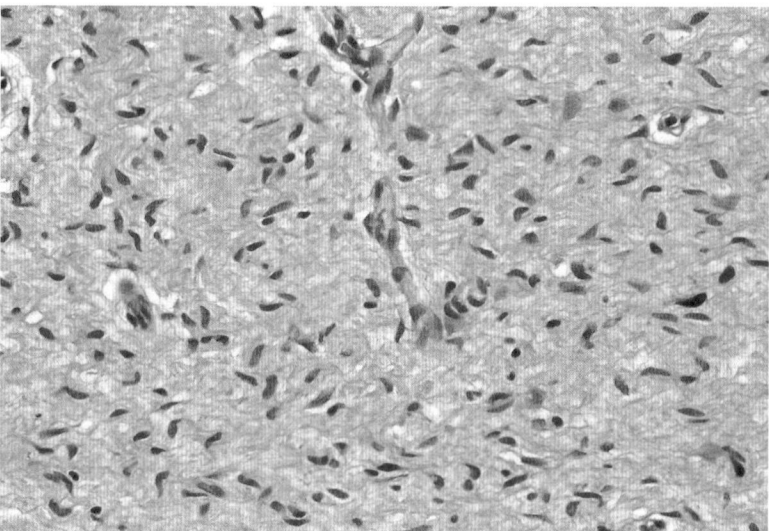

Fig. 35.327
Neurofibroma: the nuclei of the spindled cells are characteristically elongated and wavy.

in the more typical cutaneous/subcutaneous ordinary neurofibromas.[6] Local recurrence of truly benign lesions is very infrequent.

In a recent retrospective study in patients with neurofibromatosis 1, cutaneous neurofibromas were mostly located on the trunk followed by limbs and head and neck.[7] The number of tumors was found to increase with age.

Pathogenesis and histologic features

The microscopic features of neurofibroma are readily recognizable. Typically, it is a reasonably well-defined but unencapsulated dermal or subcutaneous lesion. In contrast to a schwannoma, it contains numerous small nerve fibers.

It consists of loosely arranged spindled cells with scanty pale cytoplasm and elongated wavy nuclei set in a fibrillar, collagenous and sometimes myxoid stroma (Figs 35.325–35.327). Multinucleated floret-like giant cells can be present, and in a small number of tumors are numerous.[8,9] These

multinucleated giant cells are S100 protein negative and CD34 positive and they are not a clue to the diagnosis of neurofibromatosis, as has previously been suggested.[10–12] Scattered inflammatory cells, particularly mast cells, are a prominent feature (Fig. 35.328).

The relative amounts of stromal collagen and mucin vary both within and between lesions; hyalinization of collagen may sometimes occur (Fig. 35.329). However, no recognizable biphasic appearance is seen (see schwannoma). Prominent sclerosis is present in some lesions.

Glomus-like bodies are rarely found.[13] Vascular changes may be seen in the diffuse and plexiform variants.[14]

Degenerative nuclear pleomorphism and hyperchromasia are rare features (compare with ancient schwannoma) and occasionally sporadic neurofibroma is associated with very low mitotic activity (see below) (Figs 35.330–35.332). Such pleomorphism in a lesion from a patient with neurofibromatosis type I, however, should prompt a very thorough search for mitoses. The presence of the latter in the setting of neurofibromatosis type I is regarded as evidence of malignancy. In a recent consensus the term 'atypical neurofibromatous neoplasms of uncertain biologic potential (ANNUBP)' has been proposed for these lesions (see below under Variants).[15]

Positive staining for S100 protein and SOX10 is seen in only 30–50% of cells.[16] Variable CD34 and in some cases EMA positivity is also seen.

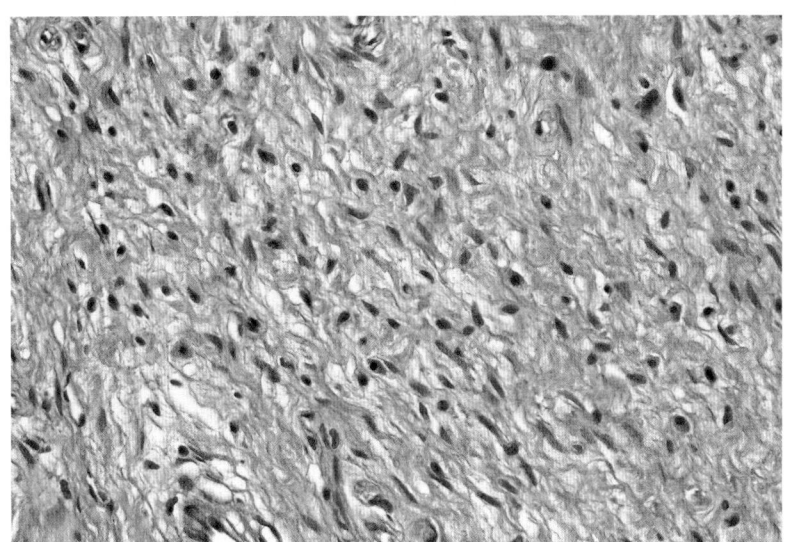

Fig. 35.328
Neurofibroma: mast cells with granular eosinophilic cytoplasm are frequently seen in these tumors.

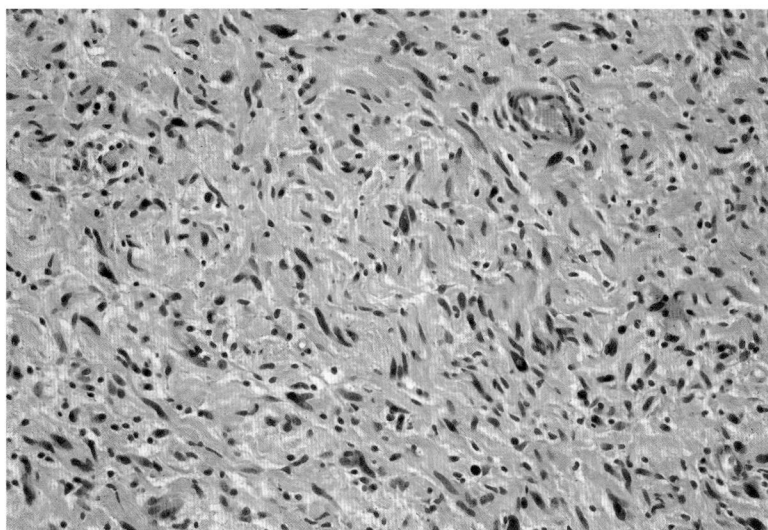

Fig. 35.331
Atypical neurofibroma: high-power view showing pleomorphic nuclei.

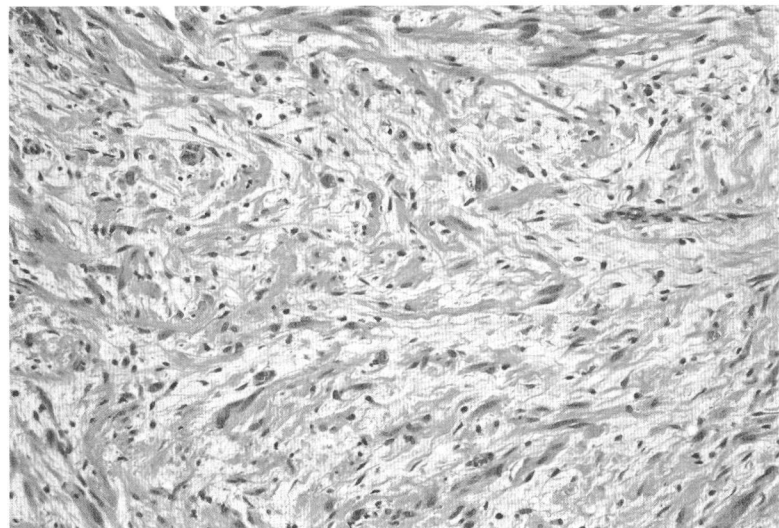

Fig. 35.329
Neurofibroma: the collagen content is highly variable, but may be prominent, as in this example.

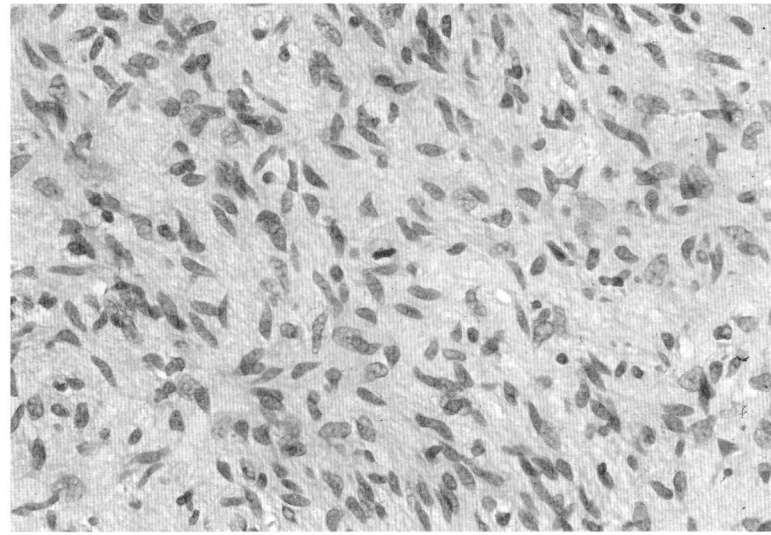

Fig. 35.332
Atypical neurofibroma: very occasionally, single mitoses may be identified.

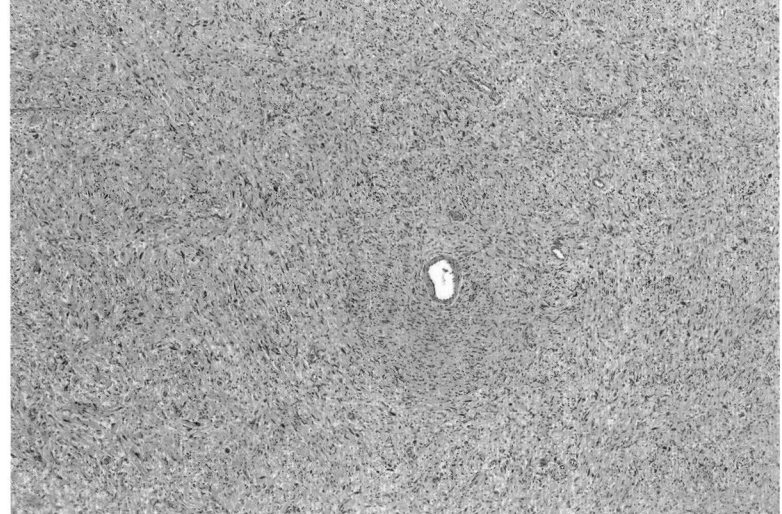

Fig. 35.330
Atypical neurofibroma: even at this magnification, hyperchromatic and enlarged nuclei are evident.

Ultrastructurally, a neurofibroma is composed of an admixture of Schwann cells, fibroblasts and perineurial cells.[17] Clonality has been demonstrated in neurofibromas, favoring a neoplastic process.[17,18] Although chromosomal imbalances are most frequently found in neurofibromas, in neurofibromatosis type I they have also been identified in sporadic neurofibromas.[19] Loss of chromosomes is the most frequent event, particularly chromosomes 17 where the NF1 gene is located and 19p.[19,20] Loss-of-function mutations in NF1 are also common and seen in multiple neurofibroma cell types.[14] More recently, mast cells, while not having NF1 mutations, have been shown to be a required component of neurofibromas in mouse models of neurofibromatosis.[15-26]

Recently it has been shown that KIR2DL5 mutation and loss is implicated in the pathogenesis of sporadic dermal neurofibromas.[27] Several gene signatures have been reported to be implicated in pathogenesis of neurofibroma and its malignant transformation.[28-30] Another study has implicated activated pericytes and smooth muscle cells of small tumor vessels in the pathogenesis of neurofibromas.[31]

Variants

- Myxoid neurofibroma is a histologic variant not necessarily associated with neurofibromatosis type I, and represents a conventional

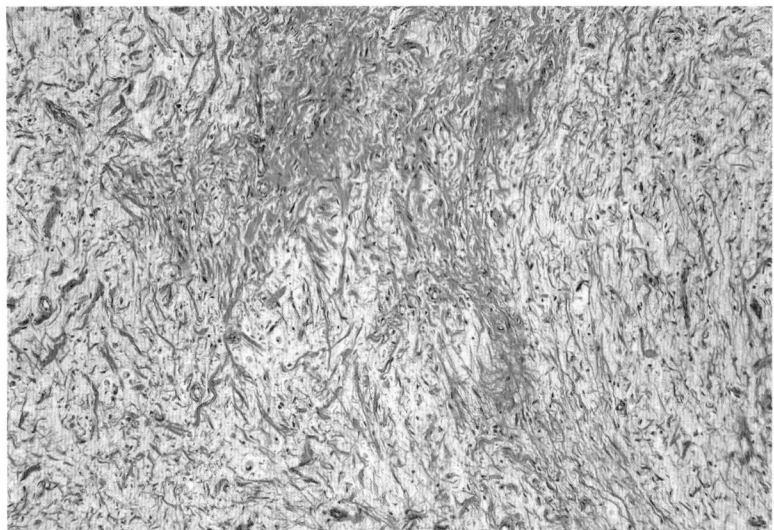

Fig. 35.333
Myxoid neurofibroma: in this variant, there is marked stromal mucin.

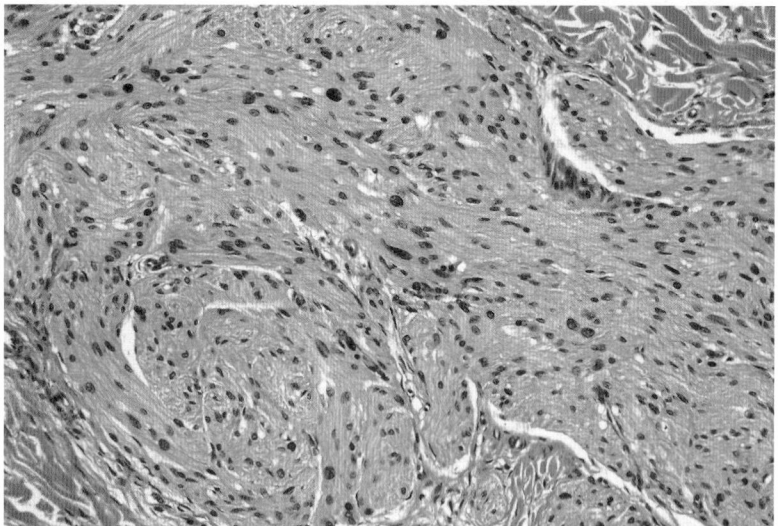

Fig. 35.335
Plexiform neurofibroma: hypertrophied nerves are seen embedded in a matrix of fibroblasts and Schwann cells.

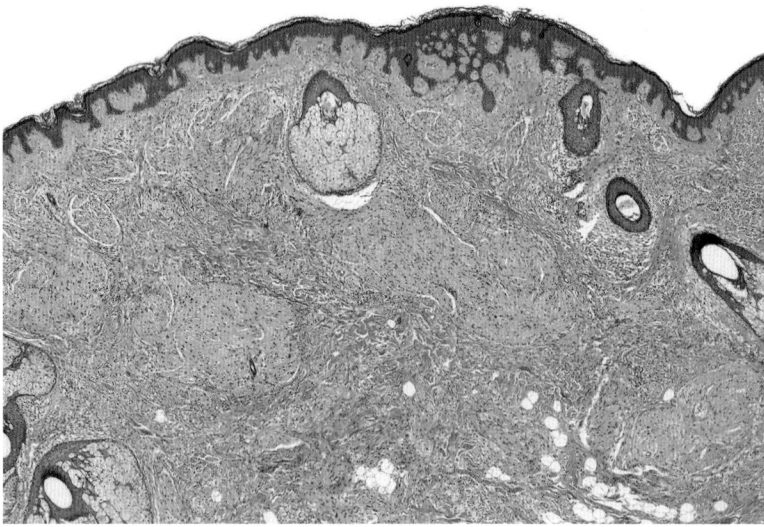

Fig. 35.334
Plexiform neurofibroma: thickened, haphazardly distributed nerve trunks are present in the reticular dermis.

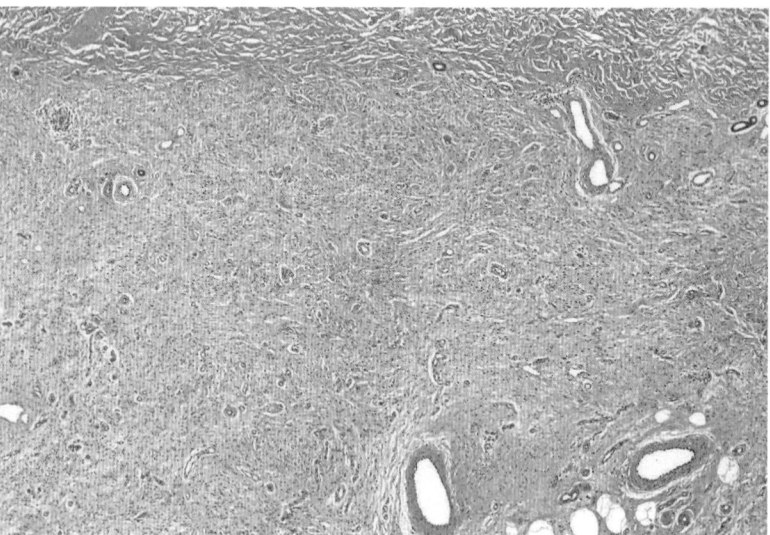

Fig. 35.336
Diffuse neurofibroma: both the papillary and the reticular dermis are extensively infiltrated by neurofibromatous tissue.

neurofibroma with extensive deposition of stromal mucin. As a consequence, the lesion may appear markedly hypocellular (*Fig. 35.333*).[1–3]

- Plexiform neurofibroma, which is considered pathognomonic of neurofibromatosis type I, most often presents in children of either sex.[1–3] Its anatomical distribution varies, but the most common site is the head and neck area. Commonly, the skin overlying the lesion shows large and redundant folds with variable hyperpigmentation; the underlying bone may be hypertrophic. The macroscopic appearance is that of a mass of nerve fibers in complex and tortuous arrangement reminiscent of a bag of worms. The histologic features consist of large thick nerves or nerve fibers often showing extensive myxoid change within a background of more typical neurofibroma (*Figs 35.334* and *35.335*). The surrounding tissue, however, may sometimes show changes of a diffuse neurofibroma. Small cutaneous lesions showing a microscopic plexiform pattern are not necessarily associated with neurofibromatosis type I. Lipoblast-like mucin filled cells may be identified.[32,33] Pseudoglandular or microcystic elements may be seen.[34]

- Diffuse neurofibroma, which is associated with neurofibromatosis type I in up to 20–30% of cases, is most often seen in young patients and generally occurs on the head, neck or trunk.[1–3] It presents as an ill-defined area of subcutaneous thickening. Histologically, it is

characterized by neurofibromatous tissue with a diffuse infiltrative growth pattern in which the stroma tends to be uniformly collagenous rather than myxoid (*Figs 35.336* and *35.337*). Meissnerian differentiation is often a prominent feature (*Figs 35.338* and *35.339*).

- Pigmented neurofibroma is characterized by whorled structures similar to Meissner corpuscles with scattered pigmented cells that are positive for melanocytic markers (*Fig. 35.340*).[35–37] In one patient, an association with hypertrichosis was documented.[38]

- Granular cell neurofibroma is focally composed of tumor cells with abundant periodic acid-Schiff-positive diastase-resistant granular cytoplasm.[3] Diagnosis is often dependent on identifying areas with more typical morphology.

- Epithelioid neurofibroma is focally composed of epithelioid cells with pink cytoplasm in a background of an otherwise typical neurofibroma.

- Dendritic cell neurofibroma with pseudorosettes is a distinctive variant of neurofibroma with a nodular growth pattern and two cell types.[39] Small round, dark, lymphocyte-like dark cells surround larger cells with vesicular nuclei, frequent intranuclear inclusions and abundant pale cytoplasm, resulting in a distinctive pseudorosette appearance (*Figs 35.341* and *35.342*). Both cell types are positive for S100 protein and CD57.[40] A case with a granulomatous. pattern has been reported.[41] An

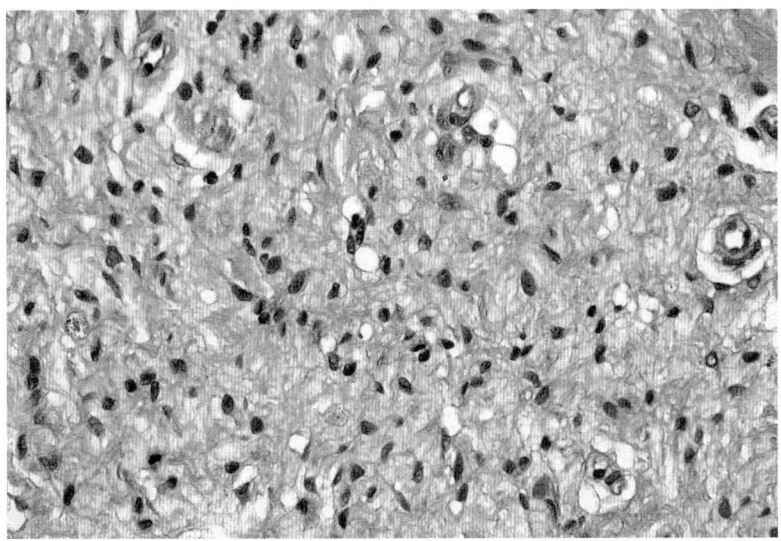

Fig. 35.337
Diffuse neurofibroma: high-power view.

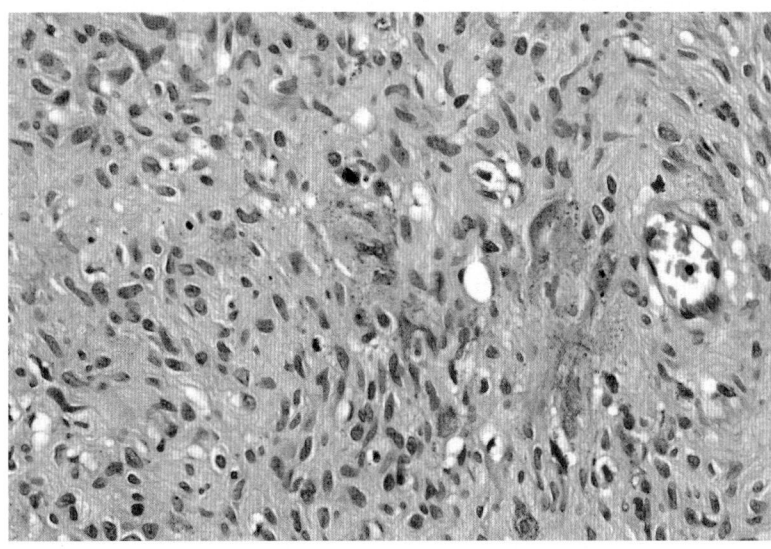

Fig. 35.340
Pigmented neurofibroma: note the pigmented dendritic cells. By courtesy of H. Diwan, MD, Houston, Texas, USA.

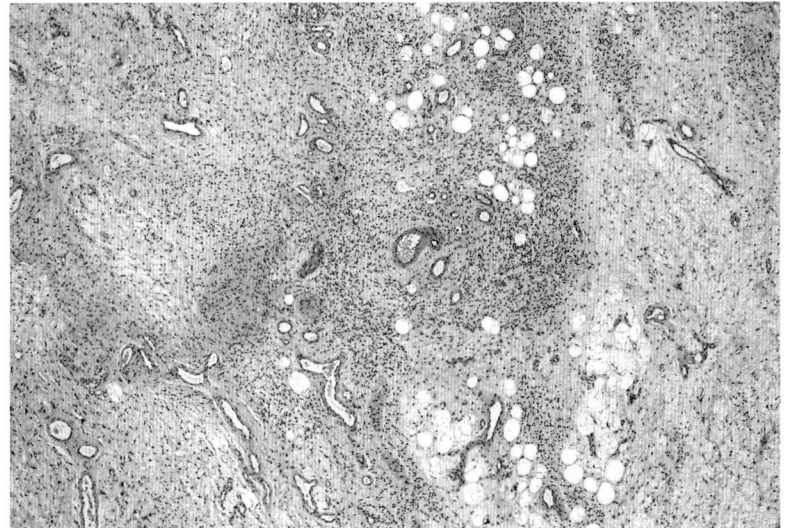

Fig. 35.338
Diffuse neurofibroma: there is marked organoid differentiation.

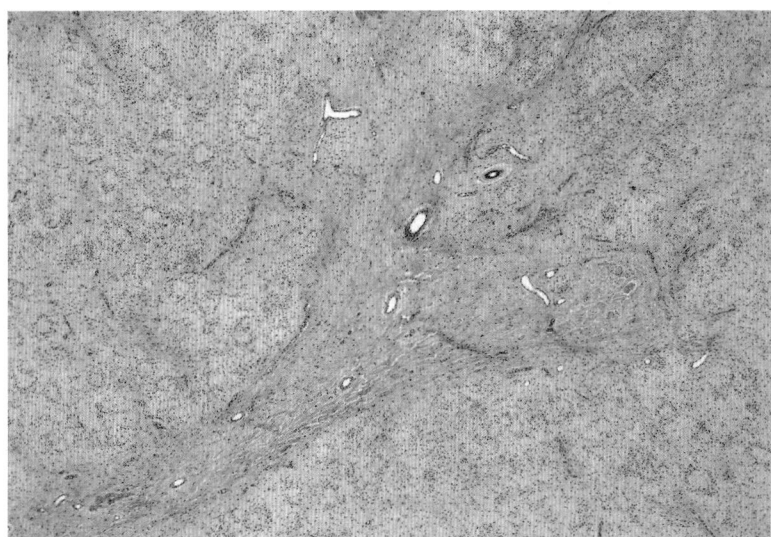

Fig. 35.341
Neurofibroma with pseudorosettes: low-power view showing conspicuous pseudorosettes.

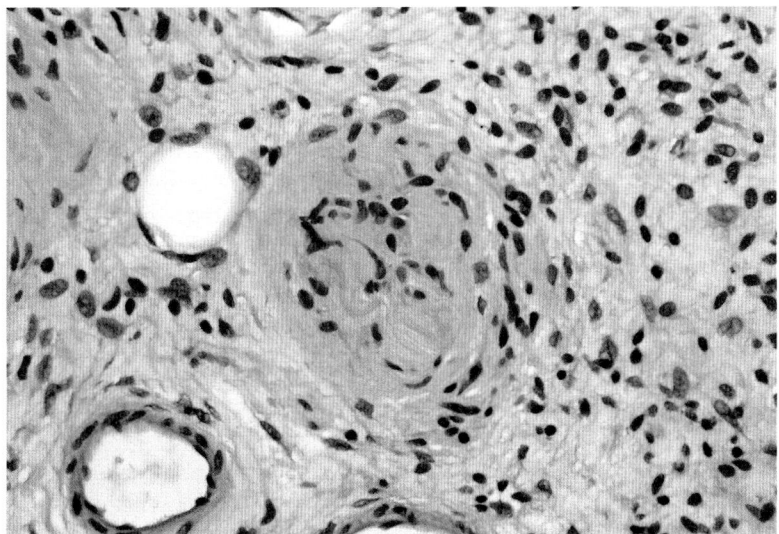

Fig. 35.339
Diffuse neurofibroma: in the center of the field there is differentiation towards a Meissner's corpuscle.

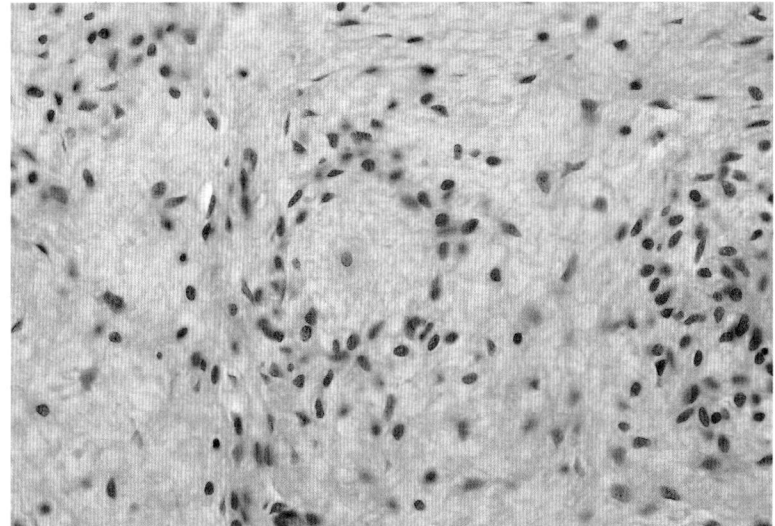

Fig. 35.342
Neurofibroma with pseudorosettes: there is a single central large pale cell surrounded by a mantle of small lymphocyte-like cells.

intraneural example of this variant has recently been documented.[42] An intraoral case has been described.[43] Similar lesions may be seen in neurofibromatosis type I.[44]

- Cellular neurofibroma with atypia (atypical neurofibroma) refers to a sporadic neurofibroma with increased cellularity, focal atypia and very low mitotic activity.[45,46] These lesions appear to have a benign behavior. Similar lesions, however, in the context of neurofibromatosis type I and in the presence of any mitotic activity, should be regarded as evidence of malignancy.
- Pacinian neurofibroma is best considered as a variant of schwannoma (see above). Examples of nerve sheath myxomas were formerly described as pacinian neurofibromas.
- Lipomatous neurofibroma refers to the presence of collections of mature fat cells within a neurofibroma.[47–49] It seems to be more common in the head and neck.[50] Distinction from a neurotized nevus with fatty metaplasia may be impossible (see differential diagnosis).
- Hybrid tumors show features of both neurofibroma and schwannoma; rarely features of perineurioma may be seen.[51–53] Perineurial differentiation and intraneural occurrence have also been documented.[54,55] Monosomy 22 has been identified in a subset of hybrid tumors.[56] In addition, it has been shown that hybrid tumors are strongly associated with neurofibromatosis and schwannomatosis.[57]
- A single case with clear cell change, one with balloon cell change and one case with prominent sclerosis mimicking sclerotic fibroma have been reported.[58–61] A variant described as angioneurofibroma has been documented.[62]
- Atypical neurofibromatous neoplasms of uncertain biologic potential (ANNUBP) is a term proposed for neurofibromas that were previously described inconsistently as atypical neurofibromas or low-grade malignant peripheral nerve sheath tumors.[14,63] According to the consensus report nuclear atypia alone is not enough for a diagnosis of malignancy. However, tumors with cytologic atypia accompanied by loss of the usual neurofibroma architecture, high cellularity, and/or mitotic activity higher than 1 per 50 HPF but less than 3 per 10 HPF are worrisome. It has therefore been proposed that when a tumor shows at least two of the above criteria the designation 'neurofibromatous neoplasms of uncertain biologic potential' should be used. Some of these tumors may show diminished S100 protein and SOX10 immunoreactivity, loss of p16/CDKN2A expression, elevated Ki67, and overexpression of TP53 as seen in malignant peripheral nerve sheath tumors. Also, as described in half of the latter, complete loss of trimethylated histone 3 lysine 27 expression, may be seen.[14]

Differential diagnosis

Small biopsies of plaque-stage dermatofibrosarcoma protuberans may be difficult to distinguish from a neurofibroma. The former, however, has a distinctive lace-like pattern of infiltration of the fat, the dermal bundles tend to be parallel to the epidermis and tumor cells are negative for S100 protein and positive for CD34. Old neurotized nevi are often indistinguishable from neurofibroma if no residual nevus cells or epidermal component are present. S100 protein will be positive in both lesions, but neurotized nevi tend to be symmetrical and are also more often NSE positive. Importantly, expression of melanocytic markers may be seen in neurofibromas (including the epithelioid variant) arising in patients with neurofibromatosis.[64]

The use of CD34 as a tool for differentiating neurofibromas (characteristic fingerprint pattern seen in neurofibroma as opposed to melanoma) from spindle cell melanomas has been reported but it is not an entirely reliable feature.[65–67]

Neurofibromatosis

Clinical features

Traditionally neurofibromatosis is classified into:
- the classic peripheral cutaneous variant or type I neurofibromatosis (NF1, von Recklinghausen disease; NF1 gene at 17q11.2),

- the central or acoustic form or type II neurofibromatosis (NF2; NF2 gene encoding merlin protein at 22q12.2).

A third variant, segmental neurofibromatosis, has also been described. This occurs as a result of mosaicism in either NF1 or NF2, more commonly the former.

Other variants of neurofibromatosis have been documented and include hereditary spinal neurofibromatosis, schwannomatosis, familial intestinal neurofibromatosis, autosomal dominant 'café-au-lait spots alone,' autosomal dominant 'neurofibromas alone,' Watson syndrome, Noonan/neurofibromatosis syndrome and multiple nevi, multiple schwannomas, and multiple vaginal leiomyomas.[1,2]

Neurofibromatosis type I is an important congenital neurocutaneous disorder with an autosomal dominant mode of inheritance, affecting about 1/3000 live births; a number of cases also arise as a result of spontaneous germline mutation.[3–12] It encompasses a constellation of signs and symptoms and may involve most systems of the body. The gene for NF1 has been cloned to chromosome 17q11.2.[13–16] The encoded protein is called neurofibromin, which helps control Ras activity in cells.[17–19] Tumors are generated with loss of heterozygosity at the NF1 wild type allele. Chromosomal imbalances are more common in NF1-associated neurofibromas than in sporadic neurofibromas.[20] Other chromosomal imbalances described in NF1 include losses in chromosomes 19 and 22q.[20] See also the neurofibroma section above.

Patients with NF1 and no evidence of cutaneous neurofibromas have a 3-bp inframe deletion in exon 17 of the NF1 gene.[21]

Recently, a neurofibromatosis type 1-like autosomal dominant syndrome lacking NF1 mutations but associated with germline inactivating mutations in SPRED1 (sprout-related EVH1 domain-containing protein 1) has been described.[22] In this syndrome, patients present with café-au-lait macules, axillary freckling and macrocephaly.

The National Institutes of Health (NIH) criteria for the diagnosis of NFI include two or more of the following:[23]
- six or more café-au-lait macules with a diameter of greater than 5.0 mm in children less than 6 years of age and greater than 15 mm in older individuals,
- two or more neurofibromas of any type or one plexiform neurofibroma,
- freckling in the axillary or inguinal regions,
- an optic nerve glioma,
- two or more Lisch nodules (iris hamartomas),
- a distinctive osseous lesion, such as dysplasia of the sphenoid bone or thinning of the cortex of long bones, with or without pseudoarthrosis,
- a first-degree relative with NF1.

Neurofibromatosis type I shows very wide clinical variability. A large study has demonstrated an association between several pairs of features in affected probands:
- intertriginous freckling and Lisch nodules,
- discrete neurofibromas and plexiform neurofibromas,
- discrete neurofibromas and Lisch nodules,
- plexiform neurofibromas and scoliosis,
- learning disability or mental retardation and seizures.[24]

Café-au-lait macules are flat, light-brown lesions which may be distributed anywhere on the integument, but are found predominantly on unexposed surfaces of the body (Fig. 35.343). Up to 10% of the population may have solitary lesions from birth. Patients may also exhibit more darkly colored macules overlying cutaneous plexiform neurofibromas (Fig. 35.344). It has been suggested that dermal fibroblast-derived stem cell factor and hepatocyte growth factor may play a role in the development of the hyperpigmentation.[25]

Neurofibromas presenting at birth are often plexiform and are located particularly around the eyes and neck; some are generalized.[26] By late childhood or adolescence, large numbers of cutaneous tumors have developed, which may be nodular, sessile or pedunculated (Figs 35.345–35.349). Neurofibromas in NFI have increased vascularity and this may result in prominent bleeding, particularly during surgical excision of large plexiform variants. The increased vascularity may result from elevated tumor cell expression of basic fibroblast and endothelial growth factors.[27]

The diffuse neurofibroma which is generally found on the head, neck and back in a proportion of cases is also associated with neurofibromatosis;

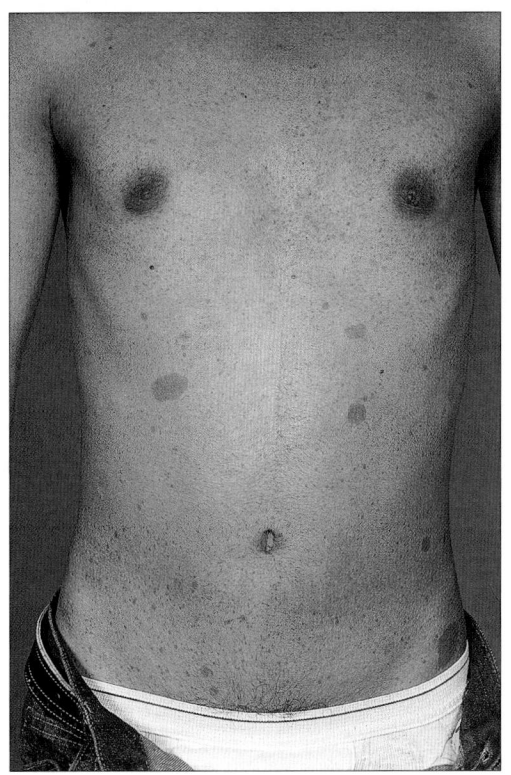

Fig. 35.343
Type I neurofibromatosis: the presence of typical café-au-lait macules is characteristic. By courtesy of R.A. Marsden, MD, St George's Hospital, London, UK.

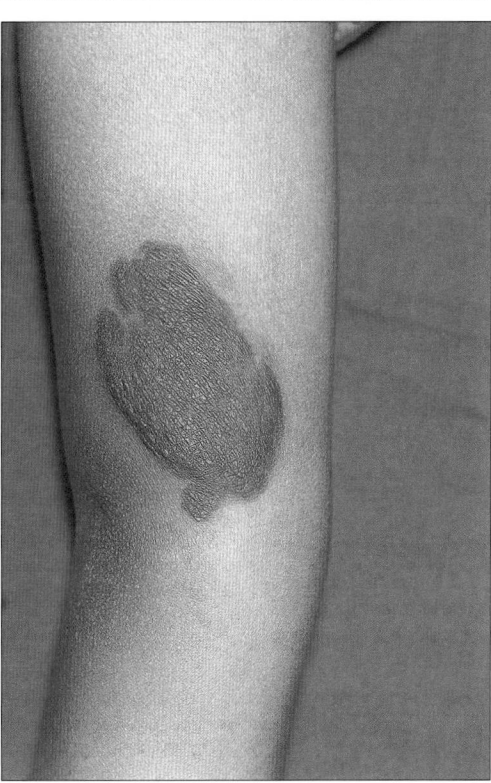

Fig. 35.344
Type I neurofibromatosis: this heavily pigmented raised lesion overlies a cutaneous plexiform neurofibroma. By courtesy of R.A. Marsden, MD, St George's Hospital, London, UK.

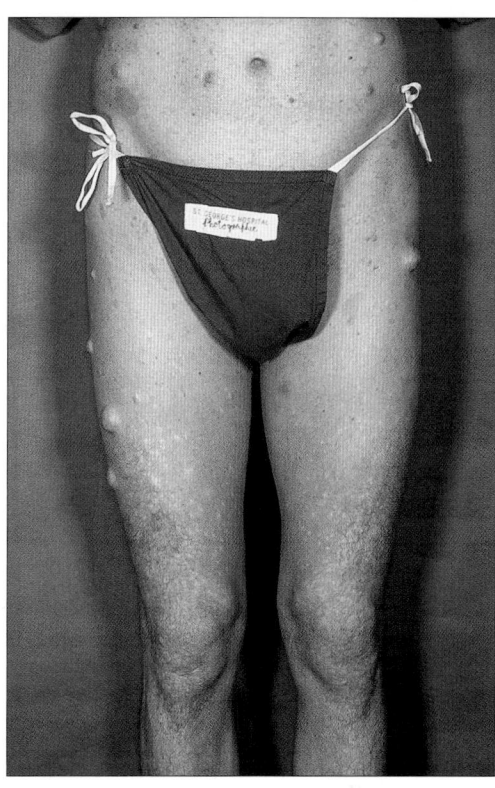

Fig. 35.345
Type I neurofibromatosis: widespread cutaneous neurofibromata are a prominent feature of the classical variant. By courtesy of R.A. Marsden, MD, St George's Hospital, London, UK.

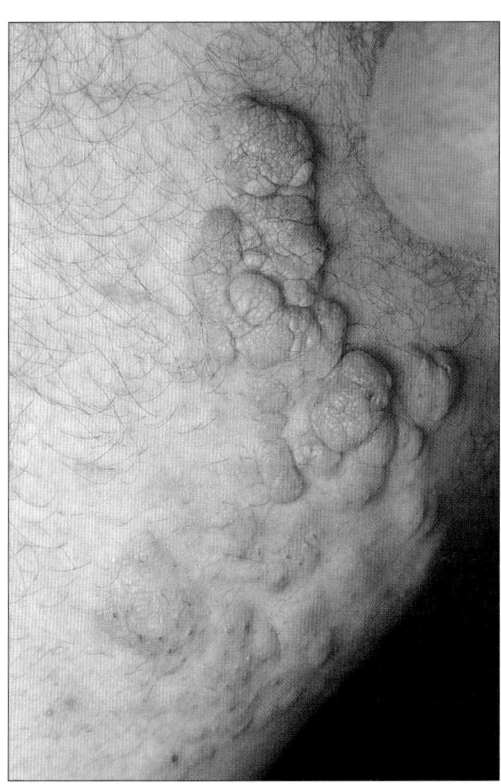

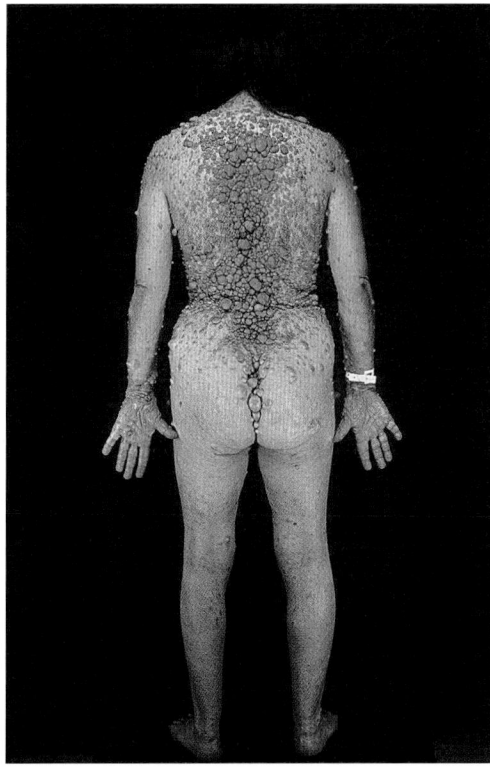

Fig. 35.346
Type 1 neurofibromatosis: lesions are often soft and appear as polypoid or sessile papules and plaques. By courtesy of the Institute of Dermatology, London, UK.

Fig. 35.347
Type I neurofibromatosis: this disease can be extremely disfiguring. By courtesy of the Institute of Dermatology, London, UK.

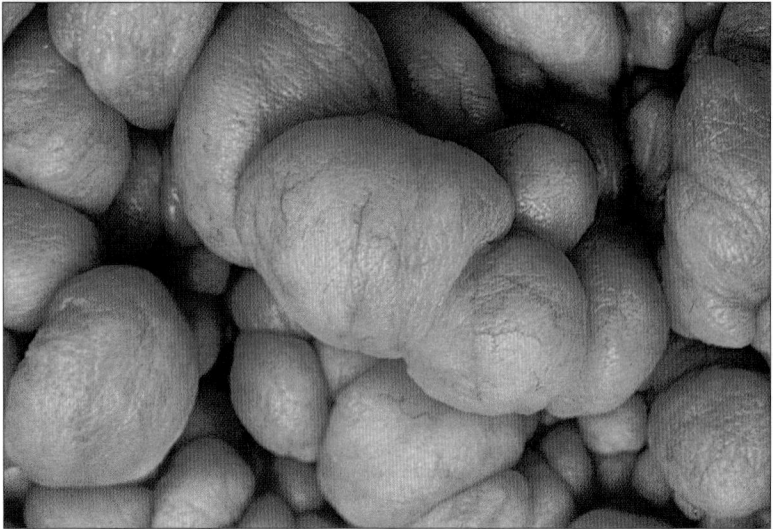

Fig. 35.348
Type 1 neurofibromatosis: close-up view. By courtesy of the Institute of Dermatology, London, UK.

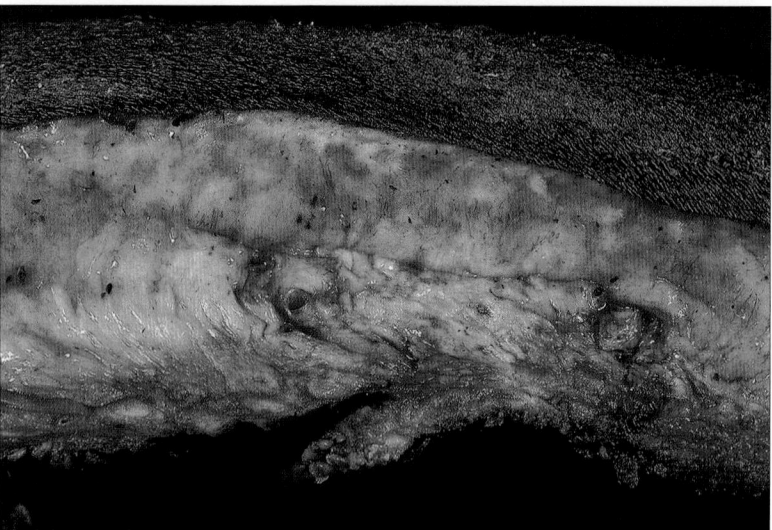

Fig. 35.350
Type I neurofibromatosis: there is extensive replacement of dermis and subcutaneous fat by a homogeneous pale yellow tumor – a diffuse neurofibroma.

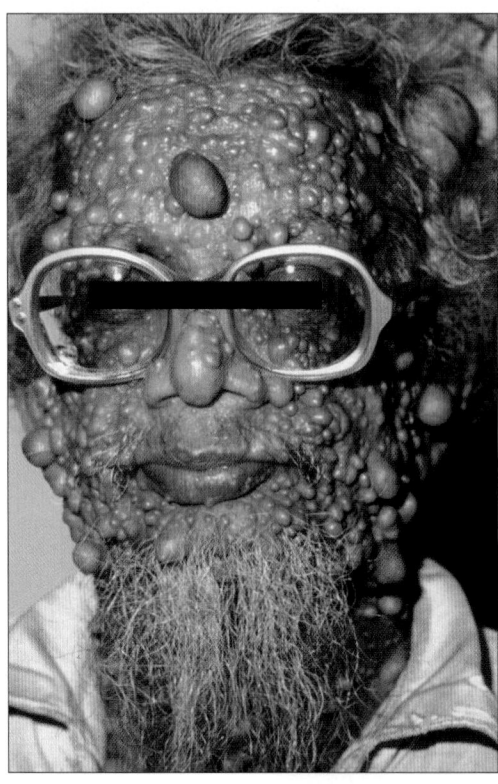

Fig. 35.349
Type 1 neurofibromatosis: there is marked facial disfigurement. By courtesy of the Institute of Dermatology, London, UK.

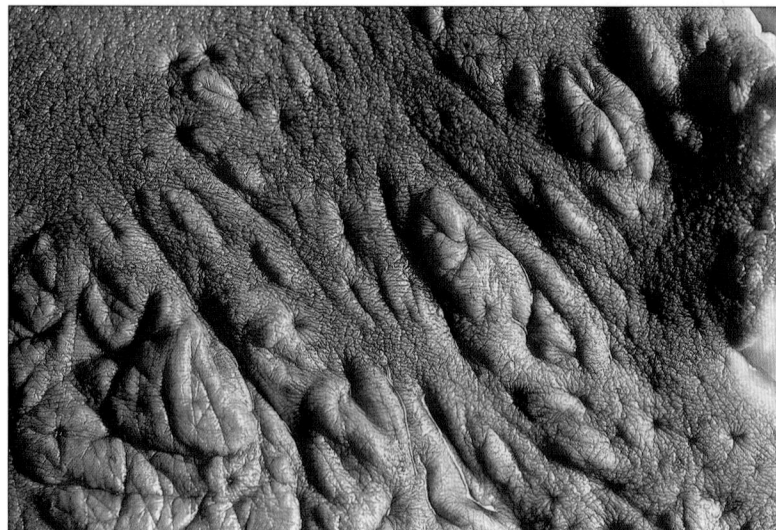

Fig. 35.351
Type 1 neurofibromatosis: the skin overlying the tumor has a wrinkled, unevenly elevated appearance.

however, in contrast to the plexiform type, it does not appear to be associated with an increased risk of malignant transformation except in rare cases (Figs 35.350 and 35.351).

Interestingly, biopsies from normal skin in patients with NF1 show an increase in the number of S100 protein-positive cells.[28]

Occasionally, large plexiform neurofibromas may be associated with excessive redundant skin folds, giving rise to the so-called elephantiasiform neurofibroma (Fig. 35.352).

Lisch nodules are pigmented hamartomas of the iris and are pathognomonic of NF1 (Fig. 35.353).[12] However, they are never found in the acoustic or segmental variants.

Patients with neurofibromatosis may develop tumors at any site in the body, including internal nerve trunks and viscera (Figs 35.354 and 35.355). As this is a progressive disorder, increasing age is associated with the acquisition of further nodules; ultimately the patient may exhibit sometimes grotesque features with accompanying psychological and social problems.

Neurofibromatosis may also be associated with a diverse range of other manifestations including short stature, pheochromocytoma, gastrointestinal neoplasms (including adenocarcinoma, carcinoid, somatostatinoma and gastrointestinal stromal tumor), mental retardation and a variety of central nervous system tumors (mainly low-grade gliomas but also high-grade tumors including medulloblastoma).[11,12,29–33] An association with juvenile xanthogranuloma and leukemia in children is also known.[34] A few cases of achondroplasia and NF1 have been documented.[35] A number of other associations have been recorded but they are likely to be coincidental. These include cutaneous T-cell lymphoma, epidermodysplasia verruciformis, urticaria pigmentosa, piebaldism, eccrine angiomatous hamartoma, segmental unilateral lentiginosis and multiple glomus tumors.[36–43]

Multiple glomus tumors of the digits, however, have been identified as an important association of NF1.[44,45] An association with Noonan syndrome is also common and both conditions are pathogenetically related.[46,47]

Factors found in a recent study to be associated independently with mortality in NF1 include the presence of subcutaneous neurofibromas, the absence of cutaneous neurofibromas and facial asymmetry.[48] Independent cutaneous predictor factors associated with internal neurofibromas include the presence of at least two subcutaneous neurofibromas, age = or less than 30, absence of cutaneous neurofibromas and fewer than six café-au-lait

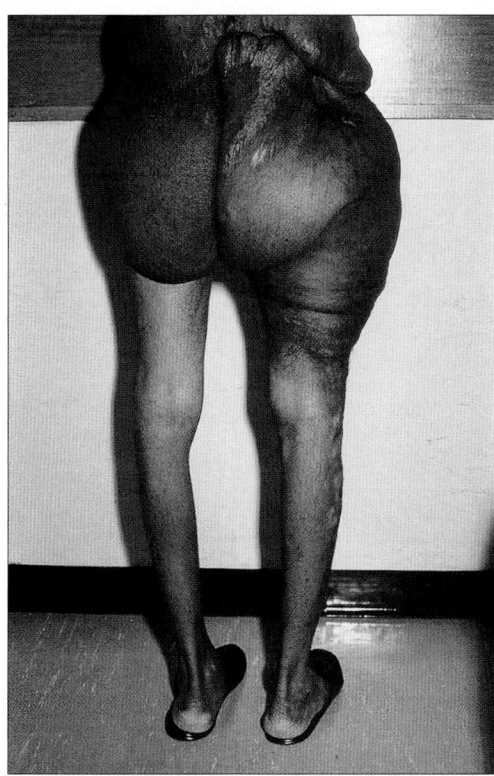

Fig. 35.352
Type I neurofibromatosis: the elephantiasiform variant. By courtesy of D. Allen, MD, St Thomas' Hospital, London, UK.

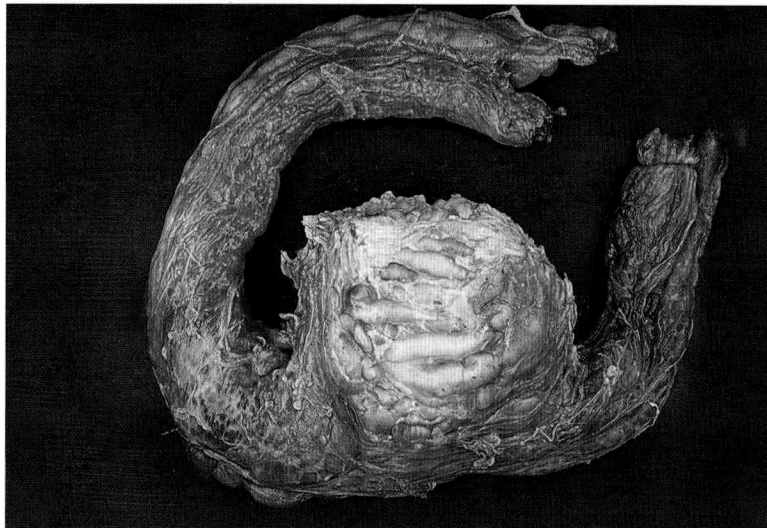

Fig. 35.354
Type I neurofibromatosis: this massive plexiform neurofibroma arose from the spermatic cord in a young man. By courtesy of H. Pambakian, MD (retired), St Thomas' Hospital Medical School, London, UK.

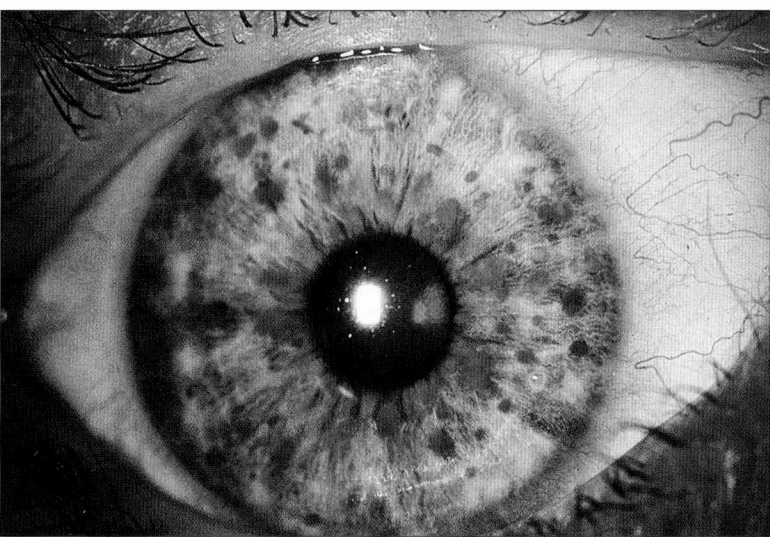

Fig. 35.353
Type I neurofibromatosis: multiple Lisch nodules (iris nevi) are a pathognomonic feature. By courtesy of D. Spalton, MD, St Thomas' Hospital, London, UK.

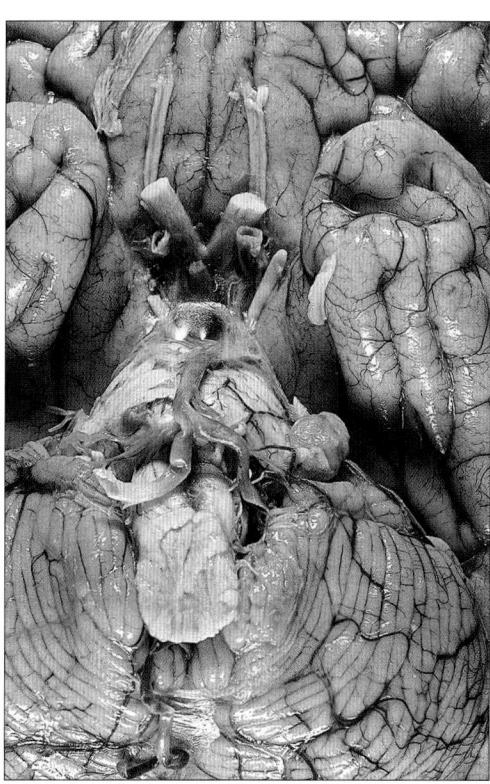

Fig. 35.355
Type I neurofibromatosis: a typical acoustic neuroma of the left eighth cranial nerve is visible in the cerebellopontine angle.

spots.[49,50] Based on the latter, a scoring system has been proposed to calculate the risk of internal neurofibromas.

Blue–red macules and pseudoatrophic macules in patients with NF1 have been shown to indicate the presence of neurofibromas.[51]

Plexiform neurofibromas in NF1 may increase in size during pregnancy but tumors do not appear to express progesterone receptors.[52,53]

As mentioned earlier, patients with NF1 have an increased risk of developing malignant peripheral nerve sheath tumors, with a lifetime incidence of between 8% and 13%.[54–59] Patients with NF1 tend to present earlier in life than those with sporadic malignancy.[59] They also tend to present with recurrences and metastatic spread at shorter intervals than patients with sporadic tumors.[60] Pain and enlargement are the most frequent signs suggesting malignant transformation. Most lesions occur in the limbs; these are highly aggressive tumors and patients have a mean survival of 18 months. Tumor volume and expression of TP53 have been found to be independent factors predictive of poor behavior.[61,62] By the use of murine models, it has been demonstrated that loss of the tumor suppressor PTEN (phosphatase and tensin homolog) combined with overexpression of the KRAS oncogene is crucial in the development of malignant transformation.[63,64]

Melanocytic differentiation has exceptionally been documented.[65]

Acoustic neurofibromatosis (NF2) comprises a syndrome of acoustic neuroma (schwannoma; see *Fig. 35.277*), which is often bilateral, and intracranial and intraspinal neoplasms, including astrocytomas, meningiomas and ependymomas. An exceptional association with a soft tissue perineurioma has been reported.[66] The gene for *NF2* has been cloned to chromosome 22.[67,68]

Segmental neurofibromatosis can occur in both NF1 and NF2 as a result of somatic mosaicism.[69–74] Segmental neurofibromatosis may occur in a patient with classic NF1 or, more commonly, in patients with no signs of neurofibromatosis other than café-au-lait spots. Most cases of segmental neurofibromatosis have no positive family history.[75,76] Involvement is usually unilateral but may be bilateral.[74]

Pathogenesis and histologic features

Neurofibromatosis type 1 results from gene mutations in the *NF1* gene. The *NF1* gene is located on chromosome 17q11.2, which encodes for the protein neurofibromin. The molecular mechanisms involved in tumorigenesis remain largely unknown; a plethora of mutations of the *NF1* gene have been investigated. Neurofibromatosis type 2 is driven by loss of function of the *NF2* gene (22q12.2) encoding the protein merlin (see also schwannoma).[77–91]

The histologic appearances of the skin and subcutaneous tumors seen in neurofibromatosis have been described under previous headings. Hypertrophy of pacinian corpuscles has been reported in a patient with NF1.[92] Increased cellularity and cytologic atypia is found in about one-fifth of cases and may represent an indicator of increased risk of malignant transformation.[93] Although it has been reported that floret-like giant cells are associated with tumors in neurofibromatosis type 1, they can also be identified in sporadic neurofibromas.[94,95] Malignant peripheral nerve sheath tumors tend to be more cellular but less pleomorphic than sporadic tumors.[60]

The café-au-lait macules show increased numbers of functionally active melanocytes with giant melanosomes.

Granular cell tumor

This has been a controversial entity for many years, particularly with respect to its histogenesis.[1–4] With the introduction of immunohistochemistry, it has become clear that most granular cell tumors represent neuroectodermal lesions.[4,5] However, it must be emphasized that the presence of granular cell change is due to an increased number of secondary lysosomes and that it can occur focally or extensively in a variety of tumors, not only in other mesenchymal neoplasms such as smooth muscle tumors, but also in epithelial tumors including basal cell carcinoma.[6,7] Additionally, a subset of granular cell tumors presenting mainly in the dermis is characterized by having a 'null' immunophenotype. The terms dermal non-neural or S100 protein negative granular cell tumor or primitive polypoid granular cell tumor have been used in the literature (see page 1879).[8–15] Based on immunohistochemical results a fibrous and root sheath origin have been postulated.[13,14] It is important to note that all granular cell tumors, regardless of their line of differentiation, are positive for NKI/C3 (which reacts with CD63, and is thus a non-specific marker of lysosomal membranes) and often a variety of immunoreagents may be necessary to establish the specific differentiation pattern.[4,8]

The following description emphasizes the more common neuroectodermal type of granular cell tumor.

Clinical features

Granular cell tumor is a comparatively common lesion, arising most often in adults of 30–60 years of age, and showing a predilection for females.[16] Occurrence in children is believed to be unusual but a study reports a 50% incidence.[17] Although it may be found at almost any cutaneous, subcutaneous or visceral site (see below), it occurs most frequently on the tongue, trunk or limbs, particularly the arms.[18,19] Less frequently, lesions may present on the feet, perianal region and genitalia including the penis, scrotum, vulva (labia and clitoris) and breast.[20–34] Tumors have also been reported in the thyroid, parotid gland, esophagus, trachea, larynx, lung, mediastinum, rectum, duodenum, pancreas, biliary tract, ureter, bladder, nerve, muscle, eye, central nervous system and within the cranium.[35–58] Up to 10% of patients have multiple tumors (which may be cutaneous, oral or visceral, particularly in the gastrointestinal tract).[59–67] Exceptional cases are familial. Lesions are slow growing, usually less than 2 cm in diameter, sometimes painful, and often have a verrucous appearance (*Fig. 35.356*). Giant tumors are rarely seen. Local recurrence is very uncommon except in the infrequent infiltrative examples. A very uncommon association with neurofibromatosis has been documented.[48,68]

The malignant counterpart is exceedingly rare in the skin and is more usually deeply seated.[69–80] A rare malignant tumor has been described in association with a nerve and a single case report of a tumor associated with polymyositis documented.[79,80]

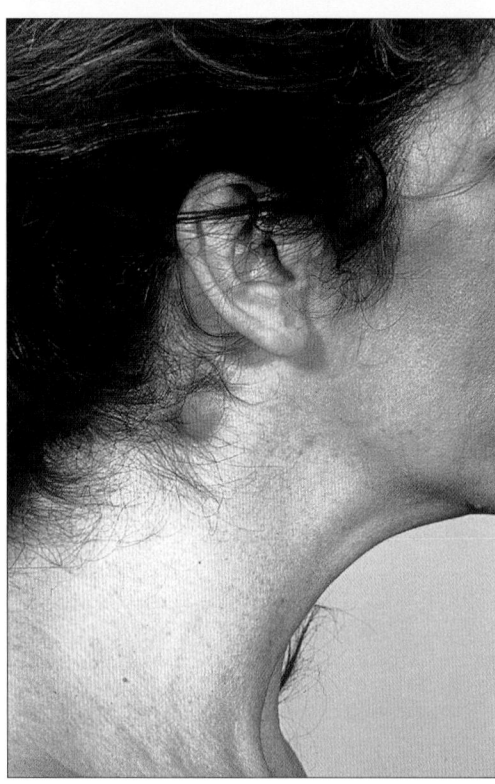

Fig. 35.356
Granular cell tumor: clinically, these tumors are not distinctive and present as slowly growing papules or nodules. By courtesy of D. Munroe, MD, St Bartholomew's Hospital, London, UK.

One patient presented with a granular cell tumor, a schwannoma and vitiligo, another with LEOPARD syndrome, yet others with Noonan syndrome, PNET and in a further case there was associated congenital deaf-mutism.[81–87]

Pathogenesis and histologic features

Cytogenetic analysis in a single malignant case showed a 46,XX,+X, dic(5;15).[88]

Monosomy 22, trisomy 10, and loss of *CDKN2A* have been reported. *PIK3CA* and *TP53* alterations have been found in malignant cases.[89]

Granular cell tumor is an ill-defined lesion composed of nests or trabeculae of large, round or oval cells with brightly eosinophilic granular cytoplasm, which in a proportion of cases stains with periodic acid-Schiff (PAS) after diastase digestion (*Figs 35.357* and *35.358*). The cell borders are indistinct, resulting in a rather syncytial appearance. Nuclei are uniformly small, round and usually centrally situated. Mitotic activity is variable. Pustulo-ovoid bodies of Milian, representing large granules surrounded by a clear halo are common.[90] Clear cell change is rare but can be prominent.[91] Uncommonly, cases with a prominent plexiform growth pattern have been reported including an intraneural lesion.[92–94] Colorectal tumors may present calcification and hyalinization.[44,95] Intravenous invasion has rarely been reported in otherwise histologically benign tumors.[96]

A distinctive and quite common finding is the presence of pseudoepitheliomatous hyperplasia of the overlying squamous epithelium in tumors of the dermis or tongue. This finding may lead the unwary to make a diagnosis of squamous cell carcinoma (*Fig. 35.359*). Exceptional cases with an overlying squamous cell carcinoma have been reported.[97] Epidermal growth factor and transforming growth factor do not appear to play a role in the induction of pseudoepitheliomatous hyperplasia.[98] Prominent perineural spread may be a feature in some lesions (*Fig. 35.360*). Rarely, prominent fibrosis is present around the tumor and in one case there was ossification.[99,100] Pagetoid spread has been documented in a single case with malignant features.[101] Tumor cells are positive for NKI/C3, NSE, CD68 and S100 protein (*Fig. 35.361*).[4,20] TFE3 is diffusely positive although it is not associated with rearrangement of the gene.[102] Tumor cells may also express calretinin, the alpha unit of inhibin, PGP 9.5, nestin and low-affinity nerve growth factor receptor.[23,103–106] With regard to other melanocytic markers, Melan-A may be focally positive and microphthalmia transcription factor is often diffusely positive but HMB-45 seems to be consistently negative.[107]

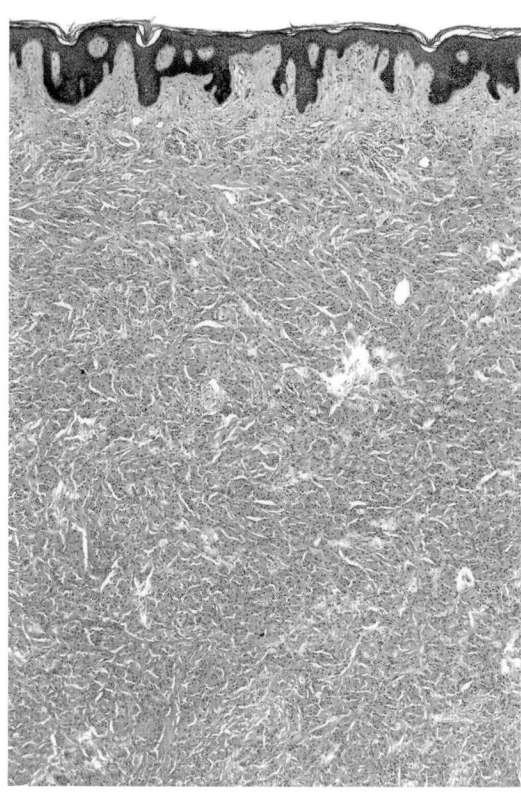

Fig. 35.357
Granular cell tumor: the lesion consists of large cells with eosinophilic granular cytoplasm.

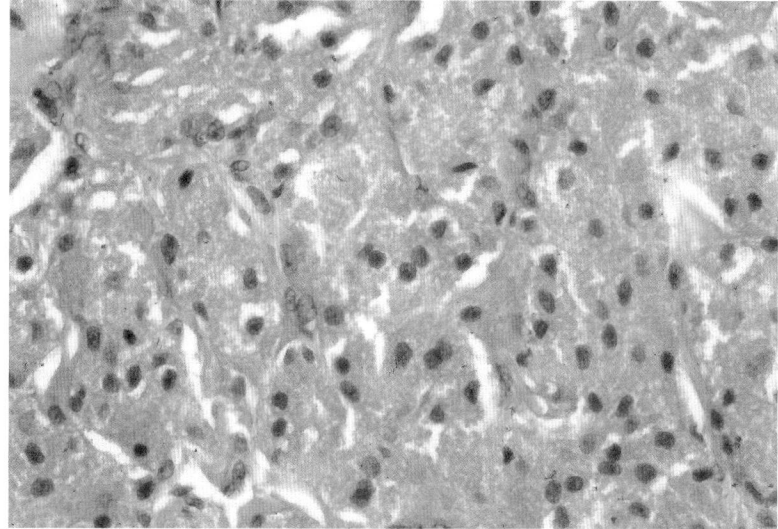

Fig. 35.358
Granular cell tumor: high-power view.

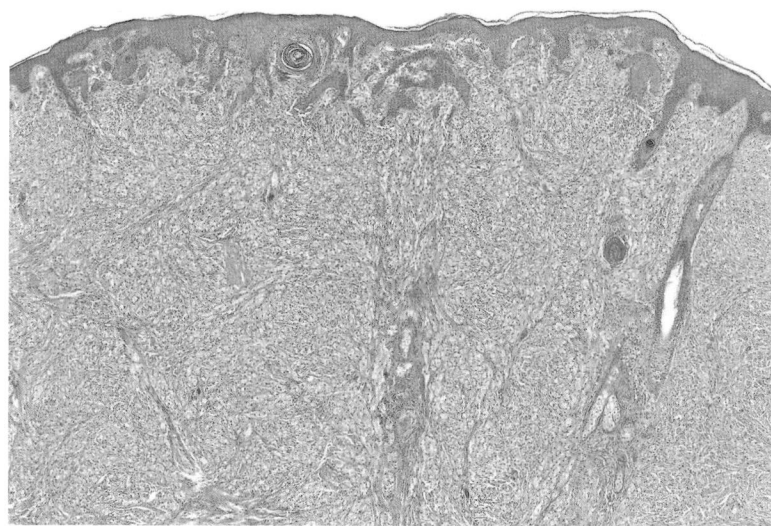

Fig. 35.359
Granular cell tumor: the overlying squamous epithelium often shows striking pseudoepitheliomatous hyperplasia, which should not be mistaken for an invasive tumor.

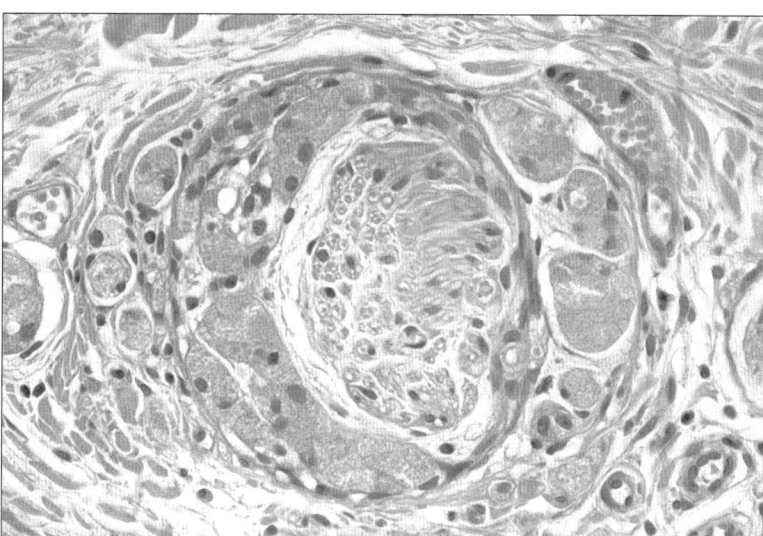

Fig. 35.360
Granular cell tumor: occasionally infiltration of the perineural space is a feature. This does not appear to be of clinical significance.

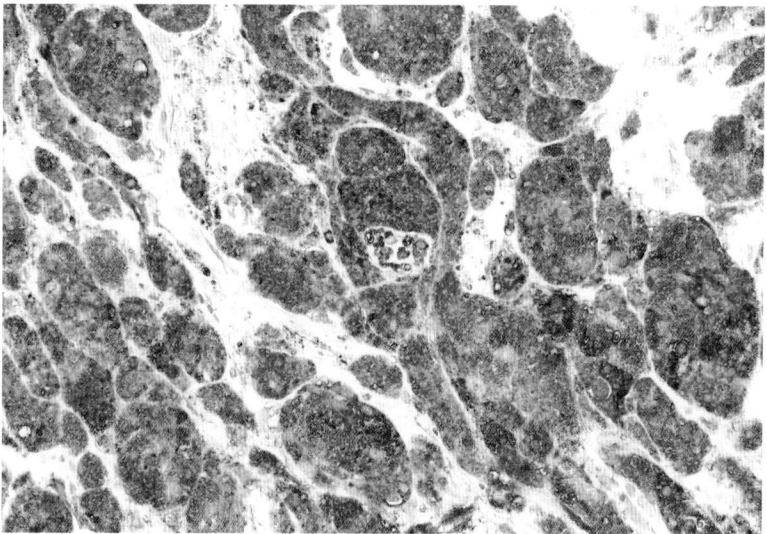

Fig. 35.361
Granular cell tumor: the tumor cells express S100 protein.

Histologic criteria for the diagnosis of malignancy are poorly defined, since cases with only mild atypia have metastasized.[69–80] However, features that should raise the possibility include large size (> 5 cm), rapid growth, vascular invasion, necrosis, high mitotic rate and increased pleomorphism.[69–71,74–77,108–111]

Electron microscopy shows that tumor cells contain numerous lysosomes correlating well with the diffuse expression of NKI/C3 on immunohistochemistry.

Differential diagnosis

The differential diagnosis is usually not problematic. Occasional cases may have to be distinguished from adult rhabdomyoma, which is desmin and myoglobin positive, and granular cell histiocytic reactions, which usually contain other inflammatory cells.

Gingival granular cell tumor of the newborn

Clinical features

Gingival granular cell tumor of the newborn (congenital epulis) is very rare and presents as a congenital polypoid lesion, most often on the lateral alveolar ridge of the maxilla.[1–5] Most cases are seen in females, and occasional patients have multiple lesions.[6–10] In the latter setting, obstructive symptoms can occur.[11,12] Tumors do not increase in size after birth and spontaneous regression is common, even after incomplete excision.[13] These features suggest a reactive pathogenesis.

Histologic features

Histologically, the features are almost identical to those of the common neuroectodermal variant, but vascularity is more prominent and there is sometimes a sparse inflammatory infiltrate composed of lymphocytes and histiocytes. There may be entrapped islands of odontogenic epithelium.

Immunohistochemically, tumor cells are negative for S100 protein, SOX10 and p75/NGFR and positive for PGP 9.5 and, as expected from the granular cell change, for NKI/C3 which stains a protein encoded by *CD63* in lysosomal membranes.[5,14] Ultrastructural studies suggest an origin from undifferentiated mesenchymal cells.

Nerve sheath myxoma (neurothekeoma)

Clinical features

Nerve sheath myxoma (neurothekeoma) arises most often on the extremities, mainly the hand/fingers, knee/pretibial region and ankle/foot, in the fourth decade of life and shows a predilection for males.[1–8] Rare cases have been reported in infants.[9] Much smaller percentage of cases presents in the head and neck including the oral cavity.[10–17] Intracranial, orbital, paravertebral, and mediastinum are rare sites of occurence.[18–22] Subungual cases are exceptional.[23,24] A single case associated with multiple angiomyxomas has been described.[25] There is no association with neurofibromatosis and typically the tumor presents as a solitary, long-standing, asymptomatic, raised, skin-colored nodule of variable duration measuring less than 3 cm in diameter.[1–7] Local recurrences, sometimes multiple, may be seen in up to 47% of patients. This tumor has no evident malignant potential.[7]

Histologic features

The appearances are distinctive; it is a well-defined, multinodular or multilobular unencapsulated mass situated predominantly in the dermis and subcutis (*Figs 35.362–35.364*).

The tumor lobules are of variable size, separated from one another by thin fibrovascular septa, and are composed of epithelioid, stellate, spindle or ring-like cells with pale indistinct cytoplasm set in an abundant myxoid matrix (*Fig. 35.365*). Tumor cells are arranged in cords, small nests or sometimes in a syncytial pattern.[7] Within some lobules are larger, more rounded cells with plump, rather hyperchromatic nuclei and eosinophilic cytoplasm (*Fig. 35.366*). Occasionally, bland multinucleate giant cells may be seen. Sparse mitotic activity is a common finding, but abnormal mitoses are not a feature (*Fig. 35.367*).

Scattered within and around the tumor are chronic inflammatory cells and mast cells. Careful examination of the small adjacent peripheral nerves may reveal tumorlike myxoid changes within them; however, nerve fibers are not identifiable within the tumor itself. Tumor cells are usually positive for S100 protein, SOX10, and low-affinity nerve growth factor receptor (*Fig. 35.368*).[7,26,27] They are also usually variably positive for glial fibrillary acidic protein (GFAP) and CD57.[7,27] All these findings support nerve sheath differentiation. Individual lobules of tumor cells are sometimes surrounded by a layer of EMA-positive cells (*Fig. 35.369*).

Typical nerve sheath myxomas in which there is a transition to more cellular lobules were described in 1986 by Rosati and coworkers as 'cellular neurothekeoma.'[28] These tumors, however, are quite different from those described by Barnhill and Mihm in 1990 under the same heading.[29]

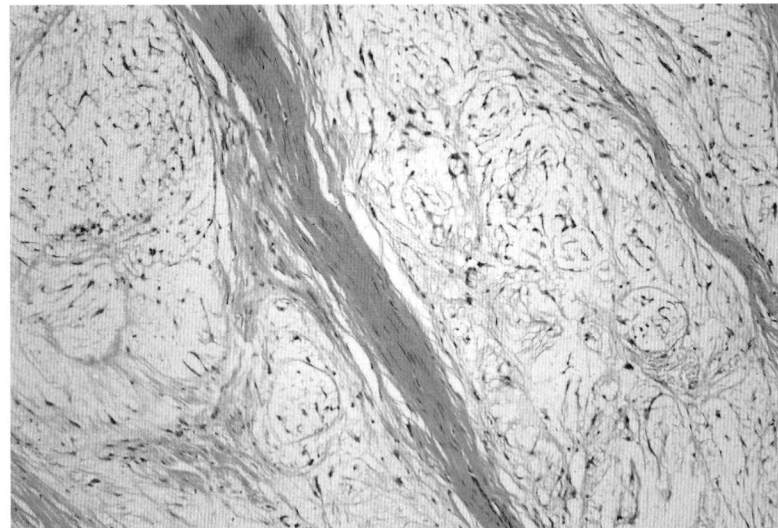

Fig. 35.363
Neurothekeoma: the lobules are composed of delicate spindled cells dispersed in a myxoid stroma.

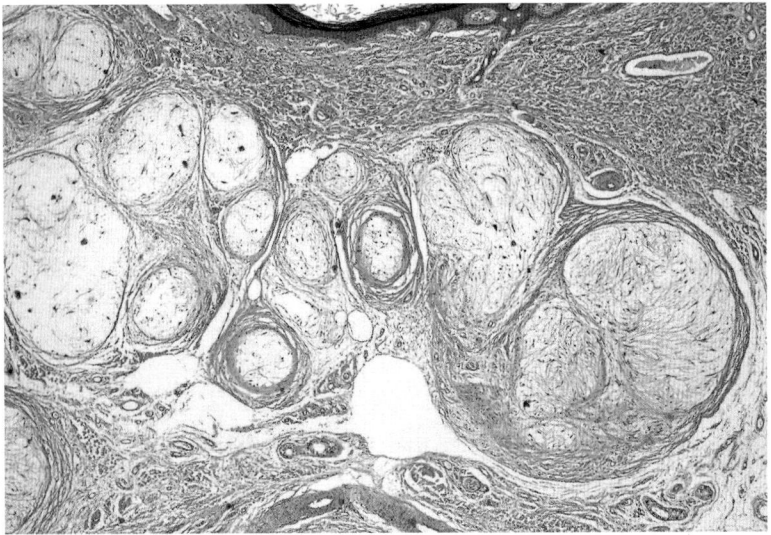

Fig. 35.362
Neurothekeoma: the tumor is composed of discrete lobules separated by fibrous septa.

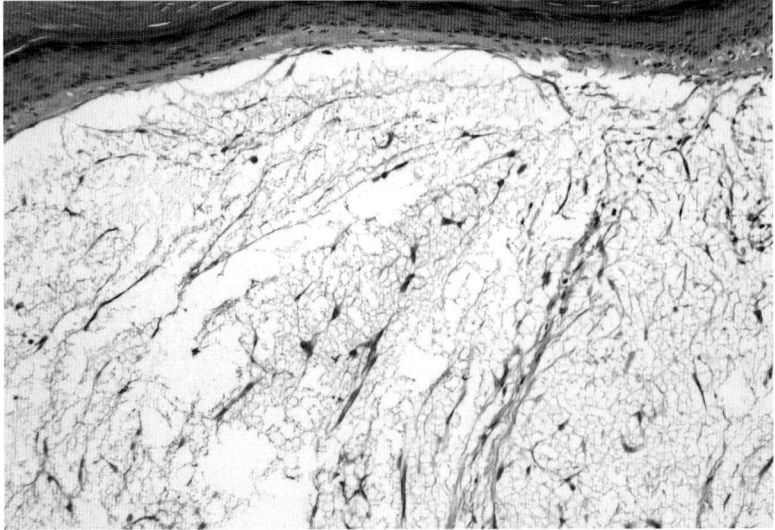

Fig. 35.364
Neurothekeoma: high-power view showing fusiform and stellate tumor cells.

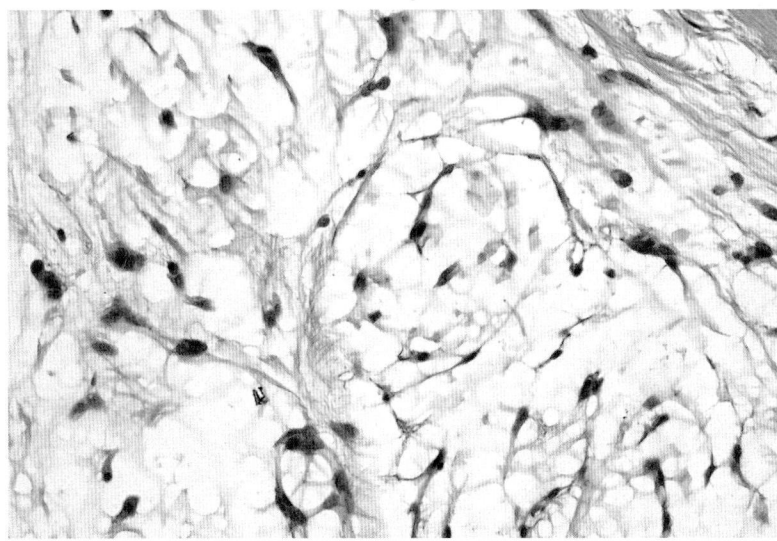

Fig. 35.365
Neurothekeoma: note the myxoid stroma.

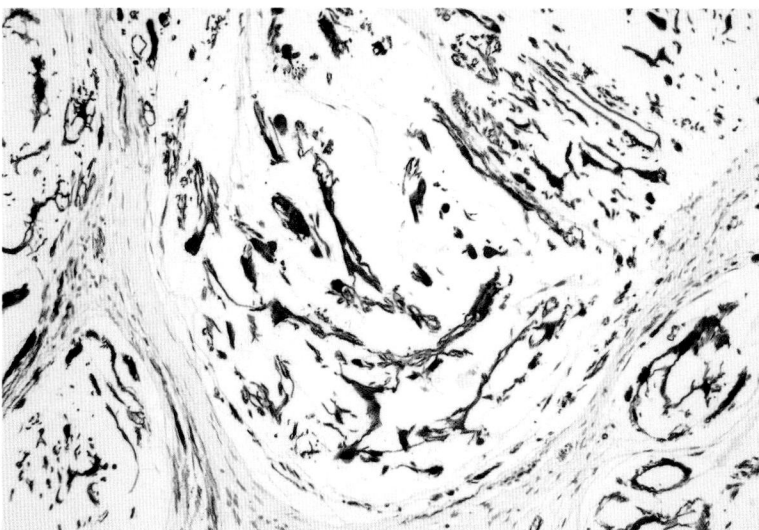

Fig. 35.368
Neurothekeoma: the tumor cells are S100 protein positive.

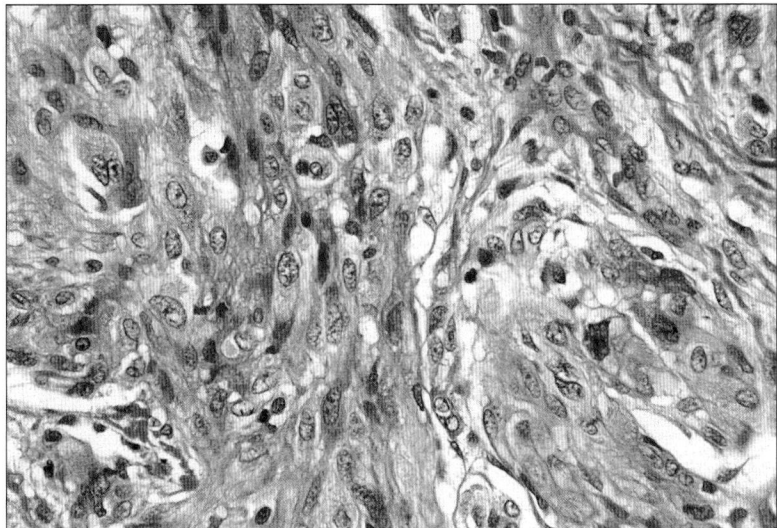

Fig. 35.366
Neurothekeoma: in this section, the cells are epithelioid with abundant cytoplasm and conspicuous vesicular nuclei.

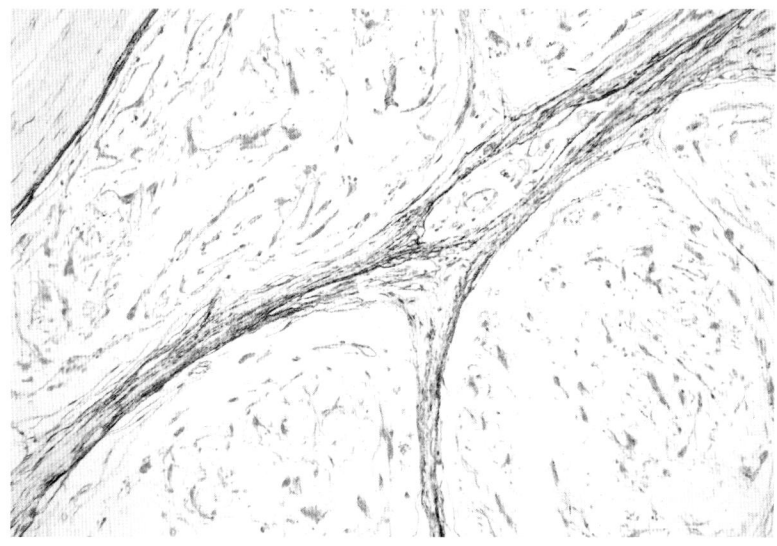

Fig. 35.369
Neurothekeoma: the perineurium is highlighted with EMA immunohistochemistry.

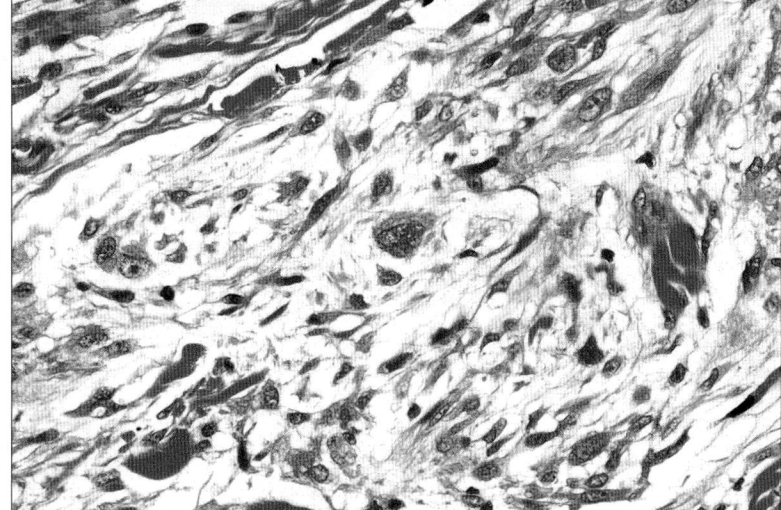

Fig. 35.367
Neurothekeoma: note the multinucleate giant cell.

Although the latter have different histologic features and immunohistochemistry that do not support a nerve sheath origin, they are nevertheless still known as cellular 'neurothekeoma' (see page 1769).

Differential diagnosis

Distinction from superficial angiomyxoma is based on the lack of circumscription, inconspicuous blood vessels, presence of scattered inflammatory cells and the common occurrence of epithelial elements in the latter tumor. Myxoid neurofibroma is poorly circumscribed and lacks a lobular architecture. Dermal myxomas are hypocellular and show few blood vessels and abundant stromal mucin. Distinction from circumscribed palisaded neuroma may be very difficult when the latter has prominent myxoid change.[30]

Perineurioma

Clinical features

Perineurioma is a neoplasm that was originally described as presenting in the subcutaneous tissue as soft tissue perineurioma or storiform perineural fibroma.[1-4] However, the spectrum of perineurioma is wide and includes other variants such as cutaneous perineurioma, intraneural perineurioma

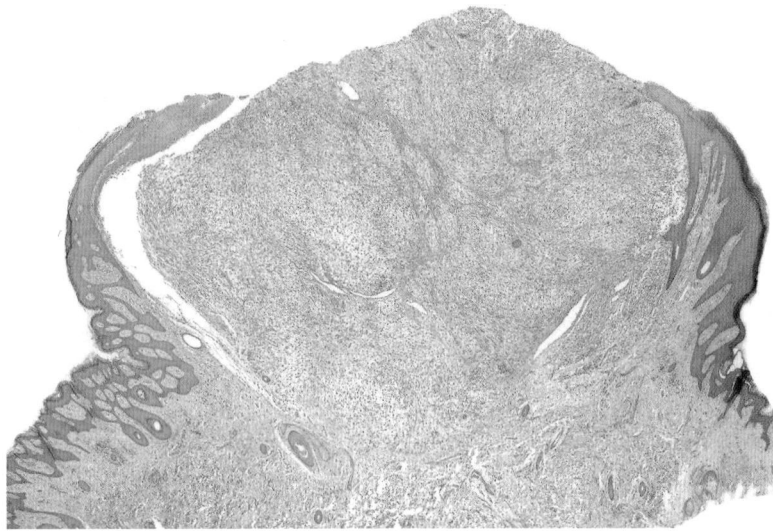

Fig. 35.370
Perineurioma: this tumor may closely resemble dermatofibrosarcoma protuberans but is generally better circumscribed.

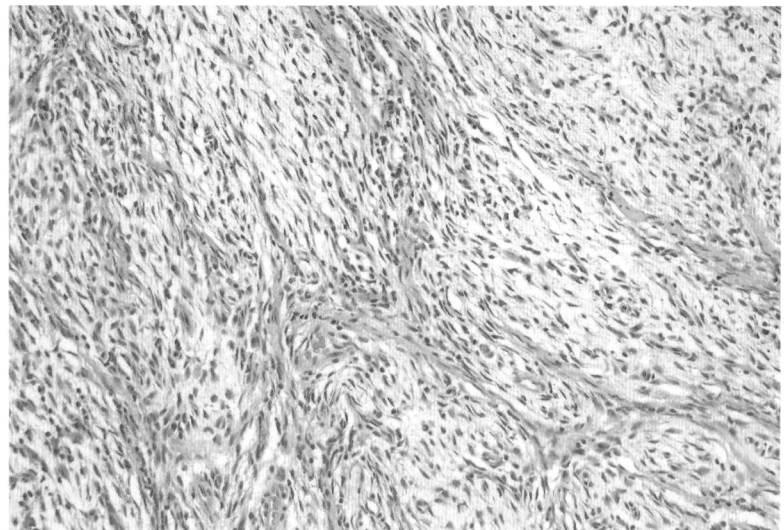

Fig. 35.371
Perineurioma: there is a whorled growth pattern.

(localized hypertrophic neuropathy) and sclerosing perineurioma.[5–12] Perineurioma usually presents in adults and rarely in children.[13] An association with neurofibromatosis has been described.[14,15] Occurrence in the gastrointestinal tract, prostate, kidney, lung, oral cavity, parotid gland, as well as orbital and meningeal cases have been reported.[16–33]

- *Cutaneous perineurioma* is relatively common and presents as a small papular lesion, mainly on the lower limbs of middle-aged adults, with predilection for females.[5–8] Behavior is benign with no tendency for local recurrence.
- *Soft tissue perineurioma* has very similar clinical features to those of cutaneous variants but lesions are subcutaneous and tend to be larger (up to 5 cm).[1–4]
- *Intraneural perineurioma* generally presents in young adults, and patients develop localized neurological symptoms as a result of intraneural growth.[9,10,34] Multiple lesions and a case associated with amyotrophy have been reported.[35,36]
- *Sclerosing perineurioma* presents in young adults, with marked predilection for the fingers and palm. Extra-acral lesions are very rare.[37–39] An exceptional case with bilateral lesions, and a patient with numerous tumors, have been documented.[40,41] Behavior is benign.[11,12]
- *Malignant perineuriomas* are exceptional.[42–48] Local recurrence has been reported but metastatic spread is rare.

Pathogenesis and histologic features

Abnormalities of chromosome 22 and specifically deletion of *NF2* have been reported in a few cases.[10,49] In addition, 10q24 rearrangements and *ABL1* gene involvement has been reported in two separate cases.[50,51]

Histologically, cutaneous perineurioma is a well-circumscribed, often dumbbell-shaped tumor composed of bland, short, spindle-shaped cells arranged in fascicles, with a focal whorling and a storiform pattern (*Figs 35.370–35.372*). Tumor cells may have focal epithelioid morphology. Variable hyalinization of the collagen is present and some cases show scattered, mononuclear inflammatory cells. Exceptional lesions with ossification, granular cell change and adipocytes or even lipoblasts have been described.[52–55] An angiofibroma -like pattern has been reported.[56] In a patient with multiple tumors, the lesions showed hybrid features of perineurioma and granular cell tumor.[57] In a further case, granular cell change was documented.[58] Soft tissue perineuriomas are very similar to those seen in the skin. Tumors are well circumscribed and generally cellular, being composed of monotonous bipolar cells with slender small nuclei in a fascicular, whorled or storiform growth pattern. Some cases are less cellular with a myxocollagenous stroma. Mitotic figures are rare and pleomorphism is absent.

A reticular variant of soft tissue perineurioma has been documented (*Fig. 35.373*).[59–61] In this variant, a lace-like or reticular growth pattern composed

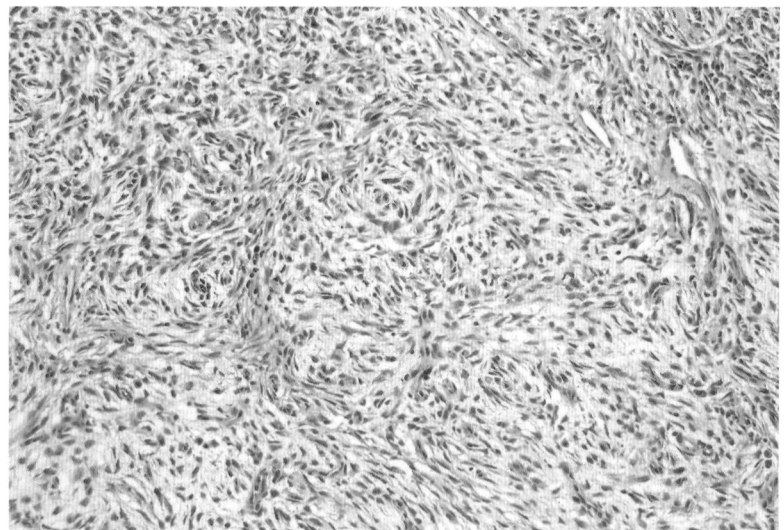

Fig. 35.372
Perineurioma: often, the tumor cells are arranged in a typical storiform growth pattern.

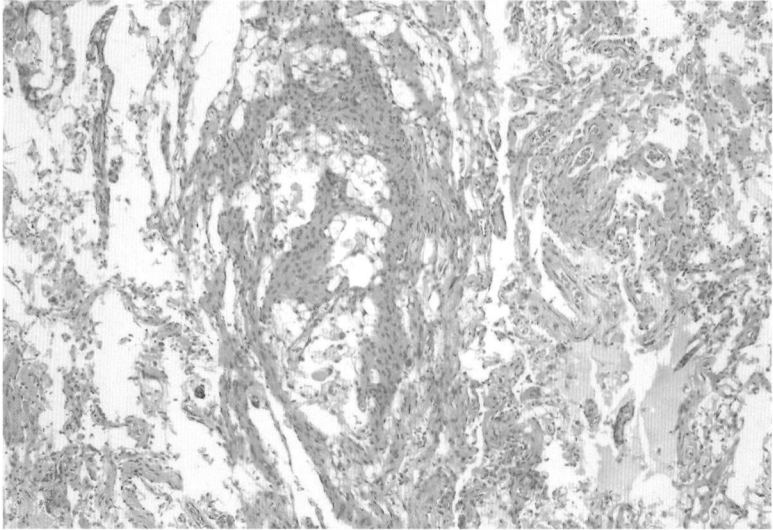

Fig. 35.373
Reticular perineurioma: note the lace-like growth pattern.

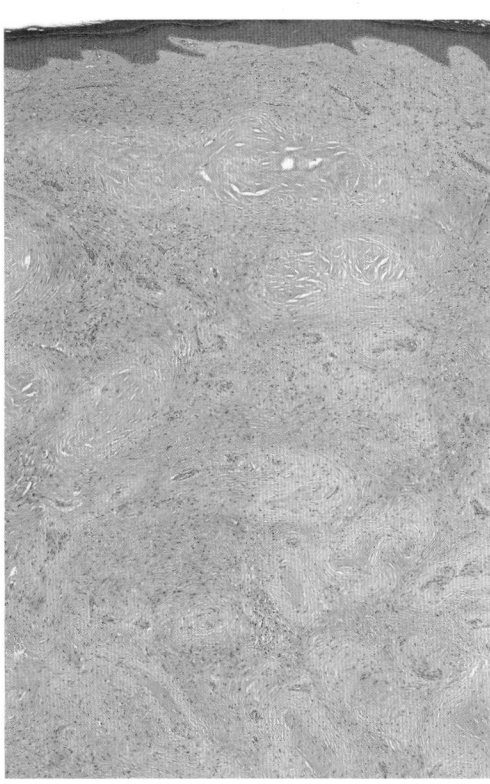

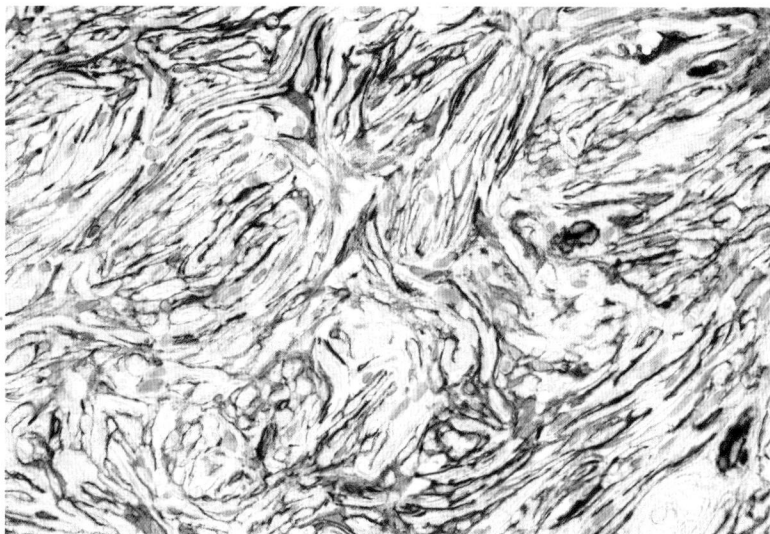

Fig. 35.376
Perineurioma: the tumor cells express epithelial membrane antigen.

Fig. 35.374
Sclerosing perineurioma: this variant is characterized by a dense fibrous stroma.

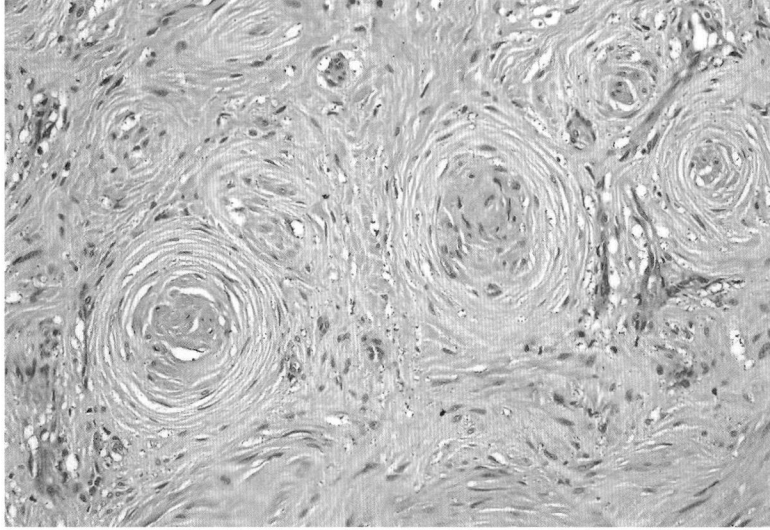

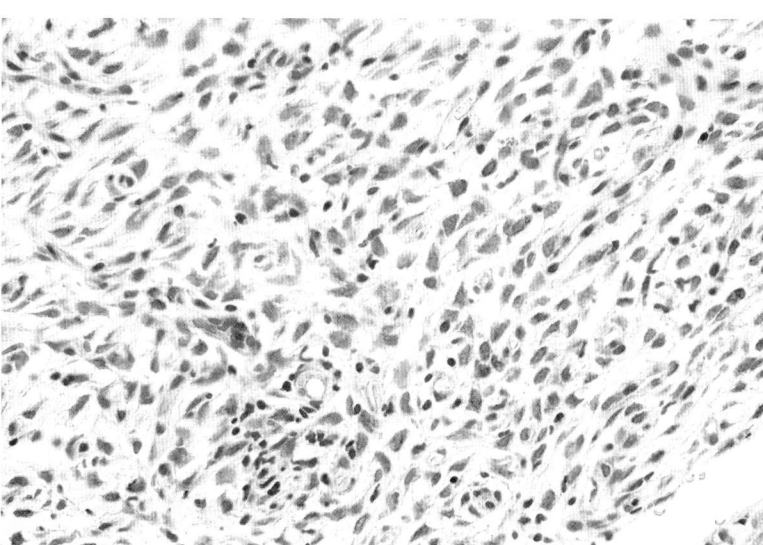

Fig. 35.377
Perineurioma: there is cytoplasmic CD34 expression.

Fig. 35.375
Sclerosing perineurioma: residual nodules are scattered throughout the lesion.

positive.[64,69] In soft tissue perineurioma and sclerosing perineurioma, rare focal positivity for keratin has been described.[11]

Differential diagnosis

Distinction from dermatofibrosarcoma protuberans is afforded by the latter's diffuse CD34 positivity and infiltrative growth pattern. Other neural tumors usually lack a storiform pattern and are generally S100 protein positive.

of anastomosing cords of spindle-shaped cells with pale pink cytoplasm and bipolar cytoplasmic processes is seen.

In intraneural perineurioma, perineurial cells proliferate around individual axons with a characteristic onion ring appearance. A reticular pattern has been documented in one case.[62,63]

Sclerosing perineurioma is characterized by prominent hyalinized collagen around the tumor cells, which are arranged in cords, bundles and whorls (Figs 35.374 and 35.375). Trabecular, reticulated and whorled patterns may be seen.[64] Cytologic atypia is absent and mitotic figures are exceptional. A single case contained mature adipocytes.[65] Xanthomatous changes have been reported.[66] A plexiform pattern and a whirling cellular variant are very rare.[58,67,68]

In all perineuriomas, tumor cells are diffusely positive for EMA, but negative for other neural markers (including S100 protein), in keeping with perineurial differentiation (Fig. 35.376).[3,4] Focal and sometimes diffuse positivity for CD34 is seen in a small number of cases (Fig. 35.377) possibly reflecting the presence of fibroblasts. GLUT 1 and claudin-1 are usually

Lipofibromatosis-like neural tumor

Clinical features

Lipofibromatosis-like neural tumor is a newly described entity which was discovered incidentally during a molecular investigation of pediatric fibroblastic- myofibroblastic tumor.[1] The tumor occurs in extremities, head and neck and flank with a maximum dimension from 1,3 to 5,4 cm and no sex predilection. The median age is 13.5 years.

Local recurrence is seen in 42% of cases albeit in patients whose excision was incomplete; a lung metastasis has been identified in a patient with prolonged duration of surgical removal and somewhat different histology.

Pathogenesis and histologic features

Lipofibromatosis-like neural tumor is characterized by recurrent *NTRK1* gene fusions.1

Histologically the tumor is infiltrative and cellular composed of spindle cells arranged in streaming fascicles. The tumor cells have indistinct cell borders and pale eosinophilic cytoplasm. The nuclei are elongated with an inconspicuous nucleolus. Nuclear atypia and hyperchromasia is mild but rare pleomorphic cells may be seen. Mitotic activity is generally low and necrosis is not a feature. A case with necrosis and increase mitotic activity has metastasized; it is postulated that long duration may lead to sarcoma-tous transformation.

By immunohistochemistry an invariable diffuse positivity for S100 protein is seen but other melanocytic markers, such as SOX10, HMB45, Melan A are negative. At least focal positivity for CD34 is seen in most cases and focal SMA positivity is detected in some. Overexpression of NTRK1 noted as cytoplasmic immunopositivity is seen in most of the cases. Desmin and GFAP are negative whereas H3K27me3 expression seems to be retained.

Heterotopias

Meningeal heterotopias

Meningeal lesions presenting in the skin are usually known as 'cutane-ous meningiomas.' The use of this term tends to imply a neoplastic origin and since most lesions in this group are probably hamartomatous or the result of developmental defect, we prefer the designation meningeal hetero-topias. It is convenient to classify cutaneous meningeal lesions into three types.[1] However, there is a great degree of overlap, especially histologically, between type I and type II lesions and they probably represent variants of a similar hamartomatous process.

Clinical features

Type I lesions have also been described as ectopic meningothelial hamar-toma and sequestrated or rudimentary meningocele.[2–9] Although they are congenital, they are sometimes only recognized during childhood and ado-lescence. There is an equal sex incidence and presentation is that of a nonde-script cutaneous or subcutaneous nodule or plaque on the scalp (especially the occipital area) or less commonly on the back along the midline (*Fig. 35.378*). Often, they are diagnosed clinically as cysts. There is no underlying bone abnormality. Alopecia and aplasia cutis can be seen.[9,10]

Type II lesions present mainly in adulthood on the head and neck mainly around mouth, nose, eyes, and ears but may rarely occur in children.[11–13] A case associated with pregnancy and one with a sinus pericranii have been documented.[14,15] Their behavior is entirely benign and it appears that they also represent hamartomas formed by remnants of meningothelial cells.[1] Cases associated with trauma have been described.[16,17]

Type III lesions represent local invasion or true metastasis from a primary intracranial meningioma.[18] The scalp is the most common site and growth through bony surgical defects is well recognized. A case of meningioma was reported after trauma due to the entrapment of meningothelial tissue in the skin [19] and another as a possible result of surgical seeding.[20]

Histologic features

Type I lesions are located in the deep dermis and subcutis and show irreg-ular, elongated, anastomosing and dilated spaces resembling vascular channels dissecting between somewhat thickened collagen bundles (*Figs 35.379–35.381*). The spaces are filled or lined by small, round eosinophilic epithelioid meningothelial cells with minimal or no atypia and showing no mitotic activity. They are consistently positive for EMA (*Fig. 35.382*).

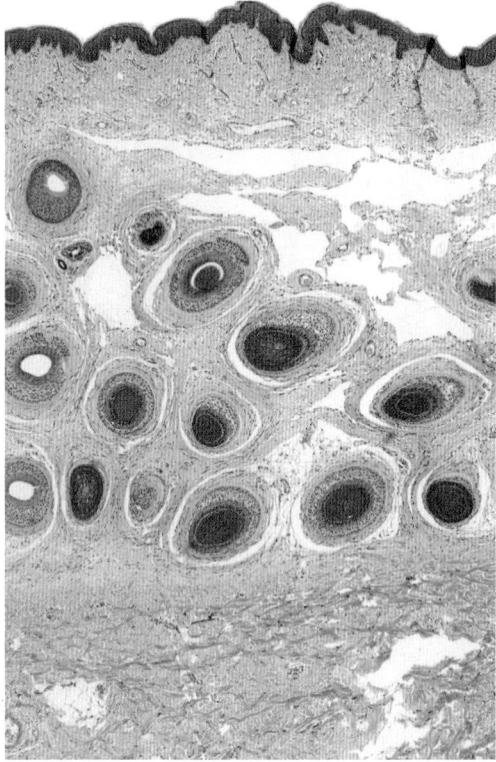

Fig. 35.379
Ectopic meningothelial hamartoma: this lesion is composed of pseudovascular clefts lined by meningothelial cells.

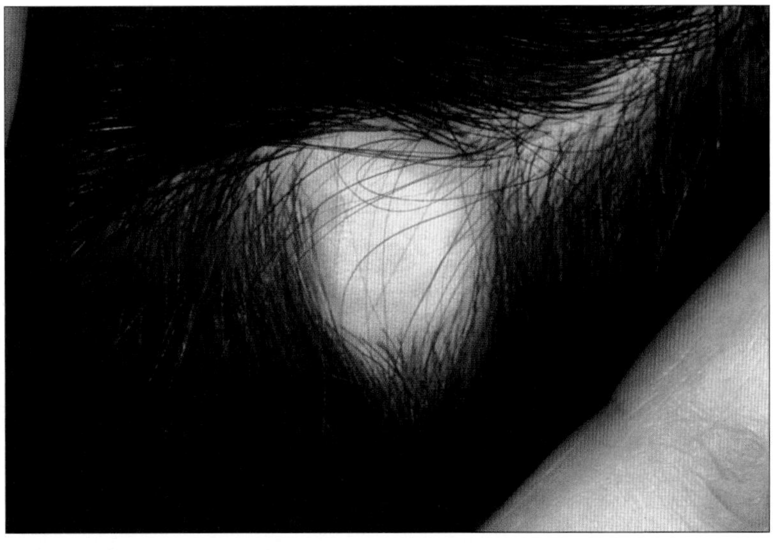

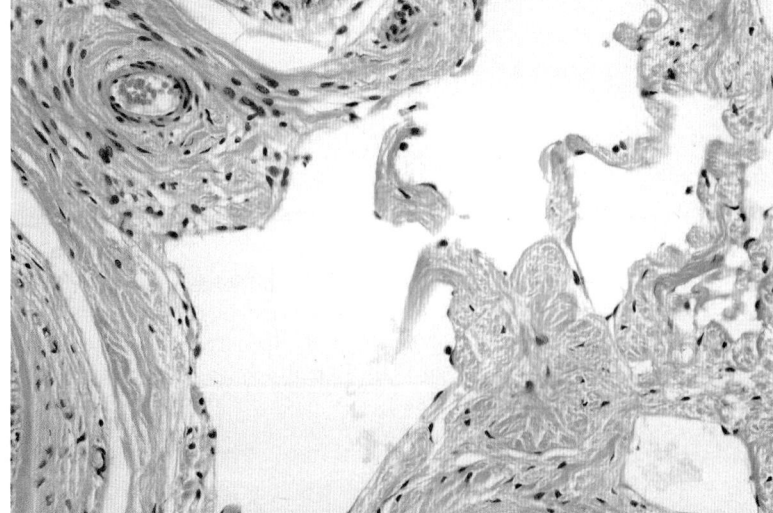

Fig. 35.378
Ectopic meningothelial hamartoma: the scalp is a commonly affected site. By courtesy of the Institute of Dermatology, London, UK.

Fig. 35.380
Ectopic meningothelial hamartoma: high-power view showing meningothelial cells lining the cystic spaces.

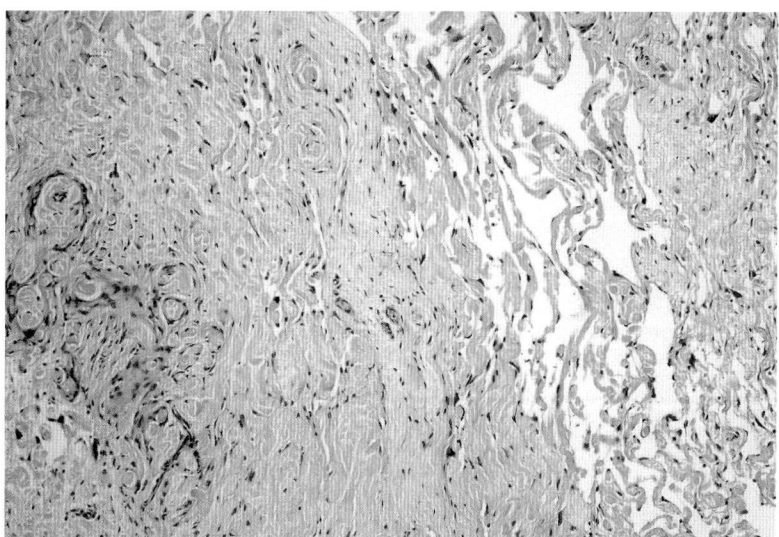

Fig. 35.381
Ectopic meningothelial hamartoma: the pseudovascular spaces are associated with dense fibrous tissue.

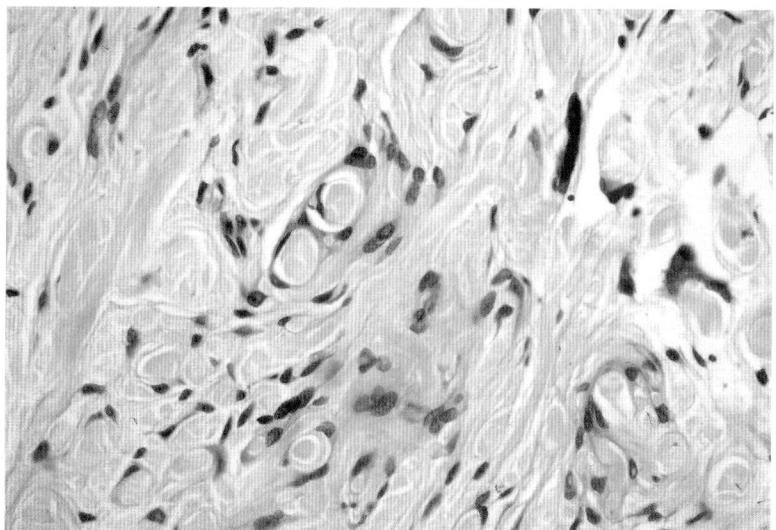

Fig. 35.383
Ectopic meningothelial hamartoma: the tumor cells characteristically entrap collagen.

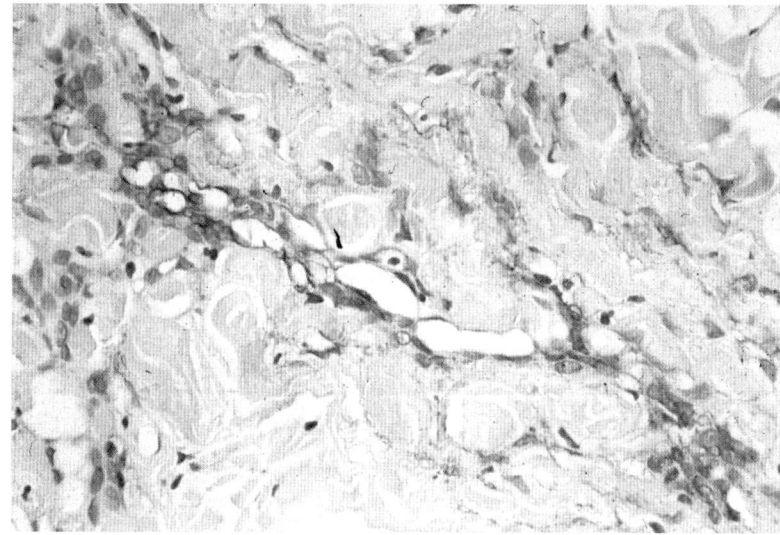

Fig. 35.382
Ectopic meningothelial hamartoma: the tumor cells express epithelial membrane antigen.

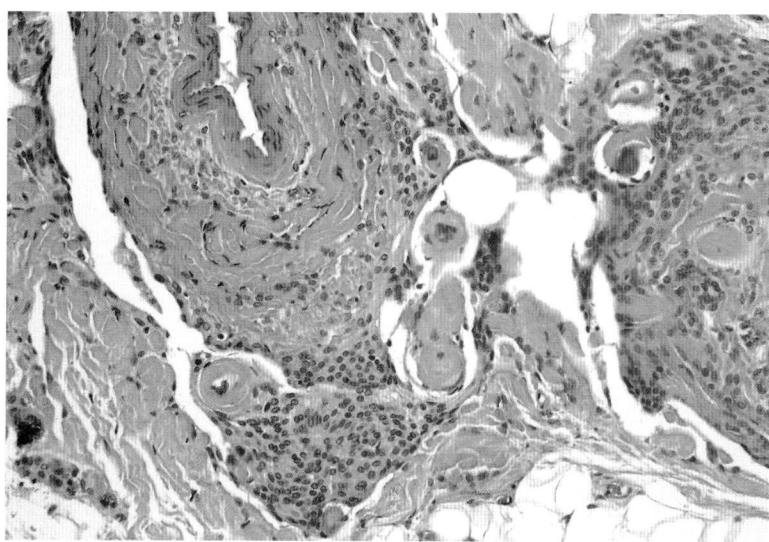

Fig. 35.384
Ectopic meningothelial hamartoma: psammoma bodies are sometimes a feature. Note the conspicuous meningothelial proliferation.

Positivity for NSE, podoplanin, NKIC3 and less commonly for Glut-1 and PR may be seen.[9] Focally, cells wrap around hyalinized collagen bundles with calcification or psammoma body formation (*Figs 35.383* and *35.384*). Occasional multinucleated cells may be a feature. A fibrotic stroma but may be prominent and in some cases the is myxoid change.[9] Throughout the tumor there is an increase in the number of normal blood vessels, and fatty tissue may be evident within the dermis. Dermal melanocytes are sometimes identified.[9] The association with brain tissue or a heterotopic ependymal cyst may be seen.[9]

Type II lesions are characterized by the presence of small numbers of more discrete and larger solid nests of meningothelial cells. A case of meningioma apparently developing from a rudimentary meningocele has been documented.[21]

A case associated with melanocytosis and a vascular malformation in an 8-year-old boy has been reported.[22]

Type III lesions show the features of an intracranial meningioma including anaplastic forms.[23] They are composed of spindle-shaped and ovoid meningothelial cells, with a variable fibrocollagenous stroma (*Figs 35.385* and *35.386*). A whorled or storiform pattern is common and sometimes the tumor cells are arranged in lobules or packets. Not infrequently, the larger

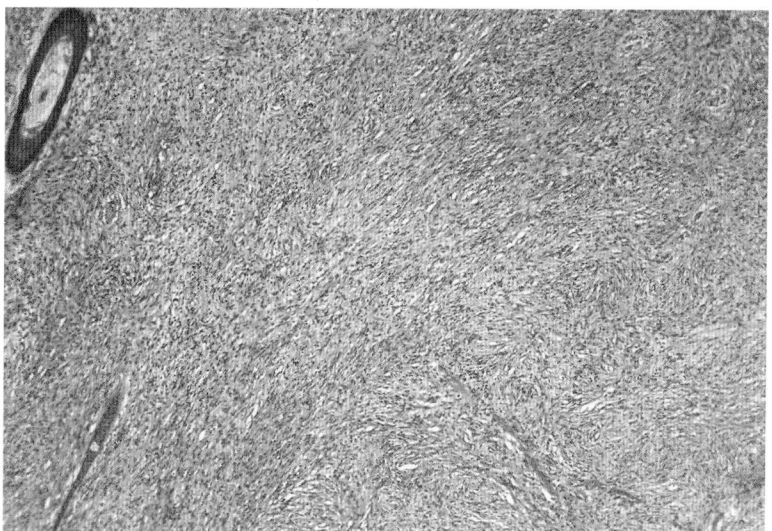

Fig. 35.385
Cutaneous 'metastatic' meningioma: the dermis is diffusely infiltrated by a spindle cell tumor.

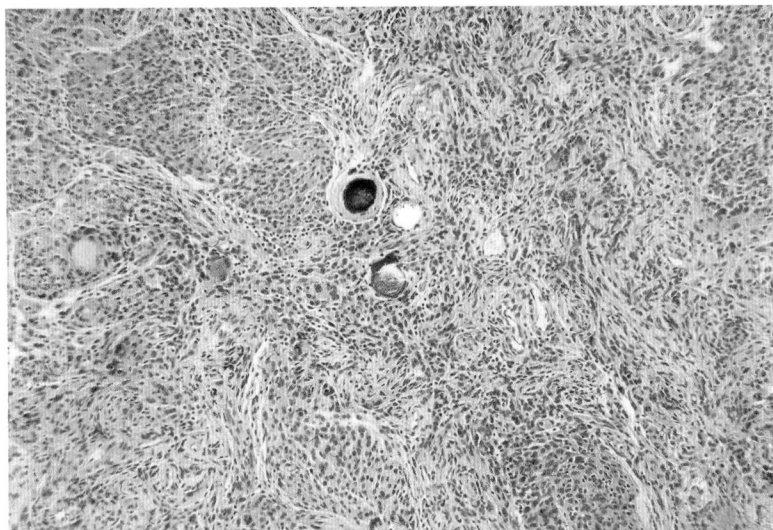

Fig. 35.386
Cutaneous 'metastatic' meningioma: in this example well-developed basophilic psammoma bodies are evident.

ovoid cells, which have indistinct cell borders, are distributed in sheets, giving rise to a syncytial appearance. Psammoma bodies are often present.

Type II and III are positive for EMA and p63 but negative for CK5/6, S100, and CD31.[24]

Differential diagnosis

Due to the pseudovascular appearance, type I lesions may be confused with angiosarcoma. The latter, however, generally occurs in older patients and typically shows cytologic atypia, multilayering, mitotic figures and positive expression for vascular markers, but not for EMA.

When a primary epithelial or adnexal tumor is considered negativity for cytokeratins and especially for CK5/6 are helpful features.[16,25]

Metastatic carcinoma can be distinguished from type I and type II lesions by a short history and the presence of cytologic atypia, mitosis and keratin positivity.

Glial heterotopias

Clinical features

Glial heterotopias are rare developmental congenital anomalies that are typically detected in infancy although very occasional cases are first noticed in adult life.[1-5] In the latter setting, a case was detected because of visual loss.[6] The majority are subcutaneous and present as a firm mass adjacent to the bridge of the nose, often with associated hypertelorism (*Fig. 35.387*). Up to one-third of cases are solely intranasal and a small proportion show both components. As most cases occur in or around the nose they are known as nasal gliomas. Lesions present as a nodule or polyp, and intranasal lesions often are accompanied by obstruction.[7] However, rare examples can arise on the lip, pharynx, oral cavity (including the tongue), scalp and even the midline of the back and the sphenoid sinus.[8-11] Multiple lesions are rare and a heterotopia and an encephalocele may occur simultaneously.[12] A case associated with agenesis of the corpus callosum has been documented.[13] A further case associated with PHACE syndrome (posterior fossa anomalies, hemangiomas of the face and scalp, arterial abnormalities, cardiac defects and eye anomalies) has also been reported.[14]

Although excision is curative, it is mandatory to preoperatively exclude the presence of a persistent communication with the frontal lobes.[15,16] Such a communication is present in about 20% of cases and although it most often manifests as a fibrous cord, it may sometimes represent a true meningocele or encephalocele.[1] Clinical and histologic features do not allow distinction between heterotopia and encephalocele, and neuroimaging studies are mandatory.[12,17]

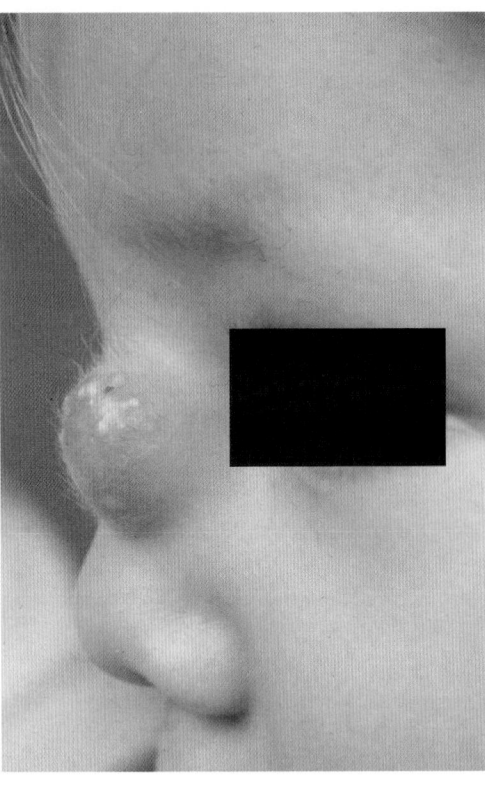

Fig. 35.387
Nasal glioma: the nose is the most commonly affected site. By courtesy of the Institute of Dermatology, London, UK.

CT and MRI scans (particularly the latter) are the preferred radiological studies but distinction from a hemangioma may be difficult. In such cases ultrasound or Doppler flow studies may afford the distinction.[18] Prenatal diagnosis may be made by ultrasound.[19,20] Incautious treatment of such patients sometimes results in leakage of cerebrospinal fluid, meningitis and cerebral abscess.

Histologic features

The microscopic appearances are characteristic, being typified by well-circumscribed nodules composed largely of well-differentiated astrocytes in a loose neurofibrillar stroma situated in the subcutaneous tissues (*Figs 35.388* and *35.389*). Oligodendrocytes may be focally identified and, in rare cases, there may be a demonstrable neuronal component (*Fig. 35.390*). Histologic distinction from an encephalocele is not possible since even heterotopias may show laminated cerebral cortex with neurons and ependymal canals (*Fig. 35.391*).[12] Focal calcifications and mild inflammation are sometimes seen.[5] Proliferation of associated eccrine sweat ducts has been described in a case.[21] In older patients, lesions may be almost completely replaced by fibrosis, making recognition very difficult.[12] Diagnosis can be confirmed by the expression of GFAP and S100 protein.[3,5]

Malignant neural neoplasms

Malignant peripheral nerve sheath tumor

Malignant peripheral nerve sheath tumor is synonymous with the terms 'neurofibrosarcoma' and 'malignant schwannoma' and is the preferred name, since the precise histogenesis of a given tumor – be it Schwann cell, perineurial cell or fibroblast – is rarely certain. Malignant peripheral nerve sheath tumors showing perineural differentiation are discussed under perineurioma.

Clinical features

Malignant peripheral nerve sheath tumor occurring in the skin is very rare and usually results from malignant change in a neurofibroma, mainly in patients with neurofibromatosis type I (50% of cases), as a complication of radiotherapy (10% of cases) or secondary to extension from a tumor arising in deeper soft tissues.[1-12] Tumors arising from a neurofibroma in patients without neurofibromatosis are exceedingly rare.[13-18]

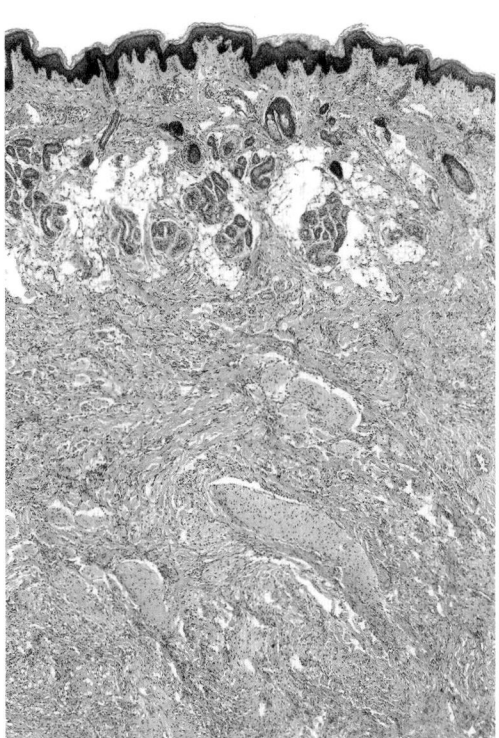

Fig. 35.388
Nasal glioma: this section from the bridge of the nose of a 2-year-old girl shows an ill-defined tumor mass deep to the compressed subcutaneous fat.

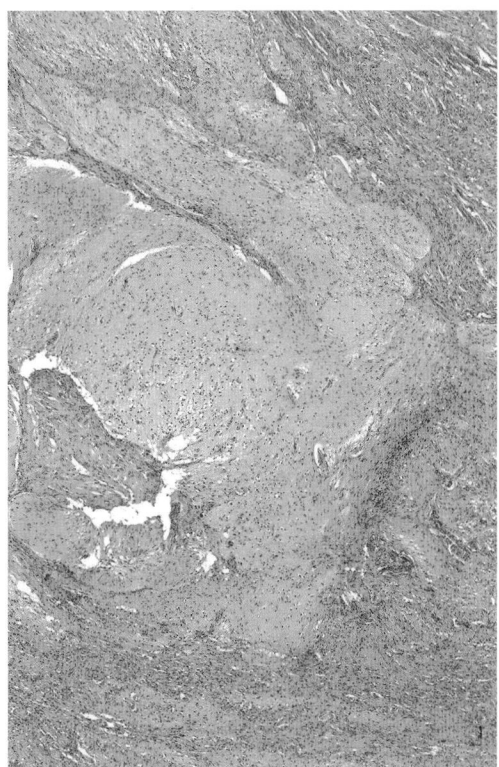

Fig. 35.389
Nasal glioma: the lesion consists of circumscribed nodules of cellular tissue dispersed within a loose glial, fibrillary stroma.

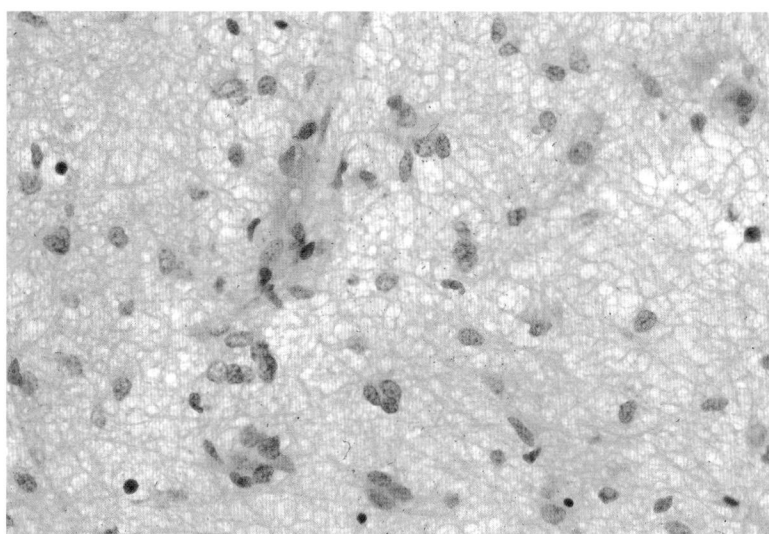

Fig. 35.390
Nasal glioma: the nodules are composed predominantly of astrocytes with round vesicular nuclei. The cells with small hyperchromatic nuclei are oligodendrocytes.

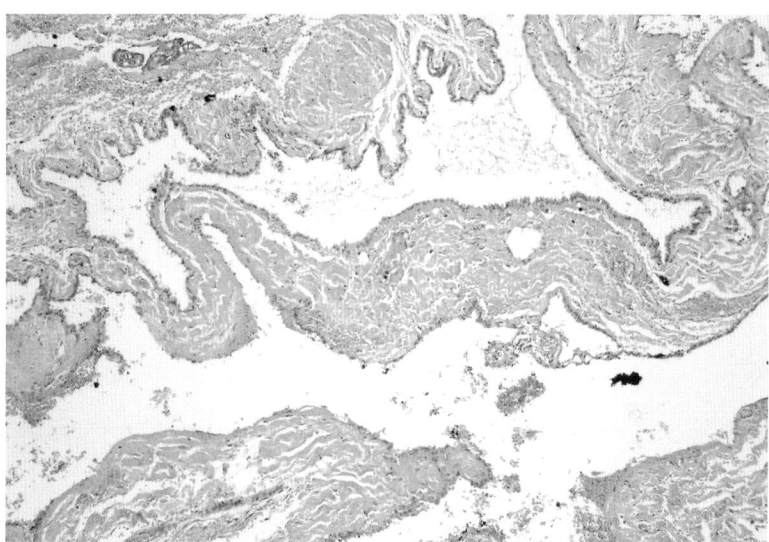

Fig. 35.391
Encephalocele: this cystic cavity is lined by ependymal cells and communicated with an intracranial component.

Additionally, the rare epithelioid variant (which is associated with a better prognosis) has a predilection for the deep dermis and subcutis.[19–21] The latter tumor, only exceptionally associated with NF1, is more common in the upper extremities of adults, with no sex predilection.[18–20,22] Cases arising in a diffuse type neurofibroma have been documented.[23]

Malignant peripheral nerve sheath tumor most often presents in adults although its age range is wide. Tumors in children are rare and may be sporadic or associated with NF1.[24] A distinctive variant – plexiform malignant peripheral nerve sheath tumor – has been reported in children.[25] This tumor tends to have a better prognosis than ordinary malignant peripheral nerve sheath tumors, with a high rate of local recurrence but low metastatic potential.

Sporadic cases show an equal sex incidence and tend to cluster in the fifth decade of life. Occurrence in elderly patients is exceptional.[26]

By contrast, tumors associated with NF1 are more common in males with a peak in the fourth decade. Anatomical distribution is wide with most lesions presenting on the limbs followed by the trunk and (less frequently) the head and neck region.

These tumors affect only 2–3% of patients with NF1.[1] They occur in either sex and most often present in the third and fourth decades; a rapid alteration in the size or symptomatology of a pre-existent neurofibroma is suggestive of malignant change. The 5-year survival for patients with NF1 and irradiation-induced tumors is around 20%, which is much lower than that for other NF1 patients.[1,8] The literature varies as to whether NF1-associated malignant nerve sheath tumors are more aggressive.[27–34] This question may be complicated by the difficulty in diagnosis of this tumor outside the context of NF1.

Cases arising from a schwannoma are exceptional and most show epithelioid morphology in the malignant component.[35–38] Examples associated with juvenile onset dermatomyositis,[39] MEN1,[40] and Cowden syndrome[41] as well as a case with PNET differentiation[42] have been reported.

Pathogenesis and histologic features

Many malignant peripheral nerve sheath tumors arise in the context of NF1 (see syndrome discussion above) and thus are associated with loss of neurofibromin, as are their neurofibroma precursors. Somatic *NF1* loss also appears to be common in sporadic tumors.[43,44] Malignant progression often proceeds with *P16* or *P53* abrogation though other genes are also involved.[45–47] Tumors often show gains in chromosomes 8q, 17q, and 7p and losses in chromosomes 9p, 11q, and 17p. Neoplasms with gains in chromosome 16p or losses in chromosomes 10q or Xq are associated with poor prognosis.[48]

In general, malignant peripheral nerve sheath tumors belong to the category of sarcomas with complex karyotype. Despite extensive research the pathogenesis is not yet clarified.[49–82] Interestingly, *EED* and *SUZ12* mutations that inactivate the polycomb repressive complex 2 (PRC2), including EZH2 methyltransferase have been demonstrated.[83–85] As a result, immuno-histochemical nuclear H3K27me expression is lost.[86–89]

Irrespective of the clinical context, the histologic features are fairly consistent, comprising alternating myxoid and cellular areas containing irregular interlacing bundles of spindled cells with scanty pale cytoplasm and wavy, usually hyperchromatic, variably pleomorphic nuclei (*Figs 35.392* and *35.393*). Myxoid change can be prominent. The degree of pleomorphism

and mitotic activity varies among cases, but correlates with the grade of the tumor (*Fig. 35.394*). Perivascular whorling by tumor cells is also a typical feature, as are hyaline nodules if present (*Figs 35.395* and *35.396*). Tumor cells quite often appear to infiltrate small vessel walls. Nuclear palisading is rare. Pigmentation and melanocytic differentiation are very rare features.[90]

It should be noted that only 50% of malignant peripheral nerve sheath tumors are S100 protein positive, probably reflecting the heterogeneity of the tumor cell population.[91–93] Lack of S100 protein reactivity may confer a worse prognosis. SOX 10 is also positive.[94]

A Ki67 higher than 20% has been found to be associated with worst prognosis.[95]

A variant of peripheral nerve sheath tumor with a prominent CD34 positive component, presenting in the endocervix, and referred to as fibroblastic MPNST has been described.[96]

Heterologous differentiation is seen in up to 15% of cases, most often as foci of malignant bone or cartilage.[97] A rhabdomyoblastic element may sometimes be apparent (malignant Triton tumor-ectomesenchymoma) (*Figs 35.397* and *35.398*).[98,99] Very rarely, gland formation is evident.[99–103] Angiosarcoma may also develop within a malignant peripheral nerve sheath tumor.[104,105]

Epithelioid malignant nerve sheath tumor comprises the small proportion of neoplasms containing, in addition to the more conventional features,

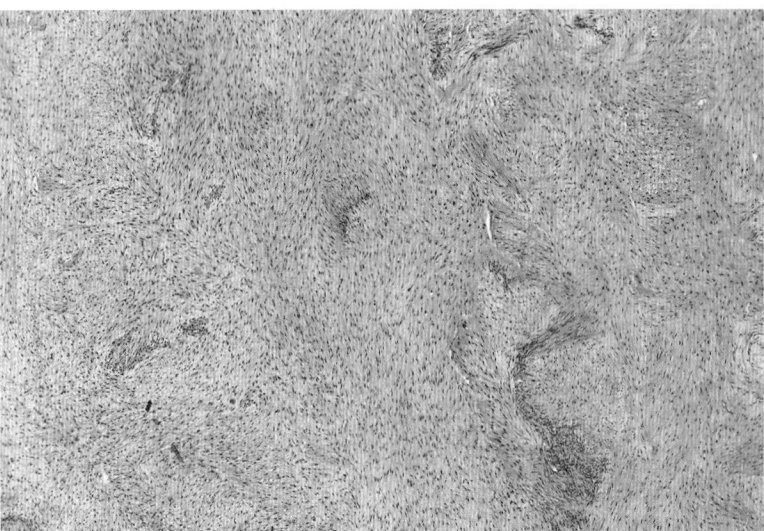

Fig. 35.392
Malignant peripheral nerve sheath tumor: this shows an infiltrate of small cells with ill-defined eosinophilic cytoplasm and focal palisading.

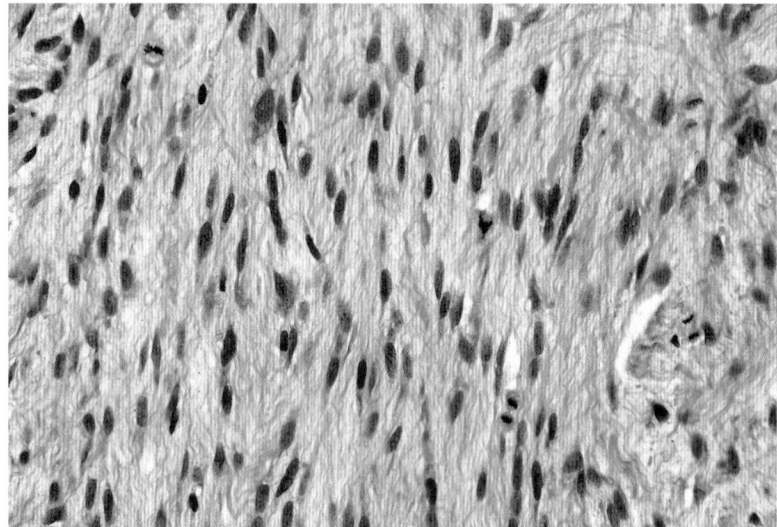

Fig. 35.394
Malignant peripheral nerve sheath tumor: note the presence of conspicuous mitotic figures.

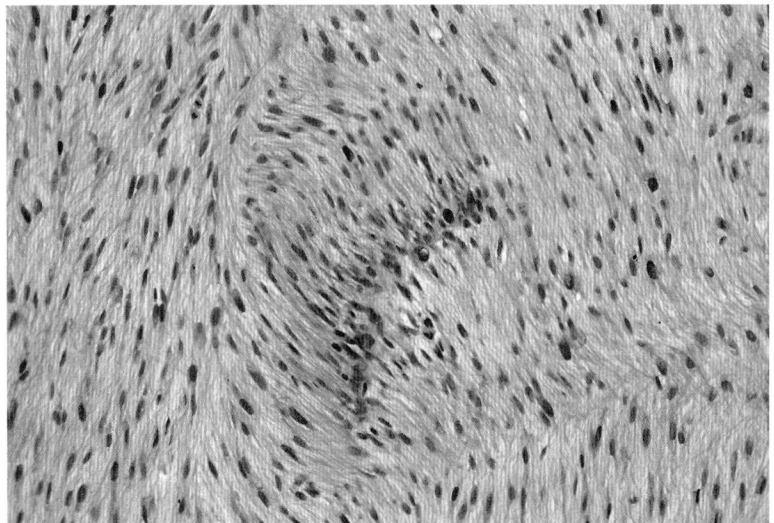

Fig. 35.393
Malignant peripheral nerve sheath tumor: nuclear palisading as seen in this field is only rarely a feature.

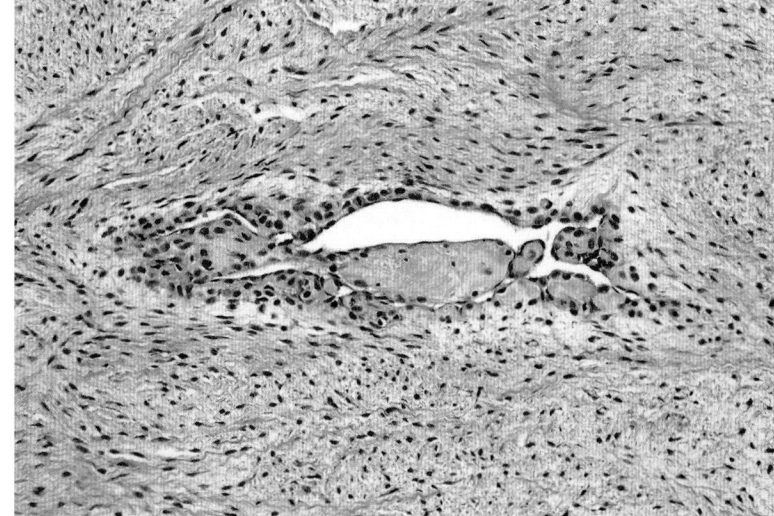

Fig. 35.395
Malignant peripheral nerve sheath tumor: the presence of focal areas of perivascular cuffing is a typical feature.

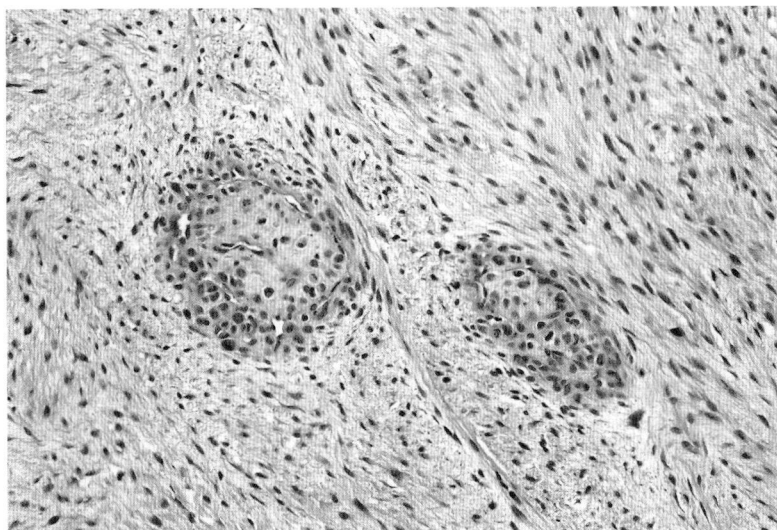

Fig. 35.396
Malignant peripheral nerve sheath tumor: hyalinized nodules, often with a peripheral ring of nuclei, are rare but characteristic.

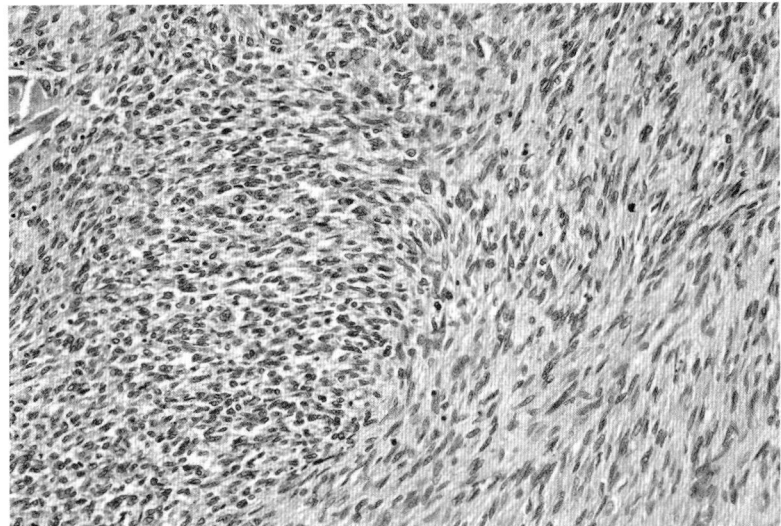

Fig. 35.397
Malignant Triton tumor: this field shows a highly cellular spindle cell tumor with nuclear pleomorphism.

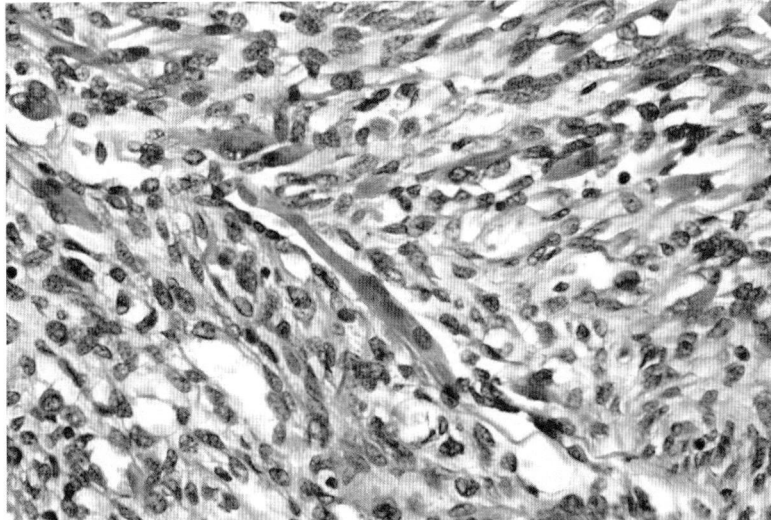

Fig. 35.398
Malignant Triton tumor: there are scattered rhabdomyoblasts with intensely eosinophilic cytoplasm within this poorly differentiated malignant nerve sheath tumor.

Fig. 35.399
Epithelioid malignant peripheral nerve sheath tumor: low-power view of an intensely cellular tumor.

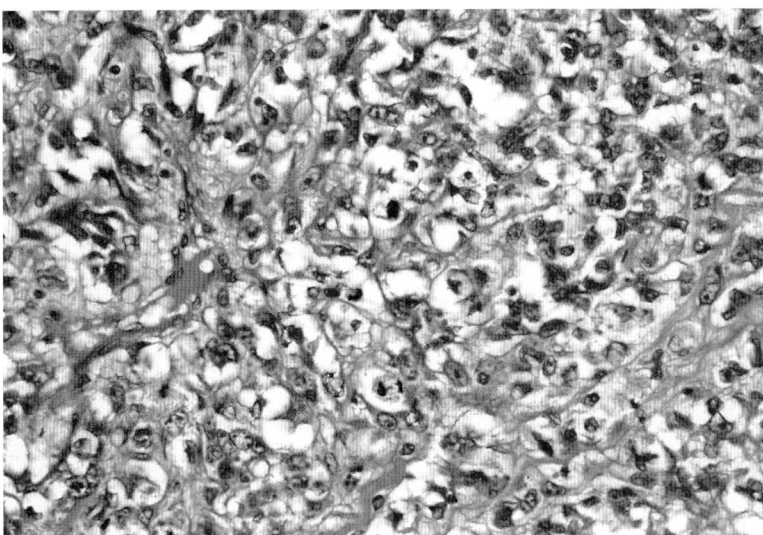

Fig. 35.400
Epithelioid malignant nerve sheath tumor: the marked nuclear and cytoplasmic pleomorphism and conspicuous eosinophilic nucleoli are reminiscent of epithelioid malignant melanoma or poorly differentiated carcinoma.

variably sized areas consisting of plump, round or oval cells with eosinophilic cytoplasm, sometimes arranged in a packeted or trabecular pattern (*Figs 35.399* and *35.400*).[18-21] These cells have an epithelioid appearance not dissimilar to amelanotic melanoma cells. Positivity for S100 protein is strong and diffuse, compared to the weak and patchy reactivity in conventional malignant peripheral nerve sheath tumor and the staining tends to be more diffuse and intense. In subcutaneous lesions, tumor cells tend to be smaller, bluer and more nevoid. INI1 nuclear expression is lost in more than 50% of cases[18,22] and can lead to an erroneous diagnosis of epithelioid sarcoma.

Plexiform malignant peripheral nerve sheath tumor is a dermal and subcutaneous lesion. It has well-defined or infiltrative margins and plexiform appearance, resembling entangled hypercellular nerve trunks.[25] Tumor cells are elongated with wavy vesicular nuclei, and mitotic activity is variable. Necrosis and vascular invasion are not seen.

Malignant melanotic schwannian tumor is discussed under schwannoma.

Differential diagnosis

Conventional malignant peripheral nerve sheath tumor must be distinguished from monophasic synovial sarcoma and fibrosarcoma: the former tends to be at least focally positive for EMA or pankeratin and usually negative for S100 protein; the latter shows a typical herring-bone pattern and is S100 protein negative. In addition, they are both negative for SOX10. The epithelioid variant of malignant peripheral nerve sheath tumor is separated from metastatic melanoma by the negativity of the former for the melanoma markers HMB-45, MelanA and MITF.[21,106] A conventional malignant peripheral nerve sheath tumor may also mimic a melanoma.[107,108] Immunohistochemical nuclear loss of H3K27me must be interpreted with caution as it can be seen in a subset of melanomas, including the desmoplastic variant.[109] CHD4 has been proposed as a potential biomarker in differentiating from cellular schwannoma.[110] It is distinguished from metastatic carcinoma by epithelial markers.

Ewing sarcoma (peripheral primitive neuroectodermal tumor/PNET)

Clinical features

Ewing sarcoma (peripheral primitive neuroectodermal tumor/PNET, Askin tumor, peripheral neuroepithelioma) is exceptionally rare in the skin, but may occur either as a primary or, somewhat more often, as a result of secondary spread.[1-19] Most cases arise in the deep soft tissues of the trunk or limbs in children and young adults, with an equal sex incidence, although the overall age range is wide.

Primary cutaneous and subcutaneous lesions have a predilection for the trunk followed by the lower and upper limbs and head and neck.[6-8,20] Most patients are children or young adults but lesions have been reported in older individuals. Prognosis is generally poor although tumors occurring primarily in the skin and subcutaneous tissue appear to have relatively indolent behavior. Although the series of primary cutaneous tumors reported so far are small and with relatively limited follow-up, recurrences and metastases have been rare.[6-8,13-21]

Pathogenesis and histologic features

The most common rearrangement is t(11;22)(q24;q12) and the fusion product of which is used for diagnostic purposes.[17,22-25] The fusion resulting from the translocation is between Ewing sarcoma *EWSR1* and *FLI1* genes and this results in overexpression of FLI1 protein.[26] While this is the most common fusion event seen in greater than 90 % of cases, more than six substitutes, all members of the ETS superfamily of transcription factors, have been described for *FLI1*, with *ERG* being the most common at around 5%.[27-29] The others are exceedingly rare.[30] Rarely *FUS* can substitute for *EWSR1*. Molecular confirmation of this diagnosis is now routine.[31-34] Non-ETS family substitutes for *FLI1* are covered in the section on Ewing-like tumor below.

Histologically, most tumors are cellular and show a lobular or (less often) trabecular growth pattern with numerous small blood vessels and little or no stroma between cells (*Figs 35.401–35.403*). Confluent areas of necrosis are common. Differences between cases reflect a spectrum of neuroectodermal differentiation.

- At the less differentiated end of the spectrum (Ewing sarcoma), tumor cells have scanty cytoplasm, round nuclei with finely distributed chromatin, and very rare or no rosettes.
- At the other end of the spectrum (neuroepithelioma), tumor cells have more abundant eosinophilic cytoplasm, nuclei have coarser chromatin with more conspicuous nucleoli, and rosettes and perivascular pseudorosettes are often seen.

Cytoplasmic glycogen detected by the PAS stain is more common in Ewing sarcoma.

By immunohistochemistry, tumor cell cytoplasmic membrane stains for an antibody against the MIC-2 protein (CD99) (*Fig. 35.404*).[26] This antibody is less specific than was previously thought and may be positive in tumors entering the differential diagnosis including lymphoblastic lymphoma. A panel of antibodies, however, usually allows accurate distinction. Other markers that may be positive in tumor cells include NSE, synaptophysin, CD57, S100 protein, chromogranin and CAM 5.2.[6] Staining for an antibody against FLI-1 protein is also present in a large number of tumors but is not specific and may be seen in lymphoblastic lymphoma.[26] Positivity

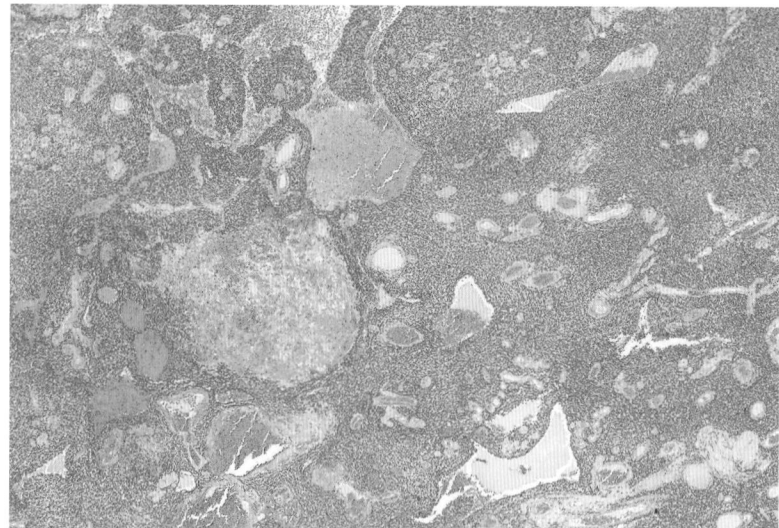

Fig. 35.401
Peripheral primitive neuroectodermal tumor: low-power view of a small blue cell tumor.

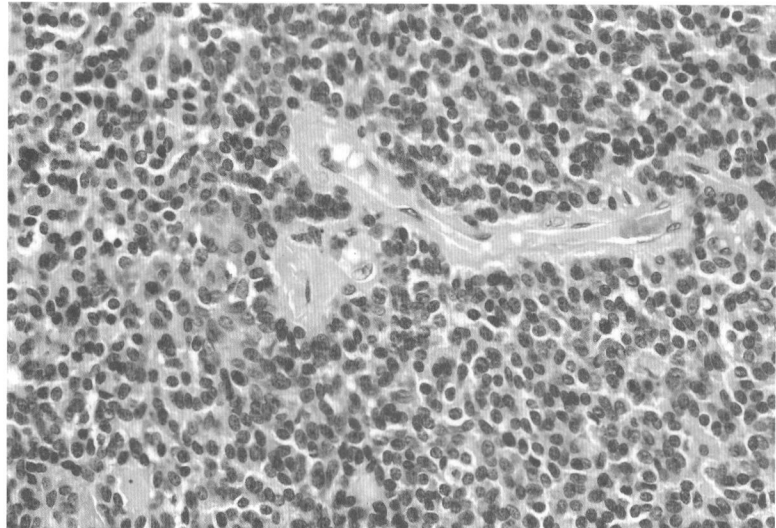

Fig. 35.402
Peripheral primitive neuroectodermal tumor: the tumor cells have hyperchromatic nuclei with ill-defined and minimal cytoplasm.

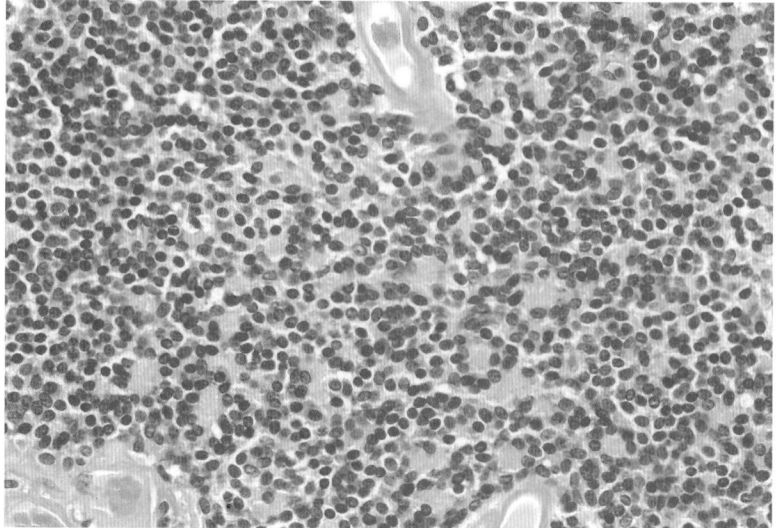

Fig. 35.403
Peripheral primitive neuroectodermal tumor: high-power view showing classical rosettes.

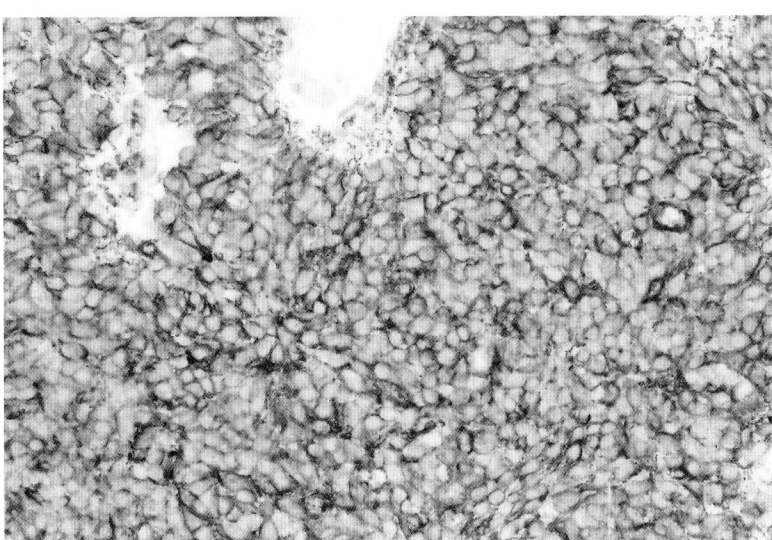

Fig. 35.404
Peripheral primitive neuroectodermal tumor: a variety of CD99 antibodies, notably O13 and MIC-2, have increased diagnostic sensitivity for this tumor. They are, however, by no means specific.

for ERG is not specific as it can be seen in some epithelial and mainly endothelial cell tumors. Variable keratin reactivity is seen in a significant subset of cases and can cause diagnostic confusion for the unwary.[31]

Differential diagnosis

Metastatic neuroblastoma is an important differential diagnosis, especially in children.[35] However, this is CD99 negative. Lymphoblastic lymphoma may on occasions be CD99 positive and leukocyte common antigen (LCA) negative. In such cases the distinction is dependent upon lymphocyte immunophenotyping.[25] A minority of cells in rhabdomyosarcoma (especially the alveolar variant) may be CD99 positive, but the tumor cells also express muscle antigens, and rhabdomyoblasts can usually be identified. Synovial sarcoma, which in the poorly differentiated or round cell variant can mimic Ewing sarcoma, is, negative for both FLI-1 and ERG and harbors an SS18-SSX1 or –SSX2 fusion.

Undifferentiated round cell sarcoma

Undifferentiated round cell sarcoma encompasses two groups of extremely rare usually skeletal, non-Ewing small round cell sarcomas.[1–24] A group in which EWSR1 is involved in non ETS fusions with genes such as NFATC2, SP3, PATZ1, SMARCA5 and POU5F1 and another group with no EWSR1 fusions but a similar molecular profile. In the latter group CIX-DUX4 and BCOR-CCNB3 sarcomas are well described. Both groups show heterogeneous clinical features. Because of their rarity it is not possible to reliably predict their biological behavior. Currently they are treated as Ewing sarcomas, but differences in response to standard therapies and their alternative molecular rearrangements suggest that CIX- and BCOR-rearranged sarcomas are likely distinct entities and could well be designated as such in the next WHO classification.

CIX-rearranged sarcoma

Clinical features

CIX-DUX4 sarcoma is the most common variant of the EWS negative round cell tumors.[3–17] It usually occurs in soft tissue, including superficial locations, particularly in trunk and extremities of young adults with no sex predilection.[8,15] Children may be affected.[6] The clinical course is aggressive and metastases, including lymph nodes are frequent.

Pathogenesis and histologic features

DUX-4 transcribes a DNA binding site that upregulates the ETS family genes.[9] In addition to DUX4, fusions with FOXO4 and NUTM2A have been documented.[3,13]

Histologically, compared to Ewing sarcoma, tumors show more abundant cytoplasm and more prominent nucleoli. Mitotic activity is high and necrosis is commonly noted. Spindle, epithelioid and rhabdoid cell morphology may be encountered. CD99 positivity is variable. WT1 is usually positive.[25] Focal reactivity for keratins and/or desmin may be seen.

BCOR-rearranged sarcoma

Clinical features

BCOR-CCNB3 undifferentiated sarcomas occur primarily in children and young adults. There is a striking male predilection in most series.[26–29] Sites of involvement are relatively evenly distributed between bone and soft tissue. Outcome appears to be similar to Ewing sarcoma and superior to CIC-DUX4 sarcomas.[27]

Pathogenesis and histologic features

The BCOR and CCNB3 genes lie very close to one another on chromosome X. A 10 Mb paracentric inversion on the short arm of this chromosome creates the fusion gene. A KMT2D-BCOR fusion has also been described. BCOR is also involved in undifferentiated sarcomas with internal tandem duplications and BCOR-MAML3 fusion.[30] The relationships of all of these fusions is ongoing, but gene expression profiles suggest relatedness relative to both Ewing sarcoma and CIC-rearranged undifferentiated sarcoma. The tumor cells can be small, round and primitive as in Ewing sarcoma, but distinct spindling is often prominent. Nuclear CCNB3 and BCOR immunoreactivity is strong in pretreatment samples.[28,31–35] The immunoprofile is otherwise not particularly distinctive. CD99 is usually weak or negative. Molecular testing is particularly helpful in diagnosis of this and CIC-rearranged undifferentiated sarcomas.[36]

Clear cell sarcoma of soft tissue/ melanoma of soft parts

Clinical features

Clear cell sarcoma (melanoma of soft parts) is a rare tumor, that usually arises in young adults, shows a predilection for females and occurs most often in the distal extremities, particularly the feet and hands and rarely on the head and neck and vulva.[1–12] Presentation in children is rare.[13] Tumors have also been rarely described in bone, gastrointestinal tract and kidney.[14–17] It presents as a slowly growing, rather deep-seated, nodular mass, often associated with an underlying tendon or aponeurosis. Superficial cutaneous (dermal) and mucosal lesions (including the tongue) are rare mostly described in small series and case reports and in such cases molecular confirmation of the diagnosis is important.[18–27]

This tumor is particularly prone to local recurrence and widespread metastases, commonly many years after the diagnosis of the primary tumor, resulting eventually in death in up to 75% of patients.[1,5,6,28] The rate of local recurrence is around 60%.

Soft tissue melanoma associated with calciphylaxis has been documented.[29]

Pathogenesis and histologic features

Cytogenetic studies in soft tissue melanoma have shown a specific t(12;22) (q13~14;q12~13).[30–33] As a result of this translocation, there is fusion of the Ewing sarcoma (EWSR1) oncogene and the activating transcription factor 1 (ATF1). Expression of the melanocyte-inducing factor – microphthalmia transcription factor (MITF) – is directly induced by the EWSR1/ATF1 fusion protein.[34–36] CREB1 t(2;22)(q33;q12) can substitute for ATF1 in a small subset of cases.[37,38] Fusions of EWSR1 and CREB1 may be more common in the gastrointestinal form of clear cell sarcoma and might be less efficient in promoting melanocytic differentiation.[39] Identical gene fusions are seen in angiomatoid fibrous histiocytoma, but MITF transcription is not induced.[40,41] Gene expression profiles confirm strong melanocytic differentiation in clear cell sarcoma.[42,43] Other neoplasms with the same gene fusions include gastrointestinal (neuroectodermal) clear cell sarcoma (which some consider a distinctive form), angiomatoid fibrous histiocytoma, primary pulmonary myxoid sarcoma, hyalinizing clear cell carcinoma of the salivary

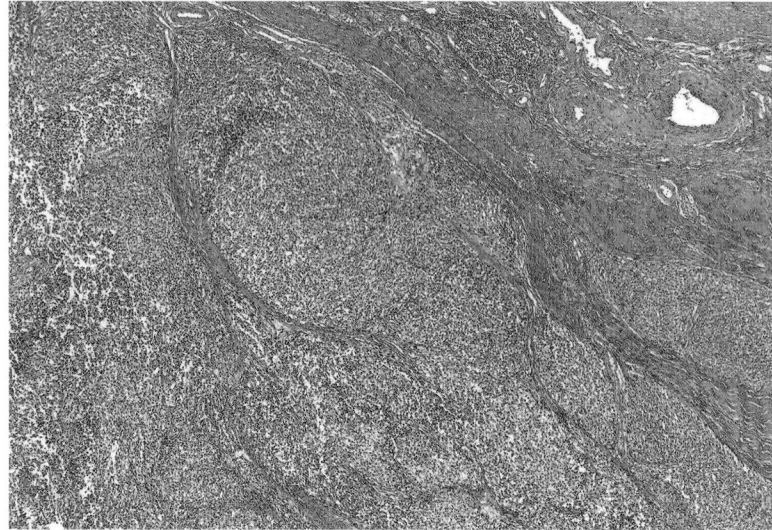

Fig. 35.405
Clear cell sarcoma: the tumor consists of nests of clear cells separated by fibrous septa.

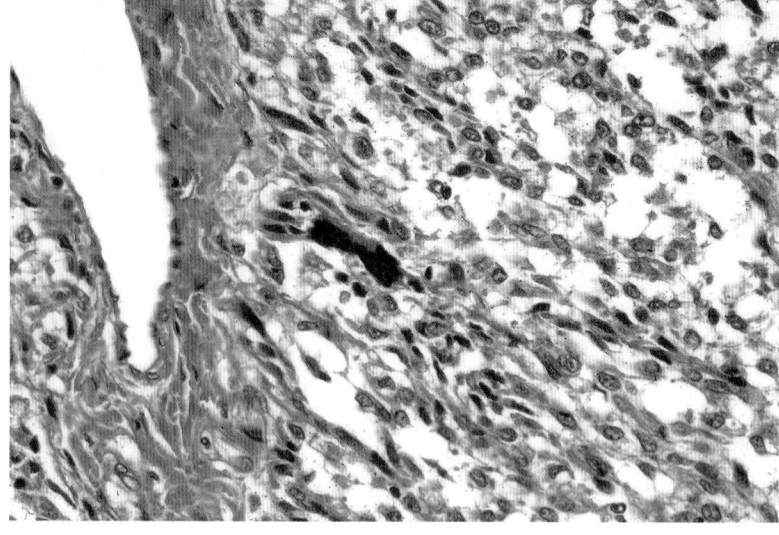

Fig. 35.407
Clear cell sarcoma: paraseptal irregular multinucleate cells are a common feature.

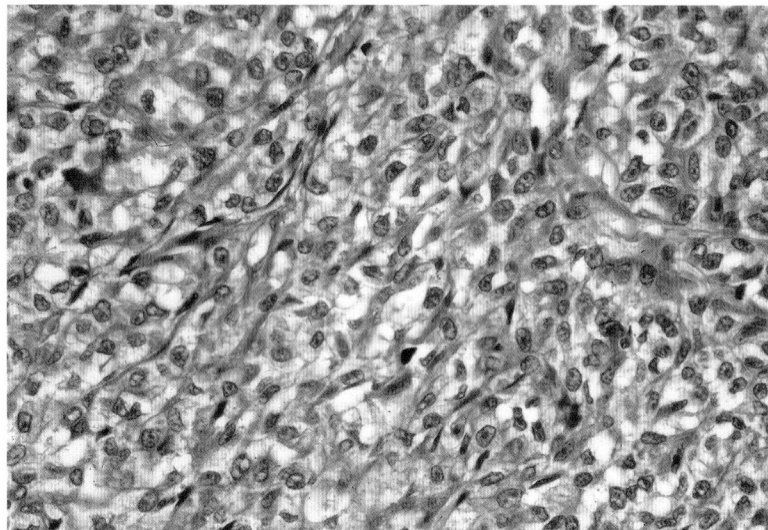

Fig. 35.406
Clear cell sarcoma: the tumor cells have clear cytoplasm and round vesicular nuclei with prominent eosinophilic nucleoli.

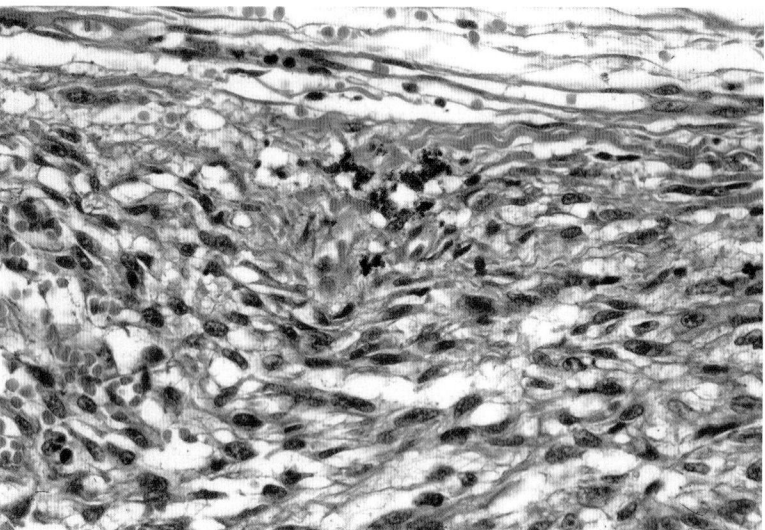

Fig. 35.408
Clear cell sarcoma: this section shows focal melanin pigmentation.

gland, clear cell odontogenic carcinoma, a subset of soft tissue myoepitheliomas, and a recently described novel myxoid mesenchymal tumor with a predilection for intracranial location.[44–46]

A cutaneous tumor with *BRAF* mutation and a subcutaneous lesion with *KIT* mutation have been reported.[47,48]

Recurrent *BCOR* internal tandem duplication (ITD) has been documented in clear cell sarcoma of the kidney which despite the name is unrelated to clear cell sarcoma of soft tissues. It is mentioned here solely for comparison. *BCOR* ITD is also reported in soft tissue round cell sarcoma of infancy.[49,50]

The tumor is typically a well-circumscribed mass composed of nests, fascicles or trabeculae of uniformly fusiform or (less commonly) rounded cells with eosinophilic to clear cytoplasm (*Figs 35.405* and *35.406*). The nuclei are usually vesicular, centrally located and have prominent nucleoli. They are relatively uniform, but otherwise appear identical to those of cutaneous melanoma. Mitotic activity is generally inconspicuous and the nests tend to be separated by delicate fibrous septa, which may impart a spurious alveolar pattern. Frequently scattered throughout the tumor are bland multinucleated giant cells with a wreath-like nuclear arrangement (*Fig. 35.407*). A rare subset of superficial dermal tumors may show an intraepidermal component, further complicating the separation from a melanocytic tumor.[18,25]

About 60% of cases contain variable amounts of melanin pigment, which can be highlighted by special stains (*Fig. 35.408*). Tumor cells are positive for S100 protein, HMB-45, Melan-A, MITF, SOX10, and NSE.[4–6,51,52]

Cyclin D1 has is positive in clear cell sarcoma of the kidney but its diagnostic utility is still uncertain.[53,54]

Ultrastructurally, tumor cells show typical features of melanocytic differentiation with melanosomes.[4]

Differential diagnosis

Occasional cases may bear a striking resemblance to a primary or metastatic melanoma and epithelioid malignant schwannoma (see above). Distinction from the former can be difficult as both tumors share the same immunohistochemical phenotype. However, cutaneous melanomas are usually more superficially located, pleomorphism is more marked and junctional activity is present. Usually metastatic melanoma also shows more mitoses, pleomorphism and necrosis, but in some patients only a careful clinical assessment will allow distinction. Epithelioid malignant schwannoma is HMB-45 and MelanA negative and does not contain melanin pigment.

Molecular confirmation of clear cell sarcoma is extremely helpful in challenging cases, as distinction from melanoma can have staging and treatment implications.

SMOOTH MUSCLE TUMORS

Smooth muscle hamartomas

Congenital smooth muscle hamartoma

Clinical features

Congenital smooth muscle hamartoma is a rare lesion that presents in infants as an indurated, often hyperpigmented macule or plaque with perifollicular papules or coarse hairs.[1–6] There is a slight male predominance and the prevalence has been estimated as 1:2600 live births.[5] Occasional cases have been reported presenting after birth.[7,8] The most frequent location is the lumbosacral area and there is also predilection for the proximal limbs, with rare cases occurring elsewhere including face, volar skin, and the oral cavity.[9–11] Unusual presentations include a linear and atrophic plaque, marked folding of the skin, a reticulate vascular nevus-like appearance, a Michelin tire syndrome-like appearance, and diffuse involvement with hypertrichosis lanuginosa.[12–18] In one case, the presenting sign was myokymia (pseudo-Darier sign).[19] In other cases, a pseudo-Darier sign can rarely be elicited.[20] Unusual sites of presentation include the conjunctival fornix.[21] Occasional patients have multiple lesions and more extensive, generalized involvement.[22,23] Familial cases may occur.[24,25] Acquired cases are exceptional.[26,27] Examples of acquired smooth muscle hamartoma of the genitalia may represent hyperplasia of smooth muscle as a result of chronic scrotal lymphedema.[28,29] Focal changes simulating smooth muscle hamartoma have been documented in a case of port-wine stain.[30]

Histologic features

Histologically, there are numerous haphazardly oriented intradermal bundles of mature smooth muscle (*Figs 35.409* and *35.410*). Hair follicles are normal in number and there is sometimes mild hyperkeratosis, acanthosis and hyperpigmentation of the basal cell layer. A rare association within the same lesion of a congenital melanocytic nevus and a smooth muscle hamartoma has been documented.[31]

Immunohistochemistry shows diffuse staining for SMA, desmin and h-caldesmon.[32]

A close relationship with Becker nevus has been suggested, but the latter is an acquired lesion that appears later in life and shows hypertrichosis, hyperpigmentation and usually only a mild increase in the amount of smooth muscle.[2,6,33]

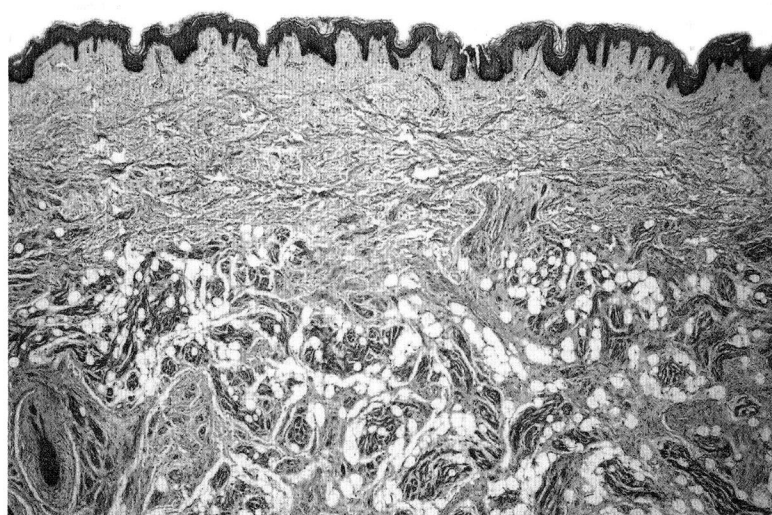

Fig. 35.409
Congenital smooth muscle hamartoma: irregular bundles of smooth muscle are present in the deeper dermis and subcutaneous fat.

Benign smooth muscle tumors

Pilar leiomyoma

Clinical features

Pilar leiomyoma usually presents in young adults, most often on the limbs or trunk (*Figs 35.411* and *35.412*).[1–5] Congenital lesions are probably variants of smooth muscle hamartoma.[6] Occurrence in children is exceptional.[7] Lesions are multiple (rarely hundreds of lesions are seen), small, slowly growing papules generally less than 1 cm in diameter, and typically painful or tender, particularly when compressed or exposed to a cold environment. In the limbs, pilar leiomyomas tend to favor the extensor surfaces. Patients

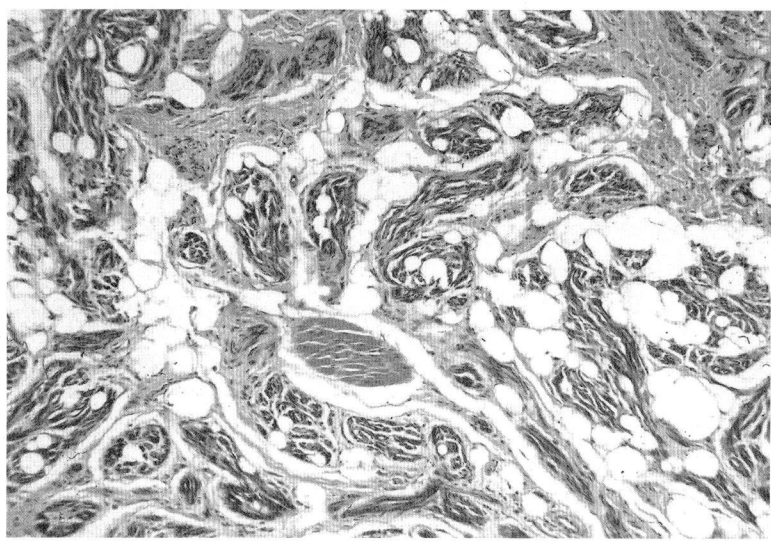

Fig. 35.410
Congenital smooth muscle hamartoma: high-power view.

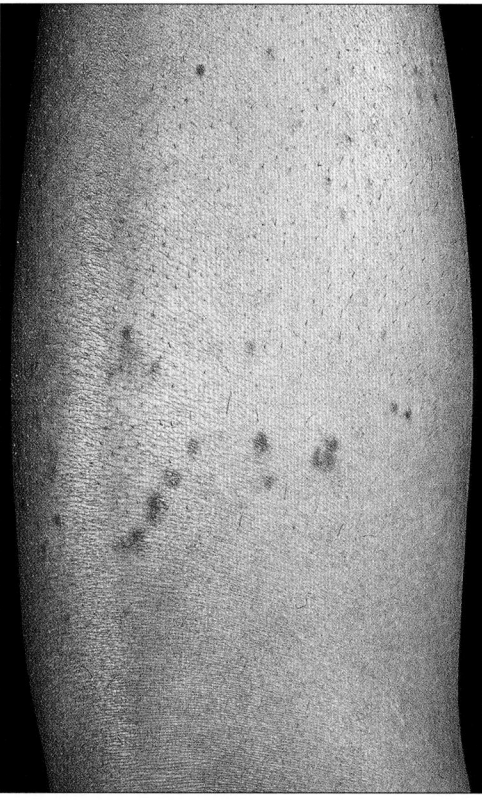

Fig. 35.411
Pilar leiomyoma: multiple erythematous papules are present. By courtesy of the Institute of Dermatology, London, UK.

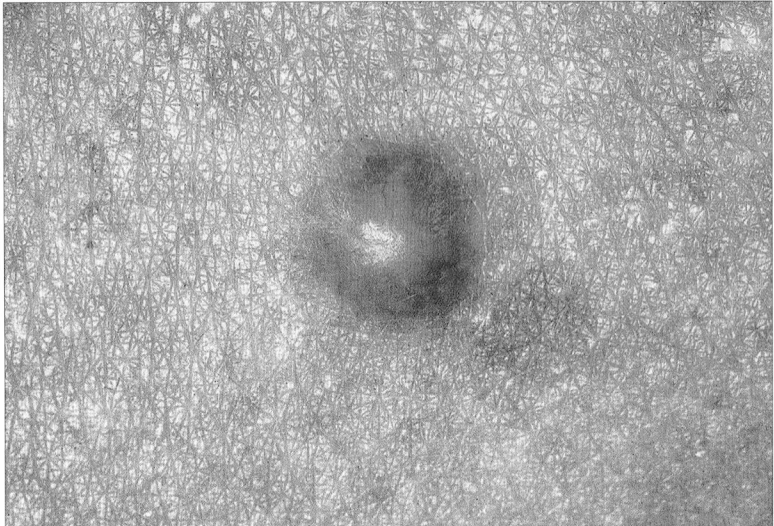

Fig. 35.412
Pilar leiomyoma: close-up view of an erythematous nodule. By courtesy of the Institute of Dermatology, London, UK.

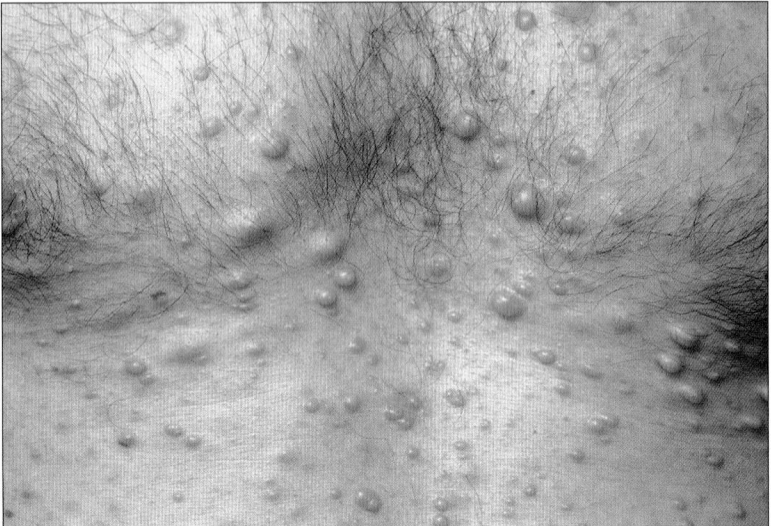

Fig. 35.413
Familial pilar leiomyomas: sometimes, hundreds of lesions may be present. By courtesy of the Institute of Dermatology, London, UK.

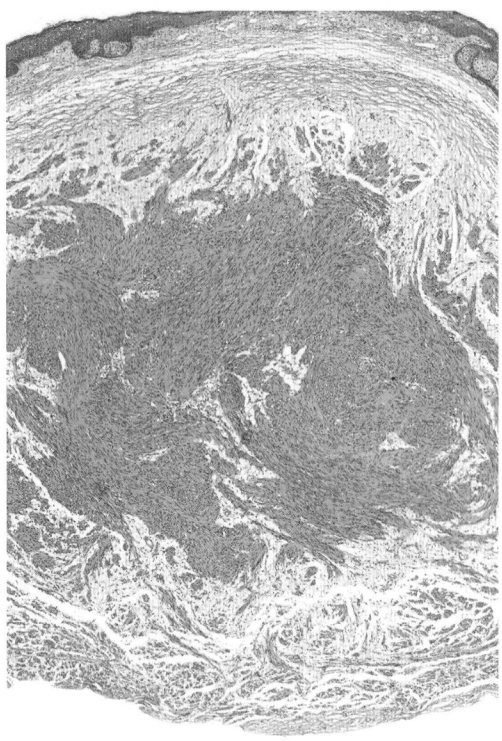

Fig. 35.414
Pilar leiomyoma: within the reticular dermis is an ill-defined tumor composed of broad interlacing fascicles of eosinophilic spindle cells.

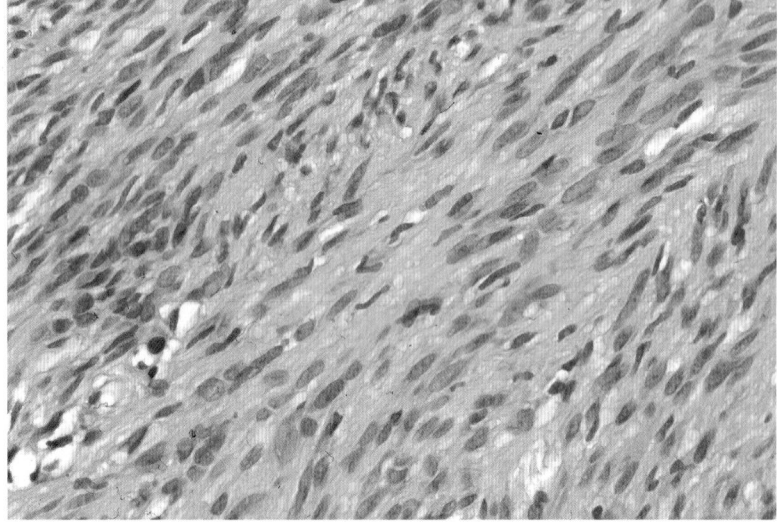

Fig. 35.415
Pilar leiomyoma: the tumor cell nuclei are characteristically cigar shaped.

may present with plaque-like variants or tumors in a zosteriform distribution.[8] Multiple leiomyomas have been described in association with HIV infection, chronic lymphocytic leukemia and erythrocytosis.[9–11]

Recurrence is uncommon after excision, but new lesions may continue to develop over the years. An eruptive case resembling spontaneous eruptive keloids has been reported.[12]

In a small proportion of cases with multiple lesions, there is a positive family history, with an autosomal dominant inheritance (*Fig. 35.413*).[13,14] A case in identical twins has been documented.[15] A segmental distribution may be seen in familial and exceptionally in sporadic cases.[16–20] For many years it was recognized that multiple cutaneous leiomyomas are associated with uterine leiomyomas (MCUL).[21–24] A further association with papillary or collecting duct renal cell cancer was been identified and the syndrome is now termed hereditary leiomyomatosis and renal cell cancer (HLRCC).[24–28] Loss of function in the gene responsible for this syndrome, *FH* (1q42.3~q43), results in fumarate hydratase deficiency.[29–36] Fumarate hydratase, a component of the tricarboxylic acid cycle, acts as a tumor suppressor gene and may be involved in DNA damage response.[37] Although most patients with the syndrome have cutaneous and uterine leiomyomas, renal cancer is only seen in a minority of patients. Interestingly, similar mutations are very rare in sporadic variants.[38,39]

Solitary pilar leiomyomas are less commonly seen and tend to be larger. There is a slight male predominance, with predilection for the limbs.[40–42]

Histologic features

Pilar leiomyomas, which are ill defined and intradermal, usually merge imperceptibly with the surrounding connective tissue (*Figs 35.414* and *35.415*). Only occasional lesions are more nodular. The epidermis is typically unaffected but elongation of the rete ridges and or hyperpigmentation may be seen.[41] Each tumor is composed of uniform interlacing bundles or irregular collections of elongated cells with brightly eosinophilic cytoplasm and blunt-ended or cigar-shaped nuclei. A mature adipocytic component is exceptional.[43] Mitotic figures are only very rarely seen.[5] Focal cytologic atypia due to degeneration may be a feature, similar to that seen in symplastic leiomyomas of the uterus (pilar symplastic or atypical leiomyoma).[44–50] Adequate sampling of these lesions is necessary as changes of otherwise typical leiomyosarcoma may be focally found.[51] Exceptionally, palisading mimicking Verocay bodies, and granular cell change may be evident.[52,53]

Tumor cells are usually uniformly positive for SMA, calponin, desmin and h-caldesmon.

Immunohistochemistry for fumarate hydratase (negative staining) has been suggested to identify patients with MCUL and HLRCC.[54] However, the sensitivity and specificity of this test in the published series was only of 83.3% and 75%, respectively.[54] In a further study by the same authors, it has been suggested that anti S-(2-Succino)-Cysteine staining (positive as opposed to negative fumarate hydratase in suspected cases) increases the diagnostic accuracy in around 19% of cases.[55]

Differential diagnosis

The clinical history, particularly in cases with multiple lesions, often makes the diagnosis straightforward. Distinction from dermatofibroma is afforded by the leiomyoma's uniform cell content and configuration in addition to desmin and SMA positivity. Cellular neurofibroma is S100 protein positive and lacks the eosinophilic cytoplasm, myofibrils and blunt-ended nuclei of leiomyoma. Differentiation from cutaneous leiomyosarcoma (atypical intradermal smooth muscle neoplasm) is based on the presence of mitoses and the usually greater nuclear pleomorphism in the latter tumor. When pyknotic nuclei are present staining with Ki67 and/or phosphohistone-H3 may be of help to identify proliferating cells or those undergoing mitosis respectively.[56] In addition S100A6 has been found to be weak or absent in leiomyoma and strongly positive in cutaneous leiomyosarcoma (atypical intradermal smooth muscle neoplasm).[57]

Genital leiomyoma

Clinical features

Genital leiomyoma originates from the superficial smooth muscle of the scrotum, vulva or nipple.[1-5] Traditionally, such cases have been classified as variants of pilar leiomyoma. This is appropriate for nipple lesions, but scrotal and vulval tumors show different pathological features. They are uncommon, tend to be larger and are better circumscribed. They usually present in middle-aged adults. Multiple leiomyomas of the vulva may be a sign of Alport syndrome.[3]

A pericentric inversion (12)(p12q13–14) has been described in a single case of vulval leiomyoma.[6]

Histologic features

Nipple leiomyoma is histologically identical to lesions arising elsewhere on the integument (*Fig. 35.416*). Scrotal leiomyomas, however, which arise from the dartos muscle, tend to be quite cellular and often show a focal mononuclear inflammatory cell infiltrate (*Fig. 35.417*). Cytologic atypia as present in symplastic leiomyoma may be seen but mitotic figures are exceptional (bizarre leiomyoma)[5,7,8] Vulval leiomyomas arise in the labia majora and commonly display myxoid change and hyalinization.[9] Epithelioid cell change may also be a feature.[6] Scrotal leiomyomas express androgen receptor.[10]

Malignant smooth muscle tumors

Leiomyosarcoma

Clinical features

Leiomyosarcoma accounts for a significant proportion of superficial soft tissue sarcomas, although it is more common in a deep location, being most prevalent in the abdomen or retroperitoneum.[1-5] The superficial tumors can be divided into two clinical groups:

- cutaneous leiomyosarcoma, which includes leiomyosarcoma of the nipple. The term atypical intradermal smooth muscle neoplasm was introduced in 2011 to include tumors previously classified as atypical (symplastic) leiomyoma and leiomyosarcoma that are primarily confined to the dermis with no or superficial extension to the subcutaneous tissue and indolent biological behavior (see below). However, this term has not been universally accepted.

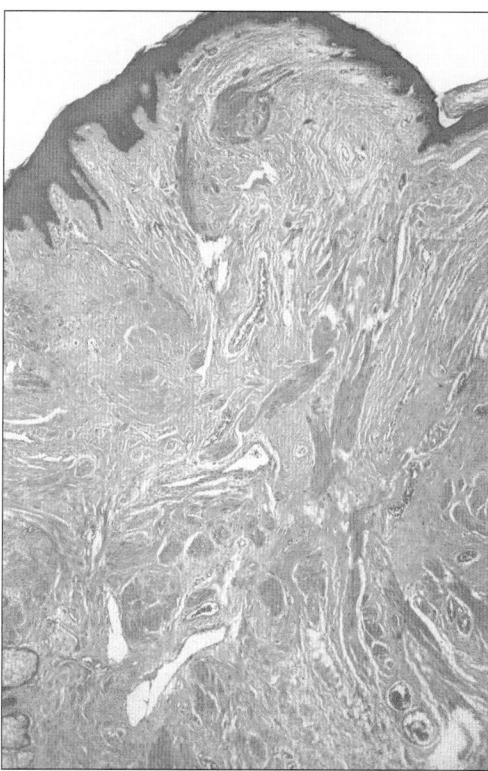

Fig. 35.416
Nipple leiomyoma: as with the pilar variant, the tumor is composed of a poorly circumscribed proliferation of mature smooth muscle cell infiltrate.

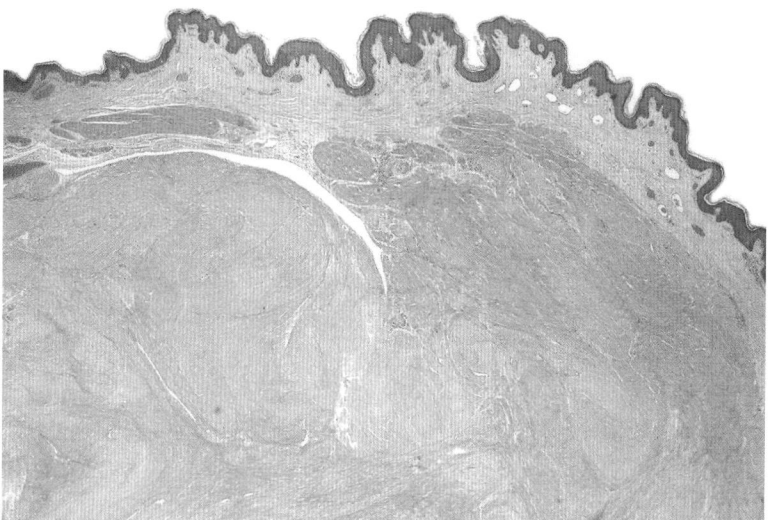

Fig. 35.417
Scrotal leiomyoma: note the circumscription and multinodularity.

- subcutaneous leiomyosarcoma, which includes vulval and scrotal variants.[7]

Cutaneous lesions are usually solitary, derived from or differentiating towards the arrector pili muscle and arise most often in young to middle-aged adults, with a predilection for males.[2-4,6,8-13] The trunk and the limbs, especially the lower leg, are most often affected, followed by the head and neck and the tumor can be painful. Local recurrence is commonly seen, but metastasis is very rare.[6,14-23] The margin status of the primary tumor seems to be the strongest predictive factor of recurrence [6,18,19] A wide excision with at least 1 cm or Mohs micrographic surgery followed by long term follow-up are considered the best treatment options.[24-31]

Subcutaneous leiomyosarcomas are very closely related to deeper leiomyosarcomas of soft tissues.[2,3,8,32] They arise most often in the fifth to seventh decades, usually in the limbs (especially the thigh) and are larger than dermal lesions. Occasional cases arise from a vein wall. There is a slight predilection for males. Local recurrence is common, and in the long term around 50% of tumors metastasize, with a mortality rate of between

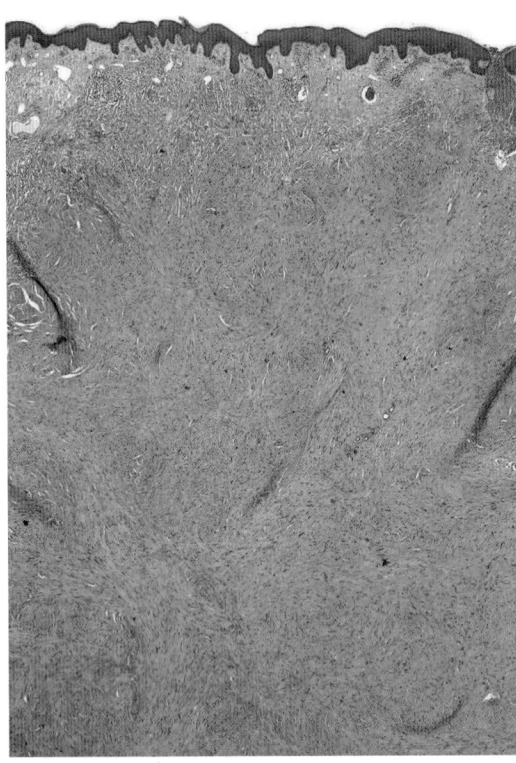

Fig. 35.418
Leiomyosarcoma: extending up to the papillary dermis is a spindled cell tumor.

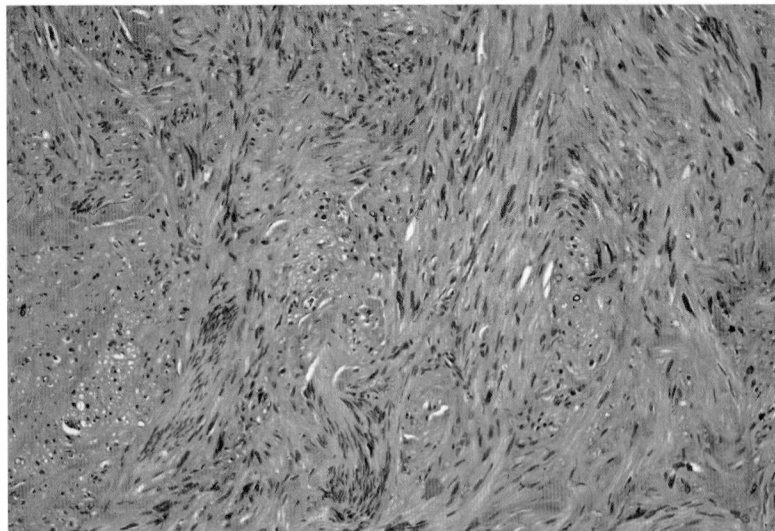

Fig. 35.419
Leiomyosarcoma: as with its benign counterpart, the spindled cells exhibit marked eosinophilia.

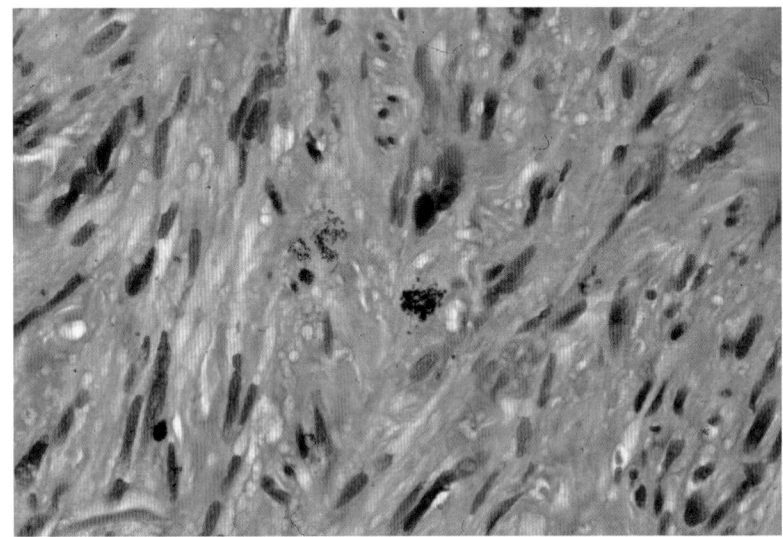

Fig. 35.420
Leiomyosarcoma: note the presence of marked mitotic activity.

30% and 50%.[11] The subcutaneous location and size are associated with aggressiveness.[33] Tumor size greater than 5 cm is associated with a poor prognosis.[11] Vulval and scrotal tumors appear to have a better prognosis than lesions arising at other sites.[6,34,35]

Exceptionally, leiomyosarcoma has been documented at the site of radiation dermatitis, in a pacemaker pocket, in a tattoo, in a scrofuloderma and in a smallpox scar, in a nevus sebaceous and in association with a chronic venous ulcer.[36–43] Giant and rapidly growing lesions may occur especially in the face.[44–46] A case with skip-lesion behavior has been reported.[47] Cutaneous leiomyosarcoma in childhood is very rare.[48]

Association with hereditary leiomyomatosis and renal cell carcinoma (HLRCC) with Li-Fraumeni (Reed) Syndrome and hereditary retinoblastoma are well documented.[6,49–54] In addition, an increased risk has been found in HIV-infected patients.[55] Epstein-Barr virus–associated cases in patients with HIV have been reported.[56–58]

Metastatic sarcoma to the skin is rare, but leiomyosarcoma is the most common sarcoma to do so and usually presents as a rapidly growing mass with predilection for the scalp and with most cases arising from the genitourinary tract rather than other soft tissues.[59–70] In a single case, the patient presented with hemorrhagic bullae.[71]

Histologic features

Cutaneous tumors tend to present as an ill-defined diffuse lesion in contrast to the well-circumscribed, more nodular subcutaneous variant. Both, however, are locally infiltrative tumors composed of interlacing bundles of smooth muscle cells with eosinophilic cytoplasm and blunt-ended, cigar-shaped, often vesicular nuclei (Figs 35.418 and 35.419). Nuclear palisading and tandem alignment are not uncommon. Significant cytological pleomorphism (even to the point of mimicking so-called pleomorphic malignant fibrous histiocytoma, MFH) is more common in subcutaneous than cutaneous variants (Fig. 35.420). Prominent pleomorphism in dermal tumors is generally a feature of metastatic lesions, particularly from the uterus.[72–74] Primary cutaneous lesions with prominent pleomorphism might be more aggressive as are those that extend into the subcutis even if the extension is minimal.[75] Most cases are usually diffusely or more uncommonly focally positive for SMA, calponin, desmin and h-caldesmon (Fig. 35.421).[8,76,77] Very focal keratin positivity has also been documented.[78] By

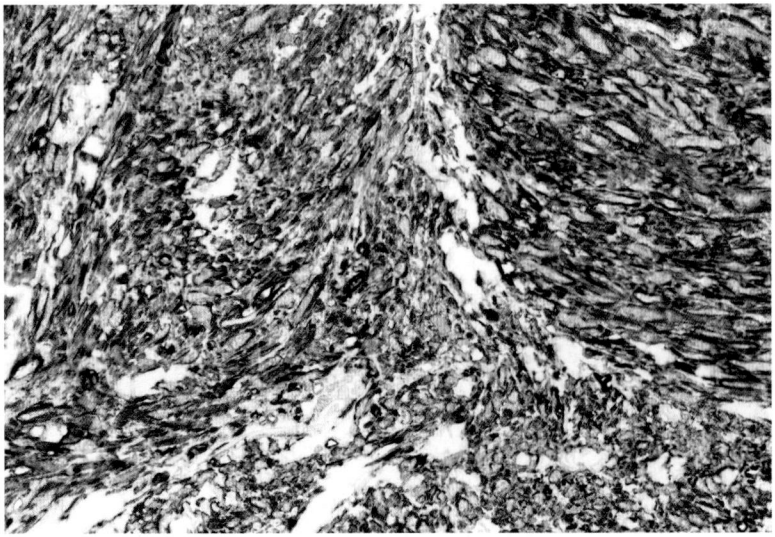

Fig. 35.421
Leiomyosarcoma: the tumor cells show strong h-caldesmon expression.

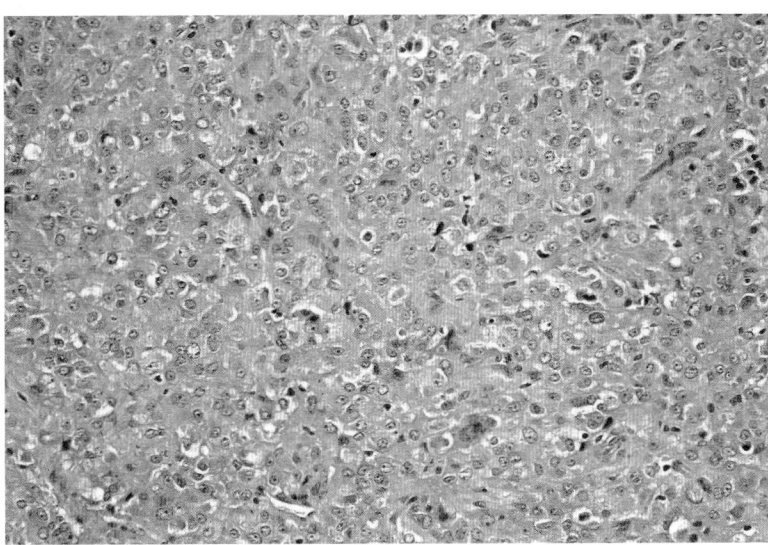

Fig. 35.422
Epithelioid leiomyosarcoma: in this variant, the tumor cells are epithelioid with abundant eosinophilic cytoplasm and vesicular nuclei with prominent nucleoli.

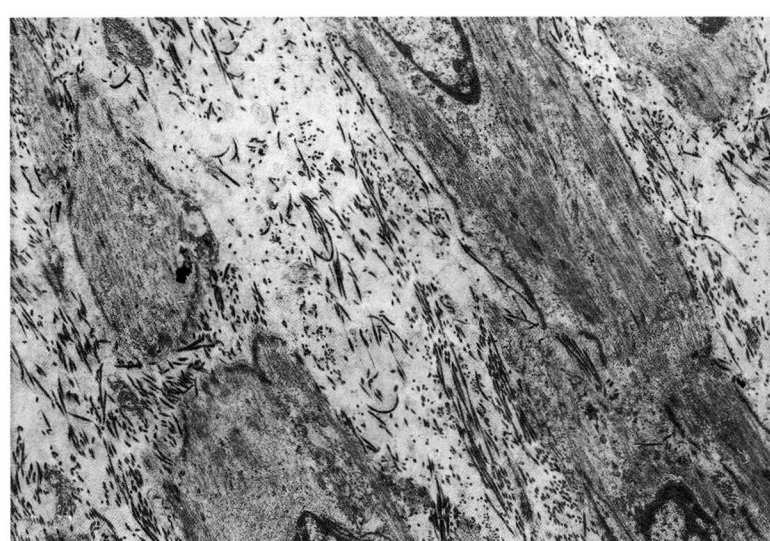

Fig. 35.424
Leiomyosarcoma: note the presence of abundant actin filaments.

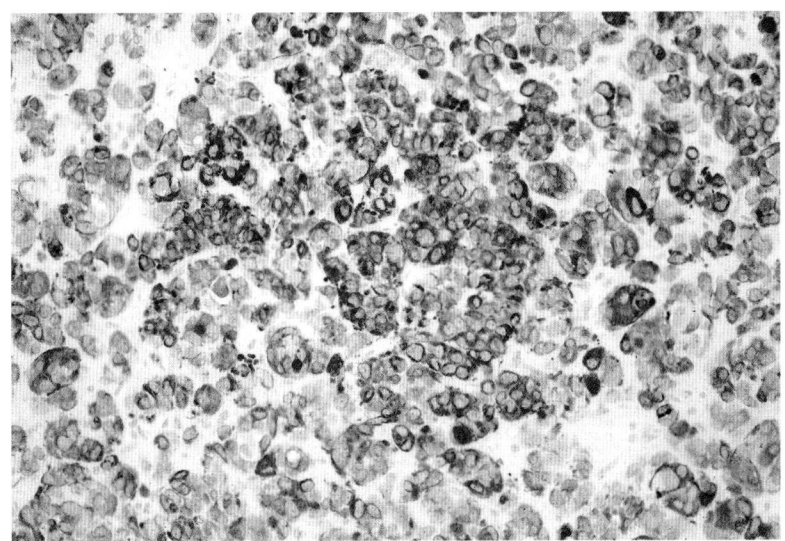

Fig. 35.423
Epithelioid leiomyosarcoma: the tumor cells express desmin.

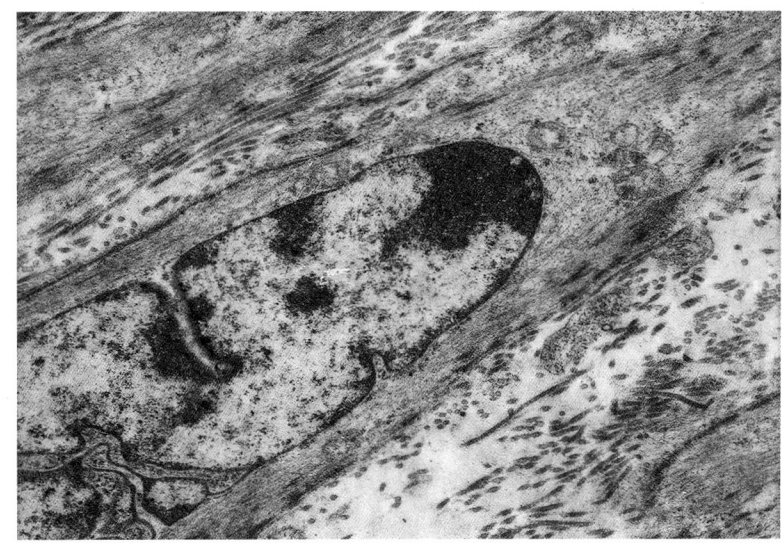

Fig. 35.425
Leiomyosarcoma: high-power view showing focal densities characteristic of smooth muscle differentiation.

immunohistochemistry, PTEN is lost in a majority of cases suggesting a possible pathogenetic molecular mechanism.[79] Periodic acid-Schiff staining may demonstrate perinuclear glycogen vacuoles. Cutaneous and subcutaneous leiomyosarcomas lesions can rarely be predominantly epithelioid or show granular cell change (*Figs 35.422* and *35.423*).[80–83] A mature adipocytic component may be seen.[84] Prominent desmoplasia has also been documented in rare cases.[85–90] In addition, subcutaneous variants sometimes display myxoid change, hyalinization, admixed osteoclastic giant cells and an inflammatory cell infiltrate.[91]

Although leiomyosarcoma may bear a close resemblance to benign leiomyoma, the former usually shows variable pleomorphism with at least mild cytologic atypia and mitotic activity. It has been suggested that positivity for p53 in a large number of cells supports a diagnosis of leiomyosarcoma.[92–95] Other markers such as Ki67 and S100A6 may be of help (see also above).[96,97] Necrosis and hemorrhage are more common in subcutaneous variants and are also suggestive of malignancy. Primary cutaneous tumors are most often grade 1 lesions. Subcutaneous extension is usually limited and superficial. Tumors either infiltrate the fibrous septa or extend into the adipose tissue typically with pushing margins. Recurrent tumors may show more cytologic atypia, and are more often associated with necrosis compared with their primary counterparts. In addition, they often show a diffuse or nodular pattern and more extensive infiltration of the subcutaneous tissue. Nevertheless, none of the histologic features seem to correlate with adverse biological behavior.[6]

The tumor cells may be identified ultrastructurally by the presence of actin filaments with focal densities (*Figs 35.424* and *35.425*).

Differential diagnosis

Differential diagnosis is usually not problematic. Spindle cell melanoma can look remarkably similar to leiomyosarcoma, especially in an acral location, but the growth pattern in the former is more infiltrative, pleomorphism is usually more prominent and S100 protein is positive whereas muscle markers are negative. Similarly, epithelioid variants of leiomyosarcoma can be distinguished from melanoma and carcinoma by immunohistochemistry. Distinction from the cellular variant of fibrous histiocytoma and cellular schwannoma has already been discussed in the representative sections. Metastatic leiomyosarcoma also enters the differential diagnosis. This typically presents as a distinct nodule showing nuclear pleomorphism and mitotic activity (*Figs 35.426* and *35.427*). Clinicopathological correlation is essential to establish the correct diagnosis.

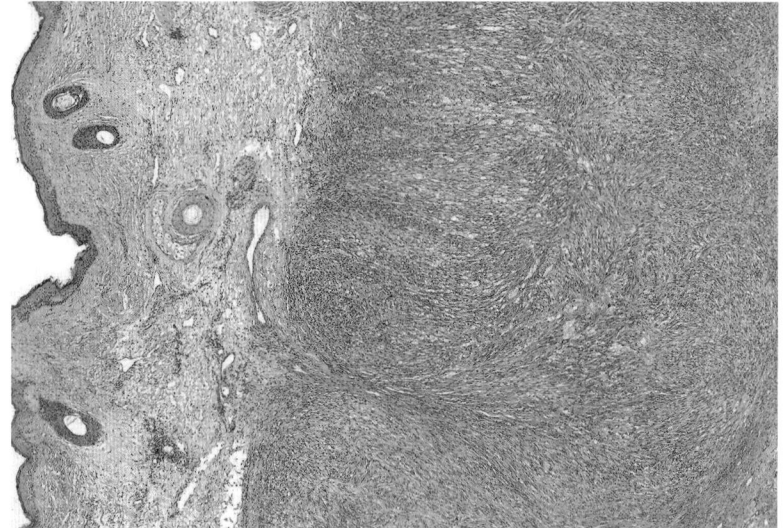

Fig. 35.426
Metastatic leiomyosarcoma: metastatic deposits are characteristically nodular and well circumscribed.

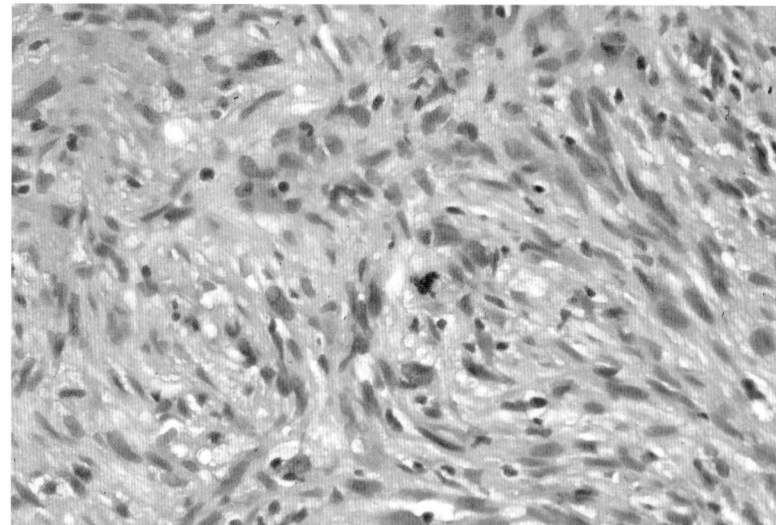

Fig. 35.427
Metastatic leiomyosarcoma: note the nuclear pleomorphism and abnormal mitosis.

STRIATED MUSCLE TUMORS

Striated muscle hamartomas hamartomas

Rhabdomyomatous mesenchymal hamartoma

Clinical features

Rhabdomyomatous mesenchymal hamartoma (also known as striated muscle hamartoma) is a very rare congenital lesion.[1–8] It presents in neonates and infants as one or more polypoid lesions simulating skin tags in the head and neck region (including intraoral lesions), especially on the central face.[9–14] Exceptional cases have been described in the perianal area, sacral area vagina, sternoclavicular area and on a digit.[15–19] Unusual clinical presentations include subcutaneous lesions, a case resembling morphea 'en coup de sabre,' one mimicking a basal cell carcinoma and another presenting as a plaque.[20–25] Multiple lesions are exceptional and a bilobulated case has been described.[26,27] Occasional cases have been associated with other congenital abnormalities including cleft lip, preauricular sinuses, sclerocorneas, low-set ears, thyroglossal sinus, colobomata, dermoid cysts, microphthalmia, spinal dysraphism, and meningocele.[7,8,28–30] It appears that some of the lesions seen in Delleman syndrome (oculocerebrocutaneous syndrome) represent rhabdomyomatous mesenchymal hamartomas.[28] Spontaneous regression has been documented.[19,31]

Histologic features

The lesions are characterized by multiple bundles of mature striated muscle admixed with variable amounts of fat and fibrous tissue in the reticular dermis.

Differential diagnosis

Distinction from accessory tragus can be made by the usual acral clinical location, histologic absence of striated muscle and the presence of cartilage in the latter condition.

Benign striated muscle tumors

Rhabdomyoma (extracardiac)

Clinical features

Extracardiac rhabdomyomas are very uncommon, usually deep-seated lesions and therefore rarely present to the dermatologist.[1–4]

- Genital type usually occurs in middle-aged women mainly in the vagina or cervix and only rarely in the vulva but may present in men most often in the spermatic cord, tunica vaginalis, and paratesticular soft tissue. The sclerosing variant seems to affect younger patients predominantly men.[5–10]
- The adult type typically arises in the head and neck region, mainly in the oral cavity and in soft tissue of the neck, and shows predilection for middle-aged or elderly males.[2,5,11–14] Occurrence in children is exceptional.[15] Laryngeal and para or pharyngeal and esophageal lesions may occur.[5,16–22] Multifocal lesions are sometimes seen.[5,23,24] Unusual sites include the lip and the extremities.[25,26] Recurrence is exceptional.[27] A case of multiple cutaneous lesions on the trunk of a child has been documented.[28] Recently, with the use of a monoclonal antibody specific for the cardiac isoform of α-actin, it has been shown that extracardiac rhabdomyomas differentiate towards mature skeletal muscle while cardiac rhabdomyomas reflect true cardiac muscle differentiation.[29]
- The fetal type presents in infants, with male predilection.[3] The great majority occur on the face and neck, with particular predilection for preauricular or retroauricular and periorbital regions. Involvement of the upper respiratory tract and intraoral lesions may also occur.[30,31] Other sites include chest, abdomen, pelvis, and extremities.[5] Genital lesions are exceptional.[32,33] There is an association with nevoid basal cell carcinoma syndrome.[34,35] A case associated with tuberous sclerosis has been reported.[36] Most tumors involve children less than 1 year of age and some are congenital. Occurrence in older children is very rare.[32] Cutaneous case have been described.[37,38]

Pathogenesis and histologic features

Genital type

A proliferation of spindle or strap-shaped cells with abundant eosinophilic cytoplasm containing cross striations embedded in a fibrous stroma is typically seen. Pleomorphism or mitotic activity are not seen. A sclerosing variant characterized by a dense collagenous stroma has been identified mainly in males in a paratesticular location, and rarely in women.[8,10]

Adult type

A case with a t(15;17)(q24;p13) has been reported.[5]

The adult type is composed almost entirely of large, round, polygonal or strap-shaped cells with plentiful eosinophilic cytoplasm (rhabdomyoblasts)[2]

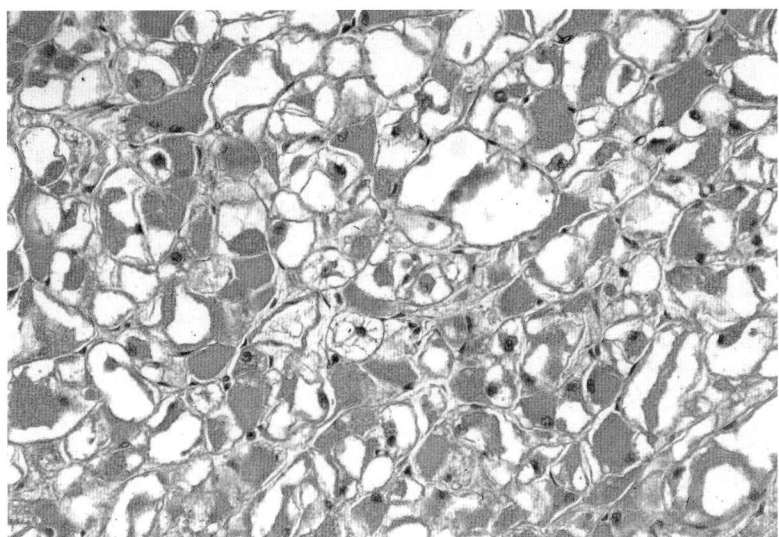

Fig. 35.428
Rhabdomyoma: the adult-type lesion is composed of large polygonal cells with copious eosinophilic cytoplasm and peripherally located nuclei without pleomorphism.

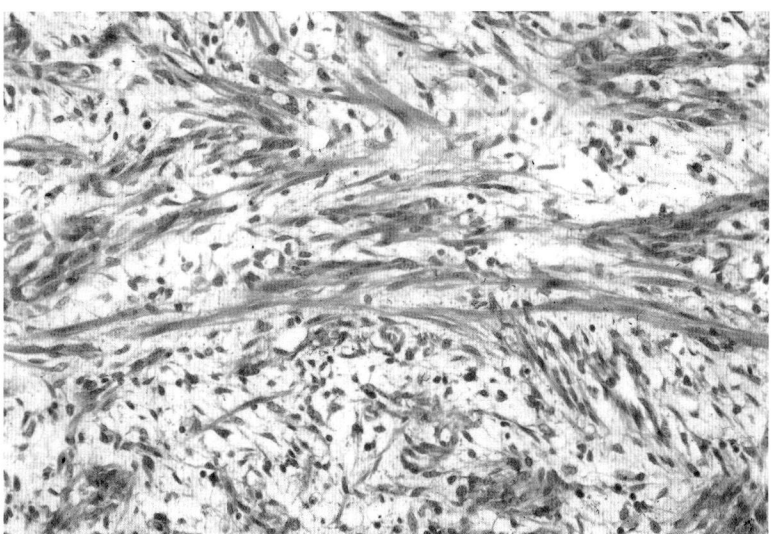

Fig. 35.430
Fetal rhabdomyoma: this example of the fetal myxoid type is composed of obvious elongated strap cells set in a loose myxoid stroma.

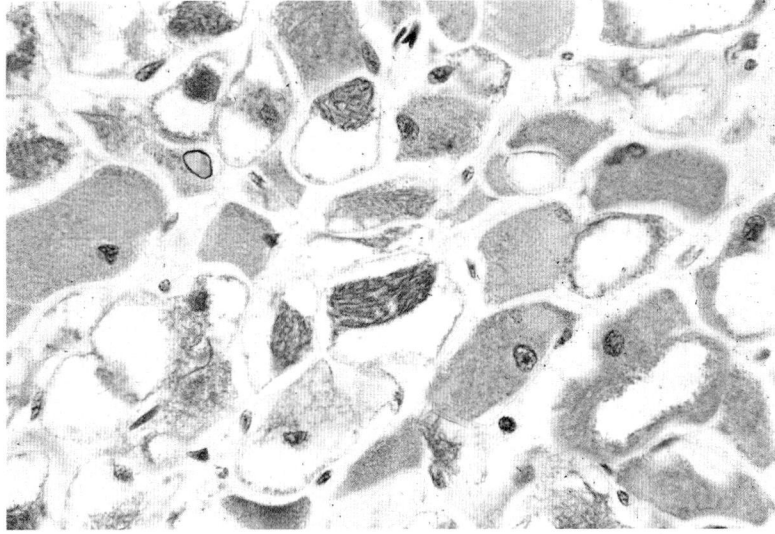

Fig. 35.429
Rhabdomyoma: in the center of the field are pathognomonic 'jack straw' intracytoplasmic inclusions.

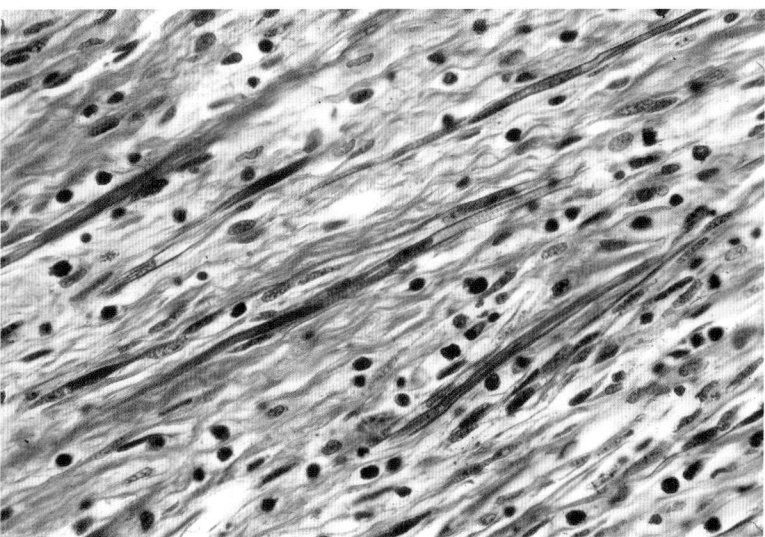

Fig. 35.431
Fetal rhabdomyoma: typical cross-striations are evident (phosphotungstic acid–hematoxylin).

(*Fig. 35.428*). Cross-striations are readily identifiable and rod-like inclusions are commonly present (*Fig. 35.429*). Oncocytic change is exceptional.[39]

Immunohistochemistry shows positivity for muscle-specific actin, myoglobin and desmin.[2] Very focal positivity for S100 protein and SMA may also be seen.[2]

Fetal type

Aberrations at the PTCH1 locus suggesting a role for the activated Hedgehog signaling in the pathogenesis of fetal rhabdomyoma have been documented.[40]

The fetal type is composed almost entirely of immature round to spindle-shaped rhabdomyoblasts in a myxoid stroma, showing progressive maturation towards more eosinophilic cells (which often show cross-striations) peripherally (*Figs 35.430* and *35.431*).

Immunohistochemistry shows positivity of tumor cells for muscle-specific actin, myoglobin and desmin.[3] Focal positivity for SMA, GFAP and S100 protein may be evident.[3]

Differential diagnosis

Distinction of any of these lesions from rhabdomyosarcoma is made possible by their lack of mitotic activity, nuclear pleomorphism or infiltrative growth pattern.

Malignant striated muscle tumors

Rhabdomyosarcoma

Rhabdomyosarcoma very rarely presents to the dermatologist, first because the tumor itself is rare, and second because it seldom arises in the dermis, albeit that occasional cutaneous metastases do occur.[1–6] Traditionally, four main subtypes have been described:[7] embryonal (including the botryoid variant), alveolar, pleomorphic and spindle cell/sclerosing. A further very rare epithelioid variant has been recently documented.[8–10] The first two, are the most common.[11–13]

Clinical features

Rhabdomyosarcoma presenting in the skin either as a primary tumor or as a metastasis is extremely rare, accounting for only 0.7% of all

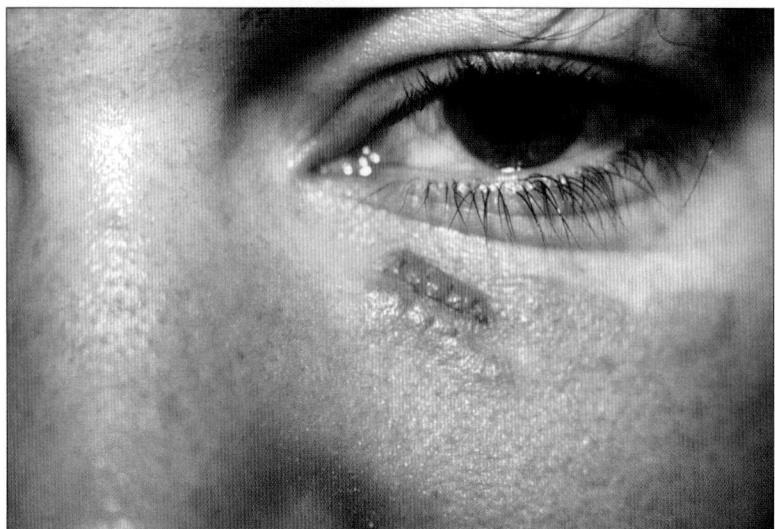

Fig. 35.432
Cutaneous rhabdomyosarcoma: presentation in the skin is exceptional and occurs in children. This was an embryonal variant. By courtesy of the Institute of Dermatology, London, UK.

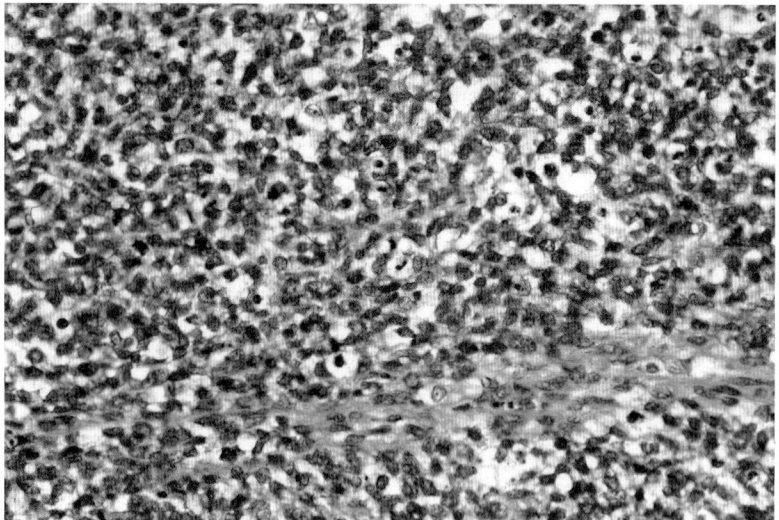

Fig. 35.433
Embryonal rhabdomyosarcoma: an example of undifferentiated rhabdomyosarcoma. The tumor cells are small and contain basophilic nuclei. Diagnosis depends upon immunocytochemistry or identifying more typical rhabdomyoblasts elsewhere in the specimen.

rhabdomyosarcomas (*Fig. 35.432*).[1–3,9,14–26] In the documented cutaneous cases there is a slight male predominance, a predilection for the head and neck, a bimodal age distribution (with a mean age of 10 years for pediatric cases and of 74 years for adult cases) at presentation. The alveolar followed by the embryonal are the most common histologic subtypes in the pediatric population whereas the pleomorphic variant is much more common in adults.[9] Cases associated with epidermal nevus syndrome have been reported.[27,28] Information about the prognosis of cutaneous lesions is extremely limited but potential for an aggressive course has been reported.[9] Although the data available for epithelioid rhabdomyosarcoma are limited, 4 of 18 cases occurred in a superficial location with an equal sex distribution and a mean age of 69.5 years.[10]

Pathogenesis and histologic features

At the molecular genetic level, the alveolar type is characterized by a t(2;13) (q35;q14) and less frequently a t(1;13) (p36;q14) fusing *PAX3* or *PAX7*, respectively, with *FOXO1A*.[13,29–32] More recently, *NCOA1* (2p23) and *AFX/FOXO4* (Xq13.1) have been shown to substitute for *FOXO1A* and pair with *PAX3* on rare occasion.[33,34] *PAX3-FOXO1* tumors seem to have a worst prognosis compared to *PAX7-FOXO1* tumors.[35] In a subset of lesions rearrangements similar to those seen in low grade liposarcoma (MDM2 and CDK4) have been identified.[36]

Embryonal lesions usually have 11p deletions amongst other cytogenetic aberrations.[11]

8q 13 rearrangements resulting in *SRF-NCOA2* and *TEAD1-NCOA2* fusion genes have been identified in spindle cell rhabdomyosarcoma.[37] A recurrent neomorphic *MYOD1* mutation correlates with worse prognosis.[38] Pleomorphic rhabdomyosarcoma shows a complex karyotype.[39,40]

Embryonal type

The embryonal type is composed largely of small round or spindle-shaped undifferentiated cells, often arranged loosely in a myxoid stroma.[11] Obvious rhabdomyoblasts are variably prominent and show eosinophilic cytoplasm with a 'strap' or 'tadpole' shape (*Figs 35.433–35.435*). Variants of this type of rhabdomyosarcoma include botryoid, spindle cell and anaplastic.

Alveolar type

The alveolar variant is typified by tumor cells arranged in discrete nests separated by fibrous septa and with an alveolar pattern of cellular dissociation at the center of the cellular aggregates (*Figs 35.436* and *35.437*).[11] Some cases, however, have an almost entirely solid growth pattern (*Fig. 35.438*). Tumor cells tend to be relatively large and rounded or readily recognizable

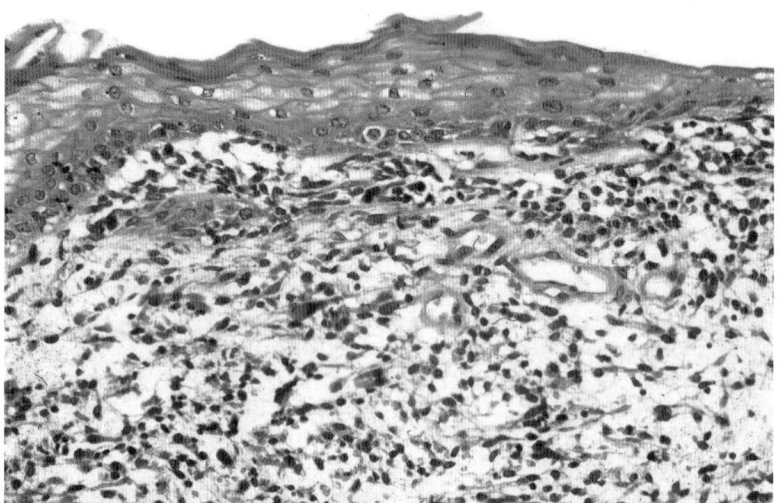

Fig. 35.434
Embryonal rhabdomyosarcoma: beneath the epithelium is an infiltrate of small basophilic cells, and there are also occasional primitive rhabdomyoblasts with more obvious eosinophilic cytoplasm.

as rhabdomyoblasts, and may be arranged as delicate papillae, solid clumps or lying free within each cell nest. Nuclei are larger and more hyperchromatic than in the embryonal type. Multinucleated (wreath-like) giant cells are a common feature (*Fig. 35.439*). Epidermotropism has been documented in a case of primary alveolar rhabdomyosarcoma.[6] Alveolar-type histology can be seen in cases lacking characteristic fusion genes. Whether these cases are more similar to embryonal or fusion-positive alveolar cases genetically and clinically is currently debated in the literature.[41–43]

Pleomorphic type

The pleomorphic type is a heterogeneous tumor characterized by bizarre spindled cells admixed with readily recognizable polygonal rhabdomyoblasts, often in large numbers (*Fig. 35.440*).[11] This variant is largely confined to adults and is almost unknown in the skin.[44]

Immunohistochemistry is very useful in the diagnosis of rhabdomyosarcoma because tumor cells tend to be at least focally positive for desmin, muscle-specific actin (HHF-35), and the more diagnostically specific myogenin and MyoD1 (*Fig. 35.441*).[11,12]

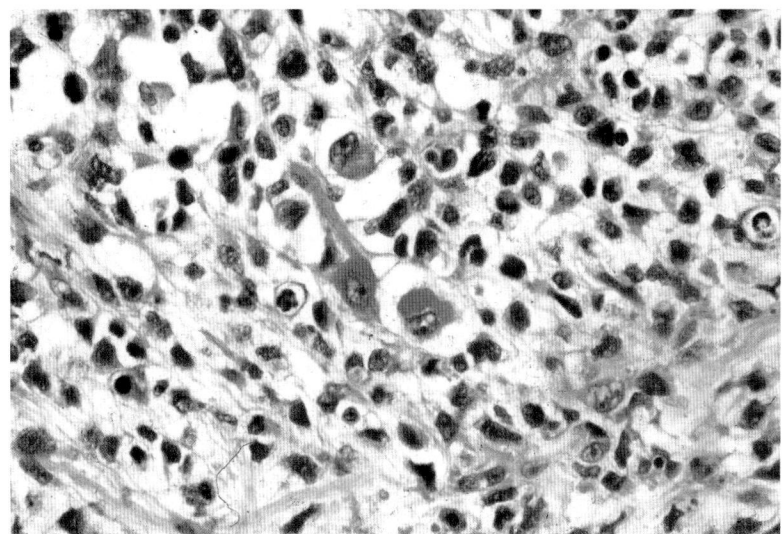

Fig. 35.435
Embryonal rhabdomyosarcoma: in the center of the field is a typical 'tadpole' rhabdomyoblast with a tapering eosinophilic, cytoplasmic process.

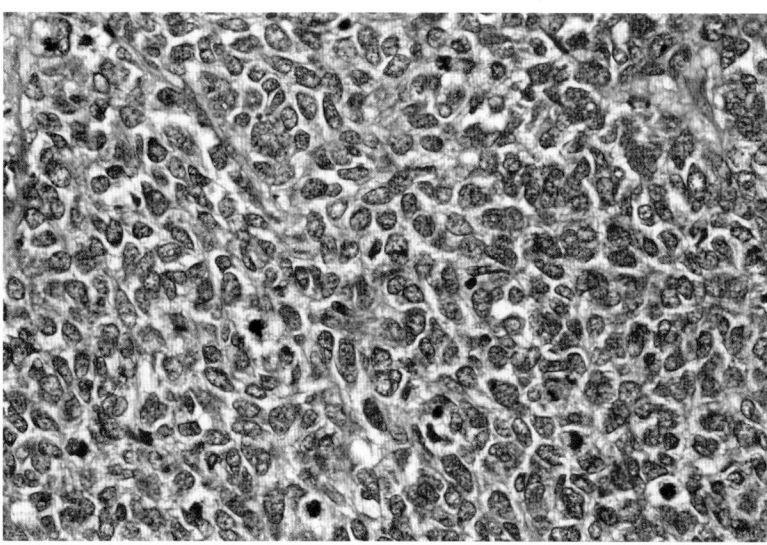

Fig. 35.438
Alveolar rhabdomyosarcoma: the tumor cells have pleomorphic nuclei and multiple mitoses are present. There is no evidence of skeletal muscle differentiation in this example. Diagnosis depends upon immunohistochemistry.

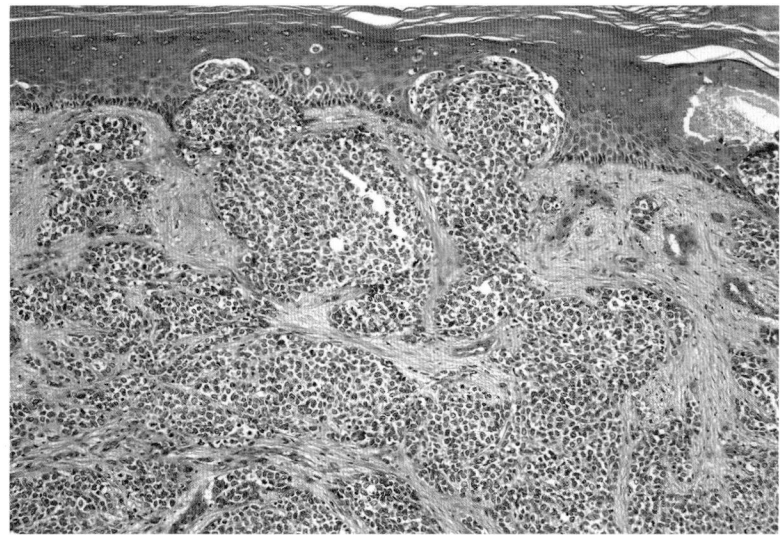

Fig. 35.436
Alveolar rhabdomyosarcoma: this is a very rare example showing epidermotropism. The features mimic neuroendocrine (Merkel cell) carcinoma.

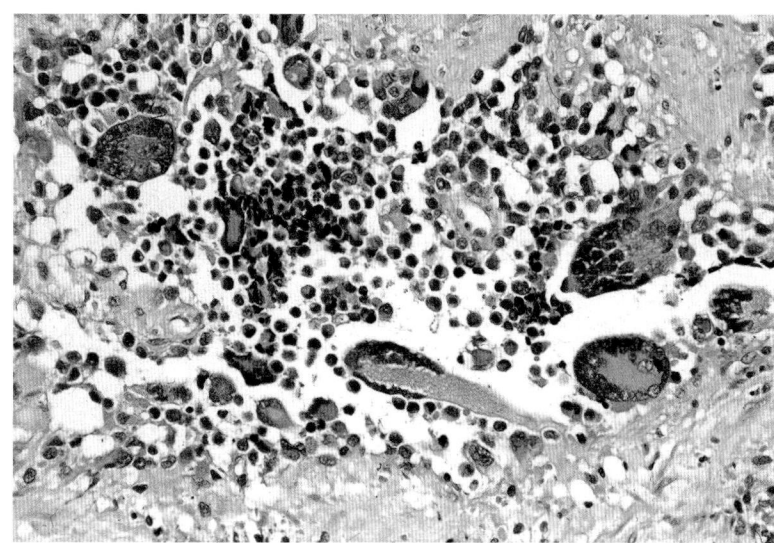

Fig. 35.439
Alveolar rhabdomyosarcoma: wreath-like giant cells are a characteristic feature.

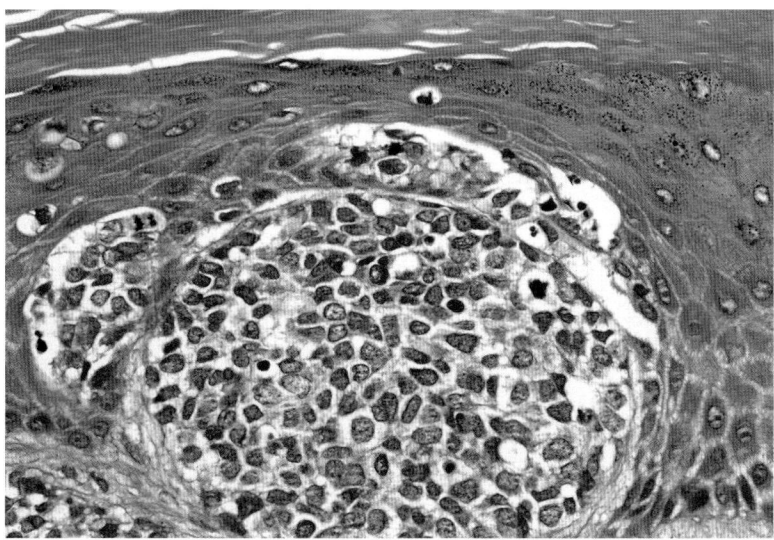

Fig. 35.437
Alveolar rhabdomyosarcoma: high-power view.

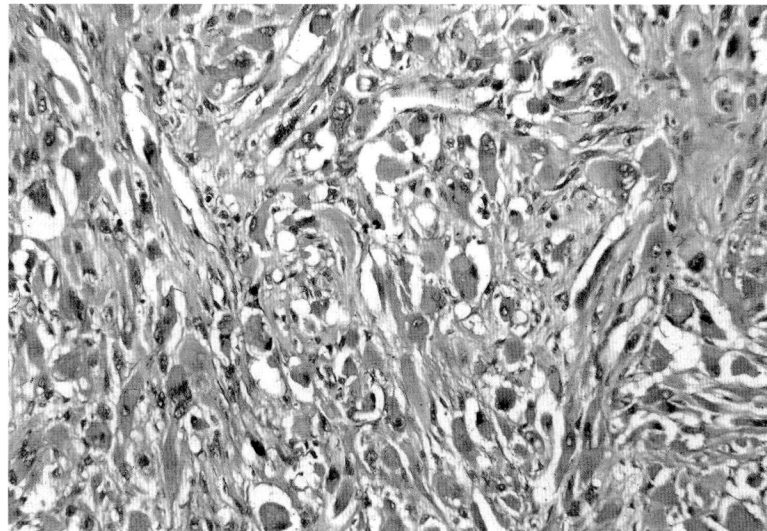

Fig. 35.440
Pleomorphic rhabdomyosarcoma: the rhabdomyoblasts are extremely pleomorphic.

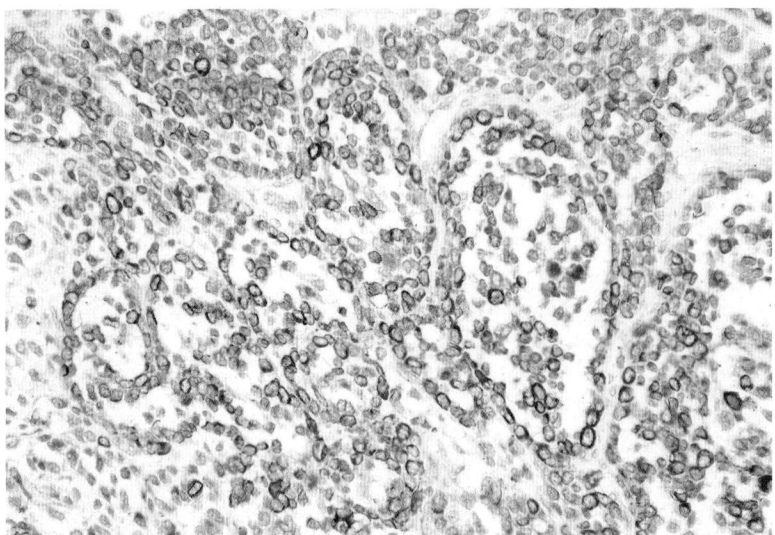

Fig. 35.441
Alveolar rhabdomyosarcoma: in this example, the tumor cells strongly express desmin.

Spindle cell type

Although embryonal rhabdomyosarcoma includes a spindle cell variant, a distinctive variant of spindle cell rhabdomyosarcoma has been described in adults. In these lesions there are atypical spindle-shaped cells intermixed with rhabdomyoblasts.[45]

Epithelioid type

This rare type is composed of uniform cells with epithelioid features (abundant cytoplasm and large vesicular nuclei) in a diffuse sheet-like growth. Nucleoli are prominent and tumor cells may resemble melanoma cells.[8] Multinucleated cells may be seen. Obvious rhabdomyoblasts are absent. Prominent necrosis is typically seen.

In all variants of rhabdomyosarcoma tumor cells are variably positive for desmin, myogenin (myf-4) and MyoD-1. Rhabdomyosarcoma may show focal positivity for cytokeratins. Furthermore, positivity for S100 may occasionally be seen focally. Myogenin, Ap2beta, NOS-1, and HMGA1 are available immunohistochemical markers that seem to correlate with fusion status.[46]

Differential diagnosis

Rhabdomyosarcomas should be distinguished from other small round cell neoplasms:

- neuroblastoma contains neurofibrils and shows rosette formation,
- primitive neuroectodermal tumor often has a packeted appearance, shows variable intracytoplasmic PAS positivity, lacks cells resembling rhabdomyoblasts and is diffusely CD99 positive,
- malignant lymphomas are most often (but not always) PAS negative and stain positively for LCA.

The pleomorphic type should be differentiated from other pleomorphic tumors by immunohistochemistry and identification of rhabdomyoblasts.

TUMORS OF VASCULAR ORIGIN

Benign tumors including reactive vascular proliferations, malformations and ectasias

Intravascular papillary endothelial hyperplasia

Clinical features

Intravascular papillary endothelial hyperplasia (Masson tumor) is a relatively common lesion that represents a distinctive pattern of organizing thrombus.[1-4] It can present as a primary phenomenon in a thrombosed normal blood vessel (usually a vein) or as an incidental finding (secondary form) in other vascular tumors, especially cavernous hemangiomas. Very rare cases are seen in an extravascular location in relation to a hematoma.[5,6] The primary form arises most often in young adults and shows a slight predilection for females. Lesions in children are rare.[7] It occurs most frequently in the head and neck region (including the oral cavity) or on the extremities (particularly the hand), presenting as a slowly or sometimes rapidly growing, elevated, rather cystic nodule that usually measures less than 2 cm in diameter. Large lesions, sometimes in unusual locations, can mimic a soft tissue sarcoma.[8] Presentation in the breast has also been described.[9] Rare cases are multiple and, in this setting, an association with treatment with interferon beta has been documented.[10,11] The behavior is entirely benign.

Histologic features

The lesion is typically well circumscribed and lies within a vessel or angioma in the dermis or subcutis. The appearances are of numerous small papillary structures covered by a single layer of flattened endothelium lying within a clearly demonstrable pre-existent vascular lumen (*Figs 35.442* and *35.443*). The papillary endothelium shows neither atypia nor mitotic activity and the core is composed of hypocellular collagen, sometimes containing tiny capillaries (*Fig. 35.444*). The papillae may be seen attached to the internal surface of the vessel wall or apparently lying free in the lumen. Adjacent associated thrombus, showing a varying degree of organization, is commonly evident.

Differential diagnosis

The principal lesion from which Masson tumor should be distinguished is angiosarcoma, from which it differs by its invariable intravascular confinement, its lack of pleomorphism, mitotic activity or endothelial multilayering, and the absence of necrosis.

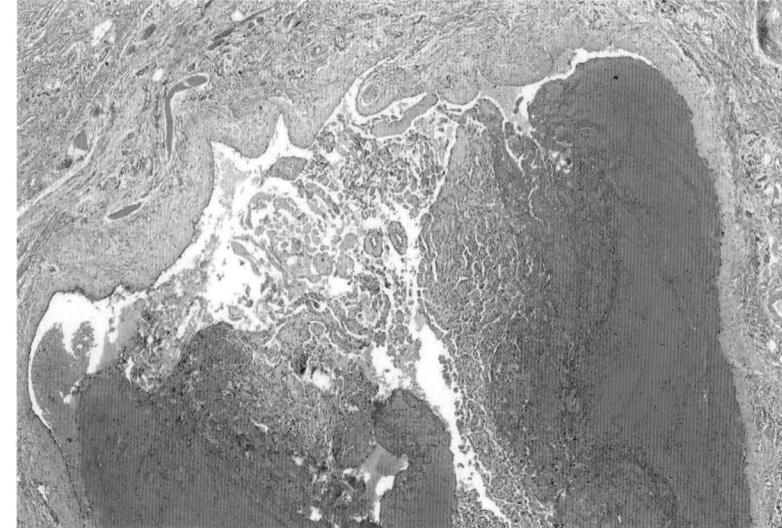

Fig. 35.442
Intravascular papillary endothelial hyperplasia: low-power view of a thrombosed hemangioma.

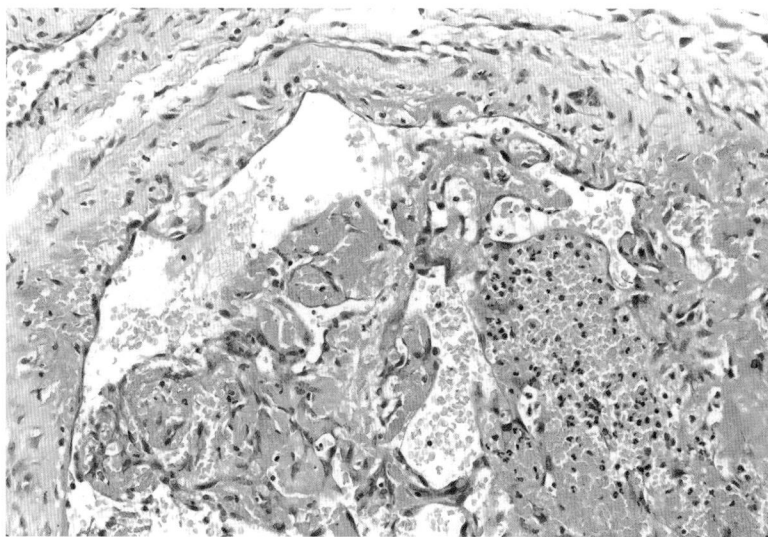

Fig. 35.443
Intravascular papillary endothelial hyperplasia: numerous small papillae are present within the lumen.

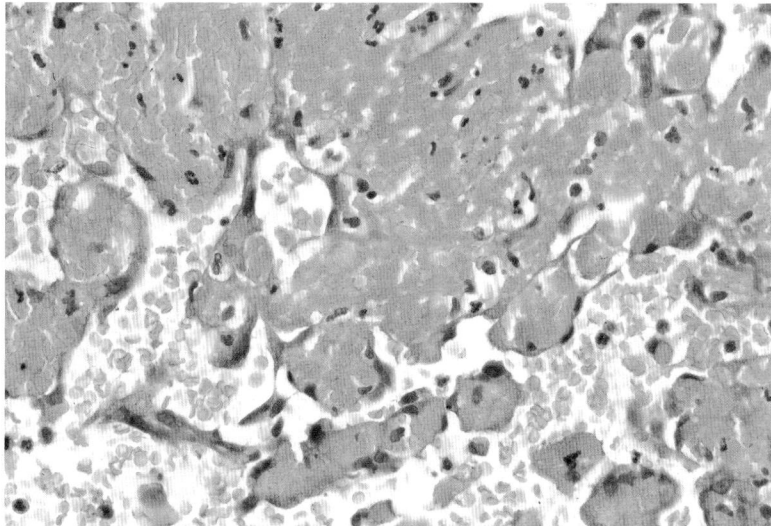

Fig. 35.444
Intravascular papillary endothelial hyperplasia: the papillae are composed of eosinophilic hyaline material covered by flattened endothelial cells. There is an absence of atypia, multilayering, and mitotic activity.

Reactive angioendotheliomatosis

Clinical features

For many years, angioendotheliomatosis was divided into benign and malignant variants, which were difficult to separate on clinical and histologic grounds.[1] With the advent of immunohistochemistry, it became apparent that the malignant type is not endothelial in nature, but is an aggressive form of systemic angiotropic lymphoma. The benign variant of reactive angioendotheliomatosis is uncommon, purely cutaneous and self-limited. It presents as erythematous macules, papules or plaques, which can occasionally be purpuric (Fig. 35.445).[1,2] Ulceration may be seen. A livedo-like pattern is sometimes observed. Anatomical distribution and age range are wide and there is no sex predilection. Presentation in children is very rare.[3]

Some cases are related to systemic infections, especially bacterial endocarditis, but this association is not as strong as was previously believed. Associations with cryoglobulinemia, paraproteinemia, renal disease, amyloidosis, antiphospholipid syndrome, rheumatoid arthritis, cirrhosis, polymyalgia rheumatica, myelodysplastic syndrome, a well-differentiated angiosarcoma and the administration of certain drugs have also been documented.[2,4–13] A case of reactive angioendotheliomatosis associated with myelodysplastic

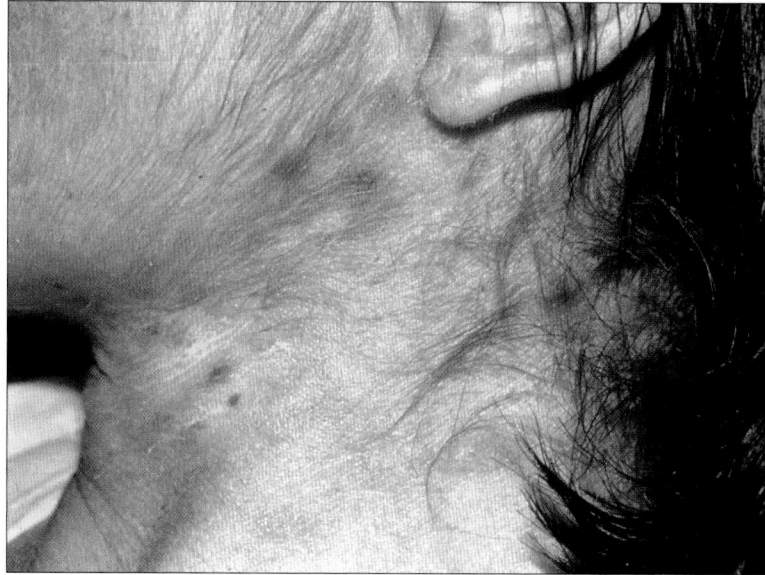

Fig. 35.445
Reactive angioendotheliomatosis: note the purpuric macular and papular lesions. By courtesy of the Institute of Dermatology, London, UK.

syndrome presented with a cellulitis-like plaque and localized lesions were described in a patient with high antiocardiolipin antibodies and subclavian stenosis.[10,14] An exceptional case localized to the intestine has been reported.[15] Simultaneous occurrence of reactive angioendotheliomatosis and leukocytoclastic vasculitis have been documented.[16,17] A number of cases are idiopathic. Localized forms of the disease are sometimes seen, may be associated with ulceration and include variants associated with peripheral vascular atherosclerotic disease and iatrogenic arteriovenous fistulas described as diffuse dermal angiomatosis.[18–22] Additional cases have been reported in association with calciphylaxis and monoclonal gammopathy.[23,24] It has also been reported in the breast of female patients with macromastia and obesity.[25–31] An association with smoking has also been reported.[25] In one case, a thrombosed artery with calcification was described in association with the disease.[28] The process may mimic an inflammatory carcinoma of the breast.[27] Rare examples of the disease can be seen in obese patients in other areas of the body particularly the abdomen.

Histologic features

Lesions are located mainly in the dermis with occasional extension into the subcutis. They consist of a multifocal, variably lobular proliferation of closely packed capillaries lined by plump endothelial cells and surrounded by pericytes (Fig. 35.446). Cytologic atypia is absent or mild and frequently the vessel lumina are obliterated by plump endothelial cells. Cases related to cryoglobulinemia show capillaries occluded by hyaline eosinophilic thrombi. In diffuse dermal angiomatosis there is proliferation of poorly canalized capillaries and endothelial cells. This proliferation may involve the whole dermis and extend into the subcutaneous tissue in a diffuse manner.

It has been suggested that intralymphatic histiocytosis and reactive angioendotheliomatosis are part of the same spectrum.[25,32] The former, however, is mainly seen in patients with rheumatoid arthritis, can be an incidental finding in skin biopsies of patients with various pathologies and is characterized by dilated lymphatics containing numerous histiocytes.[33–35] It does appear however, that the so-called intracapillary histiocytosis is better classified within the spectrum of reactive angoendotheliomatosis.[35]

Differential diagnosis

On scanning magnification, reactive angioendotheliomatosis can mimic tufted angioma. However, the clinical presentation of both conditions is different and closer histologic examination reveals the typical tufts of capillaries with a crescent-like lymphatic channel in the periphery in tufted angioma. Diffuse dermal angiomatosis may mimic angiosarcoma. In the former, although endothelial cells appear plump there is hardly any cytologic

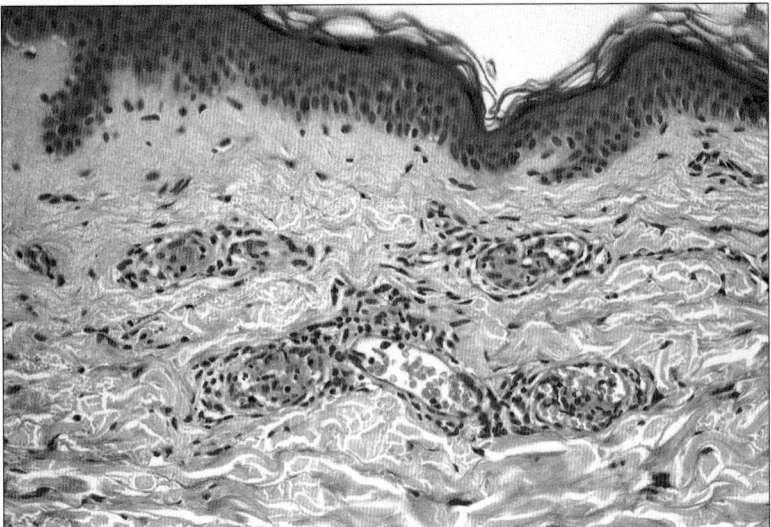

Fig. 35.446
Reactive angioendotheliomatosis: the dermis is extensively infiltrated by well-defined capillary lobules.

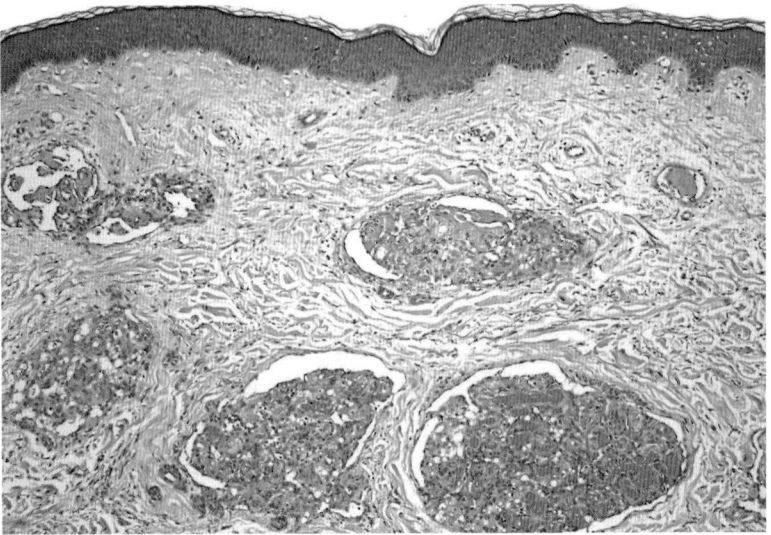

Fig. 35.447
Glomeruloid hemangioma: there is striking intraluminal capillary proliferation.

atypia, mitotic figures are rare and each vascular channel is surrounded by a single layer of SMA positive pericytes.

Glomeruloid hemangioma

Clinical features

Glomeruloid hemangioma is a distinctive reactive vascular proliferation that has been described almost exclusively in patients with multicentric Castleman disease and POEMS (polyneuropathy, organomegaly, endocrinopathy, M-protein and skin changes) syndrome (Crow-Fukase syndrome).[1-5] Patients present with numerous vascular papules on the trunk and limbs and this may be the initial presentation of the disease.[6] In one patient, intracranial hemangiomas were also seen.[7] Exceptionally, one or multiple lesions have been described in patients with no evidence of POEMS syndrome.[8-11] The latter includes a case of a single lesion presenting in the uterus.[12]

Histologic features

Histologically, appearances vary from small capillary hemangiomas (identical to cherry angiomas) to those of glomeruloid hemangioma or even a mixture of both. In the latter, there are dilated vascular spaces in the dermis, containing in their lumina clusters of capillaries surrounded by pericytes and strikingly resembling renal glomeruli (*Figs 35.447* and *35.448*). Occasional

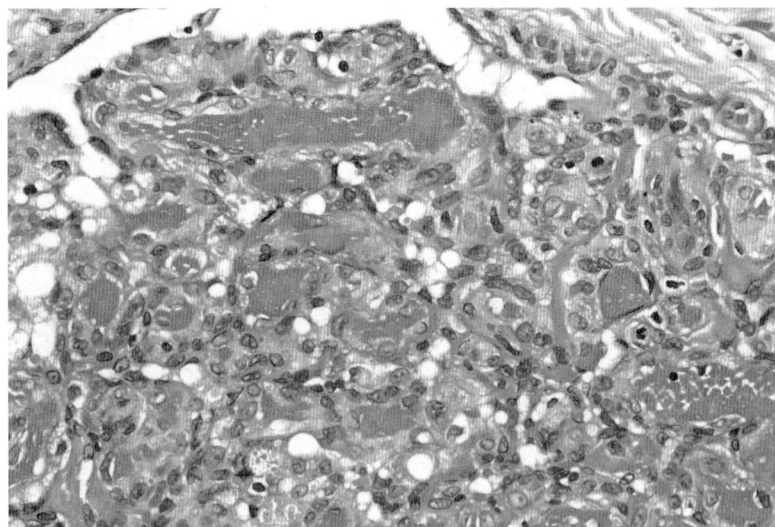

Fig. 35.448
Glomeruloid hemangioma: high-power view.

larger cells with vacuolated cytoplasm and PAS-positive hyaline globules (representing immunoglobulin) are sometimes seen. By electron microscopy, the inclusions appear to represent enlarged secondary lysosomes (thanatosomes).[13] Two types of endothelial cell with different immunophenotype have been described in glomeruloid hemangioma.[14] The endothelial cells express endothelial growth factor and its receptor.[15]

Human herpesvirus 8 (HHV-8) is not present in the lesions of glomeruloid hemangioma.[16]

Papillary hemangioma

Clinical features

Papillary hemangioma is a recently described cutaneous vascular lesion.[1] It presents as a small, long-standing papule on the head and neck with predilection for adult males. Only one of the 11 reported lesions recurred.

Histologic features

The lesion is characterized by dilated vascular spaces within the dermis. These spaces display papillary projections lined by plump endothelial cells with no cytologic atypia and containing cytoplasmic hyaline globules. The latter have been shown to represent giant lysosomes, as demonstrated by electron microscopy. These lysosomes contain cellular debris and fat vacuoles (thanatosomes).

It has been suggested that glomeruloid hemangioma and papillary hemangioma are part of the same spectrum.[2] The latter, however, is not associated with POEMS syndrome, lacks a glomeruloid architecture and is characterized by thick basement membrane-like material and pericytes within the cores of the papillary projections.[3] Whether papillary hemangioma represents a solitary variant of glomeruloid hemangioma not associated with POEMS syndrome has not been clearly established.

Nevus flammeus

Clinical features

The old term nevus flammeus encompasses both the salmon patch and the port-wine stain.[1-3] However, at present, the term nevus flammeus is only used to refer to port-wine stains.

Salmon patch

Salmon patch (nevus simplex, "angel kiss," "stork bite) is a congenital lesion that usually presents on the head and neck (forehead and nape of neck) as a reddish-purple macule and tends towards spontaneous involution. It can be seen in up to one-third of neonates, representing the most common form of vascular malformation.[4] In a study of cutaneous findings in hospitalized neonates, a salmon patch was found in 91.2% of patients.[5] In a further study in 500 newborns, a salmon patch was found in 28% of full-term infants and in 25.8% of pre-term infants.[6] A salmon patch on the nape of the neck seems to be more commonly associated with a mother greater than 35 years of age.[7]

Port-wine stain

Port-wine stain is a lateralized dark lesion that tends towards continued growth and only very rarely involutes (*Fig. 35.449*).[1-3,8] A similar lesion characterized by light-red or pale-pink color has been described as nevus roseus.[9] Rare acquired cases of port-wine stain may also be seen, often in association with trauma.[10,11]

The familial combination of port-wine stain and arteriovenous malformation appears to be related to mutations in *RASA1* (5q13.3) encoding a regulator of the Ras protein.[12-15]

Port-wine stain may be associated with ipsilateral cerebral or meningeal vascular lesions and vascular eye abnormalities (Sturge-Weber syndrome) or with hypertrophy of a limb and partial venous agenesis with varicosities (Klippel-Trenaunay syndrome)[16,17] (*Figs 35.450–35.452*). In Cobb syndrome, there is a port-wine stain overlying an underlying spinal cord vascular malformation in the midline of the back.[18,19] The cutaneous vascular lesion may also represent a verrucous hemangioma.[19]

Other vascular lesions, particularly lobular capillary hemangioma (pyogenic granuloma), vascular malformations, a combination of the latter two and even tufted angioma, may occur within a port-wine stain.[20-25] Lobular capillary hemangioma-like (pyogenic granuloma-like) lesions can occur after laser treatment.[26] Basal cell carcinoma may occasionally develop within a port-wine stain.[27,28].

Pathogenesis and histologic features

A somatic activating mutation in the GNAQ gene, located on chromosome 9, has been identified in both syndromic and non-syndromic port wine stains.[29] It has been proposed that the endothelial cells of port-wine stains

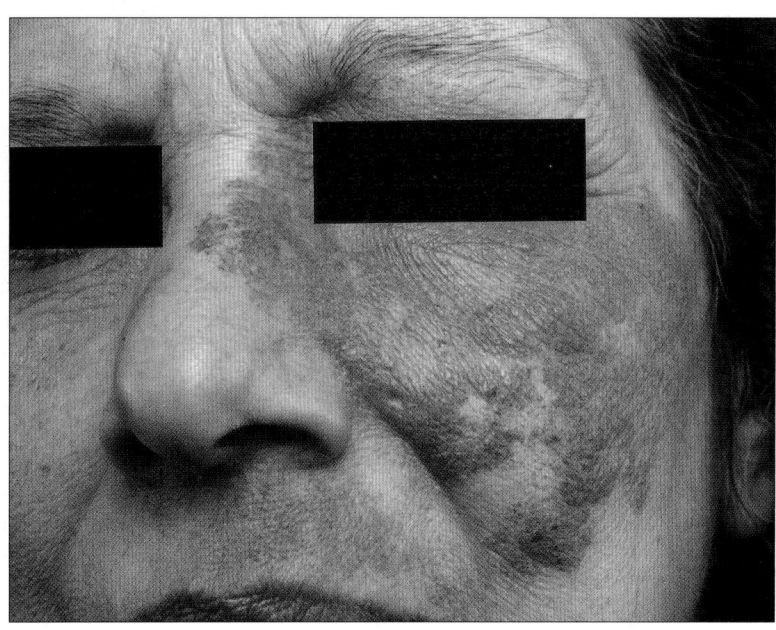

Fig. 35.449
Port-wine stain: this large red–purple lesion was present at birth and, in contrast to the strawberry nevus, shows no tendency to regress. From the collection of the late N.P. Smith, MD, The Institute of Dermatology, London, UK.

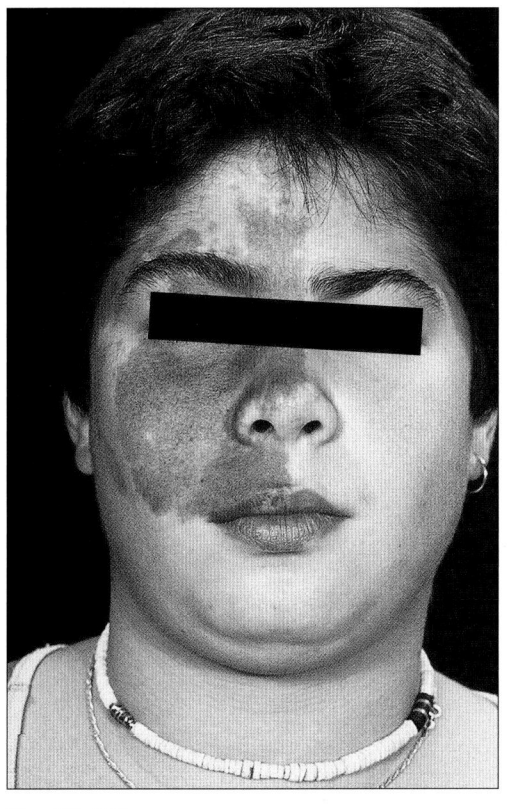

Fig. 35.450
Sturge-Weber syndrome: this 12-year-old girl presented with fits, mental retardation, and a port-wine vascular nevus affecting much of the right side of her face. CT scan showed meningeal angiomatosis. By courtesy of D. Atherton, MD, Institute of Dermatology and Children's Hospital at Great Ormond Street, London, UK.

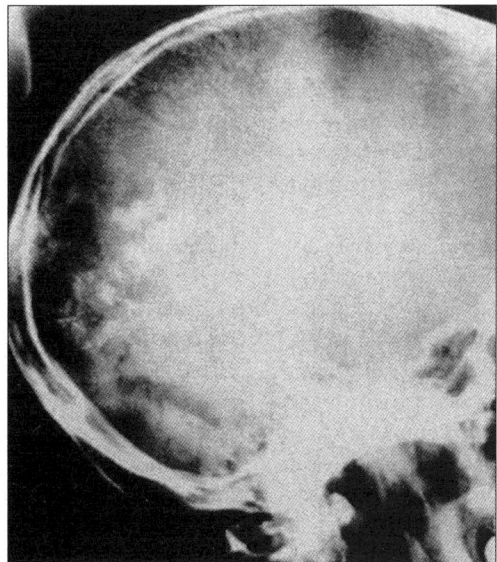

Fig. 35.451
Sturge-Weber syndrome: the intracranial moiety is often calcified, as in this radiograph. By courtesy of I. Moseley, MD, National Hospital for Nervous Diseases, London, UK.

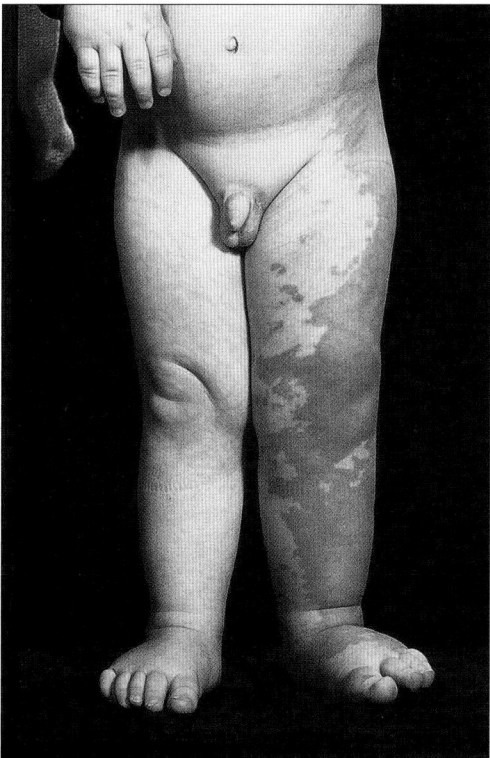

Fig. 35.452
Klippel-Trenaunay syndrome: this 2-year-old boy has a port-wine vascular nevus, affecting much of the skin of the left leg, associated with increased soft tissue growth in the leg and a slight increase in its length. By courtesy of D. Atherton, MD, Institute of Dermatology and Children's Hospital at Great Ormond Street, London, UK.

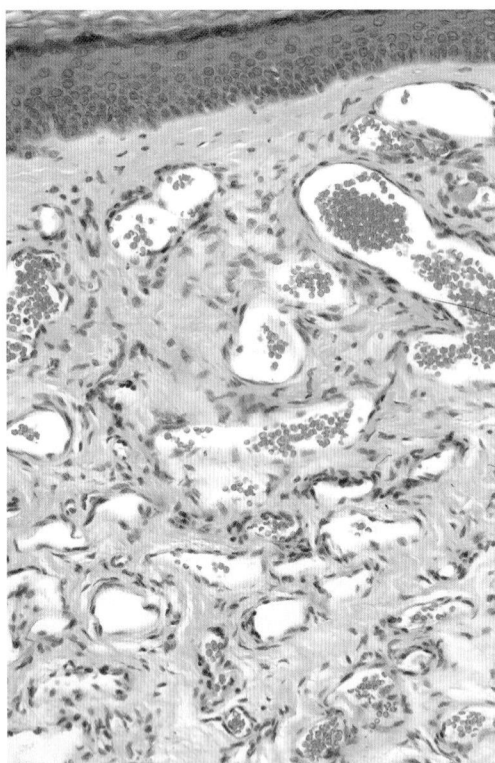

Fig. 35.453
Port-wine stain: the malformation is characterized by numerous dilated blood-filled capillaries.

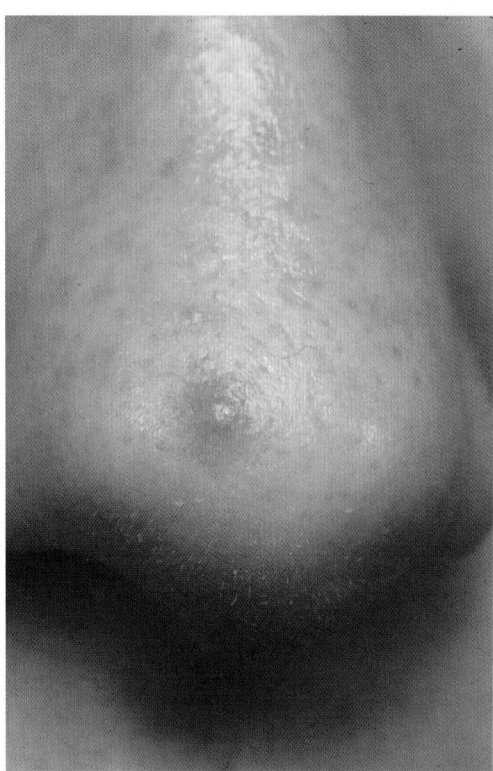

Fig. 35.454
Spider nevus: note the central macule with radiating vessels. From the collection of the late N.P. Smith, MD, The Institute of Dermatology, London, UK.

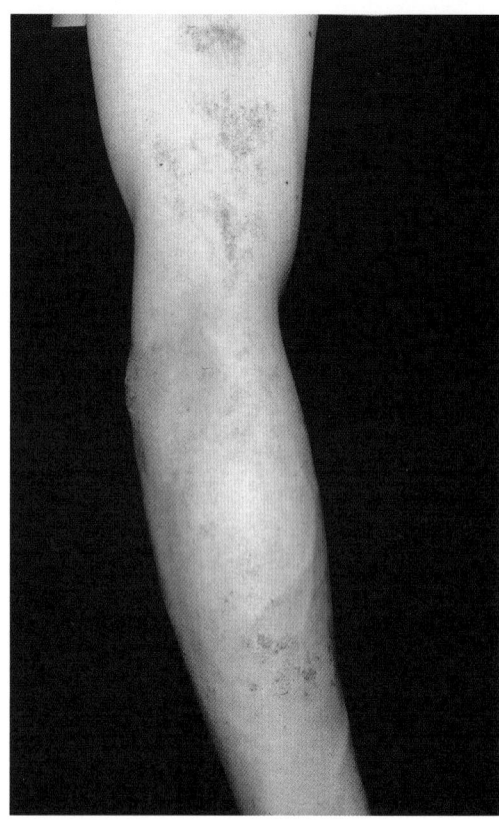

Fig. 35.455
Angioma serpiginosum: the distribution of these tiny red macules is characteristic. From the collection of the late N.P. Smith, MD, The Institute of Dermatology, London, UK.

represent differentiation impaired late-stage endothelial progenitor cells that form immature venule-like structures. As a result of disruption in the interaction between endothelial cells in these vessels (co-expressing Eph receptor B1 and ephrin B2), there is progressive dilatation resulting in the abnormality observed.[30]

Both salmon patch and port-wine stain are characterized solely by ectatic vessels of variable caliber in the dermis; designation as a true hemangioma, therefore, is probably inappropriate (*Fig. 35.453*).

Cutis marmorata telangiectatica congenita

Clinical features

Cutis marmorata telangiectatica congenita is a rare condition that presents at birth and shows an equal sex incidence.[1,2] It is characterized by cutis marmorata, telangiectasia, phlebectasia, occasional ulceration and atrophy. Lesions are more often unilateral, localized and with predilection for the limbs.[1,2] They consist of a reticulated, blue–violet vascular network. The disease is sporadic and tends to improve with age. Only rare cases persist.[3]

In two-thirds of cases, associated abnormalities – including nevus flammeus, macrocephaly, syndactyly, hydrocephalus, body asymmetry, anal atresia, hearing loss, cardiovascular abnormalities, strabismus, hypothyroidism, nevus anemicus, café-au-lait spots, lipoma and hypospadias – may be seen.[1,2,4,5] A subset of patients with cutis marmorata telangiectatica congenita were thought to be associated with macrocephaly, however, nowadays is well known that the capillary malformations in these patients represent a reticulated type of capillary malformations.[6] In the Adams-Oliver syndrome, aplasia cutis congenita and transverse limb defects are associated with other malformations in addition to cutis marmorata telangiectatica congenita.[7,8]

Histologic features

Biopsy shows dilatation of capillaries and venules in the superficial dermis. Occasionally, a true vascular proliferation may be seen.[9]

Spider nevus

Clinical features

Spider nevi are extremely common lesions of little pathological significance.[1,2] Although they may arise at any age, they are typically a cutaneous manifestation of chronic liver disease or thyrotoxicosis and may also be seen in pregnancy. The lesions manifest as pinhead-sized, deep red puncta from which tiny tortuous vessels radiate (*Fig. 35.454*).

Histologic features

A typical lesion consists solely of a dilated dermal arteriole that communicates with a network of ectatic superficial capillaries.

Angioma serpiginosum

Clinical features

Angioma serpiginosum is rare, usually arises in childhood, and occurs particularly on the extremities.[1-3] It is characterized by multiple tiny punctate red or purple lesions about the size of a pinhead, typically arranged in a gyrate or serpiginous pattern (*Figs 35.455 and 35.456*).[1-3] New papules tend to form gradually, thereby expanding the lesion. Sometimes the condition may simulate purpura.[4] A linear arrangement may rarely be seen.[5,6] Ocular and nervous system involvement has occasionally been documented.[7,8] Although most cases are localized, extensive involvement rarely occurs.[9] Occasional cases are familial.[10] In cases with a systematized segmental distribution, genetic mosaicism has been suggested.[11]

Pathogenesis and histologic features

It has been suggested that the disease is caused by deletions or mutations on chromosome Xp11 encoding for the PORCN gene.[12,13] However, this view has been challenged with the suggestion that the patients described had focal dermal hypoplasia.[14]

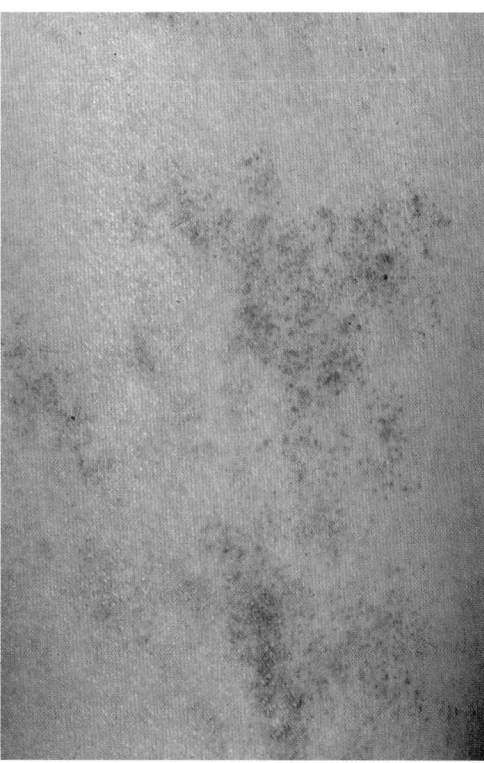

Fig. 35.456
Angioma serpiginosum: close-up view. From the collection of the late N.P. Smith, MD, The Institute of Dermatology, London, UK.

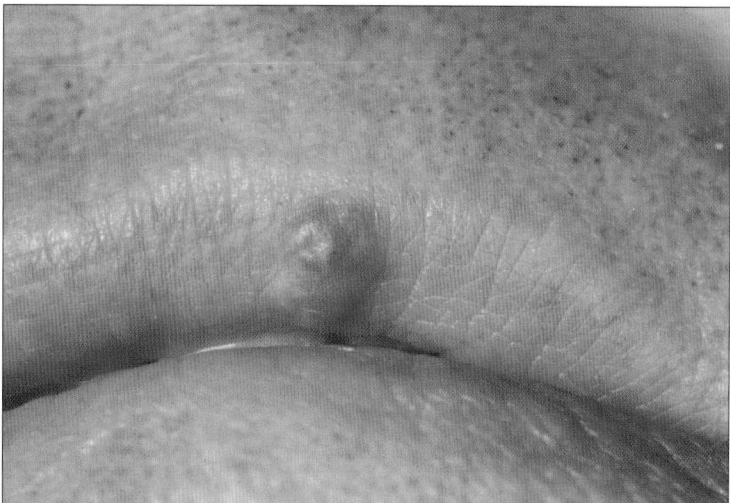

Fig. 35.458
Venous lake: there is a typical blister-like vascular lesion. By courtesy of the Institute of Dermatology, London, UK.

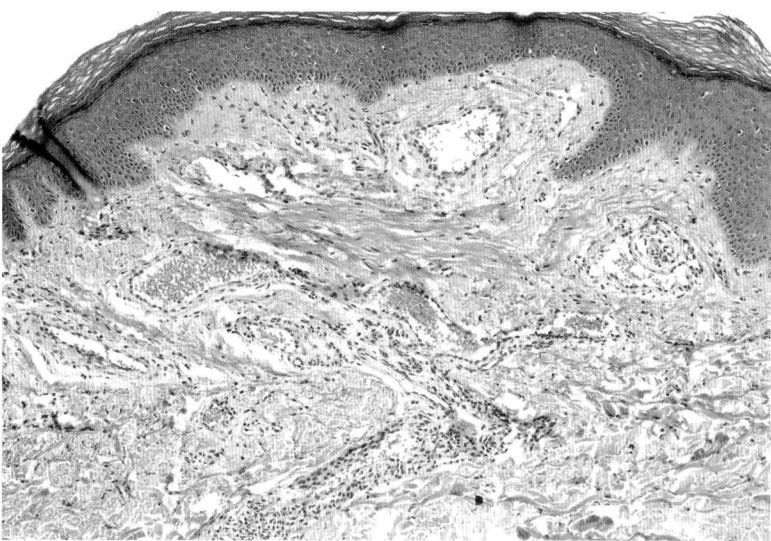

Fig. 35.457
Angioma serpiginosum: histologically, it is composed of a localized cluster of thick-walled and dilated capillaries, usually in the superficial dermis.

Each lesion is composed of a localized collection of relatively thick-walled, dilated capillaries in the superficial or mid dermis (*Fig. 35.457*).

Venous lake

Clinical features

Venous lake is a fairly common vascular ectasia that presents on the sun-damaged skin of elderly people and show a predilection for the lip (*Fig. 35.458*).[1-3] Lesions are sometimes multiple and can measure up to 1 cm in diameter.

Pathogenesis and histologic features

Histology shows a dilated and congested vein in the superficial dermis. There is no evidence of vascular proliferation (*Fig. 35.459*). The pathogenesis is possibly related to defective stromal support.

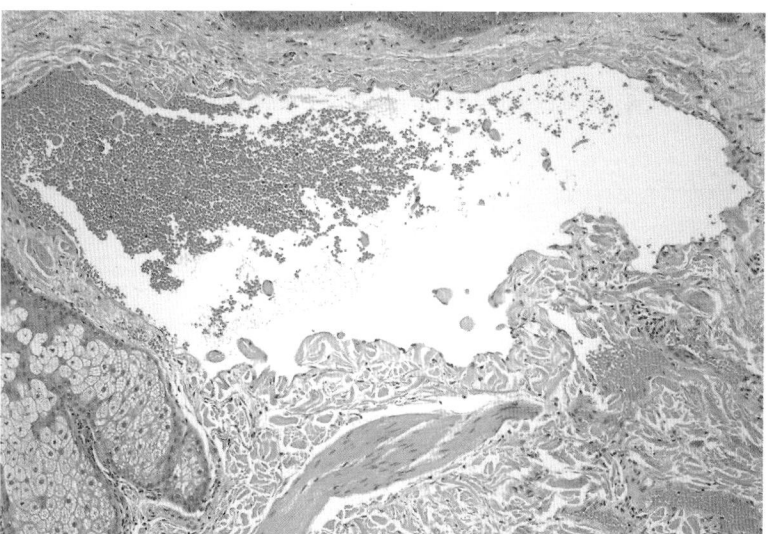

Fig. 35.459
Venous lake: there is striking venous ectasia.

Hereditary hemorrhagic telangiectasia

Clinical features

Hereditary hemorrhagic telangiectasia (Osler-Weber-Rendu syndrome) is an autosomal dominant disease. It is characterized by numerous telangiectasias involving the skin, mucosae and internal organs, especially the gastrointestinal tract and lungs.[1] The upper respiratory tract is often involved and epistaxis is a frequent finding. Lesions become more evident in early adulthood. Internal organs are often involved by vascular arteriovenous malformations and pulmonary hypertension is a frequent finding.[2,3]

Pathogenesis and histologic features

Pathogenic mutations have been found in genes at 9q33~34.1 and 12q11~14 encoding endoglin (*ENG*) and activin-like receptor type II-like 1 (*ACVRL1* or *ALK1* – which is distinct from *ALK* the anaplastic lymphoma kinase gene), respectively.[4-9] Both are related to the TGF-β receptors present on endothelial cells. A reported group of patients has combined juvenile polyposis syndrome and hereditary hemorrhagic telangiectasia with mutations in the SMAD4 on chromosome 18.[10-12] Histology shows dilated small vascular channels in the affected organs.

Generalized essential telangiectasia

Clinical features

Generalized essential telangiectasia is a rare condition characterized by multiple tiny telangiectasias arising on the limbs and trunk and shows a predilection for females.[1–3] Presentation is usually in childhood. In one case, lesions were more prominent in a surgical scar, one patient developed lesions in association with Graves disease and in a further report involvement of the conjunctiva was described.[4–6]

Histologic features

Histology shows dilated small vascular channels in the papillary dermis.

Cutaneous collagenous vasculopathy

Clinical features

This is a rare but probably underdiagnosed condition is characterized by generalized telangiectasia mimicking generalized essential telangiectasia. It presents in patients between the 5th and 9th decades of life with no sex predilection and characterized by progressive telangiectasia that often starts on the lower limbs and spreads in a progressive manner.[1–6] Occasionally, lesions are echimotic.

Pathogenesis and histologic features

The etiology is unknown. Histology shows mild dilatation of superficial dermal vascular channels with thickening of the walls associated with hyaline eosinophilic material resulting from the reduplication of the basement membrane (*Figs 35.460* and *35.461*). The material is PAS positive and stains for collagen type IV.[1–6] In a single case fibrin thrombi were identified within the lumina of vascular channels.[7]

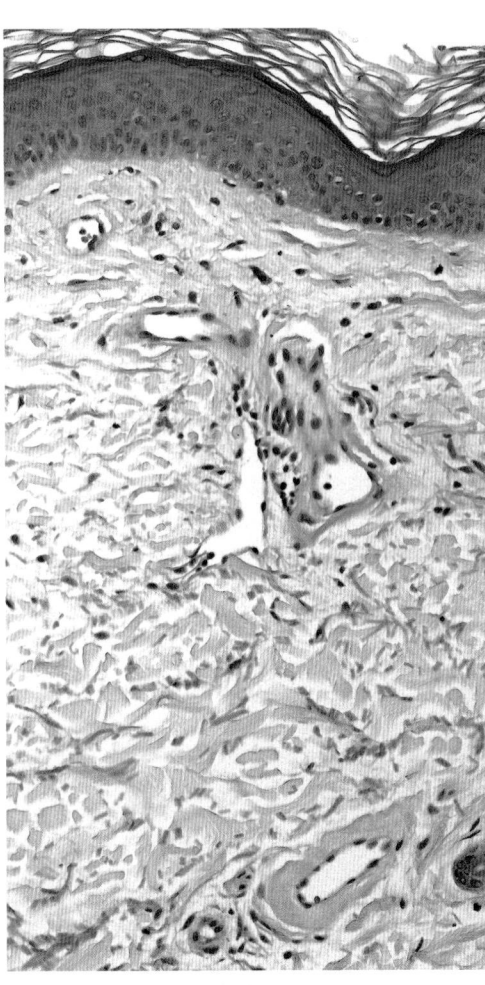

Fig. 35.460
Cutaneous collagenous vasculopathy: dilated superficial dermal vascular channels with thickened walls.

Angiokeratoma

Clinical features

Angiokeratoma represents ectasia of superficial blood vessels associated with secondary epidermal changes, especially acanthosis and hyperkeratosis.[1] Five variants have been described.

- *Angiokeratoma of Fordyce*: this develops mainly on the scrotum of elderly men as single or multiple, blue or red papules.[2] Involvement of the penis may also be seen and is sometimes prominent.[3] Similar lesions can occur on the vulva of young women.[4] Unilateral lesions are very rare.[5]
- *Angiokeratoma of Mibelli*: this presents as warty papules on the distal limbs (especially fingers and toes) of children and adolescents, showing a predilection for females.[6]
- *Angiokeratoma circumscriptum*: this is very rare and presents as grouped papules or a plaque with predilection for the upper and lower limbs of children, with a predilection for females.[7] A case associated with injury and one in a systematized band-like pattern suggesting mosaicism have been documented.[8,9]
- *Angiokeratoma corporis diffusum*: this is characterized by widespread clusters of red papules in a symmetrical distribution, especially in the 'bathing-trunk' area.[1,10] Exceptionally, lesions are seen on the palms and soles.[11] It is usually, but not exclusively, associated with Anderson-Fabry disease, an X-linked genetic disorder that results from a deficiency of the lysosomal enzyme α-galactosidase A. Treatment with the enzyme can induce regression of the angiokeratomas.[12] Patients with other enzymatic deficiencies including L-fucosidase, β-mannosidase, α-N-acetylgalactosaminidase, neuraminidase and β-galactosidase deficiency and even individuals with no detectable abnormalities, exceptionally in a familial setting, can show identical lesions.[13–21] Multiple hemangiomas without angiokeratomas in a female carrier of Fabry disease have been documented.[22]
- *Solitary and multiple angiokeratomas*: these have a wide age range and anatomical distribution and preferentially affect the lower limbs.[1] Most lesions are solitary. Multiple lesions have been reported in a zosteriform distribution.[23] Distribution along Blaschko lines can be seen.[24] Lesions can develop as a consequence of radiotherapy and angiokeratoma-like lesions can be seen in lichen sclerosus.[25–27] Injection of etanercept induced angiokeratomas in a single patient.[28] Associations with epidermal nevus, vascular malformations, nevus lipomatosus superficialis have also been documented.[29–32]

Oral angiokeratomas are seen either as an isolated phenomenon or in association with other types of angiokeratomas including Fabry disease.[33,34]

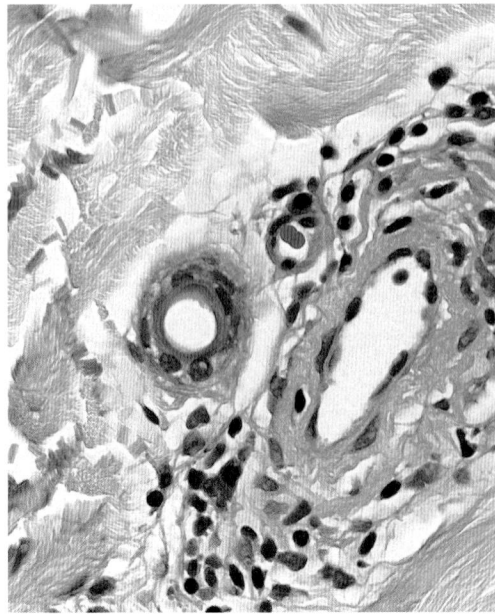

Fig. 35.461
Cutaneous collagenous vasculopathy: amorphous bright eosinophilic material around vascular channels.

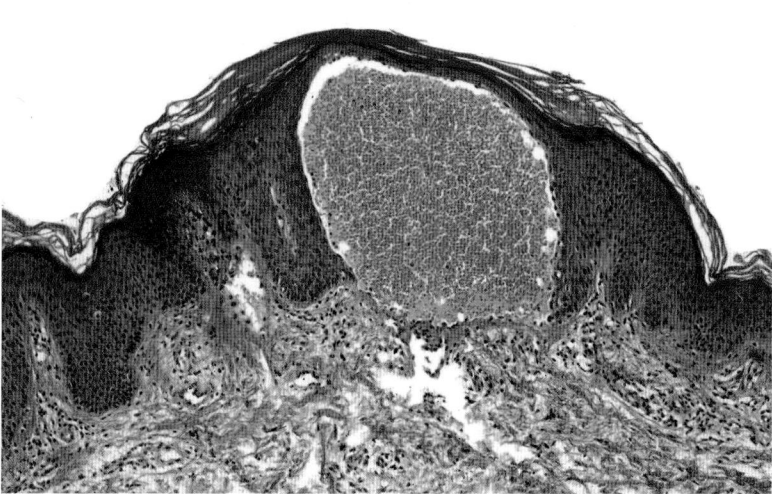

Fig. 35.462
Angiokeratoma: the lesion consists of small dilated vessels that often appear to be within the epidermis.

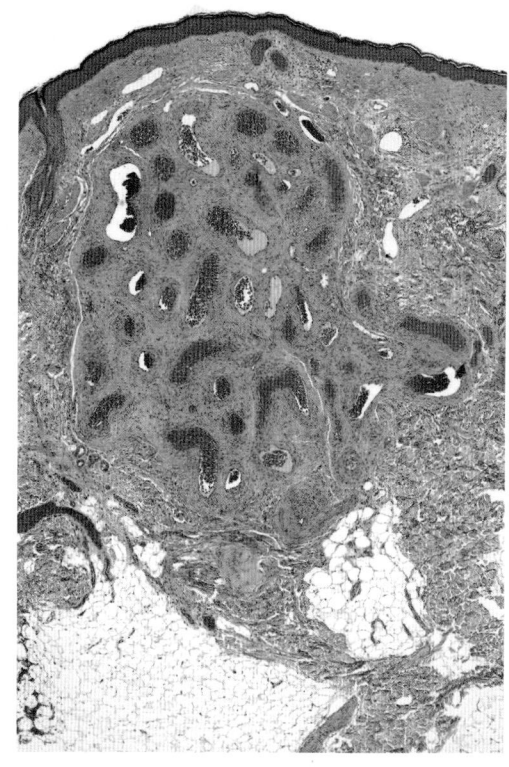

Fig. 35.463
Arteriovenous hemangioma: within the dermis is a collection of thick-walled blood vessels comprising both arteries and veins.

Histologic features

The histologic features in all variants are similar and consist of numerous dilated and congested capillaries in the papillary dermis with overlaying acanthosis and hyperkeratosis (*Fig. 35.462*). In Anderson- Fabry disease, intracytoplasmic lipid vacuoles have been described in endothelial cells, pericytes and fibroblasts.[35]

Differential diagnosis

Identical features can be seen in the superficial portion of a verrucous hemangioma, which always, however, has a deep dermal and subcutaneous component.

Verrucous venous malformation (verrucous hemangioma)

Clinical features

Verrucous venous malformation (verrucous hemangioma) typically presents as a warty dark-blue nodule mainly on the extremities, especially the lower limbs, of children.[1-5] Multiple and linear lesions are very rare.[6,7] A similar cutaneous lesion on the midline of the back associated with a spinal cord vascular malformation is known as Cobb syndrome.[8]

Pathogenesis and histologic features

Verrucous hemangioma is no longer used to refer to this entity as it is clear that it represents a form of lymphovascular malformation and therefore the proposed more accurate name is verrucous venous malformation.[9-11] Recently, a somatic MAP3K3 mutation has been described.[12]

Histologically, there are numerous dilated and congested capillaries and occasional cavernous vascular spaces involving mainly the papillary dermis, with extension into the deep dermis and subcutis. The overlying epidermis shows marked acanthosis, hyperkeratosis and papillomatosis. As the depth of the involvement is frequently overlooked, recurrences are common. WT1 is usually negative in the endothelial cells lining the vascular channels. GLUT-1 is positive in up to two third of cases.[13]

Differential diagnosis

Resemblance to angiokeratoma can be striking, but angiokeratoma lacks a deep component. Distinction between both entities in small biopsies is impossible.

Arteriovenous hemangioma

Clinical features

Arteriovenous hemangiomas (cirsoid aneurysms) present as small (less than 1 cm in diameter) reddish-blue papules, most often on the head and neck (especially the lip) or extremities.[1-4] Adults in their fifth and sixth decades are most frequently affected and there is an equal sex incidence. The papules are prone to intermittent bleeding and may sometimes be tender. Local recurrence is not a feature. Histologically comparable lesions in deep soft tissues tend to affect younger patients, may sometimes be associated with hemodynamic complications, and occasionally recur. There is an association with chronic liver disease.[5]

A distinctive variant occurring in the digits has been documented.[6]

Histologic features

Arteriovenous hemangiomas are composed of a well-circumscribed intradermal, submucosal or subcutaneous mass of numerous, fairly thick-walled vessels lined with plump endothelium (*Figs 35.463* and *35.464*). The vessels characteristically have muscular walls with variable elastic laminae and, in some cases, arteriovenous anastomoses are apparent. Luminal microthrombi are not uncommon and dystrophic calcification is occasionally seen. Frequently, it is difficult to identify the arterial component despite serial sectioning. These latter lesions are probably pure venous hemangiomas.

Congenital hemangiomas

The term congenital hemangioma is used to describe a group of hemangiomas that develop in-utero and are fully developed at birth presenting with an equal sex incidence.[1-5] These lesions were classified in the past as infantile hemangiomas, vascular malformations and cavernous hemangiomas. There is overlap with the latter entities and the concept of congenital hemangiomas is still evolving.

Congenital hemangiomas have been divided into rapidly involuting congenital hemangioma (RICH) and non-involuting congenital hemangioma (NICH).[2,3] Although they seem to represent distinctive clinicopathological entities, there is some degree of overlap not only between RICH and NICH but also between RICH and infantile hemangioma and they may be part of the same spectrum. This means that accurate diagnosis usually relies on

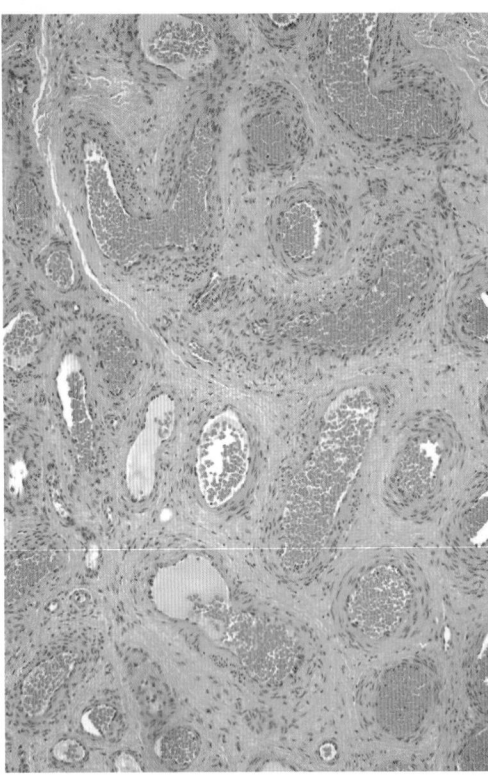

Fig. 35.464
Arteriovenous hemangioma: higher-power view showing admixture of arteries and veins.

close clinicopathological correlation. It is likely that these lesions are pathogenetically interconnected. In both types of congenital hemangiomas mutations in *GNAQ* and *GNA11* have been identified.[6]

Rapidly involuting congenital hemangioma (RICH)

Clinical features

Rapidly involuting congenital hemangioma develops fully before birth, tends to regress during the first year of life, affects males and females equally and has a wide anatomical distribution with some predilection for the head and limbs.[2] The mechanism of regression appears to be as a result of infarction. Some cases of RICH fail to involute completely and persist like NICH and have been described as partially involuting congenital hemangiomas.[7] Recently, a small group of patients with congenital hemangioma showing fetal involution have been described.[8] RICH can be associated with transient thrombocytopenia and coagulopathy.[9,10]

Histologic features

Rapidly involuting congenital hemangioma is characterized by involvement of the subcutaneous tissue and dermis. The epidermis and adnexal structures can be atrophic. The architecture is lobular, lobules are composed of capillaries, and between tumor lobules there are often bands of fibrosis with focal inflammation, dystrophic calcification, hemosiderin deposition and scattered veins, arteries, and lymphatics. Lobules are composed of variably congested, sometimes slightly dilated, capillaries, each of which is surrounded by a layer of pericytes. Larger vascular channels may be found in the fibrotic areas. Individual lobules may show variable fibrosis. Extramedullary hematopoiesis is rare and perineural extension is absent. GLUT-1 staining is usually negative or very focally positive in tumor lobules.

Non-involuting congenital hemangioma (NICH)

Clinical features

Non-involuting congenital hemangioma is fully developed at birth but does not regress; rather it tends to progress over time. Males and females are equally affected. Anatomical distribution is wide, but there is predilection for the head and limbs.[3]

Histologic features

The histologic features between RICH and NICH overlap. Microscopic distinction is often not possible on histologic grounds and therefore clinicopathological correlation is crucial to reach the diagnosis. Non-involuting congenital hemangioma is characterized by vascular lobules of variable size and often composed of capillaries and larger, sometimes thicker, blood vessels. Draining larger blood vessels are present in tumor lobules. Surrounding the latter, there are areas of fibrosis containing large blood vessels with features of veins and arteries. Arteriovenous fistulae are common and this closely mimics an arteriovenous malformation. Histologic distinction can be very difficult and close clinicopathological correlation is often necessary. As opposed to vascular malformations, NICH does not tend to recur. GLUT-1 staining is usually negative.

Differential diagnosis

Infantile hemangioma is the main differential diagnosis. Infantile hemangioma typically develops shortly after birth, grows rapidly during the first year of life and tends to involute over a period of several years. The vascular lobules of RICH and infantile hemangioma are often identical and it has been proposed that distinction between both is mainly based in the presence of bands of fibrosis around tumor lobules and lack of GLUT-1 positivity in the former. In practice, however, and especially in small biopsies, distinction may be very difficult or impossible. Clinicopathological correlation is paramount. Distinction between infantile hemangioma and NICH is easier, as the latter tends to display more variability in the size of vascular channels, GLUT-1 staining is usually negative and arteriovenous fistulae are identified. The main problem with NICH, RICH and infantile hemangioma is that there is some degree of overlap between the three entities as demonstrated by the fact that infantile hemangioma may coexist with either RICH or NICH. The problem is further compounded by the fact that some cases of RICH fail to involute completely and behave more like NICH, and in such cases the histologic appearances overlap with those of RICH and NICH. At present, the pathogenetic relation between these groups of lesions remains obscure.

Capillary hemangioma and its variants

Infantile hemangioma

Clinical features

Infantile hemangiomas (juvenile hemangioma, strawberry nevus) are the most common vascular tumors of the childhood affecting as many as 1/100 births[1-4] By definition the tumors do not present at birth but instead develop within the first weeks of life. Lesions can occur in any cutaneous region, although the head and neck are by far the most commonly involved (*Figs 35.465* and *35.466*). Females are affected more often than males.

The flat red or purple lesions, frequently less than 5 cm in diameter, gradually enlarge and develop a raised surface. Usually they are discrete but (less often) can be large, diffuse and disfiguring. Over a period of months or years, the vast majority involute spontaneously.

Histologic features

Infantile hemangiomas have a fairly uniform microscopic appearance characterized by an intradermal or subcutaneous multilobular proliferation of numerous small vascular spaces lined by plump endothelial cells, which may be mitotically active (*Figs 35.467* and *35.468*). In the early stages, vascular lumina tend to be inconspicuous and the vascular nature of the tumor might not be immediately apparent. However, a reticulin stain highlights the presence of numerous poorly canalized vascular channels. With maturation, the vessels enlarge and dilate and the endothelium appears more flattened and mature. At the deep margin of the lesion a large feeding arteriole is often apparent. An occasional entirely benign feature is the presence of perineural invasion.[5,6] Older lesions become progressively more fibrotic, showing a gradual disappearance of the vascular elements, and histologic diagnosis of largely regressed examples can be difficult.

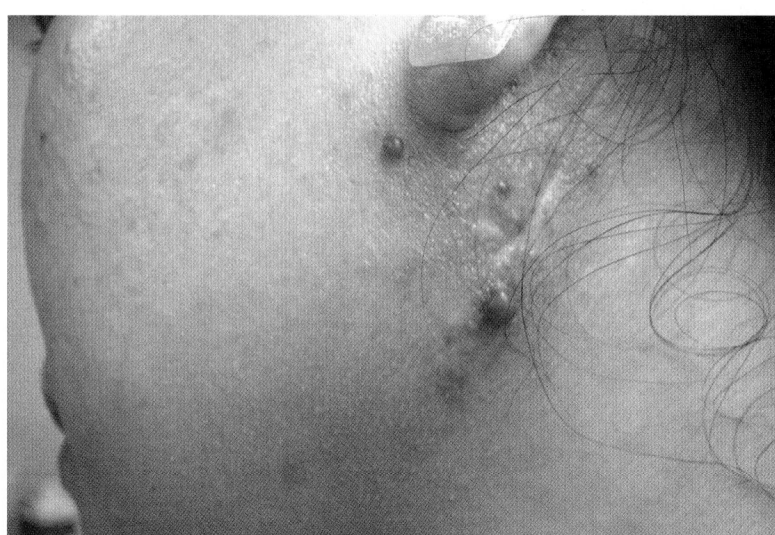

Fig. 35.465
Infantile hemangioma: multiple raised erythematous nodules are present around this child's ear and neck. By courtesy of J. Dayrit, MD, Manila, The Philippines.

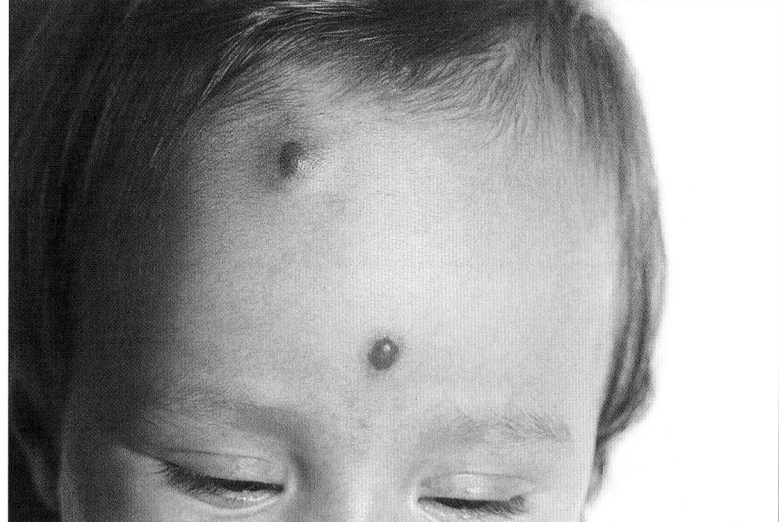

Fig. 35.466
Infantile hemangioma: two raised nodules are present on the forehead of this female infant. By courtesy of M.M. Black, MD., The Institute of Dermatology, London, UK.

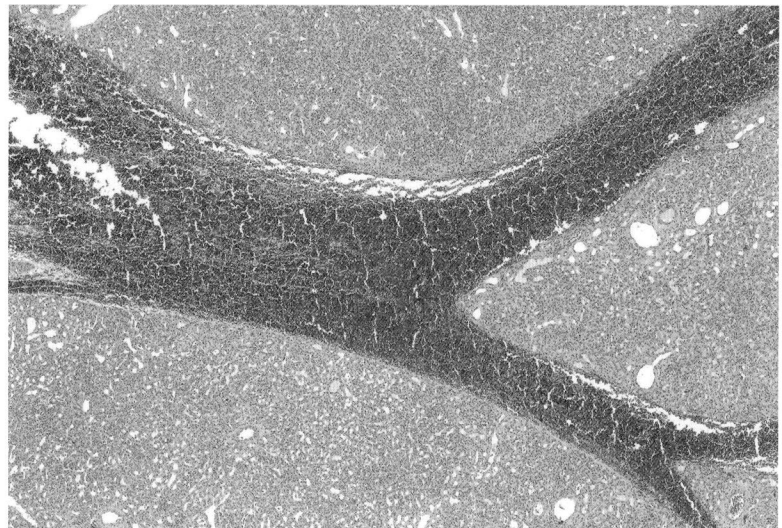

Fig. 35.467
Infantile hemangioma: this is an evolving lesion composed of lobulated aggregates of poorly canalized blood vessels.

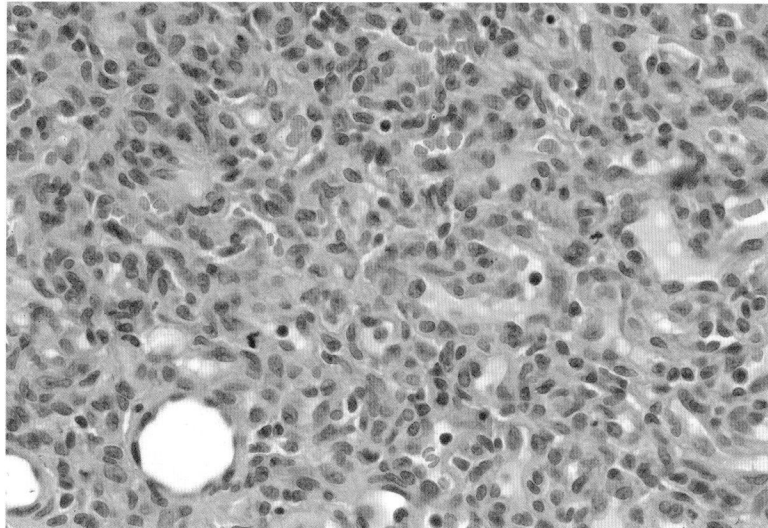

Fig. 35.468
Infantile hemangioma: the blood vessels are lined by plump endothelial cells. Note the multiple mitoses.

By immunohistochemistry and electron microscopy it has been demonstrated that the tumor cell population is heterogeneous and composed not only of endothelial cells but also of fibroblasts and pericytes.[7,8] This favors a hamartomatous process rather than a true neoplasm. It has a unique immunophenotype shared with placental microvessels expressing GLUT-1, LeY and WT-1.[9] GLUT-1, the erythrocyte-type glucose transporter protein, is expressed by these hemangiomas at all stages of their evolution.[9,10] Since GLUT-1 and WT-1 are not expressed in other vascular tumors which occur in children, the presence of this marker is a valuable aid in differential diagnosis, particularly in the setting of vascular malformations.[11,12] Endothelial cells in proliferating lesions co-express LYVE-1 and CD34 and are negative for Prox-1, while LYVE-1 is negative in involuting lesions, suggesting that endothelial cells in proliferating infantile hemangiomas are arrested early in the developmental stage of vascular differentiation.[13]. In addition, capillary hemangiomas have been shown to be clonal.[14,15]

Differential diagnosis

The differential diagnosis with congenital hemangiomas is discussed under the latter.

Infantile hemangiomas with minimal or arrested growth (abortive hemangiomas)

Clinical features

These recently described lesions are characterized by telangiectatic patches with peripheral papules and predilection for the lower body.[1-3] They are defined as vascular lesions with a proliferative component equal to or less than 25% of the total surface of the lesion.[1] Slightly less than 50% of patients have typical infantile hemangiomas elsewhere.[1] Lesions tend to persist.

Histologic features

A biopsy from the telangiectatic patch shows scattered dilated vascular channels in the superficial dermis. In the deep dermis, lobules of capillaries may be seen. A biopsy from a papule shows features of a capillary hemangioma. Endothelial cells are positive for GLUT-1. This feature, and the coexistence with typical infantile hemangiomas, confirms that they are closely related.

Cherry angioma

Clinical features

Cherry angiomas (senile angiomas, Campbell de Morgan spots), regarded as variants of capillary hemangiomas, are very common and present as multiple tiny red papules on the trunk and upper limbs of the middle aged and

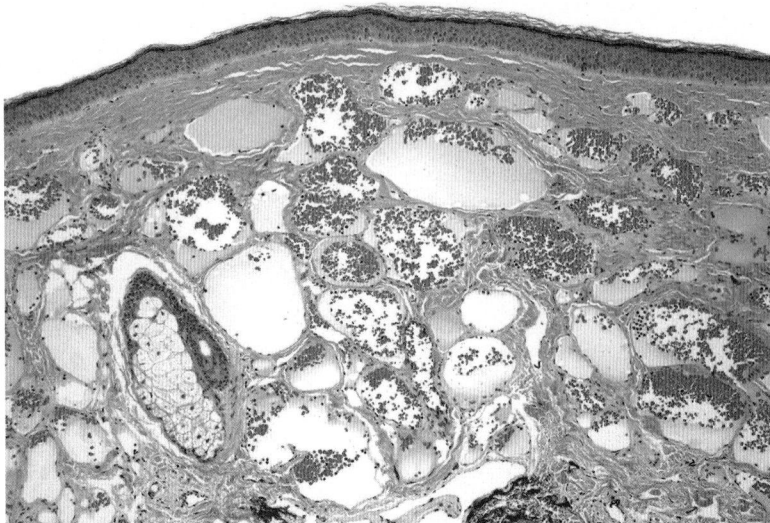

Fig. 35.469
Cherry angioma: there are widely dilated, congested vessels in the superficial dermis.

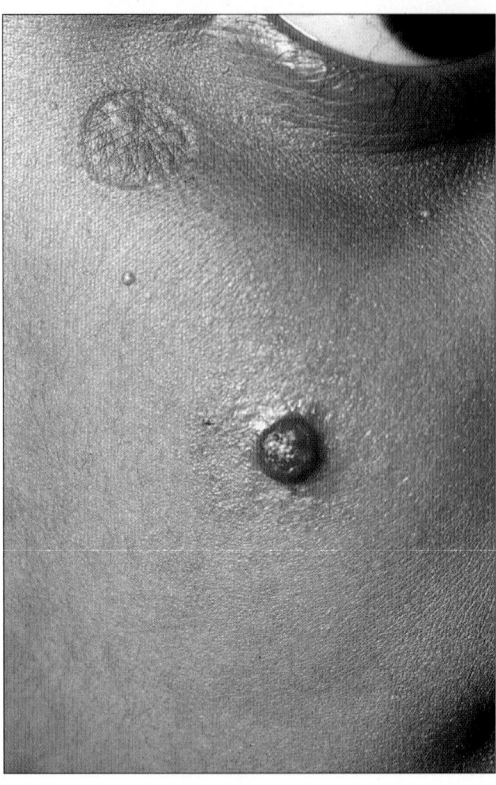

Fig. 35.470
Lobular capillary hemangioma: a typical raised red nodule on the face of a young female patient. By courtesy of M.M. Black, MD, St Thomas' Hospital, London, UK.

elderly.[1] An unusual case of cherry angiomas with segmental dyschromatosis and blue nevi has been reported.[2]

Pathogenesis and histologic features

The pathogenesis is unknown. *HRAS* and *KRAS* mutations have been found in a small number of cases indicating involvement of the ERK pathway.[3] A case of eruptive lesions associated with topical nitrogen mustard therapy, another associated with exposure to bromides, a familial nevus flammeus with early-onset cherry angiomas and a case associated with familial cerebral cavernous malformations have been documented.[4–9]

Histology shows a small polypoid lesion with an epidermal collarette and multiple lobules of dilated and congested capillaries in the papillary dermis (*Fig. 35.469*). In a single case, lesions of cherry angioma were colonized by intravascular large B-cell lymphoma.[10]

Lobular capillary hemangioma (pyogenic granuloma)

Clinical features

Lobular capillary hemangioma (pyogenic granuloma) is a very common benign vascular lesion that was regarded for many years as a reactive or infective process.[1] This assumption was based on the extensive secondary changes that are almost invariably present in these lesions. However, the underlying process is that of a lobular proliferation of capillaries, which is much more likely to be neoplastic, and therefore it has been redesignated lobular capillary hemangioma.[2] It may arise at any age in either sex and shows a predilection for the head and neck (especially the mucous membranes) and limbs (particularly the arms and hands) (*Fig. 35.470*). Oral lesions are more common in females.[3,4] Lobular capillary hemangioma also occurs in the gastrointestinal tract and other organs. Typically, the lesion evolves rapidly, reaching its maximum size (usually less than 2 cm in diameter) within a matter of months. It presents as a pedunculated red or bluish nodule, which is prone to ulceration or bleeding (*Fig. 35.471*).[5] Complete spontaneous regression does not occur and rare patients present with multiple lesions, either disseminated or localized.[6–10] Eruptive lesions have been described following a drug hypersensitivity reaction, a landmine injury, burns and associated with an acquired arteriovenous malformation.[11–13] Congenital lesions are exceptional and one case presented with disseminated lesions.[14–17] Lesions may occur within a port-wine stain and more rarely in association with unilateral dermatomal superficial telangiectasia.[18–21] Multiple pyogenic granuloma-like lesions have been documented in association with BRAF inhibitors, capecitabine, topical tretinoin, isotretinoin, gefitinib, afatinib, 5-fluorouracil, levothyroxine, EGFR tyrosine kinase inhibitors, and

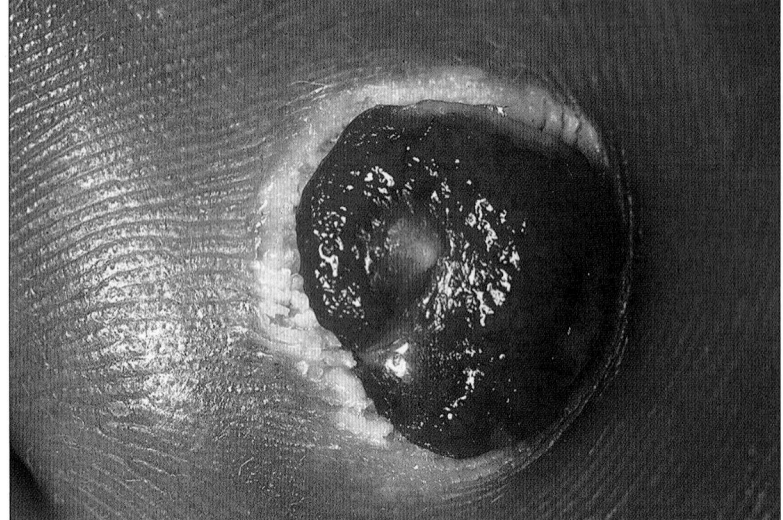

Fig. 35.471
Lobular capillary hemangioma: these lesions are characteristically ulcerated. By courtesy of the Institute of Dermatology, London, UK.

anti-TNF-alpha therapy.[22–32] In one case an association with erythropoietin was suggested.[33] Subungual lesions may occur not only in association with drugs and trauma but also after peripheral nerve injury.[34] Lobular capillary hemangiomas have also been documented as a complication of pulse dye laser used to treat port-wine stains, following orbital hydroxyapatite implants,[35,37] after bone marrow transplant[38] and in a patient with NF1 and von Hippel-Lindau syndrome.[39]

Local recurrence after excision is relatively frequent and in a small proportion of cases there is a recurrence with multiple satellite lesions that may be clinically worrying (*Fig. 35.472*).[39,40] This latter phenomenon tends to occur in younger individuals who very often have primary lesions on the trunk.

- Granuloma gravidarum is a variant that presents on the gingivae of pregnant women and involutes after delivery. Pregnancy may also induce lesions elsewhere.[41,42]

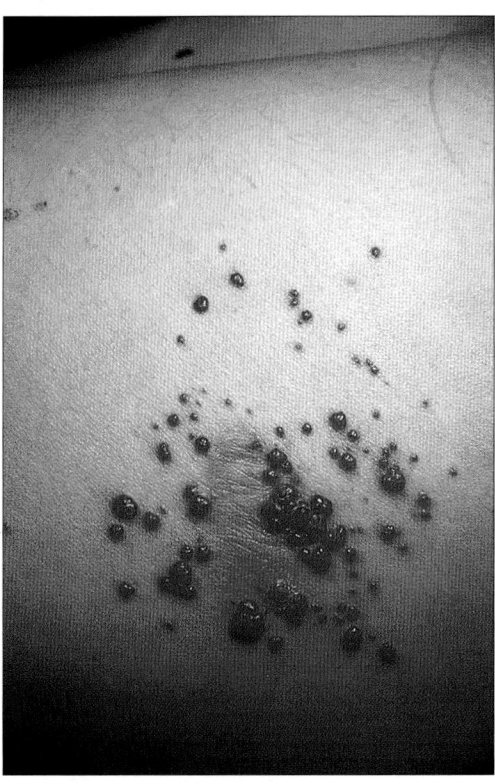

Fig. 35.472
Lobular capillary hemangioma (satellitosis): characteristic appearance of multiple satellite lesions on the trunk. By courtesy of E. Wilson Jones, MD, Institute of Dermatology, London, UK.

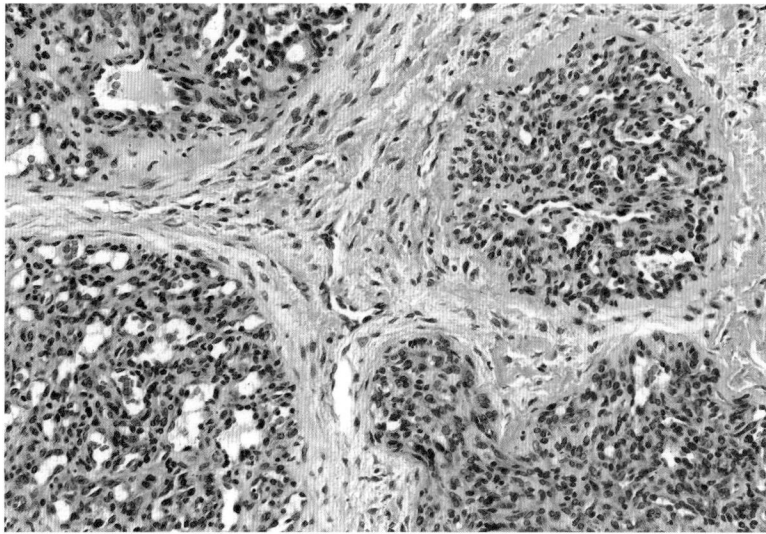

Fig. 35.474
Lobular capillary hemangioma: note the well-developed lobular architecture.

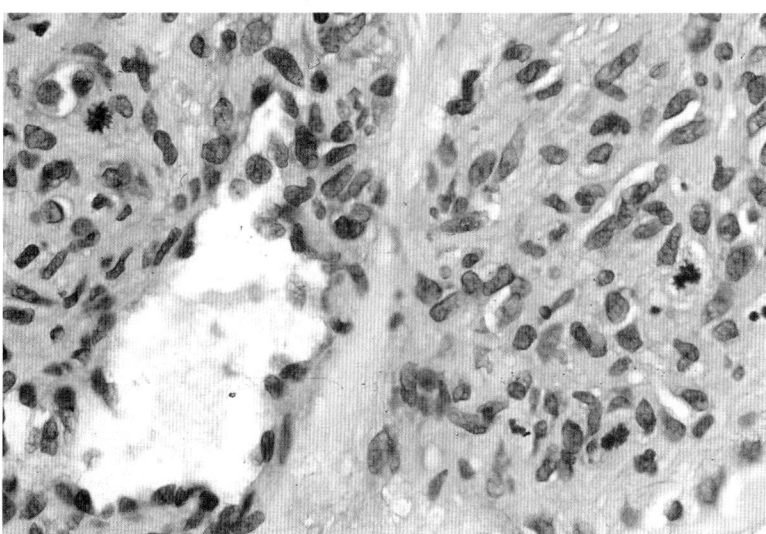

Fig. 35.475
Lobular capillary hemangioma: conspicuous mitotic activity is often present, particularly in evolving lesions.

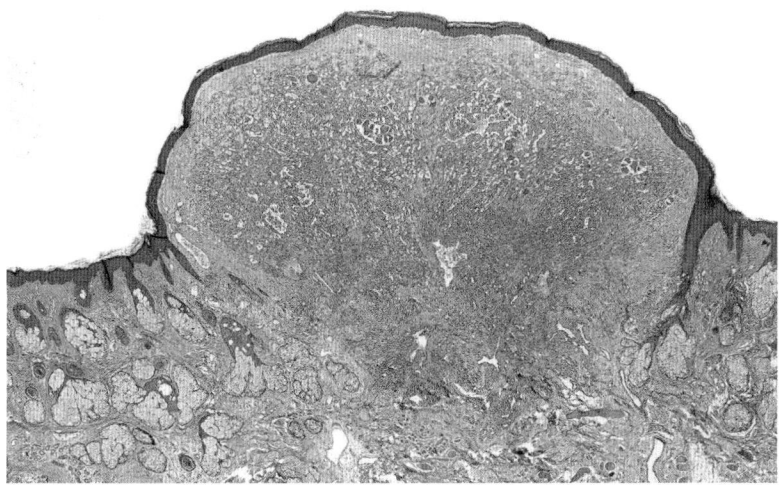

Fig. 35.473
Lobular capillary hemangioma: this scanning section shows the polypoid structure of the lesion and the well-formed collarette.

- Subcutaneous or deep dermal lobular capillary hemangioma has a predilection for the upper limb.[43,44] Since it never becomes ulcerated, it is not associated with secondary inflammatory changes.
- Intravenous lobular capillary hemangioma is uncommon, but tends to occur on the neck and upper extremity of young adults.[45–47]

Histologic features

Lobular capillary hemangioma consists of a usually exophytic, lobulated, dermal mass made up of numerous small capillaries, often radiating from larger, more central vessels set in a loose edematous collagenous matrix (*Figs 35.473* and *35.474*). Endothelial cells have variably bland to plump nuclei and may be focally epithelioid, especially in mucosal tumors.[48] Mitoses are commonly present and may be numerous (*Fig. 35.475*). Focal cytologic atypia as a result of degeneration may be seen (*Figs 35.476* and *35.477*). Metaplastic ossification is sometimes seen and extramedullary hematopoiesis has exceptionally been documented.[49,50]

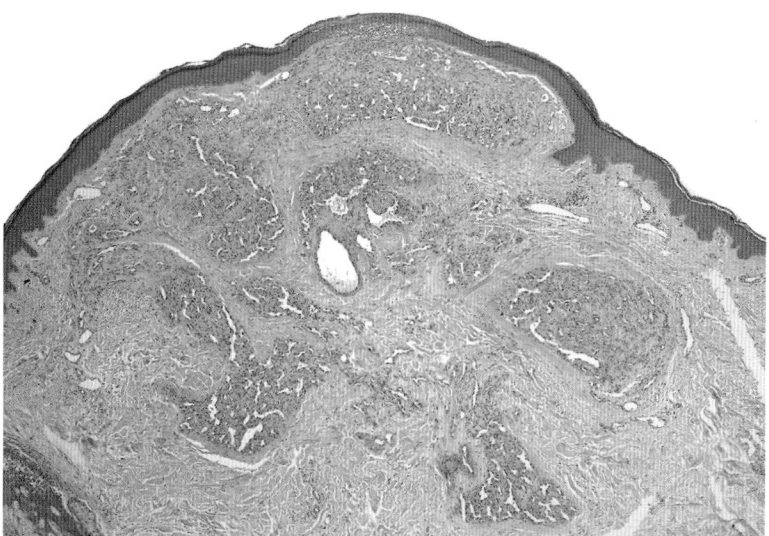

Fig. 35.476
Lobular capillary hemangioma with atypia: scanning view showing multiple lobules with an associated fibrous stroma.

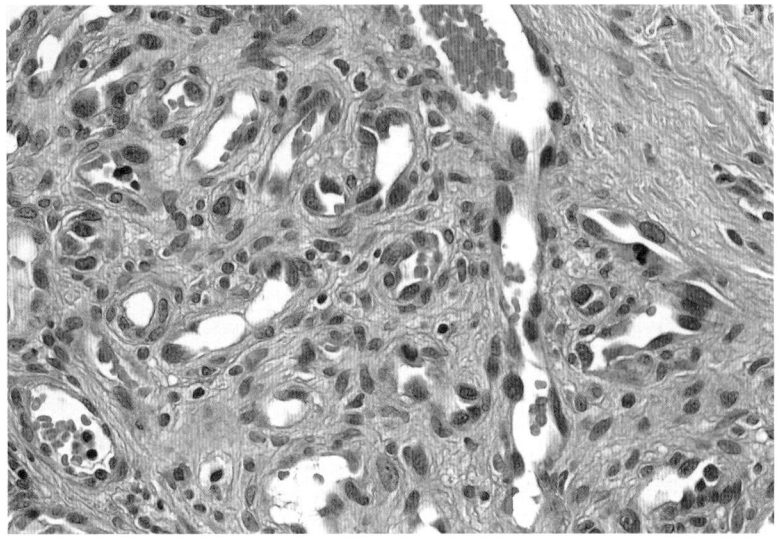

Fig. 35.477
Lobular capillary hemangioma with atypia: there is nuclear pleomorphism and an atypical mitosis is present.

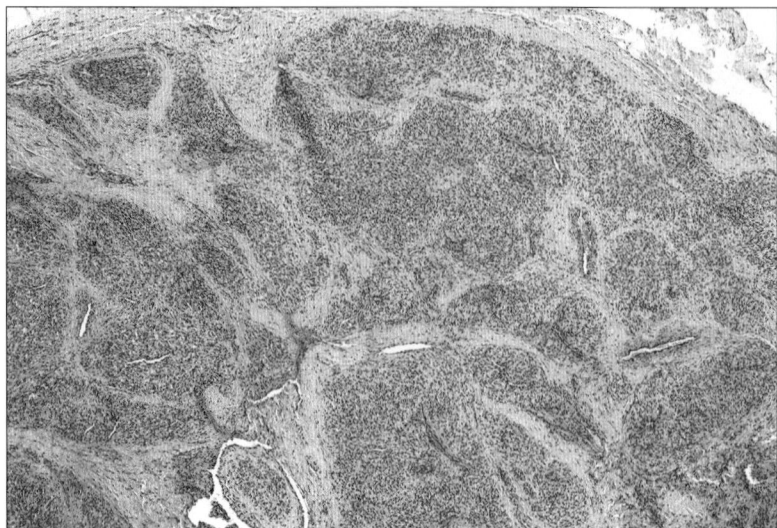

Fig. 35.479
Intravascular lobular capillary hemangioma: higher-power view showing the vascular lobules.

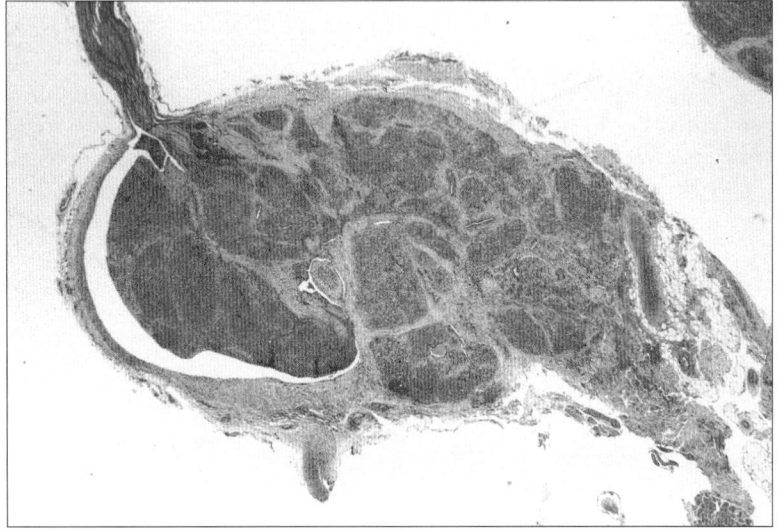

Fig. 35.478
Intravascular lobular capillary hemangioma: this is a rare lesion. Note the thin vessel wall and prominent lobularity.

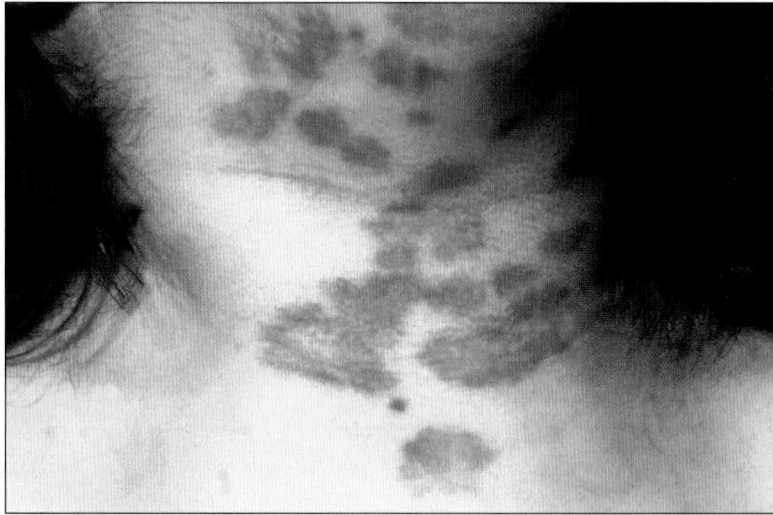

Fig. 35.480
Tufted angioma: lesions commonly present on the neck and upper trunk. Note the presence of extensive macules and plaque-like lesions. By courtesy of the Institute of Dermatology, London, UK.

Superficial infiltration by acute and chronic inflammatory cells in large numbers is a common finding, but this is seen only in ulcerated lesions. In such instances, the adjacent epidermis is often acanthotic and tends to form a well-defined collarette. When inflammation is marked, the overall features show a close resemblance to granulation tissue, except for the presence of capillary lobules in the deeper dermis at the base of the lesion.

Those cases developing satellite lesions often show extension into the subcutaneous fat.

Intravenous lobular capillary hemangioma is histologically similar to the more conventional lesion except that it lacks a significant inflammatory component (Figs 35.478 and 35.479).

Human papillomavirus type 2 has been found in some cases of lobular capillary hemangioma suggesting a possible etiological link.[51,52] RAS and BRAF mutations, particularly BRAF V600E, have been found in sporadic and lobular capillary hemangiomas associated with port-wine stains, suggesting a possible role of the RAS / ERK pathway in their pathogenesis.[52–54]

Differential diagnosis

The most important differential diagnosis is bacillary angiomatosis, an infectious vascular proliferation caused by a rickettsial organism *Rochalimaea henselae*.[55–57] The latter occurs mainly in patients with AIDS and

rarely in other immunosuppressed hosts or exceptionally in normal individuals. Although both lesions are architecturally very similar, bacillary angiomatosis is composed of pale eosinophilic endothelial cells and shows polymorphs throughout the lesion, accentuated in the vicinity of basophilic granular aggregates. The latter, when stained with Giemsa or Warthin-Starry, show clumps of short bacilli. The bacilli may also be demonstrated by immunohistochemistry.

Lobular capillary hemangioma may sometimes need to be distinguished clinically from other types of capillary hemangioma. Mucosal lesions with very plump endothelial cells and a high mitotic rate may be readily distinguished from angiosarcoma by their lobular architecture.

Tufted angioma

Clinical features

Tufted angioma (angioblastoma of Nakagawa) is a distinctive variant of capillary hemangioma which was described in the Japanese literature in 1949 as angioblastoma.[1–4] It presents most commonly in infants or children, showing an equal sex incidence and a predilection for the neck, upper trunk and limbs (Fig. 35.480).[1–8] Lesions tend to be acquired mainly during the

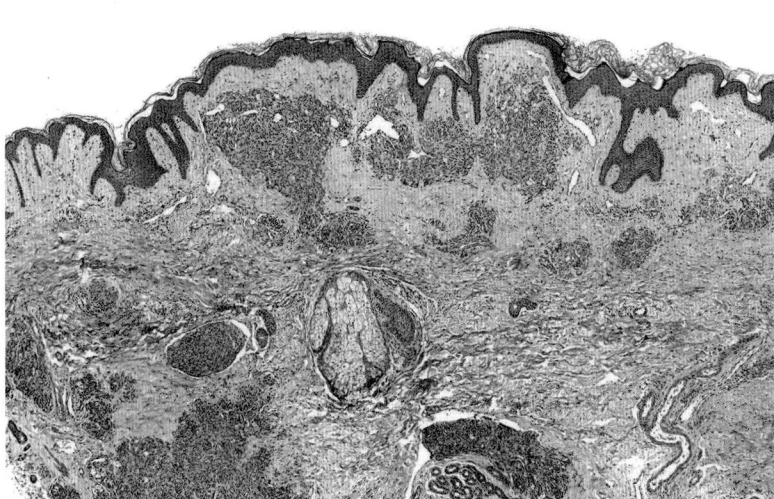

Fig. 35.481
Tufted angioma: this is a typical low-power appearance of sharply circumscribed vascular nodules in the reticular dermis.

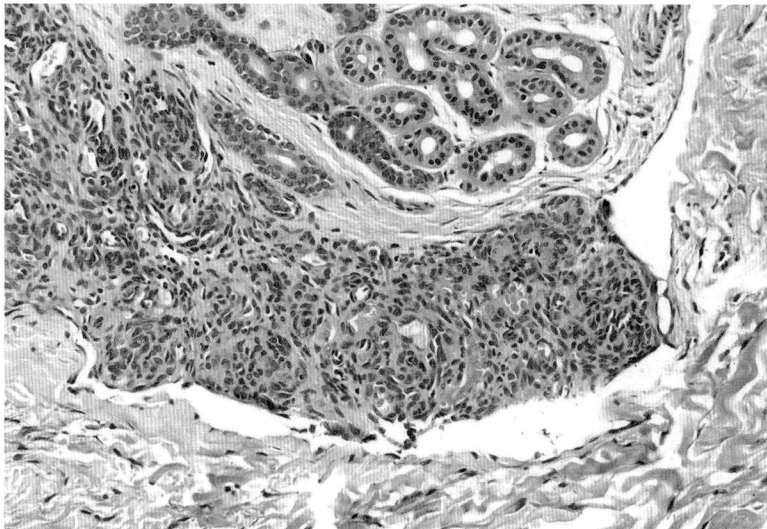

Fig. 35.482
Tufted angioma: the nodules are composed of tightly knit capillaries. Note the conspicuous lymphatic vessel.

first year of life, but congenital tumors occur in about 25% of patients.[8,9] A congenital case with disseminated lesions has been described.[10] Isolated cases occur in adults.[11,12] Familial tumors are exceptional.[13] Unusual locations of the tumor include the oral cavity, the perianal area and the palm.[14–16] A case in an intracranial location, one in the maxilla and one in the nasal cavity have been described.[17–19] The lesion grows slowly over a period of years as an erythematous macule or plaque, or as a cluster of papules attaining a size of up to 10 cm or more. An annular configuration can also be seen and multifocal lesions are rare.[20–22] In some cases hyperhidrosis and hypertrichosis are seen.[8] Kasabach-Merritt syndrome is an important complication in a very small number of cases and more rarely low-grade coagulopathy is seen.[8,23–25] Exceptional cases associated with vascular malformations, one occurring at the site of herpes zoster and one at a site of BCG vaccination have been documented.[26–29] A case of an angiomatous lesion developing in association with Ramucrimab therapy and histology mimicking tufted angioma was observed.[30] Surgical excision is difficult due to the size and extension of the tumor beyond the evident clinical margins. Spontaneous regression does occur, it is usually not complete and seems more common than previously thought.[31–34] Regression may even be seen in congenital tumors.[35]

Histologic features

At low power, the distinctive feature is the presence in the dermis and superficial subcutis of scattered, rounded, oval or elongated lobules of closely packed capillaries in a typical 'cannonball' distribution (*Fig. 35.481*). Each lobule is composed of poorly canalized capillaries lined by bland endothelial cells and surrounded by pericytes, and closely resembling the early stages of a strawberry nevus. A distinctive feature is the presence in the periphery of the lobules of dilated crescent-shaped or semilunar lymphatic channels (*Fig. 35.482*). Focal crystalline inclusions in the endothelial cell cytoplasm can be seen in some cases (*Fig. 35.483*).[36] In the dermis between the tufts of capillaries, variable number of dilated lymphatics are seen.[37] Unusual histologic features include an intravenous location and proliferation of sweat glands.[38–40] In a case with regression an increase in CD8+ lymphocytes within tumor lobules suggested a cytotoxic mediated immune response as a possible mechanism.[41] Areas of tufted hemangioma may occur in kaposiform hemangioendothelioma and it is likely that both tumors are part of the same spectrum.[42–44] By immunohistochemistry, the endothelial cells lining the capillaries are positive for ERG and CD31. The crescent-like vessels and the lymphatics in the surrounding dermis are positive for D2-40.[45] WT1 is positive.

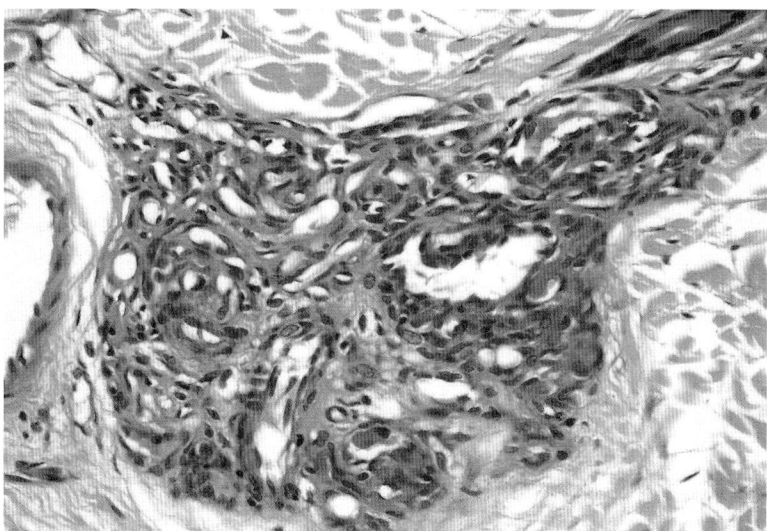

Fig. 35.483
Tufted angioma: note the eosinophilic inclusions.

Differential diagnosis

Strawberry nevus has a more diffuse, confluent and extensive involvement of the dermis and subcutis, and lacks the dilated crescent-shaped lymphatic channels at the periphery of the lobules. Distinction from nodular Kaposi sarcoma is easy because the latter lacks the 'cannonball' pattern and is composed of a uniform population of spindle-shaped cells and pseudovascular clefts. Furthermore, cutaneous involvement by Kaposi sarcoma in immunocompetent children is exceedingly rare.

Cavernous hemangioma

Clinical features

The age, sex and anatomical distribution of cavernous hemangioma are much the same as for capillary hemangioma.[1–3] However, cavernous hemangioma differs principally in its tendency to be larger and more diffuse, showing little, if any, propensity to involute (*Fig. 35.484*). These lesions are very likely to be part of the spectrum of lesions described under the rubric noninvoluting congenital hemangioma (RICH, see above). Some of them are also likely to represent vascular malformations. The overlying skin tends towards a rather more bluish-red coloration, reflecting the increased blood content of these lesions.

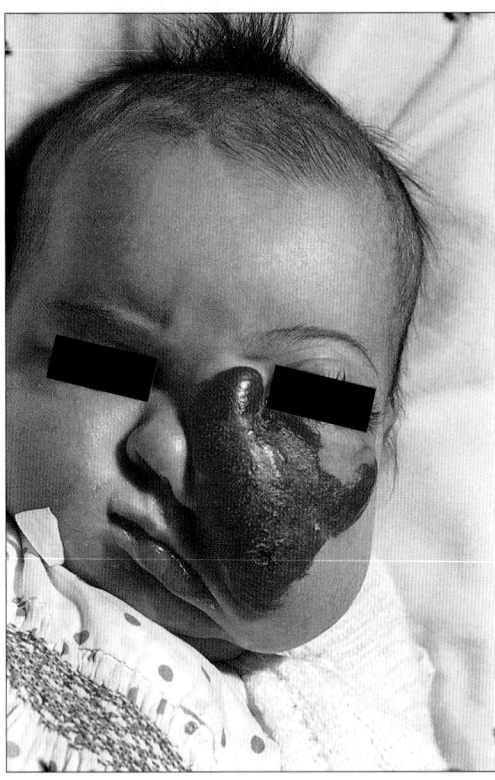

Fig. 35.484
Cavernous hemangioma: this massive lesion is distorting the nose and cheek of this female infant. Cavernous hemangiomas often involve the deeper tissues, with resultant pressure necrosis. By courtesy of M.M. Black, MD, St Thomas' Hospital, London, UK.

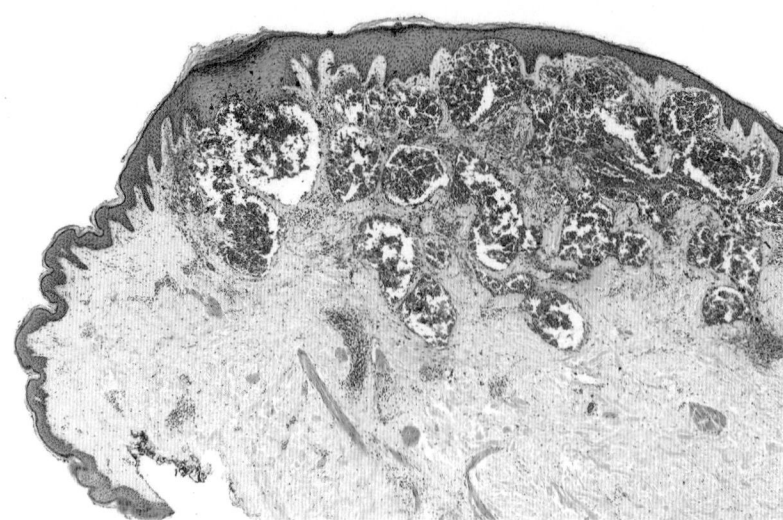

Fig. 35.485
Cavernous hemangioma: the vessels are dilated and rather thin walled.

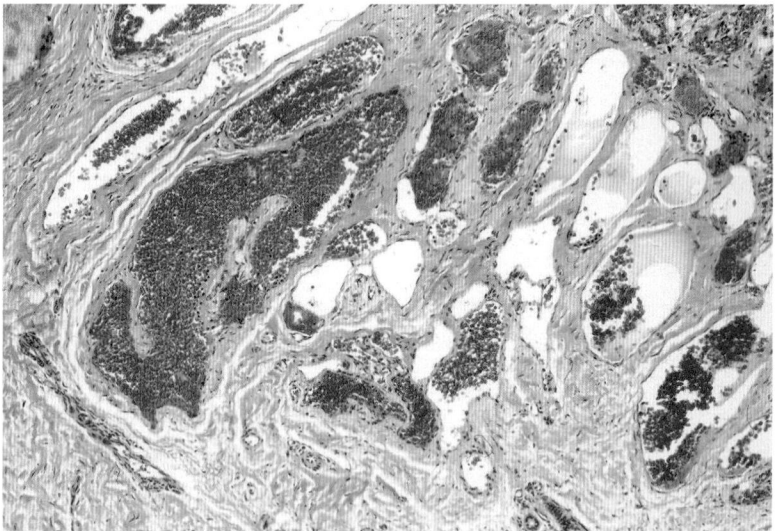

Fig 35.486
Cavernous hemangioma: higher-power view.

Cavernous hemangioma may rarely be associated clinically with multiple enchondromas (Maffucci syndrome), hemangiomas in the alimentary tract (blue rubber bleb nevus syndrome) or with a consumption coagulopathy due to sequestration of platelets within the lesion (Kasabach-Merritt syndrome).[4–7]

Sinusoidal hemangioma is a relatively uncommon variant of cavernous hemangioma.[8] This tumor shares some similarities to a distinctive hemangioma that has been described mainly in the genitourinary tract, soft tissues and other organs as anastomosing hemangioma.[9] It presents as a bluish, solitary deep dermal or subcutaneous nodule on the trunk (particularly in the subcutaneous tissue of the breast) or limbs of middle-aged adults, showing a predilection for females. Rare cases in males are associated with gynecomastia. There is no tendency to local recurrence.

Pathogenesis and histologic features

It is likely that most cavernous hemangiomas are variants of vascular malformations.

In contrast to capillary hemangiomas, cavernous lesions are composed of a nonlobular, poorly demarcated proliferation of numerous dilated vessels with flattened endothelium (Figs 35.485 and 35.486). Vessel wall thickness is variable. Moderate stromal chronic inflammation is often a feature.

The sinusoidal hemangioma is usually lobular and focally ill defined. It is composed of gaping, markedly dilated, intercommunicating, back-to-back, congested vascular channels with very thin walls, giving rise to a typical sieve-like or sinusoidal pattern (Figs 35.487 and 35.488). Cross-sectioning artifact may produce a pseudopapillary appearance reminiscent of Masson tumor. Focal thrombosis, areas of infarction, hyalinization and even calcification or ossification can be present, especially in long-standing lesions. Endothelial cells are monolayered and flat, but occasionally mild pleomorphism is a feature. Each vessel is surrounded by an attenuated layer of actin-positive pericytes.

Differential diagnosis

The diagnosis of sinusoidal hemangioma is usually straightforward, but breast lesions can sometimes be confused with angiosarcoma. The latter, however, is intraparenchymal rather than subcutaneous and shows an infiltrative growth pattern with at least focal endothelial atypia, multilayering and mitoses.

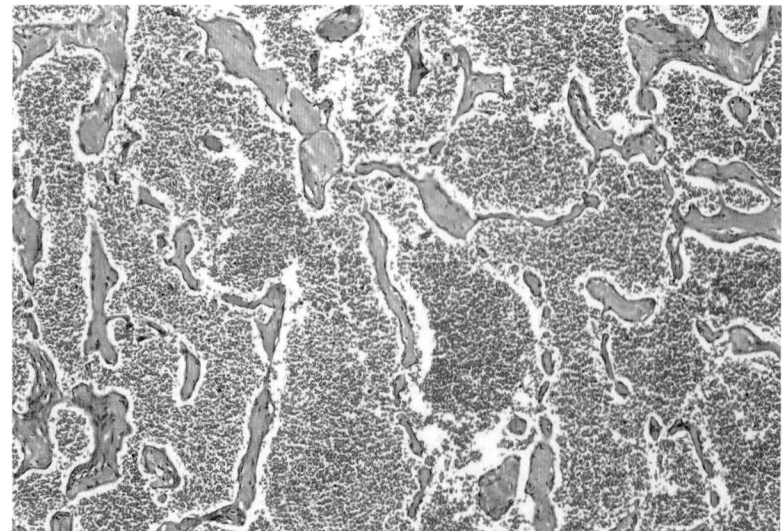

Fig. 35.487
Sinusoidal hemangioma: the back-to-back appearance is characteristic. By courtesy of C.D.M. Fletcher, MD, Brigham and Women's Hospital and Harvard Medical School, Boston, USA.

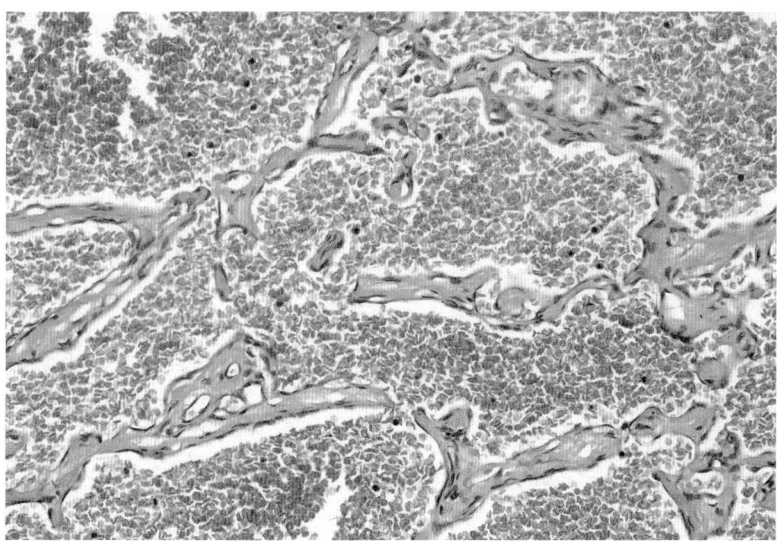

Fig. 35.488
Sinusoidal hemangioma: the presence in some cases of mild nuclear atypia combined with the thin-walled architecture may cause confusion with angiosarcoma. By courtesy of C.D.M. Fletcher, MD, Brigham and Women's Hospital and Harvard Medical School, Boston, USA.

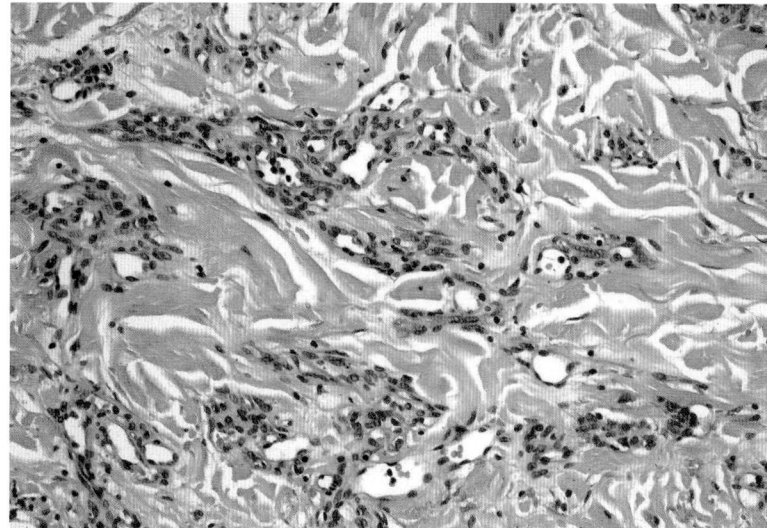

Fig. 35.490
Microvenular hemangioma: the ramifying vessels are lined by a plump endothelial monolayer and an outer layer of more spindled pericytes.

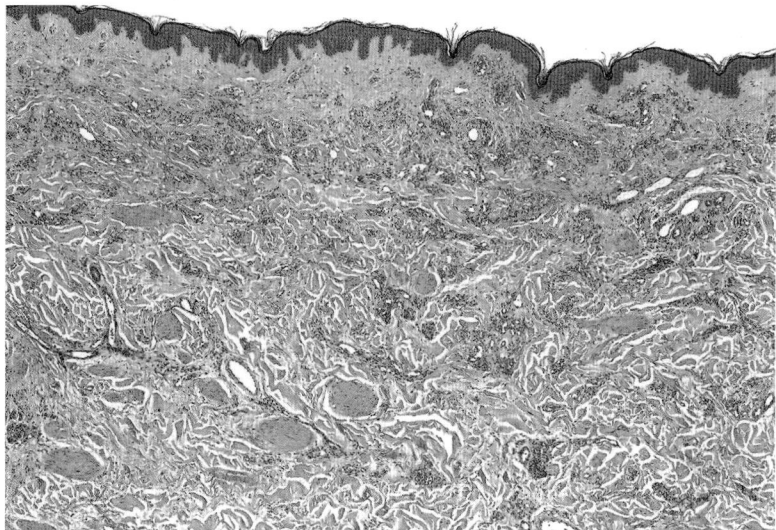

Fig. 35.489
Microvenular hemangioma: the manner in which the vessels irregularly infiltrate the dermis is sometimes mistaken for Kaposi sarcoma.

Microvenular hemangioma

Clinical features

Microvenular hemangioma is an asymptomatic lesion that commonly presents on the limbs of young adults as a red–bluish papule, nodule or plaque.[1-3] Multiple, sometimes numerous, lesions have been documented in a few patients.[3-6] In a reported case, multiple bilateral macules, patches and plaques were described.[7] Presentation in children is rare.[8,9] A case positive for human herpesvirus-8 has been documented in the context of POEMS syndrome.[10] Recurrence is exceptional.

Histologic features

Histologically, it consists of irregular, branching, thin-walled venules lined by bland endothelial cells containing plump nuclei (Fig. 35.489). The tumor extends widely throughout the dermis, dissecting between somewhat hyalinized collagen bundles (Fig. 35.490). Infiltration of arrector pili muscles by vascular channels is a frequent finding. Each channel is surrounded by a layer of SMA positive pericytes. The endothelial cells are positive for CD31, CD34, ERG and WT1 but are negative for podoplanin.[3,11,12] GLUT1 is also negative.[12,13]

Hobnail hemangioma

Clinical features

Hobnail hemangioma (targetoid hemosiderotic hemangioma) usually presents on the limbs (particularly the thigh) and trunk of young or middle-aged adults and shows a male predilection.[1-4] Lesions in infants and children are exceptional. Occasional tumors occur in the oral cavity including the tongue and gingivae.[5,6] The lesion is asymptomatic, usually less than 2 cm in diameter, and increases in size very slowly. Patients sometimes describe cyclic changes.[7] In women, lesions often become larger and darker prior to menstruation and become lighter and smaller after the menstrual period.[8-11] In pregnancy, they increase in size probably due to estrogen, and in one case two lesions developed at the same time as the secondary sexual changes.[9] Multiple lesions are exceptional. The original clinical description comprised a central red papule or macule, surrounded by successive clear and ecchymotic haloes (Fig. 35.491). Most often, however, the clinical presentation is nondistinctive and the differential diagnosis includes hemangioma, nevus or fibrous histiocytoma. There appears to be little or no tendency for recurrence.

Pathogenesis and histologic features

Based on immunohistochemical negativity for WT1 only it has been proposed that this lesion represents a superficial lymphatic malformation.[12,13]

The most striking low-power feature is the presence of a wedge-shaped vascular proliferation with the base towards the epidermis. The vascular channels are irregular, thin-walled, dilated, and lined by endothelial cells with bland protruding nuclei and scanty cytoplasm (hobnail cells) (Figs 35.492 and 35.493). Focal papillary projections are a characteristic feature. As the lesion descends into the deep dermis, the vascular channels become less conspicuous, appear to dissect between collagen bundles, and are lined by more flattened endothelial cells. Extravasation of red blood cells and hemosiderin deposition can be prominent but this depends on the stage of the lesion. Inflammation is not usually a feature but scattered lymphocytes and plasma cells may sometimes be seen.

It is likely that this tumor represents the benign end of the spectrum of a group of lesions characterized by hobnail endothelial cells, including papillary intralymphatic angioendothelioma (PILA, Dabska tumor) and retiform

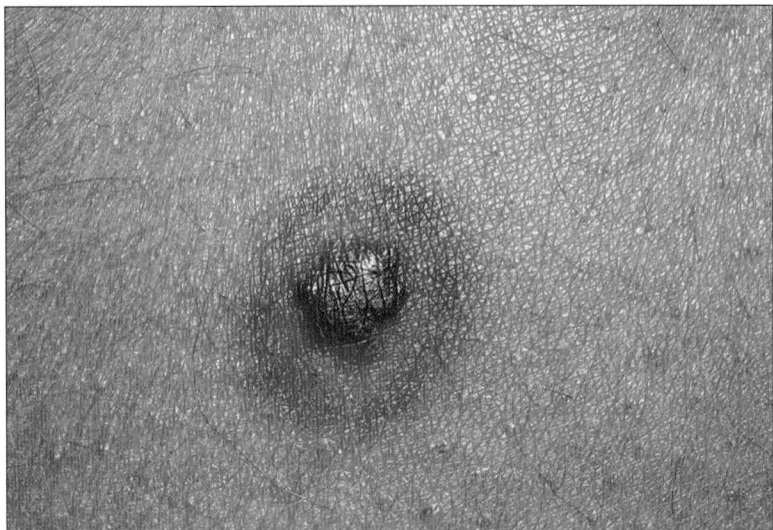

Fig. 35.491
Hobnail hemangioma: this example shows the characteristic targetoid appearance.

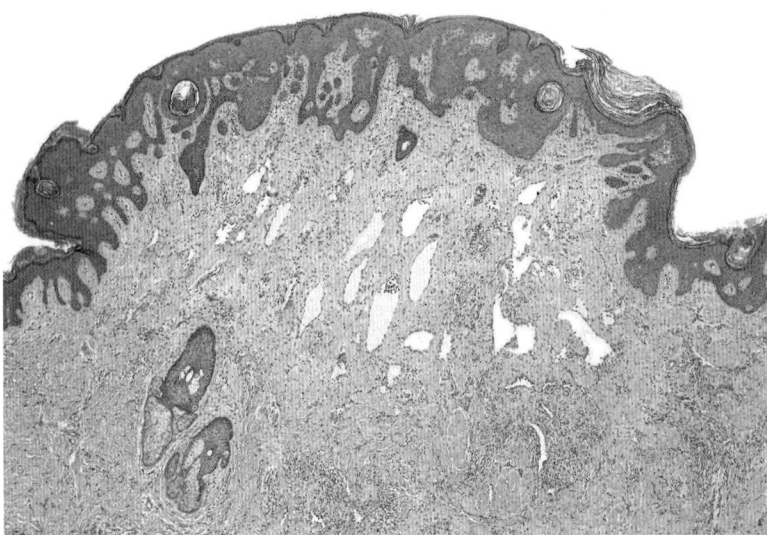

Fig. 35.492
Hobnail hemangioma: thin-walled vascular channels are present in the superficial dermis. The growth pattern is wedge shaped.

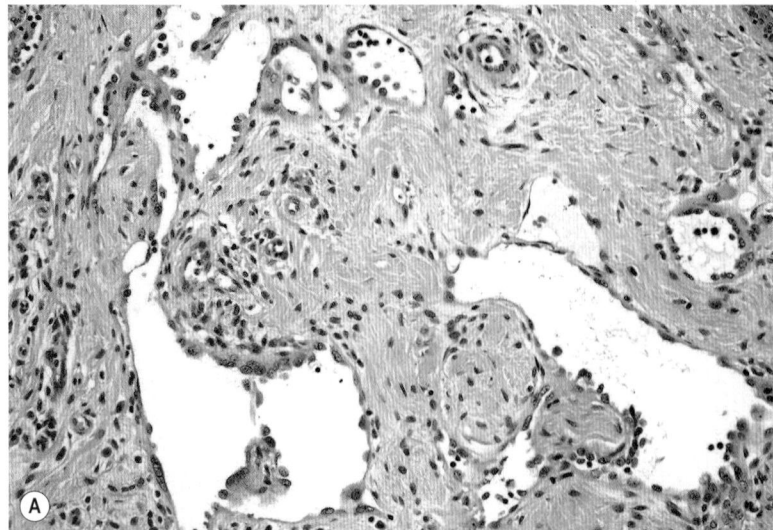

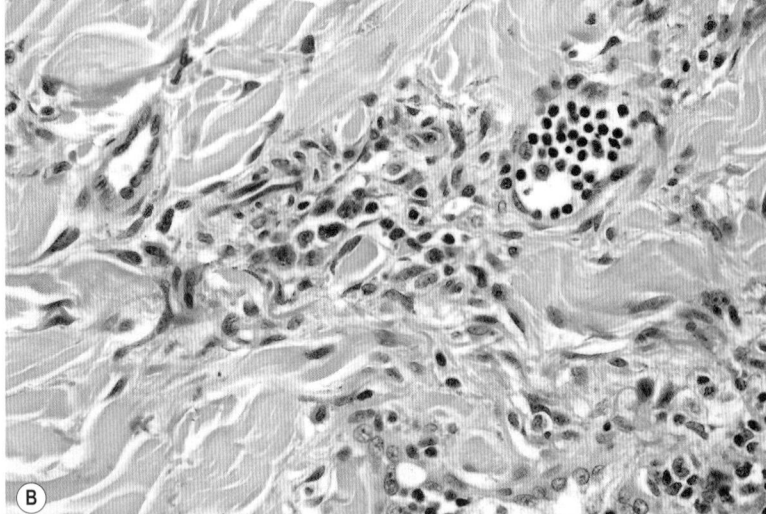

Fig. 35.493
Hobnail hemangioma: (**A**) the endothelial cells are prominent and protrude into the lumen. Note the papillary processes; (**B**) there is abundant hemosiderin pigment.

hemangioendothelioma.[14] Trauma may induce secondary changes similar to those seen in hobnail hemangioma.[15]

The endothelial cells in hobnail hemangioma stain diffusely for vascular markers including CD31 and ERG. CD34 is usually negative or only very focally positive. A layer of alpha-SMA–positive pericytes surrounds some of the vascular channels. Despite the changes associated with the menstrual cycle, endothelial cells are negative for estrogen and progesterone receptors.[9] The positive staining for vascular endothelial growth factor receptor 3 (VEGFR-3) and D2-40 has led to the suggestion that hobnail hemangioma displays lymphatic differentiation.[4,12,13,16] VEGFR-3 is, however, not entirely specific for lymphatic endothelium. Staining for HHV-8 is consistently negative.[17]

Differential diagnosis

The differential diagnosis includes retiform hemangioendothelioma and patch-stage Kaposi sarcoma: the former is diffusely infiltrative and extends into the subcutaneous tissue; the latter lacks a wedge-shaped architecture, does not display hobnail endothelial cells lining the proliferating vascular channels and plasma cells are conspicuous. Furthermore, the endothelial cells lining the vascular channels in Kaposi sarcoma are invariably positive for HHV-8.

Acquired elastotic hemangioma

Clinical features

Acquired elastotic hemangioma is a rare lesion arising in sun-exposed skin of the forearms and neck, with predilection for middle-aged and elderly women. It presents as a small, solitary, asymptomatic erythematous plaque.[1,2]

Histologic features

A band-like superficial dermal proliferation of capillaries, which are often parallel to the epidermis, is seen (*Fig. 35.494*). In the surrounding, dermis there is solar elastosis. The endothelial cells are positive for vascular markers including CD31 and ERG but are usually negative for D2-40.[3]

Cutaneous epithelioid angiomatous nodule

Clinical features

Cutaneous epithelioid angiomatous nodule is very rare and occurs as a papule or nodule in adults, with predilection for the trunk followed by the limbs and face.[1-3] Intranasal lesions rarely occur.[4,5] Multiple lesions are exceptional.[1,2,6-9] Rare cases associated with a capillary malformation and one with multiple lobular capillary hemangiomas (pyogenic granuloma) have been described.[10-12] There is no tendency for local recurrence.

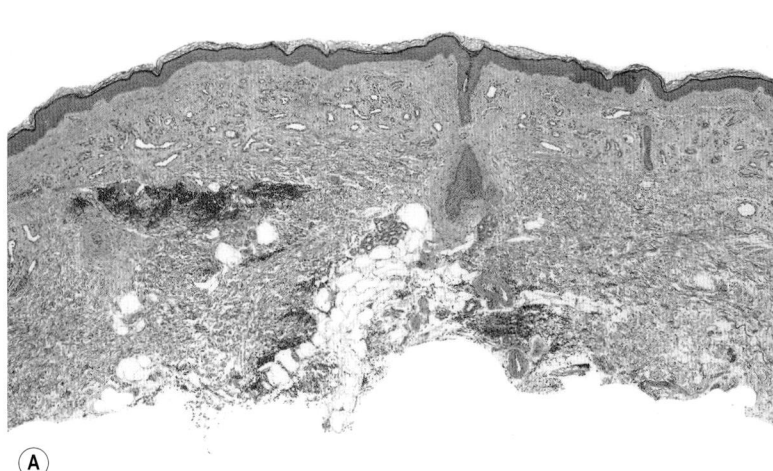

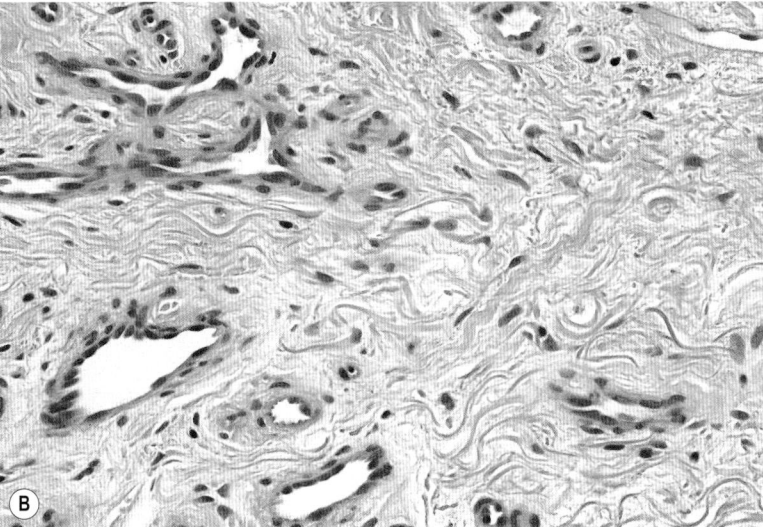

Fig. 35.494
Acquired elastotic hemangioma: (**A**) there is a superficial plaque-like proliferation of small blood vessels; (**B**) note the background solar elastosis.

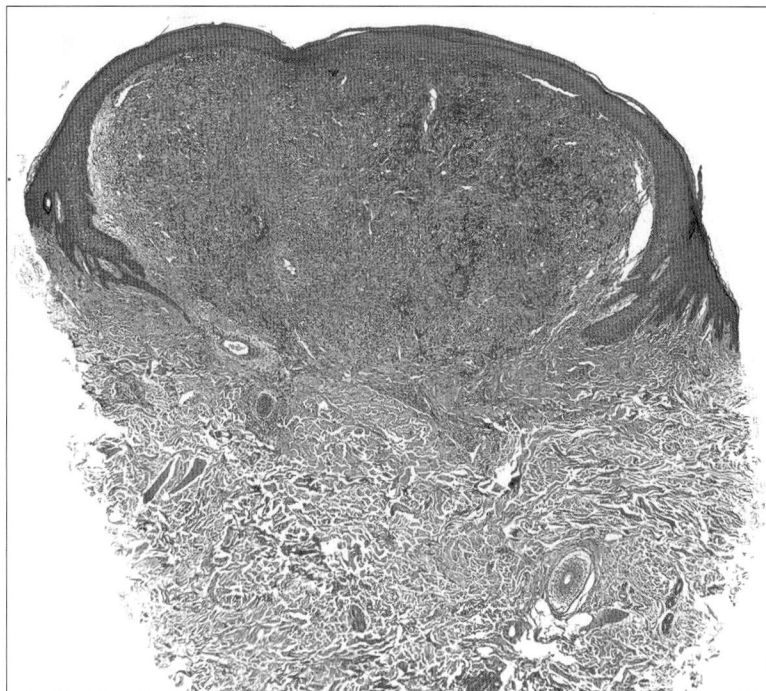

Fig. 35.495
Epithelioid angiomatous nodule: the lesion presented as a solitary nodule. It is superficially located and well circumscribed.

Histologic features

Histology shows a single small nodule composed of plump, pink, epithelioid cells with intracytoplasmic lumina and very focal formation of vascular channels (*Figs 35.495* and *35.496*). In the background there may be mild fibrosis, hemosiderin deposition and scattered inflammatory cells. Mitotic figures are usually not numerous but can be prominent in some cases. Tumor cells are positive for endothelial cell markers including CD31 and ERG and negative for keratins and EMA. Positivity for D2-40 is variable.[13] A case with expression of estrogen receptor has been described.[14]

A single case examined showed no evidence of microsatellite instability.[15]

Differential diagnosis

Distinction from epithelioid hemangioma is based on the different clinical presentation and the presence of a single lobule of epithelioid endothelial cells with very focal formation of vascular spaces other than intracytoplasmic lumina and a usually mild inflammatory cell infiltrate in cutaneous epithelioid angiomatous nodule. However, it seems likely that both lesions are related.[1–3,16,17] Epithelioid angiosarcoma is not usually circumscribed or superficial, and cytologic atypia is always seen.

Epithelioid hemangioma

Epithelioid hemangioma (angiolymphoid hyperplasia with eosinophilia) is the preferred term for a group of benign vascular tumors characterized by the presence of endothelial cells with abundant eosinophilic, sometimes vacuolated, cytoplasm that resemble epithelial cells.[1–4] An alternative name, histiocytoid hemangioma, although accurate, has been abandoned because it originally included a clinically broader group of tumors.[5,6] Other names used to describe this entity include atypical pyogenic granuloma, pseudopyogenic granuloma, inflammatory angiomatous nodule, papular angioplasia and intravenous atypical vascular proliferation.[7–9] The previously described overlap with Kimura disease was erroneous, since the latter is a morphologically quite separate immunologically mediated disorder.[10,11] It is more likely that epithelioid hemangioma is a neoplasm rather than a reactive process associated with trauma.[12,13] In some cases, there is a history of previous trauma including a burn.[14] It represents the benign end of the spectrum of a family of vascular tumors which includes epithelioid hemangioendothelioma and epithelioid angiosarcoma.

Clinical features

Epithelioid hemangioma typically arises in the third and fourth decades, shows a slight predilection for males (although purely cutaneous lesions are more common in females) and occurs most often as painless, dull red, single or multiple nodules in the head and neck region (*Fig. 35.497*).[1–4] Presentation elsewhere in the skin is rare but distribution is wide and includes the upper extremities including the palm, nail bed, the penis and the scrotum.[15–19] Lesions tend to be sessile or plaque-like and are prone to secondary ulceration and/or bleeding. Rare lesions present as a large soft tissue tumor or as a giant skin lesion.[20,21] Intravascular origin is a frequent microscopic finding but the tumor may originate from larger blood vessels including arteries.[22,23] Eruptive lesions are very rare.[24] A single case involving a nerve has been documented.[25] Tumors can present at other sites including the deep soft tissues, bone, lymph node, oral mucosa, tongue, breast, testis, ovary and colon.[2,26–36] An exceptional case presented as a giant axillary artery aneurysm.[37] Blood eosinophilia is present in up to 10–15% of cases. An association with pregnancy is probably coincidental.[38] Simple excision is often followed by recurrence, but metastasis does not occur. Spontaneous regression is exceptional.[39,40]

Transient angiolymphoid hyperplasia and Kaposi sarcoma have been documented after primary infection with HHV-8 in a patient with HIV infection.[41] However, HHV-8 is not found in lesions of sporadic epithelioid hemangioma.[42]

Lesions with features similar to those seen in epithelioid hemangioma have been documented in association with arteriovenous malformations.[43,44]

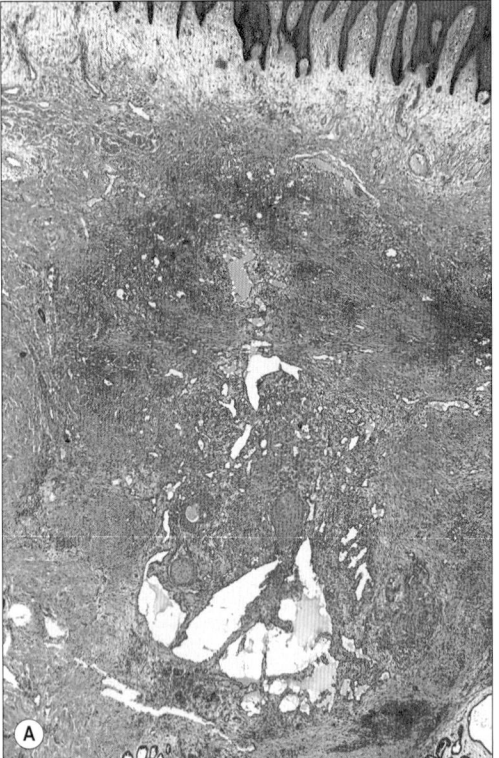

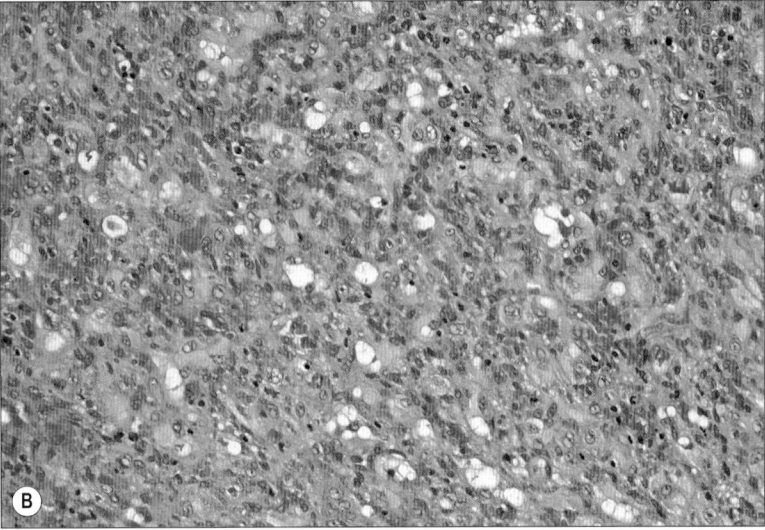

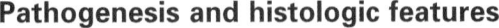

Fig. 35.496
Epithelioid angiomatous nodule: (**A**) there is a diffuse proliferation of epithelioid endothelial cells. Vascular channels may be focal or absent; (**B**) the epithelioid endothelial cells have abundant eosinophilic cytoplasm and vesicular nuclei. Note the intracytoplasmic lumina, some of which contain erythrocytes.

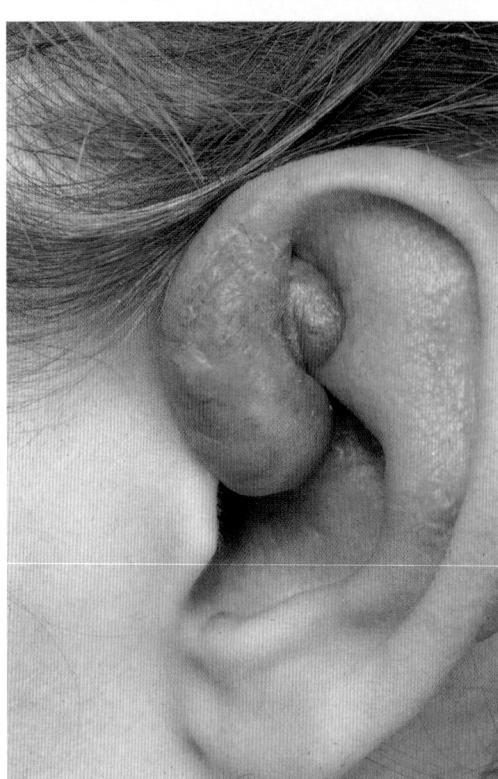

Fig. 35.497
Epithelioid hemangioma: the ear is commonly involved. There are multiple confluent lesions. From the collection of the late N.P. Smith, MD, the Institute of Dermatology, London, UK.

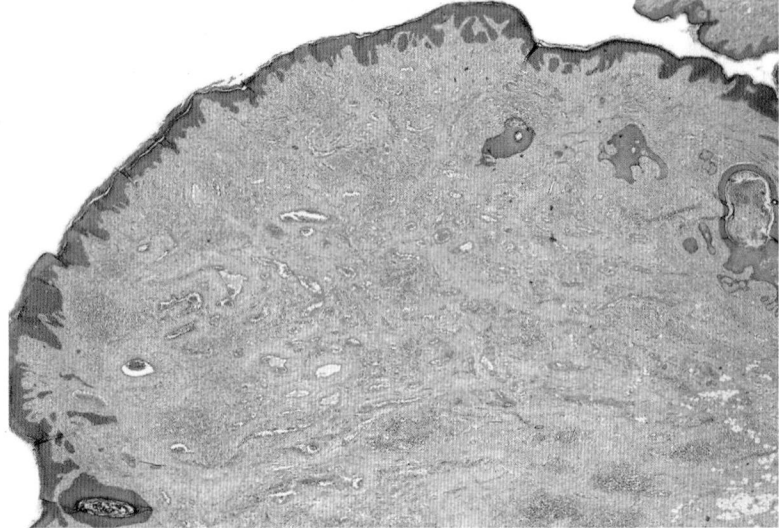

Fig. 35.498
Epithelioid hemangioma: scanning view of a vascular nodule with lymphoid aggregates at the periphery.

Pathogenesis and histologic features

FOS gene rearrangements have been found in epithelioid hemangioma of bone and soft tissue but only exceptionally in soft tissues and skin.[45–47] *FOSB* fusion has been described in a subset of intraosseous epithelioid hemangioma with some worrisome histopathological features such as higher cellularity, cytologic atypia, and necrosis.[45,46] Cases in the skin associated with the fusion are usually cellular and occur on the penis.[45,46]

Tumors are predominantly intradermal although occasionally subcutaneous variants are encountered. They present as an ill-defined, lobulated mass composed of numerous vascular spaces (*Fig. 35.498*). The latter, of varying luminal diameter, are lined by large rounded endothelial cells with copious, rather eosinophilic cytoplasm and oval vesicular nuclei (*Fig. 35.499*). Some show cytoplasmic vacuoles, representing primitive lumina (*Fig. 35.500*). Solid cords of cells may also be present. Although the endothelial cells are prominent, they do not show pleomorphism or mitotic activity. A significant proportion of cases are partially or totally intravascular, most often arising within a vein. A small percentage of skin cases are more solid with a more exuberant proliferation of endothelial cells that may be confused with malignancy and has predilection for the penis.[48]

Surrounding these small vessels is a variably prominent inflammatory cell infiltrate composed largely of lymphocytes, numerous eosinophils and histiocytes (*Fig. 35.501*). Increased lymphatic channels have been highlighted by immunohistochemistry for podoplanin.[49] Lymphoid follicles may be present in some cases (*Fig. 35.502*). Long-standing lesions show stromal sclerosis.

Unusual findings include multinucleated giant cells, a granulomatous reaction and follicular mucinosis.[50–52]

Immunohistochemically, the tumor cells are variably positive for endothelial markers but, in contrast to epithelioid hemangiomas in other locations such as bone, cutaneous lesions are cytokeratin negative except for focal positivity in penile lesions.[23,48] HHV-8 is negative.[53] Although the FOSB fusion is hardly ever found in cutaneous lesions, immunohistochemistry for this marker is positive in slightly more than 50% of cases.[24,54]

A T-cell clone has been rarely reported.[18,55] The significance of this finding is uncertain.

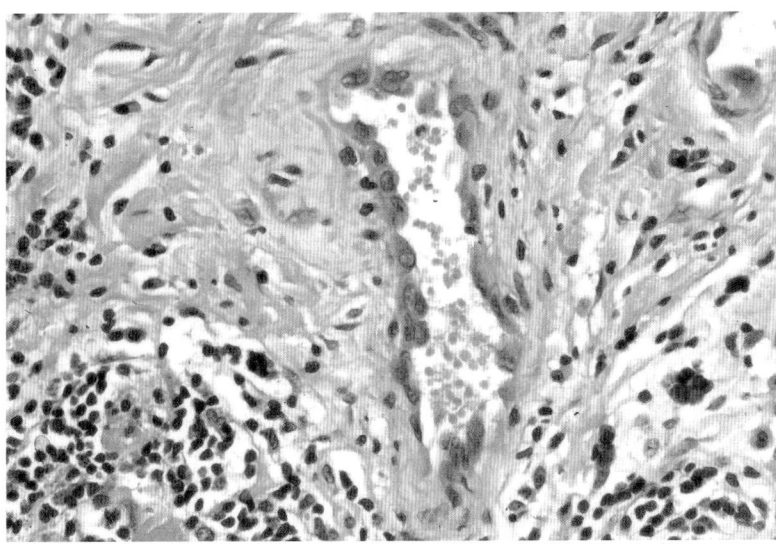

Fig. 35.499
Epithelioid hemangioma: the vessels are lined by large endothelial cells with markedly histiocytoid appearances.

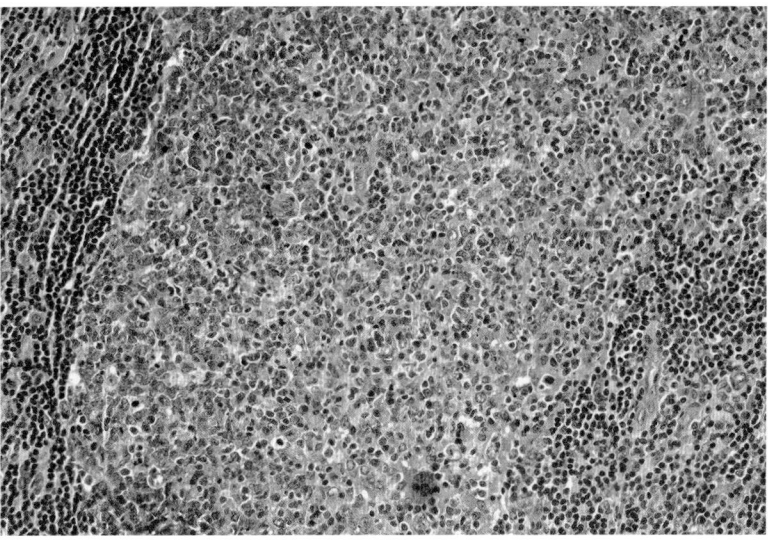

Fig. 35.502
Epithelioid hemangioma: lymphoid follicles are sometimes present

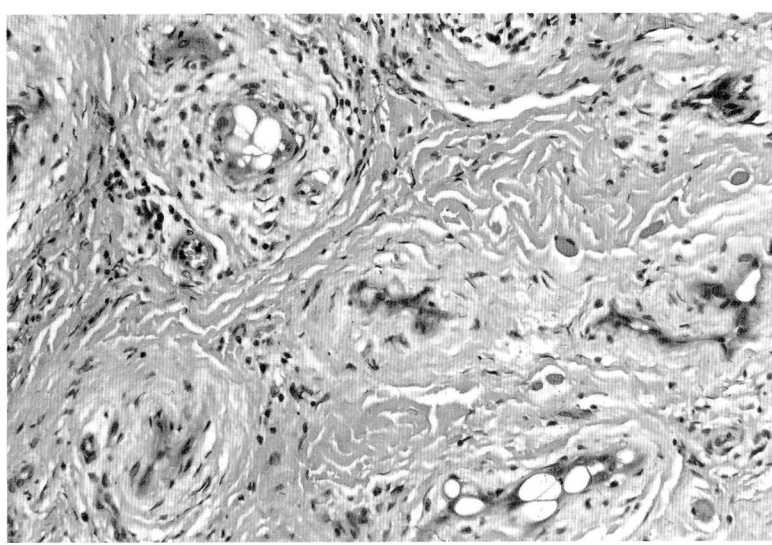

Fig. 35.500
Epithelioid hemangioma: endothelial cell intracytoplasmic lumina are a characteristic feature.

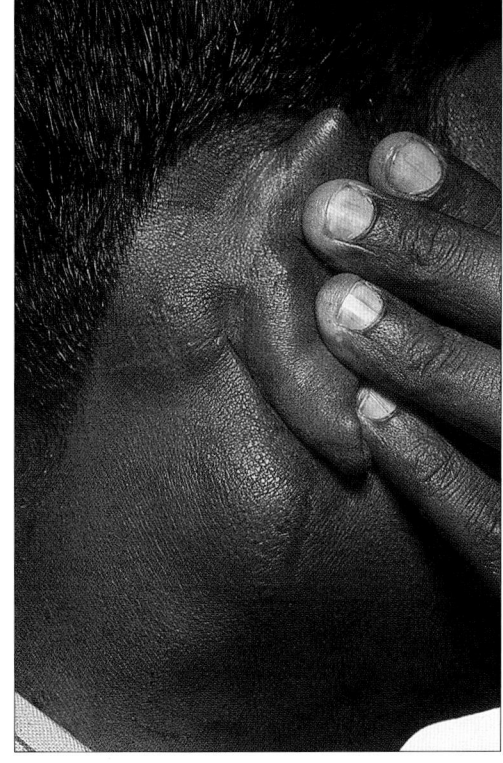

Fig. 35.503
Kimura disease: this patient presented with striking swelling of the neck. By courtesy of the Institute of Dermatology, London, UK.

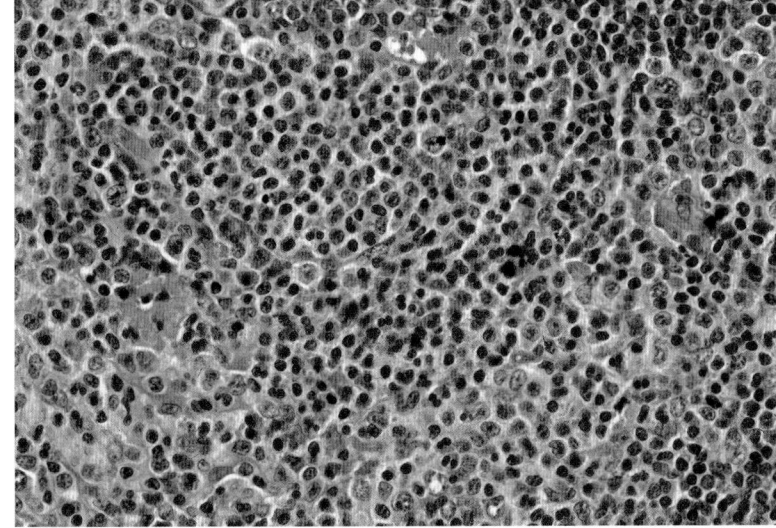

Fig. 35.501
Epithelioid hemangioma: eosinophils are conspicuous.

The *intravenous atypical vascular proliferation*[56] represent an intravenous variant of epithelioid hemangioma. They usually present as a solitary nodule on the head, neck or upper limbs with a predilection for young to middle-aged adults. Unlike, conventional epithelioid hemangioma they usually have a prominent spindle cell (pericytic) component (closely admixed with the epithelioid endothelial channels), which enhances the pseudomalignant appearance of these lesions. Although, they have no tendency to recur.[56]

Differential diagnosis

Kimura disease, with which epithelioid hemangioma is frequently confused, tends to occur more commonly in Orientals in their first and second decades. It also presents on the trunk or limbs and the lesions are frequently tender (*Figs 35.503* and *35.504*).[10,11,57] The majority of cases show a histologically distinctive lymphadenopathy, a circulating eosinophilia and raised IgE levels; some patients have associated renal disease and juvenile temporal

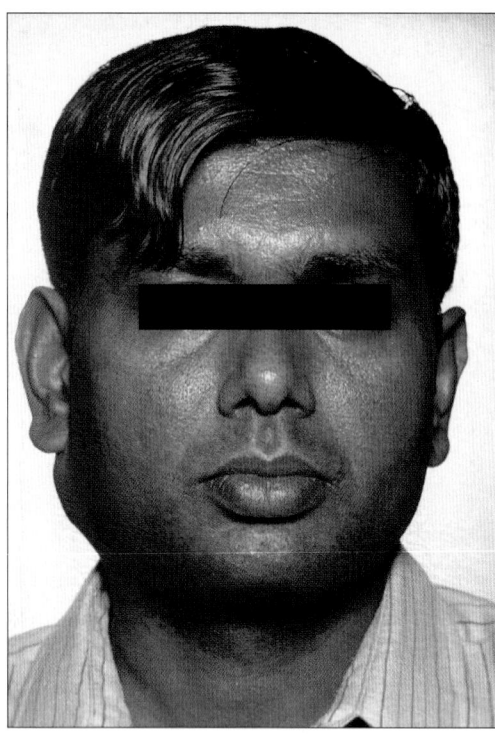

Fig. 35.504
Kimura disease: there is soft tissue and nodal involvement. By courtesy of the Institute of Dermatology, London, UK.

Fig. 35.505
Kimura disease: low-power view showing an intense cellular infiltrate.

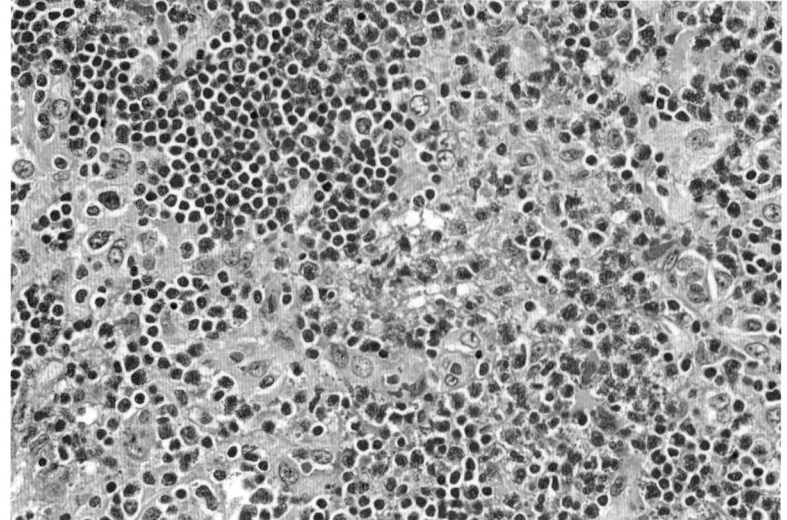

Fig. 35.506
Kimura disease: the infiltrate consists of lymphocytes and numerous eosinophils.

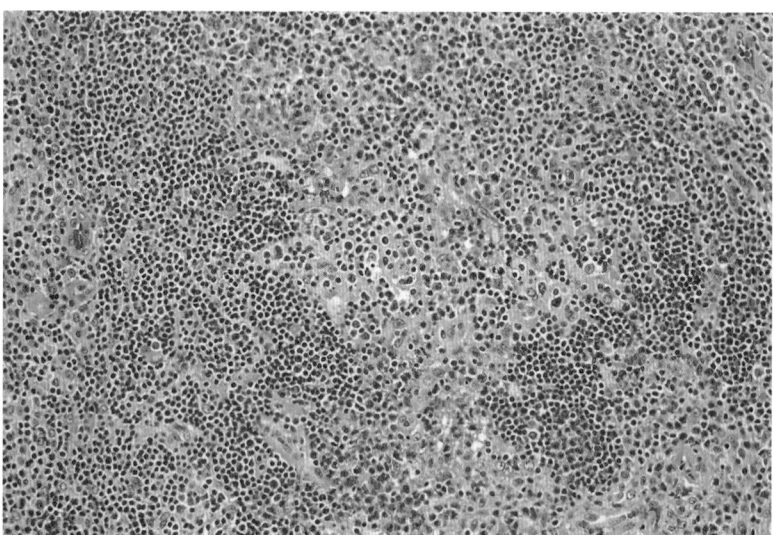

Fig. 35.507
Kimura disease: there is a background proliferation of high capillary venules.

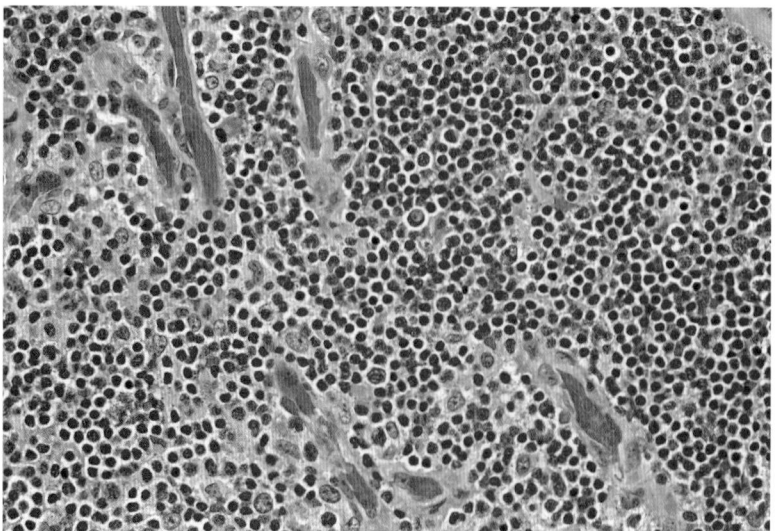

Fig. 35.508
Kimura disease: the endothelial cells are prominent but do not contain intracytoplasmic lumina.

arteritis.[58] Only one patient with epithelioid hemangioma has had associated nephrotic syndrome.[59] Histologically, Kimura disease has a prominent inflammatory cell infiltrate with numerous lymphoid follicles, eosinophil microabscesses, infiltration of germinal centers by eosinophils, proliferation of high endothelial venules (not lined by epithelioid endothelial cells) and large areas of stromal sclerosis (Figs 35.505–35.508). Rare cases of epithelioid hemangioma and Kimura disease presenting in the same patient have been reported.[60]

Cutaneous involvement by lymphoma lacks the distinctive vascular proliferation, while a persistent insect-bite reaction shows a greater number of small capillaries lined by normal flattened endothelium. In injection-site 'granuloma'" (aluminum 'granuloma'"), epithelioid endothelial cells are not a feature and histiocytes with bluish granular cytoplasmic material representing aluminum are found.[61,62] In bacillary angiomatosis, the epithelioid cells are pale and there are abundant neutrophils with nuclear dust and basophilic clumps of bacteria.

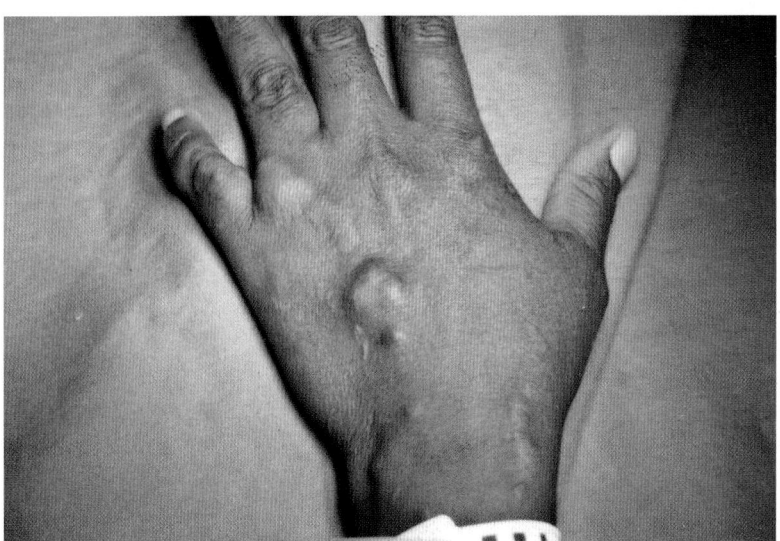

Fig. 35.509
Spindle cell hemangioma: multiple nodules are present at a characteristic site.

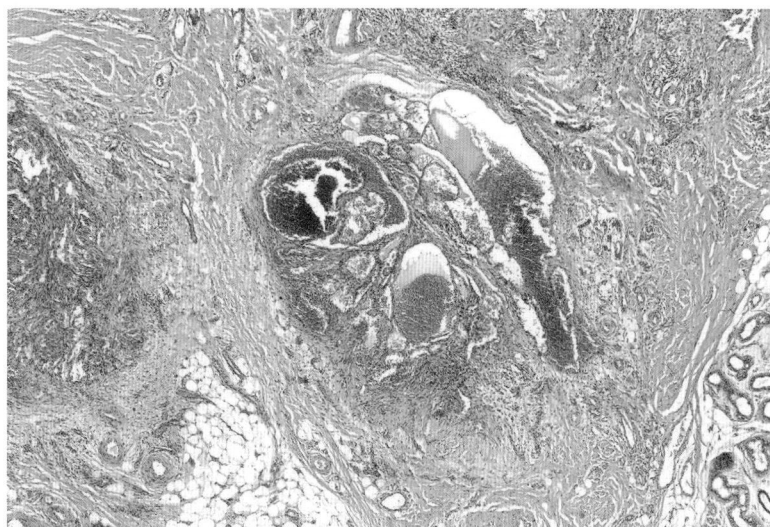

Fig. 35.510
Spindle cell hemangioma: low-power view showing conspicuous dilated vascular channels

Spindle cell hemangioma

Clinical features

Spindle cell hemangioendothelioma was first described as a variant of low-grade angiosarcoma in 1986.[1,2] This proposal was based on the fact that one of the patients in the series developed a metastasis. However, it is almost certain that this metastasis originated from a radiation-induced sarcoma and not from the original lesion. More recent evidence strongly supports the notion that this condition is probably a vascular malformation or a benign process superimposed upon a malformation (spindle cell hemangioma).[3–6]

It most commonly affects the dermis or subcutis of the distal extremities and presents as single or (in 50% of cases) multiple red–blue nodules, which are quite often painful (Fig. 35.509). Rare lesions develop in the head and neck including the oral cavity.[7,8] When multiple, lesions develop slowly over years and the clinical course is indolent. Most patients are in their first three decades and there is an equal sex incidence. Some cases are associated with early-onset varicose veins, congenital lymphedema, Klippel-Trenaunay syndrome or Maffucci syndrome.[9].

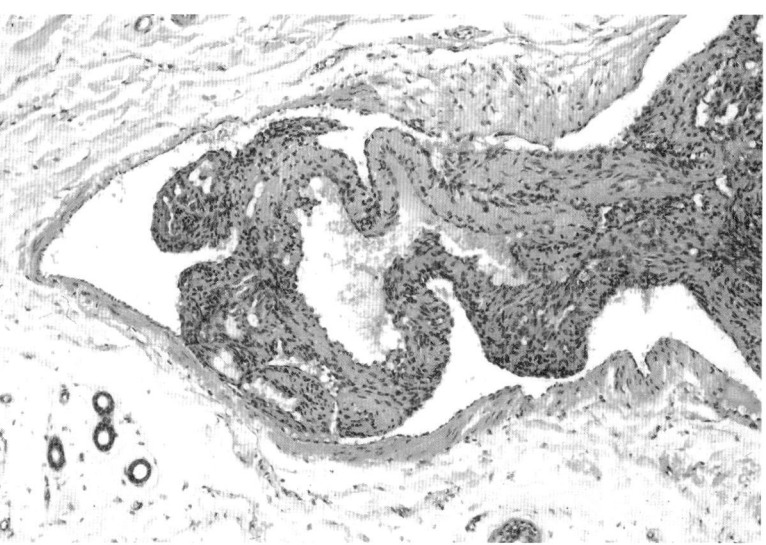

Fig. 35.511
Spindle cell hemangioma: there is an intravascular component.

Pathogenesis and histologic features

An IDH R132C mutation have been found in both sporadic and Maffucci syndrome associated lesions, confirming that this tumor represents a neoplasm.[10,11]

Lesions are poorly circumscribed and consist of thin-walled, congested cavernous vascular spaces intermixed with varying proportions of bland spindled to epithelioid cells with vesicular nuclei (Figs 35.510–35.513). Intracytoplasmic lumina are often present and are a helpful diagnostic feature (Fig. 35.514). The vascular spaces are lined by a single layer of bland endothelial cells, which can rarely show degenerative nuclear pleomorphism. Thrombosis and papillary projections resembling those seen in Masson tumor are common features. Bundles of smooth muscle are quite often present around the blood vessels and in the spindled cell areas. In the periphery of many lesions, there are thick-walled, irregular blood vessels resembling a localized arteriovenous shunt. Rare cases can be associated with epithelioid hemangioendothelioma.

Immunohistochemically, vascular markers label mainly the endothelium of the blood vessels and the more epithelioid cells in the stroma. Admixed with the latter are actin-positive pericytes.[3] Reticulin staining in the solid areas reveals a vasoformative architecture.

Differential diagnosis

In nodular Kaposi sarcoma there are usually no cavernous vascular spaces or vacuolated epithelioid cells, and hyaline globules are often present in

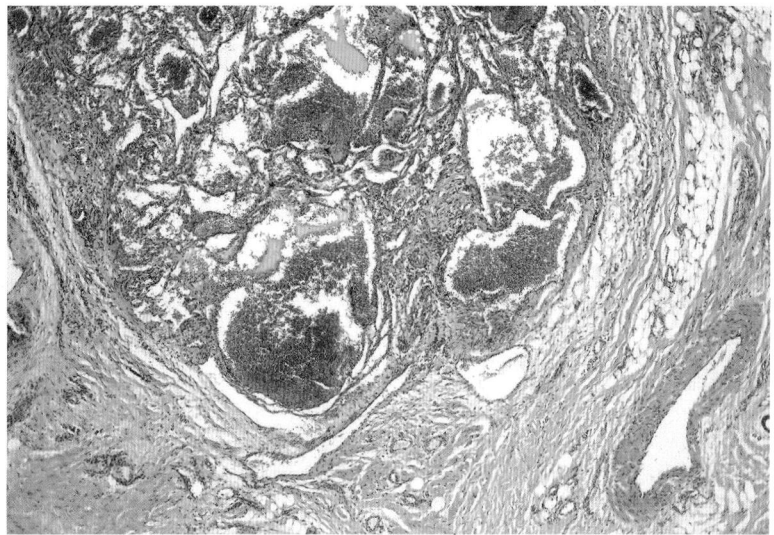

Fig. 35.512
Spindle cell hemangioma: the tumor is composed of an admixture of spindle cells and, often, cavernous vascular channels.

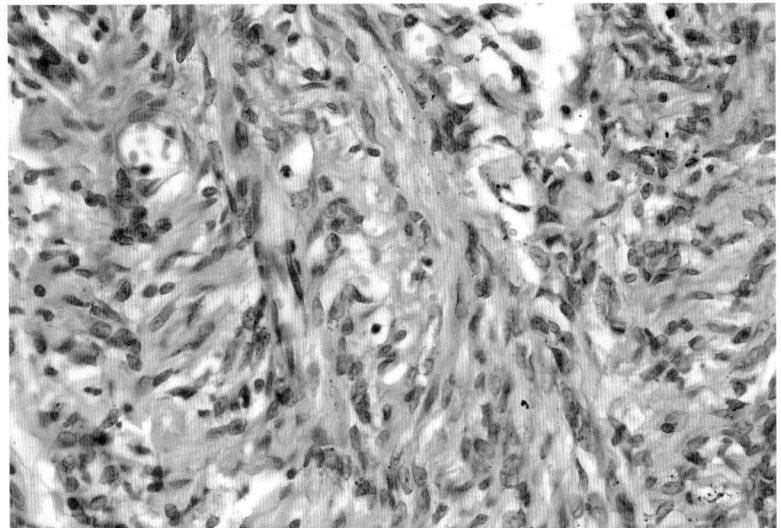

Fig. 35.513
Spindle cell hemangioma: the spindle cells are bland and have fairly regular oval or elongated nuclei.

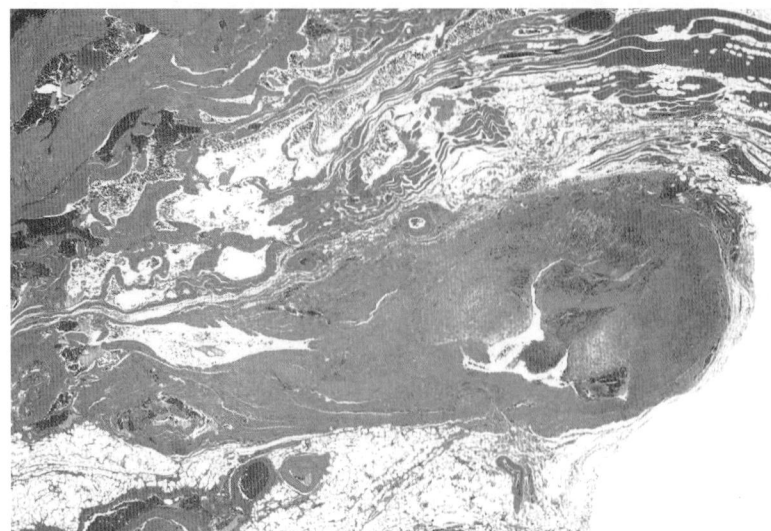

Fig. 35.515
Angiomatosis: this example consists of variably sized congested cavernous vessels.

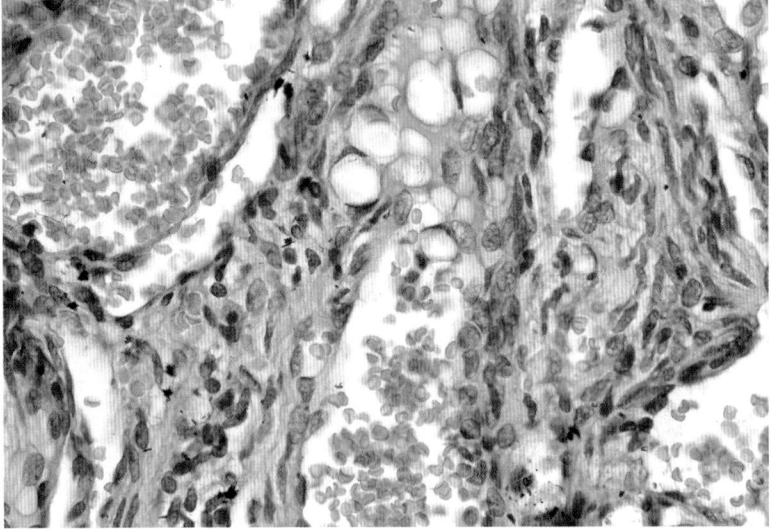

Fig. 35.514
Spindle cell hemangioma: intracytoplasmic lumina are an important diagnostic feature.

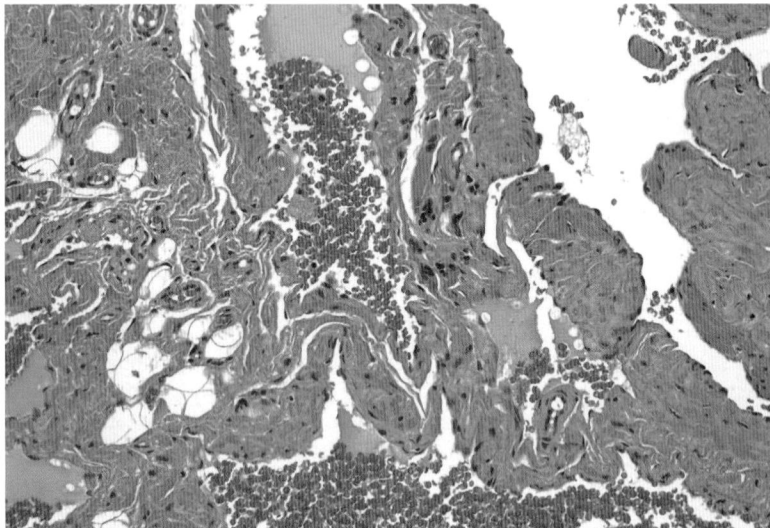

Fig. 35.516
Angiomatosis: high-power view showing dilated vessels with admixed adipocytes.

the spindled cells. The latter cells in Kaposi sarcoma are consistently CD34 positive.

Angiomatosis

Clinical features

Angiomatosis is a rare condition that presents in children and adolescents.[1–3] There is slight predilection for females. A single case involving the left forearm of an adult has been documented.[4] It is characterized by a diffuse proliferation of blood vessels affecting a large contiguous area of the body (usually a limb).[1,2] Presentation in the head and neck is rarely seen.[5] Involvement of the skin, underlying soft tissues and bone is common, and this is associated with hypertrophy of the affected limb. Lesions within parenchymal organs and the central nervous system are sometimes a feature. Due to extensive involvement, surgical treatment is often difficult.

Histologic features

Histologically, two patterns have been described:[2]
- The more common variant consists of a mixture of veins, capillaries and cavernous vascular spaces (*Figs 35.515* and *35.516*).

- The second variant consists almost exclusively of capillaries, often with a focal lobular pattern.

In both types there is an abundant admixture of mature fat. Glut-1 is negative. Perineural invasion is sometimes a feature. Osseous metaplasia has been reported in one case.[6]

Symplastic hemangioma

Symplastic hemangioma is defined as extensive degenerative changes in a pre-existing vascular proliferation, usually a vascular malformation, closely mimicking malignancy.[1–4] Only a handful of cases have been reported. The variant of pre-existing hemangioma is often not clearly identifiable.

Clinical features

It usually presents in the limbs of an adult, as a long-standing lesion that starts changing.

Pathogenesis and histologic features

The histologic appearances are likely to reflect degenerative changes within a hemangioma or more often, a vascular malformation (*Figs 35.517* and *35.518*). Tumors are often polypoid, dermal and well circumscribed. The

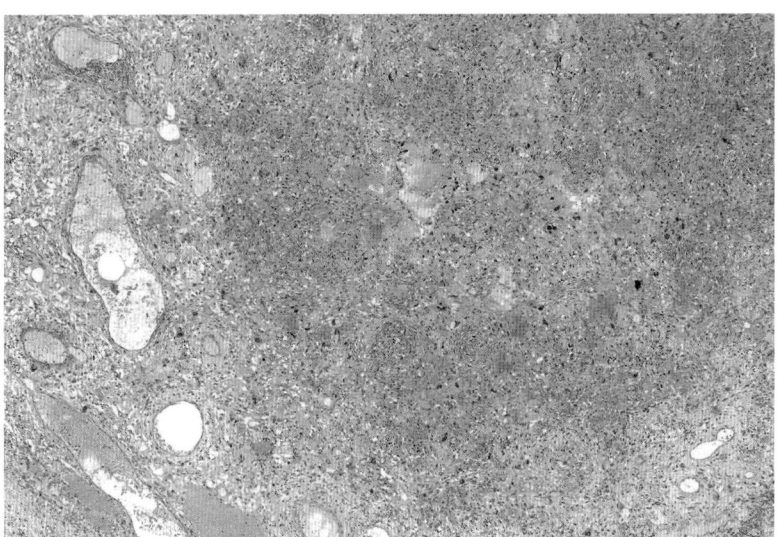

Fig. 35.517
Symplastic hemangioma: low-power view showing dilated vessels, and a cellular stroma containing conspicuous atypical cells.

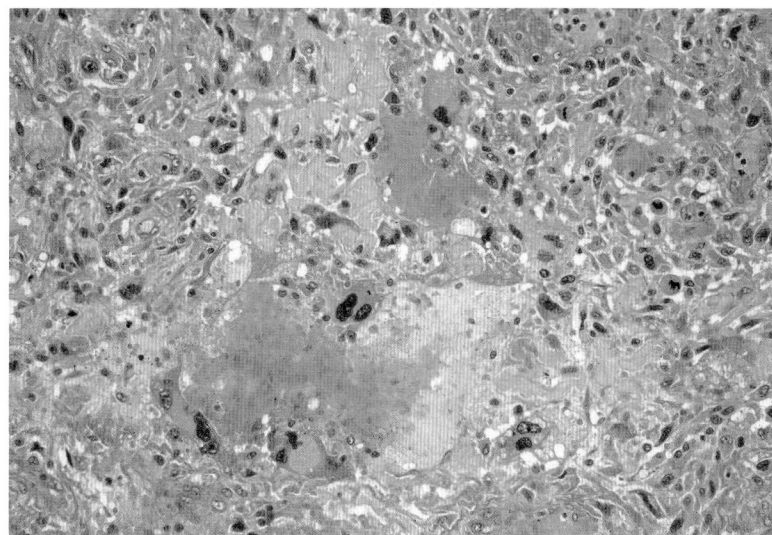

Fig. 35.519
Symplastic hemangioma: there is marked nuclear pleomorphism and hyperchromatism.

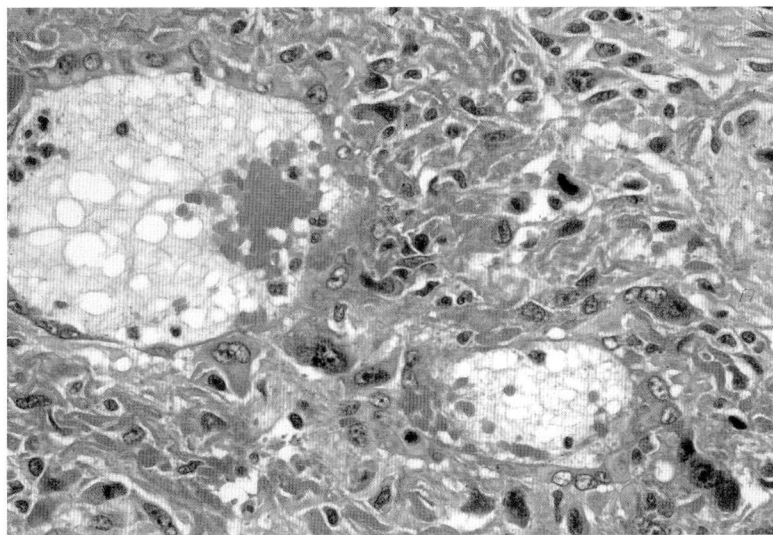

Fig. 35.518
Symplastic hemangioma: higher-power view of dilated vessels and atypical stromal cells.

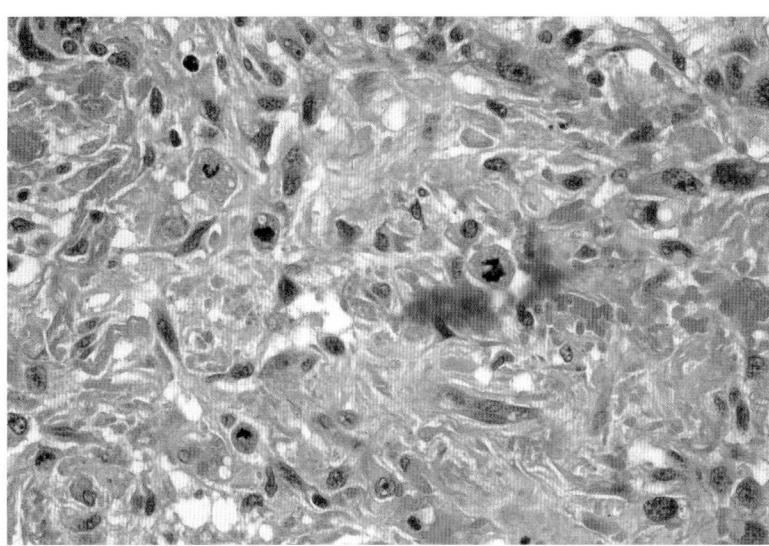

Fig. 35.520
Symplastic hemangioma: note the mitotic figures.

typical histologic picture consists of dilated and congested thin to thick-walled vascular spaces surrounded by a variable cellular stroma with frequent myxoid change and hemorrhage. Stromal cells and smooth muscle cells within the vessel walls show variable cytologic atypia consisting of nuclear enlargement and hyperchromatism (*Fig. 35.519*). Often cells have a bizarre appearance, and multinucleated cells are common. The endothelial cells lining the vascular spaces may be plump but do not display cytologic atypia, multilayering or mitotic activity, allowing distinction from an angiosarcoma. Mitotic figures may be found in the stromal component but tend to be rare (*Fig. 35.520*). Very occasional atypical mitotic figures can be a feature.

Vascular tumors of low-grade or borderline malignancy

Retiform hemangioendothelioma

Clinical features

Retiform hemangioendothelioma is a variant of low-grade angiosarcoma that is closely related to (and more common than) papillary intralymphatic angioendothelioma (Dabska tumor) (see below).[1-4] It usually presents in

young adults as a slowly growing, asymptomatic tumor and shows a predilection for the distal extremities, especially the lower leg. Sex incidence is equal. Very rarely, cases occur in association with radiation therapy or chronic lymphedema. A patient with multiple lesions and one with Milroy disease have been documented.[5,6] A case developing at the site of a cystic lymphangioma has been reported.[7] Local, often repeated, recurrences are common, but so far only two cases have metastasized to regional lymph nodes and a further case metastasized to soft tissues close to the primary tumor.[1,8,9] No distant spread or tumor-related death has been reported.

Histologic features

Lesions are ill defined and involve the dermis and/or subcutis. A striking feature is the histologic resemblance of the tumor to normal rete testis. This appearance is conferred by the presence of long, arborizing, branching blood vessels, which are lined by monomorphic bland endothelial cells with prominent apical nuclei and scanty cytoplasm (*Fig. 35.521*). These cells protrude prominently into the vascular lumina, with a typical hobnail appearance (*Figs 35.522* and *35.523*). A common but not invariable feature is the presence of numerous lymphocytes both within and adjacent to the vessels and in close relation to the endothelial cells (*Fig. 35.524*). Focally, intravascular papillae with collagenous cores are present. Most tumors show solid areas

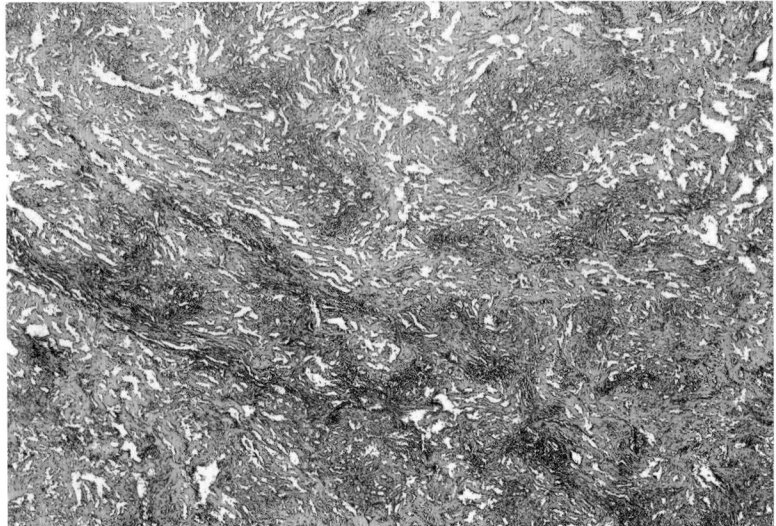

Fig. 35.521
Retiform hemangioendothelioma: low-power view showing the conspicuous vascularity.

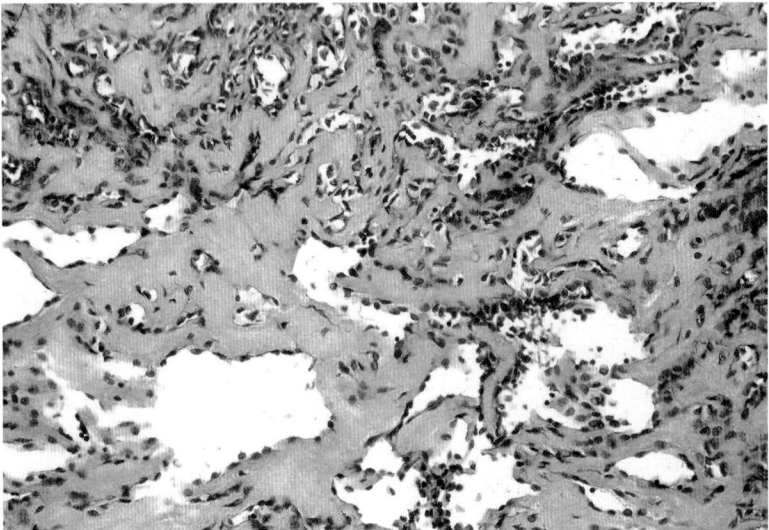

Fig. 35.522
Retiform hemangioendothelioma: protuberant (hobnail) endothelial cell nuclei are a characteristic feature.

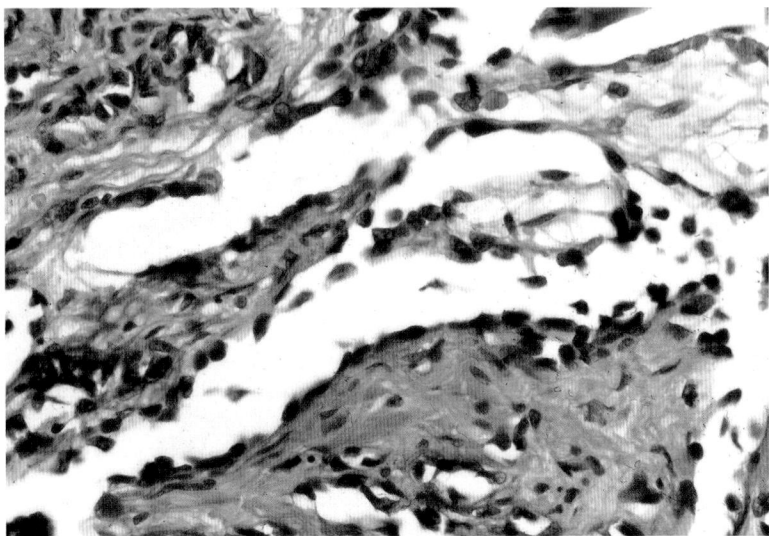

Fig. 35.523
Retiform hemangioendothelioma: intraluminal papillae are commonly present.

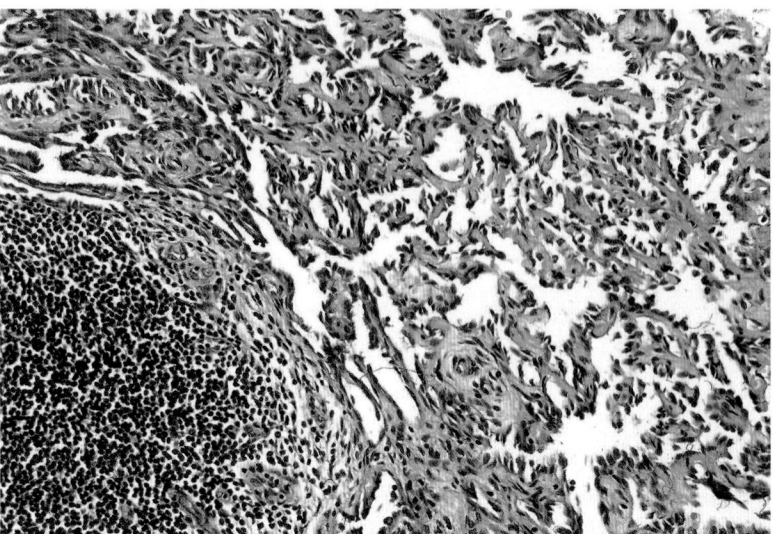

Fig. 35.524
Retiform hemangioendothelioma: aggregates of lymphocytes are frequently seen.

composed of spindled and rare epithelioid cells. The case reported in the patient with Milroy disease had solid areas with cytologic atypia raising the possibility of the tumor representing a composite hemangioendothelioma.[6]

Immunohistochemically, the cells stain for vascular markers including CD31 and CD34. Staining for lymphatic markers including D2-40 and the less specific VEGFR-3 has yielded contradictory results.[10,11]

Differential diagnosis

Retiform hemangioendothelioma has similar clinical and histologic features to papillary intralymphatic angioendothelioma (PILA) and it has been proposed that the former is an adult variant of the latter. However, in PILA, there is no retiform architecture, cavernous lymphangioma-like vascular spaces predominate and intravascular papillae with collagenous cores are prominent. Targetoid hemosiderotic hemangioma (hobnail hemangioma) is always more superficial and more localized, and hobnail endothelial cells are only focally present. Angiosarcoma usually presents in a different clinical setting and is characterized histologically by at least focal pleomorphism, mitosis, absence of hobnail endothelial cells and multilayering.

Papillary intralymphatic angioendothelioma

Papillary intralymphatic angioendothelioma (PILA) is a very rare tumor, first described by Dabska in 1969 as malignant endolymphatic angioendothelioma (Dabska tumor).[1] Since then, only very few additional cases had been reported in the literature, and there has been no consensus regarding its specific histologic features. A recent series has delineated the histologic features of this tumor more accurately and the alternative name of PILA has been proposed.[2] Tumors present mainly in infants and children but around 25% of patients are adults.[1–3] Males and females are equally affected and tumors have predilection for the limbs. Clinical presentation is that of a slowly growing, solitary, asymptomatic nodule or plaque. Single or multiple tumors have been described in bone.[4–7] Exceptional cases have been documented on the spleen, testis and tongue.[8–10] In a single case, an angiosarcoma developed within a Dabska tumor.[11]

Classification as a tumor with low-grade malignant potential is based on reports of local recurrence and rare regional lymph node metastasis in the original series.[1] However, follow-up in 8 of the 12 cases recently reported showed no evidence of either local recurrence or distant spread.[2] This finding raises the possibility that this tumor is benign but confirmation of these findings is required in larger series with longer follow-up. Until this happens, complete excision of these tumors is advised.

Pathogenesis and histologic features

Based on the close interaction between lymphocytes and endothelial cells in Dabska tumor, it has been proposed that the hobnail endothelial cells

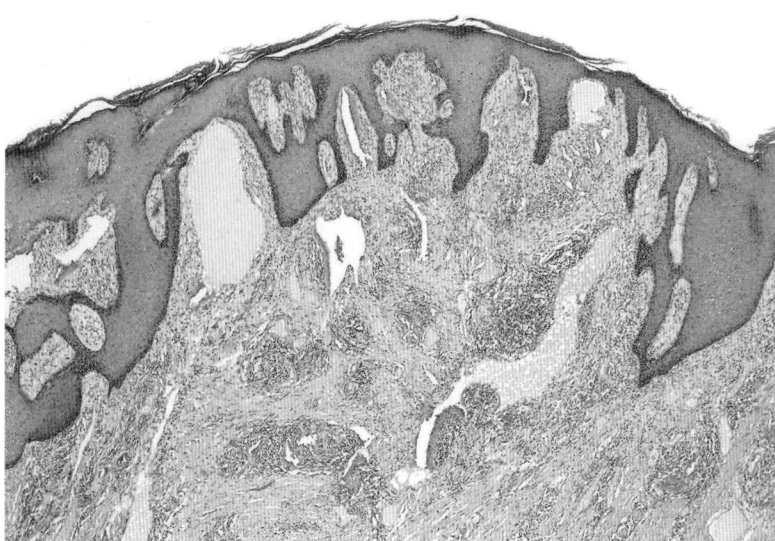

Fig. 35.525
Papillary intralymphatic angioendothelioma (Dabska tumor): tumors have dilated, thin-walled vascular spaces mimicking a cavernous lymphangioma. Note the lymphoid aggregates.

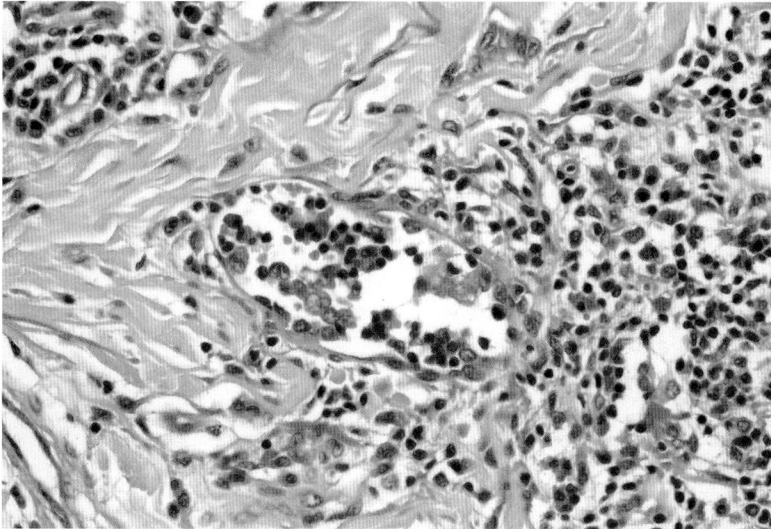

Fig. 35.526
Papillary intralymphatic angioendothelioma (Dabska tumor): high-power view showing hobnail endothelial cells.

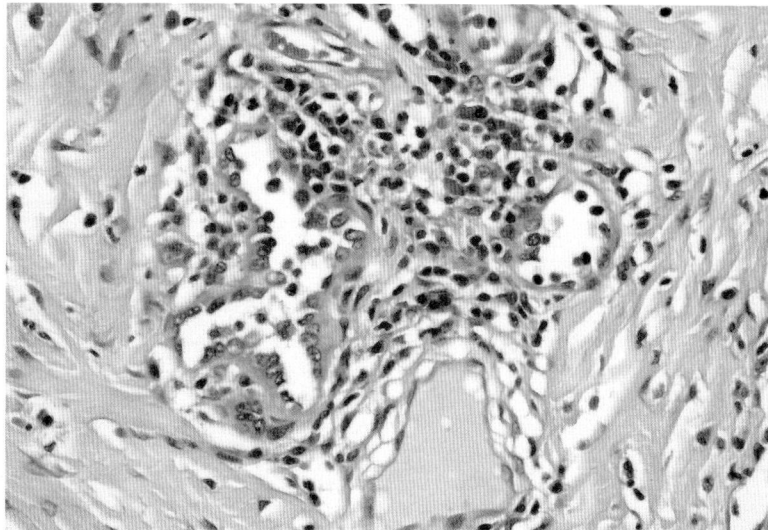

Fig. 35.527
Papillary intralymphatic angioendothelioma (Dabska tumor): hobnail endothelial cells and intraluminal papillae.

Differential diagnosis

The differential diagnosis is the same as that for retiform hemangioendothelioma. Occasionally, lesions that represent otherwise ordinary capillary hemangiomas may display focal papillary tufts which may lead to a confusion with a PILA particularly in small samples.[13]

Kaposiform hemangioendothelioma

Clinical features

Kaposiform hemangioendothelioma is a relatively rare vascular tumor that was originally described as occurring most often in the retroperitoneum or deep soft tissues of infants.[1-3] Tumors exceptionally occur in the choledocus, kidney, maxillary sinus, ethmoid sinus, mediastinum, larynx, internal auditory canal, oropharynx, thymus, spleen and lung.[4-15] Lesions involving the skin and superficial soft tissues also occur and adults may also be affected.[16,17] A case associated with trauma has been documented.[18] Cutaneous and soft tissue tumors have predilection for the limbs and head and neck. Multifocal lesions are exceptional.[19,20] Kaposiform hemangioendothelioma is characterized by locally aggressive and destructive growth. In one case, concurrent skin and concomitant pleural involvement was reported and a tumor led to fetal death due to nonimmune fetal hydrops.[21,22] An association with Kasabach-Merritt syndrome is seen in more than 50% of cases and this is an important cause of mortality.[1,3,17] Regional perinodal involvement is uncommonly seen but metastatic disease has not been reported.[17] Rarely, there is association with lymphangiomatosis.[3,23,24] A case developing in an adult patient with rheumatoid arthritis, one presenting as hydrops fetalis and one with massive fetal chylous ascites have been recorded.[25-27] An exceptional case presenting with bullae and mimicking aplasia cutis congenita has been described.[28]

It has been suggested that there is a close relationship between kaposiform hemangioendothelioma and tufted angioma.[29-31] This is based on clinical and histologic overlap and the fact that both proliferations may induce Kasabach-Merritt syndrome. This is also substantiated by both tumors sharing an identical immunophenotype with expression of PROX-1, a lymphatic endothelial nuclear transcription factor.[32] Overexpression of the latter has been shown to be associated with promotion of invasion in two murine models of kaposiform hemangioendothelioma.[33] It is likely that tufted angioma represents a more localized variant of kaposiform hemangioendothelioma.[34]

Pathogenesis and histologic features

A balanced translocation t(13;16)(q14;p13.3) has been demonstrated in a single case.[35]

differentiate towards high endothelial cells, which are normally responsible for the selective homing of lymphocytes in lymphoid organs.[12] A similar theory can be proposed for retiform hemangioendothelioma, which shares some of the histologic features of PILA. The strong expression of VEGFR-3 by tumor cells has led to suggestions that these tumors display lymphatic differentiation.[2] The specificity of this marker as an indicator of lymphatic differentiation is, however, doubtful. However, D2-40 is positive in the endothelial cells lining the vascular channels giving further support to a lymphatic lineage.

Histology shows a dermal and often subcutaneous tumor composed of markedly dilated, thin-walled vascular channels resembling a cavernous lymphangioma. These vascular channels are lined by bland hobnail endothelial cells with protruding nuclei and very scanty cytoplasm. A prominent intra- and extravascular lymphocytic inflammatory cell infiltrate is often present, and intravascular papillae with collagenous cores are a frequent finding (Figs 35.525–35.527). Commonly, the lymphocytes appear to be in close apposition to the endothelial cells. Tumor cells stain for vascular markers including ERG, CD31, CD34 and von Willebrand factor.

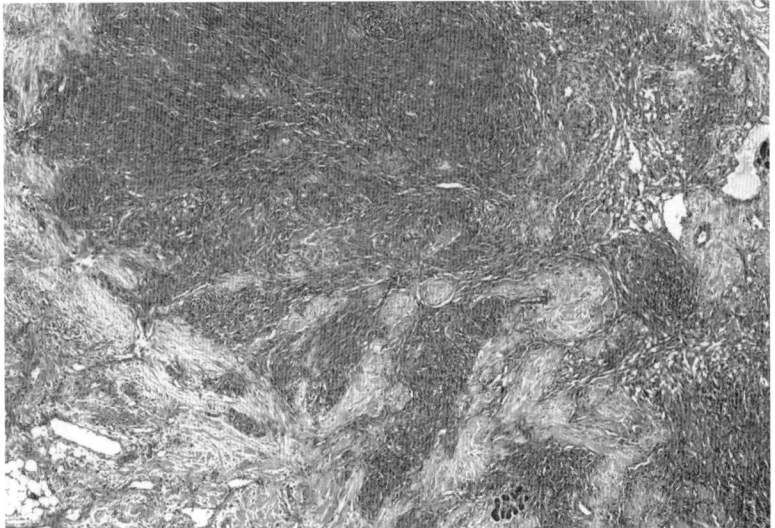

Fig. 35.528
Kaposiform hemangioendothelioma: nodular proliferation with lobular, vascular and spindle cell areas.

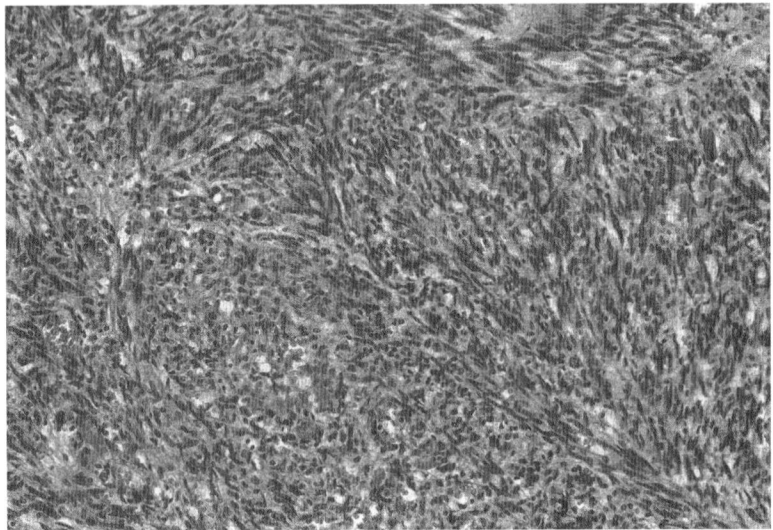

Fig. 35.529
Kaposiform hemangioendothelioma: in this field, the features are reminiscent of Kaposi sarcoma.

Histologically, tumors are lobular, infiltrative and composed of fascicles of bland endothelial cells, congested capillaries, slit-like vascular spaces and occasional pale epithelioid endothelial cells (*Fig. 35.528*). Different areas resemble either Kaposi sarcoma or capillary hemangioma (*Fig. 35.529*). Focally, the capillaries may show thrombosis, especially at the periphery of tumor lobules. Areas resembling lymphangioma are often seen.[5]

Epithelioid cells can contain hemosiderin granules, hyaline globules, and even cytoplasmic vacuoles. Rare hyaline globules can be seen in the spindle cells. Inflammatory cells are usually sparse, and mitotic figures are rare.

Biopsies of lesions after Kasabach-Merritt syndrome tend to show histologic features that resemble tufted angioma.[29] In one case, prominent telangiectasia and amianthoid-like fibrosis were described.[36] In an exceptional case, changes of lymphangiomatosis predominated and those of kaposiform hemangioendothelioma were only focal and microscopic.[37]

Endothelial cells in the tumor are positive for ERG, CD31, CD34 and FLI-1 but negative for GLUT-1 and LeY (juvenile hemangioma-associated antigens).[17,38] Podoplanin is positive in the bulk of tumor lobules but negative in the dilated blood vessels.[39] Focal actin positivity is seen in areas with epithelioid morphology. HHV-8 has not been demonstrated.

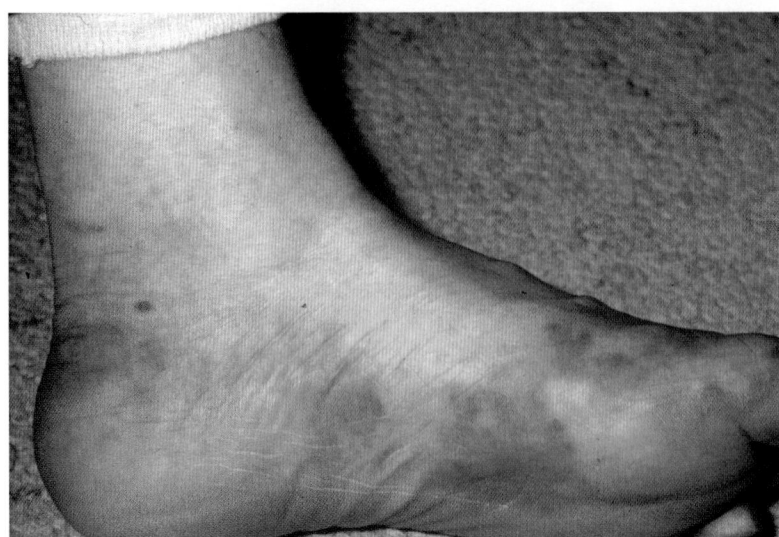

Fig. 35.530
Classic Kaposi sarcoma: the distal extremities are typically involved. From the collection of the late N.P. Smith, MD, the Institute of Dermatology, London, UK.

Differential diagnosis

Nodular Kaposi sarcoma in children usually involves the lymph nodes, has a prominent inflammatory cell infiltrate, lacks a lobular growth pattern and contains eosinophilic globules.

Kaposi sarcoma

The histogenesis of Kaposi sarcoma has been a source of debate for many years; currently, it appears most likely that it is derived from endothelial cells, particularly lymphatic endothelium.[1–3] However, some studies have demonstrated a mixed cell population. Although we include Kaposi sarcoma in the group of low-grade malignant vascular tumors, in keeping with present convention, the issue about whether it is a reactive or neoplastic process remains controversial. Clonality has occasionally been found, supporting a neoplastic process, but other studies have not confirmed this.[4–6] Although occasional cases of Kaposi sarcoma may have an aggressive behavior, at present most evidence suggests that the process is more likely to be reactive.[7] This is further supported by the discovery of DNA sequences from a distinctive new type of human herpesvirus (HHV-8, KS-associated herpesvirus) in all types of Kaposi sarcoma.[8–11] A study of multicentric advanced lesions of Kaposi sarcoma has shown that although some tumors are clonal most advanced cases represent oligo clonal proliferations, suggesting that the process is reactive rather than neoplastic.[12] Serological evidence of infection by the virus is found before patients develop the tumor.[13,14] HHV-8 is also associated with multicentric Castleman disease and primary effusion lymphoma.[15]

Clinical features

Kaposi sarcoma may be divided into four distinct clinical groups:[16–20]

- Classic (endemic) Kaposi sarcoma most often arises in elderly males and shows a predilection for the distal extremities (*Figs 35.530* and *35.531*).[16–18] Mediterranean and Jewish populations are most often affected. Familial cases are exceptional and presentation in children is very uncommon.[19,20] Lesions have been reported in children born to consanguineous parents, suggesting an autosomal recessive predisposition that facilitates induction of the tumor by HHV-8.[21] Internal lesions are distinctly uncommon and mucosal lesions are rare.[22] Disseminated disease is very rare.[23] The condition generally tends to pursue a prolonged indolent and only very rarely fatal course, but such patients have a higher incidence of lymphoreticular neoplasms, especially non-Hodgkin lymphoma.[24,25] Aggressive behavior has only exceptionally been documented.[26]

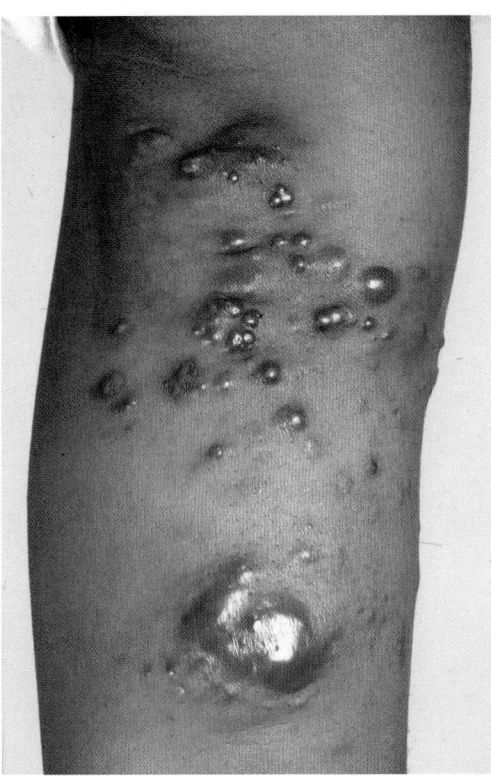

Fig. 35.531
Classic Kaposi sarcoma: numerous tumor nodules are present. From the collection of the late N.P. Smith, MD, the Institute of Dermatology, London, UK.

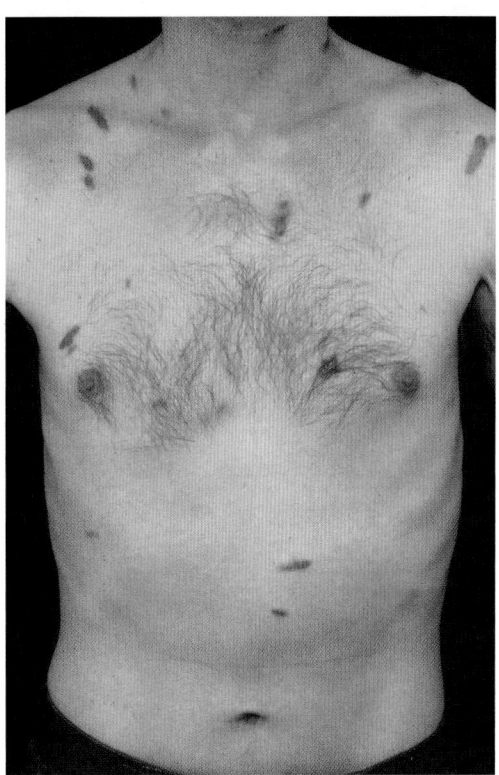

Fig. 35.532
AIDS-related Kaposi sarcoma: darkly pigmented plaques are widely distributed on this young man's chest and abdomen. From the collection of the late N.P. Smith, MD, Institute of Dermatology, London, UK.

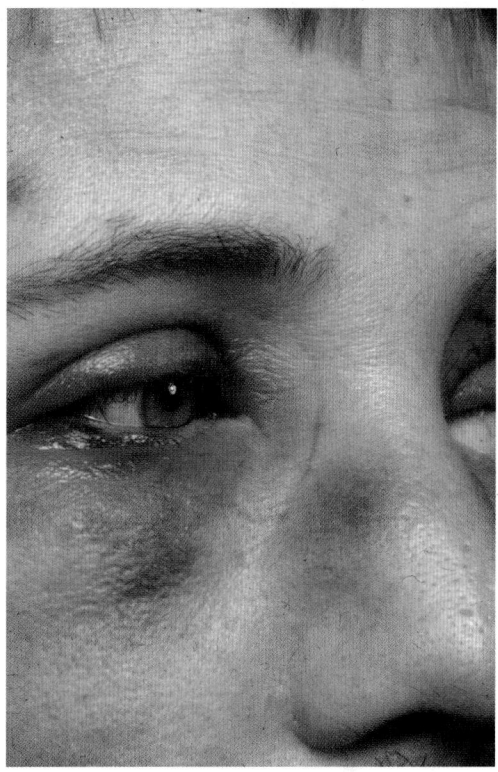

Fig. 35.533
AIDS-related Kaposi sarcoma: infraorbital and nasal purple plaques are present. From the collection of the late N.P. Smith, MD, Institute of Dermatology, London, UK.

- AIDS-related Kaposi sarcoma commonly presents in young adults, mostly males, many of whom either are homosexual or abuse drugs (*Figs 35.532* and *35.533*).[27–29] Lesions are much less common in women and children.[30] The tumor often disseminates widely and rapidly and may prove fatal. However, with the advent of highly active antiretroviral therapy, the incidence of Kaposi sarcoma has decreased dramatically, and when lesions develop they tend to be limited. The skin (especially of the trunk and limbs) and mucosae are usually extensively involved. Lesions may occur as a result of the immune reconstitution inflammatory syndrome.[31,32] The condition can also develop in association with chronic lymphedema in HIV-positive patients.[33]

- Immunosuppression-associated Kaposi sarcoma is rare and presents in patients receiving immunosuppressive therapy, especially after kidney transplantation.[34–36] Although the course of the disease tends to be indolent, it can occasionally be aggressive. Regression of the lesions sometimes occurs after immunosuppression is stopped or reduced. Kaposi sarcoma in this setting may be induced by local immunosuppression, for example after infiltration of steroids or the use of topical tacrolimus.[37,38] Chronic use of systemic steroids, leflunomide and other immunosuppressive drugs outside the setting of transplantation can also induce lesions.[39,40,41] A case associated with a hypothalamic adrenocorticotropic hormone-secreting adenoma has been documented.[42] Interestingly, although immunosuppressive drugs such as sirolimus may induce recurrence of Kaposi sarcoma, in several instances complete regression has been noted after the introduction of the drug.[43–45] Kaposi sarcoma has been described in a patient with idiopathic low CD4 counts.[46]

- African Kaposi sarcoma includes those cases arising largely in sub-Saharan Central Africa.[17,18,47,48] In this region, Kaposi sarcoma has long been endemic and accounts for up to 10% of all cases of 'malignant' disease. Within this category there are two clinical subgroups: those arising predominantly on the limbs of middle-aged

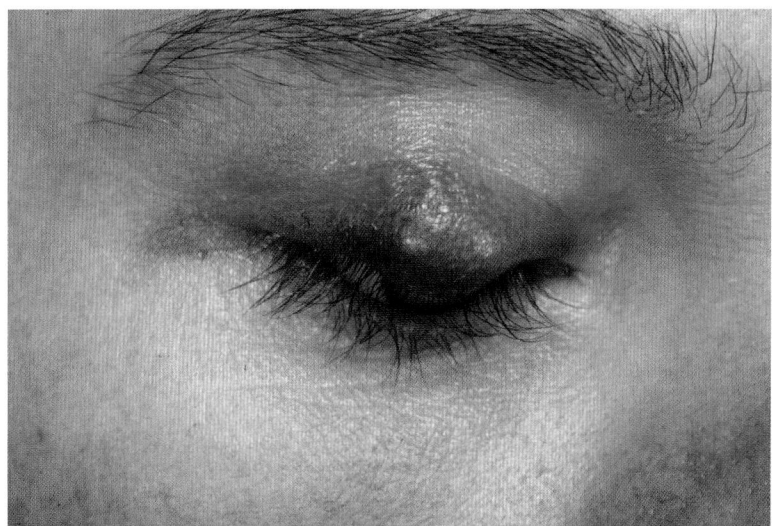

Fig. 35.534
Kaposi sarcoma: a tumor nodule is present on the upper eyelid. From the collection of the late N.P. Smith, MD, Institute of Dermatology, London, UK.

men and tending to be fairly indolent; those arising in young children who typically present with visceral or lymph node involvement and in whom the disease is usually fatal. In addition, there are a large number of AIDS-related cases in young African adults of either sex (see above). Clinically, the cutaneous lesions present similarly in all the subtypes. They commence as small, reddish-blue macules or flat plaques, which are often multiple and gradually enlarge. They may become nodular, and sometimes coalesce to form larger lesions (*Fig. 35.534*). Some may regress as new lesions continually form and others ulcerate and fungate. The rate of spread

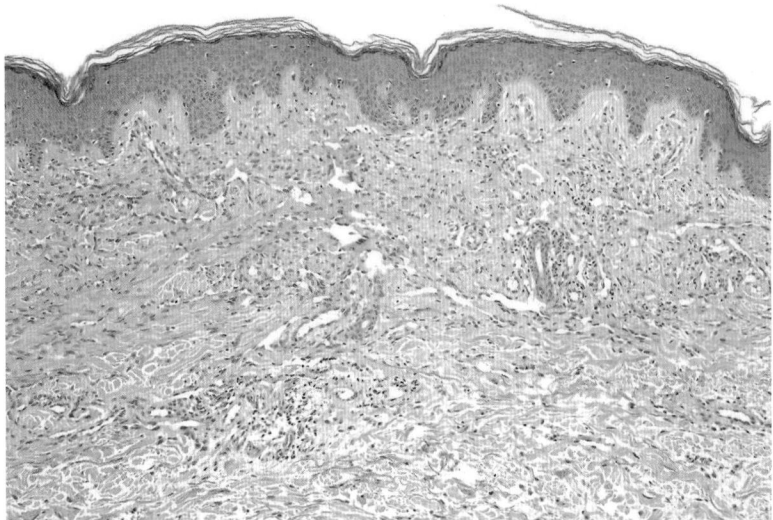

Fig. 35.535
Kaposi sarcoma (patch stage): there is increased vascularity, spindled cells and a light chronic inflammatory cell infiltrate.

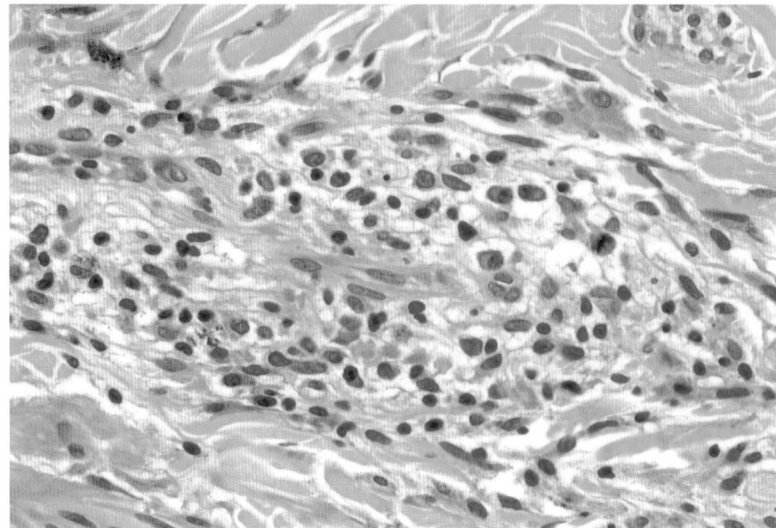

Fig. 35.537
Kaposi sarcoma (patch stage): the infiltrate consists of an admixture of lymphocytes and plasma cells.

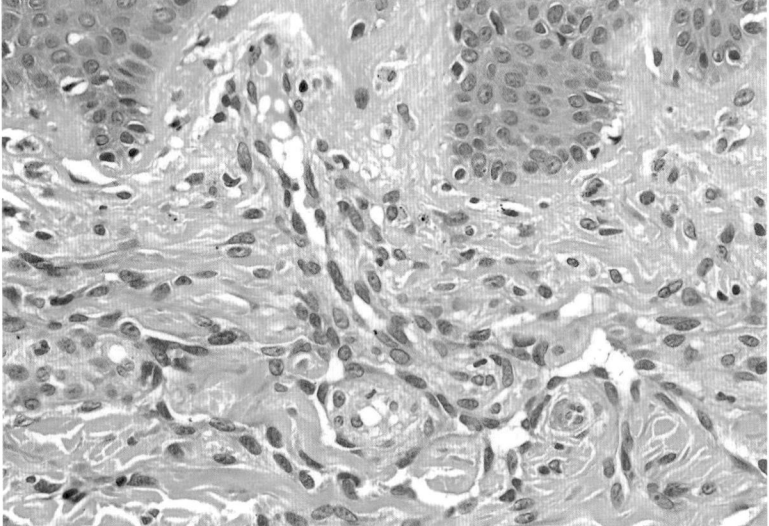

Fig. 35.536
Kaposi sarcoma (patch stage): the vessels are lined by swollen, focally hyperchromatic endothelial cells.

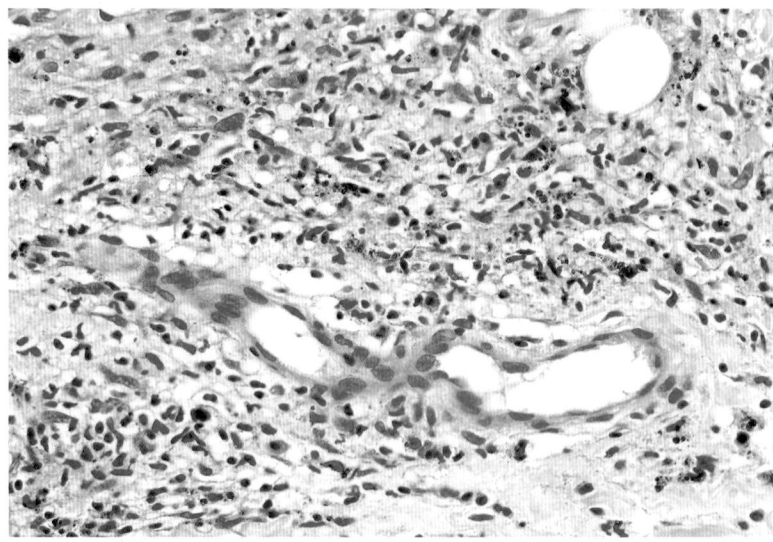

Fig. 35.538
Kaposi sarcoma (patch stage): focal hemosiderin deposition is present.

or enlargement is usually related to the clinical subgroup into which the patient falls.

Regression may occur in a number of settings, particularly after immunosuppression is stopped or reduced. Anecdotal examples of regression have been reported with imatinib and sorafenib.[49,50]

Histologic features

The microscopic appearances of Kaposi sarcoma go through three phases, apparently related to the duration of the lesion.[27–29,51] There is morphological overlap between patch and plaque phases, but nodular lesions appear distinct. Lesions usually involve the dermis and may extend to the subcutaneous tissue. Purely subcutaneous tumors are rare.[52]

- The early patch stage is characterized by a mild increase in the number of dermal vessels showing minimal endothelial atypia and characteristically surrounded by an admixture of lymphocytes and plasma cells associated with hemosiderin deposition and red cell extravasation (*Figs 35.535–35.539*). These vessels are arranged mainly parallel to the epidermis, may dissect between collagen bundles and surround adnexal structures and vessels (the promontory sign). This stage of Kaposi sarcoma is the most difficult to recognize as it bears a superficial resemblance to granulation tissue.

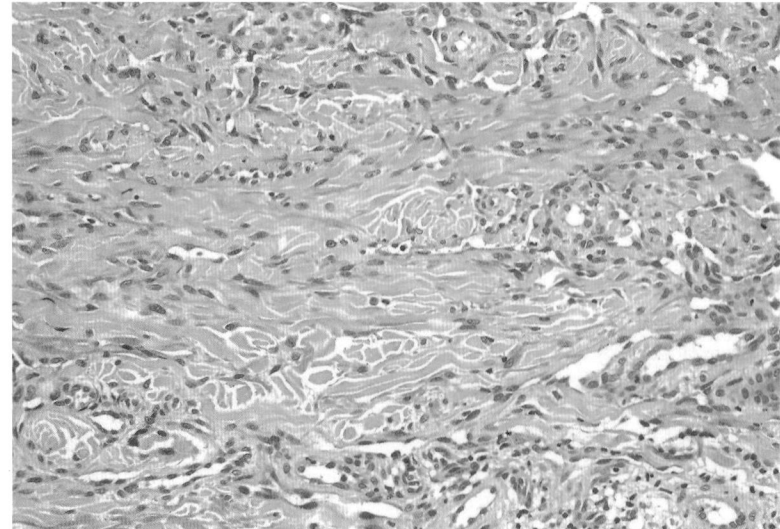

Fig. 35.539
Kaposi sarcoma (patch stage): this field shows extensive dissection of collagen (a characteristic feature).

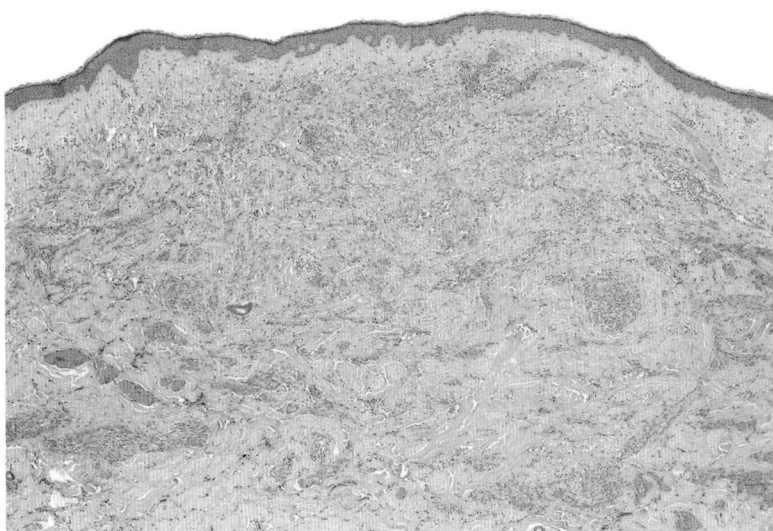

Fig. 35.540
Kaposi sarcoma (plaque stage): the changes affect the full thickness of the dermis.

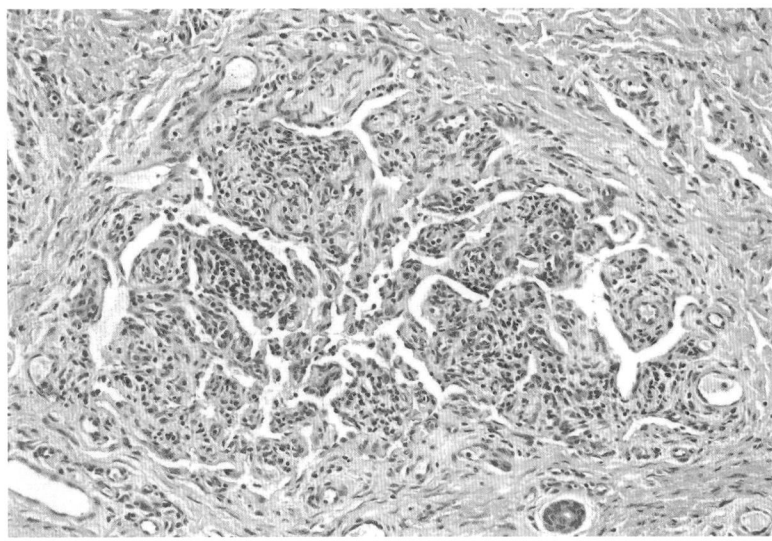

Fig. 35.542
Kaposi sarcoma: newly formed vessels sometimes ensheath pre-existent ones – the promontory sign.

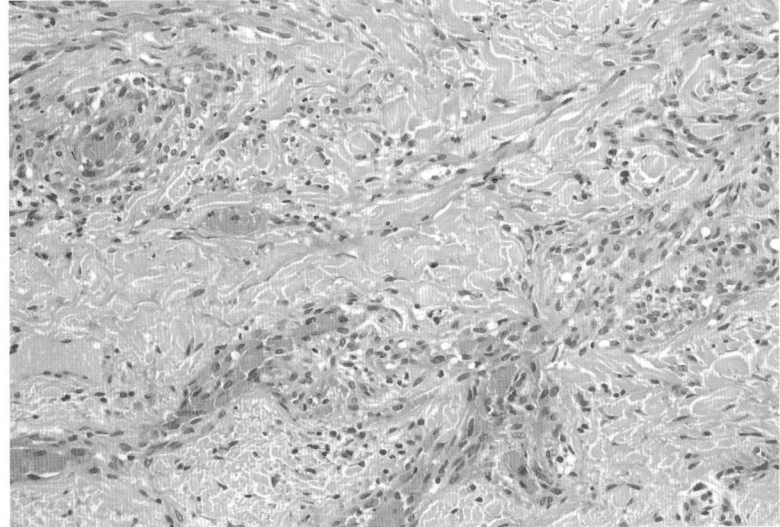

Fig. 35.541
Kaposi sarcoma (plaque stage): there is very extensive vascular proliferation.

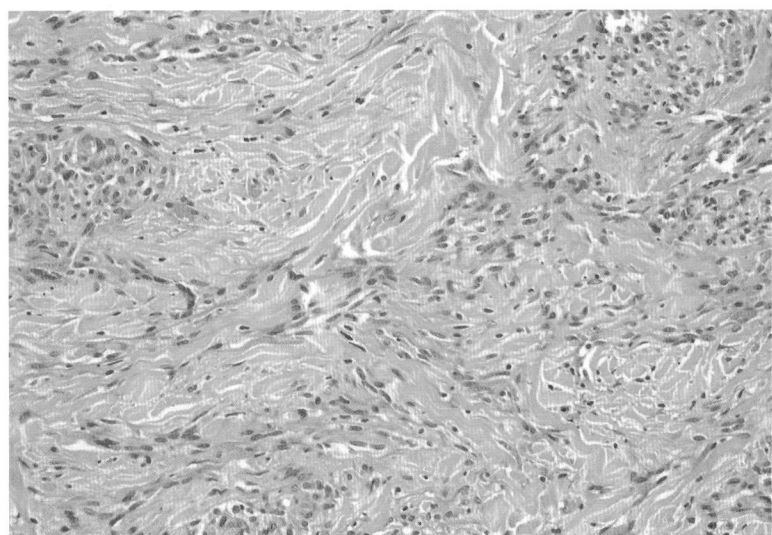

Fig. 35.543
Kaposi sarcoma (plaque stage): increased numbers of spindle cells are present. Dissection of collagen is marked.

- The plaque stage is typified by more obvious and extensive dermal vascular proliferation, the lumina of which vary considerably in caliber (*Figs 35.540–35.544*). Endothelial cells may appear plump, but remain single layered. Noticeable at this stage is the appearance of eosinophilic spindled cells in the dermis around these vessels. These cells have tapering, somewhat hyperchromatic nuclei. The margins of the lesion are ill defined and primitive vascular clefts may be apparent within the spindle cell mass. Chronic inflammatory cells remain a prominent feature.
- The nodular stage is manifest predominantly as a relatively well-circumscribed dermal mass of variably eosinophilic spindle cells (*Fig. 35.545*). Scattered between these cells are numerous irregular, slit-like, vascular spaces, which lack an endothelial lining, but often contain extravasated red cells. In cross-section these spaces resemble a sieve (*Figs 35.546–35.549*). Readily identifiable ectatic vessels may, however, still be apparent at the periphery of the nodule. Normal mitotic activity is most prominent at this stage. A chronic inflammatory infiltrate including histiocytes is variably conspicuous. The spindle cells are consistently CD34 positive and also CD31 positive (*Fig. 35.550*). Focal positivity for actin is also seen.

Rarely, nodular Kaposi sarcoma is entirely or partially intravascular.[53]

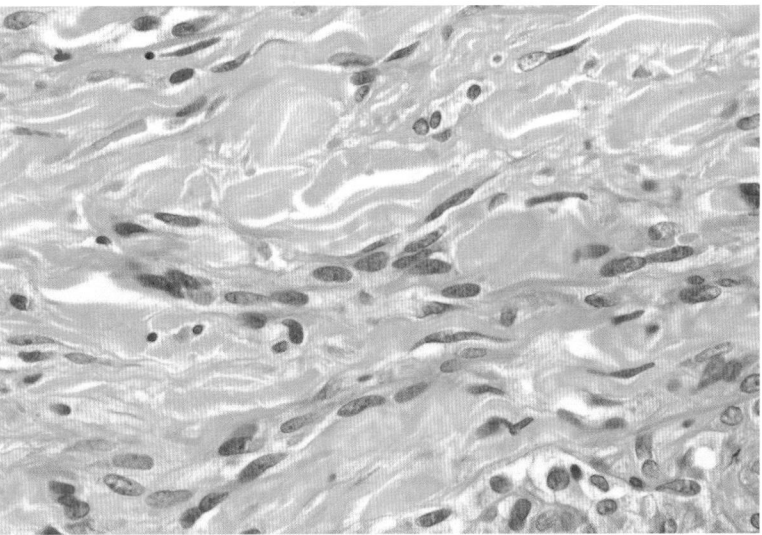

Fig. 35.544
Kaposi sarcoma (plaque stage): the spindle cells have pale eosinophilic cytoplasm with oval or elongated nuclei.

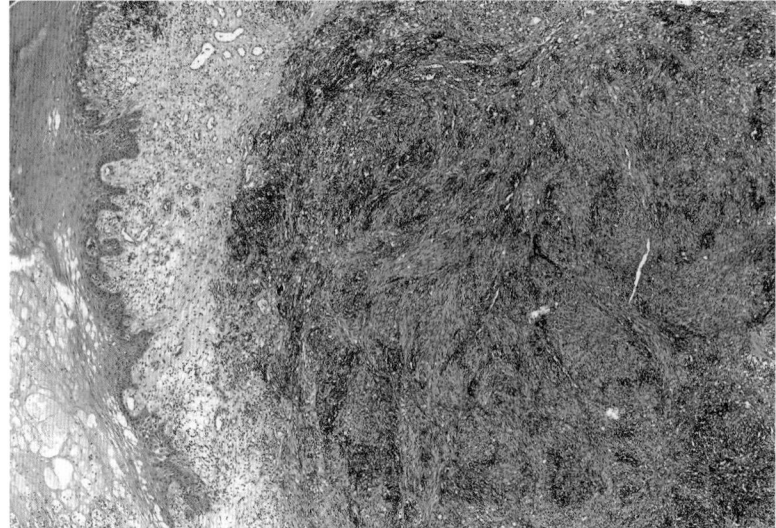

Fig. 35.545
Kaposi sarcoma (nodular stage): the dermis is diffusely infiltrated by a spindle cell tumor.

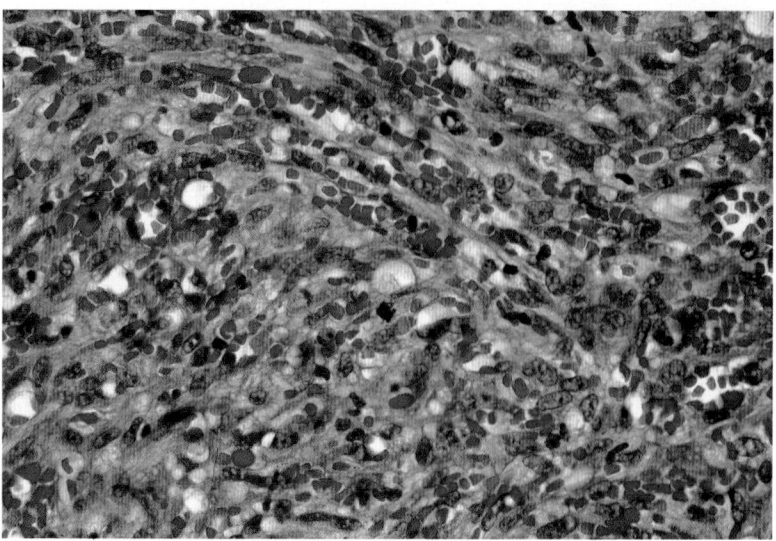

Fig. 35.548
Kaposi sarcoma (nodular stage): multiple mitoses are present.

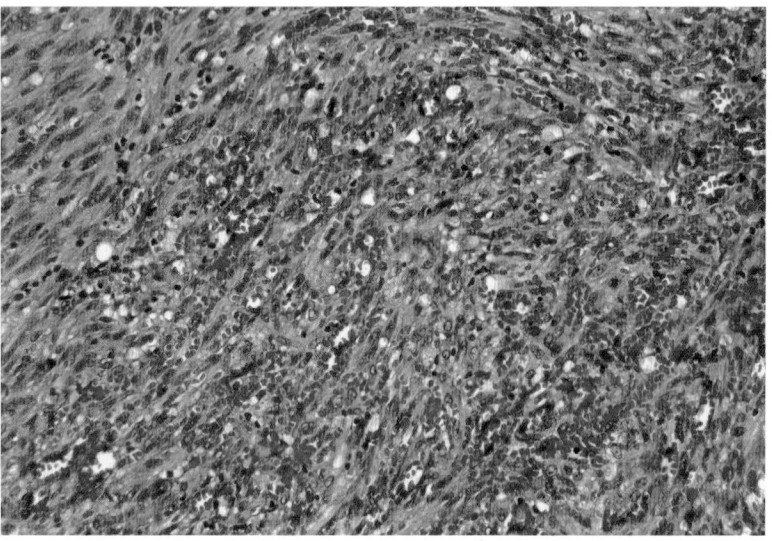

Fig. 35.546
Kaposi sarcoma: the spindled cells have eosinophilic cytoplasm. Hemorrhage is conspicuous.

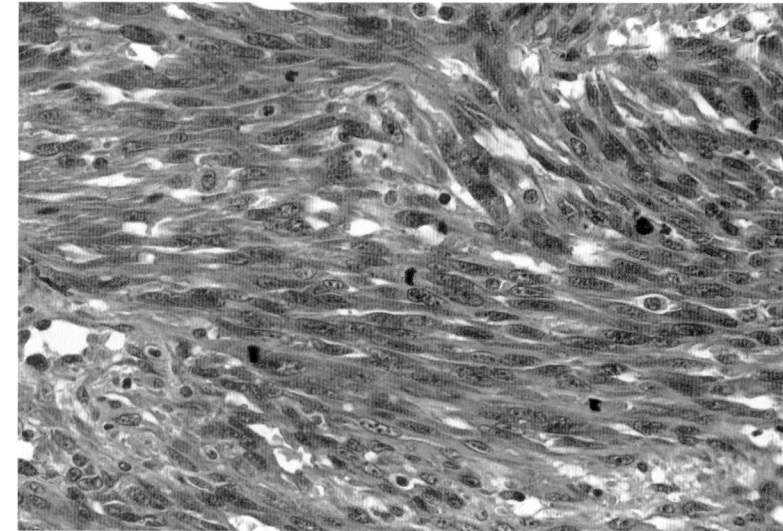

Fig. 35.549
Kaposi sarcoma: numerous mitoses are present in this predominantly spindled cell high-grade population.

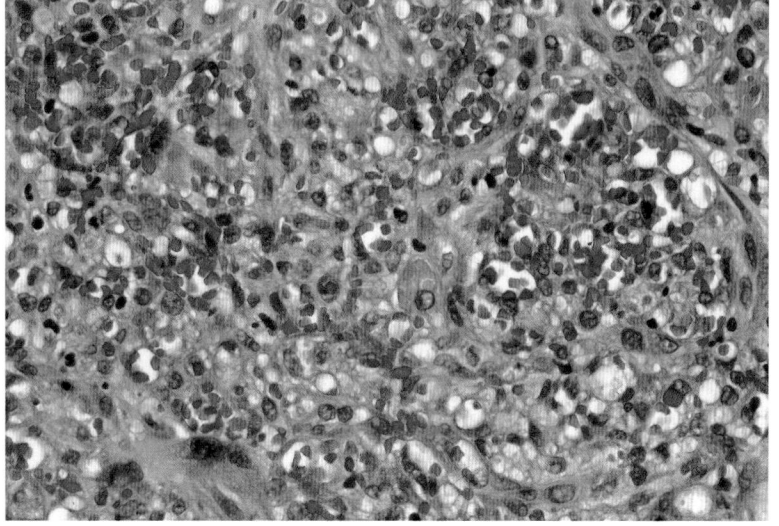

Fig. 35.547
Kaposi sarcoma (nodular stage): this sieve-like appearance is diagnostic.

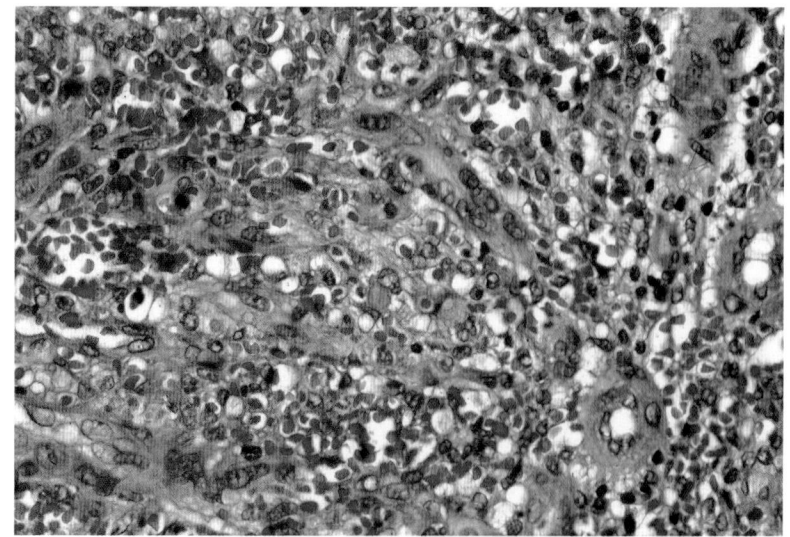

Fig. 35.550
Kaposi sarcoma: the presence of hyaline inclusions is a useful diagnostic marker.

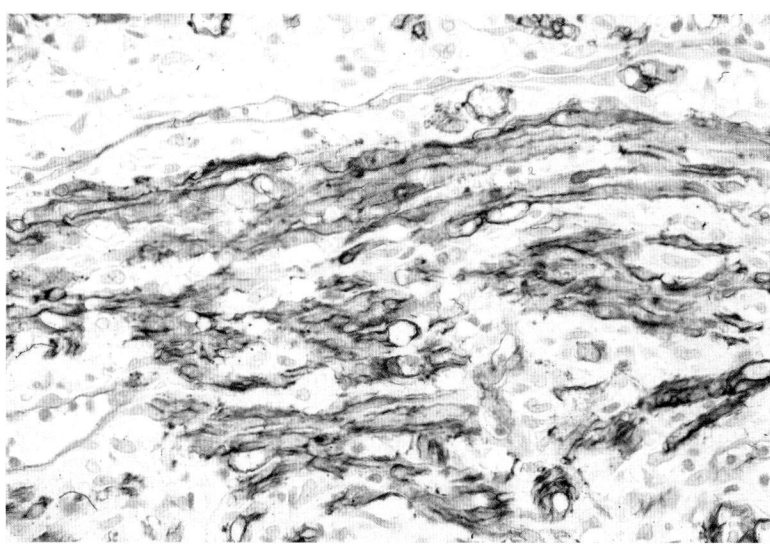

Fig. 35.551
Kaposi sarcoma: the spindled cells express CD34.

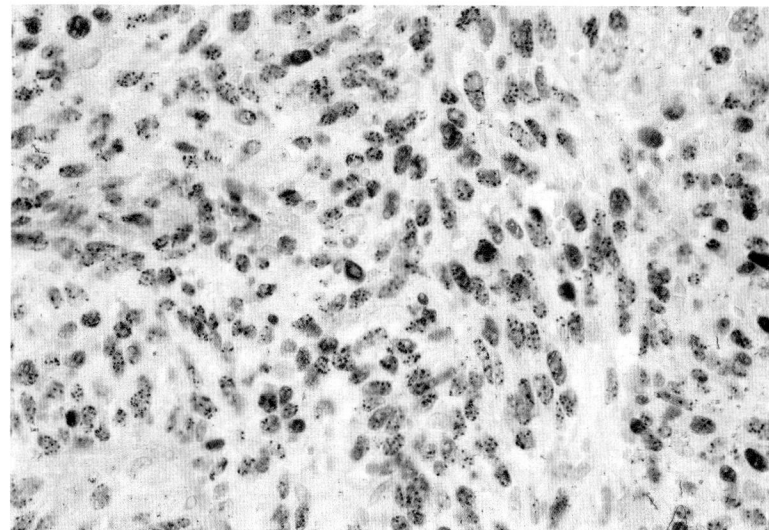

Fig. 35.553
Kaposi sarcoma: HHV-8 is regularly present.

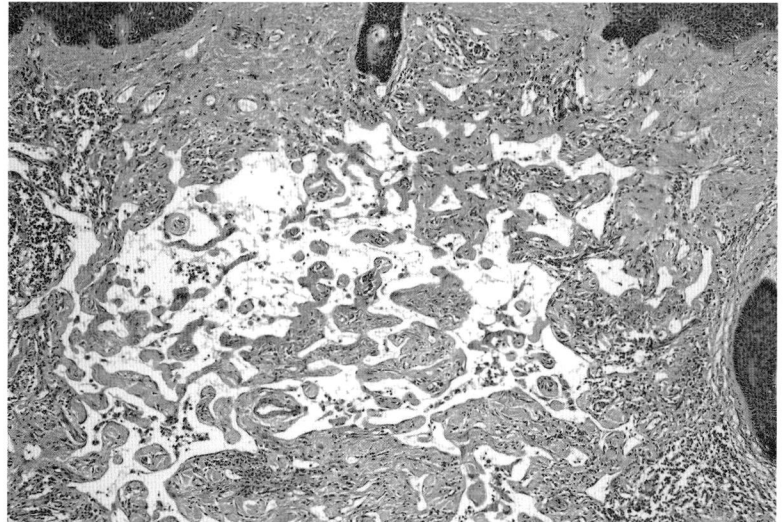

Fig. 35.552
Kaposi sarcoma: rarely, marked lymphatic dilatation gives rise to the lymphangiomatous variant.

The vascular spaces in Kaposi sarcoma are positive for D2–40, suggesting a lymphatic lineage (Fig. 35.551).[54,55]

Also noted in all forms of Kaposi sarcoma, but especially in the nodular variant, is the presence of amorphous eosinophilic hyaline globules lying free between spindle cells or intracellularly. These probably represent degenerate red blood cells.[56] They are diastase resistant and PAS positive, and stain bright red with Masson trichrome.

Lymphangiomatous Kaposi sarcoma is a variant of the patch–plaque stage in which moderately dilated vascular channels, resembling lymphatics, are prominent (Fig. 35.552).[57,58] It may be mistaken for progressive lymphangioma.

In HIV patients with chronic lymphedema, additional histologic features include fibrosis, pools of lymph fluid and fibroma-like nodules.[33] The latter may include Kaposi sarcoma spindle-shaped cells.

Anaplastic Kaposi sarcoma is very rare and characterized by cytologic atypia and variable mitotic activity.[59] Epithelioid morphology can rarely be seen.[60] Distinction from angiosarcoma is often very difficult and a helpful clue is the finding of areas typical of Kaposi sarcoma in the same sample. Many of the cases of anaplastic disease described before the advent of immunohistochemistry are probably examples of other sarcomas.

Unusual histologic variants of Kaposi sarcoma may be encountered including glomeruloid, pigmented, KS with myoid nodules, telangiectatic and ecchymotic.[61]

In HIV-positive patients with Kaposi sarcoma, treatment with paclitaxel or the angiogenesis inhibitor Col-3 induces partial or complete regression of lesions.[62] Histologically, in partial regression, there is reduction in spindled cells and fibrosis. In complete regression, there is fibrosis, lymphocytic inflammation and hemosiderin deposition. In patients on HAART, lesions can also change, becoming more circumscribed, less cellular and surrounded by a thick band of fibrosis.[63]

It is important to remember that in patients with HIV/AIDS more than one pathology can be found in a single biopsy. Kaposi sarcoma has been reported in association with cryptococcosis and tuberculosis and cryptococcosis and *Mycobacterium avium intracellulare* in the same sample.[64–66]

After the discovery of HHV-8, demonstration of virus in skin biopsies from patients with Kaposi sarcoma was done by in situ hybridization. A monoclonal antibody against the latent nuclear antigen-1 of HHV-8 is routinely used in paraffin-embedded biopsies.[67,68] This represents an invaluable tool in the histologic diagnosis of Kaposi sarcoma and its differential diagnosis as other vascular tumors are usually not positive for HHV-8 (Fig. 35.553). Exceptional cases of Kaposi sarcoma are negative for HHV-8 by immunohistochemistry and the diagnosis has to be confirmed by PCR.[69] Genomic characterization of Kaposi sarcoma to demonstrate molecular derangements has not yet been published, but might help clarify some of the debate over its neoplastic status.

Differential diagnosis

The differential diagnosis is wide and includes acroangiodermatitis, aneurysmal benign fibrous histiocytoma, progressive lymphangioma, tufted angioma, targetoid hemosiderotic hemangioma, spindle cell hemangioma, kaposiform hemangioendothelioma and angiosarcoma.[27,70]

In acroangiodermatitis, which most often affects the lower legs and complicates severe chronic venous stasis, there is proliferation of small normal capillaries in the superficial dermis associated with fibrosis, hemosiderin deposition and few inflammatory cells.[71] Aneurysmal benign fibrous histiocytoma is a more polymorphic, focally storiform lesion in which foamy histiocytes and multinucleated cells are prominent. In angiosarcoma, endothelial cytologic atypia is more prominent and endothelial multilayering is present.

Composite hemangioendothelioma

Clinical features

Composite hemangioendothelioma is a low-grade malignant vascular tumor with a tendency for local recurrence but low metastatic potential. It is defined as a neoplasm containing a mixture of histologic patterns including benign, intermediate and/or malignant.[1] It is a very rare tumor, presenting mainly

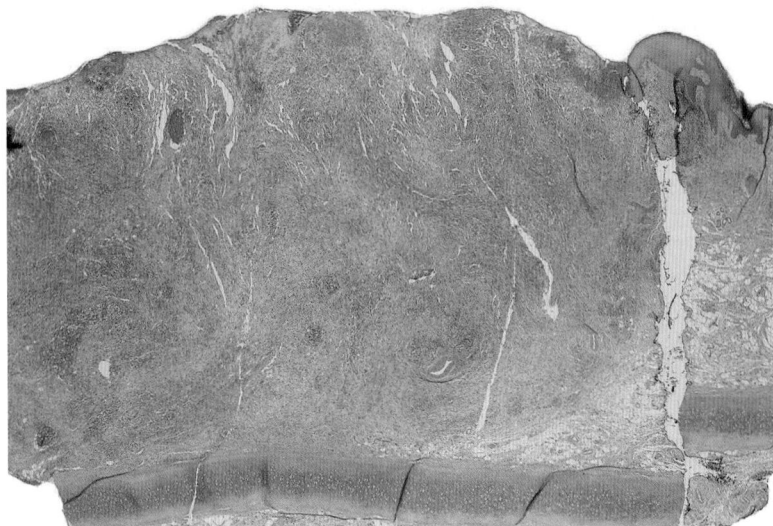

Fig. 35.554
Composite hemangioendothelioma: this lesion is characterized by various vascular patterns.

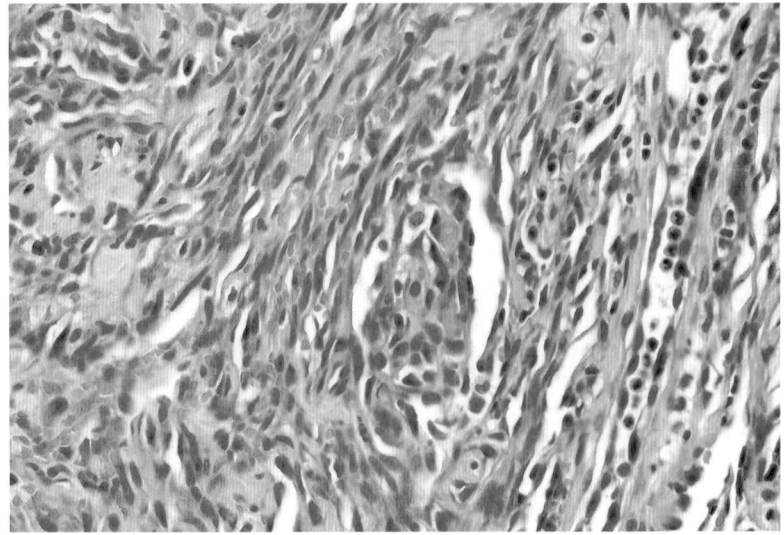

Fig. 35.555
Composite hemangioendothelioma: in this field, the features are reminiscent of spindle cell hemangioma.

in adults and only exceptionally in children.[1–6] Two congenital cases, one associated with Kasabach-Merritt and one associated with Maffucci syndrome have been reported.[3] There is no sex predilection and most tumors occur in the extremities, with a predilection for the hands and feet. A tumor arising in the mediastinum, one on the kidney, one on the spleen, one on the hypopharynx and two in the oral cavity have been documented.[3,7–10] In 25% of patients, tumors arise in association with lymphedema and present as long-standing red–blue nodules or plaques. A case presenting with alopecia has been reported.[11] The rate of local recurrence is around 50% and this may occur years after excision of the primary tumor. The metastatic rate is around 15%. Rare cases have been reported to metastasize to regional lymph nodes.[1,12,13] One of these cases was associated with satellitosis.[13] Occasionally, progression to high-grade angiosarcoma can occur over a period of many years.

The prognosis is likely to depend on the component with the highest histologic grade (see below) but this should be confirmed in larger series of cases with adequate follow-up. A handful of cases with expression of neuroendocrine markers and more aggressive behavior have been described.[14]

Histologic features

Composite hemangioendothelioma is a poorly circumscribed dermal and subcutaneous tumor, with an infiltrative growth pattern. The different components vary from lesion to lesion and may include retiform hemangioendothelioma, epithelioid hemangioendothelioma, spindle cell hemangioma, conventional angiosarcoma (low and even high grade), epithelioid angiosarcoma, lymphangioma circumscriptum and areas simulating an arteriovenous malformation (Figs 35.554–35.557).[1,3,15] Cases with expression of neuroendocrine markers are characterized by components similar to retiform hemangioendothelioma and epithelioid hemangioendothelioma, and they often have hemangioma-like areas in which channels are lined by hobnail endothelial cells.[14] These tumors display synaptophysin, less commonly CD56 and exceptionally, chromogranin.[14] Immunohistochemistry displays positive staining for vascular markers including, ERG, CD31 and CD34. D2-40 is positive in a small number of cases.

Giant cell angioblastoma

It is unclear whether this is a true vascular tumor but it is briefly described here until further reports clarify the line of differentiation. A very small number of cases have been reported, most presenting in the lower limbs of children and in bone.[1–3] Tumors are large and present with progressive growth.[1,2] A single case has been described in an adult.[4]

Histology shows aggregates of histiocyte-like cells in nodules distributed around vascular channels.

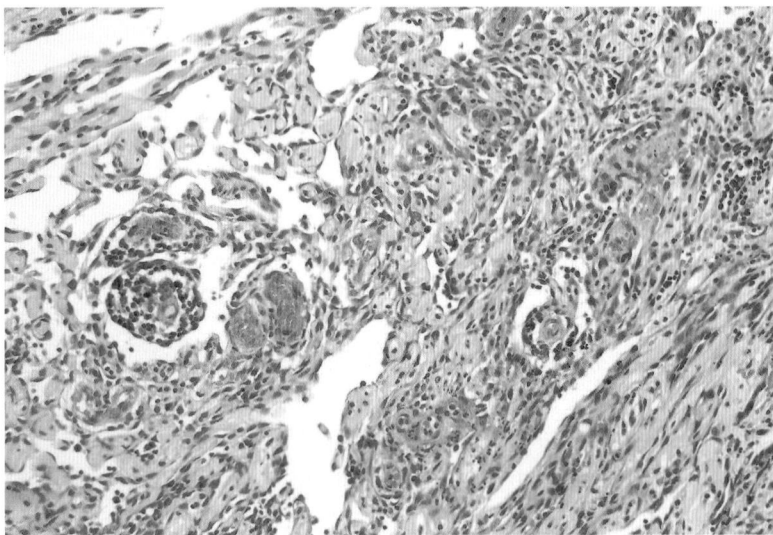

Fig. 35.556
Composite hemangioendothelioma: the appearances resemble papillary intralymphatic angioendothelioma.

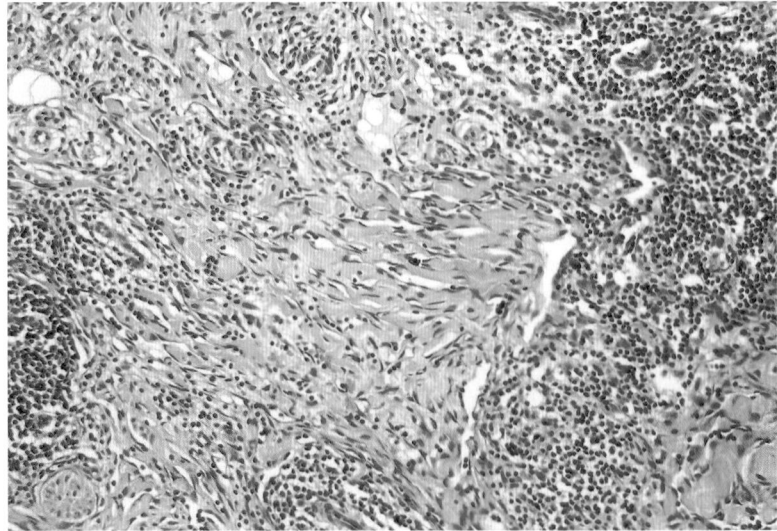

Fig. 35.557
Composite hemangioendothelioma: there is marked dissection of collagen suggestive of angiosarcoma.

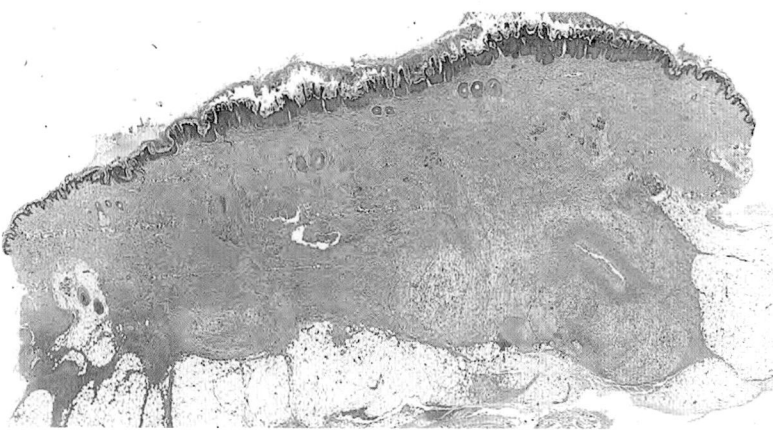

Fig. 35.558
Pseudomyogenic hemangioendothelioma: prominent involvement of the dermis and subcutaneous tissue by an infiltrative tumor.

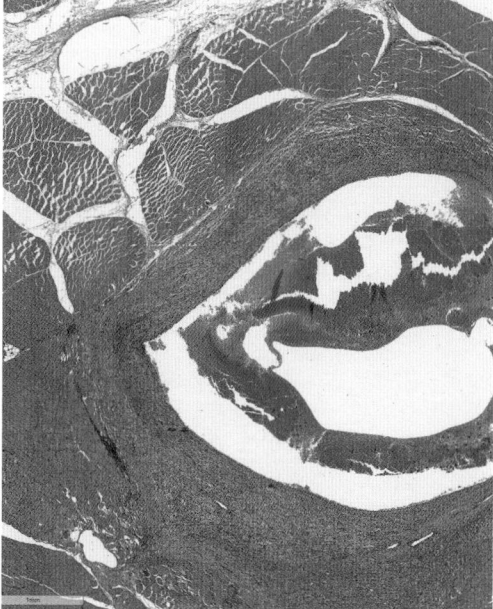

Fig. 35.559
Pseudomyogenic hemangioendothelioma: same patient as previous figure. Multifocal tumor also involving skeletal muscle.

Pseudomyogenic hemangioendothelioma

Clinical features

Pseudomyogenic hemangioendothelioma is a recently delineated low-grade malignant vascular tumor previously described under the terms fibroma-like epithelioid sarcoma and epithelioid sarcoma-like hemangioendothelioma.[1-5] Lesions usually affect children and young adults and are more common in males. Tumors present as multifocal (in up to a two thirds of cases) variably painful nodules, most often located on the limbs. Lesions usually affect multiple tissue planes of the same anatomic region, such as the skin, subcutis, and skeletal muscle, and less often bone. Involvement of the oral cavity has been described and primary osseous tumors may occur.[6-8] A tumor associated with fibrous dysplasia and a further case clinically mimicking a dermatofibroma have been reported.[9,10] The rate of local recurrence of up to 60% but aggressive behavior with metastasis to lymph nodes, distant organs and death is rare.[1,11]

Pathogenesis and histologic features

Cytogenetic studies have shown a distinctive t(7;19)(q11;q13) translocation resulting in fusion of the *SERPINE 1* and *FOSB* genes.[12-15]

Tumors are not vasoformative and consist of poorly circumscribed nodules composed of fascicles or sheets of plump, brightly eosinophilic spindle cells with vesicular nuclei intermixed with variable numbers of cells with rhabdoid appearance (pink cytoplasm and eccentric nucleus) (*Figs 35.558–35.560*). Nuclear atypia is generally mild, and mitoses are sparse.

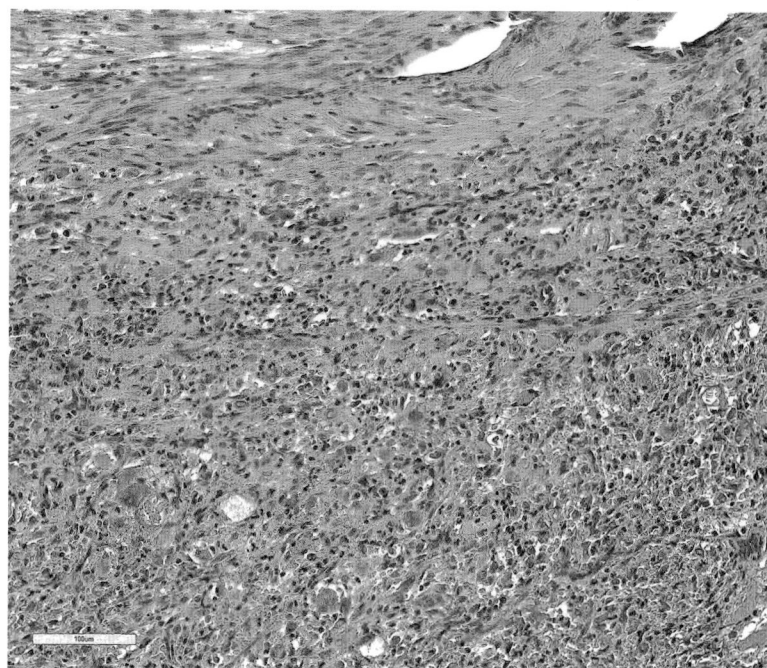

Fig. 35.560
Pseudomyogenic hemangioendothelioma: round pseudorhabdomyblast and spindle-shaped cells with no features suggestive of vascular differentiation.

A prominent neutrophilic inflammatory infiltrate identified in about 30% of cases. Necrosis and vascular invasion are rare.

Immunohistochemically, tumor cells are positive for CD31, ERG, FLI1 and keratin AE1/AE3, and negative for CD34, epithelial membrane antigen (EMA), and other keratins including MNF116.[1] Focal positivity for SMA may be seen and there is negative staining for S100 and desmin. Tumor cells display strong nuclear positivity for FOSB.[16-19] The later marker is also positive in a percentage of epithelioid hemangiomas and rarely in cases of nodular and proliferative fasciitis but not in other vascular tumors that may be confused with pseudomyogenic hemangioendothelioma.

Differential diagnosis

The most important differential diagnosis is with epithelioid sarcoma, which usually lacks rhabdoid cells, displays atypical epithelioid cells with mitotic activity and shows positivity for EMA and CD34 (50% of cases) and loss of INI1. In cases of doubt FOSB immunohistochemistry can be useful.[16]

Malignant vascular tumors

Epithelioid hemangioendothelioma

Clinical features

Epithelioid hemangioendothelioma was originally described in 1982 as a distinctive low-grade malignancy in soft tissues.[1,2] However, this tumor is now classified as fully malignant in view of its behavior with potential for metastatic spread and mortality (see below). Identical cases involving other organs (mainly lung, liver and bone) have been described in the past under different names. Most cases present in adults and only rarely in children.[3-5] Tumors can arise in any organ, as up to 50% of cases develop from a blood vessel, most often a vein. Pain is often a symptom. Multicentric disease is common, especially in the lungs, liver and bones. Involvement of the skin, which is relatively rare, may be associated with an underlying bone or soft tissue lesion and is occasionally multicentric. Cutaneous epithelioid hemangioendothelioma is rare, with wide anatomical distribution and no distinctive clinical features have been described.[6-31] Skin lesions may present in isolation or associated with lesions in other organs either simultaneously or before or after the cutaneous presentation. Intraoral lesions are very rare.[32,33] An adult patient with a hepatic tumor presented with

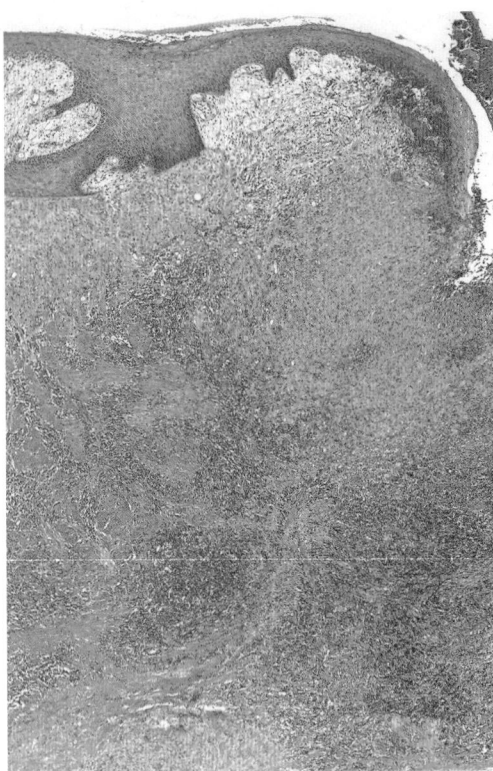

Fig. 35.561
Epithelioid hemangioendothelioma: this is the edge of an ulcerated lesion. Tumor is present superficially and is bordered by a heavy lymphoid infiltrate.

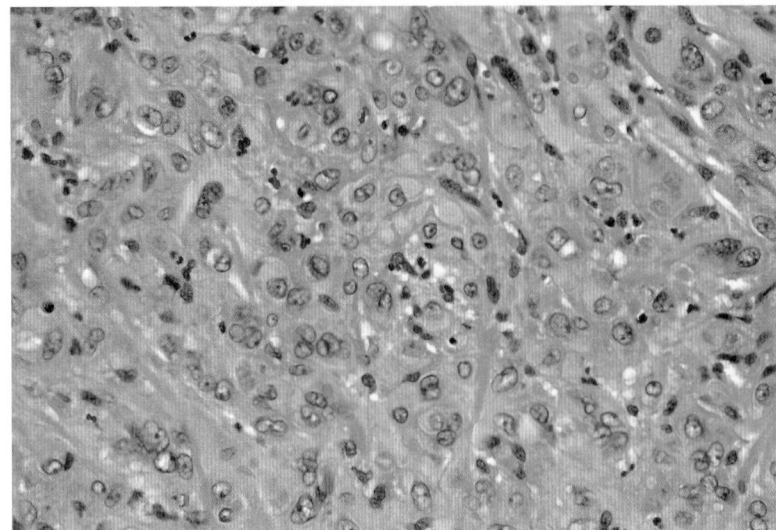

Fig. 35.562
Epithelioid hemangioendothelioma: the tumor cells have eosinophilic cytoplasm and large vesicular nuclei.

Kasabach-Merritt syndrome and in a further patient the tumor presented after radiotherapy for a congenital hemangioma.[34,35] Metastasis and mortality rates vary according to the organ involved, but it is generally believed that no more than 30% metastasize. Cases with isolated cutaneous lesions usually but not always tend to have an indolent behavior.

Pathogenesis and histologic features

The translocation t(1;3)(p36.3;q25) resulting in a *WWTR1-CAMTA1* gene fusion has been demonstrated in virtually all cases of epithelioid hemangioendothelioma.[36–41] A t(10;14)(p13;q24) producing a *YAP1-TFE3* fusion have also rarely been identified.[42,43] *WWTR1-CAMTA1* and *YAP1-TFE3* gene rearrangements can sometimes coexist.[44]

Microscopically, most tumors are ill defined, infiltrative and composed of rounded, polygonal or short spindle-shaped cells with pink cytoplasm and vesicular nuclei. They are arranged in short cords or nests and are surrounded by abundant myxoid or hyaline stroma (often with a somewhat chondroid appearance and rich in sulfated acid mucopolysaccharides) (Figs 35.561 and 35.562). Intracytoplasmic lumina with occasional erythrocytes are often prominent and resemble primitive vascular channels (Figs 35.563–35.565). Well-formed vessels, however, are not a feature of most cases or are infrequent. Calcification, ossification and (less commonly) osteoclast-like giant cells can be present.[45,46] Rare cases show significant cytologic atypia and a high mitotic rate, demonstrating a continuum with epithelioid angiosarcoma (Figs 35.566–35.568). Tumors of larger size and increased mitotic activity are associated with higher mortality. Poor prognosis is associated with tumors larger than 3 cm and more than three mitotic figures per 50 high-power fields. Necrosis, tumor site, cytologic atypia, and spindling of tumor cells do not seem to be affect prognosis.[47]

Immunohistochemically, the tumor cells label for vascular markers including ERG, CD31, CD34, podoplanin and FLI-1.[48–50] CD10 is usually positive and keratin expression is seen in up to 25% of cases.[51,52] Actin positivity may also be present.[2,53,54] CD30 expression has also been reported.[55] EMA is usually negative. CAMTA1 immunohistochemistry, which is usually expressed as positive nuclear staining helps in the differential diagnosis with other tumors with epithelioid morphology.[56,57]

Differential diagnosis

In epithelioid hemangioma, there is prominent inflammation, and well-formed blood vessels predominate. Metastatic adenocarcinoma usually

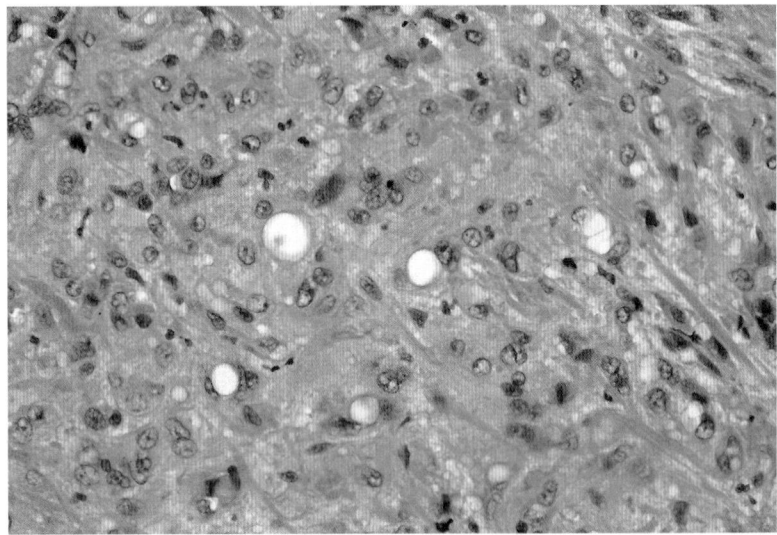

Fig. 35.563
Epithelioid hemangioendothelioma: intracytoplasmic lumina are a characteristic feature.

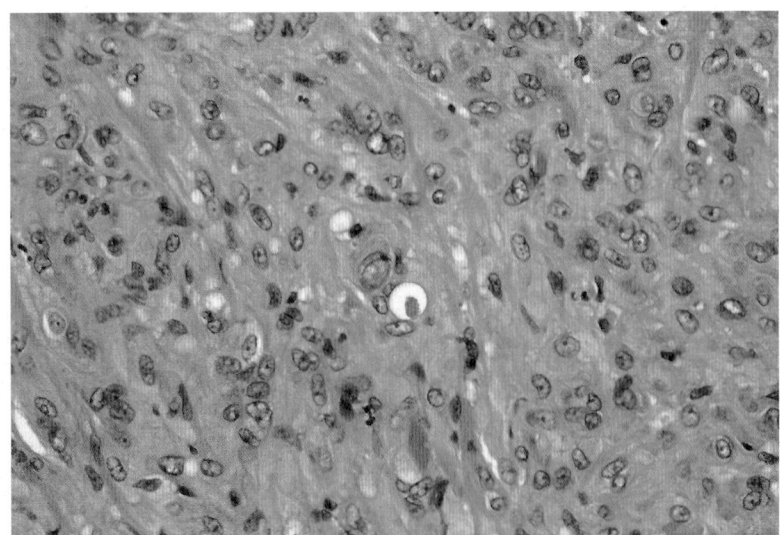

Fig. 35.564
Epithelioid hemangioendothelioma: careful scrutiny often reveals erythrocytes within the intracytoplasmic lumina.

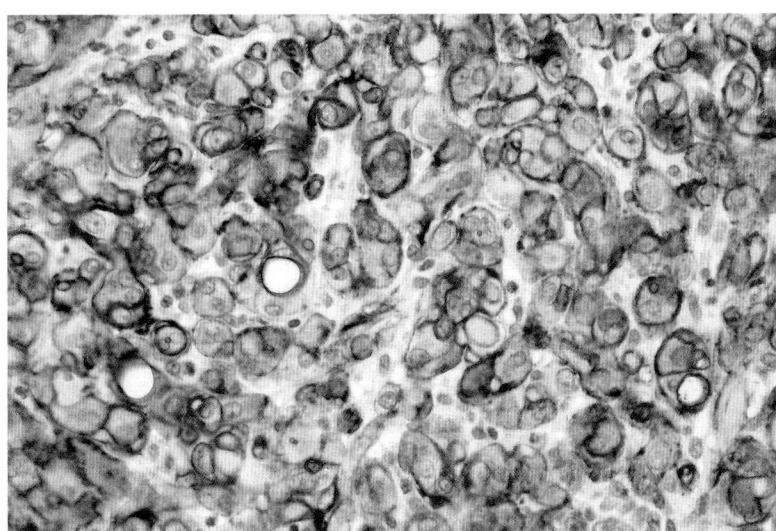

Fig. 35.565
Epithelioid hemangioendothelioma: the intracytoplasmic lumina may sometimes be highlighted with immunohistochemistry (CD31).

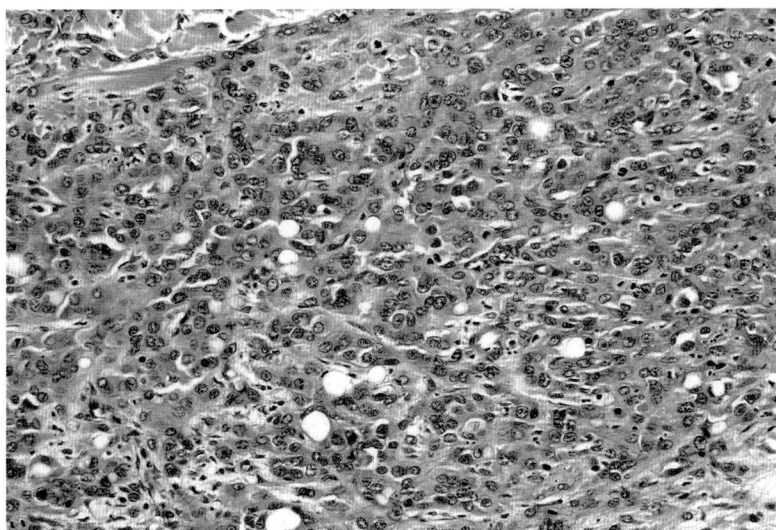

Fig. 35.566
Epithelioid hemangioendothelioma: this example is much more cellular. Intracytoplasmic lumina are still conspicuous.

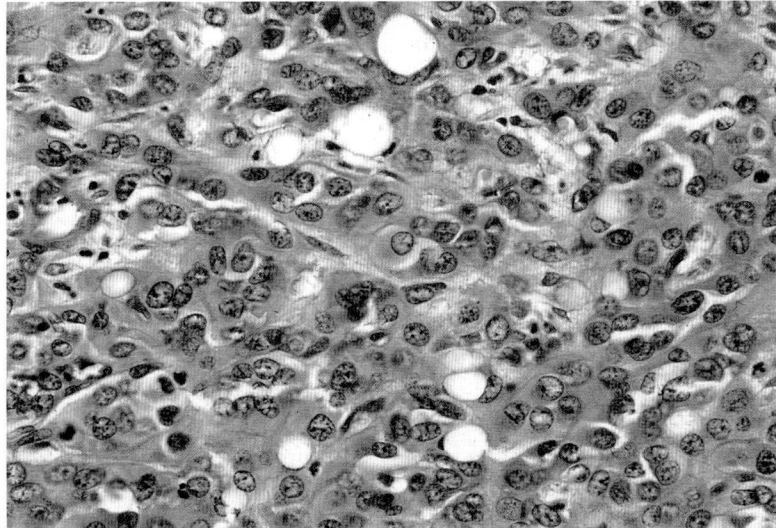

Fig. 35.567
Epithelioid hemangioendothelioma: high-power view.

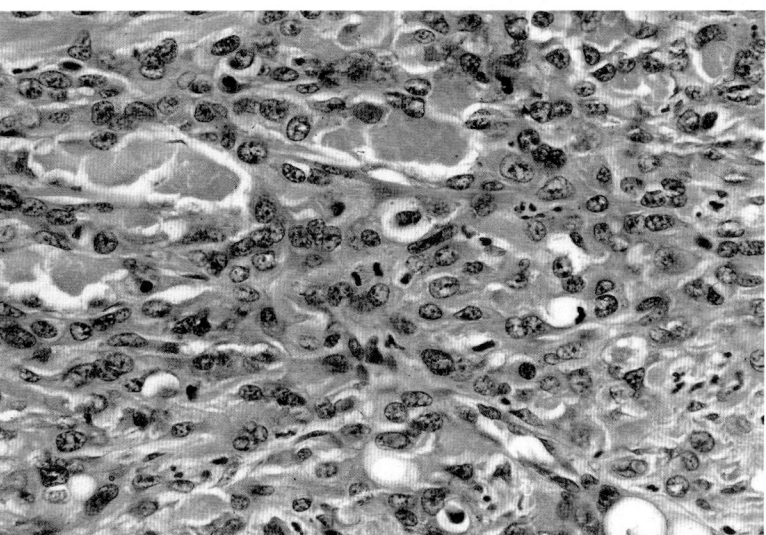

Fig. 35.568
Epithelioid hemangioendothelioma: note the mitotic figures.

shows more pleomorphism and is positive for epithelial markers including EMA and negative for vascular markers. Mucin stains are often positive in the tumor cell cytoplasm. Epithelioid sarcoma generally shows a more sheet-like growth pattern (at least in areas) and only occasional cytoplasmic vacuoles. It is positive for both keratin and EMA, often CD34 positive, but negative for ERG, CD31, von Willebrand factor, INI1 and CAMTA1. Epithelioid angiosarcoma lacks a fibromyxoid or sclerotic stroma and tends to consist of sheets of pleomorphic epithelioid cells with intracytoplasmic lumina and little tendency to form vascular channels. In addition, the latter is not associated with CAMTA1-WWTR1 fusions. Myxoid chondrosarcoma has a lobular architecture; the tumor cells are S100 protein positive and lack intracytoplasmic lumina.

Angiosarcoma

The term angiosarcoma is synonymous with hemangiosarcoma and lymphangiosarcoma.

Clinical features

Cutaneous angiosarcoma predominantly occurs in one of three clinical settings:
- idiopathic angiosarcoma of the head and neck,
- lymphedema-associated angiosarcoma,
- postirradiation angiosarcoma.[1–9]

Sporadic cases in the limbs (unassociated with lymphedema) may occur at any age. Very rare cases have been reported in association with vinyl chloride exposure, xeroderma pigmentosum, epidermolysis bullosa, stasis ulceration, a gouty tophus, as a complication of morbid obesity and in association with arthroplasty.[10–17] It has been suggested that angiosarcomas developing in the setting of xeroderma pigmentosum may not be as aggressive as other angiosarcomas.[18] A patient with Klippel-Trenaunay-Weber syndrome developed an angiosarcoma and a malignant peripheral nerve sheath tumor in the same involved limb.[19] Development of angiosarcoma in a teratoma and a congenital example have also been documented.[20,21] Angiosarcoma arising in other organs may metastasize to the skin.[22,23] Rare cases in association with chronic immunosuppression in renal transplant patients and in HIV have been reported.[24–27] Angiosarcoma in children is exceptional and tends to occur mainly in the soft tissues and internal organs, particularly the head and neck and mediastinum.[28–32] Associated conditions in children other than the ones mentioned before, include congenital lymphedema, Aicardi syndrome and congenital hemangioma.[33] The tumor may occasionally occur within a blood vessel, a hemangioma, nerve and in benign or malignant nerve sheath tumors.[34–38] A case of multiple cutaneous and visceral vascular malformations associated with hepatic disseminated angiosarcoma has been reported.[39]

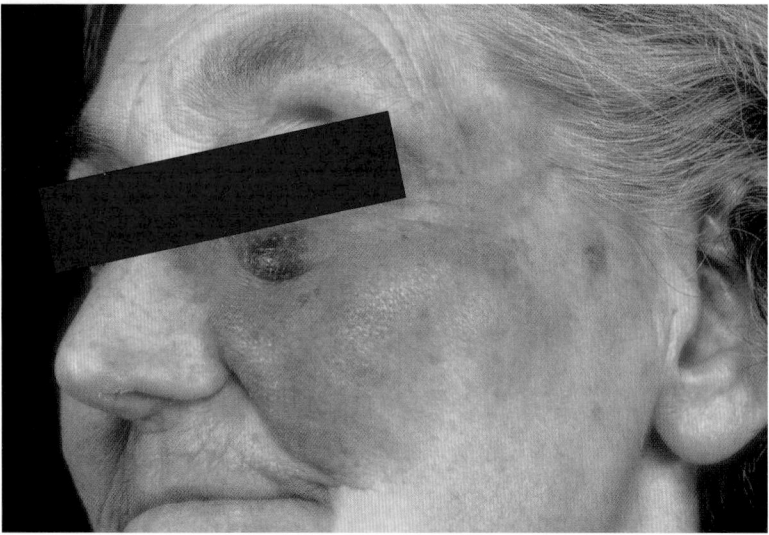

Fig. 35.569
Angiosarcoma: there is a purplish bruise-like discoloration of the face with an infraorbital nodule. From the collection of the late N.P. Smith, MD, the Institute of Dermatology, London, UK.

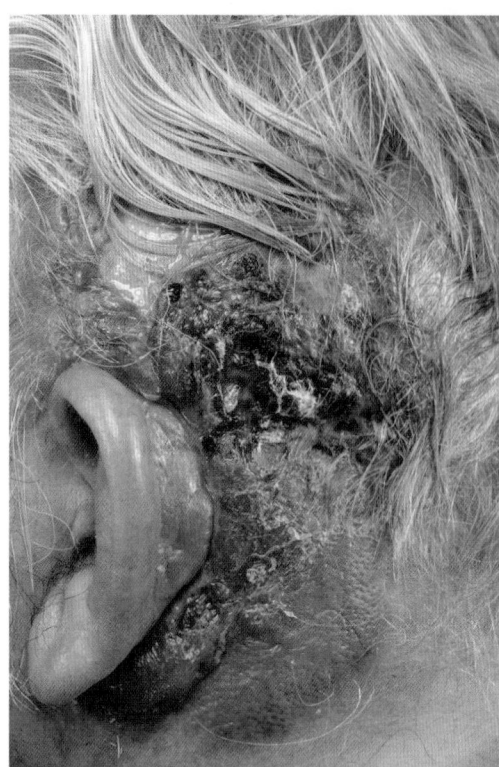

Fig. 35.571
Angiosarcoma: note this diffuse crusted and ulcerated lesion. The face and scalp are sites of predilection. From the collection of the late N.P. Smith, MD, the Institute of Dermatology, London, UK.

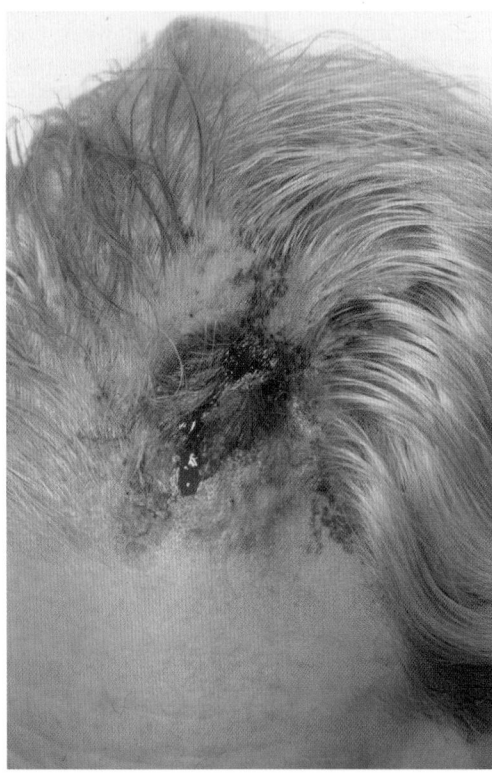

Fig. 35.570
Angiosarcoma: ulcerated and hemorrhagic plaque on the frontal scalp. From the collection of the late N.P. Smith, MD, the Institute of Dermatology, London, UK.

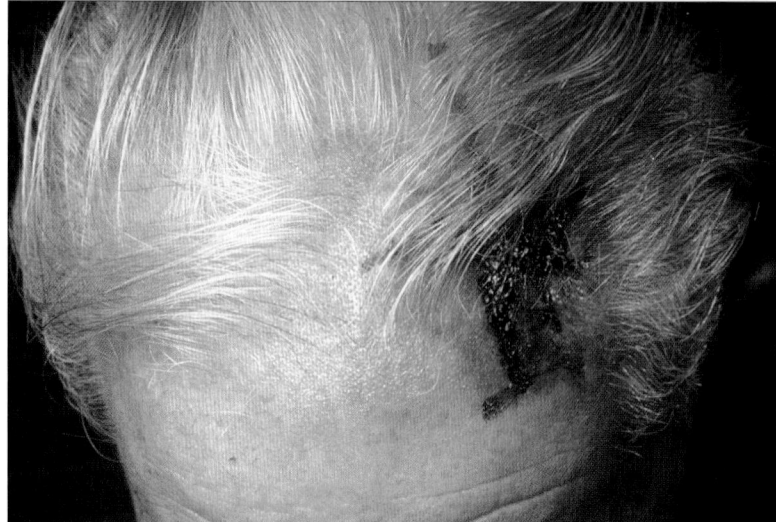

Fig. 35.572
Angiosarcoma: patients often present with a bruise-like lesion. By courtesy of the Institute of Dermatology, London, UK.

Idiopathic angiosarcoma of the head and neck

Idiopathic angiosarcoma of the head and neck is predominantly a tumor of late adulthood, with an equal sex incidence and a predilection for the scalp and central face.[1,2,8,9] Involvement confined to the eyelid has been documented.[40] It presents as single or multiple raised reddish or purple plaques, papules or nodules which may show a variable growth rate. High-grade lesions tend to ulcerate and bleed readily (Figs 35.569–35.574). The tumor is typically much more extensive than is clinically apparent. Spontaneous regression exceptionally occurs.[41,42] Rare cases may mimic other diseases including rosacea and rhinophyma.[43,44] Thrombocytopenia may rarely occur, probably as a result of platelet consumption and destruction within the tumor.[45,46] Alopecia is an uncommon manifestation.[47]

Lymphedema-associated angiosarcoma

Lymphedema-associated angiosarcoma (traditionally known as lymphangiosarcoma) classically arises on the arms of elderly females who have undergone mastectomy with axillary lymph node dissection or radiotherapy many years previously (Stewart-Treves syndrome) (Fig. 35.575).[48–51] It may also develop in other forms of iatrogenic lymphedema, congenital lymphedema, very rarely in a lymphangiomatous malformation, in association with elephantiasis, filariasis and even in areas of lymphedema secondary to morbid obesity.[52–55] A case developing in an area of lipodermatosclerosis in a lower limb with changes of stasis has been reported.[56] Lesions typically present as numerous purplish nodules or vesicles, often distributed over a wide area.

Postirradiation angiosarcoma

Postirradiation angiosarcoma is the rarest of the three variants and can develop many years after radiotherapy for benign (hemangiomas, tinea capitis) or malignant conditions.[57–62] Most cases are associated with radiotherapy from breast and gynecological cancer.[63] In cutaneous postirradiation angiosarcoma of the breast there is usually no associated lymphedema

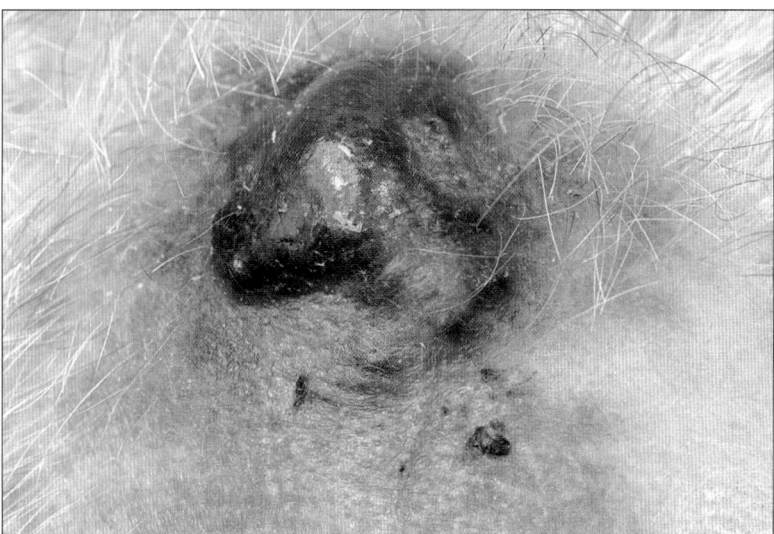

Fig. 35.573
Angiosarcoma: the scalp, particularly in bald individuals, is a commonly affected site. By courtesy of the Institute of Dermatology, London, UK.

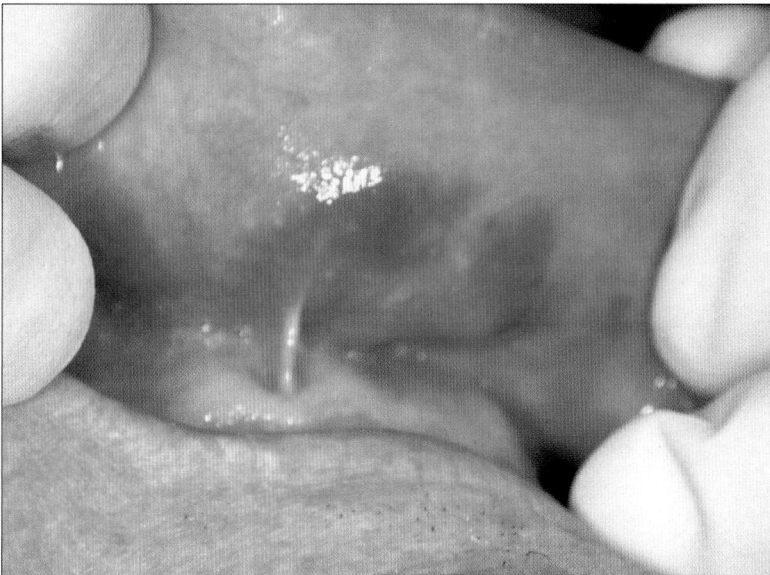

Fig. 35.574
Angiosarcoma: oral lesions in a patient with minimal cutaneous involvement highlighting the multifocality of the process. By courtesy of the Institute of Dermatology, London, UK.

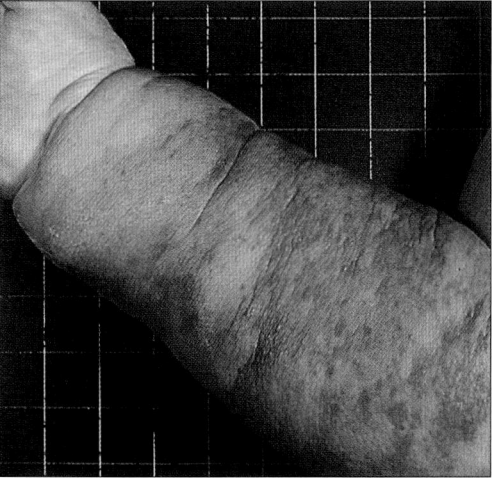

Fig. 35.575
Lymphedema-associated angiosarcoma (Stewart-Treves tumor): very marked lymphedema has complicated radical mastectomy in this elderly female patient. There is diffuse involvement of the arm by tumor.

and the latency period is shorter than that in Stewart-Treves syndrome.[64] Some cases of postirradiation angiosarcoma of the breast may be associated with chronic lymphedema and this may contribute to the development of the disease.[65] A case following treatment of metastatic melanoma has been reported.[66]

All postirradiation angiosarcomas show high-level amplification of *MYC*, reflecting gains in chromosome 8q24 and this is regarded as an early necessary alteration in the development of the tumor.[67,68] In about 25% of these cases there is co-amplification of *FLT4*, which encodes VEGFR3. Interestingly, these alterations are not found in atypical vascular proliferations associated with radiotherapy. Other types of cutaneous angiosarcomas also show *MYC* amplification.[68–70]

All forms of angiosarcoma carry a very poor prognosis, with repeated local recurrences, rapid dissemination and death in up to 80% of cases, often within a fairly short time.[71–75] A retrospective study of angiosarcoma of the scalp and face found an improved 43% 5-year survival attributed to combined modality therapy.[76] A further study including all sporadic cutaneous angiosarcomas, including those from the scalp and face and those with pure epithelioid morphology, found poor prognosis to be associated with necrosis, epithelioid morphology and old age (over 70 years).[77] Local recurrence was associated with tumor depth. This study confirms findings of a previous study in which adverse prognosis correlated with size of the tumor, depth of invasion and mitotic rate.[78] We regard pure cutaneous epithelioid angiosarcomas occurring outside the usual three clinical settings of angiosarcoma as a distinctive category of neoplasms with very poor prognosis (see below). Younger patients appear to have a better prognosis and radiation therapy appears to improve survival.[79,80] It has been suggested that increased number of CD8 positive tumor-infiltrating correlate with better prognosis.[81]

Among metastatic sites, lymph nodes and lungs are the commonest. Interestingly, complete remission of a radioresistant, an inoperable and a metastatic angiosarcoma after treatment with liposomal doxorubicin, paclitaxel or a combination of the latter and sorefenib, respectively, have been reported.[82–84]

Pathogenesis and histologic features

Cytogenetic analysis in a small number of superficial and deep angiosarcomas has shown complex chromosomal abnormalities mainly involving chromosomes 5, 7, 8, 13, 15, 20, 22, and Y.[85] Activating mutations in *KDR* and other genes which may be amenable to therapeutic targeting have been documented.[86] Mutations in *PTPRB*, *PLCG1* and the *ERK/MAPK* pathway have been recently described.[87,88] The genetic anomalies involving the *ERK/MAPK* pathway included mutations in *KRAS*, *HRAS*, *NRAS*, *BRAF*, *MAPK1* and *NF1* or amplifications in *MAPK1/CRKL*, *CRAF* or *BRAF*. Mutations in *TP53* and losses of *CDKN2A* were also found in a smaller number of cases.[88]

Microscopically, all clinical variants are largely indistinguishable other than by the presence of coexistent lymphedema and are therefore considered together. The appearances are of an ill-defined infiltrative intradermal mass of numerous anastomosing vascular channels of varying caliber (*Figs 35.576–35.579*). The endothelium, which may be single or multilayered, is typically plump, pleomorphic and mitotically active (abnormal mitoses being quite common), and may form papillae or solid nests within vascular lumina. The vascular proliferation tends to ramify through the dermis, 'dissecting' the collagen bundles (*Figs 35.580 and 35.581*). Focal epithelioid change is not uncommon and can be prominent in some instances. In some cases, the tumor adopts (focally or diffusely) a solid, undifferentiated, spindled cell appearance, which is not easily recognizable as vascular in origin (*Figs 35.582–35.584*).

A number of cases appear to demonstrate true lymphatic differentiation, mainly those located on the scalp and face.[89] These tumors are characterized by interconnecting irregular channels devoid of red blood cells lined by atypical hobnail endothelial cells, have stromal lymphoid aggregates and stain for lymphatic markers including D2-40, prox-1 and VEGFR-3. A small subset of angiosarcomas simulate Kaposi sarcoma, a feature also suggestive of lymphatic differentiation.[90,91] Distinction from the latter is very difficult in some cases, as the promontory sign which is seen in many

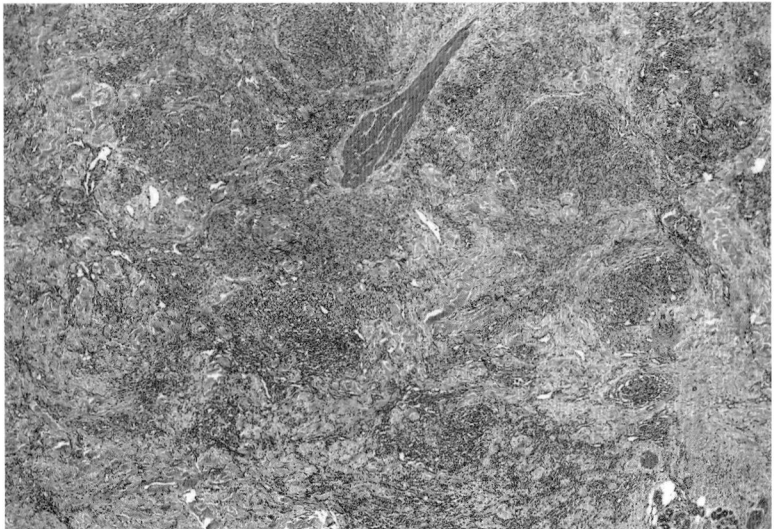

Fig. 35.576
Angiosarcoma: this low-power view shows extensive infiltration of the dermis by a vascular tumor.

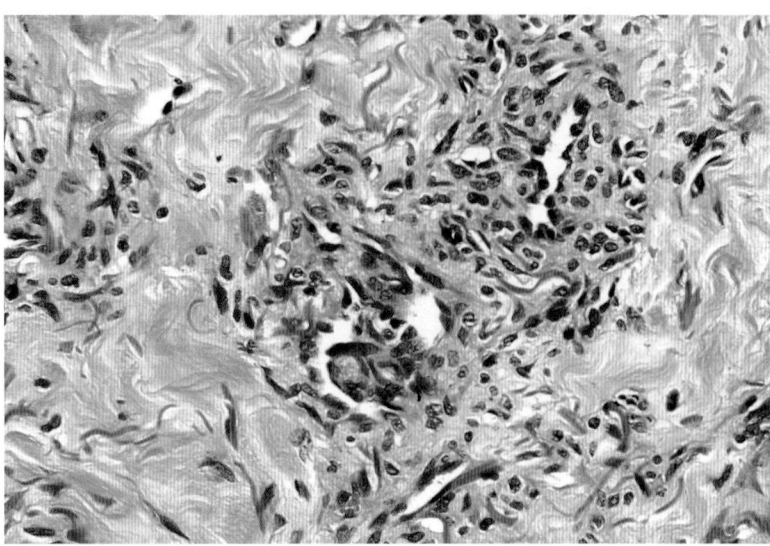

Fig. 35.579
Angiosarcoma: in this example, intraluminal papillae are present.

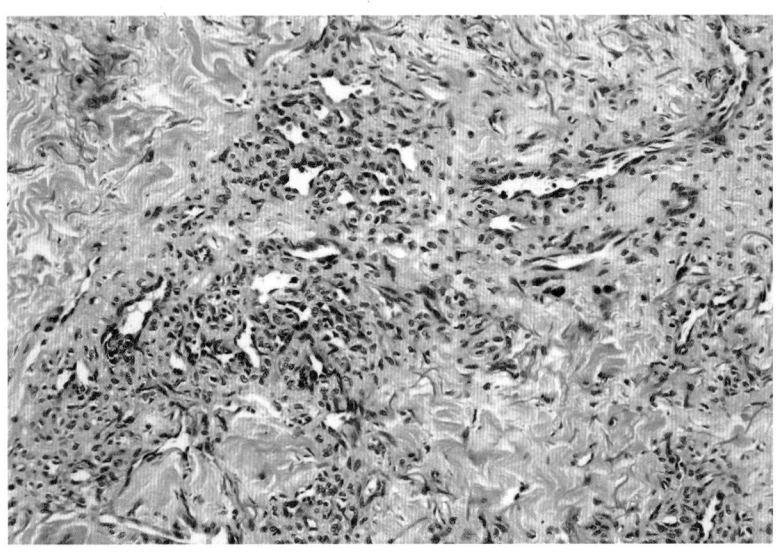

Fig. 35.577
Angiosarcoma: the endothelial cells are pleomorphic and hyperchromatic.

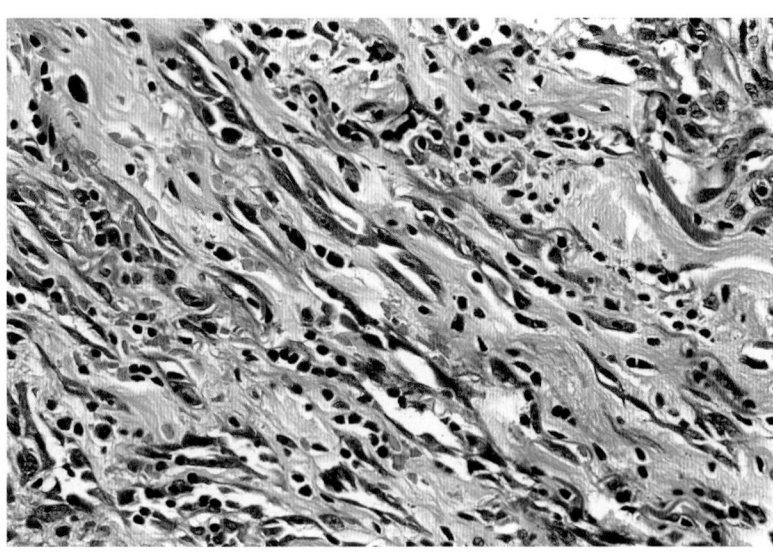

Fig. 35.580
Angiosarcoma: note the spindled cell population with vesicular nuclei and prominent nucleoli.

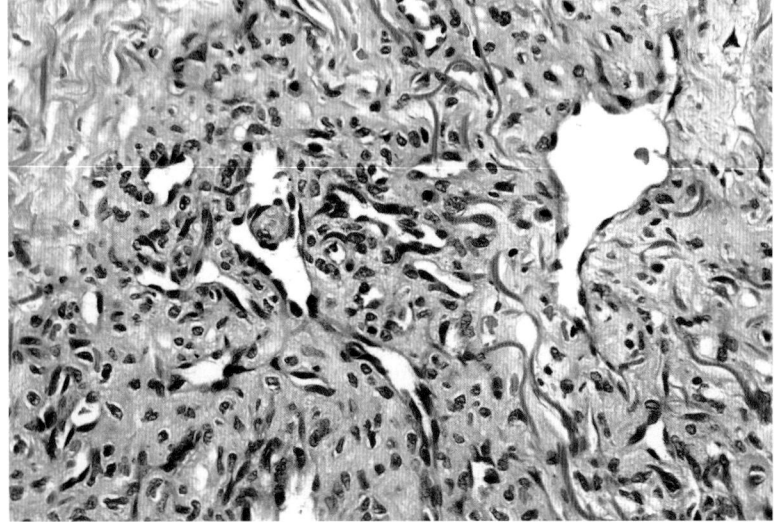

Fig. 35.578
Angiosarcoma: high-power view.

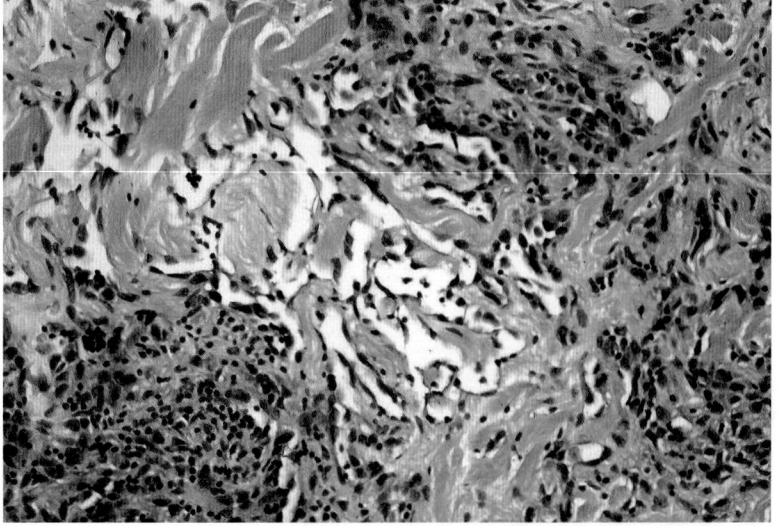

Fig. 35.581
Angiosarcoma: there is conspicuous dissection of collagen.

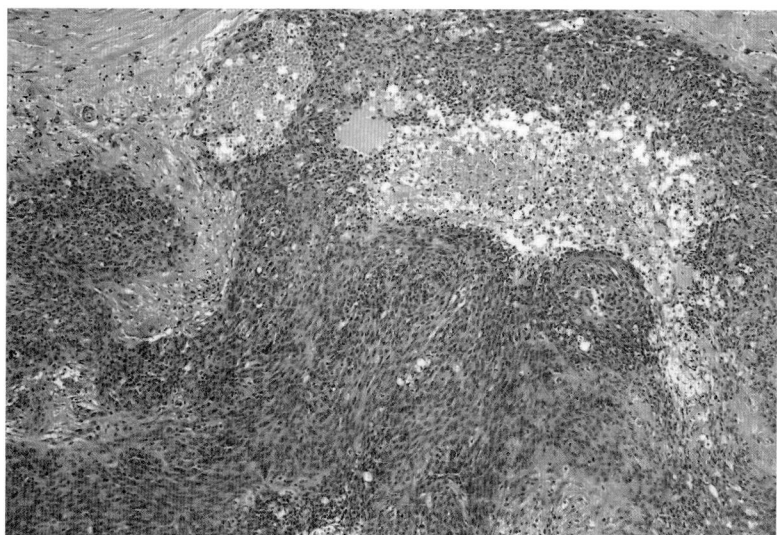

Fig. 35.582
Angiosarcoma (spindle cell variant): the dermis is extensively infiltrated by a spindled cell tumor.

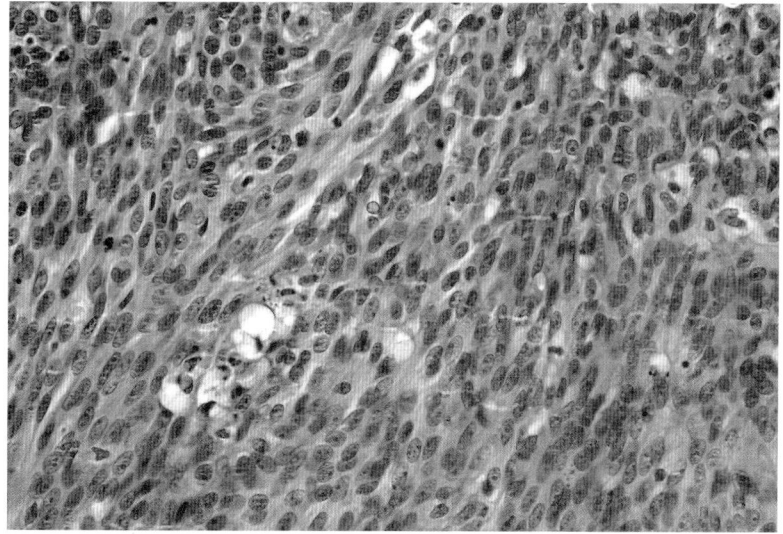

Fig. 35.583
Angiosarcoma (spindle cell variant): the spindle cells have eosinophilic cytoplasm and pleomorphic, vesicular nuclei. Intracytoplasmic lumina are apparent.

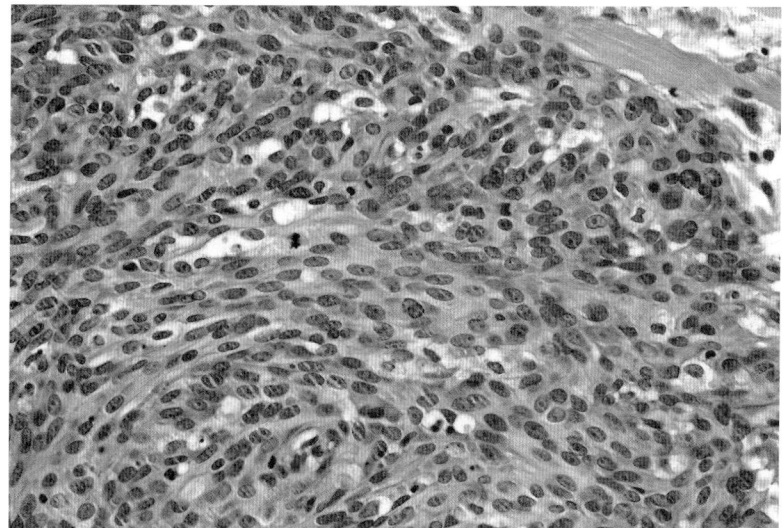

Fig. 35.584
Angiosarcoma (spindle cell variant): note the mitotic activity.

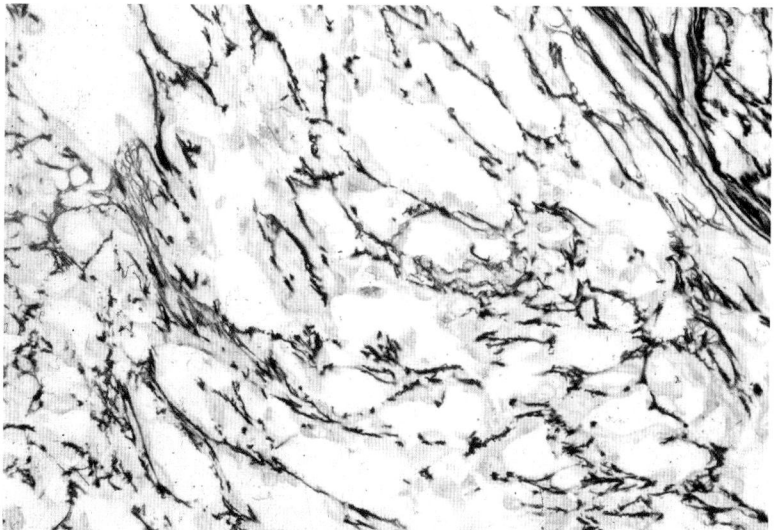

Fig. 35.585
Angiosarcoma: the tumor cells are enclosed within a reticulin sheath.

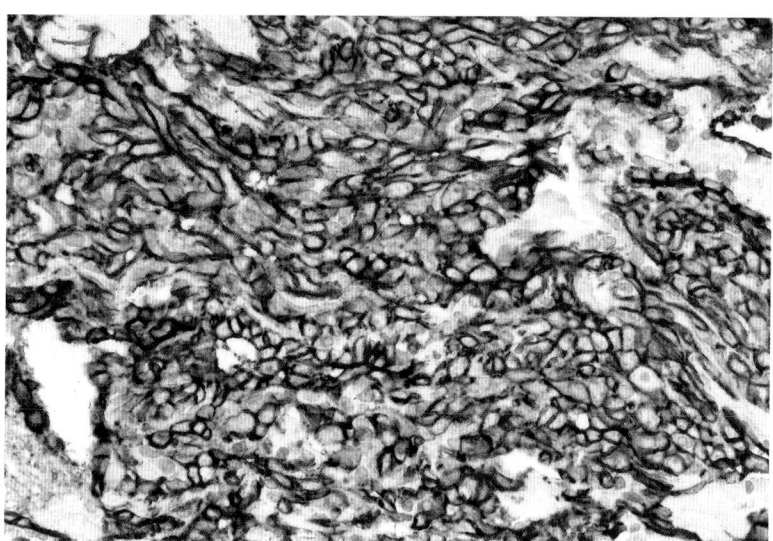

Fig. 35.586
Angiosarcoma: the tumor cells express CD31.

tumors with lymphatic differentiation particularly Kaposi sarcoma, may be seen in angiosarcoma.[92] However, in the latter there is cytologic atypia, mitotic activity and multilayering.

A useful means of identifying the vascular nature of this tumor is by reticulin staining, which will demonstrate that in the better differentiated areas the tumor cells lie within a perivascular reticulin sheath; single cells are not surrounded by the reticulin framework (Fig. 35.585). Chronic inflammatory cells scattered throughout the tumor are often a prominent feature. In exceptional cases the infiltrate simulates a lymphoma and obscure the real tumor.[93] Rare cases of angiosarcoma are mainly composed of cells with granular cytoplasm or signet ring appearance.[94–96] A variant composed of foamy cells mimicking histiocytes has also been reported.[97]

In postirradiation tumors, capillary lobules may be present, and although this has been traditionally regarded as a feature indicative of a benign proliferation, in this setting it should raise the alarm about the presence of angiosarcoma.[98,99]

In poorly differentiated cases, it is useful to assess a panel of endothelial markers because individual antibodies tend to be variably positive in different tumors. These include von Willebrand factor (factor VIII-related antigen), CD31, CD34, FLI1 and ERG (Fig. 35.586). ERG is an ETS family transcription factor now regarded as the most sensitive and specific vascular marker.[100,101] FLI1 is fairly sensitivity but less specific marker of endothelial

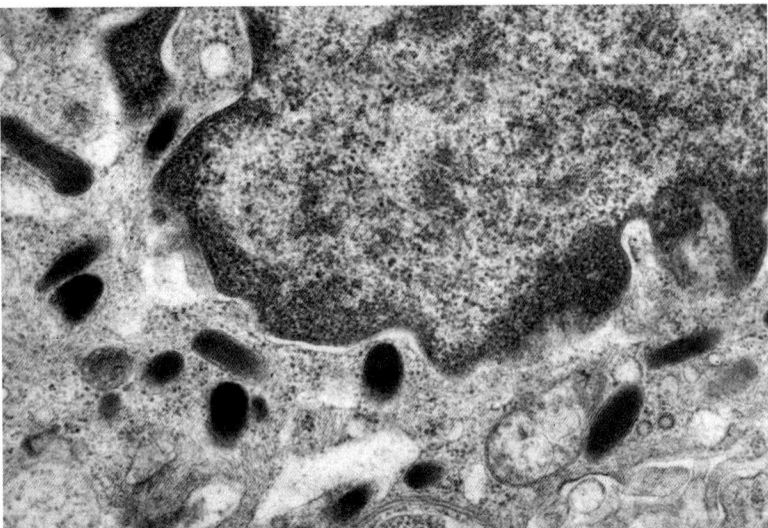

Fig. 35.587
Angiosarcoma: in spindle cell variants, the diagnosis is sometimes confirmed ultrastructurally by the identification of Weibel-Palade bodies.

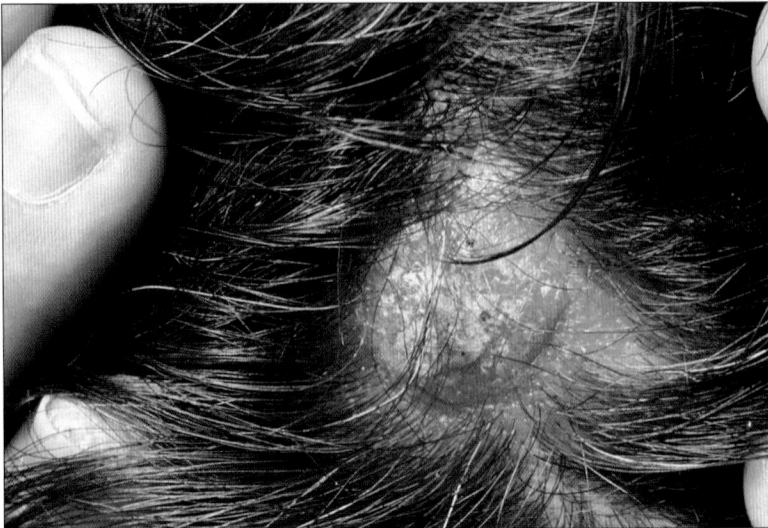

Fig. 35.588
Epithelioid angiosarcoma: presentation on the scalp is not uncommon. The lesion is less obviously vascular when compared with more typical angiosarcoma. By courtesy of the Institute of Dermatology, London, UK.

cell differentiation.[102] CD34 is variably positive and tends to be negative in angiosarcomas of the head and neck. Claudin-5 has been proposed as a good marker of angiosarcoma but it is positive in other vascular tumor and also in byphasic synovial sarcoma and carcinomas.[103] CD30 is expressed in up to one third of angiosarcomas and this may be a source of confusion in poorly differentiated tumors.[104]

Tumors lacking epithelioid morphology are usually not positive for keratin and epithelial membrane antigen.[105] It is important to remember that no antibody is entirely specific, and staining of histiocytes by CD31 may be a confounding feature in hemorrhagic atypical fibroxanthomas and my lead to a misdiagnosis of angiosarcoma.[106] CD31 staining of histiocytes is cytoplasmic and granular, while staining of cells with endothelial cell differentiation reveals not only cytoplasmic staining but also crisp cytoplasmic membrane positivity.

Angiosarcomas are usually negative for HHV-8 except in tumors occurring in patients with AIDS.[25]

Ultrastructurally, the presence of Weibel-Palade bodies confirms the vascular nature of the tumor (Fig. 35.587). However, the latter technique is hardly used nowadays.

Differential diagnosis

The presence of endothelial cell atypia, multilayering and mitotic activity allows ready distinction from a benign hemangioma (or lymphangioma) and Masson tumor. Occasional cases may need to be distinguished from spindle cell melanoma or carcinoma, in which circumstances immunohistochemistry is most helpful.

Epithelioid angiosarcoma

Clinical features

Epithelioid angiosarcoma represents the malignant end of the spectrum of epithelioid vascular neoplasms.[1-5] The term is reserved for tumors composed almost exclusively of epithelioid cells, as conventional angiosarcomas are quite often focally epithelioid. We reserve this term to tumors with epithelioid morphology occurring outside the conventional settings of cutaneous angiosarcoma described earlier. Although involvement of the skin by this tumor is rare, it appears to occur more often than was previously thought. It is likely that before it was delineated as a distinctive entity, cases were misdiagnosed as melanocytic or epithelial neoplasms. Lesions have a wide anatomical distribution and usually present in adults, with no sex predilection (Fig. 35.588). Tumors are single or less commonly multiple.[4] Tumors in the skin, soft tissues and other organs have a dismal prognosis. Early metastasis and high mortality of up to 55% is seen in primary cutaneous

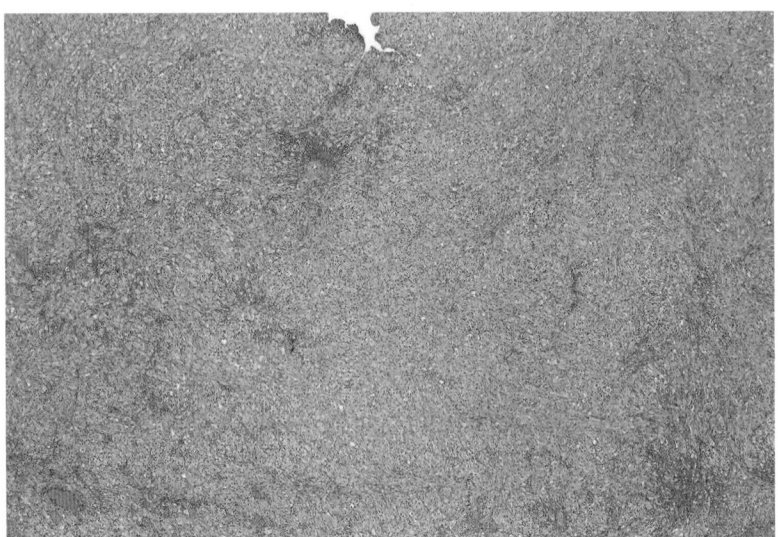

Fig. 35.589
Epithelioid angiosarcoma: there is a diffuse epithelioid cell infiltrate with multiple foci of hemorrhage.

epithelioid angiosarcoma.[4] Occasional cases have been associated with a foreign body, radiotherapy, an arteriovenous fistula, vascular dacron grafts and orthopedic joint prostheses.[1-10] One case developed at a peristomal site and one within an ovarian teratoma.[11,12]

Exceptional cutaneous metastasis from cardiac, mediastinal, bone and intravascular epithelioid angiosarcomas has been documented.[4,13,14]

Histologic features

Lesions are infiltrative and composed of sheets of large oval or round cells with abundant eosinophilic or amphophilic cytoplasm and vesicular nuclei with prominent eosinophilic nucleoli (Figs 35.589–35.591). Although cytologic atypia is present, the tumor cells are relatively monomorphic. Mitosis, necrosis and hemorrhage are common findings. Focally, a few cells show intracytoplasmic lumina containing occasional red blood cells (Fig. 35.592). Blood vessel formation can also be a feature.

A reticulin stain is useful to highlight the vasoformative architecture. Immunohistochemically, the tumor cells are consistently positive for ERG, CD31, FLI1 or von Willebrand factor (Fig. 35.593). Cytokeratin is also positive in up to 50–60% of cases and EMA is focally positive in about 25% of cases (Fig. 35.594).[1,4] INI is often focally or diffusely positive in tumor

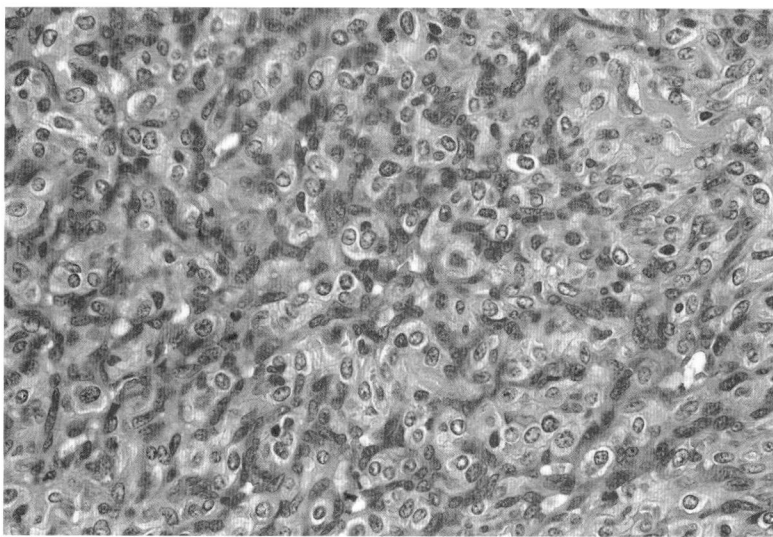

Fig. 35.590
Epithelioid angiosarcoma: the tumor cells have abundant eosinophilic cytoplasm and pleomorphic vesicular nuclei.

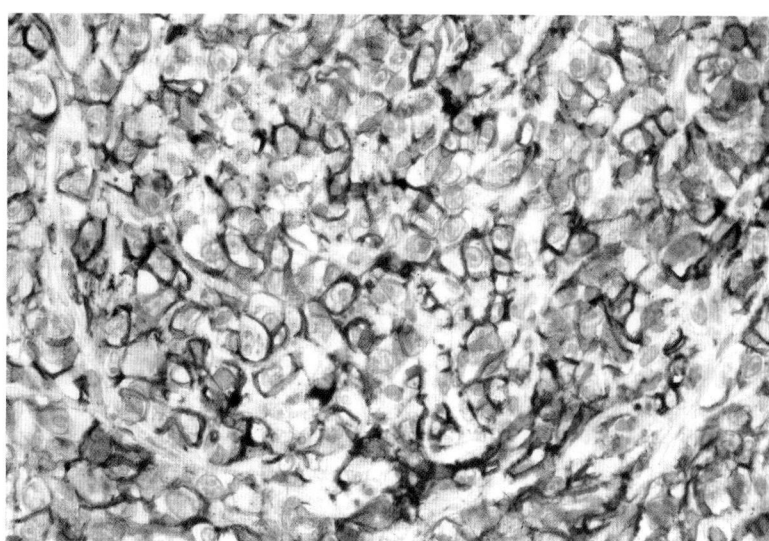

Fig. 35.593
Epithelioid angiosarcoma: the tumor cells express CD31.

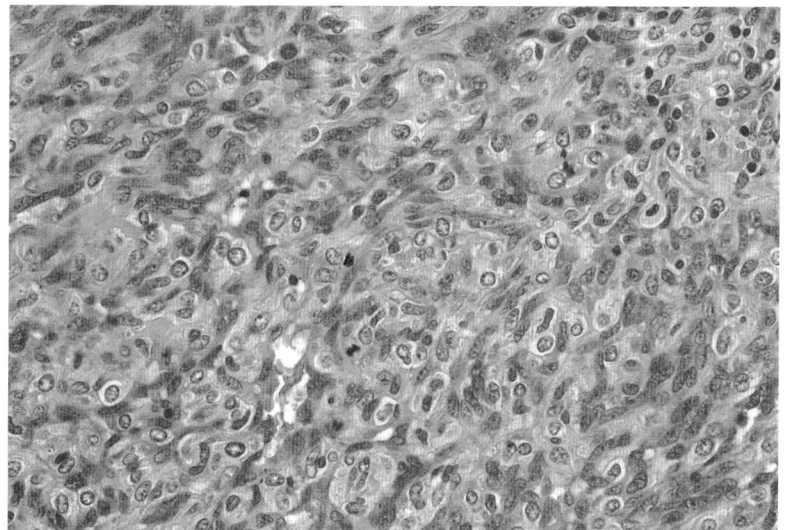

Fig. 35.591
Epithelioid angiosarcoma: note the mitoses.

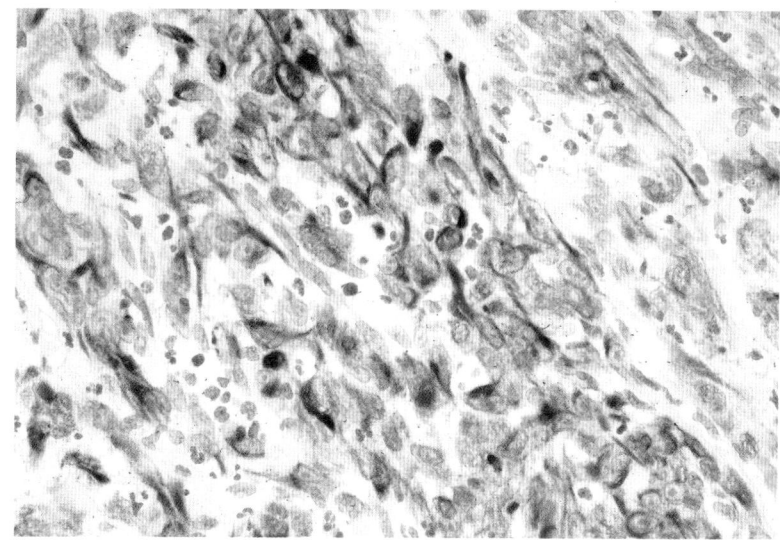

Fig. 35.594
Epithelioid angiosarcoma: this example also expressed keratin (MNF -116).

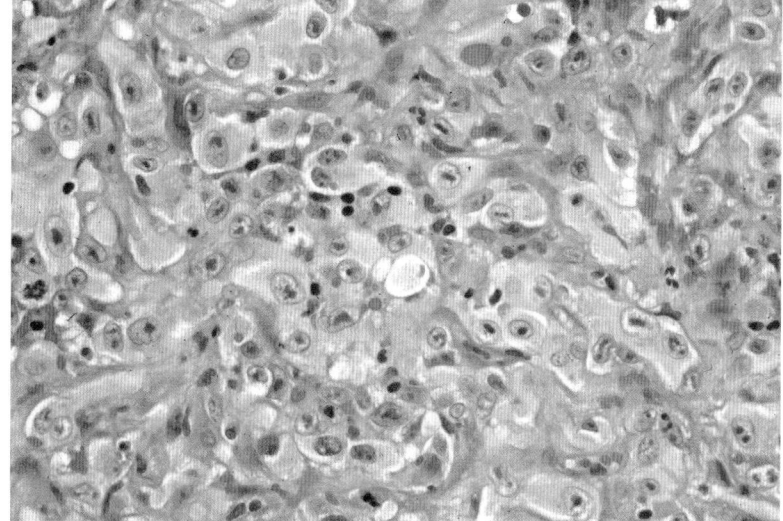

Fig. 35.592
Epithelioid angiosarcoma: intracytoplasmic lumina are present in the center of the field.

cells.[4] Exceptional focal positivity for Melan-A and smooth muscle actin can be seen.[4] A case of pure epithelioid angiosarcoma arising in the setting of radiotherapy for breast cancer was positive for CD30.[15] These important findings need to be borne in mind when considering the differential diagnosis from a carcinoma (especially metastatic) or epithelioid sarcoma.

Differential diagnosis

The differential diagnosis includes metastatic carcinoma, melanoma, epithelioid sarcoma and epithelioid malignant schwannoma, all of which are negative for endothelial markers and lack focal blood vessel formation and intracytoplasmic lumina.

Lymphangioma

Lymphangiomas take four principal forms:
- cavernous lymphangioma,
- cystic hygroma,
- lymphangioma circumscriptum,
- acquired progressive lymphangioma (benign lymphangioendothelioma).

The existence of a true capillary lymphangioma is highly questionable.

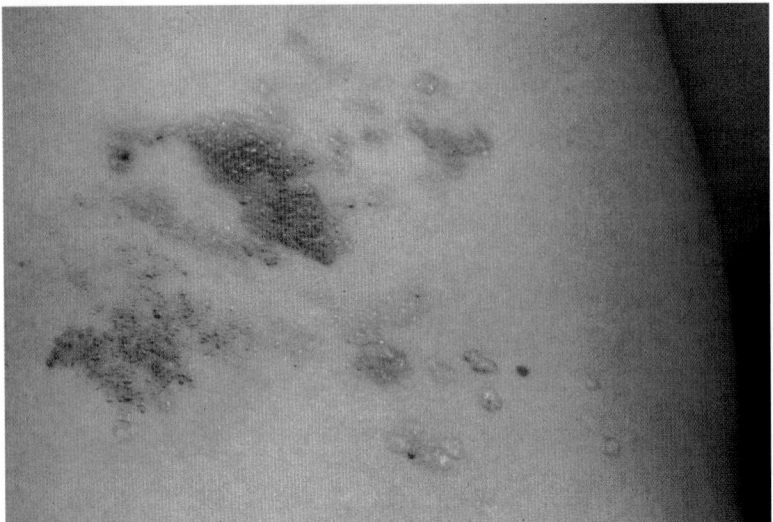

Fig. 35.595
Lymphangioma circumscriptum: the lesion presents as variable numbers of superficial fluid-filled blebs. From the collection of the late N.P. Smith, MD, the Institute of Dermatology, London, UK.

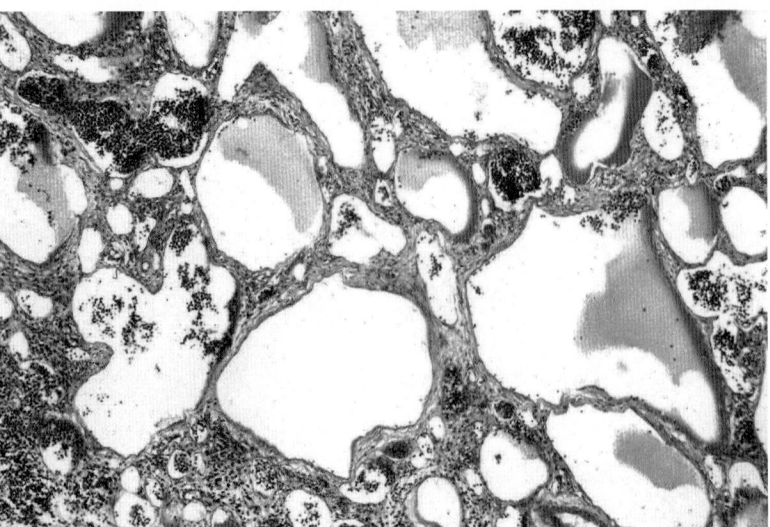

Fig. 35.596
Cavernous lymphangioma: widely dilated lymph-filled channels are characteristic.

Clinical features

Cavernous lymphangioma

Cavernous lymphangioma is a congenital or infantile lesion of equal sex incidence that arises most often in the head and neck region (particularly the tongue) and extremities.[1–5] It presents as a large diffuse, rather doughy mass and is very prone to local recurrence after simple excision. Rare cases present for the first time in adults. Coexistence with a lymphangioma circumscriptum is very rare.[6]

Cystic hygroma

Cystic hygroma is also a lesion of infancy, and presents as a large cystic mass, most often in the neck, axillae or inguinal region.[1,2,5] Scrotal lesions have also been reported.[7] Intra-abdominal and intrathoracic lesions also occur.[8,9] It is also prone to local recurrence unless widely excised, although this tendency is much less marked than with cavernous tumors. Coexistence with a port-wine stain is exceptional.[10] Lesions have been reported in adults.[11]. Cystic hygromas have been associated with trisomy 21, 13, and 18, and Turner and Noonan syndrome.[12]

Lymphangioma circumscriptum

Lymphangioma circumscriptum also presents most often in infancy, but may arise at any age and shows an equal sex distribution.[3–5] Although it develops at any cutaneous site, the proximal portions of the limbs and limb girdles are usually affected. The lesion occurs as a localized collection of numerous small vesicles or blebs which may sometimes form larger confluent masses, filled with clear fluid or blood (*Fig. 35.595*). Occasionally, solitary lesions are present. They are typically asymptomatic unless irritated by the patient.

Although the majority of these tumors probably represent developmental malformations, a small proportion are acquired, usually following block dissection of regional lymph nodes or radiotherapy.[13] Similarly, a small number of cases are associated with an underlying cavernous or cystic lymphangioma. Vulval lesions are idiopathic or have been associated with Crohn disease and radiation therapy.[14] Rare vulvar lesions associated with malignancy and hidradenitis suppurativa have been described.[15] Recurrence after excision is quite common.

Acquired progressive lymphangioma (Benign Lymphangioendothelioma)

Acquired progressive lymphangioma is a rare tumor that was originally described as more frequently seen in children.[16–22] However, the more recent literature suggests that it is more common in adults.[22] It has an equal sex incidence and particularly involves the extremities, especially the upper limbs, although the anatomical distribution is wide. It presents as a solitary, well-defined erythematous macule or plaque that gradually increases in size. Simple excision is usually curative, with only exceptional local recurrences.[22] Occasional partial spontaneous regression is rarely seen. A case has been documented after radiotherapy, a further case developed following femoral arteriography and one has been reported in an HIV-positive patient.[23–25]

Pathogenesis and histologic features

Recently, a number of lymphatic tumors presenting in isolation or as part of complex vascular malformations have been shown display somatic mutations in *PIK3CA*.[26]

Cavernous lymphangioma is typically an ill-defined lesion in the dermis or subcutaneous fat, composed of numerous dilated lymphatic channels without endothelial atypia (*Fig. 35.596*). The surrounding stroma may be inconspicuous or composed of prominent adventitial-type reticulin fibers with a chronic inflammatory cell infiltrate.

Cystic hygroma is histologically almost indistinguishable from the cavernous lesions except that its thin-walled lymphatic spaces show gross cystic dilatation. As well as a lymphocytic infiltrate, scattered lymphoid follicles are common.

In both lesions, the vascular lumina often contain proteinaceous, pale, eosinophilic lymph, and the vessel walls may contain an incomplete layer of smooth muscle.

Lymphangioma circumscriptum is usually situated in the superficial dermis. It is composed of multiple dilated lymphatic channels which often have fairly thick walls and commonly appear to extend into the overlying epidermis (*Fig. 35.597*). The latter is frequently acanthotic and a stromal lymphocytic infiltrate is sometimes evident. Cavernous spaces may be seen in the deeper dermis and occasionally a muscular lymphatic channel (often regarded as the feeding vessel) is present (*Fig. 35.598*).

In progressive lymphangioma, involvement of the superficial dermis is usually prominent, but extension into the deep dermis and superficial subcutis is not uncommon (*Fig. 35.599*). Horizontal, irregular, thin-walled vascular channels lined by a single layer of flat attenuated endothelial cells are seen dissecting the collagen bundles (*Fig. 35.600*). The channels appear empty but occasionally proteinaceous material or red blood cells are seen. Focal papillary projections are sometimes present. Some vascular spaces may have a layer of smooth muscle. Stromal inflammation is not a feature.

Differential diagnosis

Progressive lymphangioma may mimic low-grade angiosarcoma and patch-stage Kaposi sarcoma. The former has at least focal cytologic atypia and multilayering and the clinical setting is different. In the latter there are

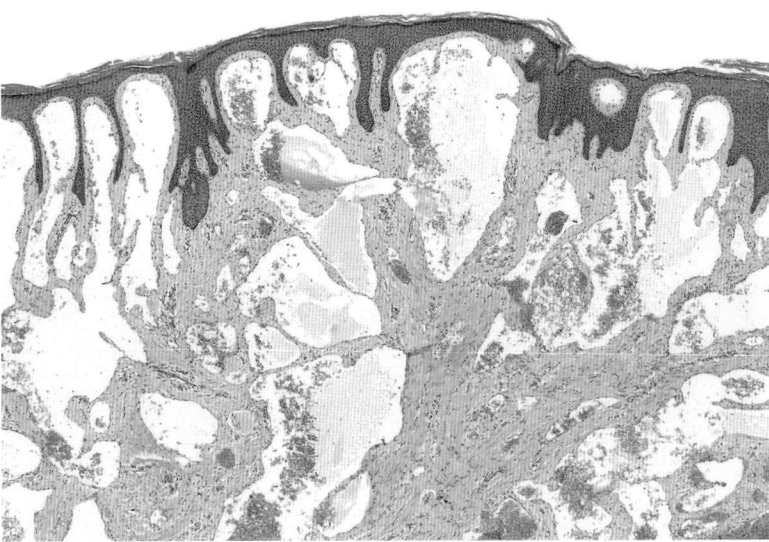

Fig. 35.597
Lymphangioma circumscriptum: thin-walled lymphatic channels are present in both the reticular and papillary dermis.

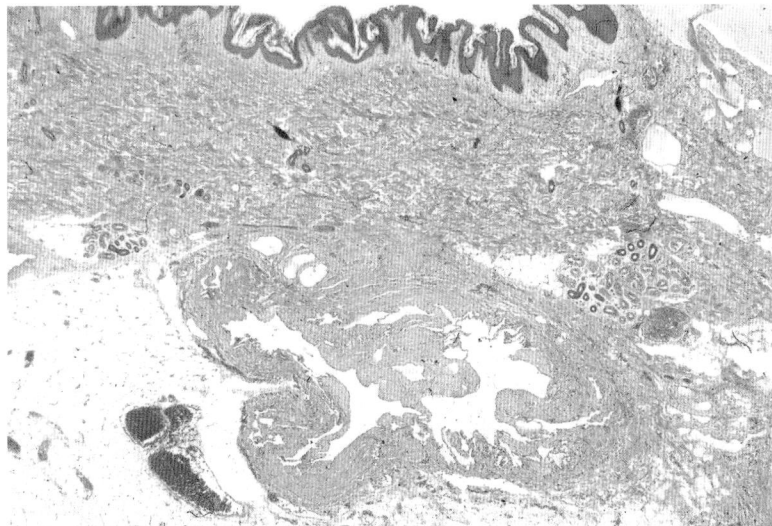

Fig. 35.598
Lymphangioma circumscriptum: within the subcutaneous fat is a large muscular 'feeder' lymphatic trunk. If this is not ligated at surgery, there is a high risk of recurrence.

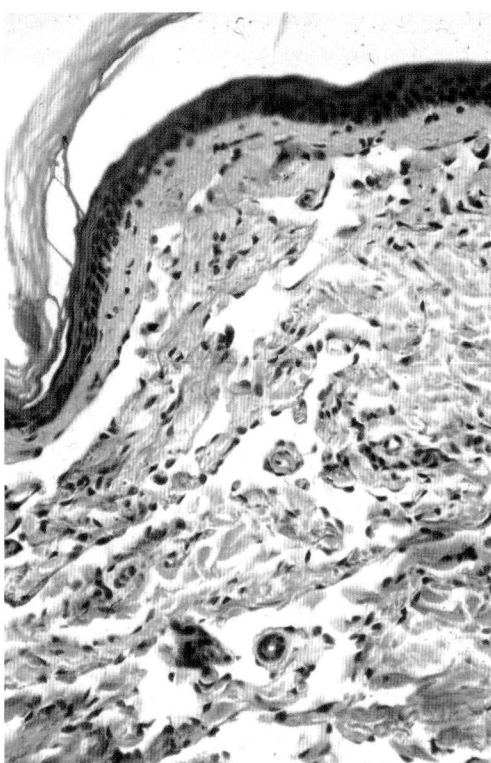

Fig. 35.599
Progressive lymphangioma: despite the architectural resemblance to angiosarcoma, there is a complete absence of endothelial multilayering or nuclear atypia.

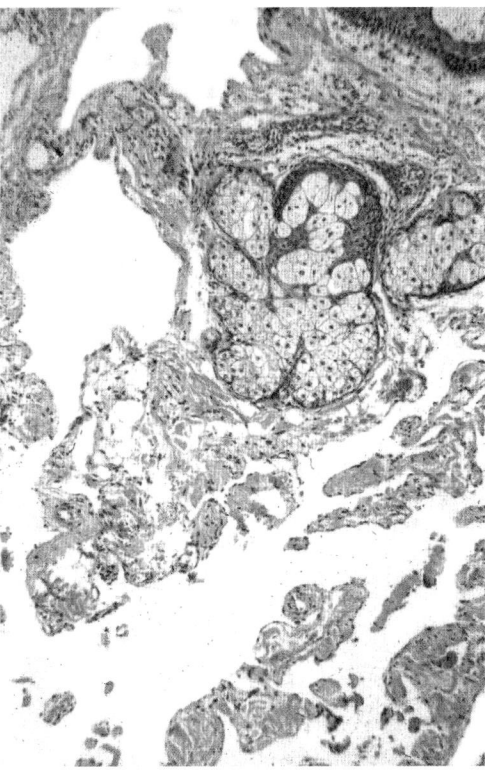

Fig. 35.600
Progressive lymphangioma: some cases show more dissection of dermal structures by the dilated lymphatic spaces.

usually multiple lesions and histologically there is hemosiderin deposition with extravasated erythrocytes and adjacent inflammatory cells, including plasma cells. Distinction from lymphangiomatosis is afforded mainly by the clinical extent of the lesion.

Kaposiform lymphangiomatosis

Kaposiform lymphangiomatosis is a rare recently delineated clinicopathological entity.[1] Most patients are children with rare cases presenting in adults. There is a slight male predominance. The majority of cases present with involvement of the thorax (lungs and mediastinum) followed by bone, spleen and intraabdominal organs. Patients present with respiratory symptoms, pleural and pericardial effusions, anemia and bleeding due to consumptive coagulopathy as a result of thrombocytopenia. Involvement of the skin and subcutaneous tissues, is very rare. Mortality is high, up to 51% at 5 years mainly due to involvement of thoracic organs. Histologically, a proliferation of dilated lymphatic channels lined by flat endothelial cells and associated with aggregates of parallel oriented spindle-shaped endothelial cells with frequent intracytoplasmic hemosiderin.

Multifocal lymphangiomatosis with thrombocytopenia (cutaneovisceral angiomatosis with thrombocytopenia)

Clinical features

This condition is also known as cutaneovisceral angiomatosis with thrombocytopenia or infantile hemorrhagic angiodysplasia, and is characterized by multiple red–brown to blue discrete papules, macules, plaques and nodules ranging in size from millimeters to several centimeters, predominantly affecting the trunk and extremities.[1-4] Many lesions are congenital but new ones continue to develop throughout childhood. Other sites involved include the gastrointestinal tract, lung, bone, liver, spleen, muscle and synovium. Thrombocytopenia is an associated phenomenon. Death from gastrointestinal bleeding and sepsis may occur. Presentation without cutaneous involvement is exceptional.[5] A case misdiagnosed as immune thrombocytopenia due to the delayed appearance of cutaneous lesions has been described.[6]

Histologic features

Microscopically, irregular dilated vascular channels involve the reticular dermis and subcutis and are lined by bland endothelial cells with hobnail morphology and focal intraluminal papillary projections.

Differential diagnosis

Benign lymphangioendothelioma, Dabska tumor and hobnail hemangioma can show similar histologic features to multifocal lymphangiomatosis with thrombocytopenia. However, the former are usually solitary lesions lacking visceral involvement or thrombocytopenia.

Atypical vascular proliferation after radiotherapy

Clinical features

Lymphangiomatous lesions rarely occur in the field of radiotherapy.[1–3] They sometimes have identical features to other lymphangiomas such as lymphangioma circumscriptum or benign progressive lymphangioma with typical histology.[2,3] However, most frequently their clinical and histologic appearances do not fit with any other vascular tumor and sometimes display atypical features, raising the possibility of a postirradiation angiosarcoma.

Lesions usually develop a few months or years after radiotherapy for breast cancer.[1–4] Similar lesions can occur at the site of radiotherapy elsewhere, mainly in relation to genital cancer, but these are rare.[3–5] The time elapsed between radiotherapy and development of the lesions is usually shorter (around 3 years) than that seen in angiosarcomas (around 6 years).[4] The former lesions tend to be smaller than angiosarcomas associated with radiotherapy. The clinical presentation is not distinctive and varies from skin colored to red, usually multiple, macules and papules.

The relationship between these lesions and postirradiation angiosarcomas is controversial and it is not clear whether the former are precursors of the latter or whether they all represent a benign process.[4–9] Although most lesions appear histologically benign, there is a wide histologic spectrum. In a few instances, overlap or even progression to angiosarcoma is seen.[4–6,10] Therefore, treatment of these lesions should be by complete excision with close follow-up.

Histologic features

Most lesions are characterized by irregular lymphatic-like vascular channels lined by a single layer of endothelial cells in the superficial and/or deep dermis (Figs 35.601–35.603). An infiltrative growth pattern is lacking and lesions are usually fairly circumscribed. The cells lining the channels often have a hobnail appearance and are usually bland although some hyperchromatism may be present. Papillary projections may occasionally be seen. Multilayering or mitotic figures are not usually found. In some cases, overlap with angiosarcoma is clearly seen. A study separated these lesions into lymphatic type and vascular type and concluded that the risk of angiosarcoma is higher in patients with the vascular type.[6] In the latter, a lymphatic component is minimal and the proliferation consists of congested capillary-like vascular channels surrounded by a layer of pericytes.

The endothelial cells lining the channels are positive for CD31 and ERG. Lymphatic markers including D2-40 are positive in the lymphatic-like channels and are usually negative in the lesions described as vascular type. MYC is usually negative (see below).

Differential diagnosis

The differential diagnosis includes a well-differentiated angiosarcoma, hobnail hemangioma and Kaposi sarcoma. As opposed to hobnail hemangioma, the lesion is asymmetrical, and the vascular channels do not have a predominant superficial dermal location. The clinical setting, the absence of inflammation and the presence of hobnail endothelial cells with focal

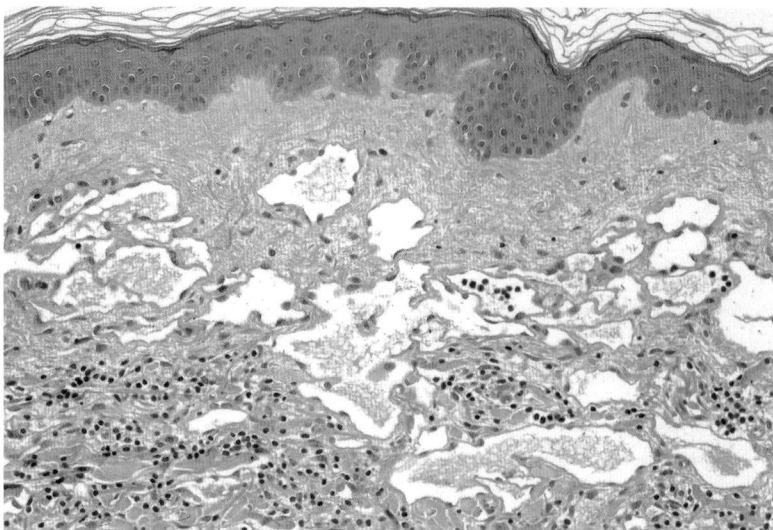

Fig. 35.601
Atypical vascular proliferation after radiotherapy: dilated vessels are evident in the superficial dermis. Nuclear atypia is minimal.

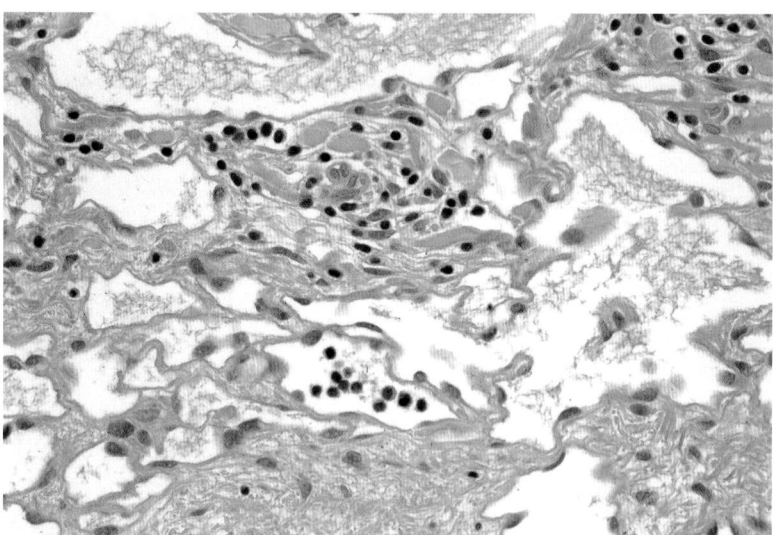

Fig. 35.602
Atypical vascular proliferation after radiotherapy: high-power view.

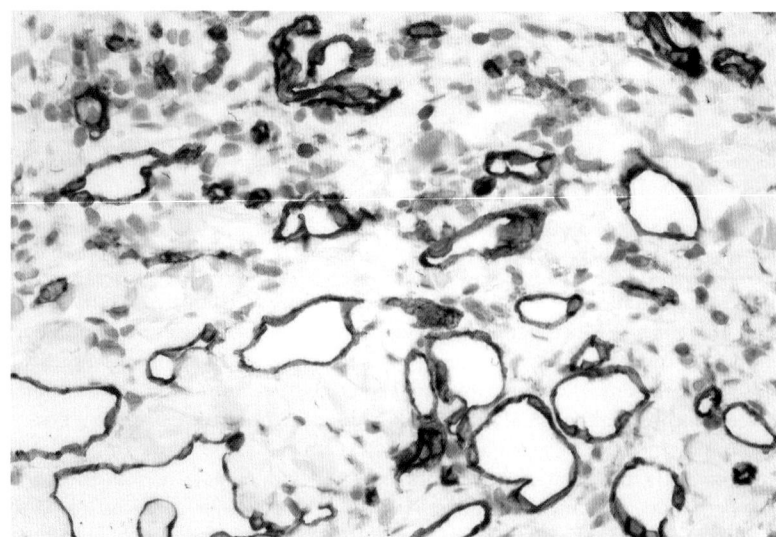

Fig. 35.603
Atypical vascular proliferation after radiotherapy: the extent of the lesion can be highlighted by immunohistochemistry (CD31).

papillary projections should allow distinction from Kaposi sarcoma. Careful examination of multiple sections is recommended to make sure that there are no mitotic figures and cytologic atypia to distinguish it from a well-differentiated angiosarcoma. This distinction can be very difficult, especially in small biopsies. In some cases, immunohistochemistry for MIB1 can be useful as this marker tends to be negative or minimally positive in benign lesions and more prominently positive in angiosarcoma. MYC amplification and expression of MYC protein has been demonstrated by FISH and immunohistochemistry respectively, and can also be useful, as is seen in post-radiation angiosarcomas, but not in atypical vascular lesions after radiotherapy.[11,12] MYC expression is usually strong in the former and can be also be seen in other types of angiosarcomas. Occasional cases of atypical vascular proliferation after radiotherapy may show focal positivity for MYC by immunohistochemistry.[12] MYC amplification however, is not seen by FISH analysis in such cases.

Lymphangiomatosis

Clinical features

Lymphangiomatosis (generalized lymphatic anomaly) is a congenital abnormality characterized by diffuse involvement of soft tissues, skin, bone, lymph nodes and (often) parenchymal organs.[1–4] The disease can be localized to the thorax or abdomen, with predilection for some organs including the kidney and spleen.[5–9] Involvement of the colon can result in protein-losing enteropathy.[10] Multifocal lymphangiomatosis has been described in association with protein-losing enteropathy in patients after palliation of complex congenital heart disease with total cavopulmonary connection.[11] An exceptional association with disseminated intravascular coagulation has been reported.[12] Extensive involvement may be associated with mortality.[13] Most cases present in children and there is no sex predilection. In rare cases, the disease affects only a limb, with or without concomitant bone involvement.[2,14] Coexistence with a cystic hygroma is exceptional.[15] Overlap with angiomatosis can occur and accurate diagnosis requires lymphangiography. Rare cases are associated with kaposiform hemangioendothelioma.[16] Gorham-Stout syndrome refers to the proliferation of lymphatic and vascular channels associated with prominent osteolytic lesions.[17] It has been suggested that this disease is mediated by monocytes that secrete cytokines, inducing angiogenesis and proliferation of osteoclasts.[18] A case of acquired lymphangiomatosis in an HIV positive patient has been reported.[19]

Pathogenesis and histologic features

A somatic mutation in *NRAS* has been reported in lymphangiomatosis.[20]

Histologically, lesions resemble a benign lymphangioendothelioma except that there is very extensive diffuse dissection of dermal structures (the 'hair-dryer effect') (*Figs 35.604* and *35.605*).[2] Long-standing lesions may show stromal sclerosis, and extramedullary hemopoiesis is evident in some cases.

The endothelial cells lining the vascular channels in lymphangiomatosis display increased expression of epidermal growth-factor receptor suggesting that this may be used therapeutically.[21]

Tumors of perivascular cells

Glomus tumor

Glomus tumor arises from the glomus body, which is a specialized arteriovenous anastomosis found most often in the fingers and palms and characterized by the Sucquet-Hoyer canal. They are thought to serve as thermoregulatory receptors. The precise cell of origin is probably a modified smooth muscle cell – the glomus cell – found scattered within the muscle coat of the Sucquet-Hoyer canal.

Clinical features

Glomus tumors are relatively common lesions and arise most often in the third and fourth decades, with an equal sex incidence.[1–3] They may occur at almost any cutaneous site, but are predominantly seen on the hands,

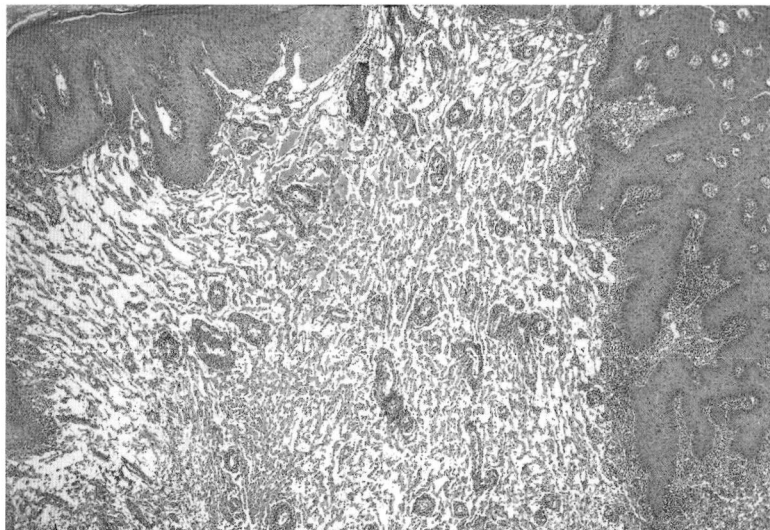

Fig. 35.604
Lymphangiomatosis: this condition shows massive dissection of the dermal collagen and is always clinically extensive.

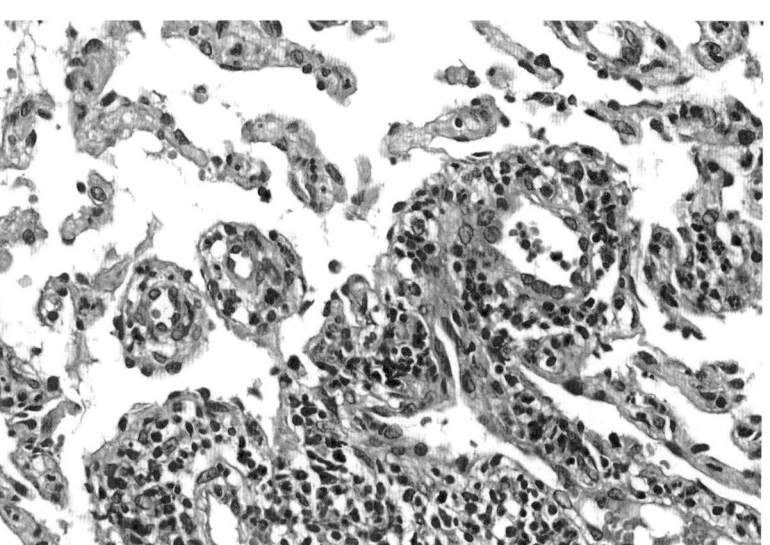

Fig. 35.605
Lymphangiomatosis: high-power view.

particularly the fingers, and especially the subungual region. Lesions can, however, occur with a wide anatomic distribution, not only in the skin but also rarely in mucosae (including oral cavity) and internal organs.[4] The latter include the esophagus, stomach, lung, trachea, bone, small bowel, colon, rectum, mesentery, pterygoid fossa, mediastinum, liver, pancreas, vagina, cervix, ovary and kidney.[5–23] A glomus tumor arising in an ovarian teratoma has been documented.[24] Typically, the tumors are small (less than 1 cm in diameter), reddish-blue nodules and classically present with paroxysmal severe pain, which is often precipitated by cold, pressure or dependency. Pain appears to be more frequent in histologically solid tumors in contrast to the more common glomangiomas.

In a small proportion of cases, the tumors are multiple and may be segmental in distribution.[25,26] Multiple lesions are usually seen in children (an otherwise unusual age group) and have an autosomal dominant inheritance (*Figs 35.606* and *35.607*).[27–29] Congenital lesions may also occur and in one there was associated hypertrichosis.[30–32] Familial glomangiomas, also known as glomuvenous malformations, are associated with inactivating mutations in *GLMN* (1p21-22), encoding glomulin which is normally expressed on vascular smooth muscle cells.[33–40] Local and systemic expression of basic fibroblast growth factor has been found in occasional patients with multiple glomangiomas, suggesting that this cytokine may play a role in their pathogenesis.[41,42]

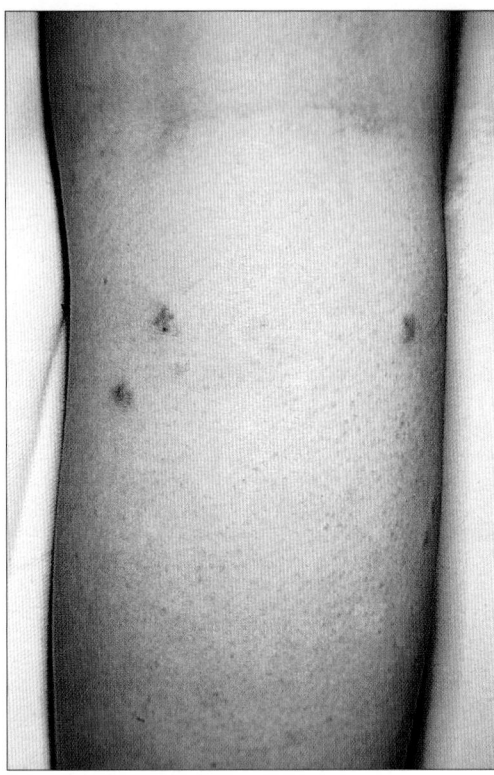

Fig. 35.606
Glomus tumor: multiple, typically small, reddish-blue papules are present on the forearm of a young male. By courtesy of the late M. Beare, MD, Royal Victoria Hospital, Belfast, UK.

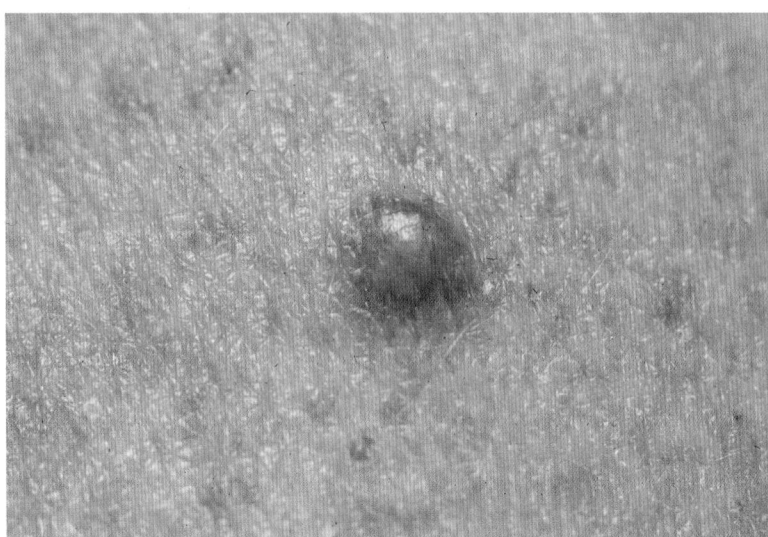

Fig. 35.607
Glomus tumor: close-up view. From the collection of the late N.P. Smith, MD, the Institute of Dermatology, London, UK.

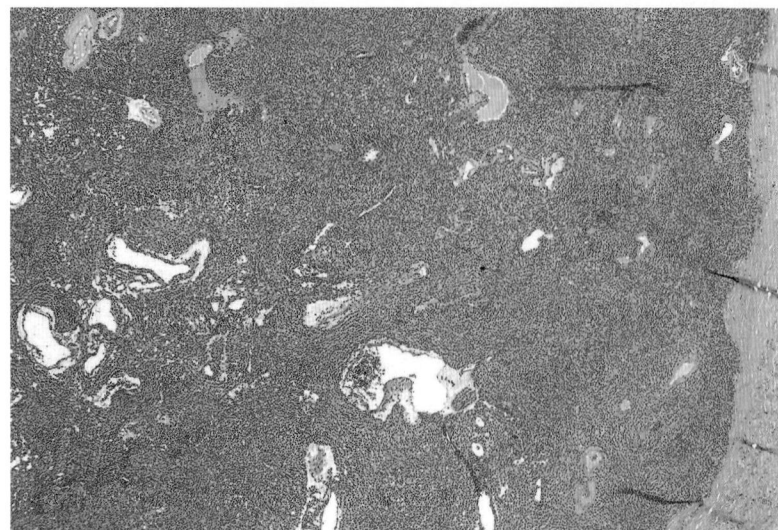

Fig. 35.608
Glomus tumor: the tumor consists of uniform small cells with eosinophilic cytoplasm associated with a conspicuous vasculature.

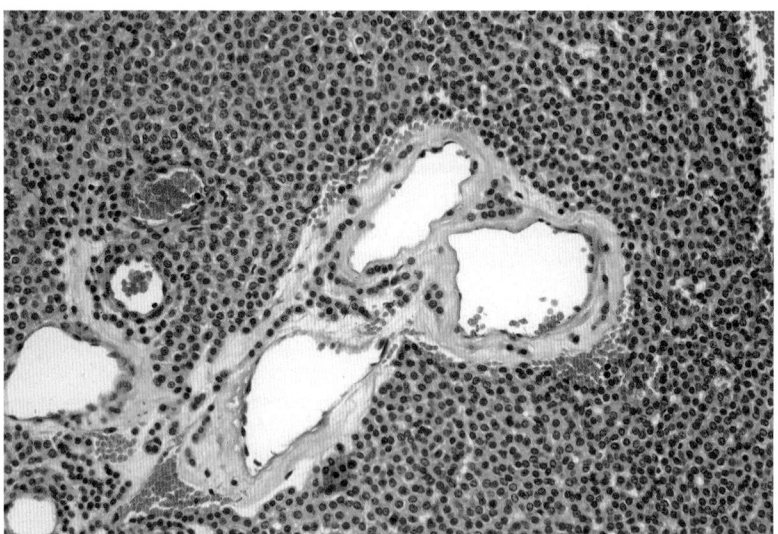

Fig. 35.609
Glomus tumor: the glomus cells have round regular small nuclei. Small numbers are present in this blood vessel wall.

Multiple or solitary glomus tumors have been described in neurofibromatosis type I.[43–45] Tumors tend to occur on the fingers and toes and they are now regarded as part of the spectrum of NF1.[46] Glomus tumors in this setting appear to be related to hyperactivation of RAS mitogen-activated protein kinase, resulting from the lack of inhibition by neurofibromin.[46]

Local recurrence, which is uncommon, only follows inadequate excision and is therefore more frequent in those rare cases (usually deep seated) with infiltrative margins.[47] Digital glomus tumors that are skin-colored or those that arise in the nail matrix appear to have a higher risk of local recurrence.[48] Rare lesions originate within a blood vessel or a nerve.[49–52] The glomus coccygeum, is a prominent glomus body located near the tip of the coccyx that can be found incidentally, and be confused with a neoplasm.[53]

Histologic features

The vast majority of glomus tumors are well circumscribed and composed of small vessels with normal endothelium surrounded by a dense, rather organoid, mantle of uniformly round glomus cells with pale eosinophilic cytoplasm, clearly defined cell margins and central nuclei (*Figs 35.608* and *35.609*). Lesional vessels have no demonstrable elastic laminae, and the glomus cells may extend to abut the endothelium or be separated from it by a thin layer of smooth muscle cells. These predominantly solid glomus tumors (the 'classic' type) are in fact less common than glomangiomas (see below). Mitotic figures, which are always normal, are only rarely seen and pleomorphism is not a feature. Small nerve fibers may occasionally be demonstrated ramifying through the tumor. Normal blood vessels adjacent to the tumors are usually surrounded by groups of glomus cells. Rare cases may show extensive oncocytic change.[54] Prominent epithelioid cell change has been documented (*Figs 35.610* and *35.611*) and in a single case there was prominent sclerosis.[55,56] Calcification is exceptional.[57]

The tumor cells are positive for SMA, muscle-specific actin and, depending on the antibody, myosin; they are only rarely focally positive for desmin.[58] CD34 may also be positive.[59] Interestingly, *BRAF* mutations have been identified in some glomus tumors.[60].

In glomangioma, the most common variant of glomus tumor (up to 60% of cases), the vascular component is more prominent and the lumina tend to be somewhat dilated or cavernous (*Figs 35.612* and *35.613*). Glomus cells may be distributed as an attenuated monolayer or bilayer in the vessel wall.

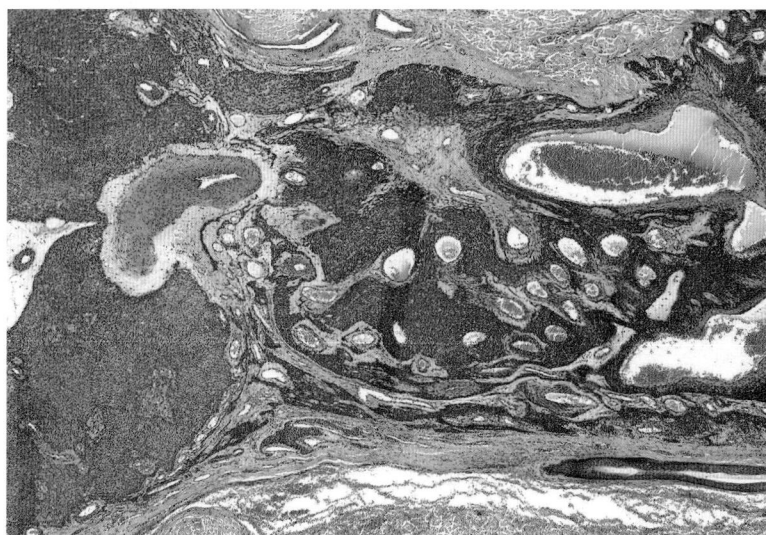

Fig. 35.610
Epithelioid glomus tumor: this field shows the transition between typical small round glomus cells and larger epithelioid variants with abundant pale pink cytoplasm.

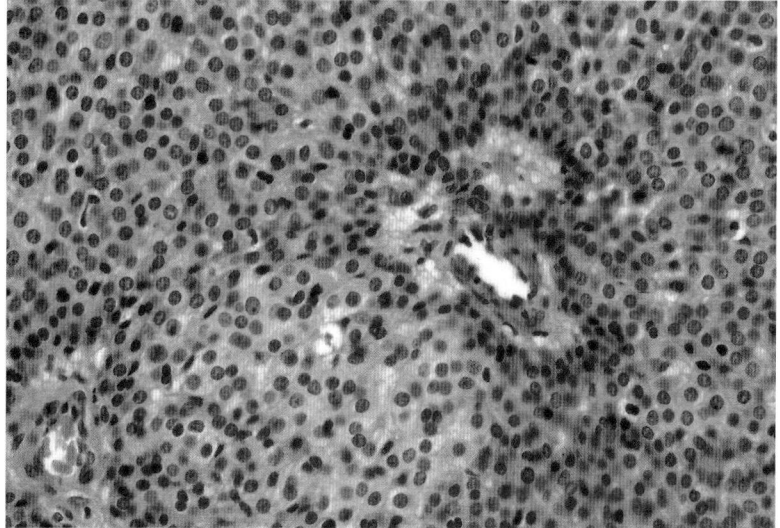

Fig. 35.611
Epithelioid glomus tumor: high-power view.

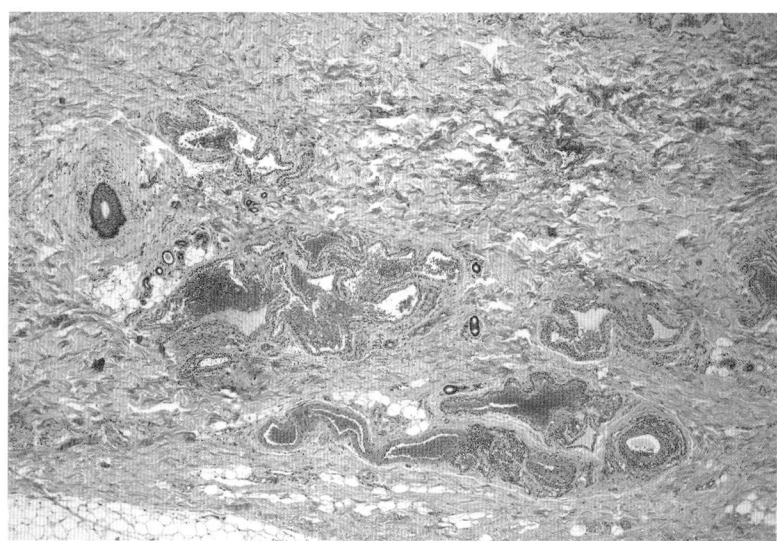

Fig. 35.612
Glomangioma: in this variant, the blood vessels predominate.

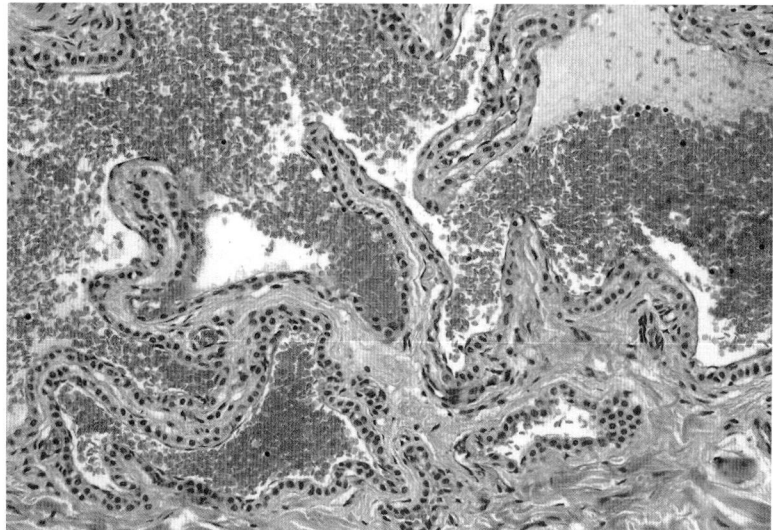

Fig. 35.613
Glomangioma: high-power view.

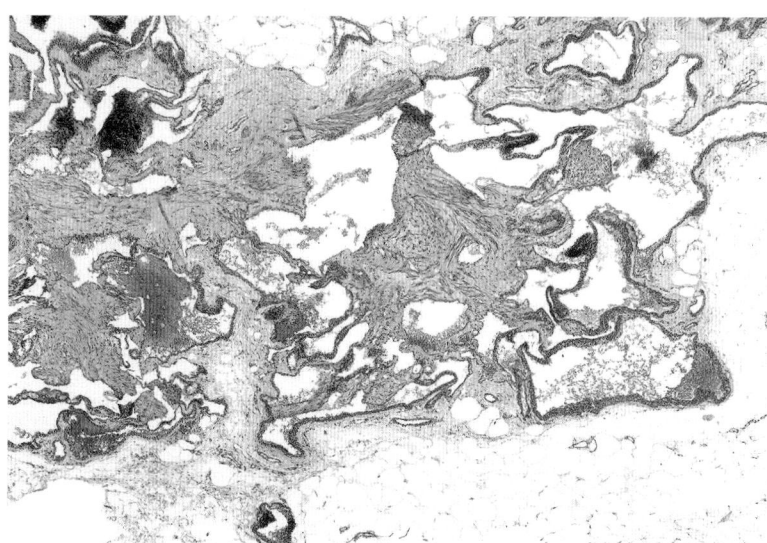

Fig. 35.614
Glomangiomyoma: in this variant, bundles of smooth muscle are present.

These cases often exhibit hyalinization of the vessel walls and may show thrombosis with the formation of phleboliths.

- Symplastic glomus tumor is defined as a tumor with high nuclear grade in the absence of any other malignant feature.[61–63]
- Glomangiomyoma, the rarest subtype (15% of cases), is characterized by a larger and more obvious number of smooth muscle cells, most often distributed adjacent to or around the vascular spaces. These muscle cells merge imperceptibly with the surrounding solid collection of glomus cells (Figs 35.614 and 35.615).
- Glomangiomatosis is defined as a tumor with features of angiomatosis and excess glomus cells.[61,64]
- Infiltrating glomus tumor is a very rare variant that usually presents in deeper soft tissues.[48,65] It is characterized by an infiltrative growth pattern and a high recurrence rate.
- Malignant glomus tumors are rare.[48,61,66–70] A single superficial case was associated with pregnancy.[71] The histologic diagnosis is difficult and only recently have refined criteria been proposed to define malignant lesions.[61] These include:
  - deep location and a size of more than 2 cm, or
  - atypical mitotic figures, or
  - moderate to high nuclear grade diagnosis and five or more mitotic figures per 50 high-power fields (HPF).[61]

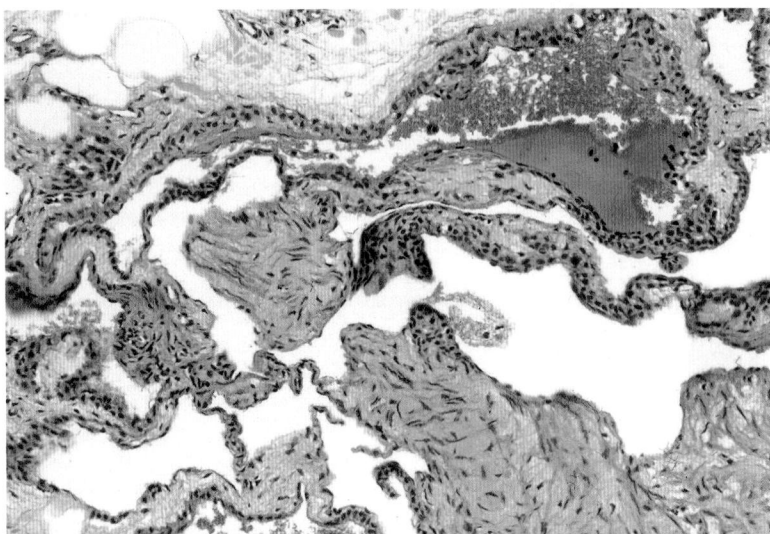

Fig. 35.615
Glomangiomyoma: high-power view.

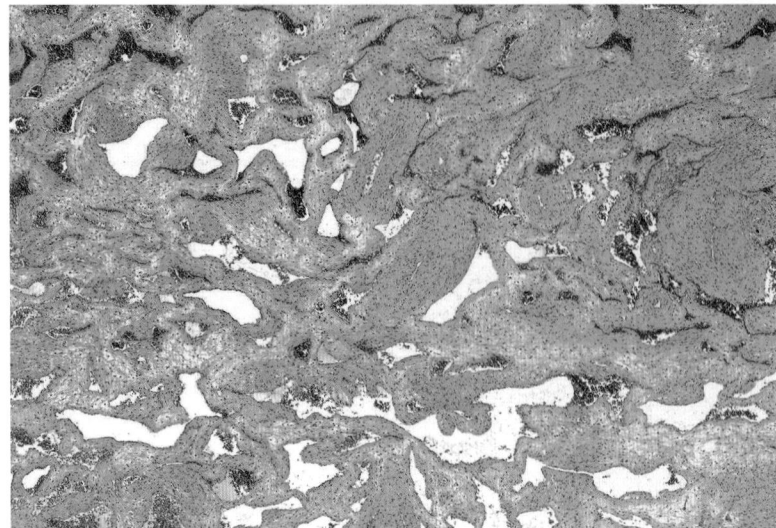

Fig. 35.616
Myopericytoma: low-power view showing dilated vessels and abundant smooth muscle.

Glomus tumors of uncertain malignant potential are defined as lesions that lack criteria for the diagnosis of malignant glomus tumor or symplastic glomus tumor but have high mitotic activity and superficial location, or large size only, or deep location only.[61] Some 38% of cases fulfilling criteria for malignancy metastasize.[61]. *NOTCH1* and *NOTCH3* fusions have been identified in visceral and soft tissue glomus tumors including malignant variants.[72]

Differential diagnosis

The classical clinical history combined with the distinctive histologic features usually prevents diagnostic confusion. Eccrine spiradenoma can be distinguished by the presence in the latter of two populations of cells, positivity for epithelial markers and focal ductal differentiation.

Myopericytoma

Traditionally, tumors thought to differentiate towards perivascular myoid cells or pericytes have been divided into two main groups: infantile hemangiopericytoma and adult hemangiopericytoma.[1,2] Both variants, however, appear to have very little in common except for the histologic presence of a pericytomatous vascular pattern. Moreover, with the combination of immunohistochemistry and electron microscopy, most tumors classified as adult hemangiopericytoma on light microscopy show other lines of differentiation including synovial sarcoma, mesenchymal chondrosarcoma, and solitary fibrous tumor.[3] The handful of cases in which the line of differentiation remains obscure are the 'true' adult hemangiopericytomas, but it is likely that they arise from an undifferentiated mesenchymal cell. These rare examples of 'true' adult hemangiopericytomas do not usually occur in the skin and will not be discussed further in this chapter.

The concept of myopericytoma was introduced to describe a spectrum of tumors composed of short oval to spindle-shaped cells with a myoid appearance and a distinctive concentric perivascular growth.[4] These tumors tend to occur mainly in the deep dermis and subcutaneous tissue and include lesions classified in the past as glomangiopericytoma, myopericytoma, myofibroma and myofibromatosis in adults. Infantile hemangiopericytoma and infantile myofibromatosis also represent part of the spectrum of tumors with true pericytic differentiation.[5–8]

Clinical features

Myopericytoma most commonly occurs in middle-aged adults (mainly in the fifth decade) with a predilection for the limbs, particularly the distal lower limb followed by the head and neck (including the oral cavity).[9] Exceptional tumors may occur in the kidney, lung, parotid gland, within the cranium, or in the thoracic spine.[10–14] Males are more frequently affected than females. Lesions are small (less than 2 cm in diameter), long-standing, usually asymptomatic, and may be single or (less frequently) multiple. Rarely, tumors are painful. Recurrence is rare and frequently represents either persistence or the development of a new tumor. Very rare malignant examples of myopericytoma have been described; these appear to have an aggressive clinical behavior.[8,15]

An association with HIV/AIDS has been reported and in this setting tumor tend to occur at sites other than soft tissue and skin (including bronchus, larynx, tongue, liver, and brain), are often multiple, and are associated with Epstein-Barr virus.[16,17] Two exceptional cases of glomangiopericytoma associated with oncogenic osteomalacia have been documented.[18,19] In two cases, trauma was suggested as a possible factor in the development of the tumors.[20]

Pathogenesis and histologic features

Recurrent *PDGFRB* alterations have been documented, similar to those seen in infantile myofibromatosis/myofibroma, supporting a close pathogenetic link between the entities.[21,22] A small number of myopericytomas show BRAF(V600E) mutations and anti-BRAF(V600E) agents have been suggested as a treatment for multifocal, infiltrative and recurrent tumor bearing this mutation.[23]

Tumors are dermal, dermal and subcutaneous, or purely subcutaneous and rarely arise in deeper soft tissues.[8] The histologic spectrum of myopericytoma is very wide and varies from lesions that are very similar to myofibromatosis to those that closely resemble glomus tumors and even an angioleiomyoma (*Figs 35.616* and *35.617*). They are well circumscribed and are composed of a mixture of solid cellular areas intermixed with variable numbers of vascular channels. The latter are often elongated and display prominent branching, resulting in a stag-horn appearance (hemangiopericytoma-like). The cells in the solid areas are round or short and spindle-shaped with eosinophilic or amphophilic cytoplasm and vesicular nuclei. Cytologic atypia is not usually a feature and mitotic figures are very rare. A common and striking feature is the presence of concentric layers of tumor cells around vascular channels, resulting in a typical 'onion-ring' appearance (*Fig. 35.618*). Myxoid change may be focally prominent. Occasional findings include hyalinization/sclerosis, cystic degeneration and bone formation. Rare examples are entirely intravascular (within a vein or an artery).[8,24–28] In some cases, tumor cells closely resemble glomus cells and are characterized by round, punched-out central nuclei and pale eosinophilic cytoplasm. These cases are referred to as glomangiopericytomas. Myopericytomatosis refers to a rare subset of tumors characterized by diffuse involvement of the dermis and subcutaneous tissue by nodules of pericytic cells.[21]

Tumors regarded as malignant display cytologic atypia and increased mitotic activity.[8,15]

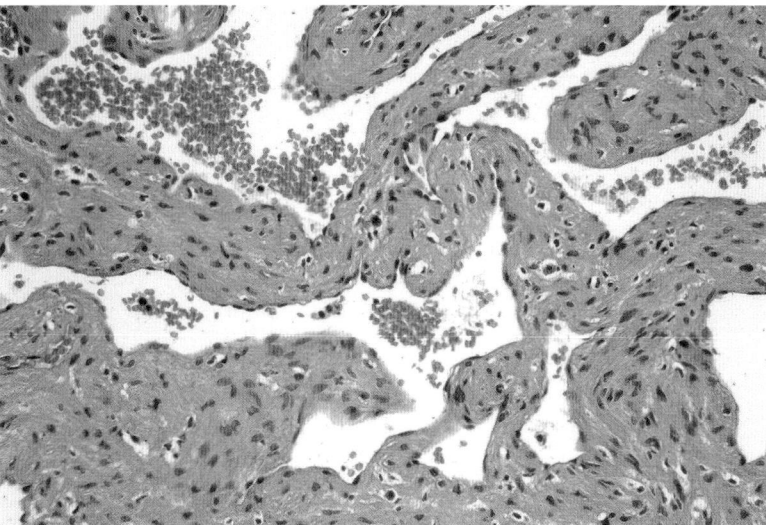

Fig. 35.617
Myopericytoma: high-power view.

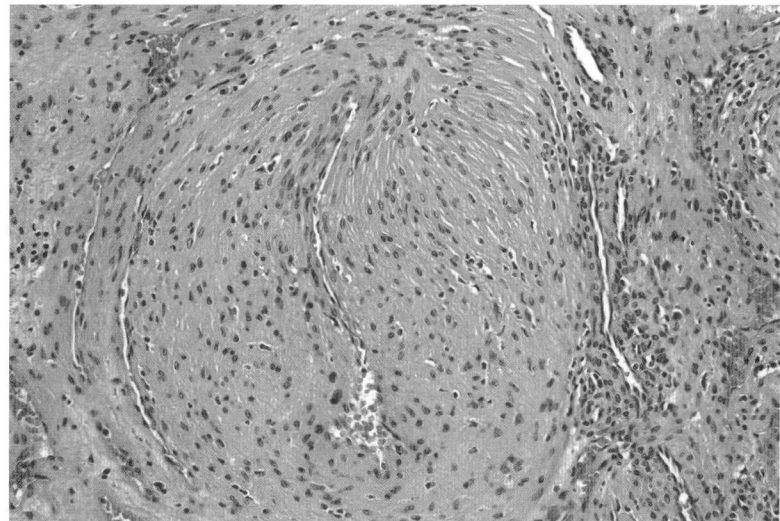

Fig. 35.618
Myopericytoma: this perivascular distribution of tumor cells in an onion ring-like appearance is characteristic.

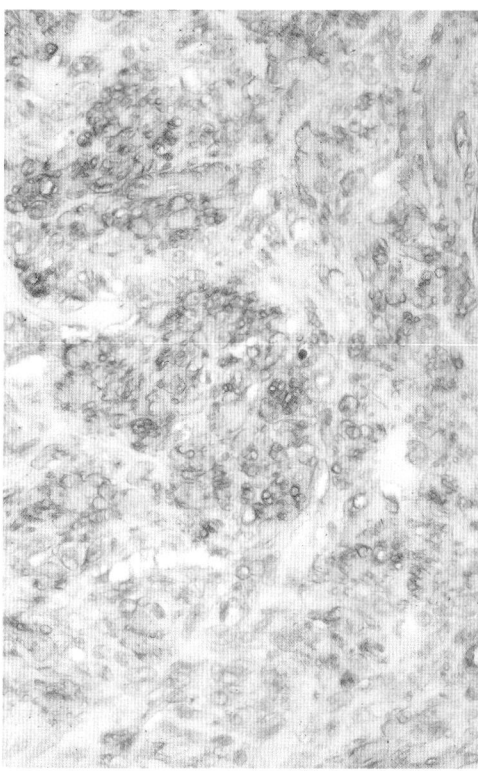

Fig. 35.619
Myopericytoma: the tumor cells express smooth muscle actin.

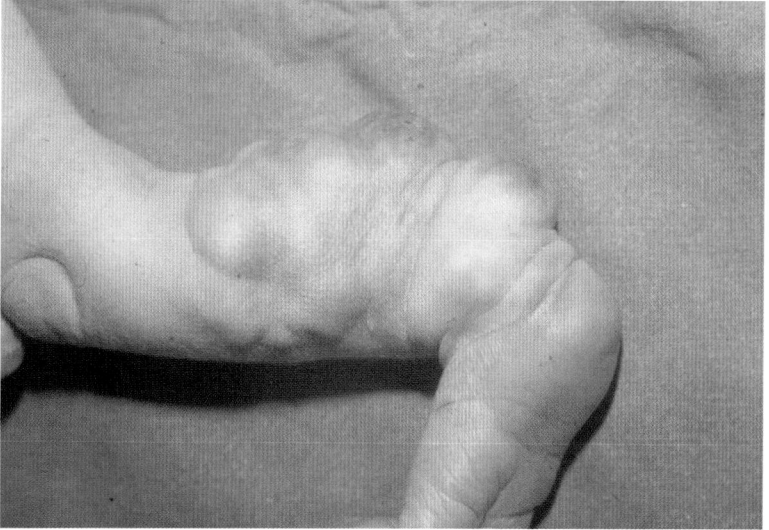

Fig. 35.620
Infantile myofibromatosis: multiple large tumor nodules are present. By courtesy of the Institute of Dermatology, London, UK.

Myopericytoma cells stain diffusely for SMA and calponin, are often positive for h-caldesmon and only very rarely focally positive for desmin (*Fig. 35.619*).[8] Focal staining for CD34 may also be seen.

Differential diagnosis

Most authors regard angioleiomyoma as part of the spectrum of myopericytoma.[29] The coexistence of both tumors in the same patient and a number of morphological features support this theory. Angioleiomyoma, however, is composed of uniform smooth muscle cells, which stain diffusely for both SMA and desmin. Furthermore, concentric arrangement of tumor cells around vascular channels is less prominent than that seen in myopericytoma.

Myofibroma and myofibromatosis

Clinical features

Solitary and multicentric myofibromas are relatively rare tumors with marked predilection for children.[1-8] Myofibroma forms part of the spectrum of myopericytoma.[9,10] Myofibroma, myofibromatosis, and angioleiomyoma along glomus tumor and myopericytoma are currently classified as tumors of perivascular cells.[11] The majority of tumors present before the age of 2 years and many of these are congenital. It appears as a usually solitary dermal, subcutaneous, intramuscular nodule or rarely intraosseous tumor, and is more frequently seen in males.[12,13] In the solitary form, the head and neck (including the oral cavity and rarely the pharynx) are most often involved, followed by the trunk and extremities.[1-8,14-17] A lesion involving the sclera has been documented.[18] Individual lesions are firm or rubbery, somewhat nodular, and rarely exceed 3–4 cm in diameter. Although most tumors are single, multiple lesions may occur in children and occasionally in adults.[19,20] Multicentric tumors in children have also been referred to as congenital generalized fibromatosis and infantile myofibromatosis (*Fig. 35.620*).[4-8,21-23] In these cases, patients are more often female and are found to have multiple soft tissue lesions with associated bony, oral or (rarely) visceral tumors of a similar nature.[24] Organs involved include the kidney, lung, pancreas, gastrointestinal tract, liver and rarely the central nervous system.[1,25-27]

A few cases appear to be inherited, most often in an autosomal dominant pattern.[5,28-30] A single case associated with porencephaly, hemiatrophy and

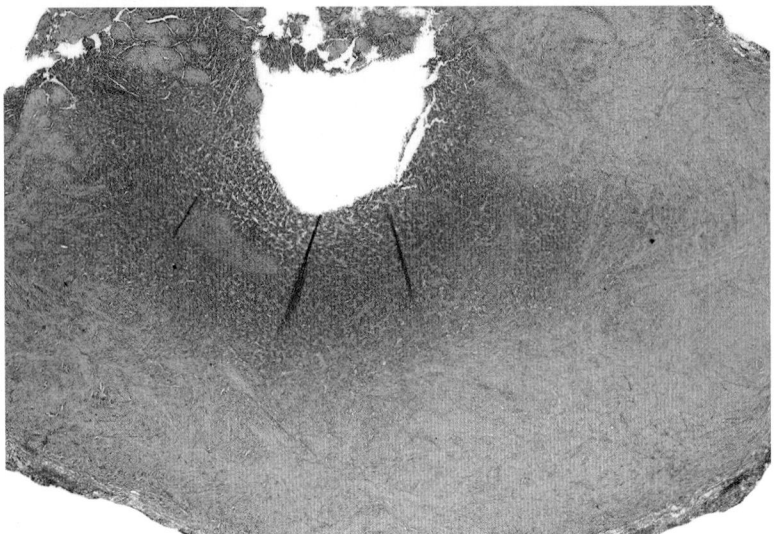

Fig. 35.621
Infantile myofibromatosis: scanning view of a circumscribed tumor showing a hemangiopericytomatous central component.

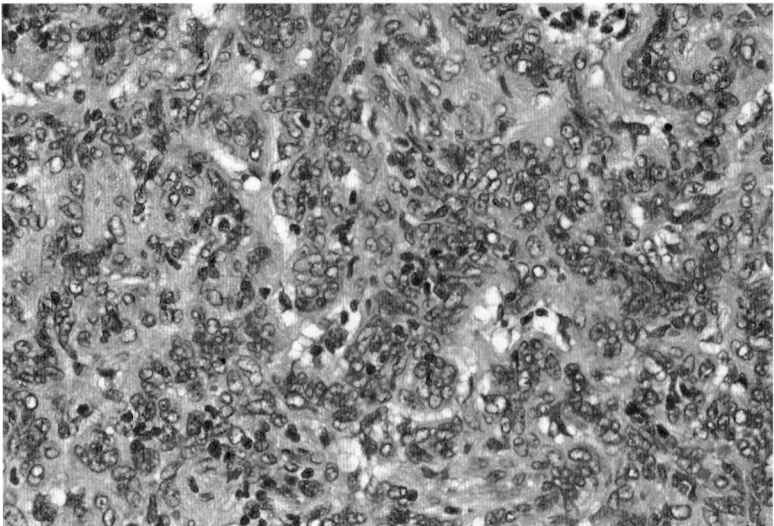

Fig. 35.622
Infantile myofibromatosis: high-power view showing primitive cells with basophilic vesicular nuclei.

cutis marmorata telangiectatica congenita has been documented.[32] A case associated with thrombocytopenia has been reported.[33]

Myofibroma in adults is almost always solitary and superficial, only exceptionally presenting as multiple lesions. A patient with multiple acral lesions had generalized morphea.[34] Usually, they affect the skin or oral mucosa, and no familial cases have been reported. Most patients are young to middle-aged adults of either sex who present with a firm superficial nodule up to 3 cm in diameter.[1–3] Lesions may be painful. Local recurrence is very rare.[35]

Solitary soft tissue or associated bony lesions may recur locally if excised; however, if these lesions are left untreated, spontaneous regression is very common. In contrast, if there is visceral involvement the course is often fatal, being associated with progressive impairment of respiratory or gastro-intestinal function.

Pathogenesis and histologic features

Recurrent *PDGFRB* alterations have been documented, similar to those seen in myopericytoma, supporting a close pathogenetic link between the entities.[36,37]

Lesions tend to be reasonably well circumscribed, but unencapsulated. A distinctive biphasic pattern is commonly produced by the presence of varying proportions of two populations of cells. These comprise:

- fascicles of bland eosinophilic myofibroblasts with tapering or vesicular nuclei,
- more primitive, smaller, round and spindle-shaped cells with scanty cytoplasm and round or oval nuclei (*Figs 35.621–35.624*).

The latter cells tend to be arranged around branching blood vessels in a hemangiopericytomatous pattern (*Fig. 35.625*). Small foci of necrosis and vascular invasion are often present. Mitotic figures may be readily found, but are never abnormal. Tumor cells in both components are usually focally smooth muscle actin positive.[6] Calponin tends to be more diffusely positive and h-caldesmon is focally positive.[38] CD34 positivity has been reported.[39]

In some cases, especially those with multicentric disease, the primitive areas with a hemangiopericytoma-like pattern predominate. These lesions are almost identical clinically and histologically to tumors classified in the past as infantile hemangiopericytoma and it has been proposed that the latter belong to the spectrum of infantile myofibromatosis.[40]

The histologic features of myofibroma are identical to those of infantile myofibromatosis, but the more primitive hemangiopericytomatous component is often not prominent and can be almost absent (*Figs 35.626 and 35.627*). The myofibroblastic nodules may undergo hyalinization with a pseudochondroid appearance. Some tumor nodules appear to be in intra-vascular locations but this mainly represents subendothelial growth. This is seen in up to 30% of cases.[1] Tumor cells are positive for muscle actin.

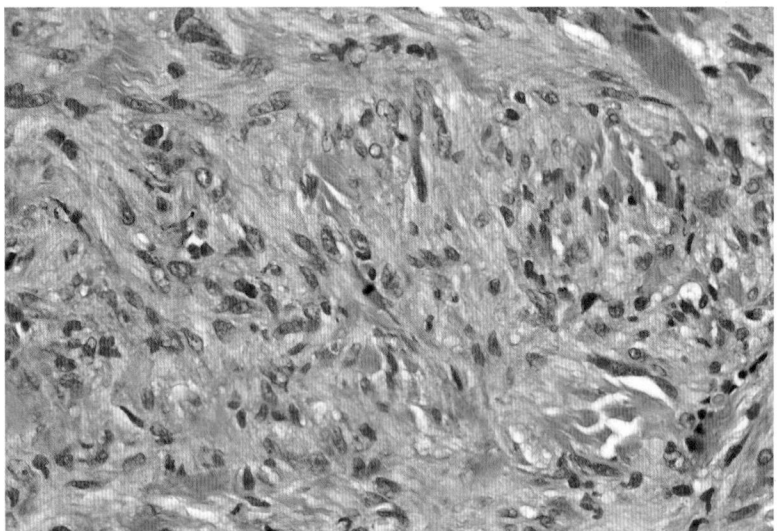

Fig. 35.623
Infantile myofibromatosis: this field highlights the myofibroblastic component.

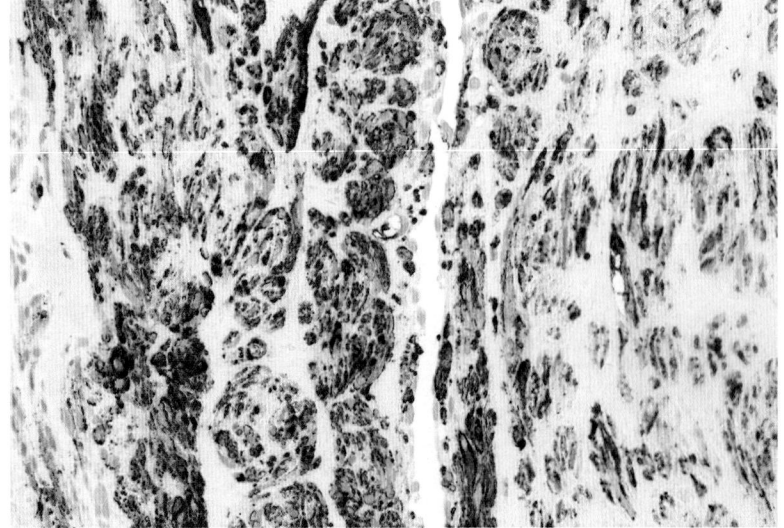

Fig. 35.624
Infantile myofibromatosis: the tumor cells express smooth muscle actin.

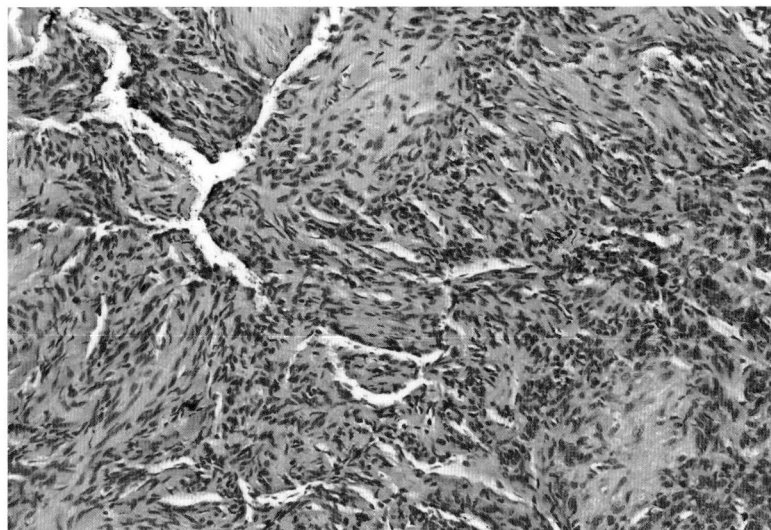

Fig. 35.625
Infantile myofibromatosis: high-power view of the center of the lesion shown in
Fig. 35.102, highlighting the hemangiopericytomatous vascular network.

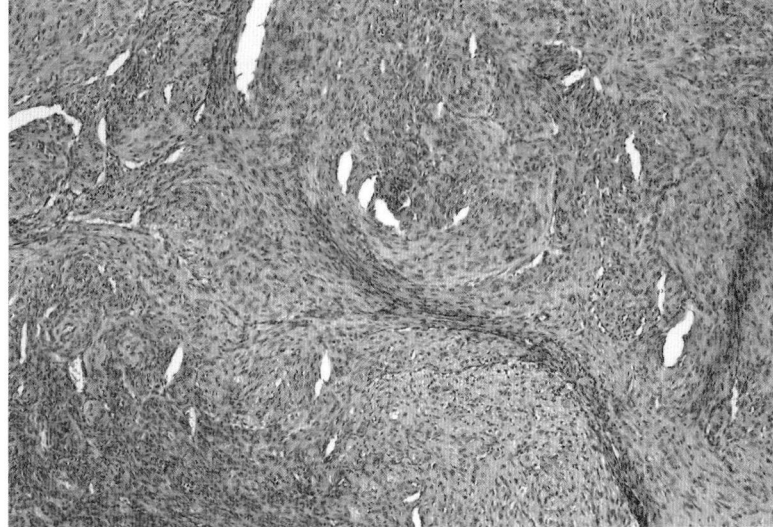

Fig. 35.626
Myofibroma: low-power view of a dermal nodule. Even at this magnification, the
biphasic nature of the tumor is apparent.

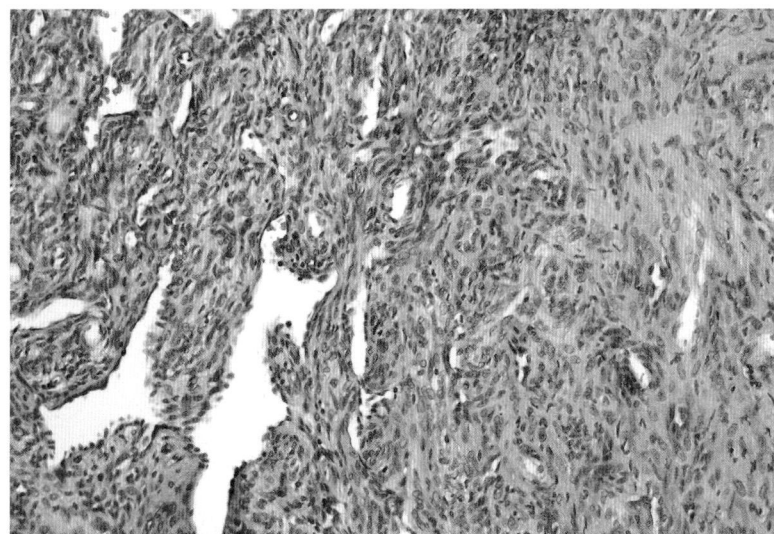

Fig. 35.627
Myofibroma: high-power view.

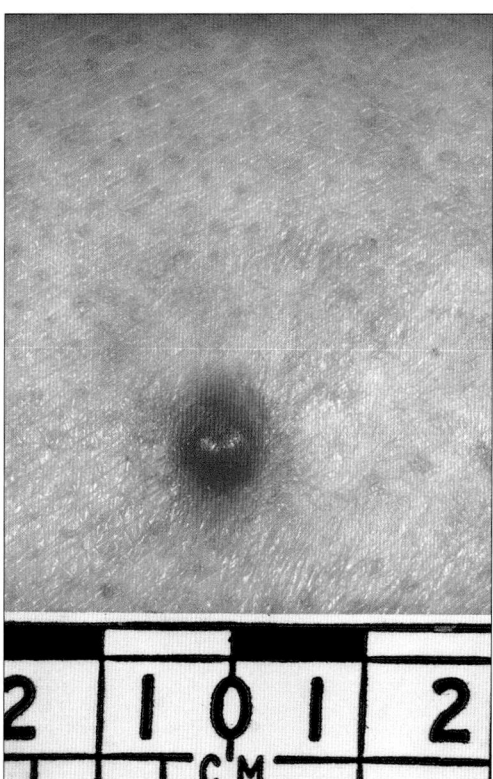

Fig. 35.628
Angioleiomyoma: lesions
are very rarely superficial,
as in this example which
presented as a vascular
papule. By courtesy of the
Institute of Dermatology,
London, UK.

Differential diagnosis

The presence of a biphasic pattern allows distinction from cutaneous
smooth muscle tumors, which are also consistently actin and desmin positive, and from fibrous histiocytoma, which is more polymorphic and less
well circumscribed.

Angioleiomyoma

Clinical features

Angioleiomyomas are common, deep dermal or subcutaneous, benign,
smooth muscle tumors that originate from vascular smooth muscle. They
are currently classified as tumors of pericytic lineage.[1] They arise most often
in adults between 30 and 60 years of age, particularly on the limbs (especially the lower legs).[2–5] Females are affected at least twice as often as males,
except in the head and neck regions where the ratio is reversed.[6] Congenital
tumors have been described.[7] Rare cases of digital (and subungual) angioleiomyoma have been documented, one with bone destruction.[8–11] Involvement of the palm is exceptional.[12] Tumors occurring on the cheek, nasal tip
and the auricle as well as a case on the scalp mimicking a dermoid cyst have
been reported.[12–16] Lesions can rarely occur in the oral cavity.[17–19] Tumors
are typically solitary, slowly growing lesions less than 2 cm in diameter,
and may be painful or tender when compressed (*Fig. 35.628*). Recurrence
after simple excision is very rare and malignant change has never been convincingly documented. An association with multiple pilar leiomyomas is
extremely rare.[20] In an HIV-positive patient, multiple lesions developed and
EBV was demonstrated by in situ hybridization within the nuclei of the
tumor cells; these likely represent cases of EBV-associated smooth muscle
tumors.[21–23]

Pathogenesis and histologic features

Cytogenetic studies vary and have revealed chromosomal imbalances and a
few nonrecurring translocations, with the most consistent loss being found
in chromosome 22.[24–26]

  Histologically, in contrast to pilar leiomyoma, these are rounded, encapsulated lesions. They are composed of interlacing bundles of uniform

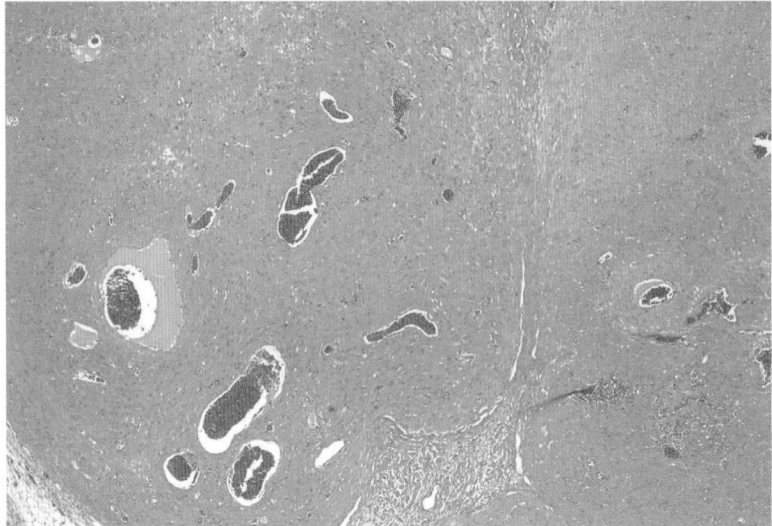

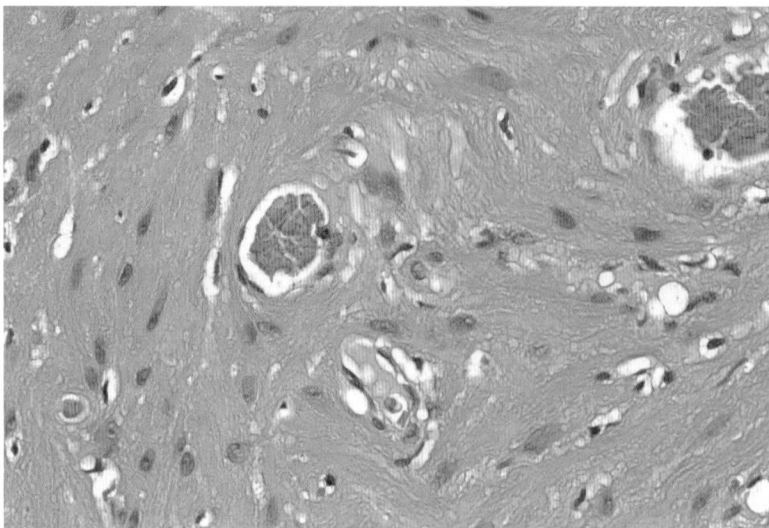

Fig. 35.629
Angioleiomyoma: the tumor is well circumscribed and shows an admixture of bundles of smooth muscle cells surrounding thick-walled blood vessels.

Fig. 35.630
Angioleiomyoma: high-power view.

smooth muscle cells, distributed around numerous small vessels with walls of variable thickness (*Figs 35.629* and *35.630*). Hyaline or myxoid degeneration, thrombosis and dystrophic calcification are frequently encountered.[27] Calcification can be very prominent and seems to be more common in acral lesions.[28–31] Some cases contain collections of mature adipocytes (angiomyolipoma, angiolipoleiomyoma) and, although they probably represent metaplastic change, it has been proposed that such variants are hamartomatous.[32–36] Such tumors are negative for HMB-45 and are not associated with tuberous sclerosis.[37] In a small proportion of cases, the vascular spaces may show marked, almost sinusoidal, dilatation. Occasionally, scattered cells with enlarged hyperchromatic nuclei are seen.[38–41] This

change is not associated with increased mitotic activity, does not indicate malignancy and is probably secondary to degeneration. Unusual findings in angioleiomyoma include epithelioid cell change, clear cell change, and prominent palisading mimicking Verocay bodies.[42–44] A case reported as intravascular angioleiomyoma overlaps with a myopericytoma giving support to the accepted proposal of the former having been part of the spectrum of tumors of perivascular cells.[1,45,46] However, tumor cells in myopericytoma are positive for actin and usually negative for desmin.

Immunohistochemical findings are identical to those for pilar leiomyoma and consist of diffuse staining of tumor cells for SMA, calponin, desmin and h-caldesmon.[47] Myosin 1B, a newly identified human pericyte marker, is negative.[48]

TUMORS OF BONE AND CARTILAGE-FORMING TISSUE

The vast majority of tumors in the skin that show ossification do so as a secondary degenerative or metaplastic phenomenon. The most common tumors showing this feature are melanocytic nevi and the calcifying epithelioma of Malherbe (pilomatrixoma). Primary bone-forming lesions arising in the skin are extremely rare. Fasciitis ossificans has already been described under fasciitis.

Benign tumors of bone

Osteoma cutis

Clinical features

Osteoma cutis is a rare benign lesion of the dermis that may be seen at any age in either sex.[1–3] Lesions are occasionally multiple and, in some cases, may be inherited or associated with diaphyseal aclasis. Microscopic osteoma cutis is not uncommonly found as a result of dystrophic ossification in association with inflammatory conditions including acne and folliculitis.[4,5] The latter is often seen in association with intradermal nevi, as the latter obstruct the hair follicle and lead to inflammation.[6] A case of Becker nevus bearing an osteoma cutis has been described.[7] Multiple miliary osteoma cutis may occur on the face of middle-aged patients with marked predilection for females.[8–13] The lesions are tiny and the etiology is unknown,

although slightly more than half of patients have a history of acne vulgaris. A cutis laxa -like presentation has been documented.[14]

Osteoma cutis is associated with Albright hereditary osteodystrophy (pseudohypoparathyroidism) a disorder caused by a mutation in *GNAS1* gene.[15–22] This is discussed further in the chapter on disorders of pigmentation (see Chapter 20). A case associated with Rothmund-Thomson syndrome and a further with Happle-Tinchert syndrome has been described.[23,24]

A case of pigmented osteoma cutis resulting from long-term tetracycline treatment and a further case after alendronate therapy for osteoporosis has been documented.[25,26]

A distinctive plaque plate-like variant of osteoma cutis can occur and it is rarely congenital.[27–33] It may be multiple and is exceptionally associated with transepidermal elimination.[34]

Perforating and eruptive and giant cases as well as a case of an extramedullary acute leukemia developing in an osteoma cutis have been reported.[18,35–38]

Osteoma cutis can be reliably identified in imaging studies sometimes as an incidental finding.[39–44]

Histologic features

Histologically, osteoma cutis is composed of a well-circumscribed nodule of mature lamellar bone, often containing marrow spaces, within the dermis (*Fig. 35.631*).

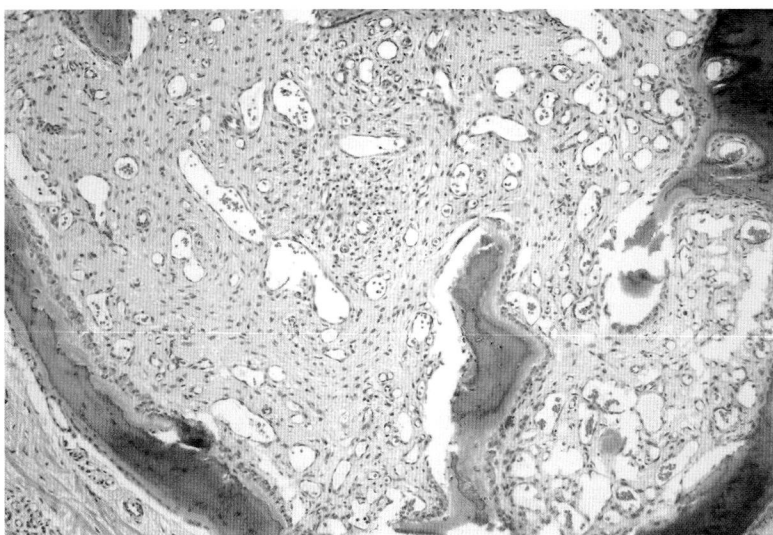

Fig. 35.631
Osteoma cutis: note the osteoid rimmed by osteoblasts and the scarred medullary cavity.

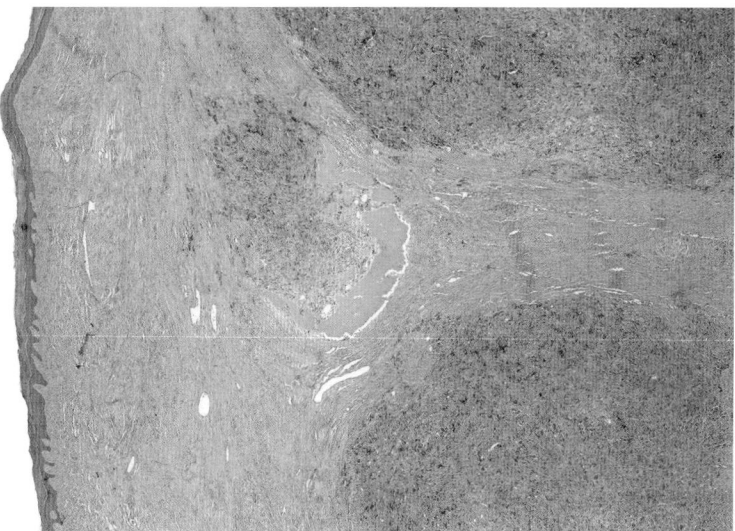

Fig. 35.632
Extraskeletal osteosarcoma: low-power view showing an osteoclast-rich cellular infiltrate with focal osteoid production in the center of the field.

Differential diagnosis

Osteoma cutis should not be confused with a benign cartilaginous exostosis. The latter condition, also known as osteochondroma, most often presents under the nail as a solitary, often painful, hard tumor nodule. Histologically, it is composed of mature cartilage overlying a layer of lamellar bone. It arises from the underlying phalanx.

Malignant tumors of bone

Extraskeletal osteosarcoma

Clinical features

Extraskeletal osteosarcoma is a rare lesion that most often arises in older adults and shows an equal sex incidence.[1-6] Occurrence in children is unusual.[7-10] It typically occurs in the deep soft tissues of the limbs, particularly the legs, but subcutaneous cases are well recognized and exceptional cases are dermal in location.[1-6,11-13] Lesion may rarely affect the hand, the breast and the penis.[8,14-19] Cases arising on a scar are exceptional.[20,21] A single case arising in a lipoma, one in myositis ossificans and a further in a recurrent ossifying fibromyxoid tumor of soft tissue have been reported.[22-24]

A case of extraskeletal osteosarcoma arising in the mediastinum metastasized to the skin.[25]

Up to 10% of lesions are associated with previous radiation to the affected site.[5,26-30]

These tumors tend towards rapid local recurrence and widespread systemic dissemination. The mortality rate is as high as 75%. Tumor size and age of the patient are the most relevant clinical prognostic factors. The role of chemotherapy and/or radiation has not been established.[31-33]

A better biological behavior, analogous to parosteal osteosarcoma, has been reported for a subset of tumors characterized by 12q amplification.[34] In a recent study, potential aggressive molecular subgroups include tumors with CDKN2A loss or biallelic simultaneous losses of RB1 and TP53.[35]

Pathogenesis and histologic features

MDM2 amplification, which correlates with protein immunoexpression, is a not an unusual finding.[35-37] Sonic Hedgehog (encoded by SHH gene) and PIK3CA mutations have been documented.[35]

The tumor is typically ill-defined and characterized by a variable admixture of pleomorphic or spindle-shaped cells associated with the production, at least focally, of an osteoid or chondroid matrix (Figs 35.632–35.634).

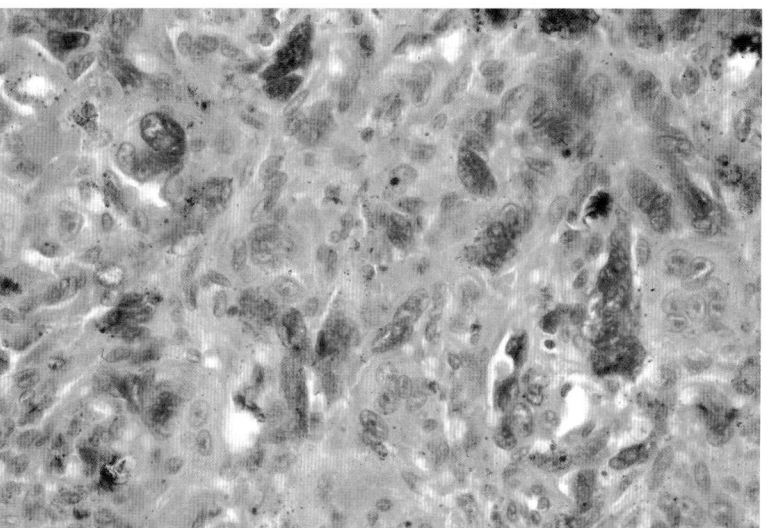

Fig. 35.633
Extraskeletal osteosarcoma: high-power view showing nuclear pleomorphism.

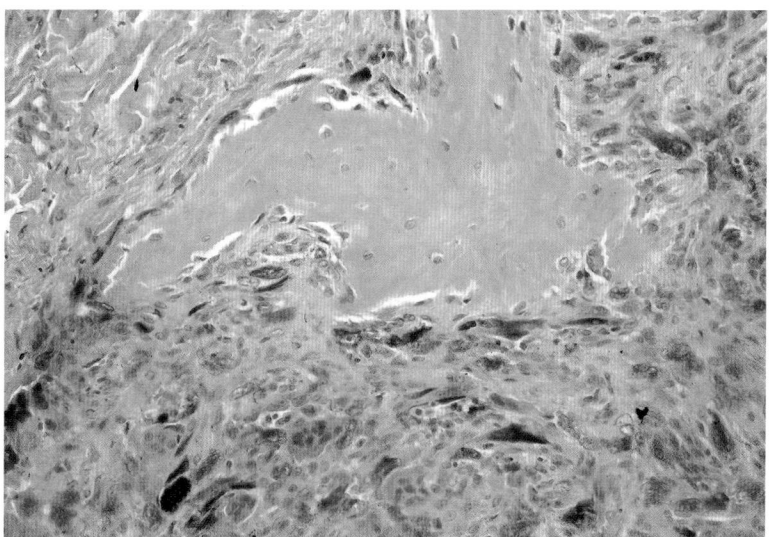

Fig. 35.634
Extraskeletal osteosarcoma: the osteoid is rimmed by malignant osteoblasts.

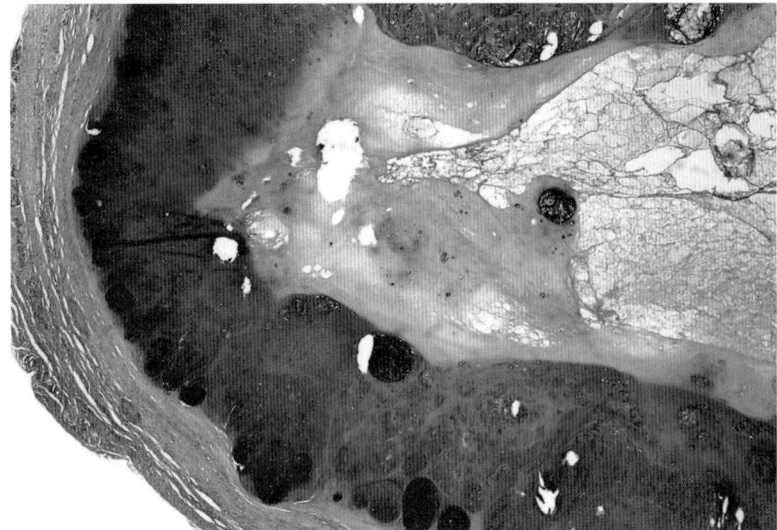

Fig. 35.635
Soft tissue chondroma: the tumor is encapsulated and composed of well-defined lobules of mature cartilage.

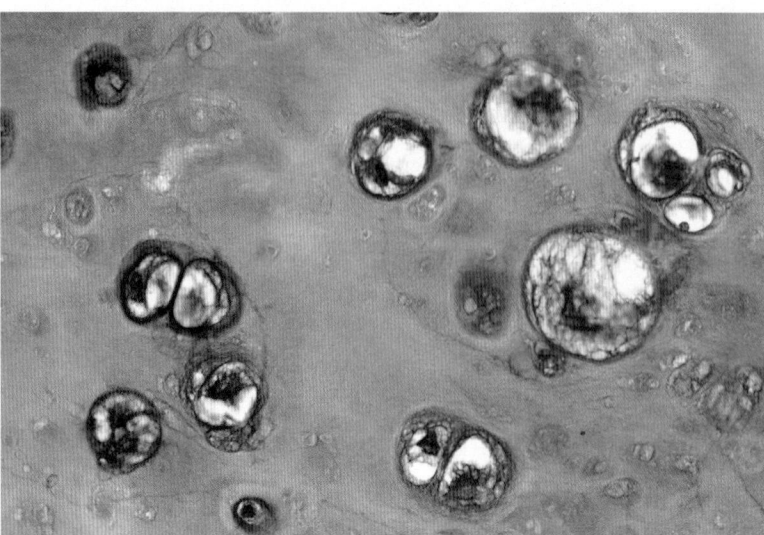

Fig. 35.636
Soft tissue chondroma: the nuclei are typically irregular. In many areas, multiple chondrocytes occupy individual lacunae.

Bizarre multinucleated giant cells are common. The diagnostic sine qua non is the presence of hyperchromatic osteoblasts within the newly formed osteoid matrix. Cases with numerous osteoclastic giant cells were often formerly labeled as so-called giant cell 'MFH'; such examples not infrequently are subcutaneous. Low-grade variants are exceptional.[38] A small cell variant has been described.[39-40] Immunohistochemical demonstration of osteocalcin and/or SATB2 may be useful in tumors with poor osteoid formation, whereas ERG may highlight areas with cartilaginous differentiation.[41-43]

Benign tumors of cartilage

Soft tissue chondroma

Clinical features

Soft tissue chondromas are uncommon tumors that arise most often in middle-aged adults, showing a slight male predominance and typically occurring on the hands or feet.[1-4] Children may be rarely affected.[5-9] A case of trigger finger caused by a soft tissue chondroma has been described.[10] True cutaneous tumors may occur.[11-12]

Rare cases develop on the face including lip, neck, oral cavity, scalp and popliteal region.[13-18] Exceptional familial cases may occur.[19] A collision tumor (chondroma- neurofibroma) has been described in the gluteal region.[20]

Lesions, which present as a slowly growing mass usually less than 3 cm in diameter, sometimes show calcification on radiological examination. Giant lesions are rarely seen.[21-23]

Up to 10% of cases recur locally after excision, but malignant change has never been reported. Bilateral chondromas have been reported, one of them occurring in association with chronic renal failure.[24,25]

Histologic features

12q 13-15 rearrangements resulting in expression of *HMGA2* gene have been documented, as well as monosomy 5 and trisomy 6.[26,27]

The tumor, which may be intradermal or subcutaneous, is composed of a well-circumscribed, lobulated mass of mature hyaline cartilage (*Figs 35.635* and *35.636*). Dystrophic or degenerative features – such as myxoid change, hemorrhage, calcification, or ossification – are commonly seen, particularly at the periphery of the tumor lobules. These features may be associated with a histiocytic and osteoclastic giant cell reaction. By immunohistochemistry ERG is frequently positive in the cartilaginous component.[28]

A typical feature, often of diagnostic concern, is the hypercellularity of the lesional cartilage, often with binucleated nuclei and focal nuclear atypia. In the context of a bone tumor, such features would be suggestive of malignancy. Some cases are composed of small, rounded, more primitive chondroblasts, often in a myxoid stroma.[29,30]

If the presence of a primary lesion in bone has been carefully excluded, the diagnosis of a benign chondroma is assured, despite the worrying features described above. The basis of this assumption is that there is no convincing evidence that a lesion such as an extraskeletal well-differentiated chondrosarcoma exists.

Distinction from a benign mixed tumor of adnexal origin is easy because the latter always shows epithelial elements.

Malignant tumors of cartilage

Extraskeletal myxoid chondrosarcoma

Clinical features

Extraskeletal myxoid chondrosarcoma is an uncommon tumor that usually arises in adulthood, shows a slight predilection for males, and occurs most often in the limbs (particularly the legs); pediatric occurrence is rare.[1-12] Although frequently of deep origin, up to 20% of cases arise subcutaneously. It presents as a slowly growing, usually painless, large mass. Unusual sites include the oral cavity and the vulva.[8,13-18] Interestingly two cases reported in the vulva showed a *PLAG1* gene activation suggesting a different molecular entity for tumors arising on the site.[19] Cases on the foot mimicking planter fibromatosis or fibroma have been described.[20,21] A spontaneous regression and a combined synovial sarcoma with extraskeletal myxoid chondrosarcoma have been documented.[22,23]

Although it was formerly believed that only 10–15% of cases recur or metastasize, it appears that most patients die of metastatic disease after long follow-up of 10–20 years.[3,4] However, in a recent study the overall 5-, 10-, and 15-year survival rates were 82%, 65%, and 58%, respectively, after combined treatment with surgery and chemotherapy.[24] Radiation therapy may be beneficial especially in localized cases.[6]

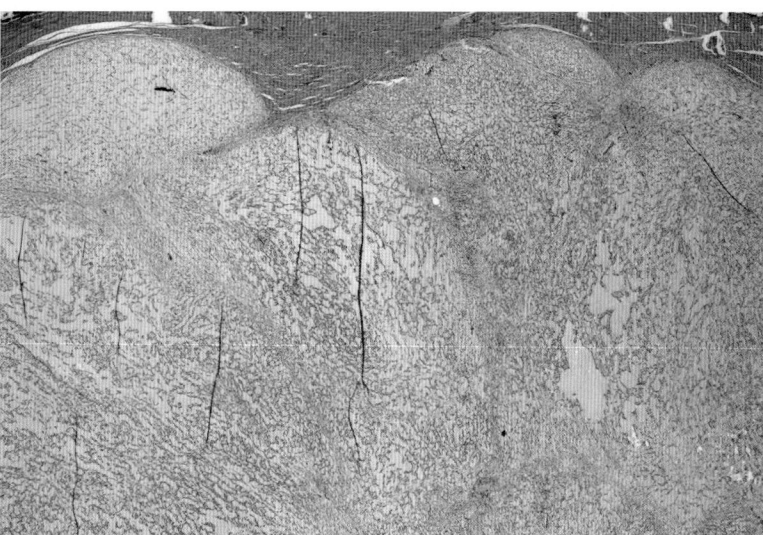

Fig. 35.637
Extraskeletal myxoid chondrosarcoma: the tumor is lobulated and shows a biphasic population. Small hyperchromatic cells at the periphery merge with a central myxoid component.

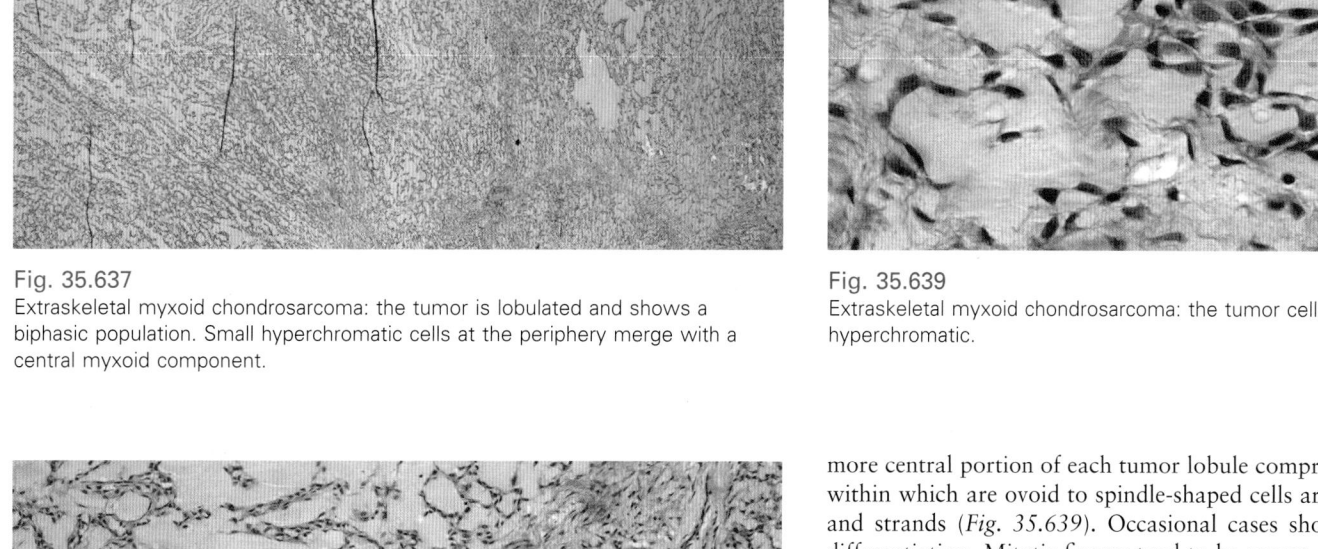

Fig. 35.639
Extraskeletal myxoid chondrosarcoma: the tumor cells are pleomorphic and hyperchromatic.

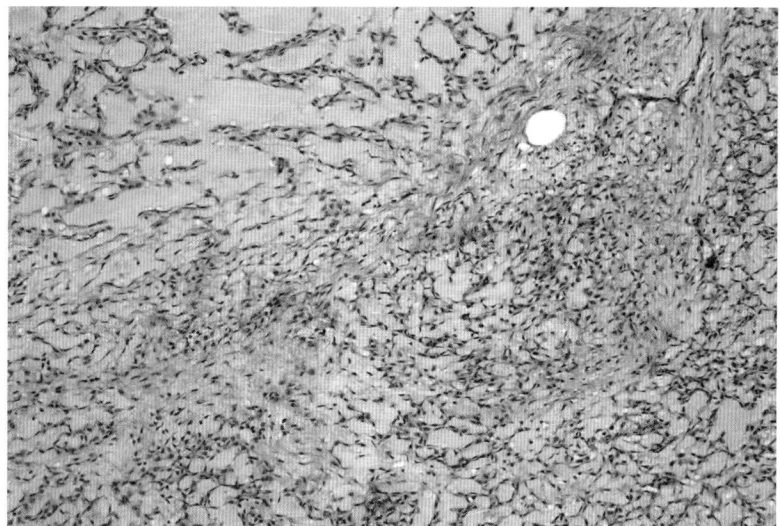

Fig. 35.638
Extraskeletal myxoid chondrosarcoma: medium-power view.

Pathogenesis and histologic features

In recent years, it has become clear that this tumor does not have chondrosarcomatous lineage as previously believed and it is more likely to represent a tumor of primitive mesenchymal cells.[7,25]

Extraskeletal myxoid chondrosarcoma is characterized in most cases by a specific t(9;22)(q22;q12) fusing NR4A3 and EWSR1.[26–29] EWSR1 can be substituted by at least three additional homologous genes in a small subset of cases. Tumors with variant NR4A3 gene fusions are related with higher grade, rhabdoid phenotype, and a less favorable outcome compared with the EWSR1-NR4A3 positive tumors.[30–45] A single case with HSPA8 as a fusion partner of NR4A3 has been recently reported.[46] Loss of nuclear INI1 (encoded by SMARCB1) expression is documented in a subset of cases, particularly those with epithelioid morphology.[47]

These tumors have a characteristic microscopic appearance consisting of irregular but well-defined lobules with peripheral closely packed undifferentiated small cells with little cytoplasm (Figs 35.637 and 35.638). The more central portion of each tumor lobule comprises a loose myxoid stroma within which are ovoid to spindle-shaped cells arranged in interlacing cords and strands (Fig. 35.639). Occasional cases show obvious chondroblastic differentiation. Mitotic figures tend to be sparse. Infrequently, there are foci of metaplastic bone formation, most often at the periphery of the lesion, and rare cases exhibit intracytoplasmic eosinophilic (rhabdoid) inclusions.

Tumor cells usually have abundant intracytoplasmic glycogen, and up to 20% of cases are positive for S100 protein; SOX 10 may also be positive.[48–50] Rarely, there may be focal positivity for EMA and keratin.[49]

Differential diagnosis

The most important differential diagnosis includes myxoid liposarcoma and malignant mixed tumors. The former has a distinctive branching vascular pattern and lipoblasts are evident, whereas the latter tumor shows epithelial elements with ductal differentiation and, often, more differentiated cartilage. In addition, it expresses keratin and actin.

Extraskeletal mesenchymal chondrosarcoma

Clinical features

Extraskeletal mesenchymal chondrosarcoma is a very rare, deep-seated tumor that tends to occur more often in younger adults than the myxoid type.[1–7] Children may be affected.8 It is more common in females and appears frequently in the head and neck region and upper trunk, and less often in the limbs. The prognosis appears to be worse than that for the myxoid variants.

Pathogenesis and histologic features

An inv(8) (q13q210) resulting in a recurrent HEY1-NCOA2 fusion gene has been identified.[9]

Extraskeletal mesenchymal chondrosarcoma has a distinctive biphasic histologic appearance characterized by undifferentiated round or spindle-shaped mesenchymal cells and variably prominent foci of generally mature, well-differentiated cartilage (Figs 35.640 and 35.641). Mitotic activity is usually prominent. Often, the undifferentiated cells are arranged around numerous slit-like vessels in a hemangiopericytoma-like pattern. Cartilaginous areas may show dystrophic calcification and sometimes ossification.

Tumor cells are positive for CD99 and Bcl-2.[10] The cartilaginous areas are S100 protein positive. ERG positivity may also be seen.[11] Nuclear Sox9, a chondrogenic transcription factor, can be detected.[4,7,12–14]

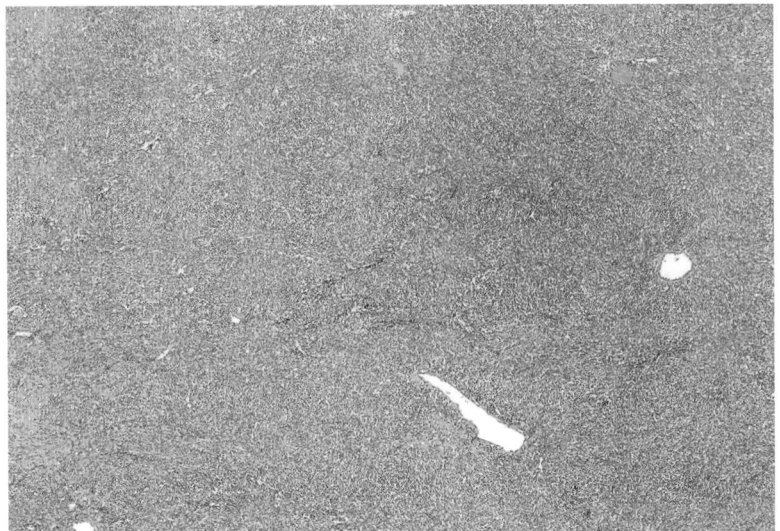

Fig. 35.640
Extraskeletal mesenchymal chondrosarcoma: low-power view showing an intensely cellular tumor.

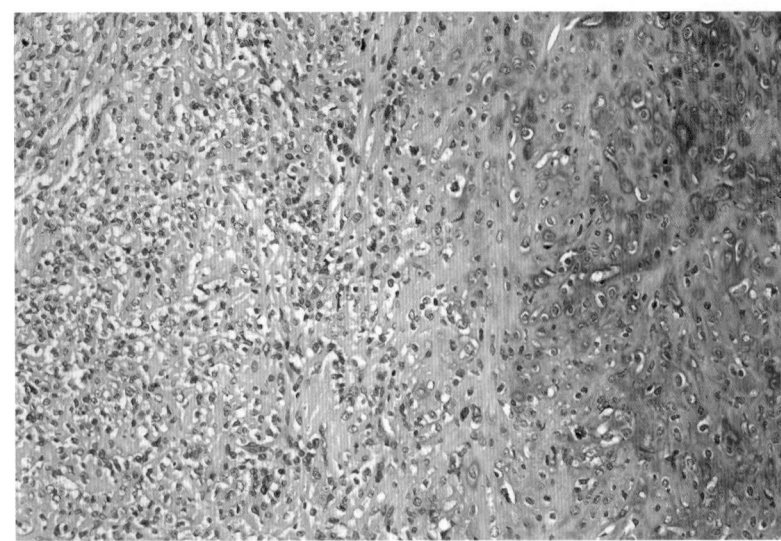

Fig. 35.641
Extraskeletal mesenchymal chondrosarcoma: malignant cartilage is present on the right of the field.

MISCELLANEOUS REACTIVE, BENIGN LESIONS AND TUMORS OF UNCERTAIN DIFFERENTIATION

Synovial metaplasia

Clinical features

Synovial metaplasia is a rare phenomenon that has no distinctive clinical features. It usually presents as an incidental histologic finding in biopsies performed at sites of previous trauma, particularly surgery.[1-5] Synovial metaplasia is not uncommon in the setting of silicone implants.[3] It may also be seen in association with the use of tissue expanders. Synovial metaplasia-like changes have also been described in oral mucoceles under the rubric papillary synovial metaplasia-like changes or myxoglobulinosis.[6-9] A single recurrent lesion has been described and a case was documented in a patient with Ehlers-Danlos syndrome.[10,11]

Pathogenesis and histologic features

It has been suggested that, at least in cases associated with foreign material, the phenomenon probably represents a specialized form of tissue repair.[12]

Histology shows a cystic cavity with a lining identical to that seen in hyperplastic synovial tissue and composed of histiocyte-like cells which are variably positive for CD68 (Figs 35.642 and 35.643).

Cutaneous myxoma

Clinical features

Cutaneous myxomas (also known as cutaneous myxoid cysts) are rare and are characterized by a solitary small painful lesion that occurs most often on the hand (especially the fingers) of adults and shows a marked predilection for females.[1] Local recurrence is common. Multiple lesions are exceptional and in one reported case there was transepidermal elimination of myxoid material.[2] A case presenting on the knee joint has been documented.[3]

Rarely, cutaneous myxomas can be associated with Carney complex (various endocrine and non-endocrine tumors and cancer) which is caused by germline mutations of *PRKAR1A* in the cyclic AMP-dependent protein kinase signaling pathway.[4] Cardiac and breast myxomas and myxomas at other sites are more common than dermal myxomas in Carney complex. The relationship of cutaneous myxomas and the superficial angiomyxomas described below is poorly delineated in the literature and likely overlap exists.

Histologic features

Histologic features consist of a poorly circumscribed dermal lesion composed of plump stellate and spindle-shaped cells with no atypia surrounded by an abundant myxoid matrix. Lesional cells are negative for S100 protein and actin. Whether these swellings are related to focal cutaneous mucinosis is uncertain.

Massive localized lymphedema

Clinical features

Massive localized lymphedema is a distinctive soft tissue lesion that arises as a complication of morbid obesity and can be confused with a neoplasm, mainly a well-differentiated liposarcoma.[1-15]

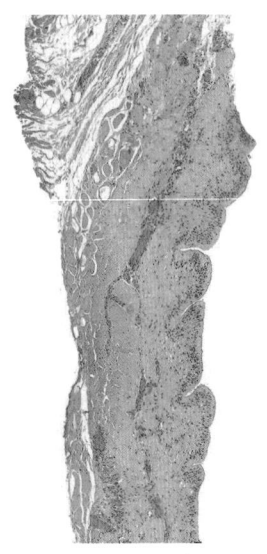
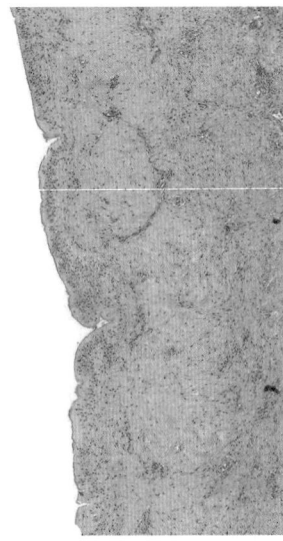

Fig. 35.642
Synovial metaplasia: low-power view of cyst lined by cells with intensely eosinophilic cytoplasm.

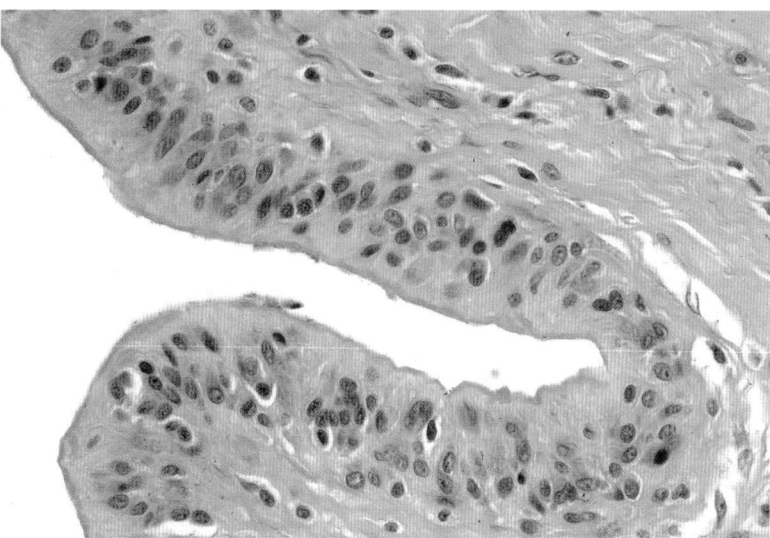

Fig. 35.643
Synovial metaplasia: high-power view.

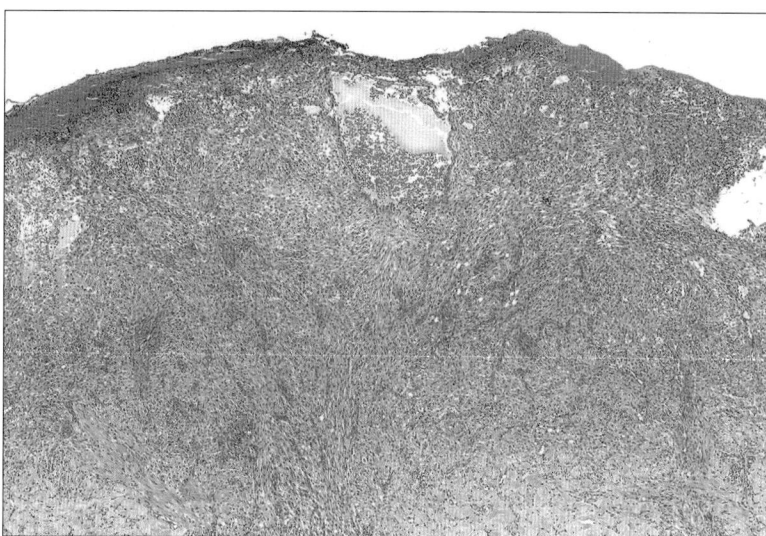

Fig. 35.644
Non-neural dermal granular cell tumor: these lesions are generally superficial and polypoid with an epidermal collarette.

Patients are grossly obese, with some predilection for females in the fifth decade of life and present with a unilateral, or rarely bilateral, large mass with predilection for the inner aspect of the proximal limbs. In some cases, multifocal presentation is seen.[13] Involvement of other areas in the limbs, scrotum, suprapubic region and rarely perianal area and flank has also been reported.[13] Lesions are long-standing, asymptomatic, ill-defined, can measure more than 50 cm, weight more than 7 kilograms and may be recurrent. The overlying skin can show a cobblestone or a verrucous appearance.[2,15] The clinical diagnosis is usually that of a lipoma or recurrent cellulitis. Cases of cutaneous angiosarcoma arising in massive localized lymphedema have been documented.[16] This might be similar to the Stewart-Treves syndrome where angiosarcoma arising in the setting of lymphedema, particularly secondary to breast axillary node dissection.

Pathogenesis and histologic features

The lesion develops as a result of localized chronic lymphedema secondary to gross obesity. The latter is complicated in some patients by other causes of chronic lymphedema including surgery and trauma. An association with hypothyroidism has been reported.[3]

Histologically, fat lobules are separated by thick fibrous and edematous septa with elongated fibroblasts. Groups of capillaries are identified at the interface between adipose tissue and the septa. Dystrophic calcifications mimicking atypical nulcei are identified in some cases and this change may raise the possibility of a liposarcoma.[13] Additional rare features include metaplastic bone formation and multinucleated cells.[13]

Differential diagnosis

The main differential diagnosis is with sclerosing atypical lipomatous tumor. In the latter, there is cytologic atypia of adipocytes, and clusters of capillaries in the interface between adipose tissue and sclerosed septa are not usually present.

Non-neural dermal granular cell tumor (primitive polypoid granular cell tumor)

Clinical features

Primitive polypoid granular cell tumor is a rare variant of granular cell tumor which usually presents as an exophytic cutaneous lesion with a wide anatomical distribution, broad age range and no sex predilection.[1-14] Oral lesions are exceptional.[5,12] A case arising at the site of a surgical wound has been reported.[13] Not all tumors are polypoid. Clinical behavior appears to be benign with only rare local recurrences.[1-4] In two cases, regional lymph node metastases have been documented.[4,6]

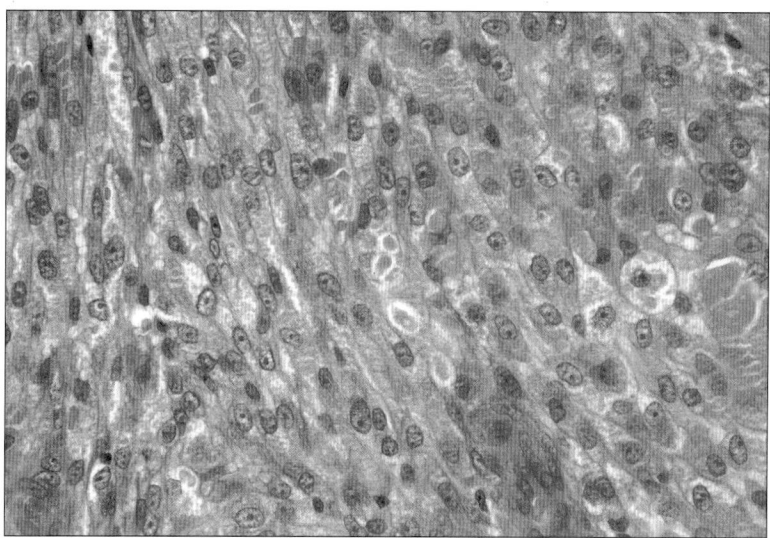

Fig. 35.645
Non-neural dermal granular cell tumor: the tumor cells have eosinophilic granular cytoplasm, similar to other granular cell tumors.

Histologic features

Histologically, lesions are often but not always polypoid, intradermal and well-circumscribed. An infiltrative growth pattern is exceptional.[7] Focal extension into the subcutaneous tissue is sometimes seen. Tumor cells are rounded or spindle-shaped cells with prominent granular cell change (Figs 35.644–35.646). Nuclear pleomorphism varies and tends to be focal. However, in some lesions, cytologic atypia may be prominent throughout. Mitotic figures may be conspicuous. Multinucleated cells are sometimes present. A desmoplastic stroma is exceptional.[9] There is diffuse positivity for NKI/C3 (a non-specific marker for lysosomes) and focal positivity for CD68. Positivity for PGP 9.5 has been documented in two cases.[8] Tumor cells do not express keratin, EMA, actin or S100 protein.[1-4]

Superficial angiomyxoma

Clinical features

Superficial angiomyxoma comprises a relatively uncommon group of lesions which present on the head, neck or trunk of adults as slowly growing,

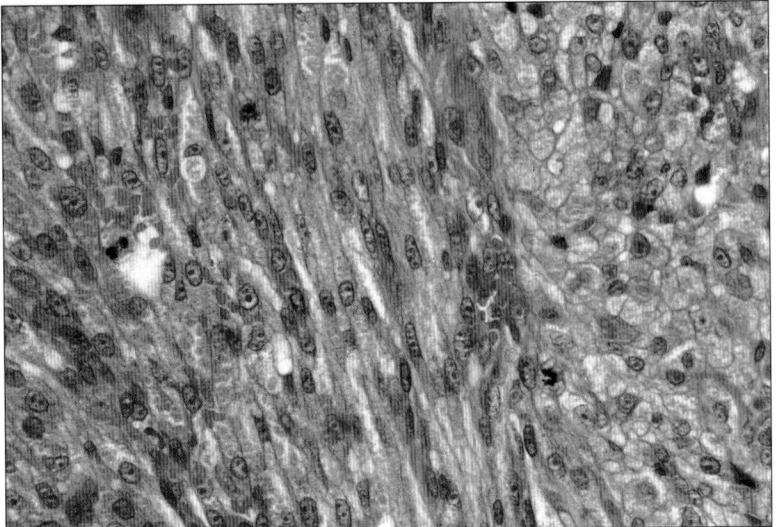

Fig. 35.646
Non-neural dermal granular cell tumor: in this example, the tumor cells are spindled and there is conspicuous mitotic activity.

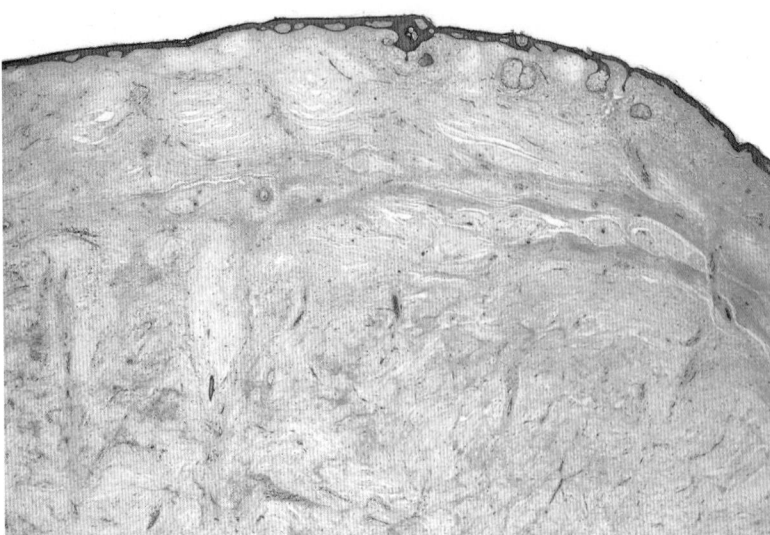

Fig. 35.647
Superficial angiomyxoma: there is massive myxoid change in the dermis associated with numerous small vessels.

solitary, asymptomatic nodules or polyps ranging in size from 1 to 5 cm.[1-3] Larger lesions rarely occur.[4] Tumors also appear to be relatively common in the genital region and are very rare in the oral cavity and pharynx.[5-15] Plantar lesions are exceptional.[16,17] Three cases associated with pilomatricomas have been documented.[18] Local recurrence is common and occurs in up to 25% of cases.

The myxomas described in the Carney complex are very similar, if not identical, to superficial angiomyxomas.[2,3,7-19] This complex, described in 1985, is an autosomal dominant disorder associated with inactivating mutations in *PRKAR1A* which encodes a regulatory subunit of protein kinase A,[20-23] consisting of myxomas, spotty pigmentation (lentigines on the face, especially the lips) and endocrine overactivity (Cushing syndrome, pituitary adenoma, and testicular tumors).[20,24,25] Additional features of the complex include blue nevi and malignant melanotic schwannoma (previously known as psammomatous melanotic schwannoma). The myxomas can present in the skin, breast, and heart. Their recognition in the skin is important because they can be the first manifestation of the syndrome. They are usually multiple, present in young adults, and have a wide anatomical distribution, with a special preference for the eyelids, ears, and nipples.[26,27]

Histologic features

Histologically, the lesions are dermal and subcutaneous, consisting of multiple, poorly circumscribed myxoid lobules containing bland spindle-shaped or stellate cells and abundant small blood vessels (*Figs 35.647* and *35.648*). Often, a sparse inflammatory cell infiltrate containing lymphocytes and neutrophils is also present. In about 30% of cases – either in the primary lesion or its recurrence – there is an epithelial component. The latter consists of epithelial strands, keratin cysts or nests of basaloid cells.[1,2,28] It may mimic a follicular tumor such as a trichofolliculoma.[29] In a single case of a vulvar tumor, necrotizing vasculitis was found within the lesion.[30]

Immunohistochemistry shows positivity of tumor cells for vimentin and variable focal positivity for CD34 and (less frequently) actin.

Differential diagnosis

Nerve sheath myxoma is composed of discrete, well-defined nodules which contain S100 protein-positive cells. Low-grade myxofibrosarcoma is also a multilobular tumor but it is more deeply located and contains pleomorphic cells with mitotic activity. Superficial angiomyxoma hardly ever occurs in the fingers, and this, together with the presence of a more prominent vascular proliferation, more cellularity and a focal inflammatory cell infiltrate, allows distinction from a myxoid cyst.

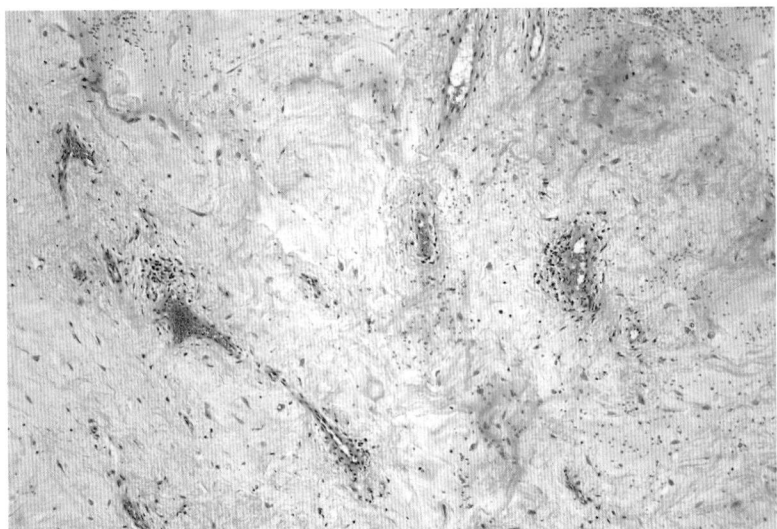

Fig. 35.648
Superficial angiomyxoma: the myxoid deposits contain stellate cells and thin-walled vessels.

Ossifying fibromyxoid tumor

Clinical features

Ossifying fibromyxoid tumor is a distinctive neoplasm that presents mainly as a small asymptomatic subcutaneous nodule usually less than 3 cm, on the trunk or proximal limbs of middle-aged adults and shows a predilection for males.[1-7] However, the anatomical distribution and age range are wide and tumors can present in the head and neck including the oral cavity and mediastinum.[8,9] Recurrence occurs in 20–30% of cases after incomplete excision, although the latter was not found to be of relevance in a large study.[3,7,8] Primary cutaneous lesions are very rare and include a malignant example.[10,11] Rare examples of atypical and malignant variants of this tumor have been described and they have metastatic potential (see below).[3,12,13] Even rarer tumors with no atypical histologic features may occasionally have an aggressive behavior. Based on this, ossifying fibromyxoid tumor should be considered as a tumor of intermediate malignancy.[3]

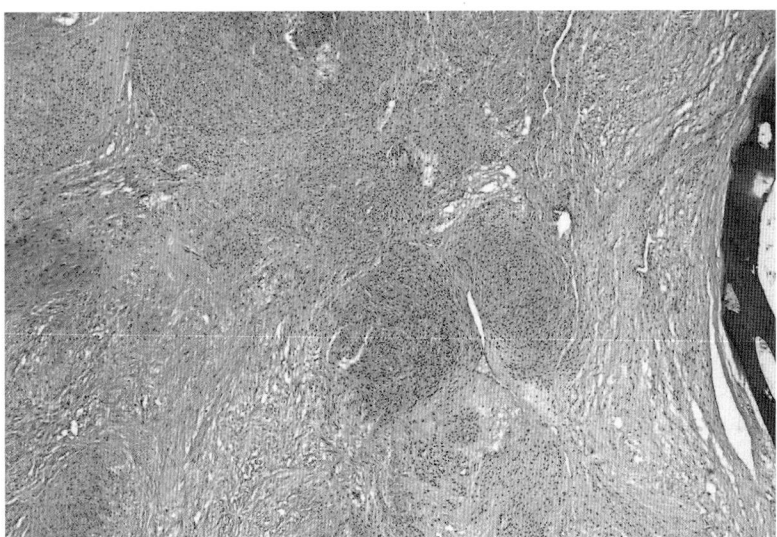

Fig. 35.649
Ossifying fibromyxoid tumor: around 60% of lesions have a distinctive outer shell of lamellar bone. Note the characteristic lobulation.

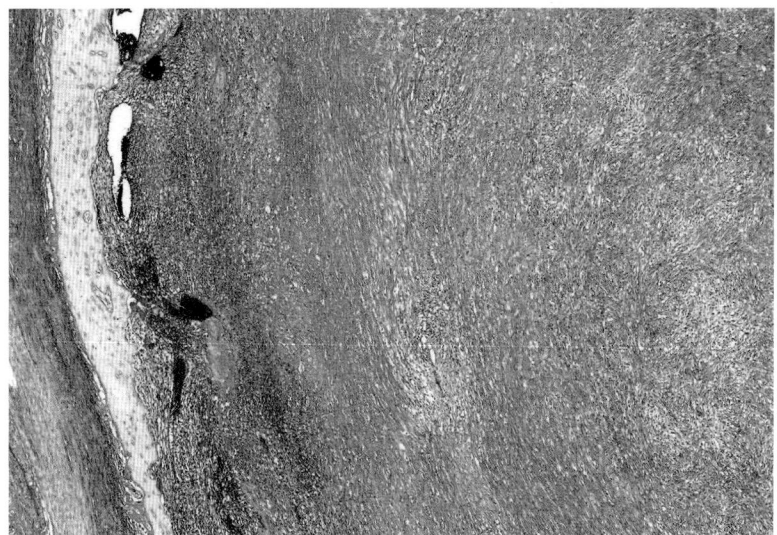

Fig. 35.651
Malignant ossifying fibromyxoid tumor: the lesion appears pseudo-encapsulated and there is a peripheral rim of osteoid. Myxoid change is present on the right side.

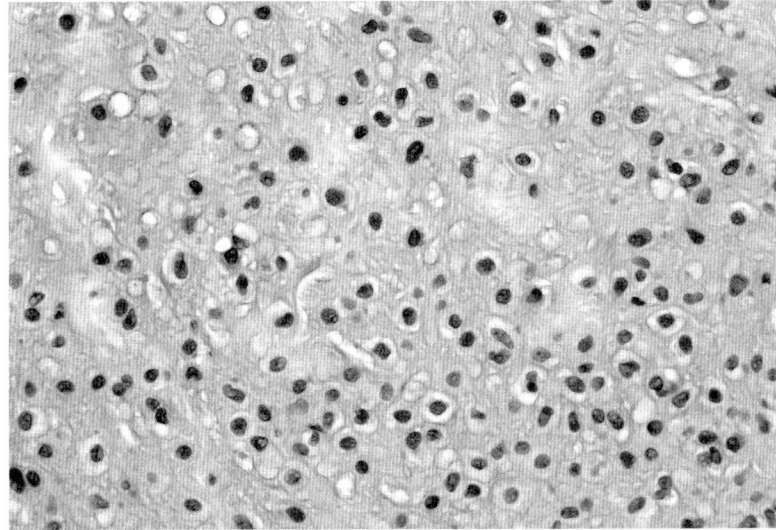

Fig. 35.650
Ossifying fibromyxoid tumor: the tumor cells are rounded and uniform with pale staining cytoplasm.

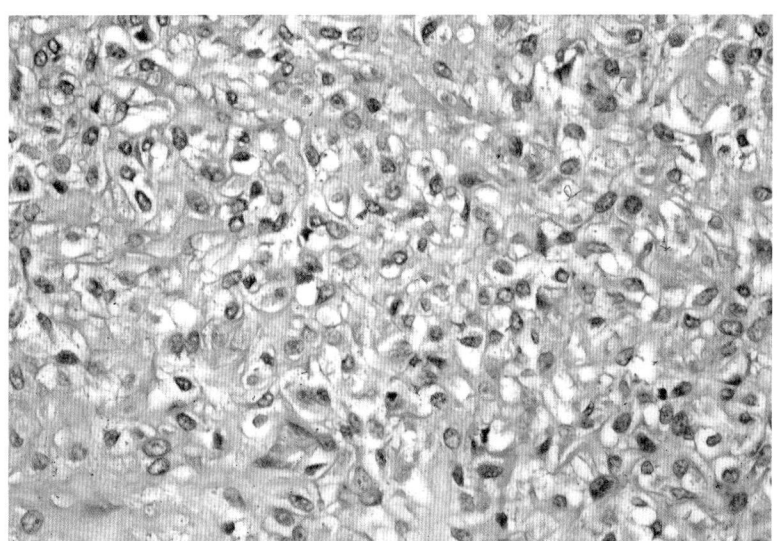

Fig. 35.652
Malignant ossifying fibromyxoid tumor: the tumor cells show nuclear pleomorphism and have pale-staining or clear cytoplasm.

Pathogenesis and histologic features

Cytogenetic studies have shown 6p21 resulting in PHF1 rearrangements or monosomy 22.[14–18] The latter is seen more often in malignant cases.[15,17] *MEAF2-PHF1* and *EPC1-PHF1* rearrangements are most common, but other variants include *ZC3H7B-BCOR*, *CREBBP-BCORL1* and *KDM2A-WWTR1*.[18,19]

The tumors are well circumscribed and lobular and consist of rounded or polygonal cells with pale or eosinophilic cytoplasm and vesicular nuclei, arranged in cords or nests, in a myxoid or hyaline richly vascular matrix (*Figs 35.649* and *35.650*). Tumor lobules are separated by fibrous septa. In up to two-thirds of cases, metaplastic bone is present within the capsule and in the fibrous septa. Nonossifying tumors may also occur (around 10% of cases). Unusual findings include microcysts, microcalcifications, satellite micronodules, epidermoid cysts, and atypical chondroid differentiation.[20,21] Rare cases with otherwise typical histologic features are more cellular, display cytologic atypia, have an increased mitotic rate, and the bone clearly originates from tumor cells (*Figs 35.651–35.653*). Necrosis (in up to 10% of cases) and vascular invasion are additional findings.[7] Histologically

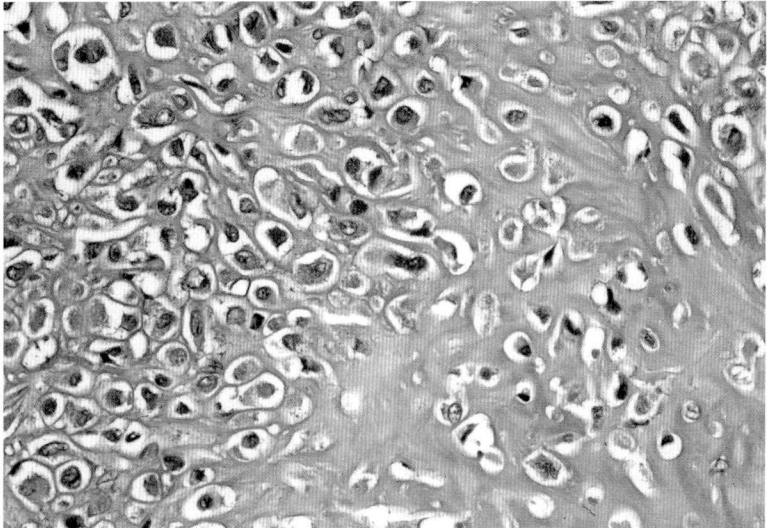

Fig. 35.653
Malignant ossifying fibromyxoid tumor: malignant cartilage is maturing into osteoid.

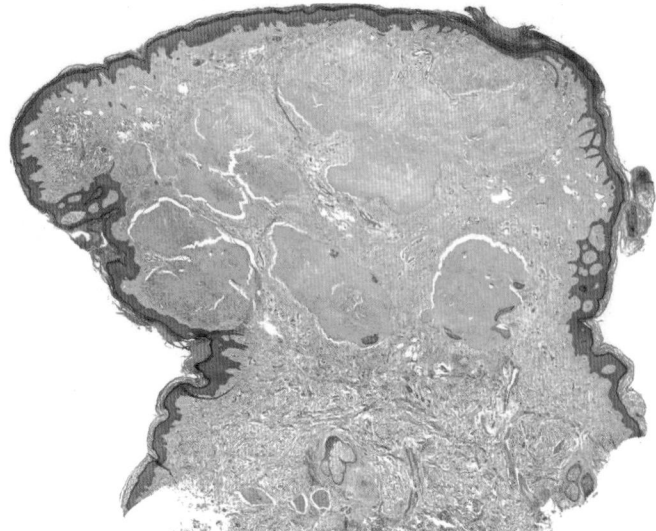

Fig. 35.654
Ossifying plexiform tumor: scanning view showing polypoid mass with multiple foci of osteoid.

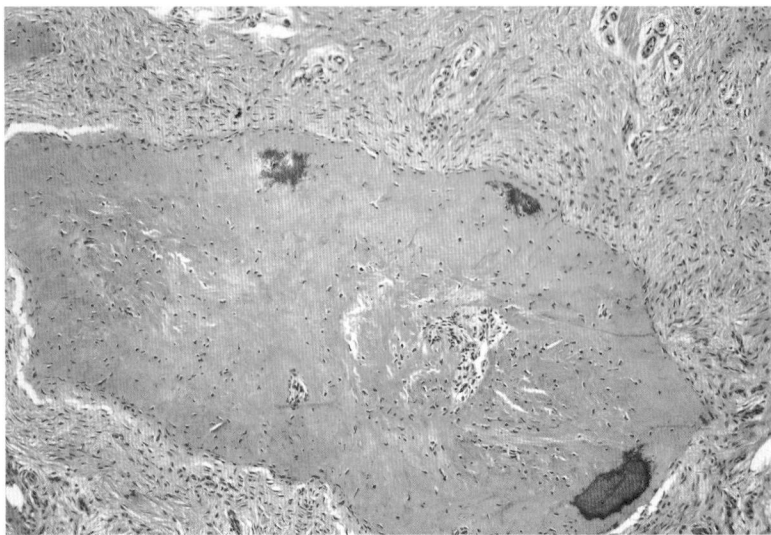

Fig. 35.655
Ossifying plexiform tumor: higher-power view showing focally calcified osteoid.

malignant cases have a high recurrence rate and pulmonary metastases and death have been reported.[3,12] It has been suggested that lesions with high nuclear grade or high cellularity and mitotic activity of more than 2 mitotic figures per 50 high-power fields (HPFs) should be regarded as sarcomas.[3] Tumors with an infiltrative growth pattern are associated with an increased recurrence rate.[3] In a more recent and larger study of 104 patients, no metastasis were noted and only a mitotic count of more than two per 50 HPFs was associated with increased risk of local recurrence.[7] Necrosis, tumor size, satellite nodules and incomplete excision were not associated with increased risk of local recurrence.[7]

The tumor cells are positive for S100 protein (in up to 94%% of cases) and desmin (up to 13% of cases).[3,4,6,7,20] Positivity for glial fibrillary acid protein, SMA, cytokeratin, EMA, collagen II, neurofilament, CD56d excitatory amino acid transporter-4 (EAAT4), MUC4, CD56 and CD99 may also be seen.[3,7,17,22] INI-1 loss of expression in a mosaic pattern is seen in an important number of cases.[17] Proposed lines of differentiation for this tumor include neural, myoid, chondroid and myoepithelial. In one case in which ultrastructural studies were performed, ribosome–lamella complexes were identified.[23]

Differential diagnosis

The differential diagnosis includes myxoid chondrosarcoma, which is usually negative for desmin and SMA, and chondroid syringoma, which in most cases shows an obvious epithelial component.

Ossifying plexiform tumor

Only three cases of this lesion with distinctive histigical features have been described.

Clinical features

All cases have presented as a firm nodule on a digit of adult females.[1,2] Behavior is benign with no tendency for local recurrence.

Pathogenesis and histologic features

It has been suggested that this tumor may represent a variant of cellular neurothekeoma. Histologically, there is a well-defined dermal lobular tumor consisting of bland epithelioid and spindle-shaped cells in a myxoid matrix. Tumor lobules are separated by fibrous bands and in the center of each lobule there is abundant mature bone often surrounded by a rim of osteoblasts (Figs 35.654 and 35.655).

Phosphaturic mesenchymal tumor (mixed connective tissue variant)

Clinical features

Phosphaturic mesenchymal tumor (mixed connective tissue variant) is a distinctive neoplasm that usually induces oncogenic osteomalacia, a paraneoplastic syndrome resulting from phosphate wasting.[1–12] Occasional identical tumors not associated with oncogenic osteomalacia are seen.[1,8,9] Lesions vary in size and arise in deep soft tissues and bone and rarely in the subcutaneous tissue.[2] Most patients are adults but the age range is wide and there is predilection for females.[1] At the time of diagnosis, patients have often had long-standing osteomalacia. In one patient, symptoms of osteomalacia only appeared 1 year after resection of the tumor.[3] Occasional malignant tumors occur and exceptionally metastases are seen.[1,4,12]

Pathogenesis and histologic features

Tumors appear to produce fibroblast growth factor-23 and this seems to be important pathogenetically, as the protein induces loss of phosphate in the renal tubules.[5] An *FN1-FGFR1* genetic fusion has been documented as a frequent event.[12–14] *FN1-FGF1* can also be demonstrated.[14]

Lesions are ill-defined and hypocellular with areas of myxoid change, bland spindle-shaped cells, hemorrhage, microcystic spaces, proliferation of blood vessels often in a hemangiopericytomatous pattern, osteoclasts and a calcified matrix (Figs 35.656–35.659). Focal ossification can also be identified. A small number of tumors display other histologic patterns including hemangiopericytoma, giant cell tumor and osteosarcoma.[1]

Tumor cells are usually positive for fibroblast growth factor-23, and this is a very useful diagnostic test. Other reported positive markers include FGFR1, CD56, actin, bcl2, and less often ERG.[12] Vascular channels in the tumor are positive for LYVE-1 and podoplanin, indicating lymphatic lineage.[6]

Superficial acral fibromyxoma

Clinical features

Superficial acral fibromyxoma (digital fibromyxoma) is a distinctive, relatively rare benign tumor with predilection for the fingers and toes, followed by the palm.[1–25] Identical lesions have been described under the rubric cellular digital fibroma.[6,7,20] Involvement of the nail region is very common. Lesions on the heel are rare.[5] Patients are usually young to middle-aged

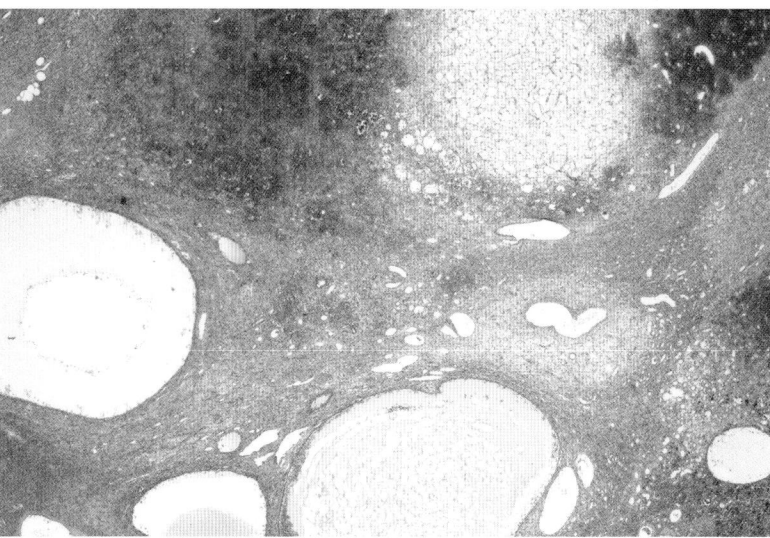

Fig. 35.656
Phosphaturic mesenchymal tumor: scanning view showing cysts, blood vessels, focal hemorrhage and a myxoid stroma.

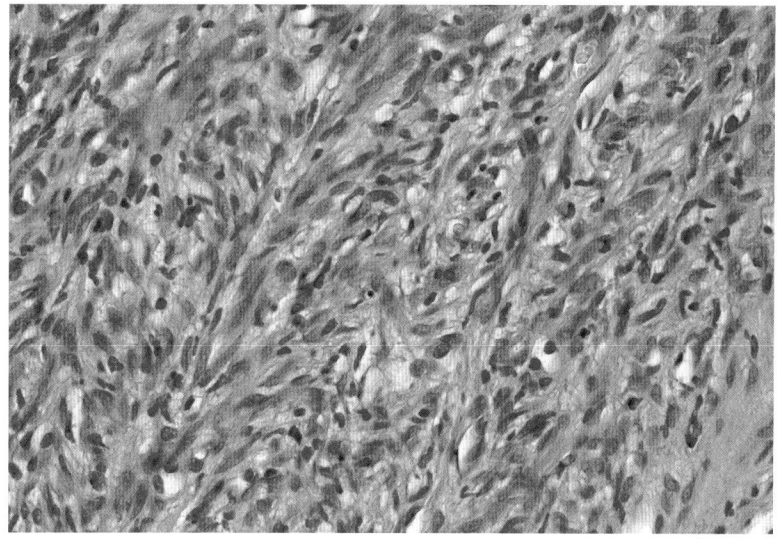

Fig. 35.659
Phosphaturic mesenchymal tumor: high-power view of spindled cells showing a vaguely fascicular growth pattern.

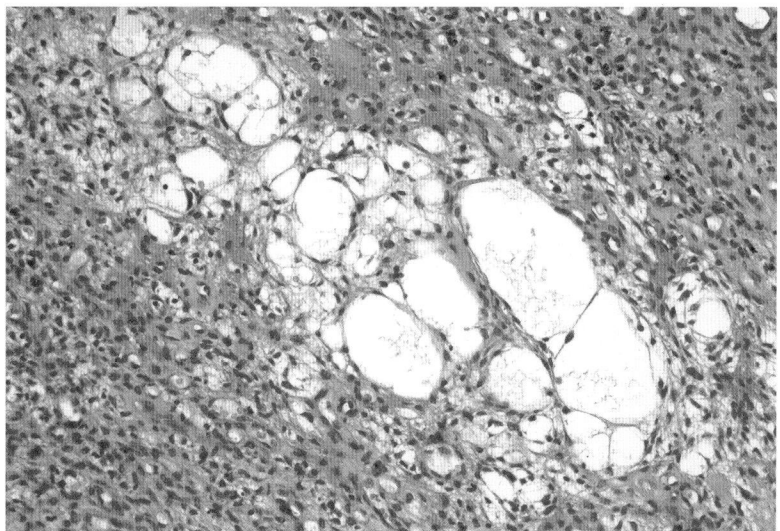

Fig. 35.657
Phosphaturic mesenchymal tumor: the tumor cells have eosinophilic cytoplasm and hyperchromatic spindled nuclei. Microcysts are present.

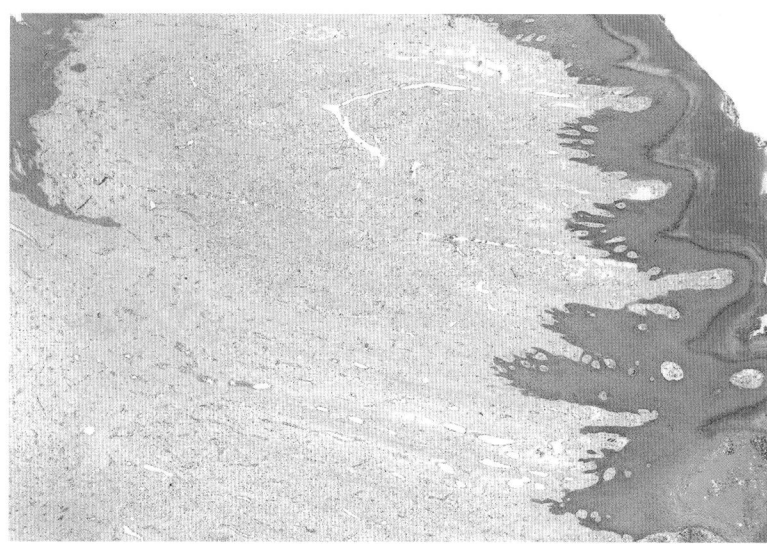

Fig. 35.660
Superficial acral fibromyxoma: low-power view of a vascular spindle cell tumor with a myxoid stroma.

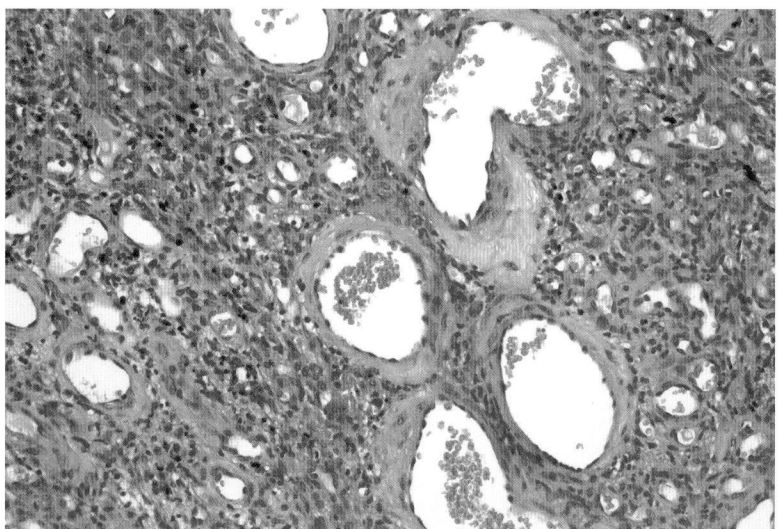

Fig. 35.658
Phosphaturic mesenchymal tumor: higher-power view showing tumor cells and blood vessels.

adults and there is predilection for males. Tumors are small, slowly growing and asymptomatic. Local recurrence after excision is rare.[8]

Pathogenesis and histologic features

RB1 gene deletions have been recently documented, suggesting a possible relationship to other *RB1*-deleted neoplasms such as spindle cell/pleomorphic lipoma, mammary-type myofibroblastoma, and cellular angiofibroma.[23]

Histology shows a fairly circumscribed dermal and/or subcutaneous tumor composed of bland, spindle-shaped or stellate cells with a focal storiform or fascicular pattern in a myxoid or collagenous stroma (*Fig. 35.660*). Lesions contain scattered small vascular channels. Some tumors are more cellular than others and in these, myxoid change tends to be very focal (*Fig. 35.661*).[3] An adipocytic component is exceptional.[9]

Mitotic figures are rare and cytologic atypia is mild or absent. Mast cells are often present.

By immunohistochemistry, tumor cells are usually positive for CD34 and may be focally positive for EMA, SMA, CD99, CD10, and nestin.[1–5,17,24] Desmin positivity has only been reported in one case.[17] There is loss of expression of RB1.[23] Ultrastructurally, tumor cells show cytoplasmic intermediate filaments and rough endoplasmic reticulum, indicating fibroblastic differentiation.[10]

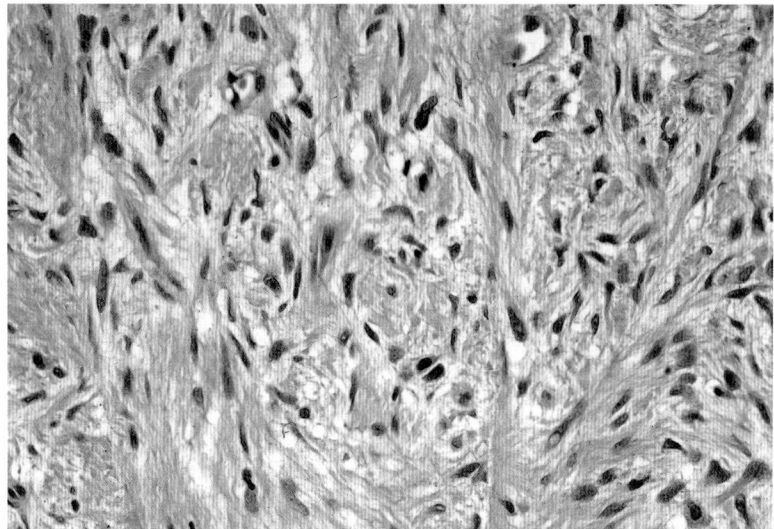

Fig. 35.661
Superficial acral fibromyxoma: high-power view of bland spindled cells in a myxoid stroma.

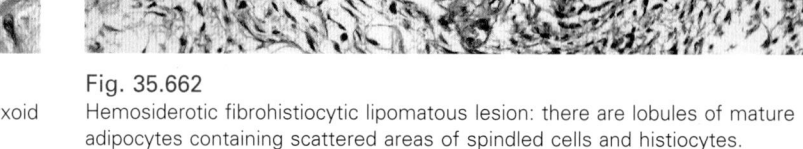

Fig. 35.662
Hemosiderotic fibrohistiocytic lipomatous lesion: there are lobules of mature adipocytes containing scattered areas of spindled cells and histiocytes.

Differential diagnosis

The differential diagnosis includes neurofibroma, onychomatricoma, dermatofibrosarcoma protuberans, minute synovial sarcoma and low-grade fibromyxoid sarcoma. Neurofibroma is rare in acral sites and, although tumor cells may be focally positive for CD34, they are also positive for S100 protein. The stromal component in onychomatricoma may be identical to that seen in superficial acral fibromyxoma with CD34-positive cells. Distinction is based in the presence of distinctive epithelial changes in onychomatricoma.[11] A focal storiform pattern may mimic dermatofibrosarcoma protuberans. However, the latter is vanishingly rare in the distal extremities, infiltrates the subcutaneous tissue diffusely and is positive for apolipoprotein D.[12] Minute synovial sarcoma of the hands and feet can have similar appearances to superficial acral fibromyxoma with myxoid stroma and bland spindle-shaped cells.[13] However, in the former there are focal areas of calcification, tumor cells are at least focally positive for keratin and cytogenetic analysis shows a tX;18 translocation. Negativity for MUC4 rules out low-grade fibromyxoid sarcoma.

Hemosiderotic fibrolipomatous tumor/hemosiderotic fibrohistiocytic lipomatous lesion

Clinical features

Hemosiderotic fibrolipomatous tumor (hemosiderotic fibrohistiocytic lipomatous lesion) develops almost exclusively on the foot, particularly the ankle, with predilection for females.[1–3] Most patients are adults but children may rarely be affected. It grows slowly and is asymptomatic. Simple excision is the treatment of choice. Local recurrence may occur.

Pathogenesis and histologic features

Hemosiderotic fibrohistiocytic lipomatous lesion was thought to be the result of trauma. It has also been suggested that the lesion may develop as a result of stasis.[4] However, it is now clear that it represents a neoplastic process of unkown histogenesis.[5,6] A consistent t(1;10) with rearrangements of *TGFBR3* and *MGEA5* have been described.[7] The same translocation is seen in a subset of myxoinflammatory fibroblastic sarcoma. It has been suggested that there is a histogenetic link between this tumor, pleomorphic hyalinizing angiectatic and myxoinflammatory fibroblastic sarcoma. This has been discussed under the latter entity. The conclusion based on a number of

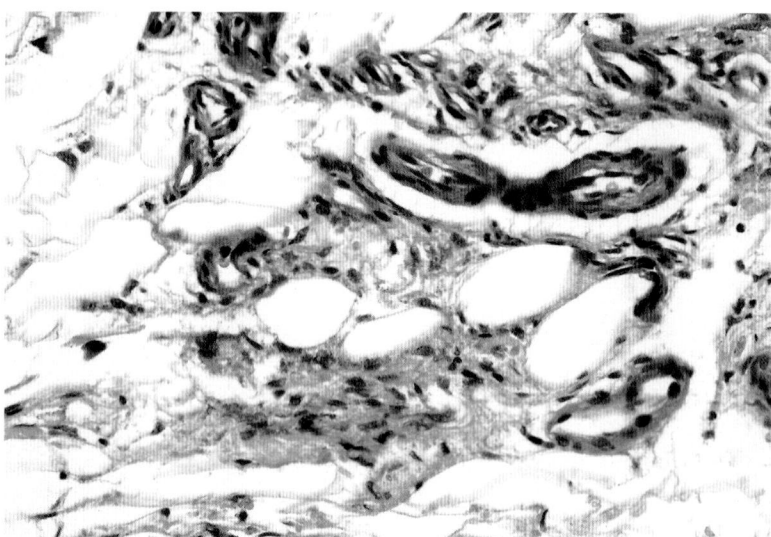

Fig. 35.663
Hemosiderotic fibrohistiocytic lipomatous lesions: there are bland spindle-shaped cells and prominent hemosiderin.

studies is that although there is a pathogenetic link between hemosiderotic fibrohistiocytic lipomatous tumor and pleomorphic hyalinizing angiectatic tumor, it is unlikely that these tumors are related to pure cases myxoinflammatory fibroblastic sarcoma.[5–24]

Histology shows a fairly well-circumscribed mass composed of abundant mature adipose tissue admixed with focal bundles of plump spindle-shaped cells with vesicular nuclei and a small inconspicuous nucleolus. Cytologic atypia is mild and mitotic figures are very rare. A striking feature is the presence of prominent hemosiderin deposition, particularly in the spindle cell areas (*Figs 35.662* and *35.663*). Focal areas of the tumor may display features reminiscent of myxoinflammatory fibroblastic sarcoma. Early lesions display histologic features that are identical to those seen in pleomorphic hyalinizing angiectatic tumor.

By immunohistochemistry, the spindle cells are positive for vimentin, calponin and CD34, and focally positive for KP1.

MISCELLANEOUS LOW-GRADE AND MALIGNANT TUMORS

Pleomorphic hyalinizing angiectatic tumor

Clinical features

Pleomorphic hyalinizing angiectatic tumor is a distinctive, rare, low-grade malignancy of uncertain line of differentiation. In the few cases reported so far, the tumor has presented in the subcutaneous tissue of adults, with the same sex incidence and predilection for the lower limbs.[1–6] Exceptionally tumors have been described in the retroperitoneum and kidney.[7,8] There is local recurrence but metastases have not so far been documented. A single case recurred with a high-grade myxofibrosarcoma component.[9]

Pathogenesis and histologic features

In one case, the translocations t(1;3)(p31;q12) and t(1;10)(p31;q25) have been described.[10] In further studies, genetic rearrangements of *TGFBR3* and/or *MGEA5* have been demonstrated in up 60% of cases.[11–13] Tumors with the latter abnormalities usually display histologic overlap with hemosiderotic fibrolipomatous tumor. The potential relationship between pleomorphic hyalinizing angiectatic tumor, hemosiderotic fibrolipomatous and tumor myxoinflammatory fibroblastic sarcoma is further discussed under myxoinflammatory fibroblastic sarcoma. Summarizing the findings in different studies, it is likely that pleomorphic hyalinizing angiectatic and hemosiderotic fibrolipomatous tumor are part of the same spectrum but myxoinflammatory fibroblastic is not related to the former entities.[10–16]

Tumors are poorly circumscribed and consist of congested, angiectatic blood vessels surrounded by spindle-shaped pleomorphic cells in a myxoid background (*Figs 35.664– 35.666*). Hemorrhage, hemosiderin deposition, and perivascular hyalinization with fibrin and collagen deposition are additional features. Mitotic activity is very low. Tumor cells are focally positive for CD34, CD99, vascular endothelial growth factor and factor XIIIa.[17,18] Early lesions of the tumor consist of spindle-shaped cells arranged in short fascicles infiltrating the fat, associated with cytoplasmic hemosiderin and with damaged blood vessels in the background.[19] There are always scattered pleomorphic cells, some of which contain intranuclear inclusions. Lipoblast-like cells and ganglion-like cells are exceptional.[20,21] This precursor lesion has been considered as identical to hemosiderotic fibrohistiocytic lipomatous lesion, a view not shared by all authors but the relationship between both tumors has been confirmed with cytogentic studies.[22–24] The presence of dilated vascular channels may reflect impaired blood circulation as a result of venous insufficiency in the vicinity of the tumor.[24]

Differential diagnosis

The differential diagnosis is mainly with an ancient schwannoma. Distinction is based on the presence of a capsule, less cytologic atypia and diffuse S100 protein positivity in the latter.

Myoepithelioma of soft tissue

Clinical features

Myoepithelioma of soft tissue is a rare tumor that presents mainly in middle-aged adults, with no sex predilection, as a subcutaneous or deep-seated, fairly well-circumscribed mass.[1,2] Lesions frequently occur in the limbs and limb girdles, followed by the head and neck and trunk. There is local recurrence in up to 20% of cases and a number of tumors with malignant histology may metastasize. It is controversial as to whether myoepithelioma represents the same tumor as parachordoma.[3,4] A case of

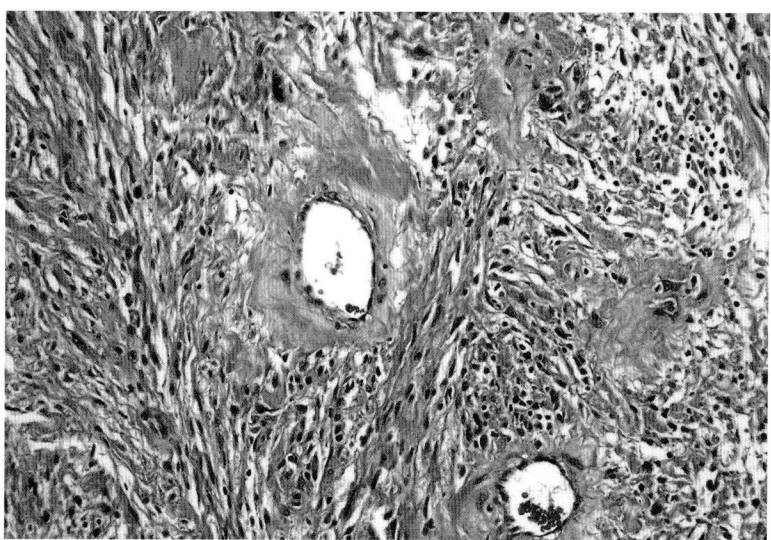

Fig. 35.665
Pleomorphic hyalinizing angiectatic tumor of soft parts: surrounding the vessels are pleomorphic spindled cells with irregular, hyperchromatic nuclei.

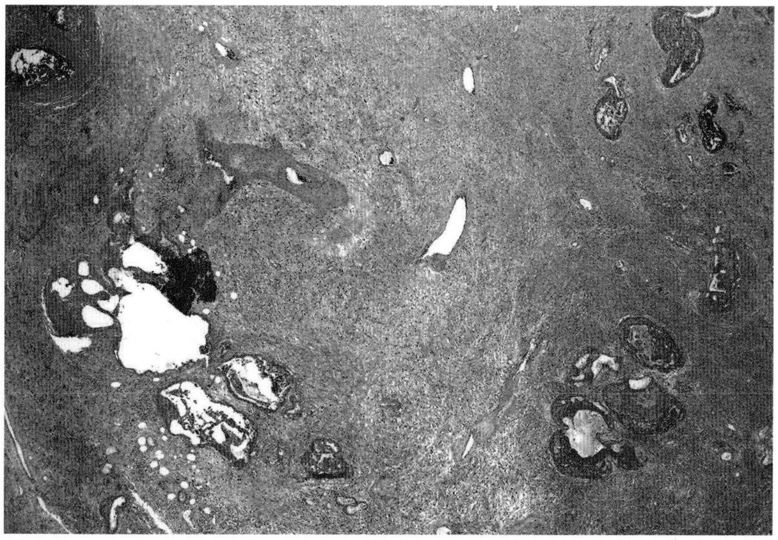

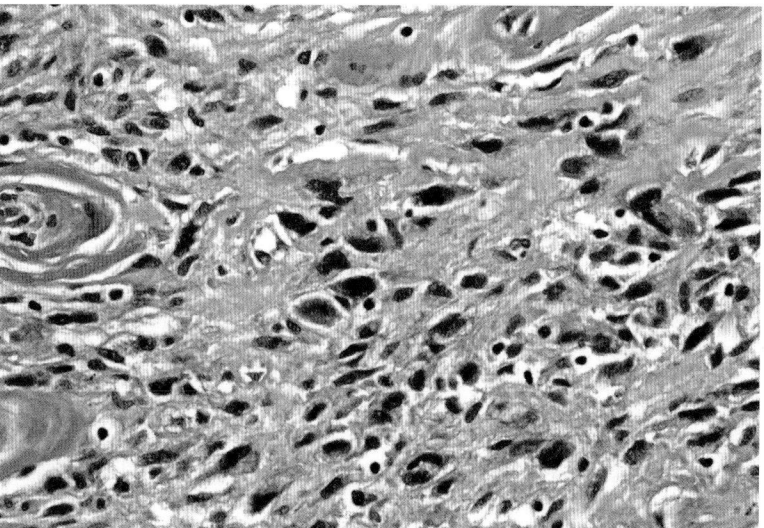

Fig. 35.664
Pleomorphic hyalinizing angiectatic tumor of soft parts: there are numerous thin-walled angiectatic blood vessels surrounded by a cellular stroma.

Fig. 35.666
Pleomorphic hyalinizing angiectatic tumor of soft parts: high-power view showing marked nuclear pleomorphism.

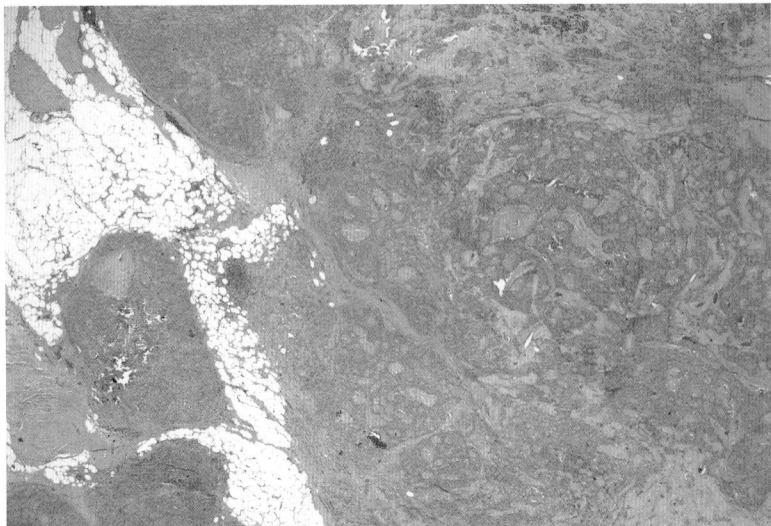

Fig. 35.667
Myoepithelioma of soft tissue: scanning view of a multilobulated tumor with conspicuous pools of mucin.

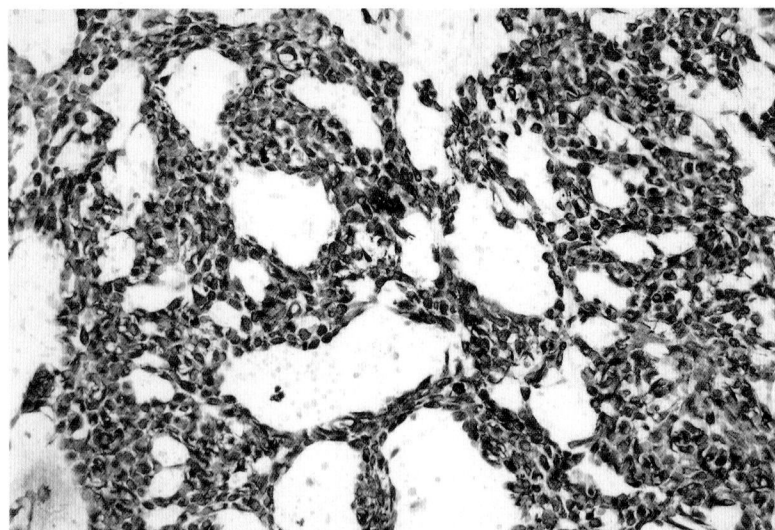

Fig. 35.669
Myoepithelioma of soft tissue: the tumor cells express pankeratin.

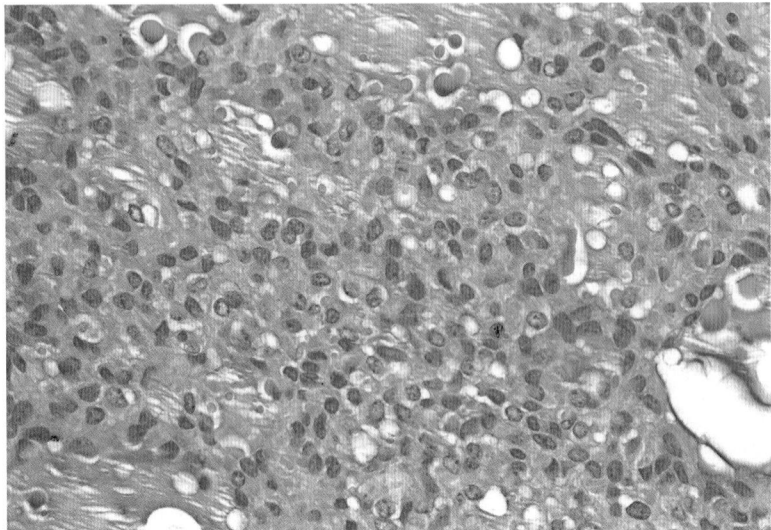

Fig. 35.668
Myoepithelioma of soft tissue: the tumor cells have eosinophilic cytoplasm and uniform round nuclei.

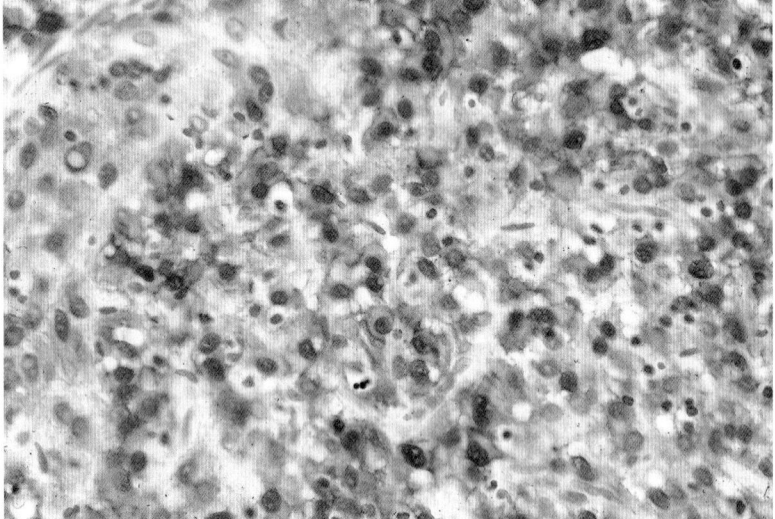

Fig. 35.670
Myoepithelioma of soft tissue: S100 protein is also expressed.

congenital myoepithelial carcinoma associated with cystic myoepithelioma has been reported.[5]

Pathogenesis and histologic features

Recently, t(19;22)(q13;q12) fusing *EWSR1* and *ZNF444* has been described in this neoplasm.[6] *PBX1* (1q23) can also pair with *EWSR1*.[6] A recent larger study demonstrated *EWSR1* rearrangements in 59% of cases and identified *POU5F1* (6p21.31) as an additional partner.[7,8] Other studies have described very heterogeneous genetic alterations in these tumors.[9–20]

Histology shows a lobulated circumscribed tumor that may have a focal infiltrative margin. Tumor cells are epithelioid, ovoid or short and spindle-shaped and are arranged in cords and nests in a variably myxoid, chondroid, hyalinized or fibrotic stroma (*Figs 35.667* and *35.668*). Solid areas may predominate and some cells may have a plasmacytoid appearance. Additional features that may be seen include ductal differentiation, squamous metaplasia and fat, bone and cartilage formation.[21] The syncytial variant is the most commonly variant encountered in the skin (see page 1631).[22]

Tumors classified as malignant have prominent atypia and variable mitotic activity. Malignant bone or cartilage may be seen.

Immunohistochemistry shows that in most cases tumor cells are positive for keratin, calponin, SOX10, and S100 protein (*Figs 35.669* and *35.670*).[2,23] Frequent staining for EMA, GFAP, and SMA is also seen, and in rare cases there is positivity for desmin (*Fig. 35.671*).[2] The syncytial variant is usually negative for keratins and most myoepithelial markers so positivity for EMA and S100 protein helps establishing the diagnosis.

Perivascular epithelioid cell tumor

Perivascular epithelioid cell tumor ('PEComa') is part of the spectrum of neoplasms that includes clear cell 'sugar' tumor of the lung, angiomyolipoma, lymphangioleiomyomatosis and clear cell myomelanocytic tumor of the falciform ligament.[1] The first three neoplasms are often associated with tuberous sclerosis. Occurrence of similar tumors in the skin and soft tissue is rare but increasingly reported and these are not associated with tuberous sclerosis.[2–9] Cutaneous lesions are more common in middle-aged females and have predilection for the limbs where they present as a slowly growing, small asymptomatic nodule. Malignant cutaneous perivascular epithelioid cell tumors are very rare.[10,11] Metastatic spread of an internal tumor to the skin is exceptional.[12]

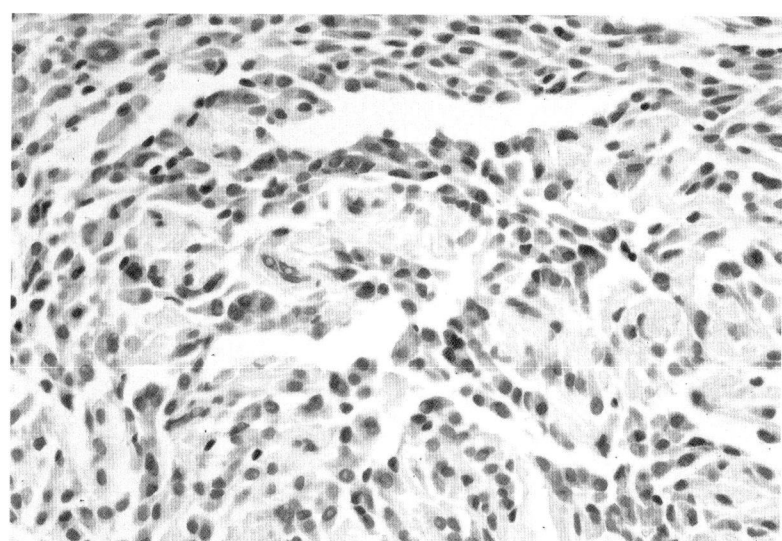

Fig. 35.671
Myoepithelioma of soft tissue: desmin is positive.

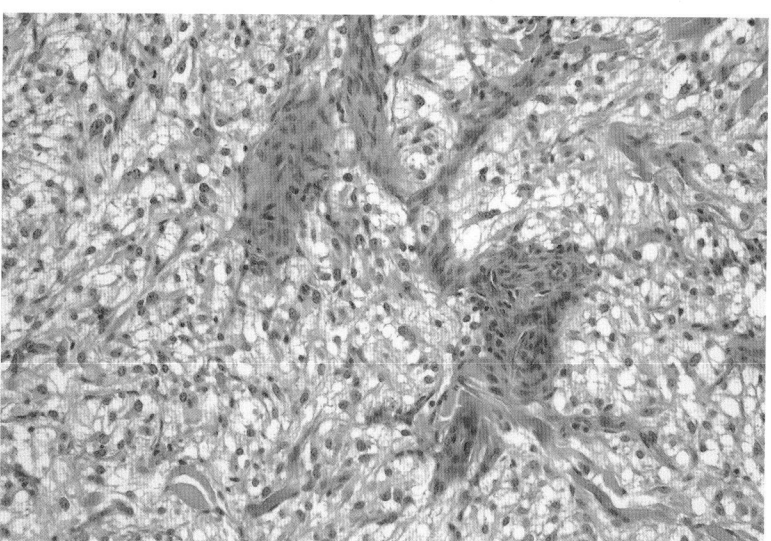

Fig. 35.673
Perivascular epithelioid cell tumor: the tumor cells are surrounded by a vascular network.

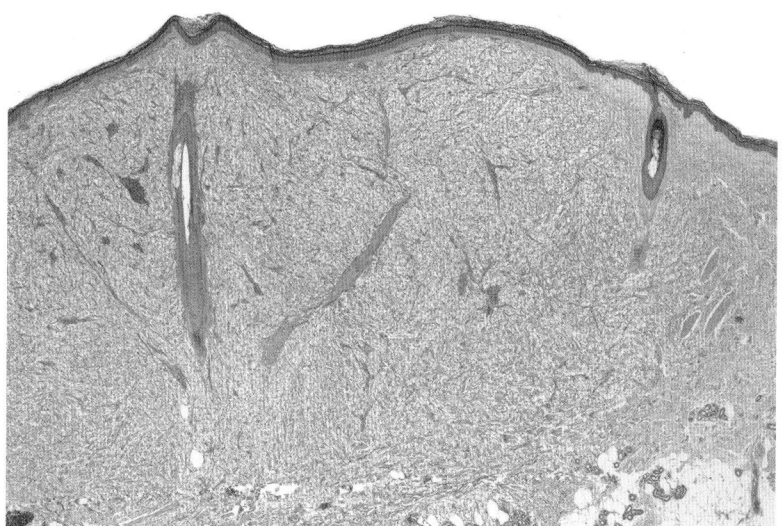

Fig. 35.672
Perivascular epithelioid cell tumor: low-power view of a clear cell tumor. Note that the appendages are spared.

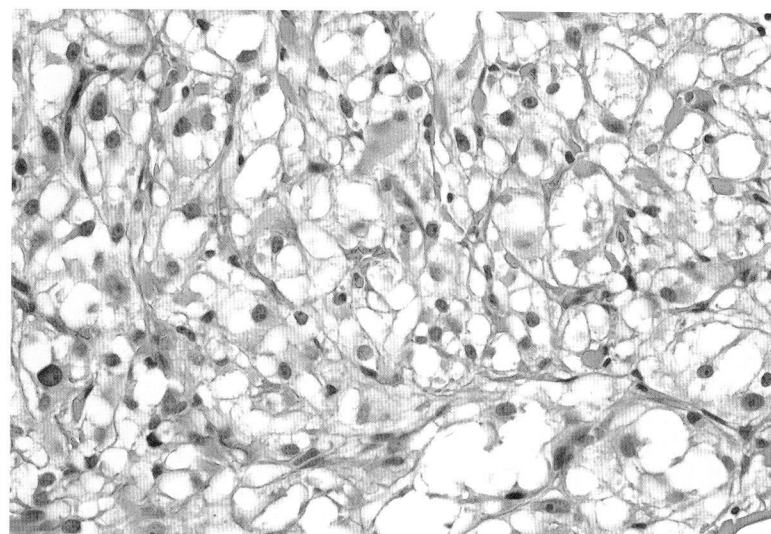

Fig. 35.674
Perivascular epithelioid cell tumor: high-power view showing clear cytoplasm and uniform vesicular nuclei with eosinophilic nucleoli.

Pathogenesis and histologic features

PEComas presenting at other sites but not in the skin have been reported to be associated with gene fusions, the most common being *TFE3*, mainly in soft tissue lesions and *RAD51B* in uterine tumors.[13–16] In skin tumors, the constant expression of 4E-binding protein suggests that the pathogenesis may be associated with the mTOR pathway.[17]

Histology shows an ill-defined dermal tumor that may extend into the subcutaneous tissue and is composed of bland epithelioid cells typically arranged radially around thin-walled vascular channels (*Figs 35.672* and *35.673*). A smaller population of spindled cells is often seen. Tumor cells have clear, granular or pale pink cytoplasm and vesicular nuclei (*Fig. 35.674*). Rare multinucleated cells may be seen. Mitotic figures are often found but are not prominent, and very focal cytologic atypia can be seen (*Fig. 35.675*). A cutaneous lesion with the presence of melanin has been reported.[18] A hyalinizing variant has been described in the retroperitoneum.[19]

The immunophenotype is distinctive, as tumor cells stain for melanocytic markers including MITF-1 and HMB45 and less commonly for Melan-A and S100. There is variable positivity for muscular markers including desmin, SMA and, less frequently, calponin. NKI/C3, bcl-1, E-cadherin and cathepsin K are consistently positive.[17] CD10 is also positive.[8,20] Cells are negative for h-caldesmon, epithelial membrane antigen, SOX-10 and keratin.

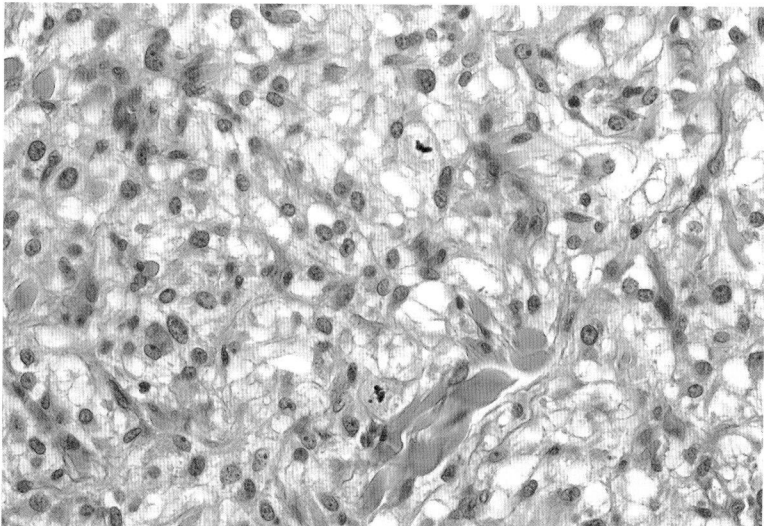

Fig. 35.675
Perivascular epithelioid cell tumor: note the mitotic figures.

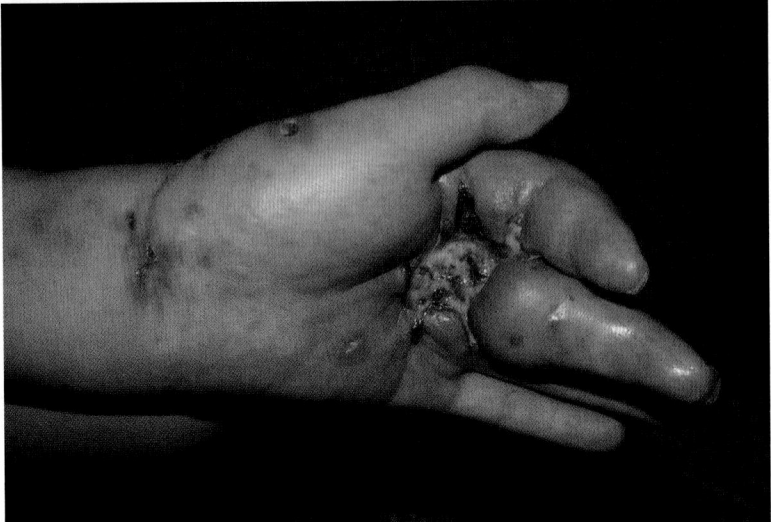

Fig. 35.676
Epithelioid sarcoma: the hand is a commonly affected site. By courtesy of Dr. Yi-Guo Feng, Xian, China.

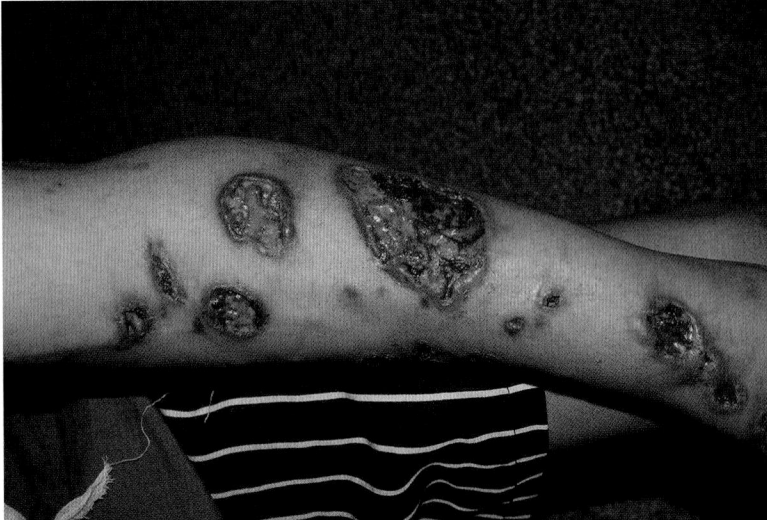

Fig. 35.677
Epithelioid sarcoma: spread along the neurovascular bundles and fascial planes commonly results in more proximal tumor deposits as seen in this patient. By courtesy of Dr. Yi-Guo Feng, Xian, China.

Differential diagnosis

Distinction from melanocytic lesions with balloon cell change is based on the presence of a junctional component and the frequent diffuse positivity for S100 in the latter. The so-called dermal clear cell neoplasm has very similar histologic features to those of perivascular epithelioid cell tumor but the former is negative for melanocytic markers. Clear cells may be focally or diffusely present in dermatofibroma but the latter is associated with epidermal hyperplasia and is negative for melanocytic markers. In metastatic renal cell carcinoma, the blood vessels are dilated and congested, there is more cytologic atypia and more prominent clear cell change and tumor cells are positive for keratins and EMA. Both tumors are positive for CD10.[20]

Epithelioid sarcoma

Clinical features

Epithelioid sarcoma is a comparatively rare tumor arising most often on the distal extremities (particularly the hand and wrist) of young adults, especially males.[1–5] Occurrence in children is uncommon.[6] The overall age range and the anatomical distribution are wide. Rare cases present in the head and even in the oral cavity and parotid gland (Figs 35.676 and 35.677).[7–10] It is predominantly a dermal or subcutaneous tumor that presents as a slow-growing, elevated, often tender nodule(s) measuring less than 5 cm in diameter. Ulceration is a common feature. Due to the distinctive tendency for extensive spread of the tumor along blood vessels, nerves, and fascia, the presence of satellite nodules at a distance from the main tumor is common. The tumor may mimic other diseases including perforating granuloma annulare and Dupuytren disease.[11,12]

Indolent and repeated locoregional recurrence is common. Metastasis to the lymph nodes, an unusual feature in other sarcomas, is quite common, followed by metastasis to the lungs. Although the overall 5-year survival is about 70%, the 20-year survival is no more than 20–25%.[2,3] Improved prognosis appears to be related to smaller tumor size.[3]

A group of epithelioid sarcomas arising in pelvi-perineal locations (including the vulva) have a very aggressive clinical course, more so than the ordinary variant, and have been described as proximal-type epithelioid sarcoma.[13–17] Similar cases exceptionally occur in other locations.[18] Independent indicators of worse biological behavior are early metastases and large tumor size.[19]

Pathogenesis and histologic features

The most consistent cytogenetic abnormality in cases studied so far has been loss of heterozygosity of chromosome 22q.[20–22] Loss of INI1 (BAF47)

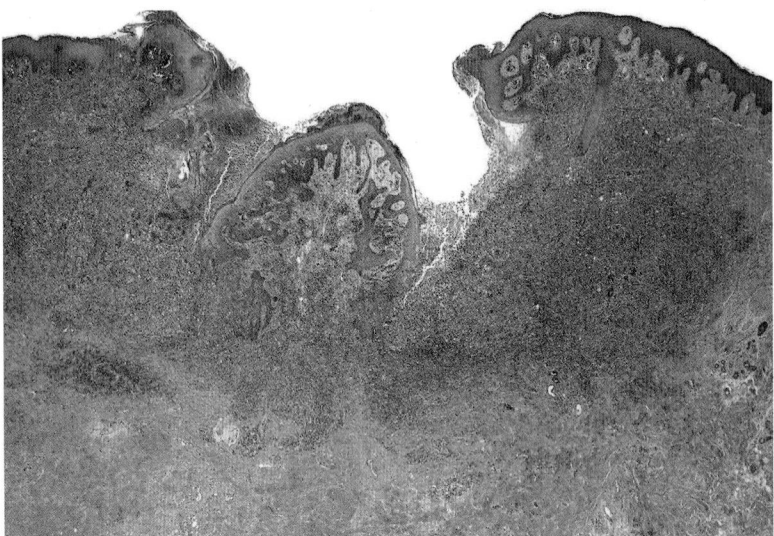

Fig. 35.678
Epithelioid sarcoma: the upper dermis is diffusely infiltrated by an ulcerated tumor.

nuclear expression encoded by SMARCB1 (INI1) at 22q11.23 is characteristic and likely critical for the pathogenesis.[23–26] Other abnormalities have been found in 8q and monosomy 21 has also been documented.[21] Overall, there are complex genomic cases and loss of CDKN2A is common, in contradistinction to the simple genomic profile of rhabdoid tumor with SMARCB1 loss.[27] Abnormalities of chromosomes 8 and 22 have also been found to be involved in the proximal-type of epithelioid sarcoma.[28]

An NRAS oncogene mutation has been described in a case of metastatic epithelioid sarcoma.[29]

The microscopic appearances are distinctive (Figs 35.678–35.680). The tumor is composed of multiple nodules of polygonal, epithelioid, or spindle-shaped cells with eosinophilic cytoplasm which show variable pleomorphism. Mitoses are often scanty. Giant cell forms are occasionally seen. At the center of these nodules, focal necrosis is a prominent feature in around 50% of cases, producing an appearance reminiscent of a granulomatous process (Fig. 35.681). Other cases show a vague fibrinoid or myxoid pattern of degeneration. The latter may predominate in rare cases. At the periphery of the nodules, the tumor cells tend to be more spindle shaped, and in rare cases this feature can be prominent (see below).[18,30] Vascular and perineural invasion is often present (Fig. 35.682). In a small number of

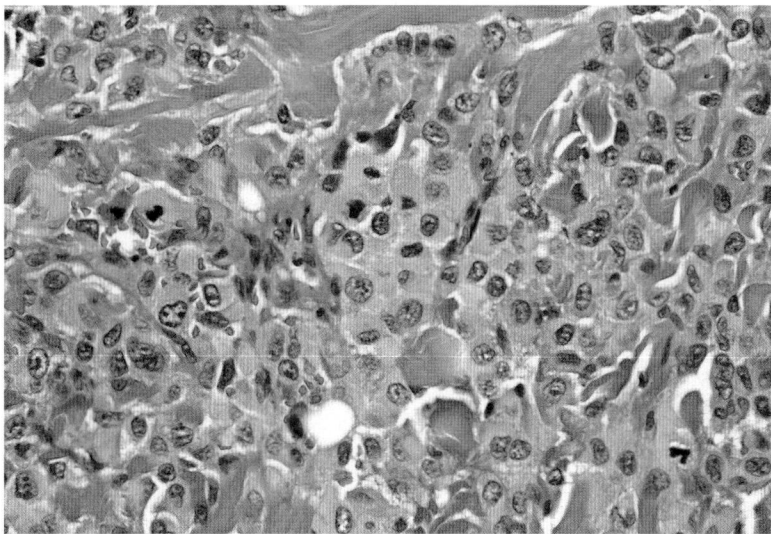

Fig. 35.679
Epithelioid sarcoma: in this field the tumor cells are epithelioid with abundant eosinophilic cytoplasm and large vesicular nuclei.

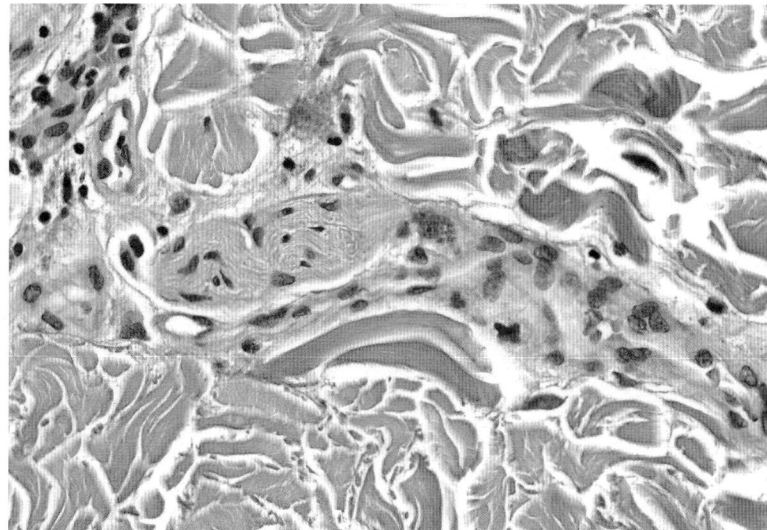

Fig. 35.682
Epithelioid sarcoma: the tumor commonly extends along nerve trunks, in part accounting for its high recurrence rate.

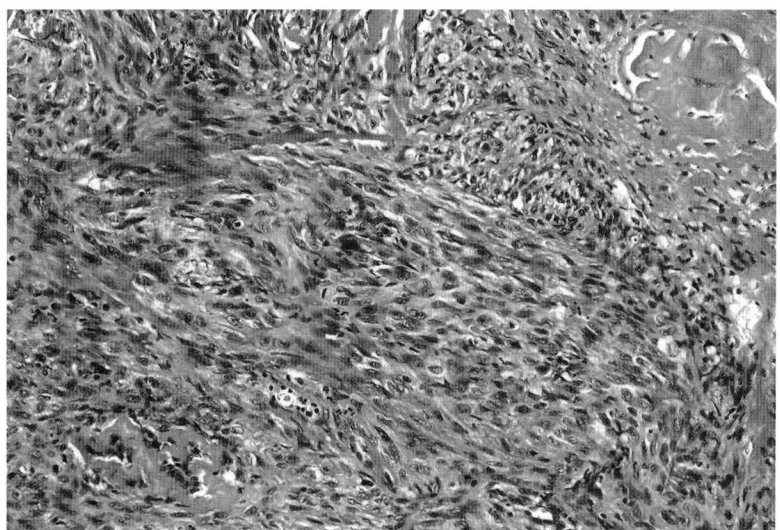

Fig. 35.680
Epithelioid sarcoma: elsewhere the tumor cells have a spindled morphology.

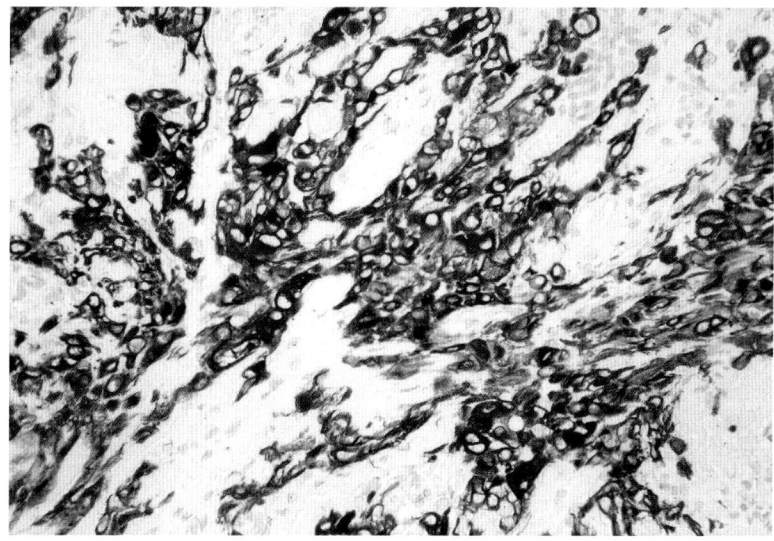

Fig. 35.683
Epithelioid sarcoma: the tumor cells characteristically express keratin, as shown in this field.

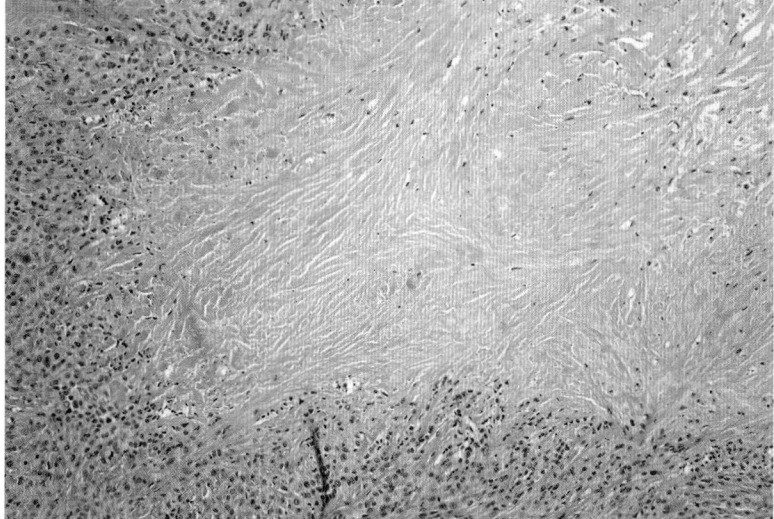

Fig. 35.681
Epithelioid sarcoma: geographical necrosis seen at low-power examination may result in diagnostic confusion with a granulomatous process.

cases, spindle-shaped cells predominate, they are arranged in bundles and necrosis is minimal or absent. This variant is known as fibroma-like.[30,31] In a few cases, an angiomatoid pattern is seen.[31] Heterotopic bone formation is exceptional.[32]

Immunohistochemically, more than 90% of cases are positive for vimentin, cytokeratin and EMA (*Figs 35.683* and *35.684*) and up to 60% are positive for CD34.[33–36] SMA is also often focally positive. The combination of vimentin, CD34 and keratin positivity is very useful in the diagnosis of epithelioid sarcoma. The immunohistochemical profile of proximal-type epithelioid sarcoma is similar to that of classic epithelioid sarcoma. Both forms show loss of nuclear INI1 expression in greater than 90 % of cases, a relatively specific finding within the reasonable differential diagnoses.[37–39] GLUT-1 is not a useful marker in the diagnosis of epithelioid sarcoma.[40] CA125 has been reportedly often positive in epithelioid sarcoma and negative in reactive and neoplastic conditions that can mimic this tumor.[41] Proximal epithelioid sarcoma is characterized by a diffuse growth pattern (*Figs 35.685* and *35.686*). Tumor cells are mainly epithelioid and mitotic activity is often brisk (*Fig. 35.687*). Focal or extensive rhabdoid change is often present (*Figs 35.688–35.690*).[17] Necrosis seems to be less common than in the ordinary variant.

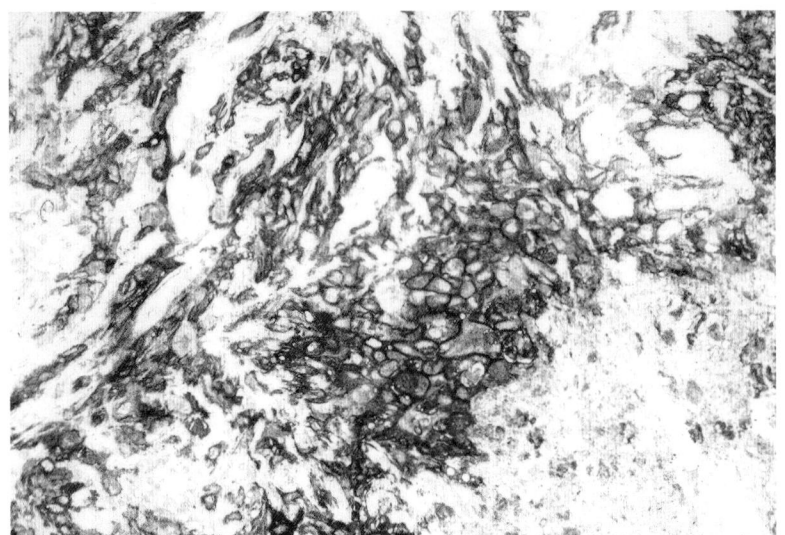

Fig. 35.684
Epithelioid sarcoma: epithelial membrane antigen positivity is usually evident.

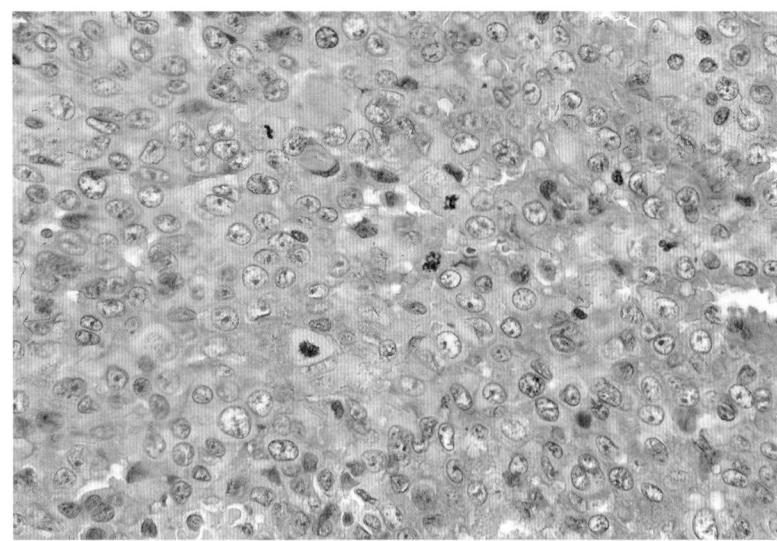

Fig. 35.687
Proximal epithelioid sarcoma: in this example, there is marked mitotic activity.

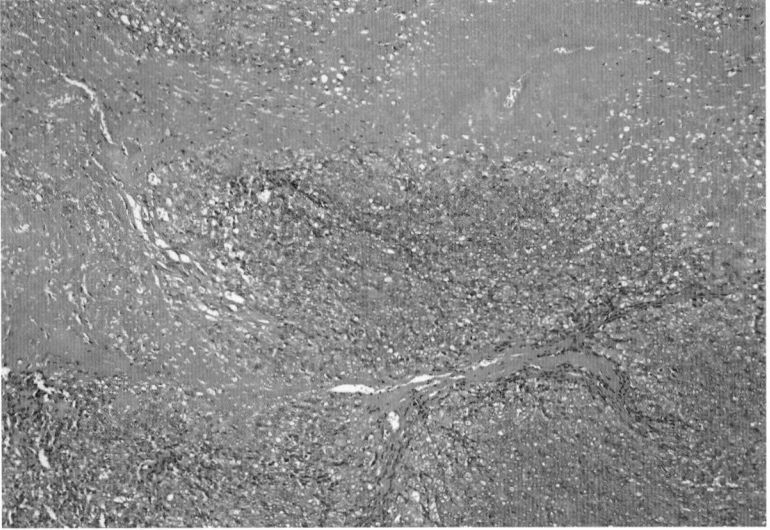

Fig. 35.685
Proximal epithelioid sarcoma: the tumor is characterized by a diffuse cellular infiltrate with widespread necrosis.

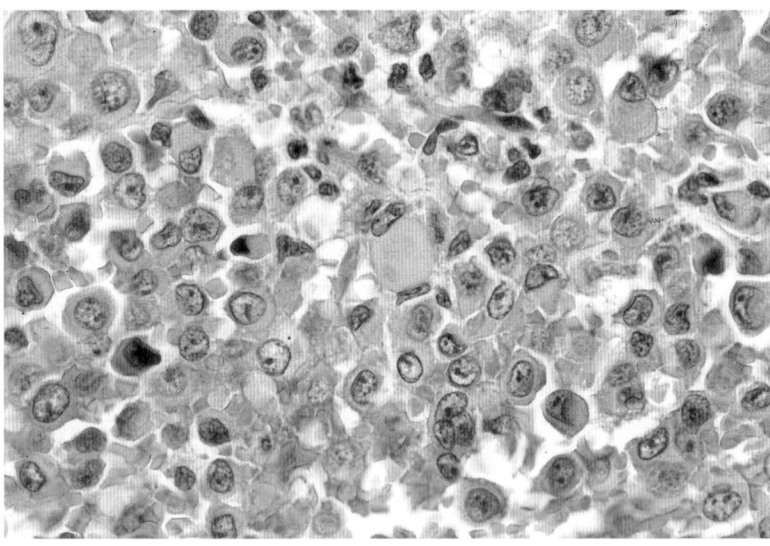

Fig. 35.688
Proximal epithelioid sarcoma: rhabdoid inclusions, as seen in the center of the field, are often present.

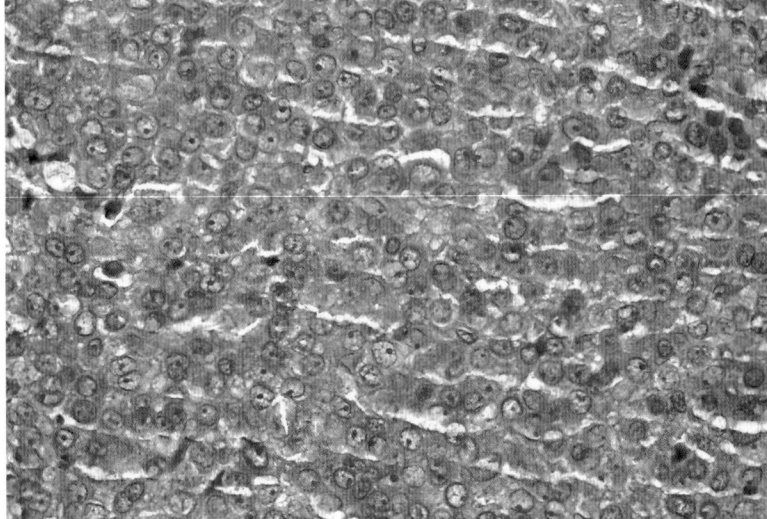

Fig. 35.686
Proximal epithelioid sarcoma: the tumor cells are epithelioid with eosinophilic cytoplasm and round vesicular nuclei containing conspicuous nucleoli.

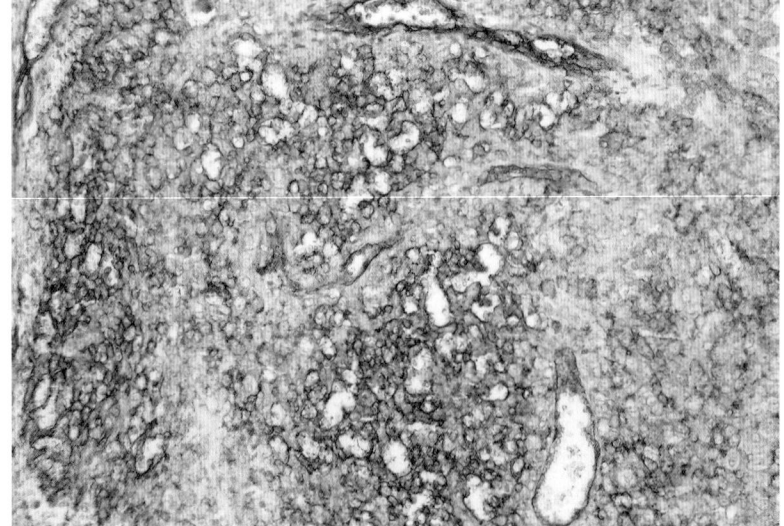

Fig. 35.689
Proximal epithelioid sarcoma: the tumor cells are positive for keratin (AE1/AE3).

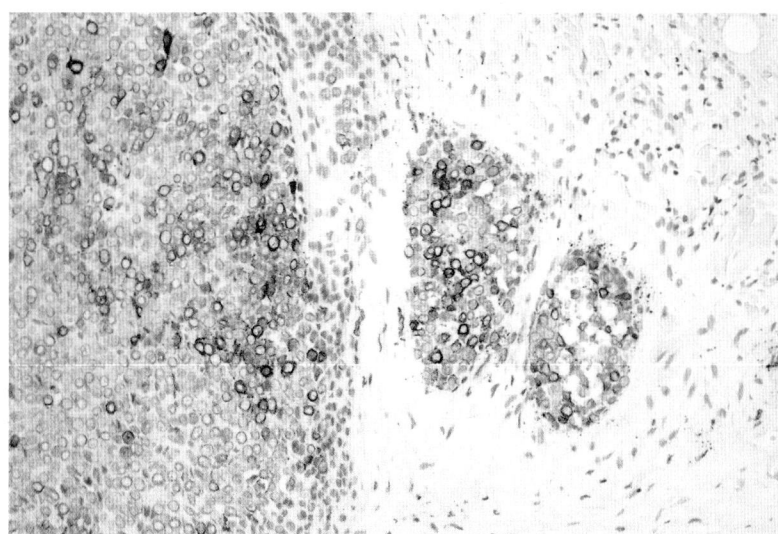

Fig. 35.690
Proximal epithelioid sarcoma: CD34 is also expressed in this example.

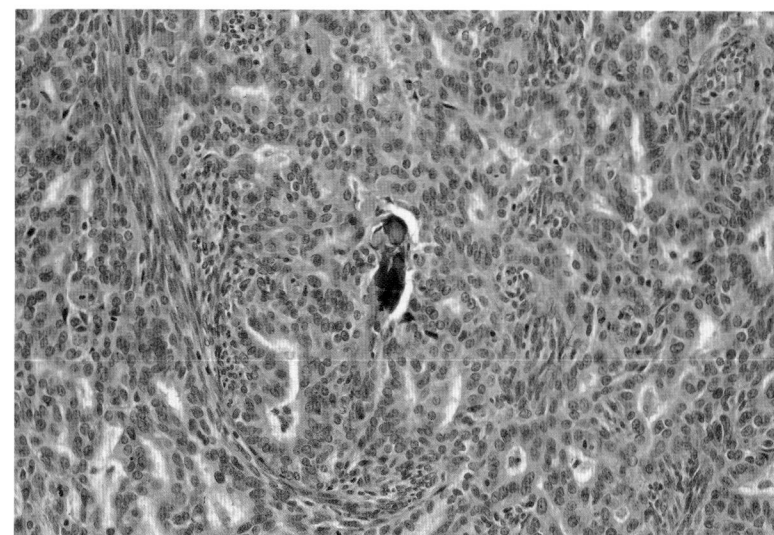

Fig. 35.691
Synovial sarcoma: this field shows the characteristic biphasic population of spindle cells and glandular spaces.

Ultrastructural studies show that the epithelioid tumor cells contain well-formed desmosome-like junctions and aggregates of intermediate filaments, often in a paranuclear location.[35] In a case of proximal-type epithelioid sarcoma immunoelectron microscopy demonstrated keratin filaments but not vimentin, suggesting a closer relation to epithelial cells than to mesenchymal cells.[42]

Differential diagnosis

The distinctive histologic features in an appropriate clinical setting usually prevent diagnostic confusion. Lack of awareness of this entity may lead to the mistaken diagnosis of necrotic metastatic carcinoma or a granulomatous inflammatory lesion. Distinction from epithelioid hemangioendothelioma or angiosarcoma can be difficult because often in epithelioid sarcoma there are pseudovascular clefts and focal cytoplasmic vacuolation. However, cells in the former tend to grow in cords, at least focally, and are often larger; they stain positively for endothelial markers and are frequently keratin positive. Malignant rhabdoid tumor shows many cells with intracytoplasmic inclusions, and although immunohistochemically the tumor cells are positive for epithelial markers, they also usually show positivity for other markers, indicating divergent differentiation. Furthermore, rhabdoid tumors have distinctive vesicular nuclei with macronucleoli. Deep granuloma annulare and rheumatoid nodule can mimic epithelioid sarcoma, particularly on low-power examination.[43] However, the former entities show neither cytologic atypia nor mitotic activity, there is absence of necrosis and presence of necrobiosis with either fibrin or mucin deposition, and histiocytes are positive for CD68 and negative for keratin and CD34.[44]

Synovial sarcoma

Clinical features

Synovial sarcoma is a relatively common, deep-seated tumor that characteristically arises in the limbs (particularly the legs) of young adults and shows a predilection for males.[1–3] Overall age and anatomical distribution is wide, including truncal and head and neck lesions. The dermis is only exceptionally involved by deep-seated tumors. Primary cutaneous synovial sarcoma is vanishingly rare.[4,5] Cutaneous metastasis of synovial sarcoma are vanishingly rare.[6] A subset of more superficial, minute synovial sarcomas measuring less than 1 cm and with predilection for the hands and feet has been described.[7,8] Histologic features are similar to those of ordinary synovial sarcoma. They seem to have a better prognosis than deep-seated lesions.[7] The name is misleading as cases show no evidence of a tenosynovial origin.

In general, the prognosis is poor, with eventual metastatic spread and death in at least 50% of patients. The tumor tends to metastasize late, and long follow-up is therefore necessary.[9]

Factors that seem to correlate with prognosis include age, size of the tumor, histologic features, stage, tumor grade, and molecular alterations.[10–21] Children and adolescents have better prognosis than adults, and tumors presenting on the limbs have better behavior than those arising on the head and neck. Histologic features associated with better prognosis proportion of poorly differentiated tumor (more than 20%), size less than 5 cm in diameter (minute synovial sarcomas have excellent prognosis), less than 5 mitoses in 1.7 mm^2 and absence of necrosis.[7,10] NY-ESO-1expression is useful to identify cases for immunotherapy targeted therapy.[11,12]

Pathogenesis and histologic features

Most cases of synovial sarcoma including monophasic and biphasic variants show a balanced t(X;18)(p11;q11) which fuses either SSX1, SSX2 or very rarely SSX4, situated together on the X chromosome, with SS18 (previously termed SYT). A t(X;20)(p11;q13) resulting in SS18L1-SSX1 fusion has also been documented.[22–24] Involvement of SSX1 is more common in biphasic tumors while any of the three can be involved in the monophasic form.[25] The prognostic value of the different fusion types is debated, but is likely small.[26–29]

When biphasic, these tumors usually have a distinctive appearance typified by an undifferentiated spindled cell component with tapering nuclei admixed with well-formed glandular spaces lined by tall columnar PAS-positive, mucin-secreting epithelium (Figs 35.691–35.693). The glandular component very rarely shows apocrine differentiation, and in superficial tumors, this may lead to a diagnosis of carcinosarcoma.[6] The relative proportions of the spindled cell and glandular components vary from tumor to tumor and most cases have a monophasic spindle cell appearance (Figs 35.694–35.696). A hemangiopericytoma-like vascular pattern and calcification are common findings, as is the presence of wiry stromal collagen and mast cells.

The glandular spaces and some of the adjacent spindled cells stain positively for epithelial markers, including keratin and EMA (Fig. 35.697).[30,31] The markers, especially EMA, are also usually positive, albeit focally, in the monophasic variant. These findings usually allow distinction from malignant schwannoma and fibrosarcoma, the latter now being regarded as extremely rare. Focal positivity for S100 protein and CD99 may also be seen.[32,33] Nuclear expression of the immunohistochemical marker TLE1 identified in a synovial sarcoma gene expression study appears to be specific and can be helpful.[34–37] Reduced immunohistochemical expression of INI1 (encoded by SMARCB1) is a helpful diagnostic feature.[38–40] This results from the SS18-SSX fusion protein perturbing the SWI/SNF BAF complex, a multiprotein complex that includes INI1.[41,42]

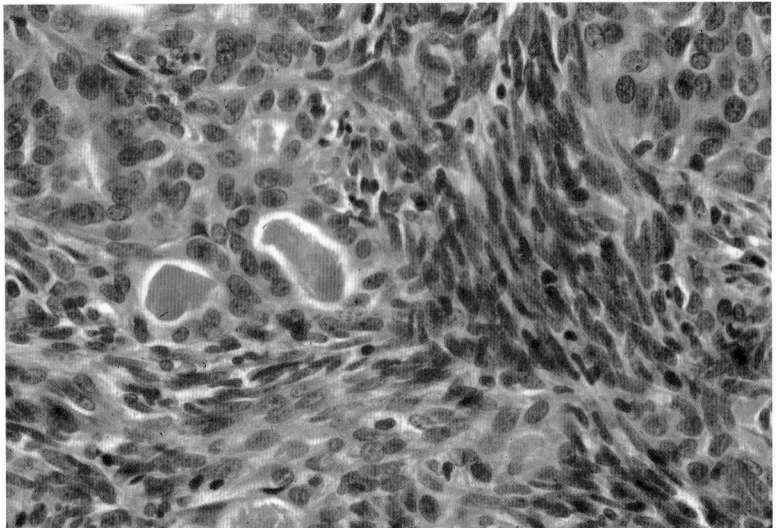

Fig. 35.692
Synovial sarcoma: the glandular spaces contain eosinophilic material.

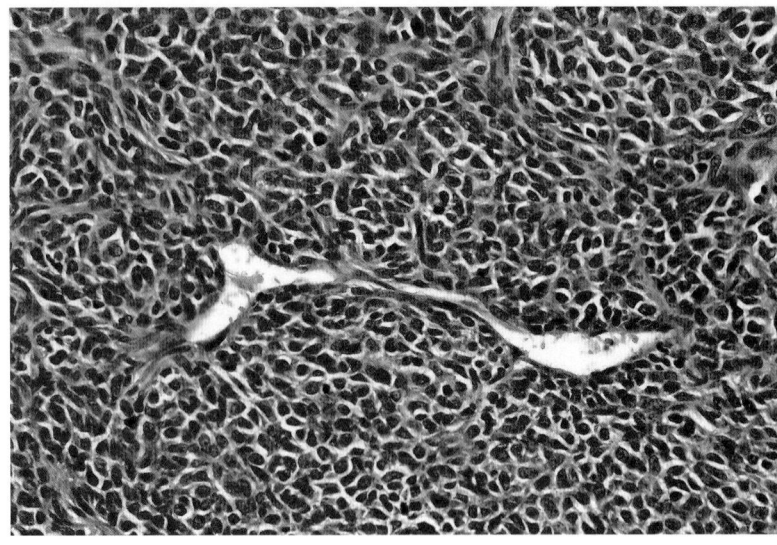

Fig. 35.695
Synovial sarcoma: high-power view showing hyperchromatic tumor cells with indistinct cytoplasm.

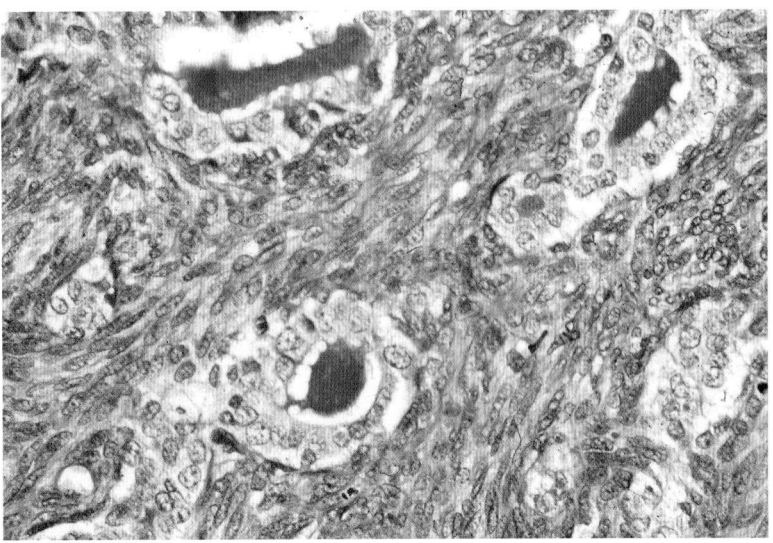

Fig. 35.693
Synovial sarcoma: the secretion is diastase–PAS positive.

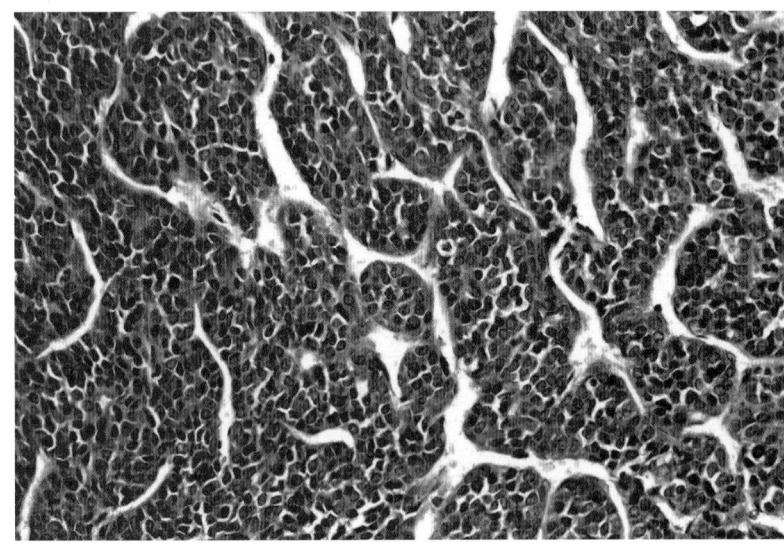

Fig. 35.696
Synovial sarcoma: this example highlights the vascular pattern.

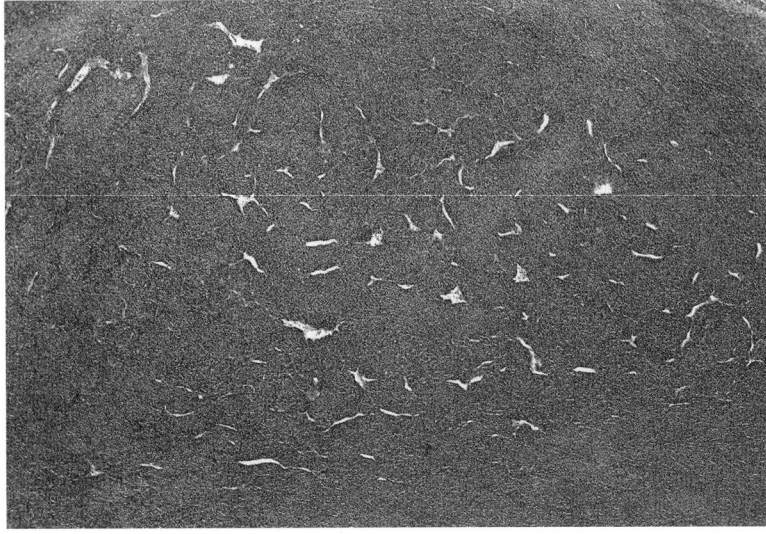

Fig. 35.694
Synovial sarcoma: low-power view of a monophasic example showing the characteristic hemangiopericytomatous blood vessels.

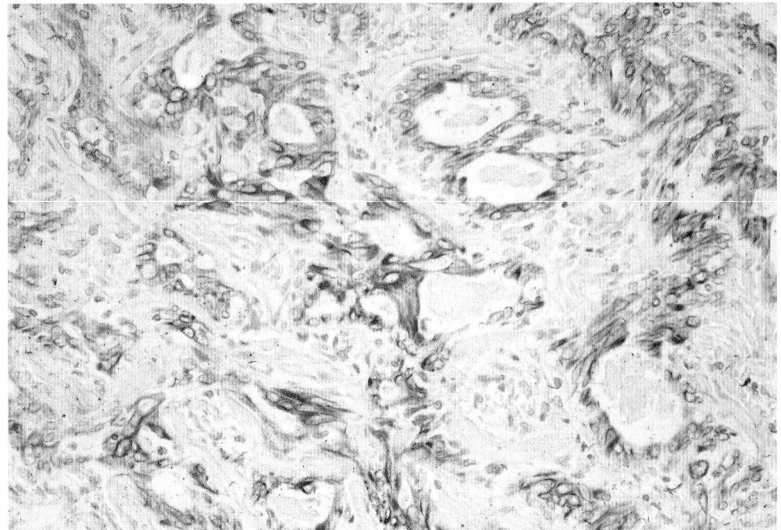

Fig. 35.697
Synovial sarcoma: the glandular component expresses keratin.

Alveolar soft part sarcoma

Clinical features

Alveolar soft part sarcoma is an extremely rare neoplasm that invariably arises in deep soft tissues and is therefore very infrequently encountered in dermatological practice.[1-5] Cutaneous metastases are, however, occasionally seen.[6-8] It presents in young adults, shows a slight predilection for females and arises most often in the extremities. The disease course can be relatively indolent, but the long-term prognosis is very poor.[3-5,7,9,10]

Pathogenesis and histologic features

Alveolar soft part sarcoma is associated with an unbalanced translocation der(17)t(X;17)(p11;q25) which fuses *TFE3* and *ASPSCR1* (*ASPL*) in virtually all cases.[7,11,12] This same translocation is present in a subset of pediatric renal tumors, though it tends to be balanced and *TFE3* is more often substituted by *TFEB*.[13-16]

Characteristically situated within skeletal muscle, this tumor is composed of large round or oval cells with eosinophilic granular cytoplasm and hyperchromatic nuclei arranged in a distinctive alveolar pattern (*Figs 35.698* and *35.699*). Some cases have an organoid pattern reminiscent of paraganglioma. Vascularity is high and vascular invasion is common. According to a study, alveolar soft part sarcoma follows an 'invasion-independent' mechanism of metastasis whereby tumor cells are shed into the circulation completely enveloped by endothelial cells.[17]

The morphological diagnostic sine qua non is the presence of intracytoplasmic PAS-positive, diastase-resistant crystals (*Fig. 35.700*) shown to be composed of monocarboxylate transporter 1 and CD147.[18] These can sometimes be difficult to demonstrate.[6] Although it has been suggested that the line of differentiation is muscular, results from different studies are not consistent. Tumors are sometimes positive for desmin and MyoD1 (often cytoplasmic and thus not meaningful) but are negative for myogenin (*Fig. 35.701*).[19-22] Immunohistochemistry demonstrating nuclear TFE3 expression is diagnostically helpful.[23-26] Intriguing for a mesenchymal malignancy, vimentin expression is absent in the great majority of cases.[27]

The crystals usually obviate the necessity of any differential diagnosis when they can be unequivocally demonstrated, but occasional cases may need to be distinguished from metastatic renal cell carcinoma or granular cell tumor (*Fig. 35.702*).

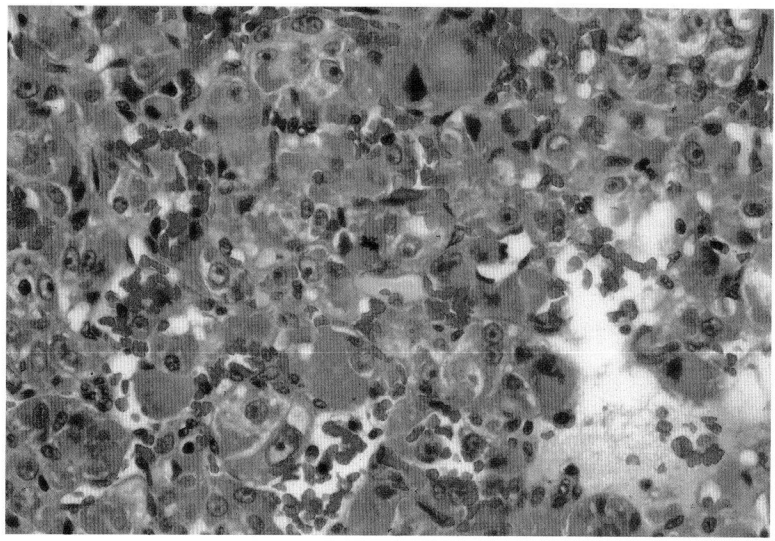

Fig. 35.699
Alveolar soft part sarcoma: the tumor cells have abundant eosinophilic cytoplasm and vesicular nuclei with large eosinophilic nucleoli. Rhabdoid forms are present.

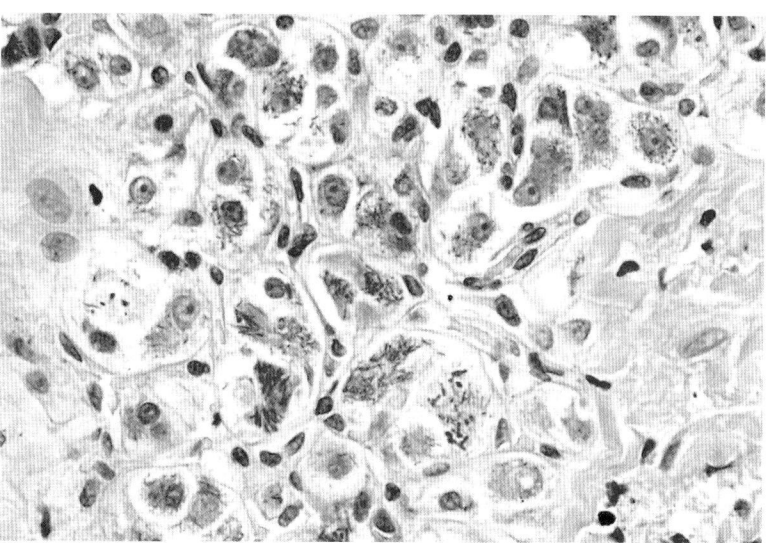

Fig. 35.700
Alveolar soft part sarcoma: periodic acid-Schiff-positive, diastase-resistant intracytoplasmic needle-shaped crystalline inclusions are a distinctive feature.

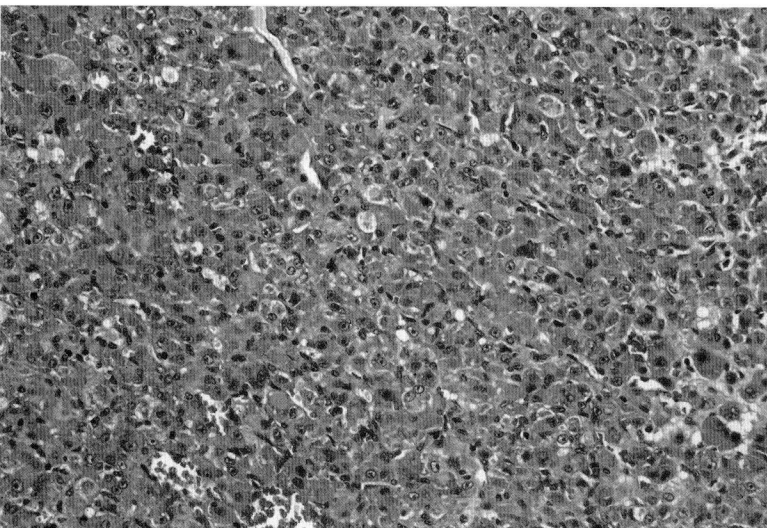

Fig. 35.698
Alveolar soft part sarcoma: this is a very rare example of a cutaneous metastasis.

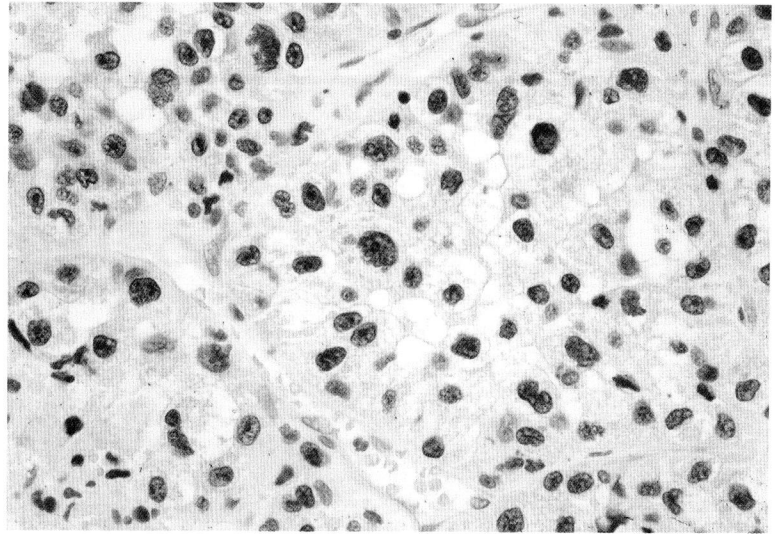

Fig. 35.701
Alveolar soft part sarcoma: there is strong nuclear expression of TFE3.

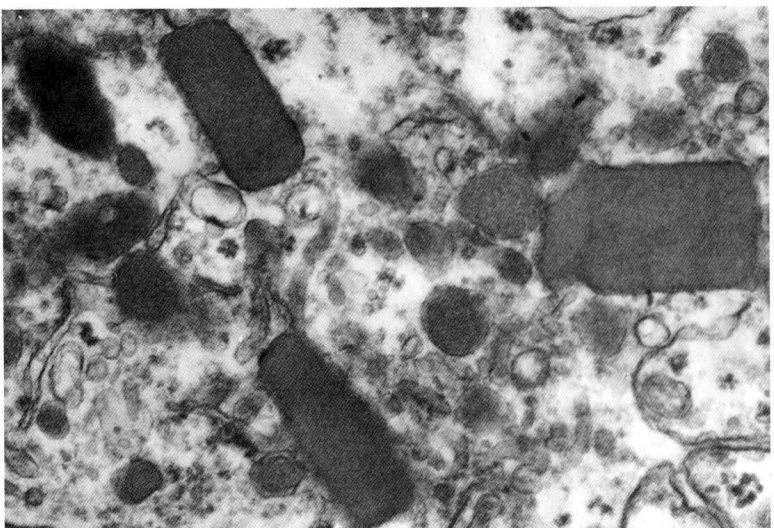

Fig. 35.702
Alveolar soft part sarcoma: characteristic partially lamellated inclusions are seen on electron microscopy. By courtesy of Nelson Ordonez MD, UT-MD Anderson Cancer Centre, Houston, Texas.

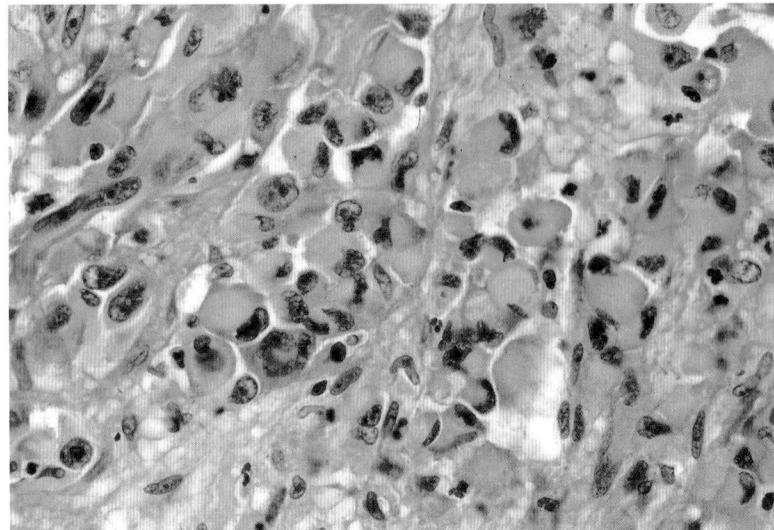

Fig. 35.703
Extrarenal rhabdoid tumor: this tumor, showing striking rhabdoid inclusions, proved to be a metastatic melanoma.

Extrarenal rhabdoid tumor

Clinical features

Extrarenal rhabdoid tumor represents a group of heterogeneous lesions that presents in almost any organ including the skin.[1–14] Most cases arise almost exclusively in infants and children, with a wide anatomical distribution (mainly the neck and paraspinal region), and the clinical course is almost invariably fatal. The best chance of longer survival is in patients with localized disease.[4] Tumors may develop in the fetus and some familial cases have been documented.[5–9,12,14]

Pathogenesis and histologic features

Cytogenetic analysis has demonstrated mutations in the hSNF5/INI1 (SMARCB1) gene located in chromosome 22q11.2.[15–18] Compared with epithelioid sarcoma with complex genomic alterations and SMARCB1 loss, rhabdoid tumor has a simple genome.[19,20]

Histologically, the tumors share the presence of globular hyaline cytoplasmic inclusions, vesicular nuclei and prominent nucleoli (Figs 35.703 and 35.704). Although the tumor cells are usually epithelioid, they vary in size and shape. The growth pattern of different tumors is not consistent and in some lesions small round blue cells may be prominent.

Immunohistochemically, the tumor cells are usually positive for cytokeratin and EMA, but positivity for a variety of other markers indicating divergent differentiation is common.[1] The relationship to their renal counterparts is uncertain as loss of nuclear INI1 expression is seen in both and can be helpful diagnostically.[21–23] Loss of INI1 is also seen in epithelioid sarcoma.[24] In addition, loss of INI1 may be seen in a variety of tumors including a subset of myxoid chondrosarcomas, synovial sarcomas, a subset

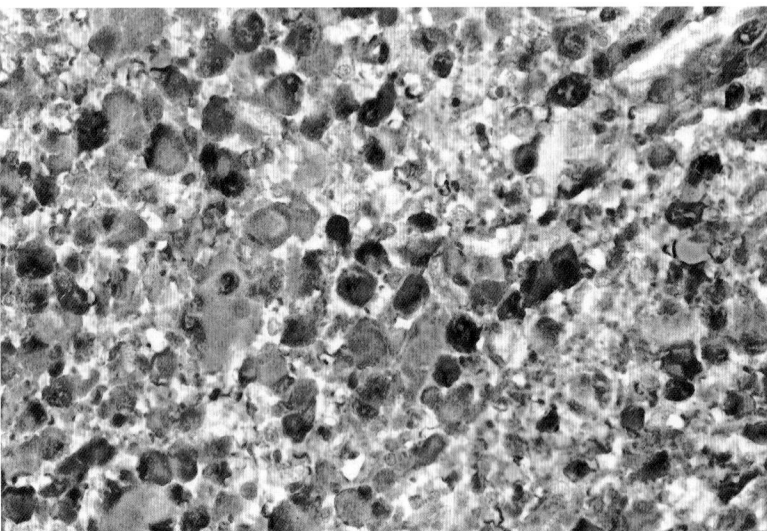

Fig. 35.704
Rhabdoid melanoma: the tumor cells were positive for S100 protein and HMB-45.

of soft tissue myoepithelial carcinomas and in epithelioid malignant peripheral nerve sheath tumor.[25,26] The schwannomas in sporadic and familial schwannomatosis show loss of expression in a subpopulation of the neoplastic Schwann cells.[25]

Secondary EWSR1 gene abnormalities have been reported in SMARCB1 deficient tumors with 22q11~12 regional deletions, including a case of extrarenal rhabdoid tumor so FISH results should be interpreted with caution.[27]

CUTANEOUS METASTASIS OF SARCOMAS

Sarcomas metastatic to the skin are rare but represent an important source of diagnostic confusion.[1–36] Usually, they occur as a late event but occasionally represent the first manifestation of the disease. Interestingly, metastatic sarcomas have predilection for the scalp sharing this feature with metastatic carcinomas. The chest, face, and arm and any other cutaneous site may rarely be affected.

The most common type of metastatic sarcoma is by far leiomyosarcoma.[2,8,12,15,20,24–26,31,34] Cutaneous metastatic leiomyosarcomas are usually much more pleomorphic than primary cutaneous dermal leiomyosarcomas

(atypical dermal smooth muscle tumor). Other sarcomas reported metastasizing to the skin include osteosarcoma,[5,6,11,13,14,17,22] angiosarcoma (especially epithelioid),[3,19,26,28] Ewing sarcoma,[4,7] chondrosarcoma,[9,30] rhabdomyosarcoma,[21,36] undifferentiated pleomorphic sarcoma,[26,33] alveolar soft part sarcoma,[16] cardiac sarcoma,[29] pleomorphic liposarcoma,[35] and gastrointestinal stromal tumor (GIST).[37]

Access **ExpertConsult.com** for the complete list of references

Animal models of skin disease

CHAPTER 36

John P. Sundberg, Lloyd E. King, Jr.,
Marcus Bosenberg, Qiaoli Li, Jouni Uitto,
Michael V. Wiles and C. Herbert Pratt

See
www.expertconsult.com
for references and
additional meterial

Introduction 1895

One gene, one disease 1896

Comparative anatomy of the human and
     mouse skin and adnexa 1896

Specialized techniques for mouse skin 1898

Creation of models of human disease 1898

Examples of mouse models for human skin
     in health and disease 1899

Infectious diseases 1900
Botryomycosis 1900
Mouse papillomaviruses 1901

Vascular changes in the skin 1901

Genetic-based skin diseases 1901

Coat color genetics 1901

A locus 1903

B locus 1904

C locus 1904

D locus 1904

P locus 1904

Mouse models of melanoma 1905

Carcinogen-induced melanoma 1905

Genetically engineered mouse melanoma
     models 1905
Transgenic approaches 1905
Conditional cre-lox models 1905

Syngeneic mouse melanoma models 1906

Humanized mouse melanoma models 1906

Anhidrotic ectodermal dysplasia: mouse
     models that helped define the
     receptor-ligand concept 1906

Hairless, rhino, papular atrichia and
     genocopies 1907

Alopecia areata 1909

Psoriasiform mouse models 1909

Xenographs: transplanting tissues from
     humans to mice 1909

Currently missing mouse models of human
     skin pathology 1911

Zebrafish as a model system to study skin
     biology and pathology 1911

Zebrafish skin development 1912

The zebrafish genome and genetic
     manipulation 1912
The zebrafish genome 1912
Forward genetics 1912
Morpholino-based knockdown of gene
     expression 1913
Genome editing in zebrafish 1913

Application of the zebrafish model for skin
     research 1913
Heritable skin disorders 1913
Wound healing and re-epithelialization 1914
Melanoma and pigmentation 1914
Small molecule and drug screening 1914

Summary 1915

Resources 1916
Accessing and using websites for mouse
     information 1916
Accessing and using websites for zebrafish
     information 1916

Introduction

The laboratory mouse has long been used as a biomedical tool. Over the past 50 years, the mouse has transformed into the standard model to study and compare their pathophysiology and genetics to a wide variety of human skin diseases and many others. These mouse models were found for many decades as naturally occurring (spontaneous), radiation, or chemical mutagen-induced genetic-based diseases. With the advent of transgenesis (moving genes from one species to another or overexpressing a gene) during the late 1970s, to gene targeted (so-called knockout) technology in the late 1980s, then inducible models, where genes could be selectively turned on or off with or without markers in the late 1990s and early 2000s, to the current state-of-the-art endonuclease modified models, that offer the possibilities of molecular correction of the germ line for genetic-based diseases, the laboratory mouse has become a singular utilitarian biological tool and powerful dermatology surrogate. Information on methods to create these mice is available elsewhere[1-4] but is summarized below. Continuing breakthroughs utilizing these mouse models have provided enlightenment on the pathogenesis of countless diseases of all organ systems including the skin and adnexa. However, mice are not the only model organism available. The zebrafish has also provided a great deal of basic information on development and genetic-based diseases of the skin. While anatomically different from the mouse, it nevertheless provides a number of advantages including serving as a second commonly used vertebrate species for genetic-based studies speed of production. This chapter provides an overview of a few of the constantly expanding types of mouse and zebrafish models for human skin diseases that exist and the context of how they can be used to dissect complex molecular pathways. While genetically engineered mice (GEMs) have opened up research to almost anyone to create and phenotype mice with targeted mutations, allowing partially or complete gene inactivation, these technologies have also caused many to question if mice can accurately model human diseases, as these types of mutations, total loss of function of a gene and the protein it codes for, are rarely found in humans. True null (total deficiency of protein production) mutations do occur naturally in humans, as in mice, but these mutations often result in embryonic lethality and fetal resorption, so no offspring are actually born to be analyzed. This has been one of the findings in the Knockout Mouse Project (KOMP), where over 20% of the null mutations result in embryonic lethality.[5] The KOMP mice are inbred while most humans are not, hence the offspring are more likely to show a lethal phenotype. Spontaneous mutations in mice often very accurately recapitulate human diseases and, in a number of cases, have provided the knowledge to correctly define new human diseases. For example, the rhinoceros (now called the rhino) mouse (a severe allele of hairless) was reported in 1859, the human homolog in 1954, and the correlation of the two in 1989.[6,7] The lanceolate hair mutant mouse (Lah), first reported in 1996,[8,9] led to the discovery of desmoglein 4 (Dsg4) in the mouse and eventually to the novel human disease, localized autosomal recessive hypotrichosis (LAH), the name of which was modified to fit the mouse locus symbol 6 years later.[10] With the advent of the CRISPR/Cas9, investigators can now make precise germline mutations in mice (and other species). When matched with mutations in patients with specific diseases, a similar if not exact duplication of the human mutation (rare variant) can now be created in mice. This duplication can be simply a point mutation in a homologous gene and location to total replacement of the mouse gene or genetic region with a human gene carrying the mutation of interest, i.e., humanization of the mouse genome. As these technologies continue to evolve, increasingly more accurate mouse models recapitulating specific subsets of human diseases will provide increasingly improved outcomes.

The second critical aspect of developing highly accurate mouse models is carefully and comprehensively defining the phenotype (i.e., accurate diagnosis) with comparison to similar human diseases to find the best match. This goes beyond simply evaluating the organ of interest in the mouse model and requires in-depth studies on all other organs in the model. Most mice used in research are inbred, meaning that within a strain all mice are essentially genetically and phenotypically identical except for their sex. This limited genetic diversity within a strain results in a highly reproducible phenotype. Such phenotypes may not represent all aspects of a specific human disease because humans are not, in general, inbred. As such, the wide genetic diversity between most humans impacts the phenotypes of many diseases creating the variability commonly seen among human patients; however, the variety and genetic diversity available in many inbred strains can allow researchers to compensate for the lack of genetic diversity within a single strain. By taking advantage of this knowledge, mouse models are increasingly becoming powerful tools to dissect the modifier genes responsible for subtypes of diseases commonly seen by dermatologists.[11]

One gene, one disease

The one gene, one enzyme hypothesis put forth in the early 1940s by George Beadle was influenced by the results of experiments looking at the inheritance of coat color differences in mice.[1] Over the next few decades, this same theory was proposed for genetic disease in general, whereby a mutation in one gene affects one disease state. Currently, we know that phenotypes, regardless of type, are not usually the result of mutations in single genes, but rather of the interaction of molecular pathways involving multiple gene products. Genes do not act in isolation, but evolved over time to both function and segregate together under natural selection to provide the organism with a related interacting set of alleles. This is illustrated by the existence of genocopies, i.e., an individual whose phenotype or disease diagnosis mimics another determined by a distinct gene or assortment of genes (http://medical-dictionary.thefreedictionary.com/genocopy). By contrast, a phenocopy is an environmentally induced phenotype (i.e., disease) mimicking one usually produced by a specific genotype (http://medical-dictionary.thefreedictionary.com/phenocopy). Laboratory mice are maintained in highly environmentally controlled rooms which can reduce environmental effects (phenocopies). The question is whether a group of interacting mutant alleles causing similar phenotypes (genocopies) is advantageous or deleterious and how to identify the genes and define their function. The mouse is the perfect tool to answer these questions regarding the linkage of genes relating to specific phenotypes. Observing mice within an inbred line allows us to study environmental inputs against a stable genetic background (phenocopies), whereas observing mice across multiple inbred lines allows the discovery of both unique and new combinations of alleles affecting a particular phenotype and molecular pathway (genocopies). Each inbred strain varies, with respect to genetics, and these variations will affect interpretation of the phenotype and more importantly, how the inbred mouse compares to a specific human disease.[2,3] This is known as the 'Cinderella effect', where knowing these differences can help fit the mouse model (like a shoe) on specific backgrounds to a specific form of a human disease.[4]

Comparative anatomy of the human and mouse skin and adnexa

At the gross, microscopic, and molecular levels, the skin, hair, and nails of most mammals, including humans and mice, are fundamentally the same.[1,2] Because of this basic anatomical phylogenetic conservation between mammals, many diseases are also, not surprisingly, very similar. However, when one first compares a mouse with a human more closely, the two species can show clear differences. Similarities and differences between mouse and human skin are summarized in *Table 36.1* and described in greater detail elsewhere.[1,2]

Table 36.1

Comparison of structures and functions of skin and adnexa between humans and mice

Criteria	Human	Mouse
Epidermis of body (thin) skin	Thick (50–100 μm)	Thin (10–15 μm)
Epidermis of thick skin (plantar/palmer surfaces)	Thick (300–400 μm) Palms of hands, soles of feet	Tail (70–80 μm), footpad (150–400 μm), muzzle (20–30 μm), eyelid (50–60 μm)
Hair types: body	Vellus Terminal	Guard Auschene Zigzag Awl
Specialized hair types	Cilia (eyelashes) Eyebrows Pubic Facial (beard, mustache) Axillary Ear hair	Cilia (eyelashes) Vibrissae (specialized somatosensory organ with blood-filled sinus around the muzzle, eyes, and feet) Perianal Tail hair Ear hair (inner and outer pinnae are different)
Emergence of hair	19–21 weeks gestation	5 days postpartum
Hair cycle	Mosaic pattern	Wave pattern of whole body as neonates Wave pattern within zones in adults
Tail and tail hairs	No (no tail)	Yes
Sebaceous glands	Yes	Yes
Modified sebaceous glands	Meibomian glands Ceruminous glands	Meibomian glands Zymbal gland Preputial gland Clitoral gland (in females) Perianal gland (in males)
Eccrine glands	Found on entire body including soles and palms	Limited to footpads
Apocrine sweat glands	Axilla, genitoanal region, ceruminous glands, mammary glands	Mammary glands present in most skin including limbs Mice do not have ceruminous glands or apocrine glands in the dermis of the body skin
Nails	All distal digits	All distal digits

Used with permission.[2]

The skin of the body (or torso) of the mouse, usually referred to as the truncal skin, is very similar to human skin. However, while the epidermis is relatively thick for the first 2 weeks of life, it thins out and remains very thin throughout adulthood. The same layers can be found in the epidermis as in other mammals, the stratum corneum, granulosum, spinosum, and basale from the most superficial layers to the basement membrane. There are no rete ridges in mouse skin. The dermis consists of dense regular collagenous connective tissue. Below the dermis is a layer of white fat (hypodermal fat layer) that varies in thickness with the hair cycle. A layer of skeletal muscle, the panniculus carnosus, is located below the hypodermal fat. The mouse truncal skin has four types of hair follicles (guard, auschene, awl, and zigzag) producing different types of hair shafts (*Fig. 36.1*).[3,4] Whole slide scans of mounted plucked normal mouse truncal hairs can be viewed online (http://eulep.pdn.cam.ac.uk/zoomify/index.php?image=288&mutant=Normal%20Plucked%20Hairs). Guard hairs are very large with long hair follicles that produce a large hair shaft. These large hair shafts extend above all others and also have a sensory function. Auschene and awl hairs are intermediate forms between guard hairs and zigzag, the last of which are most numerous

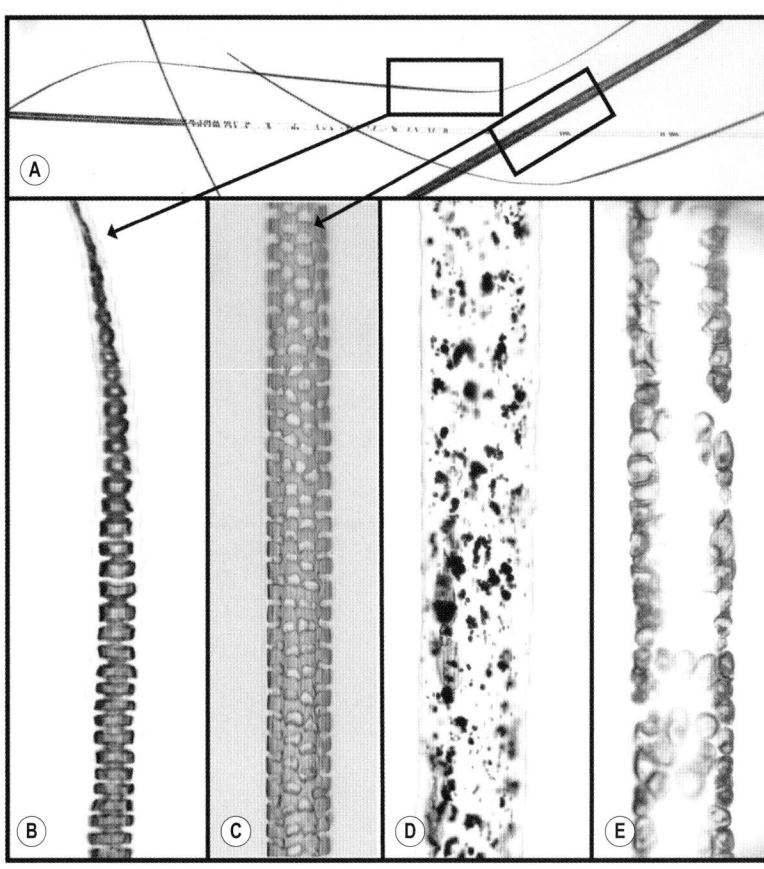

Fig. 36.1
Plucked hair from a normal mouse reveals hair shafts of various sizes and shapes: (**A**) The zigzag underhairs are thin, with a single layer of cells in a septate pattern (**B**) which thin out as the hair shaft flattens and bends (*top of frame*). (**C**) The larger guard and auschene hairs have a complex and multilayered septulated pattern. (**D**) Satin-beige mutant mice lack the septate and septulate patterns (satin mutation, *Foxq1^{sa}*) and have pigment clumping (beige mutation, *Lyst^{bg}*). (**E**) The hair interior defect mutant mice (e, *Soat1^{ald}*) also lack the normal septate and septulate patterns in their hair shafts.

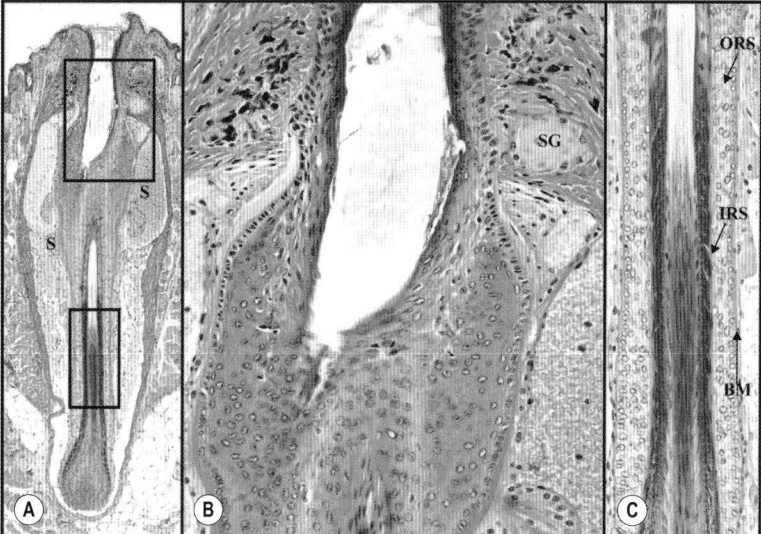

Fig. 36.2
Vibrissa follicles are common in many mammalian species but are not found in humans. These are very large compared to the truncal hair follicles, and have a thick fibrous capsule and blood-filled sinuses (S) that surround an otherwise normal hair follicle (**A**). Boxed areas illustrate the presence of sebaceous glands (SG), (**B**) as well as the inner root sheath (IRS), outer root sheath (ORS), and the basement ('glassy') membrane (BM) (**C**).

and are the underhairs that produce lift and thermal insulation. The structure of the hair shaft types is different. The medulla is well developed in mice and consists of either a single layer of cells in a septate pattern or two or more lateral rows of cells called a septulate pattern (see *Fig. 36.1*).

In addition to the four truncal hair types, mice have a variety of specialized hairs, some with human counterparts and others that are found in other mammals but not in humans. The most notable of these unique mouse hairs are called vibrissae, which are located around the muzzle, above the eyes, and just above the wrist and ankle regions on the legs. Vibrissae are most prominent along the muzzle where they form prominent rows with very long hair shafts, i.e., whiskers. These are large somatosensory organs surrounded by blood-filled sinuses (*Fig. 36.2*).[5–8]

Eyelids have a row of large follicles that produce a thick but short hair shaft, the eyelash (cilia) (*Fig. 36.3A*), which serves as a sensory organ to protect the eye, reduces deposition of airborne particles, and reduces evaporation of the tear film.[9] A row of large modified sebaceous glands (Meibomian glands) have a single duct that empties independent of this follicle at the mucocutaneous junction. This gland produces lipids to cover the cornea and which helps to reduce evaporation.[10]

The mouse nail unit is fundamentally similar to that found in humans except obviously in size and gross appearance. Distinguishing features between the species are the shape of the nail and the presence of an extended hyponychium in the mouse (*Fig. 36.3B*). Human nails form a plate while the mouse nail curves around the distal digit forming an almost tube-like structure. Both species have a proximal nail fold, cuticle, nail matrix containing stem cells, nail bed, nail plate, and hyponychium.[11–15] Gene expression patterns of most keratins are similar. These findings indicate that the mouse nail unit shares major characteristics with the human and overall represents a very similar structure, useful for the investigation of nail diseases and nail biology.[1,16,17]

Like human hands and feet, there is no hair on the footpads in the mouse, the equivalent of the human acral sites of palms and soles (*Fig. 36.3C–D*). The footpad is thicker than the body (truncal) skin and the footpad contains eccrine glands, just like humans. However, mice do not have fingerprints based on scanning electron microscopic studies.[18]

The tail is an anatomic structure not usually found on humans.[19,20] The mouse tail epidermis is thick, relative to the truncal skin, and has a regular arrangement of large follicles that produce wide, short hairs (*Fig. 36.4*). While the tail appears to be without hair in normal adults, careful examination at the gross level reveals there are fine, short hairs present. The follicles grow in triplets, and where the hair shafts emerge the epidermis is thrown into folds producing a scale-like appearance to the skin.

Ear skin in the mouse is also unique and different from human ear skin. The epidermis is thin, as it is on the trunk. However, there are uniform small short hairs and hair follicles on either side of the pinna that are different from truncal hair (*Fig. 36.5*). Ear hair shafts are very short, have a short anagen stage, and have very prolonged telogen stage. As such, ear hairs are rarely seen in anagen in histologic sections.

Hair follicles cycle in mice as they do in humans (*Fig. 36.6*); however, a major difference is that in mice the hair cycles in an anterior to posterior (A–P or head to tail) direction throughout life, in what has been described as a wave pattern as opposed to a mosaic pattern which occurs in humans. In adult mice, this wave becomes more regional but continues in an A–P direction.[21–23] This characteristic of mouse skin provides a research advantage in that one can see most, if not all, of the stages of the hair cycle in one histologic section if carefully selected. Another difference is that anagen is a relatively short part of the cycle with adult mouse follicles remaining in telogen for long periods.

Pigmentation in mice is usually not found in the interfollicular epidermis in most inbred strains of mice, but rather it is located primarily within the anagen hair follicles. This enables one to follow the hair cycle in an adult pigmented mouse by simply shaving them and watching the skin color change from pink (telogen) to light gray (early anagen) to dark gray (late anagen).[24]

The variation in skin and hair follicles at these different anatomic sites are often considered minor variations in the same anatomical structures; however, transcriptome studies of skin biopsied from different anatomic sites revealed that in mice and humans these sites are fundamentally different

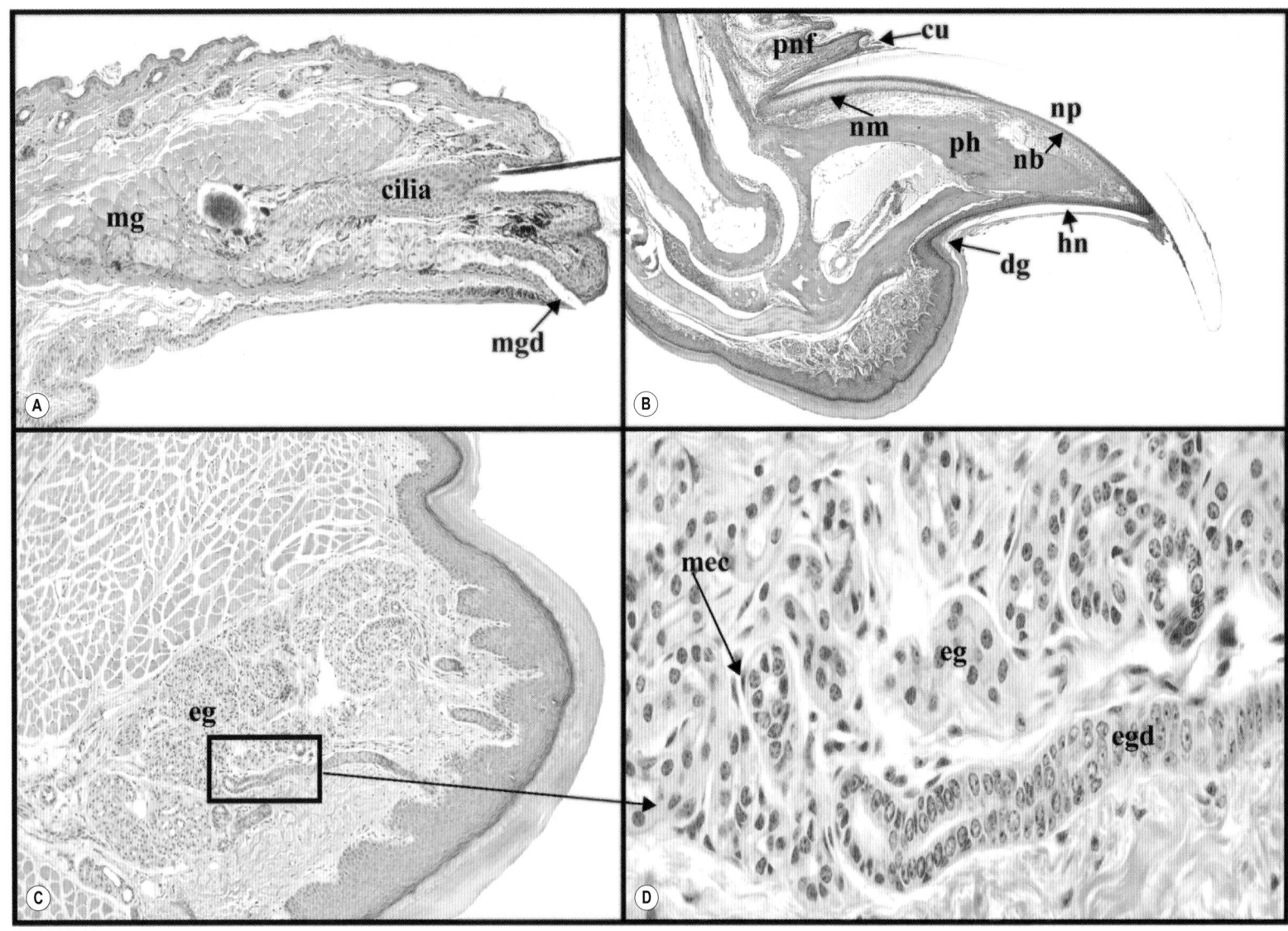

Fig. 36.3
(**A**) The eyelid has a row of large hair follicles, eyelashes (cilia) with an adjacent large modified sebaceous gland with a separate duct that empties at the mucocutaneous junction (mg, Meibomian gland; mgd, Meibomian gland duct). (**B**) Nail unit consists of the proximal nail fold (pnf), cuticle (cu), nail matrix (nm), nail plate (np), nail bed (nb), hyponychium (hn), and distal groove (dg). (**C**) The footpad has an eccrine gland (eg) and a duct that penetrates the overlying epidermis (boxed area). (**D**) Higher magnification of the boxed area in part 'C' demonstrates the cytological differences of the myoepithelial cells (mec), eccrine gland acini (eg), and eccrine gland duct (egd).

organs.[25,26] This observation is validated by the fact that several single gene mutations in mice result in skin disease at very specific anatomic sites. For example, the chronic proliferative dermatitis mutant mouse (*Sharpin^cpdm*) results in a psoriasiform dermatitis of the dorsal and ventral trunk, yet the ears, tail, and distal extremities are spared.[27] Modified sebaceous glands, such as the preputial or clitoral glands (structures not found in humans), may be completely missing in some mutant mice, such as *Hoxd13^spdh* mutant mice,[28] while all other sebaceous and modified sebaceous glands are unaffected.

Specialized techniques for mouse skin

Methods for analyzing the skin are largely applicable to all species of mammals and are well described specifically for the mouse elsewhere.[1-4] One common question is what is the best fixative for mouse tissues for histopathology? That which you are most familiar with is the best answer, as any artifacts will be similar to what you are used to. Many use neutral buffered 10% formalin, which is quite effective for mouse tissue as it is for human tissues. However, a less commonly used fixative, Fekete acid-alcohol-formalin,[5] used as an overnight fixative followed by storage in 70% ethanol, provides highly reproducible results with the added benefit of better epitope retention for immunohistochemistry than most commonly used fixatives,

including neutral buffered formalin.[6] Specific assays of value for mouse skin focus on the hair cycle. As mentioned above, the hair shaft pigmentation reflects the anagen stage of the hair cycle. This can be used as a tool to study the effects on the hair cycle of drugs or a genetic mutation by shaving the mice and watching the pink skin (telogen) change to pigmented skin (anagen).[7] The hair cycle can also be induced by wax stripping, using the same tools as humans used for cosmetic depilation.[8]

Creation of models of human disease

As detailed in *Table 36.1*, the mouse shares many characteristics with humans, making them powerful models for many human disorders. Furthermore, their use has been greatly extended in recent years with the development of genetic modification technologies allowing modification of the murine genome to be almost routine.[1] However, it is with the advent of human genome-wide association studies (GWAS) and modern sequencing methodologies allowing the identification of associated genetic variants correlating with human disease that has really empowered the mouse model in genetic research.[2,3] When these new systems are combined, i.e., human GWAS putative causal links with the ability to make similar genetic lesions in mice, it is now possible to test the genetic causal correlation and make available mouse models which presents similar disease phenotypes.[4,5] With

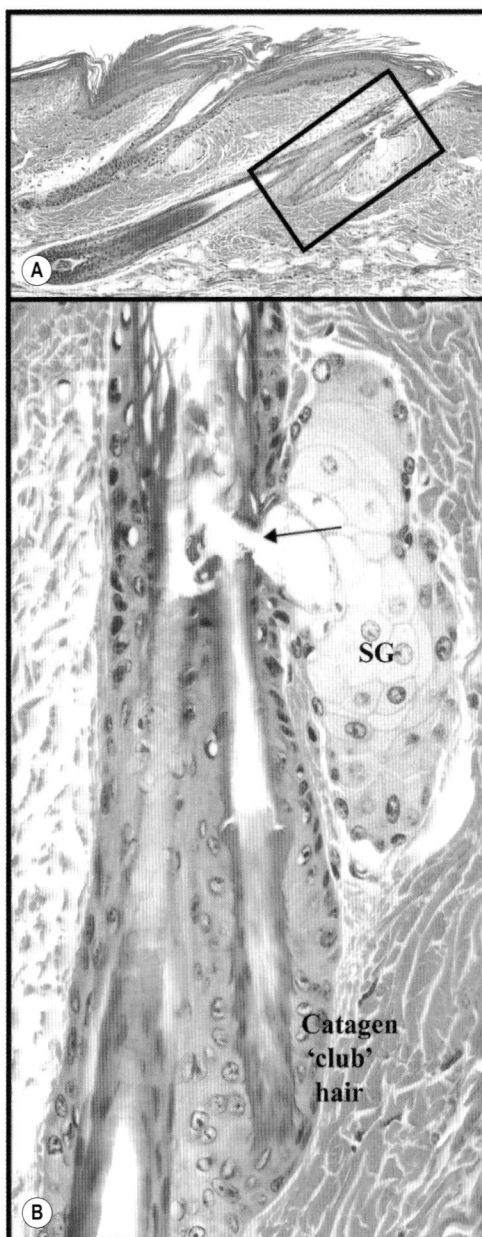

Fig. 36.4
Tail skin has large hair follicles: (**A**) this one being in late anagen. The overlying epidermis is normally thick and more cornified when compared to the truncal skin. (**B**) The boxed area shows the sebaceous gland (SG) and its duct (*arrow*) where the inner root sheath degrades allowing the hair shaft to emerge. The club hair, remnant of the last hair cycle, is pushed to the side when the new hair follicle develops.

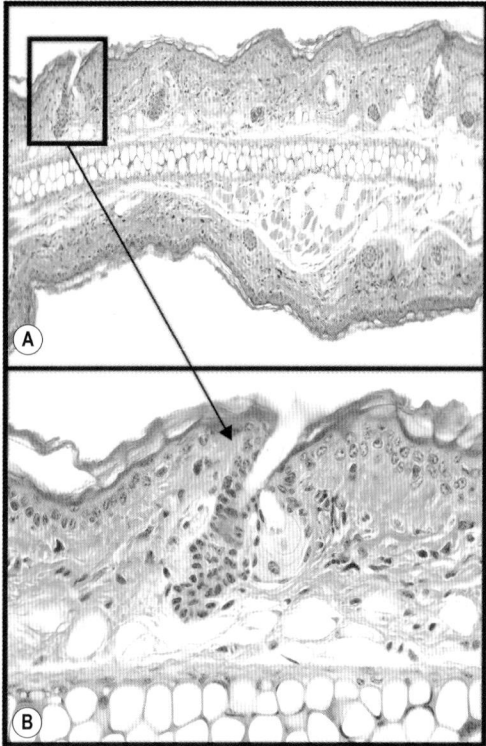

Fig. 36.5
Normal ear skin has small follicles in prolonged telogen stage. Note the auricular cartilage extending down the middle of the tissue (A). Enlargement of boxed area shows detail of the epidermis, telogen hair follicle, and auricular cartilage (B).

are created within a gene, they often lead to disruptive mutations ranging from hypomorphic to true null alleles. Upon transfer of microinjected zygotes into pseudopregnant animals, offspring are born with targeted indels at efficiencies often approaching 100% (M.V. Wiles, personal observations). More often with GWAS and other disease modeling strategies, a precision nucleotide change is desired to recapitulate a human mutation – e.g., defined, exact base change(s). Such genetic editing changes can be achieved using CRISPR/Cas9 mediated homology directed repair (HDR). For this, a zygote microinjection, consisting of approximately 100 to 200 oligonucleotide donors composed of 1–50 nucleotides of novel desired base changes, flanked by sequences homologs to the targeted region, is also introduced. Such donor oligonucleotides are often perfectly incorporated into the targeted region by HDR leading to precise genetic changes, e.g., changing a single amino acid in a gene reflecting a putative disease associated change in humans.[7,9]

As with all these approaches, there is always the wish for more complicated modifications, e.g., conditional KOs where the targeted region is flanked by LoxP sites precision insertion of reporter constructs, partial or even complete humanization of entire genes.[12–14] All of these are possible, although as the complexity and/or scale of the required genetic modifications increase so does the difficulty of achieving success.

A key aspect of using targeted nuclease methods, which is often not fully appreciated, is that it is now relatively simple to build a mouse model on any or even multiple genetic backgrounds. This opens exploration of the impact of genetic background (variation) on the penetrance of a trait. Additionally, established models can now be sequentially modified leading to a continual refinement of models and thus more sophisticated analysis.[15]

Examples of mouse models for human skin in health and disease

As with human skin diseases, there are large numbers of mouse skin diseases that occur naturally as well as those found in large-scale mutagenesis projects, be they genetically engineered (KOMP) or chemical mutagenesis methods. Mouse colonies are maintained in highly controlled environments behind barriers that minimize exposure to infectious diseases. A few examples of infectious diseases are presented. Genetic-based skin diseases, the

regard to approaches to make these precise genetic modifications, the key breakthrough leading to rapid, economic modification of mice (and other species including zebrafish) was the development of the targeting nucleases ZFN (zinc finger nuclease) and TALEN (transcription activator-like effector nuclease), with a major further reduction in cost and complexity with the more recent harnessing of the CRISPR/Cas9 system.[6–8]

At the time of writing, the method of choice in creating genetically modified mice is based on using CRISPR/Cas9. The approach is executed directly in zygotes derived from any desired mouse background.[9–11] The method uses a guide RNA (gRNA) that carries 17–20 base pairs with sequence homology to the desired genomic target. Upon introduction of the gRNA plus Cas9, generally by microinjection directly into zygotes, a complex forms leading to a double-stranded cut in the genomic DNA at the target site(s). The zygote then instigates a repair mechanism using, by an inherently error prone process, nonhomologs end joining (NHEJ) commonly leading to insertions or deletions (indels) of +1 to −1–10's of nucleotides at this region. If such indels

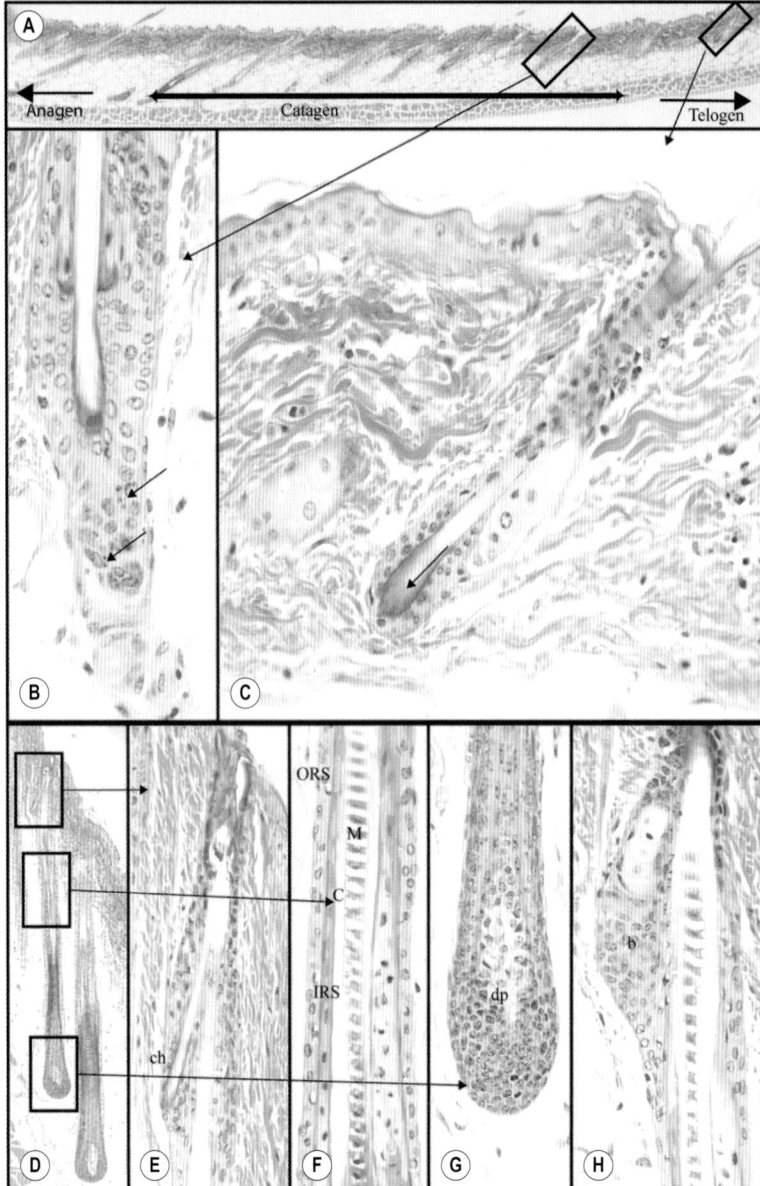

Fig. 36.6

B6(Cg)-*Tyr^c2J*/J (albino or a white black mouse) hair cycle in one section (**A**). Anagen (*left*) transitions to catagen (**B**, *middle*) to telogen (**C**, *right*). Note the marked apoptosis (*arrows*) below the club hair and redundancy of the contracting basement membrane of the catagen follicle (**B**). Telogen hair has the short residual hair club (*arrow*, **C**). Late anagen stage hair follicles (**D**). Old club hair (ch) is not pushed out by the new hair shaft but rather is pushed to the side (**E**). (**F**) Mid-level of the follicle illustrates the hair medulla (M), hair shaft cuticle (C), inner root sheath (IRS), and outer root sheath (ORS, C). Hair bulb and dermal papilla (dp, **G**). Another anagen stage follicle at a different angle illustrates the sebaceous gland and underlying bulge (b, **H**) which contains the hair follicle stem cells.

most common types of models, can be simple single gene Mendelian traits (such as coat color) or complex polygenic traits. Those with similar phenotypes due to mutations in different genes are often caused by genes that function in the same molecular pathway. As such, rather than present an encyclopedic listing of models, representative ones that fall into known or novel and evolving pathways that illustrate the power of mouse models to unravel the complexities of skin disease in mammals, which includes humans, are presented.

Infectious diseases

Laboratory mice today are usually re-derived by cesarean section or embryo transfer, raised on microbiologically defined (specific pathogen free [SPF])

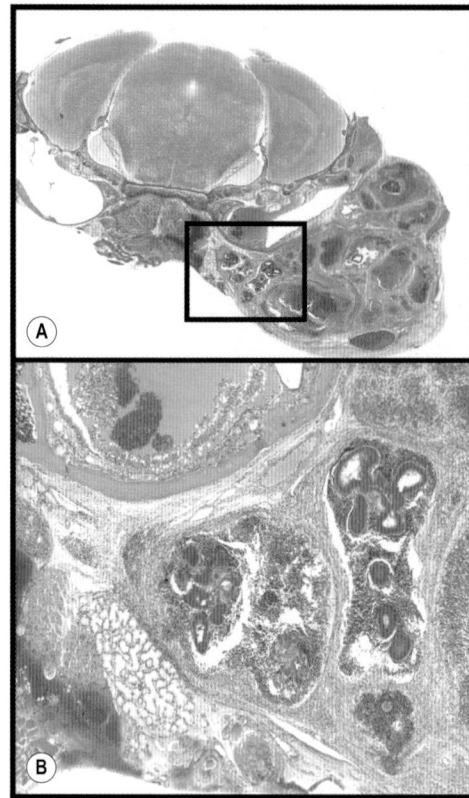

Fig. 36.7

This is a 91-day-old female mouse with botryomycosis. (**A**) Note the pink immune complexes (Splendore-Hoeppli phenomenon) surrounded by neutrophils and a wall of macrophages and fibroblasts. (**B**) Lower panel is enlargement of boxed area.

foster mothers, transferred to, and maintained in high microbiological barrier facilities to minimize exposure to opportunistic or real pathogens. In most facilities, this means no known mouse pathogens can be detected in the colony. As such, primary infections are very rare in well-run facilities making the mouse a poor model for human infectious skin diseases. Opportunistic pathogens, those considered normal commensals in a dirty environment or those carried in by animal caretakers who do not follow strict mouse handling protocols, will result in infectious disease problems, especially in mice with various types of immunodeficiencies.[1] However, infectious disease work can be done in biocontainment facilities (ABSL2 or higher facilities). Two examples affecting the skin are presented here.

Botryomycosis

Bacterial induction of disease is minimized by autoclaving or irradiating feed, treating the water (acidification or chlorination), and maintaining a high barrier. However, not all investigators follow protocols, so accidental infection of mice with human pathogens can occur. Some bacterial infections can become quite serious in the skin of mice, for example, *Staphylococcus* spp. induced botryomycosis. Here, mice can present with massive abscesses often around the head from which pure cultures of the bacteria can be isolated (*Fig. 36.7*). These infections can spread to the lungs with a miliary distribution giving the appearance of metastatic cancer. While the lesions may present as a skin lesion, entry into the body usually can be found coming through ulcerations in the epithelium surrounding the molars, which are often induced by impaction with food material and hairs (from grooming). Osteomyelitis in the maxilla spreads, resulting in prominent swelling of the face which may rupture at the skin surface. This lesion can be a major part of the phenotype of some targeted mutant mice, notably those with deficiencies in cytochrome b-245, beta polypeptide (*Cybb^tm1Din*)[2] or plasminogen activator, urokinase (*Plau^tm1Mlg*),[3] which both affect the immune system. Sentinel mice with aglobulinemia were reported to develop these lesions.[4] Staphylococcal infections have resulted in botryomycosis in cut wounds in pathogen-free colonies.[5,6]

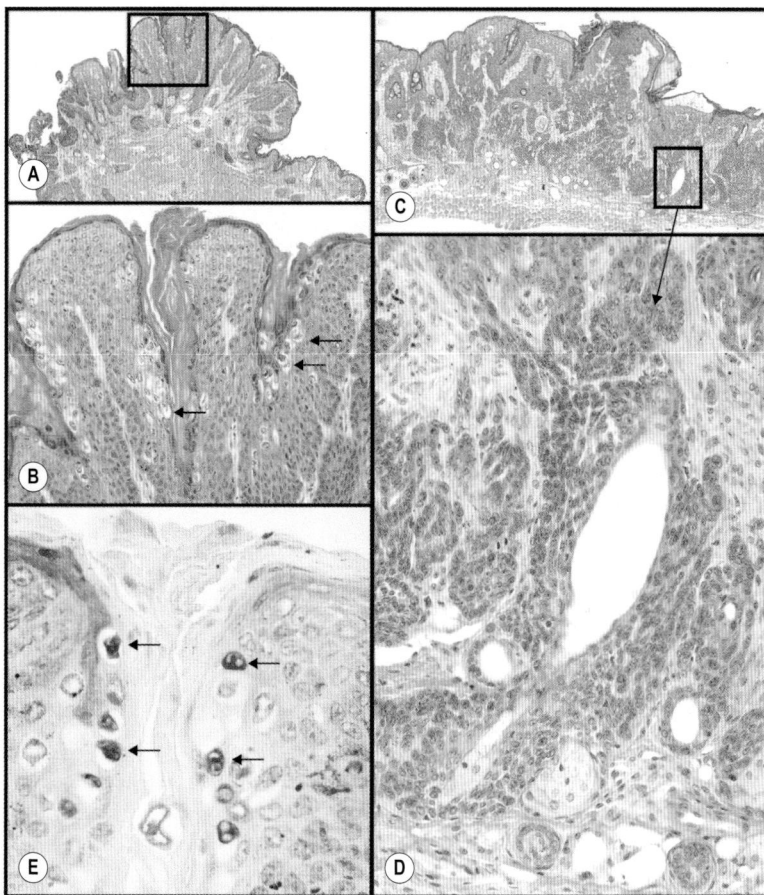

Fig. 36.8
Laboratory mouse papillomavirus infections cause exophytic papillomas on the muzzle (**A**, **B**) and tail that are productive (viral antigens can be detected in koilocytes by immunohistochemistry, **E**). However, when the virus was inoculated into the dorsal skin in the lumbar region, a slightly raised lesion developed with poorly differentiated cells that were locally invasive (**C**, **D**). These cells had a high nuclear to cytoplasmic ratio, high mitotic index, and were positive for several mouse specific keratins by immunohistochemistry.

Mouse papillomaviruses

While interest in human and nonhuman mammalian papillomaviruses has been waning since the commercialization of polyvalent recombinant vaccines, discovery of a mouse papillomavirus has opened up interesting new avenues for research. Numerous rodent papillomaviruses have been found in the past 30 years including one in a wild colony of European harvest mice.[7-10] However, only recently has a laboratory mouse papillomavirus been reported in immunodeficient nude mice that could be transmitted to other nude mice but only to a limited number of inbred backgrounds. It was noted that pan T-cell deficiencies in the mice were needed for these lesions to develop. A very similar viral subtype was found in the normal skin of immunocompetent mice, suggesting that this virus has adapted well to its host. In the immunodeficient strains, benign papillomas (warts) developed on the muzzle and tail skin, but invasive, poorly differentiated carcinomas resembling trichomatrixomas developed on the dorsal lumbar skin (*Fig. 36.8*).[11-15]

Vascular changes in the skin

Vascular changes in the skin are commonly associated with inflammation. Mice with a chronic inflammatory skin disease that resembles psoriasis, but appears more to be a form of hypereosinophilic syndrome due to a spontaneous null mutation in the *Sharpin* gene, leads to the development of chronic proliferative dermatitis.[1] Not surprisingly, there is an increase in the number and size of blood vessels in the areas of inflamed skin in these mutant mice compared to controls.[2] These vessels can be identified easily in

hematoxylin and eosin (H&E)-stained sections and confirmed using antibodies directed against smooth muscle actin for vascular smooth muscle or platelet/endothelial cell adhesion molecule 1 (PECAM1, formerly called CD31).[2]

Lymphatics are often overlooked in the mouse because in the skin, these appear as small slits below the epidermis and parallel to the angle of the hair follicle within the dermis. Once one recognizes these structures, they are easy to identify in routine histologic sections. However, antibodies directed against lymphatic vessel endothelial hyaluronan receptor 1 (LYVE1) clearly labels the lymphatic endothelial cells.[3] The C3H/HeJ mouse spontaneously develops alopecia areata,[4] which has remained the model of choice for this human disease for two decades.[5] Evaluation of skin in mice with alopecia areata as the disease progresses revealed dilation of the cutaneous lymphatics.[3]

Genetic-based skin diseases

Genetic-based skin diseases in laboratory mice have been the most useful to study the pathogenesis in great detail of many diseases. Examples are provided below to illustrate how similar phenotypes arising in mice with known genetic mutations often fall into a common molecular pathway, and actually these features help to better define and resolve the pathway(s).

Coat color genetics

In the late 1800s, Gregor Mendel, an Augustine monk, began his work in genetics with cages of mice in his room at the Abbey in Brno, Czech Republic. Although he eventually switched to studying the inheritance of traits in plants, due to political pressures from the bishop, mice – and in particular, the coat color of mice – were used in the beginning of the field of genetics. In 1902, Lucien Cuénot, along with several other investigators, rediscovered Mendel's work and demonstrated Mendelian inheritance ratios in the coat colors of mice.[1,2] The first demonstrated genetic linkage in the mouse was found between two coat color alleles, namely albino (tyrosinase [Tyr^c]) and pink-eyed dilution (oculocutaneous albinism II [$Oca2^p$]).[3] Over the next 80 years, mutant mice with coat color changes played a major role in constructing a linkage map of the mouse genome cementing the importance of the mouse in genetics.

In the mouse hair follicle, pigmentation follows a precise sequence of interactions between melanocytes and the dermal papilla.[4,5] Hair is actively pigmented only during the anagen stage of the hair cycle. Melanin synthesis is inactive during catagen and remains so through telogen[4]; thus, it is important to emphasize that follicular melanogenesis is cyclic in nature.[5]

Currently, research in the mouse has identified more genes influencing coat color than any other trait.[6] A search of Mouse Genome Informatics (www.informatics.jax.org) for the phrase 'abnormal hair/coat pigmentation' results in 1692 genotypes affecting coat color (http://www.informatics.jax.org; August 2016).[7] The most common alleles found in inbred research strains popular in research today are illustrated in *Fig. 36.9*. Although coat color genetics have been studied for nearly 100 years, the great variety of alleles affecting coat color appears to be a never-ending story. Current work in this field is actively pursuing the interconnectedness of the genes to form a genetic pathway (*Fig. 36.10*).

Mouse hair pigmentation is under complex genetic control as illustrated in the genetic pathway in *Fig. 36.10*. The genes in this pathway have a vast array of molecular targets and functions, such as enzymes (*Tyr*), scaffolding/cytoskeletal proteins (*Pmel*), transcriptional factors (*Mitf*), as well as receptors (*Kit*) and their ligands (*Kitl*).[8,9] This pathway controls hair pigmentation on the cellular (melanocyte), organ (hair follicle), and developmental (melanocyte development, migration, differentiation, proliferation, and survival) time points.[5] These genes and pathways have homologs of great importance in human tissues and disease states.

The eumelanin (black and brown) and pheomelanin (yellow) synthesis pathways share many common steps within the melanosome of the melanocytes. Melanogenesis begins with the hydroxylation of tyrosine to L-3,4-dihydroxyphenylalanine (L-DOPA) by the tyrosinase (*Tyr*) enzyme. L-DOPA is then oxidized to DOPAquinone, which can then be further processed through different enzymatic pathways to either eumelanin or

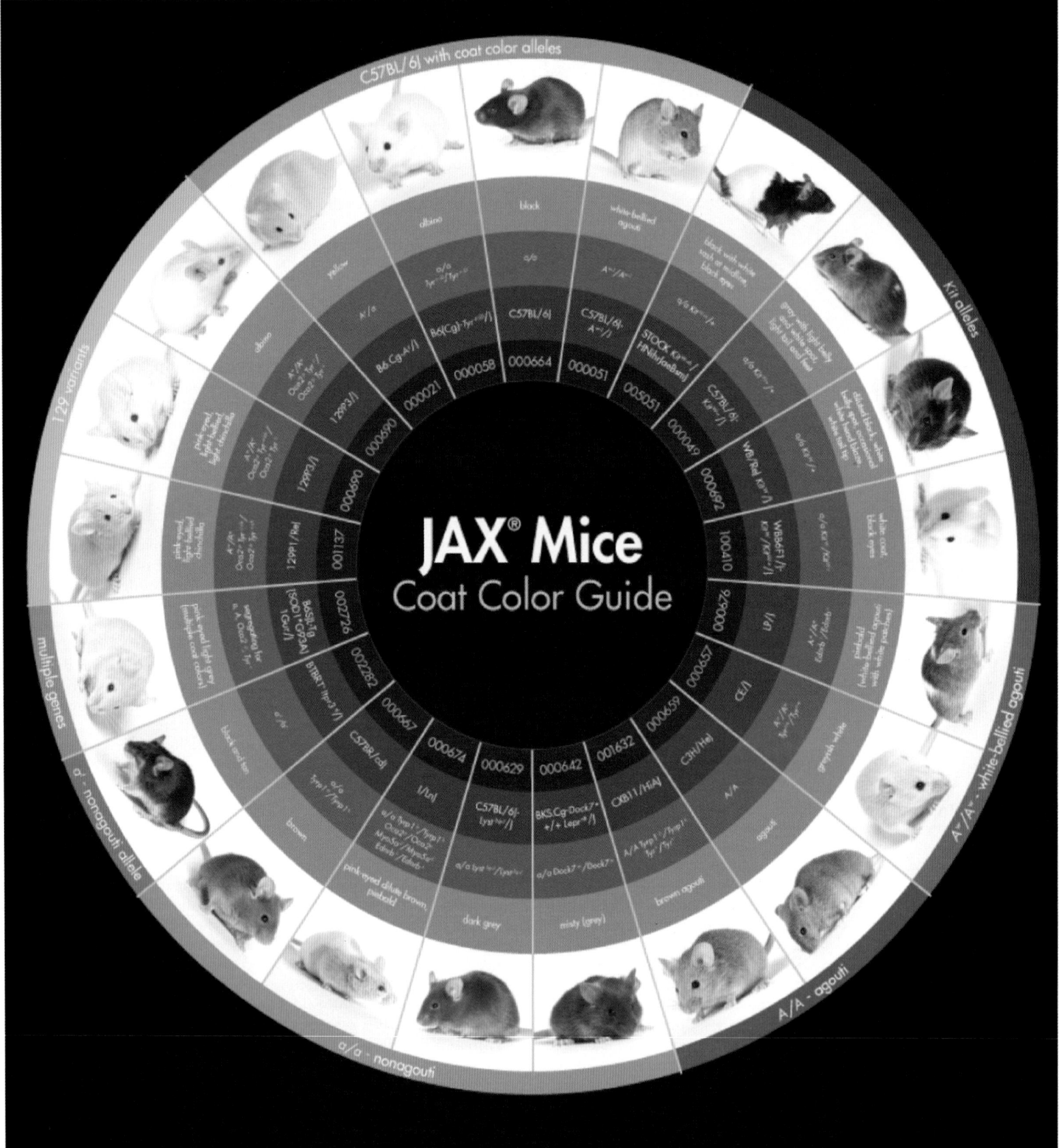

Fig. 36.9
Coat color variations in laboratory mice and the corresponding genetic mutations underlying the different colors. Stanton Short and Jennifer Torrance (JAX Creative Department, The Jackson Laboratory) are thanked for the figures and layout.

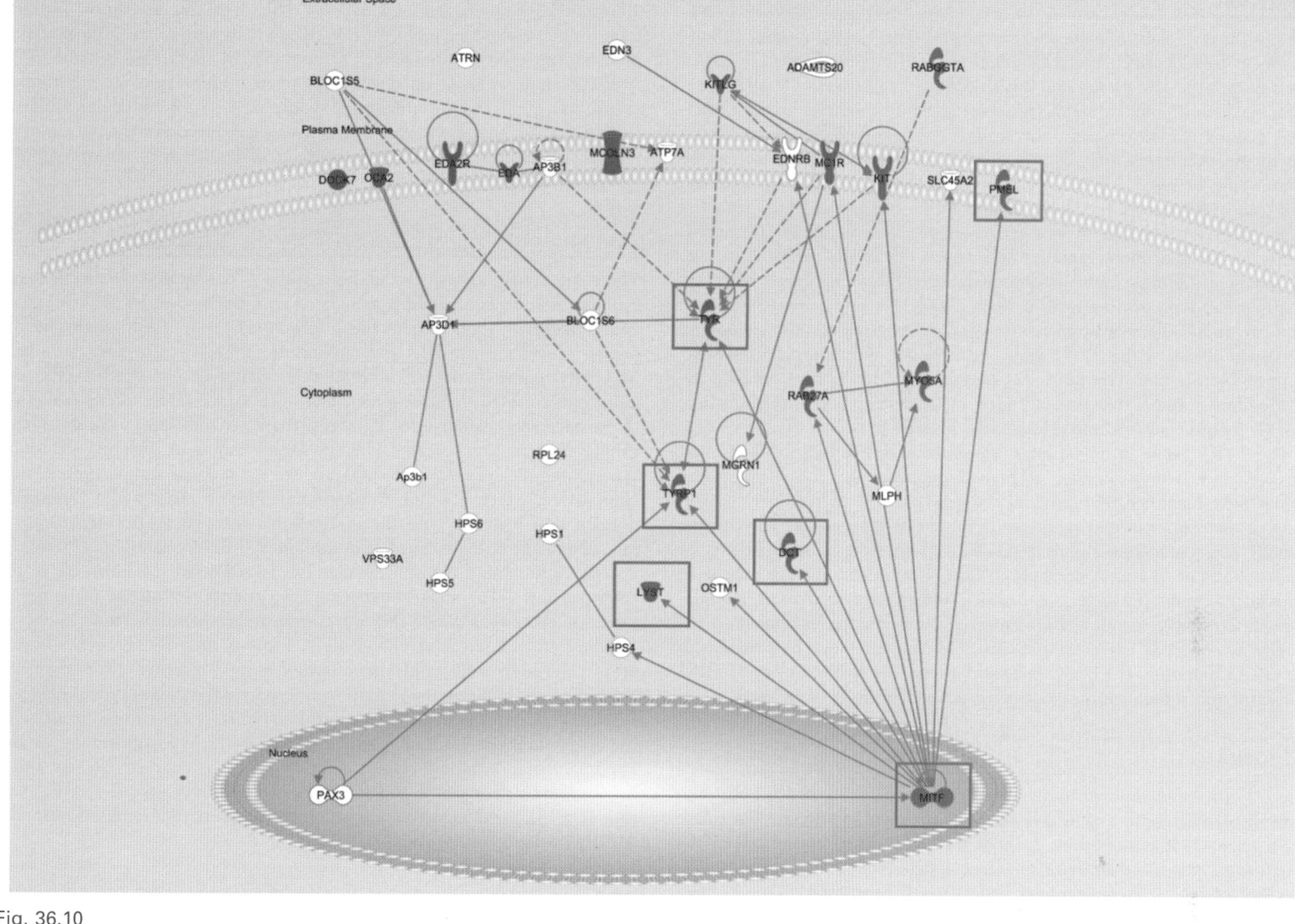

Fig. 36.10
Ingenuity Pathway Analysis Software® (http://www.ingenuity.com/) molecular pathway diagram for genes that interact in the coat color pathway. Many of the mutant mice in *Fig. 36.9* have mutations in the genes in this pathway (*red boxes*). This illustrates how variations on a common trait, coat color, help to define a molecular pathway. It also illustrates the number of other genes involved with coat color not in this pathway, which will be future goals to integrate.

pheomelanin. For eumelanin, DOPAquinone can spontaneously cyclize to produce DOPAchrome, which again can react in two ways. In the absence of DOPAchrome tautomerase (*Dct*) activity, the carboxyl group of DOPA-chrome is lost and 5,6-dihydroxyindole (DHI) is formed. DHI is further hydroxylated by tyrosinase to become indole-5,6-quinone, that is lastly oxidated to DHI-melanin. DHI-melanin is black and insoluble. In the presence of *Dct* expression, DOPAchrome is tautomerized to 5,6-dihydroxyindole-2-carboxylic acid (DHICA). Tyrosinase-related protein 1 (*Tyrp1*) catalyzes the oxidation of DHICA to indole-5,6-quinone carboxylic acid. Premelanosome protein (*Pmel*) expression functions to then polymerize indole-5,6-quinone carboxylic acid. Further oxidation forms DHICA-melanin, which is brown and poorly soluble. Synthesis of pheomelanin begins with the conjugation of DOPAquinone with cysteine or glutathione yielding cysteinylDOPA and glutathionylDOPA. CysteinylDOPA is oxidized and then spontaneously forms 1,4-benzothiazinylalanines through a tyrosinase-catalyzed oxidation and produce pheomelanin. Alternatively, DOPAquinone can be conjugated with glutathione, instead of cysteine, followed by hydrolysis of glutathionylDOPA to CysteinylDOPA.[5,8,10]

The switch from eu- to pheomelanogenesis is regulated by a number of genes, namely pro-opiomelanocortin-alpha (*Pomc/α-Msh*), melanocortin 1 receptor (*Mc1r*), nonagouti (*A*), mahogunin, ring finger 1 (*Mgrn1*), and attractin (*Atrn*). Eumelanin synthesis is promoted when POMC binds to the MC1R receptor, which in turn leads to the activation of the cyclic adenosine 3′–5′-monophosphate (cAMP) pathway and eumelanin synthesis. Meanwhile, pheomelanin is synthesized when the nonagouti signal protein is expressed and interacts with MC1R and ATRN to inhibit the cAMP pathway.[5,11,12]

A locus

The agouti locus is located on chromosome 2 of the mouse genome and is associated with the nonagouti (*a*) gene. Agouti acts in the hair follicles, primarily affecting the relative amount and distribution of yellow pigment (pheomelanin) and black/brown pigment (eumelanin) in hair. Agouti mice have banded hairs whereby a band of black melanin resides at the top of the hair followed by yellow melanin in the middle and ending with black pigment near the end of the hair shaft. Currently, there are nearly 150 known variations in the agouti locus conferring a range of coat colors and pleiotropic phenotypes (http://www.informatics.jax.org; August 2016).

The human equivalent of the nonagouti (*a*) gene in mice is the agouti signaling protein (*ASIP*) gene located at 20q11.22. Several studies using small cohorts have found single nucleotide polymorphisms (SNPs) in and around the *ASIP* gene that show a weak correlation between *ASIP* and human skin and hair pigmentation.[13,14] In addition, a melanoma risk locus was identified by three separate studies residing near *ASIP*. This locus increases the risk of early onset cutaneous melanoma and basal cell carcinoma.[15]

B locus

The B or brown locus (b) is located on chromosome 4 of the mouse genome. This locus was identified as the tyrosinase-related protein 1 gene (Tyrp1) in work during the late 1980s and early 1990s.[16,17] The wildtype allele produces black eumelanin, while the recessive allele (b) produces brown eumelanin, making a mouse harboring the Tyrp1[b/b] genotype cinnamon brown due to the occurrence of yellow-banded brown hairs. The effect on the melanosome of mice expressing the b allele versus the wildtype B allele is to change the nature of the eumelanin in the pigment granule, which is accompanied by a change in its size and shape. Brown granules are significantly smaller than black granules and display much less variation in size. The pigment granules found in the medulla of black-pigmented hairs are usually either long oval or oval in shape, while those in brown-pigmented hairs are round. Currently, there are over 60 targeted, spontaneous, and transgenic alleles of the Tyrp1 gene (http://www.informatics.jax.org/allele/summary?markerId=MGI:98881, MGI accessed 27 June 2016). Some of the most common alleles that can be found in laboratory mice strains include light (B[lt]), cordovan (b[c]), and white-based brown (B[w]).

The TYRP1 gene in humans resides at chromosome location 9p23 and has been linked to a number of human pigmentation disorders. Several studies have identified mutations in the TYRP1 gene that reduce the stability of the transcript and significantly inhibit its catalytic activity causing type III oculocutaneous albinism (OCA3)[18–21] in either single patients or small cohorts of African Americans (106delT), southern Africans (368delA, S166X), Pakistani (R373Ter), and Asian Indian (1057delAACA) populations. Interestingly, Kenney et al.[22] identified a homozygous change in the N terminus of TYRP1 (R93C) that causes Melanesian blond hair. Similar to the OCA3 mutation, the R93C mutation affects the stability of the TYRP1 transcript and subsequently the catalytic activity of the protein.

C locus

The c locus, better known as the albino locus (c), is located on chromosome 7 of the mouse and is associated with mutations in the tyrosinase (Tyr) gene.[23–28] It is important to note that albinism is epistatic (i.e., the situation in which the effect of one gene (phenotype) is dependent on the presence of one or more modifier genes) to all other coat color determinants; thus, all mice possessing a Tyr[c/c] genotype will lack pigment regardless of other coat alleles. This allele is the oldest allele that has been known and documented as far back as ancient Greek and Roman mouse fanciers.[29,30] Interestingly, albino animals do not lack normal melanocytes, but the Tyr[c] group of alleles affects the amount of tyrosinase in the melanocyte. Tyrosinase is an enzyme that catalyzes the hydroxylation of L-tyrosine to L-3,4-dihydroxyphenylalanine (L-dopa). L-dopa is then oxidized to dopaquinone, which is a common step in both the eumelanogenic and pheomelanogenic synthesis pathways.[8] Once L-dopa is formed, melanogenesis can proceed further through oxidation-reduction reactions and spontaneous transformations. Although Tyr encodes for tyrosinase, some albino mutations affect tyrosinase activity rather than structure,[31] introducing several other signaling pathways and genes that may affect albinism in mice.[32] This is illustrated in Fig. 36.10, which shows that there are a number of genes that both directly and indirectly interact with Tyr. Normal appearing melanocytes can be found in the hair and eye, but they completely lack melanin. Pigment granules within the cells are significantly smaller and fewer than in wildtype genetic backgrounds.

The tyrosinase gene is located in the human genome at 11q14.3. As with mice, humans with mutations in the TYR gene experience pigmentation disorders. Specifically, mutations in this gene have been shown to be causative in both type IA oculocutaneous albinism (OCAIA) and type IB oculocutaneous albinism (OCAIB). OCAIA, also known as tyrosinase-negative OCA,[33] presents with amelanotic melanocytes in the skin[34,35] and subsequent loss of pigmentation in the skin, hair, and eyes. Additionally, patients may also experience ocular phenotypes reducing visual acuity including strabismus and/or nystagmus.[36] OCAIB or tyrosinase-positive OCA arises from mutations in the TYR gene that affect the stability and catalytic activity of the tyrosinase enzyme. Thus, tyrosinase can still be detected in these patients

although at a significantly reduced level. OCAIB is also known as yellow albinism.[37,38] Patients with OCAIB are phenotypically similar at birth to type II oculocutaneous albinism (OCAII), yet rapidly develop normal skin pigmentation and yellow hair.[37–40] Interestingly, mutations in both TYR (R402Q) and MITF (1-bp deletion in exon 8) play roles in the autosomal recessive, digenic Waardenburg syndrome type 2 with ocular albinism (WS2-OA). Patients with WS2-OA experience reduced visual acuity, photophobia, nystagmus, strabismus, and albinotic fundus with foveal hypoplasia, along with deafness.[41–44]

D locus

The d locus, also known as the dilute locus (d), is located on chromosome 9 of the mouse genome and is associated with the myosin Va (Myo5a) gene. Mutations in this gene affect the clumping of melanin, thus reducing the overall absorbance of light and making the animals' color appear diluted. Melanin clumps in mice exhibiting this phenotype are much larger and more concentrated than those in black mice. These larger clumps decrease the surface area available for light absorbance by melanin. In practice, this can be seen microscopically whereby large clumps of melanin are found throughout the hair shaft. MYO5A is an actin-based motor protein that contains an N-terminal motor domain that binds to actin and a C-terminal domain that interacts with the melanosome through RAB27 (RAB27A, a member of the RAS oncogene family) and MLPH (melanophilin) (see Fig. 36.10). Actin-bound myosin Va functions to transport melanosomes to the cell's periphery. The melanosomes are then transported to the melanocytes dendritic extensions where they are transferred to keratinocytes.[12,45]

The human equivalent of the dilute locus is the MYO5A gene located at 15q21.12. Griscelli syndrome is an autosomal recessive disorder that is characterized by pigmentary dilution.[46] Type 1, type 2, and type 3 Griscelli syndrome are distinguished by central nervous system involvement with hypopigmentation, immunological defects with hypopigmentation, and hypopigmentation alone, respectively.[47,48] Type 3 is characterized by either homozygous deletion of the MYO5A F-exon, which is a tissue-specific exon that is transcribed in melanocytes, or by a homozygous mutation in the MLPH (melanophilin) gene.[49]

P locus

The p locus, also known as pink-eyed dilution (p), is located on chromosome 7 of the mouse genome and is associated with the oculocutaneous albinism II (Oca2) gene. Mutations in this gene affect the size, number, and composition of melanosomes. The Oca2 gene encodes a transmembrane protein that assists in regulating the pH level within the melanosome.[50] Wildtype Oca2 produces an intense pigmentation of the hair, but the mutant Oca2[p] allele reduces the pigmentation of the coat. The eyes of Oca2[p] mice resemble those of albinos, possessing a pink tint, thus the name. Oca2[p] alleles reduce both black and brown pigments (eumelanin synthesis), but has only a slight influence on pheomelanin synthesis. The melanin granules within the hair shaft of Oca2[p] mice are smaller than their normal counterparts.[51] Additionally, levels of tyrosinase are reduced within melanosomes of mice possessing the mutant allele.[52] The Oca2 gene encodes a melanosomal transmembrane protein which functions as an ion exchange protein that is similar to Na[+]/H[+] transporters.[8] The initial step in melanogenesis requires the acidification of the melanosome,[53,54] but further processing requires a rise in pH.[55] So, one function of OCA2 is to regulate the pH of the melanosome, which in turn could regulate tyrosinase activity that is dependent on the pH of the surrounding milieu.

The p locus is located in chromosomal location 15q12-q13 in the human genome. Mutations in the human OCA2 gene have been linked to both OCAII and brown oculocutaneous albinism (BOCA) in the human population. Over 50 different mutations have been reported in the literature within the OCA2 gene,[56] ranging from single nucleotide substitutions, to large deletions of entire exons, to complex rearrangements.[50,57–66] Both OCAII and BOCA are tyrosinase-positive, autosomal recessive disorders whereby pigmentation is reduced in skin, hair, and eyes, and patients have characteristic vision deficits associated with albinism, although usually less severe than those with OCAI.[40,67] As opposed to OCAI, patients with OCAII may experience darkening of their hair with age and may be freckled. In affected individuals with African and African American descent, patients may present with yellow hair and blue-gray iris. The BOCA variant of OCA has been observed mostly in African and African American populations and is characterized by light brown hair and skin color and gray irides.[40]

Mouse models of melanoma

Melanoma is a malignant disease that arises from transformation of melanocytes, the pigment producing cells of the skin and hair follicles. Spontaneous melanomas in mice are very uncommon.[1] As a result, a variety of approaches have been undertaken in order to model the complex process of melanoma formation and progression in mice. In humans, melanocytes are predominantly located at the junction of epidermis and dermis in skin as well as in the follicular bulb and bulge and dermis, but are also present in the mucosa, the central nervous system, the eye, and inner ear. Mice also have melanocytes in similar locations; however, epidermal junctional melanocytes are mainly present in tail skin and are largely absent in trunk skin. The approaches to modeling melanoma in mice have been reviewed[2,3] and are summarized below.

Carcinogen-induced melanoma

Early approaches utilizing the initiating carcinogen 7,12-dimethylbenz[a] anthracene (DMBA) were utilized to model squamous cell carcinoma and other neoplasms in mice[4] and hamsters. It was noted that hamsters also developed highly pigmented melanocytic tumors.[5] Many of these tumors grew slowly, and it was at times difficult to determine whether the lesions were benign or fully malignant. Ultraviolet (UV) irradiation is perhaps the most important environmental exposure leading to melanoma in humans, and it has been utilized to model skin cancer in non-genetically engineered mice. Chronic, repetitive exposure to UV light resulted in cutaneous malignant tumors, most of which represented poorly differentiated squamous cell carcinoma, occasional cutaneous sarcomas, and rarely resulted in melanoma.[6]

Genetically engineered mouse melanoma models

Transgenic approaches

The melanin pigment production pathway is unique to melanocytes, and definition of promoters of genes involved in this pathway has allowed for melanocyte-specific transgene expression. The tyrosinase (*Tyr*) promoter/enhancer construct has been utilized most often; however, promoter constructs from the dopachrome tautomerase (*Dct*) gene and microphthalmia transcription factor (*Mitf*) have also been utilized.[2] The first transgenic mouse melanoma model utilized a *Tyr* promoter/enhancer construct to drive SV40 early region in melanocytes. This model resulted in highly penetrant ocular and cutaneous melanoma.[7] Additional models involving transgenic expression of *Ret*, *Hras*, *Nras*, *Braf*, and *HGF* were also generated and resulted in highly penetrant melanoma formation. Several of these models utilized transgenes/oncogenes that do not appear to play a major role in human melanoma; however, collectively the models provided the opportunity to study melanoma formation and progression in genetic animal models. The models involving transgenic *HGF* expression are of note, as it was demonstrated that a single dose of perinatal UV exposure increased melanoma penetrance dramatically and altered the morphological features of resulting melanomas.[8] Of note, pagetoid spread of melanoma cells is a common feature in this model and in human melanoma, but is only rarely observed in other mouse melanoma models.

Conditional *cre-lox* models

The development of *cre-loxP* technology[9] and two melanocyte-specific inducible cre-recombinase transgenic alleles (*Tyr::creEr*) enabled conditional inducible gene recombination specifically in melanocytes.[10,11] Spatially and temporally controlled recombination of conditional *loxP*-containing alleles

could be induced by topical administration of 4-hydroxytamoxifen and resulting induction of melanocyte-specific cre activity. These alleles were utilized to generate a variety of genetically engineered mouse models of melanoma based on the most common genetic changes observed in human melanoma, including the $BRAF^{V600E}$, $NRAS^{Q61K}$, and loss of *PTEN*, *CDKN2A*, *TP53*, and/or *NF1*.[12–15] Activating mutations in the BRAF serine/threonine kinase are the most common mutations in melanoma. Two *lox*-based alleles were constructed in which the activated form of the BRAF kinase could be induced following exposure to cre activity.[12,13] These *Braf* alleles were used in conjunction with *Tyr::creEr* alleles as the basis of the vast majority of genetically engineered mouse models. Interestingly, activation of *Braf* in the absence of other genetic changes induces transient proliferation of dermal melanocytes followed by growth arrest, mimicking the growth pattern of human melanocytic nevi, 80% of which have activation of *Braf* in the absence of other genetic changes. Additional genetic changes, including loss of the *Pten*, *Cdkn2a*, or *Trp53* tumor suppressors, result in melanoma formation with complete penetrance and varying latency and multiplicity.[12,14] Constitutive activation of *Braf* and loss of *Pten* results in one of the most aggressive mouse models of cancer ever developed. Roughly 10% of melanocytes undergoing these genetic changes begin dividing within 48 hours and progress on to melanoma. Induction of these genetic changes in all melanocytes in the mouse results in innumerable melanomas (>20 000) that cover the skin of mice within 3–4 weeks. An alternative version of this model has been developed in which the *cre* induction agent (4-hydroxytamoxifen) is applied on the skin of mice. This is sufficient to induce local recombination of cutaneous melanocytes in the area of application and generally results in 40–100 distinct melanomas that grow confluently to form one cutaneous mass. This model has been widely utilized to evaluate the effects of therapeutic agents and modifying genetic changes. Histologically, the *Braf/Pten* mouse melanomas are often heavily pigmented and have unusual morphological features that somewhat resemble edematous malignant peripheral nerve sheath tumors (*Figs 36.11* and *36.12*).[12] Despite these unusual histologic features, there is little doubt that the tumors are melanomas, as all initial tumor formation/proliferation occurs in melanocytes, not peripheral nerve sheath cells.[14] The *Braf/Pten* model illustrated a previously suspected, but unproven synergy between the mitogen-activated protein kinase (MAPK) and PI3K pathways in inducing melanoma formation. The model also demonstrated that the isolated evaluation of particular combinations of genetic changes observed in human melanoma could be precisely evaluated in genetically engineered mouse models of melanoma. An additional model

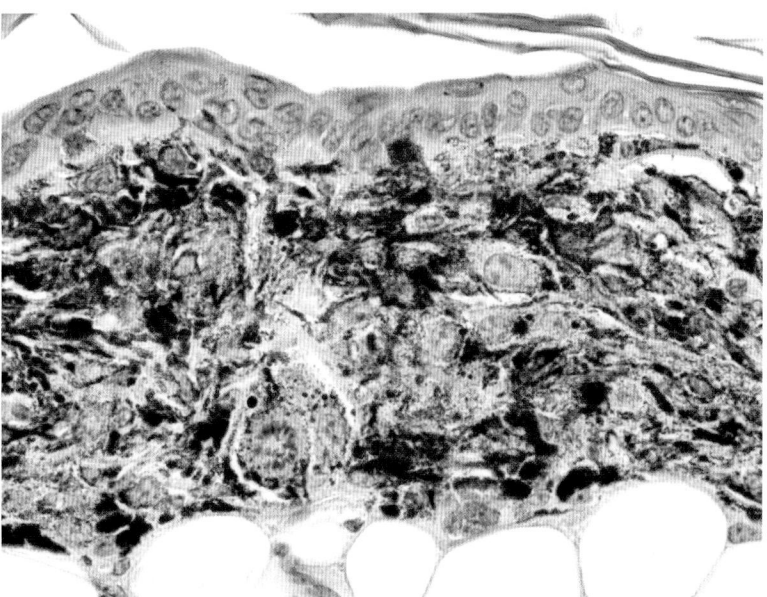

Fig. 36.11
Melanoma histology in the *Braf/Pten* genetically engineered mouse model. Pigmented junctional melanoma on the ear following perinatal 4-hydroxytamoxifen induction.

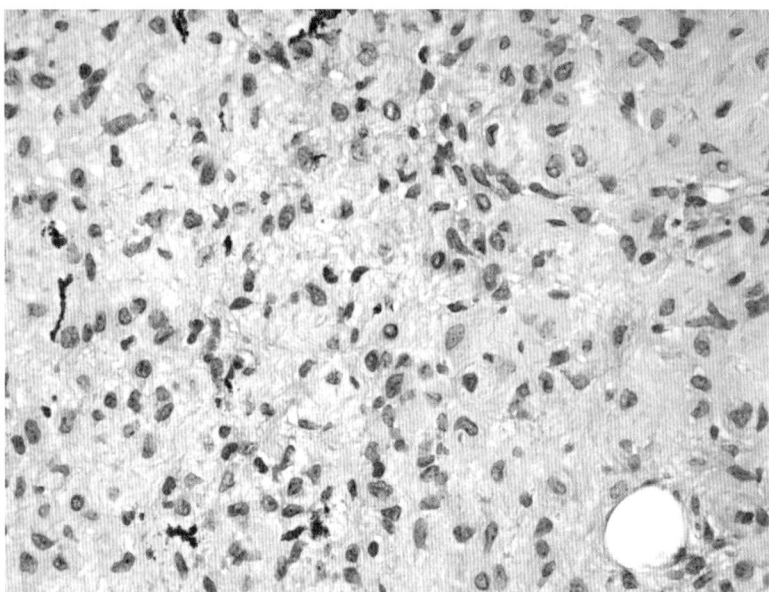

Fig. 36.12
Melanoma histology in the *Braf/Pten* genetically engineered mouse model.
Spindle and epitheliod cell melanoma in a locally induced adult mouse with
intratumoral edema and focal melanin pigmentation.

of particular interest is the combination of *Braf* activation with *Cdkn2a*
loss. *CDKN2A* is by far the most common locus for genetic changes associated with familial melanoma, accounting for approximately 40% of familial
melanoma cases. Systemic activation of *Braf* and loss of *Cdkn2a* in melanocytes resulted in completely penetrant melanoma formation. However, in
contrast to the *Braf/Pten* model, only two to four melanomas were observed
per mouse. These findings underscore the role of the *CDKN2A* locus as a
melanoma tumor suppressor, but suggest that additional stochastic changes
are required in addition to *Braf* activation and *Cdkn2a* loss in order for
progression to melanoma to occur. The combination of *Braf* activation with
Trp53 loss also resulted in melanoma formation with similar latency, penetrance, and multiplicity that were observed in the *Braf/Cdkn2a* model, also
suggesting that stochastic changes are required for full progression to melanoma in this model. Taken together, genetically engineered mouse models of
melanoma involving *cre-loxP* technology have contributed to the validation
of human candidate melanoma-relevant genetic changes and have illustrated
the specific contributions of individual genetic changes.

Syngeneic mouse melanoma models

Genetically engineered mouse melanoma models are elegant and recapitulate
many features of human melanoma, but are expensive and time-consuming
to use for scientific experiments. An alternative is the use of mouse models
that utilize melanoma cell lines that have been isolated from inbred or
congenic mice that are sufficiently isogenic to a particular reference inbred
genetic mouse strain to allow for tumor engraftment without graft rejection.
The B16 mouse melanoma cell line was isolated in 1930 and has been widely
utilized in over 17 000 publications to date.[16] This cell is highly pigmented
and has been extensively utilized to evaluate melanoma cell biology, tumor
formation, and antitumor immune responses. While the B16 model has been
widely utilized, the genetic drivers that resulted in tumor formation remain
unknown and analogous lines with similar features or behavior have not
been identified. A more recent approach has been to backcross alleles utilized to produce genetically engineered mouse models of melanoma onto a
reference genetic strain (e.g., C57BL/6J), recreate the genetically engineered
mouse model, induce melanoma, and derive congenic mouse melanoma cell
lines with the genetic features defined by the model.[17] The individual melanoma cell lines can then be tested for melanoma formation/engraftment
into immunocompetent C57BL/6J mice. Lines that form tumors/grafts are
termed syngeneic and allow for melanoma modeling with defined genetic

changes in immunocompetent hosts. The dynamic interplay between the
immune system and melanoma cells is of great interest given the high rates
of response observed in human melanoma following immune checkpoint
inhibition therapy. There is a great need for a variety of mouse models that
recapitulate the immune reactions and responses to immune-based therapies
observed in humans. The B16 model, however, is notoriously resistant to
immune therapies and generally only responds in the context of prior vaccination protocols, which are not particularly applicable to human melanoma.
A recent approach to making syngeneic mouse melanoma models more
immunogenic involves the mutagenesis and single cell-derived clonal isolation of new cell lines. The theory behind this is that the immune system can
recognize protein-coding differences between tumor and host if they exist.
Increasing the number of protein coding changes (potential neo-epitopes)
increases the chances of antitumor immune responses. This approach has
been shown to be successful, allowing for the generation of models in which
effective antitumor immune responses are generated, including the response
to blockade of immune checkpoint inhibitors PD1 and CTLA4.[18] Given that
immune-based therapies had among the highest rates of response observed
to date in a wide variety of cancers, accurate mouse models of immunogenic
tumors will be of great interest as the mechanism of antitumor immune
responses are determined and new combinations of immune therapies are
evaluated.

Humanized mouse melanoma models

While mouse melanoma models have provided great insight into the biology
of human melanoma, it is possible that humanized mouse models of melanoma will allow for the identification of biological features of melanoma
that are more specific to humans. Broadly, these models involve the engraftment of human melanoma cells or tumor pieces into immunodeficient
mouse strains that do not reject human tissue. These specific approaches
used in these models are complex and rapidly evolving, and generally strive
to recapitulate portions of the human immune system.[19] While humanized
mouse models face many challenges, the potential reward of providing more
accurate preclinical models of human melanoma is a goal that will ensure
their continued development.

Anhidrotic ectodermal dysplasia: mouse models that helped define the receptor-ligand concept

While we take the concept of gene/protein pathways and networks for
granted, it took careful observation to understand the natural biological
experiments that led to these concepts (*Fig. 36.13*). As stated above, the
prevailing concept of one gene, one disease did not explain how the same
disease could be caused by genes on different chromosomes. What was
called the tabby-crinkled-downless syndrome in mice,[1–4] a group of mutant
mice with essentially identical phenotypes due to mutations mapped to different chromosomes, helped to explain this concept. Mutations in the mouse
tabby gene (now called ectodysplasin-A, *Eda*; Chr. X; 24 allelic mutations),
crinkled (now called EDAR [ectodysplasin-A receptor]-associated death
domain, *Edaradd*; Chr. 13; eight allelic mutations), and downless (now
called ectodysplasin-A receptor, *Edar*; Chr. 10; 14 allelic mutations) (MGI;
http://www.informatics.jax.org/; 18 August 2016) resulted in very similar
phenotypes when on the same inbred background (genocopies). Phenotypic
changes in the tabby, crinkled, downless, and other allelic mutations of their
respective genes included tail skin lacking all pilosebaceous units resulting
in smooth tail skin with no scales, alopecia behind the ears, deformed teeth,
eyelids with no Meibomian glands, and lack of eccrine glands in the feet
(*Fig. 36.14*),[2–7] seen in human anhidrotic ectodermal dysplasias that are all
caused by mutations in the equivalent human genes.

These mutant mice can be used to answer specific questions, such as
confirming the site of neoplastic origination. For example, in transgenic
mice that developed mixed tumors of their eccrine sweat glands, when these
mutant mice are crossed with tabby mutant mice, no foot lesions developed
because the mice had no eccrine gland development, thus illustrating how
these types of mutant mice can be used to investigate the cellular origin of
specific cancer types.[8]

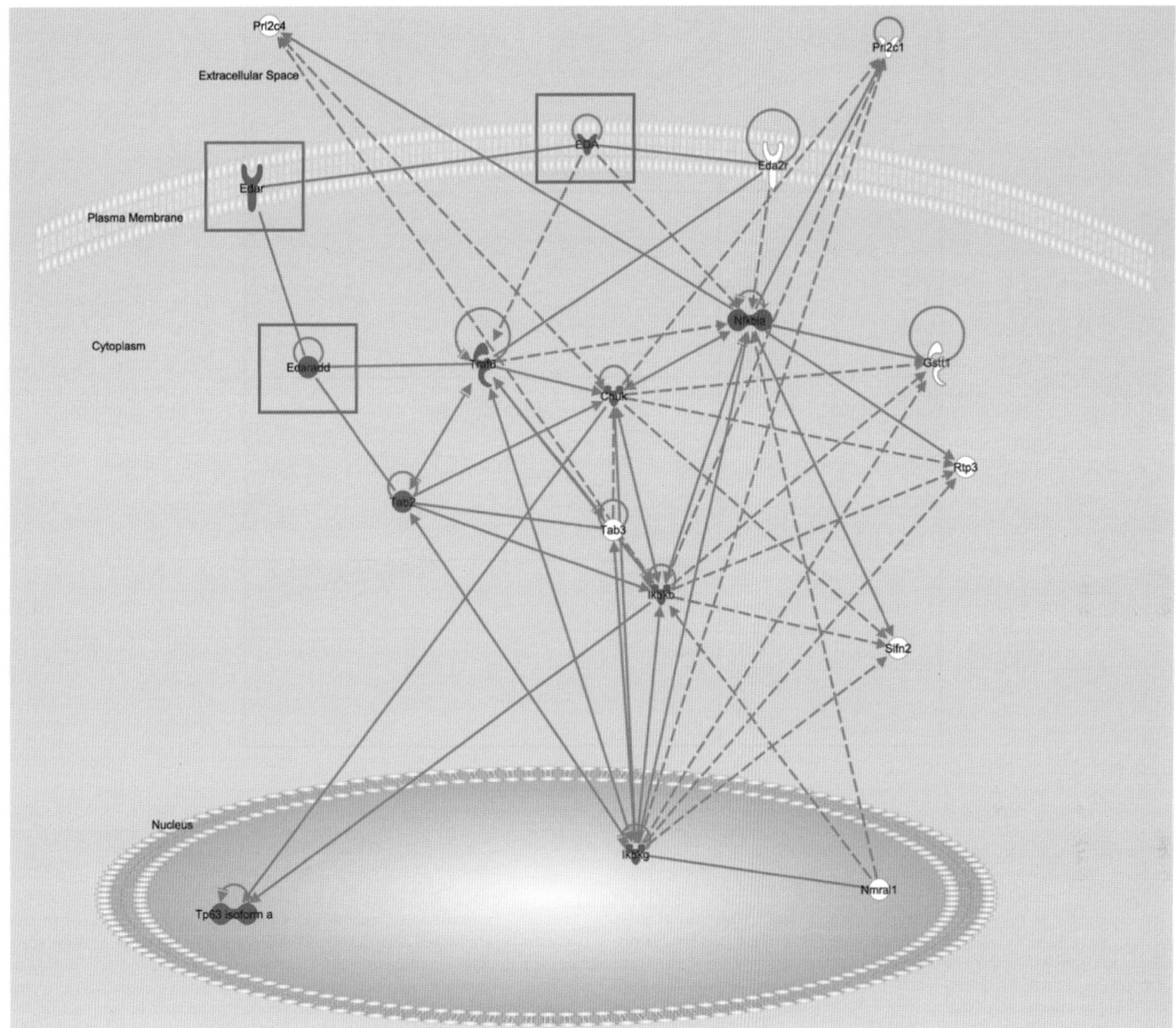

Fig. 36.13
Ingenuity Pathway Analysis Software® (http://www.ingenuity.com/) molecular pathway diagram for genes that interact with Tabby. Note that the receptor, ligand, and death domain proteins (red boxes) are part of a larger molecular pathway. Mutations in other genes in this pathway can cause some, but not all, of the lesions seen in the tabby-crinkled-downless syndrome in mice, demonstrating how linking similar or overlapping genocopies define these pathways.

Hairless, rhino, papular atrichia and genocopies

The correlation of the hairless mouse phenotype with human atrichia with papules or papular atrichia is often attributed to Ahmad[1] (http://omim.org/entry/209500); however, the correct comparison was made nearly 10 years earlier by Sundberg et al.[2,3] The underlying gene responsible has subsequently been named hairless (HR for the human gene and Hr for the mouse gene). In humans, perturbation of HR expression results in two phenotypes: when HR is absent the result is atrichia with papular lesions,[4,5] and when HR is overexpressed the result is Marie Unna hereditary hypotrichosis 1.[5] Expression studies using mouse models have shown that HR is highly expressed throughout the hair follicle during the catagen stage of apoptosis and regression; therefore, when HR is dramatically reduced, as is the case of the HR mutant mouse models, apoptosis becomes uncoordinated and

the hair follicle ceases to cycle properly.[6,7] In both humans and mice, the hairless protein is essential for re-entry into the anagen or growth phase of hair follicles.[8] This results in degenerated hair follicles and the formation of epidermal cysts that eventually take on the appearance of papules, hence the name of the disorder in humans, atrichia with papular lesions (Fig. 36.15).[9] Mutations causing greater loss of Hr expression result in a more severe phenotype characterized by both hairlessness and excessive wrinkling or skin folds (rhinoceros or rhino mice; Hr^rh).[10] Not surprisingly, mutations in the hairless gene in other primates (macaques) cause similar phenotypes.[11]

The hairless gene (HR for humans and Hr for mice) encodes a nucleoprotein that is highly expressed in the skin and brain.[12] HR protein acts as a transcriptional co-repressor for nuclear receptors, including the vitamin D receptor (VDR), thyroid hormone receptor (TR), and retinoic acid-like orphan receptor alpha.[8,13,14] Not surprisingly, null mutations in VDR result

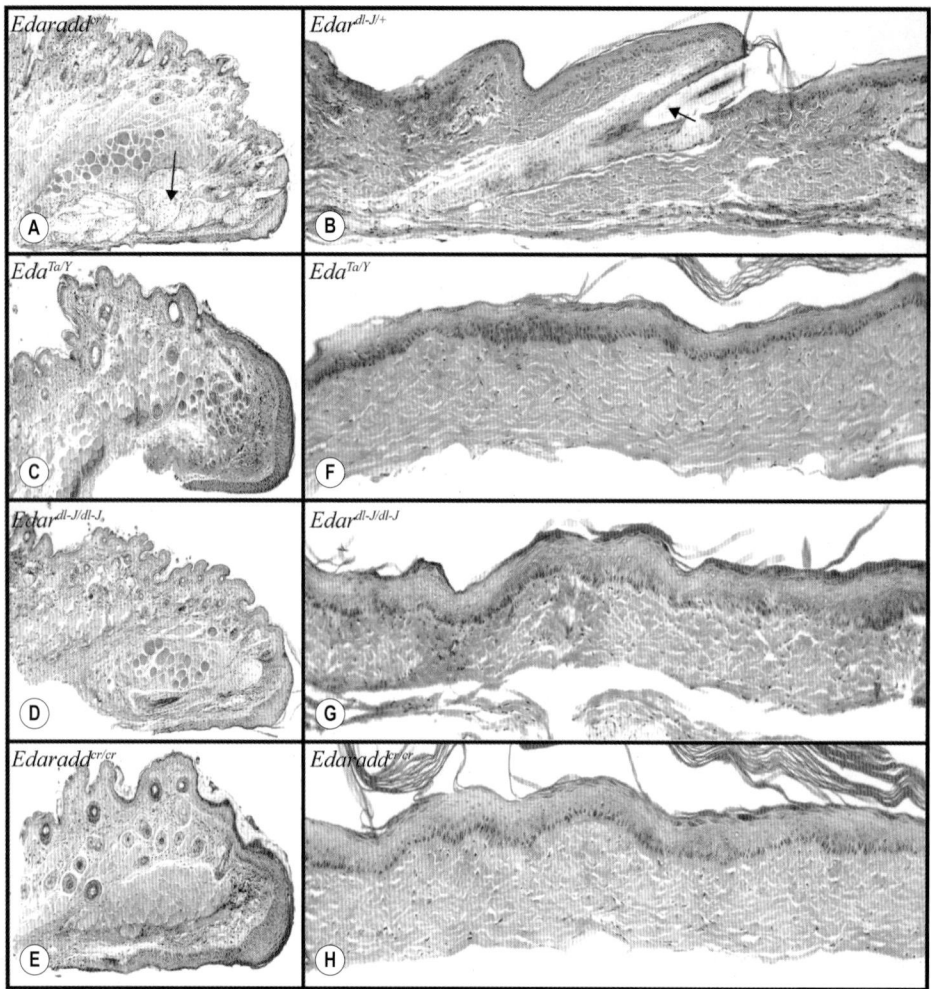

Fig. 36.14
Normal Meibomian gland (**A**, *Edaradd/+, arrow, left column*) in an eyelid and normal pilosebaceous unit in the tail skin (**B**, *Edar/+, right column*) with elevation of the epidermis forming the scale-like structure in heterozygous mice. Mutant mice on the C57BL/6J inbred background lacking the ligand (C, F, *Eda*), receptor (D, G, *Edar*), or death domain genes (E, H, *Edaradd*) all lack Meibomian glands (left column) and have no pilosebaceous glands in their tail skin (*right column*), which is relatively flat and lacks scale-like structures.

in lesions similar to those seen in humans[15] and mice[16] with mutations in their respective hairless genes. In addition, the HR protein exhibits histone demethylase activity.[12,17] *Hr* also appears to be an early UVB response gene that regulates NFKB activation, which controls cellular responses to irradiation.[18] These observations suggest that HR may interact with a number of different signaling pathways (*Fig. 36.16*).[17]

A hairless mutant that overexpressed HR (hairpoor, Hr^{Hp}) downregulated $Dlx3^{19}$, which in turn regulates *Hoxc13* (*Fig. 36.17*).[20] Targeted mutations in $Dlx3^{20,21}$ and $Hoxc13^{22}$ (*Fig. 36.18*) result in hair shaft and follicle abnormalities. *Hoxc13* regulates *Foxn1* (see *Figs 36.17* and *36.18*),[22] $Foxq1$,[23] and $Soat1^{24}$ (*Fig. 36.1*), which also have hair shaft abnormalities. Epithelial deletion of *Dlx3* impairs expression of hair keratins[21] as do mutations in the *Foxn1* gene (*Fig. 36.18*)[25–27] which are responsible for the nude mutation in mice and humans.[28] This illustrates one of the complex molecular pathways in which hairless functions result in hair shaft abnormalities that fall into different morphological types depending on where in the pathway the genes cluster (see *Fig. 36.17*).

Other genocopies appear when the key polyamine enzymes ornithine decarboxylase (ODC; *Fig. 36.15*)[29,30] and spermidine/spermine N^1-acetyltransferase (SSAT)[31] are overexpressed. Both ODC and SSAT transgenic mice have elevated epidermal levels of putrescine. HR and putrescine form a negative regulatory network, since epidermal ODC expression is elevated when HR is decreased and vice versa. Regulation of ODC by HR is dependent on the MYC superfamily of proteins, in particular, MYC, MXI1, and MXD3. Furthermore, elevated levels of putrescine lead to decreased HR expression; however, the SSAT-transgenic phenotype is distinct from that of HR

mutants. Transcriptional microarray analysis of putrescine-treated primary human keratinocytes demonstrated differential regulation of genes involved in protein-protein interactions, nucleotide binding, and transcription factor activity, suggesting that the putrescine-HR negative regulatory loop may have a large impact on epidermal homeostasis and hair follicle cycling.

The hairless $(Hr)^2$ genocopies (vitamin D receptor null $[Vdr]$,[16,32] or transgenic mice that overexpress genes in the putricine cycle, such as ornithine decarboxylase $[Odc]$ (see *Fig. 36.15*),[30,33] SSAT,[31] and others) all have, in addition to alopecia, long curved nails. A number of mice with mutations in the slug pathway also have similar nail lesions.[34] A common histologic feature in all of these mice is that the stratum granulosum of the hyponychium reflects back under the nail bed, which is associated with cornification and in so doing, loss of adhesion between the nail plate and nail bed. This may cause pain and tearing of the nail plate from the nail bed such that the mice do not wear the nails down normally. Cutaneous ulcers are often attributed to trauma from these long nails by animal caretakers; however, the ulcers are not due to scratching but to rupture of the deep dermal cysts (see hair abnormalities).

To further complicate this, nude mice $(Foxn1^{nu})$ are often confused with hairless (Hr^{hr}) because of the name. Nude mice lack a thymus, and therefore T lymphocytes, making them immunodeficient[35,36] Nude mice were the first mutant mice used heavily for xenografts. Investigators are surprised when xenographs fail on hairless mice, which are only mildly immunodeficient.[37–39] Both types of mutant mice are diffusely alopecic, but they do have hair follicles and produce hair at some time during their life, which subsequently breaks off.

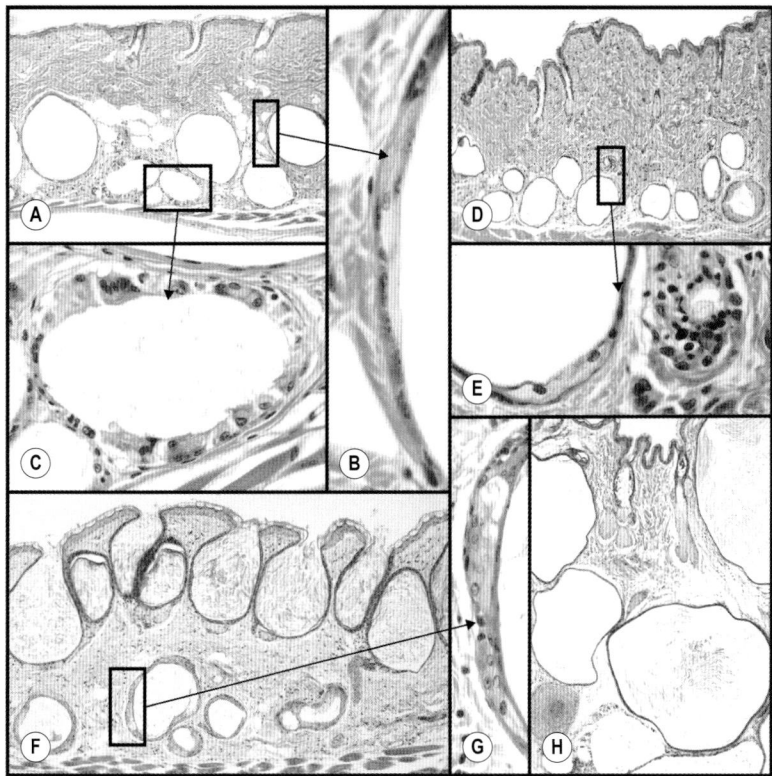

Fig. 36.15
Mutations in the hairless gene can vary between inbred backgrounds such as the SKH2/J-*Hr*^{hr} (**A–C**) and B6.Cg-*Hr*^{hr} (**D, E**). Other allelic mutations, such as the RHJ/Le-*Hr*^{rh-9J} (**F, G**), or genocopies, such as C57BL/6-Tg(K6ODCtr)55Tgo/J transgenic mice (**H**) that overexpress the ornithine decarboxylase, structural 1 gene, have large deep dermal cysts and utricles (dilation of the infundibulum) of various sizes. The deep dermal cysts have sebaceous differentiation in their walls (**B, E, G**). When the deep dermal cysts rupture, granulomas form (**C, E**) often associated around hair shafts free in the dermis. These can lead to puritis and ultimately to ulcers.

Alopecia areata

Alopecia areata is the second most common form of alopecia in humans ranging from solitary foci of hair loss, loss of hair on the head, to total loss of all body hair. While the etiology has been debated for decades, it is now clearly established that this is a cell-mediated autoimmune disease.[1] The C3H/HeJ mouse was discovered in 1991, 25 years ago, to develop patchy alopecia that waxed and waned but only occurred in 20% to 25% of the colony as they aged. The alopecia was initially observed in mice around 5 months of age, but the frequency in the colony rose and stabilized at around 12 months of age.[2] Because lesions came and either expanded or disappeared, very similar to the human disease, and only a percentage of the mice came down with alopecia areata, the C3H/HeJ model proved difficult to work with as a preclinical or basic research tool. Discovery that full thickness skin grafts onto immunodeficient mice of the same strain resulted in normal hair regrowth, but grafts onto histocompatible mice resulted not only in retention of the alopecia phenotype but also development of progressive alopecia beginning in the axillary and inguinal regions, spreading across the abdomen and eventually to the back of the mice resulting in generalized alopecia. This yielded a highly reproducible mouse model that is heavily used today.[3] Modifications of this protocol, most recently using draining lymph node derived cells, continue to be made.[4]

As with human alopecia areata, the late anagen and early catagen follicles are surrounded and infiltrated by a mixed inflammatory cell infiltrate, primarily consisting of CD4+ and CD8+ T cells. As with humans, CD8+ KLRK1 (killer cell lectin-like receptor C1 gene, previously called NKG2D) are the primary effector cells. The result is that there is a follicular dystrophy starting in the bulb region that leads to a deformity and weakness in the hair shaft, which breaks off at the skin surface when it emerges from the follicular ostium.[1]

Psoriasiform mouse models

Psoriasis is a group of human diseases with epidermal proliferation and an inflammatory cell infiltrate into the dermis. A large and ever-growing number of single or multiple mutant mouse strains and stocks have been created and proposed as psoriasis models,[1–3] as well as xenograft models.[4] Mice may not be the best mammalian model here because of anatomic differences between mice and humans; principally, mice do not develop rete ridges. The mouse stratum granulosum varies between strains, probably due to differences in the number of profilaggrin repeats in their filaggrin gene (*Flg*), which can affect whether or not those with proliferative skin disease have hypergranulosis. This was observed when the flaky skin allele of the tetratricopeptide repeat domain 7 (*Ttc7*^{fsn}) gene first arose on the A/J inbred strain, where it had almost no granular layer in the thickened epidermis. When the mutant gene was transferred to the BALB/cByJ strain to create a congenic strain, the granular layer became a prominent feature (Sundberg, unpublished data). While hypergranulosis is not considered to be a common feature in human psoriasis, it is a variation seen in some clinical cases. These issues are partial explanations as to why there is a plethora of proposed mouse models for psoriasis – but, to date, none that are well accepted. The larger issue here is that GWAS continues to indicate that human psoriasis is a very complex genetic-based disease.[5–7] Only until all or most of the genes are identified and comparable mutations made in mice and all on the same inbred strain at the same time (now possible using CRISPR/Cas9) will it be possible to recreate the disease in the mouse.

Xenographs: transplanting tissues from humans to mice

Grafting, a surgical procedure commonly used in both clinical and experimental dermatology, is the process of transferring skin from one body site to another or from another individual, without the donor's blood supply, which grows into the successful graft from the recipient host. There are four classifications of grafts: (1) autograft (tissue removed from one site and surgically implanted into another on the same individual); (2) isograft (tissue removed from an individual and surgically grafted onto a genetically identical individual, such as an identical twin or another member of the same inbred mouse strain); (3) allograft (tissue removed from an individual and grafted onto a genetically different individual of the same species, such as between different inbred strains); and (4) xenograft (tissue taken from an individual and grafted onto an individual of a different species, for example, human tissues grafted onto immunodeficient mice).[1] Allografts are commonly used for studying graft-versus-host disease in a variety of mouse models. Allografts onto immunodeficient mice, or isografts to immunocompetent or immunodeficient mice of the same inbred strain, are useful in mouse studies when the mutant mouse has an inflammatory skin disease phenotype as a tool to help determine if the inflammation is a systemic problem, or is induced by the primary skin abnormality. For example, before a congenic strain was created for the flaky skin allele of the tetratricopeptide repeat domain 7 (*Ttc7*^{fsn}) gene, skin was grafted from hybrid mice onto nude mice (which lack T cells) to demonstrate maintenance of the psoriasiform phenotype.[2] Conversely, grafting skin from C3H/HeJ mice with alopecia areata onto protein kinase, DNA activated, catalytic polypeptide mutant mice (severe combined immunodeficiency mutant mice, *Prkdc*^{scid}) on a congenic C3H/HeJ background (C3SnSmn.CB17-*Prkdc*^{scid}/J) or wildtype C3H/HeJ (immunocompetent) mice revealed that the phenotype was lost on the immunodeficient background but not only developed in the skin graft on the wildtype C3H/HeJ mice, but the mice also developed generalized alopecia universalis over a 20-week period.[3] Xenografts, moving tissues from one species to another, continue to be an experimental way to look at rare samples from endangered species, such as cutaneous fibropapillomas in sea turtles, by successfully transferring the lesions onto *Prkdc*^{scid} mice.[4] The nude mouse (forkhead box N1, *Foxn1*^{nu}) was the first immunodeficient mouse identified and used for xenografts in the 1960s. It

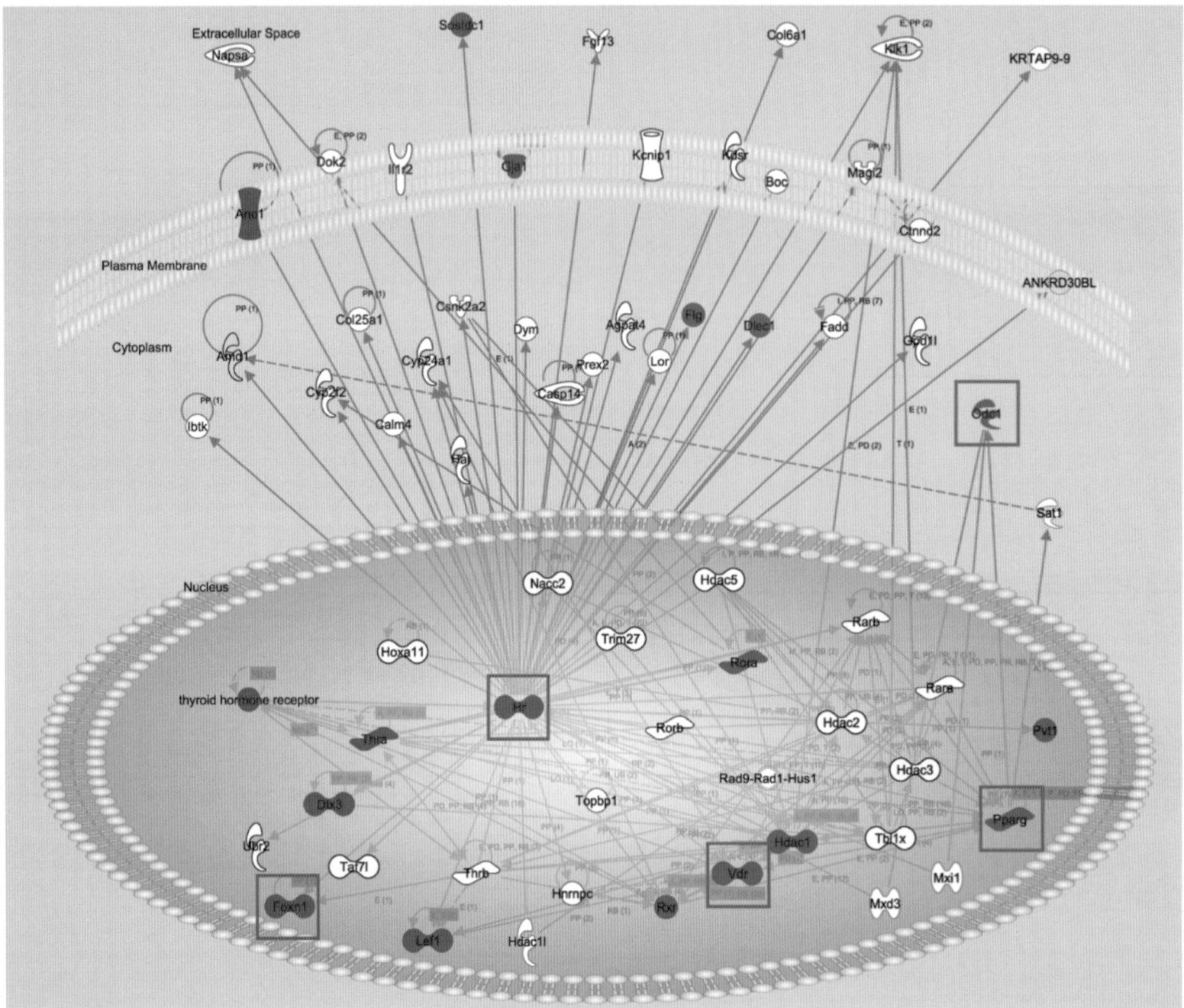

Fig. 36.16
Ingenuity Pathway Analysis Software® (http://www.ingenuity.com/) molecular pathway diagram for genes that interact with hairless (*HR*). Mutations in both mice and humans in the *Hr/HR* and *Vdr/VDR* genes result in genocopies, the same phenotypes in both groups of mutants. As these interact with other genes, it is not surprising that follicular dystrophy results, although the phenotype is different, as with *FOXN1* (nude human or mouse) or *DLX3*.

remains in use today for xenografts, isografts, and allografts, especially in dermatology because the adults are alopecic.[5] The alopecia evident in nude mice is due to a defect in the quality of their hair resulting in breakage as the hair shafts emerge from the hair follicles, and not that they do not have hair follicles.[6] One has to be careful not to confuse nude mice with hairless mice (*Hr*), which also have no hair in adulthood but have a largely intact immune system such that they will not accept xenografts or allografts.

Many more mutant mice have been discovered or created which serve as improved hosts for human tissues, especially human cancers.[7–9] Mice used for these types of studies are commonly called patient-derived xenograft (PDX) mice. Their value is that the cancers can be grafted from the patient to several recipient mice, allowed to grow, and then serially transplanted, allowing detailed molecular studies or testing with a variety of chemotherapeutic agents. The basic protocol involves mincing up fresh cancer biopsies into 3- to 5-mm³ pieces that are then surgically implanted subcutaneously into the lateral side of a NOD.Cg-*Prkdc*^{scid} *Il2rg*^{tm1Wjl}/SzJ immunodeficient

mouse, commonly referred to as an NSG mouse. Mice are monitored for 5 months. Single cell suspensions or pieces of solid cancers that develop in these recipient mice can then be implanted into additional NSG mice to expand the numbers of mice carrying the cancers for research.[10–12] A number of skin cancer PDX models are available to investigators at the time of this writing including 13 melanomas, 4 squamous cell carcinomas, and 1 Merkel cell tumor. Details can be found on these cancers in the Mouse Tumor Biology Database (http://tumor.informatics.jax.org/; 15 November 2016). A comparison between a human melanoma and the melanoma engrafted onto an NSG mouse is shown in *Fig. 36.19*; the histologic differences are negligible. Better immunodeficient mouse models are constantly being developed for these types of studies.[13] Another useful mouse tool is to use mice that have a ubiquitously expressing marker, such as enhanced green fluorescent protein (EGFP), as the donor. Using either immunofluorescence or immunohistochemistry with antibodies specific for EGFP, it is possible to follow the lineages of the cells grafted, whether they came from the host or the donor.[5]

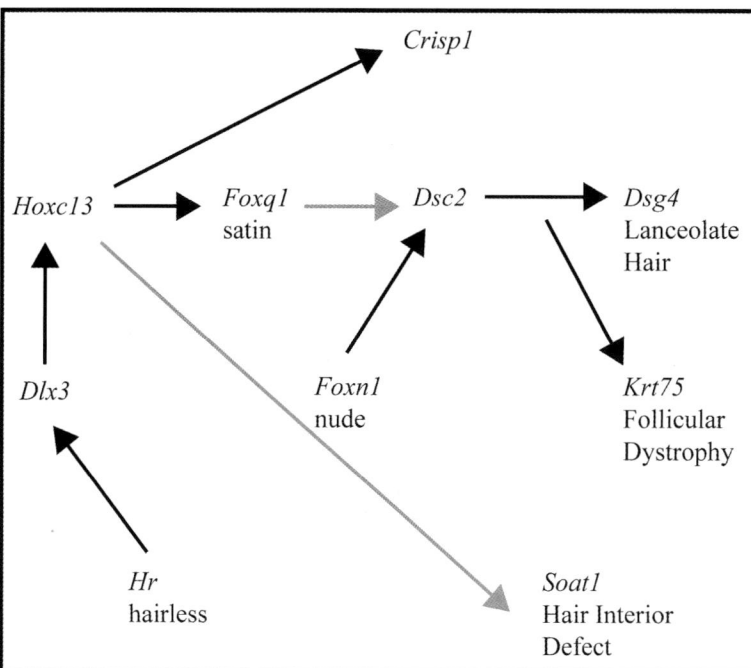

Fig. 36.17
Known and predicted molecular pathway for hair follicle development. Mice with mutations in these genes develop skin lesions that include various forms of follicular dystrophy. Some, such as *Soat1* and *Foxq1*, result in defects within hair shafts, whereas others, such as *Hoxc13* and *Foxn1*, result in weak, distorted shafts that break off. Integrating these individual mouse models for each gene in the pathway enables researchers to define their interactions and follow how defects cause clinical disease.

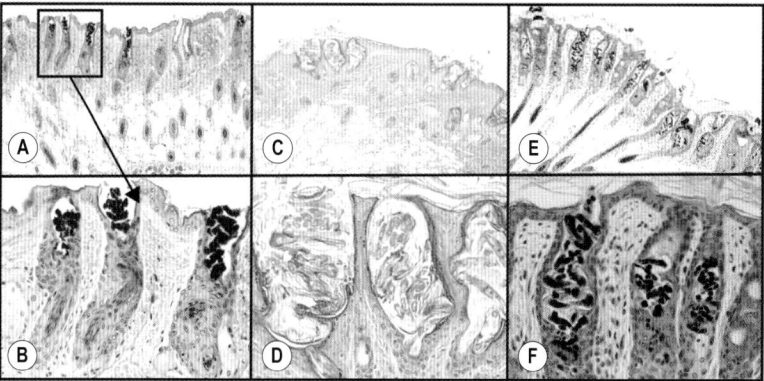

Fig. 36.18
C57BL/6J-*Hoxc13*[tm1Mrc] null adult mice (**A**, **B**) have weak hair shafts that twist within the infundibulum and break off at the skin surface. Nude mice (**C**, **D**; CByJ. Cg-*Foxn1*[nu] albino; **E**, **F**; B6.Cg-*Foxn1*[nu], pigmented) have a similar phenotype. These genes work in the same molecular pathway.

Currently missing mouse models of human skin pathology

There are large numbers of mutant mice available, and many more being created primarily in the large genetically engineered mouse programs such as KOMP, as well as the ever-expanding utilization of CRISPR/Cas9 technology. It is therefore likely only a matter of time before models become available for specific diseases currently believed to be missing. However, the needed models may be available but not accurately described or curated in databases. Alternatively, investigators focus on organs or structures of their particular interest and ignore obvious lesions in other organ systems. Using databases to search for such models can be time-consuming but sometimes rewarding. By contrast, many models have been reported as models for particular diseases that are not good or accurate models. To help remedy this situation, phenotyping standardization is being approached in the Knockout Mouse Project/International Mouse Phenotyping Consortium (KOMP/

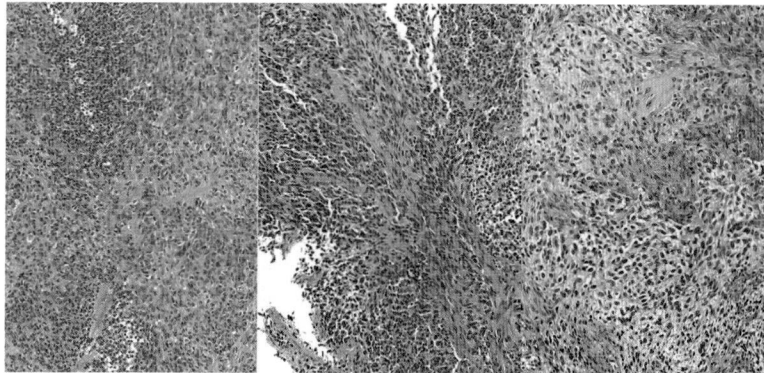

Fig. 36.19
Patient-derived xenograft (PDX) melanoma model. The left image shows the histology of a melanoma in a human patient while the two images on the right show the same neoplasm as two independent PDX in two separate immunodeficient mice. Images courtesy of Clemens Krepler and James Hayden, The Wistar Institute, Philadelphia, PA and Xiaowei (George) Xu, University of Pennsylvania, Philadelphia, PA.

IMPC) programs, but even these lack critical expertise or depth in evaluation of all organ systems.

Two examples of diseases for which models are often thought not to exist include cutaneous scarring lesions/keloids and vascular tumors.

There are numerous models for cicatricial alopecia in mice[1-3] in which scarring is limited to the hair follicles and are clearly distinct from keloids. However, a number of models are described in the literature that can be used for keloids, with most of them using PDX-type approaches.[4-11]

Vascular tumors are another disease group for which many believe mouse models do not exist. Cutaneous vascular tumors do arise spontaneously in mice, albeit very rarely. However, they are relatively common in many inbred strains but only in very old mice.[12-15] When one performs a literature search (by including terms such as hemangioma, hemangiosarcoma, and hemangioendothelioma), not surprisingly, a number of models emerge, again often based on the PDX approach.[16-24]

There are huge numbers of mouse models for most diseases already available. More are under development. As investigators continue to refine existing models, molecular pathways, or with genetic modifications, addition of more than one mutation, changing strain background, or by simply utilizing more refined and systematic phenotyping methods, better models will continue to emerge. Large biorepositories, such as the one at the Jackson Laboratory (JAX), make these mouse models available to investigators worldwide.

Zebrafish as a model system to study skin biology and pathology

Several animal models have been developed to recapitulate the features of specific skin diseases, and such model systems have provided valuable insight into the pathomechanistic details of these diseases. They have also provided useful systems for testing of treatment modalities for a number of conditions. The preferred platform for such model development has been the mouse, often through the development of 'knockout' mice or by development of transgenic mice with expression of the mutant genes. Although the mouse models have demonstrated remarkable similarity to human diseases, mice as a model system have considerable limitations, including relatively long life span, extended reproductive cycle, and high cost of development and housing. Also, the genetic background of the mouse strains can have a major influence on the development of the disease phenotype. In some cases, development of the mouse model is not feasible because of the absence of the corresponding gene in the mouse genome. These considerations, particularly in conjunction with cost-containment issues, have prompted the search for an alternative model system to study skin diseases. In fact, Vanchieri[1] suggested, 'Move over mouse: make way for the woodchucks, ferrets, and zebrafish', and Lieschke and Currie[2] said, 'Animal models of human disease: zebrafish swim into view'.

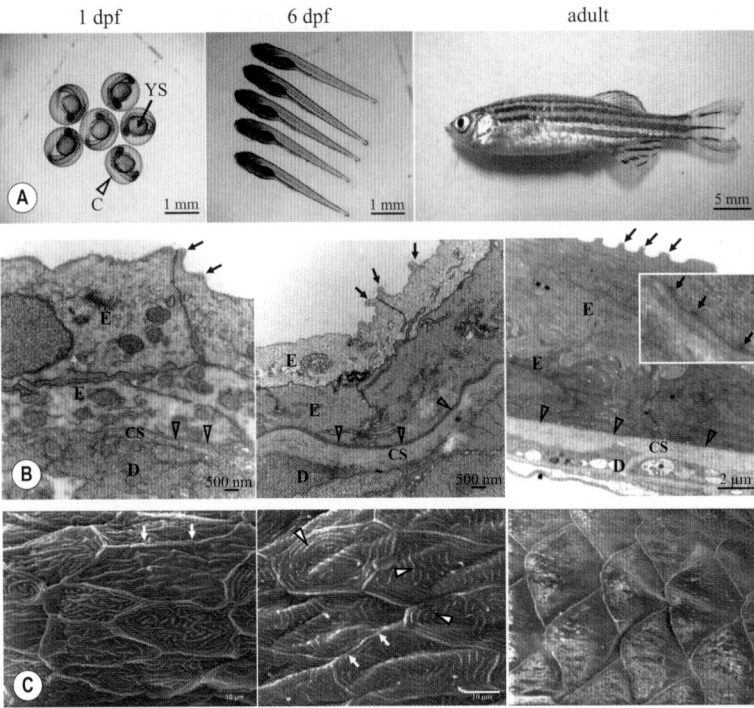

Fig. 36.20
Cutaneous biology of the developing zebrafish. (**A**) The growth of zebrafish from 1 dpf embryos, which are surrounded by a transparent chorion (C) and display a prominent yolk sac (YS), to an adult fish. At 6 dpf, pigmentation becomes apparent on the skin. (**B**) Transmission electron microscopy reveals at 1 and 6 dpf, an epidermis (E) consisting of two cell layers, and at 6 dpf, the epidermis is separated from the underlying collagenous stroma (CS) and dermis (D) by a clearly demarcated basement membrane (*open arrowheads*). In adult fish, there is a multilayered epidermis, and higher magnification of the basement membrane zone reveals the presence of hemidesmosomes (*arrows in the inset*). The spicule-like extensions of the surface of the skin (*arrows*) correspond to microridges. (**C**) Scanning electron microscopy reveals well-demarcated keratinocytes with distinct cell-cell borders (*small arrows*). In the middle of the keratinocyte surface, there are developing microridges, which at 6 dpf become well organized (*open arrowheads*). In an adult fish, the epidermis is covered by scales. dpf, days post fertilization. Adopted from reference[13].

Zebrafish skin development

There are several characteristics that favor choosing zebrafish (*Danio rerio*) for genetic and developmental studies.[2–4] Zebrafish, a small freshwater vertebrate, is easily maintained in the laboratory setting. Large number of embryos can be obtained per laying, approximately 50–100 per female, and the development of various organs in zebrafish embryos is easy to visualize in vivo because the embryos are optically transparent during the first several days of development.[5] Zebrafish have a rapid rate of maturation from embryo to fully developed fish (*Fig. 36.20A*). At 5–6 days post fertilization (dpf), all important internal organs are largely formed, and skin consists of distinct compartments, as visualized by transmission electron microscopy (*Fig. 36.20B*).

At 1 dpf, different skin layers representing the epidermis and the dermis can be recognized, although the cutaneous basement membrane zone (BMZ) at the dermal–epidermal junction is not yet developed. However, at 6 dpf, the epidermis, composed of two cell layers, is readily noticeable and clearly separated from the underlying connective tissue stroma by a basement membrane. At the surface of the epidermal contour, there are spicule-like protrusions that correspond to the microridges of epidermal cells. On the dermal side, there is a well-developed collagenous stroma with adjacent fibroblastic cells with a well-developed rough endoplasmic reticulum.[6] In the fully developed adult zebrafish skin, there is a multilayer epidermis separated from the underlying collagenous stroma by the BMZ, and at high magnification, hemidesmosomal structures can be visualized (see *Fig. 36.20B*).[7] Thus, the

zebrafish skin has a clearly demarcated dermal–epidermal BMZ, separating the epidermis from the underlying dermis.

Examination of the developing zebrafish skin surface at 1 dpf by scanning electron microscopy reveals well-demarcated keratinocytes with a surface contour containing microridges, which are well organized by 6 dpf (*Fig. 36.20C*). In adult zebrafish, the epidermis is covered by scales, which form under the control of a genetic cascade, including sonic hedgehog expression, at approximately 30 dpf.[8] However, early on, at least up to 6 dpf, the developing zebrafish epidermis has characteristic landmark features that can be altered by perturbed keratinocyte gene expression.

In addition to the structural elements of the epidermis, BMZ, and the collagenous dermis, the zebrafish skin has a neural crest-derived pigment cell system, including the presence of melanocytes, that can serve as a target to study developmental biology and pathology of pigmentation.[9,10] The zebrafish skin also has structures that are specialized for the aquatic environment, such as scales, presence of mucous secreting cells, and the lateral line. The latter organ contains 54 neuromasts that are topographically highly conserved neural elements consisting of hair cells, serving as a sensory organ regarding the rheological movements of the fish.[11] Of interest is our recent finding that the gene product of *col17a1b* is localized to neuromasts, and that 'knockdown' of the corresponding gene by morpholino abolishes the formation of functional neuromasts.[12] However, a key difference between zebrafish and human skin is the lack of mammalian appendages, including hair follicles and sebaceous glands. In addition, zebrafish lack functional stratum corneum and expression of genes necessary for terminal differentiation of epidermis.

The zebrafish genome and genetic manipulation

The zebrafish genome

The genome of zebrafish consists of 25 chromosomes and contains essentially the full repertoire of vertebrate genes. Although the zebrafish genome sequencing has not been fully completed, the most recent zebrafish reference genome assembly, GRCz11, was released. Comparison with the human genome reveals that approximately 70% of human genes have a zebrafish counterpart, and over 80% human disease genes, including oncogenes and tumor suppressors, have orthologs in zebrafish.[1]

A characteristic feature of the zebrafish genome is that a number of genes appear in duplicate, reflecting two sequential rounds of duplication of the genome before divergence of ray-finned and lobe-finned fish. In addition, there is evidence of another round of whole genome duplication near the origin of teleost fish approximately 350 million years ago.[2] Although in many cases one copy of the duplicated gene has been lost or silenced during evolution, in some cases both copies have survived in a functional state but resulted in distinct function or spatial distribution. The overall conservation in different orthologous genes between species, such as humans and zebrafish, can be determined by constructing phylogenetic trees based on precise nucleotide information. The conservation of individual genes between humans and zebrafish is variable, but certain protein domains are well conserved. Nevertheless, the overall conservation of the human and zebrafish genome forms the basis to study the role of distinct genes in cutaneous biology and pathology.

Forward genetics

One approach to study heritable skin diseases using zebrafish as a model system employs forward genetics, in which discrete point mutations are introduced into the genome with *N*-ethyl-*N*-nitrosourea (ENU), or random mutagenesis is carried out using retroviral techniques. After mutagenesis, a large number of embryos or larvae are screened for cutaneous phenotypes, facilitated by the transparency of the developing fish (*Fig. 36.21*). Large-scale forward genetics screens can also be used to identify mutated genes orthologous to those causing human heritable diseases, with phenotypic similarities.[3,4] This approach also allows identification of previously unreported genes that can be tested in patients with similar phenotypes but with no known gene defects.

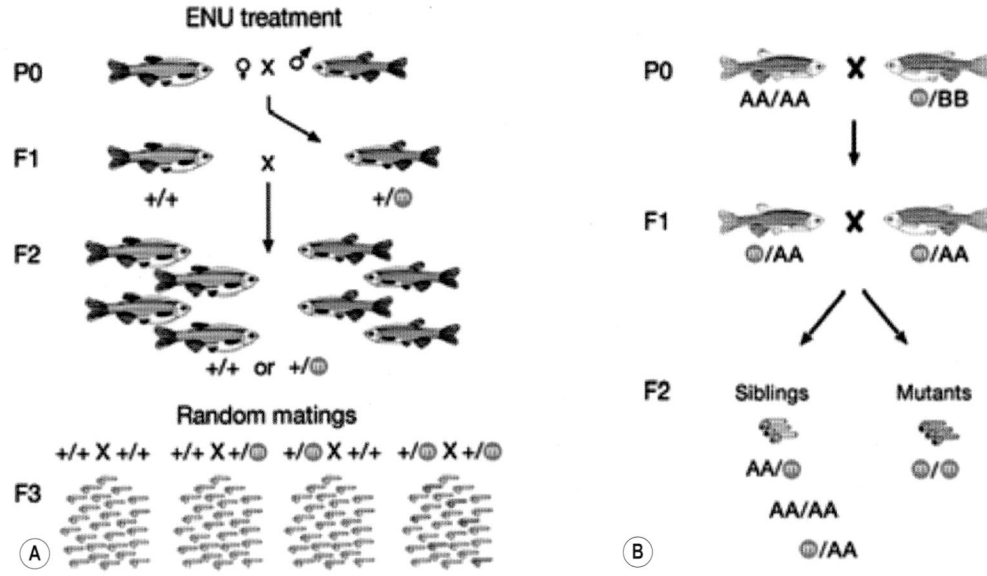

Fig. 36.21
Principles of forward genetics for identification of mutated genes in zebrafish by ethylnitrosourea (ENU) mutagenesis. (**A**) ENU treatment of male fish results in random mutagenesis (m). Mating of mutant males with normal females results in a progeny of mutant fish with a readily observable phenotype in the case of a dominant mutation in F1 and F2 generations. In the case of a recessive mutation, random matings result in a population with the phenotype (gray fish). (**B**) Identification of the recessive mutations resulting in a phenotype (gray fish). The specific mutant genes will be identified by linkage analysis and the mutations can be detected by genome sequencing. SNP, single nucleotide polymorphism; SSLP, simple sequence-length polymorphism. Adopted from reference.[23]

Morpholino-based knockdown of gene expression

Another way of utilizing zebrafish as a model system to study heritable skin diseases is to perform 'knockdown' of the expression of specific genes by stable morpholino-based antisense oligonucleotides.[5] These morpholinos can target either the sequences around or slightly upstream from the translation initiation codon (AUG) to prevent translation or splice junction sequences to prevent synthesis of a mature mRNA.[6,7] In the case of morpholinos targeting the upstream regulatory sequences, the efficiency can be monitored by co-injection of the morpholino with mRNA transcribed from an expression construct containing the 5' regulatory elements of the corresponding gene linked to green fluorescent protein reporter (*Fig. 36.22A*). In the case of splice junction morpholinos, the efficiency of the gene expression knockdown can be monitored by reverse RT-PCR (*Fig. 36.22B*).

The specificity of morpholino knockdown can be confirmed using a biologically inactive standard control morpholino without a target sequence in the zebrafish genome,[8] or by co-injection of the corresponding mRNA or protein from another species, such as mouse or humans, which counteracts the development of the phenotype,[9] the latter one being the principle of mRNA rescue assays for testing the pathogenicity of missense mutations in the corresponding human gene.[10] The specificity of morpholino knockdown can also be confirmed by injection of more than one morpholino for the same target gene. The limitation of using morpholinos in genetics studies is that morpholinos have a relatively short half-life (up to 5 days), and therefore, this approach is most suitable for evaluation of the effects of a morpholino knockdown on the early zebrafish development.[11–13]

Genome editing in zebrafish

Over several recent years, genome editing approaches have been adopted as an efficient and sophisticated approach to precisely engineer the zebrafish genome, which has further enhanced the utility of this model system.

ZFN and TALEN have been used in zebrafish to edit the genome with great success.[14–17] However, these approaches are costly and time-consuming to engineer, limiting their widespread use, particularly for large-scale, high-throughput studies. The recently discovered CRISPR/Cas9 endonuclease has the ability to create insertions or deletions at the targeted site. Alternatively, a template can be supplied, in which case homology-directed repair results in the generation of engineered alleles at the break site. CRISPR/Cas9 targeted genome editing enables inexpensive and high-throughput interrogation of gene manipulation. These changes alter the function of the targeted gene facilitating the analysis of gene function. This tool has been widely adopted in the zebrafish model.[17–22] CRISPR/Cas9 mutagenesis can be used to make conditional alleles to study tissue-specific or stage-specific gene function. CRISPR/Cas9 can also be used for whole genome forward genetic screens. This can lead to exploration of biological processes that have been intractable.

Application of the zebrafish model for skin research

The advantages of the zebrafish as a model system to study cutaneous biology and pathology are becoming widely recognized, and an increasing number of publications utilize this system.[1,2]

Heritable skin disorders

One study demonstrated the utility of forward genetic screening to identify a loss-of-function mutation in the *kindlin-1* gene in mutant zebrafish demonstrating epidermal fragility at 2 dpf.[1] The phenotype consisted of progressive rupturing and eventually of complete loss of medial fins as a result of ENU mutagenesis. Mitotic mapping positioned the causal mutation on chromosome 20 to an interval that contained *kindlin-1* (FERMT1), which encodes Kindlin-1, the zebrafish ortholog of the human protein at fault in Kindler syndrome.[2] Characterization of the zebrafish mutation in this gene revealed a G to T transversion mutation in exon 13, resulting in a premature termination mutation (p. E565X). It was noted that the fin phenotype of the *kindlin-1* mutants resembled that of knockdown embryos injected with *kindlin-1*-specific morpholino. Thus, the *kindlin-1* mutant zebrafish provides a unique model system to study epidermal adhesion mechanisms in vivo.

Other examples of zebrafish phenotype mimicking a human skin disease is the morpholino knockdown of the *col17a1a* gene expressed in the skin in hemidesmosomal complexes and knockdown of *abca12* expressed in the epidermis.[3,4] Specifically, *col17a1a*- and *abca12*-specific morpholinos were injected into zebrafish embryos to knockdown corresponding gene expression. The *col17a1a* morphant fish demonstrated skin blisters and

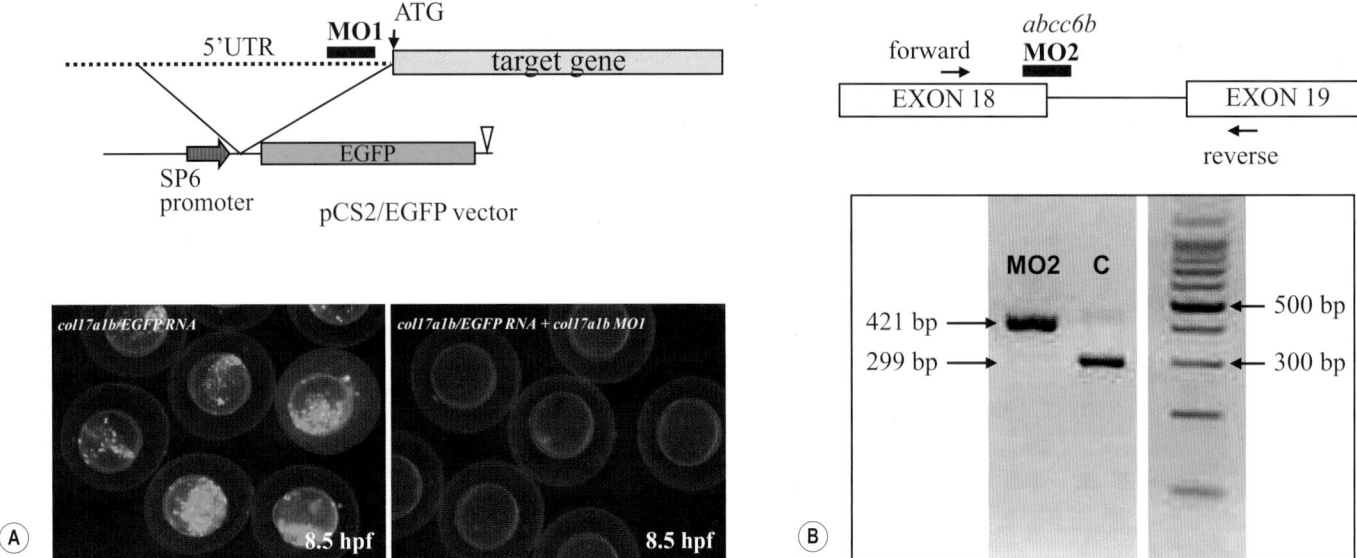

Fig. 36.22

Morpholino-mediated knockdown of zebrafish genes. (**A**) A morpholino (MO1) corresponding to the *col17a1b* gene was used to target the 5′ untranslated region of the corresponding mRNA to prevent translation. To determine the efficacy of morpholino in downregulating the translation, an expression construct consisting of SP6 promoter, 5′ UTR of the *col17a1b* gene, and downstream enhanced green fluorescent protein (EGFP) reporter gene was generated. Microinjection of mRNA transcribed in vitro from the pCS2/EGFP vector to 1–2 cell-stage embryo, shows green fluorescence at 8.5 hpf (*lower left panel*). Co-injection of this mRNA together with the MO1 morpholino completely abolished the fluorescence, indicating inhibition of the translation (bar, 1 mm). (**B**) A morpholino (MO2) corresponding to the zebrafish *abcc6b* gene was placed on the exon 18-intron 18 splice junction. Efficiency of the morpholino in preventing splicing of the *abcc6b* pre-mRNA into mature mRNA was monitored by RT-PCR using primers placed on exon 18 (forward) and exon 19 (reverse). PCR of the genomic sequence resulted in a 421-bp fragment, whereas fully spliced cDNA yields a 299-bp fragment devoid of intron 18 (122 bp). RT-PCR of morpholino (MO2)-treated zebrafish embryo reveals the presence of the 421-bp mRNA sequence only, indicating complete inhibition of the removal of intron 18 by splicing. As the intron 18 sequence is out of frame, this results in complete absence of the abcc6b protein product. dpf, days post fertilization; hpf, hours post fertilization; RT-PCR, reverse transcription-PCR; UTR, untranslated region. Adopted from Kim[6] and Li,[7] with permission.

transmission electron microscopy revealed perturbations in the BMZ (*Fig. 36.23A–B*), mimicking features in patients with a form of junctional epidermolysis bullosa due to mutations in the human *COL17A1* gene. The *abca12* morphant fish demonstrated noticeable changes in the distribution of pigment along the trunk and tail. Scanning electron microscopy demonstrated the absence of microridges and development of scale-like spicules on the surface of the skin, somewhat resembling the scales in human harlequin ichthyosis caused by mutations in the *ABCA12* gene.[4] Transmission electron microscopy suggested the presence of lipid-like vesicles in the skin (*Fig. 36.23C–D*). Similar approaches have been utilized to study congenital ichthyosis due to mutations in *capn12* gene and epidermal differentiation caused by mutations in *svep1* gene.[5,6]

In contrast, diseases that are of late onset or slowly progressing may not be evident in the zebrafish model system. An example of such conditions is pseudoxanthoma elasticum (PXE), a slowly progressive, ectopic mineralization disorder with late onset. Injection of the *abcc6a* morpholino in zebrafish resulted in an early phenotype of pericardial edema and curled tail, associated with death by 8 dpf, but there was no evidence of ectopic mineralization at this stage.[7] The mineralization phenotype, if developmentally corresponding to human or mouse pathogenesis of PXE, might occur later in life. In this context, the *abcc6* knockdown zebrafish is not an appropriate model for PXE.

Wound healing and re-epithelialization

Zebrafish are utilized as a model system for wound healing and re-epithelialization. One examined wound healing and re-epithelialization in adult zebrafish skin following full-thickness wounds inflicted onto the flank of adult zebrafish.[1] The results showed that, apart from external fibrin clot formation, all steps of adult mammalian wound repair also exist in zebrafish. Extremely rapid re-epithelialization was initiated with no apparent lag phase, followed by migration of inflammatory cells and formation of granulation tissue consisting of macrophages, fibroblasts, blood vessels, and collagen. Granulation tissue later regresses, resulting in minimal scar formation.

Further studies suggested that wound re-epithelialization occurs independently of inflammation and fibroblast growth factor signaling, essential for fibroblast recruitment and granulation tissue formation. Together, these results demonstrated that major steps and principles of cutaneous wound healing are conserved among adult mammals and adult zebrafish, making zebrafish a valuable model for studying vertebrate skin repair.

Melanoma and pigmentation

Zebrafish cancers, including melanoma, share many histopathological features with human cancers, and molecular signatures closely align with those of human cancer. In addition, zebrafish embryos and larvae are transparent, enabling tumor formation and progression to be visualized in living animals. Zebrafish cancer models have primarily depended on transgenic expression of oncogenes and ENU-induced genetic mutations in tumor suppressor genes. The zebrafish melanoma models include transgenic zebrafish expressing human $BRAF^{V600E}$ or $HRAS^{G12V}$ mutation.[1,2] The master melanocyte transcription factor MITF, a melanoma oncogene, was recently modeled in zebrafish.[3–5] A unique temperature-sensitive *mitf* mutation in zebrafish (*mitfa^{vc7}*) has recently been used to study MITF activity in the control of melanocyte proliferation and differentiation in embryogenesis, and as a cancer gene in the development and survival of melanoma. In addition, transplantation models of melanoma in zebrafish also allow assessing tumor potential, visualizing cancer homing and metastasis, and in competitive assays for tumorigenicity.[6] The advent of genome editing with CRISPR/Cas9 system now enables precise and tissue-specific genetic editing that will enable more refined genetic modeling of human melanoma.

Small molecule and drug screening

The attributes that have made the zebrafish a powerful model for genetic screening also make it well suited for small molecule screening for drug discovery. A unique feature of the zebrafish system is the ability to treat the whole organism with drug treatments by administering chemical compounds

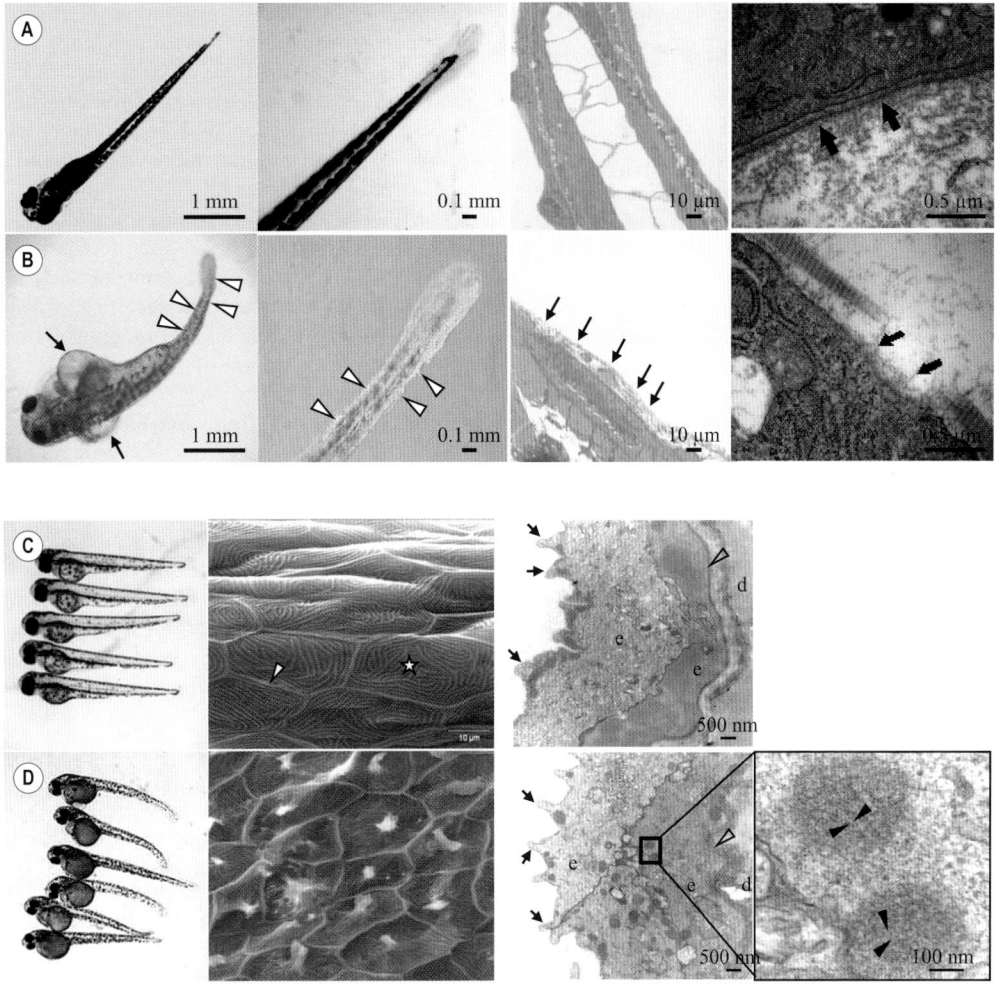

Fig. 36.23
Phenotype of zebrafish injected with scMO, *abca12* or with *col17a1a* morpholinos. Phenotype of zebrafish at 5 dpf injected with scMO (**A**) or with *col17a1a* morpholino (**B**). The morpholino-injected fish showed pericardial edema (**B**, *left panel*, arrows) and morphological changes in the skin surface contour in the tail region (**B**, *second from left*, arrowheads). Histopathological examination of the blistered skin (**B**, *second from right*) revealed vacuolization within the epidermis (*arrows*), in comparison to control fish at 5 dpf (**A**). Transmission electron microscopy revealed intact basement membrane structure (*arrows*) on the control skin (**A**, *right panel*), while the basement membrane zone structure was perturbed in the morpholino treated fish (**B**, *right panel*). (**C**, **D**) Phenotype of zebrafish larvae at 3 dpf after injection with an *abca12* MO2 morpholino (**D**) compared with larvae injected with scMO (**C**). The gross morphological changes were depicted on the left panel. Scanning electron microscopy of the skin surface is in the middle panel. The skin of the tail of the control larvae at 3 dpf shows the presence of keratinocytes with well-demarcated cell-cell borders (*arrowhead*) containing microridges (*star*, *middle top panel*). The morphant larvae injected with MO2 morpholino for *abca12* (**D**, *middle panel*) revealed perturbed microridge formation with spicules in the center of the keratinocytes. Transmission electron microscopy of 3 dpf larvae injected with scMO or *abca12* morpholinos is indicated on the right panel. Box surrounding electron dense subcellular structures was examined at higher magnification as shown in right panel in **D**. Arrows point to microridges; open arrowheads indicate basement membrane; solid black arrowheads point to the areas of accumulation of putative lipids within the electron dense granules; scMO, standard control morpholino; e, epidermis; d, developing dermis. Adopted from Kim[3] and Li,[4] with permission.

to the water.[1] This approach can be used to directly test the function of a targetable pathway in transplantation studies, to screen for new drug leads during early embryogenesis, and for testing compounds in adult zebrafish cancer models.[2] Examples include small molecule screens on the melanocyte lineage that identified 5-nitrofuran compounds, which are also effective in human melanoma,[3] and the changes caused by $BRAF^{V600E}$;$p53$ at the embryonic level that identified leflunomide, which is currently in clinical trials for melanoma treatment (Clinical trials.gov identifier NCT01611675).[4] Zebrafish have recently been established as a new in vivo model for screening melanogenesis inhibitors.[5,6] Overall, phenotypic small molecule screening in zebrafish is effective at multiple stages of the drug discovery pipeline, including hit identification, target identification, lead optimization, and preclinical animal modeling.[6–8]

Summary

Large numbers of mutant laboratory mice available in repositories worldwide with skin, hair, and nail abnormalities represent a huge biomedical resource to validate the molecular basis and pathophysiology of skin diseases in mammals, most importantly humans (see Resources section below). The latest genetic engineering technologies enable relatively rapid creations of close, if not identical, molecular defects in mice as found in human patients. What have traditionally been considered to be single gene mutation-based diseases are clearly becoming complex polygenic diseases. The most amazing feature of these mice is that they represent a living resource (or archived as frozen germ plasm). Three decades ago we perused atlases of rare skin diseases, while today this is an online catalog from which one can select mice with the desired mutation in the gene of interest or create the mouse. Basic science discoveries lead to novel, science-based therapies with better results than historical-based empirical treatments. The value of these unique animals will only continue to improve as new technologies to create genetically engineered mice or informatics algorithms are developed to define the mammalian genome.

Zebrafish is an expedient and cost-effective model system that can be exploited to explore the pathogenic mechanisms of a number of human skin diseases. It is conceivable that the zebrafish model will become increasingly popular with continued recognition of certain advantages it maintains over conventional model systems. As discussed above, the best model system is ultimately determined by a dialectic of the nature of the disease to be explored and the research questions to be asked and answered.

Resources

Accessing and using websites for mouse information

Mouse Genome Informatics (http://www.informatics.jax.org/). MGI is the number one go-to resource for information on laboratory mice. It is a massive database covering all aspects of mouse biology and genetics ranging from the rules on genetic nomenclature to an encyclopedia on all genes, details on the genes, and lists of all spontaneous, chemical mutagenized, or genetically engineered mutant mice or mutant genes in embryonic stem cells (ES cells) currently available for a particular gene. The genes & markers query (http://www.informatics.jax.org/genes.shtml) provides the most current gene name and symbol along with information on all the published mutant alleles of that gene. This information is linked to the International Mouse Strain Resource (IMSR; http://www.findmice.org/), which provides links to repositories worldwide that can provide live mice or germ plasm.

JAX® Mice Database Search (https://www.jax.org/mouse-search). The Jackson Laboratory (JAX) is a private, nonprofit research institution that serves as a large international mouse repository to distribute mice generated at JAX or obtained from investigators worldwide. Over 8000 inbred, congenic, recombinant inbred, spontaneous mutant, genetically engineered (induced mutant) mutant mice, and a large variety of specialty strains including the diversity outcross (DO) and collaborative cross (CC) mice are available from JAX and can be found by searching this website. It is impossible to maintain all of these lines as live colonies so those not in demand are available as frozen germ plasm, either as frozen embryos or sperm, which can be reconstituted to live colonies when needed. Our Genetic Resources Committee reviews 40–50 new strains per month, adding over 600 new lines per year. In addition, JAX is one of three centers in the United States that produce, phenotype, and distribute mice generated by the KOMP. Mice are maintained behind barriers in highly controlled pathogen-free colonies to maintain a high degree of microbiological consistency. Mouse strains are carefully monitored genetically to ensure that they are what they are reported to be. Genetic quality control is supported by extensive genotyping, and all protocols are available online so that end users can confirm the genotypes of their mice.

This database is relatively simple to use. One enters the gene name, symbol, or stock number or mouse strain designation, and choices show up below. Click on the specific designation of interest, and a list of mice comes up with summary information. The status of the strain, live or cryopreserved, is indicated in the upper right corner along with ordering information. Complete information is provided on the strain, gene, and allele symbol.

Other vendor websites. There are numerous commercial vendors that sell mutant mice and other species of laboratory animals. Websites include Charles River (http://www.criver.com/), Taconic (http://www.taconic.com/), and Envigo (formerly Harland Sprague Dawley; http://www.envigo.com/). These can be easily searched to find mice of interest for dermatology research. As indicated above, MGI has specific links with IMSR (http://www.findmice.org/) to find vendors and repositories where mice can be obtained from. It is emphasized that mice should be obtained from reputable sources as the use of animals of the wrong genotype can cost time and resources.

Mouse Phenome Database (MPD; http://phenome.jax.org/). The MPD is a website that has been collecting information on differences between inbred strains from researchers worldwide.[1–5] It provides a centralized resource to obtain baseline physiological data. A variety of graphic and statistical packages are integrated into the datasets to perform a wide variety of analyses on the information collected.

Pathbase (http://pathbase.net/). Pathbase is the European Mutant Mouse Pathology Database.[6–8] This database is maintained at the University of Cambridge in the United Kingdom but welcomes contributions from pathologists worldwide such as photomicrographs with annotation of lesions seen in mice that arise spontaneously or are phenotypes of

spontaneous or induced mutations in mice. There is a subsection (http://eulep.pdn.cam.ac.uk/~skinbase/index.php) that provides summaries of a number of mutant mice from a textbook[9] that have skin, hair, or nail abnormalities. There is also a section of whole slide scans of H&E-stained sections of normal skin and hair mounts as well as comparable sections from a variety of mutant mice. One can utilize medical records databases, such as MoDIS,[10,11] which can be linked to the Mouse Pathology Ontology (MPATH)[8,12] or Dermatology Ontology[13] for coding pathology reports. MPATH is integrated into and accessible from Pathbase. When using MPATH with a live link in a database such as MoDIS, one can click on the link, search for the diagnostic term, get a definition, and from that link get access to all the images on that diagnostic term in the database making this a 'virtual second opinion'.[11]

Mouse Genomes Project – Query SNPs, indels or SVs (https://www.sanger.ac.uk/sanger/Mouse_SnpViewer/rel-1303). The Sanger Institute in the United Kingdom has sequenced and annotated 18 inbred strains (the reference strain C57BL/6J and 129P2/OlaHsd, 129S1/SvImJ, 129S5/SvEvBrd, A/J, BALB/cJ, C3H/HeJ, C57BL/6NJ, CAT/EiJ, CBA/J, DBA/2J, FVB/NJ, LP/J, NOD/ShiLtJ, NZO/HlLtJ, PWK/PhJ, and SPRET/EiJ). An additional 19 inbred strains are listed but not annotated as of this writing.[14,15] The website is relatively easy to use. The gene symbol or location is entered into the search box, and a variety of criteria ranging from strains to SNP/indel types can be selected. The SNPs for the selected gene are presented in a table that is color coded with the predicted effect of the change. The only problem investigators have is when they enter obsolete gene symbols. For example, if one enters *p53* the answer is 'The gene you selected is not in the database'. The reason is that *p53* is not the official designation for the transformation related protein 53 (*Trp53* for the mouse, *TP53* for humans). When Trp53 is entered, details will be presented on 'Mouse Genomes Project – Gene: Trp53; Chr: 11:69,580,359-69,591,873'. When confronted with the gene not in the SNP database, you can go to MGI to the genes & markers query as described above. The obsolete term (listed as a synonym) will be found in the far right column with details in front of it, defining the current official name, gene symbol, chromosomal location, and position of the gene. The new symbol can then be entered into the Query SNPs, indels, or SVs in the SNP database and details on the gene found.

Accessing and using websites for zebrafish information

Penn State Bio-Atlas at the Jake Gittlen Laboratories for Cancer Research (http://bio-atlas.psu.edu/zf/progress.php). This online image database contains virtual slides on the histologic developmental anatomy of the zebrafish in different planes of section. The images of the fish are presented in coronal (dorsal to ventral), sagittal (left to right), and transverse (rostral to caudal) orientations. Images come up at 5× magnification (for young fish), which can be reduced to 2.5× or magnified up to 40×. By left clicking on the image, one can move the image around to study the skin in detail. These are images of normal zebrafish at different ages. The system features a scale bar, the ability to create web links to any specific field of view at any magnification on any slide, reference to related slides, rapid keyboard access to adjacent sections, a dynamic navigator, and micro-attribution to the source of each slide. Through the bio-atlas home page, there are also links to virtual slides of human and other animal normal and diseased tissues that have been recruited to the website.

Zebrafish Information Network (ZFIN) (http://zfin.org/). ZFIN is an online biological database of information about the zebrafish. ZFIN provides an integrated interface for querying and displaying the large volume of data in genetic, genomic, and developmental information.[16,17] To facilitate use of the zebrafish as a model of human biology, ZFIN links these data to corresponding information about other model organisms (e.g., mouse) and to human disease databases. Abundant links to external sequence databases (e.g., GenBank) and to genome browsers are included. Gene product, gene expression, and phenotype data are annotated with terms from biomedical ontologies. ZFIN is based at the University of Oregon in the United States, with funding provided by the National Institutes of Health (NIH). Information in ZFIN is tightly linked to the web resources of the Zebrafish International Resource Center (ZIRC), an independent NIH-funded facility providing a wide range of zebrafish lines, probes, and health services (http://zebrafish.org/home/guide.php). ZFIN works closely with ZIRC to connect genetic data with available probes and mutant fish lines.

Zebrafish Genome Assembly and Annotation (http://useast.ensembl.org/Danio_rerio/Info/Index). This is a website of zebrafish genome assembly.

After the previous zebrafish assembly (Zv9) was released in July 2010, the latest zebrafish genome sequence GRCz10 was released in December 2016, which is the tenth zebrafish reference assembly.

Access **ExpertConsult.com** for the complete list of references

Index

Page numbers followed by "*f*" indicate figures, "*t*" indicate tables, "*b*" indicate boxes, and "*e*" indicate online content.

McKee's

Pathology of the

VOLUME ONE | FIFTH EDITION

McKee's
Pathology of the Skin
WITH CLINICAL CORRELATIONS

Eduardo Calonje MD, DipRCPath
Director of Dermatopathology
Department of Dermatopathology
St John's Institute of Dermatology
St Thomas' Hospital
London, UK

CO-EDITORS

Thomas Brenn MD, PhD, FRCPath
Professor
Department of Pathology & Laboratory Medicine, Section of Anatomic Pathology
Department of Medicine, Section of Dermatology
Cumming School of Medicine
University of Calgary
Calgary Laboratory Services and Alberta Health Services
Calgary, AB, Canada

Alexander J. Lazar MD, PhD
Professor
Departments of Pathology, Genomic Medicine and Dermatology
Sections of Dermatopathology, Soft Tissue & Bone Pathology, and Clinical Genomics
Faculty, Sarcoma Research Center and Graduate School of Biomedical Science
The University of Texas M.D. Anderson Cancer Center Houston, Texas, USA

Steven D. Billings MD
Professor
Co-Director Dermatopathology Section
Department of Anatomic Pathology
Cleveland Clinic
Cleveland, OH, USA

For additional online content visit **ExpertConsult.com**

ELSEVIER

ELSEVIER

ISBN: 978-0-7020-6983-3 (2 volume set)
eISBN: 978-0-7020-7552-0

Content Strategist: Michael J. Houston
Content Development Specialist: Louise Cook
Project Manager: Andrew Riley
Design: Renee Duenow
Illustration Manager: Nichole Beard
Marketing Manager: Melissa Fogarty

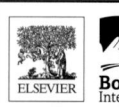

Working together to grow libraries in developing countries

www.elsevier.com • www.bookaid.org

Printed in India
Last digit is the print number: 9 8 7 6 5 4

Contents

Preface to the fifth edition

It is unbelievable that it is more than 5 years since Phillip McKee announced that he was retiring and standing down as the editor of the textbook that he started as a solo author back in the early 1990s. This book, to which he devoted a large part of his life and career, became a household name many years ago and I am very lucky that he, with his boundless generosity, invited me to be part of it when the third edition was planned. Since then, "the book" has become an intrinsic part of my life and almost my whole existence since I became the main editor three years ago when Phillip retired. It is needless to say that Phillip is sorely missed not only as a teacher and friend, but also as somebody that for so many years devoted countless hours to something that can only be described as a labour of love. Thankfully we remain close friends and in communication. However, the void that he has left is difficult if not impossible to fill. I am eternally grateful to him for putting his trust in me and can only hope that I will not disappoint him.

Although for most of the 20th century, single author books were the norm and giants in the field of pathology and dermatology produced wonderful textbooks with little outside help, the amount of knowledge and information produced at an incredible rate in all fields make it impossible to perpetuate this trend and Phillip recognized this when the third edition was planned. Thomas Brenn and Alex Lazar continue to be associate editors of this textbook, as in the past, and their help has been as always invaluable, especially as the task is daunting when one has a full-time job to take care of. In this edition we have asked Steven Billings to join the team as a third co-editor and, although I never doubted the choice, he has surpassed expectations as somebody with incredible energy, knowledge and will to help in every possible way. Many of the previous contributors have been asked to contribute again and a few new ones have joined the effort with their knowledge and expertise. To all these contributors we are deeply indebted.

In the fourth edition we made the decision to provide the references online-only to allow us to expand the text and figures facilitating a more comprehensive textbook. Unfortunately, although following the same option this time, not much extra space is available and therefore the number of new images is limited. The editors, however, have been very generous in allowing extra text to keep up to date with new developments. They have also allowed us to include a new chapter entitled 'Animal Models of Skin Disease' by John P. Sundberg and colleagues which we believe is a valuable addition to the book.

A very esteemed and famous dermatopathologist has for many years started his lectures by predicting the demise of classical dermatopathology and its almost complete replacement by molecular techniques. In his view, it is a matter of a few years before this happens and light microscopy of sections stained with H&E will be a thing of the past or limited to places where newer techniques are not available. Although there is undoubtful truth in this, as clearly demonstrated in the fields of neoplasms and inherited diseases, it is also true that light microscopy remains the gold standard and that most of the diagnoses depend at least partially on the evaluation of sections stained in routine manner with the aid of special techniques. Our view is that all these techniques complement each other. Therefore, in the fifth edition we have tried to keep a balance between traditional diagnostic techniques and recent advances, particularly in the field of molecular diagnosis. It is difficult to keep up to date with the latest developments in the field as there has been an explosion of information as never before, particularly with regards to molecular mechanisms of disease. We have tried to reflect this in the book as accurate and as extensively as possible.

During the production of this book, I have been very lucky to work with two highly professional individuals that have gone out of their way to make my life easier. They are Louise Cook and Michael Houston. I had worked with both in the past and knew that every crisis no matter how big it seems, could be resolved with patience and resolution. For more than 2 years, I have had a weekly telephone conversation with Louise to sort out even the smallest problem. I will miss this. She has never let me down and I cannot thank her enough for her patience, her resilience and for just doing an amazing job.

This preface will not be complete if I did not acknowledge the person that has been unflinchingly there for me without asking for anything in return. My wife Claudia has given her love, her time, her patience and her understanding to help me complete this project. Having to share your marriage with a book is an unenviable task and she has done wonders.

EC
2018

List of contributors

The authors would like to acknowledge and offer grateful thanks for the input of all previous editions' contributors, without whom this new edition would not have been possible.

Josette André MD
Head of the Dermatology and Dermatopathology Department.
CHU Saint-Pierre - CHU Brugmann
Hôpital Universitaire des Enfants Reine Fabiola
Université Libre de Bruxelles
Brussels, Belgium

Boris C. Bastian MD, PhD
Professor of Dermatology and Pathology
University of California, San Francisco;
Gerson and Barbara Bass Baker Distinguished Professor in Cancer
    Research, UCSF
San Francisco, CA, USA

Marcus Bosenberg MD, PhD
Co-Leader of the Genomics, Genetics and Epigenetics Program
Yale Cancer Center;
Dermatopathologist, Departments of Dermatology and Pathology
Yale University School of Medicine
New Haven, CT, USA

Chris Bunker MA, MD, FRCP
Consultant Dermatologist
University College and Chelsea and Westminster Hospitals London;
Professor of Dermatology
University College London
London, UK

Alistair J. Cochran, MD
Distinguished Professor of Pathology and Laboratory
Medicine and Surgery
Department of Pathology and Laboratory Medicine
David Geffen School of Medicine at UCLA
Los Angeles, CA, USA

Antonio L. Cubilla MD
Instituto de Patología e Investigación
Asuncion, Paraguay

Vasileia Damaskou MD
Consultant Histopathologist
2nd Department of Pathological Anatomy
National and Kapodistrian University of Athens
School of Medicine,
Attikon University Hospital,
Athens, Greece

John Goodlad MD, FRCPath
Consultant Haematopathologist and Honorary
Senior Lecturer
Department of Pathology
Western General Hospital and University of Edinburgh,
    Edinburgh, UK

Wayne Grayson MBChB, PhD, FCPath(SA)
Consultant Anatomical Pathologist and Dermatopathologist
AMPATH National Laboratories;
Honorary Associate Professor
School of Pathology
University of the Witwatersrand, Johannesburg
Johannesburg, South Africa

Lloyd E. King Jr. MD, PhD
Professor of Medicine, Dermatology and Dermatopathology
Division of Dermatology, Department of Medicine
Vanderbilt University Medical Center
Nashville, TN, USA

Fiona Lewis MB ChB, MD, FRCP
Consultant Dermatologist
St John's Institute of Dermatology
Guy's and St Thomas' NHS Trust
London, UK

Qiaoli Li PhD
Department of Dermatology and Cutaneous Biology
Jefferson Institute of Molecular Medicine
Thomas Jefferson University
Philadelphia, PA, USA

Amy Y. Lin MD
Associate Professor of Pathology and Ophthalmology
University of Illinois College of Medicine
Chicago, IL, USA

Boštjan Luzar MD, PhD
Professor of Pathology
Consultant Pathologist
Institute of Pathology
Medical Faculty University of Ljubljana
Ljubljana, Slovenia

Diego Fernando Sánchez Martínez MD
Pathologist
Instituto de Patologia e Investigación
Asunción, Paraguay

John A. McGrath MD, FRCP, FMedSci
Mary Dunhill Chair in Cutaneous Medicine
St John's Institute of Dermatology
King's College London
Guy's Hospital
London, UK

Dieter Metze MD
Professor of Dermatology
Director, Dermatopathology Unit
Department of Dermatology
University Hospital Münster
Münster, Germany

Jeffrey P. North MD
Assistant Professor
Department of Dermatology
UCSF School of Medicine
San Francisco, CA, USA

Vinzenz Oji MD
Assistant Professor
Department of Dermatology
University Hospital Münster
Münster, Germany

C. Herbert Pratt PhD
Scientific Program Manager
Department of Research and Development
The Jackson Laboratory
Bar Harbor, ME, USA

Pratistadevi K. Ramdial MBChB, FCPath(SA)
Professor and Head
Department of Anatomical Pathology
Nelson R. Mandela School of Medicine
University of Kwazulu-Natal and the National Health
Laboratory Service
Durban, South Africa

Rodrigo Restrepo MD
Director, Dermatopathology Fellowship Program
Universidad CES
Professor of Dermatopathology
Universidad Pontificia Bolivariana
Director, Laboratory of Pathology
Clinica Medellin
Medellin, Colombia

Ursula Sass MD
Assistant Professor
Dermatology and Dermatopathology Department
CHU Saint-Pierre
Université Libre de Bruxelles
Brussels, Belgium

John P. Sundberg DVM, PhD
Principal Investigator
Research and Development Department
The Jackson Laboratory
Bar Harbor, ME, USA

Anne Theunis MD
Assistant Professor
Dermatopathology and Pathology Department
CHU Saint-Pierre and Institut Bordet
Université Libre de Bruxelles
Brussels, Belgium

Jouni Uitto MD, PhD
Professor of Dermatology and Cutaneous Biology, and Biochemistry
    and Molecular Biology;
Chair, Department of Dermatology and Cutaneous Biology
Jefferson Institute of Molecular Medicine
Thomas Jefferson University
Philadelphia, PA, USA

Steve L. Walker PhD, MRCP (UK), DTM&H
Consultant Dermatologist and Associate Professor
Department of Clinical Research
London School of Hygiene and Tropical Medicine
London, UK

Michael V. Wiles PhD
Senior Director
Department of Technology Evaluation and Development
The Jackson Laboratory
Bar Harbor, ME, USA

Sook-Bin Woo DMD, MMSc
Associate Professor
Department of Oral Medicine, Infection and Immunity
Harvard School of Dental Medicine, Boston, MA, USA
Attending Dentist and Consultant Pathologist
Brigham and Women's Hospital
Boston, MA, USA
Co-Director
Center for Oral Pathology Strata Pathology Services Inc.,
Lexington, MA, USA

Acknowledgments

All the editorial team, including Louise Cook, Michael Houston, Thomas Brenn, Alex Lazar and Steven Billings have been invaluable in helping to carry this work to fruition and I am forever grateful for their efforts and hard work. My wife Claudia has never deserted me and has endured so much for the sake of my well-being that my admiration and love for her knows no boundaries. My children Matteo and Isabella have always supported me through thick and thin and I am indebted to them for this. Many people including colleagues and friends have made my life easier during these years and have helped in any way they can in order for me to complete this work. Many especially visiting fellows have had to endure lots and they have been always there for me not only with words of support but also with their help. I especially want to thank Drs Adriana Garcia Herrera, Eduardo Rozas, Fiona Lewis, Zlatko Marusic, Chao-Kai Hsu, Giri Raj, Tawatchai Suttikoon, László Fónyad, Erica Ahn, Agnes Pekar-Lukacs and Yi-Gou Feng. I am also forever grateful to my friends Celmira Manzano and Patricia Otero.

EC

The path of life is determined by the people we meet. There are many ways in which certain individuals touch our hearts, steer us in the right direction and help us achieve goals which would have been unattainable otherwise. Words aren't ever enough to really show one's true appreciation for the generosity, support and motivation received over the years.

My wonderful, loving parents, Sonja and Walter, have always been there for me and supported my every move. My professional life could have gone very wrong indeed had it not been for the kindness and gracious support from these truly unique mentors and teachers Uta Francke, Heinz Furthmayr, Ramzi Cotran and Christopher Fletcher. There is so much I owe to these two wonderful individuals who have become very close friends, Phillip McKee and Eduardo Calonje. Tinka, Yäelle and Pippa, thank you for all the color and joy you bring to my life and for keeping me humble and (relatively) sane.

TB

Our decidedly cynical postmodern outlook gives short shrift and virtually no quarter to being earnest and sincere in demeanor. Nonetheless, I find I that I am truly and greatly honored to have worked with my exceedingly talented three co-editors and the distinguished cast of chapter authors who stayed this long strange journey with us. Numerous gracious individuals have and continue to inspire and influence me and help me to find my way in life from mentors to colleagues and friends to fellows and students of various sorts and types. I am loath to attempt to name this entire cast of characters lest I neglect to list anyone in particular. Suffice it to say, you know who you are and my many glaring faults are indeed my own and exist despite what you have all tried so hard to do for me! To the many fellows and students who have endured learning with me over the years, please know that you definitely taught me at least as much if not more than I ever managed to impart to you. Your quite reasonable demands for clear, concise and reproducible diagnostic criteria and intellectual curiosity spur me to be my very best and have ignited a numerous studies and publications over the years. Truly, whatever success I have achieved is the product of intense exposure to the generosity of so many wonderfully talented and stimulating people.

AJL

I was surprised, humbled and deeply honored to be included as an editor on the book I use every day in practice. I am very grateful to Eduardo, Alex, and Thomas for including me and to Phillip McKee for his incredible contributions that are still present throughout this book. I would never have had this opportunity without the help and support of many people in my life. Notably, my parents for their support of my somewhat wandering path and my wife and daughter, Beth and Maeve, for their unending patience during the many hours spent on this book. I can never thank you enough. I am also deeply indebted to a number of mentors who have influenced me throughout my career, including Lawrence Roth, Thomas Ulbright, Thomas Davis, John Eble, Jenny Cotton, Sharon Weiss, and Andrew Folpe. I especially thank Antoinette Hood and the late William "Joe" Moores for teaching me dermatopathology. The influence of their wisdom is felt every day. Finally, I would like to thank my colleagues, residents and fellows who always teach me so much and inspire me.

SB

Dedication

To my wife Claudia, the light of my life and a person that I greatly admire in every respect.

To my children Matteo and Isabella.

EC

To Filippa.

TB

To my exceedingly patient and supportive family, Victoria, Elliott, Abigail and Sara.

AJL

To Beth, Maeve, Richard, Sally, Diane and Richard.

SB

Glossary of abbreviations

5-ARD	5-a-reductase		DIMF	direct immunofluorescence
AA	alopecia areata		DLE	discoid lupus erythematosus
ACE	angiotensin converting enzyme [inhibitor]		DNCB	dinitrochlorobenzene
AgNORS	argyrophilic nucleolar organizer regions		DSAP	disseminated superficial actinic porokeratosis
AHNMD	associated clonal hematological non-mast cell lineage disease		Dsc	desmocollin
AIDS	acquired immunodeficiency syndrome		dsDNA	double-stranded DNA
AILD	angioimmunoblastic lymphadenopathy with dysproteinemia		Dsg	desmoglein
ALA	aminolevulinic acid		DSP	disseminated superficial porokeratosis
ALK	anaplastic lymphoma kinase		EB	epidermolysis bullosa
ALK1	activin-like receptor kinase 1		EBA	epidermolysis bullosa acquisita
ALM	acral lentiginous melanoma		EBS	epidermolysis bullosa simplex
AN	acanthosis nigricans		EBS-DM	epidermolysis bullosa simplex, Dowling–Meara
ANA	antinuclear antibodies		EBS-K	epidermolysis bullosa simplex, Koebner
ANCA	antineutrophil cytoplasmic antibodies		EBS-MD	epidermolysis bullosa simplex with muscular dystrophy
API2	apoptosis inhibitor-2		EBS-WC	epidermolysis bullosa simplex, Weber–Cockayne
ARC	AIDS-related complex		EBV	Epstein–Barr virus
ATF1	activating transcription factor 1		ECE	endothelin-converting enzyme
ATLL	adult T-cell leukemia/lymphoma		ECM	extracellular membrane
BANS	back, arm, neck and scalp [sites]		EDS	Ehlers–Danlos syndrome
BB	mid borderline leprosy		EGFR	endothelial growth factor receptor
BCC	basal cell carcinoma		ELAM	endothelial leukocyte adhesion molecule
BCG	bacille Calmette–Guérin		ELISA	enzyme-linked immunosorbent assay
B-FGF	basic fibroblast growth factor		EM	electron microscopy
BIDS	brittle sulfur-deficient hair, intellectual impairment, decreased fertility and short stature		EMA	epithelial membrane antigen
			ENA	extractable nuclear antigen
BL	borderline lepromatous leprosy		ENL	erythema nodosum leprosum
BLAISE	Blaschko linear acquired inflammatory skin eruption		EPPER	eosinophilic, polymorphic and pruritic eruption associated with radiotherapy
BMP	bone morphogenetic protein			
BP	bullous pemphigoid		EPPK	epidermolytic palmoplantar keratoderma
BPA	bullous pemphigoid antigen		EPS	extracellular polysaccharide substance
BSAP	B-cell-specific activator protein		ESR	erythrocyte sedimentation rate
BSLE	bullous systemic lupus erythematosus		ETA	exfoliative toxin A
BT	borderline tuberculoid leprosy		ETB	exfoliative toxin B
C3NeF	C3 nephritic factor		EV	epidermodysplasia verruciformis
CAD	chronic actinic dermatitis		EWSR1	Ewing's sarcoma [proto-oncogene]
cAMP	cyclic adenosine 3'-5'- monophosphate		FACE	facial Afro-Caribbean childhood eruption
c-ANCA	cytoplasmic-antineutrophil cytoplasmic antibodies		FADS	fetal akinesia deformation sequence
CDC	Centers for Disease Control and Prevention		FAMMM	familial atypical multiple mole melanoma [syndrome]
CEA	carcinoembryonic antigen		FAP	familial adenomatous polyposis
CGRP	calcitonin-gene-related polypeptide		FAPA	fever, aphthous stomatitis, pharyngitis, adenitis [syndrome]
CHILD	congenital hemidysplasia with ichthyosiform nevus and limb defects [syndrome]		FHIT	fragile histidine triad
			FIGURE	facial idiopathic granulomata with regressive evolution
CK	cytokeratin		FISH	fluorescent in situ hybridization
CLA	cutaneous lymphocyte antigen		GA	granuloma annulare
CLL	chronic lymphocytic leukemia		GABEB	generalized atrophic benign epidermolysis bullosa
CMG	capillary morphogenesis protein		GCDFP	gross cystic disease fluid protein
CNS	central nervous system		G-CSF	granulocyte-colony stimulating factor
CP	cicatricial pemphigoid (mucous membrane pemphigoid)		GFAP	glial fibrillary acidic protein
CRASP	complement regulator-acquiring surface protein		GM-CSF	granulocyte–macrophage colony stimulating factor
CREST	calcinosis, Raynaud's phenomenon, esophageal dysfunction, sclerodactyly, telangiectasis [syndrome]		GSE	gluten-sensitive enteropathy
			GVHD	graft-versus-host disease
CTCL	cutaneous T-cell lymphoma		HA	hyperandrogenism
dcSSc	diffuse cutaneous systemic sclerosis		HAART	highly active antiretroviral therapy
DDEB	dominant dystrophic epidermolysis bullosa		HAIR-AN	hyperandrogenism–insulin resistance–acanthosis nigricans [syndrome]
DEB	dystrophic epidermolysis bullosa			
DH	dermatitis herpetiformis		HBV	hepatitis B virus
DIC	disseminated intravascular coagulation		HDL	high density lipoprotein

HF	hemorrhagic fever
HG	herpes gestationis
HHV	human herpesvirus
HIT	heparin-induced thrombocytopenia [syndrome]
HIV	human immunodeficiency virus
HLA	human leukocyte antigen
HMFG	human milk fat globulin
HNPCC	hereditary non-polyposis colorectal carcinoma [syndrome]
HPF (hpf)	high power fields
HPL	hyperlipoproteinemia
HPV	human papillomavirus
HRF	histamine-releasing factor
HSP	heat shock protein
HSV	herpes simplex virus
HTLV	human T-cell lymphotropic virus
hTR	telomerase RNA
HUS	hemolytic uremic syndrome
IBIDS	ichthyosis and BIDS (see BIDS above)
ICAM	intercellular adhesion molecule
ICH	indeterminate cell histiocytosis
IDL	intermediate density lipoproteins
IEN	intraepidermal neutrophilic [IgA dermatosis variant]
IFAP	ichthyosis follicularis–alopecia– photophobia [syndrome]; intermediate filament associated protein
IFN	interferon
Ig	immunoglobulin
IIMF	indirect immunofluorescence
ILVEN	inflammatory linear verrucous epidermal nevus
IMF	immunofluorescence
IP	inducible protein; immunoprecipitation
IR	insulin resistance
ISSVD	International Society for the Study of Vulvovaginal Disease
JEB	junctional epidermolysis bullosa
JEB-H	junctional epidermolysis bullosa, Herlitz
JEB-nH	junctional epidermolysis bullosa, non-Herlitz
JEB-PA	junctional epidermolysis bullosa with pyloric atresia
KID	keratitis–ichthyosis–deafness [syndrome]
KOH	potassium hydroxide
KPAF	keratosis pilaris atrophicans facei
L& H cells	lymphocytic and/or histiocytic Reed–Sternberg cell variants
LAD	linear IgA disease
LATS	long-acting thyroid stimulator
LCA	leukocyte common antigen
LCH	Langerhans' cell histiocytosis
lcSSc	limited cutaneous systemic sclerosis
LDL	low density lipoprotein
LE	lupus erythematosus
LFA	lymphocyte function-associated antigen
LH–RH	luteinizing hormone–releasing hormone
LL	lamina lucida; lepromatous leprosy
LP	lichen planus
LPP	lichen planus pemphigoides
LS	lichen sclerosus
LYVE	lymphatic vessel endothelial [hyaluronan receptor]
MAC	membrane attack complex
MAI	M. avium intracellulare
MALT	mucosa-associated lymphoid tissue
MART-1	melanoma antigen recognized by T-cells 1
MBP	myelin basic protein
MC1R	melanocortin-1 receptor
MCGN	mesangiocapillary glomerulonephritis
MCP	molecule chemoattractant protein
M-CSF	macrophage colony stimulating factor
MCTD	mixed connective tissue disease
MDR	multidrug resistance gene
Mel-CAM	melanoma cell adhesion molecule
MEN	multiple endocrine neoplasia [syndrome]

MFH	malignant fibrous histiocytoma
MGS/GRO	melanoma growth stimulatory activity
MHC	major histocompatibility complex
miH	minor histocompatibility complex
MITF	microphthalmia transcription factor
MMP	matrix metalloproteinase
MMR	mismatch repair
MSA	muscle-specific actin
MSI	microsatellite instability
NADH	nicotine adenine dinucleotide, reduced
nDNA	native [double-stranded] DNA
NEMO	nuclear factor [NF]-kappaB gene modulator
NF	necrotizing fasciitis
NFI	neurofibromatosis type I
NFII	neurofibromatosis type II
NFP	neurofilament protein
NIH	National Institutes of Health
NISH	non-isotopic in situ hybridization
NK	natural killer
NL	necrobiosis lipoidica
NRAMP1	natural resistance-associated macrophage protein 1
NSAIDs	non-steroidal anti-inflammatory drugs
NSE	neuron-specific enolase
OL-EDA- ID	osteopetrosis, lymphedema, anhidrotic ectodermal dysplasia, immunodeficiency [syndrome]
ORF	open reading frame
PAIN	perianal intraepithelial neoplasia
p-ANCA	perinuclear-antineutrophil cytoplasmic antibodies
PAPA	pyogenic sterile arthritis, pyoderma gangrenosum and acne [syndrome]
PAS	periodic acid–Schiff
PBG	porphobilinogen
PCNA	proliferating cell nuclear antigen
PCR	polymerase chain reaction
PDGFβ	platelet-derived growth factor β
PECAM	platelet endothelial cell adhesion molecule
PEComa	perivascular epithelioid cell tumor
PGL	phenolic glycolipid
PGP	protein gene product
PGWG	purely granulomatous
PI	protease inhibitor
PIBIDS	photosensitivity and IBIDS (see IBIDS above)
PILA	papillary intralymphatic angioendothelioma
PLEVA	pityriasis lichenoides et varioliformis acuta
PNET	primitive neuroectodermal tumor
POEMS	polyneuropathy, organomegaly, endocrinopathy, M-protein and skin changes [syndrome]
PPD	purified protein derivative
PPDL	pure and primitive diffuse leprosy
PPK	palmoplantar keratoderma
pRB	retinoblastoma protein
PSS	progressive systemic sclerosis
PTEN	phosphatase and tensin homolog
PUPPP	pruritic urticarial papules and plaques of pregnancy
PUVA	psoralen plus ultraviolet light of A [long] wavelength
r IL-2	recombinant interleukin 2
RBC	red blood cell
RDEB	recessive dystrophic epidermolysis bullosa
RDEB-HS	recessive dystrophic epidermolysis bullosa, Hallopeau–Siemens
RDEB- nHS	recessive dystrophic epidermolysis bullosa, non-Hallopeau–Siemens
RER	rough endoplasmic reticulum
RNP	ribonucleoprotein
RT-PCR	reverse transcription polymerase chain reaction

SA	syphilitic alopecia
SA1	slowly adapting type-1 [mechanoreceptor]
SALE	summertime actinic lichenoid eruption
SALT	skin-associated lymphoid tissue
SAPHO	synovitis, acne, pustulosis, hyperostosis, osteitis [syndrome]
SCC	squamous cell carcinoma
SCH	squamous cell hyperplasia
SCID	severe combined immunodeficiency
SCLE	subacute cutaneous lupus erythematosus
scRNP	small cytoplasmic ribonuclear protein
SEA	staphylococcal enterotoxin A
SEB	staphylococcal enterotoxin B
Shh	Sonic Hedgehog
SIBIDS	osteosclerosis and IBIDS (see IBIDS above)
SIL	squamous intraepithelial lesion
SLE	systemic lupus erythematosus
SLL	small lymphocytic lymphoma
SMA	smooth muscle actin
snRNP	small nuclear ribonuclear protein
SPD	subcorneal pustular dermatosis
SPRRs	small proline rich proteins/cornifins
SPTL	subcutaneous panniculitis-like T-cell lymphoma
SRP	signal recognition particle
ssDNA	single-stranded DNA
SSSS	staphylococcal scalded skin syndrome
STD	sexually transmitted disease
sub-LD	sub-lamina densa
TCR	T-cell receptor
TEN	toxic epidermal necrolysis
TFIIH	transcription/DNA repair factor IIH
TGF	transforming growth factor
thio-TEPA	triethylene thiophosphoramide
TIMP	tissue inhibitor of metalloproteinase
TNF	tumor necrosis factor
TORCH	toxoplasmosis, other infections, rubella, cytomegalovirus and herpes simplex [syndrome]
TRAPS	tumor necrosis factor receptor-associated periodic syndrome
TSST	toxic shock syndrome toxin
TT	tuberculoid leprosy
tTA	tetracycline transactivator [transcription factor]
TTF-1	thyroid-transcription factor 1
tTG	tissue transglutaminase
TTP	thrombotic thrombocytopenic purpura
UPS	undifferentiated pleomorphic sarcoma
URO	uroporphyrinogen
URO-D	uroporphyrinogen decarboxylase
URR	upstream regulatory region
UV	ultraviolet
UVA	ultraviolet A
UVB	ultraviolet B
UVL	ultraviolet light
VCAM	vascular cell adhesion molecule
VEGF	vascular endothelial growth factor
VEGFR	vascular endothelial growth factor receptor
VIN	vulval intraepithelial neoplasia
VIP	vasoactive intestinal peptide
VLDL	very low density lipoprotein
VZV	varicella-zoster virus
wrfr	wrinkle free [mouse model]
XP	xeroderma pigmentosum

See
www.expertconsult.com
for references and
additional material

The structure and function of skin

CHAPTER 1

John A. McGrath

Introduction

Skin is a double-layered membrane covering the exterior of the body and consists of a stratified cellular epidermis and an underlying dermis of connective tissue. In adults, the skin weighs over 5 kg and covers a surface area approaching 2 m². The epidermis is mainly composed of keratinocytes and is typically 0.05–0.1 mm in thickness. The dermis contains collagen, elastic tissue and ground substance and is of variable thickness, from 0.5 mm on the eyelid or scrotum to more than 5 mm on the back (*Fig. 1.1*).

The dermis is subdivided into a more superficial component (the papillary dermis) which is bounded inferiorly by the superficial vascular plexus and an underlying much thicker reticular dermis. Below the dermis is a layer of subcutaneous fat which is separated from the rest of the body by a vestigial layer of striated muscle.

Properties of skin

A key role of skin is to provide a mechanical barrier against the external environment. The cornified cell envelope and the stratum corneum restrict water loss from the skin while keratinocyte-derived endogenous antibiotics (defensins and cathelicidins) provide an innate immune defense against bacteria, viruses, and fungi. The epidermis also contains a network of about 2×10^9 Langerhans cells which serve as sentinel cells whose prime function is to survey the epidermal environment and to initiate immune responses against microbial threats. Melanin, which is mostly found in basal keratinocytes, provides some protection against DNA damage from ultraviolet radiation. An important function of skin is thermoregulation. Vasodilatation or vasoconstriction of the blood vessels in the deep or superficial plexuses helps regulate heat loss. Eccrine sweat glands are found at all skin sites and are present in densities of 100–600/cm²; they play a role in heat control and aspects of metabolism. Secretions from apocrine sweat glands contribute to body odor. Skin lubrication and waterproofing is provided by sebum secreted from sebaceous glands. Subcutaneous fat has important roles in cushioning trauma as well as providing insulation and a calorie reserve. Fat also has an endocrine function and contributes to tissue remodeling and phagocytosis. Nails provide protection to the ends of the fingers and toes as well as being important in pinching and prising objects. Hair may have important social and psychological value. Skin also has a key function in synthesizing various metabolic products, such as vitamin D.

Normal epidermal histology

Although the basic structure is relatively constant at various skin sites, there are often clear differences which enable one to determine the site of origin. The epidermis consists of four clearly defined layers or strata:

- Basal cell layer (stratum basale)
- Prickle cell layer (stratum spinosum)
- Granular cell layer (stratum granulosum)
- Corneocyte layer (stratum corneum)

An eosinophilic acellular layer known as the stratum lucidum is sometimes seen in skin from the palms and soles (*Fig. 1.2*).

Basal cells are cuboidal or columnar with a large nucleus typically containing a conspicuous nucleolus. Small numbers of mitoses may be evident. Clear cells are also present in the basal layer of the epidermis; these represent melanocytes. Cells with clear cytoplasm seen in the stratum spinosum represent Langerhans cells. Very occasional Merkel cells may also be present but these are not easily identified in hematoxylin and eosin stained sections. Histologically, prickle cells are polygonal in outline, have abundant eosinophilic cytoplasm and oval vesicular nuclei, often with conspicuous nucleoli. Keratohyalin granules typify the granular cell layer (*Fig. 1.3*). The granular cells typically form three tightly packed layers, with individual cells adopting a tetrakaidecahedron shape. Skin integrity is maintained by a mobile layer of tight junctions that translocate from granular layer cell surface to base as individual keratinocytes transition to the uppermost granular cell layer. Thus the main impermeability plane in skin is between the first and second granular cell layers. Further maturation leads to loss of nuclei and flattening of the keratinocytes to form the plates of the corneocyte layer (stratum corneum). Adjacent cells are united at their free borders by intercellular bridges (prickles), which are most clearly identifiable in the prickle cell layer and in disease states of the skin where there is marked intercellular edema (spongiosis) (*Fig. 1.4*).

Toker cells represent an additional clear cell population, which may be found in nipple epidermis of both sexes in up to 10% of the population.[1] Toker cells are large, polygonal or oval and have abundant pale staining or clear cytoplasm with vesicular nuclei often containing prominent, albeit small, nucleoli. The cytoplasm is mucicarmine and Periodic acid-Schiff negative.[1] The cells may be distributed singly but more often they are found as small clusters, not uncommonly forming single layered ductules.[1] They are located along the basal layer of the epidermis or suprabasally and are also sometimes seen within the epithelium of the terminal lactiferous duct.

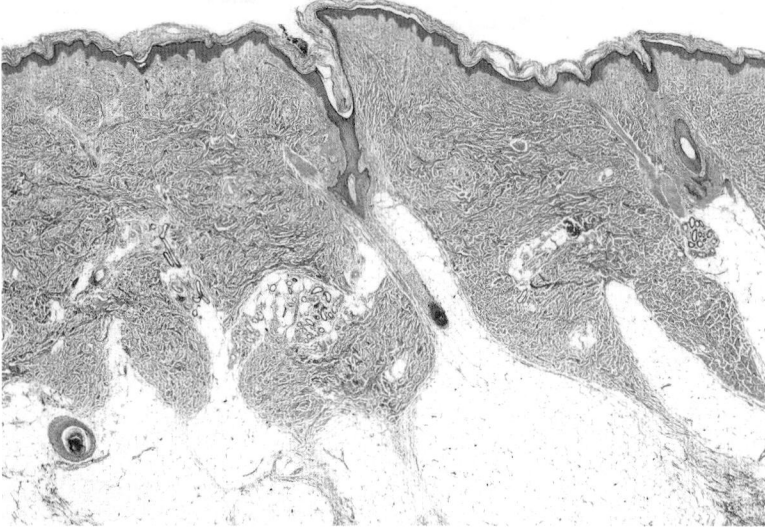

Fig. 1.1
Skin from forearm: there is a fairly thin epidermis. Compare the thickness of the dermis with that from the back (see *Fig. 1.5*).

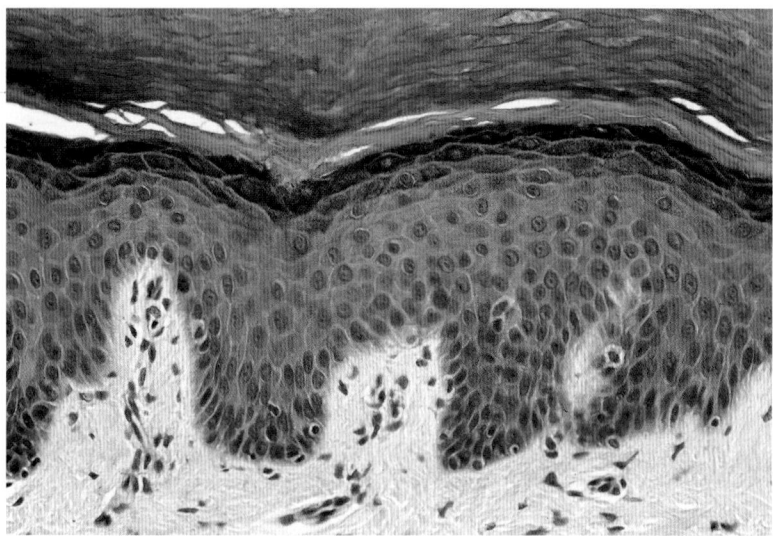

Fig. 1.2
Skin from palm: note the eosinophilic stratum lucidum clearly separating the granular cell layer from the overlying stratum corneum.

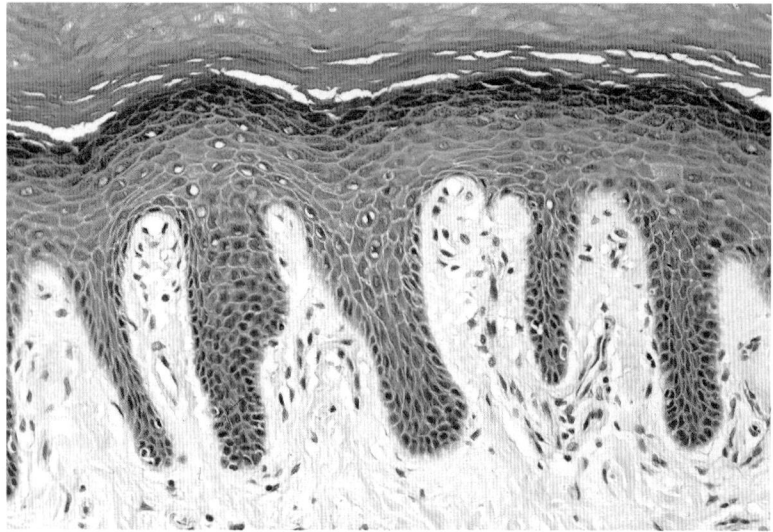

Fig. 1.3
Skin from palm: there is a conspicuous granular cell layer.

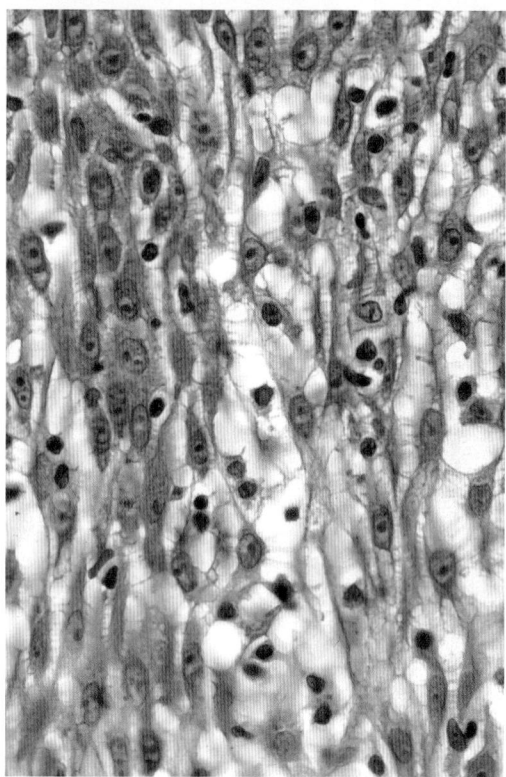

Fig. 1.4
Spongiosis: the intercellular bridges (prickles) are stretched and more visible in this biopsy from a patient with acute eczema.

Toker cells are of particular importance as they may be mistaken by the unwary as Paget cells. They are thought to be the source of mammary Paget disease in those exceptional cases where an underlying ductal carcinoma is absent.[2] Toker cells express CK7, AE1/AE3, CAM 5.2, epithelial membrane antigen (EMA), cerbB2, estrogen, and progesterone receptors.[3,4] They do not express p53 or CD138. Carcinoembryonic antigen (CEA) may also be present, albeit weakly.[4] Paget cells by way of contrast are often negative for estrogen and progesterone receptors and are p53 and CD138 positive.[4]

Regional variations in skin anatomy

There are two main kinds of human skin: glabrous skin (nonhairy skin) and hair-bearing skin. Glabrous skin is found on the palms and soles. It has a grooved surface with alternating ridges and sulci giving rise to the dermatoglyphics (fingerprints). Glabrous skin has a compact, thick stratum corneum, and contains encapsulated sense organs within the dermis but no hair follicles or sebaceous glands. In contrast, hair-bearing skin has both hair follicles and sebaceous glands but lacks encapsulated sense organs. Hair follicle size, structure and density can vary between different body sites. For example, the scalp has large hair follicles that extend into subcutaneous fat whereas the forehead has only small vellus hair-producing follicles although sebaceous glands are large. The number of hair follicles does not alter until middle life but there is a changing balance between vellus and terminal hairs throughout life. In hair-bearing sites, such as the axilla, there are apocrine glands in addition to the eccrine sweat glands. Sebaceous glands are active in the newborn, and from puberty onwards, and the relative activity modifies the composition of the skin surface lipids. The structure of the dermal–epidermal junction also shows regional variations in the number of hemidesmosomal-anchoring filament complexes (more in the leg than the arm). In the dermis, the arrangement and size of elastic fibers varies from very large fibers in perianal skin to almost no fibers in the scrotum. Marked variation in the cutaneous blood supply is found between areas of distensible skin such as the eyelid and more rigid areas such as the fingertips.

Regional variation in skin structure is illustrated in *Figs 1.5–1.20*.

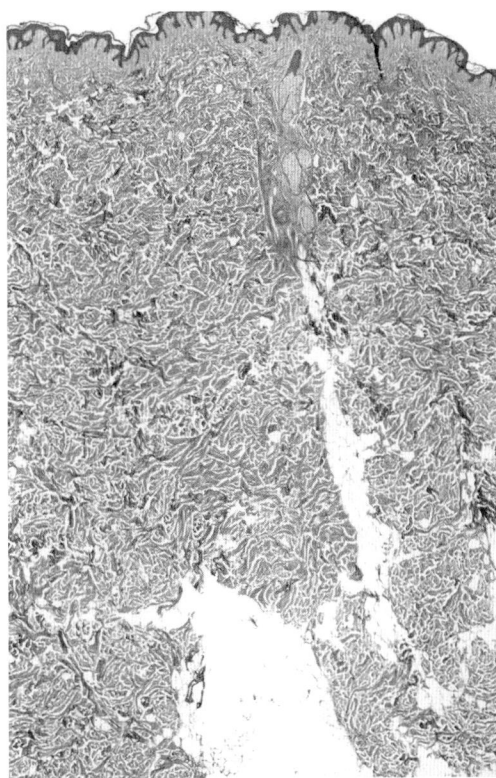

Fig. 1.5
Skin from the lower back: at this site the dermis is very thick and is characterized by broad parallel fascicles of collagen.

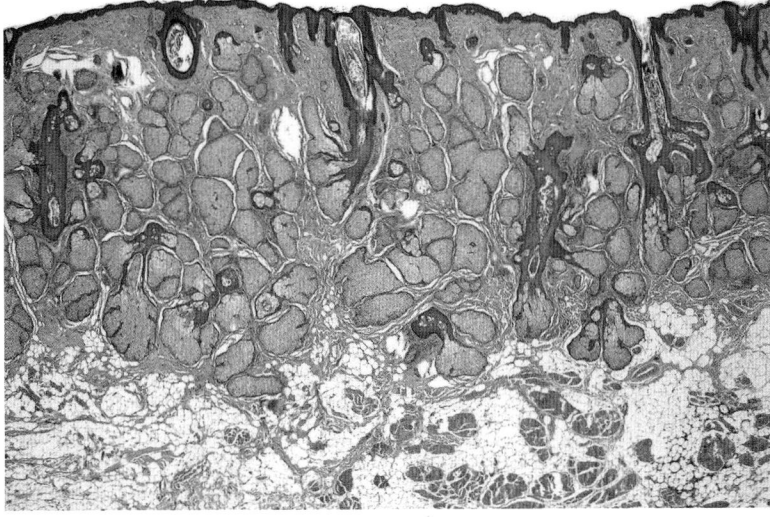

Fig. 1.6
Skin of the nose: there are conspicuous sebaceous glands: at this site, they often drain directly onto the skin surface. These appearances should not be confused with that of sebaceous hyperplasia.

Skin development

Two major embryological elements juxtapose to form skin. These comprise the prospective epidermis that originates from a surface area of the early gastrula, and the prospective mesoderm that comes into contact with the inner surface of the epidermis during gastrulation. The mesoderm generates the dermis and is involved in the differentiation of epidermal structures such as hair follicles.[1] Melanocytes are derived from the neural crest. After gastrulation, there is a single layer of neuroectoderm on the embryo surface: this layer will go on to form the nervous system or the skin epithelium, depending on the molecular signals (e.g., fibroblast growth factors or bone morphogenic proteins) it receives.[2] The embryonic epidermis consists of a

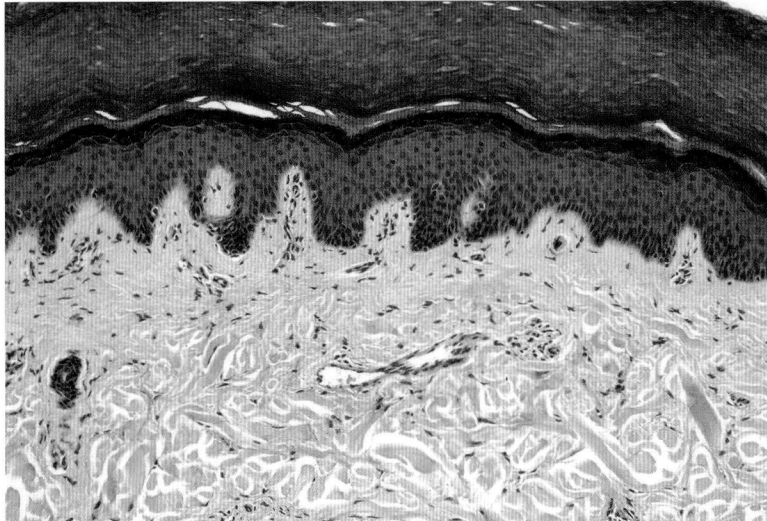

Fig. 1.7
Skin from the sole of the foot: this is typified by a thickened stratum corneum and prominent epidermal ridge pattern. The dermis is relatively dense at this site. Similar features are seen on the palms and ventral aspects of the fingers and toes.

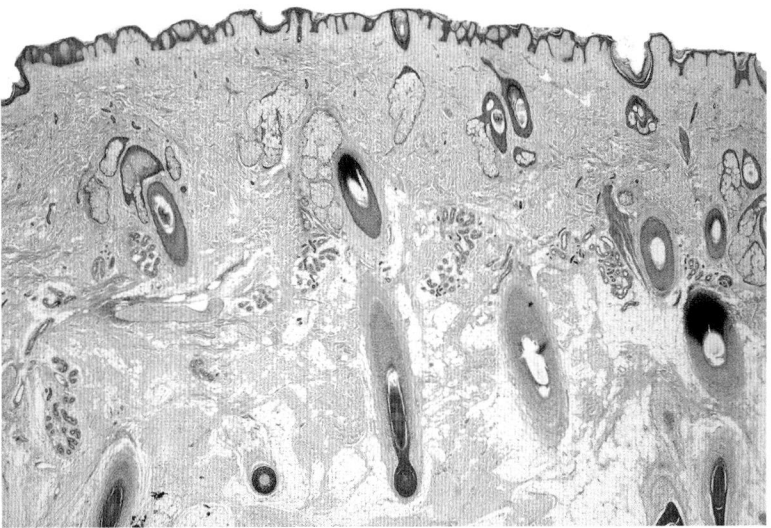

Fig. 1.8
Skin from the scalp: there are numerous terminal hair follicles with many of the bulbs in the subcutaneous fat.

single layer of multipotent epithelial cells which is covered by a special layer known as periderm that is unique to mammals. Periderm provides some protection to the newly forming skin as well as exchange of material with the amniotic fluid. During pregnancy, periderm is present until 24 weeks' gestation whereupon it is shed into the amniotic fluid. One key transcription factor in generating both an embryonic epidermal monolayer as well as a differentiated epidermis is p63.[3] Developmental signals induced by p63 occur before any keratin is generated. The embryonic dermis is at first very cellular and at 6–14 weeks three types of cell are present: stellate cells, phagocytic macrophages and granule-secretory cells, either melanoblasts or mast cells (*Fig. 1.21*). From weeks 14 to 21, fibroblasts are numerous and active, and perineural cells, pericytes, melanoblasts, Merkel cells and mast cells can be individually identified. Hair follicles and nails are evident at 9 weeks. Sweat glands are also noted at 9 weeks on the palms and the soles.[4] Sweat glands at other sites and sebaceous glands appear at 15 weeks. Touch pads become recognizable on the fingers and toes by the sixth week and development is maximal by the 15th week. The earliest development of hair occurs at about 9 weeks in the regions of the eyebrow, upper lip and chin. Sebaceous glands first appear as hemispherical protuberances on the posterior surfaces

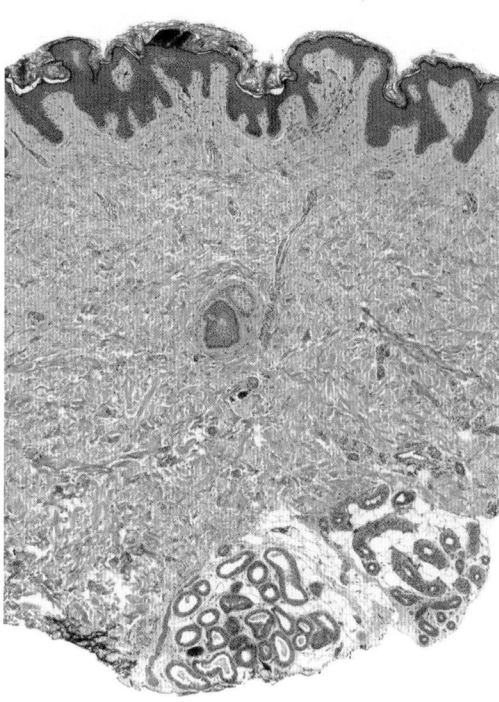

Fig. 1.9
Skin from axilla: apocrine glands as seen at the bottom of the field are typical for this site.

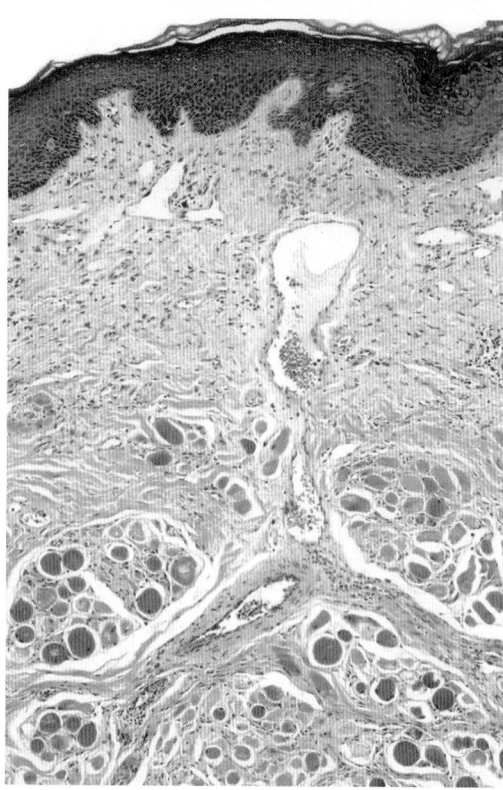

Fig. 1.11
Skin from the outer aspect of the lip: note the keratinizing stratified squamous epithelium and skeletal muscle fibers.

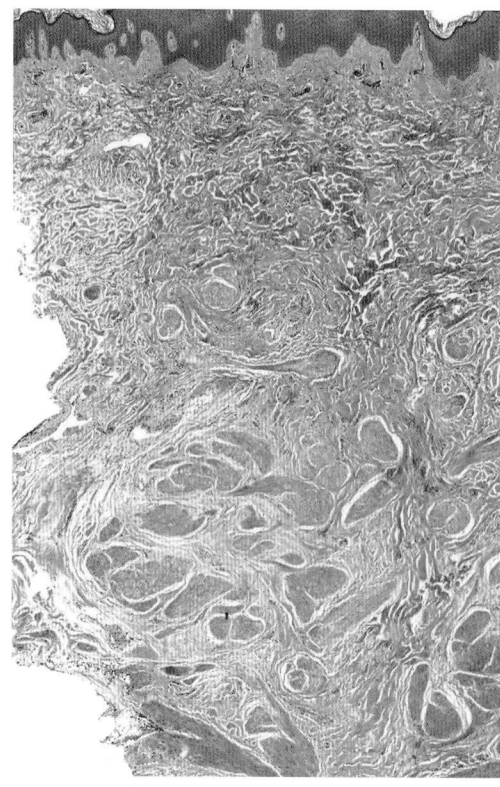

Fig. 1.10
Skin of areola: there are abundant smooth muscle fibers: lactiferous ducts may also sometimes be present (not shown).

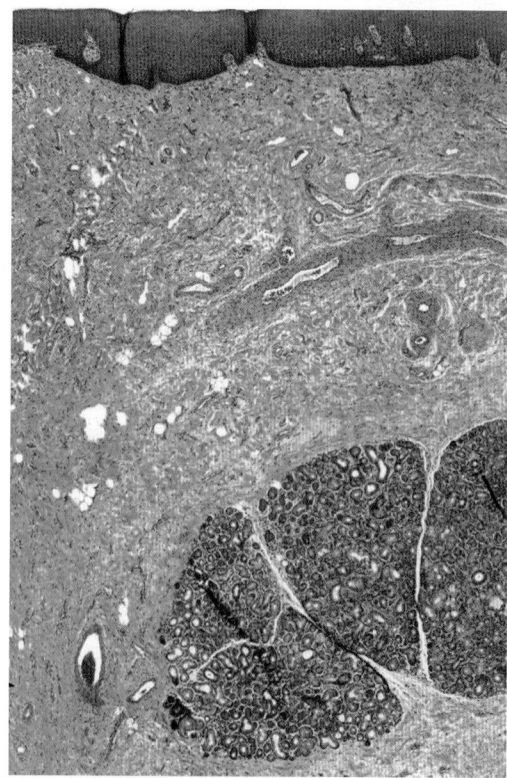

Fig. 1.12
Mucosal aspect of lip: at this site the squamous epithelium does not normally keratinize. Minor salivary glands as shown in this field are not uncommonly present.

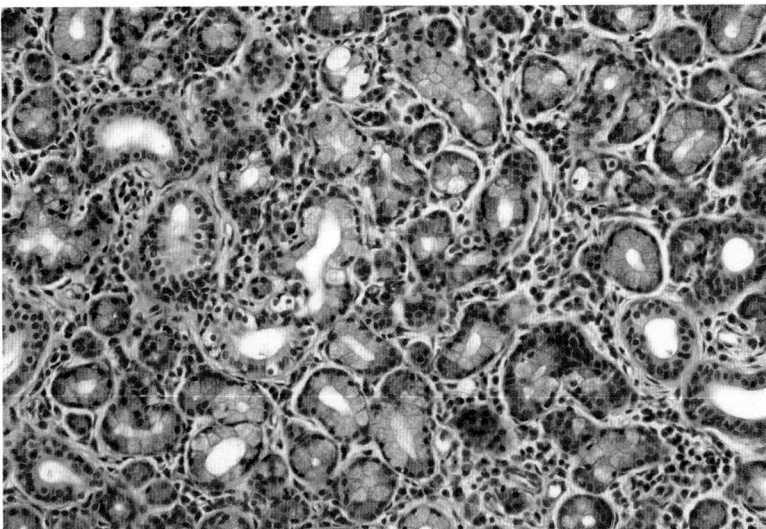

Fig. 1.13
Mucosal aspect of lip: close-up view of the salivary gland shown in *Fig. 1.12*.

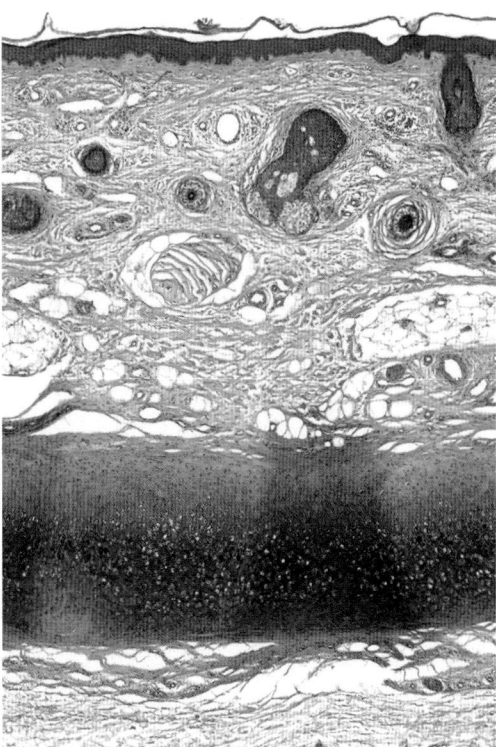

Fig. 1.15
Skin from the ear: note the vellus hairs, and a fairly thin dermis overlying the auricular cartilage.

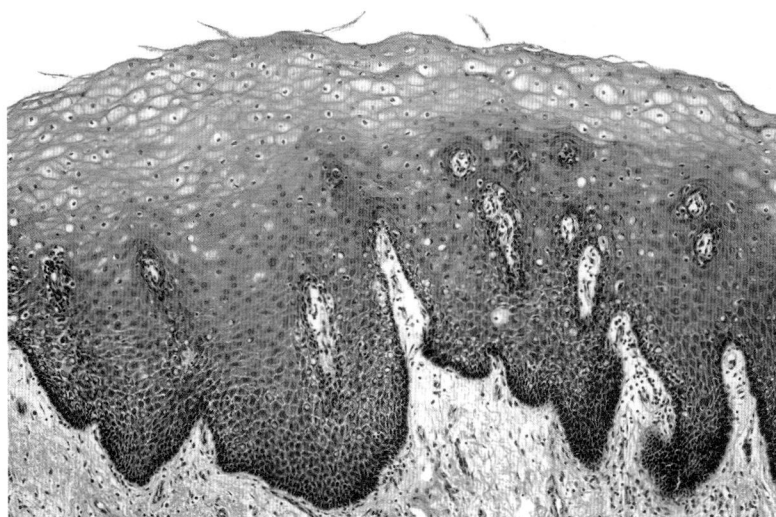

Fig. 1.14
Mucosal aspect of lip: the cytoplasm of the keratinocytes is often rich in glycogen.

of the hair pegs and become differentiated at 13–15 weeks. Langerhans cells are derived from the monocyte–macrophage–histiocyte lineage and enter the epidermis at about 12 weeks. Merkel cells appear in the glabrous skin of the fingertips, lip, gingiva and nail bed, and in several other regions, around 16 weeks. Although some cells of the dermis may migrate from the dermatome (venterolateral part of the somite) and take part in the formation of the skin, most of the dermis is formed by mesenchymal cells that migrate from other mesodermal areas.[5] These mesenchymal cells give rise to the whole range of blood and connective tissue cells, including the fibroblasts and mast cells of the dermis and the fat cells of the subcutis. In the second month, the dermis and subcutis are not discernible as distinct skin layers but collagen fibers are evident in the dermis by the end of the third month. Later, the papillary and reticular layers become established and, at the fifth month, the connective tissue sheaths are formed around the hair follicles. Elastic fibers are first detectable at 22 weeks.

Keratinocyte biology

The cytoskeleton of all mammalian cells, including epidermal keratinocytes, comprises actin containing microfilaments ≈7 nm in diameter, tubulin containing microtubules 20–25 nm in diameter, and filaments of intermediate size, 7–10 nm in diameter, known as intermediate filaments. There are six types of intermediate filaments of which keratins are the filaments in keratinocytes (*Figs 1.22, 1.23*). The human genome possesses 54 functional keratin genes located in two compact gene clusters, as well as many nonfunctional pseudogenes, scattered across the genome.[1] Keratin genes are very specific in their expression patterns. Each one of the many highly specialized epithelial tissues has its own profile of keratins. Hair and nails express modified keratins containing large amounts of cysteine which forms numerous chemical cross-links to further strengthen the cytoskeleton. The genes encoding the keratins fall into two gene families: type I (basic) and type II (acidic) and there is coexpression of particular acidic–basic pairs in a cell- and tissue-specific manner. Keratin heterodimers are assembled into protofibrils and protofilaments by an antiparallel stagger of some complexity. Simple epithelia are characterized by the keratin pair K8/K18, and the stratified squamous epithelia by K5/K14. Suprabasally, keratins K1/K10 are characteristic of epidermal differentiation (*Fig. 1.24*). K15 is expressed in some interfollicular basal keratinocytes as well as keratinocytes within the hair-follicle bulge region at the site of a population of multipotent stem cells. K9 and K2 expression is site restricted in skin: K9 to palmoplantar epidermis and K2 to superficial interfollicular epidermis.

Apart from their structural properties, keratins may also have direct roles in cell signaling, stress responses and apoptosis.[2] In epidermal hyperproliferation, as in wound healing and psoriasis, expression of suprabasal keratins K6/K16/K17 is rapidly induced.

Currently, 21 of the 54 known keratin genes have been linked to monogenic genetic disorders, and some have been implicated in more complex traits, such as idiopathic liver disease or inflammatory bowel disease.[3,4] The intermediate filament database has now recorded over 40 diseases and more than 400 mutations involving keratins (www.interfil.org). The first genetic disorder of keratin to be described was epidermolysis bullosa simplex, which involves mutations in the genes encoding K5 or K14 (*Fig. 1.25*). About half of the keratin genes are expressed in the hair follicle, and mutations in these genes may underlie cases of monilethrix as well as hair and nail ectodermal dysplasias.[5]

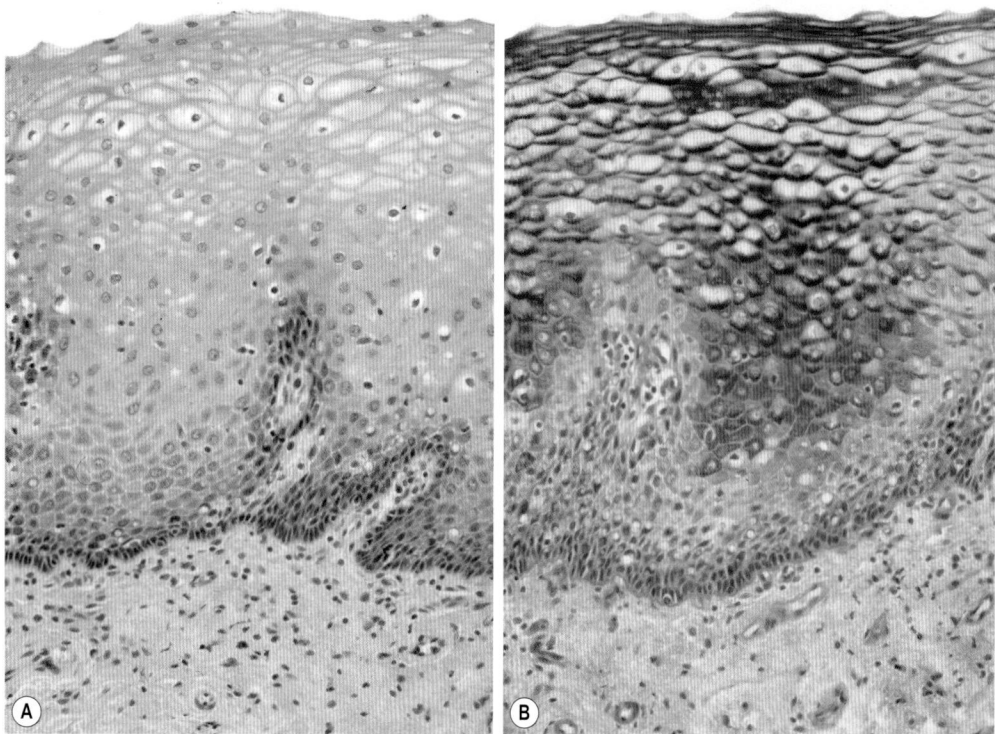

Fig. 1.16
(**A**, **B**) Vulval vestibule: at this site the stratum corneum is absent and there is no granular cell layer. The suprabasal keratinocytes have clear cytoplasm due to abundant glycogen and revealed by the periodic acid-Schiff reaction.

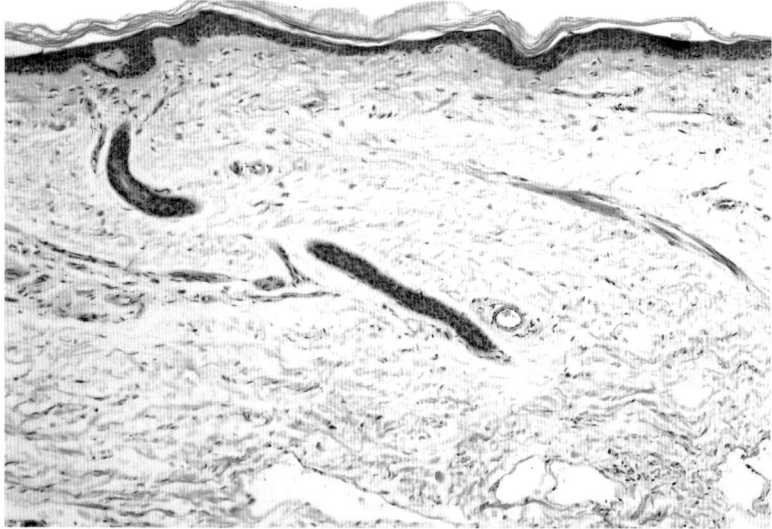

Fig. 1.17
Variation of skin: sample of skin from the forearm of a 92-year-old female. Note the epidermal thinning and dermal atrophy.

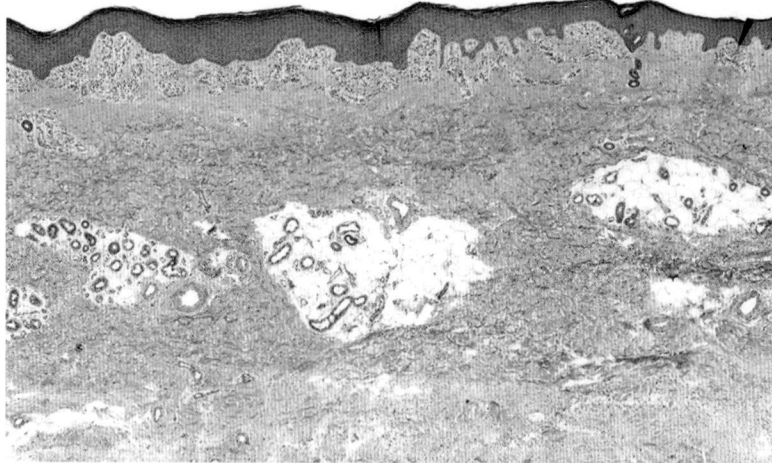

Fig. 1.18
Stasis change: skin from the lower leg. Although abnormal, the presence of stasis change characterized in this example by papillary dermal lobular capillary proliferation is a very common feature at this site.

Epidermal stem cells

To maintain, repair and regenerate itself, the skin contains stem cells which reside in the bulge area of hair follicles, the basal layer of interfollicular epidermis and the base of sebaceous glands (*Fig. 1.26*).[1] Stem cells are able to self-renew as well as give rise to differentiating cells.[2] It is not clear, however, whether every basal keratinocyte or only a proportion of cells is a stem cell.[3] Two possible hypotheses have emerged. One theory divides basal keratinocytes into epidermal proliferation units, which comprise one self-renewing stem cell and about 10 tightly packed transient amplifying cells, each of which is capable of dividing several times and then exiting the basal layer to undergo terminal differentiation.[4] This unit gives rise to a column of larger and flatter cells that culminates in a single hexagonal surface. The process of division of basal cells in this model is viewed as a symmetric process in which equal daughter cells are generated with the basal cells progressively reducing their adhesiveness to the underlying epidermal basement membrane, delaminating and committing to terminal differentiation. The alternative theory is that some basal cells (perhaps up to 70% of cells in murine studies) can undergo asymmetric cell division, shifting their spindle orientation from lateral to perpendicular.[5] Asymmetric cell divisions provide a means of maintaining one proliferative daughter while the other daughter cell is committed to terminal differentiation. Asymmetric cell divisions, therefore, can bypass the need for transient amplifying cells.

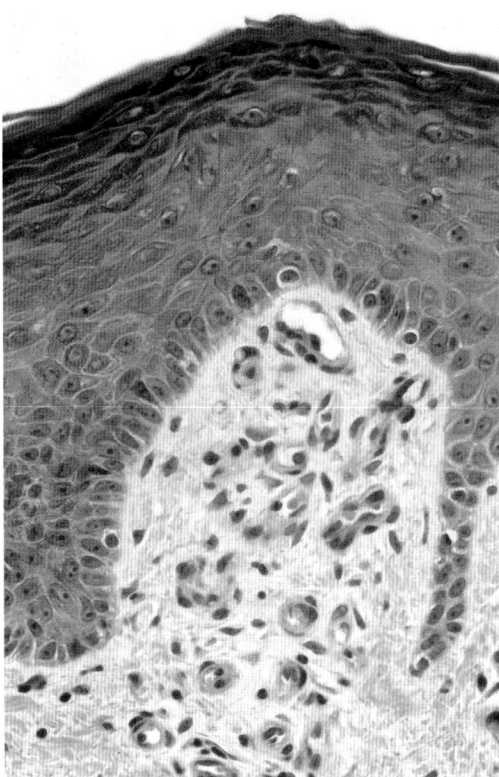

Fig. 1.19
Stasis change: high-power view.

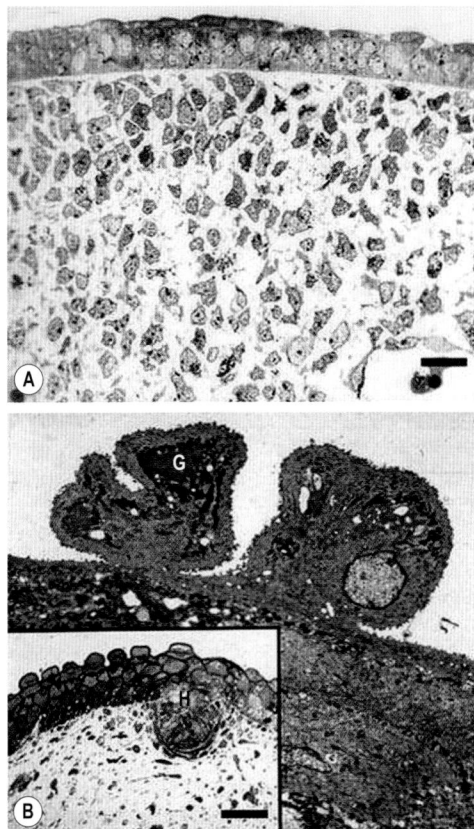

Fig. 1.21
(**A**, **B**) Development of normal human fetal skin: (**A**) at 7 weeks' gestation, the epidermis is only two cell layers thick but the dermis appears very cellular; (**B**) at 19 weeks' gestation the skin has an outer layer specific to mammals known as periderm. This contains surface blebs which are full of glycogen (*G*). Also present is a hair peg (*H*). This downgrowth of the epidermis is the first histologic step in generating a hair follicle. Bar = 25 μm.

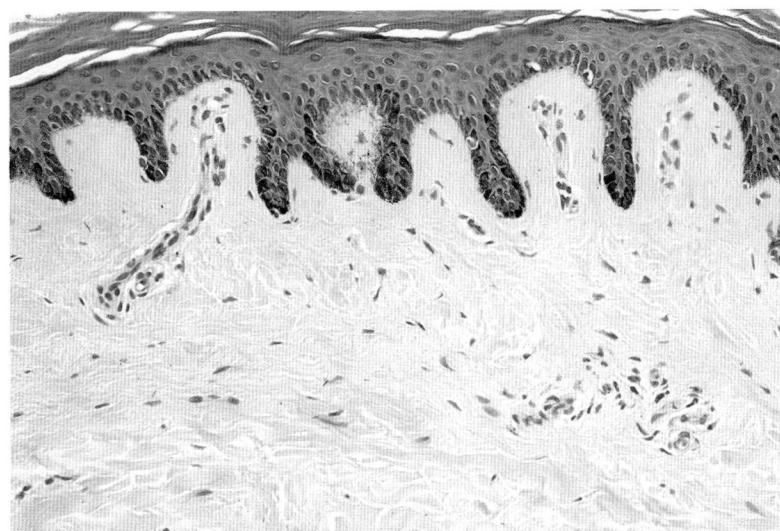

Fig. 1.20
Variation of normal skin: in dark-skinned races, the presence of intense basal cell melanin pigmentation is a normal histologic finding.

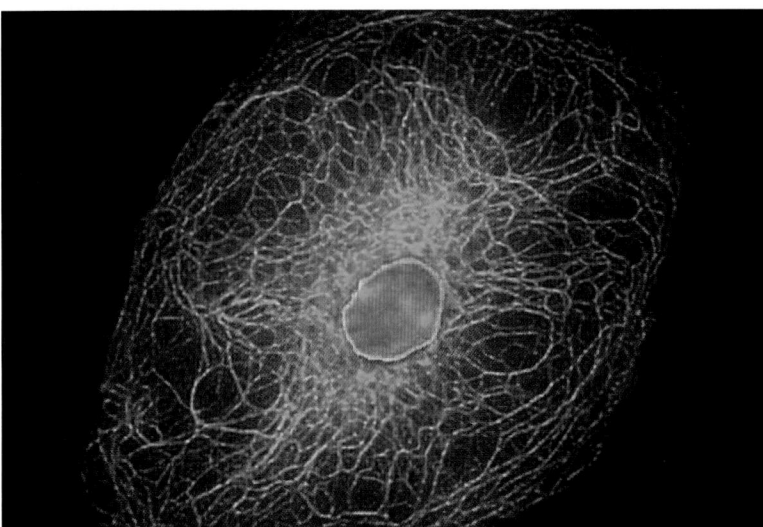

Fig. 1.22
Cytoskeleton of a keratinocyte: the major intermediate filament of a keratinocyte is keratin, highlighted in green.

Hair follicle stem cells are found in the bulge regions below the sebaceous glands (*Fig. 1.27*). The bulge area stem cells generate cells of the outer root sheath (ORS), which drive the highly proliferative matrix cells next to the mesenchymal papillae. After proliferating, matrix cells differentiate to form the hair channel, the inner root sheath (IRS) and the hair shaft. Hair follicle stem cells can also differentiate into sebocytes and interfollicular epidermis. Despite this multipotency, however, the follicle stem cells only function in pilosebaceous unit homeostasis and do not contribute to interfollicular epidermis unless the skin is wounded.[6]

Apart from stem cells in the hair follicles, sebaceous glands and interfollicular epidermis, other cells in the dermis and subcutis may have stem cells properties. These include cells that have been termed skin-derived precursors (SKPs), which can differentiate into both neural and mesodermal progeny.[7] In addition, a subset of dermal fibroblasts can have adipogenic, osteogenic, chondrogenic, neurogenic and hepatogenic differentiation potential.[8] Skin wounding can also induce mobilization and recruitment of inflammatory and noninflammatory cells (including epithelial progenitors) from bone marrow.[9]

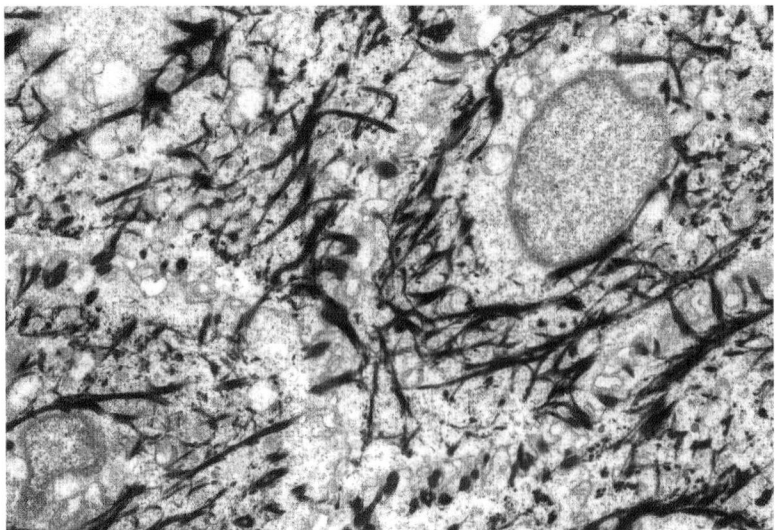

Fig. 1.23
Mid-prickle cell layer of normal epidermis: the abundant keratin filaments (tonofibrils) form a distinct interlacing lattice within the cytoplasm of keratinocytes.

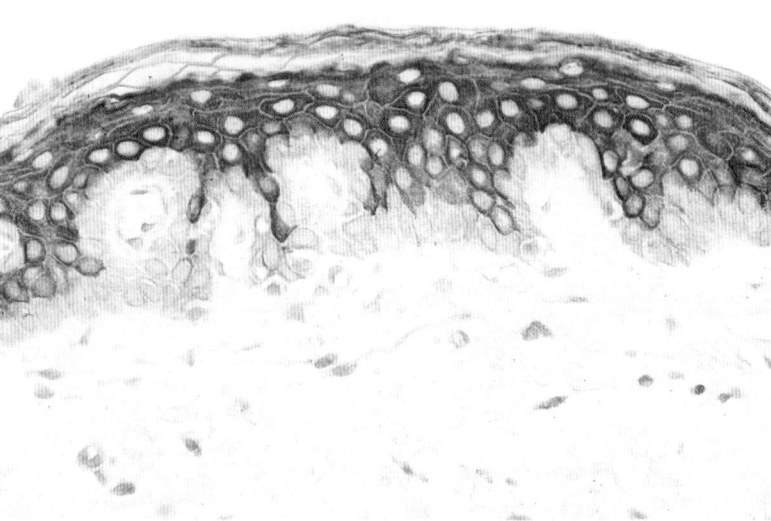

Fig. 1.24
Normal skin: suprabasal keratinocytes preferentially express keratins 1 and 10 as shown in this picture. Anti-Keratin1 antibody courtesy of I.M. Leigh, MD, Royal London Hospital Trust, London, UK.

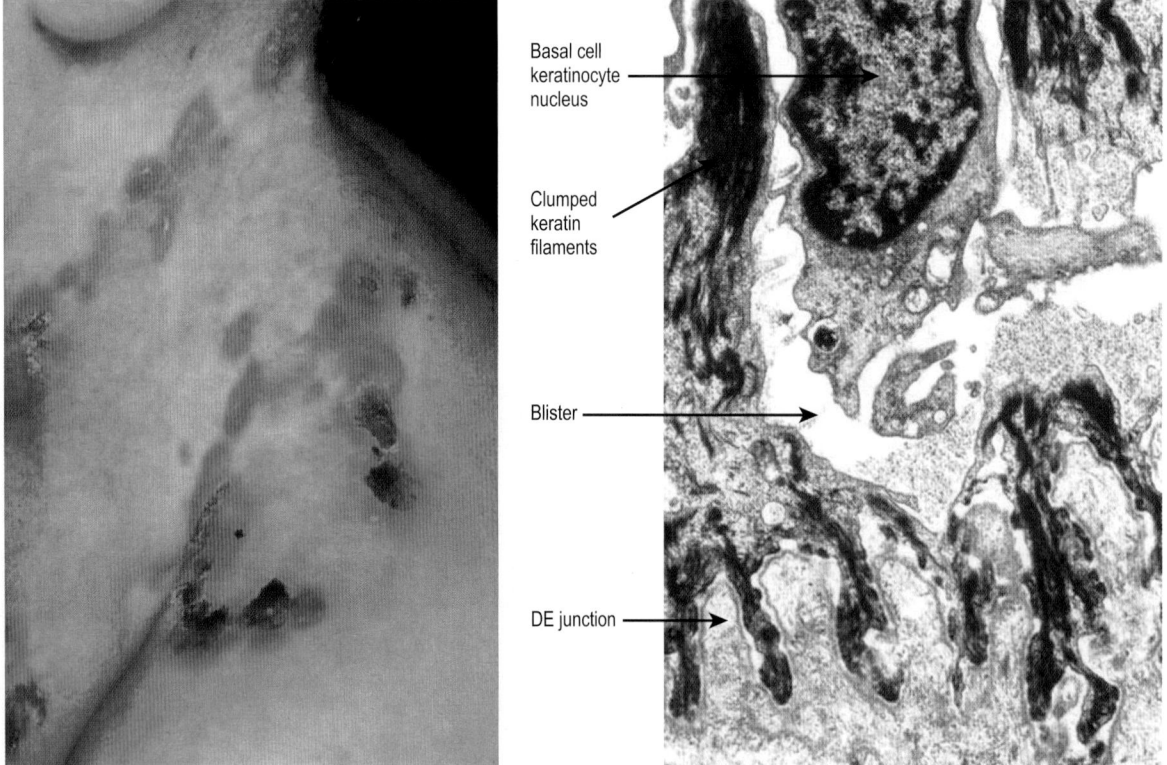

Basal cell keratinocyte nucleus

Clumped keratin filaments

Blister

DE junction

Fig. 1.25
Clinicopathologic consequences of mutations in the keratin 14 gene: (*left*) typical appearances of generalized severe epidermolysis bullosa simplex which usually results from heterozygous missense mutations in *KRT14* or *KRT5*; (*right*) ultrastructurally, there is keratin filament disruption and clumping as well as a plane of blistering just above the dermal–epidermal (DE) junction.

Skin barrier

A major function of the epidermis is to form a barrier against the external environment. To achieve this, terminal differentiation of keratinocytes results in formation of the cornified cell envelope. This physical barrier is rendered highly insoluble by the formation of glutamyl-lysyl isodipeptide bonds between envelope proteins, catalyzed by transglutaminases.[1] Several different proteins contribute to construction of the cornified cell envelope, including involucrin, and the family of small proline-rich proteins (SPR1), including cornifin or SPR1 and pancornulins. Other envelope proteins include

skin-derived anti-leucoproteases (SKALP)/elafin and keratolinin/cystatin. Some precursors of the cornified envelope are delivered by granules: small, smooth, sulfur-rich L granules contain the cysteine-rich protein loricrin, and accumulate in the stratum granulosum.[2] Loricrin is the major component of the cornified envelope. Profilaggrin in F granules may make a minor contribution to the envelope. Membrane-associated proteins that contribute to the cornified envelope include the plakin family members, periplakin, envoplakin, epiplakin, desmoplakin as well as plectin. Formation of the cornified cell envelope is triggered by a rise in intracellular calcium levels.[3] This leads to cross-link formation between plakins and involucrin catalyzed by

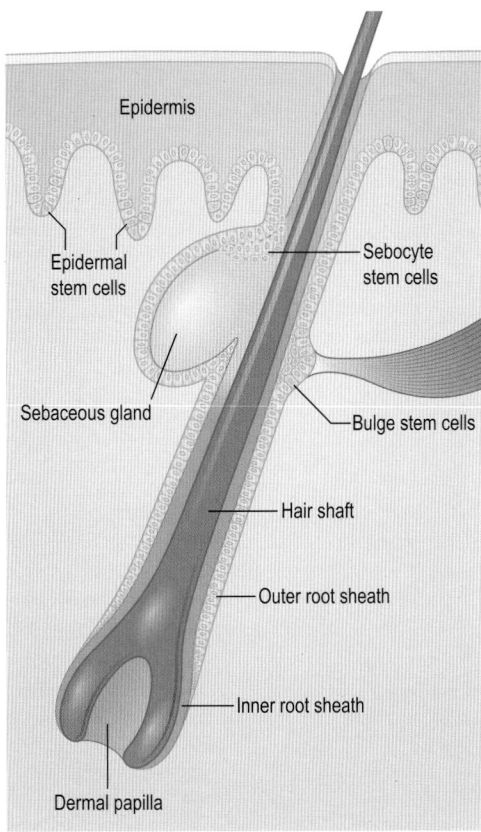

Fig. 1.26
Diagrammatic representation of the location of stem cells in human skin: stem cells are located within the bulge area of hair follicles (where the arrector pili muscle attaches) as well as in the basal keratinocyte layer in the interfollicular epidermis and at the base of sebaceous glands. Stem cells from the bulge area are capable of regenerating all parts of the pilosebaceous unit and interfollicular skin.

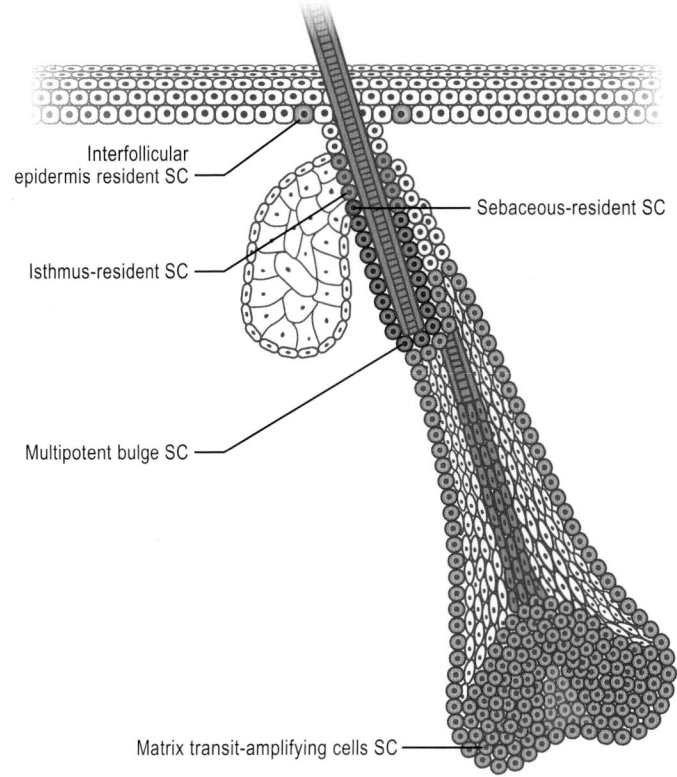

Fig. 1.27
Epidermis contains multiple resident stem cell (SC) compartments and transit-amplifying progeny. Within the bulge area of hair follicles, stem cells are multipotent, residing in the permanent portion of the hair follicle. Interfollicular stem cells reside in the basal layer of the epidermis. Resident progenitors of the hair follicle isthmus and sebaceous gland are located within the hair ORS that is above the bulge and below the sebaceous gland.

transglutaminases. Other desmosomal proteins are then also cross-linked, forming a scaffold along the entire inner surface of the plasma membrane. Ceramides from the secreted contents of lamellar bodies are then esterified onto glutamine residues of the scaffold proteins. The cornified cell envelope is reinforced by the addition of a variable amount of SPRs, repetin, trichohyalin, cystostatin α, elafin and LEP/XP-5 (skin-specific protein). Although most desmosomal components are degraded, keratin intermediate filaments (mostly K1, K10 and K2) may be cross-linked to desmoplakin and envoplakin remnants.

In the upper stratum spinosum and stratum granulosum lipid is synthesized and packaged into lamellated membrane-bound organelles known as membrane-coating granules, lamellar granules or Odland bodies (*Fig. 1.28*).[4] They are found adjacent to the cell membrane with alternating thick and thin dense lines separated by lighter lamellae of equal width, consistent with packing of flattened discs within a membrane boundary. These granules contain phospholipids, glycolipids and free sterols and move towards the plasma membrane as the cells move through the granular layer where they cluster at the cell membrane. They fuse with the plasma membrane, dispersing their contents into the intercellular space. Polar lipids from the lamellar granules are remodeled into neutral lipids in the intercellular space between corneocytes, thereby contributing to the barrier.

Within the granular layer of the epidermis, the main keratinocyte proteins are keratin and filaggrin, which together contribute approximately 80–90% of the mass of the epidermis and are ultrastructurally represented by the keratohyalin granules (*Fig. 1.29*). Filaggrin is initially synthesized as profilaggrin, a ≈500-kDa highly phosphorylated, histidine-rich polypeptide. During the post-translational processing of profilaggrin, the individual filaggrin polypeptides, each ≈35 kD, are proteolytically released. These are then dephosphorylated, a process that assists keratin filament aggregation and explains the origin of the name 'filaggrin' (<u>fil</u>ament <u>aggregating protein</u>) (*Fig.

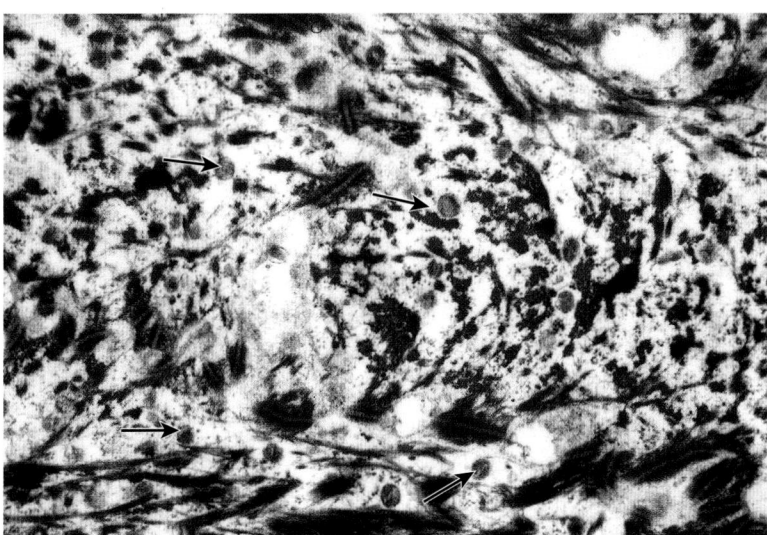

Fig. 1.28
Granular cell layer: note the keratohyalin and membrane coating granules (*arrowed*).

1.30). Typically, there are 10 highly homologous filaggrin units, although the number of filaggrin repeat units is variable and genetically determined, with duplications of filaggrin repeat units 8 and/or 10 in some individuals. Fewer filaggrin repeats leads to dryer skin. Loss-of-function mutations in filaggrin are very common, occurring in up to 10% of the European population. These mutations lead to reduced or absent keratohyalin granules, and are the cause of ichthyosis vulgaris as well as constituting a major risk factor for atopic dermatitis (*Fig. 1.31*).[5]

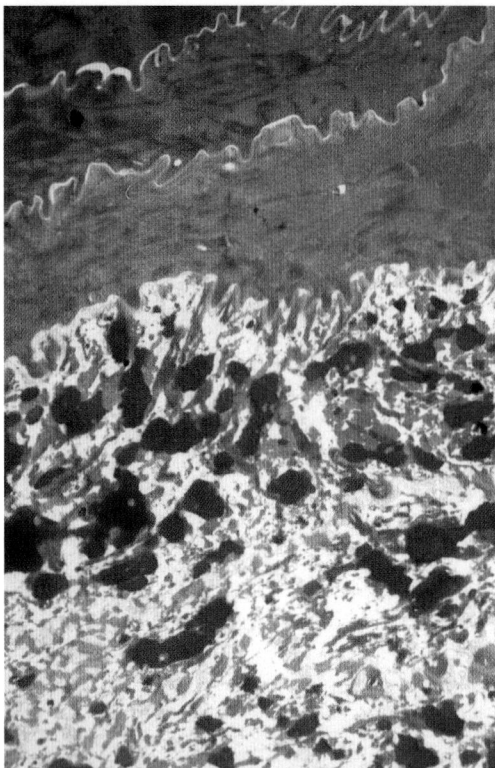

Fig. 1.29
Stratum corneum: keratohyalin granules are present just beneath the keratin lamellae.

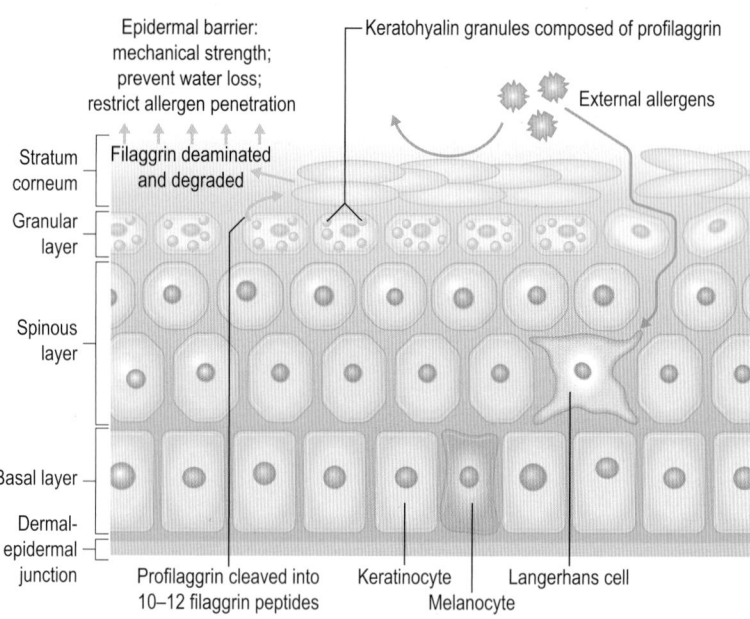

Fig. 1.30
Function of filaggrin in human skin: this is the major component of keratohyalin granules. In the granular layer profilaggrin is cleaved into filaggrin peptides subsequent deamination and degradation provides the skin with mechanical strength and restricts transepidermal water loss. Filaggrin also prevents allergen penetration. In the absence of filaggrin, for example caused by common mutations in the filaggrin gene, external allergens may penetrate the epidermis and encounter Langerhans cells. This may lead to the development of atopic dermatitis as well as other atopic manifestations and systemic allergies.

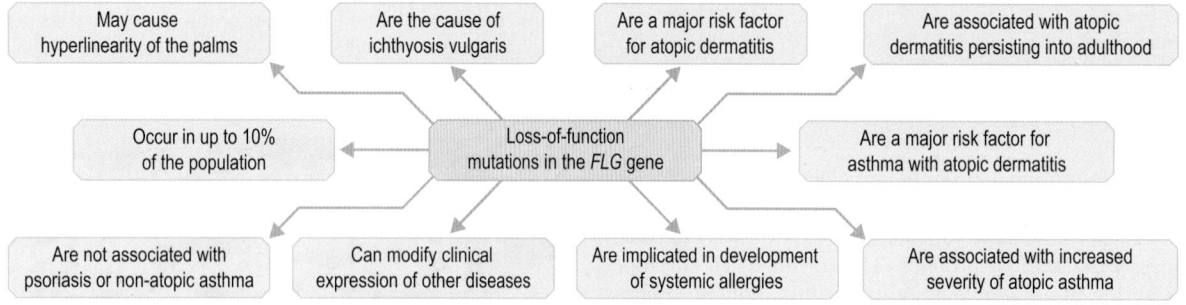

Fig. 1.31
Functional consequences of loss-of-function mutations in the filaggrin gene, which can affect up to 10% of the people in some populations.

Within the stratum corneum, the main intercellular adhesive structures are the corneodesmosomes. These complexes become modified from desmosomes at the most superficial layer of the stratum granulosum, the main difference being the presence of corneodesmosin in the extracellular portion. Corneodesmosomes are structurally different from desmosomes in that they are homogeneously electron-dense and their attachment plaques are integrated into the cornified cell envelopes. When the extracellular regions of corneodesmosomes are fully degraded, desquamation occurs. The degradation process of corneodesmosomes is carefully controlled by a number of proteases and their inhibitors. The most important proteases are the kallikrein-related peptidases, which are physiologically regulated by the lympho-epithelial Kazal-type related inhibitor. Other proteolytic regulators include matriptase, meprin and mesotrypsin. Mutations in some of these proteases or their inhibitors underlie different forms of ichthyosis, often with skin barrier impairment as well as hypotrichosis.[6]

Skin immunity

Skin possesses both innate and adaptive immune responses to defend against microbial pathogens and thereby prevent infection. Nevertheless, skin also encourages colonization by certain microorganisms to promote a cutaneous ecosystem known as the microbiome. This skin microbial community, which varies considerably with body region, interacts with host immunity to create homeostasis, with dysbiosis contributing to the pathogenesis of some skin diseases, including atopic dermatitis and rosacea.[1] One of the primary immune responses of skin is the synthesis, expression and release of antimicrobial peptides (Fig. 1.32).[2] There are dozens, possibly hundreds, of antimicrobial peptides in the skin, including cathelicidins, β-defensins, substance P, regulated on activation, normal T cell expressed and secreted (RANTES), Ribonuclease (RNase) 2, 3, and 7, and S100 calcium-binding protein A7 (S100A7). Many of these peptides have antimicrobial action against bacteria, viruses, and fungi. In the stratum corneum there is an effective chemical barrier maintained by the expression of S100A7 (psoriasin).[3] This antimicrobial substance is very effective at killing Escherichia coli. Subjacent to this in the skin there is another class of antimicrobial peptides, such as RNASE7, which is effective against a broad spectrum of microorganisms, especially enterococci.[4] Below this in the living layers of the skin are other antimicrobial peptides including the β-defensins.[5] The antimicrobial activity of most peptides occurs as a result of unique structural characteristics that enable them to disrupt the microbial cell membrane while leaving human cell membranes intact. The antimicrobial peptides can have immunostimulatory and immunomodulatory capacities as well as being chemotactic for

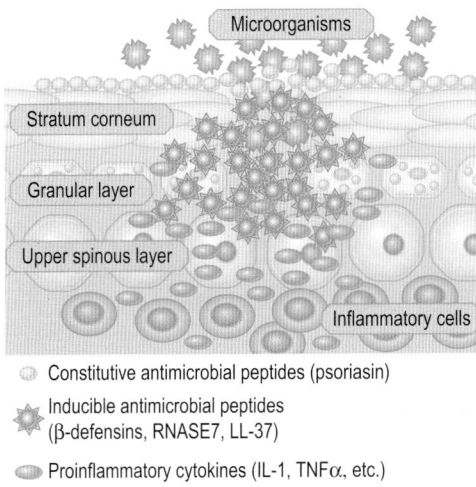

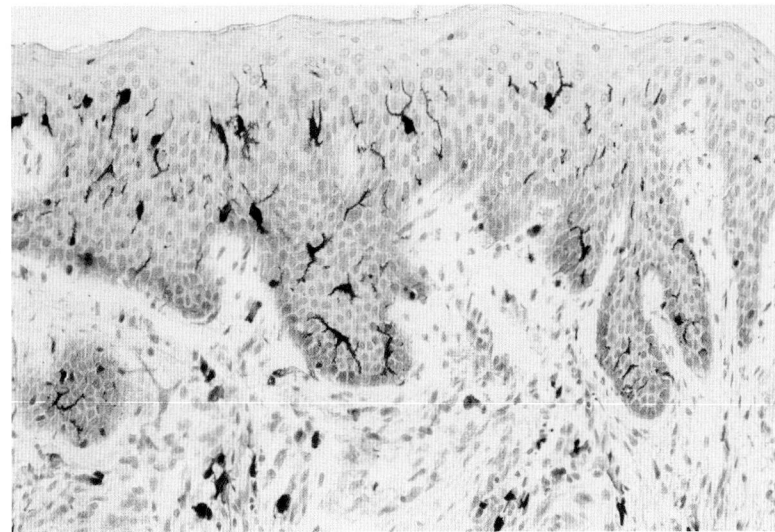

Fig. 1.32
Innate immunity in the skin: the physical barrier is complemented by an innate immune response that targets bacteria, viruses and fungi and prevents them from invading the skin. These peptides include constitutive and inducible substances against a broad range of organisms.

Fig. 1.33
Langerhans cells express S100 protein: note the conspicuous dendritic processes.

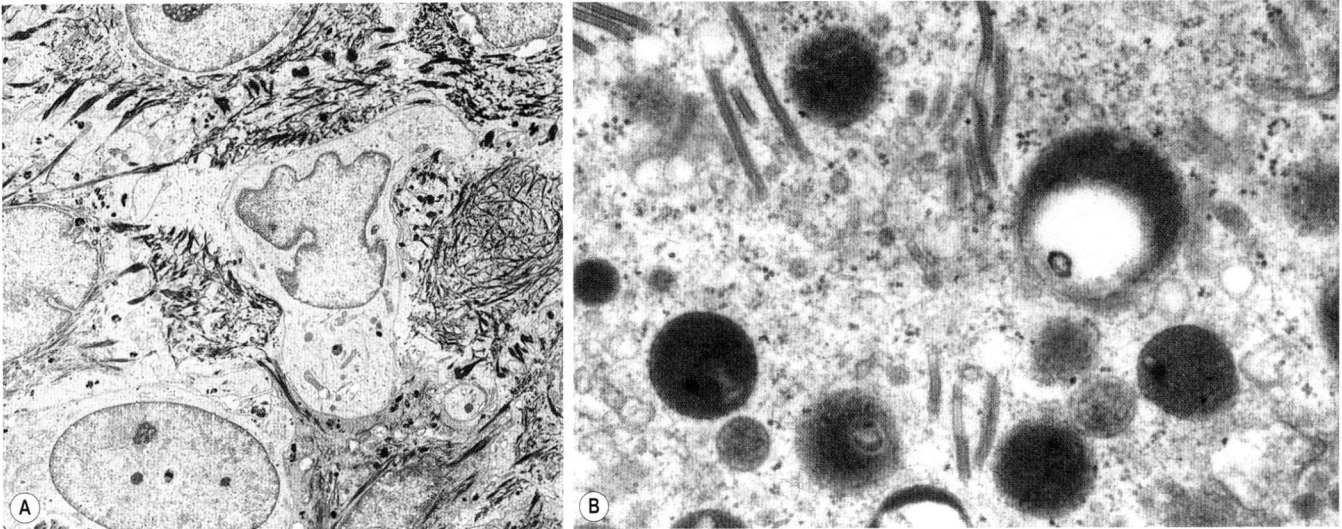

Fig. 1.34
(**A**, **B**) Langerhans cell: (**A**) note the characteristic lobulated nucleus. Dendritic processes are evident, (**B**) typical rod forms with the characteristic trilaminar structure.

distinct subpopulations of leukocytes and other inflammatory cells.[6] Some peptides have additional roles in signaling host responses through chemotactic, angiogenic, growth factor and immunosuppressive activity. These peptides are known as alarmins.[7] Alarmins may also stimulate parts of the host defense system, such as barrier repair and recruitment of inflammatory cells.

Skin immunity is also provided by a distinct population of antigen presenting cells in the epidermis known as Langerhans cells (*Fig. 1.33*). These are dendritic cells that were first described by Langerhans, who demonstrated their existence in human epidermis by staining with gold chloride. Without stimulation, Langerhans cells exhibit a unique motion termed 'Dendrite Surveillance Extension And Retraction Cycling Habitude (dSEARCH)'.[8] This is characterized by rhythmic extension and retraction of dendritic processes between intercellular spaces. When exposed to antigen, there is greater dSEARCH motion and also direct cell-to-cell contact between adjacent Langerhans cells which function as intraepidermal macrophages, phagocytosing antigens among keratinocytes. Langerhans cells can be found throughout the epidermis, extending superficially to within the granular cell layer. Stimulated Langerhans cells then leave the epidermis and migrate via lymphatics to regional lymph nodes. In the paracortical region of lymph nodes the Langerhans cell expresses protein on its surface to present to a T lymphocyte that can then undergo clonal proliferation. Langerhans cells, in combination with macrophages and dermal dendrocytes, represent the skin's

mononuclear phagocyte system.[9] By electron microscopy, Langerhans cells have a lobulated nucleus, a relatively clear cytoplasm and well-developed endoplasmic reticulum, Golgi complex and lysosomes. They also possess characteristic granules which are rod or racquet-shaped (*Fig. 1.34*). These 'Birbeck' granules represent subdomains of the endosomal recycling compartment and form at sites where the protein Langerin accumulates.

Besides antigen detection and the processing role by epidermal Langerhans cells, cutaneous immune surveillance is also carried out in the dermis by an array of macrophages, T cells and dendritic cells. These immune sentinel and effector cells can provide rapid and efficient immunologic back-up to restore tissue homeostasis if the epidermis is breached. The dermis contains a very large number of resident T cells. Indeed, there are approximately 2×10^{10} resident T cells, which is twice the number of T cells in the circulating blood. Dermal dendritic cells may also have potent antigen-presenting capacities or the potential to develop into CD1a-positive and Langerin-positive cells. Dermal immune sentinels are capable of acquiring an antigen-presenting mode, a migratory mode or a tissue resident phagocytic mode.[10]

Melanocytes

Melanocytes are pigment-producing cells and are found in the skin, inner ear, choroid and iris of the eye. In skin, melanocytes are located in the

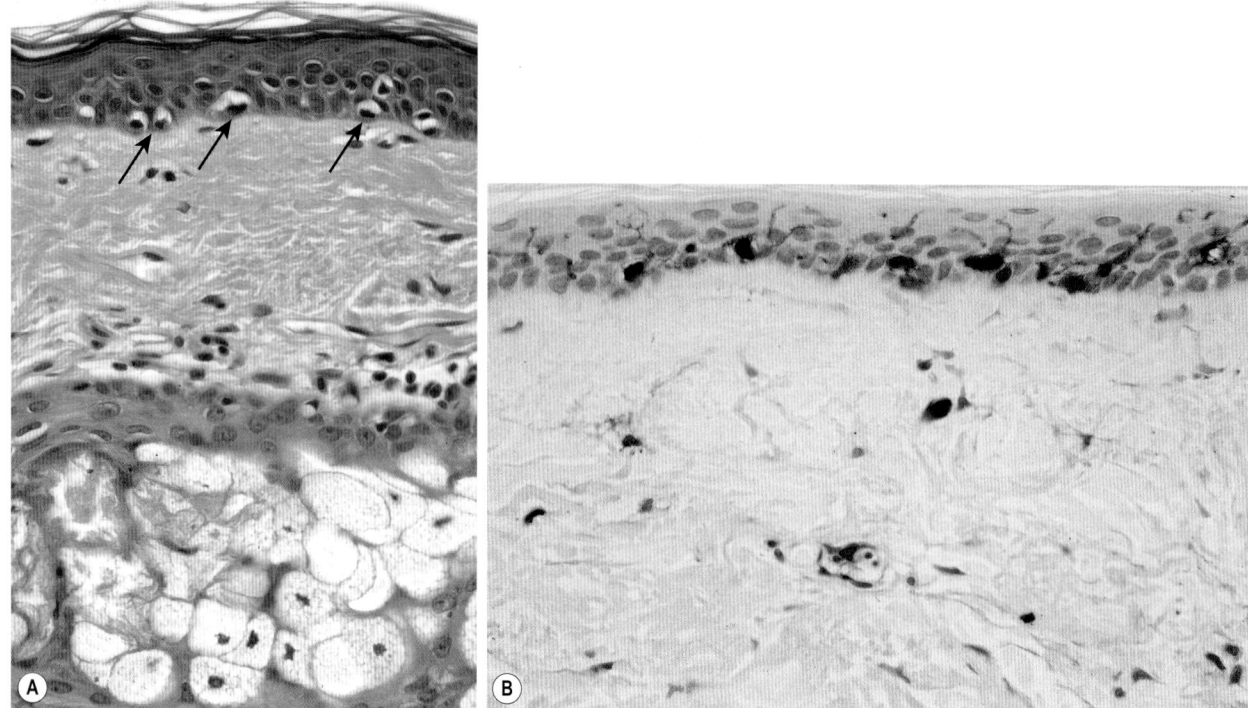

Fig. 1.35
(**A, B**) Normal epidermis: melanocytes are seen along the basal layer of the epidermis. The cytoplasmic vacuolation is a fixation artifact; (**B**) melanocytes can be highlighted with S100-protein immunohistochemistry. Note the dendritic processes.

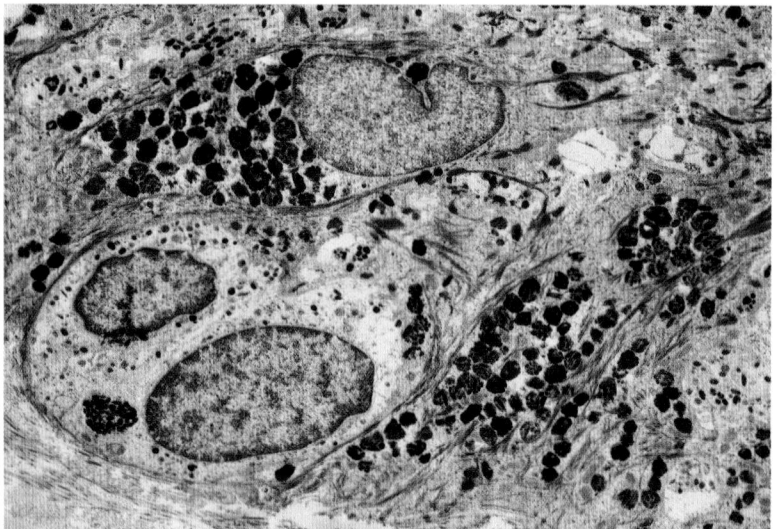

Fig. 1.36
Normal melanocyte: it has abundant pale cytoplasm and scattered solitary melanosomes. Note the absence of tonofibrils and desmosomes.

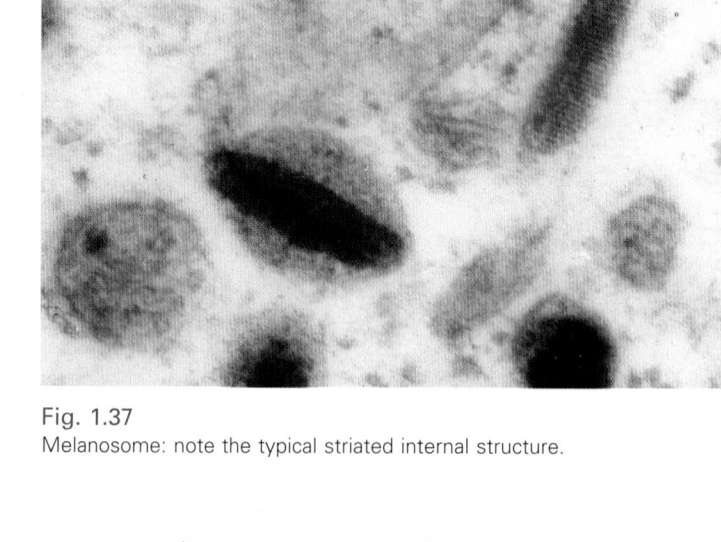

Fig. 1.37
Melanosome: note the typical striated internal structure.

basal keratinocyte layer. The ratio of melanocytes to basal cells ranges from approximately 1:4 on the cheek to 1:10 on the limbs. They appear as vacuolated cells in hematoxylin and eosin stained sections (*Fig. 1.35*). Ultrastructurally, melanocytes have pale cytoplasm and are devoid of tono-filaments, hemidesmosomes, and desmosomes (*Fig. 1.36*). They are easily recognized by their specific cytoplasmic organelles (melanosomes) which are derived from the smooth endoplasmic reticulum. Melanosomes are believed to represent a specialized variant of lysosome (*Fig. 1.37*). The function of melanocytes is the production of melanin, a complex of pigmented proteins that vary in color from yellow to red to brown or black and accounts for the various skin colors within and among races. Melanin protects the mitotically active basal epidermal cells from the injurious effects of ultraviolet light, which accounts for individuals with less pigmentation (fair-haired and light-skinned) having a much greater risk of sunburn and developing

cutaneous malignancies (squamous cell and basal cell carcinomas, and melanoma). The mechanism involves absorbing or scattering ultraviolet radiation and/or its photoproducts. Other functions of melanin include control of vitamin D_3 synthesis and local thermoregulation.

In skin and hair, two forms of melanin pigment are produced; eumelanin and pheomelanin. Eumelanin is a brown or black pigment and is synthesized from tyrosine; it is particularly found in dark-colored races, whereas, pheomelanin has a yellow-red color and is synthesized from tyrosine and cysteine; it predominates in Caucasian skin.

Melanocytes also possess melanocyte-specific receptors including melanocortin-1 (MC1R) and melatonin receptors.[1] The activation or the inhibition of melanocyte-specific receptors can augment normal melanocyte function, skin color, and photoprotection. Moreover, receptor polymorphisms are known to underlie red hair phenotypes, as well as skin pallor

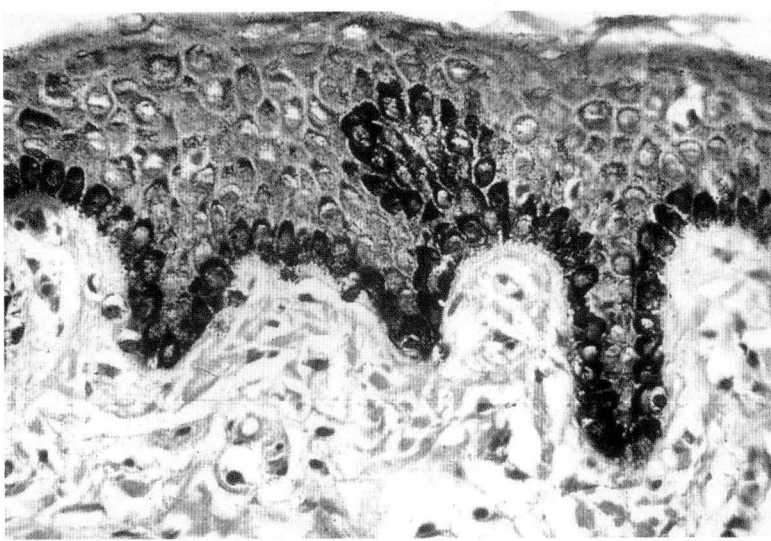

Fig. 1.38
Normal epidermis: this section of black skin has been stained by the Masson–Fontana reaction for melanin. Note the heavy pigmentation, which is present in both melanocytes and keratinocytes.

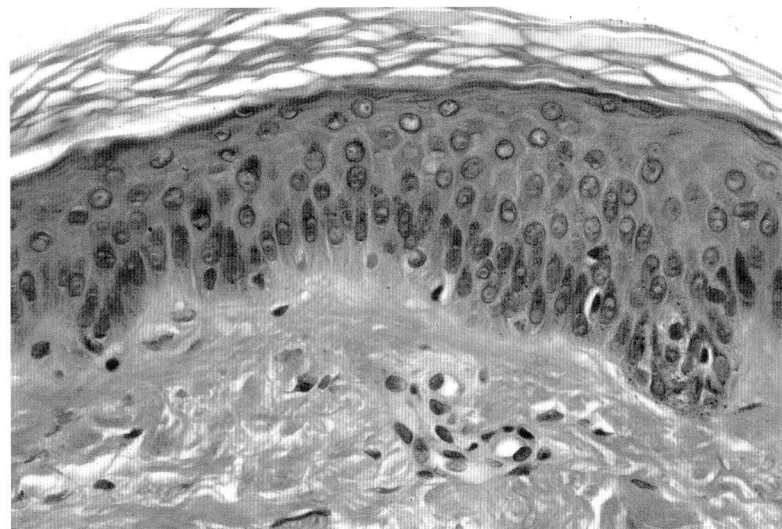

Fig. 1.39
Melanin pigment: actinically damaged skin. Note that the melanin pigment is located in a 'cap' overlying the keratinocyte nuclei.

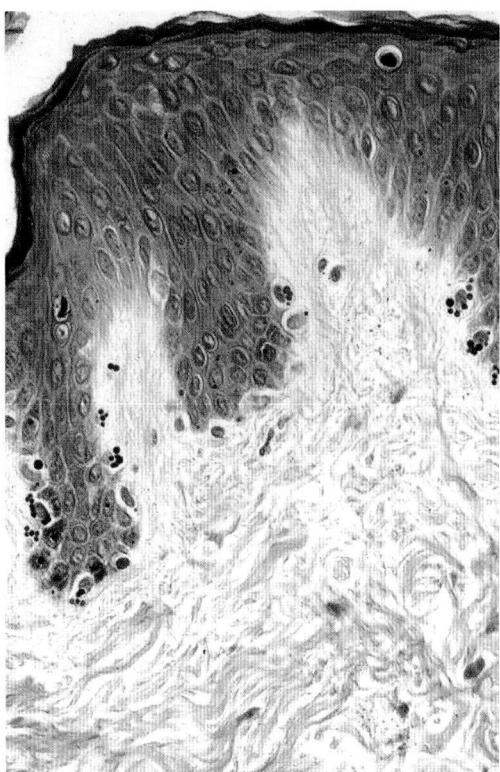

Fig. 1.40
Macromelanosomes: note the large spherical melanosomes in the cytoplasm of the melanocytes.

or freckles (ephelides).[2] Hair graying reflects abnormalities in melanocyte signaling. Notably, Notch transcription factor signaling in melanocytes is essential for the maintenance of proper hair pigmentation, including regeneration of the melanocyte population during hair follicle cycling.[3]

Melanin is transferred from melanocytes in melanosomes to neighboring keratinocytes in the epidermis and into the growing shaft in hair follicles and can be identified by silver techniques such as the Masson-Fontana reaction (Fig. 1.38). Transport occurs along the dendritic processes of the melanocytes and the melanosomes are engulfed as membrane-bound (lysosomal) single or compound melanosomes by a group of adjacent largely basally located keratinocytes (epidermal melanin unit) where they are typically seen in an umbrella-like distribution over the outer aspect of the nucleus (Fig. 1.39). A compound melanosome typically contains from three to six single melanosomes. In heavily pigmented skin and dark hair, melanosomes remain solitary and are longer than those seen in melanogenesis in paler races. Other cells that may contain compound melanosomes include macrophages (melanophages), melanoma cells and, occasionally, Langerhans cells, the other type of epidermal dendritic cell. Macromelanosomes (giant melanosomes) measure several microns in diameter and therefore are readily visible in hematoxylin and eosin stained sections (Fig. 1.40).

They may be encountered in normal skin, in lentigines, dysplastic nevi, Spitz nevi, in the café-au-lait macules of neurofibromatosis and in albinism. A key protein involved in melanosome assembly is NCKX5, encoded by the gene *SLC24A5*.[4] Loss of expression of this gene in mice results in marked changes in skin color with loss of pigment. Mature melanosomes of eumelanin are ellipsoidal in shape, while pheomelanin-producing melanosomes are spherical.

Merkel cells

Merkel cells are postmitotic cells scattered throughout the epidermis of vertebrates and constitute 0.2–0.5% of epidermal cells.[1] Merkel cells represent part of the affector limb in cutaneous slowly adapting type-1 (SA1) mechanoreceptors and are therefore particularly concerned with touch sensation. They are located amongst basal keratinocytes and are mainly found in hairy skin, tactile areas of glabrous skin, taste buds, the anal canal, labial epithelium and eccrine sweat glands. In glabrous skin, the density of Merkel cells is ≈50 per mm². Sun-exposed skin may contain twice as many Merkel cells as non-sun-exposed skin.[2] Numerous Merkel cells can be found in actinic keratoses.[3] Merkel cells cannot be recognized in conventional hematoxylin and eosin stained sections. Rather, immunohistochemistry, particularly using antikeratin antibodies (e.g., to keratin 20), or electron microscopy, is necessary for their identification (Figs 1.41 and 1.42).

Ultrastructurally, Merkel cells appear oval with a long axis of ≈15 μm orientated parallel to the basement membrane (Fig. 1.43). They also have a large bilobed nucleus and clear cytoplasm which reflects a relative scarcity of intracellular organelles. Merkel cells contain numerous neurosecretory granules, each 50 nm to 160 nm across; these are found opposing the junctions with the sensory nerve ending (Fig. 1.44). Merkel cells contain keratin filaments, particularly keratin filament types 8, 18, 19, and 20, which are characteristic of simple epithelium and fetal epidermis. Immunocytochemically, Merkel cells also express neuropeptides including synaptophysin, vasoactive intestinal peptide (VIP) and calcitonin gene-related polypeptide (CGRP).[4,5] They contain neuron-specific proteins including neuron-specific enolase (NSE) and protein gene product (PGP) 9.5.[6] In addition, Merkel cells express desmosomal proteins, membranous neural cell adhesion molecule and nerve

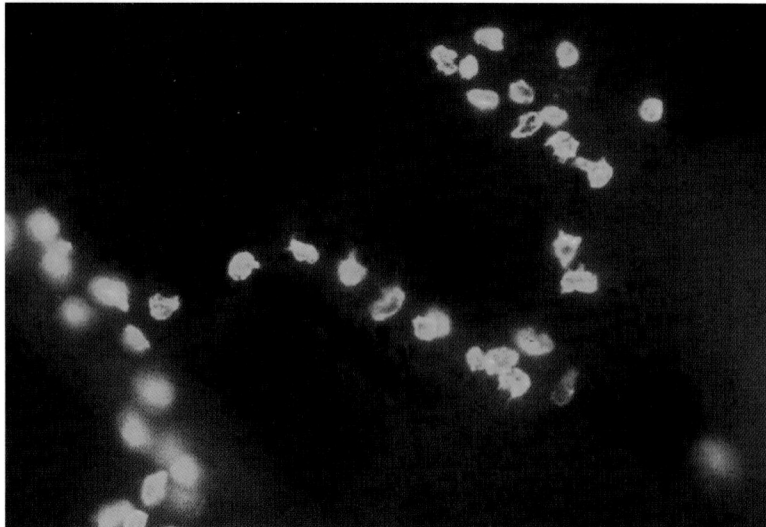

Fig. 1.41
Merkel cells: separated human epidermis showing a striking linear arrangement
(troma-1 antibody). By courtesy of J.P. Lacour, MD, and J.P. Ortonne, MD,
University of Nice, France.

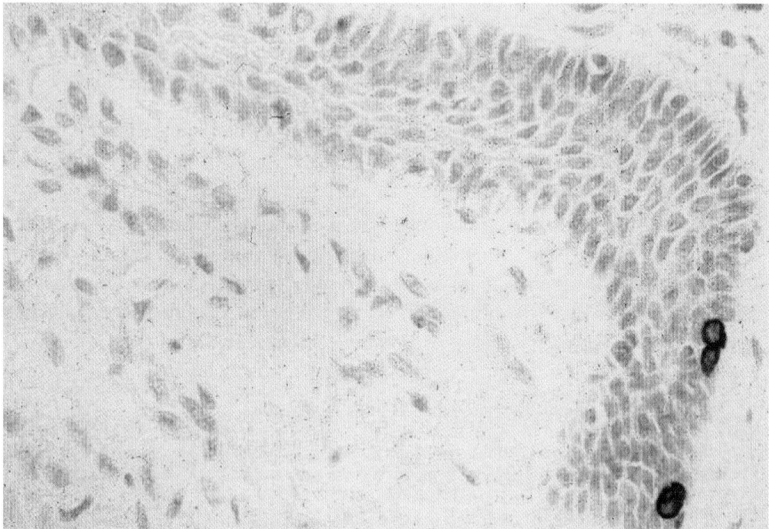

Fig. 1.42
Merkel cell: positive labeling for CAM 5.2 identifies Merkel cells in this obliquely
sectioned epidermal ridge.

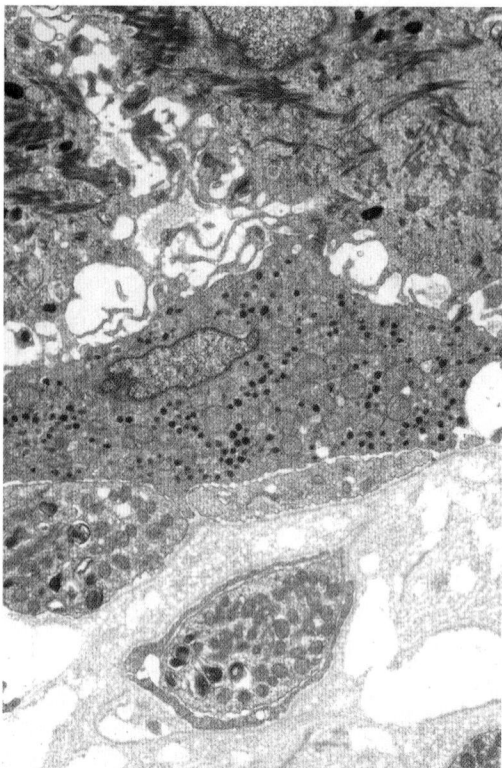

Fig. 1.43
Merkel cell: a heavily granulated Merkel cell is present in the midfield. This is
located immediately adjacent to a small nerve fiber.

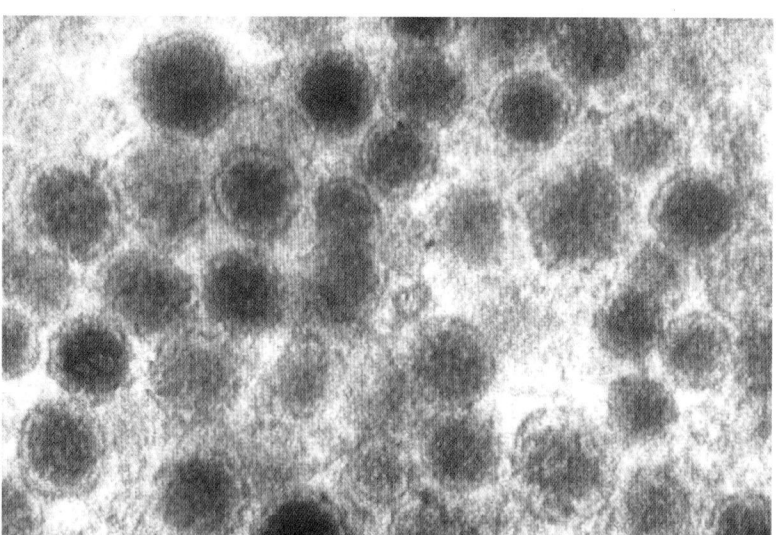

Fig. 1.44
Merkel cell granules: they are membrane bound and measure approximately
150 nm in diameter. By courtesy of A.S. Breathnach, MD (1977) Electron
microscopy of cutaneous nerves and receptors. Journal of Investigative
Dermatology 69, 8–26. Blackwell Publishing Inc., USA.

growth factor receptor.[7–9] Merkel cells show a positive uranaffin reaction.[10]
Merkel cells form close connections with sensory nerve endings and secrete
or express a number of these peptides.[11] The close contact between Merkel
cells and nerve fibers represents a Merkel cell–neurite complex, but there is
no clear evidence of synaptic transmission, although numerous vesicles can
be identified in neurons apposed to Merkel cells.[12]

Human skin contains an extensive neural network that contains cholinergic and adrenergic nerves and myelinated and unmyelinated sensory
fibers. Moreover, the skin also contains several transducers involved in the
perception of touch, pressure, and vibration, including Ruffini organs surrounding hair follicles, Meissner corpuscles, Vater–Pacini corpuscles located
in the deep layer of the dermis, and nerve endings which pass through the
epidermal basement membrane. Some of these contain Merkel cells which
form the Merkel cell–neurite complex, while others are free nerve endings.
The cell bodies for all these neurons reside in the dorsal root ganglion.
The Merkel cell–neurite complexes are thought to serve as mechanoreceptors and to be responsible for the sensation of touch via Piezo2-dependent
transmission channels.[13] They are clustered near unmyelinated sensory nerve
endings, where they group and form 'touch spots' at the bottom of rete
ridges. These complexes are also known as hair discs, touch domes, touch

corpuscles, or Iggo discs. The complex is innervated by a single, slowly
adapting type 1 nerve fiber. In hairy skin, Merkel cells also cluster in the
rete ridges and in the ORS of the hair follicle where the arrector pili muscles
attach. The function of Merkel cells in hair follicles is unclear, although they
may be involved in the induction of new anagen cycles.

There are two hypotheses for the origin of Merkel cells: one possibility is
that they differentiate from epidermal keratinocyte-like cells and the other
is that they arise from stem cells of neural crest origin that migrated during
embryogenesis, in similar fashion to melanocytes.[14] Merkel cell hyperplasia
is a common histologic finding and may accompany keratinocyte hyperproliferation as well as being frequently seen in adnexal tumors such as

nevus sebaceus, trichoblastomas, trichoepitheliomas, and nodular hidradenomas.[15] Merkel cell hyperplasia is associated with hyperplasia of nerve endings that occurs in neurofibromas, neurilemomas, nodular prurigo, or neurodermatitis.

Intercellular junctions

Desmosomes are the major intercellular adhesion complexes in the epidermis. They anchor keratin intermediate filaments to the cell membrane and link adjacent keratinocytes (*Fig. 1.45*). Desmosomes are found in the epidermis, myocardium, meninges and cortex of lymph nodes. Ultrastructurally, desmosomes contain plaques of electron-dense material running along the cytoplasm parallel to the junctional region, in which three bands can be distinguished: an electron-dense band next to the plasma membrane, a less dense band, and then a fibrillar area (*Fig. 1.46*).[1] Identical components are present on opposing cells which are separated by an intercellular space of 30 nm within which there is an electron-dense midline. There are three main protein components of desmosomes in the epidermis: the desmosomal cadherins, the armadillo family of nuclear and junctional proteins, and the plakins (*Fig. 1.47*).[2] The transmembranous cadherins comprise mostly heterophilic associations of desmogleins and desmocollins. There are four main epidermis-specific desmogleins (Dsg1–4) and three desmocollins (Dsc1–3). These show differentiation-specific expression. For example, Dsg1 and Dsc1 are found predominantly in the superficial layers of the epidermis whereas Dsg3 and Dsc3 show greater expression in basal keratinocytes. The intracellular parts of the cadherins interact with the keratin filament network via the desmosomal plaque proteins, mainly desmoplakin, plakoglobin and plakophilin.[1]

Clues to the biologic function of these desmosomal components have arisen from various inherited and acquired human diseases.[3,4] Naturally occurring human mutations have been reported in ten different desmosome genes with variable skin, hair and heart abnormalities and several desmosomal proteins serve as autoantigens in immunobullous blistering skin diseases such as pemphigus (*Figs 1.48 and 1.49*).[5] Antibodies to multiple desmosomal proteins may develop in diseases such as paraneoplastic pemphigus through the phenomenon of epitope spreading.[6] Cleavage of the extracellular domain of Dsg1 has also been demonstrated as the basis of staphylococcal scalded skin syndrome and bullous impetigo.[7]

Adherens junctions are recognized ultrastructurally as electron-dense transmembrane structures, with two opposing membranes separated by approximately 20 nm, that form links with the actin skeleton.[8] They are 0.2–0.5 μm in diameter and can be found as isolated cell junctions or in association with tight junctions and desmosomes. Adherens junctions are expressed early in skin development and contribute to epithelial assembly, adhesion, barrier formation, cell motility and changes in cell shape. They may also spatially coordinate signaling molecules and polarity cues as well as serving as docking sites for vesicle release. Adherens junctions contain two basic adhesive units: the nectin-afadin complex and the classical cadherin complex.[9,10] The nectins form a structural link to the actin cytoskeleton via afadin (also known as AF-6) and may be important in the initial formation of adherens junctions. The cadherins form a complex with the catenins (α-, β-, and p120 catenin) and help mediate adhesion and signaling. Cell signaling via β-catenin can activate several pathways linked to morphogenesis and cell fate determination.

Inherited gene mutations of the adherens junction proteins plakoglobin and P-cadherin have been reported. Plakoglobin mutations result in Naxos disease (woolly hair, keratoderma, cardiomyopathy).[3] P-cadherin mutations underlie autosomal recessive hypotrichosis with juvenile macular dystrophy as well as ectodermal dysplasia-ectrodactyly-macular dystrophy (EEM) syndrome, in which there is hypotrichosis, macular degeneration, hypodontia and limb defects, including ectrodactyly, syndactyly and camptodactyly.[11,12]

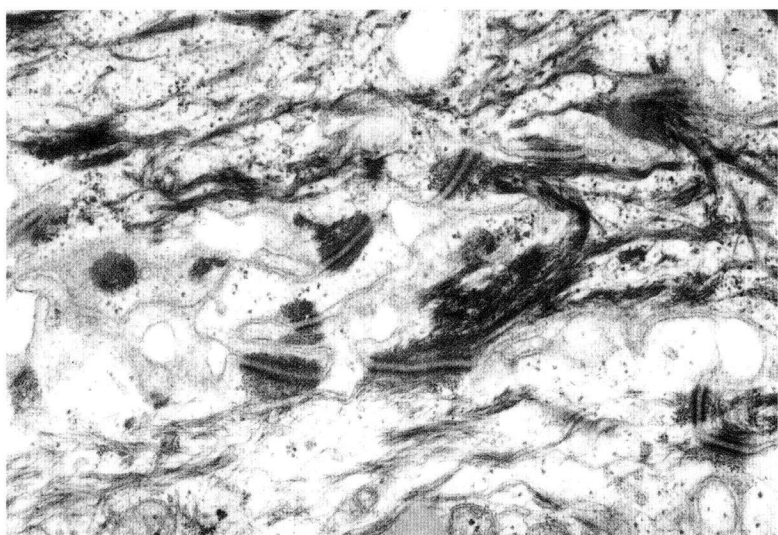

Fig. 1.45
Mid-prickle cell layer of normal epidermis: there are complex interdigitations between adjacent cell membranes with numerous desmosomal junctions.

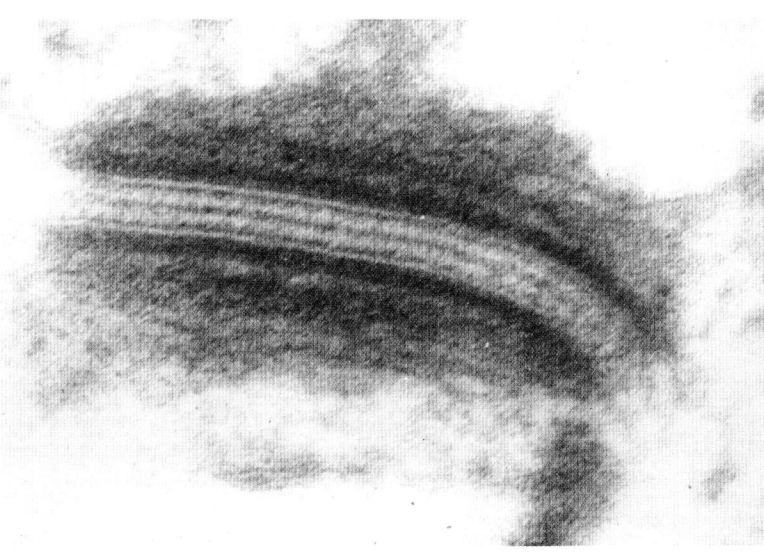

Fig. 1.46
Mid-prickle cell layer of normal epidermis showing the stratified nature of the desmosome.

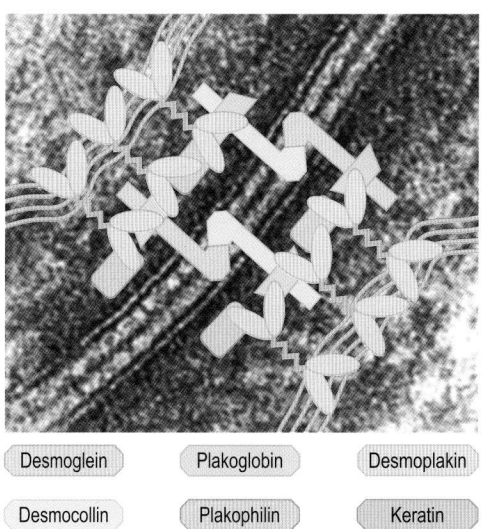

| Desmoglein | Plakoglobin | Desmoplakin |
| Desmocollin | Plakophilin | Keratin |

Fig. 1.47
Protein composition of a desmosome junction between adjacent keratinocytes. The keratin filament network of two keratinocytes is linked by a series of desmosomal plaque proteins and transmembranous molecules to create a structural and signaling bridge between the cells.

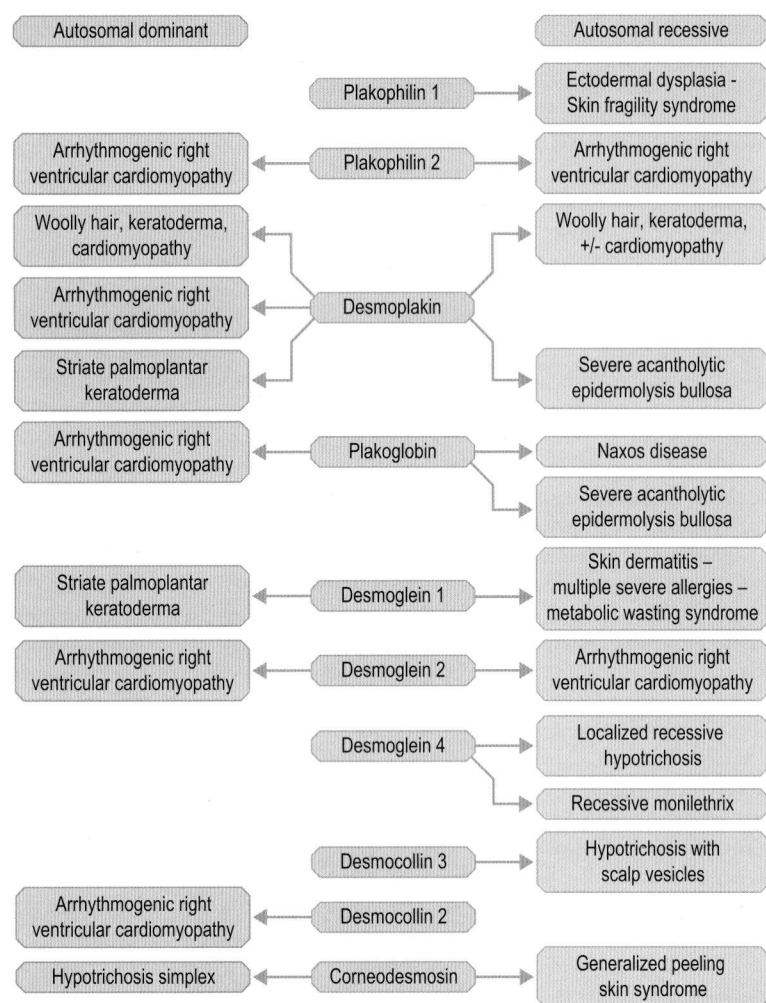

Fig. 1.48
Genetic disorders of desmosomes: autosomal dominant or autosomal recessive mutations in ten different structural components of desmosomes may give rise to specific diseases that can affect skin, hair or heart or combinations thereof.

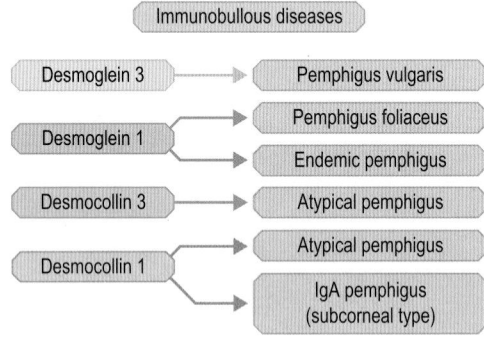

Fig. 1.49
Immunobullous diseases of desmosomes: intraepidermal blistering can arise through autoantibody disruption of four separate desmosomal proteins which leads to different clinical variants of pemphigus.

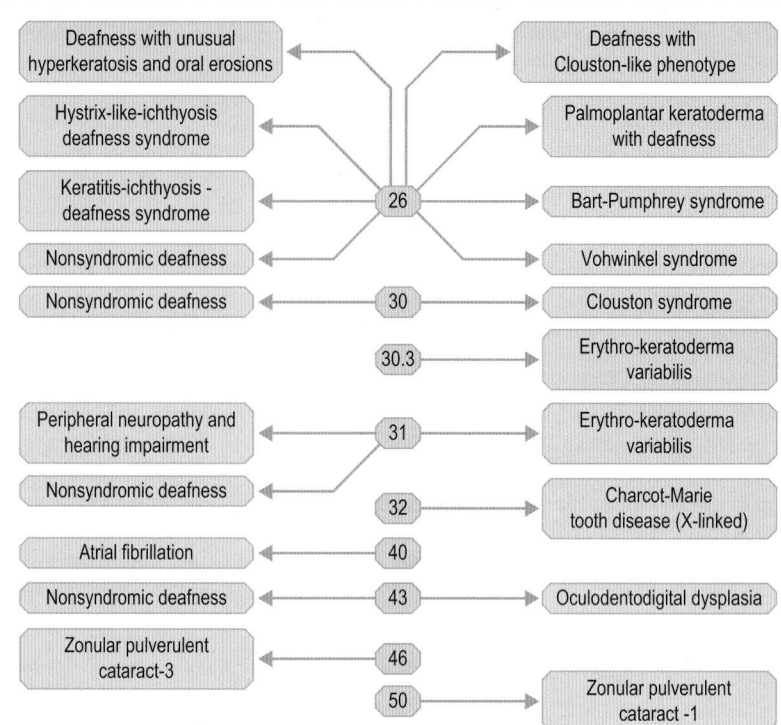

Fig. 1.50
Genetic disorders of connexins: nine different human connexin molecules are associated with different inherited diseases. Mutations in the four low molecular weight connexins shown at the top of the diagram are associated with a spectrum of skin pathology, as highlighted.

Gap junctions represent clusters of intercellular channels, known as connexons, which form connections between the cytoplasm of adjacent keratinocytes (and other cells).[13] Formation of a connexon involves assembly of six connexin subunits within the Golgi network. This complex is then transported to the plasma membrane where connexons associate with other connexons (homotypic or heterotypic) to form a gap junction. To date, 13 different human connexins have been described. The formation and stability of gap junctions can be regulated by protein kinase C, Src kinase, calcium concentration, calmodulin, adenosine 3′,5′-cyclic monophosphate (cAMP) and local pH.[14] The connexins are classified into three groups (α,

β and γ) according to their gene structure, overall gene homology and specific sequence motifs.[15] Apart from the connexins, vertebrates also contain another class of gap junction proteins, the pannexins, which are related to the innexins found in nonchordate animals. The function of gap junctions is to allow sharing of low molecular mass metabolites (< 1000 Da) and exchange of ions between neighboring cells. Gap junction communication is essential for cell synchronization, differentiation, cell growth and metabolic coordination of avascular organs, including epidermis.[14]

Inherited abnormalities in genes encoding four different connexins (Cx26, 30, 30.3 and 31) have been detected in several forms of keratoderma and/or hearing loss (*Fig. 1.50*). Nondermatologic disorders can also arise from mutations in some higher molecular weight connexins (Cx32, 40, 43, 46 and 50).

Tight junctions contribute to skin barrier integrity and maintaining cell polarity, although in simple epithelia they are major regulators of permeability.[8] An important function is to regulate the paracellular flux of water-soluble molecules between adjacent cells.[16] The main structural proteins of tight junctions are the claudins, of which there are approximately 24 subtypes, as well as the IgG-like family of junctional adhesion molecules (JAMs) and the occludin group of proteins. The principal claudins in the epidermis are claudin 1 and 4. These transmembranous proteins can bind to the intracellular zonula occudens proteins ZO-1, ZO-2, ZO-3 which interact with the actin cytoskeleton.[8,17]

Clinically, abnormalities in tight junction proteins can result in skin, kidney, ear and liver disease. Inherited gene mutations in claudin 1 have been reported in a few pedigrees with diffuse ichthyosis, hypotrichosis, scarring alopecia and sclerosing cholangitis.[18,19]

Pilosebaceous units

There are four classes of pilosebaceous unit: terminal on the scalp and beard; apopilosebaceous in axilla and groin; vellus on the majority of skin; and sebaceous on the chest, back and face. The dermal papilla is located at the base of the hair follicle and is associated with a rich extracellular matrix. Around the papilla are germinative (matrix) cells that have a very high rate of division, and give rise to spindle-shaped central cortex cells of the hair fiber, and the single outer layer of flattened overlapping cuticle cells. A central medulla is seen in some hairs, with regularly stacked condensed cells interspersed with air spaces or low-density cores. The cortical cells are filled with keratin intermediate filaments orientated along the long axis of the cell, interspersed with a dense interfilamentous protein matrix. The cuticular cells are morphologically distinct, with flattened outward-facing cells, with three layers inside the cuticle of condensed, flattened protein granules: endocuticle, exocuticle and 'a' layer.[1] Around the cuticle is the IRS, which is composed of three distinct layers of cells that undergo keratinization: the IRS cuticle, the Huxley layer and the outermost Henle layer.[2] Differentiation in the IRS involves the development of trichohyalin granules, with 8–10 nm filaments orientated in the direction of hair growth. The IRS moves up the follicle, forming a support for the hair fiber, and degenerates above the sebaceous gland. The outermost layer is the ORS, which is continuous with the epidermis and expresses epithelial keratins, K5/K14, K1/K10 and K6/K16 in the upper ORS and K5/K14/K17 in the deeper ORS.

Normal growth of the hair fiber is 300–400 μm/day. Hair growth is generated by the high rate of proliferation of progenitor cells in the follicle bulb. There are three phases of cyclical hair growth: anagen, when growth occurs; catagen, a regressing phase; and telogen, a resting phase. The follicle re-enters anagen, and the old hair is replaced by a new one.

Immediately above the basal layer in the hair bulb, cells undergo a secondary pathway of 'trichocyte' or hair differentiation, and express a further complex group of keratins, the hard keratins.[2] Two families of hair keratins, types I and II, are present in mammals, which have distinctive amino- and carboxy-terminals with high levels of cysteine residues but lack the extended glycine residues of epidermal keratins. The proteins differ from epithelial keratins in position on two-dimensional gels but form acidic and basic groups. The nomenclature for human keratins and keratin-associated proteins was updated in 2006 and 2012, respectively.[3,4]

Mutations in hair keratin genes have been found to cause autosomal dominant forms of the human disease monilethrix. More common hair variants, such as curly hair, may be explained by dynamic changes during hair growth.[5] Curvature of curly hair is programmed from the very basal area of the follicle and the bending process is linked to a lack of axial symmetry in the lower part of the bulb, affecting the connective tissue sheath, ORS, IRS and the hair shaft cuticle.

Sebaceous glands usually develop as lateral protrusions from the ORS of hair follicles, but at certain sites, such as the eyelids, lips, areolae, nipples and labia minora, they appear to arise independently and drain directly onto the skin's surface (*Figs 1.51 and 1.52*). They are widespread in distribution, being found everywhere on the body except on the palms and soles. They are particularly abundant on the face and scalp, in the midline of the back and about the perineum, and are concentrated around the orifices of the body (*Fig. 1.53*). Those of the eyelid are known as the glands of Zeis and the meibomian glands. Sebaceous glands within the areolae are known as Montgomery tubercles. The largest sebaceous glands are associated with small vellus hairs in specialized pilosebaceous units known as sebaceous follicles (facial pores).

Sebaceous glands consist of several lipid-containing lobules, usually connected to a hair follicle (*Fig. 1.54*). Each lobule is composed of an outer layer of small cuboidal or flattened basophilic germinative cells, from which arises the inner zone of lipid-laden vacuolated cells with characteristic crenated nuclei (*Fig. 1.55*). The secretions drain into the sebaceous duct, which joins the hair follicle at the level of the infundibulum (*Fig. 1.56*). The duct is lined by keratinizing stratified squamous epithelium and is continuous with the external root sheath. The glands are holocrine because their secretions depend on complete degeneration of the acini, with release of all the cells' lipid contents to become sebum.

Immunohistochemically, the sebaceous cells label strongly for EMA but they do not express CEA or low molecular weight keratin (CAM 5.2) or S100 protein (*Fig. 1.57*). Ultrastructurally, the mature sebaceous gland shows gradual accumulation of variably sized, nonmembrane-bound, lipid inclusions in differentiating cells. Numerous mitochondria, ribosomes and

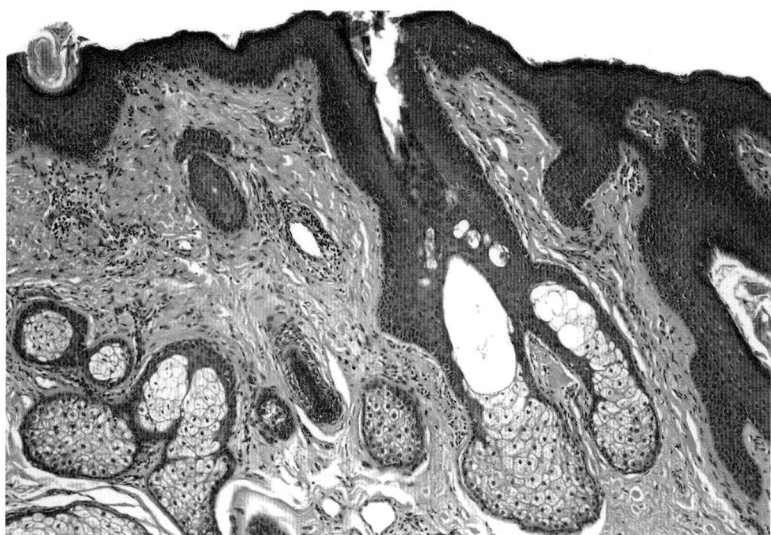

Fig. 1.52
Normal vulva: sebaceous glands are conspicuous, but arise independently of a hair follicle and open directly onto the surface epithelium.

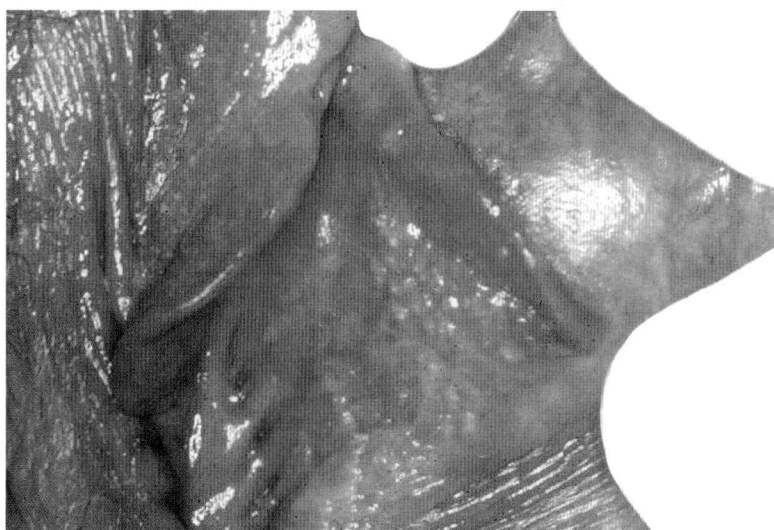

Fig. 1.51
Sebaceous glands: on the inner aspect of the labia these appear as tiny yellow papules (Fordyce spots). By courtesy of S.M. Neill, MD, Institute of Dermatology, London, UK.

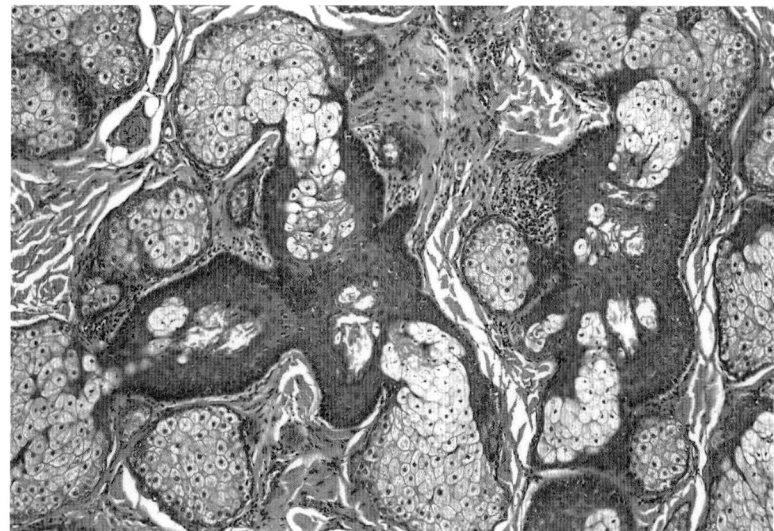

Fig. 1.53
Nose: sebaceous glands are particularly numerous at this site.

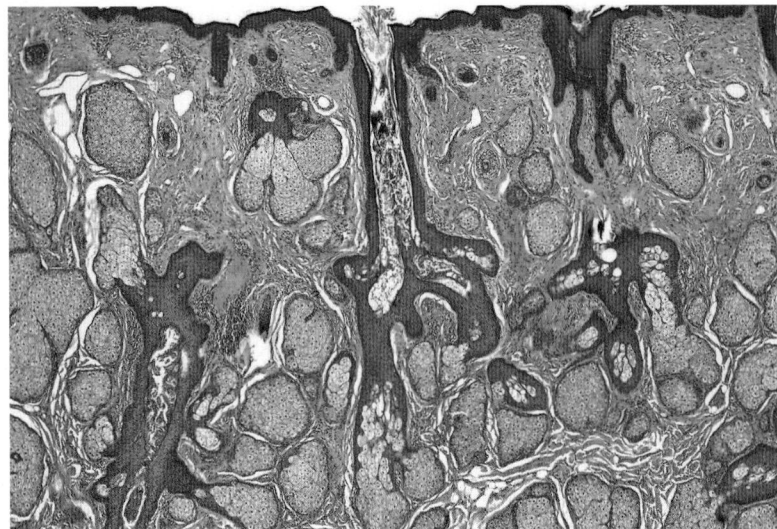

Fig. 1.54
Nose: multiple sebaceous glands are evident.

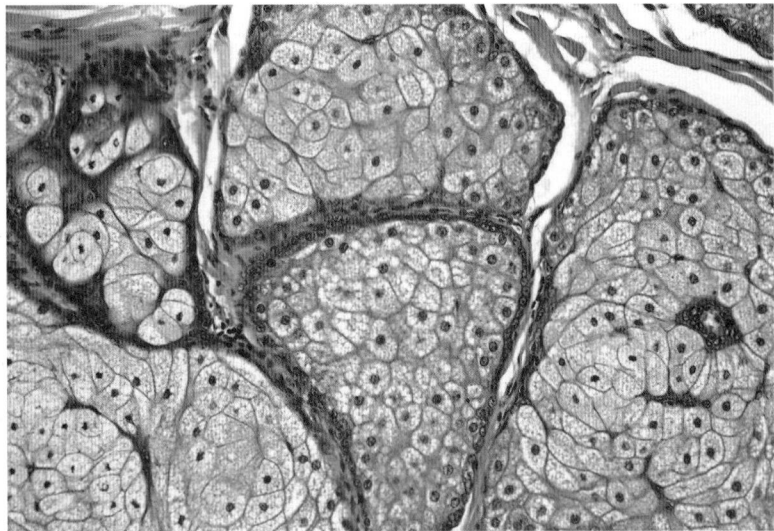

Fig. 1.55
Sebaceous lobule: germinative cells are basophilic and flattened. With maturation the cells acquire their characteristic 'bubbly' cytoplasm.

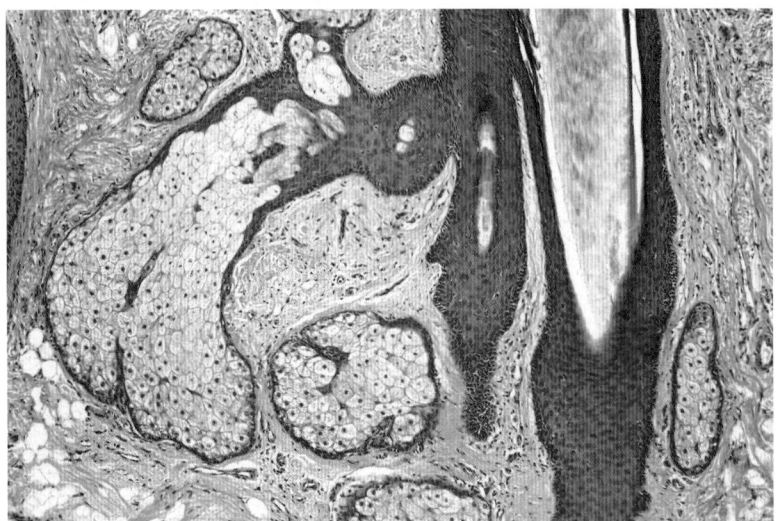

Fig. 1.56
Sebaceous duct: this is lined by keratinizing stratified squamous epithelium; it is continuous with the external root sheath.

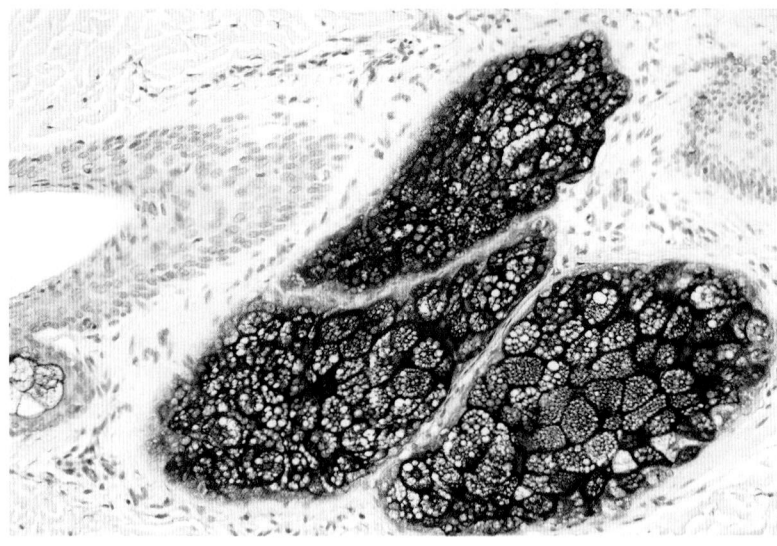

Fig. 1.57
Sebaceous gland: the epithelial cells normally strongly express EMA.

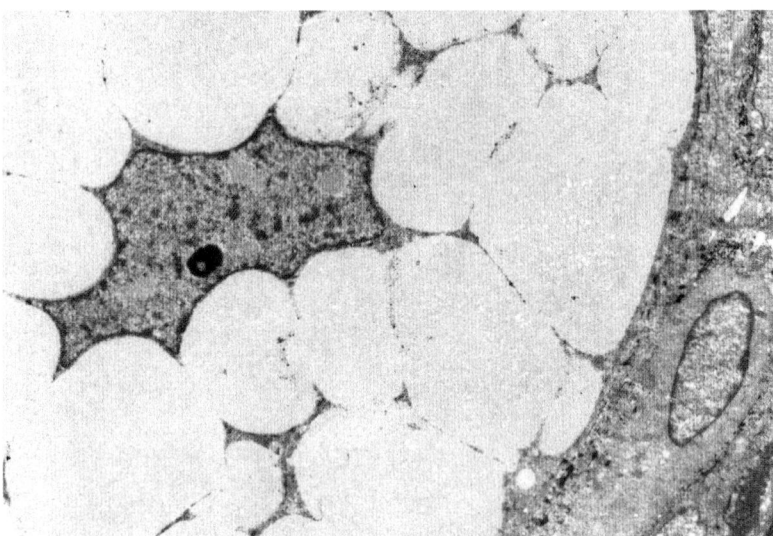

Fig. 1.58
Sebaceous gland: in this field from the center of a sebaceous lobule, the cytoplasm is completely distended with lipid droplets. Germinative cells are evident in the right-lower quadrant.

membrane-bound vesicles may also be evident. As the cells mature before their disintegration, the lipid droplets completely fill the cytoplasm and compress the centrally located nucleus (*Fig. 1.58*).

The secretion of sebaceous glands is sebum, an exceedingly complicated lipid mixture that includes triglycerides (57%), wax esters (26%) and squalene (12%). Its function includes waterproofing, control of epidermal water loss, and a protective function, inhibiting the growth of fungi and bacteria. Secreted sebum undergoes significant changes due to the presence of *Propionibacterium acnes* (triglyceride hydrolysis) within the pilosebaceous canal and *Staphylococcus epidermidis* (cholesterol ester formation) on the perifollicular skin. Skin surface lipid is composed of a mixture of sebum and epidermal lipids.

Eccrine glands

Human sweat glands are generally divided into two types: eccrine and apocrine.[1] The eccrine gland is the primary gland responsible for thermoregulatory sweating in humans.[2] Eccrine sweat glands are distributed over nearly the entire body surface. The number of sweat glands in humans varies greatly, ranging from 1.6 to 4.0 million.

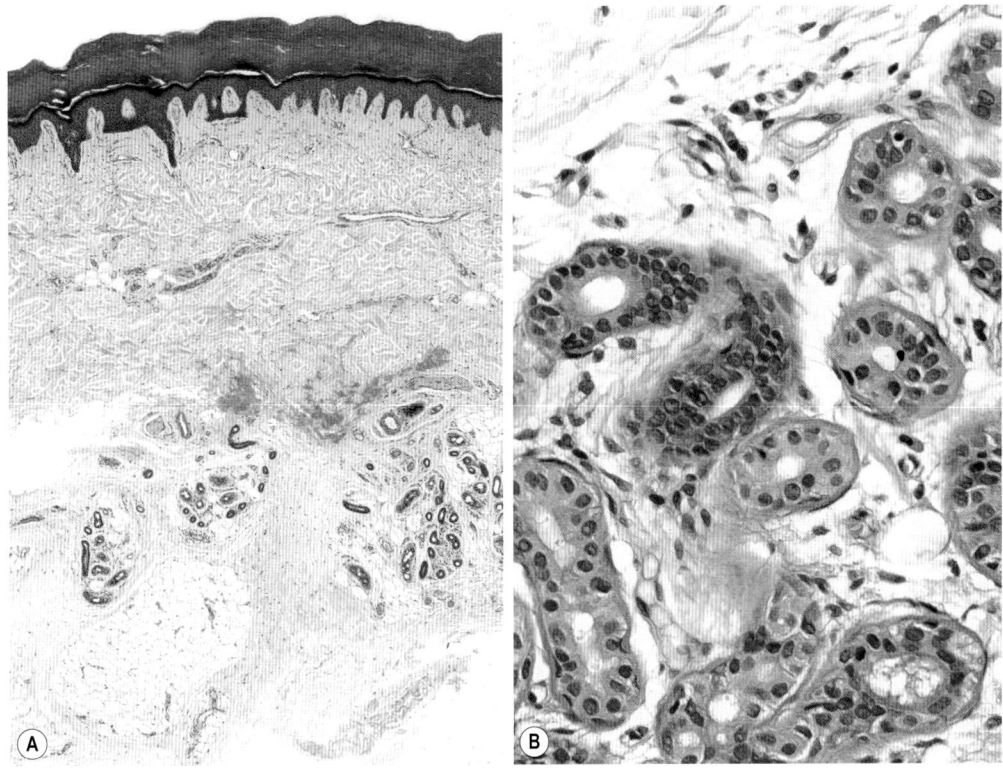

Fig. 1.59
Eccrine gland: (**A**) palmar skin showing numerous eccrine glands located in the deep reticular dermis and subcutaneous fat, (**B**) the secretory unit is in the lower field. Sections through the coiled duct are evident in the upper field. The epithelium of the duct is more darkly stained than that of the glandular component.

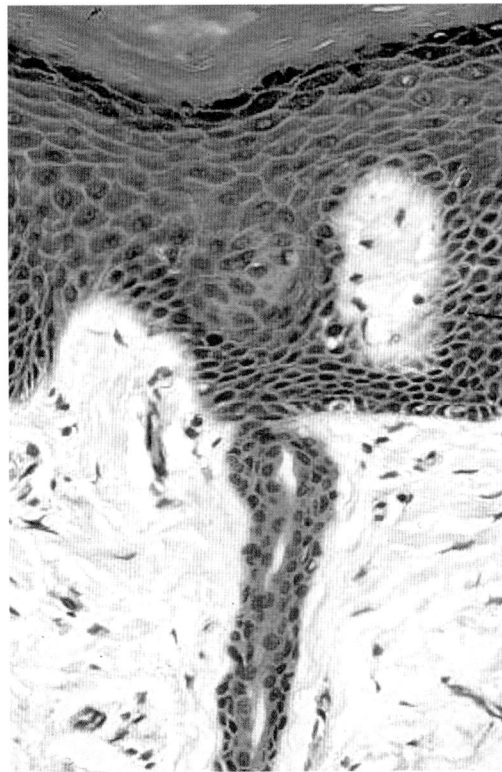

Fig. 1.60
Eccrine gland: high-power view of eccrine straight duct.

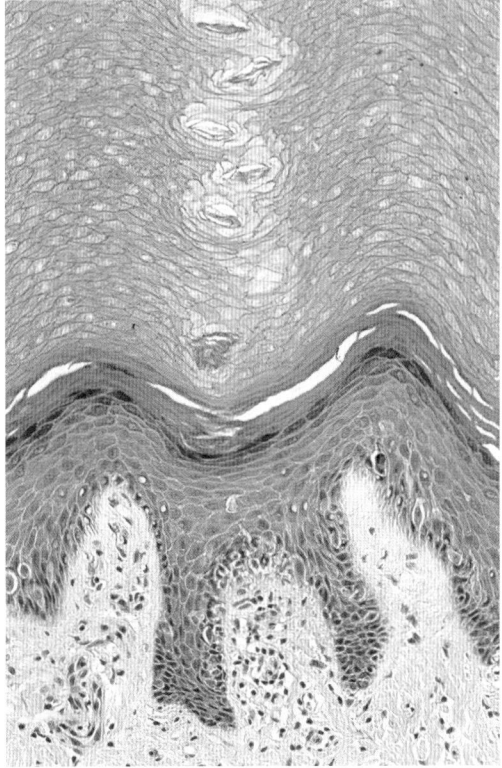

Fig. 1.61
Eccrine gland: most superficially, the duct coils through the stratum corneum.

Histologically, eccrine sweat glands are divided into four subunits: a highly vascularized coiled secretory gland, a coiled dermal duct, a straight dermal duct, and a coiled intraepidermal duct (the acrosyringium) (*Fig. 1.59*). The secretory coil is located in the lower dermis, and the duct extends through the dermis and opens directly onto the skin surface (*Figs 1.60, 1.61*). The active sweat glands are present most densely on the sole,

forehead and palm, somewhat less on the back of the hand, still less on the lumbar region, and the lateral and extensor surfaces of the extremities, and least on the trunk and the flexor and medial surfaces of the extremities. The uncoiled dimension of the secretory portion of the gland is approximately 30–50 μm in diameter and 2–5 mm in length. The size of the adult secretory coil ranges $1–8 \times 10^{-3}$ mm³. The secretory component lies in the lower reaches of the reticular dermis or around the interface between the dermis and subcutaneous fat and is surrounded by a thick basement membrane and loose connective tissue often rich in mucin. It embodies an outer discontinuous layer of contractile myoepithelial cells and an inner layer of secretory cells comprising two cell types: large clear pyramidal cells, which appear to be responsible for water secretion, and smaller, darkly staining mucopolysaccharide-containing cells (probably secreting a glycoprotein), which are much less commonly seen. Between adjacent cells are canaliculi, which open into the lumen of the tubule (see below). Sometimes the secretory lobules show striking clear cell change due to glycogen accumulation (*Fig. 1.62*). The myoepithelial cells contract in response to cholinergic stimuli. They have spindled cell morphology and are distributed in a spiral, parallel array along the long axis of the secretory tubule. On the basis of their expression of keratin filaments, they appear to be of ectodermal rather than mesenchymal derivation. They do not label for vimentin. Myoepithelial cells therefore develop from the epithelial cells of the tip of the secretory coil and not, as might be expected, from adjacent mesenchymal cells. The dermal duct components consist of a double layer of cuboidal basophilic cells. The duct is not merely a conduit, but has a biologically active function, modifying the composition of eccrine secretion and, particularly, the reabsorption of water. The intraepidermal portion of the sweat duct opens directly onto the surface of the skin. A myoepithelial layer is absent.

The secretory unit is strongly labeled by CAM 5.2 (both cytoplasmic and membranous) and Ber-EP4 and there is luminal accentuation (*Fig. 1.63*). The ductal component is completely negative. EMA can be detected along the luminal aspect of the secretory unit and outlining the intercellular canaliculi.

It is also present around the luminal border of the duct, and is often present in large quantities within the lumen. CEA is present in a similar distribution to EMA although secretory labeling tends to be rather focal and somewhat weaker while the ductal lumen is more strongly outlined. The myoepithelial cells can be identified by antibodies to S100 protein, desmin and smooth

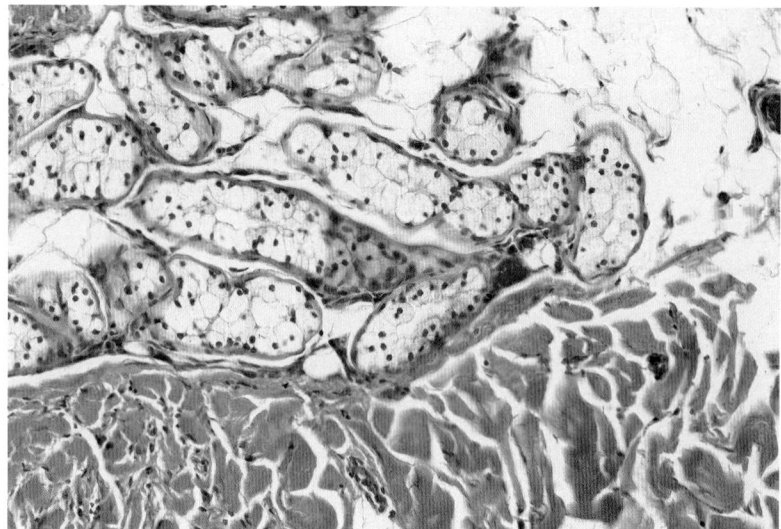

Fig. 1.62
Eccrine gland: excessive glycogen has resulted in vacuolated epithelium.

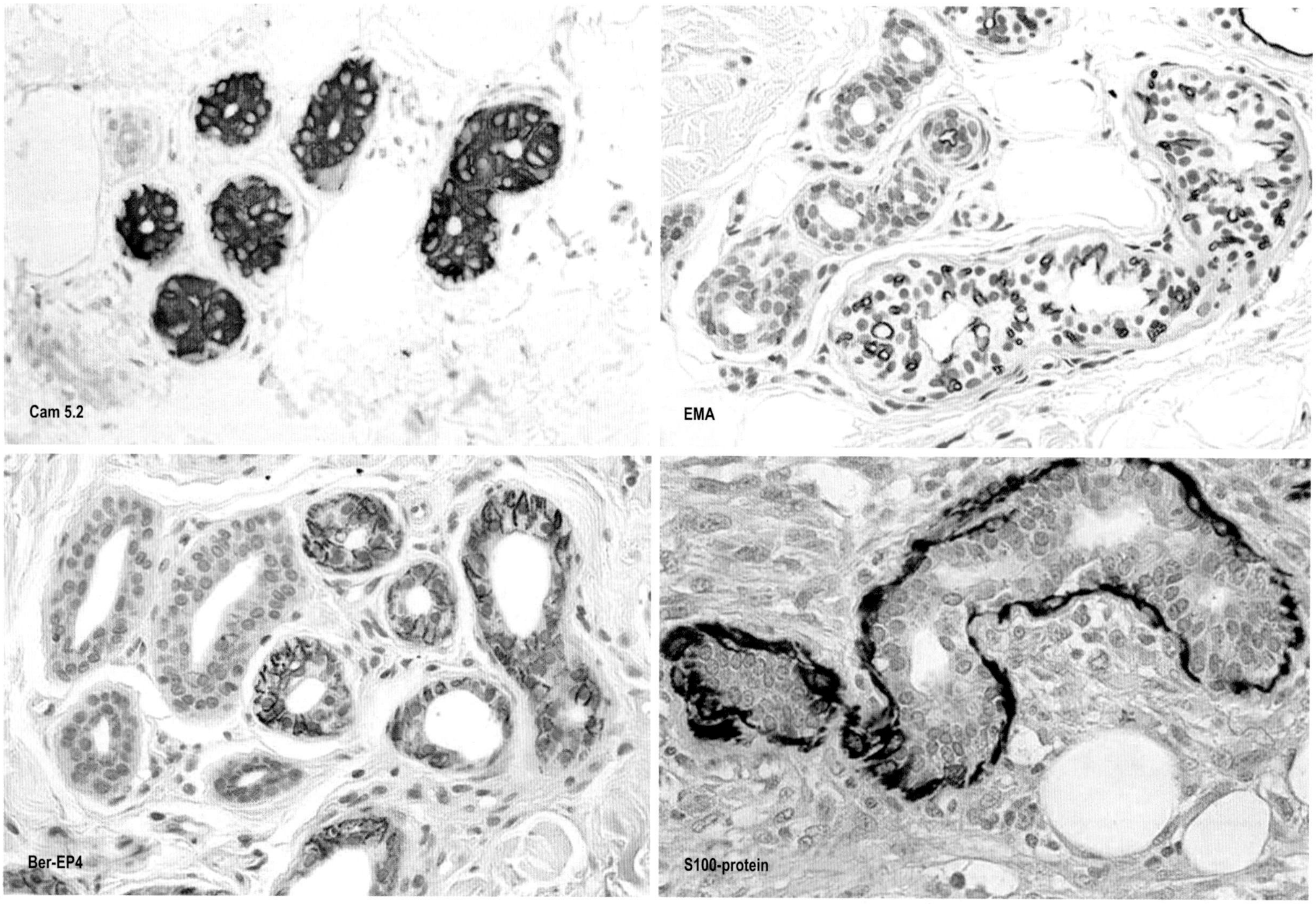

Cam 5.2

EMA

Ber-EP4

S100-protein

Fig. 1.63
Eccrine gland: immunohistochemistry.

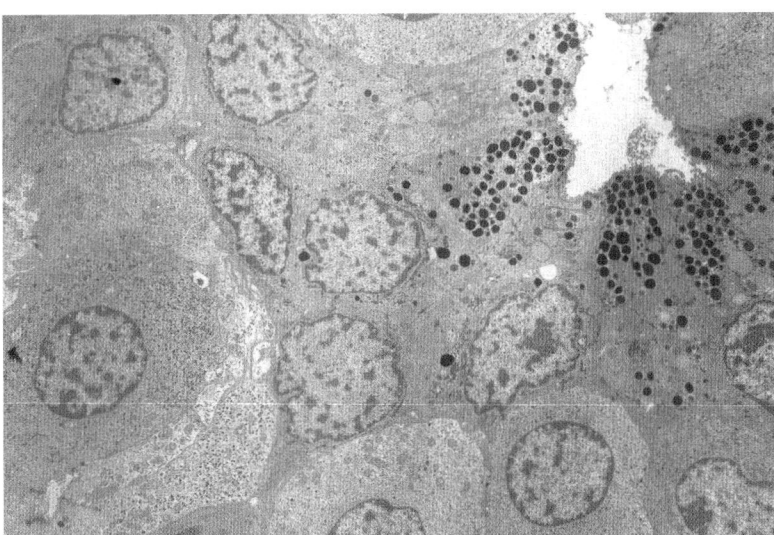

Fig. 1.64
Eccrine gland: low-power electron micrograph showing the lumen in the upper-right quadrant, granular mucous-secreting cells and serous cells.

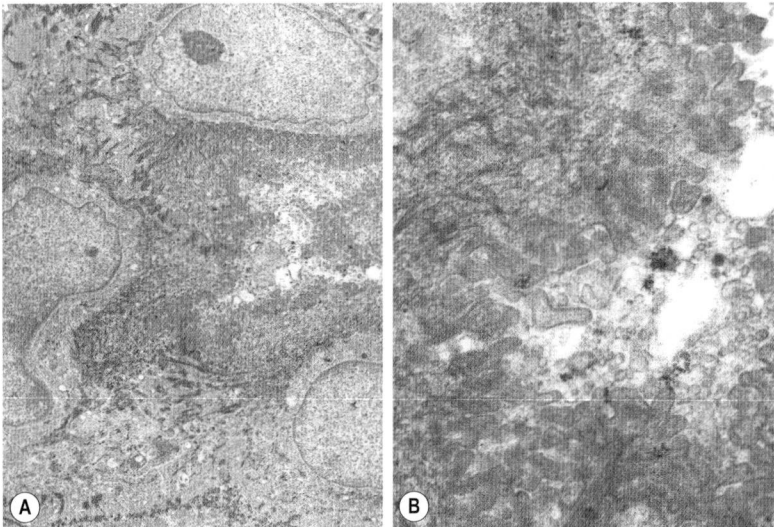

Fig. 1.66
Eccrine gland: (**A**) lumen of the eccrine dermal duct lined by conspicuous microvilli, (**B**) high-power view of eccrine dermal duct showing microvilli and circumferentially orientated tonofilaments.

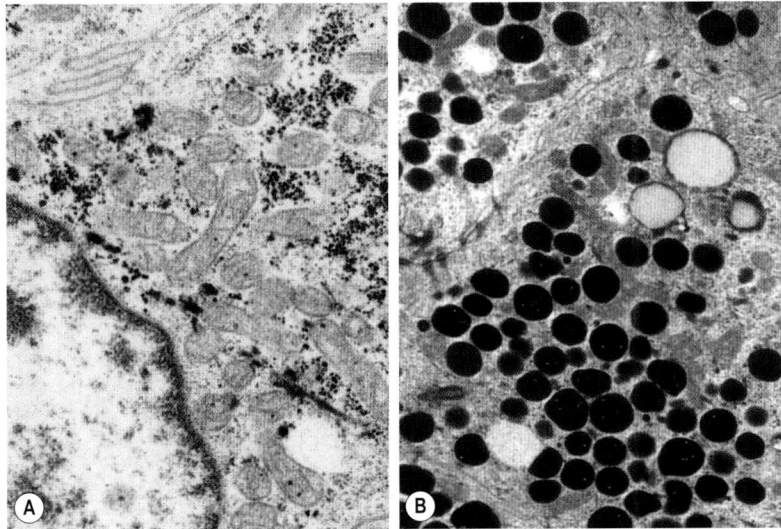

Fig. 1.65
Eccrine gland: (*left*) high-power view of clear cell showing conspicuous mitochondria and numerous electron-dense glycogen granules, (*right*) high-power view of secretory granules in a dark cell.

muscle actin. The eccrine glands show strong activity for the enzymes amylophosphorylase, leucine aminopeptidase, succinic dehydrogenase and cytochrome oxidase.[3] Weak or no activity is seen for Nicotinamide adenine dinucleotide (NADH) diaphorase, esterase and acid phosphatase.

With electron microscopy, the serous cells are characterized by abundant intracytoplasmic glycogen granules and numerous mitochondria (*Figs 1.64, 1.65*). Adjacent cell membranes, which show marked interdigitations, may separate to form microvilli-lined intercellular canaliculi. The mucous cells contain numerous electron-dense lipid droplets and lysozymes. Myoepithelial cells are present at the periphery of the secretory coil within the eccrine basal lamina (lamina densa) and contain abundant myofilaments with characteristic dense bodies. The sweat duct lumen is bordered by conspicuous microvilli (*Fig. 1.66*). The cytoplasm contains numerous clear vesicles. Tonofilaments are characteristically orientated in a circumferential manner deep to the plasma membrane, the so-called cuticle of light microscopy. This is particularly well developed in the acrosyringium.

Human perspiration is classified into two types: insensible perspiration and active sweating. Insensible perspiration involves water loss from the respiratory passages, the skin, and gaseous exchanges in the lungs. Heat, exercise and carbon dioxide can all induce active sweating in human beings.

Active sweating may be classified into two types: thermal and mental/emotional. Thermal sweating plays an important role in keeping the body's temperature constant and involves the whole body surface.[4] The secretory nerve fibers innervated in human sweat glands are sympathetic, which appear to be cholinergic in character as sweating is produced by pilocarpine and stopped by atropine.[5] VIP coexisting in the cholinergic nerve fibers has been suggested as a candidate neurotransmitter that may control the blood circulation of the sweat glands. Acetylcholine is the primary neurotransmitter released from cholinergic sudomotor nerves and binds to muscarinic receptors on the eccrine sweat gland, although sweating can also occur via exogenous administration of α- or β-adrenergic agonists. The initial fluid released from the secretory cells is isotonic and similar to plasma although it is devoid of proteins. As the fluid travels up the duct towards the surface of the skin, sodium and chloride are reabsorbed, resulting in sweat on the surface being hypotonic relative to plasma.[6] When the rate of sweat production increases, however, for example during exercise, ion reabsorption mechanisms can be overwhelmed due to the large quantity of sweat secreted into the duct, resulting in higher ion losses. The sodium content in sweat on the skin's surface, therefore, is greatly influenced by sweat rate.

Apocrine glands

Apart from eccrine glands, the skin also contains apocrine sweat glands.[1,2] Apocrine glands have a low secretory output, and hence no significant role in thermoregulation. Apocrine glands are found predominantly in the anogenital and axillary regions, but are also located in the external auditory meatus (ceruminous glands), the eyelid (Moll gland), and within the areola. They are derived from the epidermis, and develop as an outgrowth of the follicular epithelium. They first appear during the fourth to fifth month of gestation. Their function in humans is unknown, but in other mammals they are responsible for scent production and have importance in sexual attraction. As with sebaceous glands, they are smaller in childhood, becoming larger and functionally active at puberty. The secretions of the ceruminous glands are believed to lubricate, clean and protect the external ear from bacterial and fungal infections.

Apocrine glands include two distinct components: a complex secretory element situated in the lower reticular dermis or subcutaneous fat, and a tubular duct linking the gland with the pilosebaceous follicle at a site above the sebaceous duct. Microscopically, the secretory portion comprises an outer discontinuous layer of myoepithelial cells and an inner layer of cuboidal to columnar eosinophilic cells (*Figs 1.67, 1.68*). Although a histologic artifact, secretory droplets, which appear to be pinched off from

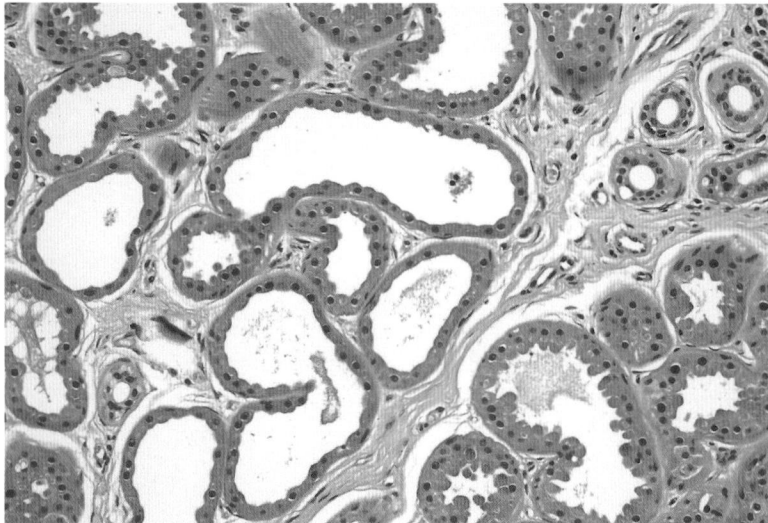

Fig. 1.67
Apocrine gland: this specimen from normal axillary skin shows apocrine secretory lobules in the subcutaneous fat. Ducts are present in the upper right of the field.

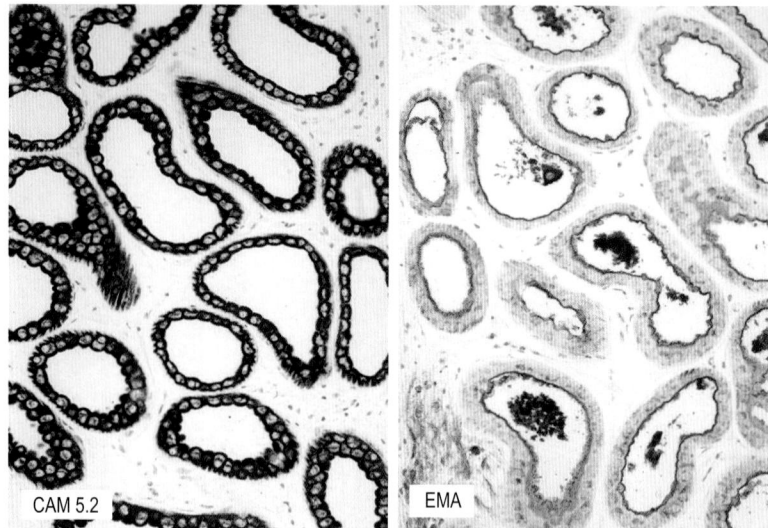

Fig. 1.69
Apocrine gland: immunohistochemistry (CAM 5.2 and EMA).

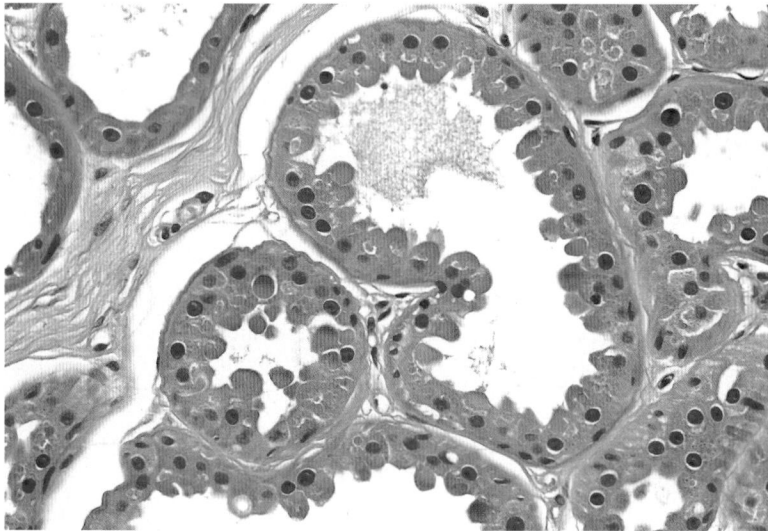

Fig. 1.68
Apocrine gland: lobules are lined by tall columnar cells with intensely eosinophilic cytoplasm. 'Decapitation secretion' is conspicuous.

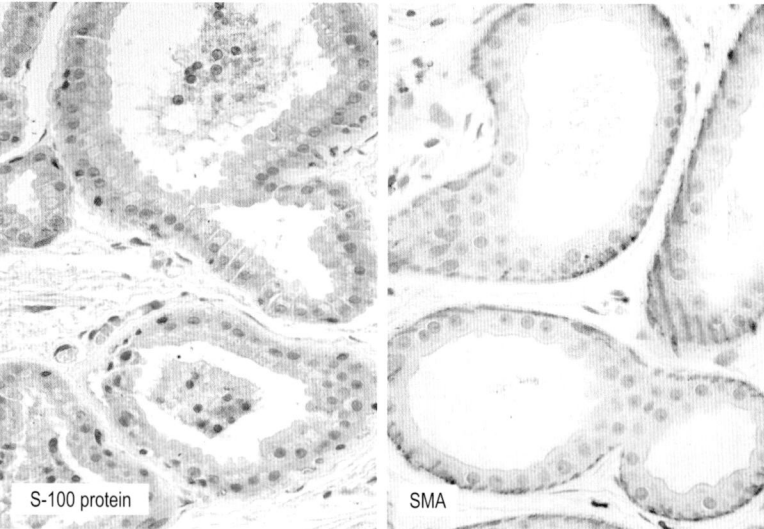

Fig. 1.70
Apocrine gland: immunohistochemistry (S100 protein and SMA).

the superficial aspect of the columnar cells (decapitation secretion), can be seen on light microscopy. The duct portion is formed by a double layer of cuboidal epithelium. It is morphologically indistinguishable from the eccrine duct. The inner layer of the secretory portion contains a single columnar secretory cell type containing numerous large dense granules located at the apical aspect, which contribute to the lipid-rich secretion produced. The inner layer is also surrounded by a fenestrated layer of myoepithelial cells but the lumen may be larger in diameter than that present in eccrine tissue. The apocrine excretory duct does not have any known reabsorptive function and consists of a double layer of cuboidal cells that merge distally with the epithelium of the hair follicle, resulting in emptying of the secretion into the hair follicle.

Immunohistochemically, the secretory unit shows very strong labeling with the antibody CAM 5.2 (both cytoplasmic and membranous), and there is luminal accentuation. The apocrine duct is negative (*Fig. 1.69*). EMA labels the cytoplasm of the secretory cells, and is accentuated along the luminal border. It is also present along the luminal aspect of the apocrine duct. With CEA, there is faint, focal staining of the secretory epithelium. The luminal aspect of the duct is strongly outlined. Cytoplasmic granules express epidermal growth factor. The myoepithelial cells of the secretory unit are reactive for S100 protein and smooth muscle actin (*Fig. 1.70*). The

apocrine secretory epithelium strongly expresses the enzymes NADH diaphorase, esterase, acid phosphatase and β-glucuronidase. There is weak or absent reactivity for amylophosphorylase, leucine aminopeptidase, succinic dehydrogenase and cytochrome oxidase. The apocrine gland also can be stained with cationic colloidal gold at pH 2.0.[3]

Ultrastructure of the apocrine reveals cuboidal to columnar secretory cells containing numerous osmiophilic secretory vacuoles. Mitochondria are present in large numbers. While some show obvious double cristae, others are so electron dense that the internal structure is obscured. The Golgi is conspicuous. The luminal border is lined by prominent microvilli (*Fig. 1.71*).

The mechanism of apocrine secretion and control of apocrine glands is uncertain, but there is adrenergic sympathetic innervation, and secretion is provoked by external stimuli such as excitement or fear.[4] The unpleasant odor of apocrine secretion, which is odorless in itself, is due to breakdown products produced by cutaneous bacterial flora.

A third type of intermediate sweat gland, the apo-eccrine gland, has also been described in axillary skin but its existence is not universally accepted.

Dermal–epidermal junction

The interface between the lower part of epidermis and the top layer of dermis consists of a complex network of interacting macromolecules that form the cutaneous basement membrane zone (BMZ) (*Figs 1.72, 1.73*).[1] Many of

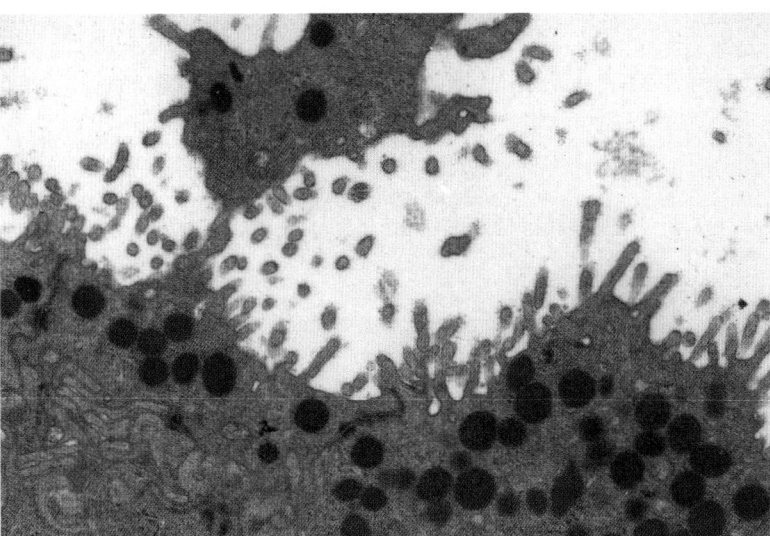

Fig. 1.71
Apocrine gland: close-up view showing microvilli and decapitation secretion.

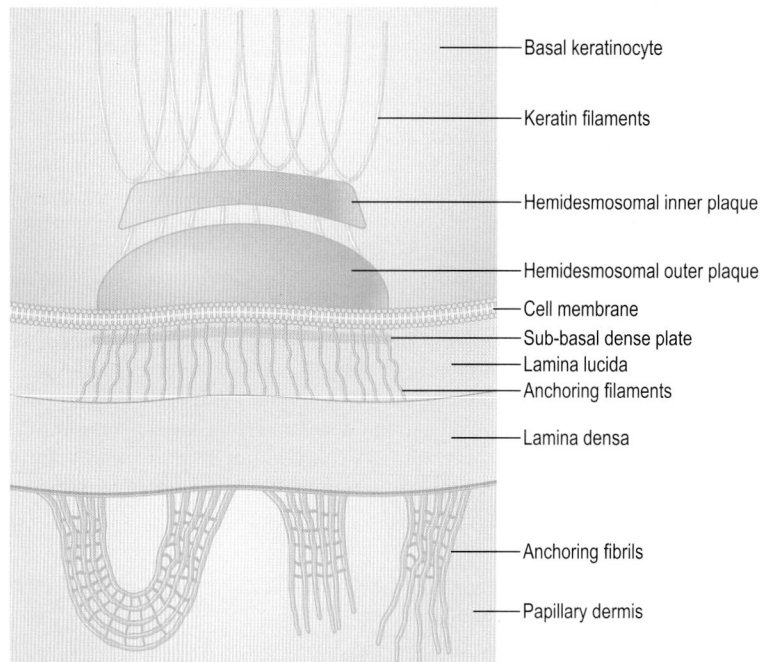

Fig. 1.73
Schematic representation of a hemidesmosome-anchoring filament-anchoring fibril complex at the dermal–epidermal junction. A continuum of adhesive proteins extends from the keratin tonofilaments within basal keratinocytes through to dermal collagen. This complex represents the main adhesion unit at the dermal–epidermal junction.

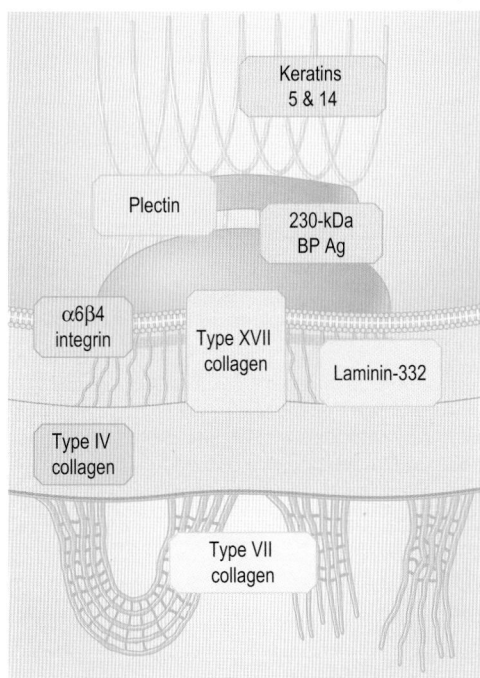

Fig. 1.72
The macromolecular components of the dermal–epidermal junction centered on a hemidesmosome-anchoring filament-anchoring fibril complex. Protein–protein interactions between these molecules secure adhesion between the epidermis and the subjacent dermis.

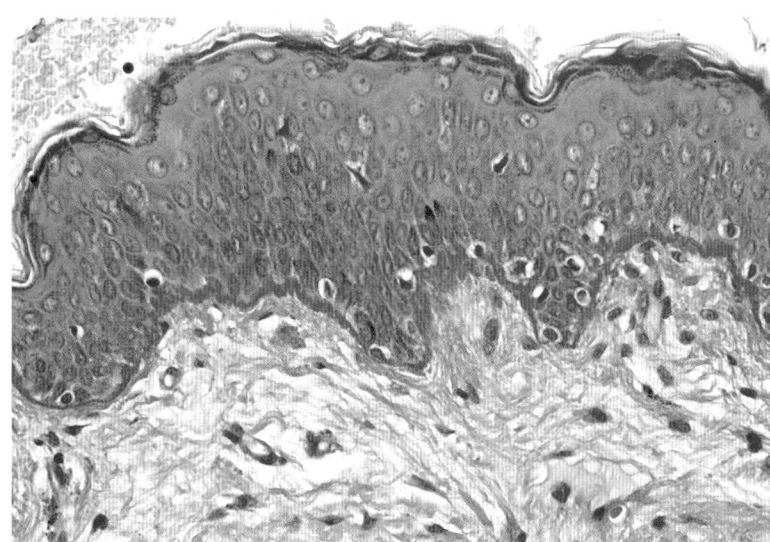

Fig. 1.74
The basement membrane region stains strongly with periodic acid-Schiff.

these components are glycoproteins and thus the BMZ can be recognized histologically as staining positive with PAS staining (*Fig. 1.74*). Ultrastructural examination of the BMZ by transmission electron microscopy shows two layers with different optical densities (*Fig. 1.75*).[2] The upper layer, the lamina lucida, is a low electron density region of 30–40 nm in breadth which is directly subjacent to the plasma membranes of basal keratinocytes. Below the lamina lucida is the lamina densa, an electron-dense region, 30–50 nm across, which interacts with the extracellular matrix of the upper dermis. Within the cutaneous BMZ distinct adhesion complexes are evident. Extending from inside the basal keratinocytes, through the lamina lucida and lamina densa, and into the superficial dermis are ultrastructurally recognizable attachment structures. The components of these adhesion units are the hemidesmosomes, anchoring filaments and anchoring fibrils.[3] The importance of these structural complexes in securing adhesion of the epidermis to the underlying dermis is highlighted by both inherited and acquired

subepidermal blistering skin diseases (*Figs 1.76, 1.77*). The precise role of individual proteins in adhesion is demonstrated by the group of inherited skin blistering diseases, epidermolysis bullosa, in which components in the hemidesmosomal structures, anchoring filaments, or anchoring fibrils are genetically defective or absent.[4] Other rare forms of epidermolysis bullosa can result from mutations in vesicle transport proteins (exophilin-5) or components of focal contacts at the dermal–epidermal junction (kindlin-1 or α3 integrin), as well as desmosomal proteins (plakophilin-1, desmoplakin, and plakoglobin) and during cornification (transglutaminase-5).[5] Collectively, these mutations lead to skin and sometimes mucous membrane fragility following minor trauma. The level of blistering in epidermolysis bullosa may vary from at or just above the dermal–epidermal junction to within the epidermis to above the granular cell layer, depending on the mutated protein.

The hemidesmosomes extend from the intracellular compartment of the basal keratinocytes to the cell membrane adjacent to the lamina lucida in the upper portion of the dermal–epidermal basement membrane. The inner plaques of hemidesmosomes serve as attachment sites for keratin filaments while the outer plaques associate with anchoring filaments that traverse the lamina lucida. Subjacent to the hemidesmosomal outer plaques in the lamina lucida are the sub-basal dense plates which contribute to the structural organization of the attachment complex. Intracellular hemidesmosomal proteins include the 230-kD bullous pemphigoid antigen 1 and the 500-kD plectin protein. Transmembranous hemidesmosomal proteins comprise the 180-kD bullous pemphigoid antigen (also known as type XVII collagen), and the α6 and β4 integrin molecules.[6] The hemidesmosomes are associated with anchoring filaments in the lamina lucida, thread-like structures 3–4 nm in diameter that span the lamina lucida to the lamina densa.

Located at the lamina lucida–lamina densa interface are the laminins. The major laminin within the cutaneous BMZ is laminin 332, previously known as laminin 5 (*Fig. 1.78*). In addition, laminin 111 (laminin 1), laminin 311 (laminin 6), laminin 321 (laminin 7) and laminin 511 (laminin 10) are also integral components of the dermal–epidermal junction.[7] The cruciform structure of laminins contains both globular and rodlike segments which contribute to interactions with other extracellular matrix molecules, as well as cell attachment and spreading, and cellular differentiation. The critical role of laminin 332 in providing integrity to the cutaneous BMZ is evident from findings that mutations in any of the three polypeptide subunits (the α3, β3, or γ2 chains) can result in junctional forms of epidermolysis bullosa.

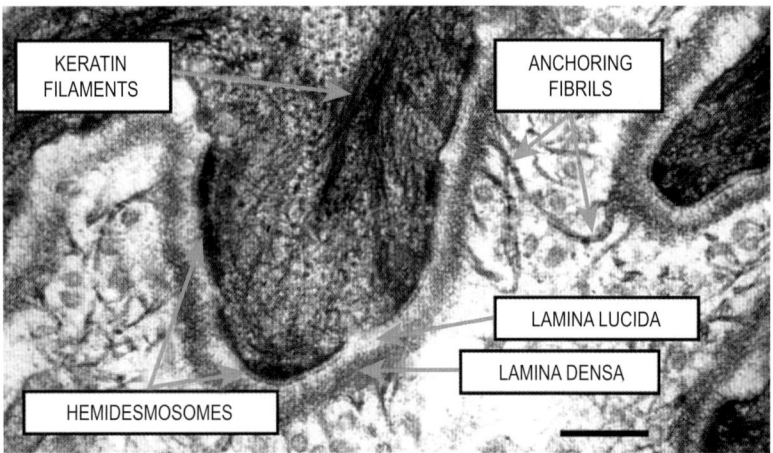

Fig. 1.75
Transmission electron microscopy of the dermal–epidermal junction. Bar = 200 nm.

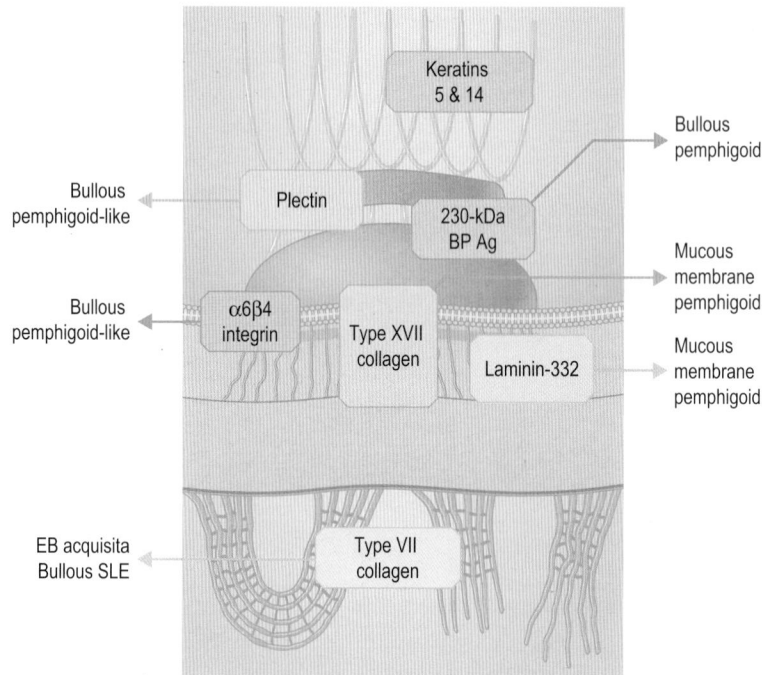

Fig. 1.77
Acquired disorders of hemidesmosomal proteins. Autoantibodies directed against components of the hemidesmosome-anchoring filament-anchoring fibril complex give rise to specific subepidermal autoimmune blistering diseases. *SLE*, systemic lupus erythematosus; *EB*, epidermolysis bullosa.

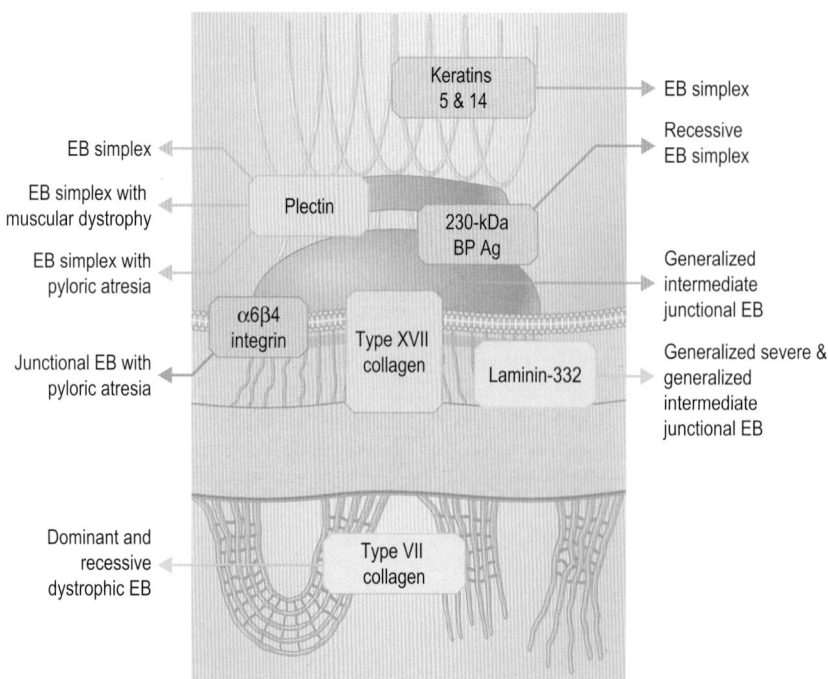

Fig. 1.76
Genetic disorders of hemidesmosomal proteins. Mutations in components of the hemidesmosome-anchoring filament-anchoring fibril network give rise to specific variants of epidermolysis bullosa (EB).

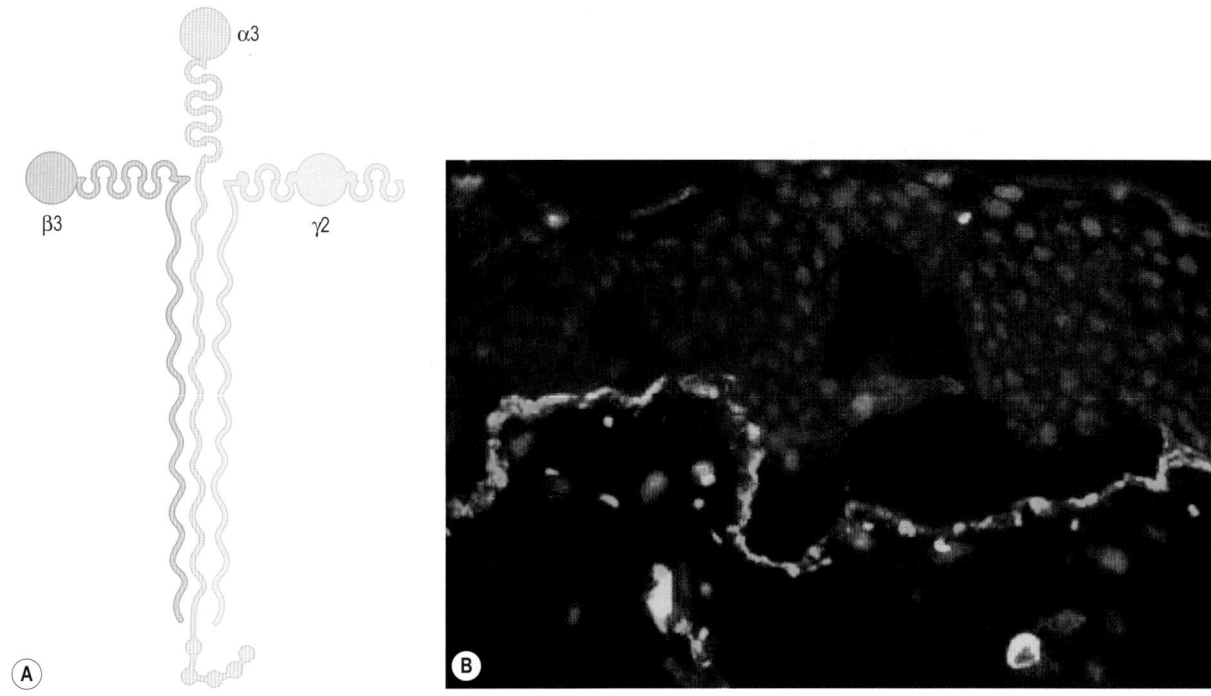

Fig. 1.78
Laminin-332 is a major adhesion protein at the dermal–epidermal junction: (**A**) the protein is composed of three polypeptide chains: α3, β3, and γ2; (**B**) Laminin-322 identified by immunofluorescence in a sample of split skin.

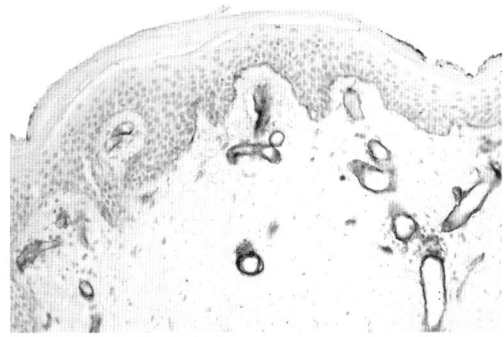

Fig. 1.79
Basement membrane: basement membrane staining with type IV collagen.

The major component of the lamina densa is type IV collagen, which in skin is mainly composed of the α1 and α2 chains.[8] Type IV collagen is assembled to form a complex hexagonal arrangement which allows high flexibility to the BMZ and facilitates interactions with other collagenous and noncollagenous proteins (*Fig. 1.79*). Other BMZ components at the dermal–epidermal junction include the glycoprotein nidogen (previously known as entactin) which interacts with type IV collagen either alone or as part of a laminin-nidogen complex. Also present are the heparan sulfate proteoglycans, which are highly negatively charged and hydrophilic and capable of interacting with a number of basement membrane components and thus contribute to the architectural organization of the BMZ.[9]

Anchoring fibrils are ultrastructurally recognizable fibrillar structures which extend from the lower part of lamina densa to the upper reticular dermis. The main component of anchoring fibrils is type VII collagen (*Fig. 1.80*).[10] Individual type VII collagen molecules are ≈450 nm long and by complexing as antiparallel dimmers and aggregating laterally, they form loops which are traversed by interstitial dermal collagens (mainly types I and III) to adhere the BMZ to the underlying dermis.[11] Type VII collagen is synthesized by both dermal fibroblasts and epidermal keratinocytes. Also inserting into the lamina densa at the dermal–epidermal junction are elastic microfibrils, containing proteins such as fibrillin. Fibrillin-containing

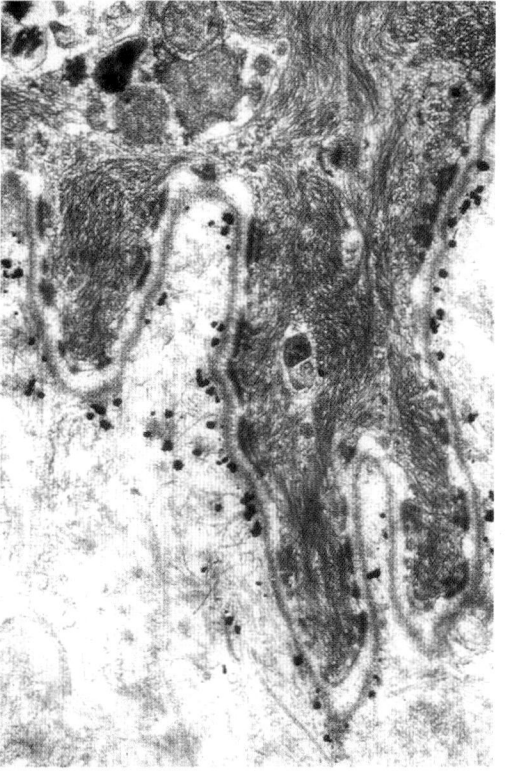

Fig. 1.80
Normal skin: the anchoring fibrils are composed predominantly of type VII collagen as shown in this pre-embedding immunogold electron microscopic preparation.

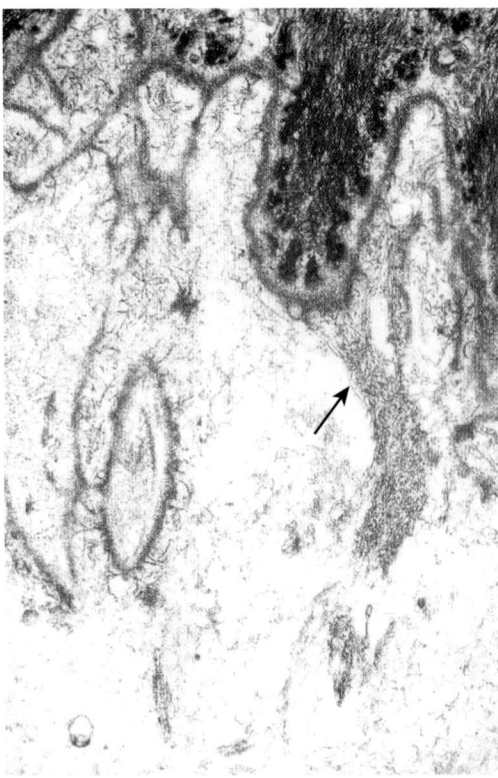

Fig. 1.81
Normal skin: this ultrastructural image shows a well-formed dermal microfibril bundle (*arrowed*).

microfibrils may exist as a fibrillar mantle surrounding an elastin core or be found independently as elastin-free microfibrils. The latter, located beneath the lamina densa, are known as the dermal microfibril bundles (*Fig. 1.81*).

Dermal collagen

The major extracellular matrix component in the dermis is collagen. Currently, 29 distinct collagens have been identified in vertebrate tissues and each is designated a Roman numeral in the chronological order of its discovery. At least eight different collagens are found in human skin. All collagen molecules consist of three subunit polypeptides which can either be identical in homotrimers or can consist of two or even three genetically different polypeptides in heterotrimeric molecules. Since the different subunits are all distinct gene products, there are well over 40 different genes in the human genome that encode the different subunit polypeptides.[1] Collagens demonstrate considerable tissue specificity and are synthesized by a number of different cell types, including dermal fibroblasts, keratinocytes, vascular endothelial cells, and smooth muscle cells. A characteristic feature of collagen is the presence of hydroxyproline and hydroxylysine residues, amino acids that are post-translationally synthesized by hydroxylation of proline and lysine residues, respectively. These hydroxylation reactions take place in the rough endoplasmic reticulum by prolyl and lysyl hydroxylases, respectively, enzymes that require ascorbic acid, molecular oxygen and ferrous iron as cofactors. The hydroxylation of prolyl residues is necessary for stabilization of the triple-helical conformation at physiologic temperatures, and hydroxylysyl residues are required for formation of stable covalent cross-links. In the rough endoplasmic reticulum, trimeric molecules are formed and following the prolyl hydroxylation reactions, triple helices are generated which are then secreted through Golgi vesicles into the extracellular space. Here, parts of the noncollagenous peptide extensions are cleaved by specific proteases, and the collagen molecules undergo supramolecular organization. To acquire fibrillar strength, the fibers are then covalently linked together by specific intra- and intermolecular cross-links. The most common forms of cross-links in type I collagen are derived from lysine and

hydroxylysine residues, and in some collagens there are also cysteine-derived disulfide bonds. On the basis of their fiber architecture in tissues, collagens can be divided into different classes. Types I, II, III, V and IX align into large fibrils and are designated as fibril-forming collagens. Type IV is arranged in an interlacing network within the basement membranes, while type VI is a distinct microfibril-forming collagen and type VII collagen forms anchoring fibrils. Fibril-associated collagen with interrupted triple helix (FACIT) collagens (fibril-associated collagens with interrupted triple-helices), include types IX, XII, XIV, XIX, XX, and XXI.[2] Many of the FACIT collagens associate with larger collagen fibers and act as molecular bridges stabilizing the organization of the extracellular matrices.

Type I collagen, the most abundant form of collagen, is the predominant collagen in human dermis, accounting for approximately 80% of total collagen. Type I collagen associates with type III collagen to form broad, extracellular fibers in the dermis. Mutations in the type I and III collagens or in their processing enzymes can result in connective tissue abnormalities seen in different forms of the Ehlers-Danlos syndrome, and mutations in the type I collagen gene lead to osteogenesis imperfecta.[3]

Type III collagen accounts for about 10% of the total collagen in adult dermis, although it is the predominant dermal collagen in the fetus. It predominates in vascular connective tissues, the gastrointestinal tract, and the uterus, and mutations in the type III collagen gene occur in the vascular type of the Ehlers-Danlos syndrome.

Type V collagen is present in most connective tissues, including the dermis, where it represents less than 5% of the total collagen. Type V collagen is located on the surface of large collagen fibers in the dermis, and its function is to regulate their lateral growth. A lack of type V collagen leads to variable collagen fiber diameters and an irregular fiber contour in cross-section. Such fibers are seen in autosomal dominant forms of Ehlers-Danlos syndrome associated with mutations in the type V collagen gene.

Mature collagen fibers are relatively inert and can exist in tissues under normal physiologic conditions for long periods. However, there is some continuous turnover of collagen that involves a number of enzymes of the matrix metalloproteinases (MMP) family. These proteinase families include the collagenases, gelatinases, stromelysins, matrilysins, and the membrane-type MMPs.[4] The MMPs are synthesized and secreted as inert proenzymes which become activated proteolytically by removal of the propeptide. The MMPs are zinc metalloenzymes and require calcium for their activity. The MMPs also have specific small molecular weight peptide inhibitors, known as tissue inhibitors of metalloproteinases (TIMPs). These proteins stoichiometrically complex with MMPs to prevent collagen degradation. In normal human skin, a number of MMPs are synthesized and secreted by fibroblasts and keratinocytes. The expression of these enzymes is enhanced in various pathologic states, including invasion and metastasis of cutaneous malignancies, as well as during dermal wound healing.

Within the papillary dermis, collagen fibers are fine and often vertically orientated whereas reticular dermal collagen consists of broad, thick bundles generally arranged parallel to the surface epithelium (*Figs 1.82, 1.83*). When longitudinal sections of collagen are examined by transmission electron microscopy they show cross-striations with a periodicity of approximately 64 nm (*Fig. 1.84*). The cross-striations are seen because of the longitudinal overlap of individual collagen molecules, which occurs during assembly of the mature fibril. Fibrous long-spacing collagen is a variant with a periodicity of 90–120 nm (*Fig. 1.85*). It is characteristically seen in peripheral nerve and central nervous system tumors. Collagen bundles exhibit anisotropy and are therefore birefringent when viewed with polarized light (*Fig. 1.86*).

Dermal elastic tissue

The elastic fiber network provides resilience and elasticity to the skin.[1] Elastic fibers are a relatively minor component in normal sun-protected adult skin, comprising less than 2–4% of the total dry weight of the dermis. The configuration of elastic fibers in the reticular dermis consists of horizontally orientated fibers which interconnect (*Fig. 1.87*).[2] Extending from these into the papillary dermis is a network of vertical extensions of relatively fine fibrils which consist either of bundles of microfibrils (oxytalan fibers) or of small amounts of cross-linked elastin (elaunin fibers) (*Fig. 1.88*).[3] Elastic

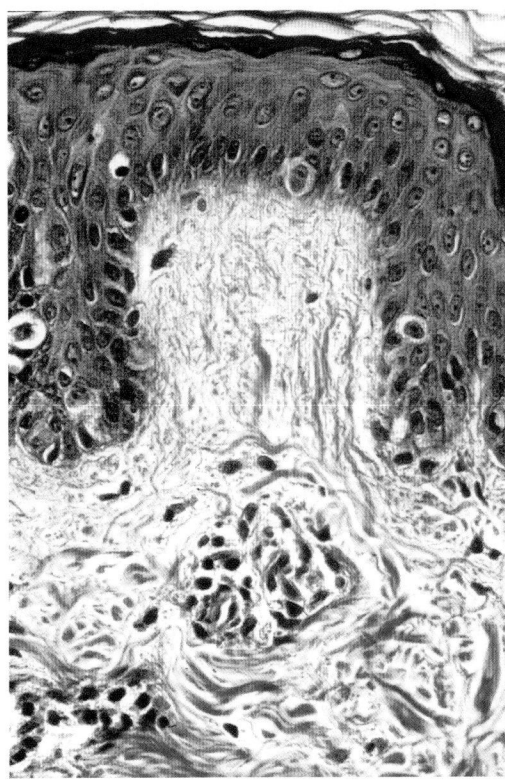

Fig. 1.82
Normal skin of forearm: in the papillary dermis the collagen fibers are fine and sometimes have a vertical orientation. Masson trichrome.

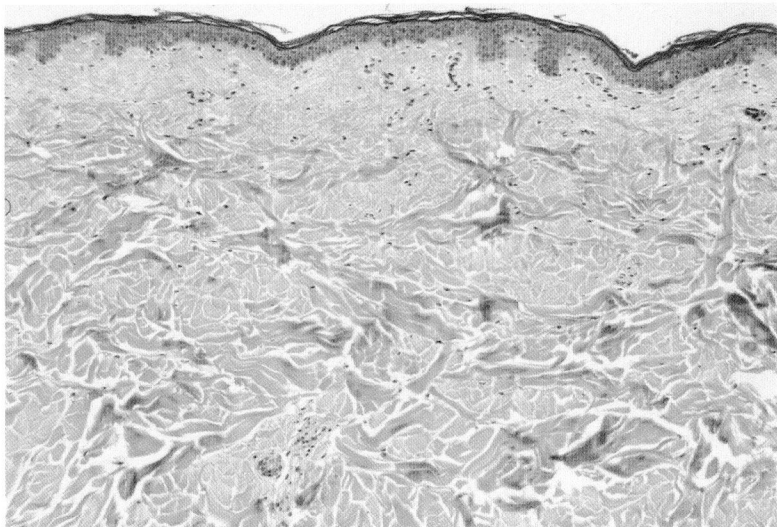

Fig. 1.83
Normal skin of back: broad bundles of collagen typify the reticular dermis. Masson trichrome.

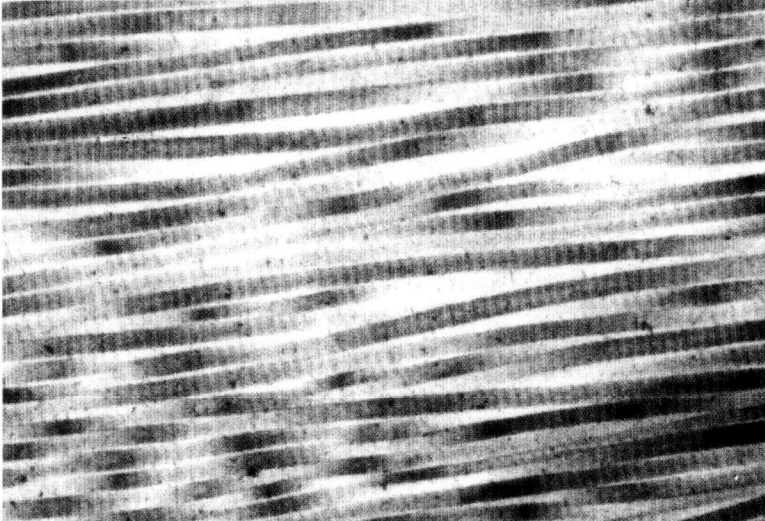

Fig. 1.84
Collagen: it is characterized by cross-striations with a periodicity of 64 nm.

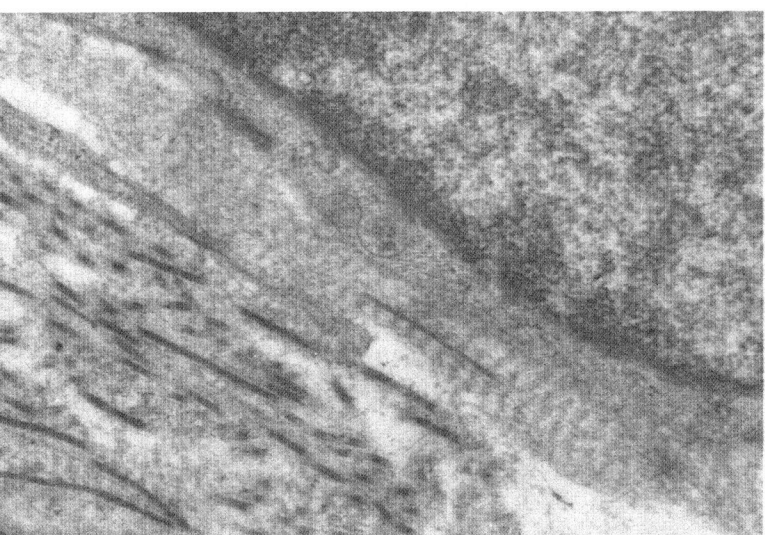

Fig. 1.85
Fibrous long-spacing collagen: compare with the adjacent conventional collagen fibers. There is a very different periodicity.

fibers have two principal components: elastin, which is a connective tissue protein that forms the core of the mature fibers, and the elastin-associated microfibrils which consist of a family of proteins. Examination by transmission electron microscopy reveals an elastin core that makes up over 90% of the elastic fiber and which is surrounded by more electron-dense microfibrillar structures (*Fig. 1.89*).

Elastin is initially synthesized as a precursor polypeptide, tropoelastin, which consists of approximately 700 amino acids with a molecular mass of ≈70 kD.[4] The amino acid composition of tropoelastin is similar to collagen in that about one-third of the total amino residues consist of glycine but the primary sequence is different, with domains rich in glycine, valine, and proline, alternating with lysine- and alanine-rich sequences: a characteristic

sequence motif is the presence of two lysine residues separated by two or three alanine residues. The lysine residues in tropoelastin are critical for the formation of covalent cross-links between desmosine and its isomer, isodesmosine, which appear to be unique to elastin. The first step in formation of these elastin-specific cross-links is oxidative deamination of three lysine residues to formaldehydes, known as allysines. These aldehydes, with additional lysine, fuse to form a stable desmosine compound which covalently links two of the tropoelastin polypeptides. Addition of desmosines to other parts of the molecule progressively converts tropoelastin molecules into an insoluble fiber structure. The oxidative deamination of lysyl residues to corresponding aldehydes is catalyzed by a group of enzymes, lysyl oxidases, which require copper for their activity. Thus, copper deficiency can lead to reduced lysyl oxydase activity and synthesis of elastic fibers that are not stabilized by sufficient amounts of desmosines. In such a situation, the individual tropoelastin polypeptides remain soluble and susceptible to non-specific proteolysis, and the elastin-rich tissues are fragile. The metabolic turnover of elastin is slow, but is increased in some forms of cutis laxa and cutaneous aging. Elastic fibers are degraded by elastases and metalloelastases.

The elastin-associated microfibrils consist of tubular structures of ≈10–12 nm in diameter. These proteins include fibrillin, the latent transforming growth factor (TGF)-β binding family of proteins, and the fibulins. Other components comprise the families of microfibril-associated

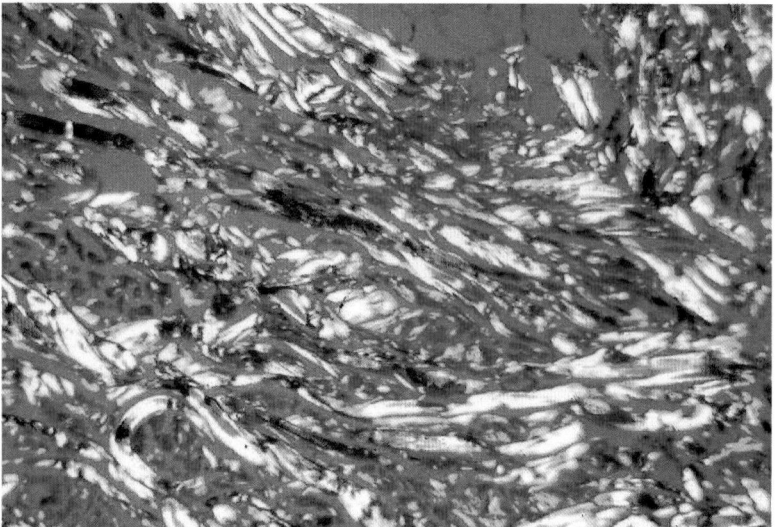

Fig. 1.86
Collagen of the reticular dermis: note the birefringence when viewed with polarized light. Masson trichrome.

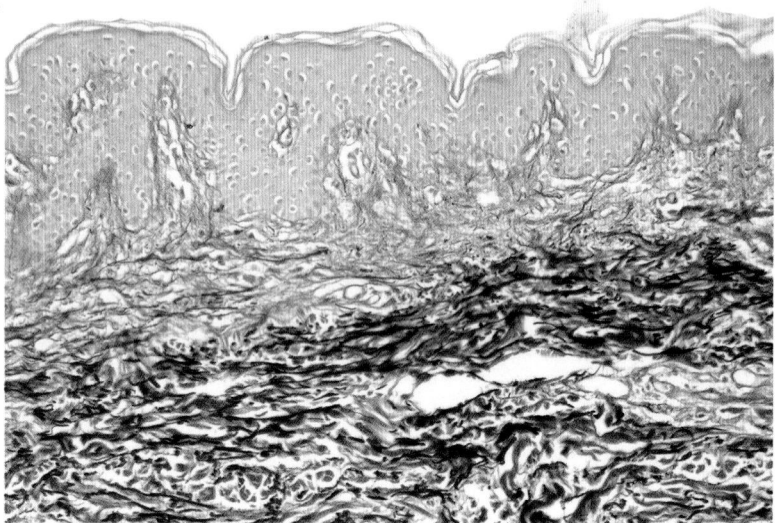

Fig. 1.87
Reticular dermis: the elastic fibers are long and fairly thick and tend to run parallel to the surface epithelium.

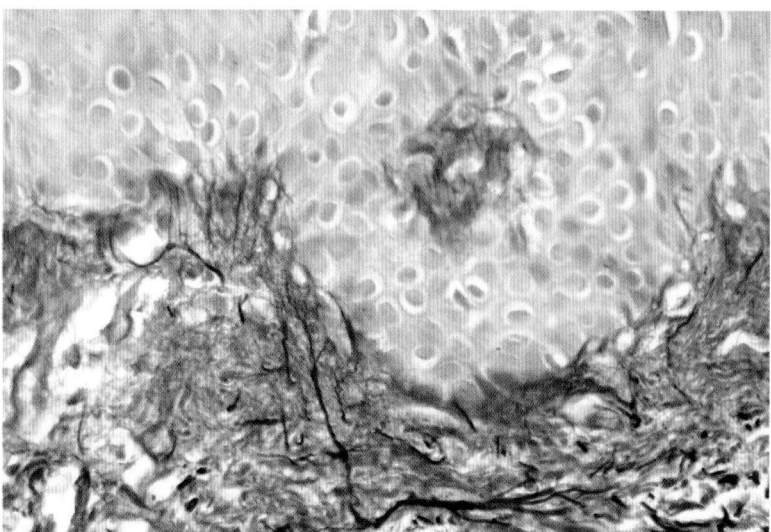

Fig. 1.88
Papillary dermis: the elastic fibers are delicate and orientated perpendicular to the epithelial surface. Weigert–van Gieson stain.

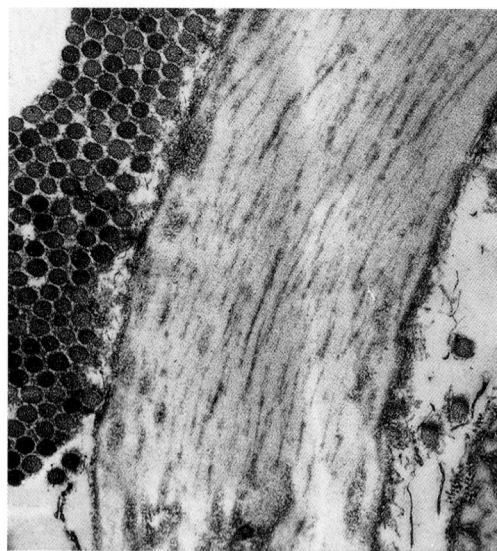

Fig. 1.89
Elastic fiber: this consists of microfibrils embedded in an electron-dense matrix called elastin.

glycoproteins and microfibril-associated proteins (MFAP), the emilins and certain lysyl oxidases. The importance of the fibrillin is illustrated by mutations resulting in Marfan syndrome with skeletal abnormalities, aortic dilatation, subluxation of the ocular lens, and cutaneous hyperextensibility.[5] Likewise, the significance of certain fibulins is evident from mutations resulting in cutis laxa, manifesting with loose and sagging skin and loss of elastic recoil.

Ground substance

Proteoglycans form a number of subfamilies defined by a core protein to which polymers of unbranched disaccharide units, glycosaminoglycans (GAGs), are linked.[1] The core proteins can be intracellular, reside on the cell surface, or be part of the extracellular matrix and the GAGs are highly charged polyanionic molecules that vary greatly in size. For example, dermal fibroblasts can synthesize versican which consists of a core protein with attachment sites for 12 to 15 GAG side chains. The GAGs in versican are primarily chondroitin sulfate or dermatan sulfate, but versican can also bind hyaluronic acid, resulting in formation of large aggregates. Proteoglycan/ GAG complexes have multiple functions. For example, the proteoglycans containing heparan sulfate and dermatan sulfate have the ability to bind extracellular matrix components, including various collagens.[2] In addition, these proteoglycans bind several growth factors, cytokines, cell adhesion molecules, and growth factor binding proteins, thereby influencing the bioactivity of these molecules. They can also serve as antiproteases. In addition to binding to a number of extracellular molecules, proteoglycans also play a role in the adhesion of cells to the extracellular matrix. For example, syndecan-4, which is selectively enriched in dermal fibroblasts, facilitates the adherence of cells in conjunction with other extracellular matrix binding molecules, such as the integrins.[3] Proteoglycans also interact with other extracellular matrix molecules besides collagen; notably, chondroitin sulfate and dermatan sulfate bind fibronectin and laminin. The largest extracellular GAG, hyaluronic acid, plays an important role in providing physical and chemical properties to the skin, mediated in part by its hydrophilicity and viscosity in dilute solutions. Of particular note, hyaluronic acid has an expansive water-binding capacity, providing hydration to normal skin. Indeed, water makes up ≈60% of the weight of normal human skin in vivo. Other properties attributed to large proteoglycans complexes, such as those formed with the versican or basement membrane proteoglycans, include their ability to serve as ionic filters, regulate salt and water balance, and provide an elastic cushion.[1]

Except when present in very large amounts, ground substance cannot be easily detected by routine hematoxylin and eosin staining (*Fig. 1.90*).

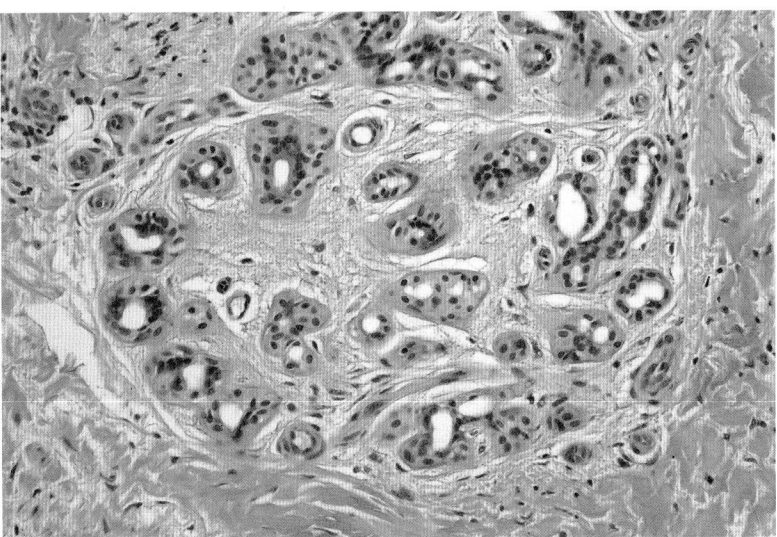

Fig. 1.90
Ground substance: an eccrine gland from the sole of the foot shows an abundance of glycosaminoglycans.

Cationic dyes, such as Alcian blue at appropriate pH and electrolyte concentration, are usually necessary for its demonstration.

Fibroblast biology

The main cell responsible for the synthesis of collagens, elastic tissue and proteoglycan/glycosaminoglycan macromolecules in the dermis is the fibroblast.[1] In the mid-dermis of postnatal skin, the number of fibroblasts ranges from 2100 to 4100 per mm³, and the cells have a limited replicative capacity ranging from 50–100 cell divisions. Fibroblasts also play a significant role in epithelial–mesenchymal interactions, secreting various growth factors and cytokines that have a direct effect on epidermal proliferation, differentiation and formation of extracellular matrix. The term fibroblast refers to a fully differentiated, biosynthetically active cell, while the term fibrocyte refers to an inactive cell.

Myofibroblasts are a specialized form of fibroblast found in granulation tissue and are involved in wound contraction. They are functionally distinct from other fibroblasts with ultrastructural, biochemical and physical features of smooth muscle cells. Moreover, myofibroblasts are characterized by the presence of intracellular bundles of α smooth muscle actin, which is the actin isoform expressed by smooth muscle cells. Currently it is thought that the evolution of myofibroblasts involves a preceding form known as the protomyofibroblast, although the latter do not always become the fully differentiated myofibroblast. In contrast to myofibroblasts, protomyofibroblasts have stress fibers but no α smooth muscle actin filaments. A biosynthetically active fibroblast has an abundant cytoplasm, well-developed rough endoplasmic reticulum, and prominent ribosomes attached to the membrane surfaces.

Fibroblasts from different anatomical sites all have similar morphology but fibroblasts in different sites have their own gene-expression profiles and characteristic phenotypes, synthesizing extracellular matrix proteins and cytokines in a site-specific manner.[2] Moreover, embryologically fibroblasts in the papillary dermis appear to be distinct from those in the reticular dermis.[3] The former contribute to hair follicle growth, whereas the latter have more prominent roles in formation of adipocytes and in wound healing.

Dermal fibroblasts have numerous functions, not only in synthesizing and depositing extracellular matrix components, but also in proliferation and migration in response to chemotactic, mitogenic and modulatory cytokines, and also autocrine and paracrine interactions. Autocrine activity includes the TGF-β-induced synthesis and secretion of connective tissue growth factor which promotes collagen synthesis as well as fibroblast proliferation. Paracrine activity affects keratinocyte growth and differentiation, specifically through fibroblast secretion of keratinocyte growth factor (KGF), granulocyte-macrophage colony-stimulating factor (GM-CSF), interleukin (IL)-6 and fibroblast growth factor (FGF)-10. Fibroblasts also contribute to basement membrane formation partly by producing type IV collagen, type VII collagen, laminins and nidogen, but also through the secretion of cytokines, such as TGF-β, that stimulate keratinocytes to produce basement membrane components.

Neovascularization and lymphangiogenesis are also important processes for the maintenance of normal skin homeostasis and wound healing, for which fibroblasts have an important paracrine role. Members of the vascular endothelial growth factor (VEGF) family include VEGF-A, -B, -C, and -D, which are produced by normal human fibroblasts and are important in regulating vascular and lymphatic endothelial cell proliferation through specific receptors.

There is, however, considerable heterogeneity within fibroblast populations. For example, fibroblasts isolated from the papillary dermis compared to the reticular dermis have higher rate of synthesis of type III collagen and there can be as much as 30-fold differences in the level of fibronectin expression within individual cells. Fibroblasts from the papillary dermis appear smaller, grow faster and have a longer replicative lifespan.[4] When co-cultured with keratinocytes, papillary dermal fibroblasts produce a more differentiated and organized epidermis with complete formation of the dermal–epidermal junction. Papillary dermal fibroblasts also produce more GM-CSF and relatively less KGF than reticular dermal fibroblasts. In addition, there are differences in the synthesis of some extracellular matrix components, such as decorin. While fibroblasts demonstrate certain variability in their gene expression profiles they are considered fully differentiated cells with relatively little plasticity. Recent observations, however, suggest that fibroblasts can be induced to become pluripotent stem cells (iPS), essentially indistinguishable from the embryonic stem cells, by transduction of cultured fibroblasts with four transcription factors, Oct4, Sox2, Klf4, and c-myc.[5]

Cutaneous blood vessels and lymphatics

The skin receives a rich blood supply from perforating vessels within the skeletal muscle and subcutaneous fat.[1] Most of the blood flow is directed toward the more metabolically active constituents of the skin, namely the epidermis, hair papillae and the adnexal structures. While the dermal papillae are richly vascularized, no capillaries actually enter the epidermis, which receives its nutrition by diffusion. The subcutaneous vessels give rise to two vascular plexuses linked by intercommunicating vessels: the deep vascular plexus lies in the region of the interface between the dermis and subcutaneous fat, and the superficial vascular plexus lies in the superficial aspects of the reticular dermis and supplies the papillary dermis with a candelabra-like capillary loop system (*Fig. 1.91*). Each loop consists of an ascending arterial limb and a descending venous limb. The vessels of the dermal papillae comprise terminal arterioles, arterial and venous capillaries, and postcapillary venules, with the last predominating. Within the deep vascular plexus are small muscular arteries, which give rise to the arterioles that supply the superficial vascular plexus (*Fig. 1.92*).

The histology of these plexuses is similar, the difference being one of size rather than structure (arterioles have a diameter of less than 0.3 mm).[2] From the lumen outwards the arteriole consists of a very thin intima resting against a conspicuous internal elastic lamina. Next to this is the media, consisting of two layers of smooth muscle, which constitutes the bulk of the vessel. The adventitia surrounding the media is composed of loose connective tissue. In small muscular arteries (but not arterioles), the adventitia often contains elastic fibers constituting the external elastic lamina. Small arterioles have an endothelium surrounded by a single layer of smooth muscle. Capillaries consist of a single layer of endothelial cells, but may have adjacent pericytes, which have less well-developed dense bodies and fewer filaments than smooth muscle cells. Endothelial cells and pericytes form tight junctions. Venous capillaries have numerous pericytes and a multilayered basement membrane in contrast to arterial vessels where the basement membrane is solitary and homogeneous. Each dermal papilla is supplied by a single capillary loop. Endothelial cells contain vimentin filaments,

Weibel-Palade bodies measuring approximately 0.1 × 3.0 μm (containing factor VIII) and numerous pinocytotic vesicles (*Figs 1.93, 1.94*). Postcapillary venules are larger, but have the same basic structure as capillaries. Their wall is devoid of smooth muscle. The small muscular venules into which the postcapillary venules drain have an intima made up of flattened endothelial cells surrounded by a smooth muscle layer one or two cells thick. They are therefore similar to small arterioles, but with much wider lumina. Veins are composed of an endothelium surrounded by a muscle coat several layers thick. Typically, an internal elastic lamina is poorly represented. There is usually a thick connective tissue adventitia, but elastic fibers are absent; only very large muscular veins have elastic tissue (*Fig. 1.95*).

Also present in the dermis are veil cells, which surround all the microvessels and separate them from the adjacent connective tissue. Veil cells are long, thin cells with an attenuated cytoplasm, and they more closely resemble fibroblasts than pericytes. They do not have a basement membrane investment and are located outside the vessel wall.

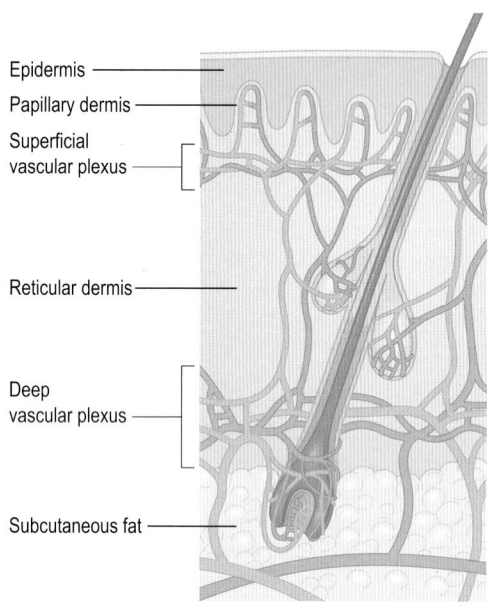

Fig. 1.91
Relationship of the superficial and deep vascular plexuses.

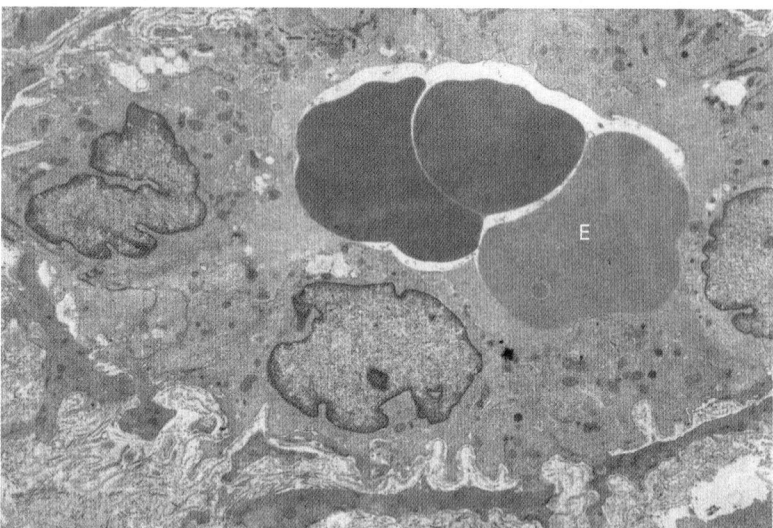

Fig. 1.93
Normal dermal capillary: note the lining of endothelial cells surrounded by a pericyte cell process and adjacent basal lamina. The lumen contains erythrocytes (*E*).

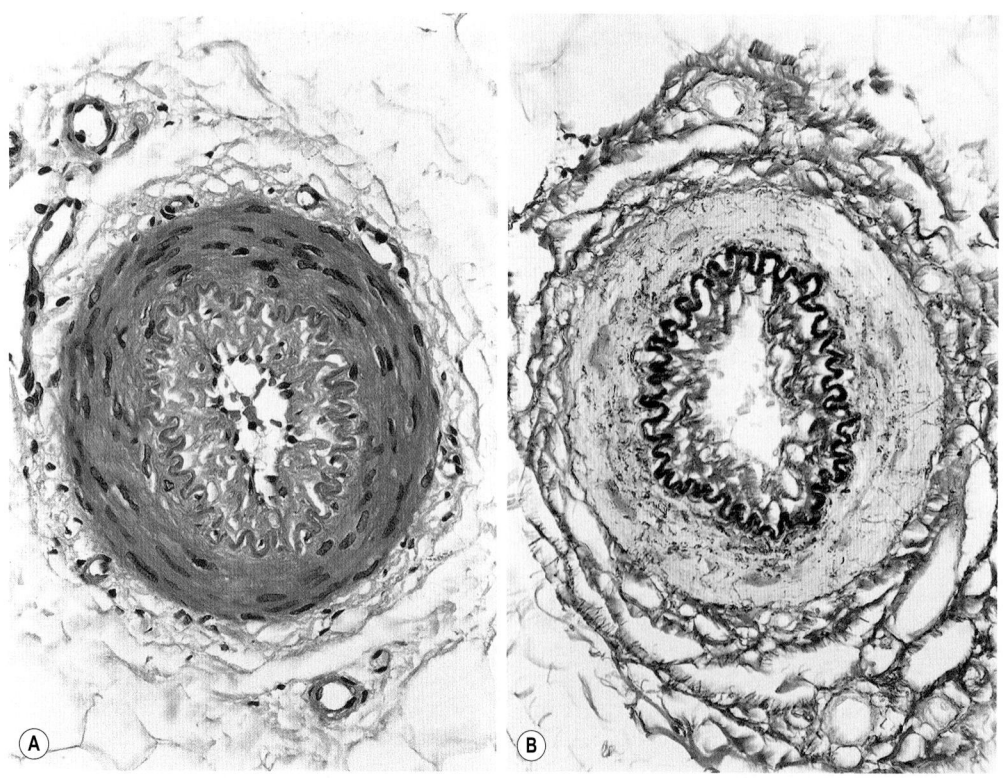

Fig. 1.92
Small muscular artery from the deep vascular plexus from the lower leg of an elderly man with endarteritis (intimal thickening): note the thick muscle coat and conspicuous internal elastic lamina, the latter accentuated by the Weigert–van Gieson reaction. (**A**) Hematoxylin and eosin; (**B**) Weigert–van Gieson.

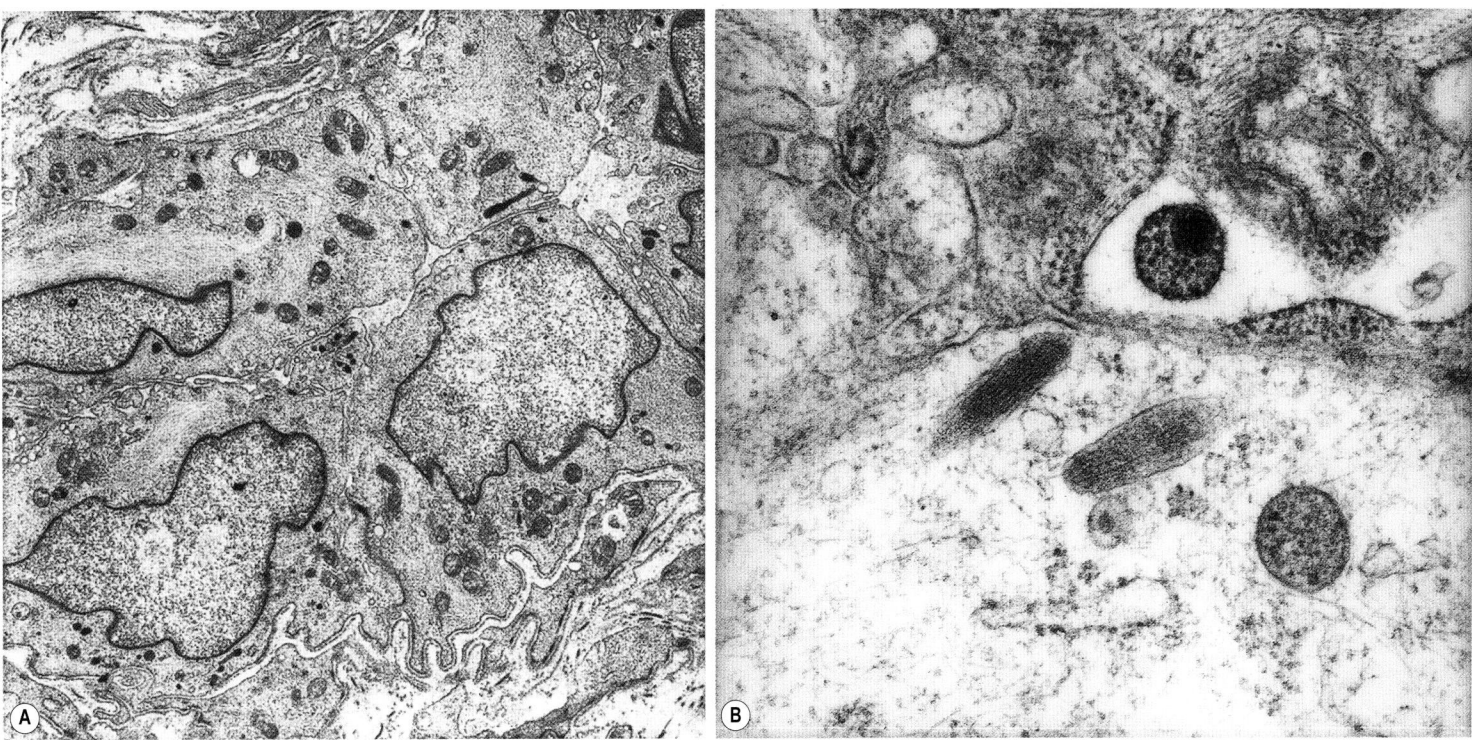

Fig. 1.94
(**A**) Small dermal arteriole: the lumen is compressed to a narrow slitlike space; (**B**) high-power view of typical Weibel-Palade bodies. These are characteristic of blood vessel endothelium.

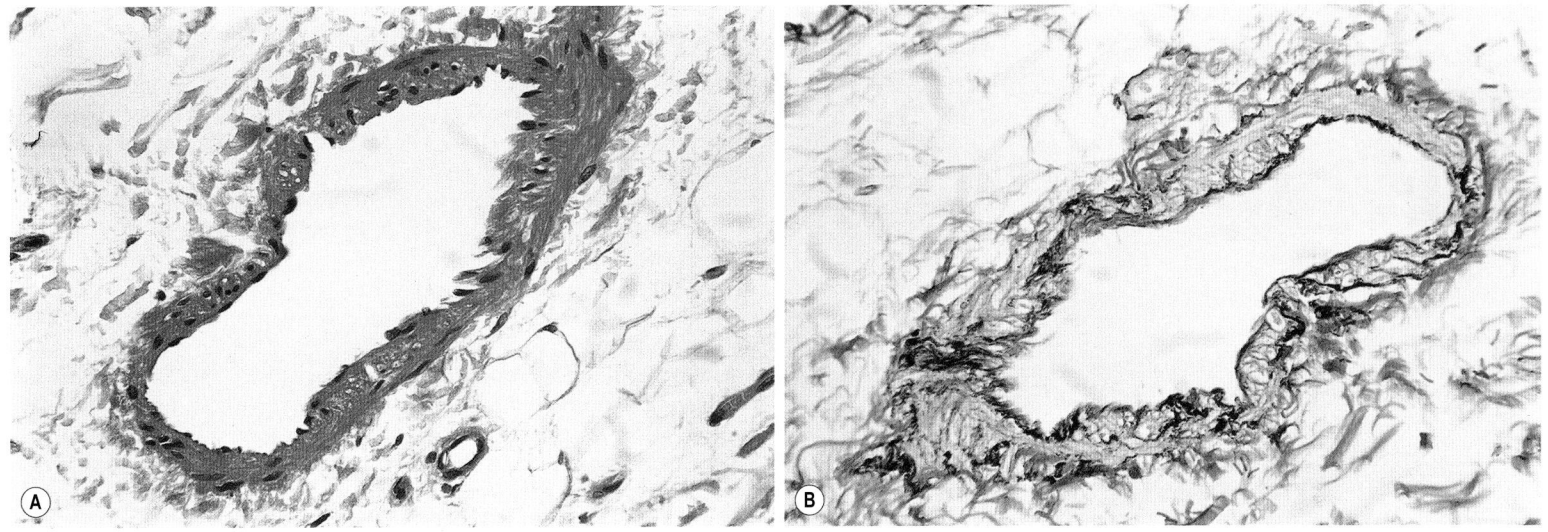

Fig. 1.95
Companion vein to *Fig. 1.92*: note the wide diameter of the lumen in comparison to the relatively thin muscle coat. There is a little elastic tissue but no discernible internal elastic lamina. (**A**) Hematoxylin and eosin; (**B**) Weigert–van Gieson.

The capillary loop in the dermal papilla has an ascending arterial component and an intrapapillary segment, which is characterized by a hairpin turn and a descending venous capillary segment. Capillary loops run perpendicular to the skin surface, except in the nail where they have a parallel orientation.

The dermis is richly supplied with arteriovenous anastomoses. Specialized shunts (glomus bodies), found primarily in the dermis of the fingertips, consist of an arterial segment (Sucquet-Hoyer canal), which connects directly to the venous limb (*Fig. 1.96*). The canal is surrounded by several layers of modified smooth muscle cells (glomus cells) with a particularly rich nerve supply. Glomus bodies function as sphincters, allowing the capillaries of the superficial dermis to be bypassed, therefore increasing the venous return from the extremities.

Cutaneous blood flow (under hypothalamic control) is of extreme importance in thermoregulation. Mediated by the autonomic nervous system, heat loss can be increased or decreased by varying the blood flow to the superficial vascular plexuses. If the environmental temperature exceeds that of the body, then the blood flow to the papillary dermis increases. A concomitant increase in eccrine sweat gland secretion, evaporation of which cools the outer parts of the body, lowers the temperature of the circulating blood and maintains a stable core temperature. Temperature control therefore depends on a delicate interplay between both vascular and sweat gland functions.

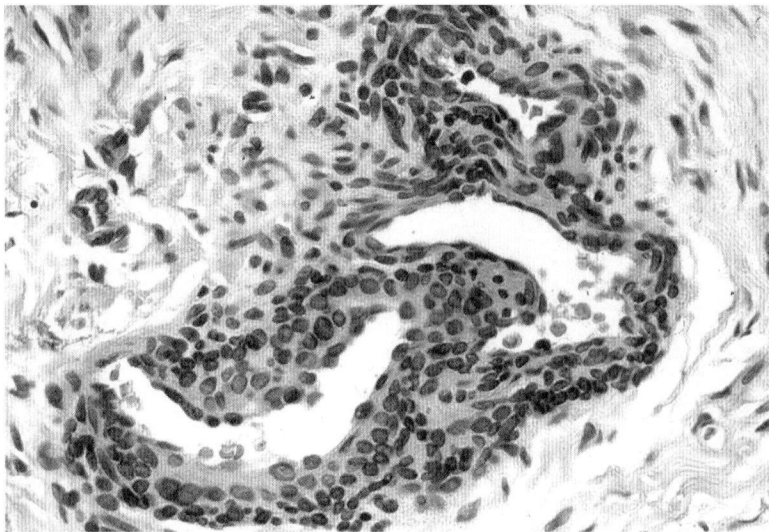

Fig. 1.96
Glomus body: note the arterial and venous limbs connected by a vascular channel rich in glomus cells.

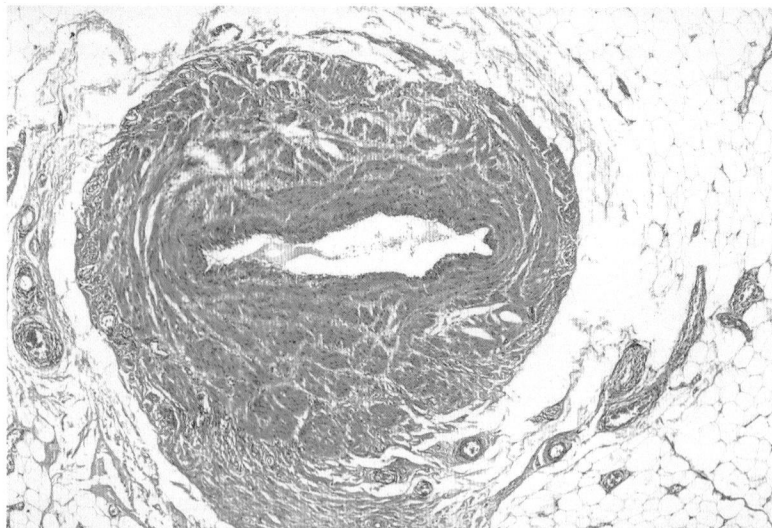

Fig. 1.98
Skin of lower leg: muscular lymphatic trunks can be readily mistaken for arteries. An internal elastic lamina is characteristically absent.

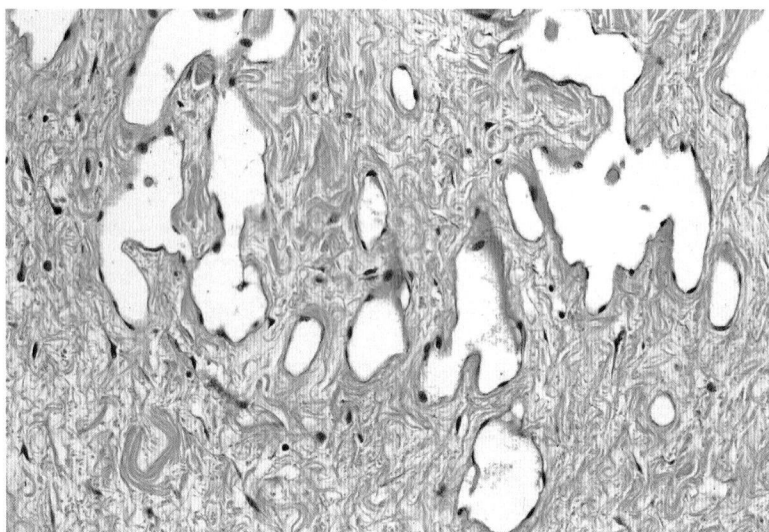

Fig. 1.97
Lymphatics: these exceedingly thin-walled channels are normally not visible in the dermis. They become readily apparent, however, when obstructed, as in this patient with lymphedema.

The dermis also contains an extensive lymphatic system, which is closely associated with the vascular plexuses.[3] Although largely disregarded except for their role in tumor spread, lymphatics are of major importance in removing the debris of daily wear and tear including fluid, cells and macromolecules (*Fig. 1.97*). They also represent the primary disposal mechanism for contaminating microorganisms. Lymphatics have been shown to supply the major route for epidermal Langerhans cells to reach the regional lymph node following antigen stimulation. Under normal circumstances these delicate vessels are collapsed and are difficult to detect. They are supported by delicate elastic tissue scaffolding and consist of a large thin-walled collapsed vessel lined by attenuated endothelium and characterized by the presence of multiple valves. Their presence is much more obvious in obstructive situations (e.g., lymphedema or due to the presence of metastases). Dermal lymphatics are loosely aggregated into a superficial and deep plexus, which drain into muscularized lymphatic trunks.[4] In the lower limbs the lymphatic trunks are very thick and muscular and can be confused with an artery (*Fig. 1.98*). The absence of an internal elastic lamina readily allows their distinction. Vascular endothelial cells may be identified by the monoclonal

antibodies CD31 and avian v-ets erythroblastosis virus E26 oncogene homolog (ERG) or by an anti-von Willebrand factor antibody. Lymphatic vessel endothelial hyaluronan receptor 1 (LYVE-1), Prox-1 and podoplanin may be useful immunohistochemical markers.[5] Recent genetic insights have demonstrated that lymphatic dysfunction is not a passive bystander in disease but in fact actively contributes to the pathophysiology of infection and immunity, malignancy, obesity and cardiovascular disease.[6]

Nervous system of the skin

The skin may be innervated with around one million afferent nerve fibers. Most terminate in the face and extremities; relatively few supply the back. The cutaneous nerves contain axons with cell bodies in the dorsal root ganglia. Their diameters range from 0.2 to 20.0 μm. The main nerve trunks entering the subdermal fatty tissue each divide into smaller bundles. Groups of myelinated fibers fan out in a horizontal plane to form a branching network from which fibers ascend, usually accompanying blood vessels, to form a web of interlacing nerves in the superficial dermis. The cutaneous nerves supply the skin appendages and form prominent plexuses around the hair bulbs and the papillary dermis. The afferent receptors consist of free nerve endings, nerve endings in relation to hair, and encapsulated nerve endings. Free nerve endings, of both myelinated and nonmyelinated types and with a low conduction speed, are mainly responsible for the appreciation of temperature, itch and pain. Hair follicles are supplied by an intricate network of myelinated fibers, some of which ramify as free nerve endings in the periadnexal fibrous tissue sheath, while others enter the epidermis to terminate as expansions in intimate association with Merkel cells in the external root sheath. The hair disc is a complex structure consisting of basally situated Merkel cells and an associated myelinated peripheral nerve fiber. Despite the name, it has an inconstant association with hair follicles. Hair discs are slowly adapting mechanoreceptors. Throughout their course the axons of cutaneous nerves are enveloped in Schwann cells but, as they track peripherally, an increasing number lack myelin sheaths. Most end in the dermis; some penetrate the basement membrane, but do not travel far into the epidermis.

Sensory endings are of two main kinds: corpuscular, which embrace non-nervous elements; and 'free', which do not. Corpuscular endings can, in turn, be subdivided into encapsulated receptors, of which a range occurs in the dermis, and nonencapsulated, exemplified by the Merkel 'touch spot', which is epidermal.

The most striking of the encapsulated receptors is the Pacinian corpuscle. It is an ovoid structure about 1 mm in length, which is lamellated in cross-section like an onion, and is innervated by a myelinated sensory axon,

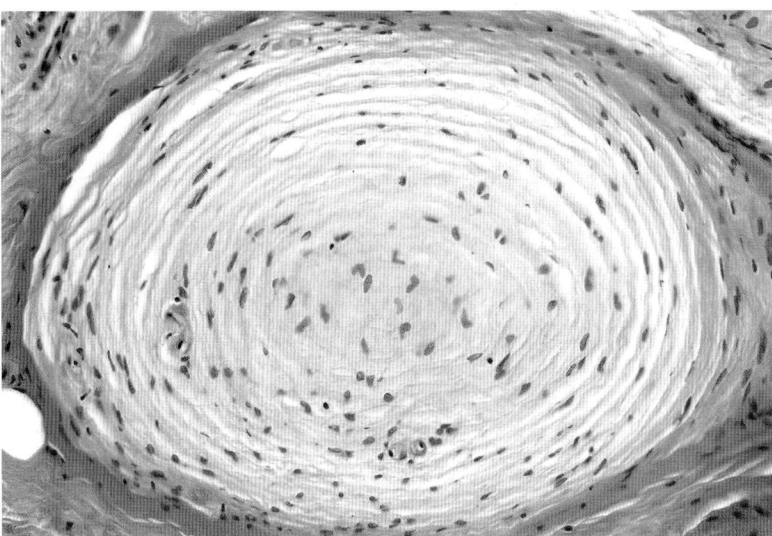

Fig. 1.99
Pacinian corpuscle: note the characteristic lamellar internal structure.

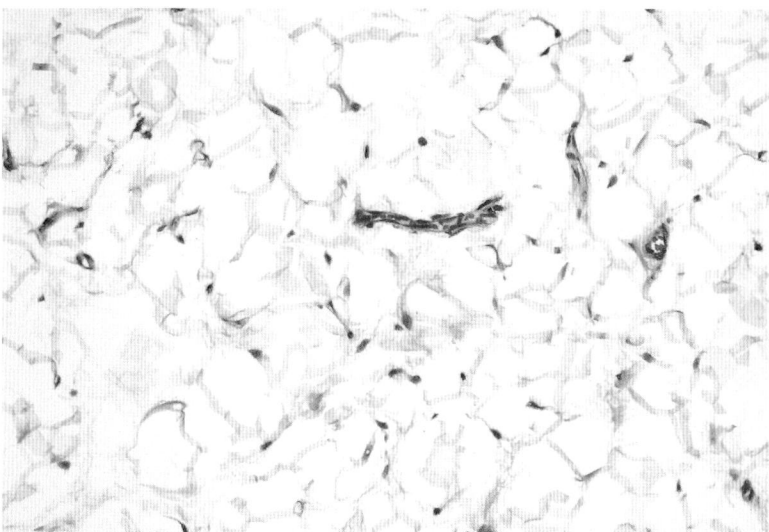

Fig. 1.101
The lipid contents of fat cells are dissolved during processing using conventional (paraffin-embedding) techniques. The cells therefore appear empty and have peripheral compressed nuclei.

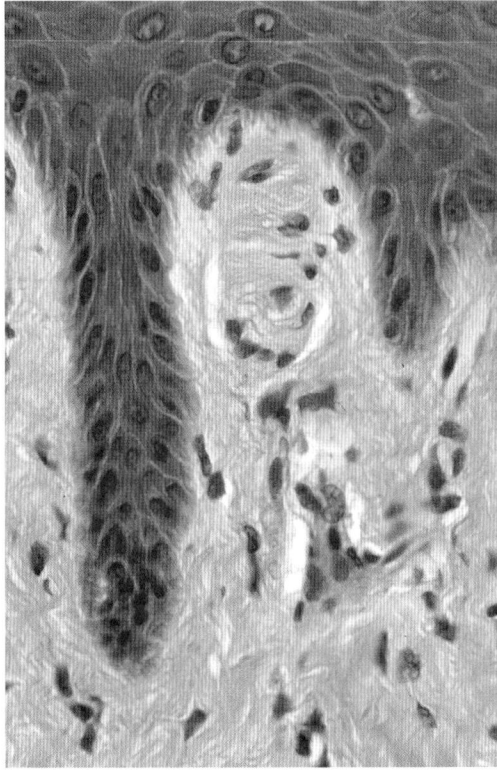

Fig. 1.100
Meissner corpuscle within a dermal papilla: with hematoxylin and eosin staining it appears as perpendicularly orientated lamellae of Schwann cells.

which loses its sheath as it traverses the core (*Fig. 1.99*). Pacinian corpuscles are responsible for the appreciation of deep pressure and vibration and are found predominantly in the subcutaneous fat of the palms and soles, dorsal surfaces of the digits, around the genitalia, and in ligaments and joint capsules.

The Golgi-Mazzoni corpuscle found in the subcutaneous tissue of the human finger is similarly laminate but of much simpler organization. Another classical receptor is the Krause end bulb, an encapsulated swelling on myelinated fibers situated in the superficial layers of the dermis.

Meissner corpuscles are characteristic of the papillary ridges of glabrous skin in primates. They have a thick, lamellated capsule, 20–40 μm in diameter and up to 150 μm long (*Fig. 1.100*).[1] Meissner corpuscles are

involved in the appreciation of touch sensation (rapidly adapting mechanoreceptors) and are found predominantly in the dermal papillae of the hands and feet, the lips, and on the front of the forearm. They comprise a perineural-derived lamellated capsule surrounding a core of cells and nerve fibers, and are supplied by myelinated and nonmyelinated nerve fibers. They make intimate contact with the basal keratinocytes. Meissner corpuscles have a multiple nerve supply and each nerve may also supply multiple corpuscles. Of somewhat different structure are the terminals first described by Ruffini in human digits, in which several expanded endings branch from a single, myelinated afferent fiber. The endings are directly related to collagen fibrils. 'Free nerve-endings', which appear to be derived from nonmyelinated fibers, occur in the superficial dermis and in the overlying epidermis.[2] Those in the dermis are arranged in a tuftlike manner and have thus been designated penicillate nerve endings.

Subcutaneous fat

Fat is a major component of the human body. In nonobese males, 10–12% of body weight is fat, while in females the figure is 15–20%. Eighty percent of fat is under the skin; the rest surrounds internal organs. Fat comprises white and brown adipose tissue, the latter being more common in infants and children and is characterized by different mitochondrial properties and increased heat production.[1] Historically, fat has been thought to provide insulation, mechanical cushioning and an energy store but recent data suggest that it also has an endocrine function, communicating with the brain via secreted molecules such as leptin to alter energy turnover in the body.[2] Adipocytes also have important signaling roles in osteogenesis and angiogenesis. Indeed, multipotent stem cells have been identified in human fat which are capable of developing into adipocytes, osteoblasts, myoblasts and chondroblasts. Biological clues to genes, proteins, hormones and other molecules that influence fat deposition and distribution are gradually being realized, from both research on rare inherited disorders (such as the lipodystrophies or obesity syndromes) as well as population studies on more common forms of obesity.[3]

The subcutaneous fat is divided into lobules by vascular fibrous septa, and its cells are characterized by the presence of a large single globule of lipid, which compresses the cytoplasm and nucleus against the plasma membrane (*Fig. 1.101*). The adipocyte is large, measuring up to 100 μm in diameter. The cytoplasm contains numerous mitochondria. Smooth endoplasmic reticulum is prominent and a Golgi is often conspicuous. Processing

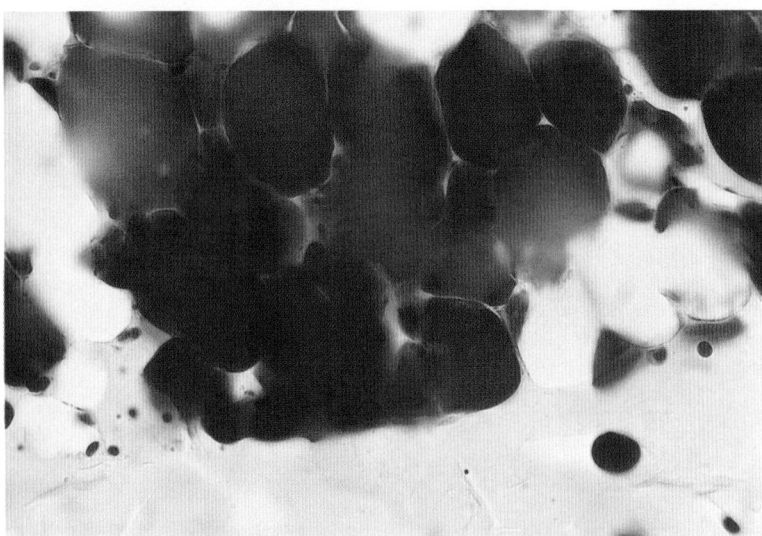

Fig. 1.102
Adult fat in frozen section stained by the Sudan IV technique.

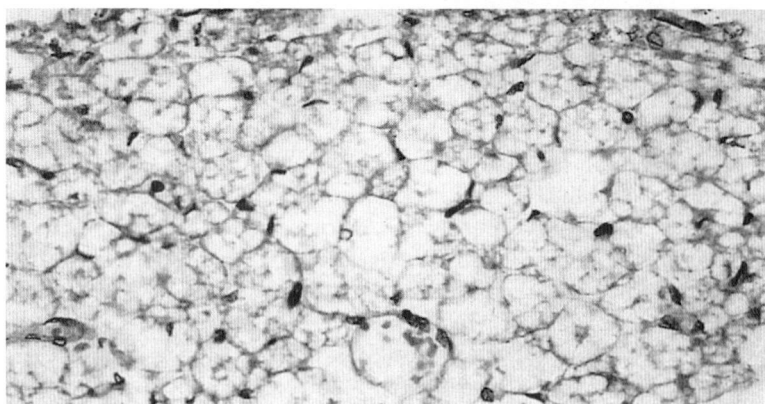

Fig. 1.103
Typical brown fat showing pink granular cytoplasm.

for routine histologic preparation dissolves the lipid, but the use of special stains on frozen sections will reveal its presence (*Fig. 1.102*). The subcutaneous fat may contain large numbers of mast cells.

Deposits of brown fat may be seen in the newborn and occasionally in adults, particularly in the interscapular region, the back, thorax and mediastinum. The brown coloration is due to the high cytochrome content. The brown fat cytoplasm contains numerous, somewhat pleomorphic, mitochondria. Endoplasmic reticulum and a Golgi apparatus are not usually visible. The adipocytes have a bubbly appearance with the nucleus located towards the center of the cell (*Fig. 1.103*).

Access **ExpertConsult.com** for the complete list of references

Specialized techniques in dermatopathology

CHAPTER

2

*Pratistadevi K. Ramdial, Boris C. Bastian, Jeffrey P. North, John Goodlad,
John A. McGrath and Alexander J. Lazar*

Specimen fixation, grossing/put-through, processing, embedding and sectioning

The aim of fixation is to maintain clear and consistent lesional features and to preserve tissue in an optimal state suitable for a range of staining and ancillary histopathological techniques.[1,2] Most fixation methods employed during tissue processing depend on chemical fixation of tissue in liquid reagents.[3] Tissue fixation may also be accomplished by physical (heat, microwave, freeze-drying, and freeze substitution) and/or chemical (coagulant and cross-linking) methods.[4] The most commonly used fixative is 10% neutral-buffered formalin solution with a pH between 7.2–7.4. It prevents the formation of formalin pigment in tissue sections. The quality of fixation is affected by:

- the size of the specimen,
- duration and temperature of fixation,
- pH,
- concentration,
- osmolality,
- ionic composition of fixatives and additives contained in the fixative.[5]

Formalin fixation occurs at an approximate rate of 1 mm per hour.[4,6,7] The volume of the fixative should ideally be at least 10 times the volume of the specimen.[7] Large specimens, such as tumors, may require sectioning into 5-mm thick slices, covering with fixative-soaked gauze or cloth and fixation overnight.[5,7]

Diagnostic dermatological biopsies may be:

- small incisional (shave, core, punch),
- excisional specimens.[8]

Prior to put-through, excisional specimens that require an appraisal of margins should be inked. If localization sutures have been inserted by surgeons then four-quadrant, four-color painting or two-color painted halves (*Fig. 2.1*) is usually appropriate. Shave biopsies are used to sample or remove lesions and, if of appropriate size, may be divided into sections, bisected or trisected and embedded on edge. Edge embedding is critical in a shave excision of a lesion such as a small melanoma so that both the width and depth of invasion can be quantified.[8,9] The main purpose of core or punch biopsies, which generally measure 2–8 mm in diameter, is for diagnostic sampling of larger lesions. Biopsies larger than 4 mm in size should be bisected and the specimens embedded with the cut surfaces down. The bisectioning and embedding cut surface down ensures that the lesion is not missed. Biopsies less than 4 mm are put through *in toto*.[9,10]

Tissue processing refers to a series of steps that effect the removal of extractable water from biopsies to ensure sections of optimal diagnostic quality.[9] These include fixation, dehydration, clearing, infiltration, and embedding in a support matrix. Use of manual and automated tissue processing achieves this goal, including:

- carousel-type processors,
- self-contained vacuum infiltration tissue processors (*Fig. 2.2*),
- microwave tissue processing.

In most laboratories, overnight processing runs are the norm.[9] However, microwave-assisted tissue processing facilitates shorter processing times of 1–2 hours. Dehydrating reagents promote the removal of unbound water and aqueous fixatives from the tissue. Clearing reagents serve as an intermediary between the dehydrating and infiltrating solutions, being miscible with both. Paraffin is the most popular infiltration and embedding medium, being suitable for the majority of routine and special stains. The important principle to be adhered to during embedding of skin biopsies is that the orientation of the skin sample should offer the least resistance to the blade during microtomy (*Fig. 2.3*). Skin biopsies are usually cut in a plane at right angles to the epidermis so as to minimize its compression and distortion.

Suboptimally processed tissue may result in incomplete tissue sections and expansion or disintegration of sections in the water bath. Incorrectly embedded tissue may result in poorly orientated incomplete sections. Faulty microtome mechanisms; loose, dull, or damaged blades; and inaccurate clearance angles may be the causes for:

- thick and thin sections,
- folds (*Fig. 2.4*),
- holes (*Fig. 2.5*),
- scores (*Fig. 2.6*),
- chatter.[10]

The presence of calcified areas and suture in skin tissue and nicks in the blade may result in chatter or splitting of sections at right angles to the knife edge.

Routine and 'special' stains

With the advent of immunohistochemistry, special stains are less commonly employed, but can still play an important role in highlighting certain tissue characteristics or for detection of infectious organisms.

Diagnostic sections are usually stained with hematoxylin and eosin (H&E), the most widely used routine stain.[1] The hematoxylin component

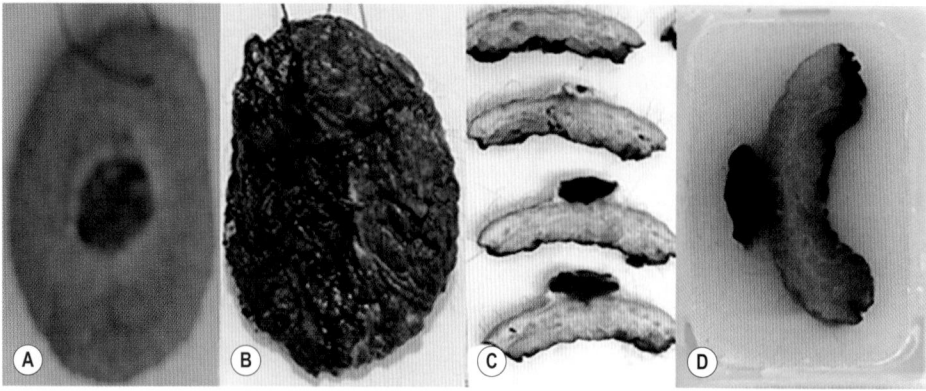

Fig. 2.1
Gross representation of pyogenic granuloma (**A**), with two-color painting of the inferior surface (**B**). 2-mm–thick gross sections demonstrating the black and blue painting at put-through (**C**) and in paraffin blocks (**D**). By courtesy of K. Nargan and K. Lumamba, Africa Health Research Institute, Durban, South Africa.

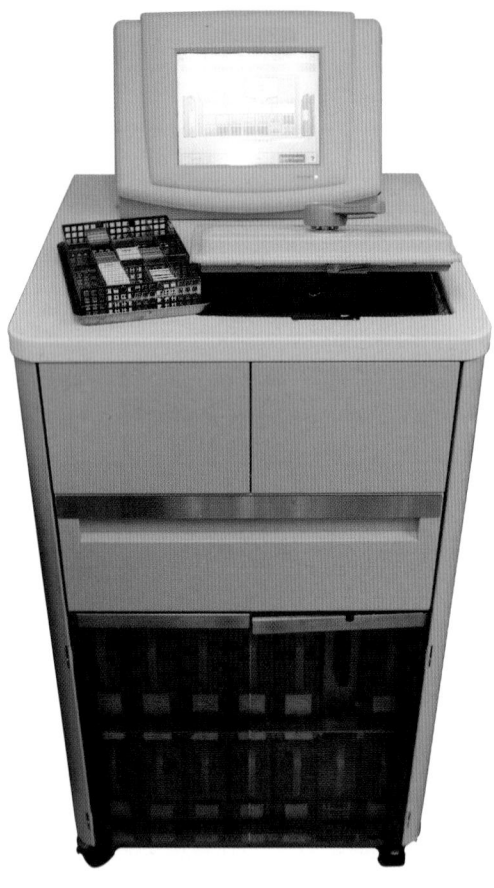

Fig. 2.2
A self-contained vacuum infiltration tissue processor of fluid-transfer type.

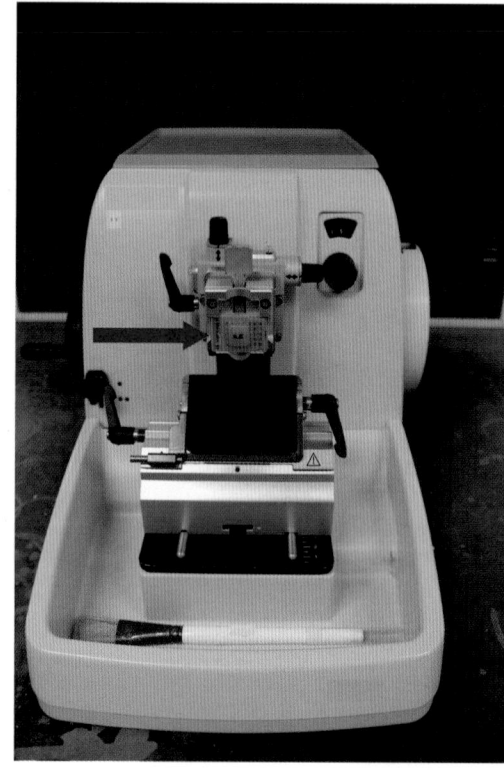

Fig. 2.3
Paraffin block containing skin tissue (arrow) on microtome.

is positively charged and thus acts as a basic dye staining the negatively charged DNA in the nucleus blue-black. Eosin is anionic and thus acts as an acidic stain of the positively charged proteins comprising the cytoplasmic compartment and connective tissue resulting in variable shades and intensity of pink, orange, and red. The periodic acid-Schiff (PAS) technique is used widely to demonstrate:

- glycogen,
- starch,
- sialomucin,
- neutral mucin,
- basement membranes,
- α1-antitrypsin,
- reticulin,
- Russell bodies of plasma cells,
- fungi.[2]

The PAS technique is employed to demonstrate basement membrane thickening in lupus erythematosus, porphyria cutanea tarda, and in some tumors. Glycogen is digested by diastase, while neutral mucopolysaccharides are not—thus these PAS-positive components can be distinguished. Mucicarmine demonstrates acidic epithelial mucins.[2] It is useful for the diagnosis of adenocarcinomas and the mucoid *Cryptococcus neoformans* capsule. Alcian blue highlights acidic mucopolysaccharides, staining the mucinous components of dermal mucinoses, granuloma annulare, scleredema of Bushke, lupus erythematosus, and metastatic adenocarcinomas among others. Alcian blue demonstrates heterogeneity of staining that is pH based: are demonstrated at pH 2.5 and sulfamucins at pH 1.0.[3]

While colloidal iron, initially described by Hale for the identification of acid mucopolysaccharides, is as sensitive as Alcian blue for this purpose, its specificity and selectivity are debatable and background staining can be problematic.[4] However, reduction of pH of the colloidal iron solution and

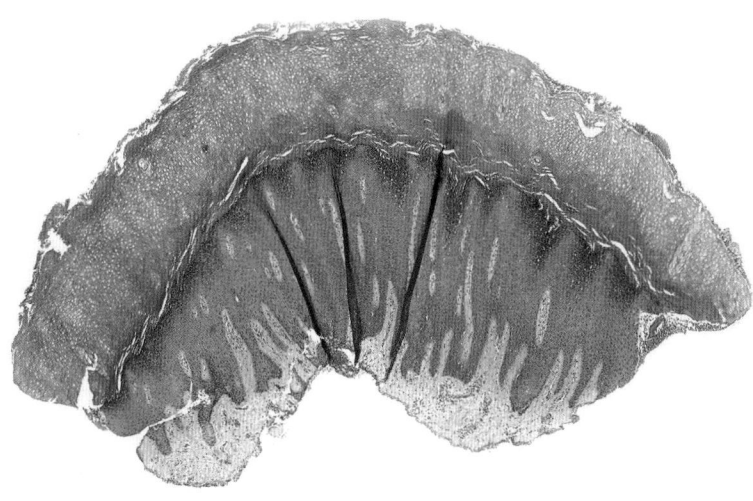

Fig. 2.4
Technical artifact: folds in tissue sections because of poor bath floating technique.

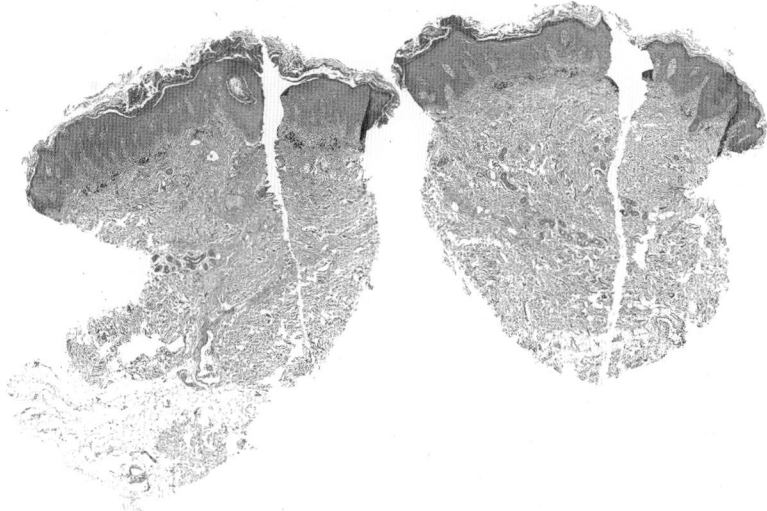

Fig. 2.6
Technical artifact: vertical scores in tissue sections caused by a damaged microtome blade. By courtesy of K. Nargan, Africa Health Research Institute, Durban, South Africa.

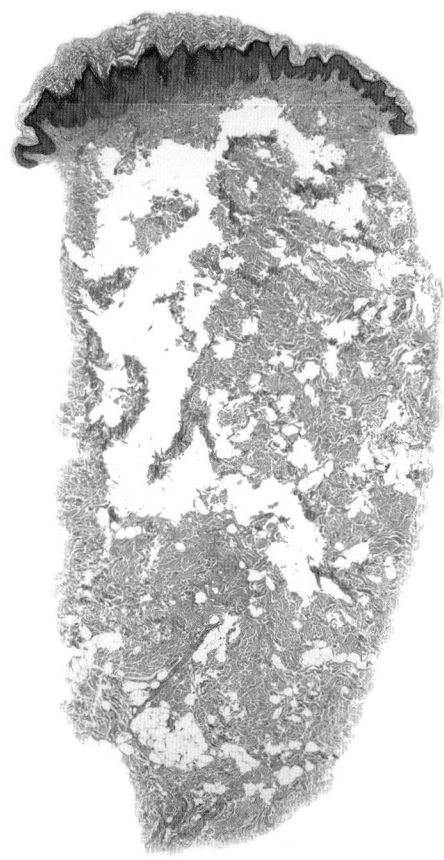

Fig. 2.5
Technical artifact: holes in tissue sections caused by excessively thin sectioning.

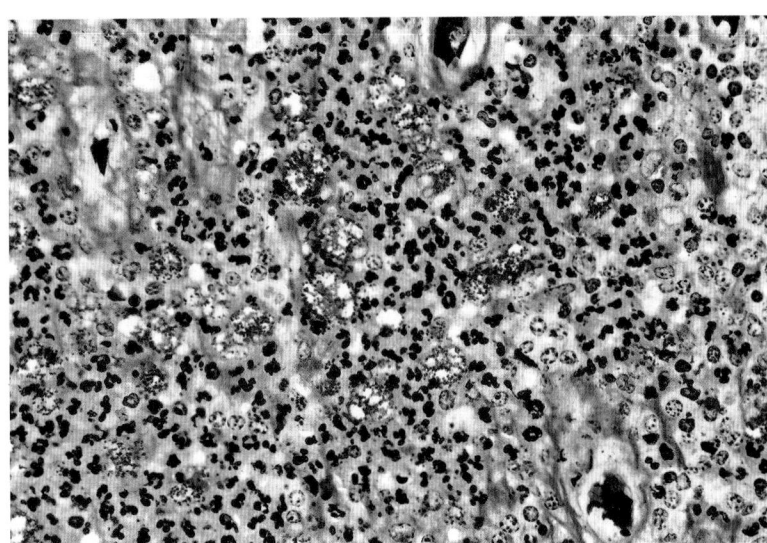

Fig. 2.7
Special stains: Warthin-Starry silver stain demonstrating Donovan bodies.

inclusion of acetic acid washes may reduce this artifact.[3-5] The high iron diamine stain, in contrast to colloidal iron, stains highly acidic sulfamucins but does not stain sialomucins or hyaluronic acid.[5-7] Connective tissue stains highlight collagen, elastic and reticulin fibers. The trichrome stain, a combination of three dyes, is employed for the differential demonstration of muscle, collagen fibers, fibrin, and erythrocytes.[8] Elastic fibers usually stain with eosin, phloxine, Congo red, and PAS stains but are demonstrated well and differentially with the Verhöeff method in the diagnosis of conditions like scleroderma, anetoderma, and pseudoxanthoma elasticum. Silver stains are useful to demonstrate reticulin fibers, melanin, and the identification of infective agents. While methenamine silver and Gomori-Grocott methenamine silver stains highlight fungi and bacteria, Warthin-Starry, Dieterle, and Steiner silver stains are particularly useful in the demonstration of spirochetes, *Bartonella* species and Donovan bodies (*Fig. 2.7*). Masson-Fontana silver staining is pivotal to the staining of the cell wall of *C. neoformans*, especially in the identification of capsule-deficient *C. neoformans*. The role of the more commonly used special stains is summarized in *Table 2.1*.

Immunohistochemical techniques

Since the first practical application of antibodies using the peroxidase-labeled antibody method on paraffin-embedded tissues in 1968, immunohistochemistry (IHC) has emerged as a powerful supplementary investigation to histomorphological assessment.[1-3] IHC has widespread dermatopathological diagnostic, prognostic, therapeutic, and pathogenetic applications, not only in a range of neoplastic (*Table 2.2*), immunobullous, and infective disease, but also in the distinction between reactive and neoplastic disorders.[4-14] Immunohistological techniques can be performed manually or in automated platforms (*Fig. 2.8*). While automation allows enhanced quality and reproducibility of staining; detailed, exact IHC protocols are critical in the many laboratories that still perform manual IHC, to achieve optimal, reproducible results.

Table 2.1
Commonly used histochemical stains

	Stain	Component	Outcome
A.	**Routine**		
	Hematoxylin-eosin	Cells, connective tissue	Nuclei: blue Cytoplasm: pink/ red Extracellular matrix: red/pink
B.	**Carbohydrates & glycoconjugates**		
	Periodic acid-Schiff (PAS)	Neutral mucins, glycogen	Magenta
	PAS-diastase	Glycogen, proteoglycans, HA resistant sialomucin	Resistant to diastase digestion
	Alcian blue, pH 2.5	Labile sialomucin	Blue
	Alcian blue, pH 1.0	Sulfomucin, resistant sialomucin	Blue
	Mucicarmine	Sialomucin, sulfomucin	Pink
	Colloidal iron	Sialomucin, sulfomucin HA, proteoglycans	Blue
	High iron diamine	Proteoglycans, sulfomucin	Blue
	Toluidine blue	Sulfomucin	Blue
	Hyaluronidase	HA	Sensitive to HA
C.	**Connective tissue fibers**		
	Masson trichrome	Collagen	Blue or green
		Muscle, nerve	Red
	Verhöeff-van Gieson	Elastic fibers	Black
	Pinkus acid orcein	Elastic	Dark brown
	Silver nitrate	Reticulum fibers	Black
D.	**Infective stains**		
	Ziehl Neelsen	Acid fast bacilli	Red
	Fite-Faraco	(weakly) acid fast bacilli	Red
	PAS	Fungi, parasites	Magenta
	Mucicarmine	*Cryptococcus* sp	Red
	Giemsa	*Leishmania* sp,	Red
		Donovan bodies	Metachromatically purple
	Methenamine silver	Fungi, bacteria	Black
	Grocott methenamine silver	Fungi	Black
	Warthin Starry silver	Spirochetes, bacteria	Black
	Dieterle and Steiner silver	Spirochetes, bacteria	Black
E.	**Other**		
	Perl potassium ferrocyanide	Hemosiderin	Blue
	Oil red O	Lipids	Red
	Scarlet red	Lipids	Red
	Von Kossa	Phosphate (often as calcium phosphate)	Black
	Alizarin red S	Calcium	Orange-red
	Alkaline Congo red	Amyloid	Apple green birefringence
	Chloro-acetate esterase	Myeloid series	Red granules

HA, Hyaluronic acid.

Table 2.2
Some diagnostic immunohistochemical applications for cutaneous tumors[4–13]

Stain	Application
	Epidermal and appendageal neoplasms
AE1/AE3	Pan-keratin. Confirms epithelial lineage
CAM 5.2	CKs 8,18. Confirm epithelial lineage. Useful to confirm glandular neoplasms
MNF 116	CKs 5, 6, 8, 17, 19. Useful in diagnosis of SCC with single cell infiltration
BerEP4	Positive in BCC. Negative in SCC
CK 7	Confirmation of mammary and extramammary Paget disease
p63	Distinguish primary cutaneous spindle SCC from mesenchymal spindle cell tumors & primary cutaneous adnexal from metastatic adenocarcinomas
CD10	Trichoepithelioma: positive in stroma and papillae, negative in epithelium. BCC: positive in epithelium, negative in stroma
bcl2	Positive in BCC, negative in SCC
	Vascular proliferations
ERG	Nuclear staining in endothelial cells. High specificity and specificity for endothelial tumors (better than CD31)
CD31	High specificity and good sensitivity for endothelial tumors
CD34	High sensitivity but low specificity for endothelial tumors
Fli-1	Nuclear staining of endothelial cells
GLUT 1	Positive in endothelial cells of all juvenile hemangiomas. Usually negative in congenital hemangiomas (rapidly involuting congenital hemangioma and noninvoluting congenital hemangioma)
	Melanocytic tumors
S100 protein	Most widely used melanocytic marker. It is highly sensitive but not as specific as other melanocytic markers
Sox-10	Newly introduced melanocytic marker also positive in neural tumors. Very useful in spindle cell melanomas including desmoplastic melanoma and in the evaluation of intraepidermal melanocytic proliferations as lentigo maligna (nuclear staining)
MITF-1	Low specificity but useful in the evaluation of intraepidermal melanocytic proliferations (nuclear staining)
HMB 45	Good specificity but relatively low sensitivity. Tends to be negative in spindle cell melanoma. Also positive in PEComa
Melan A/ Mart 1	Similar specificity to HMB45. Tends to be negative in spindle cell melanomas
Ki-67	Higher proliferation index in melanoma (13–35%) than in nevi (<5%). Useful in the evaluation of some melanocytic tumors, mainly nevoid melanoma
	Neuroectodermal and neural tumors
S100 protein	Positive in neuroectodermal, neuronal, nerve sheath, chondroid tumors, some sweat gland tumors, and myoepithelioma
NSE	Merkel cell carcinoma
CK 20	Merkel cell carcinoma
Neurofilament	Merkel cell carcinoma
Chromogranin	Merkel cell carcinoma
Synaptophysin	Merkel cell carcinoma
TTF1	Negative in most Merkel cell carcinoma
	Myogenic/myofibroblastic differentiation
MSA	Tumors of muscle origin
Desmin	Tumors of muscle origin (smooth muscle and skeletal muscle, rarely and focally in myofibroblastic tumors)
Myogenin	Positive in rhabdomyosarcoma
SMA	Positive in smooth muscle tumors, glomus tumor, myopericytoma, dermatomyofibroma

BCC, Basal cell carcinoma; *CK*, cytokeratin; *MSA*, muscle specific actin; *PEComa*, perivascular epithelioid cell tumor; *SCC*, squamous cell carcinoma; *SMA*, anti-smooth muscle actin.

Immunohistochemical techniques and trouble shooting

In many centers, IHC is now the most commonly utilized ancillary test for clinical tissue samples.

Historically, the introduction of enzymes as labels in IHC overcame difficulties associated with immunofluorescence, including the inability to assess histomorphology with the latter.[1] The peroxidase-antiperoxidase (PAP) technique was replaced by alkaline phosphatase-antialkaline phosphatase (APAAP) techniques and avidin-biotin complex (ABC) labeling.[1,2] Although the streptavidin-biotin labeling system gained popularity, the endogenous biotin-associated background staining under certain circumstances has

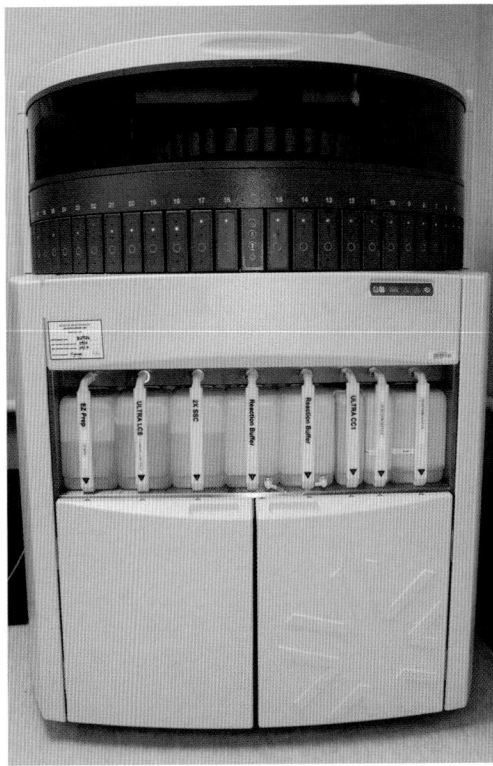

Fig. 2.8
Autostainer used for automated immunohistochemical testing.

resulted in increasing use of labeled polymer-based detection systems, suitable for manual and automated IHC platforms (*Fig. 2.9*).[3]

The direct conjugation of the primary antibody to the label formed the principle of the initial, traditional direct technique, in which the labeled antibody reacted directly with the tissue antigen.[1] In the two-step indirect technique, labeled secondary antibody directed against the immunoglobulin of the animal from which the primary antibody was obtained to visualize the unlabeled primary antibody.[4] The labeled streptavidin-biotin (LSAB) method is a three-step technique. An unconjugated primary monoclonal or polyclonal antibody attached to the tissue antigen forms the first layer, creating an antigen-antibody complex. The second layer is formed by a biotinylated secondary antibody raised against the same species of the primary animal.[1] The secondary antibody binds to the primary antibody with the biotinylated end being available for binding to a third layer. This layer may bind either to enzyme-labeled streptavidin or to a complex of enzyme-labeled biotin and streptavidin. The enzyme may be horseradish peroxidase or alkaline phosphatase. An appropriate chromogen is used for detection. In the peroxidase method, peroxidase-oriented chromogens such as diaminobenzidine or 3-amino-9 ethylcarbazole are appropriate. Indole reagents (red), naphthol fast red (red), or NBT/BCIP (blue) are the chromogens used in the alkaline phosphatase-streptavidin method.[1,4]

The presence of endogenous biotin and resultant background staining led to the introduction of the increasingly popular polymer-based immunohistochemical methods. In the new direct enhanced polymer one-step (EPOS) technique, approximately 70 enzyme molecules and 10 primary antibodies are conjugated to a dextran 'backbone.' While the entire IHC procedure is completed in one step, the method is limited to highly select manufacturer-specific primary antibodies. Other newer polymer detection systems with a dextran backbone to which multiple enzyme molecules may attach are available for manual and automated IHC. These quick, reliable, and reproducible techniques are also characterized by greater sensitivity. Single-, dual-, triple-, and multi-color staining with different chromogens is possible.[1,2,4,5]

Background staining is a common difficulty that has multiple predisposing causes.[6] While monoclonal antibodies reduce non-specific background staining, not only must antibody concentrates and prediluted preparations be optimized for usage at the correct dilution in different laboratories (*Figs 2.10* and *2.11*), diluent pH is also critical in ensuring the absence of antibody degeneration and resultant background staining. Avidin-biotin detection systems and horseradish peroxidase systems may require biotin blocking and endogenous peroxidase quenching steps to decrease unnecessary background staining. Polymer-based detection systems can effectively

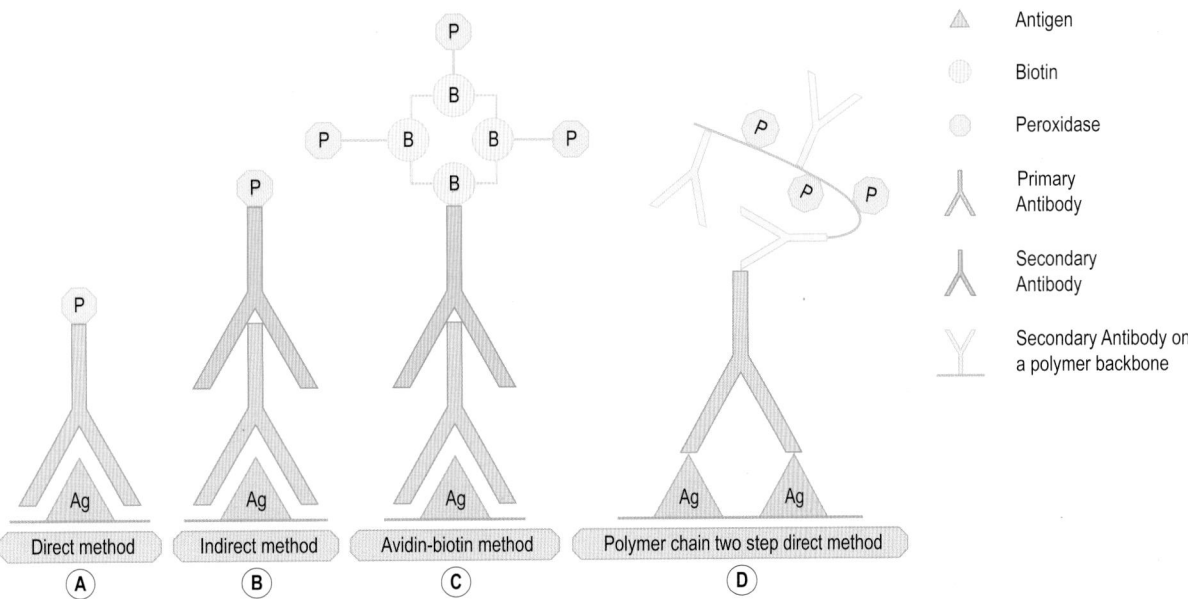

Fig. 2.9
Immunohistochemical techniques (**A**) direct, (**B**) indirect, (**C**) streptavidin biotin, (**D**) polymer chain. By courtesy of K Lumamba, Africa Health Research Institute, Durban, South Africa.

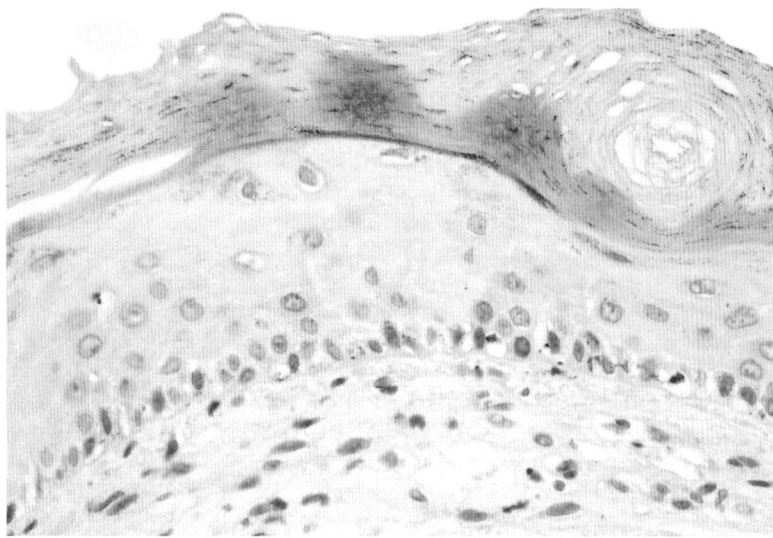

Fig. 2.10
Technical artifact: HHV8-stained sections demonstrating chromogen entrapment in stratum corneum.

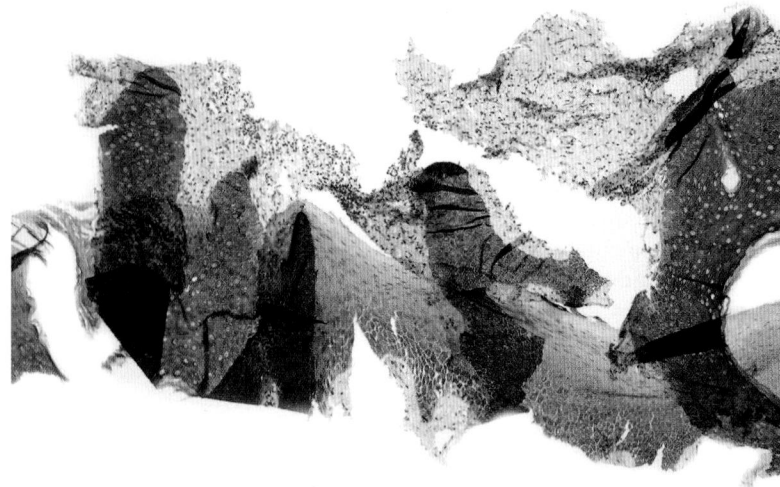

Fig. 2.12
Technical artifact: poor tissue fixation resulting in incomplete sections, fragmentation, and suboptimal AE1/AE3-stained sections.

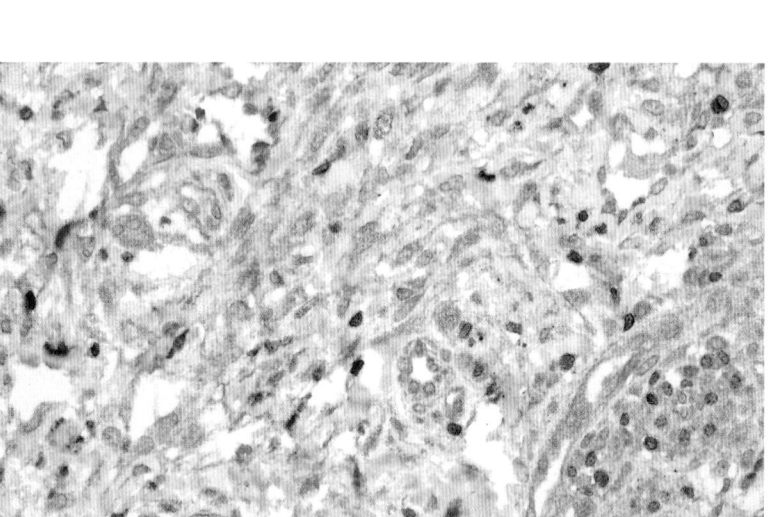

Fig. 2.11
Technical artifact: suboptimal antibody concentration of CD3 antibody resulting in background staining.

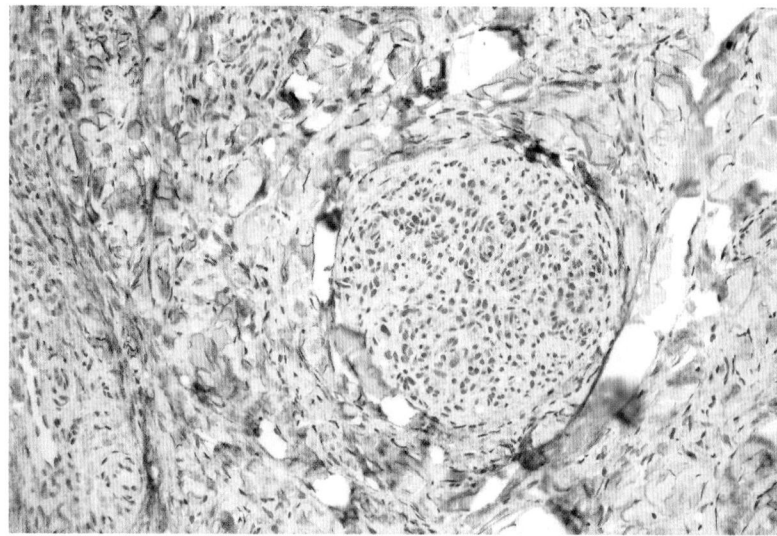

Fig. 2.13
Technical artifact p53 stain: wrinkling and background staining of tissue sections because of erroneously high temperature heat-assisted microwave antigen retrieval exposure of sections in EDTA buffer (pH 8.0).

eliminate biotin-induced false-positive staining. While antigen retrieval techniques are critical for antigen unmasking, optimal results require control of the pH and temperature of retrieval solutions and controlled enzymatic digestion.[7-10] The latter may cause variable tissue loss (Fig. 2.12), excessive background staining when sections are exposed to increased digestion time, inappropriate high temperature and inadequate rinsing, causing protein diffusion into or deposition in skin sections and background staining.

Chromogen entrapment, precipitation, and contaminants may lead to false-positive interpretation of an IHC test. Depletion of peroxidase or alkaline phosphatase chromogenic activity, a consequence of the breakdown of chromogens because of the sensitivity to light and heat, results in a background blush. A similar effect is seen when there is inadequate chromogen rinsing or prolonged chromogen time. Filtering of the chromogen is effective in preventing chromogen precipitation. Chatter, tears, folds and wrinkles and poor adhesion of sections to slides causes entrapment and suboptimal rinsing of chromogen (Fig. 2.13). Skin sections with a thick stratum corneum, dermal calcification, or sclerosis may be prone to these artifacts, requiring meticulous microtomy to prevent its occurrence. The improper handling of water baths, tissue sections, and slides with ungloved hands may cause contamination of sections with squames.[1]

False-negative immunostaining may also compromise IHC interpretation. Incomplete deparaffinization causes suboptimal or incomplete staining because of incomplete tissue penetration by the antibody. Overdigestion of tissue sections by proteolytic enzymes can destroy the tissue sections with attendant loss of antigen for antibody binding. Other causes of false-negative immunostaining include:
- incorrect temperature of reagents, including retrieval solutions,
- expired antibodies,
- inappropriate dilutions,
- suboptimal storage of antibodies.[1,3]

Immunofluorescence

Immunofluorescent techniques have the potential to define antigen-antibody interactions at a subcellular level.[1] This interaction requires the irreversible binding of a readily identifiable label for its recognition.[1,2] Fluorochromes such as rhodamine or fluorescein are labels that can absorb radiation in the form of ultraviolet or visible light.[1-5] Direct and indirect immunofluorescence (IMF) techniques demonstrate a range of tissue antigens of dermatopathological importance, including the diagnosis of infectious and autoimmune blistering disorders.[3] In the direct IMF technique, antibody is conjugated directly with a fluorochrome and is used to detect an antigen in a tissue section using ultraviolet light microscopy.[1-3] In the indirect IMF technique, patient serum (containing the antibodies) interacts with a tissue section containing the antigen. Antibody to a human immunoglobulin, conjugated to a fluorochrome, is applied thereafter.[1-7] The successful demonstration of the antigen requires the antigen to remain sufficiently insoluble *in situ*. Skin biopsies for direct immunofluorescence can be transported fresh on saline-soaked gauze in a container on ice, or in a transport medium such as Michel medium.[8] The transport medium must be maintained at a pH of 7.0–7.2.[1,3,5] The main uses for IMF in dermatopathology are in the interpretation of the autoimmune blistering diseases, lupus erythematosus, and vasculitis.[6,7] In general, immunofluorescence has the following advantages over immunohistochemistry:

- more sensitive detection of antigen.
- use of special fixation that preserves 'difficult' antigens.

Fading of immunofluorescence sections can be overcome by the use of anti-fading mountants.

Electron microscopy

Electron microscopy is much less utilized than in the past. Immunohistochemical approaches are preferred in those instances where they are a reasonable substitute.

Transmission electron microscopy offers much better resolution than light microscopy.[1] To optimize this, tissue has to be embedded in extremely rigid material to allow ultrathin sectioning at 80 nm. In most circumstances, hydrophobic epoxy resins are preferred. When a specimen requires ultrastructural examination, the portion to be examined must be treated in a suitable fixative immediately. The volume of the fixative should be 10 times the sample size. The final specimen is cubed to 1 mm portions.[1] Fixation is affected by:

- pH,
- osmolarity,
- ionic composition of buffer,
- fixative concentration,
- temperature,
- duration of fixation.

Primary fixation in an aldehyde, usually glutaraldehyde, and secondary fixation in osmium tetroxide are standard procedures. Advances in immunohistochemistry have decreased the dependence on electron microscopy for ultrastructural confirmation of cell lineage. Notwithstanding, dermatologic ultrastructural investigations are important in the diagnosis of:

- undifferentiated tumors,
- immunobullous disease,
- cerebral autosomal dominant arteriopathy with subcortical infarcts and leukoencephalopathy (CADASIL),
- amyloidosis,
- metabolic storage diseases.[2-7]

Intercellular junctions, Weibel-Palade bodies, melanosomes, and premelanosomes may help in the diagnosis of carcinomas, endothelial tumors, and melanocytic tumors, respectively.[3] In CADASIL, extracellular, electron-dense granular material is present in an indentation in vascular smooth muscle cells.[5,6] Amyloid is identifiable as randomly arranged, extracellular, nonbranching fibrils of indeterminate length and 7–10 nm diameter.[7] Transmission electron microscopy remains a valuable tool in the ongoing evaluation of the structure of normal and pathological human cell and tissue components and infective agents.[8-10] Technological advancements have enabled electronic capture of ultrastructural images (*Fig. 2.14*).

Frozen section examination of skin specimens

Although frozen section appraisal of the skin is undertaken mainly for assessment of excision margins of cutaneous tumors, it may also be used for primary diagnosis of cutaneous lesions. Frozen section evaluation of incisional (punch, shave) or excisional biopsies can be performed.[1] Frozen

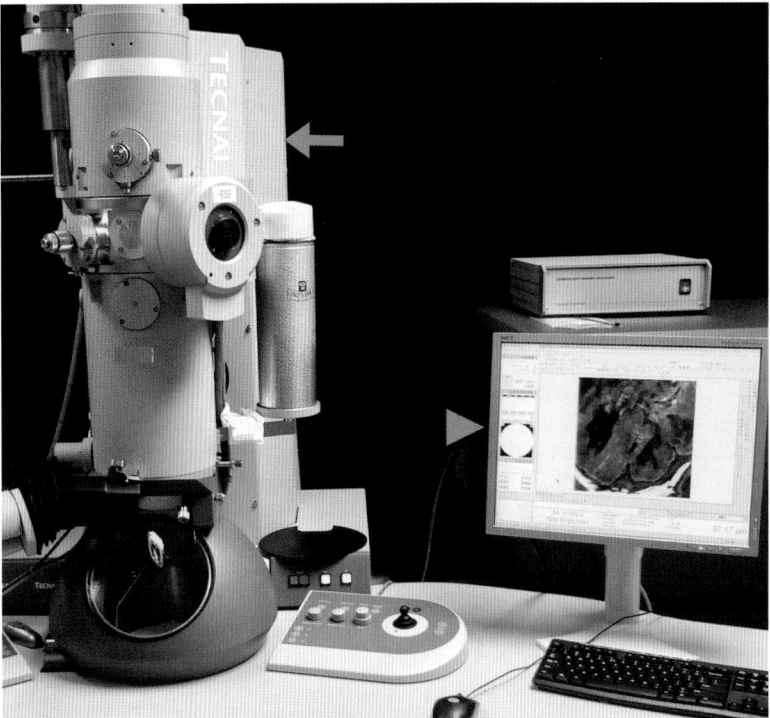

Fig. 2.14
Transmission electron microscope (*arrow*) with electronic image capture (*arrowhead*).

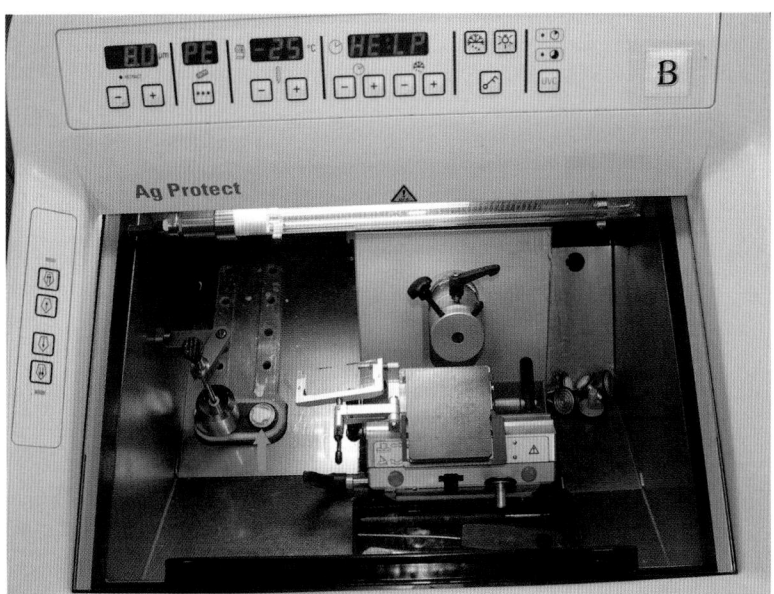

Fig. 2.15
Cryostat with tissue on freezing stage (*arrow*).

section specimen processing and sectioning is undertaken in a cryostat ('cryo' referring to cold and 'stat' referring to stationary) (*Fig. 2.15*), a refrigerated steel cabinet with a holding temperature of −5 to −30°C, containing a microtome and an anti-fogging air circulating system.[2] Commercially available freezing mixtures, e.g., optimum cooling temperature (OCT) mixture, enables rapid fixation of the skin sample on a freezing stage. Evaluation of tumor margins by conventional or Mohs micrographic surgery is expensive and time consuming; hence cases for frozen section assessment must be selected carefully.[3] Indications for frozen section evaluation include lesions with poorly defined clinical margins, infiltrative growth patterns, and long-standing and/or recurrent lesions, especially those in locations where skin preservation is necessary.

Diagnostic cytopathological techniques in dermatopathology

Cytopathological investigation of selected skin lesions has excellent outcomes in dermatopathological practice if used appropriately.[1,2] Cytodiagnostic skin testing, introduced in the previous century by way of the Tzanck test, currently encompasses exfoliative and aspirational sampling methods.[3–5] The exfoliative technique involves touch imprints or gentle scraping of a skin lesion with a straight scalpel and smearing of the scraped contents onto a slide, air drying, and staining with hematoxylin and eosin, May-Grünwald-Giemsa, or Papanicolaou stains.[6] The main indications for exfoliative cytology in dermatological practice includes autoimmune bullous disease infections and genodermatoses.[5–8] Fine-needle aspiration cytology may be used for the initial diagnosis of some superficial, palpable nodular, tumoral lesions inclusive of basal cell carcinomas, Langerhans cell histiocytosis, mast cell diseases, and adnexal tumors and infections but limitations of the technique include technical training of aspirators, poor cellular yields, and lack of assessment of tumor patterns and excision margins.[6,9] Issues related to tumor patterns and excision margins may be overcome by various cell block techniques that may be undertaken when small aspirated tissue fragments are unsuitable for cytological preparation and for processing of residual cell sediments after smear preparation.[2,5,10,11] Cell block preparations have evolved from simple sedimentation techniques to sample centrifugation and the addition of a range of cellular adjuvants for cell cohesion.[10] The fundamental steps in cell block preparation encompass fixation, centrifugation and cell pellet hardening and transfer for paraffin embedding.[10] The most popular adjuvants for manual pellet hardening include plasma thrombin and agar techniques.[10] Recent technological advances have introduced automated cell block preparation that are claimed to have shorter processing times, maintain crisp and clear cellular architecture, maximized cellularity, reduced cross-contamination risk, and minimal operator-associated result inconsistency.[12]

Diagnosis of inherited skin diseases

An efficient approach to genetic testing often relies on initial traditional histologic characterization of skin biopsies.

Recent advances in molecular genetics and gene sequencing have led to many inherited skin diseases being diagnosed or confirmed by clinical molecular biologists rather than dermatopathologists. Analysis of skin biopsies still remains vital for the accurate diagnosis of several genodermatoses, and often provides a guide for subsequent molecular analyses. Examination of the skin biopsy informs the selection of additional molecular testing. Communication between the dermatopathologist and molecular laboratory is absolutely critical for efficient use of molecular techniques.

Analysis of the inherited skin blistering disorder known collectively as epidermolysis bullosa (EB) discussed in detail in Chapter 4 demonstrates the complex, multifaceted approach to diagnosis required in such cases. EB has been shown to result from mutations in at least 18 different genes encoding different structural proteins at or close to the dermal-epidermal junction or within the epidermis (Fig. 2.16).[1,2] Clinically, the different types of EB are characterized by widely differing prognoses, from death in early infancy to blistering that may become milder in later life.[3] The clinical presentation in neonates, however, can be confusing to dermatologists and pediatricians because of the overlapping features (Fig. 2.17). In these circumstances, skin biopsy, usually a superficial shave biopsy since the key region is usually the dermal-epidermal junction, can provide critical diagnostic and prognostic information. Typically, non-blistered skin is sampled; clinicians should be discouraged from biopsying established blisters however because of the potential artifact associated with re-epithelization and misrepresentation of the true plane of cleavage. Just before the biopsy is taken, the non-blistered skin is rubbed gently in an attempt to induce fresh microsplits in the skin to facilitate the microscopic subtyping of EB (Fig. 2.18).

The most informative investigation is immunolabeling of the dermal-epidermal junction (and keratinocyte junctional proteins for more

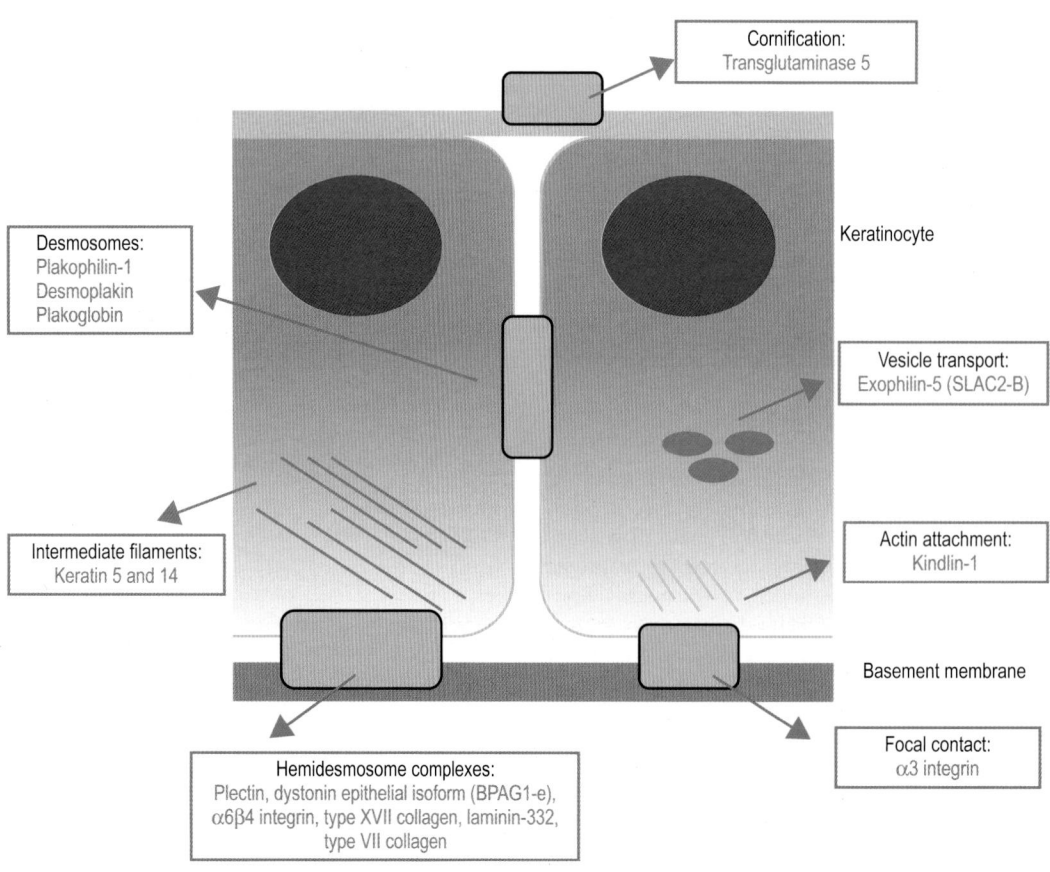

Fig. 2.16
Basement membrane region: protein components at the dermal-epidermal junction and the subtypes of EB that result from mutations in the genes encoding these proteins.

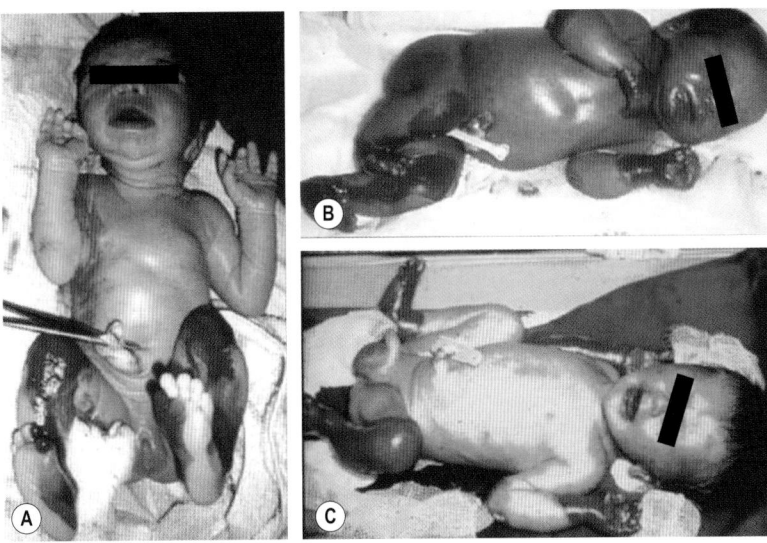

Fig. 2.17
Clinical appearances of neonates with different forms of inherited EB. All three cases have similar blisters and erosions but their respective prognoses differ considerably. (**A**) Severe, generalized recessive dystrophic EB; (**B**) Dowling-Meara EB simplex; (**C**) Herlitz junctional EB. Skin biopsy is fundamental to establishing the subtype of severe forms of EB.

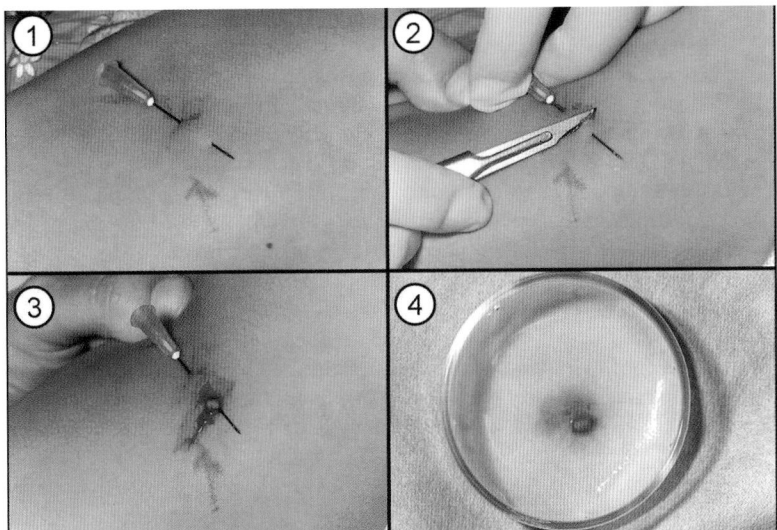

Fig. 2.18
Optimal skin biopsy for diagnosing EB: following local anesthesia, the normal-appearing skin is gently rubbed, and then a superficial shave biopsy is taken. The skin sample can then be subdivided for immunolabeling of frozen sections as well as being processed for transmission electron microscopy.

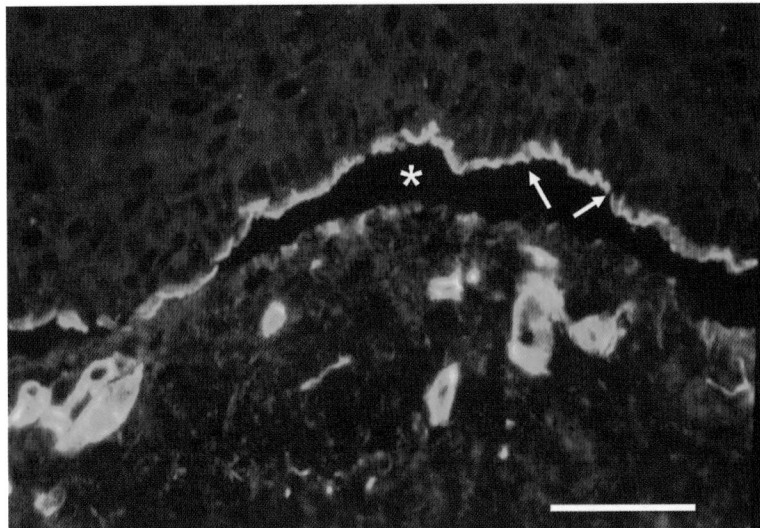

Fig. 2.19
Antigen mapping to diagnose the subtype of inherited EB: this picture shows immunolabeling of rubbed skin from an individual with EB (case illustrated in *Fig. 2.17A*) with an anti-type IV collagen antibody. Rubbing the skin induces microsplits at the dermal–epidermal junction (*asterisk*). The type IV collagen reactivity maps to the roof of the dermal–epidermal junction (*arrows*). This indicates a sublamina densa plane of cleavage and establishes a diagnosis of dystrophic EB. (Bar = 25 µm.)

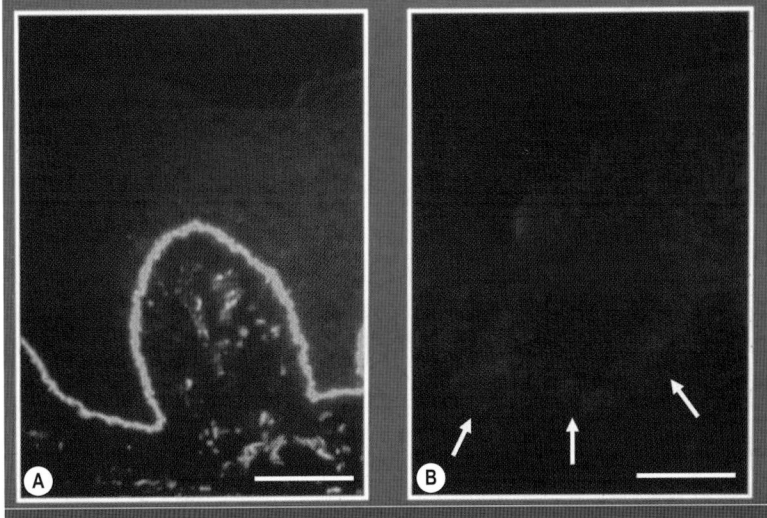

Fig. 2.20
Specific antibody probes to subtype inherited EB: (**A**) immunostaining of normal control skin with an antibody to type VII collagen shows bright linear labeling at the dermal–epidermal junction; (**B**) in contrast, the complete absence of labeling in skin from an individual with EB (case illustrated in *Fig. 2.17A*) indicates a diagnosis of severe, generalized recessive dystrophic EB. (Bar = 50 µm.)

superficial forms of EB, if necessary) using a panel of basement membrane or desmosomal antibodies. Skin biopsies can be transported in Michel medium to a diagnostic laboratory at ambient temperature: this fixative is extremely useful since basement membrane zone and desmosome immuno-reactivity is maintained for at least 6 months.[4] For the immunolabeling, frozen skin sections are used rather than formalin-fixed paraffin-embedded material because the antigenic epitopes of several transmembranous pro-teins may be lost in routine skin processing. The antibodies can be used either to determine the level of cleavage in the skin (antigen mapping) or to see if there is a reduction or absence of immunostaining for a particular antigen.[5] *Fig. 2.19*, for example, demonstrates labeling using an antibody against type IV collagen in skin from the neonate illustrated in *Fig. 2.17A*. In this example, labeling maps to the roof of the split. This indicates that the lamina densa is in the blister roof and that there is a sublamina densa plane of blister formation. These findings support a diagnosis of dystrophic EB. This diagnosis can be refined by immunolabeling with an antibody to

type VII collagen, as shown in (*Fig. 2.20*). In normal skin there is bright, linear labeling at the dermal-epidermal junction; however, in the skin from the neonate shown in *Fig. 2.17A*, there is a complete absence of type VII collagen immunoreactivity. All other antibodies show normal reactivity at the dermal-epidermal junction. These findings therefore establish a diagno-sis of generalized severe recessive dystrophic EB. Reduced or absent immu-nolabeling with specific basement membrane antibodies is an extremely useful and rapid means of diagnosing recessive forms of EB. For example, skin from the neonate shown in *Fig. 2.17C* demonstrated a lack of reactivity against laminin-332 but normal immunostaining for all other antibodies. These findings establish a diagnosis of generalized severe junctional EB.

The development of a panel of antibodies for the target proteins impli-cated in the different forms of EB, most of which are commercially available,

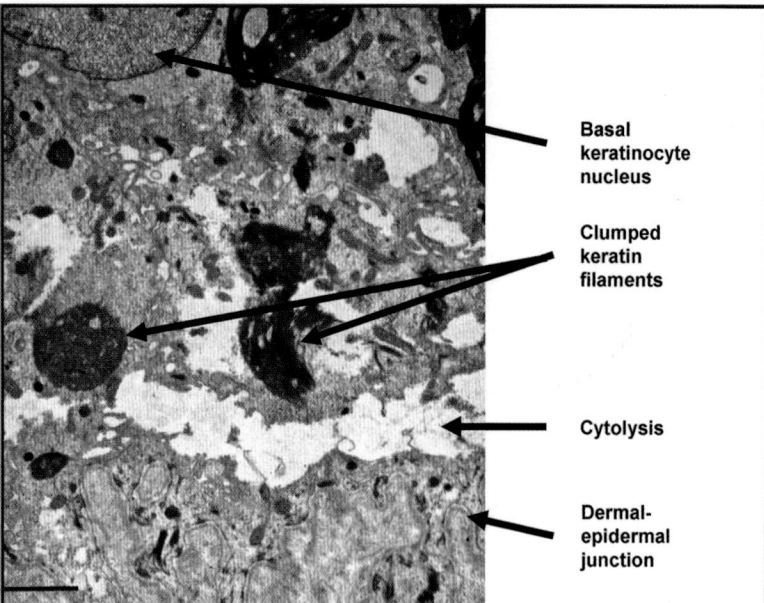

Fig. 2.21
Transmission electron microscopy of skin in Dowling-Meara EB simplex (case illustrated in *Fig. 2.17B*): within the basal keratinocyte cytoplasm the keratin filaments are condensed and form clumps and there is cytolysis that occurs just above the dermal–epidermal junction. (Bar = 1 µm.)

has led to decreased emphasis on transmission electron microscopy as a diagnostic tool in EB.[6] Ultrastructural analysis, however, can be useful in confirming the plane of cleavage and in establishing the diagnosis of certain dominant forms of EB. Skin from the neonate illustrated in *Fig. 2.17B*, for example, shows normal intensity basement membrane zone reactivity for all diagnostic probes but transmission electron microscopy (*Fig. 2.21*) identifies discrete clumps of tonofilament and basal keratinocyte cytolysis, characteristic of the generalized severe variant of autosomal dominant EB simplex. For recessive forms of EB, however, skin immunolabeling has become the most important diagnostic approach.[7] Reduced or absent staining for a particular protein provides a rapid diagnosis as well as a means of identifying the encoding gene (or genes) in which the underlying pathogenic mutations are present. Thus the skin biopsy findings, both histologic and immunohisto-chemical, provide a direct guide to molecular screening tests, most of which are PCR-based or next-generation sequencing (NGS)–based, as discussed below. For dominant forms of EB, however, skin immunohistochemistry of patient skin may be indistinguishable from normal control skin and therefore Sanger sequencing of DNA is often preferred to skin biopsy analysis as the initial diagnostic investigation.[6] Indeed, DNA sequencing is the optimal method for diagnosing the most common form of EB, localized EB simplex (blisters mainly on the hands and feet, which accounts for >70% of all cases of EB). Furthermore, the diagnosis of EB is increasingly embracing NGS technologies, including whole exome sequencing and selected gene panels, as primary diagnostic tools.[7] This molecular information can then be used for genetic counseling, carrier screening, and DNA-based prenatal testing, if indicated. Nevertheless, a clear advantage of skin biopsy diagnostics for EB is time to diagnosis: skin immunohistochemistry can be completed within 2 days and thus skin biopsy is likely to remain a key part of EB diagnostics, particularly in the diagnosis of neonates with EB, for the foreseeable future.

Molecular techniques

Chromosomal karyotyping

This technique can be used as an initial screen to demonstrate gross chromosomal aberrations associated with certain tumors. Most skin tumors are small and thus tissue is generally not set aside for karyotype analysis.

Chromosomal karyotyping is the historical gold standard for detecting chromosomal aberrations in neoplastic tissue (*Fig. 2.22*), though many

other excellent techniques now exist as well. Fresh tumor tissue is required to grow the cells and the cytogenetic preparations and interpretation require skilled personnel. Nonetheless, this technique provides an open, unbiased look at all of the chromosomes of a particular tumor. Total chromosomal gains and losses and also translocations between chromosomes can be demonstrated. Some of these chromosomal translocations are virtually diagnostic of certain tumors, particularly soft tissue and hematopoietic tumors.[1,2] Other chromosomal changes can be suggestive of certain tumor types. While most translocations are now confirmed by the other molecular methods described below, traditional chromosomal karyotyping retains a minor role as an initial examination of the chromosomal complement of a neoplasm and an important tool for discovery of new chromosomal aberrations.[3] Historically, the discovery of chromosomal translocations within specific tumor types is proportional to the number of cases karyotyped.[4] More recently, this discovery modality has been supplanted by massively parallel sequencing techniques (NGS), in particular RNA sequencing discussed further below. The interpretation of complex karyotypes can be informed by additional methodologies discussed below such as spectral karyotyping (SKY) or multiplexed fluorescence in situ hybridization (mFISH).

Allelic imbalance

Gains or losses of specific regions of DNA, often containing particular genes of interest, can provide diagnostic insight.

An allele is a variant of a particular genetic locus or region of DNA such as a gene. Detection of allelic imbalance or loss of heterozygosity (LOH) is a method that can detect the presence of deletions or gains of specific alleles in paraffin-embedded material.[5] This usually corresponds to regions of a particular gene(s) of interest. For this approach, PCR is used to amplify small genomic fragments that carry common polymorphisms and thus have a high likelihood of being present in two different variants (alleles) in an individual. Ideally, these variants are of different size so that they can easily be detected on an electrophoretic gel; DNA sequencing can be used if this is not possible. Only if two different alleles in the normal tissue of a patient are present is this technique informative. Imbalance (loss of one allele) is implied if one detects only one of the alleles in the tumor tissue, or more commonly a vast excess of one allele since normal tissue is present with the tumor cells. More detailed analysis can distinguish those that are true losses. Sites of recurrent losses are typically areas that harbor tumor suppressor genes. This method can detect losses that would not be demonstrated in a traditional chromosomal karyotype analysis and can be readily adapted to formalin-fixed, paraffin-embedded (FFPE) tissue. The limitations of LOH analysis include that it is sensitive to contamination by normal (stromal) cells that with increasing amounts can make it difficult to decide whether an allele is lost. Another drawback is its inability to determine whether the imbalance is caused by the loss of one marker or by a copy number increase of the other marker.

Fluorescence in situ hybridization (FISH)

FISH uses specific probes to determine the number of copies of a specific region of DNA that are present or whether a particular locus has been rearranged as part of a chromosomal translocation.

FISH utilizes fluorescently labeled probes that are complementary to and thus specifically hybridize a specific region of genomic DNA, allowing it to be visualized.[6,7] The labeled probe and the target genomic DNA, which can be metaphase spreads, interphase nuclei (*Fig. 2.23*), or nuclei in formalin-fixed, paraffin-embedded tissue sections (*Fig. 2.24*), are denatured and brought into contact for several hours to days. Given appropriate hybridization conditions, the labeled probes will anneal with the corresponding sequence in the target DNA. This is easiest if probes are targeted to chromosomal regions that are rich in repetitive sequences such as the centromeres. In these regions the probe can hybridize multiple times, resulting in hybridization signals that are large and easy to detect. However, these regions typically do not contain any functional genes, and while increases in chromosome copy number can be recognized, no direct information on the copy number of a specific cancer gene or locus can be obtained. Human cancers, including

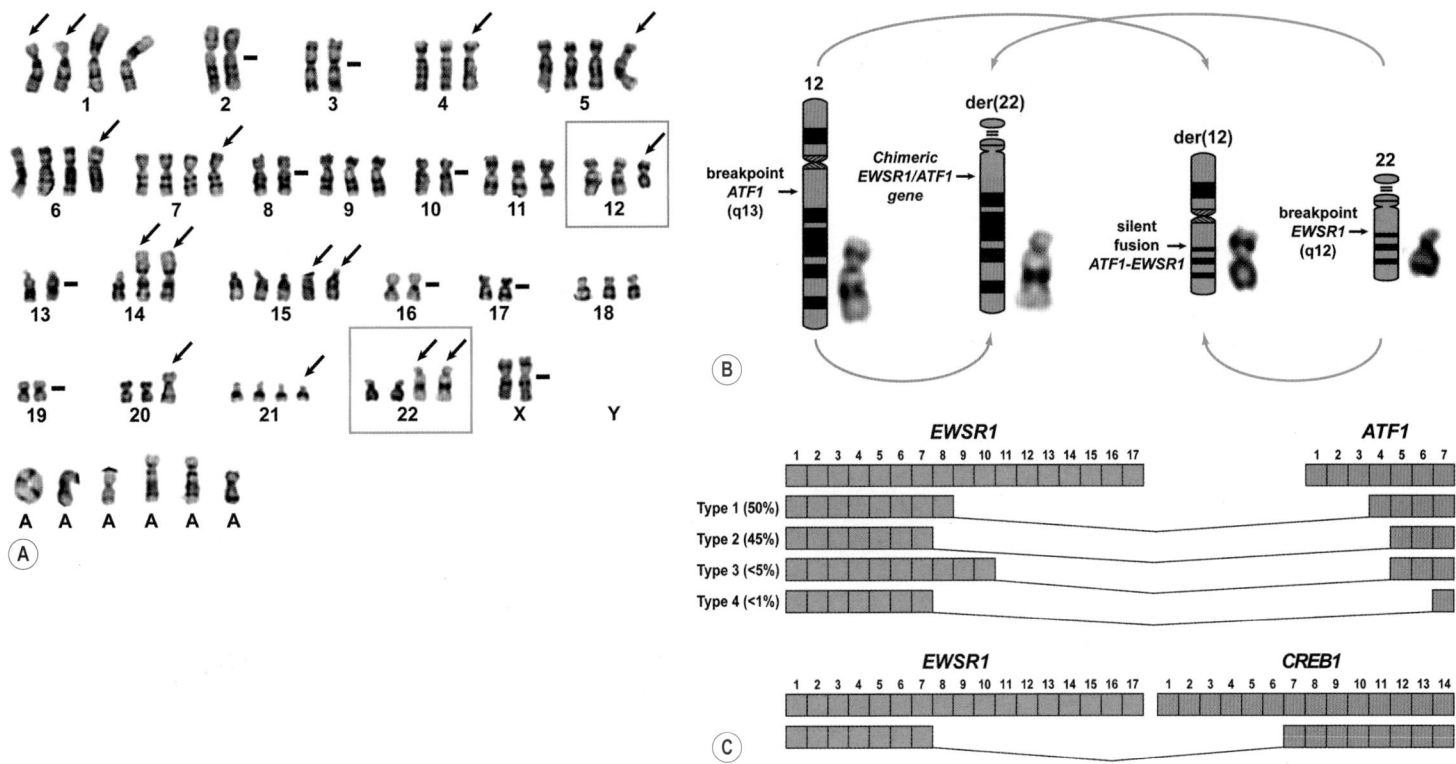

Fig. 2.22

Genetics of clear cell sarcoma: (**A**) this complicated karyotype shows derivative chromosomes 12 (*blue box*) and 22 (*orange box*). While recurrent translocation-associated karyotypes are initially simple, they can become more complex with tumor progression. (**B**) The mechanism of chromosomal translocation involves breaks in chromosomes 12 and 22 that recombine to produce novel derivative chromosomes 12 and 22. The active fusion gene (*EWSR1-ATF1*) is produced on der(22). The fusion genes can be produced by a variety of breakpoints within the introns of the involved genes making multiple exon combinations (**C**). This complicates the design of PCR-based detection methods, as does substitution of the *CREB1* gene for *ATF1* on occasion.

melanoma, frequently have aberrations that involve only fragments of the chromosome. The detection of these types of aberrations requires probes targeted to unique, i.e., nonrepetitive, sequences of DNA. Unique sequence probes give smaller hybridization signals and can be more difficult to detect. However, by using larger probe sizes of 100–300 kb, detection of unique sequences is possible in paraffin sections (see *Fig. 2.22*). The advantage of FISH is that it can detect cells with aberrations in the presence of significant numbers of normal cells, provided that the neoplastic cells can be morphologically identified in the hybridized section. Combinations of FISH and immunofluorescence have been developed to assist in the identification of the target cell population, but the compromises that have to be made to accommodate antigen preservation while maintaining acceptable hybridization efficiency restrict its application for routine use in paraffin-embedded tissue. Detection of heterozygous deletions is more difficult with FISH in tissue sections, because truncation of nuclei in tissue sections cut at normal thickness results in random loss of hybridization signals. Similarly, increased ploidy of the neoplastic tumor cell population can simulate a gain of the target locus. These problems can be compensated spatially by simultaneously hybridizing multiple, differentially labeled, probes to several loci in the genome and statistically by analyzing a larger number of cells. Comparing a probed locus to a centromeric probe on the same chromosome in an alternate color can control for cell aneuploidy. A common example of this technique is comparison of the hybridization signals for the *HER2* locus on 17q with centromere 17. This allows one to detect and distinguish both increased copy number of chromosome 17 and specific amplification of the *HER2* locus.

FISH using probes that flank a potential breakpoint associated with a chromosomal translocation can be used to demonstrate rearrangement of that locus (*Fig. 2.25*). This can be diagnostically helpful in certain hematopoietic malignancies with recurrent translocations, e.g., large cell anaplastic lymphoma and some soft tissue tumors that can involve the skin.[8,9] In this method, the flanking probes are fluorescently labeled in two different colors such as green and red, and when they are in close proximity in an intact chromosome, the spectral overlap leads to two yellow signals, one for each normal chromosome. In a cell with a rearrangement of a gene such as *EWSR1* at 22q12 in clear cell sarcoma, nuclei are seen with one intact chromosome 22 with *EWSR1* producing a yellow signal. In addition, the centromeric probe is retained on the derivative (rearranged) 22 chromosome while the telomeric probe is transferred to the recipient chromosome (12 in the case of clear cell sarcoma) leading to separate red and green signals in the nucleus. This method only indicates that a locus is rearranged, not the identity of the chromosomal partner and gene. Thus caution must be used in interpretation as different translocations seen in different neoplasms can be associated with the same probed locus. For instance, *EWSR1* is rearranged in clear cell sarcoma, Ewing sarcoma, extraskeletal myxoid chondrosarcoma, angiomatoid fibrous histiocytoma, and some cases of myxoid liposarcoma (*Fig. 2.26*). Careful correlation with the clinical and histologic features can help avoid confusion in these situations.

The disadvantage of FISH is that it can only look at a few loci at a time, and that analysis is time-consuming because signals in a large number of nuclei have to be counted. The latter restriction has been partially overcome by the development of computer-based counting algorithms.[10]

In situ hybridization can also employ chromogenic probes such that light microscopy can be used to visualize signals (termed CISH). This method is useful for detecting amplification of a genetic locus and technically can be utilized in a break-apart probe strategy to detect translocations, but in practice this latter application can be very difficult to interpret. Probably the most common use for CISH is in direct detection of nucleic acids associated with infections in cells such as human papillomavirus (HPV) or Epstein-Barr virus. In HPV, this technique can be used to type the virus and determine

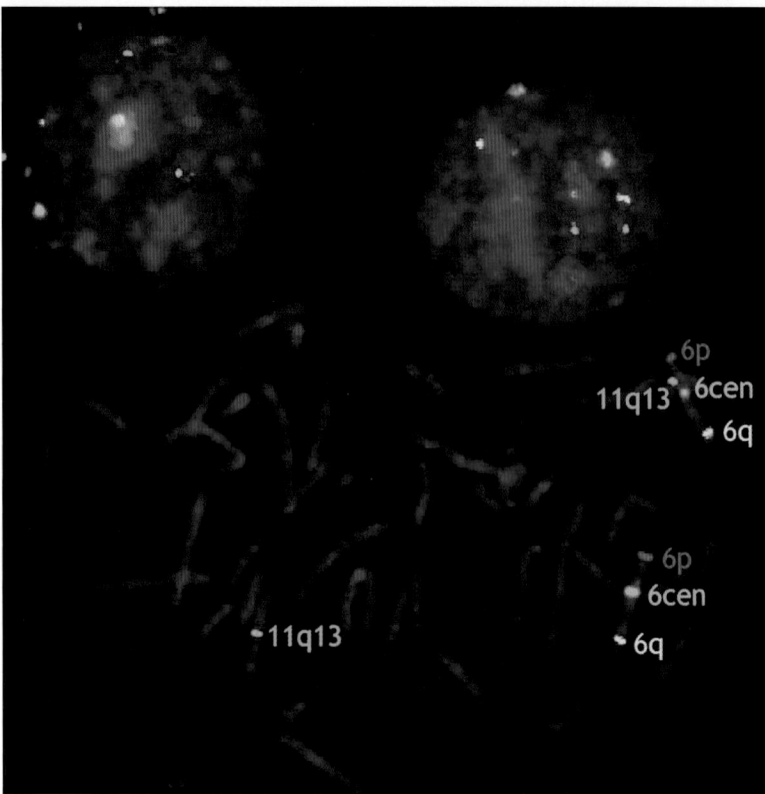

whether it is high risk (e.g., 16 and 18) or low risk (6 and 11). In this application, ISH is used to demonstrate the presence of viral DNA that is not present in a cell until infection occurs. Modifications of this technique can be used to detect messenger RNA in tissue sections as well.

In situ hybridization, fluorescent or chromogenic, is best used to demonstrate:

- amplification of a specific gene,
- rearrangement of a specific gene,
- presence of 'foreign' (infection-related) DNA or RNA.

Modifications of the FISH technique termed multiplex FISH, spectral karyotyping, or whole chromosomal painting can be used to individual color each chromosome allowing for more ready karyotyping and quickly identifying fusion or derivative chromosomes.[11] Such techniques can be very helpful in

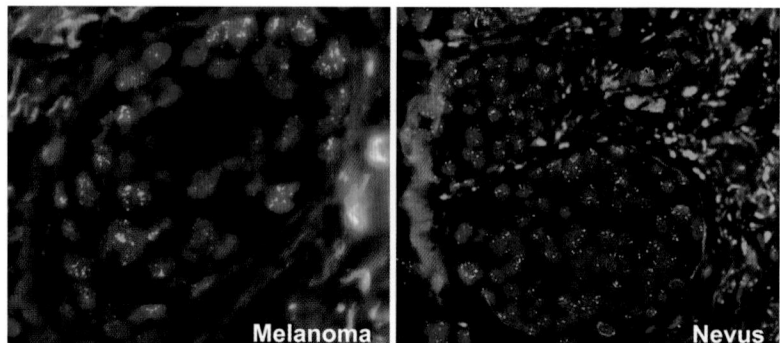

Fig. 2.24
FISH to tissue sections of a melanoma (*left panel*) and nevus (*right panel*): the panels show 400-fold magnifications of two nests of melanocytes with the nuclei stained in blue. The green probe for chromosome 11q13 shows amplification in the melanoma as evident by a marked copy number increase compared to the purple signals representing chromosome 6p. By contrast, the melanocytes of the nevus in the right panel do not show significant differences for these two loci.

Fig. 2.23
Four-color FISH to two interface nuclei and metaphase chromosomes: the upper portion shows two interface nuclei with the hybridization signals for the four colors detectable as discrete spots. In the metaphase spread underneath, the hybridization signals can be seen to map to chromosome 6p (*purple*), 6 centromere (*light blue*), 6q (*yellow*), and chromosome 11q13 (*green*).

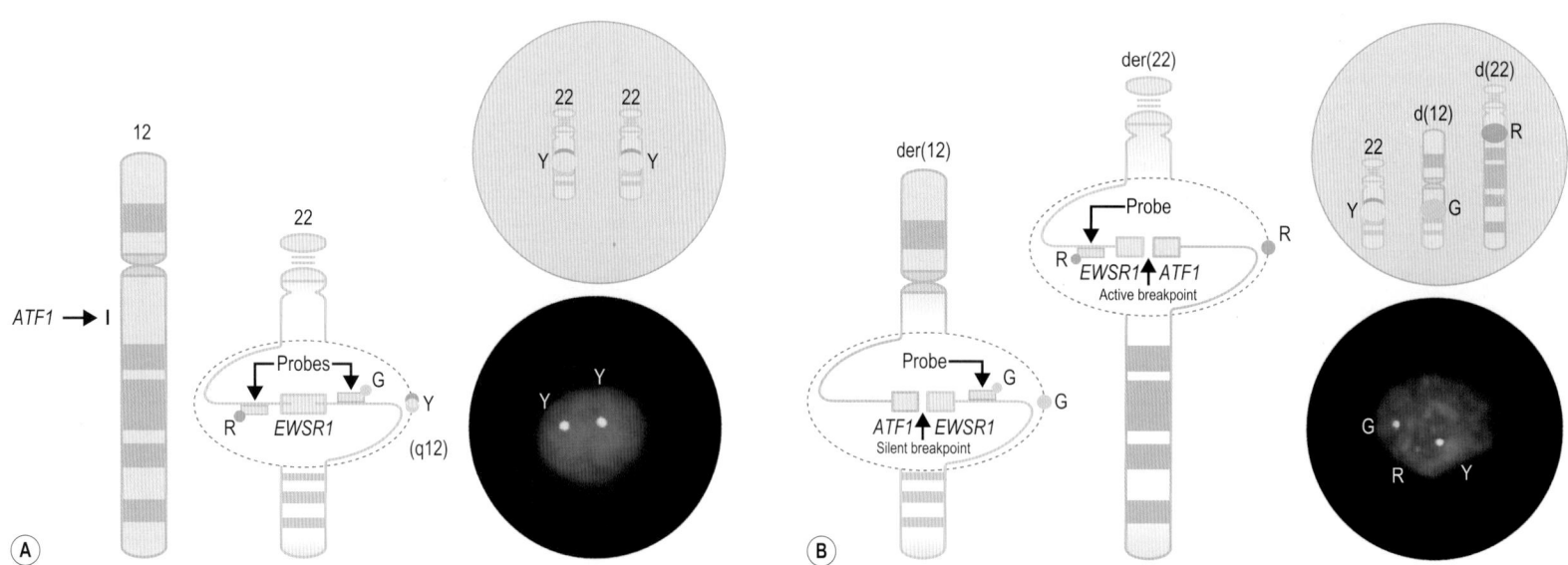

Fig. 2.25
Break-apart FISH technique: the 12;22 translocation associated with clear cell sarcoma is depicted.
(**A**) When the *EWSR1* locus is intact, the probes hybridize to the centromeric (*red*) and telomeric (*green*) regions flanking the gene. The spectral overlap of the two signals in juxtaposition produce a yellow signal. Thus in cell lacking rearrangement of this locus, two yellow signals are present, representing the two copies of chromosome 22 lacking rearrangement (*right*); (**B**) When rearrangement occurs, such as the balanced translocation with chromosome 12 depicted here, the centromeric probe (*red*) is retained by the derivative chromosome 22 while the green probe is transferred to the derivative chromosome 12. Thus in the nuclei one yellow signal indicates the intact chromosome 22 while the derivative 12 and 22 chromosomes segregate freely as single green and red signals, respectively (*right*).

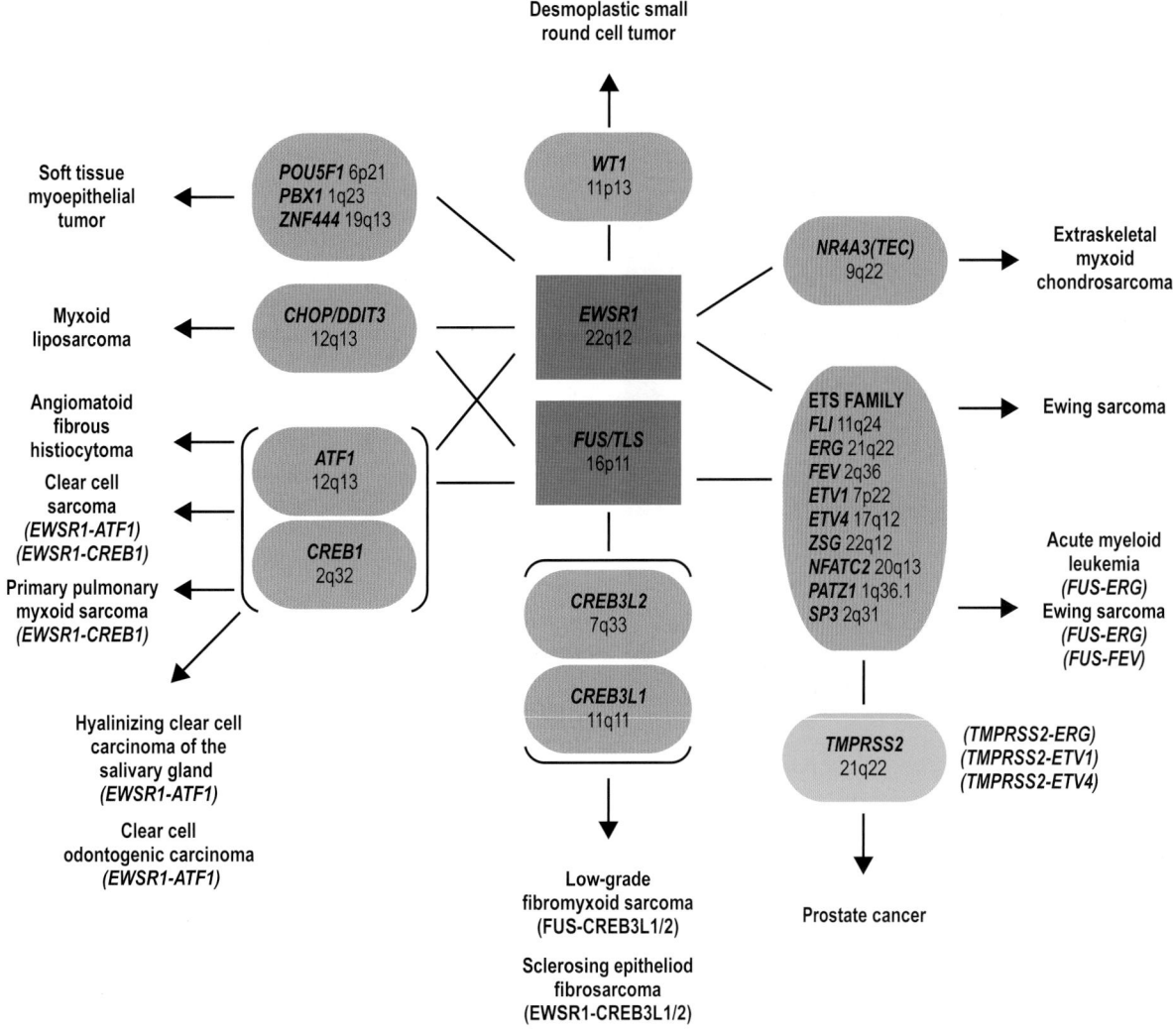

Fig. 2.26
Multiple translocations involve *EWSR1* and the homologous gene, *FUS*: both *EWSR1* and *FUS* can often substitute for one another and both are involved in balanced translocations with multiple genes resulting in a variety of neoplasms. Since FISH only indicates that a single locus, such as *EWSR1*, is rearranged and nothing about the fusion partner, results must be interpreted carefully within the clinical and morphologic context of a tested case. Sometimes techniques such as RT-PCR must be used to verify the fusion partner.

the interpretation of complex karyotypes. Computer-assisted pseudocoloration can also facilitate semi-automated karyotyping.[12]

Comparative genomic hybridization (CGH)

CGH can be used to demonstrate gains and losses of DNA through the entire genome of a tumor sample. While initially a research tool, its application has led to important discoveries that have been translated into focused genetic tests. In other cases, more global information is needed and this test is increasingly applied in the clinical setting, such as distinguishing melanoma from melanocytic mimics.[13]

CGH demonstrates for the entire genome:
- regions of chromosomal loss (often containing tumor suppressor genes),
- regions of chromosomal gains (often containing oncogenes),
- overall patterns of gains and losses (rather than just a few focused regions).

As originally described, CGH detects and maps DNA sequence copy number variation throughout the entire genome onto a cytogenetic map supplied by metaphase chromosomes (*Fig. 2.27*).[14] CGH can be regarded as a variation of FISH in which the entire genome of a sample such as DNA from a skin tumor is used as a hybridization probe. The tumor is freed as much as practically feasible from contaminating normal cells by manual dissection, the DNA extracted, and labeled with a fluorochrome (green, for example). In addition, a reference probe of normal genomic DNA from a healthy donor is labeled with a different fluorochrome (red, for example). Equal amounts of the green- and red-labeled DNA are mixed and hybridized onto a substrate, which represents the entire human genome. Originally, these were metaphase spreads of normal human chromosomes prepared from lymphocytes of a healthy donor that represented a cytogenetic map. More recently, this substrate has been replaced by manufactured microarrays composed of nucleotide probes that are printed at high density on a solid surface.[15] Depending on the number and lengths of these nucleotide probes, the entire genome can be represented on an array. By using smaller probes, higher resolution of genetic gains and losses can be achieved. During the hybridization, the red- and green-labeled DNA populations compete for binding to corresponding regional microarray targets. For each array target (or region of a chromosome in the original protocol) the ratio of red and green fluorescence intensity ratio is determined. A ratio of 1 indicates a balanced situation at this locus, i.e., no gain or loss in the tumor (see *Fig. 2.28*). In the presence of deletions in the tumor genome, less green probe will be available to hybridize to the corresponding targets, which will result in a decreased green to red fluorescence intensity ratio (<1). In the presence of increased copies, the corresponding targets still show a green to red fluorescence intensity ratio greater than 1. The ratio of red and green fluorescence intensity can be used to quantify the copy number change. A ratio of 1 indicates normal copy number, a ratio <1 indicates a loss, and a ratio >1 indicates

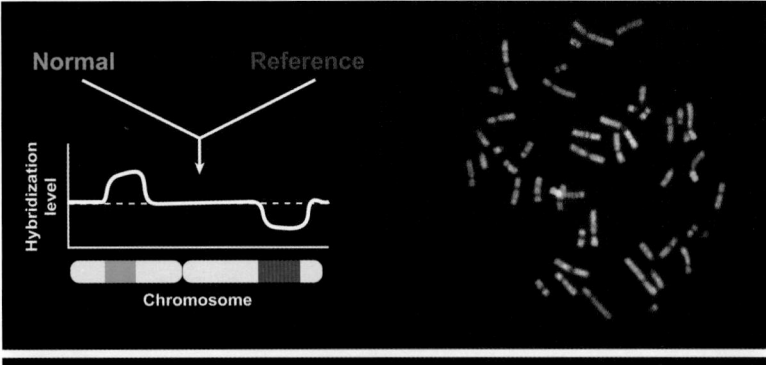

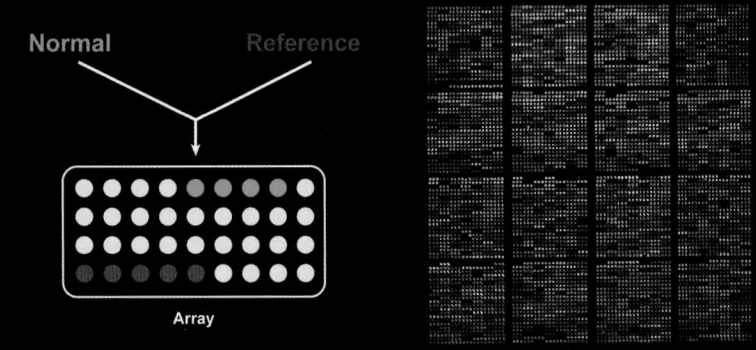

Fig. 2.27
Comparative genomic hybridization (CGH) on a metaphase chromosome spread (*upper panels*) and a microarray (*lower panels*): the regions of the chromosomes (*upper panel*) that appear red are affected by deletions, whereas the regions that appear green are affected by gains or amplifications (*bright green*). Yellow indicates an area with normal DNA complement–no gain or loss. The lower panel on the right shows a DNA microarray with approximately 2500 targets printed as triplicates spots. Triplets that appear green indicate gains whereas those that appear red indicate loss. The array targets are not printed in order of their genomic position which can help control for technical variations. The precise genomic location of the DNA copy number changes detected by the measurement only becomes apparent after plotting the average ratios of red to green fluorescence intensities corresponding to their genomic position as illustrated in *Fig. 2.28*.

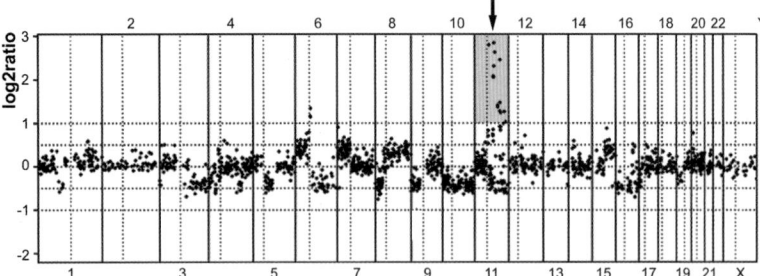

Fig. 2.28
DNA copy number changes as detected by array comparative genomic hybridization of an acral melanoma: the graph shows the $\log_2$ of the ratio of the fluorescence intensity ratios of tumor to reference DNA plotted according to their genomic position on the *x*-axis. The numbers at the top and at the bottom indicate the chromosomes. A $\log_2$ ratio of zero corresponds to normal copy number. As can be seen, multiple contiguous chromosomal regions showed losses and gains. The arrow corresponds to an amplification of chromosome 11q13 interval containing the gene that encodes cyclin D1.

a gain. Gains with a high ratio that only affect portions of a chromosomal arm are termed amplifications. They arise from multiple independent events (chromosomal breakage and fusions) that accumulate under positive selection, typically because the genomic region present in the amplicon contained an oncogene, i.e., a gene that provided a growth advantage to the tumor cells with increased copies of the gene.

The full experimental protocol for CGH is slightly more complex than outlined above. A third, unlabeled DNA population is needed to ascertain that repetitive regions that are scattered throughout the genome do not cross-hybridize and interfere with the measurement. This blocking DNA is highly enriched for repetitive regions and suppresses unwanted cross-hybridization between repetitive regions in the labeled DNA populations and the chromosomes which serve as substrate. CGH has revolutionized the cytogenetic analysis of solid tumors. Compared to conventional cytogenetic analysis, CGH does not require culture of cells for karyotypic analysis, which brings the major advantage that CGH can be performed on archival tissue. It is important to note that the DNA copy number measurement obtained with CGH represents an average of the entire cell population from which the DNA was extracted. For this reason, only the copy number alterations present in a substantial portion of the cells are detected by the method. Depending on the type and amplitude of aberration – amplifications can be detected most easily – the copy number change needs to be present in about 30% to 50% of the cells in order to be identifiable. Alterations affecting only a minority of cells remain undetected. A further limitation is that CGH only detects genomic aberrations that result in DNA copy number changes. Balanced translocations and point mutations are not detected. Copy number neutral rearrangements that arise through chromosomal recombination and LOH (see above) are also not detectable by CGH. More recent implementations that use oligonucleotides to determine single nucleotide polymorphisms (SNPs) allow the genome-wide simultaneous assessment of DNA copy number and LOH in unfixed tumor tissue.[16,17] Due to lack of sensitivity, these methods are not routinely used for clinical diagnosis.

Polymerase chain reaction (PCR)

In the diagnostic setting, PCR is used primarily to acquire sufficient DNA for analysis by sequencing or other methods, primarily to demonstrate a mutation or other genetic change or the presence of a specific gene or messenger RNA.

PCR is an extremely flexible technique and can be adapted to:
- detect mutations (base pair substitutions, insertions and deletions) in genes,
- demonstrate novel fusion transcripts (gene fusions),
- demonstrate clonality,
- demonstrate loss of heterozygosity (loss of one allele),
- detect DNA or RNA associated with infectious organisms,
- detect the levels of expression of messenger RNA.

The ability to specifically amplify and detect any segment of DNA in the human genome has opened many diagnostic doors. In this technique, a pair of short sequences of DNA (called primers) that hybridize to two sequences of genomic DNA (or RNA reverse transcribed to DNA) are designed to amplify a specific region of DNA. Using a DNA polymerase that is stable at high temperatures, a series of annealing, extending, and melting/denaturing cycles amplifies the DNA between the two probes. This technique can be used on nucleic acids extracted from formalin-fixed, paraffin-embedded tissue, although probes must be designed to amplify shorter segments of DNA since the starting material has been cross-linked and fragmented from the formalin treatment. A variety of techniques based on PCR can be used to amplify DNA and then determine its sequence. Direct sequencing of genomic DNA allows detection of point mutations in cancer, such as BRAF or NRAS in melanoma.[18] Generally, one can detect a mutation in 1 in 5 cells with this technique. More sensitive techniques such as pyrosequencing can reduce this to 1 in 10 or 20 cells by analysis for a precise mutation. Allele-specific PCR can be used to detect a known point mutation in as little as 1 in 50 or 100 cells. This technique has applications such as detecting *KIT* D816V mutation in mastocytosis in skin where the neoplastic cells may be sparse relative to the surrounding normal tissue.[19] Digital droplet PCR can also provide high sensitivity and is focused on a single precise nucleotide change.[20] Insertions and deletions in genes can also be detected, usually by Sanger sequencing.[9] Real-time PCR allows indirect visualization of the desired PCR product (amplicon) through the amplification cycles and can provide rapid assessment of a positive or negative result.[21]

Reverse transcribing RNA to DNA can allow specific detection of fusion genes produced by chromosomal translocations such as seen in clear cell sarcoma or dermatofibrosarcoma protuberans.[22,23] This technique is particularly valuable as there is no amplification product in the absence of tumor as the translocations are not seen in normal tissue or other tumors (see *Fig. 2.29*). Because the two genes involved in a translocation event can have breaks at a variety of introns (the noncoding region of DNA between the protein encoding exon segments), multiple primer pairs are often necessary to detect all of the possible translocation types. Also, since multiple genes can be involved, e.g., clear cell sarcoma can contain either an *EWSR1-ATF1* or *EWSR1-CREB1* fusion, additional primer sets will be required for detection of these as well (see *Fig. 17.18C*).[24,25] In hematopoietic malignancies, detection of fusion transcripts can be used to detect minimal residual disease in the peripheral blood or marrow to measure tumor DNA as a surrogate of tumor load to assess response to therapy or allow early detection of recurrence. This approach may be applied to solid tumors in the future.

PCR can be used to detect normal genes as well. An instance of this in dermatopathology was the attempt to detect melanocyte-specific RNA (reverse transcribed to DNA) in sentinel lymph nodes that might have been missed by histology and immunohistochemical screening.[26-28] Ultimately, this technique was not valuable, at least in part because of the presence of nodal nevi that would also be detected by this technique. While widely used in the research arena, other diagnostic approaches based on detection of gene expression will likely evolve with time.

It is often advantageous to have multiple methodologies for detecting various molecular defects, as they are used in different situations and provide slightly different information. *Fig. 2.30* depicts this for the translocation present in clear cell sarcoma.

Next-generation sequencing (NGS)

Massively parallel or next-generation sequencing (NGS) has dramatically altered both the research and diagnostic arenas in recent years. It has allowed detailed descriptions of the genomic landscapes of many cancers and helped to isolate the causative gene in many Mendelian heritable diseases.[29-31]

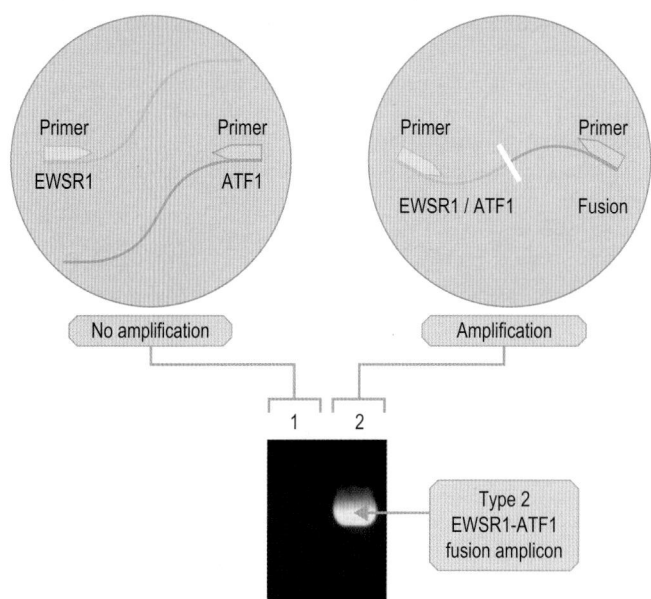

Fig. 2.29

Use of RT-PCR to detect fusion transcripts: this technique uses reverse transcription to convert RNA to cDNA that can then be amplified by PCR. This step is necessary as the breakpoints in the usually large intronic regions of genomic DNA within a gene are essentially random, making it extremely difficult to amplify such large regions to identify the breakpoints using genomic DNA as the template. When the gene is transcribed to RNA, the introns are removed during splicing and introns are directly juxtaposed (*Fig. 2.22C*) allowing more ready detection of the novel juxtaposition of exons from two different genes. When primers are designed for the exons of each of the two genes involved in a translocation, amplification only occurs of the cDNA of the fusion transcript as these introns would not be adjacent in normal tissue. This product will have a specific size and can be detected on a gel, but direct DNA sequencing or other methods should be used to confirm its identity. Amplification of normal housekeeping gene transcripts are used to ensure the quality of the cDNA.

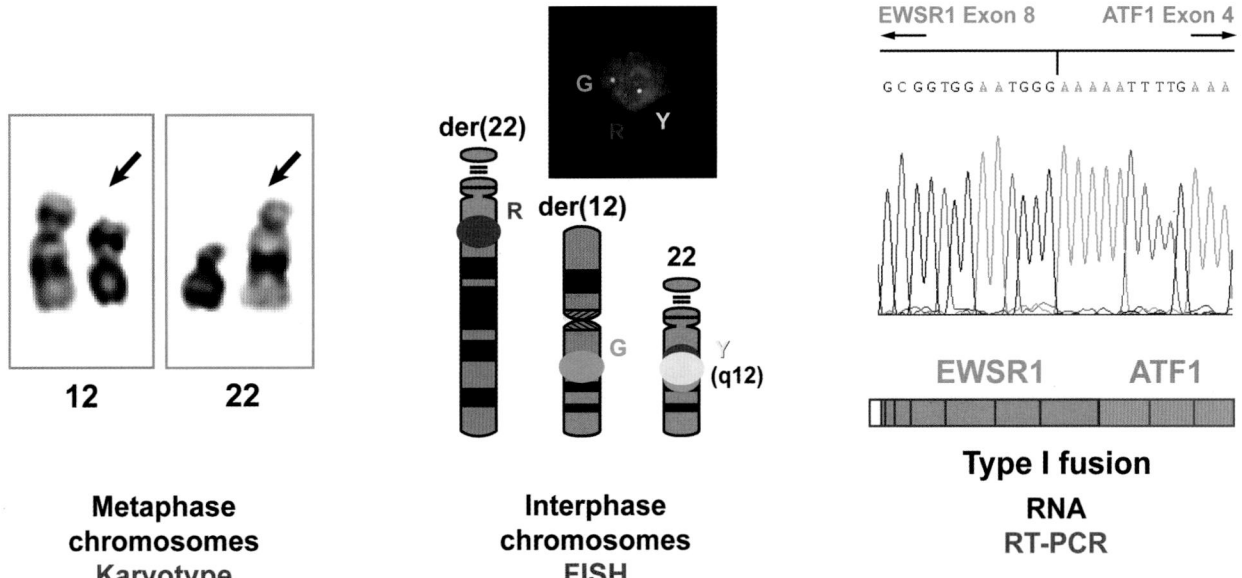

Fig. 2.30

Multiple modalities for detection of recurrent translocations. Traditional karyotypes use metaphase chromosomes spreads to detect translocations and other structural genetic aberrations using banding (staining) techniques. FISH uses less condensed interphase chromosomes to detect rearrangements or amplifications. RT-PCR can detect the precise exons involved in a fusion RNA transcript. Each is a valid method for demonstrating chromosomal translocations, but each has applicability to different sample types and provides different information.

NGS is an exceedingly flexible set of techniques and approaches and can be adapted to:

- sequence alterations in the entire genome, exome, or any subset thereof (DNA),
- provide DNA copy number information,
- sequence the entire transcriptome (transcribed RNA) or any subset thereof,
- identify translocations,
- demonstrate gene expression levels,
- use fresh or FFPE material,
- but does require complex bioinformatic interpretation and has extensive data storage requirements.

NGS uses hybrid capture or amplicon based techniques to sequence DNA or RNA (previously transcribed to cDNA). This can range from the entire genome (all ~3 billion base pairs), to all coding genes (exome; ~1% of the genome or ~30 million base pairs—that is ~20,000 genes composed of 180,000 exons), to all of the RNA transcribed from genes (transcriptome) and any subset of these. Thus it greatly outpaces prior approaches in capacity and will likely fuel molecular testing for the foreseeable future.[32] The technique uses fragmented DNA to construct a sequencing library, and then millions of individual DNA strands are sequenced simultaneously. Different chemistries can be employed depending on the approach, but all use a silicon microchip for simultaneous recording of sequences. All the determined sequences are then aligned using complex computer algorithms against an accepted reference genome to identify differences. Because individual sequenced DNA segments are aligned separately, quantification of mutations (allelic frequencies) can be very precisely determined. When extensive sequencing (beyond just a few genes) is done in cancer, it is often necessary to sequence normal (non-neoplastic) DNA extracted from lymphocytes or other normal tissue to compare and identify the changes specific to the neoplastic process.

The first human genome sequenced required many hundreds of workers at 20 centers of excellence around the world, cost $2.7 billion, and took more than a decade to finally announce completion in 2003.[33] Today, the entire genome can be sequenced in a few days, for less than $1000, essentially by a single person—though a thorough interpretation will be much more involved. In clinical practice, smaller genes sets are usually interrogated ranging from around 10 to several hundred.[34] While only a handful of genes are truly clinically actionable, examination of larger gene sets can aid the molecular classification of cancer and provide guidance for the selection of clinical trials.[35] Numerous databases are available to help interpret sequencing results, which can be very complex, and decide which results are likely to be clinically meaningful.[36] Using accepted unambiguous nomenclature is also important to communicate sequencing results for both cancer and heritable diseases.[37,38]

For cancer, NGS can detect mutations, deletions, insertions, and copy number alterations across as many genes as desired. The main clinical application of this approach in dermatopathology has been with melanoma (*Fig. 2.31*).[39-41] More specific melanoma applications will be discussed in greater detail in Chapter 26. There are balances that must be maintained between increasing the number of genes interrogated and the escalating costs and complexity of doing so. Some insight into fusion genes detection can be gained by DNA sequencing, but RNA approaches are the preferred methods as they are more sensitive and robust.[42] NGS is currently the preferred sequencing method to broadly interrogate circulating (tumor) DNA also termed liquid biopsies that may someday substitute in some situations or complement tumor tissue–based diagnostics.[43,44] RNA sequencing can also be used to determine gene expression similar to other hybridization and quantitative sequencing approaches.[45] Micro- and long- noncoding RNA can also be detected if desired. This technique can be so sensitive that RNA sequencing can be done from single cells, but there are currently no clinical applications specifically for this approach.[46] NGS has also transformed our ability to interrogate germ line DNA for variants or mutations linked to disease. These NGS-based approaches to cancer and heritable diseases are becoming widespread in the clinic and with the rapidly declining cost of NGS and improving reliability of interpretative bioinformatics algorithms, the clinical applications

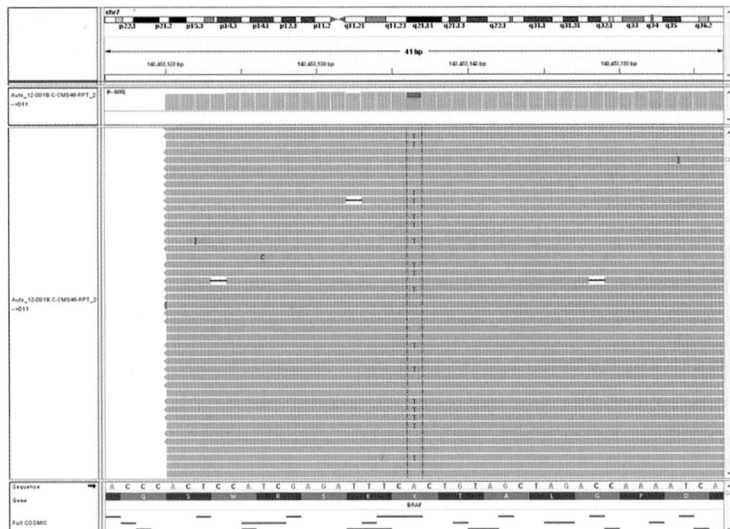

Fig. 2.31
Integrated genome viewer (IGV) depiction of a *BRAF V600E* mutation in melanoma. Note that the display shows individual DNA strands sequenced in both directions (forward and reverse strands, blue and red) by NGS sequencing. Thus the precise variant allele frequency can be determined.

of NGS will undoubtedly grow in both expected and perhaps unanticipated ways.

Diagnosis of lymphomas

The diagnosis and subclassification of lymphomas has transformed dramatically in the past three decades. Prior to this, the classifications in general use were based purely on the morphological features of the neoplastic lymphocytes.[1,2] However, modern classification systems also utilize all available immunophenotypic, genetic, and clinical information to group cases together for the purposes of treatment and prognostication.[3-7] Immunohistochemical and molecular techniques therefore form an integral part of the diagnostic process, and are routinely employed in the assessment of suspect cutaneous lymphoproliferations in order to discriminate reactive from neoplastic processes and to subclassify the latter once identified. A battery of antibodies and molecular techniques are now available to the practicing pathologist.[8-14]

This section focuses specifically on applications of the polymerase chain reaction (PCR) to diagnostic hematopathology, the molecular technique in most common usage, for the detection of antigen receptor gene rearrangement. The relevant immunophenotypic and genetic features of specific lymphoma subtypes are detailed in Chapter 29. In addition, FISH-based techniques can also be used to demonstrate translocation associated primarily with B-cell lymphomas.

PCR analysis of cutaneous lymphoid infiltrates

The diagnosis of cutaneous lymphoma relies on a constellation of morphological, immunophenotypical, and clinical features, and may be difficult, particularly in the early stages. Molecular genetic findings are increasingly incorporated into the diagnostic process. Often, their role is confirmatory, demonstrating clonality in a lesion already thought to be lymphomatous on the basis of pathological findings. However, in a significant proportion of cases, a definitive diagnosis cannot be reached with certainty on the basis of histology and immunophenotype. In such instances, the results of molecular clonality studies may provide sufficient additional information for a diagnosis to be assigned and/or to guide patient management. However, PCR analysis of skin biopsies is subject to the same limitations and pitfalls as described above. Therefore, the results of such studies must always be interpreted with caution and only following close discussions among the pathologist, molecular biologist, and clinician.

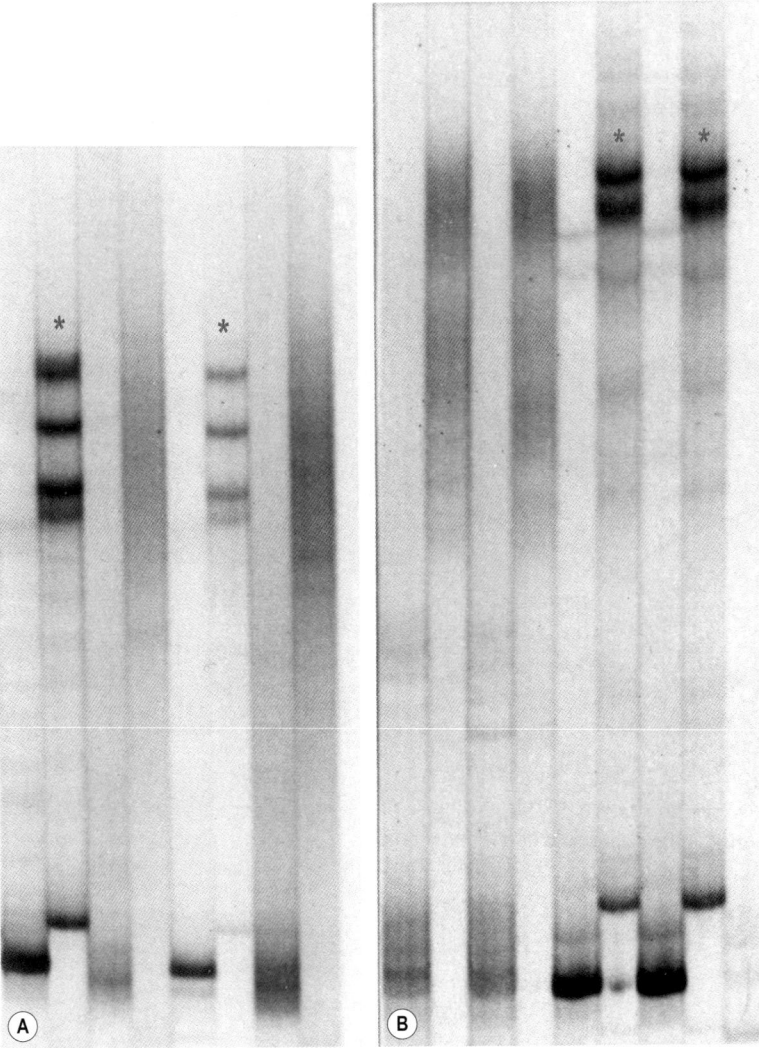

Fig. 2.32
Mycosis fungoides: TCR gene rearrangement (photo of 2 gels from different patients, A and B). *Red asterisks* indicate dominant clonal T-cell gene rearrangement shown as discrete bands rather than a smear demonstrating numerous clones and non-rearranged receptors.

T-cell receptor gene rearrangement in cutaneous lymphoproliferations

Unlike the testing of solid tumors, both PCR-based and NGS-based testing of lymphoid infiltrates can take advantage of T-cell receptor (TCR) gene rearrangements to establish clonality, although this does not always equate to malignancy.

Clonality studies may be useful in identifying the early stages of mycosis fungoides or other cutaneous T-cell lymphomas. Dominant clones can be demonstrated in the early lesions of mycosis fungoides and in cases of cutaneous T-cell lymphoma that could not otherwise be identified using conventional morphology (*Fig. 2.32*).[1-6] They have also been said to facilitate discrimination between mycosis fungoides and inflammatory dermatoses, and simulators of mycosis fungoides such as actinic reticuloid.[3-8] PCR is also useful in identifying the underlying disease in erythroderma when it is due to cutaneous T-cell lymphoma, rather than inflammatory processes such as eczema, contact dermatitis, drug reactions, pityriasis rubra pilaris, psoriasis, and pemphigus foliaceus.[5,9-12] In addition, there are certain variants and malignant mimics of cutaneous T-cell lymphoma, in which absence of a clonal TCR gene rearrangement helps confirm the diagnosis. These include extranodal NK/T-cell lymphoma of nasal type, blastic plasmocytoid dendritic cell neoplasm and leukemia cutis.

However, clonality does not always equate with a diagnosis of malignant lymphoma. Monoclonal TCR gene rearrangements have been demonstrated in otherwise typically benign dermatoses. These include:

- discoid lupus erythematosus,
- lichen planus,
- lichen sclerosus.[13-15]

Bona fide T-cell clones may also be found in examples of cutaneous T-cell pseudolymphoma, particularly those associated with reversible hypersensitivity drug reactions, and in some instances the same clone has been demonstrated in biopsies from the same patient taken at different sites.[15-19] There is also a group of disorders which generally run a benign clinical course, but can be associated with progression to cutaneous T-cell lymphoma, usually mycosis fungoides but occasionally cutaneous anaplastic large cell lymphoma or some other form of cutaneous T-cell lymphoma. These include:

- pigmented purpuric dermatosis,
- pityriasis lichenoides chronica,
- pityriasis lichenoides et varioliformis acuta,
- lymphomatoid papulosis.[20-34]

A variable, but often high, incidence of monoclonality is found when series of these conditions are analyzed by PCR for the TCRG and/or TCRB gene, and the same clone is usually found in follow-up biopsies when lymphoma ensues.[18,25,32-39]

Another similar group comprises cutaneous T-cell lymphoproliferative disorders that are currently thought to represent very indolent or prelymphomatous forms of recognized subtypes of cutaneous T-cell lymphomas including:
- large plaque parapsoriasis,[15,19,40]
- idiopathic follicular mucinosis,[15,41]
- syringolymphoid hyperplasia with alopecia,[42-44]
- hypopigmented mycosis fungoides.[45]

These are thought to be related to variants of mycosis fungoides. Idiopathic erythroderma has similarities to Sezary syndrome[46] and atypical lymphocytic lobular panniculitis to subcutaneous panniculitis-like T-cell lymphoma.[47,48] These entities are typically monoclonal and share many characteristics with the lymphomas to which they are putatively related. However, they lack full morphologic and/or phenotypic evidence of lymphoma, and although most run a recalcitrant course resistant to topical therapy, and some progress to overt malignant lymphoma, most have an innocuous clinical outcome.

It has been proposed that the following be encompassed under the rubric of 'cutaneous T-cell lymphoid dyscrasia'[49]:
- idiopathic pigmented purpuric dermatosis,
- pityriasis lichenoides,
- large plaque parapsoriasis,
- idiopathic follicular mucinosis,
- syringolymphoid hyperplasia with alopecia,
- hypopigmented mycosis fungoides,
- idiopathic clonal erythroderma,
- atypical lymphocytic lobular panniculitis.

The concept is similar to that of monoclonal gammopathy of uncertain significance, already well established for plasma cell dyscrasias.[46] 'Cutaneous T-cell lymphoid dyscrasia' is used to convey the limited but real malignant potential of these monoclonal and oligoclonal lymphoproliferations, and is preferred by the authors to terms such as 'premycotic', because evolution to overt cutaneous T-cell lymphoma is uncommon. It is hypothesized that T-cell clones develop as a result of chronic antigenic stimulation. Acquisition of genetic abnormalities by an expanded clone results in an ability for autonomous growth. This is initially held in check by the host immune cells, and only when these are overcome does the fully malignant clone emerge. Entities that occasionally harbor clonal populations of T cells, but have no malignant potential (such as drug-induced pseudolymphoma), are excluded from this category.

IG gene rearrangement in cutaneous lymphoproliferations

A number of variant gene rearrangements often involve the promoters of immunoglobulin genes to drive the expression of oncogene critical to lymphomagenesis. The current World Health Organization (WHO) classification scheme relies on these molecular results for precise classification.

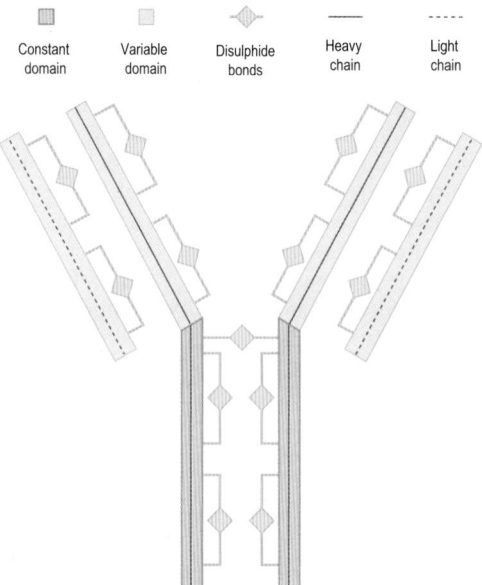

Constant domain   Variable domain   Disulphide bonds   Heavy chain   Light chain

Fig. 2.33
Structure of IG. The two epitope binding sites are formed primarily by the two variable domains.

The clonal nature of cutaneous B-cell infiltrates in both primary and secondary cutaneous B-cell lymphomas can be confirmed in a high percentage of cases using PCR and NGS techniques designed to detect IG gene rearrangements as part of the routine diagnostic work up (*Figs 2.33* and *2.34*).[1-4] However, even using BIOMED-2 and other accepted protocols, there can be a significant false-negative rate. This is particularly the case if the only primers used are for the framework regions on the IG heavy chain gene, one study detecting clonality in only 67% of primary cutaneous B-cell lymphomas.[4] This is likely to be due to the relatively high proportion of lymphomas of germinal center, or postgerminal center origin encountered in the skin, since these are associated with high levels of somatic hypermutation. Detection levels increase when assays targeting IG light chains, including the Kde, are introduced.[2] This type of increased range of detection has been more readily deployed using NGS.

Similar to analogous situations in T-cell lymphomas, clonality assays are not a reliable way of differentiating B-cutaneous lymphoid hyperplasia from cutaneous B-cell lymphoma. Monoclonal immunoglobulin gene

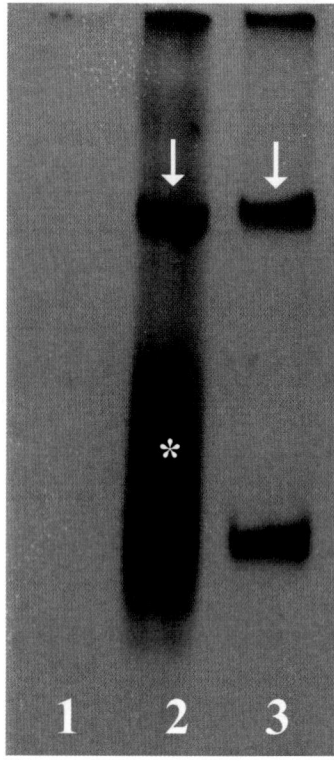

1   2   3

Fig. 2.34
B-cell lymphoma: IG gene rearrangement (photo of gel). The upper bands arrowed in lanes two and three indicate non-rearranged IG with the asterisk in lane two indicating a polyclonal IG population. The lower band in lane three shows a dominant IG clone.

rearrangements have been demonstrated in lesions designated B-cutaneous hyperplasia (or synonyms thereof), even when less sensitive Southern blotting techniques have been used.[5-9] However, in series quoting high levels of monoclonal B-CLH, relatively few cases progress to overt lymphoma.[5,7,8] These lesions may therefore be analogous to the cutaneous T-cell dyscrasias described above, in that they may run a protracted but ultimately benign clinical course, only rarely progressing to overt malignancy.

Access **ExpertConsult.com** for the complete list of references

See
www.expertconsult.com
for references and
additional material

Disorders of keratinization

Dieter Metze and Vinzenz Oji

Ichthyosis

The term ichthyosis (Gr. *ichthys*, fish) is applied to a number of heterogeneous genetic disorders characterized by permanent and generalized abnormal keratinization.[1,2] The clinical features range from mild involvement, often passed off as 'dry skin' (xerosis), through to severe widespread scaly lesions causing much discomfort and social embarrassment (*Fig. 3.1*). The scales are shed as clusters rather than as single cells as is the norm.[1] The pathogenesis of the ichthyoses is heterogeneous and ultimately depends upon abnormal differentiation resulting in impaired desquamation of corneocytes (retention hyperkeratosis) or increased corneocyte production (hyperproliferative hyperkeratosis).[3,4] In some ichthyotic diseases these alterations cause hypohidrosis with dysregulation of the body temperature, abnormal epidermal barrier function, or skin infections.[1]

Originally, ichthyotic skin disorders were classified into noncongenital ichthyoses developing 4 weeks after birth and congenital ichthyoses presenting with a collodion membrane or ichthyosiform erythroderma at birth or within 4 weeks later.[3] As too many exceptions and variations had to be notified a new classification appeared mandatory. A consensus conference on ichthyosis in Sorèz 2009 proposed a differentiation between common and rare ichthyoses, and between syndromic and nonsyndromic forms (*Tables 3.1 and 3.2*).[5,6]

Finally, hereditary ichthyoses should be differentiated from acquired ichthyosis or ichthyosiform skin conditions that do not have a genetic basis and can be caused by different underlying diseases .[7]

Ichthyosis vulgaris

Clinical features

This relatively common disorder (incidence of 1:250 to 1:1000 births) has an autosomal semidominant mode of inheritance.[1,2] The disease is usually fairly mild and becomes apparent within the first few months or years of life. It affects the sexes equally and presents as dryness (xerosis) and slight to moderate fine scaling, particularly involving the extensor surfaces of arms and legs and may spare the flexures (*Fig. 3.2A*). The light-gray scales vary in quality from thick adherent shiny plates to simply dusty accumulations which, when scratched, leave a mark just as when one touches a dusty

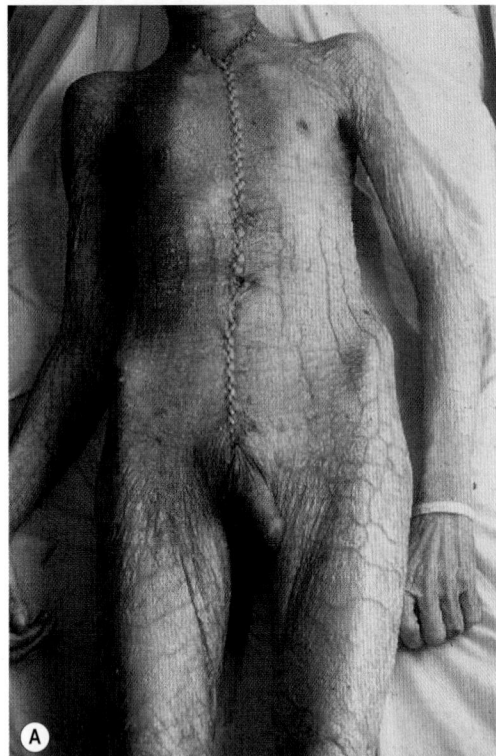

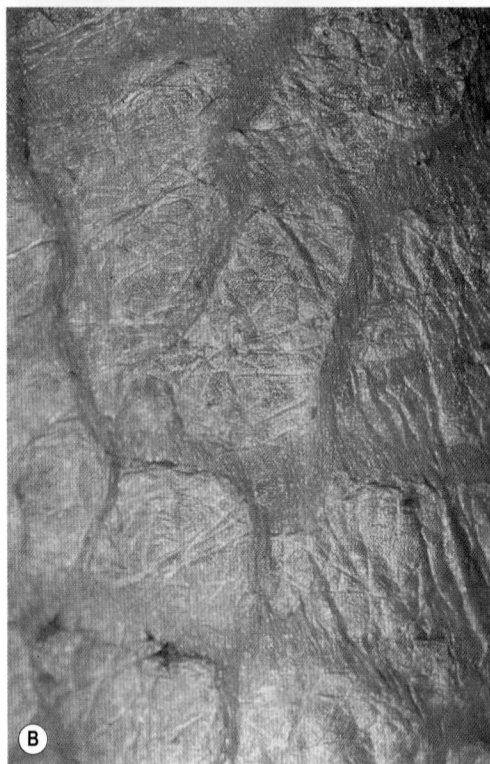

Fig. 3.1
(**A**, **B**) Severe generalized ichthyosis: this was an incidental finding at autopsy. Ichthyosis can be very disfiguring and a considerable social disadvantage. (A,B) By Courtesey Ph. McKee.

Table 3.1

Inherited ichthyoses: nonsyndromic forms

Common ichthyoses		
Ichthyosis vulgaris	semi-dominant	*FLG*
Nonsyndromic recessive X-linked ichthyosis (RXLI)	XR	*STS*
Autosomal recessive congenital ichthyosis (ARCI)		
Lamellar ichthyosis (LI)	AR	*TGM1 / NIPAL4 / ALOX12B / ABCA12 / PNPLA1 / CERS3 / LIPH*
Congenital ichthyosiform erythroderma (CIE)	AR	*ALOXE3 / ALOX12B / ABCA12 / CYP4F22 / NIPAL4 / TGM1 / PNPLA1 / CERS3 / LIPH*
Self-healing collodion baby (SICI)	AR	*TGM1 / ALOXE3 / ALOX12B*
Acral self-healing collodion baby	AR	*TGM1*
Bathing suit ichthyosis	AR	*TGM1*
Harlequin ichthyosis	AR	*ABCA12*
Keratinopathic ichthyosis (KPI)		
Epidermolytic ichthyosis (EI)	AD	*KRT1 / KRT10*
Superficial epidermolytic ichthyosis (SEI)	AD	*KRT2*
Annular epidermolytic ichthyosis	AD	*KRT1 / KRT10*
Congenital reticular ichthyosiform erythroderma (CRIE)	AD	*KRT10 (KRT 1)*
Ichthyosis Curth-Macklin	AD	*KRT1*
Autosomal recessive epidermolytic ichthyosis	AR	*KRT10*
Other nonsyndromic forms		
Loricrin keratoderma	AD	*LOR*
Erythrokeratodermia variabilis	AD (AR)	*GJB3 / GJB4*
Inflammatory peeling skin disease (PSS type B)	AR	*CDSN*
Exfoliative ichthyosis	AR	*CSTA*
Keratosis linearis-ichthyosis congenita-keratoderma (KLICK)	AR	*POMP*

AD, Autosomal dominant; *AR*, autosomal recessive; *SICI*, self-improving congenital ichthyosis.

surface. The truncal lesions tend to be thicker than those on the face and scalp. The rims of the ears are often scaly.[3] There is a mild seasonal variation, with improvement of the condition in humid climates.[2] The palms and soles show increased palmar and plantar markings (hyperlinearity), in contrast to pure X-linked ichthyosis (*Fig. 3.2B*).[3] Affected patients often present keratosis pilaris (follicular hyperkeratosis) on the arms, buttocks and thighs and suffer from hypohidrosis. An association with keratosis punctata of the palms and soles has also been documented.[4]

Pathogenesis

Ichthyosis vulgaris is caused by loss-of-function mutations of the *FLG* gene that encodes for filaggrin, the major constituent of the keratohyalin granules.[5,6] Patients may have one or two *FLG* mutations. The mutation status correlates with disease severity and ultrastructure, i.e., in line with the decreased amount of filaggrin, keratohyalin granules may be reduced, spongy or slightly crumbly.[7] Filaggrin aggregates keratin intermediate filaments in the lower stratum corneum and is subsequently proteolyzed to form free amino acids, including urocanic and pyrrolidone carboxylic acids, which are critical as water-binding compounds in the stratum corneum. The clinical severity of ichthyosis vulgaris correlates with the reduction of keratohyalin granules. Reduced immunostaining for filaggrin correlates with the severity of the defect.[8] Parents with one heterozygous filaggrin mutation may be asymptomatic, whereas affected offspring with two mutations often show classic ichthyosis vulgaris.[5] *FLG* mutations are a major predisposing factor for atopic dermatitis (AD) and related allergies.[9,10]

Histologic features

Ichthyosis vulgaris is characterized by mild to moderate orthohyperkeratosis associated with an acanthotic, atrophic or normal epidermis. The key

Table 3.2
Inherited ichthyoses: syndromic forms

	Mode of inheritance	Gene
X-linked ichthyosis syndromes		
Recessive X-linked ichthyosis	XR	STS (and others)
Ichthyosis follicularis alopecia photophobia	XR	MBTPS2
Conradi-Hünermann-Happle syndrome (CDPX2)	XD	EBP
Autosomal ichthyosis syndromes with prominent hair abnormalities		
Netherton syndrome	AR	SPINK5
Severe dermatitis-multiple allergies-metabolic wasting (SAM)	AR	DSG1
Ichthyosis with hypotrichosis	AR	ST14
Neonatal ichthyosis-sclerosing cholangitis (NISCH)	AR	CLDN1
Autosomal ichthyosis syndromes with prominent neurologic signs		
Refsum syndrome	AR	PHYH / PEX7
Multiple sulfatase deficiency	AR	SUMF1
Gaucher syndrome type 2	AR	GBA
Sjögren-Larsson syndrome	AR	ALDH3A2
Dorfman-Chanarin syndrome	AR	ABHD5
Trichothiodystrophy	AR	C7ORF11 ERCC2 / XPD ERCC3 / XPB GTF2H5 / TTDA
Cerebral dysgenesis-neuropathy-ichthyosis-palmoplantar keratoderma (CEDNIK)	AR	SNAP29
Arthrogryposis-renal dysfunction-cholestasis	AR	VPS33B
Autosomal ichthyosis syndromes with deafness		
Keratitis ichthyosis deafness (KID)	AD	GJB2 (GJB6)
ELOVL4 deficiency	AR	ELOVL4
Mental retardation-enteropathy-deafness-neuropathy-ichthyosis-keratoderma (MEDNIK)	AR	AP1S1
Autosomal ichthyosis syndromes with transient neonatal respiratory distress		
Ichthyosis prematurity syndrome	AR	SLC27A4

AD, Autosomal dominant; *AR*, autosomal recessive; *CDPX2*, chondrodysplasia punctata type 2.

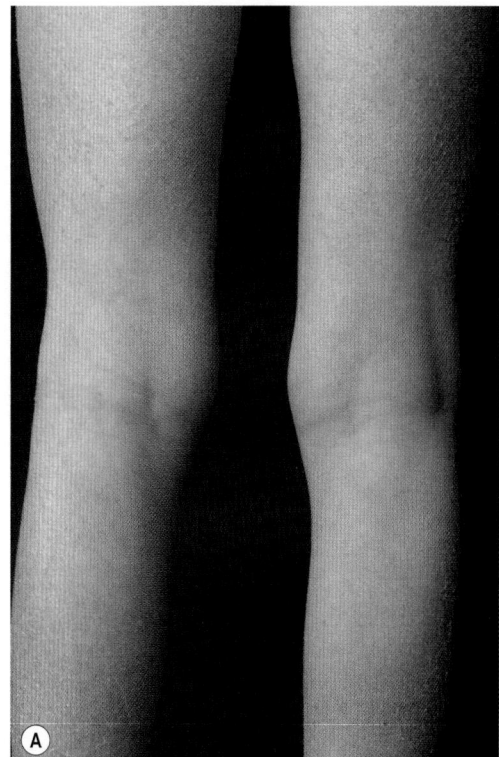

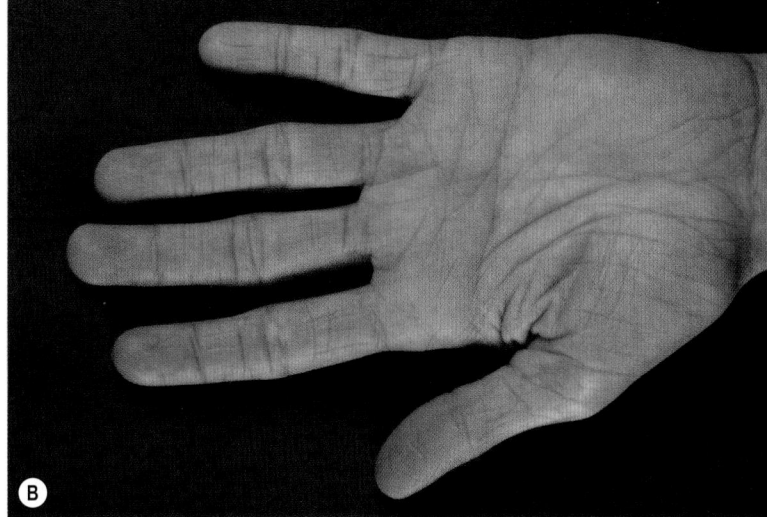

Fig. 3.2
(**A**) Ichthyosis vulgaris: fine scaling, particularly involving the extremities and characteristically sparing the flexures. (**B**) Palms show typically increased skin markings.

feature is a thin or absent granular cell layer (*Fig. 3.3*).[11,12,13] Regional variation in the thickness and/or presence of the granular cell layer may occur and therefore it is best to take the biopsy from a site of maximal scaling. The lesions of keratosis pilaris show dilated follicles containing large keratin plugs. In the upper dermis a mild perivascular lymphocytic infiltrate may be present. When ichthyosis vulgaris is associated with atopic dermatitis, parakeratosis and other signs of a spongiotic dermatitis can be found.

Differential diagnosis

The histologic differential diagnosis includes other diseases characterized by orthohyperkeratosis and a reduced or absent stratum granulosum (*Table 3.3*).

X-linked (recessive) ichthyosis

Clinical features

Also known as steroid sulfatase (STS) deficiency and ichthyosis nigricans, this X-linked, recessively inherited disorder has an incidence of 1:6000 male births.[1-3] The disease is exceedingly rarely expressed in females.[4] The disease may present at birth with dramatic but transient scaling of the skin, and this is sometimes misdiagnosed as autosomal recessive congenital ichthyosis. At the age of 2 to 6 months large and dark scales develop on the trunk, the extensor surface of the extremities, the scalp, the preauricular region, and the neck (*Fig. 3.4*).[2] Mild involvement of the flexures is present (*Fig. 3.5*),[1] but visible scaling may spare humid flexural regions of the skin.

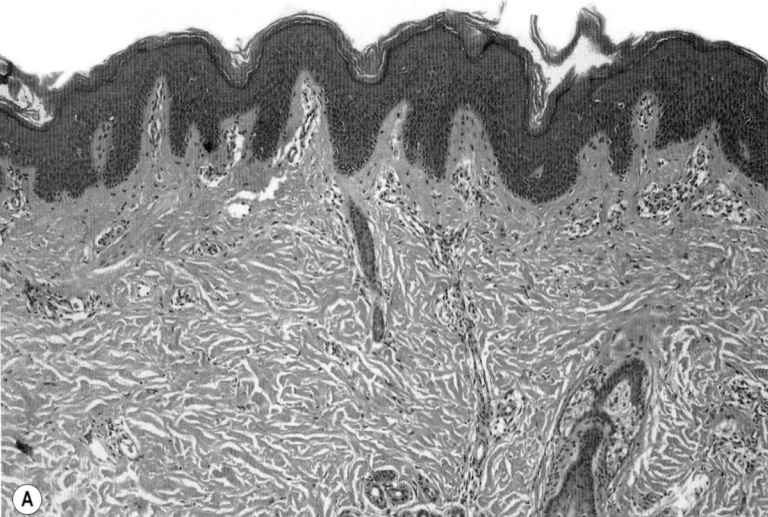

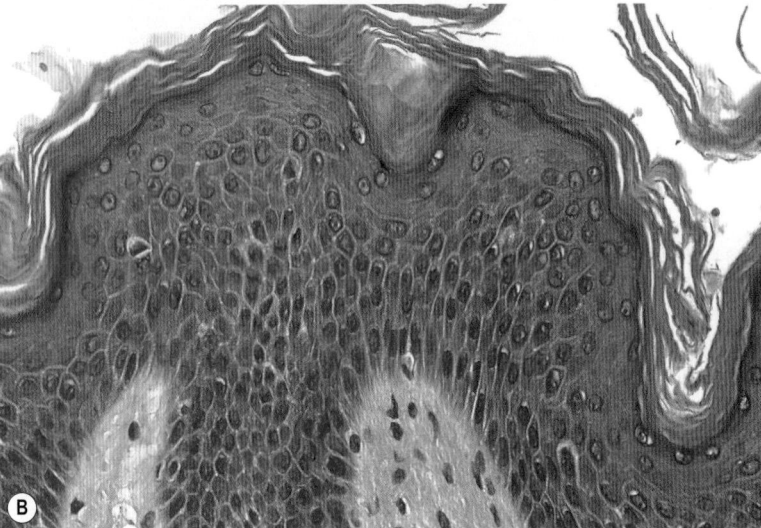

Fig. 3.3
(**A**, **B**) Ichthyosis vulgaris: there is orthohyperkeratosis with characteristic absence of the granular cell layer.

Table 3.3
Histologic patterns of ichthyotic skin disorders

Orthohyperkeratosis and stratum granulosum reduced or absent
Ichthyosis vulgaris (w/o atopic dermatitis)
Acquired ichthyosis-like condition
Pityriasis rotunda
Refsum syndrome
Dorfman-Chanarin syndrome
Trichothiodystrophy syndrome
Conradi-Hünermann-Happle syndrome
Orthohyperkeratosis and stratum granulosum well developed
XR-ichthyosis
AR-congenital ichthyosis
Harlequin ichthyosis
Acquired ichthyosis-like condition
DDx lichen simplex chronicus
Hyperkeratosis with ortho- and parakeratosis and prominent stratum granulosum
AD-lamellar ichthyosis
Harlequin ichthyosis
Sjögren-Larsson syndrome
Erythrokeratodermas and other connexin mutations (HID/KID)
Loricrin-keratoderma
KLICK syndrome
Acquired ichthyosis-like condition
DDx inflammatory skin disease
Epidermolytic hyperkeratosis
Bullous ichthyotic erythroderma Brocq
Annular epidermolytic ichthyosis
Ichthyosis bullosa Siemens
Epidermal nevi
Epidermolytic acanthoma/leukoplakia
Epidermolytic palmoplantar keratoses
Incidental finding
Perinuclear vacuoles and binucleated keratinocytes
With parakeratosis:
Congenital reticular ichthyosiform erythroderma
With orthokeratosis:
Ichthyosis hystrix Curth-Macklin
DDx epidermolytic ichthyoses (keratin clumps!)
Follicular hyperkeratosis
Keratosis pilaris, lichen spinulosus, phrynoderma
Keratosis pilaris atrophicans
Ichthyosis vulgaris with follicular keratosis
AR-congenital ichthyosis
Sjögren-Larsson syndrome
Ichthyosis follicularis with alopecia and photophobia
Congenital atrichia
HID/KID syndrome
Hereditary mucoepithelial dysplasia
Pachyonychia congenita
Ectodermal dysplasias
Darier disease
Pityriasis rubra pilaris
Psoriasis-like features
Comèl-Netherton syndrome
Peeling skin disease
Severe dermatitis-multiple allergies-metabolic wasting syndrome (SAM)
Annular epidermolytic ichthyosis
CHILD syndrome
Papillon-Lefèvre syndrome
DDx psoriasis vulgaris and dermatophytosis

Differentiation from ichthyosis vulgaris can be difficult as one-third of patients present with fine, light scales and the flexures may be spared in both diseases (*Fig. 3.6*). The palms and soles are usually unaffected and keratosis pilaris is not a feature, except if there is a concomitant deficiency of filaggrin and STS. Involvement of the trunk and neck often gives the skin a dirty appearance. Lesions may improve or disappear in warm weather.[2] The hair, nails, and teeth are not affected.

Corneal opacities due to comma-shaped deposits in the posterior capsule of Descemet membrane or corneal stroma without visual impairment (*Fig. 3.7*), are characteristic and may be detected in female carriers.[5] Inadequate cervical dilatation may lead to prolonged delivery of affected male newborns. Undescended testes and hypogonadism can be a feature in as many as 25% of affected patients.[6–9] Rarely, testicular cancer has been documented.[6] Interestingly, studies on STS deficiency have revealed an association with attention-deficit hyperactivity disorder (ADHD), and disorders within the spectrum of autism seem to occur more frequently.[10]

Pathogenesis and histologic features

The disease is associated with a deficiency of the microsomal enzyme steroid sulfatase/STS (sterol sulfate sulfohydrolase/arylsulphatase C).[11] Absence of this enzyme is associated with persistence of the sulfate moiety on a number of sulfated steroid hormones and cholesterol sulfate.[3]

X-linked recessive ichthyosis is characterized by a raised serum cholesterol sulfate.[12] The corneocytes contain excess cholesterol 3-sulfate and diminished free sterol,[13] This may lead to persistence of the lipid contents

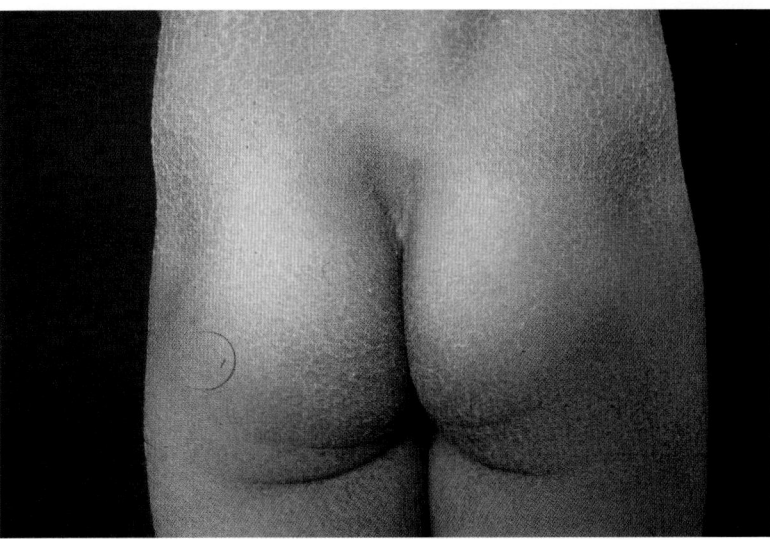

Fig. 3.4
X-linked recessive ichthyosis: many patients show large, confluent, and dark scales. By courtesy of the Institute of Dermatology, London, UK.

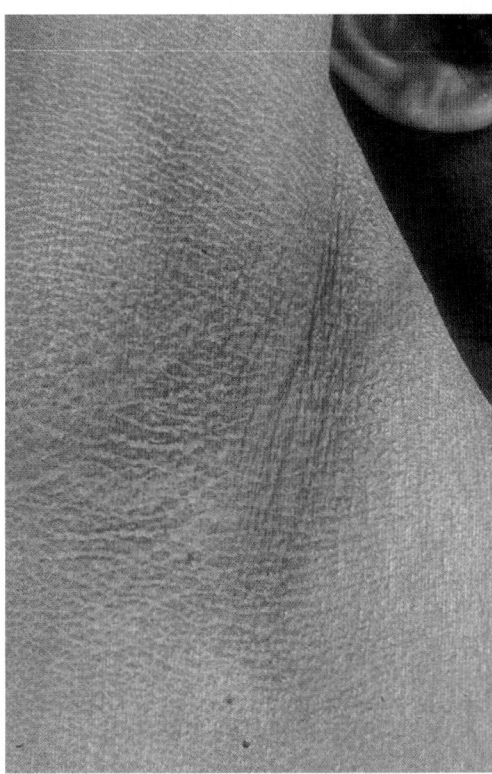

Fig. 3.5
X-linked ichthyosis: involvement of the flexures is a feature that allows differentiation form ichthyosis vulgaris. By courtesy of the Institute of Dermatology, London, UK.

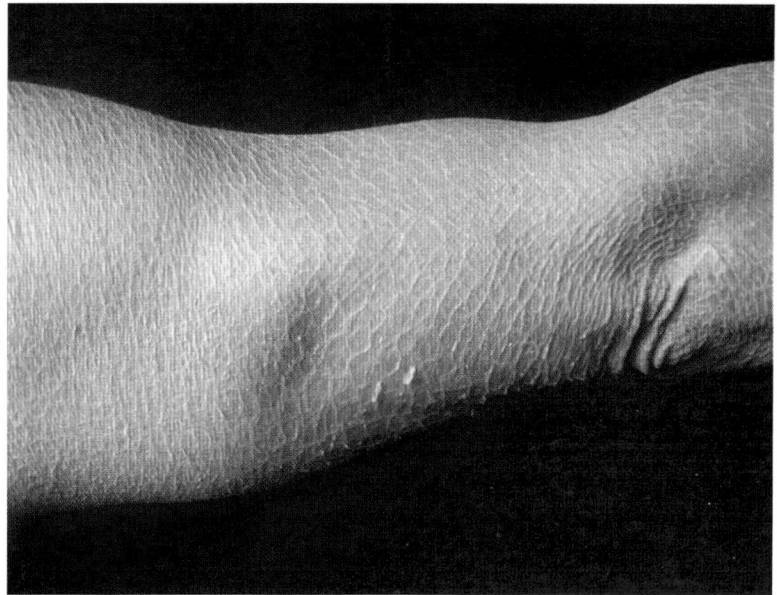

Fig. 3.6
X-linked recessive ichthyosis: some patients show light-gray scales.

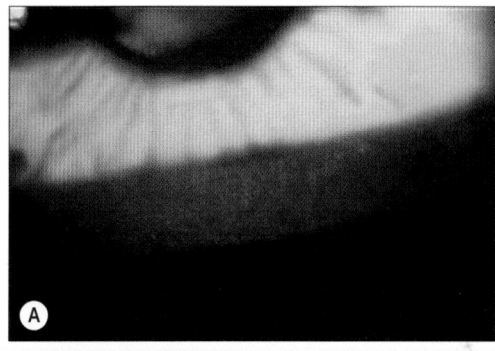

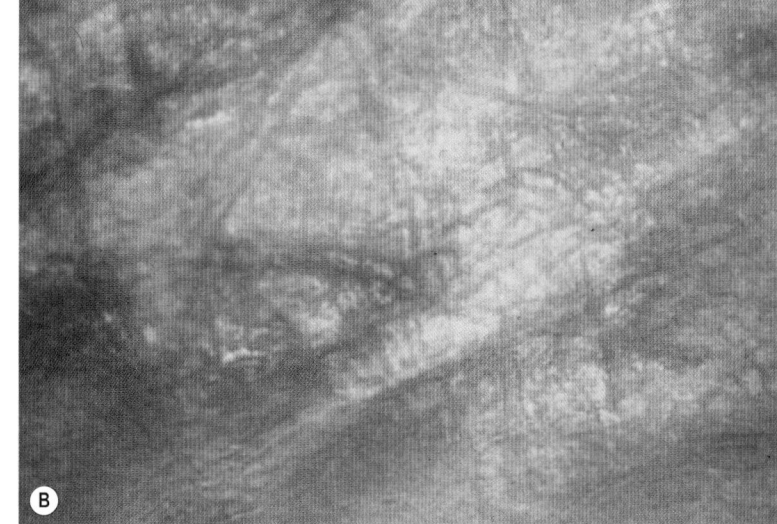

Fig. 3.7
(**A**) Sex-linked ichthyosis: characteristic linear opacities at the level of Descemet membrane. Slit-lamp photograph. (**B**) Same lesion viewed by specular microscopy. By courtesy of R.J. Buckley, MD, Moorfield's Eye Hospital, London, UK.

of the membrane-coating granules and hence increased or persistent adhesion between adjacent keratin plates in the stratum corneum. Beyond that, increased amounts of cholesterol sulfate may inhibit the epidermal serine protease activity, which results in retention of corneodesmosomes leading to less shedding of scales and retention hyperkeratosis.[14] Steroid sulfatase deficiency can be detected using the patient's peripheral leukocytes and cultured skin fibroblasts. Diagnosis may also be confirmed by lipoprotein electrophoresis, which shows increased mobility of low-density and very low-density beta-lipoproteins in addition to the steroid sulfatase deficiency.[15,16]

Technologies such as comparative genomic hybridization/comparative microarray analysis (CMA) allow rapid diagnosis in cases with large deletions.[17] Carrier status can also be confirmed by fluorescent in situ hybridization (FISH) analysis.[18] Standard sequencing techniques are used to identify a point mutation that is the cause of the disease in approximately 10% of patients. Severity of this form of ichthyosis may be aggravated by a concomitant filaggrin mutation.[19,20]

Lesional skin shows compact orthohyperkeratosis and slight acanthosis associated with a granular cell layer, which may be normal or increased in thickness (Fig. 3.8).[21,22] Keratohyalin granules show no abnormality.

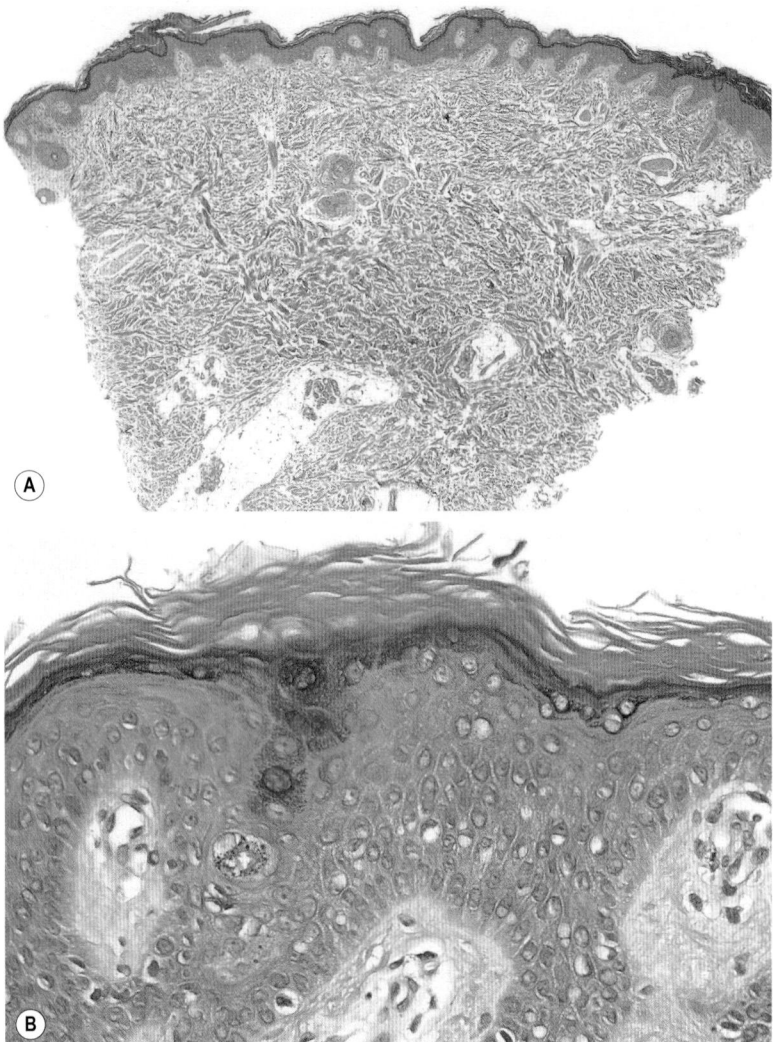

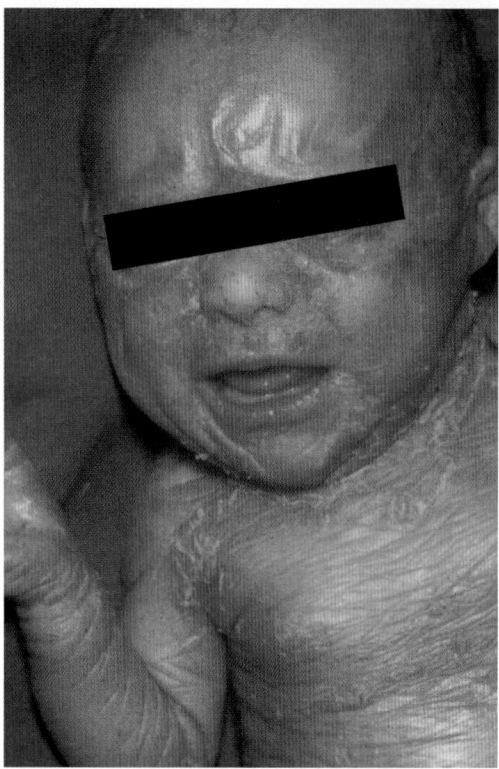

Fig. 3.8
(**A**, **B**) X-linked recessive ichthyosis: there is orthohyperkeratosis and mild acanthosis. The granular cell layer is normal.

Fig. 3.9
Autosomal recessive congenital ichthyosis: the collodion membrane is best seen on the forehead. There is scaling and erythema on the trunk. By courtesy of R.A. Marsden, MD, St George's Hospital, London, UK.

Follicular plugging is not a feature. Paradoxically, biopsies of thicker scales can show massive orthohyperkeratosis with reduction of the granular layer and a thin epidermis, causing confusion with ichthyosis vulgaris. A discrete lymphocytic perivascular inflammatory cell infiltrate may be evident.

Ultrastructural features include a high number of transitional cells and an abnormal persistence of desmosomal disks in the horny layer while keratohyalin granules are normal. An increased melanosome transfer accounts for the dark appearance of the scales.[23]

Autosomal recessive congenital ichthyoses

Autosomal recessive congenital ichthyoses (ARCI) are a group of monogenetic, nonsyndromic disorders presenting at birth with generalized hyperkeratosis and scaling (ichthyosis congenita) (see *Table 3.1*).[1] ARCI include lamellar ichthyosis (LI), congenital ichthyosiform erythroderma (CIE), bathing suit ichthyosis, self-improving congenital ichthyosis (SICI) or self-healing collodion baby (SHCB), and the most severe form, harlequin ichthyosis.[2,3] In Europe ARCI have an estimated prevalence of 1.6 : 100 000.[4,5]

At birth, most patients with ARCI are encased in a thick 'collodion', a platelike shell of keratosis (*Figs 3.9* and *3.10*) and suffer from ectropion and everted lips.[6] The shiny parchment-like membrane cracks after birth and usually peels off within the first 4 weeks of life. While the term 'collodion baby' is most often applied to cases of ARCI, similar appearances are sometimes found in a number of other disorders, such as Gaucher syndrome type 2, trichothiodystrophy, Conradi-Hünermann-Happle syndrome,

Sjögren-Larsson syndrome and sometimes Netherton syndrome. Hence, collodion baby is a clinical description but not a disease. Still, the majority of these conditions develop into one of the ARCI subtypes, including SICI or SHCB.[2,7]

In the nonerythrodermic phenotype of congenital ichthyosis, the so-called 'lamellar ichthyosis', the scales are large, dark, and platelike, and cover the entire body, including the palms, soles, scalp, and flexures (*Fig. 3.11*).[8-11] Fissuring of the hands and feet may occur and the skin around the joints may become verrucous. Many patients suffer from severe hypo- or anhidrosis with risk of hyperthermia, an important clinical symptom with great impact on the daily life of the patient.[8] Nail dystrophy, hair involvement (scarring alopecia), severe ectropion (up to 80% of patients), and eclabium are characteristic (*Fig. 3.12*). The ectropion is of the cicatricial type and develops as a consequence of excessive dryness and associated contracture of the anterior lamella of the eyelid. Complications include corneal ulceration, vascularization, and corneal scarring with eventual blindness.[11] Primary conjunctival lesions have been described including keratinization, hyper- and parakeratosis, and papilla development. The teeth are not affected.[10]

In contrast, other individuals show a more pronounced erythroderma with fine white scaling (congenital ichthyosiform erythroderma, CIE). While platelike scales may be seen on the extensor surfaces of the legs, the scalp, face, upper extremities, and trunk are covered with fine white scaling (*Figs 3.13–3.16*).[11] Mild ectropion and eclabium may be present. Some variants are associated with severe palmoplantar keratoderma (PPK), e g., yellowish focal palmoplantar keratoderma in *ichthyin* deficiency. Exceptionally, CIE has been associated with retinitis pigmentosa.[12] There is an increased risk of developing skin cancer including basal and squamous cell carcinoma.[13]

Genetics, pathogenesis, and phenotype

The most common cause of LI is transglutaminase-1 (TG-1) deficiency, which accounts for 30–40% of cases. TG-1 plays a role in the assembly of the cornified envelope by catalyzing calcium-dependent cross-linking of proteins, such as involucrin, loricrin, and proline-rich proteins and by binding omega-hydroxy ceramides to proteins such as involucrin, a major

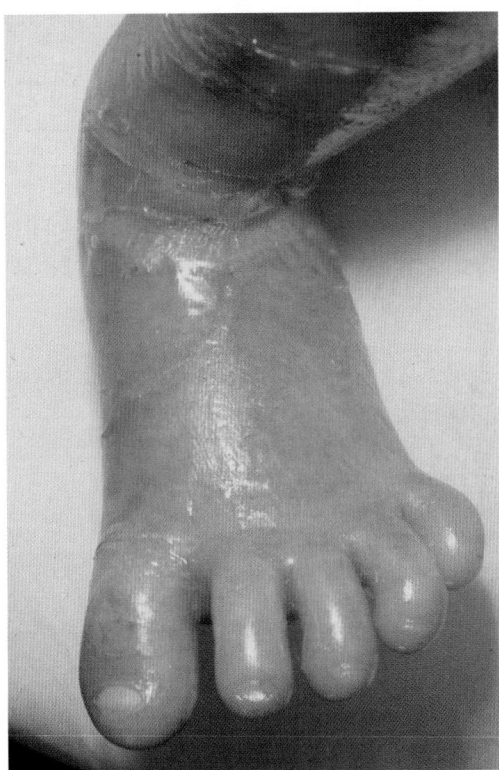

Fig. 3.10
Autosomal recessive congenital ichthyosis: note the erythema. The skin is shiny, taut, and shows fissuring around the anterior aspect of the ankle. By courtesy of D. Atherton, MD, Children's Hospital at Great Ormond Street, London, UK.

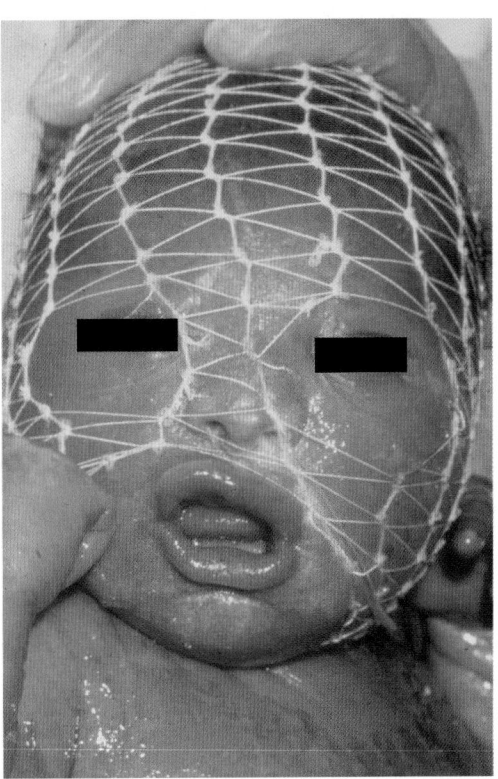

Fig. 3.12
Autosomal recessive lamellar ichthyosis: in this infant, there is gross ectropion and eclabion. By courtesy of D. Atherton, MD, Children's Hospital at Great Ormond Street, London, UK.

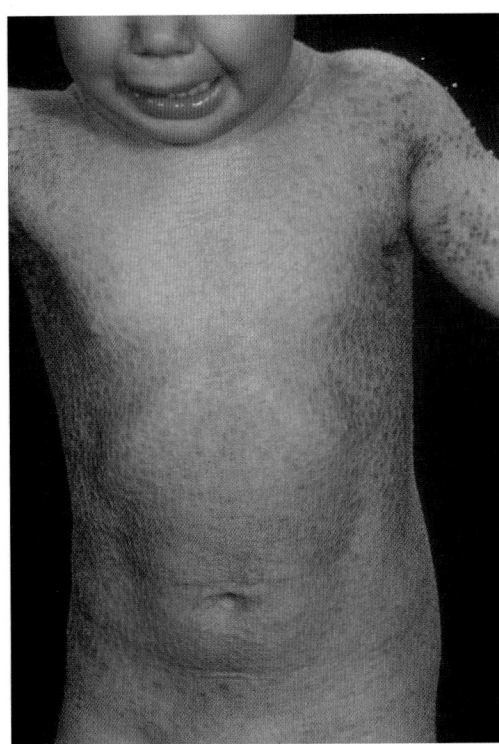

Fig. 3.11
Autosomal recessive lamellar ichthyosis: note the widespread and prominent large dark brown scales. By courtesy of D. Atherton, MD, Children's Hospital at Great Ormond Street, London, UK.

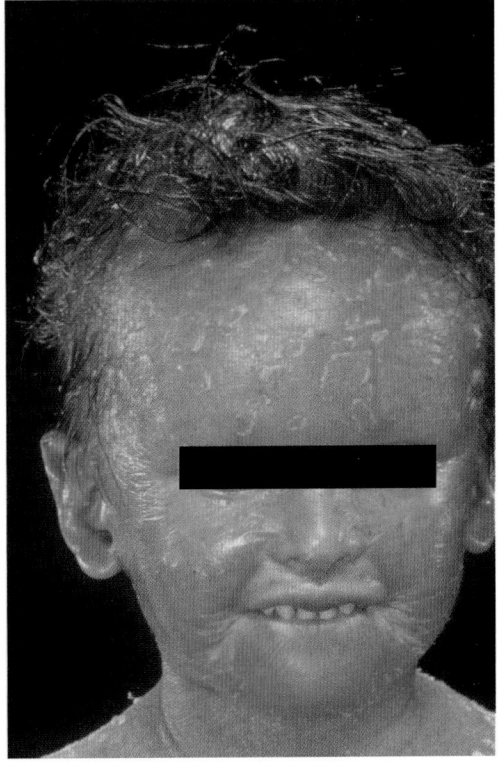

Fig. 3.13
Autosomal recessive congenital ichthyosis: there is intense erythema and fine scaling is also present. The scalp hair is sparse and the eyebrows are absent. By courtesy of D. Atherton, MD, Children's Hospital at Great Ormond Street, London, UK.

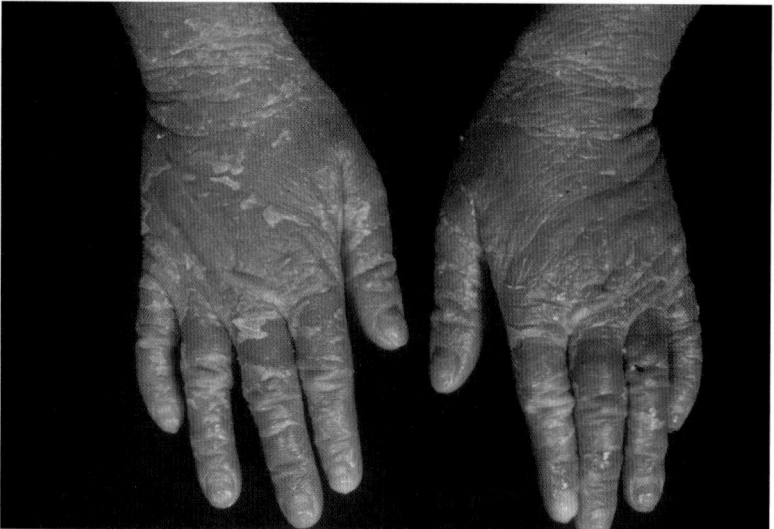

Fig. 3.14
Autosomal recessive congenital ichthyoses: there is marked erythema with severe scaling. Blistering is not seen in this variant of ichthyosis. By courtesy of D. Atherton, MD, Children's Hospital at Great Ormond Street, London, UK.

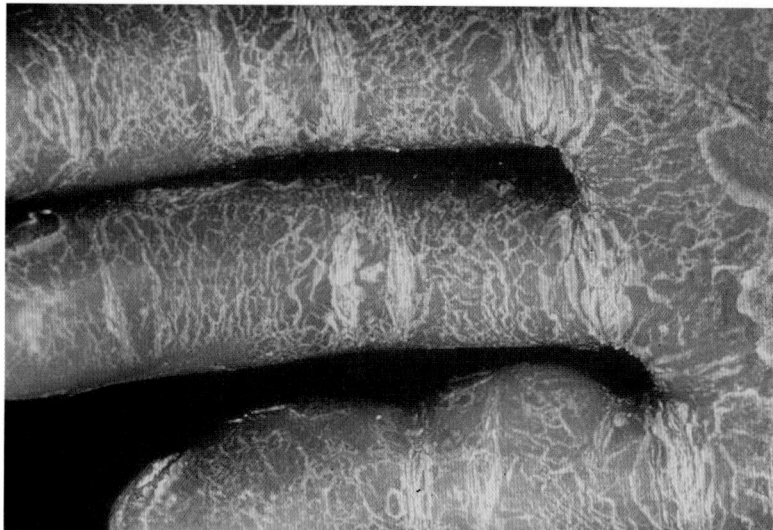

Fig. 3.16
Autosomal recessive congenital ichthyosis: there is severe palmar involvement and constriction bands are evident. By courtesy of the Institute of Dermatology, London, UK.

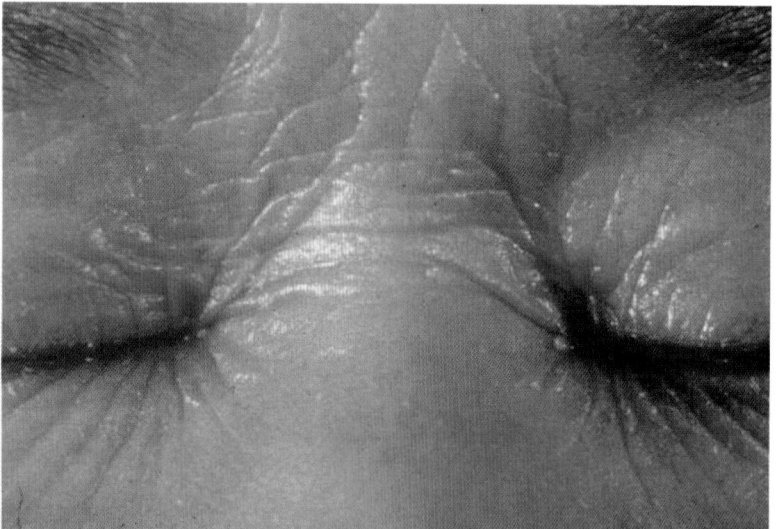

Fig. 3.15
Autosomal recessive congenital ichthyosis: there is intensive erythema and fine scaling. By courtesy of the Institute of Dermatology, London, UK.

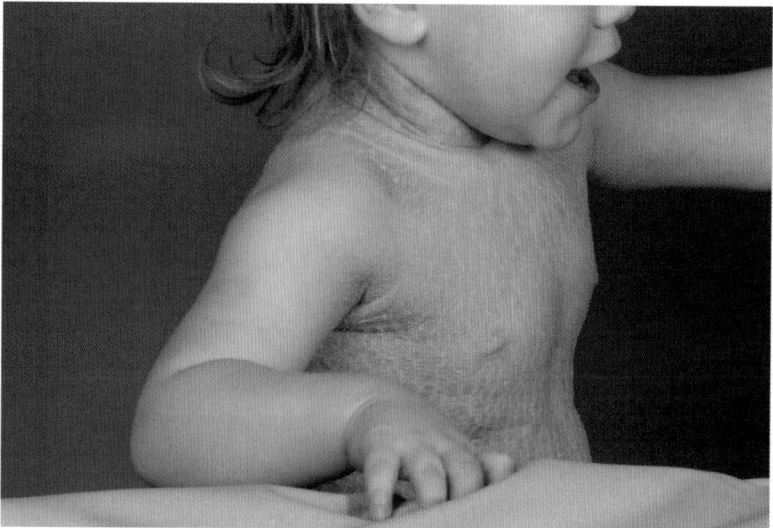

Fig. 3.17
Bathing suit ichthyosis: areas with higher skin temperature are severely affected giving a bathing suit-like appearance; those with lower skin temperature are almost completely spared.

step in connecting the lipid envelope with the cornified envelope.[14,15] Mutations in the gene of TG-1 (*TGM1*) result in markedly diminished or lost enzyme activity and/or protein.[16–20] Since conventional enzyme assays and mutational analyzes are tedious, an assay for the rapid screening of TG activity using covalent incorporation of biotinylated substrate peptides into skin cryostat sections has been developed.[21] Coupled with immunohistochemical assays using TG-1 antibodies, this allows valid identification of TG-1 deficiency.

Patients with *TGM1* mutations mostly present with classical LI including ectropion, alopecia, or small and deformed ears. Some variants of *TGM1* mutations are associated with distinct clinical features, e.g., in self-healing collodion baby the TG-1 enzyme is pressure-sensitive so that while in utero the enzyme cannot function properly, it resumes normal function after birth. About 10% of collodion babies fall into this group.[7] In bathing suit ichthyosis the mutations of TG-1 appear to be temperature sensitive so that the face and extremities are almost completely spared apart from skin areas overlying blood vessels (*Fig. 3.17*). Digital thermography has validated a striking correlation between warmer body areas and the presence of scaling, suggesting a decisive influence of skin temperature. In situ TG-1 testing in skin of bathing suit ichthyosis patients has also demonstrated a marked decrease of enzyme activity when the temperature is increased from 25 to 37°C.[22]

Two epidermal lipoxygenases associated with the genes *ALOXE3* and *ALOX12B* play a crucial role in the hepoxilin pathway. The defect is believed to have an impact on secretion of lamellar bodies (LBs) resulting in impaired formation of intercellular lipids in the stratum corneum.[23–25] Lipoxigenase mutations are often associated with the CIE phenotype, and show a striking palmoplantar hyperlinearity that should not be confused with that of ichthyosis vulgaris. Other features are pruritus and reduced sweating.[24] Biochemical measurement of lipoxygenase activity is available only in specialized research laboratories.[24]

Another common genetic subtype of ARCI affects the *NIPAL4* gene that encodes for ichthyin.[26,29] This protein has been described to localize to desmosomes and keratins and to interact with fatty acid transporter protein 4, which is defective in ichthyosis prematurity syndrome.[27,28,30] *NIPAL4* mutations may lead to a CIE/LI overlapping phenotype with mild ectropion, clubbing of the nails and – most characteristically – a focal yellowish palmoplantar keratoderma developing in childhood.[30]

Mutations in ARCI of late onset involve the acid lipase gene *LIPN* that plays a role in triglyceride metabolism of the epidermis. LIPN mutations seem to cause a late-onset form of ichthyosis at the age of 5 years, so that it is not formally a congenital ichthyosis.[31]

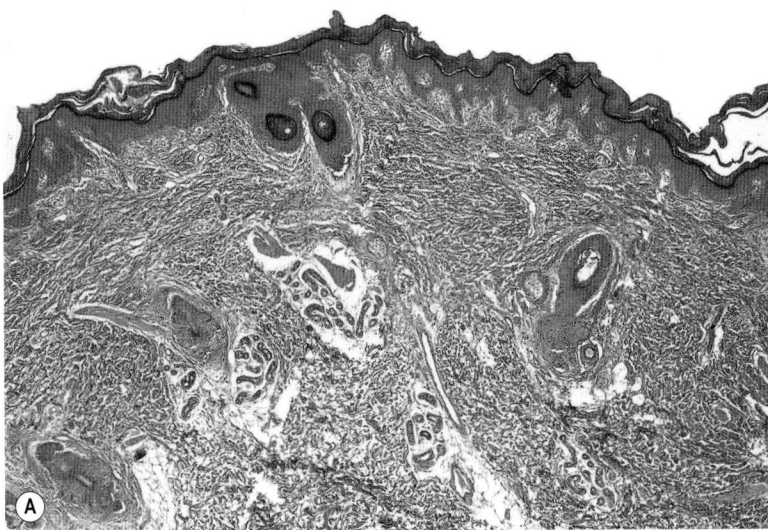
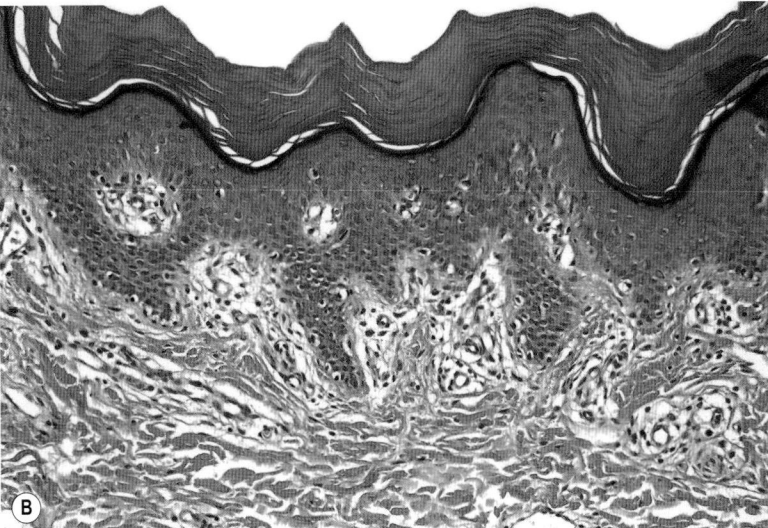

Fig. 3.18
Autosomal recessive congenital ichthyosis: (**A**) there is very marked orthohyperkeratosis and the epidermis shows papillomatosis; (**B**) the stratum granulosum is preserved. Note a mild lymphocytic infiltrate.

Other mutations in ARCI been detected in the *CYP4F2* gene encoding a cytochrome P450 polypeptide, *CERS3* gene encoding a ceramide synthase, and *PNPLA1*, a member of the patatin-like phospholipase family.[32–35] Moreover, less severe missense mutations in the *ABCA12* gene are associated with LI or CIE. Of note, nonfunctional severe nonsense mutations of the same gene are responsible for the far more severe ichthyosis form of harlequin ichthyosis (see below).[36,37]

Histologic features

Histologically, the epidermis in ARCI shows marked orthohyperkeratosis, mostly of the compact type (which may be extreme in the collodion baby) and mild acanthosis with a normal or thickened granular cell layer (*Fig. 3.18*). The hyperkeratosis is much less marked in erythrodermic than in nonerythrodermic forms. Epidermal papillomatosis associated with a psoriasiform appearance has also been documented. A perivascular lymphocytic infiltrate is occasionally a feature.[38] Dilatation and tortuosity of the dermal capillaries is sometimes evident. Follicular hyperkeratosis may rarely be seen. The histologic changes cannot be correlated with the underlying genetic defect.

Ultrastructural studies show a variety of features, including defective development of the cornified cell envelopes and electron-dense debris adjacent to the plasma membranes, lipid vacuoles, increased numbers of small and dysmorphic LBs, or membrane packages.[39] Cholesterol clefts are found in TG-1 defects.[40] Abnormal LBs and elongated membranes in the stratum granulosum indicate NIPAL4 deficiency classified as ARCI electron microscopy (EM) type III.[41] However, other ARCI subtypes lack specific ultrastructural features. Special techniques with frozen sections or osmium tetroxide and ruthenium tetroxide postfixation allow for an advanced EM diagnostic of ARCI.[42] Prenatal diagnosis of LI can be achieved by fetoscopy and biopsy.[43]

Harlequin ichthyosis

Clinical features

Harlequin ichthyosis (harlequin fetus, ichthyosis fetalis, ichthyosis congenita gravis) is a distinct severe subtype of autosomal recessive congenital ichthyosis, where babies are born with a fissured 'armor-plated' skin (*Fig. 3.19*).[1–4] Characteristically, ectropion and eclabium are very severe. Constricting bands of digits can lead to autoamputation; ears and nose may be malformed.[1] The harlequin fetus still has a high mortality due to infections, and respiratory and feeding difficulties accompanied by excessive fluid loss.[3] However, treatment with retinoids and improved intensive care have certainly improved the prognosis and quality of life. Surviving neonates develop a severe erythroderma reminiscent of CIE, and there are intermediate cases that show considerable improvement of the skin compared with the initial dramatic presentation.[5] Antenatal diagnosis is possible by genetic analysis as well as electron microscopy of fetal skin biopsy (fetoscopy).[6,7]

Pathogenesis and histologic features

This very rare form of ichthyosis is due to a dramatic loss of function of the LBs, which results from nonsense mutations in the *ABCA12* gene.[8] Less severe missense mutations are associated with LI or CIE. Intermediate forms are possible.[9,10] The *ABCA12* gene product belongs to the ATP-binding cassette (ABC) transporter family that encompass a variety of membrane proteins involved in the energy-dependent transport across membranes. In the epidermis, ABCA12 plays an important role in the LB function. As such it is responsible for the transfer of glucosylceramides, which are essential lipids for epidermal barrier formation. Moreover, it transports proteases such as kallikrein 5, 7, or 14 and secretes them into the intercellular space in the stratum corneum.[11] These proteases play an important role in desquamation by degrading corneodesmosomes, thus leading to retention hyperkeratosis.[12]

Histologically, the epidermis is pale and characterized by massive hyperkeratosis (sometimes with lipid deposits) associated with a normal or absent granular cell layer (*Fig. 3.20*). The hair follicles are usually affected first, during the second trimester.[2,7] Parakeratosis may also sometimes be evident.[13] Acanthosis is often marked and papillomatosis is sometimes a feature. A sparse mixed inflammatory cell infiltrate can be present in the superficial dermis.[7]

Ultrastructurally, the harlequin fetus is associated with deficient or morphologically abnormal LBs (including concentrically lamellated forms) and deficient intercellular lipid lamellae within the stratum corneum.[1,2,13] Small vesicles, devoid of internal lamellation, may be present in the granular cell layer (and retained in the stratum corneum), but show no association with the keratinocyte cell membranes as is typical of normal LBs.[1,13]

Immunohistochemical evidence suggests that these vesicles represent abnormal LBs characterized by an inability to discharge their lipid contents into the intercellular space. Keratin and filaggrin expression have also been shown to be defective.[2] In the harlequin fetus, the keratinocytes may display the hyperproliferative keratins K6 and K16 and show an inability to convert profilaggrin to filaggrin.[2]

Autosomal dominant lamellar ichthyosis

Clinical features

Autosomal dominant LI is characterized by generalized scaling with palmoplantar keratoderma.[1] Patients may present as a collodion baby. They are later covered by diffuse dark-gray scales that involve all areas of the body, but are most prominent on the extensor surfaces (*Fig. 3.21*). Backs of the hands and feet are characterized by lichenification. There may be massive

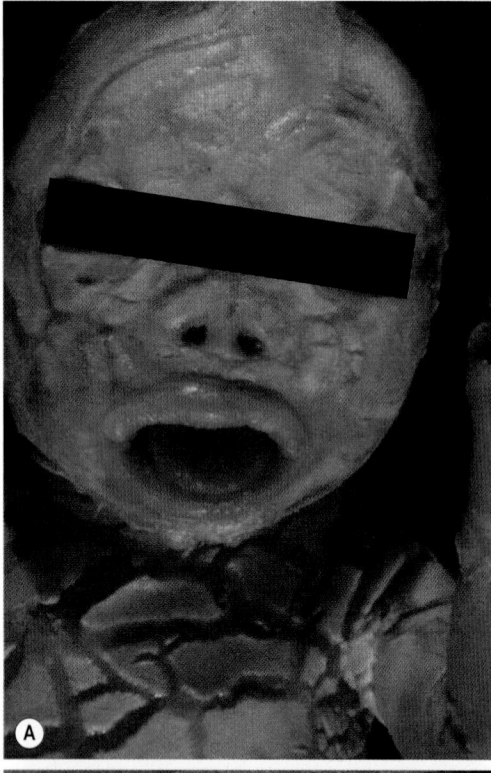

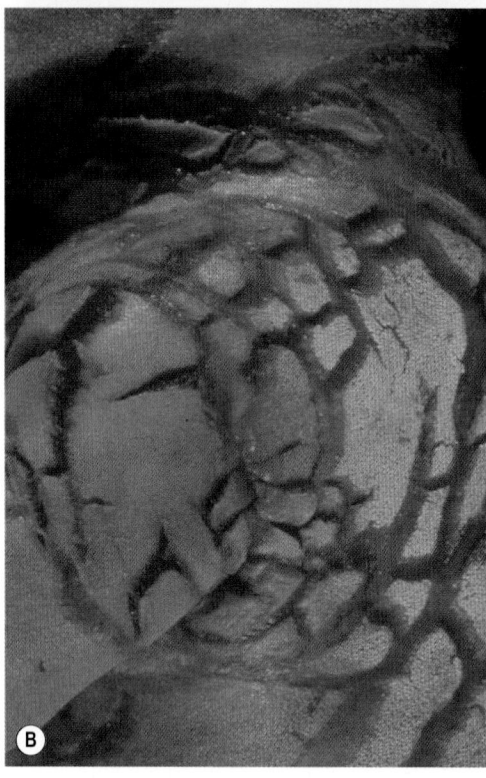

Fig. 3.19
(**A, B**) Harlequin ichthyosis: the most extreme form of congenital ichthyosis. The scales are very thick and are often referred to as armor-plating. By Courtesey of Sabine Köhler, Stanford University.

plantar hyperkeratosis with thick, yellow scales. The palms are usually only minimally involved and show accentuated markings.[1]

Pathogenesis and histologic features

This disorder appears to be genetically and clinically heterogeneous and of variable penetrance. Its genetic defect has not been identified. Biochemically, an abnormal lipid profile has been detected in the scales.[2]

Histologically, there is acanthosis, papillomatosis, and compact orthohyperkeratosis with focal parakeratosis that, paradoxically, is associated with a thickened stratum granulosum (*Fig. 3.22*).[2]

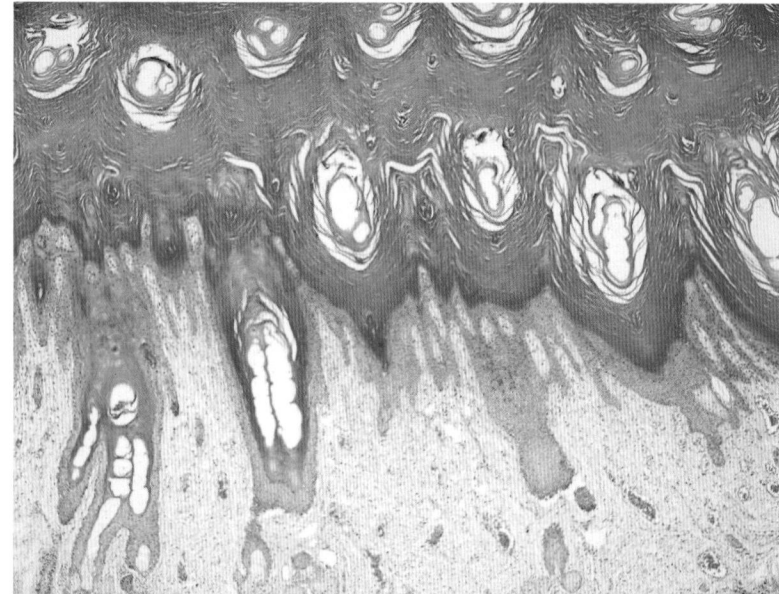

Fig. 3.20
Harlequin ichthyosis: there is massive hyperkeratosis and papillomatous and pale staining epidermis with thinning of the granular cell layer. The dilated spaces in the stratum corneum represent affected hair follicles and sweat ducts. By courtesy of S. Köhler, MD, Stanford University, USA.

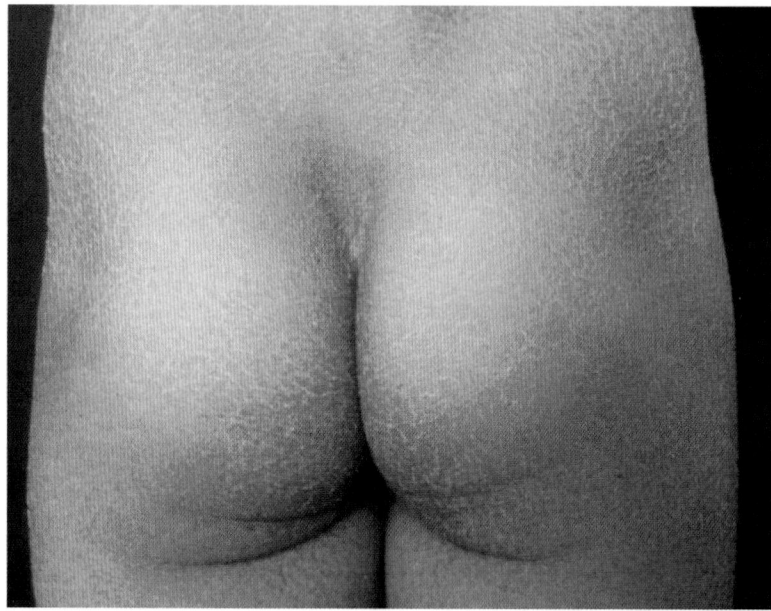

Fig. 3.21
Autosomal dominant lamellar ichthyosis: large, dark-gray scales on the entire body. By courtesy of H. Traupe, MD, Münster, Germany.

Electron microscopy shows a high number of transitional cells and a spongy appearance of the keratohyaline granules.[2]

Differential diagnosis

The differential diagnosis includes lichen simplex chronicus which, however, differs by the presence of inflammatory changes and fibrosis of the papillary dermis (see *Table 3.3*).

Keratinopathic ichthyoses

According to the Sorèze Consensus conference in 2009, keratinopathic ichthyoses have been defined as a group of rare ichthyoses, which are caused by mutations in one of the keratin genes, namely keratin 1 (*KRT1*), keratin 10 (*KRT10*) or keratin 2 (*KRT2*). The old term 'bullous congenital ichthyosiform erythroderma (of Brocq)' has been renamed epidermolytic ichthyosis

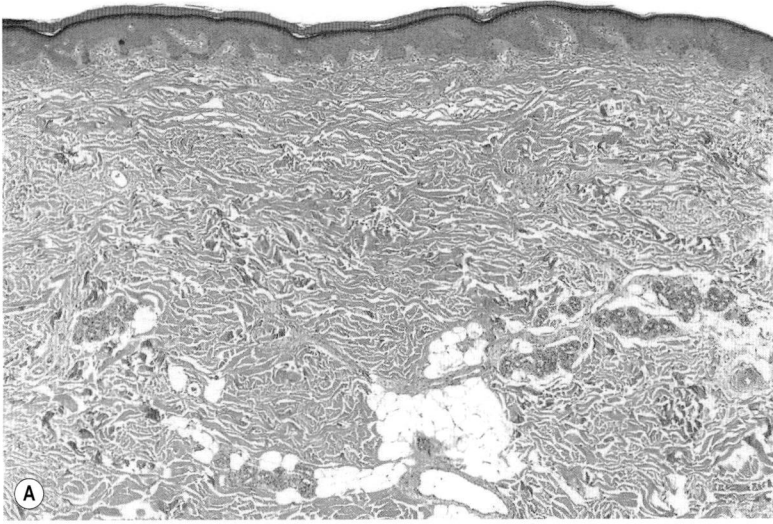

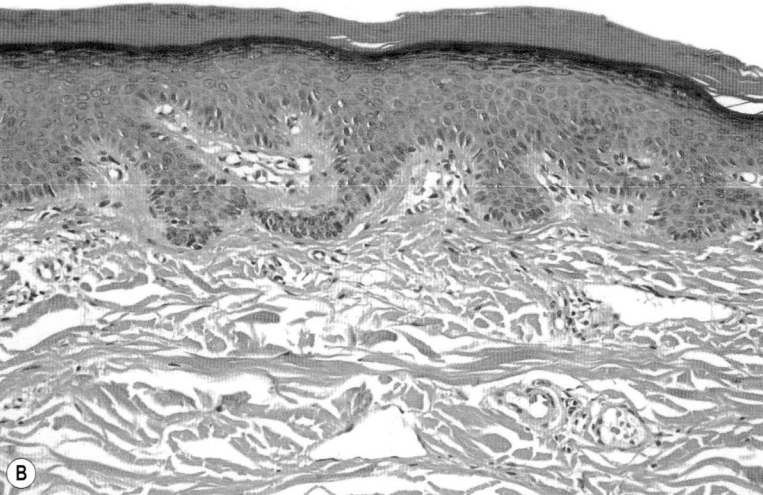

Fig. 3.22
(**A**, **B**) Autosomal dominant lamellar ichthyosis: there is a marked compact hyperkeratosis with focal parakeratosis and a prominent granular cell layer.

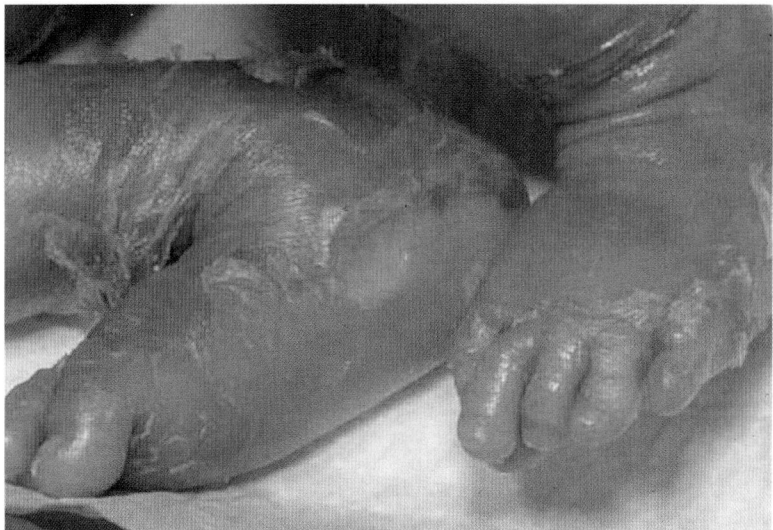

Fig. 3.23
Congenital bullous ichthyosiform erythroderma: close-up view of an infant showing intense erythema and blistering. By courtesy of M. Liang, MD, The Children's Hospital, Boston, USA.

(EI); the term superficial epidermolytic ichthyosis (SEI) refers to the *KRT2* associated subtype formerly known as 'ichthyosis bullosa of Siemens'. Moreover, there are distinct keratinopathic ichthyosis forms, such as congenital reticular ichthyosiform erythroderma (CRIE) (also known as ichthyosis en confettis), ichthyosis Curth-Macklin, autosomal recessive EI, and annular EI (see *Table 3.1*).[1]

In the skin, basal keratinocytes predominantly express keratin 5 and 14 while suprabasal cells switch to the expression of keratin 1 and 10. Keratin 2e is only expressed in the subcorneal layer. Keratin monomers form obligate heterodimers in pairs of acidic (type I) and basic (type II) keratins, which assemble into keratin intermediate filaments building a cytoskeleton for the structural stability and flexibility of epidermal cells. Mutations in the higher molecular weight keratins 1 or 10 lead to collapse of the keratin skeleton in suprabasal keratinocytes while mutations in keratin 2 affect the upper layers. As a result the keratinocytes appear pale and show perinuclear shell formation or eosinophilic clumps, the latter changes known as epidermolytic hyperkeratosis.[2–4] In these genodermatoses aggregation of the keratins is not permanent, but is inducible by pressure, high temperature, fever or skin infections. Epidermal sensitivity to hyperosmotic stress may be reduced by the chemical chaperone trimethylamine-N-oxide.[5] Keratin aggregates also induce inflammation via interaction with the ubiquitin-proteasome system, activated MAP kinases, and chaperones, such as HSP70.[7] Retinoids may interfere with collapse of the keratin skeleton in heat stressed keratinocytes with *KRT10* mutation.[6]

Epidermolytic hyperkeratosis as seen in some types of epidermal nevus is the result of somatic mutations in *KRT1* or *KRT10*.[8] A specific histologic diagnosis of this postzygotic mosaicism is mandatory as the patients risk developing full-blown keratinopathic ichthyosis.[9,10]

Differential diagnosis

Epidermolytic hyperkeratosis is a histopathologic pattern that is seen in many conditions, including keratinopathic ichthyoses, palmoplantar keratoderma of the epidermolytic type epidermal nevus (see epidermolytic epidermal nevus), epidermolytic acanthoma, and epidermolytic leukoplakia (see *Table 3.3*). Epidermolytic hyperkeratosis has been shown to be one of the many patterns in Grover disease.[11,12] It may also represent an incidental finding in normal, inflamed, and neoplastic skin (see incidental epidermolytic hyperkeratosis). Accurate clinical information is necessary to avoid diagnostic confusion.[13]

Epidermolytic ichthyosis

Epidermolytic ichthyosis (EI) is a rare autosomal dominant disease (incidence of 1 : 300 000 births), but it often arises by a spontaneous mutation.[1–3] At birth infants may show marked erythroderma and develop widespread blistering (*Fig. 3.23*). Therefore, a major differential diagnosis is epidermolysis bullosa. As the patient becomes older, the erythema and blistering become less apparent and, later, the disease is complicated by the development of verrucous hyperkeratosis, especially in the flexures (*Figs 3.24–3.28*). The descriptive word 'hystrix' (porcupine) for this cobblestone-like appearance of the skin has been abandoned. The nape, axilla, groin, and flexural folds are sites of predilection. Severe involvement of the scalp may simulate tinea capitis. Occasional blisters still arise at sites of mechanical stress, often in summer or when the patients have fever and skin infections. Many patients suffer from an offensive body odor. Neonates with EI have an increased risk of sepsis, fluid loss, and electrolyte imbalance.[1–2] Patients with *KRT1* mutation often develop severe, sometimes painful palmoplantar keratoderma. Nail dystrophy may also occur. Therapeutic administration of systemic retinoids may aggravate the complications, especially in patients with *KRT1* mutation.[3]

Pathogenesis and histologic features

First, it was shown that EI shows linkage to the keratin gene cluster either on chromosome 12q11–13 (type II keratin) or chromosome 17q21-q22 (type I keratin)[4–6] and that transgenic mice expressed a mutant *KRT10* gene.[7] This was followed by detection by direct DNA sequencing of a point mutation in *KRT1* or *KRT10* in a number of affected families.[8–14] Most mutations are missense mutations and clustered at the ends of the central helical rod domains. *KRT1* mutations typically affect palmoplantar skin. This region is

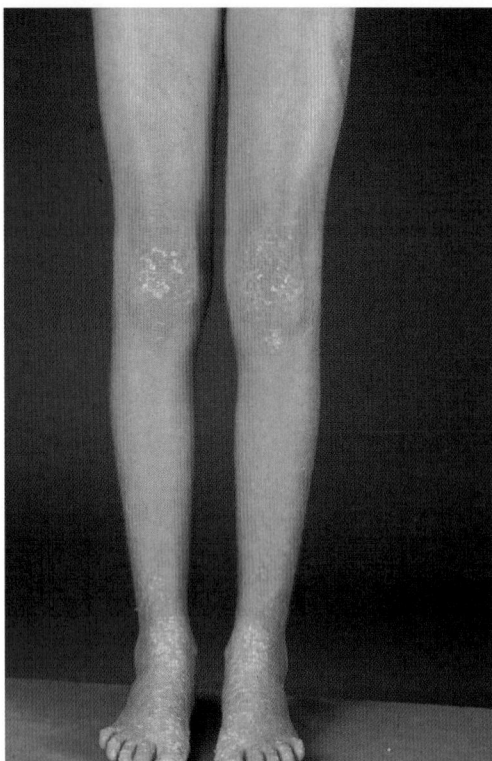

Fig. 3.24
Epidermolytic ichthyosis: hyperkeratosis and scales follow re-epithelialization of widespread blistering.

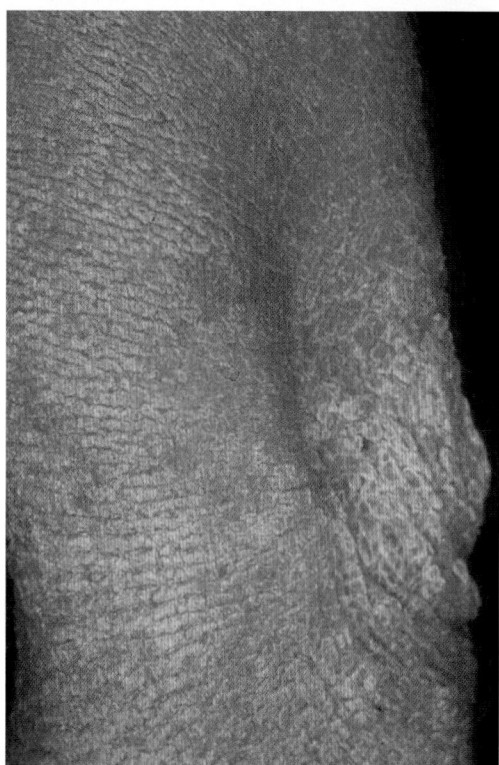

Fig. 3.26
Epidermolytic ichthyosis: same patient as *Figure 3.25*, showing elbow involvement with verrucous hyperkeratosis. By courtesy of the Institute of Dermatology, London, UK.

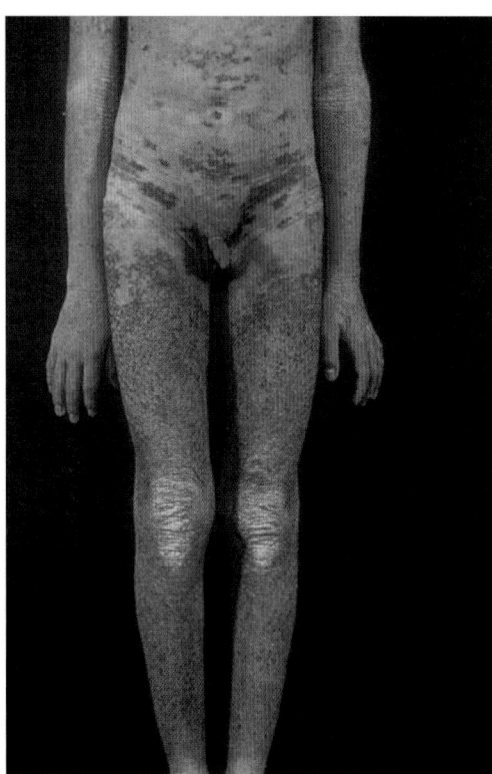

Fig. 3.25
Epidermolytic ichthyosis: adult showing very generalized scaling, particularly severe on the legs. By courtesy of the Institute of Dermatology, London, UK.

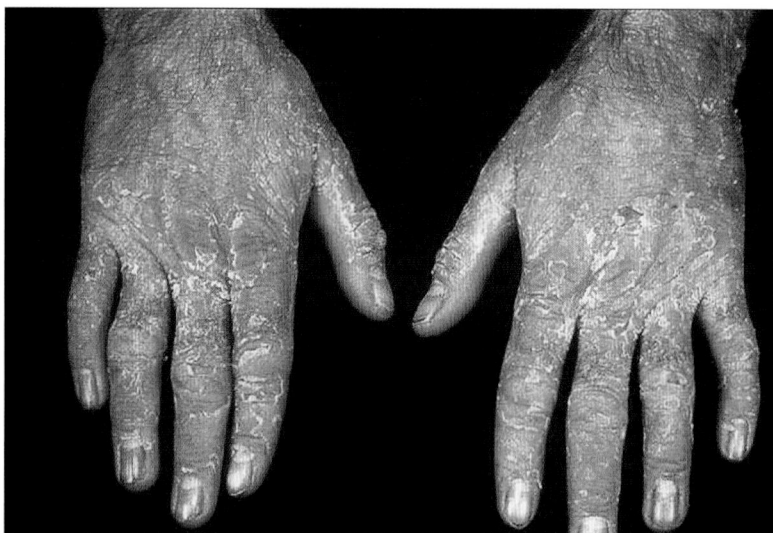

Fig. 3.27
Epidermolytic ichthyosis: the hands are particularly affected. By courtesy of the Institute of Dermatology, London, UK.

most often spared in EI with *KRT10* mutation, which can be explained by its physiological substitution of keratin 9 on palmoplantar skin.[1]

EI shows the typical features of epidermolytic hyperkeratosis.[15–17] Suprabasal keratinocytes appear vacuolated and typically contain distinct eosinophilic intracytoplasmic inclusions. The cell borders are ill defined and

intraepidermal blister formation may be present. There is massive ortho-hyperkeratosis, papillomatosis, and acanthosis. The granular cell layer is prominent and contains coarse and irregular keratoyhaline granules (*Fig. 3.29*).

By immunohistochemistry, epidermolytic hyperkeratosis shows a normal distribution pattern of keratins 5/14 and 1/10, but in addition, there is overexpression of keratin 14 in the suprabasal epithelium accompanied by quite marked labeling of the upper epithelial layers by keratin 16, as would be expected in a hyperproliferative state.[18]

Ultrastructural studies have shown that the intracytoplasmic inclusions seen on light microscopy are composed of abnormally aggregated keratin filaments. Since large areas of the cytoplasm lack a regular keratin skeleton,

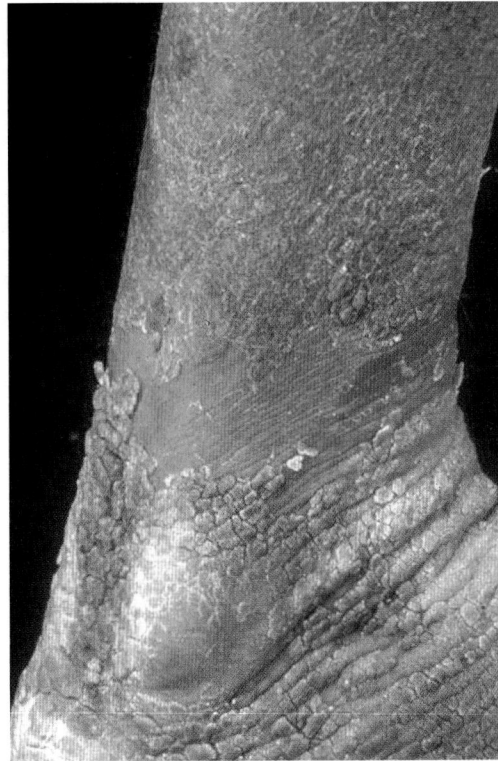

Fig. 3.28
Epidermolytic ichthyosis: blistering may sometimes be seen in adulthood. By courtesy of the Institute of Dermatology, London, UK.

the suprabasal keratinocytes appear vacuolated and contain irregular keratoyhaline granules. Impairment of desmosome-keratin complexes accounts for the fragility of the epidermis (*Fig. 3.30*). Immunoelectron microscopy has identified that the keratin clumps are composed of keratins 1 and 10.[18] These ultrastructural changes may form the basis of prenatal diagnosis including amniotic fluid squame analysis.[16-17]

Annular epidermolytic ichthyosis

Annular EI is a rare but clinically distinct form of keratinopathic ichthyosis related to a novel dinucleotide mutation in *KRT10*.[1,2] Patients have mild erythroderma and blisters at birth, but the characteristic feature is the presence of migrating annular and polycyclic, gray hyperkeratotic plaques with a peripheral erythematous border on the trunk and on the extremities (*Fig. 3.31*). High temperature in the summer, fever or pregnancy can induce recurrences.[3,4]

Histologically, epidermolytic hyperkeratosis is the dominant pattern, however a biopsy from the inflammatory border shows features of a lymphocytic, psoriasiform dermatitis with parakeratosis.[2]

Superficial epidermolytic ichthyosis

Clinical features

Superficial epidermolytic ichthyosis (SEI), formerly termed ichthyosis bullosa Siemens, is a keratinopathic ichthyosis, which is milder than EI. It presents at birth with blistering subsequently replaced by dark lichenified hyperkeratosis of the limbs, predominantly affecting the flexures and shins (*Fig. 3.32*).[1,2] The skin remains fragile and blisters on mild trauma, giving rise to characteristic superficial peeling with a molting-like appearance (Mauserung phenomenon) (*Fig. 3.33*).[2,3] Symptoms usually improve with age. Erythroderma is typically absent. Rarely, pustulation and hypertrichosis may be additional features.[3,4] There is considerable clinical overlap between SEI and EI, and their distinction can best be achieved by molecular genetic analysis.[4-10]

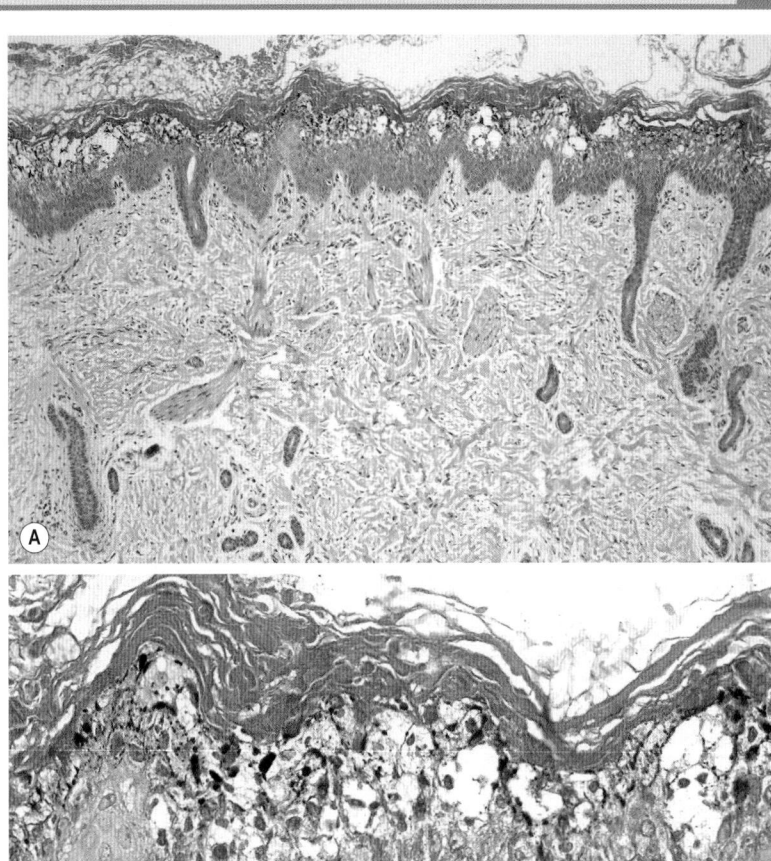

Fig. 3.29
Epidermolytic ichthyosis: (**A**) there is massive hyperkeratosis and acanthosis. The epidermis shows conspicuous superficial vacuolation, which has resulted, in vesiculation; (**B**) there is intracellular vacuolation, and irregular eosinophilic granules (representing dense abnormal aggregates of keratin filaments) are present in the superficial layers of the epidermis.

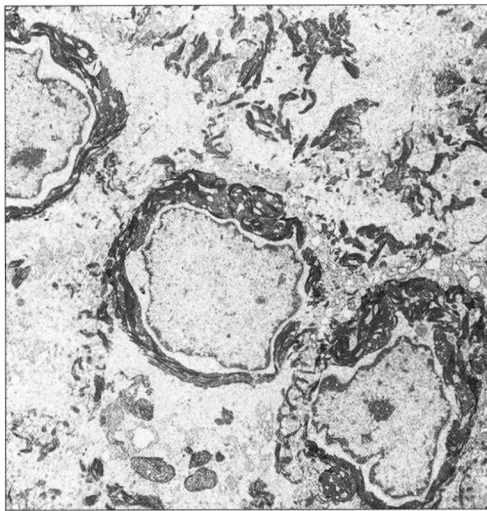

Fig. 3.30
Epidermolytic ichthyosis: striking perinuclear keratin clumping is evident. By courtesy of R.A.J. Eady, MD, Institute of Dermatology, London, UK.

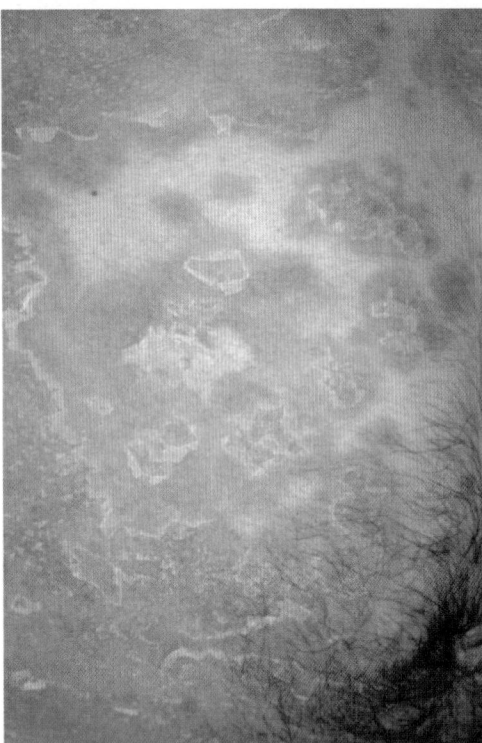

Fig. 3.31
Annular epidermolytic ichthyosis: migrating, polycyclic, gray hyperkeratotic plaques with a peripheral erythematous border. By courtesy of H. Traupe, MD, Münster, Germany.

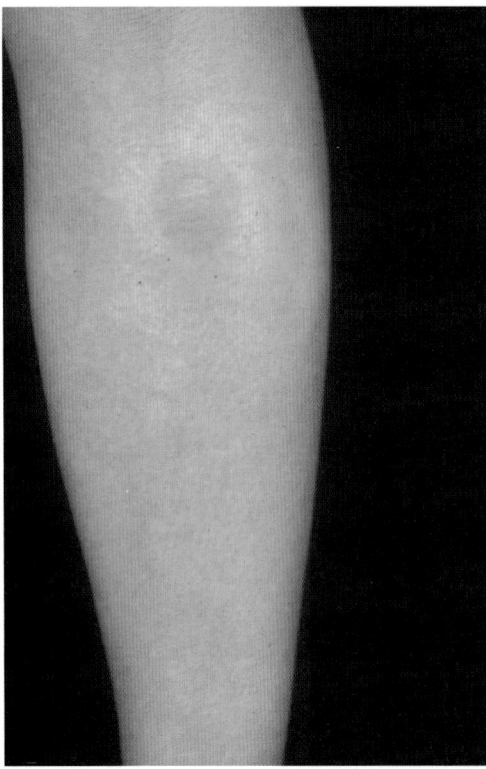

Fig. 3.32
Superficial epidermolytic ichthyosis: flexural hyperkeratosis with early blister formation. By courtesy of W.A.D. Griffiths, MD, Institute of Dermatology, London, UK.

Pathogenesis and histologic features

SEI is associated with a point mutation in the keratin 2 gene (*KRT2*) located on chromosome 12q11-q13.[4–10] Since this keratin is not expressed on volar skin, palmoplantar keratoderma does not develop.

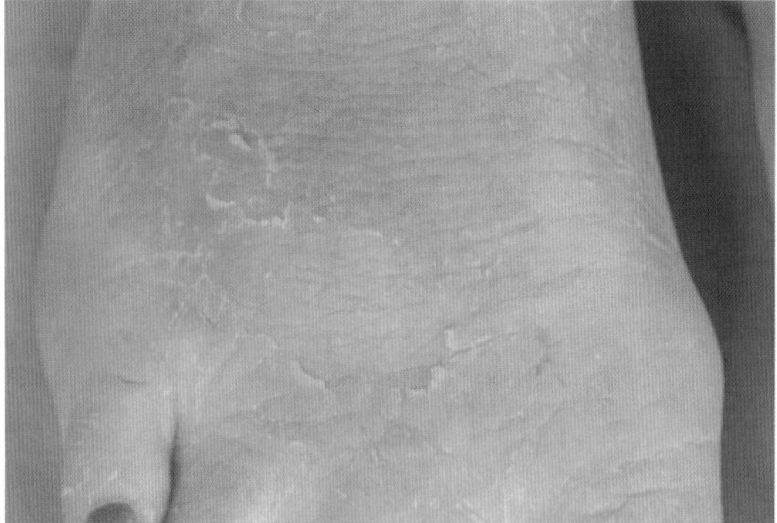

Fig. 3.33
Superficial epidermolytic ichthyosis: dark lichenified hyperkeratosis and characteristic superficial peeling with a molting-like appearance (Mauserung phenomenon). By courtesy of H. Traupe, MD, Münster, Germany.

Histologically and by electron microscopy, the features are indistinguishable from EI except that they are milder and the vacuolation of the keratinocytes and cytoplasmic inclusions are restricted to the more superficial spinous and granular cell layers. Subcorneal separation may be evident.[11]

Epidermolytic epidermal nevus

A nevoid variant of EI is the result of somatic mutations in *KRT1* or *KRT10*.[1,2] These nevi follow one or more Blaschko lines and are characterized by a prominent hyperkeratosis. The dirty-appearing verruciform aspect should raise the diagnostic suspicion of a keratin mutation (linear verrucous epidermal nevus).[3] A biopsy can easily identify the histologic pattern of epidermolytic hyperkeratosis which allows distinction from other types of epidermal nevi (*Fig. 3.34*). Since children of affected patients may develop a form of generalized EI, genetic counseling should be offered.[4]

Epidermolytic acanthoma

Clinical features

Epidermolytic acanthoma is an acquired lesion that presents as a verrucous papule or plaque approximately 1.0 cm in diameter and sometimes resembles a viral wart, nevus or seborrheic keratosis.[1–3] Caucasians and the Japanese are predominantly affected.[3] Lesions may present at any site, but the scrotum, head, neck, and lower limbs are particularly affected.[2,3] Although usually solitary, occasional patients may present with multiple localized or disseminated lesions.[4–8,11] In Japanese patients multiple depigmented flat keratotic papules following sun exposure on the shoulders and back were described as persistent actinic epidermolytic hyperkeratosis.[12] Variants affecting the mucosae of the oral cavity and female genital tract have also been documented.[9,10]

Pathogenesis and histologic features

Although it has been assumed that epidermolytic acanthoma develops as a consequence of keratin 1 and 10 gene mutation, two recent genetic studies failed to show any mutations in these keratins.[3,13,14] Still, trauma or other external triggers may interfere with the transcription or translation of the suprabasal keratins.[13] Human papillomavirus (HPV) infection has been excluded.[11]

The lesion is well circumscribed and cup shaped and only rarely polypoid. The epidermis shows hyperkeratosis, focal parakeratosis, acanthosis and papillomatosis or a flat base. (*Fig. 3.35*).[1,2] The upper prickle cell

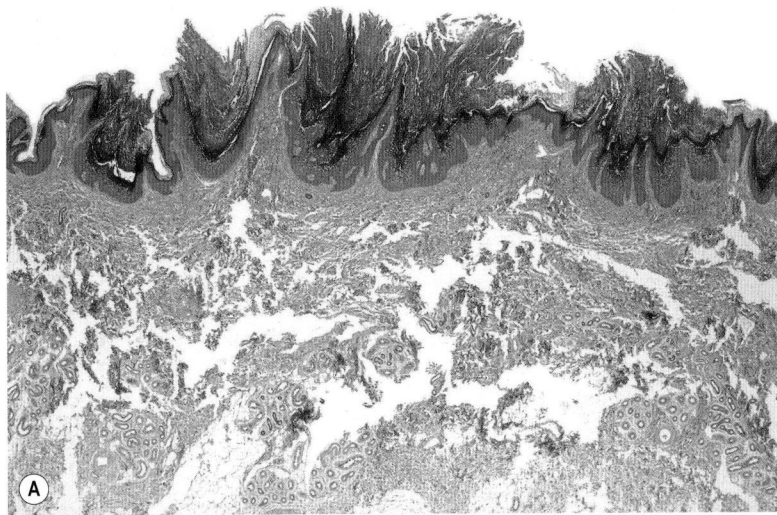

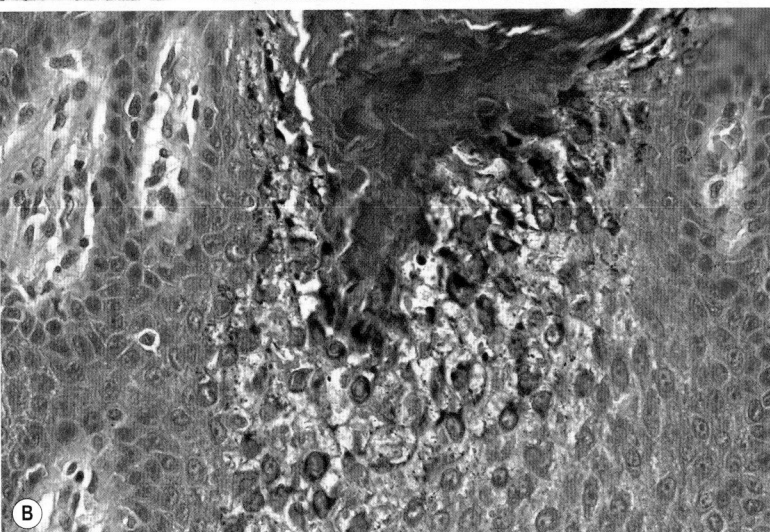

Fig. 3.34
Linear epidermolytic epidermal nevus: (**A**) low-power view showing massive hyperkeratosis and papillomatosis; (**B**) high-power view showing epidermolytic hyperkeratosis.

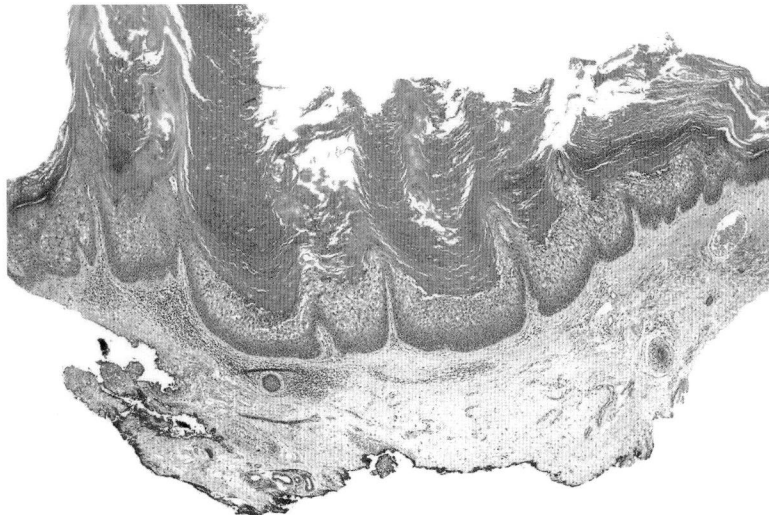

Fig. 3.35
Epidermolytic acanthoma: the lesion is papillomatous with massive hyperkeratosis. There is a superficial perivascular chronic inflammatory cell infiltrate.

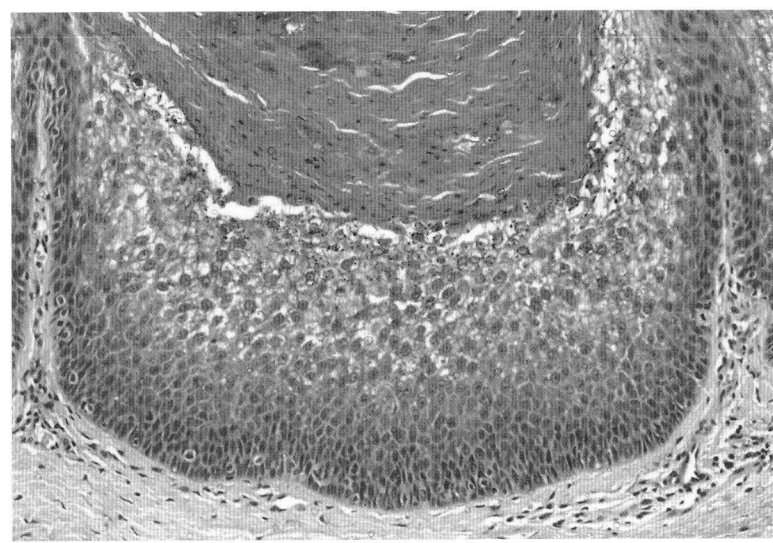

Fig. 3.36
Epidermolytic acanthoma: there is superficial cytoplasmic vacuolation and eosinophilic inclusions are conspicuous.

and granular cell layers show features of epidermolytic hyperkeratosis, i.e., marked vacuolation of the keratinocytes with eosinophilic keratin inclusions and irregular keratohyaline granules (*Fig. 3.36*). More variably, eosinophilic perinuclear keratin condensations resembling the Hailey-Hailey pattern of acantholysis are described.[11] Necrotic keratinocytes with absent nuclei can be seen in the horny layer. A perivascular lymphocytic infiltrate is often present in the papillary dermis.

Epidermolytic acanthoma displays diminished expression of keratins 1 and 10 and increased expression of the hyperproliferative keratins 6 and 16 while other differentiation markers, such as involucrin and loricrin, appear normal.[3,13]

Differential diagnosis

Identical histologic changes are seen in keratinopathic forms of ichthyosis, linear epidermolytic epidermal nevus, epidermolytic palmoplantar keratoderma, and incidental epidermolytic hyperkeratosis (see *Table 3.3*). Clinical information is usually necessary to avoid diagnostic confusion.

Incidental epidermolytic hyperkeratosis

Incidental epidermolytic hyperkeratosis represents a focal non-specific finding of epidermolytic hyperkeratosis in the epidermis overlying or adjacent to an unrelated lesion. It is very common and has been described, for example, in seborrheic keratoses, melanocytic nevi, actinic keratosis, squamous cell carcinoma, and melanoma. In such incidental cases, the changes

are limited to the epidermis overlying just one or two dermal papillae in contrast to the much more extensive involvement in other epidermolytic diseases (*Fig. 3.37*).

Incidental epidermolytic hyperkeratosis can be associated with epidermal and pilar cysts, scars and fibrous histiocytoma, It may also be seen in normal, particularly sun-damaged skin.[1-5] Incidental histopathologic reaction patterns, such as epidermolytic hyperkeratosis, acantholytic dyskeratosis, and Hailey-Hailey-like acantholysis are presumably related to field cancerization and can be regarded as a potentially premalignant change surrounding tumors.[6,7]

Beyond that, inflammatory conditions, e.g., lichen planus, nummular dermatitis, Grover disease, pityriasis versicolor, and others, may also show the incidental phenomenon of epidermolytic hyperkeratosis.[2,8]

Ichthyosis Curth-Macklin

Clinical features

Ichthyosis Curth-Macklin was originally termed ichthyosis hystrix, a descriptive name for cornification disorders with spiny and dark hyperkeratosis.

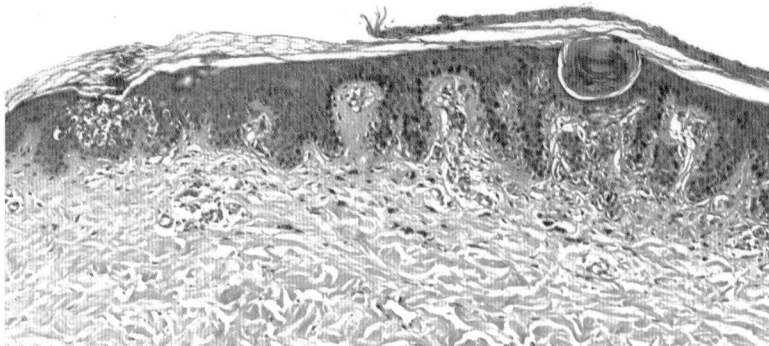

Fig. 3.37
Incidental epidermolytic hyperkeratosis: focal expression of epidermolytic hyperkeratosis in the periphery of a melanocytic nevus.

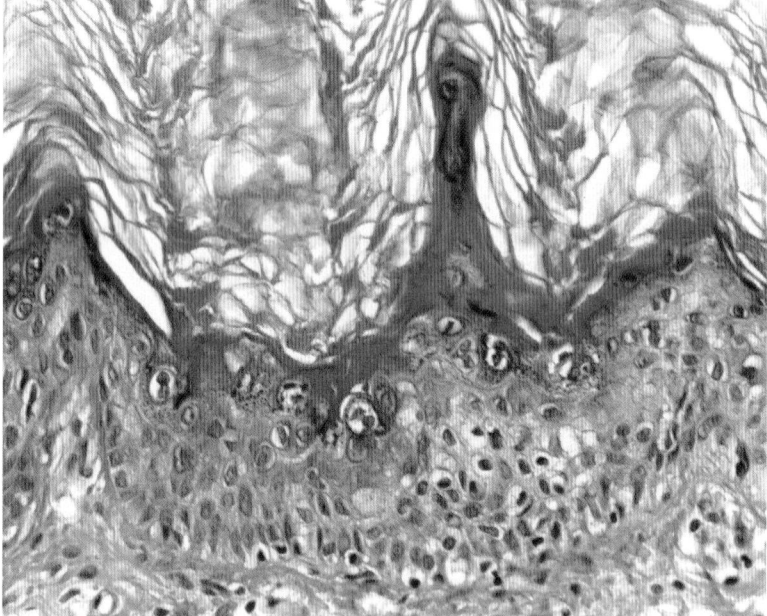

Fig. 3.38
Ichthyosis hystrix Curth-Macklin: the epidermis is acanthotic and orthohyperkeratotic. The suprabasal keratinocytes are vacuolated but lack eosinophilic intracytoplasmic inclusions and some are binucleated. By courtesy of S. Fraitag, MD, Paris

Ichthyosis Curth-Macklin is characterized by generalized verrucous plaques involving the entire trunk, the flexural surfaces of the extremities, and the palms and soles. This autosomal dominant disorder sometimes resembles EI, but there is no clinical or histologic evidence of blistering.[1–4]

Pathogenesis and histologic features

In ichthyosis Curth-Macklin the mutation affects the variable tail domain (V2) of keratin 1 which results in a failure in keratin intermediate filament bundling and retraction of the cytoskeleton from the nucleus.[2] This is the first in vivo evidence for the crucial role of a keratin tail domain in supramolecular keratin intermediate filament organization and barrier formation.[2]

Histologically, the epidermis is acanthotic and orthohyperkeratotic. The suprabasal keratinocytes are vacuolated and a few of them appear binucleated. In contrast to epidermolytic hyperkeratosis, eosinophilic intracytoplasmic inclusions are not seen (*Fig. 3.38*).[5] Ichthyosis Curth-Macklin shares many cytologic features with CRIE but lacks parakeratosis (see *Table 3.3*).

The significant ultrastructural observation in ichthyosis Curth-Macklin is the presence of perinuclear concentric shells of tonofilaments. In contrast to keratin mutations of the rod domain in epidermolytic hyperkeratosis, aggregations and clumping of keratin filaments are absent.[5]

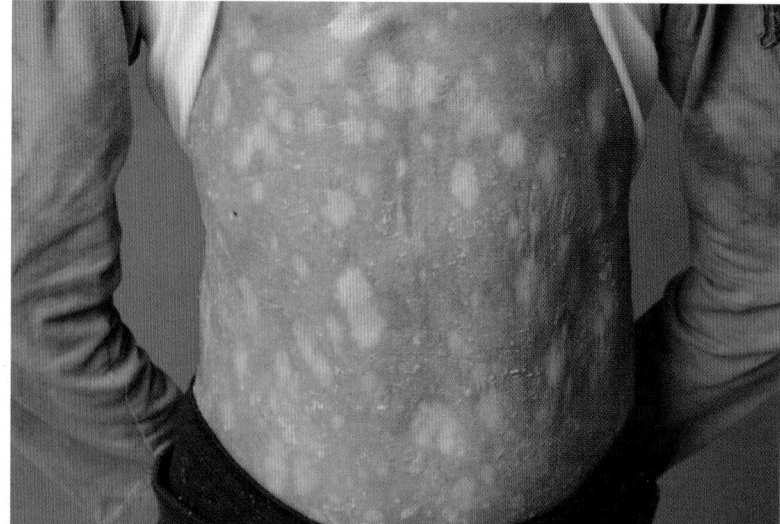

Fig. 3.39
Congenital reticular ichthyosiform erythroderma: patches of normal skin appear to be enclosed by erythrokeratotic and hyperpigmented areas in a reticular arrangement.

Congenital reticular ichthyosiform erythroderma

Clinical features

Congenital reticular ichthyosiform erythroderma (CRIE) is an autosomal dominant variant of keratinopathic ichthyosis.[1] Patients are born with erythroderma, and initially may be misdiagnosed as having autosomal recessive congenital ichthyosis, i.e., CIE. Then, during early childhood their integument develops an increasing number of small pale white spots (*Fig. 3.39*). Because of this clinical appearance the genodermatosis has also been termed ichthyosis 'en confettis' or ichthyosis variegata.[2–9] Some patients develop hypertrichosis and palmoplantar hyperkeratosis. There may be a higher risk for keratoacanthoma or squamous cell carcinoma. Although this type of ichthyosis belongs to the group of nonsyndromic ichthyoses, single cases have been described in association with hypogonadism, growth retardation, osteomalacia, or hepatomegaly.[1,5,7]

Pathogenesis and histologic features

The genetic defect in CRIE is based on specific dominant mutations in *KRT10* or in *KRT1*. The characteristic formation of white spots has a later onset in *KRT1* mutations. These mutations cause disruption of the keratin filament network and mislocalization of keratin to the nucleus.[10] The spontaneous development of multiple patches of normal skin is caused by recombination events in the mutated keratin gene. This intriguing revertant phenotype can be considered a kind of natural gene therapy.[11]

Histologically, the epidermis is pale staining and shows psoriasiform hyperplasia. The horny layer is thickened and parakeratotic. The parakeratotic corneocytes have enlarged nuclei. The keratinocytes of the upper layers show prominent perinuclear vacuolation and contain only a few keratohyalin granules. Their cell borders are well defined and intracytoplasmic eosinophilic granules are absent. Some of the vacuolated keratinocytes are binucleated (*Fig. 3.40*). While keratin 2e is missing, the other epidermal keratins are regularly expressed. The superficial dermal vessels are dilated, and there is a sparse perivascular inflammatory cell infiltrate with scattered melanophages. Biopsies from the confetti-like spots within the erythrodermic skin reveal a normal differentiating epidermis, both histologically and immunohistochemically.

At the ultrastructural level the arrangement of the keratin skeleton is highly disturbed. Immuno-electron microscopy reveals complete absence of keratin filaments in the perinuclear cytoplasm. The number of transitional cells is increased and nick end labeling (TUNEL) for DNA fragmentation shows strong labeling of the parakeratotic corneocytes consistent with an apoptotic mode of cell death. Uptake and processing of melanosomes

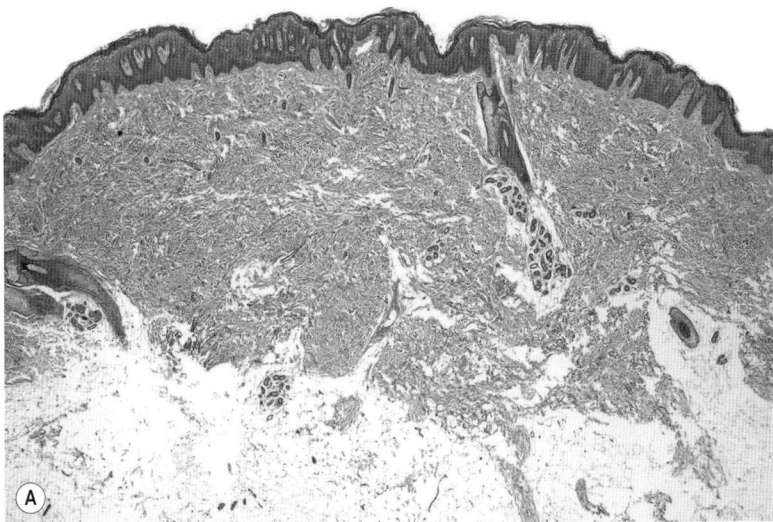

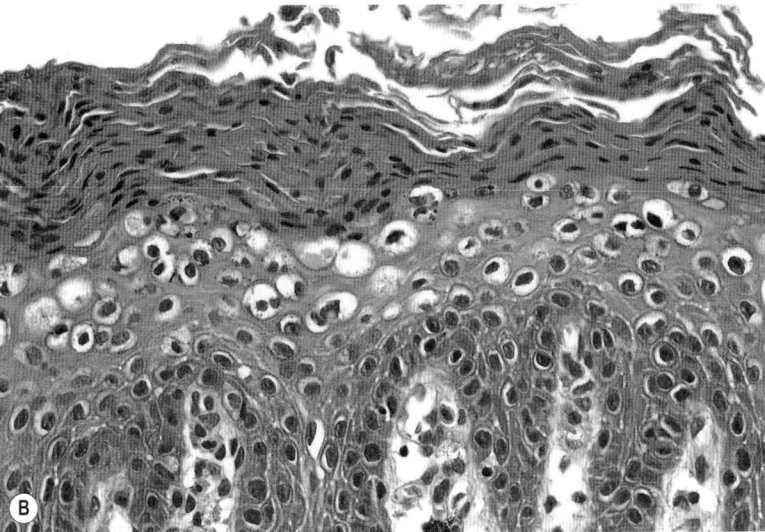

Fig. 3.40
Congenital reticular ichthyosiform erythroderma: (**A**) there is hyperkeratosis and well-developed psoriasiform hyperplasia; (**B**) parakeratosis with prominent nuclei and absence of a granular layer are also observed. Note the cytoplasmic vacuolation and binucleated keratinocytes. Eosinophilic intracytoplasmic inclusions are absent.

is irregular.[12] By immunofluorescence dotlike labelling for keratin can be demonstrated in numerous nuclei in the suprabasal epidermis.[10]

Differential diagnosis

The absence of keratin clumping clearly distinguishes CRIE from keratinization disorders characterized by epidermolytic hyperkeratosis. Ichthyosis Curth-Macklin shares the intraepidermal formation of binucleated and vacuolated keratinocytes but lacks parakeratosis and forms perinuclear shells of tonofibrils (see *Table 3.3*).

Comèl-Netherton syndrome

Clinical features

Comèl-Netherton syndrome (Netherton syndrome, ichthyosis linearis circumflexa) is a rare autosomal recessively inherited genodermatosis. It is characterized by the triad of CIE, hair shaft anomalies, and a severe atopic diathesis with high IgE blood levels and eosinophilia.[1] It is believed to affect approximately 1:200 000 of the population.[2] Generally, the CIE gradually evolves into a milder ichthyosis linearis circumflexa which is characterized by an erythematous, scaly rash predominantly affecting the trunk and limbs.[3] It is composed of polycyclic, migratory, annular and serpiginous lesions with characteristic two parallel lines of scale at the periphery, the so-called

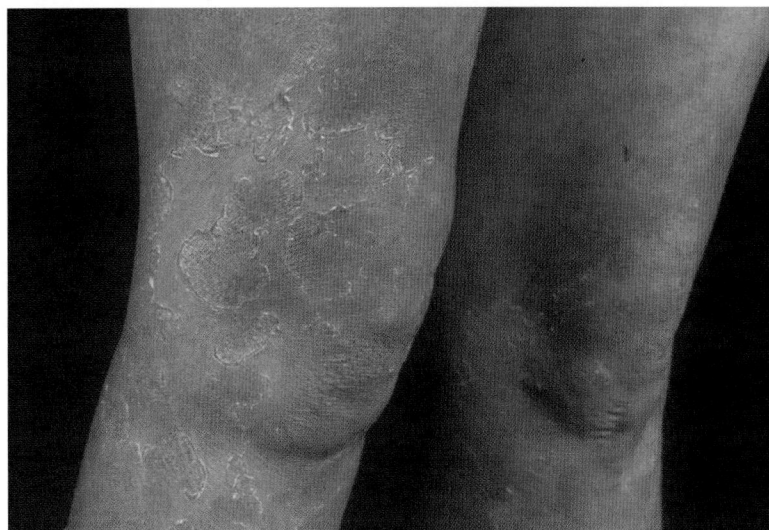

Fig. 3.41
Comèl-Netherton syndrome: ichthyosis linearis circumflexa. Note the serpiginous lesions with characteristic double border. By courtesy of M. Judge, MD, Institute of Dermatology, London, UK.

double-edged scale (*Figs 3.41* and *3.42*). In infancy, erythema and scaling may be widespread, but later the face is often predominantly affected (particularly marked around the mouth and eyes), along with the perineum, and as such the eruption can be mistaken for acrodermatitis enteropathica (*Fig. 3.43*).[1] Later the scalp, face, and eyebrows may show a yellowish scaling.[5] Comèl-Netherton syndrome is often misdiagnosed as seborrheic dermatitis, atopic dermatitis, and psoriasis vulgaris.[6]

Hairs on the scalp, eyebrows, and eyelashes may be present, sparse or absent at birth. Trichorrhexis invaginata ('bamboo hair') does not develop until childhood. These hair anomalies are caused by transient and repeated defects of keratinization, with resultant hair shaft intussusception, and present clinically as coarse and lusterless hair, which is short, brittle, and fragile (see *Fig. 3.43*). Pili torti and trichorrhexis may also occur (*Fig. 3.44*).[7]

Patients with Netherton syndrome may suffer from life-threatening neonatal dehydration with hypernatremia, failure to thrive, aminoaciduria, and recurrent skin infections often caused by *Staphylococcus aureus*.[2,9] At an older age there is a higher risk for HPV-associated papillomatous skin lesions of the groin and perineal regions, spinous cell carcinoma, and giant condyloma of Buschke-Lowenstein.[10,11] Growth retardation is due to growth hormone deficiency[8] and immune defects.[1,5] Food allergies against nuts and fish are common and lead to urticaria or angioedema. An impaired epidermal barrier is a potential risk for increased and even toxic absorption of topical medications.[1-4]

Pathogenesis and histologic features

Comèl-Netherton syndrome is caused by mutations in the *SPINK5* gene (serine protease inhibitor Kazal-type 5) encoding the serine protease inhibitor LEKTI (lympho-epithelial Kazal-type related inhibitor).[12,13] Analysis of fetal DNA from amniotic fluid in families at risk for this life-threatening disease allow for an early, rapid, and reliable method of prenatal diagnosis.[14] LEKTI is expressed in the epidermis, thymus, and oral and vaginal mucosa and controls trypsin- and chymotrypsin-like enzymes.[15] The failure of serine protease inhibition accounts for over-desquamation of corneocytes and degradation of desmosomal proteins (e.g., corneodesmosin and desmoglein 1).[16] In addition, the PAR-2 (protease-activated receptor-2) related proinflammatory response is upregulated.[17] In summary, the lack of LEKTI accounts for a unique combination of ichthyotic and inflammatory skin phenotype, which is associated with an extremely impaired epidermal barrier.

For histologic diagnosis, the biopsy should be taken from the scaly margin. A sample from this area will reveal the diagnostic psoriasiform features while biopsies from the center of the lesion show misleading features of atopic dermatitis.

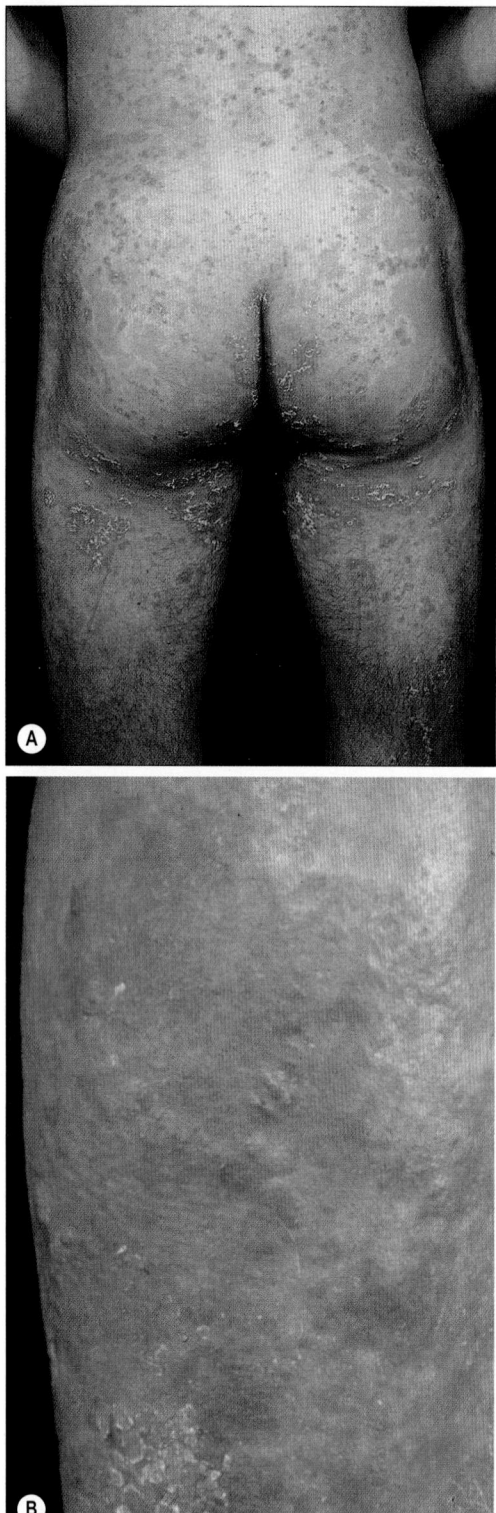

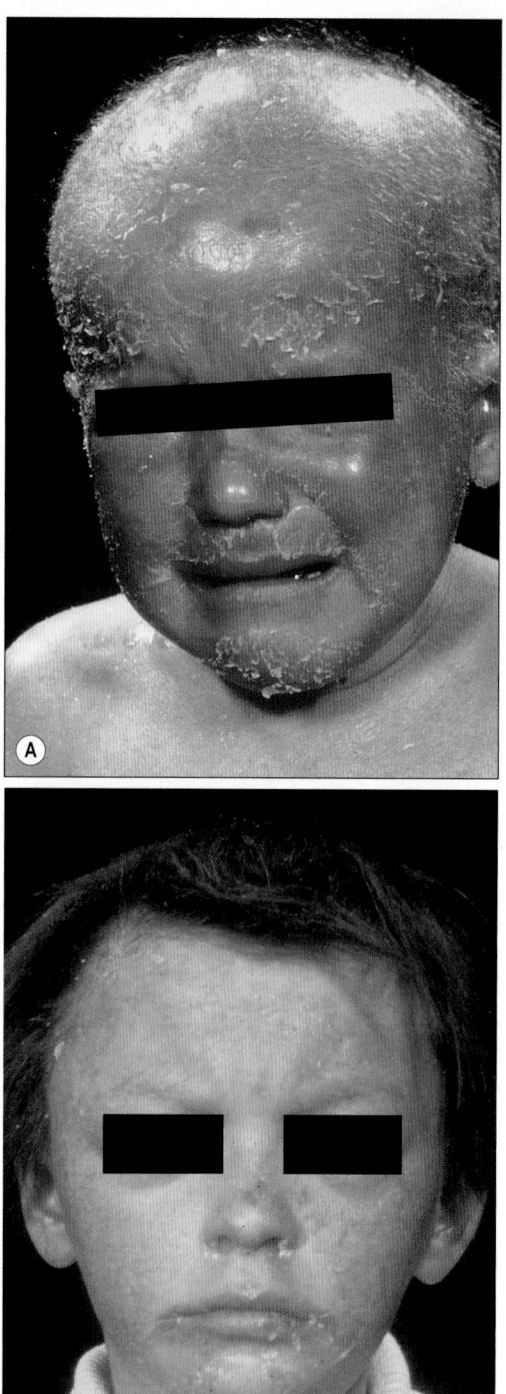

Fig. 3.42
Comèl-Netherton syndrome: (**A**) hyperkeratotic lesions may sometimes be prominent; (**B**) note the focal loss of the polycyclic pattern.

Fig. 3.43
Comèl-Netherton syndrome: (**A**) there is profound erythema with scaling; (**B**) the hair is dull and appears short and thin. The eyebrows are deficient. (**A**) By courtesy of M. Judge, MD, Institute of Dermatology, London, UK. (**B**) By courtesy of A. Griffiths, MD, Institute of Dermatology, London, UK.

Netherton syndrome shows a psoriasiform dermatitis with parakeratosis and intracorneal neutrophils (sometimes with formation of Munro microabscesses) often indistinguishable from psoriasis vulgaris (*Fig. 3.45*).[6] New findings described in a series of patients, include compact parakeratosis with large nuclei, subcorneal or intracorneal splitting, presence of clear cells in the upper epidermis or stratum corneum, dyskeratosis, elongated rete ridges without suprapapillary thinning and a superficial dermal inflammatory cell infiltrate rich in neutrophils and/or eosinophils.[18] Small, dark, round or oval granules can be identified within the stratum granulosum.[19] They are diastase-resistant, and periodic acid-Schiff (PAS) and Sudan black

positive and are thought to represent an influx of serum exudates resulting from the accompanying dermal inflammation. Similar 'inclusions' have been described in psoriasis and atopic eczema and as such they are not specific.[19]

Electron microscopy reveals reduced numbers of LBs in keratinocytes and the presence of lysosomal inclusion bodies with intercellular amorphous deposits in the horny layer.[20,21]

Immunohistochemistry can demonstrate the absence of LEKTI antigen and is highly specific for the Netherton syndrome both in neonatal

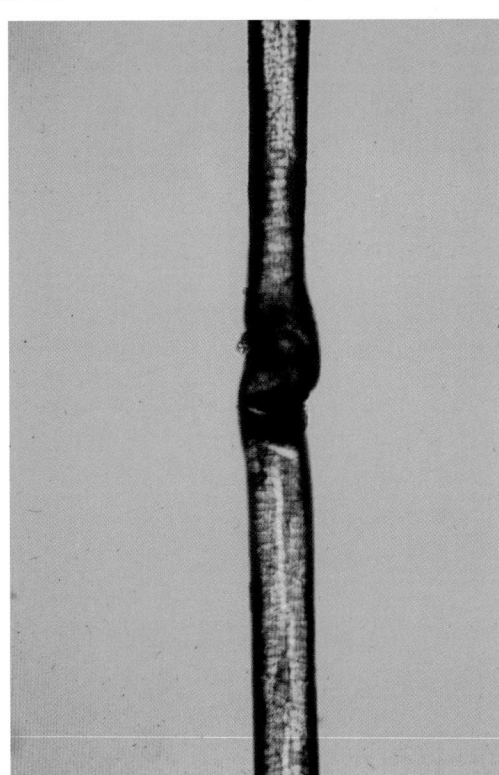

Fig. 3.44
Comèl-Netherton syndrome: bamboo hair (trichorrhexis invaginata). By courtesy of M. Judge, MD, Institute of Dermatology, London, UK.

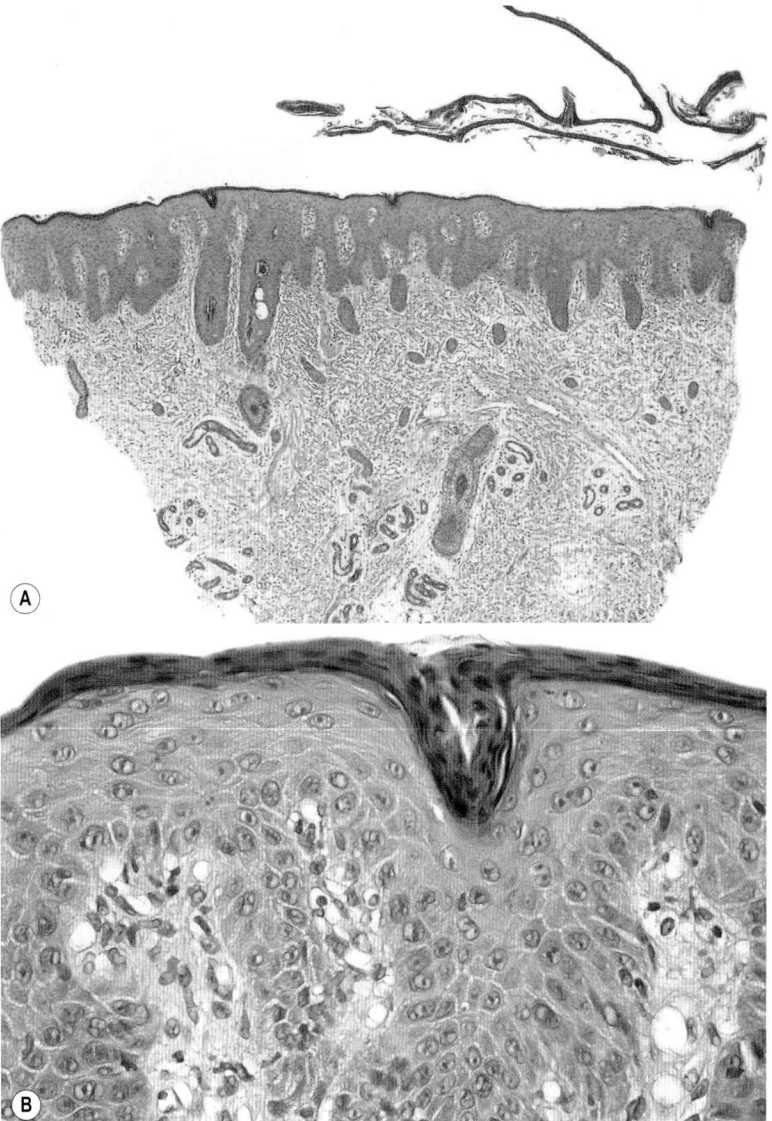

Fig. 3.45
Comèl-Netherton syndrome: (**A**) scanning view showing a detached thickened stratum corneum and psoriasiform hyperplasia; (**B**) note the marked parakeratosis and dilated vessels mimicking psoriasis vulgaris.

erythroderma and scaly rashes of adults.[22,23,24] A definite diagnosis can be made by negative staining for LEKTI in the inner root sheath of hair follicles since Netherton syndrome and other diseases may lack the stratum granulosum where LEKTI is normally expressed.[18] However, residual LEKTI expression in the outer epidermis is still demonstrable immunohistochemically in mild forms of Netherton syndrome.[25]

Differential diagnosis

Distinction from psoriasis vulgaris may be histologically extremely difficult (if not impossible) in the absence of clinical information. Other genodermatoses, dermatophytosis, and inflammatory skin diseases with a psoriasiform-like pattern must be differentiated (see *Table 3.3*). Netherton syndrome shares the distinct histologic feature of corneal splitting with other exfoliative disorders of cornification, such as peeling skin syndrome (PSS) and severe dermatitis, multiple allergies, metabolic wasting syndrome (SAM). Atopic dermatitis is another important differential diagnosis.

Peeling skin syndromes

Clinical features

Peeling skin syndromes (PSSs) are characterized by spontaneous peeling of the stratum corneum without bleeding or pain.[1,2] Different genetic and clinical entities have to be distinguished.

In **peeling skin syndrome type A** (familial continual skin peeling, keratolysis exfoliativa congenitale) a generalized lifelong and continued shedding or peeling of the entire skin starts between 3–6 years of age.[3] In contrast with the inflammatory type B, PSS type A lacks signs of inflammation or other symptoms or involvement of mucous membranes and nails. A missense mutation in *CHST8* has been described that encodes a Golgi transmembrane N-acetylgalactosamine-4-O-sulfotransferase (GalNAc-4-ST1) that may be important for epidermal homeostasis resulting in increased and continuous desquamation of the stratum corneum.[4]

Histology shows a plane of separation either within the lower part of an otherwise normal horny layer or above the granular cell layer. Ultrastructural analysis reveals an *intracellular* splitting within the corneocytes.[3]

Peeling skin syndrome type B (inflammatory peeling skin disease) presents at birth with ichthyosiform erythroderma and is characterized by lifelong patchy peeling of the entire skin with severe pruritus. Isolated erythematous lesions show flaccid peeling, leaving burning superficially denuded red patches with a peripheral collarette (*Fig. 3.46*).[5] Easy plucking of the hair and loose nail plates (onychomadesis) are further symptoms. Trigger factors are mechanical stress, low humidity or temperature changes. Pruritus and allergic symptoms of elevated IgE, food allergies, and asthma are reminiscent of Netherton syndrome.[5] Autosomal recessive loss-of-function mutations of *CDSN* encoding corneodesmosin have been identified as the molecular cause of the disease.[6]

Histologically, the epidermis displays psoriasiform hyperplasia with an absent or reduced granular cell layer and marked parakeratosis. Careful examination reveals detachment of the horny layer from the granular cell layer (*Fig. 3.47*).[5] Ultrastructurally, a loss of corneodesmosomes can be demonstrated, which is associated with *intercellular* splitting of the corneocytes from the stratum granulosum.[6] Immunostaining for corneodesmosin and LEKTI may help to distinguish between Netherton syndrome and PSS type B.[6]

Acral peeling skin syndrome is characterized by superficial painless peeling of the backs of the hand and feet (*Fig. 3.48*). In children blistering occurs on palms and soles.[7,8] Only recently it was reclassified as a form of

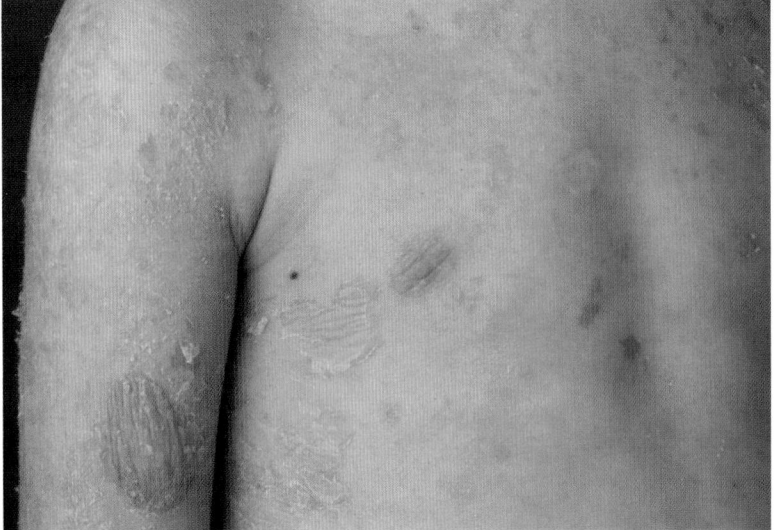

Fig. 3.46
Peeling skin syndrome type B: erythematous lesions show peeling of the skin leaving superficially denuded red patches. By courtesy of H. Traupe MD and V. Oji MD, Department of Dermatology, Münster, Germany.

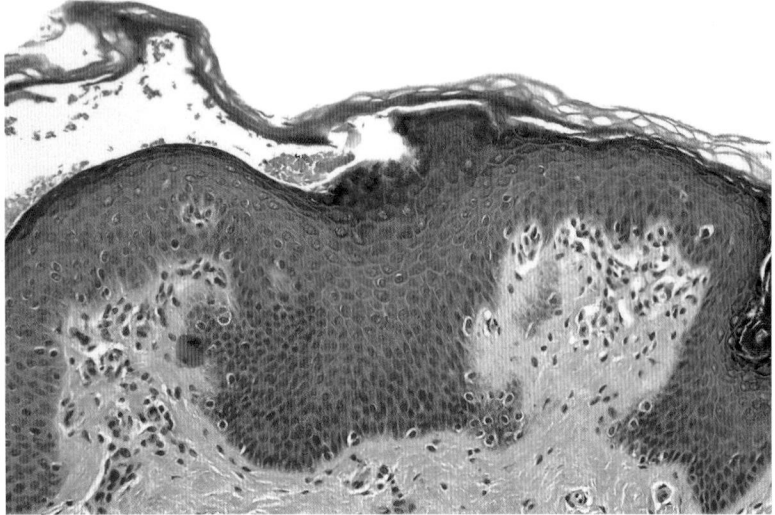

Fig. 3.47
Peeling skin syndrome type B: the biopsy is taken from the edge of the lesion. Note that the stratum corneum is clearly separated from the underlying epidermis.

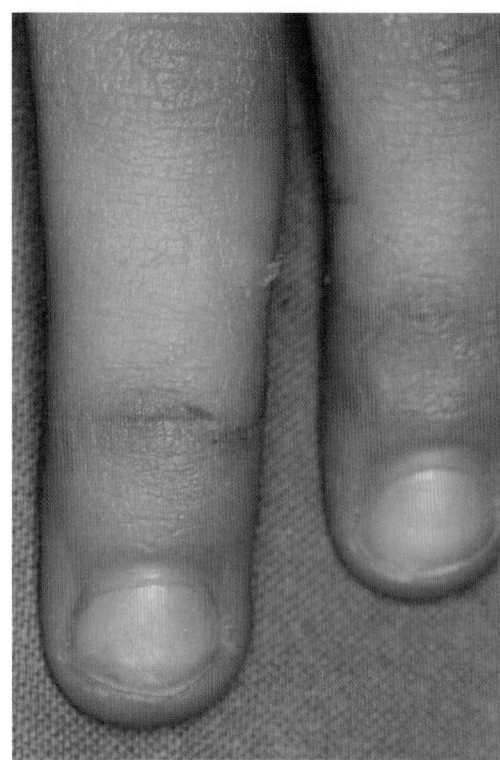

Fig. 3.48
Acral peeling skin syndrome type C: the skin of the backs of hand and feet shows reddish scaly patches. By courtesy of H. Traupe MD and V. Oji MD, Department of Dermatology, Münster, Germany.

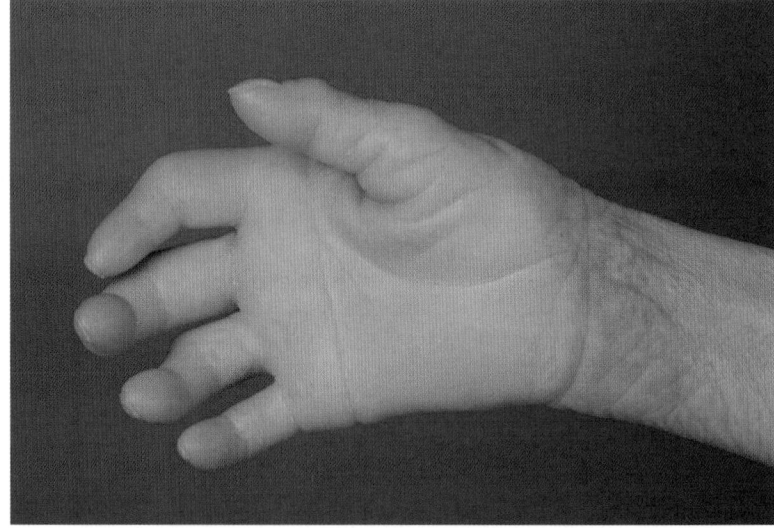

Fig. 3.49
Keratosis linearis-ichthyosis congenita-sclerosing keratoderma (KLICK): diffuse palmoplantar keratoderma and keratotic papules arranged in parallel lines on the wrist.

epidermolysis bullosa.[9] Missense mutations in the gene of transglutaminase-5 (*TGM5*) represent the molecular cause of this autosomal recessive disease— in contrast to its major differential diagnosis epidermolysis bullosa simplex (EBS), which has an autosomal dominant inheritance.[10] Other differential diagnoses of acral PSS include epidermolysis simplex superficialis[9] and keratolysis exfoliativa.[13,14] Histologically, the horny layer is detached from the stratum granulosum.[7,8]

Another type of PSS is related to the *CSTA* gene, mutations of which cause a deficiency of cystatin A. Initially, this variant was reported as 'exfoliative ichthyosis', a nonsyndromic congenital ichthyosis with dry and scaly skin associated with diffuse PPK sensitive to sweat and water exposure. The disease may display clinical features of SEI.[11,12]

Keratosis linearis-ichthyosis congenita-sclerosing keratoderma

Clinical features

Keratosis linearis-ichthyosis congenita-sclerosing keratoderma (KLICK) is an autosomal recessive genodermatosis presenting with a moderate, non-blistering ichthyosis from birth. Pathognomonic findings are keratotic punctuate plugs and papules arranged in parallel lines and circumscribed follicular keratosis around the wrists, in the folds of arms, axillae, and knees. In addition, a diffuse palmoplantar keratoderma develops including the dorsal side of hands and feet (*Fig. 3.49*). Other features include a sclerosing flexion deformity of the fingers and constriction bands.[1,2] There are no other associated features, but there is a report of an associated squamous cell carcinoma at a younger age.[3] Differential diagnosis includes loricrin keratoderma that also features palmoplantar keratoderma and a mild congenital ichthyosis but is less sclerotic and has an autosomal-dominant pattern on inheritance.

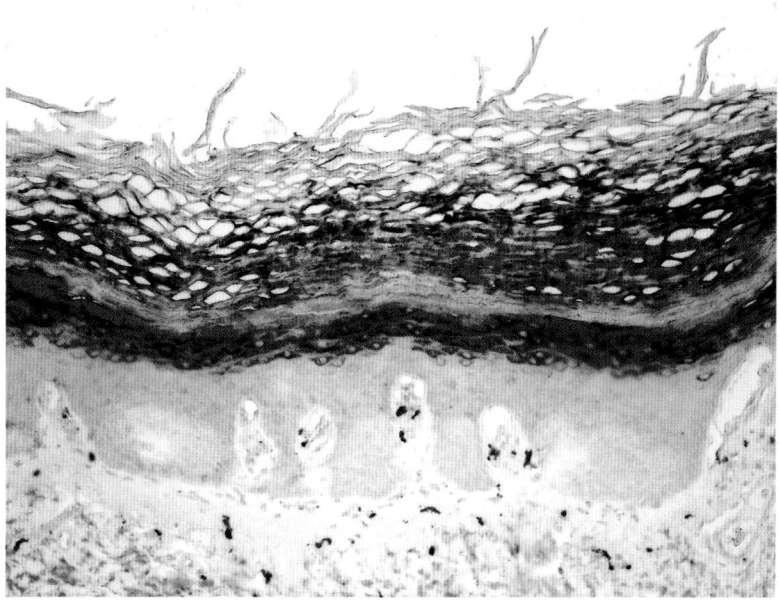

Fig. 3.50
Keratosis linearis-ichthyosis congenita-sclerosing keratoderma (KLICK): immunostaining for filaggrin shows broad immunoreactivity in the upper epidermis that characteristically extends into the horny layer.

Pathogenesis and histologic features

In KLICK a mutation of a proteasome maturation protein (*POMP*) has been identified. This protein serves as a chaperone for proteolytic enzymes degrading unneeded or damaged proteins. This proteasome insufficiency disturbs terminal epidermal differentiation and particularly interferes with processing of profilaggrin.[4]

Histologically, the epidermis is acanthotic and orthohyperkeratotic with focal parakeratosis and shows prominent hypergranulosis with irregular keratohyaline granules. This is reflected by immunohistochemistry for filaggrin which reveals extensive immunoreactivity in the upper epidermis that characteristically extends into the horny layer (*Fig. 3.50*). On non-volar skin follicular plugging is present. The papillary dermis shows papillomatosis and an inconsistent, mild perivascular lymphocytic infiltrate. Ultrastructure confirms the histologic finding of hypergranulosis and shows abnormally big keratohyaline granules.[5]

Severe dermatitis-multiple allergies-metabolic wasting syndrome (SAM)

This acronym was defined by Samuelov et al. in 2013 and refers to the cardinal features of severe dermatitis, multiple allergies, and metabolic wasting.[1] SAM is another exfoliative disorder of cornification and thus resembles Netherton syndrome or PSS type B. SAM is caused by loss-of-function mutations in *DSG1*.[1] Accordingly, apart from a psoriasiform dermatitis, subcorneal separation and acantholysis within the stratum spinosum and granulosum can be found. At the ultrastructural level half-split desmosomes are evident.[1]

Sjögren-Larsson syndrome

Clinical features

This autosomal recessive inherited disorder combines the features of ichthyosis, spastic bi- or quadriplegia and mental retardation.[1-5] It is rare, with an incidence of 0.4 per 100 000 of the population albeit it has a higher prevalence of 1:10 000 in Northern Sweden.[2,4]

The ichthyosis, which develops in the first year of life with diffuse scaling, affects the entire body with the exception of the central face and is typically intensely pruritic (*Fig. 3.51*).[3,5] Later, the skin has a brownish-yellow color and shows a cobblestone-like lichenification.[4] Hyperkeratosis around the

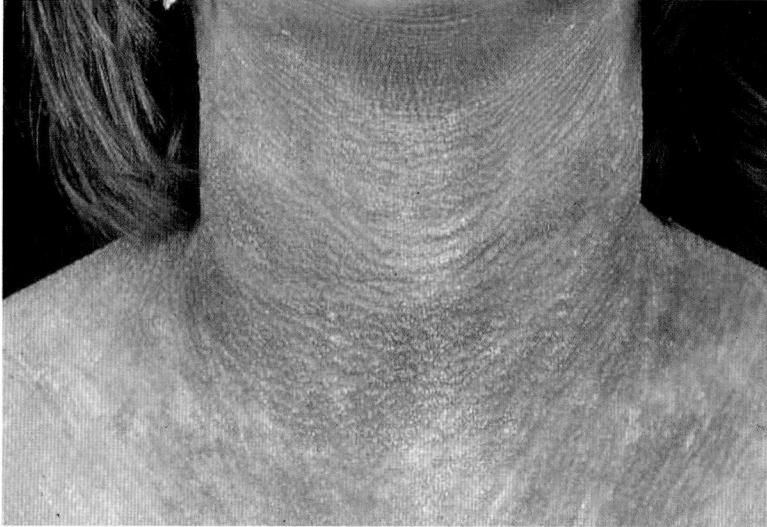

Fig. 3.51
Sjögren-Larsson syndrome: brownish-yellow color and a cobblestone-like pattern of lichenification is typical. By courtesy of M. Willemsen, MD, University Medical Center, Nijmegen, Belgium.

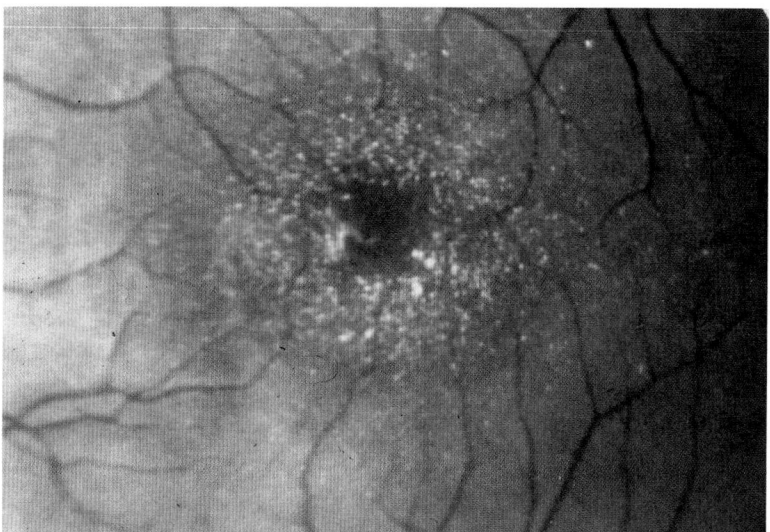

Fig. 3.52
Sjögren-Larsson syndrome: characteristic macular crystals. By courtesy of M. Willemsen, MD, University Medical Center, Nijmegen, Belgium.

umbilicus is said to be characteristic.[5] Erythroderma is not a feature and the hair, nails, and sweat glands are unaffected.[3,4] The diagnosis should be especially considered in preterm babies with congenital ichthyosis.[5]

The spasticity, which presents in early childhood, predominantly affects the legs and is often associated with contractures. The majority of patients are wheelchair bound.[4] Kyphoscoliosis may also be present.[3] Mental retardation is typically present, but is not invariable.[1] Epilepsy occurs in up to 40% of patients.[3]

Visual acuity is often impaired and photophobia is a frequent complaint. Macular degeneration associated with crystal deposition is characteristic (*Fig. 3.52*).[6]

Pathogenesis and histologic features

Sjögren-Larsson syndrome results from deficiency of microsomal fatty aldehyde dehydrogenase (*FALDH*).[7] The gene has been mapped to 17p11.2 and multiple mutations, including missense mutations, deletions, and insertions, have been identified.[8-10] In the pathophysiology of the ichthyosis a disturbed hepoxilin pathway is involved, while an abnormal lipid composition of myelin accounts for the neurological defects.[6] The abnormal level of free fatty alcohols in cultured fibroblasts, direct testing of FALDH activity, or

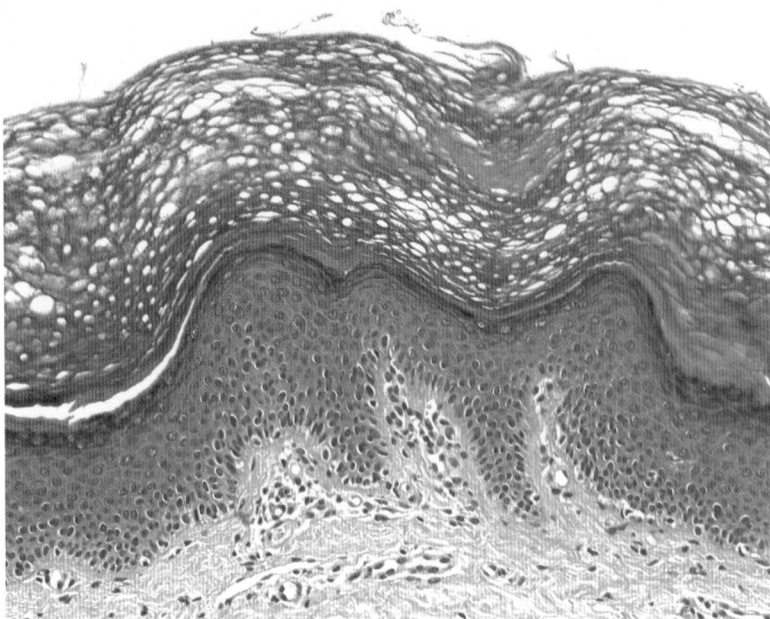

Fig. 3.53
Sjögren-Larsson syndrome: there is hyperkeratosis, with focal parakeratosis, hypergranulosis, and mild papillomatosis. A mild superficial perivascular lymphocytic infiltrate is present.

the presence of LTB4 metabolites in urine can provide biochemical screening and/or confirmation of the clinical diagnosis, prior to molecular mutation analysis of the *FALDH* gene.[5]

Histologically, there is papillomatosis, acanthosis, and basket-weave hyperkeratosis with scattered mild parakeratosis and occasional follicular hyperkeratosis (*Fig. 3.53*). Epidermal hyperproliferation has been demonstrated.[11,12] The granular cell layer may be slightly thickened. A moderate lymphocytic infiltrate is sometimes present around the superficial dermal vasculature.

Ultrastructurally, there are lamellar inclusions in the prickle and granular cell layers. Lipid inclusions are not a feature.[12]

Multiple sulfatase deficiency

Multiple sulfatase deficiency is a severe neuropediatric disorder inherited in an autosomal recessive mode. Pathophysiologically, mutations in the *SUMF1* gene block the post-translational modification of sulfatases and result in accumulation of glycosaminoglycans (GAGs) and sulfated lipids.[1] There are severe neonatal, and severe or mild infantile or juvenile forms characterized by progressive loss of mental capacity and motor abilities. Patients usually die before puberty. The ichthyosis is typically mild compared to the severity of the neurological changes.[2,3,4] Therefore, ichthyosis in a child with unexplained neurological symptoms should always prompt measurement of steroid sulfatase levels.[5]

Refsum syndrome

Clinical features

Refsum syndrome (hereditary motor and sensory neuropathy type 4, heredopathica atactica polyneuritiformis, phytanic acid deficiency) is a rare type of an autosomal recessive syndromic ichthyosis.[1] The skin changes appear in late childhood and are similar to those seen in ichthyosis vulgaris, including hyperlinear palms. Due to lipid storage, melanocytic nevi may show a yellow hue. Associated symptoms include loss of vision from retinitis pigmentosa, in which night blindness is often the first problem. Other complications are anosmia, cardiac arrhythmias, and a whole spectrum of neurological problems, including bilateral sensorineural deafness, cerebellar ataxia, and peripheral polyneuropathies.[2]

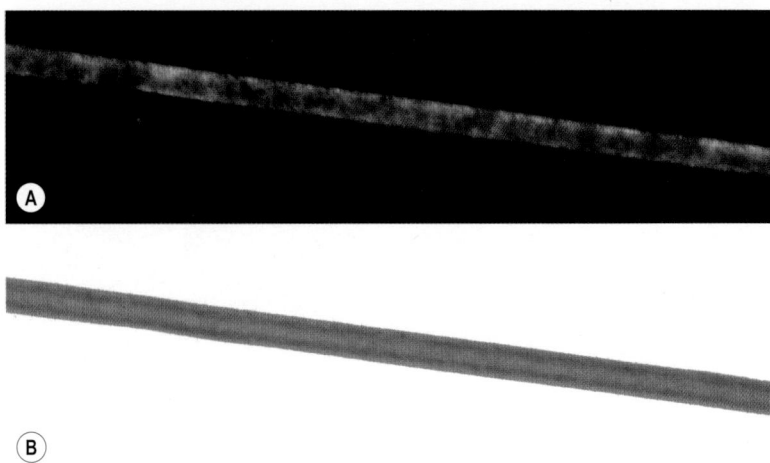

Fig. 3.54
Trichothiodystrophy: (**A**) polarizing microscopy of a hair shows an alternating light and dark banding ('tiger-tail pattern'). (**B**) The same hair without polarizing.

Pathogenesis and histologic features

Refsum syndrome is generally caused by a mutation in the *PHYH* gene encoding peroxisomal phytanoyl-CoA hydroxylase.[3,4] Mutations in the peroxisomal receptor gene *PEX7* account for adult forms.[5–7] Peroxisomes are involved in the metabolism of bile acid and cholesterol biosynthesis. Elevated levels of phytanic acid in plasma and tissue are diagnostic. Therapy includes a low-phytol diet and apharesis.[8,9]

Routine histology of a skin biopsy does not differ from ichthyosis vulgaris. When a biopsy is fixed in alcohol and a Sudan stain performed, lipid droplets are found in the keratinocytes, in particular in biopsies from melanocytic nevi. The same inclusions can be shown by ultrastructural examination.[10,11]

Dorfman-Chanarin syndrome

Dorfman-Chanarin syndrome (neutral lipid storage disease with ichthyosis) is a triglyceride storage disease with impaired long-chain fatty acid oxidation resulting in cataracts, hepatosplenomegaly, neurosensoral deafness, myopathy or developmental delay.[1] Affected neonates present as collodion babies or are erythrodermic with scaling. Later the ichthyosis resembles CIE with ectropion, flexural and neck lichenification, and palmoplantar hyperkeratosis. Pruritus and hypohidrosis are common.[2]

Pathogenesis and histologic features

The disease is due to mutations in the *ABHD5* gene product that is required by triglyceride lipase as a cofactor in the muscle, liver, and brain, but also in white blood cells.[3,4] The genetic defect leads to acylceramide deficiency resulting in ichthyosis and possibly to associated hepato-neurologic symptoms.[5,6] Histology shows orthohyperkeratosis with a possibly thinned stratum granulosum. Characteristically, intracellular lipid vacuoles can be demonstrated in the keratinocytes as well as in a variety of other cells, including circulating neutrophils (Jordans anomaly).[7] A skin biopsy fixed in alcohol is useful. Lipid vacuoles may also be found in the obligate carrier parents. Refsum syndrome patients also have epidermal lipid vacuoles, but in Dorfman-Chanarin syndrome patients, the phytanic acid levels are normal.

Trichothiodystrophy

Trichothiodystrophy (syn. Tay syndrome, IBIDS syndrome, PIBIDS syndrome, Amish brittle hair syndrome) represents a heterogeneous group of autosomal recessive neurocutaneous disorders, some of them photosensitive, that share sulfur-deficient brittle hairs.[1] Trichoschisis and brittle hairs are due to an abnormally low hair-shaft sulfur content with a decrease in cysteine. On polarizing microscopy, an alternating light and dark banding ('tiger-tail pattern') appears pathognomonic (*Fig. 3.54*).[2]

Trichothiodystrophy is associated with congenital ichthyosis: the acronym IBIDS ('Tay syndrome') refers to the clinical findings of ichthyosis (e.g., collodion membrane), brittle hair, intellectual impairment, decreased fertility, and short stature. Other features are microcephaly, dysplasia of nails, failure to thrive, 'progeria'-like symptoms, cataracts, and photosensitivity (≈ PIBIDS).[3]

In the photosensitive group, DNA-repair anomalies involving various subunits of the transcription factor TFIIH have been identified, while the non-photosensitive group, without a DNA-repair defect, exhibits mutations in the *C7ORF11* gene coding for TTDN1 protein.[4,5] Despite the DNA-repair defect and in contrast to xeroderma pigmentosum, an increased risk of malignancy is not regarded as a feature of photosensitive trichothiodystrophy.[6]

Histology of the ichthyotic skin shows acanthosis with orthohyperkeratosis and a reduced stratum granulosum (see *Table 3.3*).

Neu-Laxova syndrome

Neu-Laxova syndrome is an autosomal recessive inherited congenital ichthyosis caused by mutations leading to phosphoglycerate dehydrogenase deficiency.[1–3] It is characterized by marked intrauterine growth retardation, polyhydramnion, and congenital ichthyosis with a thin, tightly adherent, translucent skin and typical facial dysmorphology that resembles restrictive dermopathy, another neurocutaneous genodermatosis.[4] Associated syndromic features are microcephaly, central nervous system anomalies, short neck, limb deformities, and hypoplastic lungs. Histology of the skin reveals focal parakeratosis.

Ichthyosis prematurity syndrome

In ichthyosis prematurity syndrome there is polyhydramnion and the premature neonates may suffer from transient asphyxia. The infants have a thick cheesy membrane which desquamates followed by skin improvement within some weeks.[1] This syndrome is caused by mutations in the fatty acid transport protein 4 gene (*SLC27A4*).[2] The skin shows compact orthohyperkeratosis and acanthosis.

At ultrastructural level, characteristic masses of lipid membranes in lentiform paranuclear swellings of granular and horn cells can be demonstrated which has led to the designation ichthyosis congenita type 4.[3]

Other rare neuro-ichthyotic syndromes

The combination of neurologic manifestations and ichthyosis can be found in at least 16 distinct genetic disorders (see *Table 3.2*).[1] Gaucher disease type II (infantile cerebral Gaucher) is another classic neuro-ichthyosis presenting at birth with collodion membranes.[2] The diagnosis of this fetal metabolic disease can be made by measurement of glucocerebrosidase activity in peripheral blood leukocytes or in extracts of cultured skin fibroblasts.[3] Other examples are cerebral dysgenesis-neuropathy-ichthyosis-palmoplantar keratoderma (CEDNIK) syndrome[4], arthrogryposis-renal dysfunction-cholestasis (ARC) syndrome[5], and mental retardation-enteropathy-deafness-neuropathy-ichthyosis-keratoderma (MEDNIK) syndrome.[6] ELOVL4 deficiency presents with erythrokeratoderma and sensorineural deafness, thus resembling keratitis-ichthyosis-deafness (KID) syndrome.[7] Patients with Stormorken syndrome belong to the group of channelopathies affecting calcium homeostasis and is characterized with moderate thrombocytopenia, thrombocytopathia, muscle fatigue, asplenia, miosis, migraine, and dyslexia, altogether with ichthyosis.[8]

Conradi-Hünermann-Happle syndrome

Clinical features

Conradi-Hünermann-Happle syndrome is an X-linked dominant congenital ichthyosis with associated chondrodysplasia punctata. It is lethal in the majority of male embryos. Chondrodysplasia punctata is defined as a stippled calcification of the epiphyses. There are several forms but only the type 2 variant presents with severe ichthyosiform erythroderma. Later the

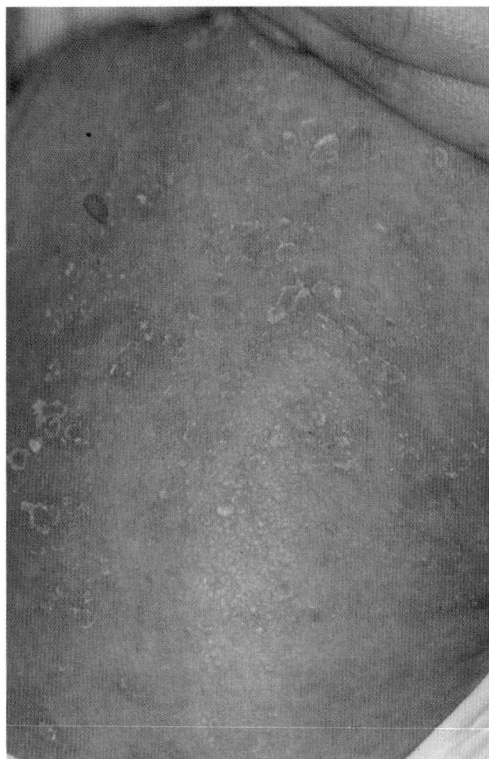

Fig. 3.55
Conradi-Hünermann-Happle syndrome: scaly erythema follows the whorled lines of Blaschko. By courtesy of H. Traupe MD, Dept of Dermatology, Münster, Germany.

erythema clears and persistent whorled scaling following the lines of Blaschko is noted (*Fig. 3.55*).[1,2]

Associated symptoms are scarring alopecia, follicular atrophoderma, localized hypo-and/or hyperpigmentation, sectorial cataracts, and skeletal dysplasia, which leads to asymmetric shortening of the long bones or severe kyphoscoliosis. Due to the individual differences in X-inactivation, expression of the disease is rather variable, even within families.[1,2]

Pathogenesis and histologic features

Biochemical analyzes using gas chromatography-mass spectrometry show elevated plasma levels of 8-dehydrocholesterol and 8(9)-cholesterol, resulting from a block of a key enzyme in sterol metabolism, namely the *8–7 sterol isomerase*. This enzyme is encoded by the emopamil-binding protein gene, which shows heterozygous mutations in Conradi-Hünermann-Happle syndrome.[3] The developmental abnormalities are presumably caused by interference of cholesterol precursors with sonic hedgehog signaling.[4] Abnormal cholesterol metabolism in the epidermis may account for the ichthyotic phenotype.[5]

The histologic features resemble those of ichthyosis vulgaris. There is hyperplasia of the epidermis, orthohyperkeratosis, a reduced stratum granulosum, and dilated hair follicle infundibula with keratin plugs. As a pathognomonic finding in newborns, von-Kossa staining demonstrates calcium deposits in the corneocytes of the stratum corneum and hair follicles. This feature allows discrimination from other ichthyoses that share the feature of a reduced stratum granulosum (*Fig. 3.56*) (see *Table 3.3*). At a later age the calcification is difficult to detect histologically but electron microscopy may reveal cytoplasmic vacuoles and electron-dense calcium crystals in the granular cell layer.[6] In addition, LBs lack their normal lamellar structure.[5]

Follicular ichthyosis

Follicular ichthyosis (ichthyosis follicularis) is an umbrella term or histologic pattern that is present in many conditions and is defined by follicular orthohyperkeratosis with or without hypergranulosis in the infundibulum.[1] For differential diagnosis see *Table 3.3*.

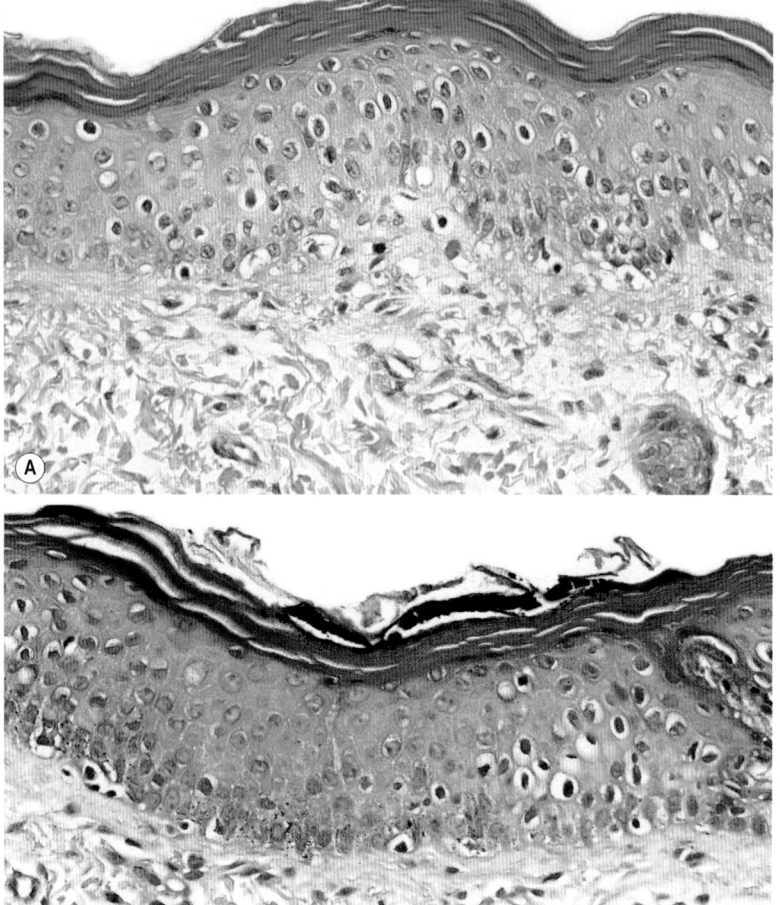

Fig. 3.56
Conradi-Hünermann-Happle syndrome: (**A**) there is hyperkeratosis, acanthosis, and a reduced granular cell layer. Note the basophilic deposits within the thickened stratum corneum; (**B**) the basophilic deposits represent calcium as seen in this von Kossa preparation.

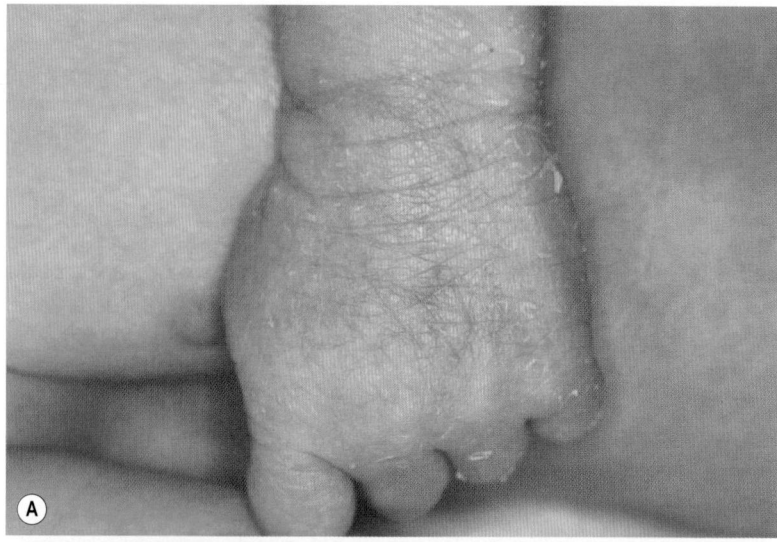

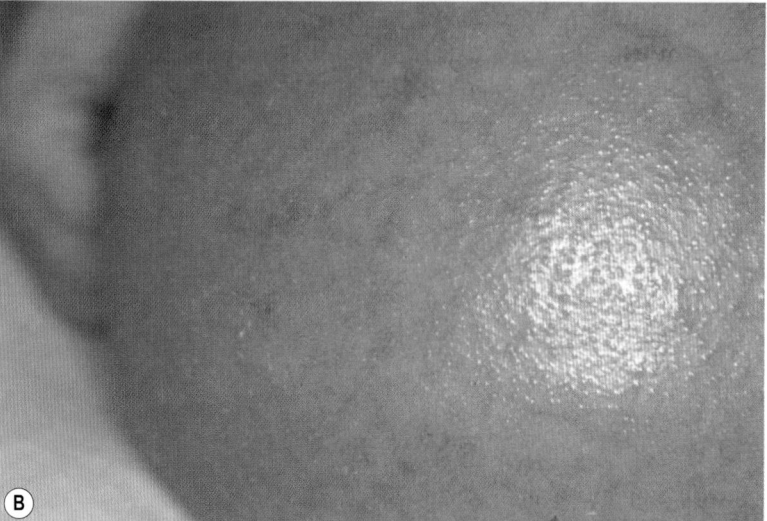

Fig. 3.57
Ichthyosis follicularis with alopecia and photophobia: (**A**) the skin is dry and ichthyosiform; (**B**) on the scalp a nonscarring alopecia with follicular hyperkeratosis is characteristic. By courtesy of H. Traupe MD, Dept of Dermatology, Münster, Germany.

Ichthyosis follicularis with alopecia and photophobia

Clinical features

Ichthyosis follicularis with alopecia (atrichia) and photophobia (IFAP syndrome) is an exceedingly rare X-linked, recessively inherited disease in males. Children can be born as collodion babies and characteristically present with generalized filiform follicular keratosis over the entire body including the scalp that often improves during the first year of life (*Fig. 3.57*).

Other features are ichthyosiform dry skin, generalized total nonscarring alopecia (with absence of eyelashes and eyebrows), and severe photophobia.[1-8] Ocular findings may include corneal deformity and opacity with surface vascularization.[7] Angular cheilitis, keratotic psoriasiform plaques on the extensor surfaces of the extremities, and nail dystrophy with periungual infection may also be present.[7] Additional findings including hypohidrosis, recurrent respiratory infections, skeletal abnormalities, growth retardation, cryptorchidism or progressive deteriorating neurologic symptoms such as generalized seizures, mental retardation, and cerebellar symptoms.[1-8] Female carriers are affected by circumscribed hairless, anhidrotic or ichthyotic areas along the lines of Blaschko.[4,5,8]

Pathogenesis and histologic features

IFAP is caused by missense mutations in the X-linked gene *MBTPS2* encoding membrane-bound transcription factor protease, site 2.[9,10] Different mutations on other sites in the *MBTPS2* gene are responsible for

keratosis follicularis spinulosa decalvans,[11] Olmsted syndrome,[12] and BRESEK/BRESHECK syndrome.[13]

Membrane bound transcription factor protease site 2 is a zinc metalloprotease essential for cholesterol homeostasis as well as for endoplasmic reticulum (ER) stress response. In cultured cells of IFAP patients, residual enzyme activity is only about a third of wild type activity.[9,10]

The follicular lesions are characterized by projecting hyperkeratotic plugs showing focal parakeratosis and associated hypergranulosis.[6] Hair follicles are atrophic and lack hair shafts and sebaceous glands (*Fig. 3.58*).[1] Sweat glands are normal, but hyperkeratosis of the acrosyringia may occlude the openings of sweat ducts (*Fig. 3.59*).[5]

The psoriasiform plaques show hyperkeratosis with parakeratosis, acanthosis, spongiosis, and a bandlike upper dermal lymphohistiocytic infiltrate.[7]

Differential diagnosis

Other forms of atrichia and follicular keratosis should be considered (see *Table 3.3*). Hereditary mucoepithelial dysplasia (HMD) may also present with photophobia and keratosis pilaris. However, it has an autosomal dominant trait and shows no mutations in *MBTPS2*.[14]

Ichthyosis with hypotrichosis

This congenital ichthyosis has two allelic variants, one characterized by a whole-body hypotrichosis without atrophoderma (autosomal recessive

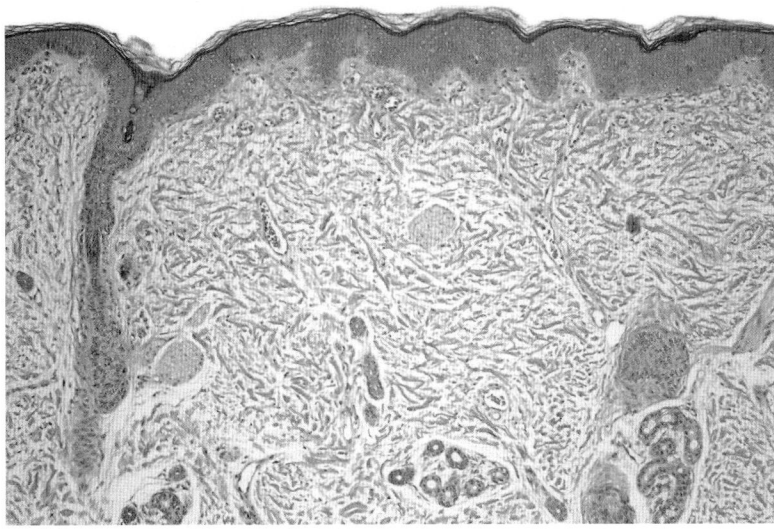

Fig. 3.58
Ichthyosis follicularis with alopecia and photophobia: The hair follicle is atrophic and lacks a hair shaft; the opening contains a keratotic plug.

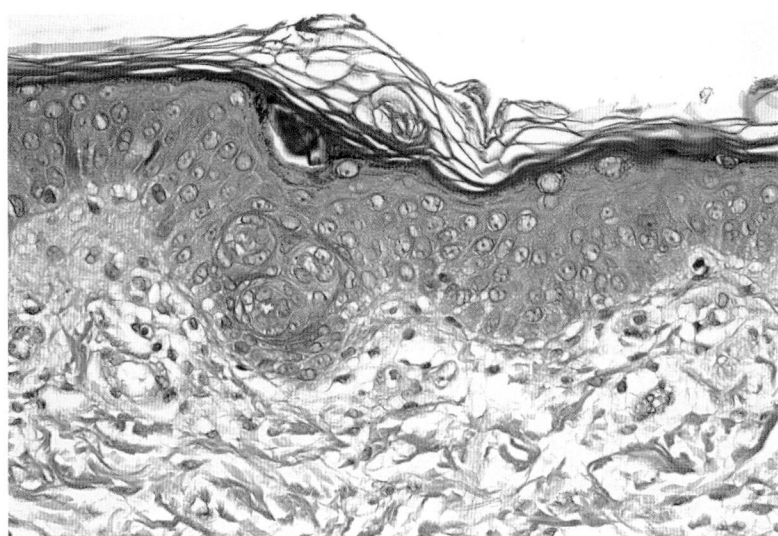

Fig. 3.59
Ichthyosis follicularis with alopecia and photophobia: there is hyperkeratosis centered on an acrosyringium.

ichthyosis with hypotrichosis [ARIH])[1,2] and one with follicular atrophoderma, i.e., follicular pitting on the dorsal aspects of the hands (congenital ichthyosis, follicular atrophoderma, hypotrichosis, and hypohidrosis [IFAH]).[3,4] Both phenotypes are associated with autosomal recessive mutations in the *ST14* gene,[1,2] which encodes a matriptase that plays an important role in the epidermal protease network.[5,6] Clinical heterogeneity may be caused by different types of *ST14* mutations.[1,4,7,8] The hair phenotype can be explained by the fact that matriptase is expressed in the cortex cells and shaft of the anagen hair.[9]

Neonatal ichthyosis-sclerosing cholangitis syndrome

Neonatal ichthyosis-sclerosing cholangitis (NISCH) syndrome is characterized by neonatal ichthyosis typically associated with jaundice due to sclerosing cholangitis of variable severity. Other features include hypotrichosis of the scalp with frontal scarring alopecia, and leukocyte vacuoles.[1–3] Autosomal recessive mutations in *CLDN1* encoding claudin-1 have been detected.[4] Claudin-1 is a major component of the tight junctions in the epidermis, cholangiocytes, and hepatocytes.[5] Dysfunctions of claudin 1 account for permeability between epithelial cells resulting in hypercholanemia or epidermal barrier defect.[6]

Table 3.4
Acquired ichthyosis-like conditions

Etiology	Diseases
Dry skin	None
Paraneoplastic	Hodgkin and non-Hodgkin lymphoma Multiple myeloma, myelodysplasia Lymphomatoid papulosis Kaposi sarcoma Various carcinomas
Infections	Leprosy Tuberculosis HIV/AIDS
Malnutrition	Pellagra Vitamin A deficiency
Drugs (examples)	Lipid-lowering agents (statins), retinoids Nicotinic acid, clofazimine, allopurinol, cimetidine, lithium, hydroxyurea
Gastrointestinal diseases	Crohn disease Celiac disease Gastrectomy
Endocrinopathies	Hyperparathyroidism Hypothyroidism Diabetes
Miscellaneous	Renal insufficiency Sarcoidosis Graft-versus-host disease Dermatomyositis and systemic lupus erythematosus Down syndrome

Acquired ichthyosis-like conditions

Acquired ichthyosis-like or ichthyosiform conditions refer to patients who develop diffuse ichthyosis-like scaling during their life (*Table 3.4*). The adult-onset renders the term 'acquired ichthyosis' inappropriate. It is an important paraneoplastic manifestation of a number of malignancies: Hodgkin lymphoma is most often encountered, but non-Hodgkin lymphoma, including mycosis fungoides and a range of carcinomas, are also associations.[1–8,17] Ichthyosiform skin changes may also accompany malnutrition, human immunodeficiency virus (HIV) and other infectious diseases, sarcoidosis, connective tissue diseases, celiac disease and other gastrointestinal diseases, renal insufficiency, hypothyroidism, and graft-versus-host disease (GVHD).[4,9–16] Ichthyosiform skin changes following kava consumption or the administration of lipid-lowering agents and other various drugs have been documented.[13,14] The features of acquired ichthyosis-like skin conditions most often resemble those of ichthyosis vulgaris both clinically and histologically (*Figs 3.60–3.63*).

Clinical differential diagnosis includes xerosis cutis, which lacks thick scales, develops at a later age, and can be easily treated by emollients.

Pityriasis rotunda

Clinical features

Also known as pityriasis circinata, this acquired disorder of keratinization was originally described in the Japanese.[1] It is also not uncommon in South Africans (Bantu) and West Indian blacks,[2,3] and has been reported in a subpopulation of Italians in Sardinia.[4–7]

Patients present with persistent, very sharply defined, circular or oval areas of hyper- or hypopigmentation associated with a fine scale (*Fig. 3.64*). Lesions, which are usually multiple and frequently numerous, are characteristically noninflammatory and asymptomatic. Often, they are confluent. They measure 0.5–28 cm in diameter and are particularly located on the trunk and limbs. The sex incidence is equal. Lesions are sometimes

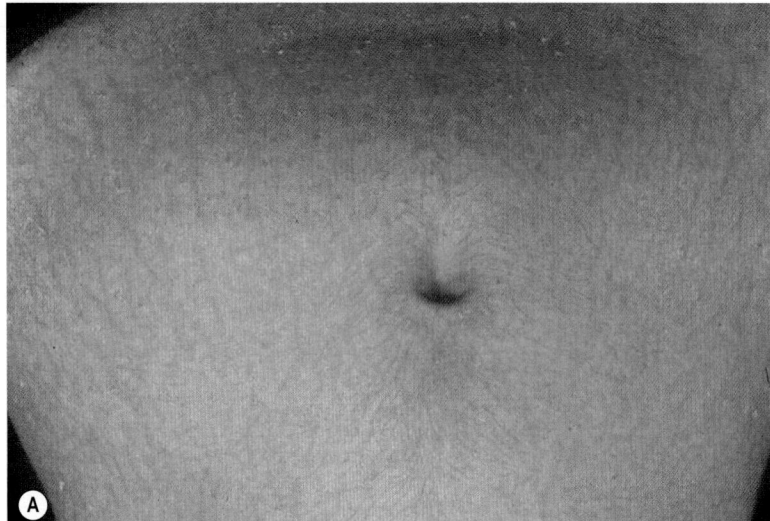

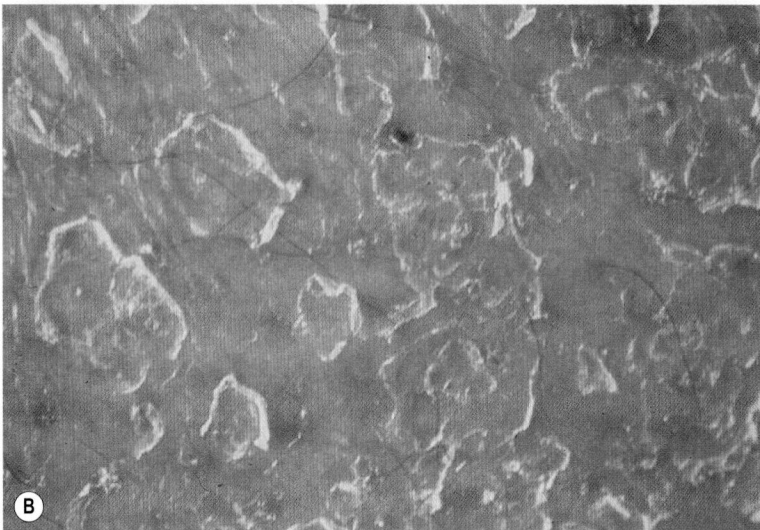

Fig. 3.60
Acquired ichthyosis: (**A**) cutaneous manifestations most often resemble ichthyosis vulgaris; (**B**) close-up view of the scale. By courtesy of the Institute of Dermatology, London, UK.

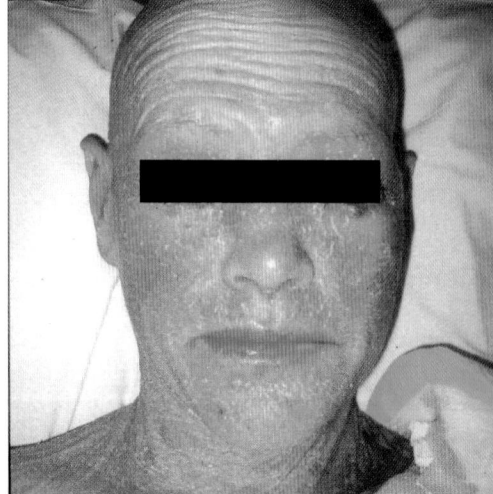

Fig. 3.61
Acquired ichthyosis: there is intense erythema and scaling. This patient also suffered from graft-versus-host disease. By courtesy of B. Solky, MD, Department of Dermatology, Brigham and Women's Hospital and Harvard Medical School, Boston, USA.

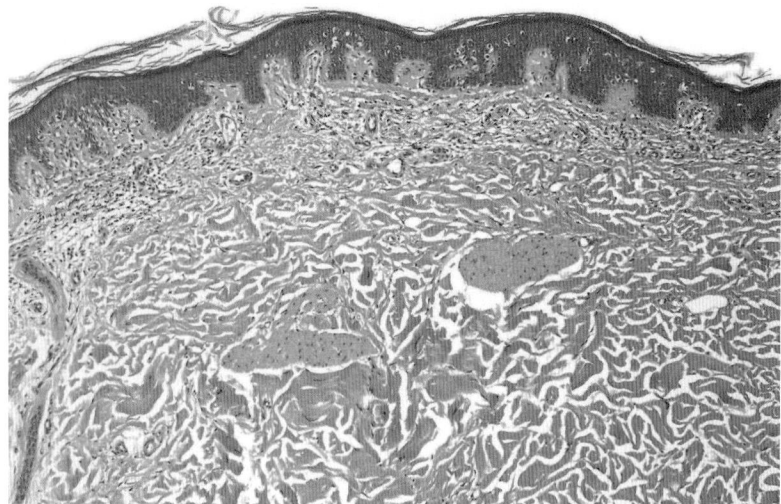

Fig. 3.62
Acquired ichthyosis: this patient developed ichthyosis in a background of mycosis fungoides. Low-power view showing marked focally compact hyperkeratosis and acanthosis.

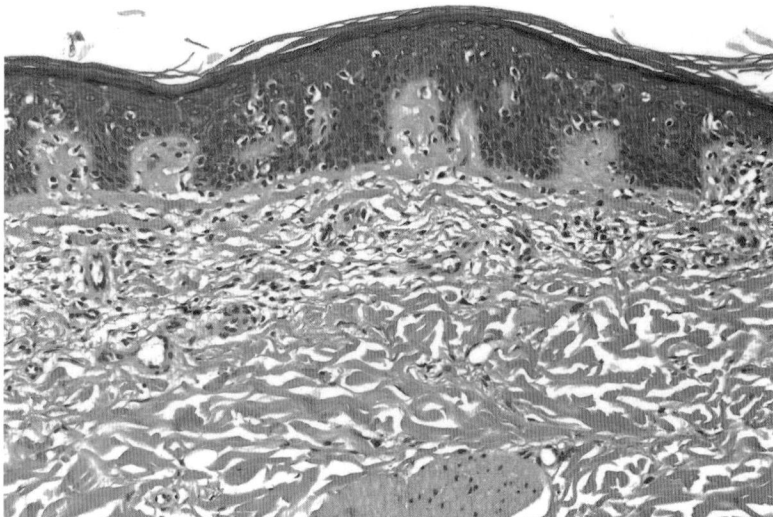

Fig. 3.63
Acquired ichthyosis: high-power view to emphasize the thinned granular layer. Mycosis fungoides as defined by an atypical lymphocyte population and epidermotropism with retraction artifact.

associated with gradual remission during the summer months and relapse in winter.[6] The maximum incidence is in the third to fifth decades. There is often a family history of ichthyosis vulgaris.[8] Familial cases may occasionally be seen.[8,9]

Pityriasis rotunda sometimes, but not always, appears to be a cutaneous marker of severe internal disease, including tuberculosis,[1] cancer (particularly hepatoma),[10,11] myeloma, leukemia,[12] cirrhosis,[6] ovarian and uterine disease,[13] malnutrition, diabetes, and favism.[8] Pityriasis rotunda is best be regarded as an acquired circumscribed variant of ichthyosis.[12]

Histologic features

The histologic features are subtle and consist of compact orthohyperkeratosis with a diminished or absent granular cell layer and loss of the epidermal rete ridge pattern. Immunohistochemistry reveals reduced expression of filaggrin and loricrin.[14,15] Increased pigmentation of the basal keratinocytes may be evident. A mild perivascular chronic inflammatory cell infiltrate is sometimes present in the superficial dermis. A superficial fungal infection, mainly pityriasis versicolor, should always be excluded.[16]

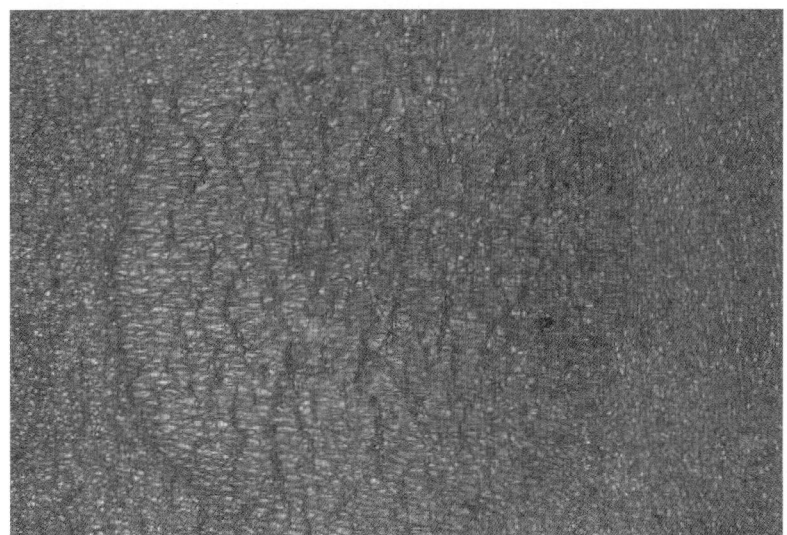

Fig. 3.64
Pityriasis rotunda: characteristic lesion showing circumscription, scaling, and hyperpigmentation. By courtesy of R.A. Marsden, MD, St George's Hospital, London, UK.

Keratosis pilaris

Clinical features

This fairly common condition, which has an autosomal dominant mode of inheritance, is probably a follicular variant of ichthyosis and, indeed, frequently accompanies ichthyosis vulgaris.[1–3] The age at presentation is most often in the first two decades of life with a peak during adolescence.[2] There is an apparent increased incidence in females, in particular those suffering from hyperandrogenism and obesity. The lesions present as pruritic small follicular keratoses, sometimes containing small, distorted hairs. They are most often found on the lateral aspects of the arms and thighs, although the face, trunk, and buttocks may also be affected (Fig. 3.65).[2] Seasonal variation, with lesions being much more severe in winter, is often documented.[2] There is an increased incidence of atopy.[2]

Although keratosis pilaris most often presents as an isolated phenomenon, occasionally it may develop in association with systemic disease, including Hodgkin lymphoma, vitamins B12 and C deficiency, hypothyroidism, Cushing disease, and treatment with adrenocorticotropic hormone.[3–5] A keratosis pilaris-like eruption has been described in BRAF kinase inhibitor therapy.[6]

Histologic features

Keratosis pilaris is characterized by follicular dilatation and keratin plugs, which may contain one or several distorted hair shafts (Fig. 3.66).[4] A mild, lymphocytic cell infiltrate surrounds superficial dermal blood vessels and sometimes also involves the hair follicles.

Keratosis pilaris atrophicans

Clinical features

Keratosis pilaris atrophicans combines the features of follicular hyperkeratosis and atrophic scarring.[1] According to different modes of inheritance, clinical presentation, and variable associations three conditions have been described, namely ulerythema ophryogenes, atrophoderma vermiculata, and keratosis follicularis spinulosa decalvans.[2]

Ulerythema ophryogenes (keratosis pilaris atrophicans faciei, KPAF) presents at birth or in early infancy with follicular papules and surrounding erythema followed by atrophic scarring affecting the lateral aspect of the eyebrows (Fig. 3.67).[3–5] The cheeks, forehead, temples, and neck may also be involved (Fig. 3.68). Later on, there may be complete loss of eyebrows. Keratosis pilaris affecting the extensor aspects of the arms and thighs is also

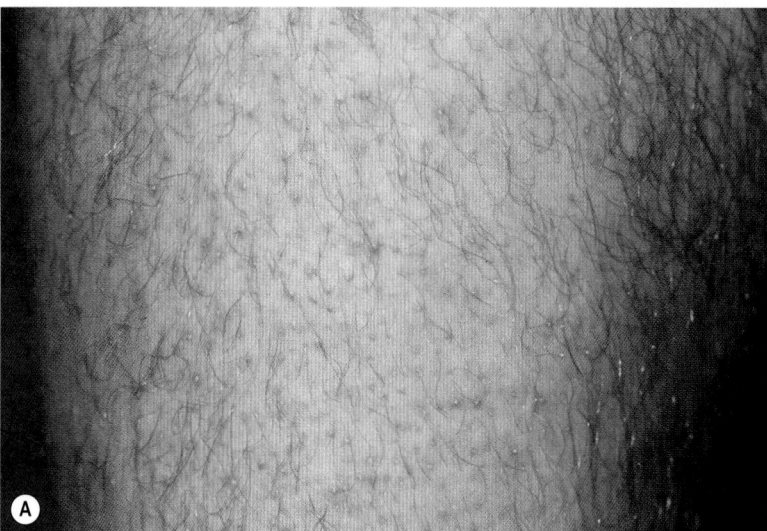

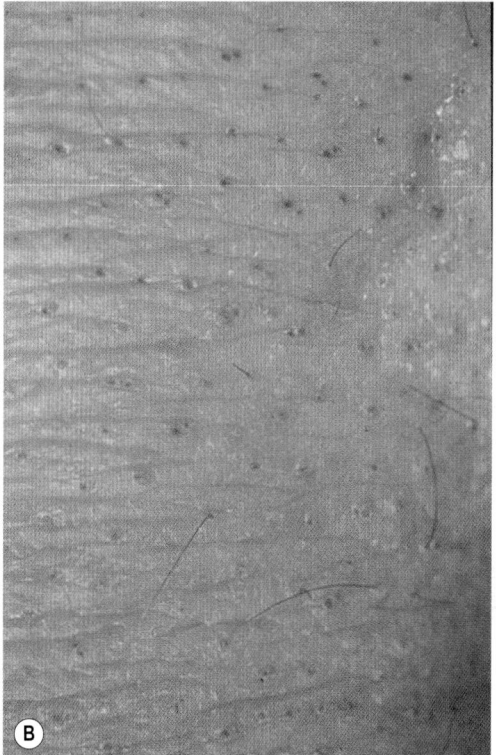

Fig. 3.65
Keratosis pilaris: (**A**) typical follicular papules and pustules on the thigh; (**B**) note the conspicuous plugged follicles. (**A**) By courtesy of R.A. Marsden, MD, St George's Hospital, London, UK. (**B**) By courtesy of the Institute of Dermatology, London, UK.

sometimes present.[3] The condition is believed to be inherited as an autosomal dominant disorder.

It may be associated with a number of other inherited disorders, including Noonan syndrome, wooly hair, cardiofaciocutaneous syndrome, Cornelia de Lange syndrome, Rubinstein-Taybi syndrome, and partial monosomy 18.[3,6–12] The association with Noonan syndrome is of particular importance since such patients suffer from potentially life-threatening congenital pulmonary stenosis. Ulerythema ophryogenes is also associated with atopy.[13]

Atrophoderma vermiculata (ulerythema acneiforme, atrophoderma vermiculatum, atrophoderma reticulata, acne vermoulante, folliculitis ulerythema reticulata, folliculitis ulerythematosa, honeycomb atrophy) is an exceedingly rare form of atrophic keratosis pilaris with an autosomal dominant inheritance. Patients present with follicular keratoses and pitted depressions separated by normal skin (moth-eaten appearance) affecting the cheeks, ears, and forehead (honeycomb atrophy).[2,14–17] The disorder presents

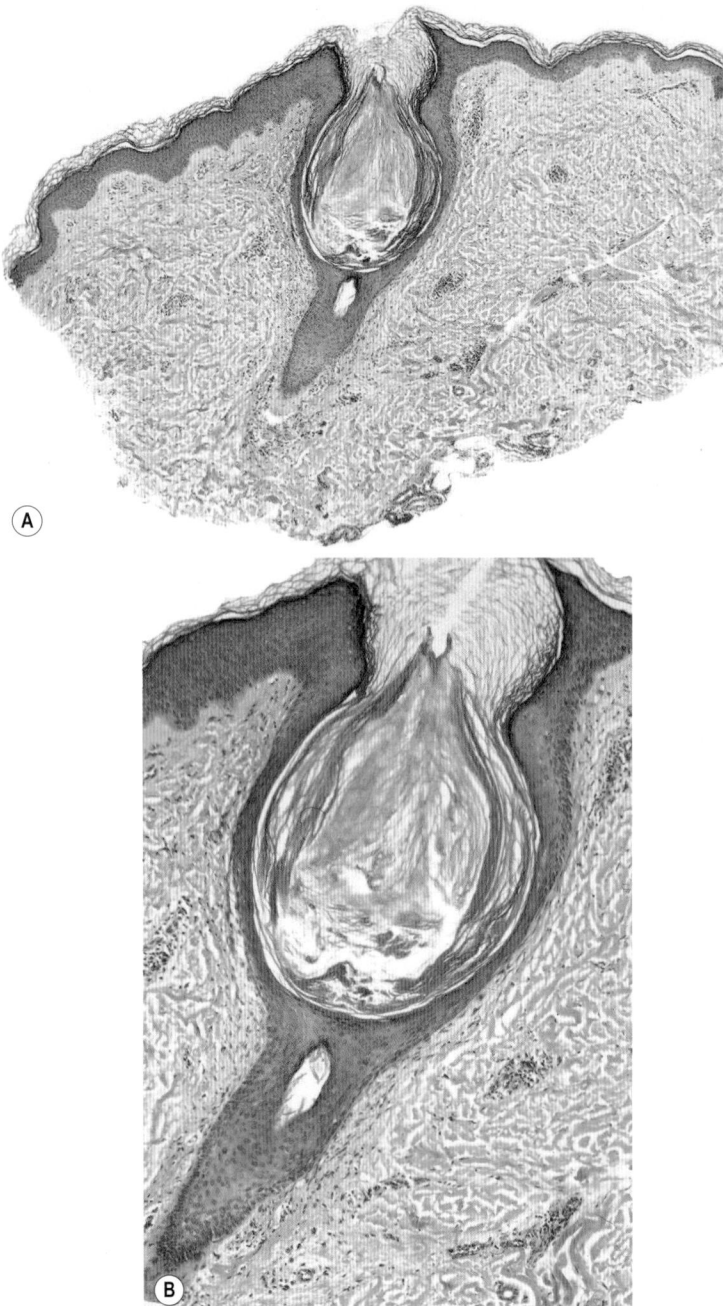

Fig. 3.66
Keratosis pilaris: (**A**) there is follicular dilatation and plugging; (**B**) note the atrophy of the infundibular epithelium.

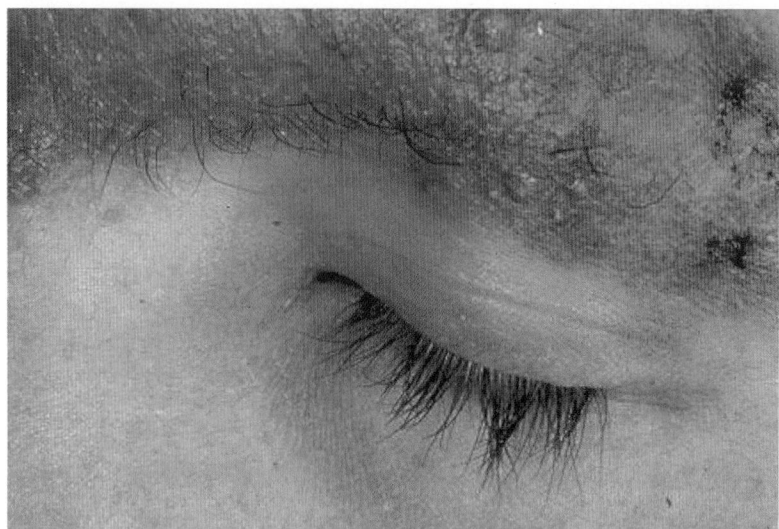

Fig. 3.67
Ulerythema ophryogenes: there is intense erythema with loss of follicles. The eyebrow is a commonly affected site. By courtesy of the Institute of Dermatology, London, UK.

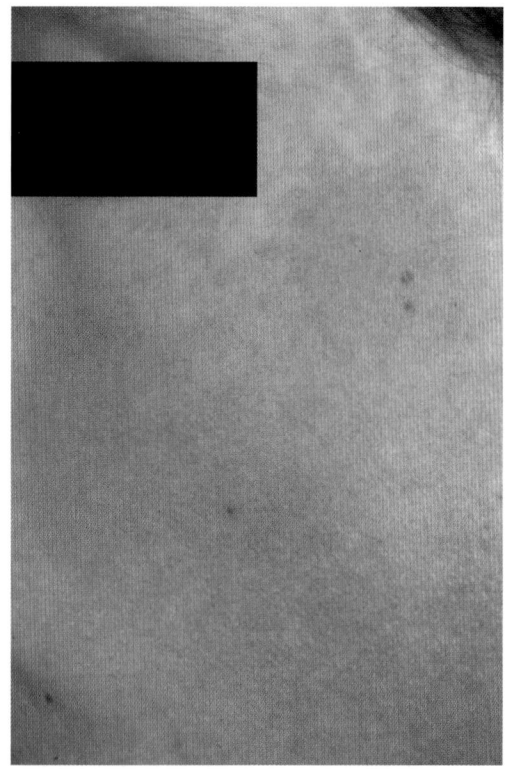

Fig. 3.68
Ulerythema ophryogenes: the cheek is also frequently involved. By courtesy of the Institute of Dermatology, London, UK.

in patients after 5 years of age.[2] Unilateral nevoid variants following Blaschko lines have also been documented.[15–17]

Keratosis follicularis spinulosa decalvans is characterized by diffuse atrophic keratosis pilaris associated with scarring alopecia affecting the scalp.[18–20] Other conditions sometimes present include atopy, palmoplantar hyperkeratosis, photophobia, and punctate keratitis.[18] In some patients it is inherited as an X-linked recessive disorder that is caused by mutations in the *MBTPS2* gene encoding membrane-bound transcription factor protease, site 2, which has been mapped to Xp21.13-p22.2.[21–23] X-linked dominant and autosomal dominant variants have also been described.[19] A pustular variant on the scalp that starts at puberty has been described as 'folliculitis spinulosa decalvans'.[24]

Pathogenesis and histologic features

The pathogenesis of keratosis pilaris atrophicans is unknown. The *MBTPS2*, as affected in keratosis follicularis spinulosa decalvans and IFAP, may interfere with sterol control and endoplasmatic reticulum stress response.[21]

All variants of keratosis pilaris atrophicans are characterized by follicular hyperkeratosis with ostial dilatation, atrophy of the sebaceous gland, and a scanty perifollicular and/or perivascular lymphohistiocytic infiltrate. Comedones and milia may be found. There is variable perifollicular fibrosis that extends into the reticular dermis (*Fig. 3.69*).[3,11,12,16]

Lichen spinulosus

Clinical features

Lichen spinulosus is a rare dermatosis of unknown etiology which particularly affects the extensor surfaces of the extremities, back, chest, buttocks,

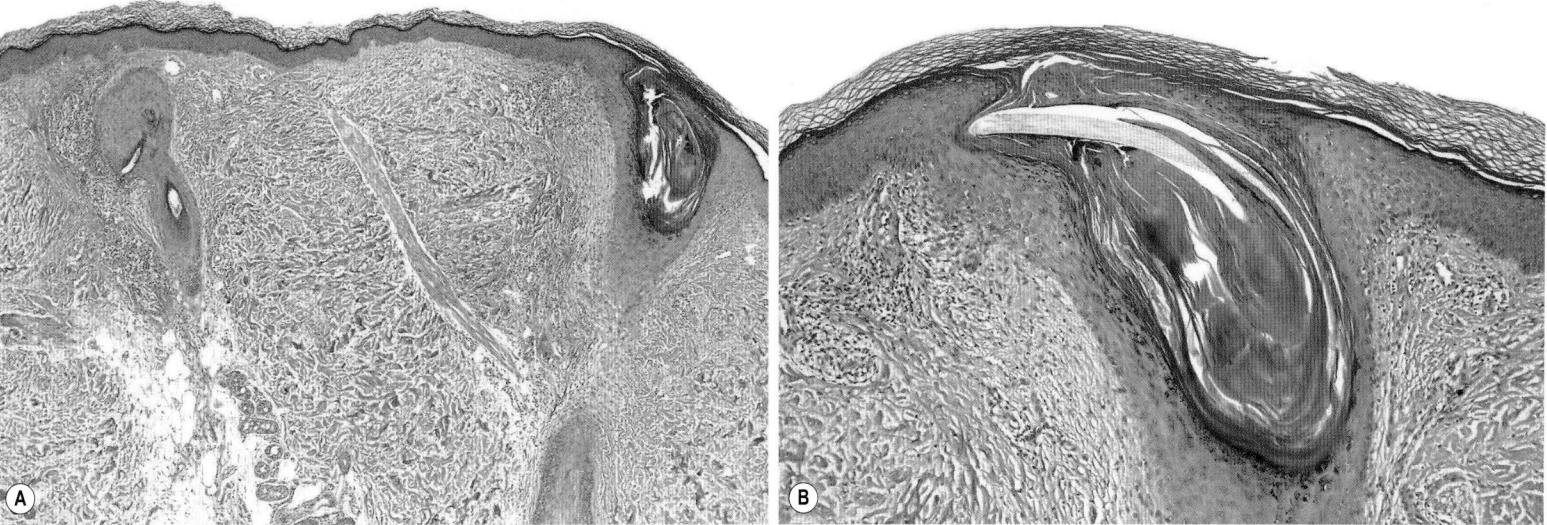

Fig. 3.69
Keratosis pilaris atrophicans: (**A**) low-power view showing gross follicular hyperkeratosis and dilatation of the ostium; (**B**) high-power view. Note the perifollicular fibrosis extending into the reticular dermis.

Table 3.5
Diseases with connexin mutations

Disease	Inheritance	Locus	Gene	Protein
Erythrokeratoderma variabilis (and progressive symmetrical erythrokeratoderma)	AD or AR	1q35.1	*GJB3*	Connexin 31
	AD	1q35.1	*GJB4*	Connexin 30.3
Erythrokeratoderma variabilis with erythema gyratum repens-like lesions	AD	1q35.1	*GJB4*	Connexin 30.3
Keratitis-ichthyosis-deafness syndrome/hystrix-like-ichthyosis deafness syndrome (KID/HID syndrome)	AD	13q11-12	*GJB2*	Connexin 26
Oculodentodigital dysplasia	AD	6q22-24	*GJA1*	Connexin 43
Vohwinkel keratoderma	AD	13q11-12	*GJB2*	Connexin 26
Hidrotic ectodermal dysplasia of Clouston	AD	13q11-12	*GJB6*	Connexin 30

face, and neck.[1] Occasionally, lesions are generalized. The condition presents in the second and third decades of life as round to oval, 2–6-cm flesh-colored and sometimes pruritic, symmetric plaques composed of multiple 1–3-mm thorny, grouped follicular papules which protrude above the surface of the skin.[1–3] The condition is of no clinical significance. Lichen spinulosus has been described in association with atopy, Crohn disease, HIV infection, and as an adverse drug reaction.[4–7]

Histologic features

Lichen spinulosus is characterized by keratotic plugging of dilated follicular infundibula and a superficial perivascular and perifollicular lymphohistiocytic infiltrate.[1] Sebaceous glands may be atrophic or absent. Perforating folliculitis-like features can be superimposed.

Differential diagnosis

There is considerable histologic overlap with keratosis pilaris and the follicular lesions of pityriasis rubra pilaris. The distinction is best made clinically.

Phrynoderma

Clinical features

Phrynoderma (toad skin) most often develops as a consequence of vitamin A deficiency.[1–4] Other proposed etiological factors include deficiencies of the vitamin B complex, riboflavin, vitamin C, vitamin E, and essential fatty acids.[4] In Western countries most cases develop as a result of malabsorption.[4,5] Patients present with xerosis, hyperpigmentation and multiple 2–6-mm, red-brown, dome-shaped papules with a central folliculocentric crater filled with laminated keratinous debris.[1,4] The elbows and knees are

predominantly affected, but lesions may extend to involve the thighs, upper arms, and buttocks.[1]

Histologic features

The papules consist of a cystically dilated follicular infundibulum filled with keratinous debris.[4]

Erythrokeratoderma

'Erythrokeratoderma' or 'erythrokeratodermia' refers to a group of genodermatoses characterized by localized erythematous lesions, hyperkeratotic plaques, and, infrequently, mild palmoplantar keratosis.[1] Many of these diseases represent connexin mutations (*Table 3.5*). Connexin genes code for transmembrane proteins that form gap junctions and are involved in epidermal differentiation. Other connexin mutations, such as the KID/hystrix-like ichthyosis-deafness (HID) syndrome and Vohwinkel syndrome are associated with sensorineural hearing loss. In others, the genetic defect has yet to be identified.[2] According to a consensus conference erythrokeratodermas are now classified as ichthyoses.[3]

Erythrokeratoderma variabilis

Clinical features

Erythrokeratoderma variabilis (Mendes da Costa syndrome) is a rare ichthyosiform dermatosis with an autosomal dominant mode of inheritance although an autosomal recessive variant has also been described.[1–5] Lesions usually present soon after birth or during the first year of life and are of two types, typically occurring simultaneously:

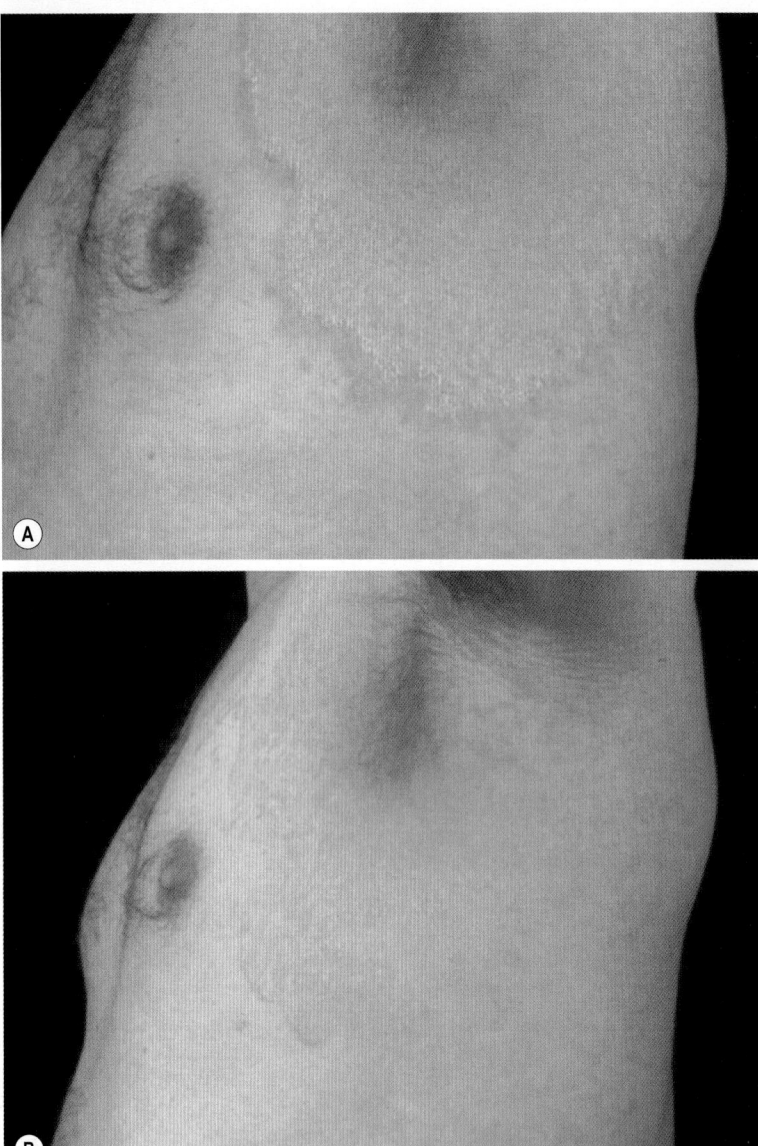

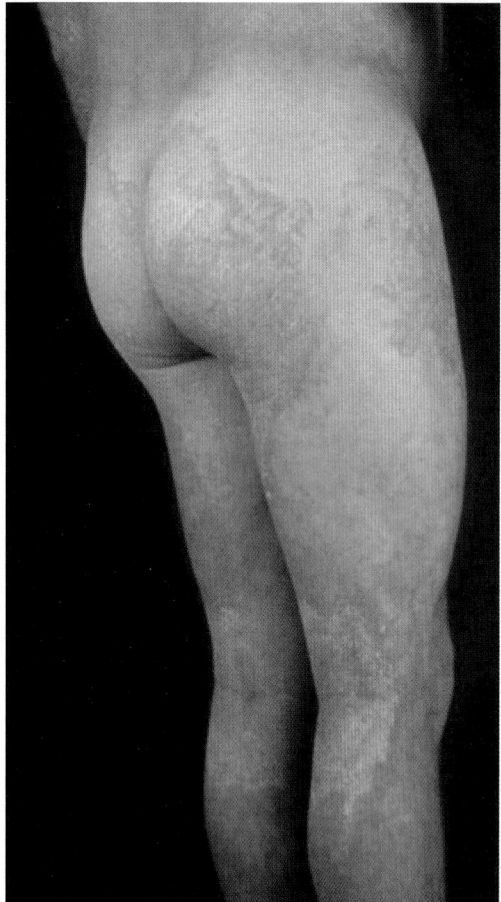

Fig. 3.71
Erythrokeratoderma variabilis: fixed geographical, reddish-yellow-brown greasy, hyperkeratotic plaques.

Fig. 3.70
Erythrokeratoderma variabilis: (**A**) annular erythematous lesions showing scaling; (**B**) migration within days.

- Type 1 lesions are symmetrically distributed, discrete figurate, and often bizarre patches of erythema, which vary in size, shape, number, and location over periods of hours and days (*Fig. 3.70*).[3]
- Type 2 lesions are well-defined, fixed geographical, reddish-yellow-brown, greasy, hyperkeratotic plaques arising either within the erythematous lesions or, more often, independently (*Fig. 3.71*).

Manifestations of the disease vary within a family and within an individual. The condition affects the face, buttocks, and extensor surfaces of the extremities. Occasionally mild pruritus or a burning sensation are a feature.[4] Cold weather in winter, stress, and estrogen-containing oral contraceptives may exacerbate the condition, while the symptoms often improve in the summer months.[1,2,4] Hypertrichosis (of vellus hairs) and mild keratoderma of the palms and soles can be present.[3,6] The mucous membranes, hair, teeth, and nails are unaffected and there are no associated systemic manifestations.[4]

Pathogenesis and histologic features

In many, but certainly not all families, dominant negative mutations in *GJB3* encoding connexin 31 or *GJB4* encoding connexin 30.3 have been found.[7–10] Autosomal recessive mutations in *GJB3* have likewise been reported.[11] A subset of patients with connexin 30.3 mutations manifest with a unique clinical feature, namely transient erythematous patches with a peculiar, circinate or gyrate border reminiscent of erythema gyratum repens, i.e., erythrokeratoderma with erythema gyratum repens-like lesions.[13–14] Connexin genes code for proteins that form intercellular channels called gap junctions that allow for transport and signaling between neighboring cells in the epidermis. In the skin, Cx31 and Cx30.3 are expressed in the stratum granulosum of the epidermis with a suggested role in late keratinocyte differentiation.[12]

The histopathological features of erythrokeratoderma variabilis are not specific, consisting of orthohyperkeratosis, variable parakeratosis, irregular acanthosis, and papillomatosis with an undulating skin surface (*Fig. 3.72*).[3,15] Dyskeratotic cells with pyknotic nuclei reminiscent of the grains of Darier have been described (*Fig. 3.73*).[6] The granular cell layer appears normal. A perivascular lymphocytic inflammatory cell infiltrate may be present in the superficial dermis.[15,16] Differentiation from psoriasis vulgaris or pityriasis rubra pilaris requires clinicopathological correlation.

Connexin immunohistochemistry discloses an irregular distribution of the epidermal gap junction proteins in erythrokeratoderma variabilis. Loss of connexin 31 seems to be compensated by connexin 43 overexpression. A cyclic up and down regulation may account for the migratory nature of some lesions.[16]

Ultrastructural observations have shown an increased number of gap junctions, some of which display four layers, suggesting a loosened connection of the keratinocyte plasma membrane through the gap junctions.[17] Other studies have revealed markedly diminished numbers of Odland bodies in the granular cell layer.[6,16] Conspicuous nonmyelinated nerve fibers and Schwann cells have been described in the papillary dermis.[6,16] These, however, are not consistent findings.[18] Nuclear encirclement by condensed keratin filaments and keratohyalin has also been recorded.[18]

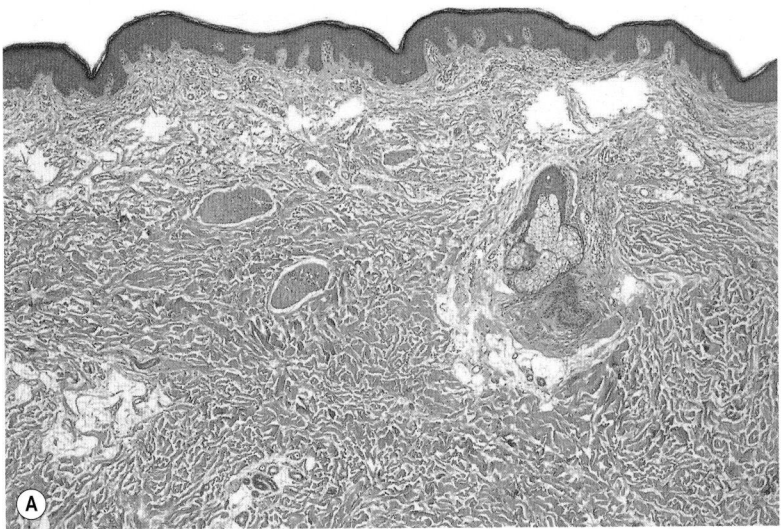

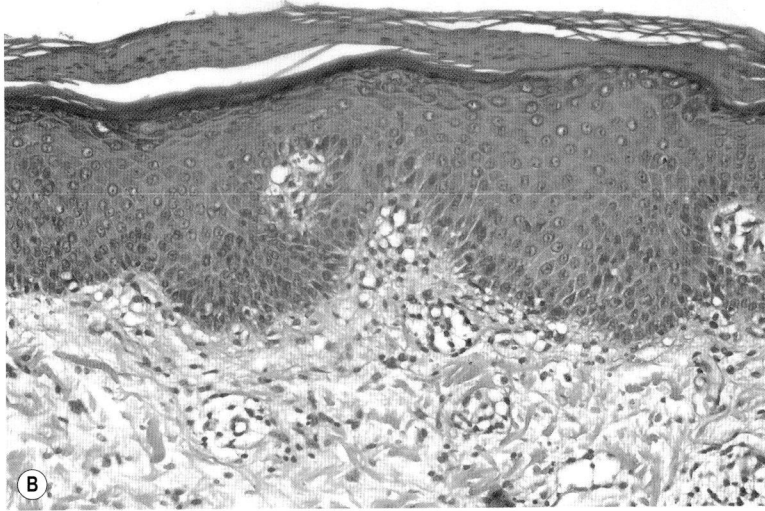

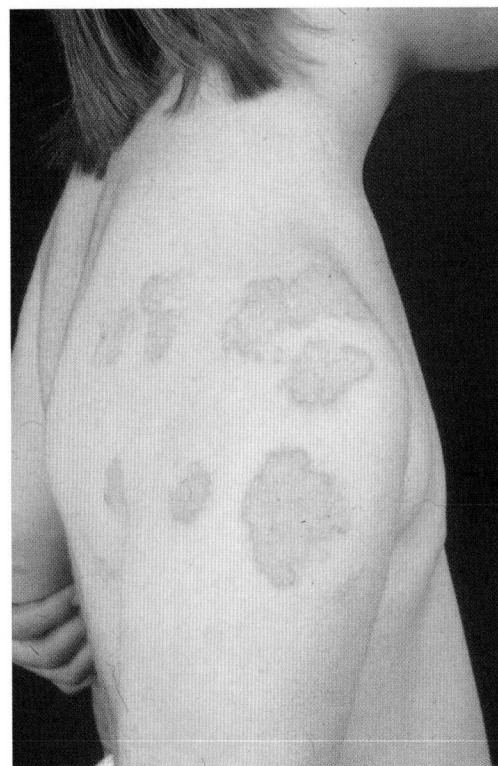

Fig. 3.74
Progressive symmetric erythrokeratodermia: erythematous scaly plaques gradually appear on the extensor surfaces on the extremities and then persist.

Fig. 3.72
Erythrokeratoderma variabilis: (**A**) low-power view showing hyperkeratosis, acanthosis with an undulating skin surface and a very mild superficial perivascular chronic inflammatory cell infiltrate; (**B**) high-power view showing marked parakeratosis overlying a thickened orthokeratotic stratum corneum. Note the presence of a granular cell layer.

Progressive symmetrical erythrokeratoderma

Progressive symmetrical erythrokeratoderma (Gottron syndrome) is a non-migratory variant of erythrokeratoderma with large, fine scaly orange-red plaques with geographic borders that are symmetrically distributed on the shoulders, cheeks and buttocks (*Fig. 3.74*).[1] Progressive symmetrical erythrokeratoderma may represent a manifestation of erythrokeratoderma variabilis as the same mutation in the gene *GJB4* has been identified in affected individuals. Some of these patients express the variable form,[2] while others develop the progressive symmetrical form of the disease.[3] In addition the coexpression of both variants of erythrokeratoderma clinically, histologically, and ultrastructurally has been reported in siblings.[4]

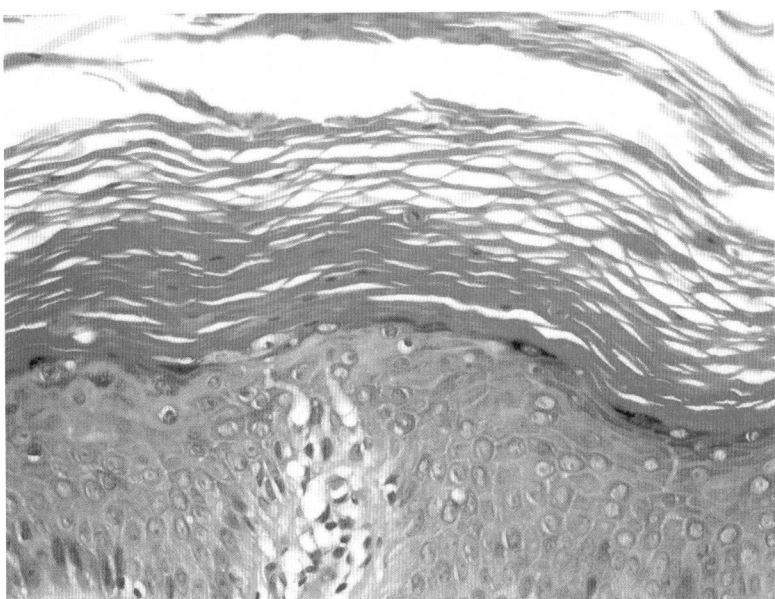

Fig. 3.73
Erythrokeratoderma variabilis: scattered dyskeratotic keratinocytes are sometimes seen.

Keratitis-ichthyosis-deafness syndrome, hystrix-like ichthyosis with deafness, porokeratotic adnexal ostial nevus

Clinical features

Keratitis-ichthyosis-deafness (KID) syndrome and hystrix-like ichthyosis-deafness (HID) syndrome are likely to represent a spectrum of phenotypic variability of the same connexin-26 mutation instead of separate entities.[1] Interestingly, a mosaicism for this mutation has been described as porokeratotic adnexal ostial nevus (PAON), also known as porokeratotic eccrine ostial and dermal duct nevus or porokeratotic eccrine nevus (PEN).[2]

Newborns with KID syndrome may present generalized erythema or a diffuse scaling and a leathery skin. During infancy patients develop spiny hyperkeratosis around the flexures, elbows, and knees, and hystrix-like scaling on the limbs. Scattered follicular hyperkeratosis can be found on the trunk. Most characteristically, symmetrical, well-demarcated hyperkeratotic and warty plaques appear on scalp, ears, face, and occasionally the trunk and limbs (*Fig. 3.75*).[3] Circumoral furrows may lead to a progeria-like appearance. Palmar and plantar involvement with accentuation of the skin markings has been likened to heavily grained leather.[4]

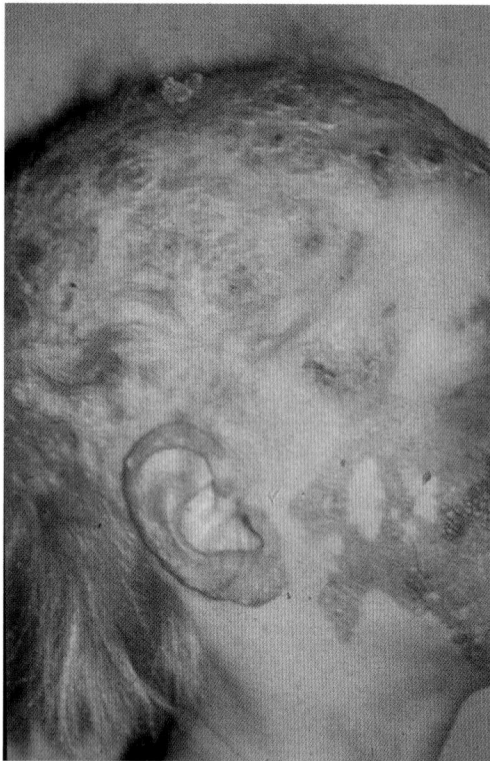

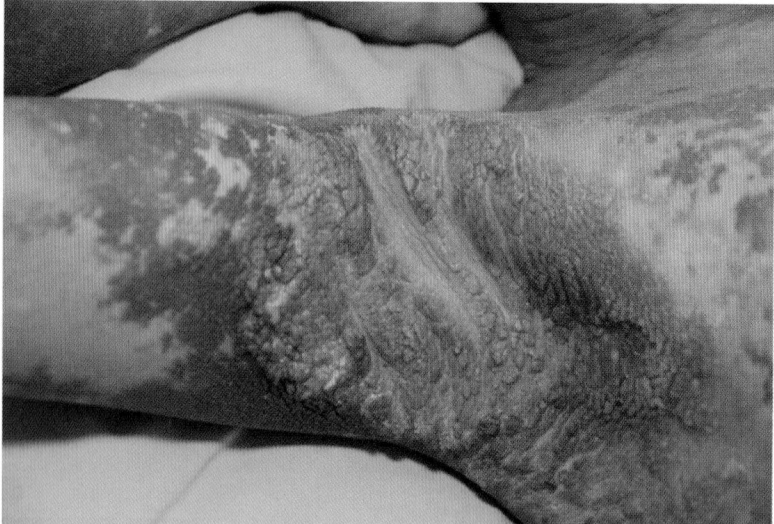

Fig. 3.76
HID syndrome: verrucous and hyperkeratotic, brownish-yellow sharply circumscribed plaques.

Fig. 3.75
KID syndrome: there is marked scaling of the scalp with alopecia. Note the facial erythema and dark plaques on the cheeks. By courtesy of R.J.G. Rycroft, MD, St John's Dermatology Centre, London, UK.

Squamous carcinoma of the tongue and skin as well as multiple hair follicle tumors including malignant pilar tumors may develop in young adults and can lead to metastases.[5–8]

Inflammation of the cornea with photophobia is usual and a vascularizing keratitis leads to severe visual impairment.[4] The end result is destruction of the cornea by a pannus of vascular or fibrous tissue (keratoconus).[3,9,10]

Deafness is of the congenital neurosensory type, but is occasionally due to recurrent otitis media; conduction defects may also be present.[3,4] It is often total and frequently present at birth.[11–13]

Ectodermal dysplasia is variably present and features include alopecia (either partial or complete, including eyebrows and eyelashes), small malformed teeth with increased caries, scrotal tongue, leukokeratosis, and a variety of dystrophic nail changes including fragility, hyperkeratosis, dysplasia, leukonychia, and aplasia.[3,4]

Additional features that may be detected include increased susceptibility to superficial and systemic chronic infections (viral, bacterial, and fungal),[14,15] neuromuscular disease, retraction of the Achilles tendon, hypohidrosis, heat intolerance, and growth deficiency.[3] Mental retardation is a rare feature.[3]

The HID syndrome shows congenital ichthyosis with hystrix-like keratosis, in particular on the trunk and on the extremities (Fig. 3.76). Keratitis of the eyes is less prominent in HID patients, but they also suffer from neurosensorial deafness, proneness to mycotic/bacterial skin infections, and skin cancer.[1,16,17]

PAON is a hyperkeratotic verrucous, hard epidermal nevus following the lines of Blaschko. Comedo-like papules and filiform keratosis have been described, as well as keratotic pits on the palms and soles. The disease is usually unilateral, but may also be bilateral with widespread distribution on the extremities, including palms and soles and, more rarely, the trunk. Focal anhidrosis, hair loss, onychodysplasia, and pruritus can occur. Noteworthy, a mother affected by PEN may give birth to a child affected by KID syndrome.[2,29,30]

Pathogenesis and histologic features

Recurrent and novel *GJB2* mutations encoding for connexin 26 have been detected not only in KID and HID syndrome, but also in many other

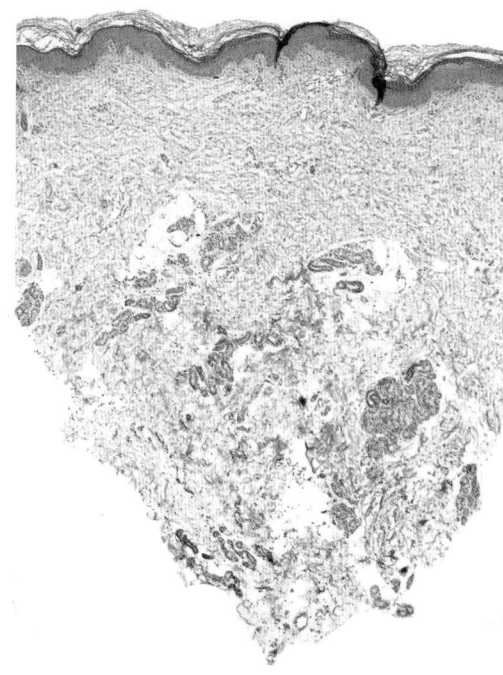

Fig. 3.77
KID syndrome: scanning magnification view showing mild hyperplasia of the epidermis. In this example the eccrine sweat glands are normal.

conditions.[18–23] Connexins are gap junction proteins that form inter- and intracellular channels for ion and molecule transfer, which is the basis for all cellular communication. Some of the *GJB2* mutations do not simply inhibit channel formation, but rather result in high conductance hemichannels at the cell surface.[24] The genotype/phenotype relationship between the various connexin 26 related conditions is not currently understood. It is important to note that the hearing deficiencies are often due to recessive mutations, whereas KID and HID syndrome are transmitted as autosomal dominant traits.[18–13]

In biopsies of HID and KID syndrome the epidermis shows psoriasiform, pseudoepitheliomatous or verruciform hyperplasia (Figs 3.77 and 3.78).[4] The granular cell layer appears partially absent or thin. A prominent and vacuolized stratum granulosum can be also observed and sometimes the nuclei of the keratinocytes are surrounded by empty spaces reminiscent of a bird's eye (Figs 3.79 and 3.80A).[25,26] The horny layer is orthohyperkeratotic or parakeratotic. Most characteristically, parakeratotic areas show tiny roundish nuclear remnants or shadow nuclei (Fig. 3.80B). The papillary

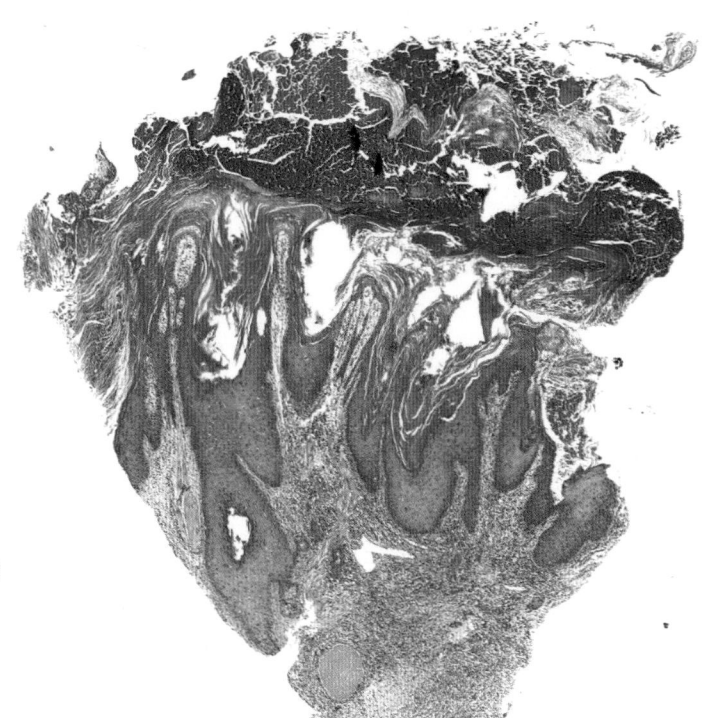

Fig. 3.78
HID syndrome: verrucous and pseudoepitheliomatous hyperplasia of the epidermis.

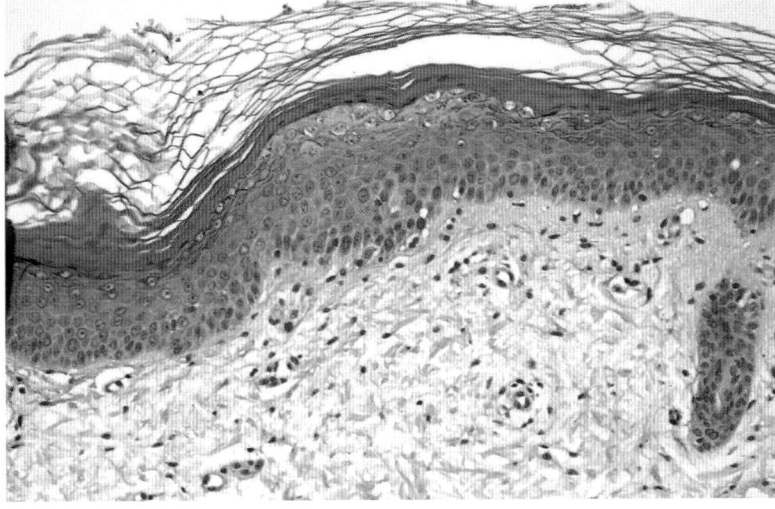

Fig. 3.79
KID syndrome: high-power view emphasizing the basket-weave keratin overlying a zone of compact keratin. There is focal parakeratosis and vacuolization of the granular layer.

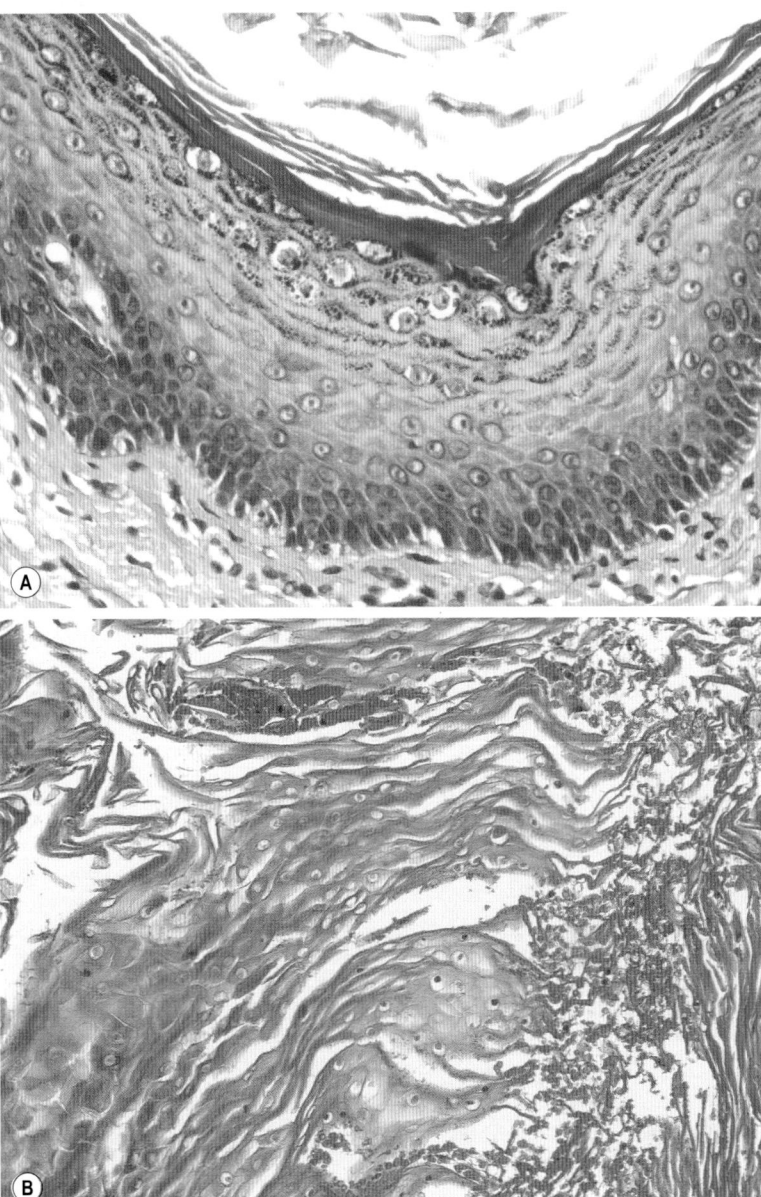

Fig. 3.80
HID syndrome: the nuclei of the keratinocytes are surrounded by empty spaces reminiscent of a bird's eye, (**A**) in the granular layer and (**B**) the horny layer.

dermis contains a mild perivascular lymphocytic infiltrate or dense mixed lichenoid infiltrate.[4] Follicular plugging is commonly present and occasionally the orifices of the eccrine ducts are similarly affected.[27] Eccrine sweat glands may be diminished in number and atrophic, with thickened, hyalinized basement membranes. Absent or atrophic hair follicles are seen in the areas of alopecia.[1,4,25]

At the ultrastructural level, keratinocytes in KID syndrome show reduction of tonofibrils and abnormal membrane-bound granules containing mucous material that is discharged into the intercellular spaces.[28]

Histology of PAON is characterized by ortho- or parakeratotic plaques or filiform keratosis protruding from dilated ostia of hyperplastic sweat glands and hair follicles (*Fig. 3.81A*). The underlying epithelium reveals vacuolated cells with pyknotic nuclei and lacks keratohyalin granules (*Fig. 3.81B*). In contrast to true porokeratosis of any type, dysmaturation and signs of interface dermatitis are absent. In the papillary dermis a sparse or lichenoid

lymphocytic infiltrate is found. The epidermis between the adnexae shows acanthosis, papillomatosis, and orthohyperkeratosis.[29,30]

Acquired symmetrical acrokeratoderma

In China a series of patients were described that developed brown to black hyperkeratotic plaques over acral regions. The lesions were symmetrically distributed particularly on the wrists and dorsum of hands, fingers, and feet, but without involvement of palms and soles. A whitish discoloration of the skin after contact with water or sweating and worsening of the symptoms during the summer has been observed.[1,2] Genetic studies have not been reported. Histopathology reveals epidermal hyperkeratosis, acanthosis, and a papillary dermal perivascular lymphohistiocytic infiltrate.[2] Ultrastructural features of a biopsy taken after immersion consist of epidermal hyperkeratosis and spongiosis with partial split of the desmosomes.[1]

Palmoplantar keratoderma

The palmoplantar keratodermas (PPKs) comprise a large heterogeneous group of acquired or inherited cornification disorders characterized by hyperkeratosis of the palms and soles.[1] Hereditary PPK may be occur in

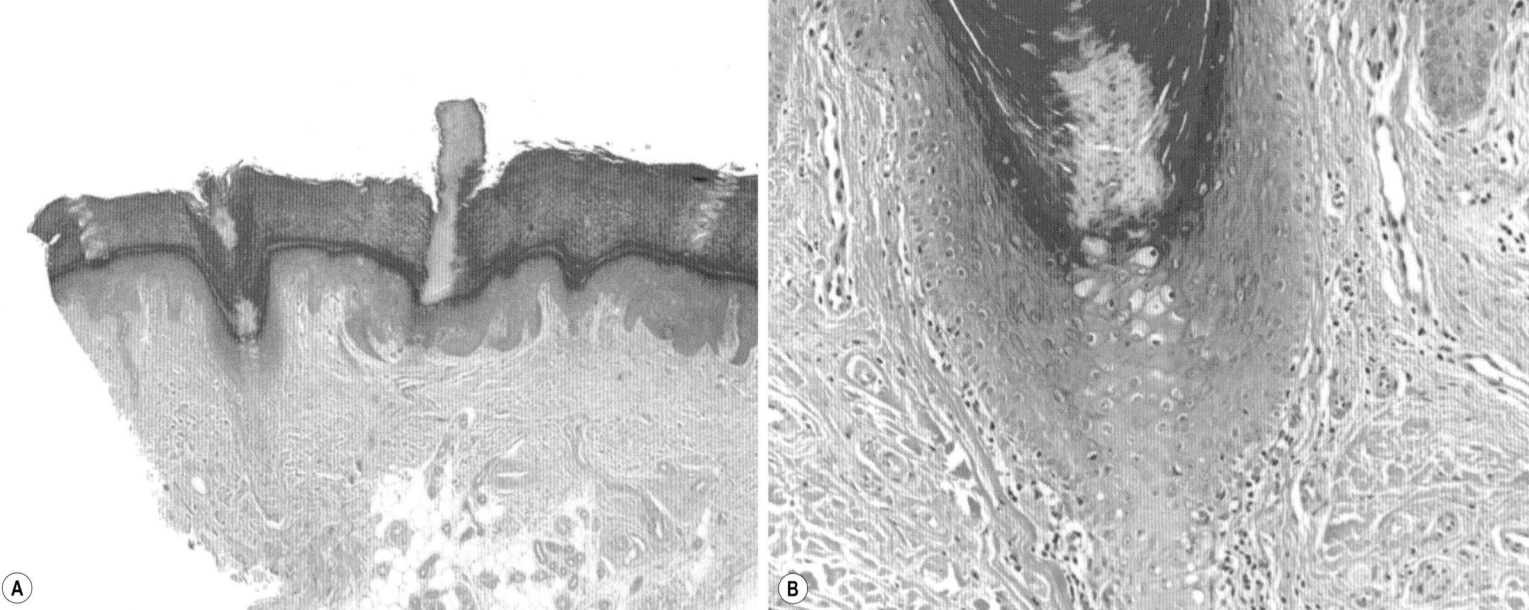

Fig. 3.81
Porokeratotic adnexal ostial nevus (PAON): (**A**) filiform keratoses, protrude from the dilated ostia of hyperplastic sweat glands and hair follicles; (**B**) the underlying epithelium reveals vacuolated epithelia with pyknotic nuclei and lacks keratohyalin granules.

Table 3.6
Palmoplantar keratodermas without associated symptoms (isolated, nonsyndromic)

Palmoplantar keratoderma	Disease	Inheritance	Gene
Diffuse	Epidermolytic PPK Vörner-Unna-Thost, (including tonotubular subtype, epidermolytic hyperkeratosis with polycyclic psoriasiform plaques, progressive palmoplantar keratoderma Greither)	AD	KRT1 or KRT9
	Non-epidermolytic PPK,		
	type Kimonis	AD	KRT1
	type Bothnia	AD	AQP5
	type Nagashima	AR	SERPINB7
	Keratolytic winter erythema	AD	Unknown
	Mal de Meleda (including Gamborg-Nielsen)	AR	SLURP1
Circumscribed	Striate palmoplantar keratoderma	AD	
	type 1		DSG1
	type 2		DSP
	type 3		KRT1
Punctate	Keratosis punctata palmoplantaris,	AD	
	type 1 (Buschke-Fischer-Brauer)		AAGAB (COL14A1)
	type 2 (Spiny keratoderma)		?
	type 3 (Marginal papular acrokeratoderma)		?

isolation or associated with other genetic diseases, such as ichthyosis, erythrokeratoderma, epidermolysis bullosa, ectodermal dysplasia, and dyskeratosis congenita (*Tables 3.6* and *3.7*).[2–6] When PPK is syndromic it may affect the heart, eyes, hearing or neural system. Acquired forms can be paraneoplastic or related to internal diseases. Therefore a specific diagnosis of PPK is mandatory for the purpose of management and genetic counseling.[2]

PKKs are classified on the basis of mode of inheritance, distribution of lesions, additional clinical features, and associated abnormalities.[1–8] Many of the inherited forms of the PPK have a late onset and show variability in one and the same family. The severity also depends on mechanical stress, e.g., exposure to pressure on the feet. The patients may suffer from maceration, blisters, malodor, and/or severe pain. Hyperhidrosis and fungal infections are common complications.

There are three major clinical categories of inherited PPK: diffuse, circumscribed, and punctate (see *Tables 3.6* and *3.7*).[4,7,8] Histologically, seven main histologic patterns have been proposed characterized by epidermolytic hyperkeratosis, orthohyperkeratosis or parakeratosis, hypergranulosis, transitional cells, widening of the intercellular spaces, intracytoplasmic eosinophilic inclusions, or depression of the epidermis with keratotic plaques (*Table 3.8*).

In many subtypes, the underlying molecular defect has been identified and can be related to structural proteins (keratins), cornified envelope (loricrin, transglutaminase), cohesion proteins (plakophilin, desmoplakin, desmoglein1), cell-to-cell communication (connexins, SLURP1, AAGAB), and epidermal proteases (cathepsin C).[5,6,9]

Epidermolytic palmoplantar keratoderma

Clinical features

Epidermolytic palmoplantar keratoderma (syn. keratosis palmoplantaris diffusa Vörner-Unna-Thost) represents the most common form of palmoplantar keratoderma with an incidence of 1:100 000. Reinvestigation of the original family with Unna-Thost PPK showed that epidermolytic forms existed within the family as had been described by Vörner. Therefore, it is not justified to separate Vörner disease from Unna-Thost disease. The unifying designation epidermolytic palmoplantar keratoderma seems more appropriate.[1,2]

This nonsyndromic PPK is inherited as an autosomal dominant and usually presents in the first years of life when the patients start running.[1–7]

Table 3.7
Palmoplantar keratodermas with associated symptoms (syndromic)

Palmoplantar keratoderma	Disease	Inheritance	Gene (Protein)	Symptoms
Diffuse	Huriez syndrome	AD	?	Sclerodactyly, nail dystrophy, squamous cell carcinomas in atrophic areas
	Vohwinkel syndrome	AD	*GJB2* (Connexin 26)	Mutilating keratoderma, sensorineural deafness
	Loricrin keratoderma	AD	*LOR* (Loricrin)	Associated ichthyosis
	KLICK syndrome	AR	*POMP*	Associated ichthyosis
	Clouston syndrome	AR	*GJB6* (Connexin 30)	Diffuse palmoplantar keratoderma, alopecia, nail dystrophies
	Olmsted syndrome	AD or XR	*TRPV3* *MBTPS2*	Diffuse mutilating palmoplantar and periorificial keratoses, ectodermal dysplasia
	Papillon-Lefèvre syndrome	AR	*CTSC* (Cathepsin)	Diffuse palmoplantar keratosis with severe periodontitis
	Naxos syndrome	AR or AD	*JUP* (Plakoglobin)	Wooly hair, cardiomegaly, tachycardia
	McGrath syndrome	AD	*PKP1* (Plakophilin 1)	Skin fragility, hypotrichosis, hypohidrosis, nail dystrophy, no cardiac complications
	Schöpf-Schulz-Passarge syndrome	AR	*WNT10A*	PPK with eyelid cysts, hypodontia and hypotrichosis
Circumscribed	Pachyonychia congenita	AD	*KRT6,* *KRT16* *KRT17*	Thickened nails, painful palmoplantar keratoderma, follicular hyperkeratosis, hair abnormalities, cysts, leukokeratosis, natal teeth
	Howel-Evans syndrome	AD	*RHBDF2*	Association with carcinoma of esophagus
	Richner-Hanhart syndrome	AR	*TAT* (Tyrosine amino-transferase)	Focal, often painful palmoplantar keratoderma
	Carvajal-Huerta syndrome	AR or AD	*DSP* (Desmoplakin)	PPK with dehiscent keratinocytes, wooly hair, arrhythmogenic left cardiomyopathy
Punctate	Cole disease	AD	*ENPP1*	Punctate keratoderma with guttate hypopigmentation, calcific tendinopathy or calcinosis cutis

Table 3.8
Histologic patterns of PPK (discarded entities in parentheses)

Epidermolytic hyperkeratosis Epidermolytic palmoplantar keratoderma Vörner-Unna-Thost, (Greither keratoderma, epidermolytic variant; hereditary painful callosities; PPK nummularis), and others
Orthohyperkeratosis, acanthosis, papillomatosis Non-epidermolytic (NEPPK) type Bothnia, type Nagashima, type Kimonis, Mal de Meleda (and variant Gamborg Nielsen), Huriez/Howel-Evans/Papillon-Lefèvre/Vohwinkel syndrome, (Greither keratoderma, non-epidermolytic variant), and others
Orthohyperkeratosis with focal parakeratosis, acanthosis, papillomatosis KLICK syndrome, erythrokeratoderma variabilis, HID/KID syndrome
Orthohyperkeratosis with parakeratosis and hypergranulosis with transitional cells Loricrin keratoderma
Widening of intercellular spaces and partial dehiscence of keratinocytes Striate palmoplantar keratoderma (type I, II), diffuse non-specified PPK with DSG1 mutation, Carvajal-Huerta syndrome, McGrath syndrome
Epithelia with pale cytoplasm and eosinophilic inclusions Pachyonychia congenita Oculocutaneous tyrosinemia

Depressed epidermis
- with overlying orthohyperkeratotic, focally parakeratotic plaque
   Keratosis punctata palmoplantaris type Buschke-Fischer-Bauer
   Keratosis punctata of palmar creases
   Marginal papular keratoderma
- with overlaying parakeratotic column
   Spiny keratoderma
- with overlying orthohyperkeratotic, focally parakeratotic plaque, fragmentation and loss of elastic fibers
   Acrokeratoelastoidosis Costa

Patients develop symmetrical, well-demarcated yellowish, smooth and waxy plaques covering the palms and soles, and, to some extent, the ventral surface of fingers and toes (*Figs 3.82* and *3.83*). The lesions reach the lateral aspects of hands and feet but not beyond. The periphery is bordered by an erythematous margin (*Fig. 3.84*).[3] Painful blisters are not uncommon. Hyperhidrosis and maceration may be present and facilitate dermatophytosis.[4,7] Rarely, associated knuckle pads or clubbed digits have been documented.[8]

The 'tonotubular' subtype of PPK is associated with disabling pain on palms.[14] Epidermolytic hyperkeratosis with polycyclic psoriasiform plaques is another distinct variant characterized by intermittent flares of fixed polycylic, erythematous, psoriasiform plaques along with diffuse palmoplantar hyperkeratosis.[17] A form of diffuse PKK where the keratosis progressively extends to the dorsum of the Achilles tendon, ankles, knee or elbows has been described as Greither keratoderma (keratosis palmoplantaris diffusa transgrediens et progrediens).[18] However, not all cases of Greither keratoderma are due to a keratin mutation. The non-epidermolytic variants are discussed below.

Identification of the epidermolytic form of PPK has therapeutic consequences since lesions become inflammatory and erosive upon systemic retinoid therapy.

Pathogenesis and histologic features

Epidermolytic palmoplantar keratoderma was initially mapped to chromosome 17q12-q21, the locus of the type I acidic keratin cluster, where different point mutations of *KRT9* encoding keratin 9 were identified. Epidermolytic palmoplantar keratoderma, however, has also been reported to be associated with keratin 1 mutations that map to chromosome 12q11–13, the site of the keratin II genes.[9–15] Keratin 1 and 9 are the major structural keratins in the suprabasal keratinocytes of the palmoplantar epidermis. Mutations in *KRT9* are associated with more severe manifestations than mutations in *KRT1*.[10]

Most of the keratin mutations affect the central regions of the protein, which are important for filament assembly and stability of the keratin skeleton. As a consequence, tonofilament clumping causes cellular degeneration and disruption, e.g., epidermolytic palmoplantar keratoderma. Mutations in the rod domain are associated with only mild focal signs of epidermolytic

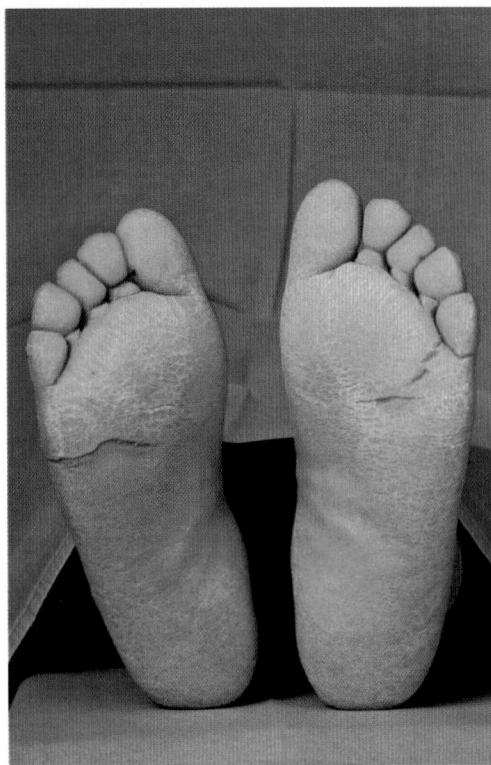

Fig. 3.82
Diffuse palmoplantar keratoderma Vörner-Unna-Thost: there is hyperkeratosis affecting the entire sole of the foot. By courtesy of W.A.D. Griffiths, MD, Institute of Dermatology, London, UK.

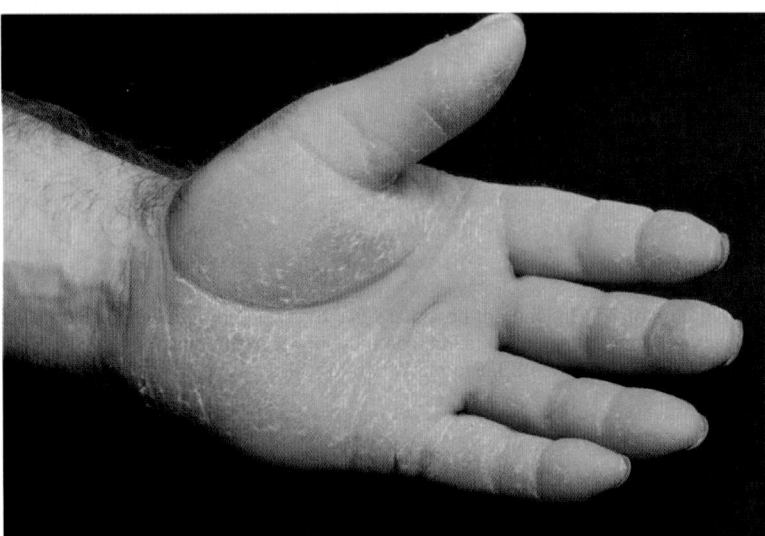

Fig. 3.83
Diffuse palmoplantar keratoderma Vörner-Unna-Thost: in this patient the palms of the hands were also affected. By courtesy of W.A.D. Griffiths, MD, Institute of Dermatology, London, UK.

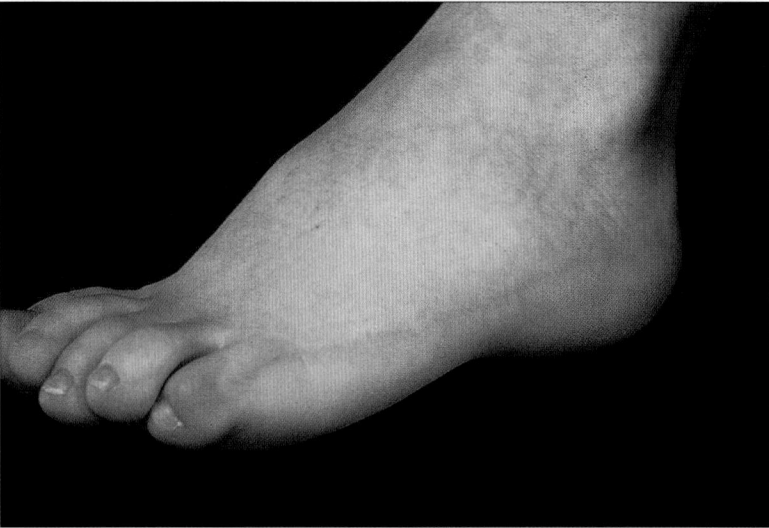

Fig. 3.84
Diffuse palmoplantar keratoderma Vörner-Unna-Thost: the border of the lesion is marked by a linear zone of erythema. By courtesy of W.A.D. Griffiths, MD, Institute of Dermatology, London.

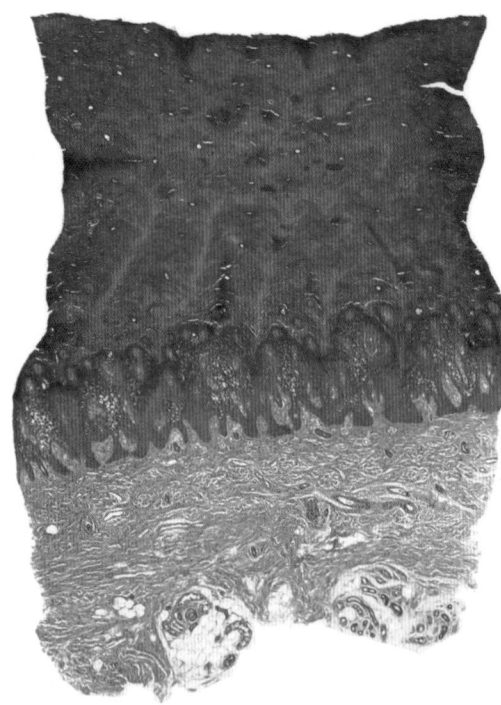

Fig. 3.85
Diffuse palmoplantar keratoderma Vörner-Unna-Thost: scanning view showing massive hyperkeratosis, papillomatosis, and acanthosis.

hyperkeratosis in the spinous layer of the palmoplantar epidermis.[13] Epidermolytic palmoplantar keratoderma with unusual formation of 'tonotubular' filaments is caused by mutations of the 1B rod domain of keratin 1.[15,16] Epidermolytic palmoplantar keratoderma is not associated with malignancy, although patients in one large kindred showed a high incidence of breast and ovarian cancer.[19] It is now believed that this represented a coincidental cosegregation of a keratin 9 mutation with a *BRCA1* mutation on 17q21.2.[20]

Histologically, there is massive orthohyperkeratosis, hypergranulosis, papillomatosis, and acanthosis accompanied by features of epidermolytic hyperkeratosis in the spinous and granular cell layers with vacuolated cytoplasm, intracytoplasmic eosinophilic granules, and coarse keratohyalin granules (*Figs 3.85* and *3.86*). A superficial dermal perivascular lymphohistiocytic infiltrate may sometimes be present. Epidermal spongiosis and vesiculation usually indicates fungal superinfection.

Electron microscopy shows aggregations of keratin filaments and keratin clumps that account for the intracytoplasmic eosinophilic granules as seen by light microscopy. Large areas of the cytoplasm that are devoid of a keratin skeleton explain the vacuolar change. Keratohyalin granules cluster in a random fashion around the keratin aggregates.

Diffuse non-epidermolytic palmoplantar keratoderma

Diffuse non-epidermolytic palmoplantar keratoderma (NEPPK) refers to a heterogeneous group of nonsyndromic keratodermas that histologically

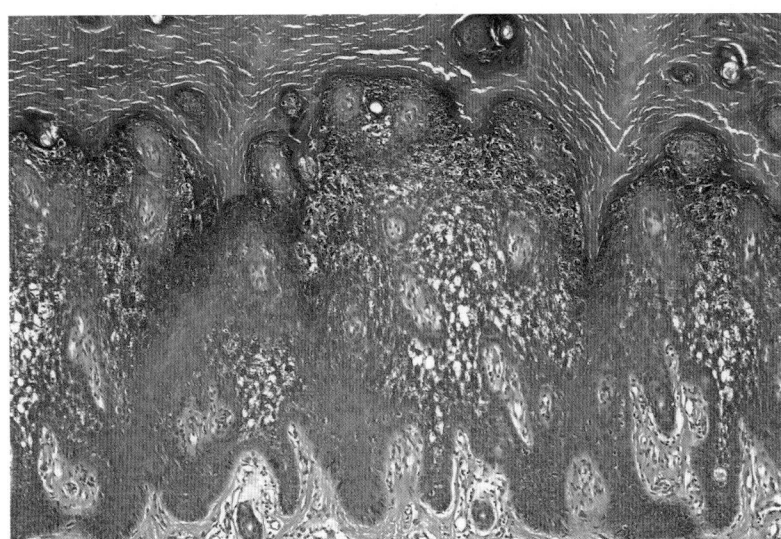

Fig. 3.86
Diffuse palmoplantar keratoderma Vörner-Unna-Thost: high-power view demonstrating the features of epidermolytic hyperkeratosis.

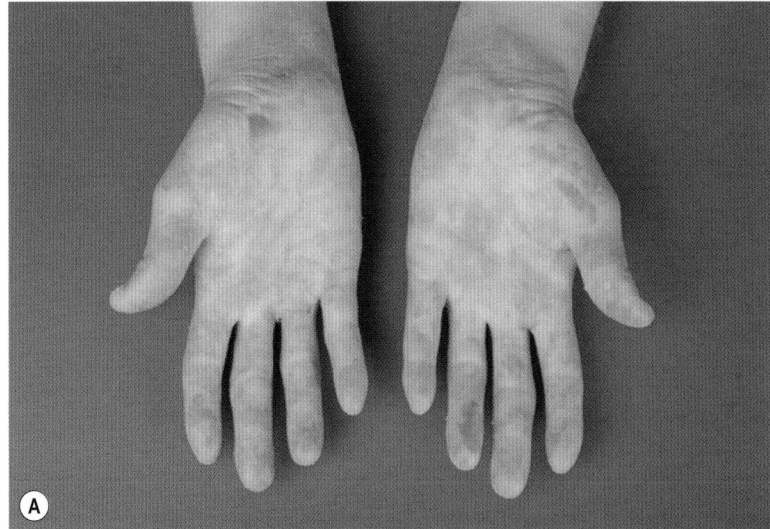

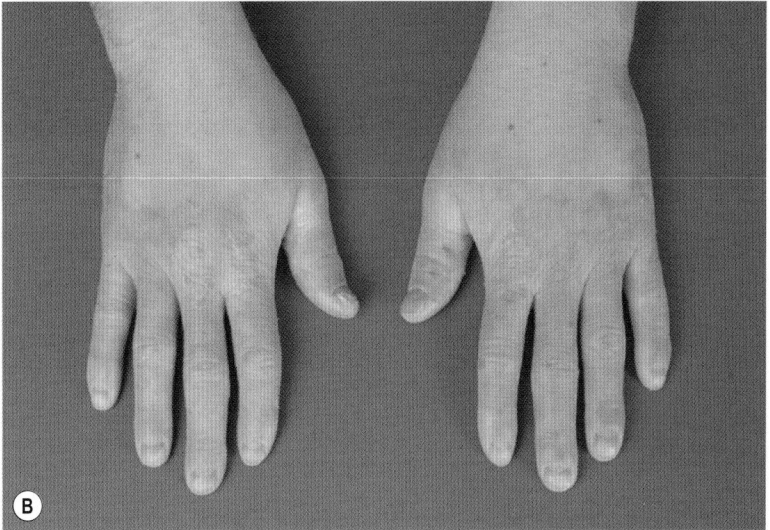

Fig. 3.87
Mal de Meleda: (**A**) hyperkeratosis is severe, waxy, diffuse, and appears macerated; (**B**) it extends on to the dorsal surfaces of hands and feet ('glove-and-socks' distribution).

lack epidermolytic hyperkeratosis (see *Table 3.6*). The following entities are included: NEPPK type Bothnia[1], Kimonis,[2] Nagashima,[3] and Mal de Meleda.[4] Greither keratoderma (PPK progrediens and transgrediens) is considered genetically heterogeneous as it shows epidermolytic and non-epidermolytic variants.[5-7] Keratoderma of Gamborg Nielsen is now regarded as a clinical variant of Mal de Meleda.[8,9]

Clinical features

The various types of NEPPK present in the first few months of life and are fully developed after 2 years of age. A variably thick, often yellow hyperkeratosis with a well-defined red border develops over the soles, followed later by involvement of the palms.[3] Hyperhidrosis is common, and dermatophyte infections and pitted keratolysis occur frequently.

NEPPK type Bothnia is additionally characterized by a white spongy appearance upon exposure to water.[1] Other conditions sensible to water contact are aquagenic palmoplantar keratoderma, acral PSS, exfoliative ichthyosis, and transient aquagenic keratoderma.

In Mal de Meleda, which has a high incidence on the island of Meleda in the Adriatic Sea, hyperkeratosis is severe and impairs the mobility of hands (*Fig. 3.87A*). The hyperkeratosis is ivory-yellow and waxy and extends across the whole surface of the palms and soles, and on to the dorsal surfaces of hands and feet ('glove-and-socks' distribution) (*Fig. 3.87B*). Keratotic lesions of the knees and elbows are highly characteristic. This PPK is often complicated by hyperhidrosis leading to an unpleasant smell, fissures, and mycotic superinfection.[10] Hyperkeratosis of the fingers can result in sclerodactyly and digital constrictions (pseudoainhum). Nails show thickening, koilonychia, and subungual hyperkeratosis. Angular cheilitis and lip involvement is variably present.[4] Hyperpigmented macules, melanoma, and Bowen disease developing in the keratotic areas have been reported.[11,12]

Greither keratoderma (syn. Greither syndrome, keratosis palmoplantaris diffusa transgrediens et progrediens, progressive palmoplantar keratoderma) is a diffuse symmetric palmoplantar keratoderma that progressively extends to the back of the hands and feet, the region of the Achilles tendon, ankles, knees or elbows where patchy hyperkeratosis develops with a tendency to improve in the fifth decade. (*Figs 3.88 and 3.89*).[5,6]

Pathogenesis and histologic features

NEPPK, as first identified in a family from Bothnia in Northern Sweden, is caused by autosomal dominant missense mutations in the *AQP5* gene, encoding aquaporin 5 (AQP5). Aquaporins are cell-membrane proteins that allow the osmotic movement of water across the cell membrane. AQP5 is localized in the plasma membrane of the keratinocytes of the stratum granulosum. The mutations lead to a gain-of-function that allows for an increased keratinocyte water uptake rather than transepidermal water loss.[1]

The NEPPK variant as described by Kimonis is caused by an autosomal dominant mutation in the V1 domain of *KRT1*. The fact that epidermolysis is missing suggests that the amino-terminal domain of keratins may be involved in supramolecular interactions of keratin filaments rather than stability.[2]

The Nagashima variant of NEPPK is an autosomal recessive disorder almost exclusively observed in Asia and caused by nonsense mutations in the *SERPINB7* gene. It encodes for a serine protease inhibitor, yet the target protease in the skin has not been identified.[13]

Mal de Meleda is caused by bi-allelic mutations in *SLURP1* (secreted Ly-6/PLAUR related protein 1) that is expressed in the granular layer of the epidermis.[14] It is postulated that SLURP1 interacts with neuronal acetylcholine receptors present in keratinocytes and sweat glands. Since SLURP1 may act as a secreted epidermal neuromodulator essential for both epidermal homeostasis and inhibition of tumor necrosis factor (TNF)-alpha release by macrophages during wound healing, this may explain both the hyperproliferative as well as the inflammatory clinical phenotype of Mal de Meleda.[14]

The previously reported cases of Greither keratoderma showed phenotypic variability suggestive of different underlying gene defects. There are epidermolytic variants with keratin mutations (see epidermolytic PPK) and non-epidermolytic variants, some overlapping with erythrokeratoderma.[5-7]

Histology of diffuse non-epidermolytic palmoplantar keratodermas (NEPPK) show orthohyperkeratosis, hypergranulosis or a normal granular cell layer and moderate acanthosis. A moderate superficial perivascular

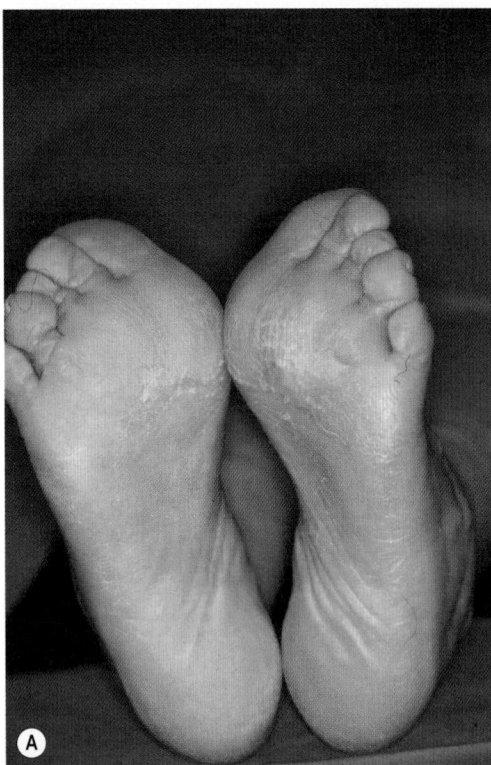

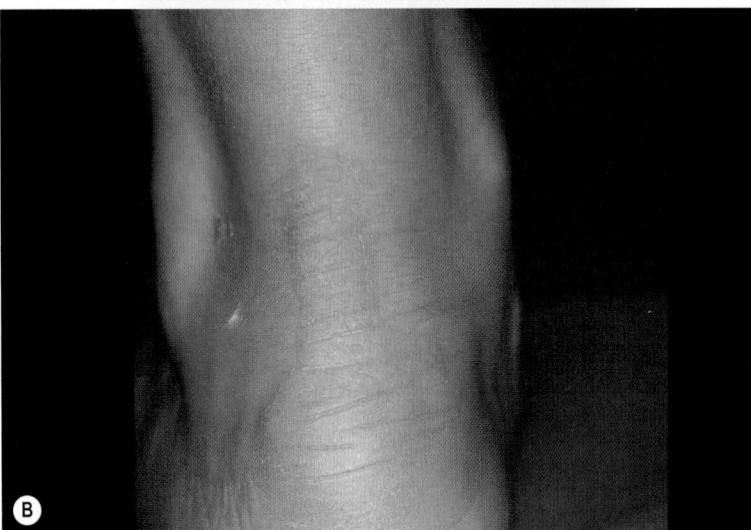

Fig. 3.88
Greither keratoderma (progressive palmoplantar keratoderma): (**A**) diffuse hyperkeratosis with fissures progressively extends to the back of the hands and feet; (**B**) affects the region of the Achilles tendon.

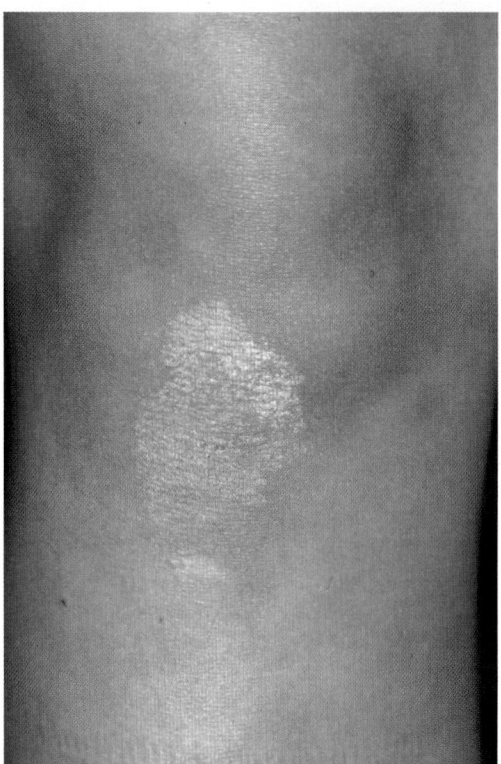

Fig. 3.89
Greither keratoderma (progressive palmoplantar keratoderma): patchy hyperkeratosis develops on the knees.

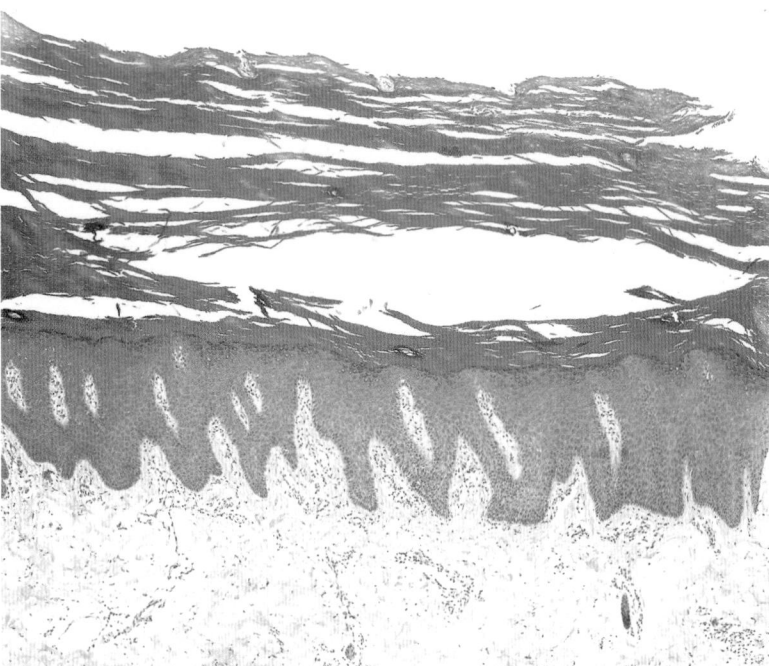

Fig. 3.90
Mal de Meleda: there is orthohyperkeratosis, hypergranulosis, and prominent papillomatosis, the latter feature is characteristic for Mal de Meleda.

lymphocytic infiltrate may be present in some cases. In Mal de Meleda, in our experience, prominent papillomatosis is a characteristic finding (*Fig. 3.90*). Otherwise, histologic changes are not pathognomonic for any type of NEPPK but exclude epidermolytic hyperkeratosis in cases of diffuse keratoderma (*Fig. 3.91*).[15,16] The presence of spongiosis and vesiculation suggests a concomitant dermatophyte infection (*Fig. 3.92*).[17] However, PAS staining is always mandatory in PPK to exclude mycotic superinfection as spongiosis and inflammation can be missing (*Fig. 3.93*).

Huriez syndrome

Clinical features

In Huriez syndrome (keratosis palmoplantaris diffusa with sclerodactyly and sclerothylosis) patients present with diffuse mild palmoplantar keratoderma, scleroatrophic skin of the limbs, hypoplasia and dystrophy of the nails, and

hypohidrosis (*Fig. 3.94*).[1-3] Aggressive squamous cell carcinoma develops in the affected skin in approximately 15% of the cases. It has an early onset with a high risk of metastasis in the third to fourth decades.[4] Huriez syndrome shares some features with a complex syndrome defined by diffuse palmoplantar hyperkeratosis with squamous cell carcinoma and sex reversal.[7-9]

Pathogenesis and histologic features

The gene responsible for Huriez syndrome has been mapped to 4q23.[5] Histology shows mild acanthosis, orthohyperkeratosis, and well developed

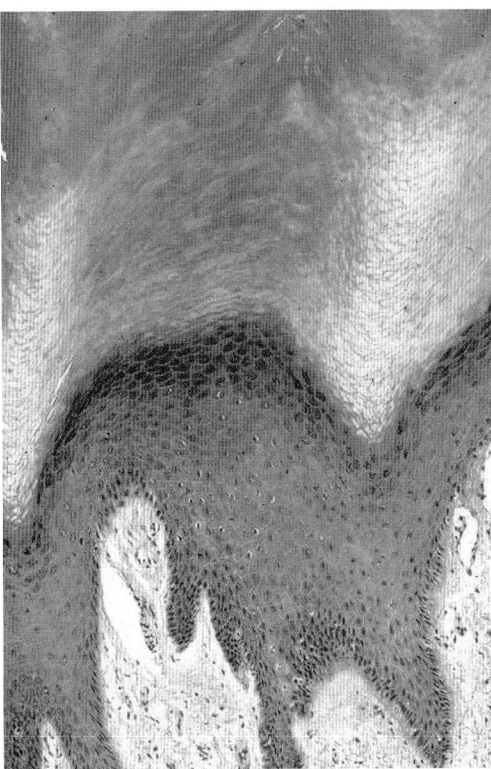

Fig. 3.91
Diffuse non-epidermolytic palmoplantar keratoderma: there is massive hyperkeratosis, hypergranulosis, and acanthosis. Absence of epidermolytic hyperkeratosis rules out diffuse palmoplantar keratoderma Vörner-Unna-Thost.

granular layer (*Fig. 3.95*). Interestingly, immunohistochemical and ultrastructural studies reveal an absence of Langerhans cells in involved skin.[4,6]

Vohwinkel syndrome

Clinical features

Vohwinkel syndrome (keratoma hereditarum mutilans, cicatrizing keratoderma with hearing impairment, keratoderma with sensorineural deafness) features palmoplantar keratoderma with a yellowish papular and honeycomb-like appearance and hyperhidrosis. Onset is in infancy or early childhood.[1,2] Other characteristics are starfish-like keratoses affecting the dorsal surfaces of the hands, feet, wrists, forearms, elbows, and knees (*Figs 3.96* and *3.97*). Flexion contractures and circumferential hyperkeratotic constriction bands (pseudoainhum) affecting the interphalangeal joints can lead to autoamputation.[3,4] A high-tone sensorineural hearing loss is probably present from birth, but may escape detection unless tested.[5] The ichthyosis-associated variant of Vohwinkel is a completely different entity (see Loricrin keratoderma or Camisa variant of Vohwinkel syndrome).[6,7] Bart-Pumphrey syndrome is an allelic condition characterized by knuckle pads and a honeycomb-like keratoderma resembling Vohwinkel syndrome, leukonychia, and mixed sensorineural and conductive deafness.[8-10] Palmoplantar keratoderma associated with hearing impairment should prompt a thorough family history as maternal inheritance suggests a rare mitochondrial type of keratoderma.[11]

Pathogenesis and histologic features

Vohwinkel syndrome is autosomal dominantly inherited and caused by mutation in *GJB2* encoding connexin 26.[12-14] Connexin 26 is expressed in the palmoplantar epidermis, sweat glands, and cochlea of the inner ear. As one of the major gap junction proteins it is crucial for signal transduction involved in epithelial differentiation and sensorineural functions.[15,16]

Histologically, the keratoderma is characterized by hyperkeratosis, hypergranulosis, and acanthosis.[4]

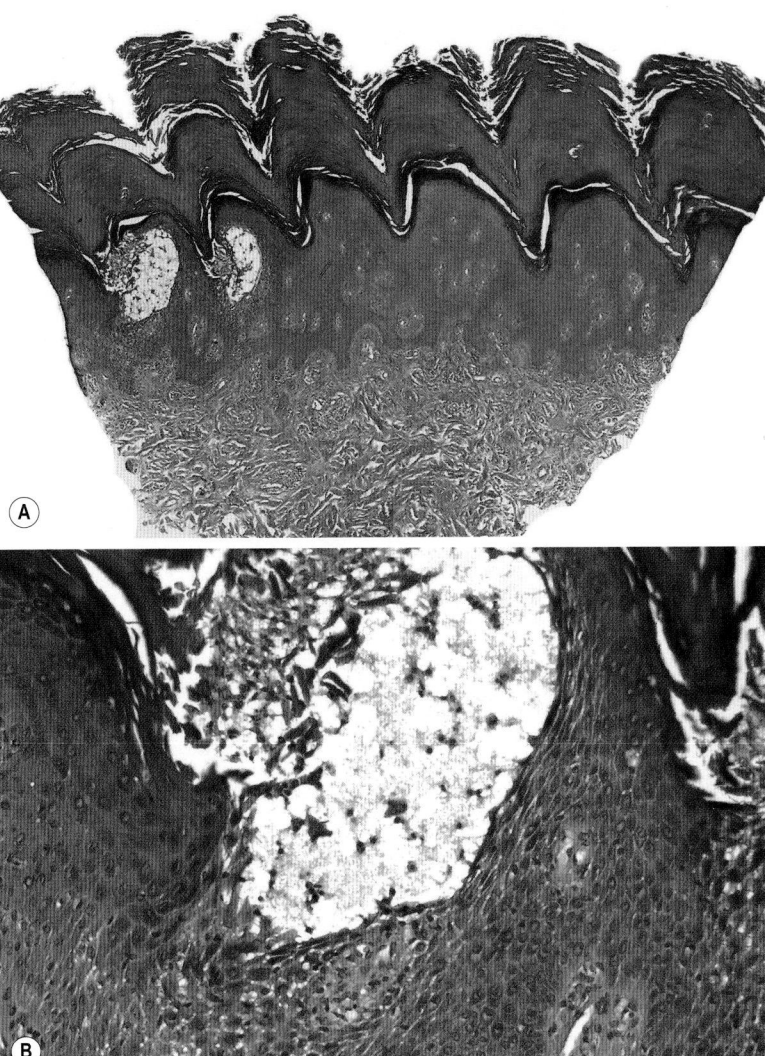

Fig. 3.92
Diffuse non-epidermolytic palmoplantar keratoderma: (**A**) in this example, there is massive hyperkeratosis with an undulating growth pattern. Intraepidermal vesiculation is apparent; (**B**) high-power view showing signs of spongiosis.

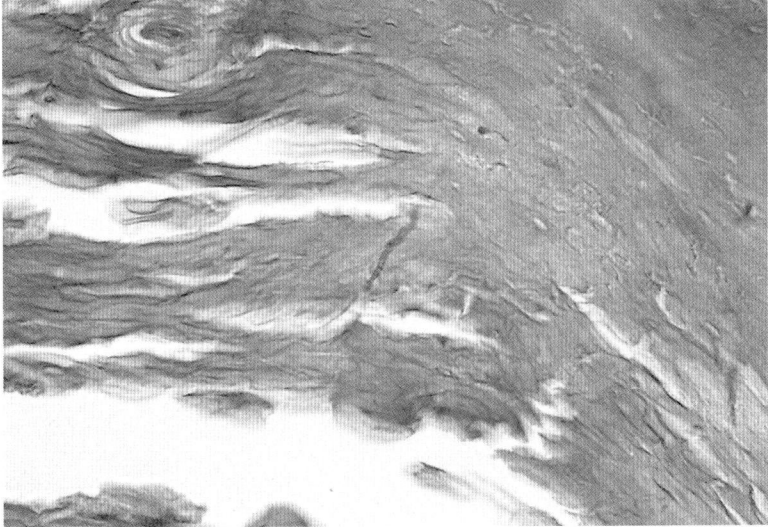

Fig. 3.93
Diffuse non-epidermolytic palmoplantar keratoderma: fungal hyphae are apparent in the thickened stratum corneum (PAS stain).

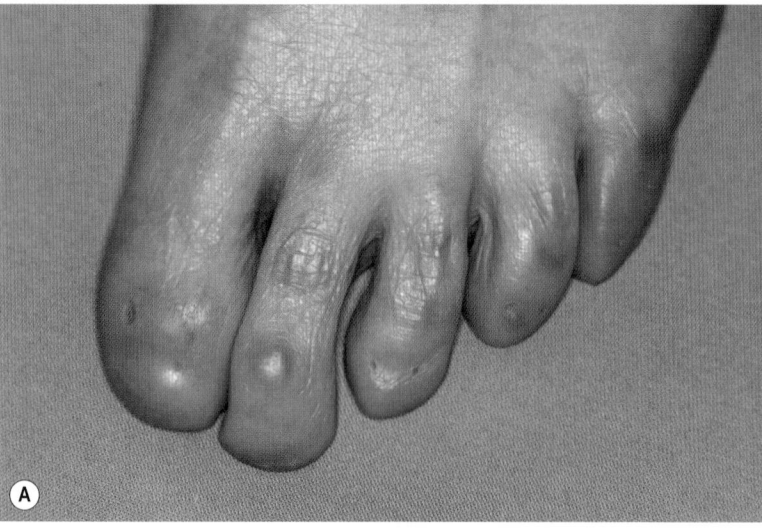

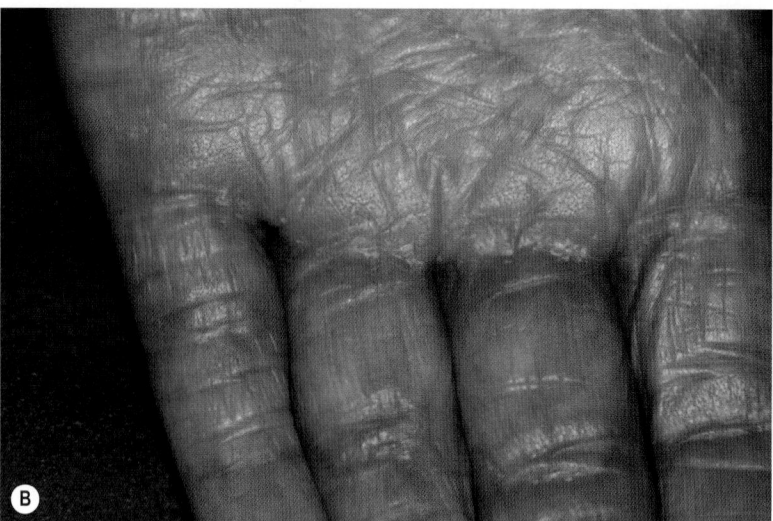

Fig. 3.94
Huriez syndrome: (**A**) the main features are sclerodactyly, hypotrophic and dystrophic nails; (**B**) there is diffuse, mild palmar keratosis.

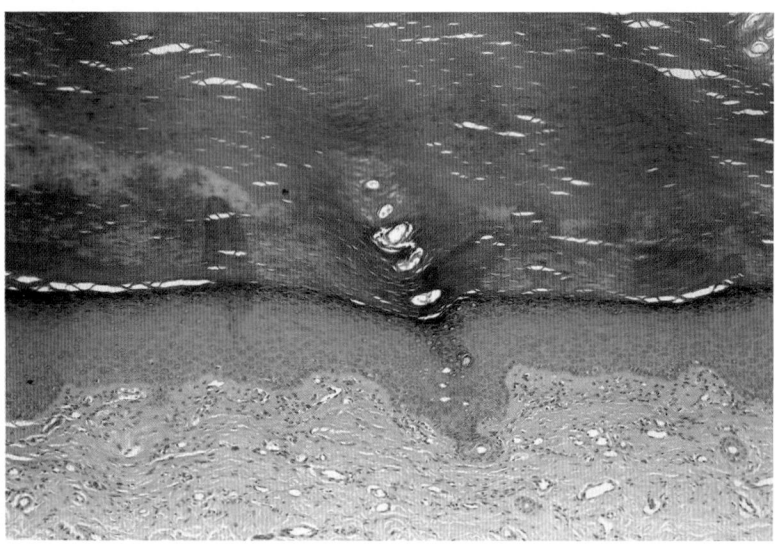

Fig. 3.95
Huriez syndrome: there is mild acanthosis, orthohyperkeratosis and a well-developed granular cell layer.

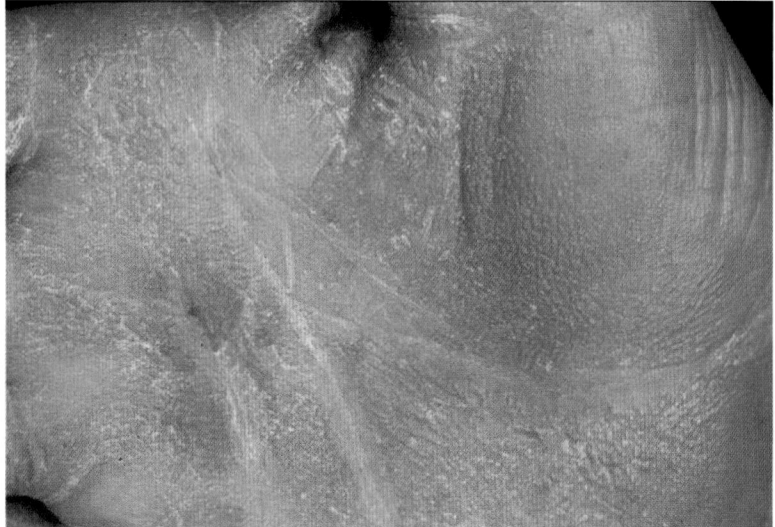

Fig. 3.96
Vohwinkel syndrome: there is marked palmoplantar keratoderma. By courtesy of W.A.D. Griffiths, MD, Institute of Dermatology, London, UK.

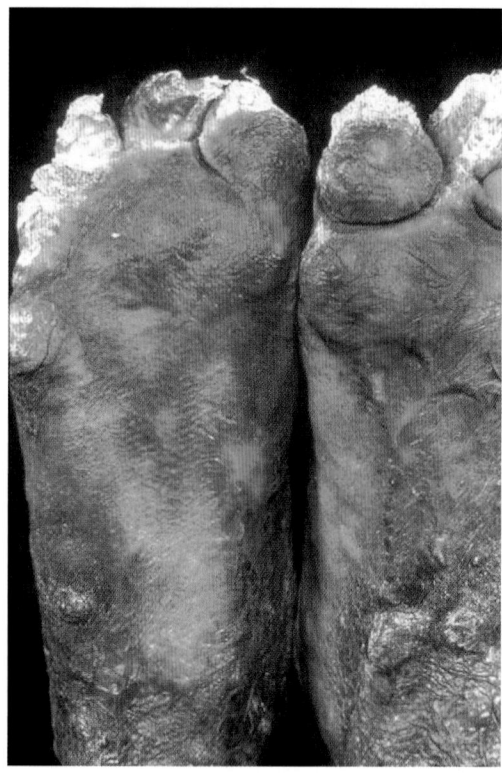

Fig. 3.97
Vohwinkel syndrome: in this example there is very disfiguring keratoderma, hence the alternative title, keratoderma hereditarium mutilans. By courtesy of W.A.D. Griffiths, MD, Institute of Dermatology, London, UK.

Loricrin keratoderma

Clinical features

Loricrin keratoderma (Camisa variant of Vohwinkel syndrome, Vohwinkel keratoderma with ichthyosis) is inherited in an autosomal dominant fashion and characterized by a diffuse palmoplantar keratoderma that is very similar to that of Vohwinkel syndrome, including the honeycomb-like appearance (*Fig. 3.98*).[1-3] In contrast to true Vohwinkel syndrome the edges of the keratoderma are diffuse, cicatricial bands (pseudo-ainhum) are less mutilating, and warty papules and starfish-like keratosis are not a prominent feature. A concomitant ichthyosis with generalized fine scaling is a constant feature and often presents congenitally prior to the development of

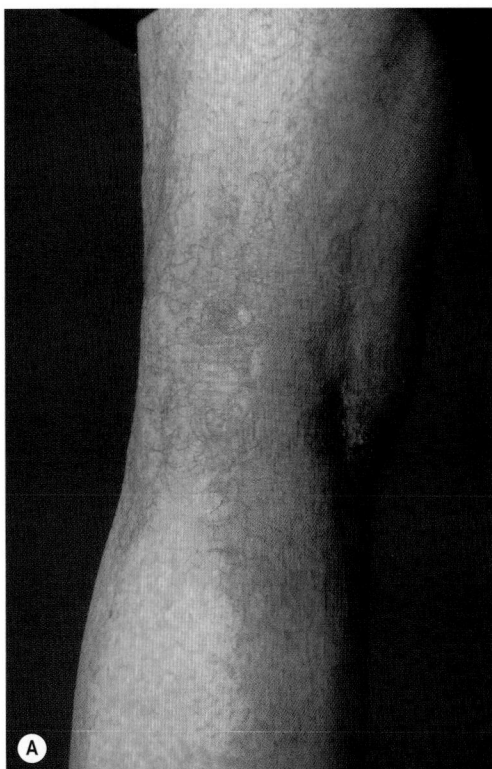

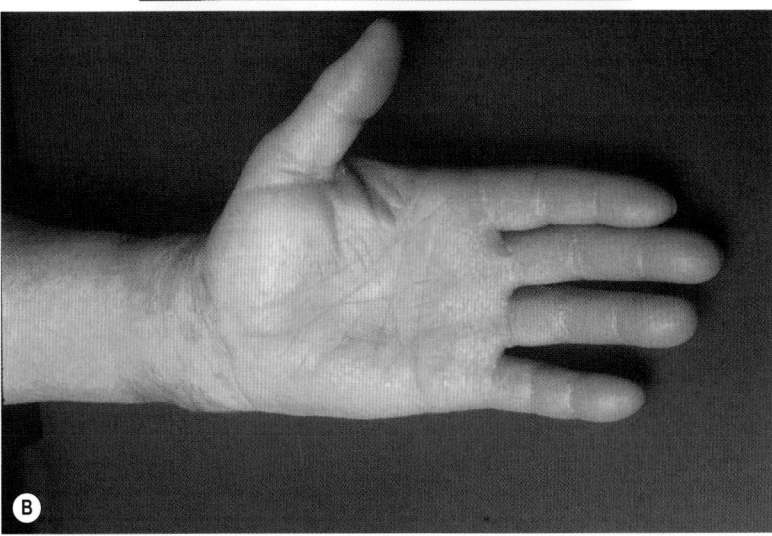

Fig. 3.98
Loricrin keratoderma: (**A**) there is a generalized fine scaling; (**B**) palmoplantar keratoderma with a yellowish papular and honeycomb-like appearance but less mutilating than in classical Vohwinkel syndrome.

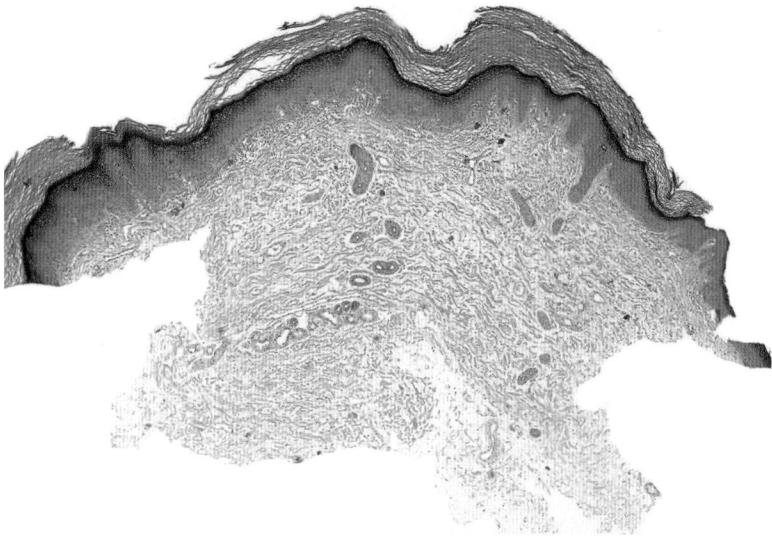

Fig. 3.99
Loricrin keratoderma: there is hyperkeratosis and mild acanthosis.

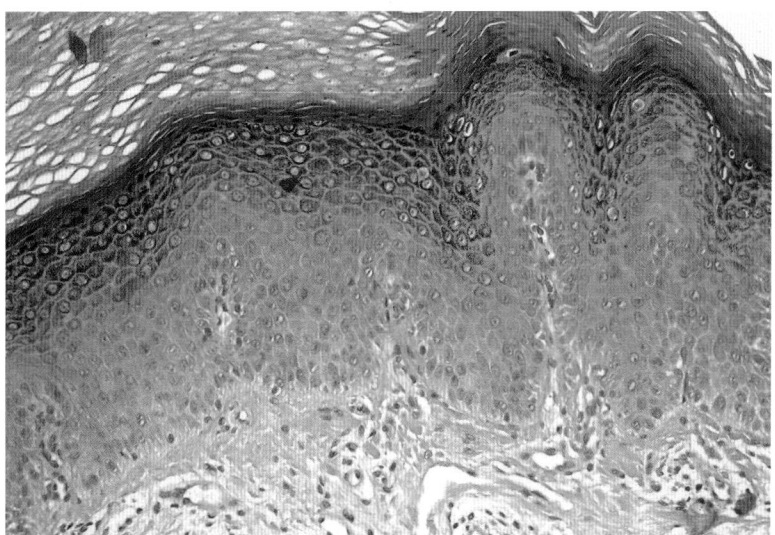

Fig. 3.100
Loricrin keratoderma: the stratum granulosum is prominent and scattered cells (on the right side of the field) show perinuclear vacuolization. The parakeratotic keratinocytes in the lower horny layer represent transitional cells. In the upper horny layers small roundish residual nuclei are preserved.

the palmoplantar keratoderma.[2] Patients do not suffer from deafness as seen in Vohwinkel keratoderma.

Pathogenesis and histologic features

Mutations on chromosome 1q21 that result in aberrant, elongated C-terminal domains of one loricrin allele may lead to abnormal loricrin expression, and impairment of cross-linking within the protein and with other cornified envelope proteins.[3–6] Mutant loricrin is segregated into the nucleus where is thought to impair the function of profilaggrin to mediate nuclear dissolution in the course of apoptosis which represents an integral part of keratinocyte terminal differentiation.[7,8] Loricrin keratoderma, and some cases of progressive symmetrical erythrokeratoderma, may share the mutation and light microscopy and ultrastructural features.[7] Therefore some authors have proposed that loricrin keratoderma should include cases of what has been formerly termed either (Vohwinkel) keratoderma with ichthyosis or progressive symmetrical erythrokeratoderma.[9]

Histologic features of loricrin keratoderma consist of psoriasiform hyperplasia of the epidermis, hyperkeratosis with small roundish nuclear debris in the upper horny layer and focally, expression of transitional cells, i.e., parakeratotic cells with prominent oval nuclei above the granular layer. The stratum granulosum is prominent and perinuclear vacuolization is sometimes seen (*Figs 3.99* and *3.100*). Inflammation is almost absent.[6] The nuclei of keratinocytes demonstrate a characteristic immunoreactivity for loricrin that is not seen in any other type of PPK.[10]

Electron microscopy characteristically reveals formation of a well-formed transitional layer, intranuclear granules in the upper stratum granulosum, and a thin cornified envelope.[7]

Clouston syndrome

Clinical features

Clouston syndrome (hidrotic ectodermal dysplasia 2) is characterized by dystrophic nails developing in early infancy with hypotrichosis in conjunction with papillomatous and fissured transgradient keratoderma.[1,2] Clouston syndrome was first documented in French Canadian families with an

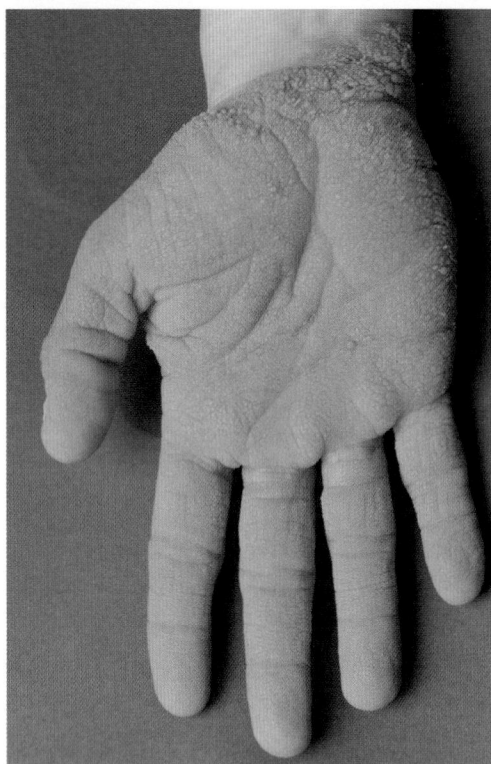

Fig. 3.101
Clouston syndrome: the keratoderma shows a typical 'pebbled' appearance.

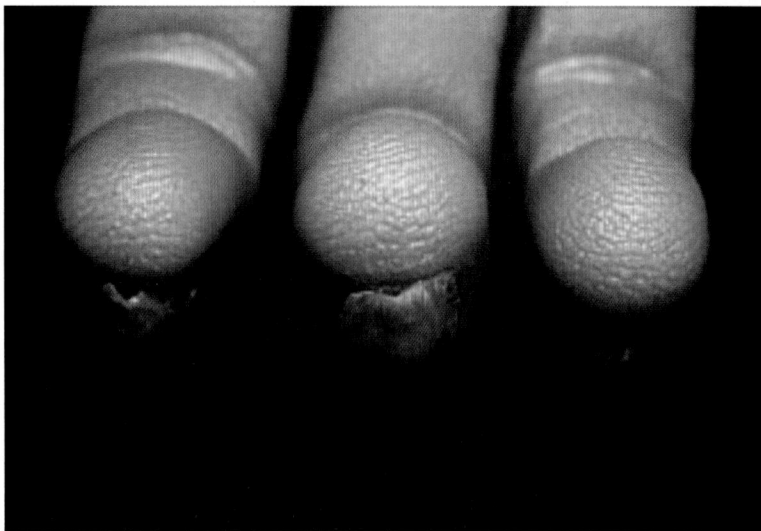

Fig. 3.102
Clouston syndrome: there is nail dystrophy accompanied by hyperkeratosis of the fingertips, thereby accentuating the epidermal surface ridges. By courtesy of D. Atherton, MD, the Children's Hospital at Great Ormond Street, London, UK.

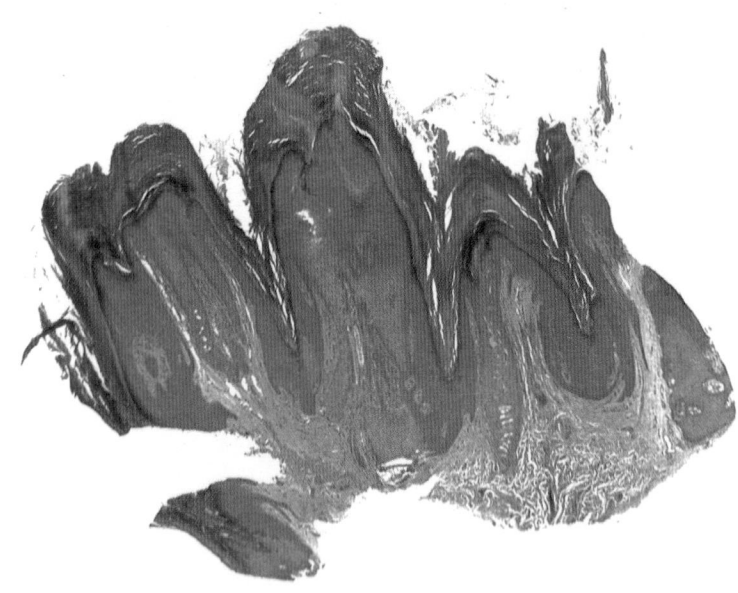

Fig. 3.103
Clouston syndrome: verruciform hyperplasia and papillomatosis of the epidermis are characteristic and should not be misdiagnosed as verruca vulgaris. The ducts of sweat glands are associated with a fibrovascular stroma.

Pathogenesis and histologic features

This autosomal dominant ectodermal dysplasia, is caused by mutations in the gap junction beta-6 (*GJB6*) gene encoding connexin 30 which is a potential target of p63.[9-13] Histologic evaluation of the thickened palms and soles shows verruciform hyperplasia and papillomatosis of the epidermis with orthohyperkeratosis and a normal granular layer. Papular lesions may demonstrate proliferation of ductal structures within a fibrovascular stroma, which is referred to as eccrine syringofibroadenomatosis (*Fig. 3.103*).[8,14] Hair follicles, sebaceous glands, and apocrine glands are reduced or absent. Ultrastructural examination of the hair shows disorganization of the hair fibers, with loss of the hair shaft cuticle.[14,15]

Olmsted syndrome

Clinical features

Olmsted syndrome combines the features of mutilating palmoplantar keratoderma with periorificial plaques.[1,2] The keratoderma is present at birth or begins in early infancy and when fully developed presents as bilateral and symmetrical massively thickened, yellow, macerated, keratotic plaques covering the whole of the soles and palms and often extending to the lateral and even the dorsal surface of the hands and feet (*Fig. 3.104*).[3,4] The heels and forearms may also be affected. The border of the plaque is sharply defined and surrounded by a pruritic erythematous border. Lesions are often fissured and extremely painful, making walking exceedingly difficult or impossible.[3,4] Blistering has occasionally been described.[5] Flexion contractures, ainhum-like constriction bands, and autoamputation are common complications.

Superinfection with bacteria and fungi, particularly *Candida albicans*, compounds the picture and as a result of this, lesions are frequently very malodorous. Development of squamous cell carcinoma or malignant melanoma has been reported.[6-9]

Affected children also develop erythematous keratotic papules and plaques around body orifices including the mouth, nostrils, ears, and anus.[3,4] The eyelids, umbilical region, inguinal region, and gluteal cleft can also be involved. The keratotic lesions are pruritic and painful causing discomfort, particularly in the gluteal cleft.[4,10,11]

Additional features include scarring alopecia, keratosis pilaris, tooth anomalies, and nail dystrophy, including ridging, transverse striae,

autosomal dominant trait.[3] The PPK initially develops over pressure points, shows involvement of the back of the hands and increases with age. The keratoderma has a 'pebbled' appearance (*Fig. 3.101*) that may also be evident on the dorsal aspects of the digits, knees and elbows. Progressive hypotrichosis leading to alopecia affects the scalp, eyebrows, eyelashes, and axillary and genital regions. The nails, which may be normal at birth, gradually become thickened and dystrophic, displaying short nail plates that are easily shed (*Fig. 3.102*).[4-6] The nail abnormalities may mimic those of pachyonychia congenita (PC) or other syndromes of 'hair–nail hypoplasia'.[7] Rare manifestations include sensorineural deafness, ocular abnormalities, skin hyperpigmentation, polydactyly, syndactyly, mental retardation, epilepsy, and dwarfism.[5,6]

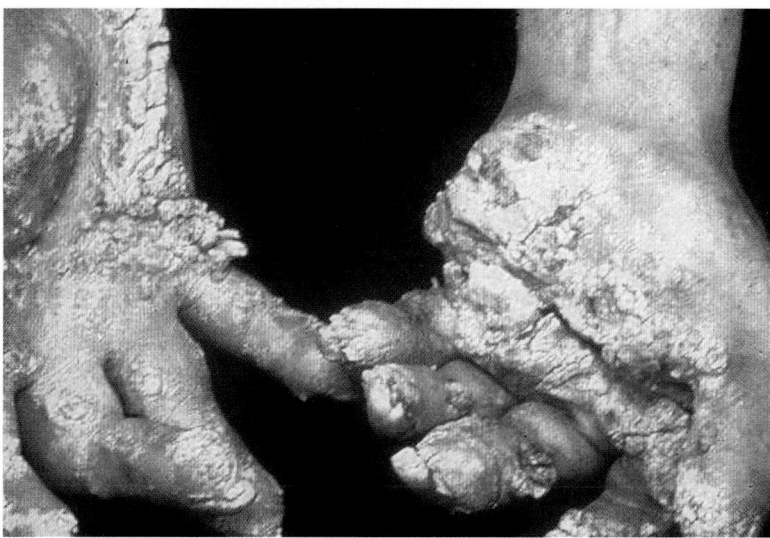

Fig. 3.104
Olmsted syndrome: in this variant, the lesions are very disfiguring. Constriction bands and autoamputation are important complications. By courtesy of W.A.D. Griffiths, MD, Institute of Dermatology, London, UK.

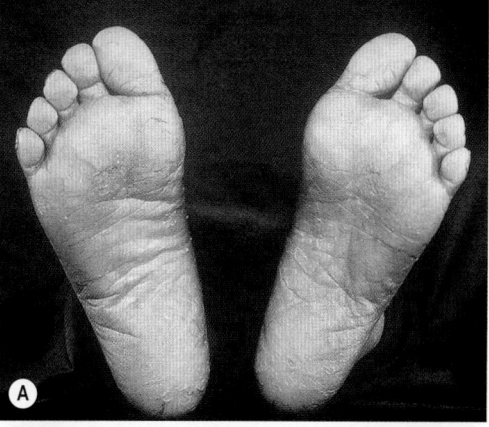

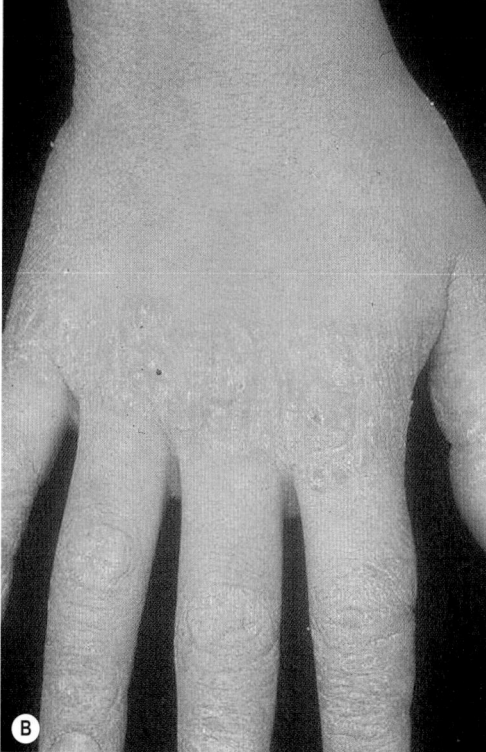

Fig. 3.105
Papillon-Lefèvre syndrome: (**A**) there is marked hyperkeratosis affecting the soles of the feet; (**B**) in this patient, the dorsal aspects of the hands, particularly the knuckles are also affected. By courtesy of W.A.D. Griffiths, MD, Institute of Dermatology, London, UK.

thickening, curvature, subungual keratosis, and infection. Hyperkeratotic linear streaks may develop in the axillae and cubital fossae. Growth retardation, laxity of the large joints, and corneal involvement are occasional manifestations.[3,4,10,11]

Pathogenesis and histologic features

Olmsted syndrome may occur sporadically and in various inherited forms. In the sporadic, the autosomal dominant and in the autosomal recessive variants gain-of-function mutations in the transient receptor potential vanilloid 3 gene (*TRPV3*) could be detected.[12,13] TRP cation selective ion channels are involved in hair growth, epidermal differentiation, and the modulation of inflammation, pain, and pruritus.[14] *TRPV3* mutations may also lead to elevated IgE levels with eosinophilia, erythromelalgia, and deafness.[15] In the X-linked variant of Olmsted syndrome with alopecia universalis and severe nail dystrophy, specific mutations in the *MBTPS2* gene have been identified. It encodes a zinc metalloprotease essential for cholesterol homeostasis, and endoplasic reticulum stress response.[16] Interestingly, mutations in the same gene account for IFAP syndrome (ichthyosis follicularis with atrichia and photophobia), KFSD (keratosis follicularis spinulosa decalvans) and BRESEK/BRESHECK syndrome.

Histologically, the plaques are characterized by massive hyperkeratosis, often with foci of vertically orientated parakeratosis.[2-5] There is hypergranulosis with large coarse granules under the former whereas the granular cell layer is absent beneath the areas of parakeratosis. The epidermis is acanthotic and shows psoriasiform hyperplasia or papillomatosis and there is edema and increased vascularity of the superficial dermis where a lymphohistiocytic infiltrate containing many mast cells is present.[17-19]

Papillon-Lefèvre syndrome

Clinical features

Papillon-Lefèvre syndrome (palmoplantar keratoderma with periodontopathia) is characterized by a diffuse, transgradient keratoderma and redness of the palms and soles (*Fig. 3.105*).[1] Pseudoainhum and hyperkeratotic lesions on elbows and knees can occur (*Fig. 3.106*). Additional features are periodontitis in childhood and premature loss of teeth (*Fig. 3.107*).[2-9] There is a predisposition to furunculosis, cerebral and liver abscesses, and other pyogenic infections.[8-10] Retinoid therapy not only improves the hykeratoses, but also diminishes oral and infectious complications.[11,12] There is a risk for development of melanoma and/or squamous cell carcinoma.[13-15] Haim-Munk syndrome is allelic with Papillon-Lefèvre syndrome and

shows additional features, such as onychogryphosis, arachnodactyly, and acro-osteolysis.[16,17]

Pathogenesis and histologic features

Papillon-Lefèvre syndrome has an autosomal recessive mode of inheritance and is associated with missense and nonsense mutations, deletions, and insertions in the gene for the lysosomal cysteine protease cathepsin C (dipeptidyl aminopeptidase I).[18-22] In homozygous patients, loss of cathepsin C activity results in impaired activation of bone marrow myeloid and macrophage granule serine proteases with resultant defective bacterial phagocytosis.[23-28] The cathepsin C gene is also expressed in squamous epithelium of the palms, soles, knees, and the oral keratinized gingiva.[19]

The histopathological features of the palmoplantar lesions show marked hyperkeratosis with acanthosis and a thickened granular cell layer (*Fig. 3.108*). Parakeratosis and epidermal psoriasiform hyperplasia have also been described. The elbow and knee lesions show epidermal psoriasiform hyperplasia with parakeratosis, elongation of the dermal papillae, and dilatation of the superficial dermal vasculature.

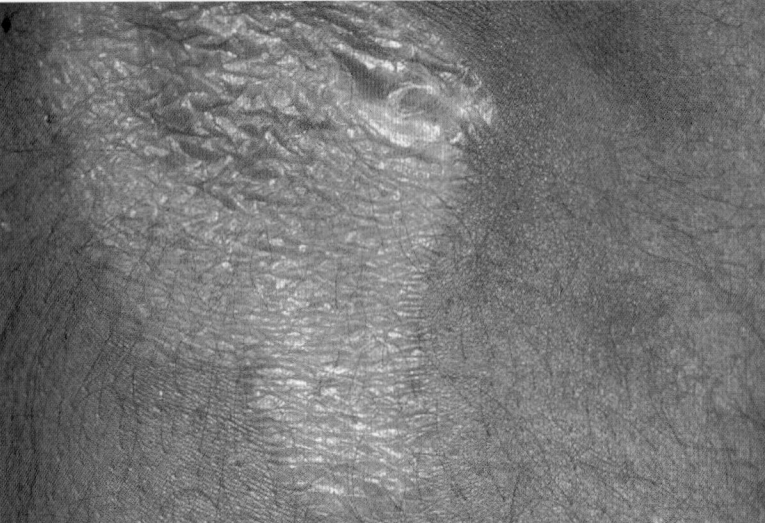

Fig. 3.106
Papillon-Lefèvre syndrome: a scaly psoriasiform plaque is present over the elbow.
By courtesy of W.A.D. Griffiths, MD, Institute of Dermatology, London, UK.

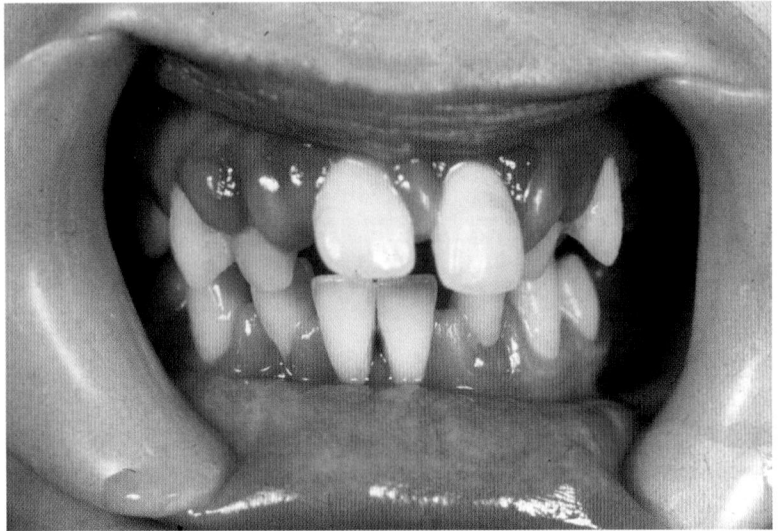

Fig. 3.107
Papillon-Lefèvre syndrome: gingival inflammation and swelling with the characteristic irregular positioning of the teeth which, as a result of destruction of supporting tissues, have shifted under the forces of mastication. This patient is a 12-year-old child, but the severity of the periodontal destruction is what might be expected in a person aged 60 years. By courtesy of R.A. Cawson, MD, Guy's Hospital, London, UK.

Howel-Evans syndrome

Clinical features

Howel-Evans syndrome (tylosis with esophageal carcinoma) is a syndromic autosomal dominant palmoplantar keratoderma that develops by 6 to 15 years of age and is associated with high risk of esophageal carcinoma.[1] Affected individuals develop painful hyperkeratoses on the pressure areas of the balls of the feet, with milder involvement of the palms, which disappear with prolonged bed rest (Fig. 3.109).[1-5] In contrast to pachyonychia nails are unaffected.[6] Other features are oral leukokeratosis, keratosis pilaris, dry rough skin, and multiple epithelial cysts. The oral leukokeratosis typically predates the onset of keratoderma and is an important diagnostic clue of early involvement in family members.[5-9] In the largest kindred reported to date, 28% developed esophageal squamous carcinoma of whom 84% died of their tumor.[4]

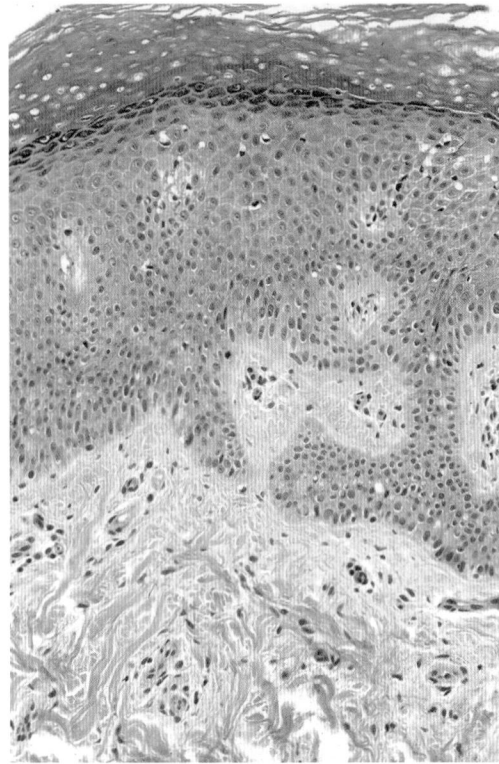

Fig. 3.108
Papillon-Lefèvre syndrome: there is hyperkeratosis, hypergranulosis and acanthosis.

Pathogenesis and histologic features

Missense mutations in *RHBDF2* (rhomboid 5 homolog 2) encoding an intramembrane protease have been identified.[10-13] Functional data suggest that mutant *RHBDF2* increases signaling through the epidermal growth factor receptor (EGFR), which promotes hyperproliferation, dysregulation of wound repair and as such predisposes to precancerous lesions.[13]

The cutaneous lesions are characterized by hyperkeratosis, hypergranulosis, and acanthosis. Features of epidermolytic hyperkeratosis are absent.

The buccal mucosal lesions are characterized by parakeratosis, acanthosis, and spongiosis accompanied by cytoplasmic vacuolation of the prickle cell layer.[4]

Schöpf-Schulz-Passarge syndrome

Clinical features

Schöpf-Schulz-Passarge syndrome is an autosomal recessive tricho-odonto-onycho-dermal dysplasia that shares dental anomalies, a diffuse palmoplantar keratoderma, and nail dystrophy (Fig. 3.110).[1-2] Schöpf-Schulz-Passarge syndrome features hypotrichosis, nail fragility, early loss of deciduous teeth, hydrocystomas of the eyelids (Fig. 3.111) or other follicular and adnexal, mostly benign, tumors occurring in older patients.[1-5] The diffuse palmoplantar keratoderma has a late onset.[1-5]

Pathogenesis and histologic features

This condition is caused by mutations in the *WNT10A* gene encoding a signaling molecule that is essential for the development of ectodermal appendages.[6] Phenotypic heterogeneity is the rule with mutations in *WNT10A* causing disorders ranging from monosymptomatic severe oligodontia to Schöpf-Schulz-Passarge syndrome.[7]

Multiple eccrine syringofibroadenomas and squamous cell carcinomas may arise on the acral surfaces in older patients. The eyelid lesions represent apocrine hidrocystomas (Fig. 3.112).[1,3,5]

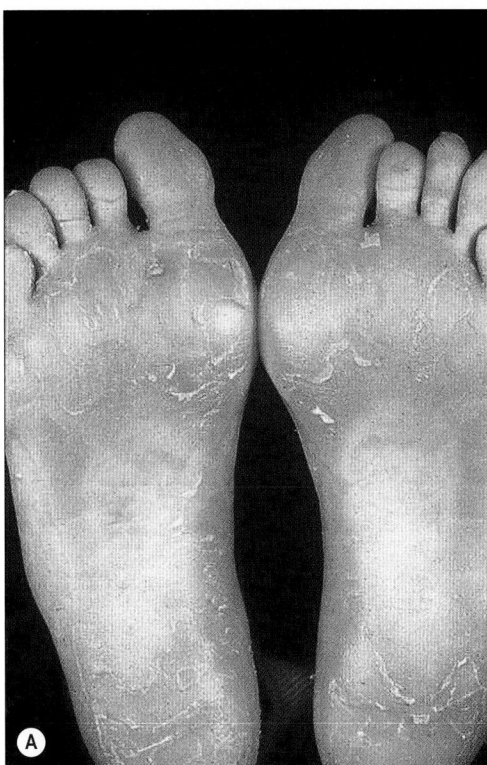

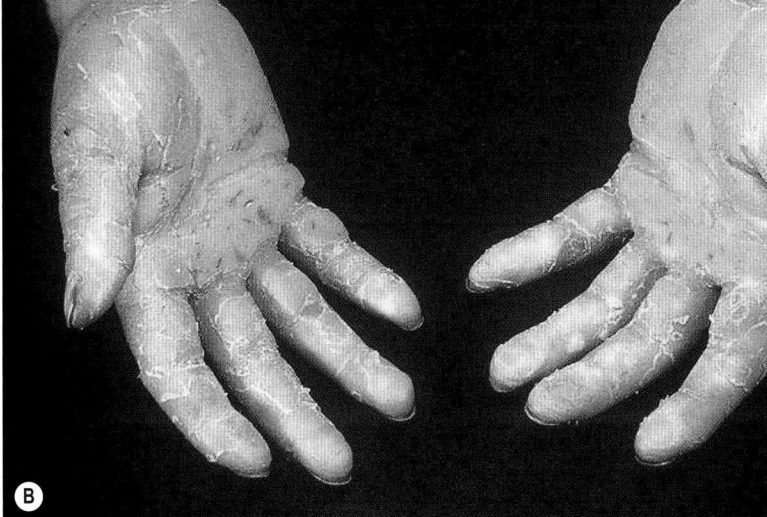

Fig. 3.109
Howel-Evans syndrome: (**A**) focal autosomal dominant palmoplantar keratoderma is associated with an increased risk of esophageal squamous carcinoma; (**B**) in this patient, the palms were also severely affected. By courtesy of the Institute of Dermatology, London, UK.

Striate palmoplantar keratoderma

Clinical features

Striate palmoplantar keratoderma (SPPK) is characterized by linear keratosis on palms and island-like areas of hyperkeratosis on soles. Although historically this form of PPK has been regarded as an entity under different designations, such as keratosis palmoplantaris varians Wachters, keratosis palmoplantaris areata et striata, or Brünauer-Fuchs-Siemens syndrome, they are genetically different.[1-4] These circumscribed PPKs show an autosomal dominant inheritance and are caused by mutations in at least three different genes coding for desmoglein, desmoplakin and keratin related to keratinocyte adhesion.[5]

The characteristic clinical features of SPPK are linear keratotic bands on palms and flexor aspects of the fingers and island-like areas of hyperkeratosis

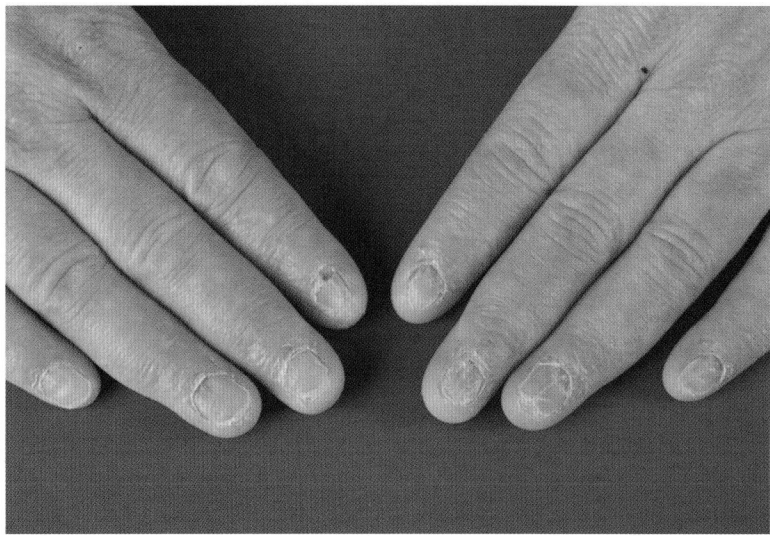

Fig. 3.110
Schöpf-Schulz-Passarge syndrome: diffuse keratoderma on palms and fingers is associated with nail dystrophy.

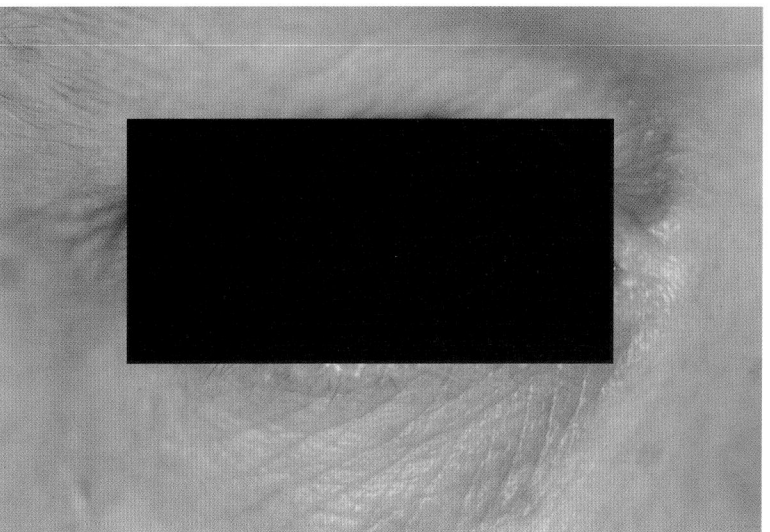

Fig. 3.111
Schöpf-Schulz-Passarge syndrome: multiple yellowish and bluish cysts on the eyelids.

on soles over pressure points (*Fig. 3.113*). Lesions evolve in adolescence or early adulthood and are exacerbated by mechanical stress. Pain and hyperhidrosis may accompany the keratoderma.[6]

Pathogenesis and histologic features

The most frequent form, SPPK type 1 is caused by mutations in *DSG1* encoding desmoglein 1. However, mutations in *DSG1* may also result in a diffuse form of PPK.[7,8] Interestingly, carriers of heterozygous mutations in *DSG1* develop striate PPK only while the offspring of two such heterozygous carriers can suffer from the SAM syndrome (severe dermatitis-multiple allergies-metabolic wasting syndrome).[9] SPPK type 2 is due to mutations in the desmoplakin gene (DSP).[10] In SPPK type 3 a frameshift mutation in the V2 tail domain of keratin 1 has been identified.[11] The mutation is similar to those being reported in ichthyosis Curth-Macklin.[12]

Histologically, striate palmoplantar keratoderma is characterized by massive hyperkeratosis, hypergranulosis, and acanthosis (*Fig. 3.114A*). Disadhesion of keratinocytes with widening of the intercellular spaces is an important histologic clue in these cell-cell junction diseases *(Fig. 3.114B).*[13] This form of incomplete acantholysis is related to the desmosomal defect and is also seen in Carvajal-Huerta syndrome, McGrath syndrome or diffuse PPK with *DSG1* mutation (see *Table 3.8*).[13] At ultrastructural level,

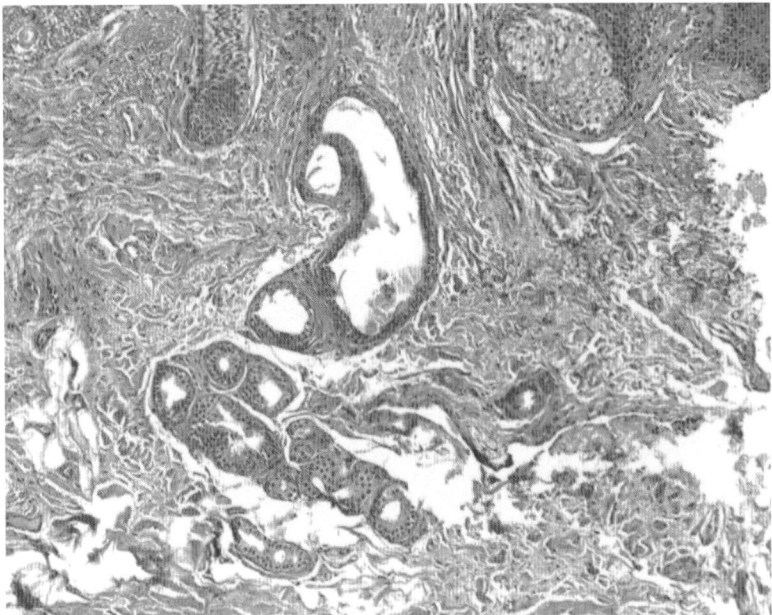

Fig. 3.112
Schöpf-Schulz-Passarge syndrome: the cysts on the eyelids represent apocrine hidrocystomas.

the size of the desmosomes appears reduced in *DSG1* related SPPK type 1, while perinuclear aggregation of keratin filaments seems more marked in DSP-associated type 2 SPPK.[14] Premature expression of involucrin and filaggrin has been described.[15]

Differential diagnosis

The absence of wooly hair and cardiomyopathy clearly rules out Carvajal-Huerta syndrome, another variant of focal or striate PPK (see below). Howel-Evans syndrome must be excluded if focal and nummular keratoderma predominate and histology lacks signs of dehiscence of keratinocytes (see Howel-Evans syndrome).

Hereditary painful callosities

Clinical features

Hereditary painful callosities (keratosis palmoplantaris nummularis) is no longer regarded as a distinctive entity but rather as a clinical symptom when plantar keratosis is prominent enough and is inevitably painful.[1-4] 'Painful callosities' may be seen in PCC,[5] desmosomal diseases[6] or oculocutaneous tyrosinemia (type II).[7] Cases with blisters correspond to epidermolytic palmoplantar keratoderma of Vörner-Unna-Thost.[3]

Naxos syndrome

Clinical features

This syndromic palmoplantar keratoderma was first identified on the Greek islands of Naxos and is characterized by keratoderma, life-threatening cardiomyopathy, and wooly hair.[1-2] Wooly hair is present from birth and this is followed by diffuse keratoderma. However, in some patients a more striate and areata type of PKK may be present.[3] Heart involvement is characterized by right ventricular cardiomyopathy and manifests by arrhythmias, insufficiency, and sudden death in adolescence with a penetrance of 100%.[4] The clinical and histologic features of Carvajal-Huerta syndrome are similar and do not allow a clear distinction.[5]

Pathogenesis and histologic features

Mutations of the *JUP* gene encoding plakoglobin, a cell junction protein found in desmosomes in the epidermis and cardiac muscle accounts for the symptoms.[6] Different mutations of *JUP* show a large phenotypic spectrum,

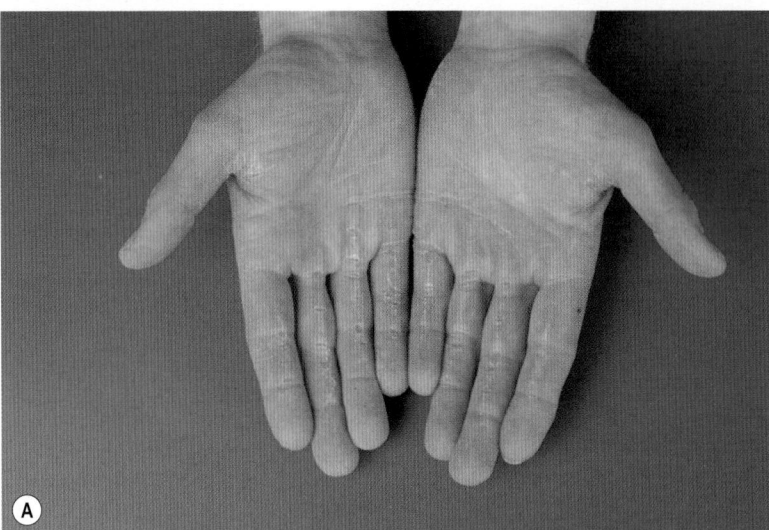

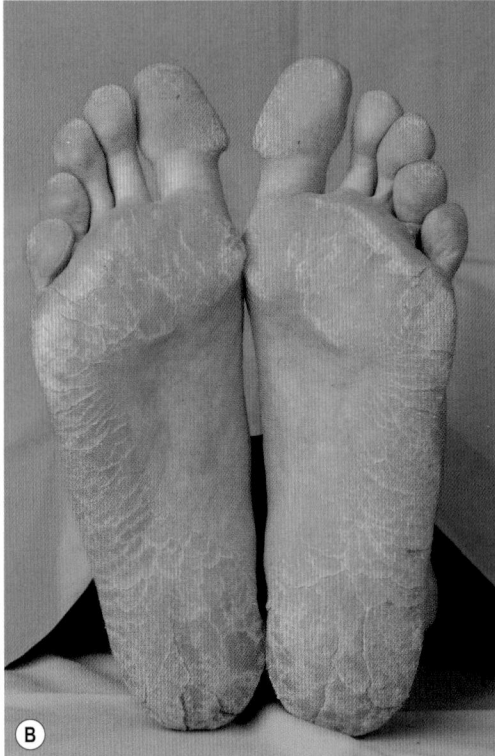

Fig. 3.113
Striate palmoplantar keratoderma: (**A**) linear hyperkeratotic bands along the palms and flexural side of the fingers; (**B**) island-like areas of hyperkeratosis on the soles over pressure points.

e.g., mutations with expression of altered plakoglobin may show mild skin fragility, keratoderma, and wooly hair only.[7,8] Of note, autosomal dominant *JUP* mutations underlie isolated arrhythmogenic right ventricular cardiomyopathy and a Naxos-variant with leukonychia and oligodontia.[9,10] Finally, complete loss of plakoglobin due to homozygous nonsense mutations may lead to 'lethal' epidermolysis bullosa.[11]

Histology shows compact hyperkeratosis, hypergranulosis, and acanthosis.[2] We are not aware if keratinocyte disadhesion is present in routine histology as evident in Carvajal-Huerta syndrome (see below).

Carvajal-Huerta syndrome

Clinical features

The Carvajal-Huerta syndrome is an autosomal recessively inherited disease with palmoplantar keratoderma, wooly hair, and dilated cardiomyopathy.[1,2] The patients are born with wooly hair (*Fig. 3.115*). Palmoplantar

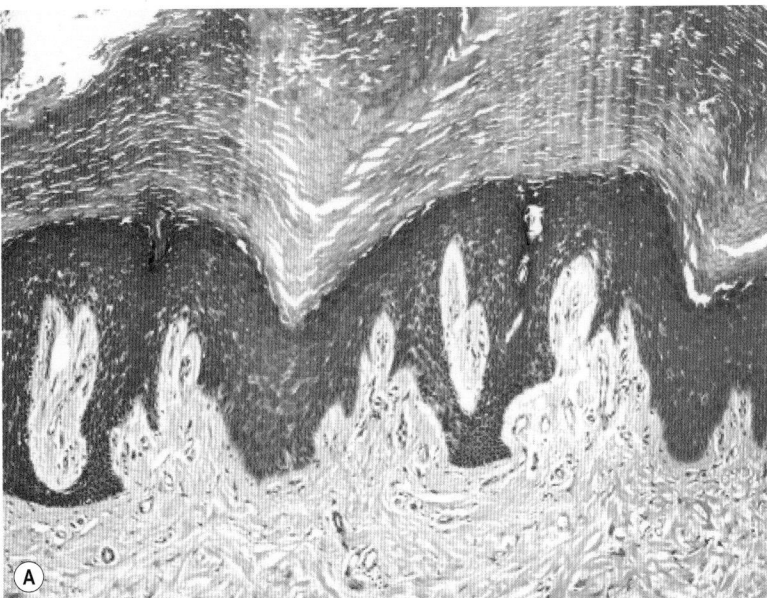

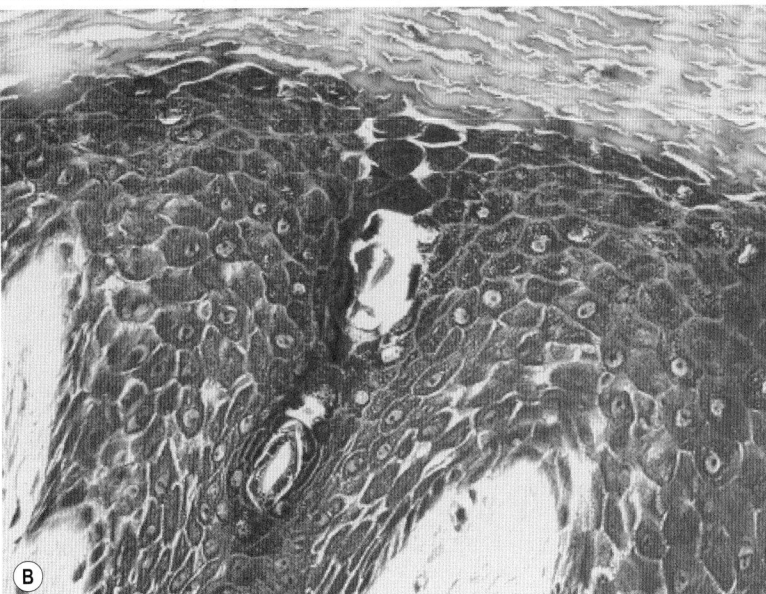

Fig. 3.114
Striate palmoplantar keratoderma: (**A**) histology reveals massive orthohyperkeratosis, hypergranulosis, and acanthosis; (**B**) loss of cohesion of keratinocytes leads to characteristic widening of the intercellular spaces.

keratoderma is striated rather than diffuse as usually occurring in Naxos disease. The first cardiac abnormalities are exclusively electrocardiographic and occur in asymptomatic patients. In these patients, dilatation of the left ventricle, together with alterations in muscle contractility, may lead to congestive heart failure with a high mortality rate at younger age.[3]

Pathogenesis and histologic features

Carvajal-Huerta syndrome is caused by mutant desmoplakin [1] (*DSP*), a major constituent of desmosomes that is responsible for the rigidity and strength of the epidermis and cardiac tissue.[4,5] Other genetic defects in desmoplakin have been found to generate a wide range of phenotypes, some of them lacking cutaneous symptoms, others lacking cardiac anomalies.[6] The residual amount of desmoplakin is critical in maintaining epidermal integrity as illustrated by compound heterozygote patients carrying one null-allele and one missense mutation, who developed pronounced skin fragility and alopecia without cardiac anomalies.[7] Complete loss of the tail domain of desmoplakin presents as 'lethal' acantholytic epidermolysis bullosa.[8]

Histology shows orthohyperkeratosis and widening of intercellular spaces and partial dehiscence of suprabasal keratinocytes (*Fig. 3.116*). For the histologic differential diagnosis of this characteristic pattern see *Table 3.8*. At

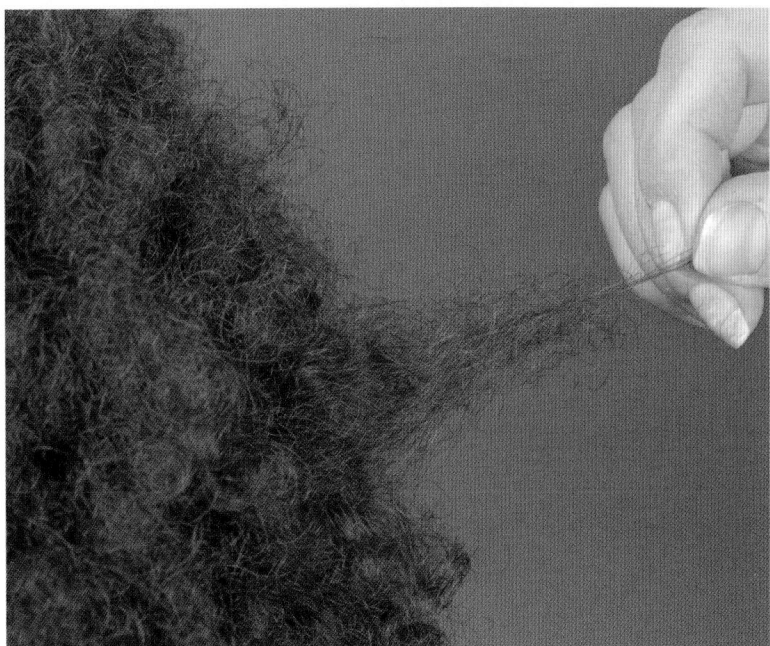

Fig. 3.115
Carvajal-Huerta syndrome: patients are born with wooly hair.

the ultrastructural level, loosening of intercellular connections, disruption of desmosome-keratin intermediate filament interactions, and rudimentary desmosomal structures can be demonstrated.[2]

McGrath syndrome

Clinical features

McGrath syndrome (ectodermal dysplasia-skin fragility syndrome) is inherited in an autosomal recessive mode and is best classified in the category of epidermolysis bullosa. Newborns present with peeling reddish skin and blisters on the soles. Thereafter, patients develop diffuse, sometimes verruciform palmoplantar hyperkeratosis with painful cracking, skin erosions, including perioral fissures, and other abnormalities of ectodermal development, such as growth delay, hypotrichosis or alopecia, hypohidrosis, and nail dystrophy.[3] In contrast to some other inherited disorders of desmosomes, there is no cardiac pathology.

Pathogenesis and histologic features

The disease has been shown to be associated with mutations in the plakophilin-1 gene (*PKP1*) leading to complete ablation of plakophilin 1, which is responsible for recruitment of desmosomal proteins to the plasma membrane and for keratin interaction.[1,2,4]

Light microscopy of the skin shows thickening of the epidermis and extensive widening of keratinocyte intercellular spaces leading to clefting and blistering.[1,2] Variable dyskeratosis of keratinocytes may also be found.[5] There is complete absence of cutaneous immunostaining for plakophilin-1.[4] Biopsies from the hypotrichotic scalp demonstrate increased number of catagen-telogen hair follicles.[5] Electron microscopy reveals loss of keratinocyte–keratinocyte adhesion. Desmosomes, particularly in the lower suprabasal layers, are small and reduced in number. The inner and outer desmosomal plaques are poorly developed.[6] Dyskeratotic keratinocytes reveal detachment of the keratin filaments from the desmosomes with perinuclear condensation.[5]

Pachyonychia congenita

Pachyonychia congenita (PC) comprises a group of autosomal dominant genodermatoses related to mutations in the genes for keratin 6A, 6B, 6C, keratin 16, or keratin 17 affecting a number of ectodermal structures, including nail bed, volar skin, oral mucosae, teeth, and pilosebaceous units.[1–3]

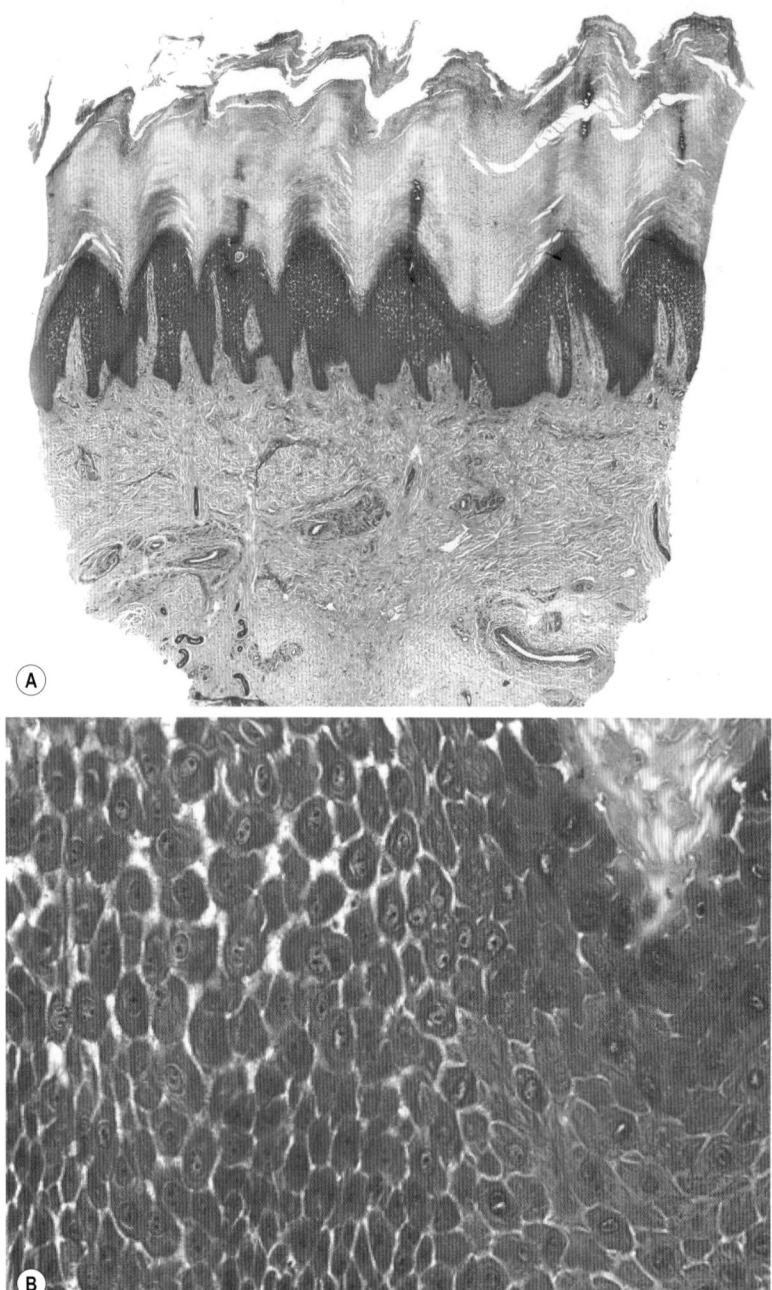

Fig. 3.116
Carvajal-Huerta syndrome: (**A**) massive orthohyperkeratosis, acanthosis, and papillomatosis; (**B**) partial dehiscence of suprabasal keratinocytes and characteristic widening of the intercellular spaces.

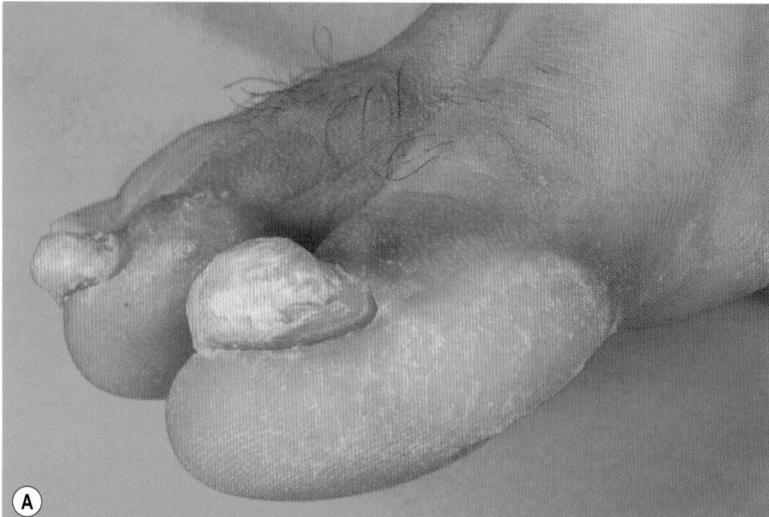

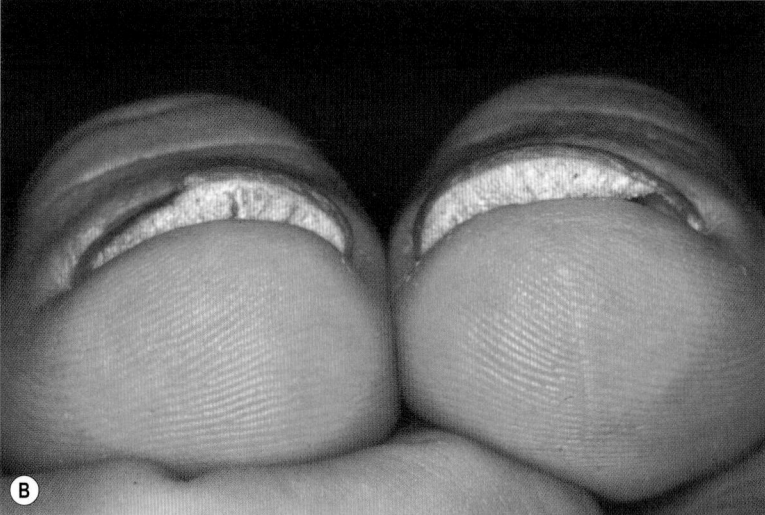

Fig. 3. 117
Pachyonychia congenita: (**A**) there is gross nail deformity with transverse arching of the distal portion. Although the nail plate appears to be thickened, most of the changes are, in fact, due to massive hyperkeratosis of the nail bed, resulting in elevation and bending of the nail plate; (**B**) in this view, the subungual hyperkeratosis is more obvious.

Historically, PC has been classified as PC type 1 (Jadassohn-Lewandowsky) and PC type 2 (Jackson-Lawler).[4–6] As originally described, PC type 1 is associated with mutations in genes encoding the dimerizing pair of K6a/ K16 and presents with PPK and oral leukokeratosis, while PC type 2 is caused by mutations of K6b/K17 and should feature pathology associated with pilosebaceous units (cysts) and neonatal teeth.[7] However, a large genotype/phenotype analysis resulted in a classification system based on the affected keratin, e.g., PC-6a, PC-6b, PC6c, PC-16, PC-17.[8] Further information on the subject is given by the International PC Consortium (IPCC) (www.pachyonychia.org).

Clinical features

Clinically, three cardinal symptoms are present in more than 90% of all patients with PC: toenail dystrophy, focal keratoderma, and plantar pain.[3,8,9] Subungual hyperkeratosis of the nail leads to elevation, thickening,

darkening, and bending of the nail plate (*Fig. 3.117*). All digits may or may not be involved and toenails and nails of the thumb and index fingers are most severely affected. Erythema of the nail bed can precede nail dystrophy in infancy. Thick yellow keratoses develop on sites of pressure forming calluses (*Fig. 3.118*), fissures, and frictional blisters, particularly during the summer. On the soles, severe pain, which makes walking difficult, is observed. Patients also suffer from palmoplantar hyperhidrosis and nail bed infections.

Additional diagnostic findings include follicular hyperkeratoses on the knees and elbows, oral leukokeratosis, palmoplantar hyperhidrosis, cysts, and natal teeth.[9] Patchy white thickened areas are seen on the tongue and oral mucosa (*Fig. 3.119*).[10] Laryngeal involvement may produce hoarseness and in infancy even fatal respiratory obstruction.[11] Patients with keratin 17 mutations develop steatocystomas and/or other forms of pilosebaceous cysts. Keratin 17 mutations are also responsible for erupted teeth present at birth.[9]

Pathogenesis and histologic features

The majority of causative mutations in PC-related keratins are heterozygous missense mutations or small insertions/deletion mutations that disrupt the cytoskeleton resulting in cell fragility.[12] The different expression patterns of the mutant keratins correlate with the variable distribution of lesions.[13–16]

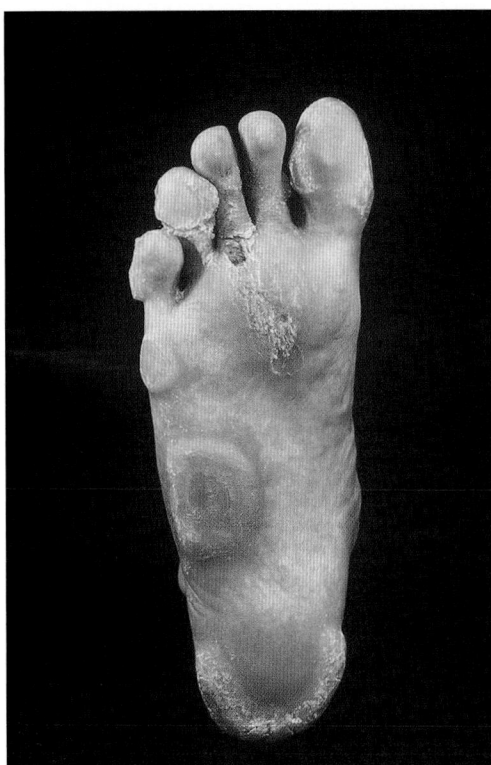

Fig. 3.118
Pachyonychia congenita: circumscribed, yellow, hyperkeratotic plaques on the soles of the feet are a common manifestation. By courtesy of R.A. Marsden, MD, St George's Hospital, London, UK.

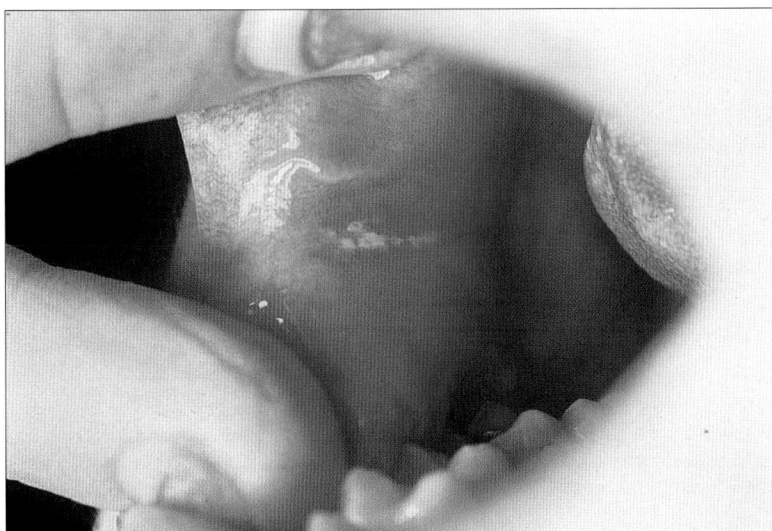

Fig. 3.119
Pachyonychia congenita: leukoplakia of the buccal mucosa is a frequent accompanying feature. By courtesy of R.A. Marsden, MD, St George's Hospital, London, UK.

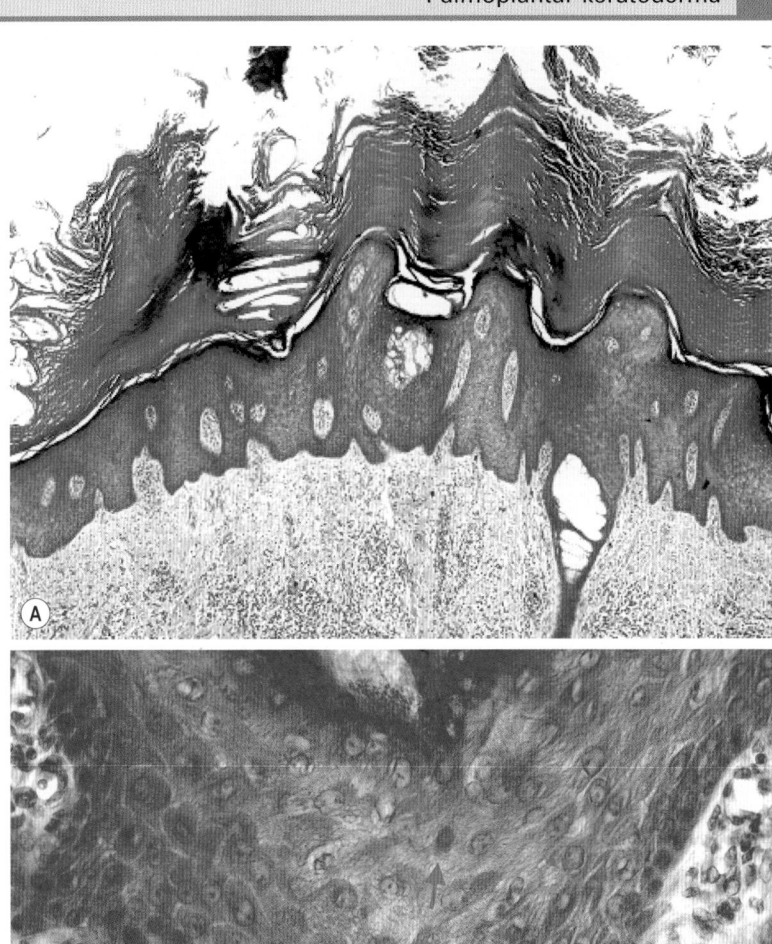

Fig. 3.120
Pachyonychia congenita: (**A**) volar skin showing massive hyperkeratosis, hypergranulosis, and acanthosis; (**B**) suprabasal keratinocytes have a characteristic pale cytoplasm and eosinophilic inclusions.

Mutations in the prominent nail keratin, keratin 6a, additionally affect the oral mucosa.[17] Keratin 17 is constitutively expressed in the pilosebaceous unit, but not to the same extent as in palmoplantar skin and mucosae.[18,19] Mutations in *KRT16* and *KRT17* have been reported in patients with isolated focal PPK or steatocystoma multiplex, respectively, without any other PC manifestations.[20] Mutations in *KRT6c* seem to be associated with a much milder focal keratoderma when compared with any other of the four PC types.[21]

Histology of the affected palmoplantar epidermis shows hyperkeratosis, acanthosis, and patchy hypergranulosis, in which large and malformed keratohyalin granules are present but epidermolysis is missing (*Fig. 3.120*).[1,15] The follicular lesions show plugging of the ostia with adjacent hyperkeratosis, parakeratosis, and acanthosis with pale keratinocytes (*Fig. 3.121*).[4] Suprabasal epithelial of the skin and oral mucosa show a characteristic pale cytoplasm and eosinophilic inclusions (*Fig. 3.122*). At ultrastructural level, these findings correlate with perinuclear condensation of mutated keratin filaments and pale staining or vacuolization of the peripheral cytoplasm.[8,22] Cysts may be keratinous epidermoid cysts, eruptive vellus hair cysts or true steatocystomas.

Differential diagnosis

The same histologic pattern of pale epithelia with eosinophilic inclusions can be also found in white sponge nevus where recurrent white plaques develop on oral and other mucosal sites as a consequence of keratin 4 and 13 mutations. Other differential diagnoses include twenty-nail dystrophy caused by autosomal recessive mutation of the frizzled 6 gene (*FZD6*).[23] In patients with pachyonychia-like nail changes devoid of any other symptoms of PC, heterozygous missense mutations in the connexin 30 have been demonstrated.[24]

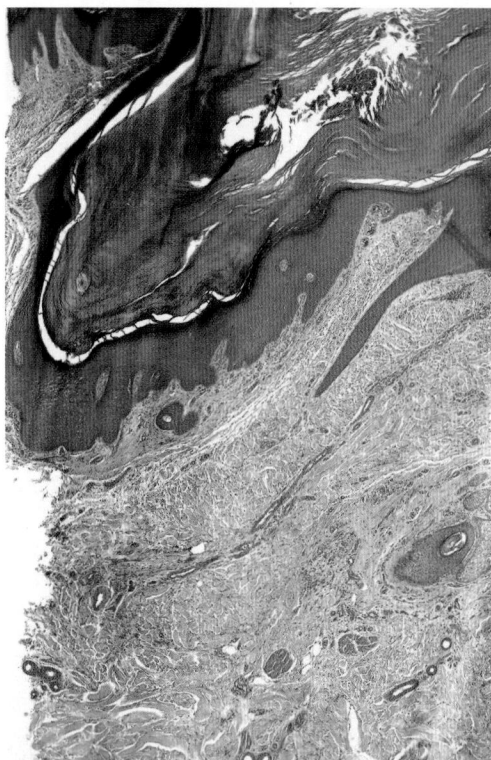

Fig. 3.121
Pachyonychia congenita: follicular lesion showing keratin plugging of the ostium with adjacent hyperkeratosis and associated acanthosis.

Richner-Hanhart syndrome

Clinical features

Richner-Hanhart syndrome (oculocutaneous tyrosinemia, tyrosine transaminase deficiency, tyrosinemia type II) is an oculocutaneous syndrome characterized by herpetiform corneal ulcers that develop during the first months of life.[1] Later painful circumscribed hyperkeratoses of digits, palms, and soles evolve, typically making the child walk on the toes. Blisters and hyperhidrosis may occur. Keratotic plaques have been described sporadically on the elbows, knees, and even the tongue. Other symptoms include severe mental and somatic retardation.[1,2]

Pathogenesis and histologic features

Tyrosinemia type II is caused by autosomal recessively inherited deficiency of hepatic tyrosine aminotransferase due to point mutations in the tyrosine aminotransferase gene *TAT*.[3,4] Tyrosine crystal deposition is seen on slit-lamp examination, and serum and urinary tyrosine levels are elevated. A tyrosine and phenylalanine restricted diet clears the keratitis and the skin lesions, and may delay or prevent cognitive impairment.[5]

Histologically the epidermis is acanthotic, the granular layer is thickened, and the keratinocytes contain eosinophilic globular inclusions similar to those seen in PC.[6]

Electron microscopy reveals clumped tonofilaments with adherent globoid keratohyalin granules suggesting enhanced microfilament aggregation due to an excessive amount of intracellular tyrosine with needle-shaped tyrosine crystalline inclusions.[6]

Keratosis punctata palmoplantaris type Buschke-Fischer-Brauer

Clinical features

Punctate palmoplantar keratoderma is characterized by small rounded papular keratoses on the palms and soles. There are three genetically unrelated entities classified as palmoplantar keratoderma punctata type 1–3.

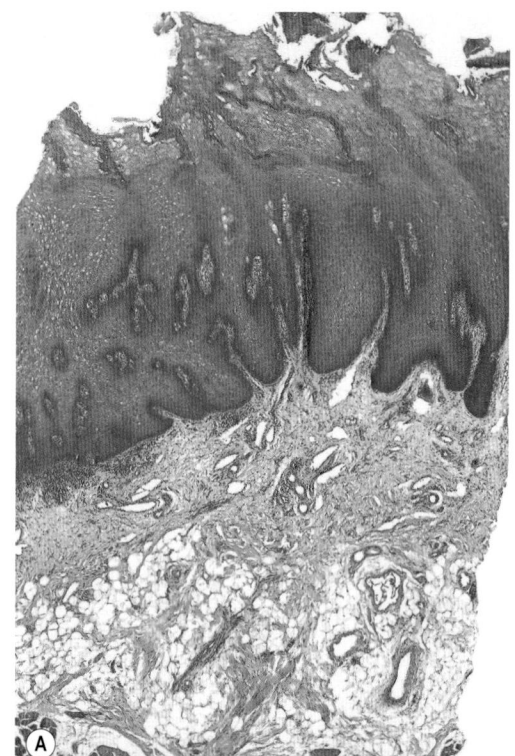

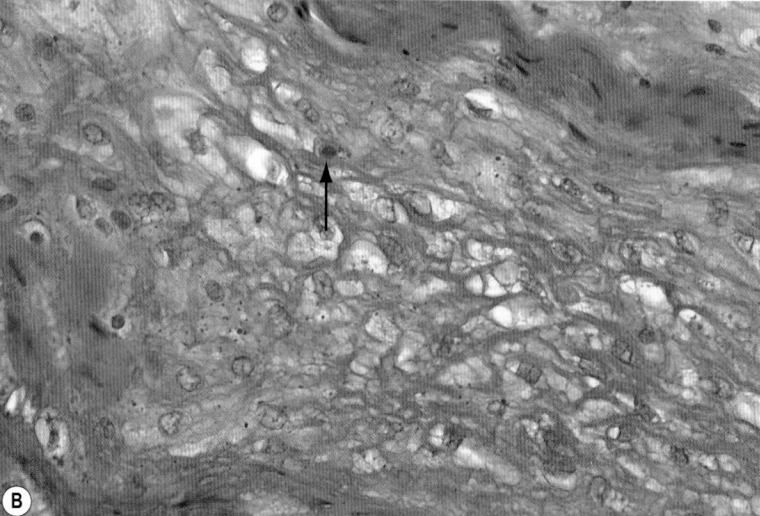

Fig. 3. 122
Pachyonychia congenita: (**A**) scanning view of the oral mucosa showing massive acanthosis with large blunt rete ridges; (**B**) high-power view showing focal parakeratosis and vacuolization of superficial keratinocytes. A single dyskeratotic cell is evident (*arrowed*).

Keratosis punctata palmoplantaris type Buschke-Fischer-Brauer (keratosis punctata palmaris et plantaris, keratoderma hereditarium dissipatum palmare et plantare, Davis-Colley disease) is now classified as palmoplantar keratoderma punctata type 1 (PPKP1).[1–4] PPKP1 is inherited in an autosomal dominant mode. Patients develop numerous tiny keratotic papules over the entire palmoplantar surfaces. The central keratotic core is translucent, may become opaque or verrucous and leaves a depressed pit after removal (*Fig. 3.123*).[5] Over pressure points of the soles the papules aggregate into large keratotic plaques (*Fig. 3.124*). Disease onset is during the first and second decade, or may be delayed up to the sixth decade of life, with large inter- and intrafamilial variability.[4] Sometimes, lesions are associated with excessive manual labor.[2] Occasionally pain, tenderness or burning may occur.[2,5] It is not clear whether PPPK1 is truly associated with malignancies.

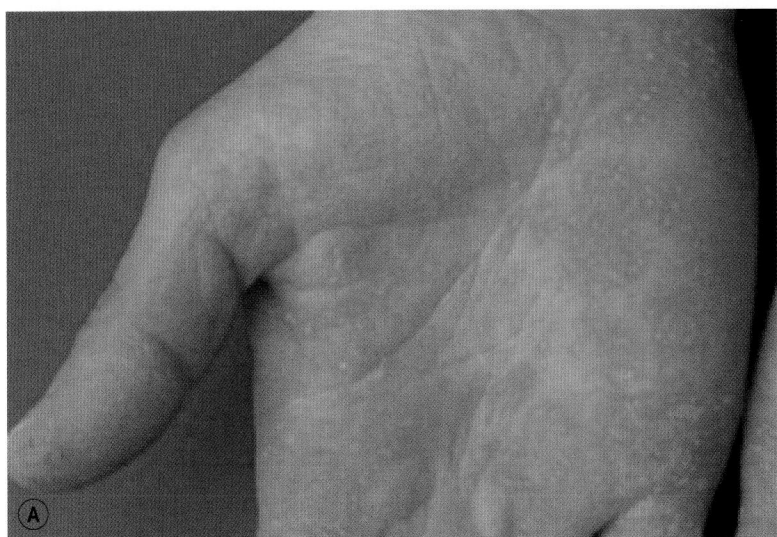

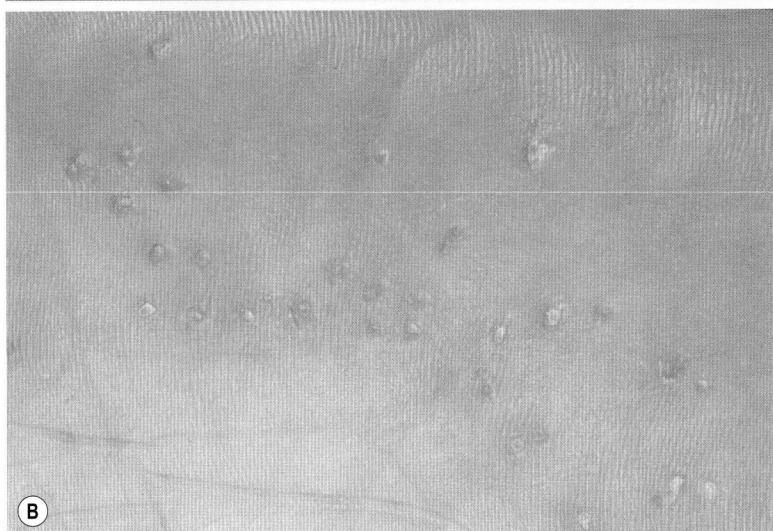

Fig. 3.123
Punctate palmoplantar keratoderma: there are tiny keratotic papules over the entire palms. The central keratotic core is (**A**) translucent and opaque or (**B**) verrucous.

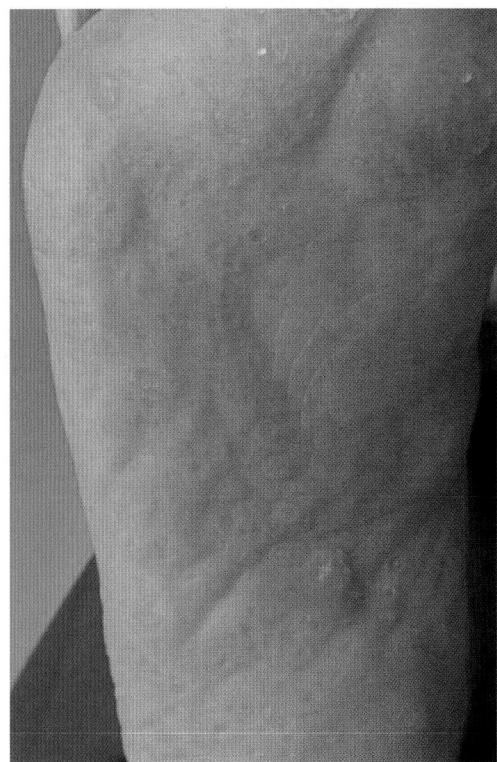

Fig. 3.124
Punctate palmoplantar keratoderma: discrete yellow keratotic papules over pressure areas coalesce into larger plaques.

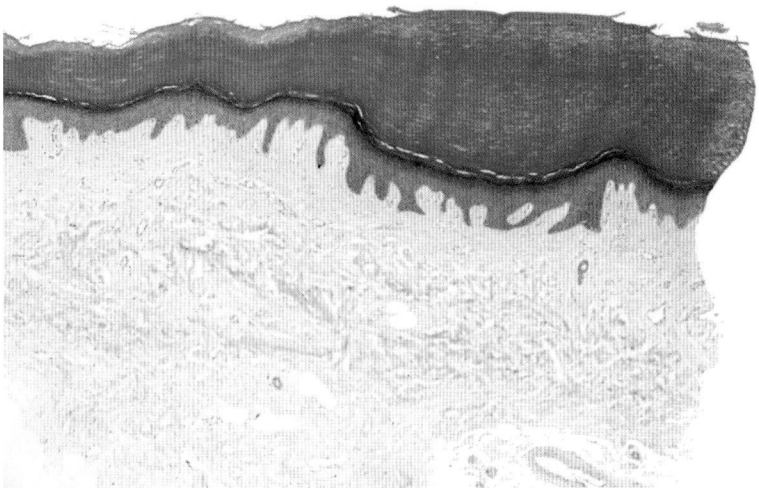

Fig. 3.125
Punctate palmoplantar keratoderma: there is massive orthohyperkeratosis overlying an epidermal depression.

Pathogenesis and histologic features

PPPK1 has been mapped to two chromosomal regions 15q22 and 8q24.13–8q24.21. The first locus harbors the *AAGAB* gene that encodes the alpha- and gamma-adaptin-binding protein p34 which is involved in the clathrin-coated vesicle trafficking.[6–8] Deficiency of p34 results in increased epidermal growth factor signaling, which in turn may drive keratinocyte proliferation.[9] The second locus on 8q was found to be associated with one missense mutation in the gene *COL14A1* in a Chinese family.[10]

Histopathologically, an epidermal depression with orthohyperkeratosis appears (*Fig. 3.125*). Underlying hypogranulosis with focal parakeratosis and elongated and curved rete ridges may be seen and are often misdiagnosed as verruca vulgaris (*Fig. 3.126*). Other cytologic features of HPV infection are lacking. Electron microscopy reveals a high number of small vesicles and dilated Golgi apparatus highlighting the dysregulation of vesicle trafficking.[9]

Differential diagnosis

Acquired forms of punctate palmoplantar keratoderma may be associated with internal malignancies, including carcinomas of the colon, kidney, breast, and pancreas, and Hodgkin lymphoma.[11,12] Punctate keratoderma-like lesions affecting the palms and the soles have been described as a complication of arsenic or dioxin exposure.[13] Keratosis punctata of the palmar creases occurs in black adults and is restricted to the creases of the digits and soles (see below).[14] Palmoplantar pits as seen in nevoid basal cell carcinoma syndrome, Darier disease or other conditions can be confused with PPK1.

Keratosis punctata of the palmar creases

Clinical features

Keratosis punctata of the palmar creases (keratotic pits of the palmar creases) is a variant of punctate keratoderma in which the lesions are confined to the palmar and digital creases.[1–5] Although very rare in white patients, it is common in young to middle-aged black adults.[3,5,6] It is characterized by sharply defined 1–4 mm warty hyperkeratoses, strictly confined to the palmar creases (*Fig. 3.127*). The development of lesions appears to be trauma related since outdoor workers are particularly affected and the condition

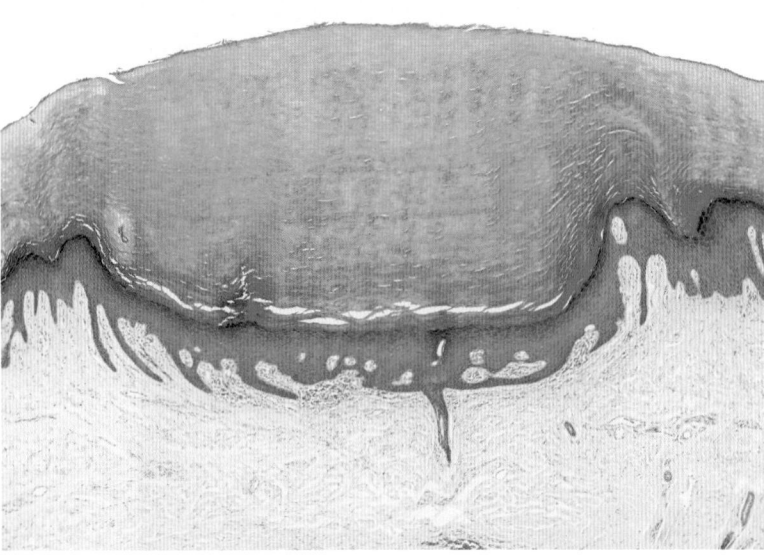

Fig. 3.126
Punctate palmoplantar keratoderma: elongated and curved rete ridges may be seen and are often misdiagnosed as verruca vulgaris.

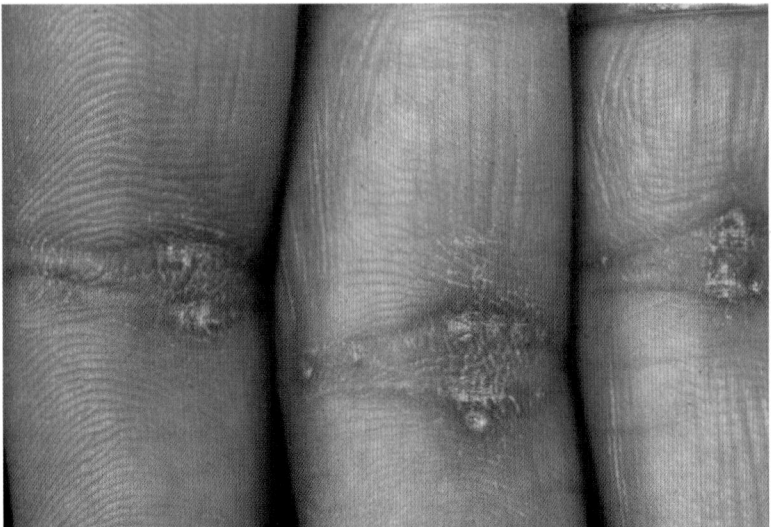

Fig. 3.127
Keratosis punctata of the palmar creases: minute punctate lesions are localized solely to the palmar creases. There is often a history of manual labor. By courtesy of the Institute of Dermatology, London, UK.

improves during holidays. Although the condition is usually sporadic, an autosomal dominant mode of inheritance has been documented.[2,4,7-9]

Histologic features

Lesions are characterized by a hyperkeratotic plug, sometimes with foci of parakeratosis below, which are deep cone-shaped depressions sometimes centered on the acrosyringium.[4] The adjacent epidermis shows acanthosis with hypergranulosis and in some cases a perivascular lymphohistiocytic infiltrate is present in the superficial dermis.

Cole disease

Clinical features

Cole disease is characterized by a punctate keratoderma with guttate hypopigmentation.[1] The disease manifests during the first year of life. Affected individuals present with a mild punctuate keratoderma. In addition, they develop sharply demarcated irregular macules with varying degrees of

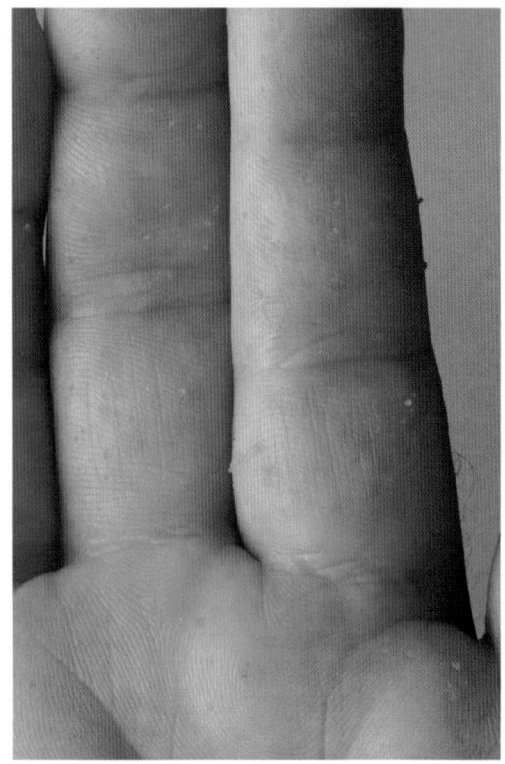

Fig. 3.128
Spiny keratoderma: multiple tiny keratotic spines project from palms, soles, and fingers.

hypopigmentation, mainly located over the extremities.[1-3] There may be an association with early onset calcifying tendinopathy or calcinosis cutis.[4]

Pathogenesis and histologic features

A missense mutation in the gene *ENPP1* encoding a cell-surface protein that catalyzes the hydrolysis of ATP to AMP has been identified. This generates extracellular inorganic pyrophosphate, which is a major inhibitor of mineralization.[4] While recessive mutations in *ENPP1* account for inherited forms of ectopic calcifications, dominant mutations in this gene cause Cole disease.

Histology shows orthohyperkeratosis, hypergranulosis, and acanthosis. Ultrastructure confirms a reduction in the melanin content of keratinocytes with disproportionately large melanosomes in melanocytes due to a defect in melanosome transfer between melanocytes and keratinocytes. The number of melanocytes is normal.[2]

Differential diagnosis

The differential diagnosis includes EBS with mottled pigmentation and Naegeli-Franceschetti-Jadassohn syndrome.

Spiny keratoderma

Spiny keratoderma is classified as palmoplantar keratoderma punctata type 2 (PPKP2) (syn. music box spine keratoderma, multiple minute palmoplantar digitate hyperkeratosis). In this autosomal dominantly inherited genodermatosis of unknown etiology multiple tiny keratotic spines project from palms and soles including the fingers beginning from the first to third decade of life (*Fig. 3.128*).[1-3] Discomfort is caused by a tendency of the lesions to catch on clothing and other objects.[4] Spiny keratoderma has to be differentiated from acquired forms of the disease that evolve after 50 years of age and are associated with neoplastic conditions (visceral carcinoma, melanoma, leukemia, and multiple myeloma) or internal diseases (hyperlipidemia type IV, diabetes, asthma, renal insufficiency, polycystic kidney with liver cysts, tuberculosis, and HIV).[2,5-8] Since there is no relation to porokeratosis, old synonyms for spiny keratoderma-like 'porokeratotic PPK', or 'porokeratosis punctata palmaris et plantaris' should be avoided.

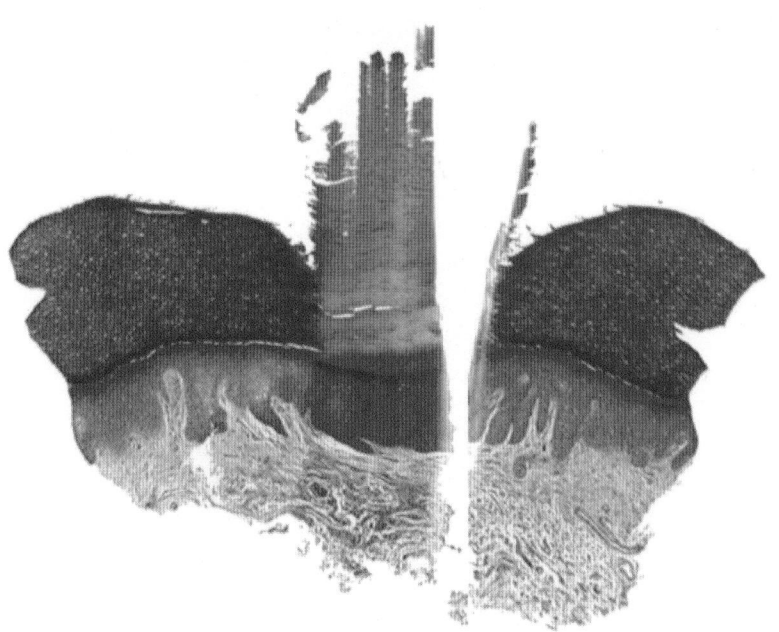

Fig. 3.129
Spiny keratoderma: a keratotic spike develops over a depressed epidermis.

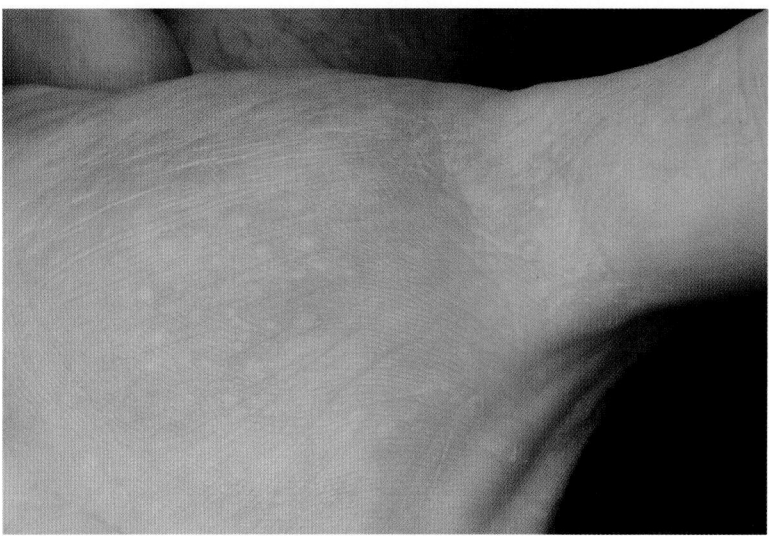

Fig. 3.130
Marginal papular acrokeratoderma: pearly papules predominantly affecting the sides of the hands, wrists, fingers.

Histology demonstrates dense keratotic spikes above a depressed epidermis. Orthokeratosis predominates over focal parakeratotic areas and the underlying stratum granulosum appears attenuated (*Fig. 3.129*).[1,3,4] The absence of dyskeratosis, pleomorphism and vacuolated keratinocytes below the parakeratotic column differentiates spiny keratoderma from porokeratosis and PAON.[1] As demonstrated by immunohistochemistry and electron microscopy, keratinization of the keratotic spikes resembles that seen in normal hair cortex suggesting that spiny keratoderma represents an attempt at ectopic hair formation of the palms and soles.[9]

Marginal papular acrokeratoderma

Clinical features

Marginal papular acrokeratoderma (palmoplantar keratoderma punctata type 3, PPKP3) refers to a complex, confusing, and overlapping group of disorders, which includes acrokeratoelastoidosis of Costa, focal acral hyperkeratosis, mosaic acral keratosis, degenerate collagenous plaques of the hands, digital papular calcific elastosis, and keratoelastoidosis marginalis of the hands.[1] All present with frequently crateriform, keratotic papules along the borders of the hands and feet (*Fig. 3.130*).[1] Although usually discrete, in some patients the papules may coalesce into plaques.

Acrokeratoelastoidosis presents in childhood and adolescence with yellowish, warty, and crateriform keratotic or pearly papules predominantly affecting the sides of the hands, wrists, fingers, and feet.[2–5] There is no racial predilection and the sexes are affected equally. Patients may also develop circumscribed keratodermatous knuckle pad-like lesions, palmoplantar hyperkeratosis, and hyperhidrosis.[1,3] Sporadic and autosomal dominant variants have been described. The disorder may be linked to chromosome 2.[6] Repeated trauma is believed to be of etiological importance.

Focal acral hyperkeratosis is clinically identical to acrokeratoelastoidosis, patients presenting with keratotic papules along the sides of the hands, fingers, and feet.[7,8] It has also been designated acrokeratoelastoidosis without elastorrhexis.[9,10] Although originally thought to be a disorder of black children, more recently it has been described in whites.[11]

Mosaic acral keratosis as reported in African patients is similar if not identical to focal acral hyperkeratosis, being characterized by keratotic papules distributed in a mosaic or jigsaw-puzzle pattern along dorsal aspects of the feet and adjacent lower limbs.[12] Hyperkeratosis may be seen on the palms and soles.[1]

Degenerative collagenous plaques of the hands affect the sun-damaged skin of the elderly and present as symmetrical yellowish, keratotic or smooth papules and plaques affecting the thumb, first web, and side of the index finger.[4,13–18] The ulnar border of the hand and volar aspect of the wrist may also be involved. Keratoelastoidosis marginalis of the hands is a similar condition described in Australians in which keratotic papules develop at sites of trauma along the index finger and thumb.[19] The skin is typically grossly sun damaged. Calcified variants of degenerative collagenous plaques are known as digital papular calcific elastosis.[20,21]

Histologic features

Acrokeratoelastoidosis is characterized by massive orthohyperkeratosis overlying a crateriform dell lined by acanthotic epidermis. Hypergranulosis may be present. The dermis shows fragmentation and loss of the elastic tissue (elastorrhexis) (*Fig. 3.131*). Collagen may be disorganized or appears homogenized and pale staining.[2,3]

Focal acral hyperkeratosis and mosaic acral keratosis are histologically identical with the exception that the elastic tissue appears normal.[7–12]

Degenerative collagenous plaques of the hands are characterized by a dense zone of thickened and distorted collagen with fragmentation of elastic fibers and overlying hyperkeratosis and acanthosis.[4,13–18] The papillary dermis is spared. Calcification is sometimes a feature (digital papular calcific elastosis).[19–21] Telangiectatic vessels may also be seen and increased dermal mucin has been described.[19]

Acquired palmoplantar keratoderma and malignancies

Acquired diffuse palmoplantar keratoderma may represent a paraneoplastic phenomenon associated with a number of internal malignancies, including carcinoma of the bronchus, esophagus, stomach, urinary bladder, and myeloma (*Fig. 3.132*).[1–6] There are also reports of acquired punctate and spiny keratoderma associated with a range of visceral cancers, including breast, kidney, colon, and lung and with lymphoma and leukemia.[7–9] 'Tripe palms' refers to velvety, thickened palmar skin with exaggerated ridges. It is often associated with acanthosis nigricans and may herald malignancies of the lung, stomach or genitourinary tract.[10] Bazex acrokeratosis paraneoplastica is discussed in Chapter 6.

Chronic ingestion of arsenic results in keratoderma and internal malignancy. Arsenical keratoses present as small, corn-like areas of hyperkeratosis on the palms and soles. Over time, the lesions enlarge, thicken, and increase in number, spreading to the dorsal surfaces of the hands and feet. The latent period between ingestion of inorganic arsenic and onset of keratoses is 10 to 30 years or longer.[11] Visceral malignancies, particularly of the

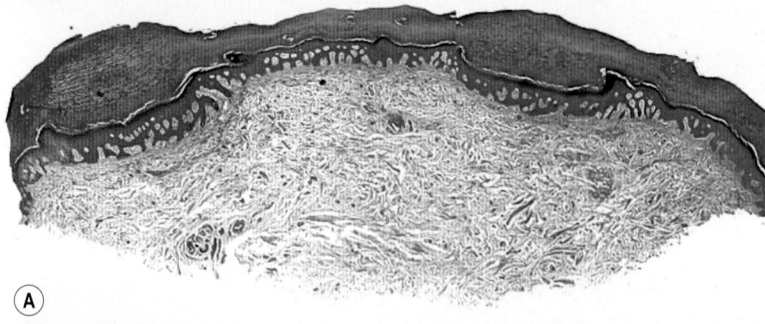

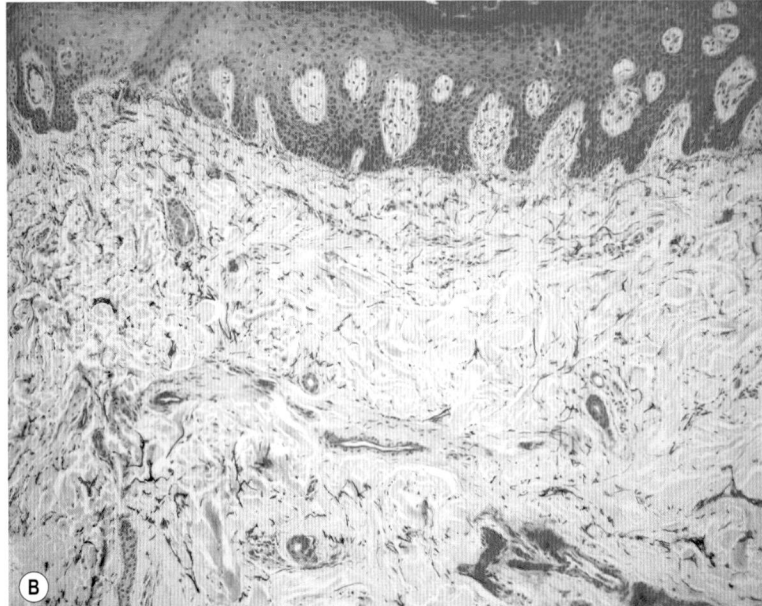

Fig. 3.131
Marginal papular acrokeratoderma, variant acrokeratoelastoidosis: (**A**) focal areas orthohyperkeratosis overlying crateriform dells lined by acanthotic epidermis; (**B**) Weigert elastic staining reveals diminution of the dermal elastic tissue.

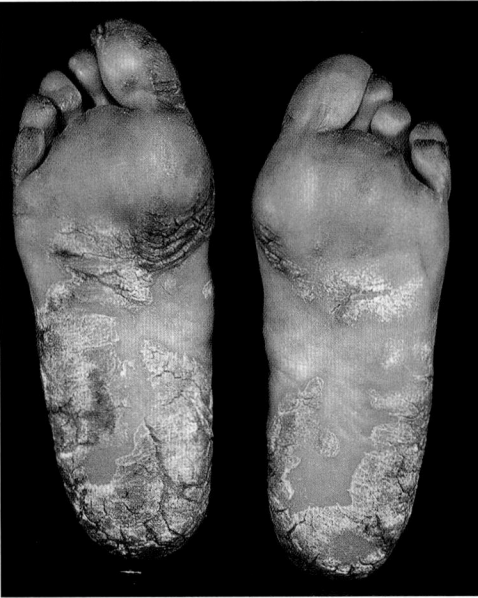

Fig. 3.132
Acquired palmoplantar keratoderma: acquired disease may be a manifestation of underlying malignancy. By courtesy of the Institute of Dermatology, London, UK.

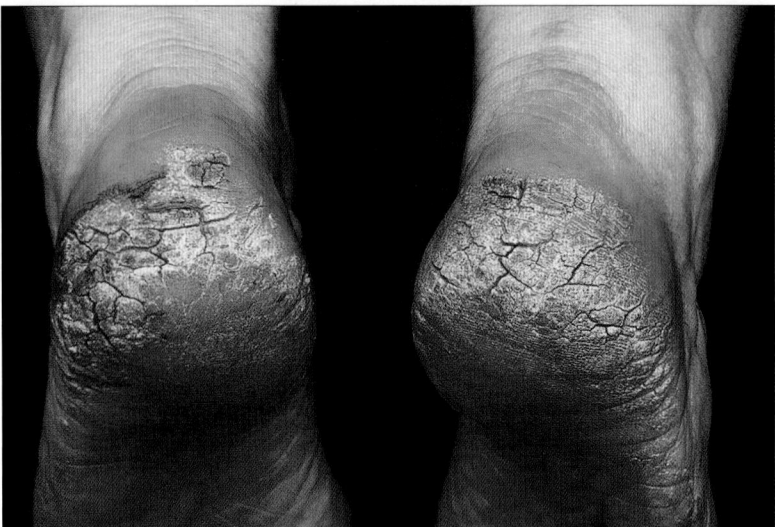

Fig. 3.133
Keratoderma climactericum: there is massive hyperkeratosis with fissuring over the heels. By courtesy of the Institute of Dermatology, London, UK.

lung and genitourinary tract, usually develop after the onset of skin tumors. Ulceration often occurs when a squamous cell carcinoma develops. On histologic examination, epidermal changes in arsenic keratosis vary from benign hyperplasia to moderate atypia or frank squamous cell carcinoma.[12]

Acquired keratodermas, others

Keratoderma climactericum (Haxthausen disease, climacteric keratoderma) is restricted to menopausal women.[1,2] Lesions present on the weight-bearing surfaces of the sole of the foot as erythematous hyperkeratotic and fissured plaques and then spread to involve the rest of the plantar skin (*Fig. 3.133*). Palmar involvement is sometimes seen with lesions affecting the area between the thenar and hypothenar eminences.[2] Similar lesions have been documented in younger women who have undergone bilateral oophorectomy.[3] The condition is distinguished from congenital palmoplantar keratoderma by its late onset. Histologically, the plantar skin shows massive hyperkeratosis, hypergranulosis, acanthosis, and spongiosis with lymphocytic exocytosis. A superficial perivascular dermal lymphohistiocytic infiltrate is present and vertically orientated dermal collagen associated with atypical myofibroblasts is often seen.[2]

Acquired palmoplantar keratoderma can be caused by myxedema associated with hypothyroidism. It improves with treatment.[4]

Patients with dermatomyositis, in particular dermatomyositis-systemic scleroderma-overlap syndrome may develop circumscribed hyperkeratoses on palms ('mechanic's hands') and soles, sometimes also on elbows and knees (*Fig. 3.134*). The diagnosis is confirmed by the presence of antibodies against aminoacyl-transfer RNA-synthetase or anti-PM-Scl-antibodies.[5] Histologically, subtle signs of interface-dermatitis may be seen.

Chronic lymphedema may also lead to keratoderma. Initially the skin thickens and this is followed by a velvety papillomatous surface, which is ultimately covered by large irregular warty projections.[6]

Several drugs, such as iodine, lithium, tegafur, and glucan as well as intoxication with arsenic, dioxin, and halogenated weed-killers may also induce keratoderma.[7,8] Drugs used for oncologic treatment not only cause palmoplantar erythema, but also keratoderma.[9]

Transient aquagenic keratoderma

Transient aquagenic keratoderma (syn. transient reactive papulotranslucent acrokeratoderma, aquagenic syringeal acrokeratoderma, acquired aquagenic palmoplantar keratoderma, aquagenic wrinkling of the palms and soles) is characterized by a mild keratoderma in the center of the palms that is triggered or exacerbated by contact with water or sweat.[1] Patients develop thickening and white to translucent, 'pebbly' changes on their palms shortly

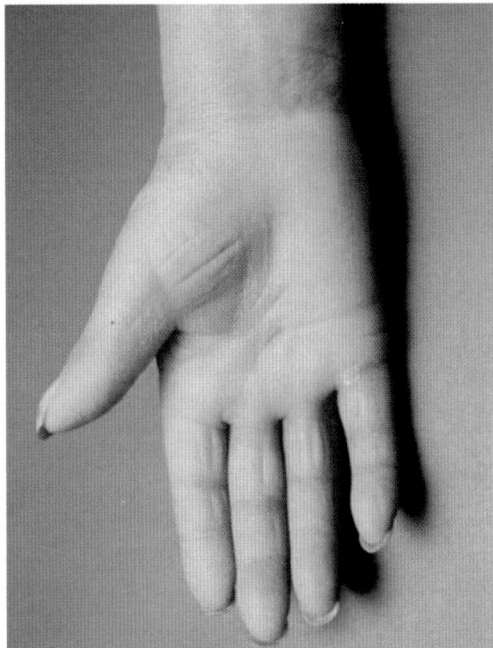

Fig. 3.134
Mechanic hands: patients with dermatomyositis, in particular dermatomyositis-systemic scleroderma-overlap syndrome may develop circumscribed hyperkeratoses on palms.

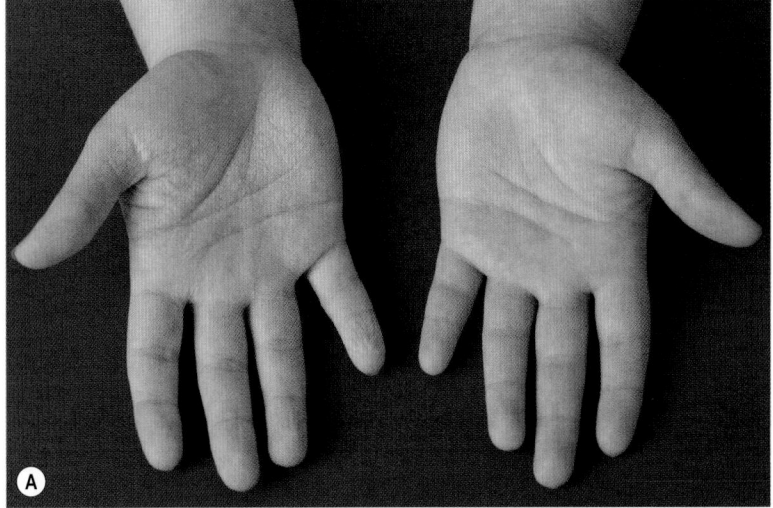

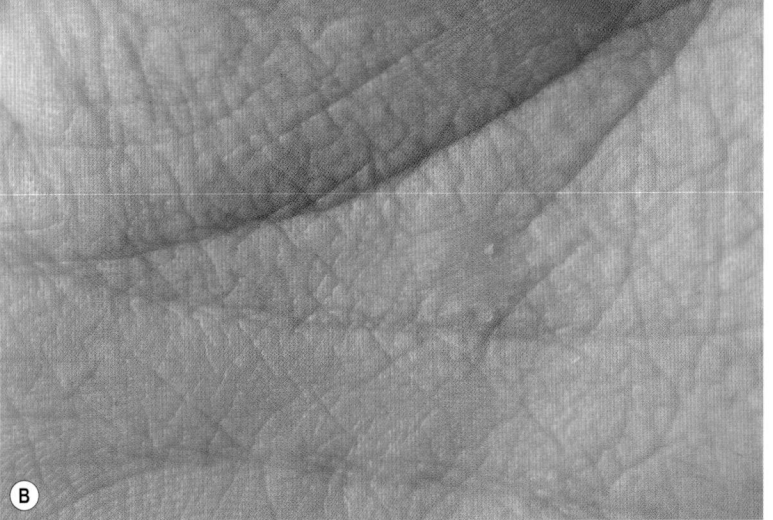

Fig. 3.135
Transient aquagenic keratoderma: (**A**) shortly after immersion of the right hand in water thickening and 'pebbly' changes developed on the palm. Left hand is the control; (**B**) the papular lesions show widely dilated acrosyringeal ostia.

after immersion in water (*Fig. 3.135A*).[2] Associated symptoms include pain, burning sensation or pruritus. Onset is typically during the second decade of life, with predilection for women. The papular lesions are associated with dilated acrosyringeal ostia (*Fig. 3.135B*).[3]

Pathophysiology and histology

Transient aquagenic keratoderma appears to be acquired, but an autosomal recessive, or dominant pattern of inheritance has been observed. It has been described after use of cyclooxygenase-2 inhibitors.[4] Aquagenic wrinkling of the palms is seen in about 50% of patients and heterozygous carriers with cystic fibrosis and in up to 10% of heterozygous CFTR gene mutation carriers.[5,6]

Histologically, normal skin or dilated eccrine ostia, hyperplasia of the eccrine sweat glands, and a mildly hyperkeratotic stratum corneum may be seen (*Fig. 3.136*).[7]

Clavus and callus

Clavi (corns) are extremely common painful keratotic lesions that develop on the dorsal or lateral aspect of the toes, often as a consequence of ill-fitting shoes. Histologically, they are characterized by a deep keratin-filled depression often associated with atrophy of the underlying epidermis (*Fig. 3.137*). The granular layer is often lost and parakeratosis is observed. A clavus can be distinguished from plantar warts by the absence of koilocytes and irregular keratohyalin granules.

A callus is a nonpainful localized focus of hyperkeratosis usually arising on the ball of the foot or heel from pressure or foot deformity.[1] Palmar lesions arise as a consequence of chronic rubbing. Extensive use of a computer mouse may lead to a 'mousing callus'.[2] Histologically, a callus is similar to a clavus consisting of a keratin-filled epidermal dell with hypergranulosis.

Keratolytic winter erythema

Clinical features

Keratolytic winter erythema (synonyms: erythrokeratolysis hiemalis, Oudtshoorn disease) is an autosomal dominant disorder first described in South Africa.[1] Sporadic cases have been reported from other countries.[2,3] The

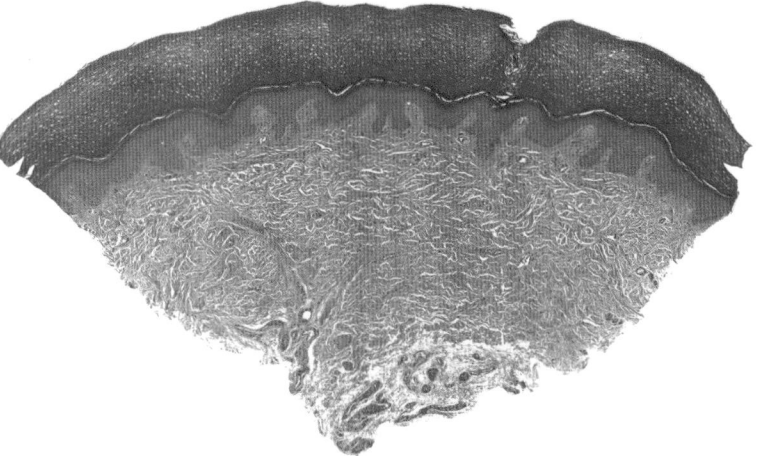

Fig. 3.136
Transient aquagenic keratoderma: note the wide opening of an acrosyringeal ostium, and the pale staining of an orthohyperkeratotic stratum corneum, otherwise there are no other histologic changes.

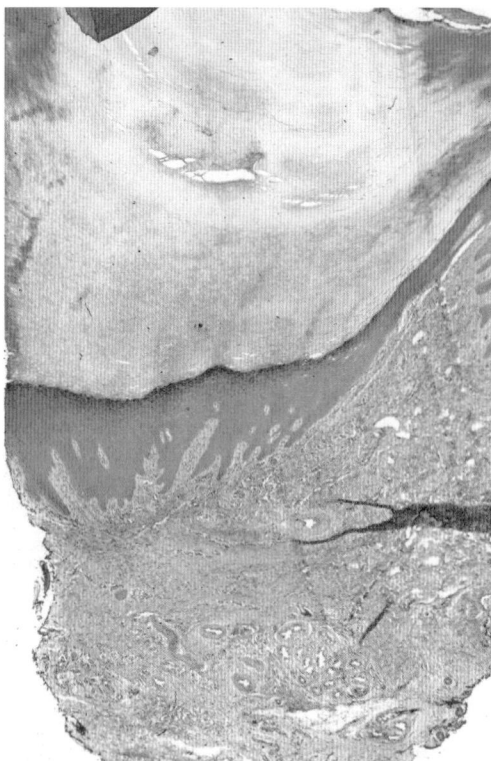

Fig. 3.137
Clavus: massive hyperkeratosis overlies an epidermal depression.

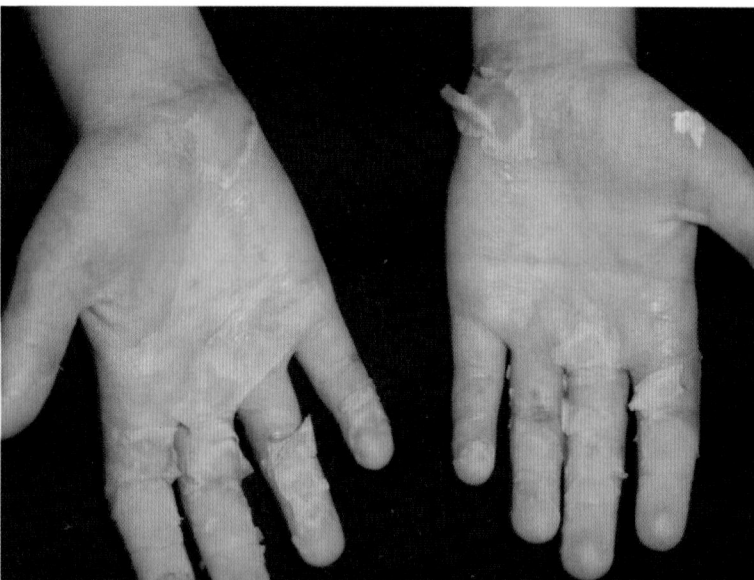

Fig. 3.138
Keratolytic winter erythema: palmoplantar erythema is followed by centrifugal peeling. By courtesy of W. Grayson, MD, University of the Witwatersrand, Johannesburg, South Africa.

disorder manifests at an early age and is characterized by recurring cycles of erythema involving the palms and soles, followed by mild hyperkeratosis and nonpruritic and nonpainful peeling (*Fig. 3.138*). In severe cases the limbs and trunk are affected with gyrate scaling erythemas. Most remarkably, the onset of symptoms occurs during cold weather.[2] Other triggers include febrile illness, surgery, stress, and menstruation. The disease improves during pregnancy and with age.

Pathogenesis and histologic features

The disorder has been mapped to chromosome 8p22–23 with some genetic heterogeneity.[4–7] Only recently, tandem duplications in a noncoding genomic

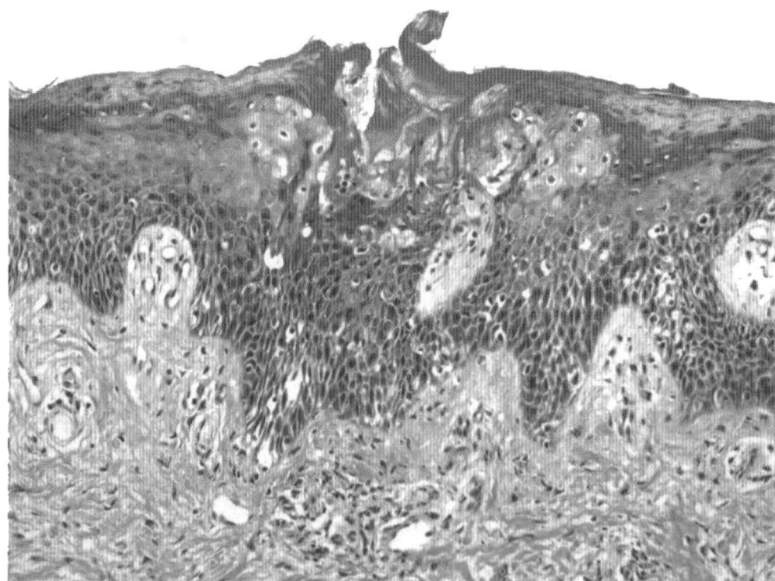

Fig. 3.139
Keratolytic winter erythema: there is hyperplasia and spongiosis of the epidermis. The stratum granulosum is absent. Keratinocytes show a pale cytoplasm, perinuclear vacuoles, and pyknotic nuclei. A parakeratotic wedge is seen within the hyperkeratotic stratum corneum. By courtesy of W. Grayson, MD, University of the Witwatersrand, Johannesburg, South Africa.

region containing an active enhancer element for CTSB, resulting in upregulation of this gene in affected individuals, have been found.[8]

Biopsy of the advancing edge of a lesion shows hyperplasia, spongiosis, and, in the upper stratum spinosum, keratinocytes with pale cytoplasm, perinuclear vacuolization, and pyknotic nuclei. In the absence of a granular layer the epidermis forms a parakeratotic wedge, which becomes sandwiched within the hyperkeratotic stratum corneum and is eventually shed (*Fig. 3.139*).[1] During regeneration undifferentiated keratinocytes are not confined to the basal layer but appear in the lower half of the epidermis.[1] A superficial perivascular lymphocytic infiltrate has been reported by some authors.[3]

Circumscribed palmar or plantar hypokeratosis

Clinical features

Circumscribed palmar or plantar hypokeratosis is characterized by the development of well-circumscribed, depressed, erythematous lesions on the thenar and hypothenar regions of the palms or the medial side of the soles (*Fig. 3.140*).[1] The lesions sometimes have an arcuate or polycyclic outline, a slightly scaling border, range in diameter from a few millimeters up to 3 centimeters, and are asymptomatic. Multiple lesions are sometimes seen. Malignant transformation has not been reported. All patients are middle aged or elderly. There is a predilection for females.[2] The clinical differential diagnosis includes Bowen disease and porokeratosis.

Pathogenesis and histologic features

The pathogenesis of circumscribed palmar or plantar hypokeratosis is controversial. Two theories have been proposed: a form of epidermal malformation favored by the long-standing nature of the lesions or a localized lesion secondary to persistent trauma.[1–4] Molecular studies failed to detect human papillomavirus except from one report that found (HPV) type 4-specific DNA.[5] In some instances, changes of circumscribed hypokeratosis have been described in epidermis overlaying a traumatized neoplasm, a verruca vulgaris, an inflammatory process, or a scar (pseudo-circumscribed palmar or plantar hypokeratosis).[6]

Histologically, lesional skin displays a sharply circumscribed loss of the cornified layer overlying an otherwise normal epidermis (*Fig. 3.141*).[1–8] There may be a thin layer of parakeratosis in the hypokeratotic zone and

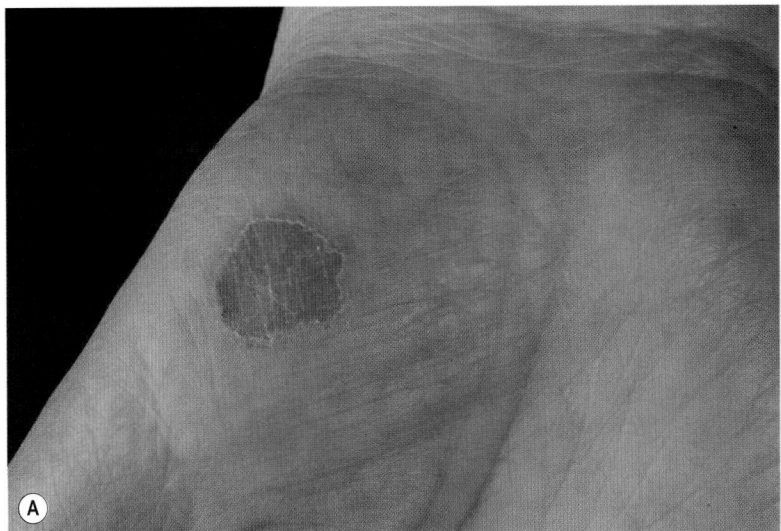

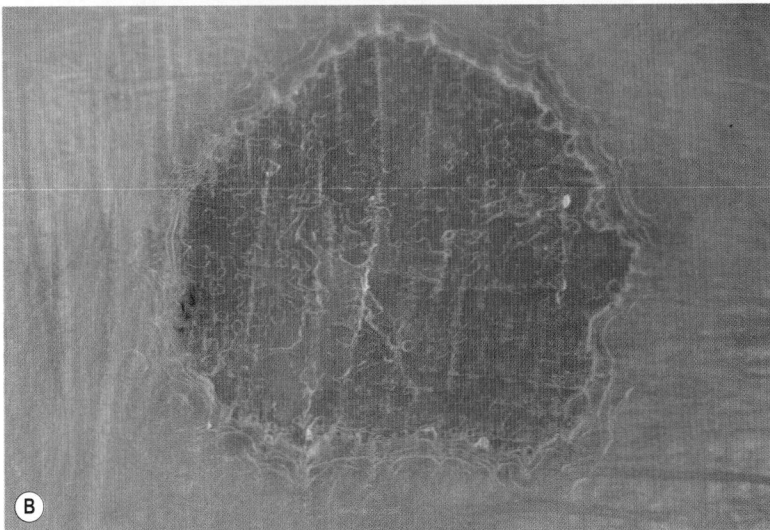

Fig. 3.140
Circumscribed palmar or plantar hypokeratosis: (**A**) on the thenar area a well-circumscribed, depressed, erythematous lesion is present; (**B**) a closer view reveals a scaly border.

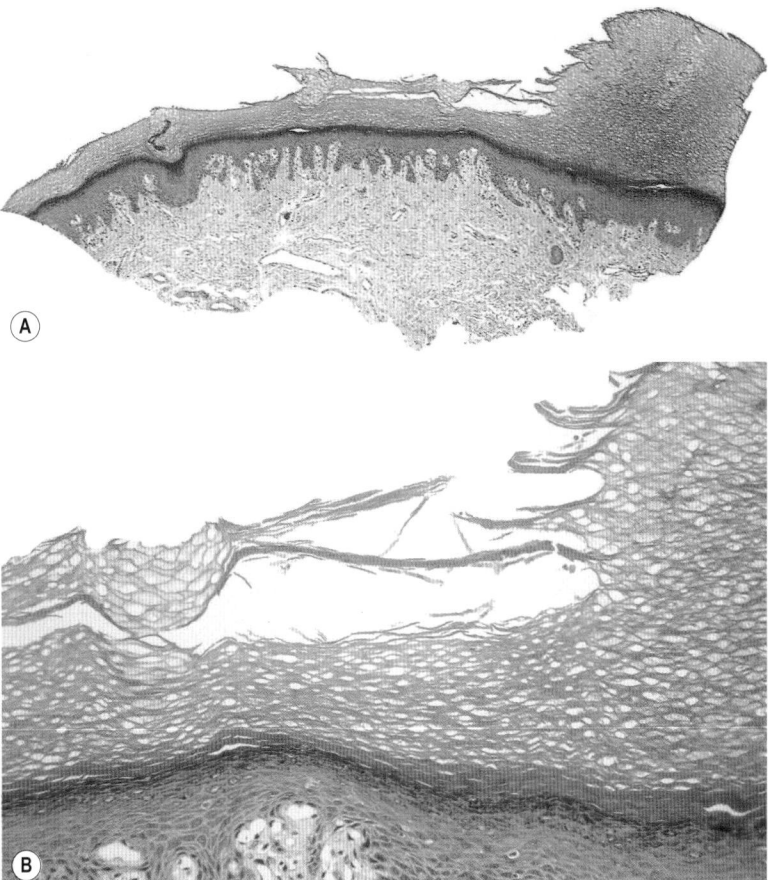

Fig. 3.141
Circumscribed palmar or plantar hypokeratosis: (**A**) there is a sharply circumscribed loss of the cornified layer and some psoriasiform hyperplasia of the epidermis; (**B**) higher view from the edge of the lesion.

some psoriasiform hyperplasia of the epidermis with expression of the hyperproliferative keratin 16.[7,8]

Additional features are hyperplasia of sweat ducts, and tortuous and elongated capillaries in the papillary dermis; an inflammatory cell infiltrate is lacking.[5]

Ultrastructurally, breakage of the corneocytes at a cytoplasmic level suggests enhanced corneocyte fragility.[7]

Acrokeratosis verruciformis of Hopf

Clinical features

This is an exceedingly rare dermatosis with an autosomal dominant mode of inheritance.[1-3] The disease presents in infancy or early childhood as dry, rough, brownish or skin-colored verrucoid, keratotic papules, located particularly on the backs of the hands (*Fig. 3.142*) and feet, and on the knees and elbows.[4] Keratotic punctate pits are found on the palms and soles. Lesions, which are clinically and histologically indistinguishable, may occasionally be seen in Darier disease.[5-7] Exceptionally, a similar association with Hailey-Hailey disease has been documented and there is a report of acrokeratosis verruciformis presenting in a patient with nevoid basal cell carcinoma syndrome.[8,9] Nail involvement, including longitudinal splitting, striations, and subungual hyperkeratosis may also be seen.[10]

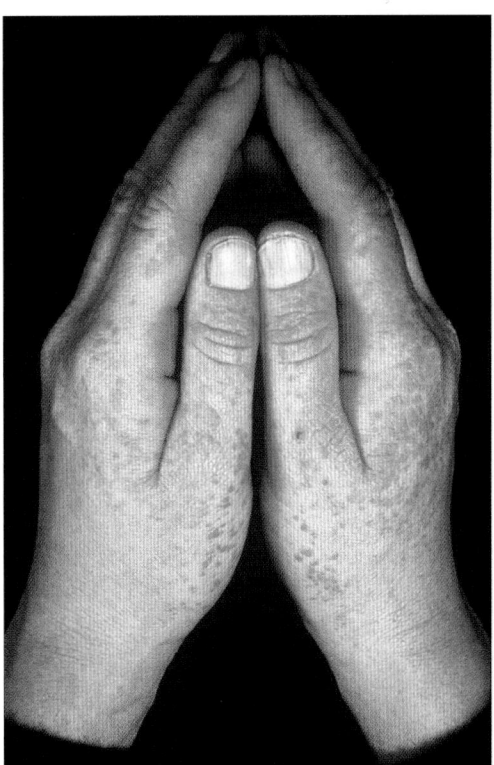

Fig. 3.142
Acrokeratosis verruciformis: numerous brown flat-topped papules are symmetrically distributed over the dorsal aspects of the hands. By courtesy of R.A. Marsden, MD, St George's Hospital, London, UK.

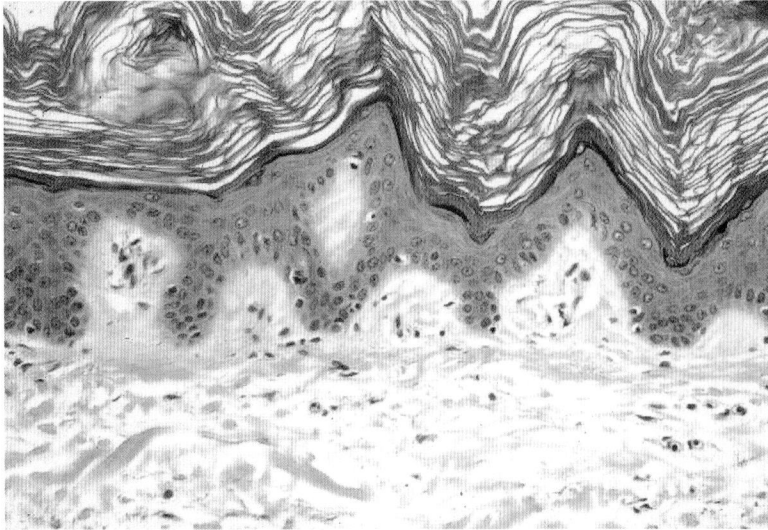

Fig. 3.143
Acrokeratosis verruciformis: there is hyperkeratosis and church-spire papillomatosis.

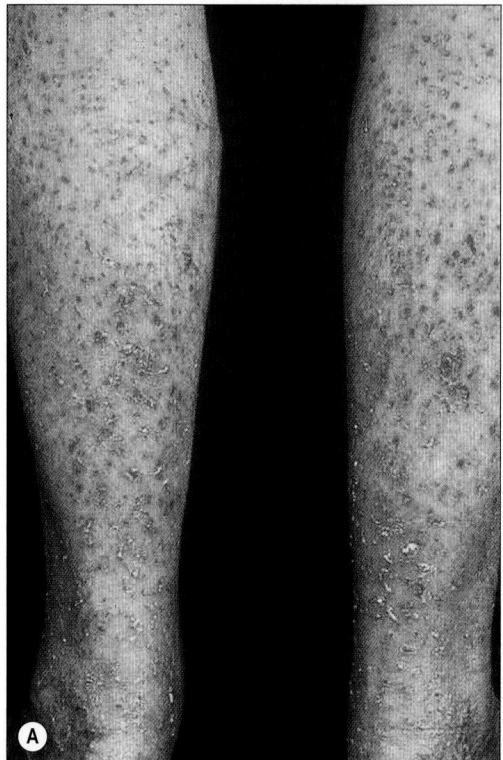

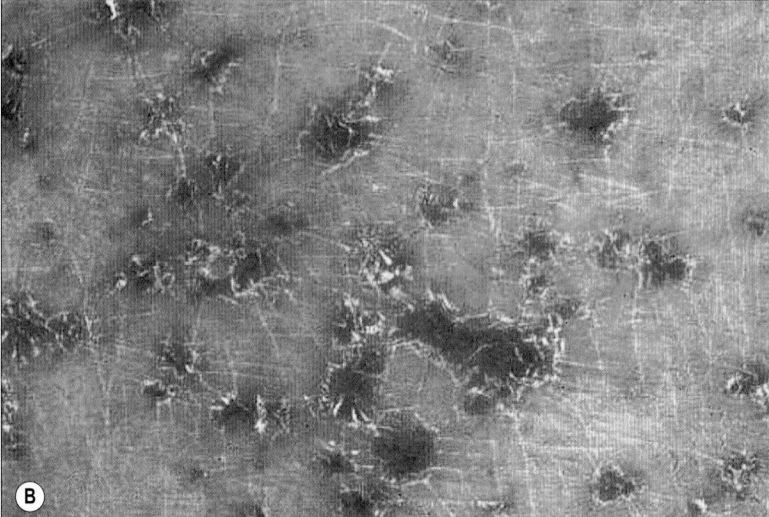

Fig. 3.144
Flegel disease: (**A**) there are characteristic disseminated erythematous scaly lesions; (**B**) the lower legs are commonly affected. Lesions are small, multiple and show irregular margins covered by a well-developed scale ('cornflake sign'). By courtesy of M. Price, MD, Institute of Dermatology, London, UK.

Pathogenesis and histologic features

Loss of function of the sarco- (endo-) plasmic reticulum Ca2+ ATPase2 mutant in acrokeratosis verruciformis provides evidence that acrokeratosis verruciformis and Darier disease are allelic disorders.[11] However, identification of mutations in genes other than ATP2A2, suggests genetic heterogeneity of acrokeratosis verruciformis.[12]

Histologically there is epidermal acanthosis with a prominent granular cell layer, typically showing a 'church spire' appearance (*Fig. 3.143*). There is usually moderate to marked hyperkeratosis. Parakeratosis is not a feature. Step sections sometimes reveal focal acantholytic dyskeratosis in cases associated with Darier disease. There is also considerable histologic overlap with stucco keratosis. Acrokeratosis verruciformis-like features may occasionally be seen in linear epidermal nevi.[13]

Flegel disease (hyperkeratosis lenticularis perstans)

Clinical features

Flegel disease (hyperkeratosis lenticularis perstans) is a rare autosomal dominant disorder of cornification presenting in older individuals, usually between the third and fourth decades of life.[1,2] A large number of discrete red-brown scaly papules with discrete irregular margins ('cornflake sign') develop over the dorsa of the feet and on the lower parts of the legs (*Fig. 3.144*). The lesions may spread to the upper part of the legs and thighs, more rarely over the arms and trunk or concha of the ear.[3–5] On palms and soles punctate keratoses have been described.[6] The lesions are either asymptomatic or mildly pruritic. Characteristically, removal of the scale is associated with pinpoint bleeding, a feature that distinguishes this disorder from stucco keratoses. Other than an isolated report of an increased incidence of both basal cell and squamous carcinoma, there is no particular associated risk of malignancy.[7]

Pathogenesis and histologic features

The causative mutation remains unknown. A low proliferation rate of keratinocytes together with downregulation of filaggrin, loricrin, and high molecular weight keratins, and loss of the keratin pattern in the horny layer, suggests a retention hyperkeratosis and complex dysregulation of epidermal differentiation.[8,9]

Histologically, there is hyperkeratosis with a focal parakeratosis overlying a thinned, flat epidermis with loss of keratohyalin granules. In the periphery of the lesions the epidermis is acanthotic with collarette-like elongated rete ridges. A lymphocytic lichenoid infiltrate with colloid body formation is displayed in early lesions (*Fig. 3.145*).[10] The lymphocytes are an admixture of CD4+ T-helper cells and, less frequently CD8+ T-cytotoxic/suppressor cells. Sézary-like cells have been described. Langerhans cells are highly reduced.[8]

Ultrastructural features consist of rudimentary keratohyalin granules, absence of, vacuolation of or abnormally lamellated membrane coating (Odland) bodies, failure to form compact keratin, and also to form a cornified envelope in the corneocytes.[9,11]

Porokeratosis

Clinical features

Porokeratosis is a heterogeneous group of keratinization disorders, most of them with an autosomal dominant inheritance characterized by a so-called 'cornoid lamella'. This is a grooved keratotic ridge, from the center of which a keratotic core (cornoid lamella) projects at an obtuse angle that borders

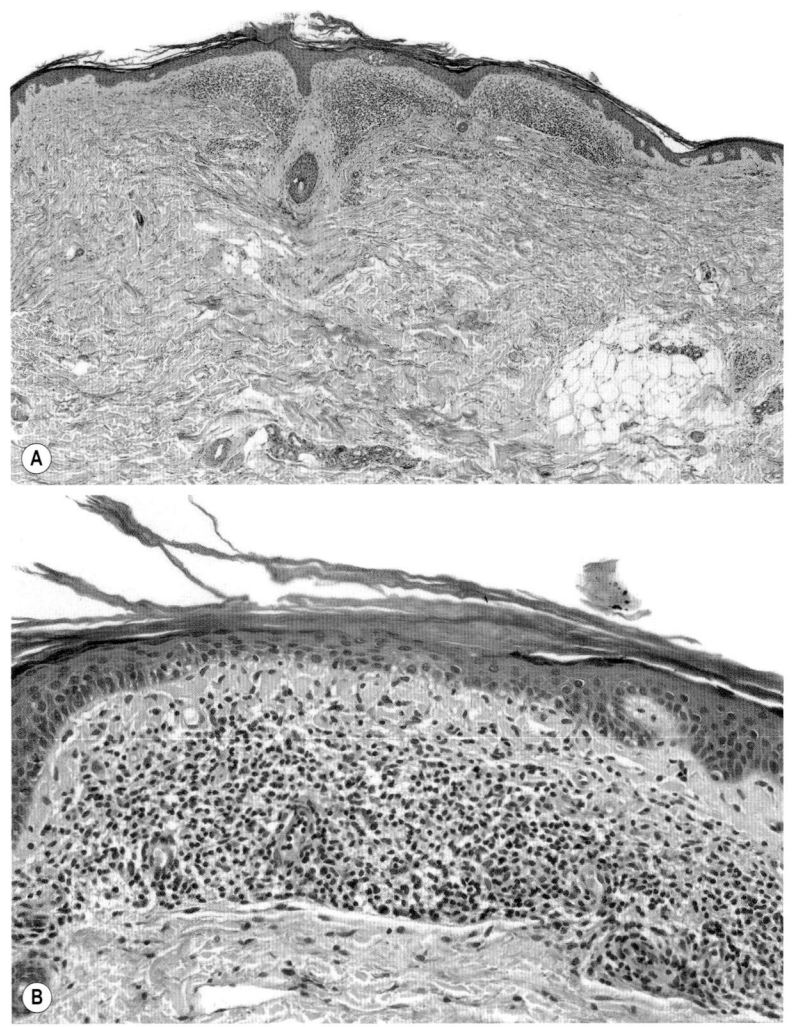

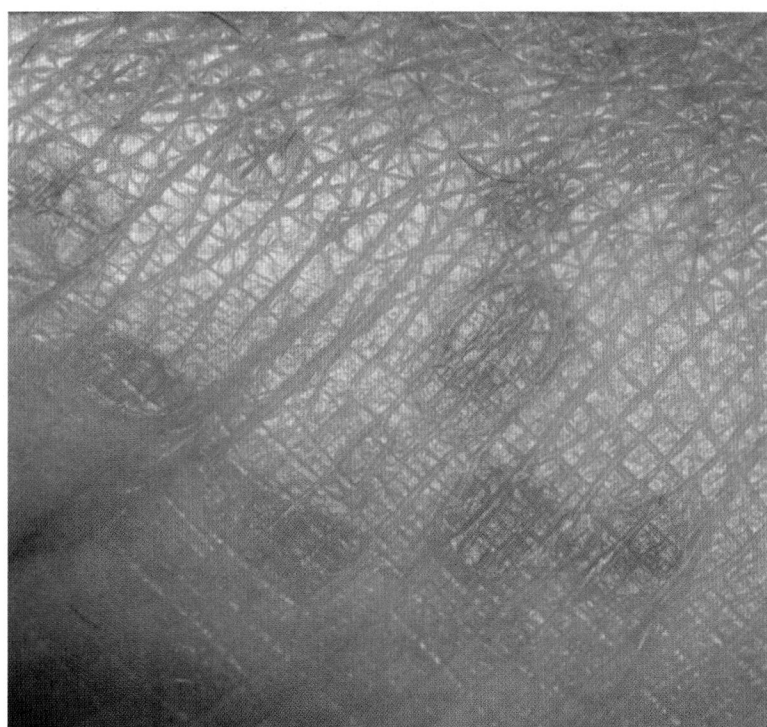

Fig. 3.146
Porokeratosis of Mibelli: the lesions are erythematous, atrophic and scaly, with a sharply defined and slightly raised keratotic rim.

Fig. 3.145
Flegel disease: (**A**) scanning view of an established lesion showing focal hyperkeratosis, and a superficial bandlike infiltrate; (**B**) there is hyperkeratosis, focal epidermal atrophy, vacuolization of the dermal–epidermal junction with many colloid bodies, below a dense lymphocytic infiltrate.

a pigmented or reddish atrophic center.[1-3] Dermoscopy, in particular when using polarized or UV-light, and in-vivo reflectance confocal microscopy, allow visualization of the cornoid lamella.[4,5] However, in punctate porokeratosis the cornoid lamella is difficult to recognize. There are various forms, which may present in an isolated or combined way, but terminology and classification are still a matter of discussion.[1-3]

In the classical variant described by Mibelli, patients develop one or several plaquelike lesions on the extremities (*Fig. 3.146*). It usually presents in adulthood as persistent lesions that are highly resistant to therapy.[6]

Giant porokeratosis presents with large lesions that may grow up to 20 cm in diameter with a surrounding elevated edge of 1 cm. This rare form is most often seen on the foot. Large lesions are said to have the highest potential for malignant transformation.[7,8]

Disseminated superficial actinic porokeratosis (DSAP), the most common variant, is characterized by numerous small, dry, shallow lesions arising on sun-damaged skin of adults (*Fig. 3.147*).[9] It may also complicate PUVA therapy and develop in the immunocompromised. Presentation is in the third and fourth decades and despite its relationship to sunlight, rarely affects the face. The legs, forearms, back, upper arms, and thighs are most commonly affected, in decreasing order of frequency.[10]

Disseminated superficial (nonactinic) porokeratosis is clinically similar to DSAP, except for a younger age of onset and involvement of both sun-protected and sun-exposed areas.[3]

In porokeratosis palmoplantaris et disseminate palms and soles are initially affected, but any site, including mucous membranes, may be involved.

The terms 'porokeratosis punctata palmaris et plantaris' or 'porokeratotic PPK' should be avoided as they are also used as synonyms for spiny keratoderma (palmoplantar keratoderma punctata, type 2) that is histologically unrelated to porokeratosis.[11]

In linear porokeratosis, the lesion is clinically reminiscent of an epidermal nevus, involves the extremities, and usually presents in infancy or early childhood (*Fig. 3.148*).[3] A zosteriform variant has also been described.[12] Nails may show fissures and pterygium.[13] The coexistence of linear porokeratoses and DSAP can be explained by loss of heterozygosity in type 2 of segmental distribution of autosomal dominant disorder.[14,15]

Eruptive pruritic papular porokeratosis is an intensely itchy eruptive variant of disseminated porokeratosis that can be easily misdiagnosed as prurigo nodularis.[16,17]

In follicular porokeratosis the cornoid lamella is limited to the follicular ostia. Persistent follicle-centered aggregated papules or erythematous or brown-colored annular plaques with a peripheral keratotic ridge develop on the trunk, limbs, genitogluteal area, and face.[18]

Porokeratosis ptychotropica (from the Greek 'ptyche': fold) presents with symmetrical brownish to reddish macules or plaques distributed on the buttocks, natal cleft, and scrotum (*Fig. 3.149*).[19] The typical presence of multiple cornoid lamellae as seen histologically (punctate type of porokeratosis) explains the clinical keratotic or verrucous appearance and expansile papular growth of the lesions. This highly pruritic disease is mostly confined to men ranging from 6 to 84 years of age.[20,21]

Reticular erythema with ostial porokeratosis a rare form of punctate porokeratosis typically missing the classic marginated rim. It is characterized by reticular erythema associated myriad papules developing in a symmetric distribution on the inner aspects of arms and legs. Histology shows cornoid lamellae within the appendageal ostia.[22]

Porokeratoma is a tumorlike hyperkeratotic nodule or plaque lacking any keratotic rim, preferentially on the distal limbs. Histology reveals an area of well demarcated verrucous epidermal hyperplasia with multiple broad cornoid lamellae. Since other manifestations of porokeratosis are missing the relationship to porokeratosis is contentious. An incidental formation of a cornoid lamella in an acanthoma of any kind may occasionally be seen.[23]

CAP syndrome is a rare autosomal recessive disorder featuring craniosynostosis, genitourinary and anal anomalies and porokeratosis-like lesions.[24,25]

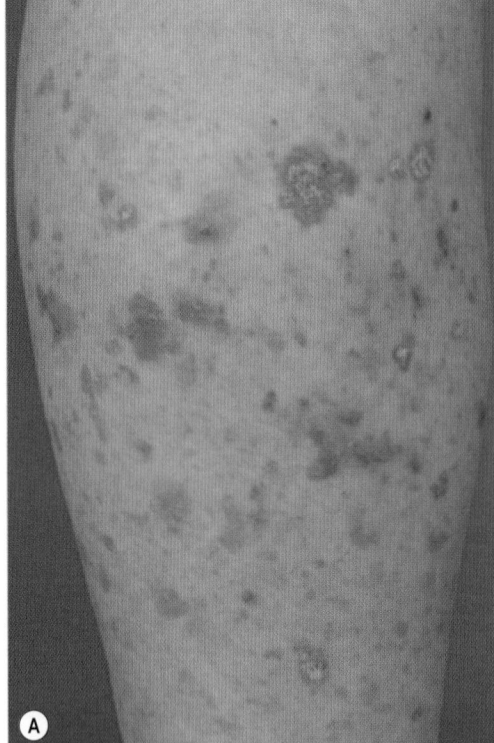

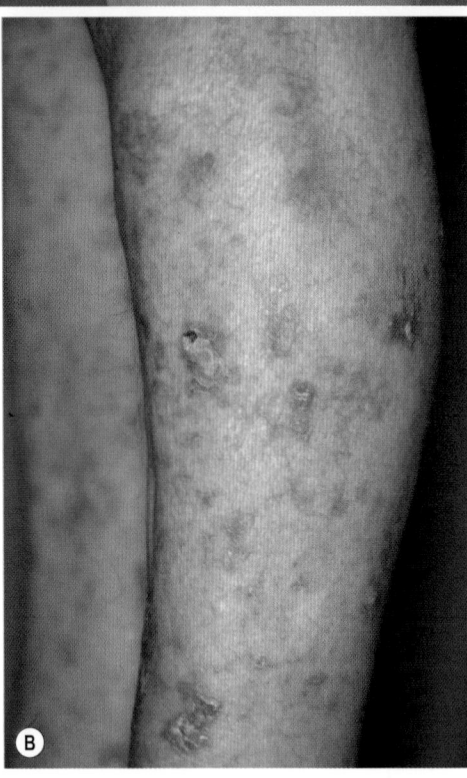

Fig. 3.147
Disseminated superficial actinic porokeratosis: (**A**) there are numerous small, reddish or brownish keratotic macules on sun damaged skin; (**B**) squamous cell carcinoma developed in the crusted and hyperkeratotic lesion.

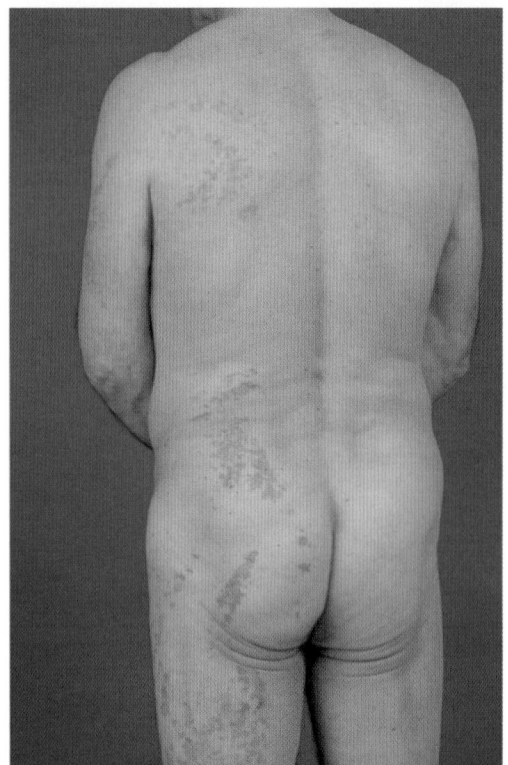

Fig. 3.148
Linear porokeratosis: in this variant, the lesions have a half-sided linear and reticulated nevoid distribution.

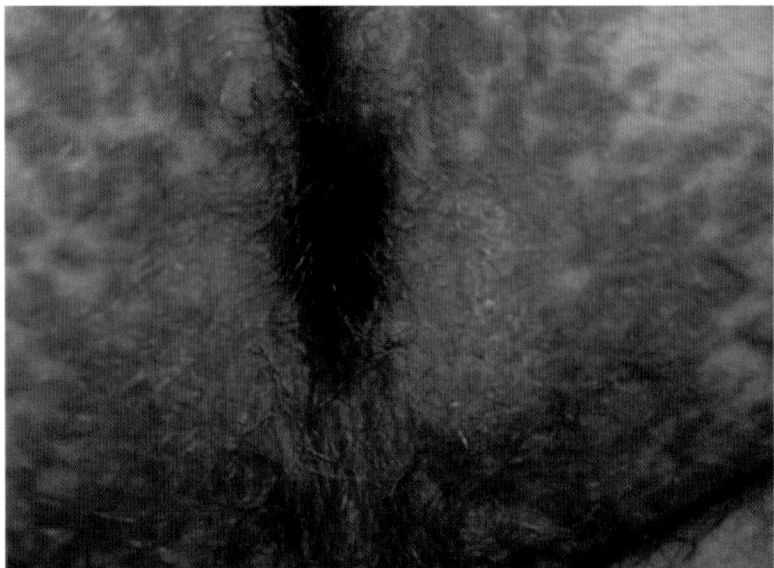

Fig. 3.149
Porokeratosis ptychotropica: brownish to reddish macules or plaques appear symmetrically distributed on the buttocks and natal cleft.

Porokeratosis has an increased risk of developing Bowen disease, and basal cell and squamous cell carcinoma.[26–32] The reported incidence varies from 6.8% to 11.6% and depends on size, duration, age of the patient, immune status, treatment with radiotherapy and the type of porokeratosis.[30,31] Tumors usually develop many years after the onset of the disease, are frequently multiple, and arise most often on large or coalescing lesions on the trunk and extremities, particularly in porokeratosis linearis and DSAP.[33]

Pathogenesis

The presence of localized dysplastic features indicates a focal, expanding clone of abnormal keratinocytes associated with the development of a cornoid lamella.[34] Porokeratotic lesions have been shown to be associated with abnormal epidermal DNA ploidy in association with increased DNA indices, midway between normal skin and Bowen disease.[35,36] Chromosomal abnormalities have been identified within cultured keratinocytes and fibroblasts derived from patients suffering from both the localized and Mibelli variants of the disease.[37,38] The mutations found in the short arm of chromosome 3 may be associated with a wide variety of malignancies.[39] Ionizing radiation, ultraviolet light, including sun tanning beds, and PUVA may be associated with the development of new skin lesions in porokeratosis.[40] The first may be of particular relevance in the development of malignancy in these lesions.[41]

Proteins p53 and pRb are overexpressed within keratinocytes immediately beneath and adjacent to the cornoid lamellae; mdm-2 and p21waf-1 are reduced.[42–45] This imbalance in cell cycle control mechanisms offers a potential explanation for the development of malignancy in porokeratosis although to date p53 mutations have not been identified.[44,46] The possibility of an infective etiology remains.[47] Some evidence of HPV infection in two patients with porokeratosis of Mibelli has been reported.[48]

DSAP has been mapped in Chinese pedigrees to chromosomes 12q, 15q,18p and 16q.[49–52] More recently, heterozygous mutations in the *MVK* gene have been reported in porokeratosis of Mibelli and in DSAP.[53–56] *MVK* encodes mevalonate kinase which is involved in regulation of keratinocyte differentiation and protection of keratinocytes from UVA-induced apoptosis.[53] For DSAP, candidate genes include *SART3* involved in regulation of messenger RNA splicing, *SSH1*, and *ARPC3* which play a role in polymerization and dynamics of actin filaments.[2] In porokeratosis Mibelli overexpression of *EMILIN2*, a pro-apoptotic gene may cause abnormal apoptosis of epidermal keratinocytes and alter the process of keratinization.[57]

Trigger and risk factors for porokeratosis, in particular porokeratosis of Mibelli, disseminated superficial actinic and nonactinic porokeratosis, and eruptive pruritic papular porokeratosis are UV-light, radiation therapy, chronic GVHD, immunosuppression (iatrogen, AIDS, hereditary deficiencies), infections (HPV, HIV, HCV, HSV), drugs (furosemide, antibiotics, TNFα inhibitor, hydroxyurea, systemic and topical steroids, immunosuppressive agents, and others). Local factors reported are lymphedema and scar formation following burns or access regions of hemodialysis.[16,17,58–62]

There are associations of porokeratosis with autoimmune and other diseases (systemic lupus erythematodes, dermatomyositis, psoriasis, vitiligo, alopecia areata, lichen planus, lichen sclerosus et atrophicus, pemphigus, diabetes, rheumatoid arthritis, Crohn disease, liver or renal dysfunction, pancreatitis, and others), neoplasms (hepatocellular-, cholangiocarcinoma, hereditary non-polyposis colorectal carcinoma, lymphoma, leukemia, myeloma, mycosis fungoides, and others), and genetic disorders (Werner syndrome, Rothmund-Thomson syndrome, cystic fibrosis, trisomy 16, erythropoietic protoporphyria, and pseudoxanthoma elasticum).[1,2]

Histologic features

The biopsy must be taken through the peripheral grooved ridge. If the long axis of the specimen does not transact the border, the diagnostic features will be missed.[63] Typical changes consist of a keratin-filled epidermal invagination with an angulated parakeratotic tier, the cornoid lamella (*Fig. 3.150*). Drawing a line perpendicular to the cornoid lamella on the surface of a punch immediately after the biopsy has been taken and before fixation, guarantees proper orientation when the specimen is bisected in the laboratory.[63] The corneocytes of the cornoid lamella express characteristic PAS-positive granules.[64] Formation of a cornoid lamella can also be seen in hair follicles or acrosyringia (*Fig. 3.151*). The involvement of the sweat pores explains the original term 'poro'-keratosis. The keratinocytes below the cornoid lamella are large, vacuolated, and pleomorphic and do not form a granular layer. Dyskeratotic cells may be present and epithelial dysplasia, ranging from mild changes through to carcinoma in situ, may occasionally be seen. Beneath, a variably dense lichenoid lymphocytic infiltrate, sometimes with features of interface dermatitis or subepidermal clefting, colloid bodies and amyloid material, is sometimes seen.[65,66] The adjacent epithelium

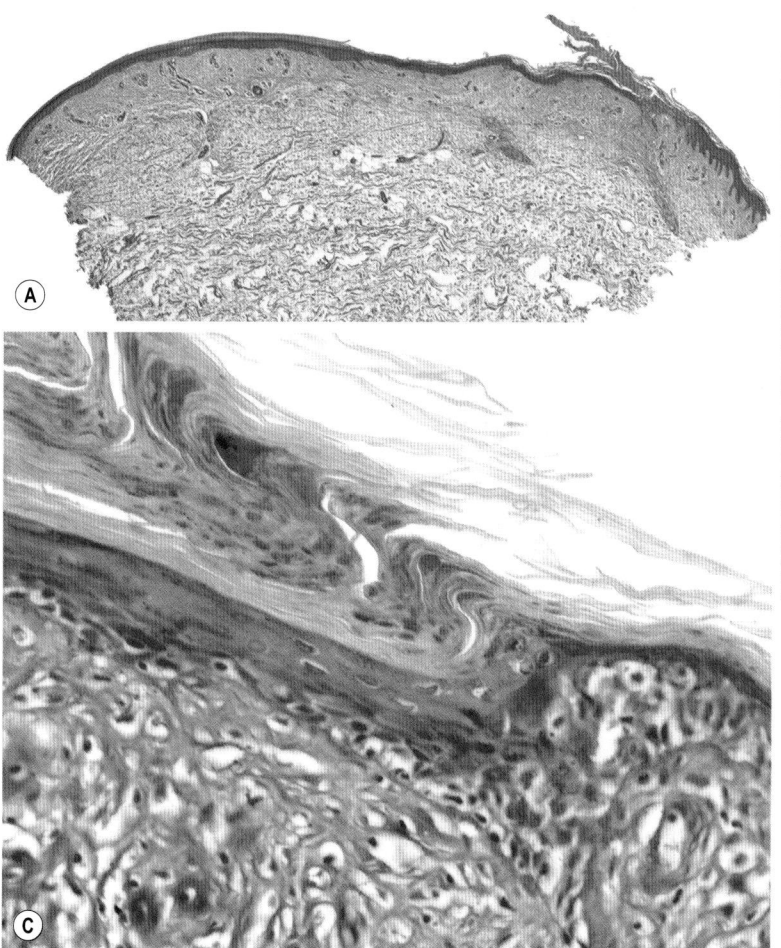

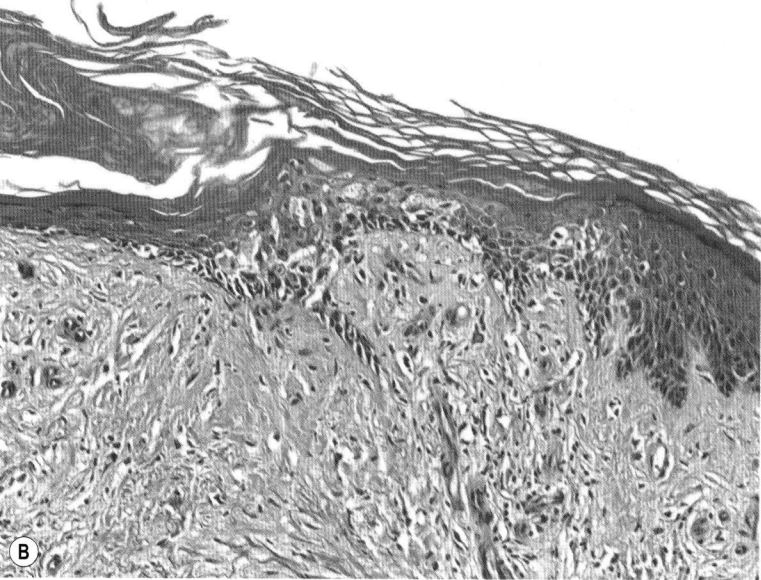

Fig. 3.150
Porokeratosis of Mibelli: (**A**) on the right side the diagnostic features is a keratin-filled epidermal invagination with an angulated keratotic tier, the cornoid lamella. The center of the lesion is atrophic. (**B**) The epidermis below the cornoid lamella expresses large, vacuolated, and pleomorphic keratinocytes and does not form a granular layer. (**C**) The corneocytes of the cornoid lamella are parakeratotic and express characteristic PAS-positive granules.

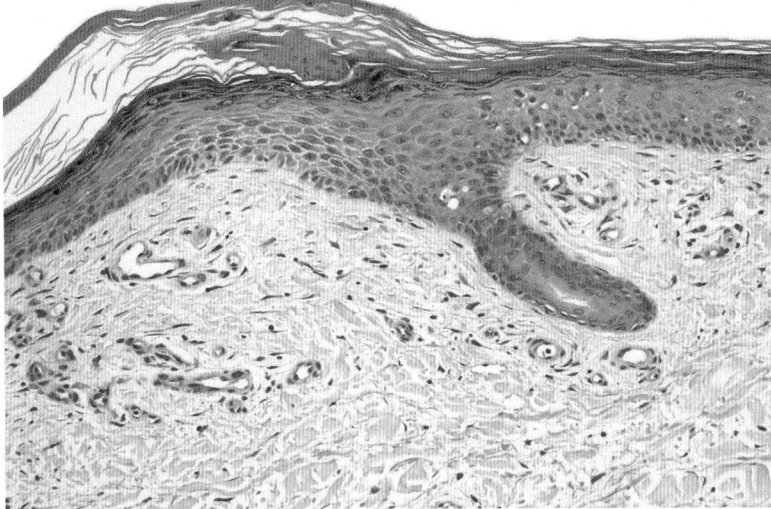

Fig. 3.151
Disseminated superficial actinic porokeratosis: in this example, the cornoid lamella has arisen overlying an acrosyringium. The epidermis towards the center of the lesion appears atrophic and the papillary dermis contains ectatic blood vessels.

towards the center of the lesion is often atrophic, but may be of normal thickness or even acanthotic with extensive hyperkeratosis (*Fig. 3.152*). The papillary dermis below is thickened and sometimes shows a lymphocytic infiltrate, melanophages, telangiectatic vessels, fibrosis, and loss of elastic fibers.[66,67] The typical features are best identified in the Mibelli variant. Changes tend to be less pronounced in the other subtypes. In the actinic variant there is often solar elastosis and atrophy of the adjacent epidermis. The pigmented variant of porokeratosis reveals melanocyte hyperplasia and pigment incontinence, which explains why it clinically mimics a melanocytic lesion.[68] In punctate types of porokeratosis there is no elevated keratotic rim but multiple focal or reticulated parkeratotic tiers above epidermal invaginations (*Fig. 3.153*).[3,19]

Differential diagnosis

PAON is a verrucous nevus due to germline mutations of connexin 26 and it is not related to porokeratosis. Histology shows an ortho- or parakeratotic filiform keratosis protruding from the dilated ostia of eccrine acrosyringia or hair follicles. PAON also features vacuolated and pyknotic keratinocytes, but lacks dyskeratosis, pleomorphism, and interface dermatitis as found in porokeratosis.[69,70]

Signs of interface dermatitis and regression may lead to the misdiagnosis of benign lichenoid keratosis when the cornoid lamella is not seen in the initial sections, therefore further deeper sections are helpful in reaching a diagnosis.[71,72]

Cornoid lamella formation, however, does occur as a non-specific, incidental finding in a variety of conditions, including psoriasis vulgaris, dermatomyositis (Wong-type), Grover disease, HIV-associated epidermodysplasia verruciformis, keratosis lichenoides chronica (Nekam disease), seborrheic keratosis, solar keratosis, verruca vulgaris, and squamous cell and basal cell carcinomas.[3,73] Cornoid lamellae are also seen in inflamed linear verrucous epidermal nevus (ILVEN), ichthyosis hystrix Curth-Macklin, and PC. They are also not uncommon in normal, and particularly actinically damaged skin.[1,3] These non-porokeratotic conditions do not feature large, vacuolated, pleomorphic or dyskeratotic keratinocytes below the cornoid lamella.

Waxy keratosis of childhood

Waxy keratosis (kerinokeratosis papulose) is characterized by development of asymptomatic hyperkeratotic papules in childhood.[1] The papules appear flesh-colored or yellowish with a waxy appearance and are generalized, e.g., on the trunk or proximal limbs.[2,3] Late presentation in adulthood has rarely been described.[4] The disorder has also been reported in a linear form.[5] The etiology is unknown. Although a familial association and the observation of

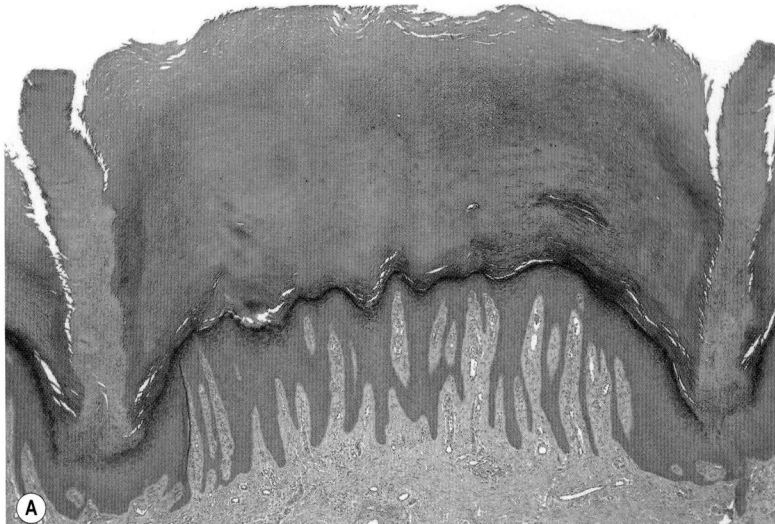

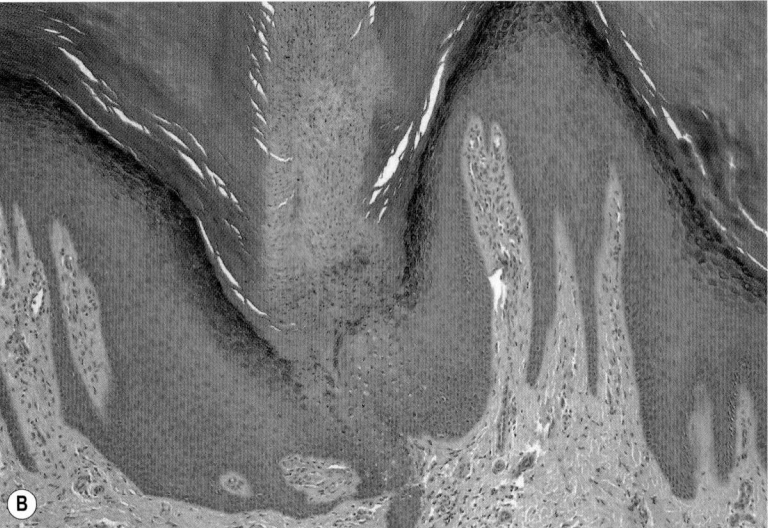

Fig. 3.152
Porokeratosis of Mibelli: (**A**) there is central orthohyperkeratosis with two well-developed cornoid lamellae on both sides. Note the epidermal depression at their bases. (**B**) The cornoid lamella can be seen to be composed of a column of parakeratosis.

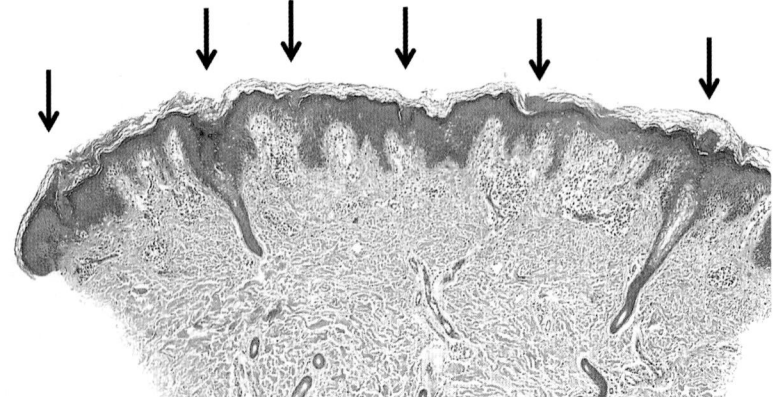

Fig. 3.153
Porokeratosis ptychotropica: there is no solitary keratotic rim on the lateral side but multiple parakeratotic tiers above epidermal invaginations (*arrows*), a characteristic feature of the punctate type of porokeratosis.

linear exacerbation in the setting of generalized disease suggest a genodermatosis, the detection of HPV type 57 has also raised the possibility of an infectious etiology.[6,7]

Histologically, waxy keratoses shows orthohyperkeratosis, a tenting surface, mild acanthosis, and papillomatosis of the epidermis. It resembles

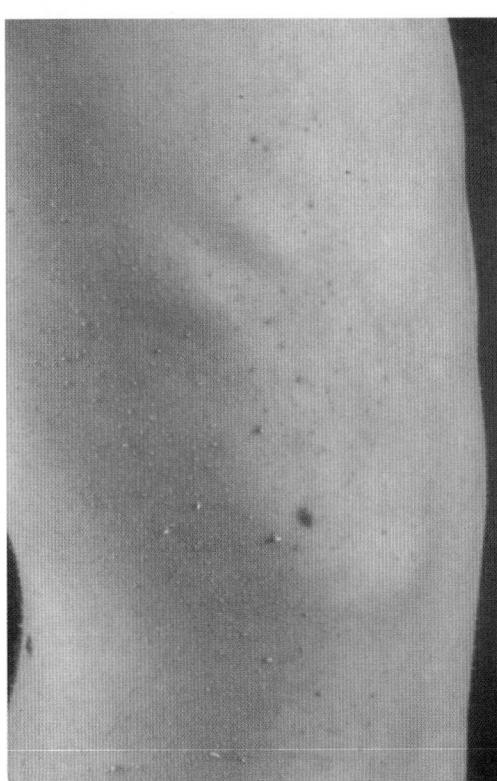

Fig. 3.154
Digitate hyperkeratosis: in this familial variant disseminated spiny keratosis developed on trunk and extremities. By courtesy of H. Traupe, Münster, Germany.

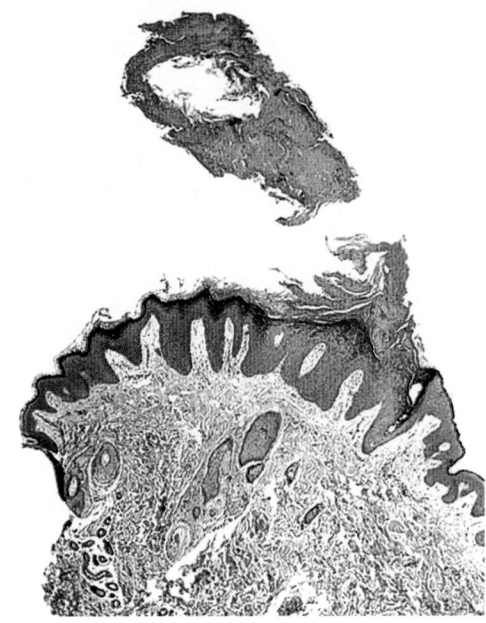

Fig. 3.155
Digitate hyperkeratosis: an orthohyperkeratotic spicule arises from a pointed epidermal elevation.

confluent and reticulated papillomatosis (Gougerot and Carteaud), but waxy keratosis displays more prominent hyperkeratosis.

Digitate hyperkeratosis

Many different hyperkeratotic conditions have been described under names such as minute and filiform keratoses, multiple minute digitate hyperkeratosis, minute aggregate keratoses, digitate keratoses or disseminated spiked hyperkeratosis.[1–4] An approach to classification proposed the unifying term multiple minute digitate hyperkeratosis.[5] Caccetta et al. proposed a useful algorithm for differentiation.[6] Myriad nonfollicular spiky keratoses develop on the trunk and limbs early or late in life and have a transient or persistent course.[6]Pathogenesis and histologic features

Familial cases of digitate hyperkeratosis have been described with a probable autosomal dominant mode of transmission.[2,3,7,8] Acquired cases may be associated with drugs, Crohn disease, and malignancy, including hematological neoplasia and radiotherapy.[4,5,8–13] Hyperkeratotic spicules on the face, particularly on the nose, are follicular and often associated with paraproteinemia, multiple myeloma, and cryoglobulinemia, but may also be idiopathic.[10,11] Filiform keratoses occur with a pityriasis rubra pilaris-like eruption and acne conglobata in association with HIV infection.[14] A familial form of filiform keratosis has been described and is associated with thickened nails, plantar hyperkeratosis, joint laxity, and long fingers (Fig. 3.154).[15]

Histologically, there are compact orthohyperkeratotic spicules mostly arising from a pointed epidermal elevation (Fig. 3.155). The stratum granulosum is usually prominent and parakeratosis may be present.[6,15–17] Hyperkeratotic spicules associated with paraproteinemia reveal eosinophilic inclusions that represent immunoglobulin deposits.[10]

Granular parakeratosis

Clinical features

Granular parakeratosis is a distinctive acquired disorder of keratinization originally reported in 1991.[1–4] The condition most often affects the axillae but it also involves other intertriginous areas including submammary and intermammary skin, groins, vulva, perianal region, and, less commonly, nonintertriginous skin including the lower back, buttocks, and flanks.[5–8] Women are affected more commonly than men. The disease mainly affects the middle aged to elderly; children are rarely involved and only one congenital case has been reported.[8–11] It presents as pruritic or burning erythematous, hyperpigmented, and hyperkeratotic patches, papules, or plaques (Fig. 3.156). Fissures and a 'cobblestone' appearance may be seen. The condition has been documented to respond to retinoids and to calcipotriene and ammonium lactate.[12,13]

Pathogenesis and histologic features

The etiology is unknown. It has been suggested that the condition develops as a result of a contact reaction to an antiperspirant or as a result of excessive use of other topical products, including creams, shampoos, and soaps.[1–6,8] However, this does not explain the involvement of areas away from the axilla. The molecular mechanism proposed to explain the disease consists of a failure to transform profilaggrin to filaggrin which interferes with the degradation of keratohyalin granules.[1,7]

The histologic appearance typically consists of a massive hyperkeratosis with parakeratosis and retention of keratohyalin granules in the stratum corneum (Fig. 3.157). The underlying epidermis may show mild acanthosis or even some degree of thinning. Hair infundibula and eccrine ostia are occasionally affected.[14,15] Necrotic areas with exocytosis of neutrophils or perforation of the epidermis are rarely found. The superficial dermis contains a sparse perivascular lymphocytic infiltrate.[1–7]

Differential diagnosis

Apart from representing a distinctive dermatosis, granular parakeratosis is a diagnostic feature in solitary keratosis, i.e., granular parakeratotic acanthoma.[16,17] Granular parakeratosis can be also found as an incidental finding in many diseases, e.g., dermatophytosis, molluscum contagiosum, dermatomyositis, solar keratosis, squamous cell carcinoma, keratoacanthoma, lymphomatoid papulosis, and basal cell carcinoma (Fig. 3.158). As such, granular parakeratosis is best considered as a histologic pattern similar to focal acantholytic dyskeratosis and epidermolytic hyperkeratosis.[18,19]

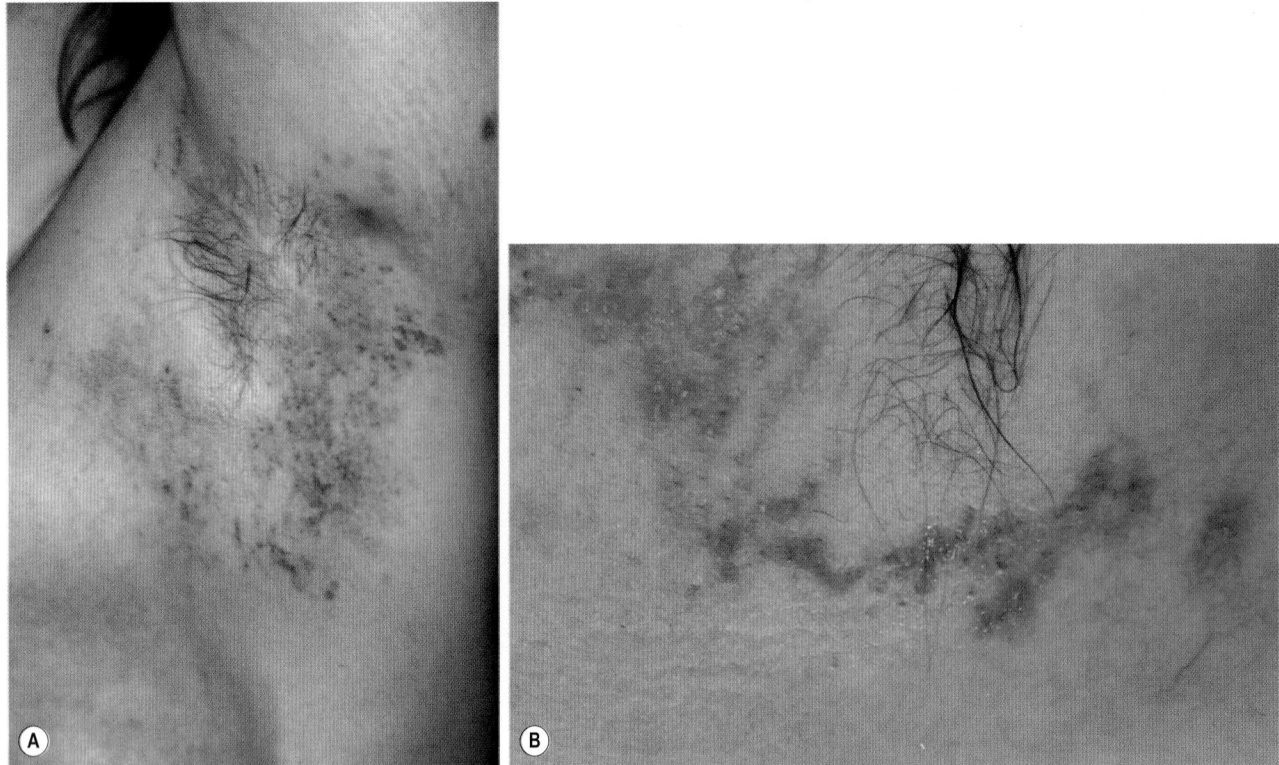

Fig. 3.156
Granular parakeratosis: (**A**) in the axilla of a middle-aged woman erythematous, hyperpigmented and hyperkeratotic papules develop in a reticulated fashion; (**B**) a few of these lesions are erosive.

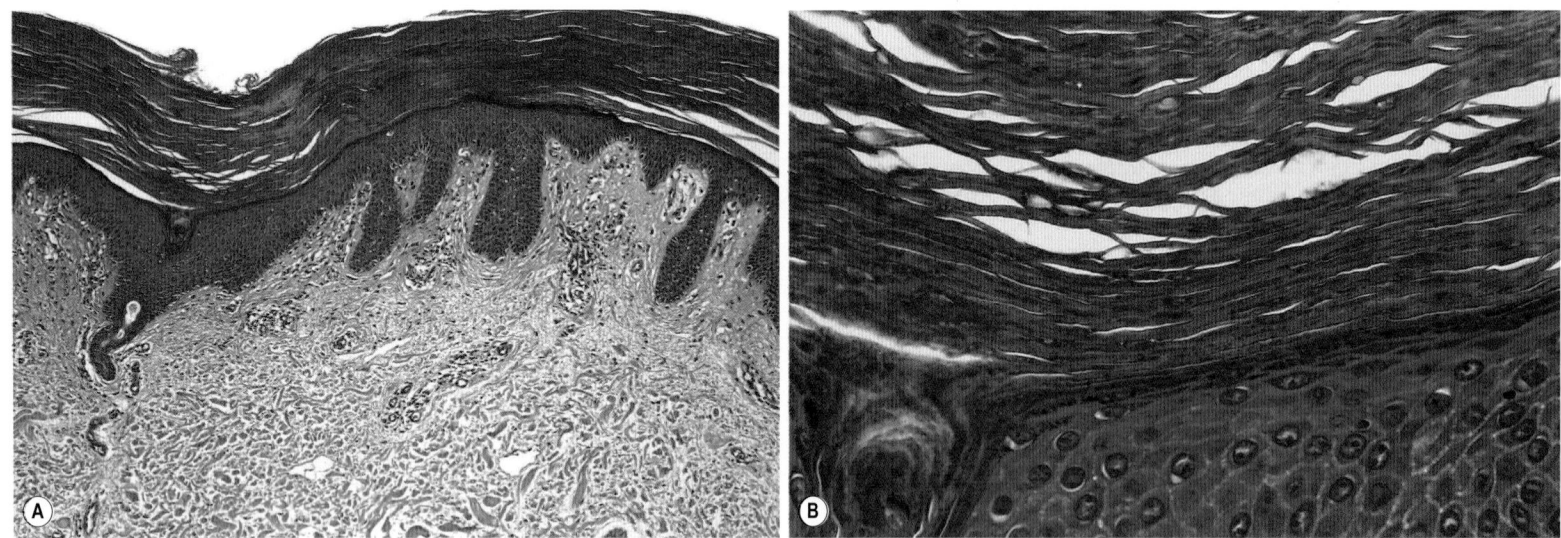

Fig. 3.157
Granular parakeratosis: (**A**) there is marked thickening of the horny layer with parakeratosis; (**B**) high-power view showing retention of keratohyalin granules.

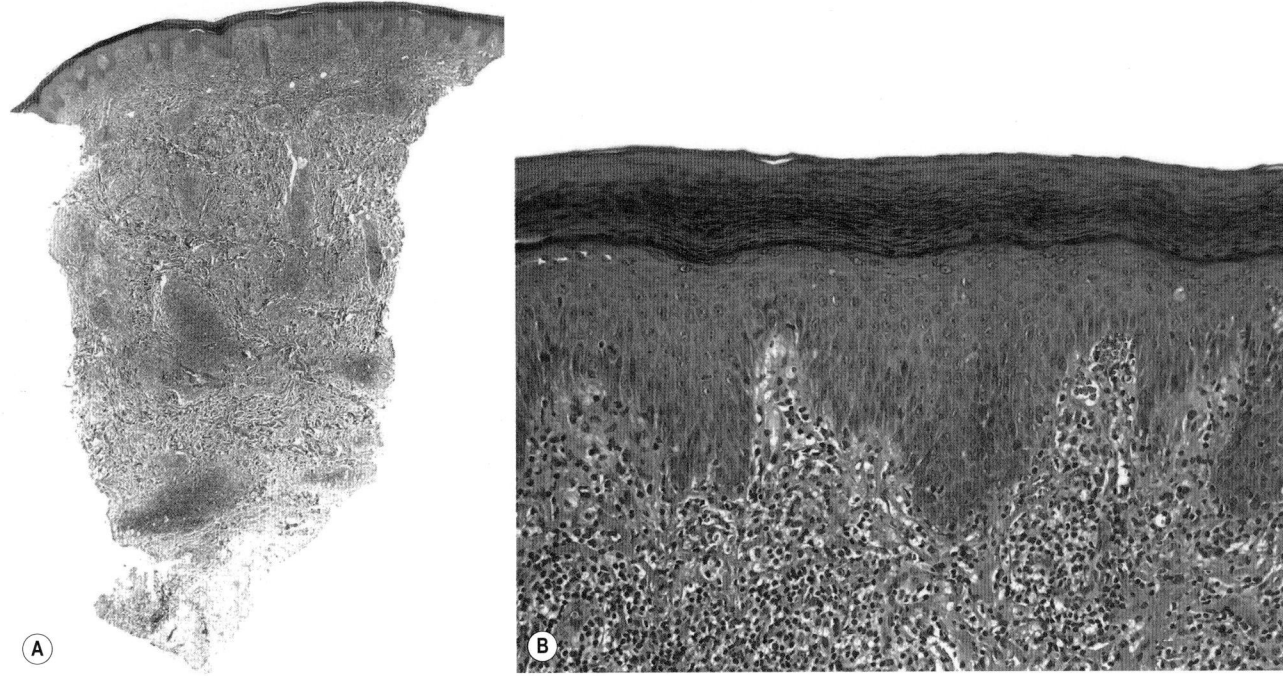

Fig. 3.158
Granular parakeratosis: (**A**) this example arose against a background of lymphomatoid papulosis; (**B**) high-power view.

Hyperkeratosis of the nipple and areola

Hyperkeratosis of the nipple and areola is bilateral and predominantly involves the top of the nipple. Lesions may cause tenderness, pruritus, or discomfort with breastfeeding.[1] The occurrence and aggravation around puberty, pregnancy or systemic hormone treatment suggests a hormonal influence.[2] Hyperkeratosis of nipple skin has also been described during sorafenib treatment and with the fungus (malassezia).[3,4] Nevoid hyperkeratosis of the nipple and areola may either appear isolated or in association with an epidermal nevus and other dermatoses, such as acanthosis nigricans,

Darier disease, chronic eczema, chronic mucocutaneous candidiasis, or cutaneous T-cell lymphoma.[5-6] Paget disease must be ruled out by histologic examination.

Keratosis of the nipple shows papillomatosis, acanthosis, and hyperkeratosis of the epidermis. The rete ridges are filiform and anastomosing and the basal layer appears hyperpigmented.[1] Intraepidermal collections of lymphocytes must not be confused with T-cell lymphoma.[7]

Access **ExpertConsult.com** for the complete list of references

Inherited and autoimmune subepidermal blistering diseases

Boštjan Luzar and John A. McGrath

See
www.expertconsult.com
for references and
additional material

Blisters, which are clinically subdivided into vesicles (L. *vesicula*, dim. of *vesica*, bladder) and bullae (L. bubble), are defined as accumulations of fluid either within or below the epidermis and mucous membranes. Although somewhat arbitrary, the term 'vesicle' is applied to lesions less than 0.5 cm in diameter and 'bulla' to those greater than 0.5 cm. Subepidermal blisters, i.e., those that develop at the epidermal or mucosal basement membrane region, include inherited variants and acquired (often autoimmune mediated) conditions. The former are usually classified as noninflammatory (cell-poor) blisters whereas the latter are commonly inflammatory (cell-rich) in nature (*Fig. 4.1*).

Subepidermal blisters may develop within the lower epidermis, the lamina lucida (e.g., bullous pemphigoid) or deep to the lamina densa (e.g., epidermolysis bullosa acquisita) (*Fig. 4.2*). In addition to clinical observations, the precise diagnosis of a blistering disorder requires careful histologic and immunofluorescence correlation. When possible, the last should include indirect studies and, in particular, NaCl-split skin should be used as substrate as a mechanism of localizing the site of dermal–epidermal separation.[1] If a sample has not been taken for indirect immunofluorescence, immunoperoxidase antigen mapping on paraffin-embedded material may on occasions be of value at least as a screening procedure. Although the results of electron microscopic investigations and, in particular, molecular studies have formed the basis of the current classification of subepidermal bullous dermatoses, such techniques are usually not essential to the everyday investigation of a patient with an acquired blistering disorder.

The mechanisms involved in the development of a subepidermal blister are variable. They include inherited mutational defects of basement membrane proteins, i.e., epidermolysis bullosa, acquired autoimmune bullous diseases such as bullous pemphigoid, cellular immunity-mediated disorders (e.g., erythema multiforme and toxic epidermal necrolysis), metabolic diseases including porphyria cutanea tarda, and profound subepidermal edema, such as may be seen in bullous arthropod bite reactions and dermal acute inflammatory processes (e.g., Sweet disease).

In this chapter, only those conditions in which subepidermal blister formation represents an inherited or autoimmune primary event are considered. Other conditions that may be associated with subepidermal blistering are dealt with in more appropriate chapters.

Split skin immunofluorescence

This technique represents a modification of indirect immunofluorescence (IIMF) where normal skin is split through the lamina lucida of the basement membrane region to produce an artificial blister cavity (with the lamina densa lining the floor) for use as substrate. Artificial separation can be achieved by the suction technique (in vivo) or by immersion of normal skin in 1 M NaCl for 48 hours at 4°C (*Fig. 4.3*). In general, the latter technique is preferred.[2] As such a split is invariably through the lamina lucida region (confirmed by electron microscopy or immunofluorescence) (*Figs 4.4* and *4.5*), the technique enables precise localization of a circulating basement membrane zone antibody to either the floor or the roof of the artificial blister cavity. In bullous pemphigoid, pemphigoid gestationis, and the majority of cases of mucous membrane pemphigoid, linear immunofluorescence is found along the roof of the artificial blister whereas in diseases characterized by a sublamina densa split (e.g., epidermolysis bullosa acquisita, antilaminin mucous membrane pemphigoid, anti-p105 pemphigoid, anti-p200 pemphigoid, and bullous dermatosis of bullous lupus erythematosus), the immunofluorescent signal is found along the floor of the blister (see references 3 and 4 for a review) (*Fig. 4.6*). In some diseases, positive immunofluorescence may be found on either the roof or the floor or even at both sites simultaneously (e.g., linear IgA disease and some variants of mucous membrane pemphigoid). Such variable labeling reflects the antigen heterogeneity in a number of bullous dermatoses.

Immunoperoxidase antigen mapping

As an alternative to split skin immunofluorescence, paraffin-embedded sections of lesional skin have been proposed in a direct immunoperoxidase antigen mapping technique to identify the level of the dermal–epidermal separation.[5–8] This procedure localizes known basement membrane region constituents such as keratins 5/14, laminin, and type IV collagen to the roof or floor of the blister cavity. The site of blister formation can therefore be characterized as intrabasal, within the lamina lucida or deep to the lamina densa. For example, in epidermolysis bullosa simplex variants, all of these immunoreactants are present along the floor of the blister cavity. In bullous pemphigoid, keratin is present along the roof of the blister while laminin and type IV collagen are found along the floor (*Fig. 4.7*). In dystrophic epidermolysis bullosa, epidermolysis bullosa acquisita, and bullous systemic lupus erythematosus, all three immunoreactants are present in the roof of the blister (*Fig. 4.8*). However, in many hereditary and acquired blistering diseases the relevant antibodies against the target antigens do not work well in paraffin-embedded material and false-positive and false-negative results are common, making this method unreliable for use in routine diagnosis. For example, antigen mapping of the group of hereditary subepidermal blistering diseases is done exclusively on frozen sections with excellent results.

Epidermolysis bullosa

Epidermolysis bullosa (EB) refers to a heterogeneous group of diseases in which the skin and sometimes the mucous membranes blister easily in response to mild trauma, hence the alternative title 'mechanobullous disease', which has sometimes been applied.[1] Indeed, the descriptive term

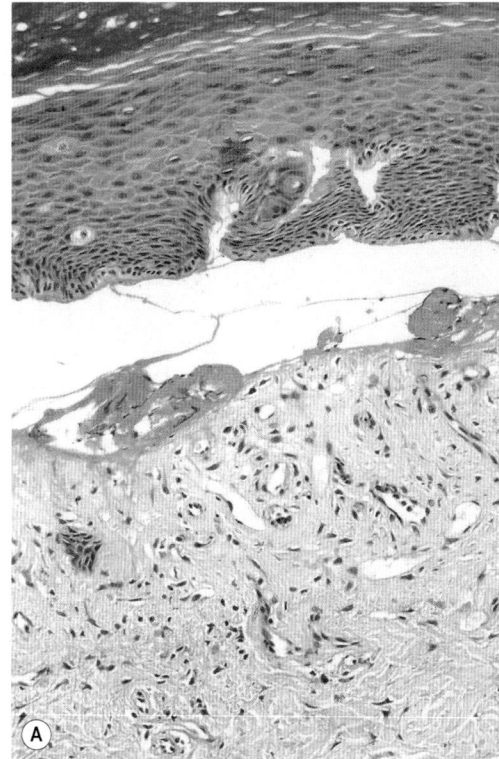

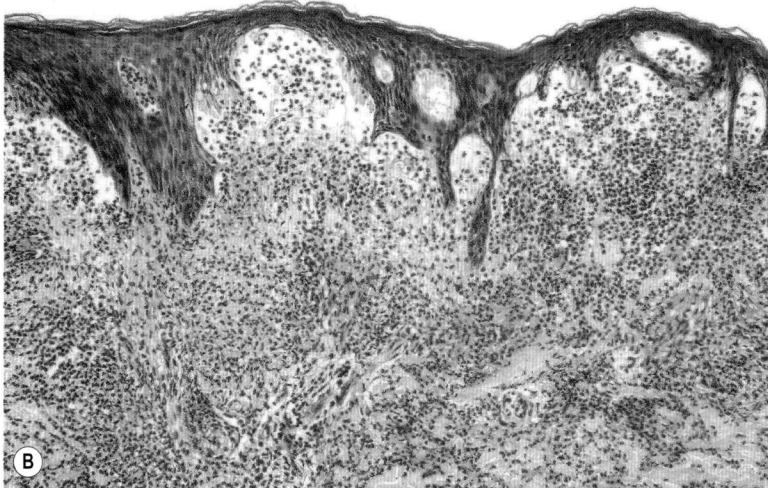

Fig. 4.1
Classification of subepidermal blisters: lesions may be subdivided into (**A**) cell-poor and (**B**) cell-rich variants.

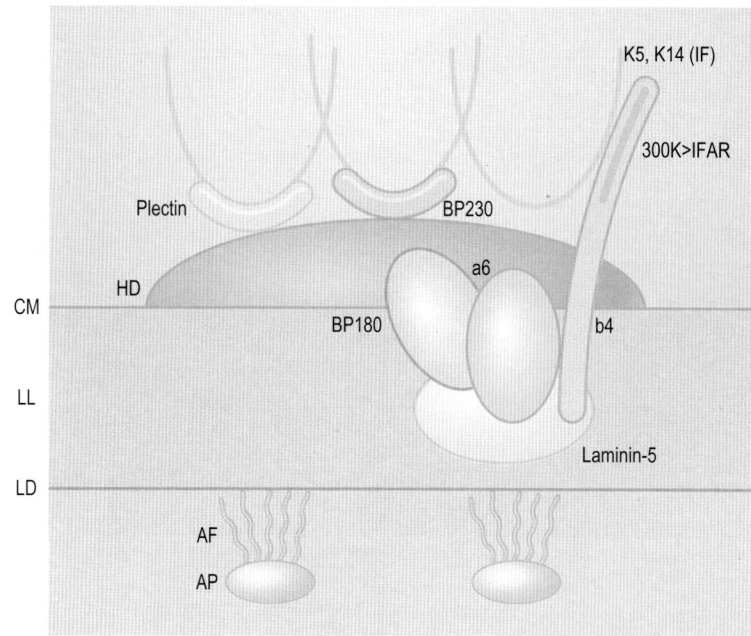

Fig. 4.2
Basement membrane constituents: blisters can be classified into those that develop within the lamina lucida (LL) and those that arise below the lamina densa (LD). (AF, anchoring fibrils; AP, anchoring plaque; CM, cell membrane.)

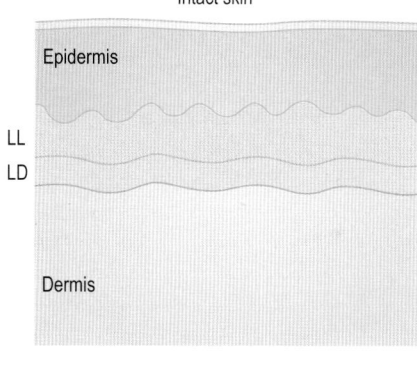

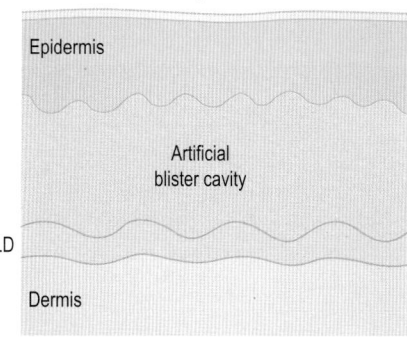

Fig. 4.3
Split skin immunofluorescence.

epidermolysis is somewhat illogical because epidermal disruption is not the primary change in several categories of EB. Nevertheless, the name *epidermolysis bullosa*, as originally used by Koebner in 1886,[2] is now so well established in the literature that it remains the accepted term. All forms of EB are rare; it is estimated that globally about 500 000 people have EB.

Classification of EB

Historically, the classification of EB has been difficult and not helped by the large variety of names and eponyms that have traditionally been used. While these early observations were important in establishing EB as an entity, a major step forward was made by Pearson in the 1960s,[3] who used transmission electron microscopy to show that the ultrastructural level of tissue cleavage (blister formation) in the skin is distinctive in the three major groups of EB: intraepidermal in EB simplex, through the lamina lucida in junctional EB, and below the lamina densa in dystrophic EB (although a separate fourth category, Kindler syndrome, has subsequently been added in which there is a variable mixed level of blistering).[4] Indeed, these different levels of cleavage still form the basis of the current classification of EB (*Table 4.1*).[1] Since Pearson's initial observations, the concept and content of EB simplex has also expanded with the addition of more superficial skin fragility disorders, including inherited disorders of desmosomes as well as cornification (*Table 4.2*). Likewise, the classification of the junctional and dystrophic forms of EB has also evolved, although the multiple variants thereof have largely been defined by clinical features (*Tables 4.3* and *4.4*). Although the clinicopathologic entities now regarded as forms of EB have expanded, most of the major forms of EB occur at or close to the dermal–epidermal junction, and a schematic of the key proteins and genes implicated in these forms of EB is shown in *Fig. 4.9*.

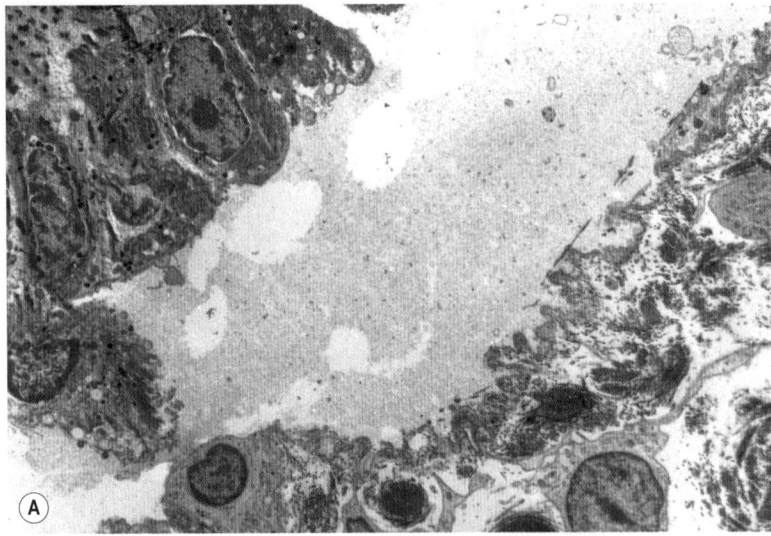

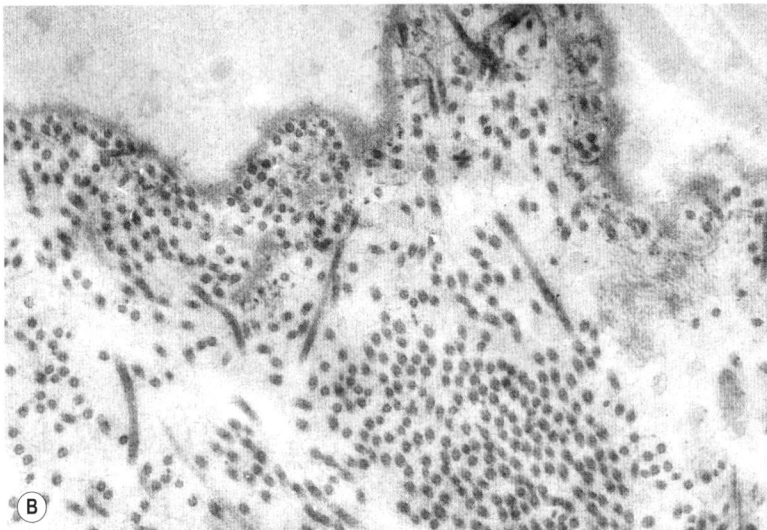

Fig. 4.4

(**A**, **B**) Split skin immunofluorescence: the split is through the lamina lucida, the lamina densa lining the floor of the artificial blister cavity.

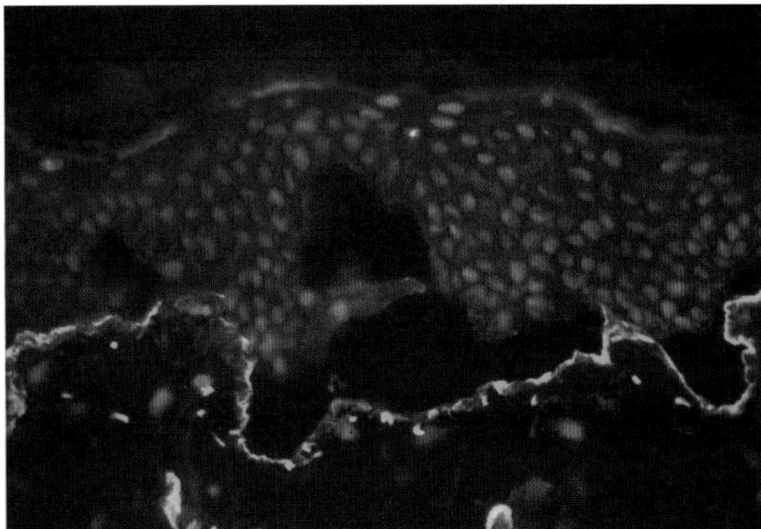

Fig. 4.5

Split skin immunofluorescence: type IV collagen lines the floor of the split skin artificial blister which therefore forms within the lamina lucida. By courtesy of B. Bhogal, FIMLS, Institute of Dermatology, London, UK.

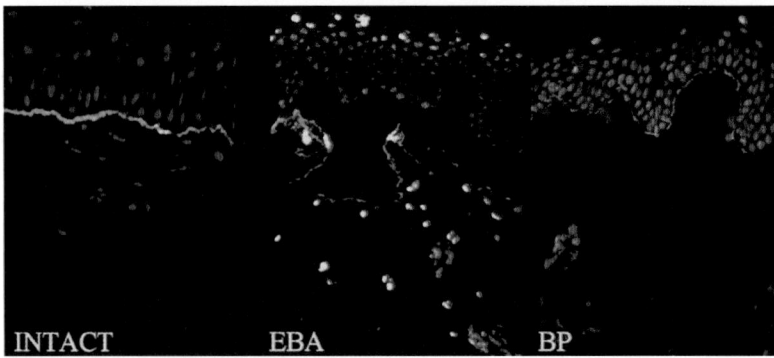

Fig. 4.6

Split skin immunofluorescence: (*left*) linear IgG at the basement membrane; (*middle*) in epidermolysis bullosa acquisita (EBA), the antibody binds to the floor of the blister cavity; (*right*) in bullous pemphigoid (BP), the antibody binds to the roof of the blister. By courtesy of B. Bhogal, FIMLS, Institute of Dermatology, London, UK.

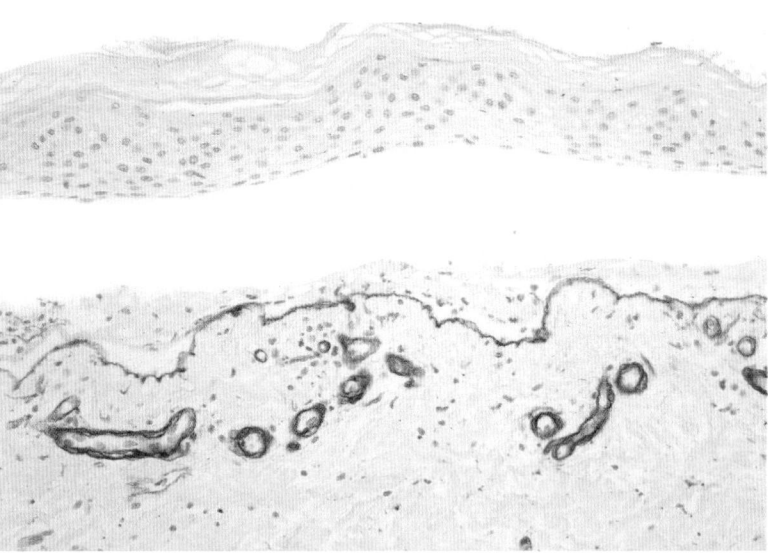

Fig. 4.7

Paraffin-embedded immunoperoxidase antigen mapping: in bullous pemphigoid, type IV collagen is present along the floor of the blister.

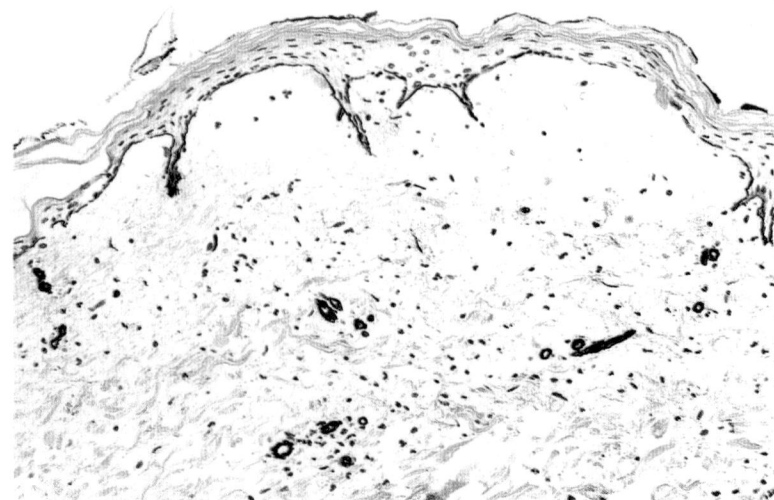

Fig. 4.8

Paraffin-embedded immunoperoxidase antigen mapping: in epidermolysis bullosa acquisita, type IV collagen is present along the roof of the blister cavity.

Table 4.1
The major forms of epidermolysis bullosa (EB)

Level of skin cleavage	EB type	EB subtype	Defective protein(s)
Intraepidermal	EB simplex	Suprabasal EB simplex Basal EB simplex	Transglutaminase-5; Plakophilin-1; Desmoplakin; Plakoglobin Keratins 5 and 14; Plectin; Exophilin-5; 230-kDa bullous pemphigoid antigen/dystonin
Intralamina lucida	Junctional EB	Junctional EB generalized Junctional EB localized	Laminin-332; Type XVII collagen α6, β4, α3 integrin subunits Type XVII collagen; Laminin-332; α6, β4 integrin subunits
Sublamina densa	Dystrophic EB	Dominant Dystrophic EB Recessive Dystrophic EB	Type VII collagen Type VII collagen
Mixed	Kindler syndrome		Kindlin-1 (Fermitin family homologue-1)

Table 4.2
Clinical subtypes of epidermolysis bullosa (EB) simplex

EB simplex type	EB simplex subtype	Targeted protein(s)
Suprabasal	Acral peeling skin syndrome	Transglutaminase-5
	EB simplex superficialis	Unknown
	Ectodermal dysplasia-skin fragility syndrome	Plakophilin-1
	Severe acantholytic EB	Desmoplakin[a], Plakoglobin[a]
Basal	EB simplex – localized[b]	Keratins 5 and 14
	EB simplex – generalized severe	Keratins 5 and 14
	EB simplex – generalized intermediate	Keratins 5 and 14
	EB simplex – mottled pigmentation	Keratin 5
	EB simplex – migratory circinate	Keratin 5
	EB simplex – autosomal recessive (K14)	Keratin 14
	EB simplex – autosomal recessive (BP230)	230 kDa Bullous pemphigoid antigen
	EB simplex – autosomal recessive (exophilin-5)	Exophilin-5
	EB simplex – muscular dystrophy	Plectin
	EB simplex – muscular dystrophy	Plectin; α6, β4 integrin subunits
	EB simplex – Ogna	Plectin

[a]Although listed as being associated with suprabasal subtypes of EB simplex, desmoplakin and plakoglobin show that pan-epidermal expression and mutations in these proteins affect basal as well as suprabasal keratinocytes.
[b]Occasionally, this type of EB simplex can also result from mutations in plectin, type XVII collagen and the β4 integrin subunit.

Table 4.3
Clinical subtypes of junctional epidermolysis bullosa (EB)

Junctional EB type	Junctional EB subtype	Targeted protein(s)
Generalized	Severe	Laminin-332
	Intermediate	Laminin-332; Type XVII collagen
	Late onset	Type XVII collagen
	With pyloric atresia	α6 and β4 integrin subunits
	With respiratory and renal involvement	α3 integrin subunit
Localized	Localized	Laminin-332; Type XVII collagen, α6 and β4 integrin subunits
	Inversa	Laminin-332
	Laryngo-onycho-cutaneous syndrome	Laminin α3a

Table 4.4
Clinical subtypes of dystrophic epidermolysis bullosa (EB)

Dystrophic EB type[a]	Dystrophic EB subtype
Dominant	Generalized Acral Pretibial Pruriginosa Nails only Bullous dermolysis of the newborn
Recessive	Generalized severe Generalized intermediate Inversa Localized Pretibial Pruriginosa Centripetalis Bullous dermolysis of the newborn

[a]The targeted protein in all types and subtypes of dystrophic EB is type VII collagen.

In addition to establishing specific levels of blistering in the different subtypes of EB, ultrastructural studies were also able to identify distinct morphologic abnormalities, such as keratin filament disruption in EB simplex, poorly formed hemidesmosomes in junctional EB, and rudimentary anchoring fibrils in dystrophic EB. During the 1980s, the immunohistochemical labeling of EB skin with basement membrane zone antibodies became a useful diagnostic addition, for example showing reduced immunostaining for proteins such as laminin-332 in some forms of junctional EB, and type VII collagen in recessive dystrophic EB, respectively. Then in the 1990s, the discovery of candidate genes and pathogenic mutations, such as mutations in KRT14 and KRT5 in EB simplex (keratins 14 and 5) and COL7A1 in dystrophic EB (type VII collagen), heralded the era of molecular diagnostics. Reflecting these advances at electron microscopic, immunohistochemical, and molecular levels, the classification of EB has evolved over the years with the most recent international consensus report (published in 2014) recommending abandonment of most historical eponyms and adoption of an "onion skin" approach to disease nomenclature – the different layers referring to the methods of diagnostic evaluation available – clinical phenotype, mode of transmission, level of split in the skin, immunohistochemistry, mutation detection, etc.[1] For example, a patient with intraepidermal blister formation, blistering confined to the palms and soles, and a family history consistent with autosomal dominant transmission would initially be classified as having localized EB simplex. Once mutational confirmation is completed, the final diagnosis, using the onion skin method, would be: EB simplex, localized, KRT5 mutation (missense mutation). It is believed that this format for diagnosing EB provides both practical and academic value in classifying EB, although it is likely to be revised further in years to come as more discoveries are made.

Molecular studies have now identified pathogenic mutations in 18 different genes in the heterogeneous clinical subtypes of EB (*Table 4.5*).[5] With regard to diagnosing EB, sequencing of patient DNA (either Sanger sequencing or next generation sequencing using whole exome sequencing or selected

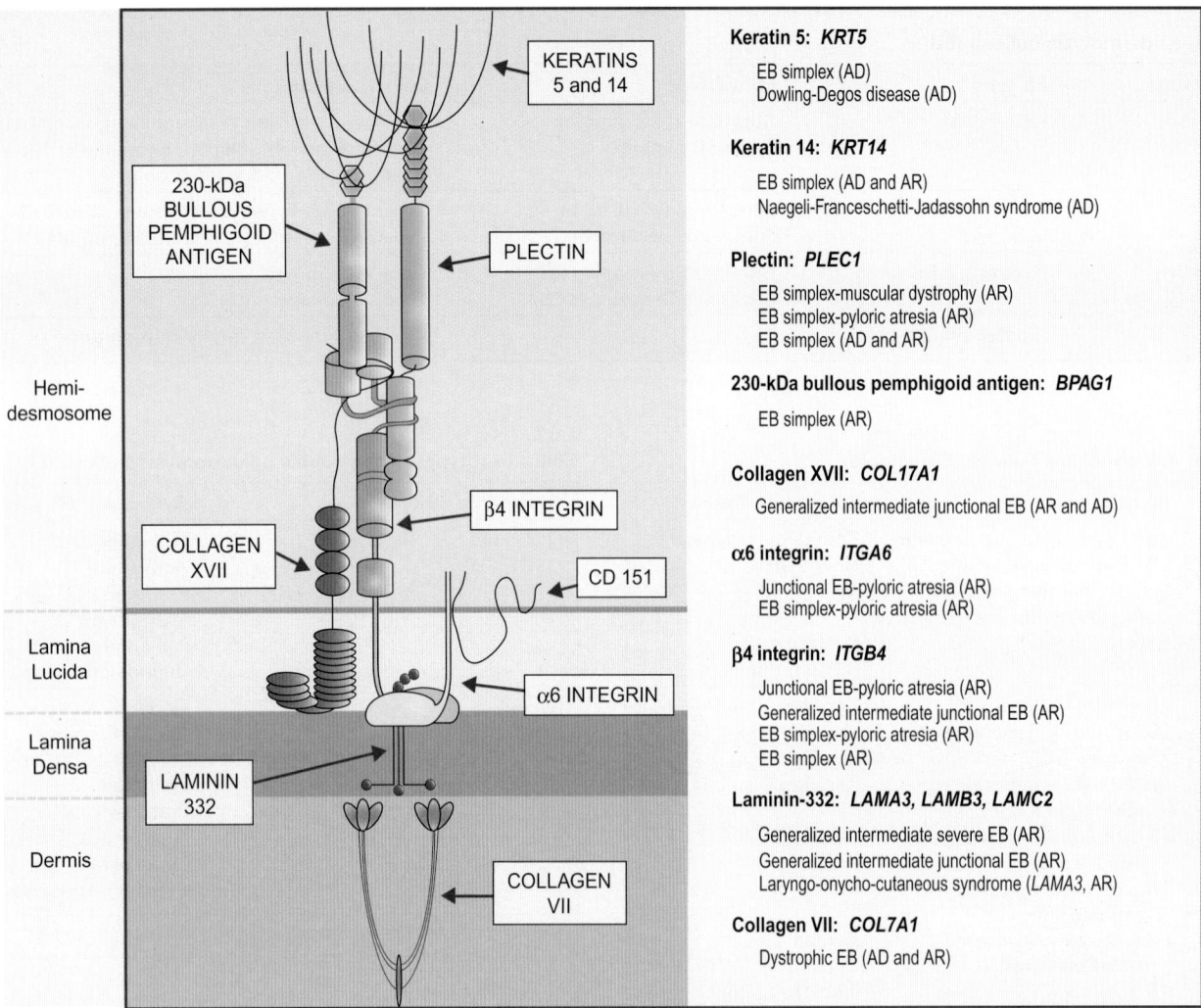

Keratin 5: *KRT5*

EB simplex (AD)
Dowling-Degos disease (AD)

Keratin 14: *KRT14*

EB simplex (AD and AR)
Naegeli-Franceschetti-Jadassohn syndrome (AD)

Plectin: *PLEC1*

EB simplex-muscular dystrophy (AR)
EB simplex-pyloric atresia (AR)
EB simplex (AD and AR)

230-kDa bullous pemphigoid antigen: *BPAG1*

EB simplex (AR)

Collagen XVII: *COL17A1*

Generalized intermediate junctional EB (AR and AD)

α6 integrin: *ITGA6*

Junctional EB-pyloric atresia (AR)
EB simplex-pyloric atresia (AR)

β4 integrin: *ITGB4*

Junctional EB-pyloric atresia (AR)
Generalized intermediate junctional EB (AR)
EB simplex-pyloric atresia (AR)
EB simplex (AR)

Laminin-332: *LAMA3, LAMB3, LAMC2*

Generalized intermediate severe EB (AR)
Generalized intermediate junctional EB (AR)
Laryngo-onycho-cutaneous syndrome (*LAMA3*, AR)

Collagen VII: *COL7A1*

Dystrophic EB (AD and AR)

Fig. 4.9
Schematic representation of the major adhesive proteins within hemidesmosome adhesion complexes at the dermal–epidermal junction and their involvement in different types of EB. (AD = autosomal dominant; AR = autosomal recessive).

gene panels) is gradually emerging as a primary investigation with the role of skin biopsy somewhat diminishing. This is certainly true for autosomal dominant forms of EB simplex or dominant dystrophic EB in which the skin pathology (both ultrastructural and immunohistochemical) may not differ significantly from normal skin, especially if no fresh blister is included in the biopsy. Nevertheless, skin biopsy remains a useful means of rapidly diagnosing autosomal recessive forms of EB, which is particularly useful in neonates with fragile skin since prompt diagnosis has important implications for optimal clinical management of affected babies and their families. Details about the most appropriate skin biopsy techniques and investigations for diagnosing EB are presented in Chapter 2.

For the dermatopathologist, a key issue will always be whether EB is best classified by skin/molecular pathology or by clinical morphology, and therefore in the sections that follow, both options are presented. Another important issue is how best to diagnose EB with the material made available. For skin that has been formalin-fixed and embedded in paraffin, successful diagnosis may depend on the presence or absence of a fresh blister. Most clinicians are aware that biopsying a blister that has been present for more than 12 hours is likely to present the pathologist with difficulties in determining the true plane of cleavage because of re-epithelialization and therefore rubbed non-blistered skin is preferentially sampled (see Chapter 2). Antigen mapping and immunoperoxidase staining is possible with antibodies to type IV collagen, which determines whether the lamina densa is present in the roof (dystrophic EB) or base (EB simplex and junctional EB) of the blister. Immunodiagnosis is also possible using selective probes, such as type VII collagen (reduced in recessive dystrophic EB). Nevertheless, the majority of the antibodies used to diagnose EB target transmembranous proteins and

therefore work suboptimally (or not at all) on paraffin-embedded skin sections. For EB diagnostics, skin immunohistochemistry is best performed on frozen sections (see Chapter 2). Part of the diagnostic skin biopsy is often fixed and processed for transmission electron microscopy although oftentimes sections are only cut if the skin immunolabeling fails to establish a diagnosis. Over the last decade, therefore, with the increasing utility of antibodies to skin basement membrane and epithelial proteins, the number of EB skin biopsies requiring transmission electron microscopy to establish a diagnosis has reduced by over 50%. This number is likely to decrease further as molecular diagnostics become more widely available, cheaper and quicker. Immunoelectron microscopy is not performed for routine EB diagnostics and is mainly used for research, including translational research when evaluating clinical trials of cell and gene-based therapies.

Clinical features of EB
EB simplex

The subtypes of EB simplex are subdivided into basal and suprabasal variants, that manifest as at least 15 distinct clinical disorders (*Table 4.2*).

Localized EB simplex

This is the most common type of EB.[6] Inheritance is autosomal dominant. The soles and palms (*Fig. 4.10*) are mainly affected. The condition is typically worse in warm weather. Hyperhidrosis of the feet is common; this increases friction, which also exacerbates blistering. The blisters usually heal without scarring or milia formation. Calluses are very common, especially in adults. Oral blistering occurs in less than 25% of cases. The hair and teeth are normal.

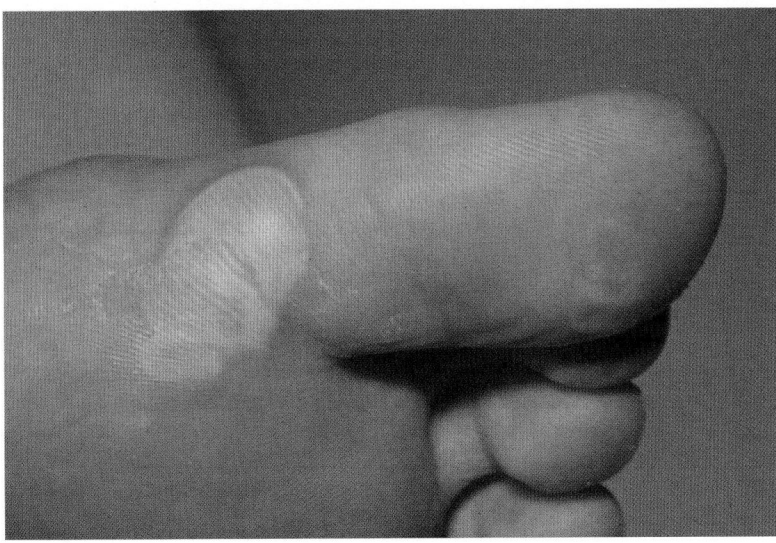

Fig. 4.10
Localized EB simplex: typical acral lesions affecting the toes. The pale color is due to the marked thickness of the roof of the blister. By courtesy of St John's Institute of Dermatology, London, UK.

Table 4.5
Genes implicated in the major epidermolysis bullosa (EB) subtypes

EB type	EB subtype	Mutated genes
EBS	EBS, suprabasal	*TGM5*
		DSP
		PKP1
		JUP
	EBS, basal	*KRT5*
		KRT14
		EXPH5
		PLEC
		DST
JEB	JEB, severe generalized	*LAMA3*
		LAMB3
		LAMC2
	JEB, generalized/localized	*LAMA3*
		LAMB3
		LAMC2
		COL17A1
		ITGB4
	JEB, late onset	*COL17A1*
	JEB with pyloric atresia	*ITGB4*
		ITGA6
	JEB with respiratory and renal involvement	*ITGA3*
	JEB-LOC syndrome	*LAMA3A*
DEB	RDEB, severe generalized	*COL7A1*
	RDEB, generalized and localized	*COL7A1*
	DDEB (all subtypes)	*COL7A1*
KS	Kindler syndrome	*FERMT1 (KIND1)*

EB, Epidermolysis bullosa; *EBS*, epidermolysis bullosa simplex; *JEB*, junctional epidermolysis bullosa; *LOC*, laryngo-onycho-cutaneous syndrome; *DEB*, dystrophic epidermolysis bullosa; *DDEB*, dominant dystrophic epidermolysis bullosa; *RDEB*, recessive dystrophic epidermolysis bullosa; *KS*, Kindler syndrome.

Acral peeling skin syndrome

A differential diagnosis of localized autosomal dominant EB simplex is autosomal recessive acral peeling skin syndrome, although both are classified as forms of EB simplex.[7] Blisters typically occur on the feet but are often more evident on the sides or dorsal aspects of the toes (*Fig. 4.11*). The level of blistering occurs above the granular layer, but because of the thicker stratum corneum in acral skin the clinical consequences may be almost identical to blistering through the basal keratinocyte layer.

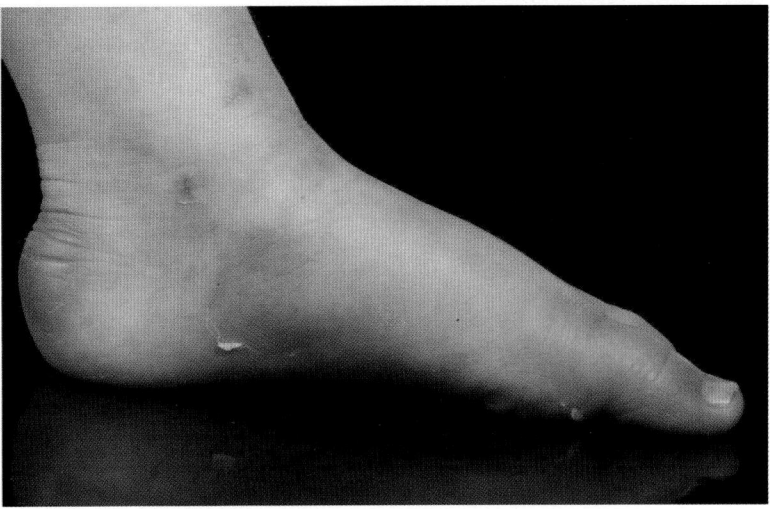

Fig. 4.11
Acral peeling skin syndrome: signs of peeling and erythema on the ankle and instep extending to the toes.

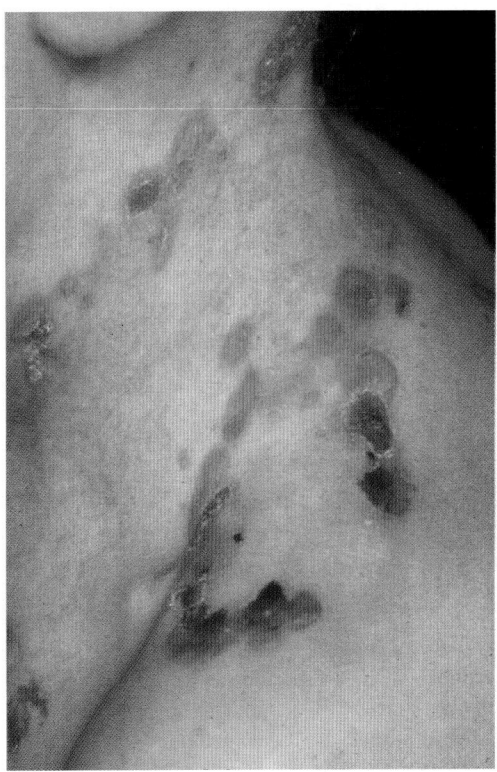

Fig. 4.12
Generalized severe EB simplex: showing characteristic grouping of blisters and erosions. By courtesy of R.A.J. Eady, MD, St John's Institute of Dermatology, London, UK.

Generalized severe EB simplex

A further common subtype of EB simplex is the generalized severe variant, previously known as Dowling-Meara EB simplex.[8] Inheritance is autosomal dominant. Blisters tend to occur in groups, hence the earlier use of the term EB herpetiformis (*Fig. 4.12*). In infancy, blistering may be severe with involvement of the mucous membranes, shedding of nails, and formation of milia. The distinctive feature is spontaneous herpetiform, annular or arcuate blistering on the trunk, limbs, and neck. Irregular hyperkeratosis of the palms and soles or keratoderma is often present. The general condition tends to improve with age.

Generalized intermediate EB simplex

This subtype of EB includes inherited blistering previously known as Koebner EB simplex.[9] Most cases are autosomal dominant. Although

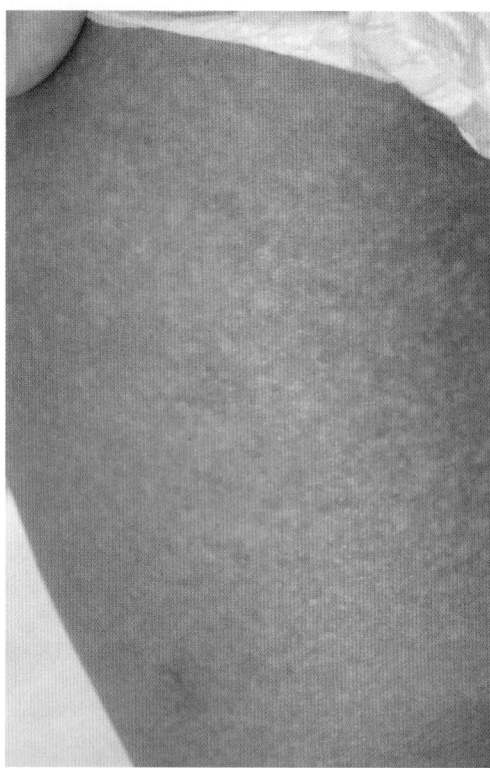

Fig. 4.13
EB simplex with mottled pigmentation: diffuse hyper- and hypopigmentation with minor small patches of erythema and occasional tiny vesicles. By courtesy of J.E. Mellerio, St John's Institute of Dermatology, London, UK

usually mild, approximately 60% of patients have localized scarring and approximately 15% have milia. The development of hair, teeth, and nails is normal. Blisters appear within the first year and may be present at birth. In infancy, they commonly appear on the occiput, back, and legs, while in childhood the hands and feet are often affected, although the palms and soles are not preferentially involved, as in localized EB simplex. In common with other forms of EB simplex, blistering is worse in warm weather.

EB simplex with mottled pigmentation

Distinction from other forms of EB simplex is made by the presence of pigmentary changes, which are present at birth or appear during infancy.[10] There is a reticulate pattern of small, tan-colored macular lesions, which may spread from acral sites to the trunk and which fade with age (*Fig. 4.13*). They may cover the entire skin surface, but preferentially involve the neck, upper trunk, or extremities. Blistering may be localized, or become more generalized. Most cases result from a specific heterozygous missense mutation in keratin 5.

EB simplex Ogna

This autosomal dominant condition was named after the village in Norway where the first affected family originated.[11] There is seasonal blistering of the hands and feet, and occasionally elsewhere. This rare subtype of EB is distinguishable clinically by a generalized bruising tendency, hemorrhagic bullae, and toenail dystrophy. The disorder results from a particular missense mutation in plectin that renders the protein more susceptible to proteolysis, thus reducing its expression and function.

EB simplex migratory circinate

This is a rare form of autosomal dominant EB simplex that is characterized by migratory circinate erythema and post-inflammatory hyperpigmentation.[12] Present at birth, blistering is generalized. The underlying cause is an atypical mutation in keratin 5 that leads to skin inflammation with a T-cell infiltrate.

EB simplex autosomal recessive keratin 14

Although much less common than autosomal dominant disease, recessive mutations in keratin 14 cases may resemble dominant generalized intermediate EB simplex.[13] Blisters are often scattered and there is usually minor palmoplantar keratoderma and varying degrees of nail dystrophy, atrophic scarring, hyperpigmentation, and oral and genital blistering. There is often a complete loss of keratin 14 expression in the epidermis, although the phenotype is typically a less severe phenotype than some dominant cases. No recessive cases involving keratin 5 have yet been reported.

EB simplex with muscular dystrophy

Inherited skin fragility can occur in association with muscular dystrophy, although myasthenia gravis and spinal muscular atrophy have also been described.[14] The blisters, which affect the skin and oral mucosa, are present at birth or soon afterwards. Muscle weakness and wasting may be severe and evident in early childhood, or milder and only detectable later in life. The blistering may be widespread, but can be limited to the hands and feet. There can be atrophic scarring, milia, nail dystrophy, and alopecia. Supraglottic scarring and hoarseness may necessitate tracheostomy. The disorder is autosomal recessive and results from mutations in plectin.

EB simplex with pyloric atresia

Pyloric atresia may rarely occur in the setting of EB simplex – most cases of which are classified as a junctional form of EB.[15] Affected infants tend to have generalized skin disease. Although only a few cases have yet been reported, this entity appears to be as severe as junctional EB with pyloric atresia and clinically impossible to differentiate from it. There are widespread blisters and erosions that increase infection risk with early demise in the neonatal period. Inheritance is autosomal recessive and involves mutations in plectin.

EB simplex autosomal recessive BP230

Mutations leading to a complete loss of the 230-kDa bullous pemphigoid antigen results in a rare form of autosomal recessive of EB simplex.[16] Blistering is lifelong and generalized but clinically is mild with only a few predominantly acral blisters that can extend to several centimeters in size, but which are noninflammatory and which heal with no scarring and only mild postinflammatory pigmentary anomalies. Oral and genital mucosae are not affected.

EB simplex autosomal recessive exophilin-5

Autosomal recessive loss-of-function mutations in *EXPH5* (encoding exophilin-5, also known as Slac2-b) result in mild, scattered, trauma-induced skin fragility, although blistering can be generalized shortly after birth.[17] In later infancy, however, the clinical features mostly comprise crusted erosions on the limbs with few intact blisters. No mucosal abnormalities are noted. Typically, the disease severity improves with age and may even remit completely.

EB simplex plakophilin-1 deficiency

This disorder represents the first inherited disorder of desmosomes; it is also known as ectodermal dysplasia skin fragility syndrome.[18] Inheritance is autosomal recessive. Widespread erosions are present at birth, with evident perioral cracking and hypotrichosis. During infancy, the skin manifestations evolve to reveal trauma-induced scale crusting, a prominent palmoplantar keratoderma with painful fissures, and nail dystrophy. Most cases have substantial loss of scalp hair and eyebrows and the perioral changes persist. Unlike some other inherited desmosomal disorders, there is no cardiac involvement in this condition since plakophilin-1 is not expressed in the heart.

EB simplex desmoplakin deficiency

Autosomal recessive mutations in the desmosomal plaque protein, desmoplakin, can result in a very severe form of inherited skin fragility. It was originally termed 'lethal acantholytic EB,'[19] although the latest classification of EB has tried to avoid using emotive terms such as 'lethal' given the impact such a devastating term can have on families as well as the possible unpredictability in disease course in some cases. Blistering is present at birth and generalized. A characteristic feature is the presence of oozing erosions rather than frank blisters. Other findings include markedly abnormal nails, neonatal teeth, intraoral erosions, and alopecia. The gastro-intestinal, genito-urinary, and respiratory tracts may also be involved.

EB simplex plakoglobin deficiency

Autosomal recessive mutations in plakoglobin, a protein found in desmosomal plaques and adherens junctions, can also result in a very severe form of inherited skin fragility. This was originally termed 'lethal congenital EB,'[20] although, as is the case for desmoplakin, the latest consensus on EB classification has avoided use of the word 'lethal' preferring to opt for skin fragility plakoglobin deficiency (or severe acantholytic EB) instead. Clinically there are widespread erosions and massive transcutaneous fluid loss leading to a poor prognosis. Cardiac involvement is possible with some inherited abnormalities of plakoglobin.

EB simplex superficialis

This autosomal dominant condition is characterized by the presence of superficial erosions rather than intact blisters, similar to those seen in pemphigus foliaceus.[21] Epidermal cleavage is typically just beneath the stratum corneum. Healing results in localized atrophic scarring or postinflammatory hyperpigmentation. The molecular basis of this subtype of EB simplex is unknown and therefore it is uncertain whether this condition is truly a discreet clinicopathological entity.

Junctional EB

Almost all clinical variants of junctional EB are characterized by autosomal recessive inheritance and by blister formation at the level of the lamina lucida. Conventionally, junctional EB is divided into two main categories: generalized and localized, each of which has a number of subtypes (*Table 4.3*). The terms Herlitz, non-Herlitz, generalized atrophic benign, cicatricial, progressive, and atrophicans are no longer used in the updated classification of EB, nor are the words 'lethal' or 'letalis' considered appropriate diagnostic labels.

Generalized severe junctional EB

This is the most severe form of junctional EB. Blistering and erosions are present at or soon after birth and rapidly become generalized.[22] The whole skin is fragile and moving the baby may cause extensive blistering (*Fig. 4.14*). Nail bed involvement is very common (*Fig. 4.15*). Eroded areas are often very slow to heal and may lead to atrophic scarring. Milia are not generally seen. Involvement of the oral and pharyngeal mucosa is frequent and may be severe; hoarseness and stridor may indicate laryngeal or supraglottic involvement, most notably potentially life-threatening stenosis or stricture. Many infants die early in infancy with overwhelming infection or from failure to thrive, but those surviving the first few months will often develop distinctive lesions characterized by non-healing, crusted erosions containing exuberant granulation tissue.

Generalized intermediate junctional EB

The early clinical course of this subtype of junctional EB may be similar to the generalized severe variant, but the patients usually survive to adulthood.[23] There is a gradual lessening in blistering severity with age. Mucous membranes are involved, and the teeth show severe enamel defects or may fail to erupt normally. Nails are often dystrophic or missing. Atrophic scarring is characteristic. There is also alopecia affecting the scalp, eyebrows, and eyelashes, and body hair is also sparse or absent. Large pigmented nevi, or acquired macular hyperpigmented lesions, are typical. In this type of junctional EB, it is common to observe small patches of skin that do not blister; this phenomenon is called revertant mosaicism (also known as natural gene therapy), and represents a spontaneous correction of one copy of the mutant gene.

Generalized late-onset junctional EB

This is a rare subtype of autosomal recessive junctional EB that overlaps with generalized intermediate junctional EB, except that the onset of

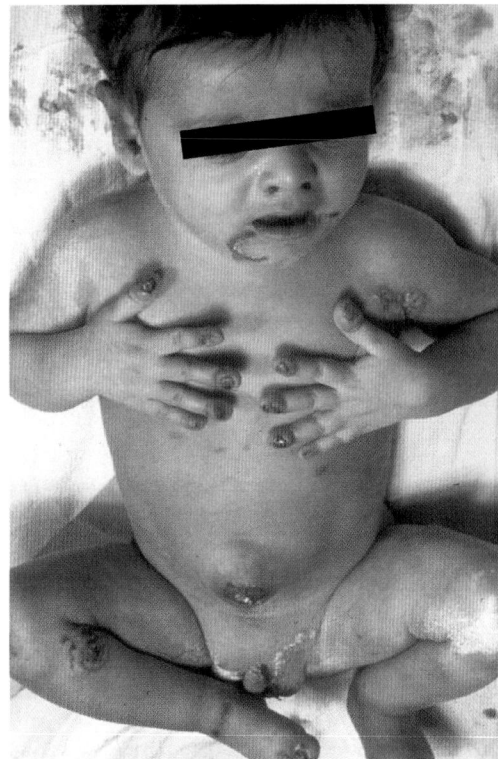

Fig. 4.14
Generalized severe junctional EB: newly born infant with blistering and nail involvement. By courtesy of J. McGrath, MD, Institute of Dermatology, London, UK.

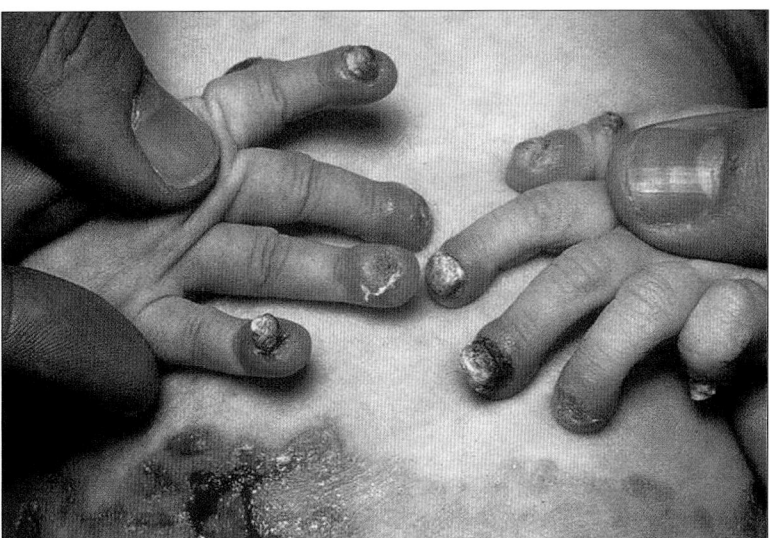

Fig. 4.15
Generalized severe junctional EB: infant showing granulation tissue at the edge of a healing blister. By courtesy of the Institute of Dermatology, London, UK.

symptoms is delayed – often not starting until childhood, typically between 5 and 8 years of age.[24] Initially, the trauma-induced blisters mainly occur on the hands and feet, although they may be preceded by nail dystrophy. Later, knees and elbows are involved. Progressive atrophic changes lead to early loss of fingerprint patterns and mild finger contractures. The tooth enamel may be defective and the tongue papillae may disappear. The oral mucosa is sometimes involved.

Junctional EB with pyloric atresia

Blistering is usually present at birth, following a pregnancy complicated by polyhydramnios. The lesions are usually widespread and can result in atrophic scarring (*Fig. 4.16*).[25] The teeth are hypoplastic, lacking normal

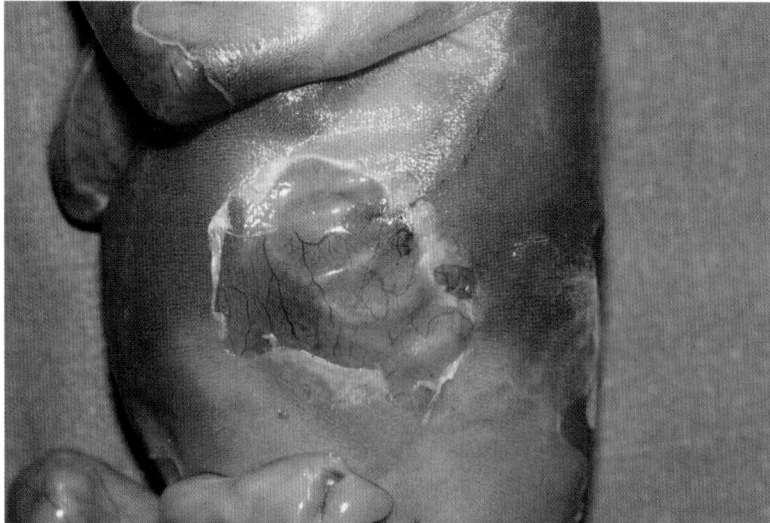

Fig. 4.16
Junctional EB with pyloric atresia: widespread blistering with deep ulceration. By courtesy of M.J. Tidman, MD, Institute of Dermatology, London, UK.

enamel, and the nails are dystrophic. Early attempts at feeding result in vomiting. The majority of cases do not survive early infancy. In those children who survive, other features include haematuria, dysuria, and recurrent urinary tract infections. The pyloric canal is often completely obliterated (*Fig. 4.17*) and requires surgical correction although the nature of the underlying molecular pathology usually influences prognosis.

Junctional EB with respiratory and renal involvement

This is a recent addition to the classification of junctional EB. The features comprise congenital nephrotic syndrome, interstitial lung disease, and skin fragility, due to autosomal recessive mutations in α3 integrin.[26] The renal and respiratory features predominate clinically, and skin blistering may be a minor feature that only occurs later. The oral mucosa is not involved. The scalp hair, eyebrows, and eyelashes are fine and sparse and nails may be dystrophic. Prognosis is poor with recurrent lung infections and multiorgan failure consistent with the known distribution of α3 integrin in several tissues.

Localized junctional EB

Localized forms of junctional EB occur: typical clinical manifestations include nail dystrophy, dental enamel changes, and blistering involving the lower legs and feet only.[27] In some individuals, chronic, painful erosions associated with hyperkeratosis develop on the soles, although it is not clear why the lower legs should be a predilection site for blistering. In some cases, blistering starts in neonates, while in others there may be late-onset disease.

Localized junctional EB inversa

In the neonatal period in the rare inversa subtype of localized junctional EB, the whole skin may be fragile with generalized blistering. Later, however, the lesions affect chiefly the groins, perineum, and axillae, hence the description of 'inversa.'[28] Healing may result in small, atrophic white streaks. Dysplastic teeth, erosions of the cornea, and feet and nail dystrophy are all features. Why there should be a preference for flexural site involvement is not known.

Localized junctional EB laryngo-onycho-cutaneous syndrome

This subtype of junctional EB starts in infancy with chronic erosions affecting the face (mainly around the nose and mouth) although erosions are also seen on the limbs, trunk, and genitalia.[29] The nails are also involved with marked periungual and subungual inflammation and a universal feature is hoarseness. The teeth may be notched. There is prominent skin and mucosal granulation tissue that can lead to delayed wound healing, laryngeal obstruction, and blindness. The disorder results from autosomal recessive mutations in a particular splice variant of the laminin α3 polypeptide.

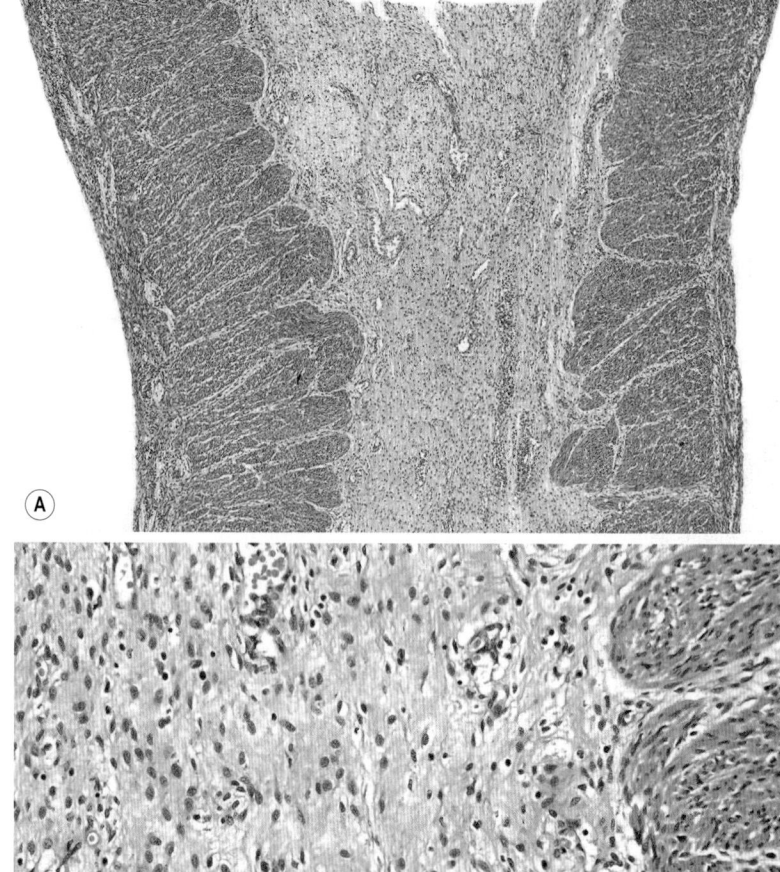

Fig. 4.17
(**A**, **B**) Junctional EB with pyloric atresia: pyloric canal is obliterated by fibrous connective tissue.

Dystrophic epidermolysis bullosa

Dystrophic EB can be autosomal recessive or autosomal dominant (*Table 4.4*). Clinically, dystrophic EB is characterized by skin fragility, blistering, scarring, nail dystrophy, and milia formation. Mucosal involvement is common and erosions and scarring can affect the mouth, esophagus, genitalia, and anus. There may be clinical overlap between some cases of recessive and dominant dystrophic EB, which can make genetic counseling difficult, particularly in sporadic cases. The most recent classification of EB no longer contains any eponymous subtypes, and also recognizes that the phenotypic appearances vary considerably between patients and that, given the spectrum of clinical appearances, diagnostic labeling within an individual category can be somewhat arbitrary in some cases.

Dominant dystrophic EB generalized

Blisters in dominant dystrophic EB mainly occur following trauma to the skin overlying the bony prominences, such as the knees and ankles, and dorsa of the hands or feet (*Fig. 4.18*).[30] The most consistent findings are localized scarring with milia formation and dystrophic nails. Nail dystrophy is probably the most important diagnostic feature of the disease, especially in adults, because many patients have only limited blistering and scarring, which becomes less noticeable with age. Blistering in the mouth is usually mild and the teeth are generally normal. However, perianal lesions may cause considerable pain, especially in children. Terms such as Bart syndrome are obsolete. Cutaneous features, such as albopapuloid lesions, once

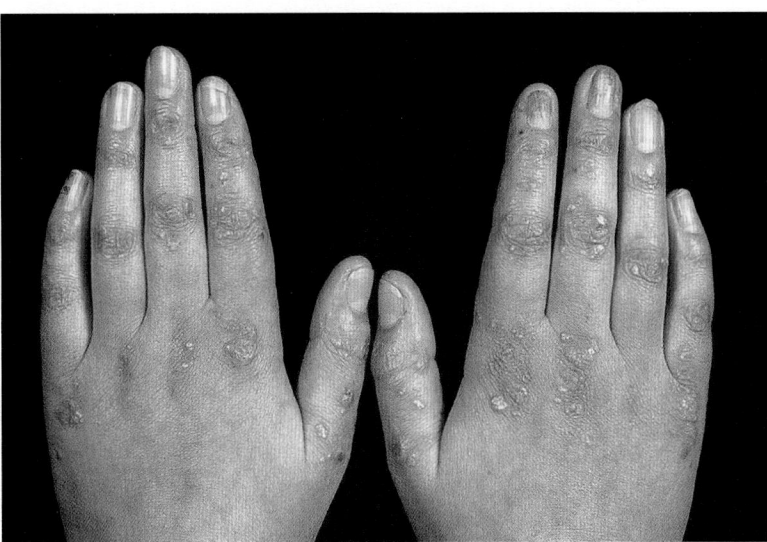

Fig. 4.18
Generalized dominant dystrophic EB: scarring, milia and nail dystrophy. By courtesy of St John's Institute of Dermatology, London, UK.

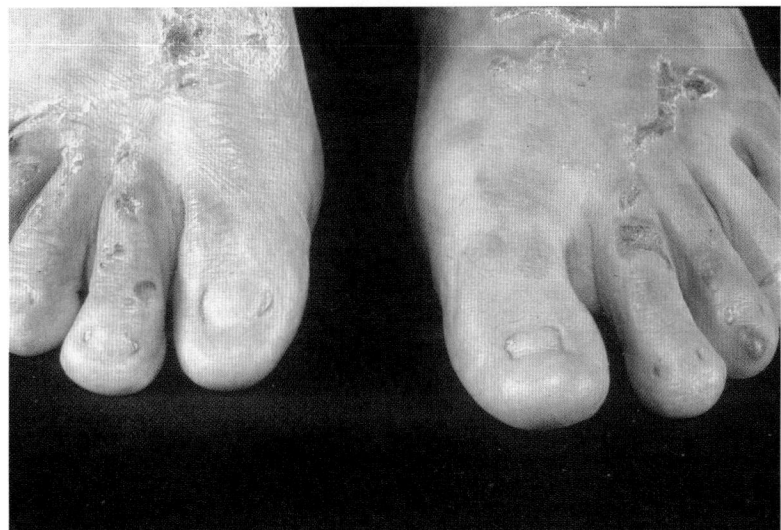

Fig. 4.19
Dominant dystrophic EB–acral: predominantly acral blisters and scarring as well as nail dystrophy. By courtesy of St John's Institute of Dermatology, London, UK.

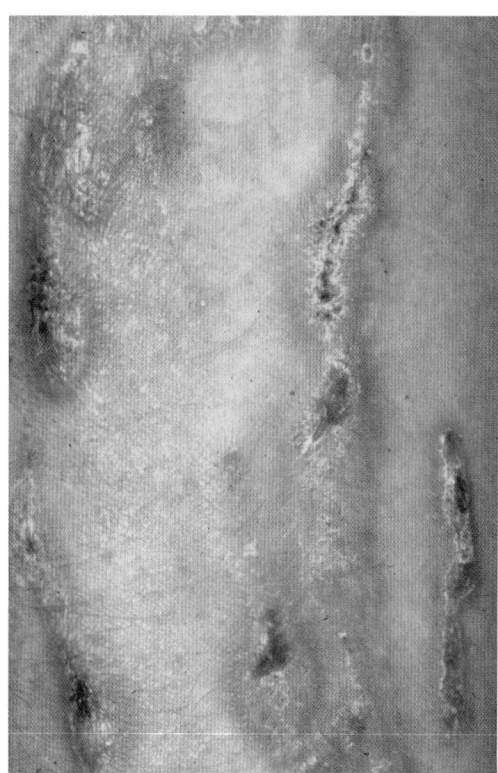

Fig. 4.20
Dominant dystrophic EB–pretibial: linear erosions with scarring localized to the front of both shins. By courtesy of St John's Institute of Dermatology, London, UK.

thought to be pathognomonic for subtypes of dominant dystrophic EB, are now recognized to occur in several forms of dystrophic EB.

Dominant dystrophic EB acral

The nature of this subtype of dominant dystrophic EB is not precisely defined as the term 'acral' is not widely used in the published literature.[31] Its inclusion in the latest classification of EB is to assist description of those cases of dominant dystrophic EB with a more localized pattern of skin involvement, usually involving the hands and feet (*Fig. 4.19*). However, the word acral is used in preference to localized because some oral or esophageal involvement can occur despite the relative lack of involvement of much of the skin. Trauma-induced blistering, scarring, and milia are typically present in acral skin.

Dominant or recessive dystrophic EB pretibial

This subtype of dystrophic EB may be inherited by either autosomal dominant (the majority) or autosomal recessive transmission with considerable overlap in appearances.[32] Clinically, there are blisters, atrophy, and scarring on the shins (*Fig. 4.20*). Lesions are usually violaceous, sometimes mimicking lichen planus. Nails on both the hands and feet tend to be dystrophic. The shins may be itchy and the phenotype can overlap with dystrophic EB

pruriginosa (see next section). Clinical signs are not exclusively confined to the shins and relatively minor skin fragility, scarring, and milia may be detected at other body sites, particularly over bony prominences.

Dominant or recessive dystrophic EB pruriginosa

This subtype of dystrophic EB overlaps clinically with the pretibial variant. The main difference is the intense pruritus, the etiology of which is uncertain.[33] Studies have excluded concomitant atopy and a range of possible metabolic, biochemical, and endocrine factors in disease pathogenesis. The clinical features can resemble hypertrophic lichen planus or nodular prurigo or autoimmune inflammatory blistering, or even dermatitis artefacta. Like the pretibial subtype, the initial onset of symptoms and signs may be delayed for several decades, often leading to a genetic cause for the skin lesions being erroneously discounted. Although the shins are often involved, pruritic skin lesions can occur at any site.

Dominant dystrophic EB nails only

This condition is often only first diagnosed when a family member presents with trauma-induced skin blistering, and a review of the pedigree reveals one or more generations of other individuals with nail dystrophy, but no history of blisters, scarring, milia, or mucosal erosions. Thus, in some individuals there are no clinical signs present apart from nail dystrophy, which can sometimes just be confined to the great toenails, and therefore in many families, a subtype of dystrophic EB is not suspected at all.[34] This variant of dominant dystrophic EB is therefore likely to be much more common than is currently appreciated.

Dominant or recessive dystrophic bullous disease of the newborn

One curious variant of dystrophic EB is when blistering in neonates shows signs of spontaneous clinical improvement over the first few weeks or months of life (*Fig. 4.21*). The amelioration in phenotype is mirrored by improvement of the underlying skin pathology with increased type VII collagen at the dermal–epidermal junction. Initial skin biopsies reveal punctate intraepidermal labeling for type VII collagen and ultrastructural signs of

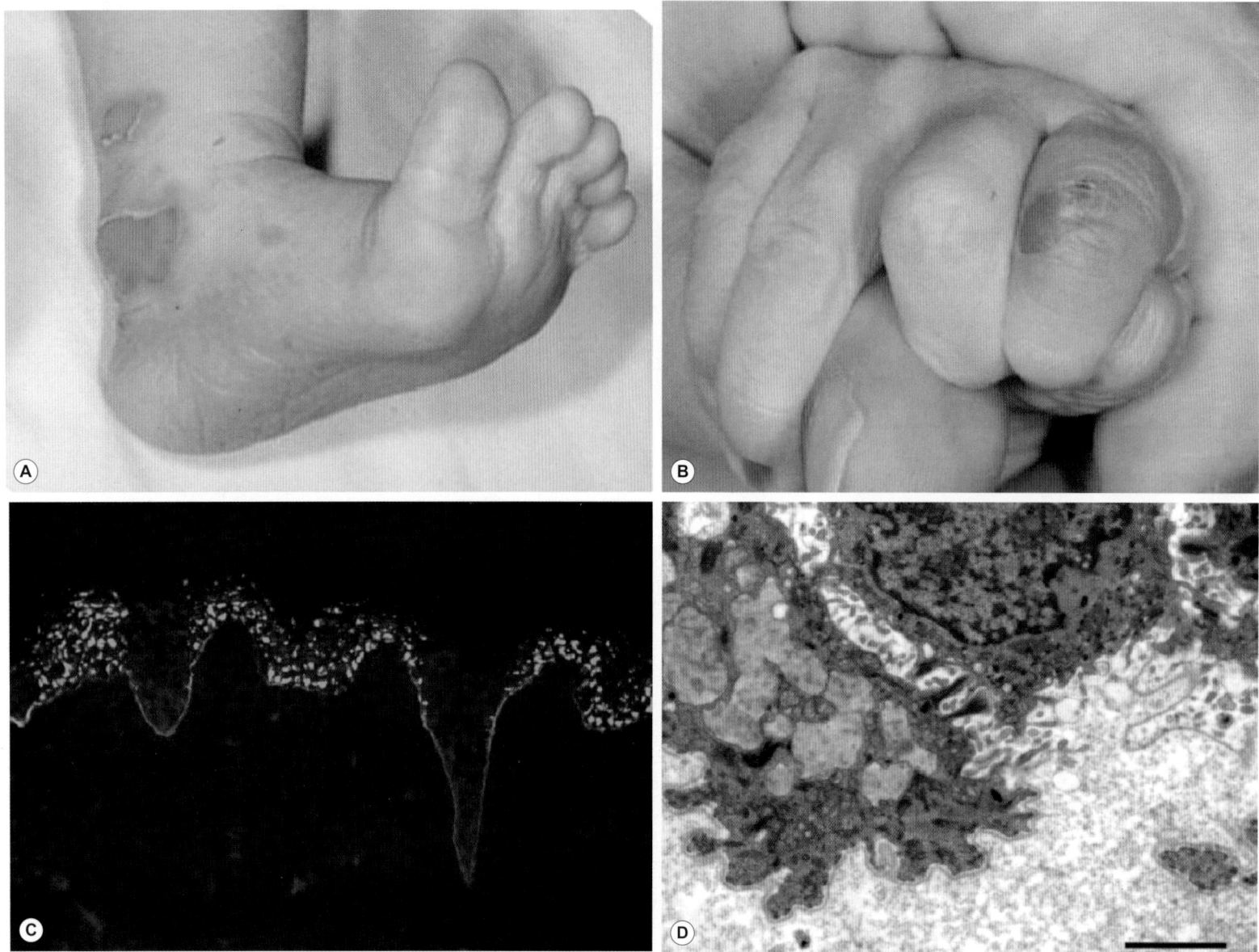

Fig. 4.21
Bullous dermolysis of the newborn: (**A**) blisters on the heel; (**B**) blisters on the fingers; (**C**) type VII collagen is present at the dermal–epidermal junction but there is also striking punctate staining within the epidermis; (**D**) ultrastructurally, in this basal keratinocyte there are numerous pale gray stellate bodies (dilated Golgi apparatus containing type VII collagen). This form of dystrophic EB usually tends to improve spontaneously during the first few months of life.

dilated perinuclear vacuoles with a granular appearance (stellate bodies). Initially, it was thought that complete correction of the type VII collagen secretion and assembly into anchoring fibrils occurred leading to the diagnostic label of 'transient bullous dermolysis of the newborn.'[35] Now, however, it is appreciated that most cases do not resolve completely and that there may be permanent stigmata of dominant or recessive dystrophic EB, albeit less severe than in early life.

Recessive dystrophic EB generalized severe

Multiple blisters are present at birth or appear in early infancy and the skin is very fragile. The clinical presentation may include localized absence of skin especially affecting the lower legs. Blisters develop spontaneously or after the mildest trauma on any part of the skin and may be hemorrhagic.[36] Milia and scarring are very common. Although any site can blister, the main areas are those subjected to repeated friction and other forms of physical trauma. These include the knees, elbows, hands, feet, back of the neck, shoulders, and over the spine. Chronic erosions and ulcers tend to become covered with a slough, often associated with heaped-up crusting and scaling, increasing the risk of secondary infection and biofilm formation. Pruritus and pain are frequent. The scalp is often involved and scarring alopecia may

occur. During childhood, repeated blistering with progressive scarring leads to fusion ('pseudosyndactyly') of adjacent fingers and toes (*Fig. 4.22*). Digits can undergo progressive contractures and gradually become encased in a cocoon-like covering of thin scar tissue, resembling a mitten.

Oral blistering and scarring can lead to ankyloglossia and microstomia. The gums are fragile, and gentle tooth brushing may induce epithelial disruption with bleeding. The lingual papillae are lost and the surface of the tongue becomes smooth. Although there is limited evidence for a primary abnormality of dental enamel in dystrophic EB, the teeth are at a high risk of developing caries. Blistering in the esophagus may cause acute pain and dysphagia, with difficulty in swallowing solids, with subsequent development of obstruction from strictures caused by scarring and fibrosis. Perianal blistering, erosions, and painful fissures are common in childhood. Eye complications include symblepharon, corneal erosions, and corneal opacity or scarring. Patients are often anemic and osteopaenia is not uncommon. Rarely, secondary amyloidosis can also develop in cases associated with persistent chronic inflammation and extensive scarring. A common and clinically very important complication of this form of EB is the development of squamous cell carcinomas, even in individuals as young as 6 years of age. Most carcinomas are on the limbs, often in areas of chronic, non-healing

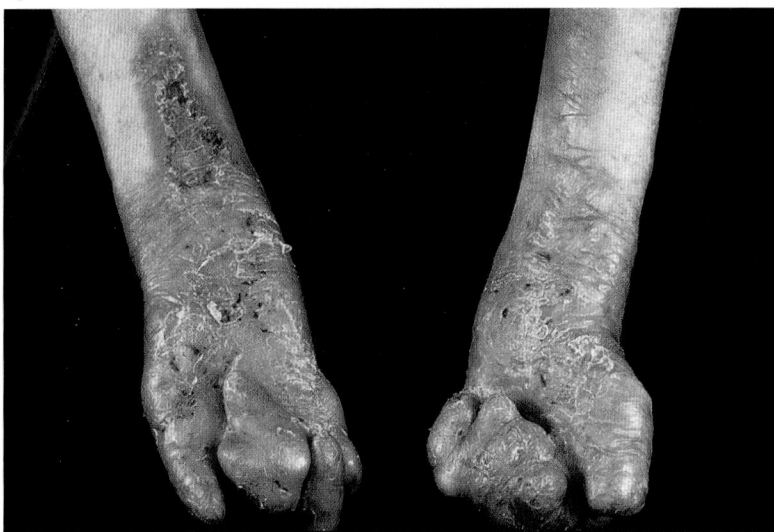

Fig. 4.22
Generalized severe recessive dystrophic EB: in addition to the gross mitten deformity, there is very severe scarring and scaling. By courtesy of St John's Institute of Dermatology, London, UK.

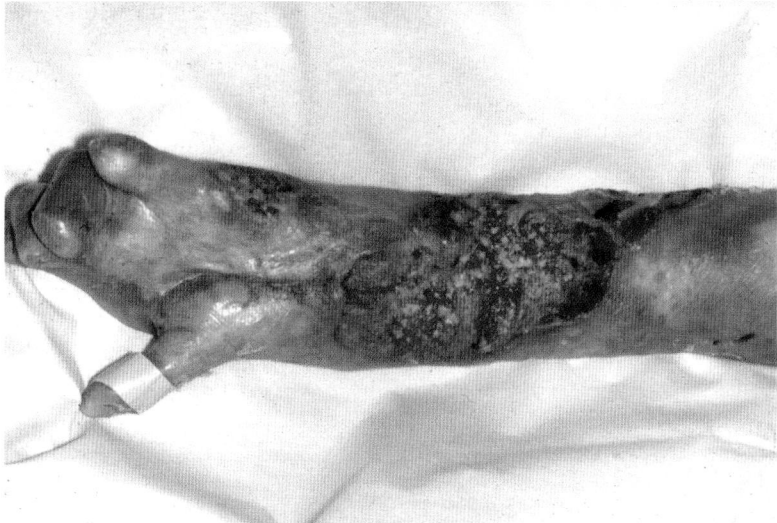

Fig. 4.23
Generalized severe recessive dystrophic EB: in this patient, numerous large keratoses are evident. Many of these progress to squamous cell carcinoma. Courtesy of R.A.J. Eady, MD, and B. Mayou, MD, St Thomas' Hospital, London, UK.

ulceration (Fig. 4.23). Multiple primary tumors, with progressive loss of differentiation for each subsequent cancer is the usual course, death typically occurs within 5 years of the first malignancy.

Recessive dystrophic EB generalized intermediate

There are milder subtypes of dystrophic EB that share several cutaneous and extracutaneous features with generalized severe recessive dystrophic EB, but to a much lesser degree.[37] The skin and mucosae are very fragile, but lesions, including nail changes, milia, and atrophic scarring, tend to be more localized and similar to those seen in many cases of dominant dystrophic EB (Fig. 4.24). Growth retardation and anemia are usually mild. Pseudosyndactyly, esophageal involvement, and squamous cell carcinoma may also occur, but these complications are usually milder, less frequent, or have a later onset compared to generalized disease.

Recessive dystrophic EB inversa

In the inversa subtype, primary areas of blistering and scarring include the groins, axillae, neck, and lumbar area, although in early life the distribution

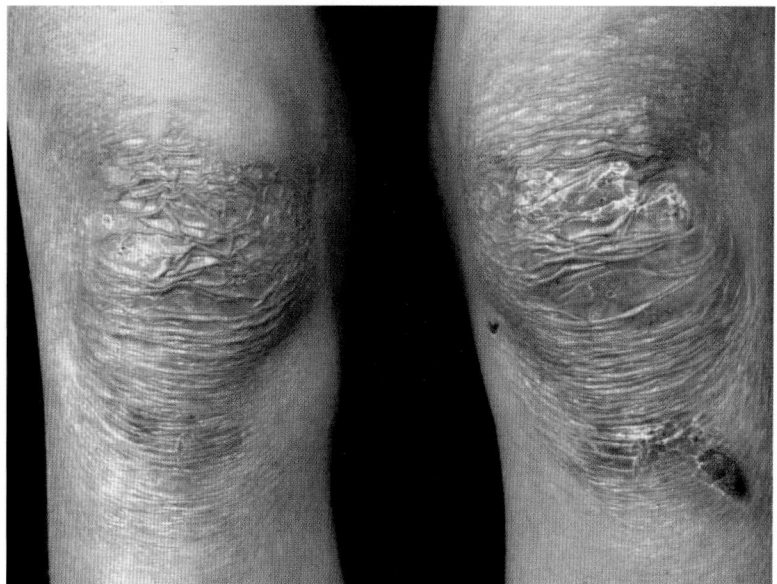

Fig. 4.24
Generalized intermediate recessive dystrophic EB: this individual has atrophic scarring and recent erosions overlying both knees.

of the blistering may be generalized and not indicative of the subsequent pattern.[38] Traumatic corneal erosions and esophageal lesions are common. Nail dystrophy, mucous membrane involvement, and dental changes are similar to those in the generalized form of the condition. Patients are also at risk of developing squamous cell carcinoma. The reason for the predominance of flexural involvement is not clear.

Recessive dystrophic EB localized

Localized forms of recessive dystrophic EB overlap with the generalized intermediate subtypes, as well as those classified as inversa, pretibial, or nails only, underscoring the spectrum of clinical features and the somewhat arbitrary goal of trying to fit all subtypes into neat, clearly defined categories. Skin fragility, scarring and milia are mostly confined to hands, feet and nails, and may be minor features.[39] In some cases, onset of symptoms may be delayed for several years after birth. Mucosal involvement is rare.

Recessive dystrophic EB centripetalis

This subtype of dystrophic EB is rare and because only one individual has been reported it is likely to be subsumed into other categories in future classifications.[40] The reported individual had generalized blistering at birth but within the first year of life her skin disease activity became confined to the hands and feet. Over several decades the blistering slowly progressed proximally, in a centripetal manner, with active blistering and milia only along the active edges with atrophic scarring and nail dystrophy distally. No systemic involvement occurred.

Kindler syndrome

Kindler syndrome is an autosomal recessive disorder. Initially it can resemble generalized or localized forms of dystrophic EB, although skin biopsy typically shows a variable plane of cleavage and a fragmented or duplicated lamina densa in contrast to the specific planes of tissue separation that underlie EB simplex, junctional EB, and dystrophic EB.[41] Thus, Kindler syndrome is classified as a separate category of EB (Table 4.1). Clinically, the initial skin blistering lessens during childhood and instead signs of a progressive poikiloderma develop (Fig. 4.25). At this stage, the differential diagnosis includes other congenital poikilodermatous disorders, including dyskeratosis congenita and Rothmund-Thomson syndrome. Other features include gingival inflammation, ectropion, corneal erosions, chronic colitis, periodontal disease, scarring of the external urethral meatus, and an increased risk of developing cutaneous squamous cell carcinoma. The hands can also show evidence of pseudosyndactyly, similar to some cases of dystrophic EB.

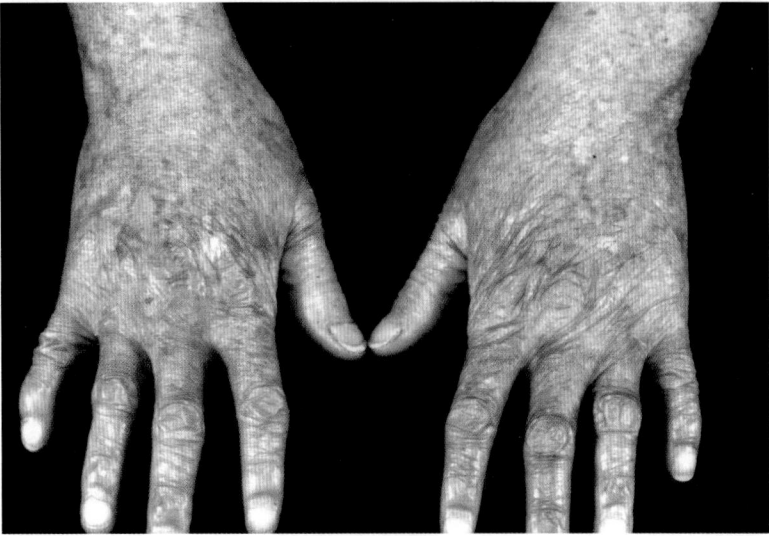

Fig. 4.25
Kindler syndrome: the hands of this 14-year-old girl show poikiloderma (hyperpigmentation, hypopigmentation, atrophy, and telangeictasias)

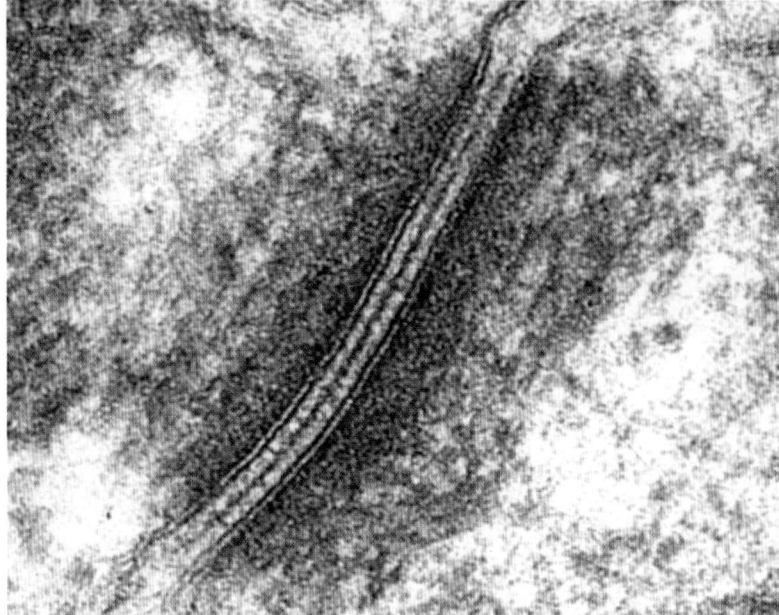

Fig. 4.27
Ultrastructural appearances of a desmosome between two keratinocytes in normal human skin.

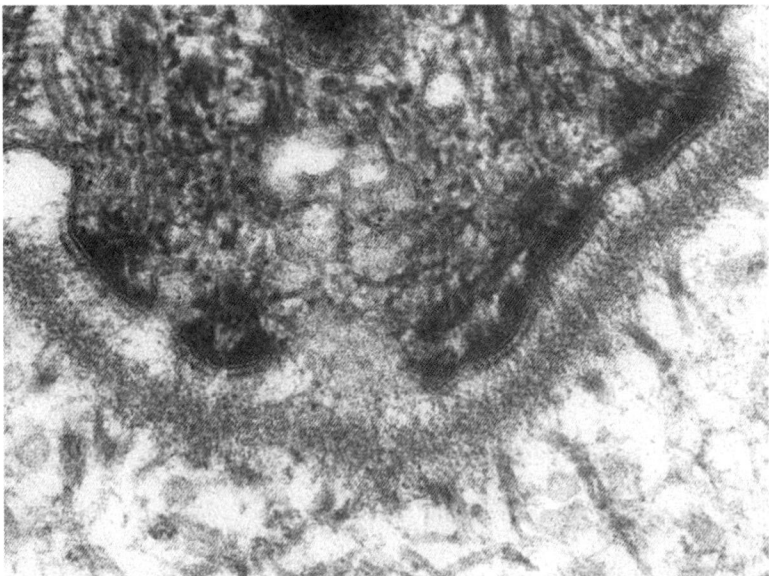

Fig. 4.26
Ultrastructural appearances of a hemidesmosome at the dermal–epidermal junction in normal human skin.

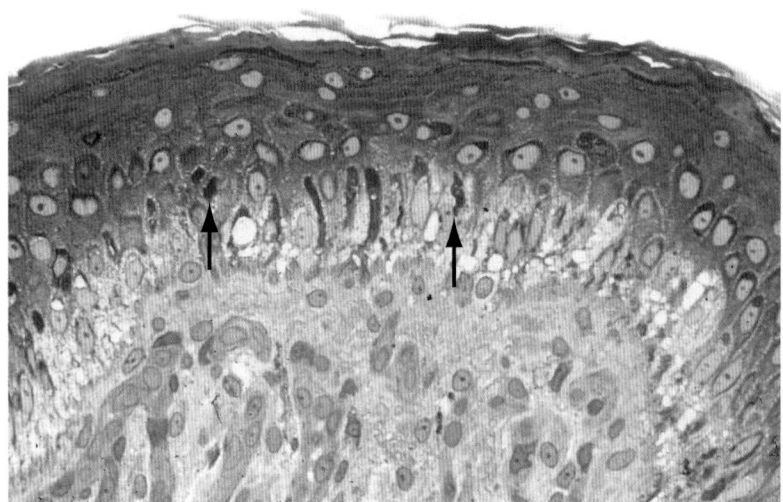

Fig. 4.28
Generalized severe EB simplex: numerous tonofilament clumps are present in the adjacent clinically normal skin (*arrowed*). By courtesy of J.A. McGrath, MD, St John's Institute of Dermatology, London, UK.

Pathologic basis of EB

The two key adhesion complexes implicated in the various subtypes of EB are the hemidesmosome (*Fig. 4.26*) and the desmosome (*Fig. 4.27*), and the 18 different genes implicated in the different types of EB are presented in *Table 4.5*.

Keratins 5 and 14: KRT5, KRT14

Keratins are the most abundant structural proteins in the cytoplasm of epithelial cells.[42] Pairs of keratin monomers polymerize to form a network of 10 nm-diameter intermediate filaments that maintain the shape of keratinocytes. Keratin 5 and 14 are the major keratins in basal keratinocytes. Autosomal dominant mutations in *KRT5* or *KRT14* underlie the most common subtype of EB, localized EB simplex, a condition affecting close to 400 000 people worldwide. EB simplex usually results in minor blistering that is typically worse in the summer months and which does not result in scarring. However, there are several other clinical variants of EB simplex that also result from *KRT5* or *KRT14* mutations (*Table 4.2*); most of these are dominant, but autosomal recessive mutations in *KRT14* can occur. Blistering typically occurs within the basal keratinocyte layer (*Fig. 4.28*), and there may

be structural alteration in the keratin filament network resulting from some *KRT5* or *KRT14* mutations (*Fig. 4.29*). The diagnosis of EB simplex by light microscopy of paraffin-embedded sections can be challenging because early changes occur very close to the dermal–epidermal junction and may be subtle (*Fig. 4.30*) whereas older lesions can appear subepidermal (*Fig. 4.31*).

Plakophilin-1: PKP1

Some forms of EB result from mutations in proteins found within desmosome cell–cell junctions (*Fig. 4.32*). Desmosomes form structural and signaling links between adjacent cells and are found in skin keratinocytes, cardiac myocytes, the meninges, and the cortex of lymph nodes. Plakophilin-1 has a restricted localization to keratinocyte desmosomes,[43] and autosomal recessive loss-of-function mutations in *PKP1* result in ectodermal dysplasia – skin fragility syndrome. Blistering and erosions result from a loss of keratinocyte adhesion within the desmosomal inner plaque just inside the keratinocyte (i.e., not true acantholysis); the ectodermal dysplasia partly results from altered epidermal differentiation and proliferation, but is also because plakophilin-1 has nuclear signaling roles in other tissues as well.

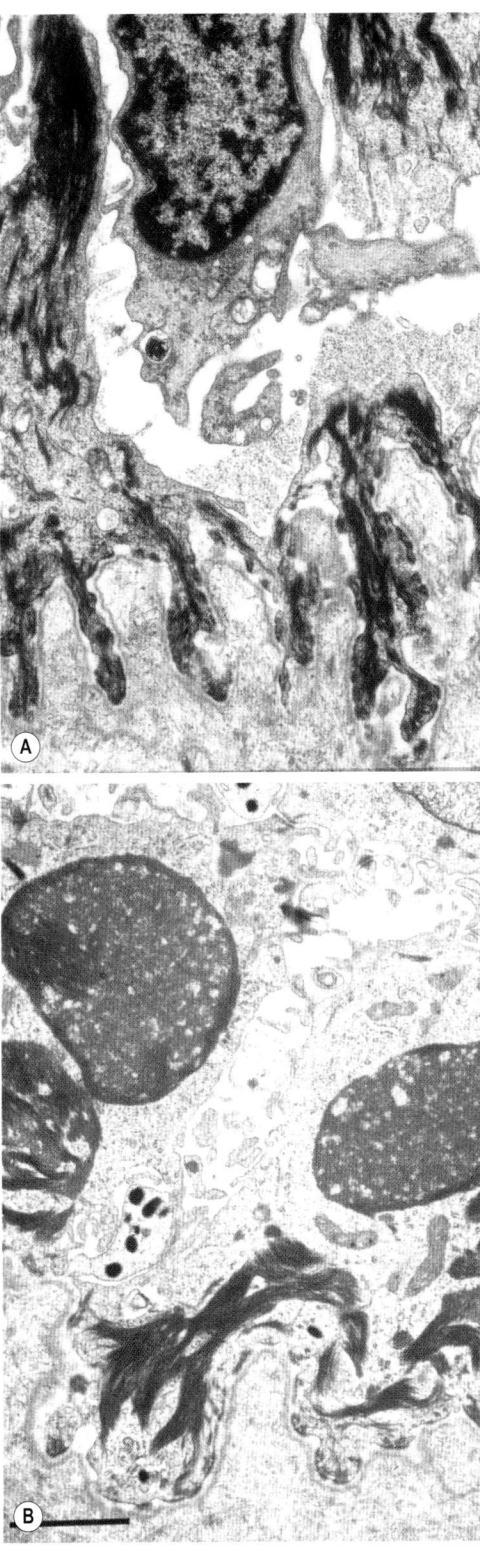

Fig. 4.29
Generalized severe EB simplex: (**A**) electron micrograph showing intrakeratinocyte splitting; (**B**) close-up view of tonofilament clumps. By courtesy of J.A. McGrath, MD, and R.A.J. Eady, MD, St John's Institute of Dermatology, London, UK.

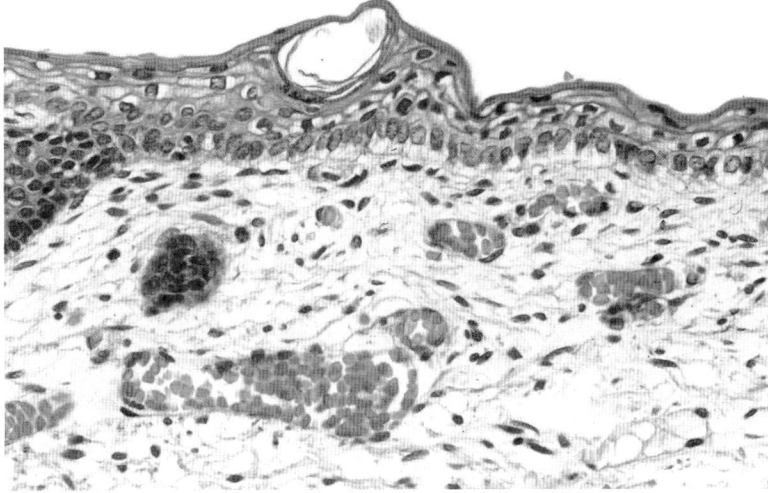

Fig. 4.30
EB simplex: the earliest histologic feature in the development of a blister is marked vacuolation of the basal keratinocytes, so-called cytolysis.

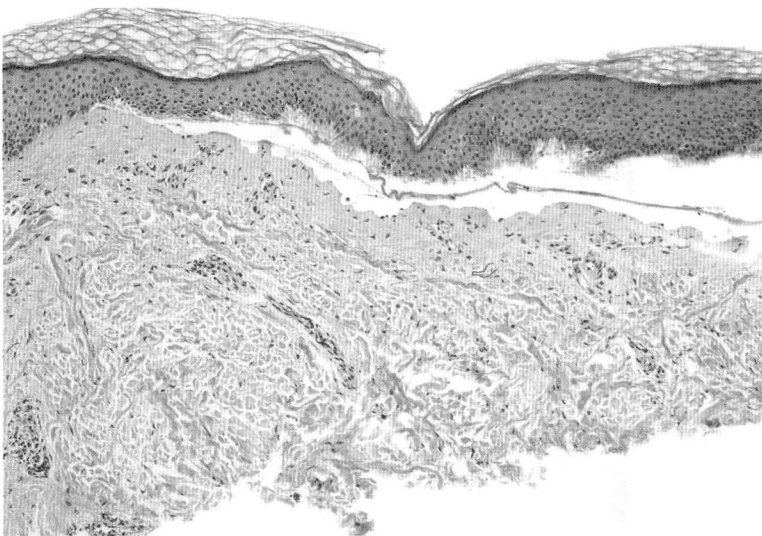

Fig. 4.31
EB simplex: old lesion; the features are those of a cell-free subepidermal blister and are not specific.

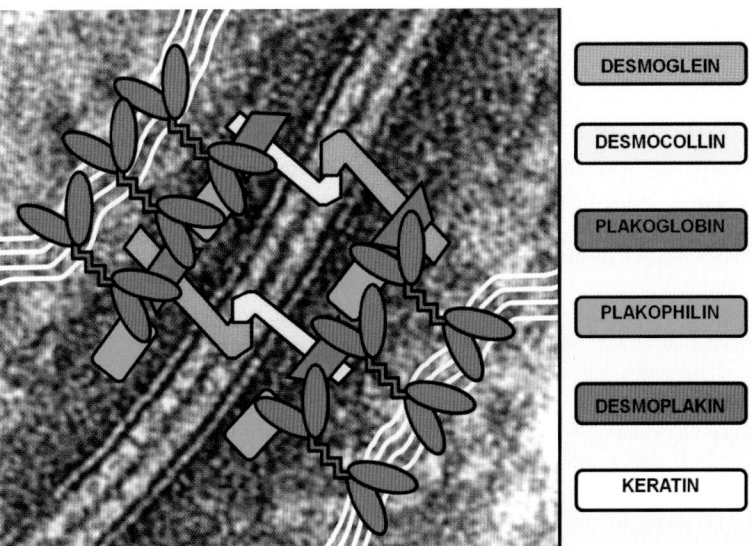

Fig. 4.32
Schematic representation of the transmembranous and intracellular components of desmosomes that provide a bridge between the keratin filament networks in adjacent keratinocytes.

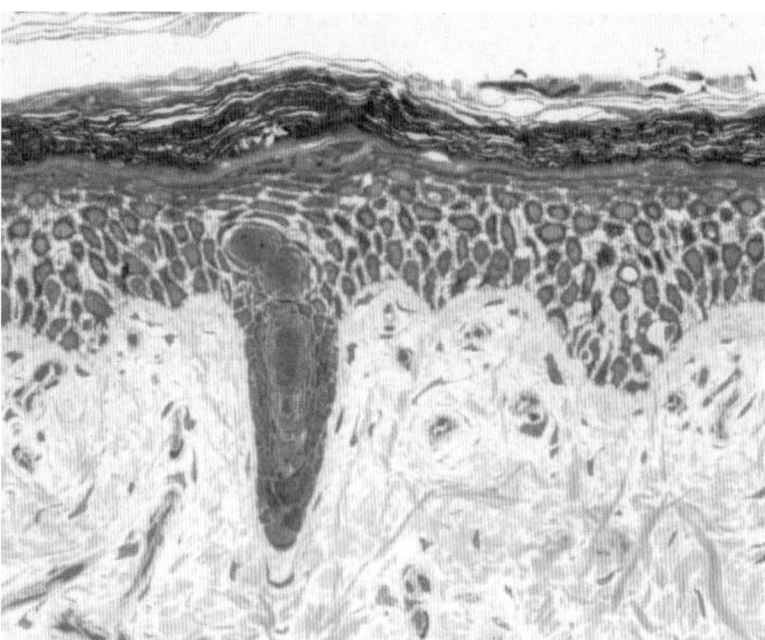

Fig. 4.33
Desmosomal EB simplex: pan-epidermal cell-cell detachment within the epidermis, here resulting from autosomal recessive mutations in desmoplakin.

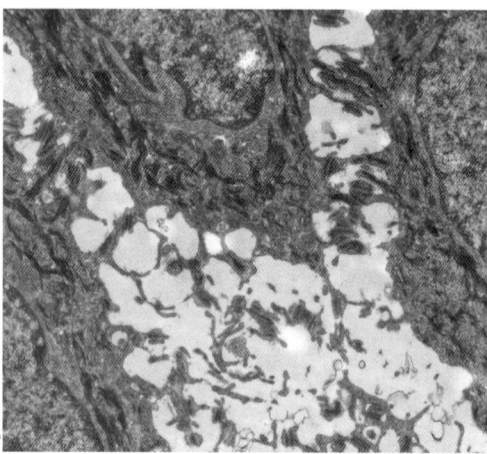

Fig. 4.34
Desmosomal EB simplex: the ultrastructural plane of cleavage leading to cell separation occurs through the intracellular desmosomal plaque consistent with the localization of the mutant desmoplakin in this case.

Desmoplakin: DSP

Desmoplakin is the major intracellular component of the desmosomal plaque.[44] Autosomal recessive mutations can result in devastating mucocutaneous skin fragility, notably in a severe acantholytic form of EB. Officially this condition is classified as a suprabasal form of EB simplex, although desmoplakin has a pan-epidermal expression and all layers of the epidermis show acantholysis (*Fig. 4.33*) with ultrastructural cleavage through the inner plaque of desmosomes (*Fig. 4.34*). Loss of desmoplakin expression in these cases leads to early death because of the profound skin loss and potential involvement of other organs, notably the heart. Other autosomal recessive mutations may result in woolly hair and keratoderma but no skin fragility, and autosomal dominant mutations in *DSP* can also give rise to striate palmoplantar keratoderma or arrhythmogenic cardiomyopathy.

Plakoglobin: JUP

Plakoglobin is an intracellular armadillo protein component of the desmosome.[45] Autosomal recessive mutations can cause an acantholytic form of EB simplex. These cases are similar to some *DSP* mutations – with the condition classified as a suprabasal form of EB simplex, but with pan-epidermal acantholysis and a poor prognosis. Autosomal recessive mutations have also been reported in individuals with Naxos disease – a combination of woolly hair, palmoplantar keratoderma, and cardiomyopathy; heterozygous carriers may also be prone to cardiac arrhythmias or heart failure. Other autosomal dominant mutations may cause cardiomyopathy.

Exophilin-5: EXPH5

EXPH5 encodes exophilin-5 (also known as Slac2-b), an effector protein of Rab GTPase Rab27B, which is thought to have an important role in intracellular vesicle trafficking along actin and tubulin networks, as well as in the transfer of vesicles to cell membranes.[46] Loss-of-function mutations in *EXPH5* lead to keratin filament clumping, cytolysis, acantholysis and increased cytoplasmic (perinuclear) vesicles. This form of inherited skin fragility has been classified as an autosomal recessive form of EB simplex.

Transglutaminase 5: TGM5

Autosomal recessive mutations in *TGM5* underlie acral peeling skin syndrome. Transglutaminase 5 is one of eight different transglutaminase enzymes expressed in the skin and has a distinct role in the formation of the cornified cell envelope.[47] The level of blister formation occurs above the granular layer, just below the stratum corneum. However, given the increased thickness of the stratum corneum in the palms and soles relative to other body sites, the clinical appearances often resemble the most common form of localized EB simplex and indeed may cause some clinical confusion, although both are included within the latest classification of EB (*Table 4.2*).

Plectin: PLEC

Plectin is an epidermal plakin protein, also found within the z-lines of striated muscle.[48] Autosomal recessive mutations in *PLEC* cause EB simplex associated with muscular dystrophy, which manifests as relatively minor skin blistering and progressive muscle weakness. Autosomal recessive mutations in *PLEC* can also cause skin blistering with pyloric atresia, or, occasionally, both manifestations, or sometimes just skin blistering. Autosomal dominant mutations in plectin may also occur in other forms of localized EB simplex (up to 10% of all cases), including one of the few eponymous variants in the current classification of EB, the Ogna subtype.

Dystonin epidermal isoform (BP230): DST-e

Autosomal recessive mutations in the epidermal isoform of dystonin, also known as the 230 kDa bullous pemphigoid antigen (BP230),[49] result in a relatively mild form of EB simplex. Ultrastructurally, there is a complete absence of the hemidesmosomal inner plaques – the sites at which keratin intermediate filaments anchor to the hemidesmosomes. Although dystonin isoforms have a wide tissue distribution, neurologic or cardiac involvement does not appear to be a clinical feature – predominantly acral skin blistering is the main abnormality.

α6β4 integrin: ITGA6, ITGB4

The α6β4 integrin is a cell adhesion dimer involved in hemidesmosome assembly and in epithelial–mesenchymal signaling.[50] Mutations in *ITGA6* or *ITGB4* (that encode the α6 and β4 integrin subunits, respectively) result in autosomal recessive junctional EB associated with pyloric atresia. The clinical severity of both the skin fragility and degree of gastric obstruction can vary, but surgical correction of the pylorus is usually required. More severe forms of the disease result from loss-of-function mutations on both alleles of *ITGA6* or *ITGB4* although missense mutations in certain critical cysteine residues may also have devastating clinical consequences. Other missense mutations can result in different forms of generalized intermediate junctional EB.

α3 integrin subunit: ITGA3

The α3 integrin subunit is a component of focal contacts at the dermal–epidermal junction, where it may dimerize with β1 integrin, and contribute to epithelial–mesenchymal signaling.[51] Autosomal recessive loss-of-function mutations in *ITGA3* have been reported in individuals with pulmonary inflammation and congenital nephrotic syndrome, reflecting the important role of α3 integrin in lung and kidney biology. Of note, skin blistering was relatively trivial and not always present. Prognosis is poor because of lung/kidney disease.

Kindlin-1: KIND1/FERMT1

Kindlin-1, also known as fermitin family homolog-1, is a component of focal contacts at the dermal–epidermal junction, and has a role in anchorage of the actin cytoskeleton and formation of a signaling platform via β1 integrin.[52] Autosomal recessive mutations in *KIND1/FERMT1* result in Kindler syndrome, a blistering genodermatosis that may resemble dystrophic EB in early life but with increasing age, the blistering often diminishes and new features of photosensitivity and poikiloderma (a combination of hyperpigmentation, hypopigmentation, telangiectases and skin atrophy), develop, mostly in sun-exposed areas. Individuals with Kindler syndrome also have an increased risk of squamous cell carcinoma.

Type XVII collagen: COL17A1

Type XVII collagen, also known as the 180 kDa bullous pemphigoid antigen, is a transmembranous protein located within the hemidesmosome and lamina lucida.[53] It is the antigenic target in the autoimmune blistering disease bullous pemphigoid, but loss-of-function mutations on both alleles result in generalized intermediate junctional EB (previously known as non-Herlitz or generalized atrophic benign EB). Some dominant missense mutations in type XVII collagen may result in defective dental enamel and occasionally skin fragility, but most pathogenic mutations in *COL17A1* are autosomal recessive.

Laminin-332: LAMA3, LAMB3, LAMC2

Laminin-332, previously known as laminin-5, is a heterotrimeric protein consisting of α3, β3, and γ2 laminin polypeptide chains located within the lamina lucida/lamina densa of the epidermal basement membrane.[54] Autosomal recessive mutations give rise to generalized severe (previously known as Herlitz junctional EB), generalized intermediate, or more localized forms of junctional EB (*Table 4.3*). The plane of tissue cleavage is through the lamina lucida at the dermal–epidermal junction (*Fig. 4.35*). Generalized severe disease is associated with widespread mucocutaneous fragility and a poor prognosis. Clinically less severe forms of junctional EB are usually associated with mutations that allow for some residual functional laminin-332 protein. Mutations in the *LAMA3A* isoform of the *LAMA3* gene are associated with laryngo-onycho-cutaneous syndrome, in which excessive granulation tissue can lead to laryngeal obstruction and blindness.

Type VII collagen: COL7A1

Type VII collagen is the major component of anchoring fibrils, adhesion complexes inserting into the dermal side of the lamina densa that are traversed by dermal collagen fibers to secure adhesion between the epidermis and dermis (*Fig. 4.36*).[55] Mutations in *COL7A1* underlie both autosomal dominant and autosomal recessive forms of dystrophic EB. Typically, loss-of-function mutations on both alleles of *COL7A1* underlie the generalized severe forms of recessive dystrophic EB in which anchoring fibrils are structurally defective or completely absent (*Fig. 4.37*). Poor wound healing results in chronic wounds, mutilating scar formation and an increased incidence of squamous cell carcinoma, often with multiple primary tumors over a few year period (*Figs 4.38* and *4.39*). Initial tumors may be well-differentiated or verrucous and difficult to distinguish from pseudoepitheliomatous hyperplasia, although successive tumors become progressively less well differentiated. However, there is a spectrum of clinical severity with less disruptive mutations giving rise to less severe intermediate or localized phenotypes (*Table 4.4*). Dominant dystrophic EB is usually clinically milder than recessive disease and most cases result from heterozygous missense mutations within the type VII collagen triple helix.

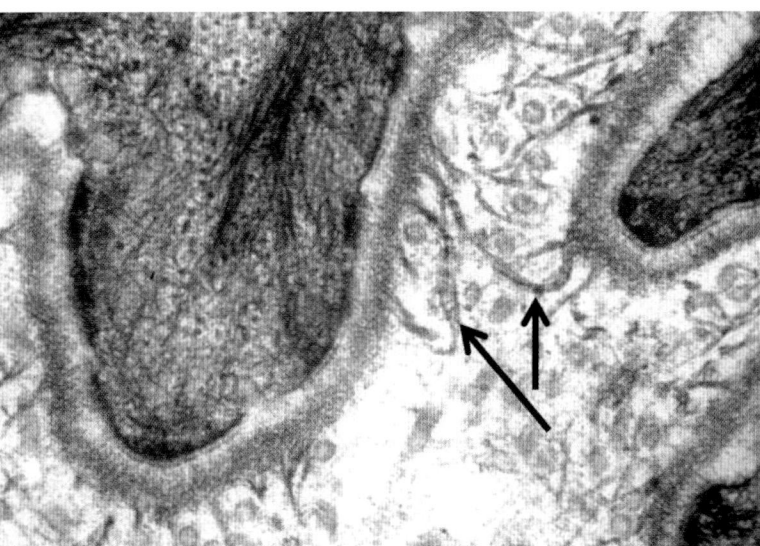

Fig. 4.36
Anchoring fibrils in normal skin: fibrillar structures with a fan-shaped appearance, central cross-banding and insertion into the lamina densa represent the ultrastructural hallmarks of anchoring fibrils in the superficial dermis (*arrows*).

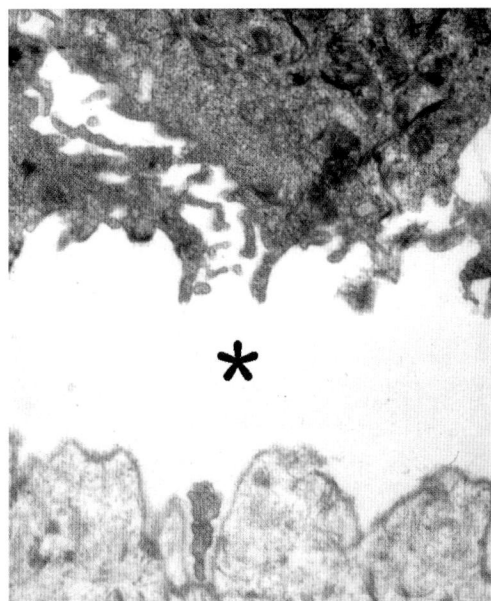

Fig. 4.35
Junctional EB: the level of blister formation at the dermal–epidermal junction is through the lamina lucida (*asterisk*).

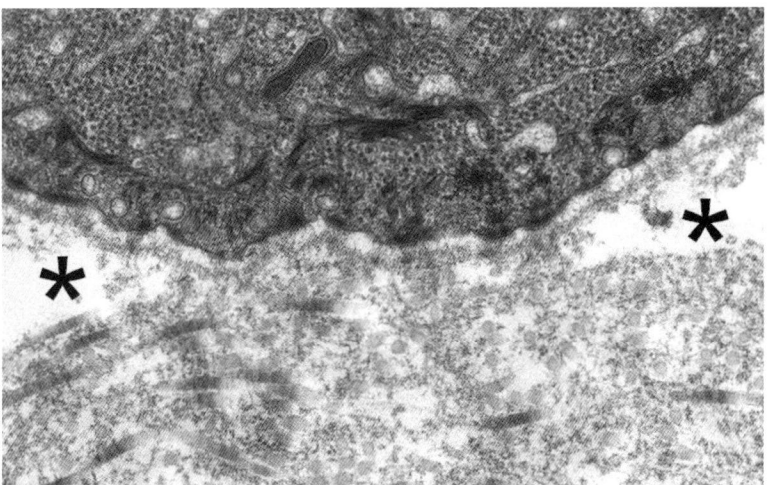

Fig. 4.37
Generalized severe recessive dystrophic EB: complete absence of anchoring fibrils below the lamina densa with onset of sub-lamina densa blistering (*asterisks*).

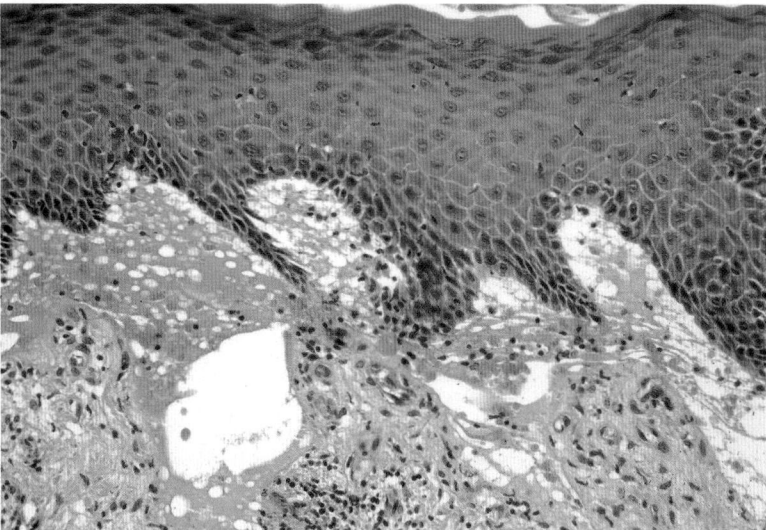

Fig. 4.38
Generalized severe recessive dystrophic EB: in addition to obvious subepidermal blistering there is dermal scarring and chronic inflammation.

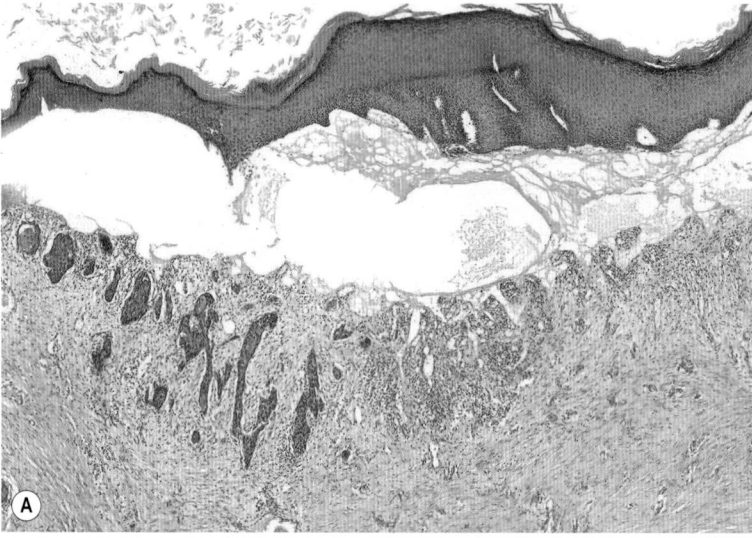

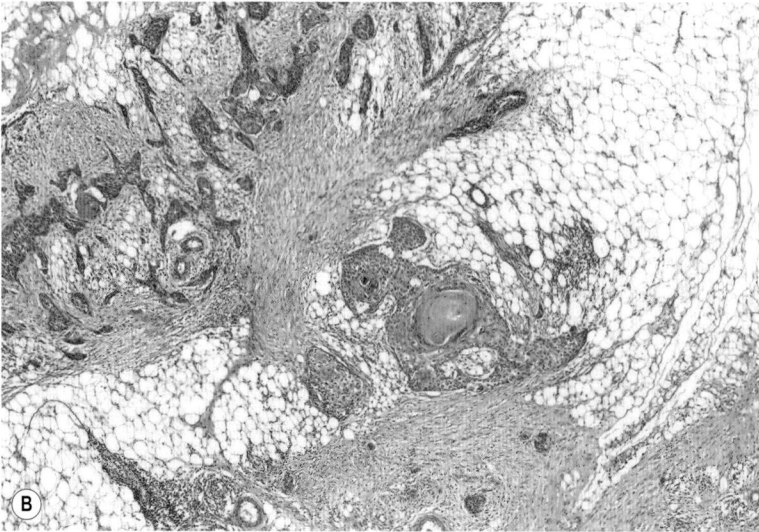

Fig. 4.39
(**A**, **B**) Generalized severe recessive dystrophic EB: biopsy from the forearm of a 30-year-old patient showing a cell-free subepidermal blister. In addition, a well-differentiated squamous cell carcinoma extends into the subcutaneous fat.

Bullous pemphigoid

Clinical features

Bullous pemphigoid is not a single disease entity. Rather, there are many subtypes, which have been classified into primary cutaneous and mucosal variants and into generalized and localized forms (*Fig. 4.40*).[1-4] Bullous pemphigoid (BP) is the most frequently encountered autoimmune bullous dermatosis with an annual incidence of 6.6 new cases per 1 million of the population.[5,6]

Generalized cutaneous pemphigoid

Any age group may be affected, but the generalized variant demonstrates a predilection for the later years of life, showing a maximum incidence in the seventh decade and over. Rarely, however, children and even infants may be affected.[7,8] The disease is associated with a worldwide distribution and shows no racial propensity. There are no significant human leukocyte antigen (HLA) associations and the sex incidence is approximately equal.

Prodromal events are numerous and include erythematous, urticarial and, rarely, eczematous phases.[9,10] Erythroderma, either preceding the bullous phase or occurring simultaneously, is a very rare manifestation (erythrodermic pemphigoid).[11,12] Similarly, patients may present with a history of generalized pruritus in the absence of visible skin lesions (pruritic pemphigoid). In such circumstances, immunofluorescence investigations are essential to establish the correct diagnosis.[13]

The characteristic lesions of established disease are tense and often intact blisters arising on normal or erythematous skin (*Figs 4.41* and *4.42*).

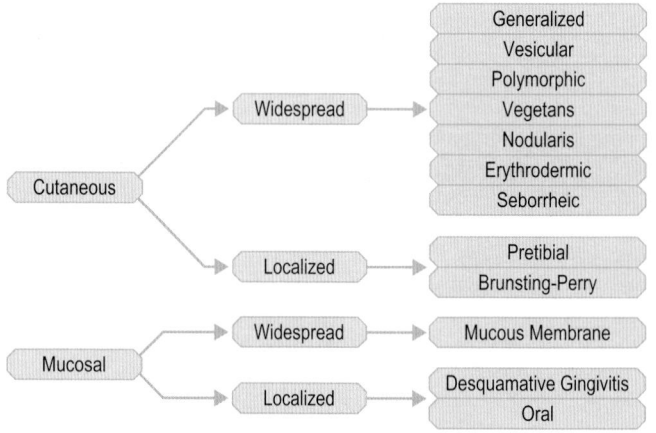

Fig. 4.40
Bullous pemphigoid: classification.

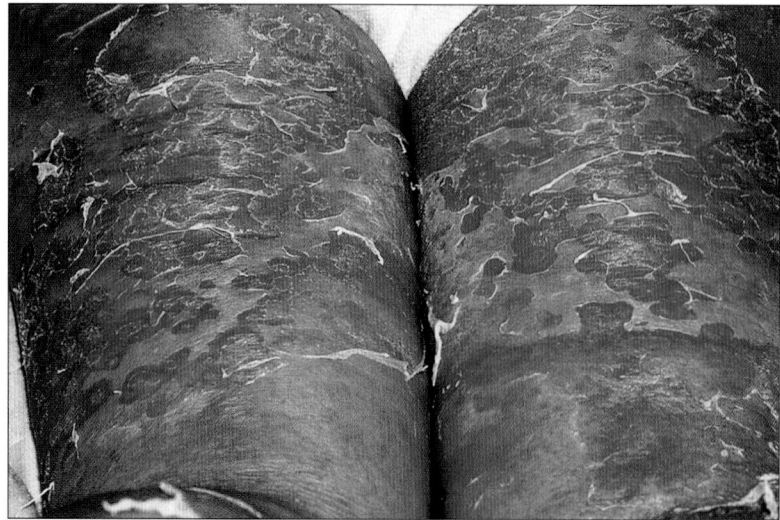

Fig. 4.41
Erythrodermic BP: blistering has developed against a background of generalized erythroderma. By courtesy of the Institute of Dermatology, London, UK.

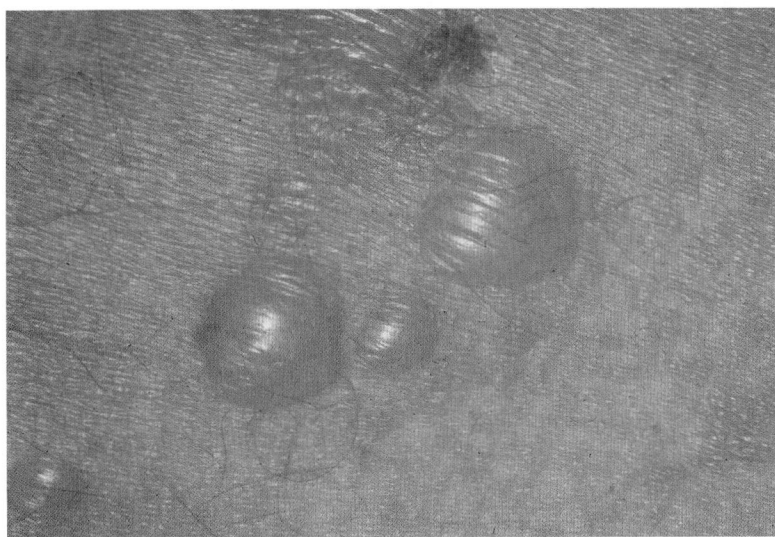

Fig. 4.42
BP: early tense blister arising on an erythematous base. By courtesy of the Institute of Dermatology, London, UK.

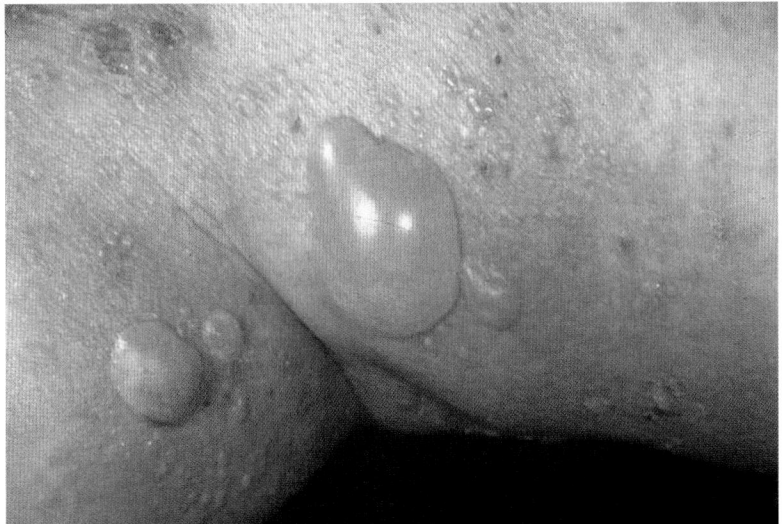

Fig. 4.43
BP: tense, dome-shaped blisters. The flexures are typically affected. By courtesy of the Institute of Dermatology, London, UK.

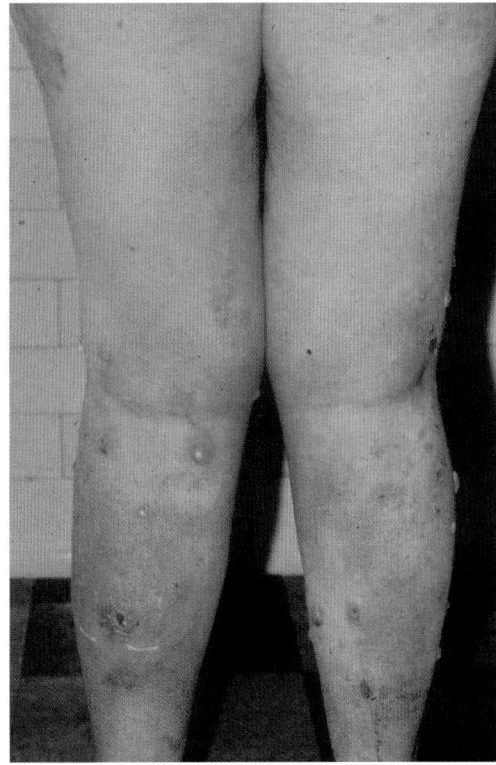

Fig. 4.44
BP: widespread, fluid-filled, hemorrhagic blisters on the arms of an elderly female. By courtesy of the late M. Beare, MD, Royal Victoria Hospital, Belfast, N. Ireland.

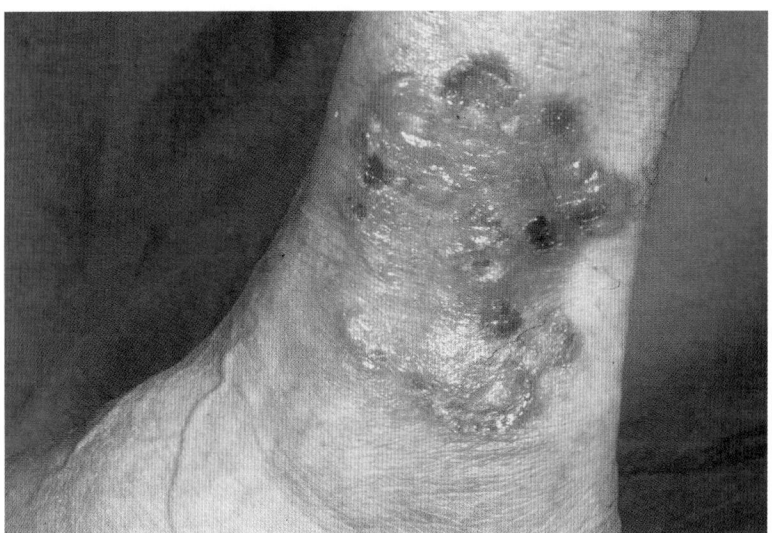

Fig. 4.45
BP: new blisters arising at the edge of a healing lesion ('cluster of jewels' sign). Although typically seen in childhood linear IgA disease, this is sometimes a feature of bullous pemphigoid. By courtesy of R.A. Marsden, MD, St George's Hospital, London, UK.

They may measure up to several centimeters in diameter and are typically dome-shaped (*Fig. 4.43*). Often, they contain clear or bloodstained fluid. Any area of the body may be affected, but the blisters are most commonly located about the lower abdomen, the inner aspect of the thighs and on the flexural surfaces of the forearms, the axillae, and groin (*Fig. 4.44*).[14] Grouping of lesions as seen in dermatitis herpetiformis is not usually a feature and symmetry is characteristically absent. A 'cluster of jewels' appearance of new blisters arising at the edge of resolving lesions as seen in linear IgA disease may, however, occasionally be a feature of bullous pemphigoid (*Fig. 4.45*).[15] The lesions are often pruritic and a burning sensation is sometimes a feature. Nikolsky sign is usually negative. In contrast to mucous membrane pemphigoid, generalized bullous pemphigoid is not associated with scarring.

Reported mucosal involvement (frequently as ulcers) is highly variable, ranging from 8% to 58%.[16–18] In a series of 115 patients, 24% had oral involvement and 7% had genital lesions.[18] Lesions are found most often on the palate, the cheeks, lips, and tongue (*Fig. 4.46*). Other sites less commonly involved include mucosae of the nose, pharynx, conjunctiva and, rarely, the urethra and vulva (see below) (*Fig. 4.47*).[17] In contrast to mucous membrane pemphigoid, mucosal involvement in generalized bullous pemphigoid is not associated with scarring.

Although bullous pemphigoid has been reported in association with a variety of internal malignancies, this may just be coincidental, merely reflecting the age incidence of these two diseases.[19] In a series of almost 500 patients from Sweden, no increased incidence of cancer was observed.[20] Other studies, however, have shown that there may be a positive correlation between internal malignancy and seronegative bullous pemphigoid patients.[21] An association with neurological and psychiatric disorders, particularly multiple sclerosis and schizophrenia, has been demonstrated.[22]

Generalized bullous pemphigoid is a serious condition with a significant mortality ranging from 10% to 20%.[1] Since the advent of steroid therapy and immunosuppressive agents, patients are more at risk of developing

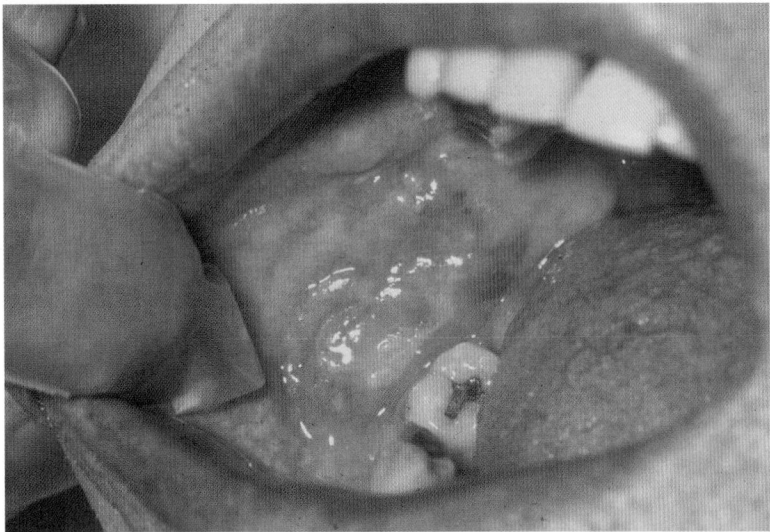

Fig. 4.46
BP: oral erosions are an occasional finding. Intact blisters are rare. By courtesy of
R.A. Marsden, MD, St George's Hospital, London, UK.

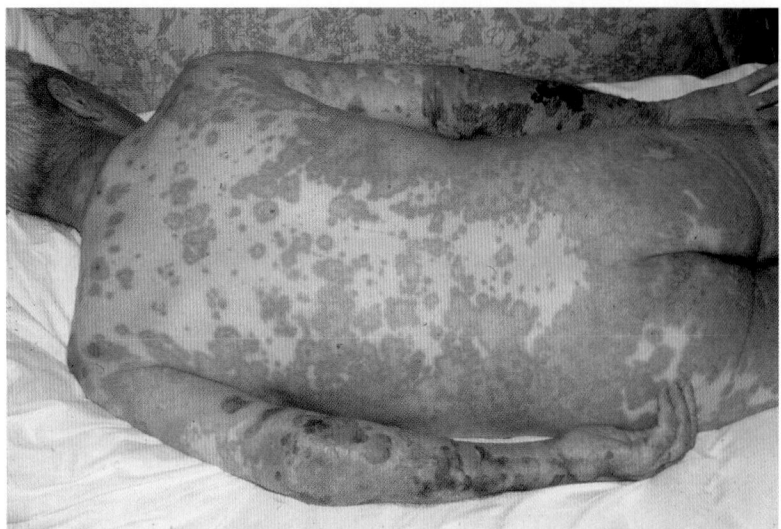

Fig. 4.48
Bullous pemphigoid: occasionally erythematous urticarial lesions may be the
presenting feature. Blisters may not evolve until several weeks later. By courtesy
of R.A. Marsden, MD, St George's Hospital, London, UK.

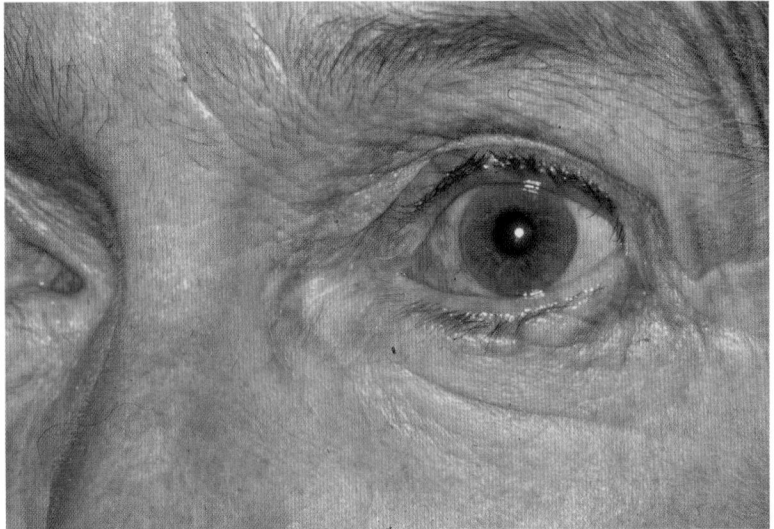

Fig. 4.47
BP: conjunctival injection is present. By courtesy of R.A. Marsden, MD, St
George's Hospital, London, UK.

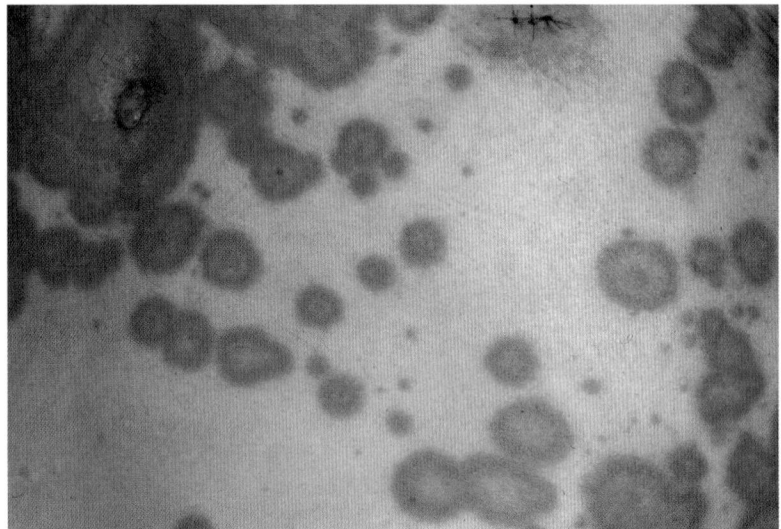

Fig. 4.49
Bullous pemphigoid: close up view. By courtesy of R.A. Marsden, MD, St
George's Hospital, London, UK.

severe iatrogenic disorders than of dying from their disease.[23] Morbidity
from this disease may be related more to the age and general state of health
of the patient than to the severity of blistering.[24] Although mortality from
the disease is low, there has been a reported increase in mortality in the last
20 years of the twentieth century.[25]

Clinical variants of generalized pemphigoid

Urticarial bullous pemphigoid presents with large persistent erythematous
plaques, which sometimes display an annular or gyrate peripheral component (Figs 4.48 and 4.49).[1] Rarely, small vesicles are also to be found.

Vesicular pemphigoid is a rare clinical variant in which the cutaneous
manifestations show a striking overlap with dermatitis herpetiformis.[26-29]
Patients present with numerous small tense vesicles that may be symmetrical,
intensely pruritic, and therefore associated with conspicuous excoriation.

Polymorphic pemphigoid is a somewhat confusing entity, which is
similar to vesicular pemphigoid, but probably shows overlap with linear
IgA disease.[30-32] Patients present with burning and itching lesions predominantly affecting the extensor aspects of the limbs, back, and buttocks. Symmetry, grouping, and a polymorphic clinical appearance of papules, vesicles,
and variably sized bullae, emphasize a similarity to dermatitis herpetiformis.

It has been suggested that polymorphic pemphigoid is not an entity sui
generis, but represents a potpourri of conditions including vesicular pemphigoid, linear IgA disease, and mixed subepidermal bullous disease in which
patients show both linear IgG and linear IgA or dermal papillary granular
IgA on direct immunofluorescence.[31]

Pemphigoid vegetans is an exceedingly rare vegetative intertriginous
variant that may be associated with chronic inflammatory bowel disease.[33-40]
Fewer than 10 cases have been documented. Patients present with vegetative, crusted, purulent, and sometimes eroded lesions in the groin, axillae,
neck, hands, eyelids, inframammary, and perioral regions (Fig. 4.50). Vesicles and bullae may also be evident. Scarring has been described.[40] The
etiology of the vegetative lesions is unknown.

Seborrheic pemphigoid is a variant in which the clinical features are suggestive of pemphigus erythematosus.[32]

Pemphigoid nodularis represents the extremely rare association of
lesions of bullous pemphigoid with intensely pruritic papules and nodules
of nodular prurigo predominantly affecting the trunk and extremities (Fig.
4.51).[41-43] The association of pemphigoid nodularis with immune dysregulation, polyendocrinopathy, enteropathy, and X-linked (IPEX) syndrome is the
subject of a single case report.[44]

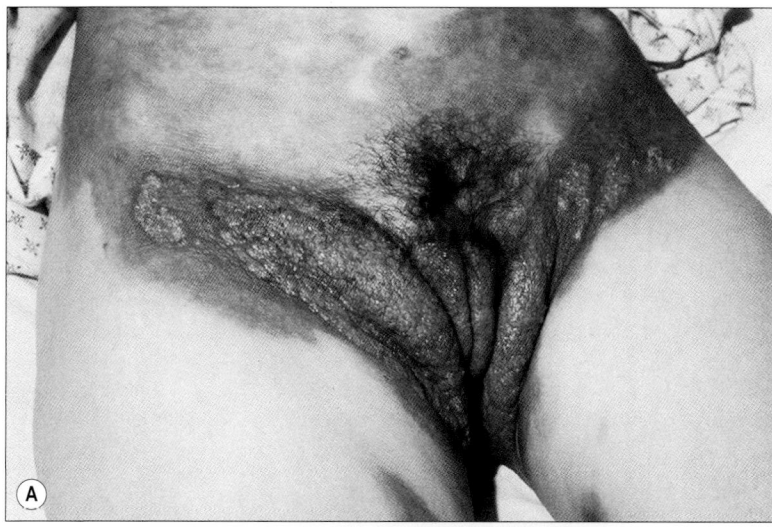

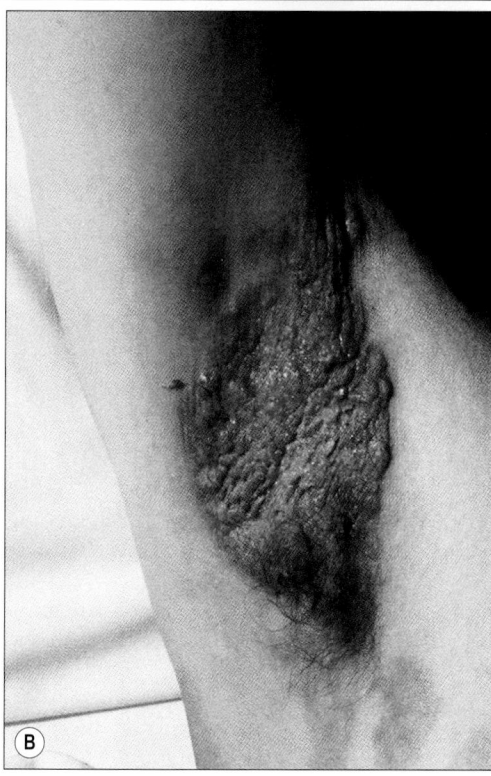

Fig. 4.50
(**A**, **B**) Pemphigoid vegetans: presentation as verrucous lesions in the flexures may result in considerable diagnostic difficulties. By courtesy of R.K. Winkelmann, MD, The Mayo Clinic, Scottsdale, Arizona, USA.

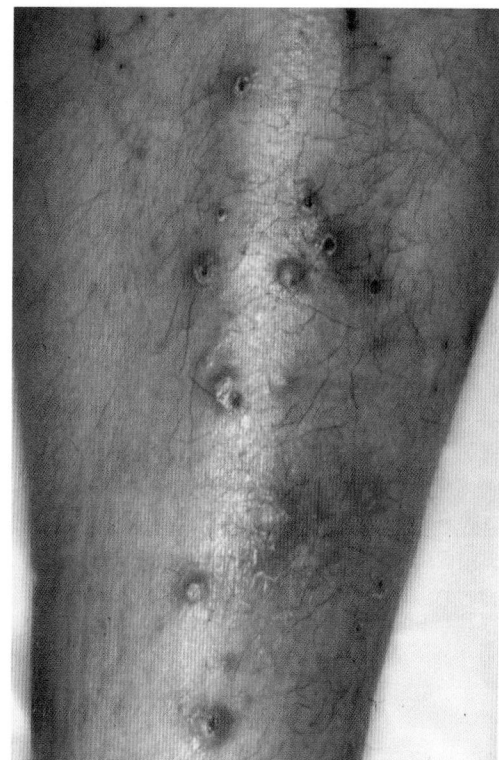

Fig. 4.51
Pemphigoid nodularis: in addition to bullous lesions, this patient also developed these pruritic nodules. By courtesy of H. Shimizu, MD, Keio University School of Medicine, Tokyo, Japan.

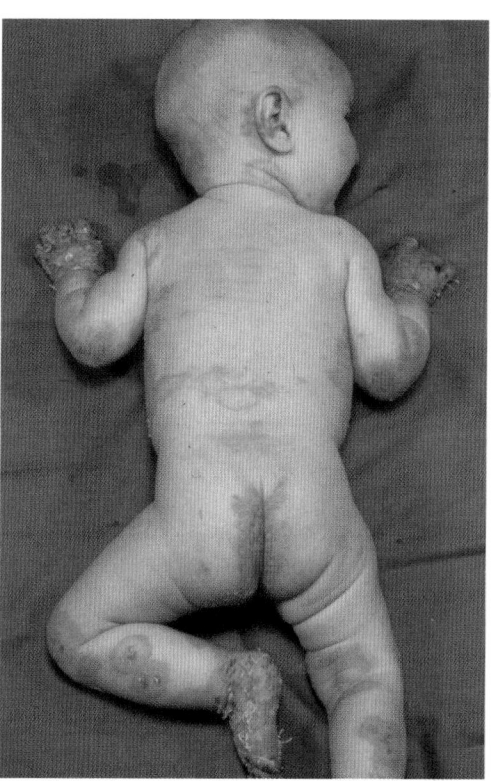

Fig. 4.52
Childhood BP: very rarely this disease affects young children and infants. There is a widespread distribution of bullae, which characteristically arise on an erythematous base. By courtesy of R.A. Marsden, MD, St George's Hospital, London, UK.

Exceptionally, patients may show immunofluorescent evidence of bullous pemphigoid in the absence of clinical blistering.[43] The cause of this unusual phenomenon is unknown, although in some patients at least, chronic scratching probably damages the basement membrane region with exposure of bullous pemphigoid antigens. There is a female predilection (2:1).[43] The age range of this variant extends from 24 to 80 years but, as with classical bullous pemphigoid, the majority of patients are elderly.

Dyshidrosiform pemphigoid is a rare variant of pemphigoid in which patients develop 1–2-mm, tense 'sago-grain-like' vesicles on the palms and soles resembling dyshidrosiform dermatitis (pompholyx).[45–51] Lesions may be localized, or precede or occur simultaneously with generalized disease. Overlap with pemphigoid nodularis has been described.[52]

Childhood pemphigoid exhibits lesions that are similar to their adult counterparts, but there is some tendency for lesions to be localized around the face, lower trunk, thighs, and genitalia, reminiscent of linear IgA disease in childhood (*Fig. 4.52*).[7,8,53–62] Similarly, a 'cluster of jewels' appearance is sometimes evident.[7] Palmar, plantar, and oral lesions are often present

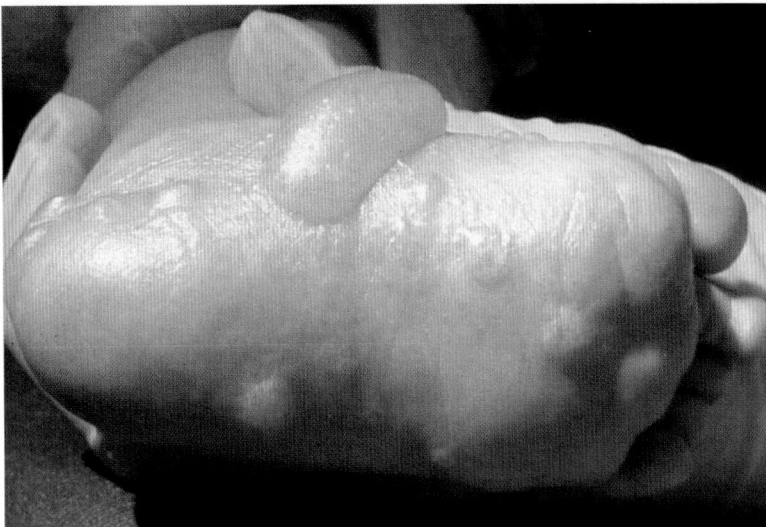

Fig. 4.53
Childhood BP: plantar involvement is sometimes the only site of disease. By courtesy of M. Liang, MD, The Children's Hospital, Boston, USA.

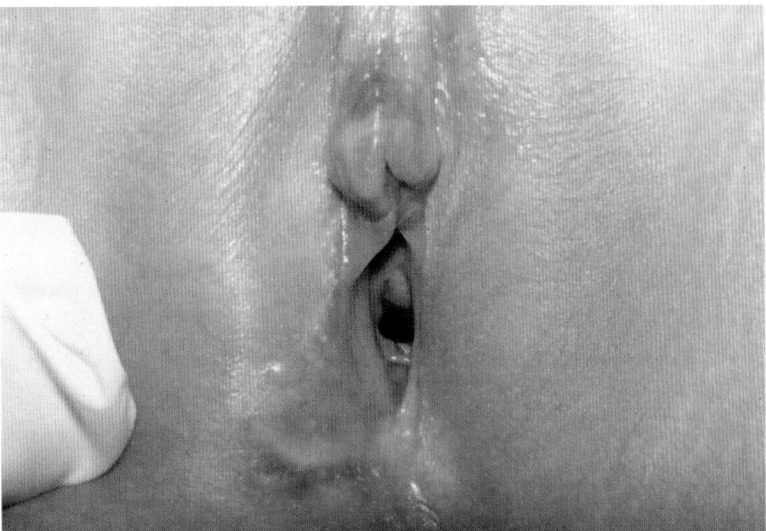

Fig. 4.54
Childhood BP: note the perineal scarring and isolated blister. By courtesy of M. Liang, MD, The Children's Hospital, Boston, USA.

and may be the sole site of involvement in infants (*Fig. 4.53*). The mucous membranes may be affected, but scarring is absent. A number of children with primary localized penile and vulval lesions have also been described (*Fig. 4.54*).[48,49,60,63,64] This is of particular clinical importance since it may be mistaken for evidence of sexual abuse. Childhood pemphigoid has a good prognosis and, as in adults, is usually self-limiting. Although the etiology is generally unknown, in some infant cases there appears to be a relationship to prior vaccination or immunization.[60,65] Presentation during infancy is often severe, with blisters on the hands and feet.[66] In this age group, the levels of anti-BP180 NC16A autoantibodies detected by ELISA are significantly higher than in adults with BP.[66] Differences between childhood and infant cases have been described, but the importance of further subdividing this group is unclear.[65]

Localized cutaneous pemphigoid

Although classical bullous pemphigoid not uncommonly presents initially as localized lesions that after a few months become generalized, occasional patients present with localized blisters that do not subsequently disseminate (localized bullous pemphigoid).[67] Traditionally, this group has been subdivided into two variants:

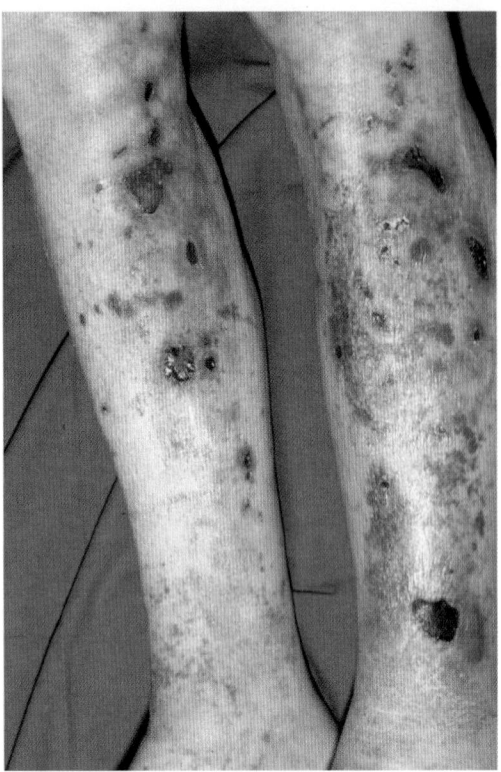

Fig. 4.55
Localized pemphigoid, nonscarring variant: lesions are found particularly on the lower legs of females. The prognosis is usually good, but occasionally the condition can become generalized. By courtesy of R.A. Marsden, MD, St George's Hospital, London, UK.

- Brunsting-Perry pemphigoid – not a true variant of bullous pemphigoid – predominantly affects the head and neck and is associated with scarring.[68]
- Localized cutaneous nonscarring bullous pemphigoid (Eberhartinger, and Niebauer variant)[69] predominantly affects the lower legs (in particular the pretibial region) of females.

The former variant is considered in the section on mucous membrane pemphigoid. Although the latter nonscarring cutaneous form particularly affects the lower legs (*Fig. 4.55*), it may also present at a variety of other sites including forearms and hands, breasts, chest, buttocks, and umbilicus. Lesions in localized bullous pemphigoid may be related to trauma.[69] It shows a peak incidence in the sixth decade. As with generalized bullous pemphigoid, patients present with tense, sometimes hemorrhagic, bullae that arise on normal or erythematous-appearing skin. Localized cutaneous nonscarring bullous pemphigoid is generally associated with a good prognosis.[69]

Rare patients present with localized bullous pemphigoid at the site of trauma without much evidence of disease elsewhere.[70]

Mucosal pemphigoid/desquamative gingivitis

Localized oral pemphigoid is described as a variant of desquamative gingivitis.[71–73] The latter, of multifactorial etiology by definition, affects the marginal and attached gingivae. It shows a female predominance (9:1) and presents most frequently in the middle aged. Desquamative gingivitis may also be a manifestation of lichen planus and pemphigus.[42] The diagnosis of localized oral pemphigoid depends upon the presence of a linear band of immunoreactants at the epithelial basement membrane region on direct immunofluorescence.[71] Clinical features include erythema, edema, erosions, and ulcers.[74] The oral lesions are nonscarring. Bullous pemphigoid-associated desquamative gingivitis may remain confined to the gingiva (the localized oral pemphigoid type), but approximately an equal proportion of patients develop full-blown cutaneous pemphigoid (*Fig. 4.56*).[71]

Pathogenesis and histologic features

The histologic features of bullous pemphigoid depend to some extent upon the age of the lesion biopsied. Early erythematous and urticarial lesions most

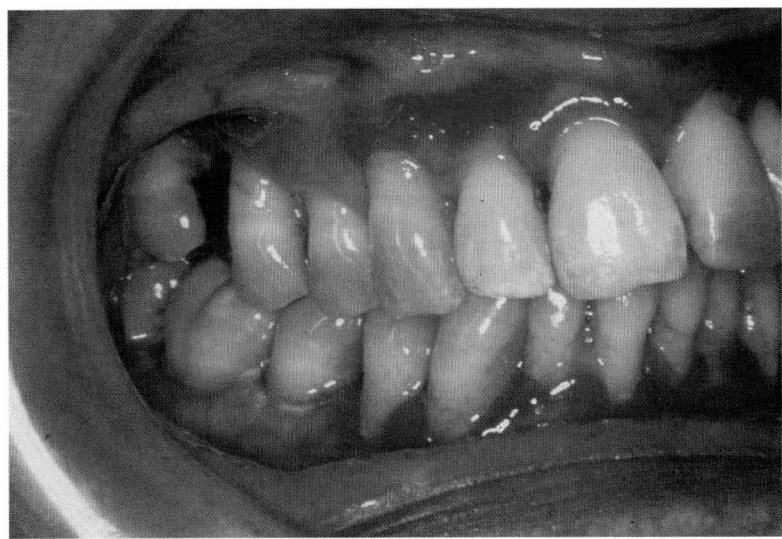

Fig. 4.56
Desquamative gingivitis: note the intense gingival erythema and retraction. Such features may also be seen in mucous membrane pemphigoid and pemphigus. By courtesy of P. Morgan, FRCPath, London, UK.

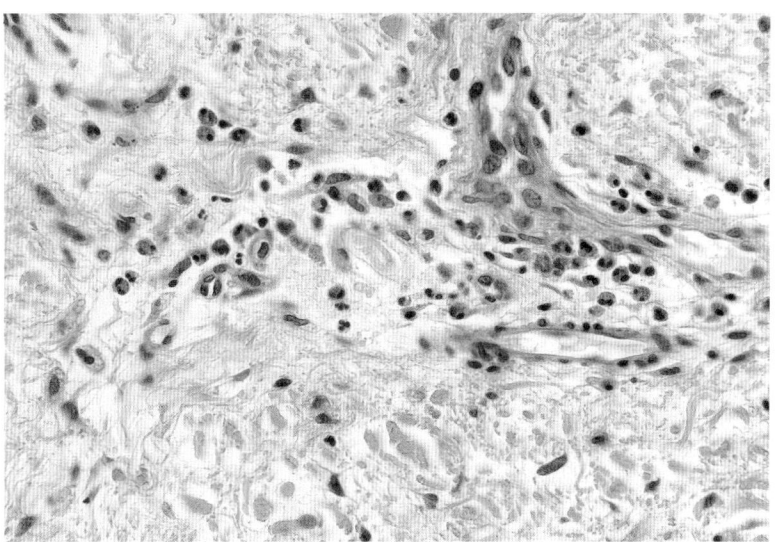

Fig. 4.58
Prebullous pemphigoid: there are numerous eosinophils.

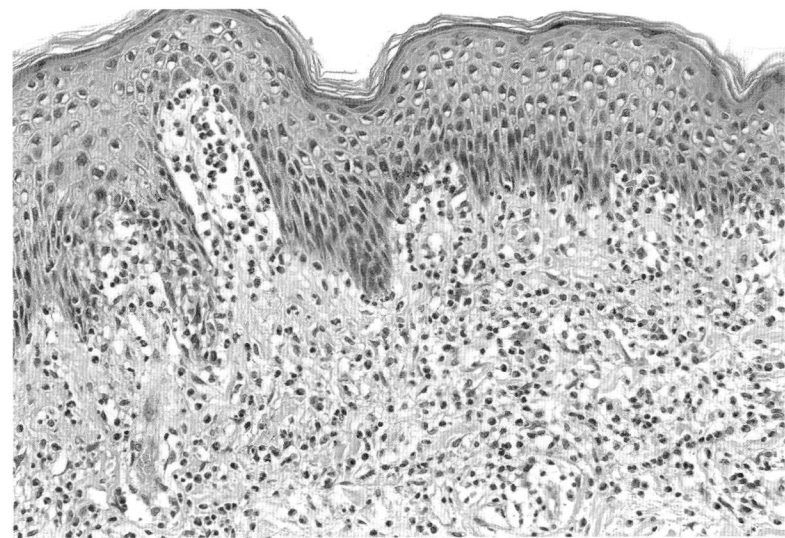

Fig. 4.57
Prebullous pemphigoid: there is upper dermal edema and a perivascular lymphohistiocytic infiltrate with conspicuous eosinophils.

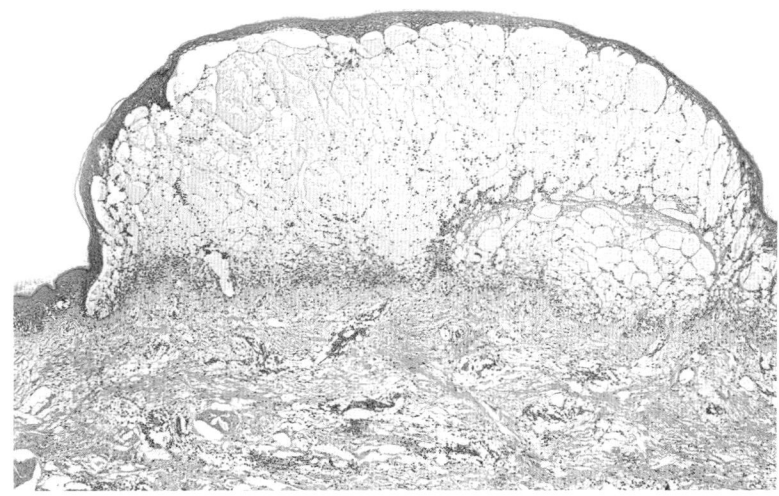

Fig. 4.59
BP: an established lesion showing a subepidermal tense, dome-shaped blister containing edema fluid, fibrin, and inflammatory cells.

often show upper dermal edema associated with a perivascular lymphohistiocytic infiltrate accompanied by usually conspicuous eosinophils (*Figs 4.57* and *4.58*). Eosinophilic spongiosis is sometimes evident and occasionally, if eosinophils are present in sufficient numbers, flame figures may be a feature. Mild interface changes characterized by basal cell hydropic degeneration can be seen in early or prodromal lesions.

If the biopsy is taken from an established blister, the changes are most often those of an inflammatory (cell-rich) variant.[75] The blister, which is subepidermal, is typically unilocular and covered by attenuated epithelium (*Fig. 4.59*). In early lesions the roof epidermis may appear unaffected or show occasional to even confluent necrotic basal keratinocytes. The blister contents include coagulated serum, fibrin strands, and large numbers of inflammatory cells including conspicuous eosinophils (*Fig. 4.60*). Variable numbers of neutrophils may be present. In cases in which an old lesion is biopsied the blister may appear at least focally, at an intraepidermal level due to re-epithelization.

A typical finding in bullous pemphigoid is retention of the dermal papillary outline (festooning) which project like sentries into the vesicle cavity (*Fig. 4.61*). The underlying dermis is inflamed and usually shows widespread severe edema. An infiltrate of eosinophils and mononuclears surrounds the

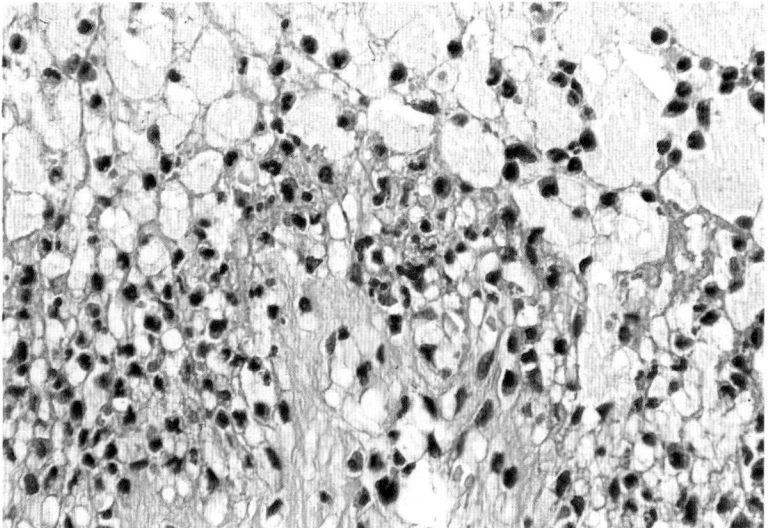

Fig. 4.60
BP: the blister cavity contains large numbers of eosinophils.

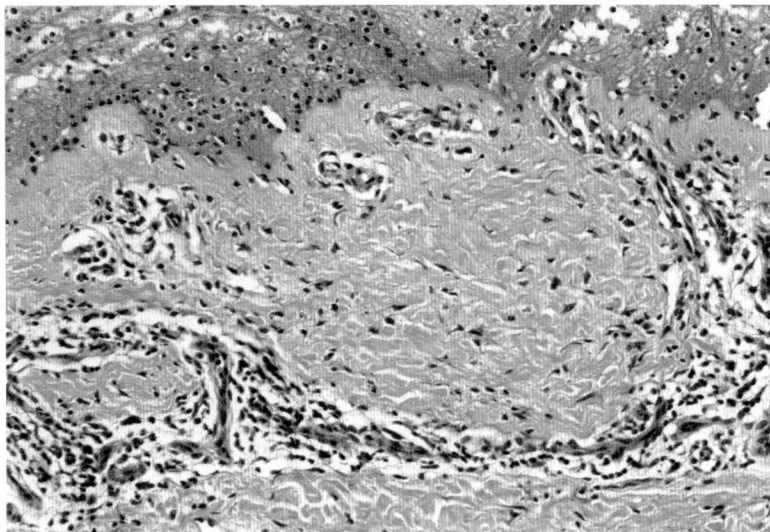

Fig. 4.61
BP: preservation of the dermal papillary outline (festooning) is a characteristic feature.

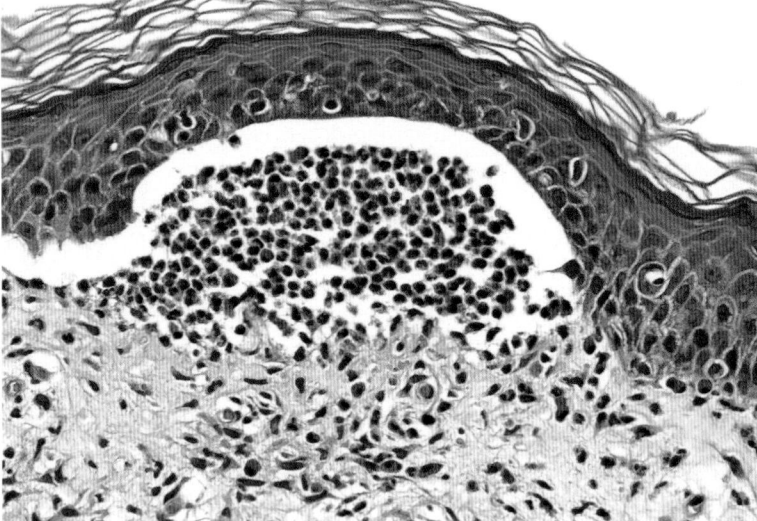

Fig. 4.62
BP: the presence of eosinophil microabscesses in the dermal papillae is a useful although rare diagnostic marker.

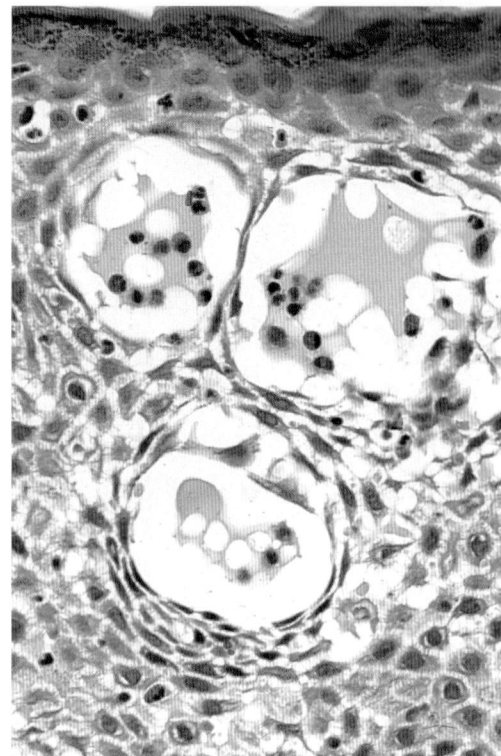

Fig. 4.63
BP: eosinophilic spongiosis is sometimes seen in the epidermis adjacent to the blister.

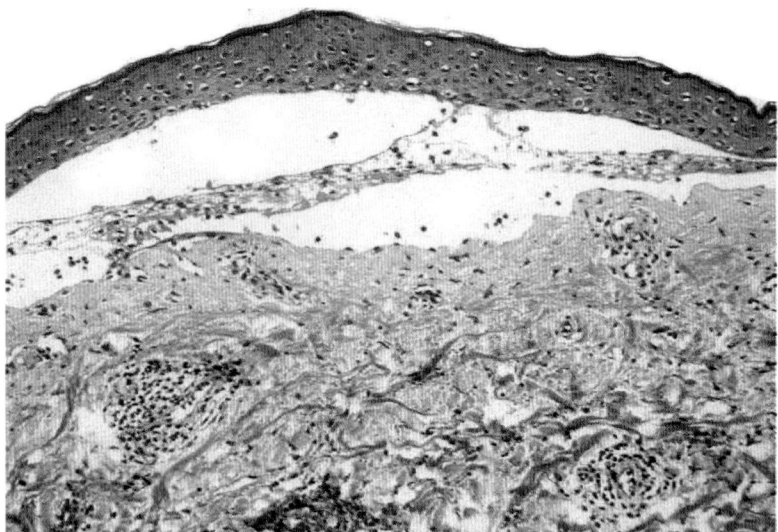

Fig. 4.64
Cell-poor pemphigoid: this is a very uncommon variant and is most often seen if a very early lesion is sampled. The blister contains only a little edema fluid and there is a light chronic inflammatory cell infiltrate in the superficial dermis.

blood vessels and extends between the adjacent collagen bundles. Leukocytoclasis is not seen and features of vasculitis are absent. The adjacent papillary dermis is often edematous and, very occasionally, eosinophil microabscesses are a feature (*Fig. 4.62*). Exceptionally rarely, neutrophil microabscesses may be seen (see vesicular pemphigoid), raising diagnostic confusion with dermatitis herpetiformis. Eosinophilic spongiosis is also sometimes evident in the adjacent epidermis (*Fig. 4.63*).[76]

Cell-poor (noninflammatory) features are occasionally seen if biopsies are taken from lesions arising on noninflamed skin (*Fig. 4.64*). Because inflammatory cells are sparse or, exceptionally, even absent in such cases, there may be considerable problems with the differential diagnosis, particularly if adequate clinical information and immunofluorescence findings are not available.

Vesicular/polymorphic pemphigoid is characterized by subepidermal vesicles with features suggesting either bullous pemphigoid or dermatitis herpetiformis or both (*Fig. 4.65*). Neutrophil dermal papillary microabscesses, which are often regarded as pathognomonic of dermatitis herpetiformis, may be seen in this variant (*Fig. 4.66*).

Pemphigoid vegetans is characterized by acanthosis, often with pseudoepitheliomatous hyperplasia, papillary dermal edema with subepidermal clefting or frank vesicle formation and an inflammatory cell infiltrate of eosinophils, lymphocytes, histiocytes, and occasional neutrophils.

Pemphigoid nodularis exhibits pruriginous lesions, which are characterized by hyperkeratosis and acanthosis, and which may amount to pseudoepitheliomatous hyperplasia and dermal fibrosis (*Fig. 4.67*). In the dermis, a perivascular infiltrate of lymphocytes and eosinophils is present. The blisters show typical features of bullous pemphigoid (*Fig. 4.68*).

Localized nonscarring (pretibial) bullous pemphigoid usually shows the histology of cell-rich bullous pemphigoid. Localized oral pemphigoid is typified by a subepithelial vesicle (when present) and cannot be distinguished histologically from oral involvement in mucous membrane pemphigoid (see below).

Ultrastructurally, in early lesions of bullous pemphigoid, the dermal–epidermal cleavage is seen to have developed between the plasma membrane of the basal keratinocyte and the lamina densa, through the lamina lucida.[77]

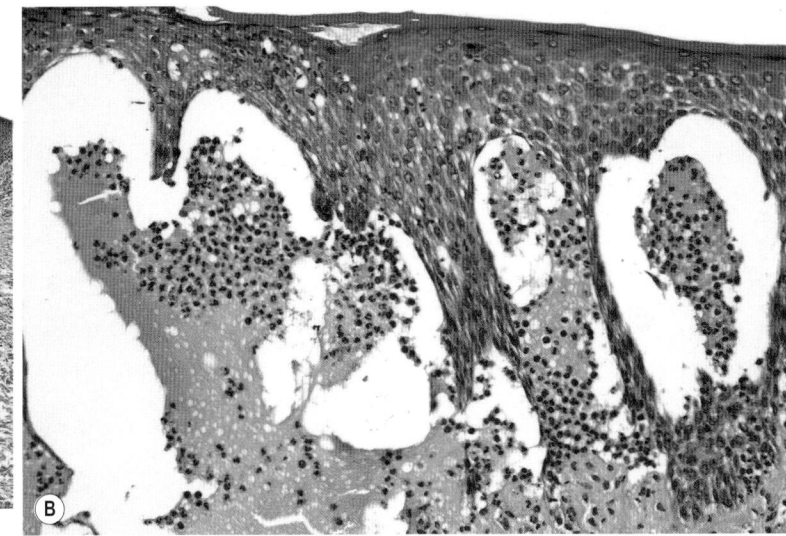

Fig. 4.65
Vesicular pemphigoid: (**A**) low-power view showing a multilocular blister; (**B**) the blister contains a neutrophil-rich infiltrate.

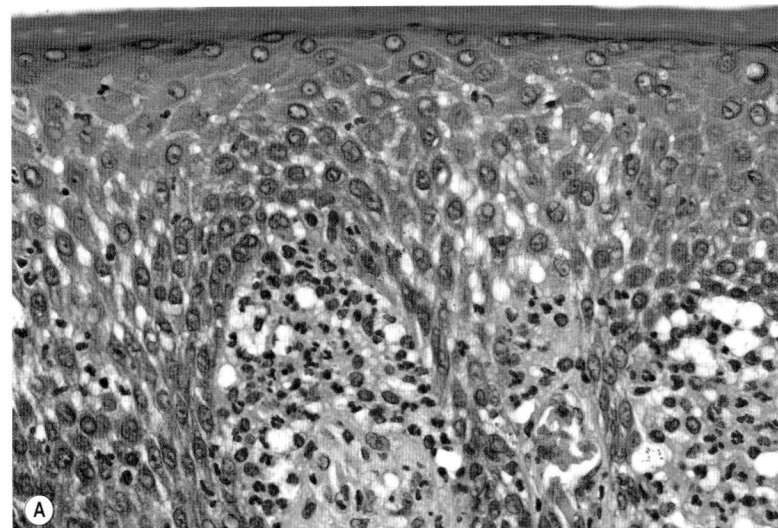
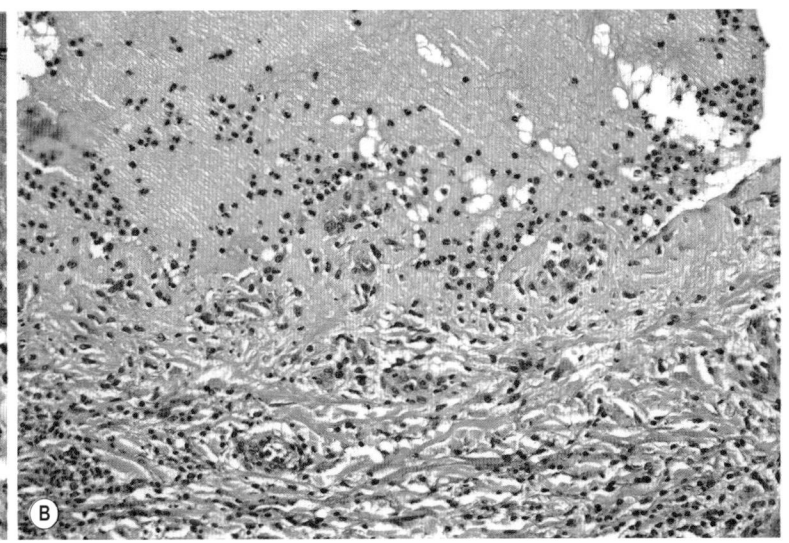

Fig. 4.66
Vesicular pemphigoid: (**A**) neutrophil microabscesses in the adjacent dermal papillae heighten the resemblance to dermatitis herpetiformis. It would be impossible to establish the diagnosis of bullous pemphigoid without appropriate immuno-fluorescent findings; (**B**) preservation of the dermal papillae may be a clue to the correct diagnosis of pemphigoid.

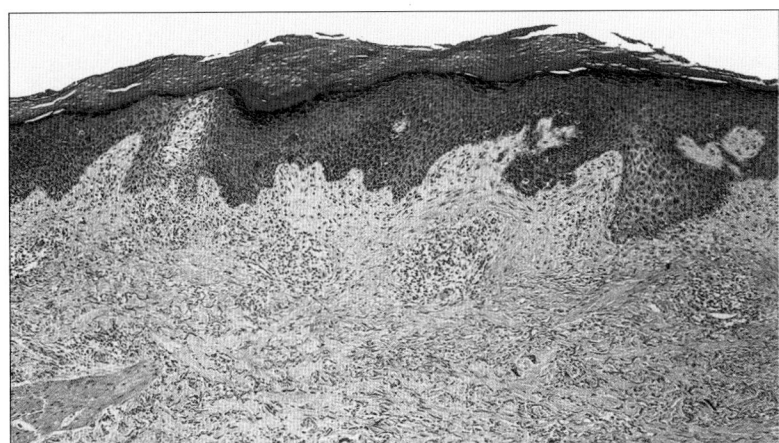

Fig. 4.67
Pemphigoid nodularis: this is a biopsy of a pruritic nodule showing hyperkeratosis, irregular acanthosis, dermal chronic inflammation, and scarring.

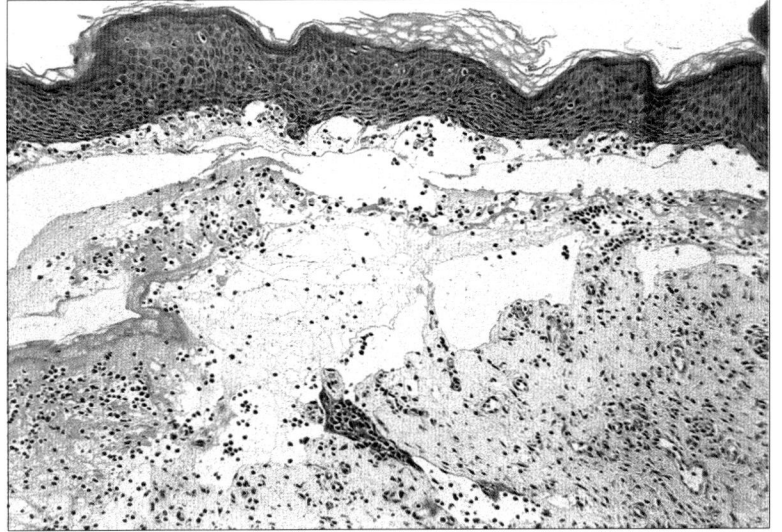

Fig. 4.68
Pemphigoid nodularis: this subepidermal blister comes from the same patient as shown in *Fig. 4.67*. Pemphigoid nodularis is of particular importance because the nodular lesions may precede clinical evidence of blistering.

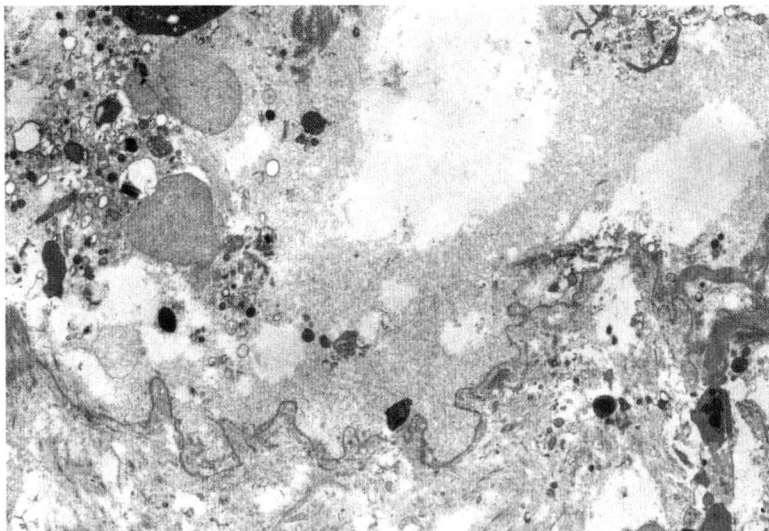

Fig. 4.69
BP: electron micrograph showing the lamina densa lying along the floor of the blister cavity.

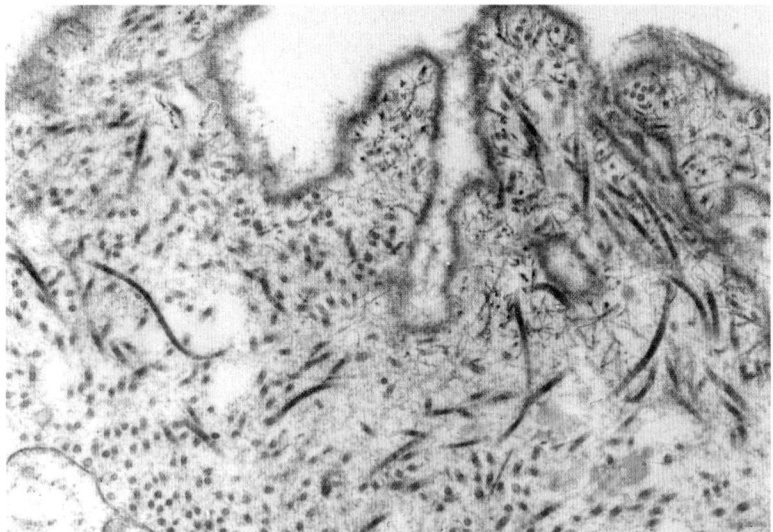

Fig. 4.70
BP: high-power view of the lamina densa.

The lamina densa is therefore located along the floor of the blister (*Figs 4.69* and *4.70*). Degenerative changes in the basal cells, including villous process formation, mitochondrial swelling, and cytoplasmic vacuolization, are frequently found. Hemidesmosomes may appear reduced in number or may even be absent.[78] Intercellular edema between adjacent basal cells is a common finding.[79] If specimens from established inflammatory lesions are examined, the lamina densa is sometimes fragmented or entirely absent.[49]

Bullous pemphigoid is characterized by a linear antibasement membrane zone antibody using the indirect immunofluorescent technique.[80] Although IgG is invariably present (and most commonly of the IgG4 subclass), other immunoglobulins, including IgE, may be represented.[81] Such antibodies are present in around 75–80% of patients.[82–85] Sensitivity can, however, be increased to 90% if split skin is used as substrate.[18] Although earlier studies failed to detect a relationship between the antibody titer and disease activity or severity, more recently it has been shown that serum antibodies to the NC16A domain of BP180 (a subunit of the bullous pemphigoid antigen) do correlate with disease activity (see below).[86–90] In addition, autoantibodies against BP180, and to a lesser degree to BP230, correlate with the clinical course of topically treated BP patients and can be used to monitor the effectiveness of the treatment.[91] Furthermore, while autoantibodies in patients with the inflammatory variant of BP generally target the NC16A domain of BP180, autoantibodies in patients with noninflammatory variant usually react with the midportion of collagen XVII.[92] Serum titers of IgE anti

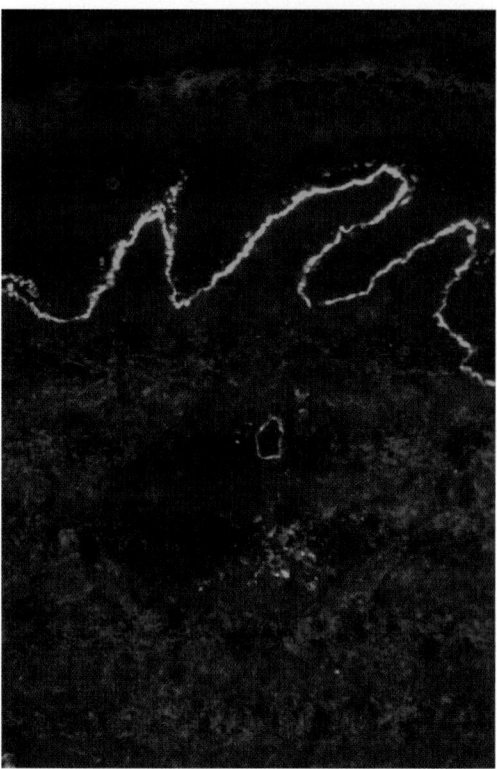

Fig. 4.71
BP: direct immunofluorescence of perilesional skin showing intense linear basement membrane zone staining (IgG).

BP180 autoantibodies correlate not only with the disease severity, but also with the formation of erythematous and urticarial lesions in BP.[93] Serum levels of IgG1 and IgG4 targeting the noncollagenous 16A domain of BP180 parallel disease activity and predict a more aggressive clinical behavior.[94]

Split skin indirect studies are essential in the investigation of a patient in whom a linear IgG antibasement membrane antibody has been detected.[95–97] Such antibodies are also characteristic of mucous membrane pemphigoid, herpes (pemphigoid) gestationis, inflammatory epidermolysis bullosa, and bullous systemic lupus erythematosus. The antibodies in pemphigoid variants (with the exception of the anti-p105 and anti-p200 variants discussed below) bind to the epidermal side of 1 M NaCl-split skin whereas those of inflammatory epidermolysis bullosa and bullous systemic lupus erythematosus bind to the floor.

In those patients in whom indirect fluorescent studies are not available, similar information may sometimes be obtained through the localization of lamina densa constituents, such as type IV collagen or laminin-1, using paraffin-embedded direct immunoperoxidase techniques. In pemphigoid, the staining is found along the floor of the blister, whereas in inflammatory epidermolysis bullosa and bullous systemic lupus erythematosus it is located along the roof (see *Figs 4.7* and *4.8*). In addition, a recent study demonstrated an immunofluorescence pattern in adnexal structures similar to that observed in the epidermis.[98] Besides serum, saliva has been reported to represent a convenient alternative for detection of BP180 NC16a autoantibodies.[99]

Bullous pemphigoid antibodies are capable of complement fixation in as many as 75% of patients.[100,101] Most of complement fixation in bullous pemphigoid antibody resides in the IgG4 subclass.[102]

Linear in vivo-bound immunoglobulin at the dermal–epidermal interface on direct immunofluorescence is present in 90% or more of patients (*Fig. 4.71*).[18,103] Complement (C3) is also usually present and is sometimes the sole immunoreactant (*Fig. 4.72*).[104] Other immunoglobulin subclasses including IgM, IgA, and IgE may be detected occasionally.[85,100,105] In addition to C3, the other components of the classical complement pathway, in particular C5b-9 (the membrane attack complex) and members of the alternative complement pathway, including properdin, factor B, and B-1H-globulin, may also be identified.[85,106] There is, therefore, evidence that both the

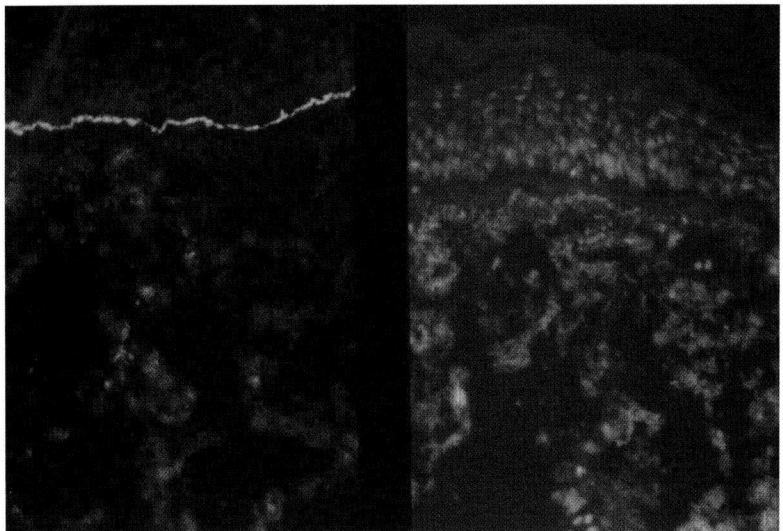

Fig. 4.72
BP: direct immunofluorescence showing C3 deposition (*left*), no staining is seen in the negative control (*right*). By courtesy of B. Boghal, FIMLS, Institute of Dermatology, London, UK.

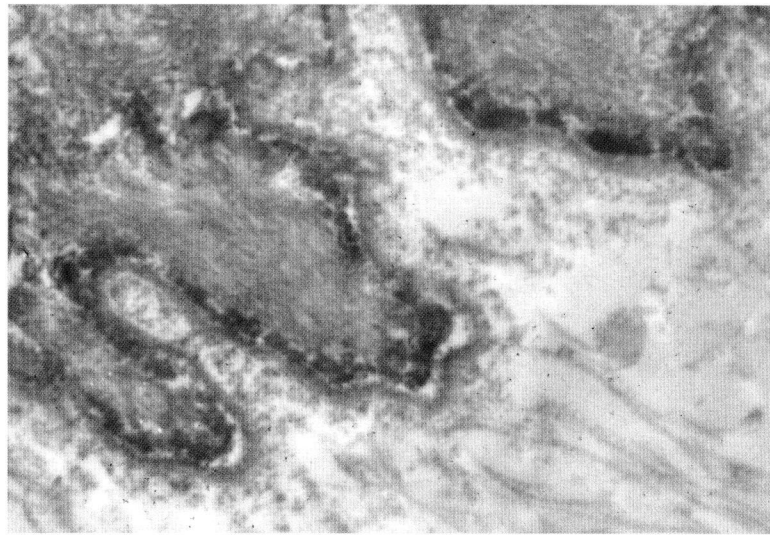

Fig. 4.73
BP: direct immunoperoxidase reaction using frozen tissue substrate showing electron-dense deposits in the lamina lucida.

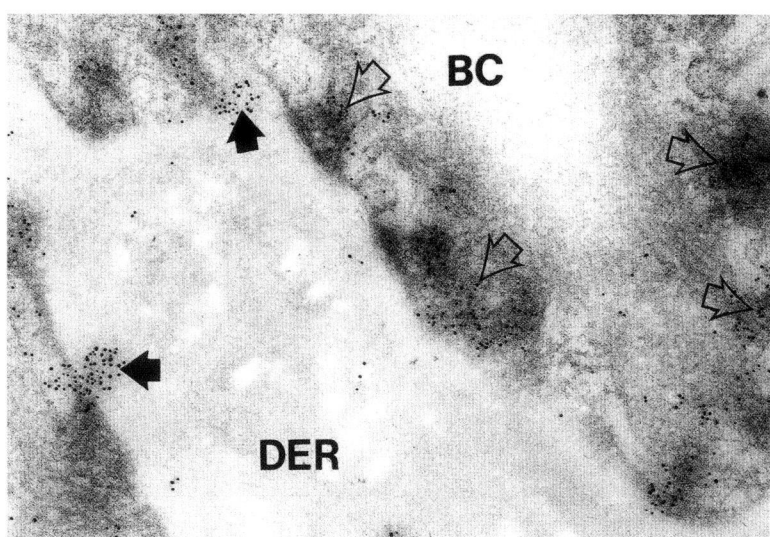

Fig. 4.74
BP: immunogold electron microscopic preparation. Note that the immunoreactant to BP180 and BP230 is particularly located on the hemidesmosomes (*open arrows*). However, deposits are also present within the lamina lucida, black arrows. (BC, basal cell; DER, dermis.) By courtesy of H. Shimizu, MD, Keio University School of Medicine, Tokyo, Japan.

classical and alternate complement pathways are involved in the pathogenesis of bullous pemphigoid.[107] The classical complement pathway, however, predominates. A recent mouse model underscores the necessity of an intact innate immune system, as the depletion of complement or neutrophils or blockage of mast cell activation prevents blister formation.[108]

The immunofluorescence findings in erythematous, pruritic, urticarial, and eczematous prodromal lesions and childhood, dyshidrosiform, vesicular, nodular, and vegetans variants are similar to those seen in the conventional generalized disease.[26-29,33-50,109,110] In polymorphic pemphigoid, either linear IgG or IgA deposits may be identified along the basement membrane region.[30-32] The serum may contain either IgG or IgA antibodies.[31]

Immunofluorescence findings in localized cutaneous disease are variable. In some reports, patients show positive direct immunofluorescence for IgG and C3 at the dermal–epidermal junction and a positive indirect immunofluorescent test for bullous pemphigoid antibody, while others may be positive for in vivo-bound complement, but negative on indirect examination.[68,69,110] One series has shown that almost 70% of patients with localized pemphigoid have circulating IgG antibodies in their sera and the presence of these can be relevant for serum-based testing, as discussed below.[69,111] A caveat is that in one study, antibodies were also detected in more than half of normal subjects who did not subsequently develop the disease.[112,113] This finding is further discussed below.

By direct immunoelectron microscopy, the immunoreactants (IgG and C3) are seen to be located within the hemidesmosomal plaque and upper lamina lucida (*Fig. 4.73*).[114-118] Indirect immunoelectron microscopic studies show that the bullous pemphigoid antigen is most often detected intracellularly in the region of the cytoplasmic face of the hemidesmosome (*Fig. 4.74*).[115,119-121]

The immunoelectron microscopic observations in childhood bullous pemphigoid, vesicular pemphigoid, polymorphic pemphigoid, pemphigoid nodularis, pemphigoid vegetans, and localized pemphigoid are identical to those of classic bullous pemphigoid.[122,123]

Two principal bullous pemphigoid antigens are recognized by Western blot and immunoprecipitation studies: one is 230 kD (*BPAG1*) and the other is approximately 180 kD (*BPAG2*) (*Fig. 4.75*).[124-130] These represent products of distinct genes.[131-134]

BP230 maps to the short arm of chromosome 6, locus 6p11-12.[132] It belongs to the plakin family and shows homology with plectin and the desmogleins.[133] It is wholly intracellular and localizes to the hemidesmosome. *BP230* is not involved in the early stages of the pathogenesis of blistering but is of importance as a secondary event; antibodies against this antigen are not required for blister formation in most cases.[135-137]

BP180 (collagen type XVII) is the major pathogenic antigen in bullous pemphigoid. The *BPAG2* (*COL17A1*) maps to the long arm of chromosome 10, locus 10q24.3.[132] It is a transmembrane adhesion molecule comprising an intracytoplasmic N-terminal fragment, a transmembrane region, and a collagenous extracellular C-terminal ectodomain.[138] The latter constitutes part of the anchoring filament and distally merges with the lamina densa. The antibodies directed against BP180 in bullous pemphigoid most commonly react with a short extracellular noncollagenous locus – NC16A (regions MCW0-MCW3) – located within the upper lamina lucida proximal to the collagenous segment (*Fig. 4.76*).[138-141] It now appears that antibodies specific to this area are generally required for blister formation and, while antibodies may also target BP180 non-NC16A domains, these latter antibodies do not appear to be pathogenic in most cases.[135-137] This finding reconciles the fact that antibodies to both BP180 and BP230 can be seen in a significant portion of the population without blister formation as these are not against the critical NC16A region of BP180.[86]

Between 50% and 90% of patients with generalized bullous pemphigoid have antibodies that react with BP230 and 35–50% have antibodies that

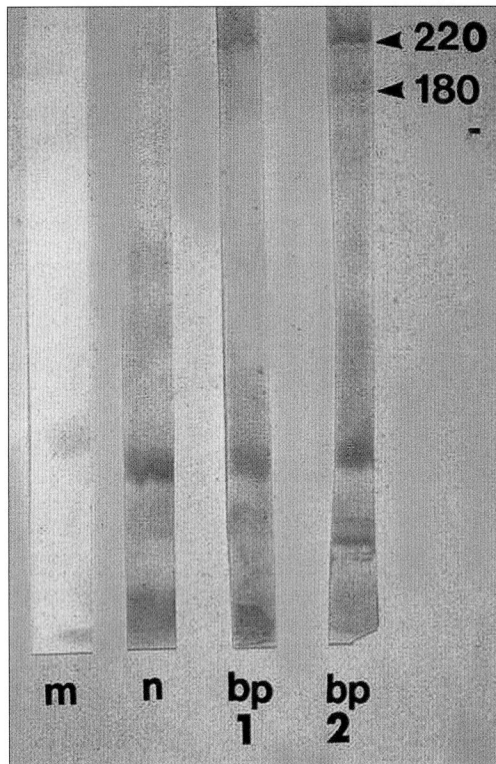

Fig. 4.75
BP: Western blot demonstrating the two quite separate bullous pemphigoid antigens. By courtesy of M.M. Black, MD, Institute of Dermatology, London, UK.

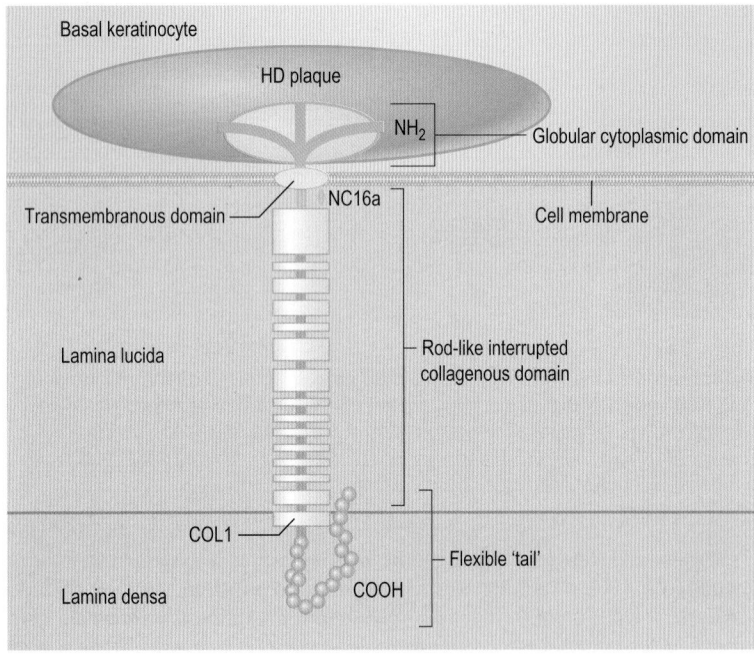

Fig. 4.76
A schematic representation of the BP180 molecule showing the globular intracellular NH2 domain, the membrane proximal NC16A domain and the flexible rod-like interrupted collagenous structure of the extracellular domain. (HD, hemidesmosome). Collagen XVII/BP180: a collagenous transmembrane protein and component of the dermal–epidermal anchoring complex. (Powell AM, Sakuma-Oyama Y, Oyama N, Black M.M. Department of Immunodermatology, St John's Institute of Dermatology, St Thomas' Hospital, London, UK.)

react with BP180 that are readily detected by immunoblotting.[142] However, the sera in 100% of patients react with BP180 NC16A domain recombinant protein.[142] This latter finding underscores the usefulness of testing for anti-NC16A domain antibodies from peripheral blood to distinguish bullous pemphigoid from other disorders.[111,143–145]

Circulating antibodies against BP180 or BP230 have also been defined in many of the other less common variants of bullous pemphigoid, including localized and vesicular forms, pemphigoid vegetans, erythrodermic pemphigoid, and pemphigoid nodularis.[142,146–150]

In childhood pemphigoid, the antibodies also react against the same antigens.[151] In addition, rarely there may also be antibodies that react with the linear IgA 120-kD antigen.[151] The BP180 antigen is most often targeted, and immunoblot analyses have shown that the antibodies react specifically with the NC16A domain as in adult patients. In some children at least, the IgG subclasses differ from adult disease, consisting of all IgG subclasses or IgG2 in isolation.[18] IgE antibodies are not a feature of childhood disease.

More recently, two patients with a nonscarring, bullous pemphigoid-like illness characterized by neutrophil-rich subepidermal blisters resembling dermatitis herpetiformis and antibodies to a unique 105-kD protein – so-called anti-p105 pemphigoid – have been documented.[152–154] This antigen localizes to the dermal side of split skin on indirect immunofluorescence. Its precise nature has not yet been determined.

Anti-p200 pemphigoid is characterized by antibodies to a lower lamina lucida basement membrane antigen.[155–157] Patients generally present with a nonscarring bullous pemphigoid-like illness although linear IgA disease-like and dermatitis herpetiformis-like variants have also been reported.[155] The disease has also been described in association with psoriasis vulgaris and only rarely with pustular psoriasis.[156,158,159] With split skin IIMF, the antibodies bind to the floor of the blister cavity.[155] With indirect immunoelectron microscopy, the antibodies bind to the lower lamina lucida.[160,161] It has been suggested, that antibodies against laminin γ1 have a pathogenetic role and that this molecule represents the autoantigen in the development of anti-p200 pemphigoid.[162,163]

Anti-p450 pemphigoid has been documented in a single patient. The antigen, which has been localized to the basal keratinocyte, belongs to the plectin family.[164] Its precise nature has yet to be determined.

Exceptionally, bullous pemphigoid may be associated with antiplectin antibody.[165]

Bullous pemphigoid has been described following PUVA therapy for mycosis fungoides. A case arising in the setting of radiation therapy and one in the setting of photodynamic therapy have also been noted, perhaps suggesting a role for tissue damage in the pathogenesis of this disease.[166,167]

A mechanism for blister development in bullous pemphigoid has been proposed by Jordon et al.[82,168] and is outlined as follows. Following antibody–antigen interaction and complement fixation, various chemotactic agents, including C3a and C4a, are produced.[169] Mast cells degranulate under the influence of the latter, or IgE, and release ECF-A, NMW-NCF, ESM, histamine, and enzymes.[170] Eosinophils and neutrophils, so recruited, bind (possibly via C3b receptors) to the basement membrane region. By direct cytotoxic action (eosinophils are capable of antibody-dependent cellular cytotoxicity) or via released proteases, particularly elastase, damage at the basement membrane region results in the development of a vesicle. Lymphocytes elaborate histamine-releasing factor (HRF), which increases mast cell degranulation and perpetuates the process. A broad range of cytokines are involved in this inflammatory reaction including interleukin (IL)-1, IL-4-IL-8, IL-10-IL-13, IL-15 and interferon gamma (IFN-γ).[171] As yet, their relative importance and time sequences are unknown.

Bullous pemphigoid is therefore a true autoimmune disease in which antigen–antibody reaction and complement fixation results in a characteristic and reproducible train of events, which is inevitably accompanied by the development of subepidermal blister formation. The etiology or initiator (other than those associated with drugs or PUVA therapy, which are the minority) is unknown. The question as to why self-tolerance breaks down with the formation of symptomatic autoantibodies in patients with this disease is an important question for further investigation.

Differential diagnosis

The inflammatory cell-rich variant of bullous pemphigoid must be distinguished from other subepidermal blistering dermatoses in which a heavy inflammatory cell component is a typical finding. These include dermatitis herpetiformis, linear IgA disease, inflammatory epidermolysis bullosa

Table 4.6
Differential diagnosis of cell-rich pemphigoid

Parameter	BP	EBA	BSLE	LAD	DHD
IMF	Linear IgG, C3	Linear IgG, C3	Linear IgG, C3	Linear IgA	Granular IgA
IIMF	IgG antibodies 75–80%	IgG antibodies 25–50%	IgG antibodies 60%	IgA antibodies 30%	Antitransglutaminase antibodies
Split skin IMF	Roof	Floor	Floor	Roof or floor or both	N/A
Type IV collagen	Floor	Roof	Roof	Roof or floor	N/A
EM: site of split	LL	Sub-LD	Sub-LD	LL, sub-LD or both	Papillary dermis
Western blot	BP180 kD BP230 kD	290 kD (type VII collagen)	290 kD (type VII collagen)	BP180 kD BP230 kD 200/280 kD 285 kD 250 kD 290 kD	Antigen uncertain

BP, Bullous pemphigoid; *BSLE*, bullous systemic lupus erythematosus; *DH*, dermatitis herpetiformis; *DIMF*, direct immunofluorescence; *EBA*, epidermolysis bullosa acquisita; *EM*, electron microscopy; *IIMF*, indirect immunofluorescence; *IMF*, immunofluorescence; *LAD*, linear IgA disease; *LL*, lamina lucida; *sub-LD*, sub-lamina densa.

acquisita, and bullous systemic lupus erythematosus (see *Table 4.6*). Successful differentiation depends upon careful clinicopathologic correlation and immunofluorescent studies or, more recently, serum-based immunologic (ELISA) testing. Split skin indirect immunofluorescence or lamina densa antigen mapping by type IV collagen or laminin-1 direct immunoperoxidase is essential to determine the level of the split. Although electron microscopy, immunoelectron microscopy, and immunoprecipitation or Western blotting provide definitive information, such techniques are not necessary in the majority of cases.

The cell-poor variant of bullous pemphigoid has a very wide range of differential diagnoses including epidermolysis bullosa (congenital and acquired), porphyria cutanea tarda, bullous amyloidosis, bullosa diabeticorum, and autolysis.

Pemphigoid gestationis

Pruritus is a very common symptom in pregnancy, occurring in up to 18% of gravid females.[1–4] When it occurs in the absence of significant cutaneous stigmata it is known as pruritus gravidarum. This may occasionally be associated with a cholestatic pathogenesis. The specific pregnancy eruptions have long been a source of considerable confusion and controversy in the literature, largely due to a diverse range of terminologies and classifications. Holmes has attempted to clarify the situation with the introduction of a new and much simplified classification and others have proposed similar schemes.[2,5] Therefore the specific dermatoses of pregnancy may be divided into:

- polymorphic eruption of pregnancy, where the predominant lesions are urticarial; in the United States, the term pruritic urticarial papules and plaques of pregnancy (PUPPP) has achieved greater popularity;
- pregnancy prurigo in which the lesions consist of itchy papules;
- pemphigoid (herpes) gestationis, an autoimmune dermatosis belonging to the bullous pemphigoid group of diseases.

Pemphigoid gestationis is a bullous dermatosis of pregnancy and the puerperium. It may be exacerbated by the use of oral contraceptives and rarely complicates hydatidiform mole and gestational (but not nongestational) choriocarcinoma. The current evidence implicates an autoimmune-mediated pathogenesis in which hormonal influences play a significant role.[6,7]

Clinical features

The term herpes (gestationis) is neither appropriate nor satisfactory. It is not of viral etiology, nor has it anything to do with creeping (Gr. *herpes*, to creep). It was originally so named because of the tendency of the disease to show 'progressive involvement by peripheral extension'.[3] Because of its intimate relationship to bullous pemphigoid, the designation pemphigoid gestationis is preferred. As the major larger series have consisted of patients derived from a variety of sources, estimates of incidence have been very variable, ranging from 1:3000 to 1:50 000 pregnancies.[4,8–10] A further study

where cases have had immunofluorescent confirmation would suggest that the latter figure is the most accurate.[3]

Pemphigoid gestationis may present in the first or any subsequent pregnancy.[3] It may first also rarely present in the postpartum period. In one series, 30% of patients were primigravidae.[9] In addition to developing in pregnant or postpartum patients, pemphigoid gestationis has rarely been described following a hydatidiform mole and gestational choriocarcinoma.[11,12] It has not, however, been reported in nongestational variants, such as those occurring in the ovary, mediastinum, and testis, or complicating malignant teratoma. Pemphigoid gestationis is predominantly a disease of white females, being exceedingly rare in blacks.[13,14] Presentation is usually in the second or third trimester, most often developing in the sixth or seventh month, but the range is variable from 2 months to 4 days postpartum.[10,15] Although the disease may rarely completely remit before delivery, most patients (up to 75%) develop an exacerbation, which is frequently severe, in the immediate puerperium when progesterone levels have fallen.[15,16] Exceptionally, the infant may show transient urticated erythema and blistering.[4]

Pemphigoid gestationis usually complicates subsequent pregnancies, frequently presenting earlier on and with more severe symptomatology.[10] Sometimes, however, it may skip intervening pregnancies.[3] This may be related to a change in paternity, or else due to compatibility at the HLA-D locus.

Pemphigoid gestationis may develop into a very protracted 'postpartum' illness associated with considerable morbidity and lasting up to 12 years.[17,18] In the majority of patients, however, the disease resolves by about 6 months postpartum.[4] The disease may first present following a change in sexual partner.[3,19] Alternatively, recurrent disease may persist even when there has been a change of sexual partner.[7] This obviously calls into question the role of specific paternal antigens.

Exacerbation following the use of the oral contraceptive is a common complication,[10,20–23] affecting 20–50% of patients.[3] Estrogens in particular have been implicated.[22] The condition may also relapse during menstruation for some weeks or months postpartum and the return of symptoms (pruritus) has also been noted to coincide with ovulation (again suggesting an estrogen influence), although this is rare.[3,10,22]

Evidence has been published relating the duration of symptoms postpartum to the practice of breast-feeding. Bullous lesions lasted only 5 weeks in those who breast-fed compared to 24 weeks in those who bottle-fed. Although hormonal factors must be implicated, the precise pathogenetic implications underlying this observation are not fully understood.[22]

Pemphigoid gestationis is associated with intense pruritus, which may be present for days or weeks before the onset of typical cutaneous manifestations.[1] The dermatosis is characteristically polymorphous, consisting of erythematous or urticarial papules and plaques, some with a polycyclic pattern, and later vesicles and bullae develop at the periphery of spreading erythematous plaques (*Fig. 4.77*).[3,10,24] When fully evolved, the blisters are tense and contain clear fluid, but at times the fluid may become hemorrhagic (*Fig. 4.78*). They typically heal without scarring.

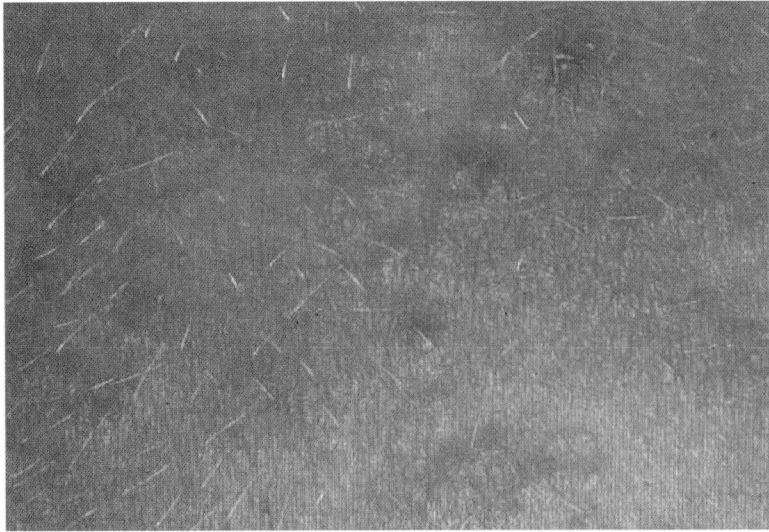

Fig. 4.77
Pemphigoid gestationis: prebullous phase showing erythema and small papules.
By courtesy of the Institute of Dermatology, London, UK.

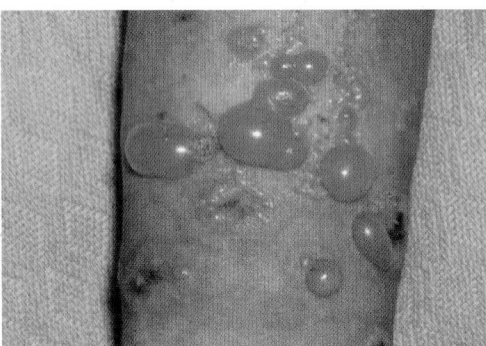

Fig. 4.78
Pemphigoid gestationis: the blisters are tense and dome-shaped. By courtesy of
R.C. Holmes, MD, Warneford Hospital, Oxford, UK.

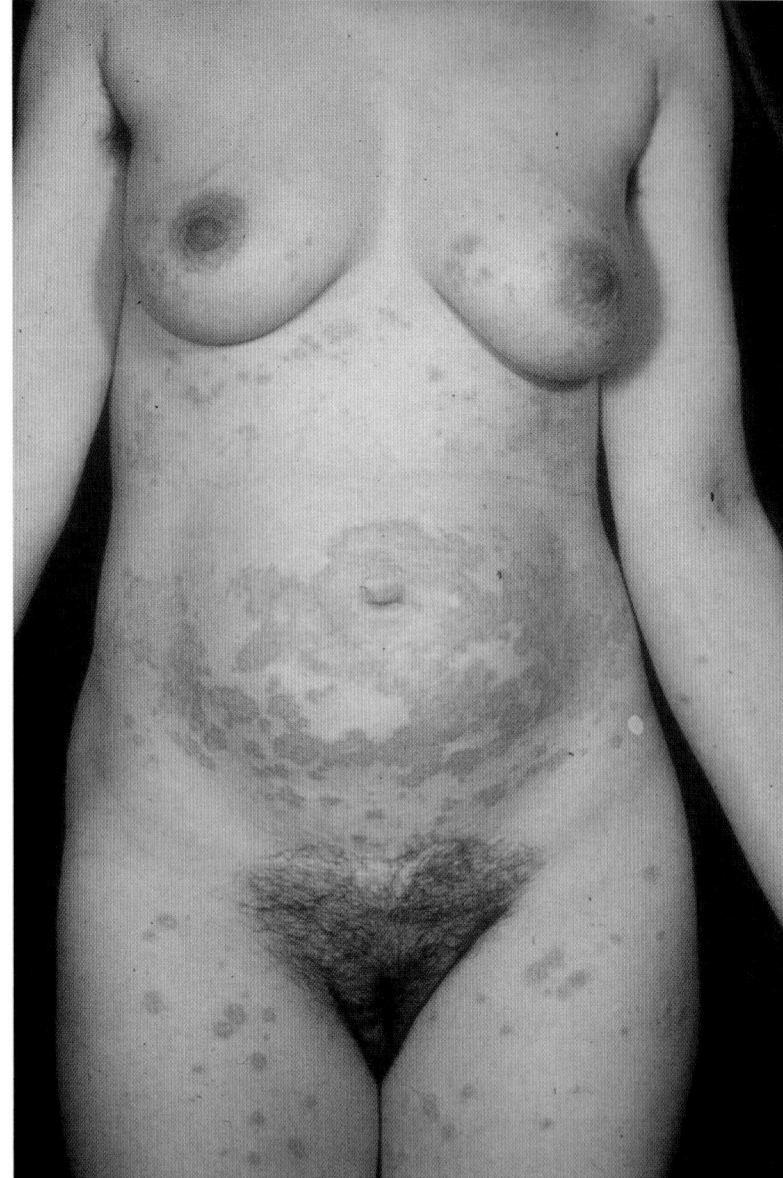

Fig. 4.79
Pemphigoid gestationis: slightly raised erythematous lesions with a propensity to
cluster on the abdomen. By courtesy of R.C. Holmes, MD, Warneford Hospital,
Oxford, UK.

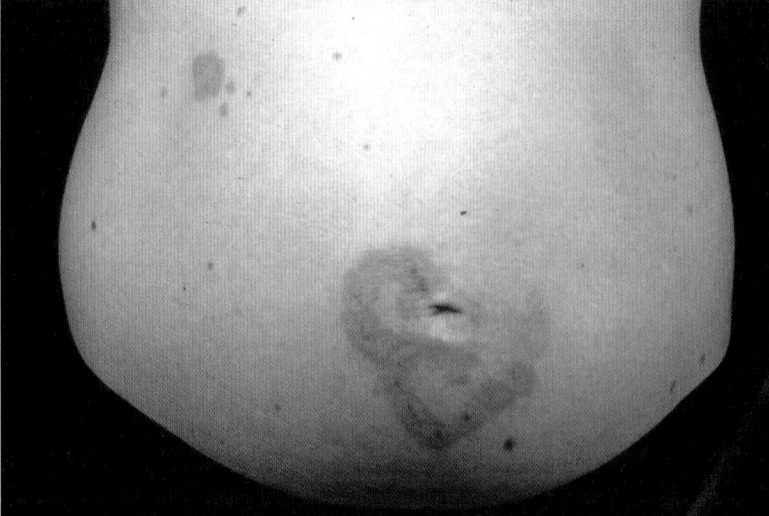

Fig. 4.80
Pemphigoid gestationis: umbilical involvement is a common mode of presentation.
By courtesy of the Institute of Dermatology, London, UK.

The umbilicus is frequently the site of initial involvement; spread to the trunk and extremities then follows (*Figs 4.79* and *4.80*).[3] Surprisingly, lesions on the face and mucous membranes are distinctly uncommon. Eventually palmar and plantar manifestations may appear. Other than pruritus, symptoms are usually mild, with stinging, burning, and pain being relatively infrequent.[10] Occasionally, the presence of target or iris lesions may mimic erythema multiforme.[25] Less commonly, features may initially suggest classical bullous pemphigoid.[25] Very occasionally, there is clinical overlap with dermatitis herpetiformis.

Pemphigoid gestationis is not associated with pre-eclamptic toxemia and there is no related maternal mortality.

Pemphigoid gestationis is accompanied by a significant increased risk of developing Graves disease, thyroiditis, pernicious anemia and an increased risk of autoantibodies,[26] likely reflecting the association of HLA-DR3 and HLA-DR4 loci with both pemphigoid gestationis and autoimmune disease.[26]

The literature concerning the incidence and nature of fetal morbidity and mortality is a source of some confusion. Kolodney therefore considered that there was no evidence of an increased incidence of stillbirths or abortions; however, his report predates the immunofluorescence era.[5] An investigation by Lawley et al.[20] of a large series of cases where immunofluorescent confirmation was available, suggested that there was an increased risk of fetal morbidity and mortality. More recently, evidence has been presented that patients with pemphigoid gestationis are liable to deliver low weight and small-for-dates infants, prematurely.[27] In contrast, however, Shornick et al. failed to show any evidence of significant fetal complications.[7] It has been shown that the onset of the disease in the first and second trimester and the presence of blisters is associated with higher morbidity including premature birth and low birth weight children.[28] Morbidity, however, still remains low.

The antibody can cross the placenta and, in approximately 5% of cases, this may be associated with a mild and transient vesiculobullous eruption.[29–32]

Pathogenesis and histologic features

The histopathologic features seen in biopsies from patients with pemphigoid gestationis are variable, depending upon whether early erythematous lesions, urticarial papular lesions, or fully established vesicles and bullae are studied.[33]

In early lesions, the major pathological features are seen in the superficial dermis where there is a perivascular inflammatory cell infiltrate consisting of lymphocytes, histiocytes, and typically very large numbers of eosinophils. This is associated with edema of the papillary dermis, which when marked may result in a 'teardrop' appearance (*Fig. 4.81*).[33] Sometimes there is accompanying spongiosis and this may be associated with large numbers of eosinophils (eosinophilic spongiosis, *Fig. 4.82*). Occasionally the infiltrate of lymphocytes, histiocytes, and eosinophils is present in a linear distribution along the dermal–epidermal junction.[3]

Vacuolar degeneration of basal keratinocytes, sometimes accompanied by individual cell necrosis, may be a feature of the early lesions, but is often more evident in the fully established vesicular or bullous stage.[33] In the latter, the blister is subepidermal in location and frequently contains large numbers of eosinophils (*Figs 4.83* and *4.84*).[33] The underlying and adjacent dermis is edematous and contains a predominantly perivascular lympho/histiocytic infiltrate with large numbers of eosinophils. Leukocytoclasis and eosinophil dermal papillary microabscesses are only rarely identified.[33,34] Ultrastructural studies show that the cleavage plane lies within the lamina lucida.[33,35]

Direct immunofluorescence of perilesional skin in pemphigoid gestationis shows a linear basement membrane zone deposition of C3 in all patients.[3,36–41] About 30–50% of cases also have an IgG band (less frequently IgM or IgA).[36] They are present in nonlesional (perilesional) as well as in lesional skin.[36] It has been suggested that demonstration of linear C3d deposition at the dermal–epidermal junction may be a useful tool in the diagnosis of the disease.[42] The authors of this study used immunohistochemistry in paraffin-embedded, formalin-fixed material with good results. Complement pathway components including properdin and properdin factor-B may also be identified.[1] IgG and complement can often be detected along the amniotic basement membrane region using direct immunofluorescence.[38,43,44] Pemphigoid gestationis antigen has been detected in the placenta from early in the second trimester onwards.[45] The antibody may also be found in the skin of infants of affected mothers.[29] Interestingly, serologic evidence of pemphigoid gestationis without manifestation of the disease may be seen. An exceptional case of neonatal pemphigus in a child whose mother had clinical and serologic evidence of pemphigus vulgaris but only serologic evidence of pemphigoid gestationis has been described.[46]

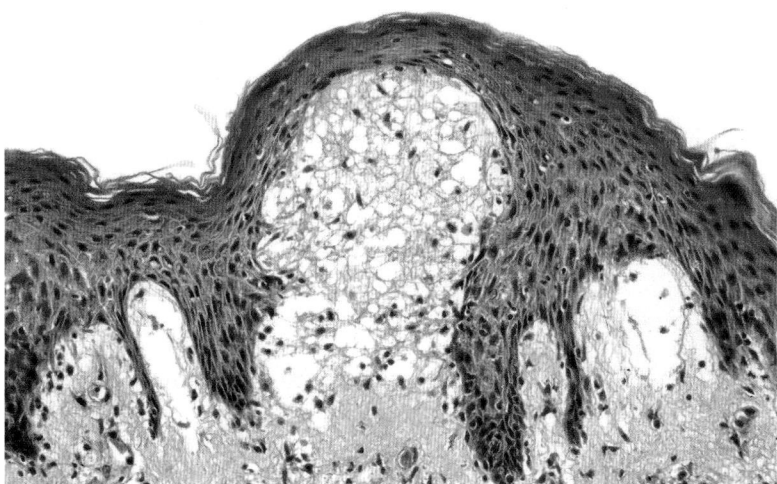

Fig. 4.81
Pemphigoid gestationis: early erythematous lesion showing marked edema of the papillary dermis and conspicuous eosinophils.

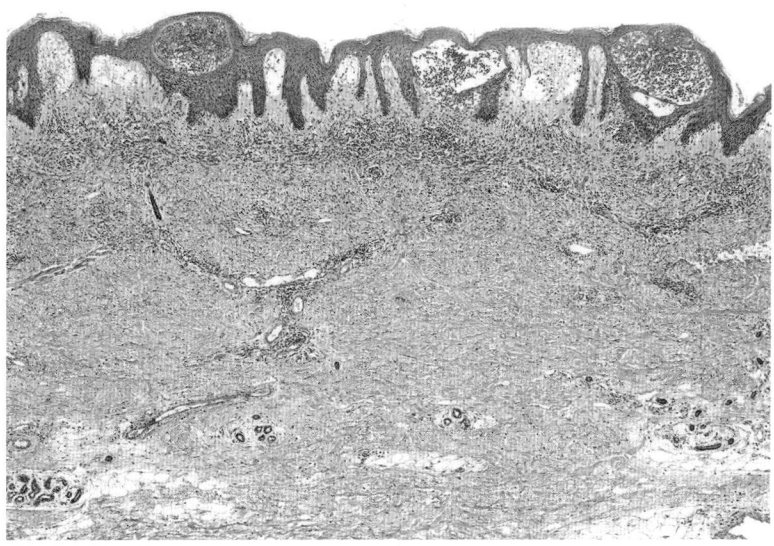

Fig. 4.83
Pemphigoid gestationis: established subepidermal blister.

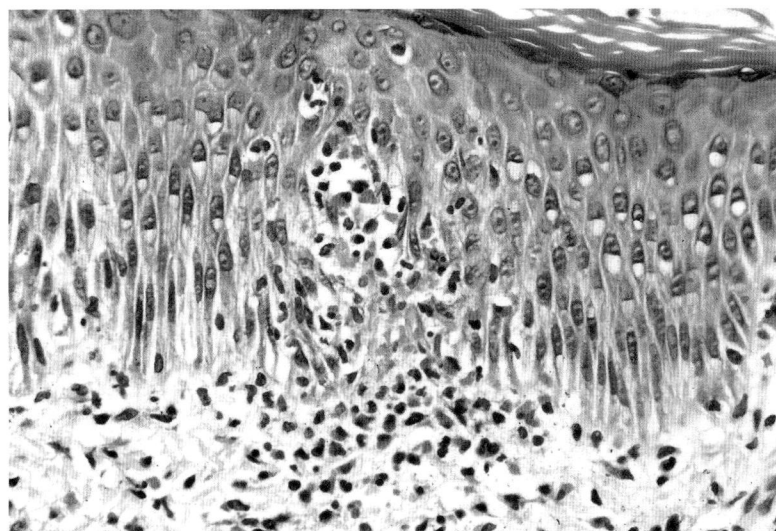

Fig. 4.82
Pemphigoid gestationis: early erythematous lesion showing eosinophilic spongiosis.

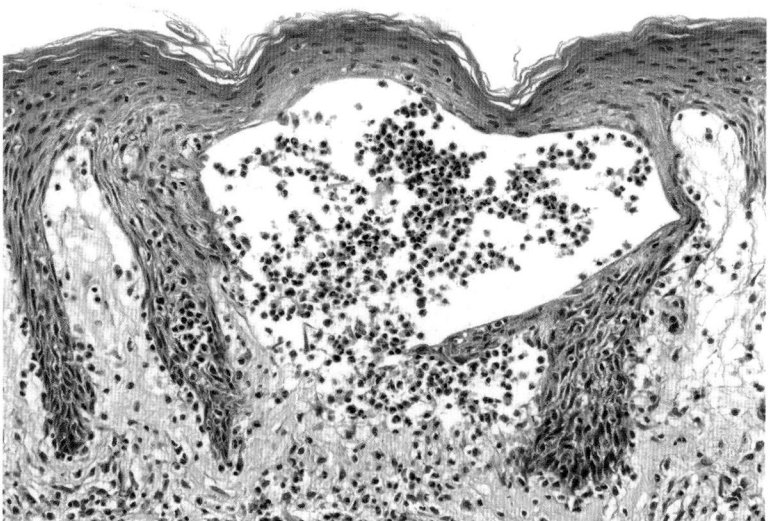

Fig. 4.84
Pemphigoid gestationis: the blister cavity contains a heavy eosinophil infiltrate.

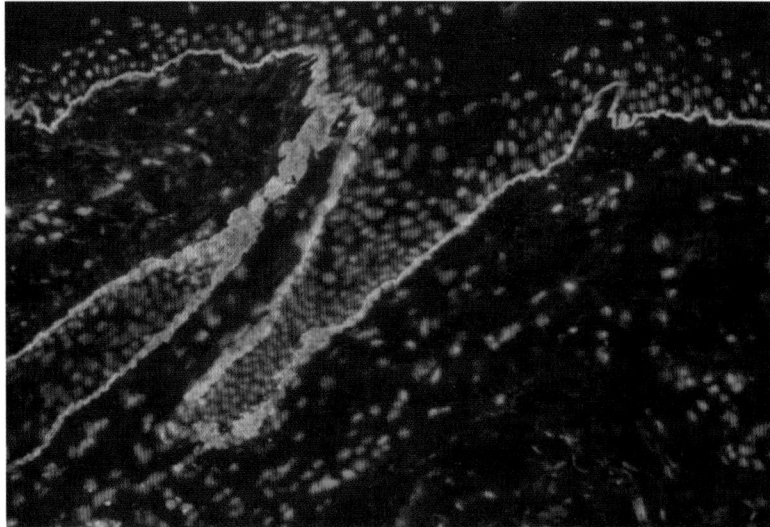

Fig. 4.85
Pemphigoid gestationis: indirect complement immunofluorescence showing linear deposition of IgG.

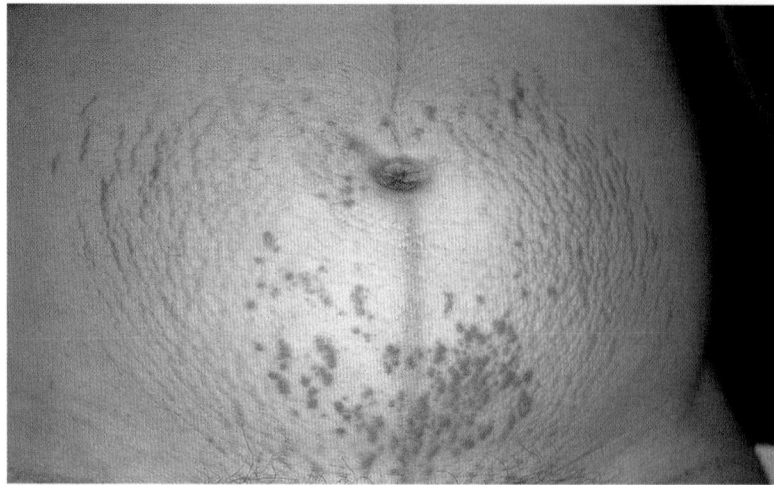

Fig. 4.86
Pruritic papules and plaques of pregnancy: note the erythematous papules particularly related to the abdominal striae, and characteristic umbilical sparing. By courtesy of R.C. Holmes, MD, Warneford Hospital, Oxford, UK.

Circulating complement-fixing (via the classical pathway) IgG antibodies (pemphigoid [herpes] gestationis [HG] factor) can be detected in 50–75% of cases by indirect complement immunofluorescence (*Fig. 4.85*).[20,36,47–51] The so-called HG factor is nothing more than a low titer IgG complement-fixing antibasement membrane antibody.[36] The antibody can be of any IgG subclass; IgG1 and IgG4 have been reported as predominant.[38,51] If monoclonal antibodies directed against IgG are used, 100% of patients can be shown to possess circulating HG factor.[38] Approximately 25% of patients have antibasement membrane zone antibodies detectable by conventional techniques.[51] These bind to the roof of 1 M NaCl-split skin.[36] The antibody also reacts with amnion and chorion basement membrane.[42,44] The autoantibodies in the disease are directed against collagen XVII which is the BP 180-kD protein (*BPAG2*). The latter plays a major role in cell adhesion and signaling. It has been demonstrated that collagen XVII is present in the epithelial cells of the amniotic membrane and in syncytial and cytotrophoblastic cells.[52] Although the exact pathogenetic mechanism of the disease is still unknown (see below), the presence of collagen XVII in these tissues seems to play a major role in the mechanism of the disease.

With immunoelectron microscopy the immunoreactants are deposited within the upper lamina lucida where they are most probably associated with the sub-basal dense plate.[53,54] In pemphigoid gestationis the antibody recognizes *BPAG2* (collagen type XVII) on Western immunoblot and localizes to the same NC16A domain as described in bullous pemphigoid.[55–62] This can be detected in serum using the same test employed for bullous pemphigoid.[60–62] Antibodies that recognize the 230-kD bullous pemphigoid antigen are present in 10–26% of cases.[56,57] Experimental models indicate that antibodies against the NC16A domain of BP180 are the pathogenic antibodies in pemphigus gestationis just as they are for bullous pemphigoid.[7,62] Serum BP180 antibody levels have been demonstrated to correlate with the disease activity and can serve as an indicator for assessment of treatment response.[60]

Patients with pemphigoid gestationis have an increased incidence of HLA-B8 (43–79%), HLA-DR3 (61–80%) and HLA-DR4 (52–53%). The paired haplotypes HLA-DR3 and -DR4 are present in 54% of patients compared with 3% in the general population.[1,3,22,63,64] The phenotype, however, does not appear to correlate with the clinical features of pemphigoid gestationis.[3,65] Patients with pemphigoid gestationis also have a high incidence (100%) of anti-HLA cytotoxic antibodies, particularly directed against the paternal antigens.[36,63–66] These are, however, found in 25% of normal multiparous women and therefore their possible role in the pathogenesis of pemphigoid gestationis is uncertain.[26]

The pathogenesis of pemphigoid gestationis relates to antibody-associated complement fixation with the production of leukocyte chemotactic factors, mast cell degranulation, and associated dermal–epidermal separation.[36]

The presence of pemphigoid gestationis antigen in both skin and amnion raises the possibility that an initial antiplacental antibody cross-reacts with skin, giving rise to the clinical features of pemphigoid gestationis.[29] Support for this theory has been the discovery that the HLA antigens -DP and -DR are consistently expressed in the placentas of patients with this condition.[64,67] The main antigen present in both the skin and placenta seems to be collagen type XVII and this, associated with genetic predisposition and specific HLA genotype, appears to trigger the disease.[68]

Differential diagnosis

The differential diagnosis includes epidermolysis bullosa acquisita, dermatitis herpetiformis, linear IgA disease, and bullous systemic lupus erythematosus (see *Table 4.6*). Pemphigoid gestationis must also be distinguished from pruritic urticarial papules and plaques of pregnancy (PUPPP) and pregnancy prurigo.

PUPPP is predominantly a disorder of first pregnancies. Lesions particularly develop around abdominal striae, and periumbilical sparing is a characteristic feature (*Fig. 4.86*). Eosinophilic spongiosis and subepidermal blistering may be seen in established lesions and therefore, in the absence of clinical details and immunofluorescence findings, distinction from pemphigoid gestationis may be impossible. Immunohistochemistry for C4d and C3d on formalin-fixed paraffin-embedded tissue can aid in the distinction between PUPPP and pemphigoid gestationis. The majority of pemphigoid gestationis cases display a linear pattern of staining along the basement membrane zone, while in cases of PUPP staining consistently negative.[42,69]

Pregnancy prurigo, which typically develops in the third trimester, presents with pruritic papules and nodules (*Fig. 4.87*). Blisters are not a feature. Histologically, the changes are those of a low-grade, non-specific spongiotic dermatitis.

Lichen planus pemphigoides

Clinical features

Lichen planus (lichen ruber) pemphigoides (Kaposi) must be distinguished from the vesicles occasionally seen in lichen planus as a consequence of severe hydropic degeneration (lichen planus vesiculosis).[1,2] Rarely, lichen planus is associated with a generally benign, bullous pemphigoid-like disease: lichen planus pemphigoides. This represents a heterogeneous condition characterized by basement membrane antibodies directed towards a number of antigens.

Clinically, the pemphigoid-like lesions are usually preceded by typical lichen planus although rarely the blisters may develop first (*Fig. 4.88*). The bullae, which are most numerous on the extremities, may arise on normal

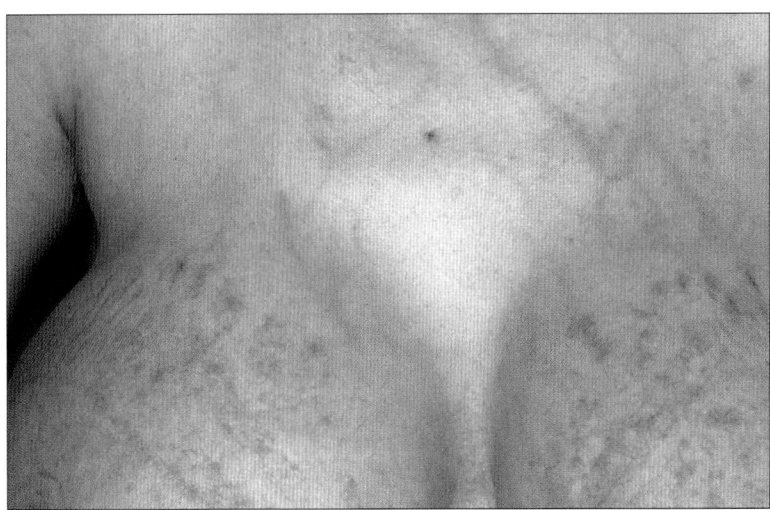

Fig. 4.87
Pregnancy prurigo: there are erythematous papules and excoriations. Blisters are not a feature of this condition. By courtesy of R.A. Marsden, MD, St George's Hospital, London, UK.

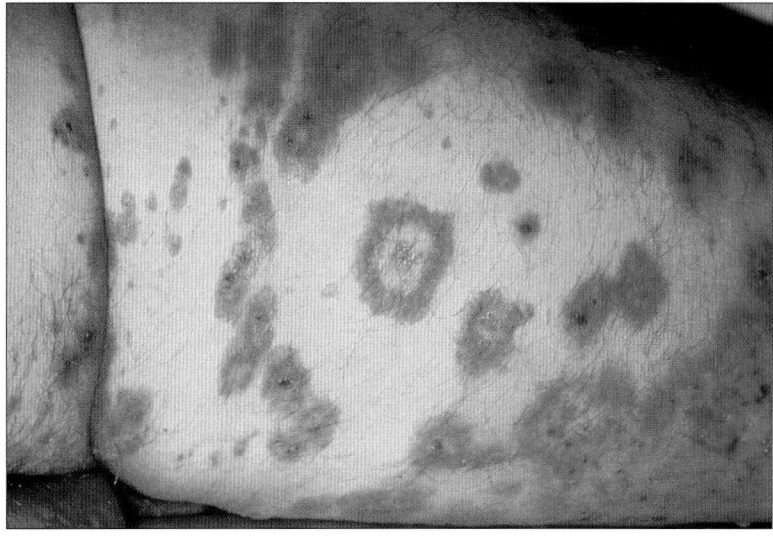

Fig. 4.89
Lichen planus pemphigoides: note the blisters and erosions arising on an erythematous base. Atypical target lesions are present. By courtesy of M.M. Black, MD, Institute of Dermatology, London, UK.

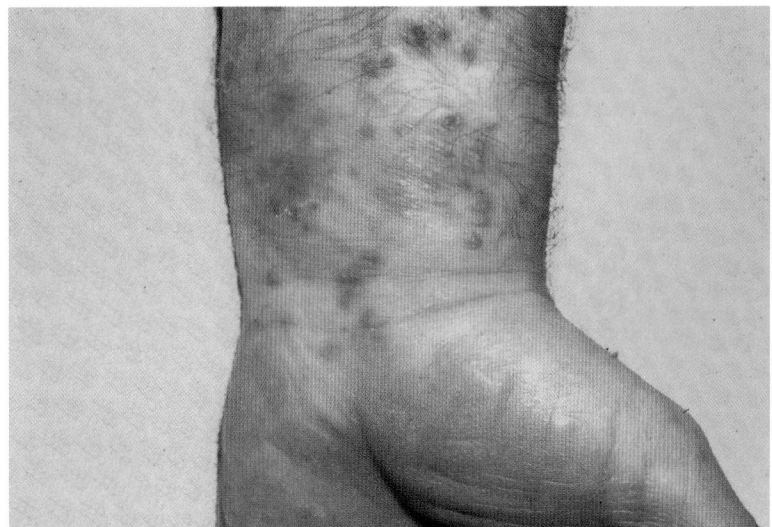

Fig. 4.88
Lichen planus pemphigoides: typical lichenoid papules are present on the anterior aspect of the wrist. By courtesy of M.M. Black, MD, Institute of Dermatology, London, UK.

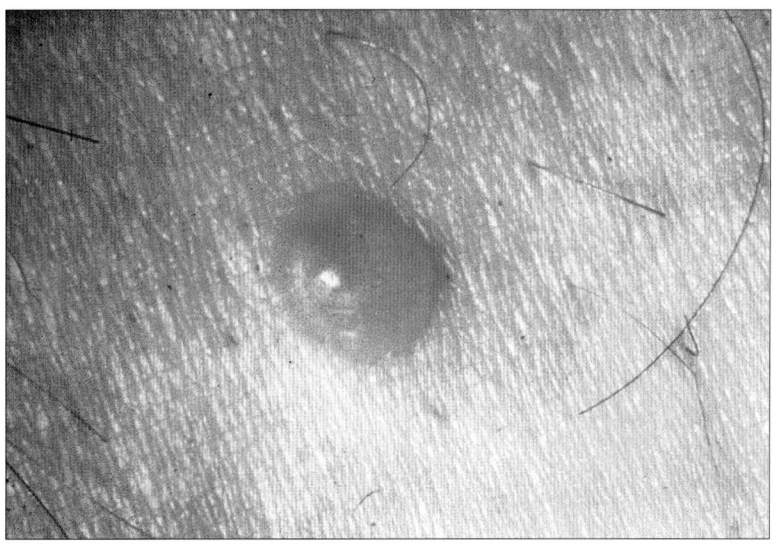

Fig. 4.90
Lichen planus pemphigoides: note the intact dome-shaped tense blister. By courtesy of M.M. Black, MD, Institute of Dermatology, London, UK.

skin, in areas of erythema or on lichenoid papules (*Figs 4.89* and *4.90*). In some patients, the blisters are generalized. Exceptionally, the blisters are localized with typical lichen planus-like lesions elsewhere. A case with single blisters on the soles has been described.[3] They are tense, dome-shaped and hemorrhagic or contain clear fluid. Evolution to pemphigoid nodularis-like lesions has been described.[4] Lichen planus pemphigoides presents most often in the fourth and fifth decades of life, shows slight female predominance and has predilection for lower and upper extremities.[5–7] Exceptionally, cases have been documented in childhood.[9–11] In contrast to presentation in adults, childhood lichen planus pemphigoides shows male predominance (M:F=2.2:1) and has higher tendency for palmoplantar involvement.[7] All races may be affected. Mucosal sites can also be involved and there is predilection for the oral mucosa.[8] Other mucosal surfaces including hypopharynx, esophagus, vulva, and conjunctiva are very rarely affected. Nail involvement is exceptional.[7] The mean time span between progression from lichen planus lesions to the vesiculo-bullous lesions of lichen planus pemphigoides is around 8 months.[7] The prognosis of lichen planus pemphigoides is usually favorable and the eruption generally resolves within a few weeks following treatment. Recurrent lesions are uncommon occurring in around 20% of cases.[7]

Pathogenesis and histologic features

The lichenoid lesions show the typical histopathological and immunofluorescent changes of lichen planus, but the bullae have features more suggestive of bullous pemphigoid (*Fig. 4.91*). A variety of findings have been described. Early erythematous lesions show intense dermal edema with a dense perivascular and an interstitial eosinophil infiltrate; eosinophilic spongiosis may also sometimes be evident. Established blisters are subepidermal and both inflammatory (cell-rich) and cell-poor variants have been documented (*Figs 4.92* and *4.93*).[5] Eosinophils are variably present, but often may be numerous.

Immunofluorescent examination of biopsies from peribullous skin reveals linear deposition of IgG and complement.[12–15] The serum contains an IgG antibasement membrane antibody in up to 50–60% of patients. With NaCl-split skin, the antibody generally labels the roof of the blister cavity. Ultrastructural investigations have shown that the level of separation is usually through the lamina lucida. By immunoelectron microscopy, the immunoreactants typically localize to the hemidesmosome and lamina lucida.[5,15,16] Mucous membrane pemphigoid and epidermolysis bullosa acquisita (EBA)-like variants have, however, also been documented.[17]

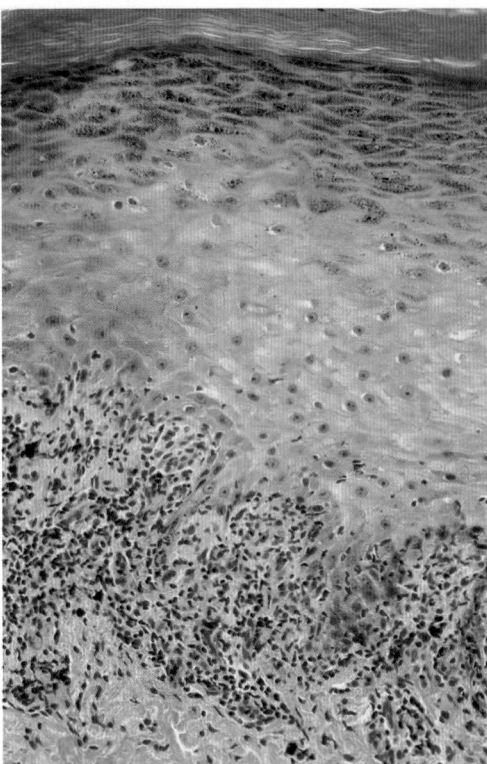

Fig. 4.91
Lichen planus pemphigoides: the lichenoid papules show typical features of lichen planus.

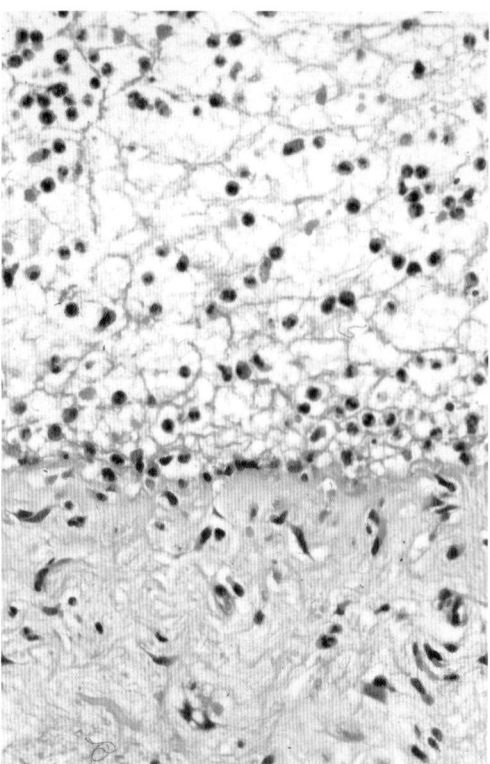

Fig. 4.93
Lichen planus pemphigoides: the blister contains eosinophils.

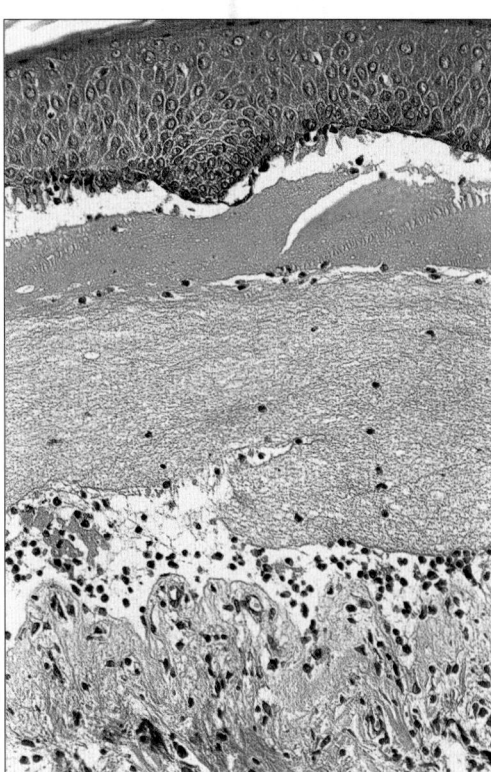

Fig. 4.92
Lichen planus pemphigoides: there is a subepidermal blister.

A number of antigens have been recognized in lichen planus pemphigoides including BP180, BP230, and an as yet uncharacterized 200-kD protein of keratinocyte derivation.[1,17–25] The segment of the NC16A domain recognized in lichen planus pemphigoides differs from BP, localizing to MCW-4 (the more C-terminal end of the domain) as opposed to MCW-0 to MCW-3.[26,27] Type VII collagen has also been implicated in the EBA-like

variant although the immunoblot was negative.[17] Although the levels of anti-BP180 autoantibodies in the serum of patients with lichen planus pemphigoides have been found to correlate with disease activity, this has not been universally proven.[28]

Although the pathogenesis of lichen planus pemphigoides has not been fully unraveled, it is likely that the basement membrane zone damage associated with lichen planus results in antigen exposure with subsequent autoantibody production and resultant bullous disease. So far, it is uncertain why only a small percentage of patients with lichen planus are affected. The pathogenesis in those patients in whom the blisters develop first is unknown although a different antigen may be involved. Exceptionally, cases have been documented as an adverse drug reaction (e.g., to angiotensin-converting enzyme inhibitors, complicating PUVA therapy, or in a patient taking paracetamol, ibuprofen, and having narrowband UVB),[29–38] following certain infections (chickenpox, hepatitis B),[39,40] or developing in the background of a henna tattoo.[41] An exceptional case of lichen planus pemphigoides developing preferentially over pre-existing scars has also been reported.[42] There has been a suggestion that lichen planus pemphigoides might be associated with internal malignancy, but the diagnosis lacked substantiation by immunofluorescence studies.[43] Two additional cases involving a patient with multiple keratoacanthomas and colonic adenocarcinoma indicating a Torre-Muir-like syndrome and association with retroperitoneal Castleman disease have also been noted.[44,45]

Differential diagnosis

Lichen planus pemphigoides differs from typical bullous pemphigoid clinically by its earlier age of presentation and predilection for the lower limbs. In those cases, associated with antibodies to BP180, epitope mapping may make the distinction.

Mucous membrane pemphigoid (cicatricial pemphigoid)

Mucous membrane pemphigoid represents a spectrum of diseases (e.g., ocular pemphigoid, oral pemphigoid, benign mucous membrane pemphigoid) which affect the mucosa and skin.[1–4] With the advent of molecular studies identifying the antigens involved, it is becoming clear that there are a

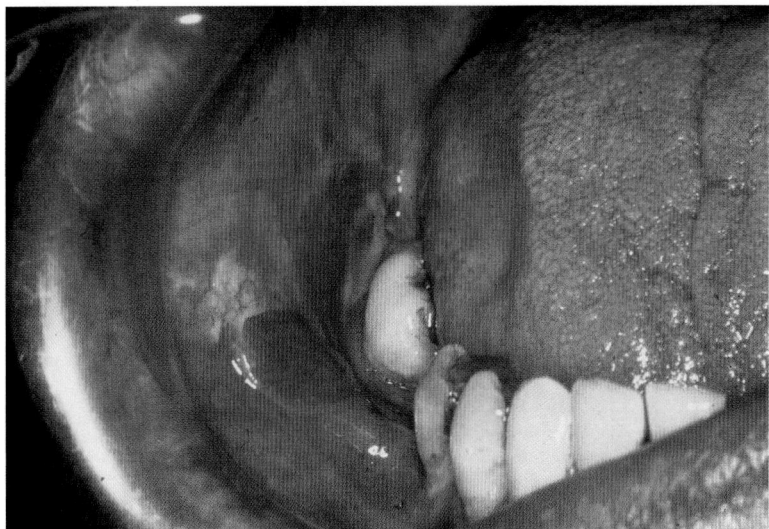

Fig. 4.94
Mucous membrane pemphigoid: there is erosion of the buccal mucosa. By courtesy of P. Morgan, FRCPath, London, UK.

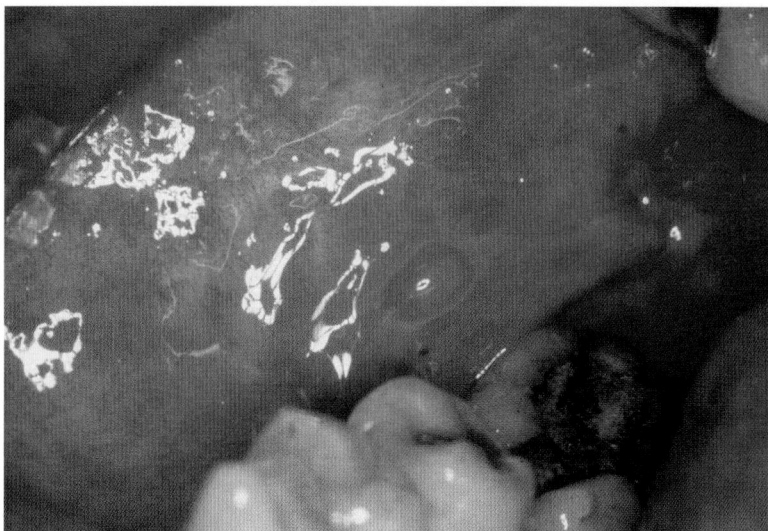

Fig. 4.95
Mucous membrane pemphigoid: in addition to erosions, intact blisters are evident. By courtesy of P. Morgan, FRCPath, London, UK.

number of relatively well-defined clinicopathological variants that arise as a consequence of autoimmune diseases directed against a number of different basement membrane antigens. Although multiple systems are often affected, pure ocular and oral variants may also be encountered.[1,2]

Clinical features

Mucous membrane pemphigoid is a rare blistering disorder in which mucosal lesions predominate and in which scarring is a characteristic feature (although not generally in the oral lesions).[1,2,5] It is often associated with severe morbidity, largely due to the effects of the scarring. As ocular and oral lesions predominate, many patients come to the attention primarily of the dental and oral surgeons or ophthalmologists rather than dermatologists.

The incidence is estimated as being between 1:12 000 and 1:20 000 of the population per year.[2] It is associated with a female preponderance (2:1) and it not uncommonly presents in the seventh decade. Very rare instances of childhood involvement have been reported.[3,6–10] Mucous membrane pemphigoid is a chronic disease and is rarely self-limiting. It shows no racial or geographic predilection.

Oral lesions occur in 85–95% of patients and commonly follow mild trauma.[11] Bullae, erosions, and erythema most commonly affect the gingival or buccal mucosa, but the hard and soft palate, tongue, and lips are also frequently involved (Figs 4.94 and 4.95). Desquamative gingivitis is the most common manifestation[12,13] and can represent an early or only presenting sign of the disease.[14] Patients with desquamative gingivitis present with painful, swollen, erythematous lesions of the gums, which may be associated with bleeding, blistering, erosions, and ulceration.[15] Most cases of desquamative gingivitis have lichen planus and only in a low percentage, around 9%, is the process a manifestation of mucous membrane pemphigoid.[16] Lesions limited to the oral cavity is a distinctive subset, usually associated with a good prognosis although characterized by chronicity.[1] Pharyngeal (19% of patients) and esophageal (4% of patients) lesions may be complicated by scarring, resulting in stenoses. Aspiration pneumonia is sometimes a fatal complication. Nasal lesions, which may occur in up to 15% of patients, lead to obstruction and occasionally cicatricial stenoses and septal perforation.[17] Laryngeal involvement occurs in 8% of patients and is sometimes complicated by such severe stricture formation and edema that tracheotomy may be a life-saving necessity.[15] Involvement of the trachea is exceptional.[18]

Ocular lesions, which occur in approximately 64% of patients, are a source of considerable morbidity.[19–21] The eye (in particular the conjunctiva) may be a sole site of involvement.[15] Early symptoms are those of a non-specific conjunctivitis. In more advanced lesions, subconjunctival fibrosis develops.[22,23] Patients may therefore present with fibrous bands (symblephara) stretching between the fornices and the globe (Fig. 4.96).

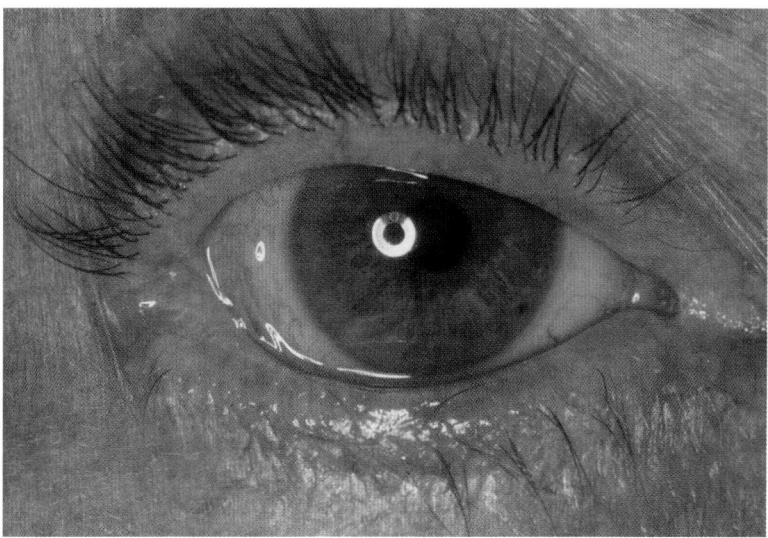

Fig. 4.96
Mucous membrane pemphigoid: there is a dense fibrous adhesion (symblepharon) between the conjunctiva lining the eyelid and that covering the globe. By courtesy of the Institute of Dermatology, St Thomas' Hospital, London, UK.

Eventually, contractures may obliterate the conjunctival sac. An essential feature of ocular cicatricial pemphigoid is the production of an abnormal tear film. This develops because of diminished lacrimal gland secretion (due to ductal stenosis), impaired goblet cell mucus secretion and ocular exposure due to impaired eye closure.[22] The end result is ocular drying and eventual keratinization of the ocular surface epithelium. Other important sequelae include entropion, trichiasis (maldirected eyelashes, which can result in corneal abrasion), erosions and perforation, corneal neovascularization and scarring with opacification (Figs 4.97 and 4.98). Primary corneal bullae have been described, but are very rare, and erosions are more typical.[11] Corneal lesions manifest as foreign body sensation, photophobia, and eventual blindness, which may be bilateral, occurring in up to 16% of patients.[9] Ocular involvement may be classified into a number of stages of progression (modified Foster staging system).[24]

Ocular involvement should not be confused with drug-induced pemphigoid (pseudo-ocular mucous membrane pemphigoid).[2] This is a self-limiting unilateral scarring disease of the eye, which most commonly develops as a consequence of long-term use of eyedrops containing pilocarpine, echothiophate iodide, idoxuridine, timolol, and adrenaline (epinephrine) in the treatment of glaucoma.[25,26]

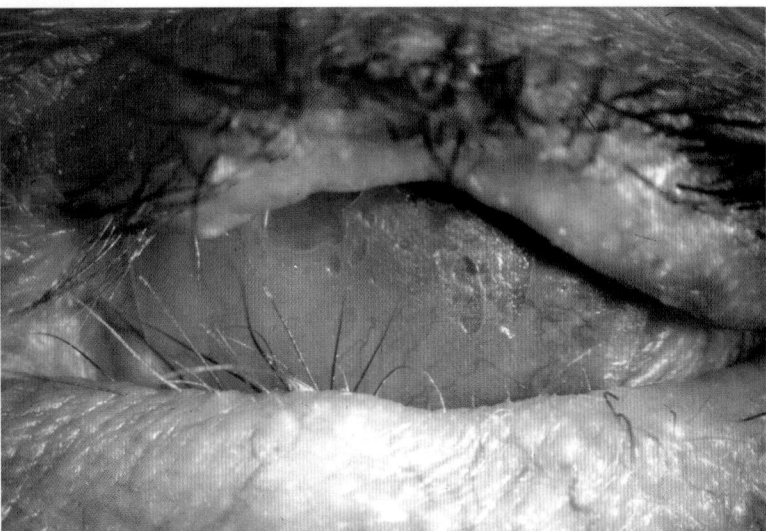

Fig. 4.97
Mucous membrane pemphigoid: in this advanced case, there is entropion and trichiasis (inwardly directed eyelashes). By courtesy of D. Kerr-Muir, MD, St Thomas' Hospital, London, UK.

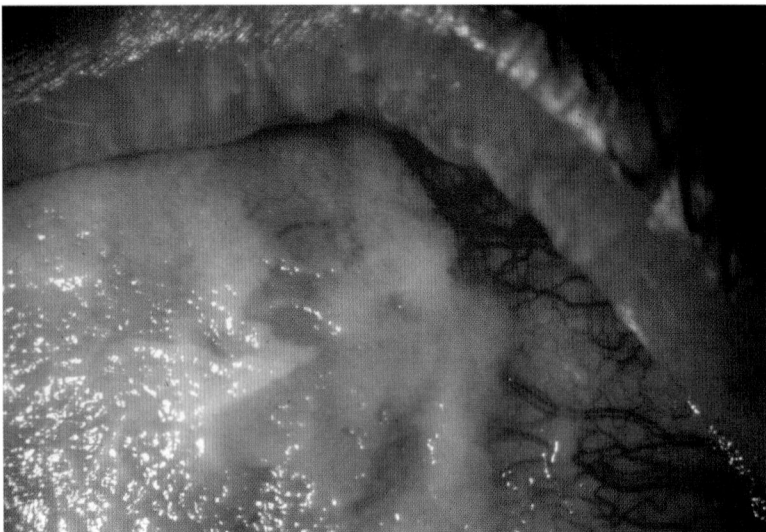

Fig. 4.98
Mucous membrane pemphigoid: here there is dense corneal scarring with complete opacification. By courtesy of D. Kerr-Muir, MD, St Thomas' Hospital, London, UK.

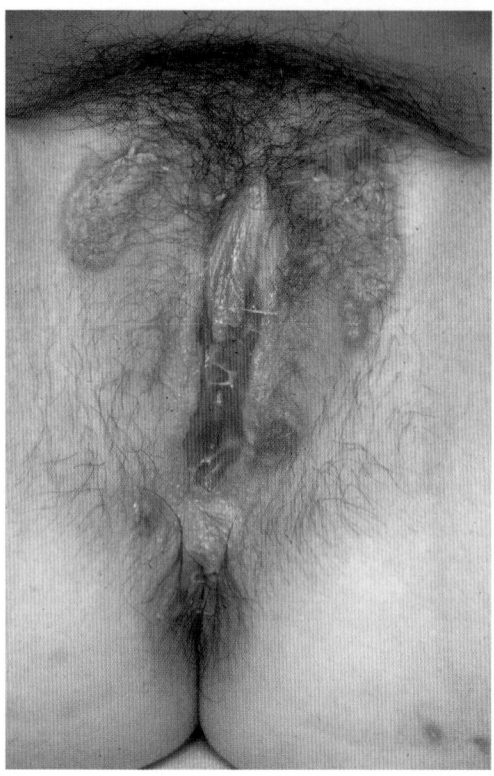

Fig. 4.99
Mucous membrane pemphigoid: in addition to erosions, marked scarring of the vulva is present. By courtesy of R.A. Marsden, MD, St George's Hospital, London, UK.

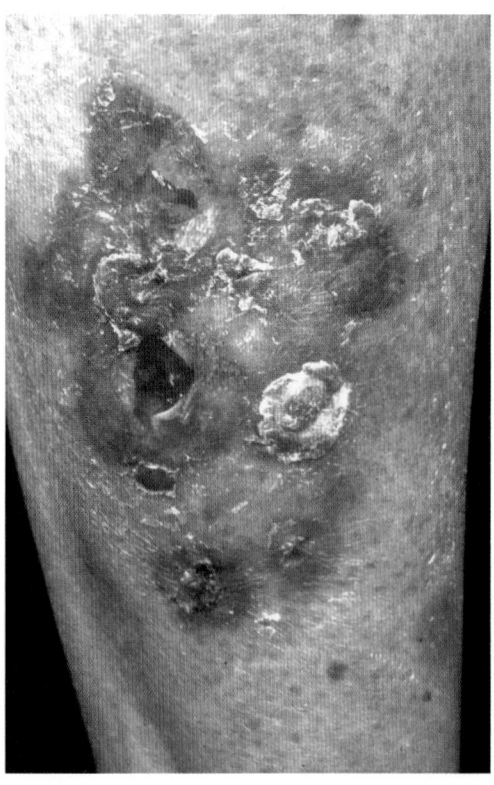

Fig. 4.100
Mucous membrane pemphigoid: note the localized blistering and erosion with scarring on the lower leg of an elderly female. By courtesy of R.A. Marsden, MD, St George's Hospital, London, UK.

Lesions of the female genitalia, which occur in 20% of patients, predominantly affect the labia majora and minora.[15] Scarring is common and may occasionally be associated with labial fusion (*Fig. 4.99*). In males, genital lesions most often affect the prepuce and the glans penis and are occasionally complicated by urethral stricture formation. Anal lesions affect up to 4% of patients and sometimes cause stenosis.[15]

Cutaneous lesions are found in approximately 25–33% of patients with mucous membrane pemphigoid and most often affect the scalp, face, and neck.[2,15,16] In some patients, presentation is similar to that of bullous pemphigoid, and fibrosis is not a feature.[2] Lesions are generally few in number and present as itchy, sometimes burning, tense bullae situated on an erythematous or urticated base (*Fig. 4.100*). They tend to recur on previously affected sites. Rarely, patients may suffer from a transient generalized bullous eruption.[15] Nikolsky sign is negative.[21]

In the Brunsting-Perry variant of localized mucous membrane pemphigoid, scarring lesions are found predominantly on the head and neck (*Fig. 4.101*).[27,28] This condition shows a male predominance (2:1) and presents most often in the sixth decade. The lesions are slowly enlarging, atrophic, or scarred plaques measuring several centimeters or more in diameter

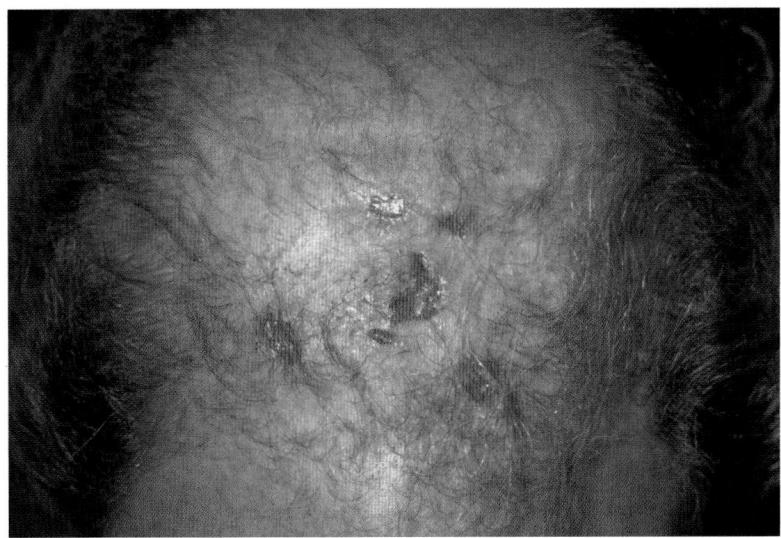

Fig. 4.101
Brunsting-Perry localized pemphigoid: there is extensive alopecia in addition to multiple erosions with scarring. By courtesy of R.A. Marsden, MD, St George's Hospital, London, UK.

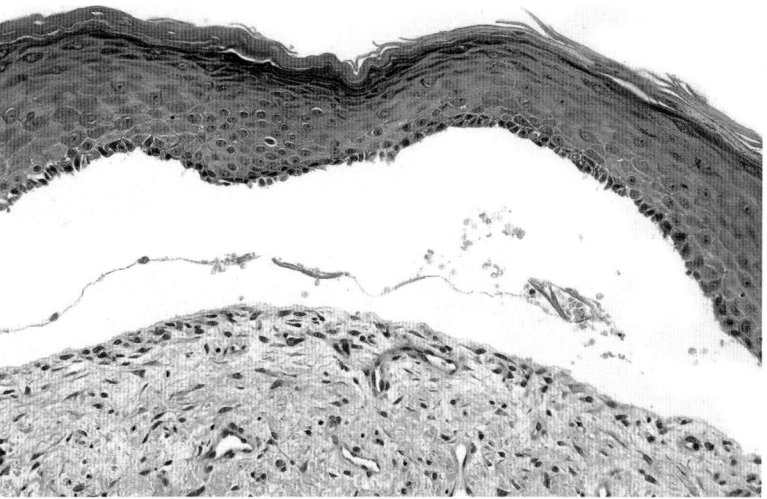

Fig. 4.102
Mucous membrane pemphigoid: in this example of a recurrent lesion, the subepidermal blister is cell free and there is dermal scarring.

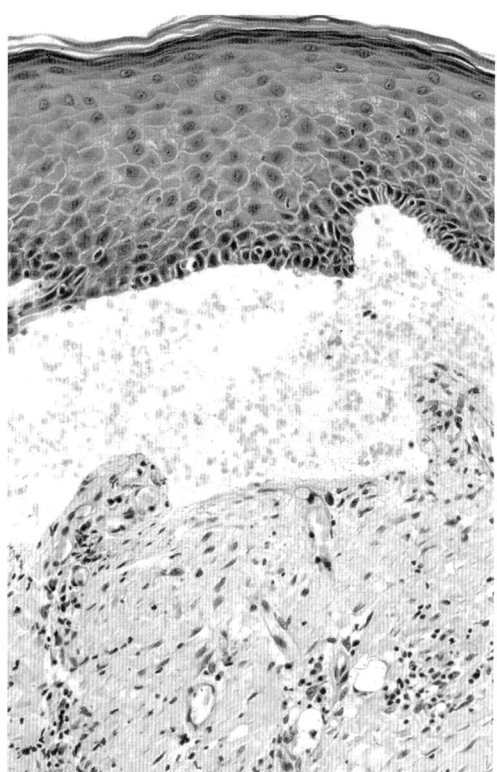

Fig. 4.103
Mucous membrane pemphigoid: high-power view of a similar lesion

and showing vesiculation and/or bullae formation, both centrally and at the enlarging margin.[29] The anterior portion of the scalp, the face (forehead, temporal regions, and cheeks), and the anterolateral aspects of the neck are most often affected.[29] In some patients, lesions are few in number and, because of crusting, they may be clinically treated as actinic keratosis, thereby delaying the diagnosis. Transient mucous membrane lesions may be a feature, but scarring is not seen.[27]

An exceptional case of anti-BP180 mucous membrane pemphigoid presenting with concomitant pemphigus vulgaris limited to mucosal surfaces has been described.[30]

Autoimmune blistering diseases are very rarely associated with HIV infection and only a single exceptional case of mucous membrane pemphigoid has been reported in association with HIV.[31]

Pathogenesis and histologic features

Mucous membrane pemphigoid has been described as a complication of D-penicillamine therapy for rheumatoid arthritis, practolol, and clonidine.[15,32] Immunologically, characteristic cicatricial pemphigoid has also been described following acute, severe ocular inflammation in patients with Stevens-Johnson syndrome.[33] Although the results of HLA associations have been variable, an increased frequency of HLA-DR4 and -DQw3 (DQB1*0301) correlates with a heightened risk of developing ocular disease.[34]

The cutaneous lesions of mucous membrane pemphigoid are often indistinguishable from those of cell-rich (inflammatory) bullous pemphigoid, comprising a subepidermal vesicle containing fibrin, edema fluid, and variable numbers of inflammatory cells. Although eosinophils are usually evident, they tend to be much less numerous than in generalized bullous pemphigoid. The dermis contains a perivascular lymphohistiocytic infiltrate, sometimes with conspicuous plasma cells and accompanied by neutrophils and eosinophils. In older or recurrent lesions, scarring may be a feature (*Fig. 4.102*). Less commonly, a cell-poor subepidermal blister is seen (*Fig. 4.103*). In late lesions, all that may be observed is a band of scarring in the superficial dermis with no inflammation and with or without a subepidermal split. If the latter is present, this is a good clue to the diagnosis, especially in localized variants where the diagnosis is not suspected on clinical grounds.

The histopathology of lesions in antilaminin 332 mucous membrane pemphigoid has been studied in a small number of cases.[35] The features are nondiagnostic and do not allow distinction from other autoimmune blistering diseases. There is subepidermal blistering and a mild to moderate, superficial mixed inflammatory cell infiltrate composed of lymphocytes, histiocytes, and neutrophils and/or eosinophils. Scarring is not often seen as biopsies are taken from early lesions.

Oral lesions may rarely be characterized by vesiculation developing between the stratified squamous epithelium (mucosa) and lamina propria (*Figs 4.104* and *4.105*). The latter is usually edematous and contains a mixed inflammatory cell infiltrate consisting of lymphocytes, histiocytes, plasma cells, and varying numbers of eosinophils and neutrophils (*Fig. 4.106*). More commonly, however, the features seen are those of erosions or ulcers lined by granulation tissue or fibrous tissue and showing non-specific acute or chronic inflammation. The histology is frequently modified by intense acute inflammatory changes due to secondary infection.

Conjunctival vesicles or bullae are very rarely seen in ocular cicatricial pemphigoid. Although erosions may be a feature, more commonly one may anticipate conjunctival squamous metaplasia with foci of hyperkeratosis and parakeratosis accompanied by goblet cell depletion (*Fig. 4.107*).[15] The lamina propria is infiltrated by a mixed inflammatory cell population consisting of lymphocytes, plasma cells, mast cells, and occasional eosinophils

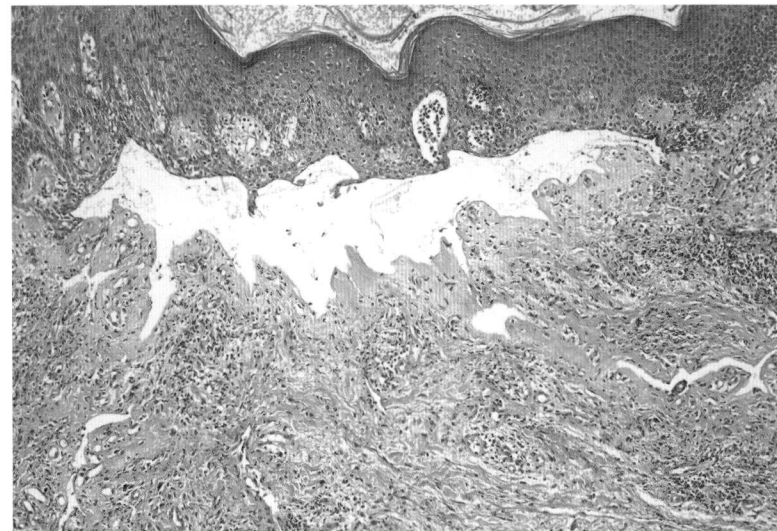

Fig. 4.104
Mucous membrane pemphigoid: oral lesion showing an intact subepithelial blister.

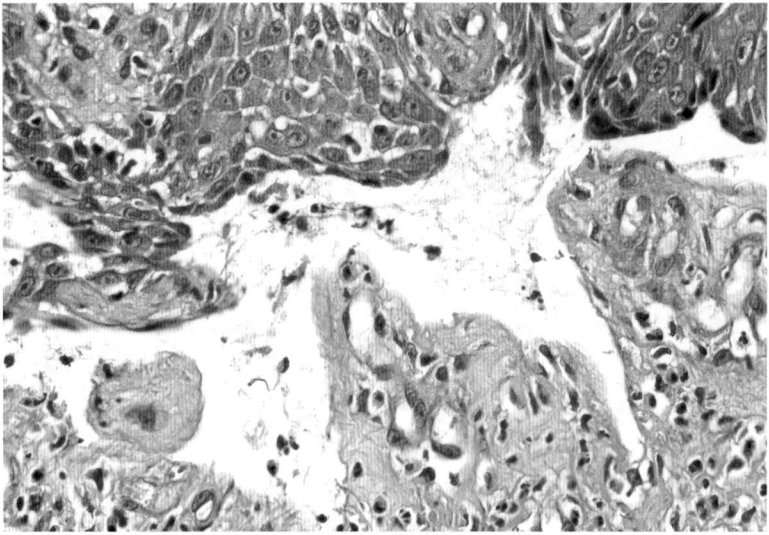

Fig. 4.105
Mucous membrane pemphigoid: note the preservation of the papillae.

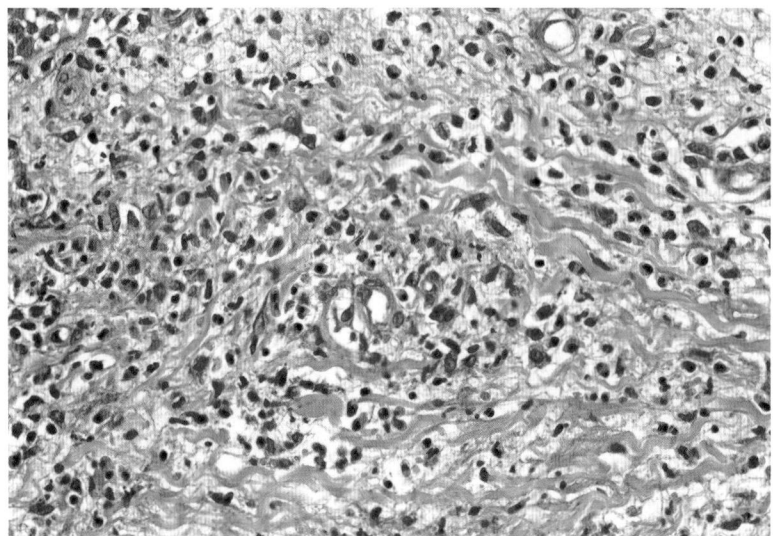

Fig. 4.106
Mucous membrane pemphigoid: in this example, the infiltrate consists of lymphocytes and histiocytes. Eosinophils are not a feature.

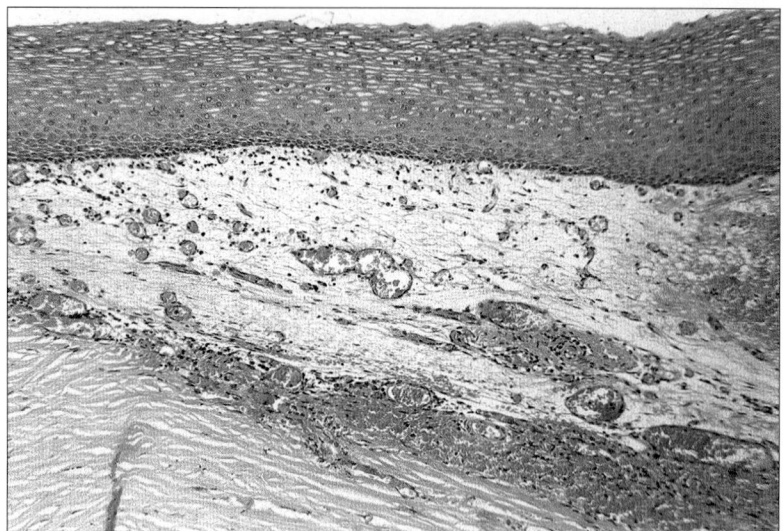

Fig. 4.107
Mucous membrane pemphigoid: this specimen of conjunctiva shows complete squamous metaplasia. Neovascularization of the lamina propria is evident. By courtesy of A. Garner, MD, Institute of Ophthalmology, London, UK.

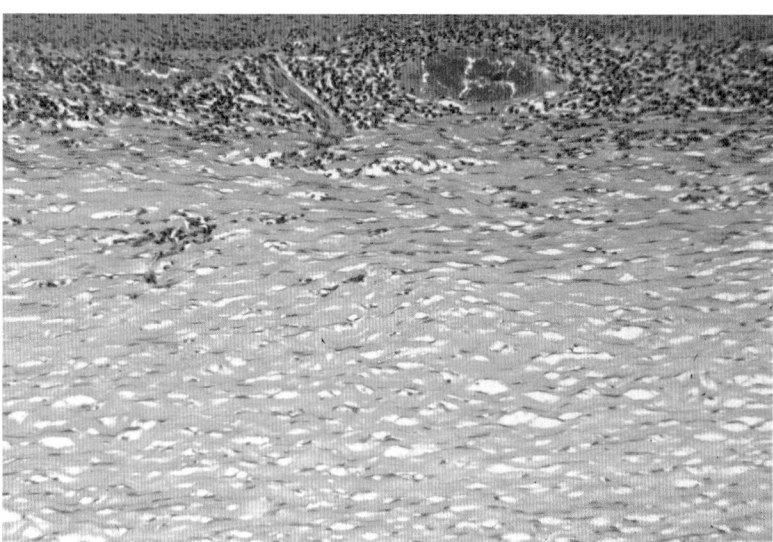

Fig. 4.108
Mucous membrane pemphigoid: section of cornea. The overlying pannus shows squamous metaplasia, chronic inflammation, and neovascularization. Blood vessels are also present in the cornea. By courtesy of A. Garner, MD, Institute of Ophthalmology, London, UK.

and neutrophils.[23] Granulation tissue may be seen in early lesions, but dense scarring is a feature of the later stage. In more severely affected patients, a variety of intraocular manifestations, including iridocyclitis, rubeosis iridis, and the development of synechiae, may be seen (*Figs 4.108–4.110*).

Laryngeal, pharyngeal, and esophageal lesions occasionally show subepithelial bullae, erosions, ulcers, inflammatory changes, and fibrosis (*Fig. 4.111*). Chronic involvement may result in serious stenosis.

The histologic features of the localized cutaneous scarring (Brunsting-Perry) variant are indistinguishable from those of mucous membrane pemphigoid.[29]

Electron microscopic observations are variable. In some patients, the split is in the lamina lucida with the lamina densa lining the floor of the blister cavity, whereas in others, lamina densa is found along the roof of the blister, and occasionally the lamina densa may be split, lining the roof and the floor.[2,36]

Direct immunofluorescent findings in mucous membrane pemphigoid are similar to those found in generalized bullous pemphigoid. Therefore a

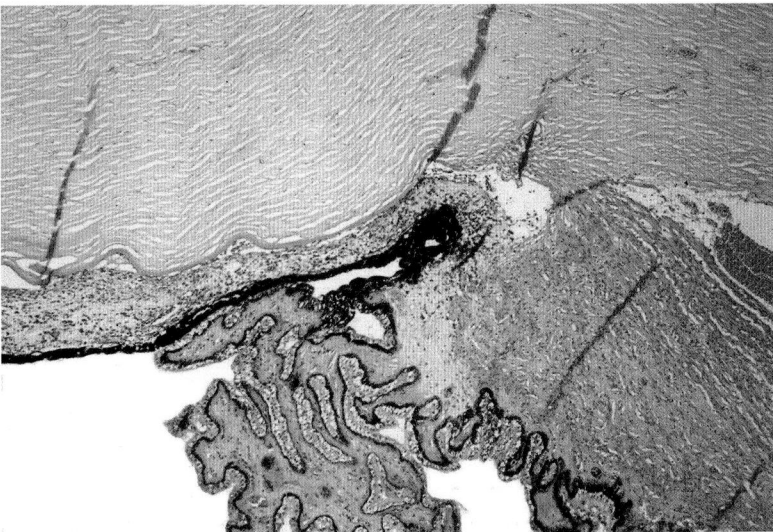

Fig. 4.109
Mucous membrane pemphigoid: this section shows iris impaction with anterior synechiae. Iritis and posterior synechiae are also present. By courtesy of A. Garner, MD, Institute of Ophthalmology, London, UK.

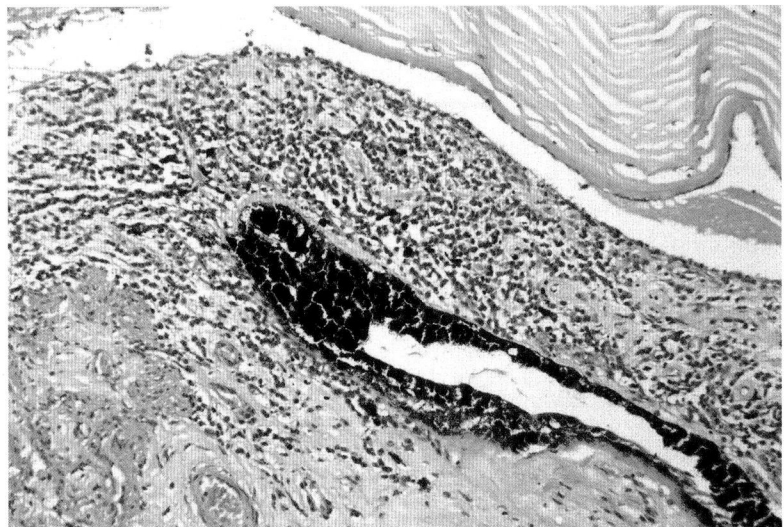

Fig. 4.110
Mucous membrane pemphigoid: this field shows anterior uveitis. There is inflammation of the iris and ciliary body. By courtesy of A. Garner, MD, Institute of Ophthalmology, London, UK.

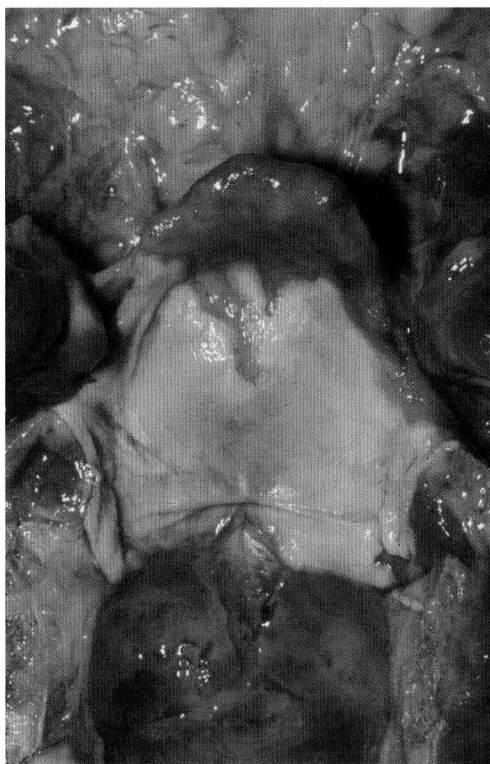

Fig. 4.111
Mucous membrane pemphigoid: postmortem specimen showing laryngeal erosion, ulceration, and scarring.

linear deposit of IgG (and sometimes IgA) and C3 is found at the basement membrane region of perilesional mucosa (the site of choice) or perilesional skin in approximately 80–97% of patients.[37–41] The presence of IgA at the basement membrane region accompanied by IgG and C3 is a diagnostic pointer towards cicatricial pemphigoid.[2] Examination of the oral mucosa is also of value in the diagnosis of ocular disease.[2] Direct immunoperoxidase of paraffin-embedded tissue has been proposed as a satisfactory alternative if a specimen has not been taken for direct immunofluorescence studies.[42]

Circulating antibasement membrane zone autoantibodies (IgG and/or IgA) are sometimes present (26–36%) and are usually of low titer.[38,43,44] Substitution of normal buccal mucosa as substrate does not increase the yield of circulating antibodies.[43] The antibody consists predominantly of IgG4 and IgG1 subclasses, the presence of the latter conferring complement-fixing ability.[45] The presence of IgA may be linked to the mucosal membrane distribution of this disease.[46]

Investigations of cicatricial pemphigoid antibodies using 1 M NaCl-split skin have yielded variable results.[47–49] Circulating antibodies may be detected in from 50% to 100% of cases with active disease.[50,51] Although the majority of sera have reacted with the epidermal side of the split, some have

labeled the floor (dermal side, subsequently shown to be due to antilaminin 332 antibodies: see below), and exceptionally both the roof and the floor have been labeled.[47–51] There is also variation in indirect immunofluorescence findings depending upon the predominant site of involvement. Thus, for example, split skin indirect immunofluorescence may be positive in up to 81% of patients with combined skin and mucosal disease, whereas much lower figures have been found in patients with mucosal disease only (18%) or isolated ocular disease (7%).[2,52]

The immunofluorescent findings in the Brunsting-Perry variant are the same as those described for mucous membrane pemphigoid.[53–56]

Immunoelectron microscopic observations in mucous membrane pemphigoid have revealed two patterns of immune reactant deposition. IgG and C3 may be localized to the lower lamina lucida and lamina densa or else identified overlying the hemidesmosome.[57–63] There is no involvement of the sublamina densa region. The variation can be explained by the different target antigens involved, i.e., BP180, laminin 332 or β_4 integrin.

In the Brunsting-Perry variant of localized chronic pemphigoid the immunoreactants are localized within the lamina lucida and on the undersurface of basal keratinocytes.[64] In a single case it was demonstrated that the antibodies in the serum reacted with the C-terminal domain of the BP180 (BPAG2) protein.[65] Additionally, however, the complement components C3 and C4 may also be detected within the lamina densa and the upper papillary dermis. It is suggested that this latter finding might account for the scarring characteristic of this disease process.[64]

A number of subsets (at least six) of mucous membrane pemphigoid have been delineated by antigen analysis and by the use of molecular techniques, including variants characterized by antibodies to bullous pemphigoid antigen of 180 kDa (BP180), bullous pemphigoid antigen of 230 kDa (BP230), both subunits of integrin $alpha_6\beta_4$, laminin-332, and type VII collagen.[45,49,59,62–78] Traditionally, this group of diseases has been classified together, but the increasing demonstration of autoimmune reactions to different cell adhesion molecules will likely ultimately lead to subtyping of this disease similar to the cutaneous forms. For now, since the clinical features are more uniform than those seen in the skin, these mucosal cases are considered together. BP180 (collagen XVII) antibodies react with at least two different sites on the extracellular domain of BP180. One is located on the noncollagenous domain NC16A; the other is located within the carboxy-terminal region.[71,79–82] Antilaminin-332 (also called epiligrin) antibodies to the γ_3 subunit (sometimes accompanied by antilaminin type-6 antibodies) are present in a minority of cases and, although the antibodies are usually IgG, IgA, and IgE, antibodies against laminin-332 may also be found in a subset of patients.[83] It has recently been demonstrated that anti-laminin-332 autoantibodies are more likely to be present in patients with severe disease.[65] Patients with antilaminin-332 antibodies have been classified as having antiepiligrin mucous membrane pemphigoid (AEMMP). Up to a third of these patients can have associated internal malignancies (including lung, colon, endometrium, stomach, ovary, pancreas, prostate, non-Hodgkin lymphoma, cutaneous T-cell lymphoma, and acute myeloblastic leukemia).[84–88] Integrin has been implicated in patients with ocular disease and an as yet unidentified 45-kD antigen, which binds to the epidermal side on split skin immunofluorescence, has been identified in some patients with IgA antibodies.[73,75,76] Presence of autoantibodies to type VII collagen is of importance in some cases of Brunsting-Perry cicatricial pemphigoid (these patients might be better classified within the epidermolysis bullosa acquisita spectrum, see below).[89]

Differential diagnosis

Apart from the presence of scarring in older lesions, mucous membrane pemphigoid is indistinguishable from bullous pemphigoid.

Epidermolysis bullosa acquisita (dermolytic pemphigoid)

Epidermolysis bullosa acquisita (dermolytic pemphigoid) is a rare, chronic blistering disease, which is characterized by variable clinical presentations and which may therefore be mistaken for a number of other blistering disorders, including congenital epidermolysis bullosa and the other acquired autoimmune bullous dermatoses.[1,2] Annual incidence figures from France and central Germany are 0.17–0.26 per million of the population.[3,4] In contrast to its congenital counterpart, epidermolysis bullosa acquisita (EBA) usually develops in adult life, although cases in childhood have been documented.[5,6] Initially, it was characterized as a porphyria cutanea tarda-like mechanobullous dermatosis. More recently, however, patients have been described in whom the disease has presented as a generalized inflammatory bullous dermatosis.[1] For many decades, the diagnosis of EBA was one of exclusion. As a result of immunofluorescence and immunoultrastructural techniques combined with immunoblotting and immunoprecipitation, EBA is now recognized as an autoimmune dermatosis, type VII collagen (290 kD) representing the target antigen.[1,7,8] Collagen VII is a homotrimer composed of identical alpha-chains (290-kDa antigen), each composed of a central collagenous triple helical rod flanked by an N-terminal 145 kDa noncollagenous domain (NC1) and 34 kDa NC2 domain.[9] The N-terminal 145-kDa NC1 domain, containing a cartilage matrix protein subdomain, nine fibronectin III-like subdomains, a collagen binding von Willebrand factor A-like subdomain, and a cysteine and proline rich subdomain, has been recognized as the immunodominant region recognized by autoantibodies in the great majority of EBA patients.[10–12] The NC2 domain and central collagenous domain are targeted less frequently.[10] Immunoreactivity against different epitopes has been suggested to be responsible for the variable clinical presentation.[13,14] Patients with EBA have increased frequency of MHC class II haplotype HLA-DR2.[15]

Clinical features

EBA was defined in 1971 by Roenigk and colleagues[5] as follows:
- clinical lesions resembling dystrophic epidermolysis bullosa (blisters developing on the hands, feet, elbows, and knees following mild trauma and complicated by atrophic scarring, milia formation, and nail dystrophy),
- an adult onset,
- a negative family history of epidermolysis bullosa,
- exclusion of all other recognized bullous dermatoses, including porphyria cutanea tarda, bullous pemphigoid, dermatitis herpetiformis, pemphigus, erythema multiforme, and bullous drug reactions.[16]

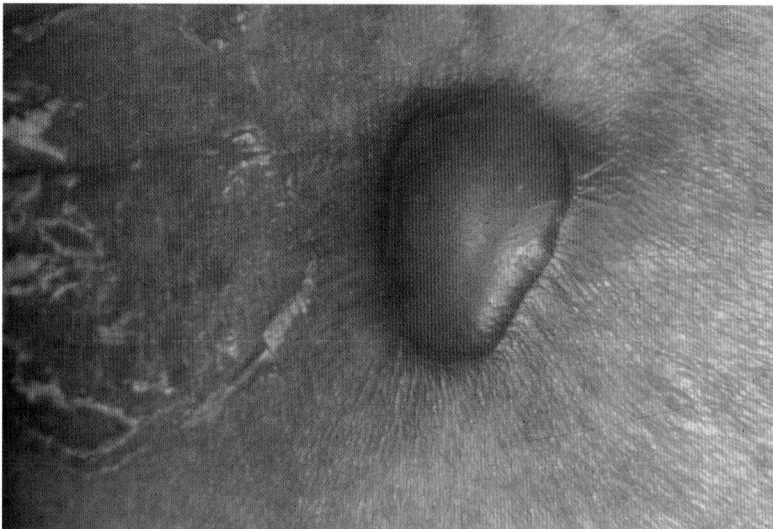

Fig. 4.112
Epidermolysis bullosa acquisita: there is a tense fluid-filled blister on the ankle. An old lesion is also evident. By courtesy of the Institute of Dermatology, London, UK.

It has a wide age incidence ranging from 11 to 77 years, with a mean age of 47 years. It is associated with a slight female predominance.

In addition to the mechanobullous classical form of EBA, inflammatory variants, including bullous pemphigoid-like, mucous membrane pemphigoid-like, and linear IgA disease-like variants, may also be encountered.[1,17,18]

A case of familial EBA has been described.[19]

Classical variant

The classical variant is the most commonly encountered variant of EBA. Patients present with a porphyria cutanea tarda-like illness showing extreme skin fragility, developing erosions, and blistering and crusting in response to mild trauma including shearing forces.[5] Lesions are located on the backs of the fingers and hands in particular and at other sites that are susceptible to trauma, including the knees, elbows, and buttocks, but virtually any site may be affected (Fig. 4.112).[1,5] The blisters are characteristically noninflammatory, painless, and tense, and may contain clear or bloodstained fluid. An exceptional example of EBA with erythroderma on initial presentation has been reported.[20]

Healing is usually associated with postinflammatory hyperpigmentation, considerable scarring, and atrophy. Milia are frequently conspicuous, and nail changes, including distal onycholysis, dystrophy, and anonychia with nail bed scarring, are common complications (Fig. 4.113). More widespread involvement may resemble dominant or more often recessive dystrophic epidermolysis bullosa. Scarring may then be extreme with resultant contractures and syndactilism. Rarely, esophageal involvement has been documented with resultant stricture formation.[17,21,22]

Bullous pemphigoid-like EBA

This is the most commonly encountered inflammatory variant.[23] On the basis of split skin indirect immunofluorescence (see below) it has been suggested that a BP presentation may account for up to 50% of cases of EBA and that 10–15% of patients diagnosed as BP, in fact, have EBA.[23] Other authors, however, have found that EBA is very rare compared to BP, the relative incidence being approximately 25–50 cases of BP for every one case of EBA diagnosed.[24,25]

Patients present with a generalized eruption of large tense blisters, which are often associated with erythema and show a predilection for the flexural and intertriginous areas.[26,27] Pruritus is common.[23] Skin fragility is typically absent and scarring and/or milia are not usually features unless the patient concomitantly shows or evolves towards a mechanobullous phase.[1,23] Infrequently, the clinical manifestations may resemble dermatitis herpetiformis (Fig. 4.114). Exceptionally, prurigo nodularis-like lesions may be seen.[28]

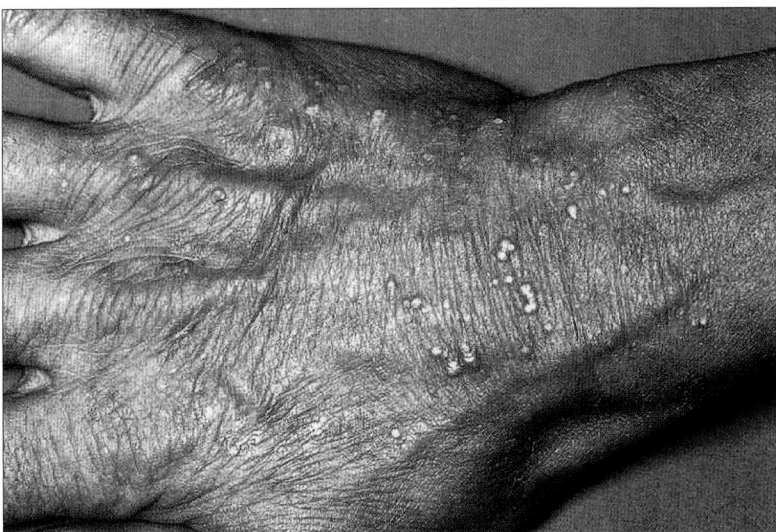

Fig. 4.113
Epidermolysis bullosa acquisita: conspicuous milia are present on the back of the hand. By courtesy of the Institute of Dermatology, London, UK.

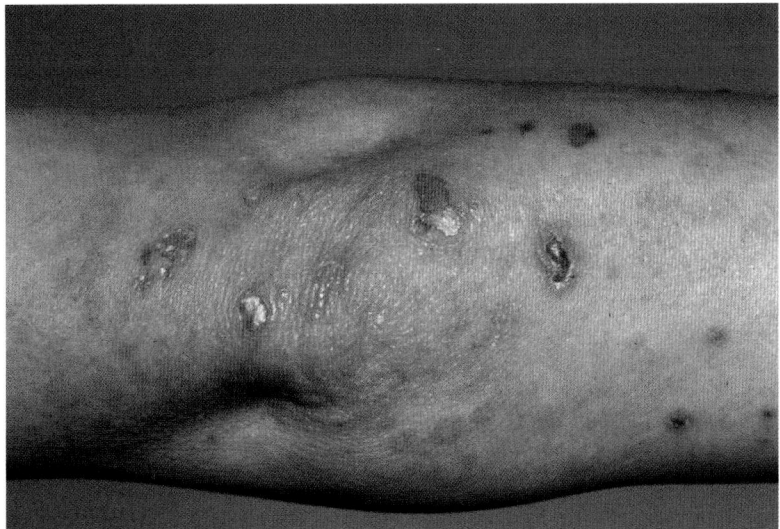

Fig. 4.114
Epidermolysis bullosa acquisita: in this patient with the dermatitis herpetiformis-like inflammatory variant, blisters, erosions, and erythematous plaques are evident on the elbow. By courtesy of R.A. Marsden, MD, St George's Hospital, London, UK.

Mucous membrane pemphigoid-like variant

Some patients present with a mucous membrane pemphigoid-like variant, characterized by mucous membrane involvement. The oral cavity is commonly affected. Erosions, ulcers, and blisters may be seen on the tongue, gums, palate, and buccal mucosa.[18] Rarely, the larynx and esophagus are affected with resultant stricture formation.[17] The anus, vulva, vagina, and bladder can very occasionally be involved.[29] Conjunctival lesions are an important, but infrequent, cause of morbidity.[17,18,30] Symblepharon, epiphora, and even blindness may occur. Alopecia is sometimes an additional feature.[7,21]

Brunsting-Perry variant

Some patients with the Brunsting-Perry variant of mucous membrane pemphigoid (characterized by blistering and scarring confined to the head and neck) have antibodies against type VII collagen and therefore might better be classified within the epidermolysis bullosa acquisita spectrum.[7,31,32] Facial involvement predominates.[32,33] A very unusual localized case with periorbital papulovesicular blisters has been reported.[34]

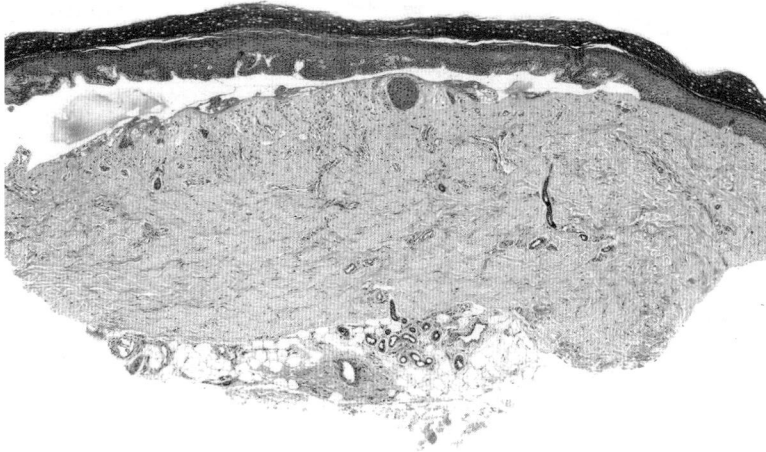

Fig. 4.115
Epidermolysis bullosa acquisita (classical variant): there is a cell-free subepidermal vesicle. Note the dermal scarring.

Linear IgA disease-like variant (IgA-EBA)

Epidermolysis bullosa acquisita may also present as a linear IgA disease-like variant in which both adult and childhood patients have IgA autoantibodies directed against type VII collagen (see below).[35-37] In adults, ocular involvement is often severe and blindness is not uncommon.[36]

Childhood EBA

Childhood EBA is extremely rare. Mucosal disease is often severe, and clinical manifestations have included classical bullous pemphigoid and linear IgA-like variants.[6,8,38-41]

Systemic disease

Epidermolysis bullosa acquisita has long been known to be associated with a number of systemic illnesses, many with an immunologically mediated pathogenesis. Most important are inflammatory bowel disease and diabetes mellitus.[2,17,23,42-53] Approximately 30% of patients with EBA manifest inflammatory bowel disease, predominantly Crohn disease.[50,54] Control of this improves the skin condition in some patients. Interestingly, although up to 68% of patients with inflammatory bowel disease have antibodies against collagen type VII, only very few develop EBA.[55] Inflammatory bowel disease, either Crohn disease or ulcerative colitis, generally predates development of EBA. Furthermore, an association with celiac disease has recently been reported.[56] Presentation as a paraneoplastic phenomenon in association with internal malignancy has also on occasion been described.[57,58]

Pathogenesis and histologic features

The histologic features are somewhat variable depending upon whether a mechanobullous or an inflammatory lesion is biopsied.

The mechanobullous lesion is characterized by a bland, 'cell-free' subepidermal vesicle containing only a few erythrocytes and a little fibrin (*Figs 4.115* and *4.116*). Usually, no significant inflammatory cell infiltrate is present either within the blister cavity or in the adjacent or underlying dermis. Sometimes, however, a small number of neutrophils, histiocytes, and eosinophils may be present. The basement membrane lines the roof of the blister. Marked scarring of the adjacent dermis is often a feature and milia are frequently identified.

The inflammatory variant is characterized by a subepidermal vesicle accompanied by a mixed inflammatory cell infiltrate comprising lymphocytes, histiocytes with prominent neutrophils, and eosinophils. Neutrophils are usually the predominant cell type and in incipient lesions they may be identified in a linear distribution adjacent to the dermal–epidermal junction.[23] Occasionally, however, eosinophils predominate.[32] Such inflammatory lesions may resemble bullous pemphigoid or dermatitis herpetiformis (*Figs 4.117* and *4.118*).[2,59] Oral lesions show similar features of submucosal vesiculation with an erythrocyte and inflammatory cell content.

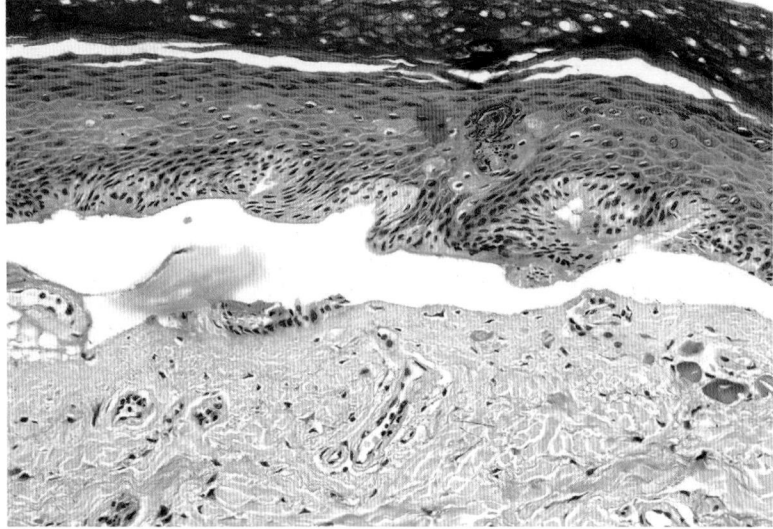

Fig. 4.116
Epidermolysis bullosa acquisita (classical variant): high-power view. There is fibrin along the floor of the blister cavity. Note the absence of inflammatory cells.

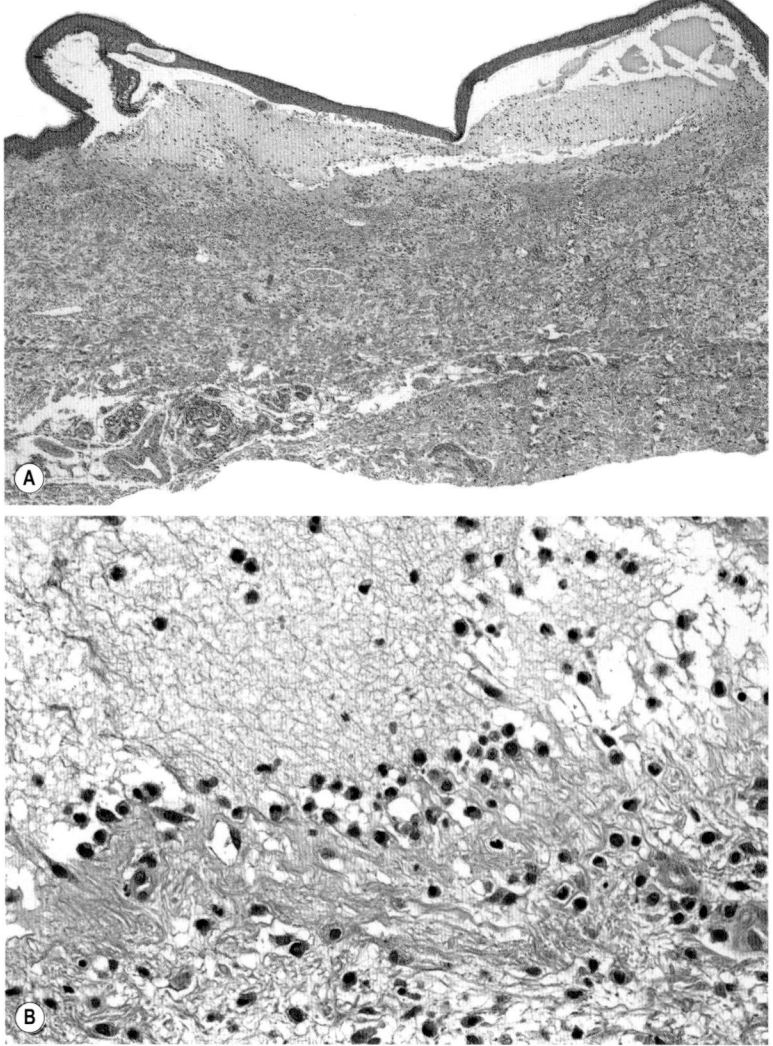

Fig. 4.117
(A, B) Inflammatory epidermolysis bullosa acquisita: in this bullous pemphigoid-like variant, subepidermal blistering is associated with an eosinophil-rich infiltrate.

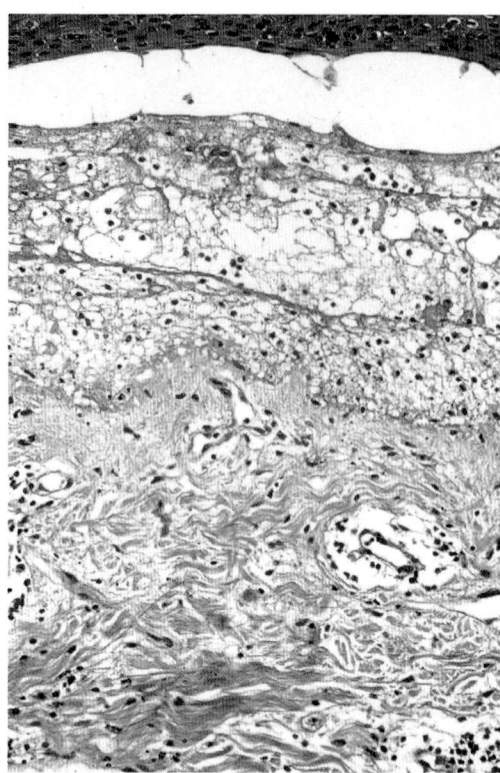

Fig. 4.118
Inflammatory epidermolysis bullosa acquisita: dermatitis herpetiformis-like variant, with a neutrophil-rich infiltrate.

By direct immunoperoxidase using paraffin-embedded material, type IV collagen is found in the roof of the blister cavity (see *Fig. 4.8*).

Ultrastructurally, the level of the split in EBA is situated within the superficial dermis immediately below the lamina densa (*Fig. 4.119*).[60–62] The basal keratinocytes appear normal. Anchoring fibrils have been variably reported as reduced in number or absent.[55–62]

An occasional finding is the presence of electron-dense, amorphous granular material within the superficial papillary dermis close to, but separated from, the lamina densa (*Fig. 4.120*).[16,43] When present, the split is usually below the electron-dense amorphous material, which is therefore located within the roof of the blister.

By direct IIMF, IgG and C3 are present in a linear distribution along the basement membrane region (identical to BP) in a very high proportion of cases of EBA (*Fig. 4.121*).[16,17,44] Less commonly, IgM, IgA, properdin, and factor B may also be identified.[1,61,62] Deposition of IgG in the absence of C3 is seen more often in EBA than BP. In linear IgA disease-like patients, IgA may be present in the absence of IgG.[35–37] Positive direct immunofluorescence has also been reported at a variety of other sites, including the oral mucosa, conjunctiva, cornea, esophagus, duodenum, and bladder.[16,36,42] In addition to a linear staining pattern of antibody deposition at the basement membrane by direct IIMF, a distinctive serrated immunodeposition pattern has also been reported; a 'u-serrated' typical of EBA and SLE, and an 'n-serrated' pattern, generally detected in other acquired subepithelial autoimmune blistering diseases, including bullous pemphigoid, mucous membrane pemphigoid, linear IgA disease, p200 pemphigoid, and antiepiligrin mucous membrane pemphigoid.[63,64] The 'u-serrated' pattern is characterized ultrastructurally by upstaining arms between the rootlets of the basal keratinocytes resulting in 'u' shapes.[63,64]

IgG antibasement membrane antibodies may be identified in 25–50% of patients, thereby increasing the similarity to BP.[2,55,60,65] Nevertheless, subtyping of IgG antibodies can aid in separation of EBA from bullous SLE. Namely, while autoantibodies in EBA are usually of IgG1 and IgG4 subclass, bullous SLE is characterized by IgG2 and IgG3 sublass of autoantibodies.[66] In many patients the antibasement membrane antibodies are associated with complement-fixing properties.[67] With split skin IIMF, which is more sensitive than conventional IIMF, the immunoreactants line the floor of the

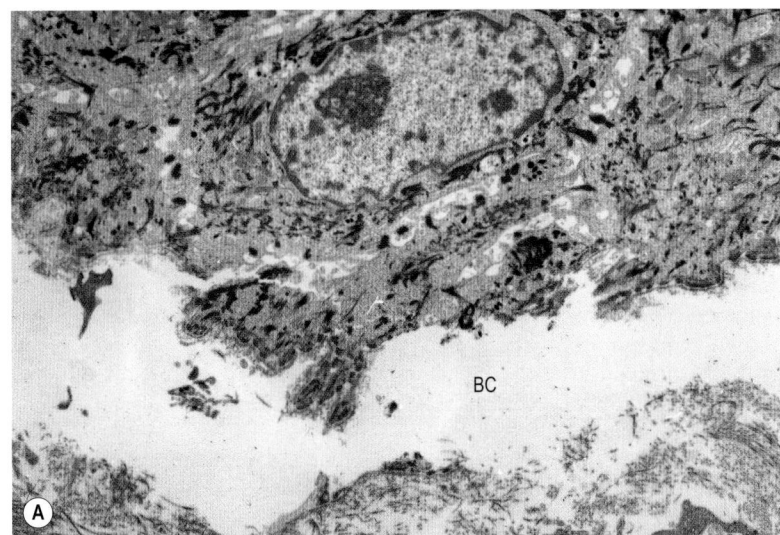

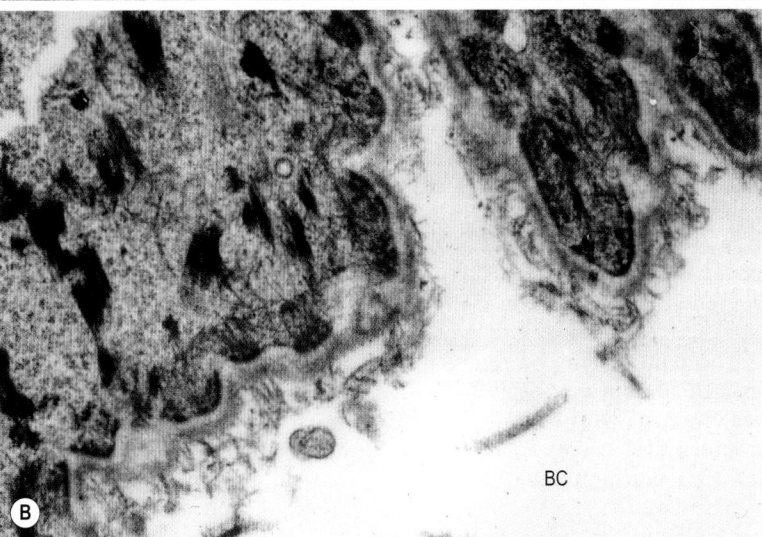

Fig. 4.119
(**A**, **B**) Epidermolysis bullosa acquisita: electron micrograph showing the lamina densa in the roof of the blister. (BC, blister cavity.)

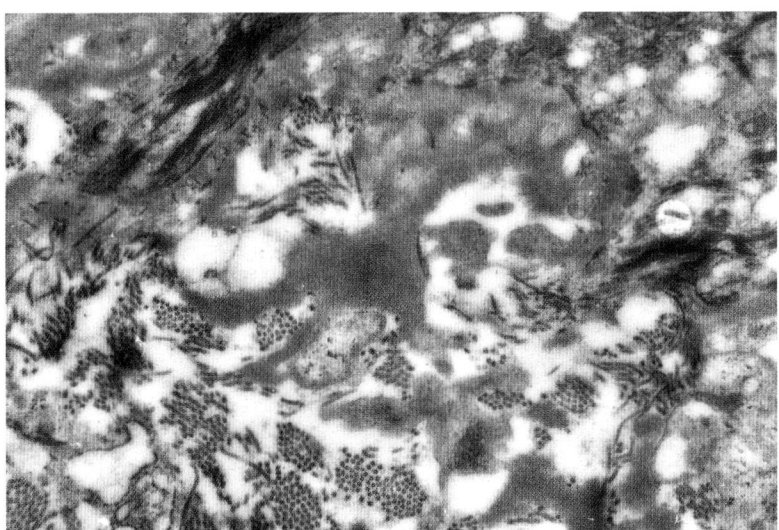

Fig. 4.120
Epidermolysis bullosa acquisita: occasional deposits of finely granular electron-dense material (immunoreactant) as seen in this field may be a useful diagnostic pointer.

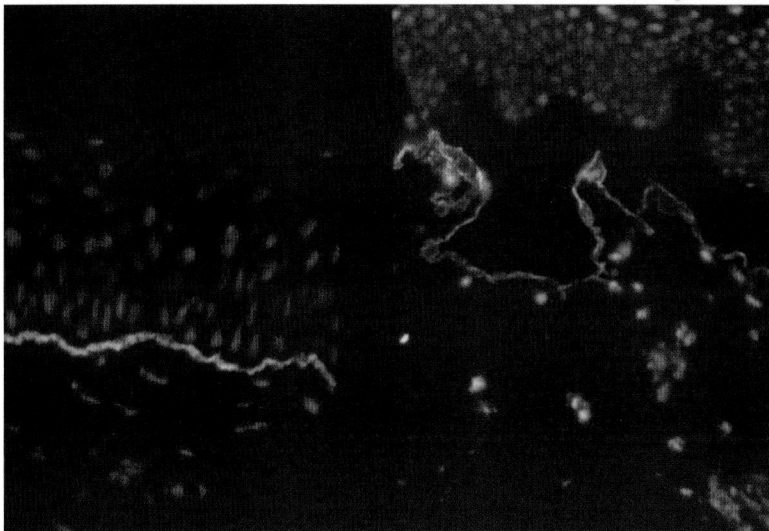

Fig. 4.121
Epidermolysis bullosa acquisita: (*left*) direct immunofluorescence shows linear IgG deposition along the basement membrane region; (*right*) with split skin the immunoreactant lines the floor of the induced lesion. By courtesy of Department of Immunofluorescence, Institute of Dermatology, London, UK.

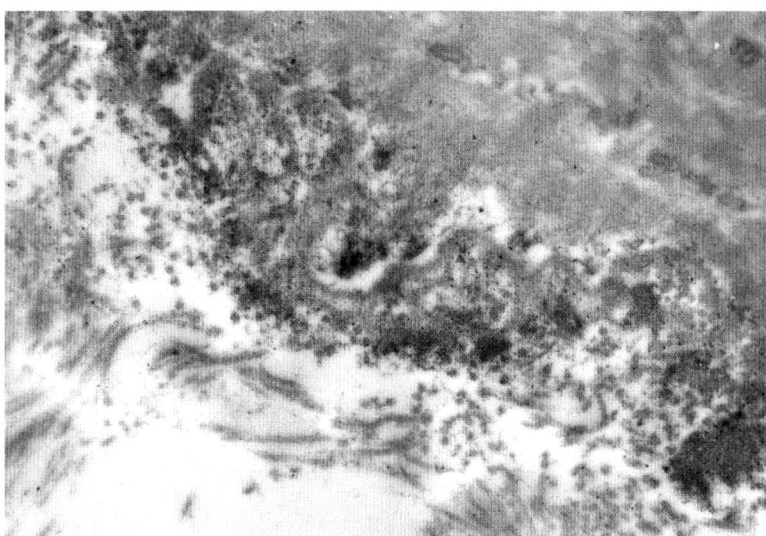

Fig. 4.122
Epidermolysis bullosa acquisita: direct immunoelectron microscopy showing reactant deposition below the lamina densa.

induced blister cavity.[68–71] ELISA-based detection and measurement of the autoantibodies against type VII collagen titers can be used as an additional diagnostic test for EBA and to monitor disease activity.[9,72–75]

Direct and indirect immunoelectron microscopic studies have determined that the immunoreactants lie on or below the lamina densa, corresponding to the site of the electron-dense amorphous material mentioned above (*Fig. 4.122*).[1,60,61,76,77] Immunogold labeling confirms that the immunoglobulin deposits are related to the anchoring fibrils (*Fig. 4.123*).[78] As a consequence of these additional observations, a modified set of criteria for the diagnosis of EBA has been recommended:[1,79]

- clinical lesions of trauma-induced bullae occurring over the joints of the hands, feet, elbows, and knees, atrophic scars, milia and nail dystrophy, or else presentation as a clinically inflammatory bullous or mucous membrane pemphigoid-like process,
- post-infancy onset of the disease,
- no family history of EBA,
- exclusion of other bullous diseases,
- IgG at the basement membrane zone on direct immunofluorescence,
- demonstration of blister formation beneath the lamina densa,

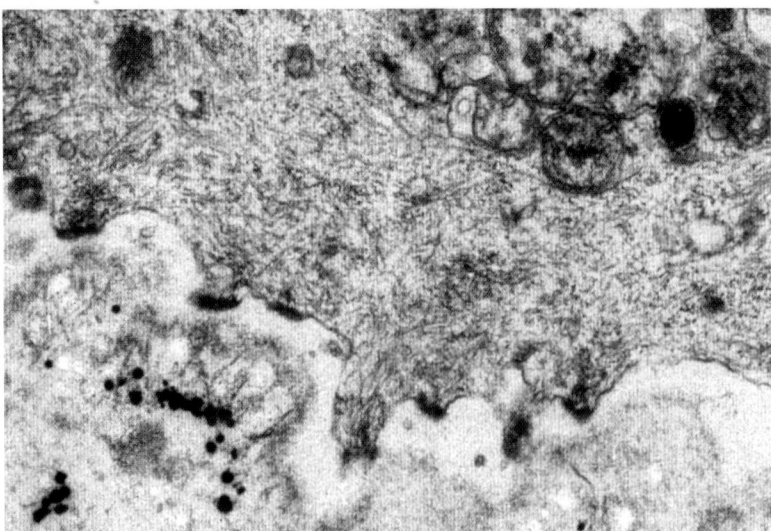

Fig. 4.123
Epidermolysis bullosa acquisita: immunogold preparation showing localization of the immunoglobulin to the anchoring fibrils. By courtesy of H. Shimizu, MD, Keio University School of Medicine, Tokyo, Japan.

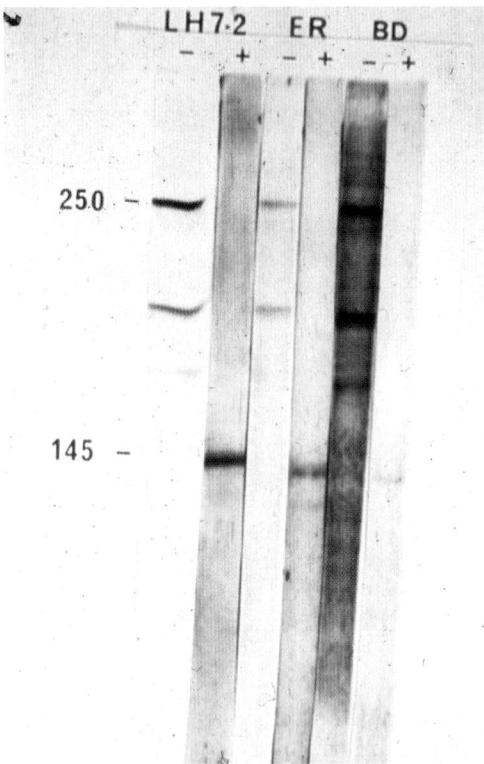

Fig. 4.124
Epidermolysis bullosa acquisita: there are two distinct antigens: one the 290-kD major antigen; the other the 145-kD minor antigen. By courtesy of I. Leigh, MD, Royal London Hospital Trust, London, UK.

- demonstration of IgG associated with anchoring fibrils beneath the basal lamina by immunoelectron microscopy,
- localization of the immunoreactants to the floor of 1 M NaCl-split skin by direct and or indirect immunofluorescence.

The EBA antigen (290 kD) is the globular (noncollagenous) carboxyl terminus of type VII procollagen (*Fig. 4.124*).[80-84] Type VII collagen is the major constituent of anchoring fibrils, which anchor the basement membrane through the lamina densa to the connective tissue constituents of the adjacent dermis, and is composed of three identical alpha-chains (each 290 kD). It is synthesized by both human keratinocytes and fibroblasts in culture, and is found in other mammalian skin, including dog, cat, guinea pig, rat, mouse, and hamster, but not in avian, reptilian, amphibian, or fish skin.[85-88] Type VII collagen has also been identified within the esophagus, mouth, colon, anus, cornea, chorioamnion, and vagina.[89] It has a high affinity for fibronectin, which is thought to be responsible (at least in part) for adhesion between cells and matrix within the dermis.[90] The interaction between the EBA antibody and type VII collagen is thought to somehow upset this delicate relationship with consequent dermal–epidermal separation.[91] Passive transfer of human EBA autoantibodies to mice and immunization of mice with type VII collagen both lead to EBA disease models, confirming the importance of this autoantibody.[92-95] An animal model and human antibody characterization indicate that the pathogenic antibodies of epidermolysis bullosa acquisita are often against the cartilage matrix protein subdomain of the N-terminal noncollagenous domain of type VII collagen.[96] In some cases of inflammatory EBA the antibodies react against epitopes in the triple-helical collagenous domain.[97]

The parallel between EBA and BP is obvious and it is tempting to extrapolate a similar downstream pathogenesis after autoantibody binds to its protein target.[98] Although the current concept for EBA points to such a similarity, additional confirmatory evidence is required. Some studies have shown that the pathogenesis is related, at least in part, to neutrophil recruitment mediated by complement activation, and the generation of complement-derived chemotactic activity (C5A) at the epidermal basement membrane region.[91] Experimental models in which immune complexes are produced by treating normal skin in organ culture with EBA complement-fixing antibodies have been shown to result in complement-dependent neutrophil migration to the basement membrane region and eventual dermal–epidermal separation.[67,99] Lack of complement-fixing function in the autoantibodies does not result in tissue injury in one model.[100] The precise mechanism whereby such blisters evolve is unknown, but it has been suggested that leukocyte-derived proteases and reactive oxygen intermediates may be important.[65]

The pathogenesis of the 'cell-free' mechanobullous variant is poorly understood. It is also associated with antibasement membrane antibody, but there is little, if any, evidence for neutrophil chemotactic activity. It has been proposed that separation at the dermal–epidermal junction may result from an abrogation of affinities between the type VII collagen and laminin-332 in addition to matrix proteins, such as fibronectin, due to a direct effect of autoantibody deposition at that site.[1,101-103] An additional potential mechanism proposed is a direct effect of the autoantibody on type collagen VII antiparallel dimer assembly leading to diminished anchoring fibril formation.[1,104] The finding of domain specificity in EBA autoantibodies will direct focus toward the function of this cartilage matrix protein subdomain.[98] It is intriguing that the pathogenetic autoantibodies in EBA are against type VII collagen, the same protein genetically interrupted in dystrophic epidermolysis bullosa, leading to nonfunctional anchoring fibrils. Nonetheless, the clinical presentation of EBA is broad and includes features not seen in dystrophic EB, such as bullous pemphigoid-like lesions.

Differential diagnosis

'Cell-free' EBA must be distinguished from congenital EB, porphyria cutanea tarda, pseudoporphyria, and cutaneous bullous amyloidosis. Diagnosis can be achieved easily by clinicopathological correlation, and particularly, with the use of immunofluorescence.

Inflammatory EBA can be distinguished from bullous pemphigoid, mucous membrane pemphigoid, and linear IgA disease by split skin IIMF and, when necessary, by Western blot (see *Table 4.6*).

It is also important that dermal–epidermal separation due to autolysis is not confused with in vivo blister formation. In autolysis, the epithelium typically shows marked eosinophilia and the nuclei are often lost.

Bullous systemic lupus erythematosus

Blisters may rarely develop as a manifestation of systemic lupus erythematosus (SLE). They can therefore arise in a background of vasculitis or complicate sunburn and photosensitivity.[1,2] Occasionally vesicles form after extreme basal cell hydropic change and consequent dermal–epidermal separation.[3]

Patients with SLE manifest a wide range of antibodies resulting in numerous complications, which include the development of autoimmune

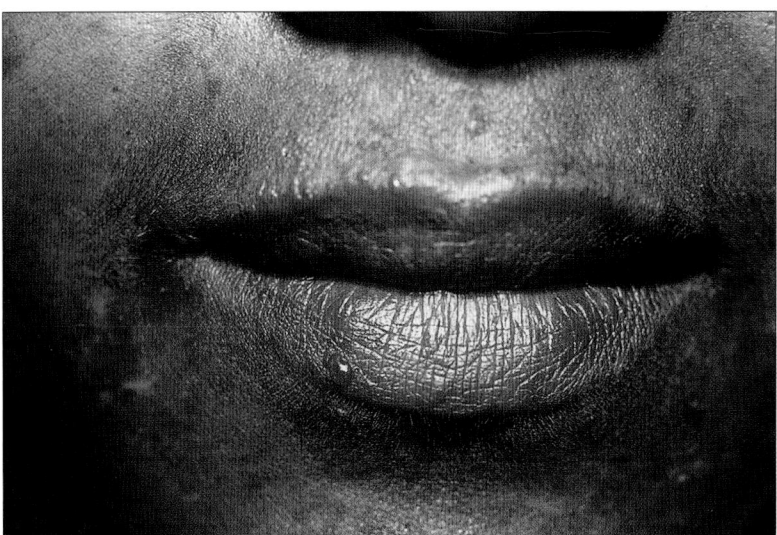

Fig. 4.125
Bullous systemic lupus erythematosus: West Indian female with perioral blistering. By courtesy of R.A. Marsden, MD, St George's Hospital, London, UK.

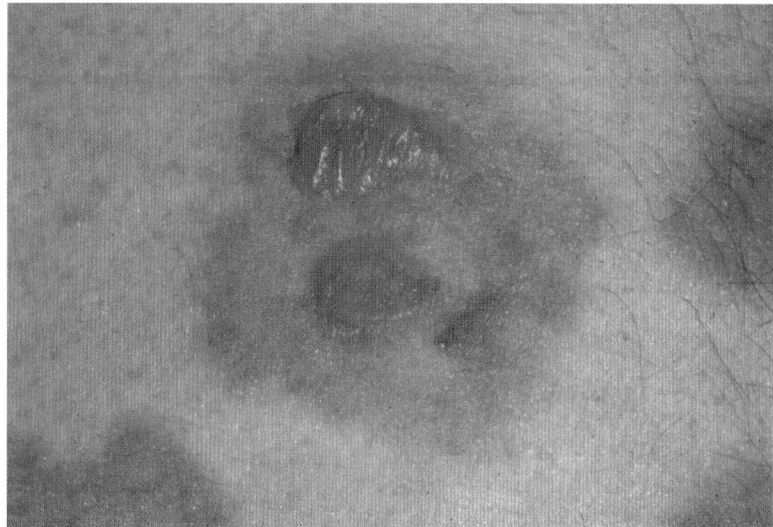

Fig. 4.126
Bullous systemic lupus erythematosus: in this example, there is a conspicuous inflammatory background. By courtesy of the Institute of Dermatology, London, UK.

bullous dermatoses, such as bullous pemphigoid, dermatitis herpetiformis, pemphigus vulgaris, pemphigus foliaceus, linear IgA disease, and epidermolysis bullosa acquisita.[4,5] In addition, a unique dermatosis comprising a widespread vesiculobullous eruption characterized by a dermatitis herpetiformis-like histology, linear and/or granular basement membrane zone antibody deposition (reacting with type VII collagen), and a striking response to dapsone, has been described in patients with SLE.[6] This constitutes bullous SLE. Importantly, and by definition, establishing the diagnosis of bullous SLE requires the diagnosis of SLE to be made according to the 1997 American College of Rheumatology revised criteria for SLE[7] (see Chapter 17 on Idiopathic Connective Tissue Diseases).

Clinical features

Bullous SLE – also termed bullous eruption of SLE, vesiculobullous SLE, and SLE with herpetiform blisters – tends to present in the second and third decades and although young black women are most often affected, all ages, races, and both sexes may develop the disease (*Fig. 4.125*).[4,8–12] Less than 5% of patients with SLE will develop blisters during the course of the disease.[13] It has been estimated that the incidence of bullous SLE does not exceed 0.2 cases per million per year.[14] Presentation in children is exceptional.[15,16]

Patients present with an acute, widespread, sometimes pruritic, tense, vesiculobullous eruption that mostly affects sun-exposed areas (*Figs 4.126–4.128*). However, non-sun-exposed skin and mucosal sites (mouth and pharynx) are also often involved.[4,9,17] Sites of predilection include the upper trunk, supraclavicular regions, upper extremities, face, vermillion border and oral mucosa.[4,13] In contrast to dermatitis herpetiformis, the involvement of the extensor surfaces of the extremities is much less frequent.[13] The vesiculobullous eruption may arise against a background of erythema or, less commonly, urticaria. The blister fluid is usually clear, and less often hemorrhagic.[13] A unique presentation of bullous SLE in a centrifugal concentric expanding pattern resembling erythema gyratum repens has recently been reported.[18] The vesiculobullous eruption can precede the onset of SLE or develop subsequently.[9,19] Unlike EBA, with which this disease has much in common, mechanobullous lesions are not seen, nor is there evidence of scarring.[4] Milia formation, although rare, has been recorded on two occasions and in both instances affected children.[10,11] Postinflammatory hyperpigmentation is a not uncommon complication. Surprisingly, patients with bullous SLE do not usually develop other cutaneous manifestations of lupus. Bullous SLE has been recorded in patients whose primary disease developed as a consequence of hydralazine, penicillamine, and methimazole therapy and identical features (including immunological) have been recorded in a patient with mixed connective tissue disease.[20–22] Although bullous SLE

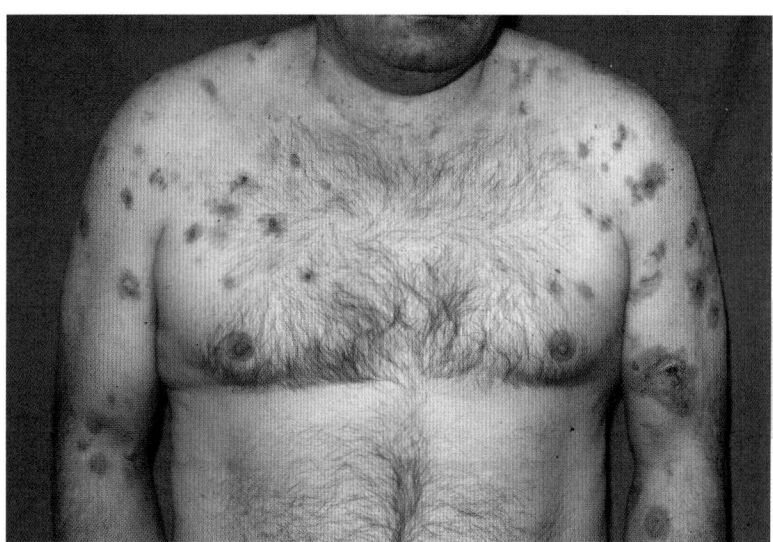

Fig. 4.127
Bullous systemic lupus erythematosus: numerous erosions are present over the chest, shoulders, and upper arms. By courtesy of R.A. Marsden, MD, St George's Hospital, London, UK.

has also been reported in patients with concomitant HIV infection, the relationship between the two diseases, if any, has not yet been elucidated.[23]

Bullous SLE is frequently associated with concurrent systemic symptoms and flares of SLE, especially with lupus nephritis reflecting the disease activity.[13,24,25]

Pathogenesis and histologic features

Patients with bullous SLE (and EBA) have a significantly higher incidence of HLA-DR2 compared to the normal population.[4] This is thought to be associated with an increased risk of developing autoimmune diseases.[18]

The histologic features of bullous SLE (BSLE) are those of a subepidermal vesicle, often indistinguishable from dermatitis herpetiformis. The roof is usually intact and the blister cavity contains fibrin with large numbers of neutrophils and karyorrhectic debris (*Fig. 4.129*). Occasionally lymphocytes, histiocytes, and eosinophils are also evident.[4] The adjacent, nonbullous skin characteristically shows subepidermal neutrophil microabscesses (*Fig. 4.130*). The upper dermis contains a perivascular mixed inflammatory cell infiltrate consisting of neutrophils, occasional eosinophils, lymphocytes,

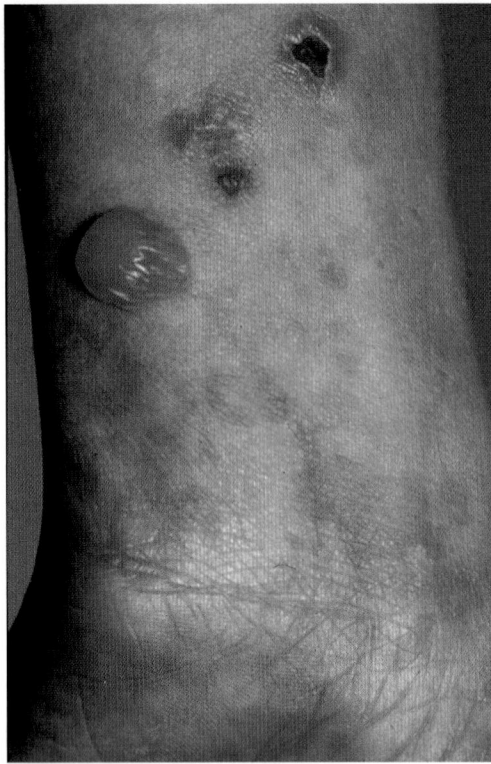

Fig. 4.128
Bullous systemic lupus erythematosus: tense bullous pemphigoid-like lesions. By courtesy of the Institute of Dermatology, London, UK.

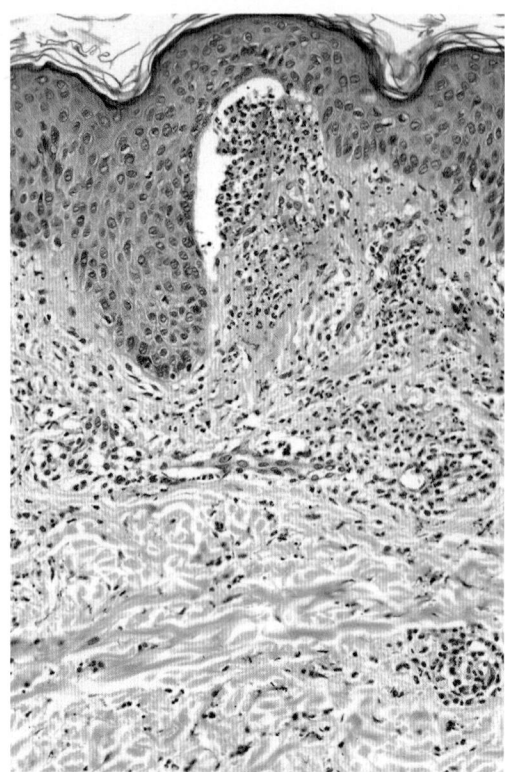

Fig. 4.130
Bullous systemic lupus erythematosus: the presence of a neutrophil abscess in the papillary dermis increases the histologic similarity of this condition to dermatitis herpetiformis.

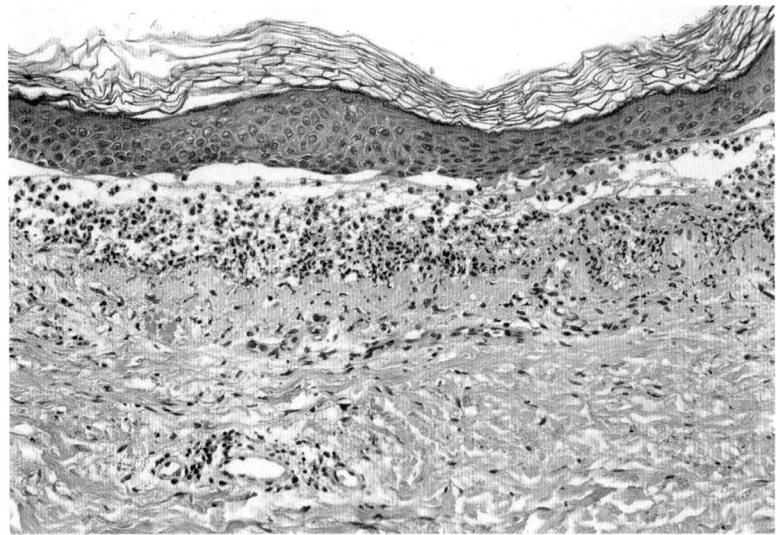

Fig. 4.129
Bullous systemic lupus erythematosus: this shows the typical features of a subepidermal, neutrophil-rich vesicle.

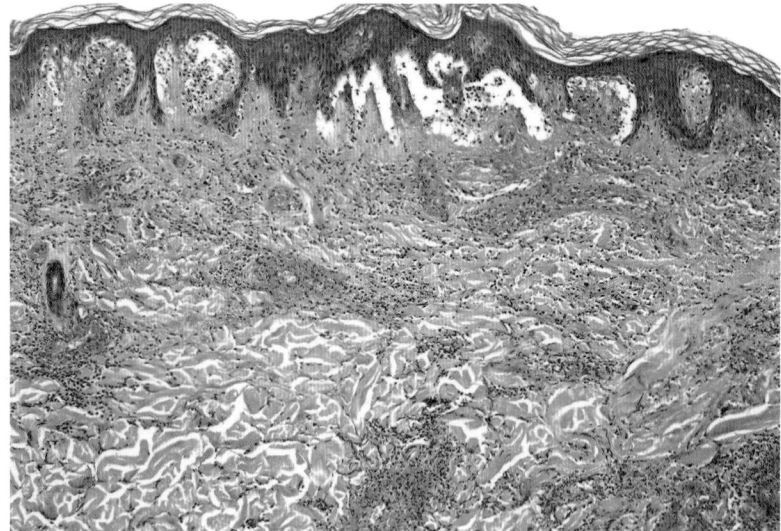

Fig. 4.131
Bullous systemic lupus erythematosus: this scanning view shows a central focus of subepidermal vesiculation. Striking inflammatory changes outline the dermal vasculature.

and histiocytes. Sometimes the features of a leukocytoclastic vasculitis are also present (*Figs 4.131–4.133*).

Electron microscopy shows that the site of the split is below the lamina densa.[4]

Using direct immunofluorescence, the disease is characterized by the presence of immunoglobulin and complement at the epidermal basement membrane region of both lesional sund perilesional skin. Immunoglobulins are frequently multiple: IgG is present in 100% of patients, IgA in 67%, and IgM in 50%.[4,8,9,26,27] Two patterns are recognized: granular in 40% of cases and linear in 60%.[9] Sometimes immunoreactants are also present within the walls of the upper dermal vasculature, particularly venules.[4] Indirect

immunofluorescence using 1 M NaCl-split skin as substrate shows the presence of a low titer antibasement membrane antibody in those patients who demonstrate linear positive direct IIMF (type 1 BSLE).[1,4,9,17,20,28–31] The antibodies generally label the floor of the blister cavity, although a roof (epidermal) variant has rarely been described.[9] Those that are negative on IIMF have been classified as type 2 BSLE.[4] Type 3 BSLE refers to those cases in which the target antigen is an epidermal, rather than dermal, epitope.[6]

Direct immunoelectron microscopy shows that the immunoreactants are present on, and immediately below, the lamina densa, obscuring the anchoring fibrils, and also occasionally somewhat deeper in the papillary dermis, similar to those seen in nonbullous SLE.[4,32–34] The antibody binds to the

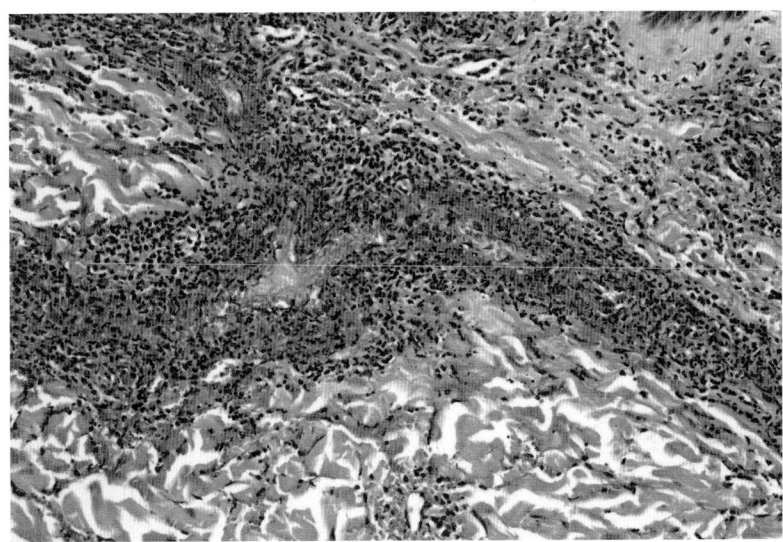

Fig. 4.132
Bullous systemic lupus erythematosus: this view shows florid leukocytoclastic vasculitis.

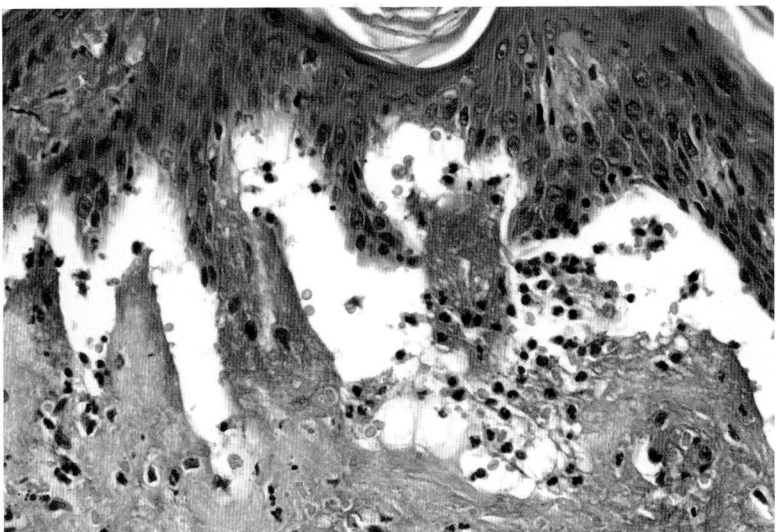

Fig. 4.133
Bullous systemic lupus erythematosus: this is a close-up view of the subepidermal vesicle shown in *Fig. 4.131*.

lamina densa and sublamina densa in a manner identical to that seen in epidermolysis bullosa acquisita.[4,33]

Western immunoblot has shown that these antibodies bind to antigens of 290 kD and 145 kD as described for EBA (i.e., directed against the non-collagenous domain type 1 (NC1) and 2 (NC2) of type VII collagen).[28] It has recently been demonstrated, albeit in a single patient, that the levels of anti-type VII collagen autoantibodies in the serum mirror disease activity.[35] Rare patients with SLE have been detected to have circulating antibodies to type VII collagen in the absence of blisters, and occasional patients with bullous SLE have been shown to have antibodies which bind to both the roof and the floor of NaCl-split skin, suggesting that a number of different basement membrane antigens may be involved.[1,4] The target antigen in the epidermal variant of bullous SLE has not yet been identified, although bullous pemphigoid antigen 1 was identified in addition to type VII collagen and laminins-332 and -311 in one patient with combined epidermal and dermal staining on NaCl-split skin IIMF, most likely representing a manifestation of postinflammatory epitope spreading.[34]

The bullous SLE antibodies are associated with complement activation activity, which results in neutrophil migration and adherence to the basement membrane region.[4] Neutrophil enzyme release is associated with basement membrane damage and subsequent dermal–epidermal separation.

Differential diagnosis

Bullous SLE shows obvious overlap with EBA. There are, however, a number of discriminatory features. Bullous SLE is not associated with a mechanobullous pathogenesis and scarring is not a feature. It develops most often in a younger age group than EBA. The dermatitis herpetiformis-like histologic features are rarely seen in EBA, and probably of greatest importance bullous SLE responds dramatically to dapsone therapy, but EBA does not.[3] Subtyping of IgG antibodies can aid in the distinction between bullous SLE and EBA. While IgG1 and IgG4 subclass of antibodies are mainly detected in EBA patients, IgG2 and IgG3 subclass of antibodies are generally present in patients with bullous SLE.[36]

Dermatitis herpetiformis

Clinical features

Dermatitis herpetiformis and celiac disease are highly interrelated conditions and best regarded as variable expressions of a common inherited tendency to autoimmune disease. Thus, dermatitis herpetiformis has been regarded as an extraintestinal manifestation of celiac disease.

Dermatitis herpetiformis (Duhring-Brocq disease) is a widespread, intensely pruritic, papulovesicular eruption affecting all ages, but particularly people in their second to fourth decades.[1-4] The male to female ratio is 2:1. Occurrence in children is much more infrequent. A recent study from Finland reported the annual incidence of childhood dermatitis herpetiformis of 0.56 per 100 000 population representing one sixth of the incidence in adults.[5]

The prevalence of dermatitis herpetiformis is highest in Northern Europe, ranging from 11.5 per 100 000 in Scotland, and 19.6 to 39.2 per 100 000 in Sweden, to as high as 75.3 per 100 000 in Finland.[2,6-10] It is less frequently seen in the United States. A recent population-based study from the UK revealed a fourfold increase in the incidence of celiac disease (from 5.2 to 19.1 per 100 000) over a period of more than 20 years, contrasting with a 4% of annual decrease in the incidence of dermatitis herpetiformis during the same period (from 1.8 to 0.8 per 100 000).[11] While the same study detected large regional variations in prevalence for celiac disease, only minimal regional variations in prevalence for dermatitis herpetiformis could be observed.[11] Interestingly, dermatitis herpetiformis with childhood onset appears to be more common in Mediterranean countries.[12] Caucasians are mainly affected, the disease being rare in Asians and blacks. Case clustering is common and familial involvement (either dermatitis herpetiformis or celiac disease), possibly autosomal dominantly inherited, has been documented in up to 10.5% of cases.[2,13] Relatives of patients with dermatitis herpetiformis have an increased risk of developing celiac disease.[2]

The lesions, which may be symmetrical, are grouped mainly on the posterior scalp, shoulders, back, buttocks, and extensor aspects of the limbs (*Figs 4.134* and *4.135*). Scratching is often severe and therefore excoriation and/or lichenification typically predominate with intact vesicles rarely being seen. However, occasionally, larger blisters similar to those found in bullous pemphigoid may be evident. Patients sometimes present with urticarial plaques and crusted erosions.[2] Oral involvement is rare.[3] Rarely, the initial presentation may be with localized lesions in areas such as the scalp.[14] The latter is not infrequently involved in more generalized disease. An uncommon presentation of dermatitis herpetiformis consists of palmoplantar purpura limited to the palms and soles with sparing of the dorsal surfaces of hands and feet, a pattern more often seen in children.[12,15-18] Petechiae may exceptionally be limited to the fingertips.[15]

The clinical response to dapsone (50–200 mg/day) is dramatic; therefore, the drug is commonly administered for diagnostic as well as therapeutic purposes. Relief from pruritus occurs within a few hours of commencing treatment and is soon followed by clearing of the rash. The eruption returns 2–3 days after dapsone is discontinued. The disease persists for many years and is usually lifelong. A gluten-free diet may result in prolonged remission in some patients or lowering of the daily dapsone requirement in others.

At least 65–75% of patients with dermatitis herpetiformis show histologic evidence of celiac disease (gluten-sensitive enteropathy, GSE). However,

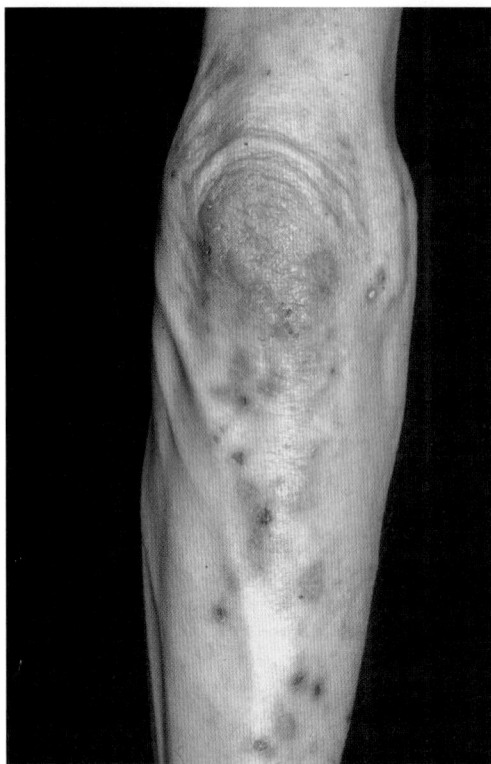

Fig. 4.134
Dermatitis herpetiformis: excoriations are present on the elbow and back of the arm. Intact blisters are uncommon in dermatitis herpetiformis because of the intense pruritus. By courtesy of the Institute of Dermatology, London, UK.

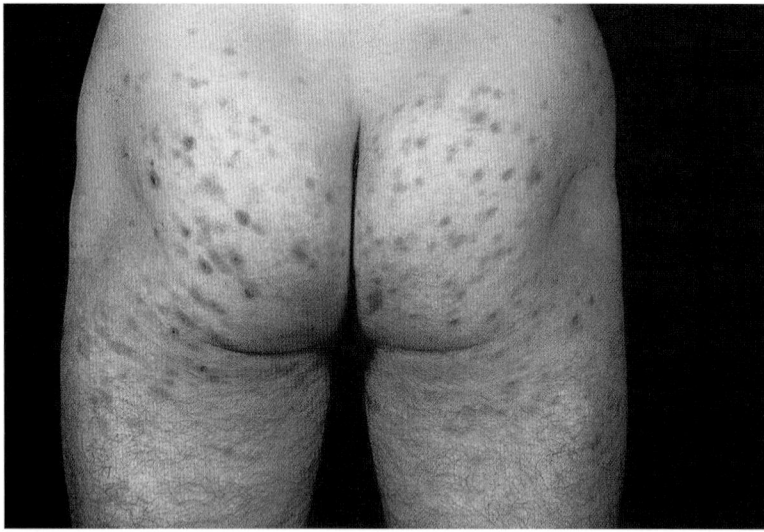

Fig. 4.135
Dermatitis herpetiformis: the buttocks are frequently affected. By courtesy of the Institute of Dermatology, London, UK.

only about 20% have clinical manifestations of malabsorption, these being usually mild.[19-24] The actual incidence of celiac disease is likely to be higher because the mucosal abnormality in dermatitis herpetiformis is patchy and may be missed unless multiple jejunal biopsies are taken.[25-27] Interestingly, patients who apparently do not have enteropathy may develop the condition when challenged with large doses of gluten (latent GSE).[22] It is therefore believed that all patients with dermatitis herpetiformis have GSE to a greater or lesser extent.[1-3] Relatives of patients with dermatitis herpetiformis may show no evidence of the skin disease, but can have subclinical or overt symptoms of the enteropathy.

Patients with dermatitis herpetiformis may have antigastric parietal cell antibody (10-25%), gastric hypochlorhydria (50-90%), and gastric atrophy

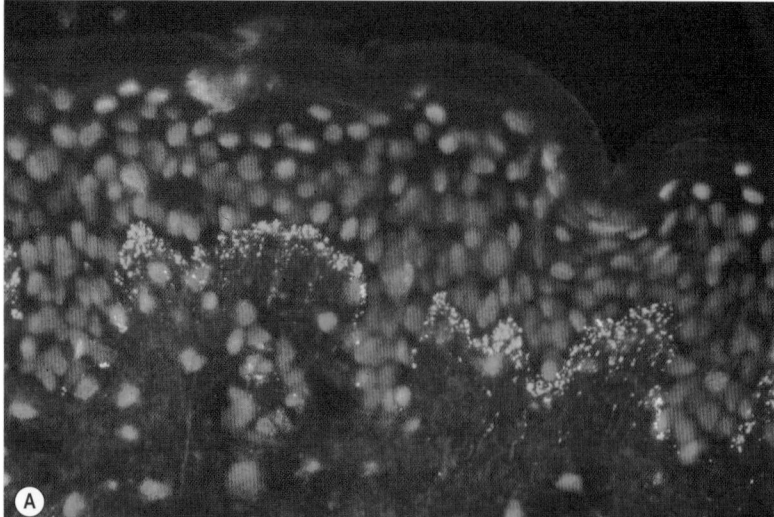

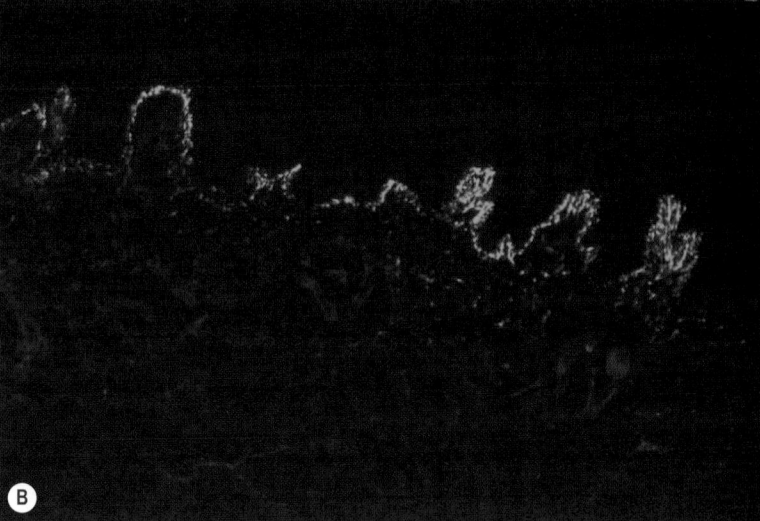

Fig. 4.136
Dermatitis herpetiformis: direct immunofluorescence showing (A) deposits of granular IgA in the dermal papillae; (B) fibrin deposition in the dermal papillae. By courtesy of the Department of Immunofluorescence, Institute of Dermatology, London, UK.

(50-70%).[3] They may also have antithyroid antibodies and show an increased incidence of thyroid disease, insulin-dependent diabetes mellitus, and connective tissue diseases including systemic lupus erythematosus and Sjögren syndrome.[28,29] As with isolated celiac disease, there is an increased risk of intestinal lymphoma.[30] Exceptionally, dermatitis herpetiformis has been associated with erythema elevatum diutinum, transverse myelitis, and bullous pemphigoid.[31-34]

Exposure to iodine may also trigger or flare the disease.[35,36]

Pathogenesis and histologic features

Patients with dermatitis herpetiformis (and celiac disease) have a high incidence of HLA-B8 (80-90%), HLA-DR3 (90-95%) and HLA-DQ2 (95-100%) compared to a normal control population (21%, 23%, and 40%, respectively).[3,37-40] More recent studies, however, have demonstrated that the increased incidence of HLA-B8 and -DR3 is due to positive linkage disequilibrium.[41] The most current data suggest that the significant positive HLA association in dermatitis herpetiformis lies with the class II antigen DQ2.[2,42] These HLA associations can be helpful diagnostically.[43] Namely, the absence of HLA-DQ2 or HLA-DQ8 haplotypes has high negative predictive value, making patients with lack of these alleles unlikely to have dermatitis herpetiformis.[44]

All patients with dermatitis herpetiformis have granular deposits of IgA in the dermal papillae of perilesional skin, and many also show in vivo-bound fibrin (Fig. 4.136).[45,46] IgA has also been identified in the oral mucosa.[47] A granular linear pattern may be seen and it seems to be more common than previously reported.[48] In patients with a linear pattern, careful attention should be paid to the presence of granularity to avoid a misdiagnosis of linear IgA disease. Recently, a fibrillar pattern has also been documented.[49] Two of the three patients reported with this pattern had clinical features of dermatitis herpetiformis but lacked antitransglutaminase and antiendomysial antibodies. In a recent study from Japan, over one third of patients displayed fibrillary IgA deposition in the papillary dermis.50 Furthermore, Japanese patients with fibrillary IgA deposits tended to have no involvement of the dermatitis herpetiformis predilection sites (e.g., extensor surfaces, buttocks) and lacked association with HLA-DQ2 and HLA-DQ8 haplotype.[50] Other immunoglobulins are not usually found in dermatitis herpetiformis, but C3 is often present.[51] This is associated with formation of the membrane attack complex (C5–C9), which is thought to result in neutrophil chemotaxis and the evolution of subepidermal vesiculation.[3,52] Cutaneous IgA deposits may still be detected after dapsone therapy. They do, however, sometimes disappear after a prolonged gluten-free diet.[2] Cutaneous IgA deposition is not seen in patients with celiac disease.[2]

Electron microscopy reveals electron-dense, amorphous granular deposits in the superficial dermis showing no particular relationship with the basement membrane region or any other specific structure.[53,54]

Immunoelectron microscopic observations initially suggested that the IgA deposits were associated with elastic-containing microfibrillar bundles, but additional published work using antifibrillin antibodies has discounted this theory.[53,55]

Antigliadin antibodies, which are often used to assess celiac disease status, are of limited value in the diagnosis of dermatitis herpetiformis.[52] They have high specificity, but low sensitivity.[22] Anti-smooth muscle endomysial antibody correlates with the gluten-sensitive state and appears before the development of any small intestinal histologic abnormality in patients with dermatitis herpetiformis.[22,56,57] Such endomysial antibodies are present in up to 70% of patients and are highly specific; they react with tissue transglutaminase (tTG) (antitransglutaminase antibodies).[58] Antibodies against epidermal transglutaminase are found more frequently than the latter. Antitransglutaminase antibodies, particularly those to epidermal transglutaminase, seem to be the most sensitive serological marker of dermatitis herpetiformis.[47,59] Patients with high levels of IgA and IgG transglutaminase antibodies usually have more prominent mucosal villous atrophy and more severe clinical disease.[60] Gliadin is an important substrate for tissue transglutaminase forming gliadin–gliadin or gliadin–tTG complexes.[61] Circulating IgA antibodies to tTG are pathognomonic of dermatitis herpetiformis and celiac disease.[62] The gut subtype of transglutaminase is TG2 while that in the skin is TG3. Cross-reactivity between these homologous proteins or antigenic drift may underlie some of the mucosal and cutaneous features of this condition.[63,64] Whatever the underlying mechanism, the IgA in some way 'fixes' in the skin, resulting in complement activation via the alternative pathway.[65–67] Neutrophil chemotaxins are then released and the ensuing inflammatory reaction leads to dermal papillary edema, fibrin deposition, and eventual vesiculation. There may be a role for cell-mediated immunity in this disease as well, perhaps involving γ/δ T cells.[68]

The histologic hallmark of dermatitis herpetiformis is the dermal papillary neutrophilic microabscess, best seen in early erythematous lesions or well away from the blister in an established eruption (Fig. 4.137).[69–71] Occasionally, many levels of the biopsy will have to be examined before a microabscess is found.

Abscess evolution depends upon the initial presence of fibrin and polymorphs within the tips of the dermal papillae (Fig. 4.138), both of which are associated with degenerative changes of the collagen and the development of edema. Development of small subepidermal microvesicles follows, leading on to the formation of multilocular subepidermal blisters.

Typically, the blister cavity contains edema fluid, a reticular network of fibrin, and numerous polymorphs (Figs 4.139 and 4.140). In contrast to bullous pemphigoid, the floor of the blister cavity usually shows effacement of the dermal papillary outline.

Within the dermis is a mixed inflammatory cell infiltrate consisting of lymphocytes, histiocytes, and abundant neutrophils. Leukocytoclasis (nuclear dust, Fig. 4.141) is characteristic. Although blood vessels frequently

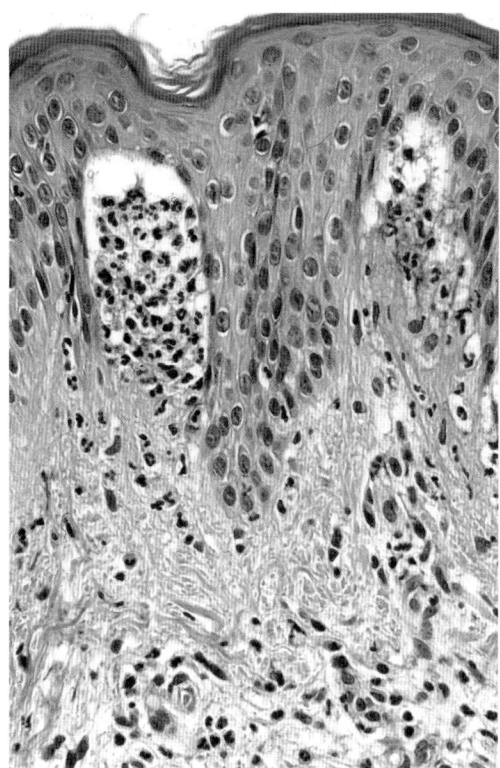

Fig. 4.137
Dermatitis herpetiformis: biopsy from an early lesion showing conspicuous neutrophil microabscesses.

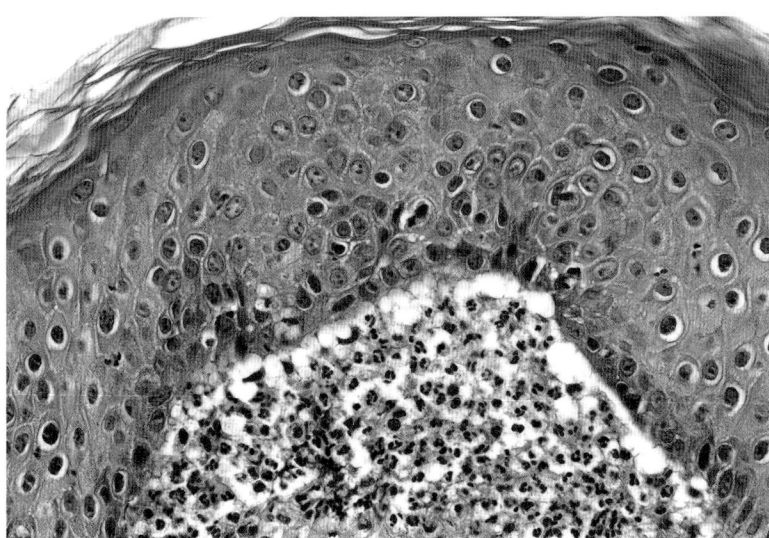

Fig. 4.138
Dermatitis herpetiformis: in this early lesion, there are thin strands of fibrin visible above the neutrophilic infiltrate.

show endothelial swelling, there is no evidence of vasculitis. Occasionally, eosinophils are quite numerous in the infiltrate, but usually they are late arrivals, appearing 24–48 hours after the neutrophils. On occasions, biopsies from typical dermatitis herpetiformis may show acantholysis, a cause of considerable confusion (Fig. 4.142).

Jejunal biopsy may reveal villous blunting, intestinal crypt elongation, flattening of surface epithelial cells with loss of microvilli, and intraepithelial γ/δ lymphocytic infiltration to a degree ranging from partial to subtotal villous atrophy.[72] If gluten is withheld from the diet, these changes revert to normal.

Differential diagnosis

A neutrophil-predominant subepidermal vesicle accompanied by neutrophil dermal papillary microabscesses in addition to dermatitis herpetiformis may

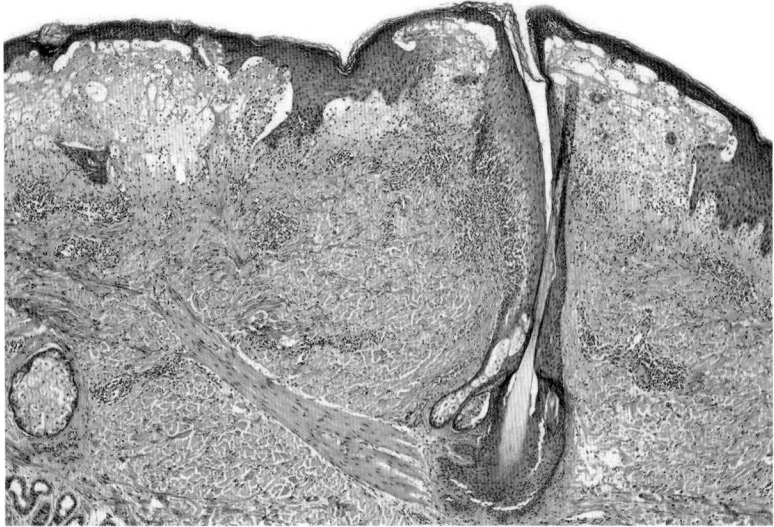

Fig. 4.139
Dermatitis herpetiformis: an established subepidermal blister. Although early lesions are usually multilocular, by 24–48 hours the lesion becomes unilocular.

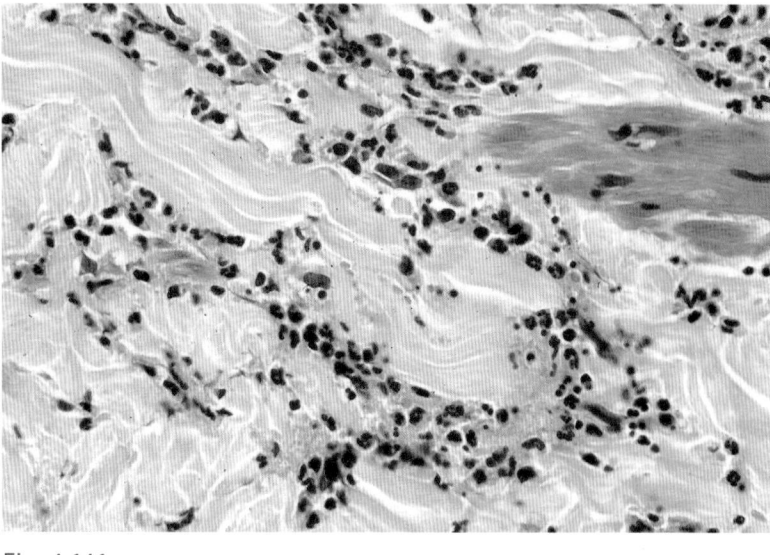

Fig. 4.141
Dermatitis herpetiformis: nuclear debris (karyorrhexis) within the dermis is a characteristic feature.

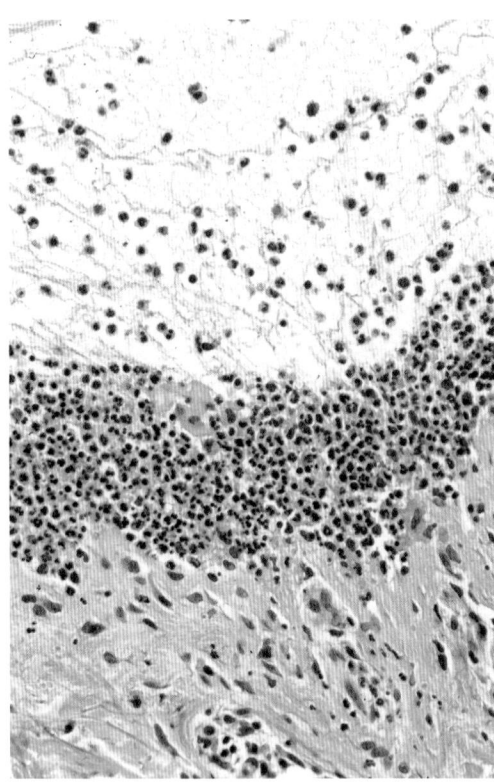

Fig. 4.140
Dermatitis herpetiformis: floor of the blister in *Fig. 4.139* showing an intense neutrophil infiltrate.

also be seen in the following conditions: vesicular pemphigoid, bullous systemic lupus erythematosus, inflammatory epidermolysis bullosa, and linear IgA disease. Distinction depends upon clinical information and the results of immunofluorescent studies (see *Table 4.6*).

Linear IgA disease

Linear immunoglobulin A (IgA) disease, also known as linear IgA bullous dermatosis, is a chronic autoimmune muco-cutaneous blistering disease characterized by the formation of subepidermal/subepithelial blisters and linear deposition of IgA along the basement membrane. Two main variants of linear IgA disease can be separated according to the age of presentation: an adult and a childhood linear IgA disease.

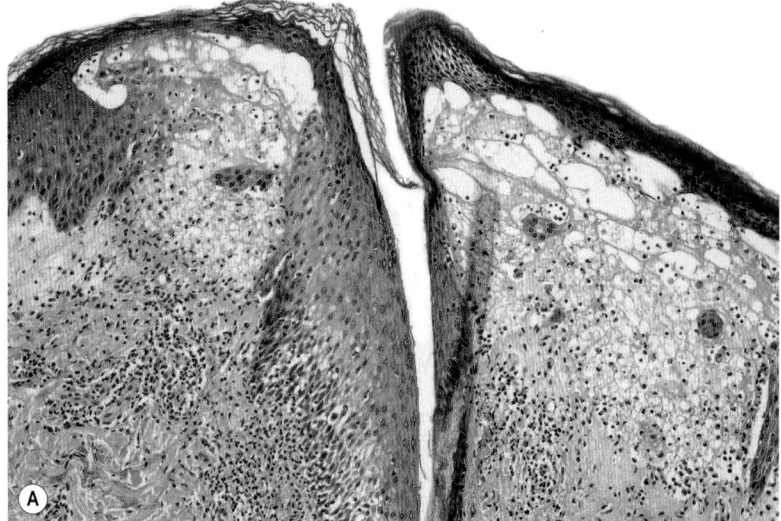

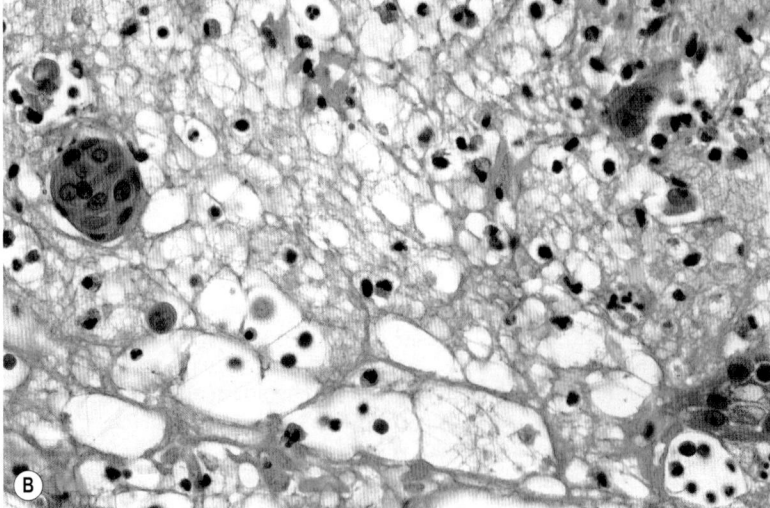

Fig. 4.142
(**A**, **B**) Dermatitis herpetiformis: in this example acantholysis may result in diagnostic confusion with pemphigus. Note that the blister is subepidermal.

Linear IgA disease of adults by definition presents after puberty. It is characterized by the development of a sometimes self-remitting dapsone or sulfonamide-responsive dermatosis typified by subepidermal vesicles and blisters in association with in vivo deposition of linear (homogeneous) IgA at the basement membrane region on direct immunofluorescence of normal or perilesional skin.[1–3] Childhood linear IgA disease (chronic bullous dermatosis of childhood) is almost identical to the adult counterpart; however, there are differences in clinical presentation and therefore these particular aspects are described separately.

Linear IgA disease of adults is a rare disease, which was originally thought to represent a variant of dermatitis herpetiformis[4–6] or bullous pemphigoid.[7,8] Some cases were reported under the rubric polymorphic pemphigoid (see above) or intermediate (mixed) forms of bullous disease.[9,10] More recently, particularly following the application of immunoelectron microscopic and immunoblotting techniques, it has been confirmed as a disease (or at least a disease spectrum) sui generis.[11–15]

Its approximate incidence in the south of England is 1:250 000.[16] In France and central Germany, the incidence is 0.5 per million of the population.[17,18] In Singapore, the incidence has been estimated at 0.26 per million population.[19] Although data for the United States are limited, the incidence in Utah has been reported as 0.6 per 100 000.[20] Some consider that this disease is underdiagnosed.

Clinical features

Linear IgA disease of adults affects the sexes equally and, while the age distribution is wide, there are peaks in teenagers and young adults and in patients in their sixties.[1] It may present as a somewhat atypical bullous eruption showing features suggestive of dermatitis herpetiformis or more commonly bullous pemphigoid (Fig. 4.143). Occasionally, it may initially resemble and be mistaken clinically for erythema multiforme.[21] Pruritus and/or a burning sensation are common manifestations and early lesions may include urticarial, annular, polycyclic, and targetoid eruptions.[15,22] The established dermatosis may be vesicular or more often frankly bullous; blisters arising at the edge of erythematous annular lesions ('string of beads' sign) are said to be characteristic.[15] Very rarely, linear IgA bullous disease can present

with widespread skin sloughing and bullae consistent with toxic epidermal necrolysis – this pattern of presentation generally represents drug-induced linear IgA bullous disease (see Chapter 14).[23]

Sites affected in decreasing order of frequency include the trunk, limbs, hands, scalp, face, and perioral region. The perineum and vagina may also be affected with erosions and blisters.[1] Mucous membrane involvement, which is common, is of particular importance because it can be associated with scarring. Important sites that may be affected include the eyes (conjunctivitis, symblepharon, trichiasis, corneal opacification, and rarely blindness; Fig. 4.144), the mouth (erosions, blisters, and chronic ulceration), nasal cavity (crusting and bleeding), and the pharynx (hoarseness).[1,24–26] When these mucosal symptoms are severe there is clinical overlap and diagnostic confusion with mucous membrane pemphigoid.

Childhood linear IgA disease (chronic bullous disease of childhood) not uncommonly develops after an upper respiratory tract illness, often following treatment with penicillin.[27–30] Females are affected more often than males (1.6:1) (Fig. 4.145). The average age of onset is 6 years, but very rare cases in neonates have been described.[31]

Lesions, which can be pruritic or burning in the early stages, may be urticated, annular, or polycyclic in appearance and usually arise on normal skin. Vesicles and large bullae (sometimes hemorrhagic) then predominate, and although the perioral regions and genitalia are particularly affected, the face, ears, trunk, limbs, hands, and feet are also often involved (Fig. 4.146). Usually, the new lesions appear around those that are resolving (the 'cluster of jewels' sign, Fig. 4.147). In older and black African children, the clinical appearances can suggest bullous pemphigoid. Healing is sometimes associated with postinflammatory hyper- or hypopigmentation. Mucous membrane lesions are common (64%). Ocular symptoms of pain, grittiness, discharge and redness are found in 40% of children; conjunctival scarring is present in approximately 21%; oral lesions are found in up to 57%.

Although linear IgA disease in children was originally thought to be self-limiting, it is now appreciated that symptoms may last over 5 years (25%) and occasionally extend beyond puberty into adult life. Exceptionally, an association with IgA nephropathy may be seen.[32]

Linear IgA disease is associated with increased expression of HLA-Cw7, -B8, -DR2, -DR3 and -DQ2.[33] The incidence of HLA-B8 association is variable, with reported figures varying from 28% to 56% (normal range 20–25%).[15,22] There is no evidence of an increase in HLA-B12.[15] Linear IgA disease is also associated with HLA-Cw7 and -DR3.[1]

Although in the earlier literature as many as 24% of patients with linear IgA disease were thought to have associated gluten-sensitive enteropathy, the incidence is almost certainly considerably lower.[1] There are, however, occasional recent references documenting occasional patients with linear IgA

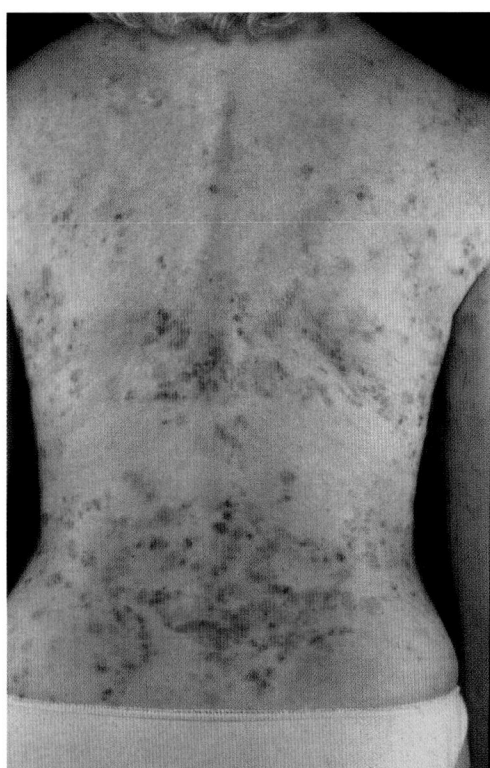

Fig. 4.143
Adult linear IgA disease: in this example, the clinical appearances of excoriated lesions are suggestive of dermatitis herpetiformis. By courtesy of the Institute of Dermatology, London, UK.

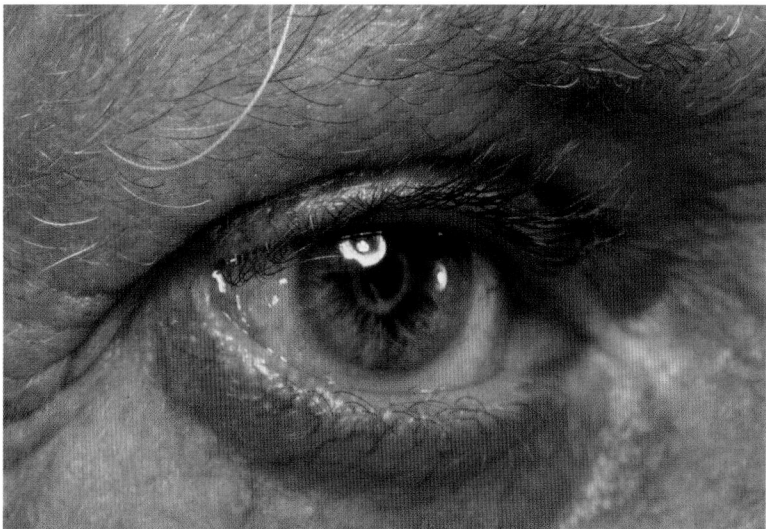

Fig. 4.144
Adult linear IgA disease: there is marked conjunctival injection and blepharitis. By courtesy of the Institute of Dermatology, London, UK.

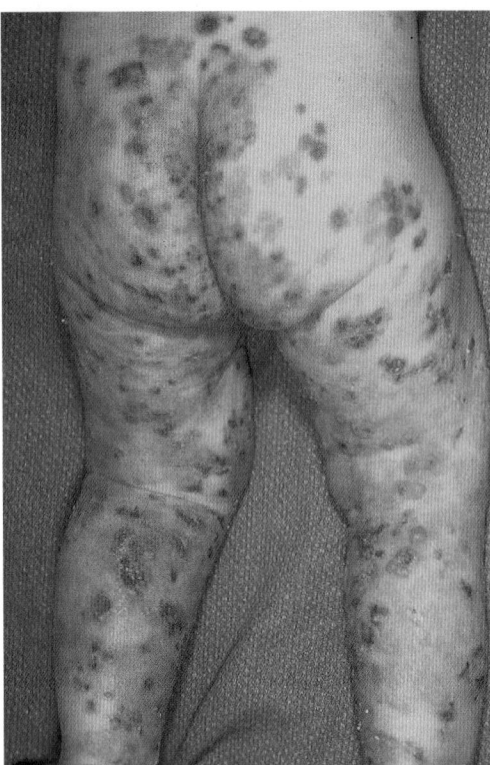

Fig. 4.145
Childhood linear IgA disease: in this case widespread erosions on an erythematous background are present on the buttocks and legs. Occasional intact vesicles are also evident. By courtesy of R.A. Marsden, MD, St George's Hospital, London, UK.

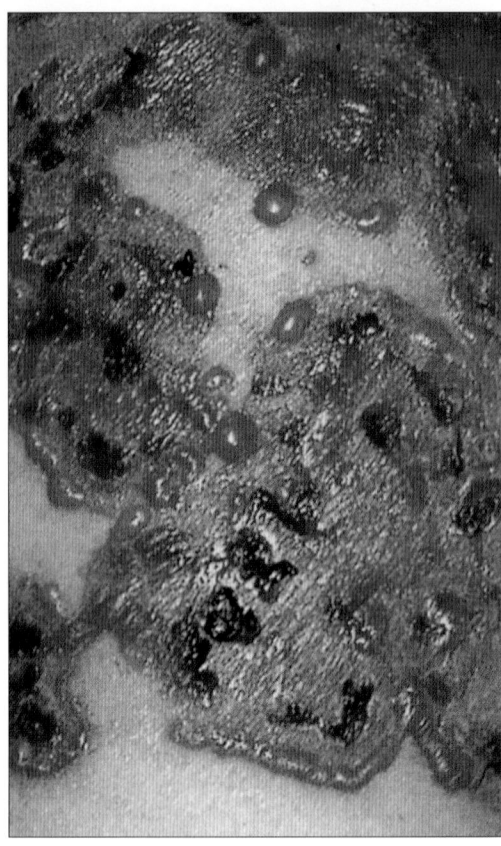

Fig. 4.147
Childhood linear IgA disease: the arrangement of blisters called the 'cluster of jewels'. By courtesy of R.A. Marsden, MD, St George's Hospital, London, UK.

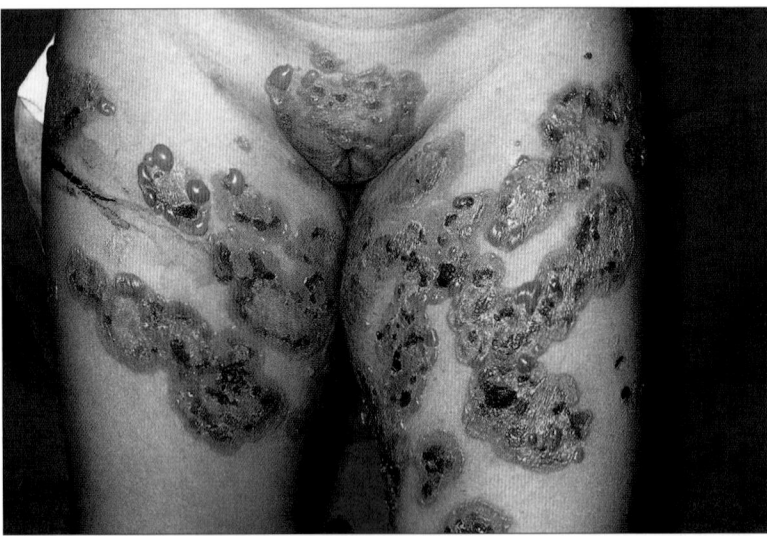

Fig. 4.146
Childhood linear IgA disease: groups of blisters are present on the vulva and inner thighs. By courtesy of R.A. Marsden, MD, St George's Hospital, London, UK.

disease with clinical and histologic evidence of gluten-sensitive enteropathy in the presence of antiendomysial and antitransglutaminase antibodies.[34,35] It is possible that these cases represent dermatitis herpetiformis with linear granular deposits of IgA in which the granularity has not been detected.

There are a number of reports documenting an association between linear IgA disease and internal malignancy, including blistering lymphoma, leukemia, carcinomas of solid organs and sarcomas, although whether this has significance is uncertain.[36–41] Other associated conditions include inflammatory bowel disease (in particular ulcerative colitis), infections, Sjögren syndrome, human papillomavirus vaccination, and drugs.[42,43] Exceptionally,

linear IgA bullous dermatosis can be induced by ultraviolet B exposure.[44,45] Drug-induced linear IgA disease is considered in Chapter 14.

Pathogenesis and histologic features

Histologically, linear IgA disease is characterized most frequently by dermatitis herpetiformis-like features (*Fig. 4.148*).[27,46,47] Occasionally, however, the histologic changes suggest bullous pemphigoid or sometimes a mixture of both diseases (*Fig. 4.149*). Eosinophilic spongiosis may rarely be a feature.[27]

Ultrastructurally, the site of cleavage may be through the lamina lucida or below the lamina densa.[21]

A homogeneous linear deposition of IgA along the basement membrane region is found by direct immunofluorescence in 100% of patients (*Fig. 4.150*).[27,48–50] Uninvolved skin (particularly of the back) is suitable.[1] Oral mucosa and conjunctiva may also show IgA deposition.[1] The linear IgA antigen is present in all stratified squamous epithelia and amnion but, in contrast to the bullous pemphigoid antigen, is not found in bladder mucosa.[49] IgG may also be demonstrable in up to 25% of cases.[12,15] IgM and C3 are occasionally present.[50]

A low titer circulating IgA antibasement membrane zone antibody is present in approximately 30% of patients.[1] Use of conjunctiva as substrate may, however, substantially increase this figure (up to 50%).[24] Circulating IgG or C3-binding antibasement membrane antibodies are seen only in those patients with overlap syndrome.[51] The IgA antibody is of pathogenetic significance since it causes dermal–epidermal separation after incubation with whole skin cultures.[52] Passive transfer of antibodies into a mouse model with human skin graft also produces characteristic lesions.[53] Blister fluid is also satisfactory for IIMF.[1]

With split skin immunofluorescence, the titer may be higher and sensitivity is increased. The IgA antibasement membrane zone antibody variably labels the epidermal side, the dermal side or both sides of the artificial blister cavity.[54–56] Immunoelectron microscopy has shown similar results, with IgA being present within the lamina lucida or below the lamina densa

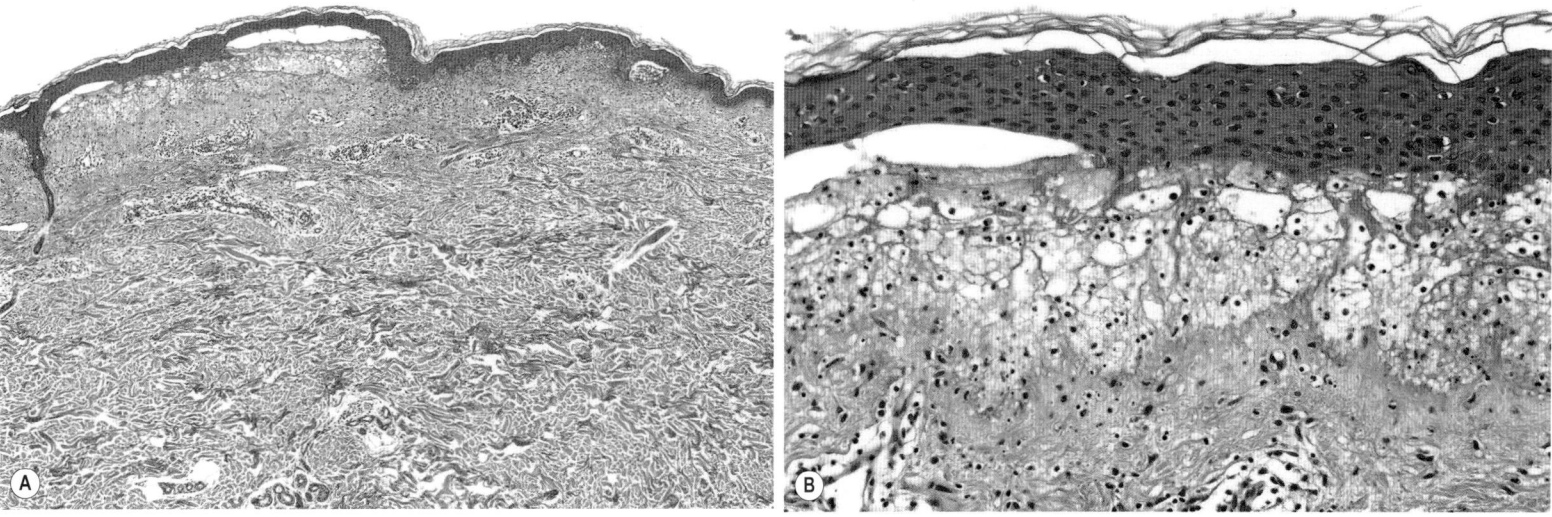

Fig. 4.148
(**A**, **B**) Linear IgA disease: in this example, the features are those of a neutrophil-rich subepidermal vesicle reminiscent of dermatitis herpetiformis.

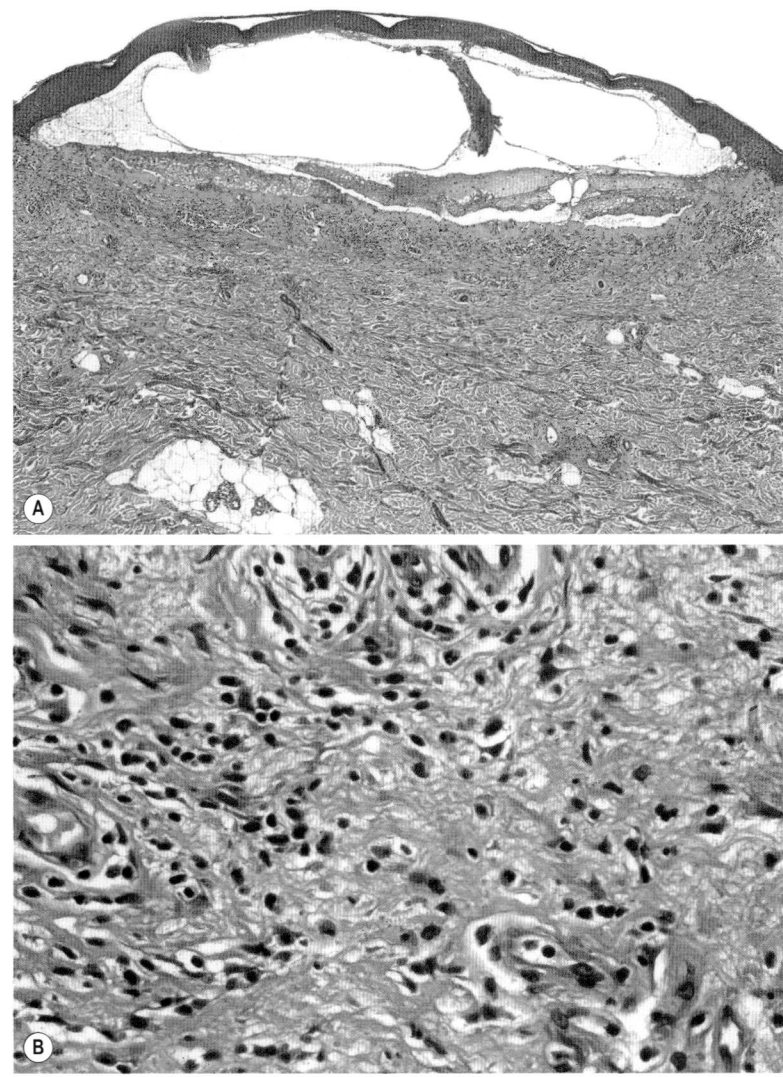

Fig. 4.149
(**A**, **B**) Linear IgA disease: in this field, the presence of eosinophils is more suggestive of bullous pemphigoid.

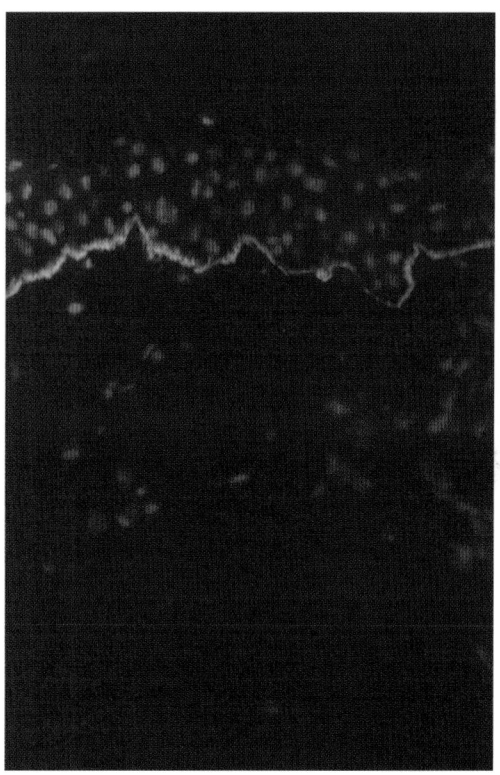

Fig. 4.150
Linear IgA disease: direct immunofluorescence showing linear IgA deposition. By courtesy of the Department of Immunofluorescence, Institute of Dermatology, London, UK.

in association with anchoring fibrils, and sometimes in both locations (*Fig. 4.151*).[57–62]

Studies by Western immunoblotting indicate that linear IgA disease is a heterogeneous condition. Thus, in those cases associated with dermal binding on indirect NaCl-split skin IIMF, the dermal antigens include 285-kD and 250-kD proteins and type VII collagen.[14,56,63,64] Epidermal binding antibodies react with BP230 (BPAG1), BP180 (*BPAG2*), and 200/280-kD antigens distinct from either of the BP antigens.[65–67] The antigens 120 kD (LAD1) and 97 kD described in earlier reports represent proteolytic cleavage products of BP180.[68–71] Linear IgA disease 180-kD antibodies recognize the NC16A domain of collagen XVII (*BPAG2*) also critical for bullous pemphigoid, pemphigoid gestationis, mucous membrane pemphigoid, and lichen planus

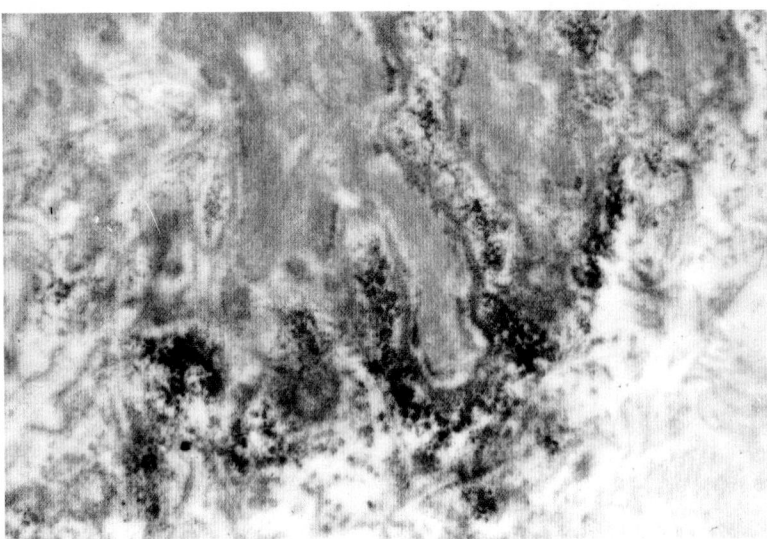

Fig. 4.151
Linear IgA disease: direct immunoperoxidase reaction using frozen tissue substrate. There is an abundance of granular IgA beneath the basal lamina.

pemphigoides described above.[72–75] This fact is remarkable considering the variable clinical features of these various autoimmune bullous disorders. LAD1 has been identified as ladinin localizing to the extracellular domain of BP180 kD.[76] Those patients with mixed IgA and IgG antibody-mediated disease also target BP180.[51] Recent reports suggest that antibodies against the NC16A domain may be more important than those against the LAD1 cleavage product of BP180, but not all cases contain the anti-NC16A antibodies.[77–79]

An immunohistochemical study detected linear staining along the floor of the blister cavity with anti-laminin 5 and anti-collagen IV antibodies in 65% and 90% of patients with adult linear IgA disease.[80]

Differential diagnosis

The diseases from which linear IgA disease must be differentiated are dermatitis herpetiformis, bullous pemphigoid, and inflammatory epidermolysis bullosa. Points of distinction are considered in *Table 4.6*.

Access **ExpertConsult.com** for the complete list of references [print tag]

Acantholytic disorders

CHAPTER

5

See
www.expertconsult.com
for references and
additional material

Introduction

The term acantholysis derives from the Greek *akantha*, a thorn or prickle, and *lysis*, a loosening. In its simplest definition, the term is used to reflect a primary disorder of the skin (and sometimes the mucous membranes) characterized by separation of the keratinocytes at their desmosomal junctions (*Fig. 5.1*). A wide range of conditions are characterized by this feature, from inherited disorders such as Darier disease and Hailey-Hailey disease, in which a calcium pump gene mutation results in desmosomal instability, through to the autoimmune pemphigus group of diseases, whereby autoantibodies directly damage desmosomes with resultant keratinocyte separation and blister formation (*Table 5.1*). Desmosomes may also be damaged by secondary phenomena, for example, following severe edema, either intercellular (spongiosis) or intracellular (e.g., ballooning degeneration as is seen in various viral infections). Such processes, however, are not included in the acantholytic category and are discussed elsewhere. The histologic features of the conditions described in this chapter show considerable overlap. The diagnosis is therefore dependent on adequate clinical information and the results of immunofluorescence investigations.

Pemphigus

Pemphigus (Gr. *pemphix*, blister) refers to a group of chronic blistering diseases which develop as a consequence of autoantibodies directed against a variety of desmosomal proteins.[1-7] The condition as a whole is rare, with an annual incidence ranging from 0.1 to 0.7 per 100 000 of the general population.[2] It is more common in the Jewish population, in which the annual incidence rises to 1.6–3.2 per 100 000.[7,8] Ashkenazi Jews are the most frequently affected.[7,8] The incidence in India also appears to be higher than in other countries.[9] There is no sex predilection.

The clinical features and, therefore, classification of these disorders depend on the level of separation within the epidermis:
- In pemphigus vulgaris (p. vulgaris) and pemphigus vegetans (p. vegetans), the blisters are suprabasal.
- In pemphigus foliaceus (p. foliaceus), pemphigus erythematosus (p. erythematosus), and fogo selvagem, the blisters are situated more superficially.

P. vulgaris is by far the most common variant, accounting for 80% of cases.[7,10,11]

In addition to affecting humans, pemphigus has been described in a variety of animals including dogs, cats, goats, and horses.[12]

Pemphigus vulgaris

Clinical features

P. vulgaris particularly affects the middle-aged (onset typically at 40–60 years of age), although occasionally (up to 2.6%) children are affected.[1-8] Self-limiting neonatal disease through transplacental transfer of maternal autoantibodies has also rarely been documented (see pathogenesis).[9-15] The disease begins in the mouth (*Figs 5.2* and *5.3*) in 50–70% of patients with painful erosions or bullae and, after a period of weeks or months, the blisters spread to involve the skin.[16-22] Oral lesions most commonly affect the buccal, palatine, and gingival mucosae.[1,19-23] P. vulgaris is only rarely confined to the skin.[24,25]

The typical skin lesion is a fragile, flaccid blister, which develops on normal or erythematous skin, and readily ruptures, leaving a painful, crusted, raw, bloody erosion (*Figs 5.4* and *5.5*). Lesions are most often seen on the scalp, face, axillae, and groin, although in some patients they are generalized (*Figs 5.6–5.8*).[1-3,26] Blisters can be induced by rubbing the adjacent, apparently normal skin – the Nikolsky sign. Direct pressure applied to the center of the blister is also followed by lateral extension – the Asboe-Hansen sign.[2] Healing is often accompanied by postinflammatory hyperpigmentation but scarring is not a feature.[2]

Before the introduction of corticosteroid therapy, the lesions usually became more extensive and in the past often led eventually to death. Treatment with high doses of corticosteroids, immunosuppressants (such as azathioprine), intravenous immunoglobulins, and, more recently, biologicals (such as rituximab) has significantly reduced the mortality to 5–15%, and prolonged remissions without treatment are now being reported.[2,27,28] A considerable proportion of the deaths that do occur, however, are due to the side effects of therapy and include staphylococcal infections and, to a lesser extent, pulmonary embolism.[2] Severe opportunistic infections due to a wide range of organisms including listeria, nocardia, enterococci, herpes virus, cryptococcus, and candida may further complicate the disease.[29-36] Patients may also suffer from Cushing syndrome, adrenal insufficiency, and myasthenia gravis, and appear to have a slightly increased risk of leukemia and non-Hodgkin lymphoma.[36]

Nail involvement seems to be more common than previously reported and may precede skin findings.[37] Patients may present with hemorrhagic paronychia, chronic paronychia, trachyonychia, onycholysis, or onychomadesis.[21,37-39] Paronychia and onychomadesis are the most common nail changes encountered. Nail involvement is more common in the nails of

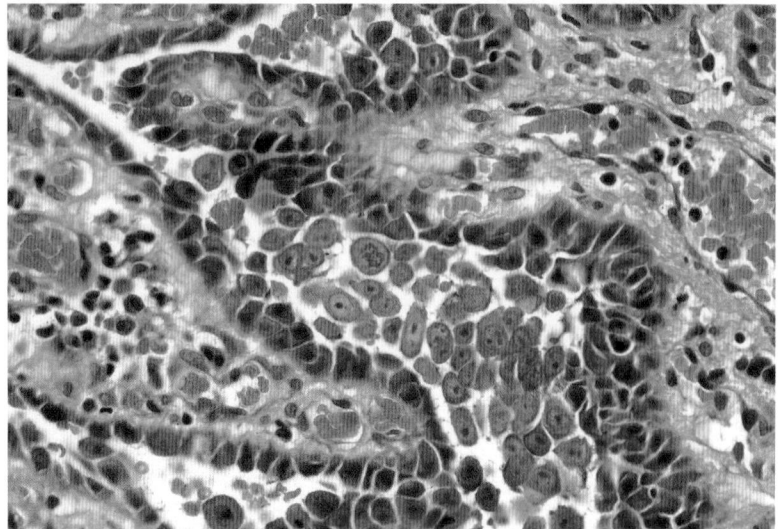

Fig. 5.1
Acantholysis: the keratinocytes are rounded and separated from each other to form an intraepidermal blister. Villi formed from the underlying dermal papillae typically project into suprabasal cavities.

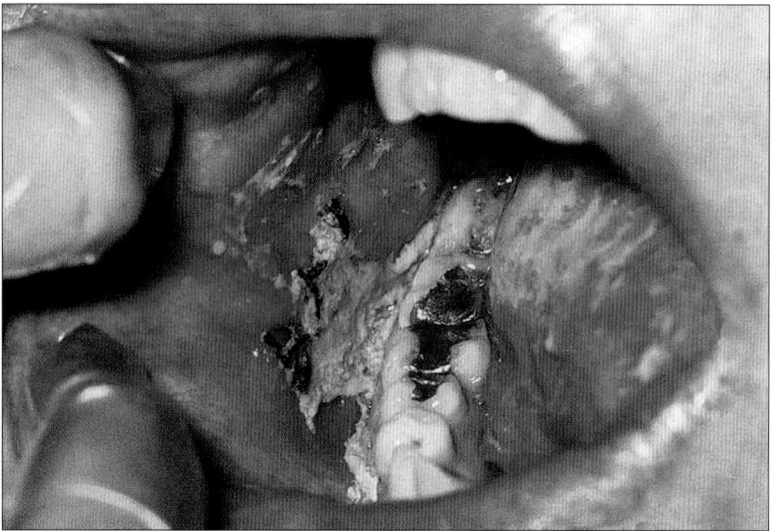

Fig. 5.2
Pemphigus vulgaris: painful erosions are present on the buccal mucosa. By courtesy of R.A. Marsden, MD, St George's Hospital, London, UK.

Table 5.1
Antigens targeted in the pemphigus variants

Pemphigus variant	Autoantigen
Pemphigus vulgaris	Dsg3 (mucosal), Dsg1 (cutaneous), desmocollins, pemphaxin, α9-acetylcholine receptor
Pemphigus vegetans	Dsg3, Dsc1, and Dsc2 in some patients
Pemphigus foliaceus	Dsg1
Pemphigus erythematosus	Dsg1
Fogo selvagem	Dsg1, rarely also Dsg3
IgA pemphigus	Dsc1, Dsg1 or Dsg3
Herpetiform pemphigus	Dsg1, rarely also Dsg3
Paraneoplastic pemphigus	Desmoplakins I and II, envoplakin, periplakin, BP230, plectin, Dsg1, and Dsg3
Drug-induced pemphigus	Dsg1 or Dsg3

Dsc, Desmocollin; *Dsg*, desmoglein.
Modified from Martel, P., Joly, P. (2001) Pemphigus: autoimmune diseases of keratinocyte's adhesion molecules. Clinical Dermatology, 19, 667.

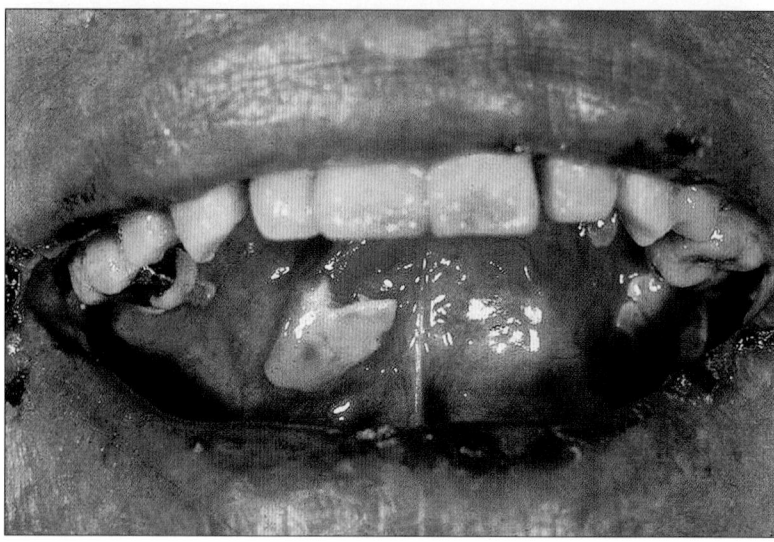

Fig. 5.3
Pemphigus vulgaris: in this patient, there is an intact blister on the floor of the mouth. Pemphigus commonly presents in the mouth. By courtesy of the Institute of Dermatology, London, UK.

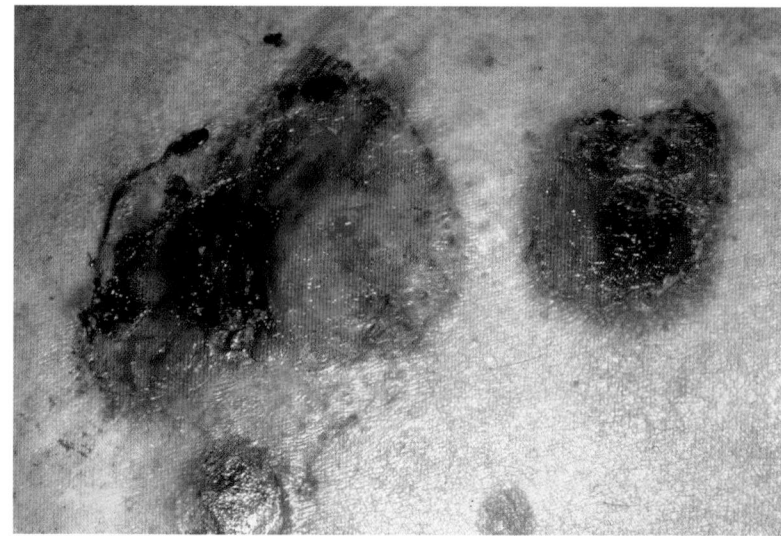

Fig. 5.4
Pemphigus vulgaris: since the blisters are superficial, erosions are more commonly encountered. By courtesy of the Institute of Dermatology, London, UK.

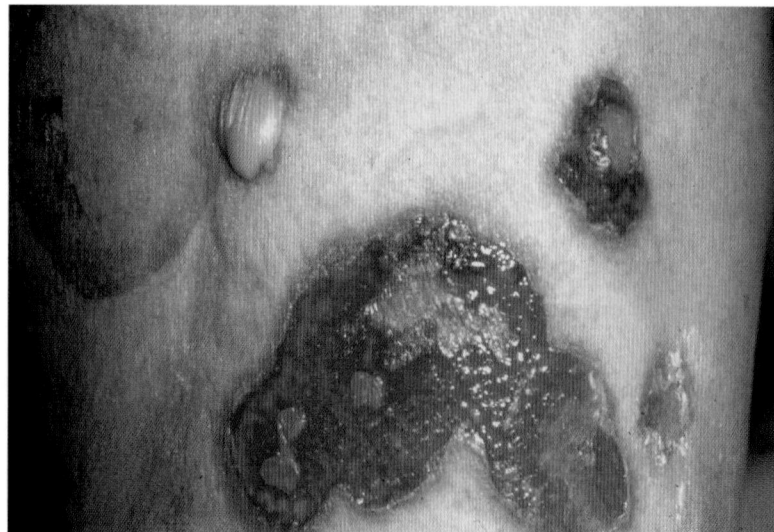

Fig. 5.5
Pemphigus vulgaris: extensive erosions and blisters are present on the shin. By courtesy of R.A. Marsden, MD, St George's Hospital, London, UK.

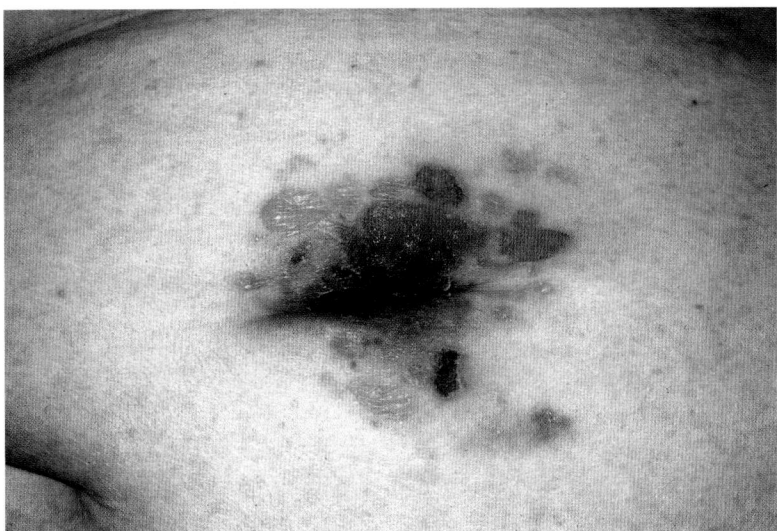

Fig. 5.6
Pemphigus vulgaris: umbilical lesions showing intact blisters as well as raw erosions. By courtesy of R.A. Marsden, MD, St George's Hospital, London, UK.

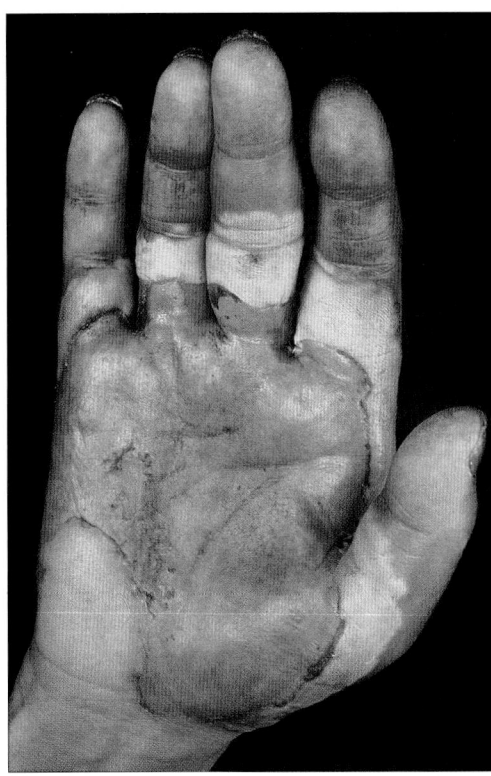

Fig. 5.7
Pemphigus vulgaris: extensive trauma-induced blisters. By courtesy of the Institute of Dermatology, London, UK.

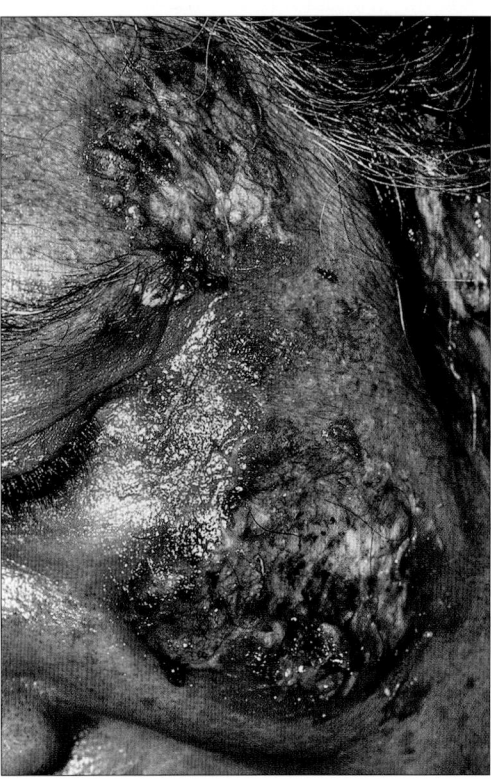

Fig. 5.8
Pemphigus vulgaris: extensive disease can be very disfiguring. By courtesy of the Institute of Dermatology, London, UK.

digits affected by periungual blisters and also in patients with large number of skin blisters.[39]

Occasional modes of presentation include linear lesions and pemphigus arising after surgery, burns, vaccination, radiation therapy, and trauma.[40–52] Development after exposure to pesticides and an association with cocaine snorting has also been reported.[53,54] A very exceptional case has been described in which blisters were initially confined to melanocytic nevi.[55] P. vulgaris may also be rarely induced by a variety of drugs, particularly angiotensin-converting enzyme (ACE) inhibitors such as captopril.[56–58]

In addition to oral and cutaneous involvement, lesions have been described at a wide variety of sites including the nasopharynx, larynx, ear, esophagus, eye, external genitalia, urethra, and anal and colonic mucosa.[1,59–61] Esophageal lesions, although originally thought to be rare, have been documented in as many as 63–87% of patients.[62,63] Erosions and ulcers are typically found, and intact blisters are rare. Exceptionally, the whole mucosa may be affected with subsequent sloughing – esophagitis dissecans superficialis.[64,65] Ocular involvement appears to be more common than previously thought, involving up to 26% of patients.[66,67] Ocular lesions are usually restricted to the conjunctiva, presenting as conjunctivitis or small vesicles that rapidly rupture.[2,66–69] Very rarely, scarring may develop, and corneal ulceration with perforation has been described.[70] Vulval, vaginal, and cervical lesions are well recognized and common.[71–77] Exceptionally, the vagina may be the sole site of involvement.[77] Penile lesions most commonly affect the glans.[78,79] They are not usually followed by any significant sequelae.

The development of pemphigus may be associated with a variety of disorders (primarily other autoimmune diseases), including bullous pemphigoid, lupus erythematosus, myasthenia gravis, Hashimoto thyroiditis, vitiligo, minimal change nephropathy, ulcerative colitis, rheumatoid arthritis, and diabetes mellitus.[80–88] It has also been described in a patient with the 1p36 deletion syndrome.[89] As in many other diseases with an immunological pathogenesis, pemphigus is accompanied by an increased incidence of internal malignancy including thymoma, lymphoma, and multiple myeloma (see paraneoplastic pemphigus).[90–93] It has also been reported in association with Kaposi sarcoma.[94]

Pathogenesis and histologic features

Pemphigus is an immunologically mediated disease.[95,96] The most reliable method to confirm the diagnosis is by direct immunofluorescence.[97] The later is more accurate than serological methods. Examination of perilesional skin by direct immunofluorescent techniques reveals in vivo-bound immunoglobulin (usually IgG) and often complement (C3) in the intercellular region of the epidermis (*Fig. 5.9*).[98] Abundant antigen in the follicular outer root sheath and germinal matrix may account for the marked scalp involvement typical of pemphigus, and plucked hair follicles may serve as an adequate substrate for direct immunofluorescence analysis.[99,100] The in vivo-bound IgG is mainly of the IgG1 and IgG4 subclasses.[101]

Indirect immunofluorescent techniques show that the serum of patients with pemphigus contains an IgG antibody that reacts with the intercellular region of normal squamous epithelium.[102] This antibody is, however, not entirely specific as it may be found in a variety of other conditions, such as severe burns and penicillin drug reactions, and following radiation

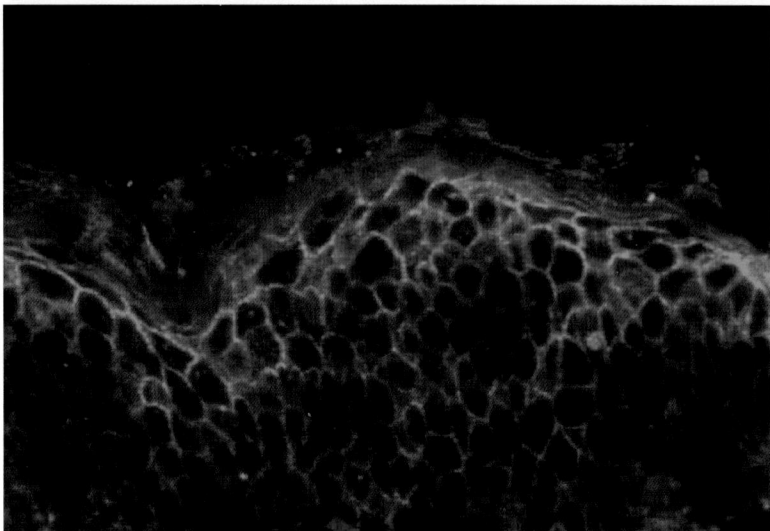

Fig. 5.9
Pemphigus vulgaris: direct immunofluorescence. By courtesy of the Institute of Dermatology, London, UK.

therapy.[103–105] Presumably, pemphigus antigens are released into the circulation following such trauma with resultant antibody production. Circulating antibodies are predominantly of the IgG1 and IgG4 subclasses; IgG3 is identified much less often.[106]

Circulating IgG is pathogenic.[96,97] The level of the antibody titer closely parallels the clinical state of the disease.[107–110] IgG4 titers diminish during remission whereas circulating IgG1 may continue to be present.[97,108] Relapse is commonly preceded by rising IgG4 antibody titers.[108]

As mentioned above, p. vulgaris rarely may be evident in a neonate born of a mother with active p. vulgaris due to passive transfer of autoantibodies across the placenta.[9–15,111,112] The condition is, however, short lived, with lesions disappearing, as the maternal antibodies are catabolized. Passive transfer of IgG4 into neonatal mice results in the development of blisters.[112] Purified IgG from pemphigus induces acantholysis in human skin explants and keratinocyte cultures.[113,114]

The pemphigus antibody binds to the full thickness of the epidermis. Compared with p. vulgaris, immunofluorescence studies on the sera of p. foliaceus patients tend to show more staining in the superficial epidermis, correlating with the level of the split.[115,116] Conversely, the sera from patients with p. vulgaris show more affinity for the lower epidermis. Despite these trends, we do not base diagnoses on these (often subtle) differences in immunofluorescence staining distribution.

The p. vulgaris antibody is directed at the extracytoplasmic domain of the 130-kD epithelial desmosomal cadherin, desmoglein 3 (Dsg3), which forms a complex with plakoglobin (85 kD).[117–123] The p. vulgaris antibody, however, does not recognize the latter. Many patients also have antibodies that bind to the p. foliaceus antigen, desmoglein 1 (Dsg1), a 160-kD polypeptide.[124,125] Dsg3 is expressed primarily in the oral mucosa and, therefore, antibodies directed against this antigen result in mucosal pemphigus. In contrast, Dsg1 is a cutaneous antigen and, therefore, antibodies directed against it result in lesions affecting the skin but not the mucosa (cutaneous pemphigus).[115] Anti-Dsg1 antibodies also show cross-reactivity against Dsg4, another member of the desmoglein family.[126,127] While patient sera contain antibodies against nonconformational epitopes of Dsg3, active disease correlates with the presence of antibodies directed against the NH2-terminal aspect of Dsg3, in particular ectodomains 2–4.[128–130] Oral disease is particularly associated with reactivity to ectodomains 1–4, which is reduced in cutaneous pemphigus.[128]

Antibodies reactive to a number of other proteins including desmoplakin, desmocollins, pemphaxin, and acetylcholine receptor have also been demonstrated in the sera of p. vulgaris patients.[130–135]

Sera from patients with p. vulgaris not infrequently contain additional IgA antibodies, in particular against Dsg1 and Dsg3.[136–138] Although the combination of both IgG and IgA antibodies has, in some instances, been referred to as IgG/IgA pemphigus in the literature, this appears to be an ill-defined and heterogeneous disease group.[136,139] In addition to p. vulgaris, the additional presence of anti-Dsg IgA antibodies has also been demonstrated in p. foliaceus, p. vegetans, pemphigus herpetiformis, and paraneoplastic pemphigus.[136,140,141] Although there is some doubt that this is a truly distinct entity, the so-called IgG/IgA pemphigus may show an atypical clinical presentation with pustules, annular lesions, or a malar rash.[139,142–150] Most do not have mucosal involvement.[151] Association with malignancy has been suggested.[151,152] Histologic features may be more reminiscent of IgA pemphigus, and the presence of IgA antibodies against desmocollins is seen in a subset of patients.[139,142–152]

The pathogenesis of the acantholysis is uncertain. Direct binding of antibody to the desmosomal cadherins is of major importance and results in internalization of Dsg3 and degradation by the endolysosomal pathway.[96,139,153] Plakoglobin has been implicated in mediating intracellular events following IgG binding to Dsg3.[154,155] In particular, the role of plakoglobin is signal transduction to the nucleus.[154,156] There is also some evidence to suggest that the process may involve, at least secondarily, the action of local proteolytic enzymes.[95] The pemphigus antibody induces expression of plasminogen activator receptor on the surface of keratinocytes.[157] Binding of plasminogen activator to its keratinocyte cell membrane receptor results in plasminogen activation with resultant production of plasmin.[158,159] This latter has non-specific proteolytic activity, which may be responsible at least in part for the dissolution of the desmosomes.[96] P. vulgaris antibodies stimulate production of keratinocyte phospholipase C and inositol 1,4,5-triphosphate and increase intracellular calcium. Protein kinase C activation results in release of keratinocyte plasminogen activator and increased expression of plasminogen activator receptor.[160–162] Other factors, however, must be of greater importance since p. vulgaris IgG can induce acantholysis in plasminogen activator knockout mice.[163] An additional phenomenon is rapid phosphorylation of heat shock protein 27 and p38MAPK, resulting in reorganization and collapse of the cytoskeleton as a result of IgG binding to Dsg3.[164,165] This process is mediated by upstream events involving EGF receptor kinase and Src.[166] Complement appears not to be essential for acantholysis, and it is thought that any involvement is secondary, perhaps accelerating or extending the process.[96] It has been suggested that apoptosis may be induced by p. vulgaris IgG, and that this mechanism may be important in the pathogenesis of the disease.[167–169] Other studies have shown that apoptosis is not a prerequisite for blistering and may be a secondary phenomenon.[170] Apoptolysis is a process whereby the autoantibodies activate the apoptotic pathway through EGFR/Src signaling through mTOR, resulting in basal cell shrinkage rather than complete apoptosis with subsequent acantholysis.[169–171]

T cells are also critical to the development of the antibody-mediated acantholysis.[95] CD4+ memory T cells are predominantly involved and both T-helper 1 (Th1) and Th2 Dsg3-specific subtypes are represented.[172,173] Th1 T cell-derived interferon-γ stimulates production of IgG1, and Th2 cells produce interleukin (IL)-4 and IL-13, which are responsible for secretion of B cell-derived IgG4.[174] Both populations are therefore of importance in stimulating production of p. vulgaris antibody.[97] In addition, there is evidence that tumor necrosis factor 1 (TNF-1), Fas-ligand, and IL-1 are also of importance in the development of acantholysis.[175] Knockout mice for both these cytokines show diminished acantholysis in passive antibody transfer experiments.[176]

There is considerable evidence of a genetic background influencing susceptibility to pemphigus as shown by strong associations with human leukocyte antigen (HLA)-DRβ1*0402, HLA-DRβ1*1401, and HLA-DQβ1*0503.[176–180] Perhaps surprisingly, however, there are only occasional documented reports of familial occurrence.[181–184]

Pemphigus blisters rupture easily. It is therefore essential to biopsy an early lesion to establish the correct diagnosis.[186a] The characteristic acantholysis develops because of damage to the intercellular bridges. Acantholytic cells are rounded and have intensely eosinophilic cytoplasm, pyknotic nuclei, and perinuclear halos.[185] An early lesion of p. vulgaris shows a slit-like suprabasal cleft or vesicle containing occasional acantholytic cells. The established blister contains acantholytic cells in clumps and in isolation (*Figs 5.10* and *5.11*). Characteristically, the floor of the cavity is lined by a single

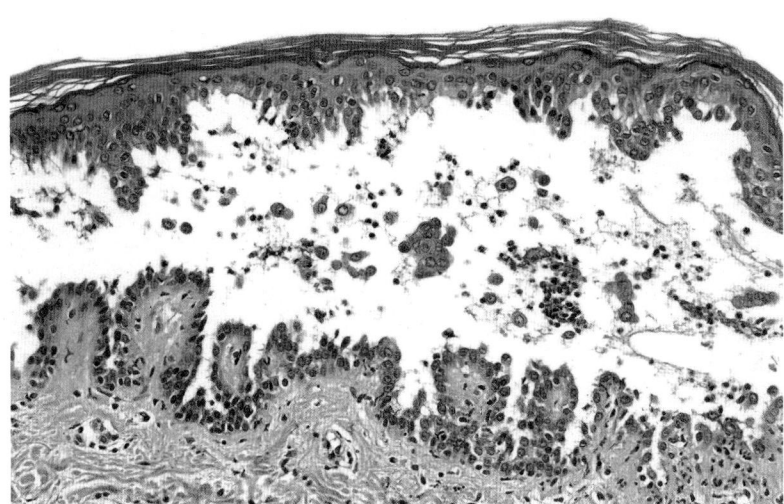

Fig. 5.10
Pemphigus vulgaris: established blister showing marked acantholysis and scattered neutrophils. The dermal papillae project into the cavity as villi.

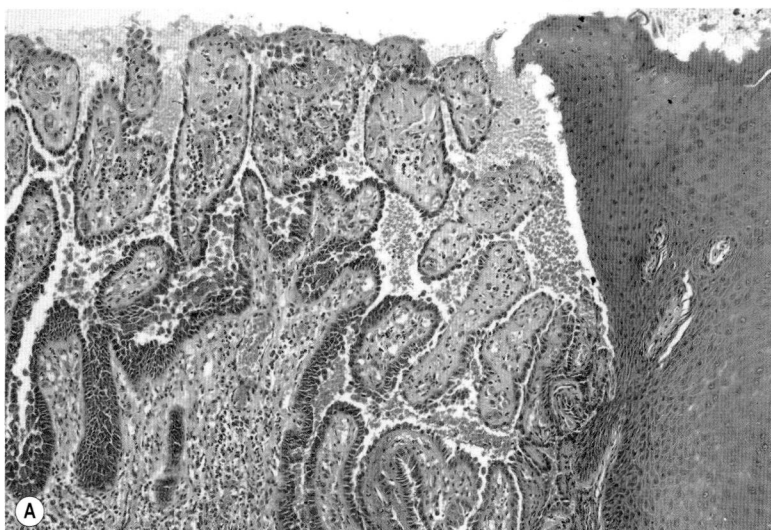

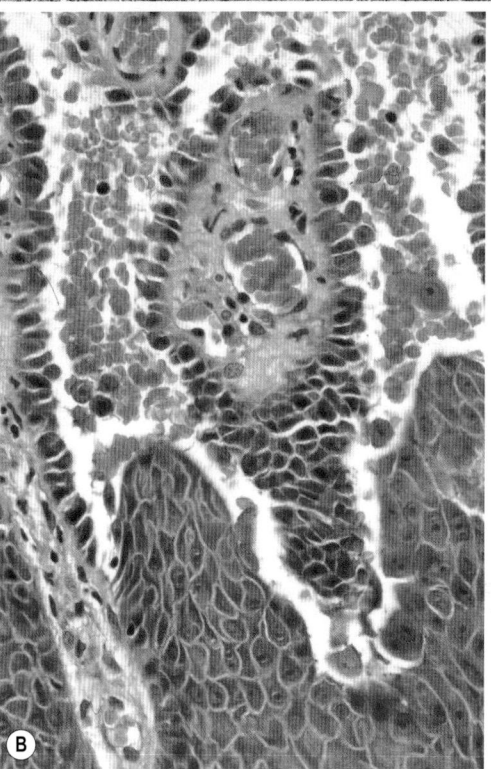

Fig. 5.11
Pemphigus vulgaris: (**A**) perianal mucosa showing acantholysis and conspicuous villi; (**B**) high-power view.

layer of intact basal cells, the so-called 'tombstone' pattern (*Fig. 5.12*).[152] The acantholytic process frequently involves the epithelium of the adnexae, which can be a useful diagnostic clue in those lesions which lack the roof of the blister (*Fig. 5.13*).[186] Acantholytic changes are also seen in epidermoid cysts. The dermal papillary outline is usually maintained, and frequently, the papillae protrude into the blister cavity. Sometimes the features of eosinophilic spongiosis are seen on biopsy, particularly in early lesions.[187] The blister cavity often contains a few inflammatory cells (notably eosinophils), and in the dermis, there is a moderate perivascular chronic inflammatory cell infiltrate with conspicuous eosinophils, although sometimes these are scanty or even absent. Mucous membrane lesions show similar histology.

The histologic features can in part be explained by the compensation theory.[120,169] This theory suggests that one Dsg type may be sufficient to maintain epithelium integrity by compensating for the loss of the specific Dsg targeted. In mucosal predominant pemphigus, the autoantibodies target Dsg3, and the relative lack of Dsg1 in mucosa explains the prominent acantholysis in the mucosa and relative sparing of the epidermis. The presence of Dsg1 compensates for the loss of Dsg3 in the skin. In p. foliaceus (see below), the primary target is Dsg1, which is primarily found in the upper epidermis. This explains the superficial nature of the split and sparing of the mucosa, which lacks significant Dsg1.

Ultrastructurally, there is dilatation of the intercellular space with consequent stretching of the desmosomal attachment points (*Figs 5.14* and *5.15*).[188] With progression, these separate and eventually disappear, with residual cell membranes often showing a pseudovillous morphology. Hemidesmosomes are morphologically normal. Immunoelectron microscopy confirms that the immunoreactants are located within the intercellular space.

Endemic pemphigus vulgaris

Patients with clinical and histologic presentation of p. vulgaris but epidemiological features of fogo selvagem were identified in the Goiania and Brasilia regions of Brazil, known endemic areas of p. foliaceus. These patients demonstrate classical mucocutaneous disease and antibodies to both Dsg1 and Dsg3, but are remarkable for early onset of disease, frequently before the age of 20.[189]

Differential diagnosis

The differential diagnosis of p. vulgaris includes a variety of conditions such as Darier disease, Hailey-Hailey disease, and transient acantholytic dermatosis (Grovers disease) (*Table 5.2*). In the absence of clinical information or without immunofluorescence studies, it may be impossible to establish a definitive diagnosis. None of these diseases has a specific pattern of immunoreactivity on direct immunofluorescence.

Dyskeratosis in the form of corps ronds and grains is typical of Darier disease, but is rarely seen in Hailey-Hailey disease, and is not a feature of pemphigus. In Hailey-Hailey disease, the perivesicular epithelium is likened to a dilapidated brick wall, an effect sometimes seen in p. vulgaris. More frequently, however, the epithelium overlying and adjacent to the blister is essentially intact.

Acantholysis involving the follicular epithelium is often seen in pemphigus, but usually not in Hailey-Hailey disease. The pemphigus-like variant of Grover disease is histologically indistinguishable from pemphigus, but the clinical history, minute size of the lesions as viewed by the microscope, and negative immunofluorescence findings make distinction relatively easy. Extreme degrees of acantholysis in acantholytic solar keratosis may on rare occasions be confused with the previously mentioned acantholytic disorders. Similarly, it is important not to misinterpret the trivial finding of incidental focal acantholytic dyskeratosis in a skin specimen removed or biopsied for an unrelated finding.

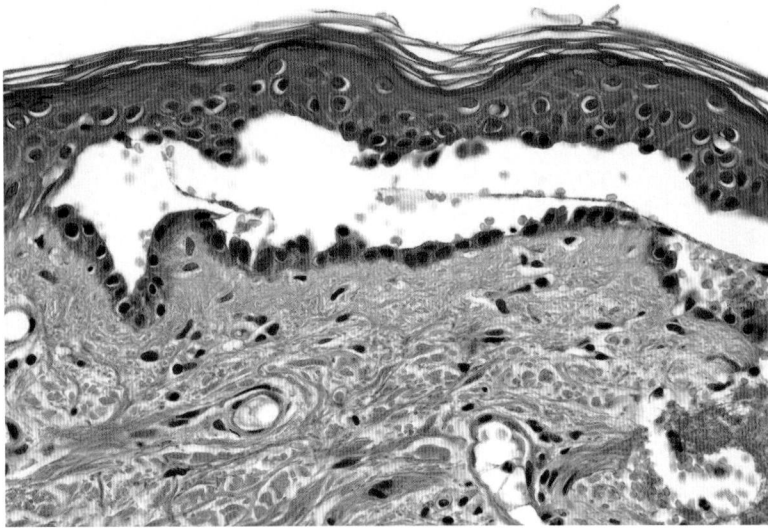

Fig. 5.12
Pemphigus vulgaris: cell-free example showing a linear palisade of intact basal keratinocytes – the so-called 'tombstone' appearance.

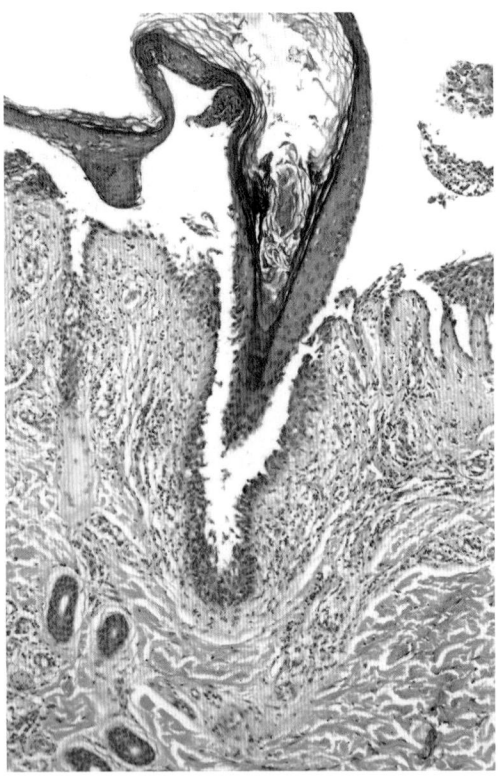

Fig. 5.13
Pemphigus vulgaris: follicular involvement distinguishes pemphigus from Hailey-Hailey disease in which it is not a feature.

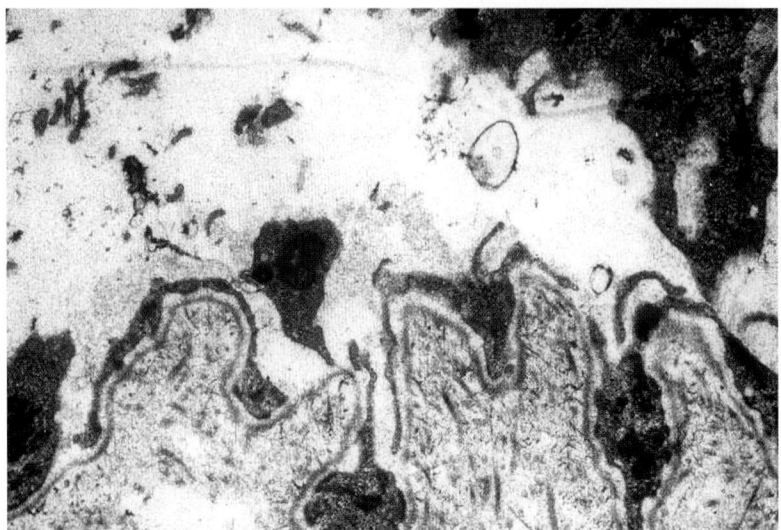

Fig. 5.14
Pemphigus vulgaris: electron photomicrograph of an early lesion showing suprabasal, intraepidermal vesiculation. Residual cytoplasm of basal keratinocytes lines the floor of the blister. The lamina densa is clearly visible.

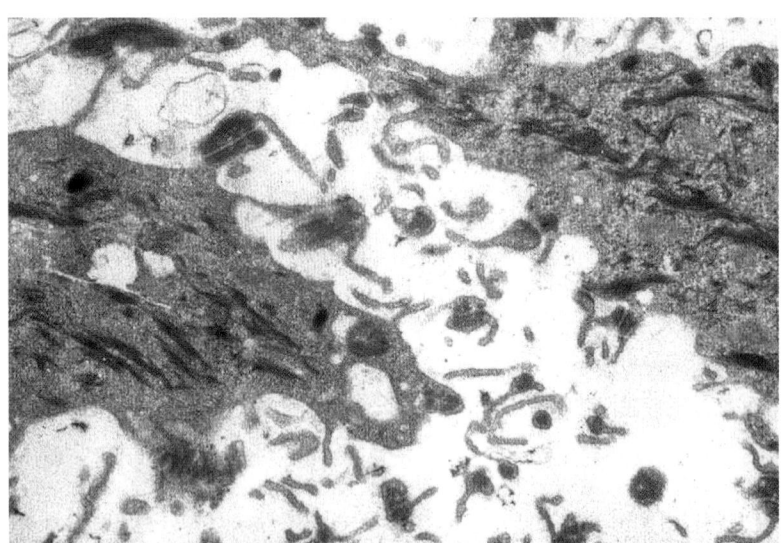

Fig. 5.15
Pemphigus vulgaris: electron photomicrograph of an early lesion showing marked dilatation of the intercellular space. Cytoplasmic 'villus' formation is conspicuous and only occasional desmosomes are apparent.

Table 5.2
Differential diagnosis of suprabasal pemphigus

	Pemphigus vulgaris[a]	Darier disease[a]	Hailey-Hailey disease[a]
Types of lesion	Intraepithelial bullae	Suprabasal clefts	Intraepithelial bullae
Adjacent epithelium	Intact	Intact	Disintegrating
Involvement of adnexae	Yes	Yes	No
Corps ronds and grains	No	Yes	Rarely
Dermal inflammation	Mononuclears, eosinophils	Mononuclears	Mononuclears
IMF	Positive	Negative	Negative

[a]The lesions of Grover disease may histologically mimic any of these and can only be distinguished with appropriate clinicopathologic correlation and/or by immunofluorescence.

Pemphigus vegetans

Clinical features

P. vegetans, a chronic variant of p. vulgaris, has a somewhat better prognosis than p. vulgaris with occasional cases associated with spontaneous remission documented.[1–3] It accounts for 1–9% of all cases of pemphigus and appears to be especially common in North Africa.[1,4] As with the vulgaris variant, p. vegetans typically presents in adults. There has, however, been a small number of cases described in childhood including a dapsone-responsive IgA-mediated variant.[5–8] The lesions, which present as blisters and erosions, are particularly prolific in the flexures, especially the axillae, the groin, the inframammary region, the umbilicus, and at the margins of the lips. The

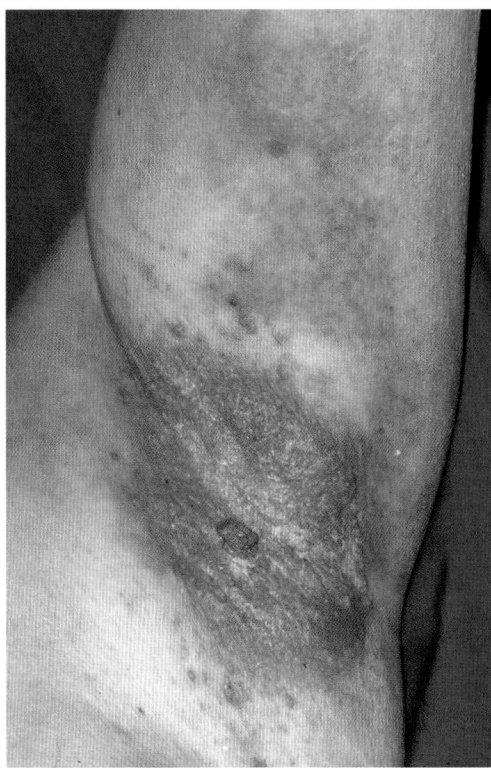

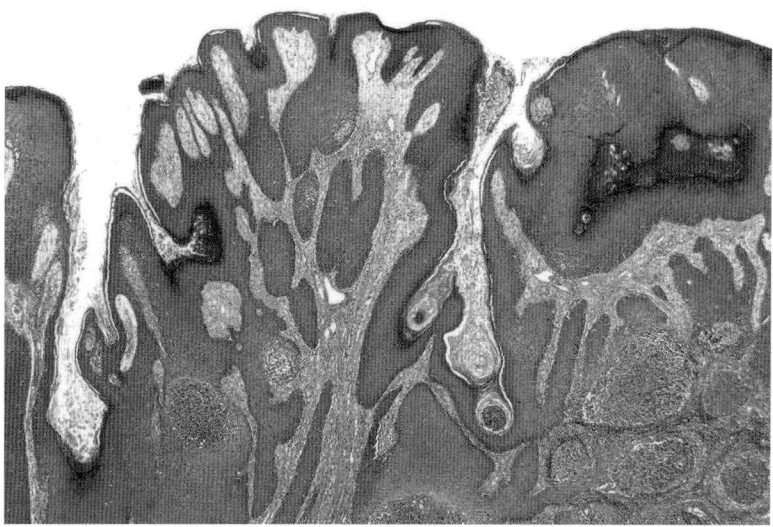

Fig. 5.17
Pemphigus vegetans: the epidermis is hyperplasic and there are scattered abscesses.

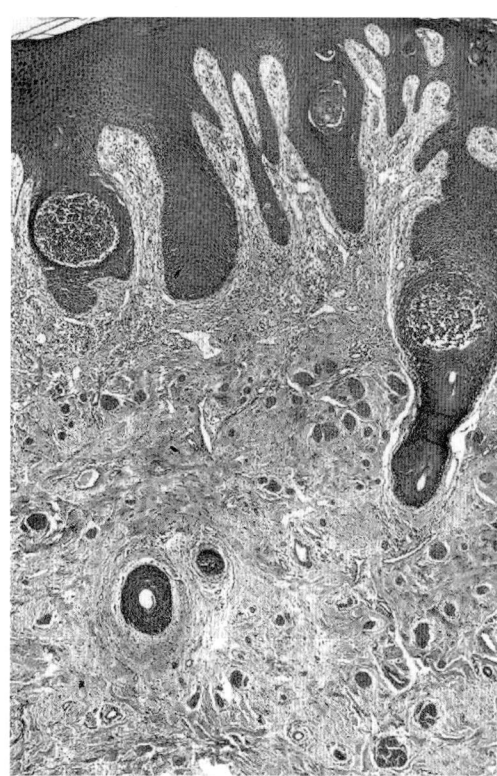

Fig. 5.18
Pemphigus vegetans: follicular involvement is seen on the right.

scalp is also said to be a site of predilection.[9,10] Soon thereafter, patients characteristically develop hypertrophic vegetations and pustules at the blistered edges (*Fig. 5.16*).[1]

The oral cavity is commonly affected, and a cerebriform or 'scrotal' tongue is said to be a diagnostic clue in cases of early involvement.[11–14] An exceptional case of the disease restricted to the tongue has been reported.[15] Esophageal involvement presenting as erosions and white plaques has been described in a number of patients, and the nasal mucosa, larynx, vulva, vagina, penis, and anus may also be affected.[8,16–20] Nail involvement including onycholysis and pustules is sometimes seen.[21] Acral involvement can clinically be mistaken for acrodermatitis continua suppurativa.[22] Peripheral blood eosinophilia is commonly present.

Two clinical subtypes are recognized:[23,24]
- In the Neumann variant (the more serious form), lesions usually begin as described in p. vulgaris, but the ensuing erosions develop vegetations. The course of this variant is similar to that of p. vulgaris.
- In the Hallopeau variant ('pyodermite vegetante'), the eruption begins as pustular lesions that rapidly evolve into verrucous vegetating plaques.[2] Bullae are usually not seen. This is a milder variant in which spontaneous remission is not uncommon.

Pathogenesis and histologic features

Support for the thesis that p. vegetans is a variant of p. vulgaris is based on the finding that both subtypes are associated with IgG and C3 deposition in the epidermal intercellular space on direct immunofluorescence, and circulating 'pemphigus' antibody.[24] P. vegetans is characterized by an antibody directed at the Dsg3.[25–27] Antibodies against desmocollins 1 and 2 as well as periplakin have also been documented.[28,29] Rarely, additional IgA antibodies to Dsg3 may also be detected.[30]

Precipitating factors for this pemphigus variant are largely unknown. A case has been described developing after and restricted to a split-thickness skin graft.[31] Exceptionally p. vegetans has been linked with the ACE inhibitors captopril and enalapril.[32,33] Further exceptional cases developed in association with intranasal heroin or cocaine abuse and HIV infection.[20,34–36] There are rare reports relating a p. vegetans-like lesion as a manifestation of paraneoplastic pemphigus and p. vegetans with underlying malignancy.[37–42]

Although a variant of p. vulgaris, p. vegetans shows strikingly different histologic features. Suprabasal acantholysis is present but is often subtle, being masked by an exuberant proliferation of squamous epithelium, which may sometimes show pseudoepitheliomatous hyperplasia (*Fig. 5.17*). The epithelial proliferation involves both the epidermis and the infundibular follicular epithelium. Characteristically, there is an intense inflammatory cell infiltrate containing numerous eosinophils, and intraepidermal microabscesses are often seen (*Figs 5.18* and *5.19*). Eosinophilic spongiosis is often a prominent feature.[43,44] The inflammatory changes and epithelial proliferation are sometimes so marked that the true nature of the lesions is obscured. Very occasionally, 10–40-µm eosinophilic hexagonal Charcot-Leyden crystals have been described within the eosinophil-rich microabscesses.[32,45] The diagnosis of p. vegetans is easily overlooked and is made only by the pathologist with a high index of suspicion.

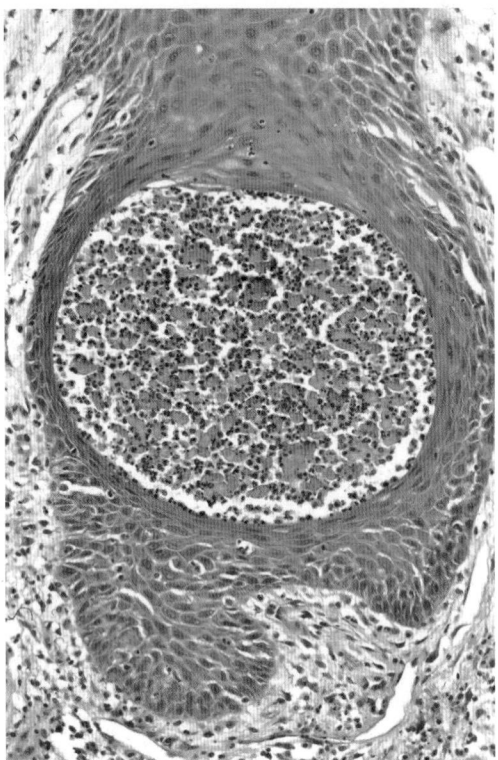

Fig. 5.19
Pemphigus vegetans: there are numerous eosinophils. Note the acantholysis.

Differential diagnosis

Given the histologic overlap with p. vulgaris, the same differential diagnosis as discussed for that variant should be considered. In established lesions associated with squamous epithelial hyperplasia, the suprabasal cleft formation is often focal and easily overlooked. Infections, particularly fungal and bacterial, that are associated with pseudoepitheliomatous hyperplasia and microabscesses may be confused with p. vegetans. In particular, pyostomatitis/pyodermatitis vegetans must be excluded in patients presenting with oral involvement. The latter is usually associated with inflammatory bowel disease, and although it may mimic p. vegetans clinically and histologically (acantholysis tends to be focal and is often absent in pyostomatitis), direct immunofluorescence is usually negative. In rare cases however, in pyostomatitis/pyodermitis vegetans direct immunofluorescence may be positive for IgA in the superficial epidermis and/or for IgG and C3 at the dermoepidermal junction. In exceptional cases there seems to be overlap between these conditions and pemphigus.[46,47] Halogenoderma (iododerma and bromoderma) may also show similar histological features with prominent eosinophilic spongiosis but in the latter acantholysis is not a feature.

Pemphigus foliaceus

Clinical features

P. foliaceus is considerably more uncommon than p. vulgaris, and although it most often affects the middle-aged and elderly, it has a very variable age of onset, sometimes affecting younger adults and even, occasionally, children.[1–8] Very exceptionally, maternal antibodies have been known to cross the placenta, resulting in neonatal disease.[9–13] In general, nonendemic p. foliaceus in children is relatively benign and of short duration.[6]

The superficial blisters of p. foliaceus are exceedingly fragile and therefore much less obvious; erosions and large leafy scales or crusts are often predominant (Figs 5.20–5.22). The lesions may remain localized to the scalp, nose, face, and trunk for many months or years, leading to a mistaken diagnosis of seborrheic dermatitis, seborrheic keratosis, or even lupus erythematosus. Sometimes the eruption involves the entire surface of the body or produces a clinical resemblance to exfoliative dermatitis (erythroderma) (Fig. 5.23).[14,15] Mucous membrane involvement is rare due to the lack of Dsg1 in oral mucosa (see below).[1,16] Exceptionally, patients may

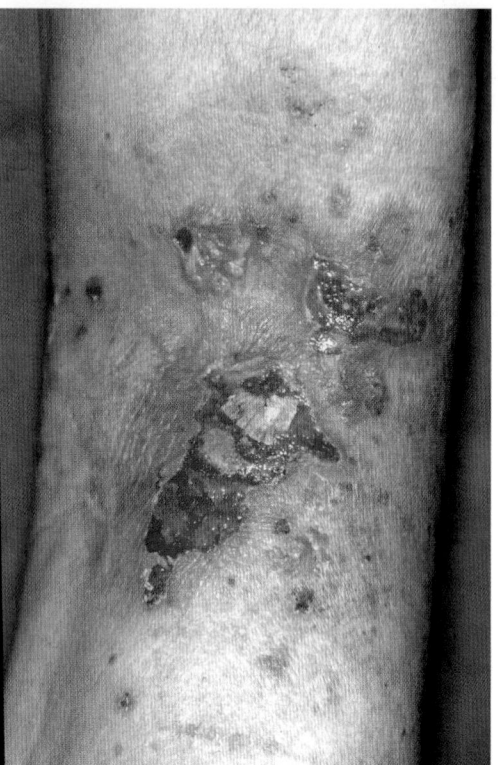

Fig. 5.20
Pemphigus foliaceus: multiple erosions are present with background erythema and postinflammatory hyperpigmentation. Courtesy of the Institute of Dermatology, London, UK.

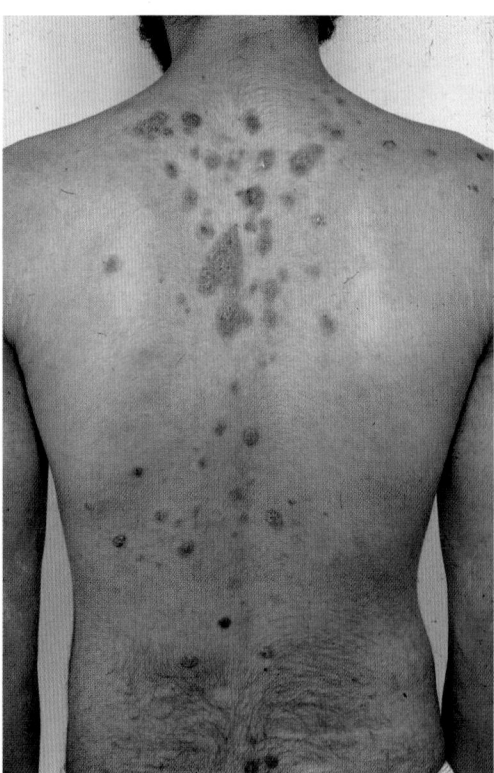

Fig. 5.21
Pemphigus foliaceus: crusted lesions are evident on the back of this young male. From the collection of the late N.P. Smith, MD, the Institute of Dermatology, London, UK.

present with localized disease, typically restricted to the face.[17,18] The development of pustular lesions is exceptional.[19] P. foliaceus often has a much more benign course than p. vulgaris, although patients with severe disease, requiring corticosteroid and immunosuppressant therapy, still have a risk of mortality. The disease may be complicated by Kaposi varicelliform eruption,

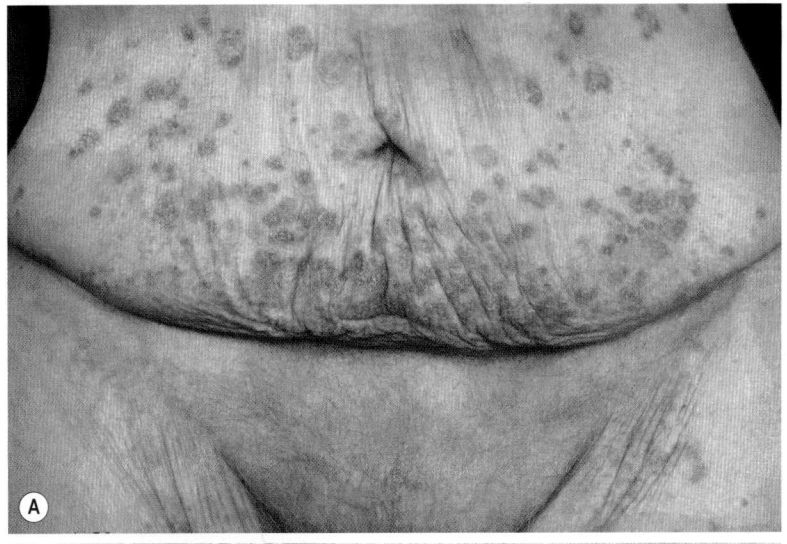

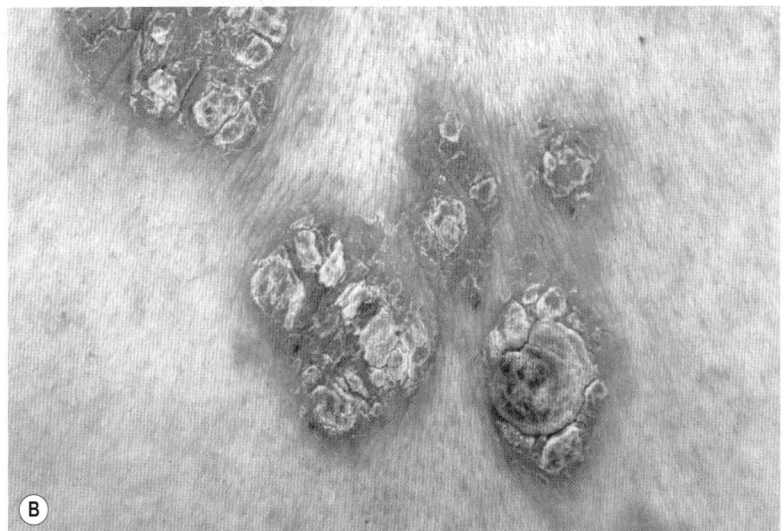

Fig. 5.22
Pemphigus foliaceus: (**A**) there are numerous crusted lesions on the lower abdomen and in the groin; (**B**) high-power view. From the slide collection of the late N.P. Smith, MD, the Institute of Dermatology, London, UK.

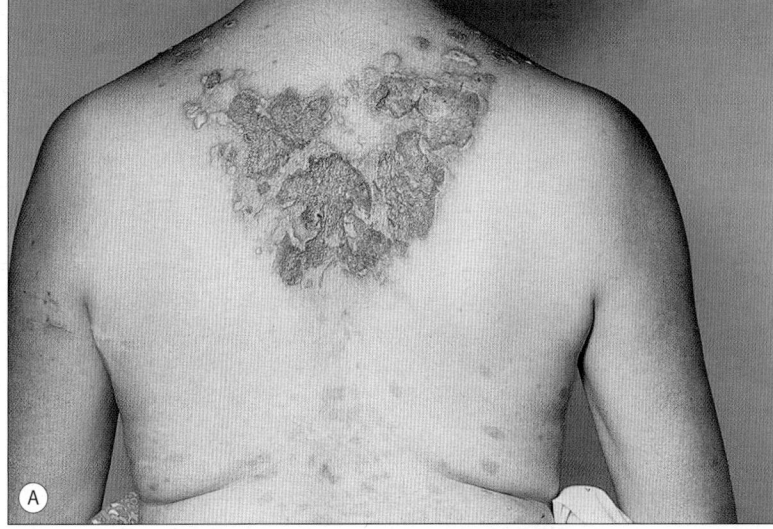

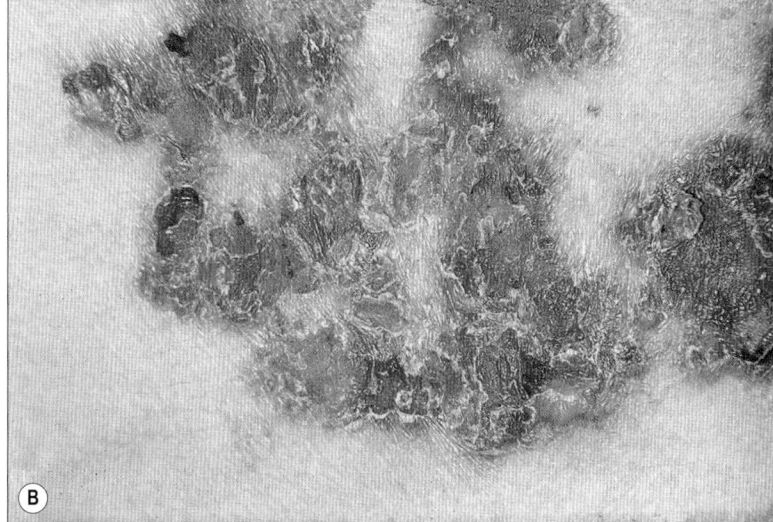

Fig. 5.24
Pemphigus foliaceus: (**A**) in this patient, the eruption was induced by penicillamine therapy; (**B**) close-up view of intact blisters, erosions, and crusting. By courtesy of R.A. Marsden, MD, St George's Hospital, London, UK.

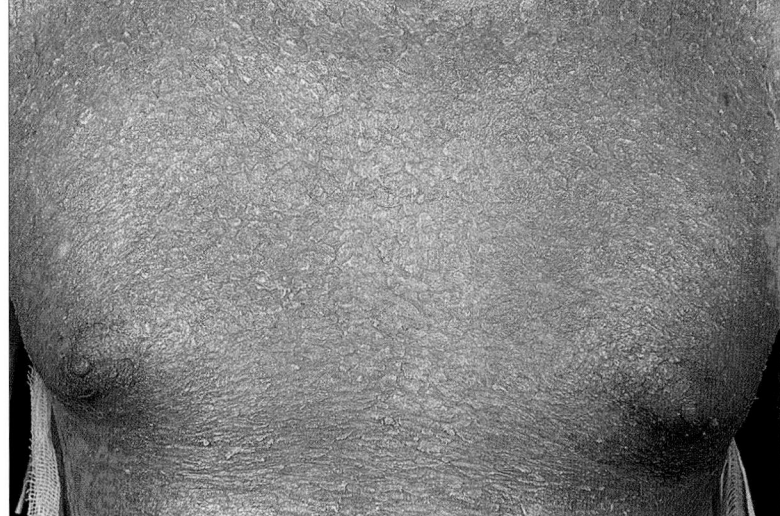

Fig. 5.23
Pemphigus foliaceus: in this patient, there is generalized erosion with scaling and erythroderma. By courtesy of R.A. Marsden, MD, St George's Hospital, London, UK.

a disseminated eruption caused by a viral infection (e.g., herpes simplex virus) superimposed on a pre-existing dermatosis.[20]

Very occasionally, patients may develop p. foliaceus during or after a previous episode of p. vulgaris and vice versa.[21-23] The development of bullous pemphigoid following an episode of p. foliaceus has also been described.[24,25] This is accompanied by an antigen shift, possibly as a result of intermolecular epitope spreading.[22,26-28] A case of a blistering disorder displaying features of bullous pemphigoid and p. foliaceus has been described in association with consumption of Spirulina algae.[29] The coexistence of both p. vulgaris and p. foliaceus in the same patient has also been reported.[30] A further case of paraneoplastic pemphigus with concomitant clinical features of p. foliaceus and the presence of antibodies against desmoglein 1 has been reported.[31]

In addition to idiopathic p. foliaceus, drug-induced variants, notably due to penicillamine, may also be encountered (*Fig. 5.24*). A localized form may also be associated with topical drugs such as imiquimod and has been reported following radiation therapy.[32-35] Recently, p. foliaceus related to an anti-TNF-α inhibitor has been reported.[36] P. foliaceus is rarely associated with an underlying malignancy including non-Hodgkin lymphoma and esophageal cancer.[37,38] An unusual case of p. foliaceus associated with myasthenia gravis and lupus erythematosus has been reported in a patient who underwent a thymectomy for a thymoma.[39]

Pathogenesis and histologic features

Similar to other variants of pemphigus, p. foliaceus is an immunologically mediated disease. Examination of perilesional skin by direct immunofluorescent techniques reveals in vivo-bound immunoglobulin (usually IgG) and often complement (C3) in the intercellular region of the epidermis.[1] Abundant antigen in the follicular outer root sheath and germinal matrix may account for the marked scalp involvement typical of pemphigus.[39]

Indirect immunofluorescent techniques show that the sera of patients with p. foliaceus contain an IgG antibody that reacts with the intercellular region of normal squamous epithelium.[40] IgG4 predominates followed by IgG1.[41,42] IgG3 is also sometimes present. This may be of importance since IgG3 is the most efficient activator of complement.[41] Some 60–70% of patients have positive indirect immunofluorescence.[43]

The p. foliaceus antibody binds to a 160-kD desmosomal cadherin, designated Dsg1.[44,45] The sera of p. foliaceus patients bind to the extracellular amino terminal domain of bovine Dsg1, whereas sera from both p. vulgaris and p. vegetans patients react with the intracellular domain of Dsg1.[46,47] Compared with p. vulgaris, immunofluorescence studies on the sera of p. foliaceus tend to show more staining in the superficial epidermis, correlating with the level of the split.[48,49] Conversely, the sera from patients with p. vulgaris show more affinity for the lower epidermis. Anti-Dsg1 antibody is pathogenic.[50] Injection of purified anti-Dsg1 antibodies from sera of patients with p. foliaceus into neonatal mice induces subcorneal acantholysis in a pattern typical of p. foliaceus.[51] Acantholysis is thought to be the result of an antibody-mediated cellular response rather than purely the result of steric hindrance.[52,53] Internalization of nonclustered Dsg1 has been put forward as a possible mechanism resulting in lack of newly formed desmosomes rather than a disruption of pre-existing structures.[48,54] Increasing evidence suggests that the blistering is the result of the activation of p38 mitogen-activated protein kinase-dependent signaling by the p. foliaceus IgG antibodies.[55] Rarely, patient sera contain additional IgG antibodies directed against Dsg3 and the presence of additional IgA antibodies against Dsg1 as well as Dsg3 has also been detected.[3,56,57] Antibodies to desmocollins may also play a role, and at least one case of childhood p. foliaceus secondary to autoantibodies exclusively directed against desmocollins has been described.[58] Patients with clinical and histologic features of p. foliaceus but direct immunofluorescence findings reminiscent of p. erythematosus have been reported. Antibodies recognizing bullous pemphigoid antigen 1 (BP230) as well as a 190-kD protein co-migrating with periplakin were detected in these patients in addition to anti-Dsg1 antibodies.[59] The use of D-penicillamine may be associated with the acquisition of a pemphigus-like antibody and the development of p. foliaceus.[60]

Since the blisters of p. foliaceus are superficial, they are therefore fragile, and it is often very difficult to obtain an intact lesion for diagnosis. Patients commonly have erosions without blisters, and frequently the clinician does not suspect a bullous disorder. Usually, the cleft or blister lies within the upper epidermis (Fig. 5.25) but may also occur in the granular layer or throughout the epidermis.[61] The roof of the fragile blister is often not present, having sloughed either before or after biopsy. Acantholysis is frequently difficult to detect, but usually a few acantholytic cells can be found attached to the roof or floor of the blister. In cases where the blister is missing, a careful inspection of the hair follicles may reveal focal acantholysis. In some cases, the acantholysis is subtle, and the biopsy may show features reminiscent of a spongiotic dermatitis (Fig. 5.26). Sometimes the blister contains numerous acute inflammatory cells (Fig. 5.27), particularly neutrophils, which can make distinction from subcorneal pustular disorders, including bullous impetigo, a dermatophyte infection, candidiasis, pustular psoriasis, and subcorneal pustular dermatosis especially difficult.[62,63] Eosinophilic spongiosis may also be seen.[64] A form with histologic and clinical overlap with psoriasis has also been described.[65]

Differential diagnosis

The histologic features in the superficial forms of pemphigus may be easily overlooked and, since bullae are often not appreciated by the clinician, the unwary pathologist may not consider a bullous disorder when evaluating the biopsy. A high index of suspicion is therefore critical. The differential diagnosis of superficial pemphigus includes bullous impetigo, staphylococcal scalded skin syndrome, IgA pemphigus, subcorneal pustular dermatosis, and psoriasis (Table 5.3). Distinction depends on a careful consideration of the clinical information, the results of bacterial culture, and immunofluorescent studies.

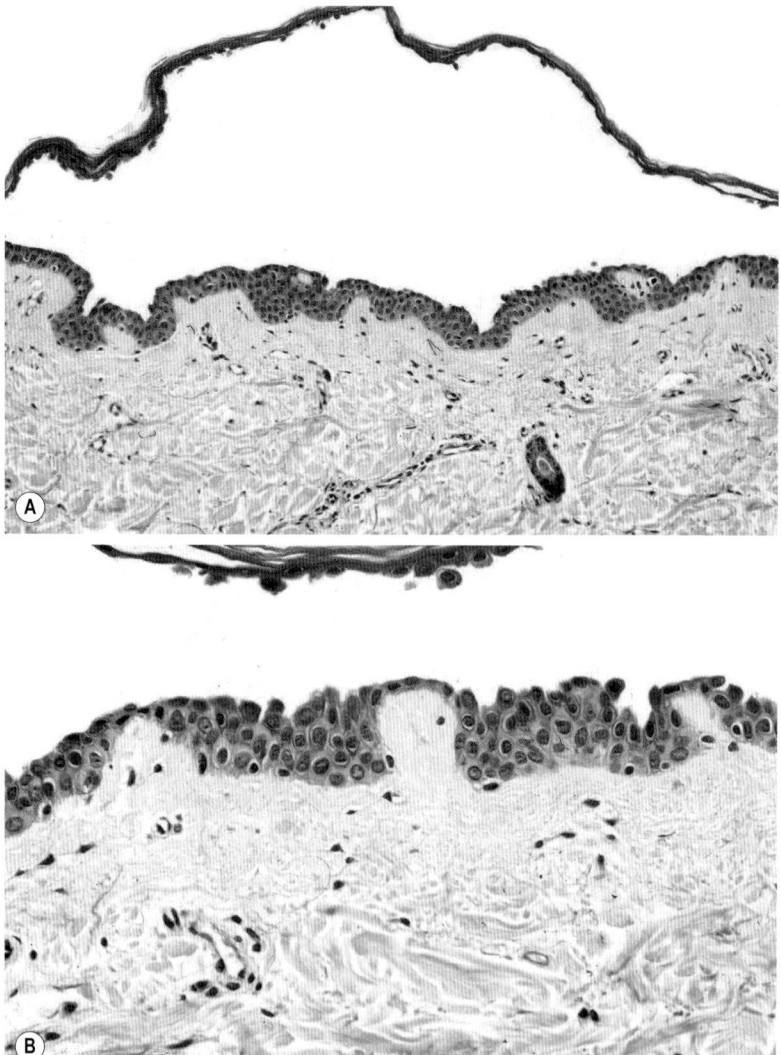

Fig. 5.25
Pemphigus foliaceus: (A) in this example, there is a cell-free, subcorneal blister; (B) occasional acantholytic cells are present adjacent to the roof.

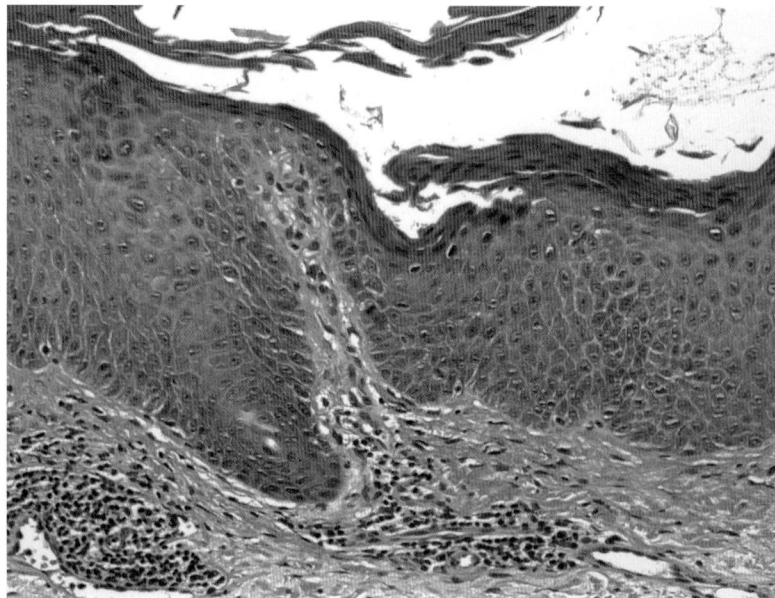

Fig. 5.26
Pemphigus foliaceus: in this example, there is spongiosis resembling a spongiotic dermatitis and only subtle, focal acantholysis.

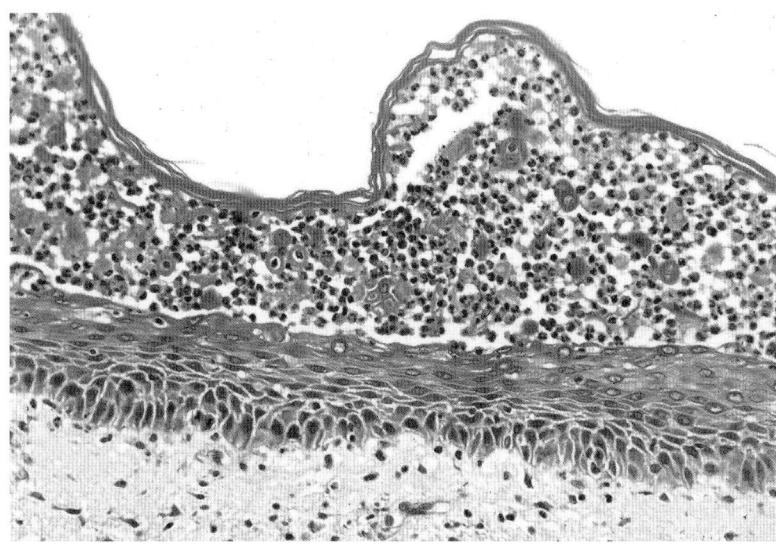

Fig. 5.27
Pemphigus foliaceus: in this example, the blister cavity contains numerous neutrophils. Acantholytic cells are conspicuous.

Table 5.3
Differential diagnosis of superficial pemphigus: conditions characterized by subcorneal pustules

Superficial pemphigus
IgA pemphigus
Subcorneal pustular dermatosis
Pustular psoriasis
Reactive arthritis
Pustular drug reaction
Bullous impetigo
Staphylococcal scalded skin syndrome
Pustular fungal infection

Endemic pemphigus foliaceus (fogo selvagem)

Clinical features

Fogo selvagem (Brazilian p. foliaceus, 'wild fire', endemic p. foliaceus) is endemic in regions of Brazil and has also been documented in other areas of Central and South America including Colombia, El Salvador, Paraguay, Venezuela, and Peru.[1–12] An endemic area has also been described in Tunisia.[13,14] The condition is associated with poverty and malnutrition and particularly affects children and young adults. Results from a more recent epidemiological study demonstrated disease manifestation also in patients of higher socioeconomic class and urban areas.[15] There is a striking familial incidence.[4] Most cases are found along major rivers, and people especially at risk include farmers and workers involved in land clearing and road construction.[2] It appears that the majority of patients live at an altitude of between 500 and 800 meters, and that their homes are generally within 10–15 kilometers of running fresh water and in the path of prevailing winds, thus suggesting an insect vector.[4,16] In support of this, a case-controlled epidemiological study has provided evidence that bites by the black fly (family Simuliidae) are a significant risk factor for development of the disease, and it has been proposed that a component of the saliva may trigger an antibody response in susceptible individuals.[17–20] *Simulium nigrimanum*, which is found in the same areas in which Brazilian fogo selvagem occurs, has been identified as being the likely species involved.[18]

The clinical presentation of fogo selvagem has been divided into a number of categories including localized and generalized forms[2,4]:

- Localized disease presents in a variety of ways including small blisters and erosions or violaceous papules and plaques distributed mainly in the seborrheic areas. Such lesions may be clinically misdiagnosed as discoid lupus erythematosus.

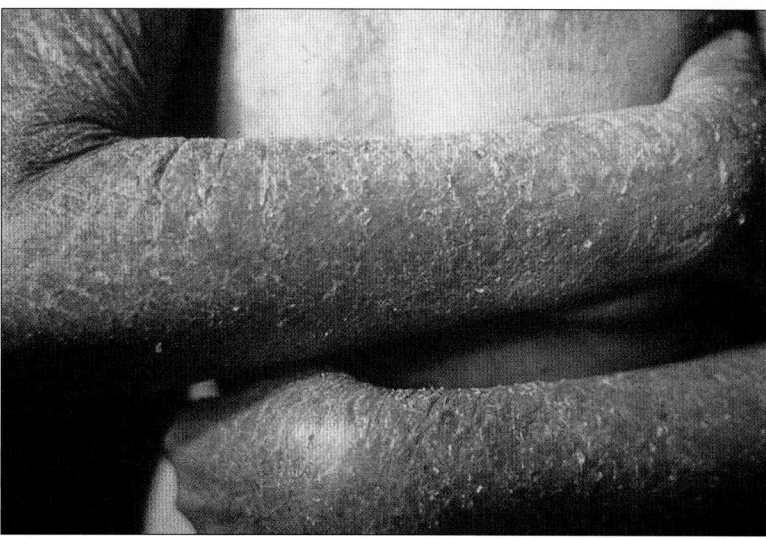

Fig. 5.28
Brazilian pemphigus foliaceus: this woman with chronic disease shows very severe scaling. Blisters are not apparent. By courtesy of S.A. Pecher, MD, Amazonas, Brazil.

- Generalized presentation includes bullous exfoliative, exfoliative erythrodermic, and disseminated plaque and nodular (resembling nodular prurigo) variants (*Fig. 5.28*).[4]

With resolution, patients may sometimes develop hyperpigmentation.[21] Rare cases of neonatal p. foliaceus have been reported, but in most patients the antibody does not cross the placental barrier.[22–24] Patients with fogo selvagem appear to rarely have other concomitant autoimmune disorders.[24–27]

In contrast to Brazilian fogo selvagem, endemic disease in the area of El Bagre, Colombia, shows several unusual and distinguishing features.[12,28] The disease affects an older population with a strong male predilection and clinical features reminiscent of p. erythematosus. In addition to the more classical presentation, patients develop hyperkeratotic plaques on the face, chest, and back reminiscent of discoid lupus erythematosus as well as an erythematous macular lesion in a butterfly-like distribution in the central face.[12,28] Active disease is also accompanied by conjunctivitis. The disease also shows characteristic immunological and histologic changes, which are discussed below.

Pathogenesis and histologic features

The immunological features of fogo selvagem are similar to p. foliaceus. Indirect immunofluorescent techniques show that the sera of patients with fogo selvagem contain an IgG4 antibody that reacts with Dsg1.[16,29] Passive transfer of this antibody to BALB/c neonatal mice results in acantholysis and subcorneal blistering clinically indistinguishable from that of human disease.[30–32] Low-titer IgG1 and IgG2 antibodies may also be present, and nonpathogenic IgG1 antibodies are present in unaffected individuals and in the preclinical stages of patients from endemic areas.[16,30] IgG antibodies may be accompanied by IgM antibodies, a finding seen more frequently in individuals from rural rather than urban areas. IgM and IgE antibodies are detected more frequently associated with fogo selvagem than p. foliaceus.[33,34] Fogo selvagem is otherwise histologically and by immunofluorescence indistinguishable from nonendemic foliaceus and, like the latter, the antibody recognizes epitopes in the ectodomain of Dsg1.[35,36] Epitope recognition is conformation specific and calcium dependent, and recently intramolecular epitope spreading has been implicated in the pathogenesis of the disease. Epitope spreading appears to be related to onset of disease as well as disease modulation with remission and relapse.[37] Specifically, it has been shown that sera from patients in the preclinical stage or in remission recognize epitopes in the COOH-terminal region of the ectodomain of Dsg1, whereas antibodies against epitopes in the NH2-terminal region of the ectodomain are detected at disease onset.[16,37] Interestingly, a study has suggested that the presence of serum IgG4 antidesmoglein-1 in asymptomatic individuals may suggest preclinical disease.[38,39] A subset of patients may

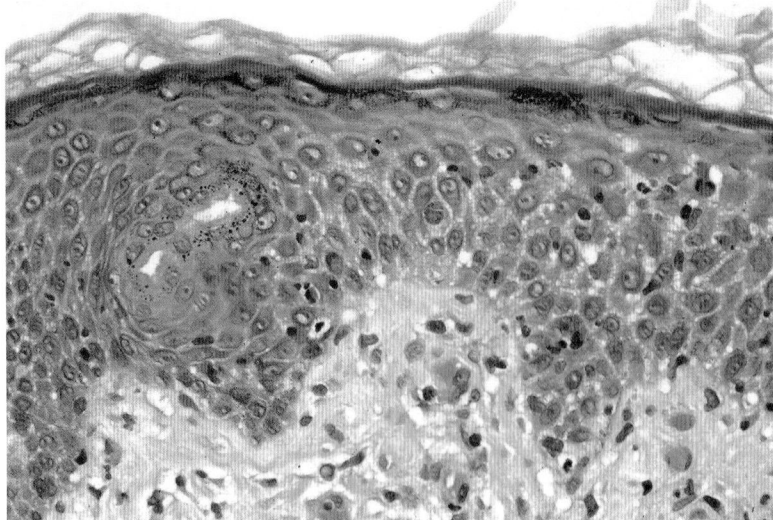

Fig. 5.29
Brazilian pemphigus foliaceus: in this example of an early lesion, the features of eosinophilic spongiosis are evident.

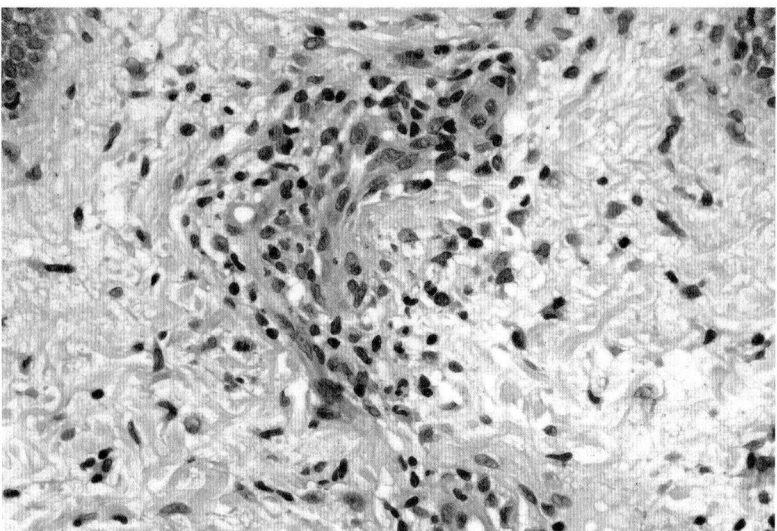

Fig. 5.30
Brazilian pemphigus foliaceus: there is superficial dermal edema and a perivascular inflammatory cell infiltrate with conspicuous eosinophils.

also have antibodies to Dsg3, ranging from <10% to 36%.[40–42] Antibodies to Dsg3 are especially common in the Terena reservation of Liao Verde, Brazil, where additional anti-Dsg3 antibodies were detected.[42] Patients have circulating CD4+ memory T cells with a Th2 cytokine profile that proliferate in response to the extracellular domain of Dsg1 and are thought to be of importance in the initiation and progression of the disease by stimulating B cell production of autoantibodies.[43–45] The systemic kinin system appears to be activated in patients with fogo selvagem, but the significance of this finding and its mechanism of action in blister formation are unclear.[46] The discussion of pathogenesis of the nonendemic form discussed above also apply to the endemic form.

Patients often share the HLA phenotype DRB1*0102 and lack DQB1*0201, which is thought to represent a dominant protective gene found in unaffected persons living in endemic regions.[38,39] HLA-DRB1*0404, *1402,*1406, or *0102 may also confer susceptibility.[4,40,47,48]

The histologic changes of fogo selvagem are identical to the other forms of superficial pemphigus (p. foliaceus and p. erythematosus).[49] Since the blisters are superficial, often only nonbullous erosions are present for histologic examination. It is very difficult to obtain an intact lesion for diagnosis. Typically, the cleft or blister lies within the upper epidermis, granular layer, or beneath the stratum corneum. Acantholysis is frequently subtle, but usually a few acantholytic cells can be found attached to the floor of the blister. The blister roof is often missing. Blisters may contain numerous inflammatory cells, particularly neutrophils. This feature may cause confusion with infection or other subcorneal pustular disorders. Eosinophilic spongiosis in association with perivascular eosinophils is also sometimes present, particularly if biopsies of early lesions are examined (Figs 5.29 and 5.30).

The verrucous plaques and nodules seen occasionally in localized or chronic fogo selvagem show acanthosis, hyperkeratosis, parakeratosis, and papillomatosis.[50] Acantholysis is invariably present.

The hyperpigmentation characteristic of remission is a direct result of pigmentary incontinence.

The histologic findings in the endemic form described in the El Bagre area in Colombia are identical to those of fogo selvagem in active disease. In addition, liquefactive degeneration of the epidermal basal cell layer is observed in a quarter of biopsies.[28] Patients may also have sclerodermoid changes, psoriasiform features, large subcorneal pustules, and hyperkeratosis of palms.[12] By direct immunofluorescence, a positive lupus band test is detected in 40% of patients in addition to IgG deposition on the surface of keratinocytes. Reactive antibodies are of the IgG4 subtype with Dsg1 being the major antigen. Sera from patients also contained additional antibodies against antibasement membrane zone as well as further IgG1 anticell-surface antibodies, which may represent desmoplakin I, envoplakin,

and periplakin.[12,51] Antibodies to pilosebaceous units and surrounding neurovascular structures have also been identified in these patients.[52]

Recently, criteria have been proposed to establish a diagnosis of fogo selvagem as distinct from nonendemic p. foliaceus[4]:

- clinical evaluation,
- presence of subcorneal acantholysis,
- positive direct and indirect immunofluorescence and/or immunoprecipitation or ELISA assays,
- confirmatory epidemiological data.

Differential diagnosis

As with p. foliaceus, the histologic features in fogo selvagem may be easily overlooked, and a high index of suspicion is critical to making the diagnosis. The differential diagnosis includes p. foliaceus, p. erythematosus, bullous impetigo, staphylococcal scalded skin syndrome, subcorneal pustular dermatosis, and, in some cases, psoriasis. Careful clinical correlation, immunofluorescence studies, and sometimes bacterial culture are necessary to establish a definitive diagnosis.

Pemphigus herpetiformis

Clinical features

Pemphigus herpetiformis (p. herpetiformis, herpetiform pemphigus, acantholytic dermatitis herpetiformis) is a variant of pemphigus which shows clinical features resembling dermatitis herpetiformis with the histology and immunofluorescent findings of pemphigus.[1–7] It is rare, accounting for only up to 7.3% of cases of pemphigus.[2,7] The sexes are affected equally, and there is a wide age range varying from newborns to 92 years, although neonatal and pediatric cases are extraordinarily rare.[3,7–9]

Patients typically present with intensely pruritic, grouped, erythematous papules and plaques, vesicles, and blisters, sometimes associated with mucous membrane involvement.[2,7] Urticaria may also be a presenting feature.[10] The Nikolksy sign is variably present. Although lesions are often generalized, there is a tendency for the extensor surfaces of the extremities to be particularly involved. Exceptionally, herpetiform pemphigus may be associated with psoriasis, systemic lupus erythematosus, or with an underlying malignancy including lymphoma, lung, prostate, and esophageal cancer, and angiosarcoma (see paraneoplastic pemphigus).[7,8,11–16] Although in some patients the clinical manifestations remain herpetiform throughout, in others, the features evolve into more typical p. foliaceus, fogo selvagem, and, less commonly, p. vulgaris.[2,4–7] Contrariwise, patients with typical p. foliaceus and p. vulgaris may go on to develop a herpetiform eruption.[17]

IgA pemphigus may also present with herpetiform lesions.[18,19]. In general, p. herpetiformis has a benign course, with most patients responding well to sulfones or steroids.[2,3,7,20]

Pathogenesis and histologic features

Immunofluorescence testing shows IgG in an intercellular pattern characteristic of the pemphigus group of disorders on both direct and indirect techniques.[1,2,4,7,20] In most patients, Dsg1 (p. foliaceus antigen) is the target autoantigen.[4,6,7,21,22] However, in some patients, antibodies against Dsg3 (p. vulgaris antigen) have also been documented.[7,22,23] A patient has been reported with both IgG as well as IgA antibodies against Dsg1 in addition to anti-Dsc (desmocollin) 3 IgG.[19] Why antibodies to Dsg1 in patients with p. herpetiformis often fail to induce appreciable acantholysis compared with p. foliaceus is uncertain. It is postulated that the p. herpetiformis antibody targets a different epitope although this has yet to be confirmed. Recently, two patients with neutrophil-rich histology were shown to co-localize pemphigus antibody and the neutrophil chemoattractant IL-8. In addition, circulating IgG antibody upregulated cultured keratinocyte IL-8 expression, thereby offering an explanation for the neutrophil recruitment.[24,25]

The biopsy findings are variable and often non-specific. Although eosinophilic spongiosis is most typical, spongiosis associated with either a mixed eosinophilic and neutrophilic, or a neutrophil-predominant infiltrate may also be encountered.[4,26] Intraepidermal vesicles and pustules, also of variable composition, are often present, and dermal papillary neutrophil microabscesses have been described.[2,6,20] Acantholytic cells are usually (but not invariably) identified. A requirement for multiple biopsies before a diagnosis can be established is a common theme in the literature.

Differential diagnosis

There is both clinical and histologic overlap with IgA pemphigus and dermatitis herpetiformis. Immunofluorescence allows for distinction between these entities. It should also be noted that, exceptionally, dermatitis herpetiformis may histologically show occasional acantholytic cells in the absence of any evidence of pemphigus herpetiformis.

In cases where eosinophilic spongiosis is the predominant histologic feature, the differential diagnosis also includes hypersensitivity reactions and infection (bacterial and fungal). Immunofluorescence studies and special stains for microorganisms will eliminate these possibilities.

Pemphigus erythematosus

Clinical features

P. erythematosus (Senear-Usher syndrome) is a mild localized form of superficial pemphigus with the histologic and immunofluorescent findings of p. foliaceus combined with features of lupus erythematosus.[1-6] In general, the latter is subclinical, being suggested only by laboratory findings, but there are also rare reports of full-blown systemic disease being present.[4] The condition shows a worldwide distribution and a slight female predominance.[5] Exceptionally, it has been described in children although immunological confirmation of the diagnosis is available in only one case.[7-10]

Clinically, it is commonly confined to the head, neck, and upper trunk, and typically resembles p. foliaceus. Lesions are erythematous, scaly, and crusted, with or without superficial vesicles, blisters, or erosions. Facial involvement often shows a butterfly distribution reminiscent of lupus erythematosus or seborrheic dermatitis (*Fig. 5.31*).[1] Mucous membrane involvement is exceedingly rare.[2]

There are reports of p. erythematosus developing after treatment with a number of drugs, notably D-penicillamine, and there are also instances attributed to therapy with propranolol, captopril, pyritinol, thiopronine, ceftazidime, cefuroxime, and atorvastatin.[11-16] P. erythematosus has also been described as a complication of heroin abuse.[17] In p. foliaceus patients misdiagnosed as having psoriasis, phototherapy can induce p. erythematosus with a positive lupus band test.[18]

P. erythematosus may rarely be associated with thymoma.[3,19-21] Typically, the thymoma precedes the onset of cutaneous lesions, which often present following thymectomy.[20,21] Most tumors have been benign, but one

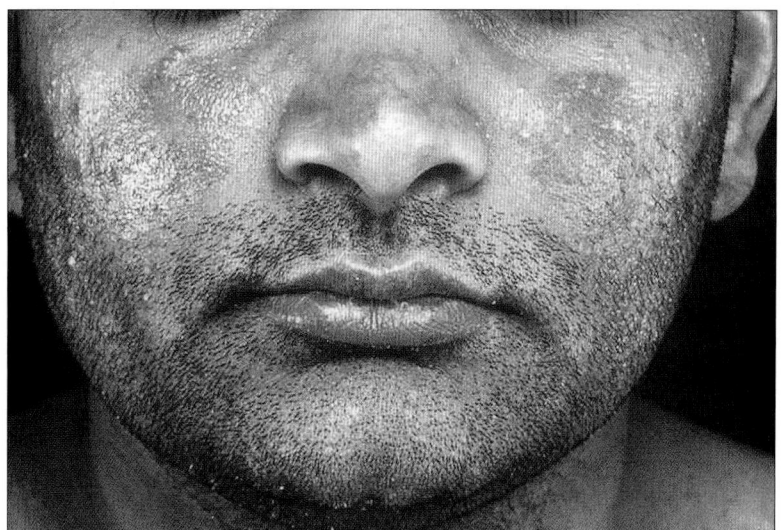

Fig. 5.31
Pemphigus erythematosus: there is scaliness and erythema affecting both cheeks. By courtesy of the Institute of Dermatology, London, UK.

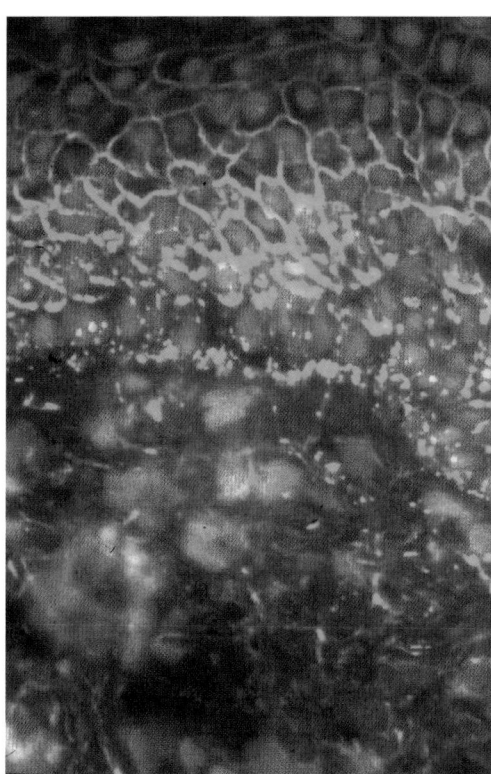

Fig. 5.32
Pemphigus erythematosus: typical intercellular immunofluorescence with granular staining (IgG) at the basement membrane region. By courtesy of B. Bhogal, FIMLS, Institute of Dermatology, London, UK.

malignant variant has been documented.[22] P. erythematosus may also be a manifestation of paraneoplastic pemphigus.[3]

Pathogenesis and histologic features

P. erythematosus, in addition to intercellular staining, also shows granular deposition of IgG and complement along the basement membrane region (positive lupus band test) (*Figs 5.32* and *5.33*).[2,23,24] Typically the latter deposits are found within sun-exposed skin, but in some patients normal, non-sun-exposed skin may also be positive.[2] Pemphigus antibody is generally present on indirect immunofluorescence, and antinuclear factor may also be identified.[23,24] Anti-DNA antibodies and antibodies to extractable nuclear antigens are negative except in those patients with features of systemic lupus erythematosus.[4] In common with p. foliaceus, the antibody

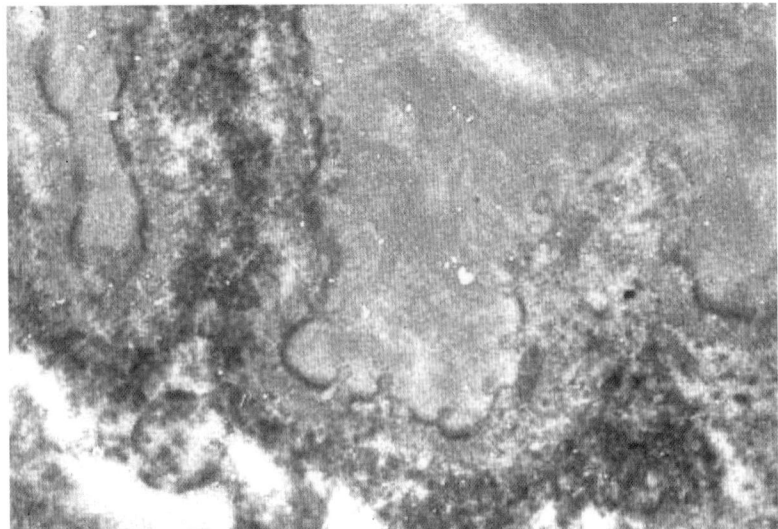

Fig. 5.33
Pemphigus erythematosus: immunoelectron micrograph showing immunoreactant beneath the lamina densa in addition to occupying the intercellular space. By courtesy of B. Bhogal, FIMLS, Institute of Dermatology, London, UK.

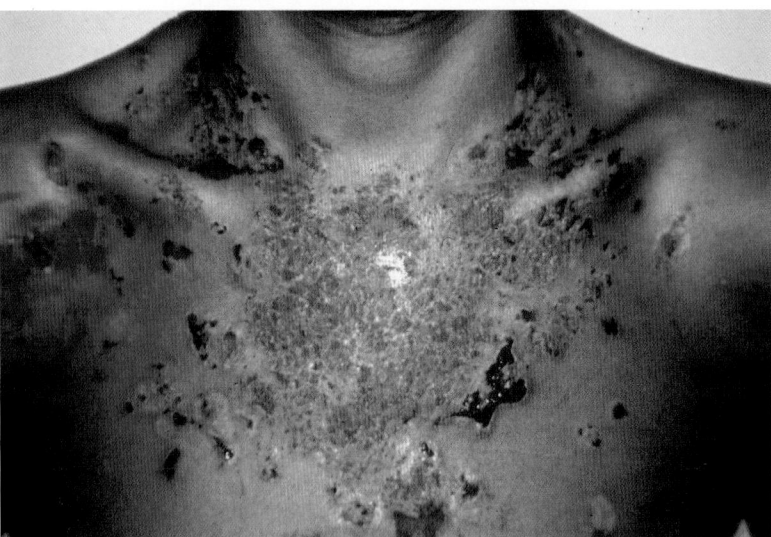

Fig. 5.34
Paraneoplastic pemphigus: there are numerous erosions and crusted lesions. Courtesy of the Institute of Dermatology, London, UK.

reacts with Dsg1.[25] In p. foliaceus patients, circulating anti-Dsg1 precipitate a cleaved off ectodomain of Dsg1 along the basement membrane.[18] This may account for the positive lupus band test in p. erythematosus.

P. erythematosus has histologic changes that are identical to those seen in p. foliaceus and fogo selvagem. As the blisters are superficial, it is often very difficult to obtain an intact lesion for diagnosis. Usually, the cleft or blister lies within the granular layer or beneath the stratum corneum. As with the other forms of superficial pemphigus, acantholysis is frequently difficult to detect, but usually a few acantholytic cells can be found attached to the roof or floor of the blister. The blister may contain numerous acute inflammatory cells, particularly neutrophils, which can make distinction from subcorneal pustular disorders especially difficult.

Differential diagnosis

The differential diagnosis includes the other forms of superficial pemphigus (p. foliaceus and fogo selvagem), bullous impetigo, and staphylococcal scalded skin syndrome, in addition to subcorneal pustular dermatosis. Distinction depends on a careful consideration of the clinical information, the results of bacterial culture, and immunofluorescence studies.

Paraneoplastic pemphigus

Clinical features

Paraneoplastic pemphigus is a variant of pemphigus, quite distinct from p. vulgaris and p. foliaceus.[1] Paraneoplastic pemphigus may be associated with a variety of tumors, such as B-cell lymphoproliferative disorders and hematopoietic malignancies, Castleman disease, Waldenström macroglobulinemia, thymoma (occasionally with myasthenia gravis), Hodgkin lymphoma, carcinomas (e.g., carcinoma of bronchus, pancreas, liver, uterus, breast, thyroid, and liver), and sarcomas (including dendritic follicular cell sarcoma, round cell liposarcoma, leiomyosarcoma, and inflammatory myofibroblastic tumor).[2–48] We have seen an exceptional association with systemic mastocytosis. Lymphoma is most often the coexistent neoplasm.[1] In a case of a patient with non-Hodgkin lymphoma, the disease developed only after six cycles of fludarabine, raising the possibility of an association with the medication.[49] Rarely, patients presented with a disease fulfilling the diagnosis of paraneoplastic pemphigus by histology, immunoblotting, and immunoprecipitation but with no underlying neoplasms have been reported.[50–54]

Paraneoplastic pemphigus has been defined by Sapadin and Anhalt as follows[55]:

- painful mucosal erosions and a polymorphous skin eruption in the context of an occult or confirmed neoplasm (*Fig. 5.34*),

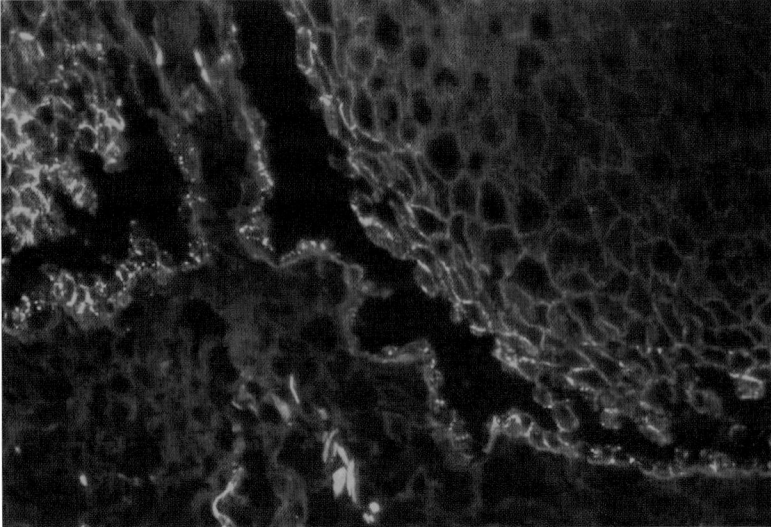

Fig. 5.35
Paraneoplastic pemphigus: IgG is evident in an intercellular distribution.

- histopathological changes of keratinocyte necrosis, intraepidermal acantholysis, and vacuolar-interface dermatitis,
- direct immunofluorescence showing intercellular IgG and complement accompanied by linear or granular complement at the dermal–epidermal junction (*Fig. 5.35*),
- indirect immunofluorescence showing circulating antibodies to simple, columnar, and transitional epithelia in addition to a more typical pemphigus pattern of binding to skin and mucosa,
- circulating autoantibodies that immunoprecipitate a high molecular weight complex of polypeptides from keratinocyte extracts weighing 250, 230, 210, 190, and 170 kD.

Although the disease may develop in a wide age range (7–83 years), the majority of patients have been in the fifth to eighth decades, and there is a male predominance.[5] Exceptionally, children may be affected.[4,56–60] Lesions are seen in both the mucosa and the skin. Patients present with refractory, painful, persistent erosions of the oral mucosa and vermilion border of the lips. In addition, the tongue, gingiva, floor of mouth, palate, oropharynx, and nasopharynx can be affected.[5] Manifestation confined to the skin or oral mucosa is exceptional.[22,61,62] Esophageal disease has been described, and the trachea and bronchi may be affected.[63–65] The latter may be accompanied by an invariably fatal bronchiolitis obliterans-like disorder in 6–29% of patients.[46,64–69] Colonic involvement is unusual.[70] Frequently, patients also have severe pseudomembranous conjunctivitis with symblephara, and eventual blindness may occur.[5,71] The vulva, vagina, and penis are sometimes affected.[4] Myasthenia gravis may be seen in up to 35% of patients with paraneoplastic pemphigus.[72] Rarely, the disease is accompanied by alopecia areata.[62]

Cutaneous lesions are typically polymorphic and often present as a pruritic papulosquamous dermatosis with subsequent blistering. The trunk, proximal extremities, palms, and soles are characteristically affected.[73] Nail involvement may occur. Although the eruption typically resembles p. vulgaris, it may also mimic p. foliaceus, IgA pemphigus, bullous pemphigoid, linear IgA disease, lichen planus pemphigoides, erythema multiforme, and toxic epidermal necrolysis.[39,74–80] P. vegetans-like lesions have been described.[50] Paraneoplastic pemphigus is associated with a very high mortality.[5,80]

Pathogenesis and histologic features

In paraneoplastic pemphigus, circulating antibodies bind to desmosomal and hemidesmosomal plakin family members including 250-kD (desmoplakin I), 230-kD (bullous pemphigoid antigen), 210-kD (desmoplakin II), 210-kD (envoplakin), 190-kD (periplakin), and 170-kD (alpha-2-macroglobulin-like-1, a protease inhibitor) antigens.[78,80–84] The presence of antibodies to envoplakin and periplakin (both cornified envelope constituents) is believed to be highly specific for paraneoplastic pemphigus, and the linker domain of plakins may be of particular significance.[85,86] Antibodies to Dsg1 and 3 are also usually present and plectin (another plakin family member) antibodies may be found.[87,88] Anti-Dsg antibodies are thought to be of particular importance in the initiation of lesions, disrupting the cell membrane and thereby exposing desmosomal and hemidesmosomal plakin proteins with resultant autoantibody formation.[81,89]

Direct immunofluorescence shows IgG deposition affecting the whole thickness of the epidermis, whereas C3 is found only on the lower layers.[80,81,90–92] Characteristically, the intercellular staining is often focal and faint.[90,91] In addition, complement C3 is present along the basement membrane region. Immunoglobulin deposition, specifically anti-epiplakin, in the respiratory epithelium has also been documented.[63–65,67] Indirect studies confirm the presence of a circulating antibody although the membrane deposition is often masked by strong cytoplasmic labeling.[81] This latter can be reduced or abolished by serum dilution.[81]

In paraneoplastic pemphigus, in addition to binding to stratified squamous epithelium, the antibody labels transitional epithelium, pseudostratified respiratory epithelium, small and large intestinal mucosa, and thyroid epithelium.[91] It also reacts with myocardium and skeletal muscle. Rat bladder epithelium is said to be highly specific for paraneoplastic pemphigus.[92] Up to 25% of cases, however, are negative.[93]

Recently, there has been accumulating evidence demonstrating considerable heterogeneity within disorders designated as paraneoplastic pemphigus in addition to overlap with other immunobullous diseases. Patients with additional IgA antibodies against Dsg1, Dsg3, desmocollins, envoplakin, periplakin, bullous pemphigoid antigens, type VII collagen, and laminin 332 have been reported.[78,93–97] Immunophenotypic variability among paraneoplastic pemphigus patients has thus been established. The documentation of patients displaying p. vulgaris-like or p. foliaceus-like features has led some authors to suggest that immunobullous disorders arising in association with malignancy would be best viewed as representing a spectrum rather than a distinct entity.[74] Included within this spectrum are other nonpemphigus immunobullous disorders resembling erythema multiforme, graft-versushost disease, and lichen planus. The description of antibodies reactive with desmoplakins I and II in some patients with erythema multiforme raises the possibility that these autoantibodies play a pathogenic role in a subset of patients.[98] However, further study will be necessary to determine the significance of this finding.

Analogous to other forms of pemphigus, recent studies have suggested a genetic predisposition. HLA typing has identified HLA-Cw*14 as the predisposing allele in a Chinese population while DRB1*03 was identified in a French study.[99,100]

The histologic findings in paraneoplastic pemphigus are highly variable but are characterized by an admixture of suprabasal acantholysis, often resembling p. vulgaris, with cleft or vesicle formation (sometimes

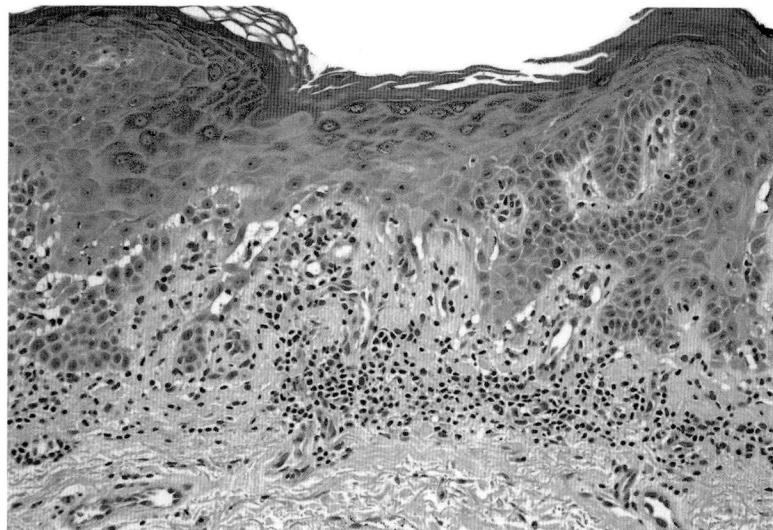

Fig. 5.36
Paraneoplastic pemphigus: this medium-power view shows suprabasal acantholysis and interface change. Note the hyperkeratosis and hypergranulosis. Courtesy of N. Brinster, MD, Virginia Commonwealth University Medical Center, Richmond, Virginia, USA.

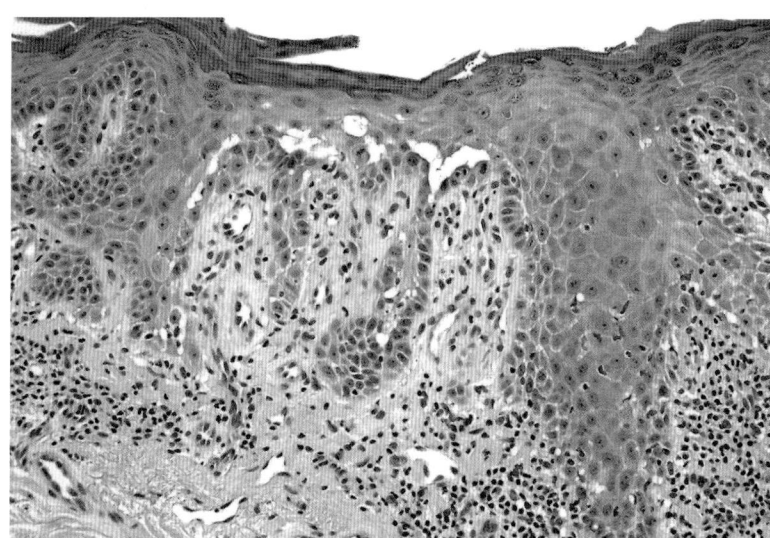

Fig. 5.37
Paraneoplastic pemphigus: higher-power view of acantholysis with suprabasal cleft formation. Courtesy of N. Brinster, MD, Virginia Commonwealth University Medical Center, Richmond, Virginia, USA.

involving adnexal epithelium), and interface changes with basal cell liquefactive degeneration, dyskeratotic keratinocytes, and lymphocytic exocytosis (Figs 5.36–5.38).[80,82,101] Spongiosis is often present.[3] A perivascular and lichenoid chronic inflammatory cell infiltrate is typically seen in the superficial dermis.[85] In some cases, the histologic features may closely simulate lichen planus. A mixture of histological patterns in different biopsies from the same patient is often seen. Eosinophils, however, are rare. Pigmentary incontinence is frequently evident.[101]

Acantholysis-like change has also been described affecting the bronchial lining epithelium and brochiolitis obliterans-like features may be seen.[63,65]

Differential diagnosis

The biopsy findings of admixed acantholysis and interface change appear to be relatively non-specific. This contention is demonstrated by skin lesions in patients with typical autoimmune pemphigus without evidence of neoplasia that have histologic features considered typical of paraneoplastic pemphigus.[92]

The differential diagnosis includes mainly interface dermatitides (e.g., drug eruption, lichen planus, erythema multiforme, graft-versus-host disease)

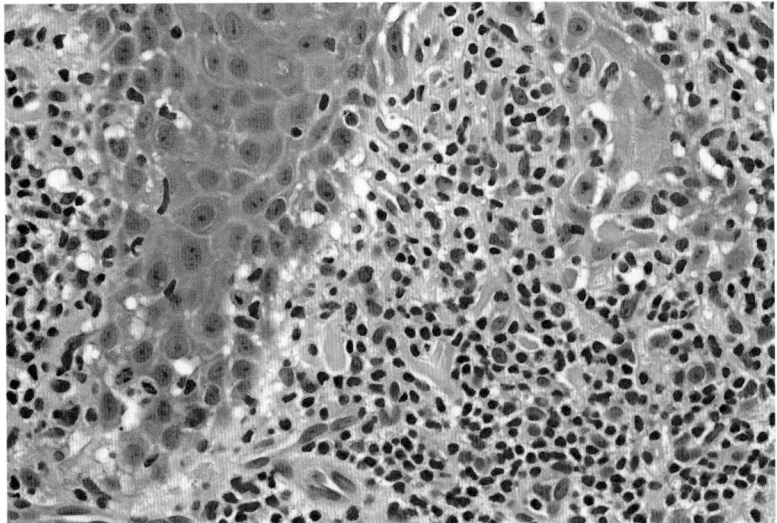

Fig. 5.38
Paraneoplastic pemphigus: note the basal cell hydropic degeneration and cytoid bodies. There is an intense lymphohistiocytic infiltrate. A single eosinophil is evident. Courtesy of N. Brinster, MD, Virginia Commonwealth University Medical Center, Richmond, Virginia, USA.

rather than other variants of pemphigus. A very high index of suspicion on the part of the pathologist and clinician alike and confirmatory immunofluorescence studies are prerequisites to achieving a correct diagnosis.

IgA pemphigus

Clinical features

IgA pemphigus is a rare dapsone-responsive variant of pemphigus that, as its name suggests, is characterized by intercellular IgA deposition and presents clinically with pustular rather than bullous or vesicular lesions.[1–6] This disease has been described under a number of different names, such as intraepidermal neutrophilic IgA dermatosis, IgA p. foliaceus, IgA herpetiform pemphigus, intraepidermal IgA pustulosis, intercellular IgA dermatosis, and intercellular IgA vesiculopustular dermatosis.[7–16] Most patients are middle-aged or elderly, but children may also be affected.[8,17–21] The sex incidence is equal. There is no racial or geographic predilection.[8,11] Drug-induced variants have occasionally been documented.[22]

IgA pemphigus is divided into two major subtypes: subcorneal pustular dermatosis (SPD) variant (IgA p. foliaceus) and intraepidermal neutrophilic IgA dermatosis (IEN) variant (IgA p. vulgaris).[7] Other less readily classifiable variants, termed atypical IgA pemphigus, may also be encountered.[23]

- Patients with SPD-like IgA pemphigus present with superficial flaccid pustular lesions, often arising on an erythematous base and typically affecting the trunk and proximal limbs, although the intertriginous sites are predilected.[11] Very uncommonly, there is exclusive involvement of the oral mucosa and perianal skin.[24] Occasionally, there is generalized skin involvement. Lesions are crusted and progress with peripheral extension to form ringlike and rosette patterns.[15] The features may be indistinguishable from classical non-IgA-associated SPD.
- Patients with the IEN IgA dermatosis variant present with generalized pustules and crusts and erythematous macules with peripheral vesicles forming the so-called sunflower-like configuration (*Figs 5.39* and *5.40*).[7] A dermatitis herpetiformis-like presentation with grouped edematous papules may also be encountered.[11,12,15]

Pruritus is common and is sometimes severe.[8]

The lesions in occasional patients resemble classic p. vulgaris or p. foliaceus. In one childhood case, a p. vegetans-like presentation associated with α1-antitrypsin deficiency was documented.[18] Mucous membrane involvement in either variant is exceptional.[17] Nikolsky sign has been reportedly negative at least in a subset of patients.[2,12,13] IgA pemphigus tends to be a chronic relapsing but relatively benign disorder.[11,12,15]

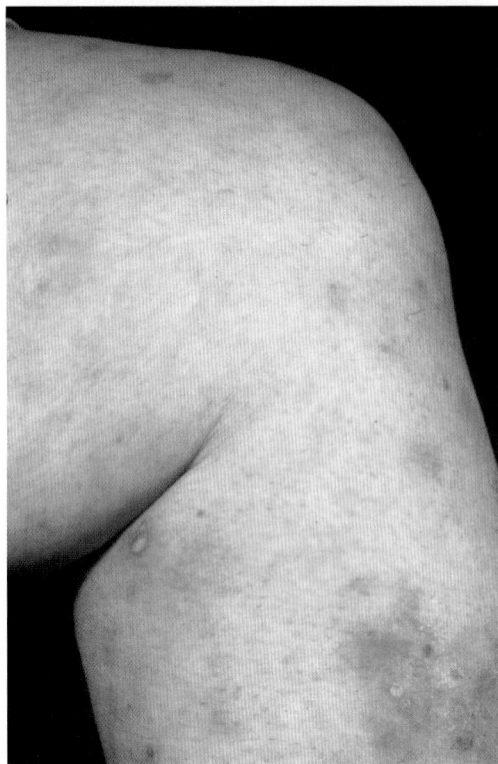

Fig. 5.39
IgA pemphigus: erythematous lesions and an intact vesicle are present. From the slide collection of the late N.P. Smith, MD, the Institute of Dermatology, London, UK.

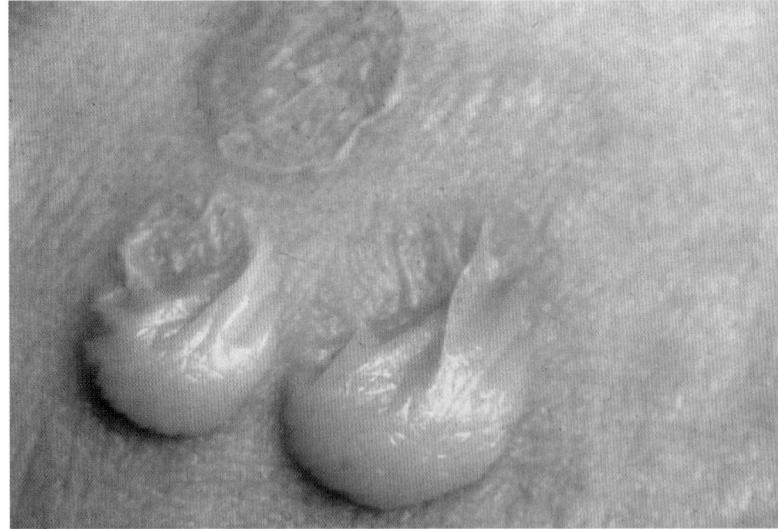

Fig. 5.40
IgA pemphigus: high-power view showing pus-filled intact blisters and an erosion. From the slide collection of the late N.P. Smith, MD, the Institute of Dermatology, London, UK.

A significant number of patients (approximately 20%) may have an associated monoclonal gammopathy, usually of the IgA class.[11,25–27] Two documented cases have been benign, and the others have represented B cell lymphoma or multiple myeloma.[11]

Pathogenesis and histologic features

SPD IgA pemphigus is characterized by intercellular IgA deposition in the upper epidermis, and circulating IgA antibodies that preferentially bind to the upper epidermis are typically present.[4] In contrast, in the IEN variant, IgA is deposited preferentially in the lower epidermis, and circulating antibodies also generally bind to the lower epidermis. In some patients, however, the IgA antibody binds to the entire thickness of the epithelium.

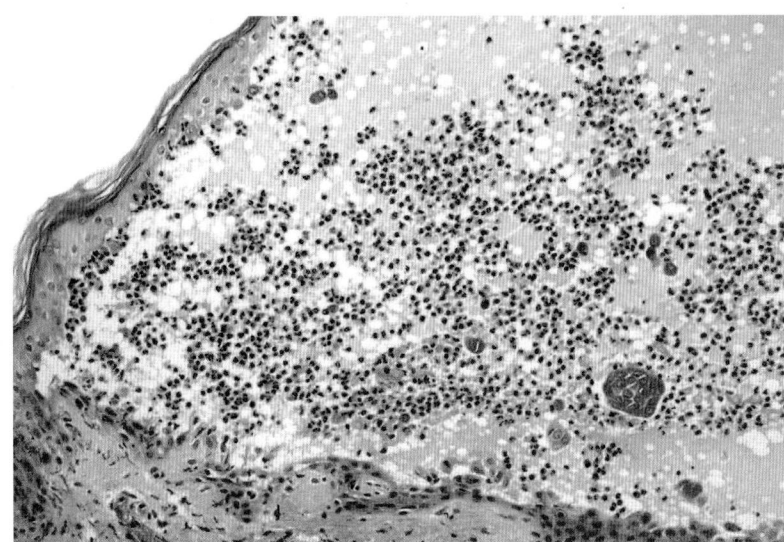

Fig. 5.41
IgA pemphigus: this biopsy is from the edge of an established blister. Note the heavy inflammatory cell infiltrate and focal acantholysis.

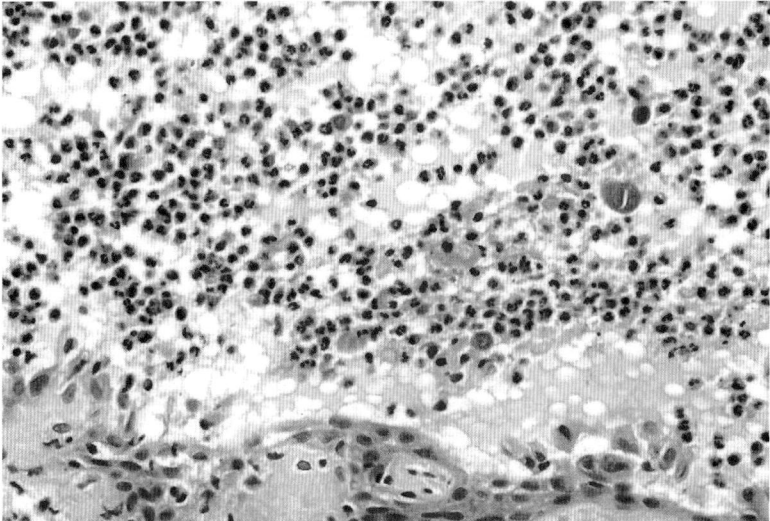

Fig. 5.42
IgA pemphigus: the blister cavity contains neutrophils and eosinophils.

A linear subcorneal distribution has also been documented.[9] Complement is not usually present and IgM is absent.[7] IgG is typically absent, but there are rare cases of atypical pemphigus with both IgG and IgA that likely represent an unusual form of IgA pemphigus.[28,29] The antibodies are of the IgA1 subclass and are usually of low titer.[4,17] They have been identified in approximately 50% of patients.[12]

By immunoelectron microscopy performed on a limited number of cases, the immunoglobulin has been identified within the intercellular space, on the keratinocyte cell membrane, in some cases showing desmosomal accentuation.[30-32] In the SPD type, labeling has been predominantly detected in extracellular spaces between keratinocytes at desmosomes, whereas labeling is mainly in intercellular spaces in nondesmosomal areas in the IEN variant.[33]

The two subtypes result from autoantibody production to different desmosomal proteins.[34] Patients with the SPD variant show reactivity with desmocollin 1.[35-38] In contrast, anti-Dsg1 or anti-Dsg3 IgA antibodies are present in the IEN variant.[19,39-41] One patient with the SPD variant showed both anti-Dsc1 as well as anti-Dsg1 IgA.[42] In some patients, however, neither desmocollins nor desmogleins appear to be involved, suggesting that IgA pemphigus is a heterogeneous group of conditions.[13,18,38,41]

Histologically, in the SPD variant, vesicles are typically found in a subcorneal location associated with a neutrophil infiltrate. It is thought that the presence of IgA is responsible for the striking neutrophil response of this disorder since IgA is associated with neutrophil chemotaxis and neutrophils bear IgA receptors.[43,44]

In the IEN variant, the pustules can be distributed throughout all layers of the epidermis and may also involve the hair follicles (Figs 5.41 and 5.42).[18] Acantholytic cells are usually (but not always) present. Typically, they are sparse and, as such, this diagnostic clue may be very easily overlooked.[11-13] Prominent dyskeratotic cells have been described in a rare case of IgG/IgA pemphigus.[45] Significant numbers of eosinophils may also be seen in occasional IEN cases.[20,46] Neutrophil dermal papillary microabscesses have also been described, sometimes accompanied by neutrophil spongiosis.[12,20] A perivascular infiltrate of neutrophils, lymphocytes, and histiocytes surrounds the superficial vascular plexus, and eosinophils may also sometimes be present. In addition to the major variants characterized by pustules, some patients with IgA pemphigus show histologic features typical of classic p. vulgaris, p. foliaceus, or even, exceptionally, p. vegetans.[4,18]

Differential diagnosis

The differential diagnosis includes subcorneal pustular dermatosis, typical p. foliaceus, and infections such as bullous impetigo. Although clinically subcorneal pustular dermatosis tends to be more restricted to the flexural sites, absolute distinction from the subcorneal variant of IgA pemphigus depends

on immunofluorescent studies. Gram stain and a periodic acid-Schiff (PAS) should always be included in the histologic workup to exclude an infective process.

Drug-induced pemphigus

There are at least 25 drugs that have been shown to be associated with the development of pemphigus.[1] Penicillamine and captopril are the most common offenders; however, bucillamine, enalapril, cetapril, ramipril, propranolol, bisoprolol, glibenclamide, cilazapril, penicillins, cephalosporins, rifampicin, pyrazolon derivatives, lisinopril, thiopronine, sulfasalazine, and antiseizure medications, among others, have also been implicated.[1-11] Some drugs such as penicillamine may elicit either p. foliaceus or p. vulgaris, but the former is much more common.

Symptoms disappear in most patients following withdrawal of causative drugs that contain a sulfhydryl group (thiol drugs). Nonthiol drugs are much less likely to be associated with remission following withdrawal.[2]

Histologically, drug-induced pemphigus resembles sporadic counterparts with positive direct immunofluorescence in most, but not all, patients.[12] As expected, given the different variants of pemphigus that drugs may induce, antibodies against both Dsg1 and Dsg3 have been documented.[9,13] It has been suggested that a monoclonal antibody against desmogleins 1 and 3 may be useful in the diagnosis and prognosis of drug-induced pemphigus.[14] Staining with this antibody is usually patchy in idiopathic pemphigus and diffuse in drug-induced pemphigus. Furthermore, cases of drug-induced pemphigus with diffuse pattern tend to have a poorer prognosis.

Contact pemphigus

Clinical features

There is a growing body of literature documenting contact with topical substances preceding the onset of pemphigus. The pathogenesis is not understood, but in some cases the exposure is thought somehow to trigger or induce pemphigus. The term 'contact pemphigus' has been proposed as a designation for this phenomenon, which has been described in the vulgaris, vegetans, foliaceus, and erythematosus variants.[1,2] Substances that have been implicated include nickel, pesticides, chromium sulfate, tincture of benzoin, phenol, diclofenac, dihydrodiphenyltrichlorethane, ketoprofen, feprazone, and imiquimod.[1-15] Clearly, further study is necessary to elucidate the relationship between exposure to topical agents and contact pemphigus.

Pathogenesis and histologic features

Whether this phenomenon relates to systemic absorption, contact allergy, or a direct 'toxic' effect on epidermal antigens is as yet unknown. It is interesting to note that in the majority of documented cases, the patient has been exposed to the offending agent for a considerable length of time before the onset of the blistering eruption.[6,15]

Biopsy of contact pemphigus shows histologic features similar to those of p. vulgaris, although one patient developed features more reminiscent of p. vegetans. Immunofluorescent studies show intercellular IgG and sometimes C3.

Differential diagnosis

The main differential diagnosis is with classic pemphigus. Only clinical information will allow distinction of contact pemphigus from other members of the pemphigus family of disorders.

Acantholytic dermatoses with dyskeratosis

Hailey-Hailey disease

Clinical features

Hailey-Hailey disease (benign familial pemphigus) is a rare, episodic, acantholytic disorder with an autosomal dominant mode of inheritance.[1,2] In only about two-thirds of patients, however, is a family history obtained. There is an equal sex incidence.[2,3]

Lesions usually present in the second to fourth decades and appear particularly at sites of minor trauma or friction, especially flexural, around the neck, and in the axillae and groin (Fig. 5.43).[1-4] However, other sites, such as the genitalia, umbilicus, inframammary regions, and scalp, may also be affected. Rarely, the disease may be generalized.[5-8] Nikolsky sign is sometimes positive.[3] Vesicles and bullae, arising on normal or erythematous skin, are soon replaced by erosions, crusting, and scaly plaques sometimes resembling impetigo (Figs 5.44 and 5.45).[2,4,9] Healing is accompanied by hyperpigmentation, but scarring is not a feature.[3,4] Lesions are frequently itchy and malodorous. Sometimes pain is a considerable problem, particularly if fissuring is present.[3] Symptoms often improve with advancing age.[1] Superinfection by *Candida albicans*, herpes simplex virus, and *Staphylococcus aureus* are frequent complications.[10-13] Segmental involvement has rarely been reported as a result of type 1 or type 2 mosaicism according to the classification by Happle, and it has now become clear that at least some of the cases of relapsing linear acantholytic dermatosis represent type 2 segmental Hailey-Hailey disease.[14-19]

The development of the lesions is related to mechanical trauma, stress, and ultraviolet radiation, and exacerbation of the disease has been reported due to scabies, contact irritation, patch testing, and multiple pregnancies.[20-25]

An exceptional case of a patient developing the disease while on efalizumab for psoriasis has been reported.[26] Symptoms often improve or even disappear during winter, but tend to worsen in summer.[1,27] Mucosal involvement is unusual. Anogenital disease, however, occasionally presents as multiple 3–5-mm-diameter warty papules.[28] This occurs most often in females, particularly blacks, and sometimes may be a presenting feature. In such instances, there is overlap with papular acantholytic dyskeratosis of the genitocrural area.[29-31]

Asymptomatic white longitudinal bands may be present on the fingernails in up to 70% of affected patients.[1,32-34] The other nail changes of Darier disease are absent.

Significant associated conditions have not been documented with the possible exception of a bipolar disorder and a patient with affective disorder (see Darier disease).[35,36] An association with supernumerary nipples has been documented in one Tunisian family.[37]

Exceptionally, squamous carcinoma has been documented as a complication in patients with Hailey-Hailey disease.[38,39] It is likely, however, that those arising on the vulva have a human papillomavirus-associated basis.[40,41] Condylomatous change and evidence of HPV infection has recently been detected in genital lesions of the disease.[42,43] Two patients with Hailey-Hailey disease and multiple primary melanomas and other malignancies have been described.[44]

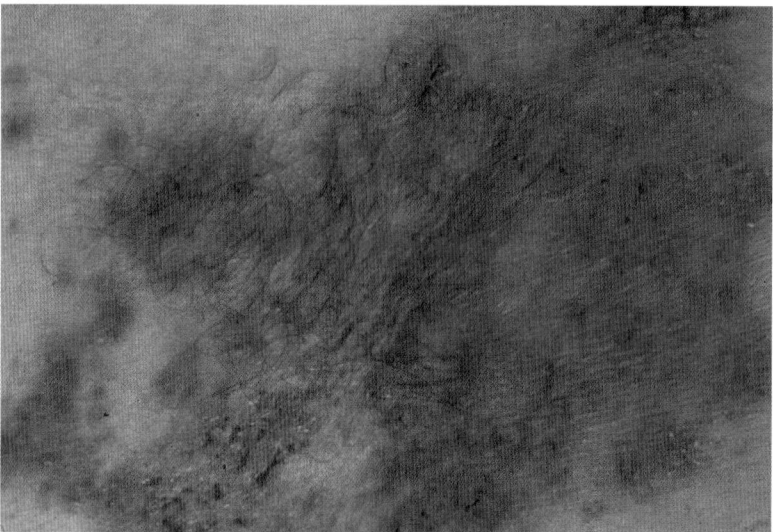

Fig. 5.44
Hailey-Hailey disease: lesions are most often seen in the flexures as a consequence of friction. By courtesy of the Institute of Dermatology, London, UK.

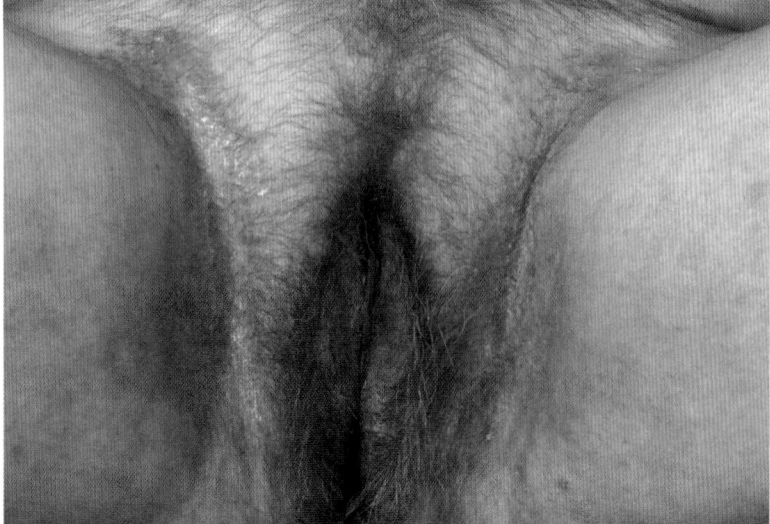

Fig. 5.43
Hailey-Hailey disease: erythematous and scaly lesions are present in the groin and on the labia majora. From the slide collection of the late N.P. Smith, MD, the Institute of Dermatology, London, UK.

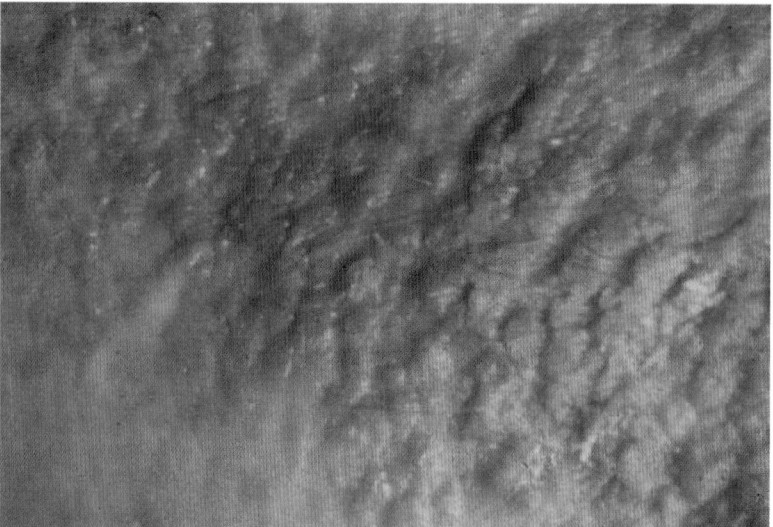

Fig. 5.45
Hailey-Hailey disease: close-up view of keratotic warty lesions. By courtesy of the Institute of Dermatology, London, UK.

Although it has rarely been reported that Darier disease may coexist with Hailey-Hailey disease, the available evidence supports the contention that these two conditions represent completely different entities.[45]

Pathogenesis and histologic features

Hailey-Hailey disease is primarily an abnormality of cell adhesion. Development of this disease has been shown to be caused by multiple mutations in *ATP2C1* on chromosome 3q21–24, a gene that encodes the calcium pump SPCA1 (type 1 sarcoendoplasmic reticulum CA^{2+}-ATPase).[46,47] SPCA1 is a Ca^{2+}/Mn^{2+} ATPase present within the membrane of the Golgi apparatus and responsible for the transport of Mn^{2+} as well as Ca^{2+} ions into the Golgi.[48,49] Over 100 mutations have been identified spanning the entire *ATP2C1* gene including missense, frameshift, splice site, as well as nonsense mutations.[5-64] However, no clear genotype–phenotype correlation has emerged as yet. Studies have shown that calcium regulation in cultured keratinocytes is impaired.[46] In addition, there is evidence that integrity of intercellular junctions may be dependent on intracellular calcium stores.[65-69] The precise mechanism by which the abnormality in the calcium pump causes acantholysis is not known. However, the addition of calcium to monolayers of squamous cells in culture elicits stratification.[66] In contrast, cells grown in low calcium medium fail to stratify.[68] It should be noted that Darier disease, another disorder showing acantholysis, is also associated with a mutation in another calcium pump – ATP2A2. That both of these disorders of acantholysis are associated with mutations in a calcium pump is strong evidence for an important role in maintaining cell–cell cohesion.

Immunohistochemical studies have confirmed that the major desmosomal proteins and glycoproteins are synthesized in Hailey-Hailey disease and distributed along the plasma membranes in uninvolved epidermis.[70] In lesional skin, there is marked cytoplasmic labeling for the desmoplakins (DpI, DpII), desmogleins (Dsg2, Dsg3), and desmocollins.[70-74] Studies on keratinocyte differentiation demonstrate premature expression and reduced levels of involucrin due to increased mRNA degradation, and it has been proposed that intact ATP2C1 is necessary for basal cell layer keratinocytes to maintain their undifferentiated state.[75,76] A number of interesting observations have been made recently in both Hailey-Hailey disease and Darier disease that provide further insight into how the alteration in the calcium gradient affects ATP receptors and keratin expression.[77] In both diseases, there is a lower level of calcium in the basal cell layer of the epidermis compared to normal skin; the ATP receptor P2Y2 is not identified at the cellular membrane in affected cells whereas P2X27, which is usually not present on the cellular membrane, is expressed in these cells probably mediating apoptosis. Furthermore, both keratins 14 and 10 are expressed in diseased cells whereas these keratins are mutually exclusive in normal keratinocytes.

While early lesions show suprabasilar lacunae, established Hailey-Hailey disease is characterized by massive acantholysis associated with suprabasal vesicle or bulla formation.[3] Typically, however, the acantholysis is incomplete, with the cell retaining some connections and giving an appearance often likened to a 'dilapidated brick wall' (*Figs 5.46–5.48*). The adnexal epithelium is usually spared. Occasionally, dyskeratotic cells resembling corps ronds and grains of Darier disease are seen.

Ultrastructural studies have primarily disclosed abnormalities of the desmosome–tonofilament units, characterized by diminished numbers of desmosomes and clumped tonofilaments.[78-81] The latter have a linear distribution in the basal keratinocytes, but develop a whorled configuration in the suprabasal layers.[79,81] The cell membranes show microvillus formation.[78] An electron microscopic study of artificially induced early lesions suggests the desmosomal splitting precedes the tonofilament clumping.[80] Dyskeratotic cells are characterized by condensed tonofilaments surrounding pyknotic nuclei.

Differential diagnosis

The histologic features of Hailey-Hailey disease must be distinguished from those of Darier disease, p. vulgaris, and Grover disease. Pemphigus is distinguished from Hailey-Hailey disease by the presence of relatively intact epithelium in the adjacent epidermis (versus disintegrating 'dilapidated brick wall') and involvement of adnexal structures. In difficult cases, positive immunofluorescence staining supports a diagnosis of pemphigus. Darier

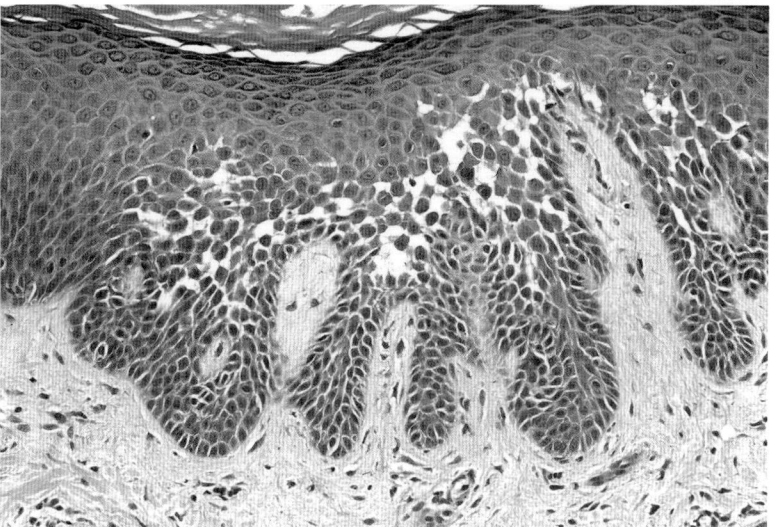

Fig. 5.46
Hailey-Hailey disease: early lesion showing the characteristic 'dilapidated brick wall' appearance.

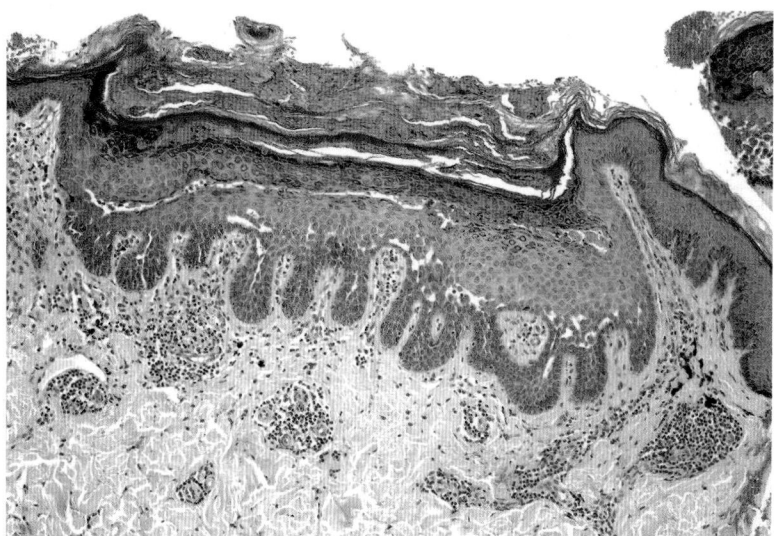

Fig. 5.47
Hailey-Hailey disease: in this example, there is marked hyperkeratosis, parakeratosis, and acanthosis. Villi project into the blister cavity.

disease tends to show prominent suprabasal cleft formation with involvement of adnexae and is associated with numerous corps ronds and grains. These points of distinction are summarized in *Table 5.2*.

Immunofluorescence studies for immunoglobulin and complement are invariably negative, aiding in the distinction from immunobullous disorders. Distinction from acantholytic dermatosis of the genital area can, however, be extremely difficult. In fact, the relationship between these disorders is not well understood. The combination of clinical features of a lesion or lesions localized to the vulvogenital area and a negative family history favors acantholytic dermatosis of the genital area.

Relapsing linear acantholytic dermatosis

Clinical features

Relapsing linear acantholytic dermatosis (Hailey-Hailey-like epidermal nevus) is an exceptionally rare nevus-like condition characterized by erythematous plaques with vesicles and erosions arranged in a linear distribution along Blaschko lines.[1-3] It typically undergoes spontaneous resolution followed by recurrence and has a chronic course. Insufficient cases have been documented to precisely determine its relationship to Hailey-Hailey disease.

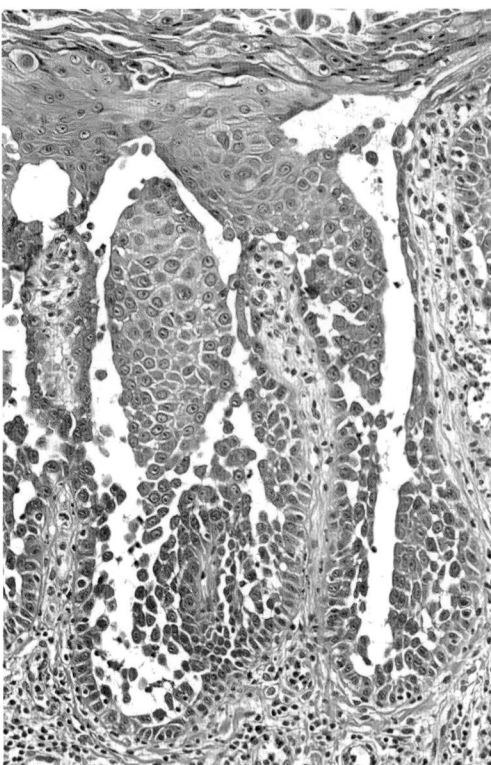

Fig. 5.48
Hailey-Hailey disease: in contrast to Darier disease, dyskeratosis is usually
minimal or even absent.

Recent data, however, demonstrate that at least some of the patients harbor
mutations in the gene responsible for Hailey-Hailey disease, *ATP2C1*. The
disease has been shown to be a type 2 mosaicism according to Happle,
resulting in homozygosity for the mutated gene and pronounced disease in
a segmental distribution superimposed on more classical disease in a heterozygous individual.[4–7]

Histologic features

The features are indistinguishable from Hailey-Hailey disease.

Darier disease

Clinical features

Darier disease (keratosis follicularis, morbus Darier), which is characterized
by abnormal keratinocyte adhesion, is a rare hereditary disorder, usually
transmitted in an autosomal dominant pattern. In a large series, however,
47% of patients had no clear family history of Darier disease.[1] Presumably,
these cases represent new mutations or evidence of incomplete penetrance.
Its documented incidence is variable. In Oxfordshire (UK), the incidence is
1:55 000, in the north of England it is 1:36 000, in the west of Scotland it
is 1:30 000, whereas in Denmark it is 1:100 000.[2–5] The sex incidence is
equal, although males appear to be more severely affected than females. The
disease usually presents in the first or second decade (with a peak around
puberty) and often follows exposure to ultraviolet light.[1] Exceptionally,
patients may not present until their sixth or seventh decade.[6] Darier disease
is a long-term illness. Remissions do not occur, although some patients
show improvement with increasing age.[6]

The lesions are frequently itchy and, less commonly, painful.[1,6,7] They
are characterized by greasy, crusted, keratotic yellow-brown papules and
plaques found particularly on the 'seborrheic' areas of the body – the scalp,
forehead, ears, nasolabial folds, upper chest, back, and supraclavicular
fossae (*Figs 5.49–5.53*).[1,5,7] There is mild involvement of the flexures in the
majority of patients although sometimes this distribution predominates.[1,6,7]
Lesions may be induced or exacerbated by stress, heat, sweating, and maceration.[1,7,8] In some areas, the lesions have a warty appearance, whereas in

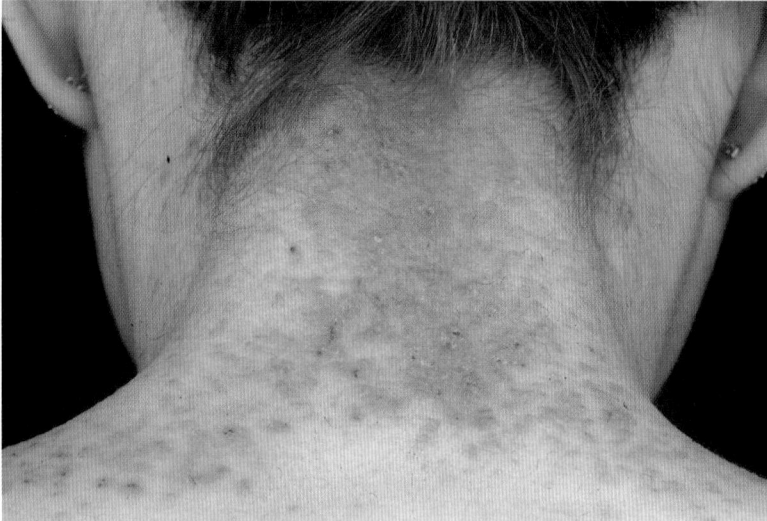

Fig. 5.49
Darier disease: in this patient, keratotic brown papules are present on the back
of the neck. From the slide collection of the late N.P. Smith, MD, the Institute of
Dermatology, London, UK.

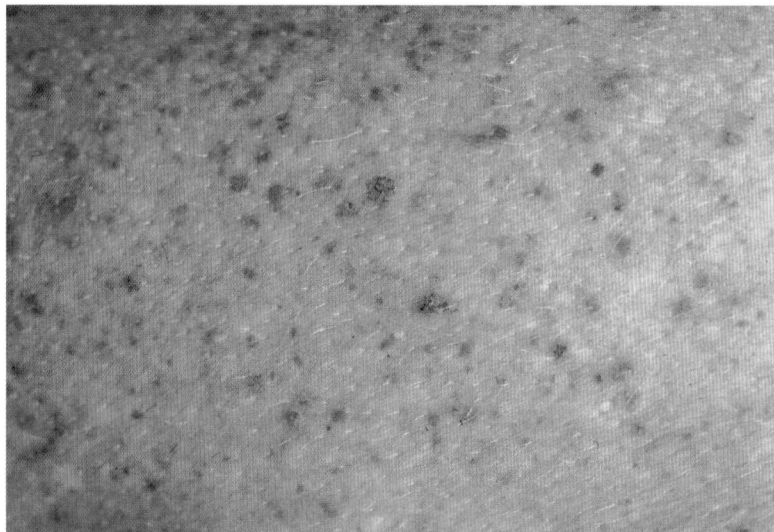

Fig. 5.50
Darier disease: close-up view of keratotic papules. From the slide collection of the
late N.P. Smith, MD, the Institute of Dermatology, London, UK.

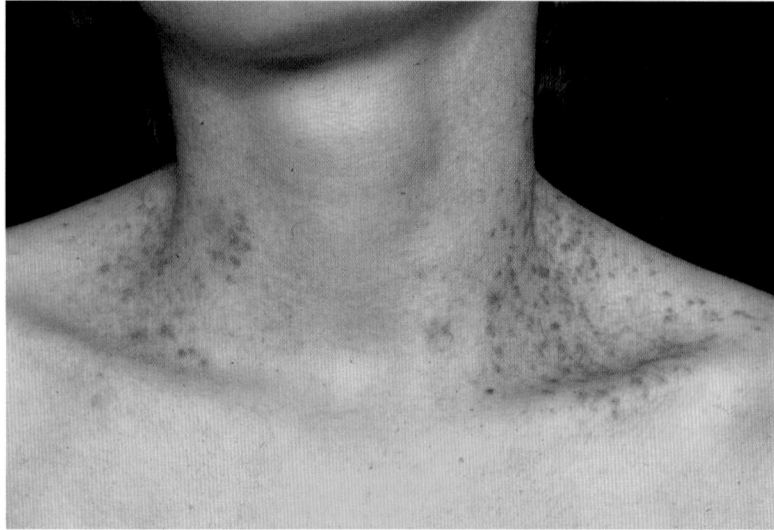

Fig. 5.51
Darier disease: this patient shows a striking symmetrical distribution. From the slide
collection of the late N.P. Smith, MD, the Institute of Dermatology, London, UK.

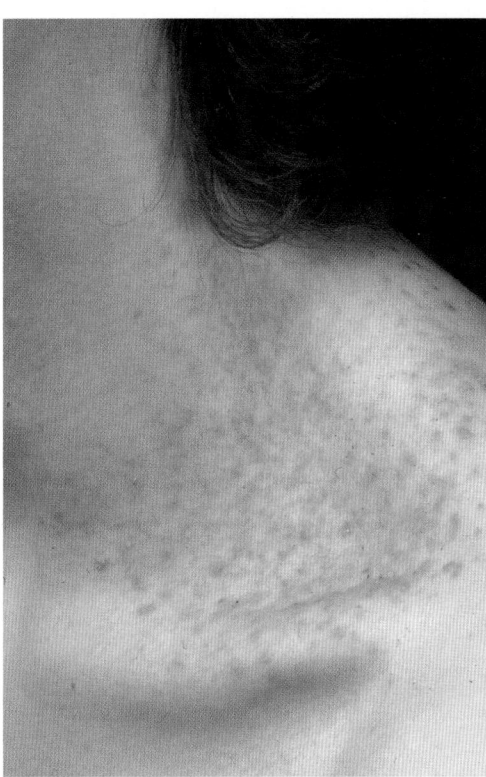

Fig. 5.52
Darier disease: lesions may be induced by heat, sweating, and maceration. From the slide collection of the late N.P. Smith, MD, the Institute of Dermatology, London, UK.

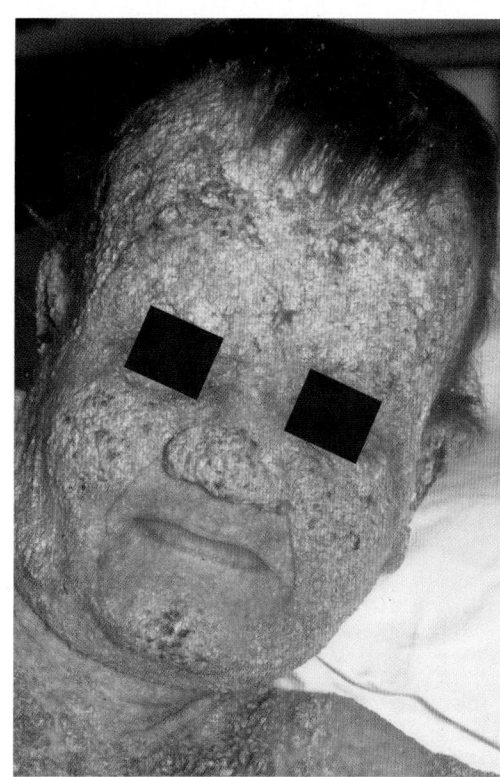

Fig. 5.54
Darier disease: skin involvement as severe as this is fortunately extremely rare. By courtesy of M. Greaves, MD, the Institute of Dermatology, London, UK.

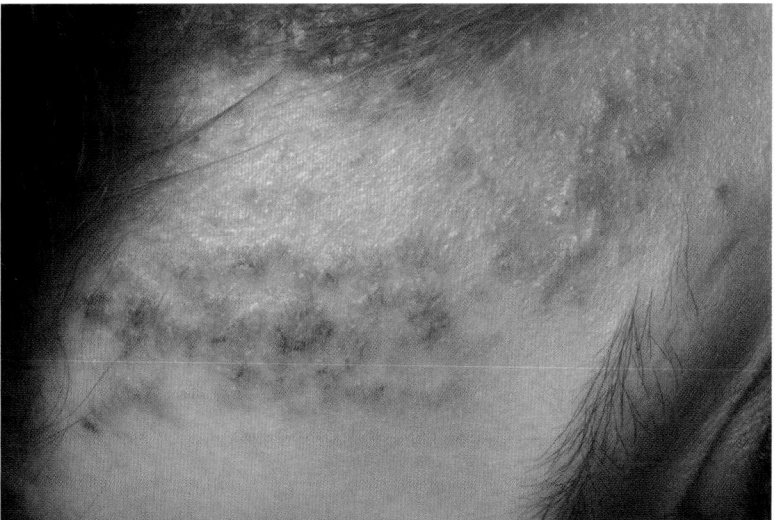

Fig. 5.53
Darier disease: close-up view. From the slide collection of the late N.P. Smith, MD, the Institute of Dermatology, London, UK.

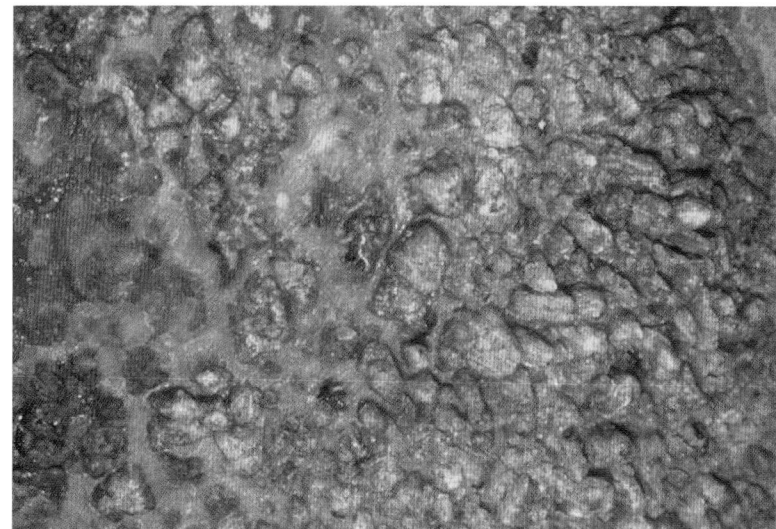

Fig. 5.55
Darier disease: severe involvement can be very disfiguring and a source of considerable disability and embarrassment. By courtesy of M. Greaves, MD, the Institute of Dermatology, London, UK.

the flexures they are often vegetative, malodorous (a particularly distressing problem), and often secondarily infected (*Figs 5.54* and *5.55*).[6,7] Bullous lesions generally following sun exposure can occur, albeit rarely.[9–12] Leukodermic macules in black patients have also been described and in the absence of more clinical typical changes of the disease, the diagnosis may be very difficult.[13–16] Additional features including cutaneous horns and hemorrhagic acrallesions have also been documented.[17–22]

Patients with Darier disease are susceptible to bacterial (particularly *S. aureus*), dermatophyte, *Candida*, and viral infections.[1,19,20,23–26] There are rare case reports of eczema vaccinatum and eczema herpeticum complicating Darier disease, and patients who developed localized anogenital and disseminated cowpox have also been reported.[27–30] Life-threatening Kaposi varicelliform eruption is a rare but important complication that is seen in severely affected patients and is usually associated with herpes simplex virus

superinfection.[31–34] No consistent abnormality of immune function has been found to explain this.[35,36] Recently, however, persistence of intracellular *S. aureus* small-colony variants in a patient with Darier disease has been shown to be of importance in chronic cutaneous infection and resistance to antibiotic therapy.[37] Lesional skin is also frequently colonized by *S. aureus*, and disease severity is correlated with extent of colonization.[26] Other cutaneous manifestations of Darier disease include unilateral, linear, or zosteriform variants, which some regard as acantholytic, dyskeratotic epidermal nevi rather than true Darier disease (see below).[38,39] It is more likely that these variants, at least in part, result from genetic mosaicism, and there is molecular evidence supporting this view.[40–42]

The hands are affected in 96% of patients.[1] Pits and punctate keratoses with focal disruptions of the skin ridges of the palms and soles are

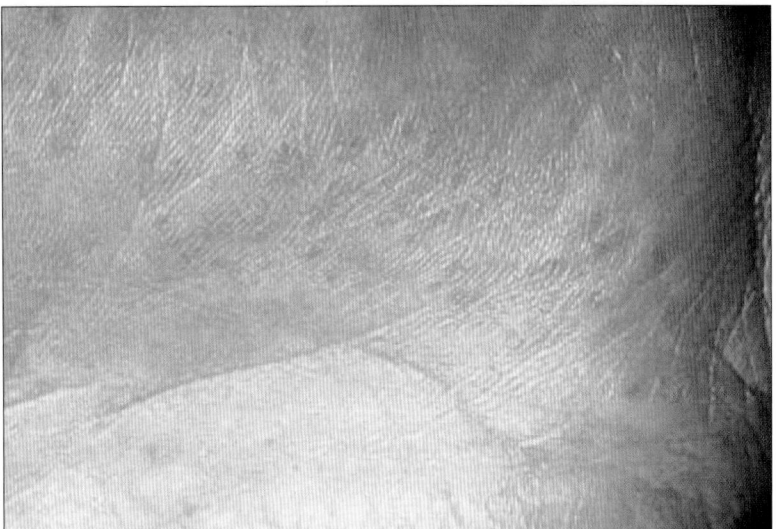

Fig. 5.56
Darier disease: palmar pits are a helpful diagnostic clue. By courtesy of J. Wilkinson, MD, Wycombe General Hospital, High Wycombe, UK.

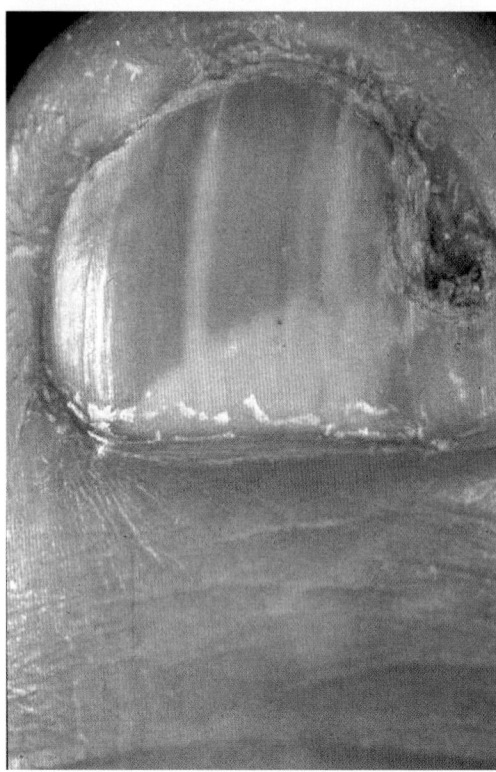

Fig. 5.58
Darier disease: notches on the free margin of the nail are common findings. By courtesy of the Institute of Dermatology, London, UK.

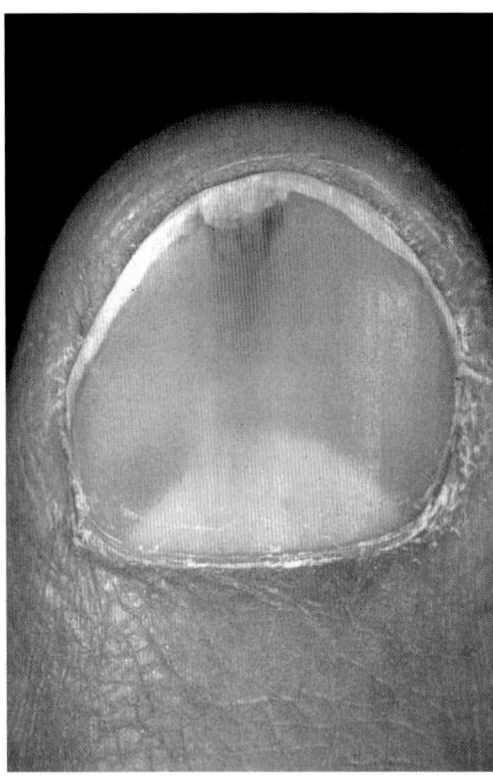

Fig. 5.57
Darier disease: parallel white and red longitudinal streaks are pathognomonic features. By courtesy of the Institute of Dermatology, London, UK.

characteristic features (*Fig. 5.56*).[1,6,43] Acrokeratosis verruciformis-like lesions are common on the backs of the hands.[1] Indeed, acrokeratosis verruciformis of Hopf, a localized disorder of keratinization of distal extremities, is closely related to Darier disease and appears to be caused by mutations in the same gene.[44,45]

Nail changes are a particularly important diagnostic feature.[1,2,6,46–48] Longitudinal white or red streaks (often both), some of which terminate in a small nick on the free margin, are typical findings (*Figs 5.57* and *5.58*).[1,48] Painful splitting and subungual hyperkeratoses are additional manifestations.[1] The toenails are affected less often (and less severely) than the fingernails.[1] Subtle hand and nail manifestations may sometimes be a presenting feature.[6]

The mucous membranes of the mouth, pharynx, larynx, esophagus, and female genitalia can also be affected.[49–58] Oral lesions are present in up to

50% of patients and consist of small white papules on the hard palate.[55,57,58] Large nodular and verrucous plaques are also sometimes present, and occasionally there are gingival, buccal mucosal, and tongue lesions.[17,56] Involvement of the salivary ducts results in salivary gland swelling with obstruction and sialadenitis.[59,60] Involvement of the parotid gland can be seen in up to 30% of cases.[57] Anal involvement may present as pruritus ani or less often as vegetating malodorous plaques.[61]

Ocular lesions, particularly affecting the cornea, are seen in up to 76% of patients.[62] Peripheral corneal opacities and central epithelial irregularity are the usual findings. Pannus formation may rarely be present. Lesions are typically asymptomatic.

Associated systemic abnormalities are unusual, but include epilepsy, pulmonary lesions, bone cysts, low intelligence, and small stature.[1] Various neuropsychiatric problems including depression and bipolar disorder have been linked with Darier disease.[6,63–65] There is some evidence to suggest that there is familial cosegregation of bipolar disorder with Darier disease, at least in a proportion of cases.[63,64]

Rare and likely incidental associations include visceral malignancy, horseshoe kidney, hemodialysis, gynecomastia, cutis verticis gyrate, and Fanconi anemia.[66–71]

Spontaneous remissions in Darier disease are rare, and in the majority of patients the disease persists throughout life.

Pathogenesis and histologic features

Positional cloning studies of different families have all shown the gene of Darier disease to be located at 12q23-q24.[72,73] Mutations in *ATP2A2*, a gene that encodes for SERCA2 (type 2 sarcoendoplasmic reticulum CA^{2+}-ATPase), cause the disease and have been identified in the majority of patients screened.[73] So far, over 100 different mutations have been reported, with new novel mutations constantly being reported. They are predominantly missense mutations, but frameshift and splice site mutations as well as mutations resulting in a premature stop codon have also been identified.[74–87] However, no clear genotype–phenotype correlation has emerged. The disease is likely a result of haploinsufficiency since only one correct copy of the *ATP2A2* gene is expressed.[88] The mutant copy may furthermore lead to enhanced proteasome-mediated degradation and/or protein dimerization resulting in complete loss of SERCA2 activity.[88,89] The precise mechanism of how mutations in the *ATP2A2* gene lead to disease is unknown although there is emerging evidence to suggest that the integrity of intercellular junctions is dependent on the intracellular calcium stores.[90] SERCA is a ubiquitously expressed calcium-ATPase, and its function is the transport of cytosolic calcium ions into the endoplasmic reticulum.[88] There are three different genes encoding these proteins, resulting in a total of nine different isoforms. Of the different isoforms, only SERCA2b appears to be expressed in keratinocytes.[91] Loss of SERCA2 function can therefore not be compensated for, explaining the severe skin manifestations in the absence of further systemic involvement in most patients with Darier disease.[88] Ultimately, intact intracellular calcium ion homeostasis has been identified as a major factor in the complex process of desmosome assembly and is necessary for intracellular interactions between desmosomal cadherins and intracellular plaque proteins such as plakoglobin.[88,92] Apoptosis in Darier disease resulting in dyskeratotic cells is likely directly related to the imbalance in calcium homeostasis, and immunohistochemical studies have revealed reduced expression of antiapoptotic proteins of the bcl-2 gene family in lesional epidermis.[93-95] It has recently been shown that mutant SERCA2 accumulates as insoluble aggregates resulting in endoplasmic resticulum stress and induction of apoptosis.[96]

No single specific ultrastructural abnormality has been identified in Darier disease. Changes described have included complete loss of desmosomes in foci of acantholysis with formation of cell membrane microvilli, cytoplasmic vacuolization, cell membrane defects, abnormal tonofilament aggregation, clumping and distribution, premature and abnormal formation of keratohyalin granules and membrane coating (Odland) bodies, and excessive lipid lamellae between the flattened keratinocytes of the stratum corneum.[97-101] Hemidesmosomes and the lamina densa usually appear morphologically normal, although discontinuities of the latter have been described. Ultrastructurally, corps ronds are characterized by large dense keratohyalin masses, numerous membrane coating granules, and tonofilament clumps.[97] They are distributed particularly around the nucleus, often surrounding a perinuclear cytoplasmic halo containing distended vesicles. Grains of Darier are composed of nuclear remnants with surrounding dyskeratotic debris.[97]

Acantholysis develops as a consequence of desmosomal breakdown and dissociation of tonofilaments, although which comes first is uncertain.

The histologic features of Darier disease depend on a variable interplay between acantholysis and abnormal keratinization (dyskeratosis), the acantholysis resulting in suprabasal cleft formation (and rarely vesicles or even blisters), and the dyskeratosis manifesting as corps ronds and grains of Darier.

- Corps ronds are large structures, usually most conspicuous in the granular layer, and consist of an irregular eccentric and sometimes pyknotic nucleus surrounded by a clear halo enclosed within a basophilic or eosinophilic 'shell' (*Fig. 5.59*). Variable amounts of highly irregular keratohyalin granules may also be evident.
- Grains are located within the horny layer and consist of somewhat flattened oval cells with elongated cigar-shaped nuclei and abundant keratohyalin granules.

In the fully established lesion, there is hyperkeratosis and often parakeratosis, sometimes arranged in a clearly defined tier (*Figs 5.60–5.62*). The epidermis may appear acanthotic or atrophic and typically shows acantholysis with suprabasal cleft formation in which the underlying dermal papillae, covered by a single layer of epithelium, project into the cavity (villus formation). The roof contains variable numbers of grains, and the adjacent epithelium has variable numbers of corps ronds. Occasionally, epithelial proliferation can be marked, resulting in pseudoepitheliomatous hyperplasia. Bullous lesions are illustrated in *Figs 5.63* and *5.64*.

There may be a perivascular chronic inflammatory cell infiltrate in the superficial dermis, although this is not a common finding.

The histologic features of the oral, pharyngeal, laryngeal, and esophageal lesions are similar to those described in the skin although dyskeratosis is said to be less conspicuous.[57] Salivary gland lesions show ductal dilatation and squamous metaplasia of the lining epithelium with acantholysis and dyskeratosis.[59,60]

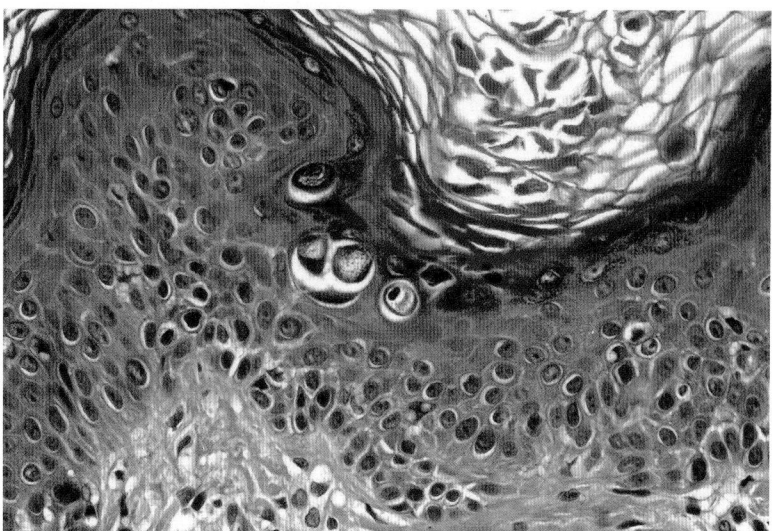

Fig. 5.59
Darier disease: very early lesion showing multiple characteristic corps ronds.

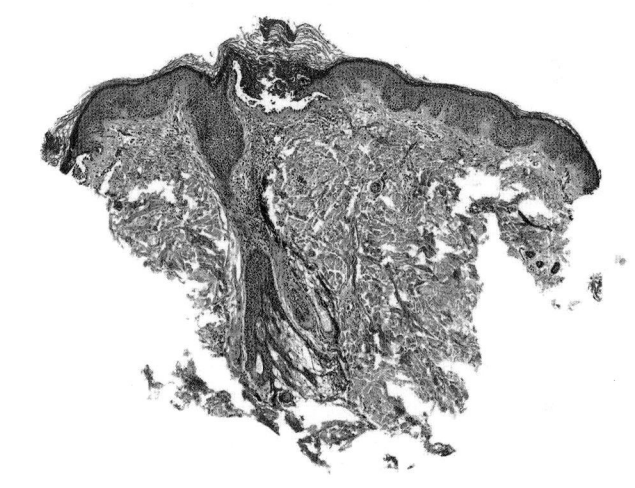

Fig. 5.60
Darier disease: scanning view through a typical lesion. Note the keratotic tier and suprabasal cleft formation.

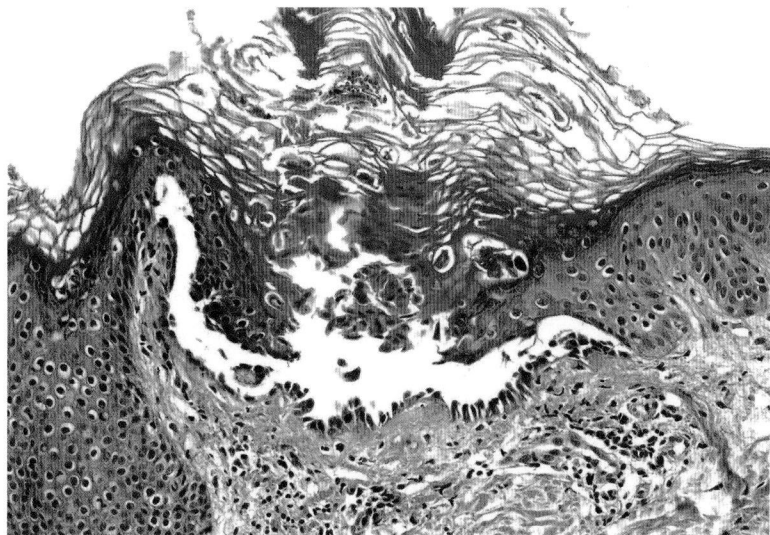

Fig. 5.61
Darier disease: higher-power view showing the well-developed vesicle with suprabasal acantholysis and well-developed corps ronds and grains.

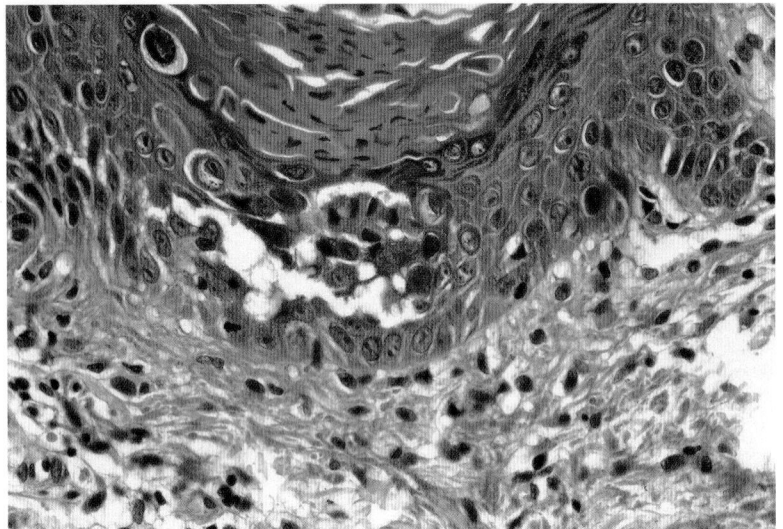

Fig. 5.62
Darier disease: in this example, both corps ronds and grain of Darier are evident.

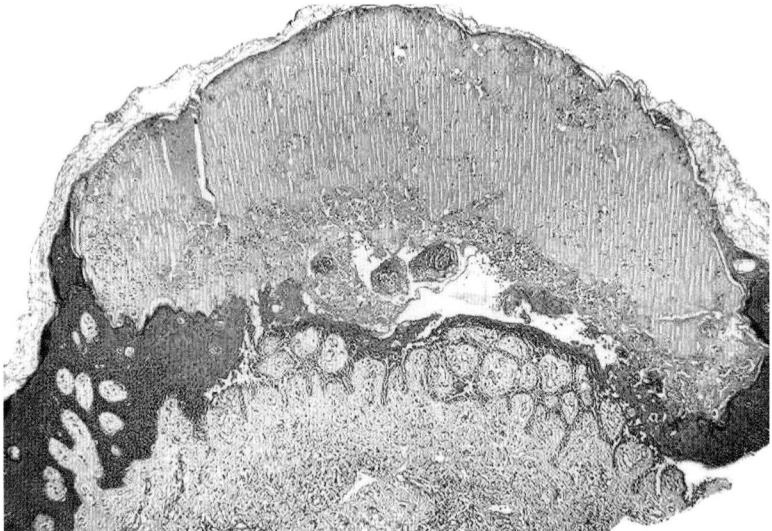

Fig. 5.63
Darier disease: bullous variant showing suprabasal acantholysis, epidermal regeneration, and a subcorneal blister.

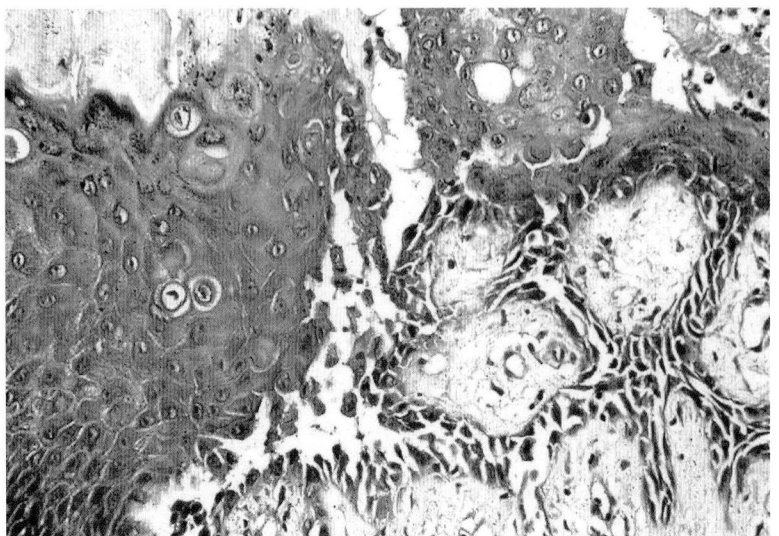

Fig. 5.64
Darier disease: high-power view of *Fig. 5.62* showing multiple corps ronds.

Corneal lesions are characterized by corneal epithelial edema, subepithelial granular deposits, and basement membrane thickening. Acantholysis and dyskeratosis are not seen.[47]

Differential diagnosis

Although warty dyskeratoma, Hailey-Hailey disease, and pemphigus are considered in the differential diagnosis of Darier disease, their distinction is not challenging when clinical information is considered. Warty dyskeratoma is a single umbilicated lesion that typically forms more pronounced papillary structures. Hailey-Hailey disease is characterized by full-thickness epidermal acantholysis and does not show extensive dyskeratosis. Grover disease may be indistinguishable from Darier disease in a given biopsy, but the lesions are usually small, spanning only a few rete ridges. The presence of some combination of spongiosis, and changes mimicking more than one of the acantholytic dermatoses, is characteristic of Grover disease. In cases that show only Darier-like changes, clinical information should allow for definitive diagnosis.

Linear Darier disease

Clinical features

Linear Darier disease (acantholytic dyskeratotic epidermal nevus, unilateral Darier disease, zosteriform Darier disease, segmental Darier disease) is a rare acquired condition characterized by the development of grouped, keratotic, sometimes pruritic, yellow-brown papules which affect the trunk, trunk and limbs, limbs, scalp, vulva, and face in decreasing order of frequency (*Fig. 5.65*).[1–9] Their linear distribution corresponds to the lines of Blaschko. Lesions may be aggravated by sunlight, heat, and sweating. Although a wide age range may be affected, the majority of patients are in the third or fourth decade. Both sexes are equally affected. There is no family history of Darier disease. Usually, patients are free from other stigmata of Darier disease, but there are very occasionally reports of patients with linear lesions associated with ipsilateral nail changes and palmar pits typical of Darier disease.[10,11]

Pathogenesis and histologic features

The precise nature of this lesion remains conjectural. Although many authors prefer to regard it as a variant of epidermal nevus with superimposed acantholytic dyskeratosis, there is an alternative school of thought which believes that many, if not all, such lesions represent localized or unilateral Darier disease, arguing that the condition develops as a consequence of genetic mosaicism. Certainly, the late age of onset is unlike a typical epidermal nevus, which usually presents in childhood. The distribution along

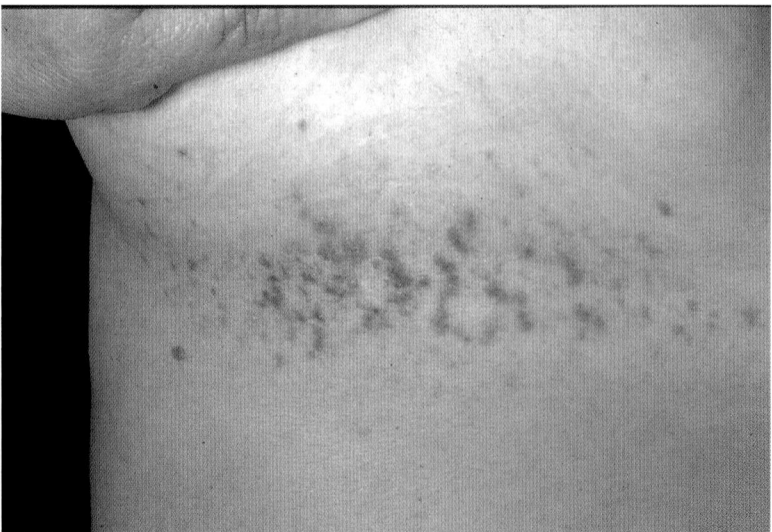

Fig. 5.65
Linear Darier disease: the trunk is a commonly affected site. Note the small papules. Courtesy of the Institute of Dermatology, London, UK.

the lines of Blaschko and the occasional reports of additional Darier-like features on the ipsilateral side of the body offers support to a concept of localized Darier disease. Recently, *ATP2A2* mutations have been identified in lesional tissue but not unaffected skin patients with linear acantholytic epidermal nevi, confirming the relationship of these lesions to Darier disease.[12,13,14]

Histologically, these lesions are indistinguishable from Darier disease.

Differential diagnosis

Very rarely, true epidermal nevus may show histologic features of acantholysis and dyskeratosis presenting against a background of a verrucous plaque characterized by marked acanthosis and papillomatosis.[15,16] Such lesions, which are present at birth, would be best classified as epidermal nevus showing acantholysis and dyskeratosis rather than being included in the spectrum of acantholytic dyskeratotic epidermal nevus.

Transient acantholytic dermatosis (Grover disease)

Clinical features

Transient acantholytic dermatosis (persistent acantholytic dermatosis) is a primary acquired, self-limiting, acantholytic disease of unknown etiology, seen predominantly in the middle-aged or elderly although there are rare reports of the disorder in children.[1-5] Males are affected more often than females (3 : 1).[2,3] Light-skinned people are predominantly affected.[5] Cases involving blacks are exceptionally rare.[6] The disease shows a predilection for the winter months in nonhospitalized patients, although some studies have not shown seasonal variation.[7,8] Although the disease is usually transient, persistent and recurring variants have also been described (persistent acantholytic dermatosis) in the literature.[9-11] The development of Kaposi varicelliform eruption is a rare and unusual complication of the disease and in one case seems to have been precipitated by vemurafenib.[12,13] Occult colonization by herpes simplex virus and *S. aureus* has also been documented.[14,15]

The skin lesions are usually rather polymorphic, consisting of 1–3-mm erythematous, red-brown or flesh-colored papules, vesicles, and eczematous plaques with a predilection for the chest, back, and thighs (*Figs 5.66* and *5.67*).[2] Superimposed excoriations are associated with the intensely pruritic eruption. Pustular, bullous, nummular, follicular herpetiform, and zosteriform variants have all been documented.[2,16-19] The mucous membranes, palms, and soles are commonly spared although there are rare reports of oral, nasal, and laryngeal involvement.[2,20,21] Postinflammatory pigmentary changes following resolution of the acute phase are common. Transient acantholytic dermatosis has been described in association with leukemia and lymphoma in addition carcinoma of kidney, renal pelvis, bladder, and prostate and melanoma.[2,22-29] In one study, 25% of patients had some form of malignancy, although that may reflect significant referral bias.[24] Other rare associations include scabies, renal failure, peritoneal dialysis, solid organ and bone marrow transplantation, and pregnancy.[30-37] It is likely, however, that the majority of these associations are coincidental. Transient acantholytic dermatosis shows a positive correlation with asteatotic eczema, allergic contact dermatitis, and atopic dermatitis.[3,38,39]

Pathogenesis and histologic features

The pathogenesis of Grover disease is incompletely understood. There are, however, a number of important known etiological factors including:

- sun exposure,
- excessive heat and sweating,
- ionizing radiation,
- adverse reaction to drugs.

Transient acantholytic dermatosis has long been known to be associated with sun exposure.[2,3,40-43] The lesions are photodistributed, and the patients commonly give a history of having recently spent time in the sun.[44] There is also a well-established relationship to excessive heat and sweating.[43,45-47] Bedridden, febrile patients are particularly at risk and as a result it has been proposed that the pathogenesis might be analogous to that of miliaria. Occlusion of sweat ducts and increased sweating resulting in acantholysis

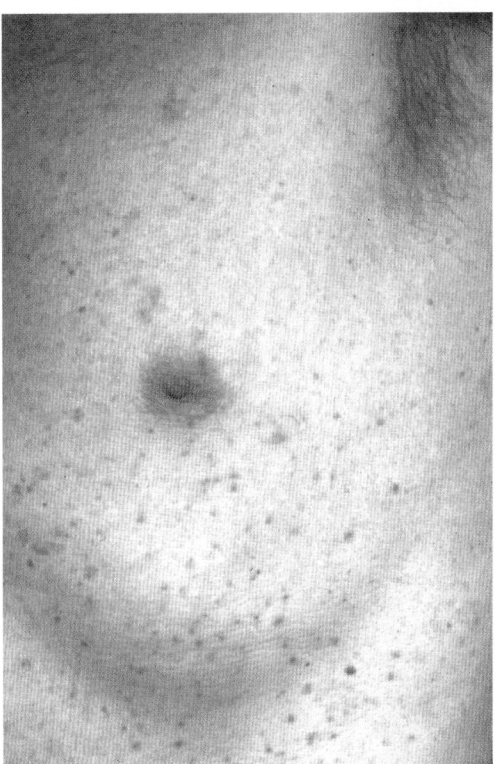

Fig. 5.66
Grover disease: innumerable erythematous papules are present on the chest wall. By courtesy of the Institute of Dermatology, London, UK.

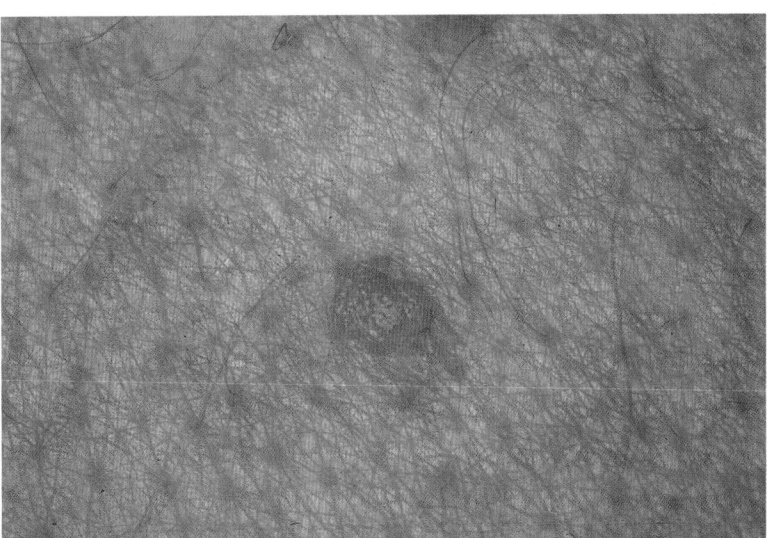

Fig. 5.67
Grover disease: close-up view. By courtesy of the Institute of Dermatology, London, UK.

mediated by high concentrations of sweat urea has been proposed, although this has yet to be proven.[48] Immunohistochemistry studies have not generally offered support for this hypothesis, although bedridden, febrile patients may occasionally show prominent involvement of the eccrine duct; this has been termed sudoriferous acrosyringeal acantholytic disease.[24,49,50] Associations with sunlamps, sun parlors, PUVA therapy, steam bath, hot tub, hot water bottle, and polyester jogging suits have also been documented.[1,2,24] Despite these well-recognized associations, there must be other important predisposing factors, since overexposure to sunlight and excessive sweating are extremely common yet this disease is rare.

Very occasional reports have described transient acantholytic dermatosis developing after radiotherapy for cancer, exceptionally with lesions confined to the area of the port.[2,25,51,52] Only a small number of drugs have been associated (rarely) with the development of transient acantholytic dermatosis.[2] There are reports of lesions following treatment with sulfadoxine–pyrimethamine, 2-chlorodeoxyadenosine, D-penicillamine, recombinant interleukin-4, cetuximab, induction chemotherapy for allogeneic bone marrow transplantation, anastrozole, and ipilimumab.[53–60] The presence of eosinophils in the dermal inflammatory cell infiltrate has raised the possibility of a hypersensitivity reaction.[24] Occasional cases arising in patients with HIV infection have been recorded.[24]

Despite the histologic similarity to Darier and Hailey-Hailey diseases, there is no evidence of a mutation in the *ATP2A2* gene.[61]

There have been a variety of both direct and indirect immunofluorescence observations including lupus erythematosus-like, bullous pemphigoid-like, and pemphigus-like findings.[24,62] These are reviewed in reference 2. A further study has shown autoantibodies in sera from Grover disease patients to a variety of proteins involved keratinocyte development, growth, adhesion, and motility.[63] The significance of these findings has not been established. Immunohistochemistry observations have included a reduction or absence of desmosomal staining with cytoplasmic redistribution of the proteins, desmoplakins I and II, plakoglobin, and desmoglein.[64–66] Redistribution and dissolution of desmosomal attachment plaques have been demonstrated as the first stage in the development of Grover disease.[66] Sera from Grover disease patients has also been shown to decrease expression of Dsg and Dsg3 in experimental models.[63]

Instead of featuring specific histopathological changes, Grover disease classically mimics three other diseases: Darier disease, Hailey-Hailey disease, and pemphigus (p. vulgaris and p. foliaceus) (*Figs 5.68–5.71*).[24] The first is by far the most commonly encountered. Thus, in the typical case, there is hyperkeratosis, parakeratosis, acanthosis, and acantholysis accompanied by corps ronds formation and grains of Darier. In the Hailey-Hailey pattern, the acantholysis is much more pronounced such that the dilapidated brick wall appearance is seen. Follicular or acrosyringeal involvement may be present.[50,67] In a subset of Grover disease, acrosyringeal involvement is quite pronounced and has been termed sudoriferous acrosyringeal acantholytic disease.[50] In the pemphigus-like variant, dyskeratosis is typically absent. Multiple specimens from any one patient may disclose differing histologic variants, and superimposed spongiosis is often present. Occasional bullae are encountered, and sometimes this can result in histologic overlap with herpesvirus infection.[68] A variable dermal mononuclear infiltrate is usual and significant numbers of eosinophils and/or neutrophils are seen in some cases.[21] The earliest changes can consist of elongation of rete ridges with focal acantholysis, mild spongiosis, and a superficial perivascular infiltrate that may be difficult to diagnose as Grover disease.[69] Additional features that have been described include porokeratosis-like columns of parakeratosis, lichenoid interface change, reactive keratinocyte atypia, papillary dermal hemorrhage, and epidermolytic hyperkeratosis.[70,71]

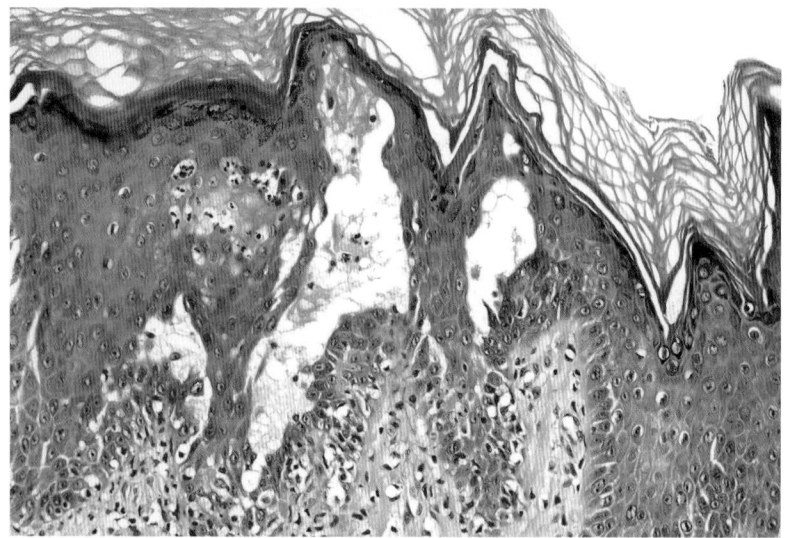

Fig. 5.69
Grover disease: high-power view showing acantholysis.

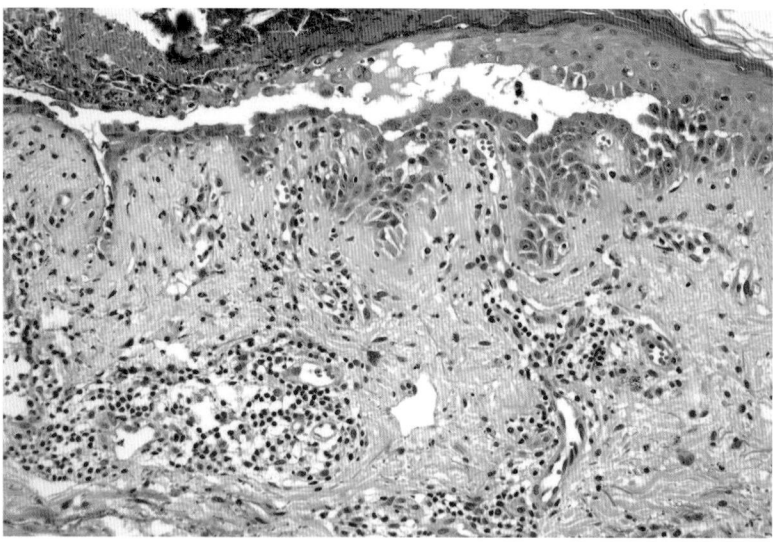

Fig. 5.70
Grover disease: this example is indistinguishable from pemphigus vulgaris.

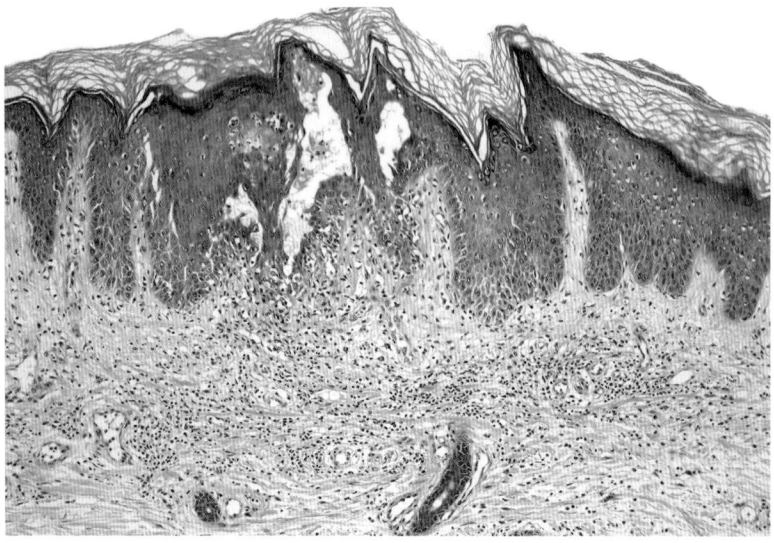

Fig. 5.68
Grover disease: low-power view showing an intact intraepidermal vesicle.

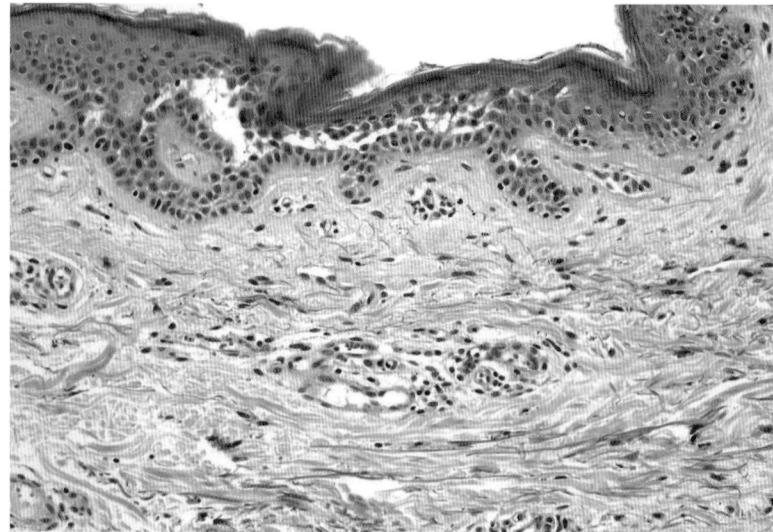

Fig. 5.71
Grover disease: early lesion showing intraepidermal vesiculation.

Differential diagnosis

Clinically, transient acantholytic dermatosis is easily differentiated from Darier disease, Hailey-Hailey disease, and pemphigus. However, the biopsy findings often mimic these diseases. A histologic clue to the diagnosis is the small size of the lesion. Usually, only one or two small discrete lesions that span a few rete ridges are noted. This is in contrast to other acantholytic dermatoses, which tend to involve the entire biopsy. Biopsies from a patient with Grover disease often show varying features mimicking more than one of the acantholytic dermatoses, and occasionally a number of patterns are seen in a single biopsy specimen. Sometimes, a biopsy will show non-specific features of spongiotic dermatitis. The association of both spongiosis and acantholysis may be a useful pointer to the diagnosis of Grover disease (see also *Table 5.2*).

Acantholytic dermatosis of the genitocrural area

Clinical features

In acantholytic dermatosis of the genitocrural area (papular acantholytic dermatosis of the vulvocrural or genitocrural area), focal dyskeratosis and/ or acantholysis may present as an isolated phenomenon on the genitocrural region, predominantly in young or middle-aged females.[1-12] Lesions sometimes extend on to the thigh and perineum.[5,13] Patients present with variably pruritic, multiple, 0.1–0.4-mm isolated or groups of white papules, solitary keratotic nodules, or, less often, with erythematous or white plaques measuring up to 1.0 cm in diameter involving the labia majora or inguinal region. Less commonly, cases with histologically similar findings have been described in males, presenting on the penis, scrotum, thigh, perianal region, and in the anal canal.[14-16]

Family history is negative for either Darier disease or Hailey-Hailey disease and, by definition, there is no evidence of similar lesions elsewhere on the body.[4] However, there may be a genetic relationship to Darier disease and Hailey-Hailey disease in a subset of patients (see below). Two cases have developed in the presence of syringomas.[1]

Pathogenesis and histologic features

The definitive pathogenesis is unknown and may be multifactorial. It is possible that the moist environment of the body folds plays a role. *C. albicans* infection has accompanied a number of cases although this may have been coincidental.[4,6] More recently, somatic mutations in *ATP2A2* have been detected in two cases, suggesting that at least some cases may represent a localized form of Darier disease secondary to genetic mosaicism.[17,18] Two other cases have been reported with mutations in *ATP2C1*, suggesting another subset may represent a mosaic form of Hailey-Hailey disease.[19] With the exception of one case showing intracellular IgG and C3 staining, immunofluorescence (when performed) has been negative.[3-5,8]

The lesions show features of hyperkeratosis, parakeratosis, acanthosis, and acantholysis, sometimes with dyskeratosis, resembling Darier disease or Hailey-Hailey disease. Warty dyskeratoma-like features associated with follicular involvement may also be encountered.[2,4] Typically, minimal or no inflammation is present.

Warty dyskeratoma

Clinical features

Warty dyskeratoma is a peculiar hyperkeratotic, umbilicated, persistent nodule that usually presents on the sun-exposed skin of the head and neck of middle-aged adults, although lesions on the trunk and extremities, and vulva have been documented (*Fig. 5.72*).[1-5] Most cases are solitary, but occasional patients with multiple tumors have been reported, particularly in Japanese patients.[3,6-9] Lesions are commonly asymptomatic but occasionally discharge and bleeding may be encountered.[2] There are conflicting data regarding gender distribution in the literature.[2,3] Although the cutaneous lesions are believed to be of follicular derivation, histologically similar nodules have been described affecting the oral and vulval mucosa.[10-15] The

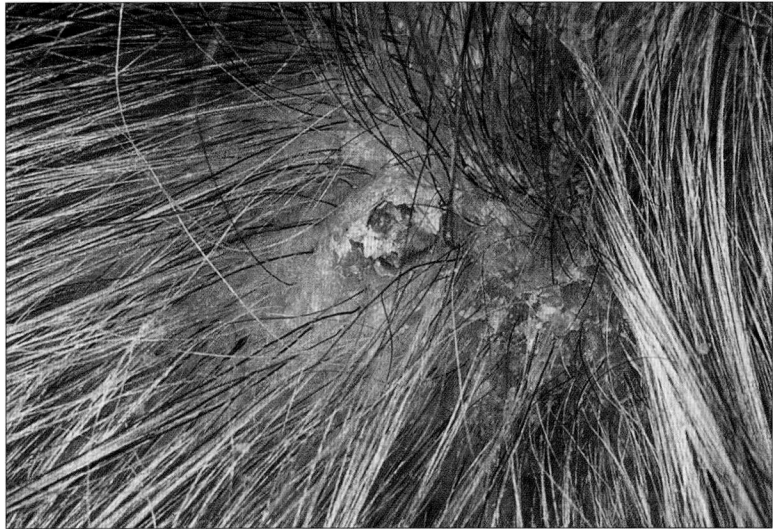

Fig. 5.72
Warty dyskeratoma: scaly nodule on the scalp, a commonly affected site. By courtesy of the Institute of Dermatology, London, UK.

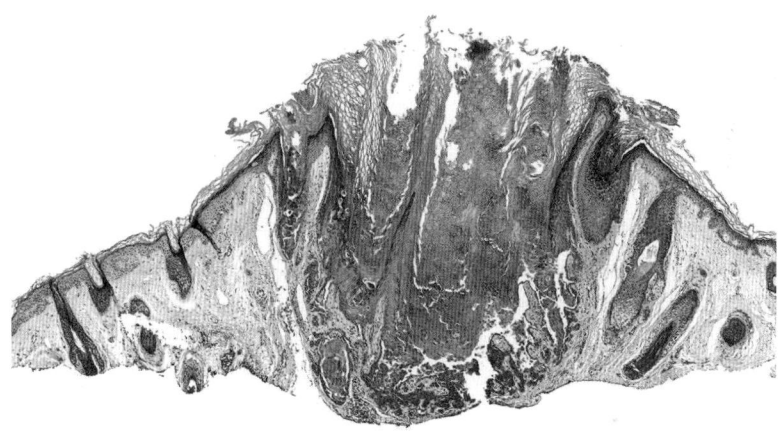

Fig. 5.73
Warty dyskeratoma: typical scanning view of a cystic nodule with acantholysis.

former occur most often on keratinized mucosa of the palate, alveolar ridge, and gingiva.[9] Subungual warty dyskeratoma-like lesions have also been documented, and an exceptional case involving the vocal cord has been reported.[16,17]

Pathogenesis and histologic features

The etiology of warty dyskeratoma is unknown, although in the past authors have suggested an effect of actinic radiation or possibly a viral infection. Neither of these has been substantiated. There is no relationship with Darier disease. Multiple lesions have been associated with chronic renal disease.[5,6] Warty dyskeratoma is most probably of follicular derivation. Thus, many examples appear in continuity with a dilated hair follicle and, less frequently, a sebaceous gland may be evident.[3,4,6] The recent observation of positive staining with antibodies directed toward cortex and inner root sheath provides additional support. Mucosal and subungual variants must have a different derivation.

Histologically, warty dyskeratoma is composed of a widely dilated cup-shaped or cystic lesion containing keratinous debris and often associated with a hair follicle (*Fig. 5.73*). Superficially, the keratinous debris contains conspicuous corps ronds and grains of Darier. The adjacent and deeper epithelium shows marked acantholysis, and suprabasal villi are a prominent feature (*Figs 5.74 and 5.75*). The underlying dermis is often infiltrated by lymphocytes and histiocytes, and sometimes plasma cells are evident.

Oral lesions can be morphologically indistinguishable although a number of cases more likely represent focal acantholytic dyskeratosis arising in a background of a benign trauma-related keratosis. A single case report has documented verruciform xanthoma-like features within a typical oral lesion.[13]

Differential diagnosis

Although there are histologic similarities with familial dyskeratotic comedones, Darier disease, Hailey-Hailey disease, and Grover disease, deeply penetrating crateriform lesions with villus formation are not associated with these entities. In addition, the clinical findings of a solitary umbilicated nodule should not be confused with any of the above disorders with the possible exception of familial dyskeratotic comedones; however, villi are not conspicuous in the latter. There is also considerable overlap with both focal acantholytic dyskeratosis and acantholytic acanthoma; however, in neither of these conditions is there a deeply penetrating crateriform lesion.

Familial dyskeratotic comedones

Clinical features

Although thought to be common, familial dyskeratotic comedones have been extremely rarely documented in the literature. To date, only a few families have been reported.[1-9] The condition is characterized by an autosomal dominant mode of inheritance. Lesions develop in childhood or adolescence and are permanent.[5] Patients present with 1–3-mm-diameter papules containing small hard keratotic plugs, which on removal leave crateriform lesions resembling comedones (*Fig. 5.76*). Cutaneous horns may also sometimes be apparent (*Fig. 5.77*).[2] Lesions are often generalized but show a predilection for the extremities, particularly the forearms and thighs. The face, scalp, palms, soles, and mucous membranes are typically unaffected. Some patients complain of pruritus or inflammation. There is no evidence of ectodermal dysplasia and systemic lesions are absent.

Histologic features

The lesions are characterized by a follicle-like crateriform cystic cavity containing laminated hyperkeratotic and parakeratotic debris and lined by squamous epithelium showing dyskeratosis and sometimes acantholysis at the base (*Figs 5.78 and 5.79*).[4] Grains of Darier are typically present, but corps ronds are sparse and poorly developed. Villi, as seen in Darier disease, are not a feature. Hair shafts and sebaceous glands are absent.

Differential diagnosis

The consistent folliculocentric nature of the eruption and absence of nail and oral mucosal changes help distinguish familial dyskeratotic comedones from Darier disease. Corps ronds, a characteristic finding in Darier disease,

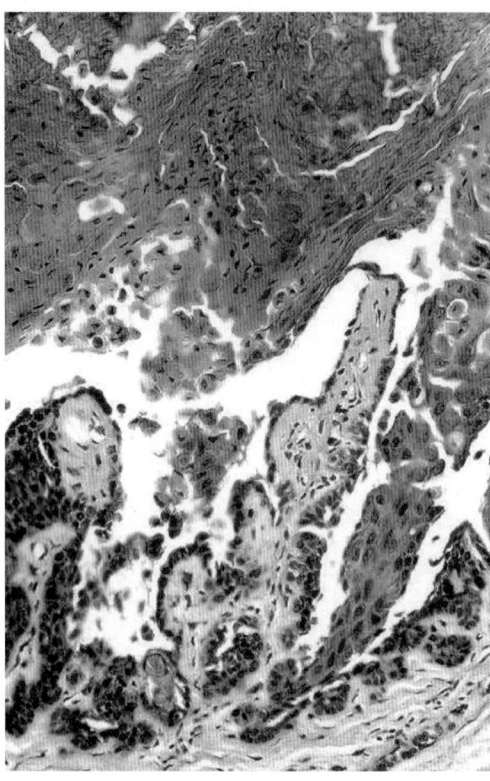

Fig. 5.74
Warty dyskeratoma: note the acantholysis and villi.

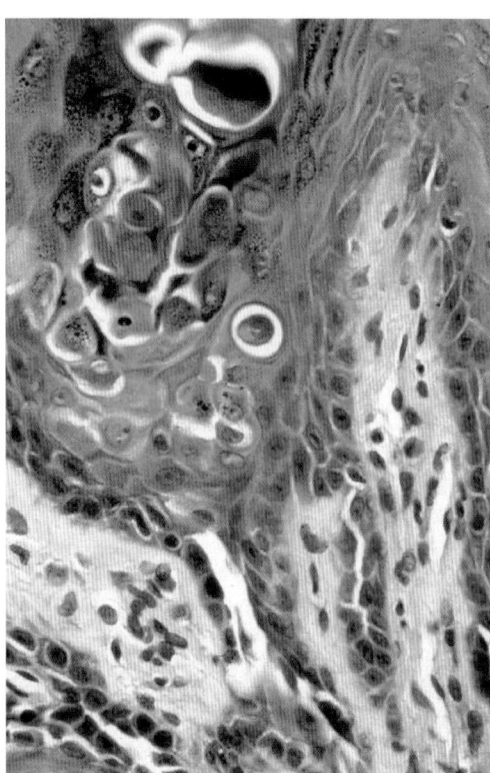

Fig. 5.75
Warty dyskeratoma: corps ronds are conspicuous.

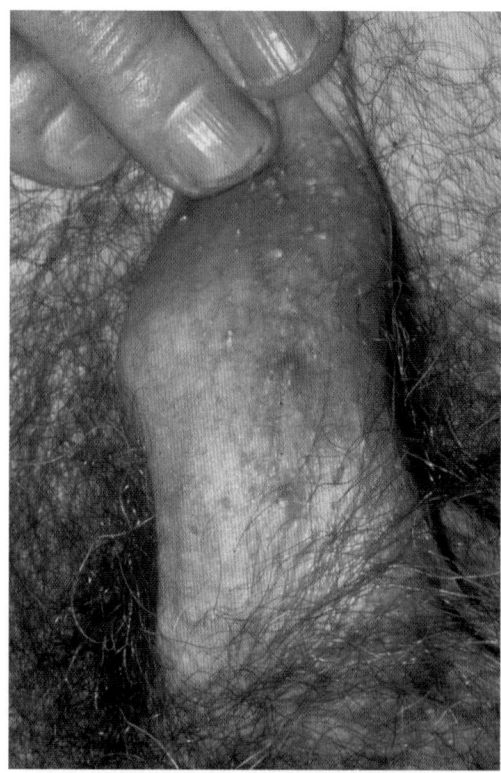

Fig. 5.76
Familial dyskeratotic comedones: numerous comedones are present on the penis and foreskin. By courtesy of B.J. Leppard, MD, Royal South Hants Hospital, UK.

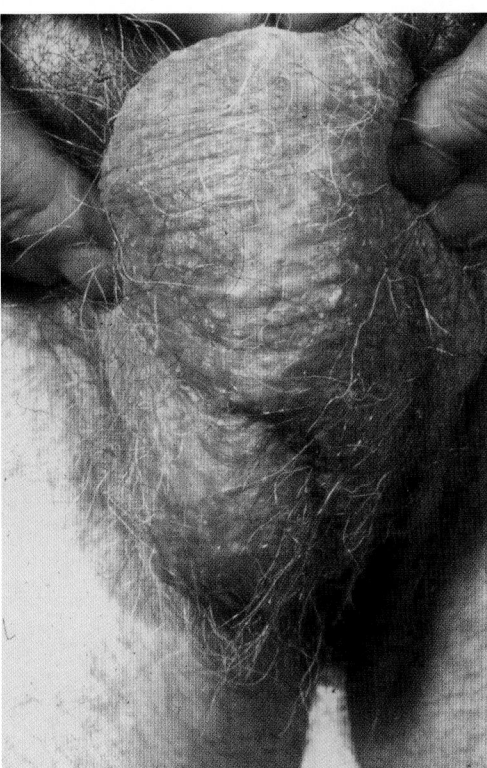

Fig. 5.77
Familial dyskeratotic comedones: a small cutaneous horn is seen arising on the scrotum. By courtesy of B.J. Leppard, MD, Royal South Hants Hospital, UK.

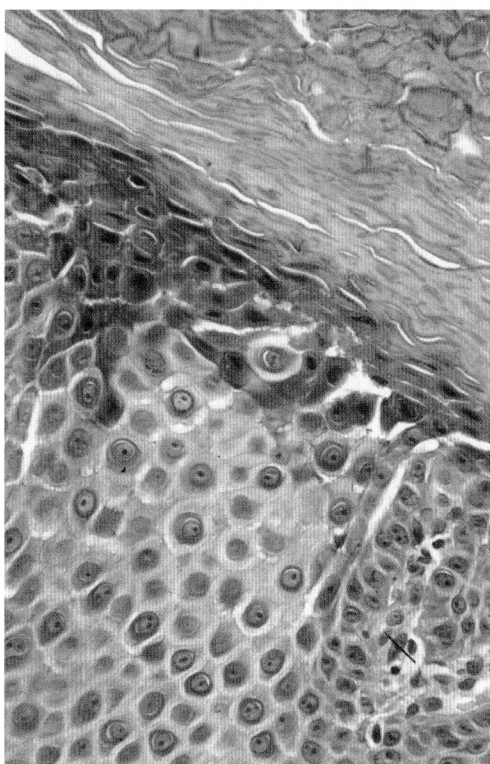

Fig. 5.79
Familial dyskeratotic comedones: note the superficial dyskeratosis. By courtesy of B.J. Leppard, MD, Royal South Hants Hospital, UK

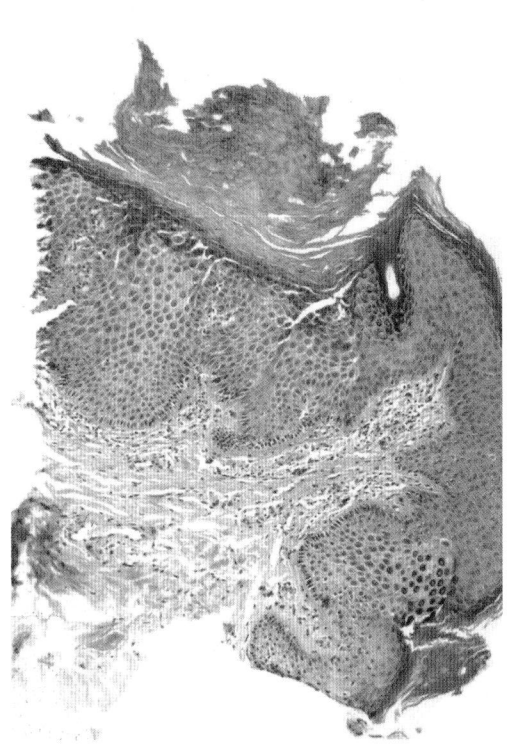

Fig. 5.78
Familial dyskeratotic comedones: this section comes from the edge of a lesion. Note the dell with associated hyperkeratosis and parakeratosis. The acanthosis is in part due to the oblique angle of the cut. By courtesy of B.J. Leppard, MD, Royal South Hants Hospital, UK.

are usually not prominent in familial dyskeratotic comedones. Villus formation and well-developed corps ronds within a solitary lesion distinguish warty dyskeratoma.

Diffuse familial comedones differ by the absence of dyskeratosis.[10–13] Familial dyskeratotic comedones may also be mistaken for Kyrle and Flegel diseases:

- Kyrle disease typically presents on the extensor aspect of the lower extremities and presents in adulthood. There is no familial incidence. Histologically, it is characterized by transepidermal elimination of parakeratotic and inflammatory debris. There is no dyskeratosis.
- Flegel disease typically presents in older adults and is characterized by prominent compact hyperkeratosis associated with marked epidermal atrophy, interface change, and dyskeratosis. A keratin-filled crateriform lesion is absent.

Perforating folliculitis presents in adults and shows a predilection for the extremities. It is characterized by a crateriform lesion containing a distorted and often curled-up hair shaft.

Acantholytic acanthoma

Clinical features

Acantholytic acanthoma is a common entity consisting of a solitary, usually asymptomatic, keratotic papule or plaque, 0.5–1.5 cm in diameter, often with overlying scale/crust. It usually presents on the trunk, arm, or neck and is clinically thought to be a seborrheic keratosis or actinic keratosis.[1–6] A case with central umbilication reminiscent of molluscum contagiosum has also been described.[7] Rare examples involving the eyelid have been reported.[8] Very occasionally, multiple lesions have been documented.[9] Some patients report pruritus. Hemorrhagic bullae may rarely be seen.[10] Patients are usually elderly (median age 60 years) and there is a predilection for males (2:1).[2,4] Lesions are not seen about the head, palms, and soles, and the mucous membranes appear to be spared.[2]

Pathogenesis and histologic features

The pathogenesis of this lesion is unknown. Although one case has been documented in association with immunosuppression, this is likely to be coincidental.[11]

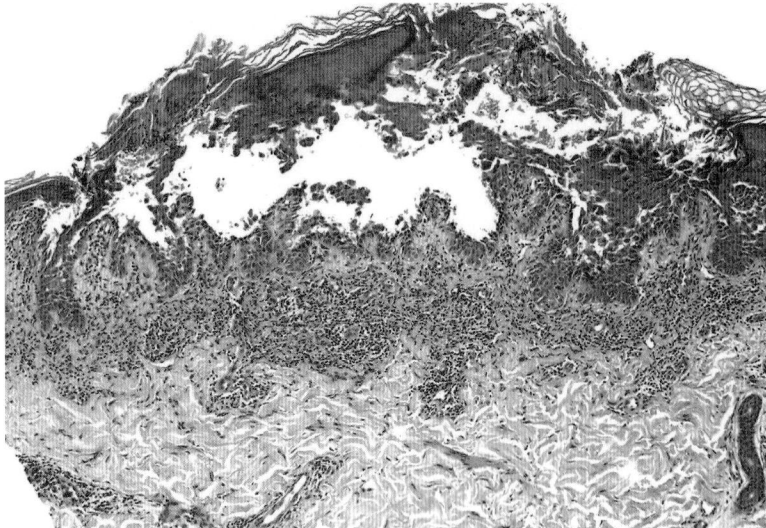

Fig. 5.80
Acantholytic acanthoma: low-power view showing hyperkeratosis, parakeratosis, intraepidermal vesiculation, and multiple foci of acantholysis.

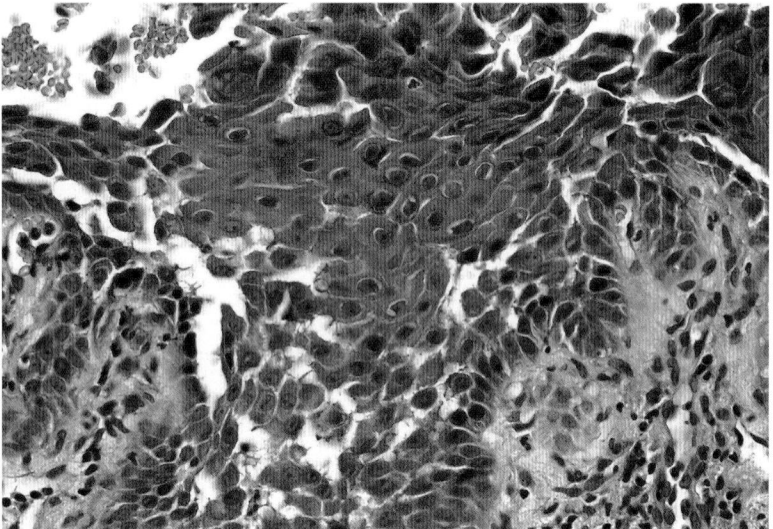

Fig. 5.81
Acantholytic acanthoma: high-power view showing acantholysis and dyskeratosis.

Diagnosis is one of exclusion and depends on the solitary nature of the lesion. The histologic features are those of hyperkeratosis, acanthosis, and papillomatosis accompanied by acantholysis affecting all or any layer of the epidermis (*Figs 5.80* and *5.81*).[1] Dyskeratosis may be evident. A perivascular lymphohistiocytic chronic inflammatory cell infiltrate, sometimes with occasional eosinophils, may be present in the superficial dermis.

Differential diagnosis

In acantholytic seborrheic keratosis, the acantholysis is typically focal and the lesion elsewhere shows the typical features of horn cysts and squamous eddies.[12] Darier disease, acantholytic dermatosis of the genitocrural area, warty dyskeratoma and pemphigus, Hailey-Hailey disease, and Grover disease may show similar histologic features but are easily distinguished clinically. Acantholytic actinic keratosis also shows dysplasia in addition to acantholysis.

Acantholytic dyskeratotic acanthoma

Clinical features

Acantholytic dyskeratotic acanthoma is a recently described entity with clinical features similar to acantholytic acanthoma. There is a predilection for the trunk of middle-aged to elderly adults with an equal gender distribution.[1] They are solitary lesions characteristically measuring less than 1 cm with a

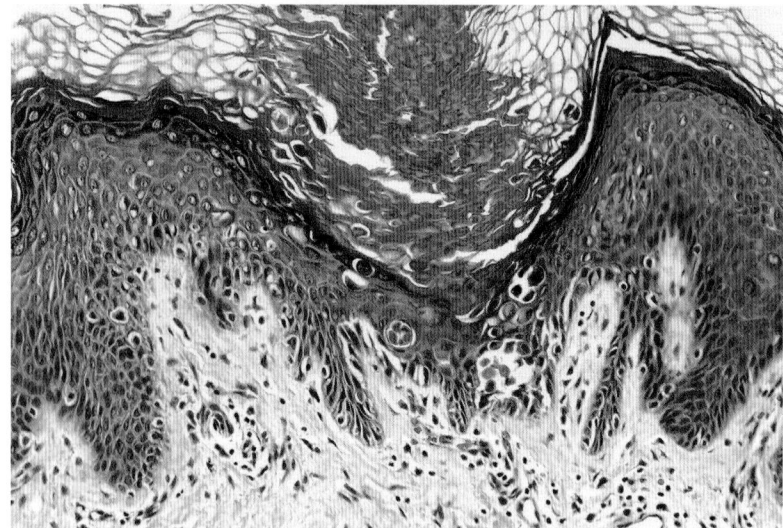

Fig. 5.82
Focal acantholytic dyskeratosis: this example showing the changes of Darier disease was an incidental finding adjacent to a completely unrelated lesion. There was no clinical evidence of Darier disease.

clinical impression of basal cell carcinoma, actinic keratosis, or squamous cell carcinoma in situ.[1,2,3] Rarely, they may present as a subungual lesion.[4]

Pathogenesis and histologic features

The pathogenesis of acantholytic dyskeratotic acanthoma is unknown.

Histologic characteristics include regular epidermal acanthosis showing acantholytic dyskeratosis with grains and corps ronds.[1-4] Acantholytic acanthosis is typically confluent, affecting varying levels of the epidermis. Occasionally, it may be confined to the granular and corneal layers or it may be nonconfluent and multifocal.[1] Cup-shaped endophytic growth and follicular involvement are not observed.

Differential diagnosis

Acantholytic dyskeratotic acanthoma differs from acantholytic acanthoma by the presence of marked dyskeratosis. Focal acantholytic dyskeratosis shows identical histologic features but is an incidental finding rather than a clinically distinct lesion. Warty dyskeratoma is characterized by its cup-shaped and endophytic growth. Pemphigus, Darier disease, and Grover disease differ in their clinical presentation.

Focal acantholytic dyskeratosis

Clinical features

By definition, this is an incidental histologic feature without a clinical correlate.

Pathogenesis and histologic features

Focal acantholytic dyskeratosis is a descriptive histopathological term referring to the finding of Darier-like features within the epidermis overlying or adjacent to an otherwise unrelated pathological lesion.[1-8] The pathogenesis is not known. The histologic features comprise hyperkeratosis, parakeratosis with suprabasal cleft formation, acantholysis, and dyskeratosis.[3] These changes may be seen in the overlying or adjacent epithelium in a variety of lesions, such as basal cell carcinoma, melanocytic nevi, chondrodermatitis nodularis helicis, malignant melanoma, dermatofibroma, condyloma acuminatum, trichofolliculoma, and as part of an epidermal nevus (*Fig. 5.82*). Focal acantholytic dyskeratosis has been described in a patient with pityriasis rubra pilaris and also in a patient with rosacea.[4,8] It has also been described in the oral cavity adjacent to squamous cell carcinoma.[9] It is important to recognize this as an incidental finding to avoid misdiagnosis as Darier disease.

Access **ExpertConsult**.com for the complete list of references

See
www.expertconsult.com
for references and
additional material

Spongiotic, psoriasiform and pustular dermatoses

ECZEMATOUS DERMATITIS

This chapter discusses a number of disorders under the rubric eczematous dermatitis, also called eczema and spongiotic dermatitis. The term eczema refers to a group of disorders that share similar clinical and histologic features but may have different etiologies. Some object to a diagnosis of eczema since it does not reflect a specific disease but is a non-specific term that simply can be used for any clinical lesion that exhibits spongiosis, which clinically manifests as moist, often 'bubbly' papules or plaques superimposed on an erythematous base. The pathogenesis of some forms is poorly understood. The histopathologist usually cannot render a more specific diagnosis other than 'spongiotic dermatitis consistent with eczematous dermatitis' and precise classification within the differential diagnosis of spongiotic dermatitis is often not possible. For these reasons, this class of disorders is discussed as a group. Distinguishing clinical, pathogenetic, and histologic features are presented in the appropriate sections.

Eczema – general considerations

Eczema encompasses a number of disorders with variable etiologies and clinical manifestations and is one of the most common complaints of patients visiting dermatology clinics.

The earliest clinical lesions are erythema and aggregates of tiny pruritic vesicles, which rupture readily, exuding clear fluid, and later become encrusted (*Fig. 6.1*). More chronic lesions become scaly and thickened (lichenification), resulting in lichen simplex chronicus (*Fig. 6.2*). Lichenification occurs if the skin is continually scratched or rubbed as, for example, in atopic dermatitis. Therefore, the clinical features of dermatitis depend upon the duration of the lesions, site(s) involved, and the amount of scratching.

For instance, in pompholyx (acute vesicular dermatitis of the hands and feet), the fluid is trapped beneath the thickened horny layer as small tense white blisters resembling rice grains. In other regions where the skin is loosely attached, as on the eyelids, scrotum, and backs of hands, tissue edema is often marked.

Eczematous dermatitis has two major etiological classifications:
- endogenous dermatitis, related to major constitutional or hereditary factors,
- exogenous dermatitis, involving environmental factors.

Endogenous dermatitis

Atopic dermatitis

Clinical features

Although atopic (infantile or flexural) dermatitis may begin at any age, it usually commences from about the sixth week onwards. It is characterized by a chronic, relapsing course.[1] In the infantile phase lesions are present mainly on the head, face, neck, napkin area, and extensor aspects of the limbs (*Fig. 6.3*). As the patient grows older and enters childhood, the eruption shifts to the flexural aspects of the limbs. Chronic atopic cheilitis may also be evident.[1] Pruritus is intense and constant scratching and rubbing leads to lichenification and frequent bouts of secondary bacterial infection (*Fig. 6.4*).[2,3] Atopic eczema is commonly associated with dry skin (xerosis). Vesiculation is uncommon. There is an increased risk of dermatophyte and viral infections.[1]

The disease improves during childhood, and in over 50% of cases clears completely by the early teens. Approximately 75% of patients with atopic dermatitis have a family history of atopy and up to 50% have associated asthma or hay fever.[4,5] The condition typically worsens in the winter months. It is associated with an increased incidence of contact dermatitis, particularly affecting the hands.[6] Other features that may be seen include

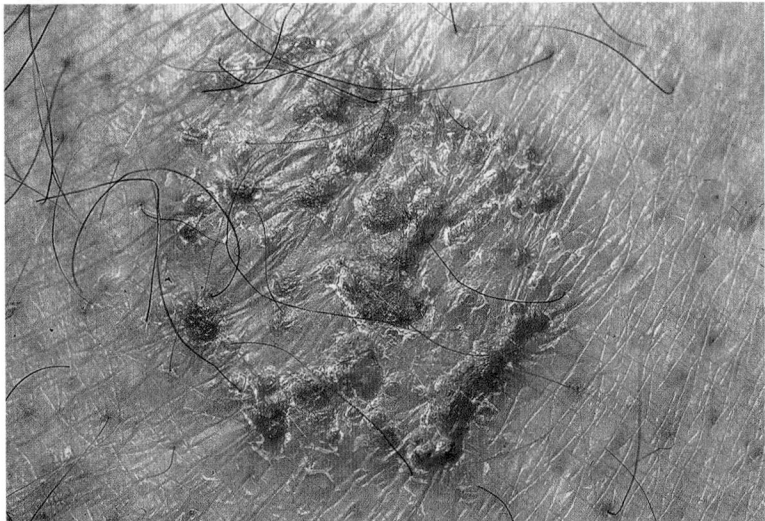

Fig. 6.1
Eczema: this is a plaque of discoid eczema. Small vesicles are present at the edge of the lesion. By courtesy of the Institute of Dermatology, London, UK.

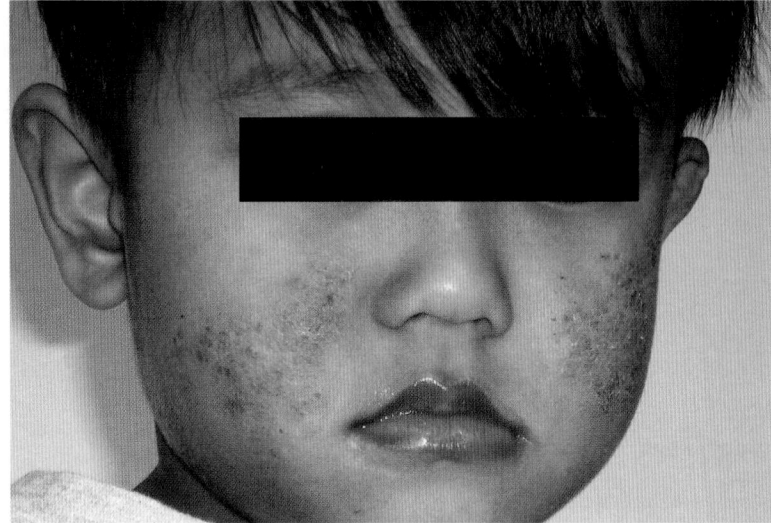

Fig. 6.3
Atopic dermatitis: lesions on the face and trunk are particularly seen in infants and young children. This child has bilateral involvement of the cheeks. By courtesy of J. Dayrit, MD, Manila, The Philippines.

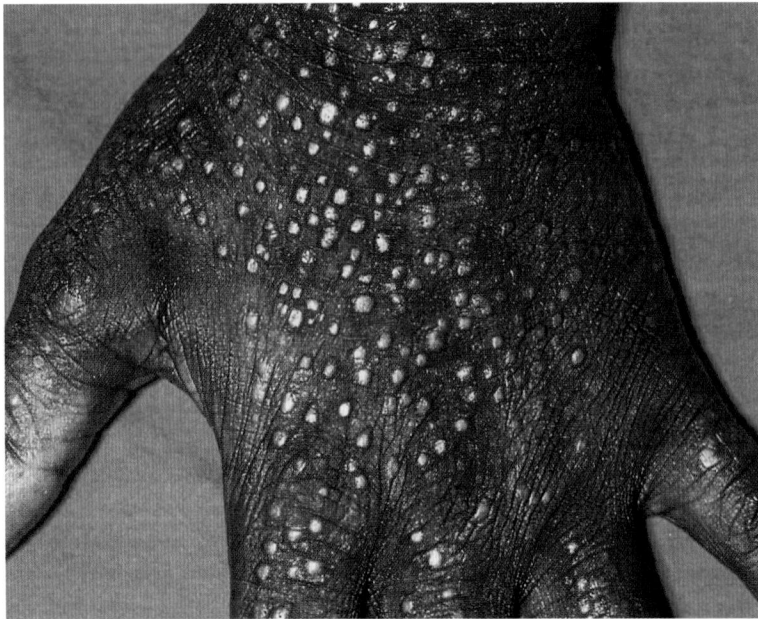

Fig. 6.2
Lichenification: pronounced pebbly lichenification on the dorsum of the hand of a patient with atopic dermatitis. Bizarre forms, as seen here, are not uncommon in black children. By courtesy of R.A. Marsden, MD, St George's Hospital, London, UK.

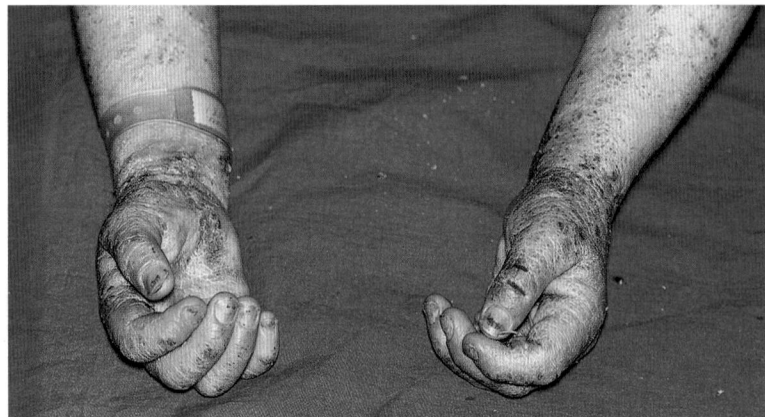

Fig. 6.4
Atopic dermatitis: these crusted, exudative and infected lesions with lichenification are characteristic. By courtesy of R.A. Marsden, MD, St George's Hospital, London, UK.

ichthyosis (50%), nipple eczema, conjunctivitis, keratoconus, bilateral anterior cataracts, sweat-associated itching, wool intolerance, perifollicular accentuation, food intolerance and white dermatographism.[5] Infraorbital folds (Dennie-Morgan folds) are said to be characteristic of atopic dermatitis, particularly when double.[1]

Pathogenesis

Atopy is defined as a genetically determined disorder encompassing dermatitis, asthma, and hay fever. It is associated with excess immunoglobulin E (IgE) antibody formation in response to common environmental antigens. A subset of patients with 'intrinsic atopic dermatitis' represents perhaps 10–30% of patients with atopy; this does not appear to be due to a response to an environmental antigen.[7] Atopic dermatitis is a multifactorial disease. Its pathogenesis is complex and, despite recent advances, only incompletely understood. In addition to a genetic susceptibility, the main elements responsible for the initiation and maintenance of the disease state include abnormal skin barrier function, and abnormal activity of the innate and adaptive immune systems, as well as environmental factors and infectious agents.[7-15]

Since patients with atopic dermatitis often have a personal or family history of asthma or allergies, a genetic predisposition to the disease has long been suspected. Studies have demonstrated that loss-of-function mutations in the *FLG* gene, encoding the cornified envelope protein profilaggrin, are present in a significant subset of patients with atopic dermatitis and represent the highest risk factor for development of the disease.[16] Together with involucrin and loricrin, filaggrin is a major constituent of the cornified envelope during terminal keratinocyte differentiation responsible for intact epidermal barrier function. Disruption of the skin barrier function appears to be of particular significance in the initiation and early stages of the disease. Nevertheless, 40% of patients with *FLG* mutations never develop atopic dermatitis and *FLG* mutations have been identified in only 14–56% of patients, indicating that other factors may also play an important role in the pathogenesis of the disease. In addition to the cornified envelope, epidermal barrier function is maintained also by other factors such as proteases and protease inhibitors as well as direct keratinocyte–keratinocyte interaction. Increased expression of kallikrein-related peptidases has been observed in the stratum corneum in atopic dermatitis and in one study a 4-bp insertion into the 3′ untranslated region of KLF7 leading to increased levels of this protease was identified in patients with atopic dermatitis.[13,17,18] However, this finding has not been substantiated in further studies.[13] Linkage has also been demonstrated to the gene SPINK5, encoding the serine protease inhibitor LEKTI. LEKTI, expressed at the granular cell layer, is an important inhibitor of the kallikrein-related peptidases KLK5 and KLK7 and is responsible for controlling desquamation. Linkage to SPINK5 is, however, significantly weaker than to profilaggrin.[13] A further mechanism involved in skin barrier function is the presence of intercellular junctions, and data have demonstrated reduced expression of the tight junction protein claudin-1 in atopic dermatitis.[15]

Many lines of evidence also implicate an abnormal immune response as pivotal in the pathogenesis of atopy. It is interesting to note that atopy is cured by bone marrow transplantation in patients with Wiskott-Aldrich syndrome, an immunological disorder characterized by susceptibility to infection and thrombocytopenia, in addition to eczematous dermatitis.[19] Wiskott-Aldrich syndrome shows an X-linked recessive pattern of inheritance and is characterized by depletion of nodal and circulating T lymphocytes. Contrariwise, patients without a prior history of atopy may develop atopic disease following transplantation of bone marrow from an atopic individual.[20]

Patients with atopic dermatitis have an abnormal immune reaction to a variety of environmental antigens leading to production of IgE antibodies and a T-cell response.[9,21–23] There is evidence that certain subpopulations of T cells selectively circulate to and perform immune surveillance for the skin and lymph nodes that drain cutaneous sites.[9,23] This subset of lymphocytes is characterized by a unique immunophenotype and is defined by expression of cutaneous lymphocyte antigen (CLA). In patients with atopic dermatitis, antigens such as dust mites and bacteria activate CLA T cells, resulting in the production of cytokines, which stimulate eosinophils to produce IgE, which, in turn, promotes mast cells and basophils to release cytokines and chemotactic factors in what has been termed the intermediate-phase response.[8] The so-called late-phase reaction is characterized by migration of eosinophils, lymphocytes, histiocytes, and neutrophils from the circulation into the dermis and epidermis.

Factors released by the various cells present in the dermis certainly play a role in the generation of the clinical appearance and induction of pruritus, leading to scratching and rubbing. In the early phase, mechanical trauma and skin barrier disruption lead to release of proinflammatory cytokines (IL-1α, IL-1β, TNF-α, GM-CSF) which activate cellular signaling and induce expression of vascular endothelial cell adhesion molecules after receptor binding to endothelial cells.[15,24,25] These steps subsequently initiate transvascular migration of inflammatory cells.[8,26] Chemokines released by inflammatory cells attract a more directed cellular immune response. In particular, CCL27, CCL22, and CCL17 are increased in patients with atopic dermatitis and levels correlate with disease activity.[14,25] Disease onset is related to Th2 cytokines IL-4, IL-5, IL-13, and IL-31, and gene variants in IL-4, IL-13, the IL-4 receptor and IL-31 have been linked to the disease.[27] In addition, the expression of thymic stromal lymphopoietin (TSLP), an IL-7-like cytokine promoting a Th2 immunoresponse, is increased in atopic dermatitis, and polymorphisms in TSLP and its receptor, the IL-7 receptor, have been linked to the disease.[27–29] Disease maintenance (chronic phase) is associated with Th1 cytokines. Other T cells, such as T$_{reg}$ and Th17, are also present in cutaneous lesions but their precise role is uncertain.[14] The demonstration that squamous cells in patients with atopic dermatitis show increased production of GM-CSF, a cytokine thought to play a role in Langerhans/dendritic cell function, further suggests that a keratinocyte defect may be involved in the pathogenesis of atopy.[30]

Another area of interest has been the role of superantigens in the pathogenesis of atopy as well as other immunologically mediated cutaneous and noncutaneous disorders.[31–36] Although superantigens have been implicated in the pathogenesis of psoriasis and Kawasaki disease, in addition to atopic dermatitis, their precise role in these and other diseases is not well understood and is controversial.[32,33] Further research is necessary to clarify the role of superantigens in immunologically mediated diseases.

Superantigens are microbiological (viral, bacterial, fungal) toxins that stimulate CD4+ T cells. They bind to T-cell receptors and to the class II major histocompatibility complex (MHC), thus stimulating lymphocyte proliferation, activation and release of cytokines, as well as T-cell-mediated tissue damage. They may also stimulate B cell activation. Superantigens are powerful mediators of the immune system by virtue of their ability to stimulate a large population of T cells in a non-specific manner. Staphylococcal superantigens have, in particular, been an area of research.[35] The skin of most patients with atopic dermatitis is colonized with *Staphylococcus aureus*. In contrast, *S. aureus* is found on the skin of only a minority of control subjects.[36] Disease severity has been shown to correlate with the presence of toxigenic *S. aureus*.[37] It is thought that staphylococcal superantigens SEA and SEB (staphylococcal enterotoxins A and B, respectively) activate T cells.[37–40] In a study of children with atopic dermatitis, there was a correlation of disease severity and presence of SEA and SEB antibodies.[38] A study has shown that application of SEB is associated with T-cell activation in both normal and atopic patients.[41] In summary, there is mounting evidence that staphylococcal superantigens play a role in the symptomatology of atopic dermatitis. Whether superantigens play a key role in the development of disease or simply exacerbate symptoms in atopic patients requires further study.

Seborrheic dermatitis

Clinical features

Seborrheic dermatitis is a common dermatosis which affects up to 1–3% of the population.[1–3] There is a male predominance. It presents in infants, with a second peak affecting adults.[4] There is often a family history of the disease. It particularly affects those areas where sebaceous glands are most numerous, i.e., the scalp, forehead, eyebrows, eyelids, ears, cheeks, presternal and interscapular areas (*Figs 6.5* and *6.6*).[5] Occasionally, the flexural regions are affected (intertrigo). Often the lesions of seborrheic dermatitis are sharply marginated, dull red or yellowish, and covered by a greasy scale.[5] They are therefore easily confused with psoriasis.

Dandruff and cradle cap are also sometimes included within the spectrum of seborrheic dermatitis.

Seborrheic dermatitis is one of the most common dermatoses seen in patients with acquired immunodeficiency syndrome (AIDS). Seborrheic dermatitis has also been associated with stress and neurological disorders including Parkinson disease, syringomyelia, and trigeminal nerve injury.[6]

Pathogenesis

The precise pathogenesis of this condition is unknown. Surprisingly, and in spite of the distribution (and the name) of the disease, sebaceous gland activity and sebum composition appear to be normal.[6]

Seborrheic dermatitis is associated with heavy colonization of the skin by the lipophilic yeast *Malassezia furfur* (*Pityrosporum ovale*) while more

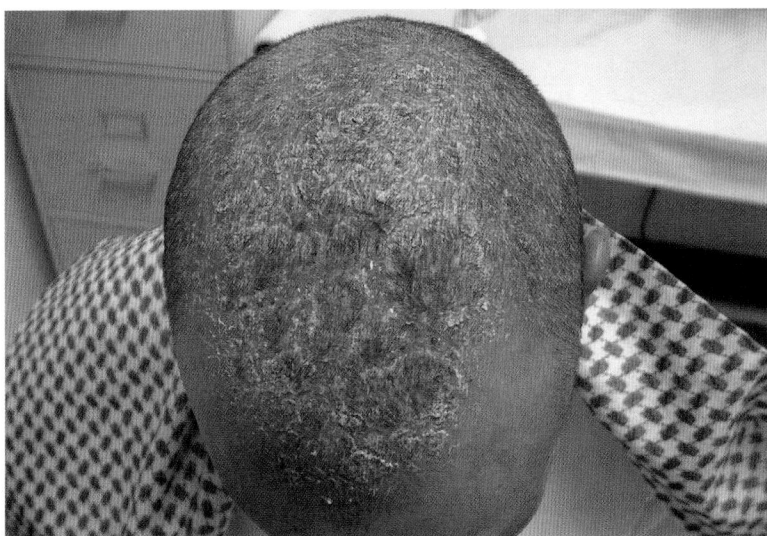

Fig. 6.5
Seborrheic dermatitis: there is diffuse erythema and scaling of the scalp. By courtesy of B. Al Mahmoud, MD, Doha, Qatar.

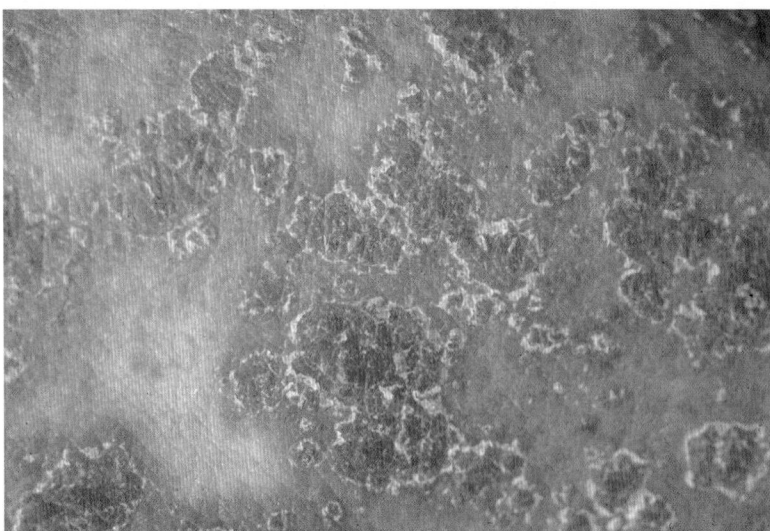

Fig. 6.6
Seborrheic dermatitis: note the marked scaling. By courtesy of the Institute of
Dermatology, London, UK.

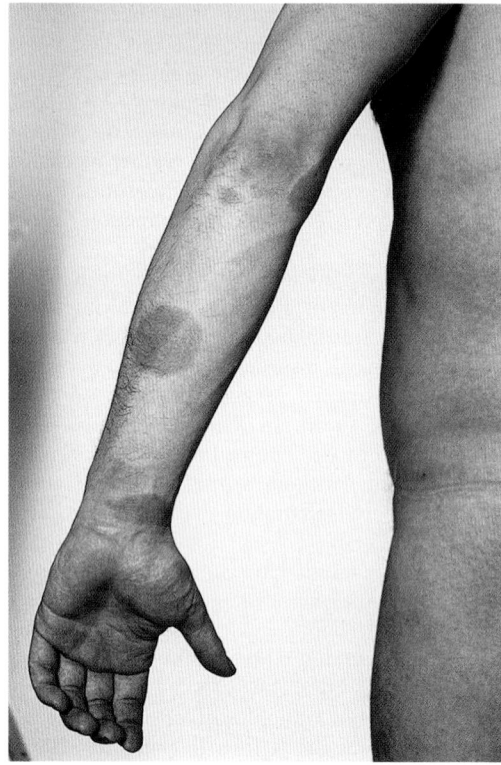

Fig. 6.7
Discoid eczema: circumscribed, erythematous lesions on the forearm, a
characteristic site. By courtesy of the Institute of Dermatology, London, UK.

recent data have identified a predominance of *Malassezia restricta* and
Malassezia globosa.[3,7–12] Although many workers in the field believe this to
be of etiological importance, an almost equal number are unconvinced. The
body of evidence favoring a significant relationship relates to the successful
treatment of seborrheic dermatitis with antifungal therapy.[1,2,13] Whether this
implies a causal relationship or merely an exacerbating factor is, however,
uncertain.

Discoid dermatitis (nummular eczema)

Clinical features

The presence of single or multiple pruritic, coin-shaped, erythematous
plaques with vesiculation, particularly involving the lower legs, forearms,
and backs of hands (*Figs 6.7–6.9*) characterize this chronic form of dermatitis.[1] The absence of a raised border clinically distinguishes it from ringworm.[1] There are two peak ages of onset: it affects young women (15–30
years of age) and middle-aged adults of both sexes. The disease tends to
chronicity.

Pathogenesis

The pathogenesis is poorly understood. A participatory role for organisms in the pathogenesis has been suggested but not been widely accepted.[2]
Discoid dermatitis may follow irritants such as soap, acids or alkalis (*Fig.
6.10*).[1] Sometimes it may be a manifestation of atopy and, occasionally, it
develops as a consequence of nickel, chromate or cobalt allergy.[3,4] Generalized disease has also been documented in the setting of interferon alpha-2b
plus ribavirin treatment for hepatitis C infection.[5]

Hand eczema (dyshidrotic eczema, palmoplantar eczema, pompholyx)

Clinical features

Hand eczema is characterized by a recurrent pruritic vesicular eruption of
the palms, soles or digits. Because of the increased thickness of the keratin
layer at these sites, the vesicles appear as small pale papules before rupturing (*Figs 6.11* and *6.12*). Occasionally, frank bullae can form. With the
passage of time, the affected parts may show scaling and cracking. The nails
sometimes become dystrophic, with discoloration and transverse ridging.[1] In
the majority of cases the cause is unknown, although heat or psychological
stress may precipitate an attack.[1] In some patients there is a personal or

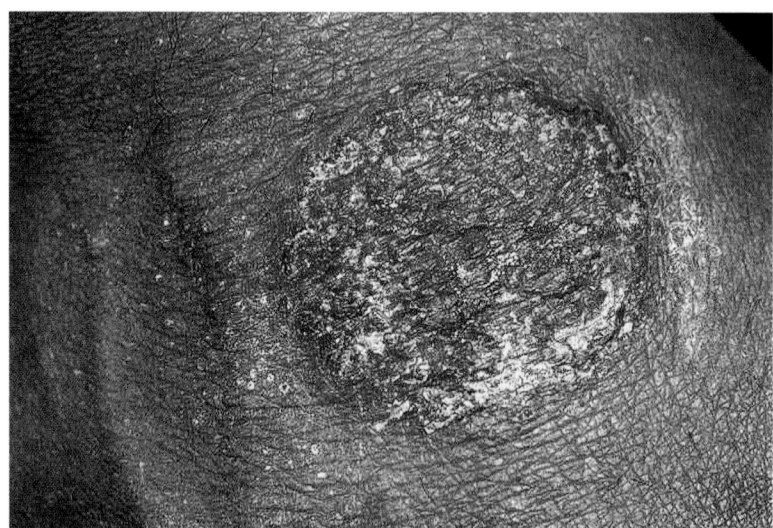

Fig. 6.8
Discoid eczema: the lesion is sharply defined and there is a pronounced scale. By
courtesy of the Institute of Dermatology, London, UK.

family history of atopy or coexisting tinea pedis. Rubber, latex, chromium,
cobalt or nickel sensitivity may be the trigger.[2–6] The condition can be exacerbated by heat and, rarely, it is photoinduced.[7]

Pompholyx is often associated with hyperhidrosis.[2] Females are
affected slightly more often than males and patients are predominantly
in the second to fifth decades.[3] A familial autosomal dominant form has
been reported where the candidate gene has been mapped to chromosome
18q22.1-18q22.3.[8]

Pathogenesis

The pathogenesis is obscure. It has been noted that serum IgE levels are
often raised.[2]

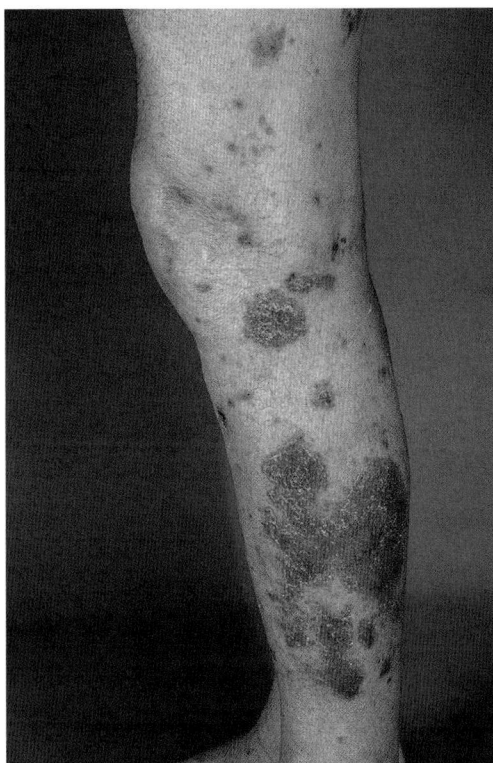

Fig. 6.9
Discoid eczema: there is extensive involvement of the leg. A sharply demarcated erythematous and scaly circular lesion is present just below the knee. By courtesy of R.A. Marsden, St George's Hospital, London, UK.

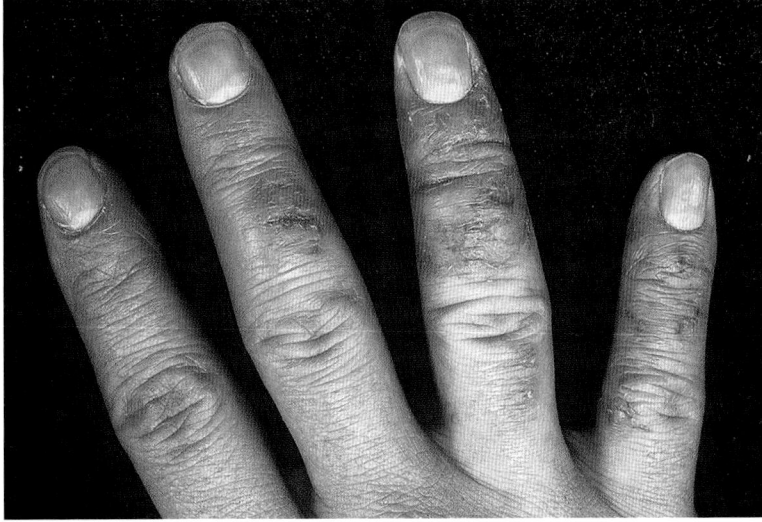

Fig. 6.10
Discoid eczema: lesions localized to the fingers most often represent a contact irritant reaction. By courtesy of R.A. Marsden, St George's Hospital, London, UK.

Autosensitization (Id) reaction

Clinical features

On occasion, patients will develop generalized spongiotic dermatitis in response to a dermatosis or infection at a distant site. The eczematous dermatitis resolves if the underlying infection or specific dermatosis is successfully treated. This phenomenon has also been designated an autoeczematization or Id reaction. The lesions that characterize the Id reaction may be a localized pompholyx-like eczematous dermatitis of the hands and feet or scattered papules on the trunk and limbs.[1-5] Disorders that may be associated with the Id reaction include fungal infection (e.g., dermatophyte infection), scabies infestation, molluscum contagiosum, tick bite, pediculosis

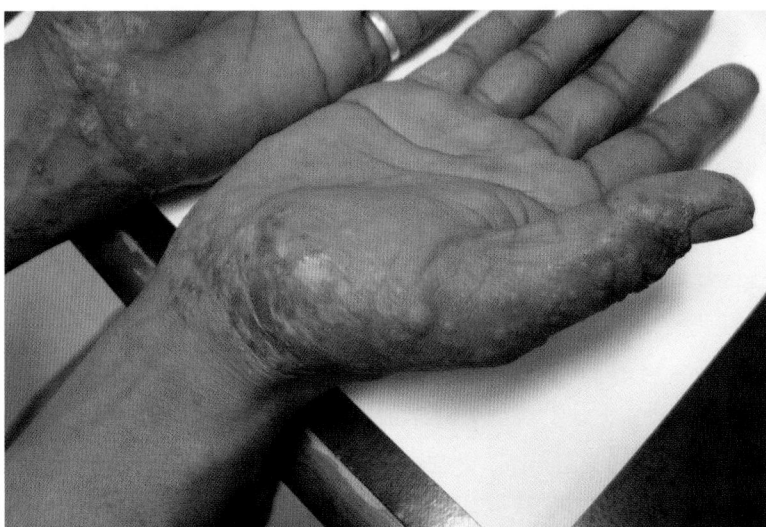

Fig. 6.11
Hand eczema: tense yellow vesicles are present. By courtesy of B. Al Mahmoud, MD, Doha, Qatar.

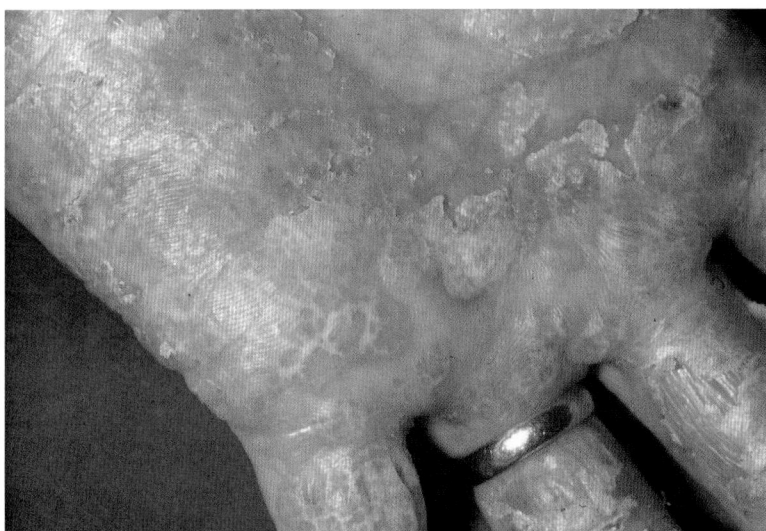

Fig. 6.12
Hand eczema: more chronic example showing marked scaling. From the collection of the late N.P. Smith, MD, the Institute of Dermatology, London, UK.

capitis, and bacterial and mycobacterial infections.[1-5] A generalized nummular dermatitis has been reported in association with localized dental infection.[6]

Pathogenesis

The pathogenesis of the Id reaction is poorly understood but some data suggest that an abnormal T-cell-mediated immune response directed against skin antigens is responsible for this curious disorder.[7]

Exogenous dermatitis

Contact dermatitis

This form of dermatitis is due to external agents and is divided into two variants: allergic contact and irritant contact.

Allergic contact dermatitis

Allergic contact dermatitis is an idiosyncratic cell-mediated immunological reaction to an environmental allergen, which may be present in very low concentration. Common examples seen in clinical practice include sensitivity to nickel (found in items such as jewelry, buttons, watches, and suspenders),

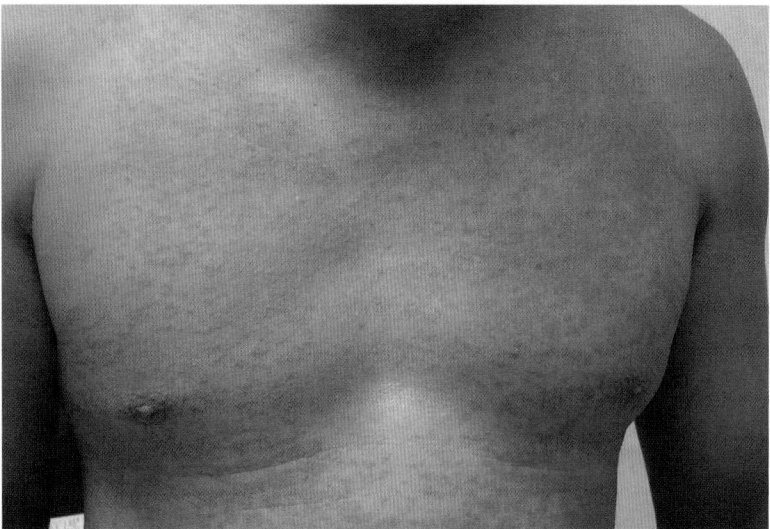

Fig. 6.13
Contact dermatitis: this early erythematous predominantly macular eruption developed as a reaction to fabric softener. By courtesy of J. Dayrit, MD, Manila, The Philippines.

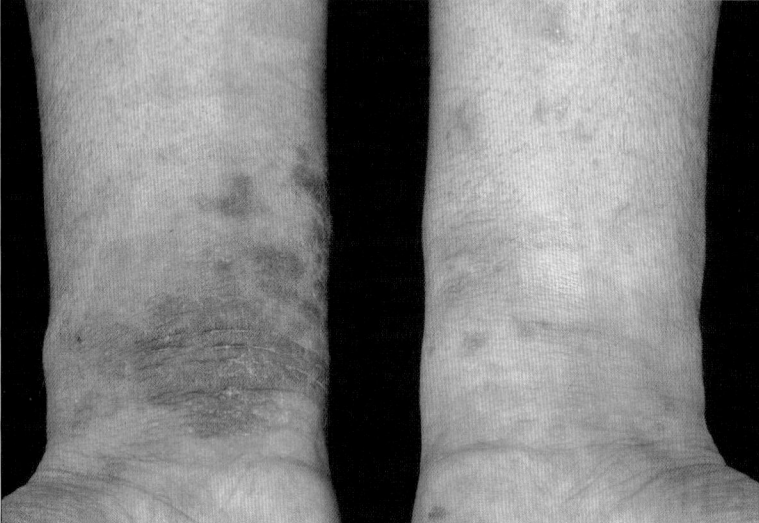

Fig. 6.14
Contact dermatitis: bilateral involvement in a patient using a watch on the right wrist and a leather bracelet on the left wrist. From the collection of the late N.P. Smith, MD, the Institute of Dermatology, London, UK.

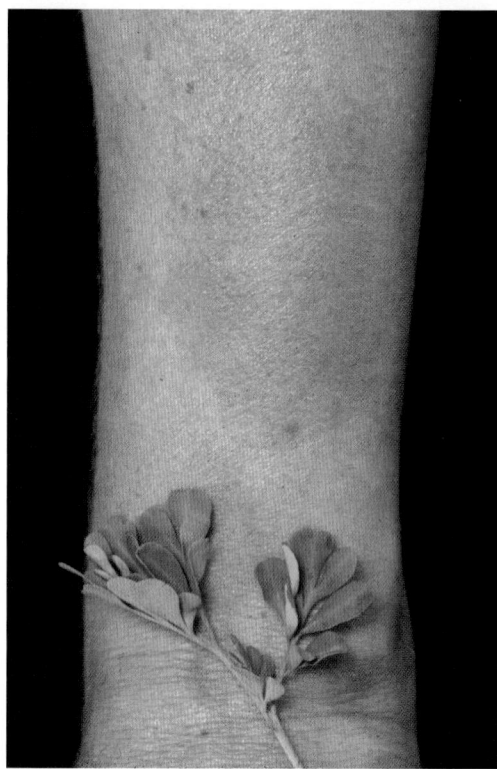

Fig. 6.15
Contact dermatitis: a severe reaction to poison ivy. From the collection of the late N.P. Smith, MD, the Institute of Dermatology, London, UK.

sites.[21] CLA-positive T cells proliferate when stimulated by the appropriate antigen or antigen–protein complex. The number of CLA-positive memory T cells increases with repeated exposures to its antigen.[1,14] When the patient is exposed to the antigen, the elicitation phase, the CLA-positive T cells are activated and release cytokines which lead to the immune reaction responsible for the clinical and histologic features associated with allergic contact dermatitis.[16] CD8+ T cells appear to be the main effector cell in the elicitation phase.[18] Keratinocytes are also thought to play a role through the release of cytokines after hapten exposure and binding.[17]

Occasionally, exposure to strong haptens may result in the development of allergic contact dermatitis in previously unsensitized individuals (primary allergic contact dermatitis).[18]

Ingested or inhaled allergens in a person who has been previously sensitized by cutaneous absorption may result in a clinical picture similar to allergic contact dermatitis (e.g., ingested nickel, chromium, or cobalt may result in the appearances of hand eczema).[22] Much less commonly, systemic allergic contact dermatitis may be histologically associated with an erythema multiforme-like eruption, vasculitis, or urticarial morphology.[22] This is thought to result from systemic exposure of a hapten via hematogenous transport to the skin.[23] It may occur with or without prior sensitization, and a large number of drugs have been implicated in the pathogenesis.[23]

Irritant contact dermatitis

Irritant contact dermatitis, which is much more common than allergic contact dermatitis, follows exposure to physical or chemical substances capable of direct damage to the skin. Mechanisms of damage are variable and include keratin denaturation, removal of surface lipids and water-holding substances, damage to cell membranes, and/or direct cytotoxic effects.[24] Acute irritant dermatitis usually results from a relatively short single exposure to a potent irritant, such as strong acid or alkali, whereas chronic cumulative insult or 'wear and tear' dermatitis is due to more prolonged contact with one or more weaker irritants, for example, soap and water, detergents or industrial oil, and plants (Fig. 6.16).[25–29]

Most forms of occupational dermatitis of the hands, including 'housewives' and 'wedding ring' dermatitis are of the irritant contact type. A diagnosis of contact dermatitis is made from the history and distribution of

constituents of synthetic rubber (e.g., thiuram in rubber gloves), primula, poison ivy, topical medicaments (e.g., neomycin, antihistamines, local anesthetics), and chromates found in cement and leather (Figs 6.13–6.15).[1–11]

Dinitrochlorobenzene (DNCB) is a potent contact sensitizer and this is used as a test of cell-mediated immunity.[12,13]

A growing understanding of allergic contact dermatitis has emerged in recent decades with the preponderance of evidence pointing to a T-cell-mediated hypersensitivity reaction.[1,14–17] It is thought that antigens causing allergic contact dermatitis are often unstable (haptens) and need to bind to epidermal host proteins.[1,14] These hapten–protein interactions are formed via covalent binding of electrophilic residues of the chemical with amino acids, especially cysteine.[18–20] In contrast, metal ions, such as nickel, are thought to form noncovalent protein–metal chelate complexes.[18] In the sensitization/initiation phase of the disease, hapten-specific T cells are generated in lymph nodes after the initial contact of the skin with a potent hapten.[20] Langerhans cells in skin and dendritic cells in lymph nodes process antigen and stimulate appropriate naive CLA T cells. CLA-positive T cells are a subset of T cells that express a skin-selective homing receptor and perform immune surveillance for the skin and lymph nodes that drain cutaneous

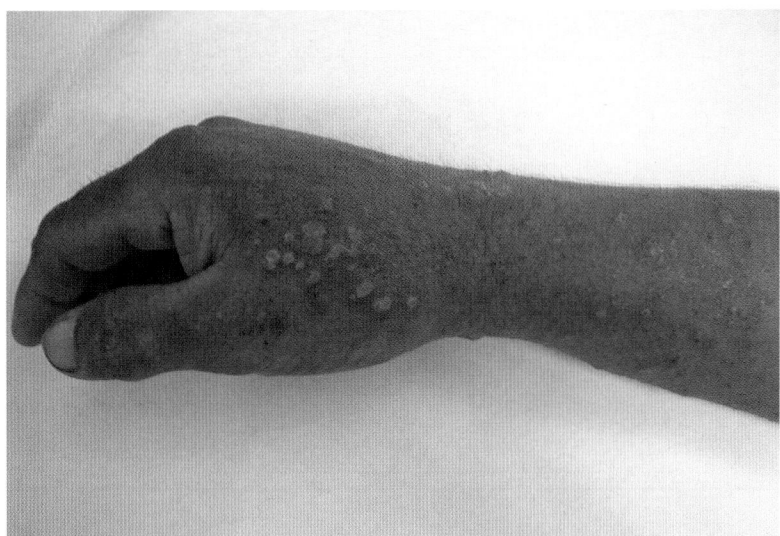

Fig. 6.16
Contact dermatitis: there is a superimposed pustular element due to an infection in this patient with a contact reaction to a domestic antiseptic. By courtesy of B. Al Mahmoud, MD, Doha, Qatar.

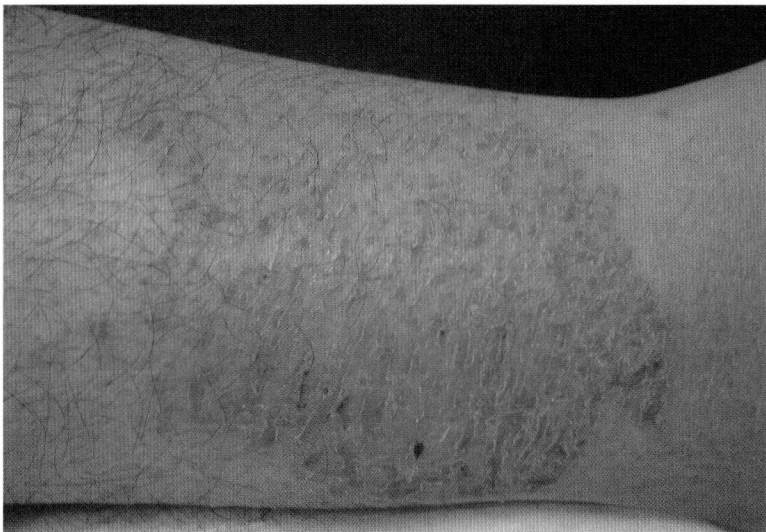

Fig. 6.18
Asteatotic dermatitis: these typical appearances are the result of scaling and fissuring. By courtesy of B. Al Mahmoud, MD, Doha, Qatar.

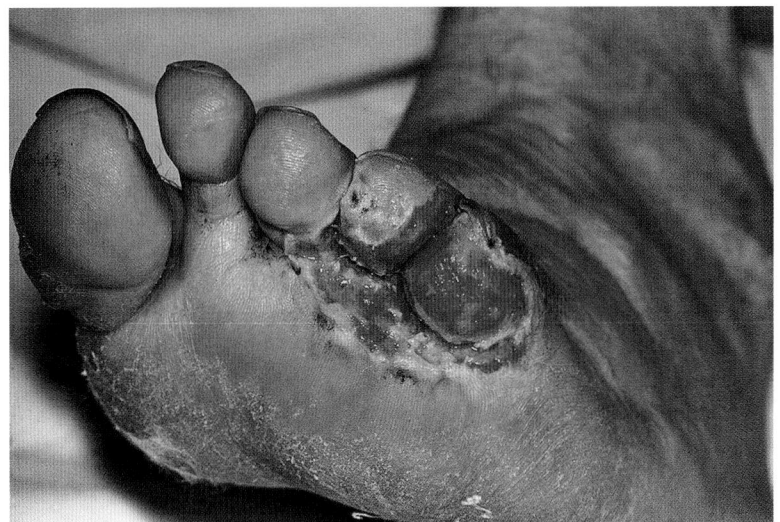

Fig. 6.17
Infective dermatitis: lesions affecting the foot web spaces are often due to staphylococci or streptococci and are associated with excess sweating. By courtesy of R.A. Marsden, MD, St George's Hospital, London, UK.

lesions and, in the case of allergic dermatitis, is confirmed by patch testing to the suspected allergen. Although both forms of contact dermatitis tend to be confined to exposed areas, the reaction may eventually spread to involve nonexposed sites and can persist even when the causative agent is removed from the environment.

Similar to atopic dermatitis, loss-of-function mutation in the *FLG* gene encoding filaggrin, may confer an increased susceptibility to chronic irritant contact dermatitis evoking an underlying skin barrier defect in the pathogenesis of the disease.[30]

Infective dermatitis

Infective dermatitis is a severe chronic and recurrent eczematous dermatitis showing pronounced exudation and crusting and presenting in children with human T-cell lymphotropic virus type 1 (HTLV-1) infection.[1–6] Adult onset is exceptional.[7–9] The disease has a predilection for the scalp, flexures, the ears and feet, and sometimes around wounds and ulcers (*Fig. 6.17*), and is frequently associated with *Staphylococcus aureus* and beta-hemolytic *Streptococcus* infection of the skin and nasal vestibule. It occurs in regions

where HTLV-1 is endemic. It has frequently been reported in Jamaica, while presentation in Japan appears relatively rare.[10] Development of the disease may be associated with a defective immune system and may be a risk factor for the development of other HTLV-1-related diseases, such as adult T-cell leukemia and tropical spastic paraparesis.[11,12]

Asteatotic dermatitis

Commonly seen in the elderly, particularly in winter and in those with minor degrees of ichthyosis, asteatotic dermatitis (eczema craquelé) may be precipitated by excessive washing, exposure to detergents, cold winds, or low humidity, all of which tend to dry the skin.[1] The affected regions are inflamed and criss-crossed by scaly lines and superficial fissures (*Fig. 6.18*). Asteatotic dermatitis may be associated with internal malignancy, including lymphoproliferative disorders and solid tumors.[2–5]

Histologic features of spongiotic dermatitis

The histopathological features of spongiotic dermatitis include both dermal and epidermal changes. Their relative proportions vary to some extent with the subtype, but perhaps more importantly, with the stage of evolution of the disease. It is essential not to consider the changes of spongiotic dermatitis as static: different features are seen at different stages.[1–3] Attempting to distinguish the various clinical subtypes based on histologic features alone is generally futile. Instead, once the disorder has been recognized as spongiotic in nature, clinical examination is a much more satisfactory method of determining the particular variant.

The histologic hallmark of spongiotic dermatitis is the presence of intercellular edema or spongiosis (L., Gr. *spongia*, sponge). Slight degrees of intracellular edema may also be evident but may easily be overlooked. In the early stages of development, spongiosis results in widening of the intercellular spaces, rendering the intercellular bridges conspicuous (*Fig. 6.19*). Further accumulation of fluid leads to the eventual development of an intraepidermal vesicle. A common finding in association with the intercellular edema is lymphocytic infiltration of the epidermis (exocytosis). In severe contact irritant dermatitis, the epidermis may be infiltrated by large numbers of neutrophil polymorphs in association with necrotic keratinocytes.[4] In addition, such reactions may be accompanied by dermal–epidermal separation resulting in a vesicle or blister. The lesions very often become traumatized and may show marked crusting.

Spongiotic dermatitides not uncommonly become infected with bacterial or fungal organisms. Superimposed infection may dramatically alter the histologic picture by causing marked acute inflammation with subepidermal, intraepidermal, and subcorneal pustules. Such changes may dominate the

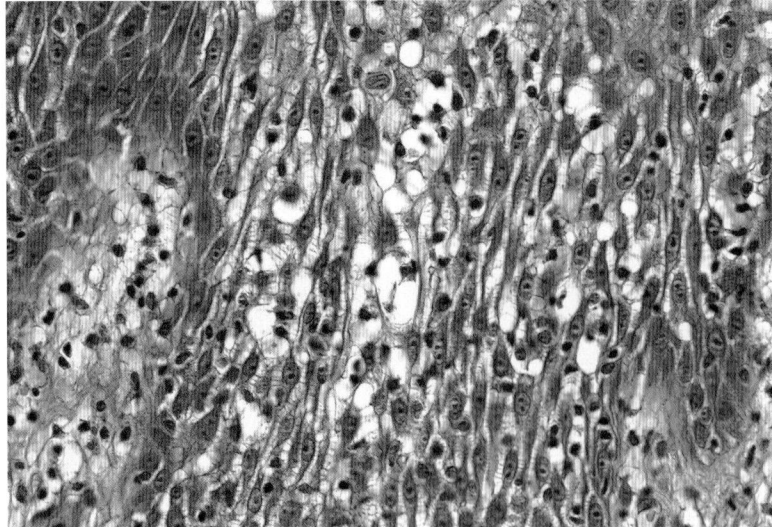

Fig. 6.19
Dermatitis: the earliest visible manifestation of intercellular edema is widening of the intercellular spaces with accentuation of the intercellular bridges.

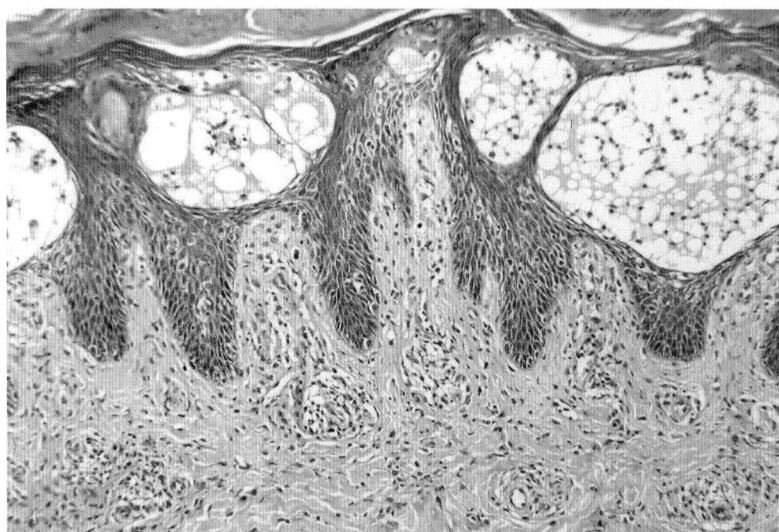

Fig. 6.20
Acute dermatitis: fluid-filled vesicle due to intense spongiosis.

histologic picture and obscure the underlying spongiotic dermatitis. Use of stains for organisms – Gram, periodic acid-Schiff (PAS) – or cultures are necessary to evaluate for infection.

Concomitant with these changes are varying degrees of epithelial proliferation, ranging from mild acanthosis in early acute dermatitis to marked psoriasiform epidermal hyperplasia in chronic variants. Parakeratosis is frequently seen overlying spongiotic foci, while hyperkeratosis is a usual accompaniment of chronic spongiotic dermatitis that has been scratched or rubbed (lichenification).

The dermis is often congested and edema is usually marked in active lesions. The vessels of the superficial vascular plexus are surrounded by a mixed inflammatory cell infiltrate composed of lymphocytes, histiocytes, and occasional eosinophils or neutrophils. The degree and composition of dermal inflammation is highly variable. Eosinophils may be numerous in allergic contact dermatitis.[4]

Traditionally, spongiotic dermatitis is subclassified histologically into acute, subacute, and chronic variants:

- In acute lesions, vesiculation and blister formation may be seen (*Figs 6.20–6.22*).
- Acanthosis and spongiosis, often with vesiculation, also characterize subacute spongiotic dermatitis (*Fig. 6.23*).
- In chronic spongiotic dermatitis, although spongiosis is evident, it may be subtle, and vesicles are uncommon. Epithelial acanthosis is marked and often shows a psoriasiform pattern (*Fig. 6.24*).

Systemic contact dermatitis may be associated with the features of vasculitis (leukocytoclastic) or erythema multiforme.[5] As with other forms of spongiotic dermatitis the histologic appearances can be divided into acute, subacute, and chronic forms. Spongiosis is more conspicuous in the acute phase although it is never marked. In contrast, the epidermal hyperplasia becomes more conspicuous and psoriasiform towards the chronic end of the spectrum.

The features of seborrheic dermatitis are often non-specific and subtle. It is characterized by hyperkeratosis and parakeratosis, the latter particularly related to hair follicles and typically associated with neutrophil exocytosis (*Figs 6.25 and 6.26*). Yeasts may sometimes be found in the stratum corneum particularly if PAS stained sections are examined. Epidermal acanthosis with thickened rete ridges is present and, although mild, may be marked in chronic lesions. It is, however, somewhat irregular in contrast to the uniform hyperplasia characteristic of psoriasis. Variable spongiosis with lymphocyte exocytosis is common. The dermis may be edematous and mild vascular dilatation is usually seen. A mixed inflammatory cell infiltrate consisting of lymphocytes, histiocytes, and small numbers of eosinophils surrounds the superficial vascular plexus.

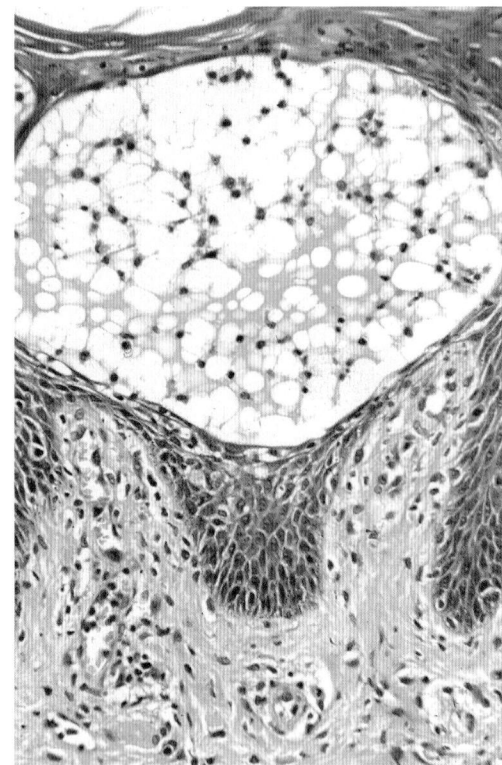

Fig. 6.21
Acute dermatitis: the vesicle contains lymphocytes and occasional eosinophils.

Differential diagnosis

Although spongiosis is a characteristic feature of spongiotic dermatitis, it is also encountered in many other inflammatory dermatoses (*Table 6.1*), particularly superficial dermatophytoses. A diagnosis of spongiotic dermatitis should never be made until a stain for fungus (e.g., PAS reaction) has been performed to exclude this possibility. This is especially important since the common treatment of spongiotic dermatitides – topical corticosteroids – would exacerbate a fungal infection (tinea incognito) (*Figs 6.27–6.29*).

Lichen simplex chronicus

Clinical features

The term lichen simplex chronicus (circumscribed neurodermatitis) refers to the development of localized areas of thickened scaly skin complicating

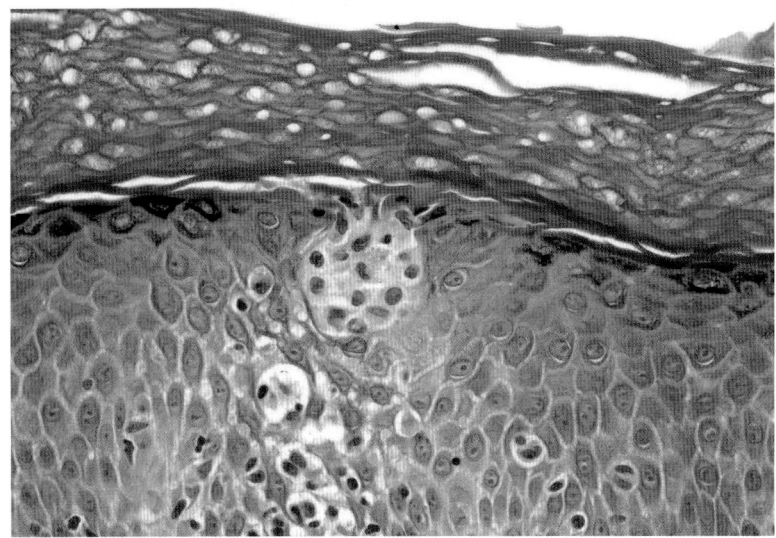

Fig. 6.22
Acute dermatitis: in contact reactions, Langerhans cell-rich vesicles are often present, as shown in this picture. These should not be mistaken for the Pautrier microabscesses of mycosis fungoides.

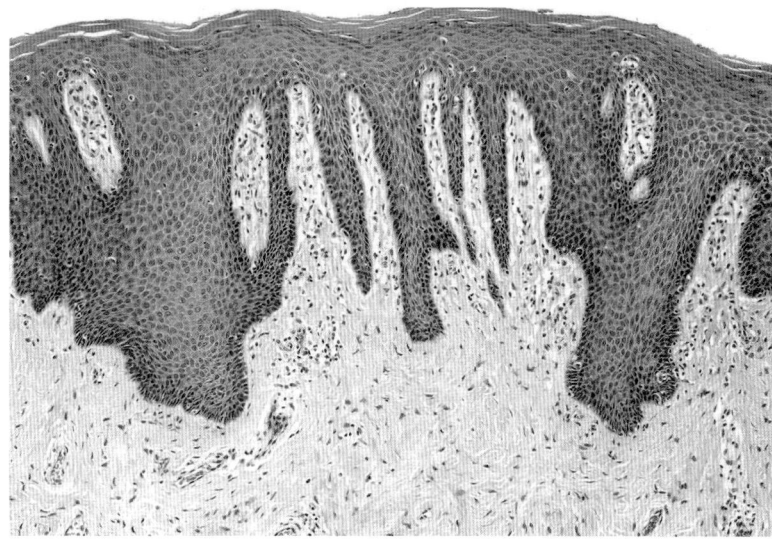

Fig. 6.24
Chronic dermatitis (lichenification): there is hyperkeratosis with hypergranulosis and psoriasiform hyperplasia. The papillary dermis is fibrosed and there is a patchy chronic inflammatory cell infiltrate.

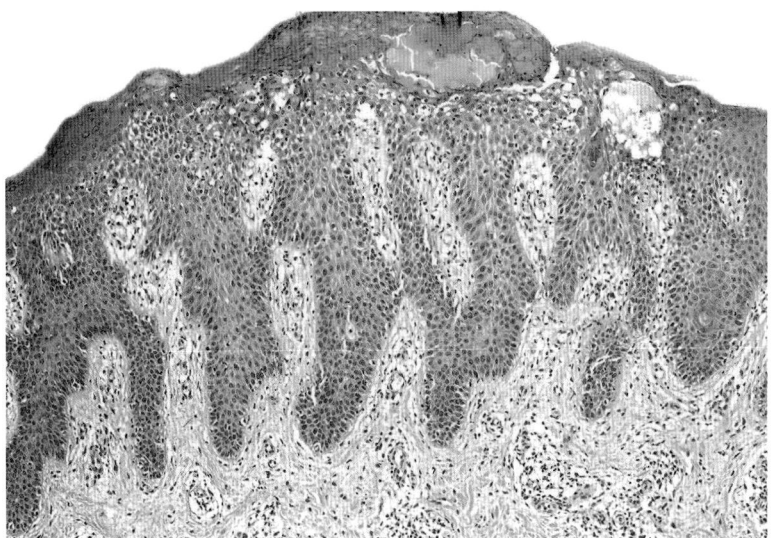

Fig. 6.23
Subacute dermatitis showing patchy parakeratosis, crusting, marked acanthosis with considerable elongation (and fusion) of the epidermal ridges, and focal spongiotic vesiculation. The dermis contains an intense lymphocytic infiltrate.

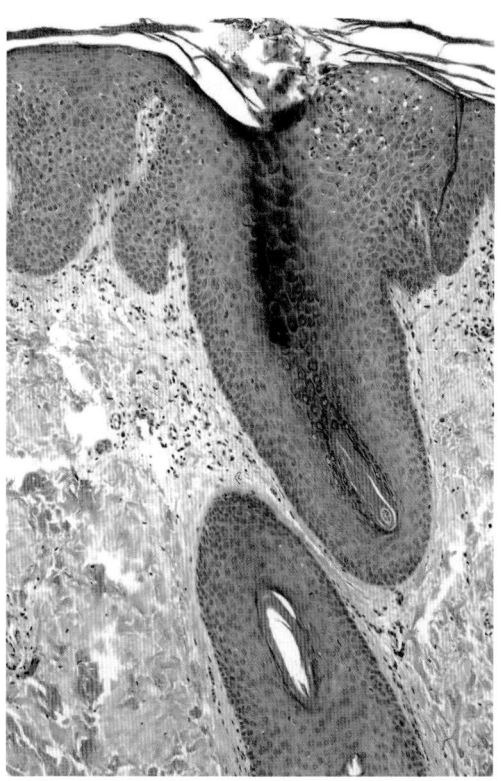

Fig. 6.25
Seborrheic dermatitis.

prolonged and severe scratching in a patient with no underlying dermatological condition (*Fig. 6.30*).[1] Lichenification is an identical process in which an underlying intensely pruritic dermatosis such as atopic eczema is present.[2] Dermatophyte infections, stasis dermatitis, and chronic allergic contact dermatitis may also predispose to lichenification. Picker nodules and nodular prurigo are related conditions (see below).[3]

Patients present with profound pruritus and localized scaly plaques with accentuated skin markings described as resembling tree bark. There is a predilection for females, and young to middle-aged adults are predominantly affected. Accessible skin is particularly affected and the nape and sides of the neck, the thighs, the lower legs and ankles, vulva, and scrotum are sites generally involved.[2]

Pebbly lichenification refers to a distinct variant in which lichenoid papules follow intense scratching in patients with inflammatory dermatoses such as atopic eczema.[2]

Histologic features and pathogenesis

Although the etiology and pathogenesis of lichen simplex chronicus remains elusive, psychological factors may play an important role.[4,5] Recent data

further suggest that an underlying neuropathy may be of importance in at least a subset of patients.[6]

Histologically, lichen simplex chronicus is characterized by marked hyperkeratosis, sometimes with small foci of parakeratosis, and a usually prominent granular cell layer (*Fig. 6.31*).[7] The epidermal ridges are elongated and irregularly thickened. Mild spongiosis is variably present depending upon the cause. A perivascular and sometimes interstitial inflammatory cell infiltrate consisting of lymphocytes, histiocytes, and small numbers of eosinophils is present in the superficial dermis. Enlarged, angulated myofibroblasts are sometimes evident and, as in many other chronic skin conditions, scattered small, multinucleated cells, so-called Montgomery giant cells, are identified. Papillary dermal fibrosis is a characteristic feature and

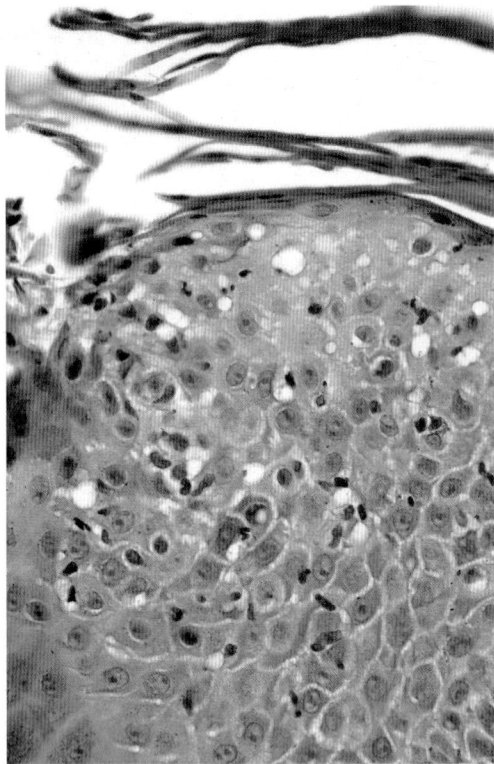

Fig. 6.26
Seborrheic dermatitis: there is parakeratosis, and occasional neutrophils are present.

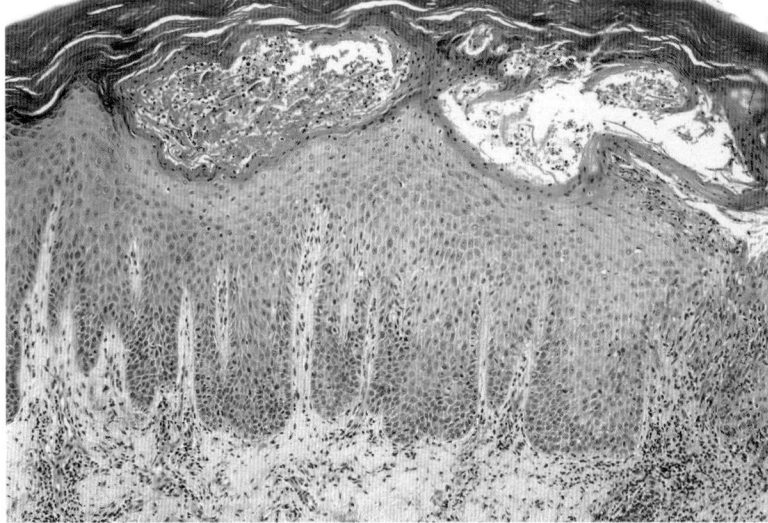

Fig. 6.27
Spongiotic superficial dermatophyte infection: there is marked subcorneal vesiculation.

Table 6.1
Conditions featuring spongiosis

- Pityriasis rosea
- Superficial fungal infections
- Herpes gestationis (early lesions)
- Polymorphic eruption of pregnancy
- Erythema multiforme
- Miliaria rubra
- Erythema annulare centrifugum
- Guttate parapsoriasis
- Acral papular eruption of childhood
- Eczema
- Lichen striatus
- Insect-bite reaction
- Prurigo nodularis

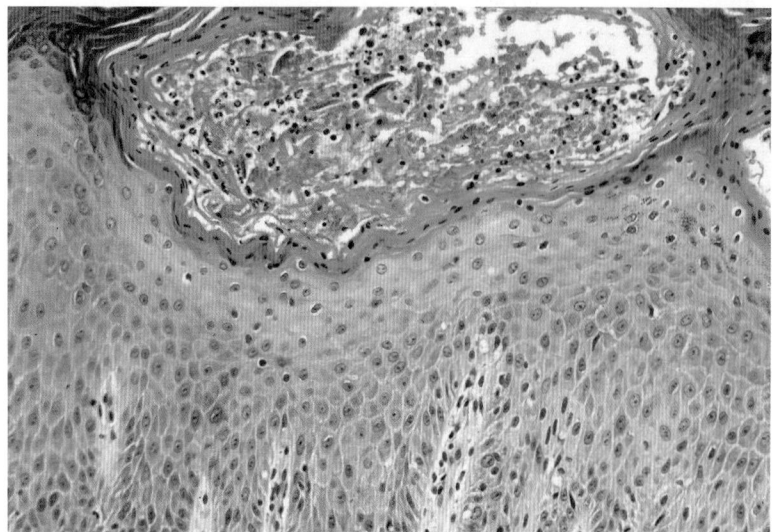

Fig. 6.28
Spongiotic superficial dermatophyte infection: higher-power view.

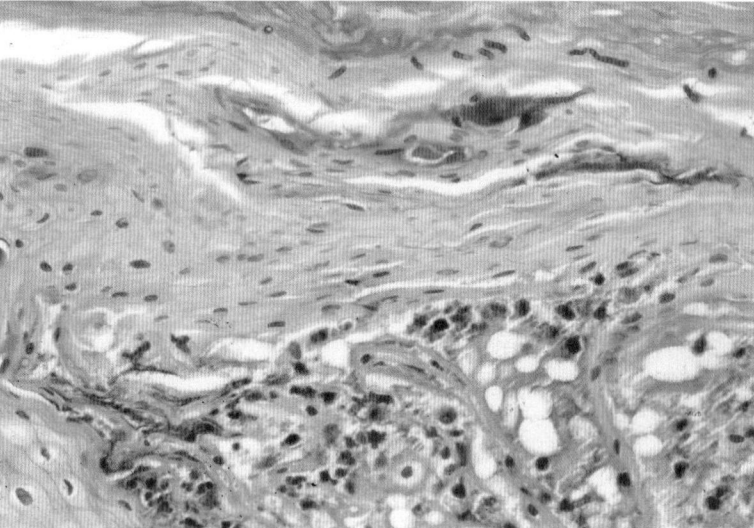

Fig. 6.29
Spongiotic superficial dermatophyte infection: numerous fungal hyphae are seen in this PAS-stained section.

in some cases nerve hyperplasia is seen (*Fig. 6.32*).[3] In our experience, however, the latter feature is distinctively uncommon.

Nodular prurigo (prurigo nodularis) and prurigo nodule (picker nodule)

Clinical features

Nodular prurigo is characterized by the development of chronic, intensely pruritic, lichenified, and excoriated nodules.[1,2] It occurs over a wide age range, from 5 to 75 years, with a mean of 40 years. Rarely, children are affected.[3] Disease duration ranges from 6 months to 33 years, with a mean of 9 years. Nodular prurigo occurs equally in men and women. It shows significant overlap with lichen simplex chronicus, although this is not uniformly accepted.[1,2]

Individual lesions are often described as globular with a warty and excoriated surface and may measure up to 2 cm in diameter (*Fig. 6.33*).[2] They are often grouped, symmetrical, and occur predominantly on extensor aspects of the (distal) limbs (*Figs 6.34* and *6.35*).[1] The trunk may also be affected.[2] Occasional disseminated cases have been described.[2] The palms and soles are typically uninvolved.[2] The intervening skin usually appears

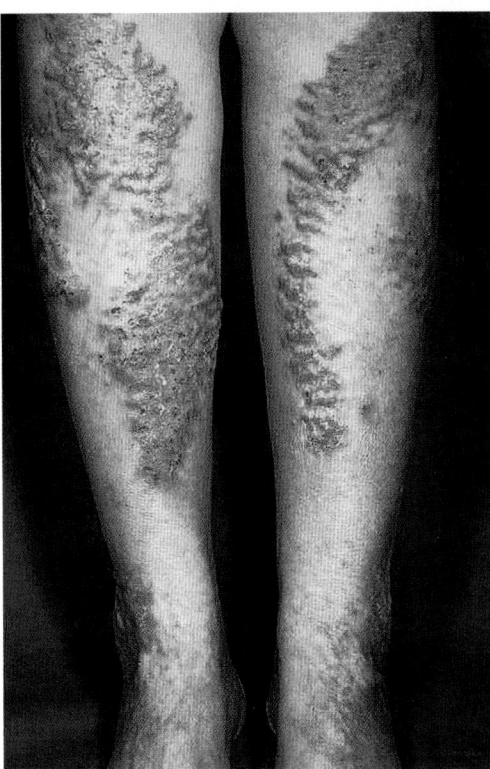

Fig. 6.30
Lichen simplex chronicus: thick, scaly erythematous plaques are present on the shins, a commonly affected site. By courtesy of R.A. Marsden, MD, St George's Hospital, London, UK.

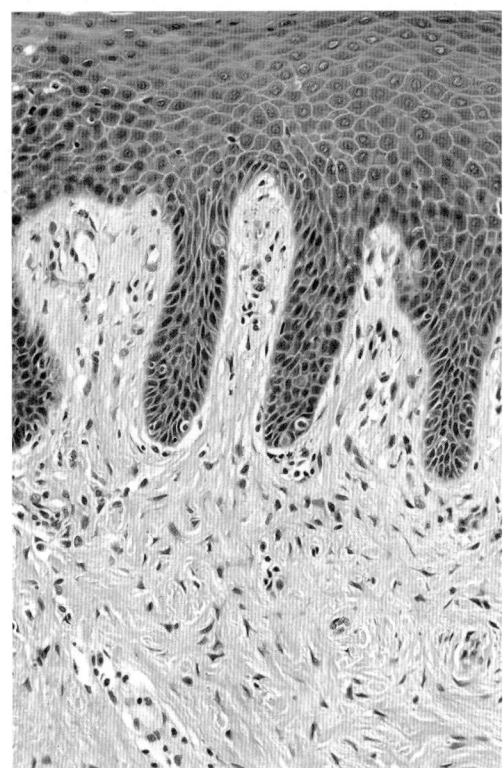

Fig. 6.32
Lichen simplex chronicus: there is hypergranulosis. Note the vertically orientated collagen fibers, a characteristic feature.

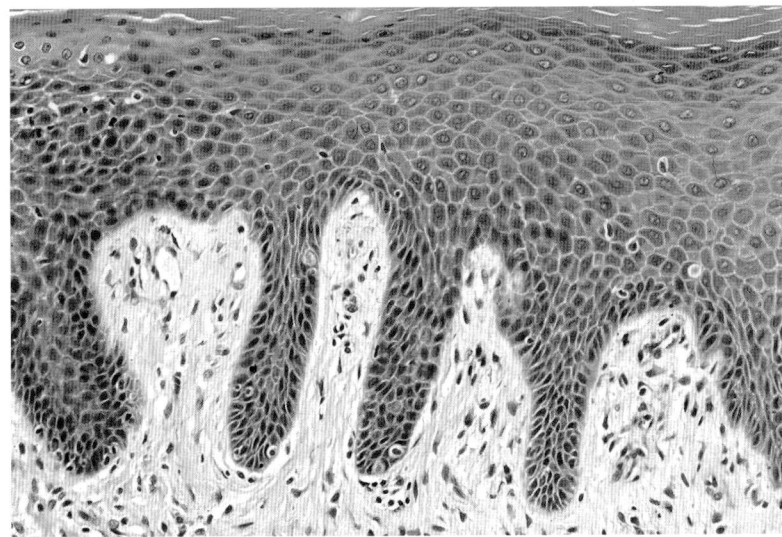

Fig. 6.31
Lichen simplex chronicus: there is hyperkeratosis, patchy parakeratosis, and elongation of the rete ridges.

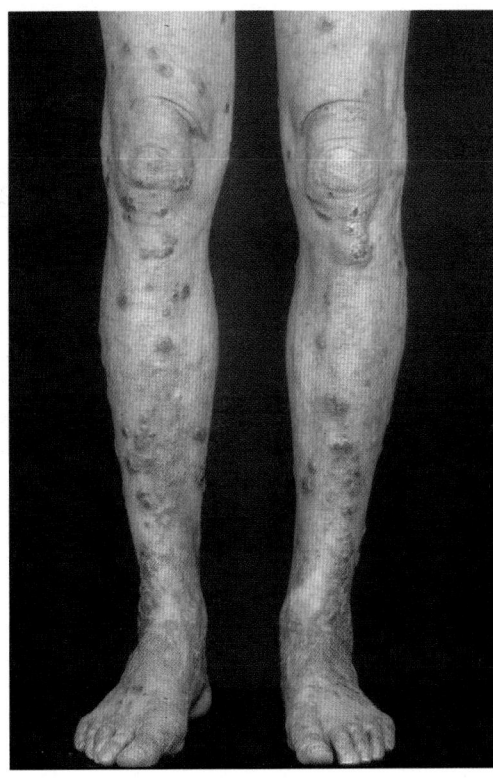

Fig. 6.33
Nodular prurigo: typical globular nodules; the intervening skin appears normal. From the collection of the late N.P. Smith, MD, the Institute of Dermatology, London, UK.

normal. Similar-looking lesions are sometimes seen in patients with eczema (see below). The majority of patients with nodular prurigo are perfectly well and investigations are unhelpful; however, occasionally nodular prurigo is found in patients with gluten enteropathy.[4] Psychosocial disorders have been reported in a high proportion of patients.[5] In some cases the eruption occurs after an insect bite, but subsequent lesions develop spontaneously.[5]

The pruritus is episodic and may be precipitated or aggravated by heat and anxiety.[5] Significant laboratory abnormalities may include anemia, eosinophilia, and raised serum IgE levels.[5]

Nodular prurigo (eczema) is defined as lesions of nodular prurigo arising on a background of overt eczema.[5] While this distinction is of academic interest it has no clinical or prognostic importance.

A prurigo nodule is a solitary variant that develops as a consequence of localized scratching and picking.

On occasion, nodular prurigo is accompanied by the features of bullous pemphigoid (pemphigoid nodularis).[6] In the latter setting, blisters are usually absent and a high degree of clinical suspicion coupled with immunofluorescence studies is necessary to confirm the diagnosis.

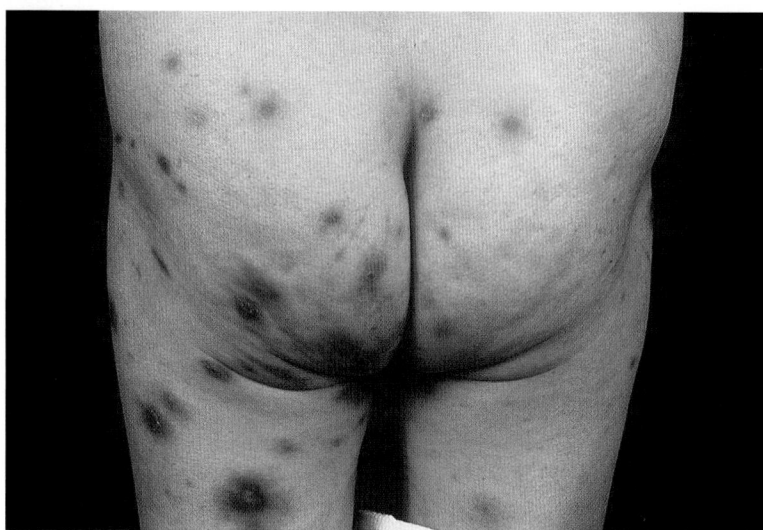

Fig. 6.34
Nodular prurigo: there are scattered, excoriated discrete nodules on the buttocks and thighs. Note the postinflammatory hyperpigmentation. By courtesy of R.A. Marsden, MD, St George's Hospital, London, UK.

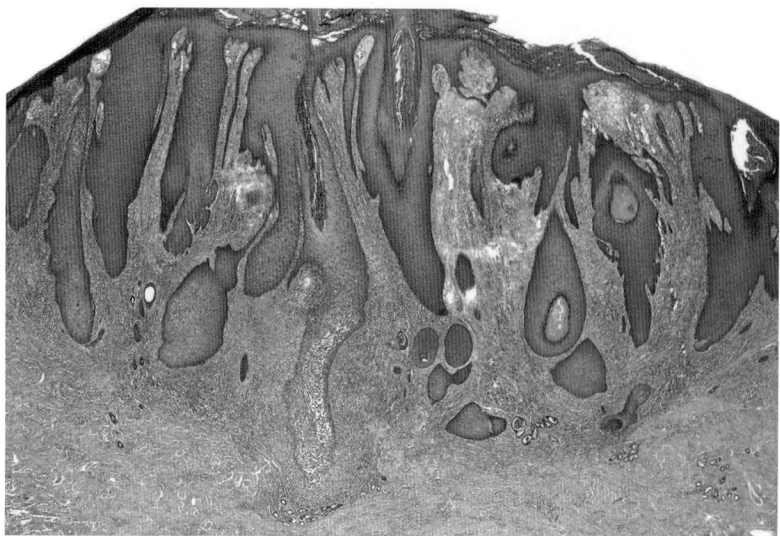

Fig. 6.36
Nodular prurigo: there is hyperkeratosis, hypergranulosis, and pseudoepitheliomatous hyperplasia. The dermis is scarred and there is a perivascular and interstitial chronic inflammatory cell infiltrate.

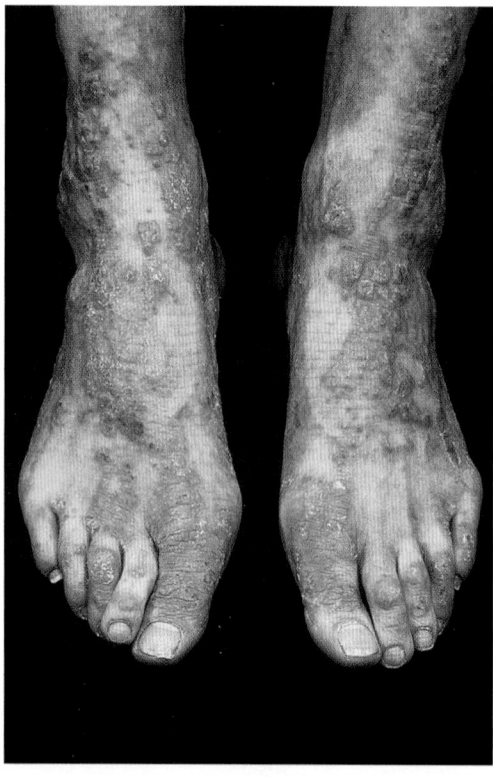

Fig. 6.35
Nodular prurigo: in this patient, there is very severe involvement of the shins and dorsal surface of the feet. By courtesy of the Institute of Dermatology, London, UK.

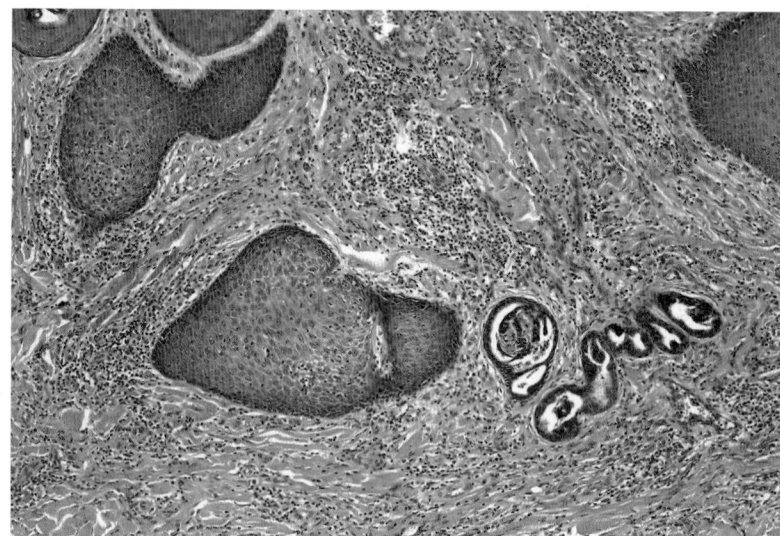

Fig. 6.37
Nodular prurigo: higher-power view.

Histologic features

Classical nodular prurigo, which is focal and characterized by hyperplasia, is particularly related to follicular epithelium.[2,7] In the epidermis this manifests as orthohyperkeratosis, hypergranulosis and acanthosis, sometimes to the degree of pseudoepitheliomatous hyperplasia (Figs 6.36 and 6.37).[8] Superficial mild spongiosis and focal parakeratosis is occasionally present and the features may resemble chronic eczema.[5] Subepidermal fibrin deposition is sometimes a feature.[9]

In the dermis there is vascular hyperplasia, with dilated vessels in both the papillary and reticular dermis. New vessel formation is apparent and there is a surrounding perivascular mild inflammatory cell infiltrate, consisting mainly of lymphocytes and some histiocytes, plasma cells, occasional

eosinophils and scattered, superficial, small multinucleated cells (Montgomery giant cells) (Fig. 6.38).[8] Mast cells are present in normal numbers.[1] The infiltrate has been described as having an inverted triangular configuration extending from the superficial dermis.[2] This has not been the present author's experience. Occasionally, the dermal features include lymphoid follicles with germinal center formation, thereby resembling a persistent insect bite reaction.[5] An additional finding is the presence of fibrosis of the papillary dermis.[8]

With light microscopy the nerves may appear normal, increased in number or occasionally hyperplastic (Fig. 6.39).[1,5] Special neural stains or S100 protein immunohistochemistry may accentuate mild proliferative changes. Nerve changes, however, do not appear to be essential for the diagnosis.[1] Studies have shown no evidence of true neuroma formation and it is thought by some authors that the neural changes are secondary to chronic trauma and scratching of the intensely pruritic nodules.[1,5,7] This intense pruritus may have been partly responsible for the large amount of attention given to neural changes in nodular prurigo in the past. Very rarely, however, hyperplastic nerve trunks are associated with Schwann cell proliferation, giving rise to small neuromata.[10]

Electron microscopy has shown vacuolation of Schwann cell cytoplasm, together with loss of definition of internal structure of the mitochondria.[5,10,11]

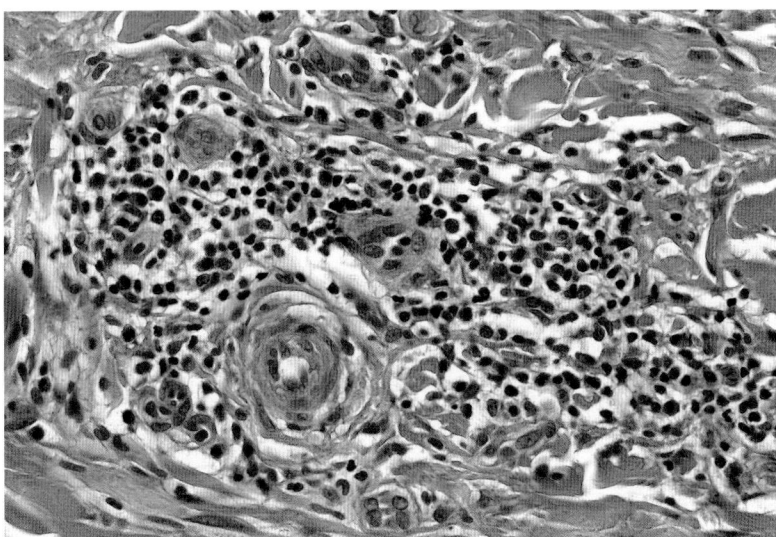

Fig. 6.38
Nodular prurigo: note the conspicuous eosinophils.

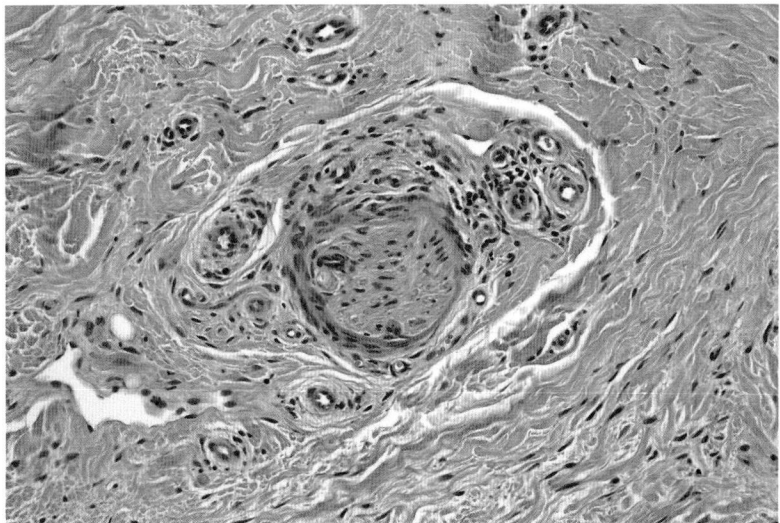

Fig. 6.39
Nodular prurigo: in our experience, nerve hyperplasia is an uncommon observation.

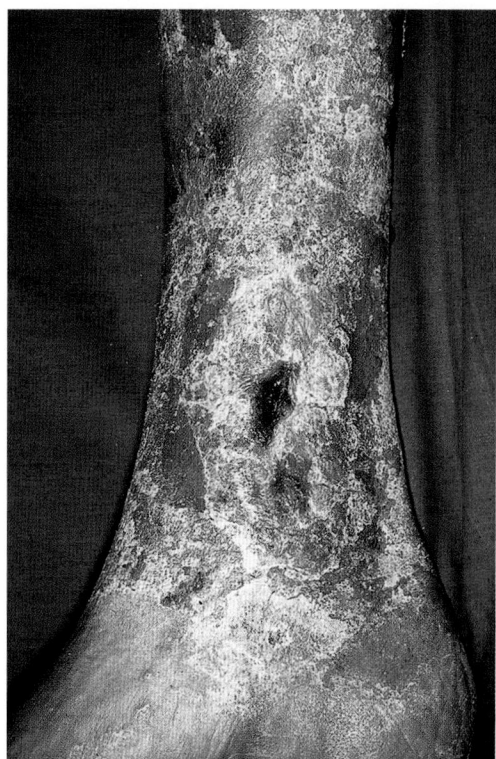

Fig. 6.40
Stasis dermatitis: there is vesiculation, exudation, and crusting on the lower leg around a stasis ulcer, which was precipitated by allergy to the antibiotic dressing. By courtesy of R.A. Marsden, MD, St George's Hospital, London, UK.

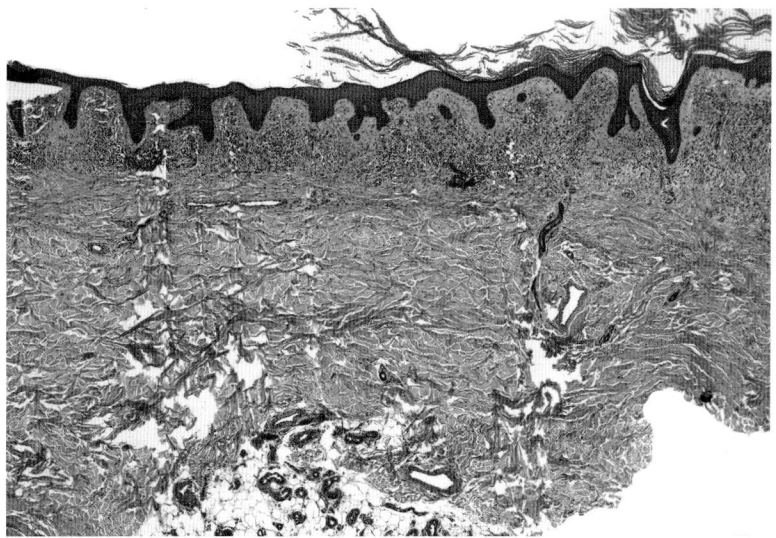

Fig. 6.41
Stasis dermatitis: there is hyperkeratosis, focal parakeratosis and marked epidermal hyperplasia. The dermis is chronically inflamed and scarred.

Stasis dermatitis and acroangiodermatitis

Clinical features

Stasis (varicose) dermatitis usually involves the medial aspect of the lower leg or ankle, but may be more widespread, and develops as a complication of impaired venous return from the lower limbs.[1] Superficial varicose veins are a frequent predisposing factor. The lesion appears as an itchy, scaly, often swollen and hyperpigmented area. Such changes are often seen around chronic stasis ulcers (*Fig. 6.40*). Malignant tumors (both squamous and basal cell carcinomas) may occasionally develop at the edge of these ulcers.[2-5] Furthermore, in the early stages of the disease, the lesion may present singly and can be clinically mistaken for a cutaneous malignancy, i.e., squamous cell carcinoma.[6]

Acroangiodermatitis (pseudo-Kaposi sarcoma, congenital dysplastic angiopathy, arteriovenous malformation with angiodermatitis) refers to the clinical manifestation of purple macules, nodules, and sometimes verrucous plaques typically developing on the dorsal aspects of the feet and toes in patients with severe and longstanding venous insufficiency.[7] Varicose veins are often present. The condition is of particular importance in that it may be clinically mistaken for Kaposi sarcoma.[8] Identical lesions have been described complicating Klippel-Trénaunay, Stewart-Bluefarb, and Prader-Willi syndromes, surgical arteriovenous fistulae as seen for example in hemodialysis patients, complicating poorly fitting suction socket prostheses on amputation stumps and on paralyzed limbs.[9-22]

Pathogenesis and histologic features

The pathogenesis of stasis dermatitis and acroangiodermatitis is unknown although it may be related to the tissue anoxia that typically results from increased venous pressure or circulatory disturbance.[13]

Stasis dermatitis shows, in addition to the epithelial changes of spongiotic dermatitis, marked hemosiderin deposition in the dermis accompanied by fibrosis and a characteristic lobular pattern of superficial and/or deep dermal neovascularization (*Figs 6.41–6.45*). Inflammatory cells – including lymphocytes, histiocytes, and variable numbers of plasma cells – are often numerous, and erythrocyte extravasation is usually prominent.

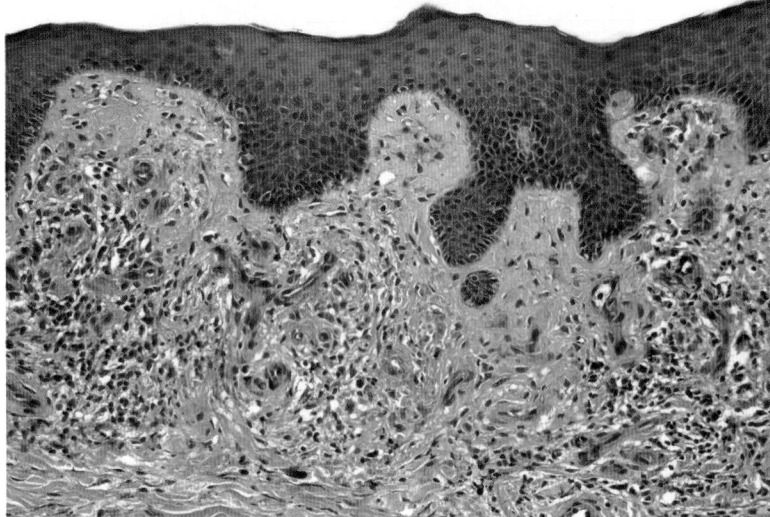

Fig. 6.42
Stasis dermatitis: note the increased vascularity.

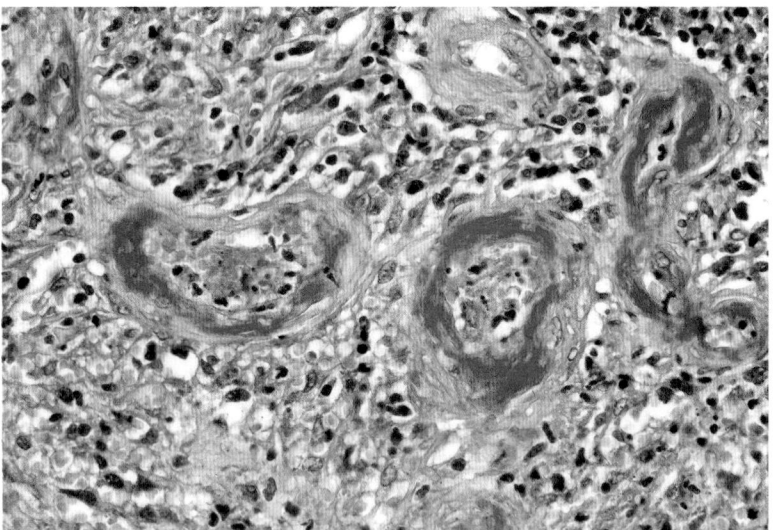

Fig. 6.43
Stasis dermatitis: there is marked mural fibrin deposition. The features often overlap with atrophie blanche.

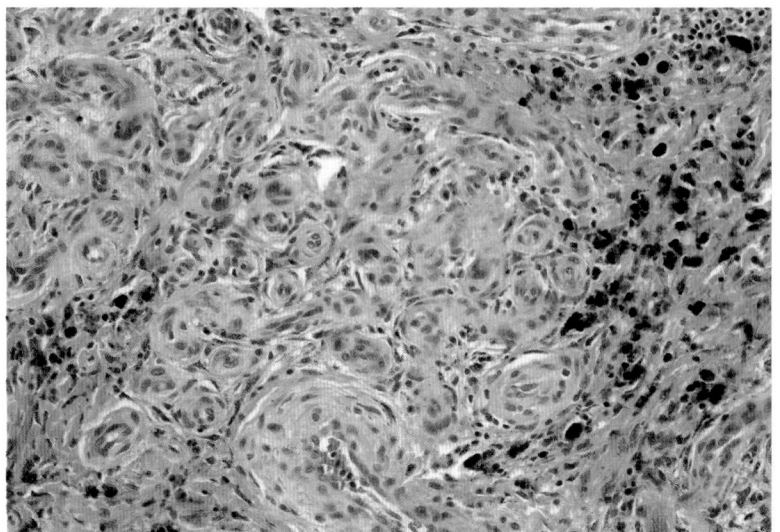

Fig. 6.44
Stasis dermatitis: in this view, there is marked new blood vessel formation and abundant hemosiderin is present.

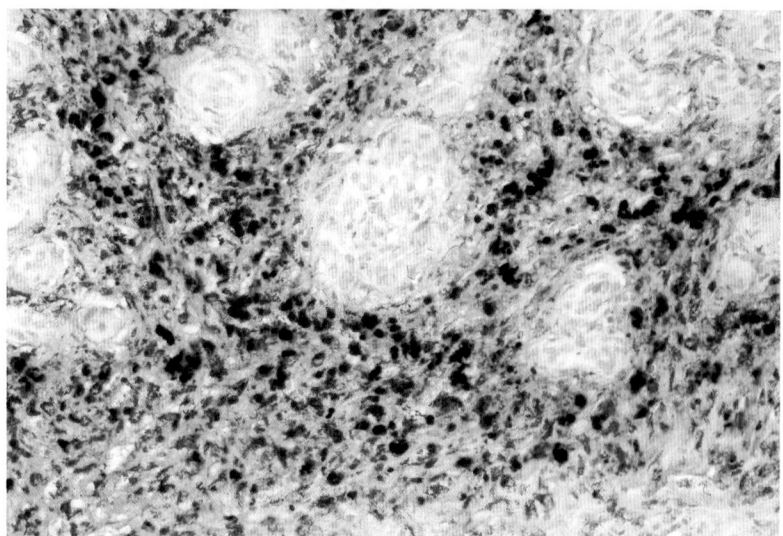

Fig. 6.45
Stasis dermatitis: the hemosiderin can be highlighted with a Prussian blue reaction for iron.

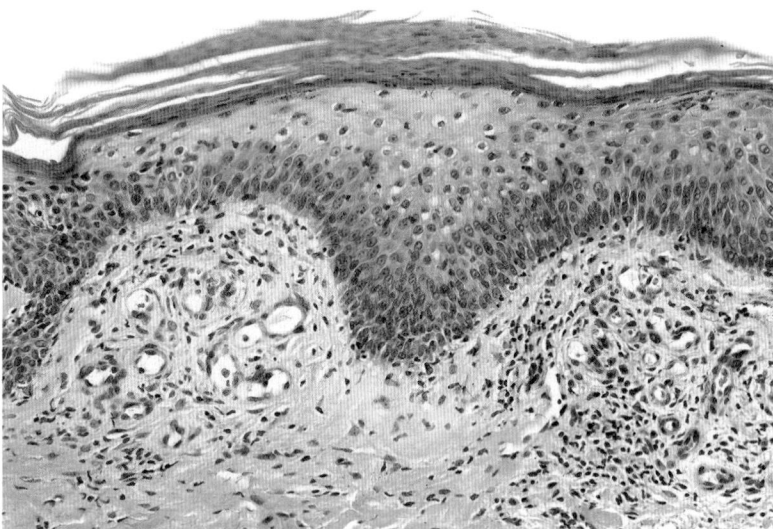

Fig. 6.46
Acroangiodermatitis showing lobular capillary proliferation, red cell extravasation, and a chronic inflammatory cell infiltrate.

In acroangiodermatitis, the vascular proliferation is often so exuberant that it may mimic a vascular neoplasm, most often Kaposi sarcoma (*Fig. 6.46*).[23]

Differential diagnosis

Acroangiodermatitis differs from Kaposi sarcoma by the absence of a spindle cell population or irregular lymphatic-like vascular channels dissecting the dermal collagen. In addition, the promontory sign (tumor vessels partially surrounding normal vessels and the adnexae) is absent. In acroangiodermatitis, the hallmark is the presence of lobular capillary proliferation.

In cases where the diagnosis is in doubt, CD34, and most importantly HHV8 immunohistochemistry is of value. The spindle cells in Kaposi sarcoma express both antigens whereas those in acroangiodermatitis do not.[24] Smooth muscle actin emphasizes the pericytes in acroangiodermatitis and a reticulin stain can be used to highlight the lobularity.

Pityriasis alba

Clinical features

Pityriasis alba is a very common form of chronic dermatitis usually affecting preadolescent children of either sex.[1] In the United States, the prevalence is

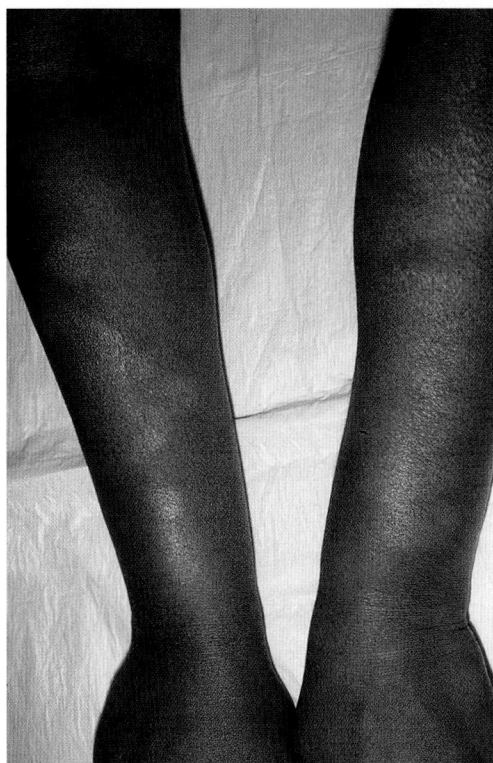

Fig. 6.47
Pityriasis alba: there are multiple hypopigmented, scaly patches on the arms. Lesions are more obvious in the colored races. By courtesy of C. Furlonge, MD, Port of Spain, Trinidad.

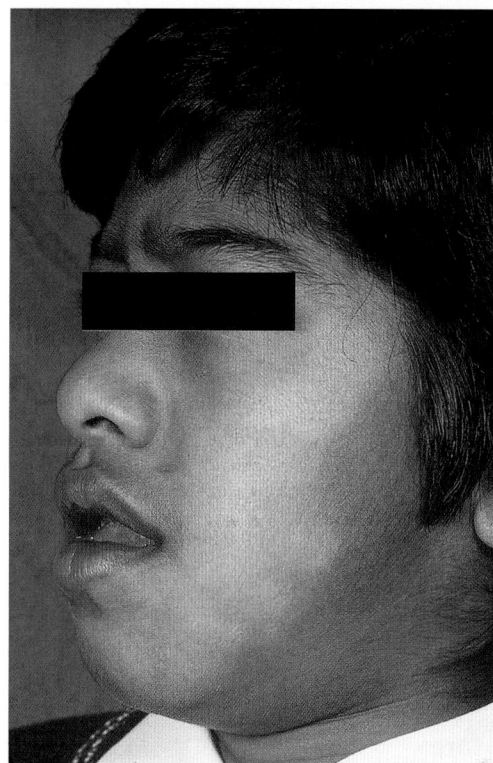

Fig. 6.48
Pityriasis alba: there is striking leukoderma on the cheek and chin, which are commonly affected sites. By courtesy of R.A. Marsden, MD, St George's Hospital, London, UK.

1.9% in a healthy population.[2] The lesions are seen on the face in particular, but the shoulders, upper extremities, and legs may also be involved (*Figs 6.47–6.49*).[1,3] Early lesions present as slightly scaly, mildly pruritic, round to oval pink plaques measuring from 0.5 to 5.0 cm or more in diameter, which later appear as scaly hypopigmented lesions.[1] The races are equally affected although lesions are more prominent in dark-skinned persons.[1,4] The condition usually resolves spontaneously after months or years.

Pathogenesis and histologic features

The etiology is unknown, although some authors believe it may be a form of atopic dermatitis since many patients also have features of classic atopic dermatitis or a family history of atopy.[5] However, some patients with pityriasis alba lack typical features of atopy. An association with xerosis has also been postulated and the condition has also been linked to copper deficiency.[6,7]

Often, biopsies taken from lesions are disappointing with subtle changes only. The histologic features of the early stage include follicular dilatation and plugging with infundibular spongiosis, parafollicular parakeratosis, and sebaceous gland atrophy accompanied by a superficial perivascular lymphocytic infiltrate and edema.[8] In the later stages, the changes are entirely non-specific and include hyperkeratosis, parakeratosis – sometimes accompanied by mild acanthosis – and slight spongiosis.[8–10] There is variable hypo- and hyperpigmentation of the basal keratinocytes with reduced or normal numbers of melanocytes and pigmentary incontinence.[8,11]

Actinic prurigo

Clinical features

Actinic prurigo is a rare familial photodermatitis with a female predilection and disease onset in childhood (4–5 years of age) although disease manifestation has also been documented in adulthood.[1–4] The disease is most commonly observed in Native Americans as well as Latin Americans. Caucasians, Asians, and Australians are less frequently affected.[1,2,4,5] The clinical presentation is varied. Patients typically present with intense

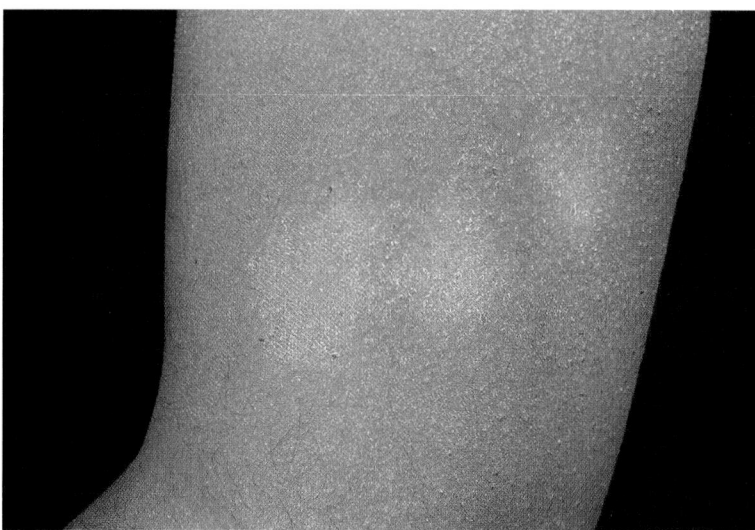

Fig. 6.49
Pityriasis alba: lesions in white-skinned patients are much more subtle. By courtesy of the Institute of Dermatology, London, UK.

pruritus and an erythematous papular eruption. Lesions may form nodules and plaques and there may be evidence of lichenification and excoriation due to repeated scratching and postinflammatory scarring.[1–3] Sun-exposed areas of the face, neck, upper chest, forearms, and hands are predominantly involved. The lips and conjunctiva are also frequently affected.[1,3,6] Associated cheilitis particularly affecting the lower lip is characterized by edema, fissuring, ulceration, and chronic dry scaling and may be the sole manifestation.[7] Conjunctival involvement results in photophobia, hyperemia, and formation of a pseudopterygium.[1,3] The disease course of actinic prurigo is chronic with significant adverse impact on the quality of life.[8] Remission may be observed in the winter months in patients living in geographic areas with significant variation of sunlight throughout the year.[1,3] In a subset of patients with childhood onset, symptoms will improve in adulthood with occasional spontaneous remission.[3]

Pathogenesis and histologic features

Using phototesting, the majority of patients show increased sensitivity to a broad spectrum of UVA as well as UVB radiation.[1,2] The disease has strong associations with HLA haplotypes, in particular DRB1*0407 (60–70% of patients) and DRB1*0401 (20% of patients).[3]

The histologic features are often nondiagnostic and areas of excoriation are frequently biopsied. In late lesions changes include regular epidermal acanthosis with overlying hyperparakeratosis and some degree of hypergranulosis. There is an associated marked superficial to mid-dermal perivascular chronic inflammatory cell infiltrate composed predominantly of lymphocytes. In the papillary dermis focal fibrosis may be seen and there is often pigment incontinence. Lymphoid follicles may be seen especially in areas of ulceration, particularly in lesions on the lip. Eosinophils are frequently noted. Biopsies from the lip show similar epidermal features in addition to spongiosis and basal cell vacuolar change. Dermal edema and prominent telangiectatic vessels are further characteristic features. An associated lymphoplasmacytic infiltrate may be bandlike or show lymphoid follicles with germinal centers. The latter is mainly seen in conjunctival biopsies.

Papuloerythroderma (of Ofuji)

Clinical features

Papuloerythroderma (of Ofuji) is a rare dermatosis first reported in 1984.[1] It affects the elderly (mean age: 73 years) and shows a strong male predilection, which appears to be most pronounced in the Asian population.[2,3,4] The disorder is pruritic and starts out as red-brown papules with little scale. The papules coalesce to form an erythrodermic eruption involving the trunk and limbs with sparing of the skin folds (so-called deck chair sign) (Fig. 6.50).[1-4] Palmoplantar keratoderma and dermatopathic lymphadenopathy is present in a subset of patients. Involvement of the face and scalp is rare and the mucous membranes, hair, and nails are spared. Peripheral blood eosinophilia and elevated serum IgE levels are frequent additional findings.[2,3] An association with an underlying malignancy is found in 22% to 54% of cases and includes mainly solid organ or hematological malignancies.[2,3] Other reported associations include an underlying infection and a drug-induced form.[2-5]

Histologic features

The histologic features are rather non-specific and may be of a subacute spongiotic dermatitis with epidermal acanthosis and focal spongiosis with overlying hyperkeratosis. There is an associated superficial to mid-dermal perivascular lymphohistiocytic inflammatory cell infiltrate containing eosinophils. The correct diagnosis depends on interpretation of the biopsy findings in the appropriate clinical setting. The clinical appearances of papuloerythroderma (of Ofuji) can also be seen in the setting of a cutaneous T-cell lymphoma, which needs to be excluded histologically, immunohistochemically, and by molecular studies.[4,6-12]

Eosinophilic spongiosis

Eosinophilic spongiosis is the histopathological term used to describe spongiosis in which eosinophils are the predominant cell type.[1-5] Eosinophilic spongiosis is a non-specific finding with which a considerable number of dermatoses may be associated. Table 6.2 lists dermatoses in which eosinophilic spongiosis is commonly encountered. Detailed discussion of each of these disorders is found in the appropriate chapters.

Erythroderma

Spongiotic dermatitis is one of the causes of erythroderma. Sometimes incorrectly called exfoliative dermatitis, erythroderma is applicable only when the entire skin surface is inflamed, erythematous, and scaly (Fig. 6.51).[1-5] The clinical features are remarkably consistent irrespective of the

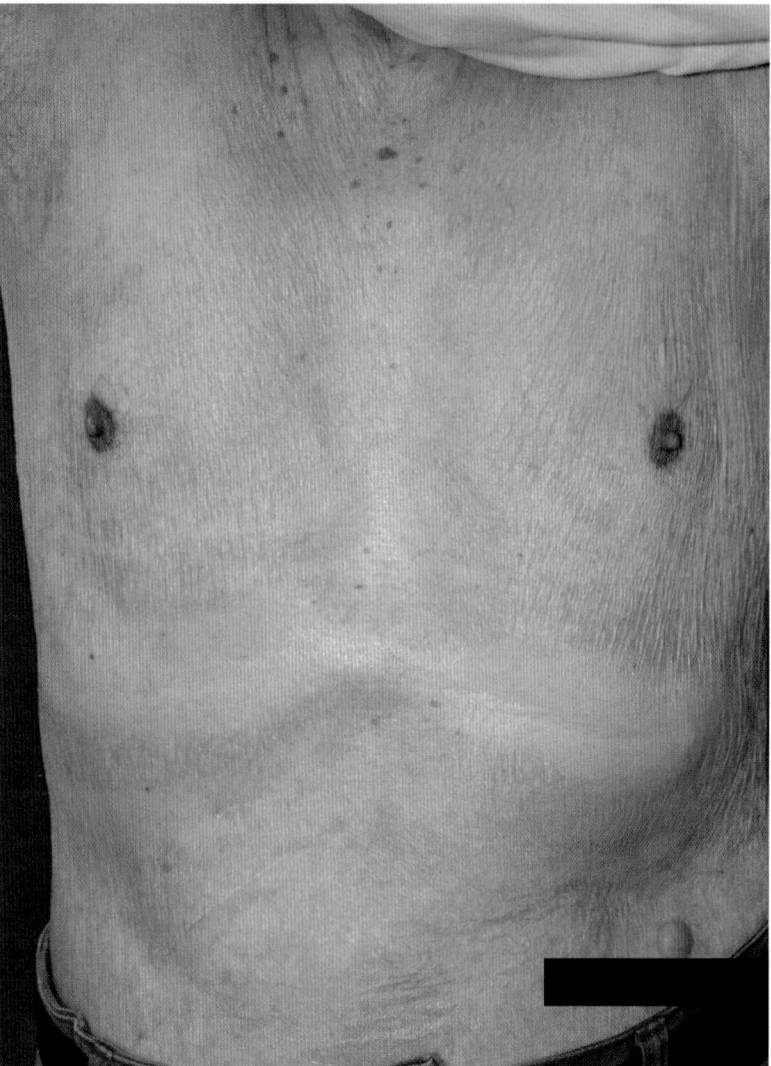

Fig. 6.50
Papuloerythrodermia of Ofuji: Erythrodermia and typical deck-chair sign. By courtesy of C.K. Hsui, MD and J.Y.Y Lee, MD, National Cheng Kung University Hospital, Tainan, Taiwan.

Table 6.2
Diseases featuring eosinophilic spongiosis

- Incontinentia pigmenti
- Pemphigus
- Bullous pemphigoid
- Linear IgA disease
- Pemphigoid (herpes) gestationis and polymorphic eruption of pregnancy
- Insect-bite reactions
- Atopic eczema
- Contact dermatitis
- Grover disease
- Drug reactions

underlying disease and therefore often pose a diagnostic challenge. Pruritus is variable, being particularly severe in the Sézary syndrome and in mycosis fungoides. Lymphadenopathy is usually present (dermatopathic lymphadenopathy). Prolonged erythroderma, particularly in the elderly, may be complicated by cardiac failure, peripheral circulatory collapse, hypothermia, and infection. Patients with erythroderma are frequently biopsied since the clinical examination findings are often non-specific. Diagnosis without clinical information is often not possible.[1] Table 6.3 lists the various causes of erythroderma. The specific diseases that cause erythroderma are discussed in detail in the appropriate chapters.

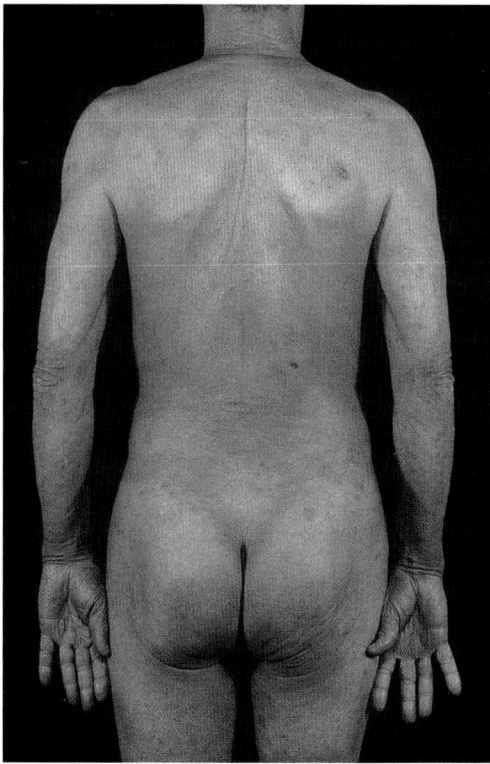

Fig. 6.51
Erythroderma: the entire skin surface is erythematous and slightly scaly. The appearances are relatively non-specific and give no indication of the cause. By courtesy of the Institute of Dermatology, London, UK.

Table 6.3
Causes of erythroderma

- Dermatitis
- Lymphoma (mycosis fungoides, T-cell leukemia, Hodgkin lymphoma)
- Drugs (gold, penicillin, etc.)
- Psoriasis
- Pityriasis rubra pilaris
- Ichthyosiform erythroderma
- Papuloerythroderma (of Ofuji)
- Scabies
- Lichen planus

Sulzberger-Garbe syndrome

Clinical features

Sulzberger-Garbe syndrome (distinctive exudative discoid and lichenoid chronic dermatosis) was originally described as a widespread pruritic eruption associated with discoid lesions in middle-aged Jewish males.[1-3] Involvement of the penis was said to be characteristic. Transformation from eczematous to lichenoid lesions and vice versa is also thought to be a typical feature. The lesions are chronic, lasting from months to years, but eventually resolving.

Pathogenesis and histologic features

The existence of Sulzberger-Garbe syndrome as a distinctive entity is controversial. Some authors consider patients classified under this designation as having nummular dermatitis.[3]

Biopsy of exudative lesions shows a non-specific spongiotic dermatitis. Biopsy of lichenoid lesions is characterized by a bandlike lymphocytic infiltrate. Variable numbers of eosinophils may be present.

Vein graft site dermatitis

Occasionally, patients undergoing coronary artery bypass develop an eczematous dermatitis in the region of the scar from the saphenous vein donor

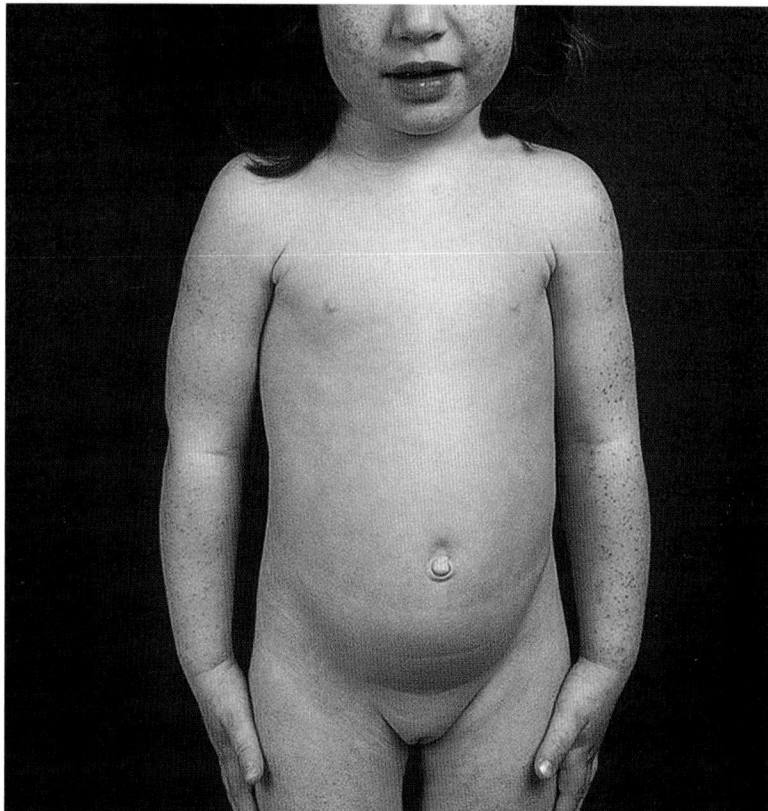

Fig. 6.52
Gianotti-Crosti syndrome: the eruption is present on the face and arms, there is sparing of the trunk. By courtesy of C. Gelmetti, MD, Milan University, Italy.

site.[1,2] The pathogenesis is unclear. Since patients often have objective evidence of neuropathy, some authors believe that the neuralgia may play a pathogenic role.[1] It is also possible that stasis changes play a role in this disorder.

Biopsy shows a non-specific spongiotic dermatitis.

Papular acrodermatitis of childhood

Clinical features

Papular acrodermatitis of childhood (Gianotti-Crosti syndrome, infantile papular acrodermatitis) is a rare disease representing a cutaneous response to a number of viral infections. It is characterized by the acute onset of monomorphic, symmetrical flat-topped papules or papulovesicles, 1–10 mm across, which range in color from pink to red or brown and are located primarily on the face (particularly the cheeks), buttocks, and extensor surfaces of the forearms and legs, with the trunk typically being spared (*Figs 6.52–6.54*).[1-4] Lesions are usually blanchable although petechial and hemorrhagic variants can be rarely encountered.[4] A positive Koebner phenomenon is sometimes elicited.[4] The lesions are occasionally pruritic and are self-limiting, lasting up to 3 weeks. Mucous membranes are not affected. Infants and children are predominantly affected although there are occasional reports of the condition developing in adults.[4-9]

Systemic signs include hepatosplenomegaly and axillary and inguinal lymphadenopathy. Sometimes a fever is evident. There may be an anicteric acute hepatitis and occasionally patients progress to chronic liver disease.

Pathogenesis and histologic features

In the original and early reports, Gianotti-Crosti syndrome was documented following infection with hepatitis B virus.[10-12] Other associations include hepatitis A virus, coxsackievirus, influenza virus, Epstein-Barr virus, cytomegalovirus, parainfluenza virus, human herpesvirus-6 (HHV-6), poxvirus, parvovirus, and rotavirus.[13-25] In addition, the disease had been associated with HIV infection.[26] Gianotti-Crosti syndrome has also been reported

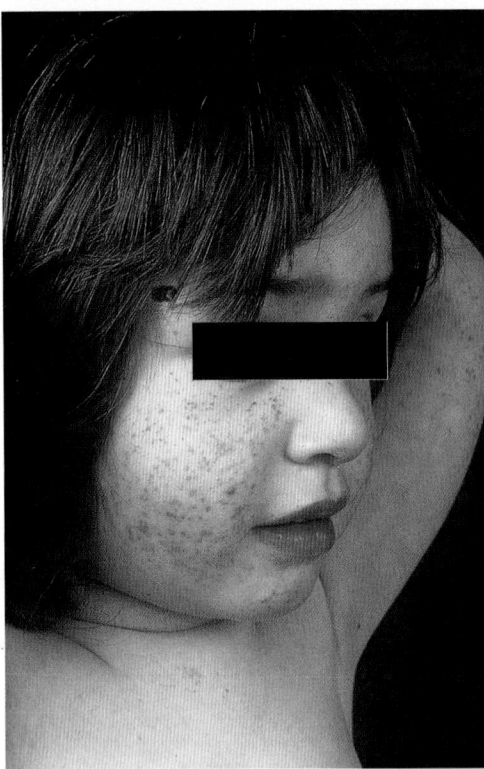

Fig. 6.53
Gianotti-Crosti syndrome: note the widespread erythematous papules on the cheeks of this young girl. By courtesy of C. Gelmetti, MD, Milan University, Italy.

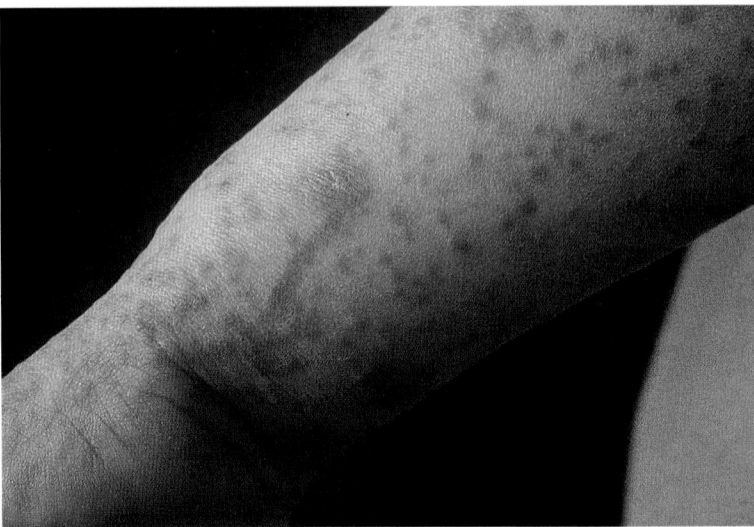

Fig. 6.54
Gianotti-Crosti syndrome: the papules are very uniform. A viral etiology is often identified. By courtesy of C. Gelmetti, MD, Milan University, Italy.

following *Mycoplasma* infection, Lyme borreliosis, and immunization.[27-35] The pathogenesis is unknown although viral antigenemia and immune complex-mediated mechanisms have been proposed.[36]

Biopsies of skin lesions show entirely non-specific histologic features. The epidermis often appears normal or it may be mildly acanthotic with parakeratosis. Lymphocytic exocytosis is usually present.[3] The upper dermis contains a lymphohistiocytic infiltrate in a perivascular distribution and there is also swelling of endothelial cells sometimes accompanied by marked papillary dermal edema.[31] Scattered eosinophils may be present.[36] Occasionally, a more lichenoid pattern of inflammation is encountered. There is no evidence of vasculitis.

Direct immunofluorescence is negative.[3]

By immunohistochemistry, the infiltrate consists of an admixture of CD4+ helper T cells and CD8+ cytotoxic T cells.[19,36,37]

In cases with hepatitis, the appearances are those of an acute viral hepatitis, which usually resolves over a period of up to 6 months. Rarely, chronic disease ensues.

Pityriasis rosea

Clinical features

Pityriasis rosea ('rose-colored scale') presents as an acute inflammatory dermatosis characterized by self-limiting oval papulosquamous lesions on the trunk and extremities.[1-3] The disease appears to be more common in females, and 75% of cases occur between the ages of 10 and 35 years.[4] It is characterized by seasonal variation, being most common in the months of December to February.[5] Although pityriasis rosea typically presents as a solitary episode, recurrent disease may occur in up to 2% of patients.[6,7]

In the majority of cases the disease first manifests itself with the appearance of a 'herald patch', a single red scaly lesion that increases in size over 48 hours up to 2–10 cm in diameter (*Fig. 6.55*).[8] A significant proportion of patients report symptoms, including pyrexia, headache, malaise, arthralgia, chills, vomiting, diarrhea, and lymphadenopathy, up to 2–3 weeks before the onset of the eruption.[9]

After the appearance of the herald patch there is a 'secondary incubation period' of 7–14 days before the generalized eruption of pink to salmon-colored elliptical scaly lesions (*Fig. 6.56*).[10] The latter are approximately 1 cm in length and their longest axes occur along the Blaschko skin tension lines, producing the characteristic 'fir' or 'Christmas tree' effect. There is usually an erythematous center, the periphery of the macule being slightly brown and scaly. In dark-skinned patients the macules tend to be darker than the surrounding skin (*Fig. 6.57*). The lesions spread from the chest to the abdomen, thighs, arms, and back, generally within 2 weeks, persist for 2–4 weeks, and fade over a further 2 weeks. Pityriasis rosea may be pruritic.

Oral lesions have been described in up to 16% of patients.[4] They may take the form of a single large erythematous plaque, bullae, multiple hemorrhagic puncta, round erythematous macules and plaques, or erythematous annular lesions.[4,11-14]

Several morphological variants may occur: a papular variant is seen in young children, pregnant women, and those of Afro-Caribbean descent; a vesicular or bullous variant may occur in infants and children; and an urticarial form has also been noted.[5,14,15] Occasionally, pityriasis rosea has a purpuric, hemorrhagic component.[5,14,16] Localized and unilateral forms, and an 'inverse' form presenting on the face and extremities, have also been documented.[17]

Pathogenesis and histologic features

The exact etiology of pityriasis rosea is unknown; however, most of the evidence points to an infectious, probably viral, cause. It sometimes complicates an upper respiratory tract infection.[18] The herald patch may develop at the site of an insect bite, particularly fleas, but patches have also occurred in areas of old trauma and scars, suggesting an isomorphic (Koebner) response.[17] Atypical pityriasis rosea has also been described in bone marrow transplant recipients and following treatment with interferon-alpha (IFN-α) as well as Hodgkin disease, and a pityriasis rosea-like eruption has been documented due to drugs such as imatinib mesylate, ACE inhibitors, and hydrochlorothiazide.[19-23] Case clustering in establishments with communal living supports an infectious etiology. HHV-7, as well as HHV-6 and HHV-8, has been identified in peripheral blood mononuclear cells in addition to plasma and skin of patients with pityriasis rosea, and herpes virus-like particles have been identified in cutaneous lesions of pityriasis rosea by electron microscopy.[24-33] Other workers, however, have failed to confirm this observation.[28,34,35] Rarely, a pityriasis rosea-like eruption may be a manifestation of HIV/AIDS.[36]

The histopathological features are those of a non-specific subacute or chronic dermatitis and comprise focal hyperkeratosis and angulated parakeratosis with slight acanthosis (*Figs 6.58–6.61*).[37] The granular cell

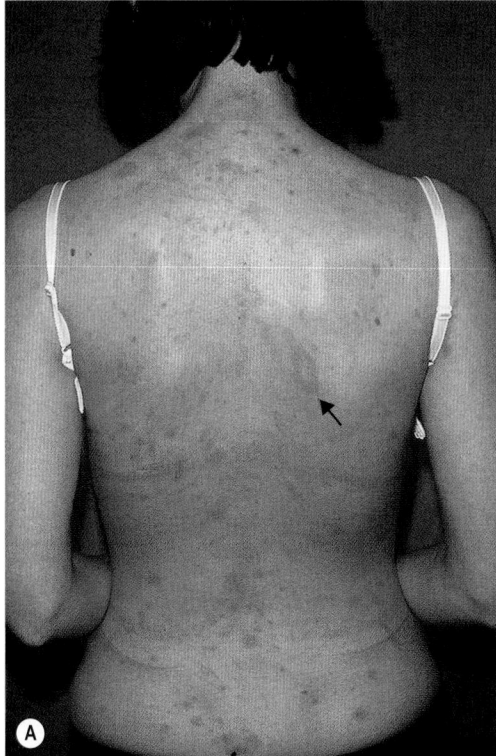

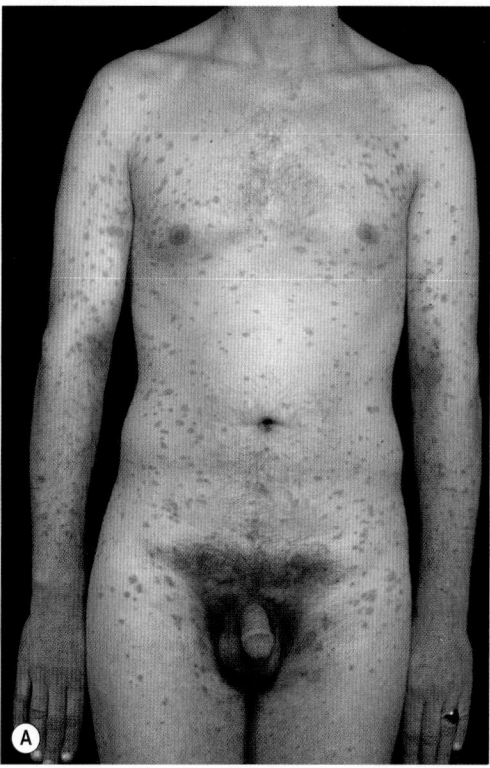

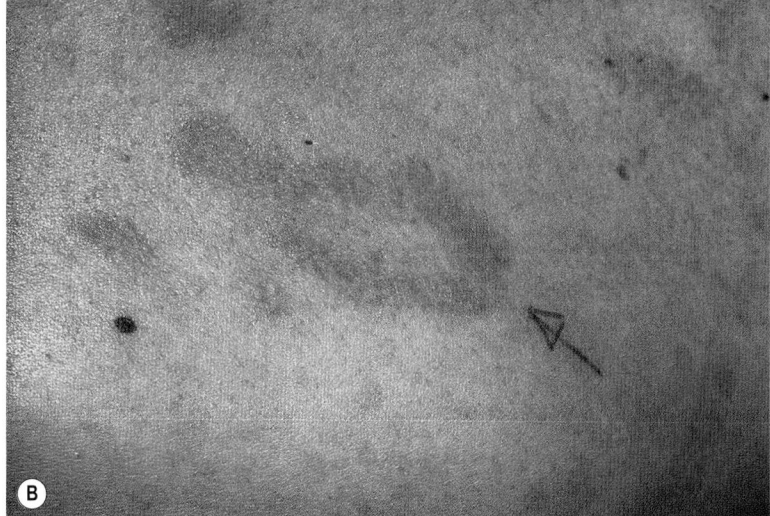

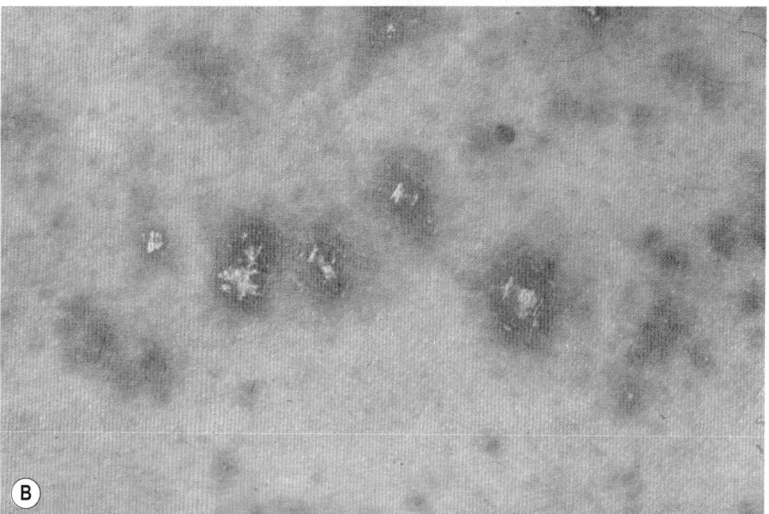

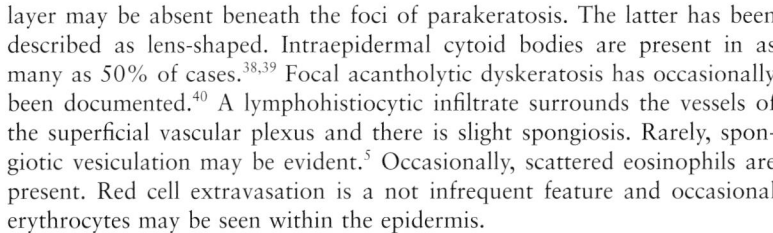

Fig. 6.55
Pityriasis rosea: (**A**) the 'herald patch' which marks the onset of this dermatosis, is marked by an arrow; (**B**) close-up view. By courtesy of R.A. Marsden, MD, St George's Hospital, London, UK.

Fig. 6.56
Pityriasis rosea: (**A**) the secondary rash presents as small pink slightly scaly macules; (**B**) close-up view. From the collection of the late N.P. Smith, MD, the Institute of Dermatology, London, UK.

layer may be absent beneath the foci of parakeratosis. The latter has been described as lens-shaped. Intraepidermal cytoid bodies are present in as many as 50% of cases.[38,39] Focal acantholytic dyskeratosis has occasionally been documented.[40] A lymphohistiocytic infiltrate surrounds the vessels of the superficial vascular plexus and there is slight spongiosis. Rarely, spongiotic vesiculation may be evident.[5] Occasionally, scattered eosinophils are present. Red cell extravasation is a not infrequent feature and occasional erythrocytes may be seen within the epidermis.

Immunocytochemical staining has demonstrated that the dermal infiltrate consists mainly of T cells, including helper and suppressor cells, together with large numbers of Langerhans cells.[41] Human leukocyte antigen DR (HLA-DR, Ia-like antigen) has been demonstrated on the surface of keratinocytes, and this has been interpreted as showing that they are taking an active role in cellular immunity.[42–44] HLA-DR antigen may also be expressed on the surface of the T-helper cells.[43]

Differential diagnosis

Guttate psoriasis shows considerable overlap with pityriasis rosea. The presence of neutrophils within the parakeratotic mounds favors a diagnosis of psoriasis.

A wide range of drugs has been associated with a pityriasis rosea-like eruption including barbiturates, ketotifen, clonidine, captopril, isotretinoin, gold, bismuth, arsenic, organic mercurials, methoxypromazine, D-penicillamine, tripelennamine hydrochloride, metronidazole, and salvarsan.[15,17] In such cases, the distinction depends upon clinicopathological correlation. The presence of large numbers of eosinophils is a clue to a hypersensitivity reaction.

Acute and subacute eczematous dermatitis may also be confused with pityriasis rosea. The presence of lens-shaped parakeratosis and limited spongiosis favors pityriasis rosea. Again, clinical findings should help make this distinction.

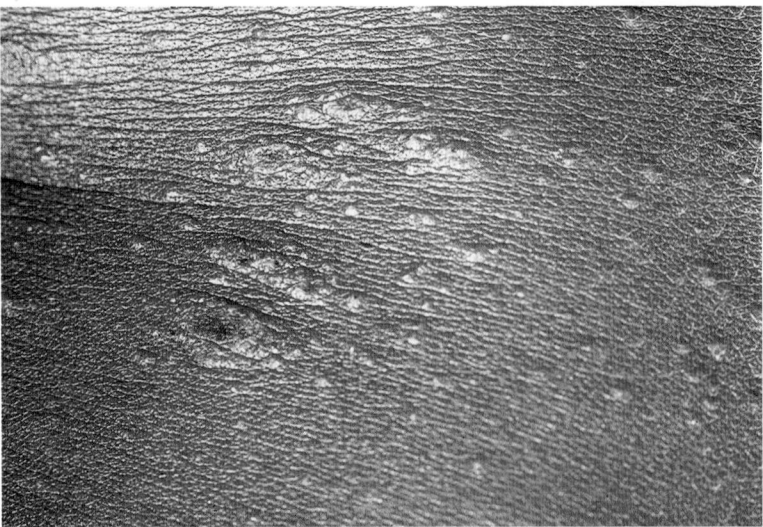

Fig. 6.57
Pityriasis rosea: in pigmented skin, there is often postinflammatory hyperpigmentation and the erythematous nature of the eruption is not apparent. By courtesy of R.A. Marsden, MD, St George's Hospital, London, UK.

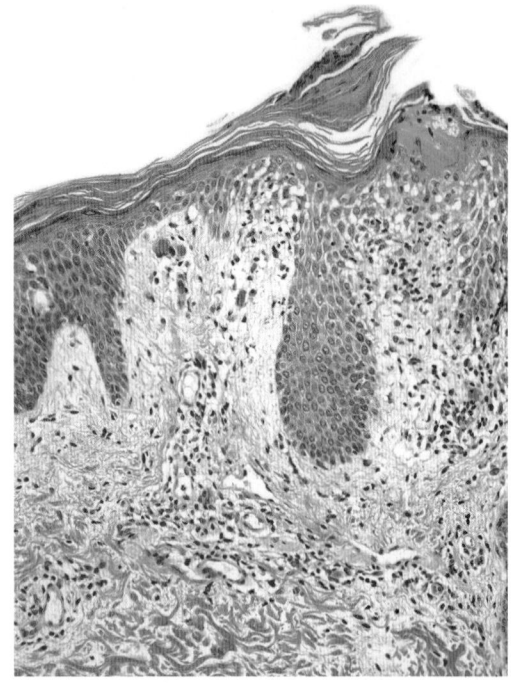

Fig. 6.60
Pityriasis rosea: there is spongiosis and a perivascular lymphocytic infiltrate. The angulated tier of parakeratosis (teapot lid sign) is characteristic.

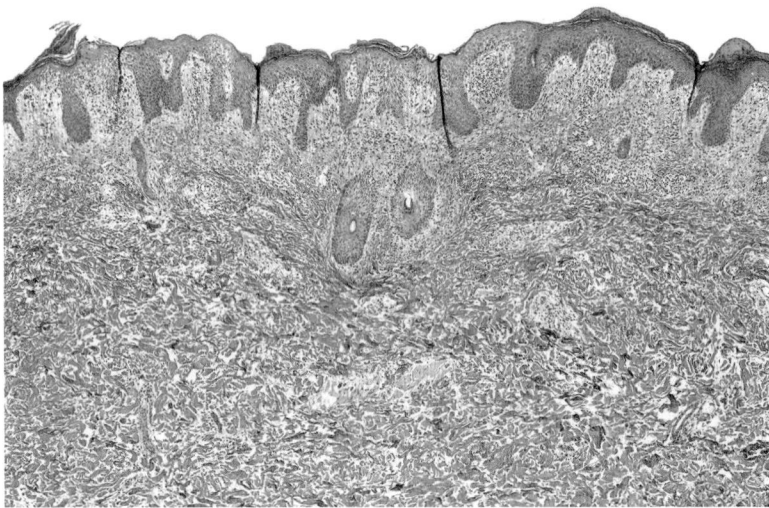

Fig. 6.58
Pityriasis rosea: low-power view showing multiple foci of scale with psoriasiform hyperplasia.

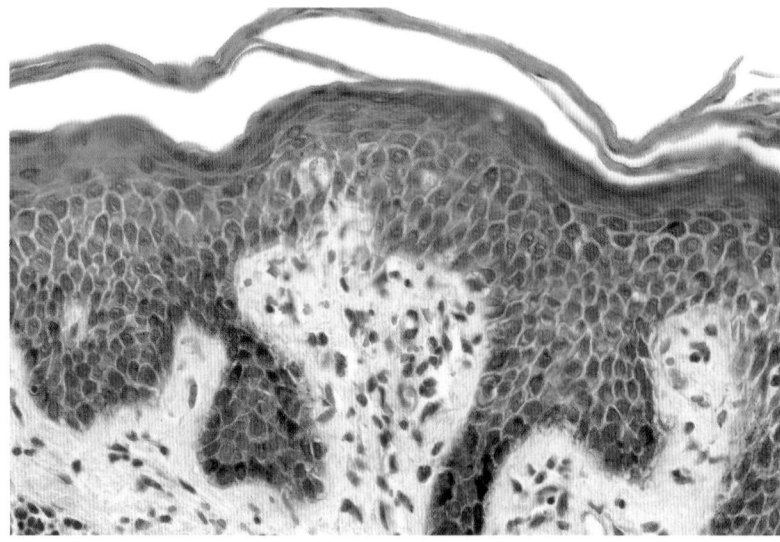

Fig. 6.61
Pityriasis rosea: in this field, there is red cell extravasation.

Pityriasis lichenoides chronica is characterized by interface change and vacuolar degeneration of the basal layer of the epidermis, features not seen in pityriasis rosea.

A PAS stain is mandatory in all cases to exclude a dermatophyte infection.

Juvenile plantar dermatosis

Clinical features

Scaly palms and soles with loss of a normal epidermal rete pattern characterize juvenile plantar dermatosis. The affected area often has a shiny red appearance with fissures (Figs 6.62 and 6.63).[1–4] As its name suggests, the disease is seen in prepubertal children with a mean age of 9.6 years.[1] The most common sites affected are the volar aspect of the great toe and the ball of the foot.[1] The hand is only rarely affected. Patients often have a personal or family history of atopy.[2,4,5] The disorder usually lasts for 6 months to

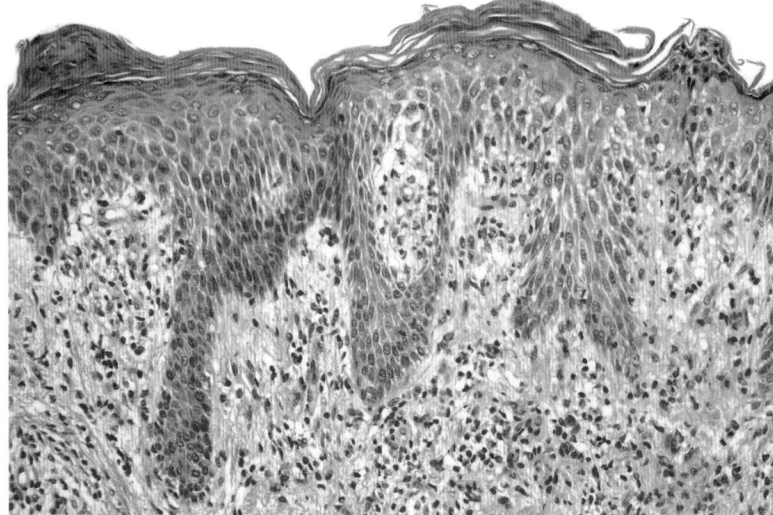

Fig. 6.59
Pityriasis rosea: small foci of parakeratotic scale are a characteristic finding. The epidermis shows mild spongiosis.

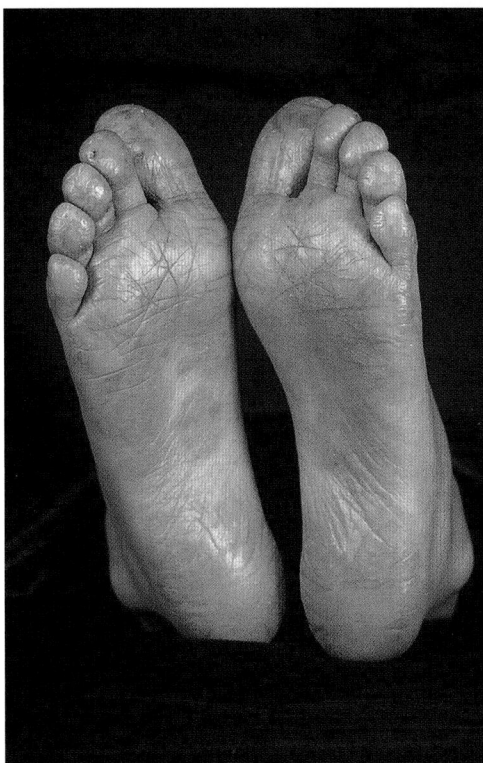

Fig. 6.62
Juvenile plantar dermatosis: multiple erythematous lesions are present on the soles of the feet. By courtesy of the Institute of Dermatology, London, UK.

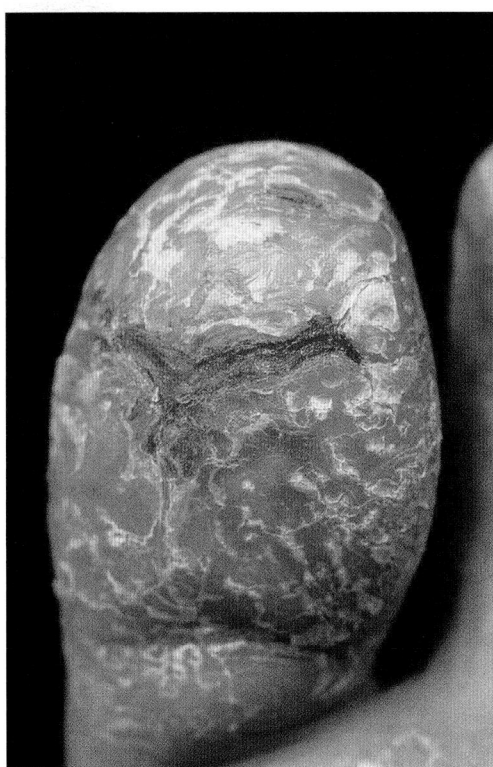

Fig. 6.63
Juvenile plantar dermatosis: close-up view showing scaling and fissuring. By courtesy of the Institute of Dermatology, London, UK.

several years before resolving.[1,3] However, many patients develop features of classic eczema of the hands later in life.[2]

Pathogenesis and histologic features

The pathogenesis of this disorder is not understood; however, it has been suggested that synthetic footwear may play a role in its development.[3]

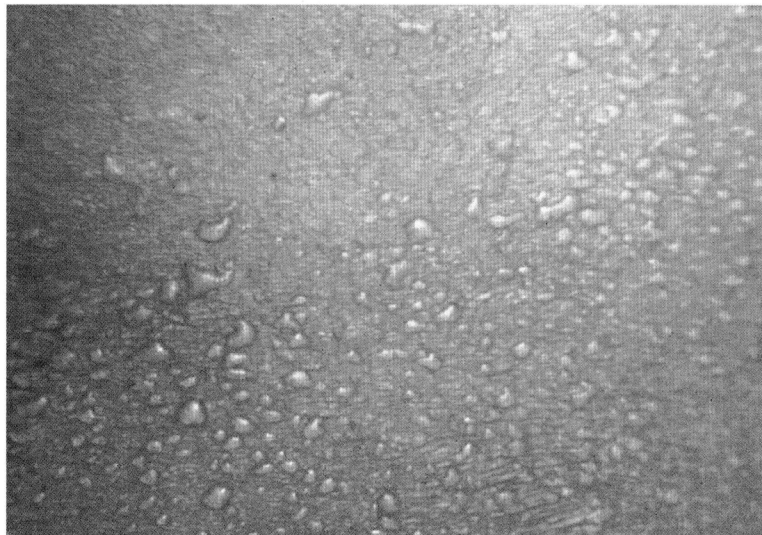

Fig. 6.64
Miliaria crystallina: tiny vesicles resembling water droplets are scattered over the abdomen of this young male. By courtesy of R.A. Marsden, MD, St George's Hospital, London, UK.

Biopsy shows epidermal acanthosis and subacute to chronic spongiosis.[1,5] Variable parakeratosis and hypogranulosis may be seen. A lymphocytic infiltrate centered on the eccrine duct is said to be characteristic.[1,5]

Differential diagnosis

The histologic changes are probably non-specific but the presence of chronic inflammation centered on the sweat duct should suggest juvenile plantar dermatosis in the appropriate clinical setting and allow distinction from other spongiotic dermatitides, which typically spare the acrosyringium. One group could not identify PAS-positive material occluding sweat ducts in multiple histologic sections of juvenile plantar dermatosis (compare with miliaria).[1] A PAS stain with diastase digestion should also be performed to evaluate for fungal infection.

Miliaria

Clinical features

This common disorder, although most often seen in children, may affect any age group but congenital presentation is rare.[1] It develops as a consequence of obstruction to the outflow tract of the intraepidermal component of the eccrine sweat duct and is associated with excessive sweating and exposure to high humidity. Traditionally, the condition is subdivided into three subtypes: miliaria crystallina, miliaria rubra, and miliaria profunda.[2,3]

- In miliaria crystallina the level of obstruction is within the stratum corneum, and results in the formation of small, clear vesicles, located particularly on the trunk (*Fig. 6.64*). There are accompanying symptoms of a high fever and pronounced sweating.
- Miliaria rubra (prickly heat) is particularly common in hot, humid climates and is due to obstruction within the prickle cell layer, resulting in erythematous papules and vesicles, usually located about the trunk and intertriginous regions (*Fig. 6.65*). This form of miliaria is particularly common in infants. The term miliaria pustulosa has been applied to the above subtypes when pustules develop. Miliaria rubra and its pustular variant have also been found in association with pseudohypoaldesteronism, type I.[4,5,6]
- In miliaria profunda, also typically seen in tropical climates, the obstruction is at level of the sweat duct. Small papules are seen on the trunk and occasionally the extremities.

Pathogenesis and histologic features

The pathogenesis of miliaria is poorly understood. It has been suggested that bacteria play a role in the development of the disease. There is evidence

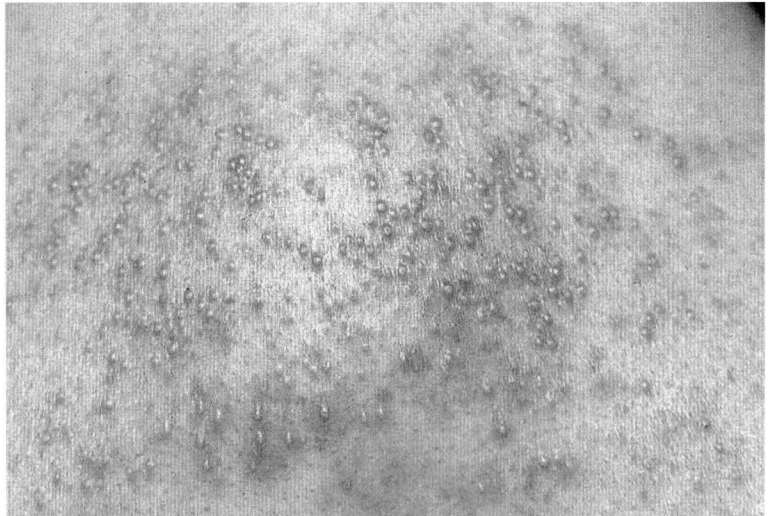

Fig. 6.65
Miliaria rubra: the characteristic appearance is of large numbers of minute papules and vesicles. By courtesy of M.M. Black, MD, Institute of Dermatology, London, UK.

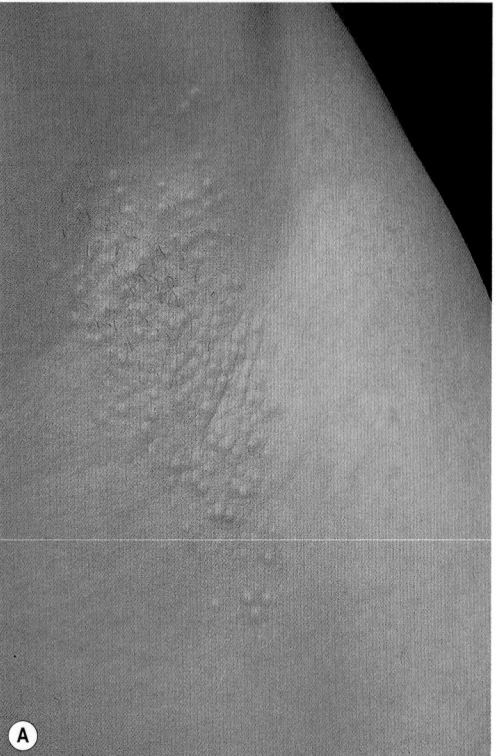

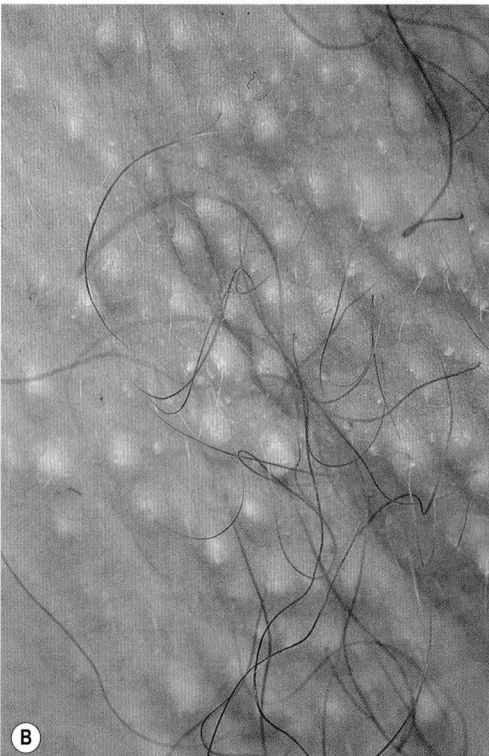

Fig. 6.66
Fox-Fordyce disease: (**A**) there are numerous white papules. The axilla is a characteristic site; (**B**) close-up view. By courtesy of the Institute of Dermatology, London, UK.

that extracellular polysaccharide substance (EPS), a PAS-positive material produced by some strains of *Staphylococcus epidermidis*, obstructs the sweat duct and causes the disease.[7] Normal controls who had *S. epidermidis* swabbed on to the volar aspect of their forearms followed by occlusion and heat developed miliaria. These results have not been replicated with other bacteria.[7] Biopsy revealed EPS in lesions from several patients.

A subcorneal vesicle containing a few neutrophils characterizes miliaria crystallina, while rubra involves an intraepidermal spongiotic vesicle. In both variants the lesions can be seen to be centered upon an intraepidermal eccrine sweat duct. Miliaria pustulosa is characterized by features of miliaria in addition to an intraepidermal or subcorneal pustule. Miliaria profunda is characterized by spongiosis of the dermal portion of the eccrine duct, often associated with dermal chronic inflammation adjacent to the affected duct.

Fox-Fordyce disease

Clinical features

Fox-Fordyce disease (apocrine miliaria, chronic itching papular eruption of the axillae and pubic region) presents as a chronic papular eruption, associated with pruritus, and located in areas containing apocrine sweat glands (i.e., the axillae, the pubic area, the vulval labia, the perineum, and areola) (*Fig. 6.66*).[1-3] The papules are discrete, firm, and flesh-colored or pigmented. Associated hair loss is often present.

The disease is uncommon and over 90% of reported cases have occurred in women, usually aged 13–35 years. Rarely, prepubescent and postmenopausal patients have been described.[4,5]

Pathogenesis and histologic features

Patients with Fox-Fordyce disease have apocrine anhidrosis. Although eccrine sweating is normal, apocrine sweating does not occur due to the keratotic plugging of the apocrine duct orifice. The continued secretion of sweat, however, causes the duct to rupture and an apocrine sweat retention cyst forms in the epithelium. The exact cause of the follicular plugging is unknown, but a hormonal link has been postulated. Occasional instances of coexistent hidradenitis suppurativa have been recorded.[6]

Follicular infundibular plugging is present in association with acanthosis, parakeratosis, spongiosis, and an underlying non-specific chronic inflammatory cell infiltrate. Dilation of the apocrine glands may be present and the presence of perifollicular foamy histiocytes is a frequent and diagnostically helpful feature.[7-9] Further reported findings include vacuolar change, dyskeratosis, and parakeratotic lamellae affecting the follicular infundibulum.[10] The keratinous obstruction prevents the outflow of apocrine secretion and

leads to the diagnostic feature of an intrafollicular sweat retention vesicle; serial sections may be needed to demonstrate this lesion.[11,12]

Transient acantholytic dermatosis with prominent eccrine ductal involvement

Grover disease (transient acantholytic dermatoses) is discussed more comprehensively elsewhere; however, since it is commonly associated with spongiosis (often in the absence of acantholysis), it deserves mention in this chapter. Studies of Grover disease have shown a strong correlation with high temperature and sweating and it has been suggested that its pathogenesis may be analogous to that of miliaria.[1-3] Supporting this concept is the development of Grover disease in bed-ridden and febrile patients. The lesions are usually present on the back. These patients often have prominent involvement of the eccrine duct and the lesions have been termed sudoriferous acrosyringeal acantholytic disease (sudoriferous Grover disease).[4] Biopsies taken from patients with sudoriferous acrosyringeal acantholytic disease often show, in addition to typical features of Grover disease, acantholysis of the superficial portion of the eccrine duct. When acantholysis is present and a clinical history is provided, the diagnosis is usually straightforward. However, not uncommonly, biopsies taken from patients with Grover disease show spongiosis only (often eosinophilic spongiosis). In these patients, a diagnosis of Grover disease may still be made in the appropriate clinical setting.

It is important to note that myriad cutaneous disorders may show some degree of spongiosis. For example, such disparate conditions as mycosis fungoides and psoriasis are not uncommonly associated with a degree of spongiosis. In this chapter, we have focused our discussion on entities for which spongiosis is a dominant and fairly consistent histologic finding. Other entities that may occasionally be associated with some degree of spongiosis are discussed in the appropriate chapters.

PSORIASIFORM DERMATOSES

The psoriasiform reaction pattern is defined by the presence of epidermal hyperplasia with fairly uniform and marked enlargement of the rete ridges. Although confluent parakeratosis with neutrophil exocytosis is characteristic of psoriasis (the prototype of this group of conditions), this feature is not included within the definition, which would otherwise become too restrictive. Diseases in addition to psoriasis which may manifest a psoriasiform pattern include reactive arthritis, pityriasis rubra pilaris, lichen simplex chronicus, psoriasiform drug reactions, subacute and chronic spongiotic dermatitis, parapsoriasis, and pityriasis rosea (herald patch). Other conditions in which psoriasiform hyperplasia may sometimes be a feature include dermatophyte infections and candidiasis, secondary syphilis, scabies infestation, inflammatory linear verrucous epidermal nevus, necrolytic migratory erythema, acrodermatitis enteropathica, and pellagra. Neoplastic conditions such as Bowen disease and mycosis fungoides, which often show marked epidermal hyperplasia, are not included in this definition.

Psoriasis

Clinical features

Psoriasis is a chronic relapsing and remitting disease of the skin that may affect any site.[1] It is one of the commonest of all skin diseases, with a reported incidence of 1–2% in Caucasians.[2,3] It is rare among blacks, Japanese, and native North and South American populations.[4] Males and females are affected equally. Although psoriasis may occur at any age, it most frequently presents in the teens and in early adult life (type I psoriasis).[5] A second peak in which the disease is often milder appears around the sixth decade (type II psoriasis).[5]

The classic cutaneous lesion of psoriasis vulgaris (plaque psoriasis), developing in about 85–90% of patients with psoriasis, is raised, sharply demarcated, with a silvery scaly surface (*Figs 6.67–6.69*).[6,7] The underlying skin has a glossy, erythematous appearance. If the parakeratotic scales are removed with the fingernail, small droplets of blood may appear on the surface (Auspitz sign); this is diagnostic. Plaques, when multiple, are often symmetrical and annular lesions due to central clearing are a common finding (*Fig. 6.70*). The scalp, the extensor surfaces (mainly the knees and elbows), the lower back, and around the umbilicus are particularly affected. The clinical features, however, show regional variation: scalp involvement often shows very marked plaque formation, whereas on the penis scaling is commonly minimal and the features may be mistaken for Bowen disease (*Figs 6.71–6.73*). Linear lesions (linear psoriasis) follow previous trauma (koebnerization) (*Fig. 6.74*).

Psoriasis may manifest in a variety of other ways.
- Guttate (eruptive) psoriasis presents as small (0.5–1.5 cm in diameter) papules over the upper trunk and proximal extremities, typically in younger patients (*Figs 6.75–6.77*).
- Psoriasis inversa is characterized by the development of plaques in the flexures (*Fig. 6.78*).
- Generalized pustular psoriasis (von Zumbusch) is an acute variant, characterized by fever of several days' duration, together with the

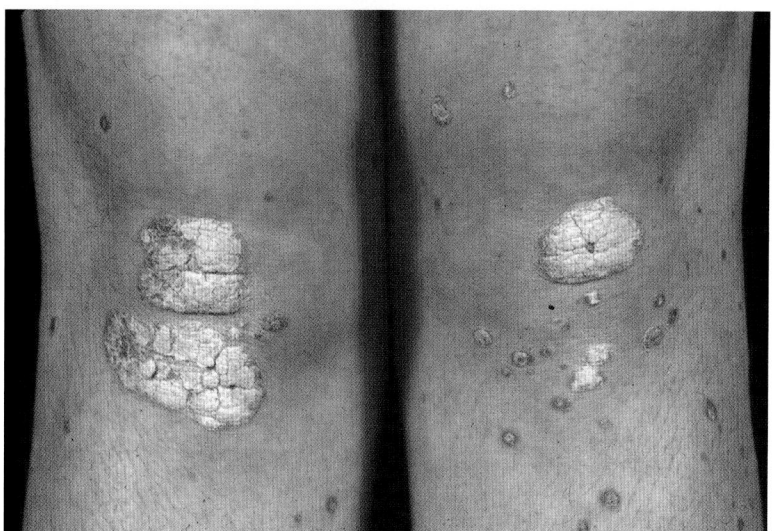

Fig. 6.67
Psoriasis: typical plaque disease showing bilateral and fairly symmetrical distribution. In this example, the silvery scale is well demonstrated. From the collection of the late N.P. Smith, MD, the Institute of Dermatology, London, UK.

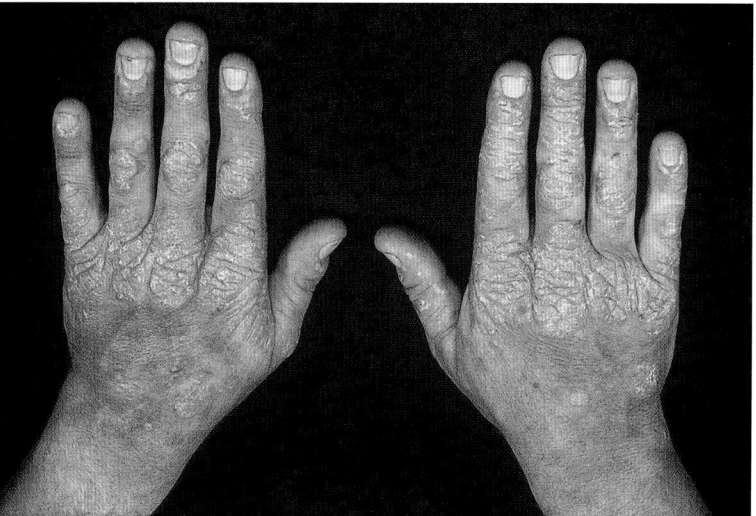

Fig. 6.68
Plaque psoriasis: note the symmetry of these lesions. By courtesy of R.A. Marsden, MD, St George's Hospital, London, UK.

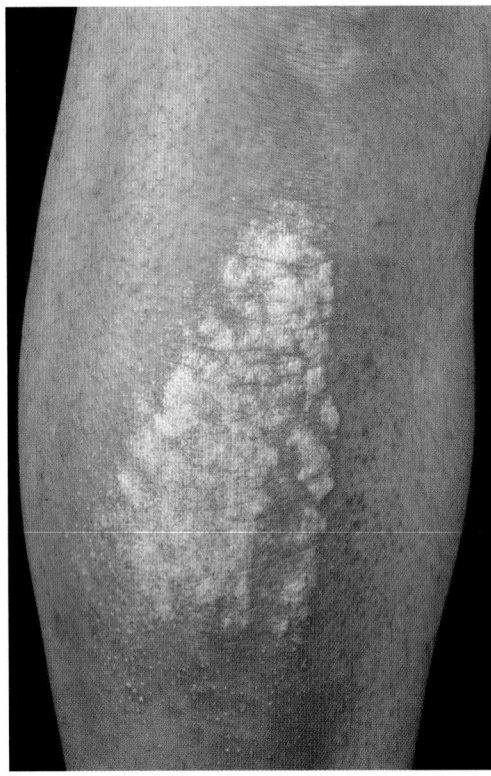

Fig. 6.69
Plaque psoriasis: close-up view showing the thick scale. From the collection of the late N.P. Smith, MD, the Institute of Dermatology, London, UK.

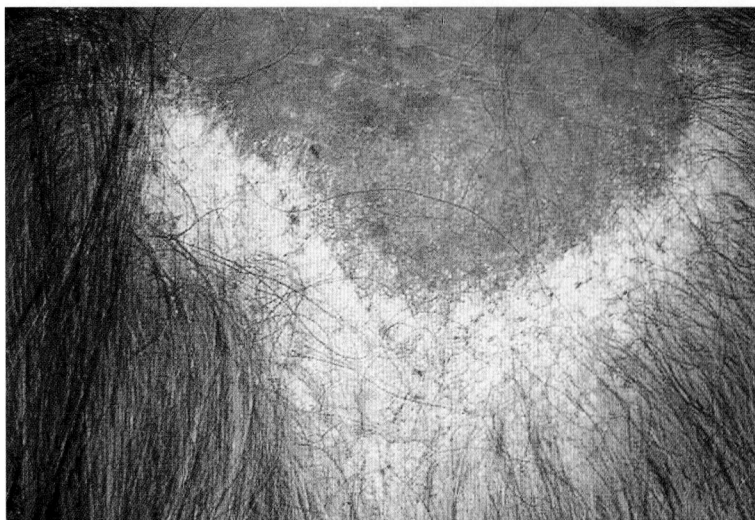

Fig. 6.71
Plaque psoriasis: the scalp is a commonly affected site. By courtesy of the Institute of Dermatology, London, UK.

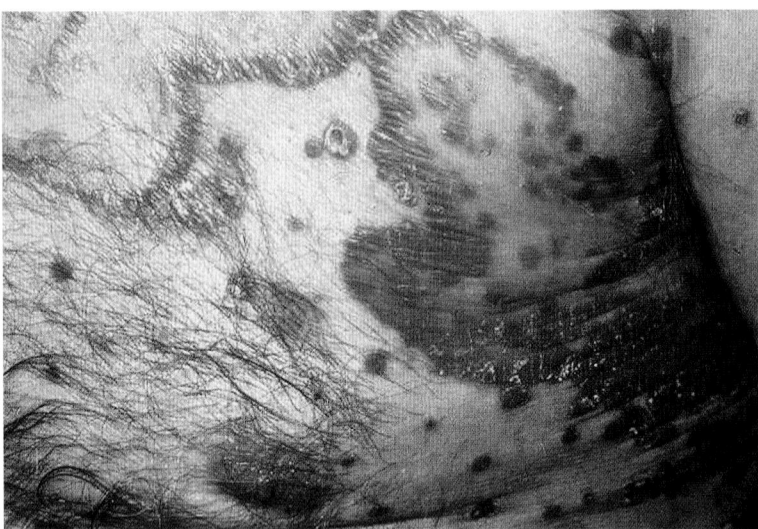

Fig. 6.70
Annular psoriasis: central clearing of plaques results in annular lesions. By courtesy of R.A. Marsden, MD, St George's Hospital, London, UK.

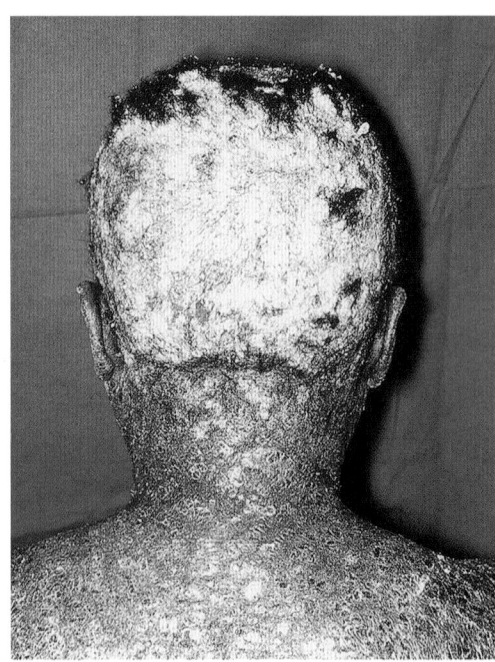

Fig. 6.72
Plaque psoriasis: in this extreme case, the initial diagnosis was Norwegian scabies. Surprisingly, alopecia is an uncommon complication. By courtesy of R.A. Marsden, MD, St George's Hospital, London, UK.

sudden appearance of sterile pustules, 2–3 mm across, over the trunk and extremities (*Fig. 6.79*).[8] The surrounding skin is erythematous and confluence may result in a generalized erythroderma (*Fig. 6.80*). Usually, recurrent episodes of fever occur, followed by fresh outbreaks of pustules (*Fig. 6.81*). Systemic signs include weight loss, weakness, and hypocalcemia, with a raised white cell count and high erythrocyte sedimentation rate (ESR). Although the precipitating factor is often unknown, pustular psoriasis may follow a streptococcal or viral infection. Withdrawal of systemic steroid therapy is also a known predisposing cause.[9] Treatment with systemic steroids or intensive topical regimens has also been incriminated.[10] Other risk factors for developing a pustular episode include drugs, pregnancy, hypocalcemia, and sunlight or phototherapy.[11] Uncommon variants of pustular

psoriasis include an annular form, exanthematous pustular psoriasis, and juvenile and infantile pustular psoriasis.[12,13] The annular variant is a somewhat less serious variant in which, due to central clearing, lesions develop an annular or gyrate morphology.[11] Often, the systemic manifestations are less florid. The exanthematous variant, which tends to develop de novo, may sometimes follow an infection or represent a pustular drug reaction.[11] Impetigo herpetiformis most probably represents pustular psoriasis of pregnancy although some authors classify it as a separate entity.[14]

- In psoriatic erythroderma, there is an intense generalized erythema affecting the entire skin surface, associated with desquamation (*Fig. 6.82*). Ectropion may be present and scalp involvement is sometimes followed by hair loss. Erythroderma may be precipitated in patients with psoriasis vulgaris by infection with *Staphylococcus aureus*, abrupt curtailment of steroid or methotrexate therapy, and sunburn.[11] Systemic symptoms including fever, chills, shortness of breath, fatigue, and

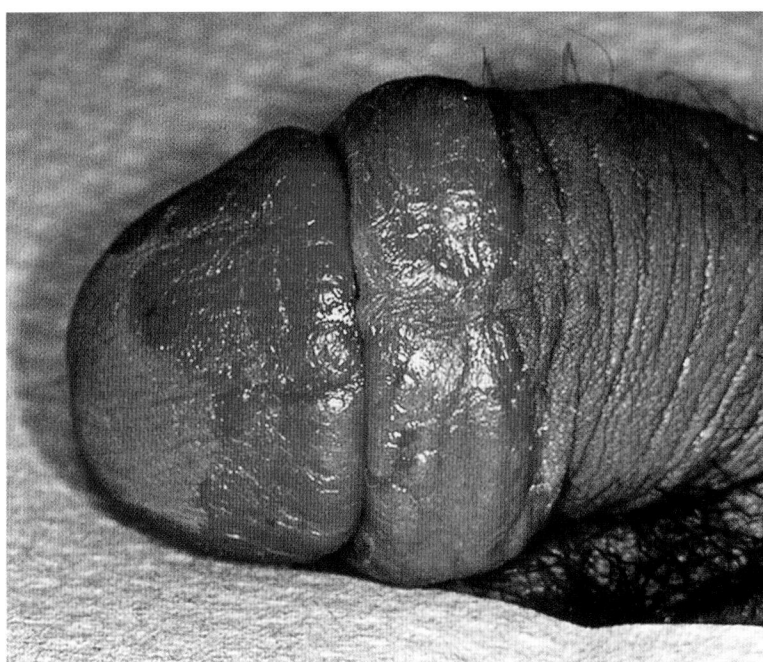

Fig. 6.73
Psoriasis: penile lesion showing a sharply demarcated, erythematous, eroded, slightly scaly plaque. By courtesy of C. Furlonge, MD, Port of Spain, Trinidad.

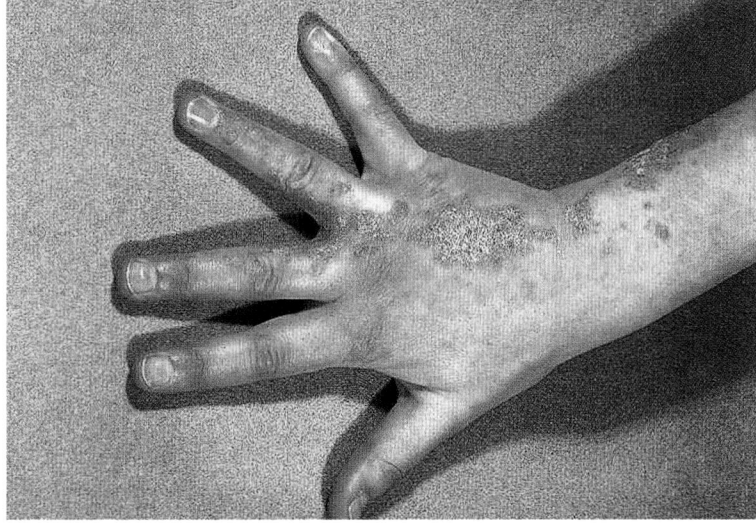

Fig. 6.74
Plaque psoriasis: linear involvement is a manifestation of koebnerization following trauma. By courtesy of the Institute of Dermatology, London, UK.

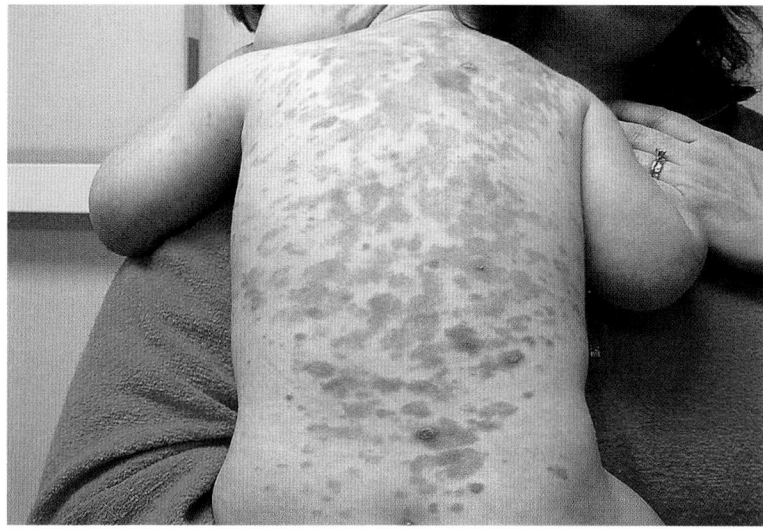

Fig. 6.75
Guttate psoriasis: this infant shows a characteristic distribution over the trunk. By courtesy of M. Liang, MD, Children's Hospital, Boston, USA.

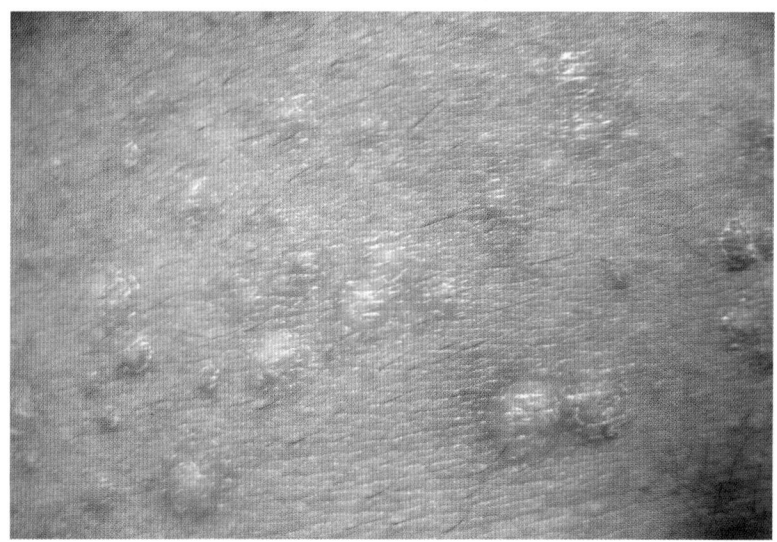

Fig. 6.76
Guttate psoriasis: this close-up view shows the erythema and scaling. By courtesy of the Institute of Dermatology, London, UK.

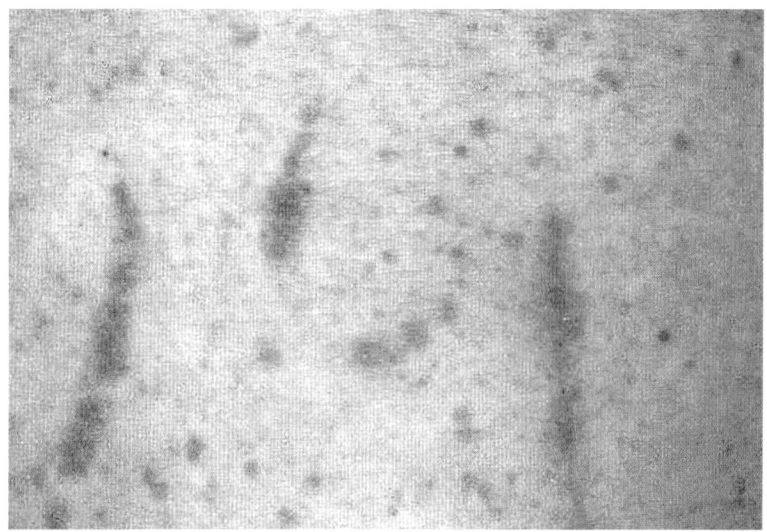

Fig. 6.77
Guttate psoriasis: as with plaque disease, guttate psoriasis is associated with a Koebner phenomenon. By courtesy of the Institute of Dermatology, London, UK.

myalgia are commonly present.[11] Biochemical abnormalities include hypoalbuminemia, anemia, and dehydration.[15] High-output cardiac failure is an important complication.

- Localized (mixed) pustular psoriasis represents the development of pustules on pre-existent plaques.[9] This variant most often develops in acute flares of psoriasis or following treatment.[11] It sometimes represents a harbinger of a more generalized process.
- Palmoplantar pustular psoriasis of Barber (pustulosis palmaris et plantaris) refers to a chronic recurrent pustular dermatosis localized to the palms and soles (*Figs 6.83* and *6.84*). It shows a strong predilection for females (9:1) in the fourth to fifth decade of life and the disease is associated with a history of smoking.[6,16,17] In about 25% of patients there is coexistent chronic plaque psoriasis.[6]
- Acrodermatitis continua (acropustulosis) of Hallopeau is a rare sterile pustular eruption of the fingers or toes, involving the nails and slowly extending proximally (*Figs 6.85* and *6.86*).

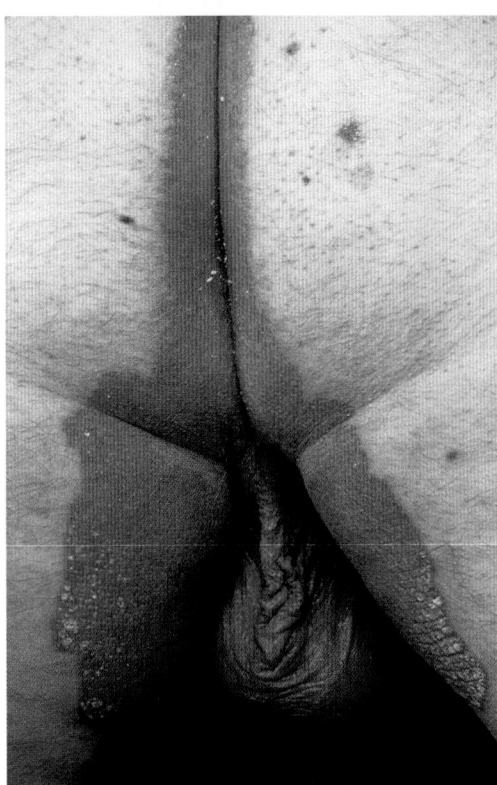

Fig. 6.78
Flexural (inverse) psoriasis: this is a rare variant in which the lesions develop on flexural skin.

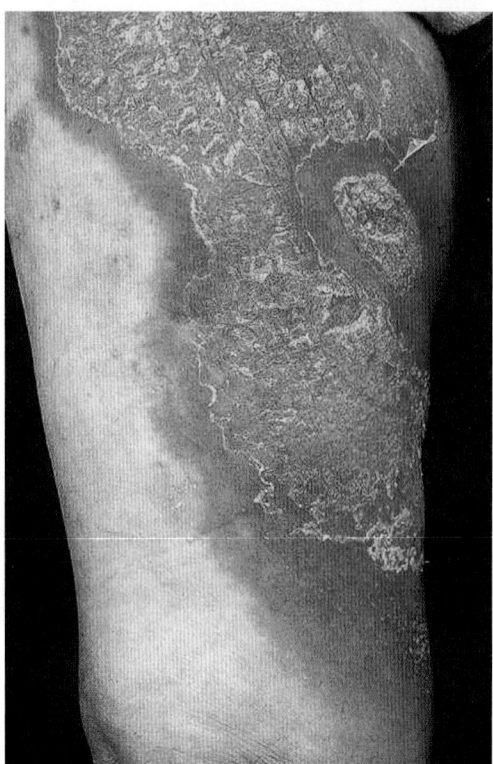

Fig. 6.80
Pustular psoriasis: early stage showing intense erythema. By courtesy of the Institute of Dermatology, London, UK.

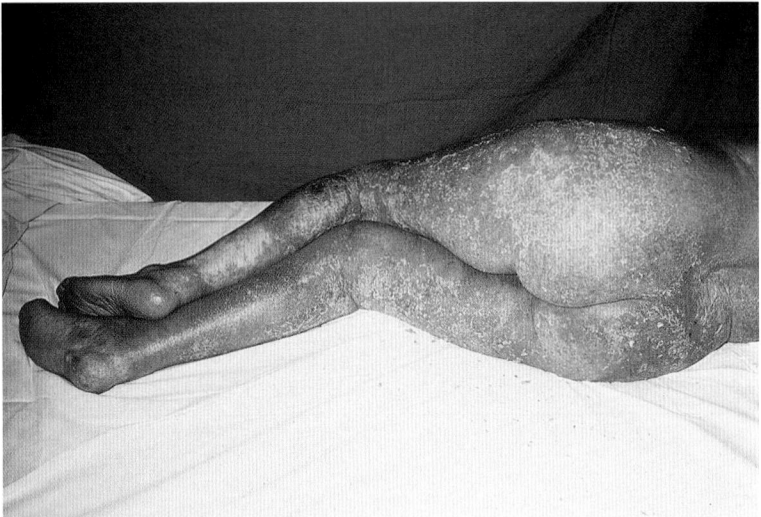

Fig. 6.79
Pustular psoriasis (von Zumbusch): note the extreme generalized erythema and pustulation. This variant is rare and may sometimes prove fatal. By courtesy of R.A. Marsden, St George's Hospital, London, UK.

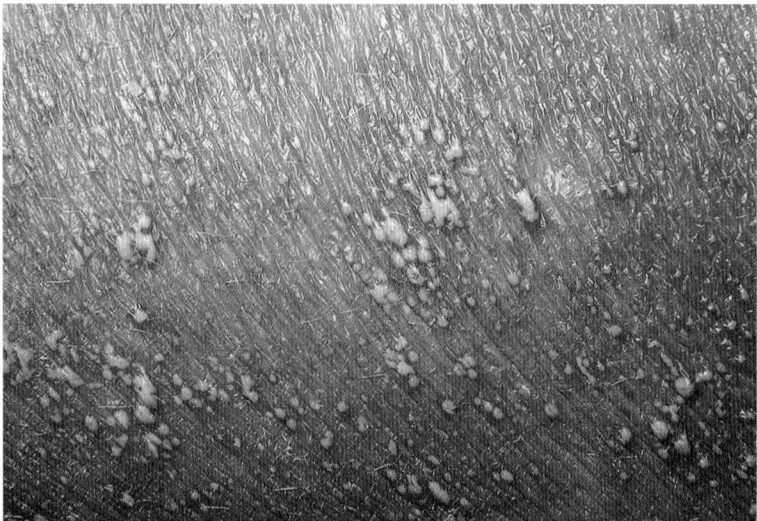

Fig. 6.81
Pustular psoriasis: close-up view showing typical pustules arising on a background of intense erythema. By courtesy of the Institute of Dermatology, London, UK.

The nail is frequently affected in psoriasis; lesions may include pitting, discoloration, onycholysis, subungual hyperkeratosis, nail grooving, and splinter hemorrhages and complete loss in pustular psoriasis.[18]

Patients with psoriasis have a higher incidence of certain comorbidities including, depression, obesity, type 2 diabetes mellitus, hyperlipidemia, hypertension, metabolic syndrome, cardiovascular disease, Crohn disease, and multiple sclerosis, as well as cutaneous and visceral malignancies.[6,19]

Psoriatic arthritis

Psoriatic arthritis has a prevalence of 0.02–7% but more recent data suggest that it could be as high as 30%.[20] It may take a number of different forms (*Fig. 6.87*):[21]

- The most common is an asymmetrical involvement of a few joints of the fingers or toes; this accounts for over 70% of cases.
- In 15% of cases a symmetrical polyarthritis, clinically indistinguishable from rheumatoid arthritis, but seronegative, is seen.
- In approximately 5% of cases the distal interphalangeal joints are involved, the classical picture of psoriatic arthropathy (*Fig. 6.88*).
- A further 5% have a destructive and severely deforming arthritis, arthritis mutilans.
- The remaining cases have ankylosing spondylitis, with or without peripheral joint involvement (*Fig. 6.89*).

Psoriatic arthritis is associated with a high incidence of mitral valve prolapse with resultant incompetence.[22] The peak age of onset is 36–45 years of age, although the destructive form may occur earlier. A high incidence

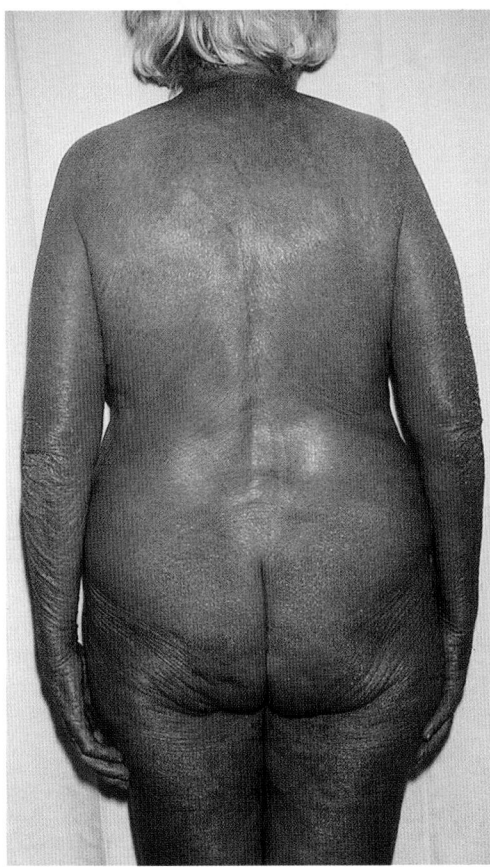

Fig. 6.82
Psoriatic erythroderma: there is generalized erythema. Patients are at risk of dehydration, hypoalbuminemia, and anemia. By courtesy of R.A. Marsden, St George's Hospital, London, UK.

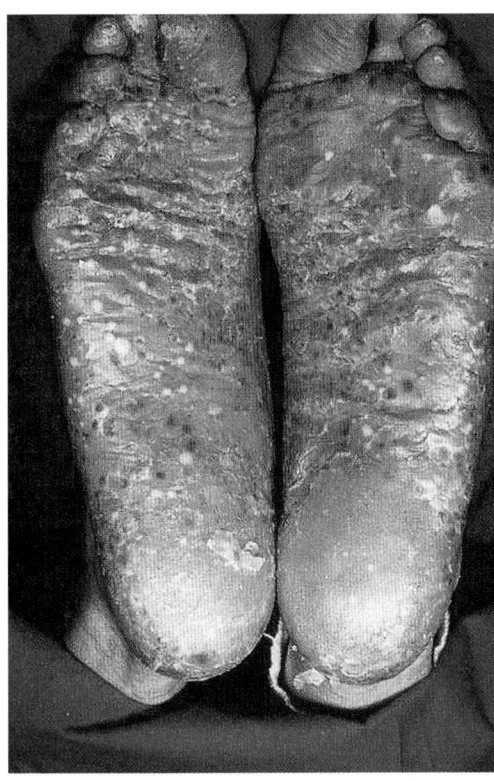

Fig. 6.83
Palmoplantar pustular psoriasis: there is intense erythema, scaling, and numerous pustules. By courtesy of the Institute of Dermatology, London, UK.

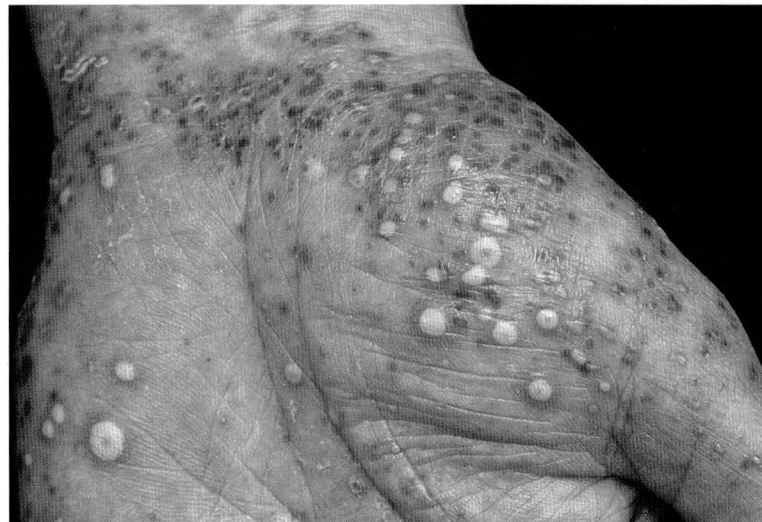

Fig. 6.84
Palmoplantar pustular psoriasis: close-up view of palmar pustules. By courtesy of the Institute of Dermatology, London, UK.

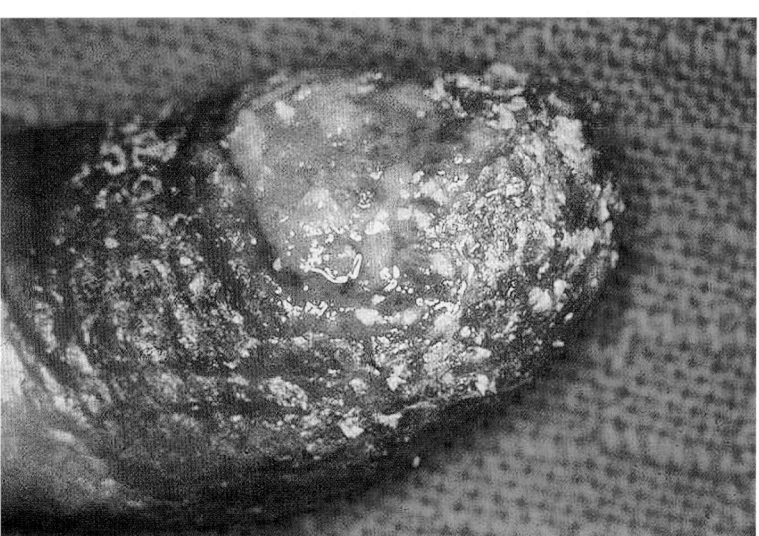

Fig. 6.85
Acropustulosis continua: there is pustulation with erythema and scaling, the nail has been shed, and there is damage to the nail plate. By courtesy of R.A. Marsden, St George's Hospital, London, UK.

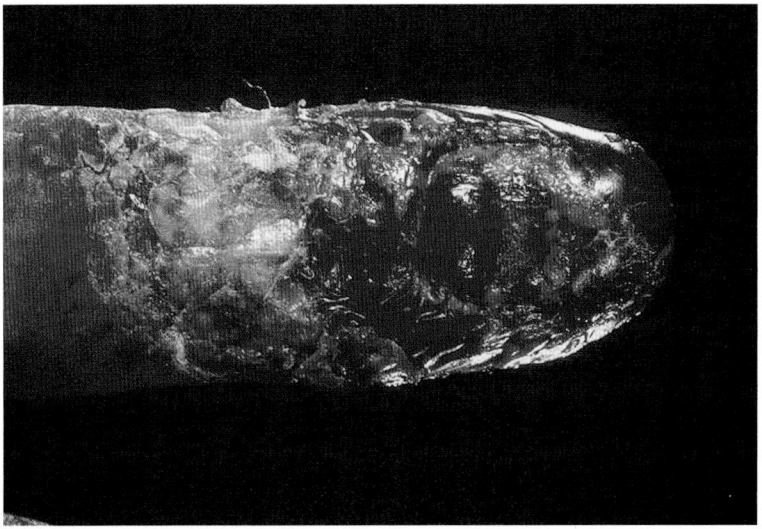

Fig. 6.86
Acropustulosis continua: a particularly severe example. By courtesy of S. Dalziel, MD, University Hospital, Nottingham, UK.

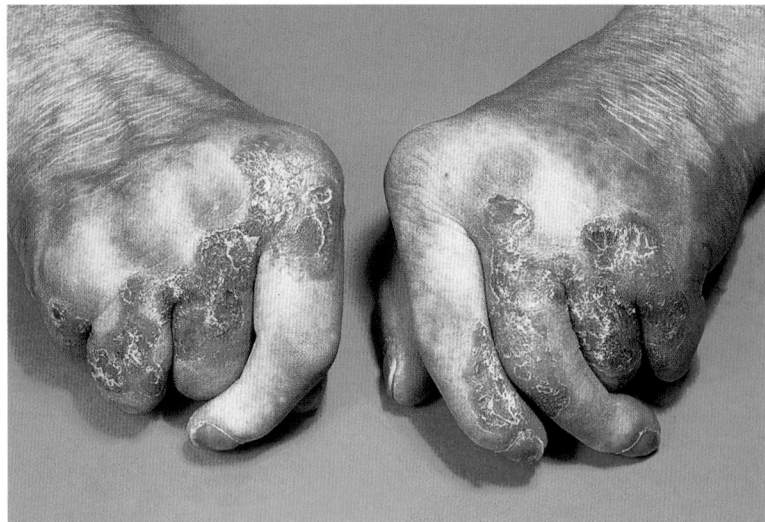

Fig. 6.87
Psoriatic arthropathy: joint involvement is a rare manifestation. Lesions of the interphalangeal joints, while said to be characteristic, are an uncommon finding. In this patient there is gross deformity. By courtesy of R.A. Marsden, St George's Hospital, London, UK.

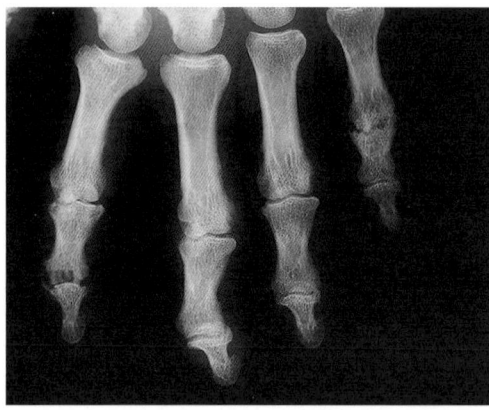

Fig. 6.88
Psoriatic arthropathy: classic type. Note the destruction of the distal interphalangeal joint of the first finger. By courtesy of the Institute of Dermatology, London, UK.

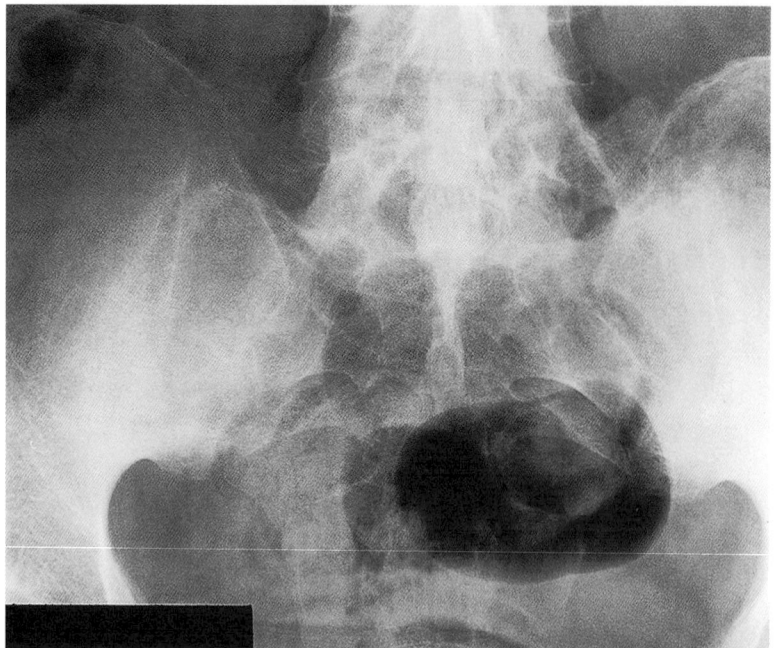

Fig. 6.89
Psoriatic arthropathy: sacroiliitis. Note the virtual obliteration of the sacroiliac joints. By courtesy of R.A. Marsden, St George's Hospital, London, UK.

of immunoglobulin gene polymorphism has been identified in patients with psoriatic arthritis, suggesting an inherited predisposition.[23]

Psoriatic arthritis in children, although uncommon, is of importance because frequently the arthritis precedes the onset of the skin lesions. A careful examination for nail changes and questioning about a family history may be of value in establishing the diagnosis.

Pathogenesis and histologic features

Although the etiology of psoriasis remains incompletely understood, considerable advances have been made in the past two decades to unravel the complex mechanisms involved in the pathogenesis of this common dermatosis. For many years psoriasis was considered to represent a primary epidermal hyperproliferative disorder. More recent studies, however, have shown that a T-lymphocyte-driven immune process is central to the development of the psoriatic plaque and, in fact, may represent the earliest stage in its evolution. Other important factors include genetic influences, the environment, and the contribution of keratinocyte-derived mediators of the inflammatory process.

The inherited predisposition to develop psoriasis has long been known. A positive family history is common. Documented prevalence rates in first-degree relatives have ranged from 7.8% to 17.6%.[24,25] Monozygotic twins have a concordance of 64–70% while that of dizygotic twins is in the order of 14–23%.[26] Linkage analysis has identified at least nine separate loci (PSORS1–9).[6,7,27–30] PSORS1 shows the strongest genetic susceptibility, being implicated in 35–50% of familial psoriasis.[6,7,31,32] The locus is present on chromosome 6p within the major histocompatibility complex and HLA-Cw6 has been demonstrated as the susceptibility allele on PSORS1.[31,32]

Genetically, psoriasis is a heterogeneous disease at the level of PSORS1 and two distinct types have been identified:[5]

- Type I disease, which affects young adults and includes guttate psoriasis, is characterized by a familial segregation involving HLA-Cw6.[5,33]
- Type II disease includes psoriasis vulgaris presenting at an older age (over 50 years) as well as palmoplantar pustulosis and shows no familial segregation and no association with the PSORS1 locus.[4,33,34] Patients with pustular psoriasis have a higher incidence of HLA-B27, as do those with psoriasis and peripheral arthritis, and this is most marked if spondylitis is present.[35] Further genes related to increased genetic susceptibility for psoriasis include the interleukin-23 receptor gene on chromosome 1p, the interleukin-12B gene on chromosome 5q, zinc finger protein 313 on chromosome 20q, the CDKAL1 gene on chromosome 6p, the PTPN22 gene on chromosome 18p, the IL-4–IL-13 cytokine gene cluster on chromosome 5q, the LCE3B/3C gene on 1q, and the PSORS2 locus on chromosome 17q.[7]

Generalized pustular psoriasis has been linked to mutations in the adaptor-related protein complex 1σ3 subunit (AP1S3) and IL-36 receptor antagonist (IL36RN) genes.[36–38]

The IL-23 receptor is of interest as it is also associated with ankolysing spondylitis and psoriatic arthritis while the CDKAL1 gene has also been associated with Crohn disease and type-2 diabetes mellitus.[7]

Certain factors are known to induce psoriasis in a person who is genetically predisposed. There is a tendency for lesions to develop at sites of previous skin trauma (e.g., mechanical friction, sunburn or childhood illnesses, such as varicella); this is termed the isomorphic or Koebner phenomenon.[39–41]

Infections are well known as predisposing factors in the onset of psoriasis. In children in particular, upper respiratory tract infections frequently trigger psoriasis, while infections with *Streptococcus pyogenes* are implicated in the development of acute guttate psoriasis, together with an exacerbation of other forms of psoriasis.[42–45] Specific streptococcal serotypes, however, do not appear to be implicated.

Other factors known to exacerbate psoriasis include stress, bereavement, HIV/AIDS, withdrawal of corticosteroids after prolonged use, and treatment with a number of drugs including lithium, antimalarials, and beta-blocking agents.[6,46]

The development of the psoriatic plaque results from a complex interplay between keratinocyte hyperproliferation with loss of differentiation, changes in the superficial dermal vasculature, and a T-lymphocyte-mediated inflammatory component.[47] The relative roles of keratinocyte hyperplasia, vascular changes, and immunological reactions have been the subject of much discussion in the literature.[48] Most recently, the focus has been particularly directed towards the importance of the innate as well as adaptive immune systems.[7]

In the skin there is an increased epidermal proliferation rate: the transit time of keratinocytes through the epidermis in normal skin is 56 days; in psoriatic skin it is shortened to 7 days.[49,50] The epidermal cell cycle is probably shortened, and there is a large increase in the number of proliferating generative cells in the basal layers, where up to three layers of proliferating cells may be seen compared with only one in normal resting epidermis.

Vascular proliferation predominantly affecting the postcapillary venules of the dermal papillae appears to be one of the earliest manifestations of psoriasis.[51] This is mediated by upregulation of $\alpha V\beta 3$ integrin and vascular endothelial growth factor (VEGF).[52–54]

The current weight of evidence suggests that a T-cell-mediated immune reaction is central to the pathogenesis of psoriasis.[47,55] Clinical studies supporting this hypothesis include the response to antilymphocyte therapies, such as ciclosporin.[56] Remission in patients with severe psoriasis has resulted from treatment with an activated T-lymphocyte selective toxin DAB389 IL-2 that interacts with the receptor-binding domain of IL-2.[57] Successful responses to therapy with monoclonal anti-CD3 and anti-CD4 antibodies adds further support.[58,59] Additional evidence has come from bone marrow transplantation studies. Unaffected patients develop psoriasis following a transplant from an affected donor whereas patients are cured of their disease following transplantation from an unaffected donor.[60] In vitro studies in which intradermal injection of T-helper lymphocytes from an affected patient into severe combined immunodeficient mice results in the development of typical psoriasis further supports a T-lymphocyte-driven pathogenesis.[61]

The innate immune system appears to play an important part in the early stages of the disease and increased numbers of activated plasmacytoid dendritic cells are present in early psoriatic lesions.[62] Production of interferon alpha by plasmacytoid dendritic cells and TNF-α and INF-γ by natural killer cells leads to activation of myeloid dendritic cells and subsequent proliferation of T cells through IL-12 and IL-23 release.[7,63]

Although CD4 Th lymphocytes are probably of importance in the earliest stages of plaque development, the major population is characterized by CD8 expression. The immunophenotype of the T cells includes CD45RO+, HLADR+, CD25+ and CLA+, indicating activated skin-specific memory cells.[64] The lymphocyte cytokine profile, which includes IL-2, IL-17, interferon gamma (IFN-γ), and absence of IL-4, IL-10, and tumor necrosis factor alpha (TNF-α), reflects a predominantly Th1-mediated inflammatory reaction as well as IL-17-A producing type 17 helper T (Th17) cells.[7,65–67] Th17 cells are of particular importance for epithelial immunosurveillance and produce IL-17 and IL-22.[68,69] IL-17 has recently been shown to play a particularly important role in the pathogenesis of psoriasis.[38,70] IFN-γ is central to the development of the plaque. In vitro studies have shown that the keratinocyte proliferation is IFN-γ dependent.[71] Also, IFN-γ injection in normal human skin results in epidermal proliferation.[72] In addition to the lymphocyte-derived cytokines discussed above, the keratinocytes themselves are a rich source of inflammatory mediators, which are likely to be of importance in initiating the inflammatory reaction and the development and maintenance of the psoriasiform plaque.[73] In particular, keratinocytes secrete IL-1α, IL-1β, and TNF-α. These cytokines play a major role in angiogenesis, in recruitment of circulating lymphocytes, and inducing expression of a number of endothelial cell adhesion molecules including E-selectin, intercellular adhesion molecule-1 (ICAM-1), and vascular cell adhesion molecule-1 (VCAM-1).[73–75] These last are of particular importance in facilitating the extravasation of lymphocytes through the endothelium.[55] Keratinocytes are also a valuable source of chemokines including IL-8, melanoma growth stimulatory activity alpha (MGS/GRO-α), gamma inducible

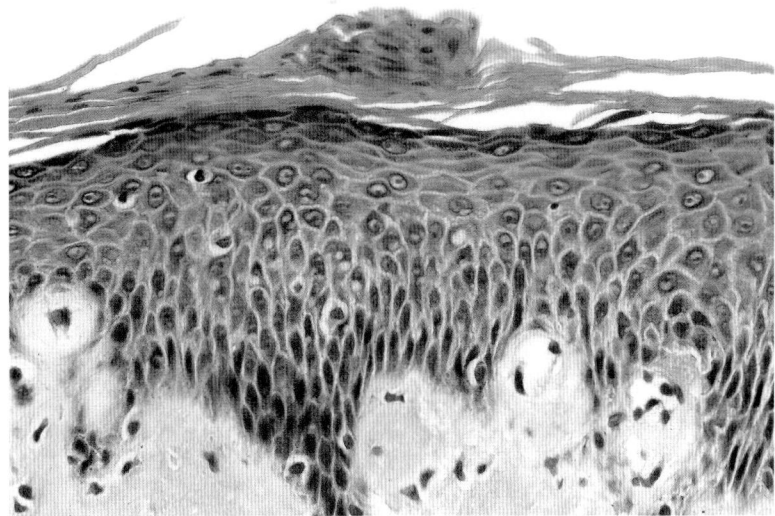

Fig. 6.90
Evolving psoriasis: in the early stages, there is capillary dilatation, with spongiosis, as shown in this field. A small parakeratotic mound is also demonstrated.

protein 10 (IP-10), and molecule chemoattractant protein 1 (MCP-1).[73] IL-8 is of importance in both neutrophil and T-lymphocyte chemotaxis.[76] It also promotes keratinocyte proliferation and induces angiogenesis.[77,78] IL-8 is predominantly derived from superficial keratinocytes and the associated neutrophils within the psoriatic plaque. MGS/GRO-α is an additional powerful neutrophil chemoattractant.[73]

The pathogenesis of psoriasis therefore involves interaction between injured keratinocytes and activated lymphocytes through the release of various cytokines developing in a background of genetic predisposition.[75] The precise relationship between the T-cell-driven immune reaction and epidermal hyperplasia, however, remains unclear. Similarly, the initiator(s) of this process are uncertain. Although autoantigens and bacterial superantigens are currently favored, the possibility of a direct consequence of lymphocyte–keratinocyte interaction has not yet been disproved.[78]

In biopsies of the early lesions, the histologic features consist primarily of dermal changes.[79–83] The evolution of the psoriatic plaque consists initially of the development of tortuous, dilated, and frequently congested capillaries in the superficial papillary dermis accompanied by edema and a perivascular mononuclear cell infiltrate (Fig. 6.90).[79] This vascular change is common to all forms of psoriasis and may even be seen in biopsies from clinically resolved lesions following treatment.[82] Lymphocytes then migrate into the lower epidermis, which becomes spongiotic. Subsequently, the upper epidermis shows focal vacuolation and eventual loss of the granular cell layer with the resultant formation of parakeratotic mounds. Migration of neutrophils from capillaries in the dermal papillae through gaps in the epidermal basement membrane and hence to the stratum corneum completes the process. Psoriasiform hyperplasia of the affected epidermis then follows.

Classical plaque psoriatic lesions show marked and characteristic acanthosis of the epidermal ridges, which are evenly elongated and club-shaped at their bases, alternating with long edematous papillae, which are club-shaped at their tips (Figs 6.91–6.94). Fusion of adjacent ridges is commonly present in established lesions. The suprapapillary plate is typically thinned and the epidermal surface is covered by confluent parakeratosis associated with diminution or loss of the granular cell layer. The lower suprabasal layers of the epidermis can frequently be seen to be actively dividing. Large tortuous capillaries are present in the papillary dermis and there is a slight perivascular lymphocytic infiltrate in the subpapillary dermis. Palmar and plantar lesions may sometimes cause diagnostic difficulty as spongiosis can be marked, and occasionally vesiculation is evident.[82]

The diagnostic features of active lesions include the 'Munro microabscess' and 'spongiform pustule of Kogoj'. Munro microabscesses represent an accumulation of polymorphs within the parakeratotic stratum corneum. Spongiform pustules are seen beneath the keratin layer and consist of small

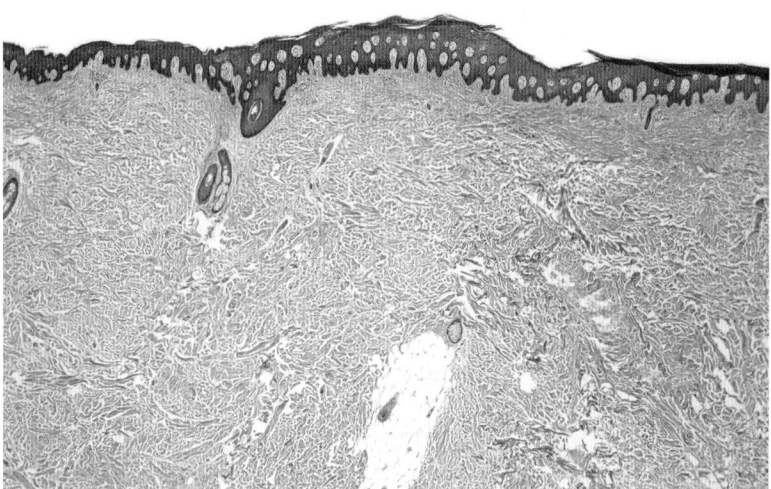

Fig. 6.91
Plaque psoriasis: scanning view showing extensive parakeratosis, regular acanthosis, club-shaped epidermal ridges, and ridge fusion.

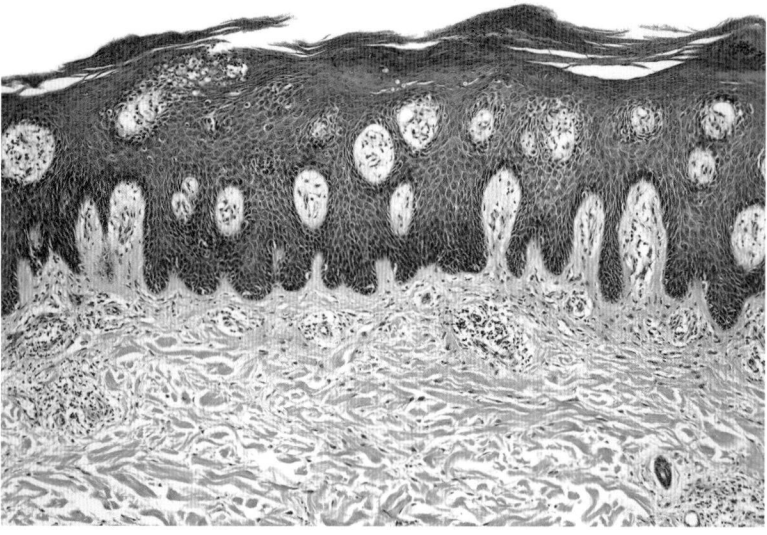

Fig. 6.92
Plaque psoriasis: closer view showing parakeratosis with neutrophil aggregates (Munro microabscess). There is marked dilatation and tortuosity of the capillaries within the dermal papillae. Spongiosis is also present.

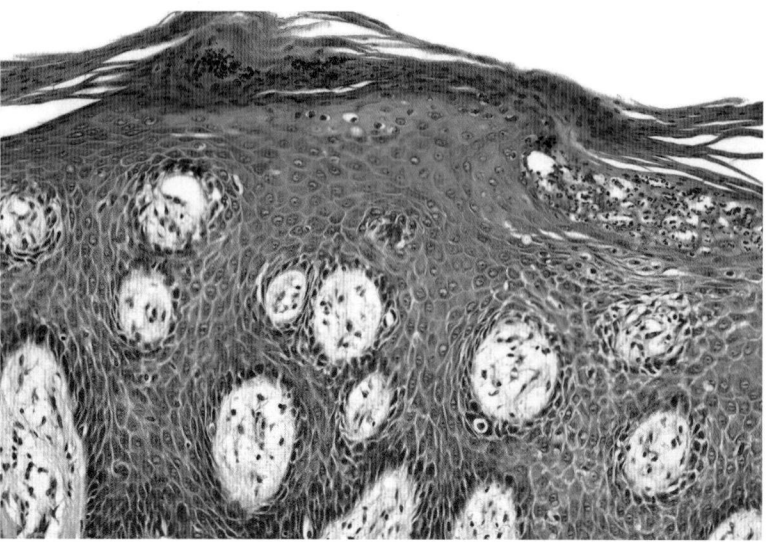

Fig. 6.93
Plaque psoriasis: Munro microabscess, spongiform degeneration, and parakeratosis.

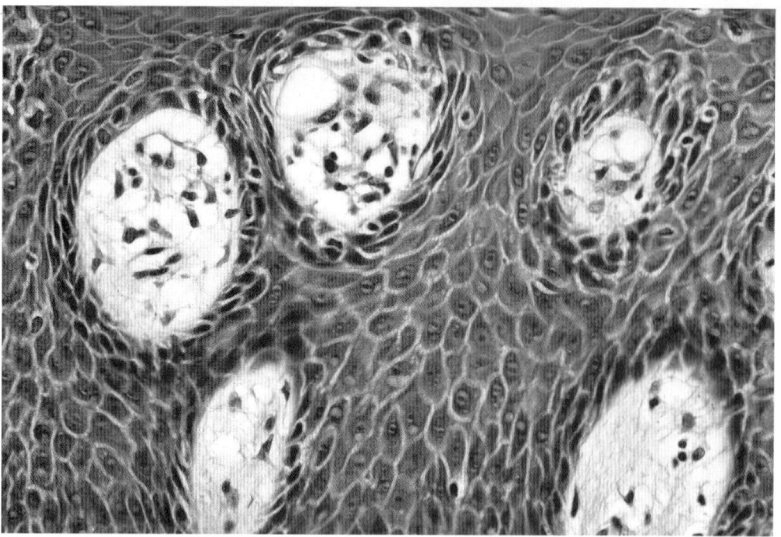

Fig. 6.94
Plaque psoriasis: tortuous and dilated capillaries.

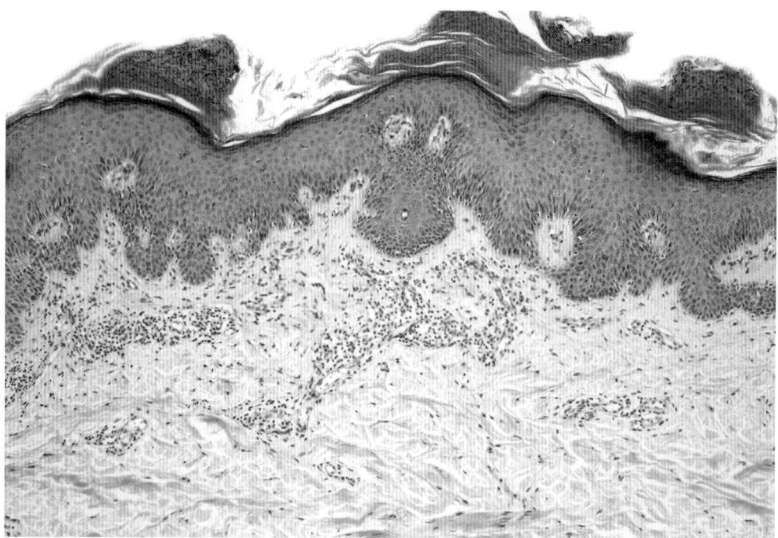

Fig. 6.95
Guttate psoriasis: the multiple discrete, parakeratotic mounds are characteristic. Hyperplasia is not as well developed as in plaque disease.

accumulations of neutrophils and occasional lymphocytes intermingled with the epidermal cells in foci of spongiosis.

In guttate psoriasis, the histologic features overlap with those of evolving disease.[82] Parakeratosis associated with loss or diminution of the granular cell layer is limited to small foci contrasting with a background of orthokeratosis (*Figs 6.95* and *6.96*). Neutrophils are seen surmounting the parakeratotic tiers. Acanthosis is much less marked than in fully established plaque disease. Neutrophils and lymphocytes are commonly present in the superficial papillary dermis and mild spongiosis is often a feature, particularly if biopsies of early lesions are examined.[84]

In generalized pustular psoriasis and its three variants the histologic picture is slightly different in that the spongiform pustule occurs as a macropustule and is the characteristic lesion (*Figs 6.97* and *6.98*).[83] As the spongiform pustule increases in size, the epidermal cells die, with resulting central cavitation. At the edges, a shell of thinned epidermal cells remains. Eventually there is migration of neutrophils into the horny layer and the picture resembles that of a large Munro abscess. Although the epidermal and dermal features may be similar to those of psoriasis vulgaris, particularly if the pustule has developed against a background of plaque-type disease, more often the features are much less well developed (*Fig. 6.99*). Frequently, therefore, there is no or only minimal epidermal hyperplasia although tortuous and dilated capillaries accompanied by a lymphocytic or mixed lymphocytic and neutrophil infiltrate are usually seen.[11]

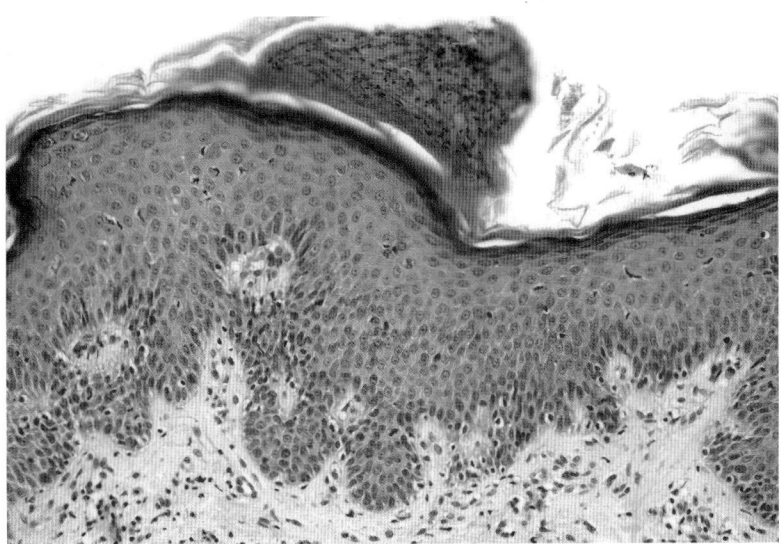

Fig. 6.96
Guttate psoriasis: close-up view.

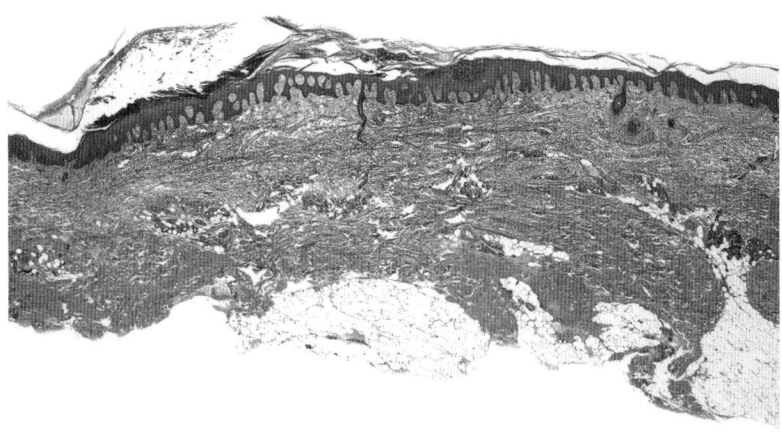

Fig. 6.97
Pustular psoriasis: a macropustule is present. Typical psoriasiform hyperplasia with parakeratosis is seen in the adjacent epidermis.

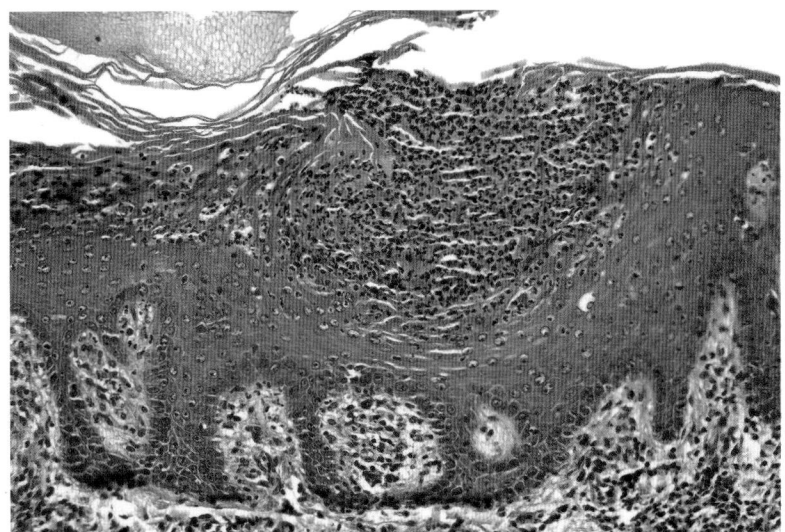

Fig. 6.98
Pustular psoriasis: close-up view.

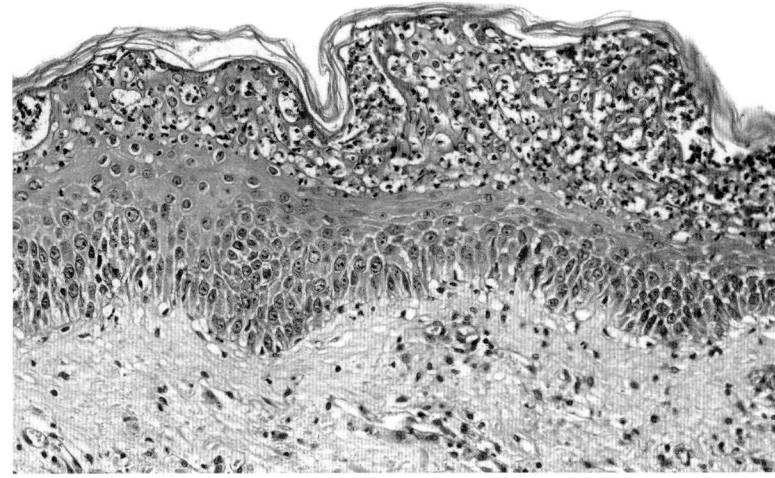

Fig. 6.99
Pustular psoriasis: in this patient, the lesions developed dramatically in the absence of significant plaque disease. There is only mild hyperplasia of the underlying epidermis.

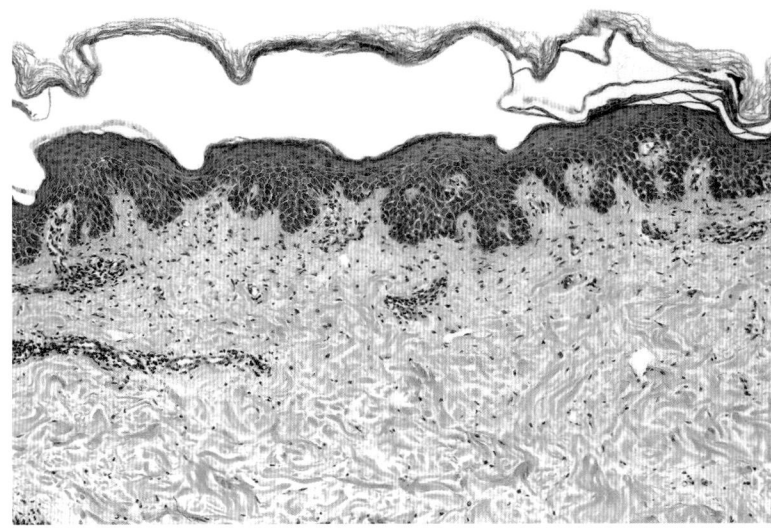

Fig. 6.100
Psoriatic erythroderma: there is only very focal parakeratosis with scattered neutrophils. The epidermal hyperplasia is only slight.

In palmar/plantar pustular lesions, the initial changes are those of spongiosis with lymphocytic exocytosis in the lower epidermis.[84] As the lesion progresses, neutrophils infiltrate the epidermis and a macropustule develops.

In psoriatic erythroderma the histologic features are variable but in the majority of cases a positive diagnosis can be established.[85] Most commonly, the features are those of evolving psoriasis similar to guttate psoriasis, i.e., slight epidermal hyperplasia, focal diminution or loss of the granular cell layer, and mild spongiosis (Fig. 6.100). Parakeratosis is often limited to slight change overlying the hyperplastic epithelium and neutrophils are variably present (Fig. 6.101). A lymphohistiocytic infiltrate is present in an edematous papillary dermis and dilated, tortuous, spiraling vessels are regularly evident. Extravasated red blood cells are a constant finding. Less commonly, the features are those of psoriasis vulgaris and sometimes the changes overlap regressing psoriasis.

In resolving lesions, foci of hyperkeratosis overlying hypergranulosis are scattered through the parakeratotic scale and the epidermal hyperplasia is less marked (Fig. 6.102).

For many years, treatment for severe widespread plaque psoriasis has included use of PUVA therapy. The latter is associated with an increased risk (albeit low) of cutaneous squamous cell carcinoma and dysplastic

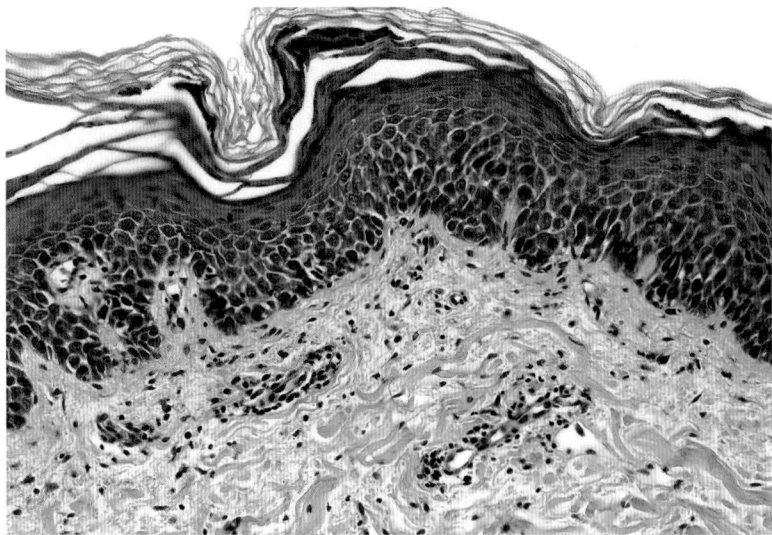

Fig. 6.101
Psoriatic erythroderma: close-up view of parakeratosis and neutrophil karyorrhectic debris.

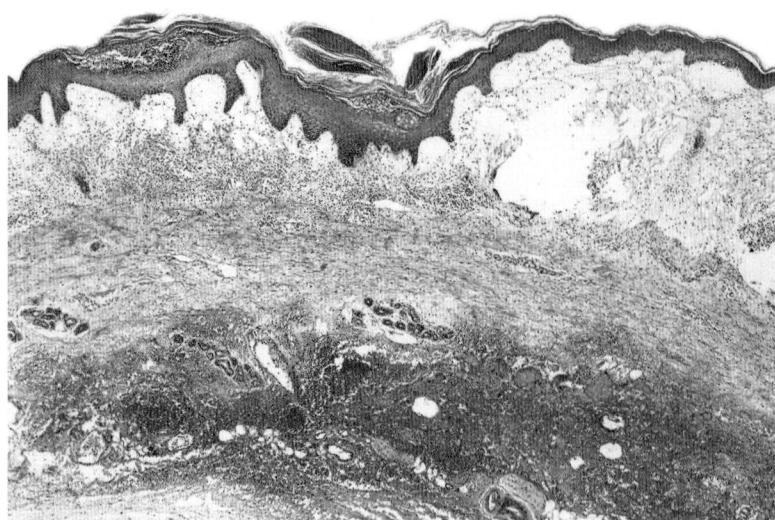

Fig. 6.103
Bullous pemphigoid and pustular psoriasis: on the left is a subcorneal pustule while on the right is a subepidermal blister.

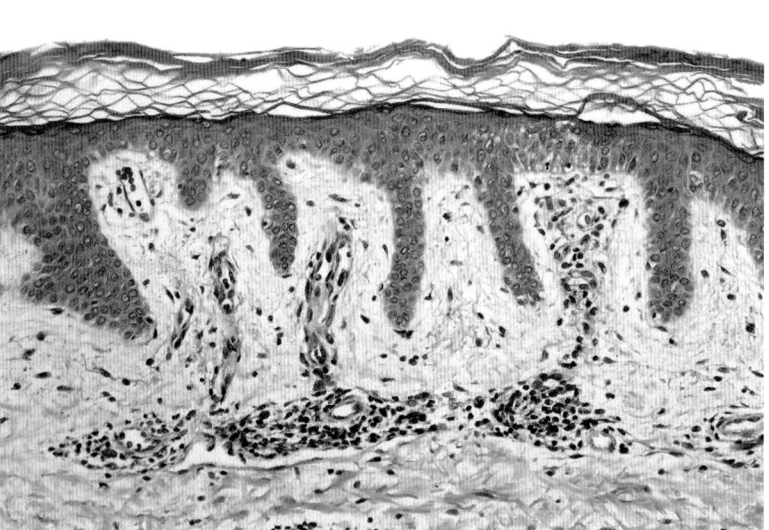

Fig. 6.102
Resolving psoriasis: newly formed basket-weave orthokeratin is seen underlying focal residual parakeratosis.

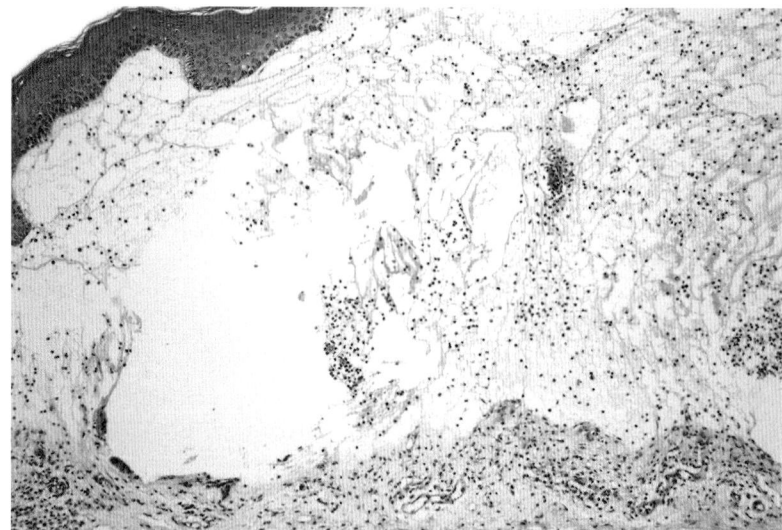

Fig. 6.104
Bullous pemphigoid and pustular psoriasis: higher-power view of the blister.

keratoses.[86–89] Patients at most risk include those who have had more than 200 PUVA treatments and/or a cumulative dose in excess of 1000 J/cm^2. There is some evidence to suggest that these tumors behave in a low-grade fashion, with little risk of metastatic spread.[89]

Psoriasis may rarely coexist with a number of autoimmune bullous dermatoses including bullous pemphigoid, pemphigus vulgaris, linear IgA disease, and epidermolysis bullosa acquisita.[90–96] Although not in all cases, there is often a relationship to treatment, particularly with PUVA therapy. In some instances, the histology may show features of both conditions (*Figs 6.103–6.105*).

Differential diagnosis

The differential diagnosis of psoriatic lesions includes a number of conditions:

- Pityriasis rubra pilaris differs from psoriasis by the presence of alternating parakeratosis and hyperkeratosis in both vertical and horizontal directions (spotty parakeratosis). Neutrophil infiltration of the stratum corneum is not a feature of pityriasis rubra pilaris unless there is secondary infection.
- Lichen simplex chronicus typically shows scarring of the dermal papillae due to persistent rubbing, and there is no thinning of the

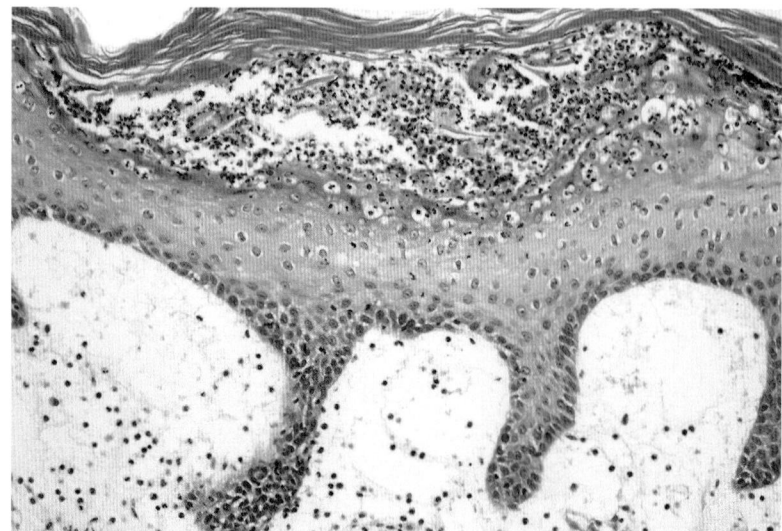

Fig. 6.105
Bullous pemphigoid and pustular psoriasis: higher-power view of the pustule.

suprapapillary plate. Hyperkeratosis and hypergranulosis are often marked and there is minimal parakeratosis unless there is a background of spongiosis.

- Papulosquamous drug eruptions (e.g., due to lithium or propranolol) may appear similar to psoriasis, but a moderate to high number of eosinophils is usually present in the infiltrate.
- Seborrheic dermatitis typically shows psoriasiform hyperplasia and corneal neutrophil infiltration may sometimes be a feature. It differs from psoriasis by the presence of a more conspicuous spongiotic component, which in psoriasis only occurs in early lesions and is usually not marked. In those cases where the distinction is not possible, the term 'sebo-psoriasis' is sometimes used.
- Pustular psoriasis and its variants are all similar; they must be distinguished from other pustular eruptions, including conditions such as pustular dermatophytoses, bacterial impetigo, and pustular drug eruptions. Pustular psoriasis may be differentiated from subcorneal pustular dermatosis by the absence of spongiform change or degeneration in the latter condition. Gram and PAS stains and culture will exclude infective conditions. Superficial pemphigus can be distinguished by the presence of acantholysis and the usual absence of psoriasiform hyperplasia. In IgA pemphigus, acantholytic cells are usually, but not always, present and this diagnostic clue may be very easily overlooked, but should allow distinction from psoriasis. In lesions of IgA pemphigus that lack acantholytic cells, immunofluorescence studies may be necessary to make the distinction from pustular psoriasis if the clinical diagnosis is in doubt.

Reactive arthritis

The skin lesions of reactive arthritis (see Chapter 12) typically show psoriasiform hyperplasia with parakeratosis. The epidermis is markedly acanthotic with elongation and hypertrophy of the epidermal ridges. The suprapapillary plates are thinned and there is infiltration of the epidermis by neutrophils, associated with the formation of spongiform pustules, microabscesses, and ultimately macropustules indistinguishable from pustular psoriasis. A perivascular lymphohistiocytic infiltrate with neutrophils is seen in the upper dermis.

Pityriasis rubra pilaris

Clinical features

Pityriasis rubra pilaris is an erythematous papulosquamous disorder characterized by follicular plugging (often best seen on the dorsal aspects of the hands and feet), perifollicular erythema that becomes confluent, palmoplantar hyperkeratosis, and pityriasis capitis.[1-3] It is an uncommon disease, accounting for approximately one of every 5000 new dermatological referrals in the United Kingdom.[3] Males and females are affected equally and the age distribution tends to peak in the first and fifth decades.[3] Although the majority of cases documented have affected Caucasian patients, occasional reports describing pityriasis rubra pilaris in black African patients have been published.[4]

Pityriasis rubra pilaris has been classified clinically into five types:[3]

- Type I, classical adult pityriasis rubra pilaris, is seen in over 50% of patients. Initially, a single erythematous patch appears on the upper half of the body (typically the face and scalp) and gradually spreads as large areas of sometimes pruritic or burning follicular hyperkeratosis with erythematous perifollicular halos (Fig. 6.106).[4] The erythematous areas coalesce and many patients develop generalized erythroderma (Fig. 6.107). Characteristically, occasional islands of unaffected skin are present (Fig. 6.108). Follicular papules on the dorsal aspects of the fingers and extensor surfaces of the wrists, arms, and thighs are said to be characteristic.[5] Fine and powdery scaling occurs on the face and scalp, with coarser scaling on the lower body (Fig. 6.109). The erythema has an orange–yellow tint, which is more noticeable on the palms and soles, together with marked hyperkeratosis (Fig. 6.110). The nails are also affected, showing distal yellow–brown discoloration,

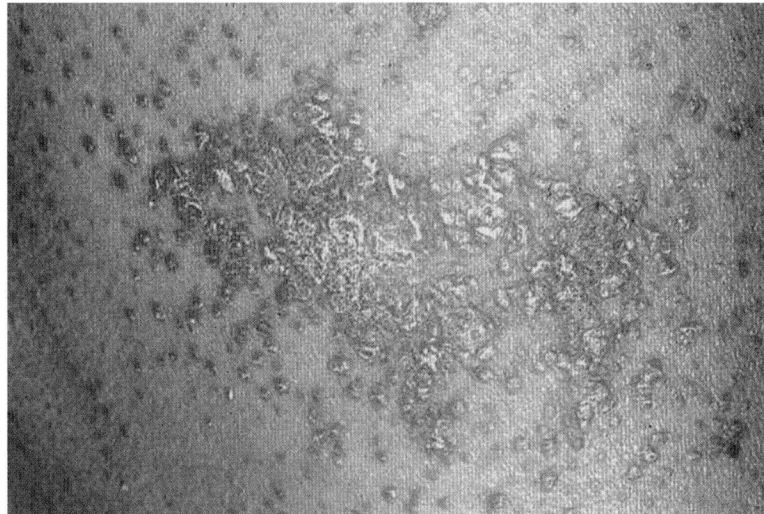

Fig. 6.106
Pityriasis rubra pilaris: there is characteristic hyperkeratosis and surrounding erythema. At the edges individual follicular lesions are evident. By courtesy of M.M. Black, MD, Institute of Dermatology, London, UK.

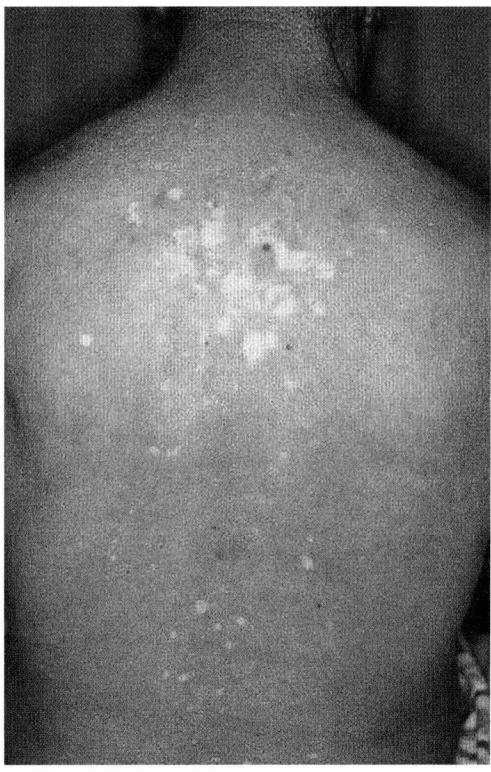

Fig. 6.107
Pityriasis rubra pilaris: confluence of lesions leads to extensive erythroderma. By courtesy of the Institute of Dermatology, London, UK.

subungual hyperkeratosis, nail thickening, and splinter hemorrhages.[6] Ectropion is often present,[7] and there may be diffuse alopecia.[8] Oral lesions are uncommon and include diffuse hyperkeratosis and macular erythema with white streaks reminiscent of lichen planus.[5] Prognosis for patients in this group is good, with up to 80% resolving within 3 years.

- Type II, atypical adult pityriasis rubra pilaris, occurs in approximately 5% of patients and is manifested by atypical morphological features and a lengthy duration, often up to 20 years. The scaling is more ichthyosiform and there are often areas of eczematous change. The prognosis in this group is poor, with only 20% resolving within 3 years.
- Type III, classical juvenile pityriasis rubra pilaris, resembles the classical adult form except for its age distribution; it affects children up to 2 years of age, accounting for approximately 10% of patients

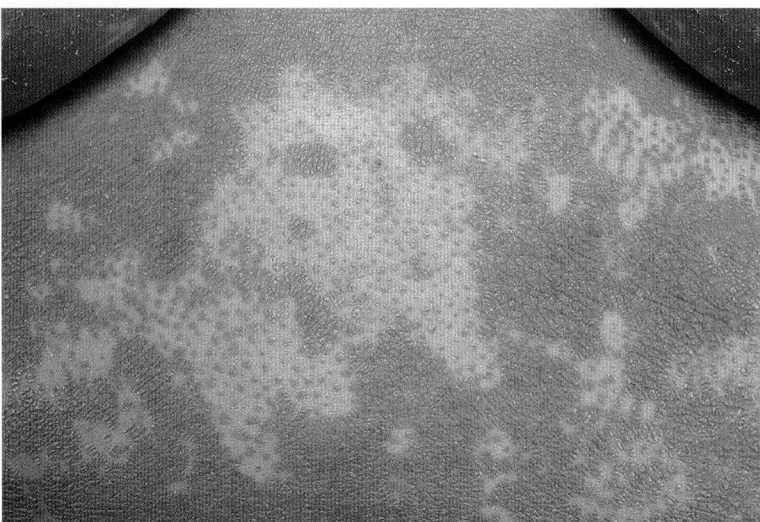

Fig. 6.108
Pityriasis rubra pilaris: characteristic, scattered islands of unaffected skin are evident. By courtesy of the Institute of Dermatology, London, UK.

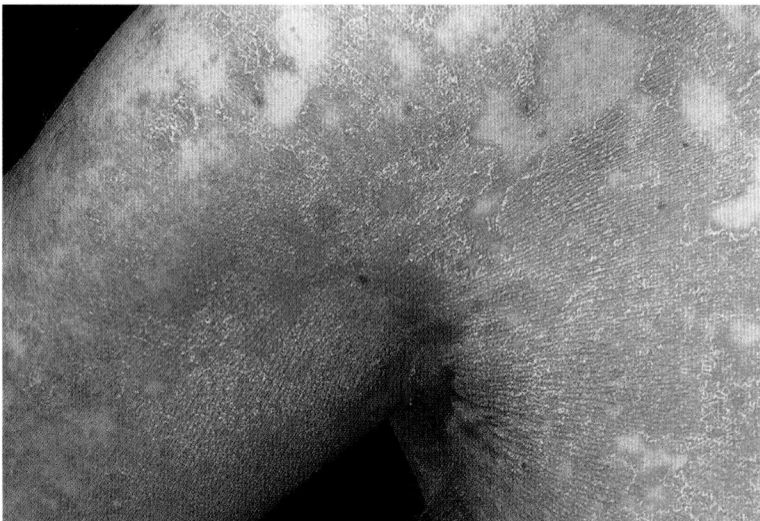

Fig. 6.109
Pityriasis rubra pilaris: in this patient, the scale is conspicuous. By courtesy of the Institute of Dermatology, London, UK.

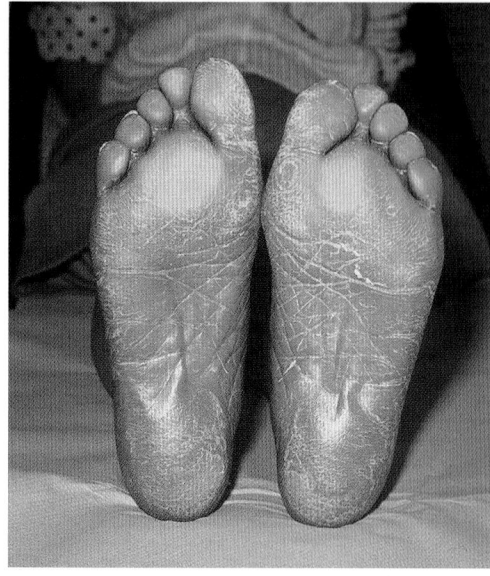

Fig. 6.110
Pityriasis rubra pilaris: palmar and plantar erythema with hyperkeratosis are frequent manifestations. Sometimes, there is an orange–yellow tint, as seen in this patient. By courtesy of the Institute of Dermatology, London, UK.

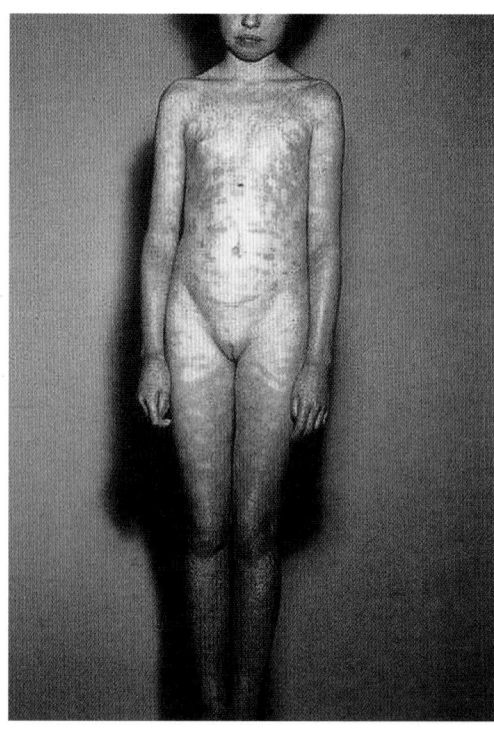

Fig. 6.111
Pityriasis rubra pilaris: classical juvenile type. Note the very extensive distribution of the lesions. By courtesy of M.M. Black, MD, Institute of Dermatology, London, UK.

(*Fig. 6.111*). More often, however, the eruption commences on the lower half of the body. The prognosis in this group is good, most patients clearing within 1 year but a recurrence rate of up to 17% has been reported.[9]

- Type IV, circumscribed pityriasis rubra pilaris, affects 25% of patients and presents in prepubertal children. Sharply defined areas of follicular hyperkeratosis and erythema are seen on the knees and elbows, together with occasional scaly erythematous patches on the rest of the body and palmoplantar hyperkeratosis.[10]

- Type V, atypical juvenile pityriasis rubra pilaris, accounts for approximately 5% of patients; presentation occurs early in life and this type has a lengthy duration. Characteristic follicular hyperkeratosis is present, together with a mild erythema. Ichthyosiform features are sometimes seen.[5] The skin of the feet and hands may become thickened and scleroderma-like.

Familial variants, which account for 0–6.5% of cases, mostly present with atypical features as described in type V pityriasis rubra pilaris.[5] In most families, inheritance has been via an autosomal dominant mechanism with variable expression and reduced penetrance although a recessive form has also been postulated.[11] The autosomal dominant form has been linked to heterozygous mutations in CARD14 on chromosome 17 and mutations have been observed in patients with type V presentation.[12,13]

Pityriasis rubra pilaris has been reported in association with HIV infection.[14,15] Nodulocystic acneiform or furuncle-like lesions and lichen spinulosus may also be present. This is a particularly severe variant, which responds poorly to therapy.[15] Further associations include rheumatological disease, in particular arthritis, dermatomyositis, and underlying malignancy possibly representing a paraneoplastic phenomenon.[16–27]

Pathogenesis and histologic features

The etiology of pityriasis rubra pilaris is largely unknown. It has been associated with abnormal vitamin A metabolism but there is little evidence in support for this other than a frequent response to vitamin A or retinoid therapy.[5] Linkage to autoimmune disease, immune dysfunction, internal

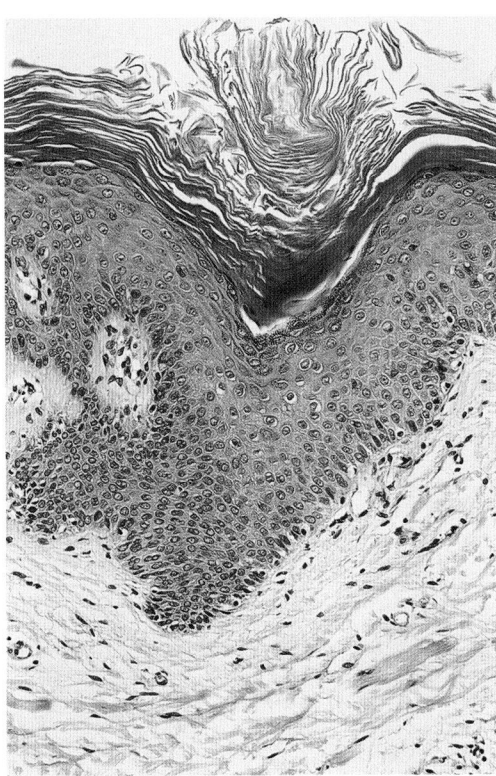

Fig. 6.112
Pityriasis rubra pilaris: follicular lesion showing the conical keratin plug. Parakeratosis is present above the adjacent epithelium.

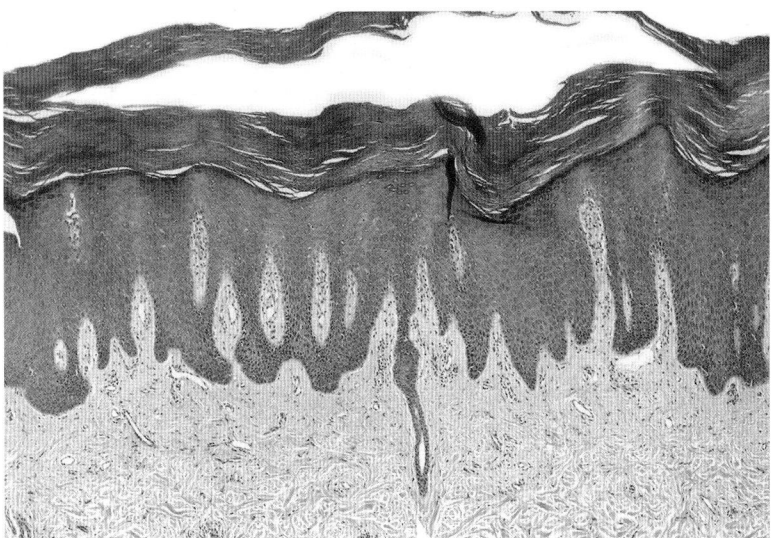

Fig. 6.113
Pityriasis rubra pilaris: there is hyperkeratosis with focal parakeratosis and psoriasiform hyperplasia.

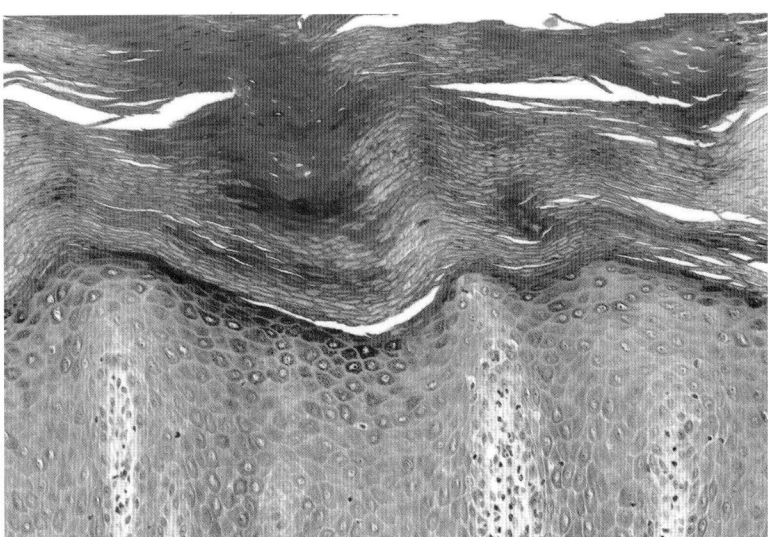

Fig. 6.114
Pityriasis rubra pilaris: alternating hyperkeratosis and parakeratosis.

malignancy, infections and, particularly in recent years, to human immuno-deficiency virus, have also been described.[5,15,28,29] In the majority of cases, however, there is no preceding or associated condition. Pityriasis rubra pilaris is associated with an increased rate of epidermopoiesis.[30-34]

Fully developed follicular papules show characteristic features comprising conical follicular plugging, with marked uniform acanthosis of the epidermis and broad epidermal ridges and dermal papillae (Fig. 6.112).[30,31,35] There is hyperkeratosis, with foci of parafollicular parakeratosis. In the dermis there is a mild to moderate inflammatory cell infiltrate and sebaceous gland atrophy.

Although the histologic features may be non-specific, biopsies from established, nonfollicular lesions comprise alternating orthokeratosis and parakeratosis in both vertical and horizontal directions, focal or confluent hypergranulosis, thick suprapapillary plates, broad epidermal ridges, narrow dermal papillae, and a perivascular lymphocytic infiltrate in the superficial dermis (Figs 6.113–6.115).[36] Small numbers of plasma cells and eosinophils are sometimes present.[28] Superficial blood vessels may appear slightly dilated. Occasionally there is also mild spongiosis with scattered intraepidermal lymphocytes.[29] Neutrophil infiltration as seen in psoriasis is not usually a feature of pityriasis rubra pilaris and its presence may indicate a bacterial or fungal superinfection. Acantholysis with or without dyskeratosis involving follicular and interfollicular epithelium has been described, and exceptionally a lichenoid infiltrate has been documented.[28,37–43]

In early lesions, the diagnosis is often problematical. Parakeratosis is usually poorly developed and lamellar orthohyperkeratosis predominates.[36] Hypergranulosis is present and the rete ridges are broadened and slightly elongated. The suprapapillary plates may be mildly thickened.

In erythrodermic lesions, the keratin layer may be thinned or lost and the granular cell layer diminished.[36]

Palmar and plantar lesions show hyperkeratosis, focal parakeratosis, and mild acanthosis (Fig. 6.116).

Differential diagnosis

Pityriasis rubra pilaris may be confused both clinically and histologically with psoriasis. Features in favor of pityriasis rubra pilaris include follicular plugging with parakeratosis of the adjacent epithelium, focal parakeratosis,

broad rete ridges, thickened suprapapillary plates, increased granular cell layer, and an absence of tortuous dilated capillaries immediately adjacent to the epidermis. In psoriasis the acanthosis is typically more marked and often strikingly regular, the rete ridges are thin and often fused, the suprapapillary plate is thinned, parakeratosis is usually confluent, and characteristic collections of neutrophils are seen in the overlying parakeratotic stratum corneum in association with spongiform degeneration of the underlying superficial epidermis.

Inflammatory linear verrucous epidermal nevus

Clinical features

Inflammatory linear verrucous epidermal nevus (ILVEN) is an uncommon condition which usually presents in infants or young children as an intensely pruritic, persistent, scaly, unilateral, linear erythematous lesion following the lines of Blaschko.[1] Individual lesions are discrete, scaly papules, which coalesce to form plaques.[2] Superimposed lichenification and excoriations are commonly present. Although lesions may be widely distributed, the leg, thigh, and buttock are sites of predilection (Fig. 6.117).[1,3] Females are more often affected than males (4:1).[2] The left side of the body is most often

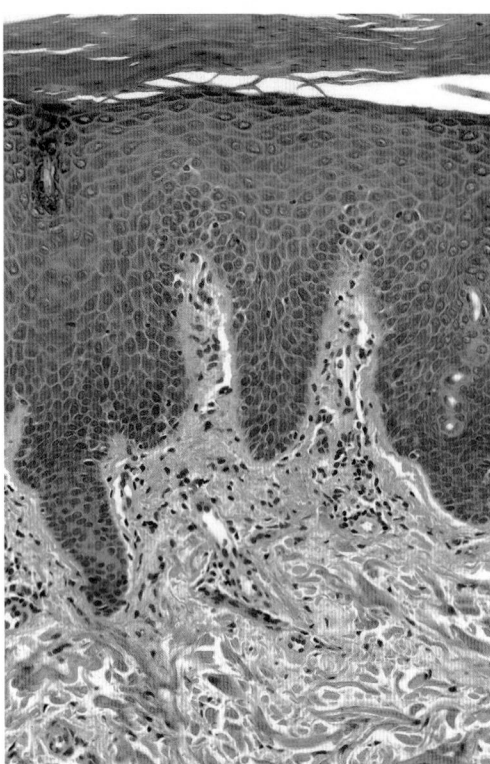

Fig. 6.115
Pityriasis rubra pilaris: close-up view.

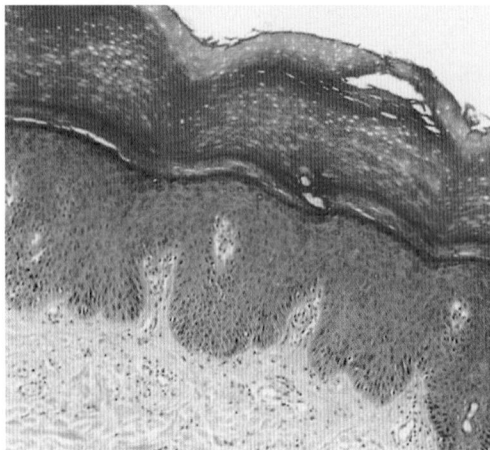

Fig. 6.116
Pityriasis rubra pilaris: plantar lesion showing hyperkeratosis, focal parakeratosis, and regular acanthosis with a rounded lower border.

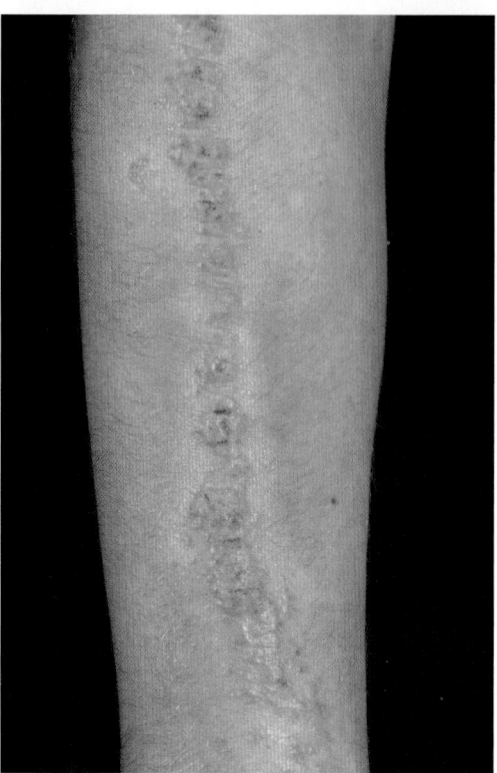

Fig. 6.117
Inflammatory linear verrucous epidermal nevus (ILVEN): patients present with scaly, erythematous, itchy papules and plaques in a linear distribution, showing a predilection for the legs. From the collection of the late N.P. Smith, MD, the Institute of Dermatology, London, UK.

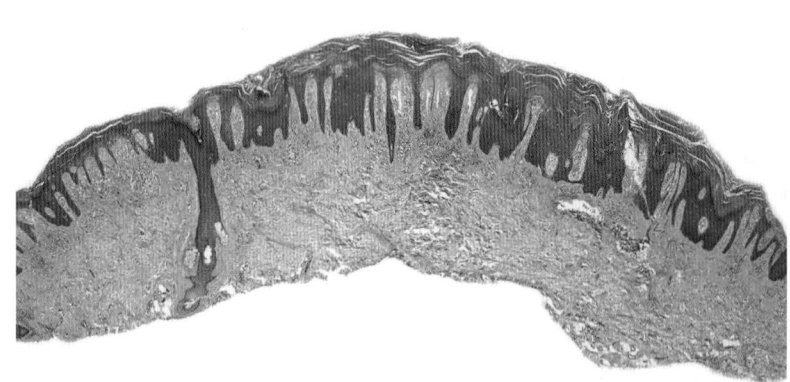

Fig. 6.118
Inflammatory linear verrucous epidermal nevus (ILVEN): in this view there is marked psoriasiform epidermal hyperplasia with massive hyperkeratosis. Mild chronic inflammation is seen in the superficial dermis.

involved.[2,4,5] Much less commonly, the disorder is bilateral and, exceptionally, the condition is generalized.[6-8] Familial cases have been documented and adults may sometimes be affected.[7-11] Occasionally inflammatory linear verrucous epidermal nevus coexists with psoriasis and rarely it presents as part of the epidermal nevus syndrome.[12,13] Exceptionally, the condition is associated with arthritis.[14]

Histologic features and pathogenesis

Recently, a somatic mutation in connexin 43 was reported in a single patient prompting speculation that inflammatory linear verrucous epidermal nevus may represent a mosaicism of erythrokeratodermia variabilis et progressiva.[15]

Histologically, the nevus is characterized by sharply demarcated, alternating parakeratosis and orthohyperkeratosis (*Figs 6.118–6.120*).[2,5,16] The epidermis shows papillomatosis with psoriasiform hyperplasia and absence of the granular layer below the foci of parakeratosis contrasting with a thickened granular cell layer underneath the orthohyperkeratosis.

Occasionally, Munro microabscesses are a feature. The rete ridges are elongated and thickened. Focal slight spongiosis is present, accompanied by lymphocytic exocytosis. A mild perivascular lymphocytic infiltrate is seen in the superficial dermis.

Differential diagnosis

ILVEN must be distinguished from linear psoriasis.[17] In ILVEN, parakeratosis alternates with orthohyperkeratosis in contrast with psoriasis where the parakeratosis is confluent. Similarly, the thickened rete ridges of ILVEN contrast with the thinned ones of psoriasis. By immunohistochemistry, in

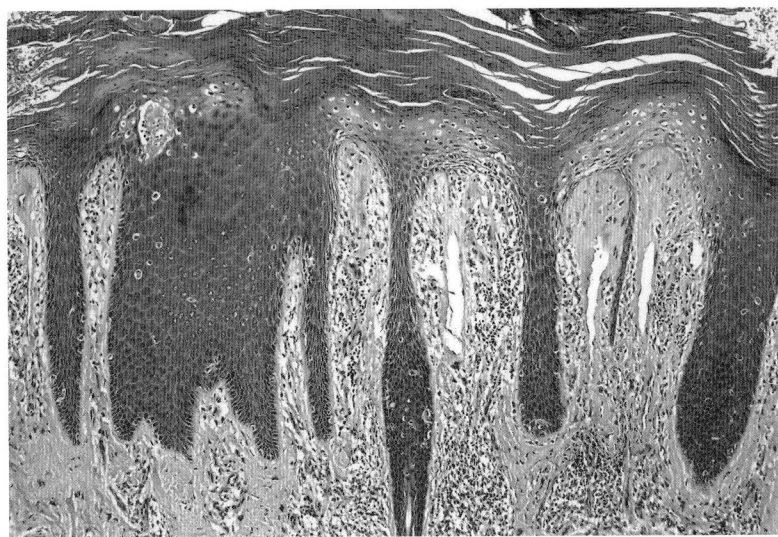

Fig. 6.119
Inflammatory linear verrucous epidermal nevus (ILVEN): alternating hyperkeratosis and parakeratosis is characteristic.

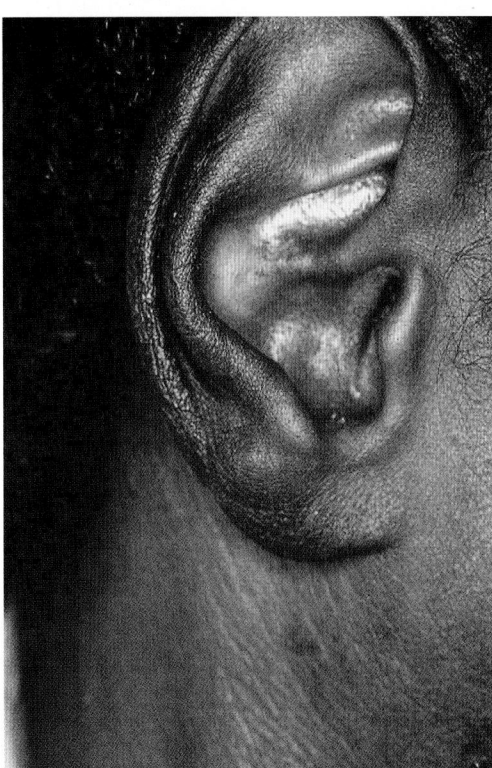

Fig. 6.121
Bazex syndrome: note the violaceous discoloration of the ear. By courtesy of J.L. Bolognia, MD, Yale Medical School, CT, USA.

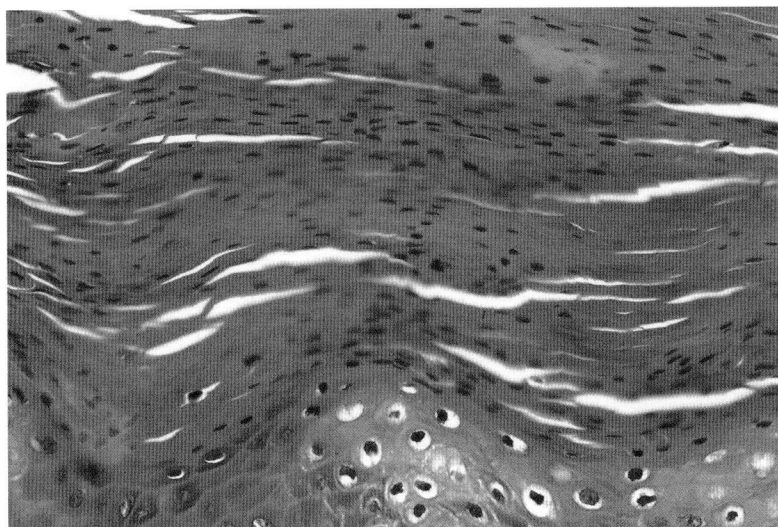

Fig. 6.120
Inflammatory linear verrucous epidermal nevus (ILVEN): close-up view.

ILVEN, involucrin expression is markedly diminished in the epithelium deep to the parakeratosis, while it is increased in the epithelium underlying the hyperkeratosis.[18] In psoriasis, there is a general increase in involucrin expression throughout the entire lesion.

Rare cases of ILVEN showing histiocyte infiltration of the underlying dermis reminiscent of verruciform xanthoma have been documented.[19–22]

Bazex syndrome (acrokeratosis paraneoplastica)

Clinical features

Bazex syndrome denotes an acral psoriasiform dermatosis in association with internal malignancy.[1–3] Elderly patients, usually males, present with a symmetric erythematous or violaceous, scaly eruption affecting the ears, nose, fingers, and toes (*Fig. 6.121*).[1,4] The knees and elbows may sometimes be involved. Vesicles and bullae are less common manifestations.[5] In patients with black or dark-brown skin, the lesions can present with hyperpigmentation.[2] Palmoplantar lesions are keratodermatous and nail involvement ranges from paronychia, horizontal or vertical ridging, yellow discoloration and thickening to onycholysis and subungual keratotic debris (*Fig. 6.122*).[1]

Patients with Bazex syndrome invariably have an associated systemic malignancy, most often affecting the oropharynx, larynx, esophagus, and

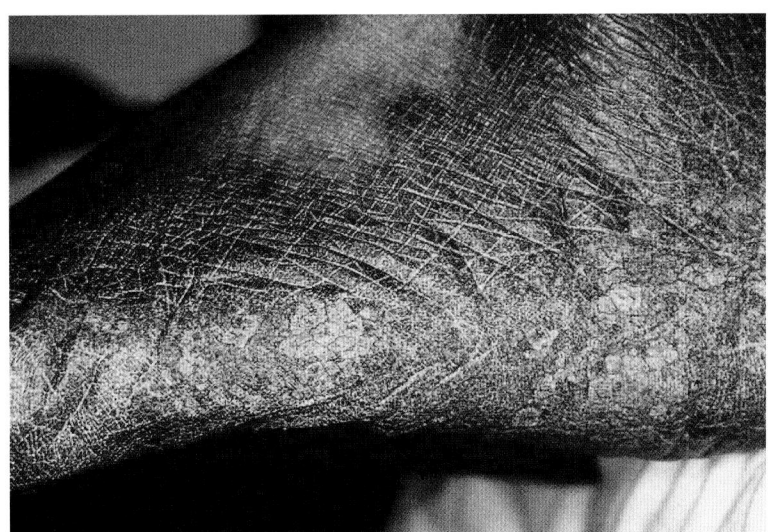

Fig. 6.122
Bazex syndrome: keratoderma. By courtesy of J.L. Bolognia, MD, Yale Medical School, CT, USA.

lung, in descending order of frequency.[1] Cervical lymph node metastases are commonly present. Persistence of the cutaneous lesions is rare and they commonly, but not always, regress following successful treatment of the underlying malignancy.[2,6]

Histologic features

Histologically, there is considerable overlap with psoriasis and chronic spongiotic dermatitis, the epidermis showing hyperkeratosis, parakeratosis, and acanthosis. In addition, however, dyskeratosis and interface changes reminiscent of lichen planus are also commonly present.[1] A perivascular or less commonly lichenoid chronic inflammatory cell infiltrate is present in the superficial dermis.

Bullous lesions may be subepidermal or, less often, intraepidermal.[1,7]

PUSTULAR DERMATOSES

Pustular drug reactions

This topic is discussed in the chapter 14.

Subcorneal pustular dermatosis

Clinical features

Subcorneal pustular dermatosis (Sneddon-Wilkinson disease) is a rare chronic, relapsing, and apparently noninfective eruption of unknown etiology.[1,2] It predominantly affects females (4:1) and is usually diagnosed during the middle years of life. Pediatric cases have, however, occasionally been described.[3,4] It may be associated with a benign or malignant IgA paraproteinemia (up to 40% of cases) or multiple myeloma, and sometimes pyoderma gangrenosum is also present.[5–15] Other associations include rheumatoid arthritis, systemic lupus erythematosus, hyperthyroidism, Crohn disease, multiple sclerosis, IgG cryoglobulinemia, bullous pemphigoid, morphea, diffuse scleroderma, Sjögren syndrome, marginal zone lymphoma, chronic lymphocytic leukemia, squamous carcinoma of the bronchus, and metastatic gastrinoma, although it is doubtful whether these are of any great significance.[15–26]

Clinically, patients present with waves of superficial flaccid pustules in circinate or serpiginous groups and sheets, particularly in the folds of the body, such as the axillae (Figs 6.123 and 6.124) and groins, beneath the breasts, and on the abdomen. Fluid levels are sometimes evident. Typically, the mucous membranes, face, scalp, and peripheries are spared. Healing is rapid, usually within a few days or weeks, and the condition responds to dapsone, although not as dramatically as dermatitis herpetiformis. Postinflammatory hyperpigmentation is common.

Canine subcorneal pustular dermatosis, particularly affecting Miniature Schnauzers, has been reported.[27]

Pathogenesis and histologic features

The etiology of subcorneal pustular dermatosis is unknown. Intercellular IgA deposits have been identified in a significant number of cases by direct immunofluorescence and many patients have a circulating IgA pemphigus antibody. These cases have been documented in the literature as IgA pemphigus.[28–34] Subcorneal pustular dermatosis should be restricted to the immunofluorescence-negative group.

The characteristic lesion is a subcorneal pustule, which appears to sit on the skin surface (Fig. 6.125). The contents of the pustules are predominantly neutrophils, although an occasional eosinophil may be identified. The epidermis beneath the pustule shows surprisingly little change except for polymorphs in transit and perhaps slight intercellular edema (Fig. 6.126).

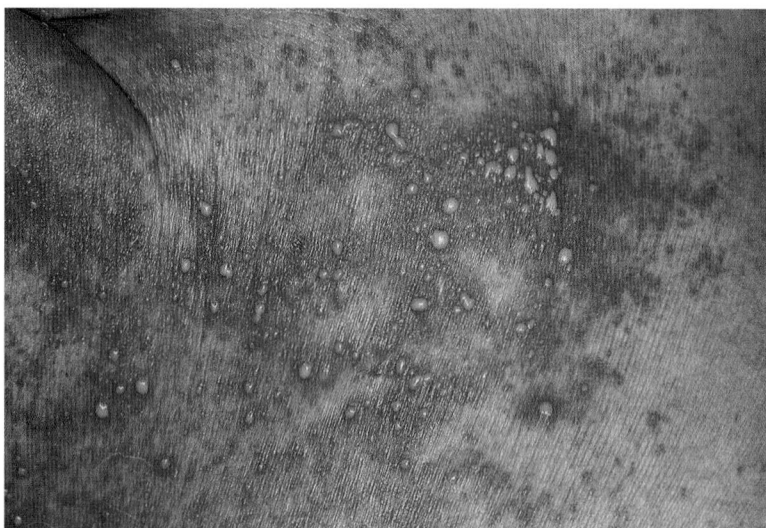

Fig. 6.124
Subcorneal pustular dermatosis: close-up view of early lesions characterized by numerous pustules arising on an erythematous background. By courtesy of R.A. Marsden, MD, St George's Hospital, London, UK.

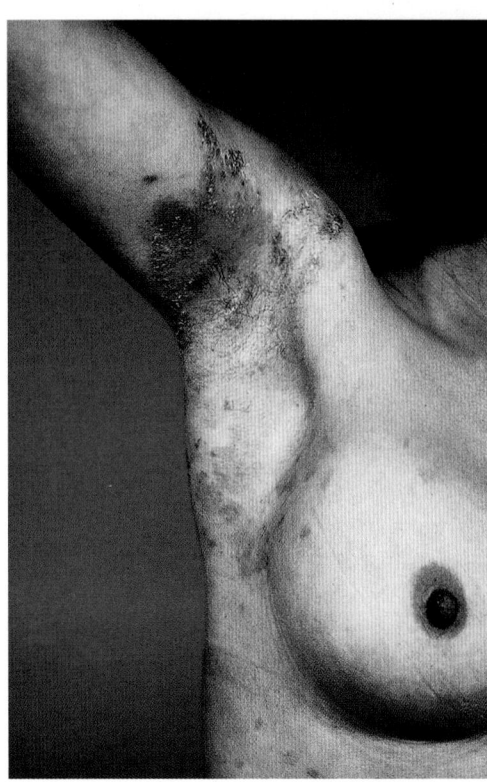

Fig. 6.123
Subcorneal pustular dermatosis: typical example showing a succession of pustules spreading outwards from the axilla. At the periphery the lesions are healing with crust formation. By courtesy of R.A. Marsden, MD, St George's Hospital, London, UK.

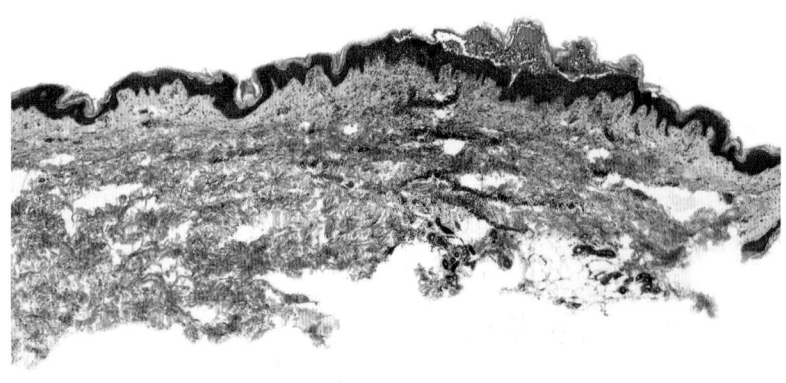

Fig. 6.125
Subcorneal pustular dermatosis: situated immediately below the stratum corneum is a blister cavity containing edema fluid and numerous neutrophils. The epidermis shows neutrophils in transit. Within the papillary dermis is a neutrophil and lymphocytic infiltrate.

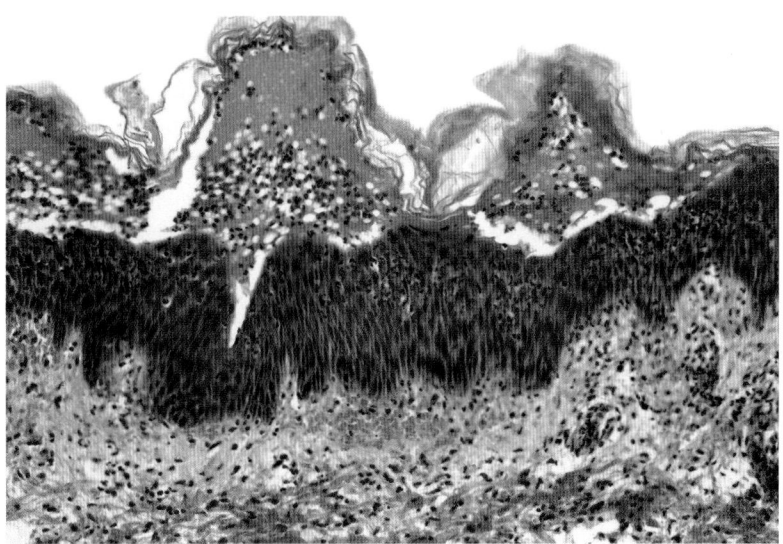

Fig. 6.126
Subcorneal pustular dermatosis: close-up view.

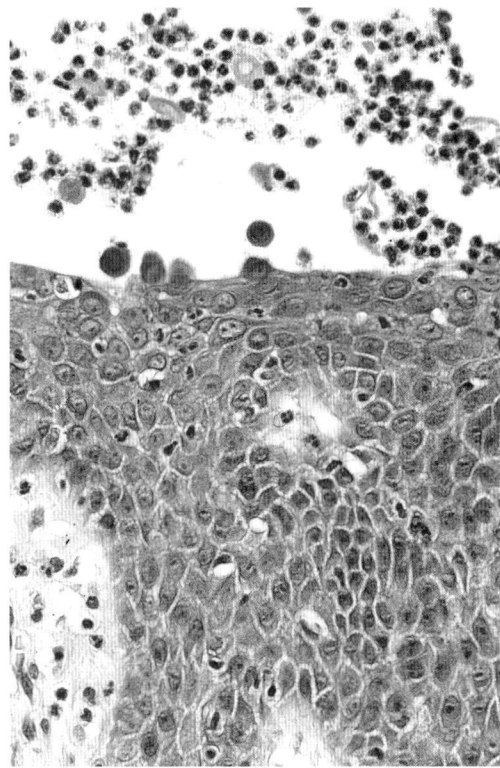

Fig. 6.127
Subcorneal pustular dermatosis: in addition to neutrophils there are scattered acantholytic keratinocytes. These features are indistinguishable from those of pemphigus foliaceus.

Older lesions may contain acantholytic cells (*Fig. 6.127*). In the dermis, superficial blood vessels are surrounded by a non-specific mixed inflammatory cell infiltrate consisting of neutrophil polymorphs and mononuclear cells.

Differential diagnosis

The histologic features of subcorneal pustular dermatosis cannot be reliably distinguished from those of bullous impetigo, staphylococcal scalded skin syndrome, pemphigus foliaceus, and IgA pemphigus. Impetigo is, however, a disease of young children and, although a Gram stain is often negative, cultures should grow staphylococci or streptococci.

The staphylococcal scalded skin syndrome (Ritter disease) is predominantly a disease of infants, but rarely it may present in adults. Clinically it is different from subcorneal pustular dermatosis, being characterized by the development of large flaccid blisters, which rupture, leaving extensive areas of denuded skin.

Although acantholysis is typical of the pemphigus group of diseases, it may occasionally be seen in impetigo, staphylococcal scalded skin syndrome, subcorneal pustular dermatosis, and pustular psoriasis. In difficult cases the demonstration of positive immunofluorescence will establish the diagnosis of pemphigus (however, see IgA pemphigus).

There has been considerable controversy in earlier literature concerning the relationship between subcorneal pustular dermatosis and pustular psoriasis, with some authors claiming them to be one and the same condition and others equally determined that they are quite different. In our view, these are two distinct diseases. Thus, in subcorneal pustular dermatosis, there is no family history and there is no evidence of more typical psoriasiform lesions elsewhere. Subcorneal pustular dermatosis responds to dapsone in the vast majority of cases and histologically spongiform change deep to the pustule (typical of psoriasis) is characteristically absent. Psoriasis is not associated with monoclonal gammopathy or multiple myeloma.

Toxic erythema of the neonate

Clinical features

Toxic erythema of the neonate (erythema toxicum neonatorum, erythema neonatorum) is a very common self-limiting disorder affecting from 48% to 72% of all newborn infants with a reported prevalence of 17–21%.[1-9] Caucasian males appear more commonly affected.[2,8-10] It presents as an asymptomatic erythematous macular rash usually in the first 3 days of life.[1,11] Occasionally, it may be evident at birth and, exceptionally, the onset is delayed until the second week after birth.[5,6,12] Sometimes there are papules and vesicles and, in some patients, pustule formation is evident. The condition most often affects the forehead, face, chest, trunk, and extremities.[1] The palms and soles are typically uninvolved. The eruption is asymptomatic and very typically transient, with lesions often lasting only a number of hours or days.[1] Full resolution is usually achieved by 1–5 days, although recurrences may occur in up to 11% of neonates.[2] Toxic erythema of the neonate is frequently associated with a peripheral blood eosinophilia.

Pathogenesis and histologic features

The etiology of this condition is completely unknown.[2] While an acute graft-versus-host type of reaction resulting from transfer of maternal lymphocytes during delivery was initially thought to be of pathogenetic importance, other data favor an immunological response to the initial colonization of the skin by commensal microorganisms.[13-18]

Early erythematous lesions show a somewhat nondescript perivascular inflammatory cell infiltrate with conspicuous eosinophils, which may be seen penetrating the epidermis in close proximity to hair follicles. In an established lesion, the pustules are follicular, lie subcorneally, and contain large numbers of eosinophils and occasional neutrophils.[19] The external root sheath of the infundibulum may also be affected.

Differential diagnosis

Toxic erythema of the neonate must be distinguished from incontinentia pigmenti. The latter, however, is characterized by eosinophilic spongiosis, a feature not seen in toxic erythema. In miliaria rubra the vesicles are related to sweat ducts rather than hair follicles and typically contain mononuclear cells rather than eosinophils. Toxic erythema of the neonate must also be distinguished from infantile acropustulosis, transient neonatal pustular melanosis, and infantile eosinophilic pustular folliculitis (see below).

Infantile acropustulosis

Clinical features

This uncommon condition usually presents in the first year of life and is sometimes evident at birth.[1-4] There is a marked male predilection. Although

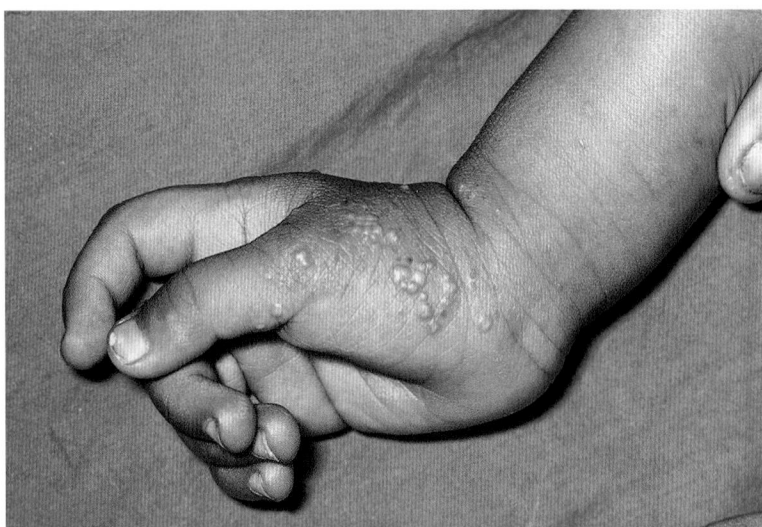

Fig. 6.128
Infantile acropustulosis: typical small pustules centered about the base of the thumb. By courtesy of R.A. Marsden, MD, St George's Hospital, London, UK.

it is most often seen in black children, it has occasionally been reported in Asians and whites.[5–8]

The disorder presents as crops of intensely itchy, erythematous papules 1–5 mm in diameter, vesicles, and pustules, which are found most often on the palms and soles, but the volar surfaces of the wrists, the ankles, the face, and scalp may occasionally be affected (*Fig. 6.128*).[6] The mucous membranes are spared.[1] Lesions are often present for 1–2 weeks and tend to recur every 2–4 weeks. With progression, the duration of the eruption diminishes and the remission lasts for gradually increasing periods of time. Spontaneous resolution has usually occurred by 2–3 years of age.

Pathogenesis and histologic features

The etiology and pathogenesis of this condition are unknown. However, infantile acropustulosis may be associated with atopy and hypereosinophilia.[6,9–11] Sometimes, a history of prior or concurrent scabies infection is present but whether this is causal is uncertain.[4]

Histology reveals a subcorneal pustule containing predominantly neutrophils, although occasionally small numbers of mononuclears and eosinophils are evident. Eosinophil-rich pustules have also been described but with hindsight most such cases probably represent eosinophilic pustular folliculitis.[11] Slight acantholysis of the adjacent epidermis has been described.[12] The underlying dermis often contains a perivascular chronic inflammatory cell infiltrate, sometimes with scattered neutrophils and eosinophils. Direct and indirect immunofluorescence tests are negative.

Differential diagnosis

The diagnosis of infantile acropustulosis depends upon careful clinicopathological correlation. Conditions that may enter the differential diagnosis include scabies, pompholyx, *Candida* and dermatophytosis, herpes simplex, juvenile dermatitis herpetiformis, toxic erythema of the neonate, bullous impetigo, eosinophilic pustular folliculitis occurring in infancy, and transient neonatal pustular melanosis.

Transient neonatal pustular melanosis

Clinical features

Transient neonatal pustular melanosis is an uncommon condition which presents with vesicles and pustules on the forehead, under the chin, on the nape of the neck, chest, back, and buttocks.[1–4] In contrast to eosinophilic pustular folliculitis of infancy, the scalp is rarely involved. It affects 4–5% of black infants and 0.1–0.3% of white infants.[2] There is no sex predilection.[3] Lesions, which present at birth or during the first day of life, heal rapidly to leave small brown macules with a peripheral scale, and have usually disappeared by 3 months of age.[3]

Histologic features

Histologically, the features are identical to those of infantile acropustulosis: i.e., a subcorneal neutrophil-rich pustule sometimes accompanied by small numbers of eosinophils.[1]

Eosinophilic pustular folliculitis of infancy

Clinical features

Eosinophilic pustular folliculitis (Ofuji disease), which is largely a condition of adults and presents as recurrent episodes of itchy follicular papules and pustules on the face, trunk, and extremities, may rarely develop in infants.[1–6] There is a predilection for males.[1,7] In the infantile form, lesions, which may be present at birth or develop during the first 24 hours, are found particularly on the scalp, hands, and feet.[1,7–11] The trunk and limbs can also be affected.[2] Patients present with 1–3-mm white to yellow crusted pustules arising on an erythematous base.[1,2] A blood eosinophilia is often present.[8,12] The condition persists from 3 months to up to 5 years.[2]

Pathogenesis and histologic features

The etiology is unknown, although in a small number of cases an association with atopy has been documented.[13] In contrast to the adult disease, HIV infection is very rarely present.[14]

The histologic features are those of an eosinophil-rich 'spongiotic' pustule related to the outer root sheath of the hair follicle from the stratum corneum to the level of insertion of the sebaceous duct.[15–19] A heavy inflammatory cell infiltrate consisting of eosinophils, lymphocytes, and histiocytes is present in the adjacent dermis. The reported histologica features are, however, less distinctive and specific compared to classic, adult-type, eosinophilic pustular folliculitis.[11,20]

Numerous other pustular dermatoses may be encountered including superficial pemphigus, particularly IgA pemphigus, pustular drug reactions, bullous impetigo and staphylococcal scalded skin syndrome, pustular dermatophyte infections, pustular lesions in pyoderma gangrenosum, and necrolytic migratory erythema. These are discussed elsewhere in this book.

Access **ExpertConsult.com** for the complete list of references

See
www.expertconsult.com
for references and
additional material

Lichenoid and interface dermatitis

The term 'lichenoid' refers to inflammatory dermatoses which are characterized by a bandlike lymphohistiocytic infiltrate in the upper dermis, hugging and often obscuring the dermal–epidermal interface. Lichen planus is the prototypic lichenoid dermatitis (*Box 7.1*). Interface dermatitis refers to the presence of basal cell vacuolization (hydropic degeneration) and is often accompanied by single-cell keratinocyte apoptosis (*Box 7.2*). These two terms are by no means mutually exclusive as lichenoid infiltrates are accompanied by interface change. However, some dermatoses are characterized primarily by interface change without a lichenoid infiltrate such as lupus erythematosus and erythema multiforme.

Lichenoid dermatoses

Lichen planus

Clinical features

Lichen planus (Gr. *leichen*, tree moss) is a common, usually intensely pruritic, symmetrical, papulosquamous dermatosis.[1,2] Its prevalence in the general population is approximately 1%, and it most often presents in the fourth to sixth decades with a slight female predominance.[3,4] It is uncommon in childhood.[5,6] Occasional familial cases have been reported.[7,8]

The disease is characterized by small, smooth, shiny, flat-topped polygonal papules measuring several millimeters to 1 cm in diameter and often having a violaceous color (*Fig. 7.1*). Delicate white lines known as Wickham striae typically cross the slightly scaly surface (*Fig. 7.2*). The lesions are found most commonly on the flexor aspect of the wrists, the forearms, the extensor aspect of the hands and ankles, the lumbar area, and the glans penis (*Fig. 7.3*). Rare cases may also have associated palmoplantar keratoderma.[9,10] Annular lesions may be seen. Lichen planus is associated with a positive Koebner phenomenon. It is a usually self-limiting although sometimes protracted disorder, patients clearing of lesions within weeks to 1 or 2 years.

Oral involvement, which is very common (affecting up to 60% of patients with cutaneous disease), shows a marked female preponderance and presents most often in the seventh decade. It may sometimes be the sole manifestation (an estimated 15–35% of patients with oral lichen planus never develop skin lesions).[11–17] The buccal mucosa, vestibule, tongue, gingivae, hard palate, fornix, lip, and soft palate may be affected, in decreasing order of frequency.[14,15] Patients frequently present with a white lacelike pattern,

but papules, plaques and erosions, ulcerated, atrophic, and bullous variants may also be found (*Figs 7.4–7.6*).[1,17,18] Lesions are usually asymptomatic, although erosions and bullae are sometimes tender and painful. Chronic ulcerated oral lichen planus is of particular importance because it has been related to an increased risk, albeit low, of developing squamous cell carcinoma (*Fig. 7.7*). The risk of developing malignancy is debated, with current literature suggesting that 0–12.5% of affected patients will develop an oral malignancy.[14,15,19–26] Oral involvement in lichen planus and its relationship to cutaneous squamous cell carcinoma is discussed in greater depth elsewhere (see Chapter 11). Involvement of the gums may present as desquamative gingivitis.[1] Other mucous membranes that may be involved include those of the pharynx, larynx, esophagus, nose, anus, and genitalia.[27] Familial cases of lichen planus limited to oral involvement are noted.[28]

Ocular involvement is rare and may include eyelid lesions, blepharitis, conjunctivitis, keratitis, punctate corneal opacities, iridocyclitis, and chorioretinitis.[29,30]

Esophageal involvement, although rare, is an important potential cause of morbidity and is the most frequently involved gastrointestinal site.[31] Concomitant oral lesions are typically present, but in rare cases esophageal involvement is the initial presentation.[32] To date, middle-aged or elderly females are typically affected.[32–36] Complications include chronic dysphagia and stricture formation affecting the mid or upper esophagus.[32,33,37–40] Patients with esophageal lichen planus may have a risk of developing squamous cell carcinoma.[31,33,35,36,41,42] Some patients may develop squamous cell carcinoma associated with esophageal lichen planus in the absence of oral or cutaneous manifestations.[43] The role of surveillance is uncertain.

Genital lesions in lichen planus are common (particularly in males), being present in up to 25% of patients, and sometimes adopting an annular configuration (*Fig. 7.8*).[1] Similar annular lichen planus may be found elsewhere on the body, including intertriginous areas.[44] Occasionally, penile lesions are the sole expression of the disease, and there is an association in uncircumcised men.[45,46] Vulval lesions may be found in up to 51% of females with cutaneous involvement.[47] Sometimes gingival and female genital lesions may coexist as a variant of erosive lichen planus, the so-called vulvovaginal-gingival syndrome.[48–51] Patients present with dyspareunia and intense burning vulval pain. The vulva appears congested, and there may be erosions, which are often surrounded by a white reticulate border. Vaginal involvement similarly presents as dyspareunia and often postcoital bleeding due to inflammatory, desquamative, and erosive changes. More typical features of lichen planus may be encountered elsewhere on the body. Squamous carcinoma is an important complication, albeit rare, of chronic vulval lichen planus and appears to be more common in nonhair-bearing mucosa.[52,53] The development of penile cancer is rare.[54] Genital involvement in lichen planus is discussed elsewhere (see Chapter 12).

The nails are affected in about 10% of patients with lichen planus; manifestations include thinning of the nail plate, longitudinal ridging, striations, pterygium formation, subungual hyperkeratosis, and, very rarely, complete destruction of the nail (Fig. 7.9).[1] Although nail involvement in children is said to be rare, some authors regard twenty-nail dystrophy of childhood as a variant of localized lichen planus, although not all accept this hypothesis.[55–59]

Most lesions heal within 6–18 months of onset. However, oral and hypertrophic variants and lichen planopilaris tend to have a chronic course.

Box 7.1
Causes of lichenoid dermatitis

- Lichen planus
- Lichenoid graft-versus-host disease
- Lichen nitidus
- Lichenoid keratosis
- Lichenoid drug reaction
- Fixed drug reaction
- Lichen planopilaris
- Lichen striatus
- Adult Blaschkitis
- Lichen aureus
- Lichenoid mycosis fungoides
- Ashy dermatoses
- Lichenoid and granulomatous dermatitis

Box 7.2
Causes of interface dermatitis

- Lichenoid dermatoses (see Box 7.1)
- Erythema multiforme
- Stevens-Johnson syndrome/toxic epidermal necrolysis
- Connective tissue disorders: lupus erythematosus, dermatomyositis, and mixed connective tissue disorders
- Graft-versus-host disease
- Poikiloderma including those related to rare inherited disorders
- Interface drug reactions
- Interface viral exanthem
- Pityriasis lichenoides

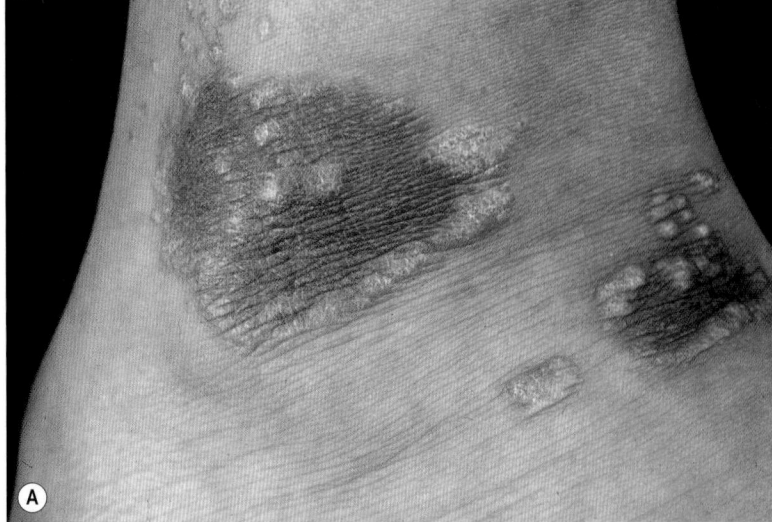

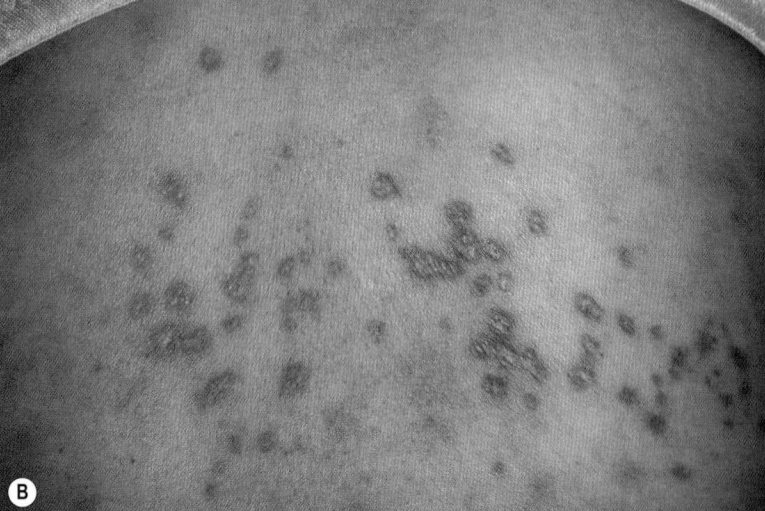

Fig. 7.2
Lichen planus: (**A**) note the characteristic Wickham striae at the edge of these pigmented lesions; (**B**) Wickham striae are evident on these lesions, which have arisen on the back, an uncommonly affected site. (**A**) From the collection of the late N.P. Smith, MD, the Institute of Dermatology, London, UK. (**B**) Courtesy of J. Dayrit, MD, Manila, The Philippines.

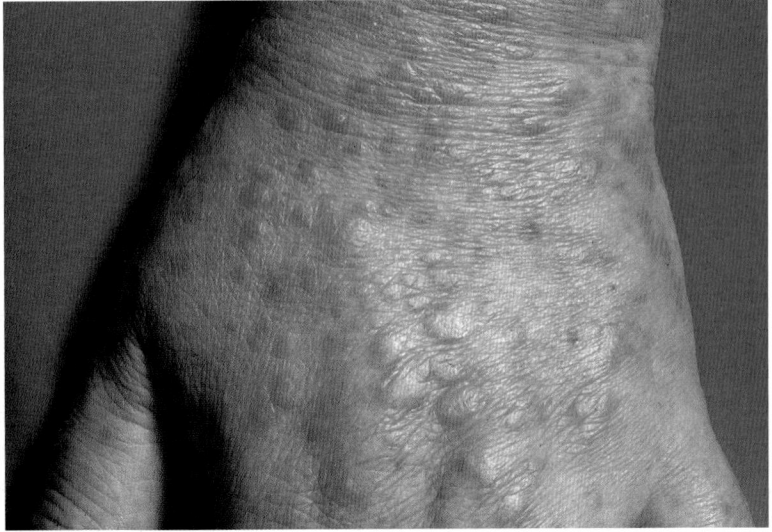

Fig. 7.1
Lichen planus: there are typical flat-topped polygonal papules on dorsum of the hand. From the collection of the late N.P. Smith, MD, the Institute of Dermatology, London, UK.

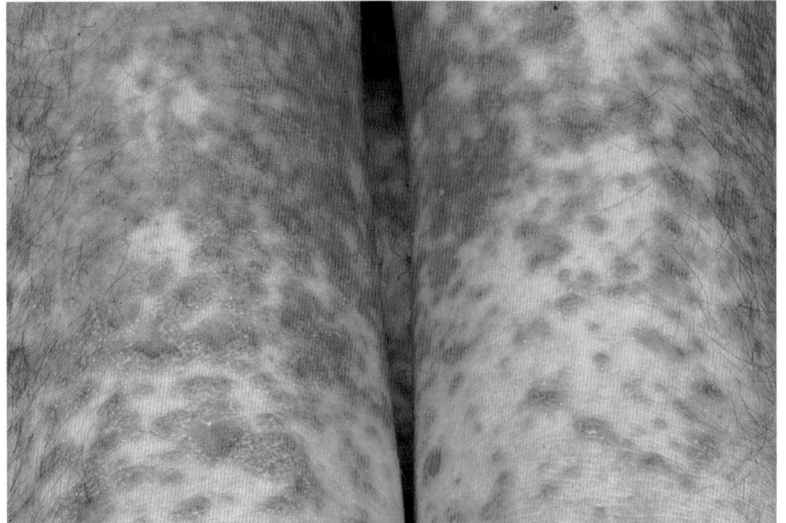

Fig. 7.3
Lichen planus: there is extensive bilateral involvement of the flexor aspect of the forearms. From the collection of the late N.P. Smith, MD, the Institute of Dermatology, London, UK.

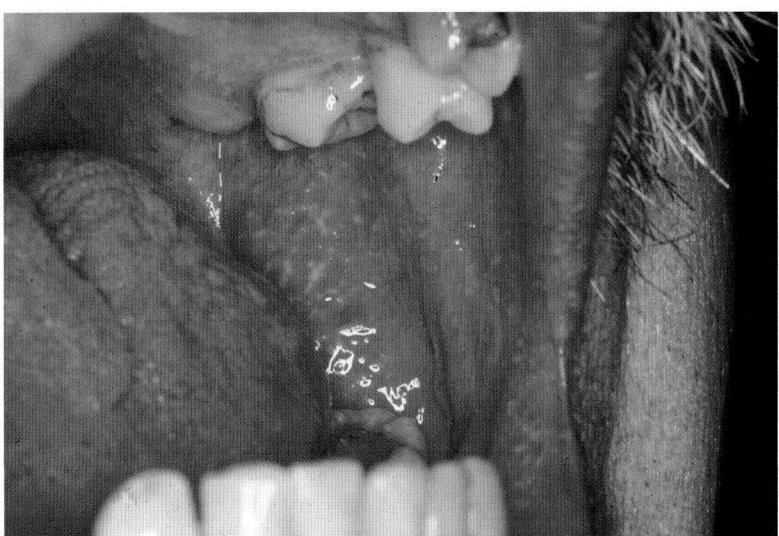

Fig. 7.4
Lichen planus: this lacelike pattern is characteristic. From the collection of the late
N.P. Smith, MD, the Institute of Dermatology, London, UK.

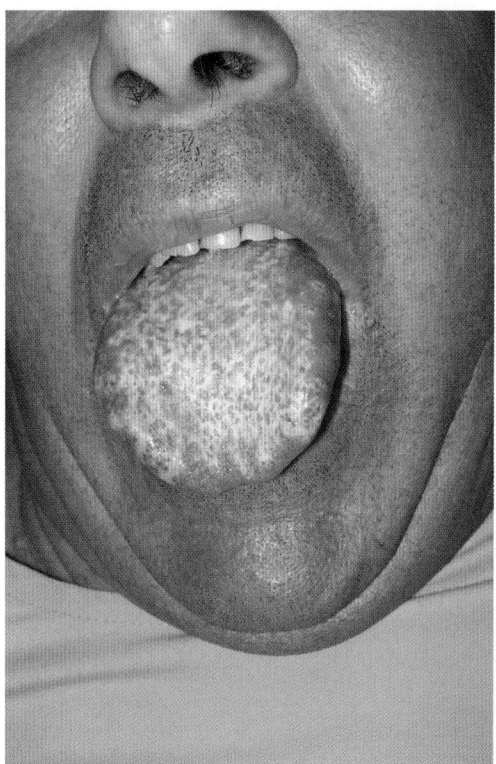

Fig. 7.6
Lichen planus: the tongue is commonly affected. By courtesy of M. Blanes, MD,
Alicante, Spain

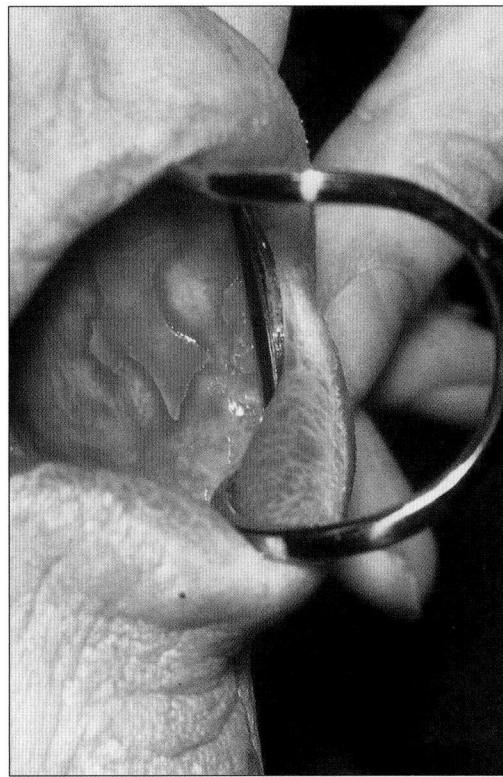

Fig. 7.5
Lichen planus: there is extensive ulceration of the buccal mucosa. By courtesy of
R.A. Marsden, MD, St George's Hospital, London, UK.

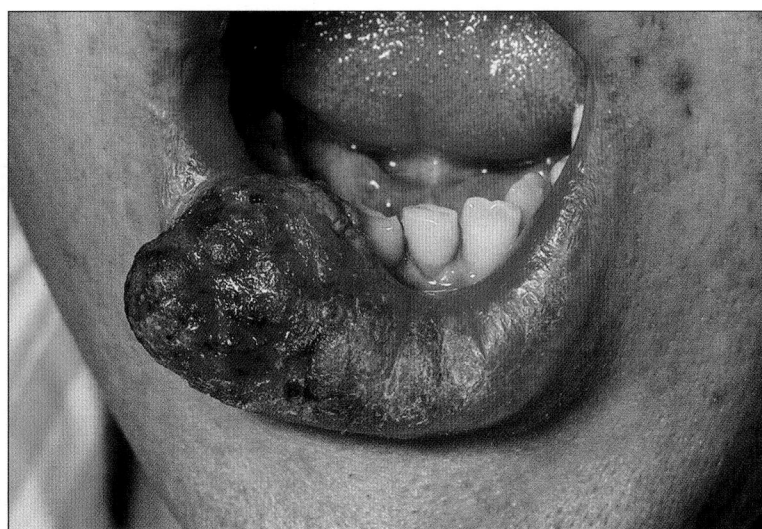

Fig. 7.7
Lichen planus: there is an ulcerated squamous carcinoma on the lower lip. By
courtesy of R.A. Marsden, MD, St George's Hospital, London, UK.

Postinflammatory hyperpigmentation is not uncommon, particularly in
darker-skinned people (*Fig. 7.10*).

A number of variants of lichen planus merit specific mention:

- Lichen planopilaris (follicular lichen planus) presents as single or
multiple plaques of scarring alopecia associated with a spectrum of
lesions including typical lichenoid papules involving the scalp to brown
or violaceous keratotic follicular papules affecting the trunk and
extremities (*Figs 7.11–7.13*).[61–63] Nonscarring plaques with prominent
follicular papules may also be present. Linear lesions have rarely been
described.[64–66] Some authors suggest that scalp lichen planus results
in some cases of pseudopélade of Brocq, although that entity likely
represents the end stage of a variety of scarring alopecias.[67–69] Children

can also be affected.[70,71] The Graham-Little-Picardi-Lasseur syndrome
refers to a variant of lichen planopilaris characterized by the following
triad: 1. multifocal scarring alopecia of the scalp; 2. nonscarring
alopecia of the axilla and groin; 3. follicular lichen planus of other
areas of the body, scalp, or both.

- Atrophic lichen planus, the clinical features of which merely reflect
resolution of the more typical active phase.
- Lichen planus actinicus [lichen planus subtropicus, summertime
actinic lichenoid eruption (SALE)] develops in patients with prolonged
exposure to sunlight and, therefore, usually manifests in spring or
summer,[72–76] with improvement or remission in the autumn or winter.
It occurs particularly in the Middle East (especially Egypt) and the Far

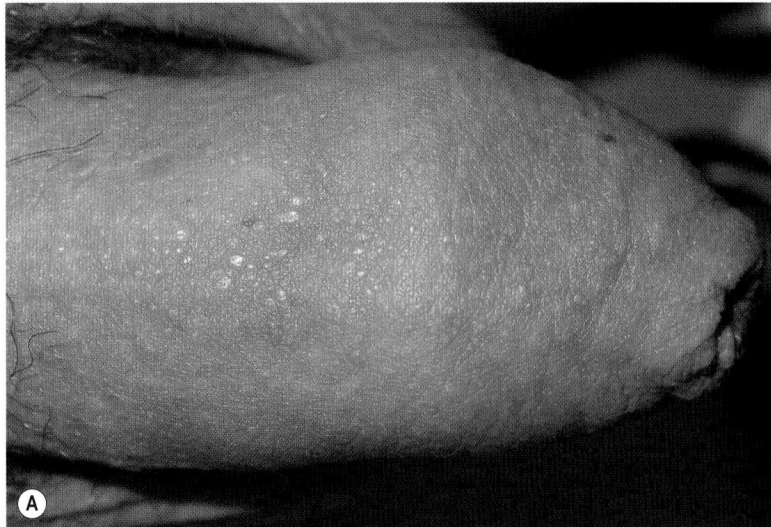

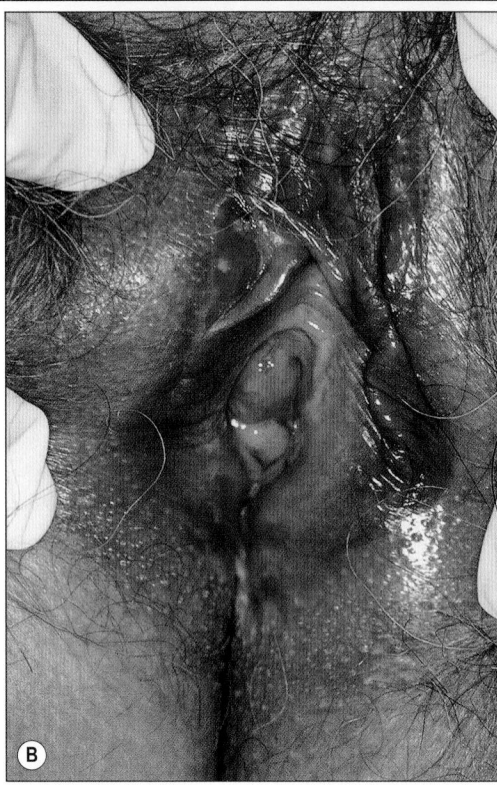

Fig. 7.8
Lichen planus: (**A**) typical papules are present on the shaft of the penis; (**B**) note the erythematous erosions around the vulval introitus and labia minora. (**A**) From the collection of the late N.P. Smith, MD, the Institute of Dermatology, London, UK; (**B**) By courtesy of S. Neill, MD, Institute of Dermatology, London, UK.

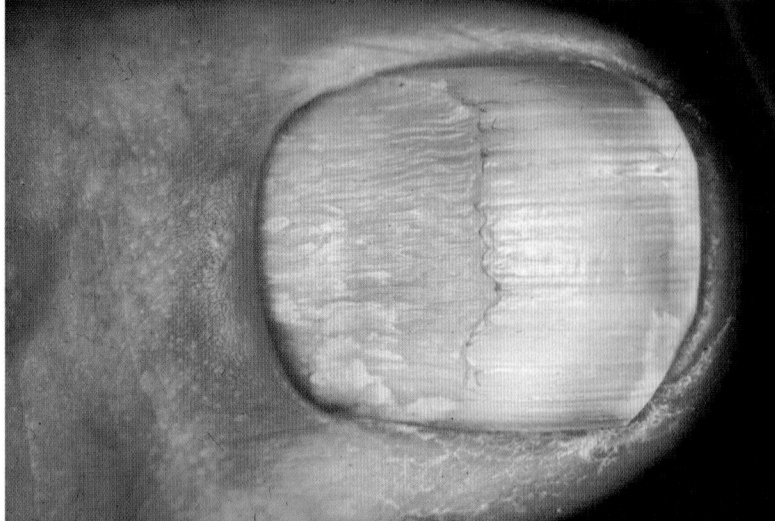

Fig. 7.9
Lichen planus: there is longitudinal ridging and striation affecting the thumbnail, with inflammatory changes in the nail folds. From the collection of the late N.P. Smith, MD, the Institute of Dermatology, London, UK.

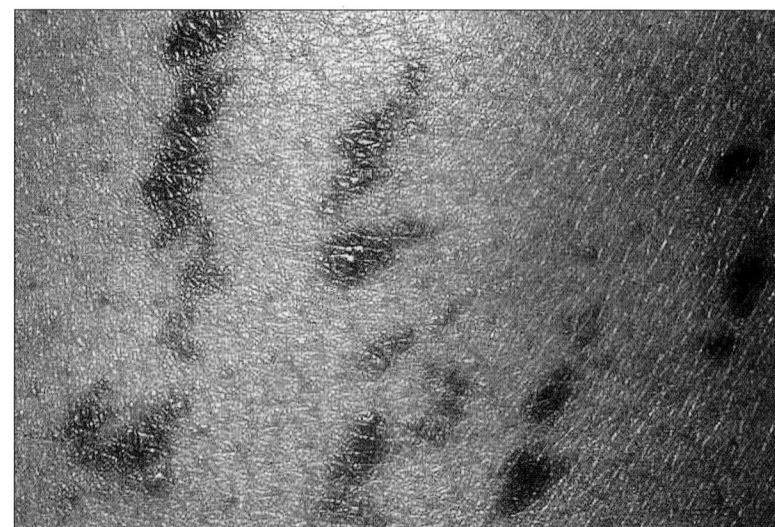

Fig. 7.10
Lichen planus: postinflammatory hyperpigmentation is a common manifestation. By courtesy of R.A. Marsden, MD, St George's Hospital, London, UK.

East and affects younger people, with a maximum incidence in the second and third decades and a slight female predominance (*Fig. 7.14*). Affected sites include the lateral aspects of the forehead, the dorsum of the hands, the forearms, face, and neck. The eruption can include a mixture of lichen planus-like and lichen nitidus-like lesions, whereas in others, the lesions appear as purely one or the other (see actinic lichen nitidus, below). Typically, the lichen planus lesions have an annular configuration with a bluish-brown, rather atrophic center and slightly raised border. They may sometimes coalesce to form circinate plaques. Occasionally, a melasma-like appearance has been documented.[76] There is usually little pruritus, and Koebner phenomenon is commonly absent. The nails are often unaffected.

- Lichen planus pigmentosus, most commonly encountered in the tropics in dark-skinned patients, is characterized by the development of variably pruritic pigmented dark brown macules predominantly affecting exposed skin and the flexures (*Figs 7.15* and *7.16*). The most common affected sites include the face and neck, but intertriginous areas may also be affected (lichen planus pigmentosus inversus).[77–83] There is no sex predilection. The disorder is characterized by periods of exacerbation and remission.[4] Exceptionally, involvement of the oral mucosa has been documented.[5]

- Hypertrophic lichen planus, which represents superimposed lichen simplex chronicus, commonly affects the lower limbs, particularly the shins, and manifests as highly pigmented warty plaques (*Fig. 7.17*).[84] Often, involvement is restricted to the shins with no other lesions elsewhere. Familial lichen planus shows an increased incidence of this variant.[85] The lesions are intensely itchy and very persistent. There is an attendant (albeit very slight) risk of neoplastic transformation.[86–88]

- Ulcerative lichen planus, a chronic variant affecting the fingers, hands, soles, and toes, is often associated with permanent loss of nails (*Figs 7.18* and *7.19*). Squamous cell carcinoma may complicate this variant of lichen planus.[89,90]

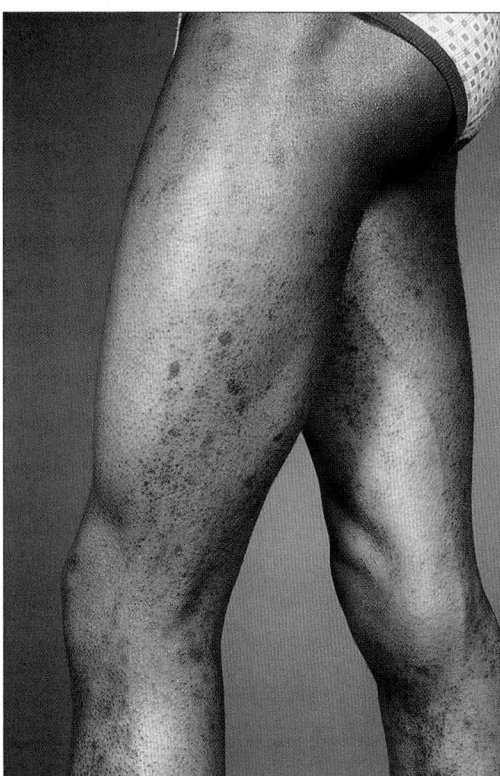

Fig. 7.11
Lichen planopilaris: there are characteristic hyperpigmented follicular papules, which are confluent in some areas. The limbs are commonly affected. By courtesy of R.A. Marsden, MD, St George's Hospital, London, UK.

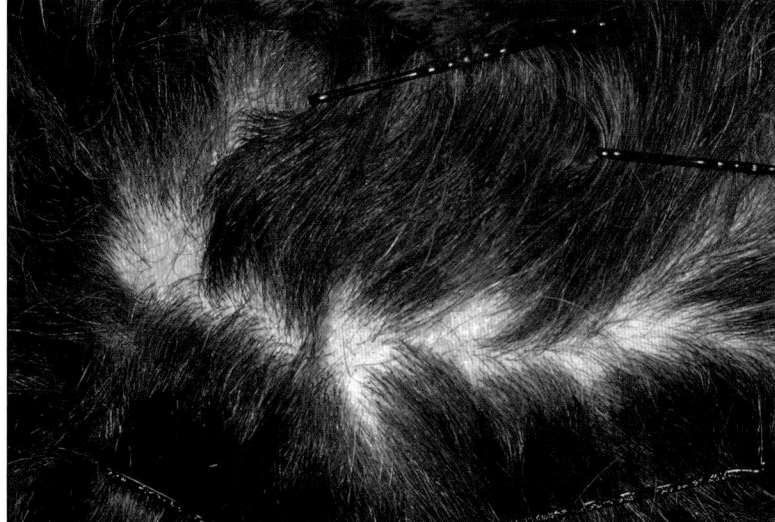

Fig. 7.12
Lichen planopilaris: marked inflammatory changes with scarring and secondary hair loss. These changes are difficult to distinguish from those of pseudopélade and chronic discoid lupus erythematosus. From the collection of the late N.P. Smith, MD, the Institute of Dermatology, London, UK.

Other variants include lichen planus linearis, which occurs predominantly in children, and the rare vesicular or bullous variants, which must be distinguished from lichen planus pemphigoides. Bullous lichen planus implies the development of vesicles or bullae on preexistent lichenoid lesions as a consequence of severe basal cell hydropic degeneration. It is more often a histologic finding rather than a clinical observation. In contrast, lichen planus pemphigoides is characterized by the development of large tense bullae arising on normal or erythematous skin in a patient with typical lichen planus elsewhere. It represents the combined expression of lichen planus and bullous pemphigoid.[91,92]

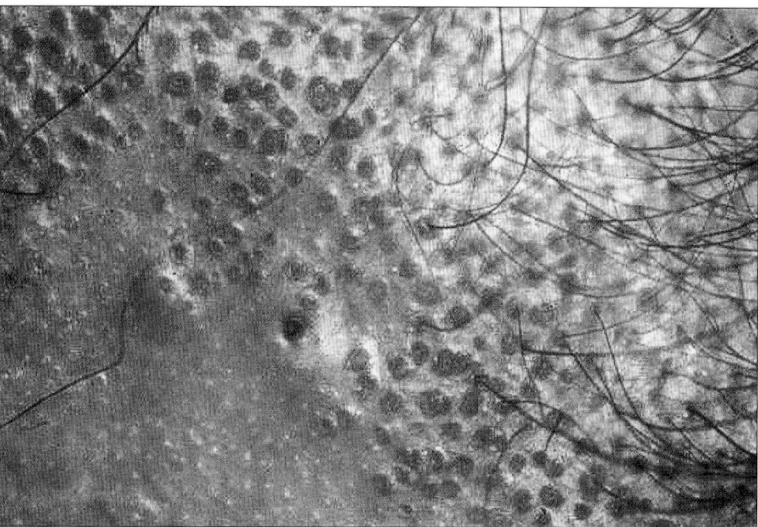

Fig. 7.13
Lichen planopilaris: follicular lichenoid papules are clearly seen in this patient. By courtesy of the Institute of Dermatology, London, UK.

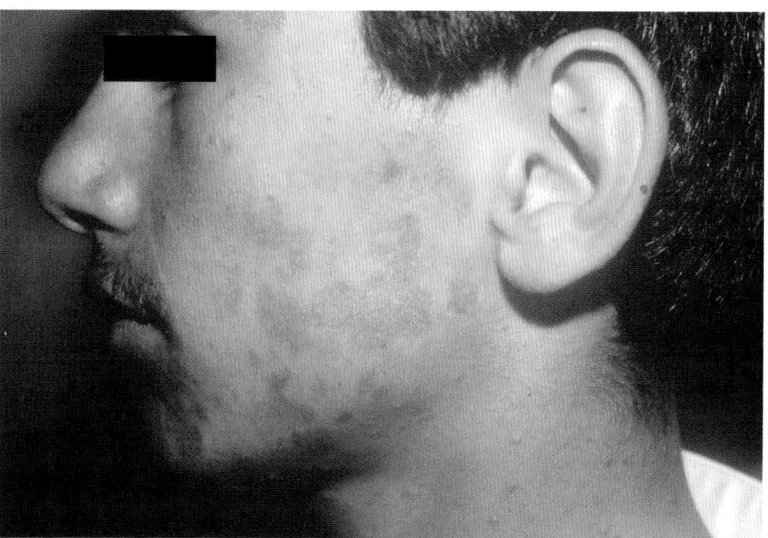

Fig. 7.14
Lichen planus actinicus: there is marked facial hyperpigmentation representing postinflammatory changes. From the collection of the late N.P. Smith, MD, the Institute of Dermatology, London, UK.

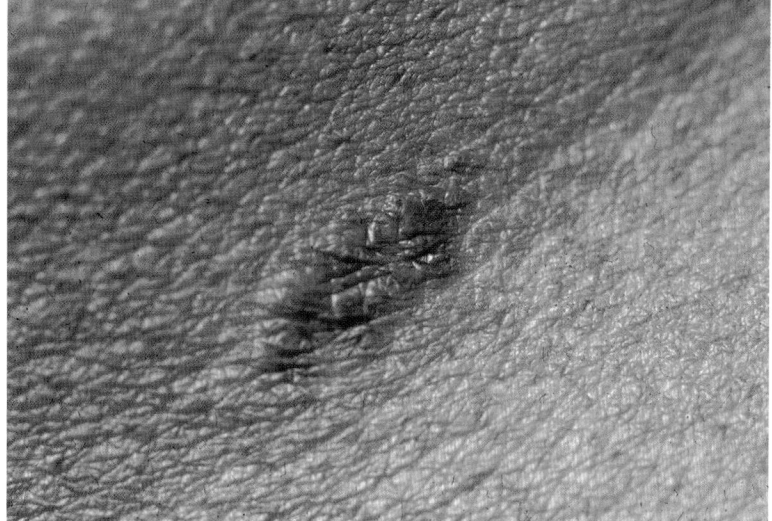

Fig. 7.15
Lichen planus pigmentosus: there are coalescent pigmented papules. From the collection of the late N.P. Smith, MD, the Institute of Dermatology, London, UK.

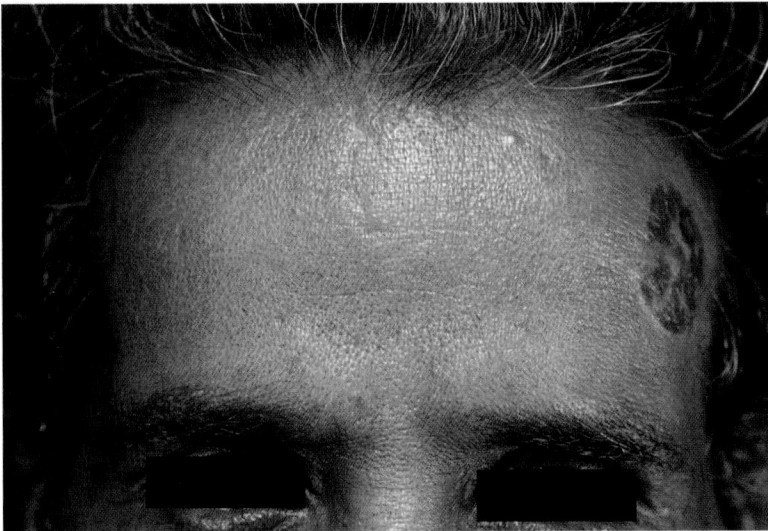

Fig. 7.16
Lichen planus pigmentosus: the face is a commonly affected site. From the collection of the late N.P. Smith, MD, the Institute of Dermatology, London, UK.

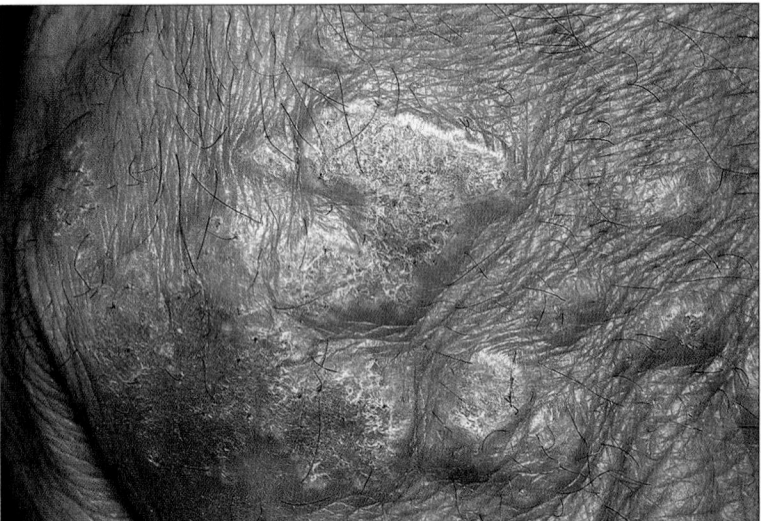

Fig. 7.17
Hypertrophic lichen planus: raised, warty, violaceous plaques on the shin of an elderly man. These lesions had been present for 30 years. By courtesy of R.A. Marsden, MD, St George's Hospital, London, UK.

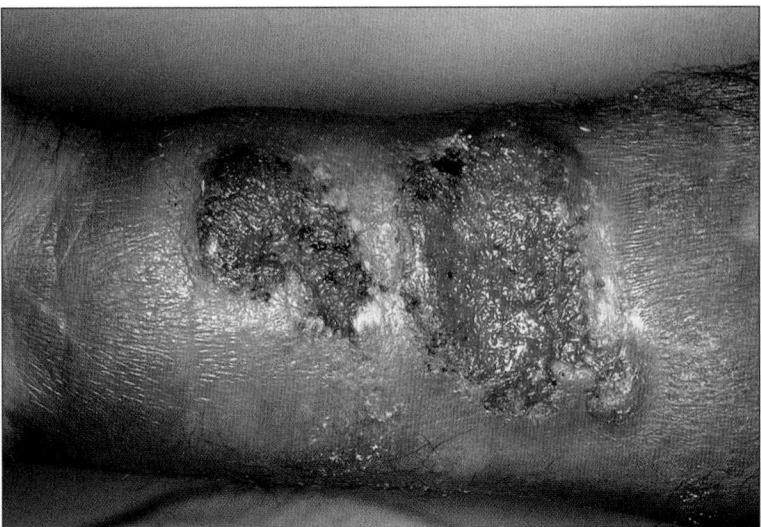

Fig. 7.18
Ulcerative lichen planus: there is marked atrophy of the skin around this crusted ulcer. By courtesy of the Institute of Dermatology, London, UK.

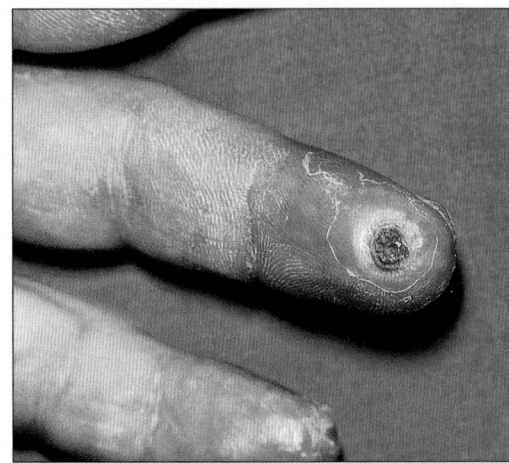

Fig. 7.19
Ulcerative lichen planus: the digits are often affected. This variant is associated with a slightly increased risk of squamous cell carcinoma. By courtesy of R.A. Marsden, MD, St George's Hospital, London, UK.

Childhood lichen planus shows a modest male predominance (2:1).[5,6,61,78] Although mucosal involvement is said to be rare, recent series report a frequency of 14–39%.[6,70,93] Hypertrophic lesions may be seen in up to 26% of cases.[6]

Pathogenesis and histologic features

The etiology of lichen planus is unknown. Theories of infectious (bacterial and viral), autoimmune, metabolic, psychosomatic, and genetic causes have all had their proponents. Currently, however, it is thought that lichen planus represents an abnormal delayed hypersensitivity reaction to an as yet undetermined epidermal neoantigen, possibly to a combination of an external antigen coupled with an internal self-antigen.[94–96] The association of lichen planus with a number of viral infections including hepatitis B and C and human immunodeficiency virus (HIV), combined with the well-recognized relationship to numerous drugs, adds support to this hypothesis.[97–99]

Lichen planus is associated with a variety of liver cell abnormalities including aberrant liver function tests and serology.[100,101] An increased incidence of chronic active hepatitis, primary sclerosing cholangitis and primary biliary cirrhosis has also been recorded.[102–107] Not all documented series, however, have confirmed these observations, suggesting that the reported relationship may be dependent on the background level of hepatitis B virus infection.[105] Lichen planus has also followed vaccination, most commonly hepatitis B vaccination but also influenza, rabies, and Tdap vaccination.[108–114] More recently, lichen planus (particularly oral disease) has been linked to hepatitis C virus and chronic liver disease. The incidence of hepatitis C virus in patients with lichen planus is, however, very variable, ranging from effectively zero in some countries, including the United Kingdom, India, Germany, and Slovenia, to as high as 100% in Japan.[115–121]

Evidence of other disorders including thyroid disease, dyslipidemia, and impaired carbohydrate metabolism including overt diabetes mellitus, has also been documented in lichen planus, particularly the oral variant.[122–131] A recent study from Japan suggests a possible association of hepatitis C infection with both diabetes and lichen planus.[129] Other studies have cast doubt on some of these associations.[132]

A significant association between lichen planus and human leukocyte antigen (HLA)-DR1, HLA-DQ1, and HLA-DQB1 has been noted by a number of authors.[133–140] This association pertains to patients with or without mucosal lesions but does not extend to patients with the drug-induced variant. It is suggested that this association relates to antigen presentation by HLA-DR1+ cells to T-helper cells with the resultant development of an autoimmune response.[133]

Although it is generally accepted that the pathogenesis of the basal cell damage in lichen planus primarily involves the cellular immune response, likely through the action of type I interferons increasing the expression of IP10/CXCR10 and recruiting CD8+ T cells via CXCR3 and CCR5,[141–143]

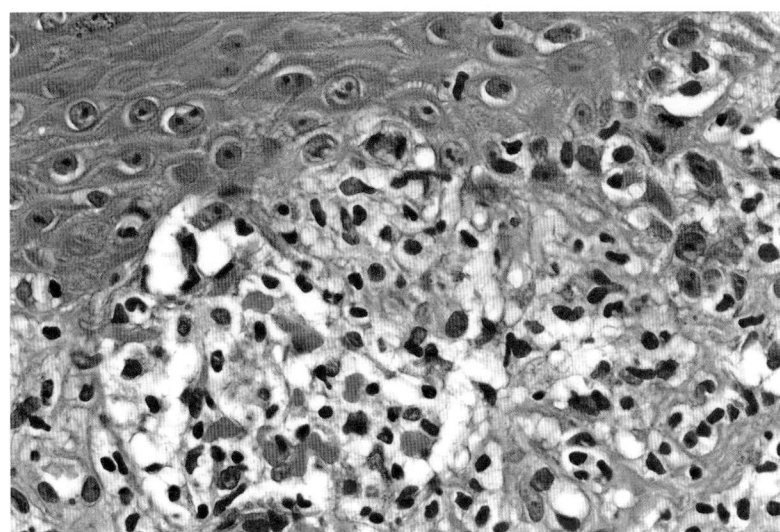

Fig. 7.20
Lichen planus: this view shows characteristic eosinophilic cytoid bodies associated with basal cell liquefactive degeneration and a lymphohistiocytic infiltrate.

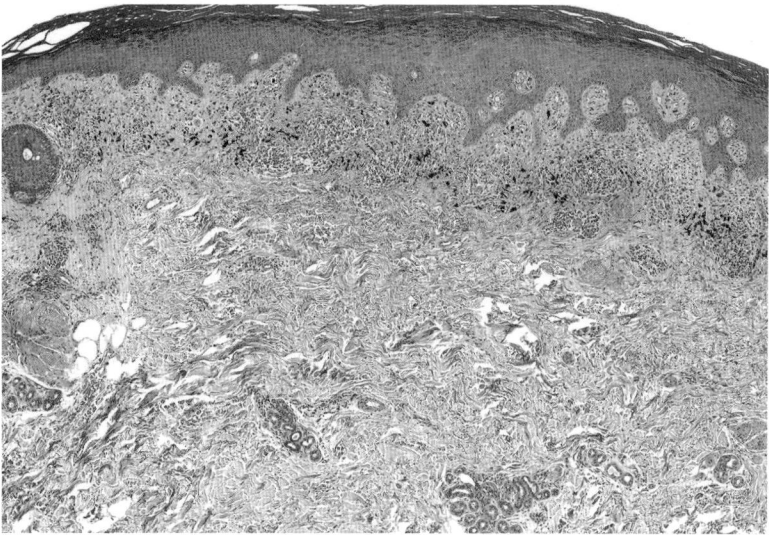

Fig. 7.21
Lichen planus: this scanning view is characteristic and highlights the hyperkeratosis, hypergranulosis, and irregular acanthosis. Note the typical bandlike inflammatory cell infiltrate and pigment incontinence.

the precise mechanism(s) require further elucidation. It is unlikely that auto-antibody and immune complex-mediated damage have a significant role in the lichenoid tissue reaction.[94,95]

The initial event in the evolution of the lichen planus papule is destruction of the basal epidermal layer (keratinocytes and melanocytes).[144,145] In the earliest stage of development, increased numbers of Langerhans cells are present within the epidermis, and it is believed that these cells process modified epidermal antigens for presentation to T lymphocytes.[146,147] Keratinocytes express HLA-DR, and this is likely to be of pathogenetic importance. Subsequent migration with resultant CD8+ T-cell activation results in basal keratinocyte death due to the combined effects of interferon-gamma (IFN-γ), interleukin (IL)-6, granulocyte-macrophage colony stimulating factor (GM-CSF), and tumor necrosis factor alpha (TNF-α).[97–99,141–143,148] The expression of FasR/FasL by the basal keratinocytes suggests that apoptosis is an important mode of cell death in lichen planus.[149] The dermal infiltrate consists predominantly of Ia+, CD4+ lymphocytes.[146,150] CD8+ lymphocytes are also present in close apposition to the dermal–epidermal junction adjacent to foci of basal keratinocyte necrosis and are said to predominate in early lesions.[148,150–152] B lymphocytes are scarce and plasma cells are characteristically absent in cutaneous lesions, except in the hypertrophic variant.

Development of the typical papule appears to be due to a combination of continued keratinocyte destruction and regenerative activity, with the latter depending upon the migration of epithelium from the edge of the lesion and from adjacent eccrine ducts, rather than from increased mitotic activity. There is little uptake of tritiated thymidine at the site of basal cell damage, but conspicuous uptake at the edges of the lesion and, as a reflection of regeneration, keratin 17 expression is also upregulated in the suprabasal epithelium.[153] The typical features of lichen planus therefore depend upon a variable interplay between basal cell liquefactive degeneration and irregular epidermal regeneration.

The earliest identifiable change in lichen planus is the presence of cytoid bodies and associated pigmentary incontinence. Cytoid bodies (colloid or Civatte bodies) are round or oval, homogeneous, eosinophilic bodies identifiable within the basal epithelium and the papillary dermis (Fig. 7.20). They display diastase-resistant periodic acid-Schiff (PAS) positivity, and may be identified within papules, perilesional skin, and even apparently uninvolved skin. Although they may be seen in a variety of dermatoses (including lupus erythematosus, graft-versus-host disease, and poikiloderma) and seemingly normal skin, where their presence, if either in large numbers or in a cluster, suggests lichen planus.

Ultrastructurally, cytoid bodies are composed of tightly arranged aggregates of filaments 6–8 nm in diameter; immunocytochemically they are composed of keratin.

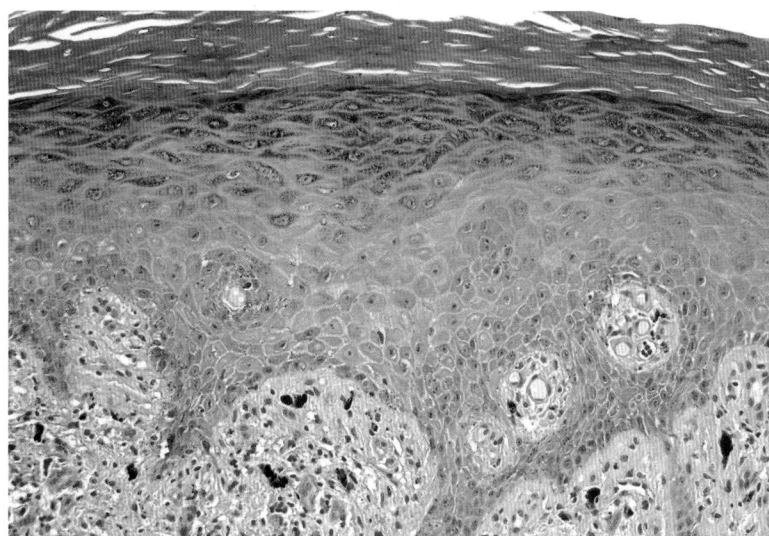

Fig. 7.22
Lichen planus: note the hyperkeratosis, hypergranulosis, and irregular acanthosis.

Characteristic histologic features of an established papule can usually be recognized at scanning magnification (Fig. 7.21). They comprise hyperkeratosis, typically wedge-shaped hypergranulosis (clinically presenting as Wickham striae) related to the intraepidermal components of sweat ducts and hair follicles, and irregular acanthosis (Figs 7.22 and 7.23). The acanthosis often has a sawtooth appearance (Figs 7.24 and 7.25). The presence of prominent parakeratosis argues strongly against a diagnosis of cutaneous lichen planus. Lymphocytes and histiocytes may sometimes be seen in the epidermis and occasionally satellite cell necrosis is a feature. Liquefactive degeneration of the basal layer of the epithelium is characteristic and often subepidermal clefts are present (Max Joseph spaces). Pigmentary incontinence is common (Fig. 7.26). A lymphohistiocytic bandlike infiltrate occupies the upper dermis and obscures the dermal–epidermal junction. Occasional eosinophils may be present.[154] Hyperkeratosis persists in resolving lichen planus, but the acanthosis regresses, leaving a flattened epidermis (Fig. 7.27); there may be focal scarring and the dermal infiltrate is less conspicuous (Fig. 7.28).

Lesions may become completely atrophic and histologically there is flattening of the epidermis, variable number of colloid bodies, and pigment incontinence with almost no inflammation. If colloid bodies are rare, distinction from poikiloderma may be very difficult.

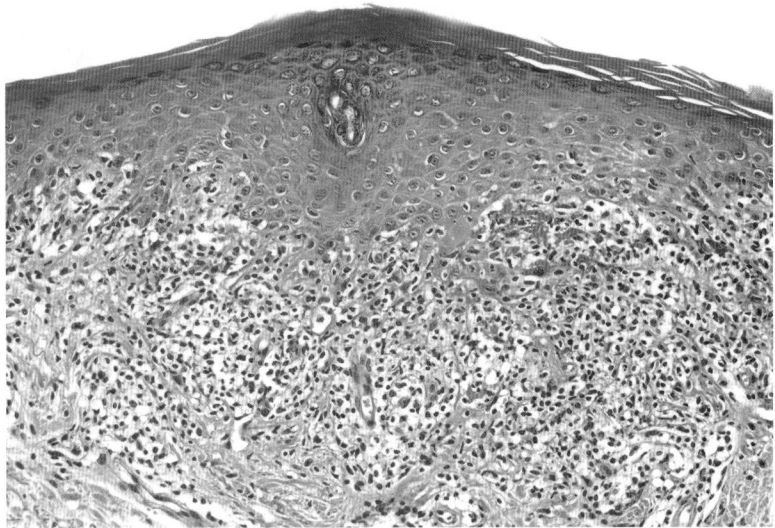

Fig. 7.23
Lichen planus: the hypergranulosis is clearly related to the acrosyringium. There is marked basal cell liquefactive degeneration. Note the fibrin deposition.

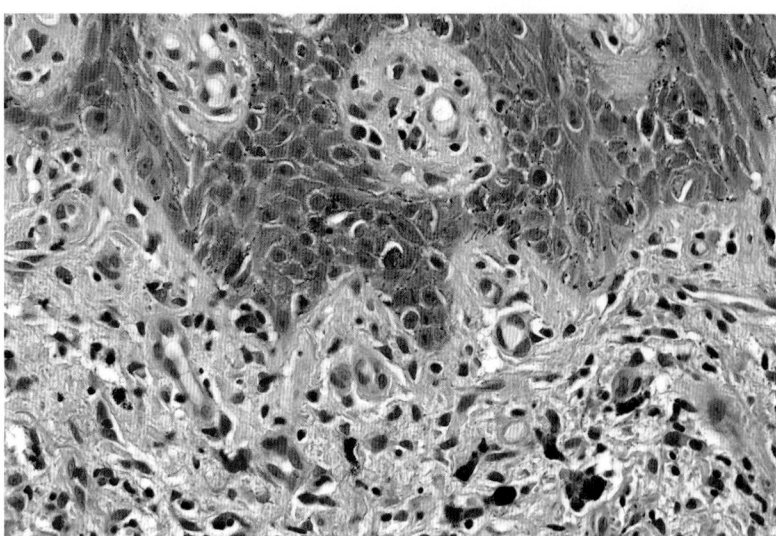

Fig. 7.26
Lichen planus: melanin pigment is present within macrophages (pigmentary incontinence).

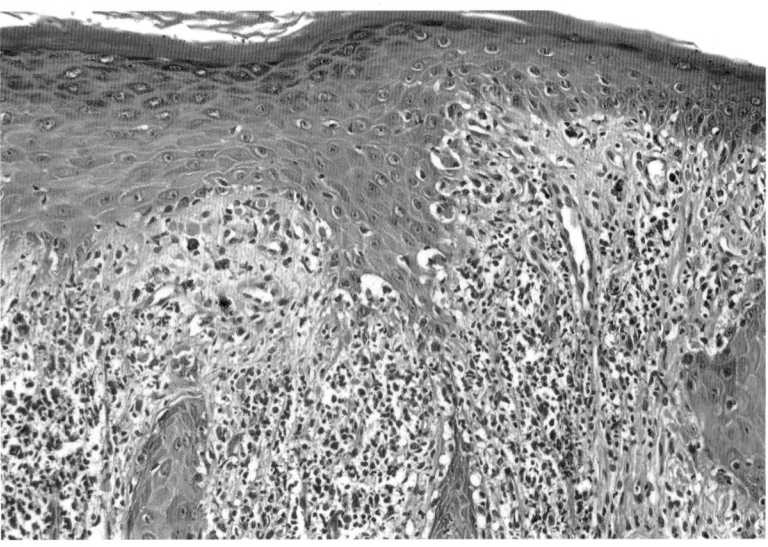

Fig. 7.24
Lichen planus: the acanthosis is irregular and often has a sawtooth appearance.

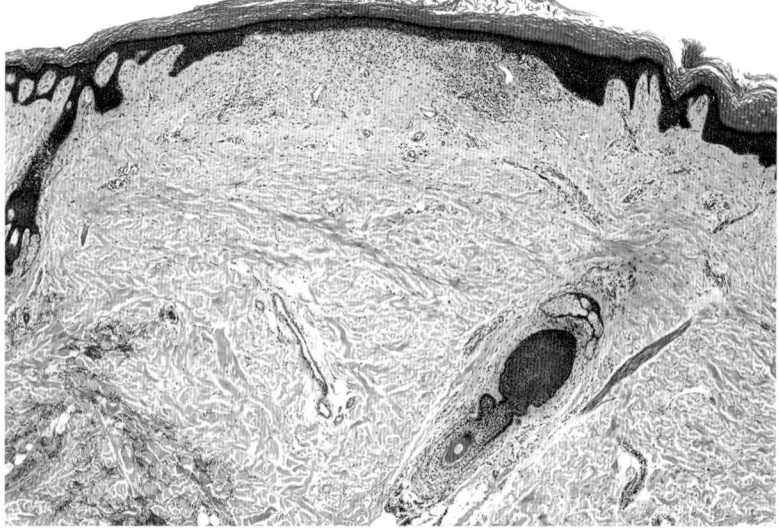

Fig. 7.27
Atrophic (resolving) lichen planus: there is hyperkeratosis, epidermal flattening, and a slight residual lymphohistiocytic infiltrate.

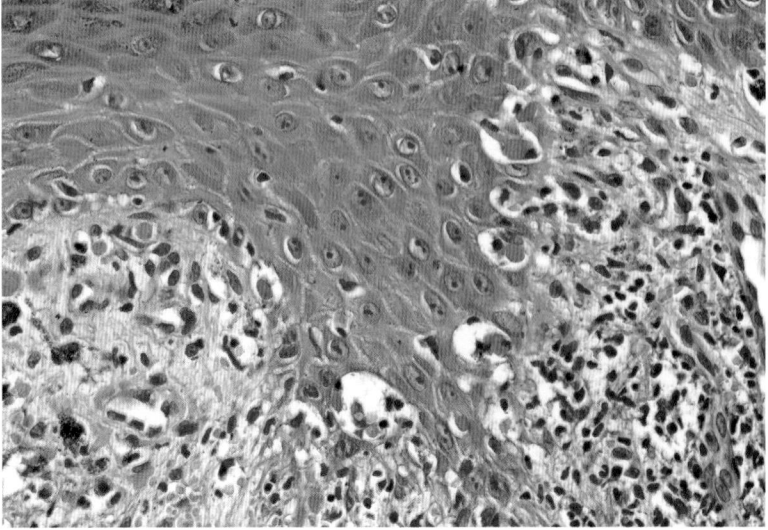

Fig. 7.25
Lichen planus: close-up view of *Fig. 7.24* showing basal cell liquefactive degeneration and cytoid bodies.

In lesions of annular lichen planus, the typical histologic features are only seen in the periphery at the advancing edge of the lesion.

In micropapular lichen planus, the changes are so focal that the diagnosis may be missed if serial sections are not examined.

Lichen planopilaris in its early stages shows an infiltrate surrounding the lower hair follicle and papilla, follicular dilatation, and keratin plugging (*Fig. 7.29*).[60,62] The adjacent interfollicular epithelium may or may not show a typical lichenoid infiltrate (*Fig. 7.30*). Basal cell hydropic degeneration, cytoid body formation, and pigmentary incontinence are also sometimes evident. In advanced scalp lesions, the hair follicles are destroyed and replaced by vertically orientated fibrous scars, reminiscent of the fibrous streamers seen in pseudopélade of Brocq.

Lichen planoporitis represents a rare variant in which lichenoid/interface changes are centered on the acrosyringium and eccrine sweat duct as it enters the epidermis. Squamous metaplasia of the ductal lining epithelium may be a feature.[155]

In lichen planus actinicus, the annular borders of the macules show typical features of lichen planus. In the center of the lesions, however, the epithelium is atrophic, thin, and flattened, although the lymphohistiocytic infiltrate remains. Foci of parakeratosis and eczematization within the

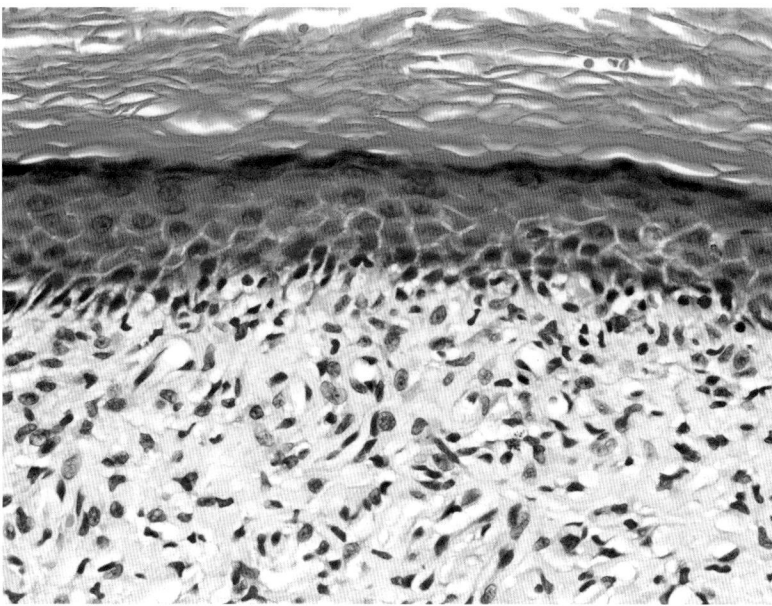

Fig. 7.28
Atrophic (resolving) lichen planus: in addition to the lymphohistiocytic infiltrate, there are excessive numbers of fibroblasts and increased papillary dermal collagen.

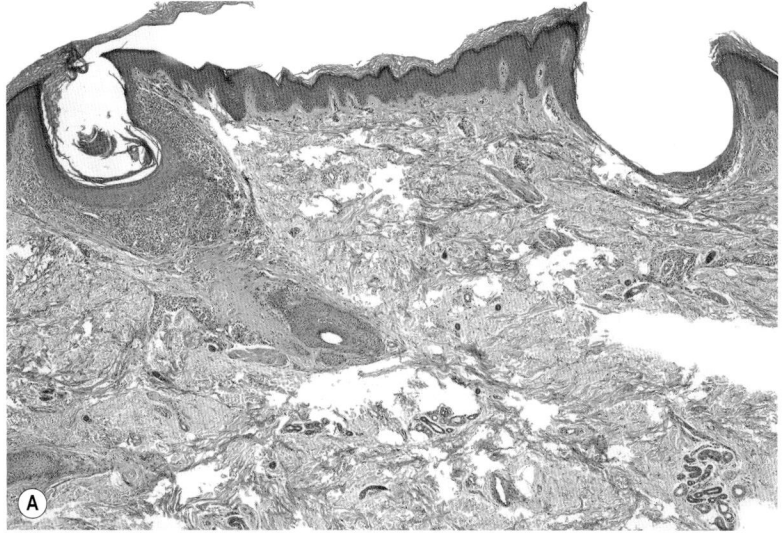

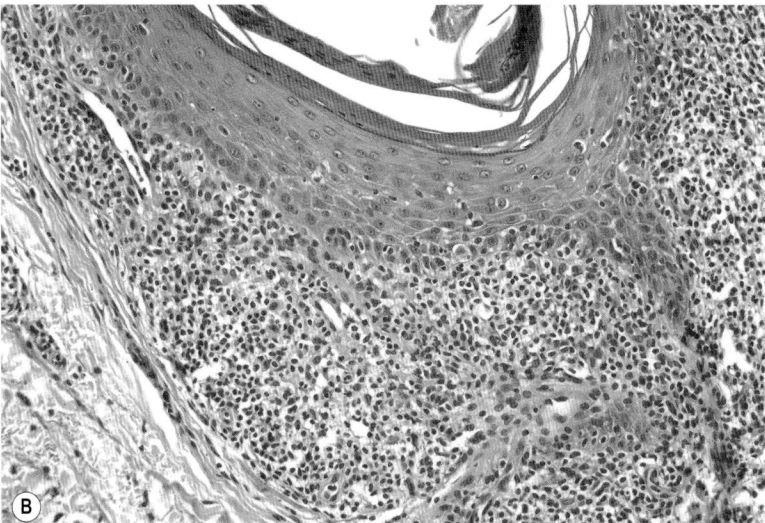

Fig. 7.29
Lichen planopilaris: (**A**, **B**) there is marked follicular dilatation and plugging accompanied by a bandlike folliculocentric infiltrate. This patient presented with scarring alopecia and typical lichen planus lesions elsewhere.

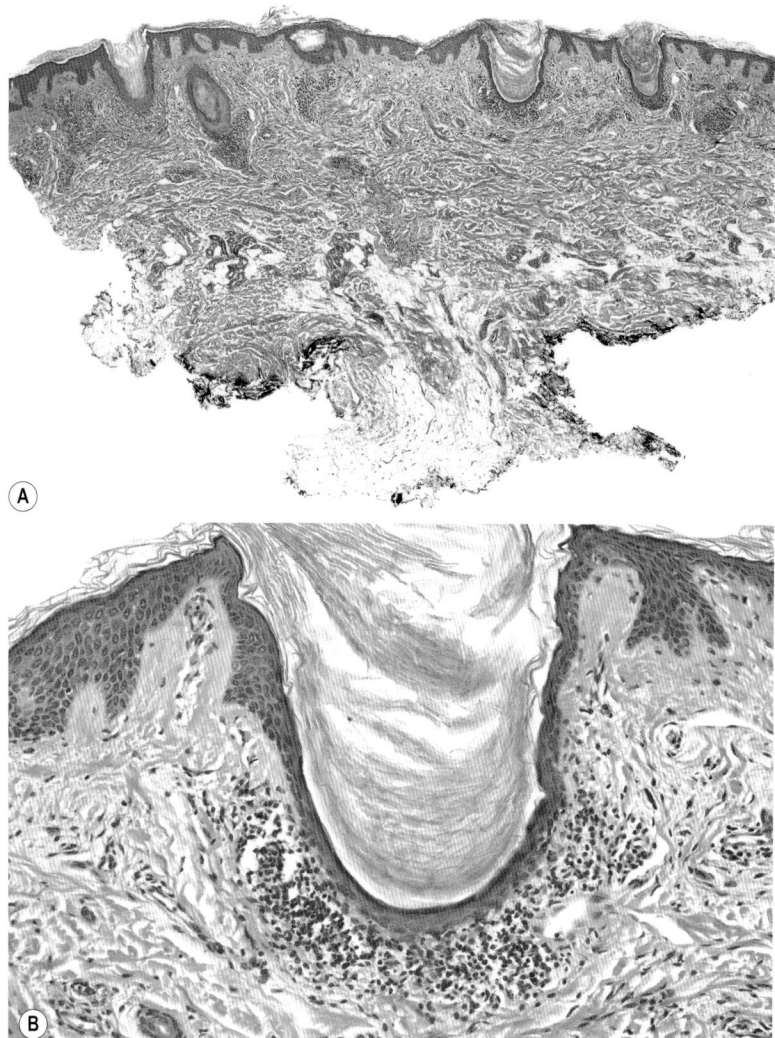

Fig. 7.30
Lichen planopilaris: (**A**, **B**) there is a strikingly folliculocentric bandlike infiltrate associated with keratin plugging. The interfollicular epidermis is unaffected.

follicular epithelium have also been described. Lichen nitidus-like lesions may sometimes be seen (see below).

Lichen planus pigmentosus is characterized by epidermal thinning accompanied by basal cell vacuolization, pigmentary incontinence, and a superficial dermal lichenoid lymphohistiocytic infiltrate.[4]

Hypertrophic lichen planus is characterized by more marked hyperkeratosis and acanthosis, with the epithelium sometimes showing pseudoepitheliomatous hyperplasia such that misdiagnosis as squamous cell carcinoma is a distinct possibility, particularly in small biopsies and if clinical information is not available (*Figs 7.31–7.33*).[84] A number of changes not seen in ordinary lichen planus may be observed and include parakeratosis, spongiosis, necrotic keratinocytes above the basal cell layer, more frequent eosinophils, and plasma cells in the dermal infiltrate. These changes may raise the possibility of a lichenoid drug eruption. The differential diagnosis is not difficult, as lichenoid drug eruptions tend to be more generalized and are not usually associated with hypertrophic changes.

The oral lesions of lichen planus, although often displaying the classical features, usually show parakeratosis; occasionally, alternate foci of both are evident.[156] In contrast to the cutaneous lesions, the epithelium is sometimes rather thin and the sawtooth pattern indistinct (*Fig. 7.34*). There is typically basal cell hydropic degeneration. Basement membrane thickening due to the deposition of fibrin-rich eosinophilic amorphous material is commonly present. The cellular infiltrate, in addition to lymphocytes and histiocytes, frequently contains plasma cells. Dysplasia may be seen.

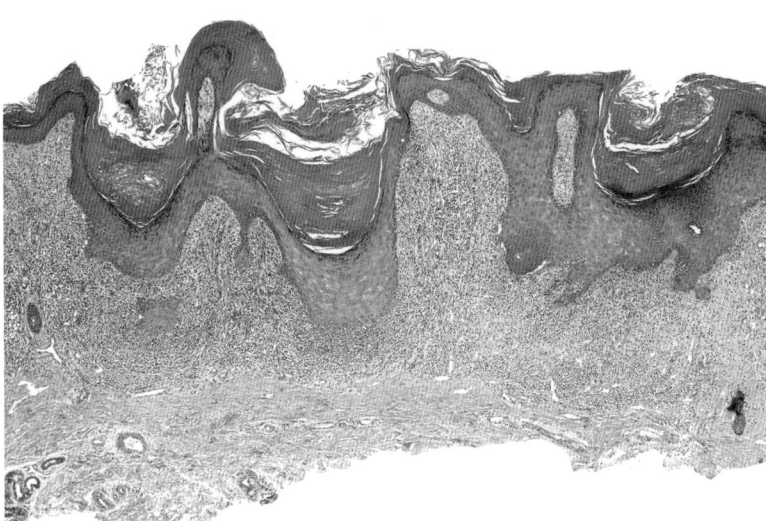

Fig. 7.31
Hypertrophic lichen planus: note the hyperkeratosis, focal wedge-shaped hypergranulosis, very marked irregular acanthosis, and superficial dense bandlike infiltrate.

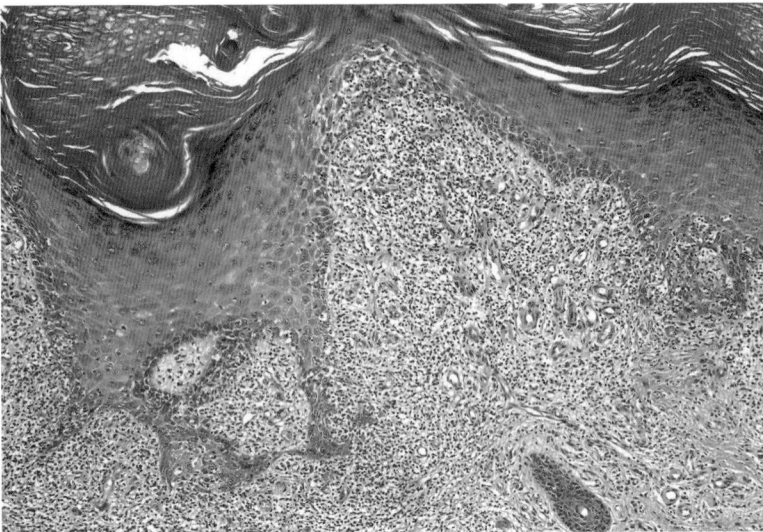

Fig. 7.32
Hypertrophic lichen planus: there is very marked irregular acanthosis. Note the hypergranulosis.

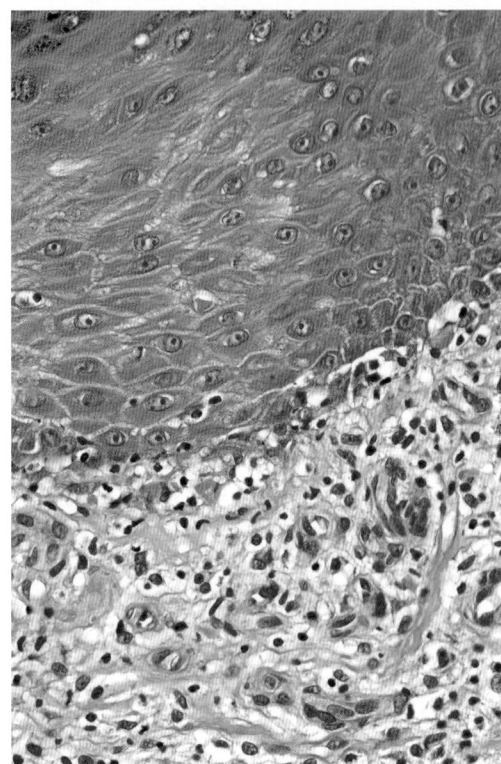

Fig. 7.33
Hypertrophic lichen planus: there is basal cell liquefactive degeneration with cytoid bodies.

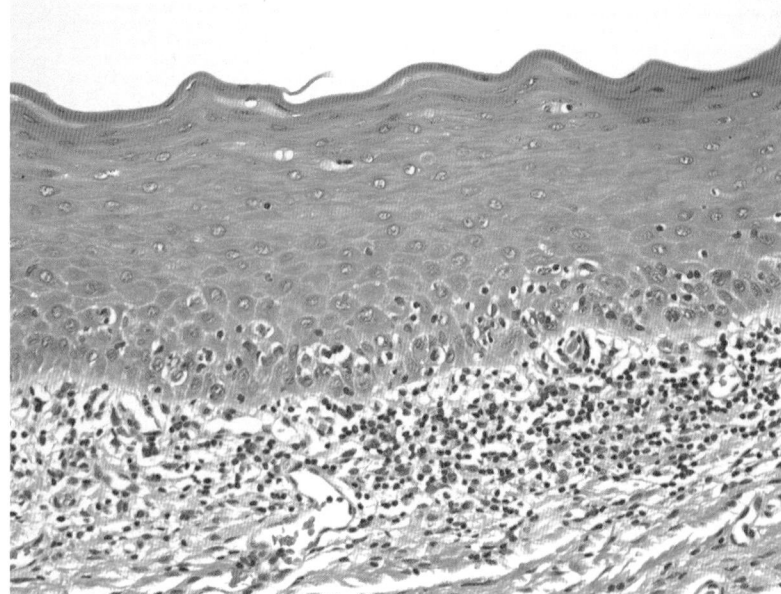

Fig. 7.34
Oral lichen planus: there is parakeratosis, a subtle granular layer, and no sawtoothing of the epithelial–subpithelial junction in contrast to cutaneous lichen planus.

Unlike skin involvement, esophageal lesions show parakeratosis. Variable epithelial atrophy and/or mild thickening are usually seen, and the sawtooth pattern of acanthosis is not a feature.[33,37–39] As with oral lesions, plasma cells often accompany the lymphocytic infiltrate.

Vesicular or bullous lesions are subepidermal and occur due to excessive edema developing in association with the basement membrane zone damage complicating basal cell hydropic degeneration (*Fig. 7.35*).

Direct immunofluorescence studies from patients with lichen planus usually reveal a linear fibrillar band of fibrin at the dermal–epidermal junction (*Fig. 7.36*). The cytoid bodies may be highlighted non-specifically, mainly to IgM, but also to IgG, IgA, and C3 (*Fig. 7.37*). A lichen planus 'specific antigen', which is present in the prickle cell and granular cell layers, has been demonstrated by indirect immunofluorescence of patients' serum with fetal skin.[157] The pathogenetic significance of this is unknown. Direct immunofluorescence of lichen planopilaris reveals follicular, linear basement membrane zone labeling with immunoglobulin (primarily IgG or IgA).[158] Fibrin may also be present. The nosological implications of this observation are uncertain. Indirect immunofluorescence for circulating antibasement membrane zone antibodies is negative.

Differential diagnosis

Lichen planus should be differentiated from other diseases showing a lichenoid infiltrate and hydropic degeneration of the basal layer of the epithelium.[159] Thus, lichen planus may be indistinguishable from lichenoid keratosis and their distinction is entirely dependent on clinicopathological correlation. In many cases of lichenoid keratoses, there are other associated changes including focal spongiosis and parakeratosis. Atrophic lesions may be confused with poikiloderma and chronic discoid lupus erythematosus. A lichen planus-like morphology is typical of the early stages of chronic

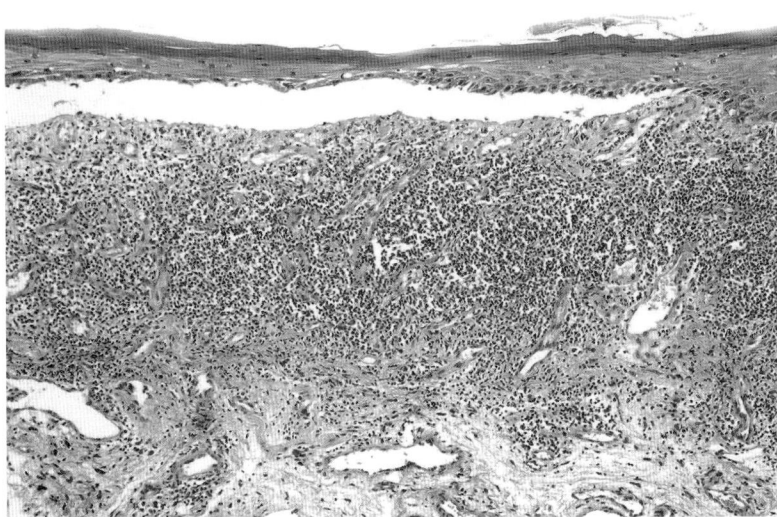

Fig. 7.35
Bullous lichen planus: oral lesion showing separation of the squamous epithelium from the lamina propria. Note the bandlike infiltrate.

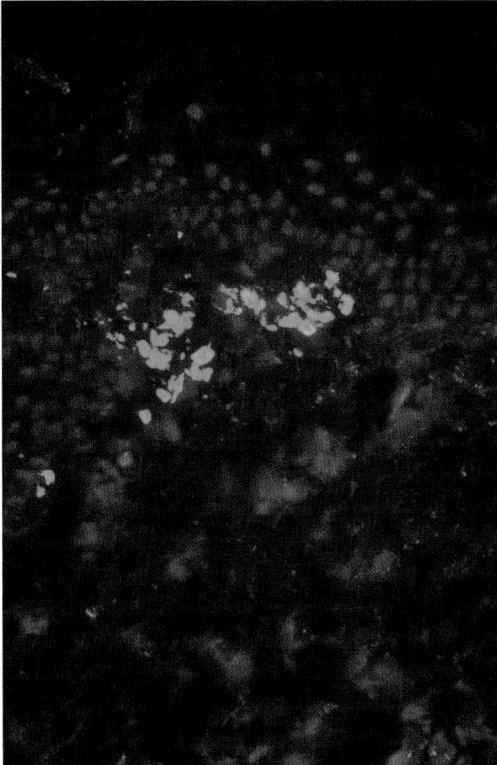

Fig. 7.37
Lichen planus: cytoid bodies labeled positively for IgM. By courtesy of the Department of Immunofluorescence, Institute of Dermatology, London, UK.

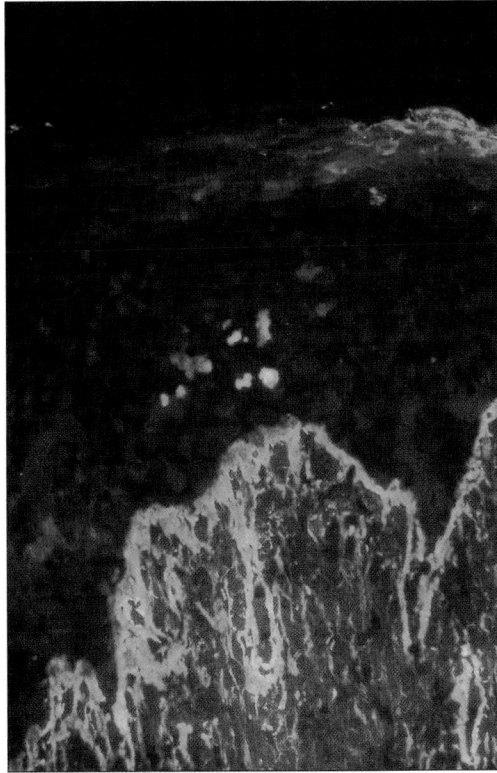

Fig. 7.36
Lichen planus: brilliant green fluorescence indicates the presence of fibrin. By courtesy of the Department of Immunofluorescence, Institute of Dermatology, London, UK.

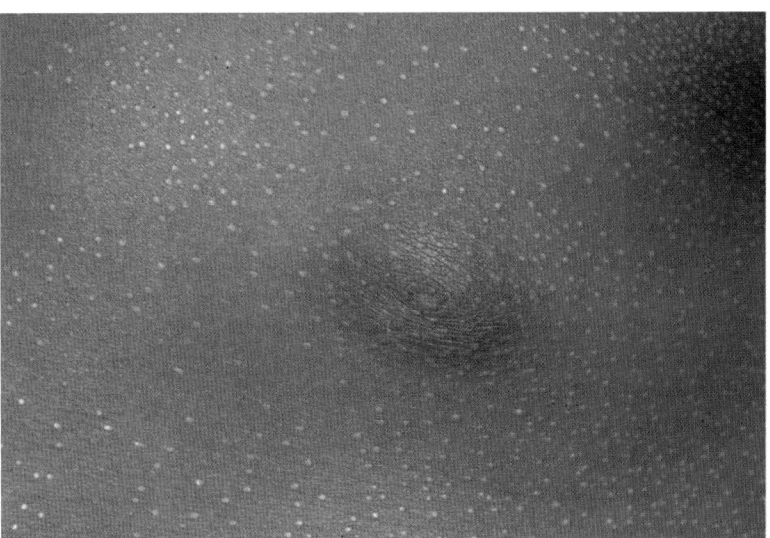

Fig. 7.38
Lichen nitidus: numerous tiny papules are present on the chest of a young child. By courtesy of R.A. Marsden, MD, St George's Hospital, London, UK.

graft-versus-host disease (GVHD), but the density of the infiltrate is typically less in this entity.

Poikiloderma shows epidermal atrophy, with loss of the ridge pattern and no tendency to a sawtooth appearance. In those examples associated with mycosis fungoides, the lichenoid infiltrate contains variable numbers of atypical lymphocytes.

Chronic discoid lupus erythematosus is associated with epidermal atrophy and follicular plugging. The inflammatory cell infiltrate is patchy with a tendency to periappendageal location with associated dermal mucin deposition. A positive lupus band test can be helpful.

Lichen planus may easily be mistaken for a lichenoid drug reaction, particularly in the absence of clinical information. Histologic features favoring

the latter include high-level cytoid bodies and frequent eosinophils within the dermal infiltrate.

Lichen nitidus

Clinical features

Lichen nitidus is a rare but distinctive dermatosis, which shows an equal sex incidence.[1] Children and young adults are predominantly affected. It presents clinically as an eruption of pinhead-sized, flesh-colored, shiny, flat-topped or dome-shaped papules and shows a predilection for the arms, chest, abdomen, and genitalia (Figs 7.38 and 7.39).[1-5] A positive Koebner

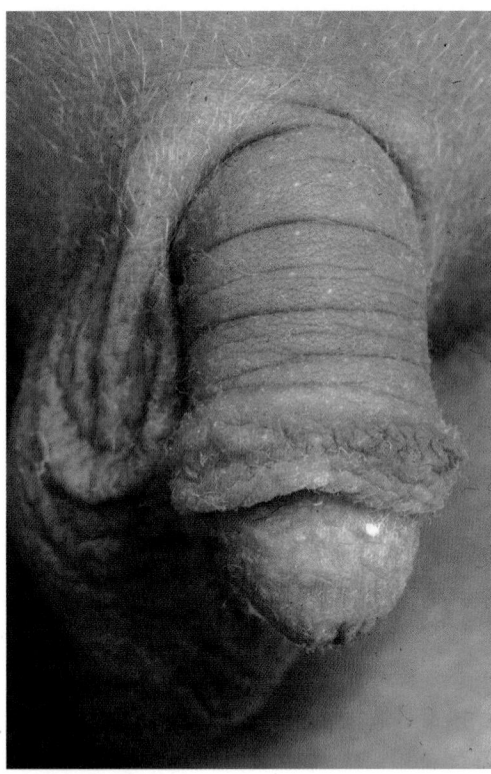

Fig. 7.39
Lichen nitidus: numerous tiny papules are present on the penis. The genitalia are commonly affected. From the collection of the late N.P. Smith, MD, the Institute of Dermatology, London, UK.

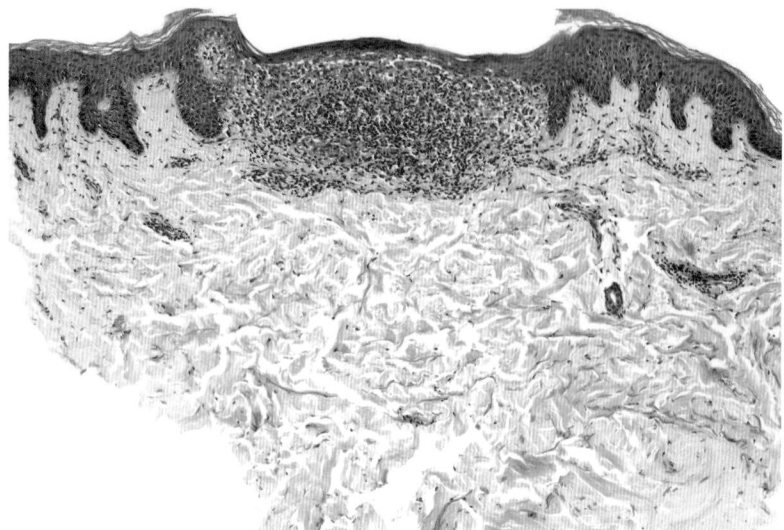

Fig. 7.40
Lichen nitidus: scanning view showing a typical small, circumscribed lesion occupying only a couple of dermal papillae. Note the clawlike epidermal lateral borders.

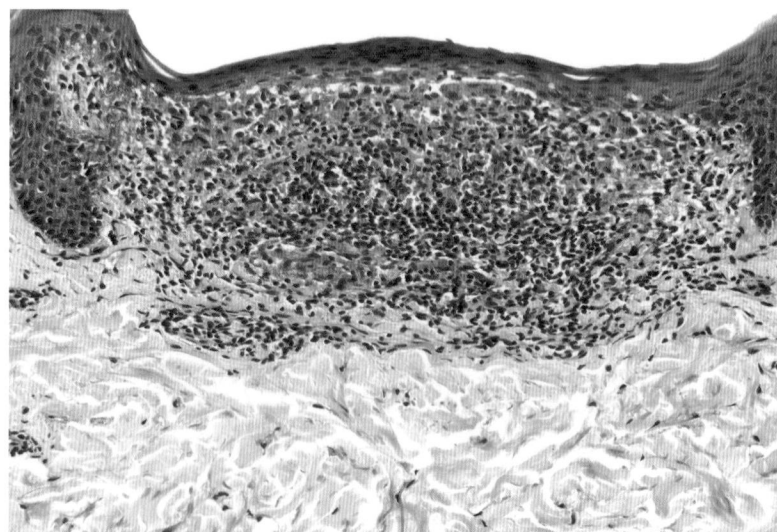

Fig. 7.41
Lichen nitidus: note the parakeratosis and bandlike infiltrate.

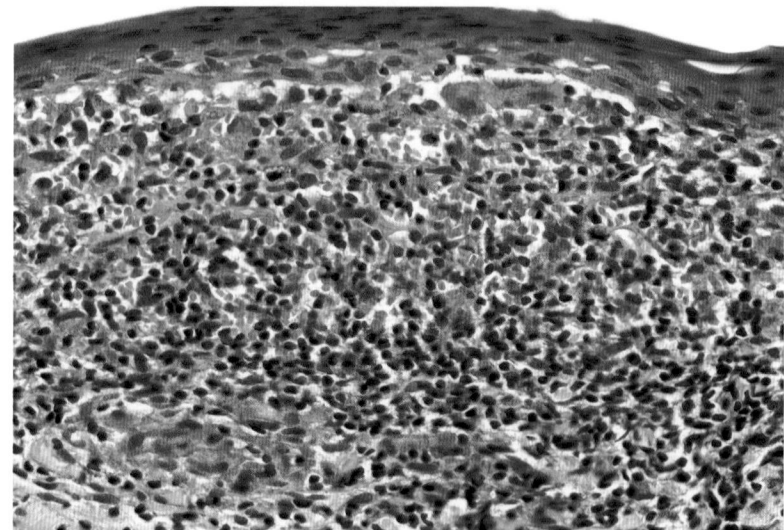

Fig. 7.42
Lichen nitidus: the infiltrate consists of lymphocytes, histiocytes, and epithelioid cells. Ill-defined noncaseating granulomata are not uncommon.

phenomenon is typically present.[5] The condition is usually localized and asymptomatic, although occasionally there may be mild or even intense pruritus.[2] Rarely, generalized lesions have been described.[2,6–9] An association with generalized lesions and Down syndrome has been documented, as has been a case after interferon-alpha therapy.[8,9] Occasionally, papules may be encountered on the palms and soles.[3–12] Familial cases have been rarely described.[13,14] Lichen nitidus can spontaneously resolve within a few months or persist indefinitely.[2]

Mucosal involvement presenting as grayish-yellow papules has also been described.[4] Nail involvement, which is rare, presents as thickening with ridges, rippling, terminal splitting, striations, and pits.[2,4]

Keratodermic, vesicular, hemorrhagic, purpuric, and perforating variants may rarely be encountered.[2,15–19] Perforating lichen nitidus shows a predilection for the forearms and fingers, and may be trauma related.[17,20,21]

Actinic lichen nitidus refers to the development of lichen nitidus on sun-exposed sites, usually during the summer months. In some cases, involvement is predominantly facial and it may present in black patients.[22] It shows considerable overlap with actinic lichen planus (see above).[23,24]

Histologic features

Lichen nitidus is recognizable by a characteristic histology in many cases. The classic papule is sharply circumscribed and occupies the space of only four or five dermal papillae. It is often depressed in the center and composed of atrophic epidermis, frequently covered by a parakeratotic tier and overlying a cellular infiltrate (*Figs 7.40–7.43*). Clawlike extensions of epidermal ridges mark the lateral boundaries of the lesion. The epithelium shows basal cell hydropic degeneration, and cytoid bodies may be a feature. The inflammatory component consists of lymphocytes, histiocytes, and variable numbers of epithelioid cells. Giant cells are sometimes a feature and true granulomata may occasionally be found, although caseation is never present.[25] A plasma cell-rich variant is exceptional. In addition to red blood cell extravasation, purpuric variants may show increased vascularity with vessel wall thickening and hyalinization.[18] In rare cases, a prominent lymphocytic inflammatory infiltrate can extend down the hair follicle and eccrine glands, making the distinction from lichen striatus challenging.[25] A

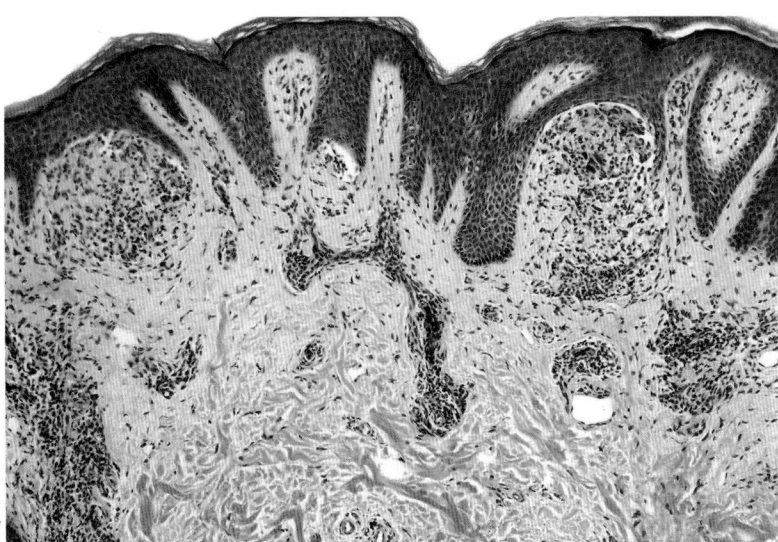

Fig. 7.43
Lichen nitidus: there are multiple lesions of lichen nitidus with an associated granulomatous component. The patient also had typical lichen planus lesions. By courtesy of R. Margolis, MD, St Elizabeth's Hospital, Boston, USA.

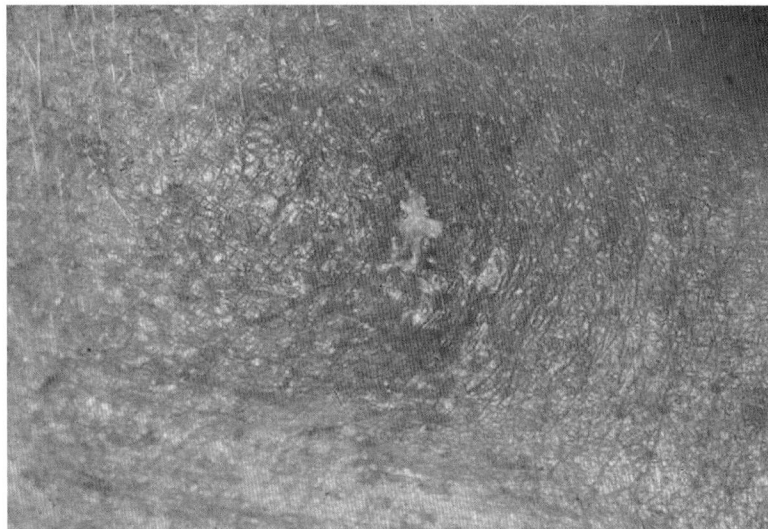

Fig. 7.44
Lichenoid keratosis: there is scaling overlying a slightly raised erythematous plaque. By courtesy of the Institute of Dermatology, London.

follicular variant of lichen nitidus may be seen and mimics lichen spinulosus histologically.[26] However, rarely, lichen nitidus and lichen spinulosus may coexist clinically.[27,28]

Palmar lesions may be identical to those seen elsewhere or show a more diffuse bandlike upper dermal lymphohistiocytic infiltrate with associated giant cells and focal parakeratosis.[3,10–12,29,30]

Fibrin can be detected at the basement membrane zone by immunofluorescent techniques, but immunoglobulin deposition is not a feature.[31,32] Immunophenotypic studies show that there is a marked excess of CD4+ cells (helper/inducer T cells) over CD8+ cells (cytotoxic/suppressor T cells).[31] Langerhans cells are conspicuous.[33] These findings are similar to those described for lichen planus.

Ultrastructural examination reveals rather non-specific findings including epidermal intercellular edema, subepidermal edema, colloid bodies, decreased numbers of desmosomes, and disruption or reduplication of the lamina densa.[34–36] Perivascular electron-dense deposits (the nature of which is unknown) have been described in purpuric variants.[8]

Comment

Lichen nitidus may coexist with lichen planus or predate it and lichen nitidus-like lesions may be found in patients with typical lichen planus, but it is unlikely that the conditions are closely related.[37,38] Wickham striae are not a feature of lichen nitidus, and mucosal involvement is exceptional.[2,4] Lichen nitidus is associated with parakeratosis and epidermal atrophy, in contrast to the orthohyperkeratosis and acanthosis seen in lichen planus. The sawtooth appearance of the lower border of the epidermis seen in lichen planus is not a feature of lichen nitidus, and immunofluorescence for immunoglobulins is negative. Epithelioid cells and giant cells are characteristic of lichen nitidus and are not typically a feature of lichen planus. Four patients with Crohn disease were reported to develop lichen niditus; however, it remains to be seen if lichen nitidus is truly an extragastrointestinal finding of this disease.[39,40] Another patient developed lichen nitidus after hepatitis B vaccine injection.[41] The significance of this is uncertain.

Lichenoid keratosis

Clinical features

Lichenoid keratosis (benign lichenoid keratosis, lichen planus-like keratosis, solitary lichen planus) is not uncommon and usually presents as a solitary, 0.3–2-cm diameter, sharply demarcated, erythematous, violaceous, tan or brown papule or plaque (*Fig. 7.44*).[1,2] Occasionally, multiple lesions may

be present.[2–4] It is usually of short duration and shows a predilection for the face (particularly the cheeks and nose), neck, upper trunk (especially the presternal area), forearm, and dorsum of the hand.[2,5–10] The surface is often scaly. Lesions are commonly asymptomatic, but mild pruritus has sometimes been documented.[9] Patients are frequently Caucasian, but occasionally blacks are affected.[2,8,9] Females develop these lesions more commonly than males, usually in their fourth to seventh decades.[2,6,10]

Lichenoid keratosis is often clinically misdiagnosed as a seborrheic keratosis, superficial basal cell carcinoma, squamous cell carcinoma, actinic keratosis, or Bowen disease.[5]

Pathogenesis and histologic features

The precise nature of lichenoid keratosis is uncertain. In the past, it was regarded as a solitary lesion of lichen planus or thought to have an actinic pathogenesis.[11–13] It was also proposed to represent an immunological or regressive response to a preexistent epidermal lesion similar to the phenomenon encountered with a 'halo' nevus.[2] The frequent association of solar lentigines or, less commonly, seborrheic keratoses in the adjacent epithelium has been cited as evidence in favor of this hypothesis.[5–7,9] Recent studies have shown the lymphocytic infiltrate in lichenoid keratosis to be immunophenotypically distinct from lichen planus. The lymphocytes in lichenoid keratosis are predominantly CD8-reactive in contrast to lichen planus. More CD20-positive B cells are usually seen in lichenoid keratosis. Furthermore, the lymphocyte infiltrate in lichenoid keratosis lacks the cutaneous lymphocyte antigen (CLA) expression, suggesting the absence of localized antigenic stimulation as seen in lichen planus.[2,14] These studies suggest that lichenoid keratosis is distinct from lichen planus despite the similarities in histology.

Histologically, as its name suggests, the features are often very similar or even identical to those of lichen planus. There is hyperkeratosis, wedge-shaped hypergranulosis, variable acanthosis, and basal cell liquefactive degeneration sometimes accompanied by lymphocytic exocytosis (*Figs 7.45* and *7.46*).[2,3,6,10] Foci of parakeratosis are also frequently seen.[1,2,10] Although the sawtooth acanthosis of lichen planus is sometimes evident, more often the epithelium merely shows broadened, widened, and irregular epidermal ridges.[5] The basal epidermal layers may sometimes show very minor degrees of cytological atypia, including cellular and nuclear enlargement with conspicuous nucleoli, but these changes represent regenerative phenomena.[3] Dysplasia as seen in lichenoid actinic keratosis is not a feature of a lichenoid keratosis. Colloid bodies are usually conspicuous in both the epidermis and dermis, and pigmentary incontinence is often marked (*Figs 7.47–7.49*).[1,2,8,10] Apoptotic keratinocytes can be prominent and may be associated with intraepidermal blister formation with subepidermal

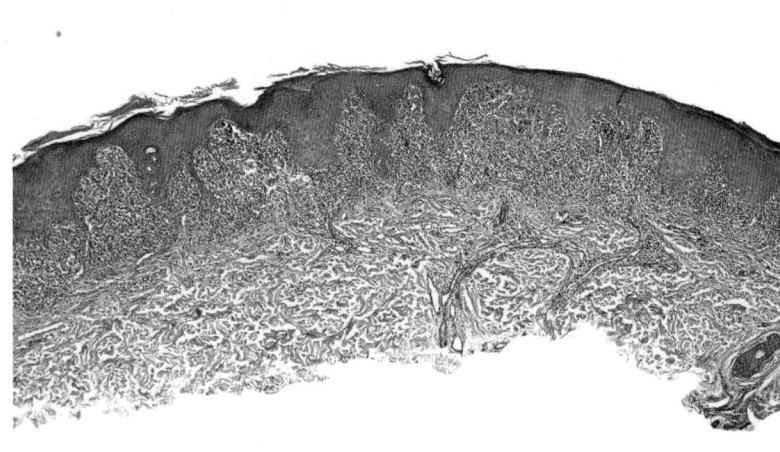

Fig. 7.45
Lichenoid keratosis: scanning view showing hyperkeratosis, hypergranulosis, irregular acanthosis, and a bandlike chronic inflammatory infiltrate.

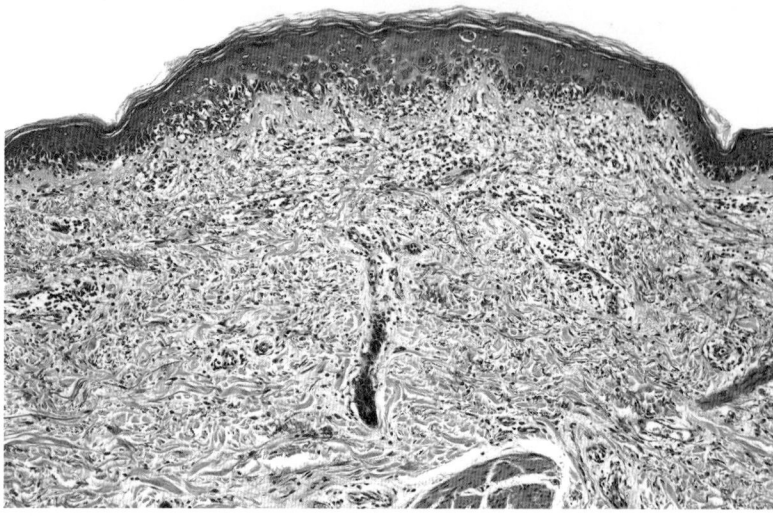

Fig. 7.48
Lichenoid keratosis: there is interface change with cytoid bodies.

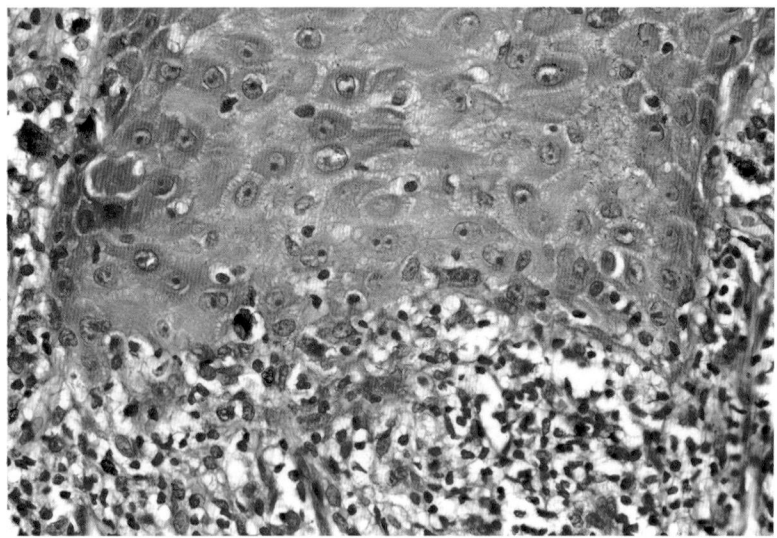

Fig. 7.46
Lichenoid keratosis: in this field there is basal cell liquefactive degeneration. Cytoid bodies are present.

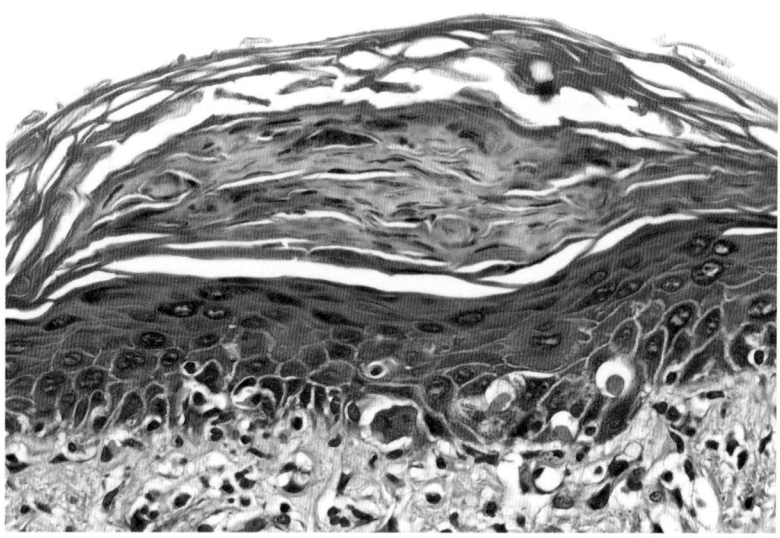

Fig. 7.49
Lichenoid keratosis: basal cell liquefactive degeneration is evident in addition to cytoid bodies. Note the parakeratosis.

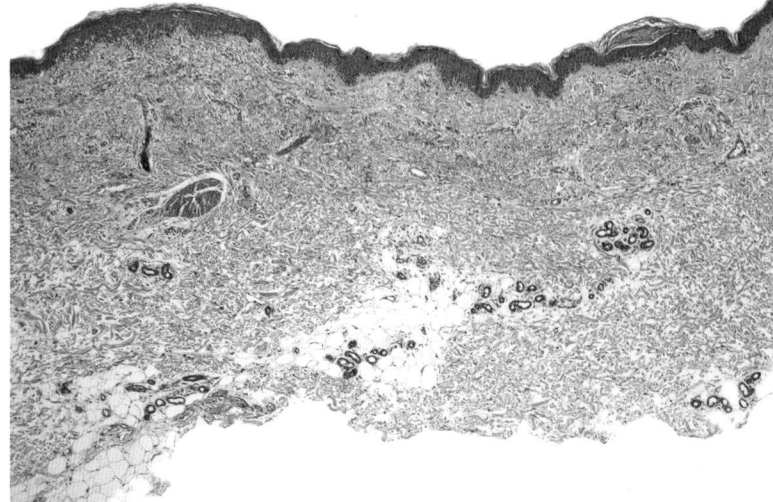

Fig. 7.47
Lichenoid keratosis: in this early lesion, there is more uniform acanthosis.

vesiculation. In such cases, the histology can mimic conditions such as sub-acute cutaneous lupus erythematosus and even erythema multiforme. Epidermal pallor and dermal edema can be seen in cases with only slight or no acanthosis and an interface population of lymphocytes along the junction with vacuolar degeneration. Foci of atrophy can be occasionally encountered.[2,10] In some cases, a combination of lichenoid and spongiotic changes may be seen.

A dense chronic inflammatory cell infiltrate is typically present in the superficial dermis. Although this characteristically has a lichenoid distribution, on some occasions it may be more discrete and predominantly perivascular in location.[4,8] The infiltrate consists largely of lymphocytes and histiocytes, but small numbers of plasma cells and eosinophils are occasionally present. Exceptionally, atypical large T lymphocytes (enlarged with hyperchromatic, irregular, contoured nuclei) which are activated CD30 positive cells can be also seen.[2] The adjacent dermis sometimes shows lentigo and solar elastosis. Features suggestive of mycoses fungoides such as Pautrier abscesses, dermal–epidermal tagging, and mild lymphocytic atypia have been exceptionally noted in benign lichenoid keratosis (lymphomatoid lichenoid keratosis).[14] Clinicopathological correlation and careful follow-up are essential in such cases to avoid misdiagnosis.

Immunofluorescence findings, which are similar to those of lichen planus, comprise deposits of IgM and, less commonly, IgG outlining cytoid bodies.[6]

Differential diagnosis

Many conditions show lichenoid histology and therefore come into the differential diagnosis. Most prominently, these include lichen planus and lichenoid drug reactions.

If clinical information is available, differentiation from lichen planus should present little difficulty. Lichen planus is characterized by large numbers of lesions in contradistinction to the single papule or plaque of lichenoid keratosis. In addition, lichen planus is usually itchy. Parakeratosis and dermal plasma cells are not usually a feature of lichen planus, but are more common of lichenoid keratosis.[8]

Both actinic keratoses and squamous cell carcinoma in situ may sometimes show a lichenoid inflammatory cell reaction. Dysplasia by definition is not a feature of lichenoid keratosis.[1,2,10] Inflamed seborrheic keratosis and porokeratosis can have a prominent lichenoid reaction. The absence of horn cyst formation, squamous eddies, and laminated stratum corneum keratin helps distinguish these lesions from seborrheic keratosis, whereas the absence of cornoid lamella excludes porokeratosis. Melanocytic lesions with halo phenomenon can become a diagnostic consideration and require examination of the dermis and dermal–epidermal junction for melanocytic nests. In difficult cases, additional step sections or immunohistochemical studies can prove useful. Finally, the presence of scattered CD30-positive lymphocytes in some cases of lichenoid keratosis may raise the histologic differential diagnosis of lymphomatoid papulosis. However, the paucity of these enlarged CD30-positive cells, the absence of a deep infiltrate, and the clinically history of a solitary lesion is reassuring for lichenoid keratosis.[2]

Lichen striatus

Clinical features

Lichen striatus [Blaschko linear acquired inflammatory skin eruption (BLAISE)] is an uncommon, usually asymptomatic, dermatosis of unknown etiology, affecting the limbs or neck in which lesions typically follow Blaschko lines.[1–9] Infrequently, the condition is pruritic.[6–8,11] It is self-limiting, normally disappearing within months to a year of onset. It shows a female predominance (2–3:1) and, although it may occur at any age, it most often presents in children aged 5–15 years.[2,5,7,8] Rarely, lichen striatus has been described in adults (adult Blaschkitis, see below).[4,10,12,13] Occurrence during pregnancy is very rare.[14] A family history is rarely encountered, suggesting a genetic predisposition and/or a common environmental etiology in such cases.[2,6,8,15,16] It is associated with seasonal variation with most series reporting the majority of patients presenting in spring and summer,[2,7] with the exception of one large series where the majority of patients presented in the winter.[8,15] Case clustering has been documented.[2]

Lesions, usually solitary and unilateral, present as erythematous or flesh-colored lichenoid or sometimes psoriasiform scaly papules, which coalesce into a continuous or interrupted linear or curved band, 1–3 cm wide and often covering the whole length of a limb, either lower or upper extremities (Figs 7.50 and 7.51).[2,8] Occasionally, multiple lesions have been recorded, as has bilaterality.[8,17,18] Presentation at two different sites and at multiple sites may exceptionally occur.[19] Nail changes, which may affect a single nail, include onycholysis, longitudinal ridging, splitting, and nail loss.[1,8,20–22] Exceptionally, lichen striatus with bilateral nail dystrophy has been described.[23,24] Lichen striatus is not associated with Koebner phenomenon. Hypo- or hyperpigmentation sometimes follows resolution, which may be marked in people with pigmented skin.[8] Lichen striatus is associated with atopy in up to 60% of patients.[1,6–8]

Pathogenesis and histologic features

The etiology of this condition is unknown although case clustering and seasonality raises the possibility of an environmental or infective basis in conjunction with an abnormal host response.[2,25] The development of lesions along Blaschko lines also raises the possibility of a cell-mediated

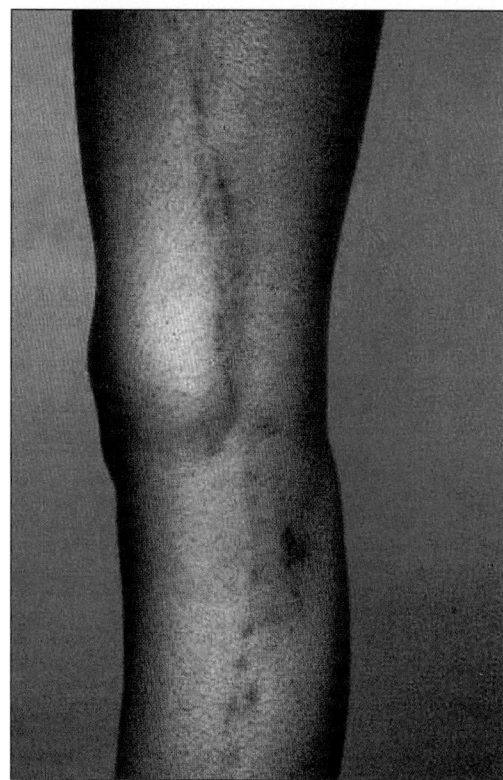

Fig. 7.50

Lichen striatus: a linear band of scaly hyperpigmented papules is present on the inner aspect of the leg, a commonly affected site. By courtesy of R.A. Marsden, MD, St George's Hospital, London, UK.

autoimmune reaction to an abnormal clone of cells. Blaschko lines are believed to represent the direction along which epidermal growth centers expand during early skin development.[1] It has been suggested that the distribution of lesions in lichen striatus may reflect a postzygotic abnormality such as somatic mutation affecting localized stem cells.[1] An intriguing case following trauma in an adult has been reported.[26] Further exceptional cases associated with solarium use, varicella and influenza infection, hepatitis B and BCG vaccine, interferon and etancercept therapy, and bee stings have been described.[27–34]

The histologic features of lichen striatus may be non-specific and show changes of mild chronic non-specific dermatitis.[35] In an established lesion, however, the changes often consist of an admixture of spongiotic dermatitis with lichenoid and interface features (Fig. 7.52).[36] Thus, there is often parakeratosis with a normal or slightly acanthotic epidermis accompanied by intercellular edema, lymphocytic exocytosis, and keratinocyte necrosis (Figs 7.53–7.55). Satellite cell necrosis may sometimes be a feature, and transepidermal elimination of keratinocyte debris (perforating lichen striatus) has occasionally been documented.[4,37] Intraepidermal Langerhans cell vesicles have exceptionally been described.[36] A heavy lymphohistiocytic infiltrate is present in the superficial dermis and also surrounds the vessels of the superficial and deep vascular plexuses and sometimes also the cutaneous adnexae (Figs 7.56 and 7.57).[4,36] Eosinophils and plasma cells are uncommon.[36]

Some biopsies may be indistinguishable from lichen planus. In those cases where there is follicular involvement, the features can resemble those of lichen planopilaris, and old lesions sometimes simulate lichen nitidus.

By immunohistochemistry, the majority of the intraepidermal lymphocytes are of a CD8+ cytotoxic phenotype.[4,36] The dermal lymphocytes consist of an admixture of CD4+ and CD8+ subtypes. CD7 is typically conserved.[29] Intraepidermal Langerhans cells may be normal, increased, or decreased.[36]

Nail changes include slight spongiosis with exocytosis, focal hypergranulosis, dyskeratosis, and a bandlike lymphohistiocytic infiltrate affecting the proximal nail fold, nail bed, and nail matrix dermis.[20]

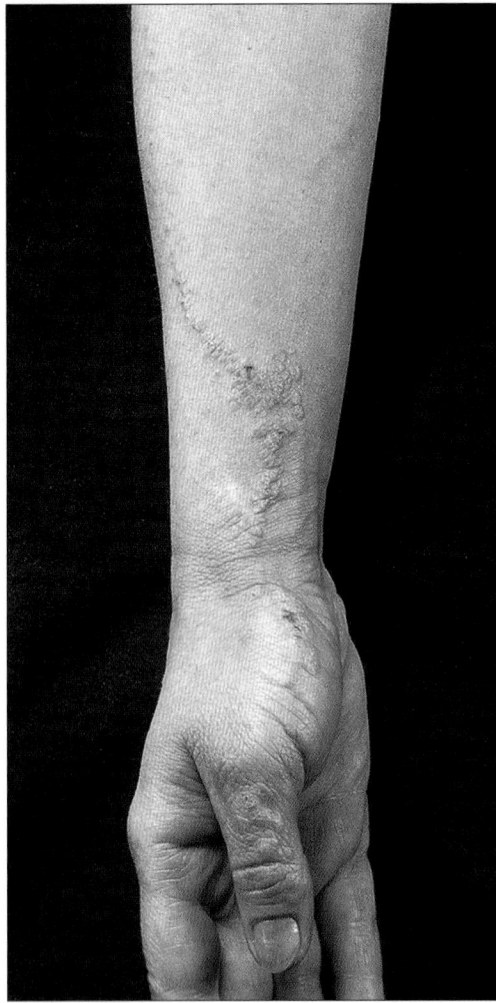

Fig. 7.51
Lichen striatus: the arms are sometimes affected. The condition most often presents in children. By courtesy of the Institute of Dermatology, London, UK.

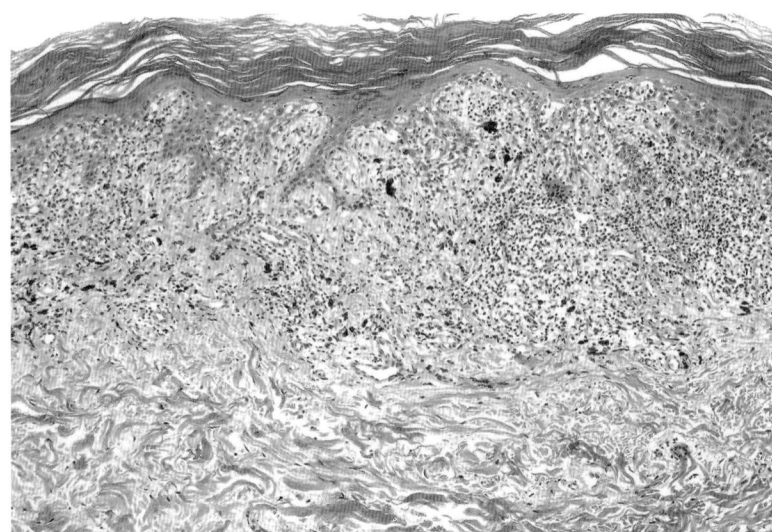

Fig. 7.52
Lichen striatus: scanning view showing hyperkeratosis, focal parakeratosis, and irregular acanthosis. A heavy inflammatory cell infiltrate is present in the upper dermis. There is conspicuous pigmentary incontinence. Case courtesy of S. Lyle, MD, Beth Israel Deaconess Medical Center, Boston, USA.

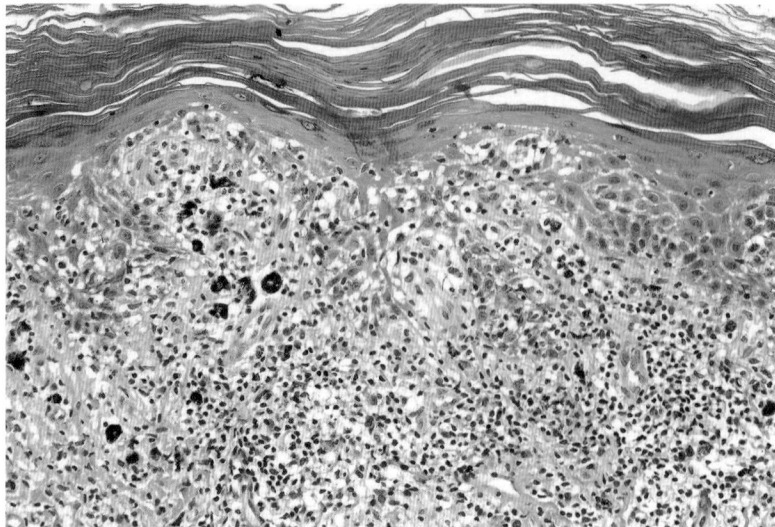

Fig. 7.53
Lichen striatus: in this field, there is parakeratosis, hyperkeratosis, spongiosis, and interface change. Note the pigment incontinence and intense chronic inflammatory cell infiltrate. Case courtesy of S. Lyle, MD, Beth Israel Deaconess Medical Center, Boston, USA.

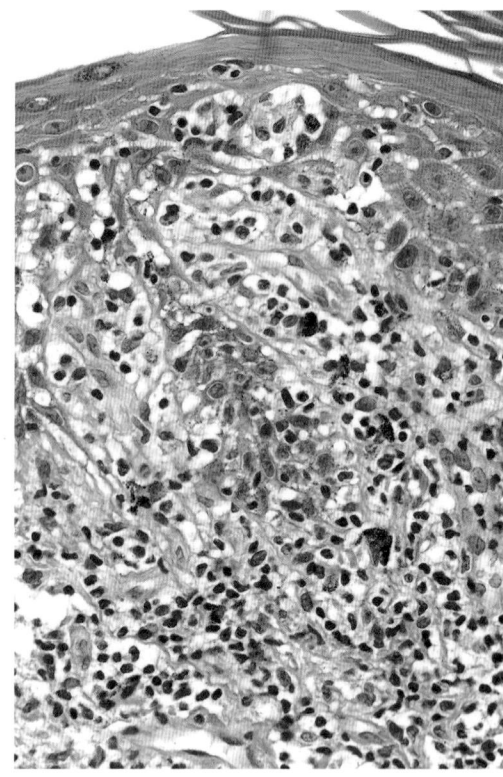

Fig. 7.54
Lichen striatus: there is spongiosis and marked lymphocytic exocytosis. Case courtesy of S. Lyle, MD, Beth Israel Deaconess Medical Center, Boston, USA.

Adult Blaschkitis

Clinical features

Adult Blaschkitis (acquired relapsing self-healing Blaschko dermatitis) is a rare, relapsing linear eruption with a mean age of onset of 40 years, predominantly affecting males.[1–14] Lesions, which are pruritic papules and vesicles, affect multiple sites, particularly the trunk, following Blaschko lines and typically resolve in days or weeks.[1] The condition, which may be unilateral or more commonly bilateral, recurs over the ensuing months or years.

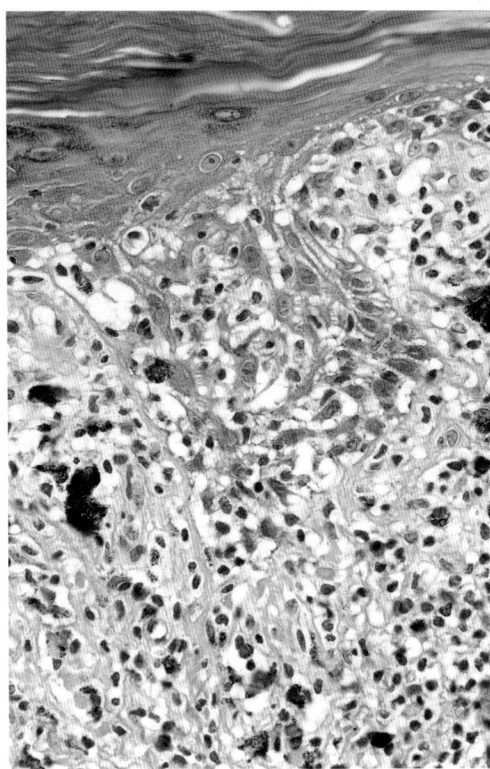

Fig. 7.55
Lichen striatus: there is spongiosis, marked lymphocytic exocytosis, basal cell liquefactive degeneration, and pigmentary incontinence. Case courtesy of S. Lyle, MD, Beth Israel Deaconess Medical Center, Boston, USA.

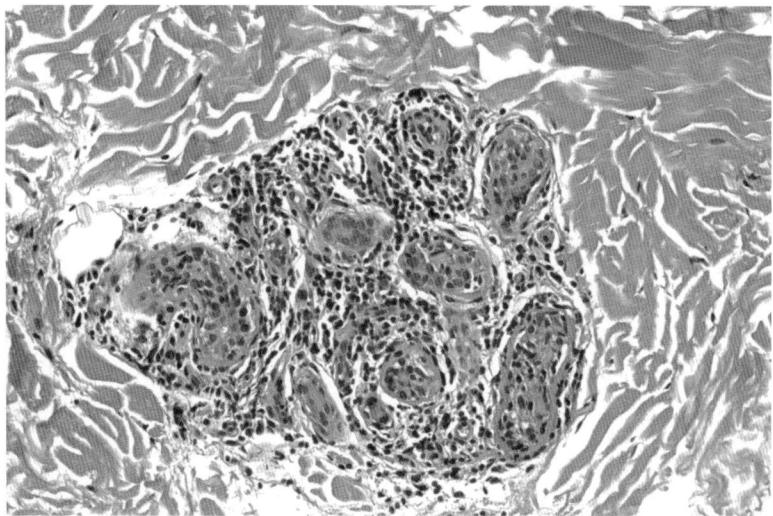

Fig. 7.57
Lichen striatus: note the perieccrine lymphocytic infiltrate.

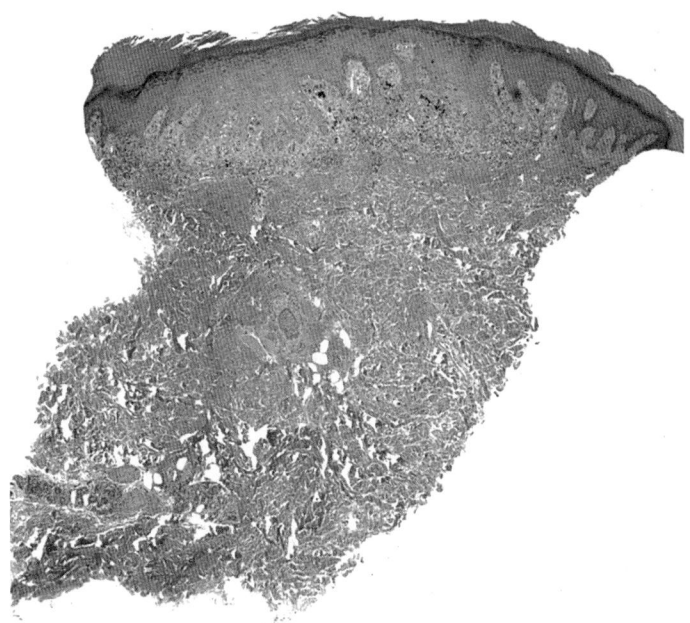

Fig. 7.56
Lichen striatus: the scanning image demonstrates a lichenoid interface dermatitis and a deeper perieccrine infiltrate.

Pathogenesis and histologic features

The etiology is unknown. Abnormalities in chromosome 18 in cells from involved skin in comparison to normal-appearing skin has been described in a female patient with adult Blaschkitis, supporting a link with cutaneous genetic mosaicism.[13] Association with drugs and emotional stress has been reported.[11,12,15,16]

Histologically, adult Blaschkitis is characterized by spongiotic changes often combined with focal interface inflammation; lichenoid features are rare, and deep involvement of adnexal structures is not often a feature.[6,8]

Differential diagnosis

It resembles lichen striatus, and it has been suggested that there is no justification for separating the two entities.[17] However, it differs clinically by the presence of vesicles, its truncal distribution, and relatively rapid resolution. Relapsing courses are typical. Pruritus is rare in lichen striatus. Lichen striatus predominantly affects young children although rare cases similar to adult Blaschkitis but affecting children have been described.

Keratosis lichenoides chronica

Clinical features

Keratosis lichenoides chronica (Nekam disease, lichen ruber verrucosus et reticularis) is a rare, chronic inflammatory dermatosis that combines the features of a seborrheic dermatitis-like eruption of the scalp and face with a progressive often reticular, lichenoid papulonodular dermatosis affecting the trunk, buttocks, and limbs.[1-6] Patients usually present in the third to fifth decades although exceptionally reports of pediatric involvement have been documented, some with possible familial association.[7-11] It may be persistent, but improvement can be seen in summer months and with phototherapy and/or systemic retinoids.[5,12,13]

Facial and scalp lesions are erythematous, greasy and scaly, and bear no resemblance to those found on the trunk and extremities, which are erythematous or violaceous lichenoid scaly papules in a confluent, reticulate, or linear distribution. The latter may suggest Koebner phenomenon (*Fig. 7.58*). Papulonodular and infiltrated plaques are sometimes also present. Lesions are typically bilateral, symmetrical, and usually asymptomatic although rarely pruritus may be intense. Scarring is not a feature. Associated features include oral papules and ulceration, ocular lesions (blepharitis, conjunctivitis, anterior uveitis, and iridocyclitis), laryngeal nodules, palmoplantar keratoderma, and nail changes including yellow discoloration and dystrophy (longitudinal ridging, nail plate thickening, onycholysis, and paronychia) (*Fig. 7.60*).[1,14-17] Genital involvement including penile and scrotal papules, chronic balanitis, and phimosis has been documented.[6,15,16]

Keratosis lichenoides chronica has been described in association with a number of systemic diseases including chronic infections (toxoplasmosis, tuberculosis, and viral hepatitis), kidney disease, and lymphoma.[3,18-21]

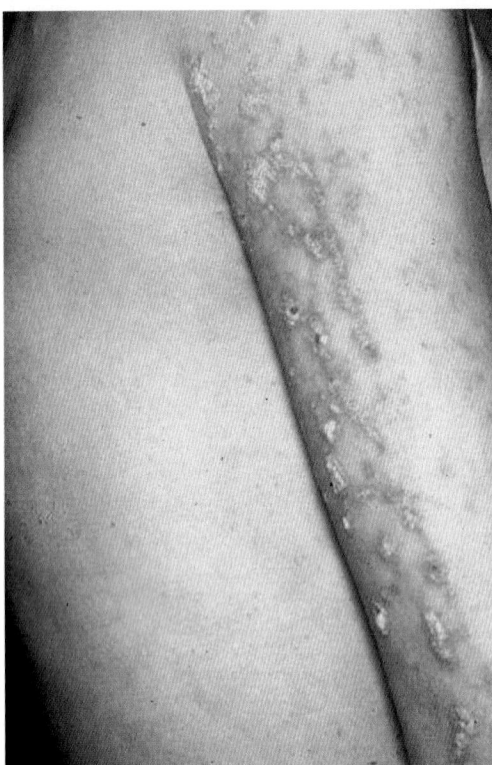

Fig. 7.58
Keratosis lichenoides chronica: there are erythematous hyperkeratotic lichenoid lesions in a linear and reticular distribution. By courtesy of R.A. Marsden, MD, St George's Hospital, London, UK.

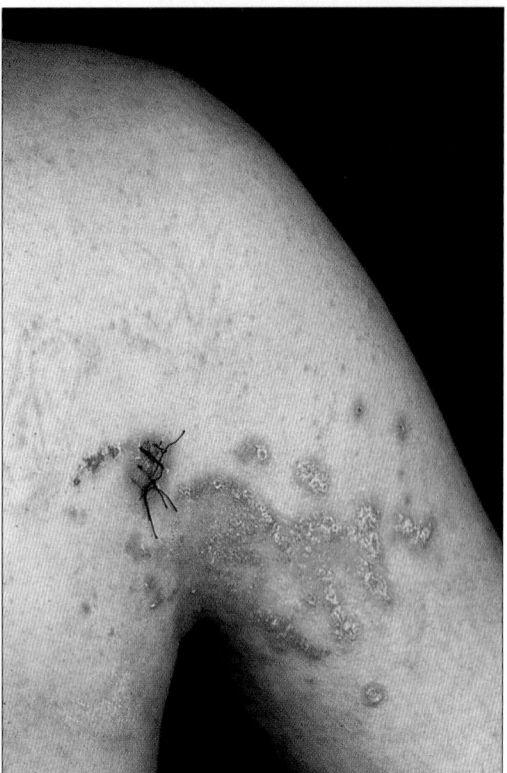

Fig. 7.59
Keratosis lichenoides chronica: close-up view of solitary lichenoid papules and a confluent plaque. By courtesy of R.A. Marsden, MD, St George's Hospital, London, UK.

Pathogenesis and histologic features

The precise nature of keratosis lichenoides chronica is uncertain. Although some authors regard it as a variant of hypertrophic lichen planus, this is unlikely.[10,22]

Histologically, the lichenoid eruption is characterized by hyperkeratosis and parakeratosis, variable acanthosis, and epidermal atrophy associated with a bandlike lymphohistiocytic infiltrate in the superficial dermis, often with conspicuous melanophages.[15] Neutrophils may be prominent in the stratum corneum. Perifollicular/acrosyringotropic and perivascular chronic inflammation may also be evident. Epidermal basal keratinocytes show hydropic degeneration, and cytoid body formation has been described.[15,22] Many necrotic keratinocytes are present.[1] Exceptionally, amyloid deposition has been documented.[23]

The dermal infiltrate consists of lymphocytes, histiocytes, and variable plasma cells and eosinophils.[15]

Direct immunofluorescence highlights the cytoid bodies.[22]

The scalp and facial lesions show the features of a chronic dermatitis, namely, spongiosis with exocytosis and patchy parakeratosis. A perivascular chronic inflammatory cell infiltrate of lymphocytes, histiocytes, and plasma cells may be present in the upper dermis.[5]

Erythema dyschromicum perstans

Clinical features

Erythema dyschromicum perstans (dermatosis cenicienta, ashy dermatosis) is an acquired, usually asymptomatic, disfiguring dermatosis which occurs particularly in Latin American (especially Mexican) populations and in Asians.[1-8] It was originally named dermatosis cenicienta after the clinical appearance of affected patients – *los cenicientos* (the ash-colored ones).[1] However, white-skinned races may rarely be affected.[9-11] It is of unknown etiology, shows a female predilection, and can develop at any age, although the majority of patients are in their first three decades.[2,8,12] Presentation in infancy has been documented.[13]

Patients develop oval, irregular or polycyclic, gray macules with erythematous, indurated, inflammatory borders of 1–2 mm. The lesions extend peripherally, show a tendency to coalesce, and often affect large areas of the integument (*Figs 7.59–7.61*). With progression, the eruption develops a gray-blue color and loses the erythematous border, which is sometimes replaced by a hypopigmented periphery. It is usually symmetrical, and particularly affects the trunk, proximal extremities, and, to a lesser extent, the face and neck.[2,8] The palms and soles, scalp, nails, and mucous membranes do not appear to be involved.[6]

Pathogenesis and histologic features

The etiology is unknown. Cases have followed HIV infection, and there is a report of simultaneous development of vitiligo and erythema dyschromicum perstans. The significance of these observations is doubtful.[14,15] Increased susceptibility with HLA-DRB1*0407 in Mexican patients has been reported.[16]

Sections from the inflammatory border show hyperkeratosis and an epidermis of normal thickness or somewhat atrophic, accompanied by basal cell hydropic degeneration and cytoid body formation (*Fig. 7.62*). Pigmentary incontinence is marked, and a mild perivascular or lichenoid inflammatory cell infiltrate is present in the superficial dermis (*Fig. 7.63*). Sections from the central gray area show epidermal atrophy, follicular hyperkeratosis, and pigmentary incontinence. Often, biopsies are obtained from late lesions, with the only feature noted that of prominent pigment incontinence. The dermal inflammatory infiltrate is composed of both CD4 and CD8 T cells, usually with CD8 forms slightly predominating.[17]

Direct immunofluorescence reveals a pattern similar to lichen planus, with non-specific staining of the cytoid bodies with IgG, IgM, and C3, and

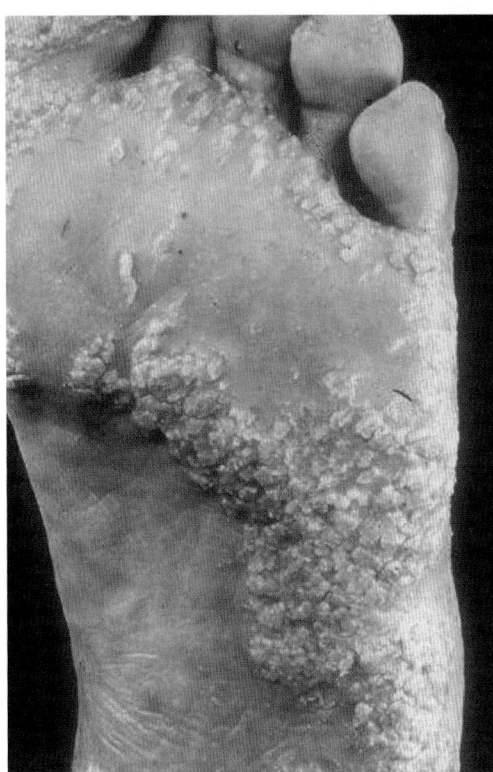

Fig. 7.60
Keratosis lichenoides chronica: plantar involvement showing disfiguring exophytic, hyperkeratotic verrucous plaques. By courtesy of R.A. Marsden, MD, St George's Hospital, London, UK.

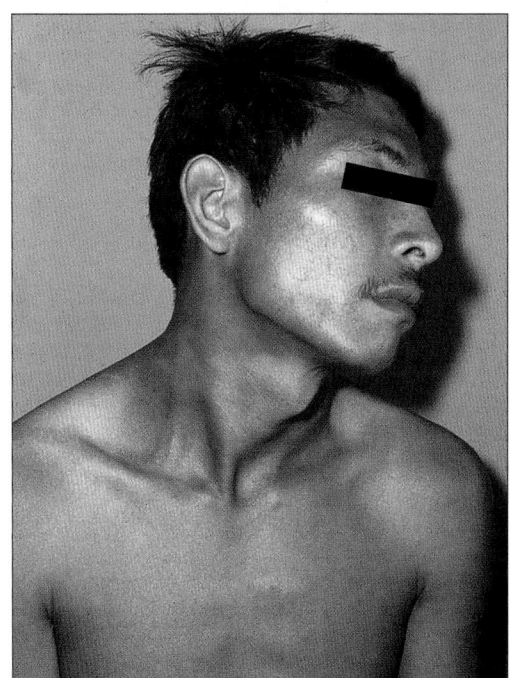

Fig. 7.62
Erythema dyschromicum perstans: in this patient, there is extensive involvement of the face, neck, and trunk. By courtesy of J. Tschen, MD, Baylor College of Medicine, Houston, USA.

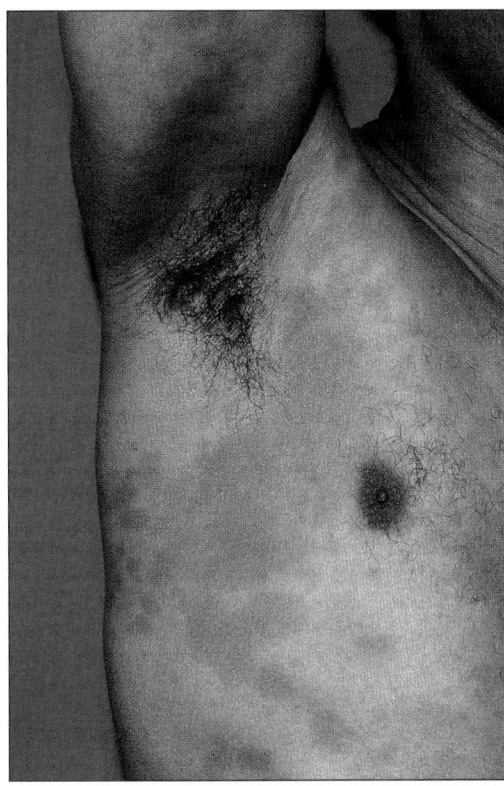

Fig. 7.61
Erythema dyschromicum perstans: this patient shows irregularly distributed gray macules. By courtesy of R.A. Marsden, MD, St George's Hospital, London, UK.

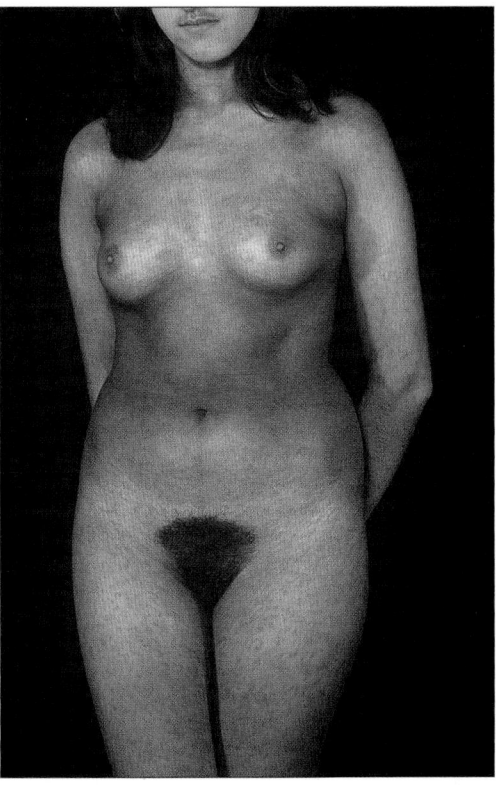

Fig. 7.63
Erythema dyschromicum perstans: in this patient with more advanced disease, there is a generalized bluish discoloration. By courtesy of the Institute of Dermatology, London, UK.

fibrinogen deposition at the dermal–epidermal junction.[18-20] The epidermal keratinocytes express Ia antigen, and the lymphocytic population comprises both helper/inducer and suppressor/cytotoxic phenotypes similar to lichen planus.[20,21]

Ultrastructural findings are non-specific, comprising intra- and interepidermal edema with cytoplasmic vacuolation, separation of keratinocytes, retraction of desmosomes, cytoid body formation, focal gaps in the keratinocyte basal lamina, and pigment-laden histiocytes in the papillary dermis.[19,22,23]

Differential diagnosis

The precise relationship of erythema dyschromicum perstans to lichen planus is uncertain. The histologic, immunological, and ultrastructural findings certainly suggests a relationship.[18,19] Typical lichen planus may precede the development of erythema dyschromicum perstans and sometimes the two conditions have presented simultaneously, although some of the documented cases may have represented lichen planus pigmentosus.[24-26]

Lichenoid and granulomatous dermatitis

Clinical features

These lesions were described in 2000 by Magro and Crowson to have features of both lichenoid and granulomatous dermatitis.[1] There is a slight female predominance (21:15) affecting a broad range of ages (5–86 years old). The extremities and trunk are most often involved, followed by the head and neck region. Clinically, the lesions present as lichenoid papules. The absence of further reports since its original description casts doubts as to whether it represents a distinctive entity.

Pathogenesis and histology

Various etiologic agents including drug, coexisting medical illnesses, and infections have been implicated. Similar to any lichenoid disorder, there is a bandlike infiltrate of lymphocytes and histiocytes.[1,2] The histiocytes are variably described as loosely aggregated and superficially located, cohesive granulomata, diffuse interstitial granulomatous inflammation, scattered solitary giant cells, and granulomatous vasculitis.[1] Cases associated with drugs also may display parakeratosis, keratinocyte necrosis, acrosyringeal accentuation, red cell extravasation, granulomatous vasculitis, eosinophils, and a plasma cell infiltrate sparing the deep dermis.[1,3] Lymphocyte atypia may also be a feature in examples associated with cutaneous lymphoma or lymphomatous drug reactions.[1]

Annular lichenoid dermatitis (of youth)

Clinical features

Annular lichenoid dermatitis of youth is a chronic condition that most commonly presents in children, with a median age of 10 years, but cases in very young children and adults have been described.[1-8] There appears to be no sex predilection, although adult cases appear to be more common in men.[4] The recognition of cases in adults have prompted the suggestion that the terminology be changed to annular lichenoid dermatitis.[4] The lesions vary from erythematous macules to the more common red-brown, annular, non-indurated patches with central hypopigmentation.[1-8] The most common sites are the groin and trunk, especially the flanks, but lesions on the buttock, abdomen, and occasionally neck have been described. Most patients have multiple patches in the involved skin, but solitary lesions have also been documented. Most are asymptomatic with occasional patients reporting intermittent pruritus.[2]

Pathogenesis and histologic features

The pathogenesis is unknown, but it does not appear to be related to parvovirus, Epstein-Barr virus, cytomegalovirus, or *Borrelia* infections, although one study has implicated Borrelia infection in Austrian patients based on serologic studies.[1,4,9] Patch testing has not revealed a contactant trigger.[1,10] A single case temporally associated with hepatitis B vaccination

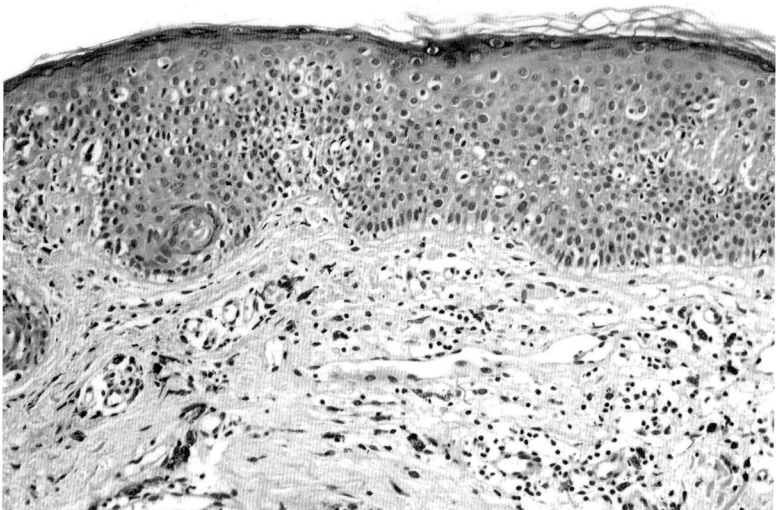

Fig. 7.64
Erythema dyschromicum perstans: there is hyperkeratosis and marked pigmentary incontinence.

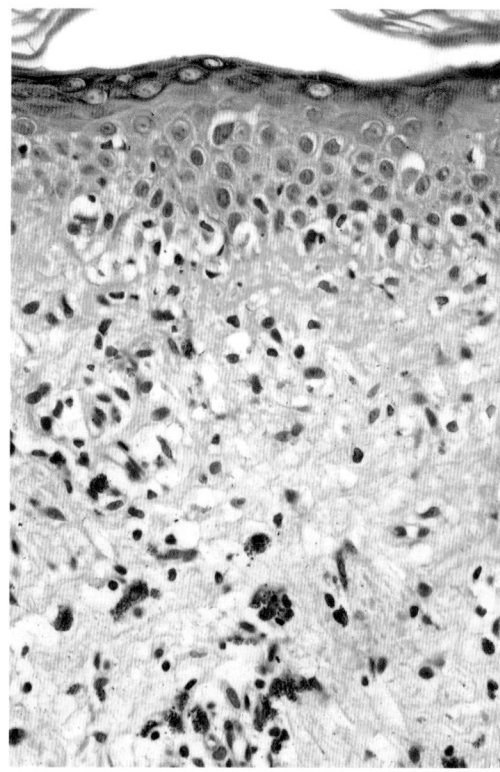

Fig. 7.65
Erythema dyschromicum perstans: note the hydropic degeneration, cytoid body, and pigment incontinence.

has been reported, but this may be coincidental, as no other reported case has been associated with vaccination.[11]

Microscopically, the epidermis is not spongiotic and has a normal to slightly hyperkeratotic stratum corneum without parakeratosis and a normal granular layer. Within the epidermis, there is a bandlike lymphocytic infiltrate with basal vacuolization and frequently numerous necrotic keratinocytes exclusively at the tips of the rete (Fig. 7.64).[1,4,7] The keratinocyte necrosis often results in a squared-off, quadrangular appearance of the rete (Fig. 7.67). Variable numbers of melanophages may be present.

In the initial description, immunohistochemical studies showed that the majority of the dermal lymphocytes are composed of CD4+ T cells, with few CD8+ lymphocytes.[1] Subsequent studies have shown that the majority of the intraepidermal lymphocytes are CD8+ cytotoxic T cells.[2,4,7,12] In some

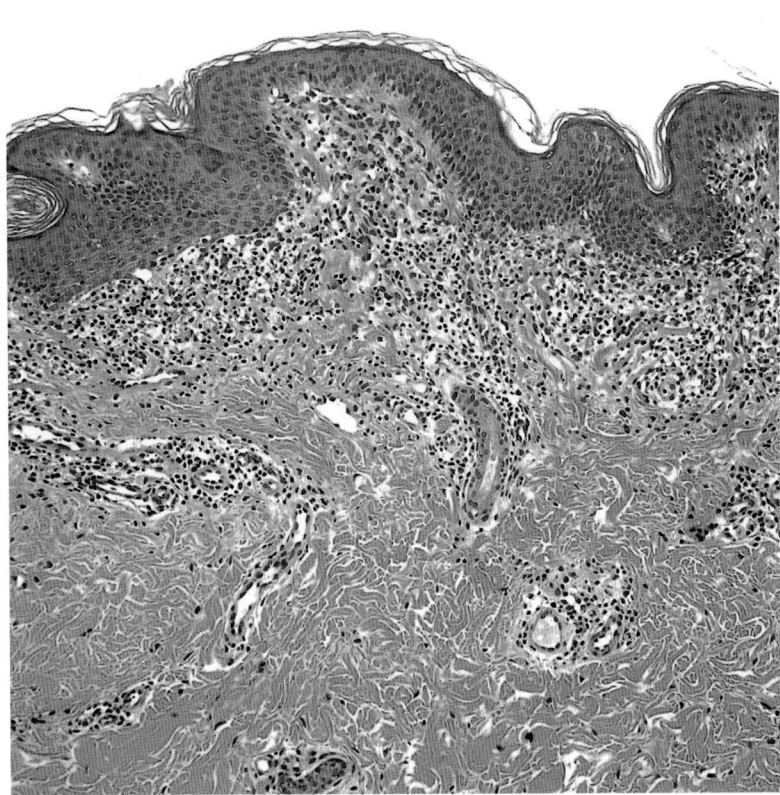

Fig. 7.66
Annular lichenoid dermatitis of youth: there is a lichenoid lymphocytic infiltrate that is concentrated at the tips of the rete. By courtesy of Dr. Carlo Tomasini, Torino, Italy.

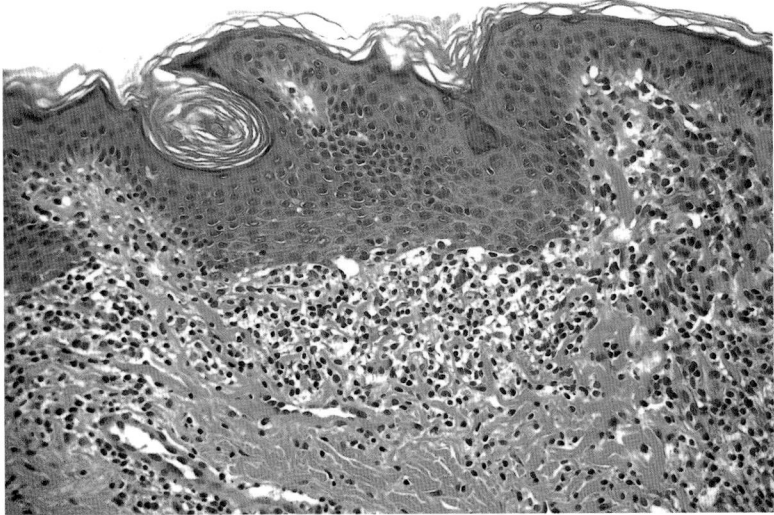

Fig. 7.67
Annular lichenoid dermatitis of youth: the infiltrate causes epidermal necrosis concentrated at the tips of the rete resulting in squared-off, quadrangular rete. By courtesy of Dr. Carlo Tomasini, Torino, Italy.

reports, the intradermal lymphocytes are also predominantly composed of CD8+ lymphocytes.[4,7,12] Immunostains for S100 protein have demonstrated an increased number of Langherans cells within the epidermis.[1] Only scattered CD20+ B-cells are present in the dermal infiltrate.

Differential diagnosis

The primary differential diagnoses include mycosis fungoides, inflammatory morphea, early lichen sclerosus, and the inflammatory phase of vitiligo. In

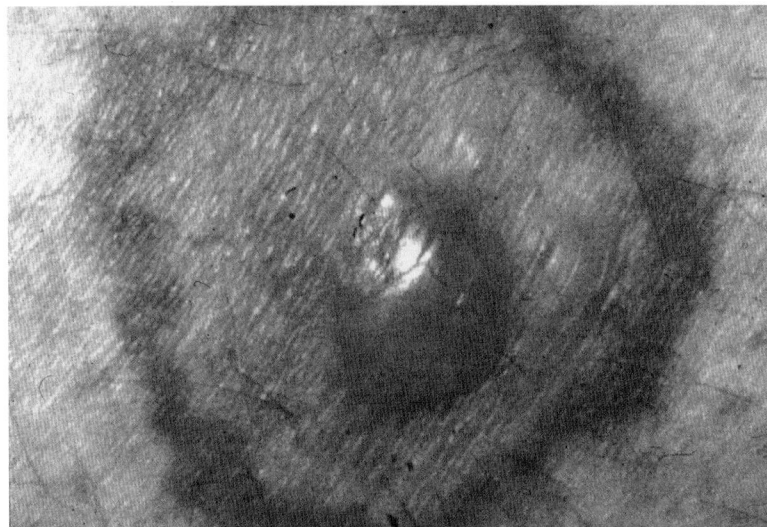

Fig. 7.68
Target lesion: characterized by a central blister surrounded by an edematous ring and an outer erythematous border. By courtesy of R.A. Marsden, MD, St George's Hospital, London, UK.

mycosis fungoides, the lymphocytes often are associated with perinuclear haloes that, with rare exceptions, are absent in annular lichenoid dermatitis of youth.[12] The lymphocytes in mycosis fungoides often demonstrate irregular nuclei. Atypia of lymphocytes in annular lichenoid dermatitis of youth is absent to only focally present. Mycosis fungoides may have necrotic keratinocytes, but does not have them concentrated at the rete tips or the quadrangular rete tips. Importantly, the infiltrate in annular lichenoid dermatitis of the youth has been polyclonal in every case tested.[1,2,4,7,12] Inflammatory morphea lacks interface change and still often shows some dermal fibrosis. Early lichen sclerosus has interface change, but not with prominent necrosis of keratinocytes at the rete tips. Early lichen sclerosus has a thickened basement membrane and does not have squared-off rete ridges. The inflammatory phase of vitiligo has a more diffuse pattern without the prominent epidermal damage concentrated at the tips of the rete.

Interface dermatoses

Definitions

There is such considerable variation in the literature as to the exact definitions and interrelationships between erythema multiforme (particularly the 'major' variant), Stevens-Johnson syndrome, and toxic epidermal necrolysis that it is often difficult or impossible to be certain to which disease the authors are actually referring![1–5] The consensus paper published in 1993 by Bastuji-Garin is used as a basis for classification because the authorship included most of the major players at that time in this difficult subject.[1]

Classification of an individual patient depends on the precise morphology and pattern of individual lesions and the extent of skin involvement (detached and detachable epidermis) as a percentage of total body surface area at the worst stage of the illness.

- Target lesions are defined as sharply demarcated and round, less than 3.0 cm in diameter, and comprising three distinct zones, namely, a central erythematous or purpuric disk with or without a blister, surrounded by a raised edematous ring, in turn bordered by an erythematous rim (*Fig. 7.68*).[1] Target lesions are typically distributed in an acral location, are often seen following a herpetic infection, and are characteristic of erythema multiforme. Typical target lesions are not seen in patients with widespread epidermal detachment.
- Raised atypical target lesions are ill-defined, round, palpable lesions with only two zones including a central raised edematous area with an erythematous border.

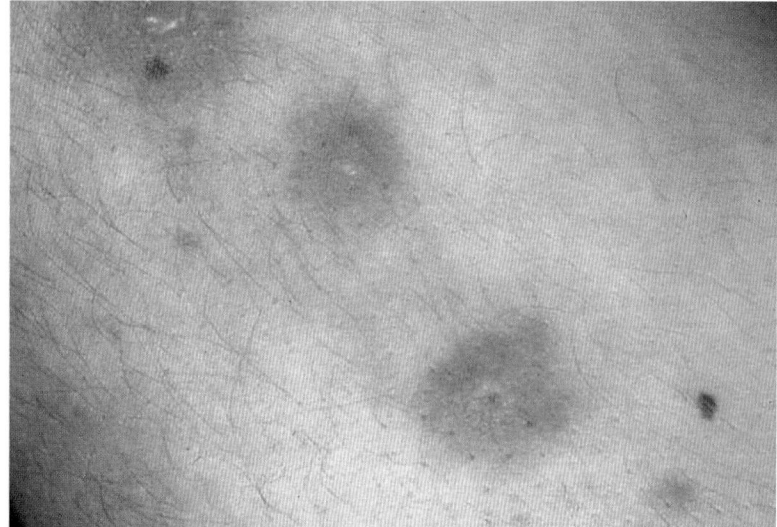

Fig. 7.69
Flat atypical target lesion: characterized by only two components, a central edematous area or blister surrounded by a zone of erythema, these lesions may be seen in erythema multiforme, Stevens-Johnson syndrome, and toxic epidermal necrolysis. By courtesy of the Institute of Dermatology, London, UK.

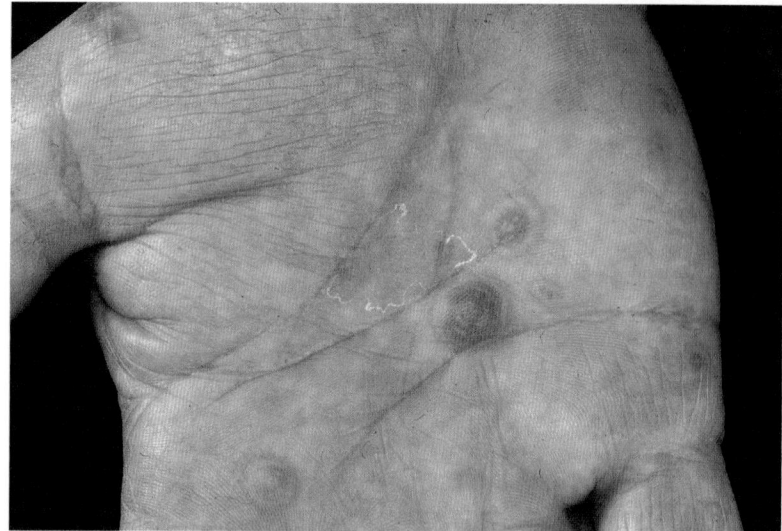

Fig. 7.70
Erythema multiforme: multiple lesions on the hand, a typical site of presentation. From the collection of the late N.P. Smith, MD, the Institute of Dermatology, London, UK.

- Flat, atypical target lesions are ill defined, round lesions with only two nonpalpable zones. The center may be blistered (*Fig. 7.69*).
- Macules with or without blisters are defined as nonpalpable, erythematous, or purpuric macules with irregular shape and size and often confluent. Blisters often occur on all or part of the macule. This lesion is characteristically seen in patients with widespread epidermal detachment who have a history of drug ingestion.

Working on this basis, the following definitions have been proposed[1]:

- Bullous erythema multiforme is characterized by <10% detachment, typical target lesions, and sometimes raised atypical target lesions.
- Stevens-Johnson syndrome is characterized by >10% detachment, flat atypical target lesions, and erythematous macules in addition to blisters and erosions affecting one or more mucous membranes.
- Overlap Stevens-Johnson syndrome/toxic epidermal necrolysis is characterized by 10–30% detachment, atypical target lesions, and flat erythematous macules.
- Toxic epidermal necrolysis is characterized by >30% detachment with flat atypical target lesions and/or erythematous macules. Rarely, toxic epidermal necrolysis may develop as large epidermal sheets in the absence of erythematous macules.

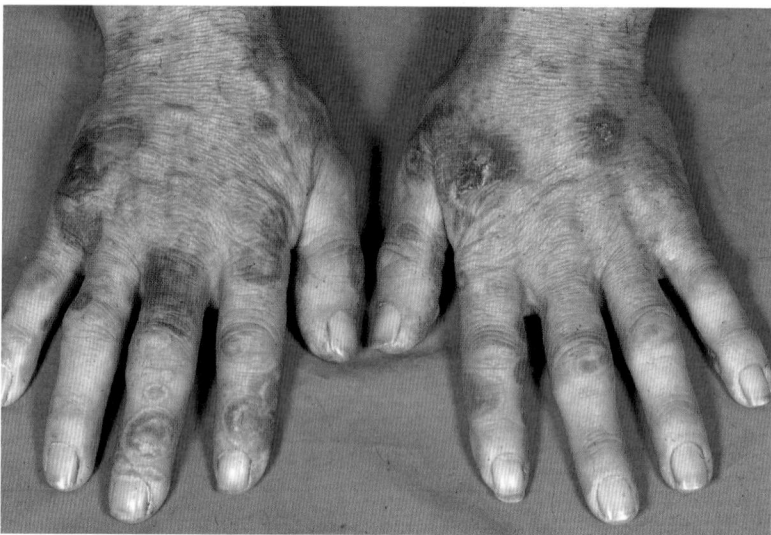

Fig. 7.71
Erythema multiforme: multiple ulcerated lesions on the hands. From the collection of the late N.P. Smith, MD, the Institute of Dermatology, London, UK.

Erythema multiforme

Clinical features

Erythema multiforme is a relatively common condition, which predominantly affects younger individuals (particularly in their second to fourth decades), including children, and shows a slight male predilection.[1–8] All races may be affected. It is self-limiting and commonly recurrent (recurrent erythema multiforme), although rarely continuous episodes of erythema multiforme have been described (persistent erythema multiforme).[9–13] Very occasionally, epidemics are seen, for example, in military camps.[4] The eruption shows seasonal variation with many patients developing the condition in spring and summer.

It presents as symmetrically distributed, fixed, discrete erythematous round maculopapules 1–2 cm in diameter which appear in crops on the acral regions, particularly the elbows, the knees, and extensor aspects of the extremities (*Figs 7.70–7.72*). Sometimes, the face, palms and soles, flexural extremities, and perineum (*Fig. 7.73*) are affected.[2] The scalp is rarely involved.[14] Typically, the center of the lesions becomes ischemic to produce a bluish discoloration (the classic iris or target lesion), which may

eventually blister. Although lesions are often present for up to 7 days, the entire episode is usually over by 6 weeks or less.[14] Lesions often number a hundred or more. Resolution may be associated with postinflammatory hyperpigmentation.

Oral lesions are common and are usually mild, typically presenting as multiple ulcers, which may involve the entire oral cavity, or predominantly affect the buccal mucosa and tongue (*Figs 7.74 and 7.75*).[15] Target lesions on the lips may also be encountered.

In many patients, episodes of erythema multiforme are recurrent, developing as often as five times each year. Such cases are almost invariably due to herpes simplex infection. Particular clinical features of this variant include a positive Koebner phenomenon, photodistribution, grouping of lesions over the elbows and knees, and nail fold involvement.[8]

In the older literature, a variant of erythema multiforme was recognized (erythema multiforme major) in which patients developed severe mucosal disease including oral, ocular, and anogenital lesions. In keeping with the current thinking on this complex topic, such cases are now included in the spectrum of Stevens-Johnson syndrome.[1,2]

Rarely, patients (usually females) may develop erythema multiforme in association with discoid or systemic lupus erythematosus – Rowell syndrome.

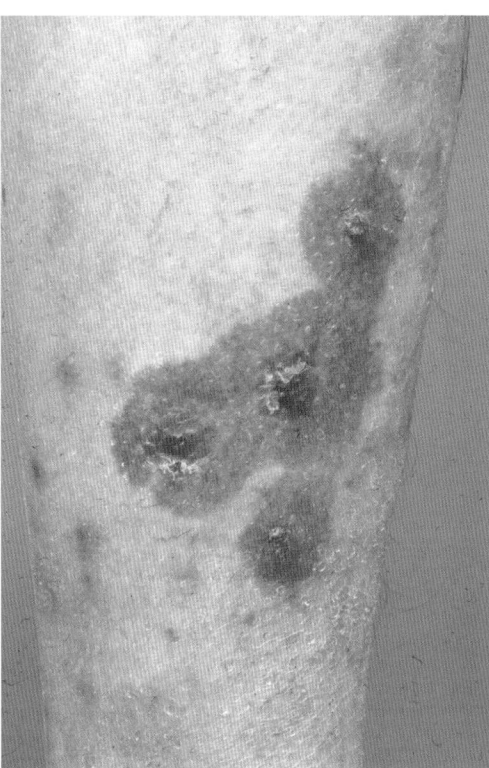

Fig. 7.72
Erythema multiforme: more extensive involvement in an adult with large erythematous lesions. The blisters have ruptured. By courtesy of the Institute of Dermatology, London.

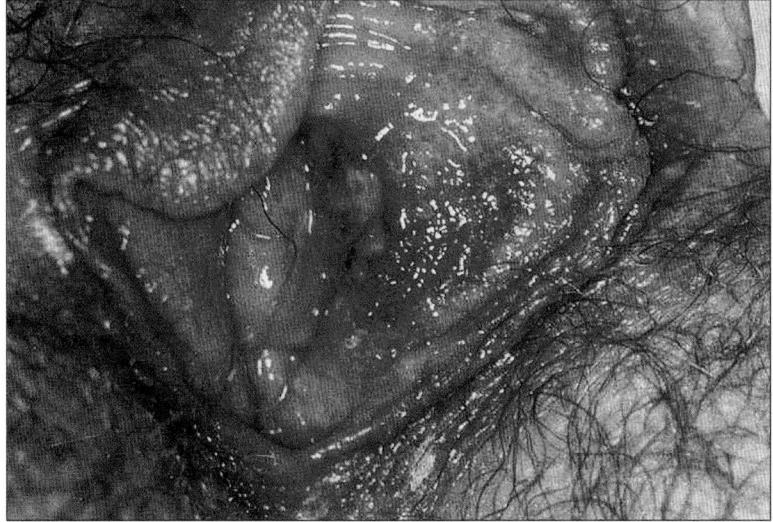

Fig. 7.73
Erythema multiforme: note the presence of erythema and erosion on the labium minus. By courtesy of P. Morgan, MD, London, UK.

Pathogenesis and histologic features

The etiology in the overwhelming majority of cases is past or present infection with herpes simplex virus (HSV) types I and II. In many patients, disease is subclinical. In some studies, the relationship is strongest in patients with recurrent disease. *Mycoplasma* infection is also of etiological importance. Many other infections have been implicated including orf, cowpox, Epstein–Barr virus, HIV, streptococcus, meningococcus, *Histoplasma*, *Leishmania*, and various vaccinations including those for meningitis, human papillomavirus, influenza, varicella, and hepatitis B.[4,14,16–27] Some of these might be better classified as some other dermatosis, including Stevens-Johnson syndrome. Erythema multiforme has also been described as a side effect of a number of drugs, an incomplete list

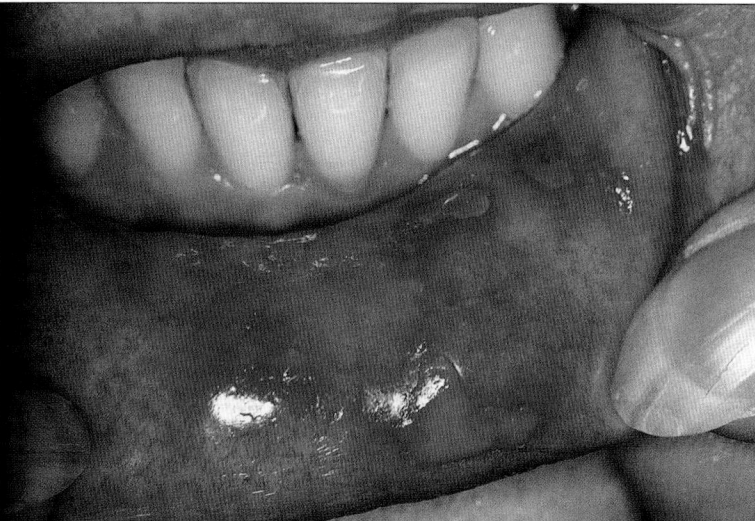

Fig. 7.74
Erythema multiforme: multiple erosions are present on the labial mucosa. By courtesy of P. Morgan, MD, London, UK.

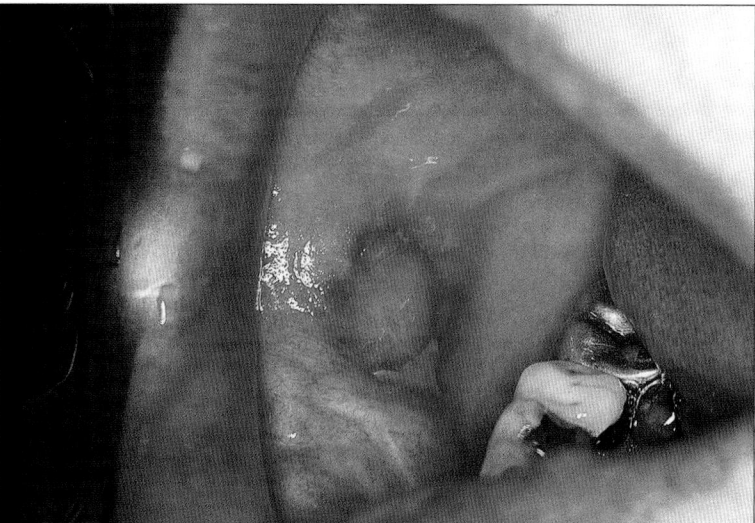

Fig. 7.75
Erythema multiforme: there is a large ulcer on the buccal mucosa. By courtesy of P. Morgan, MD, London, UK.

including sulfonamides, trimethoprim- sulfamethoxazole combinations, penicillin, barbiturates, oral contraceptives, TNF-α antagonists, bortezomib, sorafenib, antiretroviral drugs in HIV patients, ciprofloxacin, and terbinafine.[4,1,28–35] An interesting association with ciprofloxacin after alcohol ingestion has been described.[34] The antineoplastic drug paclitaxel has not only been associated with erythema multiforme but may trigger a photosensitive variant of the disease.[36] Furthermore, the eruption has also been associated with photocontact dermatitis to ketoprofen and statins and as a result of contact to hair dyes.[37–41] A localized contact dermatitis to a henna tattoo has also triggered the disease.[42] Erythema multiforme has also been associated with internal malignancy, including lymphoma, and may follow radiotherapy.[43–46]

Although cultures of skin lesions in erythema multiforme are generally negative for herpes simplex, viral DNA has been identified within the epidermis of skin lesions by polymerase chain reaction (PCR); in situ hybridization and immunohistochemistry detecting viral components are often positive.[13,16,47–54] Viral DNA is absent from healed lesions.[50] Viral gene expression correlates with lesion development.[48] As there is no evidence of a viremia, it is thought that viral DNA is transported to the skin within circulating lymphocytes rather than directly through the bloodstream or via centrifugal neuronal spread.[50,53] Why it localizes to specific sites in the skin

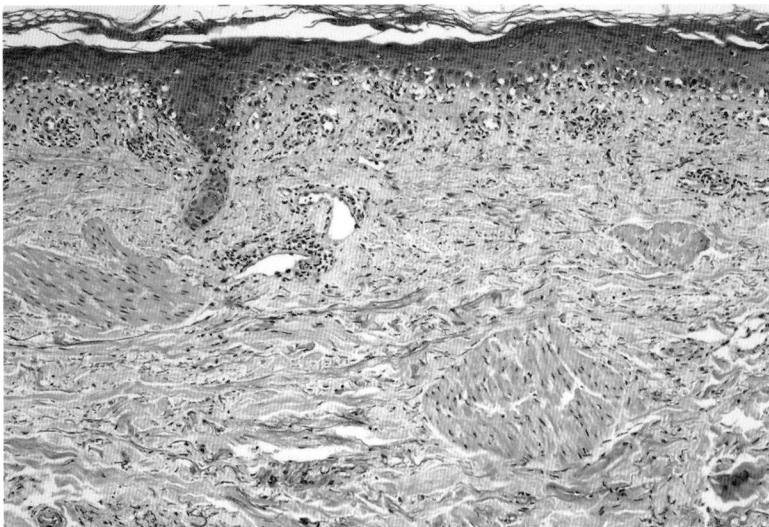

Fig. 7.76
Erythema multiforme: early lesion showing hyperkeratosis, basal cell hydropic degeneration, and occasional cytoid bodies.

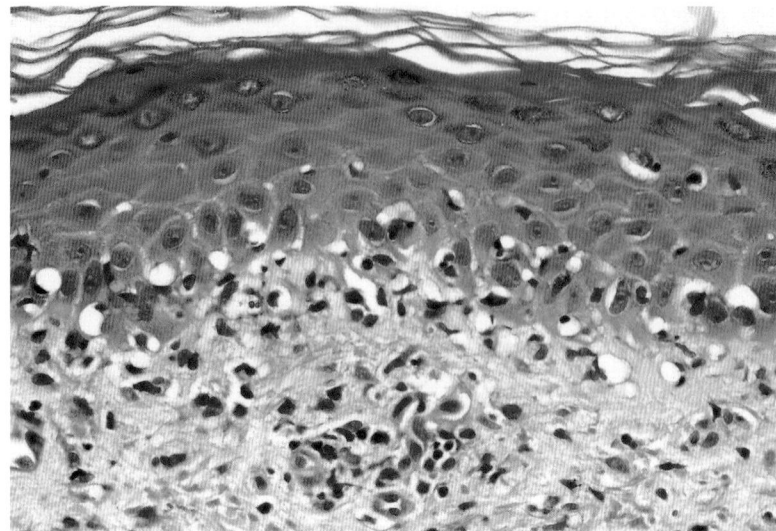

Fig. 7.77
Erythema multiforme: close-up view of basal cell hydropic degeneration.

is unknown but this may be related to ultraviolet (UV) exposure. It is likely that an episode of erythema multiforme develops as a delayed hypersensitivity (and/or cytotoxic) reaction to herpes viral antigens including DNA polymerase expressed on the surface of keratinocytes. The identification of IFN-γ in active skin lesions suggests a delayed hypersensitivity reaction with involvement of variable cytokines recruiting additional lymphocytes and macrophages to amplify the inflammatory reaction.[54,55] It has been postulated that HSV DNA polymerase might also be associated with increased expression of transforming growth factor-beta (TGF-β) and p21waf, thereby accounting for cell growth arrest and apoptosis.[56] Viral antigens do not persist in lesional skin after resolution of the eruption, and therefore in patients with recurrent disease, repeat transportation of viral DNA to the skin must occur.

Erythema multiforme is associated with an increased incidence of HLA-B15 (B62), HLA-B35, and HLA-DR53, particularly in recurrent disease.[57–60] Patients with limited mucosal involvement show an increased frequency of HLA-DQB1*0302 compared with patients in whom mucosal lesions predominate, when HLA-DQB1*0402 is more commonly identified.[60]

Erythema multiforme is characterized by a combination of basal cell hydropic degeneration and keratinocyte apoptosis accompanied by a mild to moderate superficial dermal lymphohistiocytic infiltrate associated with lymphocytic exocytosis and satellite cell necrosis.[16,61–65] Typically, the epidermis lacks parakeratosis or hyperkeratosis, and the presence of a normal stratum corneum can be a clue to the diagnosis. An exceptional case in which the predominant cells were histiocytes mimicking Kikuchi disease has been described.[66]

Apoptotic keratinocytes are rounded, intensely eosinophilic, and often anucleate, although residual pyknotic forms may be present (*Figs 7.76* and *7.77*). Their distribution may be focal, involving only an occasional and often basally located keratinocyte, or it can affect the entire epidermis, thereby resembling toxic epidermal necrolysis (Lyell syndrome) (*Fig. 7.78*). Marked basal cell hydropic degeneration sometimes results in subepidermal clefting or vesiculation (*Fig. 7.79*). Intra- and intercellular intraepidermal edema is evident and spongiotic vesiculation can be a feature (*Fig. 7.80*).

In biopsies from early lesions, the changes may be predominantly dermal with marked edema of the papillary dermis accompanied by a chronic inflammatory cell infiltrate and red cell extravasation (*Fig. 7.81*), thereby accounting for the clinical appearance of purpura. A vasculitis, however, is not seen.

The inflammatory cell infiltrate in erythema multiforme usually comprises lymphocytes and histiocytes; neutrophils are sparse or absent. Eosinophils may sometimes also be present.[67,68] Leukocytoclasis is not a feature.

Histologic features, similar to those of the skin lesions, typify involvement of the mucous membranes with spongiosis and intracellular edema.

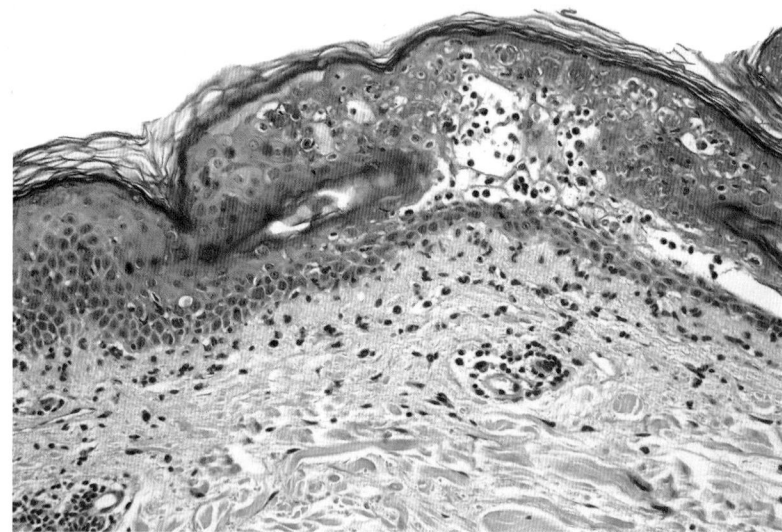

Fig. 7.78
Erythema multiforme: marked apoptosis has resulted in intraepidermal vesiculation.

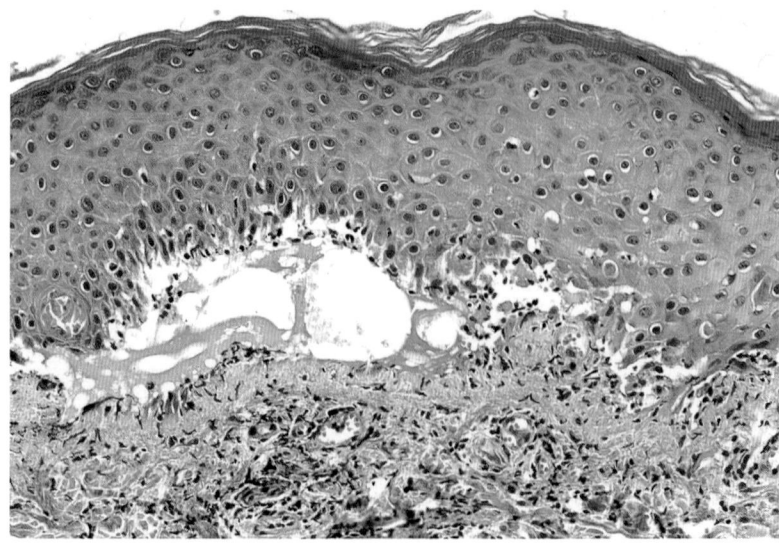

Fig. 7.79
Erythema multiforme: in this example, subepidermal vesiculation is present.

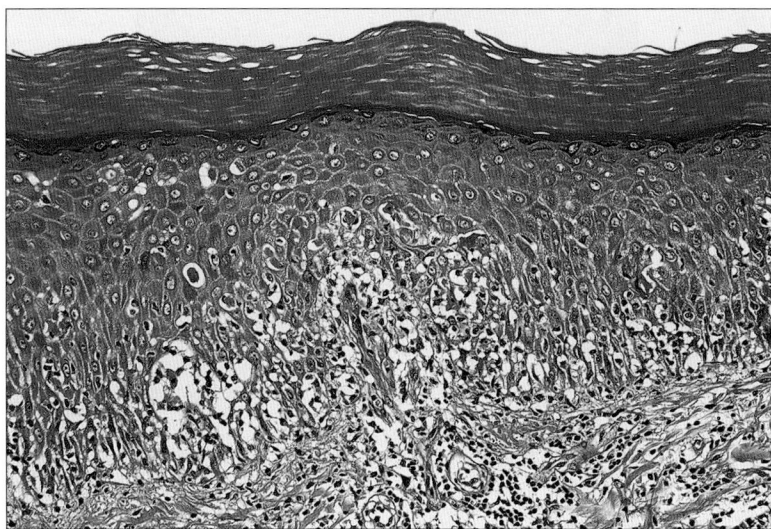

Fig. 7.80
Erythema multiforme: early lesion showing spongiosis, lymphocytic exocytosis, and cytoid bodies.

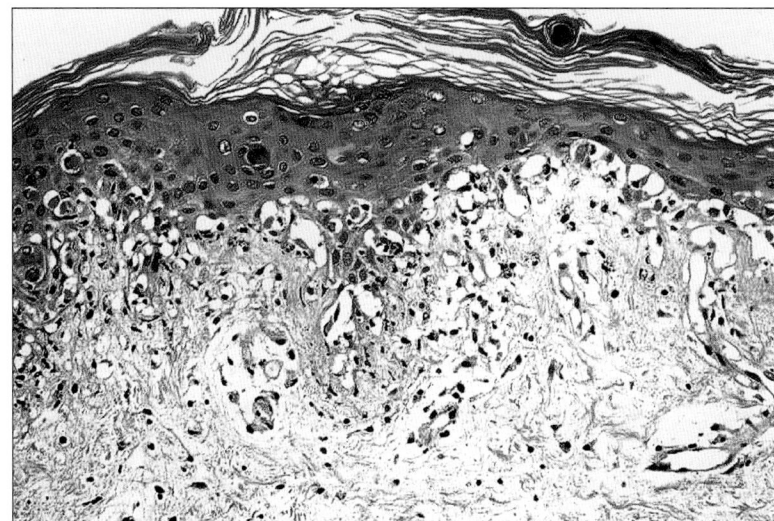

Fig. 7.81
Erythema multiforme: early lesion showing interface change and marked upper dermal edema.

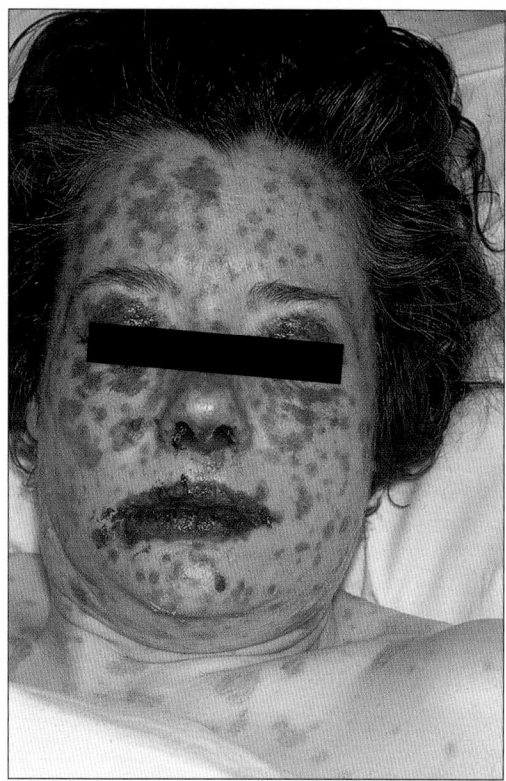

Fig. 7.82
Stevens-Johnson syndrome: this patient developed Stevens-Johnson syndrome following sulfonamide therapy. By courtesy of R.A. Marsden, MD, St George's Hospital, London, UK.

These lesions tend to be more obvious and, therefore, intraepithelial blisters are sometimes conspicuous.

With immunohistochemistry, the infiltrate consists predominantly of helper (CD4+ Vβ2+) lymphocytes with a lesser number of cytotoxic lymphocytes and admixed macrophages.[69,70] Keratinocytes express intracellular adhesion molecule-1 (ICAM-1) and HLA-DR; the latter is thought to be induced by IFN-γ of activated CD4+ T-helper 1 (Th1) cell derivation.[69,71] TNF-α is not expressed in HSV-associated lesions.[56] Circulating soluble Fas is thought to be a mediator of apoptosis, as in toxic epidermal necrolysis and Stevens-Johnson syndrome. Autantibodies to desmoplakin 1 and 2 may also play a role in erythema multiforme major.[16]

Differential diagnosis

Erythema multiforme shows considerable overlap with Steven-Johnson syndrome and toxic epidermal necrolysis. In erythema multiforme, there are commonly more marked inflammatory changes than seen in Stevens-Johnson syndrome and toxic epidermal necrolysis in which the epidermal changes of widespread apoptosis are the predominant feature. Ultimately, distinction requires clinical correlation.

Erythema multiforme may also on occasion be confused with fixed drug eruption, acute GVHD, or connective tissue diseases such as systemic or subacute cutaneous lupus erythematosus and dermatomyositis. Presence of mucin and evidence of chronicity such as hyperkeratosis and parakeratosis are useful clues for connective tissue disease. The presence of numerous eosinophils would be in favor of a drug reaction. Focal interface change combined with an absence of significant eosinophils and follicular involvement is thought helpful for distinguishing between GVHD and erythema multiforme. None of the findings is considered absolutely pathognomonic of any entity, and clinicopathological correlation will most often ensure their distinction with ease.

Toxic epidermal necrolysis and Stevens-Johnson syndrome

The original description of toxic epidermal necrolysis included two unrelated conditions[1]:
- the scalded skin syndrome seen in infants and young children and due to staphylococcal infection with toxin production,
- a drug hypersensitivity reaction, predominantly affecting adults, now regarded as the sole representative of this entity.

Clinical features

Classification of a blistering disorder as toxic epidermal necrolysis (Lyell syndrome) or Stevens-Johnson syndrome is based on the extent of detached or detachable skin at the worst stage of the illness.[2] In the former condition, 30% or more skin is involved whereas in the latter less than 10% is affected (*Figs 7.82* and *7.83*). An intermediate category where 10–30% of the skin is involved has also been recognized.[3–5]

Toxic epidermal necrolysis and Stevens-Johnson syndrome are very rare conditions, with reported incidences ranging from 0.93 to 1.3 cases per million population in Europe and 0.5 in the United States.[6–9] They represent severe drug hypersensitivity reactions except for those instances in which GVHD develops a toxic epidermal necrolysis-like appearance.[7,10] Although prior studies have shown there is no racial predilection, there is some evidence of genetic susceptibility to this condition. Patients with

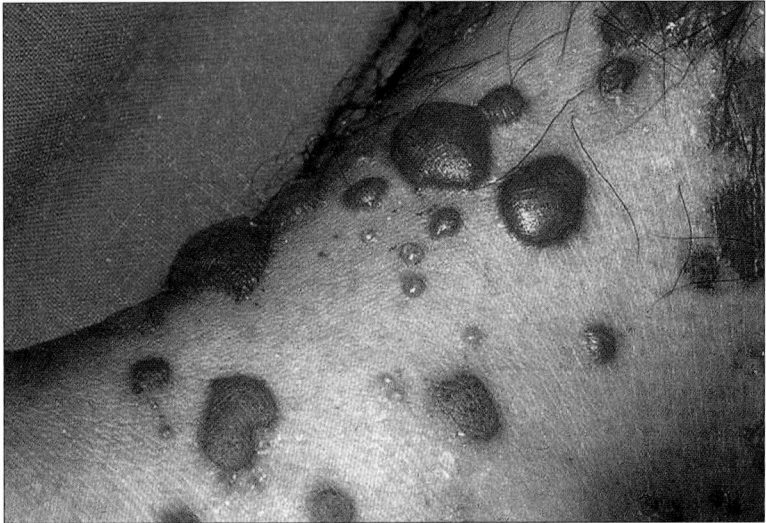

Fig. 7.83
Stevens-Johnson syndrome: this condition is distinguished from toxic epidermal necrolysis by there being less than 10% of the skin involved. Note the tense blisters. By courtesy of the Institute of Dermatology, London, UK.

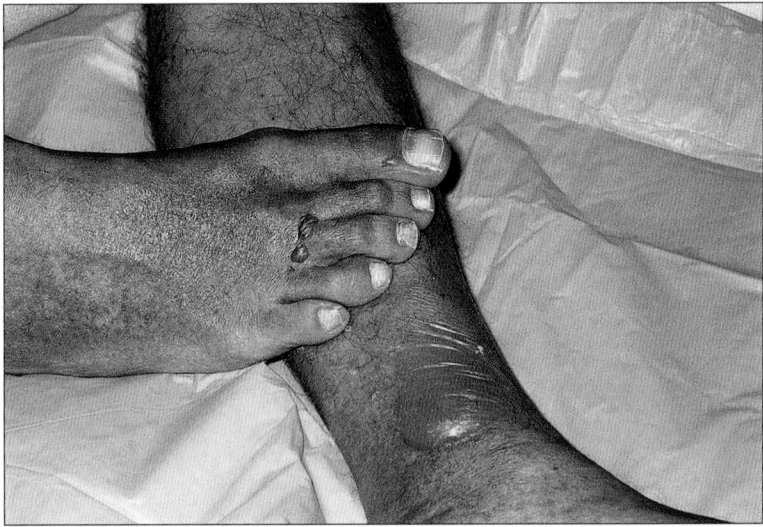

Fig. 7.84
Toxic epidermal necrolysis: early stage showing multiple large fluid-filled blisters. By courtesy of R. Reynolds, MD, Harvard Medical School, Boston, USA.

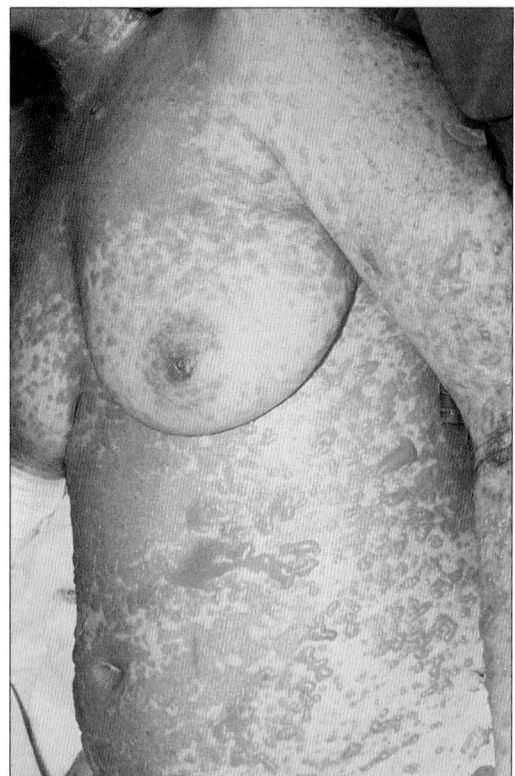

Fig. 7.85
Toxic epidermal necrolysis: there is widespread erythema and numerous blisters are evident. By courtesy of I. Zaki, MD, and S. Dalziel, MD, University Hospital, Queen's Medical Centre, Nottingham, UK.

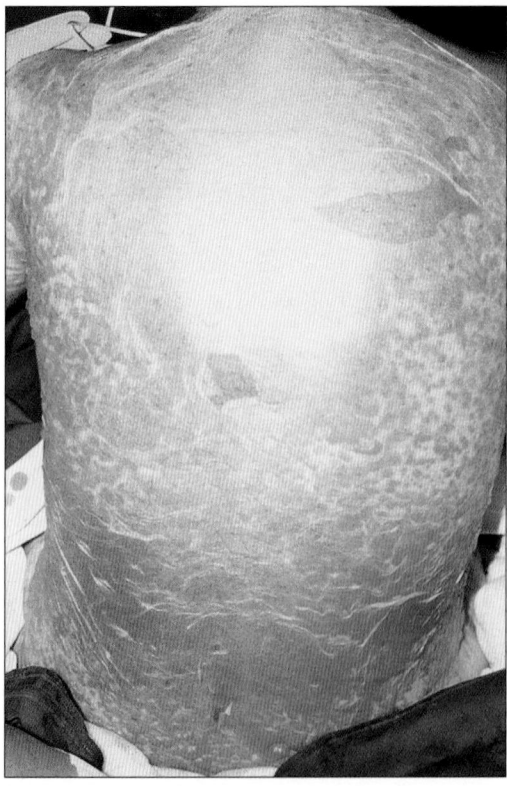

Fig. 7.86
Toxic epidermal necrolysis: note the generalized blistering resembling scalding. By courtesy of I. Zaki, MD, and S. Dalziel, MD, University Hospital, Queen's Medical Centre, Nottingham, UK.

HLA-B*1502 and HLA-B*5801 are associated with carbamazepine-induced Stevens-Johnson syndrome and allopurinol-induced Stevens-Johnson syndrome among the Han Chinese, respectively. [5,11,12] The elderly are predominantly affected, but the condition may present at any age, including children, infants, and the newborn. [13-15] In the last group, mucosal lesions may sometimes be the sole manifestation of the disease. [16] Prior studies have shown that females are affected more often than males (2:1), but more recent reports suggest that this may be changing, with more male and HIV/AIDS patients being reported. [4,15] In children, the sex ratio is equal.

Patients typically present with a short prodromal illness of pyrexia, sore throat, muscle ache, headache, anorexia, nausea, vomiting, and burning eyes, soon followed by the development of a painful rash most often starting on the face, neck, and shoulders before becoming more generalized with trunk and proximal limb accentuation. [4,5,15-18] The eruption consists of irregular, erythematous, and sometimes purpuric or necrotic, flat, atypical target lesions. In some patients, an exanthematous, morbilliform eruption is initially seen. [19] Occasionally, typical target lesions overlapping with erythema multiforme may be a feature. [9] In any event, this early stage is soon followed by the development of flaccid, fluid-filled bullae (*Fig. 7.84*). These rapidly ulcerate, leaving painful raw erosions similar to scalding (*Figs 7.85–7.88*).

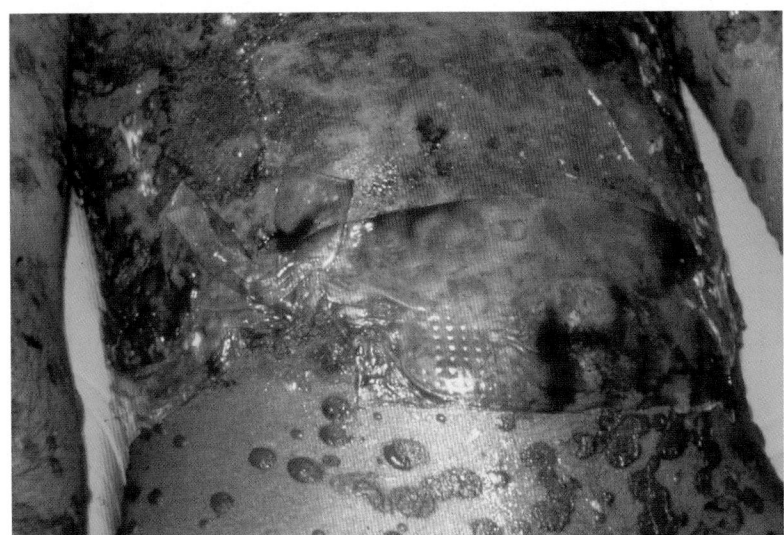

Fig. 7.87
Toxic epidermal necrolysis: this is a serious potentially life-threatening condition. This is a particularly severe example. From the collection of the late N.P. Smith, MD, the Institute of Dermatology, London, UK.

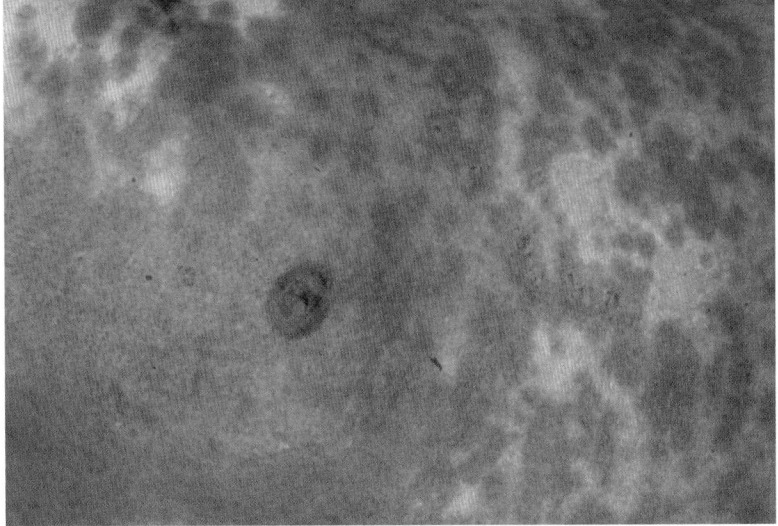

Fig. 7.88
Toxic epidermal necrolysis: healing is commonly followed by postinflammatory hyperpigmentation. From the collection of the late N.P. Smith, MD, the Institute of Dermatology, London, UK.

Nikolsky sign is positive. Eventually, the whole body, with the exception of the hair-bearing scalp, may become affected.

Toxic epidermal necrolysis/Stevens-Johnson syndrome is a multisystem disease. The mucous membranes are affected in all patients and sometimes represent the presenting manifestation.[17] The oropharynx, eyes, genitalia, and anus show particular involvement, in descending order of frequency.[4,5,19] Ocular lesions are especially important, as they are a cause of significant long-term morbidity in 40–50% of survivors and may develop months after initial presentation.[4,20,21] Patients may manifest conjunctivitis, synechiae, the sicca syndrome, trichiasis, and keratitis.[19,21] Gastrointestinal lesions, esophageal stricture, hepatitis, and pancreatitis are occasional manifestations.[22–26] Tracheobronchial involvement is fairly common and adult respiratory distress syndrome is an important and potentially life-threatening complication.[17] Anemia and leukopenia are typically seen.

The mortality of Stevens-Johnson syndrome is approximately 5%, whereas the more extensive skin involvement in toxic epidermal necrolysis is reflected in a higher mortality of up to 40%.[17,23,27–29] Causes of death include sepsis (particularly due to *Staphylococcus aureus* and *Pseudomonas*

aeruginosa), heart failure, pulmonary embolism, septic shock, disseminated intravascular coagulation, and gastrointestinal bleeding.[19] Increased age, a high proportion of skin loss, deteriorating renal function,[23] and extensive involvement of the bronchial epithelium[4] are all associated with a poor prognosis.

Pathogenesis and histologic features

Toxic epidermal necrolysis/Stevens-Johnson syndrome almost always represents an adverse drug reaction.[13,17,30] However, in children, infection with *Mycoplasma pneumoniae* has sometimes been implicated in the latter condition.[5,16] Etiological agents include sulfonamides, anticonvulsants (phenytoin, barbiturates, and carbamazepine), antibiotics (aminopenicillins, quinolones, and cephalosporins), nonsteroidal anti-inflammatory agents (phenylbutazone, oxyphenbutazone, isoxicam, and piroxicam), and allopurinol.[17,19] HIV antiretroviral agents have also been implicated.[31] Patients with such adverse reactions may show a positive patch test to the offending drug, and lymphocyte transformation may be demonstrable.[30,32]

Toxic epidermal necrolysis may also evolve in the setting of acute GVHD. Although some of these cases are undoubtedly due to an adverse drug reaction, a proportion represents a specific and severe manifestation of acute GVHD. This is associated with a very poor outlook and high mortality.[10,33]

Toxic epidermal necrolysis/Stevens-Johnson syndrome is an important complication of HIV infection and is seen in up to 1 in 1000 acquired immunodeficiency syndrome (AIDS) patients per year.[34] The high incidence relates in part to the frequent use of sulfonamides in these patients.[35] Patients with systemic lupus erythematosus are also particularly at risk.[15]

Exceptionally, toxic epidermal necrolysis has been documented in adults following an infection including hepatitis A and *Mycoplasma pneumoniae*.[4,33,34,36,37]

The precise mechanisms involved in the pathogenesis of toxic epidermal necrolysis are unclear. Affected patients in sulfonamide-related cases are commonly slow acetylators, and detoxification of resultant reactive drug metabolites is impaired.[17,39,40] Although the condition may result from a direct action in some cases, it is thought to be more likely that drug metabolites function as haptens and induce an indirect cellular immune reaction to keratinocytes. Patients with AIDS are deficient in glutathione and, as a result, persistence of such reactive metabolites may explain the increased incidence of this disease in these patients.[40] HIV patients also have decreased skin-directed CD4 lymphocytes with a relative increase in CD8+ lymphocytes, which also may contribute to the increased risk in this patient population.[41]

Toxic epidermal necrolysis is associated with an increased incidence of HLA-B12: 50% compared with 26% in the normal population.[42] As mentioned above, specific HLA types are associated with Stevens-Johnson syndrome in certain racial populations.

Although the exact pathogenesis of the disease is not clear, it has been demonstrated that the inflammatory cells in the blisters are cytotoxic T lymphocytes and natural killer cells.[43] The main cytotoxic protein expressed is granulysin, and this protein seems to be a major player in the induction of disseminated keratinocyte necrosis. When the protein is injected into the skin of mice, blisters closely simulating those seen in toxic epidermal necrolysis/Stevens-Johnson syndrome develop.[43]

The histologic features are those of variable epidermal apoptosis associated with basal cell hydropic degeneration or subepidermal vesiculation (*Figs 7.89–7.93*).[44,45] Lymphocytic exocytosis may be present, and satellite cell necrosis is sometimes apparent.[46,47] Sweat duct epithelium is also involved, and hair follicles may also be affected, although much less often (*Fig. 7.92*).[13] A light, predominantly perivascular infiltrate of lymphocytes, macrophages, and melanophages is present in the superficial dermis, which also is commonly edematous (*Figs 7.94* and *7.95*). Small numbers of eosinophils may be present.

With immunohistochemistry, the dermal infiltrate consists predominantly of CD4+ T-helper cells, whereas in the epidermis CD8+ cells are most numerous.[46,48,49] Histiocytes may be conspicuous.[50] Langerhans cells are depleted. Keratinocytes express HLA-DR. Keratinocyte cell death is thought to result from the combined effects of cytolytic enzymes including perforin and cytokines such as soluble TNF-α and IL-6.[18,44,50,51] Fas ligand-mediated

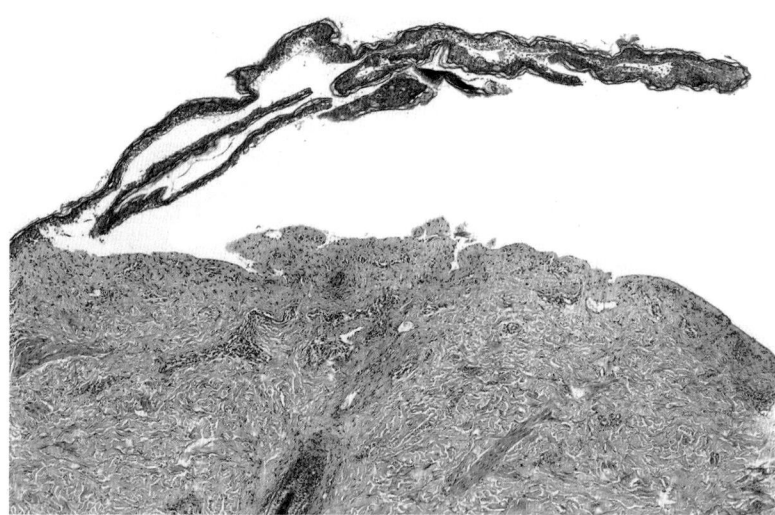

Fig. 7.89
Toxic epidermal necrolysis: low-power view showing subepidermal blistering.

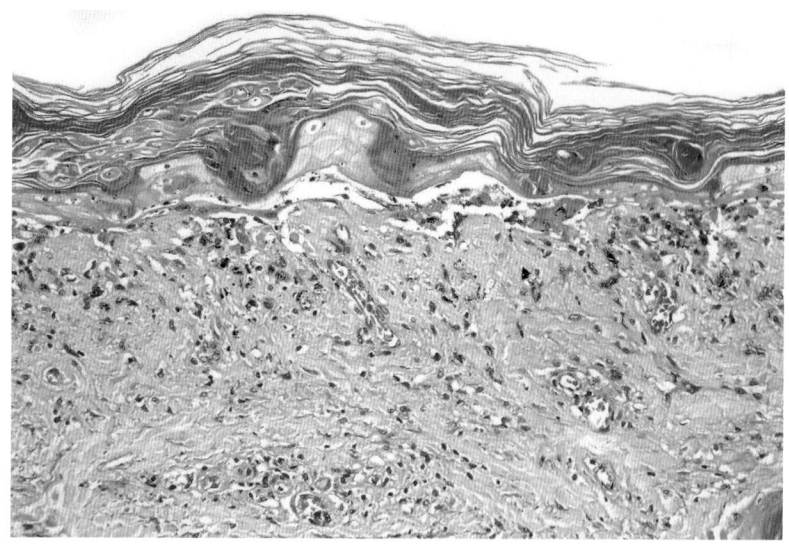

Fig. 7.92
Toxic epidermal necrolysis: medium-power view showing necrosis of the full thickness of the roof of the blister.

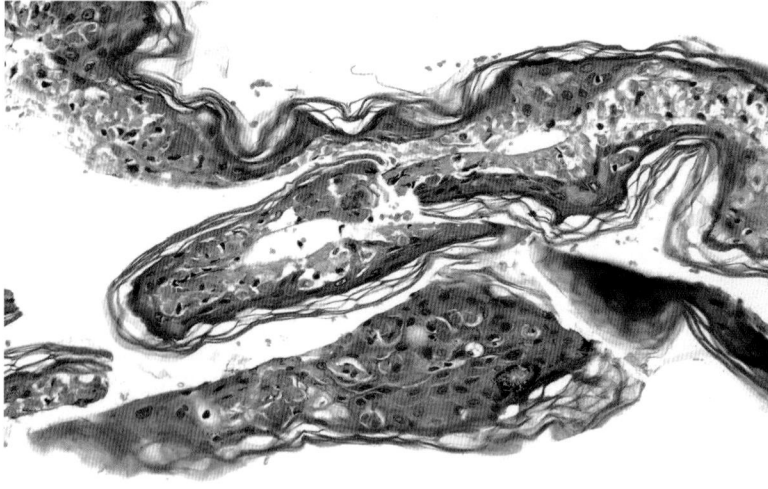

Fig. 7.90
Toxic epidermal necrolysis: the roof of the blister is completely necrotic.

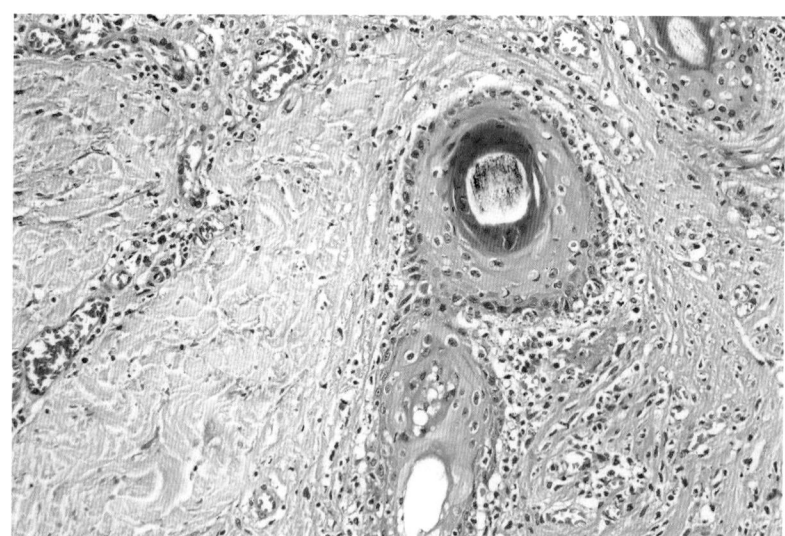

Fig. 7.93
Toxic epidermal necrolysis: follicular involvement showing basal cell hydropic degeneration and apoptosis.

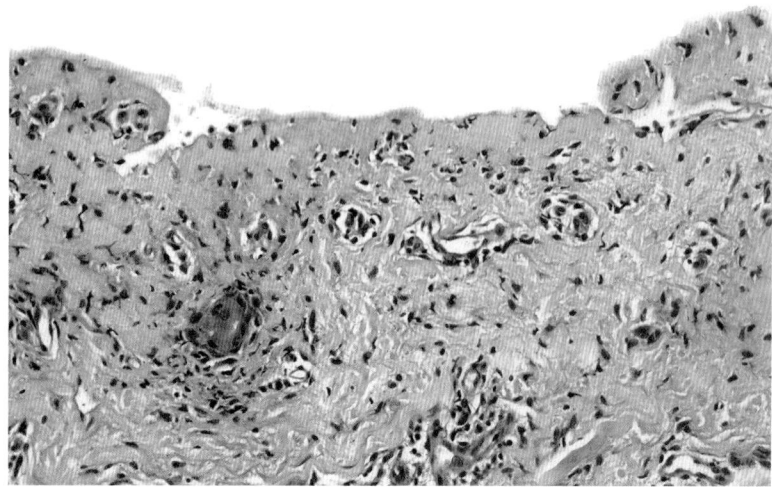

Fig. 7.91
Toxic epidermal necrolysis: this field shows the floor of the blister. There are no inflammatory cells in this example.

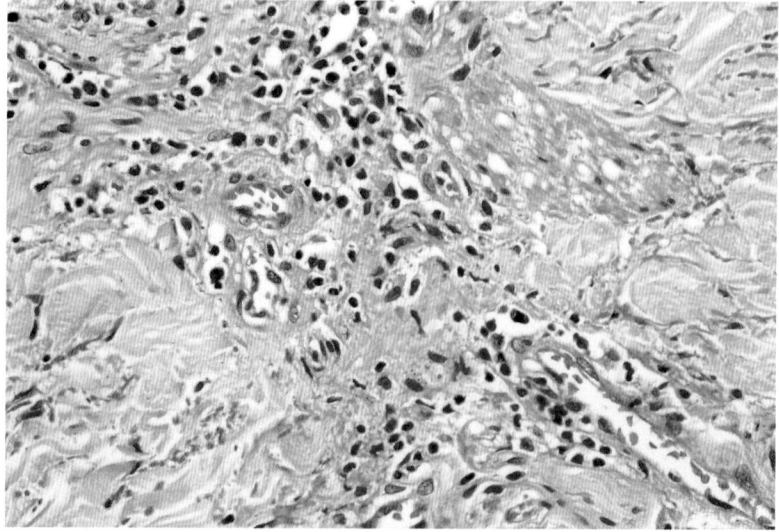

Fig. 7.94
Toxic epidermal necrolysis: there is a perivascular lymphohistiocytic infiltrate.

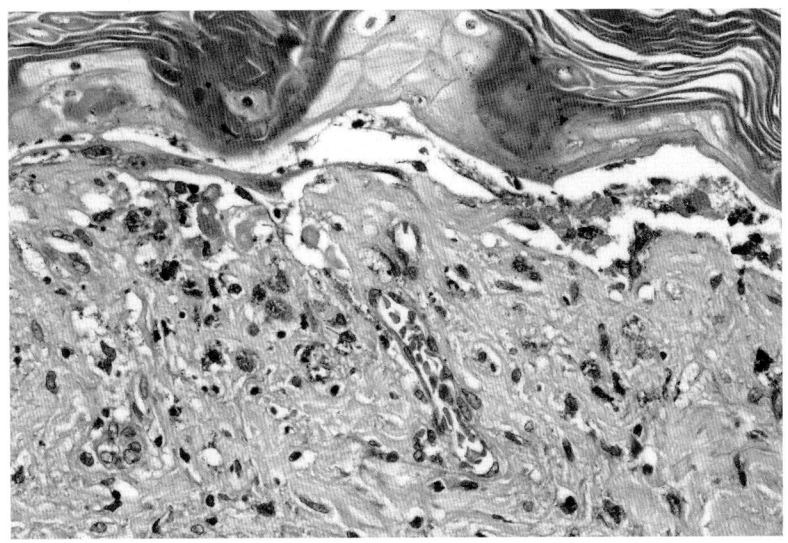

Fig. 7.95
Toxic epidermal necrolysis: note the apoptosis and pigment incontinence.

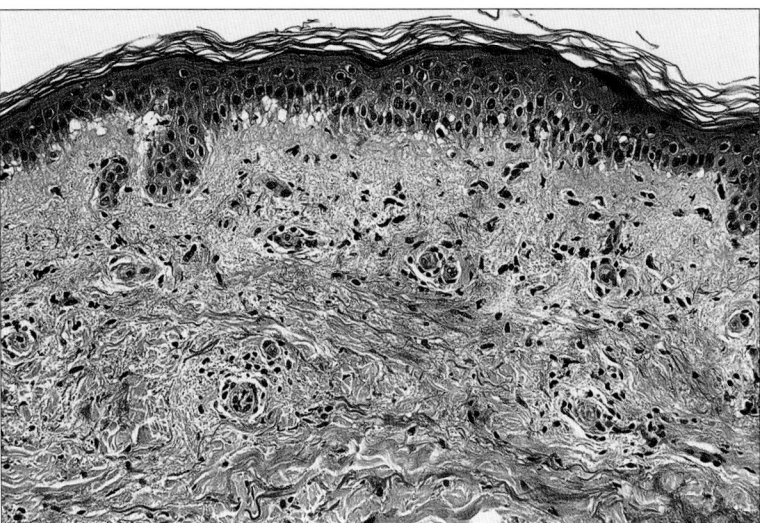

Fig. 7.96
Poikiloderma: there is basal cell hydropic degeneration and a very light perivascular lymphohistiocytic infiltrate.

apoptosis is believed to be of major importance in the final development of necrolysis.[4,5,18,44,50–52]

Differential diagnosis

Staphylococcal scalded skin syndrome is an important clinical differential diagnosis. The typical histologic finding of a subcorneal pustule or absence of the stratum corneum in this condition makes the distinction easy. In addition, staphylococcal scale skin syndrome does not demonstrate full-thickness necrosis or interface change.

Toxic epidermal necrolysis/Stevens-Johnson syndrome may sometimes be indistinguishable from severe erythema multiforme. Lymphocytic exocytosis, apoptosis predominantly affecting the lower epidermis, intense, interface dermal chronic inflammation with extension along the superficial and deep vascular plexuses, and prominent erythrocyte extravasation are more in favor of erythema multiforme.[45,53] This histologic distinction is also mirrored to some extent by the etiology. Thus, those cases that result from an infection tend to be more inflammatory than those that represent an adverse drug reaction, in which the changes are predominantly epidermal.[48] The presence of eosinophils does not seem to distinguish between drug- and infection-related causes within this histologic spectrum.[45]

Toxic epidermal necrolysis resulting from an adverse drug effect and that presenting in a background of severe GVHD are indistinguishable.

Paraneoplastic pemphigus

Erythema multiforme-like histologic features are an integral feature of paraneoplastic pemphigus (see Chapter 5).

Poikiloderma

Poikiloderma (Gr. *poikilos*, spotted, mottled, varied) is a clinical descriptive term applied to skin showing slight scaling, atrophy, variable pigmentation, and telangiectasia. It is a feature of a number of conditions including lupus erythematosus, dermatomyositis, large plaque parapsoriasis, poikiloderma of Civatte, poikiloderma congenitale, Bloom syndrome, Cockayne syndrome, dyskeratosis congenita, and DNA mitochondrial syndrome-associated poikiloderma. Histologically, poikiloderma is characterized by hyperkeratosis, epidermal atrophy with basal cell liquefactive degeneration, pigmentary incontinence, telangiectasia, and a variable superficial dermal lymphohistiocytic infiltrate (*Figs* 7.96 and 7.97).

Poikiloderma of Civatte

Poikiloderma of Civatte (poikiloderma of head and neck, Derbyshire neck) refers to a fairly common progressive and irreversible disorder in which

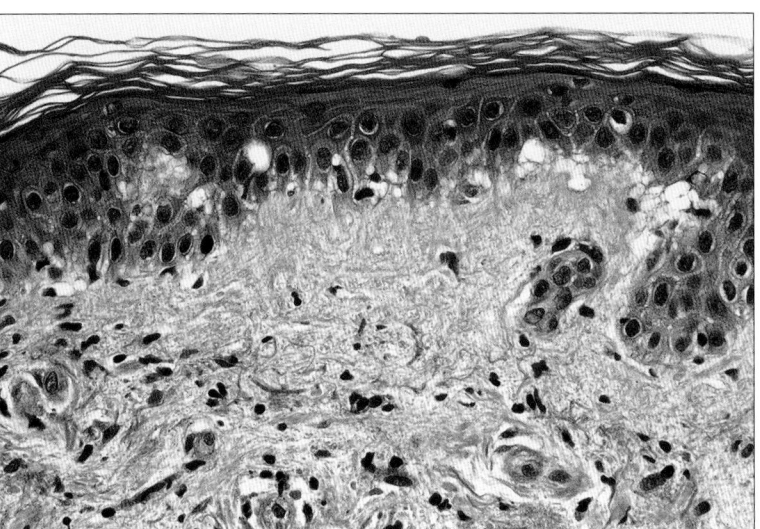

Fig. 7.97
Poikiloderma: close-up view.

typical poikiloderma presents in a photodistribution, predominantly affecting the sides of the face and neck and the 'V' of the chest (*Fig.* 7.98).[1–4] Middle-aged and elderly women, menopausal females, are predominantly affected. Possible etiological factors include hormonal effects, phototoxicity, or photoallergy possibly due to perfumes or fragrances.[4–8] Familial cases have been documented.[4]

Histologic features

In addition to solar elastosis, the epidermis is often atrophic and flattened with hyperkeratosis. In the dermis, the superficial vessels are usually ectatic with a minimal to mild perivascular lymphocytic infiltrate in association with melanophages.[3,9] Hydropic degeneration of the basal layer and follicular plugging is variably present.[9] In most biopsies, however, the changes are often mild and non-specific and do not seem to correlate well with the degree of clinical involvement.

Mitochondrial DNA syndrome-associated poikiloderma

Photodistributed poikiloderma has been documented in a number of mitochondrial DNA syndromes, particularly Pearson syndrome, which also includes failure to thrive, exocrine pancreas insufficiency, severe renal tubule dysfunction, and bone marrow suppression.[1] Other dermatological

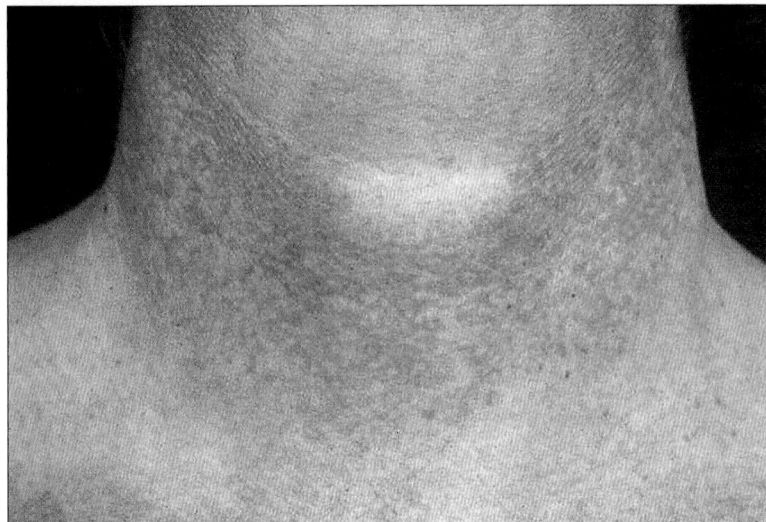

Fig. 7.98
Poikiloderma of Civatte: note the mottled hyperpigmentation in a characteristic distribution. By courtesy of the Institute of Dermatology, London, UK.

manifestations of mitochondrial DNA syndromes include acrocyanosis, dry brittle hair, vitiligo, hyperpigmentation, and anhidrosis.[2–7]

Rothmund-Thomson syndrome

Clinical features

This rare syndrome, which has been described in Asians and blacks as well as Caucasians, has an autosomal recessive mode of inheritance. In contrast to the earlier finding of an equal sex incidence, the more recent literature suggests a predilection for males (2:1).[1,2] It usually presents between the third and sixth months of life (hence the term 'poikiloderma congenitale') as a reticulated, erythematous rash – sometimes described as marmoreal (L. *marmor*, marble) – on the face, which eventually spreads to involve the extremities and the buttocks (*Figs 7.99–7.101*).[2] The trunk and flexural aspects are usually spared.[1] Affected infants are photosensitive and, therefore, there is often a history of sun exposure before the development of skin lesions.[3,4] This is later replaced by reticular, linear, or punctate foci of atrophy.[4] Telangiectasia is present and areas of hypo- and hyperpigmentation may be noted. The poikilodermatous change is seen most frequently at sun-exposed sites.[1]

A variety of other manifestations may be observed, including variable alopecia particularly involving the scalp, eyebrows, and eyelashes, and seen most often in females. This is present in up to 80% of patients.[1] Gastrointestinal problems including chronic emesis and diarrhea may be seen in infancy.[2] Juvenile, subcapsular (unilateral or bilateral) cataracts are common and skeletal abnormalities include short stature, osteopenia, pathological fractures, dislocations, irregular metaphyses, abnormal trabeculation, and stippled ossification of the patellae.[2] Small hands with shortened digits are frequently seen.[5] Frontal bossing, saddle nose, and prognathism are characteristic.[1] Absent or malformed radii are seen in 10–20% of patients and bifid or absent thumb may also be present.[1,2,6] Nail dystrophy, dental abnormalities (particularly conical-shaped teeth with caries), and hypogonadism may also be detected. Hyperkeratotic warty or verrucous lesions sometimes develop on the extensor surfaces, particularly overlying joints and especially the feet and hands.[6] While occasionally reported, mental retardation is not usually a feature of this syndrome.[1] The disease is associated with the development of cutaneous squamous cell carcinoma and more rarely basal cell carcinoma.[2,4,7,8] Multifocal Bowen disease has also been described.[8]

There is also an increased risk of internal malignancies, particularly tibial osteosarcoma and multicentric osteosarcoma (7–32%).[1,2,7,9–12] An association with duodenal stenosis and annular pancreas has been described in one patient.[13] The life span of most patients, however, is generally normal.

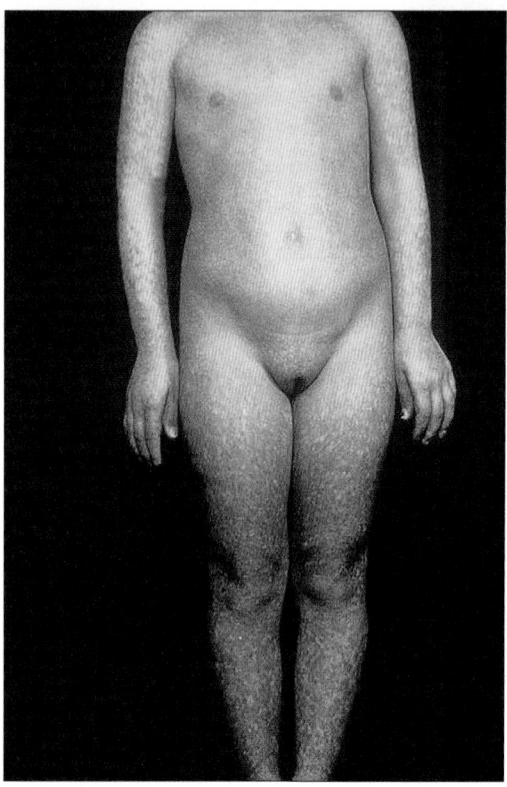

Fig. 7.99
Rothmund-Thomson syndrome: there is a marked mottled hyperpigmentation predominantly affecting the peripheries. By courtesy of the Institute of Dermatology, London, UK.

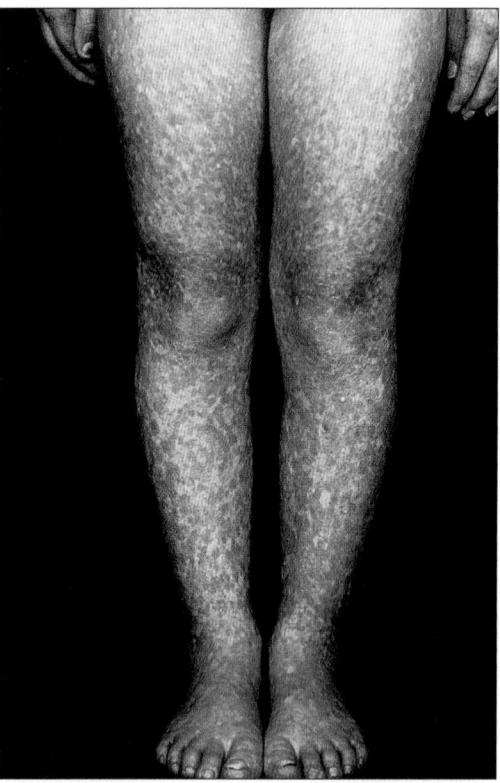

Fig. 7.100
Rothmund-Thomson syndrome: there is symmetrical involvement of the legs. By courtesy of the Institute of Dermatology, London, UK.

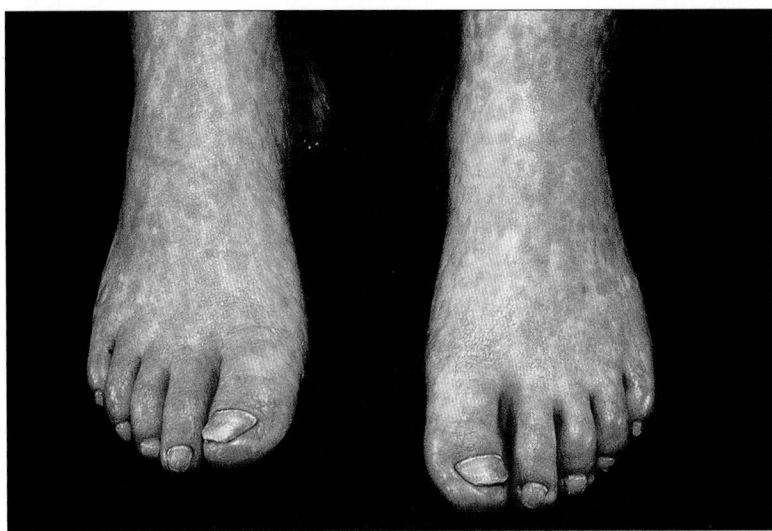

Fig. 7.101
Rothmund-Thomson syndrome: there is atrophy in addition to hyperpigmentation.
By courtesy of the Institute of Dermatology, London, UK.

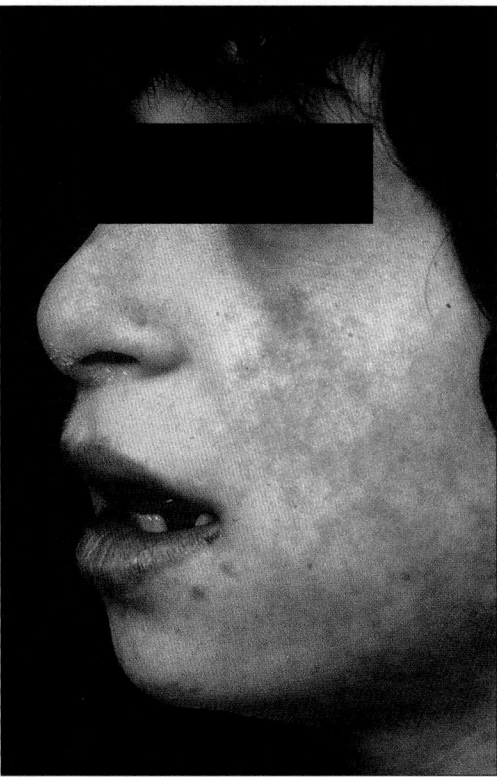

Fig. 7.102
Bloom syndrome: characteristic facies includes 'pinched' features. Marbled erythema of the cheek and crusted lesions involving the lower lip. By courtesy of D. Atherton, MD, Institute of Dermatology and Children's Hospital at Great Ormond Street, London, UK.

Pathogenesis and histologic features

Rothmund-Thomson syndrome, in some patients at least, has been shown to be associated with a mutation in the *RECQL4* gene, a member of the DNA helicase family (see Bloom syndrome).[10,14–17] Cytogenetic analysis has revealed mosaicism in a subpopulation including trisomy 8.[2] The underlying defect in Rothmund-Thomson syndrome is unknown. While most investigations have failed to demonstrate abnormal sensitivity to UVA or UVB, there have been occasional recent reports of reduced unscheduled DNA synthesis following irradiation of cultured fibroblasts with UVB and UVC.[3,18] More recent studies suggest a role for *RECQL4* in repairing DNA induced by UV irradiation.[19] Other investigations have demonstrated that *RECQL4* is also involved in DNA replication and skeletogenesis.[20–24]

No recognized diagnostic test for this disorder is available, and diagnosis is based primarily on the poioderma rash.[17] Mutational screening for the *RECQL4* gene is possible and can correlate with certain aspects of the syndrome, but additional genes such as *USB1* may also be involved.[25,26]

The histologic features of poikiloderma include hyperkeratosis, epidermal atrophy, liquefactive degeneration of the basal epidermal cells, and telangiectasia. Pigmentary incontinence may be present and a perivascular chronic inflammatory cell infiltrate is sometimes evident in the superficial dermis. The latter sometimes also shows elastic tissue fragmentation and depletion or absence of cutaneous appendages.[1] The squamous cell carcinomas show typical features.

An examination of scalp has revealed hypopigmented vellus hairs without cortices.[6]

Bloom syndrome

This rare chromosomal instability syndrome (also known as congenital telangiectatic erythema with dwarfism) has an autosomal recessive mode of inheritance and is particularly seen in East European (Ashkenazi) Jews. When found in non-Jews, there is a high incidence of parental consanguinity. It represents a genetically homogenous single locus disease without apparent heterogeneity.[1]

Clinical features

There is a characteristic appearance with microcephaly, dolichocephaly, and small, narrow 'pinched' facies, and stunted growth leading to severe dwarfism.[2,3] An erythematous rash with telangiectasia develops predominantly on the face (in particular, the 'butterfly' area) and is exacerbated by sunlight (*Fig. 7.102*).[4,5] The rash may also affect the backs of the hands and forearms and typically develops in infancy. Café-au-lait spots are a common manifestation and discrete areas of hypopigmentation are usual.[3] A peculiar high-pitched, squeaky (so-called 'Mickey Mouse') voice is sometimes a feature.[6] Male infertility is common.[3] Patients may suffer impaired concentration, short-term memory, and general mental organizational disability.[5]

Bloom syndrome is typified by an inherent propensity to chromosomal abnormalities, in particular, sister chromatid exchange. There is an associated increased incidence of most malignancies, especially acute leukemia, non-Hodgkin lymphoma, colon carcinoma, breast carcinoma, and cutaneous squamous cell carcinoma. Patients are prone to develop multiple primary tumors, which often develop at an early age (third decade). As a result, death by age 30 usually occurs due to cancer.[4,5,7] They may also suffer immunodeficiency (diminished IgG, IgA, IgM) and are therefore at an increased risk of childhood infections, pulmonary infections, and chronic lung disease.[6,8] There is also an elevated risk of adult onset-like diabetes mellitus.[9]

Pathogenesis and histologic features

The gene for Bloom syndrome, *BLM*, which has been mapped to 15q21.3, is a member of the RecQ helicase protein family, responsible for unwinding DNA and RNA.[5,10–16] It has been identified as representing part of the BRCA1-associated genome surveillance complex, which is mutated in families with hereditary breast cancer.[17] The protein functions as a 3'–5' DNA helicase and may be involved specifically in allowing sister chromatid separation during mitosis.[13,18] DNA helicases have essential roles in genetic recombination, transcription, DNA replication, and repair.[5,16] Mutation of the *BLM* gene results in genomic instability. BLM normally interacts with BRAFT and FANCOM complexes. The BRAFT complex is involved in helicase activity, whereas the FANCOM complex is crucial for sister chromatid exchange.[5] Bloom syndrome is associated with increased sensitivity to alkylating agents, increased spontaneous chromosome breakages, increased interchromatid exchange (including sister chromatid exchange, 6–10-fold), increased somatic cell mutation frequency, and reduced replication fork elongation rate.[4,5,12] Mutations include missense, nonsense, frameshift, and genomic deletions, most of which result in premature translation terminations and resultant defective Bloom syndrome protein with impaired function.[15] Multiple defective nuclear enzymes including DNA ligase I have been identified.[19] Monosomy 7 and deletions of the long arm of chromosome 7 are found in the majority of patients with myeloid leukemia.[20] A mouse model recapitulates many aspects of the human disease syndrome, including hematopoietic malignancies.[21]

The cutaneous lesions are typified by a lupus erythematosus-like histology. There is epidermal atrophy accompanied by liquefactive degeneration of the basal layer with cytoid body formation. A lymphohistiocytic infiltrate is present in the superficial dermis. Telangiectatic blood vessels are evident.

Cockayne syndrome

This is a very rare disorder with an autosomal recessive mode of inheritance and a male predominance (4:1), with the majority of cases reported to be of British ancestry. It is a multisystem disease associated with premature aging and particularly affects the skin, teeth, eyes, skeleton, and central nervous system.[1]

Clinical features

Children appear to be normal at birth and have an unremarkable early development. However, usually in the second year of life, they show photosensitivity and acquire a 'butterfly' rash (as in lupus erythematosus) on the malar region, which with time is associated with scarring and hyperpigmentary changes. These features, in association with prognathism, sunken eyes, loss of subcutaneous fat, and nasal atrophy ('beaked' nose), give the children a characteristic progeria-like or bird-headed appearance (*Fig. 7.103*).[2–4] Fine hair and anhidrosis may also be evident.[1]

Ocular lesions include corneal opacity, cataract, retinal degeneration, and optic atrophy with resultant blindness.[1] 'Salt and pepper' pigmentation of the fundus is characteristic.[2]

Patients usually suffer from progressive sensorineural deafness.[1] The patients are dwarfs and have disproportionately long limbs with enlarged hands and feet.[2] Microcephaly is common, and radiological examination reveals thickening of the skull bones. Kyphosis, ankylosis, and flexion

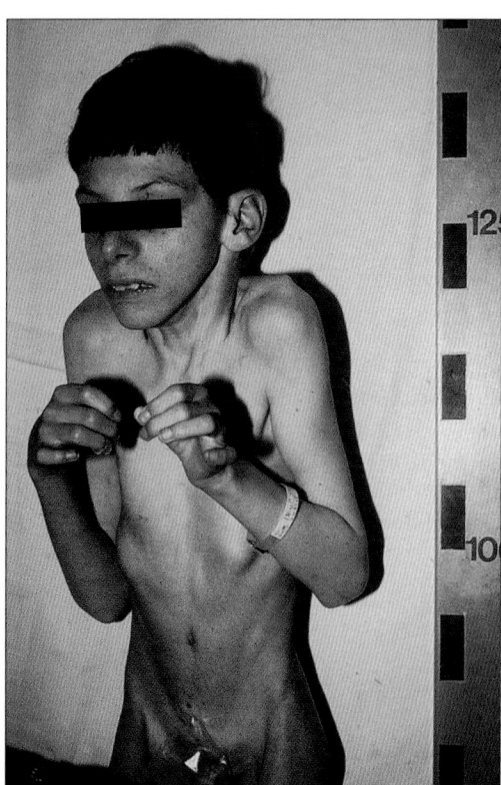

Fig. 7.103
Cockayne syndrome: the features include prominent ears, prognathism, a 'beaked' nose, and flexion contractures. By courtesy of D. Atherton, MD, Institute of Dermatology and Children's Hospital at Great Ormond Street, London, UK.

contractures are frequent complications, and dental abnormalities include malocclusions and caries. Involvement of the central nervous system presents as microcephaly, normal pressure hydrocephalus, mental subnormality, ataxia, choreoathetosis, spasticity, myoclonus, and gait disturbance.[1,2,5] Renal function is usually impaired.[6]

Patients with Cockayne syndrome have an increased incidence of infections and usually die within the third decade.

An unusually severe form with early onset and quick death associated with abnormal thymidine dimer repair (and hence showing overlap with xeroderma pigmentosum) has been described.[5,7]

Prenatal diagnosis of Cockayne syndrome is now possible.[8]

Pathogenesis and histologic features

The two genes responsible for Cockayne syndrome (*CSA/ERCC8* and *CSB/ERCC6*) have been cloned, with most cases due to mutations in *CSB*.[9–12] *CSA* encodes a WD (Trp-Asp) protein, which interacts with a number of proteins including p44 protein, a subunit of transcription/DNA repair factor IIH (TFIIH).[12,13] *CSB* belongs to the yeast SNF2/SW12 protein family, which is of importance in gene transcriptional activation.[12,13] Unlike CSA, CSB is devoid of helicase activity. CSB protein interacts with CSA and excision repair enzyme XPG. It may also have a role in response to hypoxic injury and in chromatin structure.[11,12] A mouse model of this syndrome has been developed.[14]

Patients with Cockayne syndrome have an impaired DNA excision/repair mechanism and are hypersensitive to the effects of UV radiation with an inability to promote normal levels of DNA and RNA synthesis following UV irradiation.[12,15–18] The specific defect resides within repair of mutations in transcriptionally active genes rather than in excision/repair mechanisms in general.[19,20] There are five complementation groups identifiable by cell fusion studies: CSA, CSB, XPB, XPD, and XPG.[5,11] XPB, XPD, and XPG differ from groups CSA and CSB by showing an increased incidence of skin cancer.[13] Cockayne syndrome may also coexist with trichothiodystrophy.[21]

Biopsy of the malar rash shows epidermal atrophy associated with basal cell hydropic degeneration. A chronic inflammatory cell infiltrate is present in the superficial dermis.

The cerebral lesions are characterized by loss of white matter, cerebellar cortical atrophy, hydrocephalus, and widespread calcification.[5,22] Histologically, there is demyelination and gliosis. Iron-laden neurons, neurofibrillary tangles, and giant, bizarre astrocytes have also been reported.[22,23] Severe atherosclerosis resulting in occasional strokes can occur. [22]

The kidney shows global sclerosis due to marked basement membrane (type IV) collagen deposition associated with tubular atrophy and interstitial fibrosis.[6]

Dyskeratosis congenita

Clinical features

This is a rare, but important, systemic illness with poor prognosis and high mortality. It has a predominantly X-linked recessive mode of inheritance and occurs mainly in males (6:1), although both autosomal dominant and recessive variants are also recognized.[1–5] The condition consists predominantly of a complex triad of skin pigmentation, nail, and mucosa abnormalities. There is also an increased incidence of malignancy including hematological and solid tumors.[1,2,6,7]

The skin acquires a widespread reticular pigmentation with associated poikiloderma, which at first appears most prominently on the face, neck, and the 'V' neck region of the upper chest, but later becomes generalized (*Fig. 7.104*).[1,4] During childhood, the nails become dystrophic and are often lost (*Fig. 7.105*). There may also be palmoplantar hyperkeratosis associated with hyperhidrosis, development of epiphora, early loss of dentition, caries, poor growth, sparse hair, bullous eruptions, lacrimal duct stenosis, and mental subnormality.[1–3,8,9] A reduced diffusion capacity develops from pulmonary fibrosis.[2,9,10]

Premalignant leukoplakia involving particularly the mouth and anus is an important complication, with a significant risk of squamous cell carcinoma developing in these lesions.[2,5,9,11] The urethra and vagina may also be

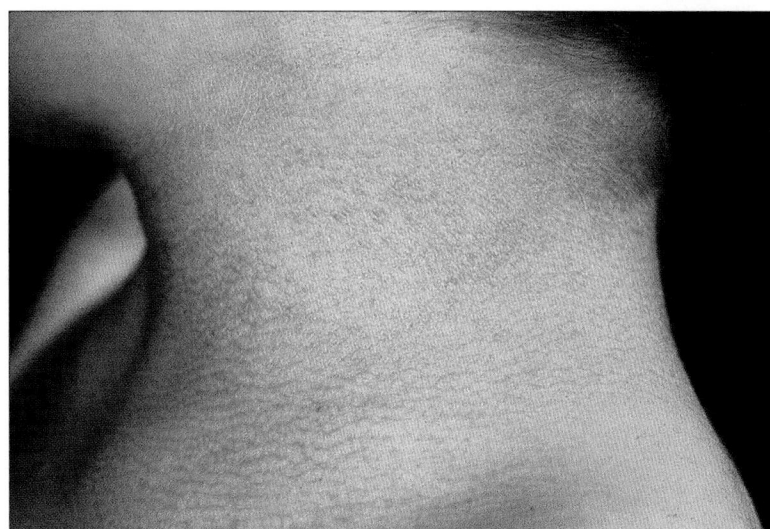

Fig. 7.104
Dyskeratosis congenita: typical poikilodermatous pigmentation on the neck. By courtesy of D. Atherton, MD, Institute of Dermatology and Children's Hospital at Great Ormond Street, London, UK.

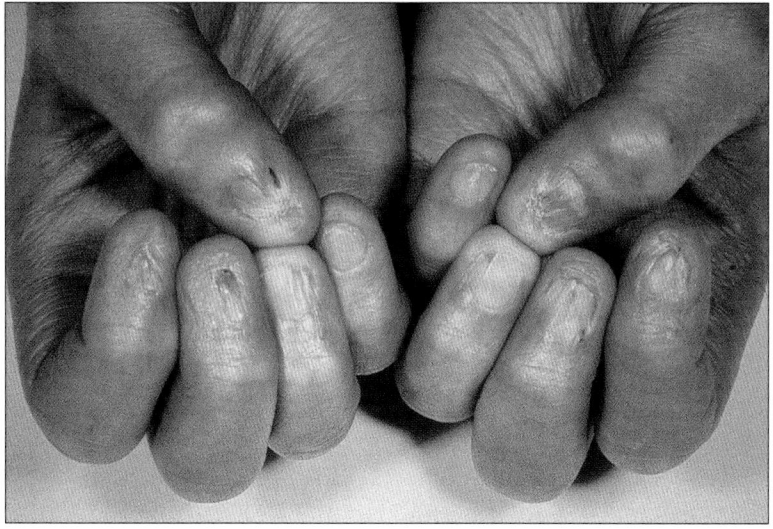

Fig. 7.105
Dyskeratosis congenita: there is dystrophy of the nails with marked atrophy of the surrounding skin. By courtesy of D. Atherton, MD, Institute of Dermatology and Children's Hospital at Great Ormond Street, London, UK.

affected. Hematological manifestations include thrombocytopenia, aplastic anemia, pancytopenia, myelodysplasia, and acute myeloid leukemia.[8,9,11–13]

The grave outlook of dyskeratosis congenita relates particularly to the development of infections complicating aplastic anemia, malignancy, and pulmonary complications.[2,9–11,14]

The clinical features of this disease are most severe in males with the X-linked variant. There is considerable variation in autosomal variants, and in some of these patients symptoms may be very mild, allowing a normal life expectancy.[2]

Pathogenesis and histologic features

Dykeratosis congenita is characterized by mutations in genes involved in telomere function, with the affected gene depending on the mode of inheritance.[6] X-linked recessive dyskeratosis congenita is due to mutations of the *DKC1* gene, which has been mapped to Xq28.[15] The mutations, which are predominantly missense, result in single amino acid substitutions in dyskerin, a nucleolar protein believed to be responsible for site-specific pseudouridylation of ribosomal RNA. It is also associated with mutations in the *ACD, CTC1, DKC1, NHP2, NOP10, PARN, RTEL1, TERC, TERT*,

TINF2, and *WRAP53* genes involved in telomere function.[9,16,17] Not all cases have a known genetic cause. There is marked chromosomal instability with a striking predisposition to develop rearrangements.[2,18] Dyskeratosis congenita therefore appears to result from defective telomerase activity with resultant impaired stem cell turnover or proliferative activity.[4,9,19] This is supported by the finding that telomeres are markedly shortened and that this develops at an early age.[6,20]

The autosomal dominant variant has similarly been shown to be associated with a mutation of the RNA component of telomerase TERC, telomerase enzyme TERT – both part of the shelterin telomere protection complex TIN2.[4,6]

Finally, the autosomal recessive variant has been associated with mutation in the *NOP10/NHP2* genes that regulate telomerase.[6]

The histologic features of the pigmentary changes are non-specific, showing only pigmentary incontinence.

Biopsies of the mucosal lesions show an acanthotic epithelium with or without dysplastic changes. In the latter case, great care must be taken to exclude the presence of squamous cell carcinoma.

Graft-versus-host disease

Clinical features

GVHD represents a complex multisystem major complication of organ transplantation, usually bone marrow, that particularly affects the skin, intestine, and liver. It develops when transplanted immunocompetent donor T lymphocytes are activated, proliferate, and respond to foreign host major histocompatibility complex (MHC)-histoincompatible antigens in a background of recipient immunosuppression.[1–9] In the context of identical class I HLA antigens, as may be seen in sibling donors, class II HLA antigens (HLA-DR, -DP, and -DQ) and minor histocompatibility antigens are of major pathogenetic significance.[1,2] These latter HLA antigens are expressed on host epithelial cells following pregraft irradiation or chemotherapy, thereby focusing the donor lymphocyte immune response on the skin, liver, and intestinal tract.[1,10,11]

GVHD is a very serious complication of allogeneic bone marrow transplantation and morbidity, and mortality is very high.[12] It may also follow solid organ transplantation, develop in severely immunodepressed patients after transfusion of nonirradiated blood or blood products, or complicate transplacental transfer of maternal lymphocytes into an immunodeficient fetus.[13–15]

The clinical features of GVHD develop as a consequence of donor T lymphocyte-mediated reactions to host tissues. Successful bone marrow transplantation is dependent on the compatibility of the ABO system blood groups and histocompatibility antigens (HLA). The D locus (HLA class II) is of particular importance; successful transplantation has occurred in the presence of identical D loci with dissimilarities at the A and B loci. However, the development of GVHD is not totally dependent on HLA incompatibility as it can develop in 35% of cases with identical A, B, and D loci, suggesting the additional importance of the minor histocompatibility antigens (miH).[2,16]

Development of acute GVHD appears to be a consequence of HLA disparity, sex mismatch, increasing patient age, and the presence of infection.[7] While the skin is a major target organ in GVHD and one of the first involved organs, the liver and gastrointestinal tract are also affected.[9,17] Manifestations include malaise, nausea and vomiting, diarrhea, malabsorption, and abnormal liver function. Additionally, patients with GVHD have an increased risk of opportunistic infections, which are an important cause of morbidity and mortality.

Historically, GVHD was conventionally subdivided into two subgroups by time after transplantation:
- Acute GVHD occurs within the first 3 months following transplantation (most often presenting between 2 and 6 weeks).[2,17–19]
- Chronic GVHD presents after the third month.

However, changing transplantation practices have resulted in delayed and even atypical presentations of GVHD. In 2005, the National Institutes of Health Consensus Development Project on Criteria for Clinical Trials in

Chronic Graft-versus-Host Disease proposed new criteria to standardize the diagnosis of chronic GVHD and also account for these new GVHD presentations, dividing it into four groups[17,19–21]:

- Classic acute GVHD: acute GVHD presenting within 100 days after hematopoietic stem cell transplant or donor leukocyte infusion,
- Persistent, recurrent, or late onset acute GVHD: acute GVHD occurring more than 100 days after transplantation without chronic GVHD symptoms,
- Classic chronic GVHD: chronic GVHD without features of acute GHVD regardless of timing from transplantation,
- Overlap syndromes: both acute and chronic GVHD features present regardless of timing from transplantation.

The classical features of acute and chronic GVHD are presented below. The other two categories show similar features and are defined by the clinical context in which they occur, that is, their timing relative to transplantation.

Acute GVHD

Acute GVHD develops in between 6% and 90% of patients who undergo bone marrow transplantation.[22,23] The incidence relates particularly to HLA mismatch, the age of the patient, and the conditioning regimen protocols used.[1,2] Additional risk factors of importance include sex mismatch, i.e., when the donor is a female (particularly if multiparous) and the recipient is male, use of radiation and/or high dosage chemotherapy prior to transplantation, prior blood transfusions, prior splenectomy, viral infections, and inadequate immunosuppression.[2]

It presents with the sudden onset of fever and malaise, which are rapidly followed by cutaneous signs including facial erythema and a generalized morbilliform, maculopapular rash characteristically affecting the palms and soles (*Figs 7.106* and *7.107*). Mucosal lesions may also be a feature (*Fig. 7.108*). The skin lesions particularly affect the upper half of the body and the back of the neck; ears and shoulders are sites of predilection.[1,7,18,19,23] Lichen planus-like features may sometimes supervene. Additional cutaneous lesions include purpura, petechiae, desquamation, and a folliculitis-like appearance.[7,19,23]

More severe variants include erythroderma or even a toxic epidermal necrolysis-like reaction. The latter has a poor prognosis and may be a manifestation of a drug reaction or represent a true component of acute GVHD. It usually affects a large surface area, shows mucosal involvement, and is associated with severe liver and gastrointestinal lesions.[23–25] Mortality is very high (50% and higher, especially if untreated), related to the effects of therapy in addition to the lesions themselves.[12,26] In the event of survival of acute GVHD, the rash may resolve completely or merge into the features of chronic GVHD. It is often difficult on clinical grounds (and histologically) to differentiate between acute GVHD, viral disorders, and cytotoxic/adverse drug reactions.

The clinical manifestations of acute GVHD are traditionally divided into four stages[1,2,17,18,23]:

- Stage I: Maculopapular eruption affecting up to 25% of surface area. Bilirubin levels of 2–3 mg/dL and diarrhea in excess of 500 mL/day.
- Stage II: Maculopapular erythema affecting 25–50% of surface area. Bilirubin levels of 3–6 mg/dL and diarrhea in excess of 1000 mL/day.
- Stage III: Generalized erythroderma. Bilirubin levels of 6–15 mg/dL and diarrhea in excess of 1500 mL/day.
- Stage IV: Toxic epidermal necrolysis. Bilirubin levels of 15 mg/dL or more and diarrhea exceeding 1500 mL/day.

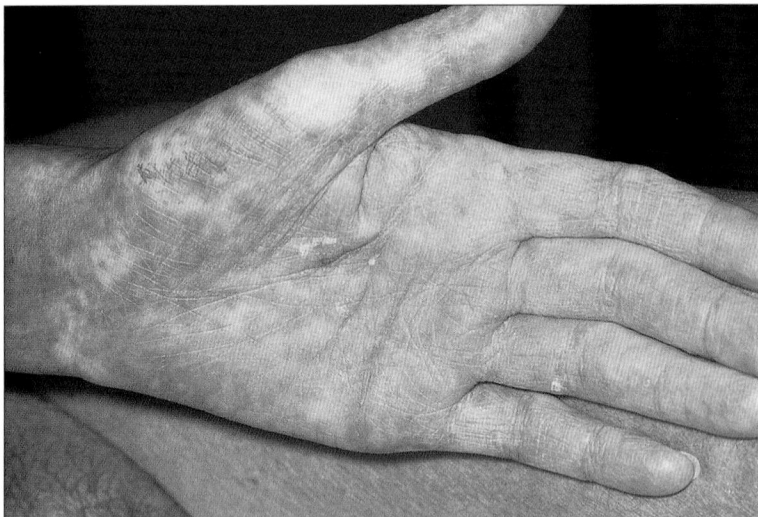

Fig. 7.107
Acute graft-versus-host disease: this vivid palmar erythema is characteristic. By courtesy of R. Touraine, MD, Hôpital Henri Mondor, Paris, France.

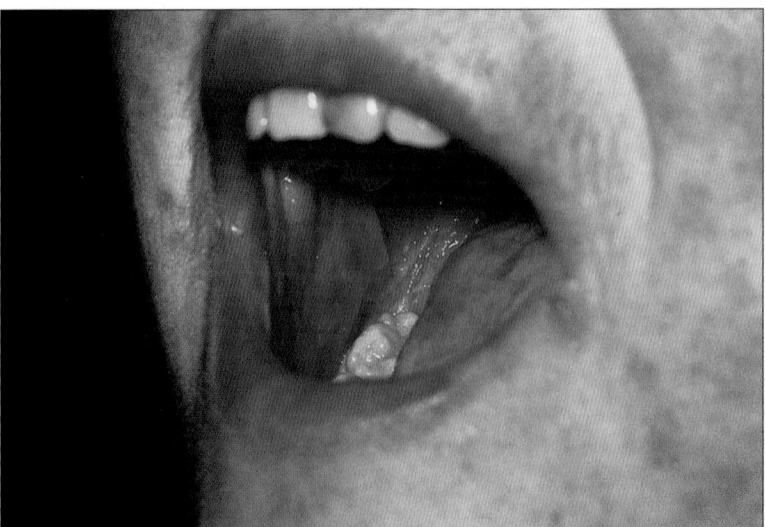

Fig. 7.108
Acute graft-versus-host disease: note the erosions on the buccal mucosa. By courtesy of R. Touraine, MD, Hôpital Henri Mondor, Paris, France.

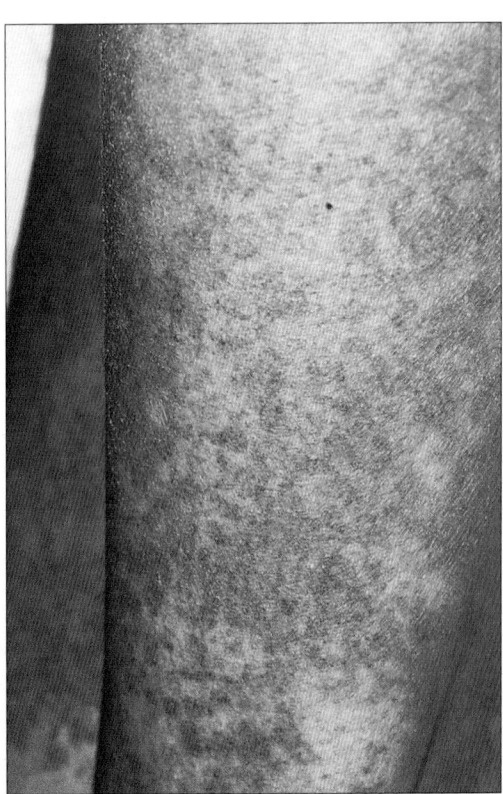

Fig. 7.106
Acute graft-versus-host disease: chest and arm showing widespread macular erythema with fine telangiectasia and mild scaling. By courtesy of R. Touraine, MD, Hôpital Henri Mondor, Paris, France.

Chronic GVHD

Chronic GVHD develops in 10% of all patients undergoing allogeneic bone marrow transplantation and in 30–70% of all long-term survivors.[27,28] Systems involved include the skin, eyes, mouth and esophagus, liver, genitalia, muscle, and peripheral and central nervous systems.[7] Virtually all chronic GVHD patients exhibit skin manifestations, and 90% develop oral lesions.[2,28,29] Some develop chronic GVHD de novo (30%); others show a gradual progression of continuous acute GVHD into the chronic variant (32%).[2] Occasionally, chronic GVHD may follow a period of resolution of acute GVHD, after an interval of quiescence (36%).[2] Chronic GVHD can occur as a lichen planus-like eruption and/or show features of a poikilodermatous or sclerodermatous reaction.[30–32] A discoid lupus erythematosus-like reaction is rare. Polymyositis and fasciitis have also been described.[33–38] In addition, a variety of presentations have been reported which can be subtle, especially in the early phase. These include xerosis, ichthyosis, follicular prominence, pityriasiform, eczematous, psoriasiform lesions, annular lesions similar to urticaria or erthyema annulare centrifugum, a morbilliform papulosquamous rash, and even erythroderma.[20] Risk factors for developing chronic GVHD include prior episode of acute GVHD, increasing age, sex mismatch, i.e., when the donor is a female (particularly if multiparous) and the recipient is male, and use of non-T-cell depleted bone marrow.[2,39]

Although early in chronic GVHD the lesions are typically lichenoid and later sclerodermatous, in some patients these features may appear simultaneously.[2] UV irradiation, trauma, and infection with herpes zoster virus or *Borrelia* can precipitate chronic GVHD.[2]

The early chronic GVHD lesion commonly has a classic lichenoid appearance with typical erythematous or violaceous polygonal papules sometimes showing Wickham striae (*Fig. 7.109*). The periorbital region, ears, palms, and soles are sites of predilection.[2] Oral mucosal lesions include typical netlike lacy white lesions, and ulcerated areas may also develop (*Figs 7.110–7.112*). The cheeks, tongue, palate, and lips are sites of predilection.[2] Symptoms of Sjögren syndrome are also often present. Onycholysis and cicatricial alopecia may be features. The rash is sometimes less typical, appearing as a desquamative active dermatitis or as follicular hyperkeratosis. As mentioned above, the findings can sometimes be subtle, such as xerosis.[20]

The late phase of chronic GVHD is typically sclerodermatous and usually presents 8–18 months after transplantation (*Figs 7.113–7.115*). The development of a poikilodermatous rash is followed by induration, atrophy, and sclerosis.[23,30] The resultant features resemble morphea or systemic sclerosis; chronic ulceration, particularly involving pressure points, can be an unpleasant complication. Blisters may occasionally develop.[23,30,33] The development of oral and cutaneous squamous cell carcinoma has occasionally been associated with chronic GVHD.[40–44]

Chronic GVHD has a mortality of up to 40%. Causes of death include infection, cachexia, and liver failure.[2]

Systemic features include chronic hepatitis, diarrhea with malabsorption, bronchiolitis obliterans, peripheral entrapment neuropathy, and polymyositis.[2] Opportunistic infections are also of major importance.

Pathogenesis and histologic features

GVHD is mediated by the combined effects of donor T lymphocytes (CD4+ T cells responding to MHC class II antigens and CD8+ T cells to class I antigens) and cytokines including IL-1, TNF-α, IFN-γ, and GM-CSF.[1,2,11,45–53] The development of acute GVHD depends on a complex interplay between

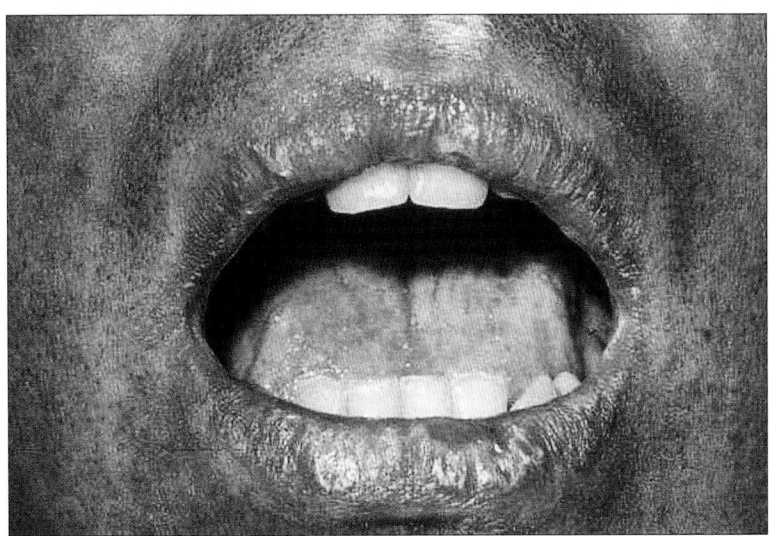

Fig. 7.110
Early chronic graft-versus-host disease: there are diffuse widespread lichenoid changes of the lips. By courtesy of R. Touraine, MD, Hôpital Henri Mondor, Paris, France.

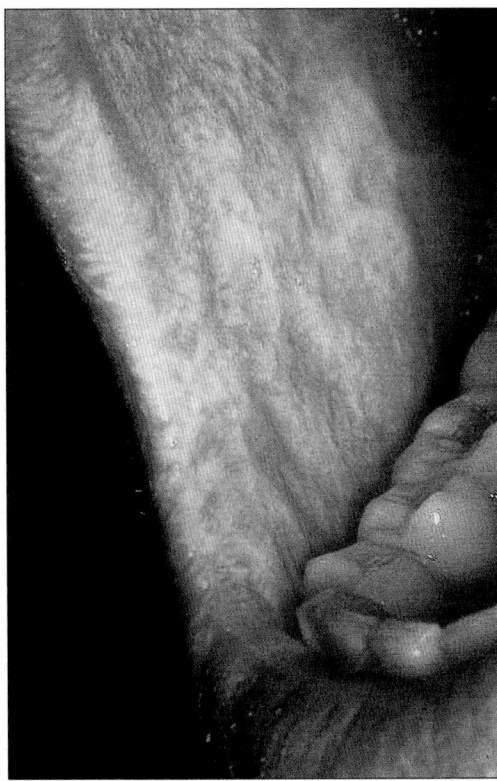

Fig. 7.111
Early chronic graft-versus-host disease: florid reticulate white striae on the buccal mucosa are evident. By courtesy of R. Touraine, MD, Hôpital Henri Mondor, Paris, France.

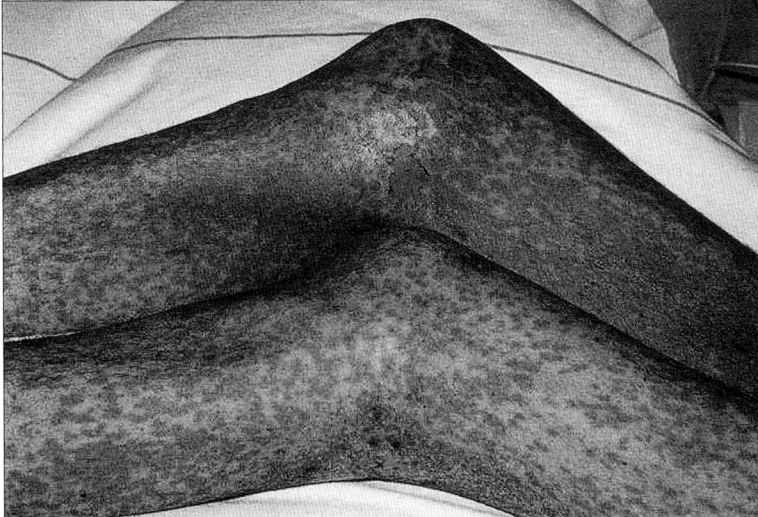

Fig. 7.109
Early chronic graft-versus-host disease: there are widespread, almost confluent hyperpigmented lichenoid papules. Associated erosion of the epidermis gives an appearance similar to toxic epidermal necrolysis (Lyell syndrome). By courtesy of R. Touraine, MD, Hôpital Henri Mondor, Paris, France.

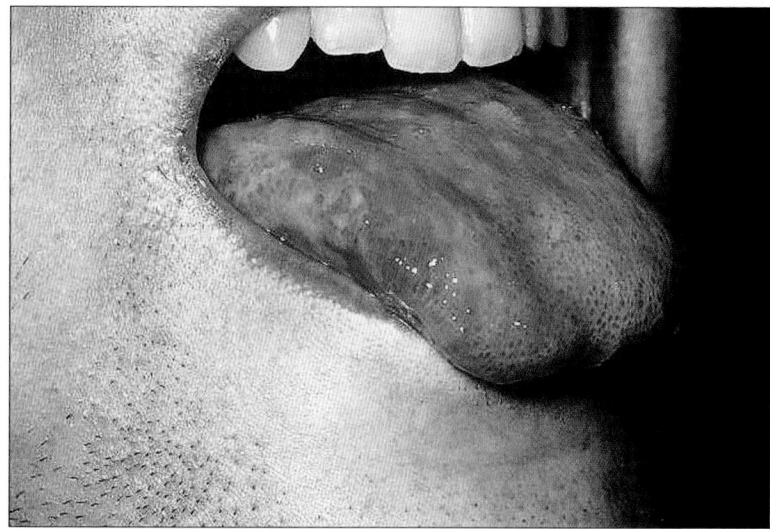

Fig. 7.112
Early chronic graft-versus-host disease: there are erosive changes on the tongue. By courtesy of R. Touraine, MD, Hôpital Henri Mondor, Paris, France.

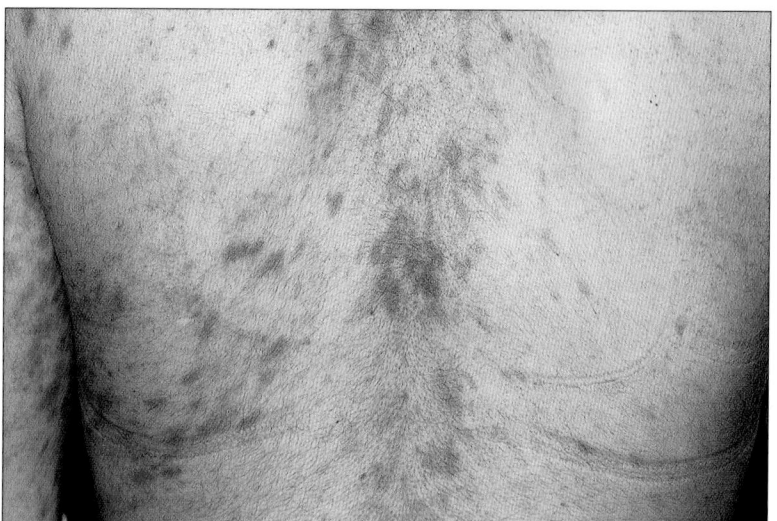

Fig. 7.114
Late chronic graft-versus-host disease: hyperpigmented sclerotic plaques are present on the back. By courtesy of R. Touraine, MD, Hôpital Henri Mondor, Paris, France.

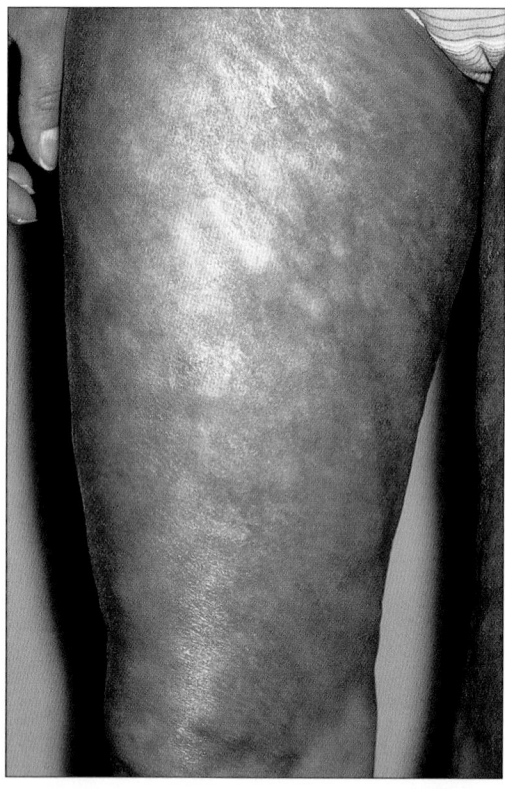

Fig. 7.113
Late chronic graft-versus-host disease: note the grossly hyperpigmented sclerotic limb. By courtesy of R. Touraine, MD, Hôpital Henri Mondor, Paris, France.

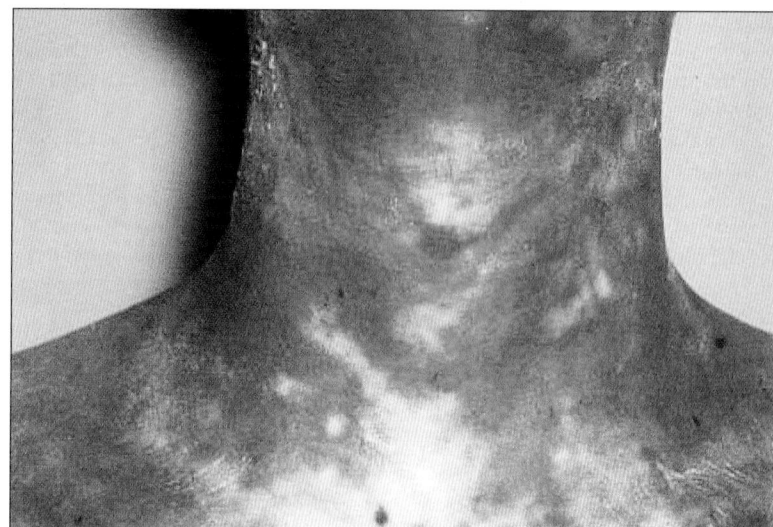

Fig. 7.115
Late chronic graft-versus-host disease: there is mottled hypo- and hyperpigmentation with gross atrophy and scaling. By courtesy of R. Touraine, MD, Hôpital Henri Mondor, Paris, France.

host immunosuppression, tissue damage as a result of pregraft induction therapy, and donor lymphocyte proliferation and activation with consequent injury and death of susceptible host tissues.[1]

The lymphocytes may be of CD4+ or CD8+ immunophenotype, and commonly there is an admixture. Both Th1 and Th2 CD4+ subtypes are represented. The former produce IL-2 and IFN-γ and are thought to promote GVHD; the latter produce IL-4, IL-6, and IL-10 and are believed to be protective, although this has been contested.[54] Natural killer (NK) cells may also be of importance although their presence appears to be variable.[55] B cells are absent. Activated keratinocytes following induction chemotherapy or irradiation produce TNF-α and IL-1 and express ICAM-1 and HLA-DR.[56] This may result in increased recognition of histoincompatible MHC antigens by donor T cells.[1] The superficial dermal endothelial cells express

E-selectin, α4β1 integrin, αLβ2 integrin, ICAM-1, platelet endothelial cell adhesion molecule-1 (PECAM-1), and vascular cell adhesion molecule-1 (VCAM-1), which mediate lymphocyte adhesion to the endothelium and facilitate recognition, activation, and response to MHC molecules.[1,57-59] The mechanisms of cell injury and death result from both cytotoxic T cell and possibly NK cell-mediated cytotoxic effects and the actions of cytokines. The former includes cytolytic actions mediated by perforin and granzyme B, and apoptosis through the Fas-Fas ligand pathway.[60,61] IL-1, IL-2, IL-6, and TNF-α are thought to be of particular importance in mediating cytotoxicity.[1] Raised serum TNF-α correlates with GVHD, and antibodies to TNF-α or its receptor protect against the disease.[1,62-64] Recently, regulatory T cells (Treg) have been postulated to play a role in GVHD. Treg are decreased in patients with GVHD, and it appears that they may inhibit tissue infiltration of CD8+ T cells into the affected skin.[17,65] Studies suggest a role for B cells in GVHD, with a possible role for targeted therapy.[66]

Deposition of IgM and C3 at the dermal–epidermal junction and around the superficial vasculature in up to 39% of patients with acute GVHD suggests that humoral responses may play a role in the pathogenesis of GVHD.[56,67]

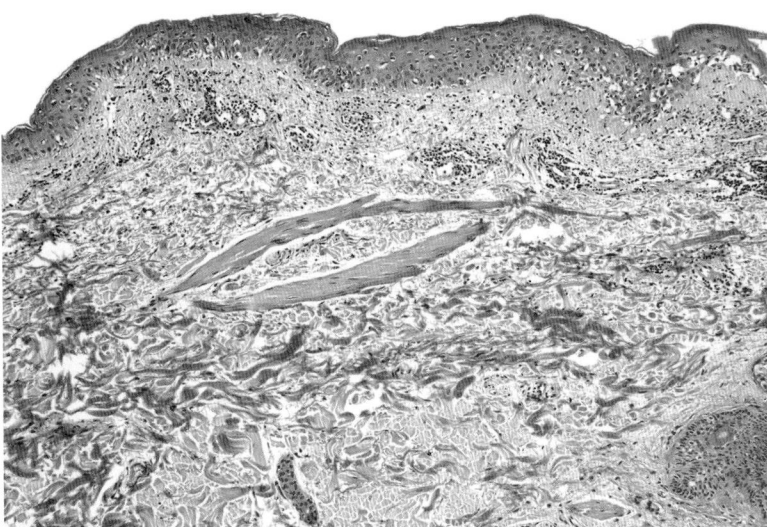

Fig. 7.116
Acute graft-versus-host disease: evolving lesion showing basal cell hydropic degeneration and scattered apoptotic keratinocytes. The dermis contains dilated blood vessels and a light perivascular chronic inflammatory cell infiltrate.

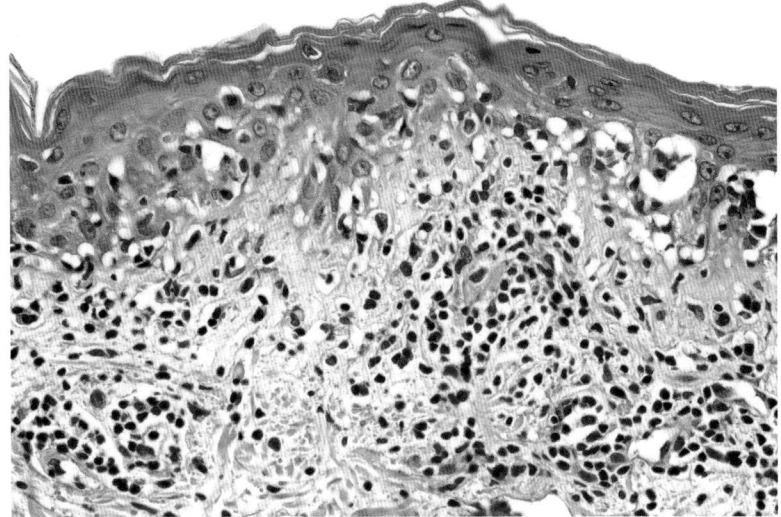

Fig. 7.118
Acute graft-versus-host disease: high-power view lesion showing parakeratosis, basal cell hydropic degeneration, and apoptosis.

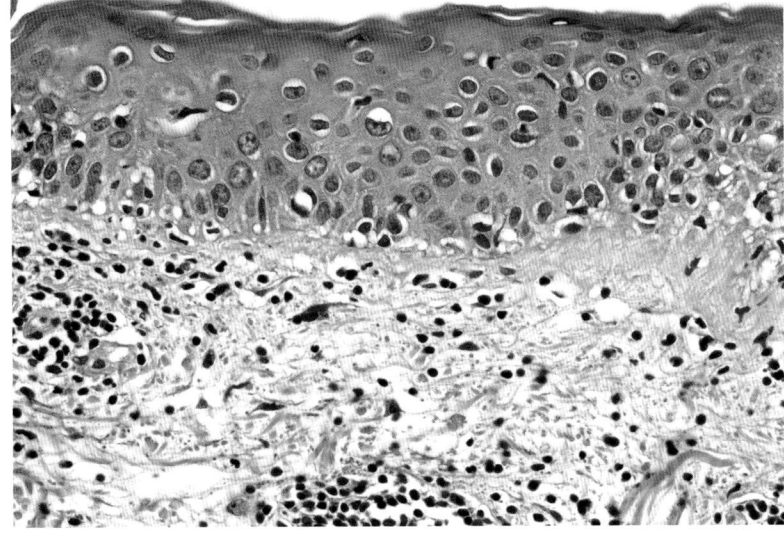

Fig. 7.117
Acute graft-versus-host disease: high-power view showing basal cell liquefactive degeneration. Diagnosis is entirely dependent on the clinical history.

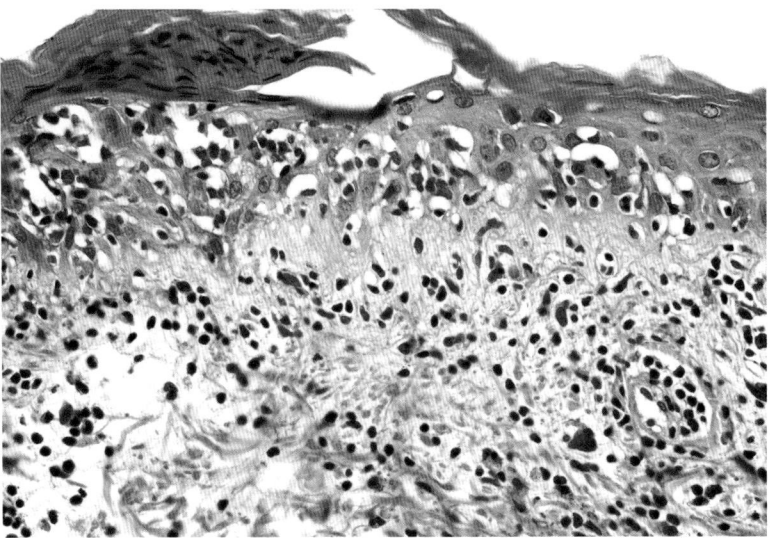

Fig. 7.119
Acute graft-versus-host disease: high-power view showing parakeratosis, apoptosis, and satellite cell necrosis.

The development of chronic GVHD is dependent on a variety of factors including, antihost tissue activity of donor T cells and the development of autoimmunity.[2,68] The infiltrate consists predominantly of CD8+ T cells; NK cells are usually absent.[2] As with acute GVHD, TNF-α and IL-1 are the major cytokines implicated.[2]

The acute lesion of GVHD is characterized by focal or diffuse basal cell hydropic change (*Figs 7.116–7.119*).[69] Apoptotic and dyskeratotic keratinocytes, at all levels of the epidermis and associated with adjacent lymphocytes (satellite cell necrosis), are characteristic.[17,70,71] Isolated cytoid bodies are also frequently evident. Lymphocytic exocytosis is invariably present, and spongiosis is sometimes a feature. Microvesiculation at the dermal–epidermal junction occasionally occurs. Follicular involvement is a common feature, and the hair bulge region is typically affected.[71,72] Langerhans cells are often reduced in number. Vascular changes include endothelial cell swelling with sloughing, and intimal and perivascular lymphocytic infiltration. Blood vessel proliferation has also been described. Perivascular edema and nuclear dust may additionally be present, and mast cells are also conspicuous.[73,74] Eosinophils are sometimes present and this finding does not necessarily indicate a drug reaction, but numerous eosinophils (≥16/10 HPFs) are indicative of a drug reaction.[75] Therefore, the histologic presentation of GVHD is broad, and no finding can be considered pathognomonic for GVHD.[12,19]

The toxic epidermal necrolysis-like lesions are characterized by severe epidermal necrosis in association with subepidermal vesiculation. Evidence of sweat gland involvement is commonly present.[76,77] Keratinous plugging of the acrosyringium may therefore be seen, and the excretory ducts often show cytopathic-degenerative and proliferative changes.[77] The former comprises basal cell hydropic degeneration, lymphocytic infiltration, and apoptosis. Follicular involvement is a not uncommon additional manifestation.[78] The histologic features of acute GVHD may be subdivided into four stages, which have prognostic significance (*Table 7.1*).[78–80]

The histology of chronic GVHD is typically lichenoid in appearance and has significant overlap with idiopathic lichen planus (*Fig. 7.120*). These features are hyperkeratosis, hypergranulosis, irregular acanthosis, basal cell hydropic degeneration, cytoid body formation, pigmentary incontinence, and a variable bandlike lymphohistiocytic infiltrate that may obscure the dermal–epidermal interface. In contrast to idiopathic lichen planus, satellite cell necrosis is often present in the early phase of chronic GVHD, and the infiltrate sometimes contains plasma cells and eosinophils and may be less dense. Squamous metaplasia of the eccrine sweat ducts has been described.[71,77]

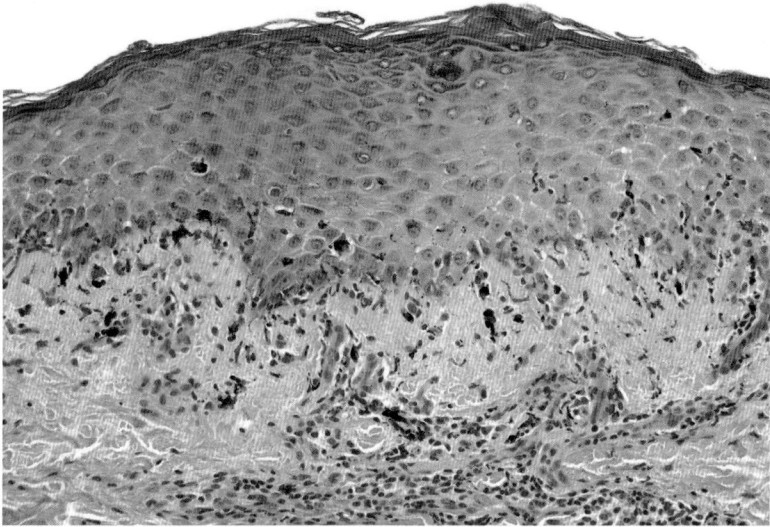

Fig. 7.120
Early chronic graft-versus-host disease: the hyperkeratosis, hypergranulosis, irregular acanthosis, and basal cell hydropic degeneration are indistinguishable from idiopathic lichen planus.

Table 7.1
Grading of acute graft-versus-host disease

Grade	Feature
I	Focal or diffuse vacuolar alteration of basal cells
II	Vacuolar alteration of basal cells; spongiosis and dyskeratosis of epidermal cells
III	Formation of subepidermal cleft in association with dyskeratosis and spongiosis
IV	Complete loss of epidermis

Reproduced with permission from Lerner et al. (1974) Transplantation Proceedings, 6, 367–371.

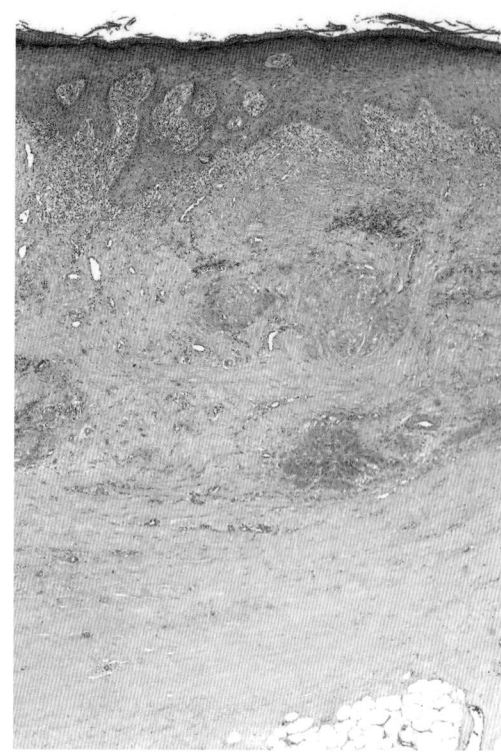

Fig. 7.121
Late chronic graft-versus-host disease: there is dense fibrosis of the dermis with tethering of the subcutaneous fat. Appendages are absent. These appearances are reminiscent of scleroderma.

The late stage of chronic GVHD is characterized by epidermal atrophy with abolition of the ridge pattern and scarring of the superficial and deep dermis, with loss of the adnexal structures (*Fig. 7.121*) imparting a sclerodermoid feature including eosinophilic fasciitis, panniculitis, morphea-like changes, and lichen sclerosus.[23,71,81,82] Features of the early stage of chronic GVHD, i.e., hydropic basal cell degeneration, cytoid body formation, and a chronic inflammatory cell infiltrate, may or may not be evident. Dermal mucin deposition has also been documented.[83] Recently, GVHD associated angiomatosis has been associated with sclerodermoid chronic GVHD.[84]

Hepatic changes include bile duct atypia with necrosis, periportal inflammation, focal hepatocyte necrosis, and cholestasis.[9] Gastrointestinal lesions show individual crypt cell necrosis accompanied by a mild chronic inflammatory cell infiltrate.[71,85,86]

Differential diagnosis

The features of acute GVHD can be reproduced by cytotoxic drugs such as cyclophosphamide and by radiotherapy. Viral infections also enter the differential diagnosis, as does an adverse drug reaction, for example, to antibiotic therapy. Although the presence of conspicuous eosinophils argues to some extent in favor of an adverse drug reaction, it may not be possible to distinguish drug reactions from acute GVHD histologically.[75,87] In short, the regular practice of skin biopsy to differentiate between GVHD, drug reactions, chemotherapy effect, and viral infection may be questionable in some cases.

Acute GVHD may be indistinguishable from erythema multiforme and, in more severely affected patients, toxic epidermal necrolysis. Bile pigment deposition may be seen in the stratum corneum of a small percentage of patients with GVHD but not in cases of erythema multiforme.[88]

The early changes of chronic GVHD may be indistinguishable from lichen planus. However, the dermal infiltrate is usually less conspicuous than that in lichen planus and sometimes contains plasma cells and eosinophils. The presence of satellite cell necrosis may be a diagnostic pointer toward chronic GVHD.

In the absence of clinical information, it is usually not possible to distinguish the features of late chronic GVHD from morphea or systemic sclerosis.

The histologic features of the eruption of lymphocyte recovery are indistinguishable from acute GVHD. The differential diagnosis of acute GVHD includes engraftment syndrome. This syndrome can occur 10–14 days after transplantation but before peripheral lymphocytes are seen. It presents with a fever, hepatitis, intestinal symptoms, and an erythematous maculopapular eruption similar to acute GVHD. Some also require the presence of weight gain and pulmonary edema. Whether or not this represents a hypoacute GVHD is uncertain. The etiology is unknown, although it is postulated that the damage may be caused by cytokines released from recovering and degranulating neutrophils. G-CSF, GM-CSF, female sex, breast cancer, and other hematopoietic drugs have been implicated as risk factors for developing this condition.[17,89]

In summary, no histologic feature is pathognomonic for GVHD, and clinical correlation is essential. Therefore, in the appropriate clinical population, a positive biopsy can be very predictive despite subtle non-specific histologic findings. A negative biopsy is less reassuring. Some have advocated the use of a four-tier diagnostic system of no GVHD, possible GVHD, consistent with GVHD, and definite GVHD, a practical proposal that reflects the realities of daily practice.[71]

Pityriasis lichenoides

Clinical features

Pityriasis lichenoides (Gr. *pityron*, bran + *iasis*; lichen; Gr. *eidos*, form) is an uncommon dermatosis of unknown etiology, although a hypersensitivity reaction to a number of infectious agents including adenovirus, toxoplasmosis, Epstein-Barr virus, and *Mycobacterium pneumoniae* have been

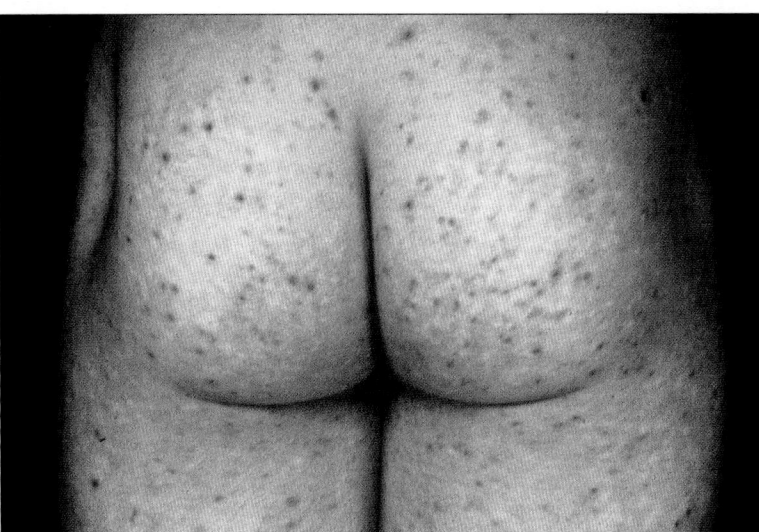

Fig. 7.122
Pityriasis lichenoides acuta: erythematous papules and crusted lesions are present on the buttocks and thighs. In severe cases, lesions may be very extensive. By courtesy of the Institute of Dermatology, London, UK.

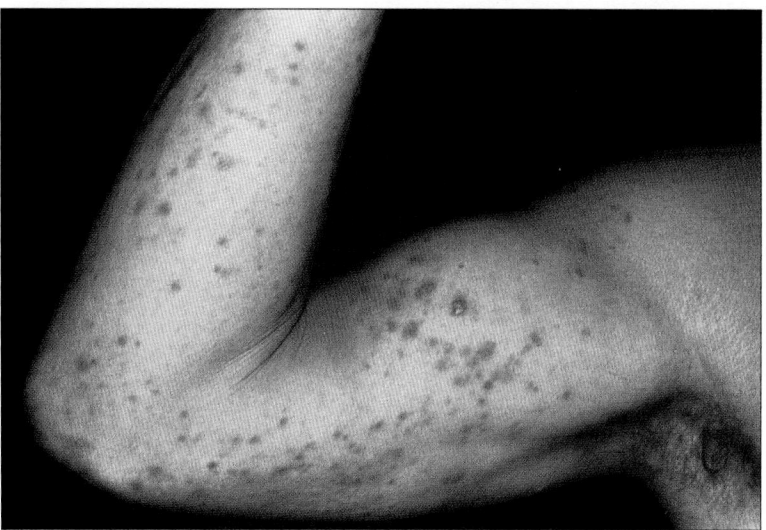

Fig. 7.123
Pityriasis lichenoides acuta: typical lesions with pustulation are present on the arm, a commonly affected site. By courtesy of the Institute of Dermatology, London, UK.

proposed.[1–4] The condition has also been documented in association with a range of autoimmune conditions such as rheumatoid arthritis, hypothyroidism, and pernicious anemia.[3,4] Two cases of pityriasis lichenoides chronica (PLC) associated with adalimumab therapy for Crohn disease and cases induced by infliximab have been described.[5,6,7] The term includes a spectrum of disease manifestations, ranging from the acute ulceronecrotic lesions of pityriasis lichenoides et varioliformis acuta (PLEVA, also known as Mucha-Habermann disease or acute guttate parapsoriasis) to the more chronic scaly papules of PLC (chronic guttate parapsoriasis); there is often clinical overlap.[8–13] In addition, a febrile, ulceronecrotic variant (febrile ulceronecrotic Mucha-Habermann disease) is recognized.[3–9,13]

Pityriasis lichenoides in more recent studies lacks strong sex predominance in adults. However, some studies have shown more of a male predominance in pediatric populations.[12,14–16] It most often occurs in childhood (5–10 years of age) and early adulthood, second or third decade.[12–16]

Lesions show a propensity to involve the arms, legs, trunk, and buttocks (Fig. 7.122). The upper limbs appear to be involved more often than the lower and the flexor more commonly than the extensor surfaces. They can begin as small macules that progress to papules. PLC is typically asymptomatic while PLEVA is associated with burning and pruritus.[10,13] The onset is usually insidious and the course fluctuating and episodic, patients experiencing recurrent crops of lesions, with the exception of the ulceronecrotic variant which is rapid. Duration of the rash is quite variable: although many patients are free of lesions by 3–6 months, others show great persistence of the disease, often for many years.[12,13] The disease shows some seasonal variation, with lesions worsening in winter and showing improvement in sunlight. Although pityriasis lichenoides is traditionally divided into acute and chronic variants, not uncommonly both types of lesions can be seen in the same patient, indicating a possible connection between PLC and PLEVA.[10]

In the more acute form of the disease, the initial lesions are crops of pink papules (Figs 7.123 and 7.124). These may become vesicular or hemorrhagic and ultimately develop necrosis and ulceration (Fig. 7.125). Healing is usually associated with the development of superficial varioliform scars. Postinflammatory hyper- or hypopigmentation is not uncommon (Fig. 7.126).[10,12,13] The rash is often polymorphic, individual patients having lesions at varying stages of evolution. Patients may be pyrexic and sometimes lymphadenopathy is present.[1]

The chronic lesions are typified by numerous, lichenoid, brownish-red, scaly papules, 3–10 mm across, the scale being most noticeable peripherally, sometimes referred to as the mica scale (Figs 7.127 and 7.128). These lesions usually heal without scarring, but are sometimes associated with hypopigmentation, which may be the most prominent feature in dark-skinned races.

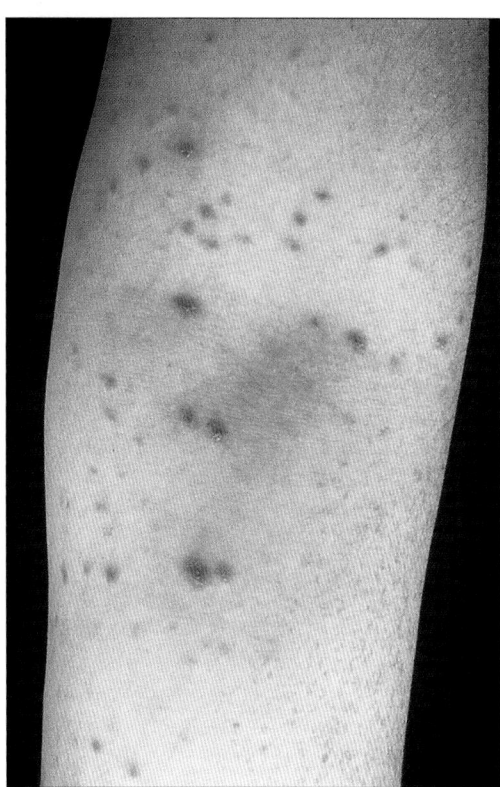

Fig. 7.124
Pityriasis lichenoides acuta: early lesions are erythematous and papular. By courtesy of the Institute of Dermatology, London, UK.

Although there are case reports of lymphoma (mycosis fungoides) developing in patients with pityriasis lichenoides, this is a rare event (see also below).[16–20]

The rare febrile ulceronecrotic variant is associated systemic features including fever, muscle weakness and pain, malaise, lymphadenopathy, arthritis, myocardial involvement, neuropsychiatric manifestations, pulmonary involvement, and even death.[3–9,12,13,21–26] Widespread cutaneous manifestations include large 2–6-cm ulceronecrotic lesions, hemorrhagic and necrotic papules, and erythema multiforme-like lesions.[3,4,12,13,21–26]

Pathogenesis and histologic features

Immunofluorescence examination of biopsies from fresh purpuric lesions commonly detects IgM and C3 in the walls of the superficial dermal blood

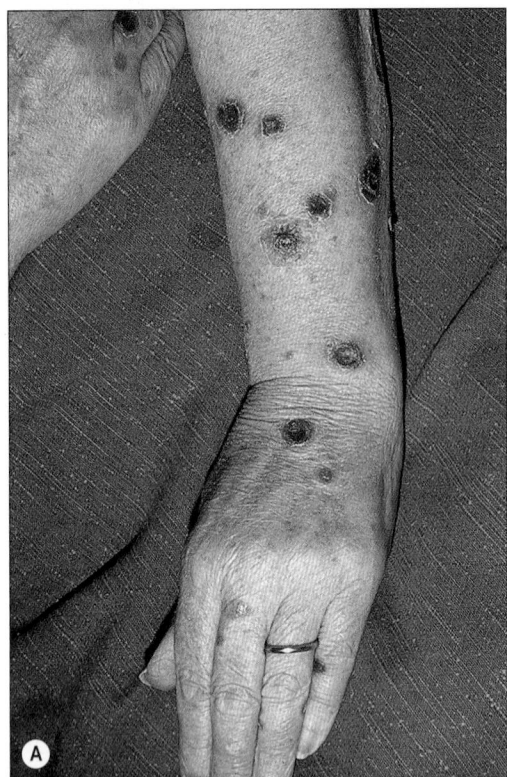

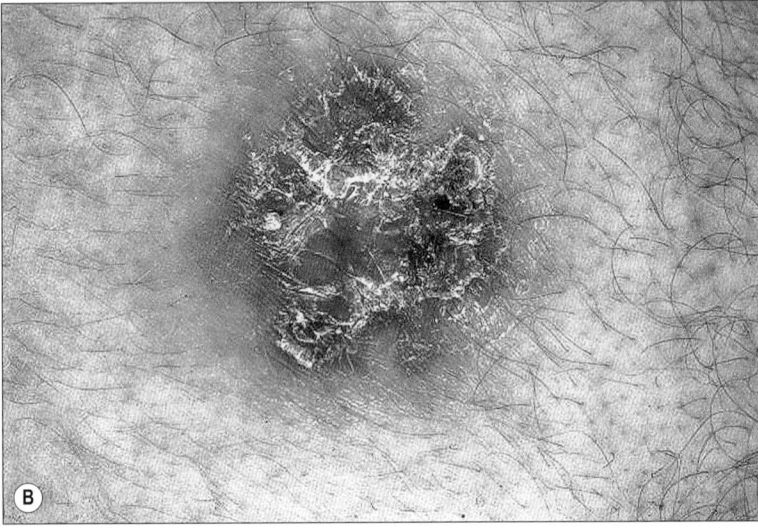

Fig. 7.125
Pityriasis lichenoides acuta: (**A**) necrotic and ulcerated lesions are present; (**B**) close-up view. By courtesy of the Institute of Dermatology, London, UK.

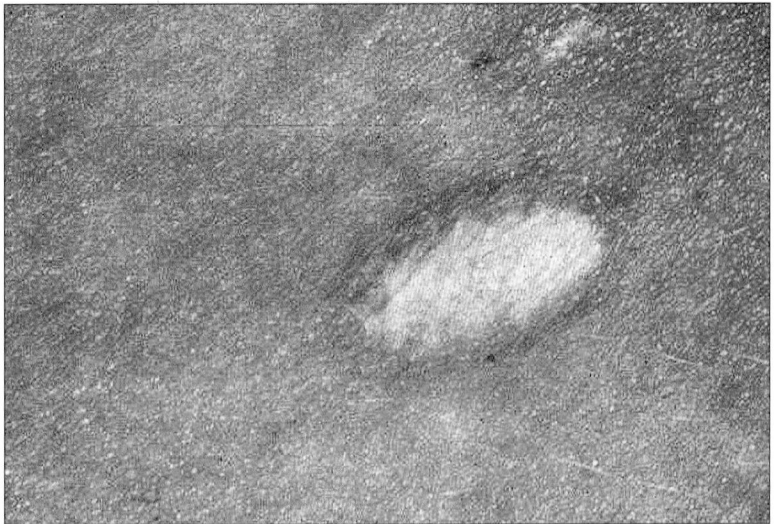

Fig. 7.126
Pityriasis lichenoides acuta: healed lesion showing scarring and hypopigmentation. By courtesy of the Institute of Dermatology, London, UK.

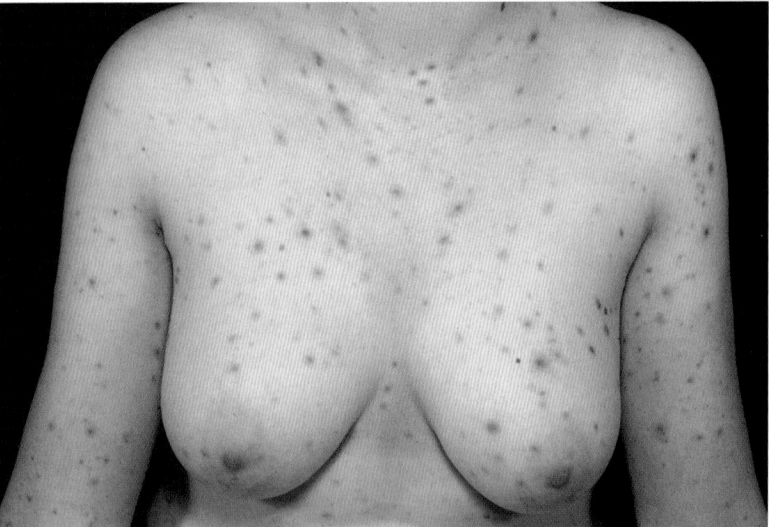

Fig. 7.127
Pityriasis lichenoides chronica: widespread scaly papules are present on the chest and arms. From the collection of the late N.P. Smith, MD, the Institute of Dermatology, London, UK.

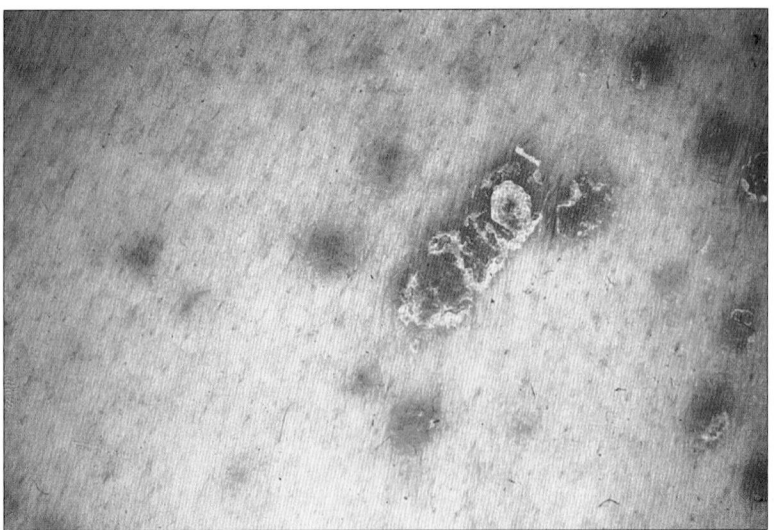

Fig. 7.128
Pityriasis lichenoides chronica: the characteristic mica scale. By courtesy of the Institute of Dermatology, London, UK.

vessels and along the dermal–epidermal junction in both the acute and chronic forms of the disease, though this is not used diagnostically.[27–29] A high proportion of patients have elevated circulating immune complexes.[30,31] Cytotoxic suppressor T cells constitute the majority of the infiltrate in pityriasis lichenoides et varioliformis acuta.[32,33] Lesser numbers are seen in PLC. These (and the overlying keratinocytes in addition to nearby endothelial cells) have been shown to express HLA-DR.[33] In contrast to lymphomatoid papulosis, CD30 is generally not expressed in pityriasis lichenoides acuta except in what has been described as overlap cases.[34,35] It is however, unlikely that the two conditions truly overlap. Macrophages are also numerous. Langerhans cells are diminished in number. Clonal T-cell receptor gene rearrangements have been described in small numbers of patients with pityriasis lichenoides acuta leading to the suggestion of a possible overlap with cutaneous T-cell lymphoma.[36,37] Exceptionally, pityriasis lichenoides acuta has been reported to progress to cutaneous T-cell lymphoma.[12,13,18–20,38,39] As a result, some have suggested that PLEVA may represent a host response to a developing T-cell lymphoproliferative disorder in

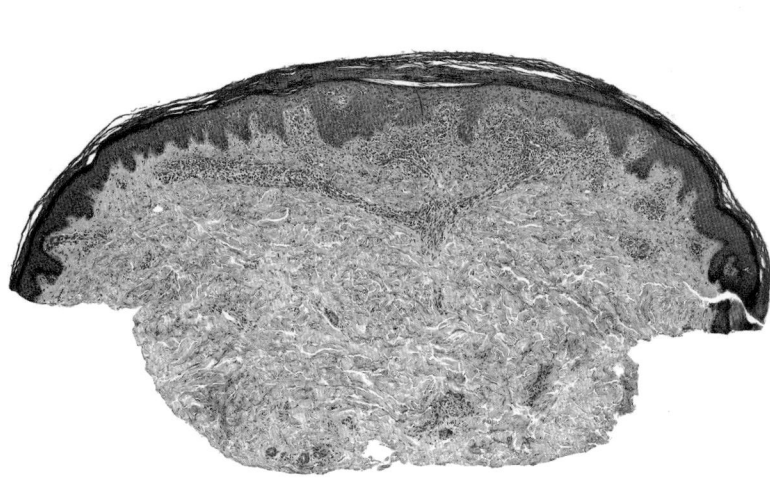

Fig. 7.129
Pityriasis lichenoides chronica: scanning view showing hyperkeratosis with parakeratosis and acanthosis.

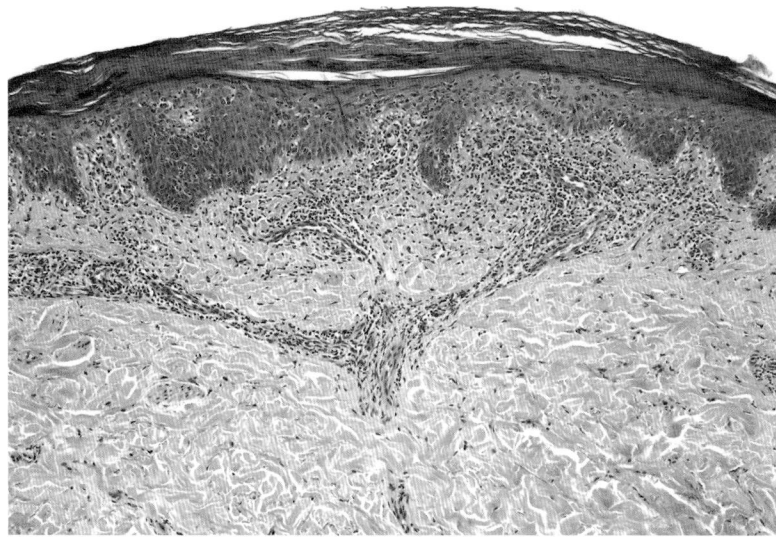

Fig. 7.130
Pityriasis lichenoides chronica: note the parakeratosis, acanthosis, and perivascular and interstitial chronic inflammatory cell infiltrate.

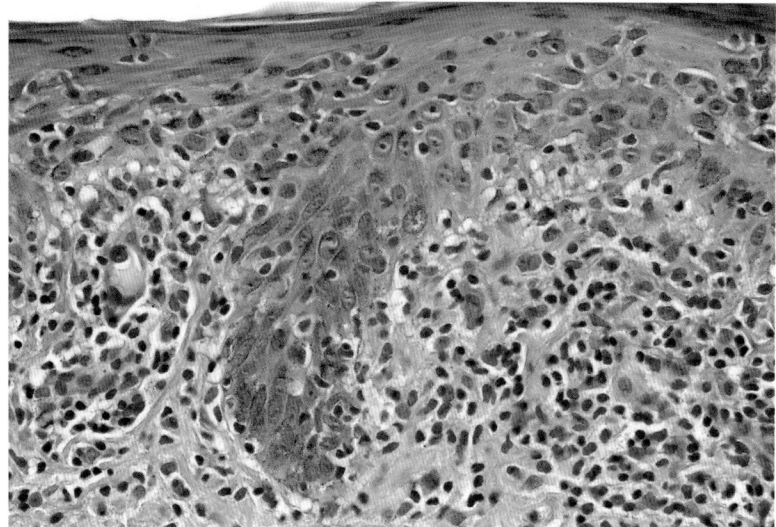

Fig. 7.131
Pityriasis lichenoides chronica: high-power view showing basal cell hydropic degeneration.

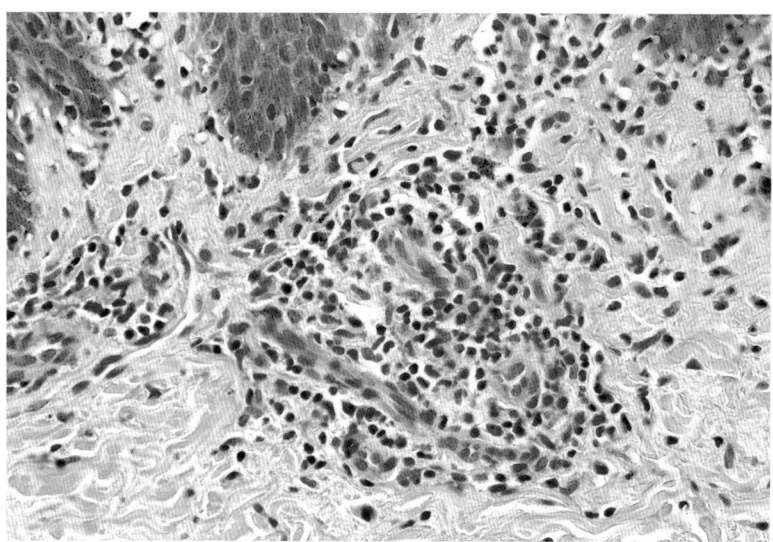

Fig. 7.132
Pityriasis lichenoides chronica: in this high-power view there is a lymphohistiocytic infiltrate and melanophages are present.

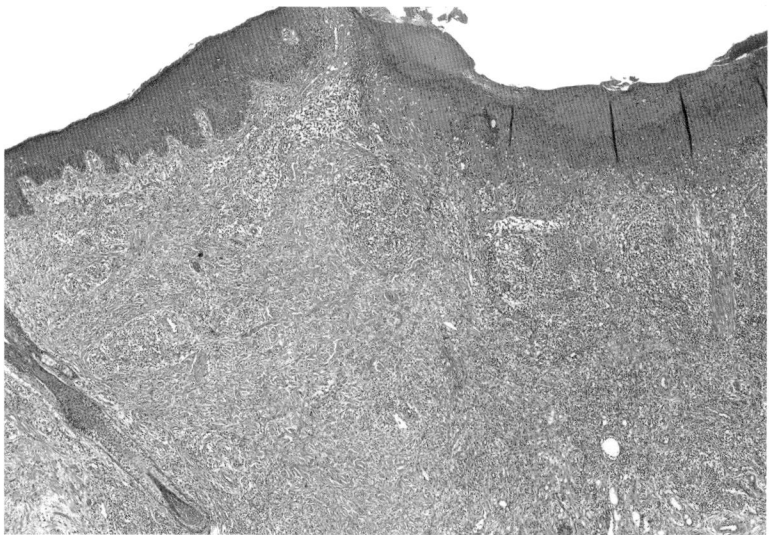

Fig. 7.133
Pityriasis lichenoides acuta: this low-power view shows an ulcerated papule with overlying crust.

some cases.[12] Complicating this issue are pityriasis lichenoides-like variants of mycosis fungoides.[40–42]

The histopathological features of pityriasis lichenoides are similar in both variants, although in the acute form the changes are usually more severe. Both are characterized by varying proportions of epidermal and dermal changes.[13,43–46]

The chronic lesions of pityriasis lichenoides are characterized by parakeratosis in which there are sometimes small collections of lymphocytes reminiscent of the Munro microabscesses of psoriasis (Figs 7.129 and 7.130). The epidermis may show slight acanthosis and usually small numbers of necrotic keratinocytes are present accompanied by multifocal but subtle interface change (Fig. 7.131). Spongiosis is often a feature. There is a perivascular, often wedge-shaped chronic inflammatory cell infiltrate in the superficial dermis (Fig. 7.132). Red cell extravasation is often present but is usually not marked.

The acute lesions of pityriasis lichenoides show similar epidermal features, but on a much exaggerated scale. Marked inter- and intracellular edema accompanied by keratinocyte necrosis and interface change frequently

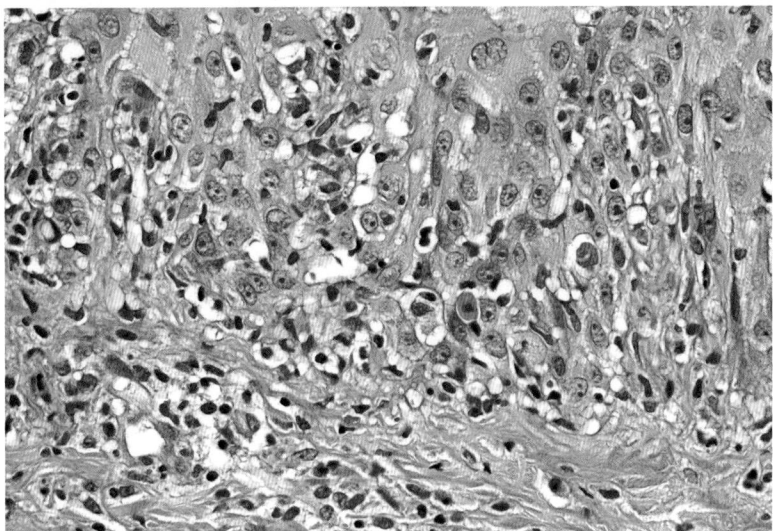

Fig. 7:134
Pityriasis lichenoides acuta: there is basal cell hydropic degeneration and apoptosis.

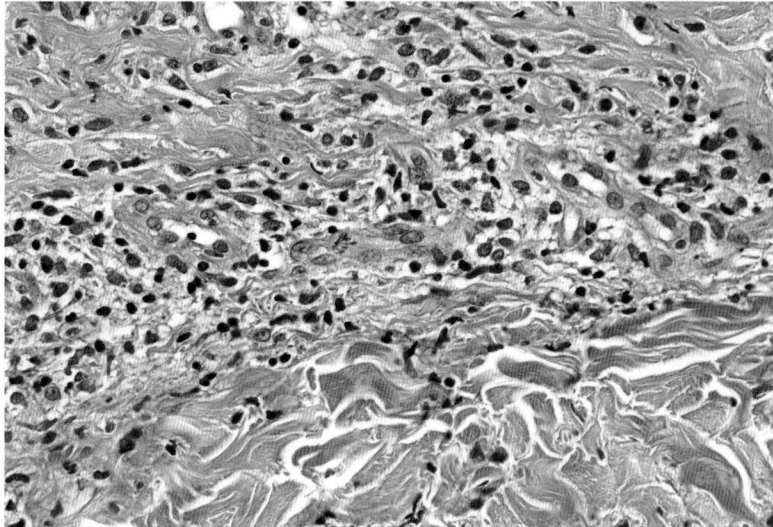

Fig. 7.135
Pityriasis lichenoides acuta: this high-power view shows a lymphohistiocytic infiltrate. Red cell extravasation can also be seen.

result in vesiculation and ulceration (*Figs 7.133* and *7.134*). Exocytosis is usually prominent and intraepidermal red blood cells are characteristic. The upper dermis is edematous and contains a chronic inflammatory cell infiltrate (*Fig. 7.135*). This is usually perivascular and varies from sparse to dense; typically, it has a wedge-shaped appearance, extending deeply into the reticular dermis, although this is only seen in biopsies from established lesions. The infiltrate consists of lymphocytes with an admixture of histiocytes. Red cell extravasation is usually conspicuous. The blood vessels of the superficial dermis are dilated and congested. Although the endothelial cells are often blurred or swollen, fibrinoid necrosis indicating necrotizing vasculitis is rarely seen (*Fig. 7.136*). The latter, if present is associated with lymphocytes and seen at the tip of the wedge in the mid to deep dermis. In febrile ulceronecrotic Mucha-Habermann disease, the features are those of very severe pityriasis lichenoides acuta and are often accompanied by changes of leukocytoclastic vasculitis.[12,13,25,47]

Differential diagnosis

The differential diagnosis includes other interface dermatitides. In lichen planus, the infiltrate is bandlike rather than wedge shaped, the epidermis lacks parakeratosis, and hemorrhage is absent. In the erythema multiforme spectrum, hemorrhage is usually not prominent, the infiltrate is less dense, and the epidermis has a normal basket weave appearance. Lupus erythematosus lacks hemorrhage and has increased dermal mucin. Lymphomatoid papulosis can have both clinical and histologic overlap with PLEVA, but has large atypical CD30+ lymphocytes. Prior reports of patients having PLEVA and lymphomatoid papulosis likely represent lymphomatoid papulosis rather than a combination.[2]

Access **ExpertConsult.com** for the complete list of references

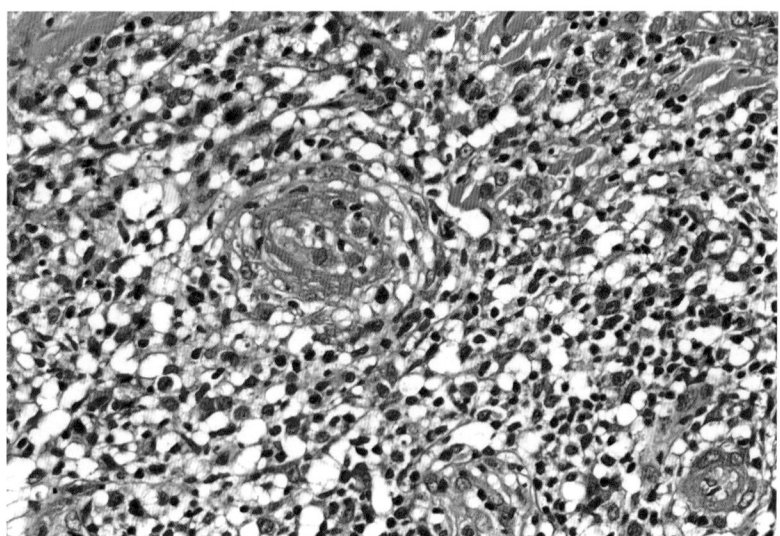

Fig. 7.136
Pityriasis lichenoides acuta: high-power view showing fibrinoid necrosis affecting the dermal vasculature.

See
www.expertconsult.com
for references and
additional material

Superficial and deep perivascular inflammatory dermatoses

Chronic superficial dermatitis

Clinical features

Chronic superficial dermatitis (digitate dermatosis, superficial scaly dermatitis, small-plaque parapsoriasis, persistent superficial dermatitis) is a not uncommon condition, which presents as erythematous scaly persistent patches, showing a predilection for the limbs and trunk. While the lesions may be round or oval, they often have a finger-like appearance, hence the alternative designation of digitate dermatosis (Figs 8.1 and 8.2).[1] The patches are usually a few centimeters in greatest dimension, but may sometimes be much larger. They are associated with a fine 'cigarette-paper' scale that often has a pale white, tan or yellowish color (Fig. 8.3). The disorder is most commonly encountered in middle-aged adults and shows a predilection for men. The patient is usually otherwise asymptomatic. Coexistence with ulcerative colitis has been reported in one patient.[2] Lesions tend to chronicity, often persisting for many years. While development of mycosis fungoides has been reported in a patient with chronic superficial dermatitis, it is most likely that these represent separate disease processes rather than disease progression.[3]

Histologic features

Biopsy shows a superficial perivascular lymphocytic infiltrate (Figs 8.4 and 8.5). The infiltrate is of variable density but is often very sparse. Cytological atypia is absent. The epidermis often shows foci of spongiosis. A confluent linear band of parakeratosis spanning multiple rete ridges is a characteristic finding.

The infiltrate is largely composed of CD4+ T lymphocytes with a minor population of CD8+ T-suppressor cells (Fig. 8.6).[2] In a small series, the CD4 to CD8 ratio ranged from 2 to 4.4. The T cells are generally reactive for CD2, CD3, and CD5 (Fig. 8.7). CD7 expression is variable and may be absent. Scattered CD68 reactive macrophages and CD1+ Langerhans cells can be seen.

Differential diagnosis

The histologic features in chronic superficial dermatitis are entirely non-specific. In fact, the constellation of histologic findings is among the most often encountered by the dermatopathologist. Certainly, the vast majority of biopsies that show the changes described above do not represent chronic superficial dermatitis. Delayed-type hypersensitivity reactions are more commonly associated with these histologic appearances. Many other diseases similarly cause such non-specific biopsy findings, including viral exanthems and drug eruptions. Therefore, clinical correlation is necessary to establish the diagnosis.

The main clinical differential diagnosis is with mycosis fungoides and, accordingly, most biopsies are obtained to exclude this possibility. The patches in chronic superficial dermatitis tend to be uniform in size, shape, and color, contrasting vividly with the greater variability of those of mycosis fungoides. The presence of spongiosis favors a diagnosis of chronic superficial dermatitis; however, mycosis fungoides may also be associated with significant spongiosis and this feature does not reliably distinguish these disorders. Diagnostic pointers favoring early mycosis fungoides include the presence of atypical lymphocytes, epidermotropism, and lymphocytes aligned along the basal cell layer of the epidermis ('tagging').

Immunohistochemistry should be viewed with caution. Loss of T-cell expression may support a diagnosis of mycosis fungoides provided there are histologic features in favor of the diagnosis and if the clinical context is appropriate. Loss of CD7 expression, however, may be seen in reactive conditions and this feature is therefore not reliable. Occasionally, only careful review of the clinical information, taken in conjunction with the histologic features of previous biopsies (if available) allows for definitive diagnosis. It is important to note that some investigators have demonstrated cases of chronic superficial dermatitis with clonal T-cell gene rearrangements by polymerase chain reaction (PCR).[4] One case with a clonal T-cell population resolved, underscoring the growing appreciation that clonality and malignancy are not necessarily synonymous.[4] Therefore, it appears that demonstration of a clonal T-cell population may not suffice to reliably distinguish chronic superficial dermatosis from early mycosis fungoides in all cases. In the past, others have concluded that chronic superficial dermatitis is mycosis fungoides.[5] The observation that chronic superficial dermatitis rarely, if ever, evolves into (or declares itself as) frank mycosis fungoides has led some authors to cast doubt on this view.[6] Other publications have asserted that chronic persistent dermatitis does not progress to mycosis fungoides.[7] It is perhaps more likely that some cases of very early mycosis fungoides cannot be reliably distinguished from chronic superficial dermatitis. Recently, clonal T-cell gene rearrangements have been demonstrated in circulating lymphocytes in blood, but not in skin of patients with digitate dermatitis.[8] Clearly, long-term follow-up studies are necessary to

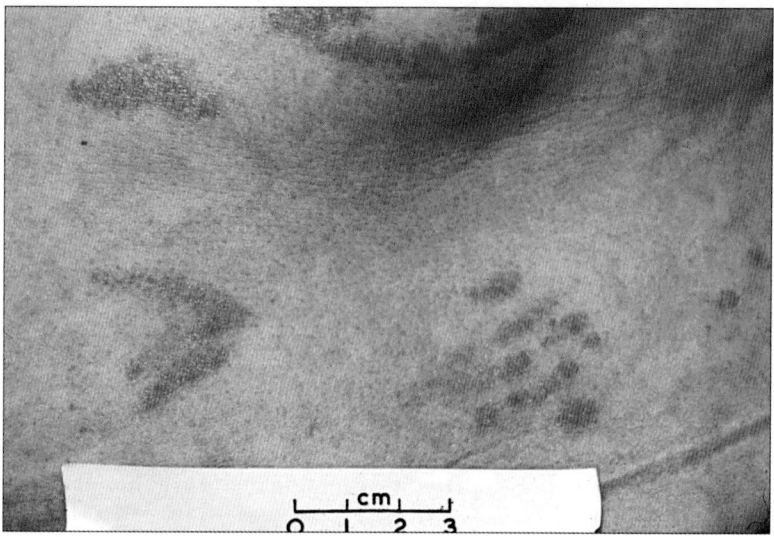

Fig. 8.1
Chronic superficial dermatitis: this patient shows digitate erythematous lesions in a characteristic distribution. By courtesy of the Institute of Dermatology, London, UK.

Fig. 8.3
Chronic superficial dermatitis: closer examination shows that the lesions appear somewhat wrinkled and have a fine scale. By courtesy of R.A. Marsden, MD, St George's Hospital, London, UK.

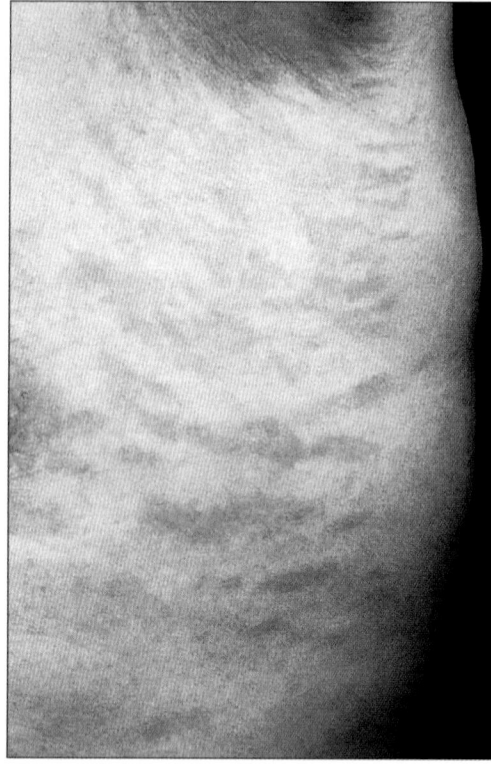

Fig. 8.2
Chronic superficial dermatitis: these uniform, linear lesions had been present for many years. By courtesy of the Institute of Dermatology, London, UK.

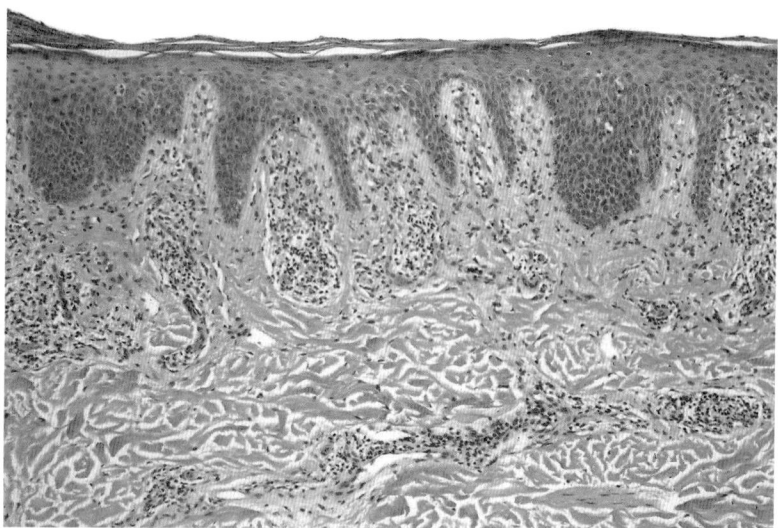

Fig. 8.4
Chronic superficial dermatitis: there is parakeratosis, acanthosis, and a superficial perivascular infiltrate.

resolve the significance of clonality in putative cases of chronic superficial dermatitis.

Pityriasis lichenoides may also be confused with chronic superficial dermatitis. Spongiosis without interface changes favors the latter. Pityriasis lichenoides is associated with either vacuolar or lichenoid interface changes in the absence of spongiosis.[9]

Toxic erythema

Toxic erythema, annular erythema, and gyrate erythema are terms used by dermatologists to describe a number of diseases that share common clinical and histologic appearances. Clinically, the terms imply annular erythematous lesions. Pathologists often also use these same terms (particularly gyrate erythema) in a generic manner to describe an inflammatory lesion with a 'cuffed' perivascular lymphocytic infiltrate. Although such nomenclature may be used as a descriptor (as one might use terms such as 'lichenoid', for example), it should not be taken to imply a specific disease. It is likely that the earlier literature frequently classified different diseases together under these appellations.[1] Therefore, to avoid confusion, it is encouraged that these terms are not used in referring to specific diseases.

Erythema annulare centrifugum

Clinical features

Erythema annulare centrifugum has an incidence of 1 per 100 000 and may be associated with certain underlying factors, including:

- Connective tissue disorders, e.g., Sjögren syndrome,[1,2]
- Drugs, e.g., penicillin, salicylates, amytriptyline, etizolam, gold, sodium thiomoalate, hydroxychloroquine sulfate, piroxicam, finasteride, hydrochlorothiazide and thiacetazone,[3–11]
- Bacterial infections, e.g., *Mycobacteria*, *Streptococcus*, *Escherichia coli*,[12]

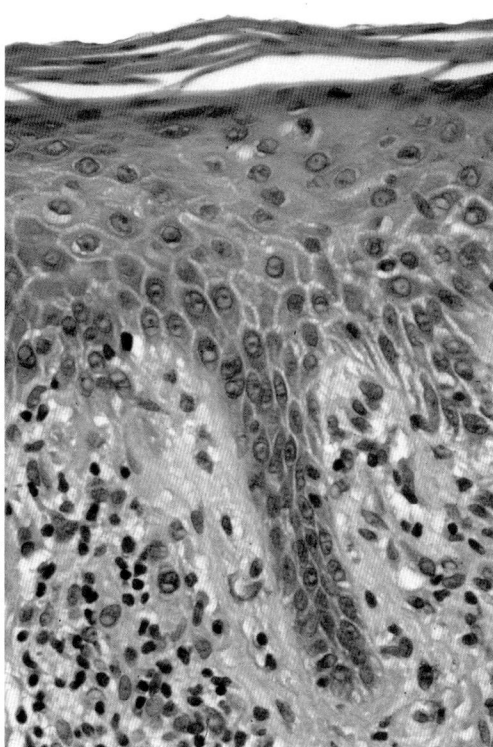

Fig. 8.5
Chronic superficial dermatitis: there is very slight intercellular edema. The infiltrate consists of lymphocytes and histiocytes.

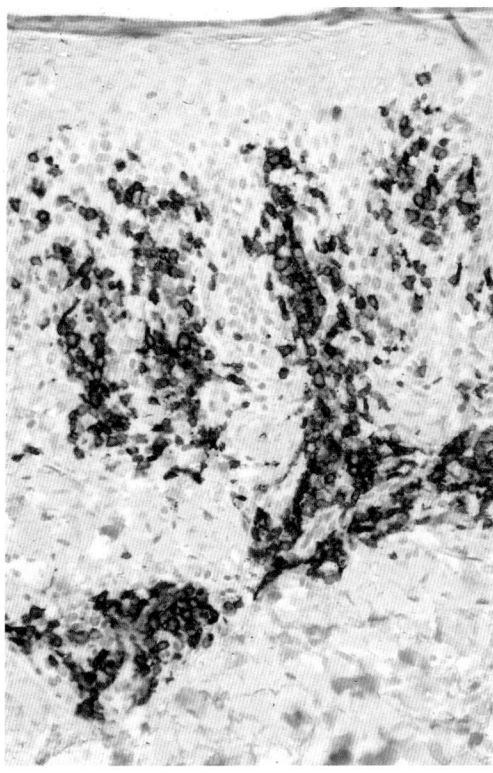

Fig. 8.7
Chronic superficial dermatitis: in this example, there is no significant loss of CD7 expression.

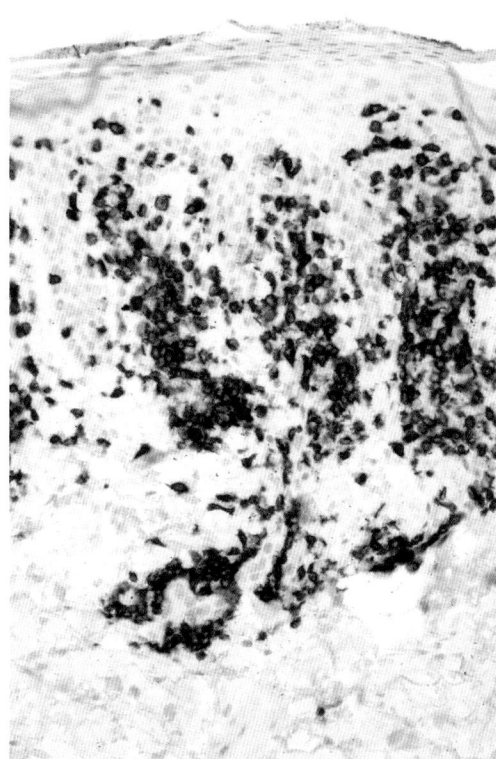

Fig. 8.6
Chronic superficial dermatitis: the infiltrate is composed predominantly of CD4+ T-helper cells.

- Viral infection, e.g., Epstein-Barr virus, HIV, herpes simplex and zoster, molluscum contagiosum,[13–16]
- Fungal infection, e.g., dermatophytoses, *Candida*,[17–20]
- Parasites, e.g., helminthes,[21]
- Arthropods,[22]

- Sarcoidosis,[23]
- Hypereosinophilic syndrome,[24]
- Bullous dermatosis, e.g., linear IgA dermatosis,[25,26]
- Autoimmune disease, e.g., polyglandular autoimmune disease type 1 as well as autoimmune progesterone dermatitis and autoimmune hepatitis,[27–29]
- Pregnancy.[20,30,31]

Many of these associations are likely to be coincidental and, in most cases, no underlying etiology is identified.[32–36] It is unclear whether erythema annulare centrifugum is a distinctive entity or simply represents the clinical expression of a number of inflammatory dermatoses, such as hypersensitivity reactions sharing common histologic features.[37]

Mahood and colleagues emphasized that many earlier reports of neoplasia associated with erythema annulare centrifugum are questionable since different subtypes of annular erythemas were often classified together.[32,38,39] However, other reports have documented erythema annulare centrifugum in patients with underlying malignancy, once again raising the issue of an association with neoplasia. Erythema annulare centrifugum in patients with non-small-cell lung carcinoma, carcinoma of breast, colon, and prostate, chronic lymphocytic leukemia, and Hodgkin lymphoma have been reported in the last decade.[14,40–45] In a recent large series, carcinoma was present in 6 of 66 (13%) patients.[46] Of these, two had leukemia (acute myelogenous and acute lymphoblastic); one patient had non-Hodgkin lymphoma; and three cases were associated with carcinoma (lung, rectal, and hepatocellular).[46]

Erythema annulare centrifugum has been reported in all age groups, including infants and neonates, but is most commonly seen in young adults.[47,48] A large series found that the lower extremities, particularly the thighs, were the most frequent site of involvement.[46] Nearly 50% of patients in this series had lower extremity involvement. The trunk was affected in 28% of patients and the upper extremity in 16%. The hands, feet, and face are usually spared. Head and neck involvement was seen in only 8% of patients. Laboratory investigation sometimes reveals a peripheral eosinophilia.[32] Although individual lesions persist for weeks to a few months before resolving, a course of relapses and remissions over months to years is common and an annually and seasonally recurring form has been reported.[49]

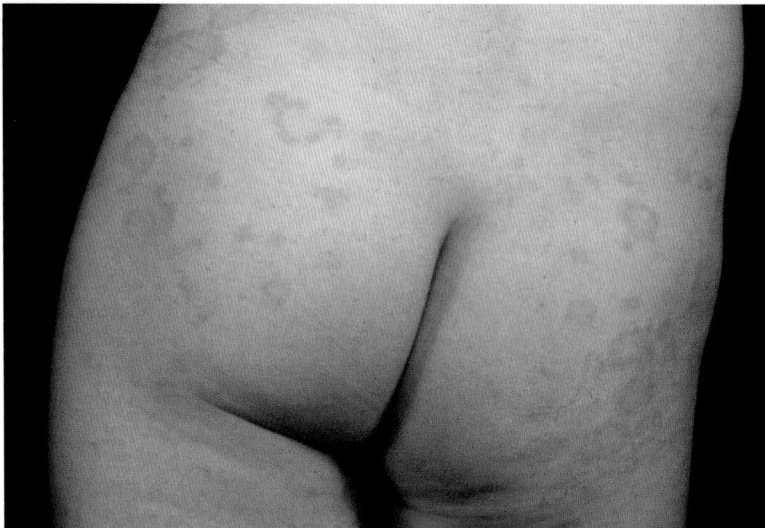

Fig. 8.8
Erythema annulare centrifugum: bilateral annular lesions are present on the buttocks. From the collection of the late N.P. Smith, MD, the Institute of Dermatology, London, UK.

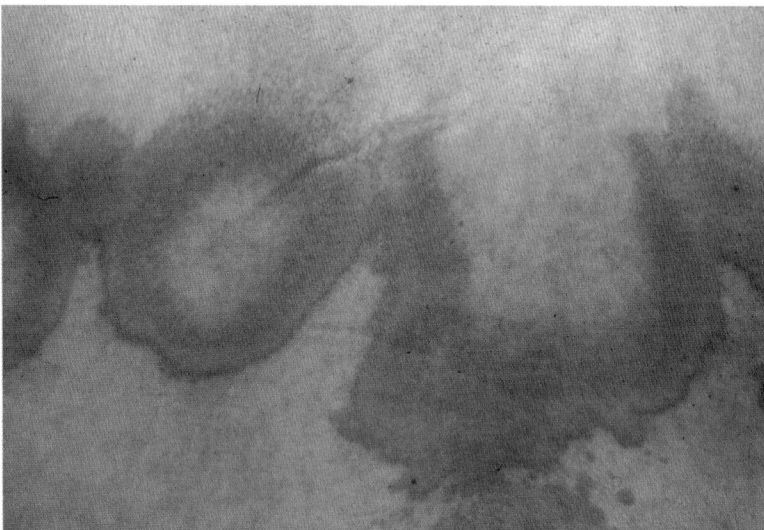

Fig. 8.9
Erythema annulare centrifugum: close-up view. From the collection of the late N.P. Smith, MD, the Institute of Dermatology, London, UK.

Kim et al. found that lesions lasted from 3 days to 18 years with a mean duration of 2.8 years.[46]

The lesions take the form of annular erythematous bands, which may spread outwards or remain stationary (*Figs 8.8* and *8.9*). They are well circumscribed with raised edges, and slight scaling that tends to trail behind the advancing margin.[50] With time, central clearing is seen. Arcuate and polycyclic variants are therefore occasionally evident.[32] Lesions may be mildly pruritic. Vesiculation is rare.[33]

Some authors have divided the disease into two distinct subtypes: superficial and deep gyrate erythema.[46]

- The superficial variant is associated with pruritus and has a trailing scale.
- The deep variant is characterized by erythematous annular lesions with indurated borders but lacking a scale.

An eosinophilic variant of annular erythema has been described.[51–53] It is not clear as to whether this entity represents a variant of Wells syndrome.

Histologic features

A spectrum of non-specific histologic findings is seen in erythema annulare centrifugum. As noted above, deep and superficial variants are recognized.[46]

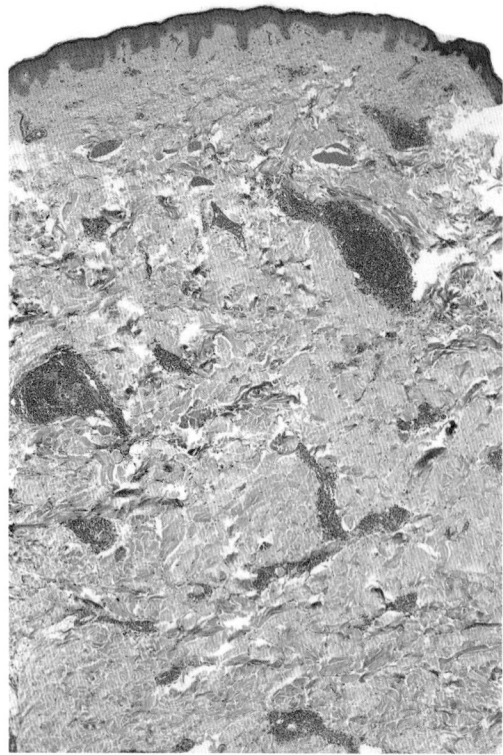

Fig. 8.10
Erythema annulare centrifugum: the superficial and deep vasculature is surrounded by a dense infiltrate.

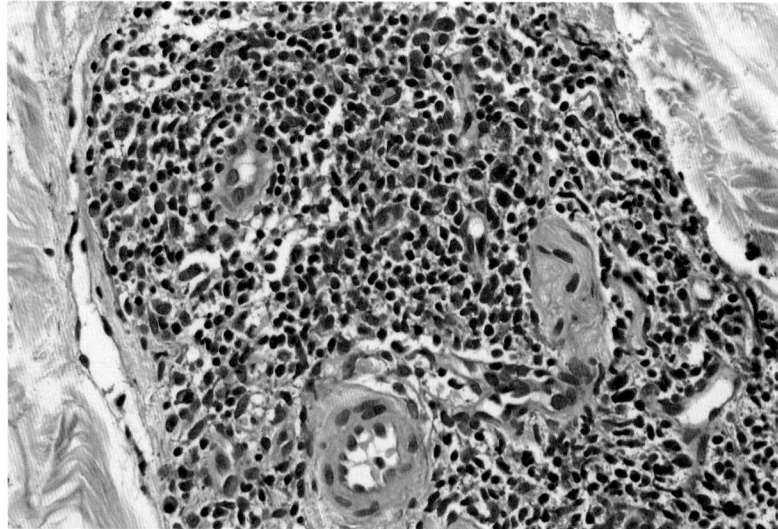

Fig. 8.11
Erythema annulare centrifugum: the infiltrate is composed of mature lymphocytes and histiocytes.

In the superficial variant, a well-demarcated perivascular infiltrate of lymphocytes and histiocytes, often described as having a 'coat sleeve' or 'pipe-stem' appearance, is confined to the superficial dermis (*Figs 8.10* and *8.11*). The overlying epidermis often may be normal; however, epidermal changes, including mild spongiosis, slight and focal basal layer vacuolar degeneration, mounds of parakeratosis or hyperkeratosis are encountered in approximately 50% of patients.[14,46]

In the deep subtype of erythema annulare centrifugum, the perivascular infiltrate involves both the superficial and deep plexuses.[14,33–35,46] Epidermal changes are usually absent or minimal.

In both variants, the degree of inflammation is variable; however, the density of inflammation tends to be greater in the deep variant. The vast majority of cells are lymphocytes; however, a minor component of histiocytes and eosinophils may be seen.

In the eosinophilic variant of annular erythema, the dermal inflammatory infiltrate is mainly composed of eosinophils and flame figure formation may be seen.[51–53]

Differential diagnosis

Given that the histologic features of erythema annulare centrifugum are not distinctive, it is critical to correlate the biopsy and clinical findings. Clinical information is necessary to distinguish this disorder from other gyrate erythemas, pityriasis rosea, hypersensitivity reactions, lupus erythematosus, viral exanthemata, and Jessner lymphocytic infiltrate. In cases with significant epidermal changes, a PAS/silver stain to exclude a fungal infection is also advised. Clinically, erythema annulare centrifugum may resemble psoriasis. The presence of parakeratotic mounds associated with neutrophils would favor a diagnosis of psoriasis. In contrast to cutaneous lupus erythematosus, interface changes are not usually well developed and immunofluorescence studies are negative. Erythema chronicum migrans also enters the differential diagnosis. The presence of plasma cells and often also eosinophils would be in favor of the latter condition. Histochemical stains for spirochetes may be positive, but are cumbersome and difficult to interpret. PCR is a more reliable and easy test to confirm the diagnosis.

Erythema gyratum repens

Clinical features

Erythema gyratum repens (L. *repens*, to crawl or creep) is an extremely rare and clinically distinctive figurate eruption mainly associated with an underlying malignancy (70%).[1] The most commonly associated neoplasm is carcinoma of the lung; other affiliated tumors include carcinoma of the uterus and cervix, esophagus, stomach, kidney, and breast as well as essential thrombocythemia.[2–12] Treatment of the cancer may be associated with remission of the cutaneous eruption, while tumor recurrence or metastases can be accompanied by a relapse.[3] Rarely, the condition develops in the absence of an underlying malignancy.[13–18] It may disclose underlying pulmonary tuberculosis. In one patient with no evidence of malignancy, the rash resolved a few days after removal of a cavitary tuberculoid lung lesion.[15]

Ichthyosis may accompany erythema gyratum repens.[19] A report of a patient with transitional cell carcinoma of the kidney who developed erythema gyratum repens and ichthyosis comes as no surprise since both conditions are associated with malignancy. The combination of ichthyosis, palmoplantar keratosis, and erythema gyratum repens, in the absence of malignancy, has also been reported.[20]

Erythema gyratum repens-like eruptions have also been described in the presence of connective tissue diseases. Typical erythema gyratum repens developed in a patient with cutaneous subacute lupus erythematosus following hydroxychloroquine treatment.[21,22] The authors of this report concluded that the patient's rash represented a peculiar pattern of involvement by subacute lupus, which they designated subacute lupus gyratum repens. An erythema gyratum repens-like eruption has also been described in association with Sjögren syndrome, neutrophilic dermatosis, leukocytoclastic vasculitis, in patients with lupus erythematosus, and in the setting of urticarial vasculitis.[23–26]

Caputo et al. reported linear IgA dermatosis, erythema, and an eruption resembling erythema gyratum repens, in a patient without malignancy.[27] Bullous pemphigoid may be associated with erythema gyratum repens and an erythema gyratum repens-like eruption has been documented in a patient with treated and resolving psoriasis and with epidermolysis bullosa acquisita accompanied by ulcerative colitis.[28–32]

Erythema gyratum repens has been described in patients with hypereosinophilic syndrome, also with no evidence of neoplasia.[33]

The eruption, which may precede the malignancy by months, takes the form of concentric bands of erythema in an annular or gyrate arrangement (*Figs 8.12* and *8.13*). These bands have been described as having a 'timber grain' or 'zebra-like' pattern and they move (up to about 1 cm) daily.[34] Scaling occurs and there may be pruritus. Lesions often commence on the

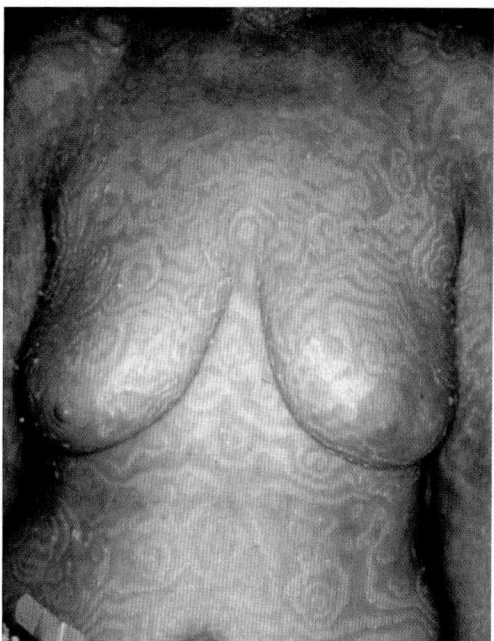

Fig. 8.12
Erythema gyratum repens: the presence of annular erythematous parallel bands with scaling is characteristic. From the collection of the late N.P. Smith, MD, the Institute of Dermatology, London, UK.

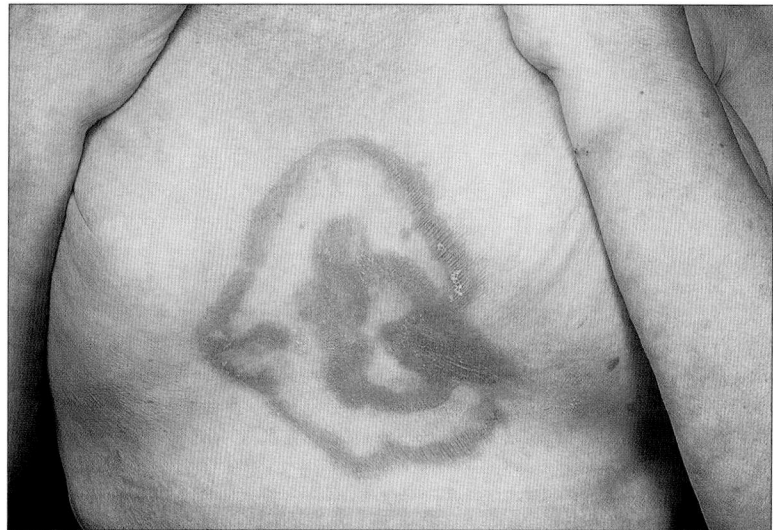

Fig. 8.13
Erythema gyratum repens: the eruption may sometimes have a bizarre appearance. By courtesy of R. Cerio, MD, The London Hospital, London, UK.

arms and legs, but frequently become generalized.[2] The hands, feet, and face are usually spared.[34] Postinflammatory hyperpigmentation may be a feature.[2] Hyperkeratosis of the palms and soles is also sometimes present.[4,13] Males are affected twice as commonly as females.[4] Patients are usually in their seventh decade.[21]

Pathogenesis and histologic features

Erythema gyratum repens may have an immunological pathogenesis, since granular deposits of IgG and C3 have been found at the basement membrane zone of both involved and uninvolved skin in a patient with associated bronchial carcinoma and in involved non-sun-exposed skin in another unassociated with neoplasia.[17,35–37] In a separate patient, although basement membrane zone immunofluorescence was negative, epidermal nuclear labeling was identified.[38] Caux et al. reported one patient with squamous cell carcinoma of the lung who had immunoreactants at the basement membrane of involved and normal non-sun-exposed skin. In addition, this patient showed

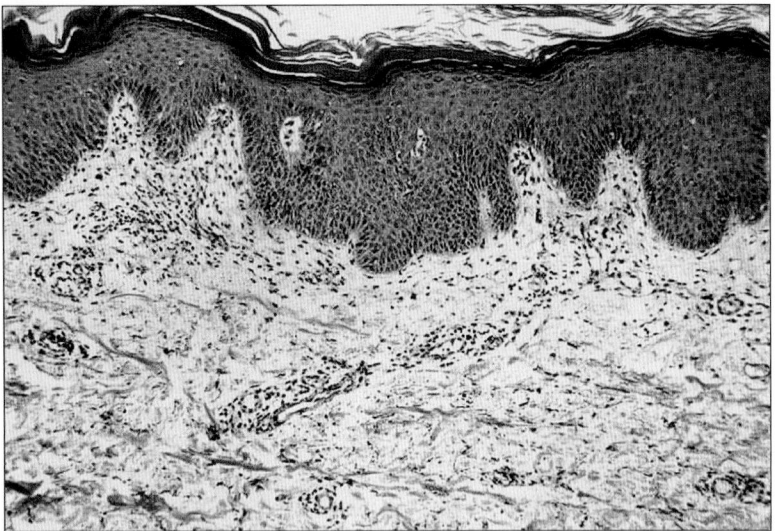

Fig. 8.14
Erythema gyratum repens: there is hyperkeratosis, acanthosis and a mild perivascular chronic inflammatory cell infiltrate.

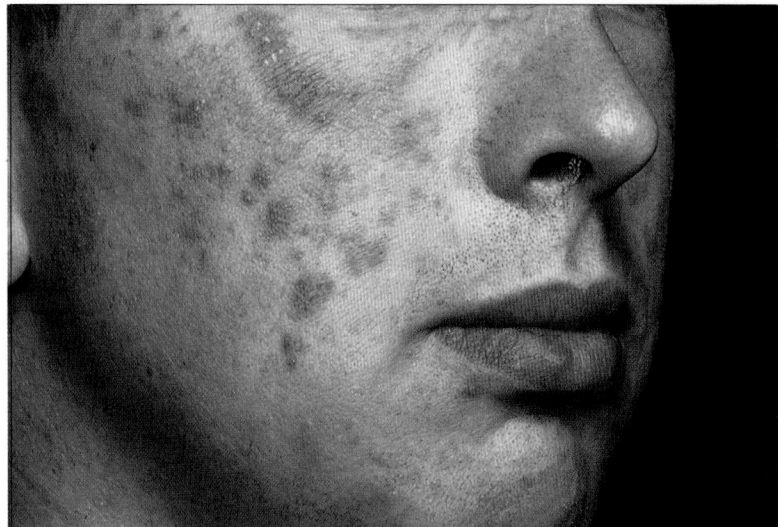

Fig. 8.16
Jessner lymphocytic infiltrate: there are multiple erythematous plaques on this young man's cheek. By courtesy of the Institute of Dermatology, London, UK.

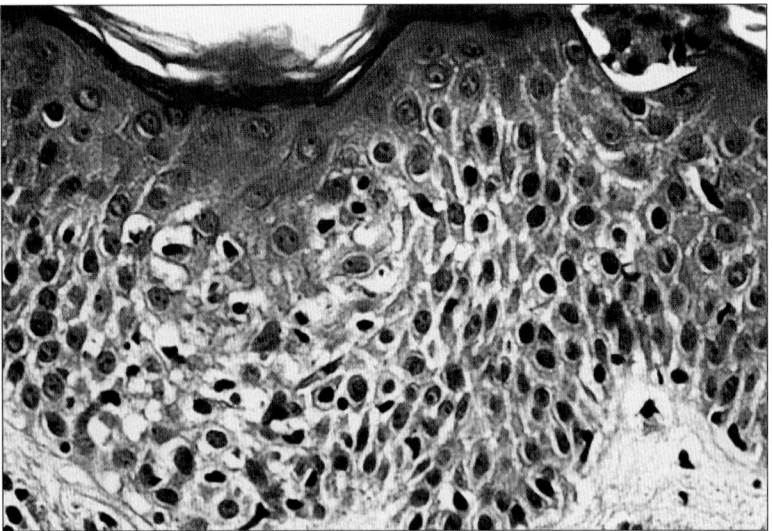

Fig. 8.15
Erythema gyratum repens: spongiosis is present.

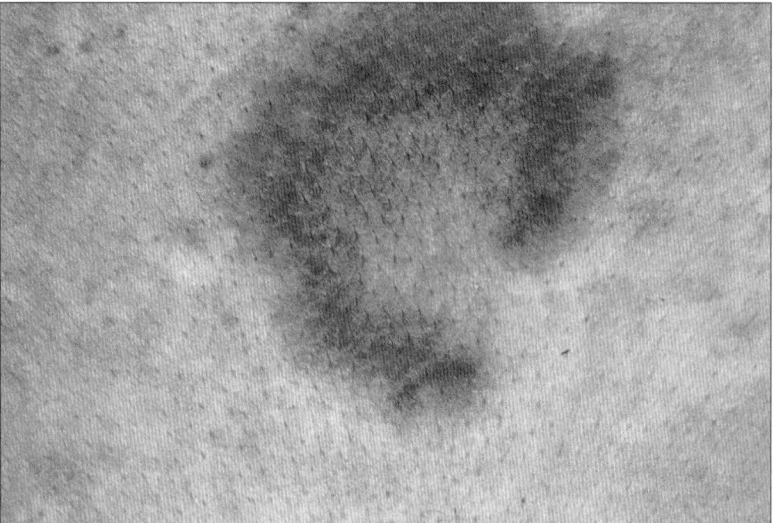

Fig. 8.17
Jessner lymphocytic infiltrate: central clearing has resulted in this circinate lesion. By courtesy of the Institute of Dermatology, London, UK.

staining of IgG, IgM, and C3 along the basement membrane of the bronchus.[36] However, the immunoreactants did not localize to the tumor.

The appearances in erythema gyratum repens are not diagnostic. They include hyperkeratosis, parakeratosis, acanthosis, and spongiosis, together with a superficial perivascular lymphohistiocytic infiltrate in the papillary dermis (*Figs 8.14* and *8.15*).[3]

Differential diagnosis

As noted above, the histologic features are non-specific and vary from patient to patient. Fortunately, the clinical features are so distinctive that confusion with other disorders is unlikely. Obviously, any patient with features of erythema gyratum repens should be very carefully evaluated for an underlying neoplasm.

Lymphocytic infiltrate of the skin (Jessner)

Clinical features

Jessner lymphocytic infiltrate of the skin is an uncommon dermatosis of unknown etiology, although a relationship with sun exposure, at least in the early stages, has been documented.[1] Lesions, which may be single or more often multiple, occur most often on the face, neck, back, and upper chest,

and present as 1–2-cm diameter, asymptomatic, discoid or annular, erythematous or brownish papules or plaques that often show central clearing to produce circinate lesions (*Figs 8.16* and *8.17*).[1-4] Familial cases have occasionally been documented.[5-8]

In contrast to discoid lupus erythematosus, with which it is sometimes confused, there is no hyperkeratosis, telangiectases or follicular plugging, and scarring is not a feature. Rarely, however, the two diseases appear to coexist.[1] The disease tends to affect adults, particularly in the third to fifth decades. Although some authors have found a predilection for males, 54% of patients in a large series were female and the overall gender distribution appears to be equal.[1,3] Rarely, the condition presents in children.[9-11] Lesions often resolve within weeks or months, but relapses are not uncommon and, in many patients, the disorder persists for years. The eruption is not characterized by seasonal variation. The evidence available suggests that lymphocytic infiltrate of the skin is a distinctive dermatosis. However, there is no universal consensus regarding this, and an association with lupus erythematosus has been suggested.

Pathogenesis and histologic features

The etiology of this curious condition is unknown. Although some patients notice a relationship with sun exposure, others do not, and lesions not uncommonly develop on covered sites.

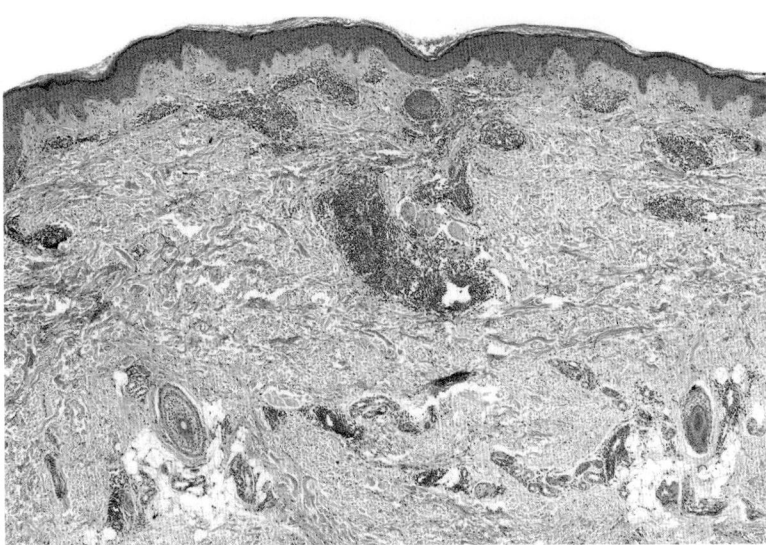

Fig. 8.18
Lymphocytic infiltrate of Jessner: a heavy chronic inflammatory cell infiltrate cuffs the vessels in the superficial and mid dermis.

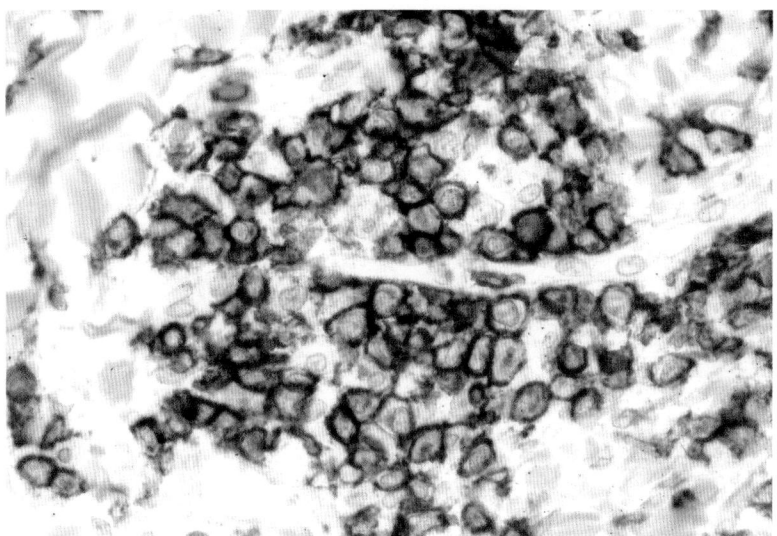

Fig. 8.20
Lymphocytic infiltrate of Jessner: the majority of lymphocytes express CD4 (T-helper cells).

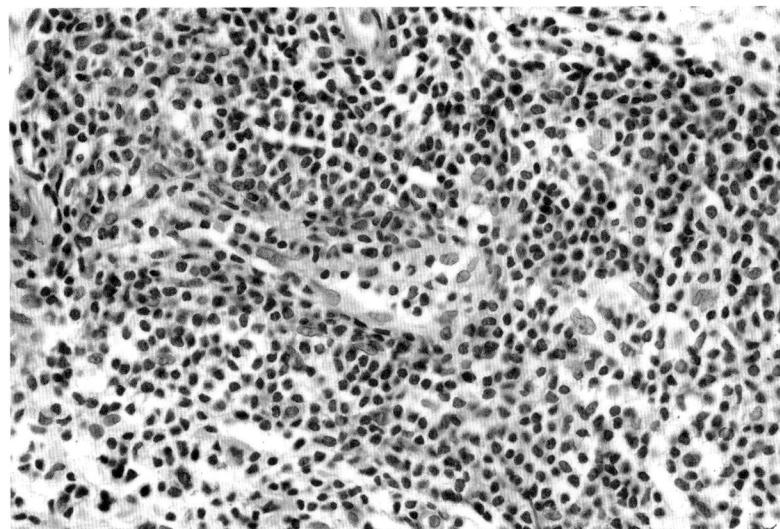

Fig. 8.19
Lymphocytic infiltrate of Jessner: the infiltrate is composed almost entirely of small lymphocytes.

Braddock and coauthors found that natural killer cell lytic activity and antibody-dependent cell-mediated cytotoxicity was decreased.[10] This same group identified increased levels of circulating immune complexes in patients with lymphocytic infiltrate of skin. In two patients, immune complexes decreased to normal levels following treatment, but became elevated during recurrence of disease following treatment.[10,11] Based on these observations, these investigators concluded that immune defects might be important in the pathogenesis of Jessner lymphocytic infiltrate. Of interest, similar findings have been observed in patients with reticular erythematous mucinosis. Clearly, further study is necessary to determine the pathogenesis of this disease.

The epidermis is typically unaffected. Within the superficial and mid dermis is a perivascular and, much less commonly, a perifollicular infiltrate of mature lymphocytes (*Figs 8.18* and *8.19*). Occasional histiocytes and scattered plasma cells may also be present and sometimes there is an increase in dermal ground substance.[12] Lymphoid follicles are not a feature.

The infiltrate consists predominantly of T cells, most often of the CD4+ helper subtype (*Fig. 8.20*). Occasionally, however, CD8+ suppressor T cells constitute the majority of cells.[3,13–16] Leu 8 is commonly expressed but human leukocyte antigen (HLA)-DR is not present. B cells are relatively sparse in number or are absent.

Differential diagnosis

Lymphocytic infiltrate of the skin differs from discoid lupus erythematosus by the absence of epidermal changes, scarring, and a negative lupus band test. Immunohistochemistry may sometimes be helpful. The infiltrate in lymphocytic infiltrate is HLA-DR negative in contrast to discoid lupus erythematosus in which the lymphocytes and often the keratinocytes are HLA-DR positive.[17] Leu 8 (immunoregulatory T-cell) expression is also more frequently seen in lymphocytic infiltrate.[13,18] In one study, the average percentage of Leu 8 positive lymphocytes was 65% in lymphocytic infiltrate of skin and only 15% in discoid lupus erythematosus.[18] The presence of CD20+ B cells favors lupus erythematosus, which tends to be composed of a mixture of B and T cells. In contrast, T cells predominate in lymphocytic infiltrate of skin.[14,19,20] One group of investigators has suggested that the presence of plasmacytoid monocytes favors a diagnosis of lymphocytic infiltrate of skin over lupus erythematosus. They found plasmacytoid monocytes to be present in 58% of patients with lymphocytic infiltrate of skin, but in only 7% of patients with discoid lupus erythematosus.[21] Others, however, have not been able to corroborate this finding.[19] The presence of significant dermal mucin would support lupus erythematosus. Reliable distinction between lymphocytic infiltrate of the skin and tumid lupus erythematosus may be difficult and frequently impossible since lymphocytic infiltrate may sometimes be accompanied by excess dermal mucin. It has therefore been speculated that these entities represent a continuous disease spectrum rather than different diseases.[22] The finding that a subset of patients with lymphocytic infiltrate of the skin also had a confirmed diagnosis of lupus erythematosus led one group to speculate whether lymphocytic infiltrate of the skin could represent a variant of lupus erythematosus.[4]

Epidermal Langerhans cells are often increased in lymphocytic infiltrate whereas they are frequently reduced in number in discoid lupus erythematosus.[13]

Lymphocytic infiltrate may often be distinguished from chronic lymphocytic leukemia/lymphocytic lymphoma by careful evaluation of cellular morphology. The benign lymphocytic infiltrate is composed of non-neoplastic lymphocytes with small, regular, and hyperchromatic nuclei. In chronic lymphocytic leukemia/lymphocytic lymphoma the nuclei are larger, irregular, and paler staining, and a nucleolus may be visible. Regardless of these subtle cytological differences, if the possibility of low-grade lymphoma exists, immunohistochemical studies should be performed. Most often, well-differentiated lymphomas are of B-cell lineage.

Lymphocytic infiltrate is usually histologically indistinguishable from polymorphous light eruption, although early lesions of the latter may show edema of the papillary dermis. It should be noted, however, that sometimes the two conditions may coexist. In cases where the diagnosis is in doubt, phototesting may be necessary. One group of investigators has found the presence of plasmacytoid monocytes to favor lymphocytic infiltrate of the skin over polymorphous light eruption.[21] However, this has not been confirmed (see above).

Histologically, lymphocytic infiltration of Jessner also shows some overlap with reticular erythematous mucinosis. Mucin deposition, however, is not generally a feature of lymphocytic infiltrate of the skin, although it may be evident. Furthermore, the inflammatory cell infiltrate in reticular erythematous mucinosis is usually mild.

Reticular erythematous mucinosis

Clinical features

This rare chronic dermatosis, which shows a female predominance (2:1), has been described worldwide.[1-3] Although it may affect a wide age range, it most frequently develops in the second to fourth decades.[2-4] Rarely, it is encountered in children.[4] Familial presentation is exceptional.[5] It usually presents as a persistent, reticulate, urticated, macular, and sometimes papular, erythema with an irregular, but well-defined border. The lesions typically occur on the central chest and upper back (*Figs 8.21–8.23*).[6-8] Less commonly, they can be found on the face, arms, abdomen, and groins, but the peripheries are spared.[1,9,10] Patients frequently notice an exacerbation in the sun, but the relationship between sunlight and the disease (if any) is not well understood.[4,8-13] Although patients are usually asymptomatic, some report pruritus or burning following exposure to sunlight. There is no evidence of systemic involvement.

Occasional patients have more infiltrated papules and plaques; this was originally described as plaquelike cutaneous mucinosis, but is now accepted as a variant of reticular erythematous mucinosis.[14-16] Of particular interest, the plaquelike form of the disease has been documented in association with carcinoma of the breast and colon and one patient suffered from essential thrombocytosis in addition to carcinoma of the lung.[15-17]

Patients with this condition have an increased risk of concomitant autoimmune disease in around 50% of cases, including thyroid disease (Hashimoto disease and hyperthyroidism), arthritis (psoriatic and rheumatoid), ulcerative colitis, and diabetes mellitus.[2-4,15,18]

Reticular erythematous mucinosis in patients with human immunodeficiency virus (HIV) infection has also been documented.[19,20] Of interest, other cutaneous mucinoses that have been described in association with HIV infection include scleredema and lichen myxedematosus.[20] Furthermore, deposition of mucin in the bone marrow of patients with acquired immunodeficiency syndrome (AIDS) is a common finding.[21] The pathogenetic

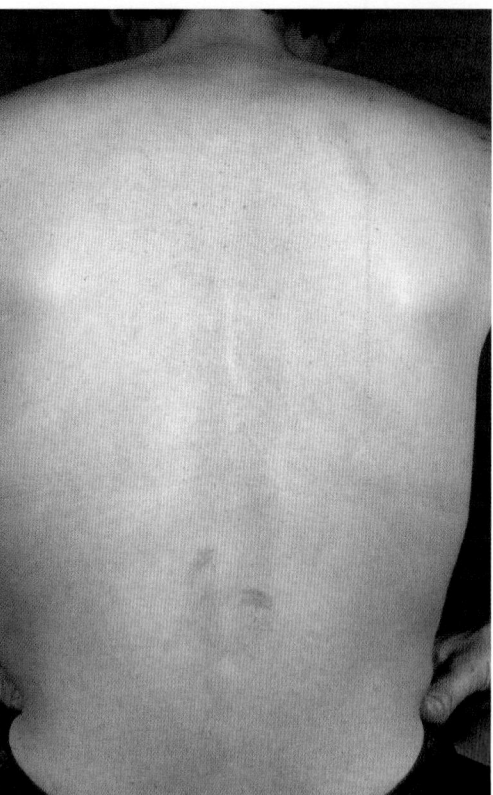

Fig. 8.22
Reticular erythematous mucinosis: location in the lower back is unusual. From the collection of the late N.P. Smith, MD, the Institute of Dermatology, London, UK.

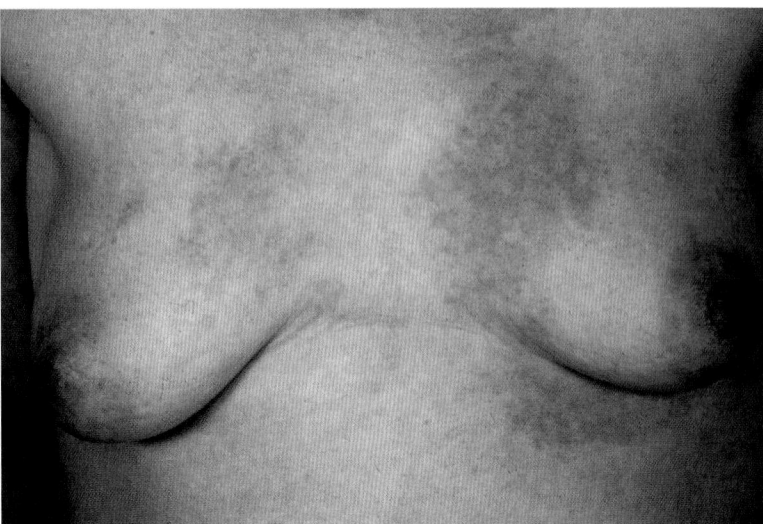

Fig. 8.21
Reticular erythematous mucinosis: erythematous reticular eruption in a characteristic distribution in a young woman. By courtesy of the Institute of Dermatology, London, UK.

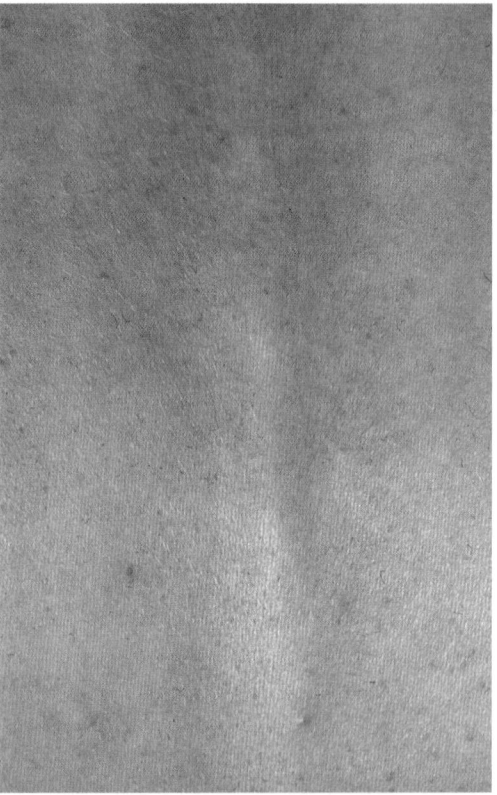

Fig. 8.23
Reticular erythematous mucinosis: closer view of previous figure. Macular elements predominate. From the collection of the late N.P. Smith, MD, the Institute of Dermatology, London, UK.

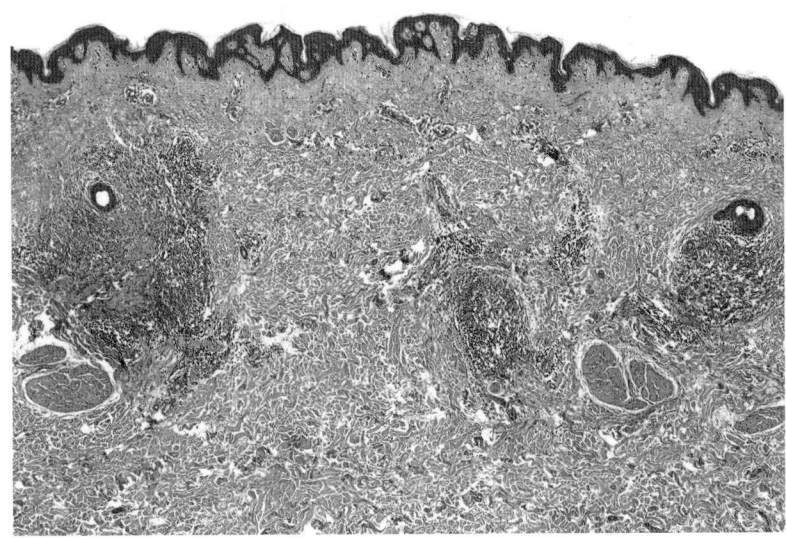

Fig. 8.24
Reticular erythematous mucinosis: there is a perifollicular and perivascular infiltrate in the upper and mid dermis.

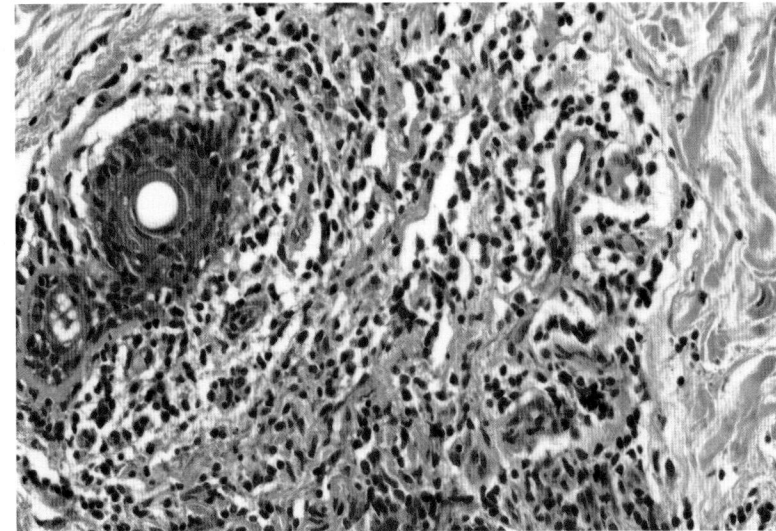

Fig. 8.25
Reticular erythematous mucinosis: the infiltrate consists of mature lymphocytes with a lesser number of histiocytes.

relationship between these various forms of mucin deposition, if any, has not been defined. It is, of course, tempting to postulate that they are related, but data to support such a conclusion are not yet established.

The presence of monoclonal IgG (kappa) paraproteinemia has been reported in one patient.[22]

Pathogenesis and histologic features

The pathogenesis of reticular erythematous mucinosis is not well understood. Phototoxicity likely plays some role in the disease, either directly or indirectly. Braddock and coauthors found that natural killer cell lytic activity and antibody-dependent cell-mediated cytotoxicity were decreased.[23] This same group found increased levels of circulating immune complexes. Of interest, two patients were observed to have circulating immune complexes that decreased with treatment only to become elevated during recurrence of disease following treatment.[23] Based on these observations, the investigators concluded that immune defects may be of importance in the pathogenesis. Of interest, similar findings have been observed in patients with Jessner lymphocytic infiltrate (see above). Clearly, further study is necessary regarding the precise pathogenetic basis of this disease.

The epidermis may be slightly flattened or appear normal. Within the dermis there is moderate vascular dilatation associated with a marked mononuclear perivascular and often perifollicular infiltrate composed mainly of T-helper lymphocytes (Figs 8.24 and 8.25).[8,15,23–26] Excess mucin (predominantly hyaluronic acid) is usually present in the upper dermis, but in more chronic lesions it is sometimes absent (Fig. 8.26). The mucin stains positively with Alcian blue (pH 2.5) and colloidal iron, but is usually not metachromatic with toluidine blue. The collagen fibers are separated, but appear morphologically normal. Fragmentation of elastic fibers is sometimes a feature.[9] There is no evidence of fibroblastic proliferation, but increased numbers of factor XIIIa-positive dermal dendrocytes have been identified by immunohistochemistry.[27]

A few cases with positive direct immunofluorescence have been reported. IgM-reactive papillary dermal cytoid bodies were documented in one case.[23] Rare examples show staining for IgM along the dermal–epidermal junction.[4,12,28] The significance of these findings is unclear, but may be further evidence of an immunological basis for the pathogenesis of this condition.[27]

Ultrastructural studies are largely unhelpful. Other than demonstrating conspicuous and dilated rough endoplasmic reticulum within dermal fibroblasts, electron microscopy merely serves to confirm the light microscopic observation of widely separated fascicles of collagen fibers.[24] A number of reports identified tubuloreticular structures within the cytoplasm of endothelial cells.[9,29,30] Although at one time these were thought to represent paramyxoviruses, other studies suggest that they may be derived from infolded endoplasmic reticulum. They have also been identified in pretibial

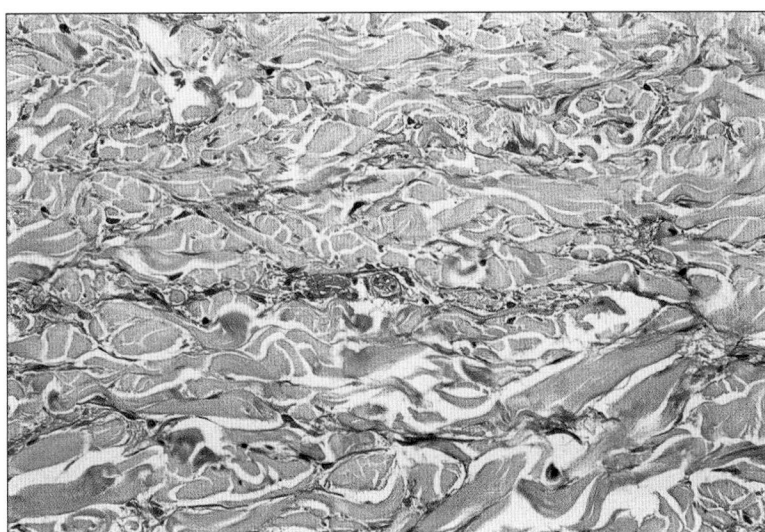

Fig. 8.26
Reticular erythematous mucinosis: increased dermal mucin (hyaluronic acid) separates the collagen fibers (Alcian blue stain).

myxedema, lupus erythematosus, dermatomyositis, malignant atrophic papulosis, and various lymphomas.[31]

Differential diagnosis

The principal clinical and pathological differential diagnoses include lupus erythematosus and polymorphous light eruption. Distinguishing between lupus erythematosus and reticular erythematous mucinosis may be very difficult, particularly as one condition may evolve into the other.[32] Histologically, reticular erythematous mucinosis lacks the epidermal changes of lupus erythematosus and the immunofluorescent findings are usually, but not always, negative.[9–11] As noted above, there are a few reports in which granular immunoglobulin deposition at the dermal–epidermal junction has been identified.[4,12,28] The presence of several immunoreactants favors a diagnosis of lupus erythematosus. Clinical and serological studies are also necessary to establish a diagnosis of lupus erythematosus.

In polymorphous light eruption, mucin deposition is much less striking and is limited to the papillary dermis.[33] Perifollicular inflammation is not a feature of polymorphous light eruption. In addition, epidermal changes of spongiosis – sometimes with vesiculation in papular and eczematous lesions and mild basal-cell hydropic change in the plaque variant – serve as further distinguishing features.[34] Polymorphous light eruption resolves once exposure to sunlight has ceased, in contrast to reticular erythematous mucinosis where the lesions persist.

Histologically, reticular erythematous mucinosis also shows some overlap with lymphocytic infiltrate of Jessner.[4] Mucin deposition, however, is not generally a feature of the latter condition and the inflammatory cell infiltrate is always more prominent.

Polymorphous light eruption (including juvenile spring eruption and lambing ears)

Clinical features

Polymorphous (polymorphic) light eruption, which is the most common photodermatosis, usually presents in young people as recurrent erythematous papules, vesicles, and/or plaques following exposure to ultraviolet (UV) light (*Figs 8.27* and *8.28*).[1–6] The face, chest, upper back, and extremities are the most common sites of involvement.[5] Most patients have multiple lesions.[5] In one study of 138 patients, the mean age at onset was 26 years.[5] There is a predilection for young women, with 89% of patients

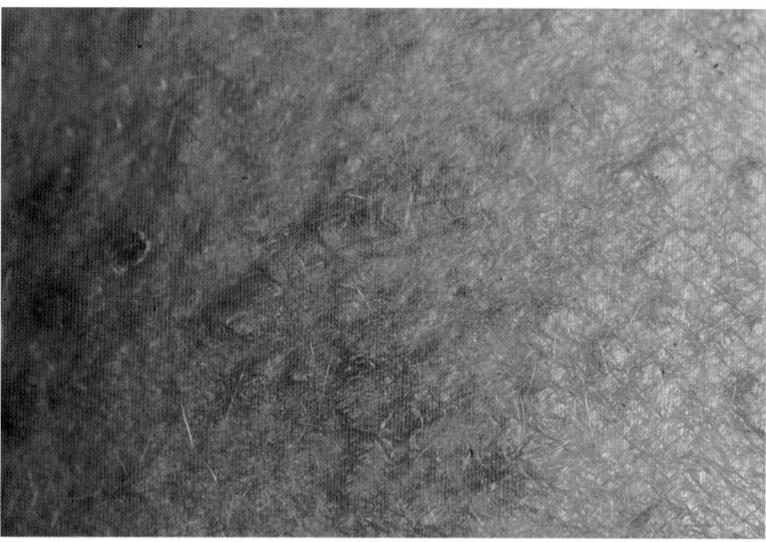

Fig. 8.27
Polymorphous light eruption: patients present with erythematous papules and vesicles on sun-exposed skin. From the collection of the late N.P. Smith, MD, the Institute of Dermatology, London, UK.

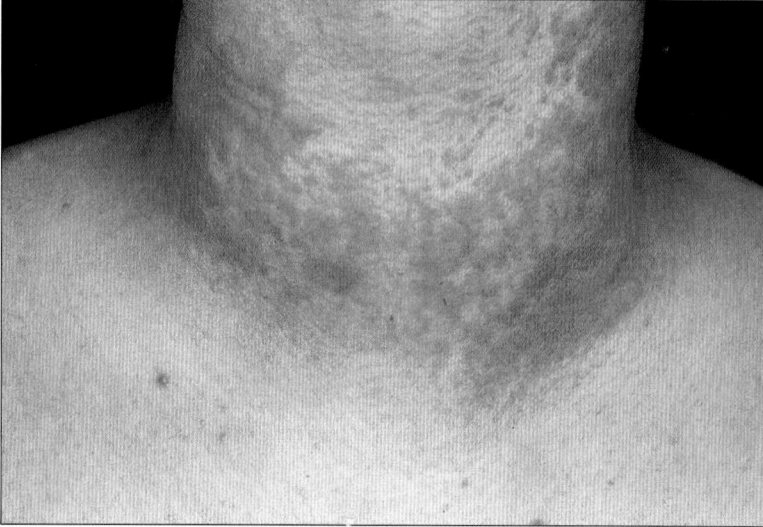

Fig. 8.28
Polymorphous light eruption: the eruption is typically symmetrical and is usually pruritic. By courtesy of the Institute of Dermatology, London, UK.

being female.[7,8] The vast majority of lesions are associated with pruritus. Most patients require less than 30 minutes of sun exposure to elicit clinical features.[5] Onset following light exposure typically takes 18–24 hours. Either the UVA or UVB part of the light spectrum may cause lesions.[2,9] Lesions are caused by UVA light in 56% of cases, UVB in 17%, and both UVA and UVB ranges in 26% of cases.[2] However, some authors have not been able to elicit lesions with UVB light.[4] Exposure resulting in sunburn is not necessary for the development of the condition.[4] Some patients report symptoms resulting from light exposure through glass.[4] Rarely, it is caused by UVC exposure, and the disease has also been observed in welders.[10]

Polymorphous light eruption most often occurs in patients with fair skin; however, dark-skinned individuals can also be affected. The disease is more common in people residing in northern latitudes. One study showed that the prevalence rates for London (UK) and Perth (Australia) were 14.8% and 5.2%, respectively.[11] In a retrospective analysis, however, the incidence of photosensitivity reactions and polymorphous light eruption in particular was found to be roughly comparable for dark-skinned and Caucasian individuals.[12] The pinpoint papular variant of polymorphous light eruption has only recently been recognized and appears to be particularly common on dark skin.[12,13] It is characterized by numerous grouped, small, 1–2-mm papules, which may be accompanied by small vesicles in the acute phase.[14]

It appears that the incidence of polymorphous light eruption is much more common than is demonstrated by contact with healthcare workers. In one survey, 21% of workers in a Swedish pharmaceutical company had symptoms consistent with polymorphous light eruption; however, only 3% had sought medical attention for their symptoms.[7]

Biopsy of experimentally induced lesions shows similar histologic features compared to clinical lesions.[4] Given the role of sun exposure in its pathogenesis, it comes as no surprise that polymorphous light eruption is most often seen in spring and summer.[4] In addition, it is not uncommon for the first sign of disease to manifest during a vacation to southern latitudes. The features, which develop after a latent period of hours to days, commonly subside completely within days and heal without sequelae.[1] However, once the disease is established, persistence for many years is common.[3] Overall, however, there is diminution of light sensitivity over time, but this process often takes years.[3] In a large study, the mean disease duration of the condition was 10.5 years.[5] Patients with a duration of up to 53 years have been studied.[7] The distribution of lesions often changes with time.[5]

One study showed that thyroid disease was present in 14% of patients.[15] This same study found lupus erythematosus in only 2 of 94 patients. The authors concluded that the risk of lupus erythematosus was not increased in patients with polymorphous light eruption. Authors of another study, however, have suggested that a subgroup of patients with polymorphous light eruption may be at an elevated risk for lupus erythematosus.[16]

Juvenile spring eruption appears to be either a variant of polymorphous light eruption or a closely related disorder.[17–22] In one study, the prevalence was 6.7% with a male predominance.[17] The lesions are characterized by erythematous papules and vesicles located on sun-exposed portions of the helix of the ear following light exposure. They tend to be pruritic. Involvement of the elbows has recently been reported.[23] In one study, 4 of 18 patients also had lesions of typical polymorphous light eruption.[18] As its name implies, the lesions tend to occur in the spring. A positive family history is present in some patients.[20] A disorder, clinically and histologically reminiscent of juvenile spring eruption, has also been reported to develop in farmers at the time of lambing and calving. It has been termed 'lambing ears'.[24]

Pathogenesis and histologic features

The pathogenesis of polymorphous light eruption is poorly understood. Study of adhesion molecule expression has led some authors to propose that polymorphous light eruption is immunologically mediated.[25] Specifically, vascular endothelial expression of endothelial leukocyte adhesion molecule-1 (ELAM-1), vascular cell adhesion molecule-1 (VCAM-1), and keratinocyte and endothelial expression of intercellular adhesion molecule-1 (ICAM-1) in biopsies of induced lesions has been documented.[25] The authors noted that their results were similar to those seen in delayed-type hypersensitivity reactions. In addition, reduced skin infiltration by neutrophils following UVB

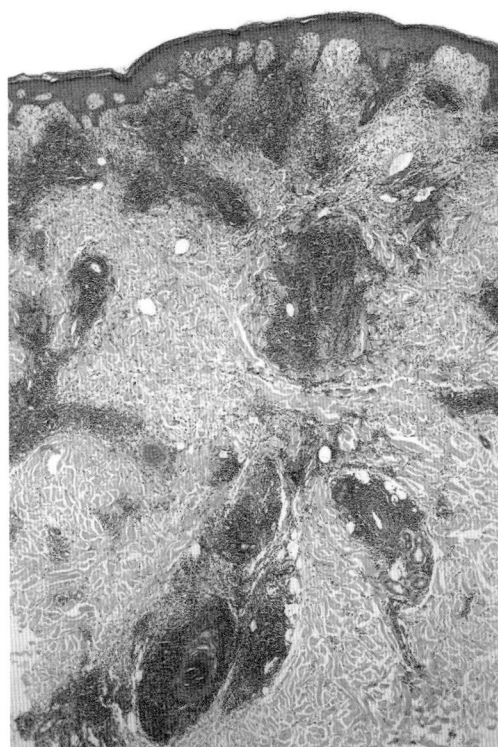

Fig. 8.29
Polymorphous light eruption: there is papillary dermal edema and a dense superficial and deep perivascular inflammatory cell infiltrate.

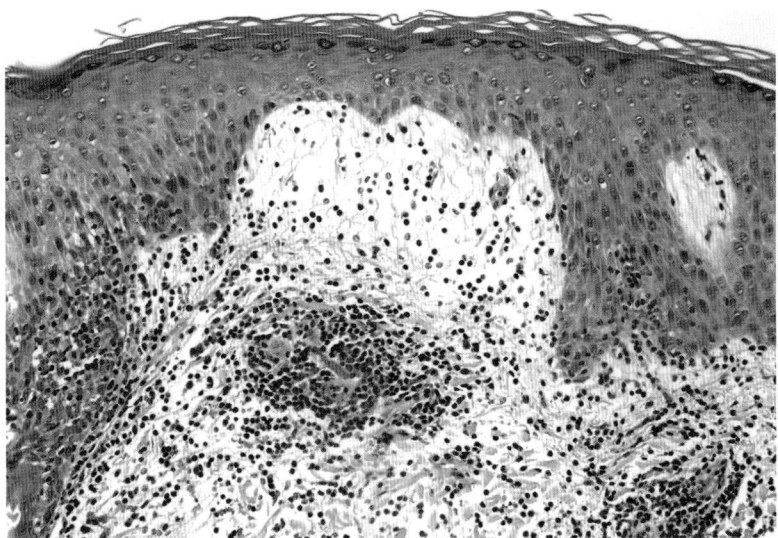

Fig. 8.30
Polymorphous light eruption: incipient subepidermal vesiculation is evident. Note the red cell extravasation and lymphocytic infiltrate.

exposure was noted.[26] However, the triggering antigen(s) are unknown.[25] It appears that polymorphous light eruption may be a heritable disorder. In one study, 46% of patients reported a positive family history.[7]

Histologically, a perivascular lymphohistiocytic infiltrate is present in the superficial and sometimes deep dermis (*Figs 8.29 and 8.30*).[27-29] A characteristic, but not uniformly present, feature is papillary dermal edema, which is often marked. The presence of massive papillary dermal edema may be associated with subepidermal or intradermal vesicle formation.

Papular and papulovesicular lesions may show epidermal acanthosis, spongiosis, occasional dyskeratotic cells, and lymphocyte exocytosis.[27,29] Spongiosis may sometimes become so severe as to lead to intraepidermal vesicle formation.[27] Other authors, however, have not found spongiosis to be a significant feature.[28] Basal cell vacuolization, usually mild, is found in

some cases.[27,29,30] Periadnexal involvement by a chronic inflammatory cell infiltrate may be present in papular and papulovesicular lesions.[27] Some authors have reported increased eosinophils and neutrophils; however, others have not confirmed this observation.[27,28] Papillary dermal erythrocyte extravasation is commonly present.[27] Finally, features secondary to scratching, such as hyperkeratosis and acanthosis, may be seen.[29]

Immunofluorescence studies have shown that immunoreactants (C3, IgG, and IgM) may be present along the basement membrane zone.[3] However, when staining is evident, it is usually weak.[3]

Juvenile spring eruption of the ears is characterized by a perivascular lymphohistiocytic infiltrate often associated with subepidermal vesicle formation.[21]

In early lesions, helper-inducer T lymphocytes predominate and increased numbers of dermal Langerhans cells are present.[28] With chronicity, cytotoxic suppressor T cells become more conspicuous.

Differential diagnosis

It should be noted that there is considerable variability in both the clinical and histologic descriptions of polymorphous light eruption. This has led some authors to suggest that polymorphous light eruption likely represents a group of related disorders rather than a single entity.[27,28] Phototesting, therefore, is probably the best 'gold standard' for establishing the diagnosis. Compared with reticular erythematous mucinosis, mucin deposition is absent or much less prominent in polymorphous light eruption. Clinically, polymorphous light eruption resolves once exposure to sunlight has ceased in contrast to the persistent lesions of reticular erythematous mucinosis.

Histologically, polymorphous light eruption also shows some overlap with other causes of gyrate erythema, such as lymphocytic infiltration of Jessner. The presence of marked papillary dermal edema, when present, favors polymorphous light eruption. A clinical history of documentation of resolution of lesions with cessation to light exposure may sometimes be the only way to distinguish these entities. In cases where the diagnosis is in doubt, phototesting may often be necessary.

The histologic features of lupus erythematosus are sometimes difficult to distinguish from polymorphous light eruption, particularly when the latter is associated with positive immunofluorescence. However, most cases of polymorphous light eruption are negative with immunofluorescence testing. When immunoreactants are present, usually only weak staining is observed. Careful clinical and serological evaluation should resolve any confusion between these conditions.

Actinic reticuloid is another eruption associated with exposure to UV light. Compared with polymorphous light eruption, actinic reticuloid is more typically associated with a dense cellular interstitial infiltrate involving the papillary and reticular dermis, and sometimes extending into the subcutaneous fat. It is composed of lymphocytes, histiocytes, variable numbers of eosinophils, and plasma cells. The presence of multinucleate stellate myofibroblasts and giant cells is a conspicuous feature that favors actinic reticuloid (chronic actinic dermatitis). Finally, the finding of some large atypical, hyperchromatic cerebriform lymphoid cells is characteristic of actinic reticuloid.

Tumid lupus erythematosus

Clinical features

Lupus erythematosus is discussed in detail in Chapter 17 and the reader is referred there for a comprehensive discussion of the disease. In this section only the tumid variant of lupus erythematosus is discussed.

Tumid lupus erythematosus (lupus erythematosus tumidus) is a rare manifestation of lupus that some authors believe to be sufficiently characteristic to justify classification as a distinctive subtype of chronic cutaneous lupus erythematosus.[1] However, the lack of an agreed-upon diagnostic gold standard makes this designation somewhat controversial. Further study and refinement of criteria for inclusion into this subtype of lupus and to allow for reliable distinction from other inflammatory dermatoses is necessary.

Raised erythematous plaques, which have been described as 'succulent', characterize the clinical lesions.[1] Follicular plugging is not a feature.[2]

Annular and gyrate forms are seen in some patients.[1] The sun-exposed areas, such as the face, chest, arms, and shoulders are most commonly affected.[1–4] In the largest series published to date, patients with this clinical appearance accounted for 16% of the total number of patients seen in a large cutaneous lupus clinic.[1] Approximately equal numbers of male and female patients are affected, in contrast to the preponderance of females affected by other subtypes of cutaneous lupus.[2,4] In this variant, young adults are most often encountered, but presentation in childhood is rare.[4,5] In most patients, lesions can be reproduced by exposure to UVA or UVB light.[1,3,6] Development of tumid lupus erythematosus has also been reported following highly active antiretroviral therapy in the setting of HIV as a manifestation of immune restoration as well as in the setting of estrogen and infliximab treatment.[7–9] Unusual and rare presentations include unilateral distribution in addition to symmetrical involvement of both elbows.[10,11]

Histologic features

Biopsy shows a superficial and perivascular 'cuffed' lymphocytic infiltrate (*Fig. 8.31*).[12] Periadnexal involvement is also seen in many cases. Abundant dermal mucin is commonly present (*Fig. 8.32*).[2,12–14] In contrast to other variants of lupus erythematosus, epidermal changes (e.g., follicular

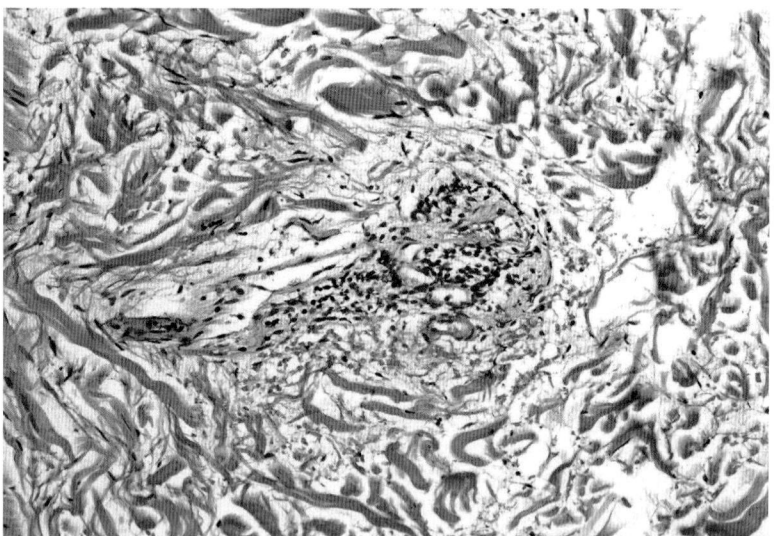

Fig. 8.31
Tumid lupus erythematosus: there is a perivascular lymphocytic infiltrate. The collagen fibers are separated by excess dermal mucin. By courtesy of J. Cohen, MD, Dermatopathology Laboratory, Tucson, Arizona, USA.

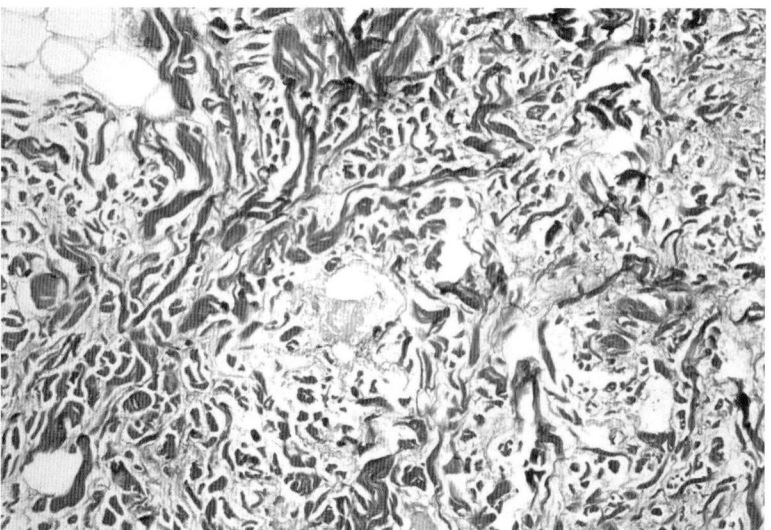

Fig. 8.32
Tumid lupus erythematosus: the mucin is Alcian blue positive. By courtesy of J. Cohen, MD, Dermatopathology Laboratory, Tucson, Arizona, USA.

plugging, vacuolar interface changes, and thickened basement membrane) are generally not apparent.[1,2,12]

Direct immunofluorescence staining fails to demonstrate reactivity.[1]

The cell infiltrate consists of a mixture of CD4+ and CD8+ reactive T lymphocytes.[2,15] Plasmacytoid dendritic cells are present in perivascular and periadnexal clusters and are highlighted by immunohistochemistry for CD123 and CD2AP.[16]

Differential diagnosis

The concept of tumid lupus erythematosus has been expanded in a large series of patients.[1] Whether there is justification for classification of the disorder in these patients as a variant of lupus erythematosus or not is debatable. None met the criteria for lupus erythematosus and most did not have significantly elevated antinuclear antibodies (ANA). However, occasional patients have been shown to develop skin lesions consistent with discoid lupus erythematosus, including prominent epidermal changes.[13,17]

In addition to patients similar to those described by Kuhn et al.,[1] patients that do fit the criteria for discoid lupus erythematosus (DLE), subacute cutaneous lupus erythematosus (SCLE) or systemic lupus erythematosus (SLE) rarely develop lesions that show a dense superficial and deep perivascular and periappendigeal infiltrate in the absence of significant epidermal changes.[18] Distinction of these subgroups of tumid lupus from lymphocytic infiltrate of Jessner and polymorphous light eruption based on histologic examination alone may be difficult if not impossible.[19] Some authors have suggested that some cases reported as lymphocytic infiltrate of Jessner or reticular erythematous mucinosis, in fact, represent tumid lupus.[20]

The histologic features of tumid lupus erythematosus may be difficult to distinguish from polymorphous light eruption. The latter condition, which is the most common photodermatosis, usually presents in young people, particularly females, as recurrent, erythematous papules, vesicles and/or plaques following exposure to UV light. Lesions, which develop after a latent period of hours to days, commonly subside completely within days and heal without sequelae.[21] A dense perivascular lymphohistiocytic infiltrate, often associated with papillary dermal edema, is present in the superficial and sometimes deep dermis.[22] The presence of significant papillary dermal edema favors polymorphous light eruption. Furthermore, the latter often has focal epidermal changes, particularly spongiosis, and lacks dermal mucin.

Lymphocytic infiltrate of the skin (Jessner) may be difficult to distinguish from tumid lupus erythematosus.[3] In such cases, immunohistochemistry may sometimes be helpful. The infiltrate in lymphocytic infiltrate is HLA-DR negative in contrast to lupus erythematosus in which the lymphocytes and often the keratinocytes are HLA-DR positive.[23] Leu 8 (immunoregulatory T-cell) expression is also more frequently seen in lymphocytic infiltrate.[23] Epidermal Langerhans cells are often increased in number in lymphocytic infiltrate whereas they are frequently reduced in discoid lupus.[24] The presence of significant amounts of dermal mucin favors a diagnosis of tumid lupus erythematosus.

Erythema annulare centrifugum differs from tumid lupus by the lack of significant dermal mucin.

As can be seen from the above discussion, tumid lupus erythematosus is a controversial entity. To some extent, the problem is a matter of semantics and definitions. Indeed, some authors have taken the position that reticular erythematous mucinosis and Jessner lymphocytic infiltrate of the skin would be more appropriately regarded as tumid lupus.[20] Clearly, further studies are necessary to more clearly define the clinicopathological features of tumid lupus erythematosus and its distinction from similar entities.

Perniosis, atypical chilblains and cold equestrian panniculitis

Clinical features

Perniosis (chilblains) is characterized by sensitivity to cold, damp weather and is therefore seen during the cold months of the year. The disease seems to be more common in environments where inadequate heating is problematical for a few months of the year and is less common in localities

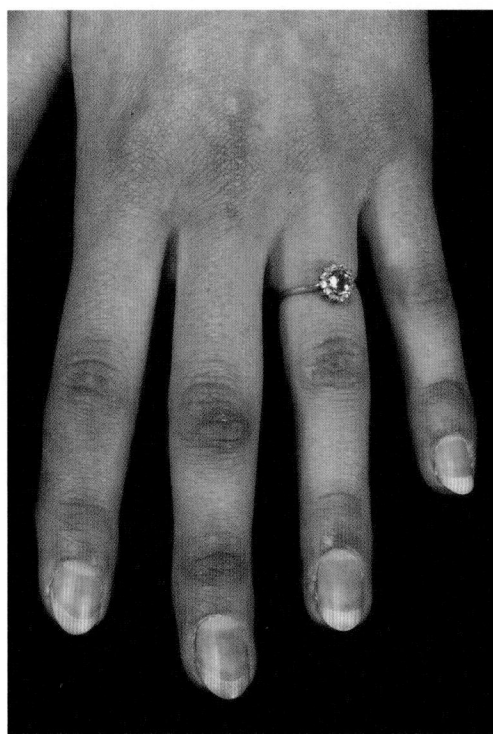

Fig. 8.33
Perniosis: erythematous nodules are present over the fingers. From the collection of the late N.P. Smith, MD, the Institute of Dermatology, London, UK.

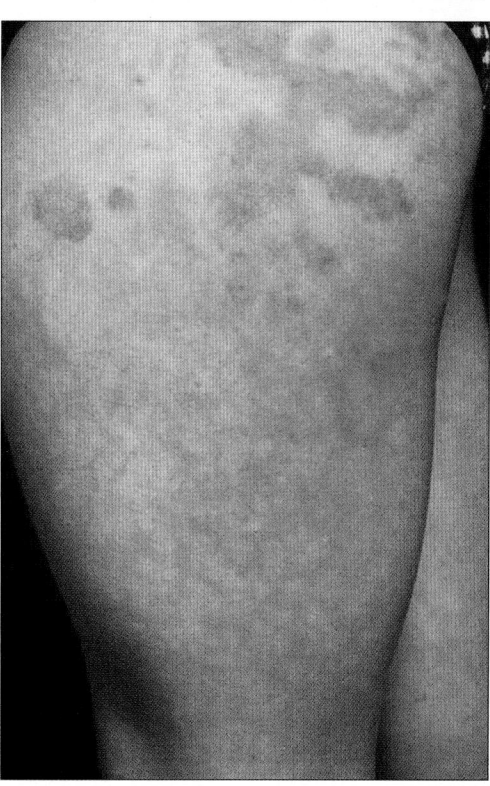

Fig. 8.35
Equestrian cold panniculitis: tender erythematous lesions on buttock and thigh. By courtesy of the Institute of Dermatology, London, UK.

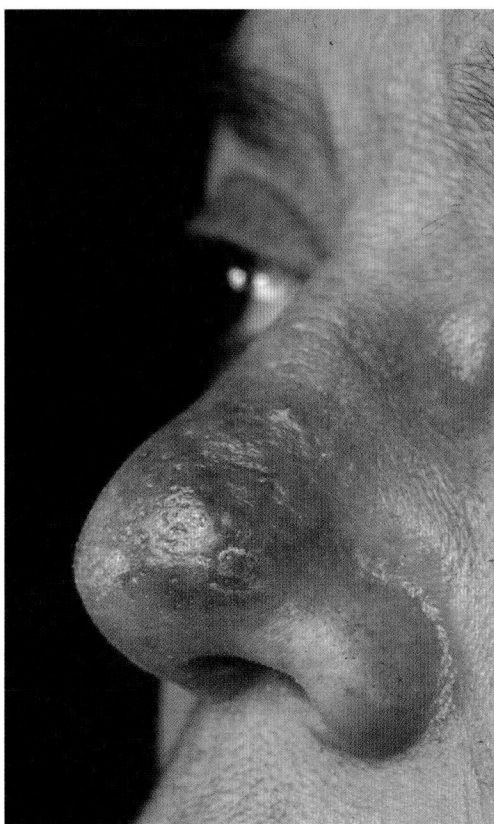

Fig. 8.34
Perniosis: in this patient, the nose is affected. From the collection of the late N.P. Smith, MD, the Institute of Dermatology, London, UK.

characterized by harsh frigid winters where adequate home heating is the norm.[1] Exposure to cold water sometimes appears to play a role.[2]

Patients present with painful, erythematous nodules on the distal extremities, especially the fingers and the toes (*Fig. 8.33*).[1,3] Other exposed sites, such as the nose and ears, may also be affected (*Fig. 8.34*). Lesions may

be complicated by blister formation or ulceration. In most patients, the condition remits during summer but often recurs during winter months. Patients with anorexia nervosa may be at increased risk of developing perniosis.[4,5]

Horse-riding enthusiasts who wear tight clothing during cold weather may develop similar lesions on the thighs (*Fig. 8.35*). This disease is associated with panniculitis and has been termed 'equestrian cold panniculitis'.[6–8] A similar presentation has also been reported after the application of ice packs for chronic back pain.[9]

Patients with lesions that persist into warmer seasons appear to be at a higher risk of developing lupus erythematosus.[10,11] Advanced age at onset and male gender are more commonly associated with an underlying systemic disease.[11,12] One group has designated patients with some criteria, but not meeting diagnostic thresholds for connective tissue diseases such as lupus erythematosus, as having 'atypical chilblains'.[10] This subset of patients appears to be at higher risk of developing unequivocal features of connective tissue disease. It is reasonable to evaluate all patients with perniosis for evidence of lupus erythematosus. Occasionally, patients with perniosis who present without clinical manifestations of connective tissue disease eventually develop SLE.[13]

Pathogenesis and histologic features

The pathogenesis of perniosis is not well understood. Clearly, cold is a requirement for development of symptoms. Tight clothing may play a role in the development of perniosis at nonexposed sites. In some patients, particularly children, the presence of cryoproteins may play a role in the disease.[14]

Biopsy reveals a cuffed perivascular lymphocytic infiltrate with variable vascular fibrinoid change (*Figs 8.36–8.38*). The inflammatory infiltrate may be superficial but often extends into the deep dermis and subcutaneous adipose tissue.[15] In some cases it is difficult to demonstrate strict criteria for lymphocytic vasculitis (*Fig. 8.39*). In other examples, however, fibrinoid vascular damage with thrombi is extensive. Papillary dermal edema, which may be marked, is often present.[16] Interface changes, either vacuolar interface, may sometimes be seen.[7,17] A chronic inflammatory infiltrate around sweat glands has occasionally been noted.[10,18]

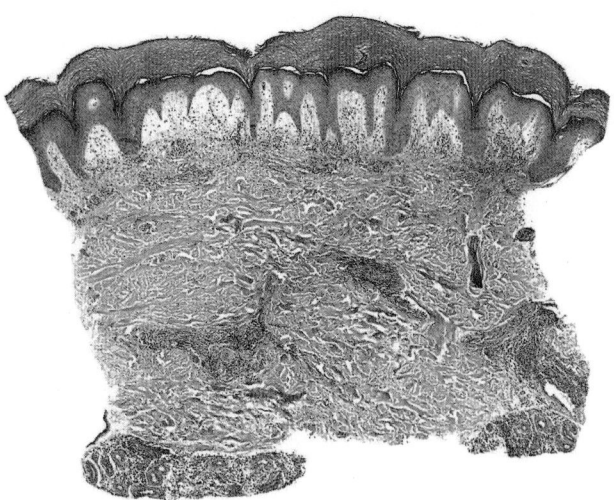

Fig. 8.36
Perniosis: there is hyperkeratosis, acanthosis, and a heavy lymphocytic infiltrate. Note the marked subepidermal edema.

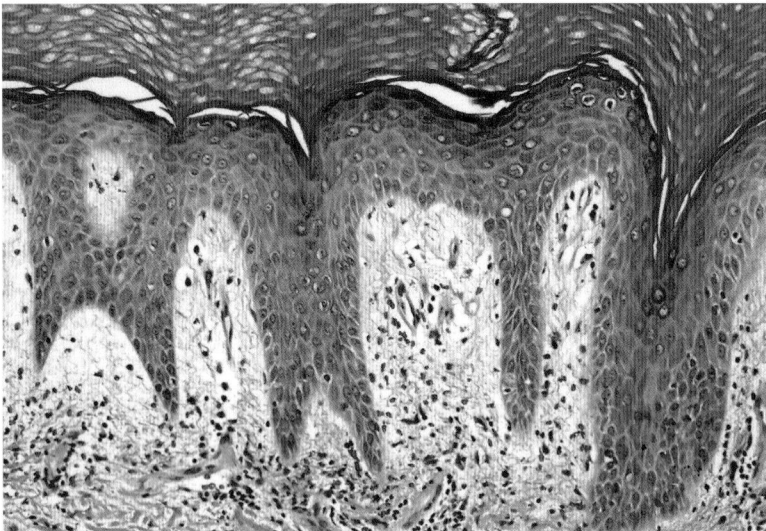

Fig. 8.37
Perniosis: there is marked subepidermal edema and red cell extravasation.

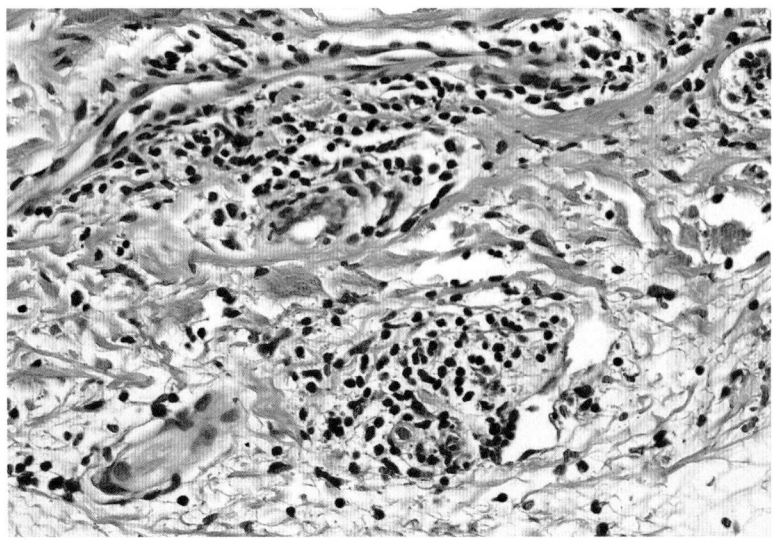

Fig. 8.38
Perniosis: the infiltrate consists largely of lymphocytes.

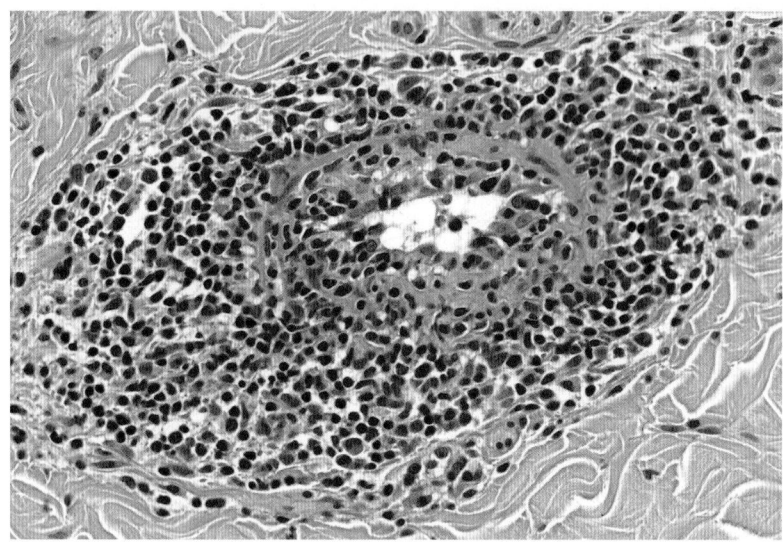

Fig. 8.39
Perniosis: this example shows a heavy mural infiltrate consistent with lymphocytic vasculitis.

Biopsy of cold panniculitis shows a perivascular chronic inflammatory infiltrate that tends to be prominent at the dermal–subcutaneous tissue junction.[6]

The inflammatory infiltrate is mostly composed of CD3+ T cells with a minor subpopulation of CD20+ B cells and scattered CD68+ macrophages.[17,19] Aggregates of CD123 positive plasmacytoid dendritic cells are also noted.[15] Rarely, atypical CD30-positive lymphoid forms may be admixed.[20]

Differential diagnosis

The biopsy findings are non-specific and other diseases causing cuffed perivascular lymphocytic reactions and lymphocytic vasculitis enter into the differential diagnosis. The diagnosis is rendered only after careful clinical correlation. Patients often have some features of, but fail to meet criteria for, connective tissue disease.[10] Also, lesions very similar, or identical, to perniosis may be seen in patients with cutaneous or systemic lupus erythematosus.[13,17,21] Frank lymphocytic vasculitis and interface changes appear to be more common in patients with chilblain lupus erythematosus than in idiopathic chilblains; however, the presence or absence of these findings may not be reliable discriminators.[10,17] A positive lupus band test or antinuclear antibodies favor a diagnosis of chilblain lupus erythematosus.[10]

Chilblain lupus erythematosus

Clinical features

Lupus erythematosus is discussed in detail in Chapter 17 and the reader is referred there for a comprehensive discussion of the disease. In this section, only chilblain lupus erythematosus (lupus pernio) will be discussed.

Chilblain lupus erythematosus may be a manifestation of either discoid or systemic lupus erythematosus and shares many clinical and histologic similarities with idiopathic chilblains (Fig. 8.40). It develops almost exclusively in females during the winter months.[1] Lesions are characterized by itchy, painful, erythematous or blue-purple papules, plaques, and nodules on the fingers, heels, and soles of the feet; the hands, calves, knees, knuckles, elbows, nose, and ears are less often affected.[2] Hyperkeratotic fissured lesions and ulcers are also sometimes present.[3] Patients may develop chilblains many years after the typical discoid rash, or lesions may develop simultaneously. Occasionally, chilblains are the sole manifestation.[3] While the majority of cases are sporadic, familial disease with an autosomal dominant inheritance has also been reported.[4–7]

Approximately 15% of patients develop SLE, particularly those who develop discoid and perniotic lesions simultaneously and those with DLE-erythema multiforme-like syndrome in addition to perniosis.[1,2,8]

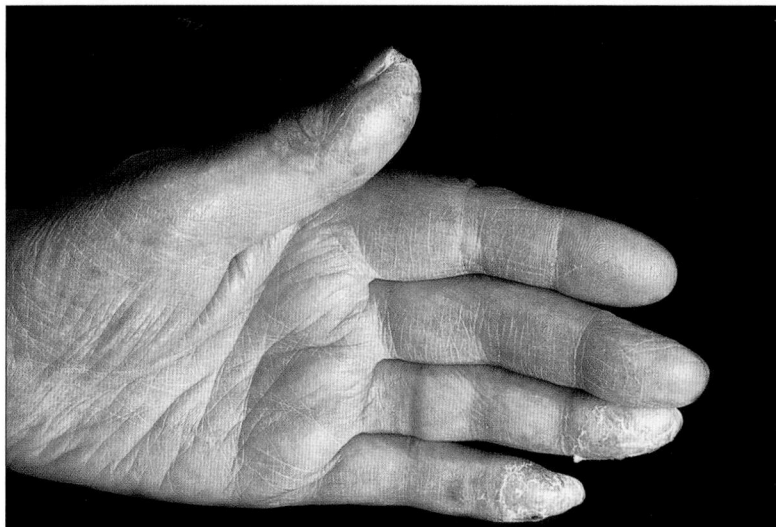

Fig. 8.40
Chilblain lupus erythematosus: resolving perniosis involving the tips of the thumb, ring, and little fingers. By courtesy of R.A. Marsden, MD, St George's Hospital, London, UK.

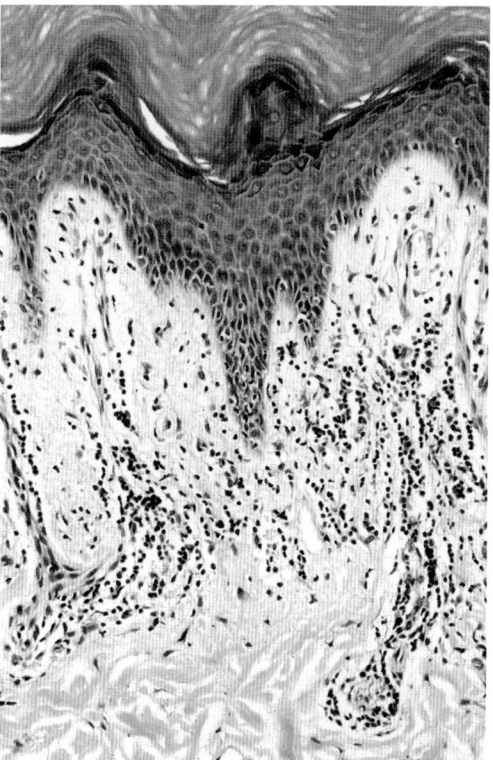

Fig. 8.41
Chilblain lupus erythematosus: there is subepidermal edema with red cell extravasation and a superficial perivascular lymphocytic infiltrate.

Patients with severe chilblains that persist into warmer seasons appear to be at higher risk of lupus erythematosus compared to those with the idiopathic form.[9] Patients with some criteria, but not meeting diagnostic thresholds for connective tissue disease, have been designated as having 'atypical chilblains'.[9] These individuals appear to be at higher risk of eventually developing frank connective tissue disease.[9] Based on the above observations, it is clear that patients with perniosis should be evaluated for evidence of lupus erythematosus.

Pathogenesis and histologic features

While the pathogenesis of sporadic disease remains elusive, mutations in the DNA exonuclease TREX1, located on chromosome 3, have been reported in the autosomal dominant familial form of chilblain lupus.[4–7] The function of TREX1 is the digestion of single-stranded DNA. Recent work has shown that lack of TREX1 function may lead to accumulation of reverse transcribed DNA with subsequent stimulation of interferon production, which ultimately may be a trigger for autoimmunity.[10,11] Mutations in TREX1 have also been reported in other autoimmune disorders such as Aicardi-Goutieres syndrome, an encephalopathy characterized by basal ganglia calcification and white matter alterations.[6,12] The development of chilblains is not infrequently seen in patients with this syndrome with clinical and histologic findings similar to chilblain lupus erythematosus.[13–15] Rarely, familial chilblain lupus is caused by mutations in the SAMHD1 (sterile alpha motif domain and HD domain containing protein1) or STING (stimulator of interferon gene) genes.[16,17]

Biopsy reveals a cuffed perivascular lymphocytic infiltrate with edema, red cell extravasation, and variable vascular fibrinoid change (Fig. 8.41). Some biopsies show frank lymphocytic vasculitis. The inflammatory infiltrate often extends into the deep dermis and subcutaneous adipose tissue. Interface epidermal changes, ranging from focal vacuolar changes to a lichenoid tissue reaction, are often present.[2,18] Chronic inflammation around sweat glands is sometimes seen.[9]

The infiltrate is mostly composed of T cells, occasional macrophages, and scattered B cells.

Differential diagnosis

Other diseases associated with a 'cuffed' perivascular lymphocytic infiltrate and lymphocytic vasculitis must be considered in the differential diagnosis. The diagnosis is rendered only after careful clinical and serological correlation. Distinction from idiopathic chilblain perniosis is not possible based on histologic features alone. The presence of lymphocytic vasculitis and interface changes appears to be more common in chilblain lupus compared with idiopathic chilblains, but these features are not reliable discriminators.[9] A positive lupus band test and the presence of antinuclear antibodies favor a diagnosis of chilblain lupus erythematosus.

Pigmented purpuric dermatoses including Majocchi disease, Schamberg disease, pigmented purpuric lichenoid dermatitis of Gougerot and Blum, and itching purpura

Clinical features

The term pigmented purpuric dermatoses (purpura simplex, chronic capillaritis) encompasses a number of clinical syndromes characterized by orange/brown pigmentation (due to hemosiderin deposition likened to cayenne pepper), interspersed with fine pinpoint purpura (due to extravasated red blood cells).[1–4] All are of unknown etiology. These disorders may show overlapping clinical and histologic features. Indeed, some authors no longer consider their classification to have nosological value. In addition to the disorders listed below, unusual clinical presentations include unilateral disease, zosteriform distribution, and concomitant morphea in addition to familial disease.[5–9]

- In Majocchi disease, the lesions tend to be discrete and annular, vary from one to several centimeters in diameter, and are associated with telangiectases (Fig. 8.42).
- Schamberg disease is characterized by purpura and petechiae with conspicuous pigmentation; there is a marked preponderance of males and presentation in childhood is unusual (Figs 8.43 and 8.44).[10] Lesions, usually irregular in shape and occurring predominantly on the lower limbs, may remain for 10 years or longer. In some cases, the findings may mimic those of chronic venous insufficiency. The lesions are asymptomatic in most cases. However, some patients complain of pruritus.
- In pigmented purpuric lichenoid dermatitis of Gougerot and Blum, patients, predominantly males, develop lichenoid papules in addition to purpuric lesions, most often on the legs.
- Itching purpura (pruriginous angiodermatitis) also shows a male predominance and is associated with an acute onset of widely

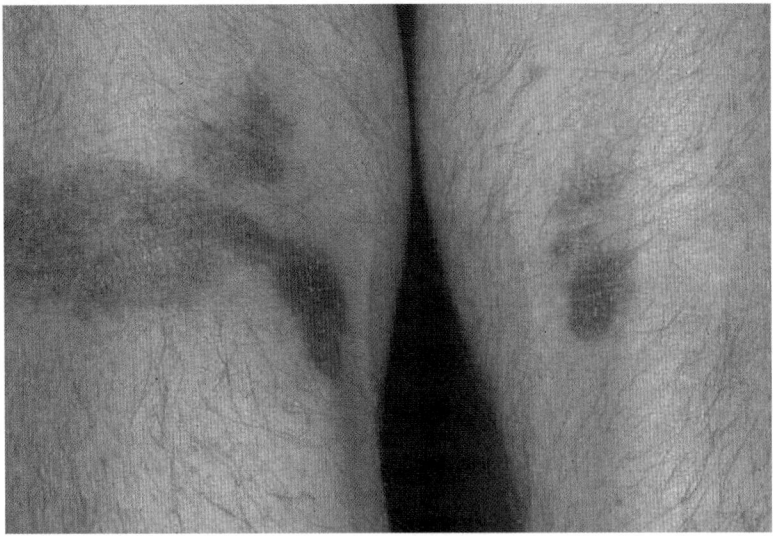

Fig. 8.42
Majocchi disease: characteristic brown plaques on the backs of the knees in a male. By courtesy of R.A. Marsden, MD, St George's Hospital, London, UK.

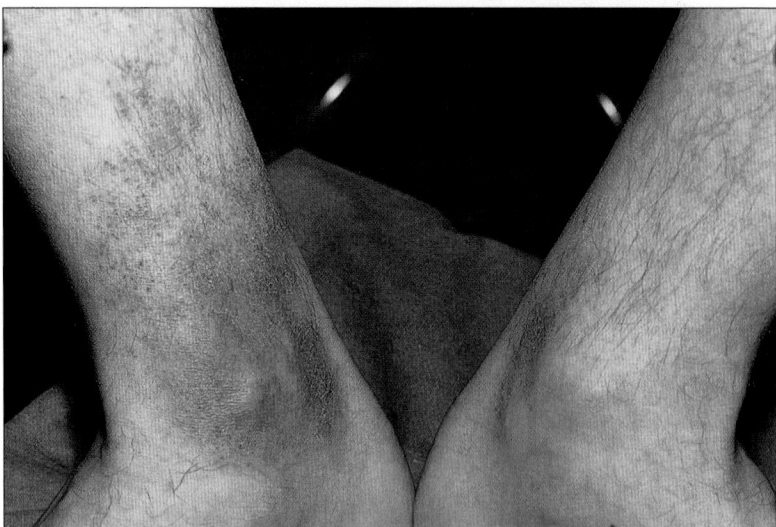

Fig. 8.44
Schamberg disease: in this patient, the bilateral distribution over the malleoli mimics the effects of venous stasis. By courtesy of R.A. Marsden, MD, St George's Hospital, London, UK.

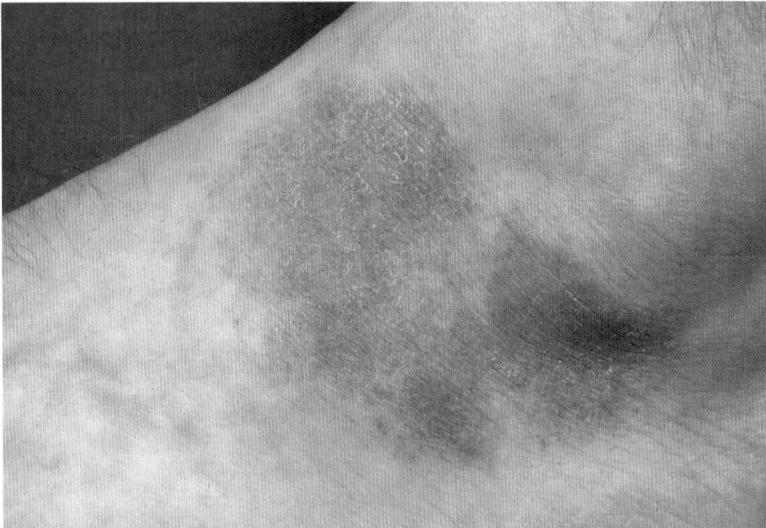

Fig. 8.43
Schamberg disease: a localized area of capillaritis showing characteristic cayenne pepper speckling over the lateral malleolus of a male. By courtesy of R.A. Marsden, MD, St George's Hospital, London, UK.

distributed orange macules (*Figs 8.45* and *8.46*). It commonly begins on the dorsal surface of the feet or ankles, but soon spreads to affect the thighs, buttocks, trunk, and arms. This variant is associated with a shorter duration than the others, with most patients being free from lesions by 1 month. The itching, which is of unknown etiology, is usually severe. Similar appearances may be caused by drug sensitivity. Since lichen aureus has more distinctive features, it is discussed separately (see below).

Histologic features

All variants show similar histopathological features. A perivascular lymphocytic infiltrate is associated with reactive endothelial changes and extravasated red blood cells (*Figs 8.47* and *8.48*).[11] The lymphocytes are predominantly of the T-helper subset.[12] The density of the infiltrate is highly variable. The Gougerot-Blum variant is often associated with a dense lichenoid lymphocytic infiltrate. Extravasated red blood cells are usually appreciated in early lesions, while in the later stages they may not be present when hemosiderin-laden macrophages become conspicuous (*Fig. 8.49*). An iron stain is useful to demonstrate hemosiderin. Cases of pigmented purpuric dermatosis associated with granulomatous inflammation

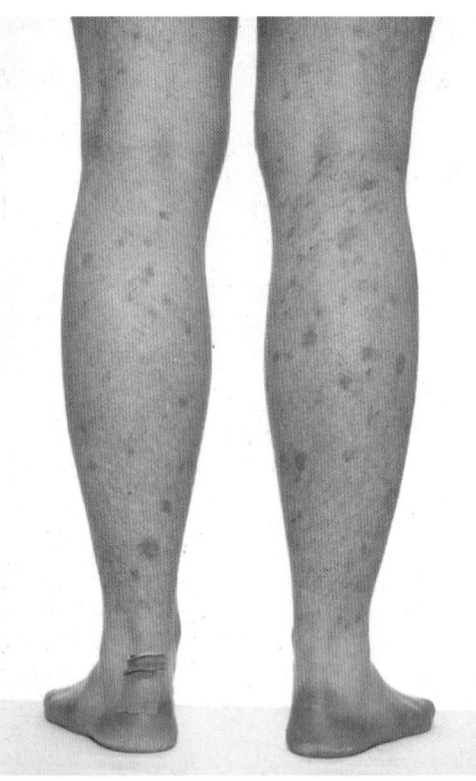

Fig. 8.45
Itching purpura: these small macules are widely distributed over both legs. By courtesy of J. Newton, MD, St Thomas' Hospital, London, UK.

have been described and designated granulomatous pigmented purpuric dermatoses.[13–18] Some cases of granulomatous pigmented dermatosis appear to be associated with hyperlipedemia.[19]

Differential diagnosis

It should be emphasized that extravasated red blood cells and hemosiderin associated with a lymphocytic capillaritis are non-specific findings. The differential diagnosis is broad and includes other forms of perivascular lymphocytic infiltrates and lymphocytic capillaritis. Careful clinical correlation is necessary to establish a correct diagnosis. Progression of lesions mimicking pigmented purpuric dermatoses to mycosis fungoides has been

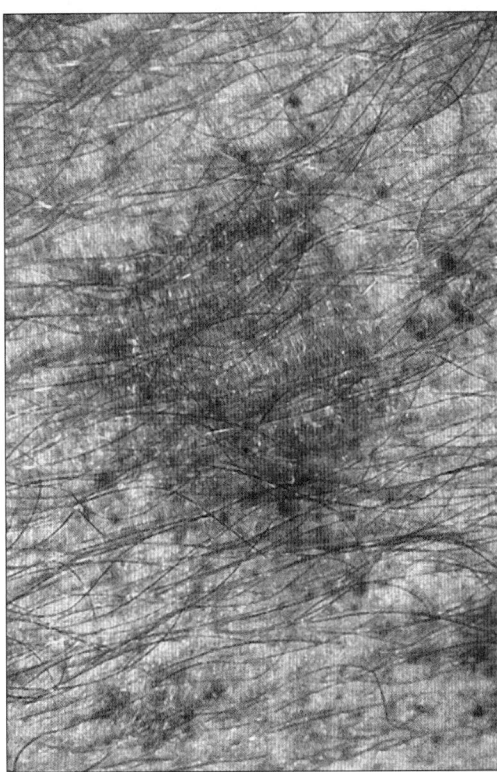

Fig. 8.46
Itching purpura: close-up view of a typical orange macule. By courtesy of J. Newton, MD, St Thomas' Hospital, London, UK.

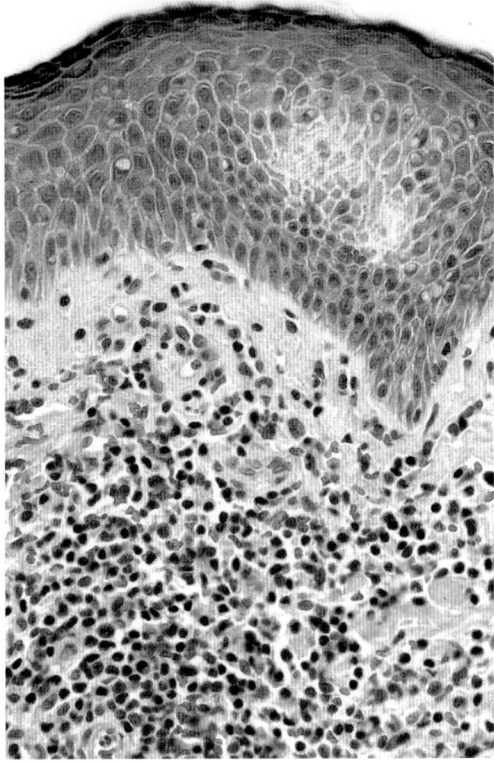

Fig. 8.48
Pigmented purpura: the infiltrate consists of lymphocytes and histiocytes. Note the red cell extravasation.

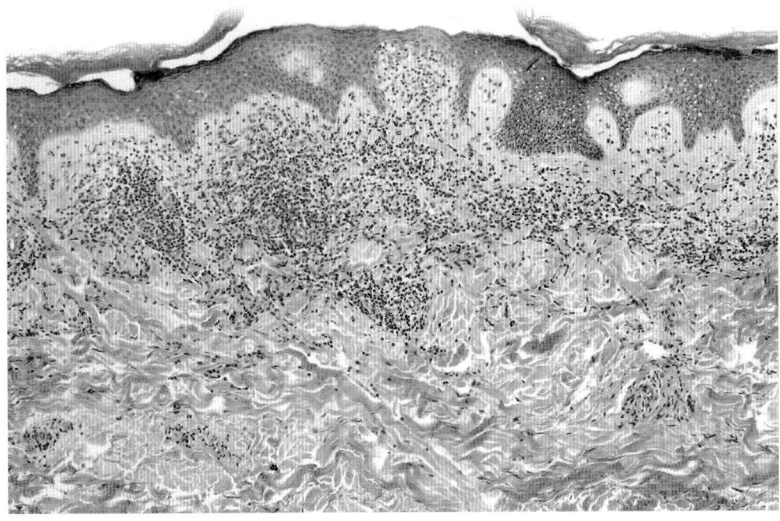

Fig. 8.47
Pigmented purpura: there is an upper dermal heavy perivascular lymphocytic infiltrate.

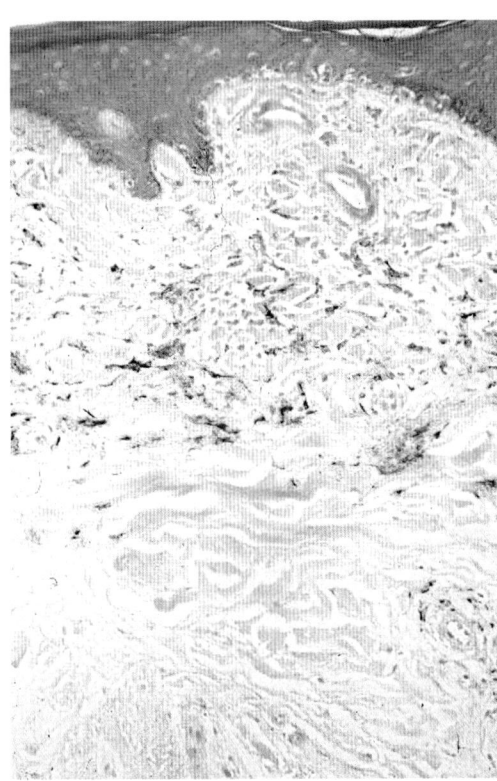

Fig. 8.49
Pigmented purpura: there is abundant hemosiderin deposition as revealed with the Perl Prussian blue stain for iron.

documented.[20,21] However, this appears to be an uncommon event and it is more likely that these cases represent examples of purpuric cutaneous T-cell lymphoma from the beginning. The absence of epidermotropism and cytological atypia favors pigmented purpuric dermatitis over a T-cell lymphoproliferative disorder. However, in rare cases, distinction may be difficult or impossible and ancillary investigations, such as immunohistological and T-cell gene rearrangement studies, may be indicated. Adding to this occasionally difficult distinction, cases of pigmented purpuric dermatoses with clonal T-cell gene rearrangements have been reported.[13,22] Therefore, it appears that the results of gene rearrangement studies may not always reliably aid in this differential diagnosis. All information – clinical, histologic, immunohistological, and genetic – should be evaluated in context.

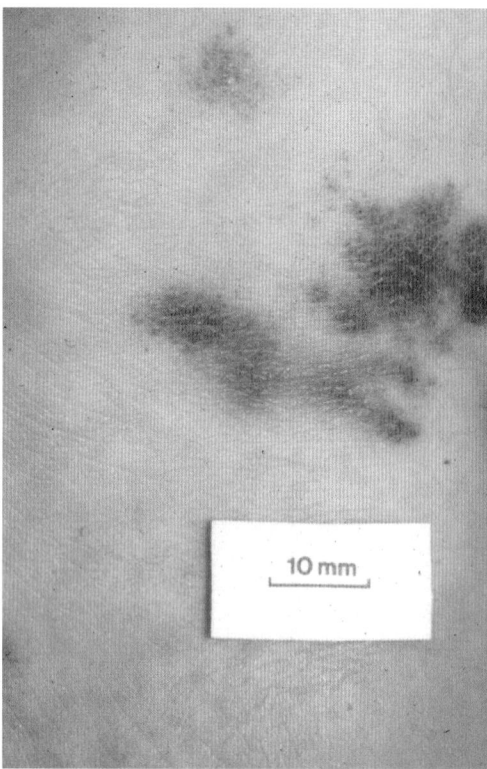

Fig. 8.50
Lichen aureus: golden-red-brown plaques on the ankle. By courtesy of M. Price, MD, St Thomas' Hospital, London, UK.

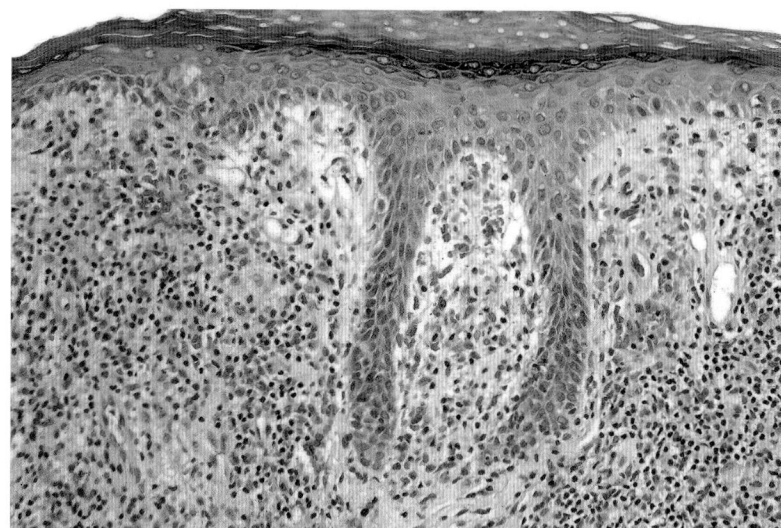

Fig. 8.51
Lichen aureus: there is a dense bandlike infiltrate in the upper dermis.

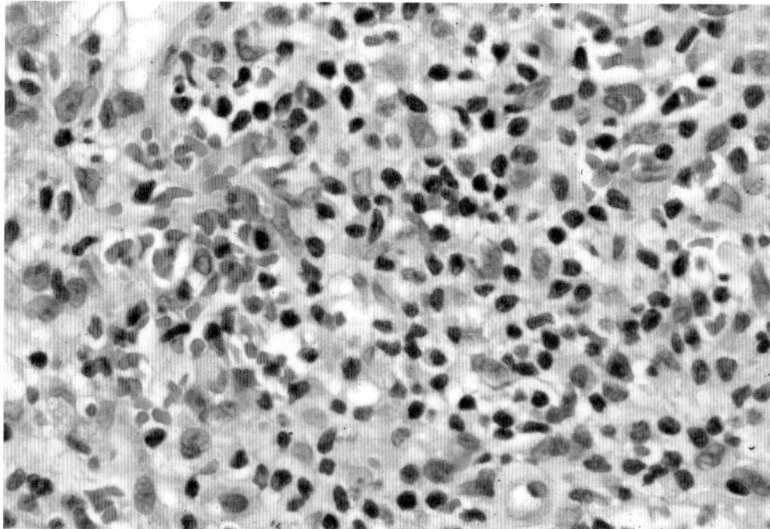

Fig. 8.52
Lichen aureus: the infiltrate consists of lymphocytes and histiocytes. Note the marked red cell extravasation.

Lichen aureus

Clinical features

Lichen aureus (lichen purpuricus) is a rare variant of the pigmented purpuric dermatoses. It may be differentiated from the other forms by virtue of its distinctive clinical and histologic features.[1-4] It is, therefore, discussed separately.

Lichen aureus shows a male predilection (2:1) and tends to affect the younger age group, with a peak incidence in the fourth decade. Children may occasionally be affected.[3] Lesions are usually asymptomatic, although pruritus is an occasional feature. The disease is characterized by discrete or confluent lichenoid macules and papules, which may be golden yellow, bronze, purple, or dark brown, and may resemble a bruise (*Fig. 8.50*). Sometimes a purpuric element is evident. The lesions of lichen aureus are characteristically very persistent, although occasionally spontaneous resolution is a feature. They occur most often on the lower legs, but may affect quite a wide variety of sites, including the arms, hands, trunk, thighs, and vulva.[5-8] Lesions are usually unilateral and limited to only one or two sites; they consist of either solitary ovoid maculopapules 3–5 cm in diameter or irregular plaques up to 20 cm across. Rarely, a zosteriform, segmental or agminate distribution, has been described.[8-11]

Histologic features

The epidermis is structurally normal. A dense lymphohistiocytic infiltrate is present in the upper dermis, usually distributed in a bandlike fashion immediately below the epidermis (*Figs 8.51* and *8.52*). In contrast to lichen planus, however, there is no evidence of basal cell hydropic degeneration and cytoid bodies are not usually found. A Grenz zone is sometimes present, although the infiltrate may abut the overlying epidermis. Lymphocytic exocytosis is sometimes present. Scattered within the infiltrate are increased numbers of blood vessels. Hemosiderin-laden macrophages are present in the deeper aspect of the infiltrate or in the adjacent noninfiltrated dermis. Purpura is a variable feature and there is no evidence of frank vasculitis.

In one study, a monoclonal T-cell population was observed in 50% of the cases studied. No progression to mycosis fungoides was seen in these cases.[7]

Differential diagnosis

There may be some histologic overlap with the Gougerot-Blum variant of pigmented purpuric lichenoid dermatitis, but lichen aureus tends to be more localized.

Pruritic urticarial papules and plaques of pregnancy

Clinical features

Pruritic and urticarial papules and plaques of pregnancy (PUPPP), also known as polymorphic eruption of pregnancy, toxemic rash of pregnancy, toxic erythema of pregnancy, and late onset prurigo of pregnancy, is a common dermatosis of uncertain etiology with an estimated incidence of 0.5%.[1,2] The disorder is most frequently seen in the primigravida.[3-5] Characteristically, it presents late in pregnancy, toward the end of the third trimester with an average time of onset in the 36th week.[3-6] Rarely, presentation during the postpartum period has been documented.[3,4,6,7] In a series, the male to female infant ratio in affected patients was 2:1.[8] In one large series, 76% of patients were primigravidas.[3,4]

As its name indicates, urticarial papules and plaques are associated with vexatious pruritus. Patients frequently complain that pruritus interferes with sleep.[3] At onset, papules are often localized to the abdomen along lines of stria distensae. This pattern is seen in approximately 50% of patients.[1,3] Small vesicles are occasionally present.[3] With time, the papules spread to involve the proximal limbs and torso and coalesce to form plaques.[4] The distal extremities are rarely affected.[4,5,9] Sparing of the face is a helpful diagnostic clinical clue. Typically, the lesions resolve shortly after delivery. Importantly (see differential diagnosis section below), PUPPP does not usually recur with subsequent pregnancies.

One group found PUPPP was associated with increased maternal weight gain and increased newborn weight compared with a control population.[10,11] Some studies suggest a relationship between PUPPP and twin gestation with two such reports documenting 10% and 16% of cases, respectively, associated with twin gestations.[10–12] These data have led some authors to postulate that abdominal distension may play a role in the pathogenesis of PUPPP.[10] Other reported association include hypertensive disorders and induction of labor.[13]

Rarely, congenital abnormalities have been noted in association with PUPPP, but this may be due to small statistical sampling. In one report, one child had hypoplastic dental enamel, while another developed congenital laryngomalacia requiring surgical intervention.[3] In this same series, another child was reported to have a ventriculoseptal defect. Most authors, however, believe that there is no direct association between PUPPP and congenital abnormalities.

Histologic features

Early lesions (urticarial papules) of polymorphic eruption of pregnancy show epidermal and upper dermal edema accompanied by a perivascular lymphohistiocytic infiltrate with variable numbers of eosinophils (*Figs 8.53–8.55*). Often, the number of eosinophils is modest and in one series only 17% of biopsies had eosinophils in the infiltrate. However, other authors report contrary experience, with most, if not all, biopsies showing eosinophils.[6] It is our experience that most biopsies show at least rare eosinophils if multiple sections are examined.

The lymphohistiocytic infiltrate is also variable in density, ranging from modest numbers of cells to a dense infiltrate with a tightly 'cuffed' perivascular distribution.[3,6] Mild papillary dermal edema is a common finding, but marked edema is rarely seen.[3] The additional feature of spongiotic vesiculation characterizes later lesions.[6] Less common manifestations include eosinophilic spongiosis.

Differential diagnosis

As can be deduced from the above histologic description, the biopsy findings are non-specific. The main differential diagnosis includes urticaria, hypersensitivity reactions, and pemphigoid gestationis. Usually, clinical examination and history will allow distinction from hypersensitivity reactions, which may show identical histologic features. Urticaria can be distinguished by the presence of neutrophils. In our experience, distinction between the prebullous phase of pemphigoid gestationis and PUPPP is the most common reason for which the clinician performs a biopsy. Distinction is important since pemphigoid gestationis, but not PUPPP, may be associated

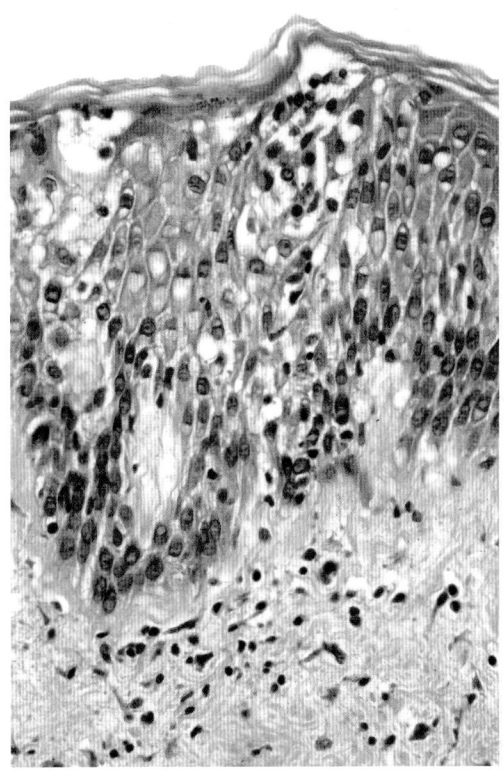

Fig. 8.54
Pruritic urticarial papules and plaques of pregnancy: high-power view showing spongiosis.

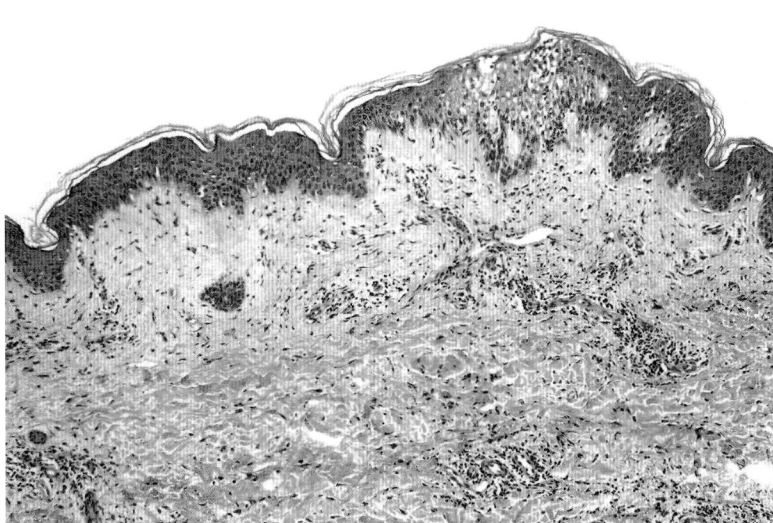

Fig. 8.53
Pruritic urticarial papules and plaques of pregnancy: there is focal spongiosis. Note the perivascular upper dermal infiltrate.

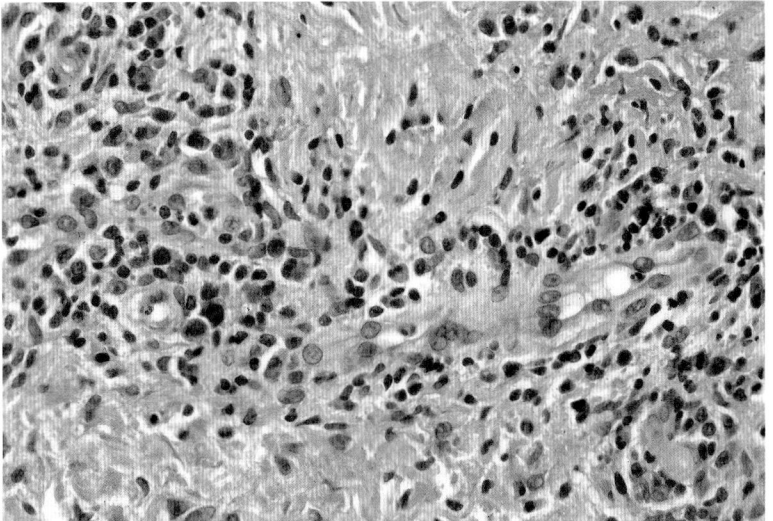

Fig. 8.55
Pruritic urticarial papules and plaques of pregnancy: the infiltrate consists of lymphocytes, histiocytes, and eosinophils.

with significant fetal morbidity. The presence of a subepidermal vesicle or marked papillary dermal edema favors pemphigoid gestationis; however, some early lesions will lack these features. Furthermore, PUPPP is frequently associated with mild papillary dermal edema. Immunofluorescence studies are often necessary for definitive diagnosis. Pemphigoid gestationis is associated with basement membrane staining for C3 and sometimes IgG. Most cases of PUPPP show negative immunofluorescence results.[14] However, it should be noted that there have been a few purported cases of PUPPP in which weak C3 staining in a linear pattern along the basement membrane was reported.[3] In some laboratories, granular deposits along the basement membrane have also been described in cases of PUPPP.[3,15] However, PUPPP is not associated with positive strong linear immunofluorescence staining or positive C4d immunohistochemical staining along the basement membrane – a result that would strongly favor pemphigoid gestationis.[15,16] As mentioned above, in contrast to pemphigoid gestationis, PUPPP does not tend to recur during subsequent pregnancies.

Pregnancy prurigo

Clinical features

Pregnancy prurigo (prurigo gravidarum, prurigo gestationis) has recently been classified under the broader disease group atopic eruption of pregnancy.[1,2] It affects 1 in 300 pregnancies, presenting as pruritic, erythematous, 0.5–1.0-cm papules and nodules with a predilection for the extensor surfaces of the extremities and the abdomen.[1,3–9] Superimposed features of excoriation with scale-crust may be seen. Lesions usually present during the third trimester, but may present at all stages of pregnancy.[1] The condition usually disappears following delivery, but in some cases, it persists into the puerperium. Blistering is not a feature. Fetal and maternal health does not appear to be adversely affected.[7]

Pathogenesis and histologic features

The pathogenesis of pregnancy prurigo is unknown. It has been suggested that the condition represents pruritus gravidarum in a background of atopic dermatitis.[3,7] Patients often have a history of atopy.[7] Serum IgE may be elevated in patients regardless of whether or not there is a positive history of atopy.[7] Of interest, eczematous dermatitis appears to be common in pregnancy.[7] Furthermore, a comprehensive analysis of dermatoses of pregnancy suggested that there is significant clinical and histologic overlap between eczema of pregnancy, pruritic folliculitis of pregnancy, and prurigo of pregnancy and that they should be regarded as a single disease complex termed 'atopic eruption of pregnancy'.[1]

The histologic features are not specific, comprising mild spongiosis, lymphocytic exocytosis, and a superficial perivascular lymphohistiocytic infiltrate with occasional eosinophils (Figs 8.56 and 8.57).[10] Frequently, histologic features of excoriation are present. Immunofluorescence studies are negative.

Differential diagnosis

The histologic features are non-specific and clinical correlation is necessary to render a firm diagnosis. The diagnosis is perhaps best approached as one of exclusion, and underlying etiologies should be sought. The major differential diagnosis includes hypersensitivity reactions (drug eruption, insect bites, etc.) with superimposed prurigo nodularis.

Urticarial vasculitis

Clinical features

Urticarial vasculitis is an uncommon condition characterized clinically by chronic urticaria and histologically by subtle leukocytoclastic venulitis.[1–3] In some patients, urticarial vasculitis is associated with antibody–antigen complexes – a type III hypersensitivity reaction.[4,5] In many patients, however, no underlying cause is discovered.

Patients may have, in addition to urticarial skin lesions, angioedema, arthralgia, gastrointestinal symptoms, and evidence of renal involvement.

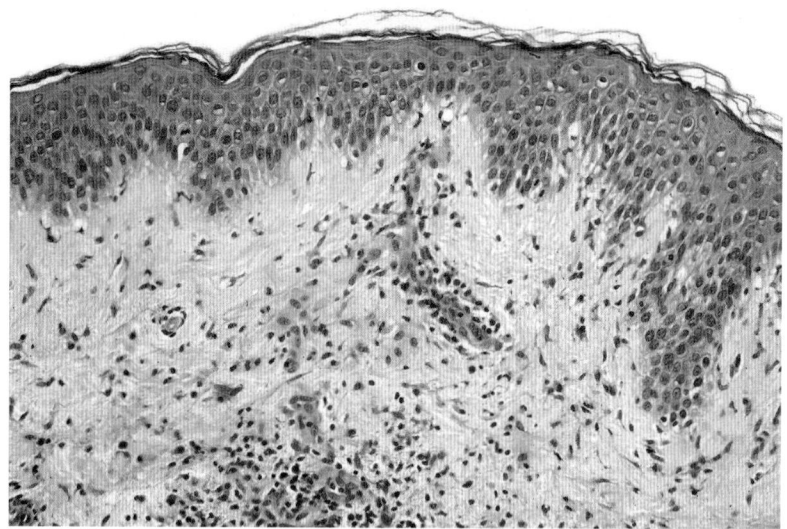

Fig. 8.56
Pregnancy prurigo: there is a superficial perivascular inflammatory cell infiltrate.

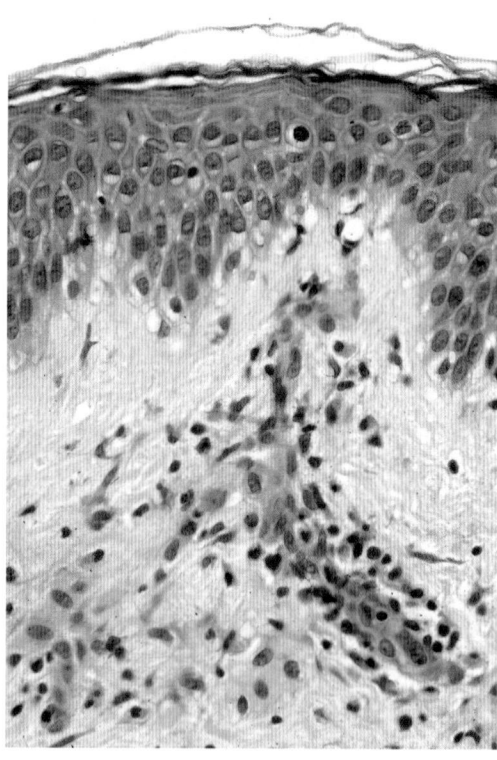

Fig. 8.57
Pregnancy prurigo: the infiltrate consists of lymphocytes with occasional eosinophils.

The spectrum of illness ranges from mild symptoms to a serious systemic illness, for which treatment with corticosteroids is sometimes necessary.[6]

The disease shows a female predominance (2:1) and is most often seen in the third, fourth or fifth decade. It is rare in children.[7] The cutaneous lesions are urticarial in appearance, but usually last 24–72 hours (Figs 8.58–8.60).[8] Pruritus, a burning sensation, or pain, are common complaints. The frequency of attacks varies from daily to monthly. The skin lesions are edematous, raised, and erythematous, and are associated with nonblanchable purpura.

Systemic manifestations/associations include joint pain, stiffness and swelling, particularly of the hands, elbows, feet, ankles, and knees. Frank arthritis is extremely rare but may be associated with the development of valvular heart disease.[9,10] Proteinuria and hematuria may be seen in some

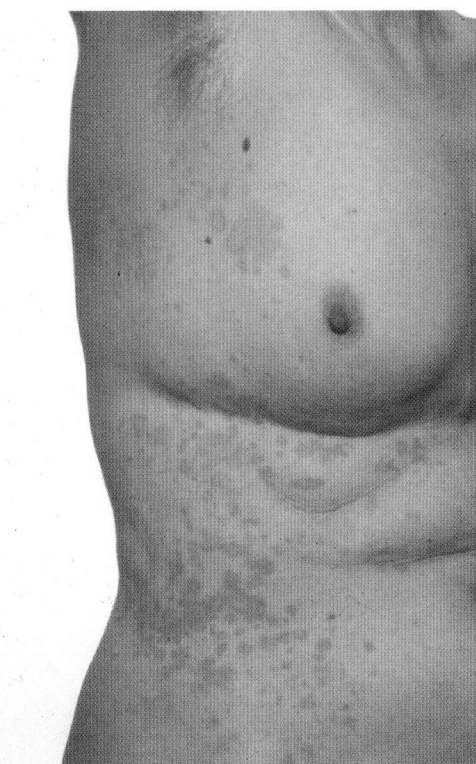

Fig. 8.58
Urticarial vasculitis: note the urticaria with a livid hue. By courtesy of J. Newton, MD, St Thomas' Hospital, London, UK.

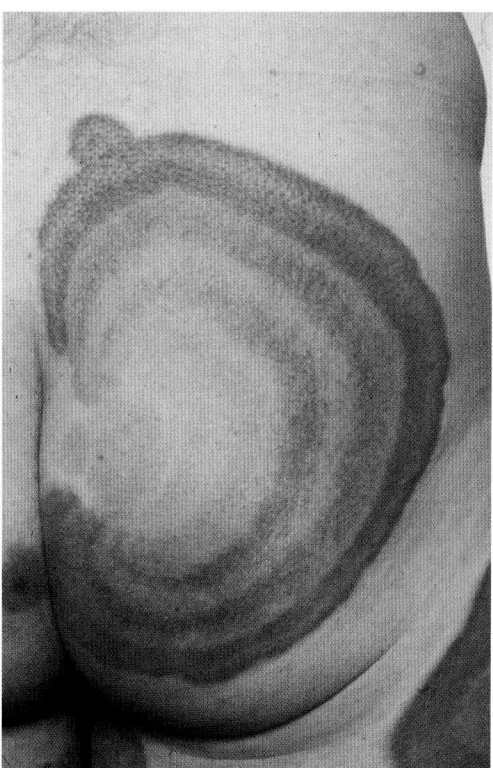

Fig. 8.60
Urticarial vasculitis: note the bizarre annular purpuric urticarial plaque. By courtesy of J. Newton, MD, St Thomas' Hospital, London, UK.

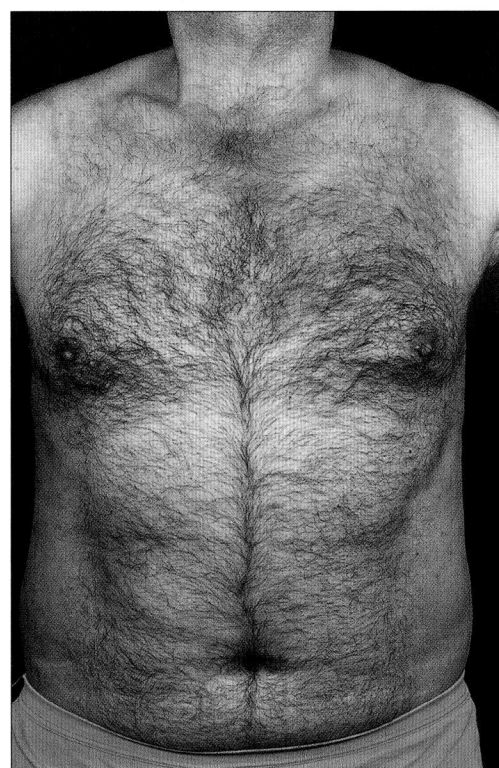

Fig. 8.59
Urticarial vasculitis: in this patient, there is an extensive urticarial plaque. By courtesy of J. Newton, MD, St Thomas' Hospital, London, UK.

patients. Many patients are hypocomplementemic.[4,11] Rarely, renal biopsy reveals the features of focal or diffuse proliferative glomerulonephritis. Crescentic glomerulonephritis, and mesangial and membranous nephropathy have also been documented.[6,12–14] Abdominal pain associated with nausea, vomiting, and diarrhea is a feature in some patients.

The erythrocyte sedimentation rate (ESR) is raised in many cases and in about 50% of patients there is hypocomplementemia. The presence of the latter correlates with systemic involvement.[6,15] There may also be depression of the early classical pathway components C1q, C4, and C2. Patients with hypocomplementemic urticarial vasculitis have a high prevalence of autoantibodies to endothelial cells and antibodies against C1q are invariably present.[16–19] The term 'Schnitzler syndrome' has been applied to patients with urticarial vasculitis and monoclonal IgM gammopathy.[20–25] Hepatosplenomegaly, elevated ESR, elevated white blood cell count, fever, and joint pain are characteristic features and renal insufficiency has also been documented.[21–23,26] An underlying lymphoproliferative disorder is present in a minor subset of patients.[20]

Importantly, urticarial vasculitis (especially the hypocomplementemic variant) is often associated with, or heralds the onset of, a variety of systemic diseases, including SLE, arthritis, interstitial lung disease, pericarditis, systemic sclerosis, mixed connective tissue disease, relapsing polychondritis, inflammatory myositis, hepatitis, inflammatory bowel disease, serum sickness, polyarteritis nodosa and Granulomatosis with polyangiitis, viral infections, Sjögren syndrome, cryoglobulinemia, polycythemia rubra vera, adverse reaction to drugs, and as a response to sunlight.[6,15,27–45] In one study, more than 50% of patients had uveitis, scleritis, conjunctivitis, or episcleritis.[6] It appears that patients with hypocomplementemia have more severe disease.[27] Some authors have postulated that hypocomplementemic urticarial vasculitis represents a form of systemic lupus erythematosus.[46] Others, however, have shown no significant difference in the association with lupus in patients with normocomplementemic compared with hypocomplementemic urticarial vasculitis.[6] A diagnosis of urticarial vasculitis in any patient should initiate an evaluation for underlying disease. Fortunately, urticarial vasculitis usually has a benign outcome.[6]

Urticarial vasculitis has been documented in association with malignancy.[6,47–52] Given the rarity of this association, it may well be coincidental.

Histologic features

In urticarial vasculitis, vascular damage is superimposed on a background of dermal edema and inflammation typical of urticaria. The vasculitis affects

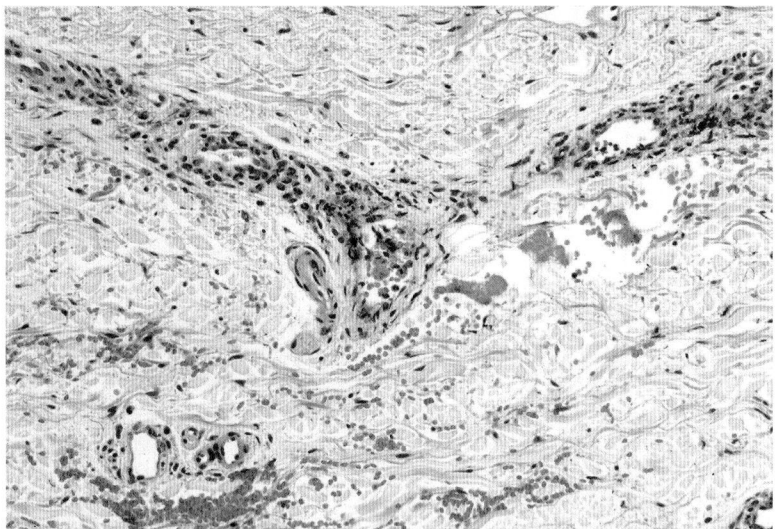

Fig. 8.61
Urticarial vasculitis: in this example of an early lesion, there is a conspicuous perivascular eosinophil infiltrate. There is no evidence of vessel wall damage.

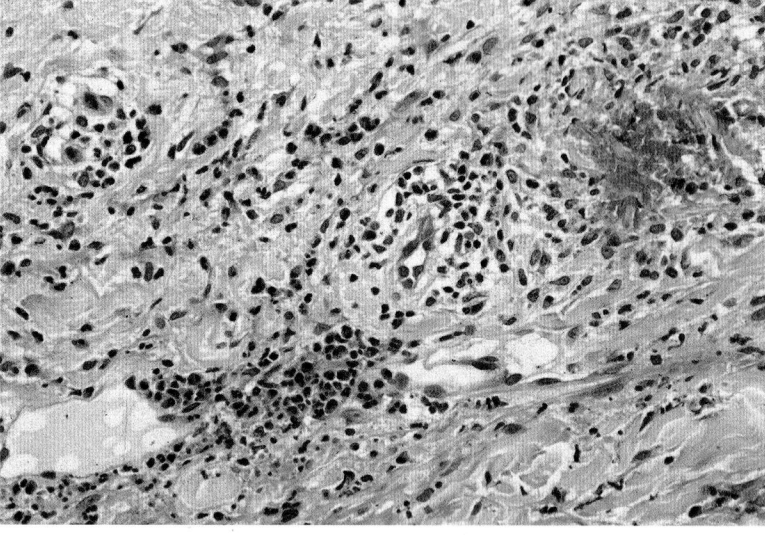

Fig. 8.63
Urticarial vasculitis: there is a heavy lymphocytic and eosinophil infiltrate. In this example, there are conspicuous flame figures.

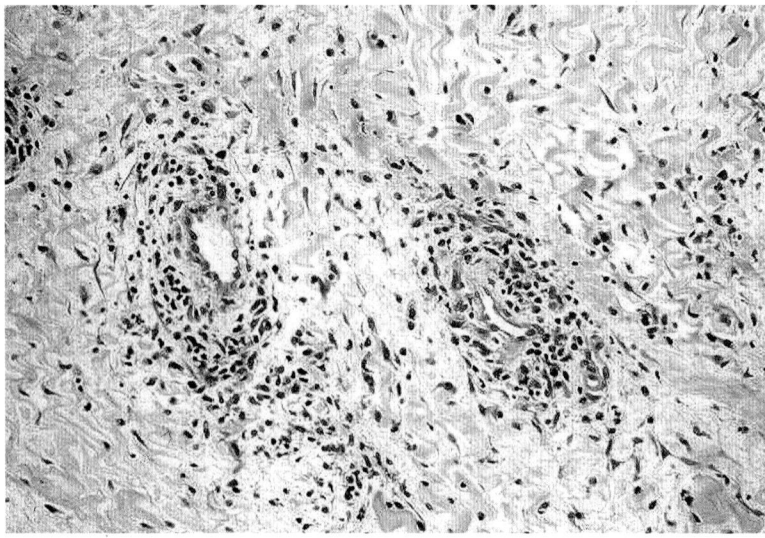

Fig. 8.62
Urticarial vasculitis: in this field, there is marked edema accompanied by a mixed lymphocytic and eosinophil infiltrate.

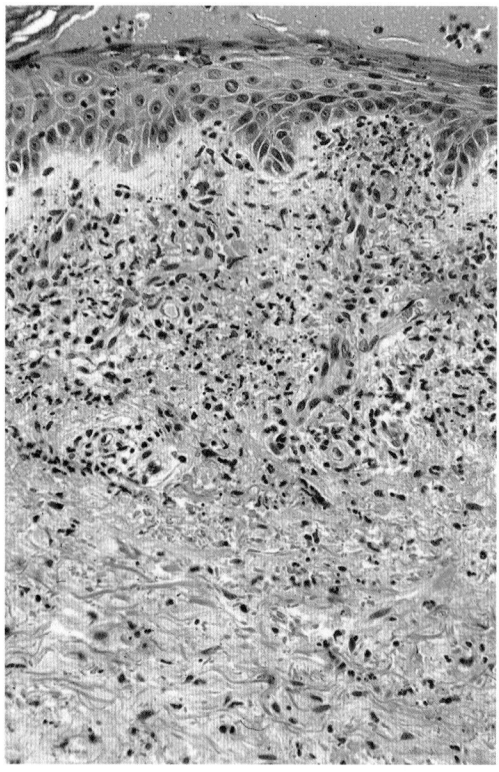

Fig. 8.64
Urticarial vasculitis: this biopsy of a purpuric lesion shows features of florid vasculitis.

the superficial vascular plexus. Extravasation of red blood cells is evidence of vascular damage. The vasculitis shows features of leukocytoclastic vasculitis except that the histologic features tend to be very subtle and are easily overlooked (*Figs 8.61–8.63*). Mild or focal fibrinoid changes associated with few neutrophils and sparse karyorrhexis are typical and eosinophils are almost always present. In our experience, the vasculitis is usually low grade in nature and often fibrinoid change is absent. Others have shown that endothelial necrosis is unusual.[53] Nevertheless, more impressive necrotizing vasculitis may sometimes be encountered (*Fig. 8.64*). Urticarial vasculitis appears to represent a spectrum of disease ranging from urticaria with very mild vascular injury to frank necrotizing vasculitis.[54–56]

Differential diagnosis

Clinical correlation is necessary to distinguish urticarial vasculitis from other forms of leukocytoclastic vasculitis. Although urticarial vasculitis is often associated with subtle, low-grade vascular injury, this pattern should not be relied upon in the distinction from other forms of vasculitis. In short, the pathologist's role in diagnosis is to confirm the presence of vasculitis.

Tumor necrosis factor receptor-associated periodic syndrome (familiar Hibernian fever)

Clinical features

Tumor necrosis factor receptor-associated periodic syndrome (TRAPS) is a rare autosomal dominant condition with a predilection for individuals of Irish and Scottish descent.[1–5] Other terms used to describe this disorder include familial Hibernian fever, benign autosomal dominant familial periodic fever, and autosomal dominant periodic fever with amyloidosis. Patients usually present in infancy or early childhood with prolonged episodes of fever accompanied by (in descending order of frequency) abdominal pain, cutaneous manifestations, myalgia, headache, arthralgia, and pleuritic chest pain.[3] Rare associations include central nervous system involvement due to a demyelinating disorder, IgA nephropathy, and small vessel vasculitis with concomitant relapsing panniculitis.[6–8]

Cutaneous manifestations include migratory asymptomatic, nonscaly erythematous macules and plaques, annular and serpiginous lesions measuring up to 28 cm in diameter.[2,3] The trunk and extremities are predominantly affected with lesions presenting proximally and migrating distally.[3] Patients may also develop conjunctivitis and periorbital edema.[2] Amyloidosis is an occasional complication.[9]

Pathogenesis and histologic features

TRAPS is due to a mutation of the TNFRSF1A gene which encodes the tumor necrosis factor receptor.[3] The gene has been localized to chromosome 12p13.[4] More than 60 mutations have been identified in the TNFRSF1A gene so far but the precise disease mechanism remains elusive.[10]

Histologically, the skin lesions are characterized by dermal edema and a superficial and deep perivascular and interstitial infiltrate of lymphocytes and a lesser number of macrophages.[1–3] There is no evidence of vasculitis. Small numbers of neutrophils or plasma cells may occasionally be present.[3]

The infiltrate consists of CD3+ T lymphocytes and CD68+ macrophages. CD4+ T-helper and CD8+ T-suppressor forms are both represented. CD20+ B lymphocytes are not present.

Eosinophilic, polymorphic, and pruritic eruption associated with radiotherapy

Clinical features

Rueda and coworkers documented a polymorphic cutaneous eruption which develops in females undergoing radiotherapy for cancer (eosinophilic, polymorphic, and pruritic eruption associated with radiotherapy, EPPER).[1–6] Although a wide spectrum of tumors may be present, cervical squamous carcinoma and breast carcinoma are by far the most common. The cutaneous lesions are intensely pruritic and include excoriations, erythematous papules, vesicles, blisters, pustules, and panniculitis-like lesions.[1–8] The extremities, particularly the legs, are predominantly affected.

Pathogenesis and histologic features

The pathogenesis of this condition is unknown.

Histologically, the eruption is characterized by a superficial and deep lymphohistiocytic infiltrate accompanied by conspicuous eosinophils. The epidermis is hyperkeratotic and there is mild acanthosis frequently accompanied by spongiosis. Other manifestations include eosinophilic spongiosis, pustules, bullous pemphigoid-like subepidermal blistering, and eosinophilic panniculitis.

Direct immunofluorescence may disclose perivascular deposits of C3 and IgM. Indirect immunofluorescence studies are negative.

The lymphocytes are of the CD3+ T-cell phenotype with a predominance of CD4+ T-helper cells over CD8+ T-suppressor cells. B cells are absent.

Table 8.1
Viruses associated with cutaneous eruptions

Cytomegalovirus
Enterovirus (coxsakievirus, echovirus)
Epstein-Barr virus
Hepatitis B virus
Human immunodeficiency virus
Paramyxovirus
Parvovirus
Roseola (human herpesvirus-6)
Rubella
Rubeola (measles)
Toga virus

Viral exanthemata

A variety of viral infections may present with cutaneous eruptions. Although some viruses are associated with an eruption with distinctive clinical features, others are affiliated with a non-specific maculopapular dermatosis (*Table 8.1*). Exceptionally, exanthemata may represent a primary cutaneous infection. More commonly, the clinical features are a manifestation of an immune response, such as an immune complex disease or a cell-mediated hypersensitivity reaction, to an infection at an extracutaneous site.

Biopsy of a viral exanthem often shows a superficial perivascular lymphocytic infiltrate. Some cases may show epidermal pathology such as interface changes with dyskeratotic cells. The histologic features are entirely non-specific, and distinction from hypersensitivity reactions (e.g., a drug eruption) is impossible without clinical (often including serological investigation) correlation. Viruses that infect cutaneous sites may be visualized by light microscopy including immunohistochemistry, or demonstrated by viral culture, immunological testing, PCR or DNA hybridization. Skin manifestations of viral infections are described in detail in Chapter 18.

Access **ExpertConsult.com** for the complete list of references

Granulomatous, necrobiotic and perforating dermatoses

See
www.expertconsult.com
for references and
additional material

Sarcoidosis

Clinical features

Sarcoidosis (Gr. *sarkos*, flesh; *eidos*, form), so named because its histologic features were originally thought to resemble a sarcoma (Boeck), is a common systemic disease of unknown etiology. It is characterized and defined by the presence of noncaseating granulomata, usually (but not invariably) affecting multiple organ systems.[1-11] Manifestations are variable. Patients may present with:

- an acute and usually self-limiting variant,
- a chronic form exclusively affecting the skin (up to between 20% and 40% of patients with cutaneous sarcoidosis do not have systemic involvement),
- a serious systemic chronic variant with widespread lesions, which affects multiple systems, is associated with high morbidity, and may occasionally be fatal.

Sarcoidosis is more commonly encountered in industrialized countries and shows particularly high incidences in northern Europe (including the UK), the USA, and New Zealand, where as many as 20/100 000 of the population may be affected. It presents particularly in people in their third and fourth decades and shows a female predominance.[12] In the USA, sarcoidosis is common among blacks, and there is a similar tendency in the UK (*Figs 9.1 and 9.2*). An epidemiological study of sarcoidosis in the Detroit, Michigan, area found that African-Americans living there had a 3.8 times greater risk of developing the disease compared with Caucasians.[13] The disease is rare in Asians.[14] First- and second-degree relatives of patients with sarcoidosis seem to have a significant risk of developing the disease compared to the normal population.[15] The disease is rare in children, presents mainly in teenagers, and although the manifestations are usually similar to those seen in adults, infants may present with symptoms simulating juvenile rheumatoid arthritis (*Fig. 9.3*).[16-18] Two forms of sarcoidosis have been identified in children. A variant affecting older children and occurring mainly during teenage years presents with a multisystemic disease similar to that seen in adults. Younger children under the age of 4 present with a cutaneous rash, arthritis, and uveitis.[19] Infantile sarcoidosis should not be confused with Blau syndrome. This disease is inherited in an autosomal dominant fashion

and is characterized by sarcoidal granulomata in the skin, uveal tract, and joints but with no pulmonary involvement.[20,21] Despite the similarities between both diseases, no genetic linkage has been identified.

Rarely, sarcoidosis presents in monozygotic twins.[22] Coexistence with common variable immune deficiency is also a rare occurrence.[23]

Cutaneous lesions occur in 20–35% of patients with systemic sarcoidosis and may be classified into non-specific (erythema nodosum) and specific (granulomatous) subtypes.[10] Cutaneous sarcoidal granulomata appear to be associated with a poorer prognosis and an increased incidence of pulmonary fibrosis and uveitis. Chronic facial lesions have been shown to be more commonly associated with involvement of the lungs, sinuses, and eyes.[24] Erythema nodosum occurs quite commonly in sarcoidosis, with reported incidences varying from 11% to 31%.[25] There is a significant female predominance (3:1). Interestingly, erythema nodosum appears to be relatively uncommon in both African-Americans and Caucasians in the USA. It presents as erythematous, tender, subcutaneous nodules, usually on the anterior tibial regions. Erythema nodosum may be associated with pyrexia, polyarthralgia (wrists, knees, and ankles), a very high erythrocyte sedimentation rate (ESR), and bilateral hilar lymphadenopathy (Lofgren syndrome). This acute form of sarcoidosis is associated with a good prognosis, with most patients experiencing resolution within 6 months of onset of symptoms.[26-28] In one study, however, 16% of patients who presented with erythema nodosum developed chronic disease.[27]

A not uncommon mode of presentation is the development of a widespread, usually asymptomatic, maculopapular eruption. Individual lesions are erythematous or violaceous, 3–6 mm in diameter, and most commonly seen on the face (particularly in a periorbital distribution), the trunk, the extensor aspects of the extremities, and the neck (*Figs 9.4 and 9.5*). In this variant, the patient may also develop acute lymphadenopathy and uveitis, and a chest X-ray examination can reveal features of early respiratory involvement. Spontaneous resolution sometimes occurs. Occasionally, micropapular lesions are seen, particularly on the face and limbs (*Fig. 9.6*). Rarely, patients develop sheets of pinhead-sized lichenoid papules on the trunk and limbs. The onset is abrupt, and lesions may appear in crops. Some patients develop nodules and plaques, which may occur anywhere on the body, but most often affect the face, extremities, buttocks, and shoulders (*Figs 9.7–9.11*). Annular or serpiginous lesions are also encountered,

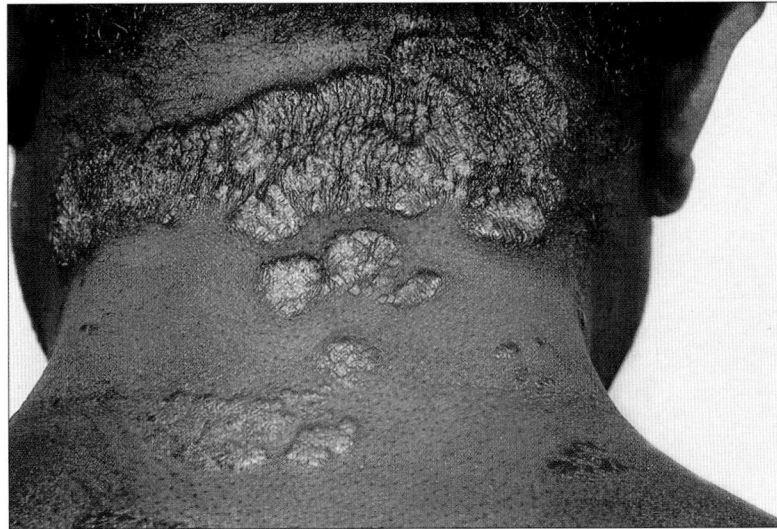

Fig. 9.1
Sarcoidosis: this patient presented with multiple plaques with raised margins on the neck. From the collection of the late N.P. Smith, MD, the Institute of Dermatology, London, UK.

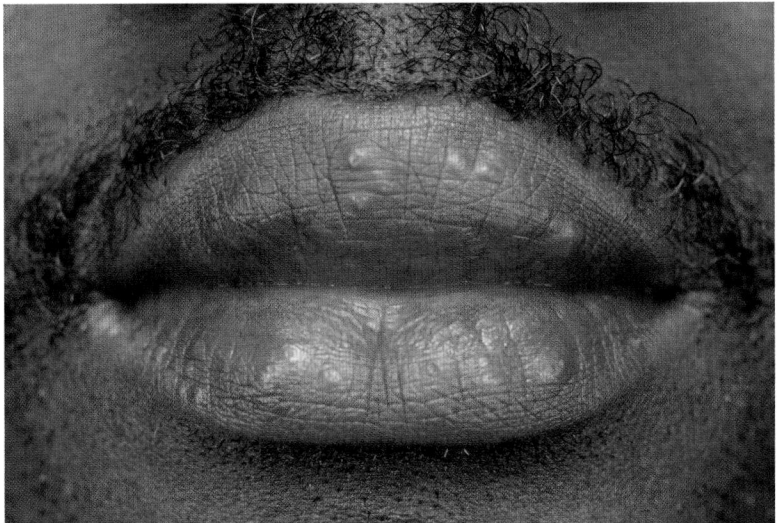

Fig. 9.2
Sarcoidosis: papules are present on both upper and lower lips. From the collection of the late N.P. Smith, MD, the Institute of Dermatology, London, UK.

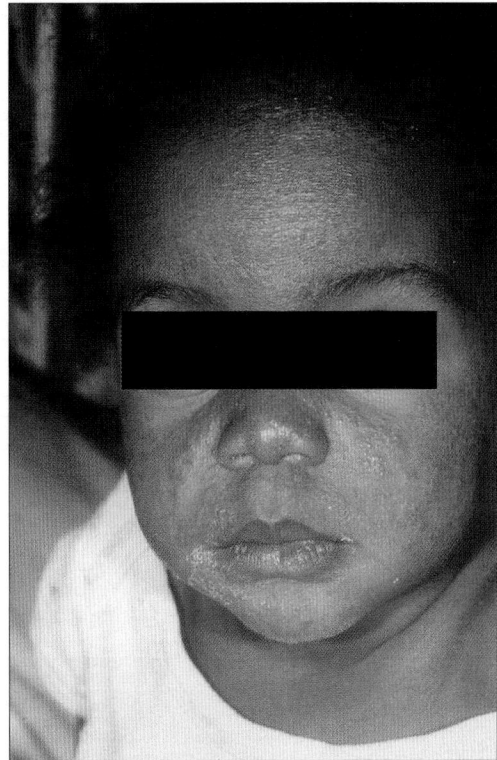

Fig. 9.3
Sarcoidosis: the condition is rare in children. There are widespread micropapules on this child's face. By courtesy of C.T.C. Kennedy, MD, Bristol Royal Infirmary, Bristol, UK.

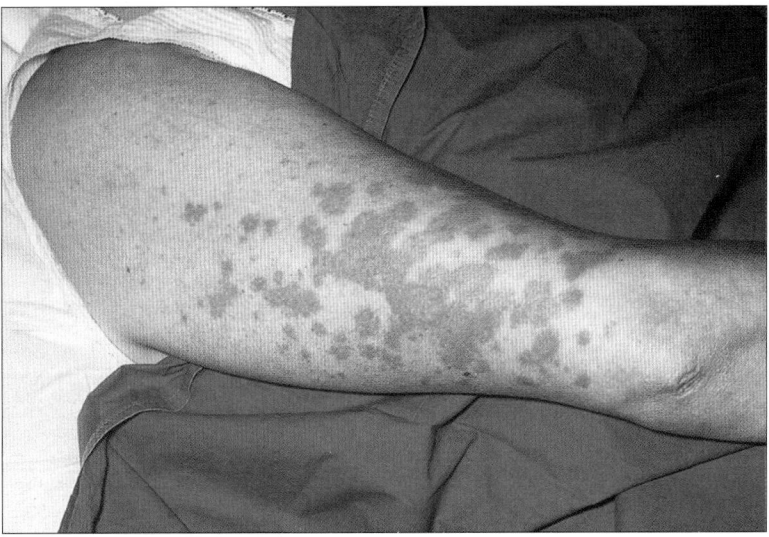

Fig. 9.4
Sarcoidosis: widespread erythematous plaques on the upper arm, some with an annular appearance. By courtesy of R.A. Marsden, MD, St George's Hospital, London, UK.

and sometimes there is a prominent telangiectatic component (angiolupoid sarcoid) (*Figs 9.12* and *9.13*).[10] Rarely, epidermal changes result in a psoriasiform or even ichthyosiform appearance.[29] An exceptional case mimicking lipodermatosclerosis has been described.[30] Chronic skin lesions are associated with pulmonary fibrosis, ocular, and bone involvement.

Most characteristic of sarcoidosis, however, is lupus pernio. This chronic violaceous plaque most often affects the nose, cheek, and ears, but lesions also sometimes affect the fingers and knees (*Fig. 9.14*). It is a particularly disfiguring variant, and resolution is especially complicated by marked scarring. Lupus pernio is often associated with lesions in the upper respiratory tract and can be followed by nasal obstruction and septal perforation. Patients also have severe pulmonary fibrosis, bone cysts, and ocular lesions. This variant has an insidious onset and is associated with a prolonged course and poor prognosis.[16]

Patients with sarcoidosis not uncommonly develop lesions in scar tissue[31,32] and also in relation to trauma at the sites of desensitizing injections, tattoos, venipuncture, surgery, laser, cosmetic fillers, and BCG (*Fig. 9.15*).[33–38] A single case attributed to copper-containing earrings has been described.[39] Sarcoidal granulomata in association with foreign bodies do not necessarily imply a diagnosis of sarcoidosis. However, a small number of patients with

sarcoidal granulomata in association with silica and tattoo pigment may have systemic sarcoidosis or the latter may develop subsequently.[40] Awareness of this problem is important as such cutaneous granulomata may be the first manifestation of the disease. Sarcoidosis has also been documented presenting in a tattoo in association with interferon-alpha (IFN-α) treatment for chronic hepatitis C.[41] Interestingly, sarcoidosis has also been reported rarely in patients receiving interferon and ribavirin for chronic hepatitis C,[42,43] and in rare patients on interferon-alpha or interferon-B therapy for melanoma.[44,45] Sarcoidosis in patients with chronic hepatitis C may present concomitantly with the disease and unrelated to medication, or more often triggered by treatment, mainly ribavirin and interferon-alpha.[46]

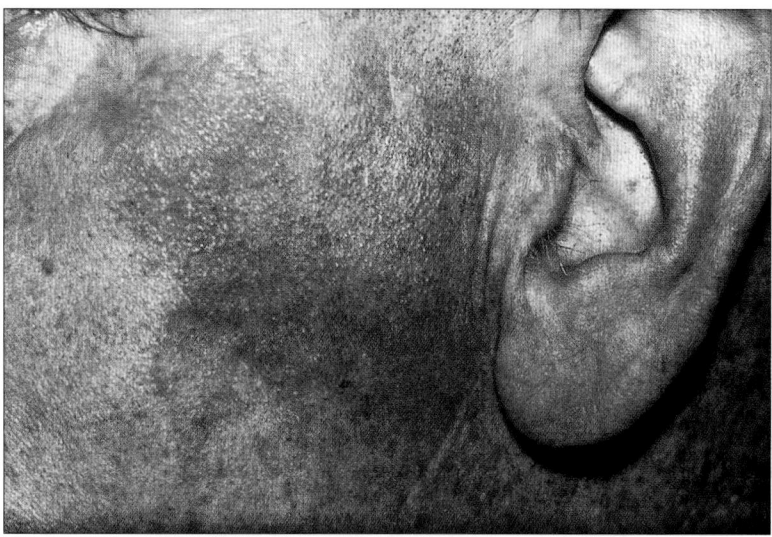

Fig. 9.5
Sarcoidosis: characteristic mauve plaque on the malar area with an infiltrative appearance. By courtesy of R.A. Marsden, MD, St George's Hospital, London, UK.

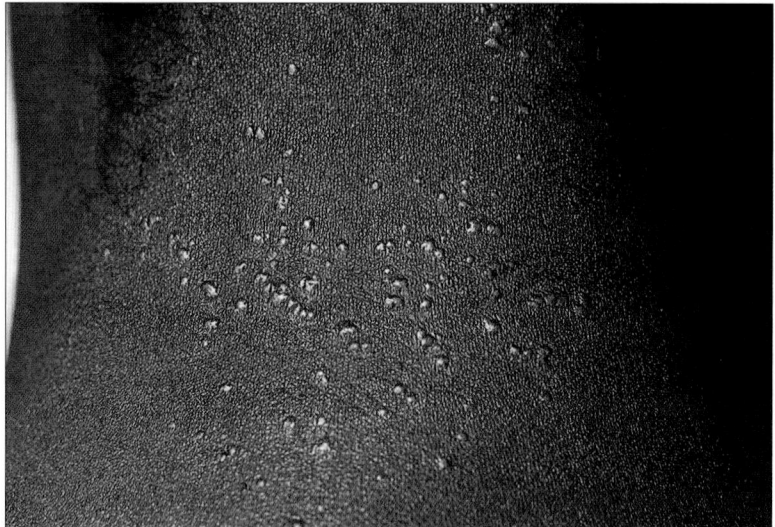

Fig. 9.6
Sarcoidosis: micropapular variant. Note the tiny lichenoid papules. By courtesy of the Institute of Dermatology, London, UK.

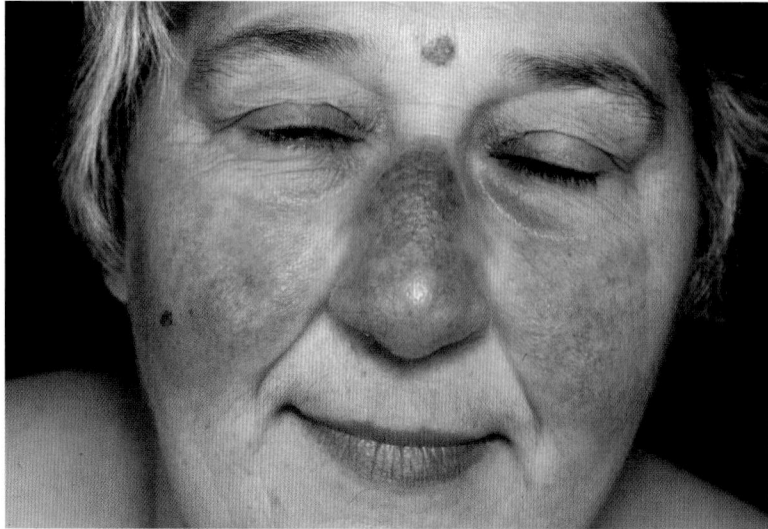

Fig. 9.7
Sarcoidosis: there is extensive facial involvement, a commonly affected site. From the collection of the late N.P. Smith, MD, the Institute of Dermatology, London, UK.

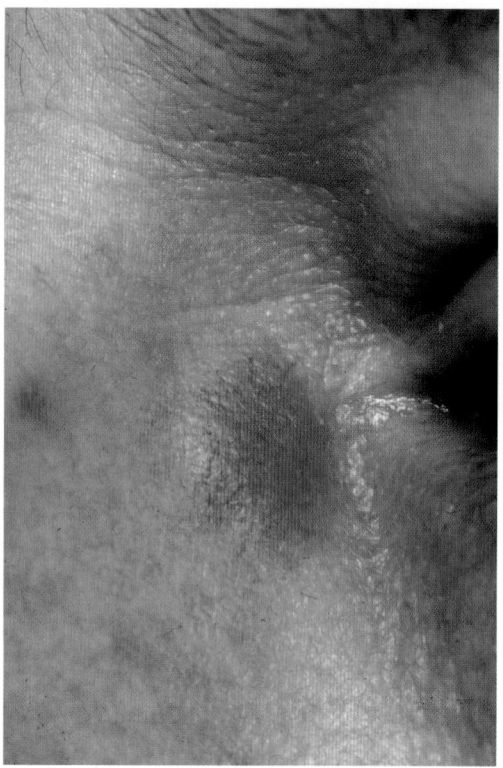

Fig. 9.8
Sarcoidosis: erythematous plaque adjacent to the eye. From the collection of the late N.P. Smith, MD, the Institute of Dermatology, London, UK.

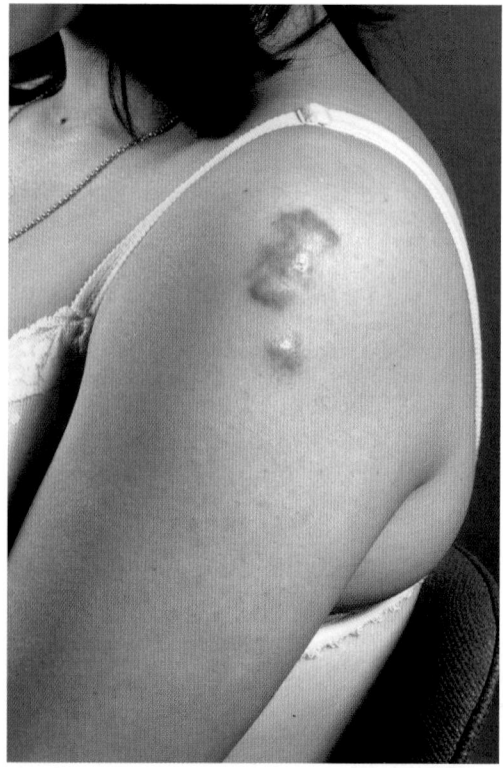

Fig. 9.9
Sarcoidosis: the extremities are commonly affected. From the collection of the late N.P. Smith, MD, the Institute of Dermatology, London, UK.

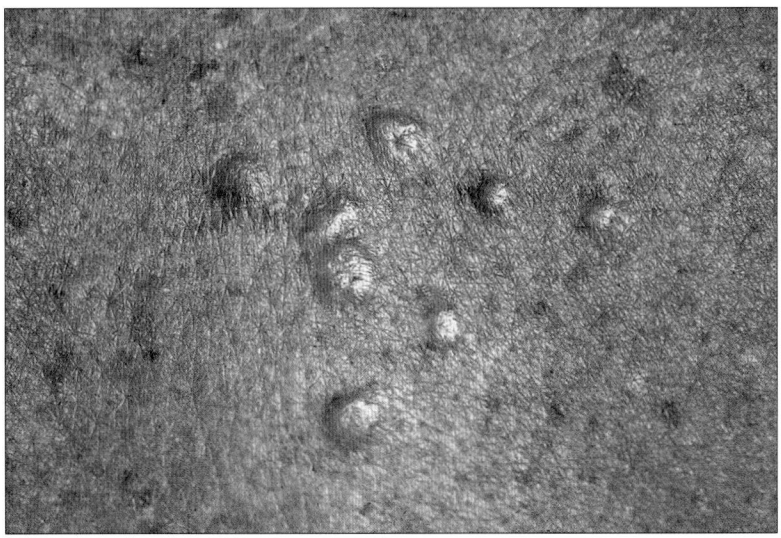

Fig. 9.10
Sarcoidosis: these grouped nodules are present on sun-damaged skin of the upper chest. By courtesy of the Institute of Dermatology, London, UK.

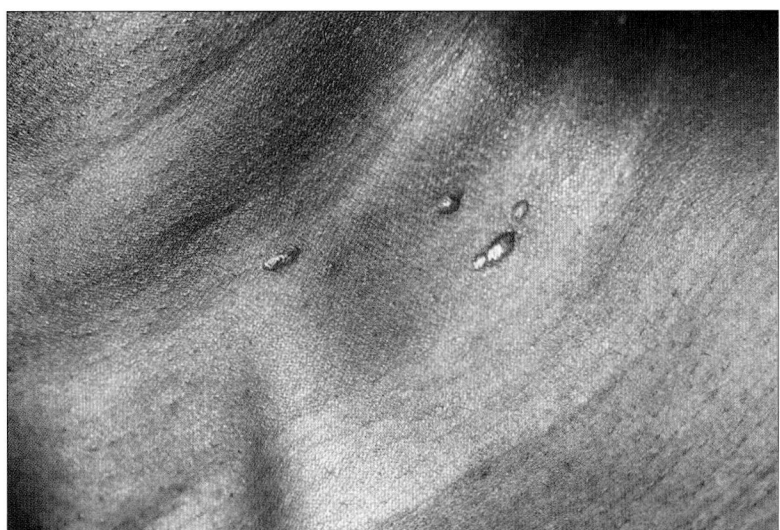

Fig. 9.11
Sarcoidosis: small nodules on the anterior aspect of the neck. By courtesy of R.A. Marsden, MD, St George's Hospital, London, UK.

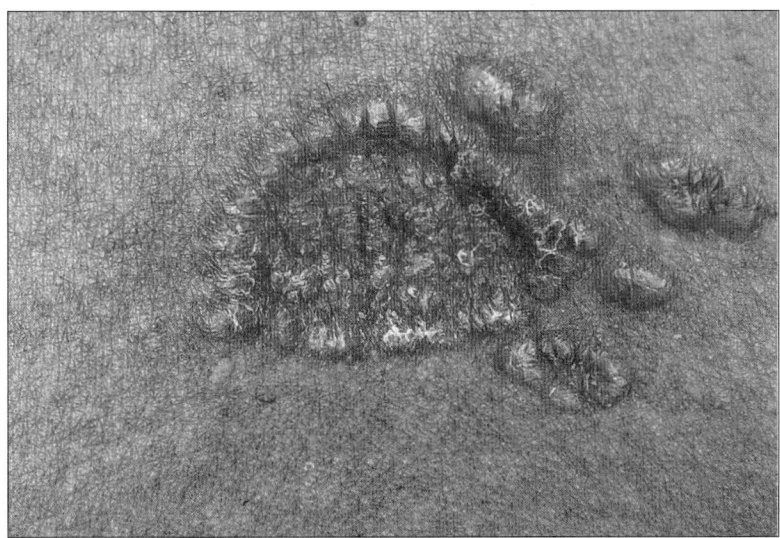

Fig. 9.13
Sarcoidosis: close-up view of an annular lesion. Note the beaded appearance. By courtesy of the Institute of Dermatology, London, UK.

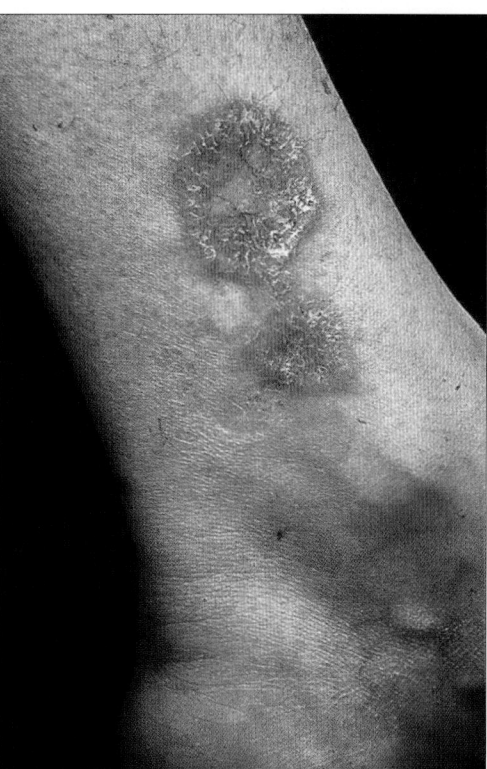

Fig. 9.12
Sarcoidosis: annular lesions on the ankle. By courtesy of the Institute of Dermatology, London, UK.

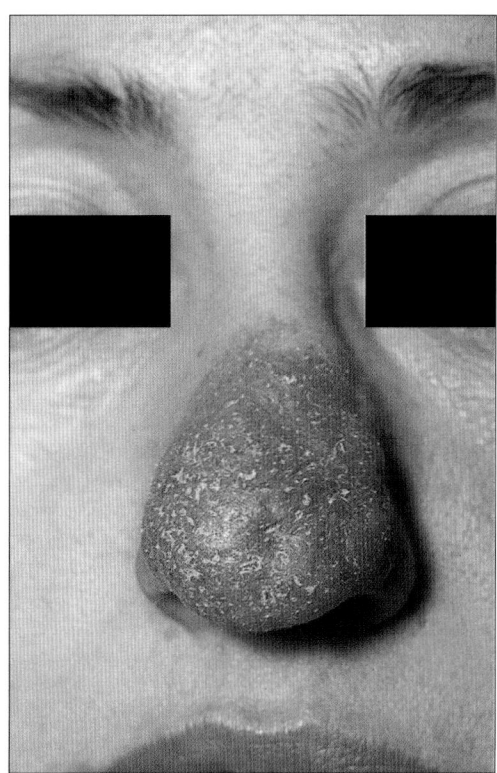

Fig. 9.14
Sarcoidosis: lupus pernio. The nose shows typical scaly violaceous swelling. By courtesy of the Institute of Dermatology, London, UK.

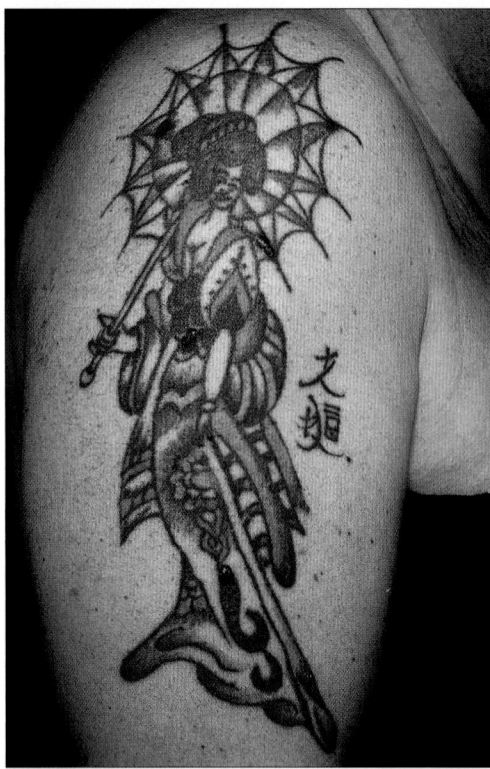

Fig. 9.15
Sarcoidosis: tattoo reaction. There are multiple dome-shaped nodules. By courtesy of the Institute of Dermatology, London, UK.

Sarcoidosis has rarely been described in patients on Vemurafenib for metastatic melanoma.[47] An association has also been occasionally reported in patients on infliximab, etanercept, adalimumab, ipilimumab, and natalizumab.[48–50] Sarcoidal granulomas occurred in a patient on nivolumab for desmoplastic melanoma.[51] The association of the disease with antitumor necrosis factor agents is paradoxical as these agents are used to treat the disease.

Hypopigmented lesions may be seen in black patients.[52] Unusual cutaneous manifestations include subcutaneous nodules, ichthyosiform lesions, erythroderma, scarring and nonscarring alopecia, lymphedema, nail dystrophy in the absence of underlying bone changes, verrucous lesions, generalized atrophy, leonine facies, palmar erythema, and leg ulcers with or without granulomatous vasculitis.[53–67] Lesions of scarring alopecia may clinically mimic discoid lupus erythematosus.[68] Subcutaneous nodules are rare and present as persistent, freely mobile, often painful lesions measuring 5–15 mm in diameter. It has been suggested that subcutaneous lesions are more often associated with systemic disease.[69] In further studies however, subcutaneous involvement does not seem to be associated with increased incidence of systemic disease or worse prognosis.[70,71] Oral and genital involvement is rare, but disease restricted to the vulva has been documented.[72–74] Sarcoidosis has also been described presenting as a testicular mass.[75] A very rare variant of seasonal photoinduced cutaneous sarcoidosis may occur.[76]

Ninety percent of patients with sarcoidosis have pulmonary involvement.[28] Bilateral hilar lymphadenopathy is the most common intrathoracic manifestation of sarcoidosis and, together with pulmonary involvement, forms the most frequent lesion. Intrathoracic manifestations in sarcoidosis are classified into five subgroups:[6,10]

- Stage 0: normal chest X-ray,
- Stage I: bilateral hilar and/or paratracheal lymphadenopathy with no pulmonary involvement,
- Stage II: lymphadenopathy with pulmonary infiltrates,
- Stage III: pulmonary infiltrates, but no lymphadenopathy,
- Stage IV: irreversible fibrosis and bullae, cysts, emphysema.

Stage I disease is frequently associated with spontaneous resolution; progression to stage II disease is uncommon. Severe pulmonary involvement as seen in stage III patients correlates with deep chronic plaque lesions and lupus pernio. Patients have interstitial fibrosis and eventual cor pulmonale, which may prove fatal.

Systemic vasculitis involving small- to large-caliber vessels has been found in some adults and children with sarcoidosis.[77] This manifestation tends to be more common in African-American and Asian patients.[77]

Ocular lesions develop in about 20% of patients with sarcoidosis. Acute anterior uveitis is the most common manifestation; it is frequently bilateral and shows a predilection for females. It correlates with a benign outcome and erythema nodosum. Chronic uveitis also affects the anterior chamber and if untreated may progress to glaucoma and blindness. Other lesions include retinal vein perivasculitis, disc edema, and neovascularization. Conjunctival granulomata may be present in up to 30% of patients; therefore, biopsy can be a useful and relatively safe method of establishing the diagnosis. The lacrimal gland is also sometimes affected.

Neurological involvement occurs in 5–15% of patients with systemic sarcoidosis. Clinical manifestations include small fiber neuropathy, facial nerve palsy, Guillain-Barré syndrome, optic nerve disease, meningitis, seizure, and encephalopathy.[6,78–80] In one study, neurosarcoidosis was the presenting symptom in 31% of patients.[79] The combination of uveitis, facial nerve palsy, fever, and swelling of the parotid gland is known as uveoparotid fever (Heerfordt syndrome). This condition is often associated with central nervous system involvement. Hypothalamic and pituitary lesions are rare and may manifest as diabetes insipidus or panhypopituitarism.

Peripheral lymphadenopathy develops in about 30% of patients. However, histologic examination of peripheral lymph nodes will reveal granulomata in about 75% of patients with sarcoidosis. Although splenomegaly is only present in 10–25% of patients, granulomata are present in about 50% of cases. Splenic disease is usually asymptomatic, but patients may have abdominal pain, hypersplenism, and, very rarely, splenic rupture. Splenic disease correlates positively with a high frequency of intrathoracic sarcoidosis. Liver function test abnormalities are quite common, and about 20% of patients have hepatomegaly; 60% of patients have hepatic granulomata on histologic examination.

Cardiac lesions are uncommon, but are of particular importance due to the associated mortality.[6] In an autopsy series, 50% of all deaths were due to cardiac disease.[81] This same study found that the clinician often does not appreciate the presence of cardiac involvement – the antemortem diagnosis of cardiac lesions was made in only 29% of patients.[81] Granulomata may occur at any site, but appear to show a predilection for the conduction system. Clinical manifestations include ventricular tachycardia, complete heart block, congestive cardiac failure, pericardial effusion, and myocardial infarction. Sarcoidal granulomata may affect small and large blood vessels, in particular the pulmonary vasculature.

Muscle involvement is usually asymptomatic. Histologic examination of random muscle biopsies reveals granulomata in as many as 50% of patients. Rare features include asymptomatic palpable nodules and a polymyositis-like syndrome.

Although a rare complication, patients with sarcoidosis appear to be more prone to develop cryptococcosis than other infections.[82]

Radiologically demonstrable bone lesions occur in about 15% of patients. Early lesions consist of osteoporosis, cortical thinning, and mottled rarefaction. Established lesions are cystic and are sometimes associated with pathological fractures. The hands and feet are predominantly affected (Fig. 9.16). Destruction of the nasal bones can result from direct infiltration in patients with lupus pernio.

Hypercalcemia and, particularly, hypercalcuria are important complications of sarcoidosis. This is possibly due to increased intestinal absorption of calcium and abnormal production of 1,25-dihydroxyvitamin D.[83] It is more often transitory, but in a small proportion of patients it is persistent and sometimes complicated by the development of renal failure due to nephrocalcinosis. Granulomata are found on histologic examination of the kidney in up to 40% of patients.

Laboratory investigations reveal a wide variety of abnormalities of the immune system (see below). Patients may demonstrate elevated levels of serum angiotensin-converting enzyme (ACE). Unfortunately, this finding is not specific for sarcoidosis, increased values also being found in patients with diabetes mellitus, alcoholic liver disease, and leprosy. It is sometimes

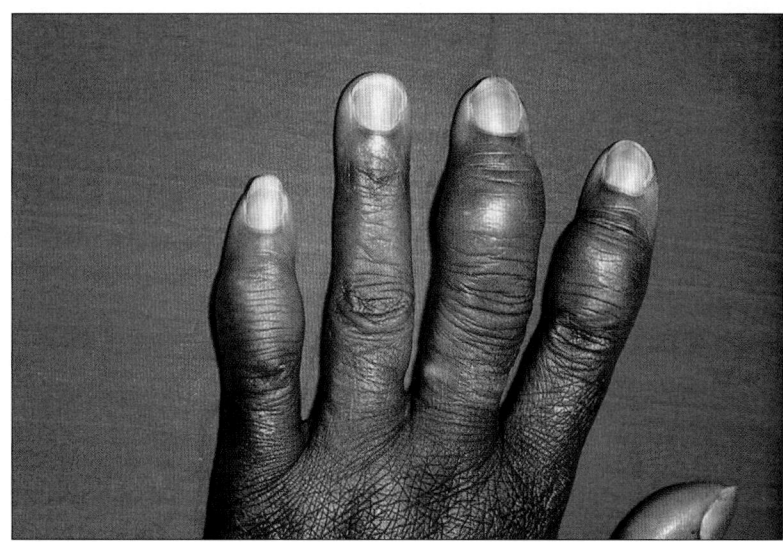

Fig. 9.16
Sarcoidosis: there is marked swelling of the distal interphalangeal joints. By courtesy of R.A. Marsden, MD, St George's Hospital, London, UK.

of value in monitoring the level of disease activity in patients known to have sarcoidosis. Patients may also display increased levels of serum and urinary lysozyme, serum beta-2-microglobulin, and collagenase.

Although sarcoidosis is associated with a high morbidity, the mortality rate is low, being of the order of 3–6%. Causes of death include cardiac involvement and respiratory or renal failure. The prognosis is better in females and appears to be improved in those with a positive purified protein derivative (PPD) skin test and normal serum immunoglobulin levels. The severity of disease is greater in blacks and Asians compared with Caucasians.[84] Of interest, despite the very marked upset in immunological phenomena, patients do not seem to have an associated greatly increased risk of opportunistic infections except as a consequence of therapy (e.g., corticosteroids).

The association between sarcoidosis and a number of systemic diseases is probably coincidental. Sarcoidosis has been documented in association with vitiligo, pernicious anemia, autoimmune thyroiditis, Graves disease, chronic hepatitis, Addison disease, Sjögren syndrome, diabetes mellitus and ulcerative colitis, lymphoma, human immunodeficiency virus (HIV) infection, and primary biliary cirrhosis.[85–96] Interestingly, patients with acquired immunodeficiency syndrome (AIDS) usually develop manifestations of sarcoidosis after antiretroviral therapy is started. This phenomenon is the result of the immune restoration syndrome.[93,97] Associations with cutaneous autoimmune disease include dermatitis herpetiformis and linear IgA disease.[98,99] A single case of trachyonychia associated with sarcoidosis has been reported.[100]

Pathogenesis and histologic features

The pathogenesis of sarcoidosis is poorly understood. The demonstration of familial clustering suggests hereditary susceptibility to sarcoidosis in at least a subset of patients.[15,101]

Despite intensive studies, the etiology and pathogenesis of sarcoidosis remains elusive.[102,103] It is likely, however, that sarcoidosis represents a reaction pattern that may develop in a predisposed patient on exposure to one or more infective agents or other antigens.

The role of mycobacteria in the pathogenesis of sarcoidosis is a controversial topic. Attempts at detection of mycobacterial DNA by polymerase chain reaction (PCR) have produced conflicting results. While some authors have failed to detect mycobacterial DNA, others have identified DNA of various strains of tuberculous and nontuberculous mycobacteria.[104–108] In one study, although amplified mycobacterial DNA was detected by PCR in 38% of sarcoidosis patients, mycobacterial DNA was also detected in tissue in 44% of control patients.[109] Furthermore, most studies published in the literature fail to report more than 6% positivity for *Mycobacterium tuberculosis* DNA in patients with sarcoidosis.[110] In another interesting study,

cell wall deficient acid-fast bacteria (L forms) were cultured from the blood of 19 of 20 patients with sarcoidosis but not from controls.[111] In summary, these mixed results between laboratories have not clarified the role of mycobacteria in the pathogenesis of sarcoidosis. It seems, however, that mycobacteria may be of etiological importance in at least a subset of cases.

Propionibacterium acnes DNA has also been identified in tissues of patients with sarcoidosis, including involved lymph nodes.[112,113] The significance of this finding remains uncertain. Human herpesvirus 8 DNA has not been demonstrated in tissues of patients with sarcoidosis.[113]

The occasional association with known autoimmune diseases, such as progressive systemic sclerosis and systemic lupus erythematosus (SLE), has inevitably led to the proposal of an autoimmune pathogenesis. Although many familial cases have been reported in the literature, no consistent pattern of inheritance has emerged. The results of human leukocyte antigen (HLA) typing have shown associations with particular features of the disease; for example, HLA-A1 and HLA-B8 are associated with arthritis, HLA-A1 is also associated with uveitis, and HLA-B13 may be associated with a chronic refractory variant.[10] Patients with HLA-DR17 have a better prognosis.[114] One study has shown that patients with sarcoidosis have an increased frequency of a glutamine residue at position 69 of the B1 chain of the HLA-DPB molecule compared with a control population.[115] This is particularly interesting since a similar polymorphism has been documented in patients with chronic beryllium disease, a disorder also characterized by granulomata and which shares some pathological features in common with sarcoidosis.

Immunological investigations in patients with sarcoidosis have produced an immense wealth of data, which reveal that there is clearly an associated state of abnormal immunological hyperactivity. There are alterations of both cell-mediated and humoral immunity. Despite great efforts to clarify the immunobiology of sarcoidosis, particularly with regard to the precise antigens that may facilitate the disease, we still do not have a clear understanding of the disease process. Sarcoidosis, at least in part, appears to be due to a hyperactive T-helper cell proliferation with lymphokine production.[11,116] Increased T-helper (Th1, Th2) cells are present in the alveolar lung parenchyma. Several studies have demonstrated selective activation of certain oligoclonal T-cell subsets.[117–122] In one study, there was a correlation between the particular oligoclonal T-cell subsets and disease activity.[117] Th1 lymphocytes (T cells expressing interleukin [IL]-2 and IFN-γ) preferentially accumulate in pulmonary parenchyma and the alveolar space compared with Th2 lymphocytes (T cells expressing IL-4 and IL-5).[121] Compared with T cells in peripheral blood, T cells obtained by bronchoalveolar lavage show greater expression of IFN-γ and tumor necrosis factor-alpha (TNF-α).[114] Of interest, patients with HLA-DR17 show a muted cytokine response, a finding that is perhaps related to the better prognosis observed in this subset of patients.[115]

T lymphocytes, in turn, stimulate B cells. Abnormalities of humoral immunity include a non-specific polyclonal hypergammaglobulinemia and circulating immune complexes in acute forms of the disease, particularly in association with erythema nodosum.

The paramount puzzle in unraveling the pathogenesis of sarcoidosis is identifying the initial event(s) that lead to the disease. Despite our increasing knowledge of the immunobiology of sarcoidosis, we seem no closer to answering this key question. It seems clear, however, that the disease is the result of a complex interaction between many different external antigens, genetic predisposition, and the immune responses.

Histologically, sarcoidosis is characterized by a dense, noncaseating granulomatous infiltrate in the dermis (Figs 9.17 and 9.18), which sometimes extends into the subcutaneous fat. The granulomata are discrete and strikingly uniform in size and shape. They are composed of epithelioid histiocytes with abundant eosinophilic cytoplasm and oval or twisted vesicular nuclei often containing a small central nucleolus (Fig. 9.19). Variable numbers of Langhans giant cells are present, and sometimes a scattering of lymphocytes is seen at the peripheral margin of the granuloma (Fig. 9.20). Discrete small central foci of fibrinoid necrosis are sometimes present but caseation necrosis is rare (Fig. 9.21).[122,123] Transepidermal elimination may be seen and seems more common than previously reported.[124,125] The epidermis is usually normal although occasional cases display acanthosis and sometimes

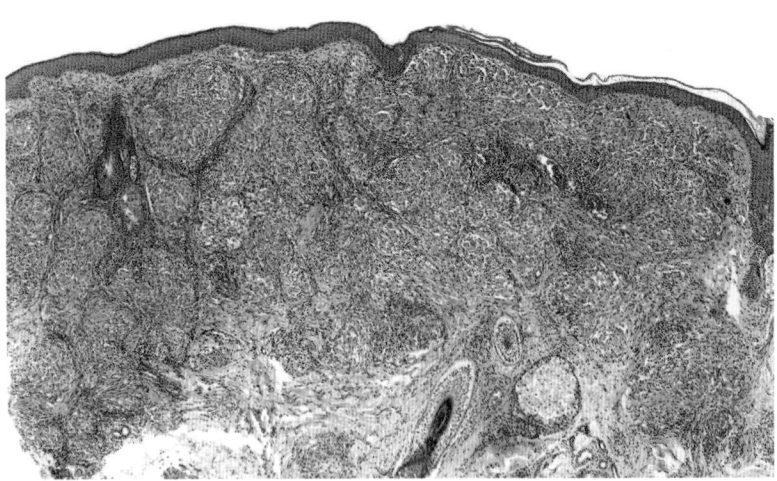

Fig. 9.17
Sarcoidosis: the dermis is replaced by uniform circumscribed nests of noncaseating granulomata.

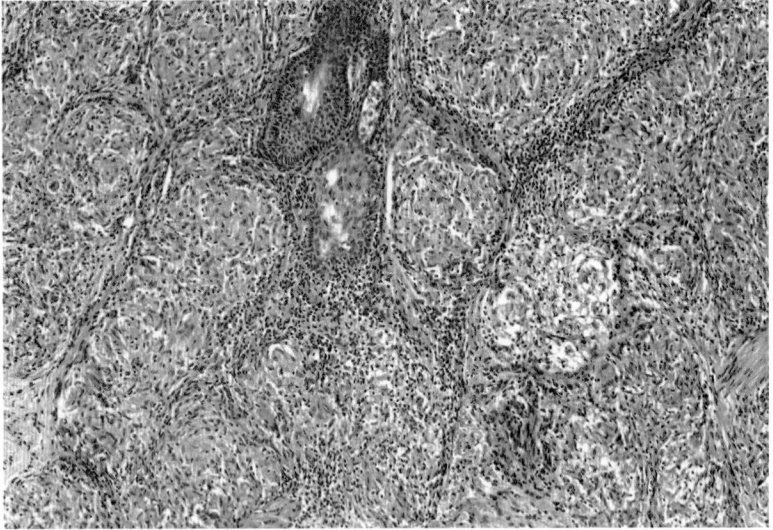

Fig. 9.18
Sarcoidosis: note the paucity of lymphocytes and absence of necrosis.

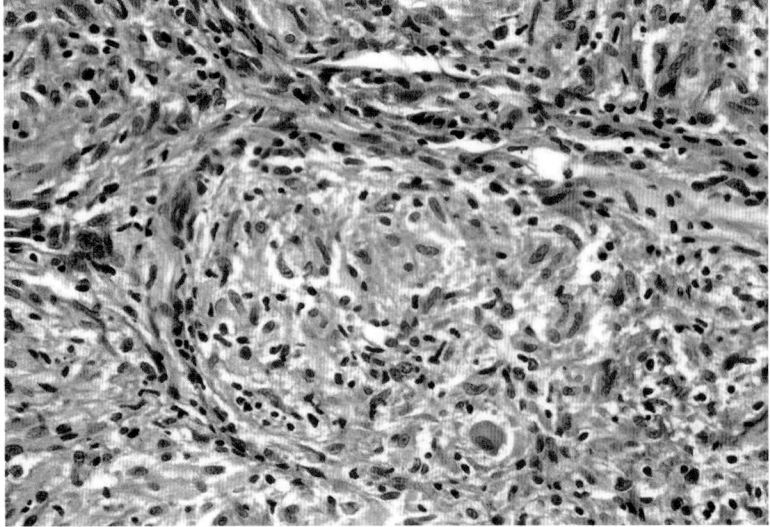

Fig. 9.19
Sarcoidosis: the epithelioid cells are composed of pink cytoplasm with a central oval or sometimes twisted vesicular nucleus containing a small basophilic nucleolus. The granuloma also contains lymphocytes and occasional fibroblasts.

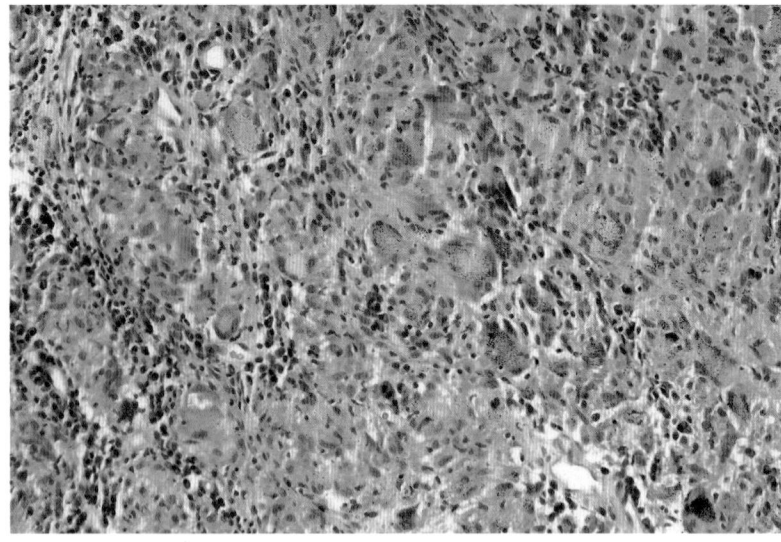

Fig. 9.20
Sarcoidosis: in this example, the granulomatous reaction is associated with abundant foreign material.

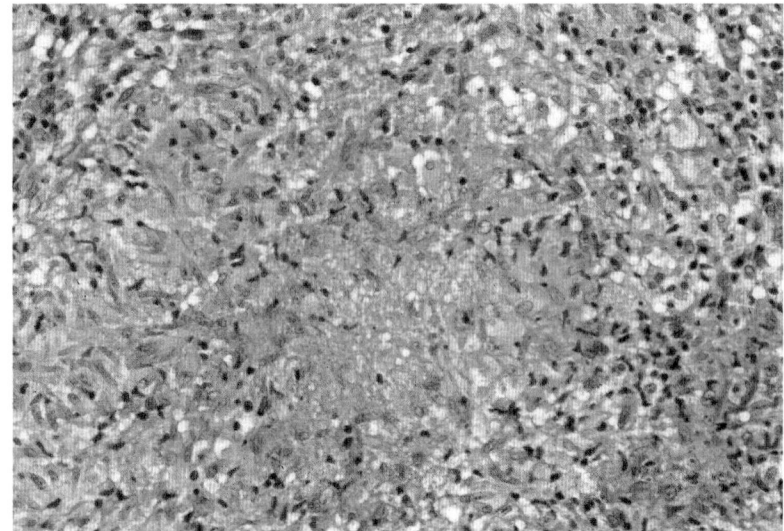

Fig. 9.21
Sarcoidosis: occasionally small foci of 'fibrinoid' necrosis may be seen in the center of the granuloma, but cellular detail is not lost.

the granulomata are focally lichenoid. A predominantly lichenoid pattern may exceptionally be seen.[126] A rare syringotropic variant with decreased sweating has been described.[127] Exceptional cases of sarcoidosis may display histologic findings that focally overlap with granuloma annulare palisading neutrophilic and granulomatous dermatitis.[128] Further histologic findings described include elastophagocytosis, perineural granulomas resembling leprosy, mucin deposition, and an infiltrate rich in plasma cells.[78,129]

In some cutaneous lesions, inclusion bodies are present, although much less frequently than in lymph nodes. The Schaumann body, a basophilic, laminated, rounded, conchoidal structure composed of calcium carbonate, calcium oxalate, phosphate, iron, and dolomite, is not specific for sarcoidosis and is seen in a number of other granulomatous conditions including tuberculosis and berylliosis (Fig. 9.22).[129–131] The asteroid body is a small intracytoplasmic eosinophilic star-shaped structure; it is not specific for sarcoidosis, being seen also, for example, in tuberculosis, tuberculoid leprosy, berylliosis, and atypical facial necrobiosis. It is also commonly found in necrobiotic xanthogranuloma.[132] Initial studies suggested that the asteroid body was composed of collagen, but more recent reports, using immunohistochemistry, suggest that it is a product of the microtubular system.[133,134] The presence of foreign material in sarcoidal granulomata does not exclude

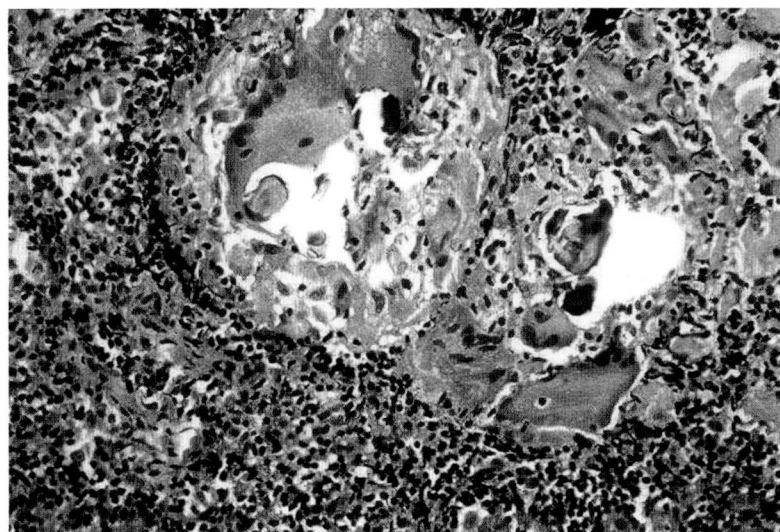

Fig. 9.22
Sarcoidosis: in this lymph node biopsy specimen, fragmented, laminated Schaumann bodies are seen. They are very rarely a feature of cutaneous sarcoidosis.

the diagnosis of sarcoidosis. In fact, polarizable material has been found in up to 5% of cases.[135-137]

It has been shown that the gli-1 oncogene is consistently and abnormally expressed in the cells forming the granulomata not only in sarcoidosis but also in granuloma annulare and necrobiosis lipoidica. This observation raises the possibility of trials using inhibitors of gli-1 signaling to treat this group of granulomatous disorders.[138]

The visceral lesions are characterized by an identical histology of noncaseating granulomata, which may be accompanied by significant scarring, for example, in the lung, where advanced cases are characterized by interstitial fibrosis and sometimes honeycomb lung formation. In the liver, granulomata are most commonly found in the portal tracts or in relation to central veins. Splenic lesions are randomly distributed and are not usually associated with significant fibrosis.

Differential diagnosis

Sarcoidosis must be approached as a diagnosis of exclusion and has to be distinguished from the numerous conditions that may be associated with a noncaseating granulomatous histology, including some forms of tuberculosis, tuberculoid leprosy, berylliosis, fungal infections, Crohn disease, and foreign body granulomatous reactions.[139] Therefore, the use of special stains, including the Ziehl-Neelsen preparation for mycobacteria and the periodic acid-Schiff (PAS) and methenamine silver reactions for fungi, is mandatory before diagnosing sarcoidosis. Depending on the clinical context, cultures may also be required to exclude an infective etiology. Tuberculoid leprosy is characterized by nerve involvement, a feature that is usually absent in sarcoidosis.

Some of the granulomata seen in a variety of primary immunodeficiency syndromes closely mimic those found in sarcoidosis, and histologic distinction may be impossible. A study comparing granulomata in sarcoidosis to those seen in primary immunodeficiencies found a much lower rate of CD4+/CD8+ cells in the former as opposed to the latter.[140]

Labial and gingival involvement may be histologically mistaken for Crohn disease and granulomatous cheilitis (Miescher). It is worth noting that in rare cases oral involvement in Crohn disease may precede systemic manifestations by several years. Metastatic Crohn disease may be difficult to distinguish from sarcoidosis. The former often shows nonsuppurative granulomata in a diffuse pattern and surrounded by a thin cuff of lymphocytes. Further frequent findings include the presence of numerous eosinophils and ulceration, findings not often seen in sarcoidosis.[141]

Granulomatous lesions that have been described in exogenous ochronosis appear to be related to sarcoidosis.[142] However, similar lesions have also been described as showing changes mimicking actinic granuloma.[143]

Granuloma annulare

Clinical features

Granuloma annulare is a common, usually asymptomatic, dermatosis of unknown etiology.[1,2] It may be divided into six clinical subsets:
- localized,
- generalized,
- perforating,
- subcutaneous,
- papular,
- linear.

Unusual clinical variants include pustular follicular lesions and presentation with patches.[3,4] A single case presenting as contact dermatitis has been reported.[5] Granuloma annulare (often with widespread disseminated lesions) has been described in patients with HIV infection and sometimes may be the presenting sign.[6-18] Granuloma annulare, mainly the generalized variant (see below), has also been reported in association with both Hodgkin and non-Hodgkin lymphoma.[19-22] Exceptionally, anterior uveitis and concomitant skin lesions have been described.[23,24] A case of oral granuloma annulare has been described.[25]

Other documented associations of granuloma annulare include morphea, chronic hepatitis C infection, autoimmune thyroiditis, secondary hyperparathyroidism, sarcoidosis, Plummer disease, myelodysplastic syndrome, metastatic carcinoma, and a bee sting.[26-34] Granuloma annulare has also been described after vaccination for tetanus and diphtheria, hepatitis B, and tuberculosis (BCG), and after mesotherapy.[35-39] It may also develop in the scars of herpes zoster.[40-43] It is important to highlight that most patients with the condition heal after variable periods of time, and long follow-up has not revealed consistent associations with any systemic diseases.[44] A further study has found no consistent relationship between malignant neoplasms and granuloma annulare.[45] However, it has been suggested that elderly patients with lesions that do not have typical features of granuloma annulare but display microscopic findings resembling granuloma annulare should be investigated for an underlying malignancy, especially lymphoma.[45]

Granuloma annulare has developed during treatment with allopurinol, amlodipine, daclizumab, antitumor necrosis factor agents, thalidomide, vemurafenib, pegylated interferon alpha and topiramate.[46-53] Interferon-alpha has been associated with generalized interstitial granuloma annulare.[54] It is most likely, however, that granuloma annulare-like eruptions secondary to drug administration often represent interstitial granulomatous drug eruptions.

Localized granuloma annulare

The localized variant is the most common type. It usually presents in the first three decades and is associated with a female preponderance (2.25:1). Lesions consist of one or several papules, which may be skin-colored, red, or violaceous, and are typically distributed to form an annular or arcuate lesion 1–5 cm in diameter (*Figs 9.23–9.27*). About 50% of patients have solitary lesions. The acral sites are most commonly affected, in particular, the knuckles and dorsum of the fingers. In a small proportion of patients, lesions are present on both the upper and lower limbs, and occasionally the trunk is affected. Lesions on the palms are exceptional.[55] Facial involvement appears to be uncommon.[56,57] In a reported case, lesions were restricted to the area involved by a Becker nevus.[58] Although lesions may be persistent, approximately 50% of patients can anticipate resolution by about 2 years from onset. However, recurrences are, unfortunately, quite common. Patients in which the disease arises earlier in life appear to have earlier resolution of lesions.[59] Interestingly, on occasion lesions regress spontaneously after biopsy.[60] Spontaneous resolution may rarely result in mid-dermal elastolysis.[61] Rarely, granuloma annulare has been reported in families and in monozygotic twins.[62] A case has been documented in which the lesions recurred seasonally with sun-exposed areas.[63] There has only been a single case report of cutaneous granuloma annulare with similar lesions in an intra-abdominal location.[64] In one case, granuloma annulare was the first sign of adult T-cell leukemia/lymphoma, in another patient it was associated with angioimmunoblastic T-cell lymphoma, and in a further patient it was

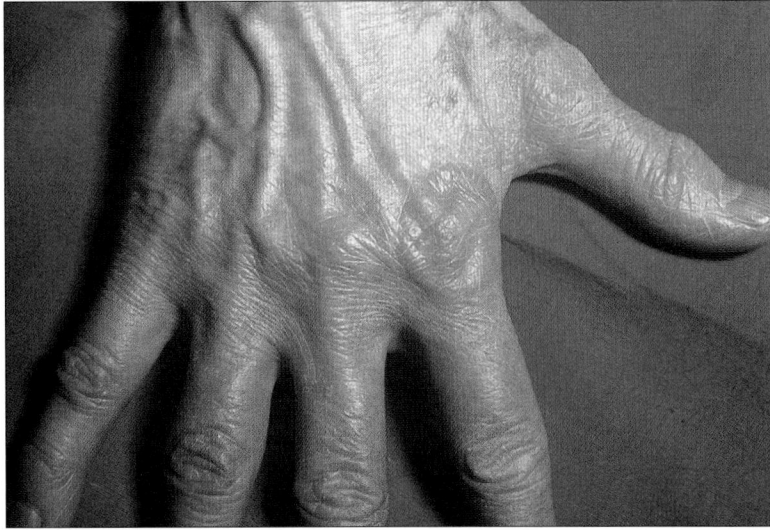

Fig. 9.23
Localized granuloma annulare: a typical annular lesion over the knuckle. Stretching of the skin reveals a translucent beaded margin. By courtesy of R.A. Marsden, MD, St George's Hospital, London, UK.

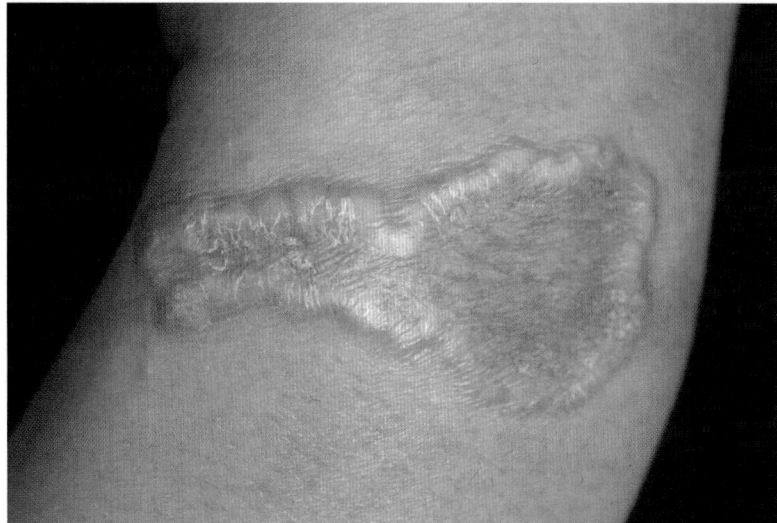

Fig. 9.25
Localized granuloma annulare: this arm lesion shows a characteristic beaded margin. From the collection of the late N.P. Smith, MD, the Institute of Dermatology, London, UK.

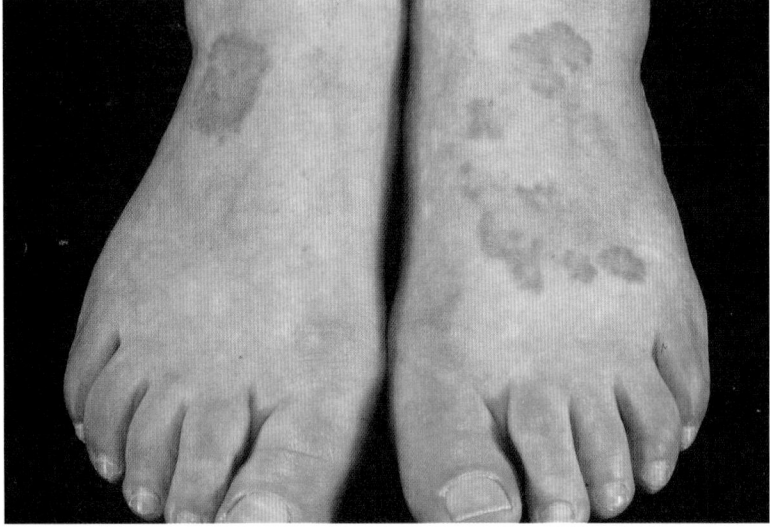

Fig. 9.24
Localized granuloma annulare: in this patient, multiple lesions are present on the feet. From the collection of the late N.P. Smith, MD, the Institute of Dermatology, London, UK.

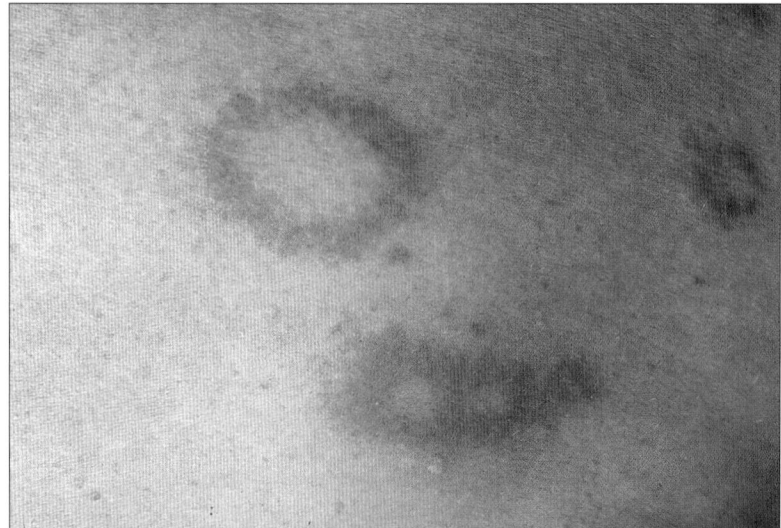

Fig. 9.26
Localized granuloma annulare: close-up view of annular lesions. By courtesy of the Institute of Dermatology, London, UK.

associated with cutaneous marginal zone lymphoma.[65–67] Very rarely, acral, localized granuloma annulare may present as an acute and painful eruption.[68] An association with penile lichen sclerosus is exceptional.[69]

Generalized granuloma annulare

Generalized lesions occur in approximately 15% of patients with granuloma annulare.[2,70] As with the localized form, there is an increased incidence in females; however, the median age differs, the majority of cases occurring in patients in the fourth to seventh decades, with the rest appearing during the first decade. Patients with generalized granuloma annulare have an increased incidence of HLA-Bw35.[71] Generalized granuloma annulare is defined as lesions occurring on at least the trunk and either upper or lower extremities, or both.[2] Most lesions are papules, which may be distributed in an annular pattern, but maculopapules and nodules also occur. They vary in hue from flesh-colored or red, to tan, brown, or yellow. Numbers vary from several dozens to hundreds (*Figs 9.28–9.30*). A single patient has been documented with generalized disease accompanied by marked swelling of the hands, and another patient developed the disease following erythema multiforme.[72,73] A further case developed after varicella zoster infection.[74] Lesions

may be asymptomatic or pruritic.[2] As with the localized form, the disease is persistent, but some patients experience resolution within 4 years. Anetoderma has been exceptionally reported as a complication of generalized granuloma annulare.[75] A remarkable association with giant cell arteritis, gastrointestinal stromal tumor, and other internal malignancies including ovarian and gastric cancer has been reported.[76–78] Tuberculous lymphadenits was an association in one case.[79] In two instances, the condition was the initial manifestation of chronic myelomonocytic leukemia.[80] An association with lymphoma, including Hodgkin disease, has also been described.[81] A patient with hepatitis B developed generalized granuloma annulare, and viral DNA was detected in the skin lesions by PCR.[82] A further case presented in a photosensitive distribution and healed with scarring and milia formation.[83] Other rare associations include hyperlipidemia and scabies.[84,85]

Perforating granuloma annulare

Perforating granuloma annulare is distinguished by the presence of transepidermal elimination of necrobiotic collagen.[10,18,86–90] Clinically, the lesion presents as a group of papules with an umbilicated crust usually located on the extremities, often the dorsum of the hands (*Fig. 9.31*). Presentation of

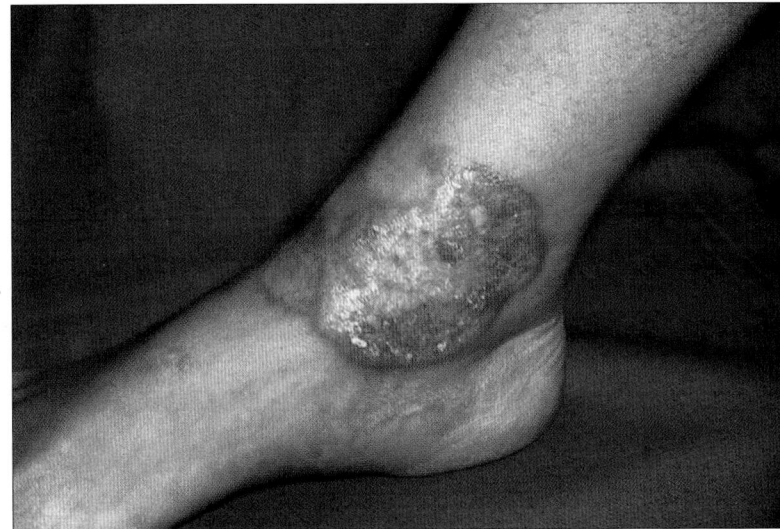

Fig. 9.27
Localized granuloma annulare: in this patient, there is a large plaque on the ankle with a hint of central clearing. By courtesy of the Institute of Dermatology, London, UK.

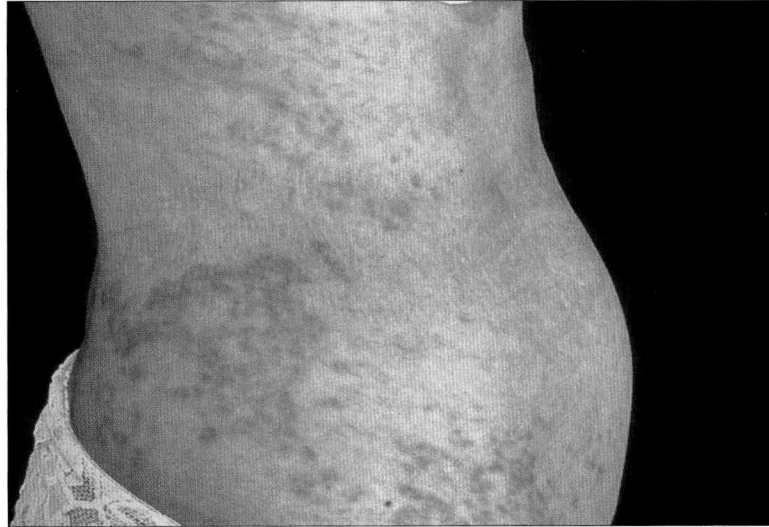

Fig. 9.29
Generalized granuloma annulare: there are widespread papules and plaques. By courtesy of the Institute of Dermatology, London, UK.

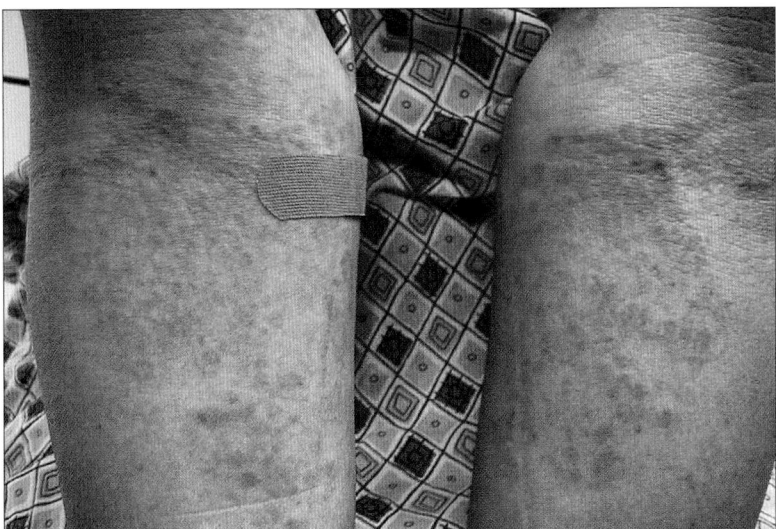

Fig. 9.28
Generalized granuloma annulare: innumerable papules are present on this patient's arms. By courtesy of J. Williams, MD, Brigham and Women's Hospital, Boston, USA.

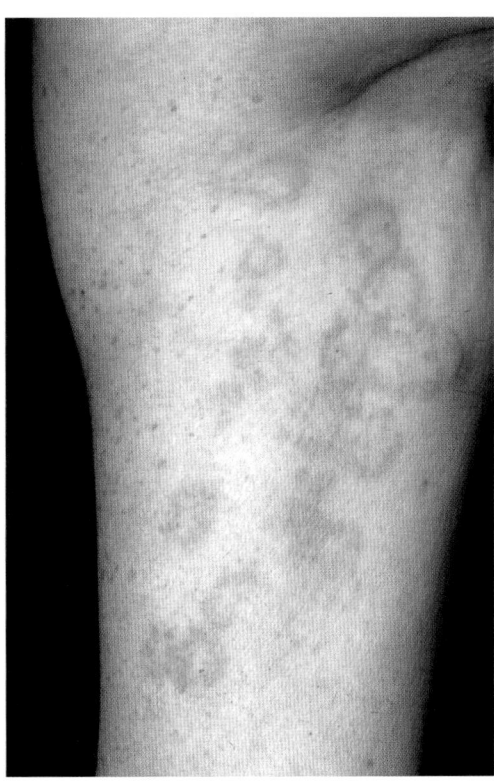

Fig. 9.30
Generalized granuloma annulare: in this patient, numerous annular lesions are present. From the collection of the late N.P. Smith, MD, the Institute of Dermatology, London, UK.

lesions on the ears has exceptionally been described, as has a generalized variant.[91–93] It may affect both children and adults, and both localized and generalized forms exist. Spontaneous resolution sometimes occurs within months or years of onset. Exceptionally, perforating granuloma annulare develops following tattooing.[94]

Subcutaneous (deep) granuloma annulare

The subcutaneous variant is synonymous with the pseudorheumatoid nodule of childhood and deep granuloma annulare.[95–98] Lesions may present de novo or arise in association with typical cutaneous papules. In about a quarter of patients, there is coexistence with dermal granuloma annulare. It occurs in childhood, often affecting the underlying periosteum and involving predominantly the lower legs (particularly the tibia), feet, buttocks, hands, and head.[99] Lesions may also present on the penis or eyelid.[100,101] An exceptional case of numerous lesions limited to the scalp of a child which regressed spontaneously has been reported.[102] A further patient presented with a periorbital subperiosteal lesion, and in another patient the lesion was congenital.[103,104] In one study of 47 patients, the mean age was 4.3 years.[99] In some instances, there is a history of trauma. By definition, such children do not have rheumatoid arthritis or rheumatic fever. The lesion

usually regresses after several years. However, recurrences appear in 19% of patients.[99]

Papular granuloma annulare

Papular granuloma annulare presents as flesh-colored or hypopigmented, 1–3-mm-diameter papules on the dorsal aspect of the hands, usually in male children. Involvement of the palms and soles may be seen, and rarely lesions are painful.[105] Occasional lesions may be umbilicated or generalized (Figs 9.32 and 9.33).[106]

Linear granuloma annulare

The linear variant is very rare and may have a bilateral distribution.[107,108] Rarely, it may follow Blaschko lines.[109] This variant overlaps and may in

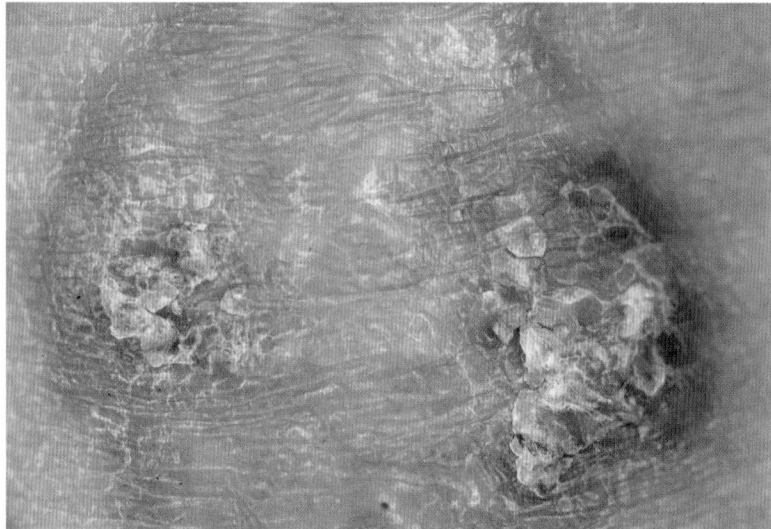

Fig. 9.31
Perforating granuloma annulare: the extremities are most often affected. Necrotic debris and crust can be seen. From the collection of the late N.P. Smith, MD, the Institute of Dermatology, London, UK.

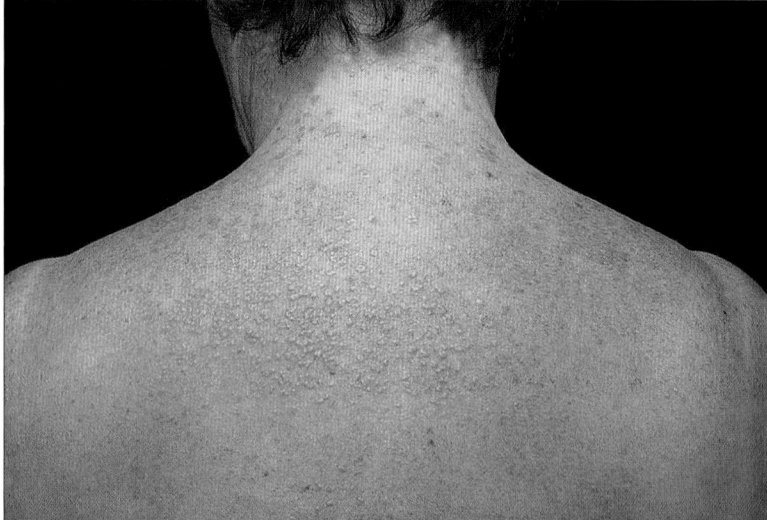

Fig. 9.32
Papular granuloma annulare: widespread papules are present on this patient's back and shoulders. By courtesy of the Institute of Dermatology, London, UK.

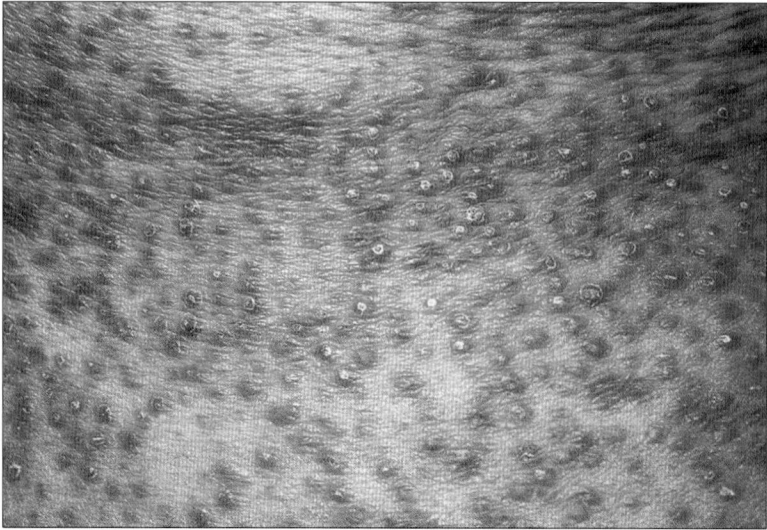

Fig. 9.33
Papular granuloma annulare: numerous small, scaly papules are present. By courtesy of the Institute of Dermatology, London, UK.

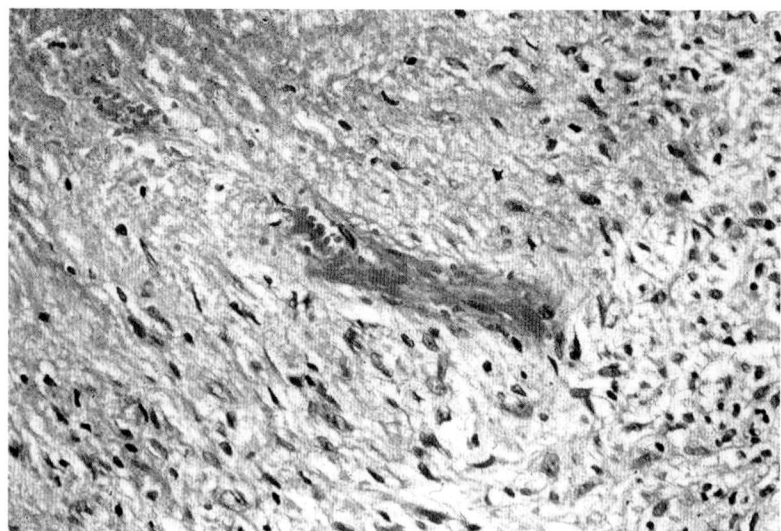

Fig. 9.34
Granuloma annulare: view through the edge of a necrobiotic focus. In the center, a small blood vessel shows fibrinoid necrosis with occlusion. This is an uncommon finding.

some cases be the same as the condition described as palisading neutrophilic and granulomatous dermatitid.

Pathogenesis and histologic features

The cause of granuloma annulare is unknown. The original concept that it represented a tuberculid has long since been discounted. Although it has been reported at the site of previous herpes zoster infection and verruca vulgaris, it is unlikely that an infectious pathogenesis exists. *Borrelia* has been demonstrated by focus-floating microscopy in a number of biopsies of patients with granuloma annulare, raising the possibility of a pathogenetic role for the organism in some cases of the disease.[110] However, a study based on PCR found no association between granuloma annulare and *Borrelia* infection.[111] There is a wide variety of currently possible pathogenetic mechanisms, most of which have some merit, but none of which satisfactorily clarifies the precise mechanism by which the lesions of granuloma annulare develop.[112] Particularly popular are an immune complex vasculitic process and a cell-mediated delayed hypersensitivity reaction. Evidence in favor of the former has been the detection, by direct immunofluorescence, of immunoreactants (IgM and complement) in blood vessel walls in some patients.[112] Elevated levels of circulating immune complexes have also been recorded.[113] The histology may reveal features suggestive of a vasculitic process, including endothelial swelling, vessel wall thickening (due to the deposition of PAS-positive material), vascular occlusion, and necrosis (*Fig. 9.34*).[114] All of the latter changes may, of course, develop as a consequence of the inflammatory process rather than cause it. A study of serial sections of 38 biopsies in 35 patients found no evidence of a vasculitic process in any of the cases.[115]

In favor of a cell-mediated delayed hypersensitivity reaction are:
- the finding of activated T lymphocytes in lesions of granuloma annulare on electron microscopic examination,
- the predominance of T-helper inducer cells in the infiltrate,
- the histopathological resemblance of the infiltrate to that of conditions of known delayed hypersensitivity pathogenesis, including sarcoidosis and tuberculosis.[116]

It has been suggested that Th1 lymphocytes expressing interferon-gamma induce a delayed hypersensitivity reaction leading to macrophages becoming aggressive effector cells that express tumor necrosis factor-alpha and matrix metalloproteinases.[117] If tumor necrosis factor alpha plays a role in the induction of the disease, then agents that block this cytokine may be useful in treating the condition. Although some patients respond to these agents, others do not, and the reason for this is not clear. Monozygotic twins with generalized granuloma annulare and the 8.1 ancestral haplotype,

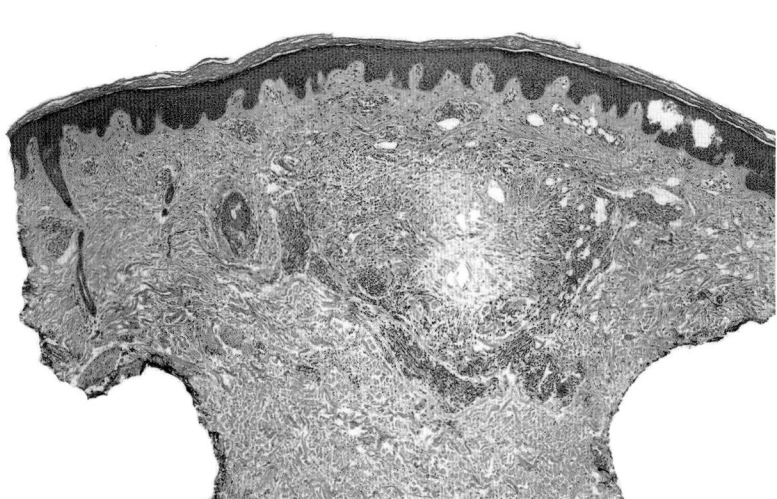

Fig. 9.35
Localized granuloma annulare: the characteristic appearance of a well-circumscribed palisading granuloma consisting of a necrobiotic center surrounded by a cellular infiltrate.

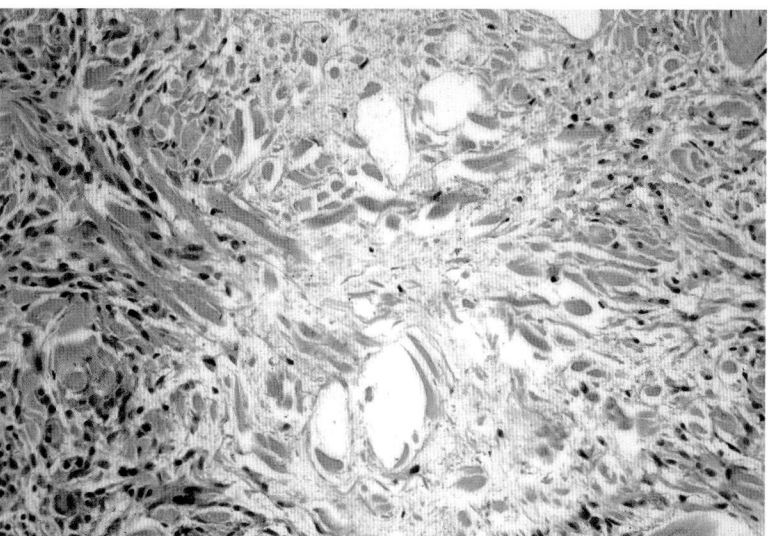

Fig. 9.36
Localized granuloma annulare: the collagen is fragmented and in part granular. Note the peripheral palisade of histiocytes, occasional lymphocytes, and fibroblasts.

a genotype that leads to increased production of tumor necrosis alpha, have responded well to adalimumab.[118]

Patients with granuloma annulare may have raised serum migration inhibition factor activity.[98] Defective neutrophil migration has also been reported.[119,120] Other proposed pathogenetic mechanisms include collagen damage by macrophage lysosomal hydrolytic enzymes as the initial event, or a primary disorder of collagen leading to an allergic or nonallergic tissue reaction. The increased incidences of diabetes mellitus and HLA-B8 may also be of pathogenetic significance (compare with necrobiosis lipoidica).[121] In a study of a group of pediatric patients with multiple lesions of granuloma annulare, it was found that they had significantly lower serum insulin values than the control group and showed mild impairment of glucose tolerance.[122] However, these children often had a family history of diabetes mellitus.

Although there are reports of generalized granuloma being associated with sunlight, this appears to be of doubtful significance.[2]

It has been shown that the glioma-associated oncogene homologue gli-1, a member of the vertebrate zinc finger transcription factor genes of the gli superfamily, is highly expressed in a number of granulomatous disorders including granuloma annulare.[123] The relevance of this in the pathogenesis of granuloma annulare is not clear, but it raises the possibility of using inhibitors of gli-1 signaling in the treatment of granulomatous noninfectious diseases.

The most characteristic histologic lesion seen in granuloma annulare is the palisading granuloma (*Figs 9.35–9.38*). This consists of a central core of degenerate (necrobiotic) collagen, surrounded by an often radially arranged infiltrate of lymphocytes, histiocytes, and fibroblasts. Elastic tissue may be absent within these foci and there can be phagocytosis of elastic fibers by giant cells at the periphery of the granuloma (*Fig. 9.39*).[124] However, altered elastic fibers are not a constant finding. Solar elastosis is not a feature of granuloma annulare. In some lesions, the altered collagen has a somewhat basophilic appearance due to the presence of acid mucopolysaccharides, but more commonly there is eosinophilia, due in part to fibrin deposition (*Fig. 9.40*). Heparin sulfate is an important component of the mucin in granuloma annulare but not of other cutaneous diseases associated with mucin deposition (*Fig. 9.41*).[125]

Occasionally, sparse karyorrhectic debris is present in the center of the lesion and sometimes the necrobiotic foci contain lipid droplets. More often, however, the collagenous degeneration is not organized into a nodular pattern, but affects isolated fibers in a random pattern, an appearance often best appreciated on low-power examination (*Fig. 9.42*).[126] In this so-called diffuse or interstitial form of granuloma annulare, affected fibers, which are swollen and intensely eosinophilic, alternate with apparently normal fibers

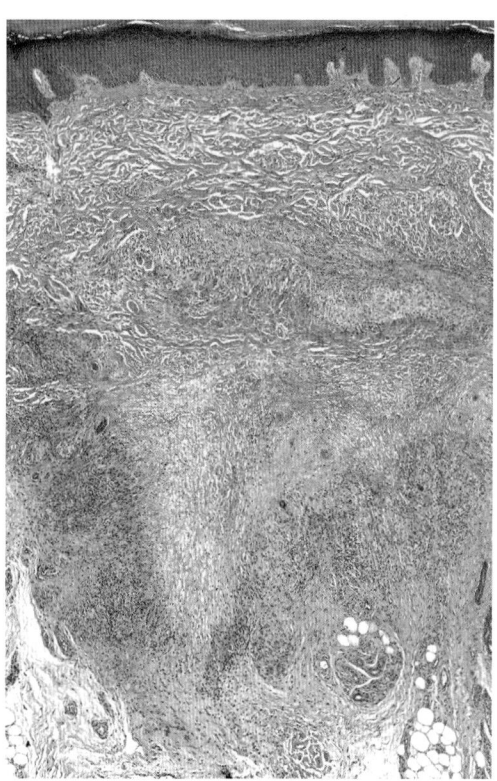

Fig. 9.37
Localized granuloma annulare: this lesion is from the palm of the hand, an uncommonly affected site. There is a sharply delineated focus of necrobiosis in the deep reticular dermis.

to give a rather disorganized appearance (*Figs 9.43* and *9.44*). Necrobiosis is minimal or absent. Characteristically, the collagen fibers are separated by mucin, which stains positively with Alcian blue at pH 2.5. Histiocytes are often seen infiltrating around and between affected fibers, and this feature may be a helpful clue to the diagnosis in early cases when the collagen changes are inconspicuous and should, therefore, encourage examination of additional sections to detect more typical features (*Fig. 9.45*).

An almost inevitable feature of granuloma annulare is the presence of a perivascular chronic inflammatory cell infiltrate, both within the lesion and in the adjacent tissue. Well-formed sarcoidal granulomata with associated giant cells are seen in some cases. Significant numbers of eosinophils may be

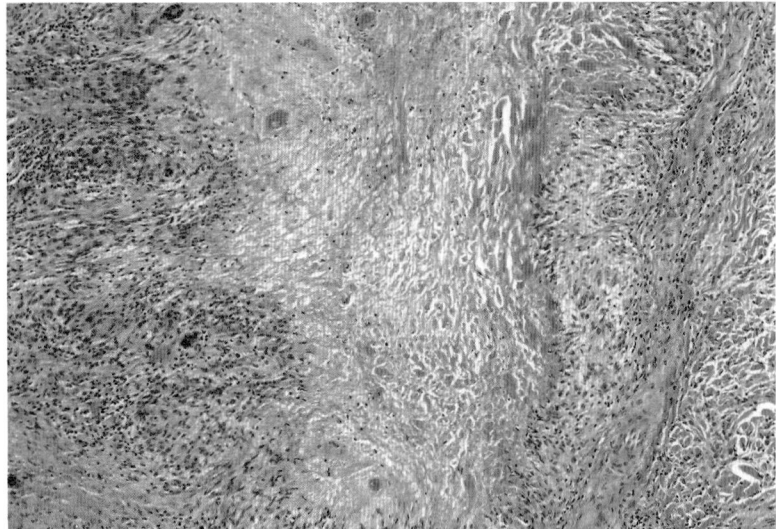

Fig. 9.38
Localized granuloma annulare: the necrobiosis is advanced, presenting as eosinophilic granular debris. The histiocytic palisade is well established.

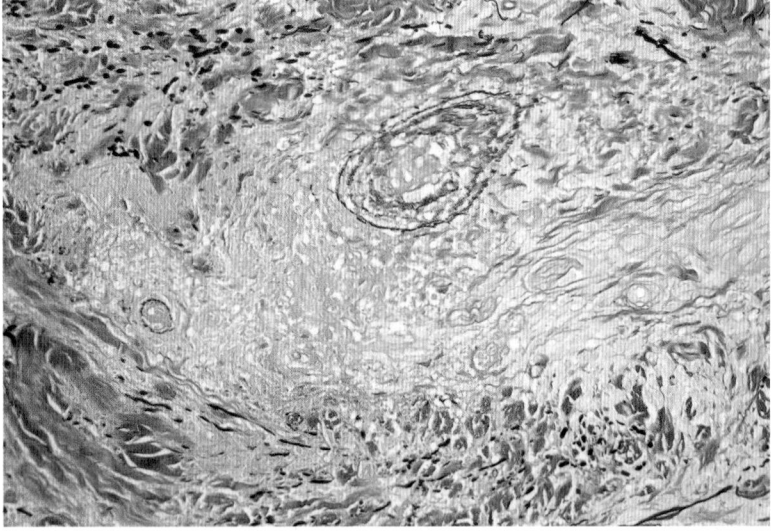

Fig. 9.39
Localized granuloma annulare: there is loss of elastic tissue within the granuloma. Elastic-van Gieson.

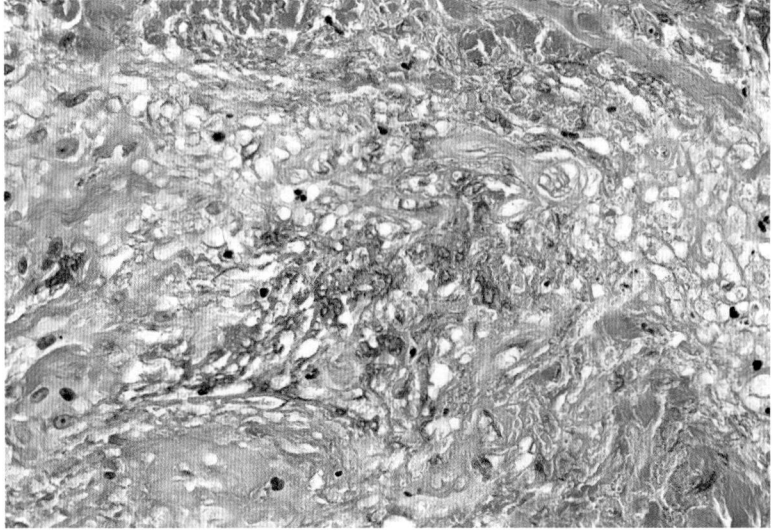

Fig. 9.40
Localized granuloma annulare: the red-staining material in the center of the granuloma is fibrin. Martius scarlet blue.

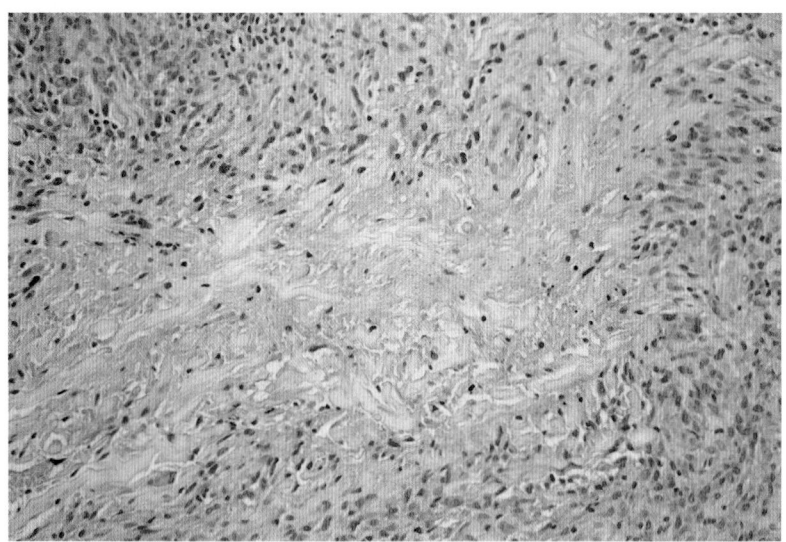

Fig. 9.41
Localized granuloma annulare: in this example, there is abundant mucin in the center of the necrobiotic focus. Alcian blue stain.

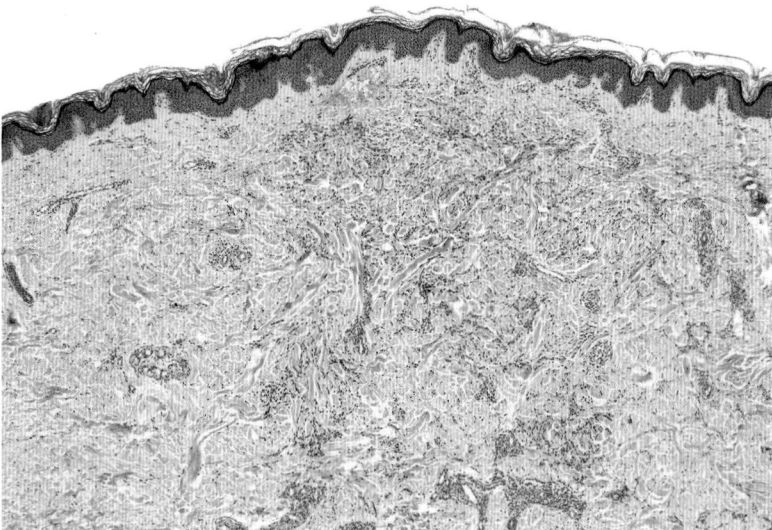

Fig. 9.42
Diffuse granuloma annulare: the collagen bundles are arranged haphazardly. Note the circumferential lymphocytic infiltrate.

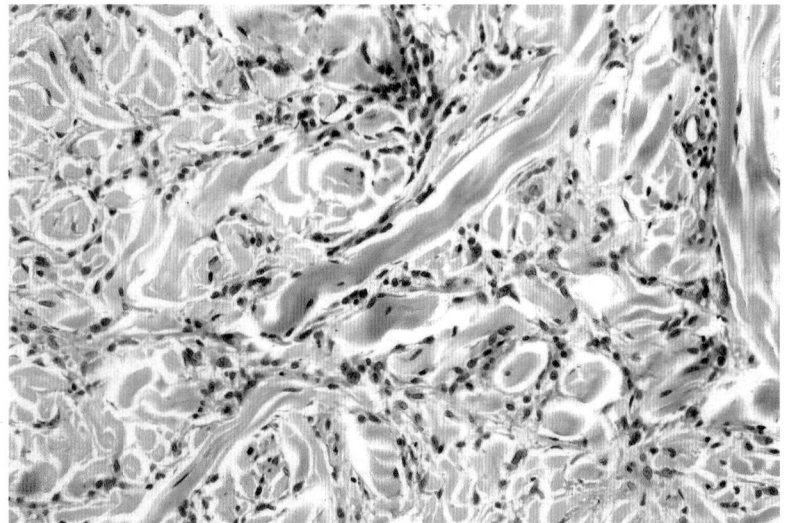

Fig. 9.43
Diffuse granuloma annulare: individual fibers are swollen and intensely eosinophilic. The apparent separation of the fibers is due to increased mucin.

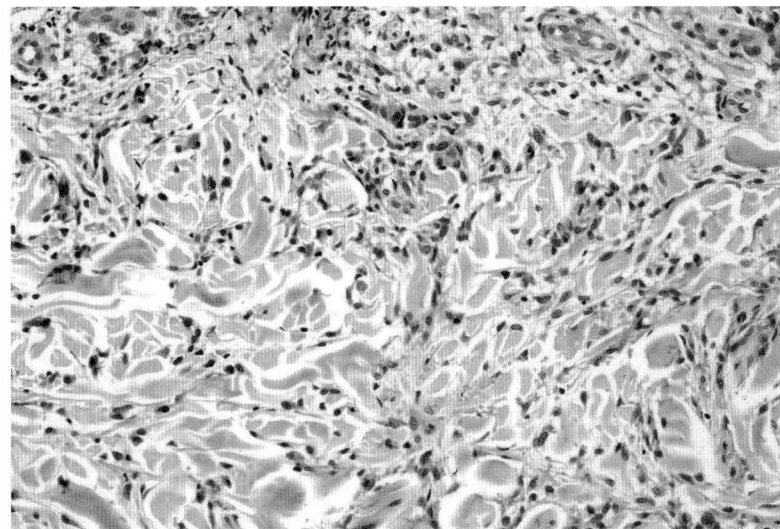

Fig. 9.44
Diffuse granuloma annulare: higher-power view showing the dense interstitial histiocytic infiltrate.

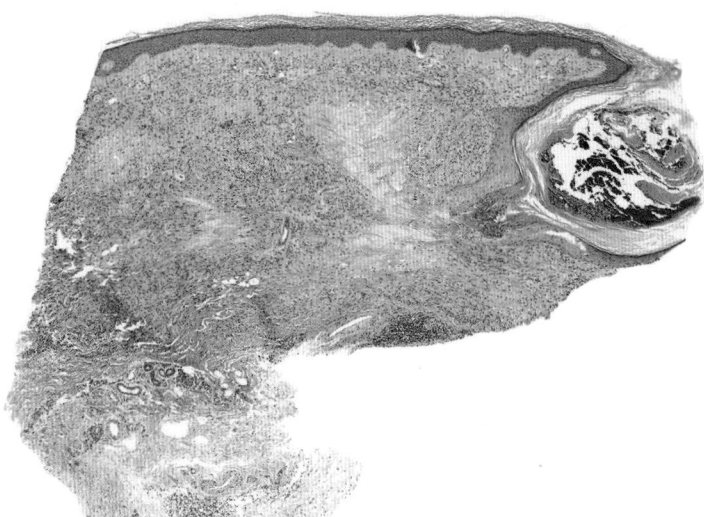

Fig. 9.46
Perforating granuloma annulare: scanning view showing widespread typical granuloma annulare (in the upper-right quadrant, degenerate collagen is undergoing transepidermal elimination).

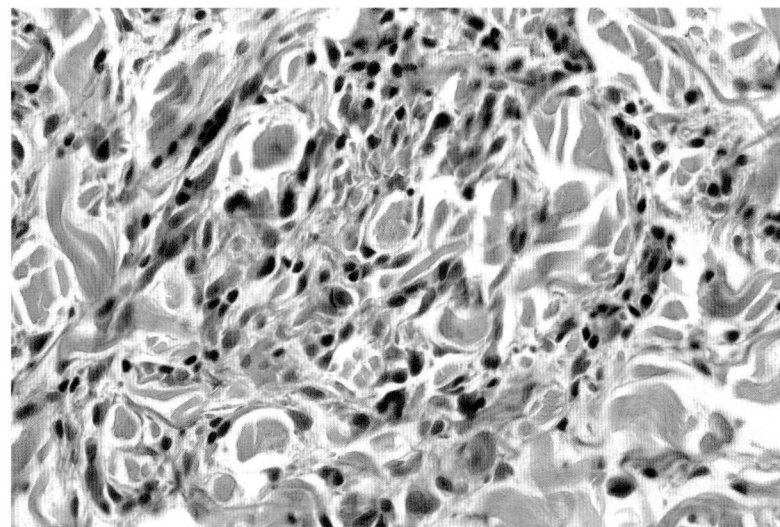

Fig. 9.45
Diffuse granuloma annulare: high-power view.

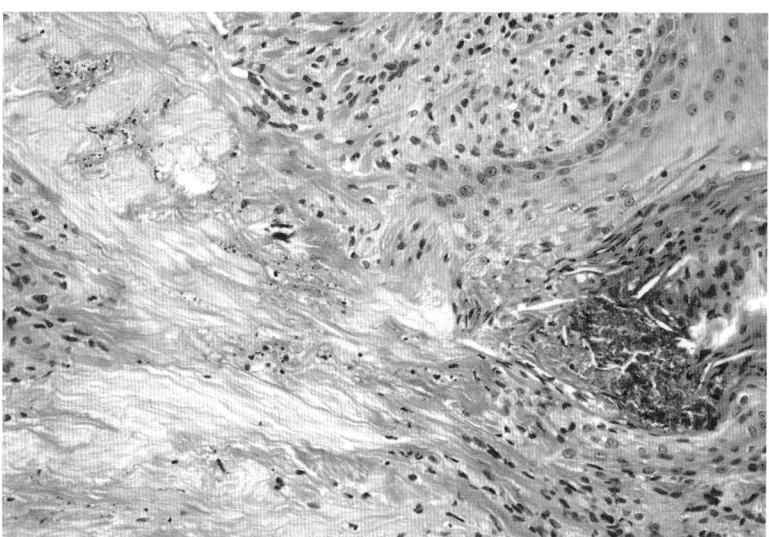

Fig. 9.47
Perforating granuloma annulare: close-up view showing the dermal perforation and transepidermal elimination of collagenous debris.

encountered.[127] In one study, eosinophils were present in 66% of biopsies, of which 14% showed more than 10 eosinophils per high-power field.[126] Plasma cells are rare, and this is useful in the differential diagnosis with necrobiosis lipoidica (see below). Neutrophils are a rare finding and when present, particularly in association with changes of vasculitis, it is likely that there is an association with systemic disease.[128] Rarely, an associated prominent lymphocytic infiltrate mimicking a lymphoma may be encountered.[129]

Although the relationship with *Borrelia* infection is debatable, it has been suggested that formation of pseudorosettes in granuloma annulare may suggest infection with the organism.[130]

In perforating granuloma annulare, the necrobiotic debris is present in close proximity to the epidermis and may be seen to be engulfed by the latter to form a perforating channel by which the necrotic material is extruded to the surface (*Figs 9.46* and *9.47*). If serial sections are performed, the perforation is often shown to occur through a hair follicle.

The subcutaneous lesions are much larger than the superficial ones (*Figs 9.48* and *9.49*) and are frequently composed of multiple nodules. There is usually massive necrobiosis and abundant mucin; on occasions, lipid droplets are evident. Mucin, however, may be minimal or not apparent and if fibrin deposition is present, distinction from rheumatoid nodule is impossible. A dense rim of lymphocytes, histiocytes, and fibroblasts surrounds the necrobiotic center. Multinucleate giant cells are common and eosinophils

are often present. The latter appear to be more common in this variant than in ordinary granuloma annulare. Fibrosis of the surrounding tissue may be marked. In up to 25% of cases of subcutaneous granuloma annulare, changes of classic granuloma annulare may be seen in the dermis.[131]

Papular and linear variants show histologic features similar to those described for typical granuloma annulare.

Differential diagnosis

Granuloma annulare must be distinguished from necrobiosis lipoidica, rheumatoid nodule, actinic granuloma, and granuloma multiforme. Points of distinction are summarized in *Table 9.1*.

The pattern of adipophilin expression has been reported as useful in the histological distinction between granuloma annulare, necrobiosis lipoidica, and sarcoidosis. In granuloma annulare, adipophilin staining pattern is both intra- and extracellular in relationship with the histiocytes in the infiltrate. In necrobiosis lipoidica the staining pattern tends to be exclusively extracellular in areas of abnormal collagen, and in sarcoidosis the staining pattern is usually exclusively intracellular within histiocytes.[132]

Occasionally, granuloma annulare may display epithelioid cell granulomas mimicking sarcoidosis. However, the presence of mucin in the

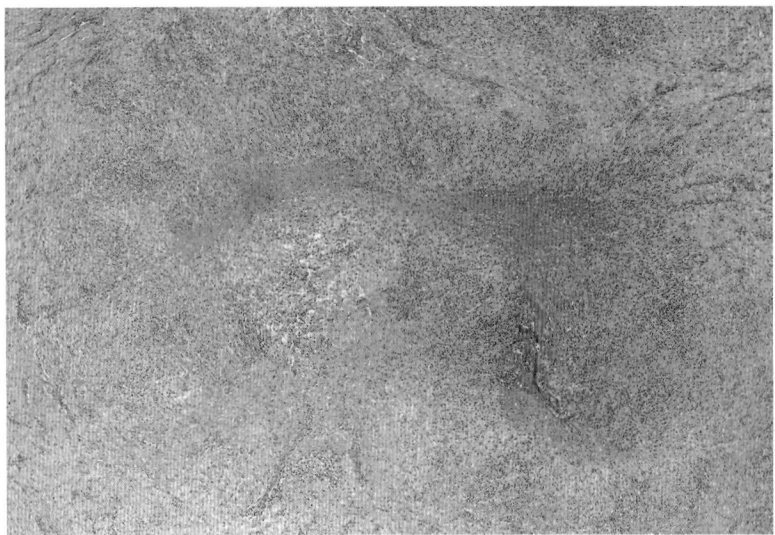

Fig. 9.48
Subcutaneous granuloma annulare: within the subcutaneous fat and involving the fascia is a massive necrobiotic nodule.

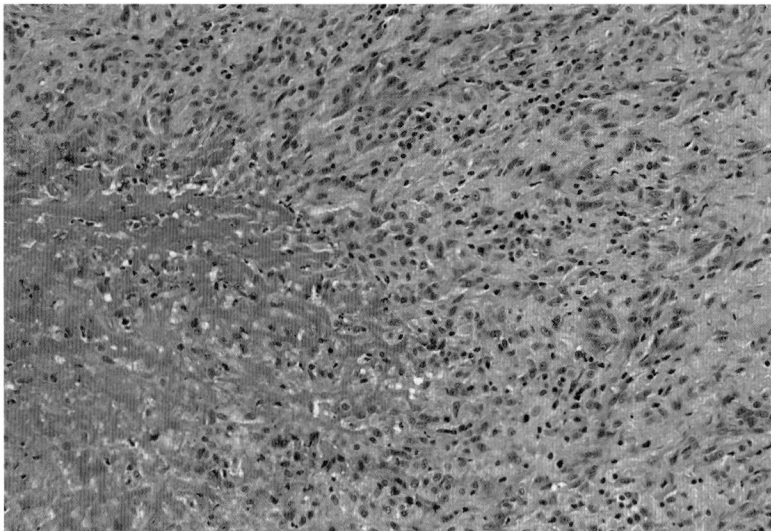

Fig. 9.49
Subcutaneous granuloma annulare: note the intensely eosinophilic necrobiosis and surrounding fibrosis.

Table 9.1
Differential diagnosis of palisading granulomata and variants

	Granuloma annulare (GA)	Subcutaneous GA	Perforating GA	Necrobiosis lipoidica (NL)	Atypical NL	Rheumatoid nodule	Actinic granuloma	Granuloma multiforme
Epidermis	Normal	Normal	Transepidermal elimination	Normal or atrophic or acanthotic	Normal	Normal	Normal or atrophic	Normal
Location of lesion	Superficial dermis	Deep dermis and subcutis	Superficial dermis	Deep dermis and subcutis	Upper and mid dermis	Deep dermis and subcutis	Upper and mid dermis	Upper and mid dermis
Necrobiosis	Circumscribed or ill defined	Massive sharp border	Circumscribed	Diffuse and marked	Rarely present	Massive sharp margin	Absent	Focal
Mucin	Common	Abundant	Common	Variable	Absent	Common	Absent	Present
Lipid	Occasional	Variable	Variable	Common	Absent	Variable	Absent	Absent
Fibrosis	Absent	Marked	Absent	Common; may be marked	Absent	Common	Usually absent	Slight
Loss of elastic	Yes	Yes	Yes	Yes	Yes	Yes	Very marked	Yes
Vascular thickening	Common	Variable	Minimal	Common	Absent	Variable	Absent	Absent
Capillary hyperplasia	Absent	Common	Absent	Variable	Absent	Common	Absent	Absent
Giant cells	Relatively few	Common	Relatively few	Common	Common	Relatively few	Abundant; contain elastica	Common
Asteroid bodies	Absent	Absent	Absent	Absent	Present	Absent	Not uncommon	Absent
Palisading of histiocytes	Common	Common	Common	Variable degree in	Absent	Common	Infrequent	Inconspicuous

Reprinted from Muhlbauer JE. Granuloma annulare. J Am Acad Dermatol 3:217–230; Copyright Elsevier 1980, with permission from the American Academy of Dermatology, Inc.

background along with other more typical changes of granuloma annulare allows distinction in challenging cases.[133]

Granuloma annulare-like lesions with the added features of vasculitis and a significant component of acute inflammatory cells may be encountered in the setting of systemic disease.[129,134] This pattern of disease is discussed in detail in the section on palisaded neutrophilic and granulomatous dermatitis and related disorders.

Granuloma annulare-like drug eruptions have been reported. The presence of associated interface changes favors a drug eruption.[10,135]

Very rarely, scleromyxedema may focally mimic interstitial granuloma annulare histologically.[136] However, the changes simulating granuloma annulare are focal, and elsewhere in the biopsy there are more typical features of scleromyxedema including fibrosis and increase in fibroblasts.

Occasionally, infection by *Mycobacterium marinum* may mimic interstitial granuloma annulare. The microscopic features may be so similar that the diagnosis can only be made by special stains and culture.[137]

Although epithelioid sarcoma, with its associated geographic necrosis, may bear a superficial resemblance at low-power examination to granuloma annulare, the degree of nuclear atypia and pleomorphism in the former condition should afford their distinction in the majority of cases. In addition, epithelioid sarcoma often shows perineural tumor infiltration. It should be noted, however, that mitotic activity may be encountered in granuloma annulare.[138] In difficult cases, keratin, epithelial membrane, in up to 60% of cases, CD34 antigen immunoreactivity and loss of INI1 expression in epithelioid sarcoma should assist in this differential diagnosis.

Rare cases of mycosis fungoides may be associated with a tissue reaction resembling granuloma annulare.[139–141] Although interstitial mycosis fungoides may show histiocytes between collagen bundles, the predominance of interstitial lymphocytes with nuclear atypia and epidermotropism, a feature not seen in granuloma annulare, should resolve this differential diagnosis. Most patients with interstitial mycosis fungoides have other classical clinical features of the disease. Of interest, interstitial tumor cells in cutaneous T cell lymphoma often have a cytotoxic phenotype.[141]

Acrodermatitis chronica atrophicans can rarely display histologic changes resembling granuloma annulare.[142] However, clinicopathological correlation and the presence plasma cells in the former usually allows distinction to be made.

Necrobiosis lipoidica

Clinical features

Necrobiosis lipoidica is a disease of unknown etiology which shows a strong association with diabetes mellitus.[1–6] Although the affiliation is likely to have pathogenic implications, the precise mechanism by which the lesions of necrobiosis lipoidica develop is, nevertheless, unknown, and the nature of the relationship between the two diseases is unclear. Therefore, although the diagnosis of diabetes is most often established before the onset of the skin lesions (in up to 62% of cases), in a number of cases, typical plaques present simultaneously (in up to 24% of cases) or may precede (in up to 14% of cases) the apparent onset of diabetes mellitus by several years.[2,7,8] The course of the cutaneous disease does not appear to be related to the hyperglycemia, and treatment of diabetes does not affect the outcome of the cutaneous lesions. In one study, proteinuria, retinopathy, and smoking were more common in patients with necrobiosis lipoidica compared with patients with diabetes but no skin disease.[9] In another study, patients with diabetes type I and necrobiosis lipoidica tended to have higher levels of glycemia, and the duration of the diabetes was longer compared to patients without necrobiosis lipoidica.[10] Interestingly, however, only a minority of patients with necrobiosis lipoidica has diabetes mellitus. It has been shown that 11% of patients with necrobiosis lipoidica have diabetes mellitus and a further 11% develop the disease or altered glucose tolerance on follow-up.[11]

Necrobiosis lipoidica may develop in both juvenile (type I) and maturity-onset (type II) diabetes. Interestingly, the condition improves or even resolves in diabetic patients after pancreatic transplant.[12,13] Necrobiosis lipoidica has been documented in patients with endocrine disorders other than diabetes such as hypo- and hyperthyroidism, and also in association with inflammatory bowel disease and vasculitis.[14] One nondiabetic patient with necrobiosis lipoidica and ataxia telangiectasia has been reported.[15] Exceptionally, necrobiosis lipoidica and granuloma annulare have presented simultaneously.[16,17] The disease has also been documented in association with sarcoidosis.[18,19]

Necrobiosis lipoidica shows a marked female preponderance (3.3:1), and although a wide age range may be affected, patients present most often in the fourth decade (those associated with diabetes mellitus) or fifth decade (those not associated with diabetes mellitus). The condition is rare in childhood and is often associated with diabetes mellitus. It also appears to be related to underlying renal and retinal disease.[20–24] Familial cases may also occur, with or without diabetes.[25–27] A case of monozygotic twins with diabetes mellitus type II and necrobiosis lipoidica has been reported.[28]

The characteristic lesion, sometimes referred to as a sclerodermatous plaque, is round or oval, circumscribed, and often has a slightly elevated rim. It is typically a few millimeters to several centimeters in diameter. Newly acquired lesions are often red-brown in color, but with progression the center of the lesion becomes yellowish and the peripheral border may acquire a violaceous hue. Larger plaques are usually irregular and more variably shaped. Scaling and telangiectasia may become evident. Dermoscopy shows elongated serpentine telangiectasias with a whitish structureless background.[29] Ulceration appears to be relatively frequent and has been

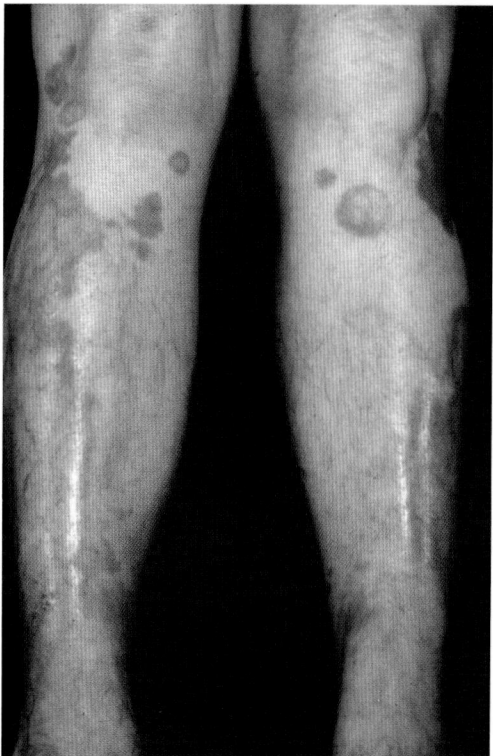

Fig. 9.50
Necrobiosis lipoidica: characteristic, bilateral, symmetrical lesions. From the collection of the late N.P. Smith, MD, the Institute of Dermatology, London, UK.

reported in up to 13% of patients.[30–32] It is more common in males and in those with diabetes mellitus.[33] Perforating necrobiosis lipoidica is very rare and may be seen very exceptionally in children.[34,35] In perforating cases, the clinical appearance may consist of a focal scaly depression or comedone-like lesions. Atypical forms may also be found: patients sometimes manifest papules and nodular lesions, and occasionally plaques resembling granuloma annulare are seen. (It should be noted, however, that rarely these two conditions appear to coexist.)[16,36] Clinical presentations with papulonecrotic and noduloulcerative lesions mimicking gummata or erythema induratum have been documented, albeit exceptionally.[30] The lesions may be solitary or multiple, often symmetrical, and show a predilection for the lower extremities, in particular, the pretibial area (Figs 9.50–9.53). They can also occur on the arms, hands, fingers, abdomen, nipples, and back; rarely, the face or scalp is affected, in which case diabetes is seldom present.[37] Generalized lesions may exceptionally occur.[38]

The so-called atypical necrobiosis lipoidica of the face and scalp does not represent a variant of necrobiosis lipoidica, and it is more likely to represent a variant of elastolytic granuloma (see page 329). The name was chosen because of the coexistence of typical lesions of necrobiosis lipoidica on the shins of one of the patients in the original series. However, most patients do not present with classic lesions of necrobiosis lipoidica elsewhere and the microscopic findings do not resemble the latter entity.[39]

Involvement of the penis with lesions resembling chronic balanitis has been described.[40–42] Exceptional involvement of the scrotum has also been described.[43] Rarely, lesions are associated with Koebner phenomenon.[44–46] Necrobiotic and silicotic granulomata developing within phlebectomy scars have also been reported.[47] The condition may also occur in association with surgical scars after appendicectomy and breast reconstruction surgery, exceptionally at the site of a burn and in association with a tattoo.[8,48–50]

The disease tends to chronicity. It is of interest that necrobiosis lipoidica has been reported to be associated with cutaneous hypo- or complete anesthesia in both diabetic and nondiabetic patients.[51,52] One study found loss of nerves within lesions and, based on this finding, the authors postulated that destruction of nerves might explain the sensory loss that is observed in some patients.[52,53] Hypohidrosis and partial alopecia have also been reported.[54]

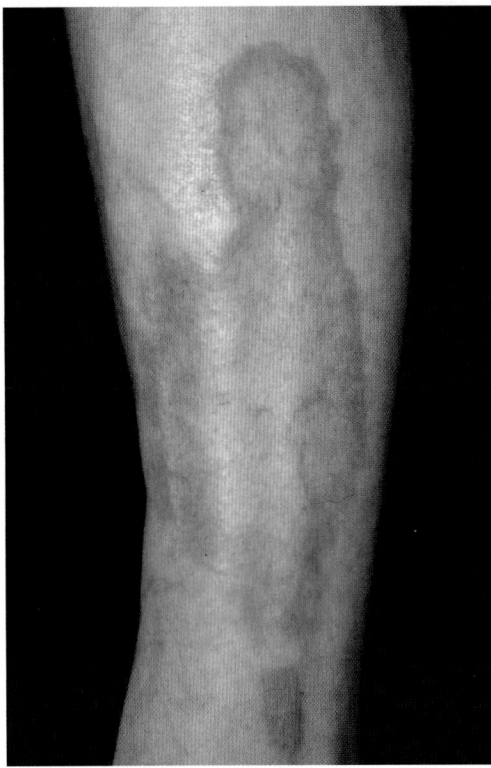

Fig. 9.51
Necrobiosis lipoidica: typical lesion with an erythematous border. From the collection of the late N.P. Smith, MD, the Institute of Dermatology, London, UK.

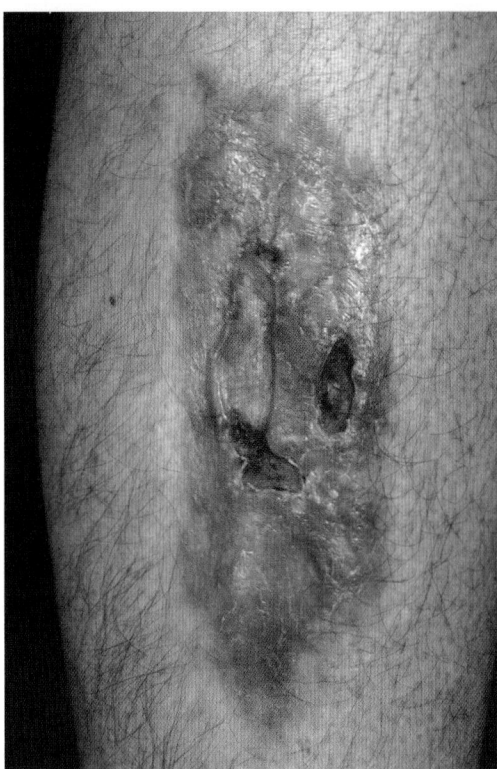

Fig. 9.53
Necrobiosis lipoidica: chronic lesion with ulceration and crusting. From the collection of the late N.P. Smith, MD, the Institute of Dermatology, London, UK.

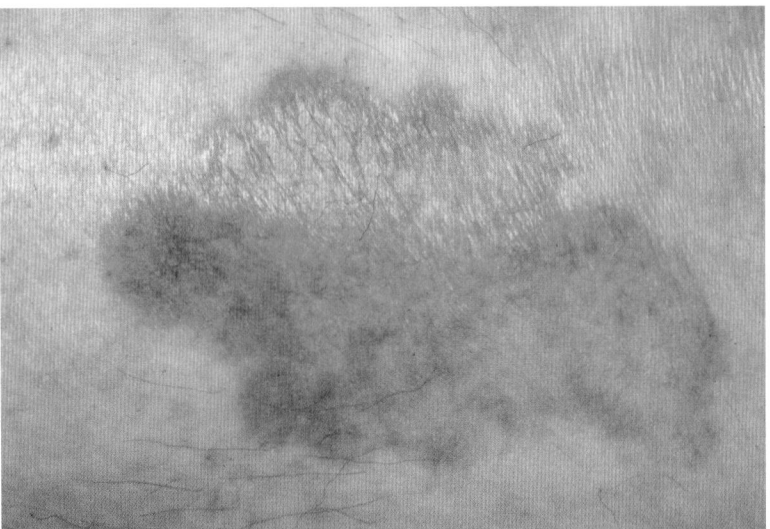

Fig. 9.52
Necrobiosis lipoidica: lesion on shin showing atrophy and telangiectasia. From the collection of the late N.P. Smith, MD, the Institute of Dermatology, London, UK.

Rarely, squamous carcinoma may arise in long-standing lesions.[55-59] One such case developed in association with perforating necrobiosis lipoidica.[60]

Pathogenesis and histologic features

The precise pathogenesis of necrobiosis lipoidica is unknown. Of primary importance is the temporal relationship between collagen degeneration and the inflammatory infiltrate.[61] The close association of necrobiosis lipoidica and diabetes mellitus suggests a causal relationship, but the exact mechanism is uncertain. In the past, some 60% of patients with necrobiosis lipoidica were reported as having coexistent diabetes mellitus.[2,4,62,63] However, its reported prevalence in diabetes is only of the order of 3/1000.[61] Furthermore, a recent study has found that only a minority of patients with necrobiosis lipoidica have diabetes.[11]

It has been suggested that the lesions develop as a consequence of diabetic microangiopathy: the vessel walls in lesions of necrobiosis lipoidica are typically thickened by a diastase-resistant PAS-positive material. This does not explain the development of necrobiosis lipoidica in nondiabetic patients or the absence of the disease in patients with established microvascular lesions. An association with venous insufficiency and hypercholesterolemia has been suggested in a very small group of patients.[64] The significance of this finding is therefore unclear. Study of microcirculation by Doppler flowmetry and oxygen partial pressure in necrobiosis lipoidica lesions in nondiabetics has demonstrated an altered microcirculation.[65] Low oxygen and high carbon dioxide pressures, presumably reflecting ischemia, characterize necrobiotic plaques.[66] Such vascular changes, although possibly causal, could equally well develop as a consequence of the necrobiotic changes. Aberrant platelet aggregation may also play a role in pathogenesis. Platelet survival times are markedly reduced in patients with necrobiosis lipoidica.[67] Whether this is of pathogenic importance is uncertain.

Autoantibodies against cytoskeleton proteins have been observed in sera from patients with necrobiosis lipoidica. These autoantibodies (IgG antitroponin, antidesmin, antikeratin, anti-insulin, antitrinitrophenol, and IgA and IgM antikeratin) were found to be elevated in patients with necrobiosis lipoidica compared with diabetic patients without evidence of necrobiosis lipoidica.[68] What role, if any, these autoantibodies play in the pathogenesis of necrobiosis lipoidica is unclear. Synthesis of collagen by fibroblasts cultured from lesions is decreased compared with fibroblasts from normal skin.[69]

Also of uncertain significance is the reported detection, by immunofluorescence, of immunoreactants (IgM and C3) in blood vessel walls in some cases of necrobiosis lipoidica.[70,71] Epidermal dendritic S100-positive cells are increased in number.[72] Whether this reflects an immunological aspect to the development of necrobiosis lipoidica has yet to be determined.

Glut-1 (the human erythrocyte glucose transporter) is expressed by the fibroblasts in areas of sclerotic collagen from biopsies of patients with necrobiosis lipoidica.[73] This raises the possibility of an altered transport of glucose in the affected areas contributing to the histopathological features seen in this disease.

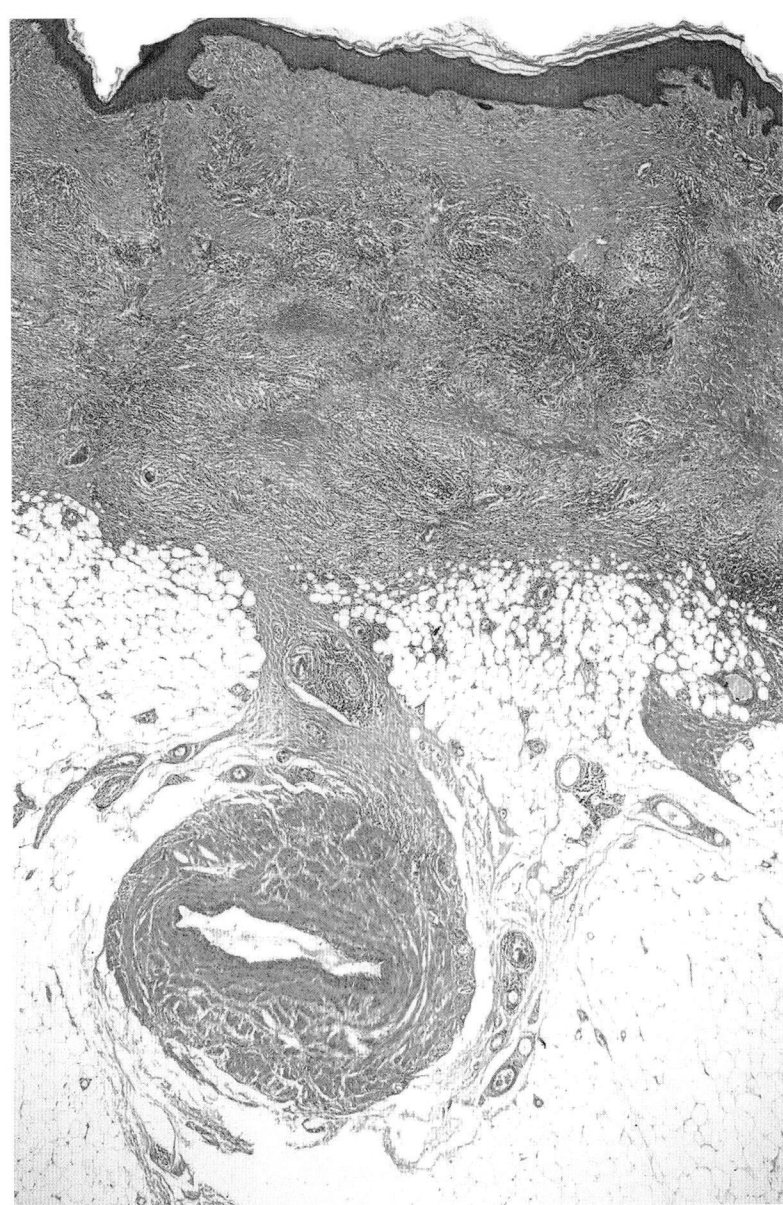

Fig. 9.54
Necrobiosis lipoidica: the epidermis is unaffected; there is extensive necrobiosis in the reticular dermis. A heavy chronic inflammatory cell infiltrate is present.

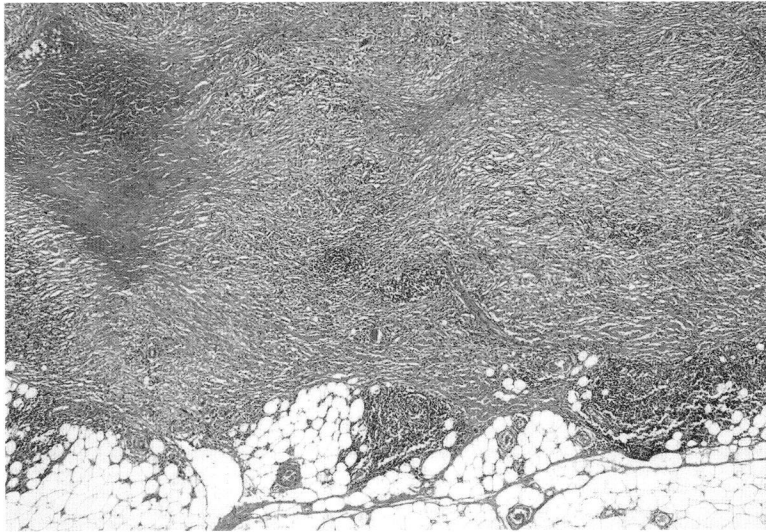

Fig. 9.55
Necrobiosis lipoidica: the lesion extends down to the subcutaneous fat.

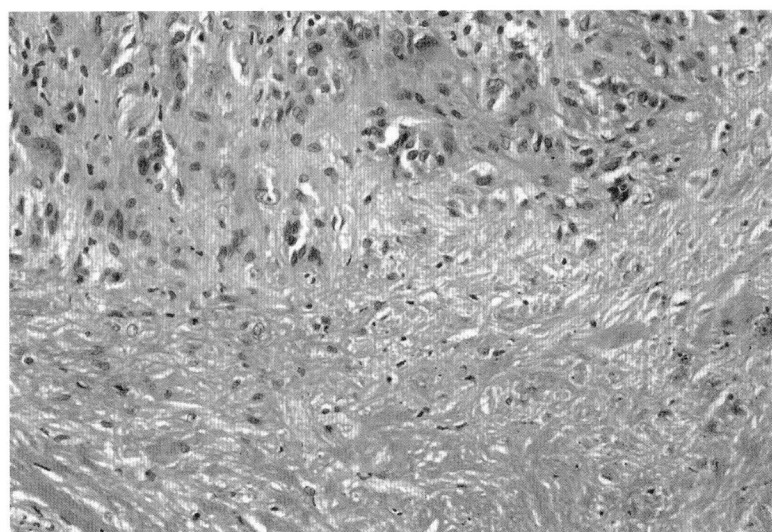

Fig. 9.56
Necrobiosis lipoidica: high-power view of *Fig. 9.54*.

Gli-1, the glioma-associated oncogene homologue, has been found to be expressed in a number of granulomatous skin disorders including necrobiosis lipoidica.[74] The explanation for this is not clear, but it suggests that inhibitors of gli-1 may be used in the treatment of the disease.

Recently, spirochetal microorganisms, likely to be *Borrelia*, have been identified in lesions of necrobiosis lipoidica in patients from central Europe.[75] The significance of this finding is unclear.

The histopathological features are variable, depending to some extent on the presence or absence of coexistent diabetes mellitus.[76,77] The palisading granuloma with necrobiosis is more typical of the diabetes-related variant, whereas a granulomatous sarcoidal type of reaction is more often a feature of nondiabetes-related necrobiosis. Nevertheless, there is very considerable overlap and in the majority of cases one cannot predict, on histologic grounds alone, which cases are, and which are not, diabetes-related.

The epidermal changes are usually inconspicuous or absent. There may, however, be acanthosis or atrophy, and hyperkeratosis is not uncommon.

The hallmark of necrobiosis lipoidica is the palisading necrobiotic granuloma. Large, often confluent areas of necrobiosis are present, usually centered in the lower dermis, although the superficial dermis and subcutaneous fat may also be affected (*Figs 9.54–9.56*). When the subcutaneous fat is involved, the changes are seen mainly in the septa. The foci of necrobiosis consist of eosinophilic, swollen or degenerate collagen, often appearing hyalinized with a surrounding infiltrate of variable numbers of lymphocytes and histiocytes (*Fig. 9.57*). Aggregates of lymphoid cells, with or without germinal center formation, are frequently found.[78] Plasma cells are almost invariably present. In a single case, the plasma cell infiltrate was monoclonal, and further investigations revealed an underlying monoclonal gammopathy.[79] The necrobiotic foci sometimes contain mucin. Palisading is variable, being more conspicuous in those instances associated with a heavy inflammatory cell infiltrate. The areas of necrobiosis are associated with loss of elastic tissue (*Fig. 9.58*). Usually, epithelioid histiocytes and giant cells are evident and sometimes there are well-formed granulomata resembling the sarcoidal type of necrobiotic histologic reaction (see below) (*Fig. 9.59*). Very rarely, asteroid bodies are identified.[80] Lipid droplets, best seen with oil red O or Sudan IV staining on frozen tissue, are almost invariably present in the necrobiotic foci. Usually, a mild to moderate perivascular lymphocytic infiltrate is seen in the adjacent dermis. Cholesterol clefts are rare and only exceptionally may be prominent.[81,82]

A careful search often reveals vascular changes in necrobiosis lipoidica. These consist of blood vessel wall thickening, with intimal proliferation and narrowing of the lumen. Occasionally, thrombi are noted. Sometimes increased numbers of vessels are a feature. The vascular changes are more obvious in patients with associated diabetes mellitus or other systemic disease. These changes are particularly severe in those cases where

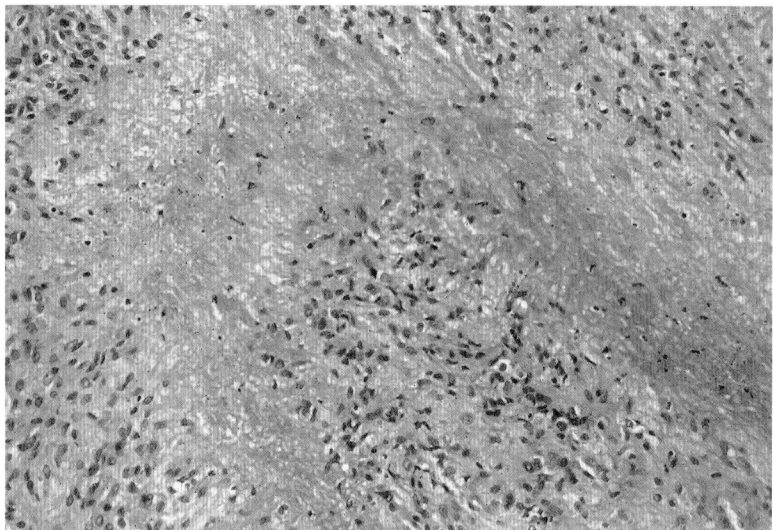

Fig. 9.57
Necrobiosis lipoidica: the degenerate collagen is surrounded by a palisade of histiocytes, lymphocytes, and fibroblasts.

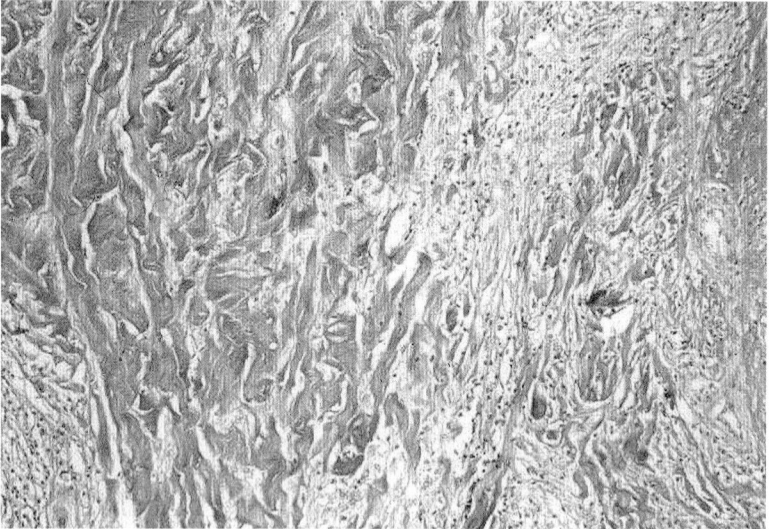

Fig. 9.58
Necrobiosis lipoidica: note the complete absence of elastic tissue. Elastic-van Gieson.

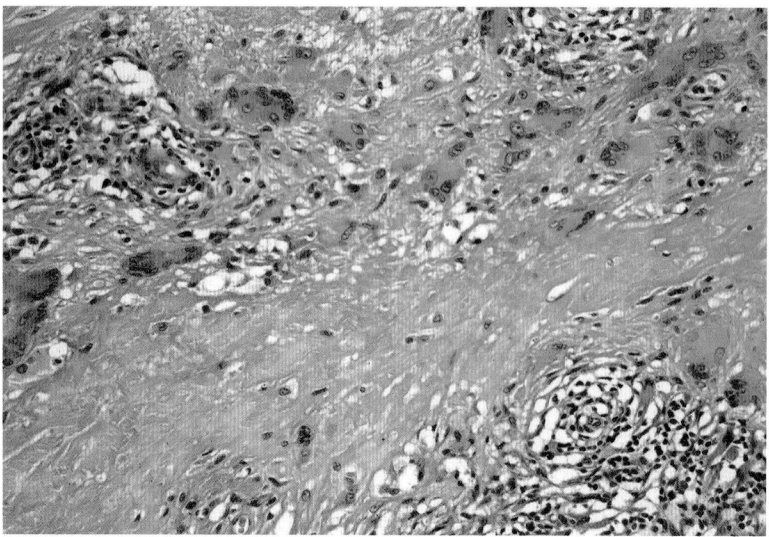

Fig. 9.59
Necrobiosis lipoidica: there is a granulomatous infiltrate with conspicuous multinucleate giant cells.

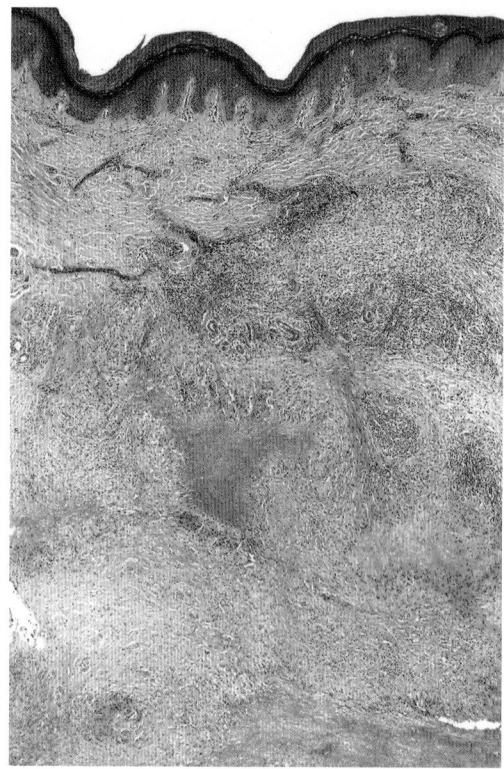

Fig. 9.60
Necrobiosis lipoidica (diffuse variant): a broad band of confluent necrobiosis has destroyed the entire reticular dermis.

necrobiosis is very marked. One study also showed that neutrophilic and granulomatous vasculopathies correlated with systemic disease.[83] In addition, telangiectatic superficial venules are a common feature. Cases with necrobiosis-like features and significant vasculitis and neutrophilic infiltrates in the setting of systemic disease are discussed in detail in the section on palisaded neutrophilic and granulomatous dermatitis associated with systemic disease (p. 334). In lesions with anesthesia, S100 shows destruction of nerve fibers in the areas of necrobiosis.[52,53]

In the diffuse variant, there is very widespread necrobiosis with a minimal inflammatory cell response; such cases are usually associated with diabetes (*Fig. 9.60*). Sometimes linear infiltrates of histiocytes between collagen fibers are a feature, as in granuloma annulare. Lipomembranous fat necrosis is noted in occasional cases.[84]

In the sarcoidal type of necrobiosis lipoidica, which is more often noted with the nondiabetes mellitus-associated variant, the appearances are those of naked epithelioid cell granulomata, particularly in the lower dermis (*Fig. 9.61*). Langhans and foreign body giant cells are usually conspicuous, and a lymphocytic and plasma cell infiltrate may be evident (*Fig. 9.62*). Necrobiosis is usually minimal; multiple levels may have to be examined before its presence is confirmed (*Fig. 9.63*). The sarcoidal type of necrobiosis lipoidica in patients without diabetes mellitus has in the past been described as Miescher granuloma.

Perforating necrobiosis lipoidica is associated with transepidermal elimination of necrobiotic collagen and also degenerated elastotic material (*Figs 9.64–9.66*).[81,85,86]

Exceptionally, skin changes at the sites of intravenous drug abuse and leishmaniasis may mimic necrobiosis lipoidica.[87,88] Histologic changes of both necrobiosis lipoidica and granuloma annulare may exceptionally coexist in a tattoo reaction.[89] A small number of patients reported in a series presented with pretibial lesions suggestive of necrobiosis lipoidica, but on histology, only features of venous insufficiency were observed. The name of pretibial angioplasia has been proposed for this entity.[90]

Differential diagnosis

Necrobiosis lipoidica must be distinguished from granuloma annulare, rheumatoid nodule, actinic granuloma, and granuloma multiforme. Points of

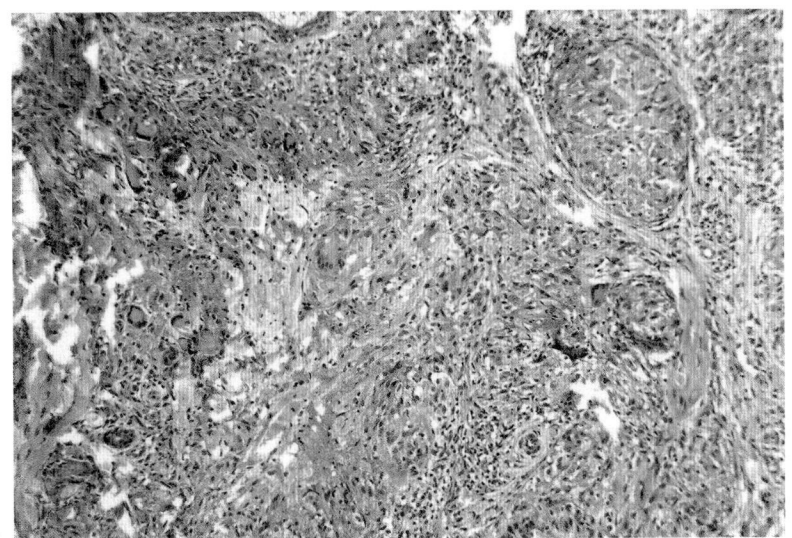

Fig. 9.61
Necrobiosis lipoidica (granulomatous variant): well-defined noncaseating granulomata replace the reticular dermis. Necrobiosis is present to the left of center.

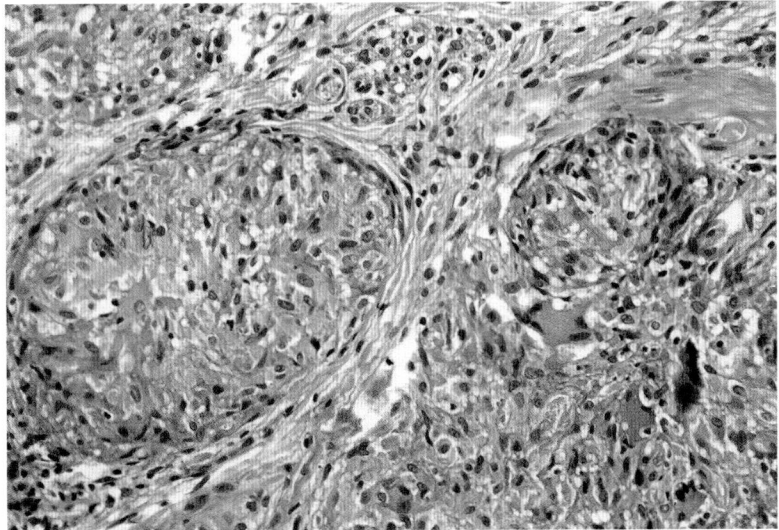

Fig. 9.62
Necrobiosis lipoidica (granulomatous variant): the naked granulomata are very reminiscent of sarcoidosis. Note the multinucleate giant cells.

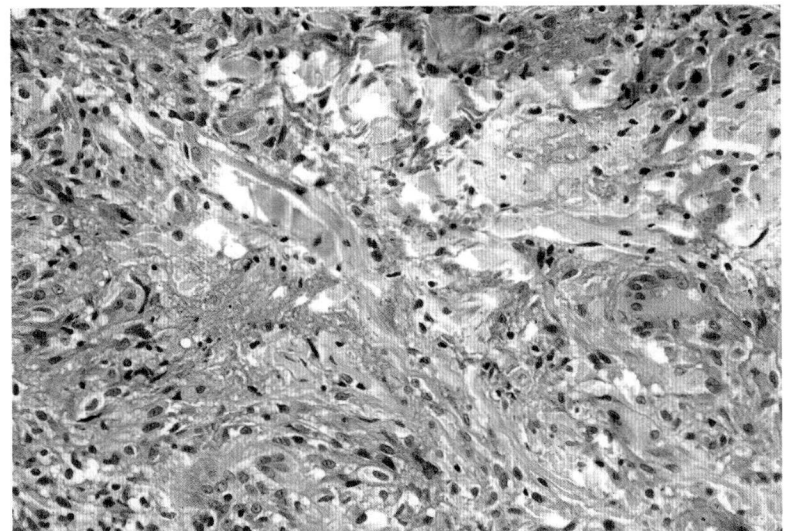

Fig. 9.63
Necrobiosis lipoidica (granulomatous variant): higher-power view of the necrobiotic focus seen in *Fig. 9.61*.

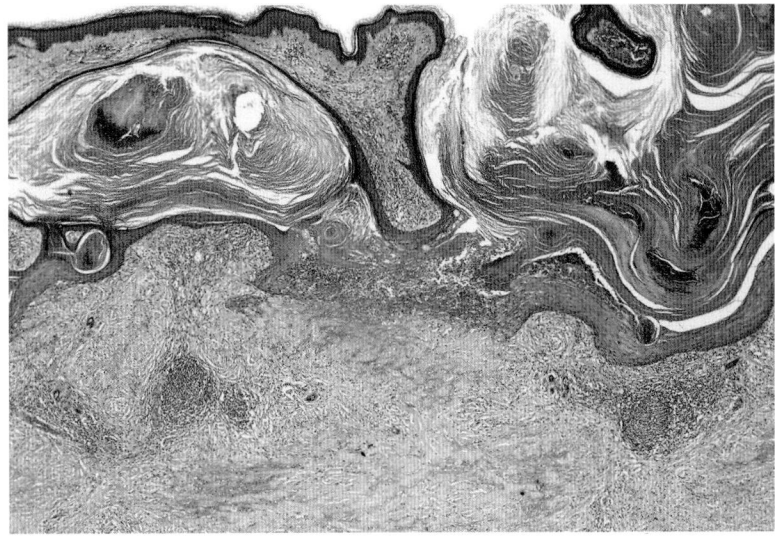

Fig. 9.64
Perforating necrobiosis lipoidica: there is widespread hyperkeratosis and crusting. A perforating channel is seen on the right side of the picture.

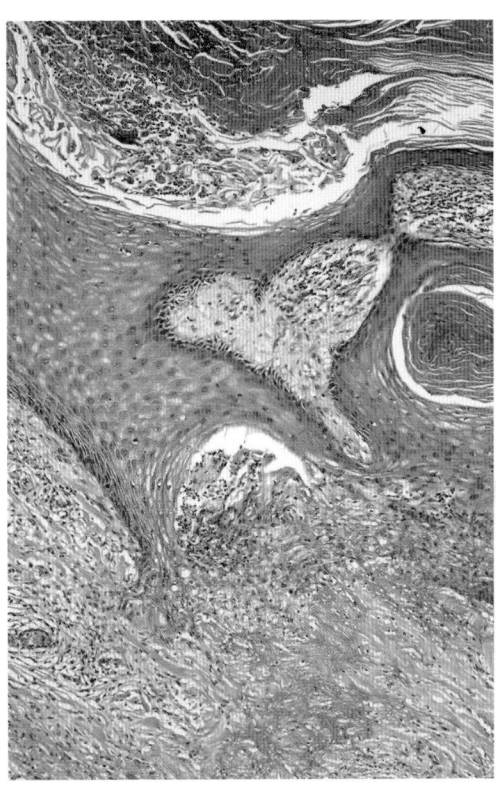

Fig. 9.65
Perforating necrobiosis: close-up view of the perforating channel.

distinction are summarized in *Table 9.1*. The presence of massive necrobiosis associated with numerous cholesterol clefts, bizarre multinucleated giant cells, and Touton-type giant cells distinguishes necrobiotic xanthogranuloma from necrobiosis lipoidica. As noted above, prominent cholesterol cleft formation, which is a feature that usually suggests necrobiotic xanthogranuloma, may rarely be seen in necrobiosis lipoidica.[76,77] Small punch biopsies may not be adequate for definitive evaluation, and sampling bias may be misleading. Clinical correlation should be taken into consideration before making a final diagnosis. It has been proposed that the pattern of immunostaining with adipophilin may be of use in the differential diagnosis of granulomatous dermatitis. In necrobiosis lipoidica adipophilin staining is usually limited to extracellular areas in zones of damaged collagen, whereas in granuloma annulare there is extracellular and intracellular staining and in sarcoidosis the staining tends to be intracellular.[91]

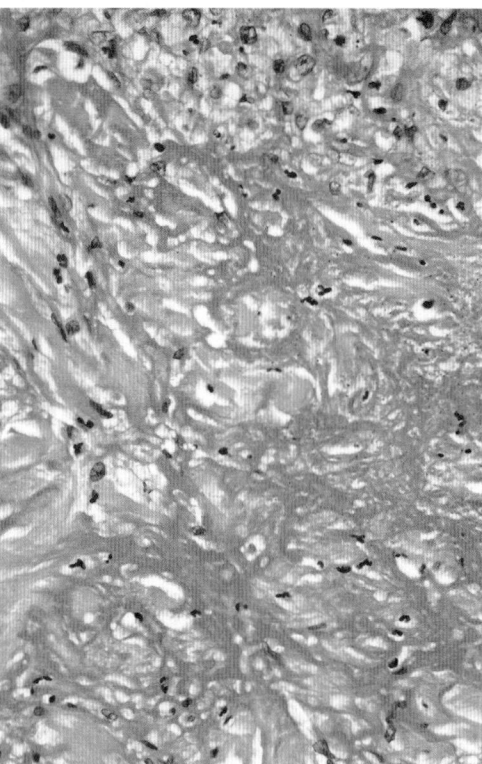

Fig. 9.66
Perforating necrobiosis: the dermis immediately beneath the site of perforation shows severe necrobiotic change.

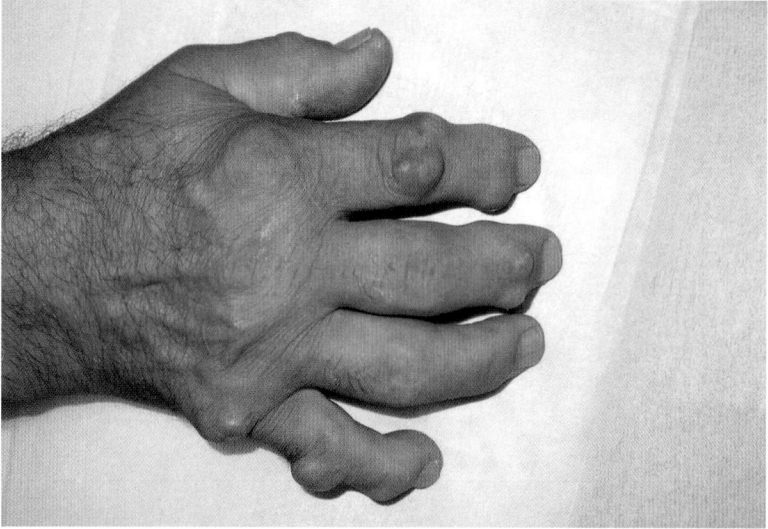

Fig. 9.67
Rheumatoid nodules: lesions on the knuckles are commonly seen in rheumatoid arthritis. By courtesy of Dr J.C. Pascual, MD, Alicante, Spain.

Rheumatoid nodule

Clinical features

Rheumatoid nodules are subcutaneous lesions that develop at sites of trauma or at pressure points in approximately 30% of adults with rheumatoid arthritis.[1-4] They are most commonly found on the extensor aspect of the forearms and elbows (particularly the olecranon process), the feet, knees, knuckles, buttocks, scalp, and back (Figs 9.67 and 9.68).[5] They have also been described involving a wide variety of other sites, including the abdominal wall, heart (pericardium, myocardium, and valves), larynx, lungs, pleura, splenic capsule, peritoneum, mesenterium, eye, bridge of nose, pinna, ischial tuberosity, thyrohyoid membrane, Achilles tendon, oral mucosa, leptomeninges, lymph nodes, vagina, breast, and conjunctiva.[6-14]

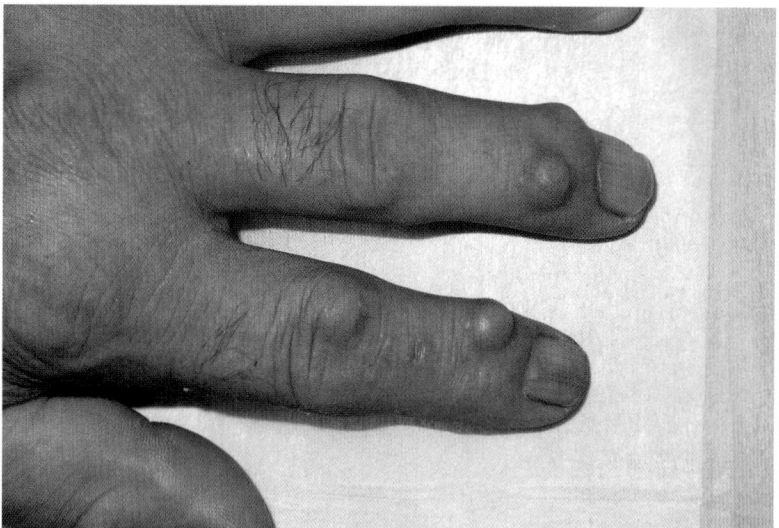

Fig. 9.68
Rheumatoid nodule: close-up view. By courtesy of Dr J.C. Pascual, MD, Alicante, Spain.

Lesions are often fixed to the underlying periosteum or deep fascia. They present as firm, asymptomatic, dome-shaped masses in the subcutaneous fat or deeper tissues and measure from several millimeters to 5 cm in diameter. Numbers may vary from one to over a hundred. Ulceration sometimes occurs. Intrapulmonary rheumatoid nodules have been exceptionally associated with leflunomide in a patient with rheumatoid arthritis.[15] A rare association with anti-tumor necrosis factor alpha treatment for rheumatoid arthritis has been described.[16] A case of large cavitary pulmonary lesions in a patient with HIV has been reported.[17]

Rheumatoid nodules are more commonly found in patients with severe rheumatoid arthritis and are associated with a high titer of rheumatoid factor, joint erosions, and an increased incidence of rheumatoid vasculitis.[18] They are not, however, specific for rheumatoid arthritis, being found in approximately 5–7% of patients with SLE (although in this condition they tend to be localized about the hands) and occasionally in seronegative ankylosing spondylitis.[19,20] Clinically similar lesions have also been reported in patients with scleroderma. Presentation of multiple rheumatoid nodules on the fingers in association with little or no arthritis has been described as rheumatoid nodulosis.[21-23] This, however, can be associated with destructive arthritis.[24] A similar name (cutaneous nodulosis) has been given to the development of multiple small nodules at different sites during methotrexate therapy for rheumatoid arthritis.[25] Etanercept has been linked to the exceptional development of extensive pulmonary nodulosis, while infliximab and the aromatase inhibitor letrozole are associated with accelerated cutaneous nodulosis.[26-28]

Pathogenesis and histologic features

Although these lesions develop at sites of pressure and trauma (implying pathogenetic significance), there is some evidence in support of an immune complex-mediated pathogenesis, as both IgG and IgM have been detected by immunofluorescence in the walls of blood vessels adjacent to rheumatoid nodules.[29] Similarly, both rheumatoid factor and complement have been demonstrated within the substance of rheumatoid nodules. Localization of IgM rheumatoid factor and terminal complement complexes C5b-9 has been demonstrated on the luminal surface of endothelial cells in rheumatoid nodules.[30] C4d has been shown in association with palisading macrophages and in areas of fibrinoid necrosis, further supporting the role of complement activation in the pathogenesis of the lesions.[31] Proinflammatory cytokines and cell adhesion molecules (TNF-α, IL-1β, IL-Ra RNA, E-selectin) have been shown in rheumatoid nodules and are likely to play a role in mediating injury.[32] The expression of cytokines in the rheumatoid nodule is very similar to that in the synovial lining in rheumatoid joints and suggests that the pathogenesis of both is very similar and driven by Th1 lymphocytes.[33] The cytokines involved include IFN-γ, IL-1beta, TNF-α, IL-12, IL-18, IL-15,

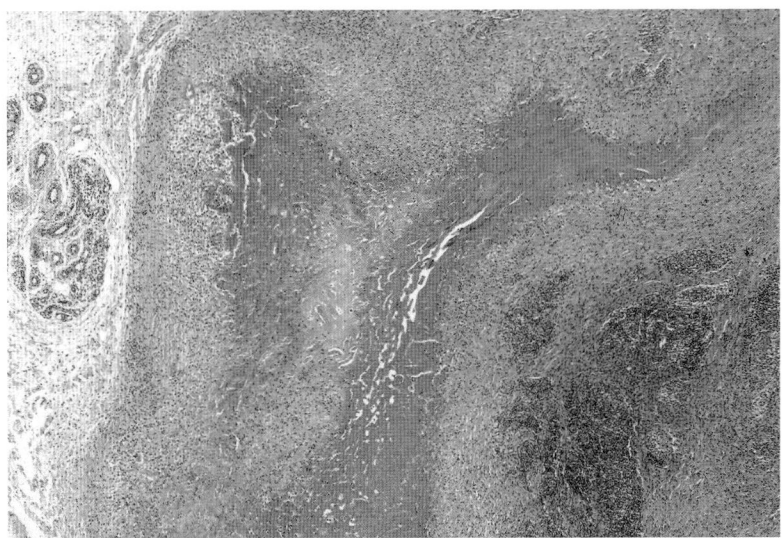

Fig. 9.69
Rheumatoid nodule: there is massive necrobiosis with adjacent scarring and a dense lymphocytic infiltrate. Rheumatoid nodules characteristically occur in the soft tissues.

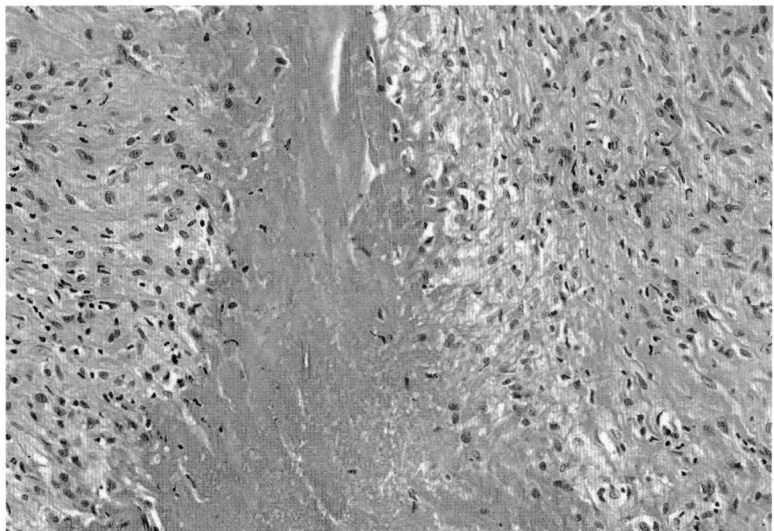

Fig. 9.71
Rheumatoid nodule: the necrobiotic connective tissue is surrounded by a well-developed histiocytic palisade.

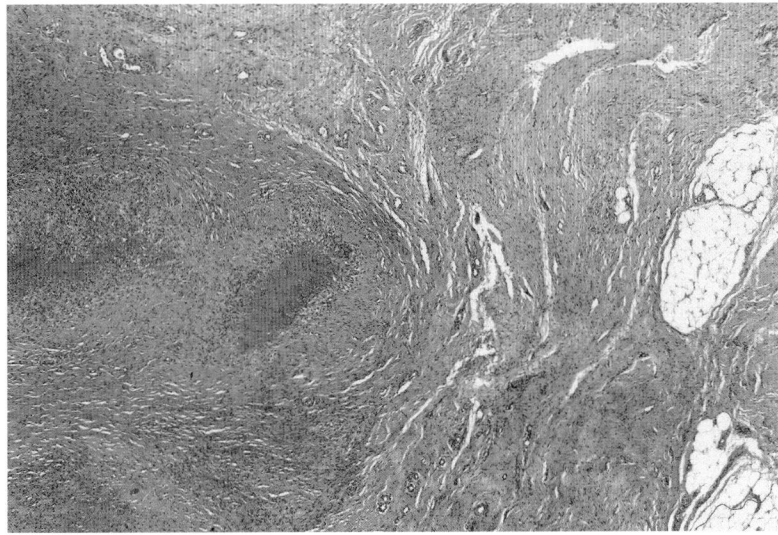

Fig. 9.70
Rheumatoid nodule: in this example, tendon can be seen on the right side of the field.

and IL-10.[32] Although massive central necrosis is predominant, apoptosis has been demonstrated throughout the nodule.[34]

Rheumatoid nodules are typically located in the subcutaneous fat or soft tissues although they may extend into the deeper reticular dermis. This is in contrast to the more superficial location of both granuloma annulare and necrobiosis lipoidica. They are multinodular and associated with very extensive necrobiosis (Figs 9.69 and 9.70). Fibrin deposition is often seen in the center of the nodule.[35] Immunoglobulin, lipid, glycosaminoglycans, and nucleoproteins may also be present. Old lesions are sometimes associated with cyst formation due to liquefactive degeneration of the contents of the nodules. A well-developed palisade of histiocytes and occasional giant cells characteristically surrounds necrobiotic foci and fibrinoid material (Fig. 9.71). Asteroid inclusions are not a feature. The outer layer is composed of vascular granulation tissue, and in older lesions marked fibrosis is a frequent accompaniment. An inflammatory cell infiltrate of lymphocytes, plasma cells, and eosinophils is often present. Leukocytoclastic vasculitis has occasionally been reported to affect the blood vessels in and around early nodules. A rare case with perforation of the epidermis has been documented.[36]

Differential diagnosis

In some cases of deep granuloma annulare, the histologic changes are similar to rheumatoid nodule. Deep granuloma annulare ('pseudorheumatoid nodule') tends to have more mucin deposition and less fibrin than typical rheumatoid nodules.[37] Therefore, the latter are referred to as 'red' granulomas and the former as 'blue' granulomas.[38] However, some rheumatoid nodules do contain mucin. Clinicopathological and serological correlation is advised before establishing a definitive diagnosis.

Compared to rheumatoid fever nodule, rheumatoid arthritis nodules tend to be better circumscribed and surrounded by a well-defined palisade of histiocytes. In addition, the fine fibrinoid strands that form the center of a rheumatic fever nodule contrast with the more dense sheet-like areas of necrobiosis and fibrin deposition in the rheumatoid arthritis nodule.

Patients combining the features of severe rheumatoid arthritis with palisading granulomata accompanied by a neutrophilic infiltrate and leukocytoclastic vasculitis have been described.[18] These lesions are discussed under the rubric of palisaded neutrophilic and granulomatous dermatitis with vasculitis. In short, lesions showing these features may be associated with a number of systemic diseases, including rheumatoid arthritis.

Although epithelioid sarcoma, with its associated geographic necrosis, may bear a superficial resemblance at low power to rheumatoid nodule, the degree of nuclear atypia and pleomorphism in the former should allow easy distinction between these conditions (Fig. 9.72). However, in difficult cases, expression of keratin and epithelial membrane antigen and loss of INI-1 expression in epithelioid sarcoma should assist in the differential diagnosis.[39]

Elastolytic granulomata

This is a controversial group of diseases, the prototype of which is the actinic granuloma. Other entities that very likely belong to this group include atypical facial necrobiosis lipoidica, Miescher facial granuloma, and granuloma multiforme (see below). It has been suggested that all these conditions represent examples of granuloma annulare occurring in different clinical settings.[1–4] However, the clinicopathological features are distinctive and the pathological process clearly relates to the primary destruction of elastic fibers by a granulomatous infiltrate. In granuloma annulare, as in diseases such as sarcoidosis, destruction of elastic fibers does not always occur and when it does, it tends to occur focally, developing as a secondary phenomenon.[5]

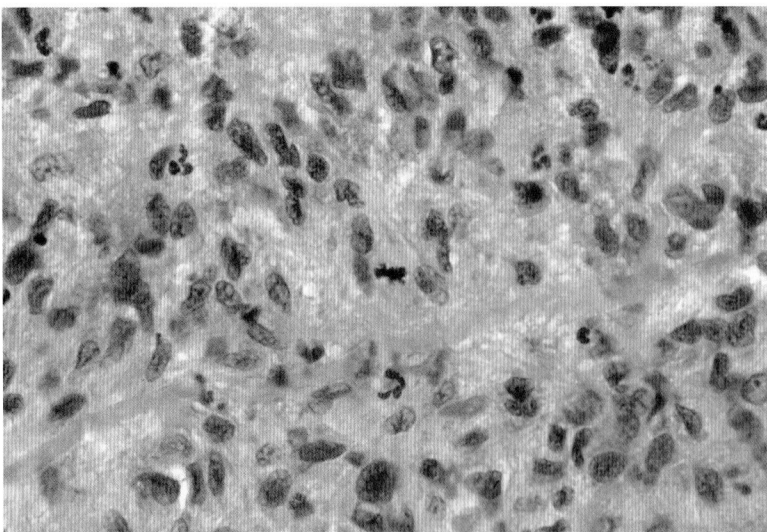

Fig. 9.72
Rheumatoid nodule: the palisading histiocytes may sometimes show mitotic figures which may lead the unwary to consider epithelioid sarcoma.

Annular elastolytic giant cell granuloma (annular elastolytic granuloma)

Clinical features

The term 'annular elastolytic giant cell granuloma' has been used to describe not only cases of actinic granuloma but also lesions in which destruction of elastic fibers occurs in the absence of solar elastosis.[6] In fact, some cases present at sites with little sun exposure and the disease may also occur in children.[7] Thus, although the terms actinic granuloma, elastolytic giant cell granuloma, and even elastolytic actinic giant cell granuloma have been used interchangeably in the literature, the latter term should be reserved for elastolytic granulomata occurring in skin without solar elastosis but not restricted to covered skin.[8,9]

Lesions usually present on the trunk and neck and rarely on proximal limbs. They vary in size but tend to be large. Despite the name annular, some cases present with papules or reticular erythema.[10] In those that are annular, there is an advancing raised border which may be papular. Rarely, lesions are generalized and in one of such cases, the lesions spared the striae distensae.[11,12] Spontaneous resolution is rare.[10] A reported case describes a lesion that developed at the site of an old burn scar and spread after trauma.[13] In a single report, repigmentation of the gray hairs within the affected area of the scalp has been described, and in a further case the granulomas developed on lesions of vitiligo.[14,15]

Elastolytic granulomata have rarely been described in association with adult T-cell leukemia lymphoma, primary cutaneous CD4-positive small/medium-sized pleomorphic T-cell lymphoma, acute myelogenous leukemia, monoclonal gammopathy, Hashimoto thyroiditis, temporal arteritis in one case following herpes zoster infection, squamous cell carcinoma of the tonsil, late-onset X-linked dominant protoporphyria, diabetes mellitus, and prostate cancer.[16–24] A unilateral lesion developing in a hemiplegic stroke patient has been reported, and in a further patient the lesion developed after the implantation of a pacemaker.[25,26] Elastolytic granulomata have also been documented in internal organs.[27] The latter, however, probably represents sarcoidosis with prominent elastolysis.

Pathogenesis and histologic features

Elastic fibers become altered through an unknown mechanism and appear to induce factor XIIIa-positive cells and CD68-positive macrophages to form granulomata.[28]

Histologic features may be identical to those of actinic granuloma (see below) except for the absence of solar elastosis. Ideally, in annular lesions the biopsy should be a wedge including the center, the advancing edge, and normal skin for comparison purposes. This is not always possible, particularly in lesions that do not have an annular configuration. The center of the lesion is completely devoid of elastic fibers, and there is usually no inflammation. The loss of elastic fibers appears to be irreversible.[29] In the advancing margin, there is a granulomatous reaction with fragmentation and phagocytosis of elastic fibers. In one case, histology showed features of mid-dermal elastolysis leading the authors to suggest that annular elastolytic giant cell granuloma may possibly represent a prodromal or inflammatory stage of the disease.[30] Rarely, sarcoidal granulomas may be a prominent feature.[31]

Differential diagnosis

Many granulomatous reactions, including infections, often display elastophagocytosis. However, in these conditions the change is mild and focal. In granuloma annulare, there is usually very little or no elastophagocytosis, while in annular elastolytic giant cell granuloma there is no necrobiosis, mucin, or palisading granuloma.[32] Although a necrobiotic variant of the condition has been described, it is likely that these represent variants of necrobiotic disorders rather than true elastolytic granulomas.[9]

Actinic granuloma (O'Brien)

Clinical features

Actinic granuloma develops on the sun-damaged skin of the neck, face, upper chest, or arms of middle-aged patients.[1–5] It may also affect the conjunctiva, and a single case affecting the upper lip has been reported.[6–9] Lesions restricted to the conjunctiva of young women are exceptional.[10] A further case presented as alopecia.[11] The incidence is equal in men and women, and individuals with blond hair and freckled skin are predisposed, particularly those living in sunny climates. An association with the long-standing use of sunbeds and with doxycycline phototoxicity has also been described.[12,13]

Lesions present as one or more skin-colored or pink papules, which enlarge to form annular or arcuate plaques up to 1 cm in diameter. The edge of the lesion is somewhat raised, forming a border 0.2–0.5 cm in width. These annular plaques enlarge slowly, and the center may gradually clear to appear relatively normal or slightly atrophic with variable depigmentation. Lesions are asymptomatic and there is no evidence of anesthesia. However, there is usually clinical exacerbation associated with sun exposure.[14] They do not develop on non-sun-damaged skin. Spontaneous resolution may take place after months or years.

Bilateral periocular actinic granulomata have been documented in a patient with renal failure.[15] Other rare associations likely to be coincidental include relapsing polychondritis, cutaneous amyloidosis, giant molluscum contagiosum, chronic lymphocytic leukemia, and erythema nodosum.[16–20]

Pathogenesis and histologic features

The pathogenesis of actinic granuloma is poorly understood. It has been suggested that the antigenic stimulus for the formation of granulomata in both actinic granuloma and temporal arteritis is actinically degenerated elastic tissue.[21,22] Interestingly, phototesting in a single case failed to reproduce the lesions of actinic granuloma.[23]

The features are best appreciated by examination of a radial biopsy through the edge of a lesion and including uninvolved skin.[24,25] The epidermis may be normal or atrophic. The peripheral unaffected skin shows gross solar (actinic) elastosis (Figs 9.73–9.75). Within the rim of the lesion there is a foreign body giant cell reaction in association with, and engulfing, fragmented elastotic material (elastoclasis) (Figs 9.76 and 9.77).[24,25] The granulomatous reaction is centered in the zone of solar elastosis and, accordingly, tends to be confined to the superficial dermis.[26] The giant cells may contain asteroid bodies. There is an accompanying chronic inflammatory cell infiltrate composed of histiocytes, lymphocytes, and plasma cells. Necrobiosis is not a feature of this condition. Palisading of histiocytes is either absent or minimal and, if present, is related to the elastotic debris. Dermal mucin does not appear to be increased.[24] Fibroblasts are scant and fibrosis is minimal. In the actinic granuloma, blood vessels appear normal. Within the central zone the collagen appears relatively normal, although it is more obviously

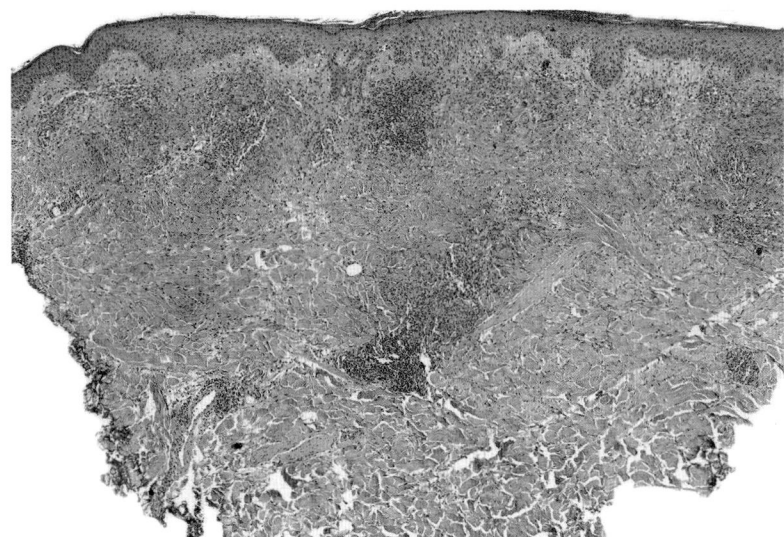

Fig. 9.73
Actinic granuloma: a granulomatous reaction is present the superficial dermis surrounding an ill-defined necrobiotic process. Solar elastosis is evident.

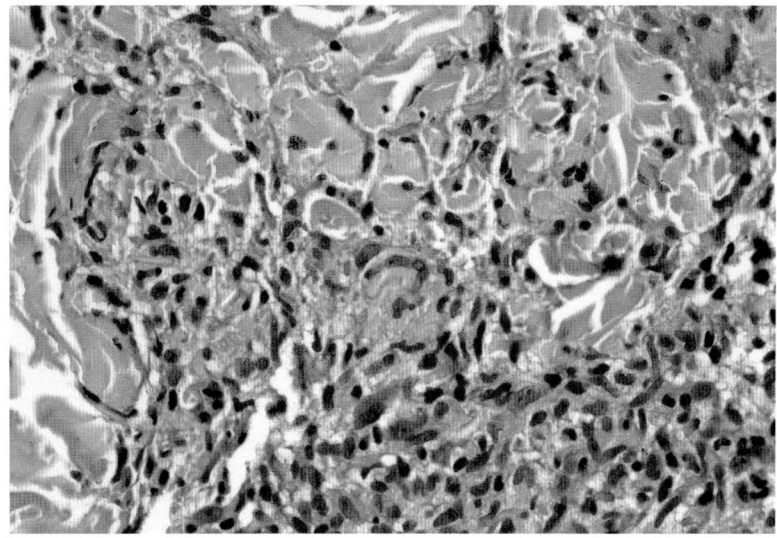

Fig. 9.76
Actinic granuloma: elastotic material is seen in the cytoplasm of the giant cell in the centre of the field.

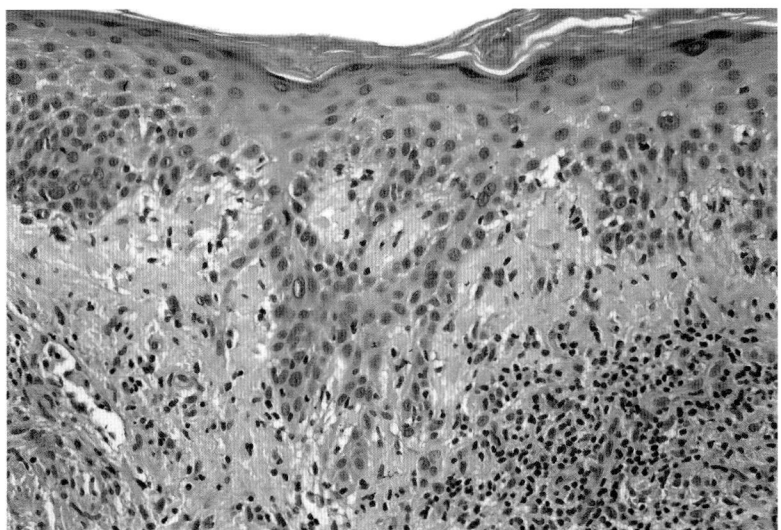

Fig. 9.74
Actinic granuloma: in addition to solar elastosis, this example also shows interface change with conspicuous cytoid bodies.

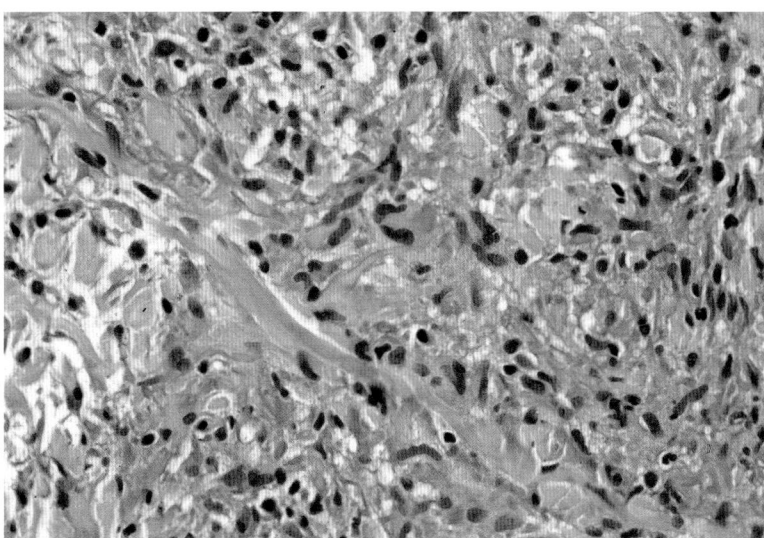

Fig. 9.77
Actinic granuloma: high-power view of basophilic degenerate elastic fibers.

horizontally aligned and may appear more closely packed than normal. Slight scarring is present in the central area where elastic tissue is absent.[26]

Differential diagnosis

The facial location, presence of elastophagocytosis, and absence of necrobiosis aid in distinguishing actinic granuloma from other granulomatous lesions. The absence of dermal mucin, necrobiosis, and palisading granuloma and the presence of marked elastoclasis and mild scarring help to distinguish actinic granuloma from granuloma annulare, the disorder that it most resembles.[16,27]

Atypical facial necrobiosis lipoidica

Clinical features

Despite its name, this is not a variant of necrobiosis lipoidica and deserves separate mention because of its unusual clinical features and distinctive histology.[1-5] Atypical facial necrobiosis lipoidica, which predominantly affects females (9:1), usually develops in the absence of diabetes mellitus, and manifests most often in the fourth decade. Patients present with one or more annular, nonscaling plaques on the upper face and scalp, which typically have slightly raised, relatively uniform borders and measure 1–5 cm in

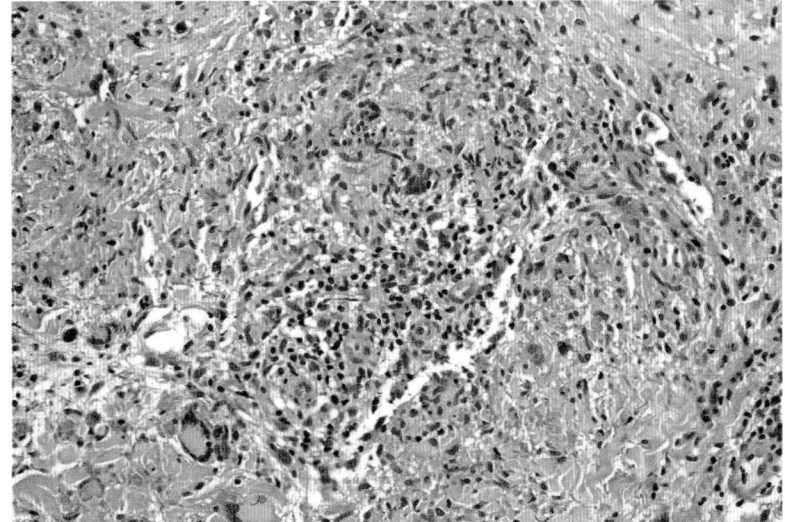

Fig. 9.75
Actinic granuloma: the granulomatous infiltrate is associated with degenerate elastic fibers.

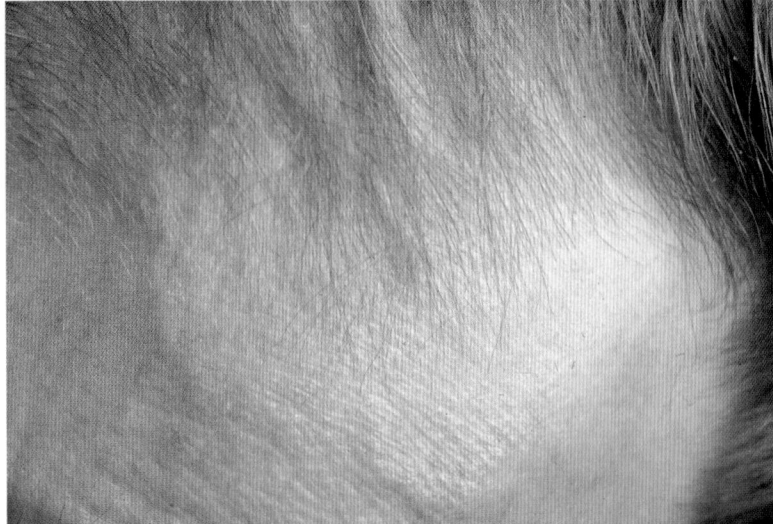

Fig. 9.78
Atypical facial necrobiosis lipoidica: atrophic plaque on forehead with a well-defined edge. From the collection of the late N.P. Smith, MD, the Institute of Dermatology, London, UK.

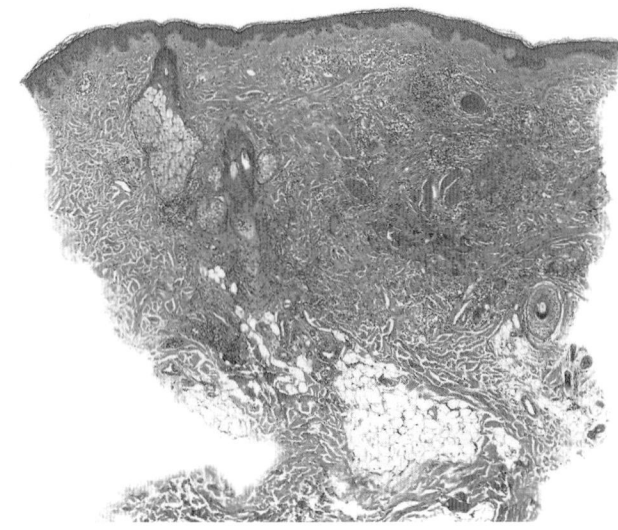

Fig. 9.79
Atypical facial necrobiosis lipoidica: a dense granulomatous infiltrate occupies the dermis.

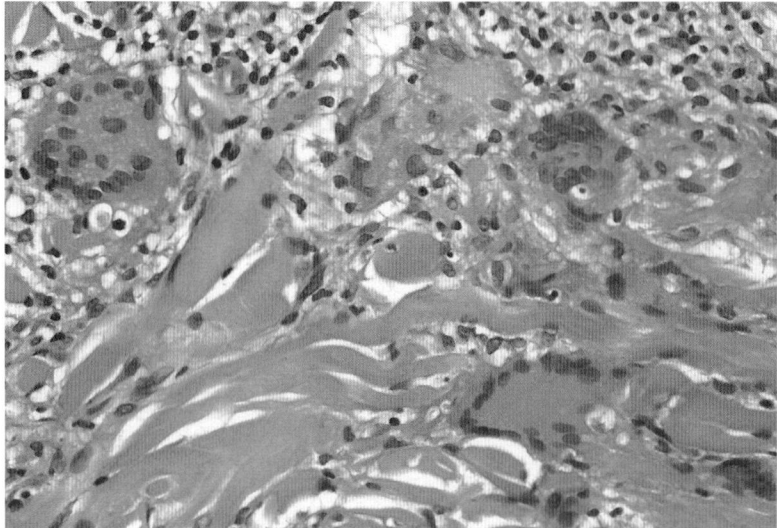

Fig. 9.80
Atypical facial necrobiosis lipoidica: close-up view of the granulomata. Note the conspicuous giant cells.

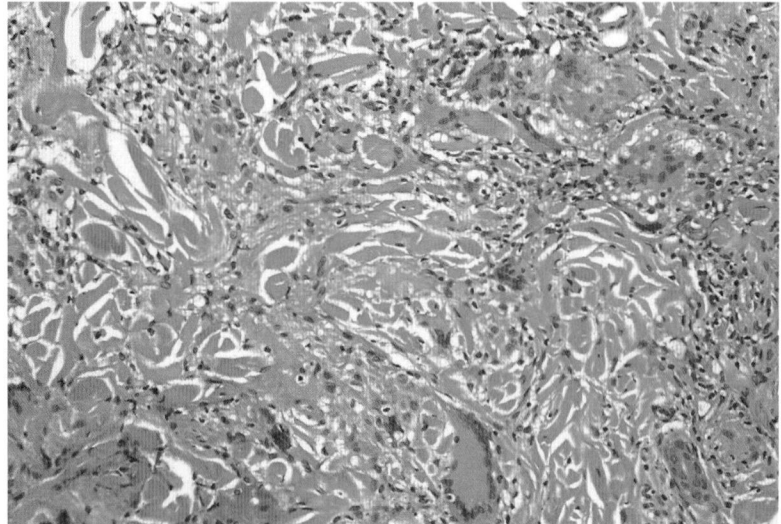

Fig. 9.81
Atypical facial necrobiosis lipoidica: an ill-defined focus of necrobiosis is present.

diameter (*Fig. 9.78*). Although early lesions are erythematous with a brown border, older lesions are characterized by central depigmentation. Atrophy, however, is minimal or absent. Patients may, in addition, show involvement of other sites, including the arms, hands, and trunk. Very rarely, patients have concomitant typical necrobiosis lipoidica on the shins. It is for this reason that the name was originally coined. We now believe, however, that the condition probably has no relationship whatsoever to necrobiosis lipoidica. It is much more likely that it represents a variant of an annular elastolytic granuloma.

Histologic features

The condition is characterized by a dense granulomatous infiltrate, with conspicuous giant cells, involving the dermis (*Figs 9.79* and *9.80*). The infiltrate has a rather irregular distribution, being dispersed between individual collagen bundles. Occasional circumscribed granulomata may sometimes be a feature. Asteroid bodies are often found in the cytoplasm of giant cells. Typically, there is loss of elastic tissue in the areas of granulomatous inflammation. Rarely, ill-defined foci of necrobiosis are noted (*Fig. 9.81*), but well-defined palisading granulomata are not present. In cases with coexistent necrobiosis lipoidica, biopsies from the affected areas on the shins show the typical histologic features of this condition.

Differential diagnosis

In contrast to actinic granuloma with which this condition is often confused, the surrounding skin does not show evidence of significant solar elastosis and elastoclasis.

Granuloma multiforme

Clinical features

This dermatosis of unknown etiology is of particular importance because clinically it can be confused with leprosy; however, it is not associated with cutaneous anesthesia.[1,2] Granuloma multiforme, which shows a marked female predominance, is seen most often in Central Africa, especially eastern Nigeria. It has also been documented in the Congo, Uganda, India, and Tunisia.[3–6] The disease is very common in some villages. It particularly affects patients over 40 years of age. Lesions, which tend to chronicity, are found on the upper and exposed parts of the body. They commence as small, flesh-colored, indurated, pruritic papulonodules, 1–8 mm in diameter and raised 1–3 mm above the skin surface, which extend peripherally and coalesce to form annular lesions and plaques (*Figs 9.82* and *9.83*). Very large lesions become irregular and develop scalloped or gyrate borders. Central healing may be associated with residual hypopigmentation.

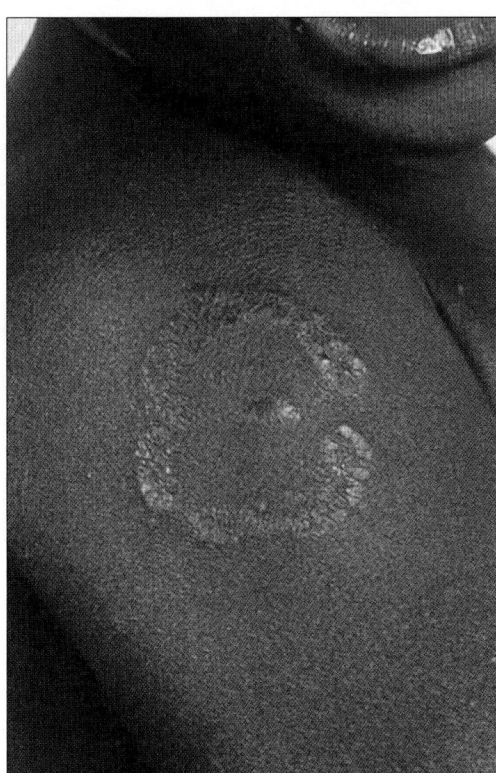

Fig. 9.82
Granuloma multiforme: typical annular lesions with raised borders in a child. By courtesy of R.A. Marsden, St George's Hospital, London, UK.

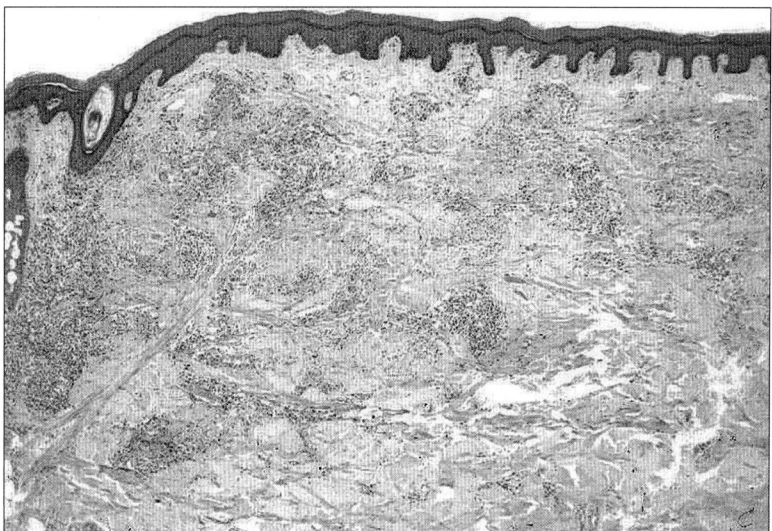

Fig. 9.84
Granuloma multiforme: there is extensive necrobiosis.

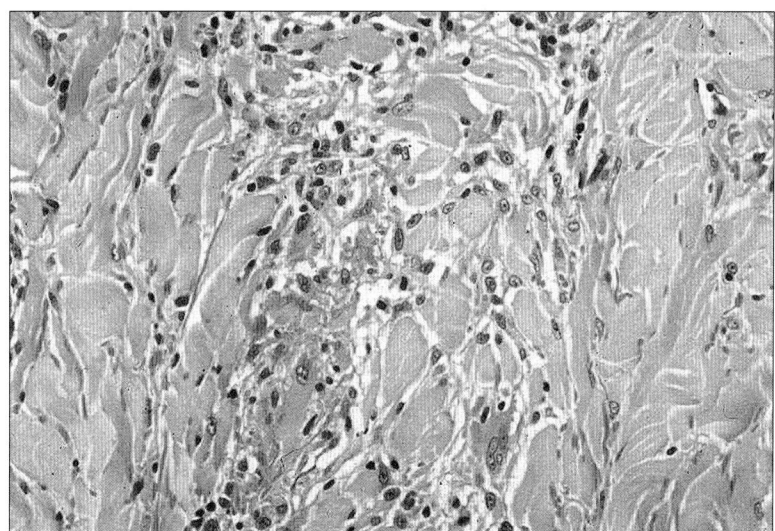

Fig. 9.85
Granuloma multiforme: necrobiosis is seen in the center.

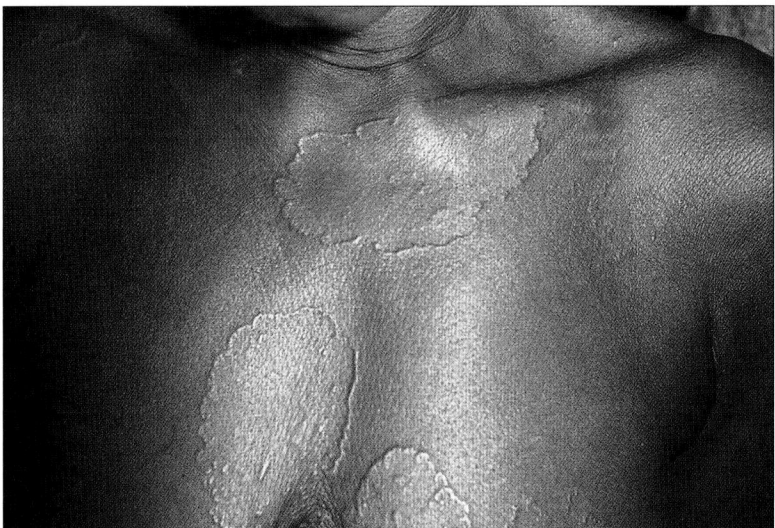

Fig. 9.83
Granuloma multiforme: there are multiple large irregular plaques. By courtesy of the Institute of Dermatology, London, UK.

Histologic features

The epidermis is normal. Situated within the dermis is an ill-defined, irregular, necrobiotic lesion (*Fig. 9.84*).[7] In general, this affects individual collagen fibers, producing a rather haphazard picture of abnormal fibers interspersed with unaffected ones and associated with a histiocytic infiltrate (*Fig. 9.85*). Only rarely is a well-defined palisading granuloma seen. In addition to histiocytes, giant cells are commonly found and the tissues show a perivascular lymphocytic infiltrate with variable numbers of plasma cells and eosinophils. The giant cells do not contain asteroid bodies. Perineural involvement is not a feature.[1] The adjacent vasculature is normal. Loss of elastic tissue is typical in relation to the inflammatory infiltrate, and healed areas are characterized by absence of elastic tissue and mild superficial scarring (*Fig. 9.86*).[1]

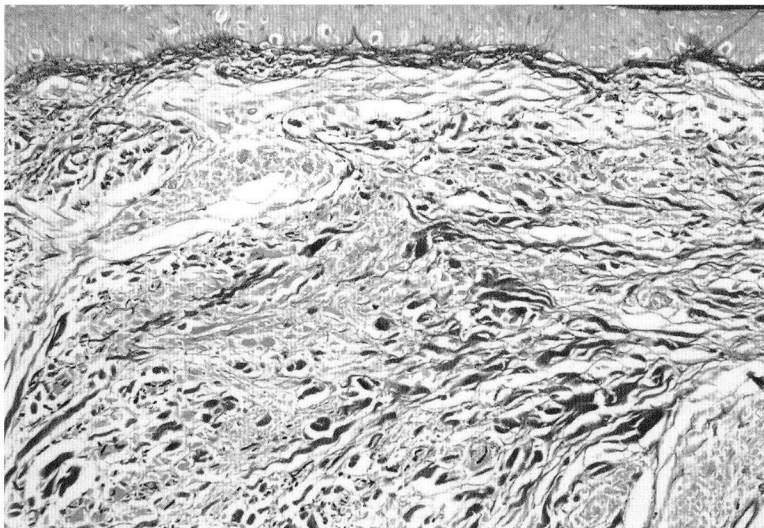

Fig. 9.86
Granuloma multiforme: note the complete loss of elastic tissue. Elastic-van Gieson.

Differential diagnosis

The exact nosological position of granuloma multiforme is unknown. It is probably a clinicopathological variant of elastolytic granuloma. An association with sun exposure has been suggested.[8] The granulomata do not show a perineural distribution, thus helping to distinguish granuloma multiforme from leprosy. Nevertheless, since infection must be excluded before giving a definitive diagnosis, stains for organisms (especially mycobacteria and fungi) must be performed to exclude this possibility. Culture should also be performed when clinically appropriate.

Rheumatic fever nodule

Clinical features

Fortunately, effective antimicrobial therapy has relegated rheumatic fever to a rare pediatric infection. As a consequence, complications of rheumatic fever are only rarely encountered in dermatology practice. In older studies, approximately one-third of patients with rheumatic fever develop papules that had a tendency to occur over bony prominence of the knee, elbows, fingers, ankles, spine, scalp, and rarely at other sites.[1–3] Most patients had multiple nodules. In one report, the number of nodules ranged from 1 to 108.[1] Lesions persisted from days to several months. Although in a more recent study of 44 patients with rheumatic fever, only one had a single subcutaneous nodule, a further larger study of 60 patients confirmed the presence of subcutaneous nodules in slightly more than a third of patients with a first episode and in almost half of the patients with recurrent episodes of the disease.[4,5] All patients with nodules had associated carditis.

Histologic features

Biopsy shows central gossamer fibrin associated with variable numbers of neutrophils, lymphocytes, plasma cells, and karyorrhexis. The lesions are often not well circumscribed and histiocytes surround the lesion, forming a poorly defined palisade.

Differential diagnosis

The histologic features of the rheumatic fever nodule are not pathognomonic. Clinical correlation is required to establish a definite diagnosis. The rheumatic fever nodule can be classified under the rubric of 'palisaded neutrophilic and granulomatous dermatitis associated with systemic disease'. Rheumatic fever nodule is discussed separately, however, because of its historic interest and its long-standing recognition as a distinct clinical entity. The differential diagnosis is therefore that of palisaded neutrophilic and granulomatous dermatitis. Other systemic diseases, including connective tissue disease, infection, vasculitis, neoplasia, and inflammatory bowel disease, may be associated with lesions with similar histology. The reader is referred to this section for a more detailed discussion of this group of disorders (p. 334). In short, a diagnosis of rheumatic fever nodule should only be made in the setting of confirmed rheumatic fever. In the absence of such history, a careful search for other underlying systemic diseases is necessary.

Rheumatoid arthritis nodules tend to be better circumscribed and surrounded by well-defined palisade of histiocytes. In addition, the fine fibrinoid strands that form the center of a rheumatic fever nodule contrast with the more dense sheetlike areas of necrobiosis in the rheumatoid arthritis nodule.

Necrobiotic xanthogranuloma

Clinical features

Necrobiotic xanthogranuloma (necrobiotic xanthogranuloma with paraproteinemia) is an extremely rare condition of unknown etiology.[1–3] It occurs equally in men and in women, in the late middle aged and elderly (average age at presentation is 56 years). The disease is characterized by the development of nodules and plaques, which show a predilection for the face, neck, trunk, and, less commonly, proximal limbs. Lesions limited to single body site are rarely seen. The facial lesions are characteristically periorbital (most

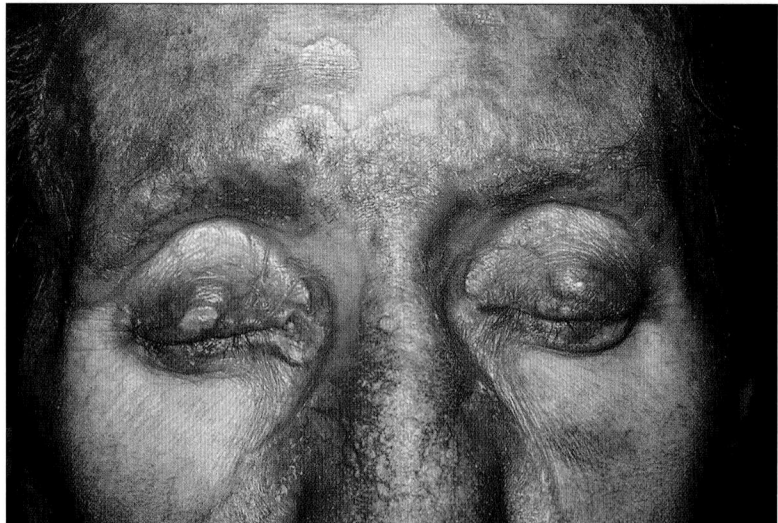

Fig. 9.87
Necrobiotic xanthogranuloma: indurated yellow plaques are present around both eyes and on the eyelids. By courtesy of the Institute of Dermatology, London, UK.

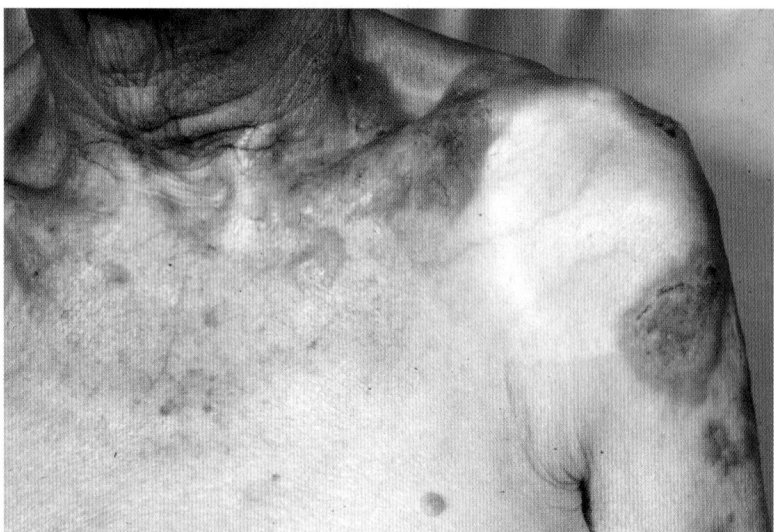

Fig. 9.88
Necrobiotic xanthogranuloma: there are multiple yellow plaques around the shoulders and overlying the clavicles. By courtesy of the Institute of Dermatology, London, UK.

often infraorbital) in distribution and consist of papules that progress to nodules, and plaques that may form irregular ulcers (Fig. 9.87). Although periorbital involvement is fairly constant (in up to 80% of patients), in some patients this feature is absent.[4,5] Scarring and telangiectasia are common. Lesions are sharply demarcated and have a distinctive xanthomatous appearance. Ocular complications are common and include episcleritis, necrotizing scleritis, keratitis, proptosis, uveitis, and iritis.[6,7] Some patients report pain but this is not a usual feature.[2]

The lesions on the trunk and limbs are irregular, well-demarcated, bright yellow, dermal and subcutaneous plaques measuring up to 25 cm across (Fig. 9.88). They may be complicated by ulceration, hemorrhage, scarring, central atrophy, and telangiectases, and typically have a peripheral inflammatory border. Violaceous and flesh-colored nodules are sometimes present, particularly over the trunk. Unusual presentations include a solitary nodular lesion mimicking a tumor and, exceptionally, the absence of skin involvement.[8,9] A lesion presenting at the site of a blepharoplasty scar and a further lesion presenting in the scar of a burn have been reported.[10,11]

Involvement of myocardium, lung, larynx, kidneys, salivary gland, skeletal muscle, oral mucosa, and vulva has been documented.[12–19] Patients may have arthritis, chronic obstructive pulmonary disease, neuropathy, or hypertension.[2] Other reported cases include one associated with Graves disease, another with linear morphea, one with scleroderma, and one with lichen sclerosus.[2,20–22] In rare patients, there was an association with syncitial giant cell hepatitis and with autoimmune immunoglobulin G4-related pancreatitis.[23–25] Nodular transformation of the liver is a feature noted in rare patients.[15,26] A single patient also had associated normolipemic xanthomatosis.[18]

Laboratory investigations reveal anemia, leukopenia, and a raised ESR. Most patients with necrobiotic xanthogranuloma have an associated monoclonal paraproteinemia of uncertain significance (MGUS), usually IgG kappa type (60% of cases). Few present with a lambda paraprotein and an exceptional case has been documented with two monoclonal paraproteins. An association with Waldenström macroglobulinemia is exceptional.[27] There is an important association with multiple myeloma, and the latter can develop many years after the diagnosis of the disease.[28] Other associations include B-cell lymphoma and chronic lymphocytic leukemia.[29–34] A case with associated Hodgkin lymphoma has also been reported.[35] Diabetes mellitus is sometimes present and occasionally, hyperlipidemia. Other associations that may be encountered include low serum complement levels and cryoglobulinemia.

Pathogenesis and histologic features

The pathogenesis of necrobiotic xanthogranuloma is unknown. The plasma cells in the infiltrate are consistently polyclonal, supporting a reactive process.[3] Direct immunofluorescence has shown IgM, C3, and fibrinogen deposition in blood vessel walls.[6] It has more recently been suggested that activation of monocytes is responsible for the intracellular accumulation of lipoprotein-derived lipids and the hypocholesterolemia.[36] Focus-floating microscopy of six cases demonstrated the presence of *Borrelia*.[37] The significance of this finding is unclear, but it is unlikely that the bacteria plays a pathogenetic role in the disease.

Necrobiotic xanthogranuloma has a very distinctive histologic appearance.[8,33] Large areas of marked necrobiosis alternate with foci of xanthogranulomatous infiltration throughout the reticular dermis with extension into the subcutaneous fat (*Fig. 9.89*).[4] Exceptionally, necrobiosis is absent.[38] Involvement of the subcutaneous fat is predominantly in a septal distribution and can mimic panniculitis.[39] The necrobiotic collagen appears as amorphous eosinophilic debris (*Fig. 9.90*). The granulomatous infiltrate is composed of epithelioid and foamy histiocytes in addition to conspicuous giant cells, many of which are of the Touton type (*Figs 9.91* and *9.92*). Foreign body giant cells are also present. Lymphocytes and plasma cells are often prominent and formation of germinal centers is sometimes seen. A characteristic feature is the presence of large and bizarre angulated giant cells with considerable numbers of nuclei irregularly grouped together

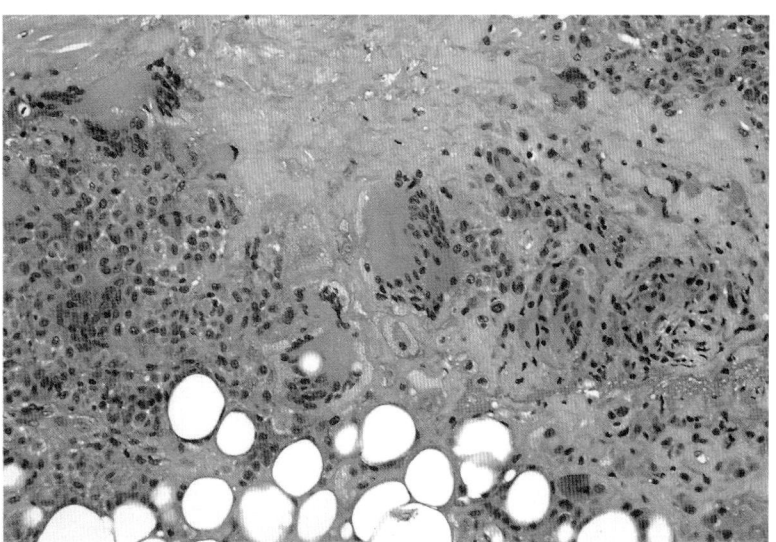

Fig. 9.90
Necrobiotic xanthogranuloma: there is extensive necrobiosis and a dense histiocytic infiltrate with conspicuous giant cells.

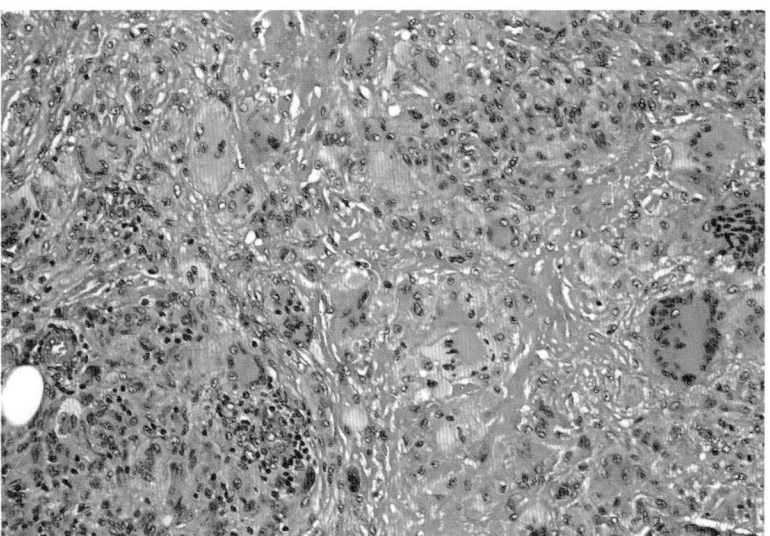

Fig. 9.91
Necrobiotic xanthogranuloma: in this field, there are conspicuous xanthomatized histiocytes.

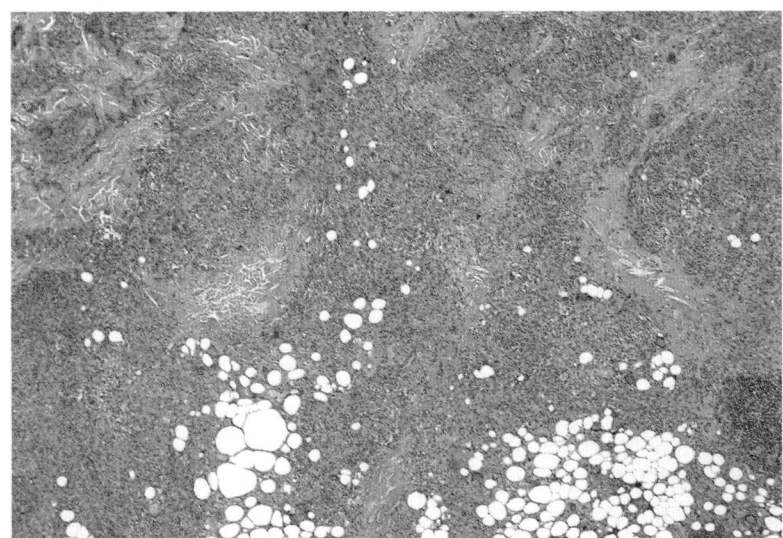

Fig. 9.89
Necrobiotic xanthogranuloma: there is a dense infiltrate extending throughout the dermis into the subcutaneous fat.

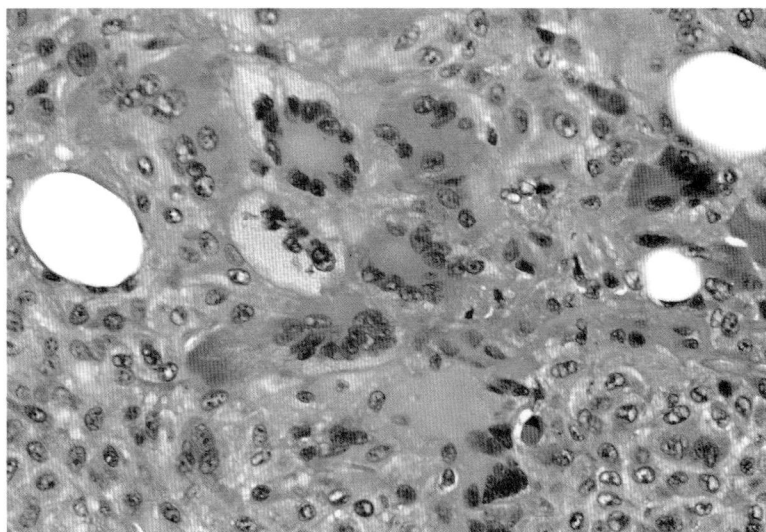

Fig. 9.92
Necrobiotic xanthogranuloma: Touton giant cells are sometimes prominent.

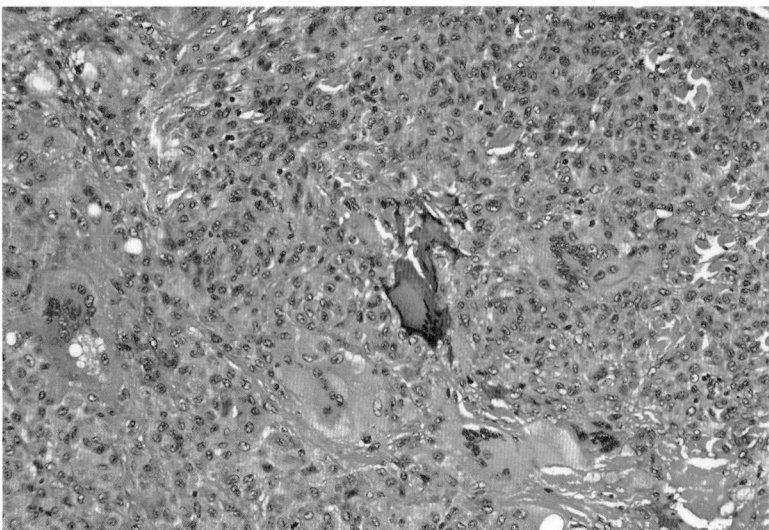

Fig. 9.93
Necrobiotic xanthogranuloma: angulated giant cells with darkly staining nuclei are commonly present.

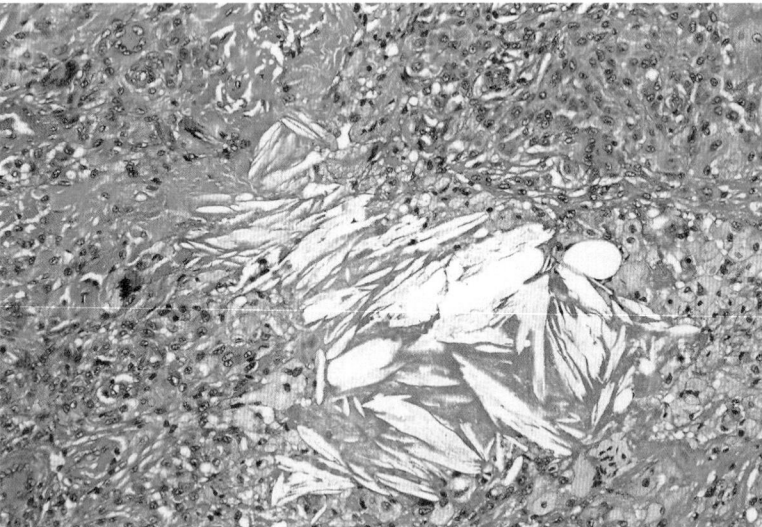

Fig. 9.94
Necrobiotic xanthogranuloma: cholesterol clefts are a characteristic feature.

within copious eosinophilic cytoplasm in the tissue immediately adjacent to foci of necrobiosis (*Fig. 9.93*). Asteroid bodies, which are often found in the cytoplasm of giant cells, have been suggested as a useful diagnostic finding.[40] Frozen sections and oil red O staining for fat may reveal focal lipid droplets. Staining for adipophilin also highlights the lipid deposits (see below). Cholesterol clefts and lipid vacuoles are sometimes seen within the foci of necrobiosis and xanthogranulomatous inflammation (*Fig. 9.94*). In rare cases, however, lipid deposition and giant cells are inconspicuous.[41] The granulomatous and necrobiotic process may affect muscular arteries. Staining for elastic fibers reveals their absence in the necrobiotic areas; Alcian blue staining may reveal small amounts of interstitial mucin. As with most necrobiotic disorders, transepidermal elimination of necrobiotic collagen is sometimes a feature.[42] A case with prominent elastophagocytosis has been described.[43] The lungs and heart may show giant cells, granulomata, necrobiosis, or a combination of these features in patients with systemic disease.[13] In very rare cases, some of the most characteristic histologic findings of the disease including necrobiosis may be missing and the diagnosis may be very difficult.[44,45]

Differential diagnosis

The clinical and histologic features are distinctive: the presence of massive necrobiosis associated with numerous cholesterol clefts, bizarre multinucleated giant cells, and Touton-type giant cells distinguishes necrobiotic xanthogranuloma from necrobiosis lipoidica and other necrobiotic dermatoses. It should, however, be noted that prominent cholesterol cleft formation may rarely be seen in necrobiosis lipoidica.[46] Adipophilin staining has been reported as being of use in the differential diagnosis between both conditions. In necrobiotic xanthogranuloma, the staining pattern is diffuse, highlighting the necrobiotic and cellular areas. In necrobiosis lipoidica, however, the staining is restricted to necrobiotic areas.[47,48] Small punch biopsies may not be adequate for definitive evaluation and sampling bias may be misleading. Clinical correlation should be taken into consideration before making a definitive diagnosis.

Palisaded neutrophilic and granulomatous dermatitis

Clinical features

Palisaded neutrophilic and granulomatous dermatitis (interstitial granulomatous dermatitis) is a term that has been applied to a reaction pattern of necrobiotic and granulomatous inflammation encountered in the setting of systemic disease.[1] Other terms that have been applied to similar, overlapping, and, in some cases, probably identical lesions, include interstitial granulomatous dermatitis with arthritis, rheumatoid papules, superficial ulcerating rheumatoid necrobiosis, cutaneous extravascular necrotizing granuloma, and Churg-Strauss granuloma.[1–6] Myriad underlying systemic diseases, mainly autoimmune and autoinflammatory diseases, have been purported to be associated with these lesions including rheumatoid arthritis, lupus erythematosus, systemic sclerosis, Sjögren syndrome, thyroiditis, Raynaud syndrome, hepatitis, inflammatory bowel disease, lymphoproliferative disorders, myelodysplastic syndrome, vasculitis (Granulomatosis with polyangiitis, Churg-Strauss syndrome, Takayasu arteritis, periarteritis nodosa), hemolytic uremic syndrome, thrombotic thrombocytopenic purpura, mixed cryoglobulinemia, drug reactions (especially sulfonamides), carcinoma, diabetes, and infections (streptococcal, HIV, Epstein-Barr virus, parvovirus, Lyme disease).[1–4,7–14] In most cases an underlying systemic disease is found, and it is rare that an underlying disease is not detected.[15]

The lesions are mainly located on the extremities and less commonly the trunk in an adult.[1] Children are seldom affected.[16,17] The disease is characterized by papules and nodules, which are often arranged in a linear pattern. These linear lesions may be confluent and have been described as linear bands or cords with a 'ropelike' consistency (the so-called rope sign). Plaques have also been described.[6]

Pathogenesis and histologic features

The pathogenesis of palisaded neutrophilic and granulomatous dermatitis most likely depends on the associated/underlying disease. In a number of cases, autoantibodies, particularly anti-DNA in type, are found.[18] It has been suggested that the disease is mediated by immune complexes.[19] Direct immunofluorescence studies have demonstrated fibrin and IgM in the vasculature of some patients.[1]

A variety of histologic patterns have been described. These patterns may be seen in the same or different biopsies from the same patient, emphasizing the fact that they are not separate diseases.[20,21] Some biopsies resemble the interstitial variant of granuloma annulare without a well-defined palisade, loosely organized histiocytes, and variable numbers of neutrophils with nuclear dust. Histiocytes often wrap individual collagen bundles. Fibrin is also seen. In fact, some would label these lesions as falling within the spectrum of granuloma annulare.[4] However, mucin deposition is not as marked as seen in granuloma annulare, and the changes are more ill defined. In other samples, palisaded histiocytes surround individual collagen bundles and in the background there is a neutrophilic infiltrate with karyorrhexis (*Figs 9.95* and *9.96*). In late stages, fibrosis may be seen. The various changes described are more likely to represent the evolution of the lesions. Variable numbers of eosinophils may be noted and, when present, appear to occur mostly in patients with a peripheral eosinophilia. Frank leukocytoclastic vasculitis is present in some cases.[20] A few cases may resemble necrobiosis lipoidica.[4]

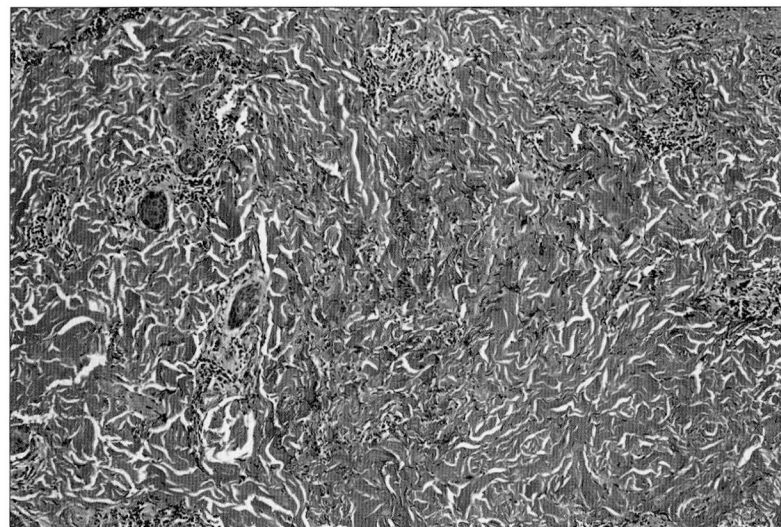

Fig. 9.95
Palisaded neutrophilic and granulomatous dermatitis: an interstitial inflammatory cell infiltrate is present in the center of the field, mimicking diffuse granuloma annulare.

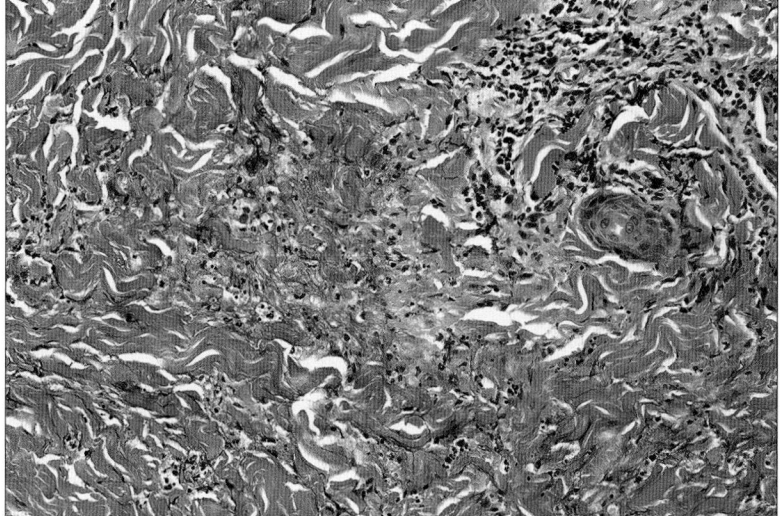

Fig. 9.96
Palisaded neutrophilic and granulomatous dermatitis: close-up view showing necrobiosis, histiocytes, and neutrophils associated with karyorrhexis.

Differential diagnosis

From the above discussion, it can be seen that a number of different terms have been proposed to describe lesions resembling granuloma annulare or, rarely, necrobiosis lipoidica but with the added features of acute and eosinophilic inflammation, karyorrhexis, and neutrophils with leukocytoclasia and rarely with leukocytoclastic vasculitis. Some authors include these changes within the spectrum of granuloma annulare and necrobiosis lipoidica.[4] The precise terminology preferred by the dermatopathologist is probably not important. More significant than any nosological nuances is issuing a report that alerts the clinician to the possibility that the patient may have underlying systemic disease and that, when such lesions are encountered, appropriate clinical evaluation is necessary.[12]

'Metastatic' Crohn disease

Clinical features

Patients with Crohn disease may present with cutaneous and oral lesions, the most frequent of which are aphthous stomatitis, pyoderma gangrenosum, and erythema nodosum.[1] Metastatic cutaneous lesions in Crohn

disease are rare and defined as the presence of sterile granulomatous lesions that occur at sites not contiguous with the gastrointestinal tract. They predominantly involve the skin of the lower limbs, genitalia, perineum, perianal region, and lips. One review of the literature showed that approximately 50% of patients with cutaneous Crohn disease have involvement of the lower extremities.[2] Most affected patients are adults especially young adults, but lesions may rarely be seen in children.[3,4] Genital involvement is more common in children. Both sexes are affected equally. The lesions present as single or multiple papules, plaques, nodules, and ulcers, and can be localized or more uncommonly disseminated.[2–13] Papules, some of which are lichenoid, pustules, and abscesslike masses may be seen.[4] Ulcerated lesions are more common on genital skin and on the vulva, and fissures resembling knife cuts may be seen.[4] Condylomatous lesions, fibroepithelial polyp-like lesions, and lymphedema are rarely seen and may represent the only manifestation of the disease.[14,15] Vulval tumorlike masses, vulval or penile and scrotal swelling, and herpes virus-like lesions have occasionally been described.[11,16–18] Penile lesions may sometimes occur.[19] Colostomy site involvement has also been documented. One patient has been reported as presenting with an erysipelas-like eruption involving the lip and nasolabial region, and a further patient presented with involvement of the nipple.[6,20] Most affected patients have a diagnosis of gastrointestinal disease when lesions develop. However, rarely, metastatic lesions may precede the diagnosis of gastrointestinal disease even by long periods of time.[8,21,22] Of uncertain significance is the finding that cutaneous Crohn disease seems to be highly associated with involvement of the large bowel.[16] The duration of lesions is variable, typically lasting from months to years. There is no clear correlation between disease activity of cutaneous lesions and gastrointestinal lesions.[4,17]

Pathogenesis and histologic features

The pathogenesis of mucocutaneous Crohn disease is not understood. Histologically, lesions are usually manifest as ill-defined, noncaseating, and nonsuppurative granulomata present in the superficial (often papillary) dermis; however, granulomata may also involve the deep dermis and even subcutaneous adipose tissue.[23,24] The granulomata are surrounded by a small cuff of lymphocytes.[24] They may mimic closely the granulomas seen in sarcoidosis. In addition, there is a superficial and deep, perivascular, mixed inflammatory cell infiltrate. The granulomata resemble those seen in the bowel. Necrobiotic collagen has been described in a number of cases.[23] Lymphocytes and plasma cells are also commonly present and eosinophils can be prominent.[24] Ulceration of the epidermis may be seen.[23] Recently, the histologic features of metastatic Crohn disease have been expanded to include the findings of significant necrobiosis with leukocytoclasis, and vasculitis (see palisaded neutrophilic and granulomatous dermatitis, above).[23,25]

Differential diagnosis

Since the histologic features of cutaneous Crohn disease are non-specific, a definitive diagnosis requires clinical confirmation of the presence of associated bowel disease. Therefore, endoscopy, evaluation of gastrointestinal biopsies, and review of clinical findings all play a role in confirmation of this diagnosis. Sarcoidosis may be indistinguishable from metastatic Crohn disease; however, the granulomata of the former tend to be more discrete and compact. Eosinophils may be prominent in metastatic Crohn disease and are rare in sarcoidosis.[22] Mycobacterial infection is also an important differential diagnosis; therefore, liberal use of special stains for microorganisms is essential. Culture should be performed as deemed clinically appropriate.

As noted above, cutaneous granulomata may precede evidence of bowel involvement.[8,20,21] Therefore, patients with granulomatous skin disease of uncertain etiology should be followed up carefully for evidence of bowel disease.

Granulomatous cheilitis may also show identical histologic features. Studies have documented patients presenting with granulomatous cheilitis who subsequently developed clinical manifestations or pathological evidence (without gastrointestinal symptoms) of Crohn disease.[24,26–31] One group study described a patient in whom granulomatous cheilitis antedated development of Crohn disease by 7 years.[32] It appears, therefore, that some patients with granulomatous cheilitis are at risk for development of Crohn disease and require gastrointestinal evaluation and careful clinical follow-up. Similarly, vulval Crohn disease precedes development of bowel involvement in 25% of cases.[16]

Granulomatous cheilitis

Granulomatous cheilitis (cheilitis granulomatosa, Meischer cheilitis, orofacial granulomatosis) is discussed in Chapter 11.

Acne agminata

Clinical features

Acne agminata (lupus miliaris disseminatus faciei, acnitis, papular tuberculid) is a rare condition originally thought to be a form of tuberculid, but an association with tuberculosis has since been excluded.[1–4] Some authors consider this disease to be synonymous with granulomatous rosacea. However, the distinctive clinical presentation, and the absence of typical rosacea in patients affected by the disease, argue against this. Recently, a new name has been suggested for the disease: facial idiopathic granulomata with regressive evolution (FIGURE).[5]

Clinical presentation is characterized by fairly monomorphous yellowish-brown papules typically involving the central face with predilection for periocular areas (*Fig. 9.97*). The disease is limited to the eyelids and canthus in rare cases.[6,7] Involvement of axillae or upper limbs is an exceptional finding.[8–11] There is no sex predilection, and the age range is wide although most cases occur in young to middle-aged adults.[12] An exceptional case during pregnancy has been documented.[13] Response to conventional treatment for rosacea is often ineffective, but lesions tend to regress spontaneously over a period of months or even years, leaving mild scarring.[14]

Pathogenesis and histologic features

As suggested by some synonyms, infection by mycobacteria has been favored by certain authors as a potential etiological factor. This theory is no longer tenable due to the absence of past or present systemic tuberculosis and the constant failure of isolation of bacilli. In a study from Israel, mycobacterial DNA was not detected by PCR.[1] It has been suggested that the development

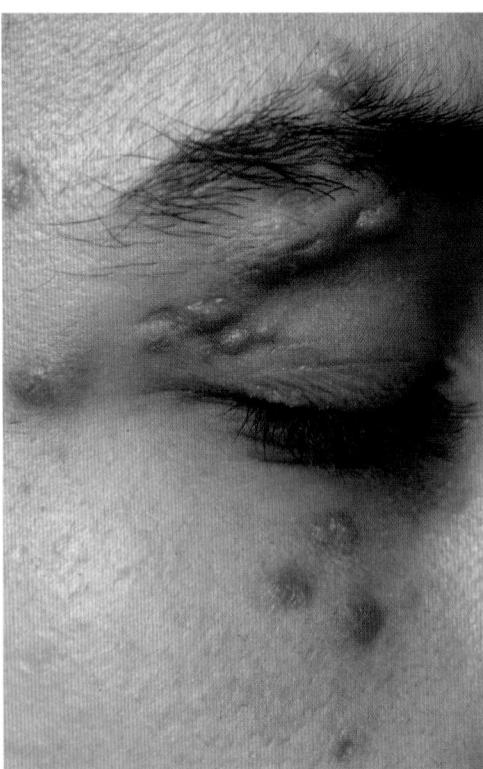

Fig. 9.97
Acne agminata: note the characteristic distribution of papules on the cheek and around the eyes. From the collection of the late N.P. Smith, MD, the Institute of Dermatology, London, UK.

of lesions is due to an unusual granulomatous reaction to ruptured hair follicles.[15]

The histologic features vary with the stage of evolution and may be entirely non-specific.[16] A biopsy from a well-established lesion shows a central area of well-defined caseous necrosis surrounded by multinucleate giant cells and epithelioid cells (sometimes indistinguishable from tuberculous infection) (*Figs 9.98* and *9.99*). Serial sections often reveal a relationship of the necrosis to a destroyed hair follicle. Sarcoidal granulomas may be a feature. Special stains may demonstrate a ring of elastic fibers in the center of the necrotic focus, possibly representing the isthmus of the hair follicle. The granulomata are not usually related to *Demodex folliculorum* as is often the case in granulomatous rosacea. Lymphangiectasia is often a feature.[7] Focal vasculitis is only exceptionally seen.

Differential diagnosis

The diagnosis is fairly easy in the presence of granulomata surrounding an area of caseation necrosis since the latter is not usually a feature of either granulomatous rosacea or perioral dermatitis. In biopsies showing only focal granulomatous inflammation, establishing the diagnosis may require very careful clinicopathological correlation. In idiopathic facial aseptic granuloma which is a self-limited condition that may related to granulomatous rosacea and presents in children as one or several facial papules/nodules, the granulomas are of the foreign body type and necrosis is not seen.[17,18]

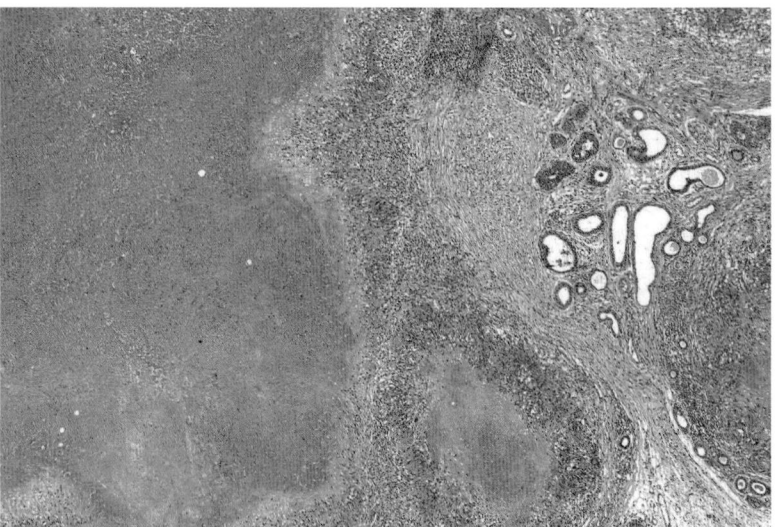

Fig. 9.98
Acne agminata: there are multiple caseating granulomata.

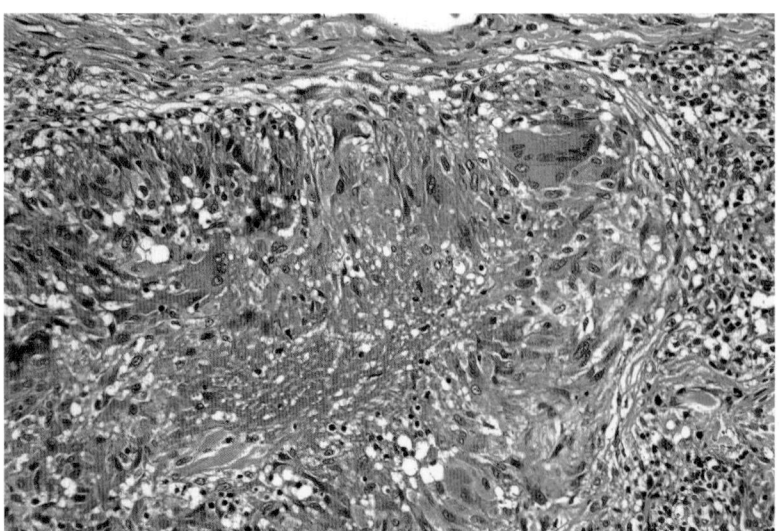

Fig. 9.99
Acne agminata: close-up view. The condition is not a tuberculid. Special stains and culture for tubercle bacilli are invariably negative.

Periorificial (perioral) dermatitis

Clinical features

Perioral dermatitis (perioral granulomatous dermatitis, periorificial dermatitis) is a common dermatosis that may represent a variant of rosacea.[1–6] It is discussed in this section since it can, on occasion, be associated with granulomatous histology. Patients are usually young women but the condition can occur in children.[1,7] Presentation in identical twins is exceptional but has been documented.[8] A granulomatous variant of periorificial dermatitis has been described in children.[9–11] It tends to be more common in Afro-Caribbean children, tends to be characterized by a more monomorphous eruption of papules, and has been labeled facial Afro-Caribbean childhood eruption (FACE).[9,12] Typically, periorificial dermatitis consists of erythematous papules and pustules with a characteristic distribution on the chin and nasolabial folds (*Fig. 9.100*). Involvement of the inner cheeks, the skin around the nose, forehead, or periocular area is unusual. Based on the fact that some cases show perinasal and periocular involvement, the name periorificial dermatitis has been suggested.[13] Extrafacial and generalized involvement has also been documented.[14] Very rarely, the disease may present initially as a rash mimicking chalazion and blepharitis.[15] The clinical appearances may mimic acne but comedones are absent.[16]

Pathogenesis and histologic features

The pathogenesis of periorificial dermatitis is not clearly understood, but the condition seems to be etiologically linked in some cases to the use of potent topical steroids, the application of cosmetics, certain toothpastes, epoxy diacrylates in dental composite resins, contraceptive pills, some moisturizing creams, and propolis.[17–27] In rare patients, the disease appears during pregnancy and may flare up before the menstrual period.[27,28] Even inhaled and systemic corticosteroids have triggered perioral dermatitis.[29–31] Physical sunscreens with high sun protection factor have also been blamed for causing the disease in children.[32] Multiple dental fillings with a mercury-containing amalgam induced perioral dermatitis in a girl, and in a further case the disease appears to have been triggered by orthognathic surgery.[33,34] An association has also been reported in renal transplant patients on systemic steroids and azathioprine.[35] Fusobacteria have also been suggested as having a possible role in the disease.[36]

Biopsy shows mild acanthosis, focal spongiosis, and hyperkeratosis with parakeratosis and a mild perivascular and periadnexal lymphohistiocytic infiltrate. The appearances are almost indistinguishable from those found in rosacea.[37] Ruptured hair follicles with microabscess formation are occasionally seen. Sometimes granulomata with sarcoidal features are present.[38]

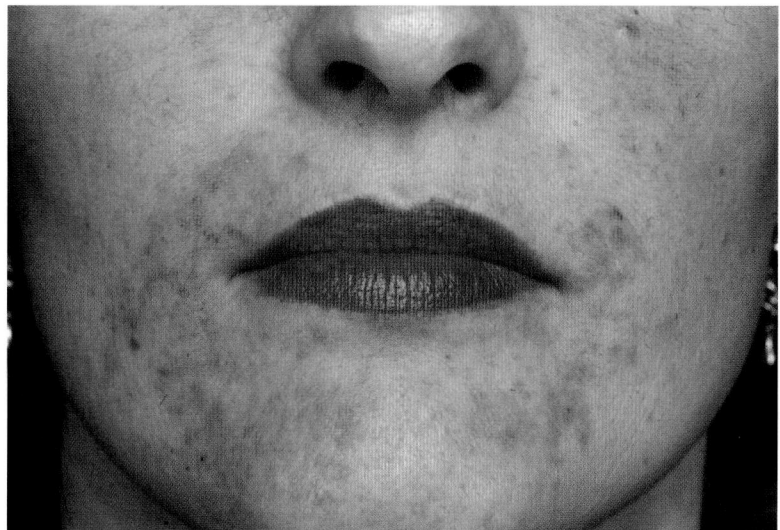

Fig. 9.100
Perioral dermatitis: erythema and papules in a characteristic distribution. From the collection of the late N.P. Smith, MD, the Institute of Dermatology, London, UK.

Giant cells have also been documented, in which case distinction from sarcoidosis may be difficult.[1,39] In most cases, clinical correlation resolves any diagnostic difficulties.

Demodicosis

There are two species of *Demodex* that live in a symbiotic relationship in human hair follicles. The mites are *D. folliculorum* and *D. brevis*. The former is mainly found in the infundibulum of the hairs and the latter in the sebaceous glands. They are ubiquitous in the skin but there is a predilection for the face. Their pathogenetic role in skin diseases has always been controversial and they are often regarded as innocent bystanders. However, it does seem that in a small number of cases, particularly in immunocompromised patients, they have an important role in causation of disease.[1–4] The mites do not appear to be a primary factor in the development of rosacea although they may play a part in the granulomatous form of the disease. Traditionally, three facial forms of involvement have been described: pityriasis folliculorum, rosacea-like demodicosis, and demodicosis gravis. Recently, a classification of the disease into primary and secondary forms has been proposed. The latter is associated with immunosuppression. The primary form has been divided into: 1. spinulate demodicosis or pityriasis folliculorum not usually associated with inflammation; 2. papulopustular/nodulocystic or conglobate demodicosis presenting with inflamed lesions with predilection for skin around the eyes and mouth; 3. ocular demodicosis; and 4. auricular demodicosis.[5] Skin eruptions attributed to the mites have variable manifestations and include a rosacea-like eruption, a perioral dermatitis-like eruption, follicular plugging, and erythema, and a disseminated form in immunocompromised patients.[1–13] Localized pustules and even abscesses have also been reported.[14] An unusual case of a patient with demodicosis presenting as a facial plaque after ophthalmic herpes zoster has been described. In a further case, the disease mimicked favus in a child.[15] Eye involvement usually presents with chronic blepharitis or chalazion and more rarely with keratoconjunctivitis. Ear involvement is mainly associated with otitis externa or myringitis. Adults are mainly affected but cases in children have been reported.[10–12,16]

Pathogenesis and histologic features

The pathogenetic link between the mites and cutaneous disease is a matter of controversy. In cases where there seems to be a clear link, the density of mites is very high.[4] A role for the symbiotic relationship between the mites and bacteria has been suggested but remains to be proven.

Histologically, the findings combine suppurative and granulomatous changes. Dilated hair follicles with multiple mites are seen and there is formation of neutrophilic pustules. This is associated with a variable, perifollicular mononuclear cell infiltrate composed of lymphocytes and plasma cells. When the hair follicle ruptures, focal granulomata are seen and often contain fragments of the mites.

Infective granulomata

Infections, particularly fungal and mycobacterial, are often associated with granulomatous inflammation. Conversely, the vast majority of routine biopsies showing granulomatous inflammation are not due to an infection. However, when faced with a specimen showing granulomatous inflammation, the pathologist must maintain a low threshold for performing stains for organisms and for issuing recommendations for microbiology culture. If such an approach is not taken, the vast majority of infectious causes of granulomatous inflammation will be misdiagnosed. In addition, although pathologists tend to associate certain patterns of granulomatous inflammation with infection by specific organisms (e.g., caseating granulomatous inflammation and *M. tuberculosis*), it should be remembered that the same organism can cause several different patterns of granulomatous inflammation (e.g., *Mycobacterium leprae*). Similarly, mixed suppurative and granulomatous inflammation may result from both atypical mycobacteria and deep fungal infections. A practical corollary to this is that the pathologist should order several special stains to evaluate for a variety of organisms rather than relying on a single stain for the most likely culprit.

Specific infectious causes of granulomatous inflammation are discussed in detail in Chapter 18.

Foreign body granulomata

A wide variety of substances when present within the dermis may result in a foreign body giant cell reaction and can mimic primary granulomatous disorders. These are summarized in *Table 9.2* and examples are shown in *Figs 9.101–9.106*. Therefore, when examining specimens with granulomatous inflammation of uncertain etiology, all sections should be examined with polarized light to exclude foreign material. Most foreign body granulomatous reactions occur as a result of external foreign matter, particularly suture material. It can also occur as a result of injury from sea urchin spines, particularly on acral sites.[1–4] The granulomata formed are often foreign body and sarcoidal, but other types of granulomata including necrobiotic, suppurative, and tuberculoid have been described.[4] Interestingly, a study found *M. marinum* DNA using PCR in a number of sea urchin granulomata, raising the possibility that the organism may be involved in the pathogenesis of the disease.[5] Foreign body granulomatous reactions secondary to internal foreign bodies are mainly secondary to hair shafts within the dermis after folliculitis or to fragments of keratin as a result of ruptured epidermoid or trichilemmal cysts. Another source of foreign body granulomatous reaction to internal material is gout.

The pathologist should be particularly aware that beryllium and zirconium may be associated with granulomata that mimic sarcoidosis, the so-called sarcoidal 'naked' granuloma. It is especially important to think of these agents as rare possible causes of granulomata since neither is visible with routine or polarization microscopy. Beryllium was once used in the manufacture of fluorescent light bulbs. Following exposure to beryllium, patients may develop either systemic berylliosis or have cutaneous involvement only. Pulmonary lesions follow inhalation.[5] Skin involvement, in the form of papules, follows direct inoculation.[6] Diagnosis of chronic beryllium disease is based on demonstration of a cell-mediated response to beryllium by patch testing.[6] Diagnosis may also be established by laser microprobe mass spectrometry.[6,7]

Zirconium was once added to antiperspirants.[8] Patients developed papules at sites where the substance was used, and interstitial lung disease

Table 9.2
Important causes of foreign body granulomata

Endogenous	Exogenous		
Keratin	Silica	Graphite	Cactus spine
Hair shaft	Beryllium	Paraffin	Vegetable oil
Ruptured cyst contents	Zirconium	Shrapnel	Mineral oil
Released lipids	Talc	Sutures	Food particles
Urate crystals	Silicone	Arthropods	Wood splinters
	Tattoo pigment	Sea urchin spine	

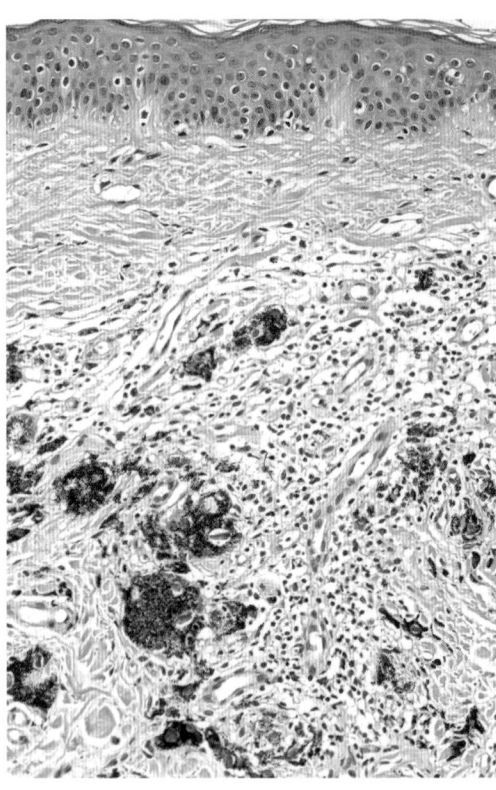

Fig. 9.102
Tattoo site: foreign body and sarcoidal responses may occasionally be seen in tattoo reaction.

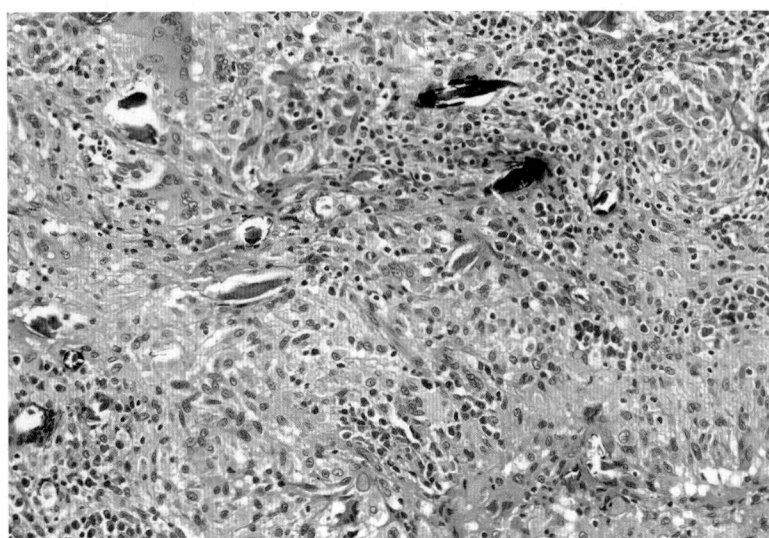

Fig. 9.101
Foreign body granuloma: there is a florid granulomatous reaction to shrapnel.

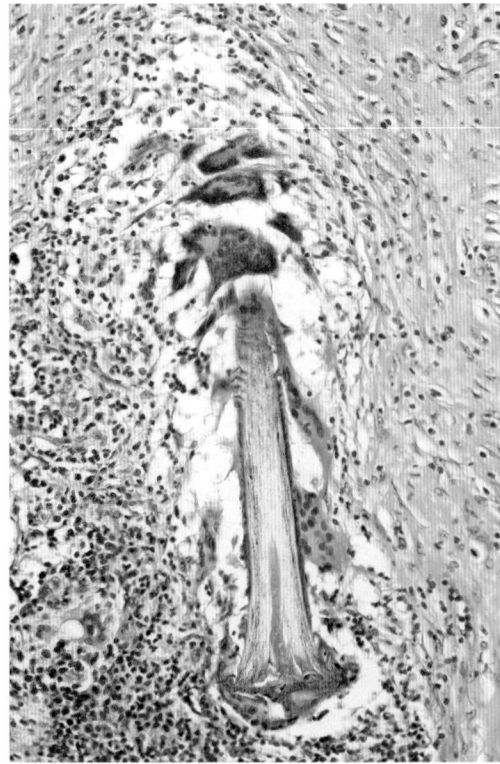

Fig. 9.103
Foreign body granuloma: this free hair shaft has been partially engulfed by foreign body giant cells.

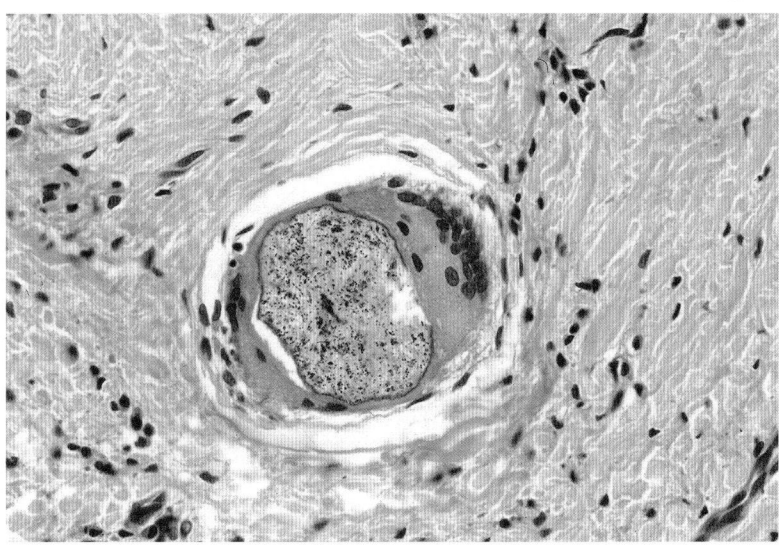

Fig. 9.104
Foreign body granuloma: high-power view

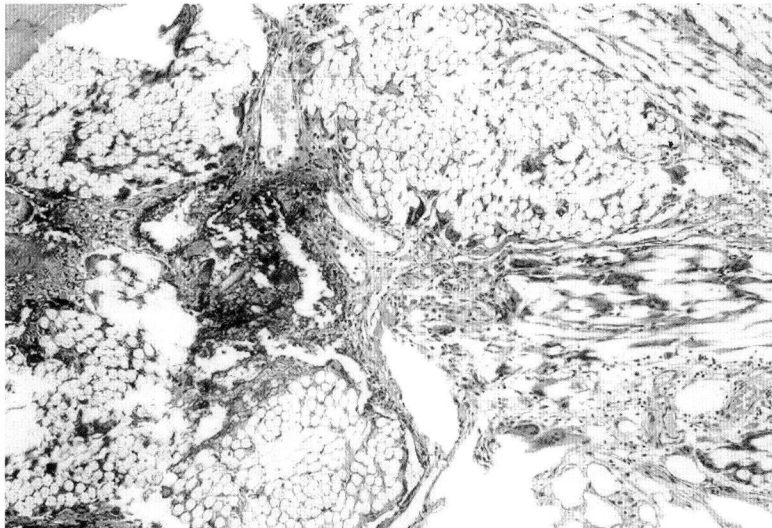

Fig. 9.105
Suture granuloma: suture fragments are present; note the multinucleate giant cells.

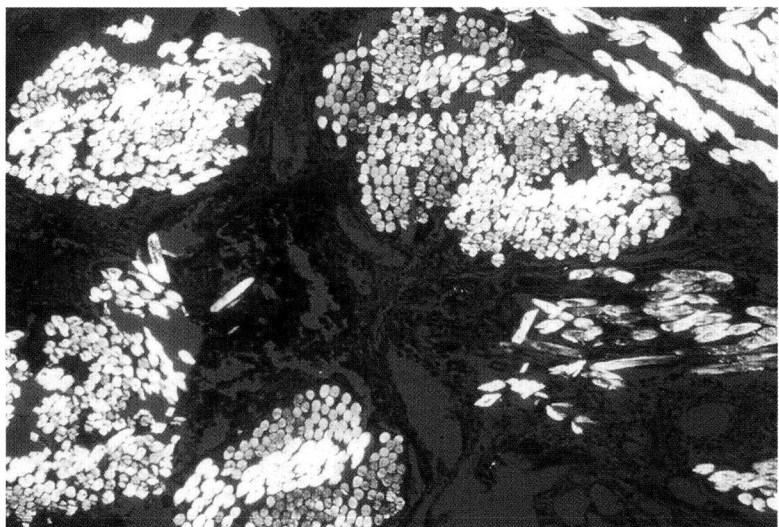

Fig. 9.106
Suture granuloma: when viewed with polarized light, suture fragments show birefringence.

also occurred.[9] More recently, elephantiasis following nodal involvement has been described in patients with beryllium and zirconium exposure from mineral-rich soil (podoconiosis).[10] Diagnosis may be made using spectrographic analysis.[6,7,11]

Foreign body granulomata following esthetic microimplants are relatively uncommon nowadays, as the material used is greatly improved. Silicone granulomata are sometimes found and occasionally one encounters foreign body granulomata to cosmetic microimplants such as Dermalive (hyaluronic acid and acrylic hydrogel), artecoll (PMMA-microspheres), bioplastique (polymethylsiloxane), and bioalcamid.[12,13] Foreign body granulomata to iron oxide after permanent pigmentation of the eyebrows have also been reported.[14] Reactions to cosmetic implants are discussed in more detail in Chapter 14.

A metastatic silicone granuloma mimicking acne agminata and associated with the sicca complex has been reported in a silicone breast implant patient.[15]

Granulomatous contact dermatitis

Clinical features

There are rare reports of a granulomatous reaction to metals, mainly palladium and less commonly gold and a titanium alloy, particularly at the site of ear piercing but also in relation to piercing at other body sites.[1-9] Granulomata induced by titanium have also been reported after implantation of a titanium-containing pacemaker.[10] Areas of swelling, induration, or red papules and/or nodules develop at the site of piercing, and this may occur shortly, weeks after or even months after the patient starts wearing earrings. Most cases have been reported in adults, but similar lesions may be seen in children.[11]

A granulomatous contact dermatitis to propolis has also been described.[12]

Pathogenesis and histologic features

The pathogenesis is likely to be a delayed hypersensitivity reaction to the metal. This is proven by the fact that patients usually have a positive patch test to palladium or less frequently gold. A positive reaction to zinc has also been found.

Throughout the dermis and sometimes extending into the subcutis, there is a prominent, diffuse granulomatous inflammatory cell infiltrate. This comprises epithelioid histiocytes and scattered giant cells surrounded by lymphocytes, and sometimes plasma cells are present. Necrosis is not usually seen. In rare cases granulomas are absent and difficult to find, and the picture is mainly that of a pseudolymphoma that may mimic cutaneous marginal zone lymphoma.[13] In a case report of a reaction to titanium alloy (containing titanium, aluminum, and vanadium), brown-black particles were demonstrated histologically within the cytoplasm of macrophages.[8] In another example triggered by gold earrings, intracytoplasmic crystalline inclusions were found within macrophages.[6]

Differential diagnosis

The differential diagnosis from sarcoidosis and other granulomatous processes may be difficult. The clinical history of piercing and the sites affected are useful in achieving a correct diagnosis.

Granulomata in congenital immunodeficiency syndromes

A number of inherited immune deficiency diseases may rarely present with noninfectious granulomata involving different organs including the skin.[1-8] These diseases include combined immune deficiency, chronic granulomatous disease, ataxia telangiectasia, common variable immunodeficiency, X-linked infantile hypogammaglobulinemia, cartilage hair hypoplasia syndrome, Ommen syndrome, and Blau syndrome (*Figs 9.107–9.110*).[1-8]

The mechanism of granuloma formation is not clearly understood. It has been proposed that it results from immune dysregulation of cell of the monocyte/macrophage lineage. This is the result of absence of naïve T cells

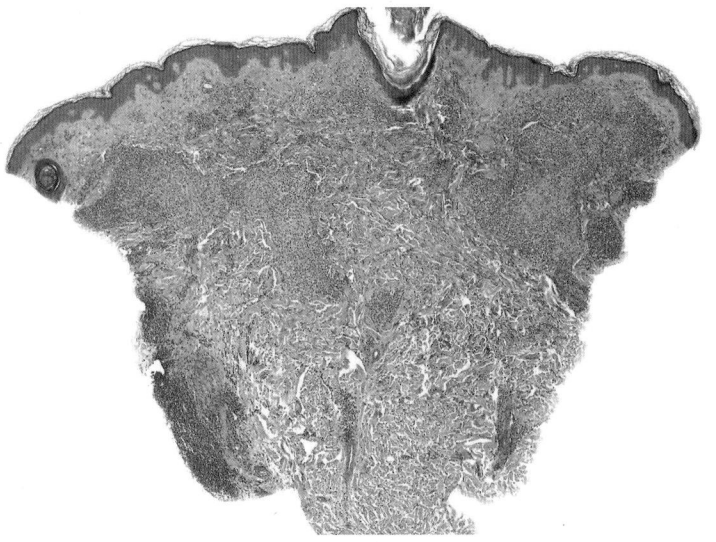

Fig. 9.107
Tuberculoid granulomata in agammaglobulinemia: there is a diffuse granulomatous infiltrate throughout the dermis.

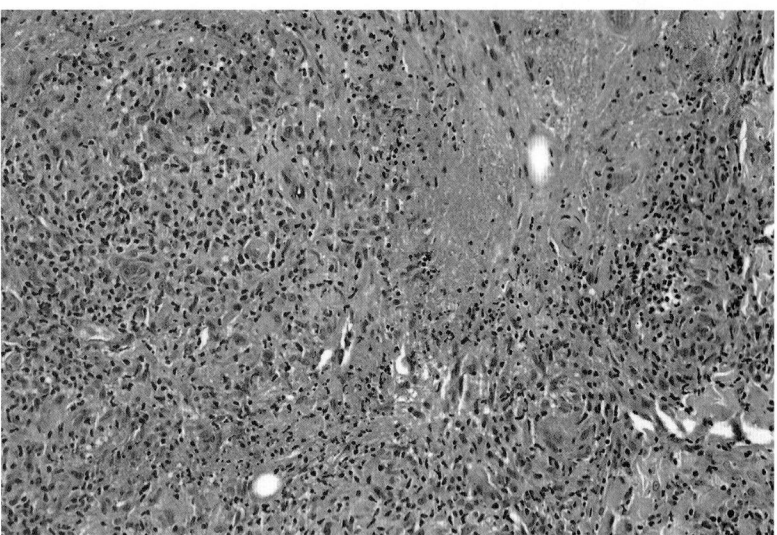

Fig. 9.110
Necrotizing granuloma in agammaglobulinemia: high power view.

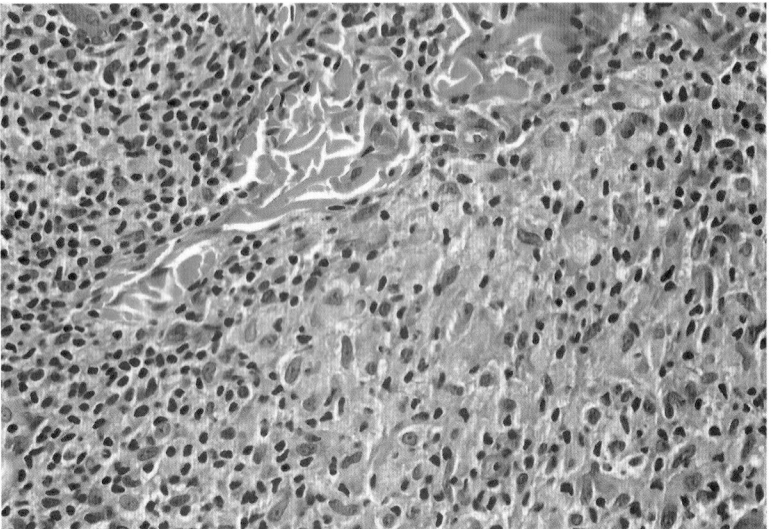

Fig. 9.108
Tuberculoid granulomata in agammaglobulinemia: high-power view.

Fig. 9.109
Necrotizing granuloma in agammaglobulinemia: there is very extensive dermal necrosis with a surrounding granulomatous infiltrate.

and the unopposed activity of gamma delta T cells and/or natural killer cells.[9]

In combined immune deficiency, cutaneous tuberculoid and necrobiotic granulomata may occur, and in a single instance perineural invasion was identified, closely mimicking tuberculoid leprosy.[10,11] Cutaneous granulomata in chronic granulomatous disease may show caseation necrosis without a detectable trigger and can also be associated with foreign bodies.[12,13] In ataxia telangiectasia, patients present with either necrobiotic or tuberculoid granulomata.[14–16] In common variable immunodeficiency, tuberculoid, sarcoidal, and caseating granulomata have been documented.[17–19] In X-linked infantile hypogammaglobulinemia, caseating granulomata have been reported.[20] In cartilage hair hypoplasia syndrome granulomas may be tuberculoid, sarcoidal, or necrotizing, whereas in Ommen and Blau syndromes granulomas are more commonly sarcoidal.[6,8] An unusual perforating neutrophilic and granulomatous dermatitis has been reported in a patient with agammaglobulinemia.[21] Granulomas can rarely masquerade a rare variant of CD8 positive lymphoma in primary immunodeficiencies.[22] It is important to highlight the fact that affected patients have an immunodeficiency; therefore, every effort should be made to rule out an infectious process with special stains and cultures. Differential diagnosis between granulomas associated with sarcoidosis and those seen in primary immunodeficiencies is extremely difficult, and clinicopathological correlation is paramount. Immunohistochemistry may be of help in distinction as in the inflammatory cell infiltrate in sarcoidosis, the ratio between CD4 and CD8 positive cells tends to be more than 2, while in the inflammatory infiltrate associated with primary immune deficiencies the ratio is usually less than 1.[23]

Perforating disorders

Reactive perforating collagenosis

Clinical features

This is a very rare disorder of uncertain etiology in which patients are predisposed to develop an unusual skin reaction to mild trauma, causing damaged collagen to be extruded through the epidermis.[1–4] Although sporadic cases do occur, in many instances reactive perforating collagenosis appears to be an inherited condition, autosomal recessive and dominant variants having been described.[5–8] Reactive perforating collagenosis has been documented in association with the Treacher Collins syndrome.[9] The disease shows an equal sex incidence, with most cases presenting in childhood, although lesions tend to persist into adult life. In familial cases, the expression of the disease is variable and can sometimes be mild and subtle.[10] Lesions may be precipitated by sun exposure.[10] An acquired variant occurring in adulthood

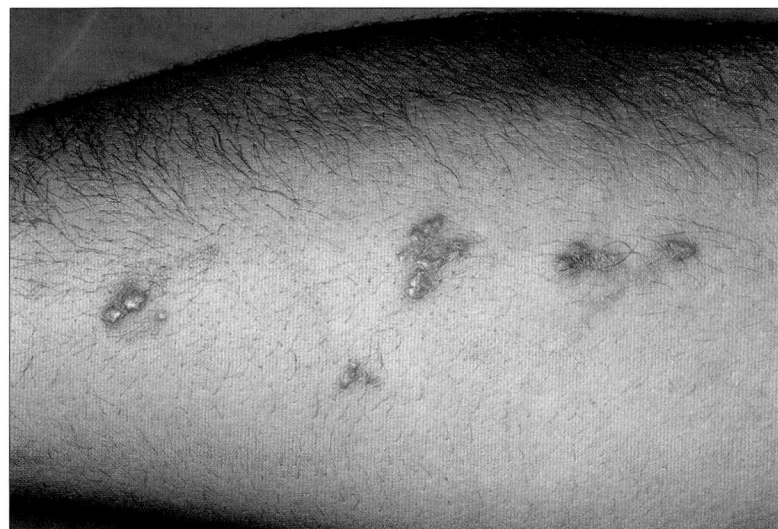

Fig. 9.111
Reactive perforating collagenosis: there are multiple pink papules, some showing central umbilication with crusting. By courtesy of D. McGibbon, MD, St Thomas' Hospital, London, UK.

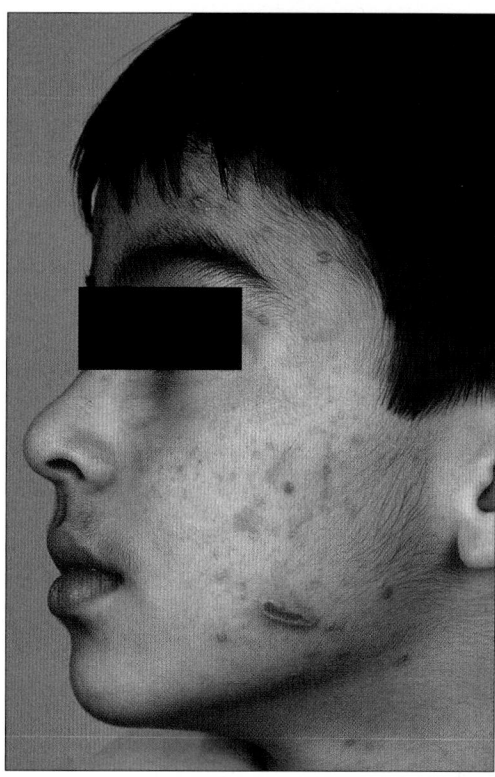

Fig. 9.112
Reactive perforating collagenosis: an example on the cheek of a young boy. By courtesy of E. Young, MD, Wycombe General Hospital, High Wycombe, UK.

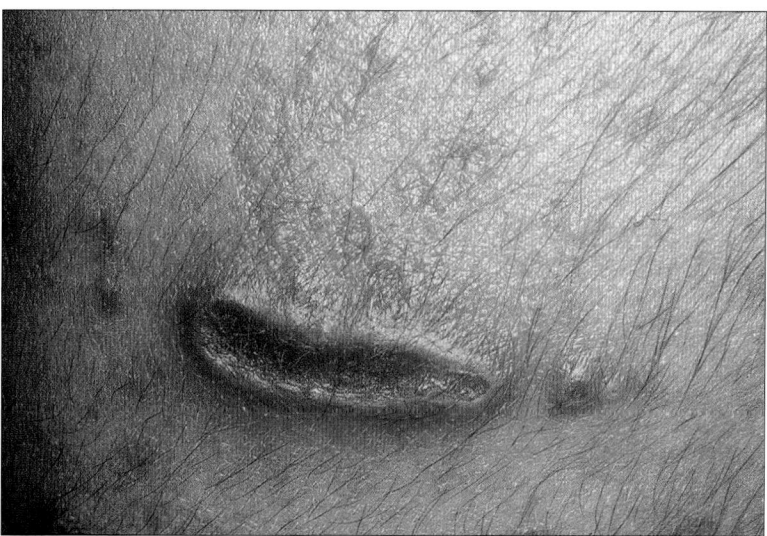

Fig. 9.113
Reactive perforating collagenosis: close-up view. By courtesy of E. Young, MD, Wycombe General Hospital, High Wycombe, UK.

is mainly associated with diabetes mellitus and renal failure.[11,12] Other associations include insect bites, Down syndrome, lupus erythematosus, dermatomyositis, leukocytoclastic vasculitis, urticarial vasculitis, IgA nephropathy, hydronephrosis, lung fibrosis, herpes zoster infection (Wolf isomorphic phenomenon), cytomegalovirus, scabies, lymphoma, leukemia, and carcinoma (including papillary thyroid carcinoma, breast carcinoma, hepatocellular carcinoma, and lung adenocarcinoma).[13–39] In a single patient with Mikulicz disease, the condition showed histologic features of IgG4-related sclerosing disease in the same biopsy.[40] A case developing at a tattoo site has been described.[41] Drugs including sirolimus, indinavir, and erlotinib have also been associated with the disease.[42–44] The inherited cases are not associated with any systemic disorder. Reactive perforating collagenosis has also been reported in a patient with HIV/AIDS in association with end-stage renal failure.[45] Perforating collagenosis is seen in approximately 10% of patients with renal failure.[1,2,46] Patients may develop lesions either before or after dialysis treatment.[2] In most cases, underlying diabetes mellitus is also present.[1,2,46] Affected individuals suffer generalized pruritus and crusting papules. A single case with a zosteriform distribution has also been documented.[47]

Following mild trauma, such as a scratch or insect bite, patients develop flesh-colored papules 1–2 mm in diameter. These enlarge, become umbilicated, and, over the course of about 4 weeks, grow to reach a diameter of some 5–10 mm (Figs 9.111–9.113). Rarely, giant lesions are observed.[48] The umbilicated area contains keratinous debris, which is dark brown, hard, and leathery. It is also very densely adherent, and bleeding results if detachment is attempted. This is followed by regression. The papules flatten, and by 6–8 weeks from onset all that remain are residual scars or hypopigmented areas. It is of interest that lesions develop only after mild superficial trauma, with deep penetrating wounds healing normally. A positive Koebner phenomenon is characteristic, and lesions may be induced by gentle needle scratching. Lesions tend to be rather polymorphic: as old lesions heal, new ones develop. They are distributed primarily on the upper and lower extremities and face, although the trunk may be affected.[49,50] Rarely, the palms and soles may be involved. Mucosal involvement has also been described in one patient.[51] The severity of this condition seems to increase in cold weather, whereas there is a reduction in the number of lesions in summer. Exceptionally, secondary bacterial infection within the lesions may occur.[52]

Pathogenesis and histologic features

The pathogenesis of reactive perforating collagenosis has not been elucidated.[53] Transepidermal elimination of type IV collagen has been demonstrated, but the mechanism that triggers the process is not clear.[54]

A broadened dermal ridge containing degenerate, basophilic collagen characterizes early, nonumbilicated lesions. The overlying epithelium is atrophic and centrally is composed of a thin layer of parakeratotic material. At the lateral margins, there is typically acanthosis. In the fully established umbilicated lesion, the central plug is composed of parakeratotic debris, degenerate collagen, and inflammatory cells (Figs 9.114 and 9.115).[55] The epidermis deep to the plug is markedly thinned and is traversed focally by vertically orientated collagen fibers (Figs 9.116 and 9.117). Elastic fibers are not present within the extruded connective tissue debris. On either side of the cup-shaped deformity, the epidermis is acanthotic and hyperkeratotic. A lymphohistiocytic infiltrate is present in the superficial dermis. The histologic appearances in reactive perforating collagenosis and acquired perforating collagenosis are identical. Distinction between these disorders requires clinical correlation (Figs 9.118 and 9.119).

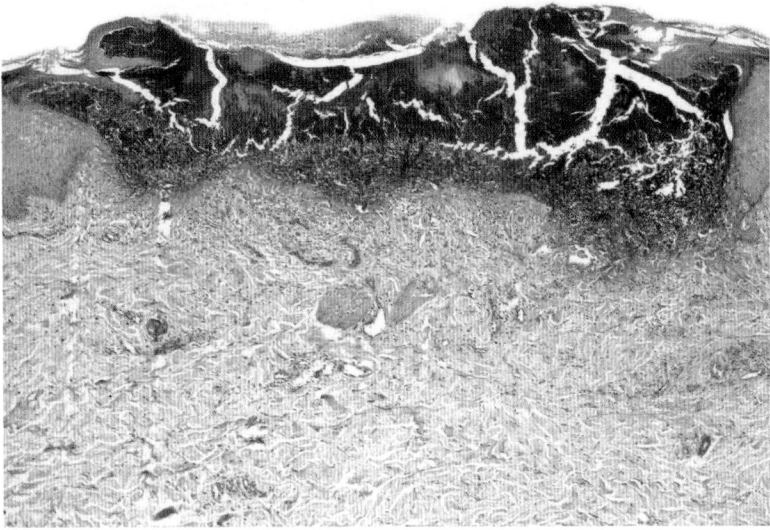

Fig. 9.114
Reactive perforating collagenosis: this is a transverse section through the center of a lesion. Note the crust overlying multiple points of incipient perforation.

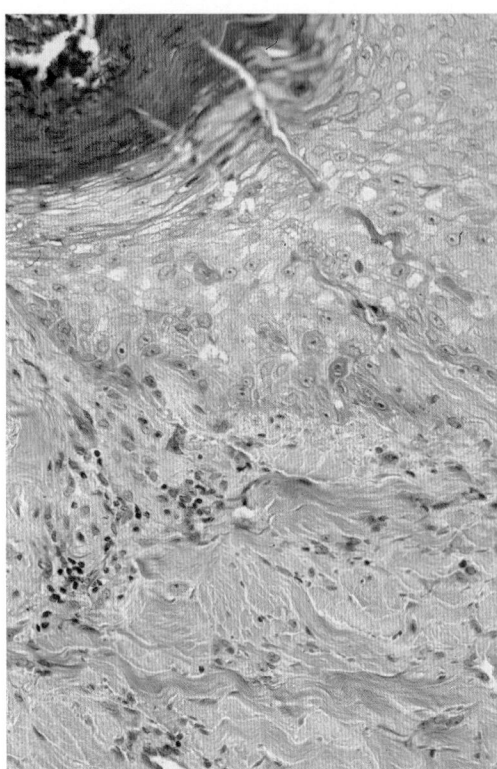

Fig. 9.116
Reactive perforating collagenosis: close-up view of collagen fibers within the epidermis.

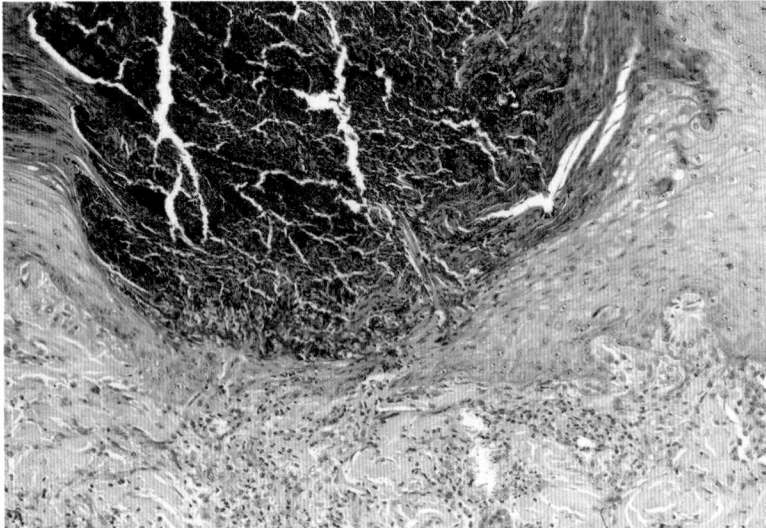

Fig. 9.115
Reactive perforating collagenosis: irregular, swollen collagen fibers have penetrated the epidermis.

Differential diagnosis

Changes identical to those seen in reactive perforating collagenosis may be seen following trauma in 'normal' patients without stigmata of the disease. Not uncommonly, biopsies of patients with prurigo nodularis/lichen simplex chronicus (but who do not meet clinical criteria for reactive perforating collagenosis) show transepidermal elimination of collagen in a pattern similar to that seen in perforating collagenosis. *Table 9.3* highlights points of distinction among the perforating disorders.

Perforating folliculitis

Clinical features

Perforating folliculitis is a not uncommon, usually asymptomatic, dermatosis of unknown etiology that superficially resembles Kyrle disease.[1–4] It shows a female predominance (2 : 1) and, although a wide range of age groups may be affected, the majority of patients present in the third decade. The disease is characterized by the development of discrete, erythematous follicular papules, 2–8 mm in diameter, each containing a small central white keratotic core. Lesions most often affect the extremities, with a predilection for the hairy portions of the arms, forearms, and thighs. The buttocks may

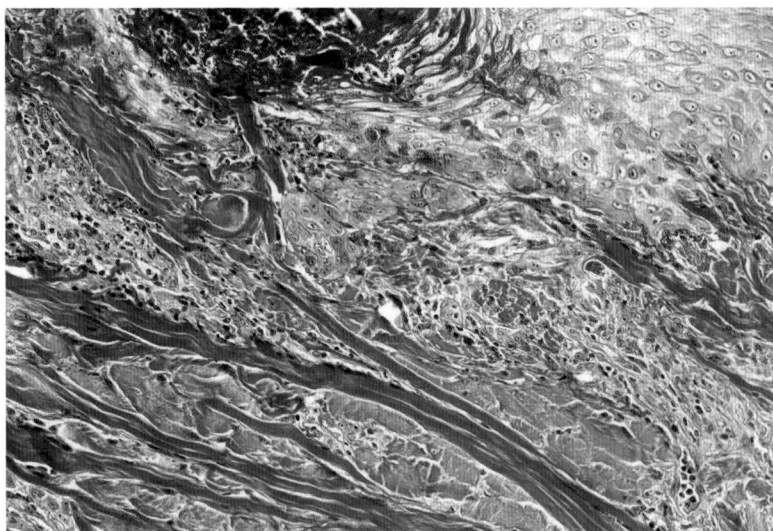

Fig. 9.117
Reactive perforating collagenosis: transepidermal elimination is seen to better advantage with this Masson trichrome stain.

also be involved (*Figs 9.120* and *9.121*). Koebnerization is not usually a feature. Duration of the rash is variable, ranging from several months to years and remissions, and exacerbation may punctuate the course. Some patients present with features of more than one perforating disease (i.e., perforating folliculitis and elastosis perforans serpiginosa).[5]

Perforating folliculitis is associated with renal failure and diabetes mellitus.[6–8] It has also been reported in the setting of HIV infection, in two dialysis patients with markedly elevated serum silicon levels, in a patient with antisynthetase syndrome, and in a case of cystic fibrosis.[9–12] Primary sclerosing cholangitis may rarely be associated with perforating folliculitis.[13,14] A number of medications have been associated with perforating folliculitis including sorafenib, infliximab, etanercept, lenalidomide, and nilotinib.[15–19]

Table 9.3
Differential diagnosis of perforating disorders

	Kyrle disease	Reactive perforating collagenosis	Elastosis perforans serpiginosa	Perforating folliculitis
Age of patient	Average 30 years (20–60)	Childhood	Second decade	Third decade
Sex distribution	♂ = ♀	♂ = ♀	4 ♂ = ♀	2 ♀ = ♂
Site	Extensor lower extremities; upper extremities; head, neck and trunk	Upper and lower extremities; face	Side and back of neck; upper extremities; face; lower extremities	Hair-bearing portions of arms, forearms, thighs
Koebner phenomenon	Occasionally positive	Positive	Occasionally positive	Negative
Associated diseases	Diabetes mellitus; renal failure; hepatic insufficiency; congestive cardiac failure	None; (acquired variant renal failure)	Down syndrome; Ehlers-Danlos syndrome; osteogenesis imperfecta; pseudoxanthoma elasticum	None
Mode of inheritance		? autosomal recessive ? autosomal dominant		
Histology	Transepidermal elimination of degenerate parakeratin and inflammatory debris	Transepidermal elimination of collagen	Transepidermal elimination of abnormal elastic tissue	Intrafollicular curled-up hair; transepidermal elimination of degenerate connective tissue

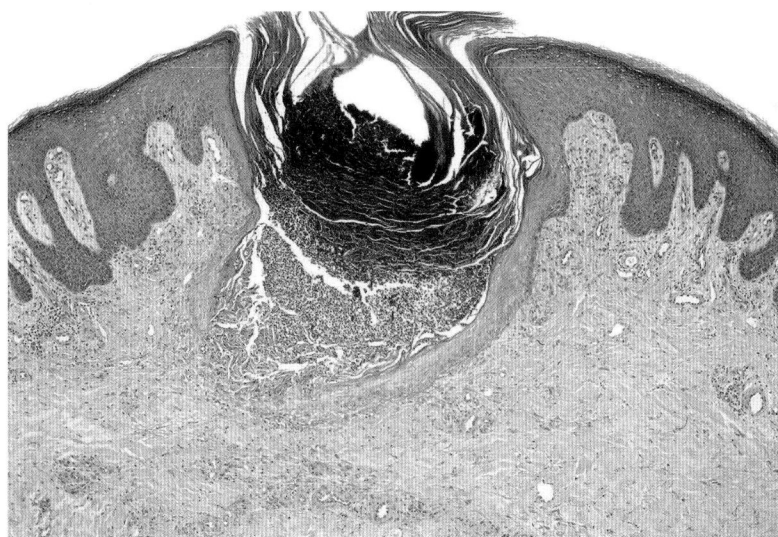

Fig. 9.118
Reactive perforating collagenosis: this example developed in a patient with chronic renal failure.

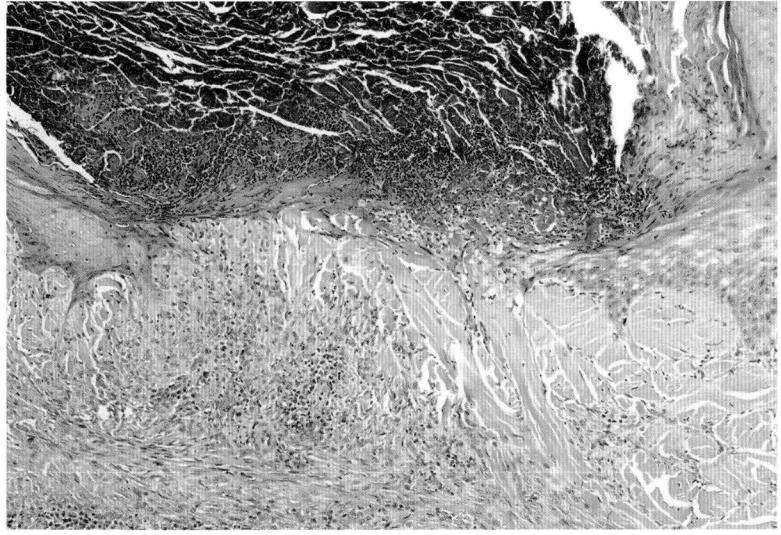

Fig. 9.119
Reactive perforating collagenosis: higher-power view.

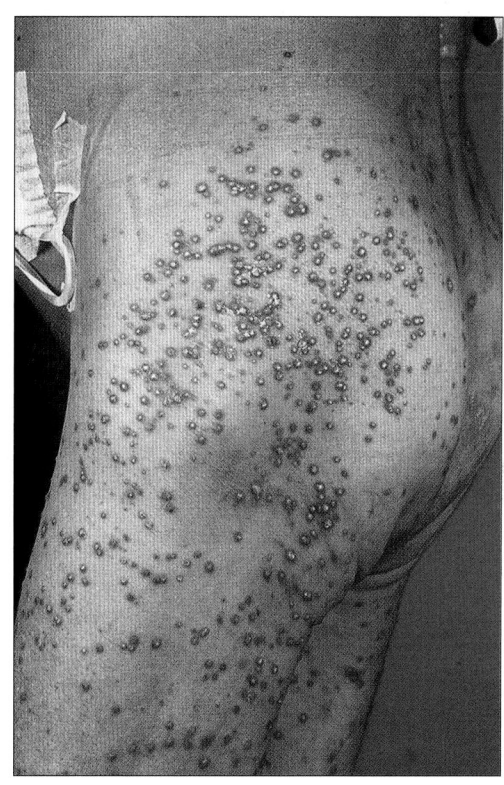

Fig. 9.120
Perforating folliculitis: discrete scaly lesions on the buttocks and thighs. By courtesy of K. Green, MD, Lister Hospital, Stevenage, UK.

Pathogenesis and histologic features

Although the exact etiology is unknown, the frequent finding of a distorted, curled hair within the dilated follicle, often associated with disruption of the epithelium, and the occasional presence of hair fragments within the adjacent dermis suggest that mechanical disruption of follicular epithelium by hair may be the cause of this condition. The lesions of perforating folliculitis occur most commonly on the extensor aspects of the extremities, suggesting that trauma may be implicated. It has been proposed that, as with Kyrle disease, chronic friction leads to abnormal keratinization of the follicular epithelium, which eventually results in follicular perforation. The subsequent exposure of the follicular contents to the underlying dermis results in necrosis of connective tissue and subsequent transepidermal elimination.

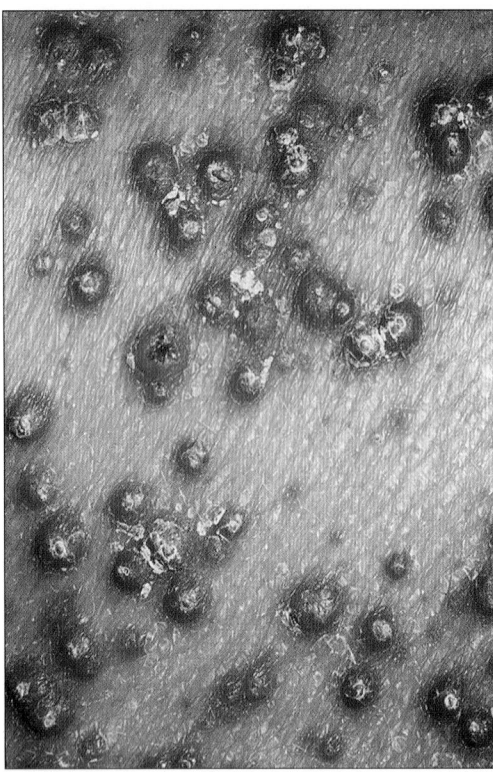

Fig. 9.121
Perforating folliculitis: close-up view. By courtesy of K. Green, MD, Lister Hospital, Stevenage, UK.

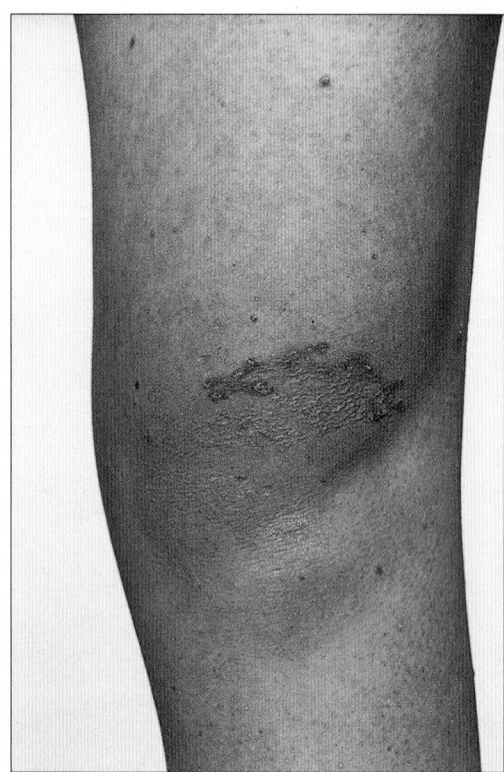

Fig. 9.123
Elastosis perforans serpiginosa: typical scaly serpiginous eruption on the elbow. By courtesy of M.M. Black, MD, St Thomas' Hospital, London, UK.

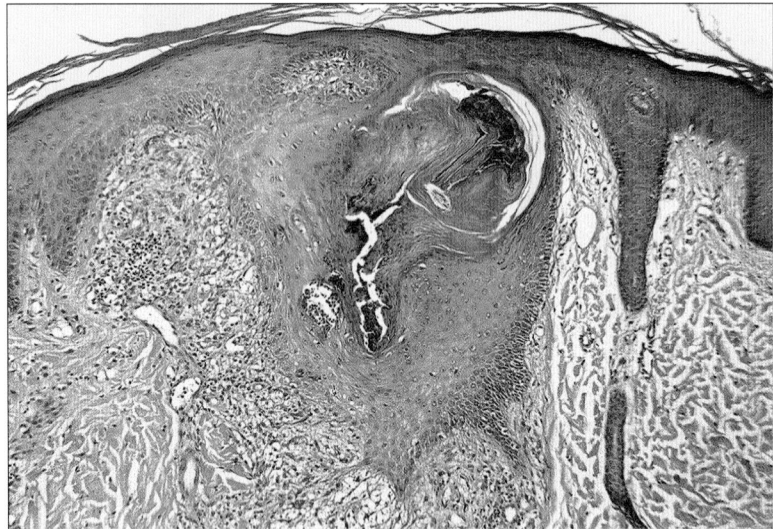

Fig. 9.122
Perforating folliculitis: this field shows a dilated hair follicle containing keratinous and basophilic debris. A hair shaft is visible.

The histopathological features of perforating folliculitis are those of a widely dilated hair follicle containing ortho- and parakeratotic keratin, basophilic necrotic debris, connective tissue elements, and degenerate inflammatory cells (*Fig. 9.122*).[2] A curled-up hair is sometimes found within the keratinous plug or extruded into the perifollicular dermis. Typically, the infundibular follicular epithelium is disrupted at single or multiple foci. The underlying degenerate dermis, including collagen and elastic fibers, may be seen to impinge upon the perforated follicle. The adjacent epidermis often shows pseudoepitheliomatous hyperplasia. A foreign body giant cell reaction is sometimes found within the superficial dermis.

Differential diagnosis

Perforating folliculitis is differentiated from Kyrle disease by uniform follicular involvement associated with infundibular epithelial perforation (compared with perforation at the base of the lesion in Kyrle disease) and the presence of tortuous hairs. Although elastic fibers may be found within the dilated follicle, they are neither abnormal in appearance nor increased in quantity as seen in elastosis perforans serpiginosa. *Table 9.3* highlights points of distinction among the perforating disorders. Keratosis pilaris is associated with keratotic plugs that tend to be folliculocentric, but perforation and inflammation are not features.

Elastosis perforans serpiginosa

Clinical features

Elastosis perforans serpiginosa (L. *serpere*, to creep) is a rare dermatosis associated with transepidermal elimination of abnormal elastic tissue.[1-3] It shows a male predominance (4:1) and presents most often in the second decade. A case with simultaneous onset in two sisters has been reported.[4] Another unusual case has been documented in an individual with a 47 XYY karyotype and unilateral atrophoderma of Pasini and Pierini.[5]

The primary lesion is a 2–5-mm flesh-colored or red keratotic papule containing an adherent plug, the removal of which is associated with bleeding. Classically, the papules are arranged in an arcuate or serpiginous pattern, although sometimes they are randomly distributed (*Fig. 9.123*). Most often the lesions are confined to one site, with the back and sides of the neck being most frequently affected. Symmetrical involvement is very rare.[6] Other sites include the upper extremities, face, lower extremities, and abdomen, in decreasing order of frequency. The penis is very rarely involved.[7] In those cases where multiple sites are involved, symmetrical distribution is characteristic. Rarely, lesions are widely disseminated. The eruption is usually asymptomatic, although mild pruritus is sometimes a feature. Koebnerization is occasionally noted.

Although elastosis perforans serpiginosa may occur as an isolated phenomenon, in quite a high proportion of cases it develops in association with other conditions including Down syndrome, Ehlers-Danlos syndrome, osteogenesis imperfecta, Marfan syndrome, pseudoxanthoma elasticum, cutis laxa, acrogeria, the Rothmund-Thomson syndrome, and Moyamoya disease.[8-17] Rarely, elastosis perforans serpiginosa may develop

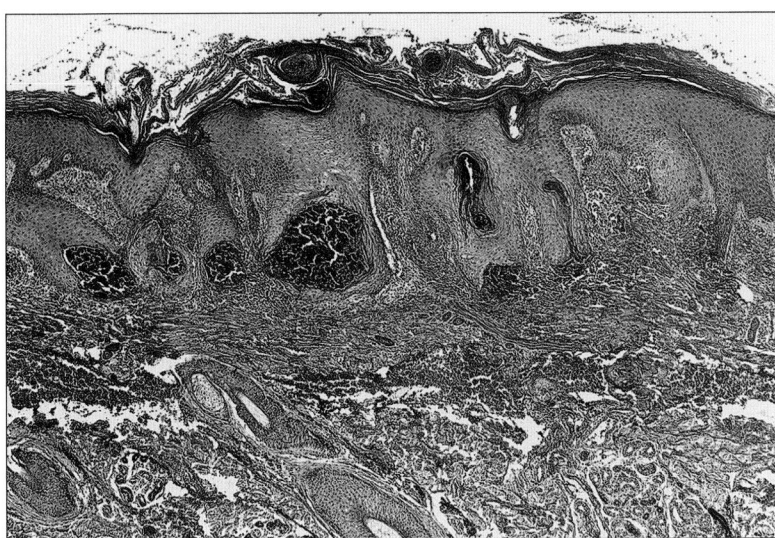

Fig. 9.124
Elastosis perforans serpiginosa: the epidermis is markedly thickened. Multiple perforating channels containing basophilic debris are present.

as a complication of penicillamine therapy for Wilson disease and cystinuria.[9,18-23] In patients treated with penicillamine, it may be associated with pseudoxanthoma elasticum and cutis laxa.[24,25] It has also been described in a case of juvenile rheumatoid arthritis and a further case of Behçet disease.[9,26] A single case associated with a scabies mite has been described but this is likely to be coincidental.[27]

Pathogenesis and histologic features

The pathogenesis of elastosis perforans serpiginosa is not entirely understood. The documentation of familial cases suggests that a genetic component plays a role in a subset of patients.[28] The common association of elastosis perforans serpiginosa with a variety of connective tissue disorders raises the possibility of an elastic tissue defect as being of pathogenetic significance. Histochemical and enzyme studies have confirmed that it is the elastic tissue that is undergoing transepidermal elimination: electron microscopic studies have shown that the elastic fibers are increased in size and have a convoluted and branched pattern.[29] It appears that these abnormal fibers have an irritant effect, resulting in epidermal proliferation and their eventual engulfment by the epidermis. Following epidermal growth with consequent upward migration, the abnormal elastic tissue is expelled via perforating canals. Recently, it has been demonstrated that the 67-kD elastin receptor is present in the keratinocytes associated with the elimination of elastic material in elastosis perforans serpiginosa.[30,31] This expression varies with the stage of the disease and suggests that the elastin-keratinocyte interaction plays an important role in the transepidermal elimination of elastin.[30,31]

It is of particular interest that this condition has been described following the use of the copper chelating agent D-penicillamine.[9,18,19] This medication can be demonstrated in the affected dermis even many years after therapy.[32] Tissue copper deficiency is known to be associated with damage to the elastica of arteries in experimental animals. The Blotchy mouse, which develops fusiform aortic aneurysms, has a copper metabolism defect that includes reduced activity of the copper-dependent enzyme lysyl oxidase, which is essential for cross-linking the elastin molecules. In Menkes syndrome, there is an abnormality of copper metabolism associated with reduced numbers of elastic fibers in arterial walls. It may be, therefore, that penicillamine locally depletes the dermis of copper, resulting in abnormally formed elastic tissue and the subsequent development of elastosis perforans serpiginosa.

In the established lesion, there is a marked increase in elastic tissue in both the reticular and papillary dermis (*Fig. 9.124*). The vertically oriented fibers of the latter are thicker than normal and can be seen to penetrate the epidermis. A section through the center of the lesion shows characteristic transepithelial perforating canals, which may be transepidermal,

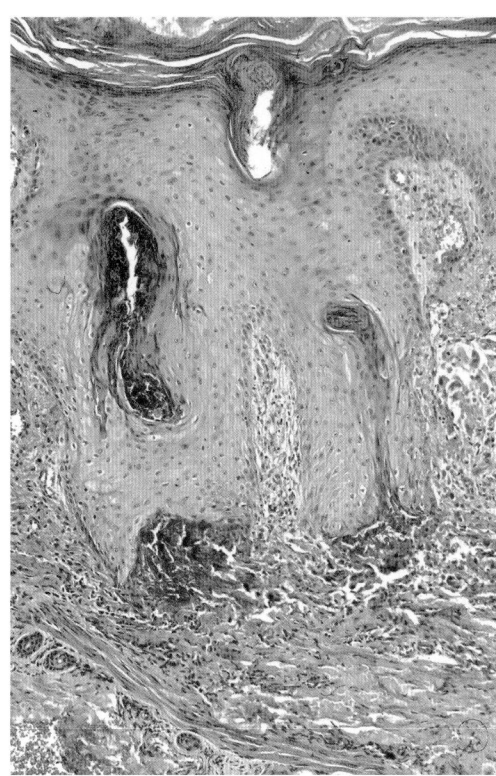

Fig. 9.125
Elastosis perforans serpiginosa: this picture is taken through the center of a characteristic tortuous perforating canal. Note the degenerate elastic tissue at the base of the lesion.

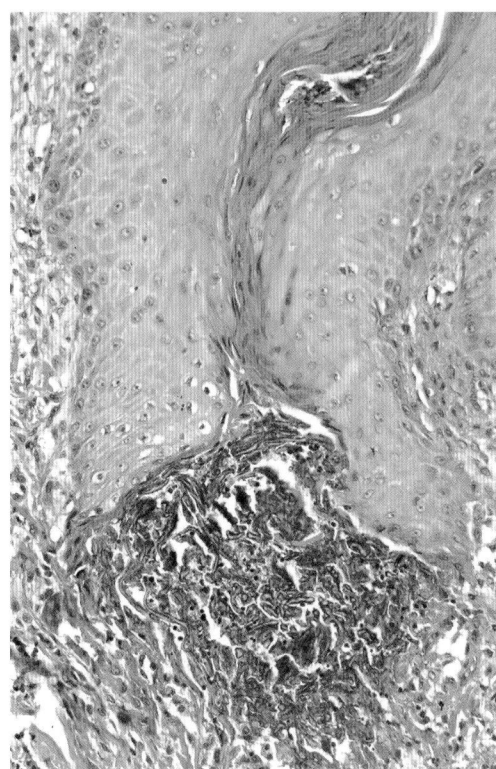

Fig. 9.126
Elastosis perforans serpiginosa: high-power view.

parafollicular, or transfollicular in location and straight, wavy, or screwlike in configuration (*Figs 9.125* and *9.126*). The canal contents consist of a basophilic mass comprising degenerate epithelial cells, inflammatory debris, and numerous elastic fibers (*Fig. 9.127*). The superficial plug is composed predominantly of keratinous material and basophilic debris. Sometimes

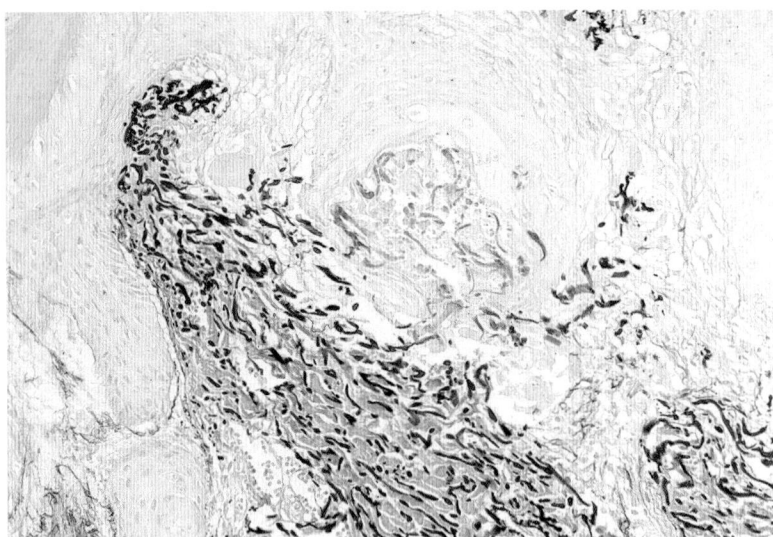

Fig. 9.127
Elastosis perforans serpiginosa: the elastic fibers stain strongly with elastic-van Gieson in the superficial dermis, but less strongly as the fibers undergo transepidermal elimination.

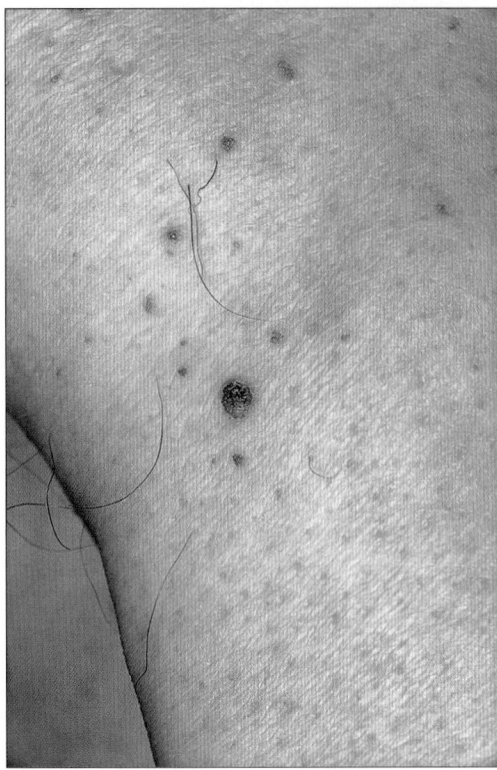

Fig. 9.128
Kyrle disease: multiple umbilicated lesions are present on the thigh. The largest contains a keratin plug. By courtesy of M.M. Black, MD, St Thomas' Hospital, London, UK.

elastic fibers are identified in the stratum corneum. The epithelium on either side of the perforating canal is acanthotic and may manifest pseudoepitheliomatous hyperplasia. Commonly, a foreign body giant cell reaction is present in the superficial dermis and occasionally elastophagocytosis is evident.

In the penicillamine-induced variant, the elastic fibers characteristically have an irregular, serrated, sawtooth border ('lumpy-bumpy' elastic fibers).[7] Similar changes may be seen in the elastic fibers in noninvolved skin.[33] Ultrastructurally, this gives the lateral borders of the affected elastic fibers a 'lumpy bumpy' appearance.[5]

Differential diagnosis

Although elastic fibers may be found within the dilated follicle in perforating folliculitis, they are neither abnormal in appearance nor increased in quantity as seen in elastosis perforans serpiginosa. Keratosis pilaris is associated with keratotic plugs that tend to be folliculocentric, but perforation and inflammation are not features. Kyrle disease is differentiated from elastosis perforans serpiginosa by perforation of a keratin plug at the base of the lesion associated with curled hairs in the former. *Table 9.3* summarizes the points of distinction among the perforating disorders.

Hyperkeratosis follicularis et parafollicularis in cutem penetrans (Kyrle disease)

Clinical features

Hyperkeratosis follicularis et parafollicularis in cutem penetrans (Kyrle disease) is a very rare dermatosis of unknown etiology.[1-4] It has an equal incidence in men and women and an age of onset ranging from 20 to 60 years, with an average of 30 years. Presentation in children is exceptional.[5] The disorder is characterized by a widespread, asymptomatic, and typically bilateral eruption of 1–8-mm papules, each containing a central cone-shaped keratotic plug. Although lesions are located most often on the extensor aspect of the lower extremities, they may also affect the upper extremities, head, neck, and trunk (*Figs 9.128* and *9.129*). They may or may not be related to hair follicles. The mucous membranes, palms, and soles are characteristically spared. Ocular changes have been documented in a single kindred with the disease.[6] In a further patient, there was involvement of the conjunctiva and oral mucosa.[7] Lesions may coalesce into plaques, and occasionally, a Koebner-like appearance is present. There is no evidence to suggest that Kyrle disease has a genetic etiology. However, the disease exceptionally can be seen in siblings and families.[6,8,9] It is sometimes associated with diabetes mellitus, renal failure, hepatic insufficiency, and congestive cardiac failure.[10,11] It is unclear whether Kyrle disease is a

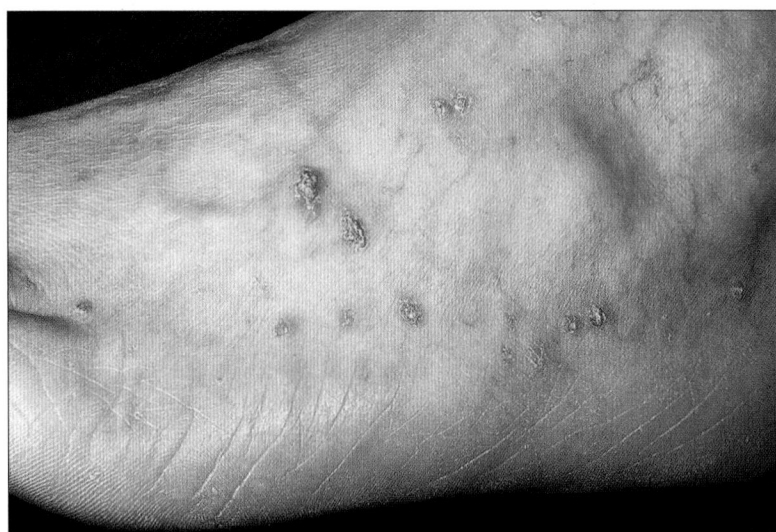

Fig. 9.129
Kyrle disease: multiple keratotic lesions are present on the dorsum of the foot. By courtesy of the Institute of Dermatology, London, UK.

distinct entity. Some cases clearly overlap with a perforating folliculitis, and reports of examples in patients with diabetes and renal failure may actually represent examples of the latter condition. An overlap with Flegel disease has also been described.[12]

Pathogenesis and histologic features

The precise pathogenesis of Kyrle disease is unknown; however, it has been suggested that the lesions develop as a consequence of rapid and abnormal keratinization, which proceeds at a faster rate than epidermal proliferation, with consequent premature and abnormal differentiation of all the epidermal layers. In most instances, this is complicated by dissolution of the epidermal basement membrane region, with extrusion of keratinous debris into

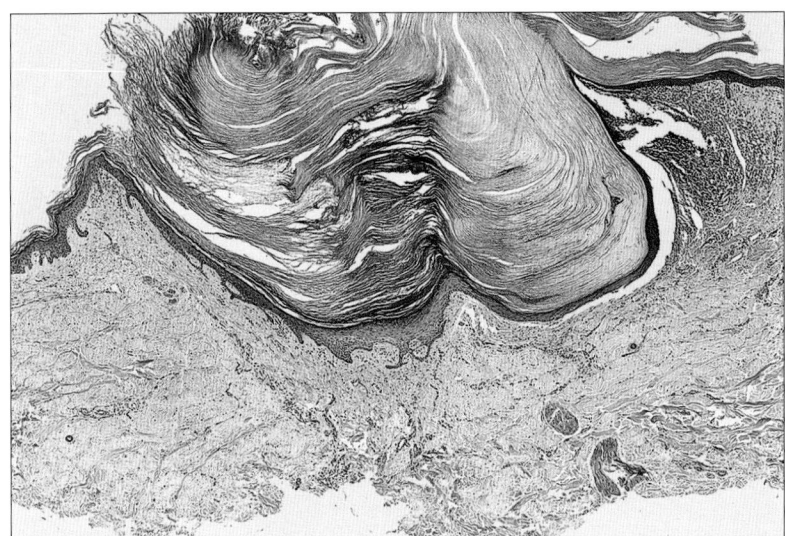

Fig. 9.130
Kyrle disease: scanning view through the center of an established lesion showing the keratin plug.

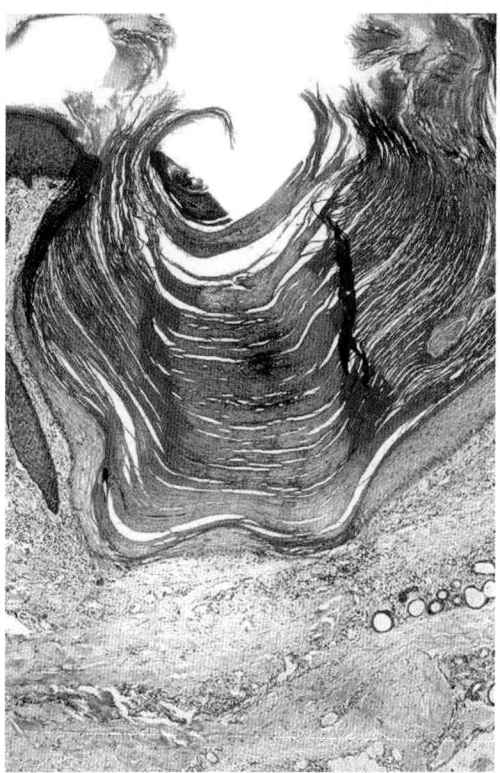

Fig. 9.132
Kyrle disease: a somewhat earlier lesion in which perforation has not yet occurred. Note the thinning of the epidermis basally. Where parakeratosis is evident, there is absence of the granular cell layer.

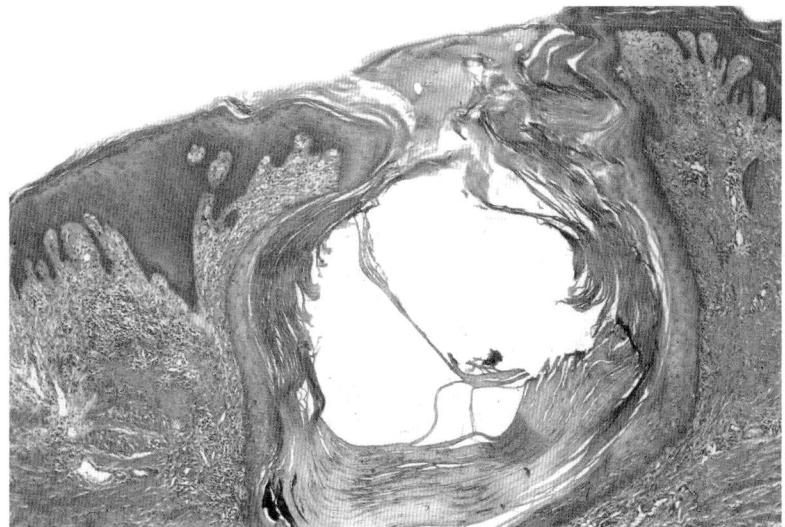

Fig. 9.131
Kyrle disease: this lesion shows a flask-shaped epidermal invagination containing parakeratotic debris. In the lower-left corner of the lesion is a laminated focus of basophilic degenerate material.

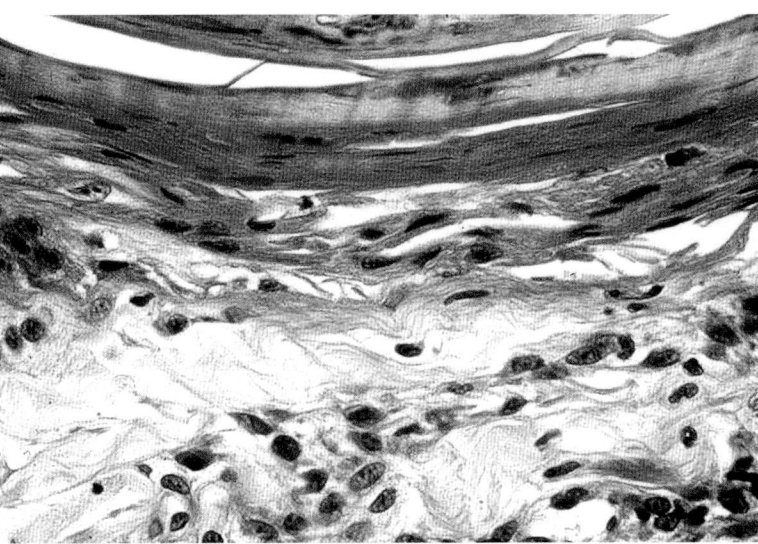

Fig. 9.133
Kyrle disease: this high-power view shows parakeratosis of the residual epithelium.

the dermis and subsequent development of a foreign body granulomatous reaction. Following this, the epithelium adjacent to the site of the breach proliferates downwards and, by fusion medially, eventually walls off the inflammatory debris. Subsequent epidermal proliferation deep to the debris results in eventual transepidermal elimination. Transepidermal elimination or perforation, it seems, is of secondary rather than primary importance in this disorder. From this description, it follows that in early lesions there may be no evidence of an epidermal breach.

In a single case, reported regression of the lesions was seen after treatment with clindamycin, raising the possibility of a bacterial agent in the etiology of the disease. However, there is very little additional evidence to suggest that the process may be triggered by bacteria.[13]

The histologic features of an established lesion consist of a keratotic plug filling an epidermal invagination.[14-16] The keratinous plug shows parakeratosis and contains basophilic cellular debris (Figs 9.130 and 9.131). Elastic tissue is absent. The epithelium deep to the plug shows parakeratosis, which extends to the point of epidermal disruption (Figs 9.132–9.135). Where the keratinous debris is in contact with the dermis, there is often a granulomatous infiltrate. In more advance cases, downward epidermal proliferation

and encirclement results in incorporation of the basophilic keratotic debris into the lower reaches of the epidermis and hence subsequent elimination. A lymphohistiocytic infiltrate is often seen around the epidermal downgrowth and the superficial blood vessels. An exceptional case with acantholytic dyskeratosis mimicking Darier disease has been described.[17]

Differential diagnosis

Kyrle disease must be distinguished from reactive perforating collagenosis and elastosis perforans serpiginosa. In the former, collagen bundles may be seen entering the lesion from the dermis; in the latter, the basophilic material is elastic tissue. Kyrle disease must also be distinguished from perforating

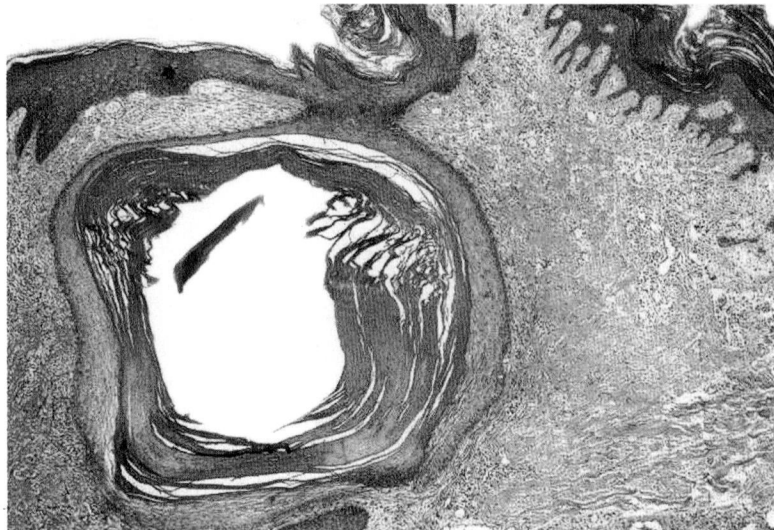

Fig. 9.134
Kyrle disease: in this example, there is incipient perforation.

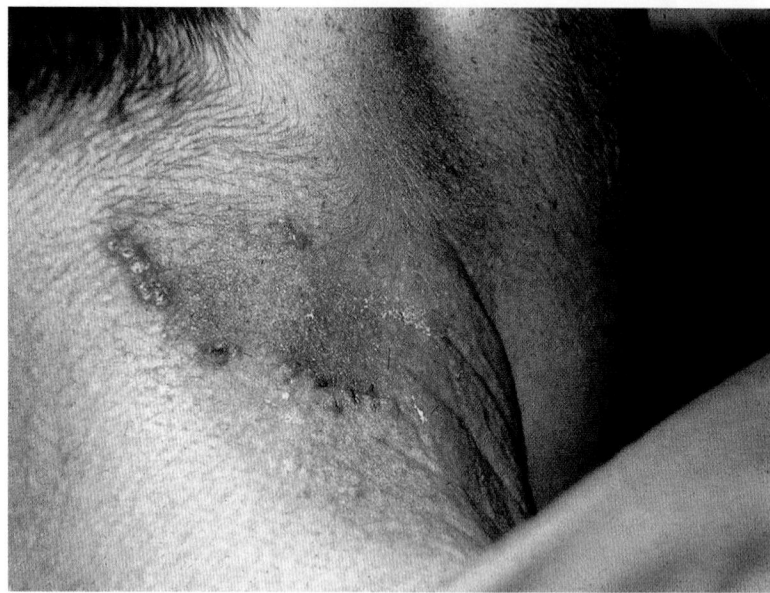

Fig. 9.136
Perforating pseudoxanthoma elasticum: multiple small crusted lesions are seen in a background of typical yellow papules. By courtesy of the Institute of Dermatology, London, UK.

Necrotizing infundibular crystalline folliculitis

Clinical features

Only few of this distinctive entity have been reported. The first two cases were described as a perforating disorder under the rubric transepidermal elimination of urate-like crystals, but it has more recently been suggested that it represents a form of folliculitis.[1–6] Males appear to be involved more frequently than females, and the disease has predilection for the face particularly the forehead and cheeks and the back. Patients present with multiple umbilicated papules with waxy keratinous material in the center. The lesions are asymptomatic and transient, and usually resolved spontaneously without any treatment.

Pathogenesis and histologic features

The etiology of the process remains unclear. However, an association with *Malassezia* species and *P. acnes* has been suggested based on the presence of yeasts and bacteria in the infundibula of some of the involved hair follicles and in the clinical response to antifungal agents.[6]

Although the material within the umbilicated craters resembles urate crystals (monosodium urate monohydrate), none of the patients had evidence of gout or hyperuricemia.

Histology is characteristic and consists of a crater full of eosinophilic filamentous material surrounded by an amorphous matrix and bulging into the dermis (*Figs 9.137* and *9.138*). Focally, the filaments are distributed in a parallel fashion mimicking urate crystals. The crystals are negatively birefringent. It is important to highlight that identical histologic features may be observed rarely as an incidental finding in skin biopsies obtained for other pathologies.[6] A single case associated with perforating mucinosis has been described.[4] Although in the first two cases a relationship with the hair follicles was not described, in the most recent case partially destroyed hair follicles were demonstrated. The residual infundibular portion of the hair follicles showed vacuolar and filamentous degeneration. By electron microscopy, the filamentous material appears to represent tonofilaments.

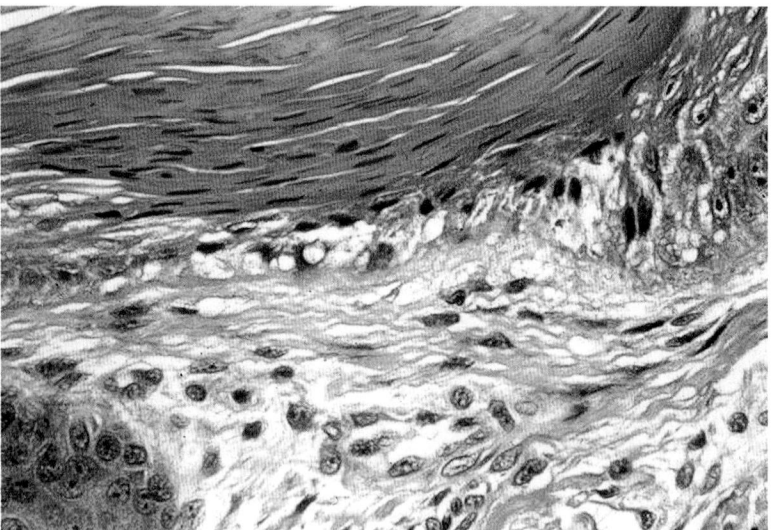

Fig. 9.135
Kyrle disease: high-power view showing liquefactive degeneration of the basal layer.

folliculitis (see above). *Table 9.3* highlights points of distinction in the differential diagnosis of perforating disorders.

Perforating pseudoxanthoma elasticum

Pseudoxanthoma elasticum (Grönblad-Strandberg syndrome) is an inherited generalized degenerative disease of elastic tissue of which there are autosomal dominant and autosomal recessive variants. The disease is briefly discussed in this section since a perforating variant is recognized.

Perforating pseudoxanthoma elasticum is seen predominantly in multiparous, obese, middle-aged, and frequently hypertensive black women who present with isolated abdominal, periumbilical involvement.[1–6] Whether this represents a forme fruste or a distinct entity is not yet known (so-called acquired pseudoxanthoma elasticum). In some cases, however, transepidermal elimination is seen in patients with systemic manifestations (*Fig. 9.136*).[7] The perforating variant may be associated with renal failure.[6]

In a single case, the confocal microscopy appearance of the lesion has been described.[7] The altered elastic fibers appeared hyperreflective.

The perforating subtype is characterized by transepidermal elimination of the degenerate elastic tissue.[8,9]

Chondrodermatitis nodularis chronica helicis

Clinical features

Chondrodermatitis nodularis chronica helicis presents as a small, usually solitary, painful dome-shaped nodule on the helix of the ear, most commonly

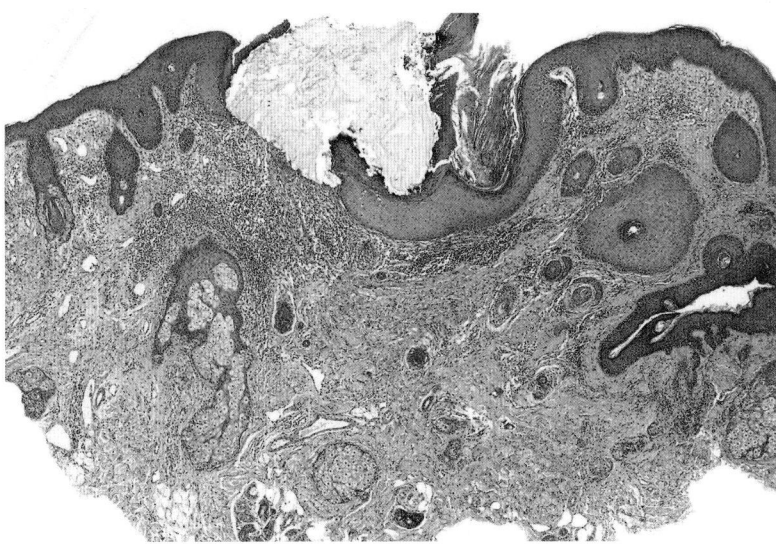

Fig. 9.137
Necrotizing infundibular crystalline folliculitis: note a craterlike area containing filamentous material.

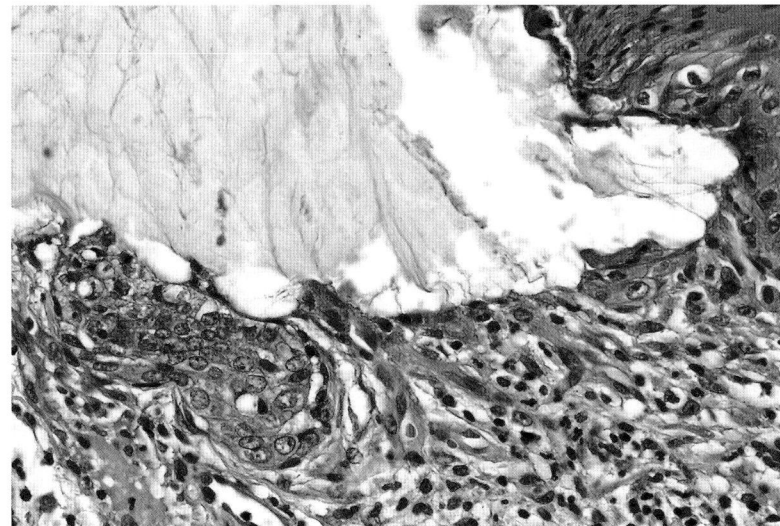

Fig. 9.138
Necrotizing infundibular crystalline folliculitis: filamentous material mimicking urate crystals.

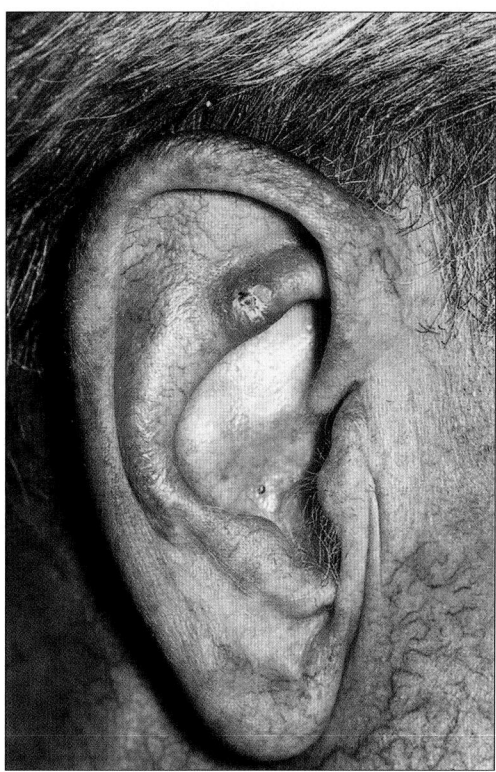

Fig. 9.139
Chondrodermatitis nodularis: this presents as a crusted lesion on the helix and may be clinically misdiagnosed as an epithelial neoplasm. By courtesy of R.A. Marsden, MD, St George's Hospital, London, UK.

in males over 40 years of age (mean age 60 years) and develops as a consequence of chronic trauma (*Fig. 9.139*).[1–3] Bilateral involvement is very rare.[4,5] The process is less common in women, when it is usually located on the antihelix. Cases in children are exceptional.[6] The pain is typically severe enough to wake the patient at night if the affected ear touches the pillow. In the majority of patients, symptoms are present for 2–3 years.[3]

On close examination, a firm crust with a small erosion or tiny channel underneath usually covers the nodule. Lesions measure 3–15 mm in diameter.[7] After surgical treatment, there is a recurrence rate of 20%. Chondrodermatitis is frequently mistaken for squamous cell or basal cell carcinoma, but the clinical history and auricular location should allow the diagnosis to be made without difficulty. Nevertheless, histologic confirmation is often necessary. An association with systemic sclerosis and childhood dermatomyositis has been reported.[8,9] A further study described an association with systemic vascular diseases and connective tissue diseases including lupus erythematosus and rheumatoid arthritis in a group of younger patients, with a predilection for females.[10]

Pathogenesis and histologic features

The etiology is multifactorial, but trauma is likely to be of primary importance. The exposed position of the ear, together with a known history of solar or physical trauma, appears important as many patients have outdoor jobs and evidence of solar damage elsewhere. Of historic interest, in the past there appeared to be a high frequency of cases in telephonists and nuns (wearing a wimple), again supporting the role of physical trauma to the ear. Other factors including cold, anatomical aberrations of the ear (such as a poor vascular supply), and senile degeneration of the cartilage may play a role in its development.[3] Recently, it has been suggested that the process is due to arteriolar narrowing in the perichondrial region of the pinna.[11] It is most unlikely, however, that the cartilaginous changes described below are anything other than secondary. An exceptional case described the simultaneous occurrence of the disease in middle-aged monozygotic twins.[12]

The pathogenetic mechanism of chondrodermatitis nodularis has been interpreted as representing the process of transepidermal elimination.[3] This phenomenon occurs when a disturbance in the dermis initiates an epidermal response. Foreign material in the dermis may elicit one of three responses:
- If the material is inert, there is no response.
- If the material is an irritant, either a superficial abscess or necrosis will develop.
- The material (in this case degenerate collagen) may be eliminated by a gradual process of transepidermal elimination.

Ulceration, although usual, may not be seen in early lesions.[3,7] The epithelium on either side of the ulcer is hyperplastic and shows features of lichen simplex chronicus (*Figs 9.140* and *9.141*). Pseudoepitheliomatous hyperplasia is occasionally evident.[7,13] Lesions have sometimes been shown to be related to the follicular infundibulum.[7] The crateriform ulcer contains keratinous and epidermal debris superimposed on a focus of fibrinoid necrosis of the underlying dermal collagen (*Fig. 9.142*). The base and radial edges of the lesion contain granulation tissue and a variable chronic inflammatory cell infiltrate, comprising lymphocytes, histiocytes, and occasional plasma cells (*Fig. 9.143*). Vascular thromboses and hair shaft fragments are sometimes evident.[7] Nerve hyperplasia may be found, and it has been suggested that this may explain the pain experienced by pressure.[14]

It is thought that the pathogenetic process at advanced stages of this disease represents the transepidermal or, occasionally, transfollicular

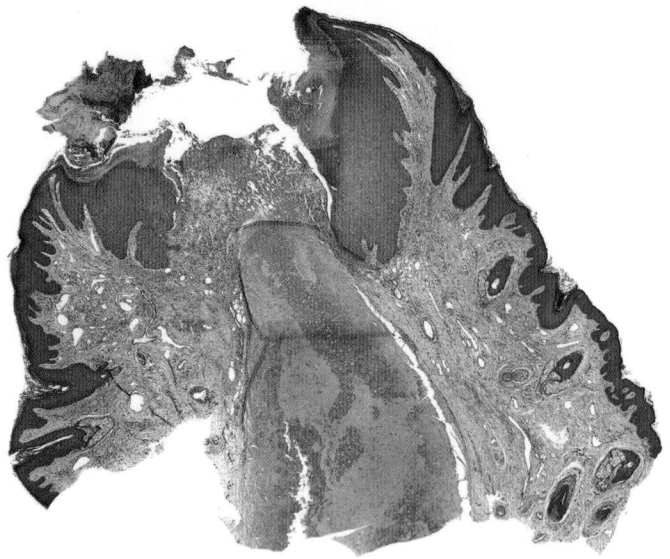

Fig. 9.140
Chondrodermatitis nodularis: this is a section through the center of the lesion showing ulceration. The adjacent epithelium is hyperkeratotic, parakeratotic, and acanthotic. There is chronically inflamed granulation tissue at the base of the lesion. Cartilage is evident in the center field.

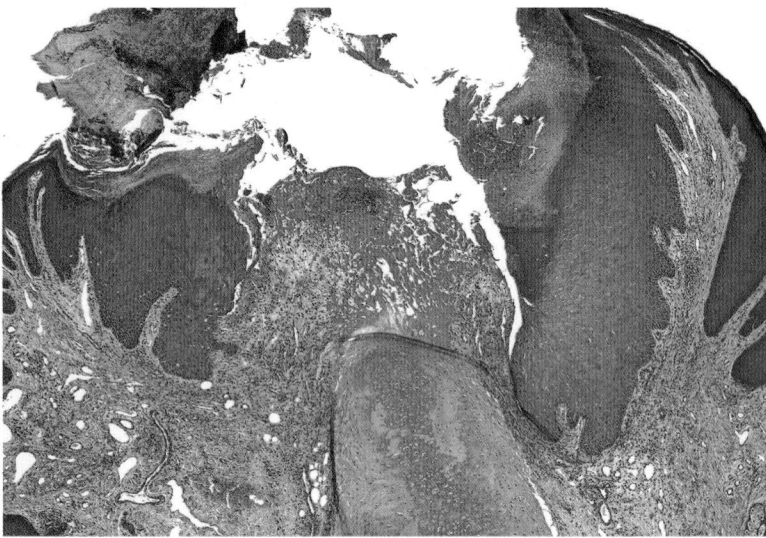

Fig. 9.141
Chondrodermatitis nodularis: there is abundant granulation tissue at the base and adjacent to the ulcer.

elimination of damaged collagen.[3,15] There are often degenerative changes present in the underlying cartilage, including hyalinization, tinctorial changes, and perichondritis. Occasionally, degenerate and fragmented cartilage may also be seen undergoing transepidermal elimination. The adjacent dermis often shows marked solar elastosis.[3]

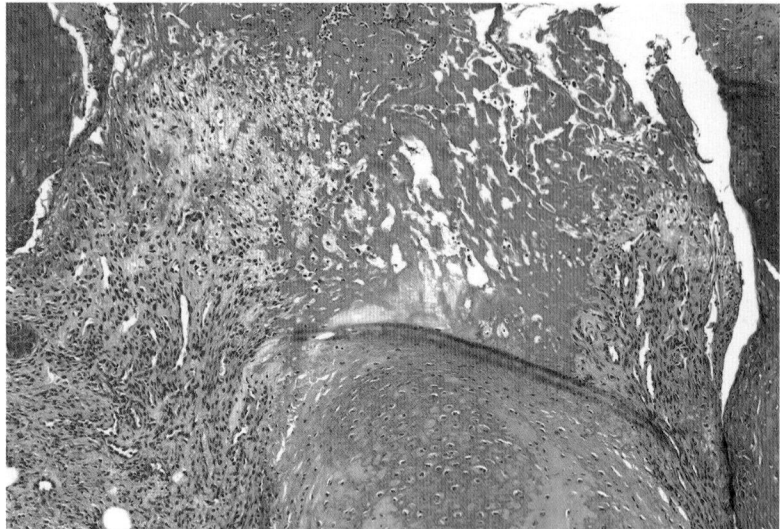

Fig. 9.142
Chondrodermatitis nodularis: note the fibrin and intensely eosinophilic degenerate cartilage.

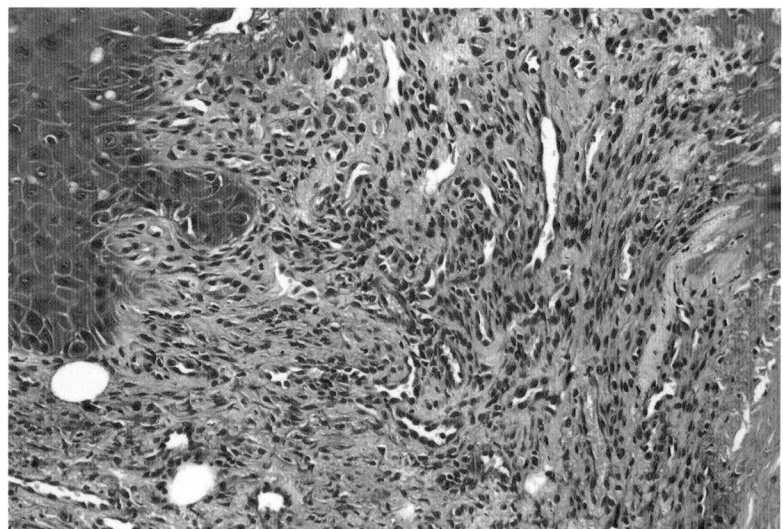

Fig. 9.143
Chondrodermatitis nodularis: high-power view of granulation tissue and inflammation.

Differential diagnosis

Punch biopsies, which show the characteristic layering of fibrin, granulation tissue, and degenerating cartilage, are diagnostic and distinctive. Often, superficial shave biopsies sample only fibrin and granulation tissue without cartilage. Nevertheless, if the clinical setting is appropriate, the diagnosis can still be suggested.

Access **ExpertConsult.com** for the complete list of references

See
www.expertconsult.com
for references and
additional material

Inflammatory diseases of the subcutaneous fat

Boštjan Luzar and Eduardo Calonje

CHAPTER

10

Inflammatory diseases of the subcutaneous fat are a source of considerable confusion and often cause diagnostic difficulty to clinicians and pathologists alike. This stems in part from the use of classifications and clinical descriptions based on time-honored but outdated literature.[1–4] Inadequate biopsy specimens are also a source of considerable difficulty, particularly the punch biopsy specimen, which often yields no subcutaneous fat at all. Similarly, histologic subdivision into diseases that affect the lobule and those that affect the septa is to some extent artifactual and sometimes unrewarding since most disorders affect both.[2,3,5] There is also a somewhat monotonous clinical presentation, with most patients complaining of deep-seated, variably tender or painful nodules, often affecting the lower extremities.

The subcutaneous fat has a limited repertoire of responses to noxious stimuli. Fat necrosis is a common manifestation of many forms of panniculitis and, as a consequence, there is often considerable histologic overlap. Although there are many variants of fat necrosis – including enzymatic, crystalline, suppurative, hyalinizing, and microcystic – lipophagic fat necrosis is the subtype most commonly encountered and is often a secondary feature in many forms of panniculitis (*Fig. 10.1*). This is characterized by a lobular infiltrate of histiocytes, xanthomatized cells, and foreign body giant cells, frequently accompanied by granulomata (*Fig. 10.2*).

It is important to remember that the subcutaneous fat may be involved in a secondary manner, for example, in the vasculitides, the deep cutaneous fungal infections, by metastatic tumor, and following surgery or radiotherapy (*Figs 10.3* and *10.4*). In this chapter, the panniculitides are classified, where possible, on an etiological basis (*Table 10.1*).

There is considerable histologic overlap in the various types of panniculitis, and one must take into account all the clinical information before attempting to reach a definitive diagnosis. In patients in whom the diagnosis of panniculitis is suspected, a deep surgical incisional biopsy is essential (*Fig. 10.5*). The punch biopsy has no role whatsoever in the diagnosis of panniculitis.

Erythema nodosum

Clinical features

Erythema nodosum represents the most common form of nodular panniculitis and is the prototype of septal panniculitis.[1,2] It is, of course, a clinical syndrome rather than a specific disease in its own right, representing a complex of symptoms and signs with multiple and very variable etiologies.[3,4] It typically affects young adults and shows a marked predilection for women (as high as 9:1 in some series). Children are only rarely affected.[5] Patients present with a sudden onset of bright red, warm, tender nodules; these typically affect the anterior and lateral aspects of the lower legs, but the arms, face, calves, and trunk are occasionally involved (*Figs 10.6* and *10.7*).[6,7] Involvement of the soles of the feet is rare, although it appears to be more often encountered in children.[8,9] The lesions are usually multiple, bilateral, symmetrically distributed, elevated above the skin surface, and measure 1–15 cm in diameter.[7] Ulceration and scarring are not features. Subsequently, the erythema fades to a bluish or livid hue and then to a yellow discoloration, reminiscent of a bruise (*Fig. 10.8*). The duration of the illness is 3–6 weeks. Patients sometimes also have pyrexia, malaise, and vague aches and pains in the joints. Laboratory findings may include a raised erythrocyte sedimentation rate (ESR), leukocytosis, and mild anemia.[3]

Two clinical variants have been described.

- Erythema nodosum migrans (subacute nodular migratory panniculitis, migratory panniculitis) is similar to classic erythema nodosum, but the lesions appear to migrate due to central clearing of established lesions and the development of new nodules at the periphery.[10–13] The lesions, which may persist for months or years, are usually associated with only mild symptoms.[10] Recurrences are sometimes encountered. Scarring is not a feature. This variant is typically asymmetrical, unilateral, and distributed solely on the leg. It also shows a marked female

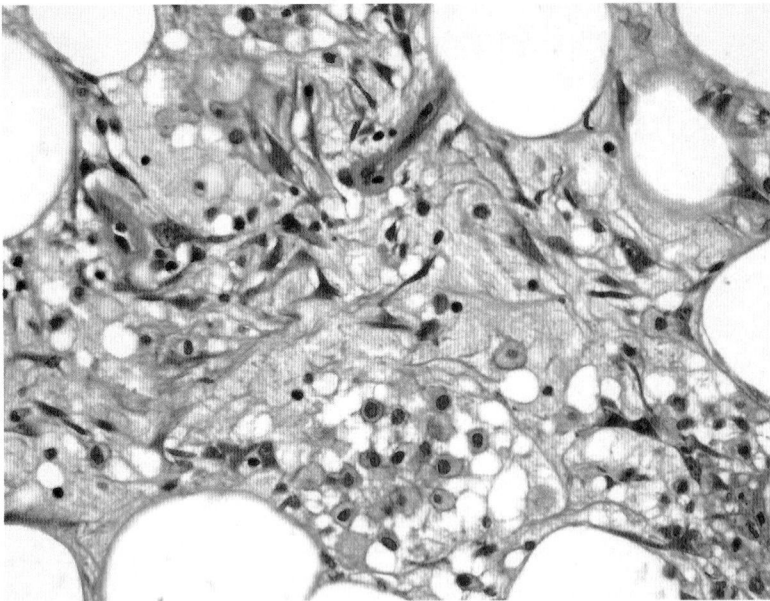

Fig. 10.1
Lipophagic fat necrosis: numerous xanthomatized histiocytes have engulfed free lipid following fat necrosis.

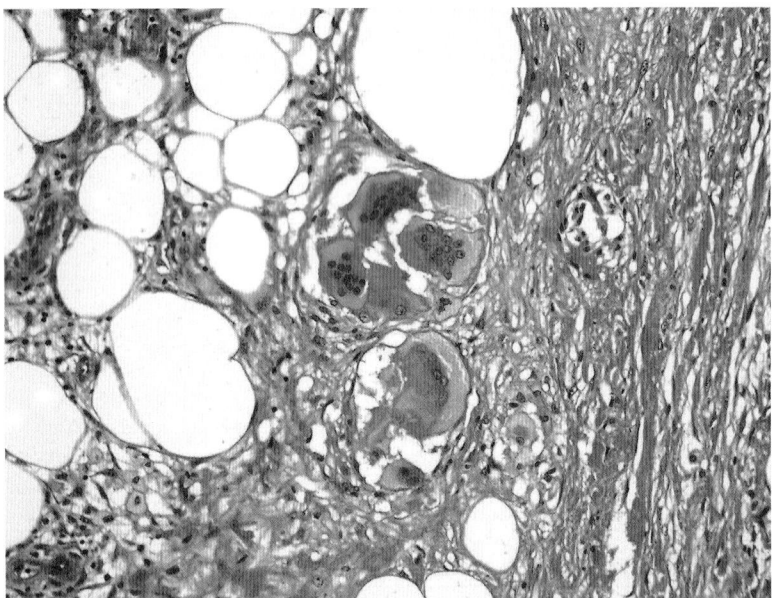

Fig. 10.2
Lipophagic fat necrosis: in this field xanthomatized multinucleated foreign body giant cells are present. Such an infiltrate is a common manifestation of many forms of panniculitis and merely reflects the presence of fat necrosis.

predominance (approximately 9:1), but tends to affect an older age group than classic erythema nodosum (mean age, 50 years).[11]

- Chronic erythema nodosum, a somewhat controversial entity, is characterized by the presence of nodules over a course of months or even years.[14] Otherwise, the clinical features appear indistinguishable from the more typical condition.

Pathogenesis and histologic features

The etiology and pathogenesis of erythema nodosum are unknown. Despite the very occasional finding of immunoreactants (IgM or IgG, and C3) in the blood vessel walls, an immune complex-mediated vasculitis is not considered likely.[6] It is probable that erythema nodosum represents a non-specific hypersensitivity reaction that involves delayed hypersensitivity mechanisms in addition to a type 3 component.

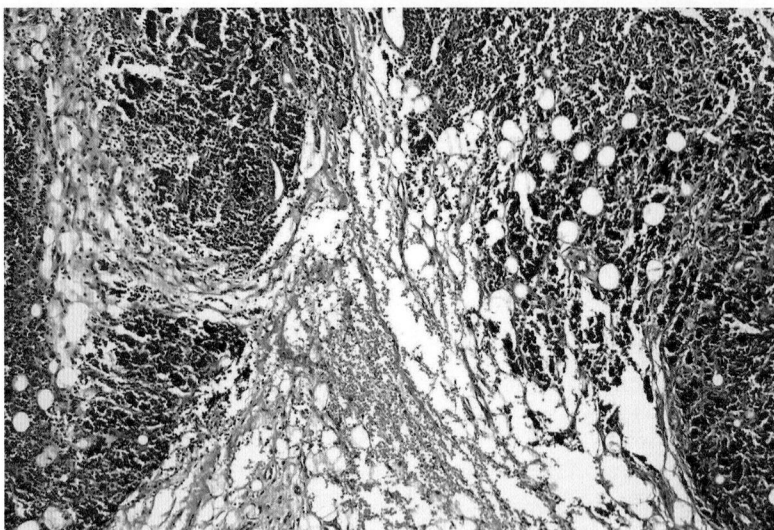

Fig. 10.3
'Malignant' panniculitis: this patient had a known history of bronchial small cell carcinoma and presented with a subcutaneous nodule on the chest wall.

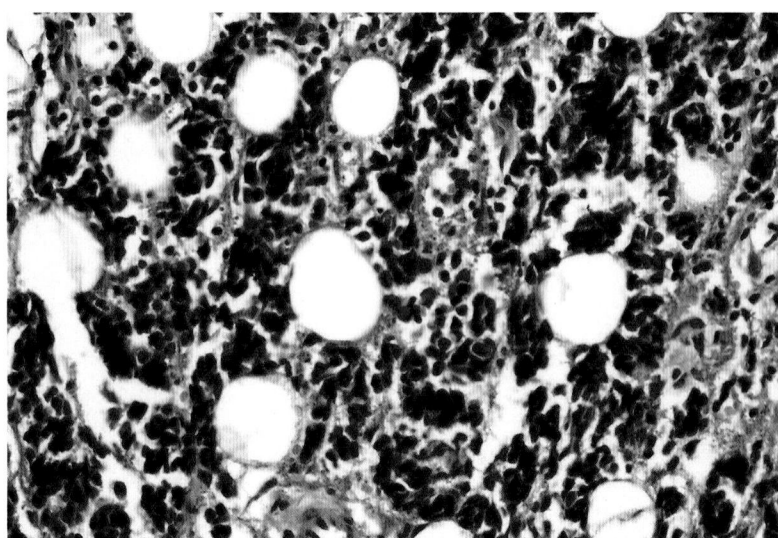

Fig. 10.4
'Malignant' panniculitis: high-power view showing basophilic tumor cells with hyperchromatic nuclei. Note the crush artifact.

There are many known associations. Although some are certainly of significance in the etiology of this dermatosis, many are probably coincidental (Table 10.2).[15–28] In the earlier part of the twentieth century, tuberculosis was noted in up to 90% of adult patients with erythema nodosum, but this is now found in less than 1% of cases. Today, the more frequent associations include streptococcal infections, sarcoidosis, ulcerative colitis and Crohn disease, Sweet syndrome, Behçet disease, menstruation, pregnancy, estrogens and the oral contraceptive, cat scratch disease, and various drug treatments (e.g., bromides, antibiotics, and sulfonamides). Other infectious conditions that have been described in association with erythema nodosum include cytomegalovirus, Epstein-Barr virus, parvovirus b19, *Yersinia*, *Mycoplasma*, *Brucella*, *Bartonella*, *Rickettsia*, *Cryptococcus*, *Salmonella*, *Shigella*, *Chlamydia*, *Chlamidophila pneumonia*, *Helicobacter pylori*, hepatitis B, atypical mycobacterial infections (e.g., swimming pool granuloma), meningococcal septicemia, Q fever, leptospirosis, syphilis, human immunodeficiency virus (HIV), kerion, histoplasmosis, blastomycosis, amebiasis, ascaris, *Staphylococcus xylosus*, *Sporothrix schenckii*, *Trichophyton mentagrophytes*, and giardiasis.[15,25–27,29–56] Simultaneous occurrence of erythema nodosum in monozygotic twins following streptococcal pharyngitis has also been reported.[57]

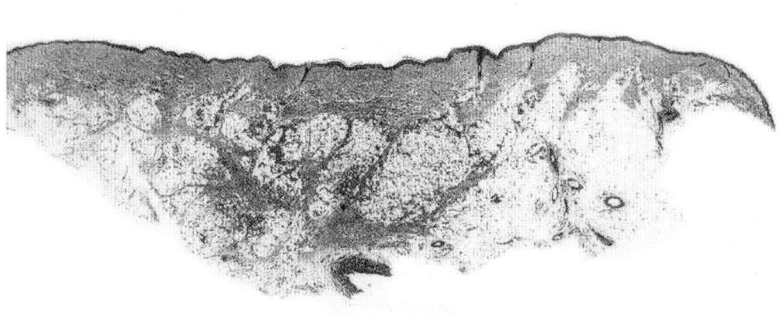

Fig. 10.5
Panniculitis: a deep surgical biopsy is essential in all cases where panniculitis is suspected.

Table 10.1
Classification of panniculitis

Mostly septal panniculitis
With vasculitis
Superficial thrombophlebitis
Cutaneous polyarteritis nodosa
Without vasculitis
Eryhtema nodosum
Necrobiotic xanthogranuloma
Rheumatoid nodule
Subcutaneous granuloma annulare
Necrobiosis lipoidica
Deep morphea
Whipple disease
Mostly lobular panniculitis
With vasculitis
Erythema nodosum leporosum
Lucio phenomenon
Erythema induratum of Bazin
Necrobiotic lobular panniculitis associated with rheumatoid arthritis
Crohn disease
Without vasculitis
Sclerosing panniculitis
Calciphylaxis
Sclerema neonatorum
Cold panniculitis
Lupus panniculitis
Pancreatic panniculitis
Alpha$_1$ – antitrypsin deficiency panniculitis
Infective panniculitis
Factitial and traumatic panniculitis
Subcutaneous sarcoidosis
Lipomembranous fat necrosis
Lipodystrophy/Lipoatrophy
Subcutaneous fat necrosis of the newborn
Poststeroid panniculitis
Sclerosing postirradiation panniculitis
Gout panniculitis
Oxalosis
Cytophagic histiocytic panniculitis
Others
Eosinophilic panniculitis

Adapted from Segura S and Requena L. (2008). Anatomy and histology of normal fat, necrosis of adipocytes and classification of panniculitis. Dermatol Clin, 26, 4119–424.

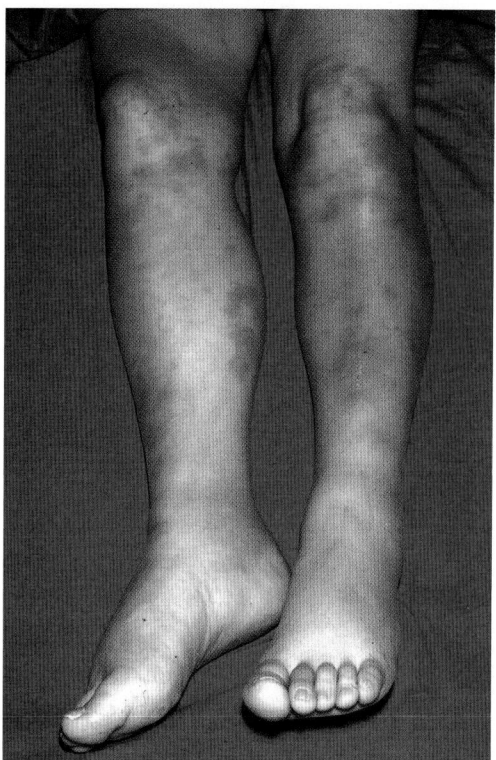

Fig. 10.6
Erythema nodosum: typical erythematous nodule on the shins of a young woman. From the collection of the late N.P. Smith, MD, the Institute of Dermatology, London, UK.

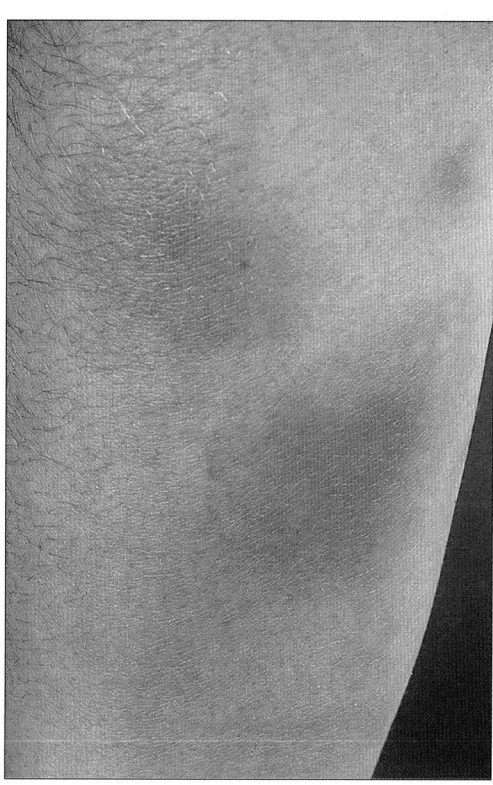

Fig. 10.7
Erythema nodosum: the lesions are raised and erythematous. By courtesy of the Institute of Dermatology, London, UK.

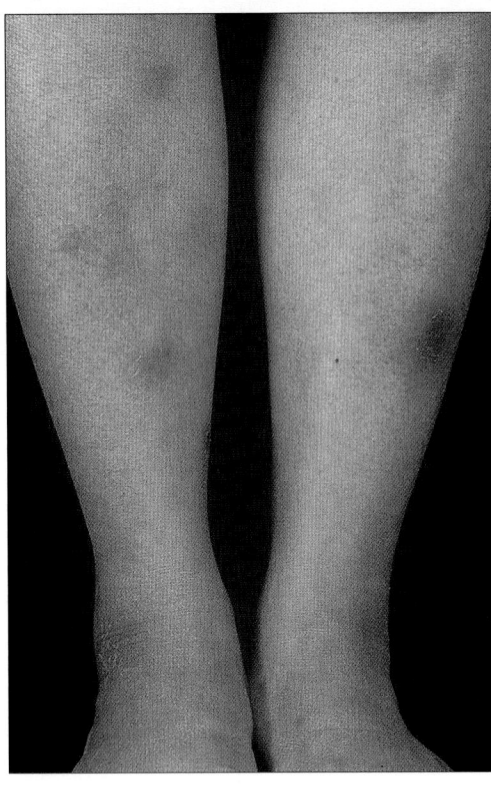

Fig. 10.8
Erythema nodosum: in this patient, the lesions are healing and show a characteristic bruiselike appearance. By courtesy of the Institute of Dermatology, London, UK.

Table 10.2
Erythema nodosum: etiology

Streptococcus	Sarcoidosis
Tuberculosis	Sweet syndrome
Chlamydophila psittaci	Cat scratch disease
Crohn disease	*Yersinia* infection
Drugs	Ulcerative colitis
Behçet disease	Malignancy

Additional drugs that have been implicated in the development of erythema nodosum include isotretinoin, interleukin (IL)-2, minocycline, thalidomide, echinacea, gold salts, vaccines (hepatitis B, tetanus-diphtheria-pertussis, cholera, human papillomavirus, malaria, rabies, small pox, tuberculosis, typhoid), all-*trans*-retinoic acid, capecitabine, azathioprine, aromatase inhibitors, cabergoline, valproate, terbinafine, BRAF inhibitors (vemurafenib, dabrafenib), sulfasalazine, anti-TNF therapy, and lidocaine.[16,58–78] Erythema nodosum has also been reported following a variety of malignancies including Hodgkin lymphoma, myelodysplastic syndrome, hairy cell leukemia, acute myeloid leukemia, acute myelomonocytic leukemia, diffuse large B-cell lymphoma, hypernephroma, non-small cell lung carcinoma, pheochromocytoma, carcinoid tumor, hepatocellular carcinoma, carcinomas of the colon, pancreas, and uterine cervix, and after radiotherapy.[79–96] In 20–30% of patients, no obvious cause is identified (idiopathic erythema nodosum).[2] Erythema nodosum in renal transplant recipients can be related to infections, malignancies, drugs, inflammatory bowel disease, or autoimmune diseases.[97]

Erythema nodosum has rarely been described in association with other diverse conditions, including idiopathic granulomatous mastitis, diverticulitis, pernicious anemia, Gianotti-Crosti syndrome, and autoimmune hepatitis.[98–107]

Erythema nodosum migrans seems to be particularly related to pregnancy, the oral contraceptive, streptococcal infection, and thyroid disease.[10–12]

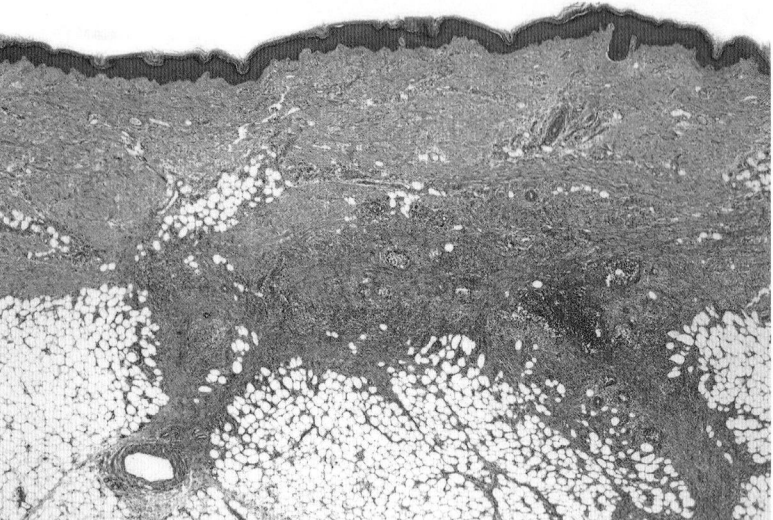

Fig. 10.9
Erythema nodosum: this example shows the classical appearance of septal inflammation with spread into the immediately adjacent lobule, giving rise to a lacelike appearance.

Many cases, however, have no obvious associated predisposing factors or conditions.

Histologically, erythema nodosum represents the prototype of septal panniculitis. It is characterized by a combination of features, including vascular change, septal inflammation, hemorrhage, and a variable degree of acute or chronic panniculitis (*Fig. 10.9*). Although it is often said that erythema nodosum characteristically affects the septal component of the panniculus, it should be noted that there is not infrequently involvement of the lobule, in part or in whole, particularly if older lesions are biopsied. In the past, cases of the latter might have been diagnosed as Weber-Christian disease.

Frank vasculitis is only very exceptionally encountered. When present, it involves the small veins, and very occasionally medium-sized vessels within the connective tissue septa.[108] It may be acute and necrotizing, associated with thrombosis and hemorrhage, or may manifest as chronic venular inflammation associated with endothelial cell swelling (*Figs 10.10* and *10.11*). The overlying dermis typically shows a perivascular and periadnexal chronic inflammatory cell infiltrate.

In the early stages, the septal inflammation may be acute, characterized by an infiltrate of neutrophil polymorphs, but this is soon replaced by lymphocytes and histiocytes (*Figs 10.12–10.14*).[109,110] Eosinophils are sometimes found, and rarely they can be conspicuous. Septal collections of histiocytes surrounding a cleftlike space (so-called Miescher radial granuloma) are said to be a characteristic feature, although they have been reported in Sweet syndrome, nodular vasculitis, and necrobiosis lipoidica (*Figs 10.15–10.17*).[2,111,112] Further progression leads to the development of a frankly granulomatous infiltrate in which giant cells may be conspicuous. Coagulation and caseation-like necrosis are never seen in erythema nodosum (compare with nodular vasculitis below). Sometimes the connective tissue in the fibrous septa shows fibrinoid necrosis, and hemorrhage is almost invariably present (*Figs 10.18–10.20*).

Characteristically, the septal infiltrate (lymphocytes, histiocytes, and granulomata) spills over to affect the periphery of the fat lobule to give a delicate lacy appearance, but fat necrosis is not usually present. On occasion, however, otherwise typical erythema nodosum may be associated with fat necrosis and a neutrophil inflammatory cell infiltrate (*Fig. 10.21*).[108,113]

If an older lesion is biopsied, septal fibrosis can sometimes be quite marked. Residual granulomatous inflammation is usually present.

Erythema nodosum migrans is characterized by densely scarred and thickened interlobular septa accompanied by a conspicuous granulomatous infiltrate (*Figs 10.22* and *10.23*). Numerous giant cells may be seen, and often they form a palisade along the septal borders. Granulation tissue-like vascular proliferation is often a conspicuous feature. Vasculitis is absent and hemorrhage is not usually seen.

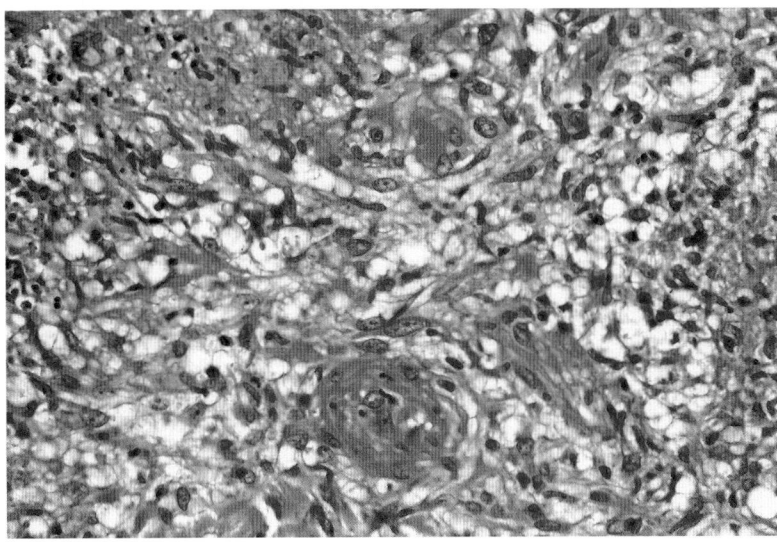

Fig. 10.10
Erythema nodosum: in the acute phase, venulitis is very occasionally present although many sections or levels must be examined before its presence is detected.

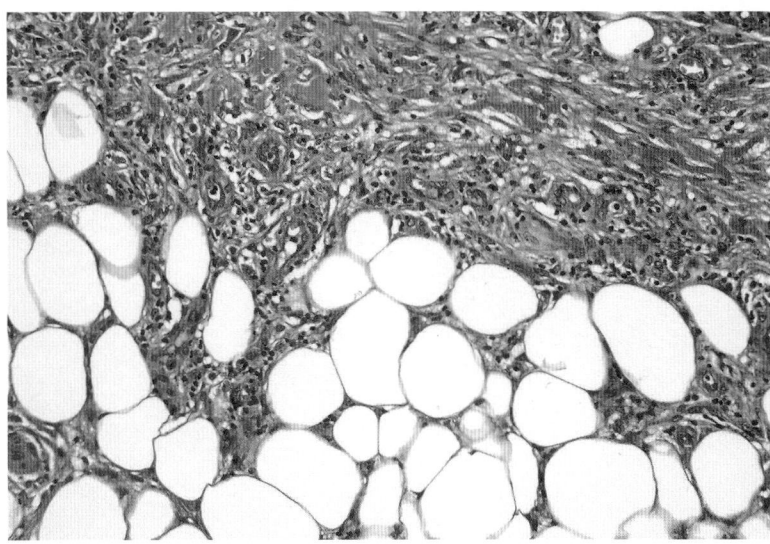

Fig. 10.13
Erythema nodosum: this view shows the interface between the septum and the lobule.

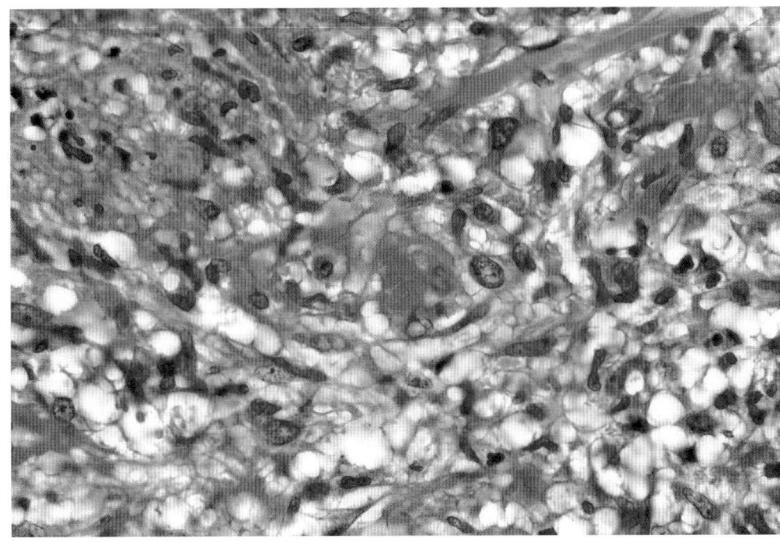

Fig. 10.11
Erythema nodosum: in this field there is a thrombosed venule associated with marked hemorrhage.

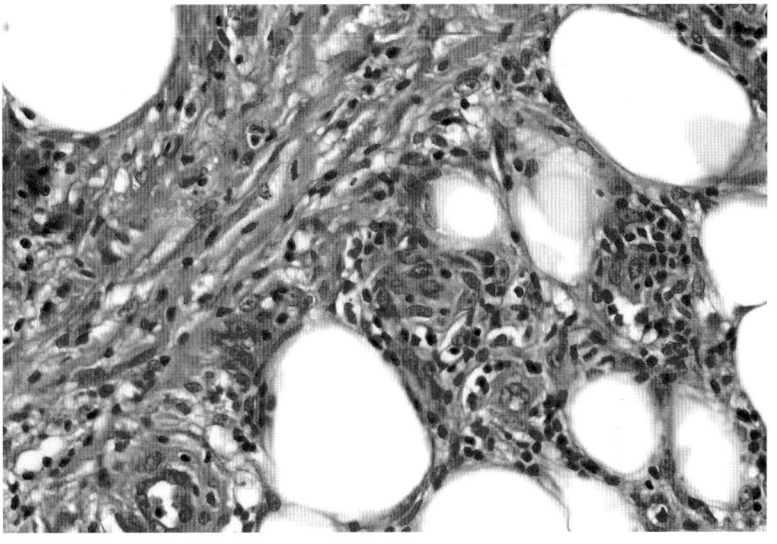

Fig. 10.14
Erythema nodosum: close-up view of cellular infiltrate.

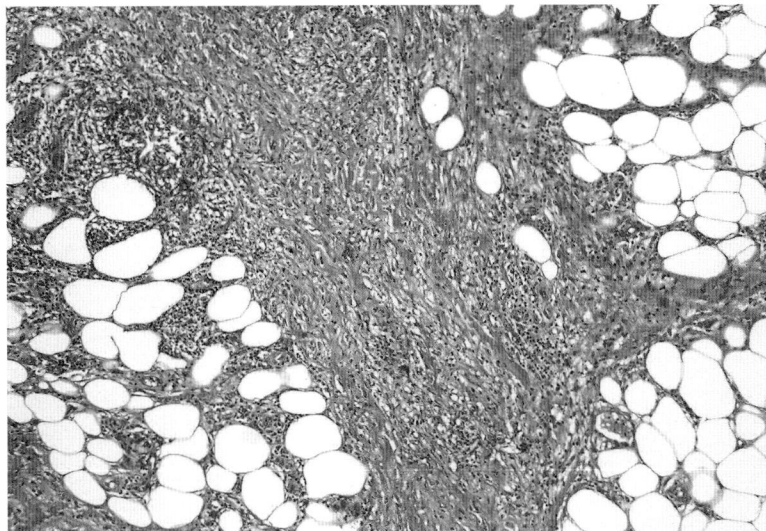

Fig. 10.12
Erythema nodosum: there is septal thickening with a lymphohistiocytic infiltrate.

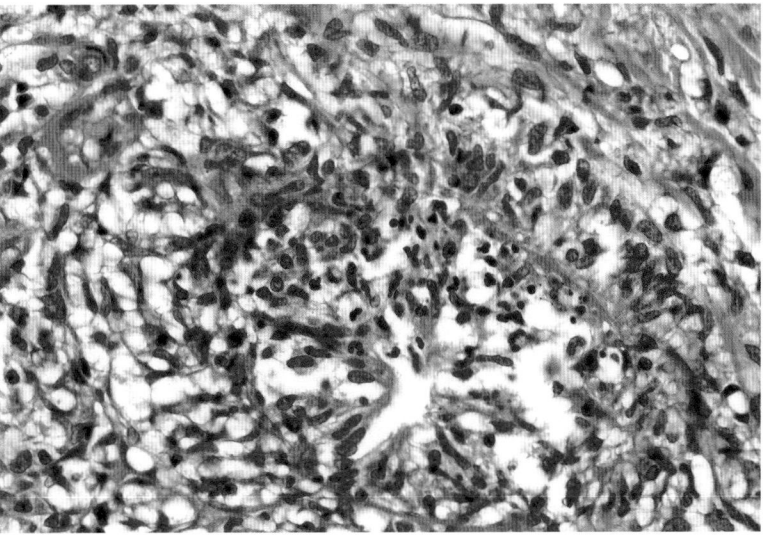

Fig. 10.15
Erythema nodosum: collections of histiocytes known as Miescher granulomata are a common finding. Fibrinoid necrosis affecting a small venule is also present.

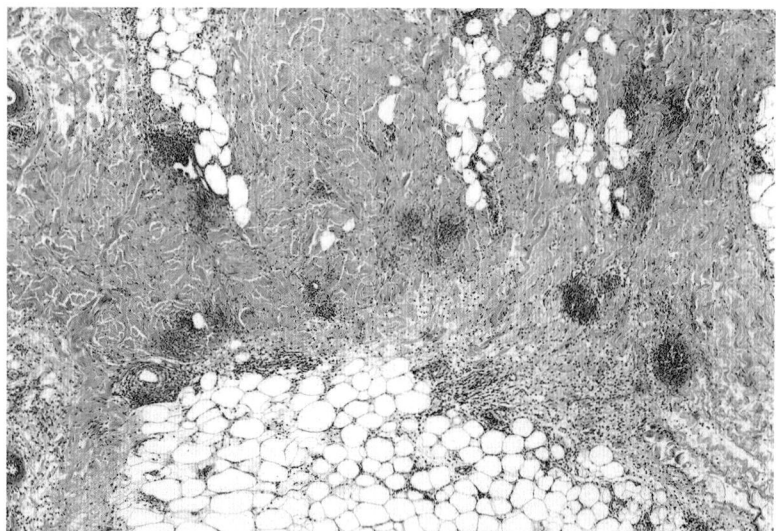

Fig. 10.16
Erythema nodosum: in this example, multiple small granulomata are evident in the thickened septa.

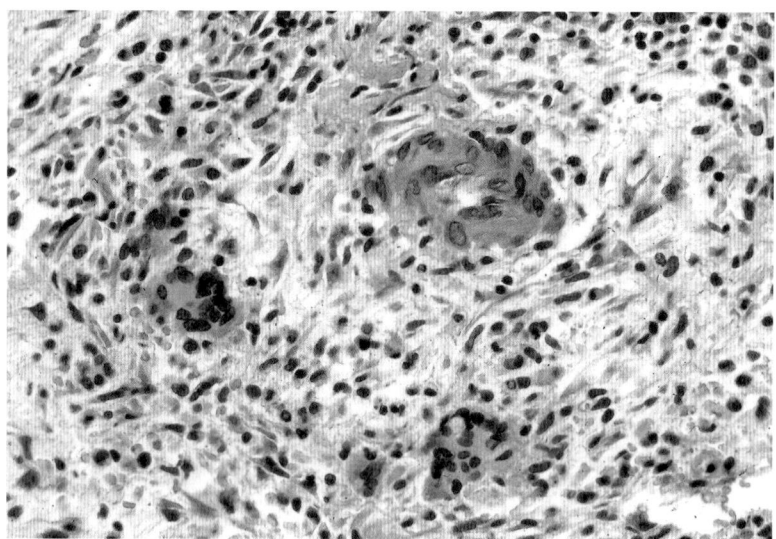

Fig. 10.17
Erythema nodosum: high-power view of granulomata.

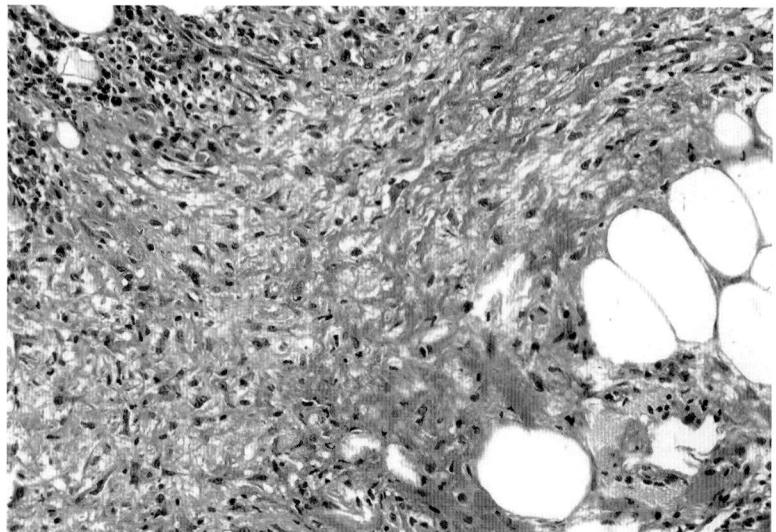

Fig. 10.18
Erythema nodosum: fibrinoid necrosis of the connective tissue septa is an occasional feature.

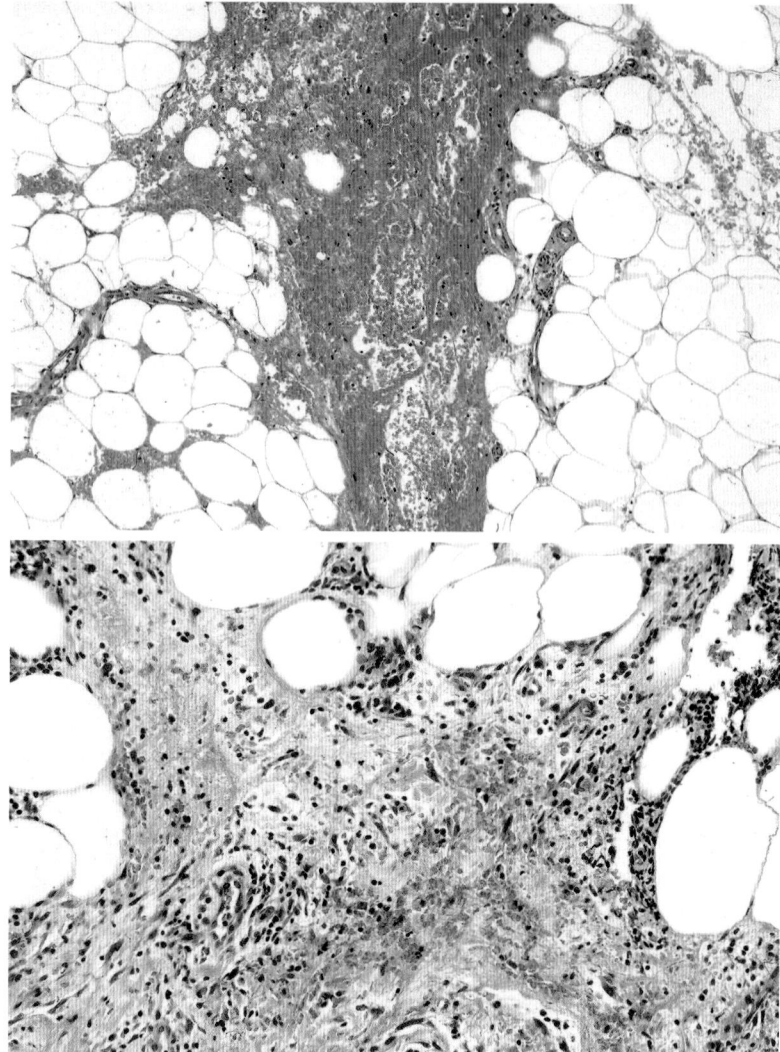

Fig. 10.19
Erythema nodosum: there is marked red cell extravasation.

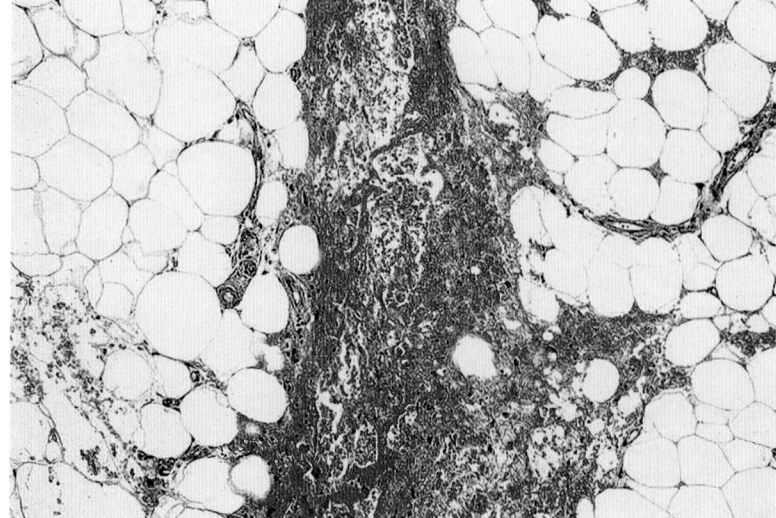

Fig. 10.20
Erythema nodosum: in this example there is massive hemorrhage. Subsequent breakdown with hemosiderin formation accounts for the clinical appearance of bruising.

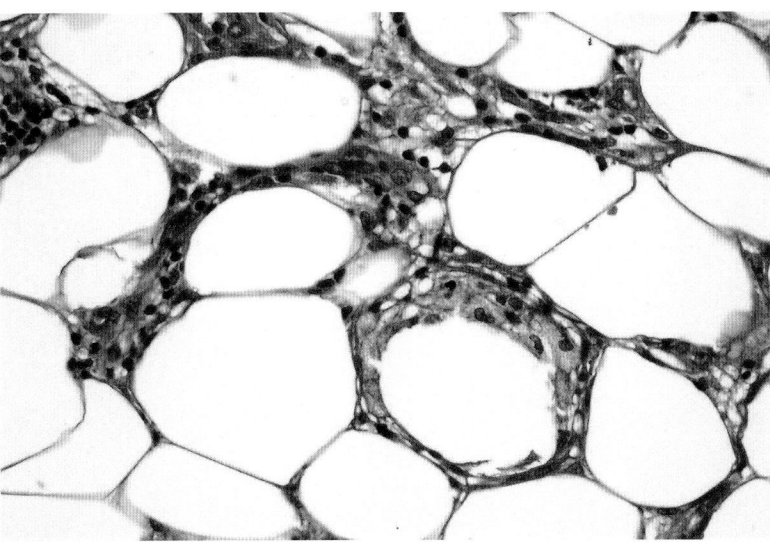

Fig. 10.21
Erythema nodosum: focal fat necrosis associated with lipid-laden histiocytes.

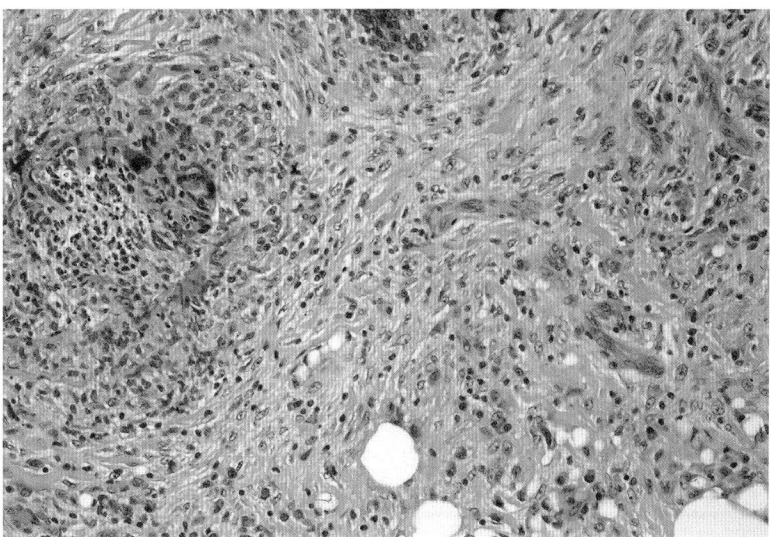

Fig. 10.23
Erythema nodosum migrans: close-up view showing granulomata and newly formed blood vessels.

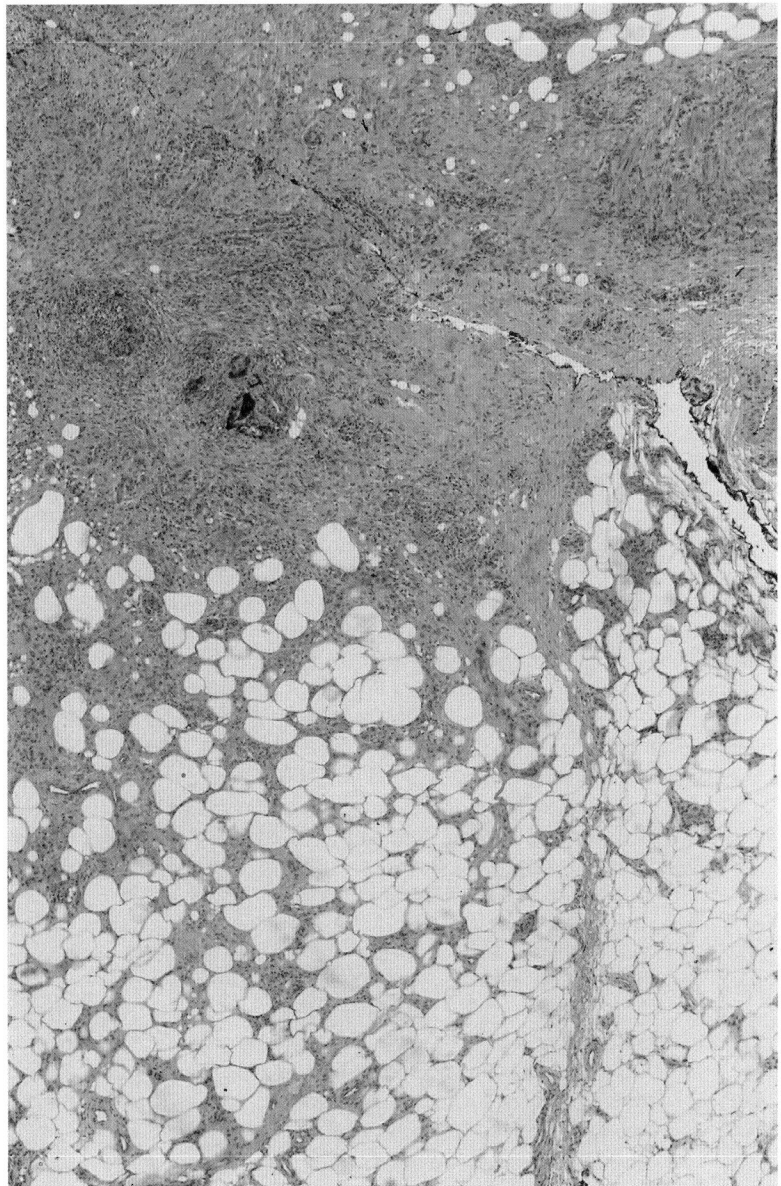

Fig. 10.22
Erythema nodosum migrans: there is marked septal thickening with conspicuous granulomata. Granulation tissue extends into the adjacent lobule.

In chronic erythema nodosum, the histologic changes are similar to, but usually milder, than those of the acute variant.[11]

Differential diagnosis

At scanning magnification, vasculitic processes affecting the septa of the subcutaneous fat may be mistaken for erythema nodosum. Occasionally, the features of leukocytoclastic vasculitis are seen within the septa in the absence of the more usual superficial dermal involvement.[114] Such instances present as erythematous nodules, usually affecting the lower legs. Similarly, superficial thrombophlebitis presents within the subcutaneous fat septa. In this condition, however, the vein is the focus of the inflammatory process with associated thrombosis, and there is little or no involvement of the lobule. Cutaneous polyarteritis nodosa affects muscular arteries within the lower dermis and subcutaneous fat septa and, therefore, should not be confused with erythema nodosum.[114] Nephrogenic systemic fibrosis can rarely be associated with mild septal mononuclear cell infiltrates and granulomata, thereby simulating erythema nodosum.[115]

Erythema nodosum-like lesions in Behçet disease

Recurrent erythematous, tender, nodular lesions on the lower extremities (clinically reminiscent of erythema nodosum) are a common manifestation of Behçet disease.[1-6] Erythema nodosum-like lesions develop in more than 40% of the patients during the course of the disease.[7] Erythema nodosum-like lesions and superficial thrombophlebitis could represent predictive markers for visceral involvement.[8] Furthermore, male patients with erythema nodosum-like lesions in Behçet disease have an increased risk for deep vein thrombosis.[9]

The fronts of the shins are most often affected, but lesions may also occur on the arms, face, neck, and buttocks.[2] Although histologically they have been described as showing erythema nodosum-like features, more commonly they are characterized by a lobular or mixed septal and lobular panniculitis associated with a neutrophil-rich infiltrate, neutrophilic vasculitis (affecting arterioles and venules), and associated fat necrosis.[2,10] Less often, a lymphocytic vasculitis and, exceptionally, polyarteritis nodosa-like features are encountered. Miescher granulomata may sometimes be present.[2,11]

A recent study of 26 patients with Behçet disease and erythema nodosum-like lesions classified histologic changes into those indistinguishable from conventional erythema nodosum (27% of the lesions), and erythema nodosum-like lesions with vasculitis (venulitis or phlebitis).[12] In contrast to previous reports, arteries or arterioles were not involved in the vasculitic process.[12] Patients with lesions indistinguishable from erythema nodosum were associated with a mild clinical course of Behçet disease, while those with severe vasculitis were at risk to develop gastrointestinal tract involvement.[12]

Weber-Christian disease

As originally defined by Christian in 1928 (relapsing febrile nodular non-suppurative panniculitis), this disorder was characterized by recurrent attacks of fever associated with the development of subcutaneous tender nodules (particularly over the extremities), which were histologically characterized by the presence of nonsuppurative panniculitis which healed to leave a depressed scar.[1-4] Lesions were said to affect mainly young white females, and although the lower extremities were predominantly affected, the upper extremities, buttocks, abdominal wall, breasts, and face could also be involved. Arthritis, arthralgias, and myalgias were often present.[3] A systemic variant – which was potentially fatal and affected the intestines, mesentery, lungs, heart, and kidneys – was also recognized.[3,5-11] A presumed case of Weber-Christian disease developing during pregnancy has also been reported.[12]

Since 1928, there have been many case reports in the literature dealing with this so-called 'specific disease'. In general, however, many of the (particularly earlier) studies used imprecise clinical and histologic diagnostic criteria. Some were certainly examples of erythema nodosum. In the light of current knowledge of the panniculitides, many cases would now be reclassified. A Weber-Christian-like disease may be seen in erythema nodosum, factitial panniculitis, lupus panniculitis, pancreatic fat necrosis-associated panniculitis, α1-antitrypsin deficiency-associated panniculitis, connective tissue diseases, infectious panniculitis (e.g., *Mycobacterium chelonae*), subcutaneous panniculitic T-cell lymphoma, and gamma-delta T-cell lymphoma.[13-23] The term has also been applied to cases of infective panniculitis, and panniculitis following jejunoileal bypass surgery.[24-27]

It seems unlikely, therefore, that Weber-Christian disease represents a distinct entity in its own right. It is proposed, therefore, to take this opportunity to bury it once and for all. As suggested by Patterson, 'a clinical diagnosis of Weber-Christian disease should signal the beginning of a search for the true cause of the disorder'.[16] Likewise, the term Rothmann-Makai syndrome should be abandoned.[28] More often than not, it probably represents erythema nodosum.

α1-Antitrypsin deficiency-associated panniculitis

Clinical features

Deficiency of α1-antitrypsin is associated with a severe and particularly intractable form of panniculitis.[1-14] Patients have recurrent episodes of painful or tender nodules which are particularly resistant to therapy. The disease shows a slight male predominance (3:2), and although a wide age range can be affected (7–73 years), most patients are in their fourth or fifth decade.[5,7] Children, however, may occasionally be affected.[5] The nodules, which are often precipitated by trauma, develop most often on the trunk and proximal extremities, but the buttocks, chest, back, and abdomen are sometimes also affected (*Fig. 10.24*). Occasionally, the disease spreads to the genitalia, and involvement of the abdominal fat has been described. Panniculitis can exceptionally be the presenting sign of α1-antitrypsin deficiency.[15]

The nodules may be erythematous and are frequently associated with ulceration and the spontaneous discharge of clear, serosanguinous, or oily fluid.[5] Deeply penetrating sinuses associated with liquefaction of the subcutaneous tissues are an important complication. Extensive necrosis with development of a polycyclic ulcer mimicking pyoderma gangrenosum has also been reported.[16]

Fever is a common accompaniment, and patients often have pulmonary problems including panacinar emphysema, chronic obstructive pulmonary disease, effusions, and embolic phenomena.[5,17] Peripheral edema and anasarca are occasional manifestations. This is a particularly severe form of panniculitis, which has been successfully treated by the use of infusions of commercial α1-antitrypsin concentrate or liver transplantation.[5,9,18,19] It is thought that many of the previously reported cases of Weber-Christian disease belong to this group.[20]

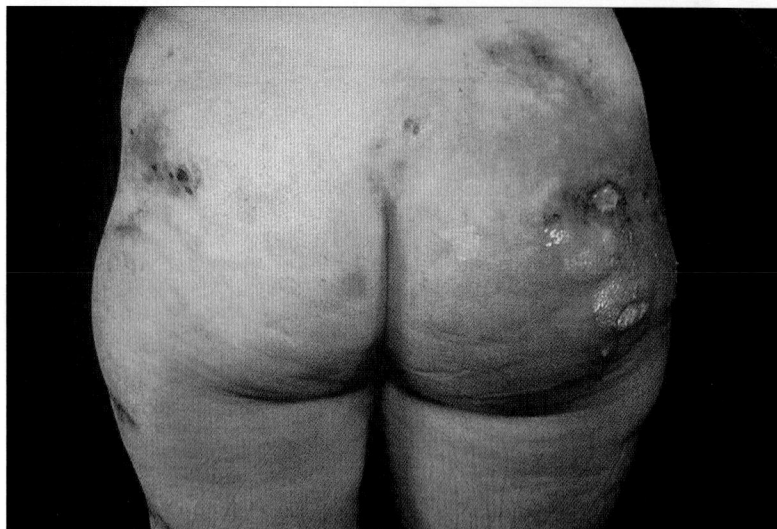

Fig. 10.24
α1-Antitrypsin deficiency-associated panniculitis: note the extensive involvement of the buttocks in this young female. By courtesy of M.R. Pittelkow, MD, Mayo Clinic, Rochester, Minnesota, USA.

Panniculitis in association with α1-antitrypsin deficiency has been induced by cryosurgery,[21] pregnancy, cesarean section delivery, and clarithromycin leak at the site of intravenous application.[19,21-23] In one patient with the enzyme defect, Sweet syndrome was followed by the development of acquired cutis laxa (Marshall syndrome).[24] An acquired α1-antitrypsin deficiency panniculitis following liver transplantation has been reported, which was successfully treated with retransplantation of the liver.[25]

Pathogenesis and histologic features

α1-Antitrypsin (a glycoprotein of hepatic derivation) is a serine protease inhibitor (PI) that greatly modifies the effects of proteolytic enzymes, accounting for at least 90% of serum proteolytic enzyme inhibition. In addition to antitrypsin inhibition, it is also responsible for inhibition of proteinase 3, cathepsin G, α-defensins, chymotrypsin, collagenase, elastase, granzyme B, plasmin, thrombin, plasminogen activators 1 and 2, factor VIII, factor Xa, and kallikreins 7 and 14.[7,26] Its deficiency has been associated with panacinar emphysema, noninfective (neonatal and adult) hepatitis, and cirrhosis. More recently, associations have also been described with cutaneous vasculitis, atopic dermatitis, psoriasis, nodular prurigo, and cold urticaria.[27] It has been proposed that absence of the protease inhibitor is associated with unrestrained complement activation with increased inflammatory cell activity, endothelial injury, and resultant autolytic tissue damage.[28]

Immunoglobulin (IgM) and complement (C3) have been identified in blood vessel walls in patients with this variant of panniculitis.[6] The significance of this is uncertain.

The gene for α1-antitrypsin on chromosome 14 has in excess of 100 alleles and is inherited as an autosomal dominant.[7,15] Deficiency occurs in between 1:3000 and 1:5000 of white North Americans.[29] The genotypes are classified based on the speed of migration on electrophoresis gel (M = median, S = slow, and Z = very small).[15] The MM genotype is most common, and individuals with normal activity are coded PiMM. The ZZ genotype is associated with deficient α1-antitrypsin activity and the panniculitis is usually found in PiZZ individuals.[30] Instances of panniculitis in PiMZ, PiSZ, PiMS, PiSS, and Null patients, however, have also been recorded.[31-34] Panniculitis may also develop as a consequence of dysfunctional α1-antitrypsin.[34,35] Recognition of this particular form is of importance as serum α1-antitrypsin levels are normal and therefore the diagnosis can easily be missed.

The earliest changes consist of necrosis of the connective tissue in the reticular dermis and septa of the subcutaneous fat accompanied by a neutrophil polymorph inflammatory cell infiltrate (*Fig. 10.25*).[36] The histologic features of an established lesion are those of a predominantly acute panniculitis (*Fig. 10.26*). The changes, which affect the septa and the paraseptal

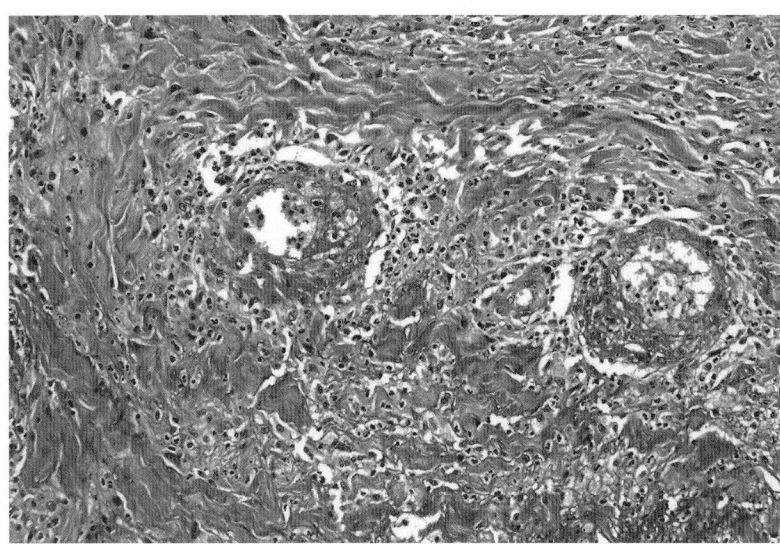

Fig. 10.25
α_1-Antitrypsin deficiency-associated panniculitis: early lesion showing necrosis and acute inflammation of the deep reticular dermis. Blood vessels are also affected. By courtesy of M.R. Pittelkow, MD, Mayo Clinic, Rochester, USA.

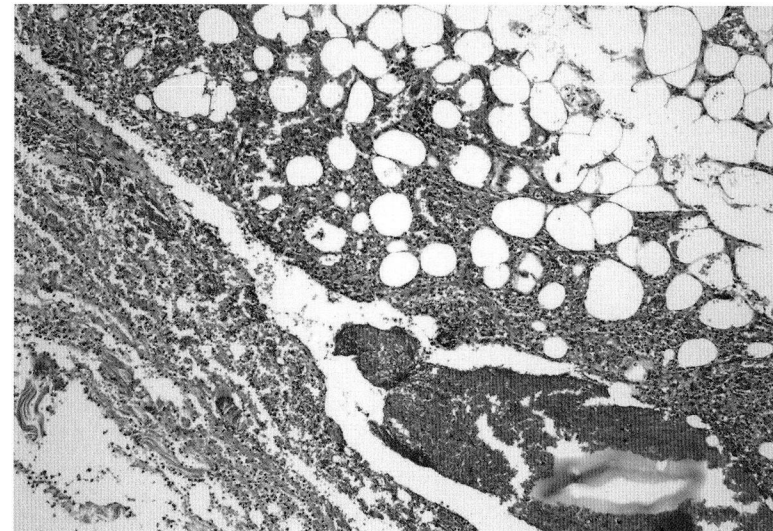

Fig. 10.27
α_1-Antitrypsin deficiency-associated panniculitis: in this field hemorrhage is evident in addition to the inflammatory changes. By courtesy of M.R. Pittelkow, MD, Mayo Clinic, Rochester, USA.

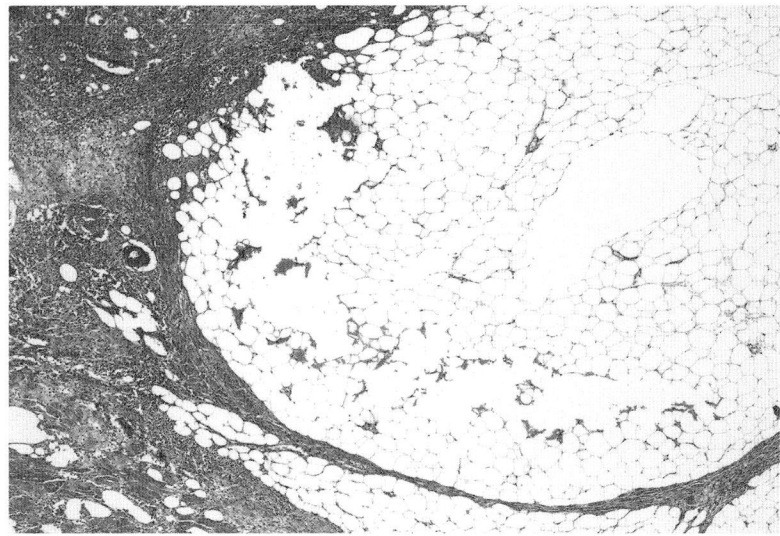

Fig. 10.26
α_1-Antitrypsin deficiency-associated panniculitis: there is intense acute inflammation extending from the septum into the edge of the lobule. Note the necrosis of the adjacent dermal connective tissue. By courtesy of M.R. Pittelkow, MD, Mayo Clinic, Rochester, USA.

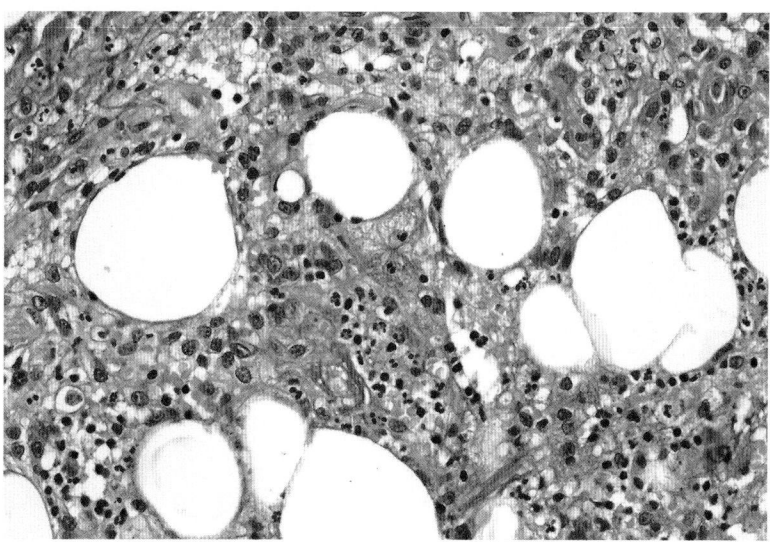

Fig. 10.28
α_1-Antitrypsin deficiency-associated panniculitis: high-power view showing an intense neutrophil infiltrate. By courtesy of M.R. Pittelkow, MD, Mayo Clinic, Rochester, USA.

aspect of the lobule, are characteristically focal in nature. In acutely inflamed areas, large numbers of neutrophil polymorphs infiltrate the lobule. Fat necrosis is common, and a characteristic feature is said to be the presence of normal fat adjacent to necrotic and inflamed fat (*Figs 10.27* and *10.28*).[6,37] Special stains often show fragmentation and loss of elastic tissue.[6] Z-type α_1-antitrypsin polymers have been demonstrated in the lesional as well as unaffected fatty tissue by immunohistochemistry in a single patient.[38] Foci of hemorrhage associated with vascular thrombosis may be present, but there is no evidence of active vasculitis (*Fig. 10.29*).[6] Elsewhere, a histiocytic infiltrate is conspicuous, involving both the deep vasculature and adjacent panniculus. Lipid-laden foamy macrophages are sometimes evident and multinucleate giant cells are occasionally found. Healing is by scarring.

Differential diagnosis

The clinical features may suggest traumatic or factitial panniculitis. The heavy neutrophil infiltrate can cause diagnostic confusion with an infectious etiology.[10] In cases of doubt, special stains for microorganisms should be performed.

Factitial and traumatic panniculitis

Clinical features

Factitial panniculitis is by definition self-induced and vigorously denied, and may be caused by mechanical, physical, or chemical means. The diagnosis is always worth considering in those patients with bizarre clinical lesions and inflammatory changes in the subcutaneous fat that defy ready classification. It should be particularly sought in those patients with panniculitis who have a known history of psychiatric illness or drug or alcohol abuse. Lesions are most commonly found on the more accessible sites including the buttocks and thighs.

Mechanical causes include local pressure and repeated blunt trauma; the latter may be readily recognized by the presence of obvious bruising. Cold is another possible cause of factitial panniculitis.

By far the most common etiology is the subcutaneous injection of chemical substances including drugs, oily materials, and organic matter.[1-4] Panniculitis has been described as a complication of morphine and tetanus antitoxoid injections. Similarly, repeated injections of pentazocine cause a

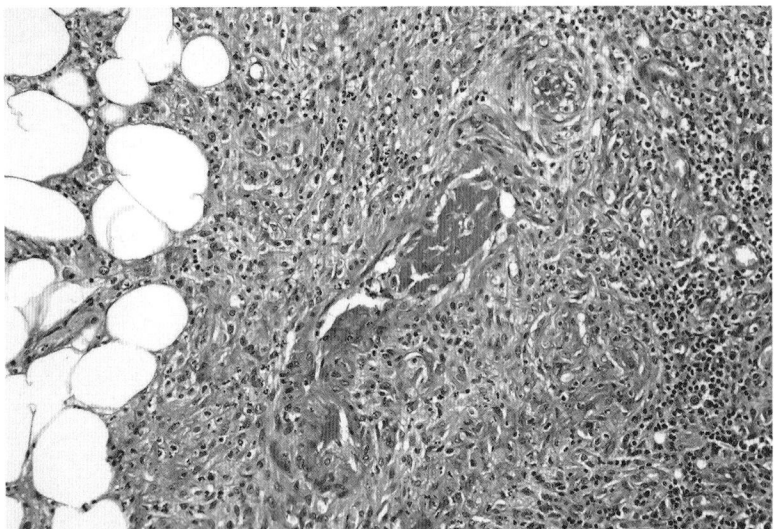

Fig. 10.29
α_1-Antitrypsin deficiency-associated panniculitis: note the organizing thrombus. By courtesy of M.R. Pittelkow, MD, Mayo Clinic, Rochester, USA.

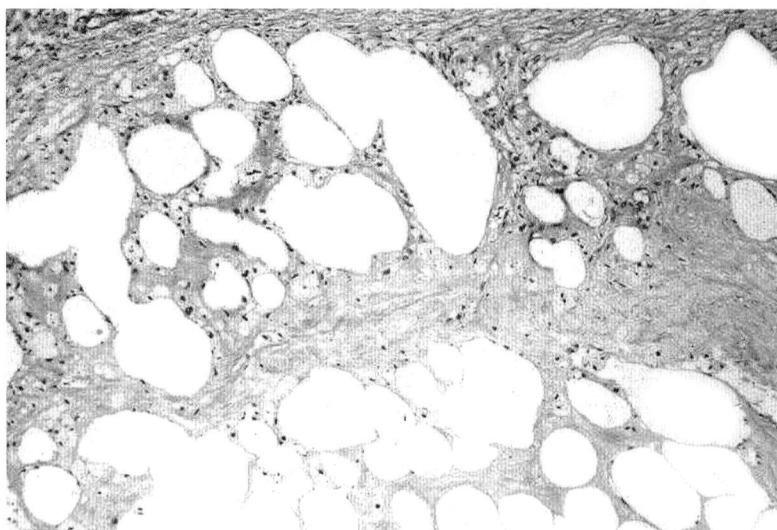

Fig. 10.31
Paraffinoma: empty spaces of variable size (due to the removal of lipid during processing) characterize this lesion. The appearance is often likened to Swiss cheese.

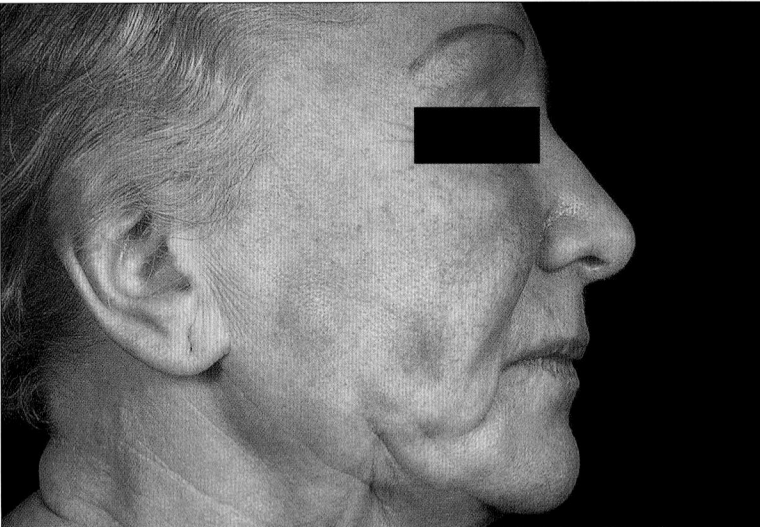

Fig. 10.30
Paraffinoma: note the infiltrated plaque with foci of retraction. By courtesy of the Institute of Dermatology, London, UK.

characteristic woody fibrosis of the skin and subcutaneous fat accompanied by deeply penetrating ulcers and hyperpigmented halos.[5–7] Pentazocine abuse has been described, particularly in members of the medical profession.[5] There appears to be a relationship with a personal or family history of diabetes mellitus. It has been suggested that peripheral ischemia may be the pathogenetic link.[7] A similar problem has been described following injections of the opioid ketobemidone.[8]

An important cause of factitial panniculitis is the repeated injection of oily materials including paraffin and liquid silicon (paraffinoma, sclerosing lipogranuloma, lipogranulomatous panniculitis) (*Fig. 10.30*).[1,2,4,9–13] Sclerosing lipogranuloma was a condition usually seen in the male genitalia that developed as a consequence of the injection of paraffin oil and related compounds into the penis in the mistaken belief that this would enhance erections. Povidone (polyvinylpyrrolidone), a synthetic dispersing or suspending agent which has been used in both pharmaceutical products and hair sprays, may result in a particular characteristic histologic variant of panniculitis.[14,15] Associated features have included pulmonary lesions, lymphadenopathy, and hepatosplenomegaly. Organic substances that have been implicated in the etiology of factitial panniculitis include food matter, milk, and even feces.

Nodular cystic fat necrosis is a distinct posttraumatic lesion that is seen predominantly in adolescent boys and middle-aged women. Lesions, which are usually found on the legs, are often associated with a history of trauma.[16] A freely moving nodule(s) is often found on clinical examination.

Traumatic fat necrosis is a not uncommon condition and occurs predominantly in middle-aged or elderly females with large pendulous breasts. Its importance is that it may be clinically mistaken for a malignancy. In addition, it can be seen to involve the arms, trunk, buttocks, and thighs of the very obese.

A number of therapeutic injections have been associated with the development of panniculitis including interferon-beta (IFN-β),[17–21] glatiramer acetate,[22–24] nadroparin calcium,[25] and granulocyte-colony stimulating factor.[26] Aluminum granuloma may present as a panniculitis (see Chapter 14). Panniculitis has also been documented following vitamin K₁ injections.[27] Two patients with factitial panniculitis caused by electroacupuncture have been described.[28]

Pathogenesis and histologic features

The histologic features of factitial panniculitis are not usually specific and depend to some extent upon the cause. In some instances, therefore, the changes are those of acute lobular inflammation associated with fat necrosis and a neutrophil polymorph infiltrate. In older lesions, mononuclear cells, lipid-laden histiocytes, and foreign body giant cells become predominant and sometimes the response becomes frankly granulomatous. On other occasions the septa may be primarily affected, thereby mimicking erythema nodosum.[2] Calcification is occasionally evident.[2] It is sometimes rewarding to view the sections with polarized light, as birefractile material may be identified, raising the possibility of the factitious nature of the condition.

Paraffinoma is characterized by the presence of round or oval spaces within the dermis and subcutaneous fat ('Swiss cheese' pattern) (*Fig. 10.31*); careful examination may reveal foamy histiocytes or giant cells lining the edges of these cystic cavities (*Fig. 10.32*).[9] There is often associated dense fibrous scarring. Early lesions sometimes show a marked granulomatous component.[9] Similar features have been described following a grease gun injury.[29]

In panniculitis due to pentazocine abuse, the histologic features include dense dermal fibrosis accompanied by variable scarring of the subcutaneous fat.[5] A 'Swiss cheese' appearance may be evident. Small-vessel thrombosis is frequently present.[5]

Povidone panniculitis is characterized by histiocytic accumulation of gray-blue, Congo red-positive foamy material accompanied by necrosis and hemorrhage.[14]

Lesions caused by blunt trauma show the features of an organizing hematoma. Granulomata and foci of hemosiderin pigment may additionally be present.[30]

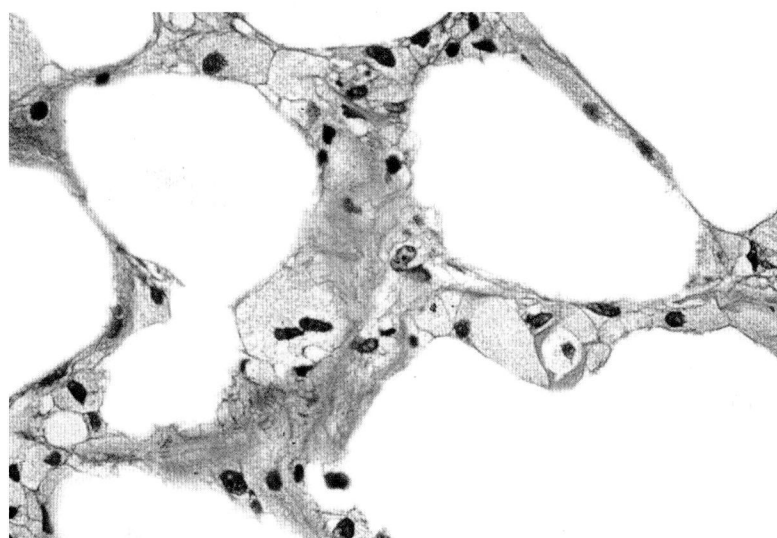

Fig. 10.32
Paraffinoma: on high-power examination, the cystic spaces can often be seen to be lined by lipophages.

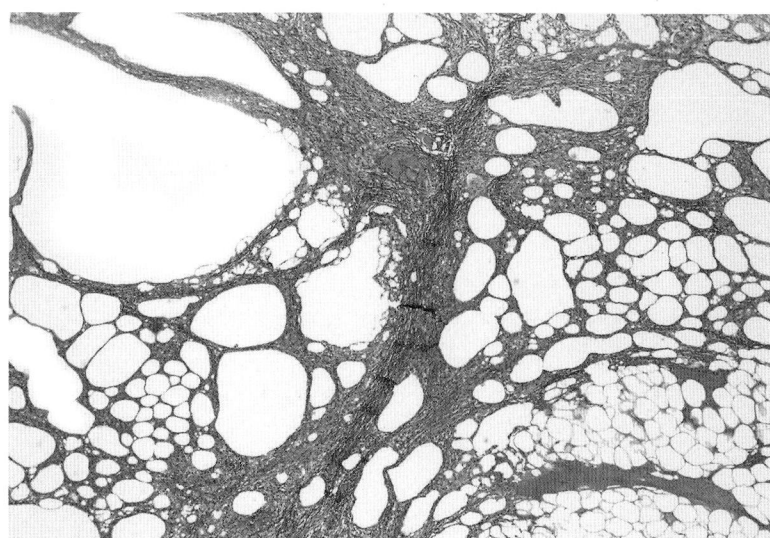

Fig. 10.34
Traumatic fat necrosis: there is intense lobular inflammation with septal fibrosis and hemorrhage.

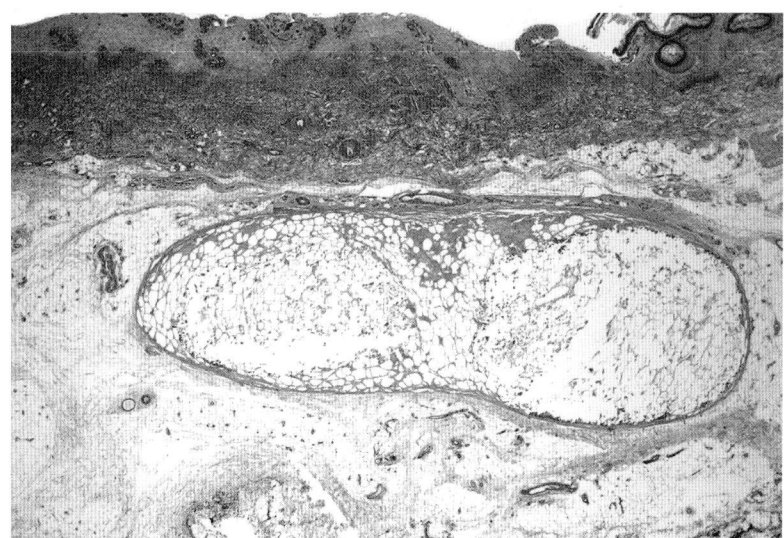

Fig. 10.33
Nodulo-cystic fat necrosis: typical low-power appearance; note the encapsulated fatty cyst, scarring, and chronic inflammation.

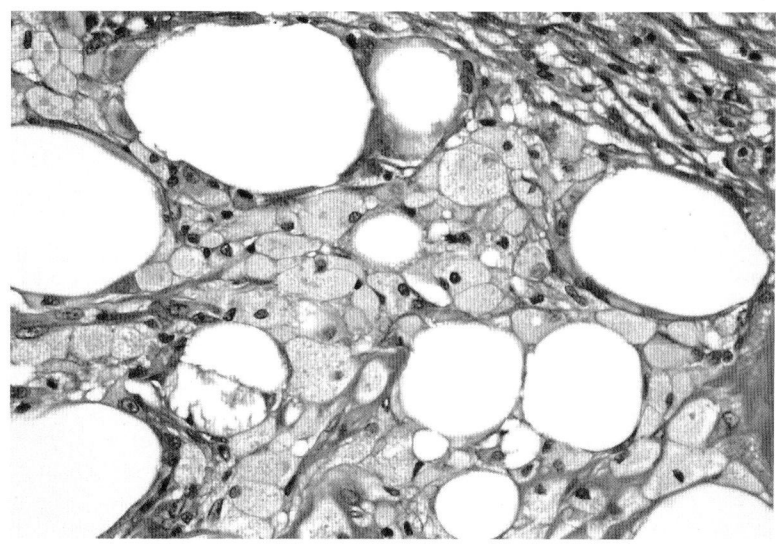

Fig. 10.35
Traumatic fat necrosis: collections of lipophages are characteristic.

Nodular cystic fat necrosis is thought to have an ischemic pathogenesis. Histologically, it is characterized by an encapsulated nodule of necrotic (anucleate) fat cells (*Fig. 10.33*).[31,32] Variable inflammation is present.

Post-surgical panniculitis is a variant of traumatic panniculitis developing at sites of previous surgical excision. It represents a variant of lobular panniculitis and is characterized histologically by pseudocystic degeneration and necrosis of adipocytes, the presence of foamy cells (lipophages), extravasation of erythrocytes, and deep-seated phlebitis.[33] Fat necrosis with histiocytes (lipophages) and giant cells is a common histologic finding in specimens taken from sites of previous surgery of the subcutaneous fat (or deeper). Zelickson and Winkelmann have described this as lipophagic panniculitis.[31] Hemosiderin deposits are also commonly found and, in many instances, fragments of suture material may be identified.

The histologic features of traumatic fat necrosis are not specific and are characterized by fat necrosis accompanied by a variable inflammatory cell infiltrate (*Figs 10.34* and *10.35*). In early lesions this is predominantly composed of neutrophils, later replaced by lymphocytes and monocytes. Aggregates of lipophages are seen frequently and often the reaction becomes frankly granulomatous. Fat cysts are a common feature. With resolution, fibrosis takes place (*Fig. 10.36*). As evidence of the traumatic nature of

the lesion, foci of hemosiderin deposition are not uncommon (*Fig. 10.37*). Occasionally, the presence of fat necrosis is complicated by focal calcification (*Fig. 10.38*).

Panniculitis after subcutaneous injection of interferon-beta can mimic histologically erythema nodosum, lupus panniculitis, and pancreatic panniculitis.[18–20]

Glatiramer acetate-induced panniculitis is characterized histologically by a predominantly lobular inflammatory infiltrate composed of lymphocytes, plasma cells, and scattered neutrophils and eosinophils in the background of lipophagic granulomata.[23] Reactive germinal centers may also be seen.

Interferon-beta-induced panniculitis and glatiramer acetate-induced panniculitis are frequently associated with subsequent lipoatrophy.[18,22]

Cold panniculitis

Clinical features

This rare condition was originally described in infants and young children who developed tender, warm, erythematous plaques on exposed sites, namely, the cheeks and submental region, after experiencing low

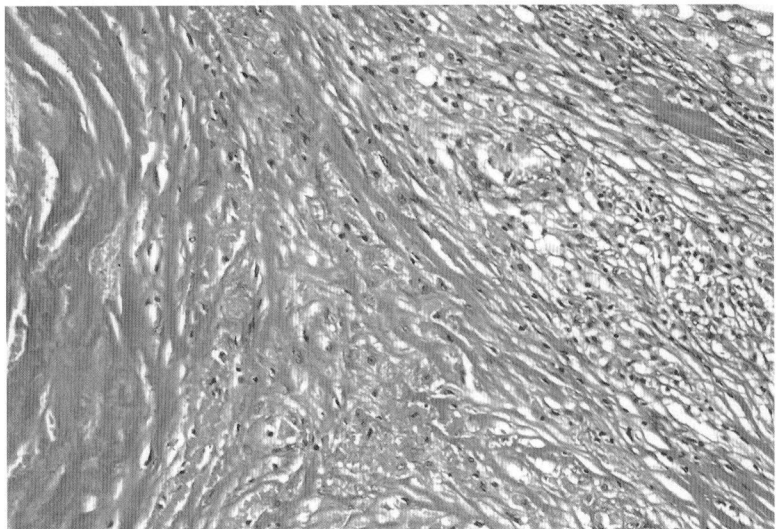

Fig. 10.36
Traumatic fat necrosis: scarring is a feature in more chronic lesions.

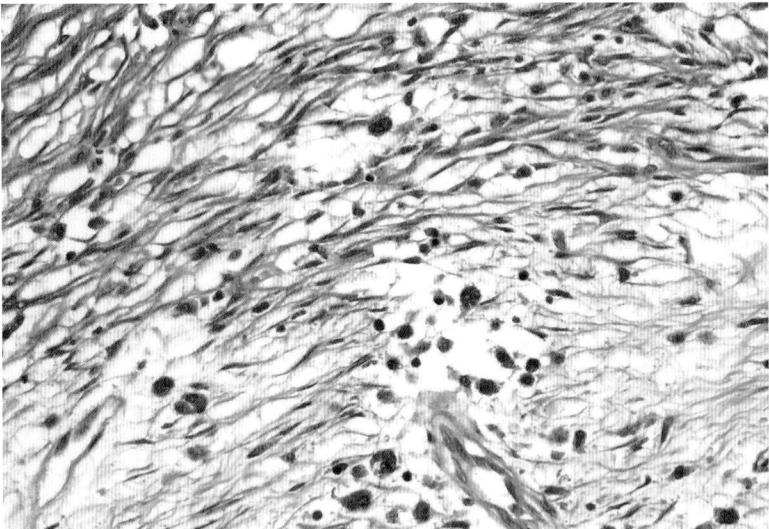

Fig. 10.37
Traumatic fat necrosis: there is marked hemosiderin deposition.

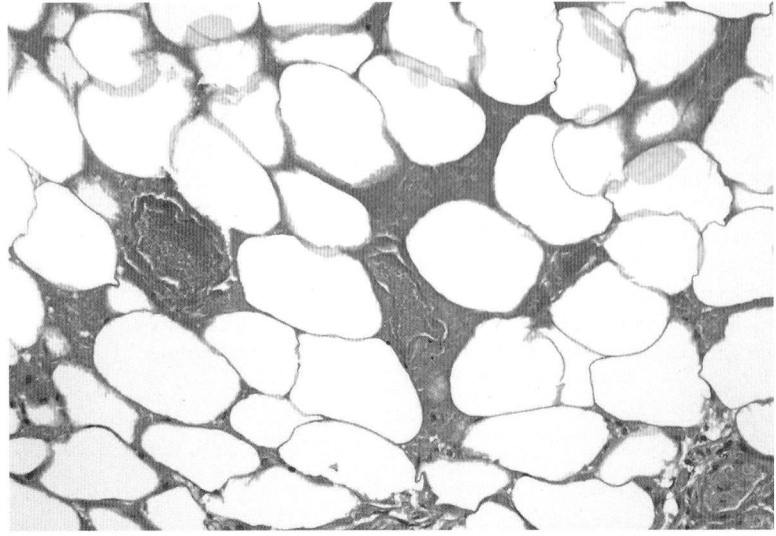

Fig. 10.38
Traumatic fat necrosis: in this example there is marked granular calcification.

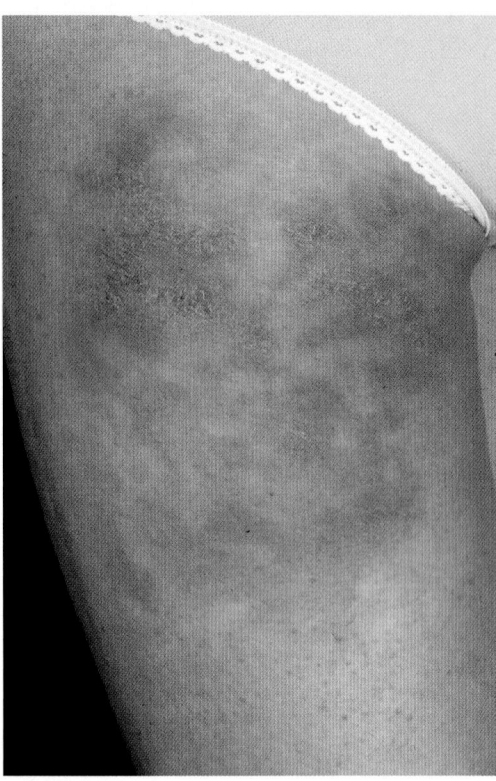

Fig. 10.39
Cold panniculitis: there are ulcerated lesions on this patient's thigh. From the collection of the late N.P. Smith, MD, the Institute of Dermatology, London, UK.

temperatures,[1–6] and usually appeared within the first 72 hours after exposure.[7] These plaques resolved spontaneously after 2–3 weeks, with no residual sequelae. The application of an ice cube to a child's skin may result in the development of similar lesions. Identical changes have also been described in infants following the sucking of ice lollies (popsicles; 'popsicle panniculitis').[8–11] Increased saturated fat content having a higher melting point may precipitate the development of panniculitis in children. Furthermore, cold-induced panniculitis has also been reported in adult patients at sites of ice pack application (or cold therapy) to relieve local pain due to various conditions.[12,13]

A similar phenomenon has been described in young women following horseback riding in cold weather (equestrian cold panniculitis); these patients develop indurated red-violaceous plaques on the superolateral aspect of the thighs following prolonged riding in freezing conditions (Fig. 10.39).[14–17] There is a tendency to ulcerate; healing is associated with post-inflammatory hyperpigmentation and the development of depressed scars. It is thought that these lesions occur as a result of extremely cold temperatures combined with the effect of noninsulated, but tight-fitting, clothes which impair the circulation around the thighs. Risk factors for the development of equestrian cold panniculitis include young age, active smoking, tight clothing, and long periods of riding.[18] Two patients with cold agglutinins and this condition have also been described.[15]

Chilblains (perniosis) also represent localized, abnormal inflammatory responses to the cold.[19] They have an acral distribution (e.g., dorsal surfaces of the fingers and toes) and present as pruritic erythematous lesions, which may blister or ulcerate.

Histologic features

The features of cold panniculitis are most noticeable at the interface between the dermis and subcutaneous fat (Fig. 10.40).[3,8] The infiltrate, which contains lymphocytes, histiocytes, and neutrophils, extends from a perivascular location into the adjacent fat, where it is associated with adipocyte necrosis and the development of small cysts (Fig. 10.41). Excess hyaluronic acid may sometimes be present. Granulomata are not usually conspicuous.[20] The blood vessels show thickening of their walls and endothelial swelling, but frank vasculitis is not a feature. The combination of a superficial and

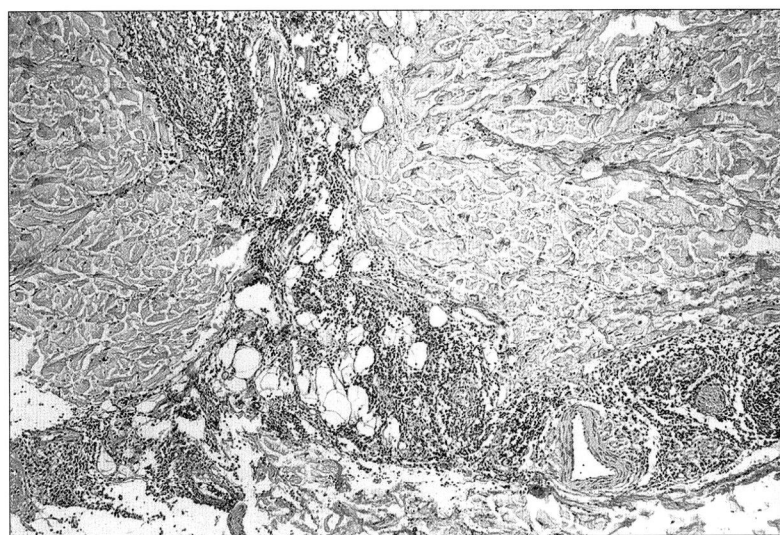

Fig. 10.40
Cold panniculitis: an intense inflammatory cell infiltrate is present at the junction between the dermis and subcutaneous fat. By courtesy of P.H. Cooper, MD, University of Virginia Medical Center, USA.

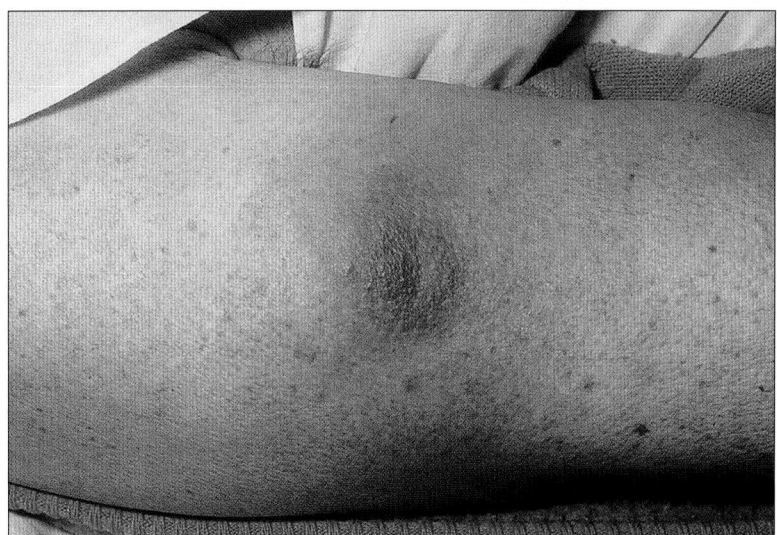

Fig. 10.42
Cytophagic histiocytic panniculitis: an extensive, erythematous, indurated plaque is present on the upper arm. By courtesy of M. Cook, MD, St George's Hospital, London, UK.

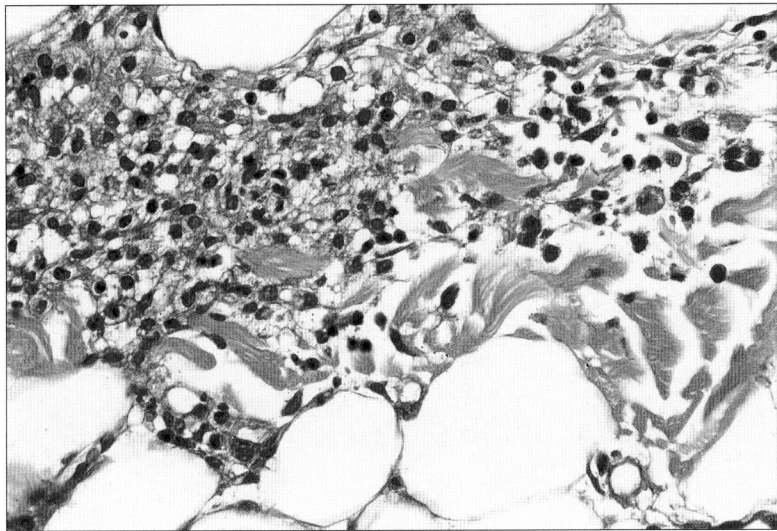

Fig. 10.41
Cold panniculitis: the infiltrate consists of lymphocytes and histiocytes.

deep perivascular and periadnexal lymphocytic inflammatory cell infiltrate coupled with mucin deposition and superficial lobular lymphocytic panniculitis can mimic lupus erythematosus.[12]

The histologic features of perniosis include intense papillary dermal edema and a superficial perivascular mononuclear infiltrate. The blood vessel wall characteristically shows very marked edema and often there is fibrin deposition.[19]

Cytophagic histiocytic panniculitis

Clinical features

Cytophagic histiocytic panniculitis (panniculitis associated with hemophagocytic syndrome) was originally described as a serious disorder of immune dysregulation.[1–3] It may develop in association with a number of underlying conditions including viral infections such as cytomegalovirus and Epstein-Barr virus.[4–8] HIV infection has also rarely been incriminated.[7] Bacteria, fungi, and parasites are sometimes of etiological significance.[9–12] The condition has been described as a complication of phenytoin therapy, following bone marrow transplantation, in systemic lupus erythematosus

(SLE), and as an adverse reaction to interferon-alpha (IFN-α) therapy.[13–17] Some examples in the earlier literature were described as Weber-Christian disease.[18]

Of particular importance, the hemophagocytic syndrome may also be associated with a number of malignancies, most commonly T-cell lymphoma (nodal or cutaneous).[8,18–20] It is likely that many of the cases of the entity described in the past represent examples of lymphomas including subcutaneous panniculitis-like T-cell lymphoma, nasal-type extranodal natural killer/T-cell lymphoma, and, particularly, gamma delta T-cell lymphoma. Rarely, an underlying systemic B-cell lymphoma has been incriminated.[21] Most patients are immunosuppressed; however, very exceptionally, the cause is unknown (idiopathic histiocytic cytophagic panniculitis).[19,22] It is, therefore, of particular importance that all patients diagnosed with this condition are investigated to exclude an underlying lymphoma, particularly of T-cell lineage.

Clinically, the cutaneous manifestations of cytophagic histiocytic panniculitis include erythematous to violaceous or hemorrhagic nodules, which particularly affect the lower limbs and trunk (Figs 10.42 and 10.43). In many patients, however, the distribution is much more widespread. Ulceration is sometimes seen. Severe localized or generalized edema may also be a feature.[18] Constitutional symptoms including pyrexia, malaise, weight loss, fatigue, and myalgia may be present. Patients commonly develop hepatosplenomegaly, lymphadenopathy, hypertriglyceridemia, anemia, leukopenia, thrombocytopenia, and disseminated intravascular coagulopathy.[2–4] Steatohepatitis may complicate exacerbation of cytophagic hemorrhagic panniculitis.[23]

The course of the disease is variable and to some extent depends on the underlying cause.[24–33] Some patients have a prolonged indolent disease over many years before progressing to clinical evidence of systemic hemophagocytosis. Rarely, patients may present with cutaneous lesions and a relatively benign illness[22,27,32,34]; others have a rapidly progressive condition with hemophagocytosis and its sequelae from the outset. The mortality rate for these last patients is high. In addition to the direct effects of bone marrow failure and disseminated intravascular coagulation, systemic infections including opportunist bacteria and fungi are important causes of death.[8]

Pathogenesis and histologic features

Hemophagocytosis appears to develop as a consequence of excess T-cell cytokine production, either virally induced or as a consequence of neoplastic transformation. Tumor necrosis factor-alpha (TNF-α) and IL-2 may be of particular importance.[8] Perforin gene mutation has been detected in a child with cytophagic lymphocytic panniculitis associated with fatal hemophagocytic lymphohistiocytosis.[35] In addition, a missense mutation in the *STX11*

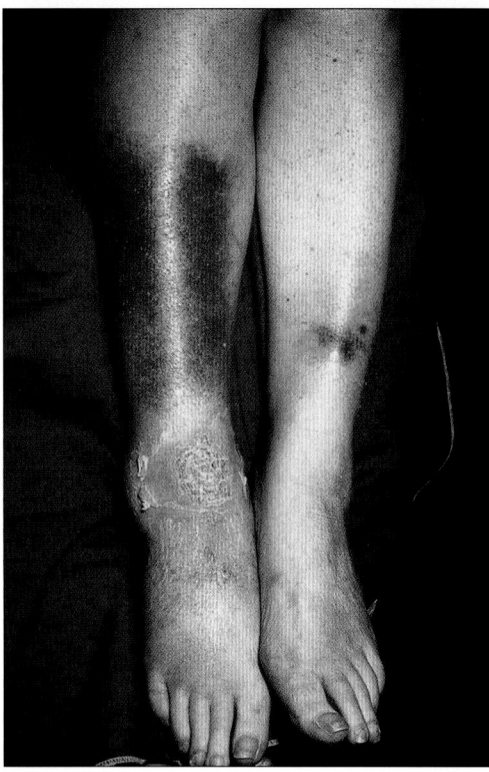

Fig. 10.43
Cytophagic histiocytic panniculitis: in this example the lesions are hemorrhagic and ulcerated. By courtesy of M. Cook, MD, St George's Hospital, London, UK.

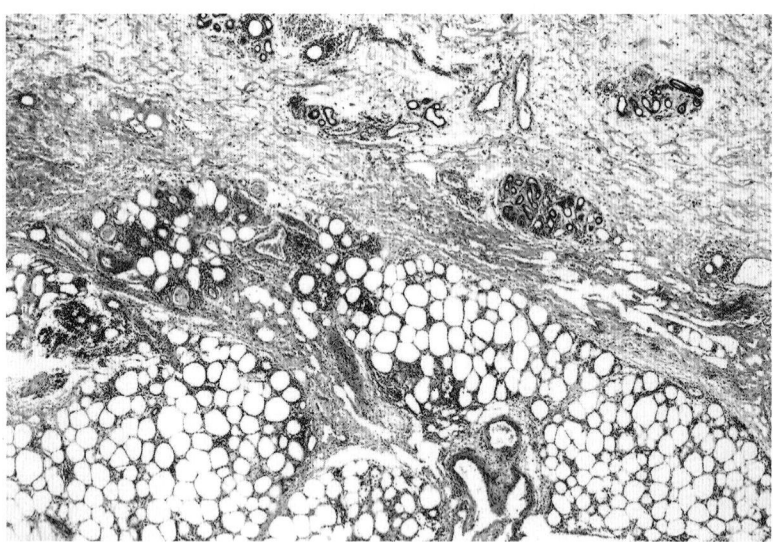

Fig. 10.44
Cytophagic histiocytic panniculitis: there is a cellular infiltrate associated with fat necrosis.

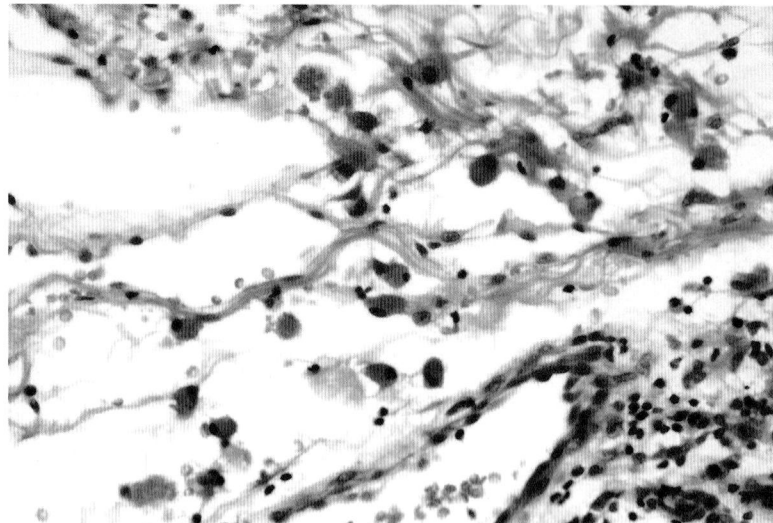

Fig. 10.45
Cytophagic histiocytic panniculitis: note the histiocytes with abundant eosinophilic cytoplasm, some of which show erythrophagocytosis.

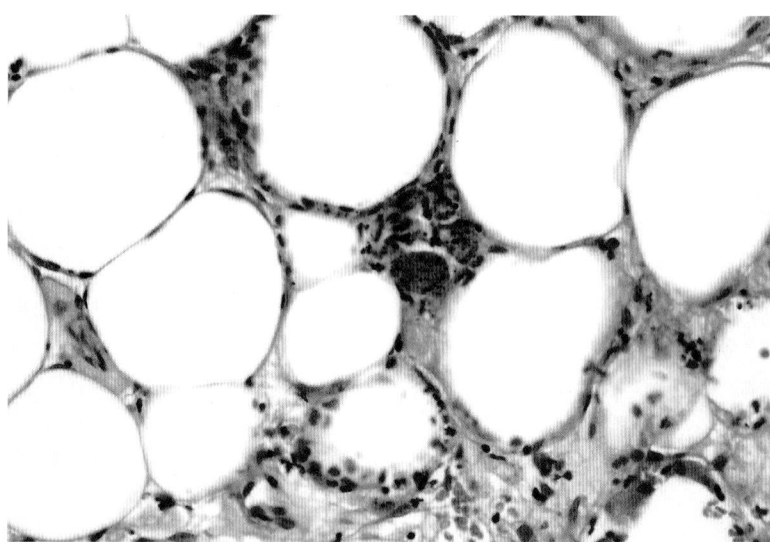

Fig. 10.46
Cytophagic histiocytic panniculitis: in the center of the field are several multinucleated giant cells containing phagocytosed nuclear debris ('bean-bag' cells).

gene was detected in another child with cytophagic histiocytic panniculitis with a relapsing familial form of hemophagocytic lymphohistiocytosis.[36]

Histologically, the lesions are characterized by an infiltrate of histiocytes with abundant eosinophilic cytoplasm and uniform, variably hyperchromatic or vesicular nuclei containing small nucleoli. Variable numbers of lymphocytes and neutrophils are also present. Although the distribution is predominantly lobular, septal involvement is usually apparent and the lower dermis is also often involved (*Fig. 10.44*). Red cell extravasation is typically present, and frequently the lesions are frankly hemorrhagic. Erythrophagocytosis is invariably a feature and phagocytosis of lymphocytes or nuclear debris is also often evident (*Fig. 10.45*). The enlarged and distended histiocytes are sometimes described as 'bean-bag' cells (*Fig. 10.46*).[2,3] Giant cells

and granulomata are not usually a feature unless there is concomitant fat necrosis. Lymphoid nuclear atypia is evident in those cases in which a T-cell lymphoma is present (see below).

Differential diagnosis

Cytophagic histiocytic panniculitis must be distinguished from other conditions in which erythrophagocytosis or hemophagocytosis may be a feature including subcutaneous T-cell panniculitic lymphoma, angiocentric lymphoma, and cutaneous Rosai-Dorfman disease.

In subcutaneous panniculitic T-cell lymphoma, the lymphocytes show cytological atypia with karyorrhexis and mitotic activity (*Fig. 10.47*). In children with cytophagic histiocytic panniculitis, a clonal reactive T cell proliferation mimicking panniculitis-like T cell lymphoma has been reported in exceptional cases, likely following a viral infection.[37] Angiocentric T-cell lymphoma is characterized by an angioinvasive and frequently angiodestructive atypical lymphoid infiltrate usually accompanied by widespread coagulative necrosis. In cutaneous Rosai-Dorfman disease, the infiltrate is usually centered on the dermis. Lymphophagocytosis is often marked, but erythrophagocytosis is not usually present. The histiocytes are characteristically S100 protein positive.

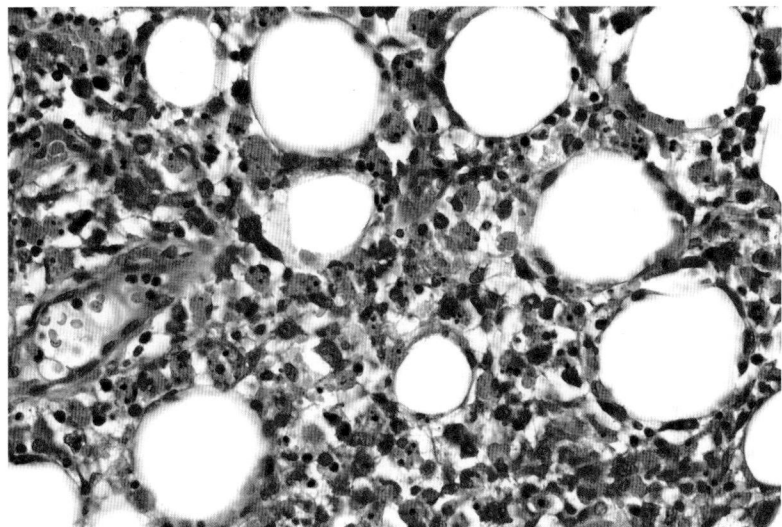

Fig. 10.47
Subcutaneous panniculitic T-cell lymphoma: numerous histiocytes showing hemophagocytosis are present. In addition, however, there are conspicuous hyperchromatic and irregular atypical lymphocytes.

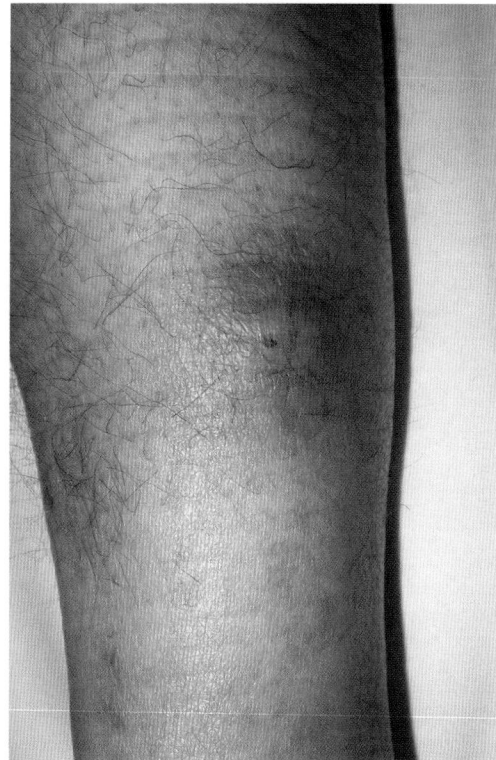

Fig. 10.48
Pancreatic panniculitis: early lesions are often erythematous. By courtesy of J.C. Pascual, MD, Alicante, Spain.

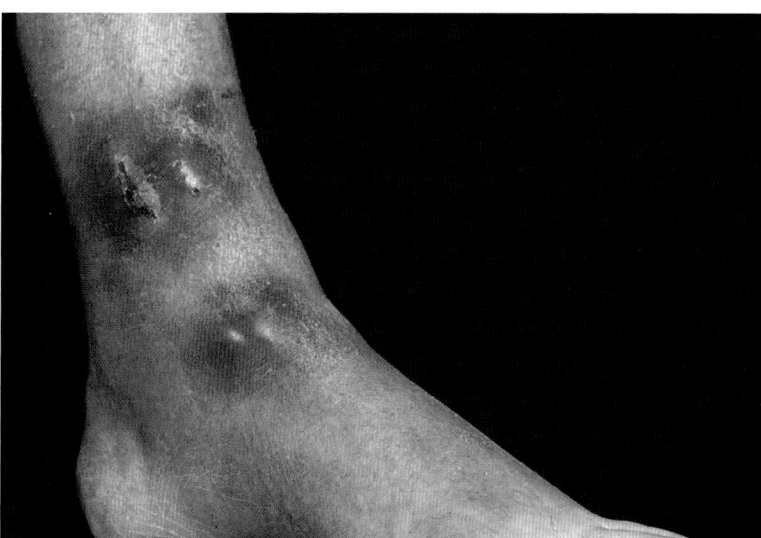

Fig. 10.49
Pancreatic panniculitis: a more advanced lesion. From the collection of the late N.P. Smith, MD, the Institute of Dermatology, London, UK.

Subcutaneous Whipple disease

Clinical features

Whipple disease is a rare condition which most often affects males and is due to infection with the bacillus *Tropheryma whippeli*.[1,2] It is characterized by small intestinal involvement leading to malabsorption accompanied by fever and arthritis, although virtually any organ system may be affected. Cutaneous lesions include hyperpigmentation, erythroderma, purpura, vasculitis, erythematous and urticarial lesions, eczematous dermatitis, and lichenoid granulomatous lesions.[3,4] Exceptionally, subcutaneous nodules have been described[3,5–8] with occasional symmetrical distribution on inner thighs and forearms.[9]

Histologic features

Involvement of the subcutaneous fat presents as a predominantly septal 'panniculitis' characterized by a mixed inflammatory cell infiltrate consisting of lymphocytes, neutrophils, and foamy periodic acid-Schiff (PAS)-positive histiocytes,[4,9] occasionally accompanied by formation of granulomas. Similar changes can also be present in the dermis.[8]

Electron microscopy reveals degenerate bacilli within membrane-bound vesicles in the cytoplasm of the histiocytes.[3]

Polymerase chain reaction (PCR) and immunohistochemical techniques can be used as a diagnostic aid.[10]

Pancreatic panniculitis

Clinical features

Pancreatic panniculitis is rare, occurring in 1–3% of patients with underlying pancreatic disease.[1–24] Recognizing the association of subcutaneous fat necrosis (metastatic fat necrosis) with pancreatic disease is of particular importance because sometimes the underlying pancreatic process is clinically silent. Furthermore, pancreatic panniculitis can be the presenting sign of an underlying pancreatic disorder in as many as 35% of the patients. The pancreatic diseases include acute pancreatitis, chronic pancreatitis, pancreatic pseudocyst, pancreatic divisum, and pancreatic neoplasms (mostly acinar cell carcinoma, but also ductal carcinoma, neuroendocrine carcinoma, intraductal papillary mucinous neoplasm, and mucinous adenocarcinoma).[1–29] Pancreatic panniculitis can also develop as a complication of endoscopic retrograde cholangiopancreatography.[30,31] In addition, pancreatic panniculitis has been described as a possible adverse drug reaction following renal transplantation for SLE, simultaneous pancreas-kidney transplantation for type I diabetes, and following liver transplantation.[32–35] Pancreatic panniculitis has been reported following L-asparaginase treatment for acute lymphoblastic leukemia, peginterferon/ribavirin/telaprevir combination treatment for hepatitis C, but also in a patient with nephrotic syndrome due to rapidly progressing glomerulonephritis and in a patient with DiGeorge syndrome.[36–39] There are two additional reports of the disease developing in a background of lupus erythematosus.[40,41]

Patients present with multiple, exquisitely tender nodules, which are erythematous or violaceous in appearance (*Figs 10.48* and *10.49*). The lower extremities, buttocks, and trunk are most often affected, although occasionally the upper arms, thorax, and scalp are involved. Occasionally, the nodules ulcerate and release a creamy or oily discharge (*Fig. 10.50*).

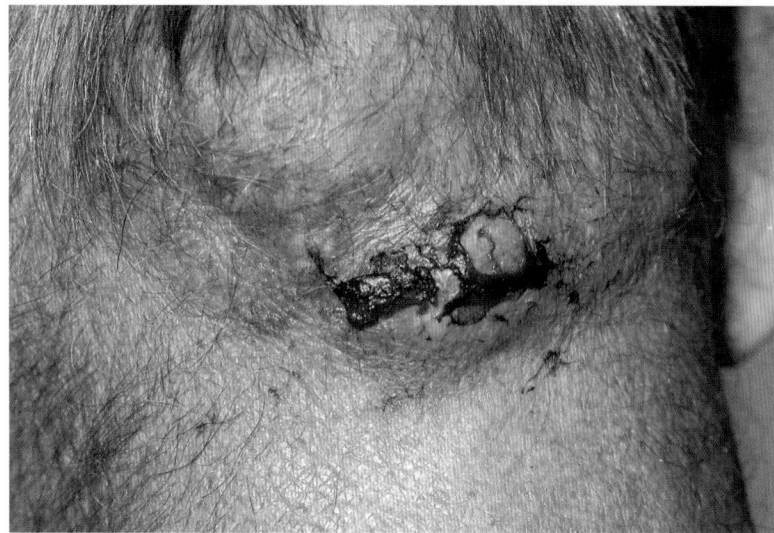

Fig. 10.50
Pancreatic panniculitis: the nodules may ulcerate and release blood-stained fluid.
By courtesy of J.C. Pascual, MD, Alicante, Spain.

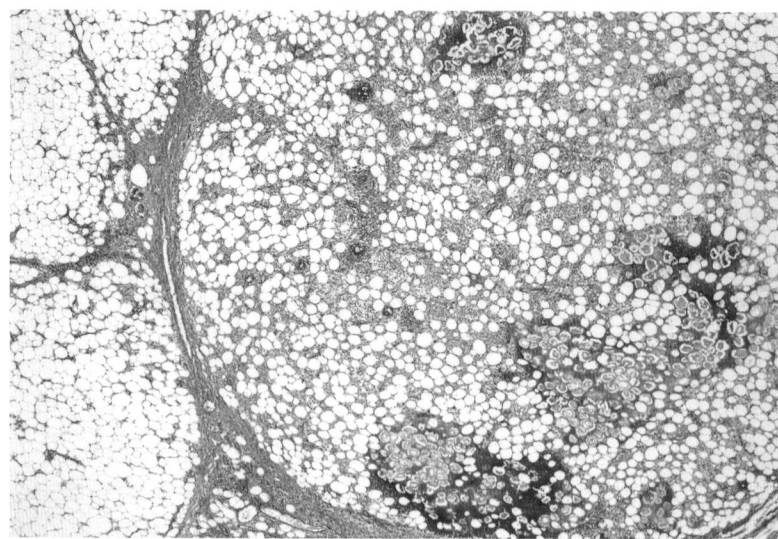

Fig. 10.51
Pancreatic panniculitis: the changes predominantly affect the lobules.

Joint manifestations (pain and swelling) are an important feature of this syndrome (also designated pancreatitis panniculitis polyarthritis syndrome), occurring in approximately 54% (pancreatitis-associated) to 88% (pancreatic carcinoma-associated) of patients.[5,42–49] The ankles are most often affected, but the knees, elbows, wrists, metacarpophalangeal, and metatarsophalangeal joints are occasionally involved. A single case with chondronecrosis and osteonecrosis has been reported.[50] Additional features include pleural effusions (in 25%), ascites (in 30%), and very occasionally, pericardial effusion.[4] Intramedullary fat may also be affected and intestinal involvement has rarely been documented.[1,46] Peripheral blood eosinophilia is quite a common laboratory finding (19% in pancreatitis-associated; 65% in pancreatic carcinoma-associated). Males are affected more often than females (pancreatitis 2 : 1; carcinoma 7 : 1), and patients are most often in the fourth, fifth, or sixth decade. This disease is associated with a high mortality, 42% in pancreatitis-associated variants and up to 100% in those cases presenting with an underlying carcinoma.[4]

Pathogenesis and histologic features

The development of subcutaneous fat necrosis in association with pancreatic disease is due to the release into the peripheral circulation of trypsin, lipase, phospholipase, and amylase.[7,51] It has been postulated that trypsin damages the vasculature, particularly in dependent sites, thereby permitting lipase to enter the surrounding tissues. In vivo evidence suggests that this may be too simplistic a viewpoint.[9] Serum lipase levels do not always correlate with subcutaneous fat necrosis, and examples of patients with fat necrosis and normal serum lipase levels have been documented.[10] The reports of Wilson et al. and Simkin et al., however, provide striking in vivo evidence to support a pathogenetic role for released pancreatic enzymes.[42,43]

Histologically, the features are very distinctive and are identical to those seen in the peripancreatic adipose tissue following an episode of acute hemorrhage pancreatitis (Fig. 10.51). Although very early changes can show features of septal panniculitis without fat necrosis or vasculitis, most frequently, however, the changes are lobular in distribution and are characterized by the presence of ghost cells (Fig. 10.52).[52] The latter are anucleate, composed of amorphous granular debris, and often show a rim of eosinophilia (Fig. 10.53). Stippled basophilia due to calcification is commonly found (Fig. 10.54). Ghost-like adipocytes can be surrounded by peripheral eosinophilic striations consistent with the Splendore-Hoeppli reaction.[53] A neutrophil polymorph response is usually evident around the foci of fat necrosis, and hemorrhage is an almost invariable feature (Fig. 10.55). The uninvolved surrounding fat is heavily infiltrated by acute and chronic inflammatory cells including large numbers of macrophages, many of which have foamy cytoplasm due to ingested lipid, and occasional multinucleate giant cells (Fig. 10.56). Birefringent crystals have been described in the mesenteric

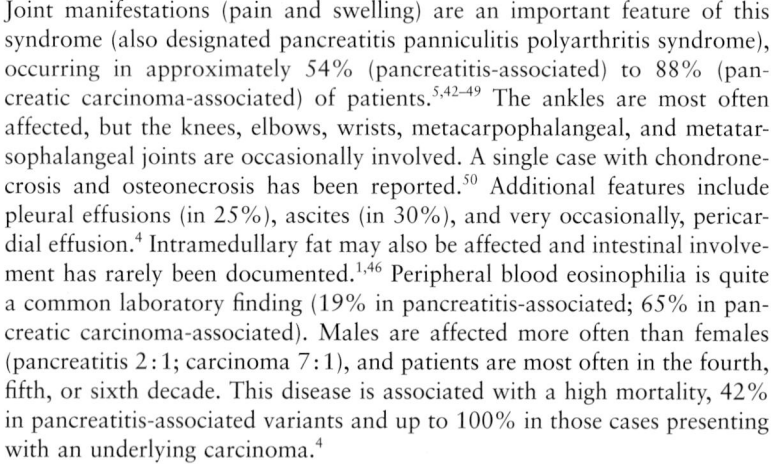

Fig. 10.52
Pancreatic panniculitis: there is extensive enzymatic fat necrosis. Note the characteristic ghost cells.

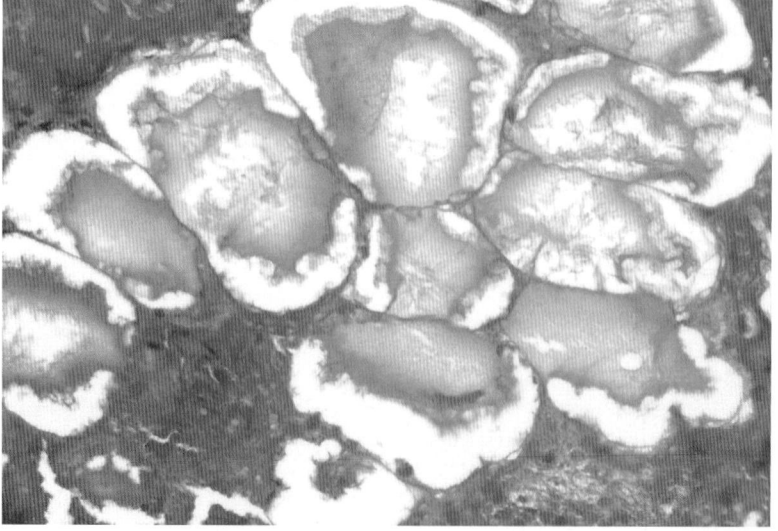

Fig. 10.53
Pancreatic panniculitis: close-up view of ghost cells.

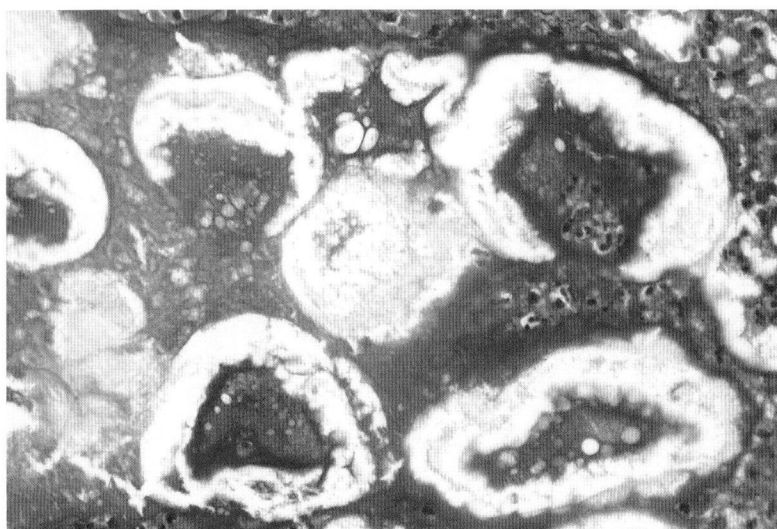

Fig. 10.54
Pancreatic panniculitis: the stippled basophilia represents calcification.

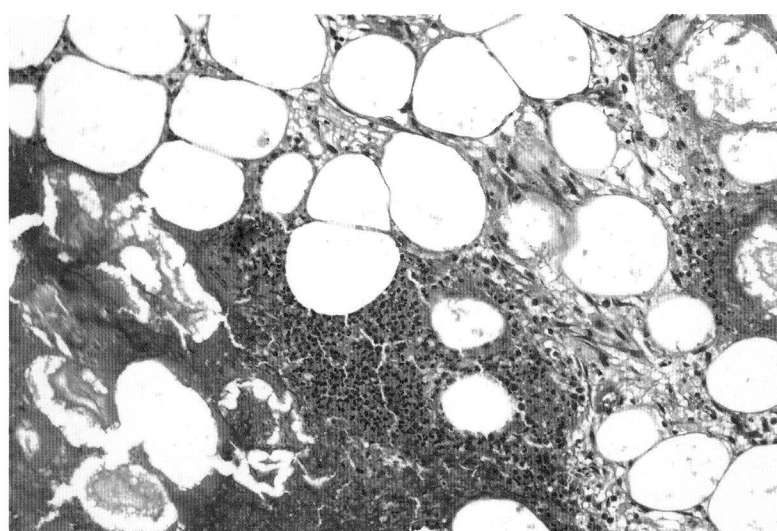

Fig. 10.55
Pancreatic panniculitis: there is a heavy neutrophil infiltrate.

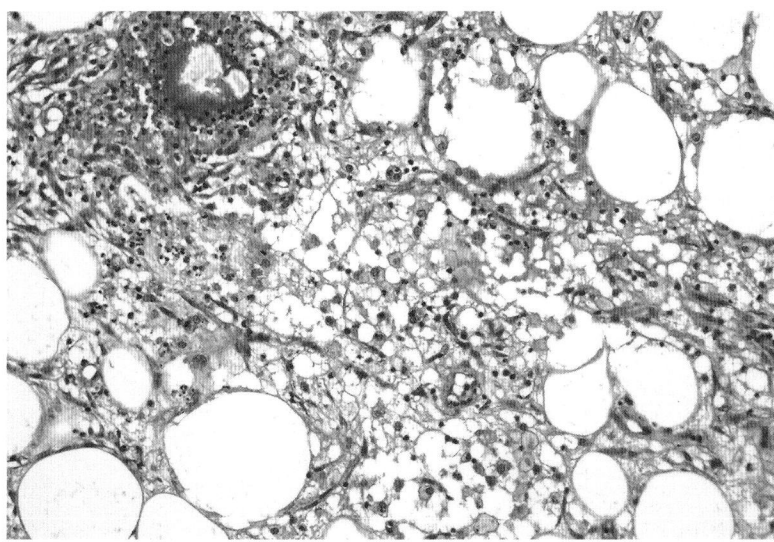

Fig. 10.56
Pancreatic panniculitis: as with other forms of fat necrosis, lipophages are often evident.

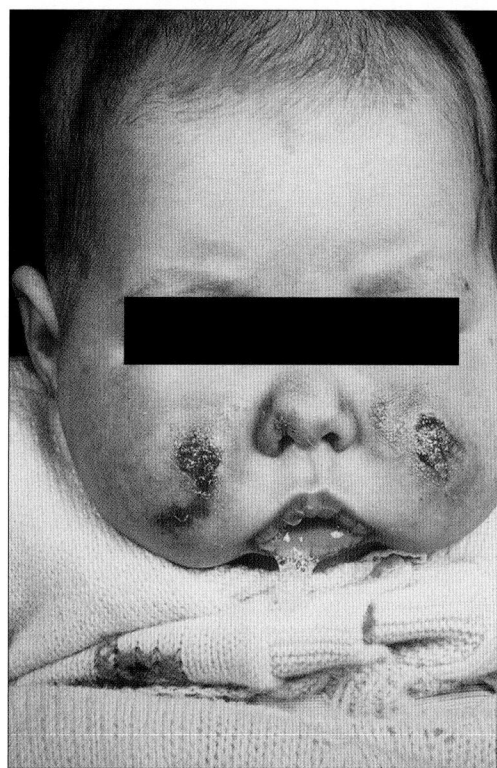

Fig. 10.57
Subcutaneous fat necrosis of the newborn: crusted, ulcerated nodules on both cheeks. By courtesy of the Institute of Dermatology, London, UK.

fat and within affected joints but not in the subcutaneous fat.[54,55] Generally, there is no evidence of a vasculitis. However, the presence of muscular arteritis in the connective tissue septa at the periphery of inflamed fat lobule has exceptionally been reported.[53]

Pancreatic panniculitis can be complicated, albeit in isolated cases by infection with *Corynebacterium tuberculostearicum*.[56]

Differential diagnosis

Some deep fungal infections including aspergillosis and subcutaneous injections of interferon beta can induce a histologic picture mimicking pancreatic fat necrosis.[57,58] Special stains for microorganisms and close clinicopathological correlation usually allow distinction to be made.

Subcutaneous fat necrosis of the newborn

Clinical features

This uncommon disease presents in full-term or post-term neonates in the first few weeks of life.[1–4] Affected babies develop painless subcutaneous nodules measuring from a few millimeters to several centimeters in diameter. The overlying skin may appear normal or be erythematous or violaceous. Lesions are symmetrical and distributed over bony prominences, the arms, shoulders, buttocks, thighs, and cheeks (*Fig. 10.57*). The nodules frequently soften and become fluctuant, occasionally liquefying. The disease is usually self-limiting and benign, with spontaneous resolution occurring within a period of weeks to months in the majority of cases. An exceptional example of a recurrent subcutaneous fat necrosis of the newborn, developing several weeks after the clearance of initial lesions at distant sites, has been reported.[5]

Subcutaneous fat necrosis of the newborn is associated with hypercalcemia from 29% to 69% of the patients, and much less frequently with dyslipidemia, thrombocytopenia, hyperglycemia, and lactic acidosis.[4,6–14] Hypercalcemia may be asymptomatic and associated with failure to thrive, fever, vomiting, irritability, and seizures.[1,15] Calcium deposits have been described in the kidneys, liver, inferior vena cava, and heart.[4,16] Delayed onset of hypercalcemia up to 6 months after occurrence of the subcutaneous fat necrosis of the newborn is also possible.[17] Exceptionally, this disease can prove fatal.

Pathogenesis and histologic features

The pathogenesis of the hypercalcemia is unknown. A number of theories have been proposed including calcium release from resolving plaques, elevated parathormone and prostaglandin E2 levels, increased vitamin D sensitivity, and most recently, lesional histiocytic production of excessive 1,25-dihydroxyvitamin D_3 with resultant increased intestinal absorption of calcium.[18–26]

The cause of subcutaneous fat necrosis of the newborn is unknown, but most cases are related to some form of fetal distress, including obstetric or other birth trauma, cord accidents, meconium aspiration, infections, hypothermia, placenta previa, cesarean section, and neonatal asphyxia.[2,4] Pre-eclampsia and maternal diabetes have also been associated with this condition.[4,8] A recent prospective study established higher birth weight to be an independent risk factor for subcutaneous fat necrosis in asphyxiated newborns.[27] A primary abnormality of subcutaneous fat may also be of some importance.[28] Neonatal fat is characterized by elevated levels of saturated fatty acids which have a high melting point and are therefore susceptible to precipitation as a consequence of neonatal hypothermia. Deficiency of brown fat has also been proposed as a potential etiological factor.[29] Although not histologically confirmed, a case of simultaneous development of sclerema neonatorum and subcutaneous fat necrosis of the newborn was described in an infant following cesarean section for fetal distress, hypothermia, neonatal respiratory distress, and hypoglycemia.[30]

Subcutaneous fat necrosis has also been described after hypothermic cardiac surgery, as a complication of congestive heart failure in an infant with ventricular septal defect and patent ductus arteriosus, associated with maternal diabetes, increased blood pressure, smoking, thrombosis-related risk factor, a possible complication of cocaine abuse, following the in partum use of calcium channel blockers, and as a consequence of prolonged exposure in very cold weather.[4,31–37]

The histologic changes are characteristic.[24,38–40] The subcutaneous fat is the scene of intense necrosis. Individual adipocytes are swollen and contain abundant radially arranged eosinophilic crystalline spaces resulting from dissolved lipid (Figs 10.58 and 10.59). The crystals are largely composed of triglycerides.[39] There is a heavy inflammatory cell infiltrate comprising polymorphs, lymphocytes, histiocytes, and numerous foreign body giant cells (Fig. 10.60). Neutrophilic granulocytes are usually absent or form a minor fraction of the inflammatory cell infiltrate. Nevertheless, a neutrophil-rich variant of subcutaneous fat necrosis of the newborn has been reported with neutrophilic granulocytes representing the predominant cell type (over 75%) in the inflammatory infiltrate.[41] Such examples mimic infective panniculitis

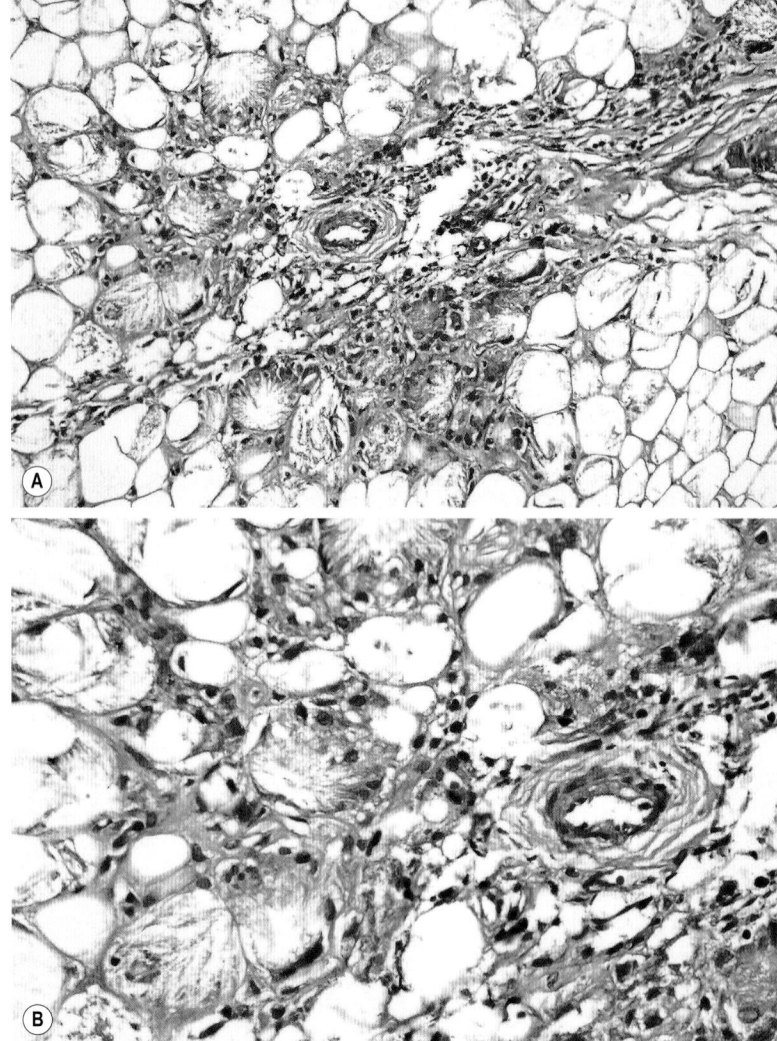

Fig. 10.59
(A, B) Subcutaneous fat necrosis of the newborn: individual adipocytes are swollen and contain characteristic, radial, eosinophilic crystals.

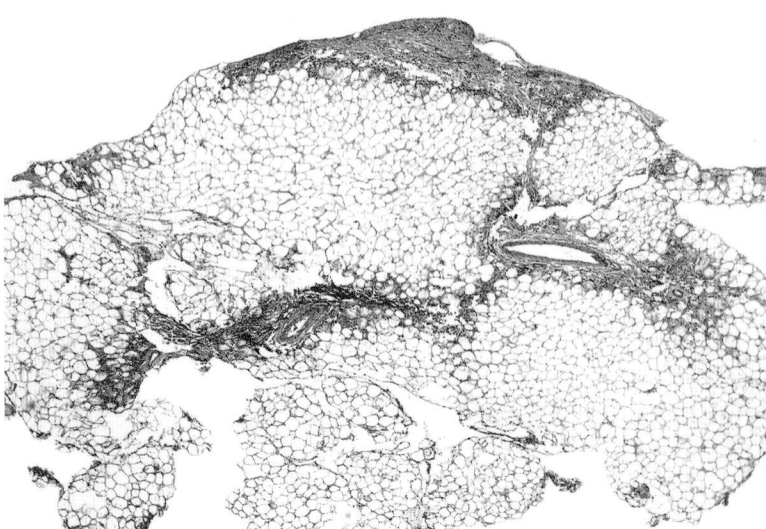

Fig. 10.58
Subcutaneous fat necrosis of the newborn: multiple foci of fat necrosis with chronic inflammation are present.

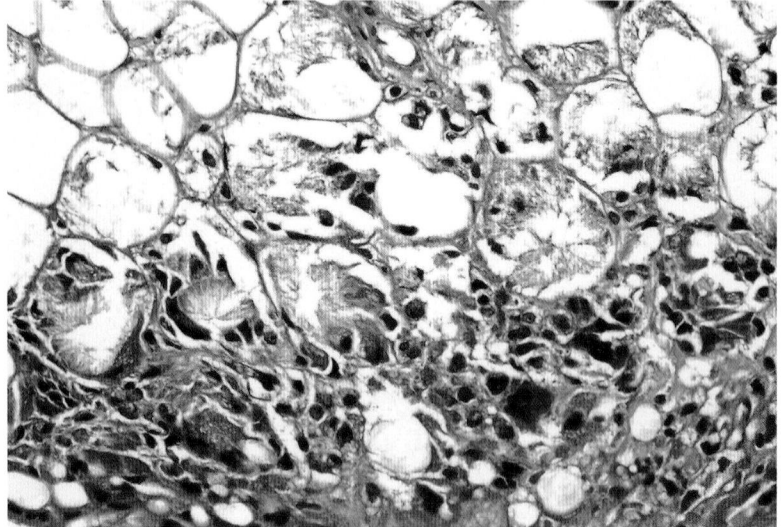

Fig. 10.60
Subcutaneous fat necrosis of the newborn: surrounding the foci of fat necrosis is a chronic inflammatory infiltrate containing numerous foreign body giant cells.

and require exclusion of infection by special stains and/or cultures.[41] Large numbers of eosinophils have been described in two cases.[24] Multinucleated giant cells containing eosinophilic granules in their cytoplasm have also been reported.[42,43] The significance of these granules is unknown, and their origin from degranulating eosinophils has been postulated.[42] Older lesions may show fibrosis and foci of calcification. Systemic involvement is sometimes present.[40]

Differential diagnosis

It is of interest to note that identical histologic features were seen a number of years ago in the poststeroid panniculitis syndrome.[44–49] This condition occurred in children who had been treated for rheumatic fever or glomerulonephritis with very large doses of steroids; sudden withdrawal of the steroids resulted in the development of subcutaneous swellings up to 4 cm across on the cheeks, arms, and trunk. The disease is now of historic interest only due to the standard practice of steroid taper when withdrawing the drug. The skin overlying the nodules was erythematous, warm, and itchy. In mild cases, the panniculitis resolved spontaneously; in more severe examples, it subsided following the reintroduction of steroids. Poststeroid panniculitis has also been reported in an adult patient.[50]

Sclerema neonatorum

Clinical features

Sclerema neonatorum is a very rare condition associated with high morbidity and mortality (75–90%).[1] It is sometimes confused with, and therefore must be distinguished from, subcutaneous fat necrosis of the newborn.[2–4] Infants present in the first week of life (average age of onset, 4 days; range, birth to 70 days) with a diffuse, rapidly spreading, waxlike thickening, and induration of the subcutaneous fat, resembling lard. This usually commences about the buttocks, thighs, and trunk, and often spreads to involve the whole body, excluding the palms, soles, and genitalia. The fat is typically tethered to the underlying fascia and the skin cannot be grasped between the fingers. Pitting edema is not a feature. A delayed onset of sclerema neonatorum several months after delivery is exceptional.[5]

Affected infants are usually hypothermic, but body temperature may be normal or, rarely, raised.[6,7] Some of the infants are premature, but they are a minority. The children commonly have some other associated illness, such as septicemia, pneumonia, diarrhea, dehydration, intestinal obstruction, congenital heart disease, or other congenital malformations.[8] A patient with both sclerema neonatorum and concurrent subacute fat necrosis of the newborn has been described.[9]

Pathogenesis and histologic features

The etiology and pathogenesis of this condition are uncertain. It is thought that the structural alterations of the subcutaneous fat probably predate the development of the clinical features. Neonatal subcutaneous fat is characterized by a higher content of saturated fatty acids (palmitic and stearic) and a lower content of unsaturated fatty acids (oleic) than adult subcutaneous fat.[2] It also has higher melting and solidification points. It has been suggested that infants with sclerema neonatorum have an inadequately developed enzyme system for converting saturated to unsaturated fatty acids.[2] It is thought that this, in association with stress, might result in the precipitation of triglycerides and consequent solidification of the subcutaneous fat. It has been proposed that redistribution of blood flow to the systemic circulation with resultant relative ischemia of the subcutaneous fat may be of pathogenetic importance.[10] Sclerema neonatorum is characterized by increased blood lipid peroxidation and diminished superoxidase dismutase activity, which raises the possibility that free radicals may play a role in its pathogenesis.[11] There is no evidence of vasculitis.

The histologic features are surprisingly bland. The subcutaneous fat is greatly thickened and the fibrous septa are broader than normal. The adipocytes, which are increased in size, may contain radially orientated fine crystals identical to those described in subcutaneous fat necrosis of the newborn although often they are inconspicuous.[1,12] In contrast to the latter condition, however, there is no necrosis or significant inflammatory cell infiltrate.

Calcification is rarely a feature.[1] The dermis may appear sclerotic with hyalinization and the epidermis atrophic with loss of the rete ridges.[12]

Changes in the subcutaneous fat similar to sclerema neonatorum, characterized by the radial arrangement of nonpolarizable needle-shaped crystals within adipocytes, have been reported in an adult patient as an adverse reaction to gemcitabine treatment for metastatic pancreatic cancer.[13]

Cutaneous oxalosis

Clinical features

Oxalosis, in which there is widespread deposition of calcium oxalate in the tissues, may represent a primary metabolic disease or a secondary phenomenon due to increased intake of oxalate precursors or defective excretion.[1–5] Secondary oxalosis can also result from pyridoxine deficiency, glycerol infusion, methoxyflurane anesthesia, excessive ascorbic acid, extensive hemodialysis, peritoneal dialysis, and ethylene glycol poisoning.[2]

Primary oxalosis, which is associated with overproduction of oxalate, is an autosomal recessive condition and includes three subtypes:
- Type I, which is most often encountered, develops as a result of deficiency of the hepatic enzyme alanine:glyoxylate aminotransferase with resulting increased urinary excretion of oxalate, glycolate, and glyoxylate.[1–3]
- Type II (L-glyceric aciduria) results from cytosolic D-glycerate dehydrogenase and glyoxylate reductase deficiencies with associated increased urinary excretion of L-glycerate and oxalate accompanied by normal glycolate and glyoxylate excretion.[4]
- Type III develops as a result of primary small intestinal disease associated with excessive oxalate reabsorption.[5]

Calcium oxalate crystal deposition occurs most commonly in the kidneys (calcium oxalate stones and chronic renal failure).[4] With the onset of the latter, hyperoxalemia develops with resultant deposition of oxalate crystals in the blood vessels, retina, myocardium, cardiac conducting system, central nervous system, peripheral nerves, bones, and joints.[6]

Cutaneous manifestations may occur in both primary and secondary forms.[6–24] Lesions most often result from vascular involvement, patients presenting with acrocyanosis, livedo reticularis, Raynaud phenomenon, and distal gangrene (Fig. 10.61).[7–12] Ulceronecrotic lesions reminiscent of calciphylaxis have also been documented.[13–15] Less often, crystals are deposited in the skin of the face and the fingers as miliary deposits, as dermal/subcutaneous nodules or as painful subungual nodules.[16–21] Exceptionally, generalized cutaneous nodules have been documented.[22] Vascular involvement is said to be more common in patients with primary disease whereas

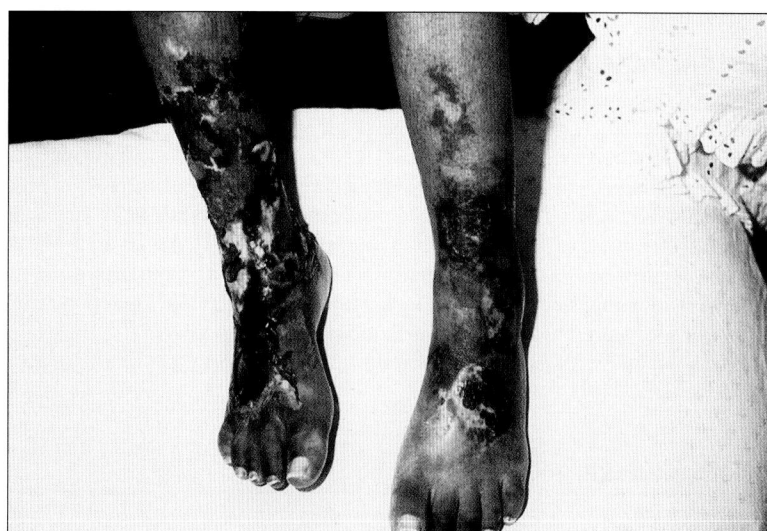

Fig. 10.61
Cutaneous oxalosis: this child shows gangrene with ulceration. By courtesy of N. Saxe, MD, Groote Schuur Hospital, Cape Town, South Africa.

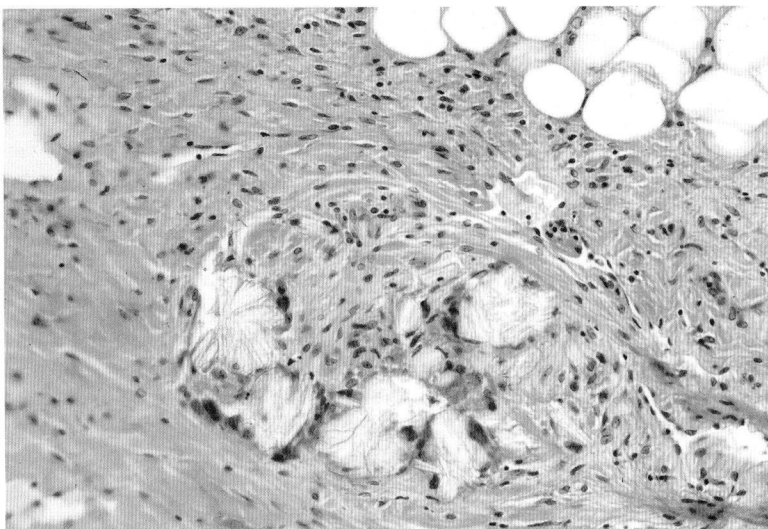

Fig. 10.62
Cutaneous oxalosis: note the radially orientated, needle-shaped crystals.

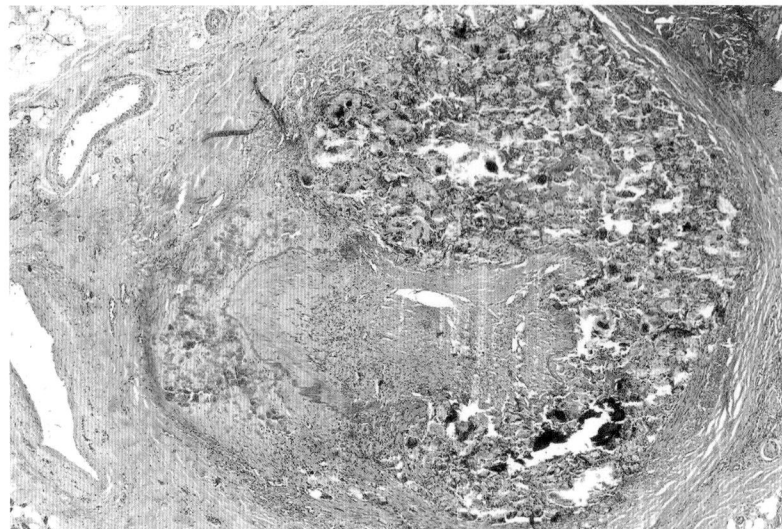

Fig. 10.64
Cutaneous oxalosis: in this field there is dramatic vascular involvement with destruction of the media and massive intimal thickening.

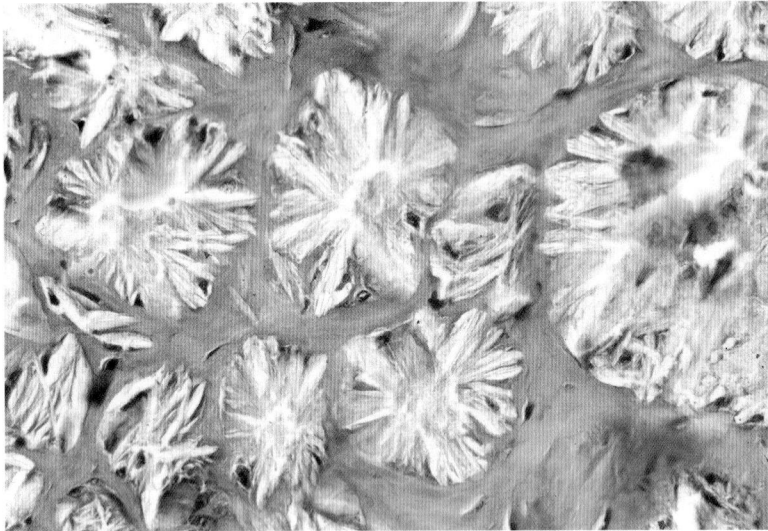

Fig. 10.63
Cutaneous oxalosis: note the radial crystals viewed under polarized light.

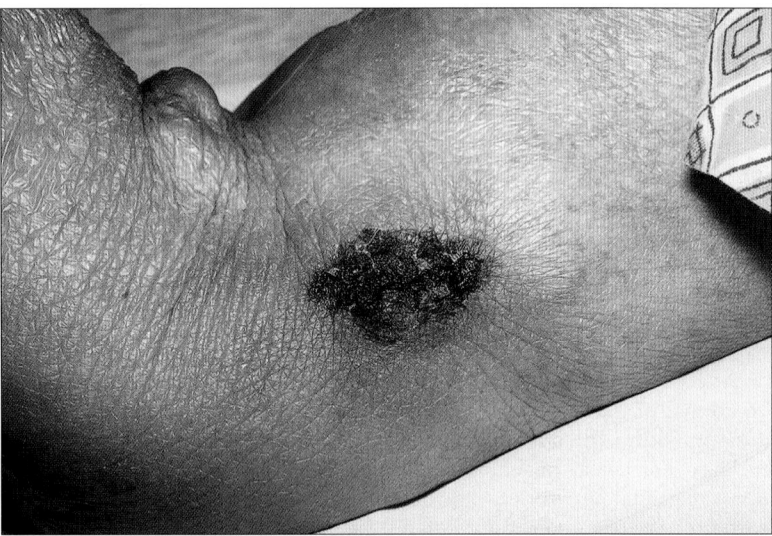

Fig. 10.65
Calciphylaxis: ulcerated gangrenous lesion with surrounding erythema. By courtesy of A. Qureshi, MD, Department of Dermatology, Brigham and Women's Hospital, Boston, USA.

cutaneous extravascular lesions are predominantly seen in patients with secondary disease.[21]

Histologic features

Calcium oxalate crystals are yellow to brown, radially arranged, needle-shaped or rectangular in shape (*Figs 10.62* and *10.63*). In the skin, they may be found in the reticular dermis or within the subcutaneous fat. Vascular involvement may also be seen where the media of arteries is predominantly affected (*Fig. 10.64*). Less commonly, crystals may be seen within the lumina of smaller arteries or arterioles.[1,11,12] The crystals show striking yellow or blue birefringence when examined in polarized light. They are sometimes accompanied by a foreign body giant cell reaction, particularly when present as dermal or subcutaneous deposits.[8,18,22–24] In those cases associated with gangrene or livedo reticularis, fibrin thrombi may also be detected.[8]

Calciphylaxis

Clinical features

Calciphylaxis was originally defined by an experimental model in rats, in which sensitization with parathormone or dihydrotachysterol followed by the injection of a challenging agent such as a metal salt resulted in localized necrosis and calcification.[1] The term was subsequently adopted to describe a condition in which an abnormality of calcium/phosphate metabolism is followed by calcification of the vasculature of the subcutaneous fat with subsequent thrombosis accompanied by extensive skin necrosis.[2–7]

Calciphylaxis presents clinically as an often bilateral and symmetrical, pruritic, and frequently painful/tender eruption most often affecting the lower limbs (*Fig. 10.65*). Less often, lesions may affect the breasts, buttocks, abdomen, and penis.[8–24] Calciphylaxis shows female predominance (about 2:1) and most commonly develops in the fifth decade of life.[25] Lesions are often well-delineated, livedoid, violaceous plaques and nodules associated with ischemic necrosis of the underlying tissues, sometimes extending down to the fascia. Ulceration is typically present, and sometimes bullae are a feature. Gangrene and autoamputation may accompany acral involvement.[6] Intestinal involvement with massive hemorrhage has exceptionally been documented.[16]

Calciphylaxis is associated with considerable morbidity and a high mortality of up to 60%.[4,14,26] The majority of patients succumb to secondary infection. Calciphylaxis due to the end-stage kidney disease can exceptionally develop in children.[27]

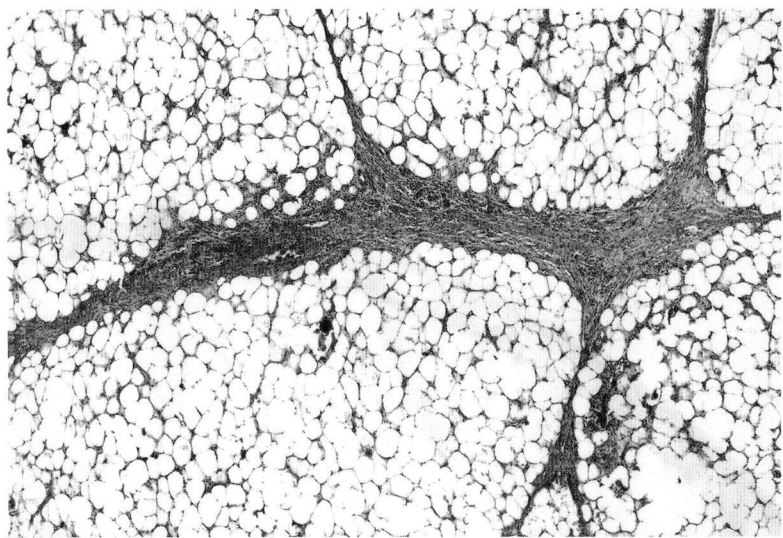

Fig. 10.66
Calciphylaxis: there is focal fat necrosis and widespread calcification affecting the small vessels. Note the thickened and fibrosed septa.

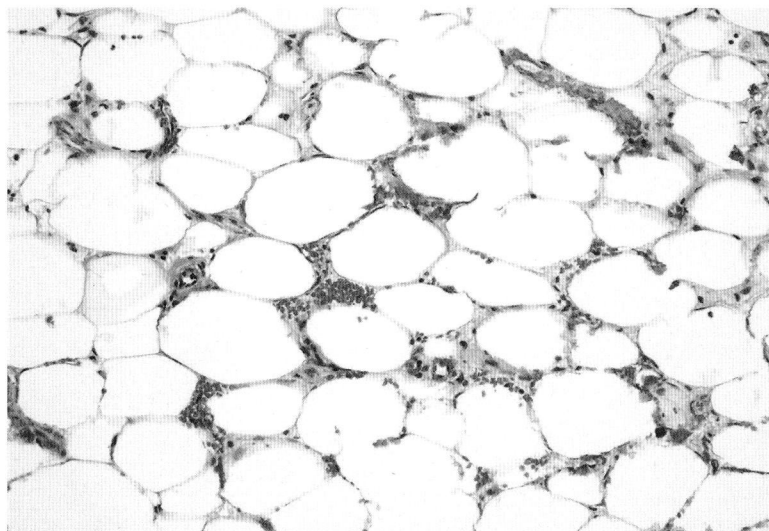

Fig. 10.67
Calciphylaxis: calcification of the small vessels and capillaries within the subcutaneous fat is evident.

Pathogenesis and histologic features

The precise mechanism by which the subcutaneous vasculature undergoes calcification is uncertain but is probably multifactorial. In the majority of patients, however, sensitization occurs as a consequence of abnormal calcium/phosphorus metabolism in a setting of chronic renal failure and secondary or tertiary hyperparathyroidism. Frequently, the patients are undergoing dialysis. Less often, there is a background of primary hyperparathyroidism or hypervitaminosis D.[4,12,14,17] Although in many patients calcium deposition occurs in association with an increased calcium-phosphorus product, in a significant proportion of patients calcium and phosphorus levels are normal.[4] It has been suggested that in such patients the calcification develops as a direct response to excess parathormone or vitamin D. Challenging agents resulting in the vascular precipitation of calcium salts are unknown, but a number of substances (including albumin, corticosteroids, warfarin, and immunosuppressives) have been incriminated.[12,28–30] Calciphylaxis has also been described in association with decreased functional protein C.[13] Rarely, the condition has presented in a patient with no evidence of a renal disorder or increase in parathormone level.[17] Diabetes, obesity, autoimmune diseases (rheumatoid arthritis, systemic lupus erythematosus, antiphospholipid syndrome), malignant tumors, giant cell arteritis, as well as alcoholic liver disease have been implicated in these patients.[25,31–38]

Histologically, the characteristic feature is calcification of the small- to medium-sized arteries and arterioles (Figs 10.66 and 10.67). Calcified debris may sometimes be present within the lumina, and occasionally the vessels are thrombosed (Fig. 10.68). Intimal fibroblastic proliferation with luminal narrowing has also been described (Fig. 10.69).[9] Hemorrhage within the subcutaneous fat may be seen and fat necrosis accompanied by a lobular lymphohistiocytic infiltrate has been documented in a number of cases (Fig. 10.70). Interstitial calcification is only rarely a feature.[9] Exceptionally, pseudoxanthoma elasticum-like changes have been documented.[39] In a related phenomenon, epidermal and follicular calcification have been described in the absence of vascular lesions in a patient with toxic epidermal necrolysis in a background of hyperparathyroidism.[40]

Differential diagnosis

Calcification involving small arteries and arterioles not accompanied by thrombosis has been described in patients with nephrogenic systemic fibrosis.[41] Furthermore, incidental vascular calcifications can also be found in patients with peripheral vascular disease, renal insufficiency, and diabetes mellitus.[42]

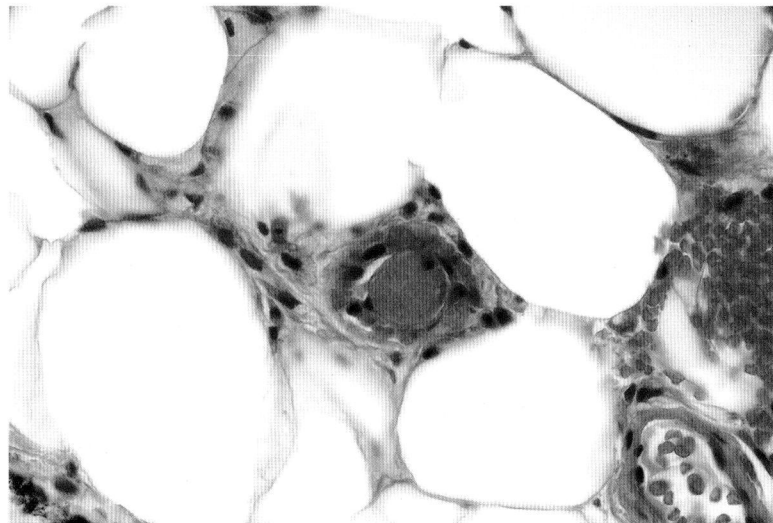

Fig. 10.68
Calciphylaxis: note the thrombosed vessel in the center of the field.

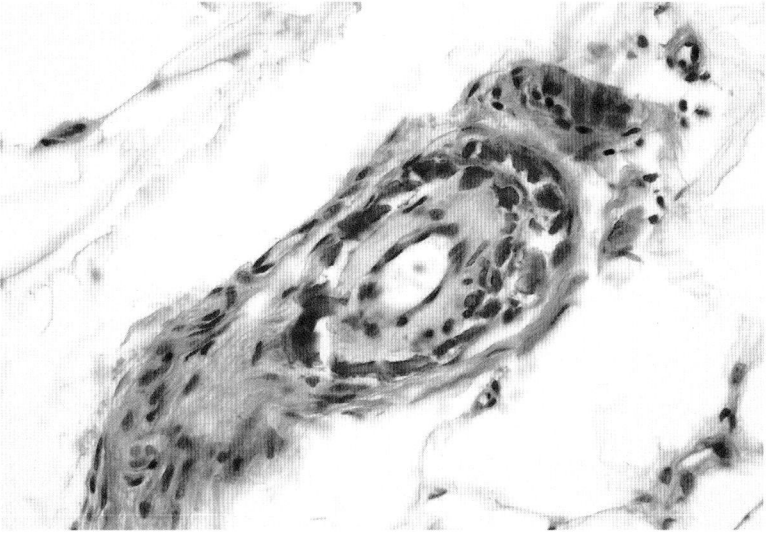

Fig. 10.69
Calciphylaxis: in addition to mural calcification, there is marked intimal fibroblastic proliferation.

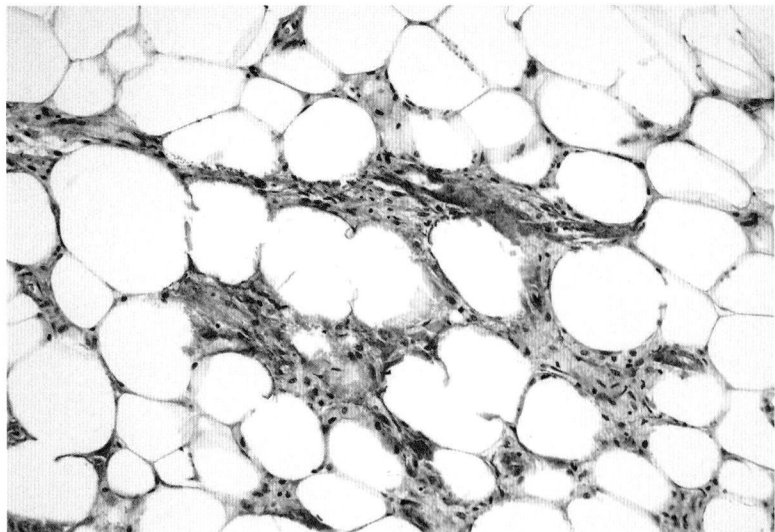

Fig. 10.70
Calciphylaxis: fat necrosis with conspicuous lipophages. In addition, there is widespread calcification.

Gouty panniculitis

Gouty panniculitis is an exceedingly rare cutaneous manifestation of gout characterized by the deposition of monosodium urate crystals in the subcutis.[1-9] The most common presenting features are indurated, occasionally painful plaques or nodules with a tendency to ulcerate with subsequent drainage of chalky material.[7,8] Although any site can be affected, there is a predilection for lower extremities. A disseminated variant has been reported.[7] Gouty panniculitis is more common in males (M/F, 5:1) and typically develops in the fifth decade of life.[9] Although generally a late manifestation of chronic gout, gouty panniculitis can also be an initial manifestation of the disease.[9] Hyperuricemia is present in the vast majority of patients.[5]

Histologic features

On histology, gouty panniculitis presents as a crystalline lobular panniculitis.[1-5] In formalin-fixed specimens, amorphous material surrounded by variably abundant granulomatous inflammation can be appreciated in a lobular distribution.[7,9] Extension into the deep dermis is not uncommon. Direct detection of crystals using polarized light requires either ethanol fixation or touch imprint slides.[9] For a more detailed description of gout, including differential diagnosis, see Chapter 13.

Nodular vasculitis

Clinical features

Nodular vasculitis (erythema induratum) is a rare condition which usually presents in young or middle-aged women, often in those with an erythrocyanotic circulation.[1] Males are only rarely affected.[2] Patients present with painful, tender, violaceous, indurated nodules particularly affecting the calves although the shins, feet, ankles, thighs, and upper limbs may sometimes be involved (*Figs 10.71* and *10.72*). Lesions are often bilateral, and the overweight with fat calves are most often affected. Seasonal variation has been noted with an increased incidence being recorded in the cold winter months. Skin lesions often recur over many years. Ulceration is common and scarring with hyperpigmentation frequently accompanies healing (*Figs 10.73–10.75*).

In those cases that represent a manifestation of underlying tuberculosis, the term erythema induratum (Bazin disease) is frequently applied. In this condition, there is invariable hypersensitivity to intradermal injection of purified protein derivative (PPD) at a dilution of 1:10 000 and a complete clearing of all skin lesions following treatment with antituberculous chemotherapy.[3-6]

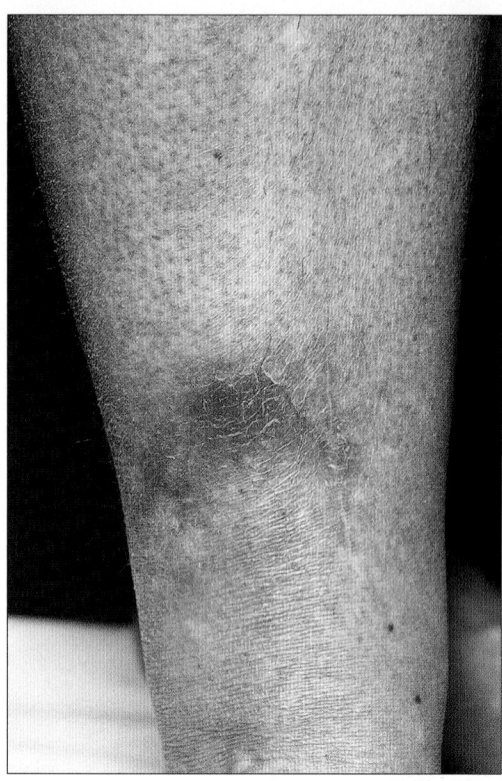

Fig. 10.71
Nodular vasculitis: early lesion presenting as an erythematous nodule on the calf of a middle-aged female. By courtesy of M.M. Black, MD, St Thomas' Hospital, London, UK.

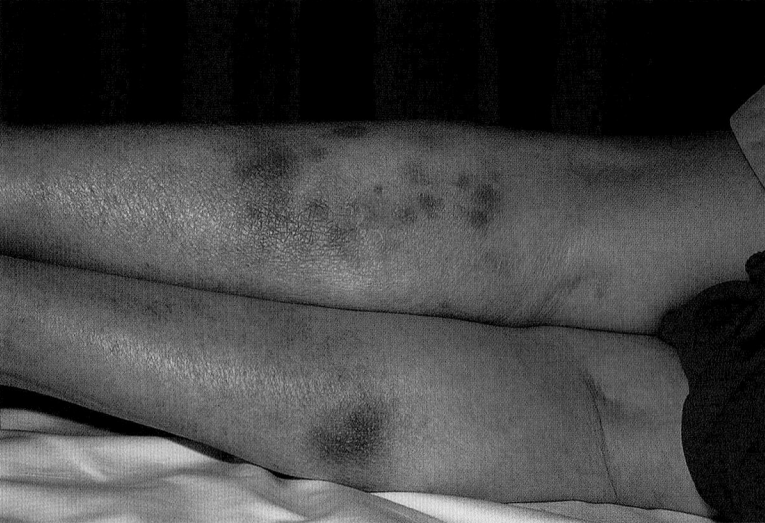

Fig. 10.72
Nodular vasculitis: typical bilateral involvement of the calves. By courtesy of the Institute of Dermatology, London, UK.

Pathogenesis and histologic features

The relationship between erythema induratum and nodular vasculitis has for many decades been the subject of controversy. Similarly, the association of the former condition with an underlying tuberculous infection has been the subject of prolonged debate.

As outlined above, the more recent literature gives considerable support to the notion that occult tuberculosis is present in many patients with erythema induratum and that the two terms are, therefore, synonymous in a substantial proportion of cases. Thus, erythema induratum may be associated with evidence of active tuberculosis.[7-14] Although cultures of lesions are invariably negative, the demonstration of *Mycobacterium tuberculosis* DNA

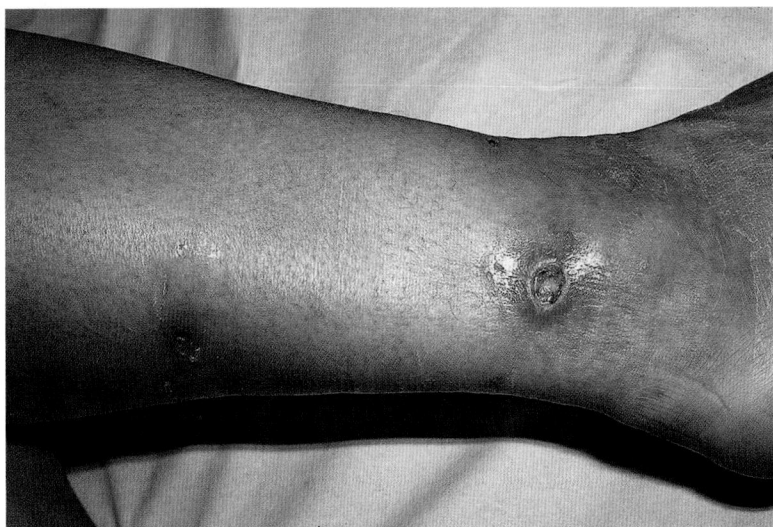

Fig. 10.73
Nodular vasculitis: the nodules frequently ulcerate. By courtesy of R.A. Marsden, MD, St George's Hospital, London, UK.

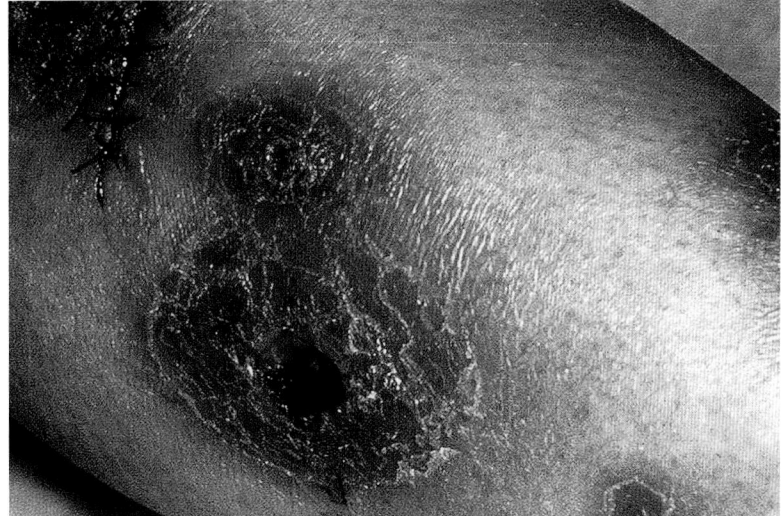

Fig. 10.74
Nodular vasculitis: in this severely affected patient, ulcerated lesions are present on the shins in addition to the calves. By courtesy of R.A. Marsden, MD, St George's Hospital, London, UK.

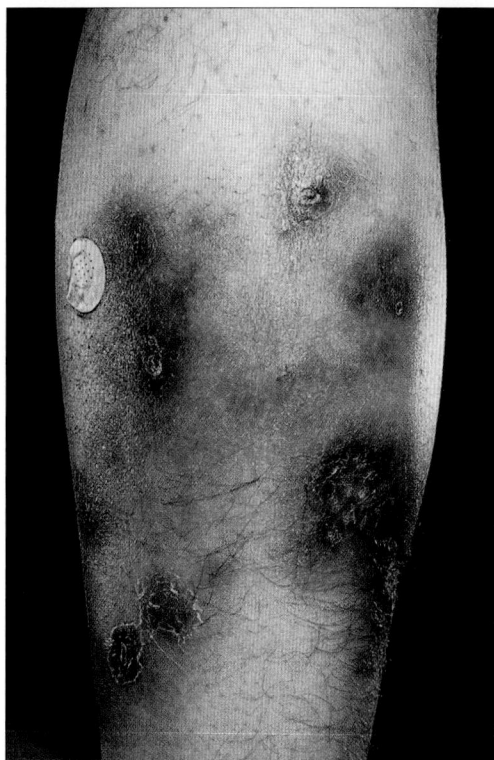

Fig. 10.75
Nodular vasculitis: multiple scarred lesions. Note the marked hyperpigmentation. By courtesy of the Institute of Dermatology, London, UK.

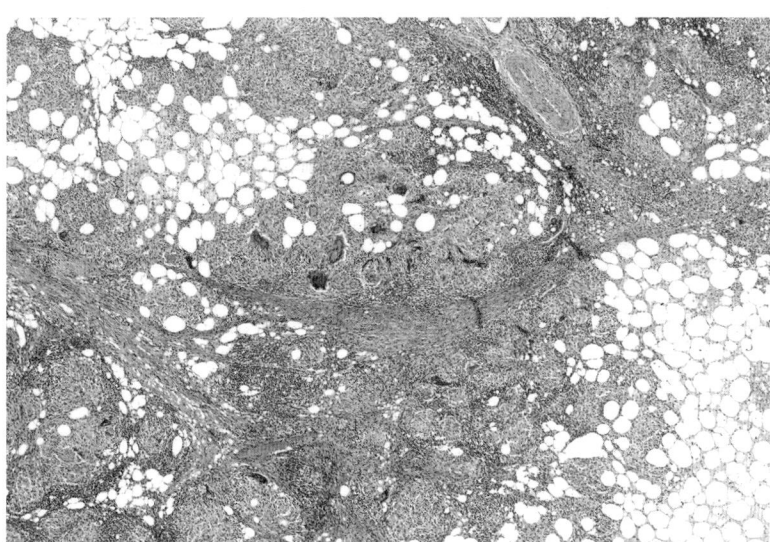

Fig. 10.76
Nodular vasculitis: note the distinct nodules of granulomatous inflammation at the periphery of the lobule.

by PCR in lesional tissue adds strong additional support to the proposal of an underlying tuberculous etiology.[15-25]

Nodular vasculitis can, therefore, be regarded as a hypersensitivity reaction in which mycobacterial antigens are one important cause. Immune complex and delayed hypersensitivity mechanisms have both been proposed.[16] Other predisposing factors for this condition have not yet generally been identified, although nodular vasculitis has been described in association with different infections (hepatitis B and C, *Nocardia*, *Pseudomonas*, *Fusarium*, *Mycobacterium avium*, *M. chelonae*, and *Chlamydia*), acute and chronic myeloid leukemia, ulcerative colitis, Crohn disease, rheumatoid arthritis, systemic lupus erythematosus, superficial thrombophlebitis, hypothyroidism, and as an adverse drug reaction to propylthiouracil and etanercept (tumor necrosis factor alpha inhibitor).[23,26-37] Bacille Calmette-Guérin (BCG) vaccination, distal painful peripheral neuropathy, and granulomatous aortic valve stenosis may on occasion be associated with erythema induratum of Bazin.[38-41]

The histologic features combine septal and lobular changes (*Fig. 10.76*). The presence of vasculitis has traditionally been regarded as a sine qua non for the diagnosis of nodular vasculitis (erythema induratum). Nevertheless, a study analyzing 101 biopsy specimens from 86 patients with clinical features of erythema induratum failed to detect the presence of vasculitis in 9.9% of specimens, even after examination of multiple serial sections.[31]

In a biopsy from an established lesion, the septa are widened and chronically inflamed (*Fig. 10.77*). Acute vasculitis (affecting septal and lobular veins and venules) with a heavy inflammatory cell infiltrate consisting of neutrophils, lymphocytes, and histiocytes is typically present, sometimes accompanied by vessel wall necrosis and thrombosis (*Fig. 10.78*). The most frequently affected are small lobular veins, followed by both septal veins and lobular venules.[31] In addition, septal arteries may also be involved by the vasculitic process.[31]

Occasionally, septal granulomatous inflammation can also be evident.

Lobular inflammation may occasionally be limited to a focal element adjacent to an acutely inflamed vessel.[42] More frequently, however, it presents as

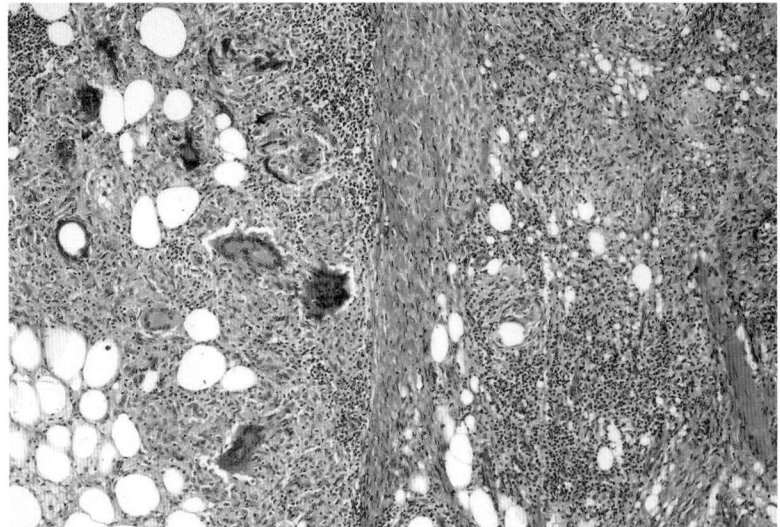

Fig. 10.77
Nodular vasculitis: well-formed epithelioid granulomata and multinucleate giant cells are present.

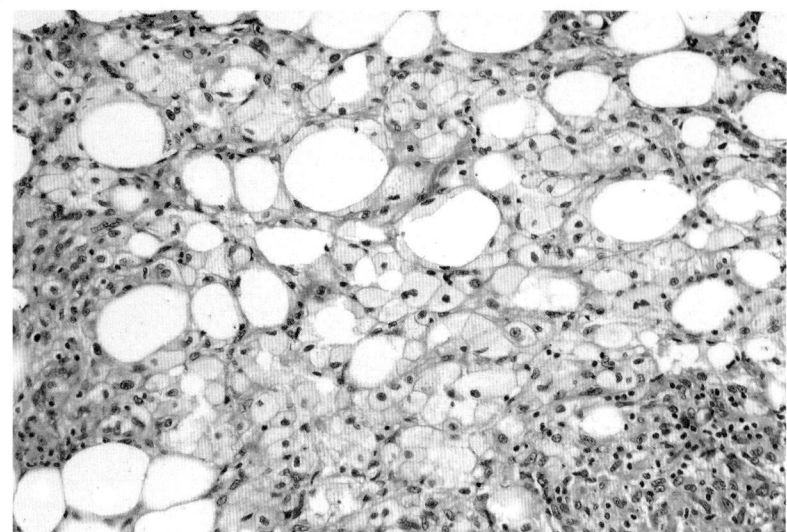

Fig. 10.79
Nodular vasculitis: note the presence of numerous lipophages.

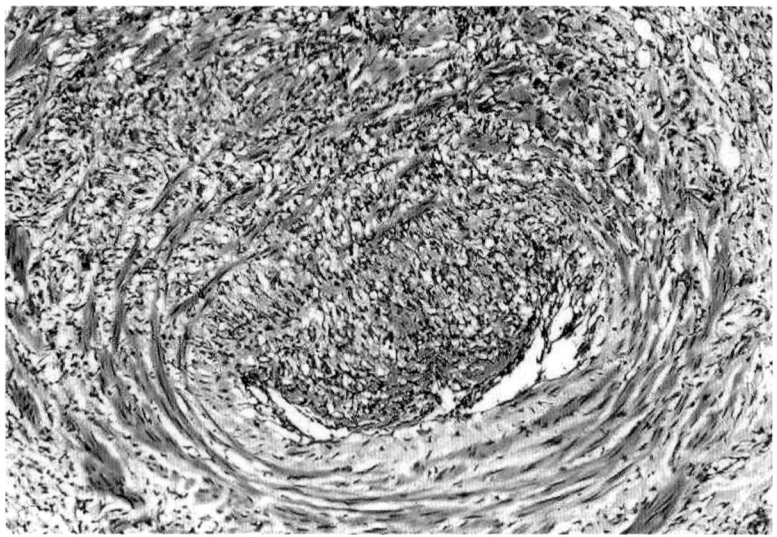

Fig. 10.78
Nodular vasculitis: vascular involvement as seen in this field is a characteristic feature.

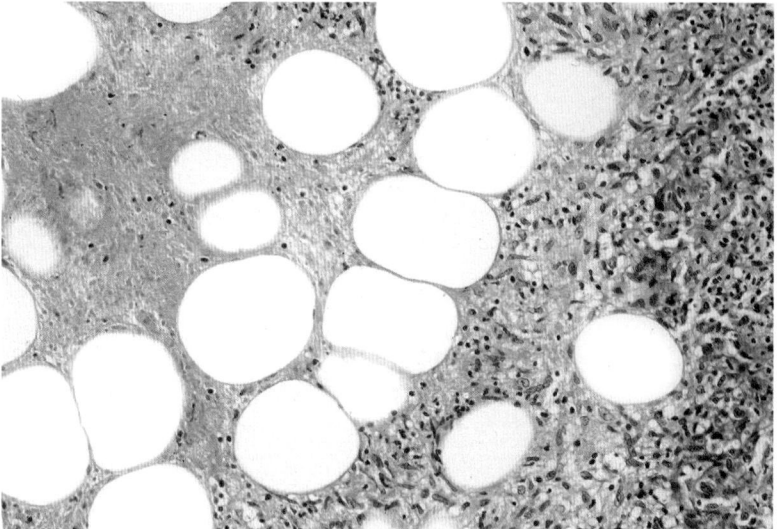

Fig. 10.80
Nodular vasculitis: the eosinophilic necrotic debris reminiscent of caseation is a typical feature.

nodular lesions scattered throughout the whole lobule or affecting multiple lobules. Fat necrosis is invariably present and is often florid. The features are varied and range from typical lipophagic fat necrosis to coagulative or, more rarely, caseation-like necrosis (*Figs 10.79* and *10.80*).[43] Neutrophils, lymphocytes, and histiocytes with xanthomatized forms are typically seen. Granulomata are often present, and giant cells of both foreign body and Langerhans type are frequently a feature (*Fig. 10.81*).

In biopsies from chronic or resolving lesions, fibrosis of both the septa and lobules is often present. Giant cells and granulomata may still be present.

Differential diagnosis

Due to the frankly granulomatous nature of the histology, it is mandatory to exclude infective causes of panniculitis, particularly mycobacterial and fungal infections, including cryptococcosis, mycetoma, chromomycosis, sporotrichosis, and aspergillosis. Subcutaneous sarcoidosis should also be considered, although in this condition granulomata are also seen in the dermis. Asteroid inclusions and Schaumann bodies, which are both features of sarcoidosis (see below), are not characteristic of erythema induratum.

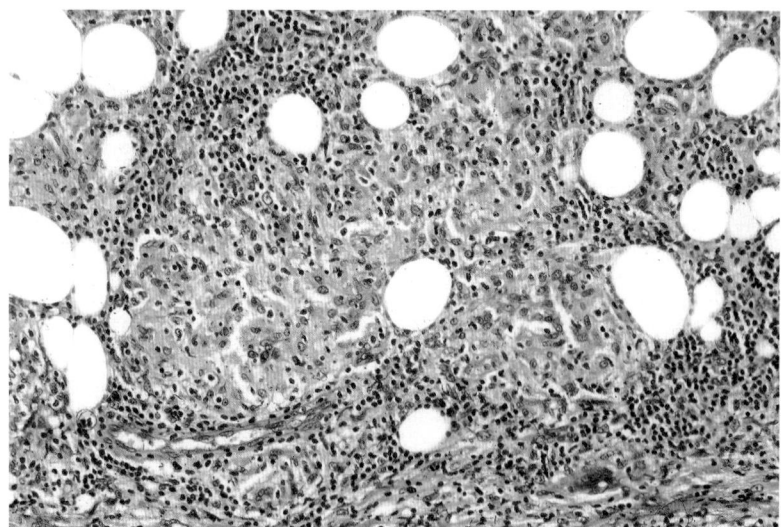

Fig. 10.81
Nodular vasculitis: granulomata may be seen within the lobule and also in the septa.

Subcutaneous sarcoidosis

Clinical features

A recent population-based epidemiological study from Minnesota, USA, revealed an incidence of cutaneous sarcoidosis of 1.9 patients per 100 000 population with female predominance.[1] Nevertheless, the frequency of subcutaneous sarcoidosis in patients with systemic sarcoidosis has been reported in different studies to be from 1.4% to as high as 16%.[2-5] Subcutaneous sarcoidosis most often presents as asymptomatic or tender, flesh-colored to erythematous, mobile, round to oval subcutaneous nodules with frequent clustering, principally affecting the extremities, although a more generalized distribution has also been documented.[3,4,6-12] Exceptionally, subcutaneous involvement may be the initial or even the only feature of sarcoidosis.[8,13,14] Isolated subcutaneous sarcoidosis has also been reported following interferon treatment for melanoma, and following treatment with adalimumab (a tumor necrosis factor alpha inhibitor) for pulmonary sarcoidosis.[15-17] It can also develop at sites of previous scar.[18] More commonly, however, subcutaneous lesions are associated with visceral disease, particularly bilateral hilar lymphadenopathy. In these patients, subcutaneous sarcoidosis tends to develop early in the course of the disease and generally follows an indolent clinical course.[5]

Subcutaneous sarcoidosis shows a predilection for females and the majority of patients are in the fifth and sixth decades.[8]

Histologic features

The changes, which predominantly involve the lobule, consist of well-formed, noncaseating granulomata, sometimes associated with fibrosis, which may extend into the septa. Typically, the granulomata are of the 'naked' type, i.e., devoid of a peripheral rim of lymphocytes, and giant cells of both foreign body and Langerhans types are usually present. Exceptionally, caseation and calcification have been described.[19,20] Noncaseating granulomas in the subcutaneous fatty tissue are rarely associated with granulomatous vasculitis.[21]

Differential diagnosis

Subcutaneous sarcoidosis is a diagnosis of exclusion; other causes of granulomatous inflammation – including mycobacterial and fungal infections, foreign body reactions, and so-called 'metastatic Crohn disease' – must be considered in the differential diagnosis.[22,23]

Neutrophilic lobular panniculitis associated with rheumatoid arthritis

Clinical features

Also known as pustular panniculitis, this rarely described entity has been documented in middle-aged females who presented with painful nodules predominantly affecting the lower legs.[1-5] Similar changes have also been reported on the back, upper arms, forearms, and nasal bridge in an infant with juvenile rheumatoid arthritis.[6] Blister formation, pustulation, ulceration, and discharge of oily, necrotic debris may occur.[3-5]

Pathogenesis and histologic features

The pathogenesis may be related to circulating immune complexes since high levels have been identified in patients with this condition.[3,4]

The lobules and septa are infiltrated by neutrophils with central lobular necrosis accompanied by a histiocytic and giant cell response.[2-5] Small numbers of eosinophils are sometimes present.[4] Nuclear dust can be conspicuous and cyst formation with membranous change has been described.[4,5] Leukocytoclastic vasculitis affecting the dermal arterioles and venules may be seen.[4] Endothelial swelling, hemorrhage, and fibrin deposition may also be present.[7]

Neutrophilic lobular panniculitis has also been reported in a patient with nonrheumatoid arthritis.[8]

Differential diagnosis

Factitial disease and infections must always be excluded in neutrophil-rich panniculitides. Similarly, pancreatic disease-associated panniculitis and α_1-antitrypsin deficiency-associated panniculitis are typically linked with a lobular neutrophil-rich infiltrate. The lobular panniculitis associated with bowel bypass is also typically neutrophil rich.[9,10]

Eosinophilic panniculitis

Clinical features

Eosinophilic panniculitis is not a disease in its own right, but represents a reaction pattern that may be found under a variety of circumstances.[1] It is seen more often in females than males (3:1). Although a wide age range is affected, there are two peaks: one in the third decade and the other in the sixth decade and above. Occurrence in children is exceptional.[2] Patients present predominantly with nodules and plaques, although papules and pustules are sometimes seen.[3-6] Lesions, which may be single or multiple, affect the legs, arms, trunk, and face in decreasing order of frequency.

Eosinophilic panniculitis may be found in association with erythema nodosum, immune complex-mediated vasculitis, atopic dermatitis, refractory anemia, chronic recurrent parotitis, artifact, leukocytoclastic vasculitis, drug reactions, eosinophilic cellulitis, insect bites, toxocariasis, gnathostomiasis, Fasciola infection, human immunodeficiency virus (HIV), specific immunotherapy with aqueous lyophilized bee venom, injection site reactions, trauma, and in patients with lymphoma.[6,7,22] On rare occasions, no obvious underlying condition can be detected.[2,20] Other than in those patients with an associated neoplasm, eosinophilic panniculitis appears to be a self-limiting and benign condition.[8]

Histologic features

The histologic features affect the lobules and the septa and are characterized by an intense infiltrate of eosinophils, which may be accompanied by variable numbers of other inflammatory cells including neutrophils, lymphocytes, and monocytes (*Figs 10.82* and *10.83*). Vasculitis is usually not seen. Fat necrosis is sometimes present. On occasion, typical 'flame figures', as seen in eosinophilic cellulitis, may be noted (*Fig. 10.84*). The changes sometimes extend into the reticular dermis, and occasionally the underlying fascia is involved.

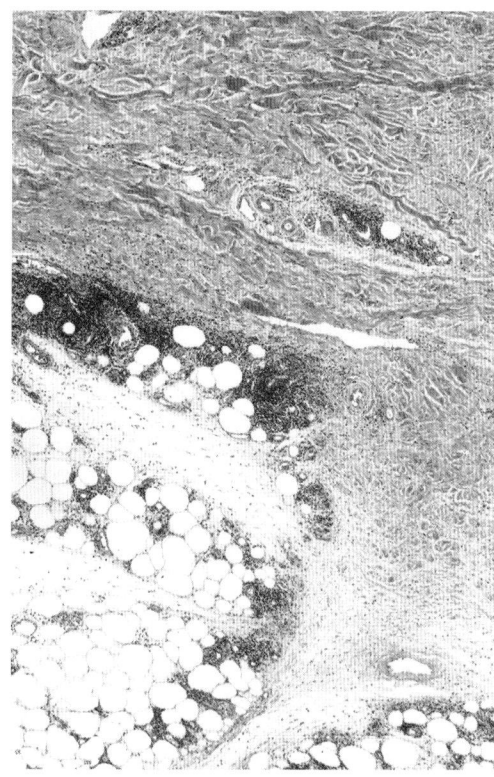

Fig. 10.82
Eosinophilic panniculitis: there is a heavy, predominantly lobular inflammatory cell infiltrate.

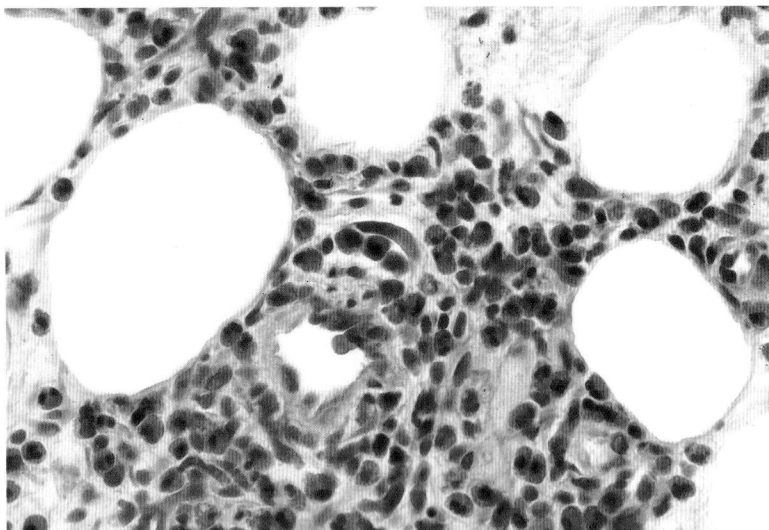

Fig. 10.83
Eosinophilic panniculitis: note the massive eosinophilic infiltrate.

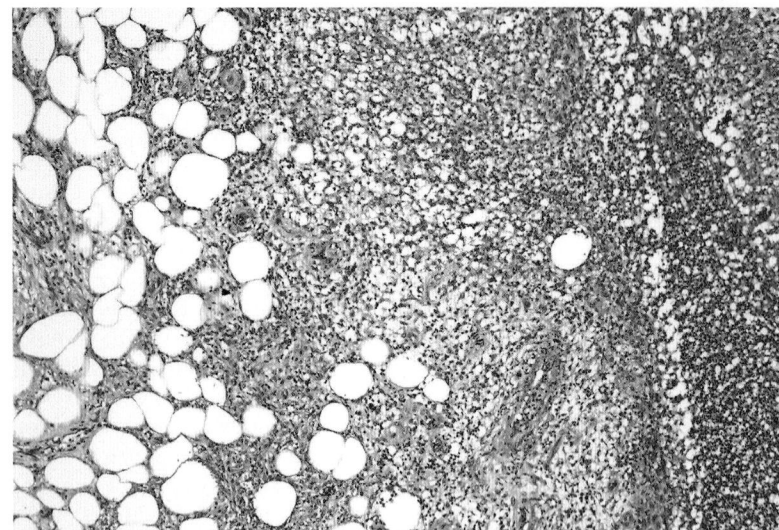

Fig. 10.85
Infective panniculitis: there is intense acute inflammation with abscess formation.

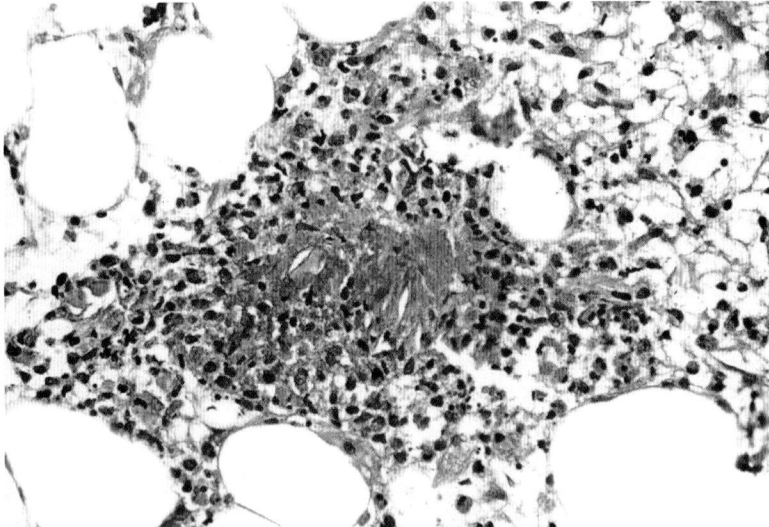

Fig. 10.84
Eosinophilic panniculitis: note the flame figure in the center of the field.

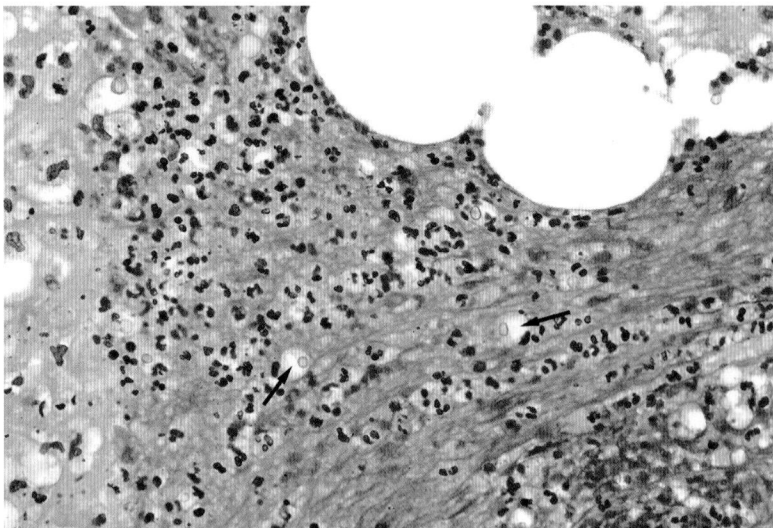

Fig. 10.86
Infective panniculitis: this example is due to cryptococcal infection. Note the typical yeast forms (*arrowed*).

Infective panniculitis

Clinical features

The clinical features in patients with infective panniculitis are not specific and include nodules, ulcerated lesions, abscesses, and erythema nodosum-like lesions.[1] Patients are usually, but not invariably, immunosuppressed. The legs and feet are the sites most often affected. Specific infections, which have presented with panniculitis, include *Histoplasma capsulatum*, *Pseudomonas aeruginosa*, *Candida albicans*, *Aspergillus* spp., *Zygomycetes*, *Cryptococcus neoformans*, *Fusarium* spp., *M. avium intracellulare*, *Mycobacterium ulcerans*, *Mycobacterium marinum*, *M. chelonae*, *Mycobacterium massiliense*, *Brucella* ssp., *Neisseria meningitidis*, *Streptococcus pyogenes*, *Staphylococcus aureus*, *Actinobacillus*, *Actinomyces* spp., *Coxiella burnetii*, and cytomegalovirus.[2–30]

Histologic features

Epidermal changes may include parakeratosis, acanthosis, and spongiosis.[1] The dermis is edematous and often shows a perivascular and interstitial inflammatory cell infiltrate containing many neutrophils. Hemorrhage is sometimes present.

Most commonly, the subcutaneous fat shows features of a mixed septal/lobular panniculitis (*Figs 10.85–10.89*).[1] Erythema nodosum-like or erythema induratum-like features may be evident.[1,29] Changes suggestive of an infective etiology include a prominent neutrophilic infiltrate, hemorrhage, basophilic necrosis and necrosis of sweat glands, vascular proliferation, and discrete abscess formation.[1,31]

Granulomata are sometimes conspicuous in atypical mycobacterial infections. On other occasions, acute inflammatory changes with abscess formation are seen (e.g., *M. chelonae* infection). In the latter condition, organisms may be identified in microcysts lined by neutrophil polymorphs.[1] Small cystic spaces may mimic adipocytes. Mycobacterial infection may also occasionally manifest as phlebitis.[32] Deep fungal infections commonly involve the subcutaneous fat, presenting as granulomatous or mixed suppurative and granulomatous inflammatory processes.

From the above description, it is obvious that special stains for bacteria and fungi should be performed in all cases of panniculitis where the etiology is uncertain. Culture may also be necessary in some instances.

Acute infectious id panniculitis – panniculitic bacterid

This is a variant of lobular neutrophilic panniculitis, which likely represents an id reaction to infections other than *M. tuberculosis*.[1]

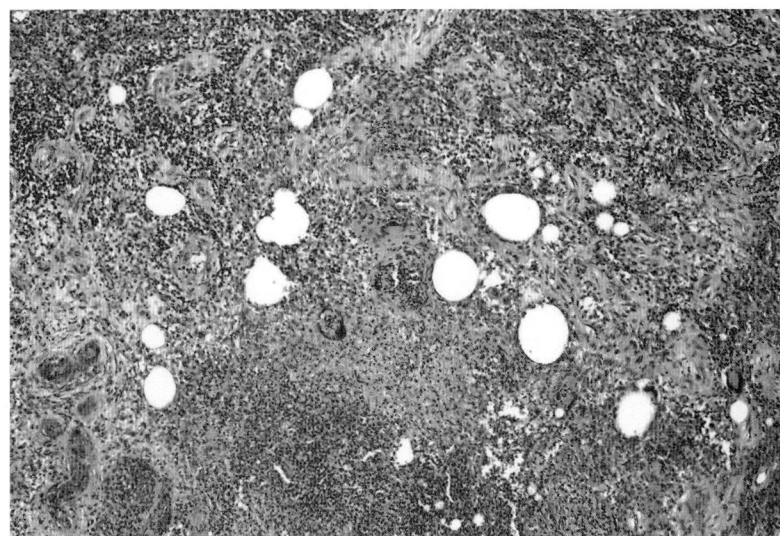

Fig. 10.87
Infective panniculitis: in this example, there is a granulomatous infiltrate.

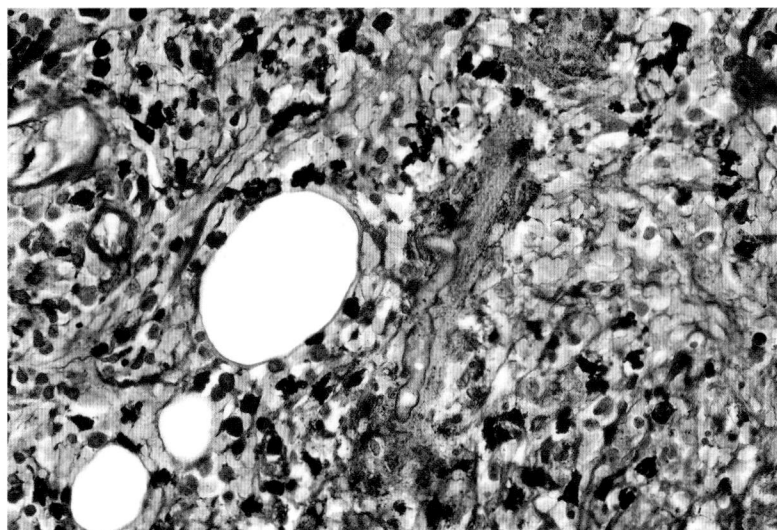

Fig. 10.88
Infective panniculitis: a twisted hypha typical of zygomycosis is present.

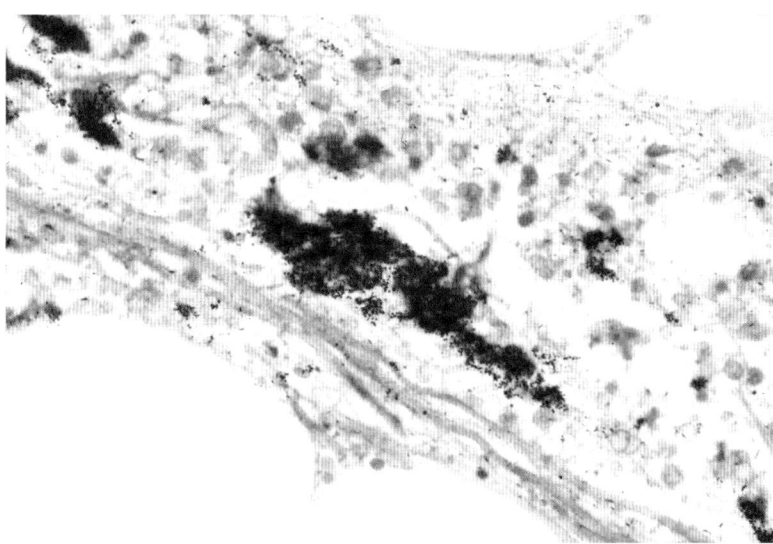

Fig. 10.89
Infective panniculitis: numerous cocci are present in this section from a patient with necrotizing fasciitis.

Clinical features

Following primary infection elsewhere (sinusitis, breast and dental abscess, impetigo, cellulitis, viral pharyngitis, *Pseudomonas pneumonia*, and ulcerative colitis), all 10 described patients (4 males, 6 females) presented with sudden development of tender nodules on the lower extremities, with additional involvement of the upper extremities in three patients. The lesions resolved completely after adequate therapy of the primary focus. Hyperviscosity conditions were present in three patients.

Histologic features

Fat lobules and septa were infiltrated by a prominent inflammatory cell infiltrate composed predominantly of neutrophils forming small microabscesses, accompanied by fat necrosis. Lymphocytes and histiocytes were also present in the infiltrate, with occasional granuloma formation. Spilling of the inflammation into the dermis was seen. Vascular changes consisted of necrotizing vasculitis involving arterioles and venules in the fat lobules and lower dermis, but also of thrombotic microangiopathy of the capillaries in the subcutaneous fat.

Special stains for microorganisms were negative in all cases. Infection with *M. tuberculosis* was excluded in all patients.

Differential diagnosis

Infection should be excluded with appropriate stains. Neutrophilic lobular panniculitis associated with rheumatoid arthritis can have a similar morphology, and clinicopathological correlation is vital.

Sclerosing panniculitis

Clinical features

Sclerosing panniculitis (stasis-associated sclerosing panniculitis, hypodermatitis sclerodermaformis, lipodermatosclerosis, lipomembranous change in chronic panniculitis) is a relatively common condition which most often develops in middle-aged or elderly, overweight females with a history of peripheral venous disease including varicose veins, thrombophlebitis, and deep venous thrombosis.[1–8] Less often, the condition follows arterial ischemia. Although early changes are characterized by painful erythematous and swollen plaques, the majority of patients present with indurated, woodlike, sclerodermiform plaques affecting the lower legs in a stocking distribution and characteristically resembling an inverted bottle appearance (*Fig. 10.90*).[1,3] Often, the changes are bilateral and symmetrical.[2] The overlying skin may show additional changes of venous stasis including atrophy, ulceration, hyperpigmentation, and telangiectasia. Patients with sclerosing panniculitis and systemic sclerosis frequently have associated pulmonary hypertension.[9] Changes similar to lipodermatosclerosis have also been reported following treatment with gemcitabine and pemetrexed.[10,11]

Pathogenesis and histologic features

The pathogenesis of sclerosing panniculitis is venous stasis within the centrilobular capillaries leading to ischemia and eventual infarction of the subcutaneous fat. Increased interstitial fibrinogen as a result of excessive capillary permeability due to venous hypertension is thought to be of importance.[4] Fibrin deposition around the dermal capillaries results in hypoxia. In addition, there is some evidence to suggest that increased matrix metalloproteinases and urokinase-type plasminogen activator may be of importance in the pathogenesis.[12,13]

The histologic features are variable depending on whether the biopsy represents an early stage in the development of this disorder or an established lesion.[5,14]

Within the subcutaneous fat, early lesions are characterized by centrilobular ischemia with infarction of fat cells and vascular congestion/hemorrhage.[5] Vascular thrombosis may also be seen, but there is no evidence of vasculitis. A lymphocytic infiltrate is present in the septa and this may spill over to affect the edge of the lobule. Histiocytes are often part of the inflammatory cell infiltrate.[8] Hemosiderin deposition is commonly present, but is usually more pronounced in established lesions.[8]

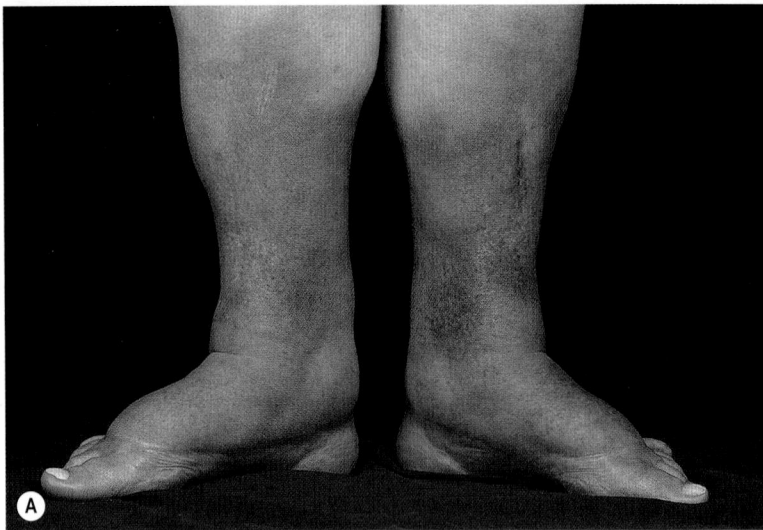

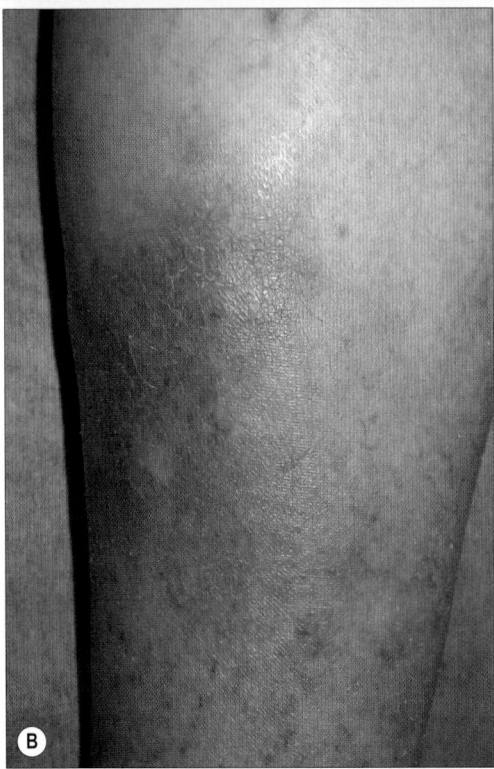

Fig. 10.90
Sclerosing panniculitis (**A**, **B**): (**A**) the skin shows features of stasis. Dense fibrosis has resulted in this inverted bottle appearance. Note the characteristic symmetry; (**B**) close-up view of an early lesion showing an indurated, markedly erythematous plaque. (**A**) By courtesy of the Institute of Dermatology, London, UK; (**B**) By courtesy of J.C. Pascual, MD, Alicante, Spain.

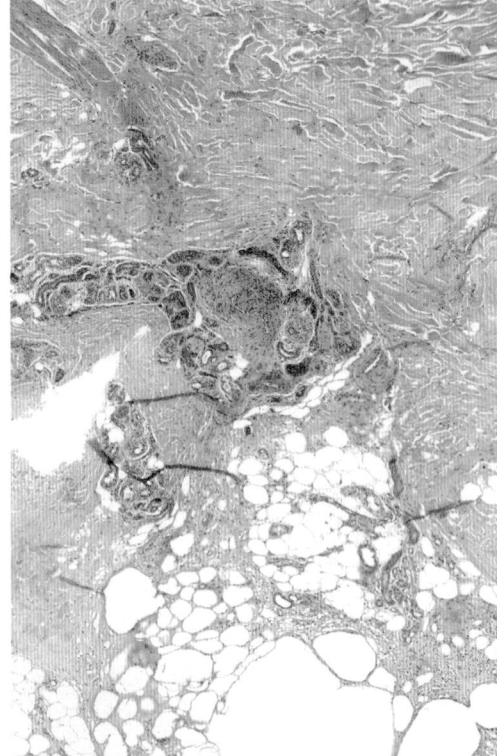

Fig. 10.91
Sclerosing panniculitis: there is typical microcystic change.

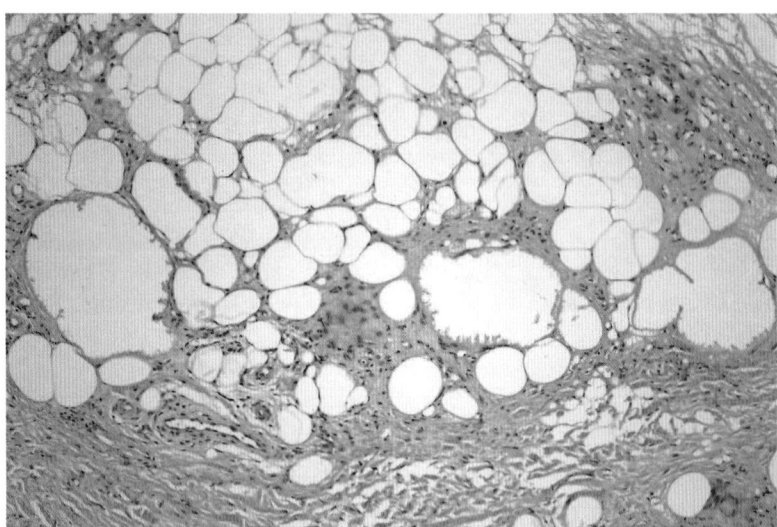

Fig. 10.92
Sclerosing panniculitis: close-up view of microcysts.

In established lesions, ischemic changes may still be evident but more often there is microcystic change with hyalinization within the fat lobule (*Figs 10.91–10.93*). Membranous fat necrosis is often present and lipophagic changes may be evident. Septal scarring is present, which in advanced lesions can be marked with resultant atrophy of the subcutaneous fat.

The dermis typically shows the features of stasis including chronic inflammation, fibrosis, vessel-wall thickening, lobular capillary proliferation, and hemosiderin deposition. Acanthosis, spongiosis, and lichenification may be evident.

Differential diagnosis

The absence of sclerodermiform dermal changes and the presence of features of venous stasis distinguish end-stage sclerosing panniculitis from morphea profunda, scleroderma, and acrodermatitis chronica atrophicans (a late manifestation of Lyme disease).

Membranous fat necrosis

Clinical features

Membranous fat necrosis is a non-specific change found predominantly in the subcutaneous fat. It was first described, however, in patients with progressive sudanophilic leukoencephalopathy (Nasu-Halola disease).[1-3] This is a rare condition in which cystic lesions develop in subcutaneous fat and bone marrow associated with pathological fractures and cerebral lesions resulting in seizures and presenile dementia.

Subsequently, membranous change has been recognized as a common manifestation of venous stasis-associated disease.[4-7] It has, however, also been observed in association with numerous other conditions including arterial insufficiency, diabetes mellitus, erythema nodosum, nodular vasculitis,

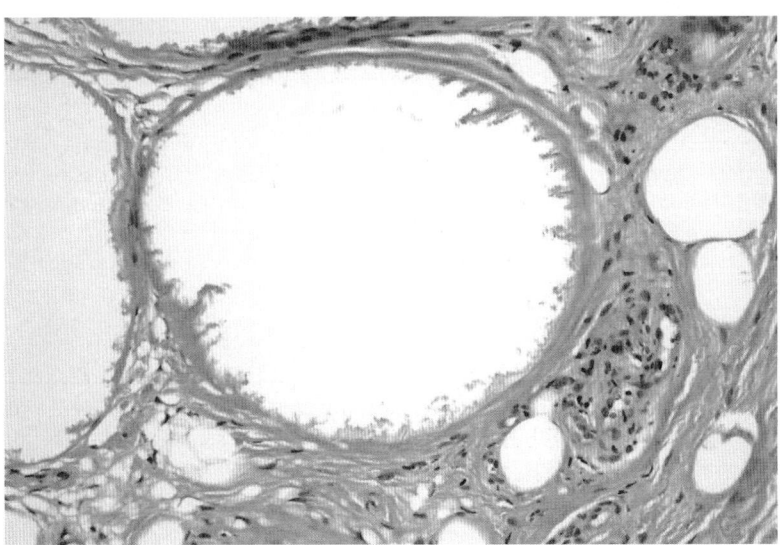

Fig. 10.93
Sclerosing panniculitis: membranous fat necrosis is evident.

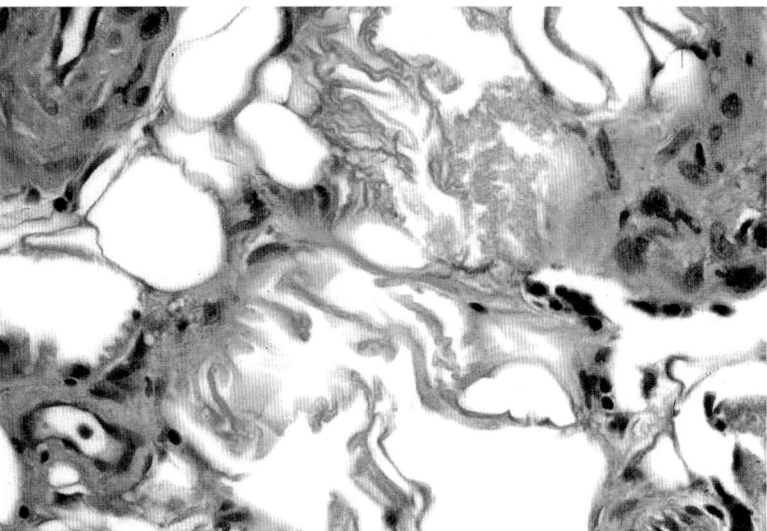

Fig. 10.95
Membranous fat necrosis: close-up view.

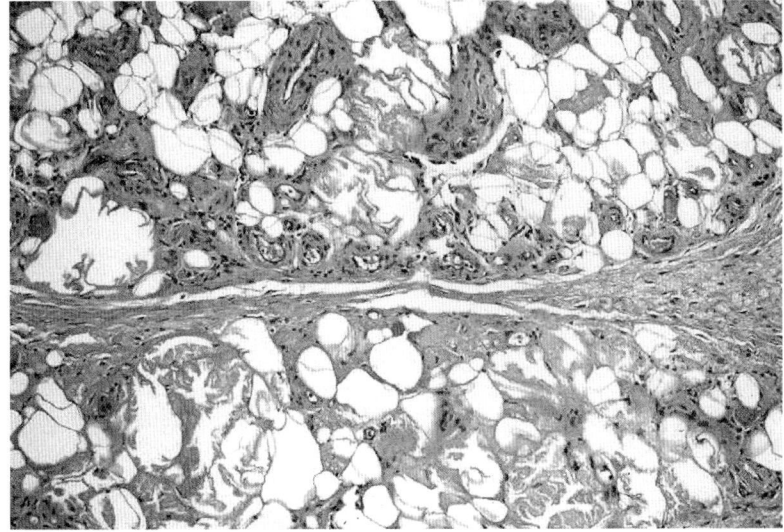

Fig. 10.94
Membranous fat necrosis: note the delicate membranes lying within small cystic spaces.

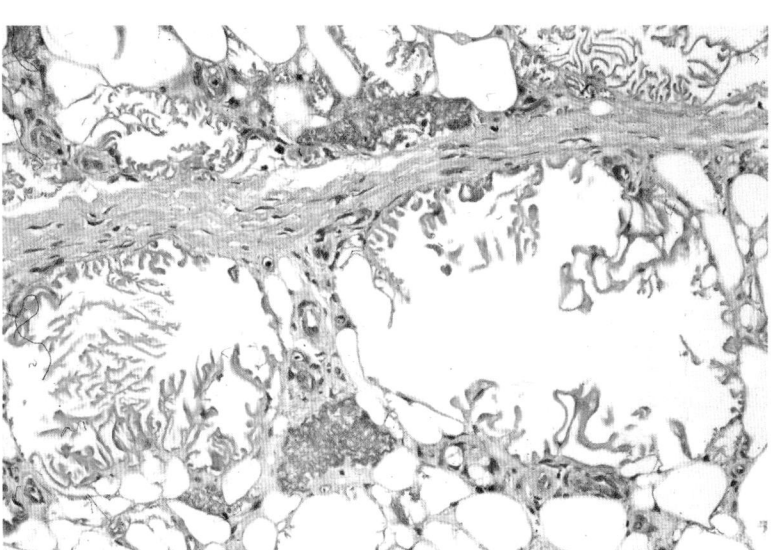

Fig. 10.96
Membranous fat necrosis: the features are highlighted with a Masson trichrome stain.

infective panniculitis, pancreatic disease-associated panniculitis, subcutaneous sarcoidosis, morphea, morphea profunda, cytophagic histiocytic panniculitis, dermatomyositis, systemic sclerosis, lupus panniculitis, necrobiosis lipoidica, and nodular cystic fat necrosis.[6–16] It has also been described in the breast, testis, in appendices epiploicae, within an ovarian cystic teratoma, and following subcutaneous elemental mercury injections.[17–23] Membranocystic change accompanied by myospherulosis has also been documented.[24]

Clinical presentation of membranous fat necrosis is variable. Patients can present with nonpainful or tender nodules, ecchymotic lesions, ulcerated or atrophic plaques, but also with diffuse swelling of the affected area.[25]

Pathogenesis and histologic features

Although in the majority of cases an ischemic pathogenesis is likely, its presence following trauma and in a background of infection suggests that other mechanisms are sometimes responsible. The membrane change likely represents altered adipocyte cell membranes although a contribution by histiocytes has been postulated.[5–7]

Histologically, it presents as amorphous, autofluorescent, eosinophilic, PAS-positive membranes outlining cysts within the lobules of the subcutaneous fat (Fig. 10.94). Pseudopapillary and arabesque patterns are commonly present (Figs 10.95 and 10.96). The membrane also stains for lipid using Sudan black and is luxol fast blue positive.[5] This is thought to represent ceroid, at least in part.[26]

Ultrastructurally, the membrane is composed of perpendicularly orientated microvilli alternating with dilated tubular crypts reminiscent of smooth endoplasmic reticulum with adjacent electron-dense material.[5]

LIPODYSTROPHY

Classification and clinical features

The lipodystrophies are a complex group of disorders characterized by a familial or acquired, complete or partial loss of subcutaneous fat.[1–4] They have been classified as follows[1]:

- Familial lipodystrophy including:
  - generalized lipodystrophy (Berardinelli-Seip syndrome)
  - partial lipodystrophy (Dunnigan and Köbberling variants)
- Acquired lipodystrophy including:
  - generalized lipodystrophy (Lawrence syndrome)
  - partial lipodystrophy (Barraquer-Simons syndrome)
  - HIV-associated lipodystrophy
- Localized lipoatrophy (localized lipodystrophy) including:
  - drug-induced lipoatrophy
  - pressure-induced lipoatrophy
  - panniculitis-associated lipoatrophy
  - centrifugal variant lipoatrophy
  - idiopathic lipoatrophy.

Familial lipodystrophy

Congenital generalized lipodystrophy (Berardinelli-Seip syndrome)

This exceedingly rare variant of lipodystrophy is inherited in an autosomal recessive mode and is usually recognizable at birth.[1–4] Its prevalence varies among different ethnic groups; from 1:200000 in Lebanon to 1:12000000 in the United States, with the worldwide prevalence somewhere in the range of 1:10000000.[1,5] The sex incidence appears to be equal, although some recent studies demonstrated female predominance.[6,7]

Congenital generalized lipodystrophy is characterized by a complete or near-complete absence of metabolically active subcutaneous fat in association with insulin resistance, hyperinsulinemia, hypertriglyceridemia with normal or slightly raised cholesterol, and nonketotic diabetes mellitus.[4] Mechanical fat such as is found in the orbits, on the palms and soles, and around the external genitalia is unaffected.[1] Patients also have a voracious appetite associated with a hypermetabolic state and marked hyperhidrosis. Additional features include an anabolic syndrome with increased height velocity, advanced bone age, muscular hypertrophy, masculine body build, acromegaloid stigmata, hepatomegaly, enlarged external genitalia in childhood, abundant curly hair on the scalp, hypertrichosis, umbilical hernia, acanthosis nigricans, mild mental retardation with hydrocephalus, cardiomyopathy, cardiac arrhythmia, muscular dystrophy, phlebomegaly, anemia, breast enlargement, steatorrhea, pancreatitis, achalasia, intraventricular hemorrhage, nephrolithiasis, epilepsy, pilocytic astrocytoma, and hypothalamic–pituitary dysfunction.[4,5,8–16]

Diabetes is thought to develop as a consequence of extensive pancreatic amyloid deposition with loss of β cells.[17] Postmortem studies have demonstrated fatty liver with cirrhosis.[18]

Congenital generalized lipodystrophy has currently been classified into four types according to the type of mutations. In about 95% of the patients, the genes for congenital generalized lipodystrophy have been mapped to human chromosome 9q34 and 11q13, and are designated 1-acylglycerol-3phosphate O-acyltransferase 2 (AGPAT2) gene and Berardinelli-Seip congenital dystrophy 2 (BSCL2) gene or SEIPIN gene, respectively.[19–23] Mutations in the AGPAT2 gene are a defining feature of congenital generalized lipodystrophy type 1 while mutations in the BSCL2 gene define congenital generalized lipodystrophy type 2. Calveolin 1 (CAV1) is mutated in congenital generalized lipodystrophy type 3 and polymerase I and transcript release factor (PTRF) gene in type 4 congenital generalized lipodystrophy.[23–28] Not all patients have mutations in these genes, suggesting the presence of additional yet unidentified genetic loci.[29] In agreement with this, a de novo variant of congenital generalized lipodystrophy associated with mutation in the promoter of the FOS gene has recently been reported.[30] The genes involved in the pathogenesis of congenital generalized lipodystrophies are responsible for the synthesis of triacylglycerol, fusion of lipid droplets, as well as development and maturation of adipocytes.[7]

Diagnostic criteria as outlined in Table 10.3 have been recommended.[1]

Familial partial lipodystrophy (Dunnigan variant, type 2 FPLD)

This is another exceedingly rare condition with an estimated prevalence of less than 1 in 15000000 of the population.[1] The original cases were all females, and therefore a sex-linked dominant mechanism, lethal in hemizygous males, was postulated.[31,32] The more recent publication of families with affected male members suggests, however, that an autosomal dominant mechanism is at play.[33]

Patients are normal at birth, but at puberty they lose subcutaneous fat from the extremities and to a lesser extent from the trunk.[34] The face is spared and, indeed, in some patients, excessive fat deposition on the face and neck has been documented giving the patients a cushingoid appearance. Diabetes mellitus, hypertriglyceridemia, and low serum high density lipoprotein (HDL) cholesterol levels become manifest in early adulthood.[1,35,36] Patients may develop chylomicronemia and pancreatitis.[1] Acanthosis nigricans, hirsutism, steatosis of the liver, nonischemic and ischemic cardiomyopathy, heart conduction defects, menstrual abnormalities, polycystic ovaries, and fertility problems are also sometimes evident.[1,37] The extent of subcutaneous fat loss has been associated with the severity of associated metabolic complications.[37]

The gene responsible for familial partial lipodystrophy has been mapped to chromosome region 1q21-22.[38–40] It has been identified as the lamin A/C (LMNA) gene, which codes for a nuclear envelope protein lamin.[41–43] More than 85% of the patients harbor mutation in a single allele encoding the arginine residue at position 482.[44]

Diagnostic criteria as outlined in Table 10.3 have been recommended.[1]

Familial partial lipodystrophy (Köbberling variant, type 1 FPLD)

This is an exceedingly rare variant in which only a small number of affected pedigrees have been documented.[1,45–47] The majority of patients display an autosomal dominant mode of inheritance.[48] Sporadic variants have also been described.[1,47,49] In these patients, loss of fat is limited to the extremities. There may be increased truncal fat, in particular, subcutaneous and visceral abdominal fat.[1,47,48] Less often, fat accumulates in the face and neck.[48] Recognizable lipodystrophy generally develops before the adolescence.[48] The severity of metabolic abnormalities is inversely correlated to the percentage of fat in the lower extremities and directly proportional to the amount of visceral fat.[48] Hypertriglyceridemia, arterial hypertension, insulin resistance, or diabetes mellitus are usually present, and the patients have increased risk for premature cardiovascular disease and pancreatitis.[1,47] Acanthosis nigricans has been described in a single patient.[47] To date, documented affected patients have been female.

Familial partial lipodystrophy associated with mandibuloacral dysplasia

This autosomal recessive variant of lipodystrophy is characterized by the presence of a variety of bony defects including mandibular and clavicular hypoplasia, acroosteolysis, delayed closure of cranial sutures, and joint contractures associated with cutaneous hyperpigmentation.[50,51] Some patients also show progeroid characteristics. Genetically, it is a heterogeneous disorder. Mutations in genes encoding nuclear lamina proteins and zinc metalloproteinase have been detected.[52–55] Lipodystrophy varies from loss limited to the extremities (type A) through to generalized loss (type B). Patients also

Table 10.3

Lipodystrophies: diagnostic criteria

Disorder	Essential criteria	Confirmatory criteria
Congenital generalized lipodystrophy	Generalized lack of body fat Extreme muscularity from birth	Acanthosis nigricans Acromegaloid features Umbilical hernia Clitoromegaly and mild hirsutism Severe fasting or postprandial hyperinsulinemia Onset of diabetes or impaired glucose tolerance test in teenage years Hypertriglyceridemia with low HDL cholesterol concentration Characteristic body fat distribution on MRI
Familial partial lipodystrophy (Dunnigan variant)	Normal physical appearance at birth Loss of subcutaneous fat of the extremities commencing at puberty Muscular-appearing extremities commencing at puberty	Normal or excessive facial adipose tissue Acanthosis nigricans Mild to moderate fasting or postprandial hyperinsulinemia Onset of diabetes or impaired glucose tolerance after age 20 years Hypertriglyceridemia with low serum HDL cholesterol concentrations Characteristic body fat distribution on MRI
Acquired generalized lipodystrophy	Generalized loss of subcutaneous fat developing in childhood or later Extreme muscularity appearing in childhood or later	Loss of fat from palms and soles Severe fasting or postprandial hyperinsulinemia Impaired glucose tolerance or diabetes Hypertriglyceridemia with low serum HDL cholesterol concentrations Nodular panniculitis preceding onset of lipodystrophy Coexistence of autoimmune diseases
Acquired partial lipodystrophy	Gradual loss of subcutaneous fat of the face, neck, trunk, and upper extremities developing in childhood or adolescence	Normal or excess fat on hips and lower extremities Proteinuria Biopsy-proven mesangiocapillary glomerulonephritis Low serum C3 levels Presence of C3 nephritic factor Absence of insulin resistance Presence of other autoimmune diseases Characteristic body fat on MRI

HDL, high density lipoprotein; MRI, magnetic resonance imaging. Derived from Garg, A. (2000) American Journal of Medicine, 108, 143–152.

have insulin-resistant hyperinsulinemia and hypertriglyceridemia and diminished serum HDL cholesterol levels.[51]

Acquired lipodystrophy

Acquired generalized lipodystrophy

Acquired generalized lipodystrophy (Lawrence syndrome, lipoatrophic diabetes, lipoatrophic panniculitis, lipodystrophic diabetes) can be subclassified into three variants:

- Type 1: the panniculitis variant,
- Type 2: the autoimmune disease variant,
- Type 3: the idiopathic variant, and affect 25%, 25%, and 50% of the patients, respectively.[56]

Acquired generalized lipodystrophy is similar to the congenital form although there is a predilection for females (3:1).[1,56–59] Patients present in childhood or adolescence with fat loss, which progresses over a period of months or years.[1] The entire body is affected, particularly face, arms, and legs. The muscles of the extremities appear unduly prominent. Children with this disorder may have a voracious appetite.

Features of an inflammatory nodular panniculitis appear to have preceded the onset of lipodystrophy in a number of cases (lipoatrophic panniculitis).[56,60,61] These patients appear to have less severe fat loss and lower prevalence of hypertriglyceridemia and diabetes in comparison with patients having the autoimmune or idiopathic variant of the disease.[56]

Autoimmune diseases associated with acquired generalized lipodystrophy include juvenile dermatomyositis in particular, followed by Hashimoto thyroiditis, juvenile rheumatoid arthritis, juvenile and adult-onset dermatomyositis, systemic lupus erythematosus, systemic sclerosis, Sjögren syndrome, Graves disease, autoimmune hemolytic anemia, non-thrombocytopenic purpura, chronic urticaria, angioedema, type I diabetes, and vitiligo.[1,62–66]

Liver involvement may be marked with steatosis, autoimmune hepatitis, and cirrhosis supervening in a substantial number of cases.[4,67] Additional features include severe insulin resistance, diabetes, hyperinsulinemia, and hypertriglyceridemia accompanied by low serum HDL cholesterol concentrations.[1,56] Acquired generalized lipodystrophy can also be associated with cerebellar degeneration, unicameral bone cysts, and proteinuric nephropathy.[68–70]

A preceding viral illness has frequently antedated the development of acquired generalized lipodystrophy, although whether this is causal or not is unclear.[1,4] A case of panniculitis of the acquired generalized lipodystrophy variant was reported recently, presumably triggered by pulmonary tuberculosis.[71] Patients with acquired generalized lipodystrophy are at increased risk for lymphoma development, in particular, peripheral T-cell lymphoma.[72,73] Additional lymphomas reported in these patients include ALK-positive anaplastic large cell lymphoma, mycosis fungoides, and Burkitt lymphoma.[73]

Diagnostic criteria as outlined in *Table 10.3* have been recommended.[1]

Acquired partial lipodystrophy

Acquired partial lipodystrophy (Barraquer-Simon syndrome, progressive lipodystrophy, cephalothoracic progressive lipodystrophy) is one of the more common variants of lipodystrophy. Females are affected three times more often than males.[1] Patients present in late childhood or adolescence with gradual loss of the subcutaneous fat of the face followed by the neck, shoulders, arms, thorax, and upper abdomen (*Fig. 10.97*).[1,74–76] The distal subcutaneous fat is typically spared and sometimes, in contrast, there is even excessive fat deposition around the pelvis and on the legs.

Mesangiocapillary (membranoproliferative) glomerulonephritis (MCGN II) and hypocomplementemia often accompany this variant.[77–79] C3 levels are usually low in contrast to C1q, C4, C5, C6, factor B, and properdin, which are normal.[80,81] The glomerulonephritis and low C3 have been shown to be due to an IgG autoantibody, the C3 nephritic factor (C3NeF).[82] It has been shown that the latter has the capacity to induce adipocyte lysis.[83] Three patients have been described that presented with low C4 complement levels, widespread acquired lipodystrophy, and chronic autoimmune hepatitis.[84]

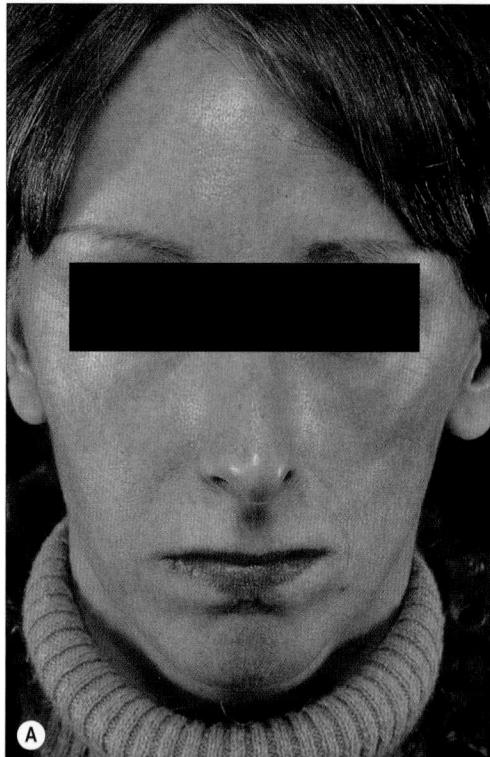

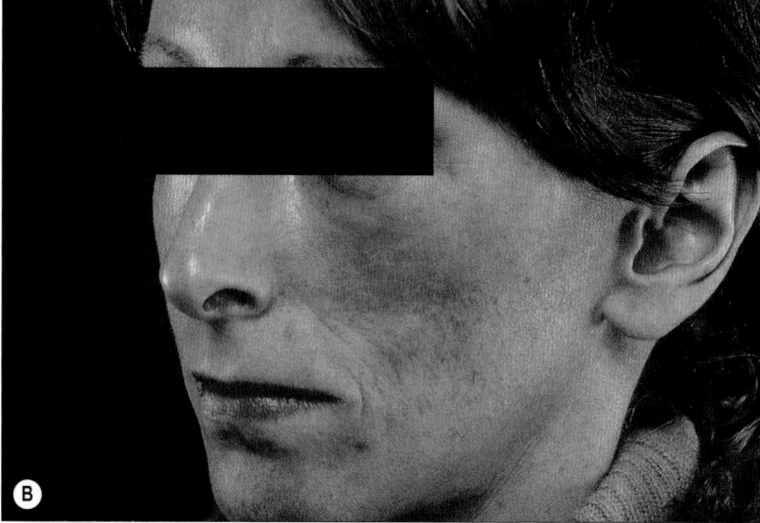

Fig. 10.97
(**A, B**) Partial lipodystrophy: note the striking loss of symmetry due to diminished fatty tissue of the left side of the face. By courtesy of the Institute of Dermatology, London, UK.

An association with a number of other autoimmune diseases including Sjögren syndrome, dermatomyositis, hypothyroidism, SLE, autoimmune hepatitis, rheumatoid arthritis, vitiligo, scleroderma, and idiopathic thrombocytopenic purpura has also been documented.[85–92] Patients may in addition develop hyperlipidemia, hypertriglyceridemia, low HDL holesterol levels, nonketotic diabetes mellitus, acanthosis nigricans, and hirsutism.[1,6] A recent study from Turkey demonstrated that about three-fourths of patients with acquired localized lipodystrophy display at least one metabolic abnormality, most commonly hypertriglyceridemia.[6] Furthermore, 28% of patients developed diabetes at a young age.[6] Hepatomegaly due to fat accumulation is occasionally present. Extrinsic allergic alveolitis has been reported in a single patient.[93] Ocular changes have rarely been described and include retinal pigment alterations, drusen, and choroidal neovascularization.[94–96] Acquired partial lipodystrophy with a distribution similar to Dunnigan-type familial partial lipodystrophy has been reported in five patients following hematopoietic stem cell transplantation to treat leukemia or neuroblastoma.[97] In addition, a single case of acquired partial lipodystrophy after bleomycin treatment has also been described.[98]

Expression gene analysis in a single patient with acquired partial lipodystrophy demonstrated downregulation of the *PPARγ* gene, which is normally associated with adipocyte differentiation, as well as reduced expression of mitochondrial genes.[99] In addition, heterozygous mutations of the *LMNB2* gene have been detected in some patients.[100,101]

Diagnostic criteria as outlined in *Table 10.3* have been recommended.[1]

Localized lipoatrophy

Clinical features

Localized disease (lipoatrophy) is a much more common phenomenon. The subject has, however, been made extremely complicated by virtue of the large number of synonyms that have been used to describe the same disease process over the years (e.g., lipodystrophy, annular lipoatrophy, annular lipodystrophy, semicircular lipoatrophy, postinjection lipoatrophy, involutional lipoatrophy, lipodystrophia centrifugalis abdominalis infantilis, centrifugal lipodystrophy). Essentially, localized lipodystrophy may result from a range of injurious stimuli and present at a wide variety of sites but essentially all of the subtypes listed above are variations of the same disease process. In general, localized lipoatrophy can be classified as primary (idiopathic) or as secondary due to trauma, injections of various drugs and vaccines, connective tissue diseases, or malignant neoplasms.[102,103]

Lesions affecting the proximal extremities or buttocks should raise the possibility of infection or trauma. Localized lipoatrophy has been described following subcutaneous injections of insulin, penicillin, amikacin, methotrexate, corticosteroids, glatiramer acetate, triamcinolone acetate, and iron dextran, and following vaccinations.[102,104–113] It has also been described as a complication of idiopathic connective tissue diseases including systemic lupus erythematosus (profundus), dermatomyositis, polymyositis, linear morphea, facial hemiatrophy, lichen sclerosus, and progressive systemic sclerosis.[114–116]

Other types of localized lipodystrophy include annular lipodystrophy and a variant that affects only half the circumference of an extremity (lipoatrophia semicircularis). These distinctive annular lesions are likely to result from a localized pressure effect such as that which may occur with tight clothing or persistent localized trauma.[117–120] Idiopathic variants are also recognized including lipoatrophy associated with Becker nevus and lipodystrophia centrifugalis abdominalis infantilis.[121–124]

Pathogenesis and histologic features

The exact pathogenesis of lipodystrophy is unknown. A variety of theories has been proposed, including hypothalamic–pituitary dysfunction (overproduction of fat-mobilizing peptides and amines), disordered fat metabolism, infection, and heredity. A favored area of research is directed towards the role of abnormal insulin receptors on fat cells. It has been postulated that abnormal insulin receptors are associated with diminished uptake of lipid by fat cells with resultant lipodystrophy, hyperlipidemia, and hyperinsulinemia.

In general, the histopathology of lipodystrophy is noninflammatory in nature.[125–127] There is a progressive diminution of adipocyte lipid accompanied by a decrease in cell size so that the cells become separated from one another (*Fig. 10.98*). The stroma becomes hyalinized or myxomatous and contains clusters of tortuous capillaries. As the end result resembles embryonic fat, this process of atrophy is sometimes called 'reversal of embryogenesis'.

Patients with multiple areas of localized lipoatrophy may show mild inflammatory changes comprising perivascular and periseptal lymphocytic infiltration accompanied by minor septal fibrosis.

Lipoatrophic panniculitis

Clinical features

Lipoatrophic panniculitis (atrophic connective tissue panniculitis) represents a very rarely documented inflammatory form of localized lipoatrophy.[1–7] In

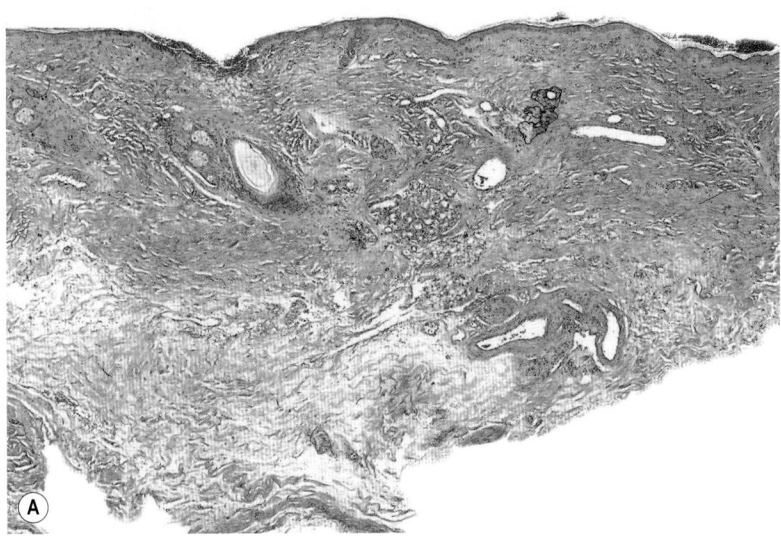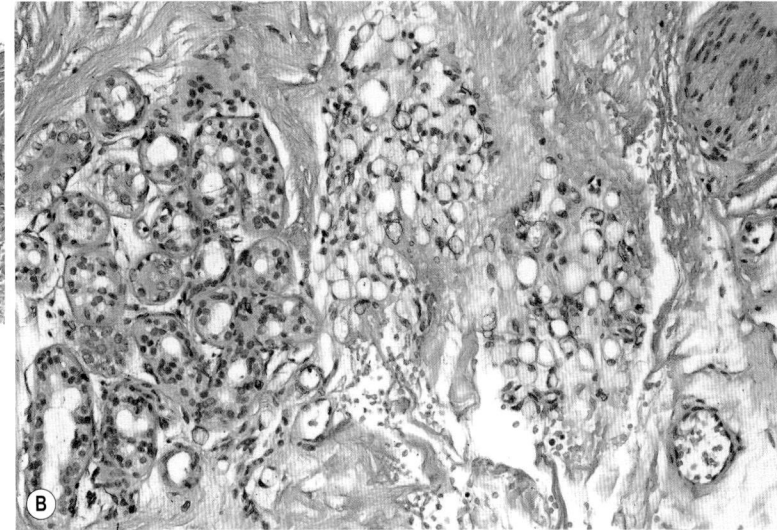

Fig. 10.98
Lipodystrophy: (**A**) there is only a very small residual amount of subcutaneous fat in the center of the field; (**B**) these tiny adipocytes are reminiscent of embryonic fat. By courtesy of W.P.D. Su, MD, Mayo Clinic, Rochester, USA.

the original report, three children developed centrifugally enlarging erythematous nodules and plaques with atrophic centers on the lower extremities. Healing of the lesions resulted in the clinical appearances of localized lipoatrophy. The areas of lipoatrophy coalesced to give an appearance resembling partial or total lipodystrophy.[1] All three patients had elevated ESRs. Two patients had associated diabetes mellitus (one with coexistent Hashimoto thyroiditis), and one developed juvenile rheumatoid arthritis. Peters and Winkelmann described a similar condition under the rubric 'atrophic connective tissue disease panniculitis'.[2] Nowadays, this entity would probably be best included in the spectrum of acquired total or partial lipodystrophy.

Histologic features

In atrophic connective tissue panniculitis, the histologic features are those of a lobular panniculitis.[1,7] The deep dermis may manifest a perivascular lymphocytic and histiocytic infiltrate. Lymphocytes and mononuclear phagocytes extensively infiltrate the fatty lobules. Eosinophils and multinucleate giant cells are uncommon. In more advanced lesions, there is fatty atrophy accompanied by an infiltrate composed mainly of foamy macrophages.[3] Vasculitis is not a feature of this disorder.[1]

Lipophagic panniculitis of childhood

Clinical features

Lipophagic panniculitis of childhood (lipophagic granulomatous lipoatrophy) is exceedingly rare and presents in children as recurrent erythematous asymptomatic or tender plaques and nodules affecting the arms or legs, which are later associated with lipoatrophy.[1-7] There is striking predilection for girls.[3] Fever is common and the children usually have a raised ESR, thrombocytosis, and microcytic anemia, but frequently also malaise, abdominal pain, and hepatosplenomegaly.[2] Laboratory abnormalities can persist beyond the febrile attacks.[2] Antinuclear factor may be present.[1] A similar disorder has rarely been described in adults (adult lipophagic atrophic panniculitis).[8] Winkelmann postulates that many cases of Weber-Christian disease documented in the earlier literature belong to this disorder (literature summarized in reference 1).

Histologic features

Histologically, lipophagic panniculitis is characterized by panlobular inflammation with histologic features of lipoatrophy.[1] The inflammatory cell infiltrate consists of histiocytes and Touton-like lipophages. In addition, lymphocytes, neutrophils, plasma cells, and myeloid cells may be evident. Eosinophils are sometimes numerous.

The composition of the infiltrate depends on the stage of the process. Early lesions typically contain numerous neutrophils surrounding individual necrotic adipocytes but are also seen dispersed more diffusely within the fatty lobules. Myeloperoxidase positive myeloid cells are also frequently present around necrotic adipocytes in the early stages.[2] Lymphocytes are frequent during all stages of the panniculitis. Nevertheless, late stages are characterized by the predominance of macrophages, often containing foamy cytoplasm and giant cells, forming lipophagic granulomas.[2] There is no evidence of vasculitis.[1] The epidermis and dermis are usually unremarkable.[2]

Connective tissue panniculitis

Clinical features

This extremely rare chronic condition, originally described in two female patients by Winkelmann and Padilha-Goncalves, comprises recurrent tender subcutaneous nodules mainly on the shoulders and upper arms, but the cheek, breast, trunk, neck, or leg may also be affected.[1] Healing is sometimes associated with lipoatrophy and hyperpigmentation, which can be particularly disfiguring (*Fig. 10.99*).[2]

Laboratory findings include leukopenia, anemia, a raised ESR, positive antinuclear antibody, and an unclassifiable antibody to extractable nuclear antigen.[3]

Histologic features

A lymphohistiocytic panniculitis associated with both acute and caseation necrosis characterizes the lesions. Lipophagic histiocytes and giant cells may be present, but granulomata are not a feature and there is no evidence of septal involvement or vasculitis.[1,2]

At present, this variant of chronic panniculitis has defied further classification.

Lupus erythematosus profundus

Clinical features

Lupus erythematosus profundus (lupus panniculitis) is an uncommon variant of panniculitis, which may develop in association with either discoid lupus erythematosus (DLE) or systemic lupus erythematosus (SLE).[1-8] The incidence of lupus panniculitis in SLE ranges from 2% to 10%[4,9-11]; DLE is present in from 33% to 70% of cases.[4,5] Lupus panniculitis may, however, also present in the absence of any other manifestations of lupus erythematosus.[9] In a series from the Mayo Clinic, 50% of patients had no evidence of any autoimmune-associated disease.[4] Lupus panniculitis shows a

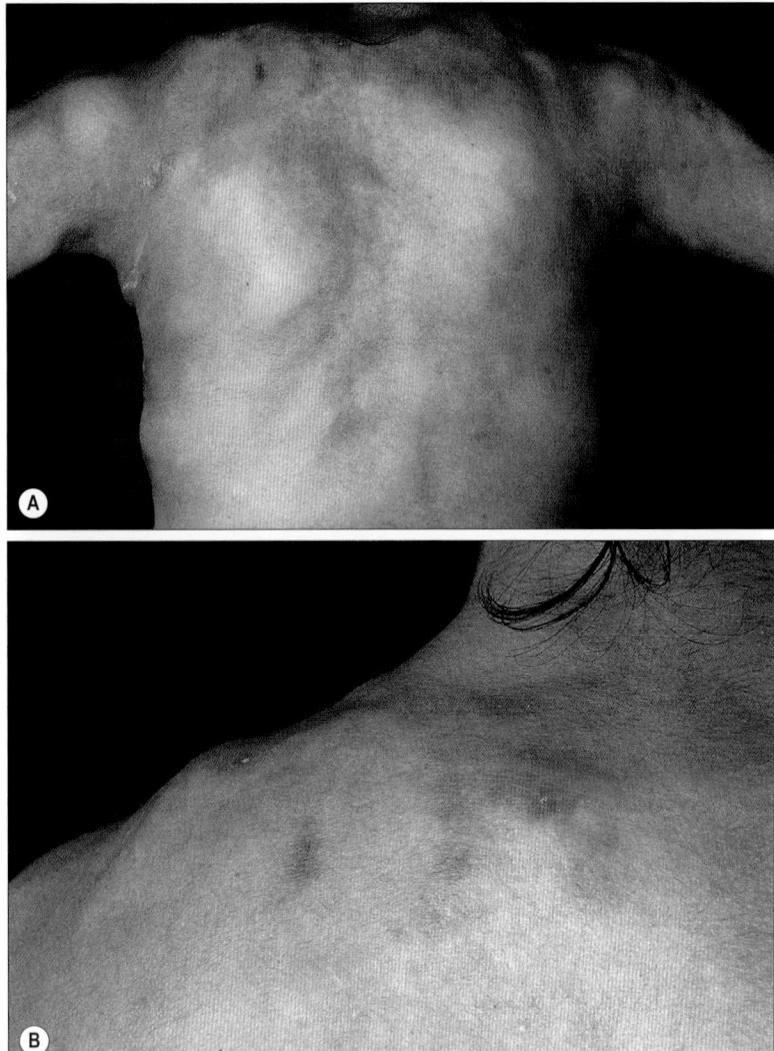

Fig. 10.99
(A, B) Connective tissue panniculitis: this patient shows diffuse hyperpigmentation associated with generalized scarring and deformity. By courtesy of M.M. Black, MD, London, UK.

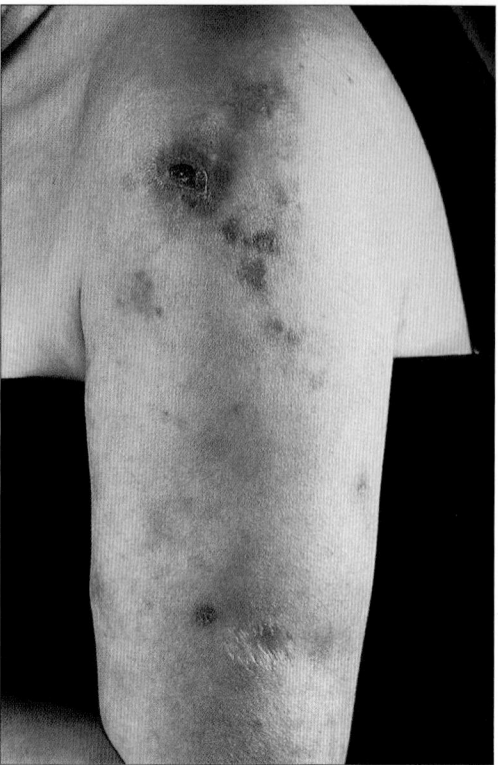

Fig. 10.100
Lupus erythematosus profundus: erythematoviolaceous plaques showing focal ulceration at the characteristic site. By courtesy of the Institute of Dermatology, London, UK.

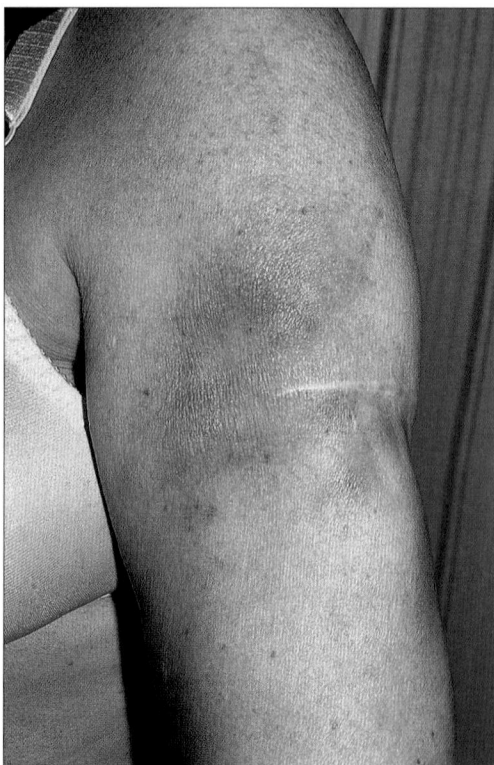

Fig. 10.101
Lupus erythematosus profundus: a depressed scarred area due to end-stage lipoatrophy. By courtesy of the Institute of Dermatology, London, UK.

predilection for females (4:1), and most patients are middle aged.[4] Rarely, however, children (including infants) may be affected.[7,12] A recent study from Brazil found 0.7% of children and adolescents with juvenile systemic lupus to have associated lupus panniculitis.[13] Rarely, lupus panniculitis may signify recurrence of SLE.[14]

Patients develop discrete, firm, asymptomatic, or painful nodules, one to several centimeters across, in the subcutaneous fat; the nodules are often associated with trauma.[9] Linear distribution of lupus panniculitis has rarely been reported and is likely associated with a more aggressive clinical behavior.[15–18] Linear lupus panniculitis of the scalp is even more infrequent and presents clinically as alopecia distributed along the Blaschko lines.[19–21] The overlying skin may appear clinically normal or show discoid lupus plaques, poikiloderma, erythema, atrophy, or ulceration (*Fig. 10.100*).[10,22] Anetodermic lupus panniculitis has been associated with antiphospholipid antibodies.[23] Lupus erythematosus profundus is characteristically chronic, with patients developing recurrent crops of lesions. Spontaneous resolution may occur and leave depressed atrophic disfiguring scars (lipoatrophy) (*Fig. 10.101*). Sites of predilection include the face, upper and outer parts of the arm, the breasts, back, and buttocks. Breast involvement with scarring and calcification may be clinically mistaken for carcinoma (so-called 'lupus mastitis').[24,25] Salivary gland and primary periorbital lesions have also been documented.[26–30] Rarely, the disease may present with generalized lesions.[8] Lupus panniculitis following treatment with interferon, antitumor necrosis factor alpha, adalimumab, and human papillomavirus quadrivalent vaccination has exceptionally been reported.[31–34]

In cases with associated SLE, patients frequently manifest arthralgia and Raynaud phenomenon; there appears to be a relatively low incidence of renal and neurological involvement.[10] Positive serology may include antinuclear antibody, anti-DNA antibody, anti-extractable nuclear antigen (ENA) antibodies, and rheumatoid factor.[9,22] In those patients in whom there is

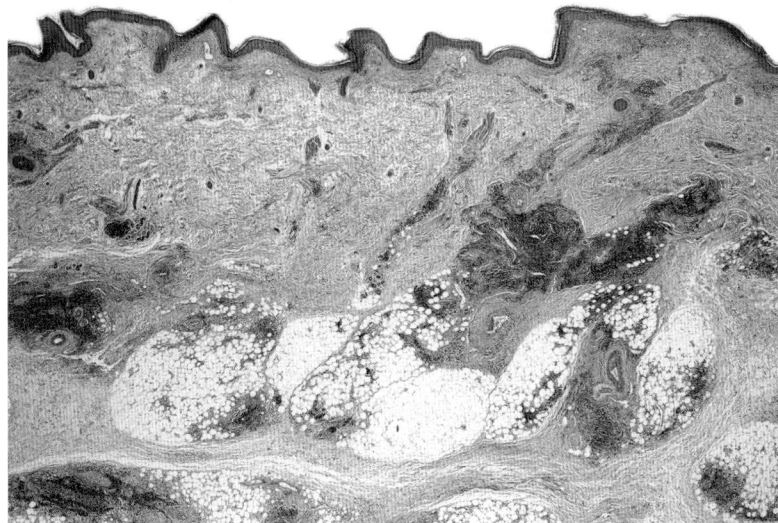

Fig. 10.102
Lupus erythematosus profundus: low-power view showing epidermal atrophy with hyperkeratosis and a dense dermal lymphocytic infiltrate with extension into subcutaneous fat.

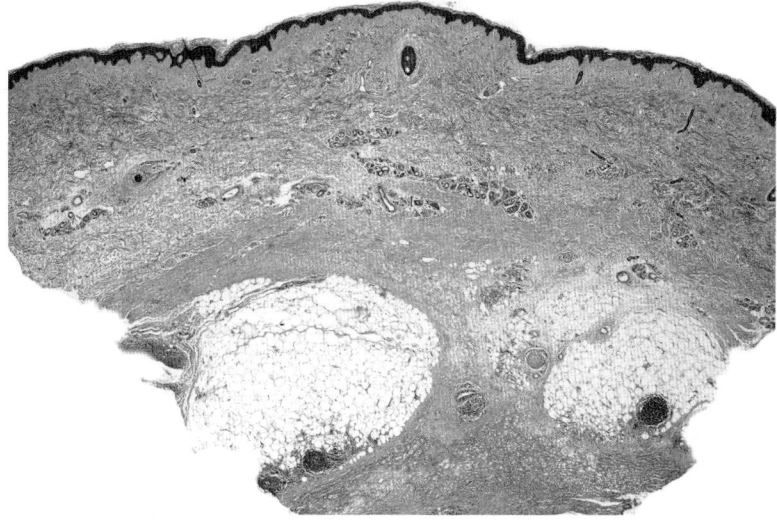

Fig. 10.104
Lupus erythematosus profundus: in contrast, this patient showed disease limited to the subcutaneous fat.

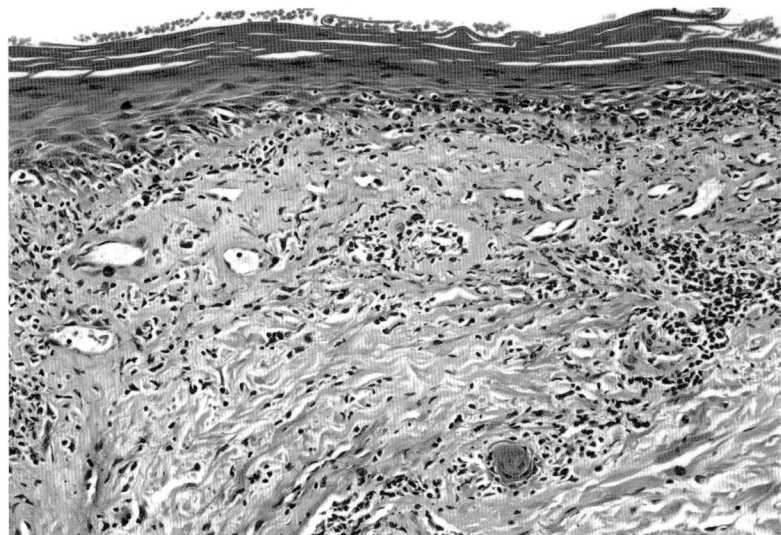

Fig. 10.103
Lupus erythematosus profundus: in this example, there are typical features of discoid lupus erythematosus.

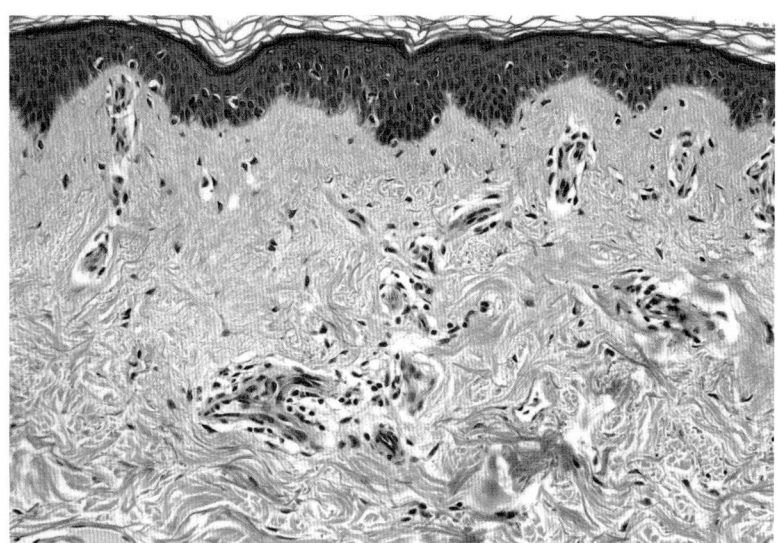

Fig. 10.105
Lupus erythematosus profundus: the epidermis appears normal.

no evidence elsewhere of lupus erythematosus, a raised antinuclear factor may be the only serological abnormality.[4] Although in these latter patients the prognosis is generally thought to be good, in some patients there is considerable mortality and the disfigurement is a source of considerable distress.[35,36] Partial C4 deficiency has been described in a patient with lupus erythematosus profundus.[37]

Histologic features

In an established lesion, the histologic features of lupus erythematosus profundus are virtually diagnostic. The overlying epithelium and superficial dermis may show features of DLE, poikiloderma, or be unaffected (*Figs 10.102–10.105*).[38,39] Within the deep dermis, and extending into the widened septa of the subcutaneous fat, is a dense chronic inflammatory cell infiltrate consisting predominantly of nodules of lymphocytes with lesser numbers of plasma cells (*Figs 10.106–10.108*).[11,14,39] Lymphocytic nuclear debris or dust within a lymphoplasmocytic infiltrate is frequently seen.[14] Occasionally, lymphoid follicles with germinal centers are evident (*Fig. 10.109*). The infiltrate may surround and permeate the walls of blood vessels and sweat glands; involvement of the perineural sheath is occasionally a feature (*Fig. 10.110*).[38,40] Less often, frank lymphocytic vasculitis with mural fibrinoid necrosis and luminal thrombosis is seen (*Fig. 10.111*).

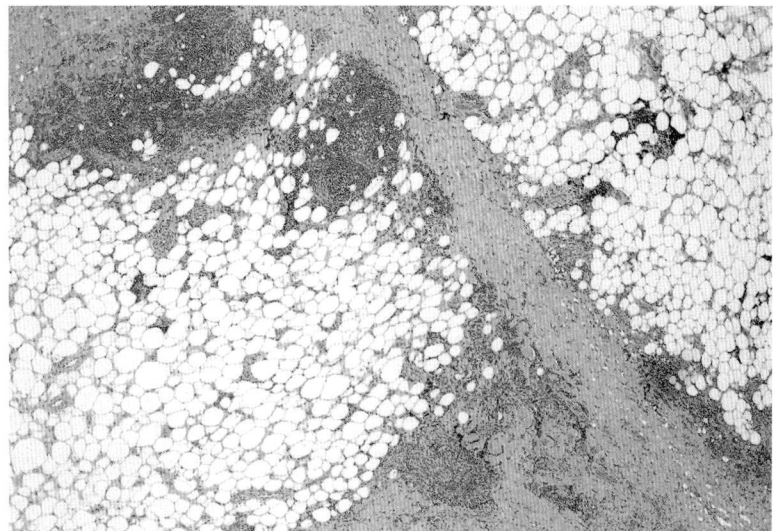

Fig. 10.106
Lupus erythematosus profundus: the septa are thickened and there is a dense infiltrate.

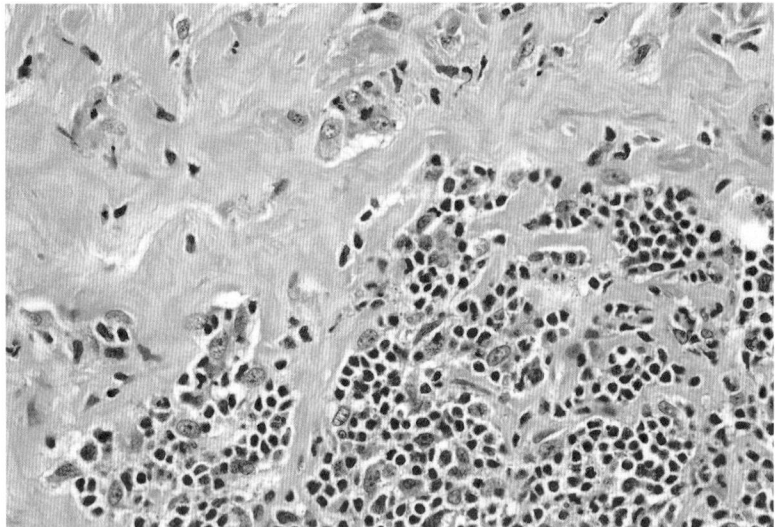

Fig. 10.107
Lupus erythematosus profundus: the infiltrate is largely lymphocytic.

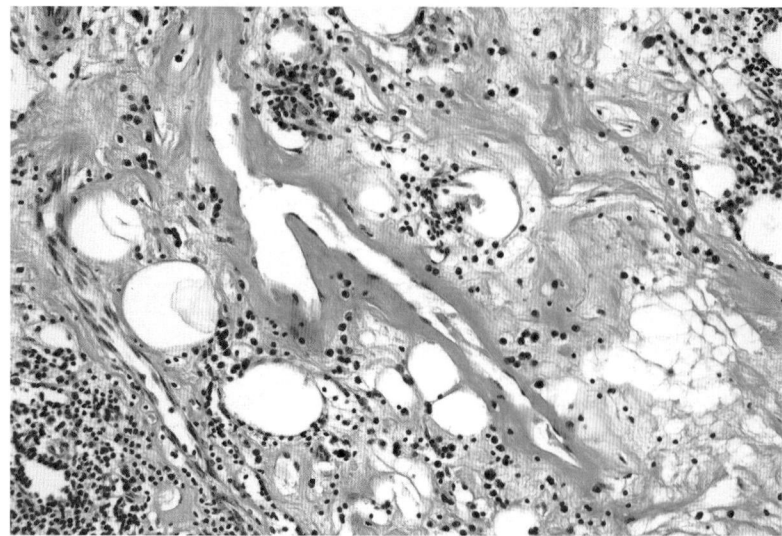

Fig. 10.110
Lupus erythematosus profundus: blood vessel walls are commonly thickened and hyalinized.

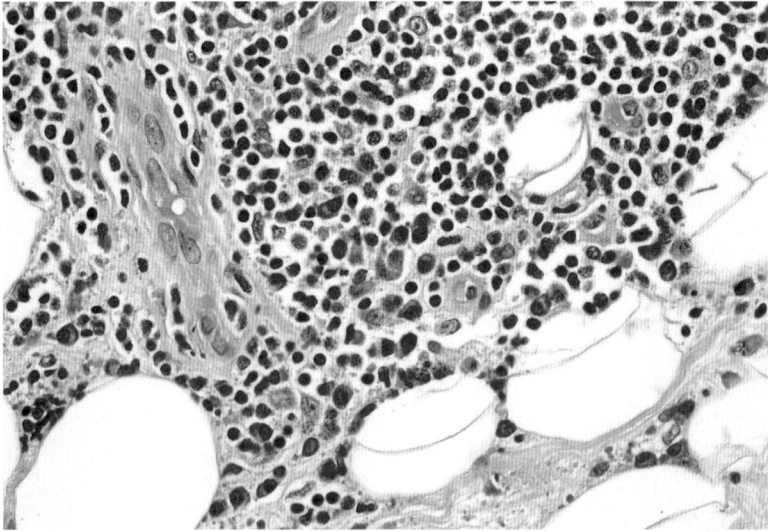

Fig. 10.108
Lupus erythematosus profundus: plasma cells, as shown in this field, are sometimes conspicuous.

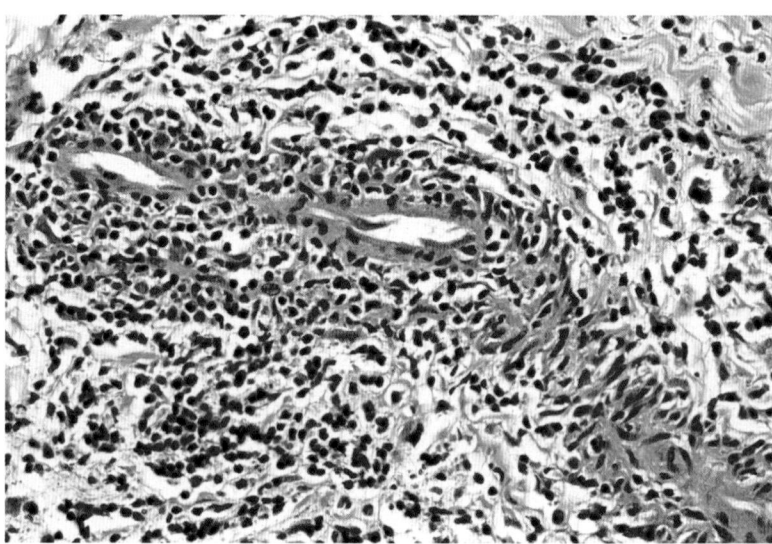

Fig. 10.111
Lupus erythematosus profundus: lymphocytic vasculitis, as noted in this field, is not uncommon.

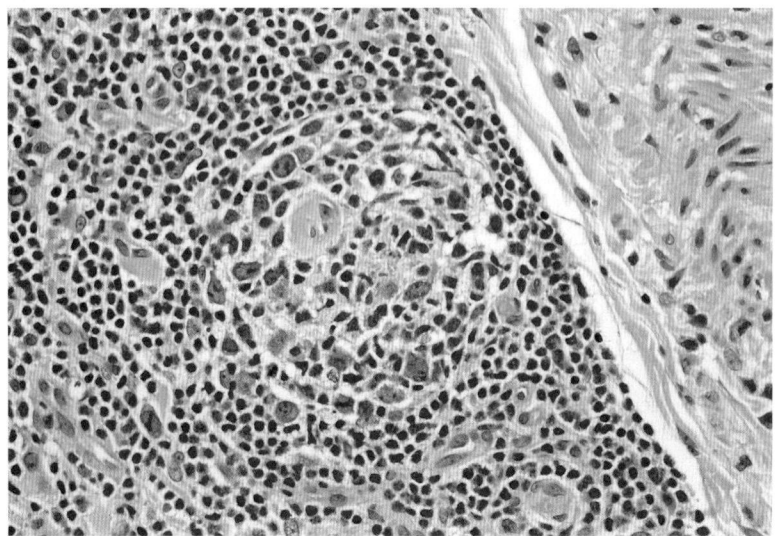

Fig. 10.109
Lupus erythematosus profundus: lymphoid follicles, as shown in this field, may be a prominent feature.

The infiltrate often extends into the periphery of the fat lobules and when associated with fat necrosis there may also be moderate numbers of neutrophil polymorphs. The collagen of the deep dermis and the fibrous septa of the subcutaneous fat show striking fibrinoid degenerative changes. Fibers may be markedly swollen and intensely eosinophilic, or fragmented into amorphous granular debris. Similar changes are seen surrounding individual adipocytes. In more advanced examples, glassy eosinophilic necrosis gives a diffusely hyalinized appearance to the subcutaneous fat (*Fig. 10.112*). The foci of collagenous degeneration are sometimes associated with mucin deposition, and foci of calcification, which may on occasion be very prominent.[10,14,22,38,39,41] Extensive endarteritis obliterans has been reported in a single case of lupus panniculitis, which was associated with membranocystic changes and dystrophic calcification.[42]

By immunohistochemistry, the predominant cells are α/β T-helper lymphocytes, intermingled with B lymphocytes.[14] Molecular analysis by polymerase chain reaction generally reveals a polyclonal phenotype.[14]

Immunofluorescence commonly reveals immunoglobulin and complement at the dermoepidermal junction and sometimes around the superficial blood vessels.[22,38]

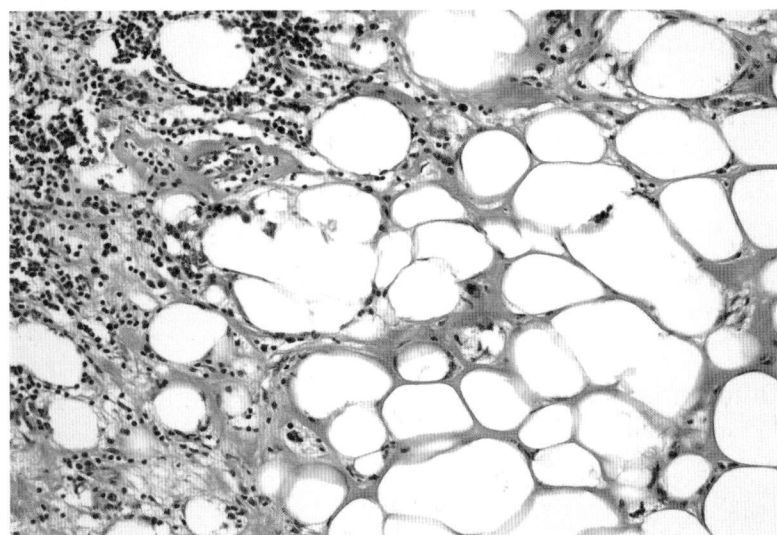

Fig. 10.112
Lupus erythematosus profundus: hyalinization of the fat is a characteristic feature.

Differential diagnosis

Similar histologic features may be seen in other connective tissue diseases including linear morphea, morphea profunda, systemic sclerosis, dermatomyositis, mixed connective tissue disease, and polymyositis.[43–46] Sjögren syndrome has been added to the causes of so-called plasma cell panniculitis.[47] Lobular panniculitis with sclerosis reminiscent of lupus panniculitis has also been described in a patient with Degos disease (malignant atrophic papulosis).[48] Distinction between lupus profundus and subcutaneous panniculitis-like T-cell lymphoma can, on occasion, be extremely difficult on clinical as well as on histologic grounds.[49–52] The presence of atypical lymphocytes with immunohistochemical features of cytotoxic T cells (CD3+,CD8+) accompanied by high proliferation rate and monoclonal TCR-γ gene rearrangement is suggestive of lymphoma.[49] On the other hand, clusters of CD123 positive plasmacytoid dendritic cells are more suggestive of lupus panniculitis.[53] Nevertheless, lupus profundus and panniculitis-like T-cell lymphoma may coexist in the same patient.[49] Overlapping histologic features with characteristics of both lupus profundus and subcutaneous panniculitis-like T-cell lymphoma are seen in these patients.[49,54–58] It has recently been suggested that lupus erythematosus profundus and panniculitis-like T-cell lymphoma may represent two ends of a spectrum.[56] Cold panniculitis and ice-pack dermatosis can closely resemble the pattern of lupus profundus, and close clinicopathological correlation is essential for correct recognition of the underlying condition.[59]

Scleroderma panniculitis

Clinical features

Sclerosis and chronic panniculitis have been recorded as main features in both generalized morphea and progressive systemic sclerosis.[1–3] In addition, morphea profunda has been described as a sclerosing variant of morphea, which primarily affects the subcutaneous fat analogous to lupus erythematosus profundus.[4,5] This condition, which shows a female predominance (3:1), affects a wide age range (9–62 years) and presents primarily as subcutaneous sclerosis.[6] The sclerosis may be generalized and extend to the digits, or present as solitary or multiple, localized, inflamed, hyperpigmented or erythematous, asymmetrical and ill-defined plaques with a predilection for the shoulders, upper arms, and trunk.[6–8] A variant localized to the paraspinal region in children has also been described.[9,10] Patients with systemic sclerosis can also develop sclerosing panniculitis. These patients have systemic sclerosis associated with pulmonary hypertension.[11]

Histologic features

The significant features include thickening and hyalinization of the connective tissue of the deep dermis, subcutaneous fat, and muscular fascia.[3] Lipomembranous fat necrosis can also be a feature.[12] A perivascular and focal interstitial lymphocytic and plasma cell infiltrate is present in the subcutaneous fat. Exceptionally, plasma cells may be very numerous – so-called plasma cell panniculitis.[13–15] Lymphoid nodules (usually without germinal center formation) are evident and mast cells may be increased in number.[6] Scattered eosinophils are occasionally seen. Mucin deposition is sometimes a feature, and diminished elastic tissue is a frequent finding, although in some cases it appears increased in quantity.[8] Localized osseous metaplasia with transepidermal elimination has been documented.[16] The changes in the fascia are similar to those described in the subcutaneous fat.

Differential diagnosis

Morphea profunda differs from conventional generalized morphea by the deeper involvement of the sclerotic process and the more intense chronic inflammatory cell infiltrate.[6] Some authors regard eosinophilic fasciitis as part of the spectrum of morphea profunda.[6]

Dermatomyositis panniculitis

Clinical features

Panniculitis has been described as a non-specific incidental finding in biopsy specimens of skin or muscle from patients with dermatomyositis.[1–3] Rarely, however, it presents as a symptomatic disorder, with patients complaining of indurated, erythematous, tender, painful plaques and nodules, located about the arms, thighs, abdomen, and buttocks.[3–11,12] In some cases, the panniculitis precedes the onset of the myositis.[3] With chronicity, patients can develop lipoatrophy and calcification.[13,14] Both children and adults may be affected.[15,16] Panniculitis has exceptionally been reported in dermatomyositis patients with associated malignant tumors.[14,17,18]

Histologic features

Dermatomyositis panniculitis is characterized by a predominantly lobular infiltrate of lymphocytes and plasma cells, sometimes accompanied by lymphoid follicles with germinal centers.[4,5] Focal fat necrosis may be present and lymphocytic vasculitis has occasionally been documented dermal mucin deposition is a frequent finding..[6] The septa of the subcutaneous fat become progressively thickened and hyalinized. Membranocystic changes have been described in a number of cases, particularly in Japanese patients.[1,13,19] Calcification is a late change, but can be very prominent.[1,20] Aggregates of CD123 positive cells may be seen.[21]

Mild inflammatory changes may be seen in the subcutaneous fat in patients with dermatomyositis in the absence of panniculitis including focal lymphocytic infiltration, fibrosis, and calcification.[5]

The overlying epidermis may show interface change with basal cell vacuolation and lymphocytic exocytosis.[1,7]

Immunofluorescent findings are variable. In the majority of cases it is negative, but C3 was found at the dermal–epidermal junction in one case and, in another, C3 and IgM were identified within the blood vessel walls in the superficial dermal vasculature.[6,7]

Differential diagnosis

An association of childhood dermatomyositis with subcutaneous panniculitic T-cell lymphoma has been described in a single case report.[22]

Postirradiation pseudosclerodermatous panniculitis

Clinical features

This is a rare complication of high-dose radiotherapy. Postirradiation pseudosclerodermatous panniculitis has predominantly been reported in female patients who have received this treatment modality for breast carcinoma either following conservation surgery or after radical mastectomy.[1–6] In

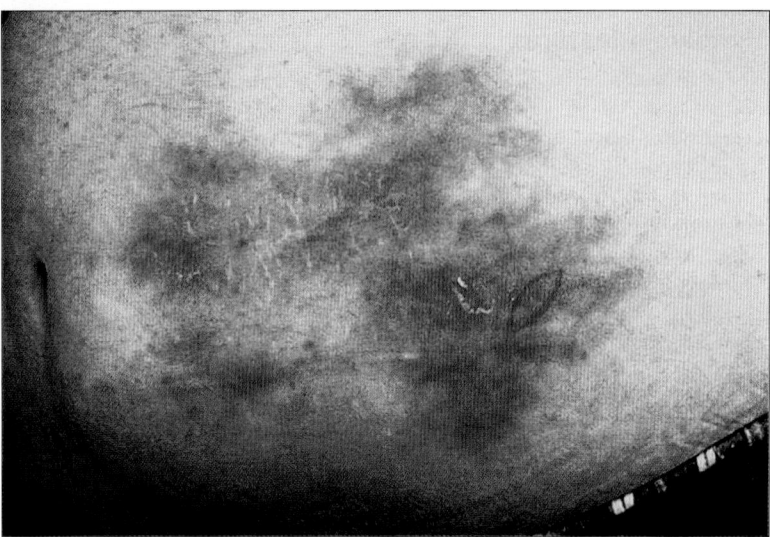

Fig. 10.113
Postirradiation pseudosclerodermatous panniculitis: erythematous irregular plaque.
By courtesy of the Institute of Dermatology, London, UK.

addition, similar changes have been described following radiotherapy for myxoid liposarcoma, non-small cell lung cancer, and metastatic breast carcinoma.[7,8] Patients present with deep-seated and progressive induration of the subcutis in the area of previous irradiation (*Fig. 10.113*), usually within the first 5 years after radiation therapy.[1–3,5]

Histologic features

The main histologic features are localized to the subcutaneous fat where there is a lobular panniculitis characterized by fat necrosis with foreign body (lipophagic) granulomata and a lymphocyte and plasma cell infiltrate.[1,2] The septa are grossly thickened by hyalinized collagen. In addition, coexisting changes of chronic radiodermatitis are present in the dermis in a subset of patients, characterized by vessels with hyalinized/sclerotic walls, fibrosis, perivascular and interstitial lymphocyte and plasma cell infiltrate, and scattered atypical bizarre (myo)fibroblasts.[1,5,6] Dilated lymphatics may also occasionally be found in the dermis.[3] Epidermal changes of radiotherapy are absent.[2]

Differential diagnosis

In patients with this condition, sections should be very carefully scrutinized for evidence of recurrent/metastatic breast carcinoma. Immunohistochemistry may prove invaluable.

Postirradiation pseudosclerodermatous panniculitis can be histologically confused with both morphea profunda and lupus erythematosus profundus.[2] Clinicopathological correlation should readily establish the correct diagnosis.

Access **ExpertConsult.com** for the complete list of references [print tag]

Diseases of the oral mucosa

CHAPTER

11

See
www.expertconsult.com
for references and
additional material

Sook-Bin Woo

Introduction

Oral and maxillofacial pathology is the specialty of dentistry that is involved in the histopathological and clinical diagnosis, as well as management of diseases of the oral mucosa and supporting bone and soft tissues, teeth, salivary glands, lip vermilion, and perioral skin. It would be impossible to discuss diseases affecting all of the above entities in one chapter. As such, this chapter is confined to the more common and distinctive mucosal lesions that are often seen and biopsied by the oral and maxillofacial surgeon, dermatologist, or otorhinolaryngologist. If a condition presents on the skin in addition to the mouth (such as pemphigus), only a brief mention of the oral manifestations is made since the topic will have been covered in detail elsewhere in this book.

From a histologic perspective, the oral mucosa is divided into nonkeratinized and keratinized sites. The former include the lip mucosa (wet inner surface of the lip), buccal mucosa, maxillary and mandibular sulcus/vestibule, ventral tongue, floor of mouth, soft palate, nonattached gingiva, and crevicular epithelium. The crevicular epithelium is the continuation of marginal gingival epithelium where it turns to face the tooth. Any keratin on these surfaces is considered abnormal and should be reported as such. The linea alba ('bite line') which is located on the buccal mucosa where the upper and lower teeth meet may be thinly parakeratinized, and this is considered within the realm of normal (*Fig. 11.1*).

Normally, orthokeratinized sites include the hard palatal mucosa and the attached gingiva (extending from the cervix of the tooth for a band of 2–5 mm) while the tongue dorsum is normally parakeratinized. The tongue is a specialized structure because of its role in taste sensation, and has filiform, fungiform, circumvallate, and foliate papillae, with the last three containing taste buds (*Fig. 11.2*). The taste buds are innervated by the subgemmal neurogenous plaque best seen in the posterior lateral tongue (*Fig. 11.3*).

The oral mucosa consists of epithelium and underlying lamina propria that can be arbitrarily divided into superficial and deep portions, and underlying muscle or bone. Because there is no muscularis mucosa, there is no true submucosa. The epithelium of the oral mucosa is thickest on the tongue dorsum (20–25 cells thick), moderately thick on the buccal and lip mucosa (15–25 cells thick), and thinnest on the floor of mouth, ventral tongue, and soft palate (8–15 cells thick) (*Fig. 11.4*). Pathologists not familiar with this feature tend to diagnose normal buccal, lip, or tongue epithelium as being acanthotic or exhibiting psoriasiform hyperplasia. The attached gingiva and the hard palatal mucosa abut the periosteum so that the deep lamina propria appears densely fibrotic (*Fig. 11.5*). A diagnosis of 'fibrosis' is therefore inappropriate since this feature is normal for the site.

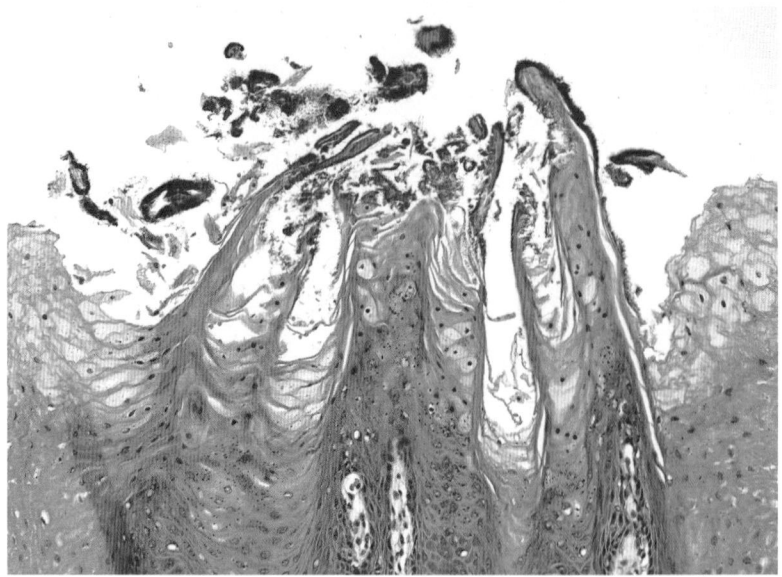

Fig. 11.2
Normal tongue dorsum: there are four ovoid fungiform papillae and many filiform papillae on the left of field also (inset) composed of spires of parakeratin associated with bacterial colonies.

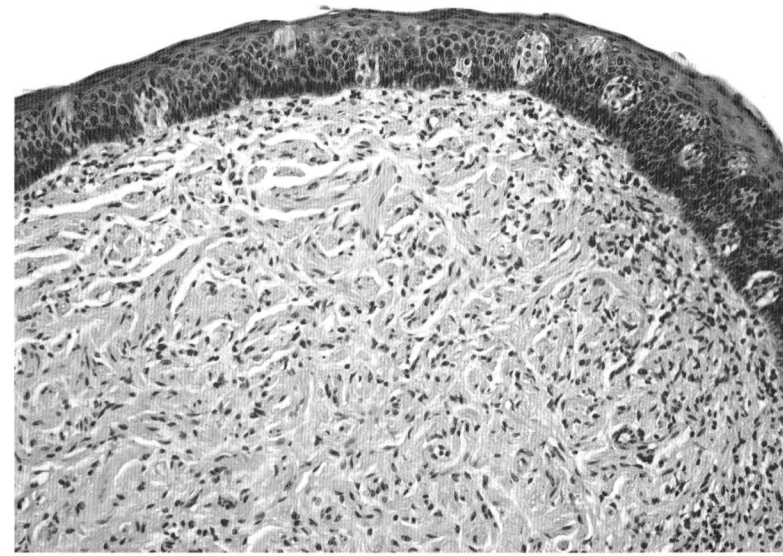

Fig. 11.3
Subgemmal neurogenous plaque: this is a neural plexus located beneath taste buds and commonly seen on the posterior lateral tongue.

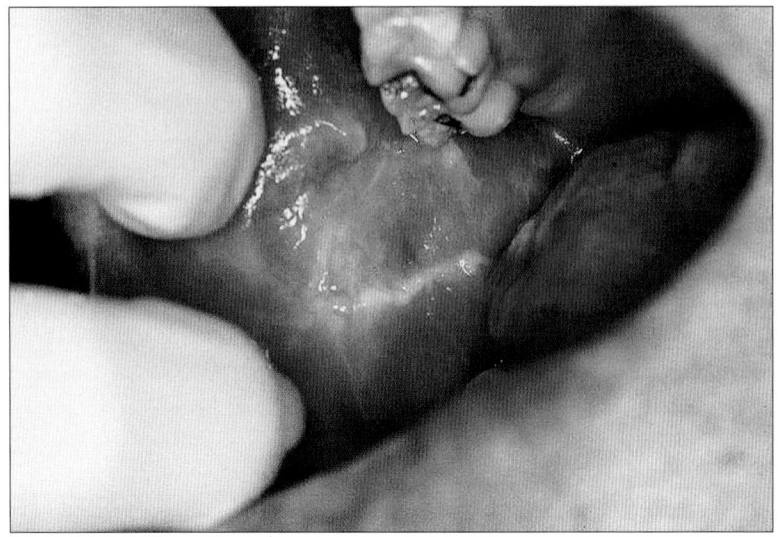

Fig. 11.1
Linea alba on the buccal mucosa: this keratotic linear lesion is caused by friction from teeth and exhibits parakeratosis and keratinocyte edema.

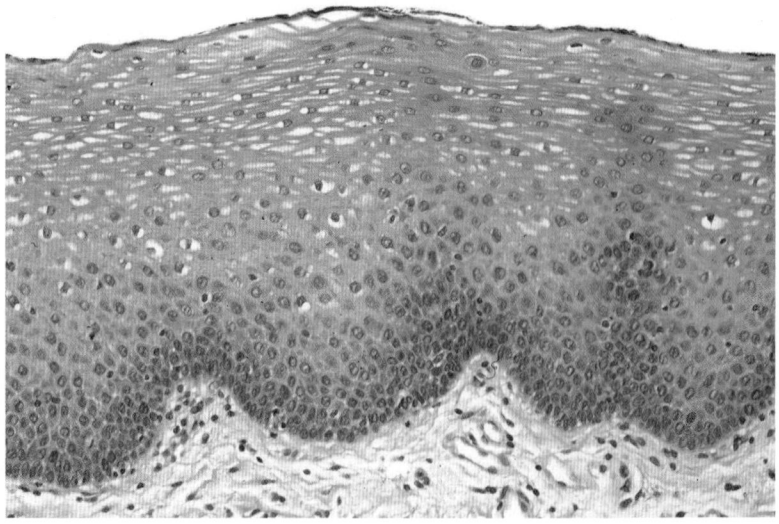

Fig. 11.4
Normal buccal mucosa: the epithelium is nonkeratinized and is 15–25 cells thick.

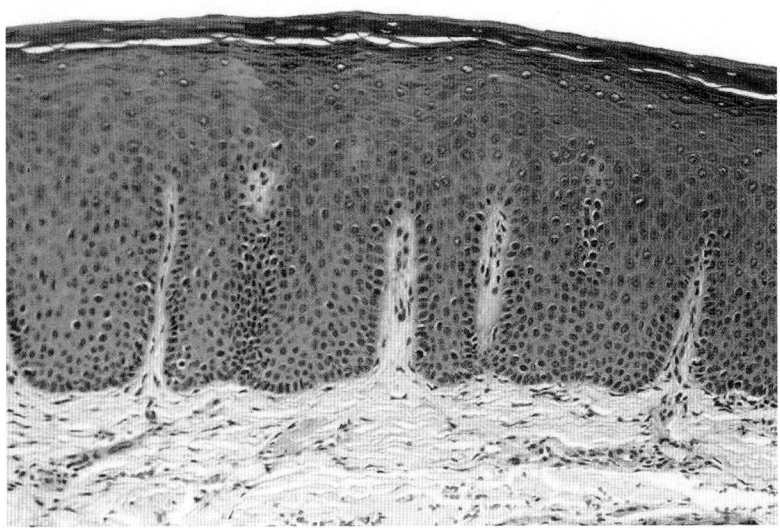

Fig. 11.5
Normal palatal mucosa: the palatal mucosa and gingiva both are thinly orthokeratinized. The dense fibrous tissue in the lamina propria is normal for these sites.

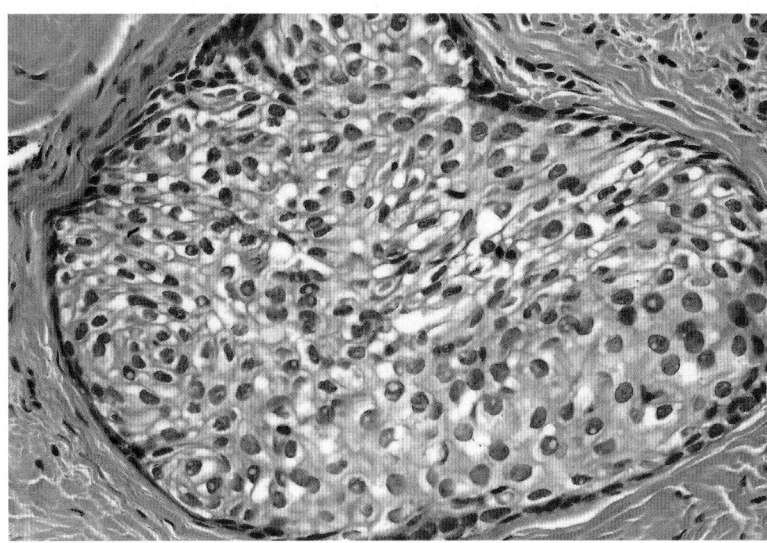

Fig. 11.6
Odontogenic rest of Serres in the gingiva: this is composed of mainly clear cells (inset).

The tooth is composed of an outer highly calcified thin shell of enamel on the visible crown of the tooth; the non-visible portion within the bone is covered by cementum, which is similar in composition and appearance to bone. The bulk of the tooth consists of tubular dentin and the dental pulp containing fibrovascular and neural tissues (the source of most toothaches)

courses through the length of the tooth. Odontogenic rests of Serres are common within the gingiva, and these consist of nests of squamous epithelium that may exhibit clear cytoplasm and sometimes show palisading of the basal cell nuclei (*Fig. 11.6*).

HEREDITARY CONDITIONS

Macular lesions

White sponge nevus

Clinical features

White sponge nevus (Canon white sponge nevus) is an autosomal dominant condition with high penetrance and variable expressivity. Onset is in early childhood, with 50% of patients diagnosed before age 20.[1-3] The buccal mucosa is almost invariably affected, and other commonly affected sites are the lip mucosa, tongue, alveolar mucosa, and the floor of mouth. Nasal, esophageal, vaginal, anal, and penile mucosae may be involved, but not that of the conjunctiva, although there is one report of associated colobomas.[4] Lesions appear as painless, diffuse, white–gray, spongy, folded plaques (*Fig. 11.7*).[2,5,6]

Pathogenesis and histologic features

White sponge nevus is caused by a mutation in the helical domain of mucosal-specific keratins K4 (on chromosome 12q) and K13 (on chromosome 17q). The mutations are in the form of amino acid deletions, substitutions, and insertions resulting in keratin filament instability and abnormal aggregation of tonofilaments.[7-9] Cases reported to have resolved with antibiotic therapy are not likely to represent this condition but rather reactive/frictional keratoses.[10,11]

There is parakeratosis and acanthosis with the formation of broad, blunt rete ridges (*Fig. 11.8*). Dyskeratotic cells exhibit dense peri- and paranuclear eosinophilic condensations, with vacuolation of cytoplasm at the periphery of the keratinocyte resulting in a falsely 'spongiotic' appearance on low magnification; there is insignificant inflammation (*Fig. 11.9*).[5,12,13] Parakeratin plugs and streaks have been noted beneath the superficial keratinocytes.

One case that exhibited foci of epidermolytic hyperkeratosis has been documented.[14]

The eosinophilic condensations correspond to tonofilament aggregates in a peri- and paranuclear location.[1,12,13,15] Organelles tend to segregate and are absent in vacuolated areas. Odland bodies are abundant within keratinocytes, but few are present in the intercellular spaces, suggesting a lack of acid phosphatase leading to retention, rather than normal shedding, of superficial cells.[1]

Hereditary benign intraepithelial dyskeratosis

Clinical features

This autosomal dominant disorder of the eye and oral cavity was first described in a tri-racial isolate (Caucasian, Native American, and African) in North Carolina called the Halowar, Haliwa, or Haliwa-Saponi Native Americans.[1] Because of migration, cases have been reported in descendants living now in New York, Pennsylvania, Virginia, and Washington, DC.

The eye lesions, which usually present by the first year of life, are gelatinous plaques in the bulbar conjunctiva in a perilimbic distribution both nasally and temporally. Patients experience eye irritation often with a sensation of foreign material in the eye, and photophobia, and there may be exacerbations in spring. Corneal vascularization sometimes leads to visual loss.[2]

Oral involvement is asymptomatic and is therefore generally not noticed until the second decade. Lesions involve the buccal and lip mucosa, floor of mouth, lateral and ventral tongue, and gingiva, but not usually the dorsum of tongue or uvula.[3-5] The mucosa is white, opalescent, spongy, macerated, folded, and shaggy, often resembling white sponge nevus (*Fig. 11.10*). There is generally no involvement of genital, nasal, or rectal mucosa.

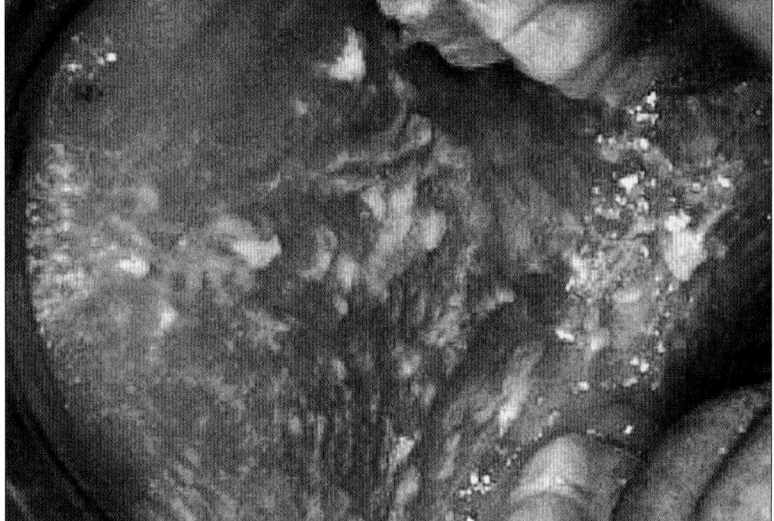

Fig. 11.7
White sponge nevus: typical white, thickened, spongy-appearing mucosa. By courtesy of C. Allen, DDS, Columbus, USA.

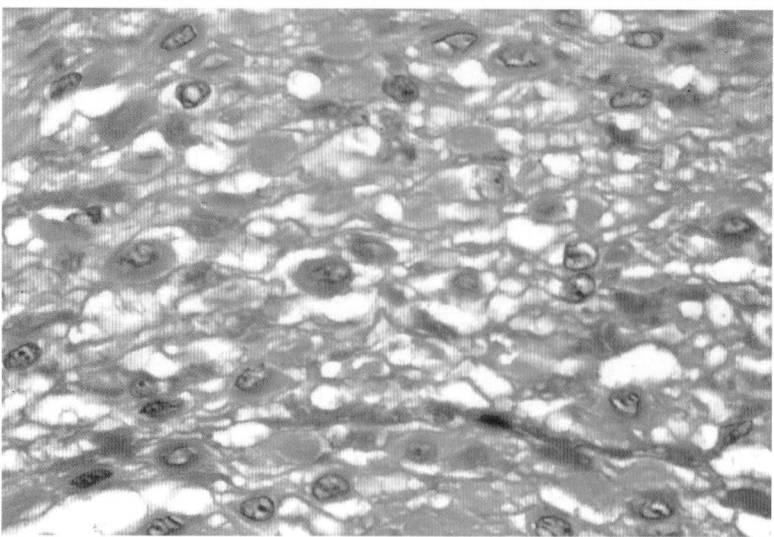

Fig. 11.9
White sponge nevus: there are perinuclear eosinophilic keratin condensations and cytoplasmic vacuolation.

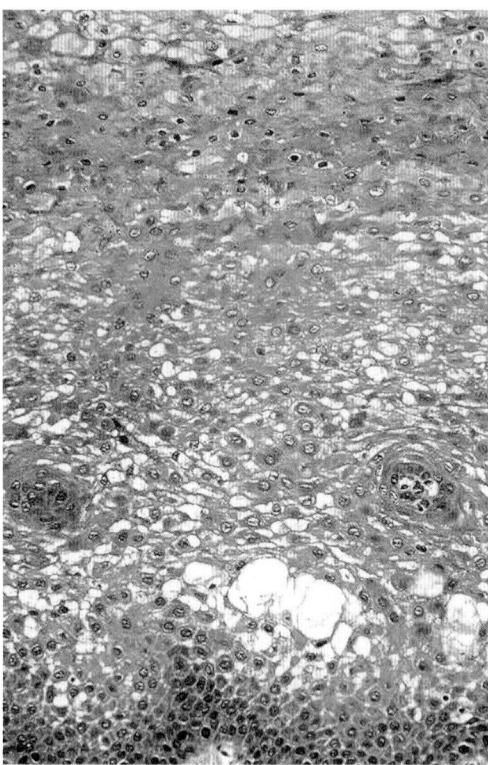

Fig. 11.8
White sponge nevus: the epithelium exhibits vacuolation, acanthosis, and dyskeratosis.

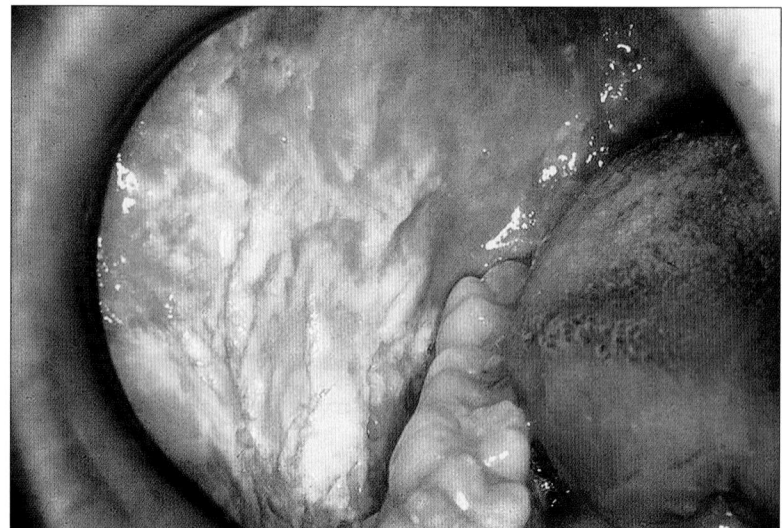

Fig. 11.10
Hereditary benign intraepithelial dyskeratosis: the mucosa appears white and thickened. By courtesy of J. McDonald, DDS, Cincinnati, USA.

Pathogenesis and histologic features

Genetic studies have localized the gene for this condition to chromosome 4q35 with a duplication segregating in affected individuals.[6]

There is parakeratosis and acanthosis (*Fig. 11.11*). Dyskeratotic cells (also called 'tobacco cells' because of their orange-brown color on Papanicolaou-stained smears) are present in the mid to upper one-third of the epithelium, appearing engulfed by adjacent normal keratinocytes; this 'cell-within-a-cell' appearance is a characteristic feature and is well seen in cytological smears (*Fig. 11.12*)[4,7,8,9]

The dyskeratotic cells are packed with tonofilaments and vesicular bodies that may represent Odland bodies.[7] Some keratinocytes also show loss of cellular interdigitations and desmosomes.

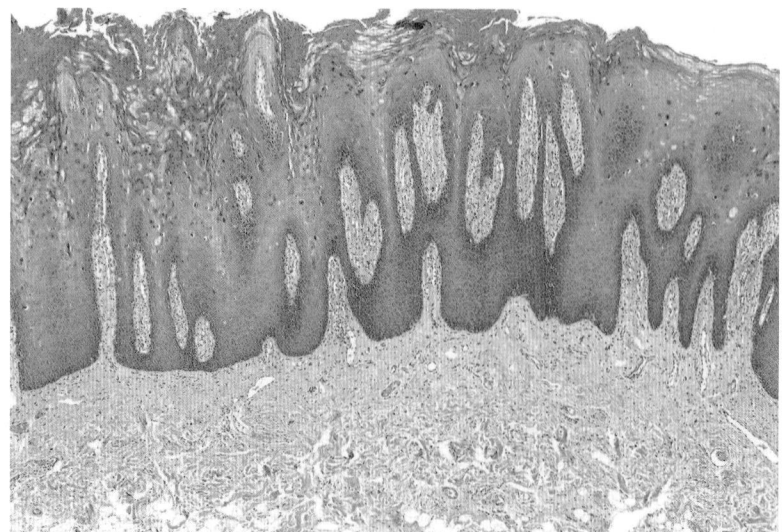

Fig. 11.11
Hereditary benign intraepithelial dyskeratosis: there is parakeratosis, dyskeratosis, and acanthosis. By courtesy of J. McDonald, DDS, Cincinnati, USA.

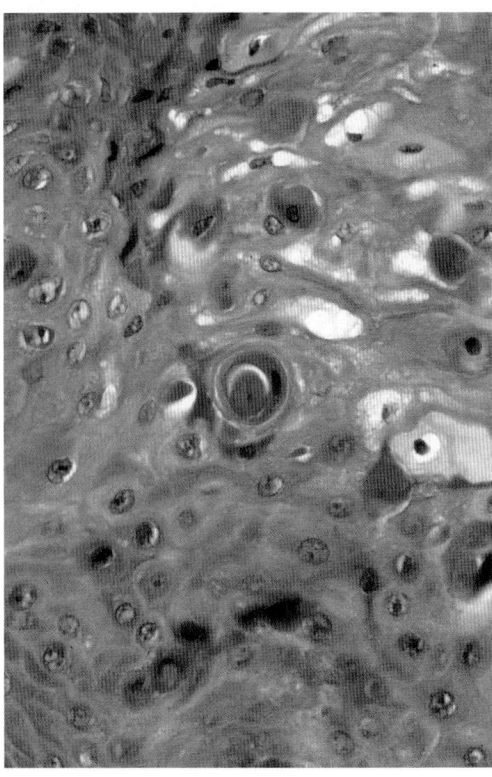

Fig. 11.12
Hereditary benign intraepithelial dyskeratosis: note the dyskeratotic cell apparently surrounded by a keratinocyte forming the typical 'cell-within-a-cell' structure. By courtesy of J. McDonald, DDS, Cincinnati, USA.

Pachyonychia congenita

Clinical features

This rare genodermatosis is characterized by nail dystrophy, palmoplantar keratoderma, follicular keratoses, epidermoid cysts, and keratotic oral plaques; other findings include hyperhidrosis, hoarseness, angular cheilitis, and dental findings such as natal teeth. Nomenclature for this condition has been revised and is now based on molecular and genetic data. For example, patients with mutations in *KRT6a* and *KRT16* are now designated pachyonychia congenita (PC)-K6a and PC-K16, respectively, rather than jointly as having Jadassohn-Lewandowsky syndrome (see below).[1,2] The oral findings, usually noted within the first two decades of life and often at birth, are characterized by focal or generalized white keratotic plaques on the dorsum and lateral borders of the tongue, and buccal mucosa and are present in almost all patients with PC-K6a and in 40–50% of patients with PC-K6b and PC-K16.[1,3–6] Natal teeth are seen in over 80% of patients with PC-K17.

Pathogenesis and histologic features

Pachyonychia congenita is inherited as an autosomal dominant disorder characterized by mutations in five main keratin genes expressed in the nail bed, palmoplantar epidermis, and oral mucosa. These genes are *KRT6a*, *KRT6b*, *KRT6c*, *KRT16*, and *KRT17*,[2,6] and nomenclature for this condition now reflects these genetic mutations and have replaced Jadassohn-Lewandowsky and Jackson-Lawler syndromes.[7,8] There is a defect in the association of protein subunits in the assembly of keratin filaments leading to fragility of epithelial cells, and reduced strength and resilience to trauma.

There is parakeratosis or hyperkeratosis, acanthosis, intracellular vacuolization, and perinuclear eosinophilic condensations (likely tonofilaments).[4,8–11] Because pachyonychia congenita and dyskeratosis congenita are generally diagnosed on skin biopsy, there are few detailed reports on the histology of oral lesions. Unlike true leukoplakia that develops in dyskeratosis congenita, the oral keratotic plaques of pachyonychia congenita have no malignant potential.

Differential diagnosis

Cannon white sponge nevus also exhibits perinuclear eosinophilic condensations because of abnormal tonofilament aggregation, but does not exhibit skin or nail involvement.

Dyskeratosis congenita

Clinical features

Dyskeratosis congenita (Zinsser-Engman-Cole syndrome) is a genodermatosis that is associated with nail dystrophy, poikiloderma, oral leukoplakia, and development of pancytopenia and bone marrow failure, often requiring hematopoietic stem cell transplantation. The mucosa of the conjunctiva, urethra, and genital tract may also be involved.[1–4] Oral leukoplakia, particularly of the tongue, presents in the second decade of life in at least 65% of cases, and has a high propensity for developing dysplasia and/or squamous cell carcinoma at an early age; teeth have short roots and are mildly taurodontic.[5–7] Early oral lesions on the gingiva may be erythematous and erosive.[8,9]

Pathogenesis and histologic features

Dyskeratosis congenita is considered a premature aging syndrome or telomeropathy caused by poor telomere maintenance with mutations in *DKC1*, *TERC*, *TERT*, *TINF2*, and other genes.[10]

The lesions of leukoplakia exhibit parakeratosis, and/or hyperkeratosis with variable dysplasia or invasive squamous cell carcinoma. Early lesions may exhibit only hyperkeratosis or parakeratosis but are still likely to represent 'keratosis of unknown significance' with the potential to subsequently develop dysplasia, unlike the keratoses noted in pachyonychia congenita or other genodermatoses (see earlier).

Darier disease

Clinical features

Oral findings occur in approximately 50% of patients with Darier disease (Darier-White disease, keratosis follicularis) and does not occur in the absence of skin findings. Mild involvement comprises minute white or pink keratotic papules, while more extensive disease results in larger plaques or a cobblestone mucosal surface. Lesions are generally asymptomatic.[1–5] The palatal mucosa is the most common site affected, perhaps because of its normally keratinized nature, followed by the gingiva, tongue, buccal mucosa, and floor of mouth; the lips are rarely involved.[6,7] Recurrent parotid or submandibular swelling may be reported in up to approximately one-third of cases and is most likely the result of strictures in the main duct causing obstruction.[4,6] In general, the degree of oral involvement parallels the extent of skin lesions.[2,6]

Pathogenesis and histologic features

This disease is associated with a mutation of *ATP2A2* on chromosome 12q that encodes a sarcoendoplasmic Ca^{2+}-ATPase isoform 2 (SERCA) that is involved in cytoplasmic calcium transport which is required for post-translational processing and proper functioning of desmosomes and keratin.[8]

There is hyperkeratosis, acanthosis, and suprabasal clefting with acantholysis forming villous-like projections that protrude into the cleft. Corps ronds and grains may not be as prominent as in skin lesions.[2,6] Papanicolaou-stained smears show an orange-brown staining of the dyskeratotic 'grains' and refractile concentric perinuclear rings and granular bands in corps ronds.[9] Excretory salivary ducts may become metaplastic or be involved by the same process leading to stricture formation and obstruction.[1,10,11]

Differential diagnosis

Oral warty dyskeratoma has similar histopathological findings although usually with few or no corps ronds or grains; it occurs as a solitary papule, plaque, or umbilicated nodule on the hard palatal mucosa or gingiva in the fifth and sixth decades of life, and as such, is distinguished from Darier disease by its clinical presentation.

Pemphigus vulgaris and pyostomatitis vegetans both exhibit acantholysis but not generally dyskeratosis; pemphigus shows intercellular IgG deposits on direct immunofluorescence while pyostomatitis vegetans exhibits intraepithelial eosinophilic abscesses.

Tumorlike lesions

Choristomas and heterotopias

Clinical features
Osseous choristoma

The majority of these lesions (93%) occur as sessile or pedunculated masses on the posterior dorsum of the tongue, near the foramen cecum, although it may occur at other sites such as the buccal mucosa.[1-5] Most develop in the second and third decades, and females are three to five times more likely to be affected.[2,4] There may be dysphagia.

Pathogenesis and histologic features

Theories of origin include ossification of branchial arch remnants, metaplastic bone formation secondary to trauma, and osteogenesis of unknown cause from multipotent mesenchymal cells in the area.

The lesion consists of a well-circumscribed mass of viable lamellar bone with haversian systems and variable osteoblastic rimming, surrounded by fibrous connective tissue; hematopoietic and fatty marrow or even cartilage may be present (*Figs 11.13* and *11.14*).[1,6-8]

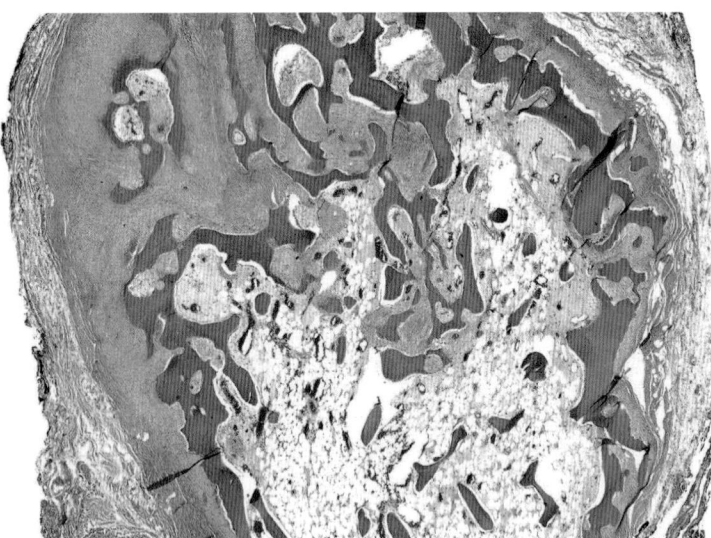

Fig. 11.13
Osseous choristoma from the tongue: there is a discrete nodule of bone and fatty tissue.

Differential diagnosis
Osseous metaplasia may be noted within pleomorphic adenoma or lipoma, and within myositis ossificans.

Clinical features
Cartilaginous choristoma

Cartilaginous choristomas present as discrete nodules, usually on the lateral border of the tongue (85% of cases) and less often on the buccal mucosa and soft palate.[1-3] Most occur in adults.[4,5]

Pathogenesis and histologic features

They may represent developmental malformations that arise from multipotent mesenchymal cells of the tongue, metaplastic change secondary to trauma or cartilaginous rests.

Cartilaginous choristoma consists of a mass of benign mature hyaline cartilage surrounded by perichondrium; loose myxoid tissue containing spindle cells reminiscent of primitive mesenchyme, or even mature fat may also be present.[2,4,6] Some cases show ossification.[2,3,7] Rare cases of chondrosarcoma have been reported.[8]

Differential diagnosis

Metaplastic cartilaginous nodules are often seen in cases of denture-associated fibrous hyperplasia (Cutright tumor), but these occur in the maxillary and mandibular vestibules associated with denture flanges. Cartilaginous rests are also common in the area of the nasopalatine canal. Some authors believe that cartilaginous rests of the soft palate/tonsillar area are a metaplastic phenomenon, occurring in 20% of tonsils examined.[9] A pleomorphic adenoma with extensive chondroid metaplasia should be considered in the differential diagnosis, but this would contain ductal structures and myoepithelial cells.

Clinical features
Fordyce granules, sebaceous hyperplasia, adenoma and choristoma

Oral sebaceous glands or Fordyce granules occur as 1–3-mm yellow macules or papules in the buccal and lip mucosa, and vermilion in approximately 80% of the adult population (*Fig. 11.15*).[1] However, these may become hyperplastic (sebaceous hyperplasia) or adenomatous (sebaceous adenoma), forming painless papules, plaques, or nodules; rarely, these may be associated with Muir-Torre syndrome.[2-4] They occur in the same sites as Fordyce granules.

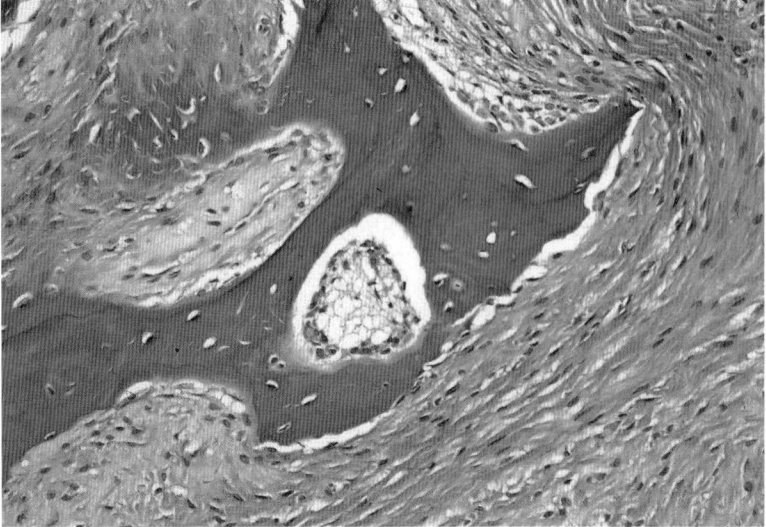

Fig. 11.14
Osseous choristoma from the tongue: the woven bone exhibits focal osteoblastic rimming and is deposited by the surrounding mesenchymal spindle cells.

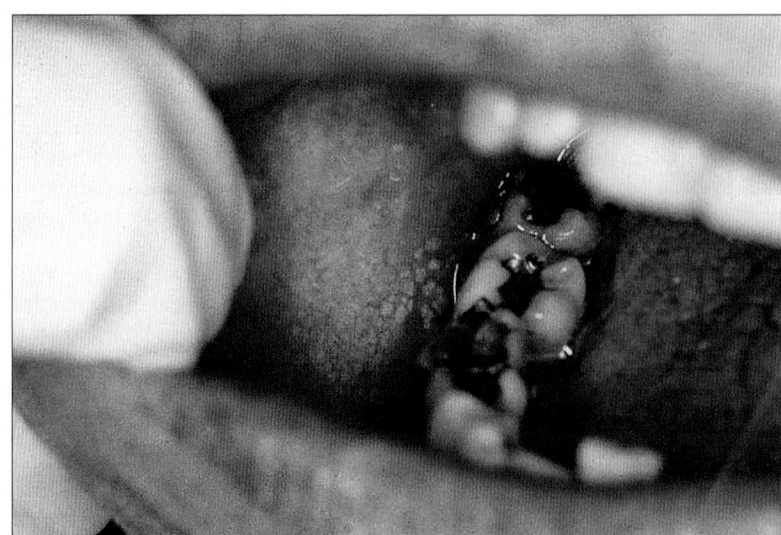

Fig. 11.15
Fordyce granules: typical yellow papules of the buccal mucosa.

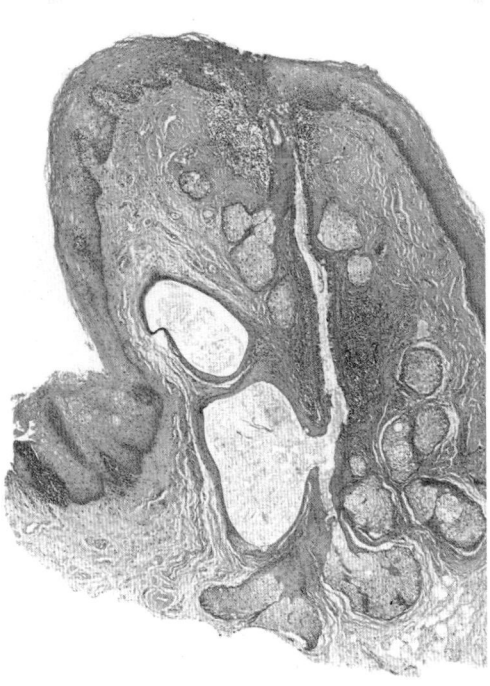

Fig. 11.16
Sebaceous hyperplasia: numerous lobules of sebaceous glands empty into a central dilated duct.

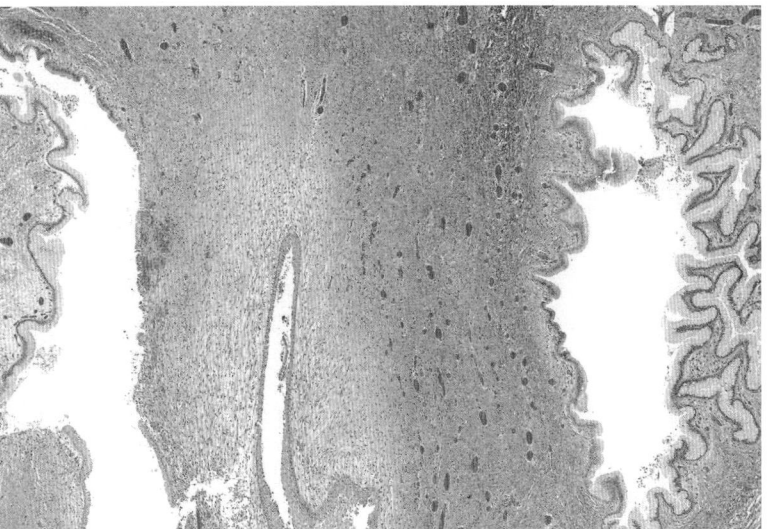

Fig. 11.17
Heterotopic gastrointestinal tissue: cystic structures are lined by squamous epithelium and colonic-type epithelium.

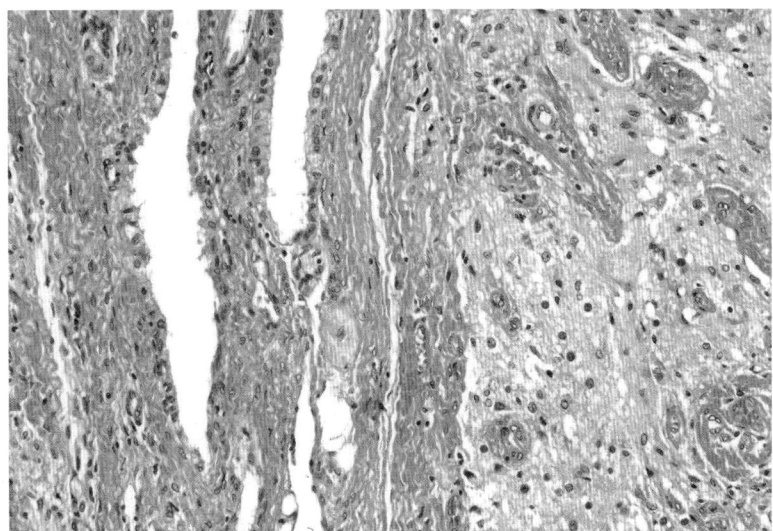

Fig. 11.18
Heterotopic brain tissue: note the presence of glial and ependymal tissue.

Rare cases of sebaceous choristomas have been reported in adults or infants. They present as dome-shaped masses in the midline of the dorsum in the area of the middle or posterior one-third of the tongue.[5,6]

Pathogenesis and histologic features

Fordyce granules are generally considered a variation of normal anatomy and consist of mature lobules of sebaceous glands that may communicate with the surface epithelium via a duct. There may be pseudocyst formation with retention of secretions; the rare occurrence of hair follicle and *Demodex* within a Fordyce granule has been reported.[7–9]

In sebaceous hyperplasia, at least 15 lobules (a somewhat arbitrary number) of mature sebaceous glands empty into ducts that communicate with the surface (*Fig. 11.16*).[2] Sebaceous adenomas, in addition, show a proliferation of basaloid germinative cells at the periphery of the lobules.[9–12] Some of these may represent sebaceous adenoma of the minor salivary gland.[13] The term sebaceous choristoma has been used to described mature sebaceous units usually in the midline present in infants.[14] However, if it is associated with eccrine glands, hair follicles, and apocrine glands, it is more appropriately termed epidermal choristoma.[6,15,16] Rarely, sebaceous carcinoma develops intraorally.[17]

Clinical features
Gastrointestinal choristoma/heterotopia

Almost all of these are cystic lesions that present as swellings of the tongue, usually ventral midline, or the floor of mouth.[1–3] Sometimes they appear as sinus tracts.[4] They are most often seen in infancy or early childhood and may be associated with orofacial malformations.[3]

Pathogenesis and histologic features

Theories of pathogenesis include epithelial entrapment, displacement, or persistence of intestinal epithelial buds that subsequently proliferate and differentiate.[4,5]

The cystic lesions are lined by epithelium typical for the cardiac, fundic, or pyloric regions of the stomach with parietal and Paneth cells.[4,6] However, some are lined by squamous, colonic, and/or ciliated epithelium (*Fig. 11.17*).[5] Smooth muscle is usually identified, and the presence of pancreatic tissue has also been reported.[7] If ectodermal and mesodermal elements are also present, the lesion should be considered a teratoma.

Heterotopic brain tissue

Clinical features

This uncommon condition presents in the first year of life, most often affecting the palatal mucosa, tongue (especially the foramen cecum area), or oropharynx presenting as a nodule or mass. Some patients have associated palatal defects.[1] Respiratory obstruction is a major cause of morbidity, and feeding difficulties are common if lesions are large.[2]

Pathogenesis and histologic features

It occurs as a result of displacement of primitive neural elements in an early stage of development, or neuroglial differentiation from multipotent cells.[3,4]

Mature elements of the central nervous system including astrocytes, oligodendrocytes, ependymal tissue, and choroid plexus-like tissue, and, rarely, neuronal tissue may all be identified (*Fig. 11.18*).[3–7]

Oral lymphoepithelial cyst

Clinical features

Oral lymphoepithelial cysts generally occur in the fourth decade of life with a 2 : 1 female predilection.[1–3] These also occur in the parotid gland, in

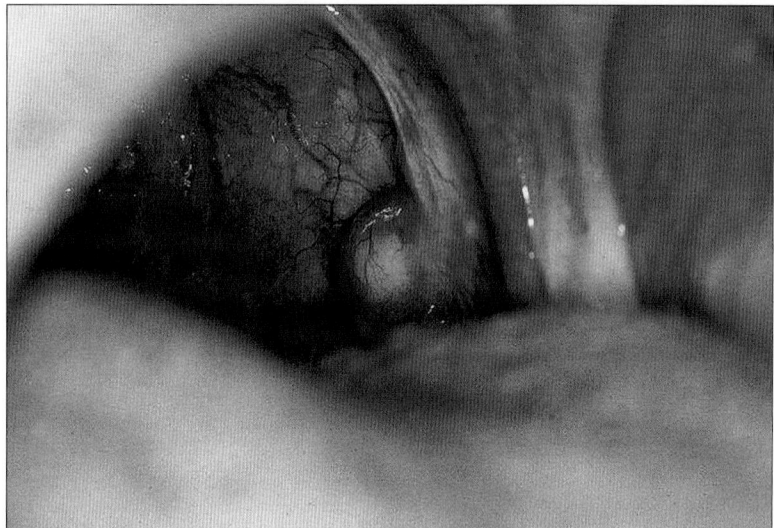

Fig. 11.19
Oral lymphoepithelial cyst: note the yellow nodule located behind the anterior faucial pillar.

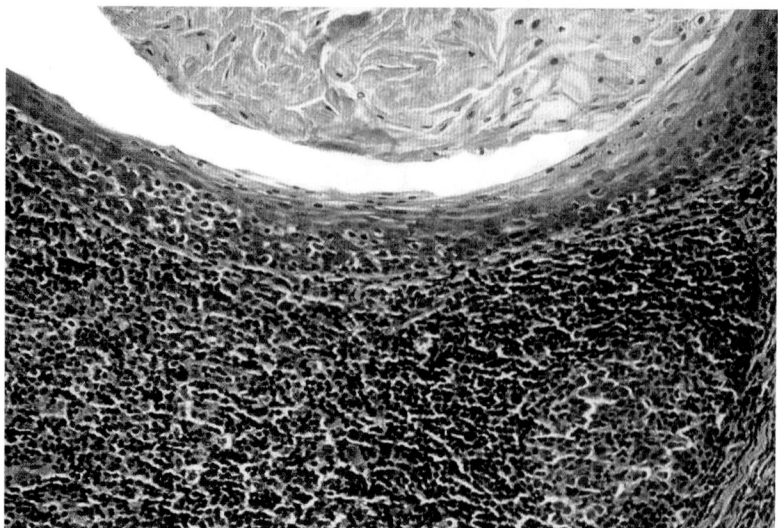

Fig. 11.21
Oral lymphoepithelial cyst: there is lymphocyte exocytosis through the reticulated lymphoepithelium and a small germinal center is present.

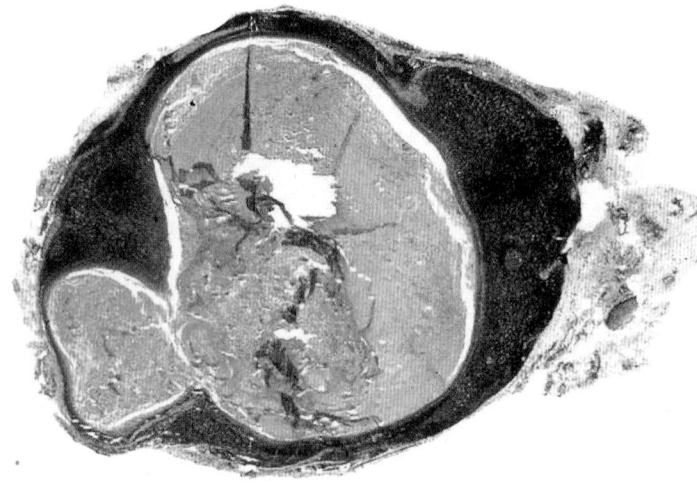

Fig. 11.20
Oral lymphoepithelial cyst: the cyst is filled with keratin debris and completely encircled by lymphoid tissue.

particular, in human immunodeficiency virus (HIV)-positive individuals.[4,5] They present as painless, yellowish nodules, usually less than 1 cm in diameter, most commonly affecting the floor of mouth followed by the posterior ventral tongue, soft palate, and tonsillar fauces (*Fig. 11.19*).[4,6,7] They are commonly filled with cheesy, keratinaceous material. Some authorities believe that lesions that present at sites where tonsillar tissue is normally found represent blocked tonsillar crypts with retention of secretions.[6]

Pathogenesis and histologic features

Three theories of pathogenesis have been proposed:
- There is enclavement of epithelium within oral lymphoid tissue during embryogenesis and subsequent proliferation and cystic degeneration.[1]
- Such lymphoid aggregates are ectopic oral tonsils, where the crypt openings have been blocked, resulting in retention of secretions.[7,8]
- The epithelium represents squamous metaplasia of excretory salivary ducts, and the lymphoid tissue is a reaction to inflammation or immunological stimulation.[4]

The last theory is particularly pertinent in floor of mouth lesions, a site where tonsillar/lymphoid tissue is not normally found.

The cyst is lined by parakeratotic stratified squamous epithelium and the lumen is filled with desquamated keratinaceous material (*Fig. 11.20*).[4,6,9]

Rare cases may be lined by pseudostratified columnar epithelium with or without mucous cells.[7] The epithelium usually demonstrates lymphocytic exocytosis and resembles the reticulated lymphoepithelium of the tonsils. The surrounding lymphoid tissue may encircle the cyst epithelium completely or partially, and germinal centers may be well formed or absent (*Fig. 11.21*). Some cases demonstrate communication with the overlying surface epithelium, often through a narrow opening.

Salivary glands and ducts may be present in the vicinity, especially floor of mouth lesions.[1,4]

Differential diagnosis

Salivary duct cysts are lined by stratified squamous, columnar, oncocytic, or respiratory epithelium, sometimes with mucous cell prosoplasia. They may show foci of chronic inflammation but not usually the thick mantle of lymphocytes with germinal centers. Dermoid and epidermoid cysts lack the lymphoid mantle and produce orthokeratin, and dermoid cysts contain adnexa in the wall.

Epidermoid, dermoid and teratoid cysts

Clinical features

This usually occurs in children and young adults, and there may be a slight male predilection. The midline floor of the mouth is the most common site of presentation, and some cases are congenital.[1-3] Classification of these lesions is based on anatomical location such as lingual, submental or submandibular, and on the histologic appearance.[1,2,4] The term 'congenital germline fusion cyst" has been proposed for these lesions.[4]

They present as dome-shaped, yellow masses with a rubbery or doughy consistency. Intraoral lesions cause feeding, swallowing, and speech difficulties while extraoral variants below the myohoid muscle lead to a noticeable submental mass. Dumbbell-shaped cysts have both intra- and extraoral swellings.[5]

Pathogenesis and histologic features

One theory suggests that these cysts arise from entrapped epithelial rests in the line of fusion of the first and second pharyngeal arches. Another proposes that the lining develops from displaced embryonic rests or traumatic implantation, possibly occurring even in utero.[3] Some authorities suggest a single term, 'congenital germline fusion cyst', for epidermoid, dermoid, and teratoid cysts.[6]

Both epidermoid and dermoid cysts are lined by orthokeratinized squamous epithelium, and the lumen is filled with keratinaceous material. Epidermoid cysts (also called epithelial inclusion cysts) have no adnexa in the wall, while dermoid cysts always have hair follicles, sebaceous glands, and/ or eccrine or apocrine structures in the wall. Oral dermoid cysts are three times more common than epidermoid cysts.[2] Some cysts also contain gastrointestinal mucosa or respiratory mucosa.[7-9] If tissues from all three germ layers are represented, the term 'teratoid cyst' is applied.

Differential diagnosis

Gingival cyst of the adult is generally nonkeratinized and is lined by low cuboidal to columnar or stratified squamous epithelium, with occasional epithelial plaques containing clear cells.[10] Gingival cysts of the newborn, which are not biopsied because they exteriorize on their own, are filled with keratinaceous material.[11] Both can be differentiated from epidermoid cysts by their location on the gingiva.

Dermoid tumor (dermoid), teratoma and epignathus

Clinical features

These rare conditions generally present congenitally or in infancy as masses protruding from the mouth, causing respiratory distress and feeding difficulties. They have been classified as follows:

- dermoid tumor ('hairy polyp') where only ecto- and mesodermal structures are present,
- teratoid tumor and teratoma with tissue from all three germ layers represented; the tissues in teratoid tumor are not as well organized as in a teratoma,
- epignathus where there is recognizable organ and limb formation; however, this term is also often applied to any teratoid tumor or teratoma that arises from the nasopharyngeal or palatal areas with epignathus being the most mature variant.

Of these, the dermoid is the most common.[1]

Dermoids tend to occur in females (six to seven times more often than in males) as pedunculated masses in the nasopharynx, oropharynx, and soft palate.[2,3] The mass is covered by skin, hence its other name, 'hairy polyp'. It may also grossly resemble an accessory auricle.[4]

Teratomas, teratoid tumors, and epignathi present as masses that may protrude from the mouth, and airway obstruction is a frequent presenting symptom; there is a female predilection and most are present at birth.[5] Unlike dermoids, these tumors are often associated with other malformations and findings such as elevated alpha fetoprotein and polyhydramnios.[6,7]

Epignathi in particular may be associated with severe congenital malformations, and stillbirth is a common occurrence. They most often arise from the hard palatal mucosa (hence its name), although the posterior nasopharynx and upper lip can be involved, and there may be palatal clefts and cranial extension.[7-9] Grossly, the tumor sometimes contains rudimentary limbs, or even a head resembling an incomplete twin or fetus in fetu.[10]

Lingual (tongue) teratomas are generally not associated with such developmental defects.[11]

Histologic features

Dermoids are covered by skin with its constituent adnexa. In addition, cartilage, bone, muscle, and adipose tissue may be present (*Fig. 11.22*).[3,7,12,13] Teratomas contain tissue derived from all three germ layers to include ectoderm, mesoderm, and endoderm. As such, neural, brain, lung, gastrointestinal, and respiratory tissues may be present.[6,11]

Epignathi is a form of duplication and consist of tissues organized to form grossly recognizable specific organ systems such as limbs, a head, or eyes.[7,10,14]

Congenital granular cell tumor/epulis

Clinical features

The congenital granular cell tumor presents as a pink, pedunculated mass, usually on the anterior alveolar ridge mucosa with an intact surface (*Fig. 11.23*). There is a 10:1 female predilection, and it is three times more common in the maxillary mucosa.[1,2] It may cause problems with nursing.

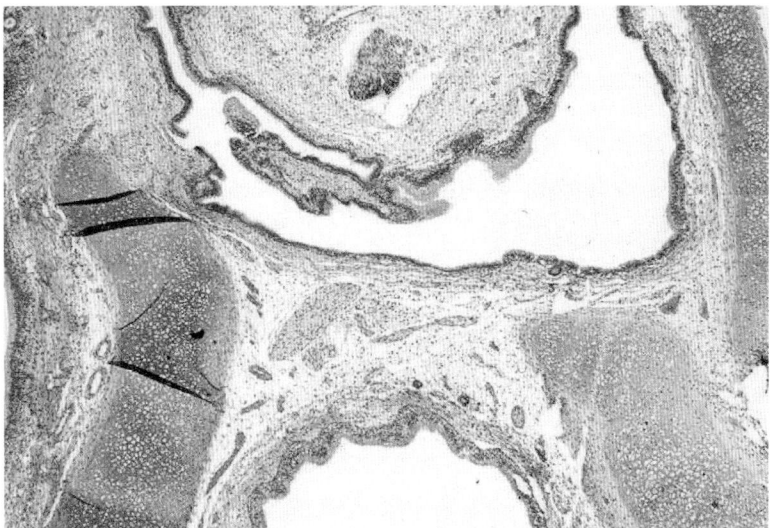

Fig. 11.22
Dermoid tumor: note the presence of cartilage and cystic spaces lined by intestinal-type epithelium. By courtesy of the Registry of Oral Pathology, AFIP, Washington, DC, USA.

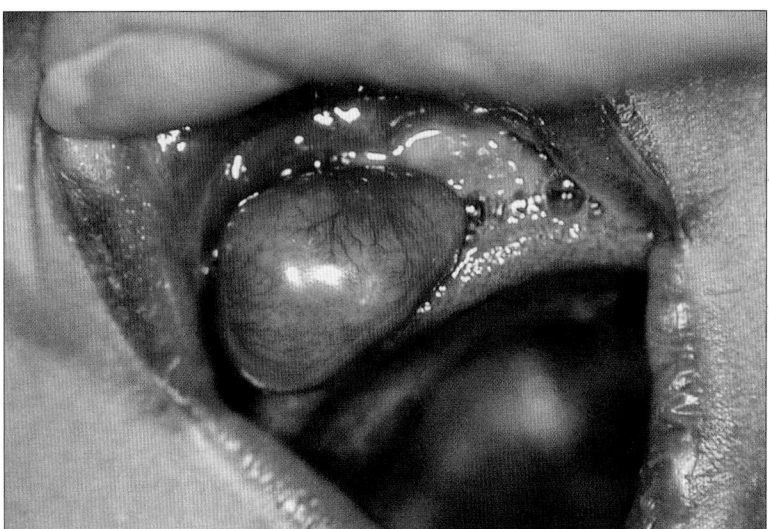

Fig. 11.23
Congenital granular cell tumor: there is a firm nodule on the maxillary alveolar ridge mucosa, which is a typical location for this tumor. By courtesy of B. Padwa, MD DDS, Boston, USA.

Approximately 9% of patients have multiple tumors and some may have concurrent tongue lesions.[3-5]

Pathogenesis and histologic features

Theories of histogenesis have included pericytic, myofibroblastic, and neural differentiation. The current hypothesis is that it represents a mesenchymal tumor with degenerative change. This is supported by lack of growth after birth of the infant, resolution of some cases over time, histologic evidence of degeneration, and lack of recurrence in spite of incomplete removal.[1,6-8]

Histologically, a Grenz zone may or may not be present and the overlying epithelium is typically atrophic without pseudoepitheliomatous hyperplasia. The cells are round or polygonal with distinct borders, abundant eosinophilic granular cytoplasm, eccentric small nuclei, and inconspicuous nucleoli; a prominent delicate and arborizing capillary network is usually evident (*Fig. 11.24*).[4,7,9] The granules are periodic acid-Schiff (PAS) positive and diastase resistant; odontogenic rests may also be present.[5,10]

The granular cells do not express S100 protein but are always vimentin positive and CD68, NK1C3, and PGP9.5 positive; 40% are also positive for neuron-specific enolase (NSE).[7,11-13] Studies for smooth muscle actin (SMA),

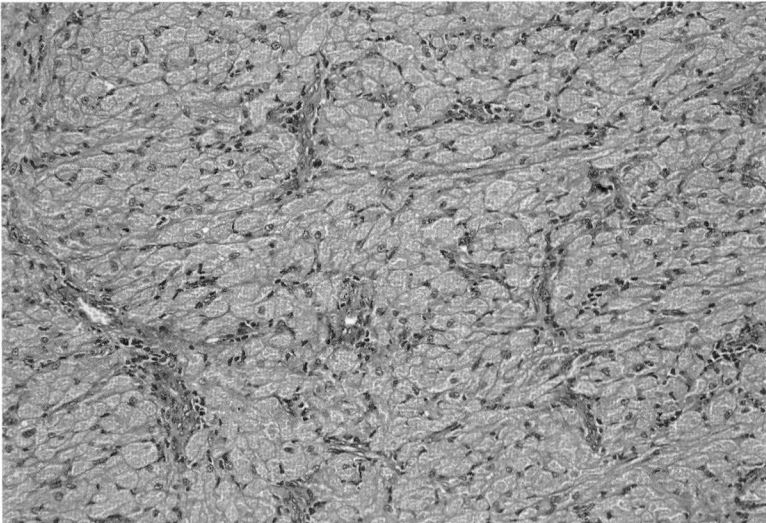

Fig. 11.24
Congenital granular cell epulis: note the large pale cells with distinct cell borders and granular cytoplasm; arborizing vessels are present.

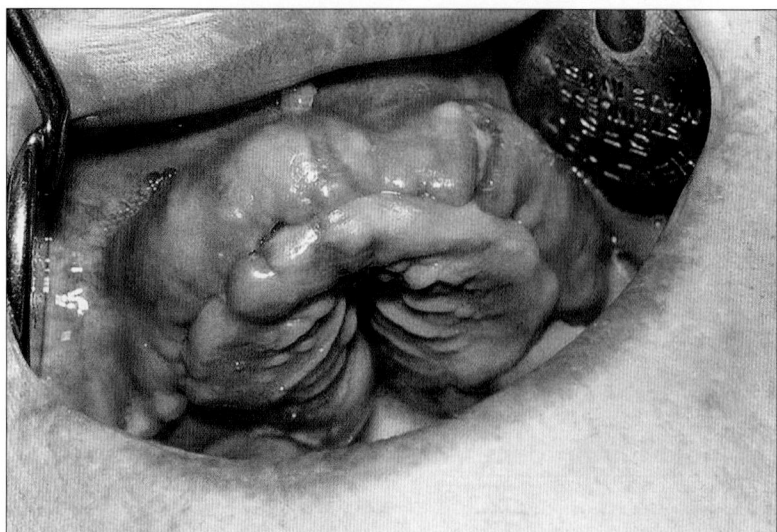

Fig. 11.25
Hereditary gingival fibromatosis: there is extensive overgrowth of dense fibrous tissue in the maxillary mucosa. By courtesy of G. Gallagher, DMD, Boston, USA.

estrogen and progesterone receptors, glial fibrillary acidic protein (GFAP), myelin basic protein (MBP), and neurofilament protein are negative.[1,7,]

Ultrastructural studies reveal the presence of membrane-bound granules with electron-dense contents that most likely represent phagolysosomes.[1,4,11,14] The presence of subplasmalemmal dense bodies, pinocytotic vesicles containing precollagenous material, and intracytoplasmic laminin and fibronectin suggests myofibroblastic differentiation.[4,10,11]

Differential diagnosis

The cells of conventional granular cell tumor are histologically indistinguishable from those of congenital granular cell tumor. However, in congenital granular cell tumor, there is no pseudoepitheliomatous hyperplasia and there is a prominent arborizing delicate vascular network; importantly, the cells are S100 negative. Angulate bodies, seen ultrastructurally in conventional granular cell tumor, are absent.

Congenital gingival leiomyomatous polyp/hamartoma has a similar clinical presentation (usually in the midline of the maxillary mucosa) but histologically contains a nonencapsulated proliferation of fusiform and spindle smooth muscle cells that, as expected, express HHF-35, SMA, and desmin but not S100 protein.[15-18] This condition may also occur at other sites.[19-21]

Lingual thyroid

Clinical features

Approximately 10% of cadaveric tongues contain nests of thyroid tissue, with no sex predilection.[1,2] However, when thyroid tissue occurs as a mass in the tongue, the term 'lingual thyroid choristoma' or 'ectopic lingual thyroid' is used. Since approximately 86% of such tumors consist of the only thyroid tissue in the body, the terms 'lingual thyroid' or 'ectopic lingual thyroid' are more accurate.[3]

Females are three to seven times more likely to be affected than males and there are two peaks of presentation, i.e., the first and second decades and the fifth and sixth decades, probably related to hormonal influences.[4-6] The lesion presents as a rounded, soft-to-firm mass within the base of the tongue between the foramen cecum and the epiglottis. It may cause dysphagia, dyspnea, dysphonia, or a globus sensation, and hemorrhage may occur.[2-4] One-quarter of patients may be hypothyroid.

Pathogenesis and histologic features

The thyroid anlage develops in the area of the foramen cecum and descends from there into the neck. As such, failure to descend or persistence and proliferation of remnants of the anlage results in a noticeable mass.[7] In most

cases, a biopsy is not indicated if imaging studies are positive for thyroid tissue. However, difficulty swallowing may necessitate excision.

The tissue consists of thyroid follicles that contain mature or embryonic thyroid epithelium and exhibit microfollicular, macrofollicular, or adenomatous changes.[1,5] There may be an associated thyroglossal duct.[2] Follicular and papillary carcinomas can sometimes occur, in the same frequency as one would expect in the normal thyroid gland[8-10]; even medullary carcinoma has been reported.[11]

Lymphangioma of the alveolar ridge

Clinical features

Lymphangioma has been identified in approximately 4% of infants, all of whom were black. Females are twice as likely to be affected as males, and 74% of subjects have more than one lesion.[1-4] They present as dome-shaped, bluish, fluid-filled vesicles usually affecting the posterior maxillary and mandibular alveolar ridge mucosa and are typically 3–4 mm in diameter.[3,5] Many (if not most) regress by 6 months of age.[1,6,7]

Histologic features

Lymphangioma is characterized by slit-like spaces lined by flattened endothelial cells and filled with sparse, fibrillar, eosinophilic material consistent with lymph, and often red blood cells.[1,2] Odontogenic rests sometimes may be present.

Differential diagnosis

Lymphangioma circumscriptum has an identical histology but is seen in older patients.

Gingival fibromatosis

Clinical features

In this condition, there is a benign, diffuse, nonhemorrhagic, and fibrotic gingival enlargement, often occurring bilaterally and involving the maxillary and mandibular gingiva, sometimes to the extent that it may reach the occlusal/incisal edges of the teeth.[1,2] Several forms are recognized. The inherited form (usually an autosomal dominant trait, but occasionally autosomal recessive), which is less common, tends to present congenitally or in the first decade of life, coinciding with eruption of teeth, and often exhibits generalized gingival involvement. The gingival growth is densely fibrotic and covered by normal-appearing mucosa (*Fig. 11.25*). There is a strong

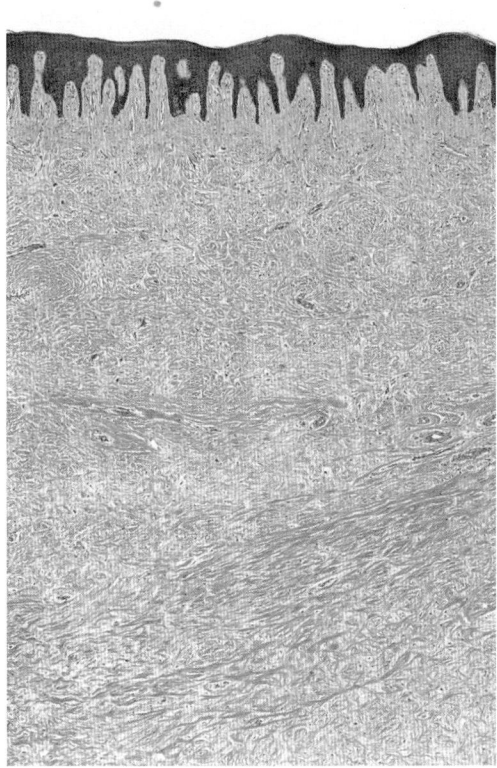

Fig. 11.26
Hereditary gingival fibromatosis: there is a marked proliferation of fibrous tissue and ground substance.

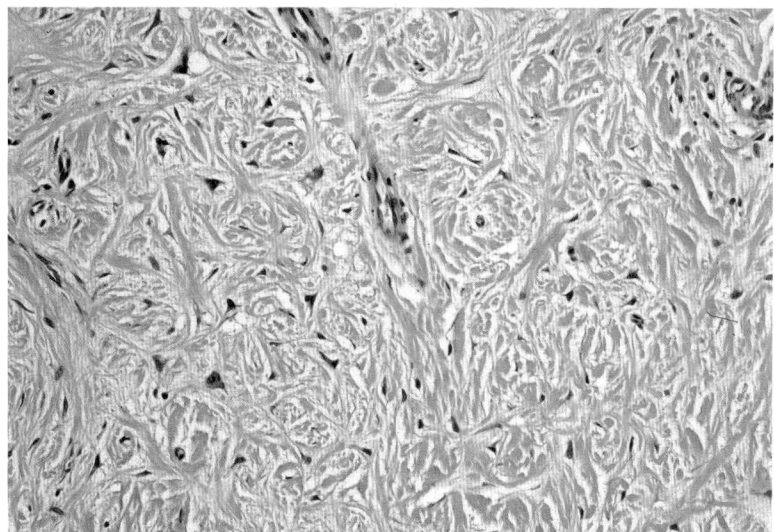

Fig. 11.27
Hereditary gingival fibromatosis: plump, stellate-shaped fibroblasts are seen in a densely collagenous stroma.

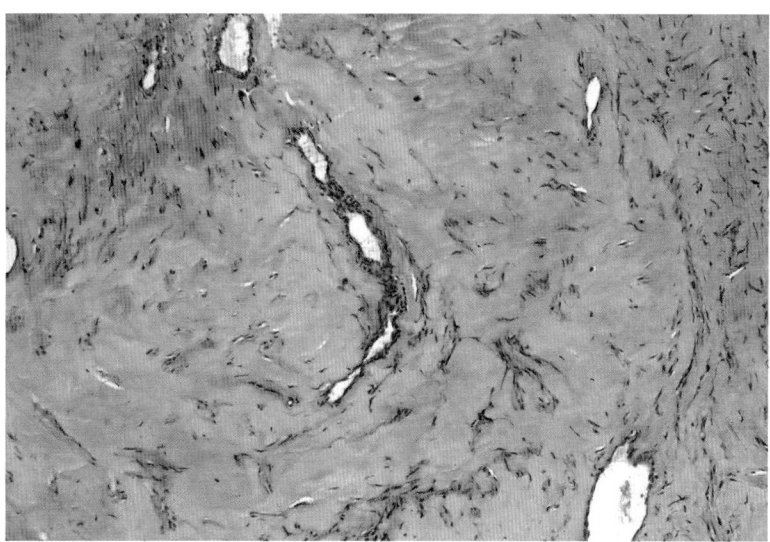

Fig. 11.28
Juvenile hyaline fibromatosis: there is diffuse deposition of eosinophilic, hyalinized fibrocollagenous material with scattered fibroblasts. By courtesy of J. Sciubba, DDS, Baltimore, USA.

association with hypertrichosis and mental retardation and/or seizure disorders, and medications such as phenytoin taken to control seizures aggravate the gingival hyperplasia. Gingival fibromatosis is also a feature of Zimmerman-Laband, Ramon, Rutherford, Cross, and other syndromes.[2,3] An idiopathic form occurs later in life usually with limited involvement of the gingiva by similar fibrotic masses often confined to just one quadrant, or to the maxillary tuberosity or lingual mandibular mucosa bilaterally. There is no tendency for regression.[1]

Pathogenesis and histologic features

The nonsyndromic, autosomal dominant form of the disease is caused by a mutation in *SOS1* on chromosome 2p21–22.[4–6]

The gingival overgrowth is caused primarily by an increased production and reduced metabolism of connective tissue. Native fibroblasts show elevated rates of proliferation and increased synthesis of fibronectin and type I collagen.[7] Reduced matrix metalloproteinase levels, possibly mediated by increased production of transforming growth factor beta-1 (TGF-β1), results in excess accumulation of extracellular matrix.[8]

Histologically, there is a diffuse proliferation of collagenous tissue within a background of excessive ground substance (*Fig. 11.26*). Some lesions contain plump, stellate-shaped fibroblasts (*Fig. 11.27*). Dystrophic calcification may be seen in up to 43% of cases.[2] The overlying epithelium is variably acanthotic, and there are few inflammatory cells.

Differential diagnosis

Generalized gingival hyperplasia caused by local irritation or systemic influences (such as medications or hormones) is distinguished from gingival fibromatosis on clinical grounds and by more prominent inflammation.

Hyaline fibromatosis (hyaline fibromatosis syndrome)

Clinical features

Hyaline fibromatosis is an autosomal recessive condition with two distinct subgroups, although both exhibit joint contractures, skin papules and nodules, gingival hyperplasia, and osteopenia. In the less severe form referred to as juvenile hyaline fibromatosis, patients exhibit pearly papules and larger fibrotic nodules on the skin (around the face, ears, scalp, neck,

and trunk) and survive for several decades, while the more severe form referred to as infantile systemic hyalinosis exhibits systemic involvement, skin hyperpigmentation, perianal nodules, protein-losing enteropathy with diarrhea, recurrent infections, and survival of less than 2 years.[1–6]

Pathogenesis and histologic features

Mutations of capillary morphogenesis factor 2 gene, *ANTXR2*, on chromosome 4q21 causes defects in basement membrane matrix assembly resulting from compromised cell-matrix or cell-cell interactions.[5,7–10]

The gingival and skin lesions of juvenile hyaline fibromatosis show extensive deposits of PAS-positive, diastase-resistant, and Congo red-negative homogenous, eosinophilic, hyalinized material in the connective tissue (*Fig. 11.28*).[3,5] Fibroblasts are round and chondrocyte-like, lying within lacunae-like spaces and exhibit large vesicular nuclei.[3,11] The hyaline material consists of glycoproteins, glycosaminoglycans, and collagens.

Ultrastructurally, there are prominent Golgi complexes, dilated rough endoplasmic reticulum, and multivesicular bodies and vesicles filled with fibrillogranular material that resembles collagen.[12]

REACTIVE CONDITIONS

Leukoedema

Clinical features

This is a benign, painless condition of adults, usually affecting the buccal mucosa bilaterally, and occasionally the tongue; it is not symptomatic. The mucosa has a diffuse gray-white hue with faint reticulations that disappear on stretching (*Fig. 11.29*).[1,2]

The prevalence ranges from 20% to 36% among those who do not use tobacco or chew coca leaves, to 51–68% in those who use tobacco, coca, or cannabis.[3-8] Its incidence increases with age.[9] A prevalence of 51% was reported in African-Americans but without mention of tobacco habits.[10] Another study found a prevalence of 93% in a Caucasian population, leading the author to question whether this condition is merely a variation of normal.[2]

Pathogenesis and histologic features

A low-grade topical injury, such as occurs with the use of smoked tobacco or coca leaves, gives rise to this condition. As such, most changes are limited to the superficial layers of keratinocytes.

There is acanthosis with little or no parakeratosis. The characteristic feature is keratinocyte edema where degenerated and swollen cells are present in the superficial and mid-epithelial layers (*Fig. 11.30*).[11] The most superficial cells have abundant pale, watery cytoplasm, sometimes pyknotic nuclei and prominent collapsed cell membranes, forming a jigsaw puzzle pattern; anucleate forms are caused by plane of section of these swollen cells (*Fig. 11.31*). There is usually no inflammation in the lamina propria.

Ultrastructural studies show abnormal keratohyaline granules and loosely dispersed tonofilaments with fragmented organelles in the superficial degenerated cells. The mid-level swollen cells contain abnormal swollen mitochondria.[11,12] These features support the theory of limited cell damage with keratinocyte edema and swelling. Similar features have also been reported in the sucking pads of neonates.[13]

Differential diagnosis

In morsicatio mucosae oris, there is shaggy parakeratosis associated with many bacterial colonies without inflammation; keratinocyte edema is often present beneath areas of such factitial keratosis (see below).

Smokeless tobacco lesion presents with keratin chevrons and shows a band of coagulated and degenerate cells with anucleation similar to leukoedema. The transition zone from normal to degenerate is often abrupt in smokeless tobacco lesion (see below). This should also be considered a severe form of keratinocyte edema caused by contact irritation.

Hairy leukoplakia may exhibit leukoedema and concomitant morsicatio mucosae oris, but will also exhibit viral cytopathic change caused by Epstein-Barr virus.

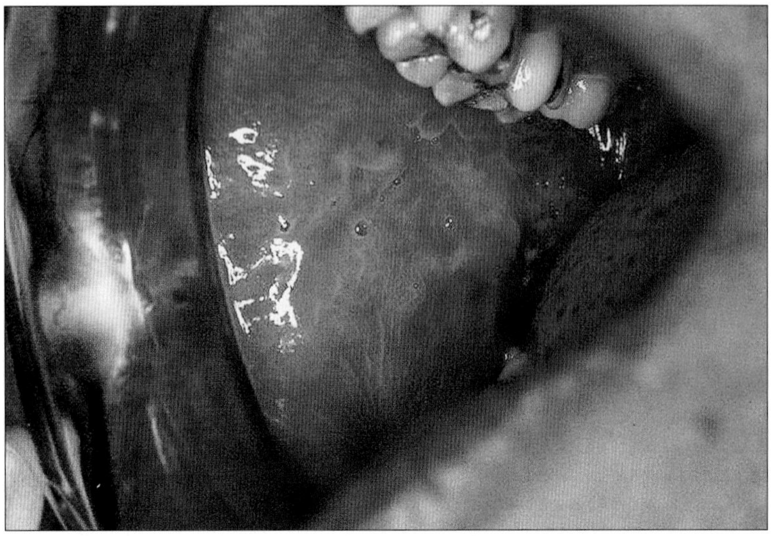

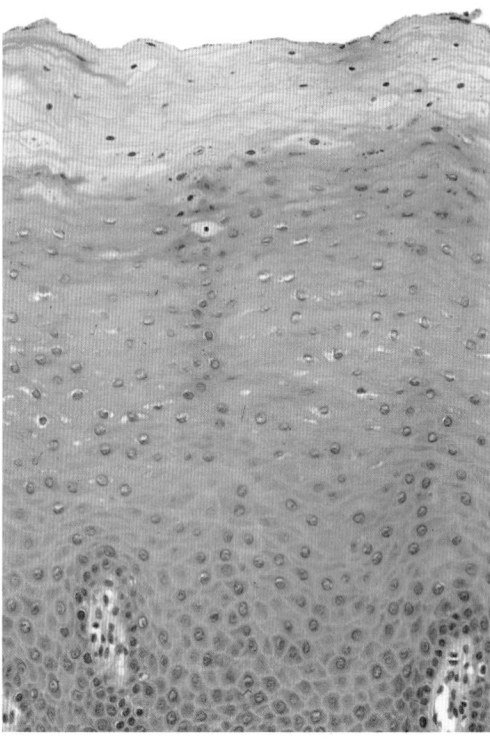

Fig. 11.30
Leukoedema: there is acanthosis and keratinocyte edema of superficial cells.

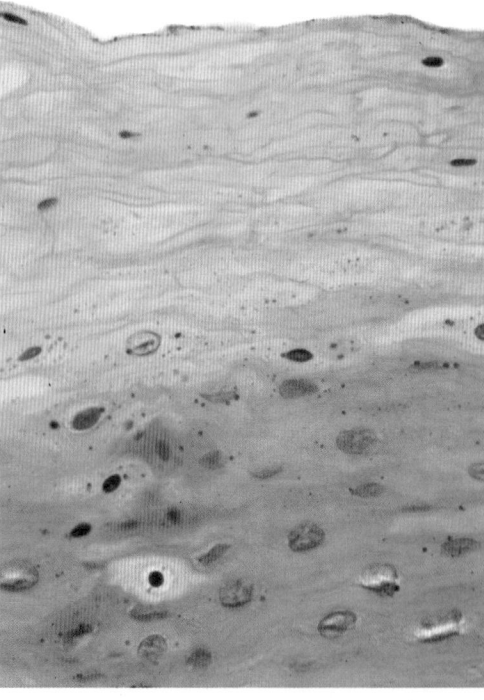

Fig. 11.31
Leukoedema: the superficial cells characteristically have pale cytoplasm and are anucleate with a 'jigsaw-like' pattern of cell membranes.

Fig. 11.29
Leukoedema: the buccal mucosa has a pale, milky white appearance.

Morsicatio mucosae oris/factitial keratosis

Clinical features

This is usually seen in adults, is often bilateral, and may involve the buccal mucosa (most common), lateral tongue, and lower lip mucosa.[1-3] The site of injury exhibits shaggy white papules and plaques that have a peeling, thready, macerated surface; erosions are sometimes present, and occasionally ulcers are seen (*Figs 11.32* and *11.33*). Similar lesions have been noted in areca nut chewers and glass blowers.[4,5] This has no malignant potential.

Pathogenesis and histologic features,

In morsicatio mucosae oris, buccal mucosa, lip, or tongue chewing habits occur either subconsciously at night or as a conscious parafunctional habit, leading to keratosis and maceration of the mucosa.

There is shaggy, irregular parakeratosis, which may be severe, and acanthosis. Characteristically, the keratin is thrown into papillations with fissures and clefts, rimmed by bacteria, but this is not invariably present (*Fig. 11.34*).[2,6,7] Spongiosis or leukocyte exocytosis are usually absent although plasma pooling may be present within superficial keratinocytes. Superficial cells are ballooned and degenerated, typical for keratinocyte edema. Inflammation in the lamina propria is insignificant unless there is erosion and ulceration. In betel nut chewers, there is a yellow-brown pigment on the surface of the keratin and within epithelial cells, representing fragments of the betel quid.[5,7] Biopsy of the linea alba (the white line on the buccal mucosa bilaterally where the upper and lower teeth meet) essentially reveals identical histologic features confirming the frictional/factitial nature of this condition.

Differential diagnosis

Morsicatio mucosae oris may occur as a primary mucosal disorder such as has been described above, or it may present as a secondary finding related to chronic injury of protuberant plaques and nodules, such as fibromas.

Hairy leukoplakia may show similar shaggy parakeratosis from trauma. However, the typical changes of chromatin condensation, amphophilic Cowdry inclusions, and the presence of Epstein-Barr virus easily afford their distinction.

Smokeless tobacco lesion shows sharply demarcated coagulation of the superficial cells, sometimes accompanied by hyalinized, amorphous eosinophilic material in the lamina propria.

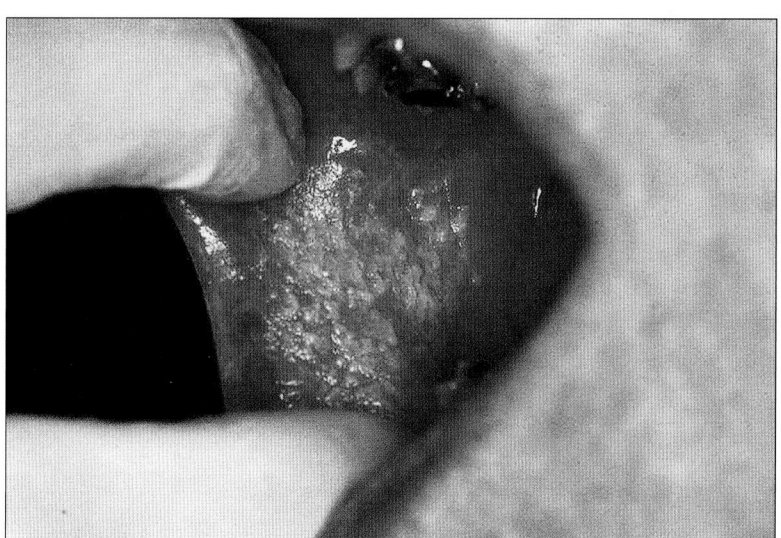

Fig. 11.32
Morsicatio mucosae oris (chronic bite/factitial keratosis): there are rough, shaggy, poorly demarcated papules and plaques on the buccal mucosa.

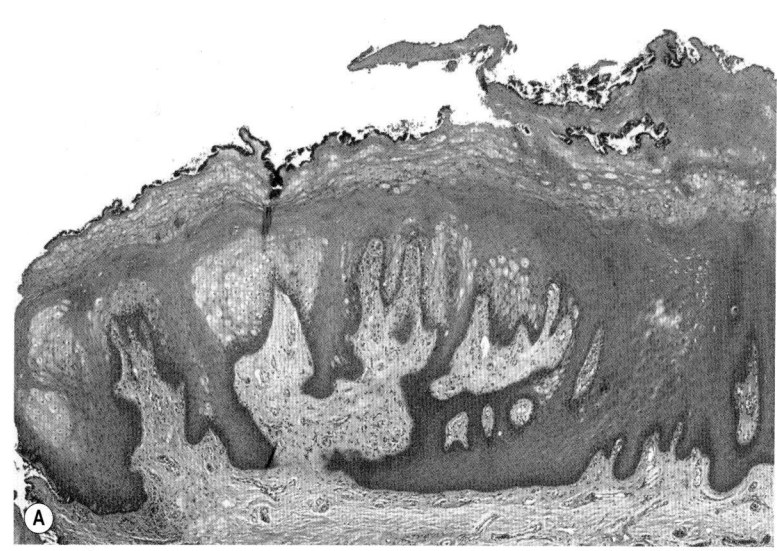

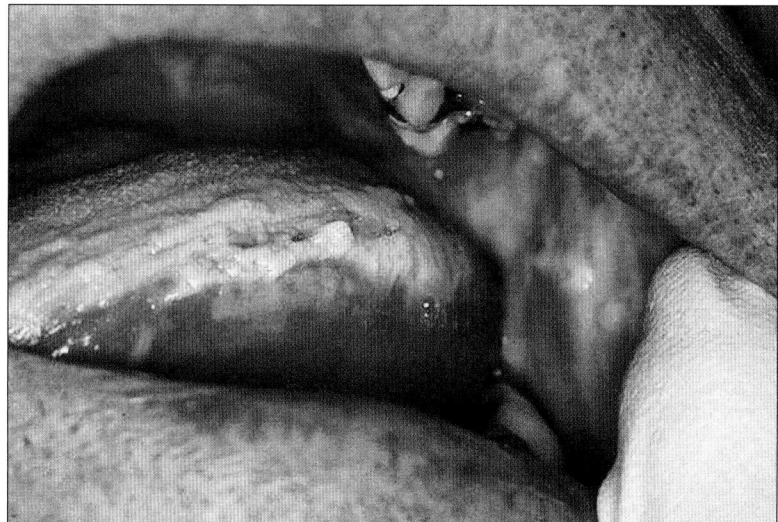

Fig. 11.33
Morsicatio mucosae oris (chronic bite keratosis): there are macerated, poorly demarcated shaggy plaques on the buccal mucosa and lateral border of the tongue.

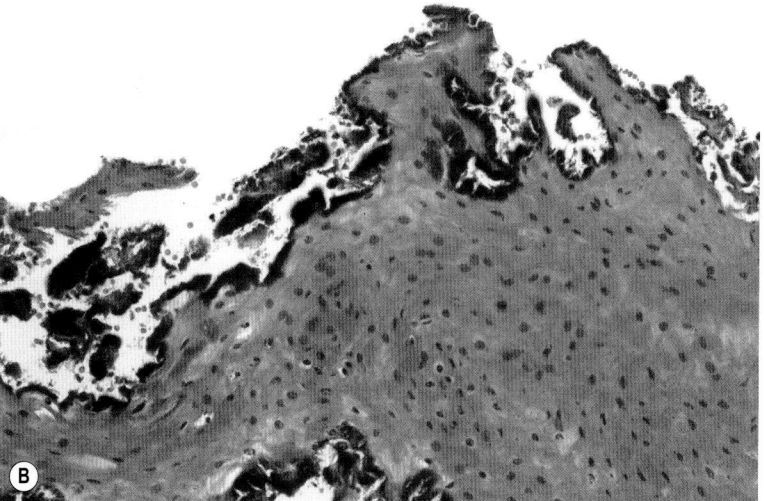

Fig. 11.34
Chronic bite/factitial keratosis: (**A**) there is marked shaggy parakeratosis with acanthosis and keratinocyte edema but little inflammation; (**B**) the characteristic fissures and clefts in the parakeratin are rimmed by bacteria with little or no inflammation.

Benign alveolar ridge keratosis/oral lichen simplex chronicus

Clinical features

This is a condition seen in adults on the keratinized mucosa. This presents as nontender, white, rough plaques that occur on the crest of the alveolar ridge mucosa, in particular in the area of the mandibular retromolar pads, often bilaterally (*Fig. 11.35*).[1] It may occur in any other part of the ridge mucosa where a tooth has been extracted. It has no malignant potential.

Lesions reported as merely 'alveolar ridge keratosis' are any white lesions on the alveolar ridge and gingiva with no histologic connotations and include both benign and dysplastic/malignant keratotic lesions of the gingiva and alveolar ridge; they are not synonymous with benign alveolar ridge keratosis, which has the specific histologic appearance of lichen simplex chronicus.[2]

Pathogenesis and histologic features

These lesions are caused by chronic frictional trauma to the ridge, not necessarily by direct tooth-to-ridge contact, but by food being crushed by teeth against the opposing edentulous ridge mucosa.

They have the typical histopathology of skin lesions of lichen simplex chronicus. There is hyperkeratosis often with wedge-shaped hypergranulosis, surface undulations or papillomatosis, and acanthosis (*Fig. 11.36*).

Rete ridges are tapered and generally uniformly elongated and often confluent at the tips. There is usually minimal to insignificant chronic inflammation in the lamina propria. Lesions from the retromolar pad often contain stellate-shaped fibroblasts, which are normal for that site.

Differential diagnosis

Verrucous hyperplasia may have a similar histology and often occurs on the gingiva or alveolar ridge mucosa; this is a form of architectural dysplasia (see later). However, the papillomatosis is usually more marked and other features include epithelial atypia, bulky epithelial hyperplasia, and an endophytic growth pattern. This must be correlated with clinical findings especially with a clinical lesion known as 'proliferative verrucous leukoplakia', where lesions are extensive, multifocal, and highly associated with malignant transformation.

Smokeless tobacco lesion/keratosis

Clinical features

In smokeless tobacco lesion (snuff dipper's keratosis), tobacco placed in the mandibular and less often, maxillary sulcus is associated with the

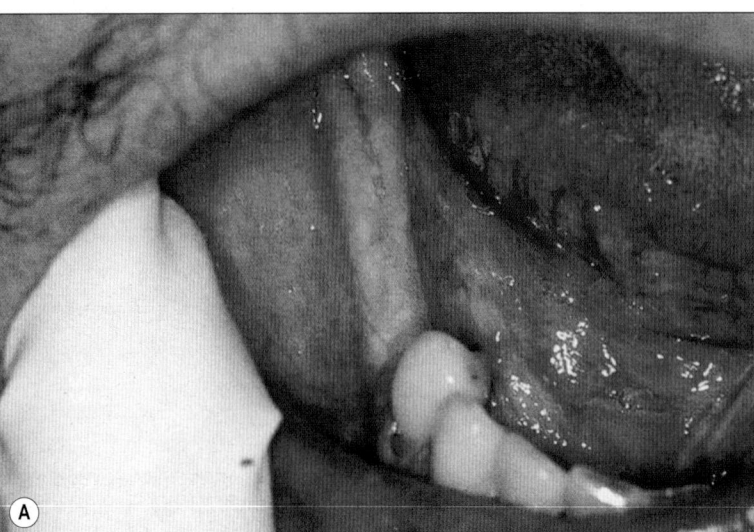

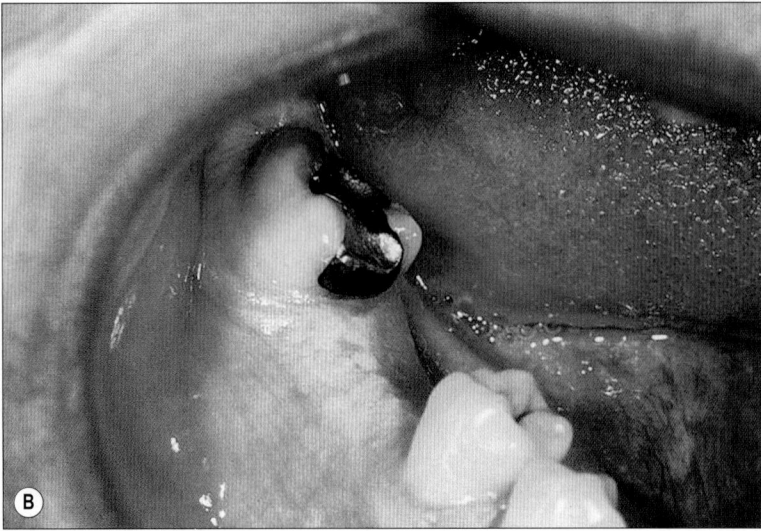

Fig. 11.35
Benign alveolar ridge keratosis: (**A**) the retromolar pad is a typical location for this condition; (**B**) the mucosa of the crest of the alveolar ridge, site of a previous tooth extraction, is another typical location for this condition.

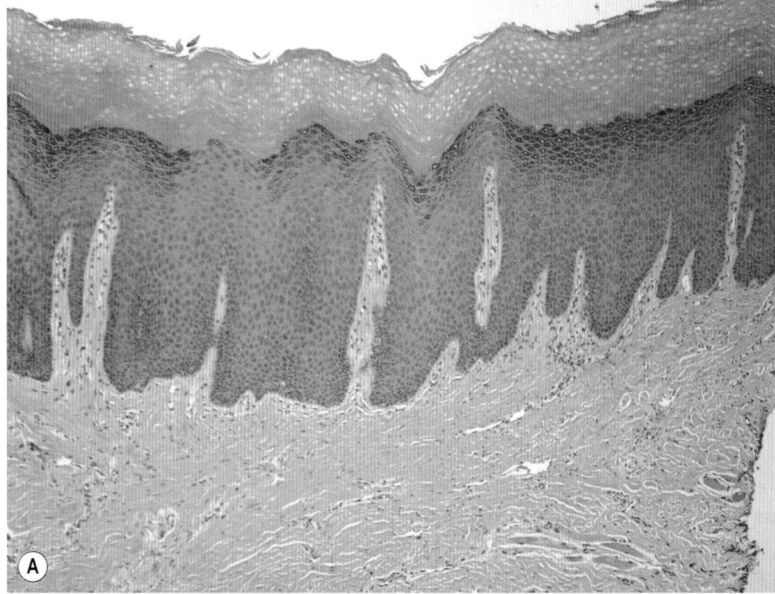

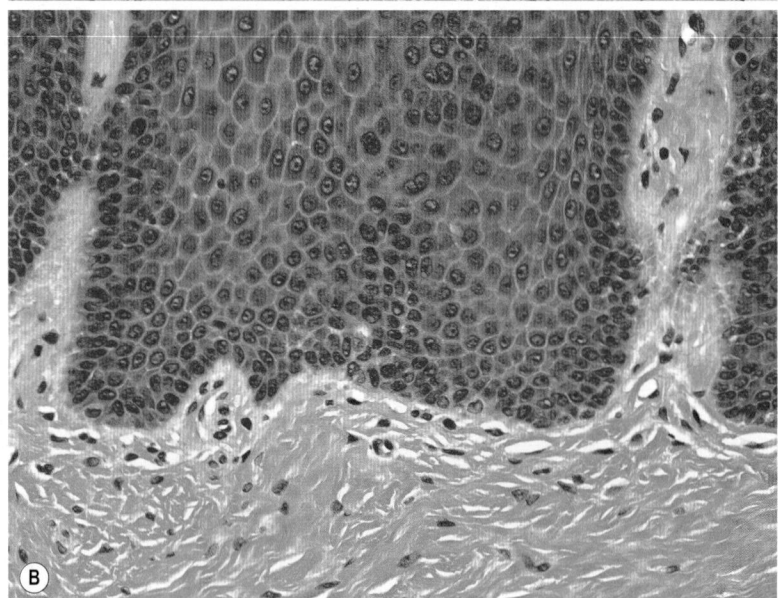

Fig. 11.36
Benign ridge keratosis: (**A**) there is hyperkeratosis, wedge-shaped hypergranulosis, slight papillary acanthosis, tapered rete ridges, and minimal to no inflammation; (**B**) there is no evidence of cytological atypia.

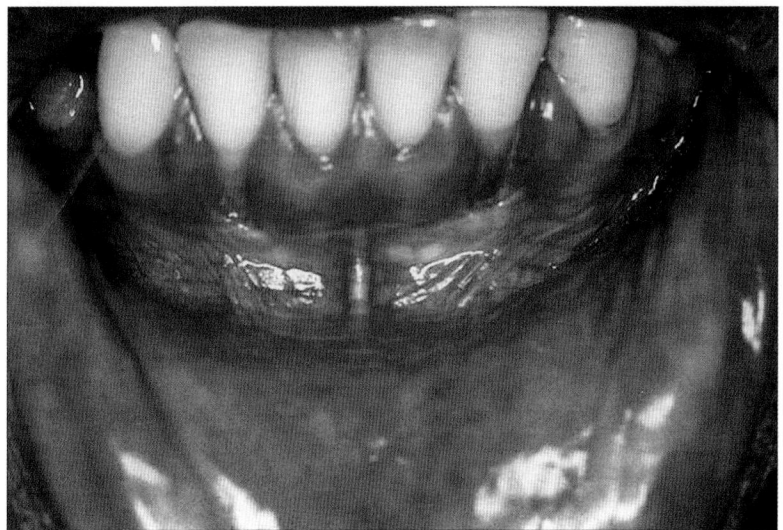

Fig. 11.37
Smokeless tobacco keratosis: note the gray white, pale, wrinkled mandibular vestibular mucosa.

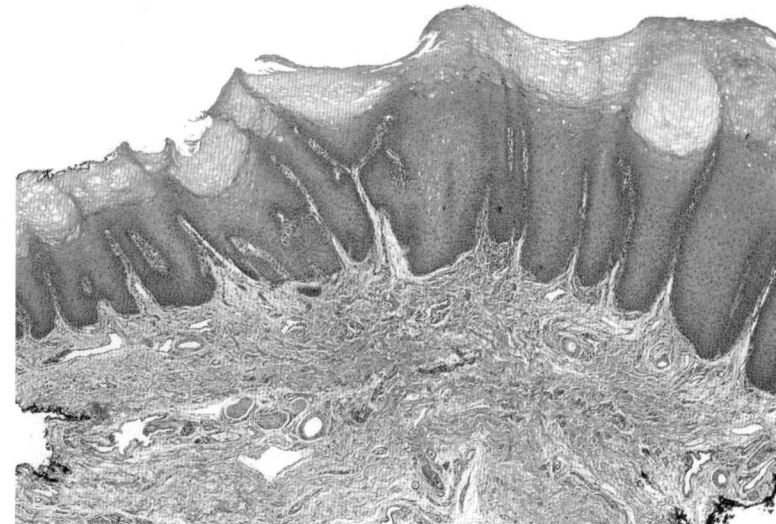

Fig. 11.38
Smokeless tobacco lesion: the superficial edematous keratinocytes are sharply demarcated from the underlying acanthotic epithelium, and there are parakeratin chevrons.

development of white lesions at the site of contact in 13–46% of cases.[1–4] The severity of oral lesions is proportionate to the duration of use and the amount of smokeless tobacco in contact with the mucosa.[2]

This is a condition seen in teenagers and adults depending on acceptability of this habit within the culture. Early and mild lesions show slight wrinkling and pallor of the mucosa and discontinuation of the habit leads to resolution of lesions (Fig. 11.37).[5] Advanced lesions develop after many years of use and are well-demarcated white plaques with fissures, typical for leukoplakia, a premalignant condition (see later). Such leukoplakias are irreversible and have the same connotations for dysplasia and carcinomatous transformation as at other sites. Patients are prone to develop gingival recession and periodontal disease in the area of placement of tobacco.[2]

Pathogenesis and histologic features

Smokeless tobacco takes the form of chewing tobacco (cured, shredded, and flavored tobacco leaves) or snuff which may be moist or dry. Moist snuff (known as snus in Scandinavia) is by far the more popular and is composed of finely cut or ground, cured, and flavored tobacco often available in pre-portioned pouches, while dry snuff, which has waned in popularity, is fermented, powdered tobacco rubbed onto the gingiva or inhaled. Snus has greater alkalinity (pH 8–9) and as such, better mucosal penetration, and a greater propensity to cause lesions compared with dry snuff.[1,2] Sudanese snuff (toombak) is a mixture of tobacco and sodium bicarbonate and is highest in tobacco-specific nitrosamines.[6] In general, the risk of developing oral cancer is less with smokeless tobacco than with cigarette smoking, although much depends on the composition of the product.[7,8]

There is disturbed differentiation of keratin as evidenced by increased expression of K13 and K14 in patients using toombak as compared with those using Swedish snuff.[9] Mutations in the p53 gene have been described.[10]

The term 'smokeless tobacco keratosis' is somewhat of a misnomer because early lesions are not significantly keratotic. Rather, the clinical appearance of whiteness is a result of edema of the superficial keratinocytes from direct contact injury and is a form of irritant contact stomatitis.

Early lesions (before the development of leukoplakia) show a characteristic pale-staining surface layer of ballooned and edematous keratinocytes occasionally covered by a thin layer of parakeratin (Fig. 11.38). Typically, this superficial pale layer is sharply demarcated from the underlying viable epithelium, which shows acanthosis and variable chronic inflammation. In addition, spires of parakeratin 'chevrons' are usually present within this pale surface zone although this finding is not specific to this lesion and may be seen in frictional or other reactive parakeratosis; there is nuclear pyknosis (Fig. 11.39).[11–13] Mild reactive epithelial atypia may be present, and lesions resolve on discontinuation of the habit.[5,14] Sialadenitis of minor

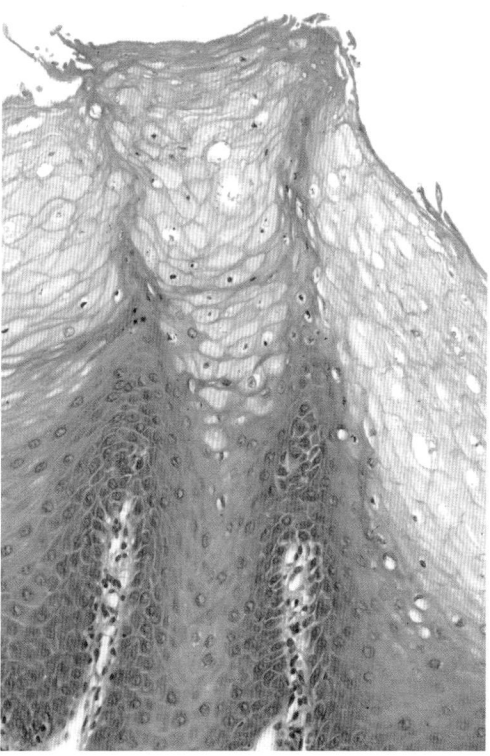

Fig. 11.39
Smokeless tobacco lesion: note the parakeratin chevrons and anucleate and edematous superficial keratinocytes with pyknotic nuclei.

salivary glands has been reported in up to 42% of cases, and there is a reduction in the number of intraepithelial Langerhans cells.[15,16]

Hyaline deposits may be seen as a dense homogenous, eosinophilic band in the lamina propria in 8–17% of cases, and sometimes involving the gland parenchyma and surrounding ducts (Fig. 11.40).[15,17,18] This PAS-positive, noncongophilic material is not amyloid and is thought to represent altered collagen.[19]

When leukoplakia develops, lesions should be evaluated for dysplasia in the same fashion as leukoplakias elsewhere (see later).[12] Squamous cell carcinoma is an infrequent complication of smokeless tobacco use in the absence of cigarette smoking and/or excessive alcohol consumption.[3,4,12,18,20]

Differential diagnosis

Hyaline deposits resemble amyloid but are not congophilic.

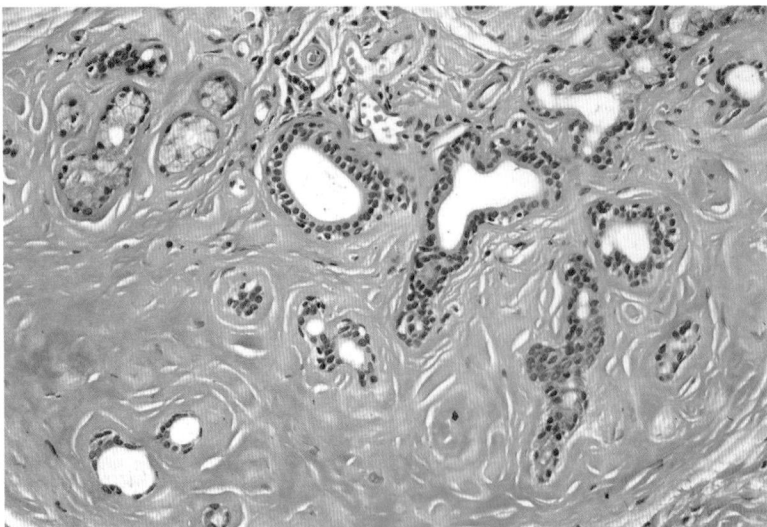

Fig. 11.40
Smokeless tobacco lesion: eosinophilic amyloid-like material is often seen within underlying salivary gland parenchyma.

Benign migratory glossitis

Clinical features

Benign migratory glossitis (geographic tongue, geographic stomatitis, stomatitis/erythema areata migrans) occurs in 1–2% of the population (usually adults), although this figure may be low because of the evanescent nature of the condition.[1,2] Pain, burning or sensitivity, may or may not be present. Lesions present as recurrent, erythematous, and atrophic areas with a serpiginous white, slightly raised border that may appear annular or scalloped (*Fig. 11.41*).[2,3] These 'map-like' areas migrate and change in shape over the tongue dorsum as the condition resolves at one edge and involves another. Some lesions, however, are stationary. Overall, 20–60% of patients have concurrent fissured tongue[1–3]; more than half the patients are atopic.[3,4]

'Ectopic geographic tongue' or, more appropriately, migratory stomatitis, refers to a similar-appearing lesion at other sites, in particular the buccal and lip mucosae.[5–7] Only 0.5% who present with benign migratory glossitis have psoriasis, but 5–14% of patients with psoriasis are affected by this condition.[8–10] This prevalence is likely higher in patients with pustular disease.[11,12] The condition also occurs in patients with reactive arthritis.[13] Lithium carbonate (which can exacerbate psoriasis) has also been reported to precipitate migratory glossitis.[14]

Human leukocyte antigen (HLA)-Bw62 and Bw63 are seen with higher frequency in affected patients and atopic individuals (odds ratio of 6.5), as well as in patients with associated type II diabetes mellitus lesions[15–19]; however, the association with diabetes mellitus has been refuted. There is also an increased incidence of HLA-C*06 and HLA-B13 in addition to a reduced incidence of HLA-Cw4.[20] Other authors have shown increased incidences of HLA-DRw6, and -DR5 with reduced incidences of -B51 and -DR2.[21] An increase in polymorphism in the interleukin (IL)-1β gene has been reported.[22]

Histologic features

The tongue dorsum exhibits loss of the filiform papillae (*Fig. 11.42*). There are spongiotic pustules and microabscesses (often involving up to half or more of the thickness of the epithelium) in the absence of *Candida* infection (*Fig. 11.43*).[2,5,23] The epithelium shows variable spongiosis and neutrophilic exocytosis, psoriasiform epithelial hyperplasia with broad rete ridges, edema of the lamina propria, a variable lymphocytic infiltrate, and dilated capillaries.

Differential diagnosis

Candidiasis, which must always be excluded, more typically presents with spongiotic pustules affecting only the top two to three layers of

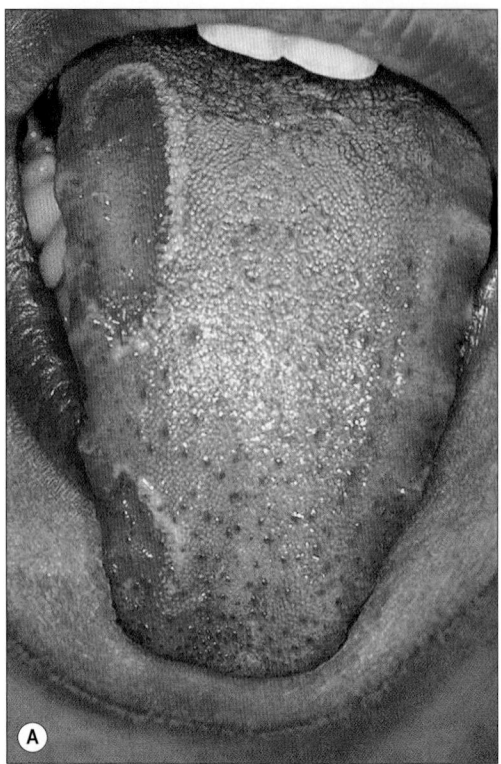

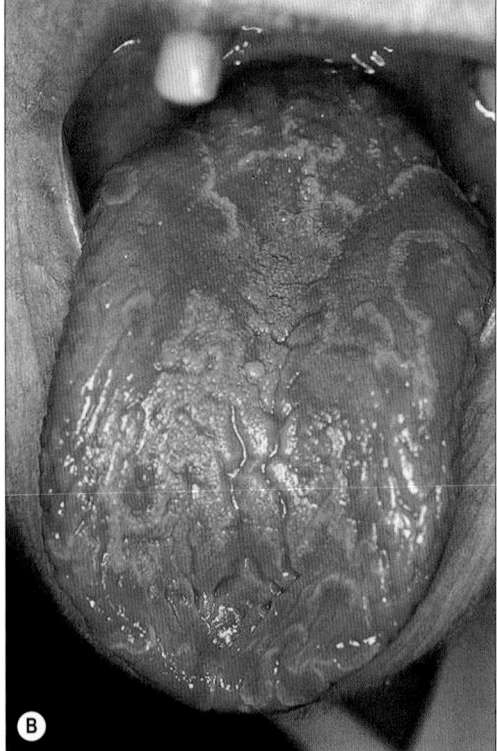

Fig. 11.41
Benign migratory glossitis: (**A**) note the erythematous depapillated area with a white rim; (**B**) more extensive involvement of the tongue which is fissured.

keratinocytes. A PAS stain should be performed routinely for all oral lesions with spongiotic pustules. Median rhomboid glossitis, a form of candidiasis, also enters the differential diagnosis since it may have a somewhat similar clinical presentation with atrophy of filiform papillae, although the area does not 'migrate' (see below).

The epithelium at the edge of a healing ulcer or at sites of trauma often shows spongiotic pustules devoid of *Candida* accompanied by neutrophilic exocytosis.

Oral psoriasis is histologically indistinguishable from lesions of benign migratory glossitis, and up to 10% of patients with psoriasis develop migratory glossitis.[24,25]

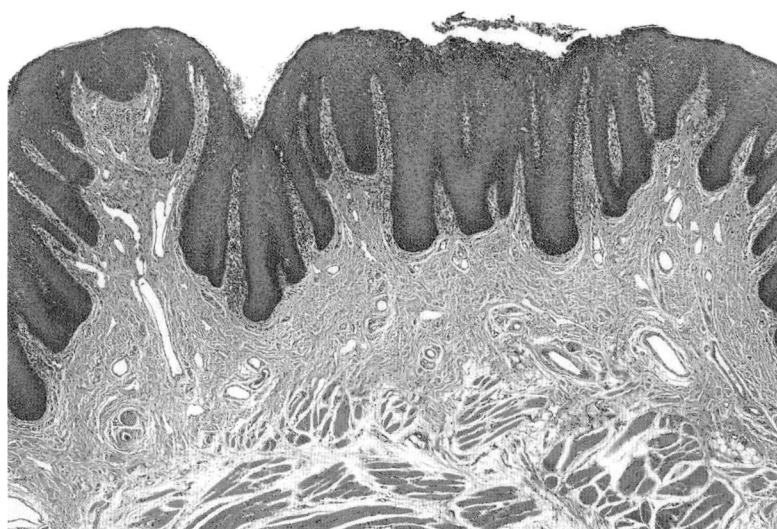

Fig. 11.42
Benign migratory glossitis: note the absence of filiform papillae (filiform papillary atrophy) and psoriasiform epithelial hyperplasia.

Foreign body gingivitis

Clinical features

This condition occurs more often in females than in males (4:1), usually in the fifth decade. The gingiva presents with multifocal or diffuse erythema that is sensitive or painful in the majority of patients and often, there is a recent history of dental treatment. Some lesions are ulcerated.[1–3]

Pathogenesis and histologic features

Energy dispersive X-ray microanalysis have revealed Si, Al, Fe, Cu, and Ti in the majority of cases, and in many lesions, the analyses match those of dental abrasives. It is therefore thought that some of these cases result from such abrasives forced into the gingiva during professional dental cleaning. Some analyses also match those of amalgam.[3,4]

The epithelium is acanthotic or atrophic, and basal cell degeneration is present in up to 50% of cases. The inflammatory infiltrate varies in severity and is lichenoid (bandlike and lymphocytic) in half the cases (*Fig. 11.44*). In one-quarter of cases, granulomatous inflammation may be seen, sometimes accompanied by foreign body giant cells.[1,2,5] Plasma cells may be abundant. Foreign bodies, ranging from 1 to 5 microns in diameter, are present in all cases, and 44% are refractile (*Fig. 11.45*).

Differential diagnosis

Plasma cell gingivitis, a contact hypersensitivity reaction, exhibits an intense polytypic plasmacytic infiltrate, usually in sheets, and foreign material is not identified.

Pyostomatitis vegetans

Clinical features

This is the oral counterpart of pyoderma vegetans.[1,2] Men are two to three times more commonly affected than women.[2,3] The most common associations are ulcerative colitis (approximately 70%), Crohn disease (10–15%), and liver disease (21%).[3–6] Patients present with numerous painful, shallow ulcers and erosions, miliary abscesses, and pustules that coalesce to form linear 'snail track' lesions (*Fig. 11.46*).[7–10] These develop on erythematous mucosa in which vegetations may be a feature. There is sometimes folding and fissuring of the buccal mucosa. The dorsal surface of the tongue is usually spared.[11,12] Peripheral blood eosinophilia is present in 90% of cases.[3]

Histologic features

There is acanthosis, sometimes accompanied by papillomatosis, and spongiosis. Suprabasilar clefting with acantholysis is usually seen (*Fig. 11.47*).

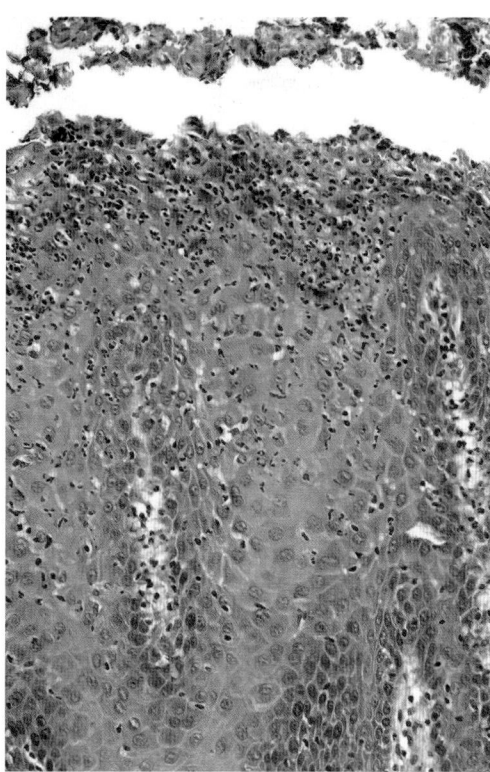

Fig. 11.43
Benign migratory glossitis: many spongiotic pustules are present and there is neutrophilic exocytosis.

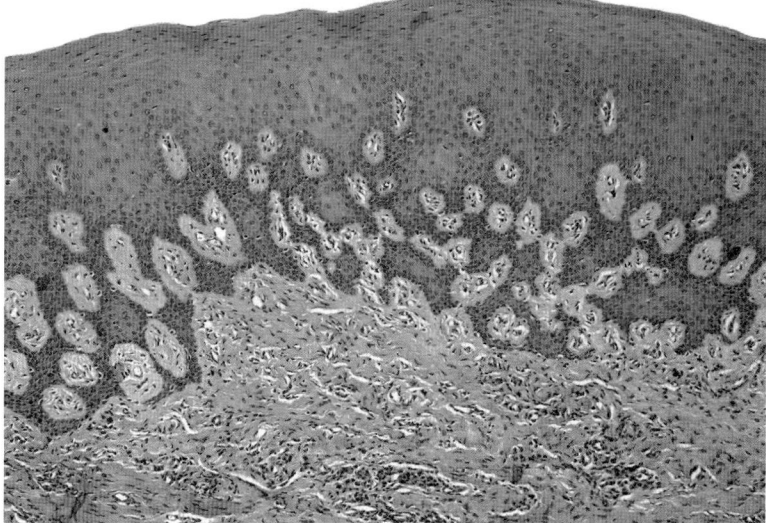

Fig. 11.44
Foreign body gingivitis: there is non-specific mild chronic inflammation in the lamina propria.

Characteristically, neutrophilic and eosinophilic abscesses are present in the connective tissue papillae at the interface, and sometimes within the epithelium (*Fig. 11.48*).[3,7,11–13] Eosinophils and neutrophils permeate the epithelium, and a mixed inflammatory infiltrate of lymphocytes, plasma cells, neutrophils, and eosinophils is present in the lamina propria.

Direct immunofluorescence studies for IgG and C3 are negative. When positive, the staining is usually weak and represents a secondary reaction to epithelial inflammation and damage rather than a primary autoimmune phenomenon.[3,14]

Differential diagnosis

Pemphigus vulgaris exhibits acantholysis, but neutrophilic and eosinophilic abscesses are absent and papillary epithelial hyperplasia is not usually a feature. Pemphigus vegetans shows considerable histologic overlap although oral lesions are rare. Distinction from both of these conditions is readily made by direct immunofluorescence studies which show intercellular IgG deposition.

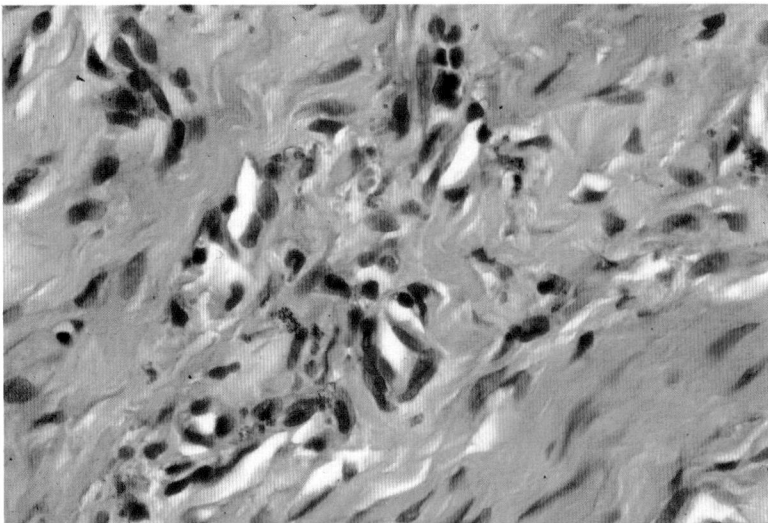

Fig. 11.45
Foreign body gingivitis: small granules of foreign material that are refractile in polarized light are present.

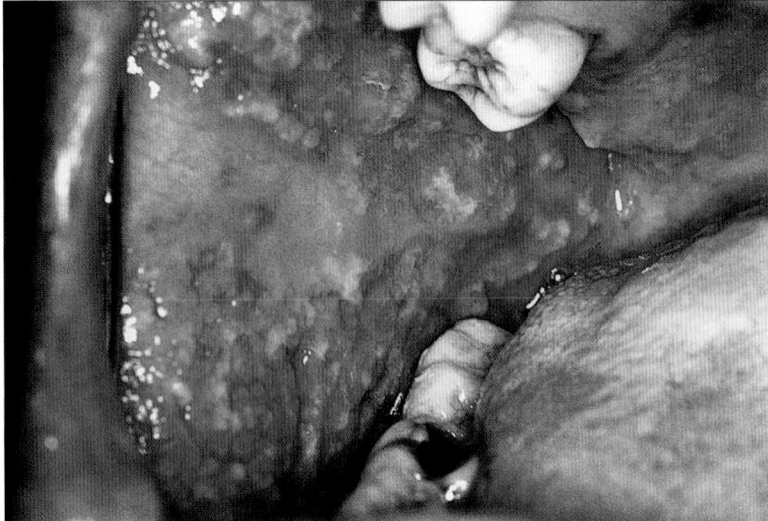

Fig. 11.46
Pyostomatitis vegetans: note the yellow pustular papules and linear lesions on the buccal mucosa. By courtesy of B. Neville, DDS, Charleston, USA.

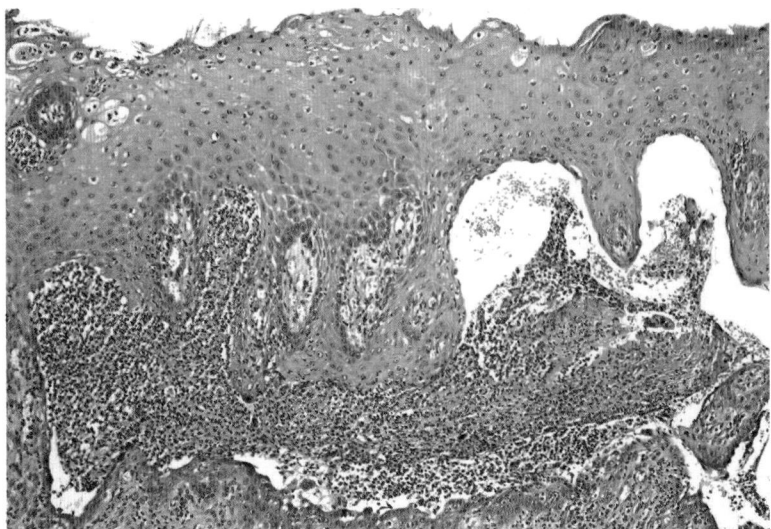

Fig. 11.47
Pyostomatitis vegetans: note intraepithelial clefting and abscesses.

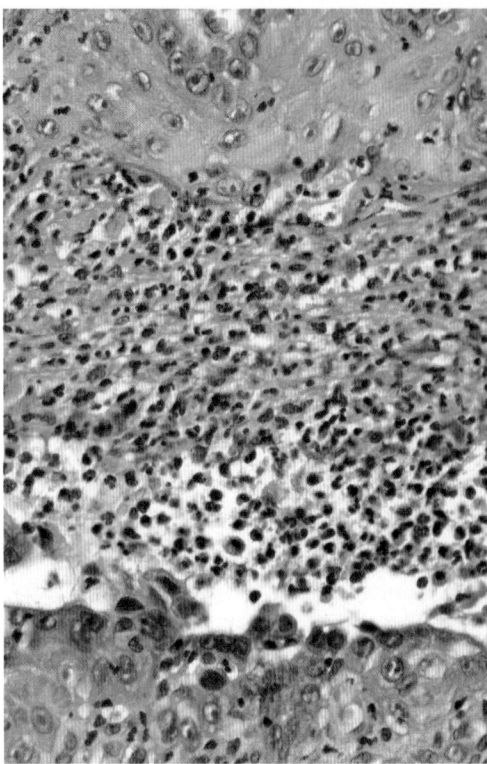

Fig. 11.48
Pyostomatitis vegetans: there is acantholysis and many neutrophils and eosinophils are present suprabasally.

Warty dyskeratoma may exhibit the presence of corps ronds and grains without eosinophilic abscesses and negative direct immunofluorescence studies; clinically, it is a solitary keratotic papule or nodule.

Warty dyskeratoma

Clinical features

This usually solitary lesion, sometimes referred to as oral focal acantholytic dyskeratosis, resembles Darier disease histopathologically, generally occurs in the fifth or sixth decade, and almost always arises on the keratinized and attached mucosa of the palatal mucosa or gingiva on the left side (buccal mucosa and tongue are much less frequently affected) with a 2:1 female predominance.[1-5] Almost all are less than 1 cm in size; the papular variety appears as a white papule or plaque, while the nodular variety has an umbilicated or crateriform appearance. There is an association with tobacco use.[3,6]

Histologic features

Similar to Darier disease, oral warty dyskeratoma is characterized by suprabasilar clefting, villous-like projections, and less often, corps ronds and grains; there may be papillary epithelial hyperplasia.[3,7,8] In the nodular form, there is central umbilication filled with parakeratin.[9]

Differential diagnosis

Pemphigus vulgaris can be readily distinguished by the clinical history and the characteristic presence of intercellular IgG deposition on direct immunofluorescence. Pyostomatitis vegetans exhibits diffuse and not solitary lesions, with many eosinophils and neutrophils.

Nicotinic stomatitis

Clinical features

Nicotinic stomatitis (stomatitis nicotina) is associated with pipe smoking and its severity is proportional to the duration of the habit. Early lesions are reversible on habit cessation.[1-3]

This is a condition seen in adults. Early lesions appear as small red punctate areas associated with diffuse and symmetric whiteness of the palatal

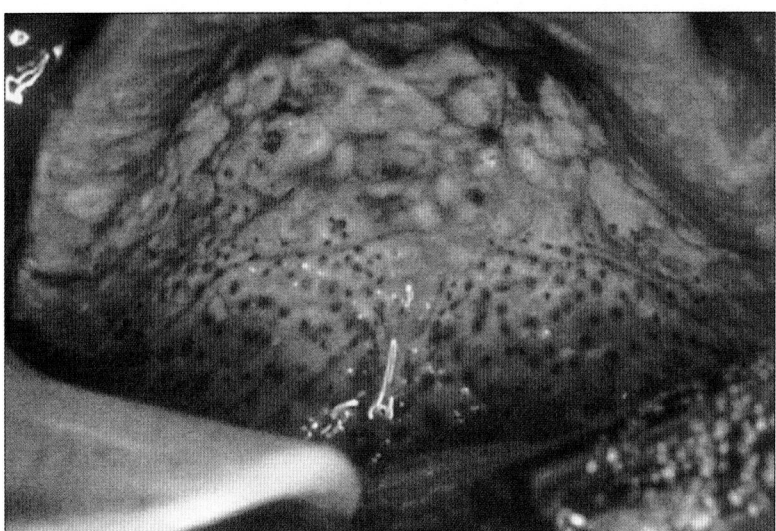

Fig. 11.49
Nicotinic stomatitis: note the cobblestone, multinodular appearance of the hard palatal mucosa, with interspersed red puncta, in a patient who reverse smokes. By courtesy of L. Lee, DDS, Toronto, Ontario, Canada.

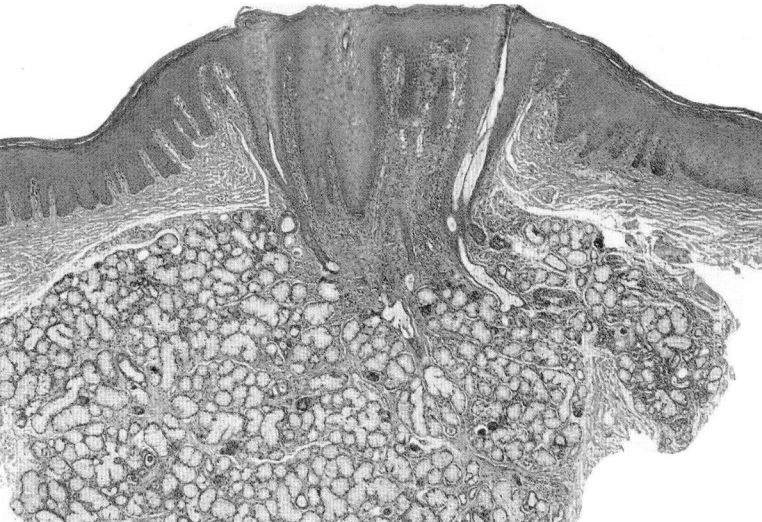

Fig. 11.50
Nicotinic stomatitis: each nodule consists of metaplastic excretory salivary ducts and surrounding chronic inflammation; there is hyperkeratosis.

mucosa. As lesions progress, the palatal mucosa takes on a cobblestone appearance with raised red and white papules having slightly umbilicated central puncta (*Fig. 11.49*).[1,3] The red puncta represent the inflamed ostia of the excretory salivary ducts.

Pathogenesis and histologic features

This condition is caused by the heat from the pipe smoke, and not nicotine. Similar changes have been described in patients who practice reverse smoking (smoking with the lighted end of the cigarette in the mouth as is common in parts of Asia) where the heat in the mouth is intense.[4,5] This condition has also been noted in patients who consumed hot beverages.[6,7]

There is parakeratosis or hyperkeratosis, and acanthosis. The papules represent openings of the excretory salivary ducts that have undergone squamous metaplasia, and the ductal epithelium exhibits leukocyte exocytosis and is surrounded by variable numbers of plasma cells and lymphocytes (*Figs 11.50* and *11.51*).[2,8]

Dysplasia or even invasive squamous cell carcinoma may be present in patients who reverse smoke, but in general malignant change is not a feature in pipe smokers.[3]

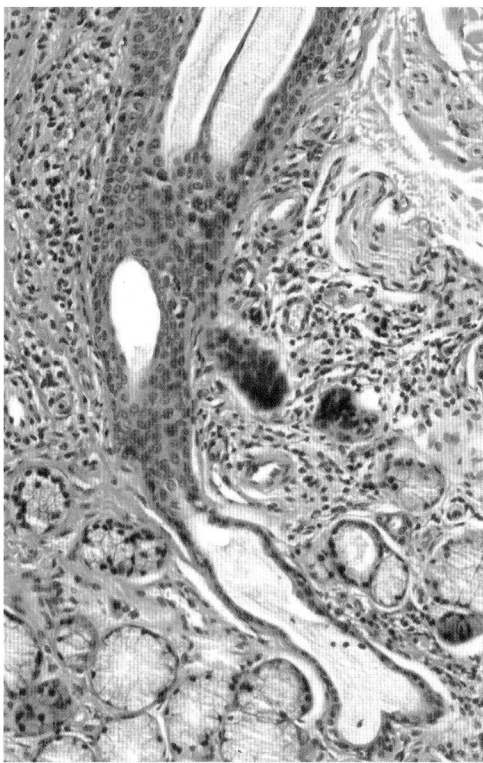

Fig. 11.51
Nicotinic stomatitis: there is chronic inflammation in the surrounding fibrous tissue and lymphocyte exocytosis through the duct epithelium.

ULCERATIVE CONDITIONS

Recurrent aphthous stomatitis

Clinical features

Recurrent aphthous stomatitis occurs in 15–20% of the adult population, with a slight female predilection. It first manifests in teenage years and early adulthood.[1,2] It is a chronic, painful, relapsing, ulcerative condition of the nonkeratinized mucosa (*Fig. 11.52*). There are four variants: minor, major, herpetiform, and severe.

- Minor aphthous ulcers (the most common variant) are less than 1 cm, last 7–14 days, and heal without scarring; episode frequency varies and 10% of females report coincidence with the menstrual cycle.
- Major aphthous ulcers are usually greater than 1 cm, last many weeks, and heal with scarring.
- Herpetiform aphthous ulcers are less than 1 cm, and occur in small crops of 10–100 ulcers in any one episode.[2,3]
- Severe aphthous ulcers are similar to minor aphthous ulcers but patients have ulcers continuously without significant ulcer-free periods.

Most aphthous ulcers are idiopathic in nature although there is usually a strong family history of such ulcers. Ulcers become less frequent with age and will often resolve by middle age. It does not represent herpes simplex virus infection or any other infection although some believe *Helicobacter* plays a role.[4–7]

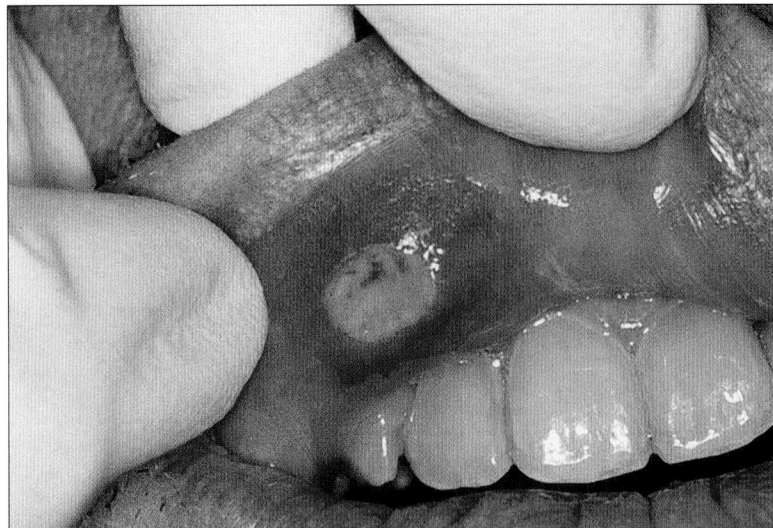

Fig. 11.52
Recurrent aphthous ulcer: a typical aphthous ulcer covered by yellow fibrin membrane with surrounding erythema on the upper lip mucosa.

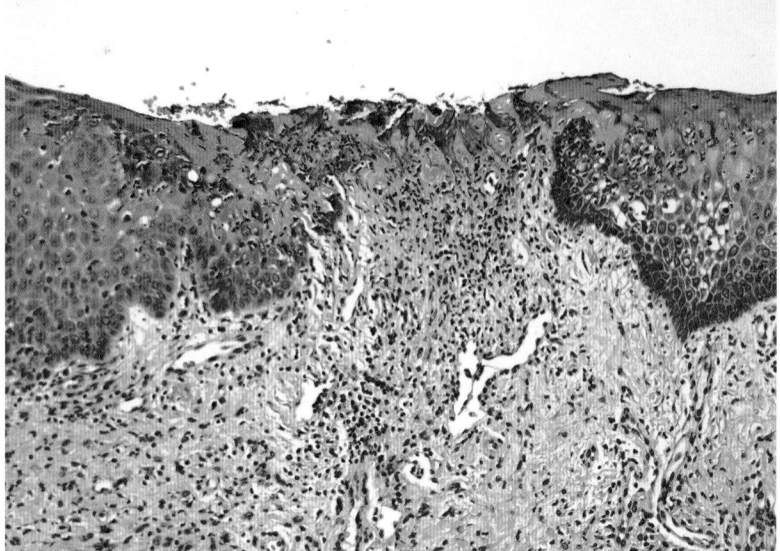

Fig. 11.53
Recurrent aphthous ulcer: there is a fibrin membrane with underlying acute and chronic inflammation and vascular ectasia; the adjacent epithelium exhibits spongiotic pustules and intraepithelial hemorrhage.

Some conditions frequently associated with aphthous-like ulcers include Behçet disease, hematinic deficiency (especially iron and vitamin B_{12}), inflammatory bowel disease, gluten-sensitive enteropathy, food hypersensitivity, HIV/acquired immunodeficiency syndrome (AIDS), neutropenia, and adverse effects of medications (such as nonsteroidal anti-inflammatory medications or mTOR inhibitors).[8–10] Aphthous stomatitis presenting in association with rheumatological or mucocutaneous disorders is sometimes referred to as complex aphthosis.[11] In children, aphthous stomatitis may be syndromic and associated with periodic fever, lymphadenopathy, and pharyngitis (PFAPA syndrome, a periodic fever syndrome).[12–15] Interestingly, such patients often show complete response after tonsillectomy and/or adenoidectomy.[16]

Pathogenesis and histologic features

Cross-reaction of antigens of *Streptococcus mutans* with a mitochondrial heat shock protein may play an important role in the pathogenesis of this condition.[17] Others believe there is reduced expression of heat shock protein 27 and IL-10.[18] Expression of HLA class I and class II antigens on epithelial cells may result in targeting for cytotoxic attack.[19] There is no evidence of increased circulating immunoglobulins or immune complexes.

The ulcerative process results from activation of the Th1 response leading to destruction of the epithelium. Early lesions show a predominance of T-helper cells followed by an increase in T-suppressor cells during the ulcerative phase; T-helper cells reemerge during the healing phase.[20–22] Increased numbers of peripheral gamma-delta cells have been noted, suggesting that antibody-dependent cell-mediated cytotoxicity may play a role in the immunopathogenesis of this disease.[23] Cell lysis may be mediated through tumor necrosis factor-alpha (TNF-α).[24]

The histologic features are those of non-specific ulceration composed of a fibrin clot with enmeshed neutrophils and underlying granulation tissue with acute and chronic inflammation (*Fig. 11.53*).[25] The adjacent epithelium may exhibit reactive atypia, spongiotic pustules, and intraepithelial hemorrhage; viral cytopathic effect is not seen. Inflammation and degeneration of superficial skeletal muscle fibers may also be evident, but this should not extend into the deep muscle.

Differential diagnosis

Traumatic ulcers and the ulcers of Behçet disease are histologically indistinguishable, and their distinction is dependent on clinical findings Sometimes, marked parakeratosis with superficial bacterial colonization is noted adjacent to the ulcer in traumatic ulcers. If there is inflammation of the muscle associated with a histiocytic infiltrate and eosinophils, a diagnosis of traumatic ulcerative granuloma is more appropriate (see below). If the fibrin clot and underlying granulation

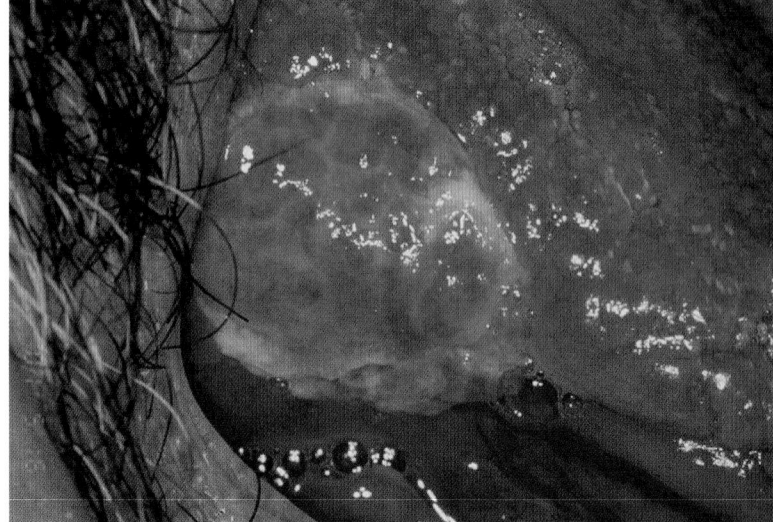

Fig. 11.54
Traumatic ulcerative granuloma: this indurated ulcer had developed after a tongue biopsy at that site.

neutropenia-associated ulceration, such as is seen in HIV disease and cyclic neutropenia, must be considered.

Traumatic ulcerative granuloma

Clinical findings

Traumatic ulcerative granuloma (traumatic ulcerative granuloma with stromal eosinophilia, eosinophilic ulcer/granuloma of the tongue, Riga-Fede disease) occurs in two age groups. The less common form – and one that is not usually biopsied – occurs in infants in the first year of life. Painful ulcers occur on the ventral tongue or lower lip as a result of the child rubbing the mucosa against the developing lower anterior deciduous teeth (Riga-Fede disease).[1] The second presentation, and the more common, is in the fifth and sixth decades of life, with ulcers occurring in males twice as frequently as females[2]. The lateral tongue (up to 64% of cases), followed by the buccal mucosa, are most often affected.[3–6] An ulcer or indurated area develops and persists for weeks or months (*Figs 11.54* and *11.55*).

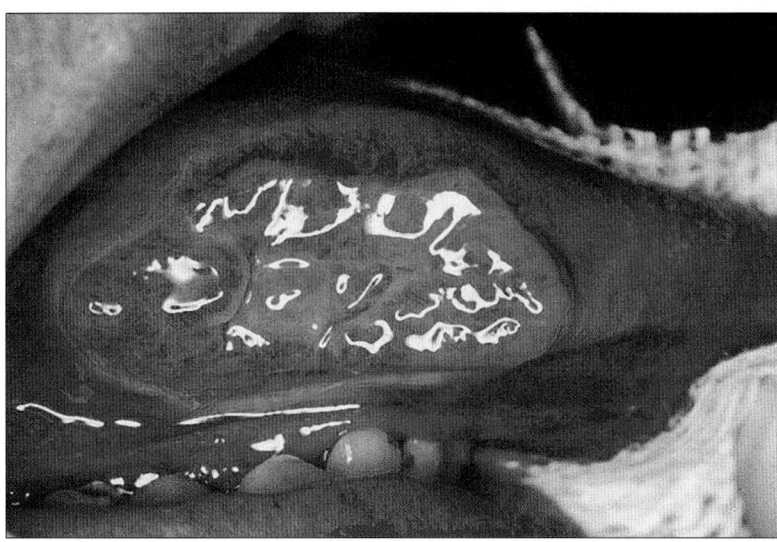

Fig. 11.55
Traumatic ulcerative granuloma: this patient had bitten her tongue during a seizure and the indurated mass developed over a few days.

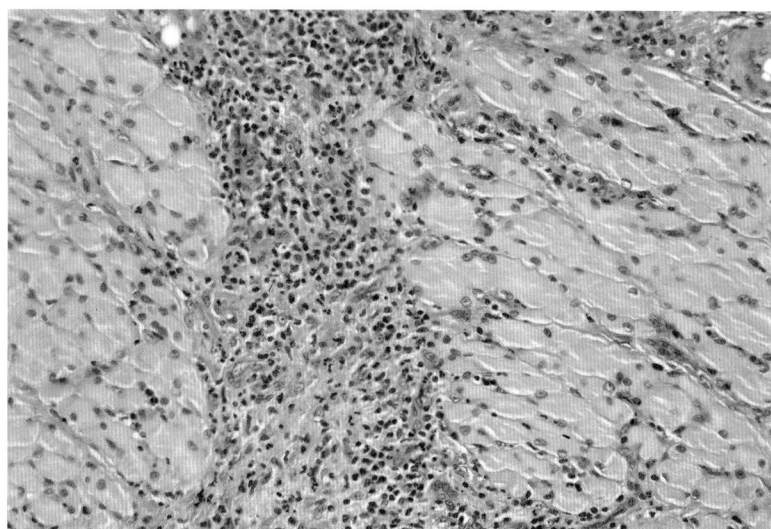

Fig. 11.57
Traumatic ulcerative granuloma: there is prominent interfascicular inflammation and muscle degeneration.

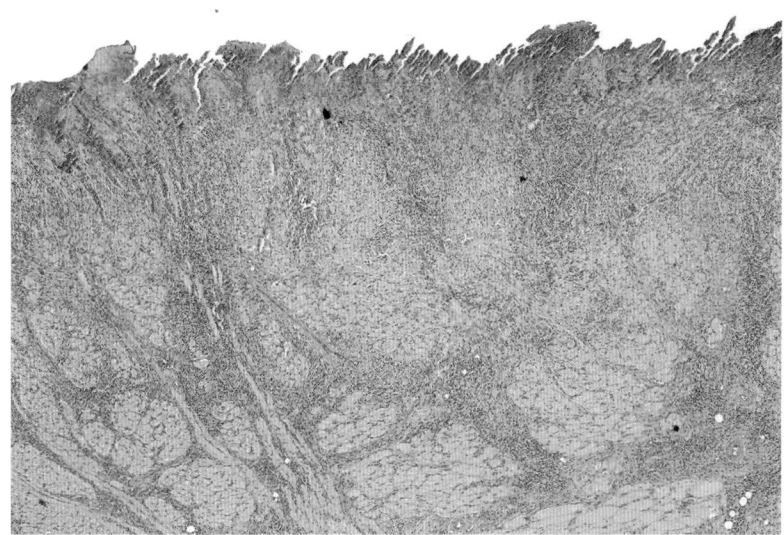

Fig. 11.56
Traumatic ulcerative granuloma: note the ulcerated surface and the penetrating inflammation that separates muscle fascicles.

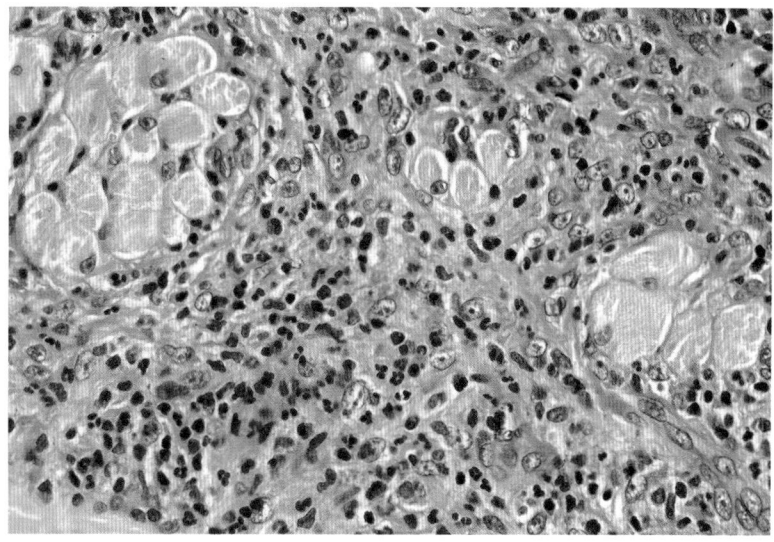

Fig. 11.58
Traumatic ulcerative granuloma: note the presence of histiocytes and many eosinophils.

The lack of pain, often a feature of this condition, raises the clinical suspicion of squamous cell carcinoma.[5] A history of trauma is elicited in only 50% of cases.[3,4] Lesions are often multifocal, and up to 30% of lesions recur.[6]

Pathogenesis and histologic features

Lesions similar to this condition can be experimentally induced in animals by crush injury.[7] It is likely that this is caused by penetrating inflammation that causes myositis whether this is brought on by chronic and repeated trauma (most common etiology) or some other ulcerative process (such as major aphthous ulcer) that is untreated or inadequately treated and becomes deep and penetrating.[3,4] Infectious agents and foreign material have not been identified in these lesions.

There is an ulcer with abundant granulation tissue at the ulcer base accompanied by a polymorphous inflammatory infiltrate of lymphocytes and plasma cells, which extends into the underlying muscle (Figs 11.56 and 11.57). The presence of many histiocytes and eosinophils in between degenerated and fragmented muscle fibers is characteristic (Fig. 11.58).[3,4,7–10] The muscle sometimes has a 'checkerboard' pattern from fragmentation. Lack of eosinophils especially in older lesions, does not preclude this diagnosis.

The large histiocytes express either CD68 and CD163, and some cells are positive for factor XIIIa.[8] Scattered CD30+ cells may be present in this lesion but they should not be plentiful.[5,11]

Differential diagnosis

Conventional aphthous ulcers or traumatic ulcers may show inflammation of the superficial myocytes, but not deep penetrating inflammation noted in this condition.

Epstein-Barr virus-associated mucocutaneous ulcers are ulcers of the skin, oral or gastrointestinal mucosa that occur in immunocompromised patients (such as those on immunosuppressive therapy for autoimmune diseases), post-organ transplantation, in elderly, immunosenescent patients, or in patients with HIV/AIDS. They are also deeply penetrating with a polymorphous infiltrate, and exhibit atypical immunoblast-like lymphocytes and Reed-Sternberg-like cells (Figs 11.59 and 11.60). They are positive for CD20, CD30, MUM-1, PAX-5, and Epstein-Barr virus (Fig. 11.61).[12–14] Some of these may have been referred to in the past as CD30+ traumatic ulcerative granuloma, atypical histiocytic granuloma, or pseudolymphoma.[15–18] These may heal spontaneously, with reduction of immunosuppression or with definitive therapy. Rare cases represent CD30+ lymphoma.[11]

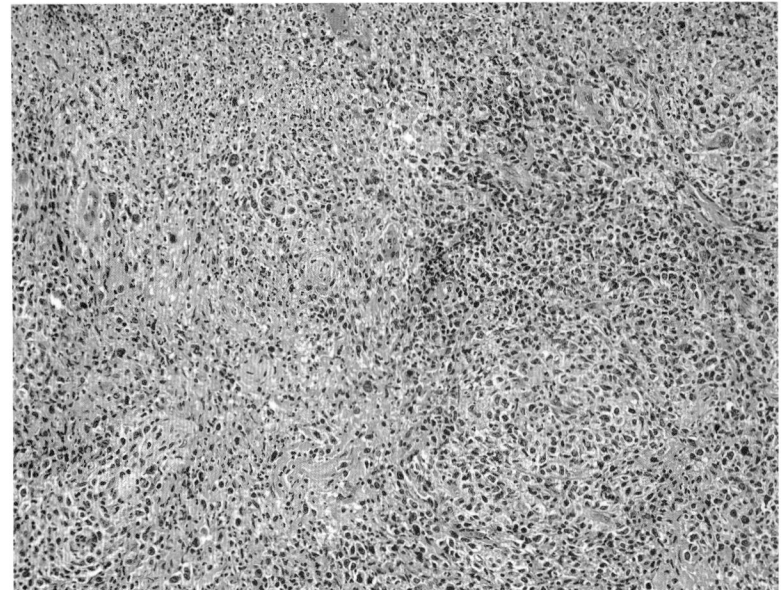

Fig. 11.59
Epstein-Barr virus mucocutaneous ulcer: there is a diffuse and dense atypical lymphocytic infiltrate.

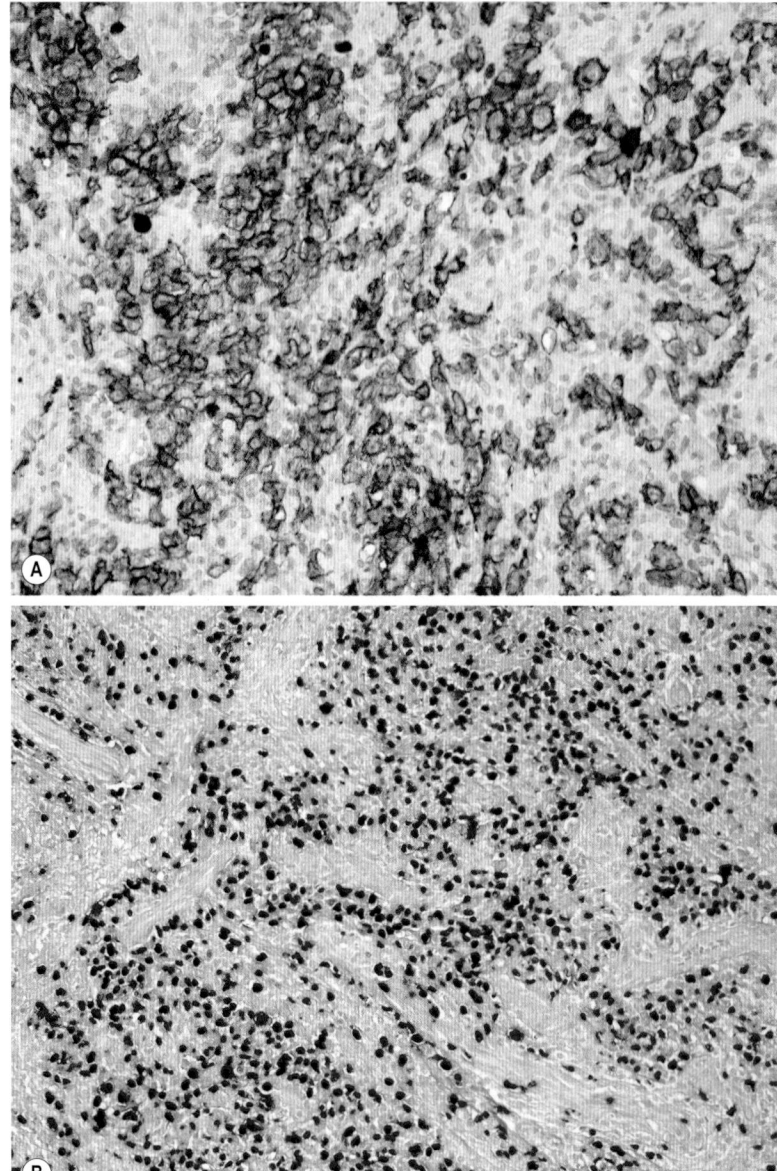

Fig. 11.61
Epstein-Barr virus mucocutaneous ulcer: (**A**) positivity for CD30; (**B**) positivity for EBER.

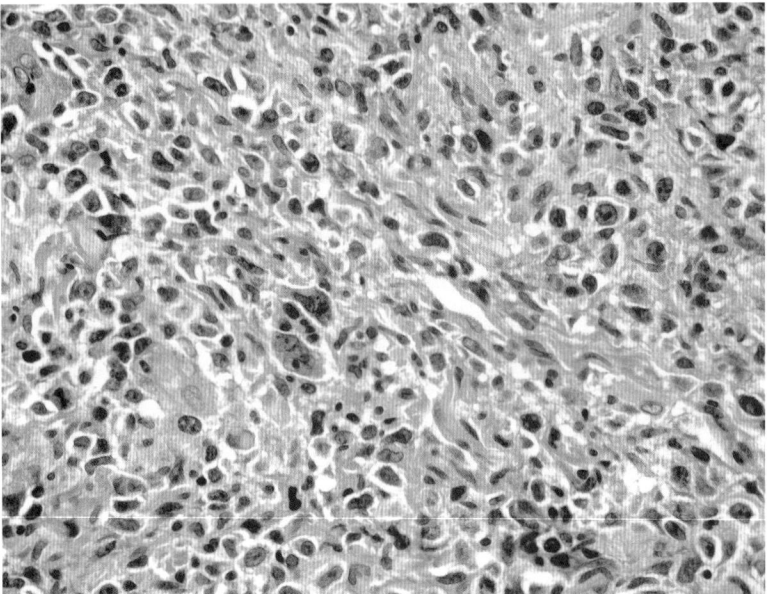

Fig. 11.60
Epstein-Barr virus mucocutaneous ulcer: many atypical lymphocytes with pleomorphic nuclei with irregular contours (Reed Sternberg-like) are present

Epithelioid hemangioma (previously known as angiolymphoid hyperplasia with eosinophilia) may sometimes present in the lip and tongue.[19,20] There is a proliferation of epithelioid endothelial cells forming vascular channels and intracytoplasmic lumina, that are positive for vascular markers. Lymphocytes, plasma cells, and eosinophils are commonly seen, and occasional lymphoid follicles with germinal centers are present (*Figs 11.62* and *11.63*).[21,22]

Histiocyte-like cells and eosinophils are a feature of Langerhans cell histiocytosis. However, Langerhans cells have the characteristic grooved nuclei and are positive for S100 protein, CD1a, and langerin (CD207) by immunohistochemistry.

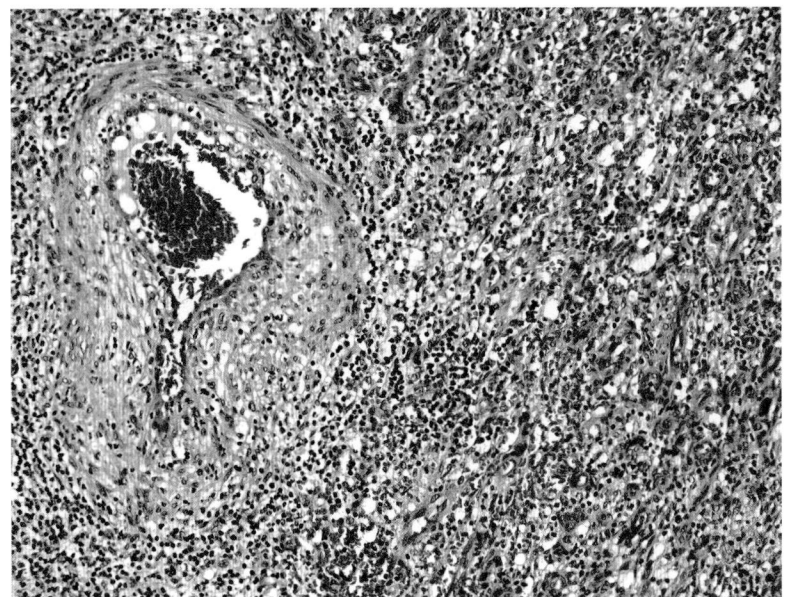

Fig. 11.62
Epithelioid hemangioma: there is a proliferation of epithelioid endothelial cells in sheets, with many lymphocytes and fresh hemorrhage.

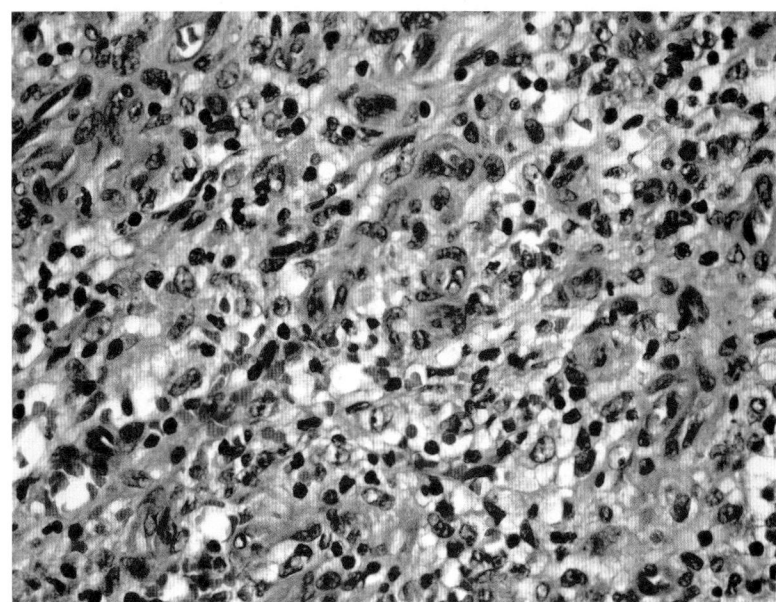

Fig. 11.63
Epithelioid hemangioma: the epithelioid endothelial cells are positive for vascular markers, and they form small vascular channels; there is abundant fresh hemorrhage and hemosiderin.

PAPILLARY LESIONS

Squamous papilloma

Clinical features

Squamous papilloma generally presents in children and young adults in the second to fourth decades. Sites of predilection include the soft palate-uvula complex and the tongue, although any region in the oral cavity may be affected. Lesions may be white or mucosal-colored with a rough surface and finger-like projections (Figs 11.64 and 11.65).[1,2]

Etiopathogenesis and histologic features

Lesions are caused by human papillomavirus (HPV) and in situ hybridization and polymerase chain reaction (PCR) studies have identified HPV (usually -6 and -11) in up to 67% of cases; HPV-2 is occasionally present.[3–5]

The epithelium is thrown into uniformly thin papillary folds, and parakeratosis or hyperkeratosis is variably present. In general, papillomas arising from the uvula or soft palate tend to be nonkeratinized or only thinly keratinized with prominent keratinocyte edema (Fig. 11.66).[1] Koilocytes are not usually apparent. The connective tissue cores contain dilated capillaries, and there may be hyalinization. Inflammation and reactive basal cell hyperplasia and atypia may be present if the lesion has been traumatized.[1,2]

Differential diagnosis

Verruca vulgaris may occasionally occur in the oral cavity and, as in the skin, it is characterized by marked hyperkeratosis with prominent coarse keratohyaline granules and axial inclination of epithelial papillary projections. HPV-2 is identified in up to 20% of cases of intraoral and up to 100% of lip verruca vulgaris.[6–8]

Oral condyloma acuminatum shows large, bulbous rete ridges and prominent koilocytosis, and HPV-6 and -11 are often identified (Figs 11.67 and 11.68).[9–11] This condition occurs most frequently in patients who are on long-term immunosuppression such as organ transplant recipients.

Focal epithelial hyperplasia (Heck disease), which is associated with infection by HPV-13, HPV-32, and HPV-55, is usually papular exhibiting acanthosis and uncommonly, papillary epithelial hyperplasia. Importantly, 'mitosoid' figures (cells exhibiting karyorrhexis) and apoptotic cells are characteristic features (see later)

Rare cases of oral acanthosis nigricans have been reported, and these are generally associated with gastrointestinal malignancy while the benign form is associated with diabetes mellitus, obesity, and hepatitis B.[11,12]

Papillary hyperplasia caused by dentures consists of hyperplasia of both epithelium and fibrovascular tissue (see later).

Verruciform xanthoma

Clinical features

Verruciform xanthoma affects adults in the fourth and fifth decades with no significant sex predilection.[1–5] It presents as an asymptomatic, well-circumscribed rough, granular or pebbly, raised or depressed, yellowish or reddish plaque (Fig. 11.69). Seventy percent occur on the hard palatal mucosa, gingiva, or alveolar ridge mucosa. Lesions on the skin (especially of the anogenital area) and other mucosal sites have also been reported.[6] Although there is one report of a patient with multiple lesions and lipid storage disease, most patients do not exhibit hypercholesterolemia or disorders of lipid storage.[7]

Pathogenesis and histologic features

It has been postulated that verruciform xanthoma is a reaction to damaged and degenerated epithelial cells which release lipid that becomes engulfed by macrophages. Neutrophils are recruited to the area by the degenerating cells.[6,8] The gingiva and palatal mucosa are constantly traumatized by mastication, and these are the common sites of occurrence for this condition. Verruciform xanthoma also occurs in association with other conditions where epithelial damage occurs such as lichen planus, pemphigus vulgaris, discoid lupus erythematosus, epidermolysis bullosa, and chronic graft-versus-host disease, as well as in dysplastic lesions and invasive carcinoma.[9–15]

Histologically, there is parakeratosis with the parakeratin exhibiting a bright orange hue. Loose keratin squames are present on the surface or within epithelial crypts, and spongiotic pustules are common. The surface of a verruciform xanthoma generally has a papillary configuration although some lesions are flat.[1] Rete ridges are uniformly long and sometimes coalesce at their bases (Figs 11.70 and 11.71). Large, foamy, lipid-laden macrophages are found within the connective tissue papillae (Fig. 11.72);

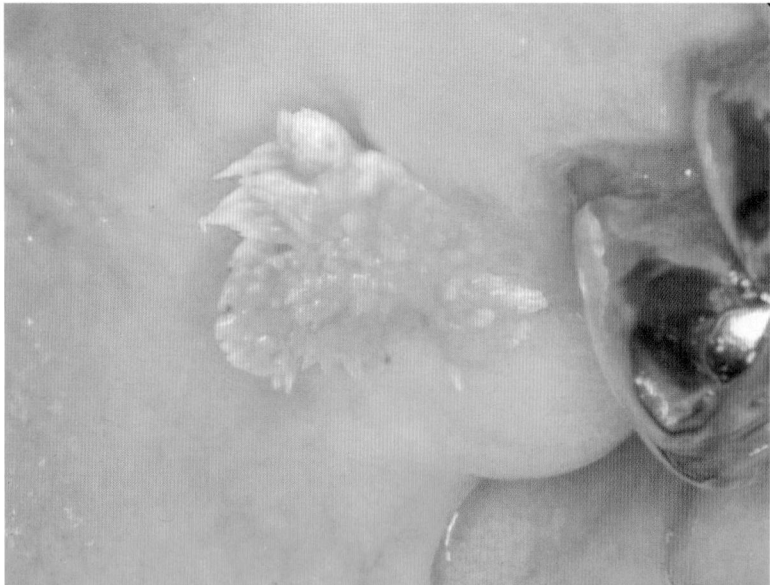

Fig. 11.64
Squamous papilloma: there is a rough, warty lesion of the palatal mucosa.

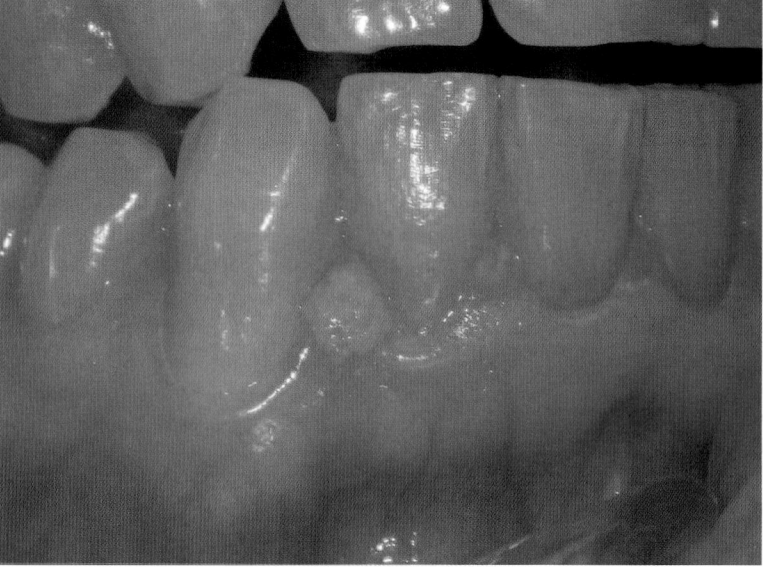

Fig. 11.65
Squamous papilloma: there is a rough, white warty lesion of the gingiva.

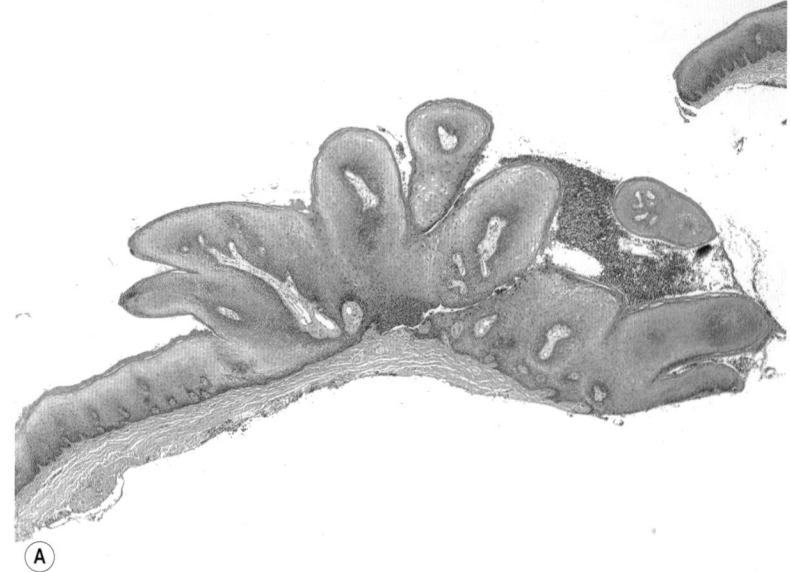

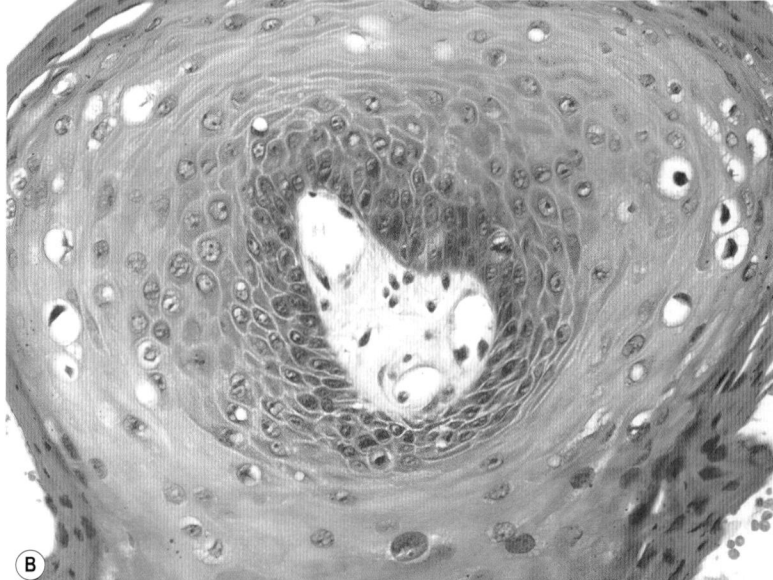

Fig. 11.66
Squamous papillomas of palatal mucosa: (**A**) there is a benign papillary proliferation of parakeratotic stratified squamous epithelium exhibiting keratinocyte edema; (**B**) dilated capillaries are present within fibrovascular cores.

occasionally, such cells extend beyond the deepest portion of the rete ridges or are seen within the epithelium.[16–19] Rarely, nonmucosal cases may show a cystic and inverted, crateriform configuration.[6,20]

The xanthoma cells express CD68, CD163, and NK1C3 and are negative for S100 protein.[18,19,21] Most of the xanthoma cells represent reparative (RM3/1) and resident (25F9) foam cells.[22] Slight granular positivity for keratin within the foam cells also supports the presence of epithelial fragments.[6] HPV immunohistochemistry is negative.[6,19]

Ultrastructurally, the xanthoma cells contain membrane-bound granules consistent with lysosomes, myelin figures, and fragments of desmosomes, the last supporting the theory of phagocytosis of epithelial cell debris.[8,16,23] There is fragmentation of the basal lamina and hemi-desmosomes.[24]

Localized juvenile spongiotic gingival hyperplasia

Clinical features

This occurs most frequently in the second decade of life with 90% occurring below age 20 with a 2:1 male predilection. More than 80% occur on the

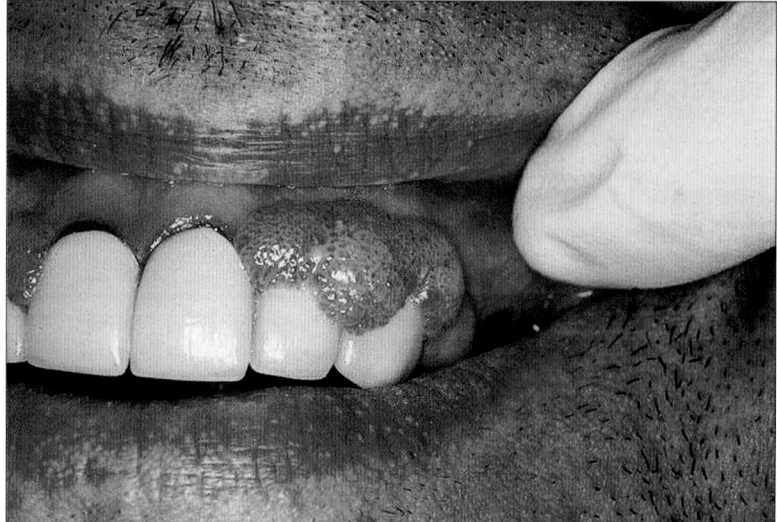

Fig. 11.67
Condyloma acuminatum: this larger warty lesion on the gingiva occurred in a patient on long-term immunosuppression after lung transplantation.

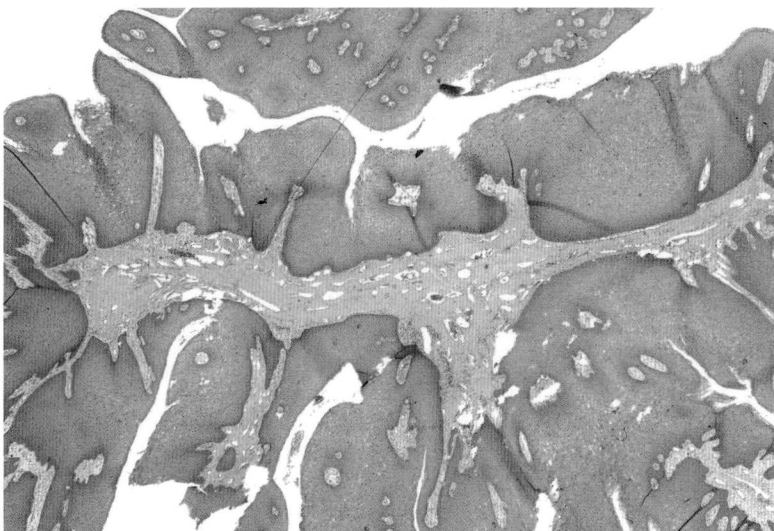

Fig. 11.68
Condyloma acuminatum: unlike squamous papilloma, the rete ridges are large and bulbous and koilocytes are readily identified.

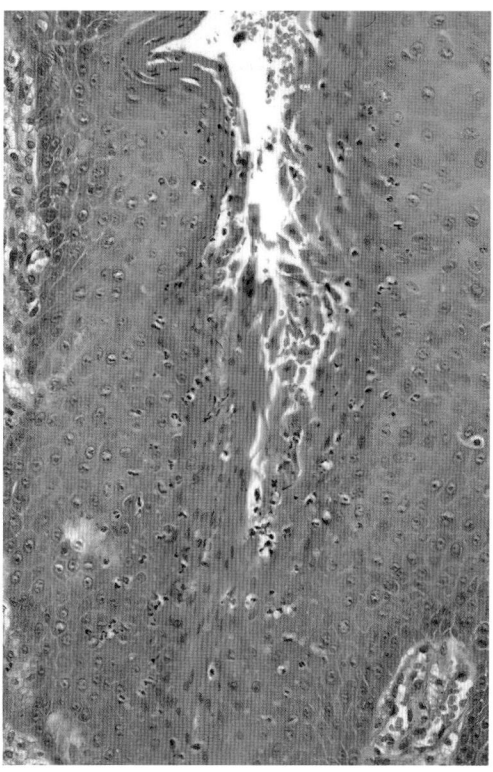

Fig. 11.71
Verruciform xanthoma: parakeratotic squames on the surface of the keratin and in the crypts are a characteristic feature; spongiotic pustules are often present.

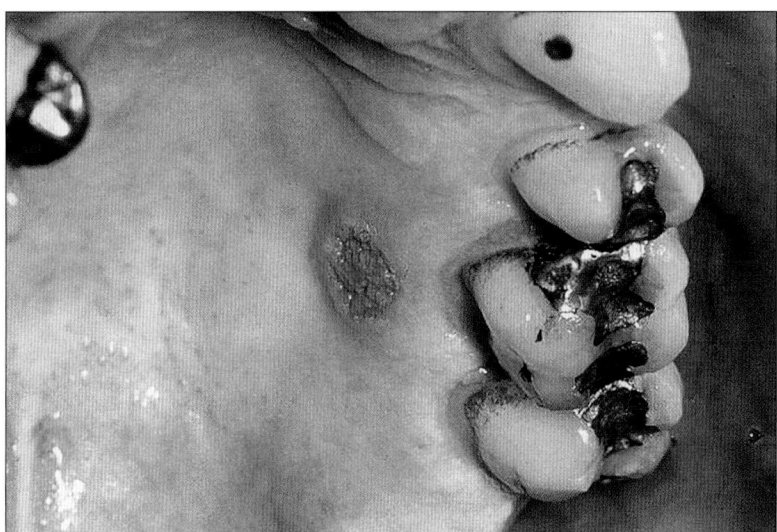

Fig. 11.69
Verruciform xanthoma: note the warty sessile lesion on the left hard palate. By courtesy of C. Allen, DDS, Columbus, USA.

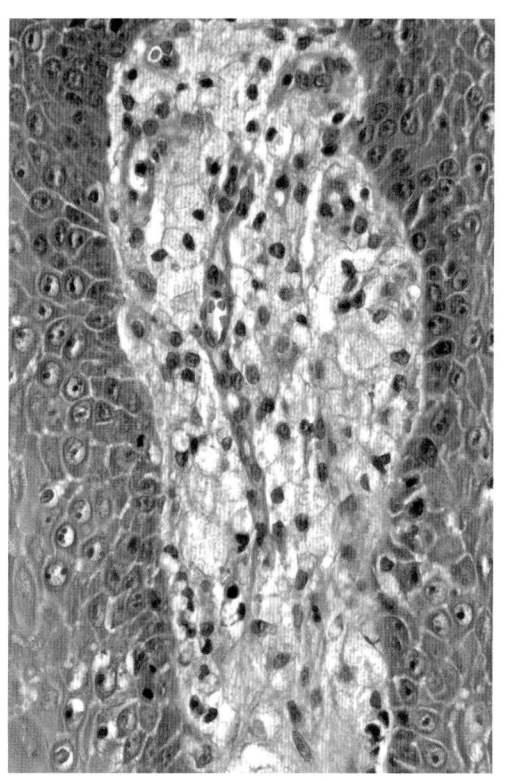

Fig. 11.72
Verruciform xanthoma: the lamina propria contains numerous foamy macrophages.

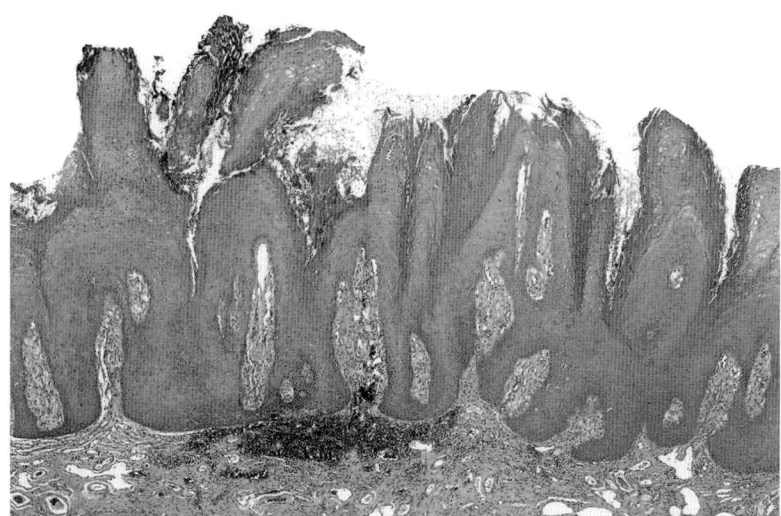

Fig. 11.70
Verruciform xanthoma: there is marked brightly eosinophilic parakeratin and papillomatosis with confluence of rete ridges at the tips.

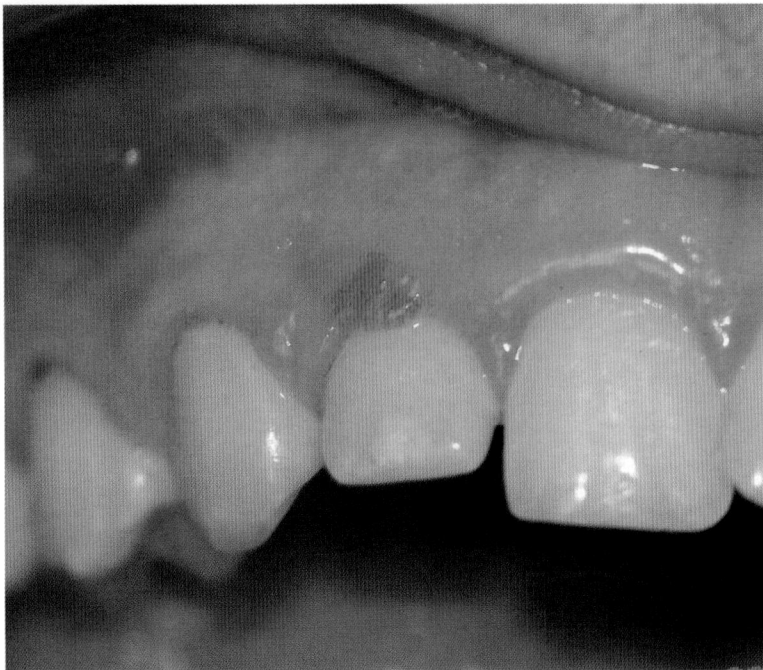

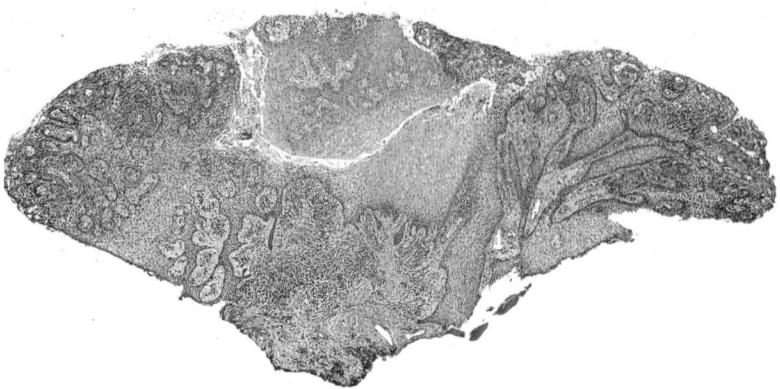

Fig. 11.74
Localized juvenile spongiotic gingival hyperplasia: there is a benign papillary proliferation of nonkeratinized stratified squamous epithelium with marked spongiosis.

Fig. 11.73
Localized juvenile spongiotic gingival hyperplasia: there is an erythematous papule on the gingiva with a slightly papillary surface.

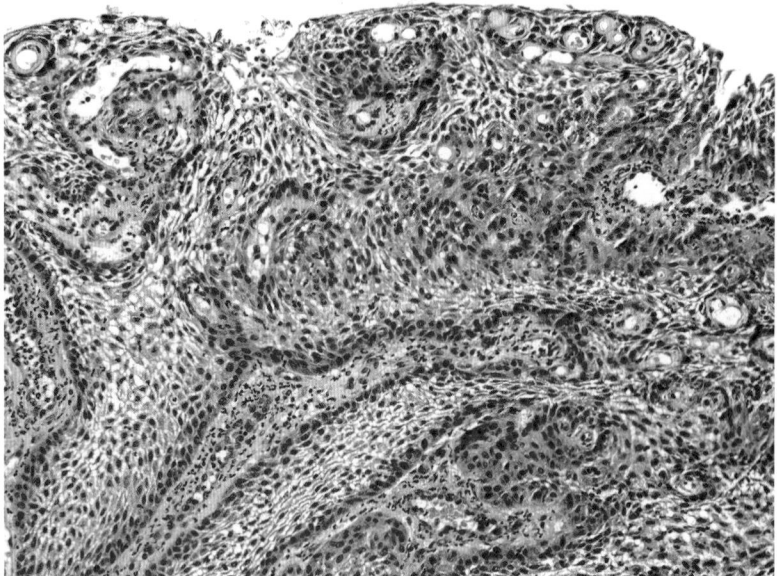

Fig. 11.75
Localized juvenile spongiotic gingival hyperplasia: there is marked spongiosis, neutrophilic exocytosis and congested capillaries within fibrovascular cores, with focal hyalinization.

maxillary marginal gingiva, and 15% are associated with orthodontic hardware. Lesions appear as nontender, erythematous, pebbly, sessile papules and plaques on the gingiva that infrequently are multifocal (*Fig. 11.73*).[1,2]

Pathogenesis and histologic features

This is a reactive condition related to trauma and local irritation, and it has been suggested that the epithelial proliferation arises from the crevicular or junctional epithelium of the gingiva.

There is a pedunculated or sessile papillary proliferation of squamous epithelium with marked spongiosis and neutrophilic exocytosis with loss of surface keratin. Many dilated and congested capillaries are present within fibrovascular cores, sometimes with hyalinization (*Figs 11.74* and *11.75*).[1,2] HPV has not been consistently identified.[3]

TUMORLIKE CONDITIONS

Fibroma

Clinical features

Fibroma (fibrovascular polyp, fibroepithelial polyp, irritation/bite fibroma) is the most common tumor-like (but non-neoplastic) condition in the mouth. It is usually located at sites of trauma, namely, the buccal mucosa at or near the linea alba, the lateral borders and tip of the tongue, the lower lip mucosa, and the gingiva.[1,2] It presents as a fleshy, pedunculated, or sessile dome-shaped nodule that may be mucosal-colored, ulcerated or keratotic (*Figs 11.76* and *11.77*).

Pathogenesis and histologic features

The fibroma is not a true neoplasm but rather a nodule of scar tissue caused by bite trauma.

The fibroma consists of a mass of fibrocollagenous tissue with variable vascularity and usually mild to insignificant inflammation unless there is overlying ulceration (*Figs 11.78* and *11.79*). On occasion, the lesion may resemble a hypertrophic scar or keloid. The epithelium may be hyperkeratotic, acanthotic or atrophic. If adipose tissue is present, the term 'fibrolipoma' or 'lipofibroma' is sometimes applied.

Differential diagnosis

Sclerotic fibroma (storiform collagenoma) has been reported in the oral cavity, and the collagen in these lesions has a storiform appearance with clefts between hyalinized collagen and stellate or multinucleated fibroblasts with dendritic processes; multiple such lesions are seen in Cowden syndrome. The cells are sometimes positive for CD34.[3]

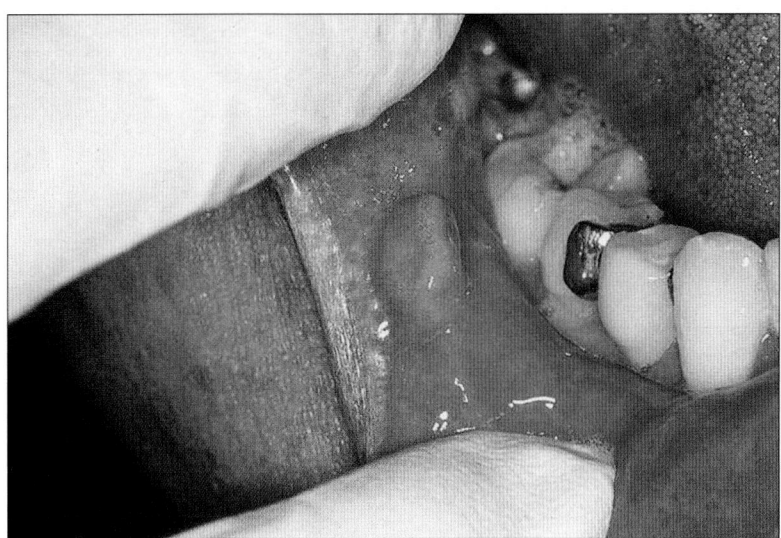

Fig. 11.76
Fibroma: there is a fleshy pink sessile mass on the lower lip mucosa.

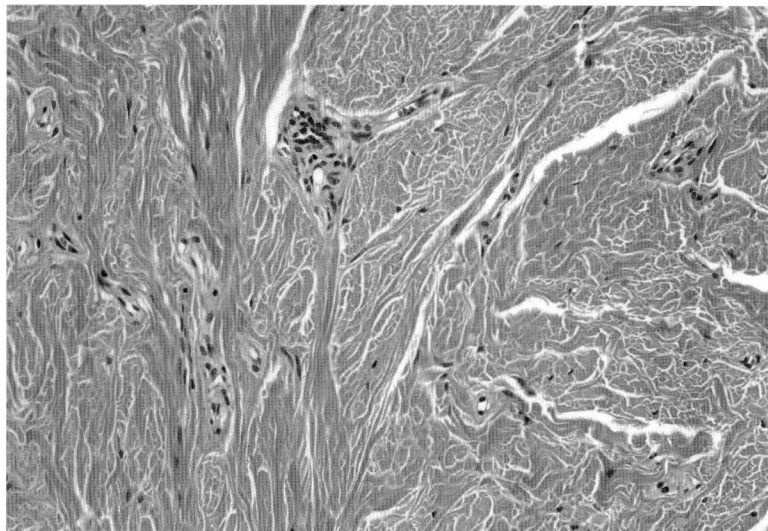

Fig. 11.79
Fibroma: the fibrous tissue is densely collagenous with a few scattered capillaries.

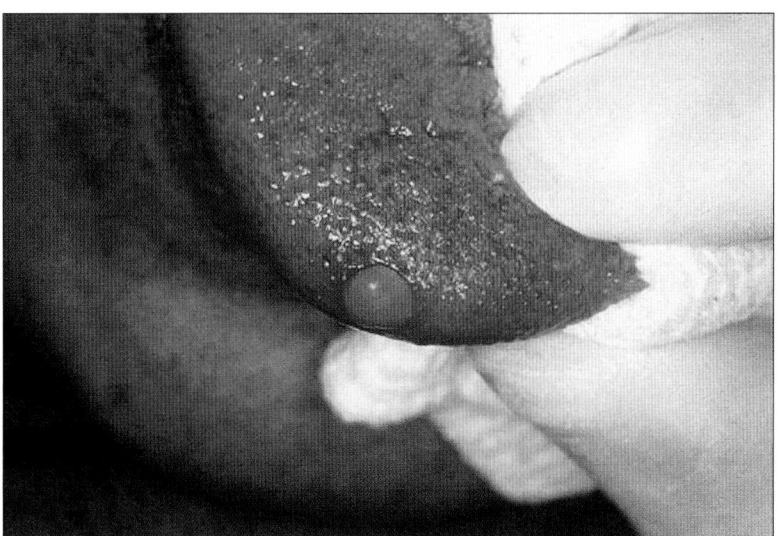

Fig. 11.77
Fibroma: there is a fleshy, polypoid nodule on the lateral border of the tongue.

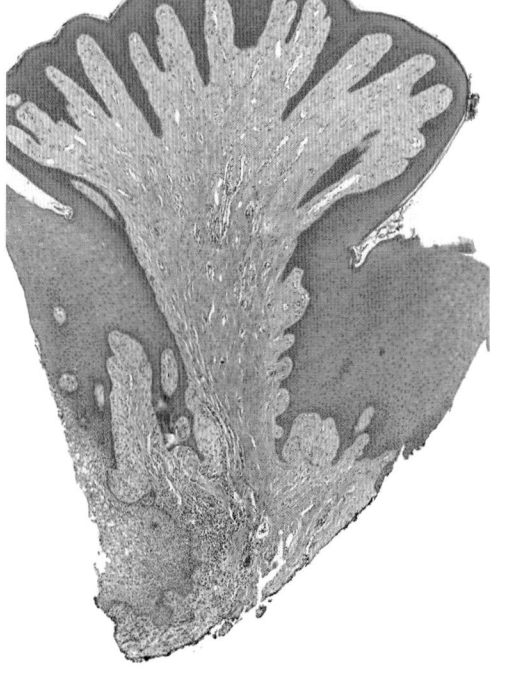

Fig. 11.80
Giant cell fibroma: note the undulating surface and spiky rete ridges.

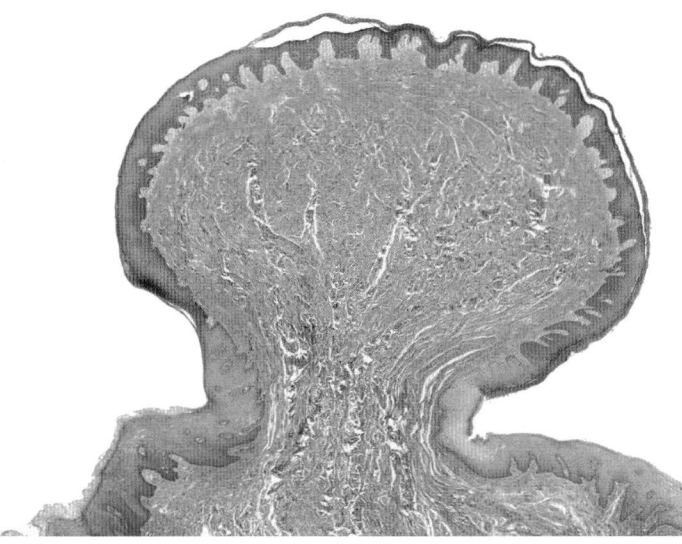

Fig. 11.78
Fibroma: there is a mass of densely collagenous tissue with hyperkeratosis of the epithelium.

Giant cell fibroma

Clinical features

Giant cell fibroma occurs in the first three decades of life, and the most common sites affected are the keratinized regions of the gingiva (44–49%), tongue (17–22%), and palatal mucosa (15–18%).[1,2] It often has a papillary or bosselated surface. It bears some resemblance to the fibrous papule of the nose, angiofibroma, and the pearly penile papule.[3] The retrocuspid papilla has a similar histology and is located on the lingual mandibular gingiva in the area of the cuspid.[4–6]

Histologic features

The most characteristic feature of the giant cell fibroma is the presence of giant, stellate-shaped fibroblasts within densely collagenous stroma (*Figs 11.80* and *11.81*).[1,2,7] Multinucleated, stellate-shaped giant fibroblasts ('manta ray cells') are common. The overlying epithelium is usually

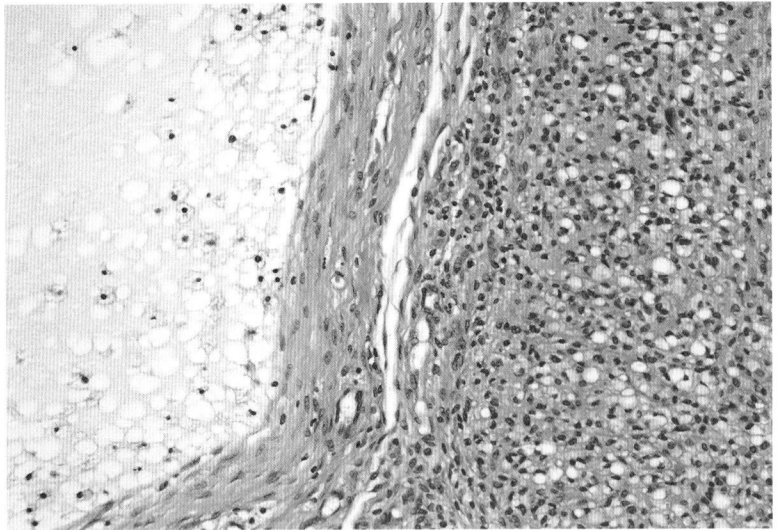

Fig. 11.81
Giant cell fibroma: note the stellate-shaped and multinucleated cells.

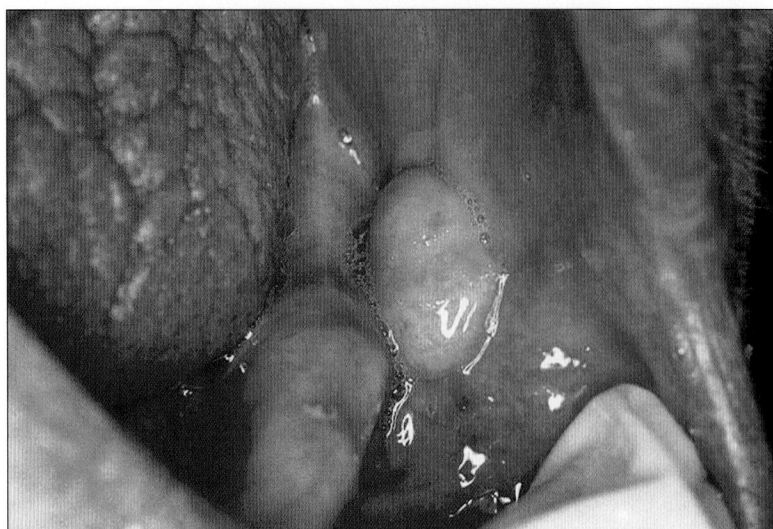

Fig. 11.82
Lipoma: note the yellowish, sessile nodule on the buccal mucosa.

hyperplastic, forming spiky, sawtooth-shaped rete ridges, and there may be surface papillomatosis.

The cells express vimentin, occasionally factor XIIIa, but not S100 protein or CD68.[7,8]

Differential diagnosis

The multinucleate cell angiohistiocytoma occurs rarely in the oral cavity and contains multinucleated giant cells, branching capillaries, and myxoid stroma.[9,10]

Lipoma and atypical lipomatous tumor

Clinical features

Lipoma usually occurs in adults in the sixth and seventh decades.[1–3] It presents as a yellowish, soft and doughy, painless, sessile or pedunculated nodule that generally occurs on the buccal mucosa, tongue or oral vestibule (*Fig. 11.82*). Other sites include the lips and floor of mouth. Infiltrating or intramuscular lipomas tend to occur two decades earlier and generally involve the tongue.[2,4,5]

Many lipomas of the buccal mucosa are not true tumors but represent herniation of the buccal fat pad from trauma.

Histologic features

Lipomas represent circumscribed proliferations of mature adipocytes identical to normal adipose tissue, with regularly sized vacuoles and benign nuclei.[3,6] Often bands of fibrous tissue separate lobules of adipocytes, and the term 'fibrolipoma' is applied (*Fig. 11.83*). Cartilaginous and osseous metaplasia have occasionally been reported.[7,8] Similar benign adipocytes are present within skeletal muscle fibers in an infiltrating (intramuscular) lipoma.[4]

Differential diagnosis

Distinction must be made between a traumatized lipoma and an atypical lipomatous tumor that generally occurs on the tongue of adults, and that represents a superficial variant of well-differentiated liposarcoma. These are infiltrative tumors containing lipoblasts with atypical, hyperchromatic, and indented nuclei (*Figs 11.84* and *11.85*); cells are usually positive for MDM2 and CDK4, unlike traumatized lipoma.[8–12] Some of the vacuolated cells of traumatized lipomas are histiocytes and they do not exhibit nuclear atypia seen in true lipoblasts. Foci of spindled cells and dedifferentiation have also been reported.

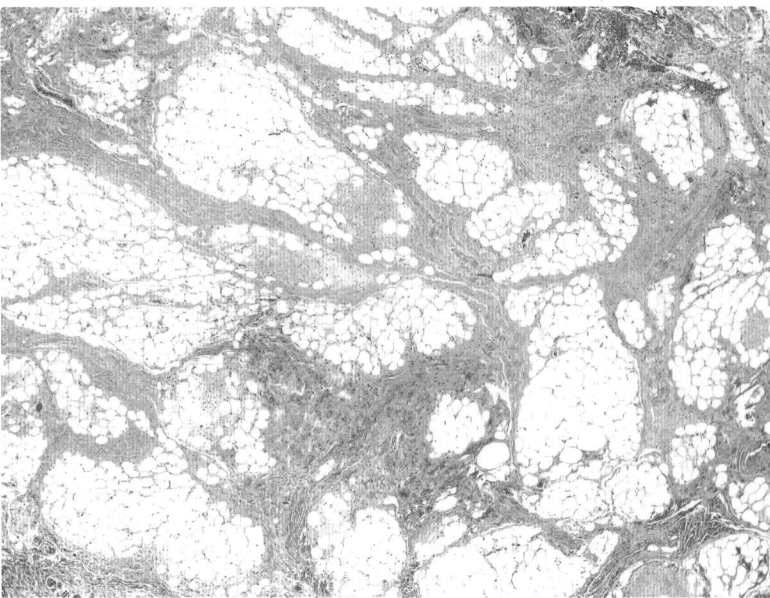

Fig. 11.83
Fibrolipoma: there are many mature adipocytes with regularly sized vacuoles separated into lobules by dense fibrous bands.

Oral spindle cell lipoma has also been reported, and this consists of spindle cells showing slight nuclear pleomorphism within a myxoid stroma with ropey collagen and mast cells (*Fig. 11.86*).[3,13]

Denture-associated fibrous hyperplasia

Clinical features

Denture-associated fibrous hyperplasia (inflammatory fibrous hyperplasia, epulis fissuratum, denture hyperplasia, papillary hyperplasia, inflammatory papillary hyperplasia) occurs in older patients and presents as a linear mass of tissue arising in the mucobuccal sulcus around the flange of a poorly fitting denture. A fissure is present into which the denture flange fits, hence the moniker 'epulis fissuratum'. The anterior maxillary and mandibular sulci are the preferred sites of involvement (*Figs 11.87* and *11.88*).[1–4]

Papillary hyperplasia or inflammatory papillary hyperplasia of the palatal mucosa appears as erythematous, edematous and pebbly, multinodular excrescences usually in a symmetric fashion (*Fig. 11.89*).[5,6]

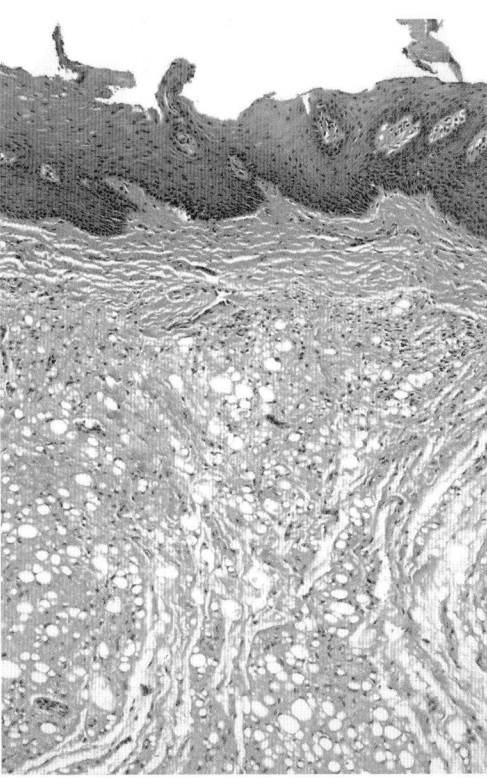

Fig. 11.84
Traumatized lipoma the tumor has infiltrative margins and cells with variably sized vacuoles.

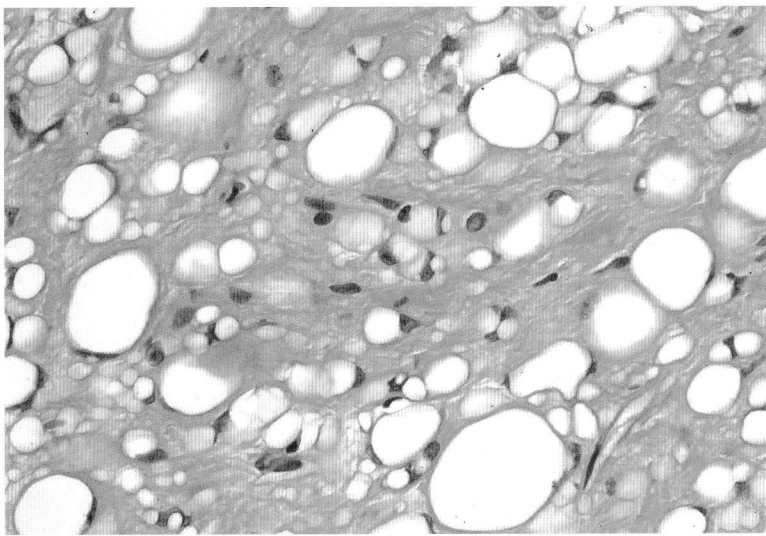

Fig. 11.85
Traumatized lipoma: note variably sized and multiple vacuoles, and indented nuclei without significant atypia or hyperchromasia.

Pathogenesis and histologic features

The redundant tissue cushions the mucosa against ongoing trauma caused by a poorly fitting denture sliding on the mucosa.

Denture-associated fibrous hyperplasia is characterized by proliferation of dense fibrous tissue with variable vascularity. Lymphocytes are generally diffusely dispersed at the interface of epithelium and fibrous tissue; the epithelium is hyperplastic and is usually thrown into papillary folds (*Fig. 11.90*). Pooling of plasma on the surface of the mucosa from trauma is common. Osseous and chondroid metaplasia (Cutright tumor) are seen in approximately 5% of cases, particularly in the anterior maxilla.[7,8] Salivary glands are present in 43% of cases and traumatic neuromas are often present.

In palatal lesions, the histopathology is that of multiple small nodules of fibrovascular tissue containing chronic inflammatory cells that are typically removed piecemeal (*Fig. 11.91*).[5] If spongiotic pustules are present, *Candida* infection should be excluded.[9]

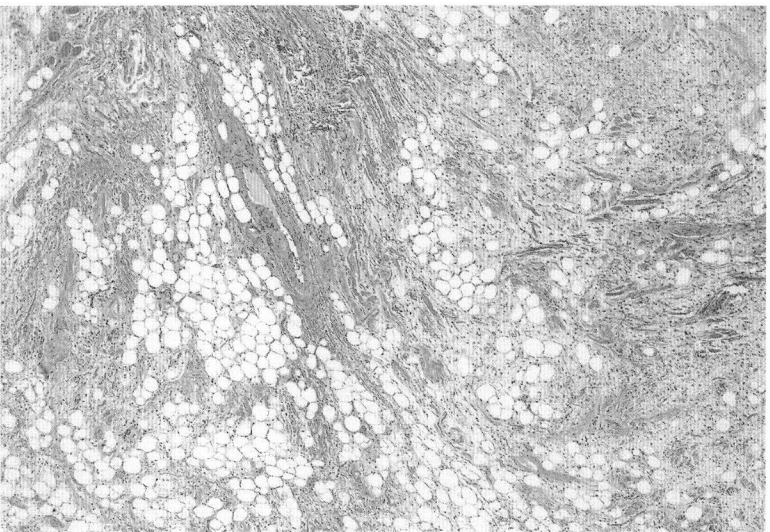

Fig. 11.86
Spindle cell lipoma: this is composed of a proliferation of adipocytes and spindle cells in a stroma of delicate and ropey collagen, often with mast cells.

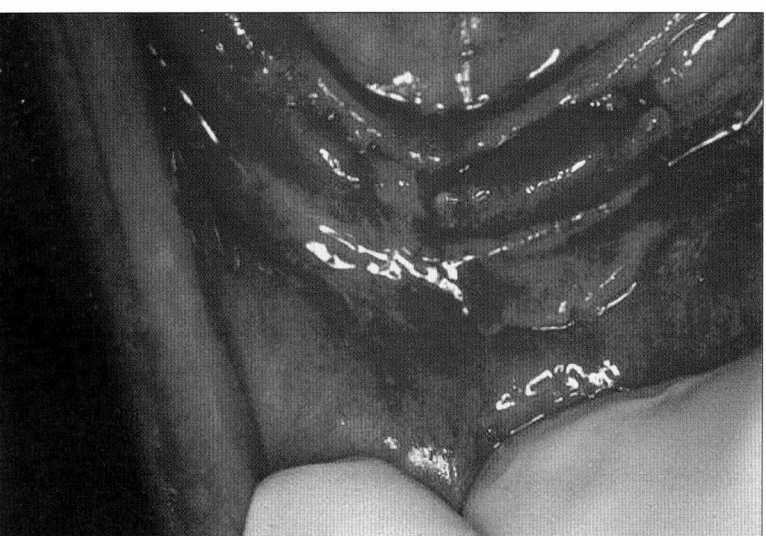

Fig. 11.87
Denture-induced fibrous hyperplasia (epulis fissuratum): there is an elongated mass of soft tissue in the mandibular sulcus with a fissure running through it.

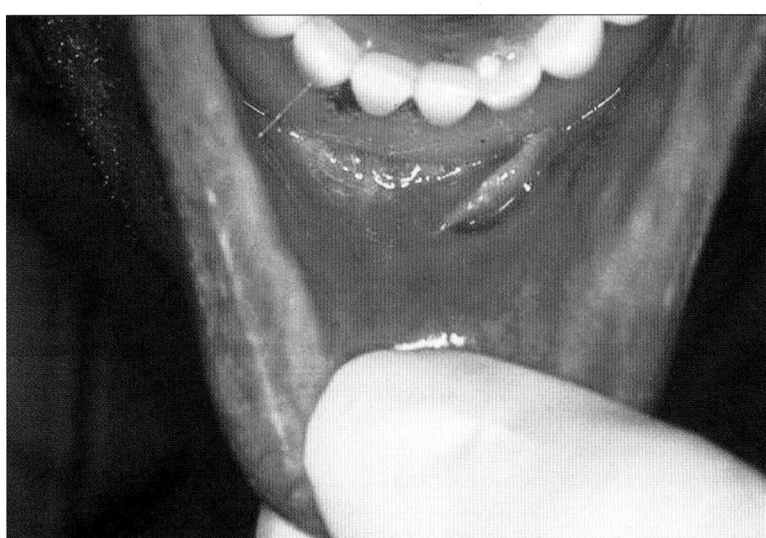

Fig. 11.88
Denture-induced fibrous hyperplasia (epulis fissuratum): the denture flange (edge) fits into the fissure.

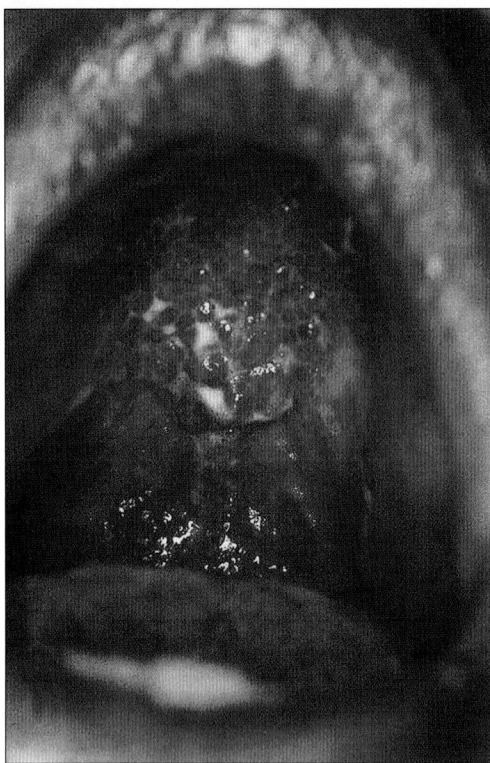

Fig. 11.89
Denture-induced papillary hyperplasia of the palatal mucosa: note the typical pebbly papillary structures on the palate.

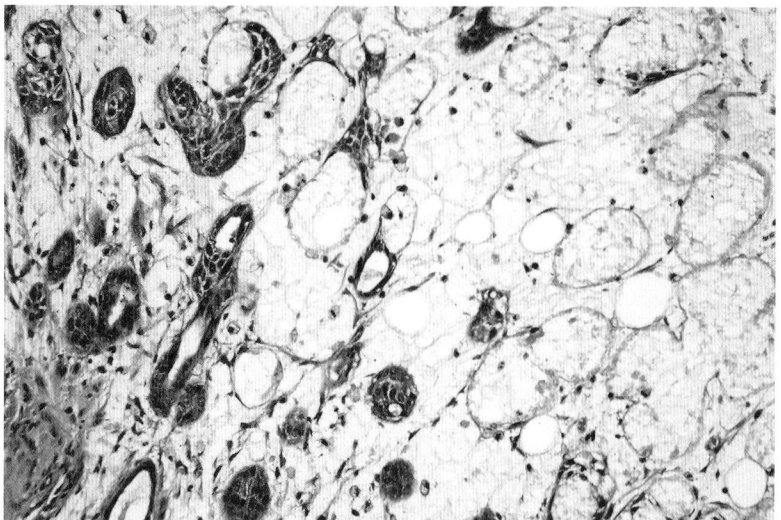

Fig. 11.91
Denture-induced papillary hyperplasia: there is a multinodular proliferation of fibrovascular tissue with a moderate lymphocytic infiltrate.

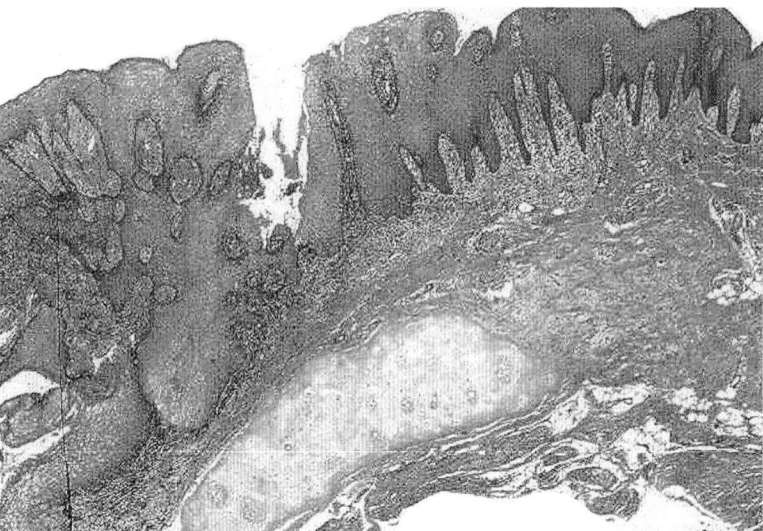

Fig. 11.90
Denture-induced fibrous hyperplasia: there is papillomatosis and hyperplasia of epithelium and fibrous tissue. A mass of mature cartilage is present in this lesion from the anterior maxillary sulcus (Cutright tumor).

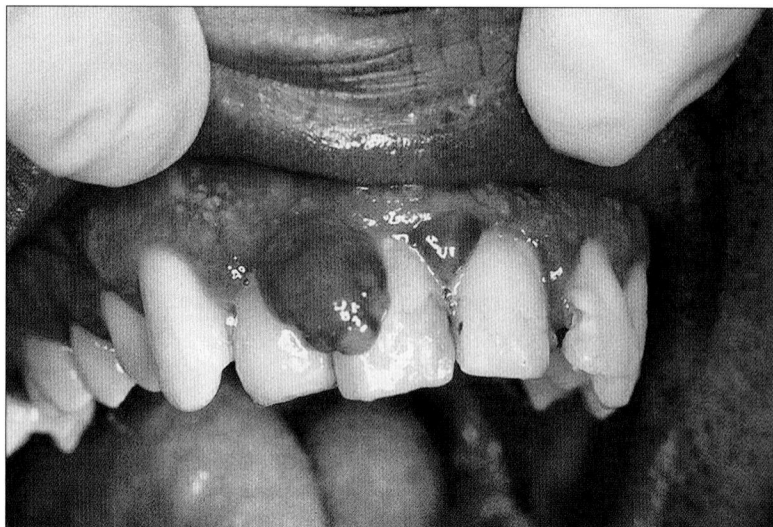

Fig. 11.92
Gingival nodule: there is a fleshy mass arising from the marginal gingiva; note a small mass between the central incisors.

Gingival nodules

Clinical features

The term 'epulis' refers to any mass or nodule on the gingiva or alveolar ridge mucosa and should be avoided if possible. The exception is epulis fissuratum (see above).

Most solitary gingival nodules represent one of the following conditions: reactive tumor-like proliferations, odontogenic cysts, primary odontogenic and nonodontogenic neoplasms, and metastatic neoplasms. Lesions in the first group are by far the most common and consist of the following entities:

• fibroma or fibrous hyperplasia with or without inflammation,
• giant cell fibroma,
• lobular capillary hemangioma (pyogenic granuloma),
• peripheral ossifying fibroma,
• peripheral giant cell granuloma.

These lesions are located on the marginal gingiva adjacent to teeth. Depending on the degree of vascularity, inflammation, and/or ulceration present, they may be mucosal-colored, erythematous, or ulcerated and painful (Figs 11.92 and 11.93).[1]

These fibrous and vascular reactive nodules develop as a response to irritation from dental plaque and calculus, often exacerbated by the presence of defective restorations. Multipotent mesenchymal cells in the connective tissue proliferate and differentiate into cells that form native tissues in the area such as fibroblasts (fibroma), endothelial cells (pyogenic granuloma), bone- and cementum-producing cells (peripheral ossifying fibroma), or osteoclasts (peripheral giant cell granuloma). It is therefore not uncommon to see features of all four entities present to varying degrees within any one lesion. Unless the source of irritation is removed completely, these lesions often recur.

Dental plaque is often present as clumps of Gram-positive filamentous bacteria that morphologically resemble actinomycotic colonies. Unless surrounded by a mantle of neutrophils, such colonies are surface colonizers and do not represent Actinomycosis infection.

Other gingival nodules and masses include the gingival and periodontal abscess and the parulis.

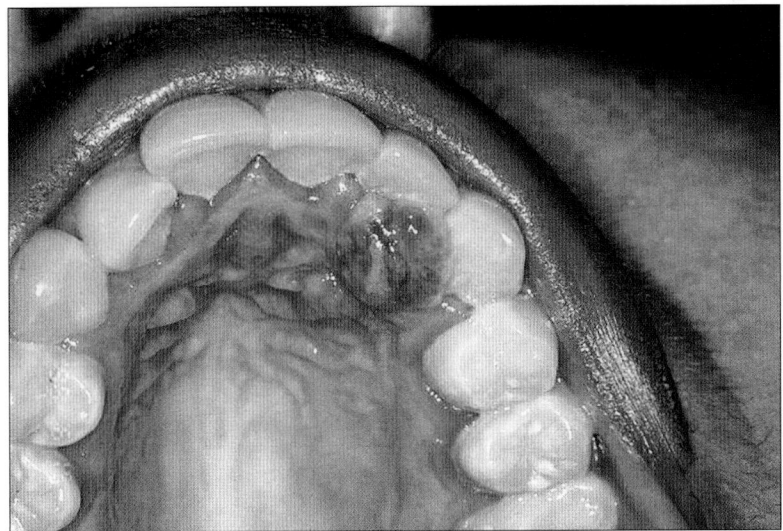

Fig. 11.93
Gingival nodule: there is a fleshy ulcerated mass on the palatal gingiva.

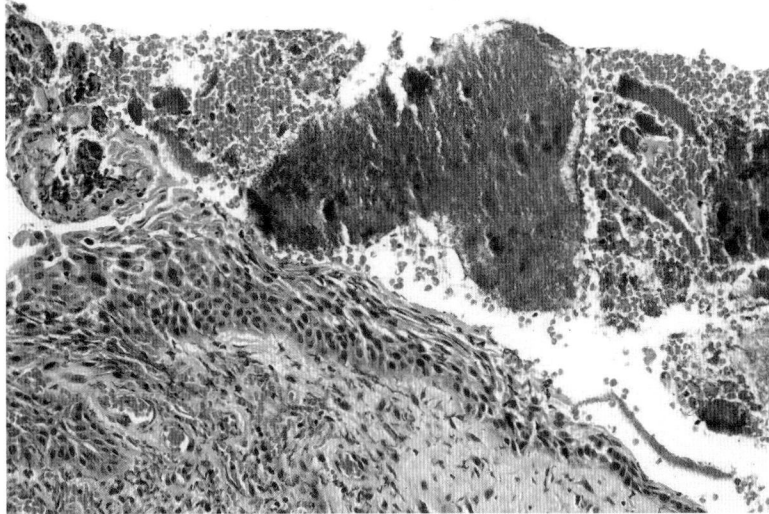

Fig. 11.95
Inflammatory fibrous hyperplasia of the gingiva: note the crevicular epithelium with spongiosis and the piece of dental plaque that morphologically resembles a mass of actinomycotic organisms.

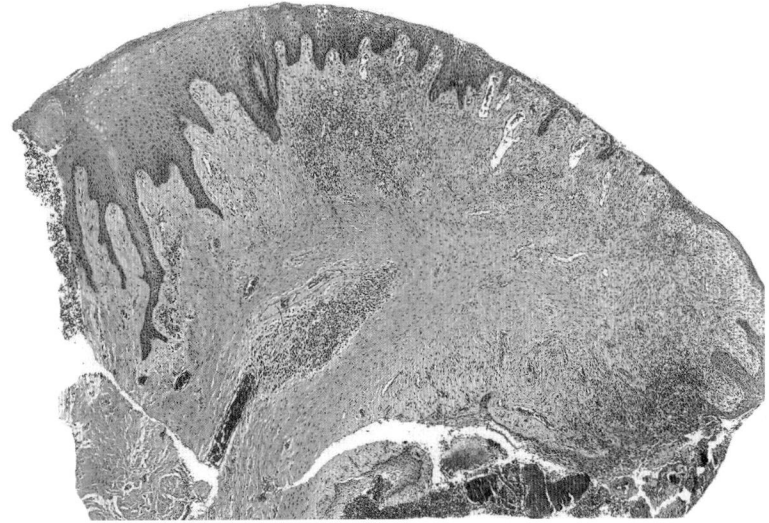

Fig. 11.94
Inflammatory fibrous hyperplasia of the gingiva: this consists of a mass of fibrovascular tissue with chronic inflammation; the surface keratinized epithelium is in continuity with the nonkeratinized crevicular epithelium (lower right), where inflammatory cells and bacterial colonies are present.

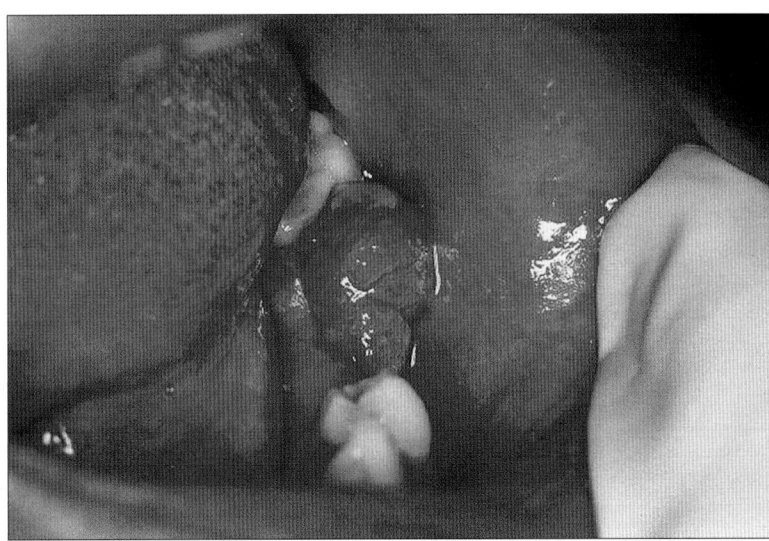

Fig. 11.96
Granuloma gravidarum: this nodule occurred in an edentulous part of the mandible.

Gingival fibroma (inflammatory fibrous hyperplasia)

Clinical features

Some fibromas represent the scarred remnants of pyogenic granulomas and unlike nongingival fibromas, most gingival fibromas are inflamed. A variant is the giant cell fibroma, which often has a papillary surface and may be clinically mistaken for a papilloma (see above).

Histologic features

Gingival fibroma is composed of a mass of densely or delicately collagenized tissue with variable vascularity and generally a variable lymphoplasmacytic infiltrate (*Fig. 11.94*).[1,2] If there is significant chronic inflammation, the stroma may be edematous. The overlying epithelium is sometimes hyperkeratotic and is in continuity with crevicular epithelium, the latter exhibiting spongiosis, neutrophilic exocytosis, and an underlying plasmacytic infiltrate (*Fig. 11.95*). It is common to see plaque bacteria close to the crevicular epithelium, composed mostly of Gram-positive filaments and cocci, morphologically similar to *Actinomyces*. However, these are surface colonizers only

and not to be confused with actinomycosis where suppuration is present as well as the Splendore-Hoeppli phenomenon. Edema and mucinous change when extreme warrants a diagnosis of oral focal mucinosis.

Lobular capillary hemangioma (pyogenic granuloma)

Clinical features

These nodules tend to occur in the second to fourth decades, and are dark red or purple and bleed readily. One variant of this lesion is the granuloma gravidarum which occurs in the second and third trimester of pregnancy (*Fig. 11.96*).[1] The recurrence rate is 16%.[2]

Although the majority of intraoral lesions occur on the gingiva, the lip mucosa (especially the upper), buccal mucosa, and tongue may be affected.[3–6]

Pathogenesis and histologic features

Many if not all gingival pyogenic granulomas are reactive. They have a gene signature that involves the nitric acid pathway, hypoxia-induced angiogenesis, and vascular injury.[7] In pregnancy-related lesions, there is no increase

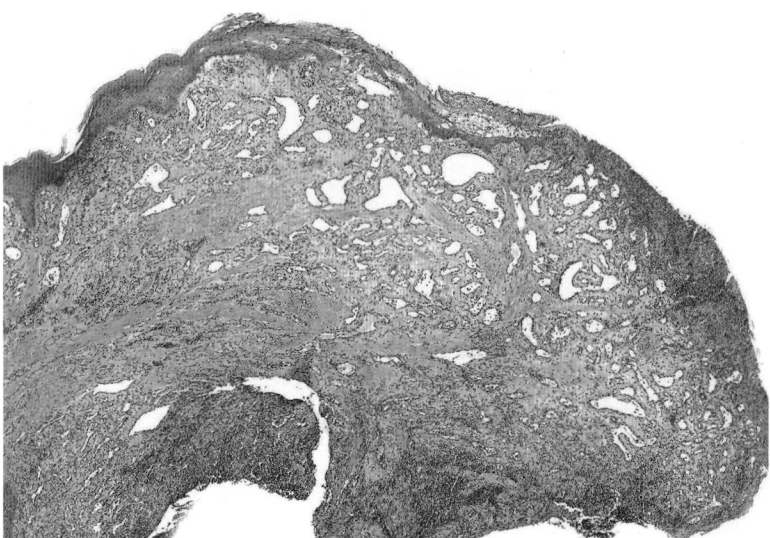

Fig. 11.97
Gingival pyogenic granuloma: there is a vaguely lobular proliferation of endothelial cells and capillaries with overlying ulceration.

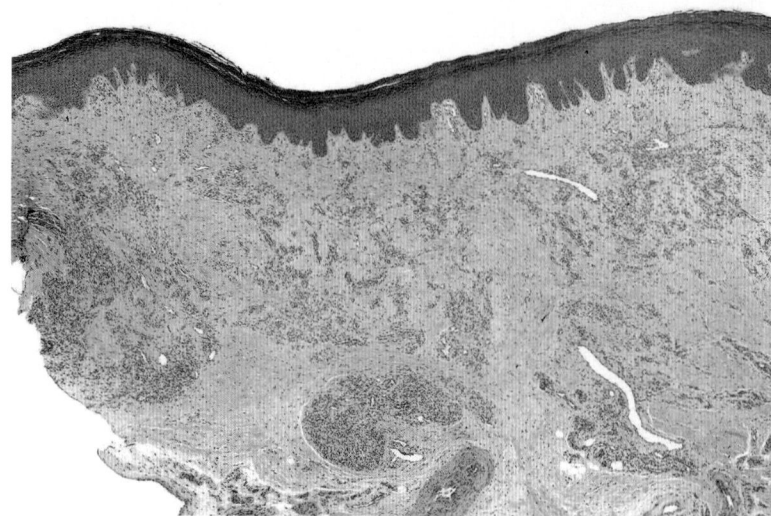

Fig. 11.99
Sclerosing pyogenic granuloma: note the effacement of lobular architecture by fibrous tissue.

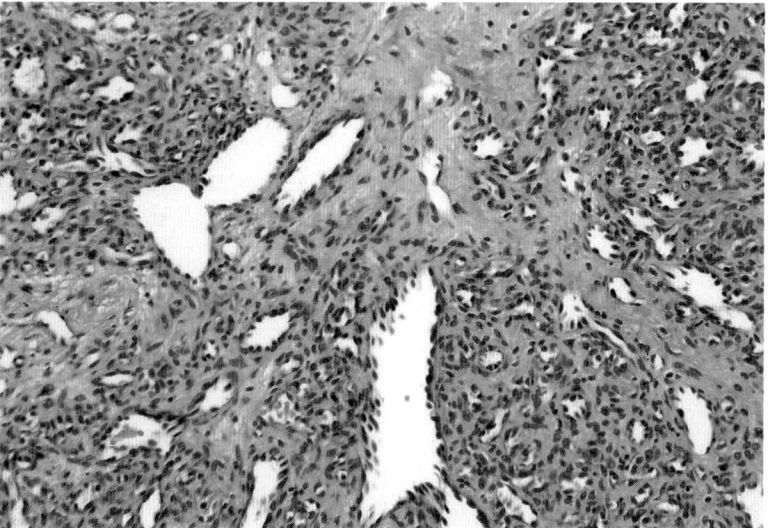

Fig. 11.98
Pyogenic granuloma: note benign-appearing endothelial cells and dilated capillaries.

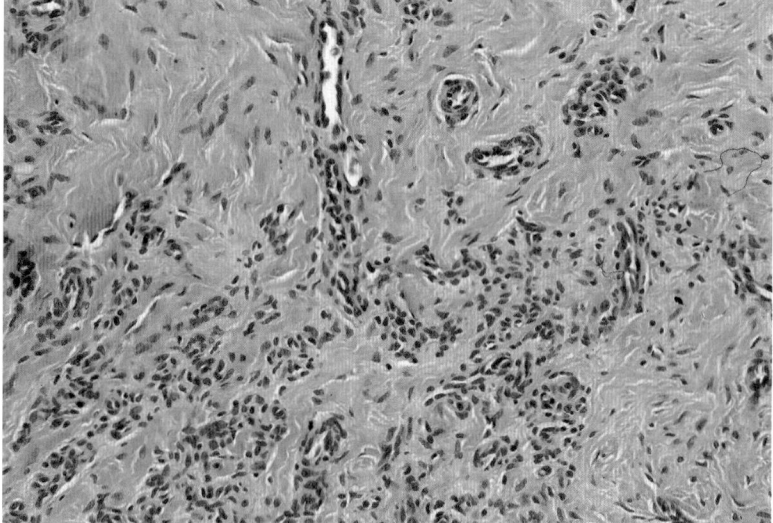

Fig. 11.100
Sclerosing pyogenic granuloma: note marked sclerosis and corresponding reduction in the number of vessels.

in the number of estrogen receptors on the endothelial cells of such lesions compared with controls, although they may express more vascular endothelial growth factor and other angiogenesis-enhancing factors, and fewer inhibitory factors.[8–10]

Gingival pyogenic granuloma is characterized by a diffuse or lobular (more common on nongingival sites) proliferation of endothelial cells and congested capillaries (*Figs 11.97* and *11.98*).[5] Dilated, branching vessels are usually present in the center of lobules.[3] The overlying epithelium is ulcerated in 75% of cases, and there is a variable neutrophilic, lymphocytic, and plasmacytic infiltrate.[2] Some lesions become increasingly sclerotic and may eventuate in gingival fibrous hyperplasias after the bulk of the vasculature is replaced by fibrous tissue (*Figs 11.99* and *11.100*). Unlike infantile hemangiomas, these tumors are GLUT-1 negative.[11]

Peripheral ossifying fibroma

Clinical features

This tumor, also known as calcifying fibrous epulis or calcifying fibroblastic granuloma, occurs in the second and third decades, and women are affected up to two times more often than men (1.5–2:1). Up to two-thirds occur in the maxillary gingiva.[1,2] Lesions may be pale and fibrotic or red and inflamed, and a giant variant exists that is generally >2 cm.[3] The recurrence rate is 8–16%.[1,2]

Histologic features

This lesion is not a true neoplasm but rather a fibrous hyperplasia that forms metaplastic bone, and cementum-like droplets ('cementicles') that may resemble psammoma bodies. The lesion presents as a nonencapsulated cellular proliferation of plump, spindled fibroblast-like cells with fusiform-to-ovoid vesicular nuclei with deposition of varying amounts of cementum droplets, osteoid, and woven and lamellar bone, often rimmed by osteoblasts (*Figs 11.101* and *11.102*). Droplet calcifications ('cementicles' or cementum droplets) and less commonly, globular masses of cementum are sometimes seen (*Fig. 11.103*).[1,4] Even if calcifications are not clearly identified, a cellular proliferation of such spindled fibroblast-like cells should raise the suspicion of this entity, and deeper sections will usually reveal the presence of osteoid or cementum droplets. Foci of osteoclast-like multinucleated giant cells are occasionally present in addition to areas resembling pyogenic granuloma (*Fig. 11.104*).[1,2]

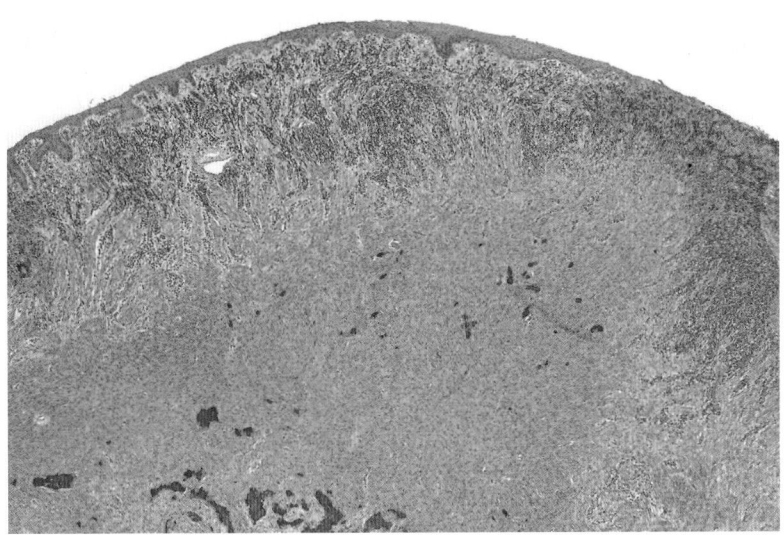

Fig. 11.101
Peripheral ossifying fibroma: there is a cellular proliferation of spindled fibroblast-like cells with deposition of osteoid (lower left) and cementum droplets (upper right).

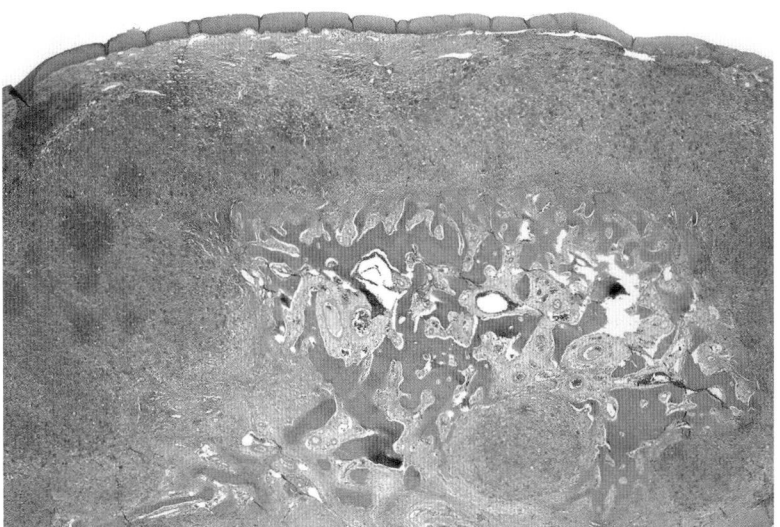

Fig. 11.102
Peripheral ossifying fibroma: there is a cellular proliferation of spindled fibroblast-like cells with deposition of osteoid, and multiple foci of multinucleated giant cells.

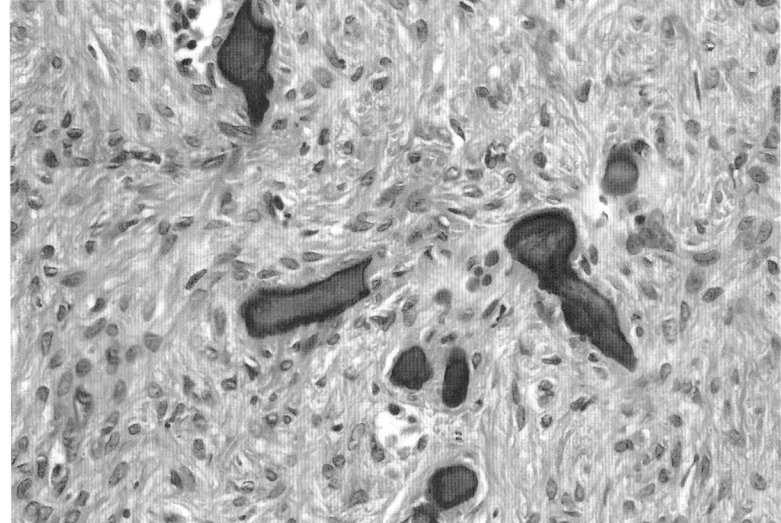

Fig. 11.103
Peripheral ossifying fibroma: the spindle cells have plump ovoid nuclei and they deposit cementum droplets.

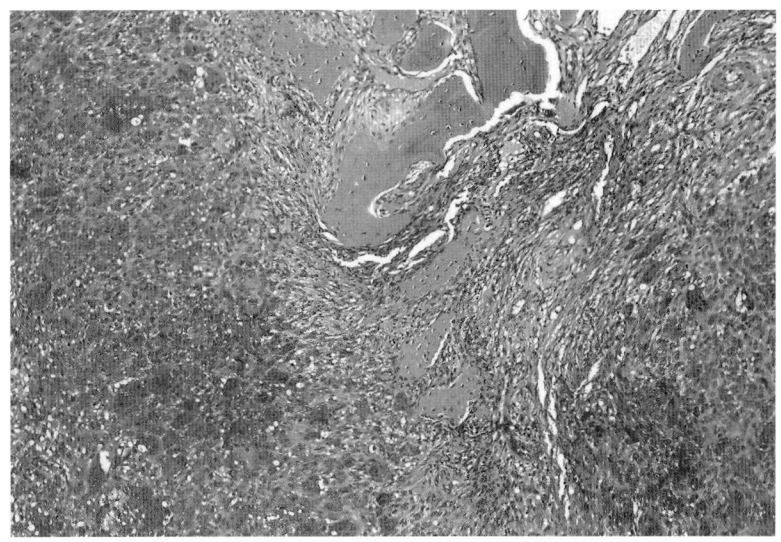

Fig. 11.104
Peripheral ossifying fibroma: there is deposition of woven bone and clusters of osteoclast-like giant cells.

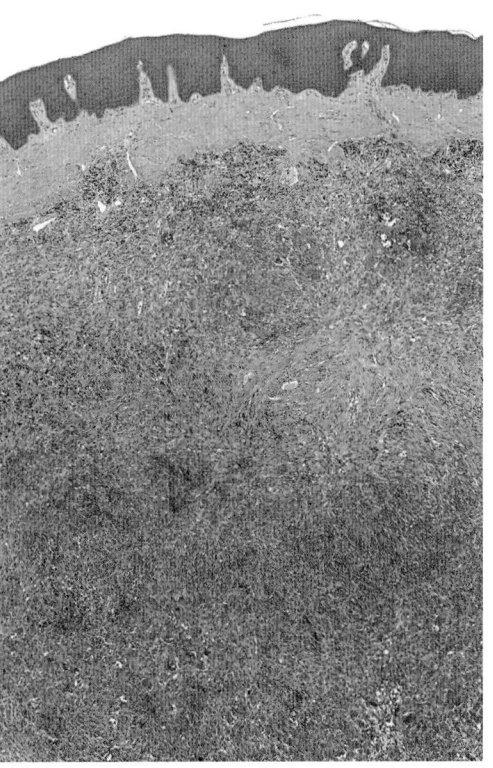

Fig. 11.105
Peripheral giant cell granuloma: a Grenz zone separates the giant cells from the epithelium and many siderophages are noted in this area.

Peripheral giant cell granuloma

Clinical features

This lesion usually occurs in the fourth and fifth decades of life, and the mandibular gingiva is two to three times more often involved than the maxilla. It often resides in a saucer- or cup-shaped depression within the underlying bone, with 19–22% occurring in edentulous areas; the recurrence rate is up to 22%.[1-4] One must rule out gingival extension of central giant cell granuloma particularly if peripheral lesions are detected in patients with hyperparathyroidism.[5,6]

Histologic features

Peripheral giant cell granuloma is characterized by a discrete but unencapsulated diffuse or lobular proliferation of osteoclast-type multinucleate giant cells and mononuclear/monocytic cells in a vascular stroma with abundant fresh hemorrhage and hemosiderin deposition (*Figs 11.105* and

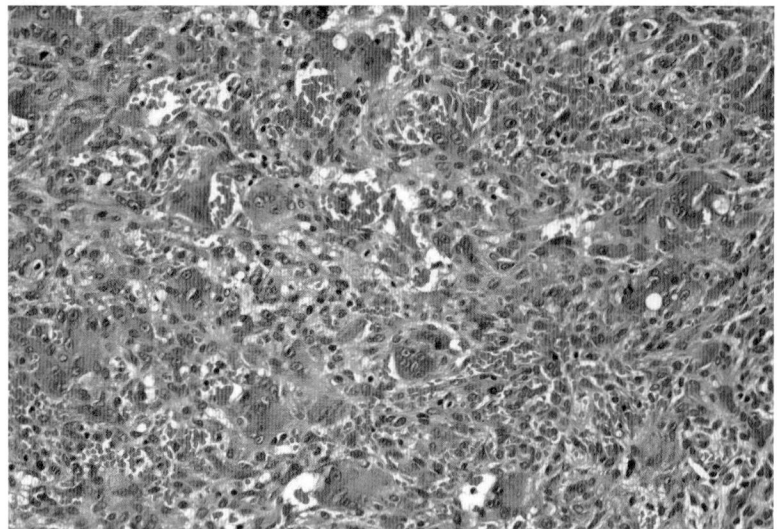

Fig. 11.106
Peripheral giant cell granuloma: there is a cellular proliferation of mononuclear/monocytic cells and multinucleated giant cells in a vascular and hemorrhagic stroma.

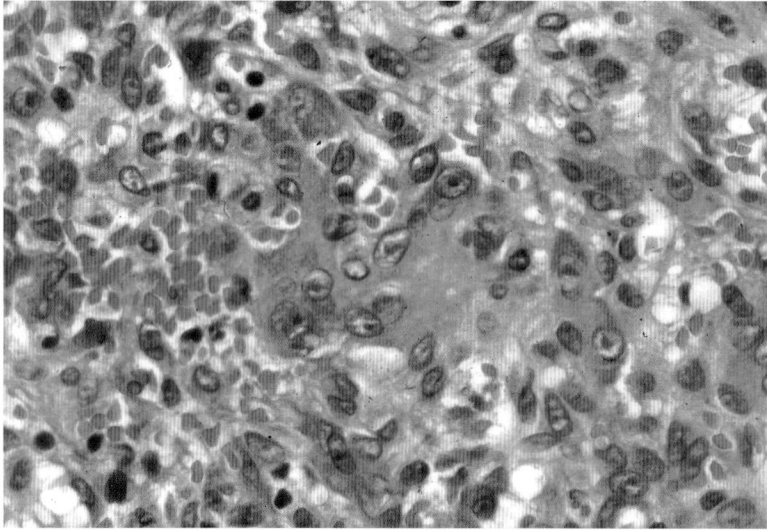

Fig. 11.107
Peripheral giant cell granuloma: multinucleated osteoclast-like giant cells, and mononuclear/monocytic cells are present.

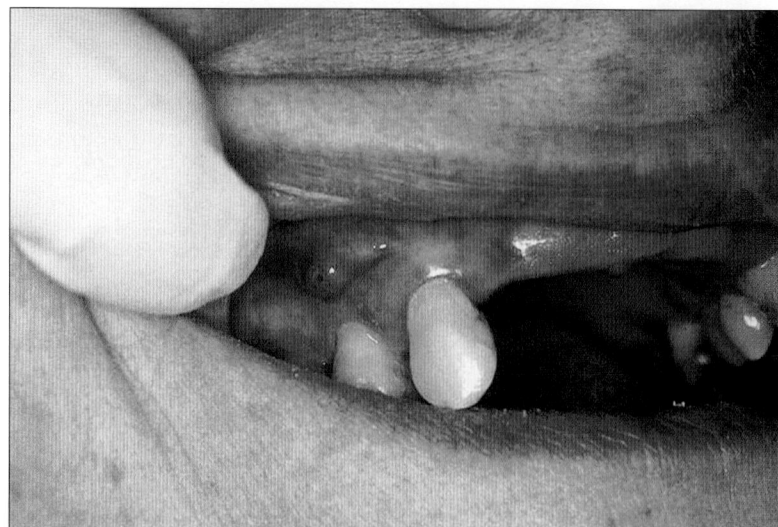

Fig. 11.108
Parulis: note the small papule with a punctum located on the nonattached gingiva, at some distance from the gingival margin.

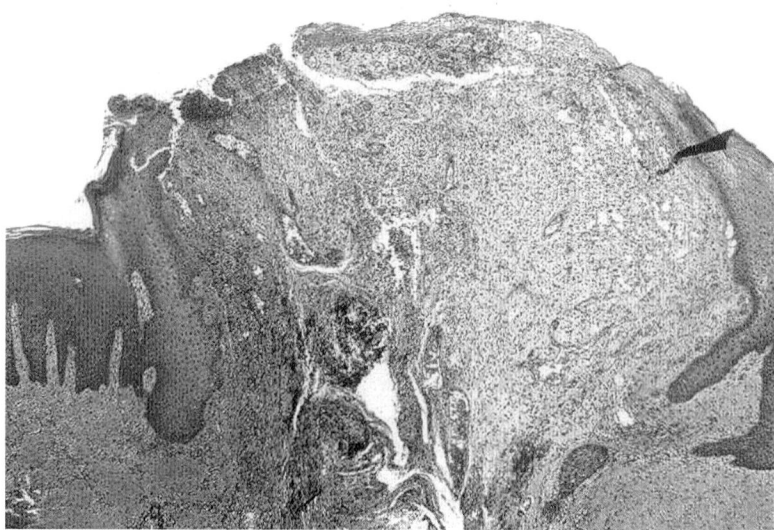

Fig. 11.109
Parulis: the papule is composed of edematous granulation tissue; a tract leads from deep in the tissues to the surface.

11.106).[7,8] The mononuclear cells have large vesicular nuclei with prominent nucleoli, and mitoses are common (*Fig. 11.107*).[9] A Grenz zone containing siderophages often separates the giant cells from an overlying intact or ulcerated epithelium.[2] A variable lymphoplasmacytic infiltrate is present. Myofibroblasts have been demonstrated, supporting the reactive nature of this lesion.[10] Foci of cemento-osseous metaplasia (peripheral ossifying fibroma) are present in one-third of cases.[9,11,12]

The giant cells and mononuclear cells express vimentin, muramidase, α_1-antitrypsin, α_1-antichymotrypsin, and CD68, typical for monocyte-phagocyte lineage.[8,13] Other studies have shown that the multinucleated giant cells stain for MBI, an osteoclast marker, as well as for receptor activator of NF-kappaB ligand and osteoprotegerin.[14,15] Estrogen but not progesterone receptors have been identified in both mononuclear and giant cells.[16]

Parulis

Clinical features

The parulis/sinus tract (or gum-boil) is a red or pink, painless papule, usually with a central punctum. It is located away from the gingival margin, usually overlying the apex of a tooth, and represents the opening of a draining sinus tract from an intraosseous odontogenic infection (*Fig. 11.108*).

Histologic features

The nodule consists of a proliferation of edematous granulation tissue containing many acute and chronic inflammatory cells and microabscesses; a tract is present usually lined by neutrophils and this may open onto the surface (*Figs 11.109* and *11.110*).

Differential diagnosis

Although this lesion bears a superficial resemblance to a mucocele, no mucin or muciphages are present. Mucoceles almost never occur on the gingiva since salivary gland tissue is absent at this site.

Gingival cyst of the adult

Clinical findings

This lesion occurs in the fifth decade with an equal sex distribution. Three-quarters occur in the mandibular buccal gingiva, mainly in the cuspid/

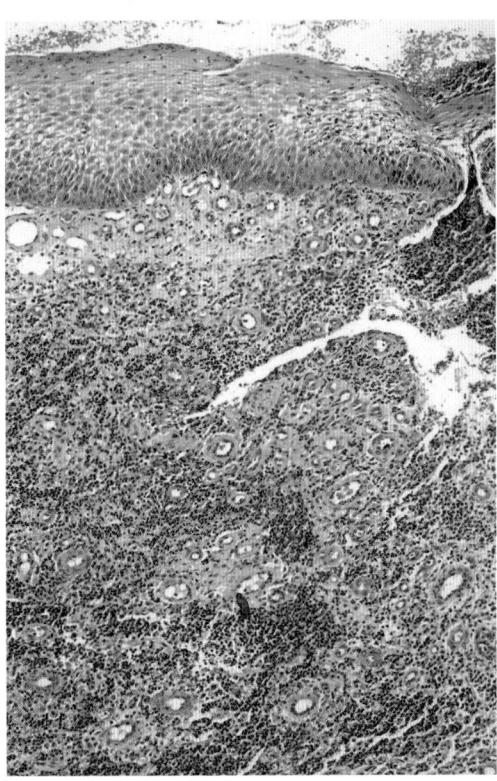

Fig. 11.110
Parulis: there is granulation tissue containing many acute and chronic inflammatory cells and a tract lined by and containing neutrophils.

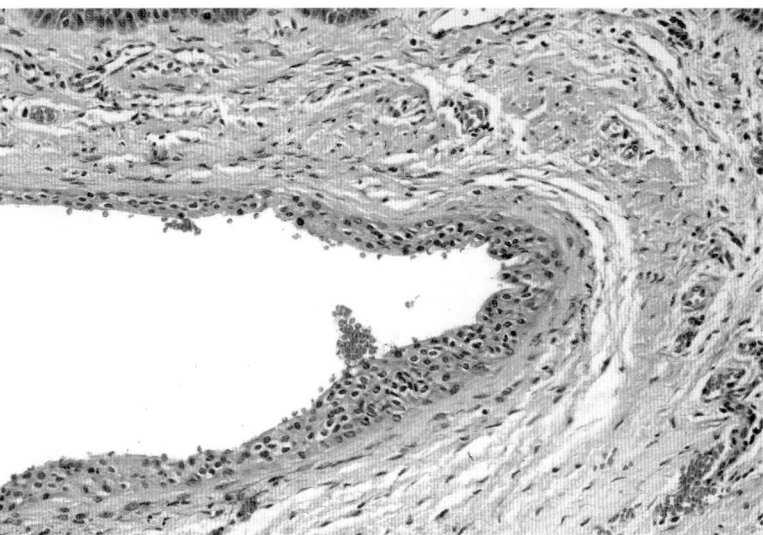

Fig. 11.112
Gingival cyst: the cyst is lined by three to ten layers of squamous or low cuboidal cells.

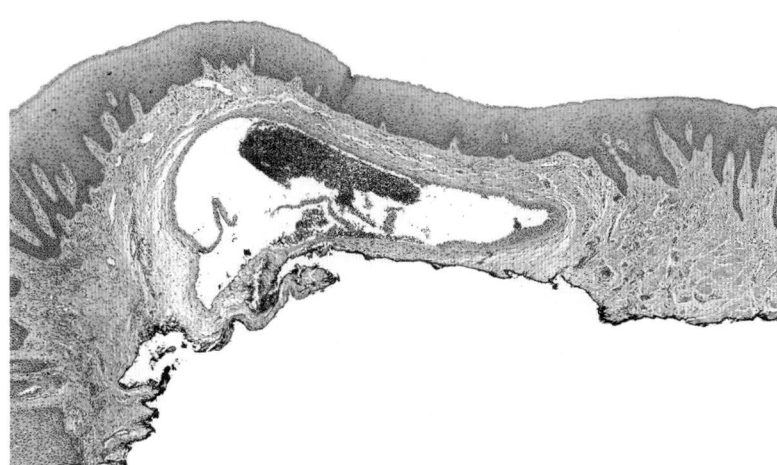

Fig. 11.111
Gingival cyst: note thinly lined cyst in the lamina propria.

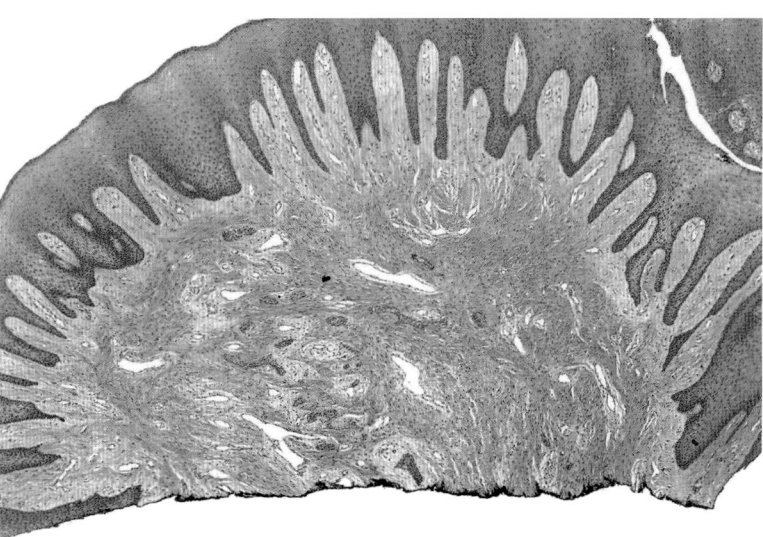

Fig. 11.113
Peripheral odontogenic fibroma: islands and strands of odontogenic epithelium are present in a mass of fibrous tissue.

bicuspid region. It presents as a bluish nodule, usually measuring less than 1 cm in diameter.[1–3]

Pathogenesis and histologic features

The gingival cyst is likely to arise from stimulated rests of dental lamina (a residuum of odontogenesis) that undergo cystic degeneration.[2,4,5]

The cyst is usually lined by nonkeratinized epithelium, either low cuboidal or squamous, 2–5 cells thick (*Figs 11.111* and *11.112*). Focal epithelial plaques (sometimes with a morular appearance) are present in approximately one-third of cases, some of which contain clear cells.[1–3] Occasional lesions represent peripheral odontogenic keratocysts with a thin epithelial lining 5–10 cells thick, corrugated parakeratin, and palisading of the basal cell nuclei.[6,7] Extraosseous extension of an intraosseous keratocyst must be ruled out.

Differential diagnosis

In children, dental lamina cysts of the newborn occur on the alveolar ridge (especially maxillary) and are almost always filled with keratin, resembling

milia.[8] If the cyst contains oncocytic cells, it is much more likely to be a salivary duct cyst. Salivary gland lesions do not occur in the gingiva (which does not contain salivary gland tissue), although they may extend onto the gingiva from the maxillary or mandibular vestibule.

Peripheral odontogenic fibroma

Clinical features

The preferred site for this tumor is the gingiva of the mandibular premolar/cuspid and anterior maxillary regions.[1] It mainly occurs in adults in the third decade with an equal sex predilection. Recurrence varies from 3% to 50%.[1–3]

Histologic features

The nodule consists of a proliferation of fibrous tissue that may be densely or loosely collagenous and variably hypercellular or hypocellular. More typically, the stroma has a whorled, streaming, or fasciculated pattern.[2,4,5] Islands, strands, and nests of odontogenic epithelium are present to a variable extent (*Figs 11.113* and *11.114*). Epithelial cells may have clear cytoplasm or be squamous, and hyaline cuffs are sometimes seen around the

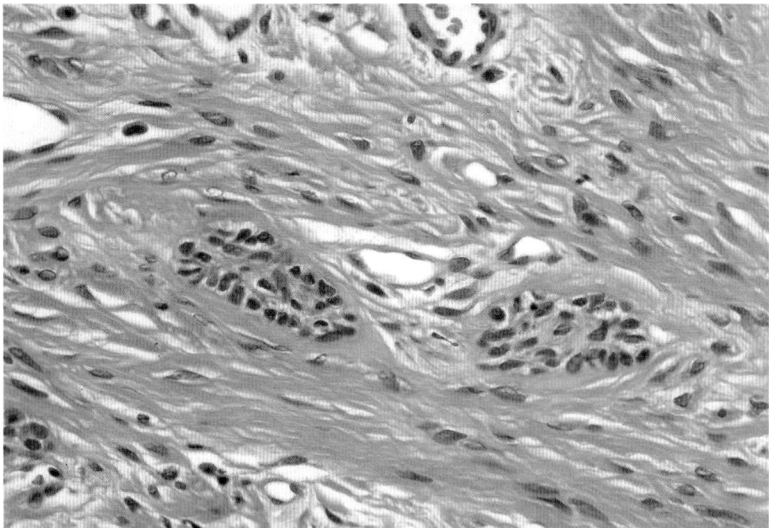

Fig. 11.114
Peripheral odontogenic fibroma: islands of squamous epithelium show a hint of palisading of the peripheral nuclei, typical for odontogenic epithelium.

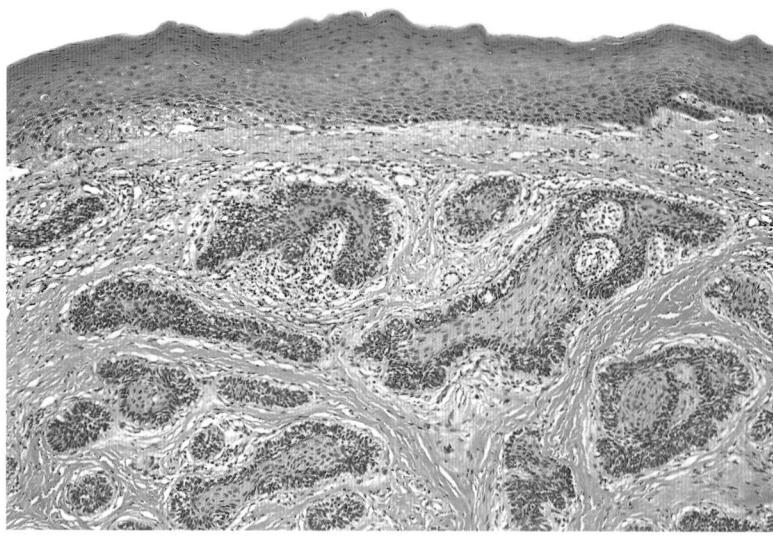

Fig. 11.116
Peripheral ameloblastoma (follicular pattern): islands or follicles of epithelium with palisading of the basal cells are present in the lamina propria without continuity with the overlying epithelium.

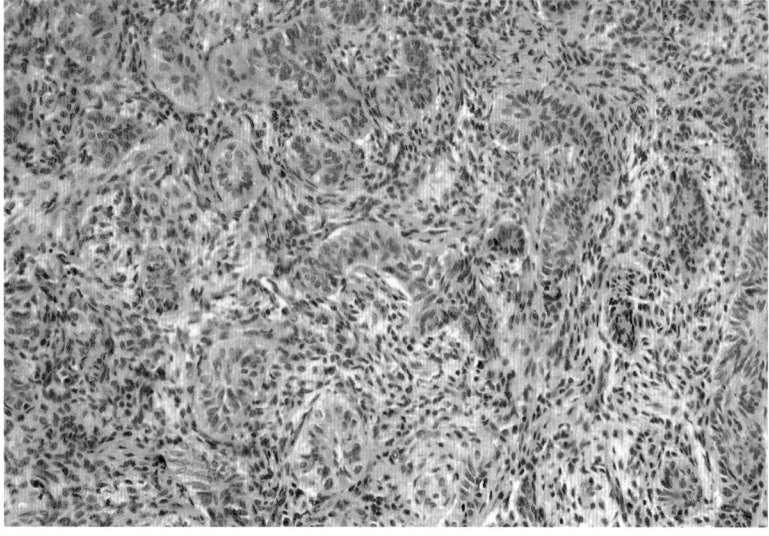

Fig. 11.115
Peripheral odontogenic fibroma: note the abundance of epithelium in this lesion. By courtesy of T. Daley, DDS, Winnipeg, Ontario, Canada.

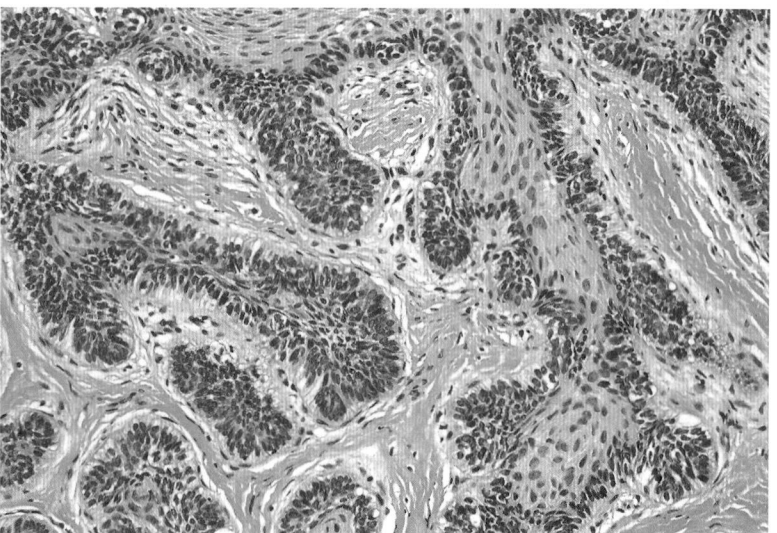

Fig. 11.117
Peripheral ameloblastoma (follicular pattern): the tumor islands exhibit palisading and reverse polarization of the basal cell nuclei; the center of the islands contain squamous cells.

epithelium (the so-called 'inductive effect'). Calcifications are present in 33–60% of cases and take four forms: dentinoid, globular cementum-like calcifications, osteoid, or dystrophic calcifications.[1–3,5,6] When epithelium is abundant, the term 'odontogenic gingival epithelial hamartoma' has been applied (*Fig. 11.115*).[7] The presence of giant cells has also been reported in up to 8% of cases.[3,8] If the stroma contains granular cells, the diagnosis is more appropriately peripheral granular cell odontogenic tumor.[9]

Differential diagnosis

Lack of significant atypia distinguishes this lesion from metastatic carcinoma, although it must be borne in mind that many malignant glandular and/or adnexal tumors can sometimes show minimal pleomorphism.

Peripheral odontogenic fibroma is the most common peripheral odontogenic tumor and should also be distinguished from other odontogenic tumors that may present on the gingiva.[10] The peripheral ameloblastoma is usually follicular in pattern and contains many large islands of odontogenic epithelium with palisading and reverse polarization of the basal cell nuclei, resembling a basal cell carcinoma; the tumor islands may show stellate

reticulum-like cells or be acanthomatous (*Figs 11.116* and *11.117*).[11,12] Mutations of *BRAF V600E* and SMO are seen in approximately 60% and 40% of cases of mandibular and maxillary intraosseous ameloblastoma, respectively[13]; tumors are also often calretinin positive.[14] It is unclear if these findings apply to peripheral lesions.

Peripheral calcifying odontogenic cyst is a cyst lined by basaloid cells; ghost cells, sometimes with dystrophic calcification, are a hallmark of this lesion, and there is usually deposition of dentinoid, an eosinophilic amorphous material resembling osteoid (*Figs 11.118* and *11.119*).[15,16] Expression of β-catenin is present in 90–100% of cases.[17,18] The counterpart of this lesion on the skin is the calcifying epithelioma of Malherbe (pilomatrixoma). A solid variant called the dentinogenic ghost cell tumor has a predominance of ghost cells and dentinoid with similar basaloid cells but is not cystic.[19]

Peripheral calcifying epithelial odontogenic tumor consists of large polyhedral cells with eosinophilic cytoplasm associated with amyloid deposits and usually, but not invariably, dystrophic calcification; nuclear pleomorphism is a frequent finding, and a clear cell variant exists (*Fig. 11.120*).[20–22]

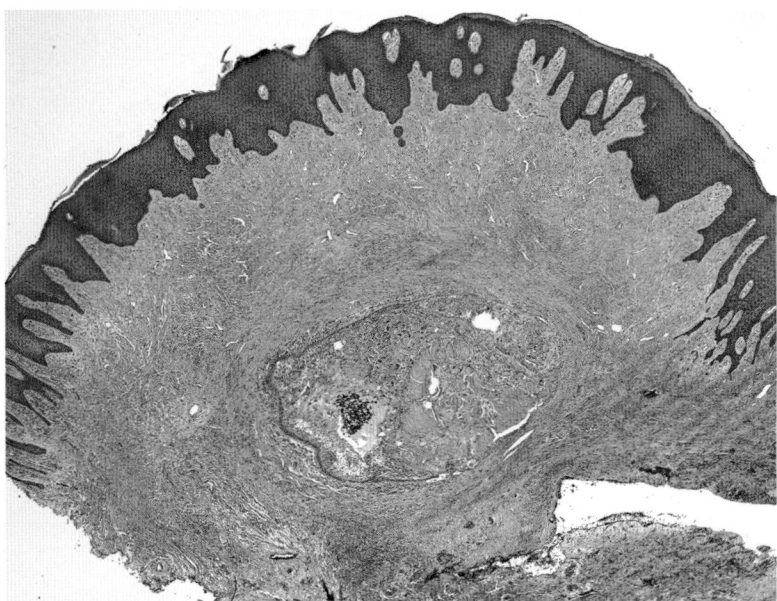

Fig. 11.118
Peripheral calcifying cystic odontogenic tumor: the tumor is composed of basaloid cells and calcified material within the lamina propria of the gingiva.

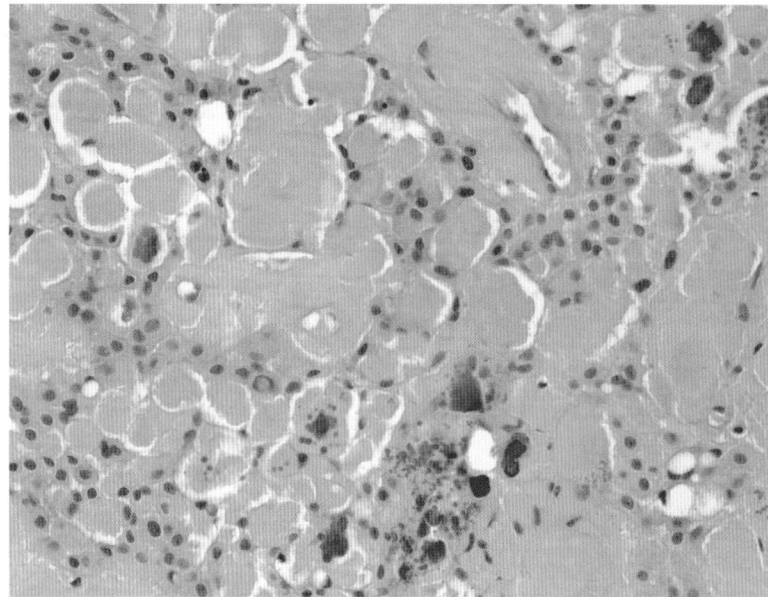

Fig. 11.120
Calcifying epithelial odontogenic tumor: there are strands of epithelium with slightly atypical nuclei, amyloid, and dystrophic calcifications.

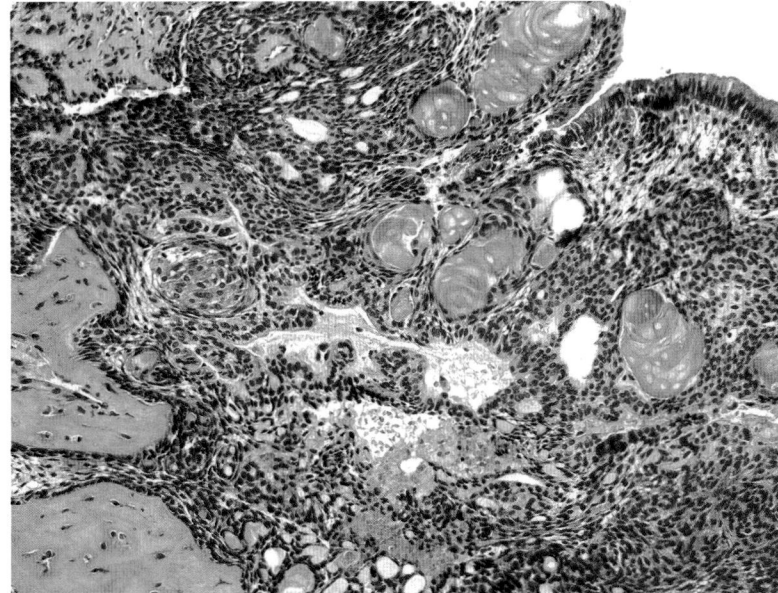

Fig. 11.119
Peripheral calcifying cystic odontogenic tumor: there is a proliferation of basaloid cells with ghost cells and dentinoid (left)

Generalized gingival hyperplasia

Clinical features

In this condition, multiple and usually all quadrants of the upper and lower gingiva are involved, initially by nodular hyperplasia in the interdental areas, which then become coalescent to form diffuse nodular/papillary masses. The gingiva may be edematous, boggy, and erythematous, or it can be firm, fibrotic, and so proliferative as to reach the biting surfaces. Most cases are inflamed and bleed readily such as with toothbrushing. Aggravating factors include:

• poor oral hygiene (*Fig. 11.121*),
• hormonal influences (during puberty and pregnancy),
• ingestion of medications, in particular phenytoin, valproic acid, calcium channel blockers, and ciclosporin (*Fig. 11.122*).

Such overgrowths are rare in edentulous patients, and if the teeth are extracted, the lesions do not recur, pointing to the role plaque bacteria plays

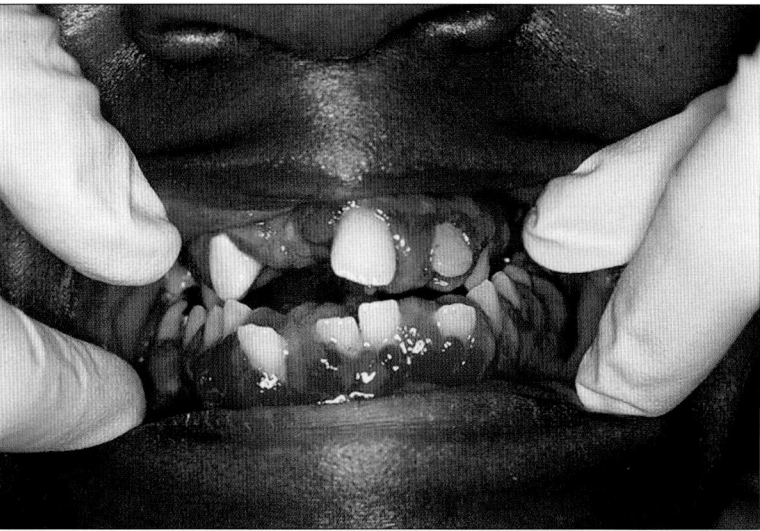

Fig. 11.121
Generalized gingival hyperplasia: this overgrowth of gingiva was caused by poor oral hygiene.

in their pathogenesis.[1–3] In general, good oral hygiene measures reduce the severity of disease.

Gingival hyperplasia occurs in approximately 50% of patients taking phenytoin,[4,5] 15–40% of patients taking nifedipine,[3,6] and 25–70% of patients on ciclosporin.[7–9] Renal transplant patients taking both ciclosporin and nifedipine show greater gingival overgrowth than those taking ciclosporin alone.[10] Of all calcium channel blockers, nifedipine and those of the hydropyridine class are most likely to cause gingival hyperplasia. Verapamil causes hyperplasia in 4% and amlodipine in 3% of cases, which is probably not significantly different from patients not taking these medications.[11,12]

Several cases of ciclosporin-induced fibrous hyperplasias/pyogenic granulomas of extragingival sites have been reported in patients treated for chronic graft-versus-host disease (*Fig. 11.123*).[13–15] It is, however, unusual to see significant gingival hyperplasia in patients taking ciclosporin for treatment of chronic graft-versus-host disease.

Pathogenesis and histologic features

Gingival hyperplasia caused by ciclosporin (the most widely studied of all the drugs) results from accumulation of collagen and extracellular matrix

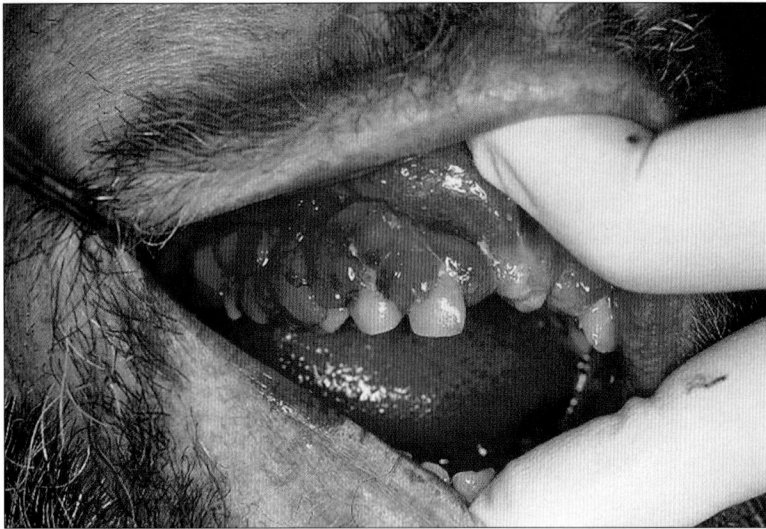

Fig. 11.122
Ciclosporin-induced gingival hyperplasia: this patient was taking ciclosporin to prevent rejection of a renal allograft as well as nifedipine, a calcium channel blocker, for hypertension.

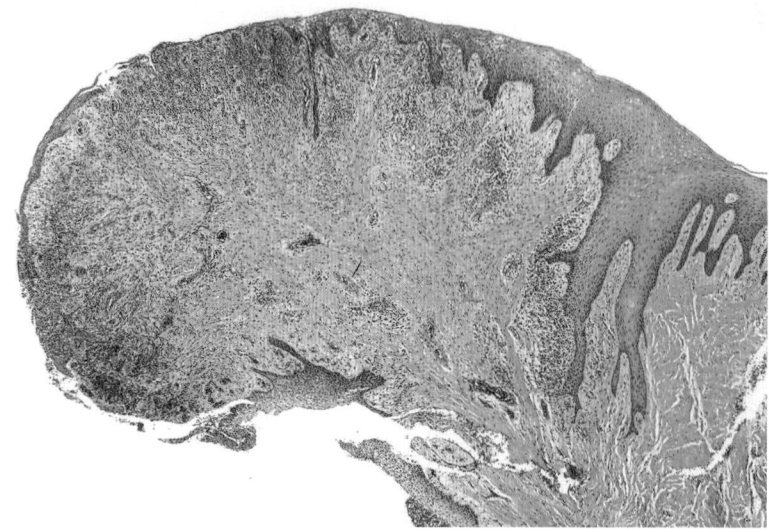

Fig. 11.124
Inflammatory fibrous hyperplasia: the histology is similar to that of the solitary gingival nodules of similar etiology.

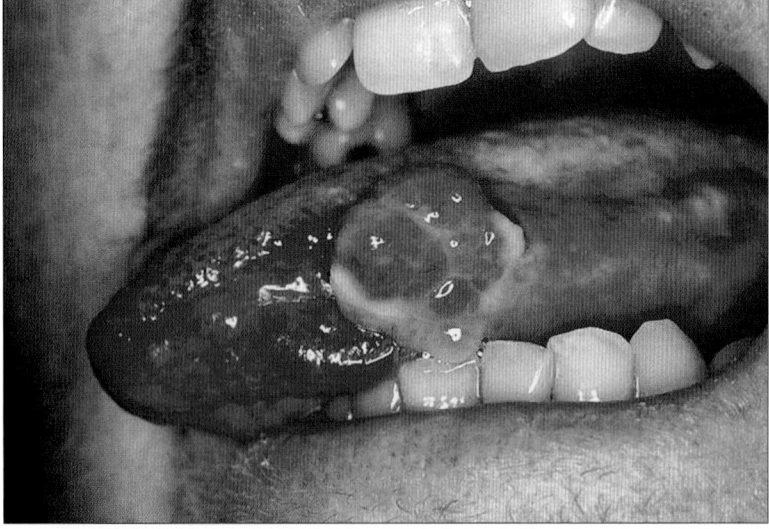

Fig. 11.123
Ciclosporin-induced nongingival hyperplasia: this patient was taking ciclosporin for treatment of chronic graft-versus-host disease after allogeneic bone marrow transplantation.

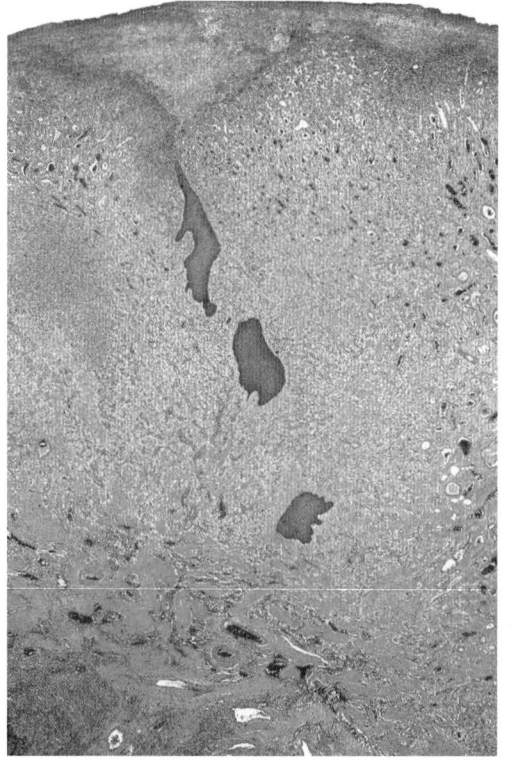

Fig. 11.125
Ciclosporin-induced nongingival hyperplasia: these are essentially polypoid masses of granulation tissue similar to pyogenic granuloma.

as a consequence of either increased production from susceptible subpopulations of fibroblasts in the gingiva, or else, decreased degradation.[16,17] Calcium homeostasis is an important pharmacodynamic feature of these drugs, and it has been postulated that impairment of calcium-dependent mechanisms (such as collagenase and metalloproteinase activity) plays an important etiological role. Ciclosporin upregulates the activity of TGF-β1, a potent cytokine involved in collagen homeostasis.[18,19] A recent study suggest that medications inhibit cellular folate uptake resulting in decreased collagenase activity and matrix degradation.[20]

Histologically, there is proliferation of fibrous tissue and ground substance with variable hyperplasia of fibroblasts. The epithelium may also be hyperplastic, and there is often a lymphoplasmacytic infiltrate and vascular ectasia (*Fig. 11.124*). Straight-sided 'test tube' rete ridges have been reported in such drug-induced gingival hyperplasias but this is not a specific finding.[6,7,21] There may also be foci that appear myxoid/mucinous.

In ciclosporin-induced nongingival lesions, the tumors are essentially inflammatory fibrovascular polyps that are extensively ulcerated and composed of edematous granulation tissue with varying degrees of inflammation; some resemble pyogenic granulomas (*Figs 11.125* and *11.126*).[13–15]

Ultrastructural studies show an increase in cytoplasmic volume of fibroblasts with more extensive rough endoplasmic reticulum and Golgi complexes, reflecting increased synthetic activity and concomitant reduction in phagocytic activity of fibroblasts.[22,23] Increased numbers of fibroblasts exhibiting secretory granules filled with sulfated mucopolysaccharides have been noted.[24] Myofibroblasts are present in increased numbers.[25]

Differential diagnosis

One unusual form of gingival hyperplasia is seen in ligneous (pseudomembranous or membranous) conjunctivitis, an autosomal recessive disorder leading to functional plasminogen deficiency and compromised extravascular fibrin clearance during wound healing, resulting in pseudomembranes of fibrin in the conjunctiva, gingiva, and other mucosal sites.[26–28] The gingiva and other mucosal sites develop painless coalescent waxy nodules similar to those on the conjunctiva.[29–31] This condition may occur after systemic

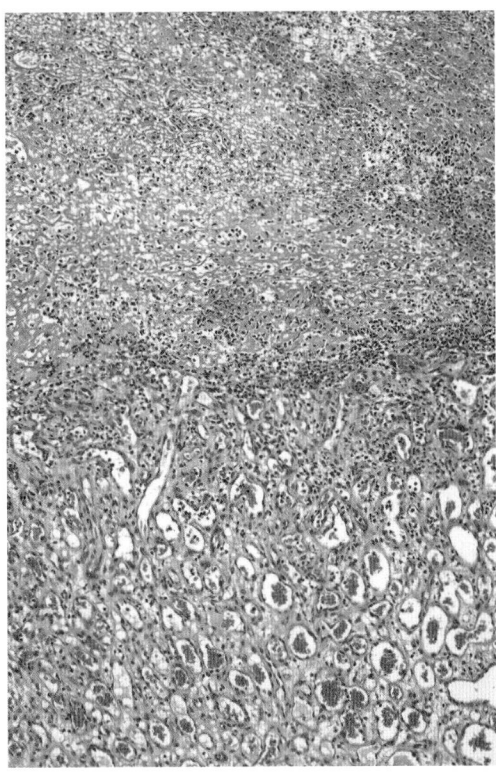

Fig. 11.126
Ciclosporin-induced nongingival hyperplasia: note the edematous granulation tissue and inflammation.

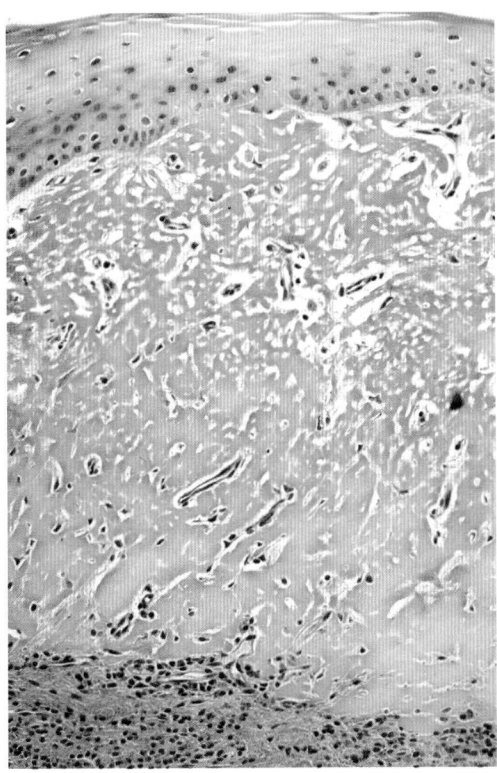

Fig. 11.127
Ligneous gingivitis: there is abundant fibrinous eosinophilic material that fills the lamina propria.

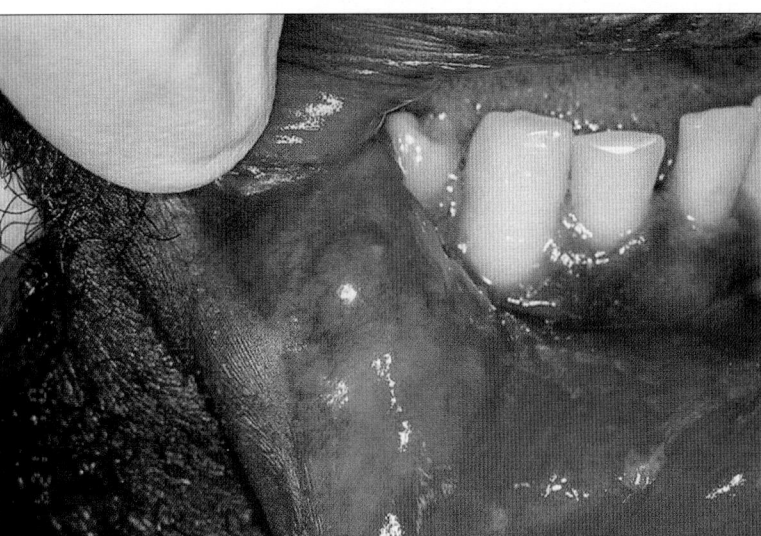

Fig. 11.128
Varix: note the blue bleb on the lower lip mucosa.

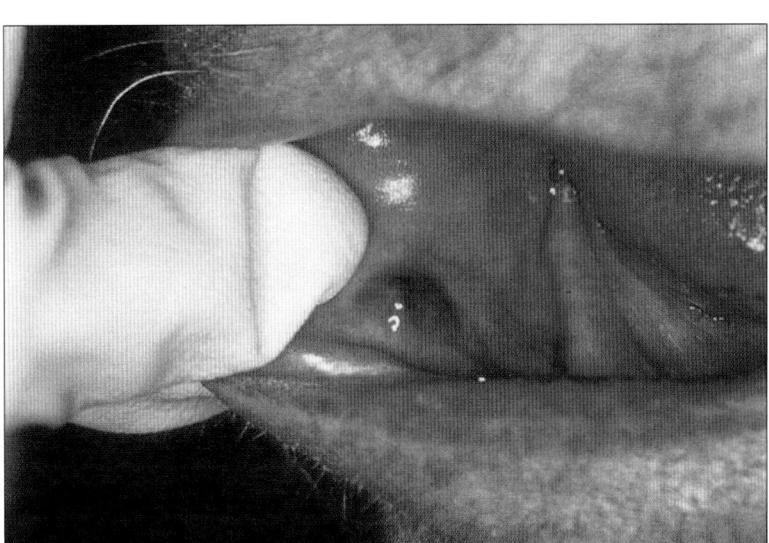

Fig. 11.129
Varix: note the blue bleb on the buccal mucosa.

tranexamic acid (an antifibrinolytic agent) therapy.[32] In ligneous or membranous gingival hyperplasia, the lamina propria is filled with eosinophilic, PAS-positive amorphous material that stains with MSB phosphotungstic acid-hematoxylin typical for fibrin (*Fig. 11.127*).[28,29] Stains for amyloid are negative. Early lesions show fibrin deposits around blood vessels.

Accumulations of eosinophilic material in the gingiva may be seen in lipoid proteinosis (hyalinosis cutis et mucosae); these deposits do not stain for fibrinogen or fibrin, and there is usually involvement of the skin and other sites.[33,34] Similar amyloid-like material may sometimes be seen in the buccal mucosa (but not usually in the gingiva) of patients who use snuff.

Varix and vascular malformation

Clinical features

Varices (or venous lakes) are most commonly seen in older individuals on the ventral surfaces of the tongue (sublingual varicosities) and on the lower lip and buccal mucosa (*Figs 11.128* and *11.129*).[1-3] They are bluish-purple blebs that are usually less than 1 cm in size, that may become firm and painful if thrombosed.

Histologic features

A varix represents a dilatation of an endothelium-lined venule (usually post-capillary) with a muscular wall of variable thickness, usually confined to the lamina propria (*Figs 11.130* and *11.131*).[4] Some develop thrombi or even a Masson tumor (intravascular papillary endothelial hyperplasia) (*Fig. 11.132*).[5] Larger lesions that present within deeper structures such as the muscle of the tongue are likely to represent small venous malformations although in the past, they have been referred to as cavernous hemangiomas.[6]

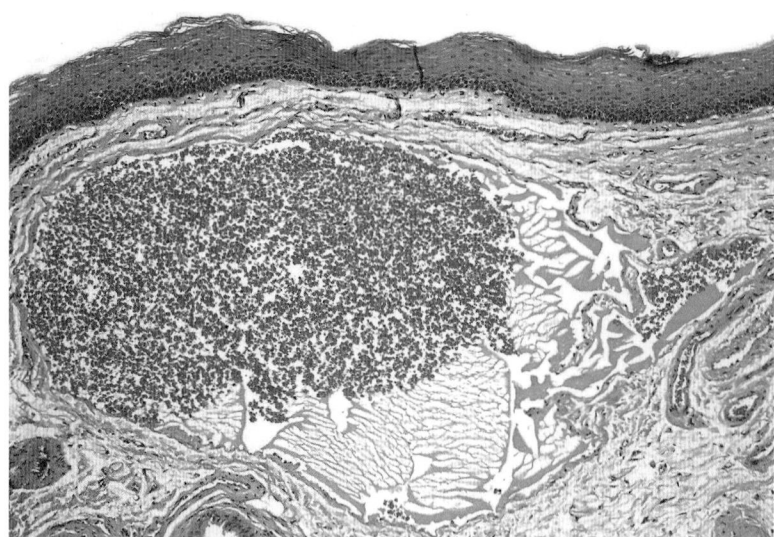

Fig. 11.130
Varix: there is a grossly dilated venule in the lamina propria.

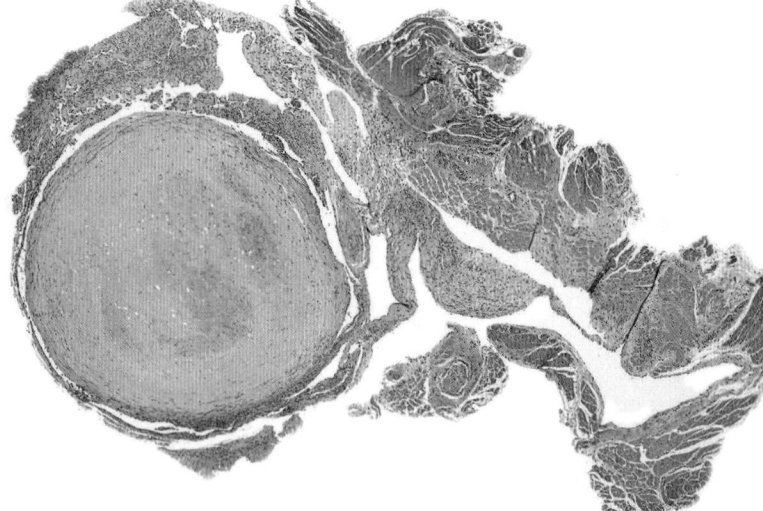

Fig. 11.131
Varix with thrombus: thrombosis is frequently seen within a varix.

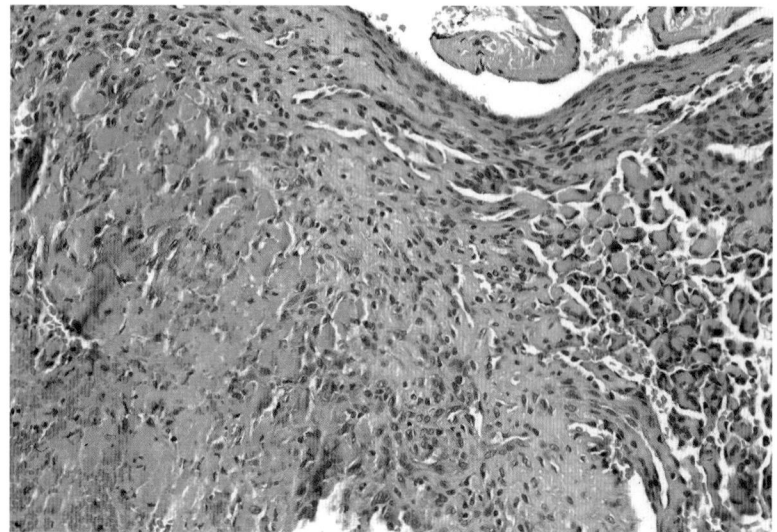

Fig. 11.132
Varix with organizing thrombus: there is intravascular papillary endothelial hyperplasia (right) within this organizing thrombus.

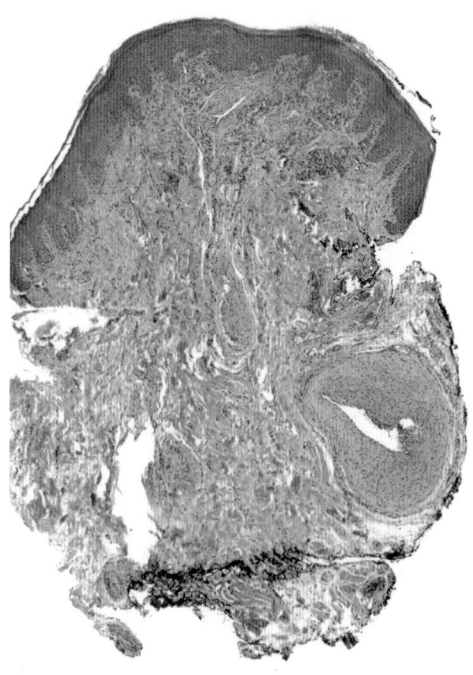

Fig. 11.133
Caliber-persistent artery: this labial artery is superficially located.

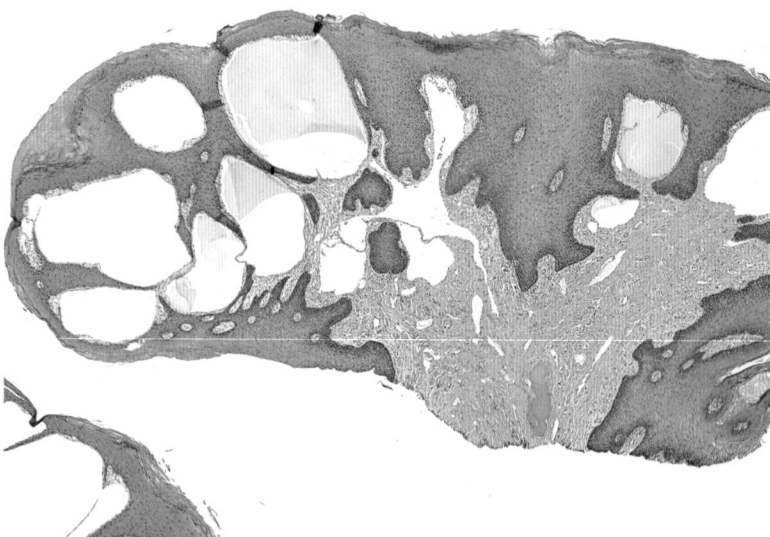

Fig. 11.134
Lymphangioma circumscriptum: there are dilated lymphatic channels filled with lymph that abut the surface epithelium.

Differential diagnosis

The caliber-persistent labial artery (a pulsatile lesion more often of the lower lip) consists of an artery that lies close to the surface epithelium with an artery diameter/depth ratio of less than 1.6 (*Fig. 11.133*).[7,8] These putatively represent arterial branches from the labial artery that are present within the superficial mucosa without loss of caliber.[8,9] Lymphangioma circumscriptum or lymphatic malformations are lined by a single layer of endothelial cells and are filled with lymph, and usually abut the surface epithelium (*Fig. 11.134*).

INFECTIONS

Median rhomboid glossitis

Clinical features

Median rhomboid glossitis is a form of oral candidiasis that occurs specifically in the midline of the tongue just anterior to the circumvallate papillae (*Fig. 11.135*).[1-3]

It is unclear why this particular area of the tongue is predisposed to candidiasis.

Histologic features

There is parakeratosis and psoriasiform epithelial hyperplasia with spongiotic pustules associated with candidal organisms (*Figs 11.136* and *11.137*). The identification of the median raphe, a densely hyalinized fibrous band within the lamina propria, confirms that the tissue is from the midline of the tongue (*Fig. 11.138*).

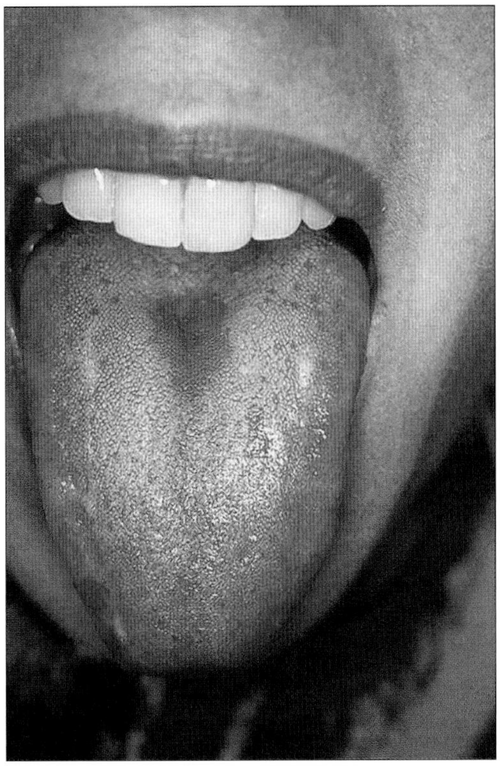

Hairy leukoplakia

Clinical features

Hairy leukoplakia is an Epstein-Barr virus infection of the oral epithelium that was first described in the HIV-infected population.[1] It may also be seen in other immunocompromised patients who are susceptible to opportunistic viral infections or reactivations, such as organ transplant recipients,[2-5] as well as increasingly, in apparently healthy individuals.[3,6] Although the term is now entrenched in the scientific literature, 'hairy leukoplakia' as used in

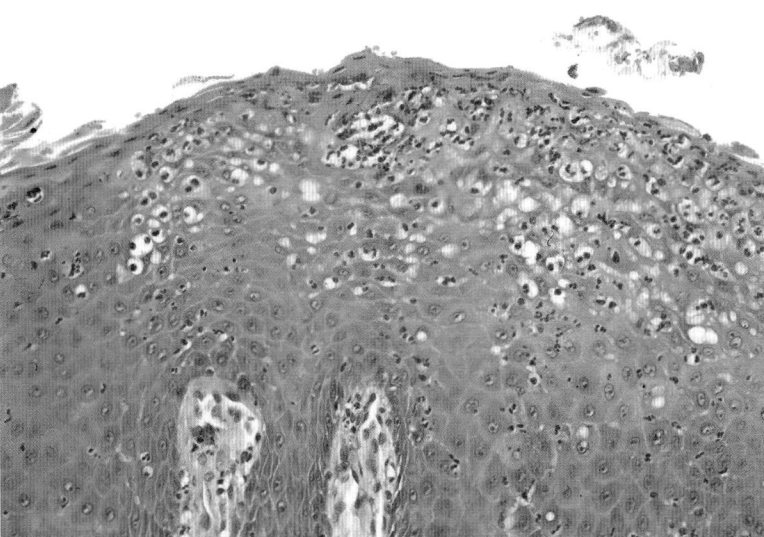

Fig. 11.135
Median rhomboid glossitis: there is an ovoid/rhomboidal-shaped area in the posterior midline of the tongue.

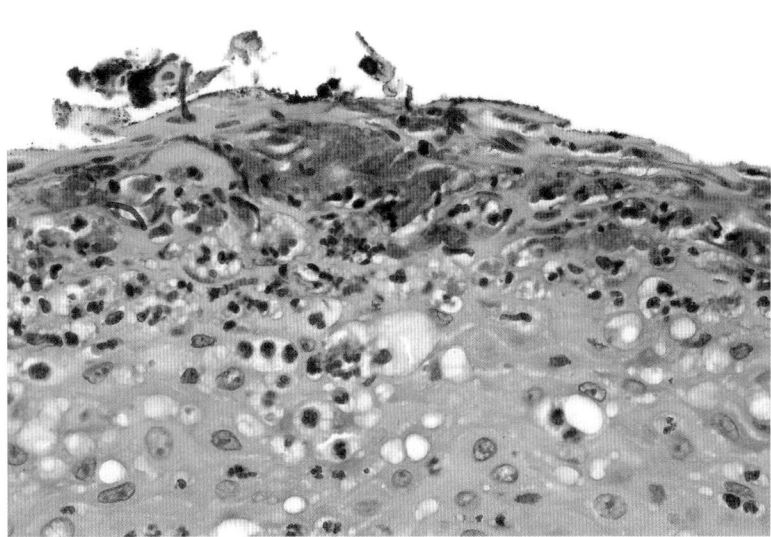

Fig. 11.137
Median rhomboid glossitis: *Candida* pseudo-hyphae are present with the PAS stain with diastase digestion.

Fig. 11.136
Median rhomboid glossitis: many spongiotic pustules are present.

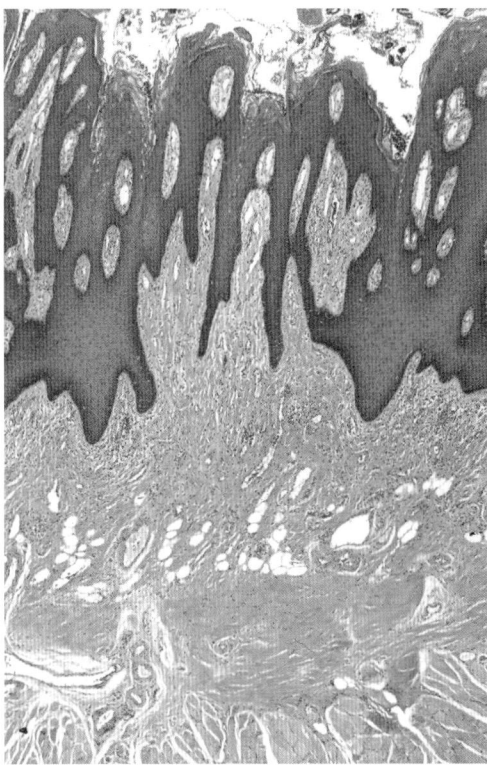

Fig. 11.138
Median rhomboid glossitis: there is psoriasiform epithelial hyperplasia and a dense median raphe just above the muscle fibers.

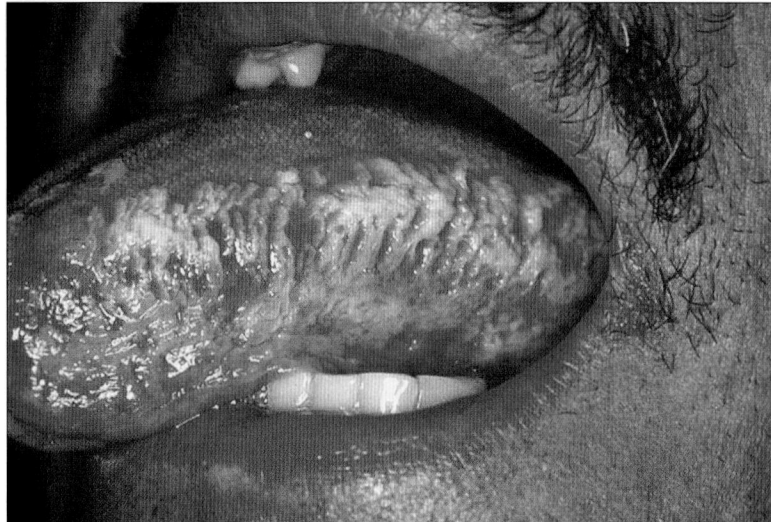

Fig. 11.139
Hairy leukoplakia: there is a thick white plaque on the lateral border of the tongue with vertical fissures.

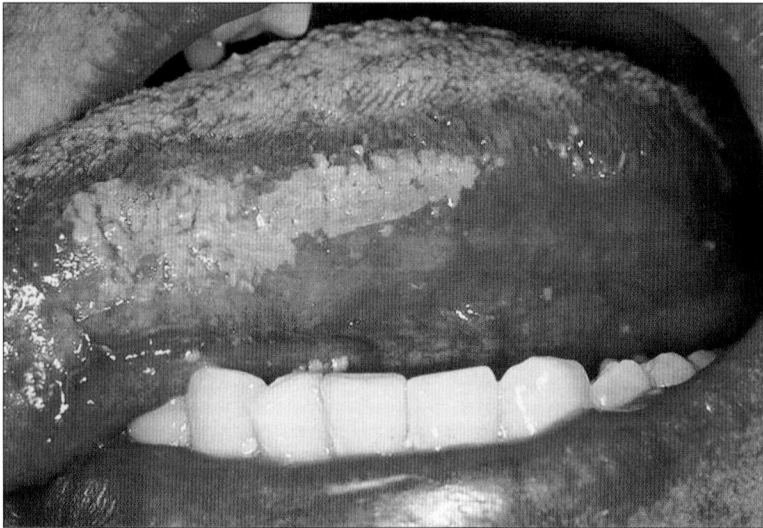

Fig. 11.140
Hairy leukoplakia: this white plaque does not have vertical fissures.

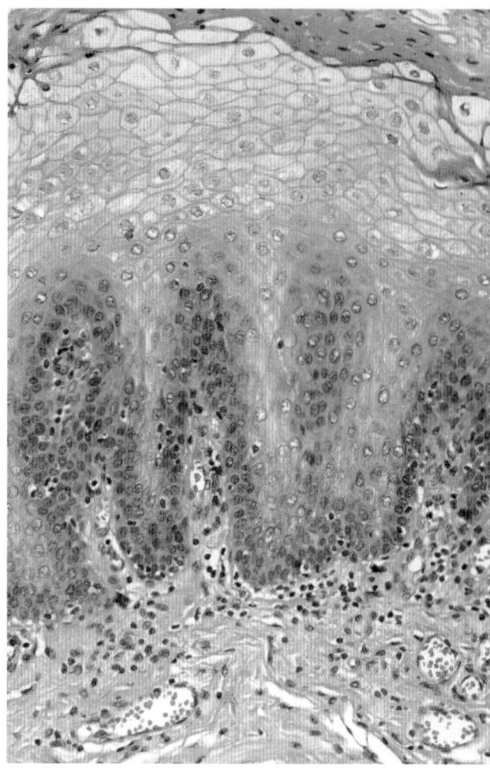

Fig. 11.141
Hairy leukoplakia: note the thick parakeratin and, importantly, the vacuolated virally infected cells just beneath.

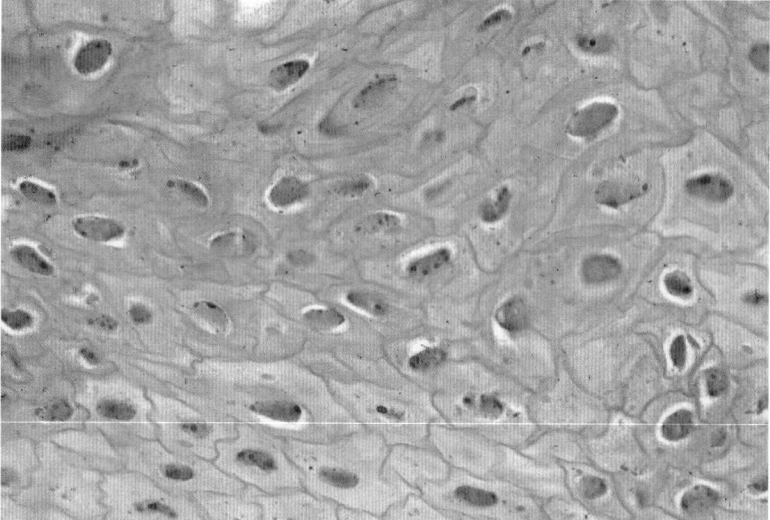

Fig. 11.142
Hairy leukoplakia: note condensation of chromatin in a beaded pattern against the nuclear membrane and central amphophilic Cowdry inclusion.

this condition does not connote an increased risk for development of dysplasia or squamous cell carcinoma as is the case for true leukoplakia.

The majority of cases (>70%) occur bilaterally on the lateral border of the tongue as a white, corrugated (hence 'hairy') plaque that in early lesions has vertical fissures running perpendicular to the long axis of the tongue (*Figs 11.139* and *11.140*).[7,8] In the HIV positive population, appearance is associated with the development of AIDS within 3 years in one-third of patients and is an AIDS-defining lesion.[9,10]

Pathogenesis and histologic features

The oropharyngeal epithelia and lymphoid tissue are sites of persistent latent Epstein-Barr virus infection and reactivation of the virus results in hairy leukoplakia.[11,12]

Oral hairy leukoplakia is characterized by parakeratosis with a slightly shaggy surface. *Candida* hyphae are present in 80% of cases, usually unassociated with spongiotic pustules.[7,8,13,14] Beneath the keratin is a distinct band of vacuolated and ballooned cells (*Fig. 11.141*). These pale cells contain Cowdry type A amphophilic inclusions that fill the nucleus and characteristically exhibit condensation of chromatin against the nuclear membrane ('beaded effect') (*Figs 11.142* and *11.143*).[15] This morphology is readily

seen even on exfoliative cytology.[16,17] In situ hybridization studies localize Epstein-Barr virus within keratinocyte nuclei (*Fig. 11.144*).

PCR in situ hybridization studies demonstrated proteins that disrupt Epstein-Barr virus latency in all layers of the epithelium including basal cells, supporting the concept of reactivation of latent Epstein-Barr virus infection. HIV has also been identified within the keratinocytes.[12]

Although HPV was identified in hairy leukoplakia in earlier studies, more recent studies have disputed this observation.[7,12,18] Even if present, they are not likely to be transcriptionally active.

Differential diagnosis

Lesions of chronic bite keratosis may resemble hairy leukoplakia because of keratinocyte edema, but identification of Epstein-Barr virus establishes the diagnosis.

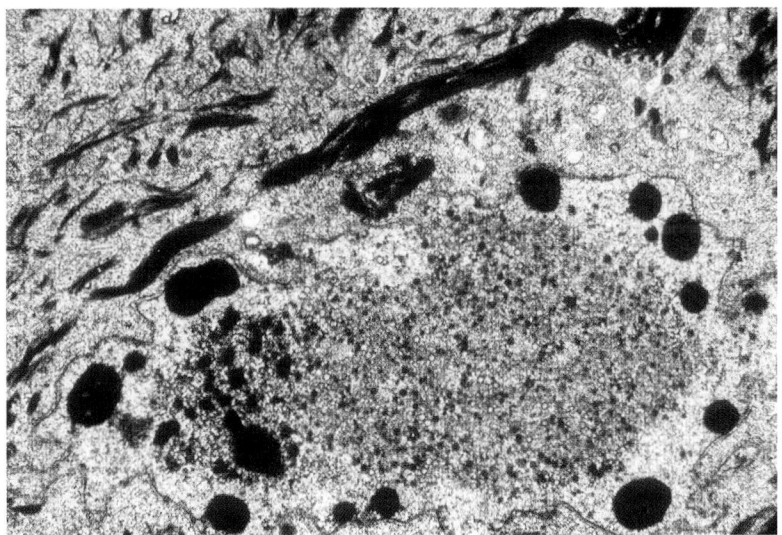

Fig. 11.143
Hairy leukoplakia: ultrastructurally, the center of the nucleus is filled with herpes virus (Cowdry inclusion) and chromatin condenses against the nuclear membrane in a bead-like pattern.

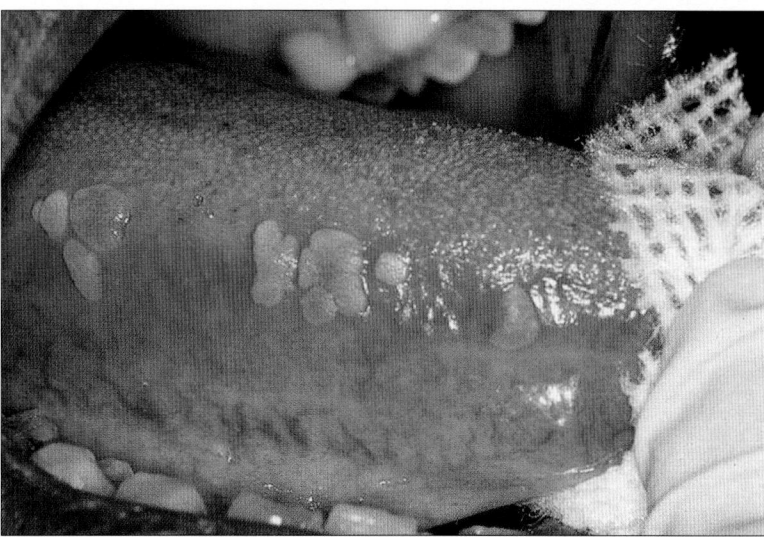

Fig. 11.145
Heck disease: the lesions present as pale, fleshy papules.

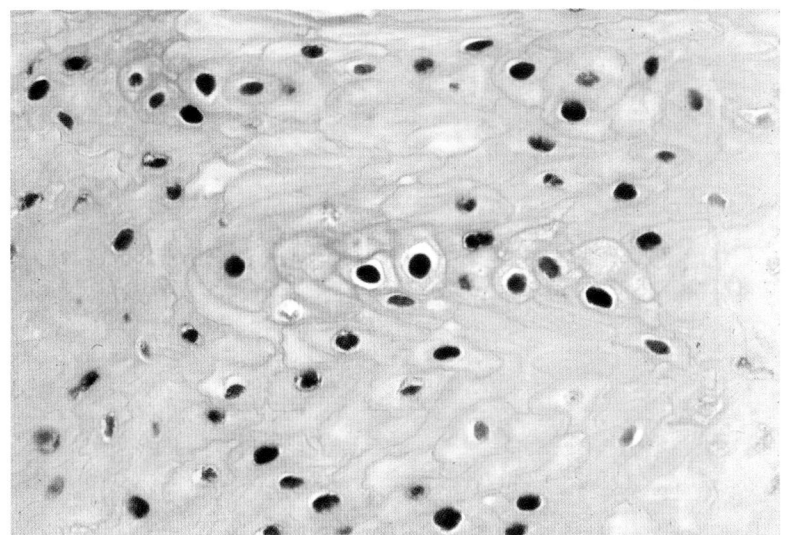

Fig. 11.144
Hairy leukoplakia: in situ hybridization reveals the presence of intranuclear Epstein-Barr virus.

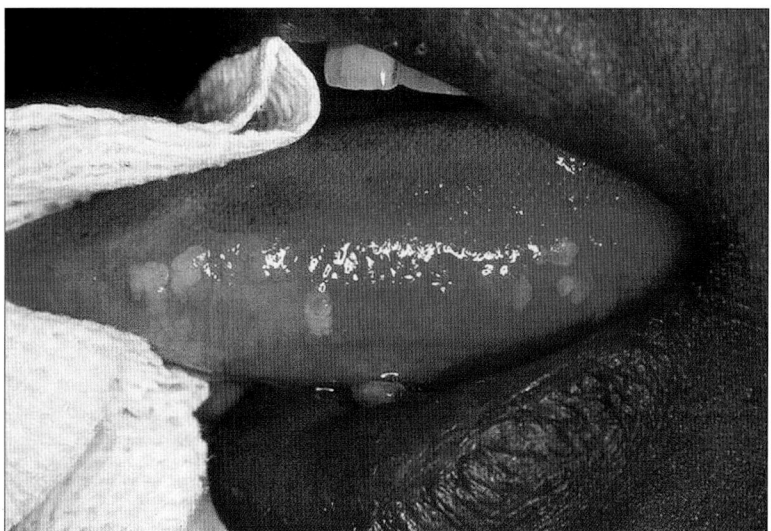

Fig. 11.146
Heck disease: typical multiple coalescent papules on the lateral tongue in this native of East Africa.

Focal epithelial hyperplasia (Heck disease)

Clinical features

Although any racial group may be affected, there is a predilection of focal epithelial hyperplasia (Heck disease, multifocal papillomavirus epithelial hyperplasia) for Native Americans of Central and South America, Inuits, and Africans. Over 90% of cases occur in the first two decades of life, and there is a prevalence of 7–13% in predisposed populations.[1-3] The condition tends to regress over time. Focal epithelial hyperplasia also occurs in patients infected with HIV.[4]

Lesions are almost always multiple and multifocal, favoring the labial mucosa, lips, buccal mucosa, and lateral tongue (*Figs 11.145* and *11.146*). They are mucosal-colored papules or nodules that sometimes appear papillary.[2]

Pathogenesis and histologic features

HPV-13 has been identified in 50–100% of cases while HPV-32 was found in 60% of cases; HPV-55 has also been identified.[3,5-7]

The papule exhibits benign epithelial hyperplasia with slight parakeratosis and broad interconnected rete ridges without evidence of atypia or dysplasia; papillary architecture is not a frequent finding (*Fig. 11.147*). Koilocytes are usually present superficially. 'Mitosoid' figures are a characteristic finding within the epithelium (*Fig. 11.148*). These represent degenerated and karyorrhectic nuclei resembling mitoses and are evidence of viral cytopathic effect. They may be identified in up to 50% of original sections and are almost always present in deeper levels.[2,5,8] Brightly eosinophilic apoptotic cells with pyknotic nuclei are often present.

Differential diagnosis

Condyloma acuminatum may appear similar clinically and histologically, but generally this lesion does not contain HPV-13 and HPV-32 and 'mitosoid' bodies are not usually present. HPV-associated oral epithelial dysplasia will also exhibit 'mitosoid' bodies and apoptotic cells, but there is surrounding severe epithelial dysplasia; dysplastic epithelium is positive for p16 in a continuous band and in situ hybridization studies are positive for high-risk HPV, mainly HPV-16 (see later).

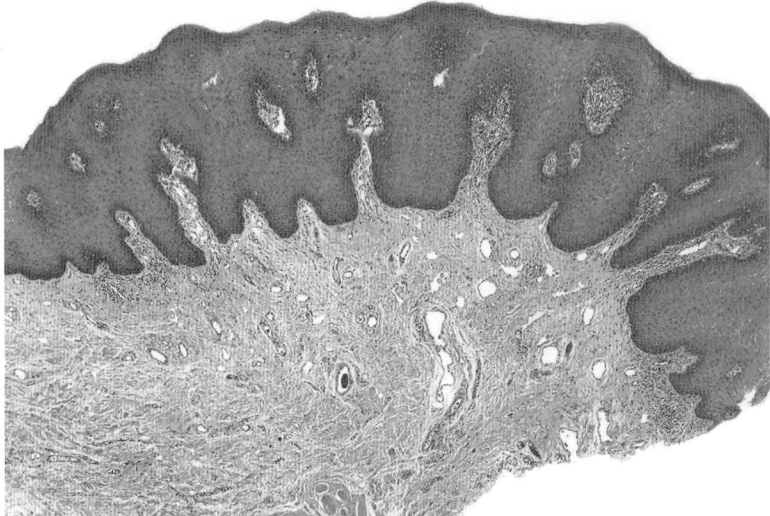

Fig. 11.147
Heck disease: there is epithelial hyperplasia with the formation of broad rete ridges, somewhat similar to a condyloma.

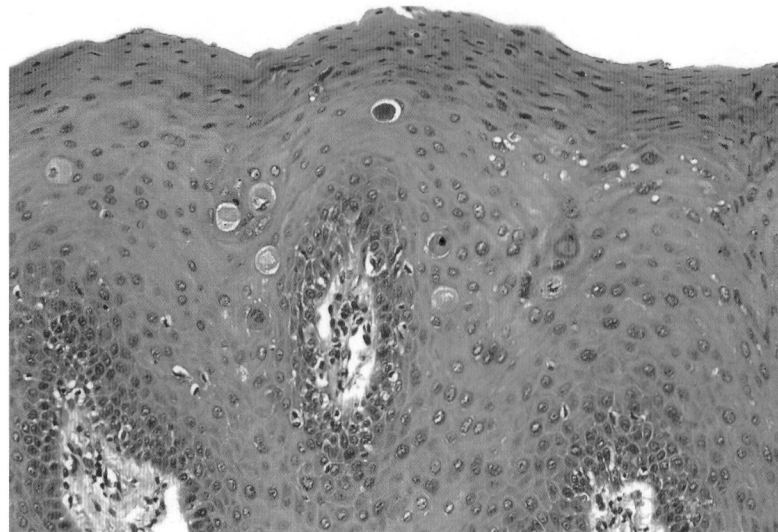

Fig. 11.148
Heck disease: there are 'mitosoid' bodies (karyorrhectic cells) and apoptotic cells.

LICHENOID AND HYPERSENSITIVITY REACTIONS

Oral lichen planus and lichenoid stomatitis

Clinical features

Oral lichen planus is a chronic inflammatory mucocutaneous disorder that affects the mouth in 1–2% of the population (range, 0.08–4.0%).[1] There is a 1.5- to 3-fold predilection for women, and most patients are in the sixth decade of life.[2-4] The buccal mucosa is affected in 80–90% of cases, followed by the tongue and the gingiva.

While the older literature described five to six clinical variants, they can be grouped simply into three main categories:

- Keratotic reticular and/or papular oral lichen planus presenting with classic lacy white keratotic striations (Wickham striae). Annular, papular, and linear variants may also be seen. This variant tends to be non or only mildly symptomatic (*Fig. 11.149*).
- Erythematous (or erosive) oral lichen planus presenting as variably symptomatic reddened mucosa. Because the mouth is a trauma-intense environment, bullae or vesicles of bullous lichen planus are rarely seen. Any blisters that develop rupture quickly giving rise to erythematous and erosive lesions. An important erythematous variant presents clinically as 'desquamative gingivitis' with a diffusely red/eroded gingiva (*Fig. 11.150*).[5-7]
- Ulcerative lichen planus presents with a yellow fibrinous exudate on the surface and is almost always painful (*Fig. 11.151*).

Oral lichen planus often presents with a combination of the above clinical manifestations and may also change from one presentation to another over time.[8] From epidemiological studies, reticular lesions are the most common, especially on the buccal mucosa, whereas in studies from referral centers, the erythematous and ulcerative forms predominate because they tend to be symptomatic. Similarly, the skin is reportedly involved in approximately 5% of cases in epidemiological studies and 20–40% at referral centers.[2,3,9] Concurrent involvement of the gingiva with erosive oral lichen planus and lesions affecting the female or male genitalia is known as the gingival-genital syndrome associated with a HLA-DQB1*0201; these patients may also experience involvement of other mucosal sites such as the esophagus, and scarring is often a feature.[10-13] Spontaneous remission occurs in approximately 7% of cases.[2]

Plaque-type lesions resembling leukoplakia should be considered conventional leukoplakia arising in association with oral lichen planus. The rate for malignant transformation varies from 0% to 12.5%, but many reports with the higher rate did not correct for tobacco usage as a confounding factor.[2,3,14,15] The true risk is probably in the order of 0.1–1.5%.[16] Some authors believe that plaque-type disease has a higher association with malignancy while others believe erosive lesions are particularly susceptible. One explanation for the confusion is that erythro-leukoplakia, also a red and white lesion (see below) which has a high prevalence of dysplasia and high malignant transformation rate, often shows a lichenoid inflammatory infiltrate on biopsy, and clinicians equate this lichenoid infiltrate in the pathology report with clinical lichen planus. Lesions of proliferative leukoplakia and proliferative erythroleukoplakia have also been misdiagnosed clinically as lichen planus for the same reasons. As such, correlating the clinical presentation of bilateral, symmetric, and reticulated lesions with the histopathology is essential.

Pathogenesis and histologic features

Local factors that may induce oral lichen planus or oral lichenoid lesions include contact lichenoid reactions to mercury in amalgam restorations. Between 16% and 91% of patients have a positive patch test to mercury, especially those with lesions in direct contact with the restoration.[17-19] These lesions regress when the restorations are replaced. Similar reactions have been reported to composite restorations, possibly representing a reaction to formaldehyde.[20,21] In the Saudi Arabian population, chewing of *deram* has been reported to cause oral lichen planus.[22]

Oral lichenoid drug eruptions and oral lichen planus are clinically and histologically indistinguishable. The classes of drugs that have been implicated include antihypertensive agents (in particular thiazides), antimalarials, gold, nonsteroidal anti-inflammatory drugs (NSAIDs), hypoglycemic agents, penicillamine, allopurinol, carbamazepine, and new biologic agents to name but a few.[23-26] Patients previously diagnosed with Grinspan syndrome (oral lichen planus, diabetes mellitus, and hypertension) were probably exhibiting a lichenoid mucosal reaction to their medications. Patients with autoimmune conditions such as lupus erythematosus and chronic graft-versus-host disease often present with oral lesions that are clinically and histologically indistinguishable from lichen planus (*Figs 11.152* and *11.153*).[27-29] There is also an increased prevalence of oral lichen planus in patients with hepatitis, in particular hepatitis C, and especially in Southern European and Japanese populations associated with an increase in HLA-DR6 (*Fig. 11.154*).[30-32]

Patients with oral lichen planus show an increased incidence of HLA-Bw57 in the white British population, HLA-DR9 in the Chinese and Japanese, and HLA-DR3 in the Swedish, with a decrease in incidence

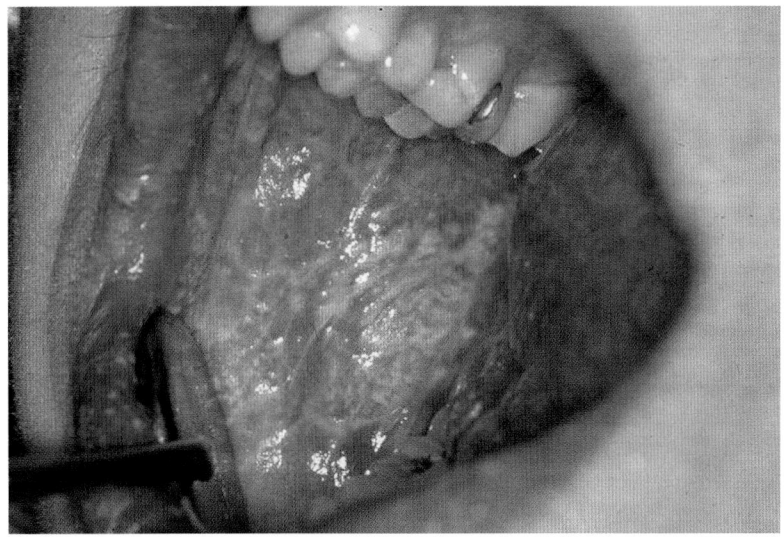

Fig. 11.149
Oral lichen planus: Wickham striae of reticular lichen planus with mild erythema.

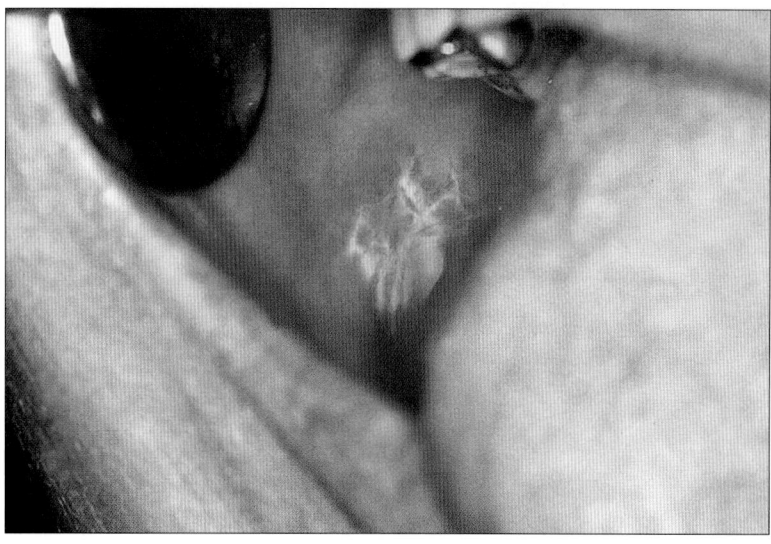

Fig. 11.152
Oral lesions of discoid erythematosus: keratotic reticulations in a patient with systemic lupus erythematosus.

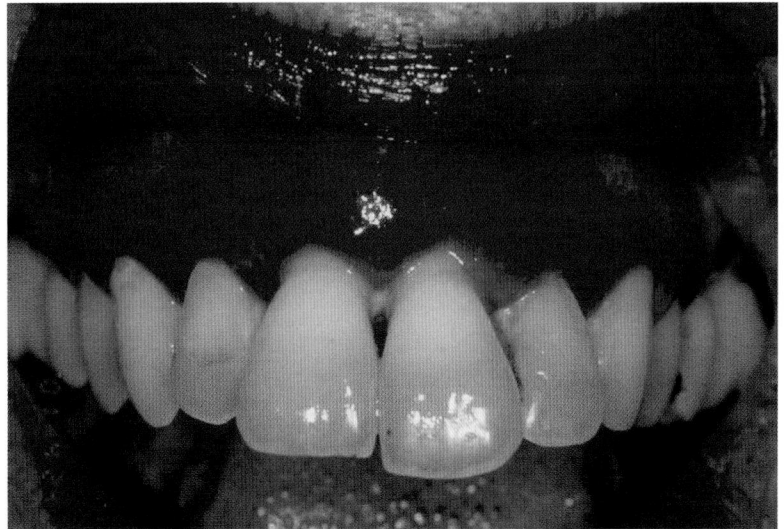

Fig. 11.150
Oral lichen planus: desquamative gingivitis is one manifestation of erythematous lichen planus.

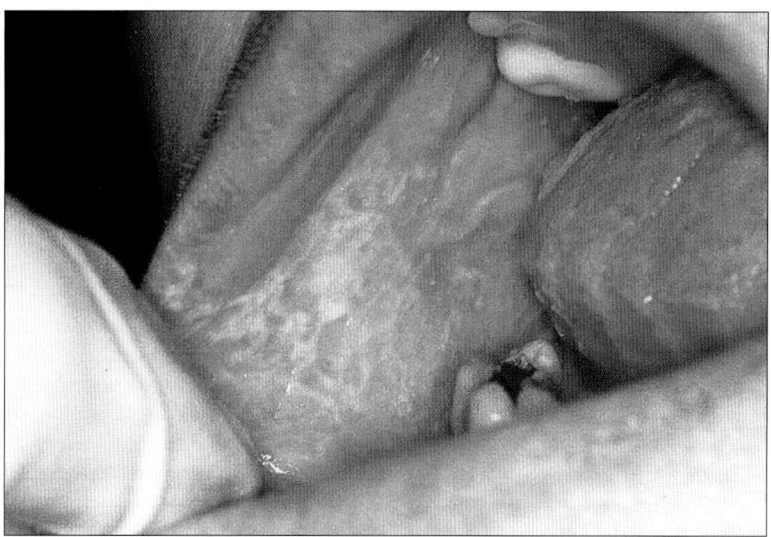

Fig. 11.153
Chronic oral graft-versus-host disease: keratotic reticulations in a patient with chronic oral graft-versus-host disease.

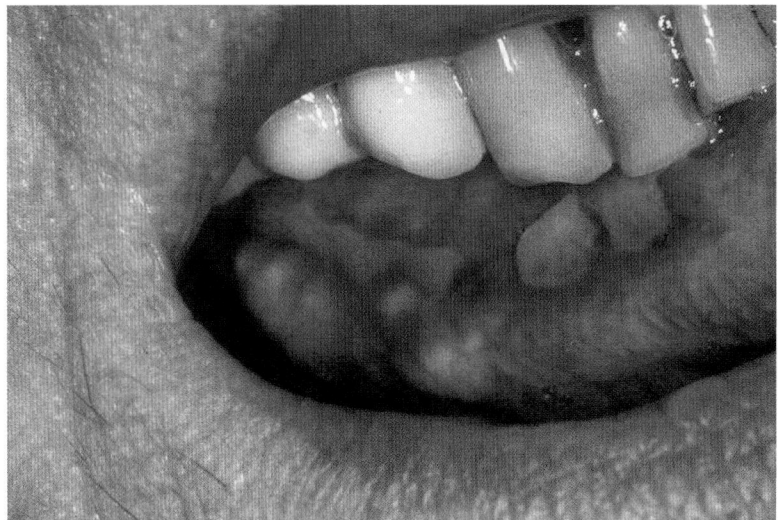

Fig. 11.151
Oral lichen planus: note the presence of faint white striations, erythema, and ulcers.

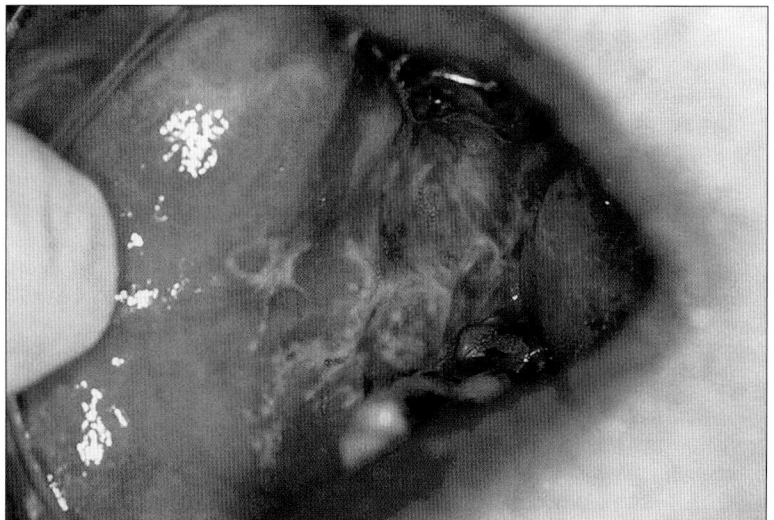

Fig. 11.154
Oral lichen planus: keratotic reticulations in a patient with hepatitis C.

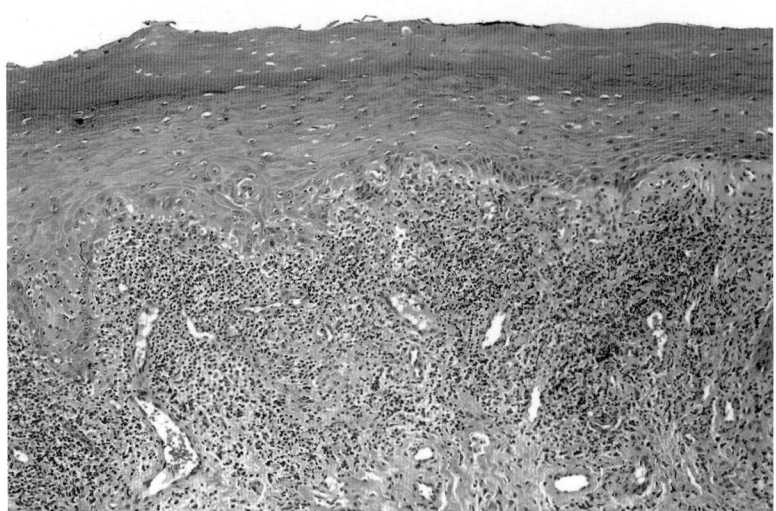

Fig. 11.155
Oral lichen planus: typical features of hyperkeratosis, acanthosis or atrophy, squamatization of basal cells, and a lymphocytic band at the interface.

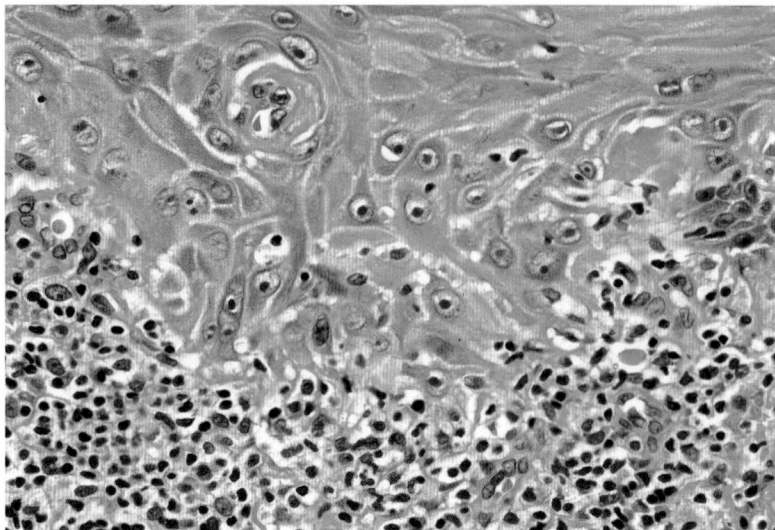

Fig. 11.156
Oral lichen planus: high-power view emphasizing the interface stomatitis with basal cell destruction; note the presence of colloid bodies.

of HLA-DQ1 in the white British population.[33–36] The Israeli population showed a significant association with HLA-DR2 and a decrease in DR4.[37] Interferon-gamma (IFN-γ) and IL-4 gene polymorphisms influence disease susceptibility and progression of oral lichen planus in a Chinese cohort.[38]

Because so many different conditions can lead to the clinical appearances of oral lichen planus – contact phenomena, hypersensitivity to medications, and autoimmune diseases – it is more appropriate to view oral lichenoid lesions as the final common pathway of expression of the mucosa to local or systemic antigens. In the idiopathic form, it represents a T-cell reaction to basal cells resulting in basal cell lysis.

The pathogenesis of oral disease has been reviewed in several publications, and only a summary – albeit somewhat simplistic – is presented here.[24,39,40] The initiating event is alteration of the keratinocyte either from antigen bound or unmasked on the cell surface (e.g., drugs, major histocompatibility complex [MHC] or viral antigens). Keratinocytes and antigen-presenting cells secrete chemokines that attract lymphocytes. Antigen-presenting cells in the epithelium present antigens via MHC II molecules to CD4 cells while basal cells present antigens via MHC I molecules to CD8 cells. A Th1 response mediated by CD4 cells results in secretion of IL-2 and IFN-γ that bind receptors on CD8 cells that become activated and trigger basal keratinocyte apoptosis.[40] In the meantime, local mast cells are activated and secrete TNF-α, which induces endothelial cell adhesion molecule expression, priming the vasculature for lymphocyte adhesion and transmigration.[41] The chemokine RANTES and intercellular adhesion molecule (ICAM)-1 are both expressed in lesions of oral lichen planus and amalgam-induced lichenoid reactions, but not IL-8.[42]

The reticular/papular type exhibits either parakeratosis or hyperkeratosis with hypergranulosis, and variable acanthosis (Figs 11.155 and 11.156). The erythematous form is non or thinly keratinized and exhibits epithelial atrophy or erosion (Fig. 11.157). In both manifestations, there is variable lymphocyte exocytosis, mild spongiosis, and increased numbers of Langerhans cells. Common to all variants is destruction of the basal cell layer with blurring of the epithelial-connective tissue interface, and a superficial band of lymphocytes.[39] Early lymphocytic infiltrates contain mainly CD4 cells while older lesions consist predominantly of CD8 cells. Sawtoothed rete ridges and apoptotic cells (cytoid, colloid, or Civatte bodies) may be present, and the basement membrane zone is sometimes thickly eosinophilic due to fibrinogen deposition. Subepithelial clefting is occasionally present but may be artifactual from basal cell loss (albeit a reliable one) (Fig. 11.158).[43] Although lymphocytes predominate, plasma cells may be seen, particularly in hypersensitivity lichenoid reactions, if an ulcer or erosion is present or in gingival lesions which are always plasma cell-rich. The phrase 'lichenoid stomatitis/mucositis consistent with lichen planus in the appropriate clinical context' is sometimes used when a lesion has only

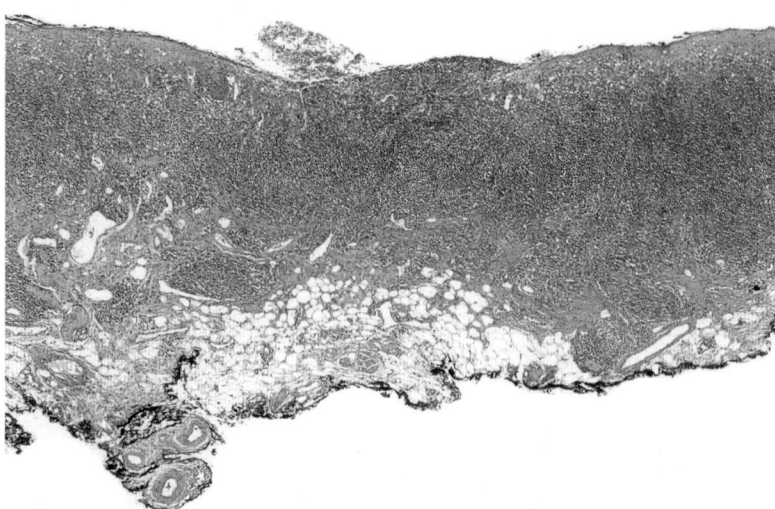

Fig. 11.157
Oral lichen planus: erosive and ulcerative lichen planus without hyperkeratosis.

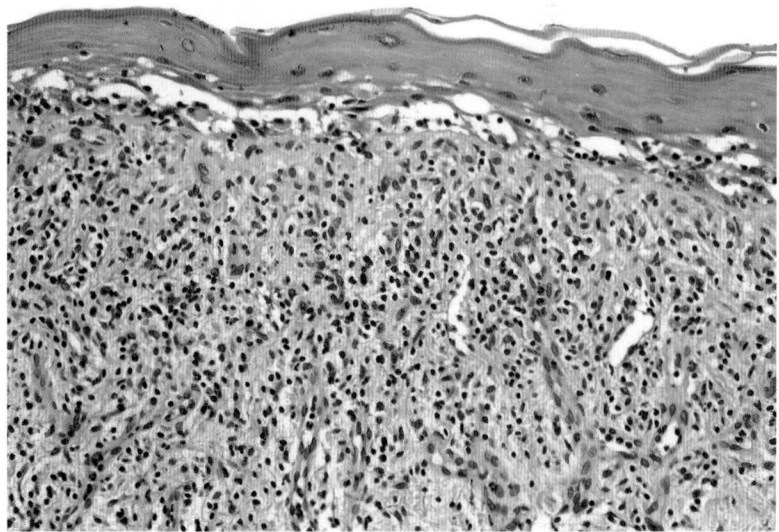

Fig. 11.158
Oral lichen planus: subepithelial clefting occurs to varying degrees and is well demonstrated in this case.

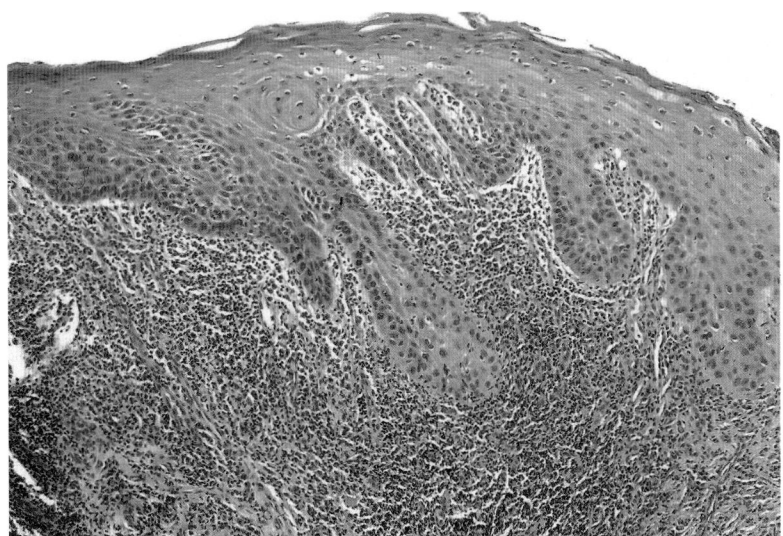

Fig. 11.159
Epithelial dysplasia with lymphocytic band at the interface: note that there is basal cell prominence and maturation disarray.

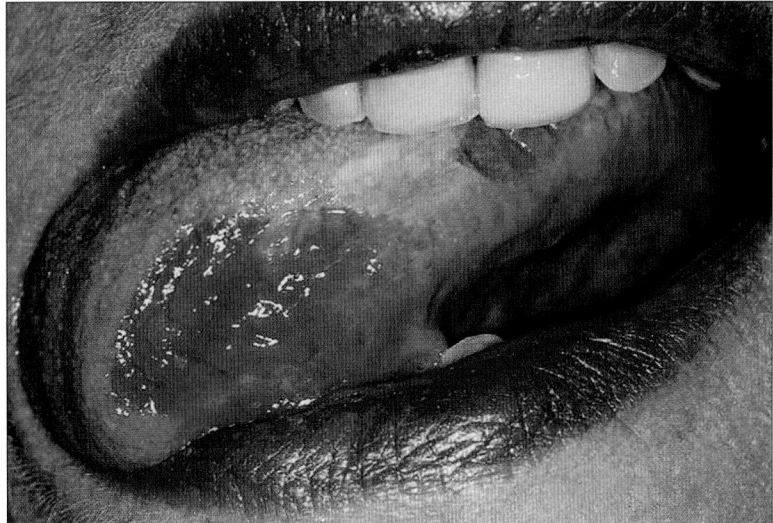

Fig. 11.160
Cinnamaldehyde-associated contact stomatitis: erythematous area on the tongue caused by cinnamon gum contact hypersensitivity reaction.

some of the above features, in particular, only focal basal cell degeneration or a sparse lymphocytic band at the interface. The diagnosis in such cases depends largely on the clinical presentation. Lesions of amalgam-induced oral lichen planus, banal lichen planus, and lichenoid lesions seen in lupus erythematosus and chronic graft-versus-host disease are histopathologically indistinguishable.[44]

Although reactive epithelial atypia may be present, unequivocal epithelial dysplasia should be reported as such. The term 'lichenoid dysplasia' was originally coined to denote epithelial dysplasia associated with a lymphocytic band at the interface, which subsequently progressed to squamous cell carcinoma.[45,46] This band is likely analogous to the tumor-associated lymphocytic response noted within invasive carcinomas (Fig. 11.159). Such lesions are no different from conventional oral epithelial dysplasia and should not be classified separately. An important feature in true dysplasia is basal cell hyperplasia and atypia rather than basal cell degeneration, although it may be sometimes difficult to distinguish reactive atypia from dysplasia. In one report, dysplastic lesions with a lichenoid histologic character were seen more commonly in clinically 'lichenoid lesions' rather than reticulated oral lichen planus.[47] Such lichenoid histologic and clinical lesions (rather than typical histologic and clinical lesions of lichen planus) also showed a higher rate of malignant transformation.[48] This again underlines the importance of correlating the histopathology with clinical findings of bilateral, symmetric, and reticulated lesions for a diagnosis of lichen planus.

Contact lichenoid hypersensitivity reactions to cinnamic aldehyde show peri- and paravascular nodular lymphocytic infiltrates (Figs 11.160 and 11.161).[49,50] The absence of eosinophils does not rule out an oral hypersensitivity reaction.

Direct immunofluorescence demonstrates fibrinogen at the basement membrane zone, often in a fibrillar, shaggy 'stalactite' pattern with occasional presence of C3 and IgM. Cytoid bodies also stain with IgM or C3.[51] Indirect immunofluorescence studies have shown that there may be circulating antibodies directed against basal cells although this is controversial.[52–54]

Loss of heterozygosity on chromosome arms 3p, 9p, and 17p is not a feature of oral lichen planus, a finding that supports the hypothesis that this disease is not intrinsically premalignant; however, a high frequency of loss was found in dysplastic lesions with a lichenoid infiltrate.[55] Telomerase activity has been detected in up to 70% of patients.[56] A high rate of TP53 mutations has also been reported in oral lichen planus.[57] However, the role of p53 in the development of malignancy is still unclear.[58]

Differential diagnosis

Biopsies of patients with chronic ulcerative stomatitis (an erosive-ulcerative condition of the mouth that clinically resembles erosive oral lichen planus) show histopathological features of lichen planus or lichenoid

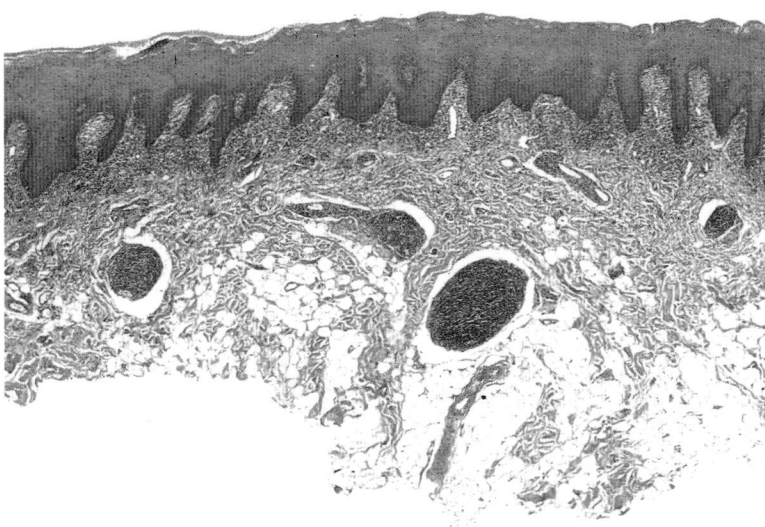

Fig. 11.161
Cinnamaldehyde-associated contact stomatitis: there is a lymphocytic band at the interface with peri- and paravascular nodular lymphocytic aggregates; in this case, the basal cells are intact.

mucositis. However, direct immunofluorescence studies show stratified epithelium-specific antinuclear IgG in a speckled pattern primarily affecting the lower epithelium.[59–61] Indirect immunofluorescence using guinea pig esophagus demonstrates nuclear reactivity particularly well. The putative antigen is δNp63α, an isoform of p63.[62] However, it is still unclear what the relationship is between these two conditions.[63,64]

Lichenoid and granulomatous mucositis presents as diffuse erythema of the lip mucosa (mostly upper lip) without striations, and is likely a contact hypersensitivity reaction. The histopathological features are similar to lichen planus except that the infiltrate is predominantly histiocytic with subtle or well-formed granulomas within the papillary lamina propria and in a peri- and paravascular location[65] (Fig. 11.162).

Lesions of discoid lupus erythematosus may also show a lichenoid lymphocytic band at the interface and peri- and paravascular nodular lymphocytic infiltrates (Fig. 11.163). Direct immunofluorescence studies are usually positive for the lupus band test in lesional tissue. Lesions of chronic graft-versus-host disease resemble lichen planus except that the lymphocytic infiltrate is often sparse because of immunosuppression. An intense chronic inflammatory infiltrate at the interface is seen in plasma cell gingivitis

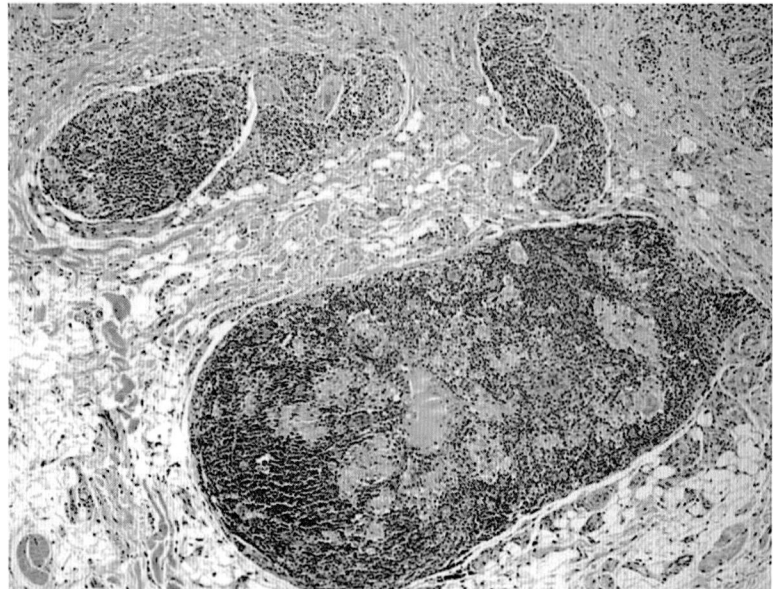

Fig. 11.162
Lichenoid and granulomatous contact stomatitis.

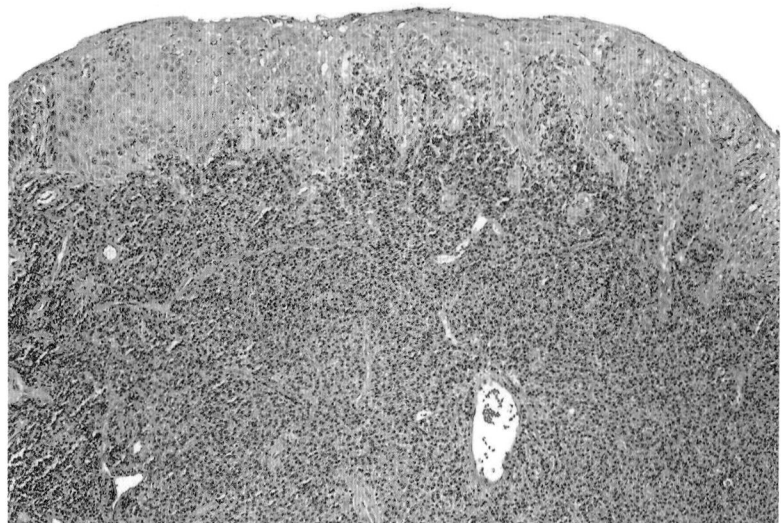

Fig. 11.164
Plasma cell gingivitis: there are sheets of plasma cells that fill the lamina propria; the epithelium exhibits spongiosis, leukocyte exocytosis and apoptosis.

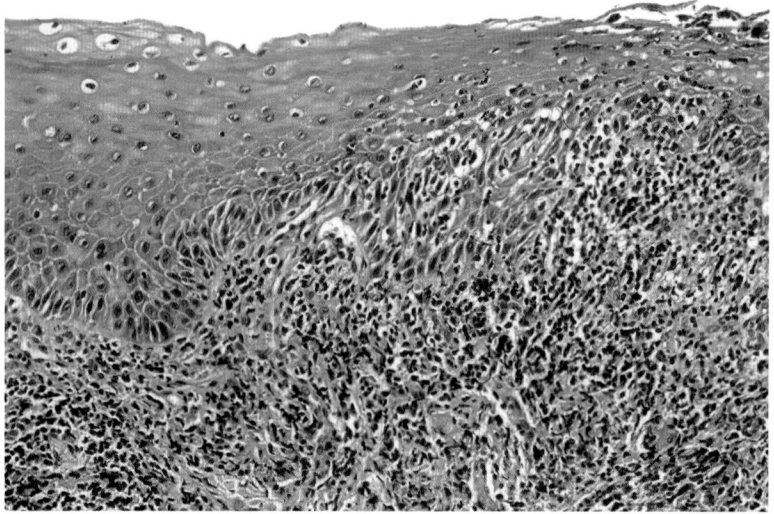

Fig. 11.163
Oral lupus erythematosus: there is variable epithelial atrophy and acanthosis, spongiosis, leukocyte exocytosis and a lymphocytic band at the interface.

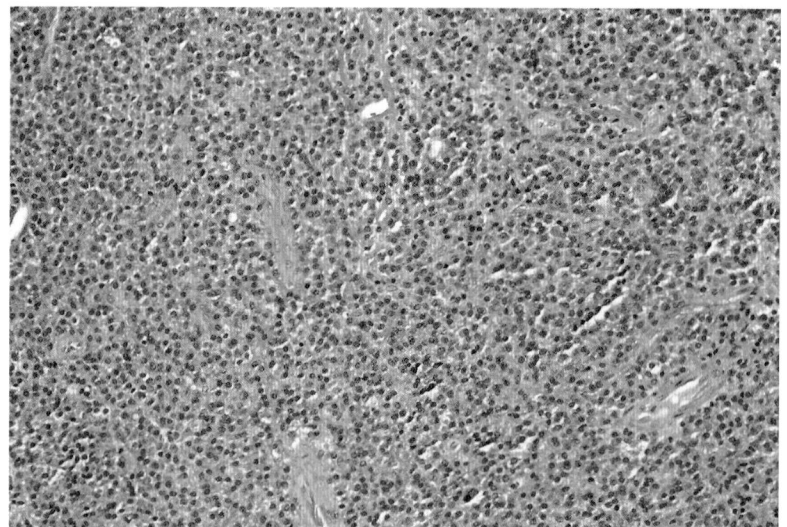

Fig. 11.165
Plasma cell gingivitis: the lamina propria is packed with plasma cells.

although the cells in this condition are predominantly plasmacytic. Rare cases of lichen planus pemphigoides have been reported.[66,67]

Plasma cell gingivostomatitis

Clinical features

In the 1960s and early 1970s, patients presented with symptoms of soreness and burning of the oral mucosa following the use of chewing gum. There was angular cheilitis with fissuring, dry atrophic lips, and occasional desquamation. The tongue was often fissured, edematous, with scalloped borders, and the gingiva (free and attached) was fiery red, often with extension onto the palatal mucosa.[1,2] Some patients had drug allergies while others were atopic. The gingiva was sometimes the only site of involvement.[3]

Discontinuation of gum chewing led to resolution of lesions in most, but not all, cases, and it was postulated that this condition represented a hypersensitivity reaction to some component of chewing gum or some other unidentified antigen.[1,2] Since that cluster of cases and reformulation of chewing gum, only occasional cases occur now in response to a variety

of putative topical irritants such as cinnamicaldehyde-flavored toothpastes and khat.[4,5]

Subsequent to these reports, patients were identified who not only presented with oral symptoms of pain but also with hoarseness, dysphagia, and airway obstruction. On endoscopy, the larynx showed thickened, red, velvety, and edematous mucosa; the lips were thickened and fissured with angular cheilitis and fissured tongue.[6–9] The soft palate and gingiva were sometimes concurrently involved. It is unclear whether this widespread involvement of the mucosa of the upper respiratory tract indicates a more severe and extensive form of plasma cell gingivostomatitis. No obvious allergen has been identified. Equivalent lesions occur on the penis (Zoon balanitis) and the vulva.

Pathogenesis and histologic features

As mentioned above, this is a form of contact hypersensitivity reaction.

Plasma cell orificial mucositis and plasma cell gingivostomatitis have similar histology. There is psoriasiform epithelial hyperplasia with spongiosis, spongiotic pustules, and leukocyte exocytosis (Fig. 11.164).[1,3,10] Apoptosis is often present in more severe cases.[6,8] Characteristically, the lamina propria is filled with sheets of plasma cells with expression of both kappa and lambda light chains (Fig. 11.165). Russell bodies may be present, but Dutcher bodies are not seen. Occasional lymphocytes are also present.[1,3]

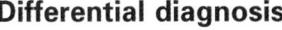

Fig. 11.166
Chronic periodontitis: note the pockets of plasma cells separated by bands of collagen.

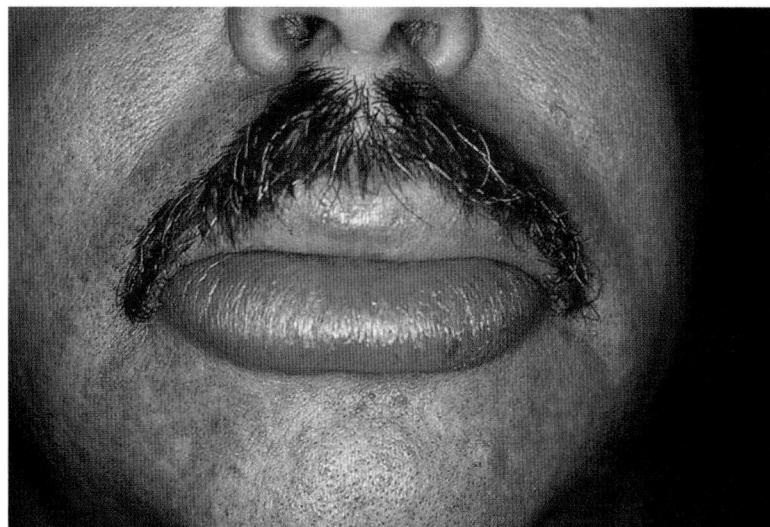

Fig. 11.167
Orofacial granulomatosis: there is diffuse rubbery swelling of the lower lip.

Differential diagnosis

An intense plasma cell infiltrate is characteristic of banal chronic gingivitis and periodontal disease. However, in these lesions, the plasma cells are not generally present in sheets but have a compartmentalized, slightly lobular character (*Fig. 11.166*).

Plasma cell granuloma, a rare lesion in the oral cavity, is histologically similar to plasma cell orificial mucositis except that the lesions are clinically tumorous masses or nodules.[11-14] Cases of plasma cell granuloma reported from the periodontal space most likely represent chronic periodontitis or banal inflammatory fibrovascular hyperplasias with the usual intense plasma cell infiltrate.[15]

Lack of light chain restriction excludes plasmacytoma.

Orofacial granulomatosis

Clinical features

Orofacial granulomatosis (cheilitis granulomatosa, granulomatous cheilitis) is a chronic, non-necrotizing, granulomatous, and inflammatory condition, likely a delayed-type hypersensitivity reaction. It occurs mostly in teenagers and young adults and is characterized by firm, occasionally tender, swelling and edema of the lips and/or face, often but not always accompanied by swelling of the gingiva (usually around the anterior teeth), and cobblestoning, folding, and erythema of the buccal mucosa. There may be angular cheilitis, ulcerations, and prominent vertical fissures in established lesions.[1]

In general, the swelling of the lips is the most important clinical sign, and is initially soft and relapsing (*Fig. 11.167*). However, swelling may involve other sites such as the periorbital, zygomatic, or mental regions.[2] Over the years, it becomes persistent and rubbery. The gingiva is affected in 20–30% of cases.[3,4] Gingival swellings extend onto the alveolar mucosa and become increasingly fibrotic over time (*Fig. 11.168*).[4] Facial nerve palsy is present in 13–47% of cases and may be due to either direct granulomatous involvement of the nerve or edema leading to nerve compression. It predates facial/lip swelling in 57–100% of cases, and these two signs together with fissured tongue constitute Melkersson-Rosenthal syndrome.[3-6] Fissured tongue is present in 40–50% of cases although its significance is uncertain since this is a relatively common oral finding.[3,6] Spontaneous improvement or resolution occurs in approximately one-third of patients.[3] Some patients exhibit staghorn swelling of the distal portions of the submandibular duct.

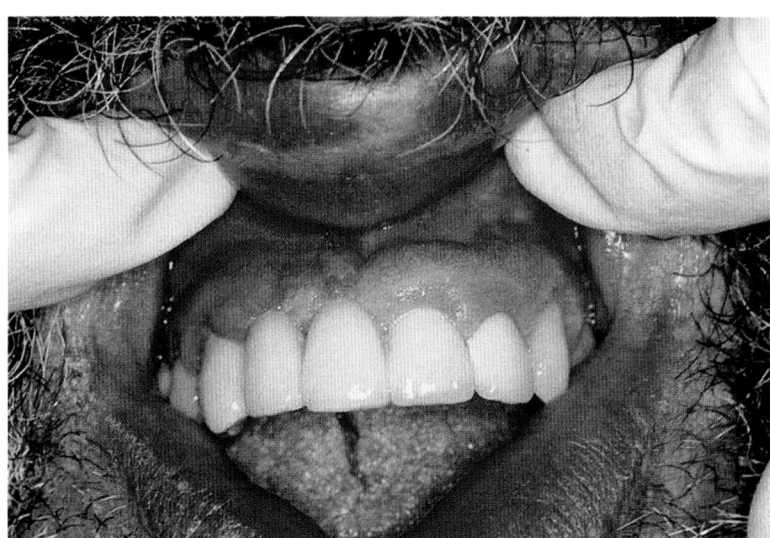

Fig. 11.168
Orofacial granulomatosis: note the thickened anterior maxillary gingiva.

Ten percent of patients have associated Crohn disease while only 3% have associated sarcoidosis.[7] Pediatric patients who develop this condition (as opposed to adults) are more likely to develop Crohn disease in adulthood.[8] Vulval and eye lesions have been reported in addition to more extensive neurological involvement. Of interest, patients with orofacial granulomatosis without gastrointestinal symptoms were found on ileocolonoscopy and biopsy to have intestinal pathology and granulomata in 54% of cases.[9]

Pathogenesis and histologic features

Hypersensitivity to foods (such as eggs, chocolate, and dairy products), flavorings, antioxidants (such as octyl butylated hydroxyanisol and cinnamaldehyde), preservatives (such as benzoate and metabisulfites), and fragrances have been demonstrated in up to 20% of cases; there is often a strong history of atopy.[1,10-13] Elimination diet, especially a low-phenolic diet, may result in significant improvement of symptoms.[14,15] Investigations targeting an infectious etiology with emphasis on *Saccharomyces cerevisiae*, *Mycobacterium tuberculosis*, and *Borrelia burgdorferi* have yielded variable results.[16-18] Genetic influences may play a role because of a high prevalence in the United Kingdom. Orofacial granulomatosis is associated with increased HLA-A3, B7, DR2, and HLA-B*44 expression.[19,20] The cytokine profile (such as increased production of IFN-γ) is consistent with a predominantly Th1 response, similar to that seen in gut lesions of Crohn disease.[21]

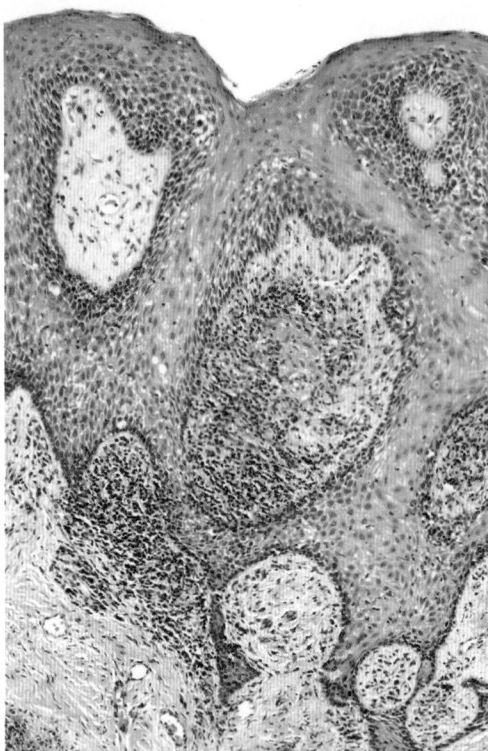

Fig. 11.169
Orofacial granulomatosis: this was the only granuloma present in the multiple sections examined.

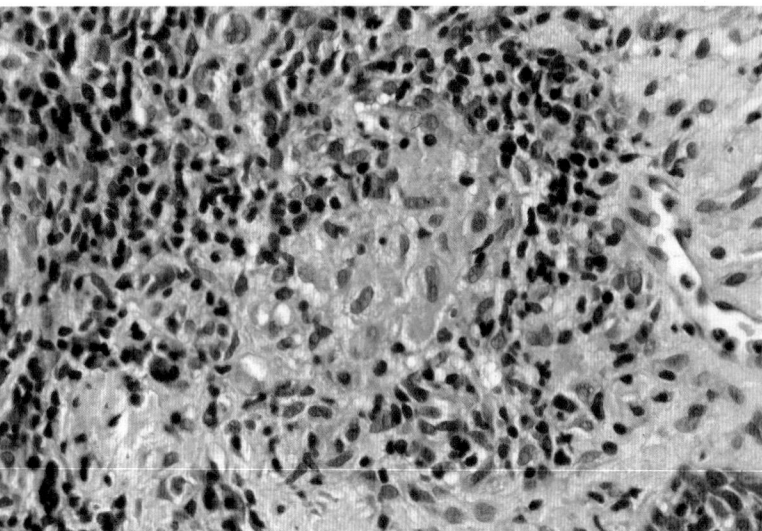

Fig. 11.170
Orofacial granulomatosis: there is a subtle non-necrotizing granuloma.

Non-necrotizing granulomata are present in the lamina propria, sometimes adjacent to vessels with variable numbers of lymphocytes and plasma cells (*Figs 11.169* and *11.170*).[2,6] The granulomata may be subtle and poorly formed and often require serial sectioning to be identified with certainty. They may bulge into and obstruct vessels.[22] Edema and vascular dilatation has also been reported but such features in the absence of granulomata are insufficient for a diagnosis of orofacial granulomatosis. Foreign material within the granulomata effectively excludes a diagnosis of orofacial granulomatosis. As with any granulomatous infiltrate, special stains for microorganisms should always be performed.

Differential diagnosis

Granulomata in this clinical setting are histologically indistinguishable from those of extragastrointestinal Crohn disease; clinical differences help to differentiate between the two. In general, the granulomata of sarcoidosis tend to be larger and more conspicuous. Angioedema and hypersensitivity reactions may present with edema and vascular ectasia in the absence

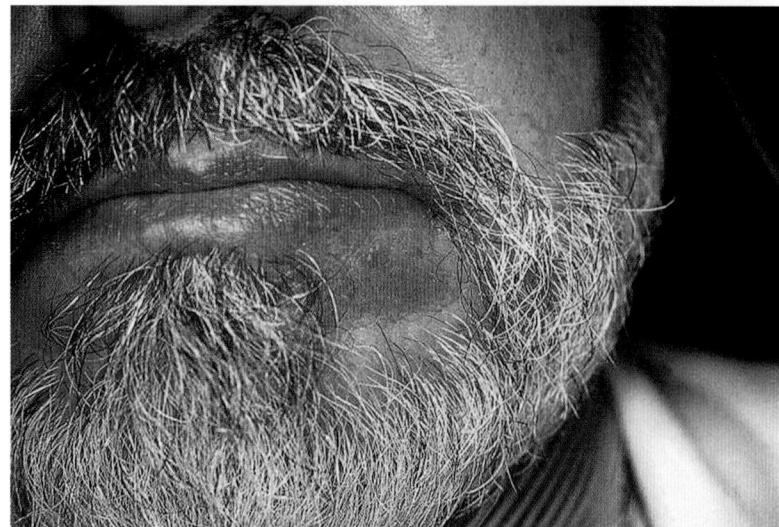

Fig. 11.171
Oral Crohn disease: there is swelling of the lips and an erythematous, indurated area of skin adjacent to the lower vermilion typical for skin involvement by Crohn disease.

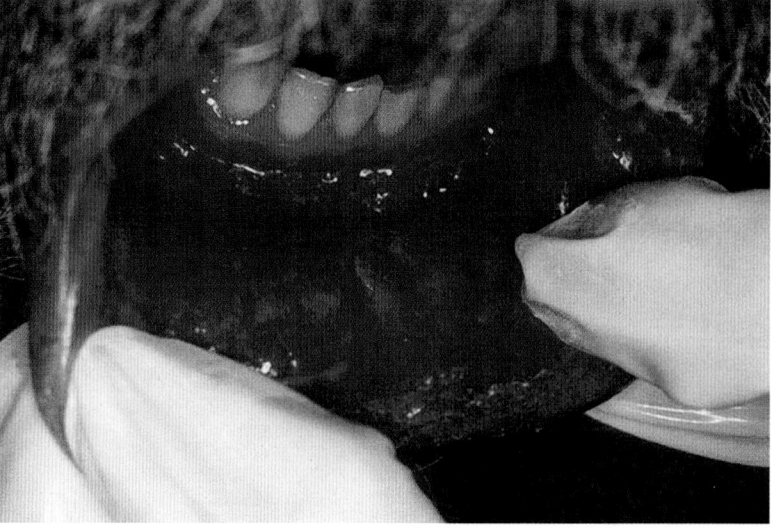

Fig. 11.172
Oral Crohn disease: note the fissures and cobblestoning of the lower lip mucosa.

of granulomata. Oral granulomatosis with polyangiitis is accompanied by pseudoepitheliomatous hyperplasia and a mixed acute and chronic inflammatory infiltrate with abscesses, hemorrhage in the papillary lamina propria, necrosis, and eosinophils. Foreign body granulomatous gingivitis occurs in response to dental polishing pastes (see above).

Oral Crohn disease

Clinical features

Crohn disease usually presents in the second decade, with a male predominance.[1,2] In one study, 37% of patients had asymptomatic gastrointestinal disease.[3] There is usually swelling of the face or lips and peri-vermilion induration; additionally, there may be linear vestibular aphtheiform ulcers, angular cheilitis, papulous and polypoid masses, mucosal tags, lip and gingival swelling, gingival erythema, and cobblestoning of the mucosa (*Figs 11.171* and *11.172*).[1,3-5] Some patients present with pyostomatitis vegetans and 'snail-track ulcers'.[6] In 22–60% of cases, oral symptoms precede intestinal symptoms.[1-3] Adhesions may lead to limitation in mouth opening.[2] Some patients present with staphylococcal panstomatitis.[7]

Pathogenesis and histologic features

It is believed that patients with mutations in the *NOD2/CARD15* and autophagy genes are predisposed to Crohn disease and that the disease represents a dysregulated proinflammatory immune response and impaired defense to gut commensals or other organisms.[8,9]

Granulomata, which are seen in up to 88% of mucosal lesions, are typically noncaseating, often subtle, and usually located in the superficial lamina propria, similar to orofacial granulomatosis.[1–3,6] They are found within the papulous folds, mucosal tags, ulcers, and salivary glands. Eosinophils are often noted within these granulomas.

Differential diagnosis

Granulomatous diseases associated with specific infections or foreign material must always be excluded. The histologic features of oral Crohn disease are indistinguishable from those of idiopathic orofacial granulomatosis (see above).

AUTOIMMUNE CONDITIONS

Desquamative gingivitis

Desquamative gingivitis is a chronic condition of adults, usually women (4:1), affecting either the gingiva diffusely or multifocally. It presents as friable, fiery red, painful, eroded, denuded attached gingiva, primarily on the facial or buccal aspect, with occasional areas of ulceration.[1,2]

Desquamative gingivitis represents a distinct clinical manifestation of autoimmune blistering diseases, hypersensitivity reactions, or oral lichen planus.[2–4] Large studies of desquamative gingivitis have shown that mucous membrane pemphigoid and lichen planus together accounts for approximately 80–85% of cases (with lichen planus accounting for the majority of cases depending on referral patterns), and pemphigus vulgaris representing 10–15% of cases.[5–7] Occasional cases of epidermolysis bullosa acquisita present as desquamative gingivitis. Cases of linear IgA confined to the mouth likely represent IgA-type mucous membrane pemphigoid.[8]

Mucous membrane pemphigoid

Clinical features

Mucous membrane pemphigoid is the most common autoimmune blistering disease presenting in the mouth. Several subsets of mucous membrane pemphigoid exist, with variable antigenic characteristics, but all are characterized by predominant involvement of the mucous membranes by a subepithelial blistering disorder.[1–3]

Mucous membrane pemphigoid usually occurs in the sixth decade and upward with a female predilection.[1,4–11] The oral cavity is affected in 84–96% of cases, and the conjunctiva in 52–81%.[4–6,12] Other sites of involvement in order of frequency are the upper airway (40–50%), skin (20–25%), and (less frequently) genitalia (9–17%), anorectal area (3–4%), and esophagus (3–4%).[4–6,12] Compared with patients with oral mucosal involvement alone, patients who exhibit involvement of the conjunctiva, genitalia, nasopharynx, esophagus, and the larynx have higher morbidity because of life-threatening airway obstruction, stricture, and scarring that may lead to blindness.[3]

The oral cavity is the only site involved in approximately 60% of cases and is the first manifestation of the disease in 48–96% of patients.[4,13,14] In many cases, it is the only site of involvement such that oral mucous membrane pemphigoid may represent a subset of this condition. The gingiva is the most frequent site of involvement affecting anywhere from 64% to 94% of cases and takes the form of desquamative gingivitis.[1,6,8,9,14] Desquamative gingivitis may be the sole manifestation of pemphigoid in at least 60% of cases (*Fig. 11.173*).[10] The buccal mucosa, lip mucosa, and tongue are less often affected. Lesions present as painful areas of erosion, erythema, and ulceration, and intact blisters are rarely seen. The collapsed blister roof may take the form of a yellow-white membrane that readily peels off the mucosa. Unlike cases with ocular involvement, cicatrization is an uncommon finding and was noted in only 9% of cases in one series.[4]

Paraneoplastic pemphigoid has been reported in association with lymphoma and lung cancer and likely represents paraneoplastic autoimmune multiorgan syndrome (see below).[15,16]

Oral and ocular pemphigoid is associated with increased frequency of HLA-DQB1*0301.[17–19]

Pathogenesis and histologic features

Mucous membrane pemphigoid is a heterogenous disease, and immunoblotting and immunoprecipitation studies on mucosal specimens demonstrate autoantibodies directed against BP180 (BPAg2 or type XVII collagen) and less often BP230 (BPAg1), laminin-332, laminin-6, β4 subunit of α6β4 integrin, and a 120-kDa undefined epithelial antigen. Those with antibodies against laminin-332 have more severe disease.[3,12–33,34]

Mucous membrane pemphigoid is characterized by subepithelial clefting with preservation of the basal keratinocytes (*Figs 11.169* and *11.174*).[8–10]

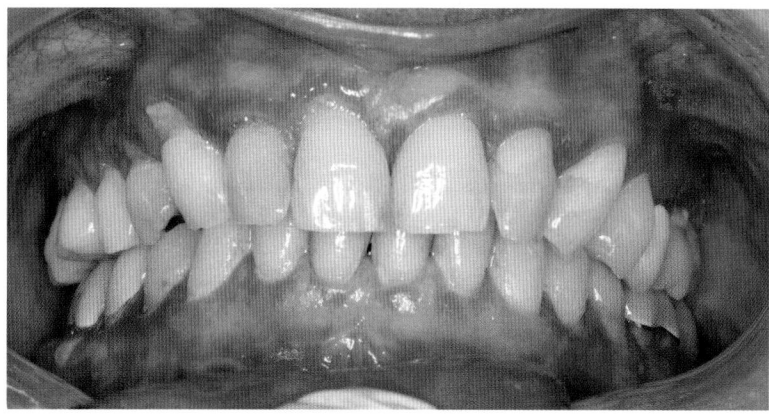

Fig. 11.173
Mucous membrane pemphigoid: this case presented with desquamative gingivitis characterized by erythematous gingiva and white epithelial sloughs.

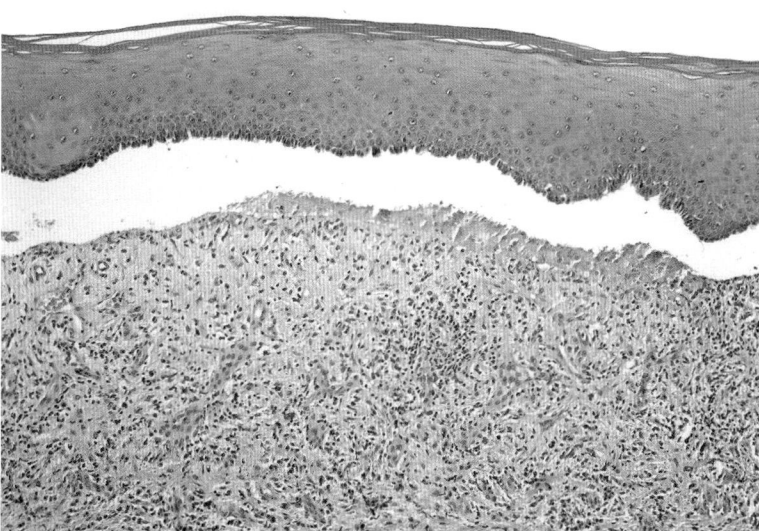

Fig. 11.174
Mucous membrane pemphigoid: there is preservation of the basal cells with subepithelial clefting, and a mild lymphocytic infiltrate in the lamina propria.

A variable lymphoplasmacytic infiltrate is usually present in the lamina propria. Unlike bullous pemphigoid, eosinophils are rarely seen.

Direct immunofluorescence studies reveal basement membrane zone antibodies in a smooth, continuous linear fluorescence pattern in 67–96% of cases.[12,20,21] IgG is present in 39–96% of cases, C3 in 43–97% of cases, and IgA in 20–30% of cases; cases with IgG and IgA may have more severe refractory disease.[3,7,9,20–22]

Indirect immunofluorescence studies for circulating autoantibodies (usually IgG) are present in approximately 20% of cases.[9,12] However, one study using oral mucosa as a substrate elicited a 36% positivity rate.[20] There is no consistent correlation between antibody titer and disease activity.

Indirect immunofluorescence studies in salt-split skin reveal circulating IgG or IgA in 84–100% of cases.[21,23,24] The majority (57–82%) show epidermal binding (roof of the split) with 9–22% showing dermal (floor of the split) or both epidermal and dermal localization. Those with both circulating IgG and IgA are virtually certain to need systemic immunosuppressive therapy.[21]

Differential diagnosis

Oral lesions in mucous membrane pemphigoid must be distinguished from other subepithelial and autoimmune bullous dermatosis, and lichen planus. The latter shows destruction of basal cells, colloid body formation, a dense lymphocytic infiltrate, and shaggy fibrinogen only on direct immunofluorescence studies. Cases of pure oral disease with positive direct immunofluorescence positive for IgA represent IgA mucous membrane pemphigoid because linear IgA disease always affects the skin.[8,35]

Pemphigus vulgaris

Clinical features

Oral pemphigus vulgaris typically begins in the sixth decade of life with a female predilection, and patients are often of Ashkenazi Jewish descent. The mouth is involved in up to 87% of cases.[1–4] Lesions in the oral cavity precede those at other sites in up to 80% of cases.[5] It presents as large ulcers with a pseudomembrane (from collapsed roof of the blister), and often shallow erosions (especially of the palatal mucosa, a site of frequent trauma) affecting any mucosal site; it may present as desquamative gingivitis (*Figs 11.175* and *11.176*).[5] Patients with pemphigus vegetans (a vegetating and pustular variant of pemphigus vulgaris) infrequently demonstrate oral lesions.[6,7] Mucous membrane involvement in pemphigus foliaceus and pemphigus erythematosus is exceedingly rare. Paraneoplastic pemphigus almost always involves the oral cavity (see below).

Histologic features

Pemphigus vulgaris exhibits autoantibodies directed against desmoglein-3. Biopsies of lesional tissue of pemphigus vulgaris reveal suprabasilar acantholysis and clefting.[4,8] Pemphigus vegetans, in addition, shows papillary epithelial hyperplasia and eosinophilic abscesses.[6]

Direct immunofluorescence studies in pemphigus vulgaris and vegetans reveal characteristic staining of the epithelial intercellular space in a 'netlike pattern' with IgG in all cases with active untreated disease.[4,8] This differentiates pemphigus from pyostomatitis vegetans, which also shows suprabasilar acantholysis and negative direct immunofluorescence findings.

Paraneoplastic pemphigus (paraneoplastic autoimmune multiorgan syndrome)

Clinical features

In paraneoplastic pemphigus, the oral mucosa is involved in all cases with persistent, painful, treatment-resistant erosions and ulcers of the oropharynx and lips; the crusting vermilion lesions are reminiscent of Stevens-Johnson syndrome.[1–6] More recently, the concept of paraneoplastic autoimmune multiorgan syndrome has been proposed.[4,7] This syndrome is characterized by an autoimmune blistering mucocutaneous disease with positive immunofluorescence findings, characteristic immunoprecipitation findings, presence of malignancy (most often lymphoproliferative in nature), and involvement of other organ systems such as the lungs (leading to bronchiolitis obliterans, and often the major cause of mortality) and kidneys. The mucocutaneous disorder may resemble pemphigus vulgaris, erythema multiforme, or be lichenoid.

Pathogenesis and histologic features

It is believed that either dysregulation of the immune system caused by the neoplasm leads to production of autoantibodies or host antitumor response produces antibodies that cross-react with native antigens.[4]

Histologically, there is suprabasilar acantholysis identical to pemphigus, in addition to individual keratinocyte necrosis and vacuolar interface change, suggestive of a lichenoid inflammatory process.[1,4]

Direct immunofluorescence shows deposition of IgG and/or complement in the intercellular space, and along the basement membrane zone.[1,5] Indirect immunofluorescence is positive in a large number of cases if rat bladder is used.[4] Antibodies against envoplakin and periplakin are consistently present, although antibodies against desmoplakin, desmogleins, and plectin are also present.[4,7,8]

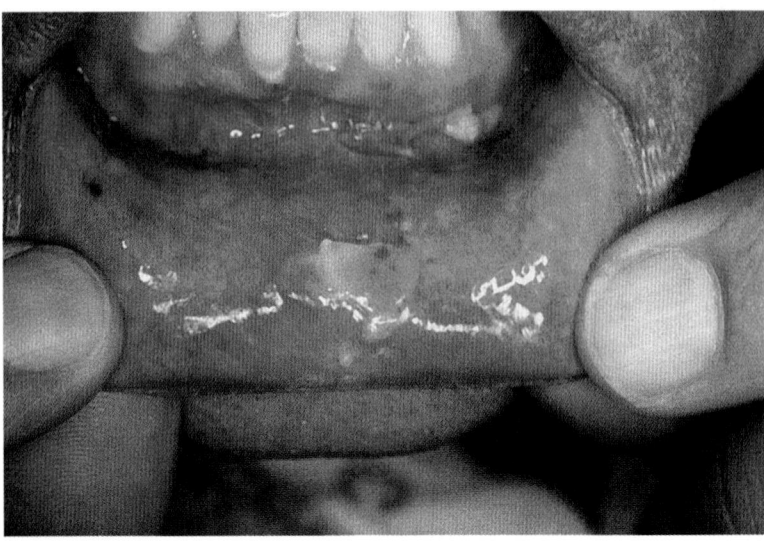

Fig. 11.175
Pemphigus vulgaris: this presented as an ulcer on the lower lip mucosa.

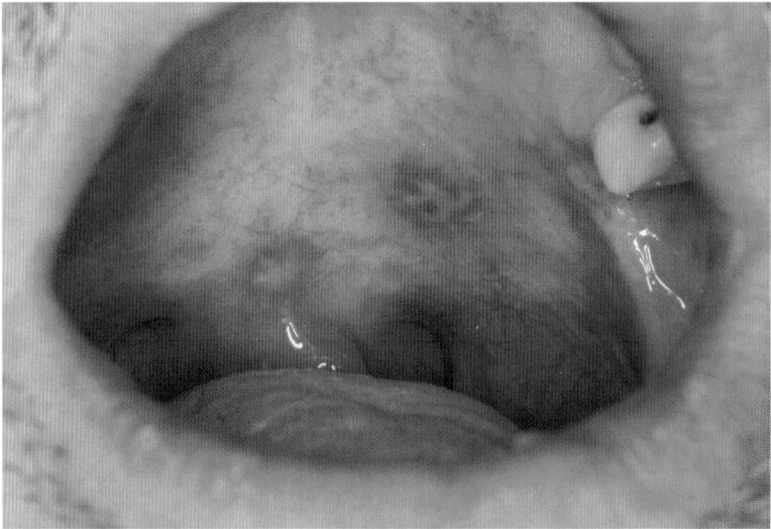

Fig. 11.176
Pemphigus vulgaris: erosions and ulcers on the palatal mucosa are characteristic for oral pemphigus.

Linear IgA disease

Clinical features

Oral mucosal lesions associated with linear IgA disease occur in 26–100% of cases and present as vesicles, bullae, erosions, or ulcerations.[1-4] They may be located on the palatal mucosa, buccal or lip mucosa, and oropharynx.[3,5-7]

Histologic features

The antigen is a 97-kDa that localizes in the basement membrane zone. There is a subepithelial vesicle or bulla with neutrophil or eosinophil predominance.[5,6] In many lesions, the infiltrate is mixed neutrophilic and eosinophilic.

Direct immunofluorescence studies reveal linear deposits of IgA along the basement membrane zone.[1,5,6] Currently, it is thought that cases of desquamative gingivitis alone (without skin lesions) that are positive for linear deposition of IgA represent mucous membrane pemphigoid, although some believe that pure oral linear IgA disease exists.[8,9]

Dermatitis herpetiformis

Clinical features

Oral involvement in dermatitis herpetiformis, a condition associated with celiac disease, presents as erythematous, pseudovesicular, purpuric, or erosive lesions in 70% of patients.[1,2] Aphthous-like ulcers accompanied by mucosal erythema and atrophic glossitis have been described in up to 22% of patients.[3]

Histologic features

The antigen is epidermal transglutaminase. Mucosal biopsies reveal neutrophil microabscesses at the epithelial-connective tissue interface, occasional evidence of subepithelial blistering, and eosinophils and lymphocytes in the lamina propria.[1,2] Extravasated erythrocytes are often conspicuous.

Direct immunofluorescence studies reveal granular deposits of IgA in the basement membrane, particularly at the tips of the papillae.[1,2,4]

Epidermolysis bullosa acquisita

Clinical features

The oral mucosa is involved in 53–64% of cases, although in many reports the nature of the lesions is not documented.[1,2] Ulcers and erythema of the buccal mucosa as well as desquamative gingivitis are common.[3] Scarring is a common sequela and may lead to laryngeal stenosis.[4]

Histologic features

Autoantibodies are directed against type VII collagen. The histologic features are variable. In some lesions, there is a cell-free subepithelial blister, whereas in others, a neutrophil-rich or eosinophil-rich lesion is seen.

Direct immunofluorescence studies show linear deposits of IgG and C3 at the basement membrane zone similar to lesions of pemphigoid.[5] Circulating antibasement membrane antibodies localize exclusively to the floor of the blister in salt-split skin.[6]

Lupus erythematosus

Clinical features

Oral involvement in the form of ulcers, erythema with or without white striations and keratotic plaques, is seen in 26–45% of patients with systemic and discoid lupus erythematosus, presenting primarily on the hard palatal mucosa, buccal mucosa, and lips. Some lesions cause burning or soreness while others are asymptomatic.[1-7] Patients with bullous and subacute lupus erythematosus have similar lesions.[8-10]

Histologic features

Oral lesions of both systemic and discoid lupus erythematosus exhibit parakeratosis or hyperkeratosis, epithelial hyperplasia or atrophy, vacuolar degeneration of the basal cells, PAS-positive thickened basement membrane zone, perivascular inflammatory infiltrates (with some cases showing a bandlike lichenoid infiltrate), and interstitial mucin.[2,6,11,12]

Direct immunofluorescence studies show granular/linear deposition of IgG, IgM, IgA, and/or C3 at the basement membrane zone (lupus band test); cytoid bodies stain for IgM.[6]

Granulomatosis with polyangiitis (granulomatosis with polyangiitis)

Clinical features

Granulomatosis with polyangiitis (granulomatosis with polyangiitis) is a small- and medium-sized vessel necrotizing vasculitis affecting mainly capillaries and venules and represents one of the three conditions that comprise antineutrophil cytoplasmic antibody (ANCA)-associated vasculitis. Characteristically, there is noninfectious granulomatous inflammation of the upper and lower respiratory tract, and glomerulonephritis.[1] Involvement of the heart and lungs can have serious consequences. Although almost all patients show upper and/or lower airway disease, some cases with isolated skin and mucosal disease have been reported. In some patients, the disease runs a protracted course limited to the upper airways before progressing to multiorgan involvement.[2,3]

Approximately 5–10% of patients have oral involvement, and patients are in the seventh decade of life. The gingiva is hyperplastic, often with a friable, granular, erythematous-to-magenta appearance, the so-called 'strawberry gingivitis' (Fig. 11.177).[4] Milder disease manifests with pinpoint gingival hemorrhage. Ulceration and necrosis are often present, and when affecting the palatal mucosa this is referred to as midline destructive disease.[5-7] The dentition in the affected sites becomes mobile, and extraction sockets heal poorly.

Pathogenesis and histologic features

Patients' sera demonstrate the presence of ANCA directed against cytoplasmic proteinase C (also known as c-ANCA) present in 80% of cases, or against perinuclear myeloperoxidase (p-ANCA) in 20% of cases. Some patients exhibit antibodies against lysosome-associated membrane protein-1. However, disease limited to the upper airway may be negative for such antibodies.[8] There is ANCA-induced activation of primed neutrophils and monocytes that activates the alternative complement pathway leading to degranulation and the secretion of additional cytokines, resulting in apoptosis and necrosis of endothelial cells.[9]

Oral mucosal biopsies show marked pseudoepitheliomatous hyperplasia with edema, a mixed acute and chronic inflammatory cell infiltrate and

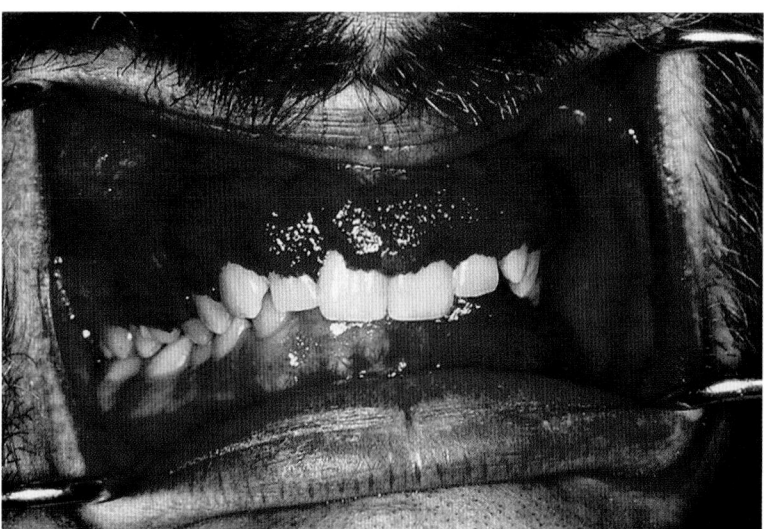

Fig. 11.177
Oral granulomatosis with polyangiitis: note the typical 'strawberry gingivitis'. By courtesy of S. Zunt, DDS, Indianapolis, USA.

hemorrhage especially in the papillary lamina propria; many eosinophils may also be present. Granulomata are usually poorly formed or absent, although scattered multinucleated giant cells are sometimes present (*Fig. 11.178*).[5,9] Vasculitis with fibrinoid necrosis is sometimes a feature.[6,10] The typical geographic necrosis with palisaded granulomata is not usually a feature in oral mucosal biopsies, although it is occasionally evident in the major salivary glands.[11]

Direct immunofluorescence studies may show immune deposits of IgG or IgA around blood vessels in skin biopsies.[12]

Differential diagnosis

Infectious processes must be excluded in the setting of a mixed inflammatory infiltrate. The presence of pseudoepitheliomatous hyperplasia with eosinophils and scattered giant cells raises the possibility of a deep fungal infection, such as blastomycosis. Other vasculitides should also be considered although sole presentation in the oral cavity is rare. Pyostomatitis vegetans and pemphigus vegetans do not show vasculitis or granulomata and typically show acantholysis, although both may exhibit pseudoepitheliomatous hyperplasia and eosinophils.

Cocaine-induced midline destructive disease may resemble granulomatosis with polyangiitis, particularly if obvious granulomas are not seen, and they may also be ANCA positive; diagnosis is established by the history and sometimes the presence of talc or other foreign material in the biopsy.[13] Nasal natural killer (NK)/T-cell lymphomas of the palate and nasal cavity is characterized by the absence of an atypical lymphocytic infiltrate (see below).

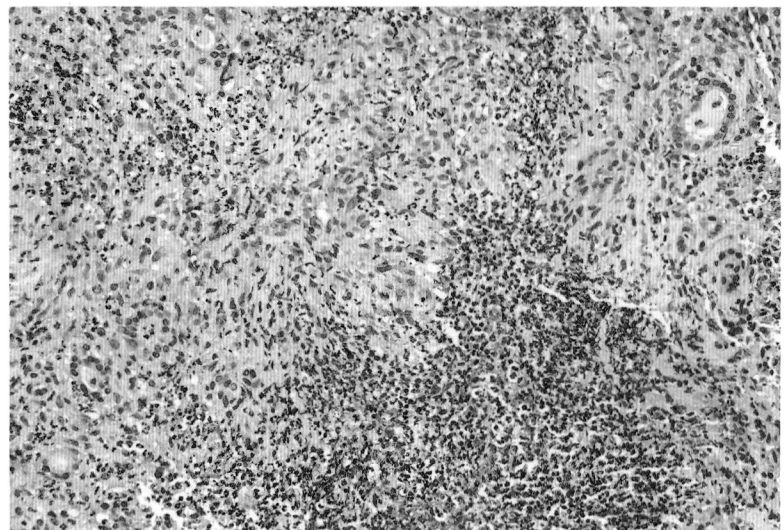

Fig. 11.178
Oral granulomatosis with polyangiitis: there is necrosis, acute and chronic inflammation involving salivary glands and granulomatous inflammation.

SALIVARY GLAND DISEASE

Reactive conditions

Mucocele and salivary duct cyst

Clinical features

This usually arises in children and young adults, and the most common locations are the lower lip mucosa (59–73%), buccal mucosa (11–17%), floor of mouth (7–12%), and ventral tongue (4%) (*Fig. 11.179*).[1-6] It presents as a dome-shaped, fluctuant, bluish, and sessile lesion, which often increases and decreases in size. Some sclerose to form fibromas.

Superficial mucoceles are distinctly vesicular or dewdrop-like, raising the suspicion of a herpetic infection or autoimmune vesiculobullous disease and occur in older adults, particularly on the hard palatal mucosa, retromolar pad, and buccal mucosa. They occur often in patients with chronic graft-versus-host disease likely as a result of hyposalivation but may also be associated with other inflammatory mucosal disorders.[7-10]

Floor of mouth mucoceles, when large, are also called ranulas, and these may extend below the mylohyoid muscle presenting extraorally as a 'plunging ranula'.[11] There is recurrence in approximately 2% of cases.[1]

Salivary duct cyst occurs in the sixth decade and the most common site is the floor of mouth (approximately 25%), and unlike extravasation mucoceles, the lower lip mucosa is only affected in 16% of cases.[12]

Pathogenesis and histologic features

A mucocele (mucous extravasation type) is a pseudocyst caused by a discontinuity in the excretory duct and spillage of mucin into the connective tissue. Salivary duct cyst or sialocyst results from dilatation of the excretory duct, caused by a distal obstruction and is therefore a true retention cyst.

Mucous extravasation mucoceles consist of pools of mucin containing muciphages and often many neutrophils surrounded by condensed granulation tissue with associated muciphages (*Figs 11.180* and *11.181*).[1,2,13] Some specimens consist only of the collapsed wall of granulation tissue or even a solid mass of granulation tissue containing muciphages or clear cells (*Fig. 11.182*). Synovium-like papillary structures may be present[14] (*Fig. 11.183*).

Mucin may be dispersed in the inter- and intralobular connective tissue, and portions of a metaplastic duct are seen in 20% of cases.[2] Occasionally, eosinophilic globular masses are present within the mucin pools, a condition referred to as myxoglobulosis (*Fig. 11.184*).[15-17]

Superficial mucoceles exhibit pools of mucin that are bordered superiorly by surface squamous epithelium only that is often atrophic, with the adjacent epithelium forming a collarette around the mucin pool (*Fig. 11.185*).[8,18]

Salivary duct cysts are lined by cuboidal or columnar epithelium, sometimes with an undulating luminal surface, often with squamous metaplasia, and also variably mucous, oncocytic, ciliated, or apocrine cell metaplasia (*Figs 11.186* and *11.187*).[7,12,19] In many cases, smaller dilated ducts with similar histopathology are present within gland parenchyma, confirming the reactive and not neoplastic nature of this condition. The associated minor salivary glands exhibit varying degrees of acinar atrophy, ductal dilatation, and interstitial chronic inflammation with fibrosis.

Differential diagnosis

Parulides or sinus tracts of the gingiva may be mistaken for extravasation mucoceles because edema fluid is interpreted as mucin. However, neither pools of mucin nor muciphages are present, and microabscesses and sinus tracts are almost always evident. Mucoceles do not occur on the gingiva.

Papillary cystadenomas are uncommon neoplasms consisting of a benign adenomatous proliferation of salivary ductal cells in a cystic configuration (see below). Only a single case of papillary cystadenoma lymphomatosum (Warthin tumor) has been reported in the minor glands, and this may represent a salivary duct cyst that is inflamed.[20]

Sialolith

Clinical features

Sialoliths or salivary gland calculi affect patients in their sixth or seventh decade. Those in the minor glands are generally asymptomatic unless infected, while those in the major glands, especially in Wharton duct (the most common site for sialoliths), cause symptoms of pain, pressure, and

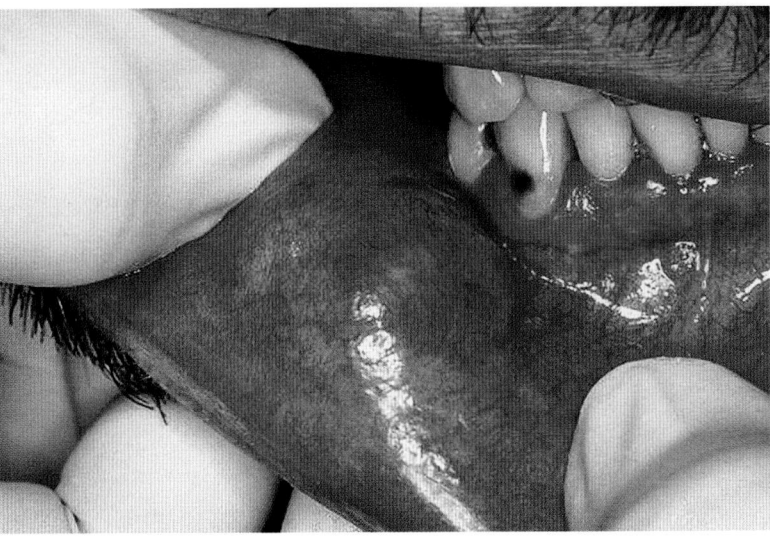

Fig. 11.179
Mucocele: note the bluish sessile nodule on the lower labial mucosa, a typical site.

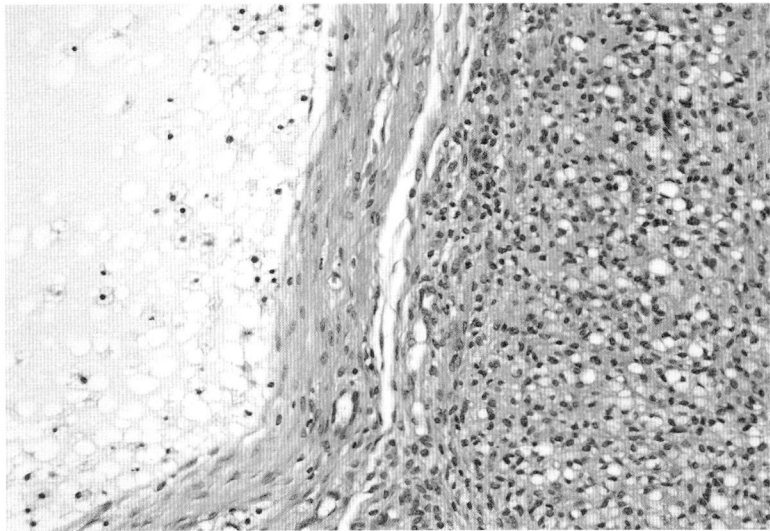

Fig. 11.181
Mucocele: the mucocele contains mucin and muciphages and is surrounded by granulation tissue containing muciphages and inflammatory cells; there is no lining epithelium present.

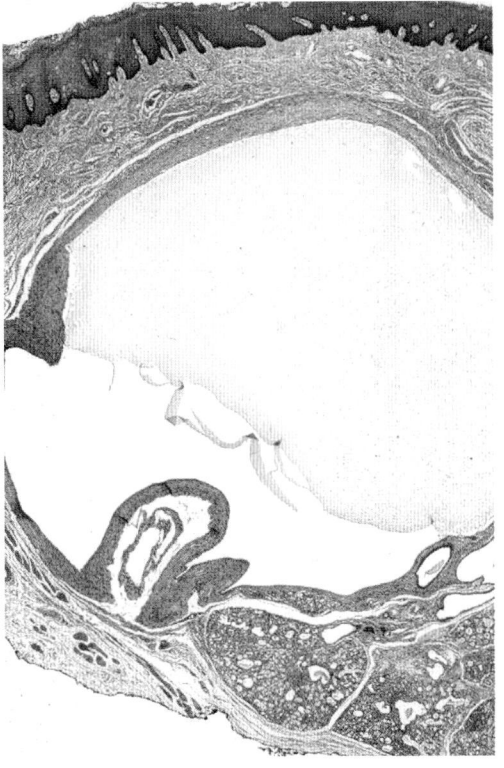

Fig. 11.180
Mucocele: there is a cyst-like cavity filled with mucin surrounded by granulation tissue without lining epithelium.

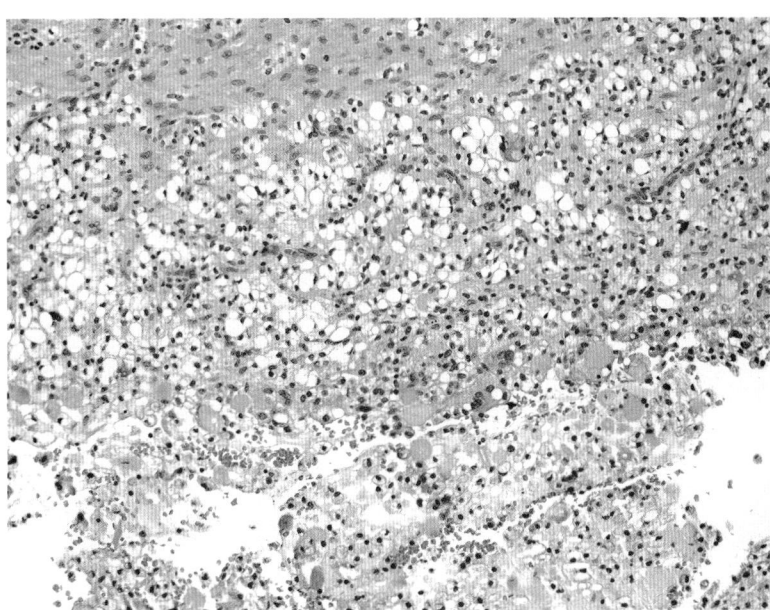

Fig. 11.182
Mucocele: the wall of a mucocele may contain clear cells

swelling just before meals. The most common sites for minor gland sialoliths are the upper lip mucosa and buccal mucosa, which together account for 75–90% of all minor salivary gland lithiasis.[1–3] They present as hard nodules and may drain if infected.

Pathogenesis and histologic features

Sialoliths form around a central nidus of bacteria, cell debris, and/or mucous plug. It is most common in the Wharton duct in the floor of mouth because of the long and tortuous nature of the duct.

The sialolith consists of concentric lamellar and globular calcifications within a cystically dilated excretory duct that exhibits squamous, mucous cell or ciliated cell metaplasia, and periductal inflammation (*Fig. 11.188*).[1,2] Bacteria, inflammatory cells and cellular debris may be present within or around the lith. Rupture can lead to acute and chronic inflammation and/or a foreign body reaction. Approximately one-quarter of calculi are unmineralized.[1]

Differential diagnosis

Phleboliths and calcified thrombi are generally not lamellated and occur within vascular lumina lined by endothelial cells.

Necrotizing sialometaplasia

Clinical features

This is a self-healing inflammatory condition of salivary glands that may be clinically and histologically mistaken for a malignancy because of its rapidly progressive, ulcerative nature and the lack of associated pain in a substantial proportion of cases.

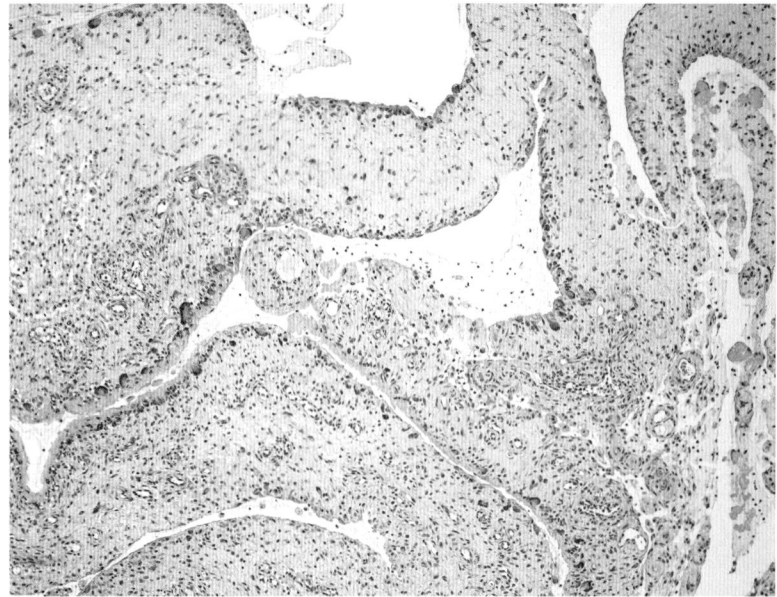

Fig. 11.183
Mucocele: the granulation tissue around the mucocele may throw into folds resembling synovium.

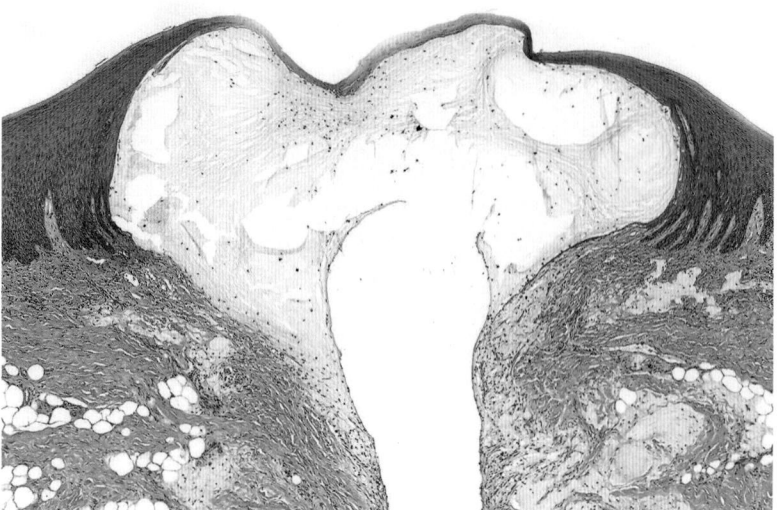

Fig. 11.185
Superficial mucocele: pools of mucin abut thinned epithelium, which forms a collarette at the periphery.

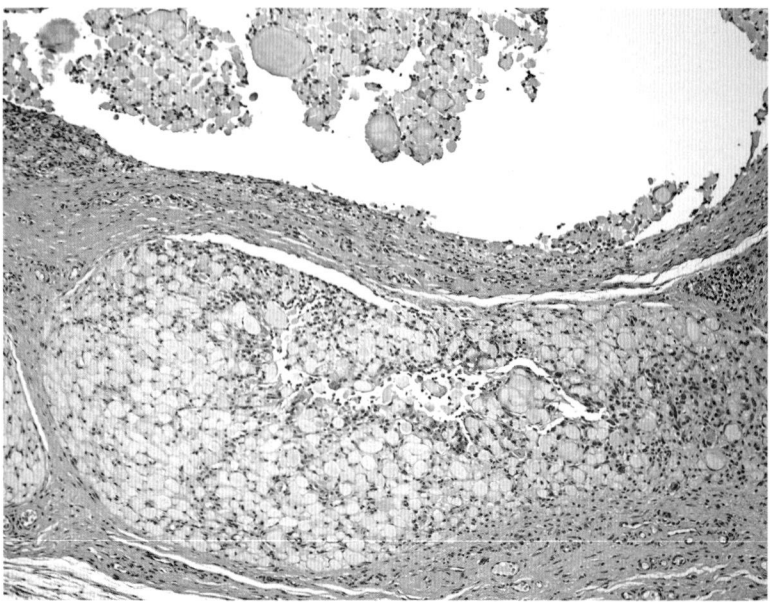

Fig. 11.184
Mucocele: there are eosinophilic globules of condensed mucin within the pseudocystic cavity and within the wall.

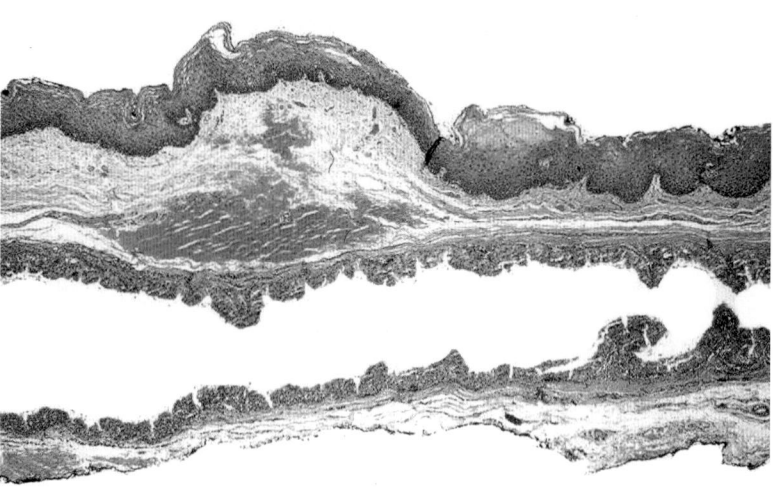

Fig. 11.186
Salivary duct cyst: this retention cyst consists of a grossly ectatic excretory salivary duct; intraluminal papillary projections are evident.

Adults are mainly affected with a mean age of onset in the fifth decade, with a 2:1 male:female ratio. It usually presents as a painful or painless ulcer or, less often, as a swelling, with the majority (approximately 80%) occurring on the hard palatal mucosa (*Fig. 11.189*). Approximately 10% of cases affect the major glands and less frequently, the mucous glands of the nose, maxillary sinus, and larynx.[1] One-third of patients give a history of recent surgery at the site. Other predisposing factors include a history of trauma, injection of local anesthetics, or alcohol and tobacco use, and there is sometimes an association with tumors.[1,3,4] Cases have been reported in bulimic patients and chronic cocaine users.[2,5,6] Generally, healing occurs spontaneously within several weeks of diagnosis.

Pathogenesis and histologic features

The etiology is vascular compromise leading to infarction of the glands and reactive squamous metaplasia of the ducts and acini. This has been experimentally produced by ligation of salivary ducts and injection with local

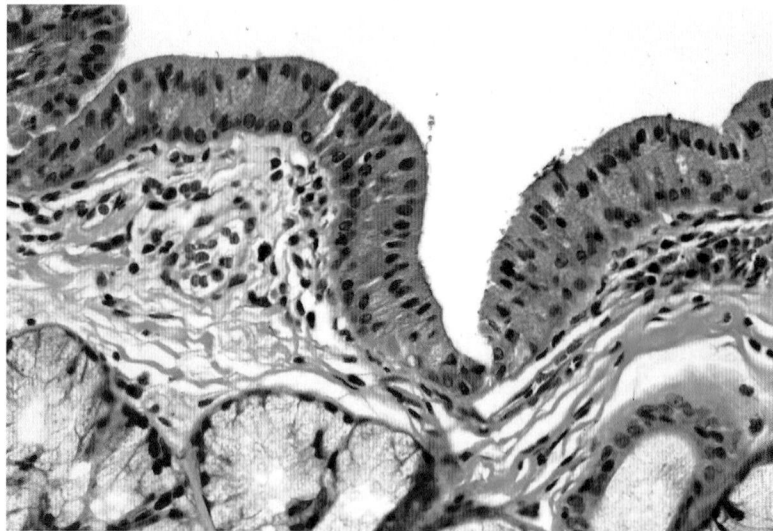

Fig. 11.187
Salivary duct cyst: the lining cells are oncocytic (oncocytic sialocyst).

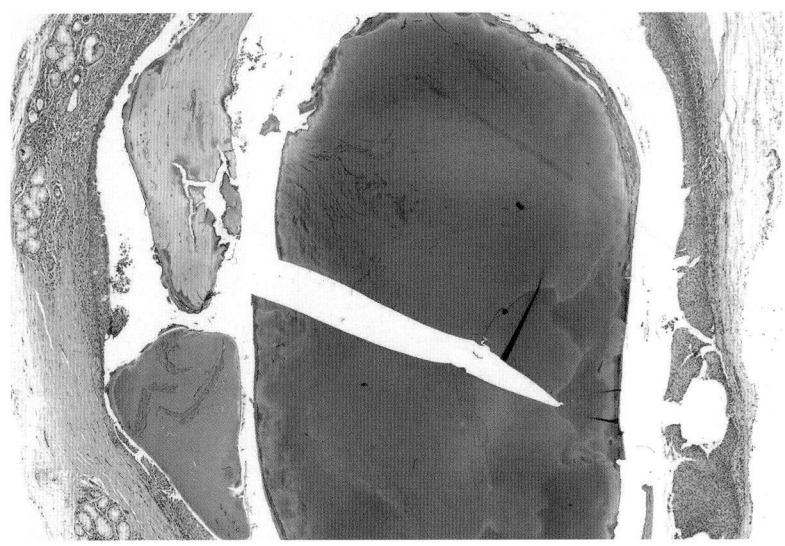

Fig. 11.188
Sialolith: the sialolith is present within an ectatic salivary duct, the lining of which exhibits squamous metaplasia.

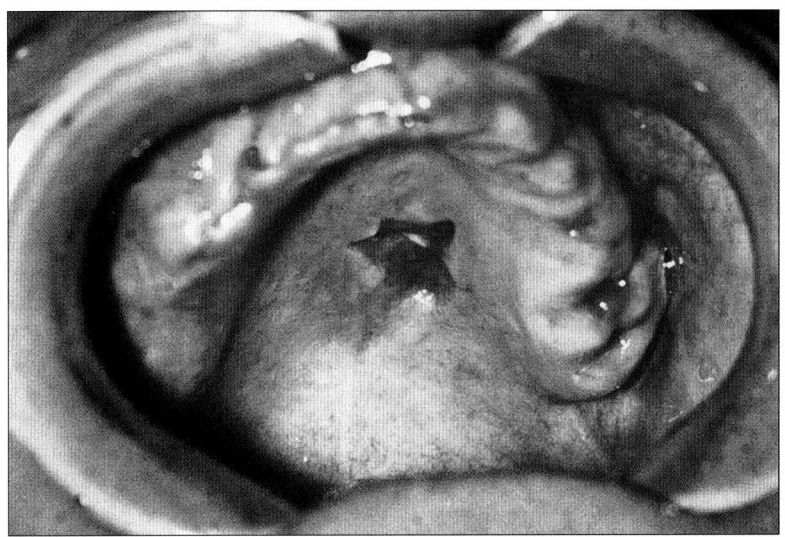

Fig. 11.189
Necrotizing sialometaplasia: there is punched-out ulcer on the hard palatal mucosa. By courtesy of C. Allen, DDS, Columbus, USA.

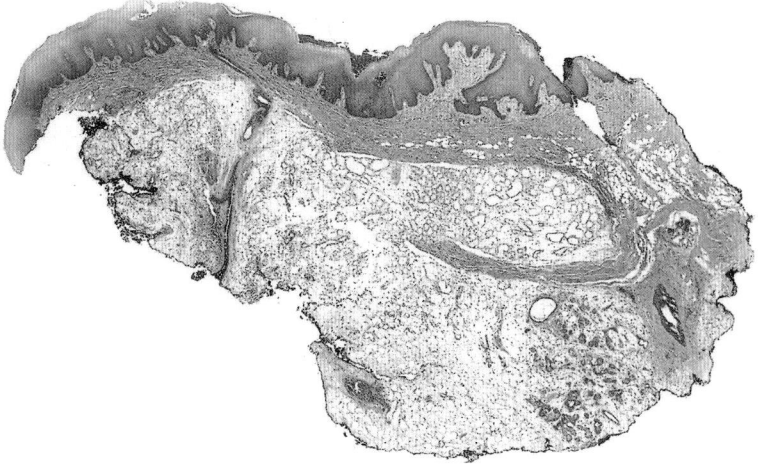

Fig. 11.190
Necrotizing sialometaplasia: there is extensive infarction necrosis with mucous extravasation; in this case, lobular architecture has been effaced.

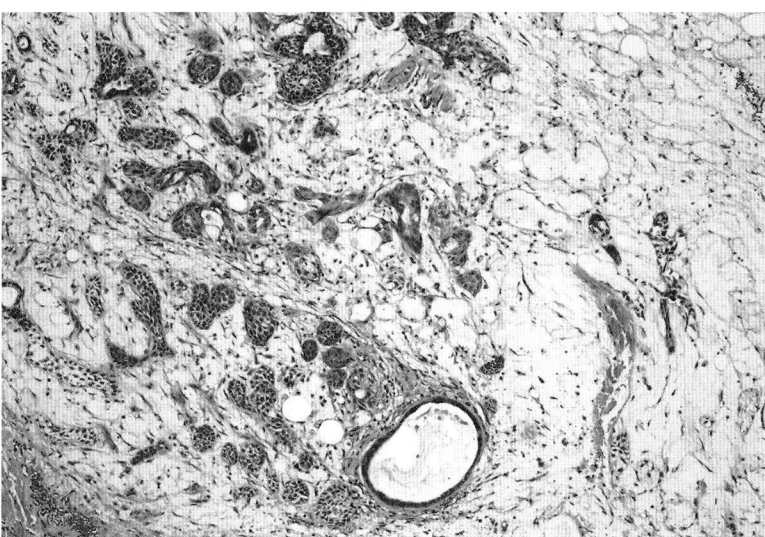

Fig. 11.191
Necrotizing sialometaplasia: there is preservation of the basement membrane of acini with acinar atrophy, and squamous metaplasia of ducts.

anesthetics.[7,8] This hypothesis is supported by the development of necrotizing sialometaplasia in a patient with Buerger disease.[9] Hypoxia-inducible factor-1-α has been identified within gland parenchyma, the endothelium, and stromal cells.[10]

There is generally preservation of lobular architecture, although sometimes this may be effaced. Very early lesions may show predominantly mucus spillage. Early lesions show infarction of acini and loss of acinar cells resulting in outlines of acinar units from preservation of the basement membrane and necrosis; more advanced lesions show pseudoinvasive islands of benign-appearing metaplastic squamous epithelium (*Figs 11.190* and *11.191*). There is generally a prominent inflammatory infiltrate with granulation tissue formation in later stages.[1,11–13]

Variable features include pseudoepitheliomatous hyperplasia, reactive epithelial atypia, and vascular occlusion. Serous and mucoserous glands are less likely to show the necrosis and infarctive changes.[1]

Differential diagnosis

The preservation of lobular architecture, lack of infiltration of the surrounding tissues by the epithelial elements, infarction necrosis, and generally bland nuclear morphology of the metaplastic islands distinguish this condition from squamous cell carcinoma. Mucoepidermoid carcinoma exhibits a proliferation of epidermoid, intermediate, and mucous cells often forming cystic and ductal structures and solid sheets, with infiltration of surrounding structures (see later).

Subacute necrotizing sialadenitis characteristically develops in younger patients (second and third decades), with an almost exclusive location on the palatal mucosa. Presentation, which is typically acute and occurs over a matter of days, is characterized by a painful, nonulcerated mass, with rapid resolution within 2 weeks.[14] Since most cases have been reported in the military, there is speculation that this may represent a viral infection that is transmitted between individuals living in close quarters. There is multifocal acinar necrosis with little ductal metaplasia (*Fig. 11.192*). The glands are diffusely infiltrated by a mixed inflammatory infiltrate of neutrophils, lymphocytes, histiocytes, and occasionally eosinophils.[15,16]

Cheilitis glandularis (stomatitis glandularis)

Clinical features

Cheilitis glandularis (stomatitis glandularis, cheilitis glandularis apostematosa) is a rare chronic, recurrent, inflammatory, and, in some cases, suppurative condition of the minor salivary glands, usually of the lower lip. Simple, deep, and deep suppurative forms have been identified. Because

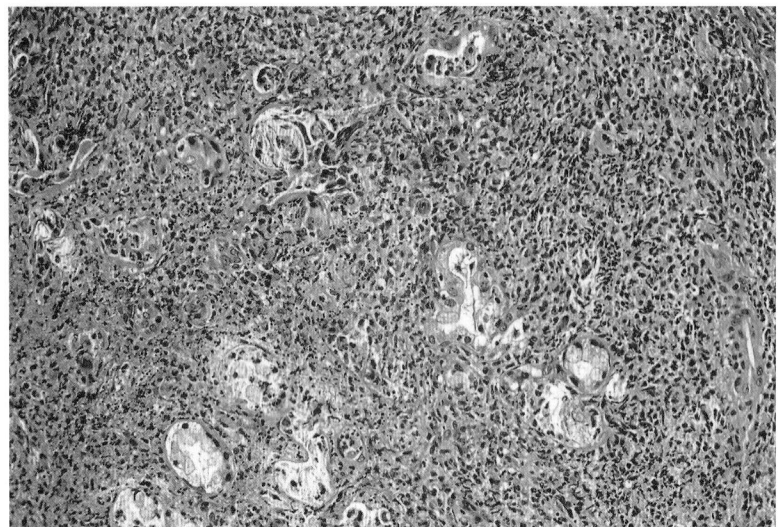

Fig. 11.192
Subacute necrotizing sialadenitis: there is marked acute and chronic inflammation with destruction of the acini.

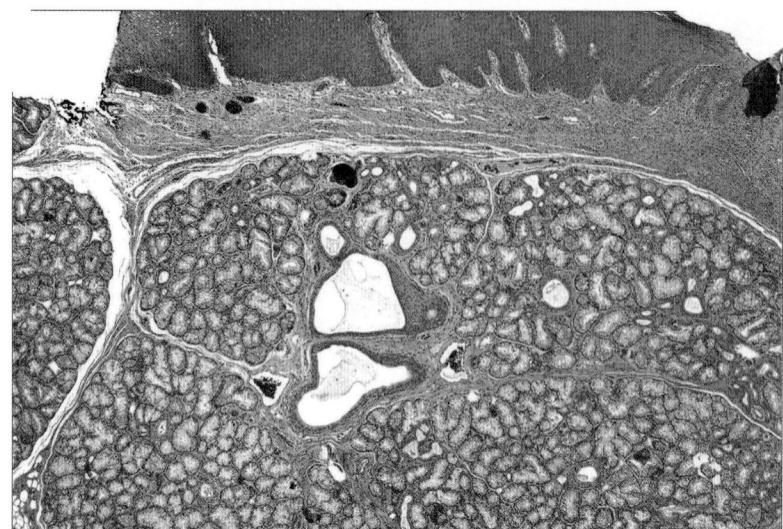

Fig. 11.194
Salivary gland adenomatoid hyperplasia: there is benign hyperplasia of mucous acini.

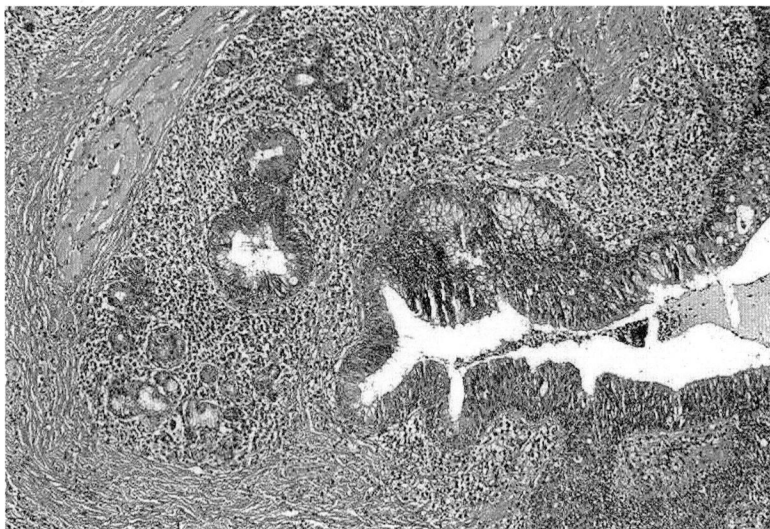

Fig. 11.193
Cheilitis glandularis: there are dilated excretory ducts with mucous cell metaplasia, intraluminal suppuration, and surrounding chronic inflammation.

salivary glands at other mucosal sites may be affected, the alternative term 'stomatitis glandularis' has been proposed.[1]

This condition affects older adults with a 3 : 1 male predilection. There is a painless or painful swelling and eversion of the lip, often with a mucous or mucopurulent discharge through duct ostia.[1-3] The lip exhibits photodamage.

Pathogenesis and histologic features

The etiology is unknown, but the condition is likely to represent an inflammatory response to either actinic damage extending down the salivary ducts, and/or to local irritants. Cases of carcinomatous transformation have occurred in older male patients who smoke, and who have been engaged in outdoor activities for decades; it is postulated that eversion of the lower lip increases its exposure to actinic damage.[4,5] Familial examples have been reported.[6,7]

There is dilatation and metaplasia (squamous, mucous cell and/or onco-cytic) of the excretory ducts with variable periductal acute and chronic inflammation. Intraluminal suppuration is almost always present.[1,2,8-10] The minor salivary glands exhibit non-specific inflammatory changes of acinar atrophy, ductal ectasia, interstitial fibrosis, and interstitial inflammation (*Fig. 11.193*).[2,9] Cases should always be evaluated for dysplasia and carcinoma.

Differential diagnosis

Similar histologic changes are seen in glandular obstruction such as occurs in glands draining into a mucocele and, in particular, in glands that have been plugged by thick mucinous secretions or by small calculi with subsequent inflammation. The clinical presentation of diffuse lip involvement separates this condition from mucocele or sialolithiasis, both of which are localized and discrete phenomena.

Salivary gland neoplasms

Clinical features

Here, only the more common salivary gland neoplasms affecting the minor glands will be discussed. Approximately half of intraoral salivary gland neoplasms are benign and half are malignant, and there is a female predilection.[1-4] The most common sites are the mucosa of the hard and soft palate, lip mucosa (especially upper), and buccal mucosa, although any site may be involved. As expected, lesions present as a firm swelling at the site. Benign lesions tend to have a long history of gradual enlargement, while malignant lesions tend to grow more rapidly and ulcerate. Over the past two decades, much progress has been made in identifying gene rearrangements and fusion products associated with both benign and malignant tumors.[5]

The ensuing discussion will focus on the histopathology of only five lesions which present with some frequency in the oral cavity:
- pleomorphic adenoma,
- canalicular adenoma,
- mucoepidermoid carcinoma,
- polymorphous adenocarcinoma,
- adenoid cystic carcinoma.

There may be some variation in prevalence of some tumors over others based on racial differences.[3,4]

Pleomorphic adenoma (with its variant, myoepithelioma) and canalicular adenoma comprise the two most common benign neoplasms.[1,3,4] The canalicular adenoma has a particular predilection for the upper lip in females and lesions are often multifocal.

The most common malignant neoplasm is mucoepidermoid carcinoma, the second most common tumor overall after pleomorphic adenoma.[1,3,4] Polymorphous adenocarcinoma and adenoid cystic carcinoma occur with approximately equal frequency.[6-8] Adenomatoid hyperplasia of the minor glands consists of a lobular proliferation of normal-appearing mucous acini. This condition is often seen adjacent to, and possibly as a reaction to, an adjacent salivary gland neoplasm and should prompt a search for the primary tumor (*Fig. 11.194*).[9-11]

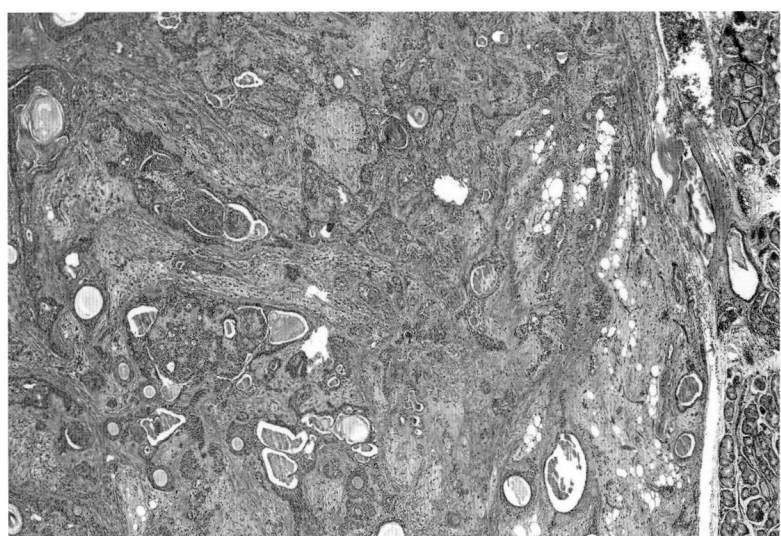

Fig. 11.195
Pleomorphic adenoma: the tumor consists of a discrete proliferation of ducts and myoepithelial cells in a myxo-chondroid stroma.

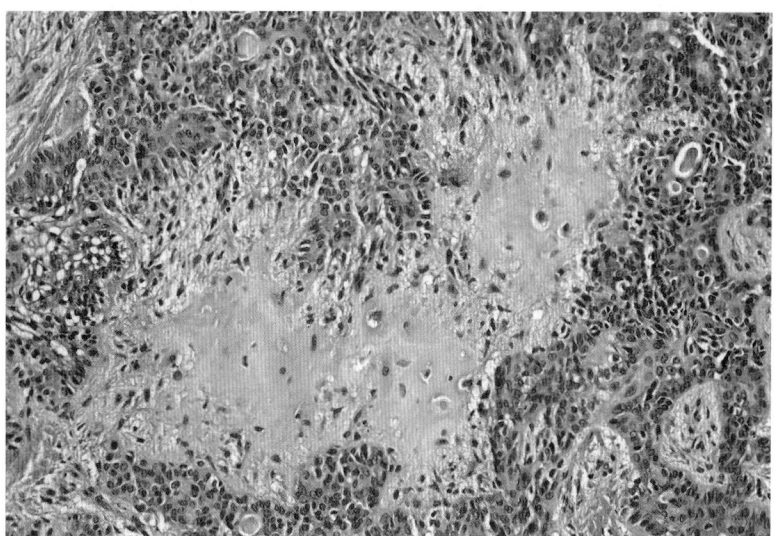

Fig. 11.197
Pleomorphic adenoma: there is a focal chondroid stroma and myoepithelial cells are epithelioid, spindled and stellate-shaped.

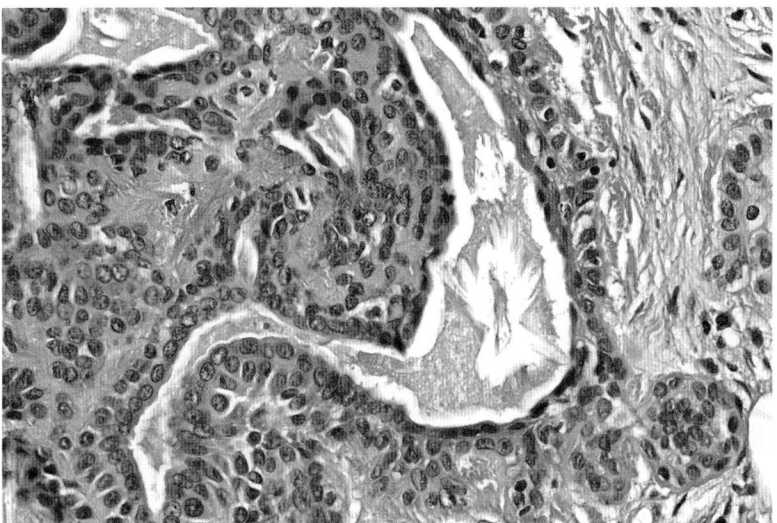

Fig. 11.196
Pleomorphic adenoma: the ducts are lined by uniform cuboidal cells surrounded by multiple layers of myoepithelial cells.

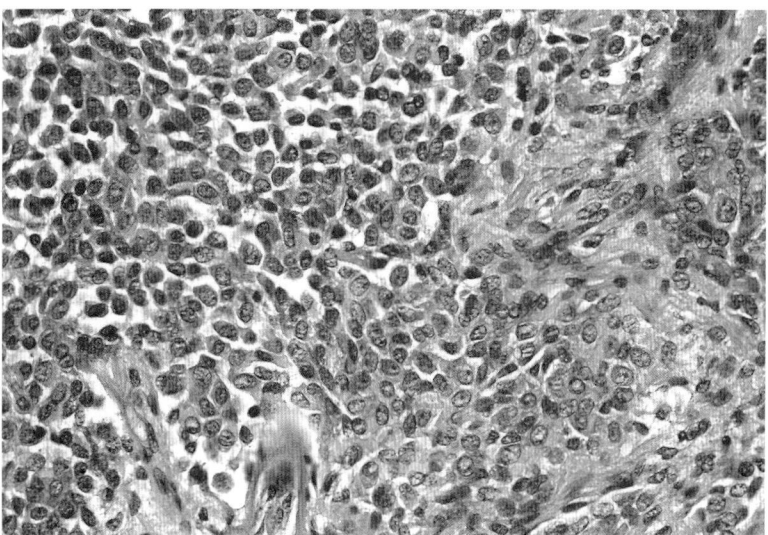

Fig. 11.198
Myoepithelioma: there are many plasmacytoid myoepithelial cells with eccentric nuclei and abundant eosinophilic cytoplasm.

Pleomorphic adenoma

This term is preferable to the old term of 'benign mixed tumor'. It is believed to arise from intercalated duct reserve cells with differentiation towards ductal and myoepithelial cells. Over 90% of pleomorphic adenomas and myoepitheliomas are positive for *PLAG1* or *HMGA2* rearrangements.[12,13]

In its classic presentation, it comprises a discrete and usually unencapsulated proliferation of ductal and myoepithelial cells within a myxochondroid matrix.[14] Ducts are lined by eosinophilic cuboidal cells and surrounded by a cuff of epithelioid myoepithelial cells that become spindle or stellate-shaped within the stroma which is hyalinized and/or myxochondroid, sometimes with bone or adipose tissue formation (*Figs 11.195–11.197*).[15] Tyrosine crystals may be present and keratin pearl formation is not infrequent and should not be misinterpreted as a sign of malignancy, and neither should focal capsular involvement by tumor. Many variations of this classic histology may be seen including cellular and myxoid variants and, importantly, the myoepithelial predominant variant, or myoepithelioma.[2–4]

Myoepitheliomas are a variant of pleomorphic adenoma where the myoepithelial element predominates and where ductal structures may be minimal or altogether absent. Most lesions occur on the palatal mucosa and consist of spindled cells, plasmacytoid or 'hyaline' cells (large round or polyhedral cells with abundant eosinophil cytoplasm, eccentric nuclei, and nuclear pleomorphism), clear cells, epithelioid cells, or a combination (*Fig. 11.198*).[16] Clusters of such plasmacytoid myoepithelial cells may be seen in banal pleomorphic adenoma. Differentiation of myoepitheliomas from plasmacytoma is based on the myoepithelial cells not exhibiting a zone of Hopf, the lack of a clumped chromatin pattern, and negative studies for B-cell markers.

Ductal cells are immunopositive for epithelial membrane antigen (EMA), AE1/AE3, CK7, CK8, CK19, and SOX10. Myoepithelial/basal cells are immunopositive for pankeratin, K14, S100 protein, vimentin, calponin, SMA, smooth muscle myosin long chain, GFAP (in neoplastic cells), p63, p40, and SOX10.[14,17,18]

Malignant transformation in intraoral pleomorphic adenomas occurs but it is uncommon, and the pre-existing pleomorphic adenoma is identified from rearrangements of *PLAG1* or *HMGA2*.[14,19]

Canalicular adenoma

This tumor also likely arises from the intercalated duct reserve cell with differentiation towards ductal structures without a myoepithelial component.[20] There is an encapsulated proliferation of interconnected ribbons,

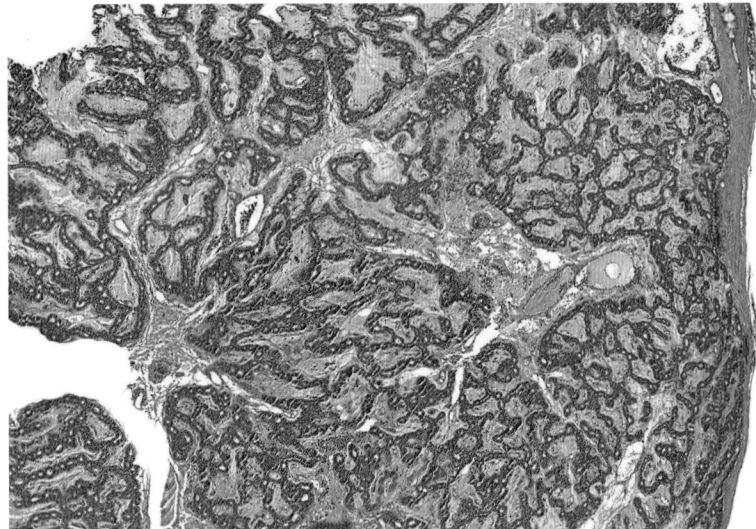

Fig. 11.199
Canalicular adenoma: the tumor is encapsulated and composed of interconnected strands and trabeculae of basaloid cells in myxoid stroma.

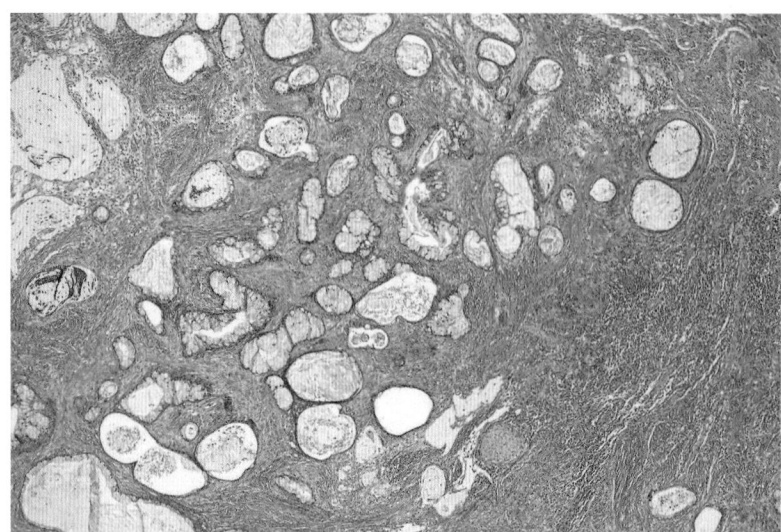

Fig. 11.201
Mucoepidermoid carcinoma: the tumor consists of ducts and cystic spaces lined by mucous and epidermoid cells with stromal infiltration.

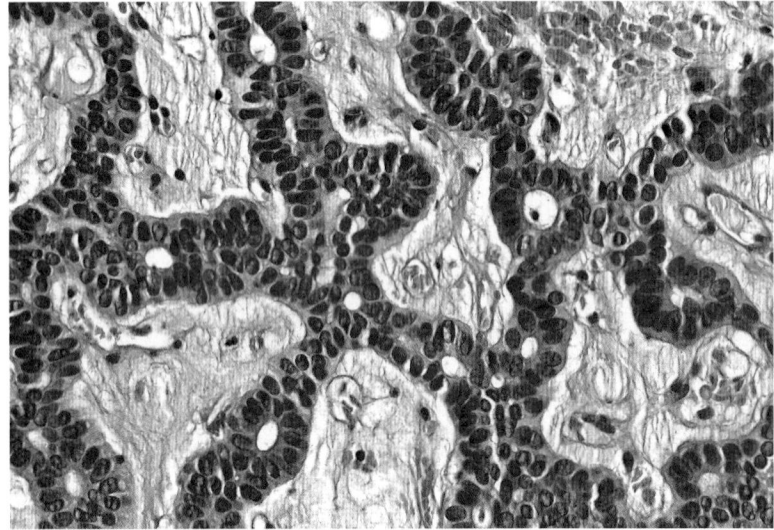

Fig. 11.200
Canalicular adenoma: the tumor strands are two cells thick and form small knots where they bulge; ductal structures are present, and the stroma is myxoid with dilated capillaries and little collagen or fibroblasts.

strands and trabeculae of basaloid cells, often in a double layer; beads or knots of cells form where there is bulging of the epithelial strands. Solid and trabecular forms are also recognized.[21,22] The nuclei are fusiform with small nucleoli and dispersed chromatin, and are palisaded. Clusters of mucous cells and oncocytes may be seen. The stroma is generally mucinous/myxoid and contains ectatic capillaries with scant collagen. Multifocality is not uncommon and should not be mistaken for infiltration (*Figs 11.199* and *11.200*).[23,24] Tumor cells are immunopositive for AE1/AE3, CAM 5.2, CK7, CK19, EMA, S100 protein, vimentin, CD117, and SOX10, but not SMA or other myoepithelial markers although GFAP is often positive at the tumor-capsule interface.[14,22,25,26]

Mucoepidermoid carcinoma

This tumor is believed to arise from the excretory duct reserve cell. It is associated with the fusion oncogenes *MECT1/3* (*CRTC1/3*)-*MAML2* in 40–60% of cases, which correlates with younger age, lower grade lesions, and better prognosis.[27,28] Mucoepidermoid carcinoma consists of a proliferation of mucous, epidermoid cell, and intermediate cells with variable duct and cyst formation (*Figs 11.201* and *11.202*).[14,29,30] The epidermoid

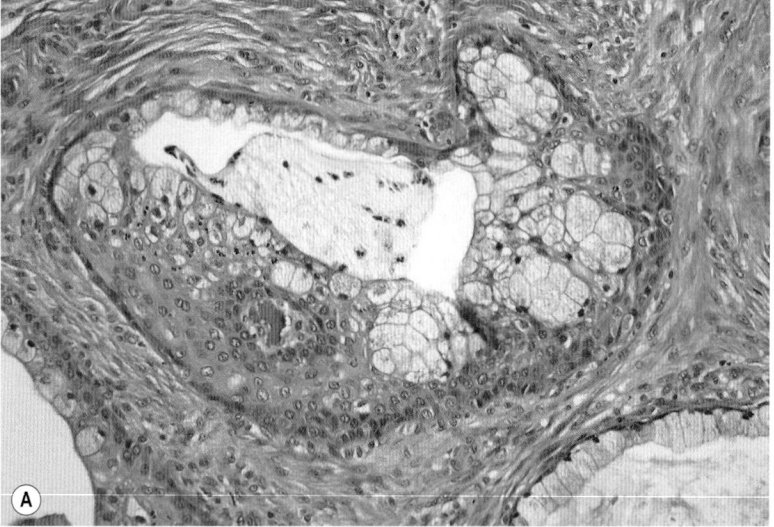

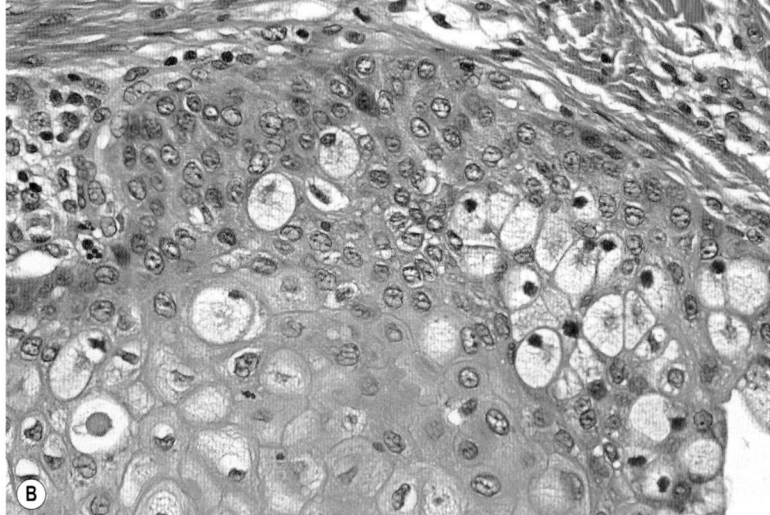

Fig. 11.202
Mucoepidermoid carcinoma: (**A**) this tumor island consists of mucous, intermediate and epidermoid cells; (**B**) this tumor island contains mostly squamous and intermediate cells with scattered mucous cells.

cells have ample, pale eosinophilic cytoplasm and medium-sized nuclei with dispersed chromatin, while intermediate cells have less cytoplasm. Cystic structures are often lined by all three cell types, often with luminal proliferation of the same cells forming ducts and complex architecture. Some tumors have a preponderance of clear cells. Invasion of the stroma occurs as small islands of cells, and these may not always be readily identified. Mucous cells are mucicarmine positive, and most tumor cells are immunopositive for p63 and membrane-bound mucins MUC1 and MUC4 (>70%), and are negative for S100 protein and SOX10.[31-34] A sclerosing variant that exhibits sclerosis and stromal eosinophilia, and an oncocytic variant exist.[35,36]

For many decades, grading into low, intermediate, and high grades was based on the presence of cystic spaces and the proportion of mucous to epidermoid cells. Studies have proposed grading schemas using point systems based on the proportion of cystic structures, necrosis, anaplasia, mitotic activity, stromal and bone invasion, and neural and vascular invasion.[37,38] However, in the 2017 fourth edition of the World Health Organization (WHO) Classification of Head and Neck Tumors, no particular grading system was adopted.[39] Expression of p27 and high Ki-67 index may negatively impact prognosis; however, the presence of *MECT1/3* (CRT-C1/3)-*MAML2* fusion genes is associated with lower clinical stage and improved prognosis.[28,40,41]

Secretory carcinoma is usually microcystic or papillary, lacks significant numbers of mucous cells, and is immunopositive for S100 protein, vimentin and mammoglobin, and negative for p63; it is positive for *ETV6* rearrangement.[42,43] Low-grade cystic lesions may be mistaken for papillary cystadenomas.[14,44] In cystadenoma, there is no luminal proliferation of mucous and epidermoid cells, complex ductal architecture and invasion of the surrounding stroma are not present, and p63 is positive in a single layer of myoepithelial/basal cells rather than throughout the tumor in mucoepidermoid carcinoma.[45]

Mucoepidermoid carcinoma may also share similarities with a mucinous papillary cystadenocarcinoma which has prominent luminal papillae, shows hobnailing of cells into the lumen, and more cytological atypia and mitotic activity, but this too will show p63 positivity only in the basal/myoepithelial cells in a single layer.[46]

Polymorphous adenocarcinoma

Two tumors previously named polymorphous low-grade adenocarcinoma (PLGA) and cribriform adenocarcinoma of salivary gland (CASG) have now been combined into a single entity in the recent WHO update with the CASG considered the rare cribriform variant of polymorphous adenocarcinoma.[47,48] However, for the sake of discussion, the old terms of PLGA and CASG will be used here because there are histopathological and prognostic differences between the two.[48] One clinical difference is that more than 80% of PLGAs occur in the palatal mucosa while more than 60% of CASG occur in the tongue. PLGAs also tend to behave less aggressively thatn CASG.

An activating hotspot mutation in *PRDK1* has been identified in over 70% of tumors previously classified as PLGA,[49] while CASG shows tranlocations involving *PDRK1* and *ARID1A* and *DDX3X*. PLGA is an unencapsulated tumor is characterized by two features: a marked variation in the pattern of the tumor cells with solid, ductal, cribriform, cordlike, trabecular, cystic, or fascicular patterns, and isomorphism of the cells themselves (*Figs 11.203* and *11.204A*).[8,14,50] The cells are ovoid to spindled with moderate amounts of pale cytoplasm and medium-sized nuclei with finely dispersed chromatin, and small nucleoli. Nests of oncocytes, clear cells, mucous cells, and crystalloid bodies may be present. Mitotic activity and necrosis are infrequent. A helpful feature is the presence of cells 'in single file' at the periphery or near the mucosal surface of the tumor, and a swirling or 'targetoid' appearance of tumor cells especially around nerve fibers (*Fig. 11.204B*); perineural invasion is common in spite of the tumor being of low grade, but this has no effect on prognosis. The stroma is hyalinized and/or myxoid, but cartilaginous and osseous elements are not seen. It may be difficult to identify areas of true stromal invasion in curetted specimens. Tumor cells are positive for p63, S100 protein, and vimentin, weakly reactive for GFAP and CD117, and negative for p40.[50,51]

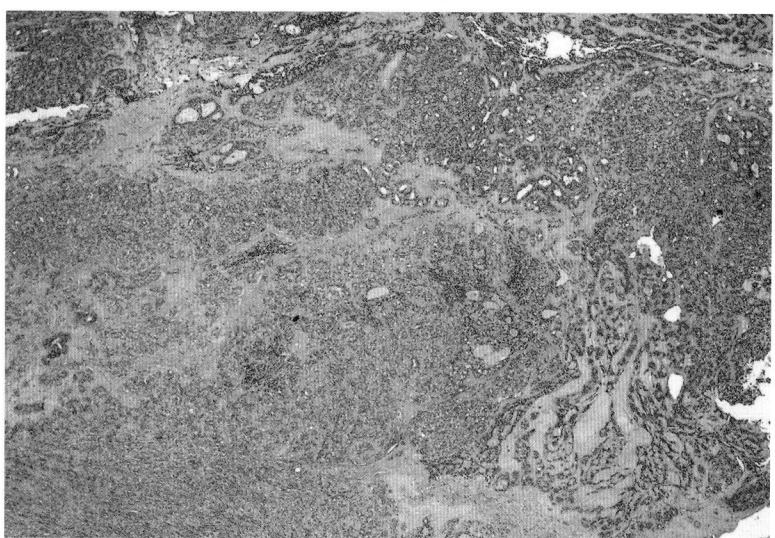

Fig. 11.203
Polymorphous low-grade adenocarcinoma: this tumor exhibits solid areas, ductal differentiation, and focal myxoid stroma.

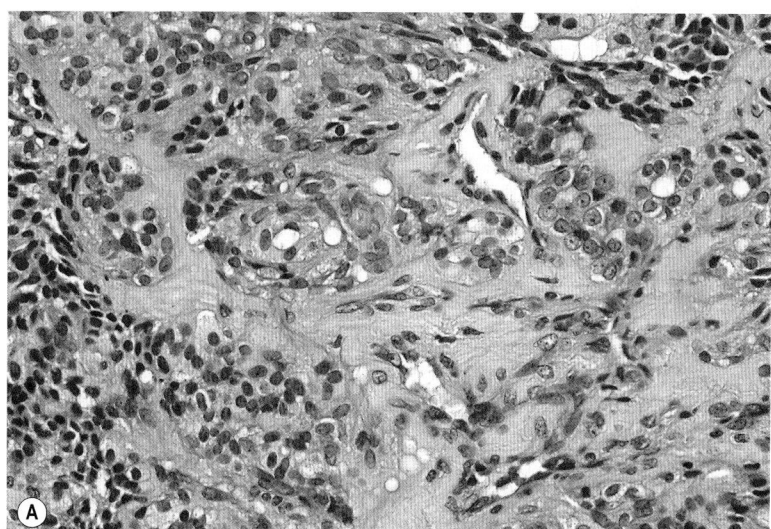

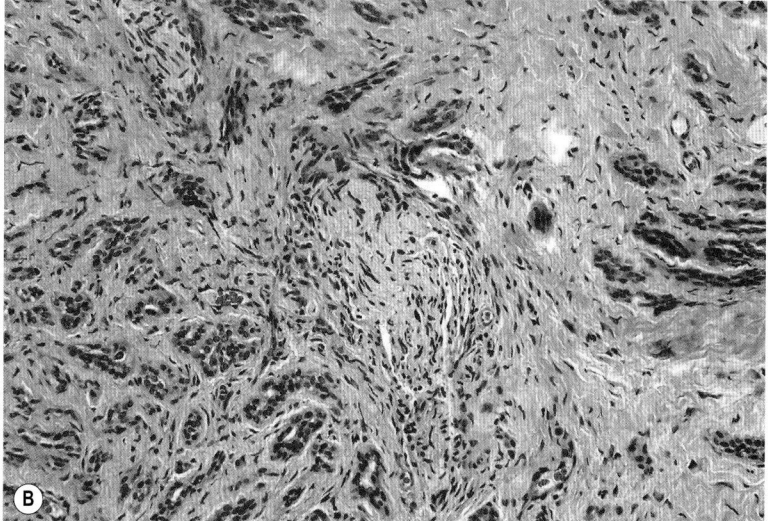

Fig. 11.204
Polymorphous low-grade adenocarcinoma: (**A**) the tumor cells are isomorphic, ovoid or spindled with pale cytoplasm, vesicular nuclei and small nucleoli; the stroma is myxoid (**B**) perineural invasion is a frequent occurrence.

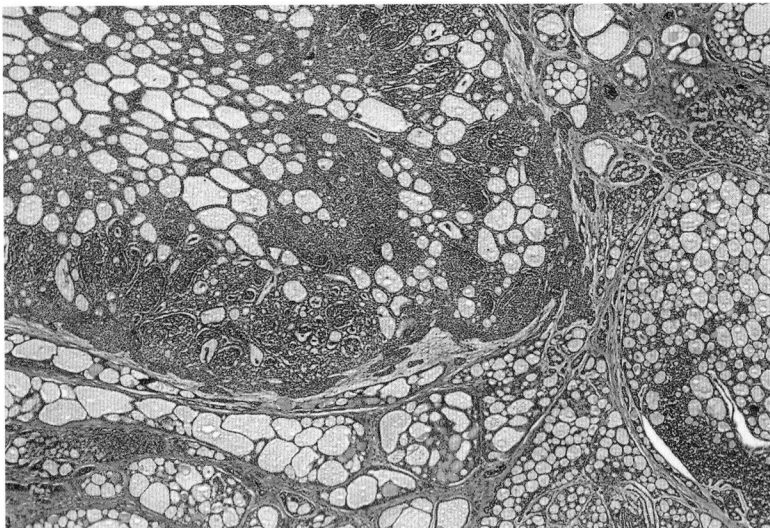

Fig. 11.205
Adenoid cystic carcinoma: this tumor has cribriform and solid patterns.

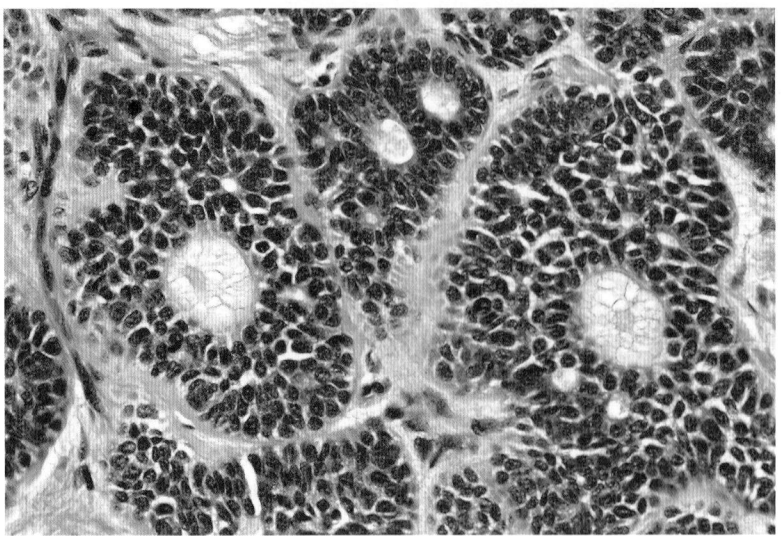

Fig. 11.206
Adenoid cystic carcinoma: tumor cells form true ducts and pseudoducts, and have pleomorphic, hyperchromatic, angular nuclei.

CASG, a rare tumor, has a monophasic cell population similar to PLGA and a solid or lobular proliferation of tumor cells with a cribriform, solid, papillary, or glomeruloid pattern.[52] The characteristic feature is in the nuclei which are clear or ground glass and overlapping similar to those of papillary thyroid carcinoma. Lymphovascular invasion is frequently seen. Lymph node metastasis occurs in up to 65% of cases,[52] and these may be misdiagnosed in lymph node biopsies as metastatic papillary thyroid carcinoma. However, tumors are negative for TTF and thyroglobulin and positive for S100 protein, p63, CK14, and other cytokeratin markers, as well as CK117 in many cases.[53]

Differentiation of PLGA from a pleomorphic adenoma may be difficult if there is no evidence of perineural invasion since it shares many features with pleomorphic adenoma such as variable pattern, bland cytology, and myxoid stroma. The presence of plasmacytoid myoepithelial cells and the cuffing of ductal structures by a layer of myoepithelial cells are features of pleomorphic adenoma not seen in PLGA which has a single tumor cell population. Pleomorphic adenomas are positive for both p63 and p40.[51,54]

The tumor may also resemble adenoid cystic carcinoma, which is a biphasic tumor and tends to have more nuclear pleomorphism, hyperchromasia and angulated nuclei. Ductal cells are positive for CD117 while periductal cells are positive for both p63 and p40.[51,55,56]

Adenoid cystic carcinoma

This tumor is positive for *MYB-NFIB* gene fusion in over 85% of cases using frozen sections and in approximately 50% of cases using formalin-fixed tissue.[57,58] It takes three forms: the classic type that has a prominent cribriform pattern, the tubular type, and the solid type which forms few ductal or cribriform structures and carries the worst prognosis.[14,21,59]

Adenoid cystic carcinoma is an invasive tumor. The cribriform pattern (so-called 'Swiss cheese' appearance) is the most common and characteristic pattern and consists of lobules of tumor cells with pseudoducts and true ducts (*Fig. 11.205*). The former consists of glycosaminoglycans surrounded by myoepithelial cells, while the latter consists of cuboidal cells with eosinophilic cytoplasm around a lumen. The tubular type consists of simple true ducts surrounded by myoepithelial cells while the solid variant consists of basaloid cells present in sheets. The tumor cells have large, ovoid or irregularly-shaped, angular, hyperchromatic nuclei (*Fig. 11.206*) The stroma is variably myxoid or hyalinized, and perineural and intraneural invasion is a frequent finding (*Fig. 11.207*). Perineural and intraneural invasion of major nerves is associated with higher local recurrence and lower survival rates as are tumors with high Ki-67 index and >30% solid component although some argue that any solid component heralds a worse prognosis.[60,61]

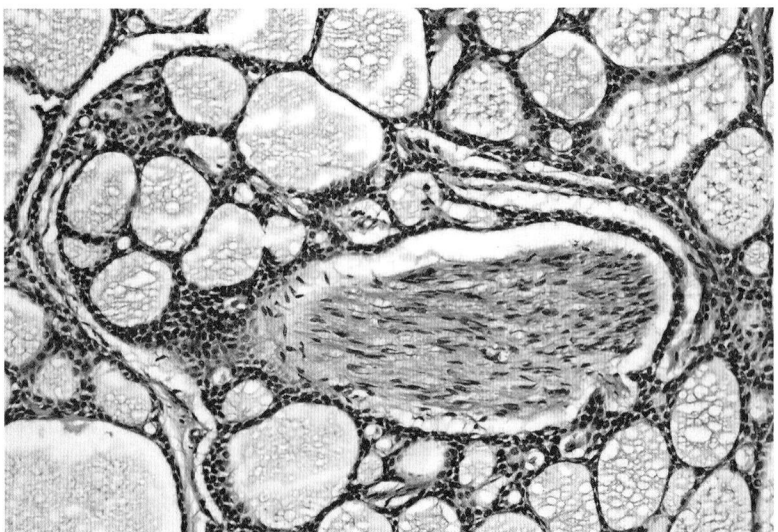

Fig. 11.207
Adenoid cystic carcinoma: this tumor has a cribriform pattern with pseudoducts, and perineural invasion.

More than 80% of adenoid cystic carcinoma are positive for myb protein.[57] The cells forming true ducts are CD117 positive, while the rest of the cells are positive for p63 and p40, distinguishing this tumor from PLGA, which is p63 positive and p40 negative.

Adenoid cystic carcinoma-like HPV-associated squamous cell carcinoma of the sinonasal tract lacks *MYB-NFIB* gene fusion, exhibits dysplasia of the overlying epithelium, and positivity for p16 and usually presence of HPV-33.[62]

Papillary ductal lesions

Three conditions deserve mention: intraductal papilloma, inverted papilloma, and sialadenoma papilliferum.[1] They are all likely reactive papillary and metaplastic lesions and not true neoplasms.

The intraductal papilloma and inverted papilloma present as mucosal nodules or masses. The intraductal papilloma occurs within a cystically dilated salivary duct and presents as a papillary proliferation of columnar and squamous epithelium and usually mucous cells overlying fibrovascular cores (*Fig. 11.208*).[1] The inverted papilloma presents as an endophytic

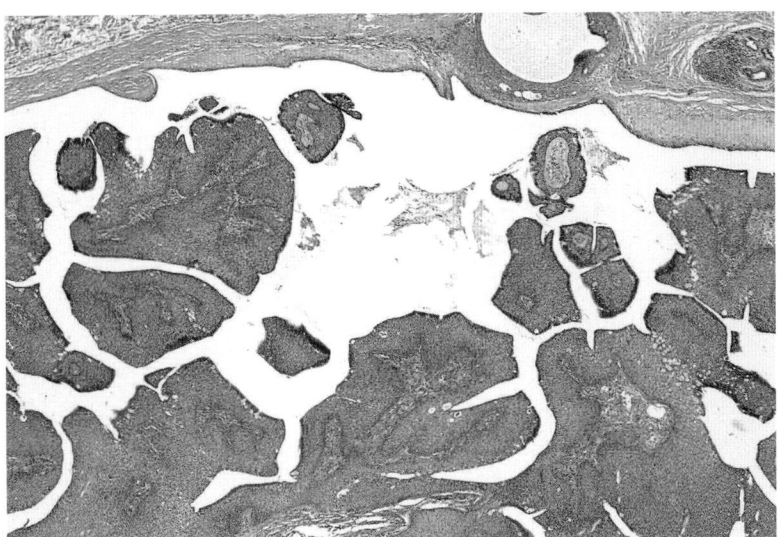

Fig. 11.208
Intraductal papillomas: there is a papillary proliferation of squamous and cuboidal epithelium with fibrovascular cores, within the lumen of the duct.

papillary proliferation of epithelium forming lobules of benign ductal epithelium with clefts that represent extensions of the lumen.[2] The epithelium is columnar on the luminal aspect and squamous or slightly basaloid within the lobules. Mucous cells and microcysts are present. There is minimal mitotic activity and usually no atypia. HPV 6 and 11 have been identified in rare cases.[3]

Sialadenoma papilliferum is the mucosal counterpart of syringocystadenoma papilliferum.[4,5] These lesions are usually located on the palatal mucosa and clinically present as an exophytic papillary growth. Microscopically, there is an exophytic benign proliferation of squamous cells resembling a squamous papilloma, and an endophytic adenomatous hyperplasia in the depth of the lesion with cystic structures. This deep component often has a complex branching architecture and luminal papillary projections of columnar and mucous cells.[4]

PREMALIGNANT CONDITIONS

Leukoplakia, erythroplakia and epithelial dysplasia

In the oral cavity, cytological changes alone are insensitive for the diagnosis of epithelial dysplasia, and correlation with clinical findings greatly improves diagnostic sensitivity and specificity. Furthermore, multiple biopsies should be obtained if the lesion is large, multifocal, and/or nonhomogenous.

Clinical features

Leukoplakia, a clinical term, is defined as a white plaque of questionable risk having excluded (other) known diseases or disorders that carry no increased risk for cancer; it excludes all frictional keratoses and is a clinical term only, modified after histopathological evaluation.[1-4] Its prevalence is 1.5%.[5] There is a strong association between the appearance of leukoplakia and the use of tobacco products.[6,7] Conversely, of all patients who have leukoplakia, 70–90% have a tobacco history and prevalence increases with age.[8,9]

Clinically, lesions may appear homogeneous (in color and texture, often with fissures) or nonhomogeneous. If the latter, they may be referred to as erythroleukoplakia (or speckled leukoplakia if red and white), verrucous leukoplakia, or nodular leukoplakia (*Figs 11.209* and *11.210*).[1,2,10] The most common sites are the tongue, buccal mucosa, and gingiva/alveolar mucosa.[6,10-12] However, sites with a higher prevalence of dysplasia and carcinoma, or 'high-risk' sites, are the floor of mouth, tongue, and soft palate (*Fig. 11.211*).[10,11,13]

Dysplasia, carcinoma in situ, or invasive squamous cell carcinoma is present in 20–43% of leukoplakias overall, although this figure is lower in subcontinental Indians.[8,10,12,14] The malignant transformation rate of leukoplakia is 3–5%.[15] If epithelial dysplasia is present, the rate increases to 12–19%, and may be as high as 27–37%.[8,10,16–20] Risk factors for malignant transformation include the presence of and degree of dysplasia, size of lesion, and verrucous/papillary architecture.

Verrucous leukoplakia represents a precursor lesion of verrucous carcinoma or papillary squamous carcinoma. Clinically, this presents as a rough white plaque on the gingiva or alveolar mucosa in patients in the sixth decade and older, with a roughly equal sex distribution.[21] More extensive and/or multifocal lesions are referred to as proliferative verrucous leukoplakia. The latter is a persistent and progressive form of leukoplakia that tends to affect women (3:1), with a tobacco habit present in only 20–30% of cases.[22–26] It starts as an innocuous leukoplakia that subsequently spreads

or develops multifocally, becoming increasingly verrucous and sometimes erythematous over one or two decades before it is recognized (*Figs 11.212* and *11.213*). Initial biopsies of these lesions show only hyperkeratosis and epithelial atrophy or verrucous epithelial hyperplasia without dysplasia, while biopsies taken years or decades later show dysplasia, and often aneuploidy.[27–29] Malignant transformation to squamous cell or verrucous carcinoma occurs in at least 70 of cases.[25,26]

Erythroplakia (similar to erythroplasia) presents as a velvety or granular red papule or plaque that is usually painless. It is much less common than leukoplakia (*Fig. 11.214*). Dysplasia, carcinoma in situ, or invasive carcinoma is present in 69–91% of cases at the time of biopsy.[30–32]

Pathogenesis and histologic features

The majority of oral squamous cell carcinomas arise in leukoplakia and the less common lesion, erythroplakia. As with other malignancies, development of invasive tumor is a multi-step process involving a series of mutational and likely epigenetic events, and these start within the visible lesions of leukoplakia or erythroplakia.[33] Oral epithelial dysplasia should be considered intraepithelial neoplasia similar to cervical intraepithelial neoplasia, and terms such as squamous intraepithelial neoplasia/lesion and oral intraepithelial neoplasia have been introduced but have not been universally accepted.[34,35] Genomic and epigenetic alterations such as loss of heterozygosity, and copy number gains (by far more common) and losses and driver mutations have been reported in leukoplakias and dysplasias; in particular, loss of heterozygosity in 3p and 9p are strongly associated with malignant transformation.[36–41] There is increased expression of p53 in moderate and severe dysplasia and carcinoma in situ.[42,43] The presence of p53 in suprabasal cells correlates with the development of oral squamous cell carcinoma even when clear evidence of dysplasia is not present.[44] Other studies have demonstrated increasing aneuploidy with increasing grades of dysplasia.[45] However, the current 'gold standard' for the evaluation of dysplasia is still routine histology.

Leukoplakias should be evaluated for dysplasia for architectural (low power objective), organizational (intermediate power objective evaluating the relationship of cells to each other within the epithelium) and cytological changes (high power objective and are changes seen on cytological smears) (*Table 11.1*). Architectural changes may be associated with only very mild cytological atypia, and verrucous hyperplasia (mainly exophytic squamous proliferation) and verrucous carcinoma (bulky exo- and endophytic

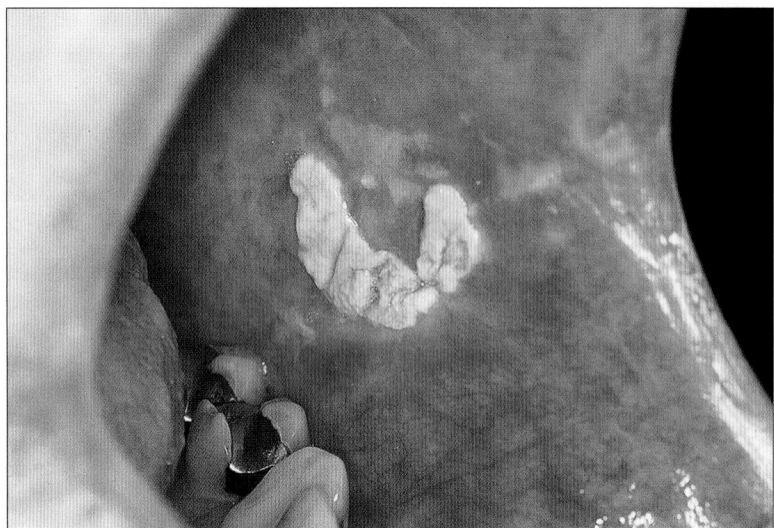

Fig. 11.209
Leukoplakia: nonhomogeneous sharply demarcated and fissured white plaque on the buccal mucosa. This exhibited moderate dysplasia.

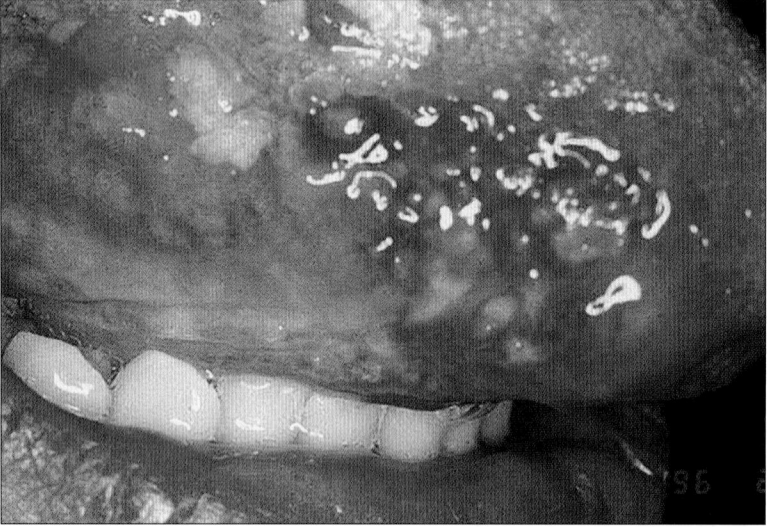

Fig. 11.210
Leukoplakia: erythroleukoplakia on the lateral tongue. This exhibited moderate dysplasia.

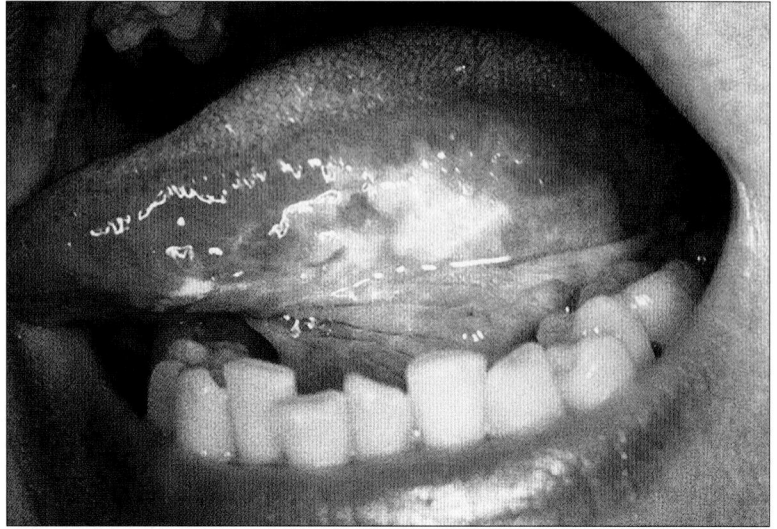

Fig. 11.211
Leukoplakia: this red and white plaque exhibited severe epithelial dysplasia.

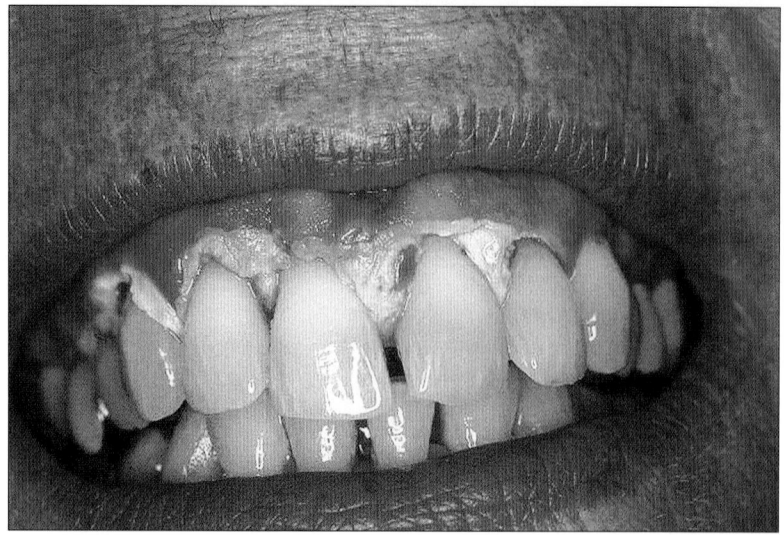

Fig. 11.212
Proliferative verrucous leukoplakia: this patient had been aware of this progressive lesion for approximately 10 years. This was a verrucous carcinoma arising from proliferative verrucous leukoplakia.

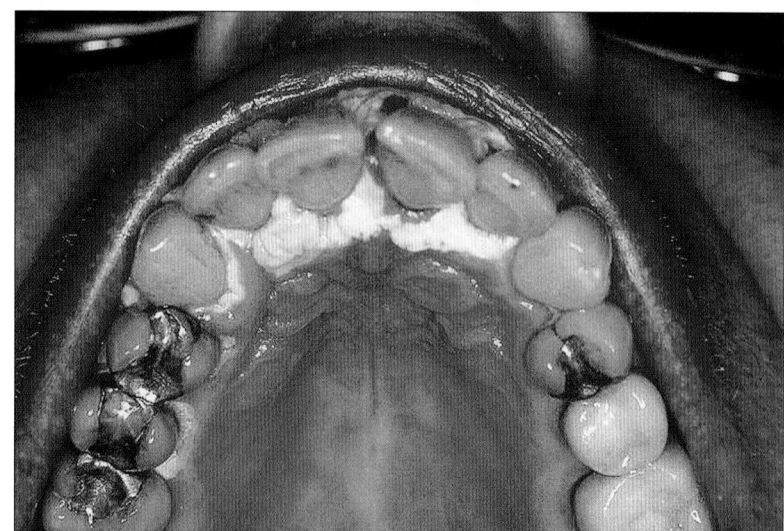

Fig. 11.213
Proliferative verrucous leukoplakia: this is the same patient depicted in *Fig. 11.212*, showing palatal involvement.

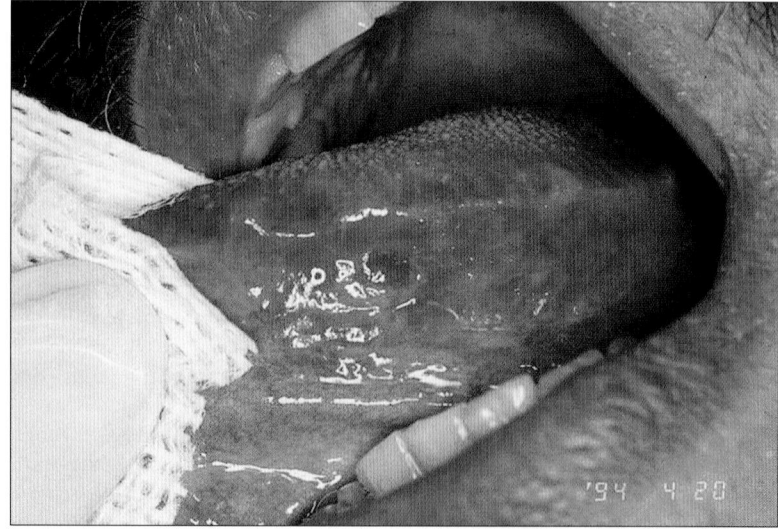

Fig. 11.214
Erythroplakia: this innocuous-appearing red macule on the lateral tongue was an invasive squamous cell carcinoma histologically.

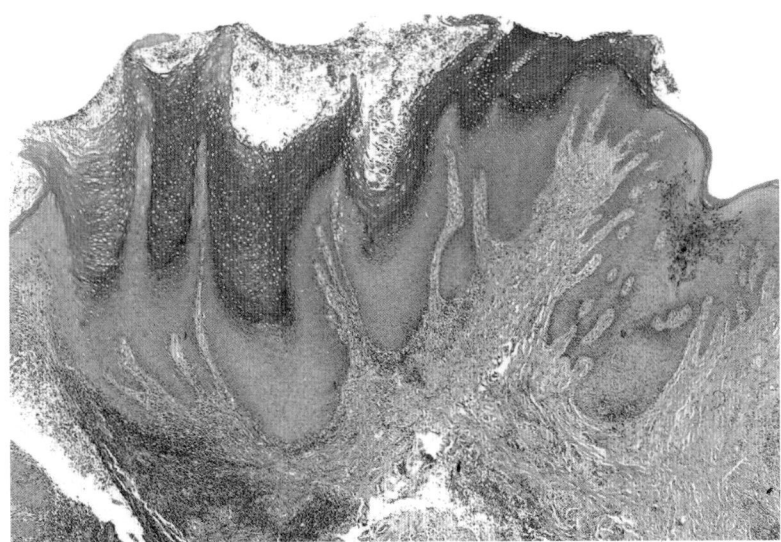

Fig. 11.215
Verrucous hyperplasia: note the bulky exo- and endophytic squamous proliferation with marked hyperkeratosis; normal epithelium is present at the right edge.

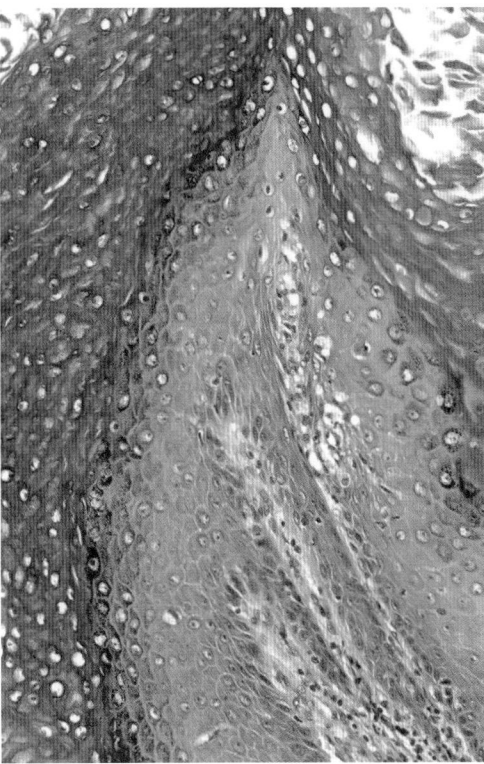

Fig. 11.216
Verrucous hyperplasia: there is hyperkeratosis and minimal cytological atypia.

Table 11.1
Criteria for diagnosis of oral epithelial dysplasia

Features	
Architectural features	• Verrucous/papillary architecture • Bulky endophytic squamous proliferation (at least three times the thickness of the normal epithelium for that site in the absence of significant spongiosis, leukocyte exocytosis or other inflammatory changes • Skip areas of keratosis and nonkeratosis • Bulbous, drop-shaped or festooned rete ridges • Hyperkeratosis with epithelial atrophy in the absence of significant inflammation, usually demarcated
Organizational features	• Dyscohesion (not spongiosis) • Basal cell hyperplasia* • Basal cell crowding • Mitotic figures beyond the basal and parabasal layer • Keratin pearl formation especially at the tips of rete ridges
Cytological features	• Basal cell hyperplasia* • Dyskeratosis • Pleomorphism of cells and nuclei • Increased nuclear:cytoplasmic ratio • Hyperchromasia • Coarse chromatin • Prominent nucleoli • Abnormal mitoses • Cells with 'glassy' cytoplasm • Multinucleate epithelial cells with increased nuclear/cytoplasmic ratio
*This feature is is both an organizational and cytologic feature of dysplasia.	

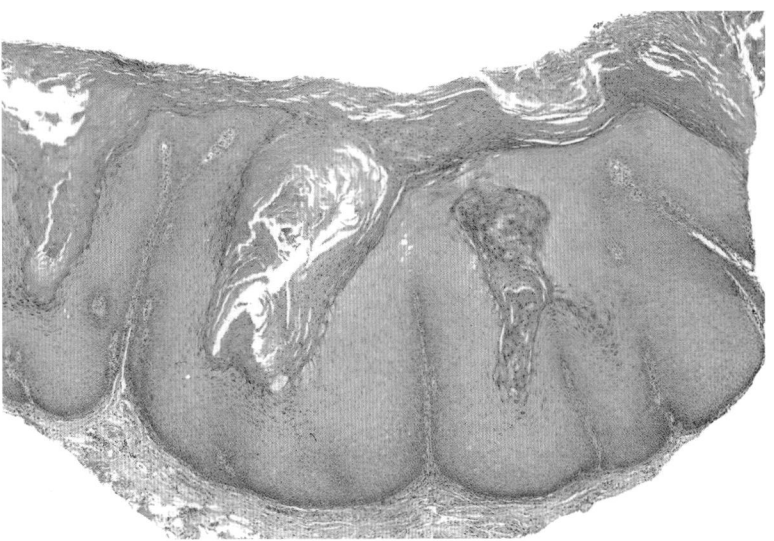

Fig. 11.217
Verrucous hyperplasia/early verrucous carcinoma: note the bulky exo- and endophytic squamous proliferation with bulbous pushing rete ridges.

squamous proliferation) are examples of how the diagnosis of dysplasia and carcinoma are established based on architectural changes in spite of minimal cytological atypia (Figs 11.215–11.218).

Dysplastic lesions are characterized by parakeratosis or hyperkeratosis if they are leukoplakias, and are nonkeratinized if erythroplakic. By convention, the terms mild, moderate, and severe dysplasia are applied if less than one-third, between one- and two-thirds, and greater than two-thirds of the epithelium is affected, while carcinoma in situ connotes full thickness involvement (Figs 11.219–11.221). However, a two-tiered grading system of low-grade and high-grade dysplasia is also in use. Importantly, neither system takes into account architectural changes.

Extension and spread of dysplastic cells from the surface epithelium down excretory salivary ducts (particularly in floor of mouth dysplasias)

without evidence of stromal invasion is accompanied by the same recurrence rate as for invasive squamous cell carcinoma (Fig. 11.222).[46] This may, in part, explain recurrences in the floor of mouth after superficial excision or laser ablation.

If 20–43% of all leukoplakias are dysplasia, carcinoma in situ, or invasive carcinoma, then 57–80% of cases are hyperkeratotic lesions without dysplasia or 'keratosis of unknown significance'[14]; many of these exhibit epithelial atrophy (Figs 11.223 and 11.224). While some of these lesions may be reactive, they do not have the characteristics of frictional/reactive keratoses or other specific keratotic disease such as lichen planus. This condition has been referred to in the literature as 'benign hyperkeratosis' or other similar terms; however, 3–16% of such cases when followed, subsequently develop dysplasia or invasive carcinoma, a rate similar to cases of dyplasia.[8,15,17,18,47] Using the phrase 'keratosis of unknown significance' or 'hyperkeratosis, not reactive') distinguishes this group of lesions from frictional/reactive keratoses, which also show hyperkeratosis and parakeratosis without dysplasia.

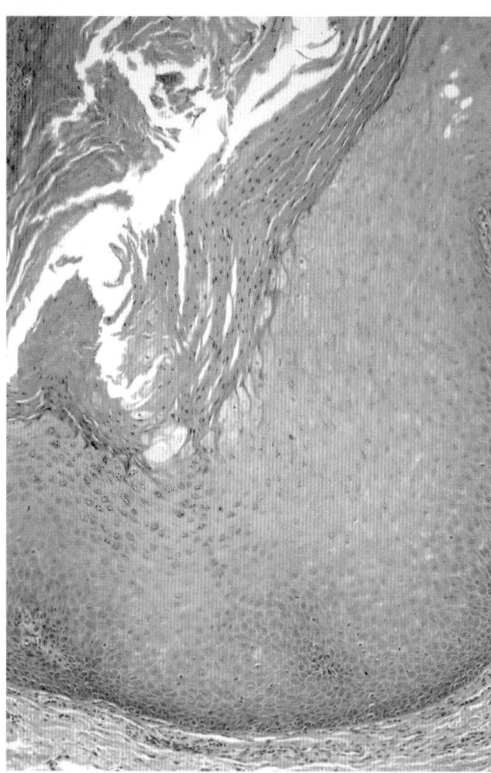

Fig. 11.218
Verrucous hyperplasia/
early verrucous carcinoma:
there is parakeratin
plugging, minimal atypia,
and a broad endophytic
front.

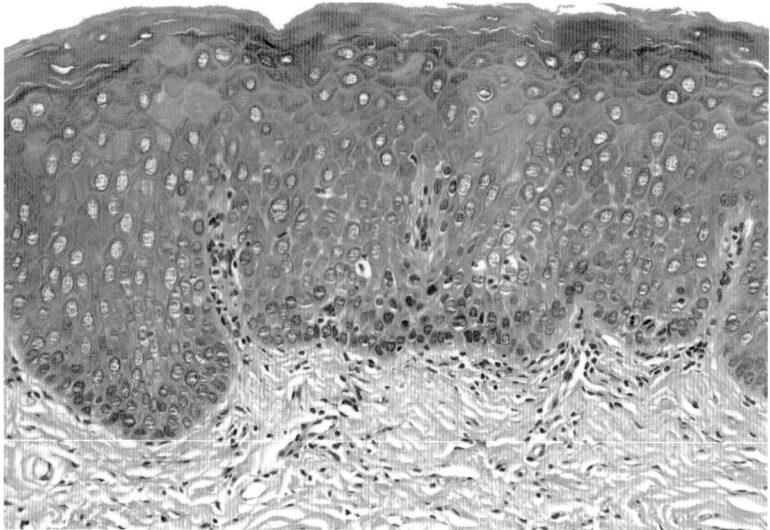

Fig. 11.219
Mild epithelial dysplasia: there is budding of the rete ridges; dysplastic cells
involve less than one-third of the thickness of epithelium.

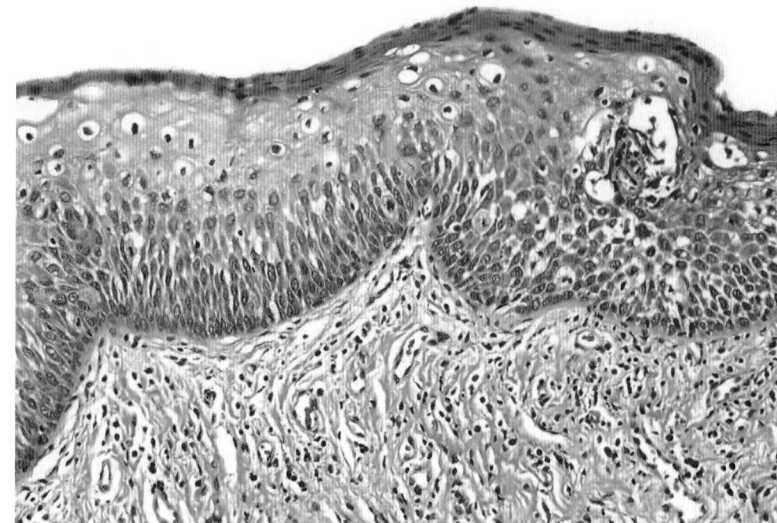

Fig. 11.220
Moderate epithelial dysplasia: dysplastic cells involve greater than one-third but
less than two-thirds of the epithelium and there is dyscohesion.

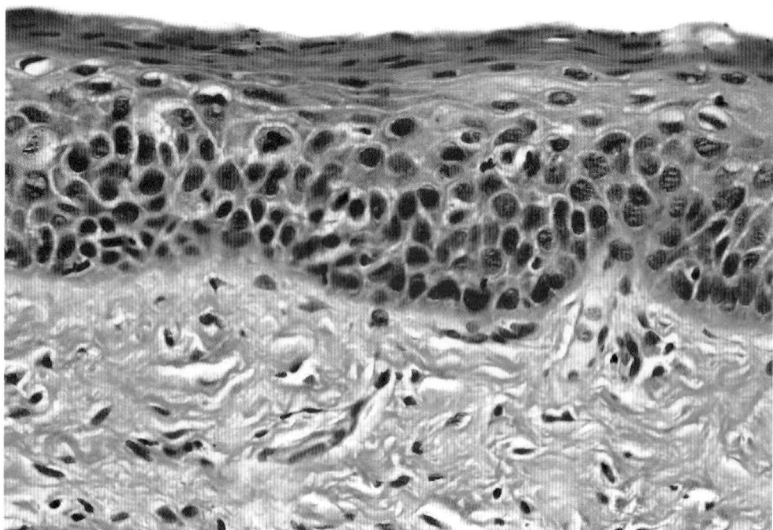

Fig. 11.221
Severe epithelial dysplasia: dysplastic cells involve less than the full thickness of
the epithelium.

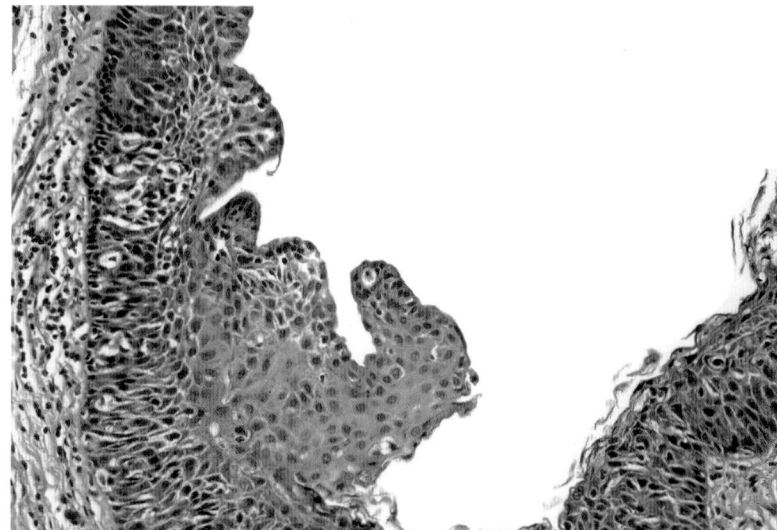

Fig. 11.222
Carcinoma in situ: dysplastic cells involve the excretory salivary duct; this has
important prognostic implications.

The presence of p53 in dysplastic epithelium varies greatly depending on the antibody that is used, but in general, high positivity is associated with higher grades of dysplasia, as are proliferation markers (*Fig. 11.225*).[42–44,48,49]

The histopathological features of the clinicopathological entity, proliferative verrucous leukoplakia are variable and usually those of verrucous hyperplasia. They all show hyperkeratosis or parakeratosis and papillomatosis. Epithelial dysplasia may be absent to mild in early lesions. As they spread relentlessly over the mucosa, lesions may show increasing cytological evidence of dysplasia, more marked exophytic papillomatosis, and finally, an endophytic and/or frankly invasive growth pattern of conventional squamous cell carcinoma, papillary squamous cell carcinoma or verrucous carcinoma.[25] HPV has been identified in both proliferative verrucous leukoplakia and conventional localized leukoplakia in approximately 25% of cases, but it may be a passenger.[50] DNA aneuploidy has also been reported especially as lesions progress to dysplasia.[27,28]

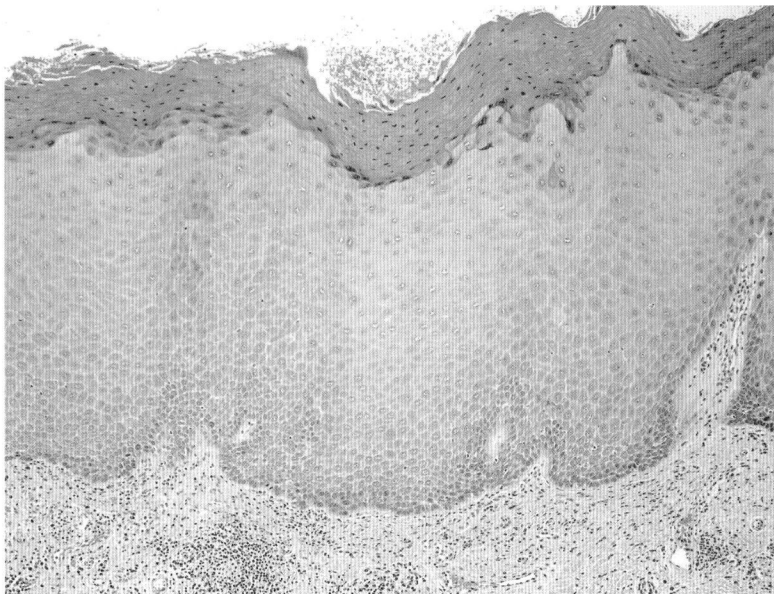

Fig. 11.223
Keratosis of uncertain significance: there is parakeratosis, acanthosis, minimal-to-no cytological atypia, and mild chronic inflammation.

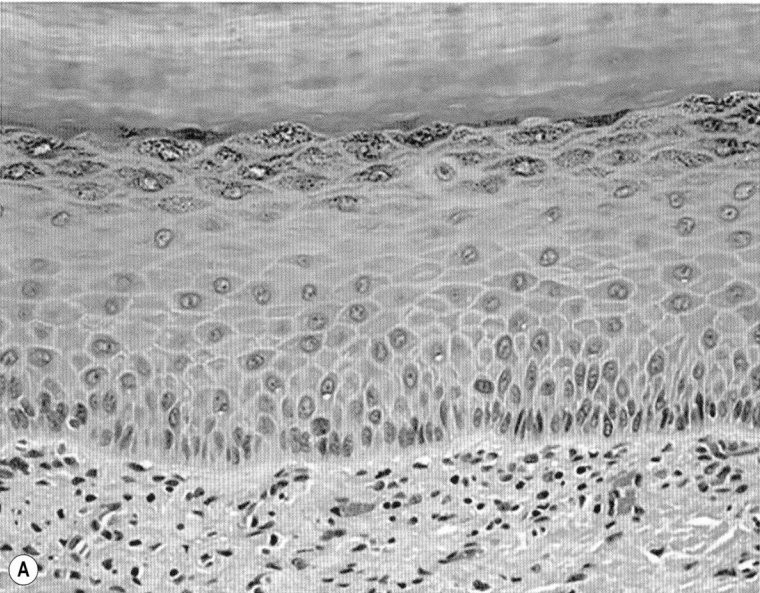

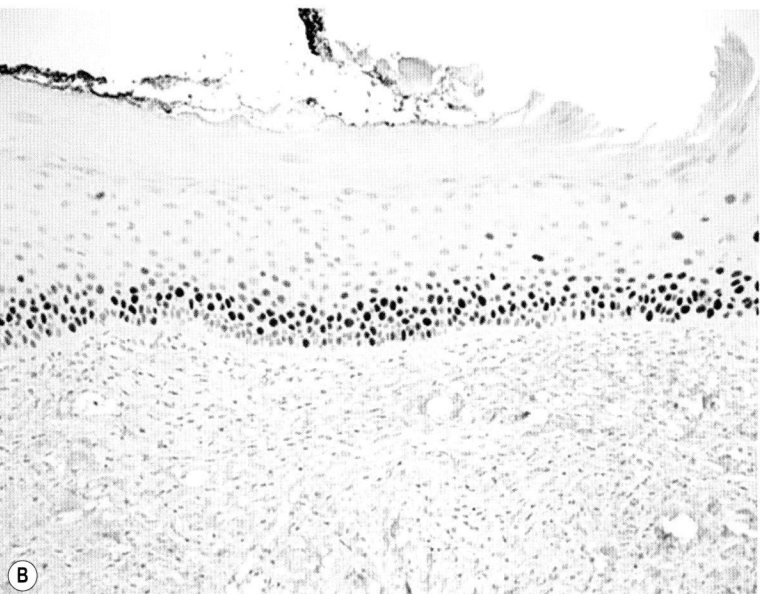

Fig. 11.225
Dysplasia and p53: (A) mild epithelial dysplasia exhibiting basal cell hyperplasia; (B) p53 present in a continuous band in basal cell nuclei.

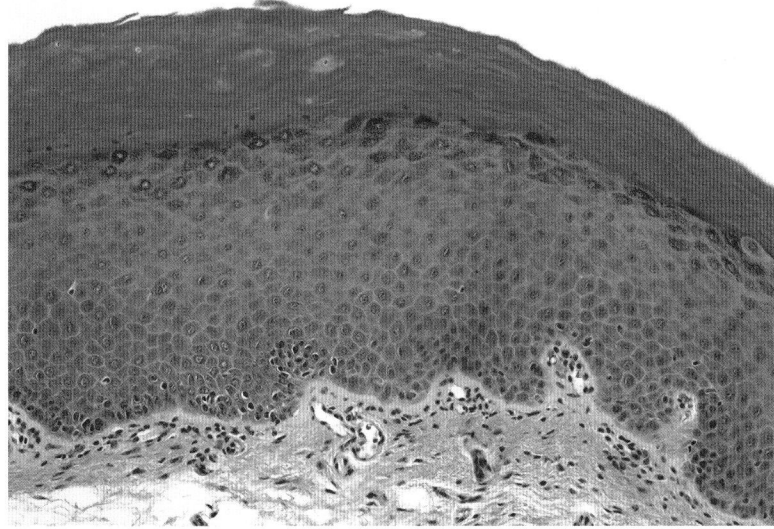

Fig. 11.224
Keratosis of uncertain significance (gingiva): there is hyperkeratosis, epithelial atrophy, minimal-to-no cytological atypia, and mild chronic inflammation.

HPV-associated oral epithelial dysplasia has a 6:1 male predilection and specific histopathological features. These are brightly eosinophilic parakeratosis, karyorrhectic cells similar to the 'mitosoid' bodies seen in Heck disease, apoptotic cells with brightly eosinophilic cytoplasm and pyknotic or absent nuclei, pericellular halos, and a background of basaloid carcinoma in situ (*Fig. 11.226*)[51]. All show continuous positivity for p16, and high-risk HPV (*Fig. 11.227*). Some of these cases had been reported in the past as 'koilocytic dysplasia' or bowenoid lesions.[52–54]

Differential diagnosis

The term 'lichenoid dysplasia' has been used to denote epithelial dysplasia associated with a band of lymphocytes at the interface. In such instances, it may be less confusing to use the term 'epithelial dysplasia with lichenoid inflammatory infiltrate' because the lymphocytic band is likely a host response to dysplastic cells. Otherwise, clinicians may erroneously conclude that the dysplasia arose within a clinical lesion of lichen planus.

Reactive epithelial atypia may be difficult to distinguish from dysplastic changes. If changes occur in the presence of ulceration, spongiosis, leukocyte exocytosis, and substantial inflammation in the lamina propria, it is more likely to be reactive, but always bear in mind that dysplastic lesions may become ulcerated and inflamed. In such cases, the use of p53 and, more importantly, the clinical features of the lesion may be helpful: true leukoplakias tend to be demarcated lesions often with fissures.

Submucous fibrosis

Clinical features

This condition affects adults of usually Asian descent (subcontinental Indians in particular but also southeast Asians) who chew areca nut by itself, as a component of betel quid (areca nut and slaked lime in betel leaf) with or without tobacco, or gutka (sachets of powdered areca nut, flavoring agents, and tobacco).[1,2] Patients develop progressive pallor, fibrosis, and a marble-like rigidity of the buccal mucosa, soft palate and fauces, lips, and tongue. Palpable fibrous bands run vertically within the buccal mucosa in advanced lesions and lead to reduction in mouth opening. Ulcers, areas of

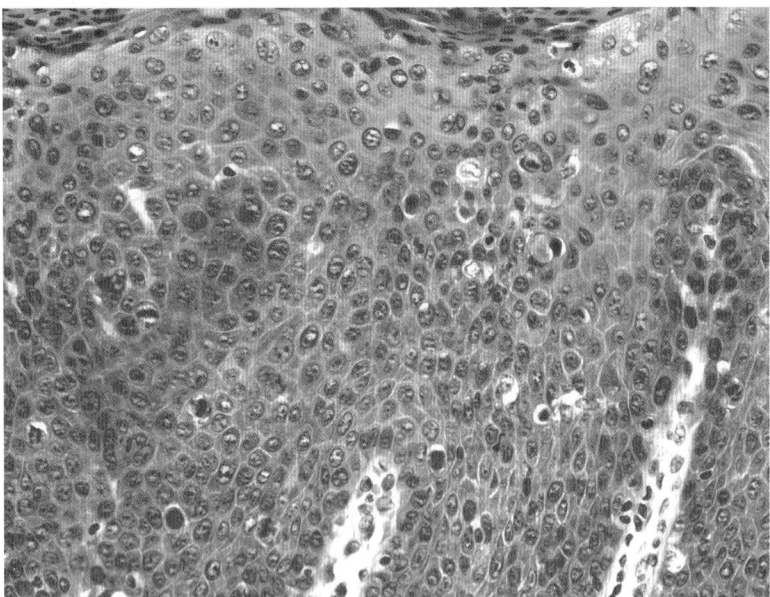

Fig. 11.226
Human papillomavirus-associated severe epithelial dysplasia: there are many karyorrhectic cells (mitosoid bodies) and apoptotic cells.

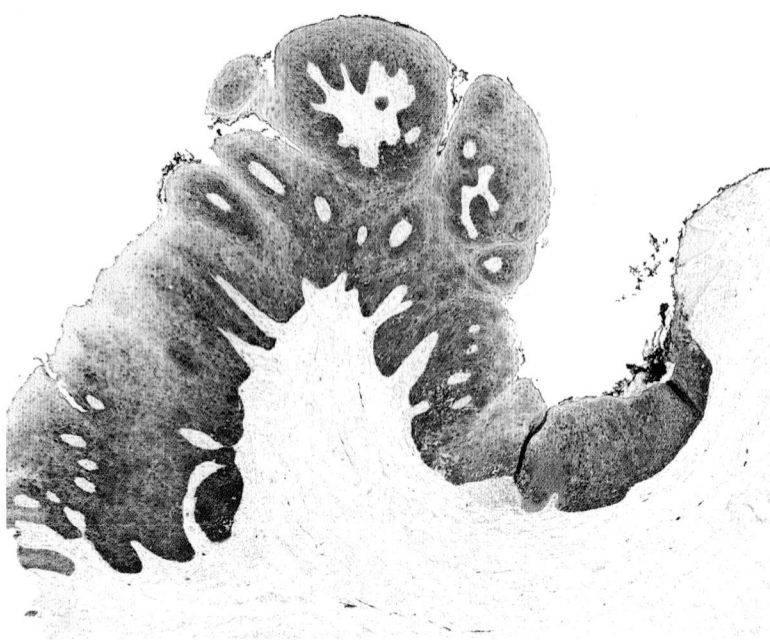

Fig. 11.227
Human papillomavirus-associated severe epithelial dysplasia: the study for p53 is positive in a continuous band involving the full thickness of keratinocytes.

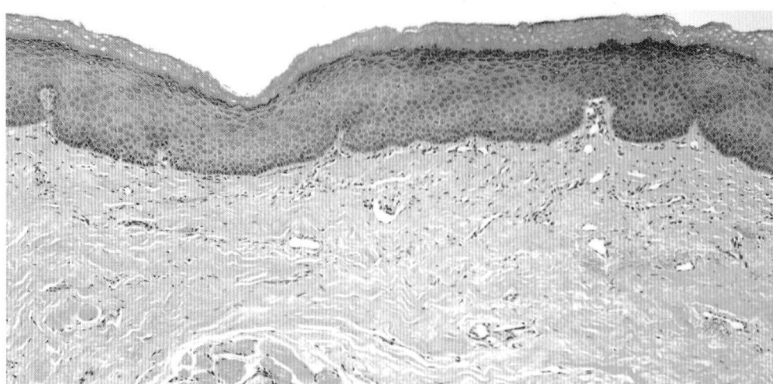

Fig. 11.228
Submucous fibrosis: there is hyperkeratosis, mild epithelial dysplasia, and dense fibrosis that surrounding skeletal muscle fibers.

erythema, and symptoms of burning are common.[2,3] This is a premalignant condition, as squamous cell carcinomas develop in 2–8% of cases.[4,5]

Pathogenesis and histologic features

Arecoline (areca nut alkaloid) dysregulates the cell cycle at G1/S and G2/M phases, and also inactivates tumor suppressor genes, among its many functions.[6] Hypoxia-inducible factor-1-α is also upregulated, which in turn leads to increased angiogenesis. Increased collagen synthesis and reduced matrix degradation mediated through TGF-β and tissue inhibitor of metalloproteinase leads to fibrosis.[7,8] Destabilized chromosome loci and loss of heterozygosity at loci associated with oral squamous cell carcinoma have been identified in almost half of cases of submucous fibrosis in one study, as well as inhibition of *TP53* and DNA repair, and impairment of T-cell function.[6,9–11]

The epithelium is hyperkeratotic and either acanthotic or atrophic with loss of rete ridges. The subepithelial connective tissue first shows edema, vascular dilatation, and chronic inflammation. Progressive thickening of collagen bundles occurs with increasing degrees of hyalinization proportionate to exposure (*Fig. 11.228*). In severe cases, hyalinized bands of collagen are devoid of cells.[3,12,13] Half of cases may show a lichenoid pattern of inflammation.[13] Epithelial dysplasia was noted in 9% of cases, but this increases with exposure.[13]

Differential diagnosis

The eosinophilic bands of collagen are not congophilic. Smokeless tobacco keratosis may exhibit similar eosinophilic bands of altered collagen, but in addition, there is edema and coagulation of superficial keratinocytes and parakeratin chevrons. Involvement of the oral mucosa by systemic sclerosis is an important differential diagnosis that can be excluded on clinical grounds and with serological tests.

Lichen sclerosus is a rare oral condition. In addition to the hyalinized eosinophilic subepithelial band, there is basal cell degeneration and a lymphocytic band beneath the area of hyalinization.[14–17]

SQUAMOUS CELL CARCINOMA AND VARIANTS

Squamous cell carcinoma

Clinical features

Squamous cell carcinoma is the most common malignancy in the oral cavity, accounting for more than 90% of all oral cancers. In the United States, cancer of the oral cavity and pharynx is the eighth most common malignancy in males, and oral cavity cancer accounts for approximately 42 000 cancer cases diagnosed annually.[1,2] The two most significant risk factors are cigarette smoking (by far the most important) and excessive alcohol consumption, with these two risk factors acting synergistically.[3–5] In Asian countries, tobacco use and areca nut chewing in its various forms are a major cause of oral cancer, and it is the most common form of cancer among men in India, where such habits are prevalent.[5] Other risk factors include a history of a previous oral squamous carcinoma, history of cancer elsewhere in the body, history of immunosuppression, family history of cancer, and age.[6–8] Lip carcinoma is generally not included in the discussion on oral lesions because of its different etiology (sunlight) and its better prognosis.

In the United States, HPV is identified in only 4% of carcinomas of the anterior oral cavity but is found in approximately 70% of oropharyngeal

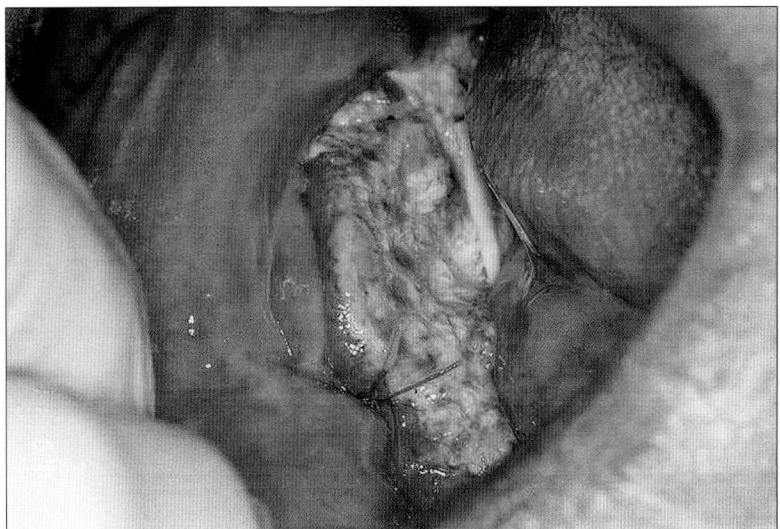

Fig. 11.229
Squamous cell carcinoma: there is a fungating mass on the buccal mucosa.

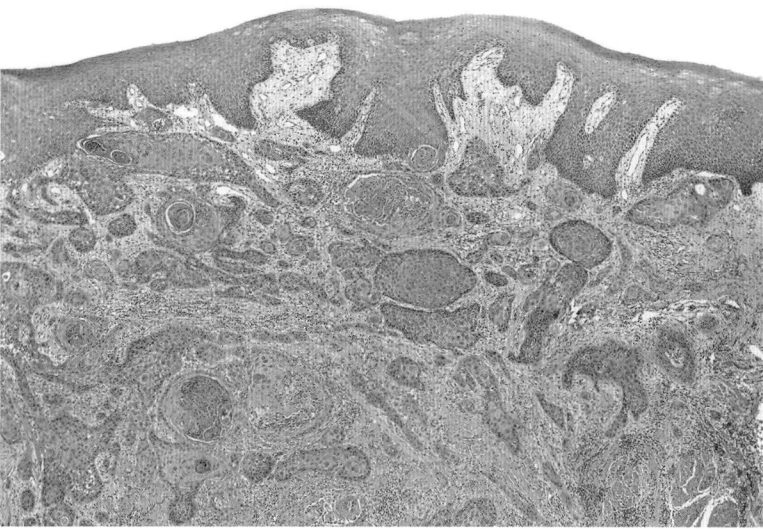

Fig. 11.230
Squamous cell carcinoma: conventionally invasive well-differentiated squamous cell carcinoma.

carcinomas, 80% of tonsillar carcinomas, and 70% of base of tongue carcinomas.[9,10] There is a 3:1 male predominance, and patients are generally younger than those with smoking-associated cancer. Many also present initially with cervical lymph node metastases. The vast majority are caused by HPV-16 and importantly, such patients exhibit improved survival.[11-14]

Oral squamous cell carcinoma presents in the seventh decade of life or older, and there is a 2:1 male:female predilection. The tumor may present as plaque lesions of leukoplakia, erythroplakia, and proliferative verrucous leukoplakia, or as nonhealing ulcers, masses, or nodules (*Fig. 11.229*); the most common sites are tongue and floor of mouth.[1] Up to 25% of patients present with synchronous or metachronous tumors of the upper aerodigestive or digestive tract.[15,16] Prognosis is still highly dependent on staging and is negatively impacted by positive resection margins. Overall 5-year survival is approximately 64% with localized tumors showing 83% 5-year survival, while those with regional and distant spread exhibit 63% and 38% 5-year survival, respectively.[1]

Pathogenesis and histologic features

Similar to other malignancies, acquisition of sequential driver mutations result initially in abnormal cell proliferation and eventually in invasive tumor.[17] HPV-negative tumors (usually smoking-related) are associated with mutations in *TP53*, *PIK3CA*, *CDKN2A*, *HRAS*, *CASP8*, and *NOTCH1*, while HPV-positive tumors are associated with mutations in *PIK3CA*, *FGFR2/3*, and *KRAS*, loss of *TRAF3*, and amplification of *E2F1*.[18,19] MiRNAs such as miR-196a and HOXB9 are al highly expressed in head-and-neck squamous cell carcinoma.[20] Copy number alterations involving losses in 3p and 9p, and gains in 3q, 5p, and 8q chromosomal regions are common.

Histologically, these tumors are similar to squamous cell carcinoma arising at other sites (*Fig. 11.230*). The overlying epithelium shows varying degrees of dysplasia, and histologic grade ranges from well to poorly differentiated. Well-differentiated tumors contain large cells with abundant eosinophilic cytoplasm, intercellular bridges, and keratin pearl formation, while poorly differentiated tumors produce minimal keratin and cells have only scant cytoplasm; well-differentiated stage I and II tumors are associated with better survival.[21] Conventional invasive squamous cell carcinoma infiltrates the stroma as small and large islands of tumor cells often with a tumor-associated lymphocytic response with or without desmoplasia. Unfavorable pattern of invasion (tumor islands containing <15 cells, or satellite islands away from the main tumor mass) and depth of invasion (>4 mm for tongue tumors) have been shown to correlate with locoregional recurrence and poor survival.[22,23] Studies have shown that tumor thickness in the tongue or floor of mouth ranging from 2 to 5 mm are associated with poor prognosis.[24-29] More recently, depth of invasion (measured from the basement membrane zone of the adjacent noninvasive portion of the epithelium) has been added as a new criterion to the tumor (T) stage, and both

tumor thickness and depth of invasion must be reported.[30] Perineural and lymphovascular invasion also adversely affect prognosis, and their presence or absence must always be reported in the pathology report.[31] A 'blunt' or 'pushing border' pattern of invasion is considered to be the most favorable type of invasion.[22] The infiltrative pattern is associated with a significantly higher incidence of lymph node metastasis compared to bluntly invasive tumors.[32,33] Two groups of investigators have applied a point system to various histopathological criteria to prognosticate risk of recurrence and survival.[22,28]

The use of molecular markers for prognostication is under investigation.[34] High epidermal growth factor receptor gene copy number is seen in approximately 60% of patients and is associated with a poorer prognosis.[22,35]

Sentinel node biopsy in patients without clinical evidence of cervical metastases has disclosed metastatic disease in approximately 25-50% of cases.[36,37]

Intraoral keratoacanthomas are rare and more commonly seen on the lip and peri-oral skin.[38-40] They typically have a crateriform architecture with the cup-shaped depression filled with keratin; there may be papillomatosis. This is a well-differentiated tumor and cells exhibit abundant 'glassy' cytoplasm, and the underlying stroma is usually infiltrated by tumor cells exhibiting cytological atypia. Oral keratoacanthomas do not tend to regress and is best regarded (and treated) as a variant of well-differentiated squamous cell carcinoma, keratoacanthomatous pattern. Interestingly, oral squamous cell carcinomas in the pediatric population tend to exhibit this pattern.[41-43]

Sarcomatoid squamous cell carcinoma

Clinical features

Sarcomatoid carcinoma (spindle cell carcinoma, carcinosarcoma, metaplastic carcinoma) is a tumor of the sixth to eighth decades with male predominance.[1,2] The most common sites are the lower lip, tongue, and alveolar ridge mucosa and a polypoid, exophytic configuration is a common presentation.[1,3] A history of radiation to the site has been noted in 13-67% of cases.[1,3,4] Oral cavity tumors tend to be deeply invasive with 5-year survival of 40% and overall survival of 24%, which is substantially lower than that in conventional squamous cell carcinoma[5,6]; polypoid lesions may have a better prognosis.[3,7]

Histologic features

The tumor, which is typically ulcerated, is biphasic with a conventional squamous cell carcinoma usually present at the base of the polypoid lesions, and a malignant spindle cell component in the main body of the tumor.[1,6] Tumor cells are seen to stream from the surface epithelium as spindle cells

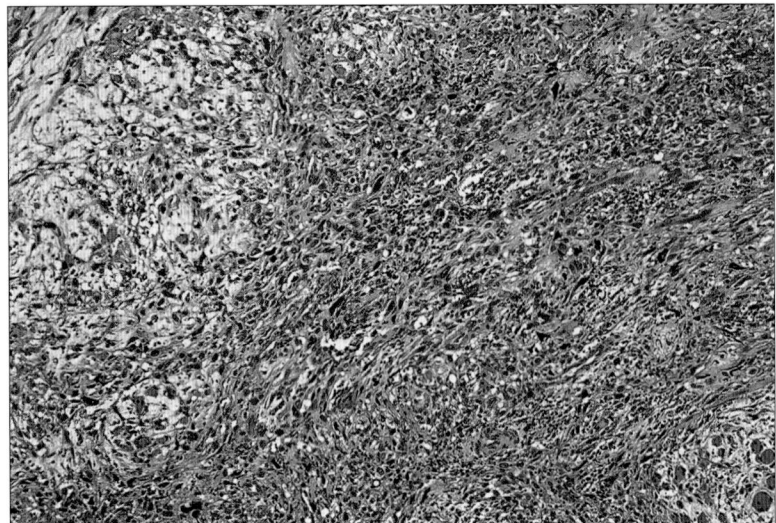

Fig. 11.231
Sarcomatoid carcinoma: there is a mass of pleomorphic epithelioid and spindle cells with hyperchromatic nuclei.

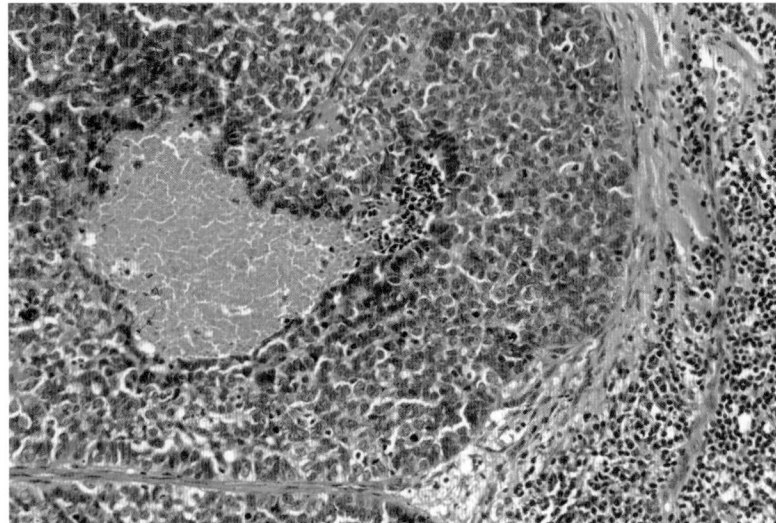

Fig. 11.233
Basaloid squamous cell carcinoma: there is comedo-necrosis and lobules of malignant basaloid cells.

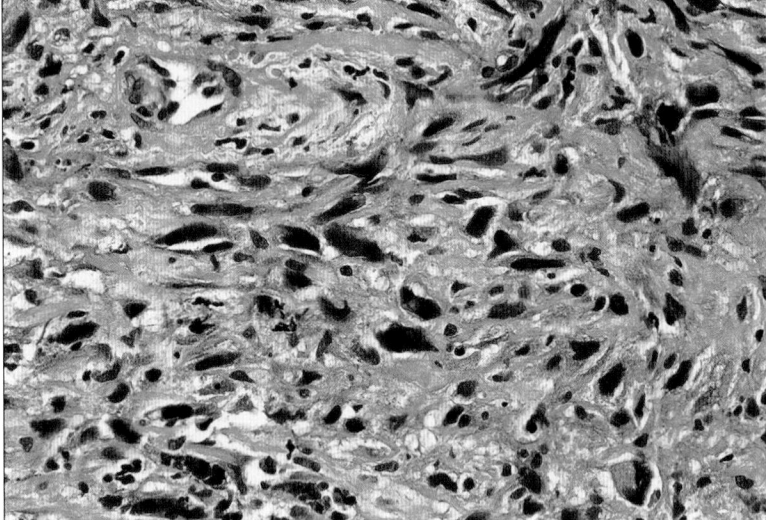

Fig. 11.232
Sarcomatoid carcinoma: the spindled cells have hyperchromatic, pleomorphic nuclei.

into the underlying stroma. The spindle cells form fascicles and storiform patterns, and have a prominent myxoid stroma (reminiscent of granulation tissue) (*Fig. 11.231*).[1,3,8] The cells may have bipolar processes, or be stellate-shaped and epithelioid; nuclei are generally pleomorphic with prominent nucleoli (*Fig. 11.232*). There are usually abundant mitoses, and pleomorphic tumor giant cells as well as osteoclast-like giant cells are sometimes present. Osteoid is present in 7% of cases and malignant cartilage has been reported.[1,7,9]

Tumor cells are usually positive for AE1/AE3, CAM 5.2, CK 5/6, EMA, and p63 in 36–62% of cases, with p63 within spindle cells being the most useful and diagnostic marker; spindled cells may also coexpress vimentin, and S100 protein and GFAP are typically negative.[2,4,7,10,11] Unlike conventional oral squamous cell carcinoma, sarcomatoid tumors express epidermal growth factor receptor at a lower rate, mostly in the squamous and not in the spindle cells.[6]

Differential diagnosis

Sarcomatoid carcinoma is the most common spindle cell malignancy in the oral cavity.[12] The diagnosis is not usually difficult when a spindle cell malignancy is present in association with typical squamous cell carcinoma, although the latter may be only evident focally at the base of polypoid lesions. Important differential diagnoses include radiation-induced fibroblastic atypia, nodular fasciitis, spindle cell melanoma, sarcoma, and malignant myoepithelioma. In difficult cases, immunoperoxidase studies will usually enable distinction with p63 confirming the epithelial nature of the spindle cells.

Basaloid squamous cell carcinoma

Clinical features

Most (76%) of basaloid squamous cell carcinomas of the oropharynx and base of tongue are caused by high-risk HPV, usually HPV-16, while this is true for only 6% of nonoropharyngeal sites.[1,2] HPV-positive tumors have a better prognosis than HPV-negative tumors. At this time, it is unclear to what extent basaloid squamous cell carcinomas that occur in the oral tongue and anterior oral cavity are caused by transcriptionally active HPV, because the old data comprised a combination of HPV-positive and HPV-negative tumors.

Nevertheless, basaloid squamous cell carcinoma is considered to be an aggressive variant of squamous cell carcinoma that primarily affects men in the sixth and seventh decades, with a predilection for the tongue and floor of mouth; 60–80% develop local and/or distant metastases.[3–5]

Histologic features

This unusual tumor is characterized by a minimally keratinizing squamous cell carcinoma composed of lobules and interconnected trabeculae of basaloid cells. The tumor lobules often exhibit comedo-like necrosis and microcystic spaces filled with PAS-positive material (*Fig. 11.233*). A cribriform pattern may be present, and hyalinized material, sometimes globular, surrounding tumor cells is an important feature; there may be peripheral palisading of tumor cells, and the basaloid tumor cells have dark hyperchromatic nuclei and indistinct nucleoli (*Fig. 11.234*).[3,6] Focal spindle cell morphology is sometimes seen.[7] Mitoses are often abundant and perineural invasion is frequently conspicuous.[5] There is usually an area of recognizable conventional squamous cell carcinoma.

The cells express cytokeratin (in particular, AE1/AE3, CAM 5.2, and 34βE12), EMA, and NSE (weakly). Carcinoembryonic antigen (CEA) and S100 protein are present in approximately 50% of cases.[4] Others report vimentin in a perinuclear rim in the basaloid cells, and the absence of NSE and S100.[5,6,8] Chromogranin and synaptophysin are absent.[4,5] Approximately 50% of tumors are aneuploid, although this may not have prognostic significance.[9,10] These tumors show marked proliferative activity (proliferating cell nuclear antigen [PCNA] studies) and expression of p53 protein and Bax.[11–13]

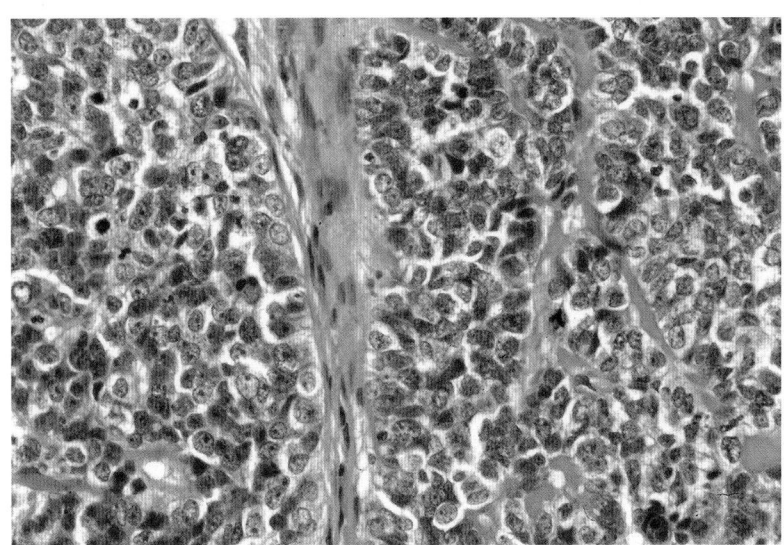

Fig. 11.234
Basaloid squamous cell carcinoma: tumor cells have hyperchromatic nuclei and small amounts of cytoplasm; there are many mitotic figures and trabeculae of hyalinized material.

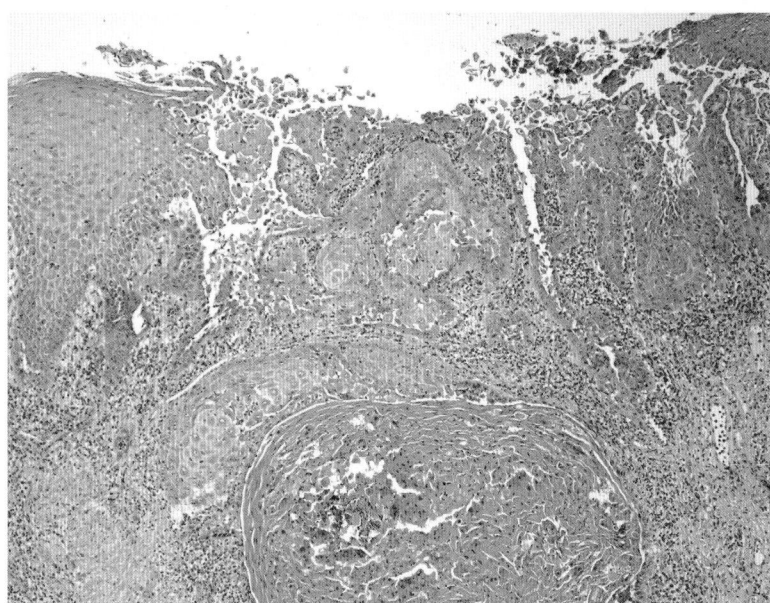

Fig. 11.235
Adenoid (acantholytic) squamous cell carcinoma: there is a keratinizing squamous cell carcinoma with areas of acantholysis.

Differential diagnosis

Nonkeratinizing HPV-associated squamous cell carcinoma of the oropharynx and base of tongue tends to affect males at a younger age than conventional squamous cell carcinoma. The histopathology appears very similar to that of basaloid squamous cell carcinoma and is composed of trabeculae and large lobules of tumors cells often with comedonecrosis, and many mitotic figures and apoptotic cells similar to HPV-associated oral dysplasia. Cells have indistinct cell borders, spindle hyperchromatic nuclei, and small-to-indistinct nucleoli.[14,15] They are almost always p16 positive and positive for high-risk HPV in 69–75% of cases. Distinguishing HPV-associated carcinoma from conventional squamous cell carcinoma is very important because of the better prognosis of HPV tumors.[13,16] Furthermore, many cases present initially with metastatic disease to a cervical lymph node with a cystic tumor that may be mistaken for 'malignant' branchial cleft cyst, which is often also p16 positive, but would be negative for high-risk HPV.[17]

Adenoid cystic carcinoma can be differentiated from basaloid squamous cell carcinoma because of the presence of true as well as pseudoducts, a more prominent cribriform pattern, negative p16 studies, and positive studies for CD117 within ductal epithelium with a surrounding rim of p63 positive abluminal cells (see earlier). If the study is p16 positive, then it is likely that the tumor is HPV-related carcinoma with adenoid cystic-like features, almost all of which present in the nasal cavity and paranasal sinuses; they are positive mostly for HPV-33.[18]

Merkel cell carcinoma has a trabecular or solid growth pattern and is positive for NSE, chromogranin and synaptophysin. Keratin expression is characterized by CK20 positivity presenting as paranuclear punctate dots.[19,20]

Adenoid squamous cell carcinoma

Clinical features

In adenoid squamous cell carcinoma (acantholytic squamous cell carcinoma, pseudoglandular squamous cell carcinoma), the majority of tumors present on the lower lip with a five-fold male predilection.[1–3] Approximately 21% occur on the upper lip, an unusual site for conventional squamous cell carcinoma.[4] While lip lesions generally have a good prognosis, intraoral tumors have a mortality of up to 75% for stage 4 lesions.[2,4,5]

Histologic features

Conventional squamous cell carcinoma must be identified. Pseudoglandular structures with central 'lumina' lined by two to three layers of

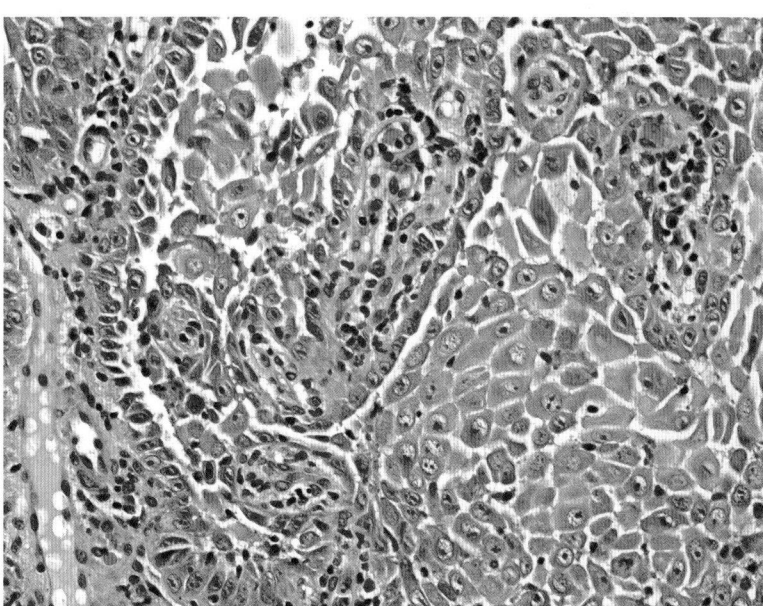

Fig. 11.236
Adenoid (acantholytic) squamous cell carcinoma: note acantholysis, marked cytologic atypia and dyskeratosis.

atypical squamous epithelium are seen within the tumor islands, and rounded acantholytic tumor cells are noted within the 'lumina' (Figs 11.235 and 11.236).[1,2,4–6] In most lesions, the acantholysis appears to begin in the immediate suprabasal cells.[7] In lip lesions, there is typically a background of solar elastosis, and sometimes acantholytic actinic keratosis is present, supporting the association with sun damage.[8] Clear cell change may also be seen.[9] The epithelial cells stain for keratins and EMA but not for mucin.[2,4,9] Tumor cells are also positive for vimentin but show minimal positivity for E-cadherin, suggesting acquisition of an epithelial-mesenchymal transition phenotype.[10] The lesion may appear as anastomosing pseudovascular spaces lined by epithelioid cells, mimicking angiosarcoma.[11] The lining cells are positive for keratin and do not express vascular antigens.

Differential diagnosis

These lesions must be differentiated from adenosquamous carcinoma in which true glandular differentiation occurs (see below).

Adenosquamous carcinoma

Clinical features

Only a few cases have been reported in the oral cavity, although the larynx and paranasal sinuses are common sites for this tumor.[1,2] It occurs in older men (male:female of 3:1) with a predilection for the floor of mouth, tonsil, and palatal mucosa.[3] At least half the cases show metastasis to regional and distal sites, and 40–50% of patients are dead of disease within 2 years.[1,4–6]

Histologic features

Two distinct components are present: there is a conventional squamous cell carcinoma which generally forms the bulk of the tumor and an adenocarcinoma composed of well-formed ducts, tubules, and alveolar structures; ductal carcinoma in situ may be present (*Figs 11.237* and *11.238*).[7] Mucin is present within lumina or intracellularly.[1,2,4,5,8] High molecular weight

keratins are present in the squamous cell carcinoma component and low molecular weight keratins in the adenocarcinoma.[4] CEA and CAM 5.2 are often present in the adenocarcinoma but not in the squamous areas; most tumors are positive for p53 with high Ki67 index.[9] A subset of cases (39%, usually non-oral) are p16 positive and positive for high-risk HPV (16%).[7] A ciliated variant that is HPV positive exists, and this is p16 positive and positive for high-risk HPV by in situ hybridization.[10]

Differential diagnosis

High-grade mucoepidermoid carcinomas tend to have a less conspicuous cystic and mucous cell component and may be mistaken for adenosquamous carcinoma. In general, the malignant epidermoid component does not show the degree of pleomorphism, atypia, and keratinization of a conventional squamous cell carcinoma. Importantly, mucoepidermoid carcinoma is generally positive for *MECT1/3* (CRTC1/3)-*MAML2* translocation, which is absent in adenosquamous cell carcinoma.[11]

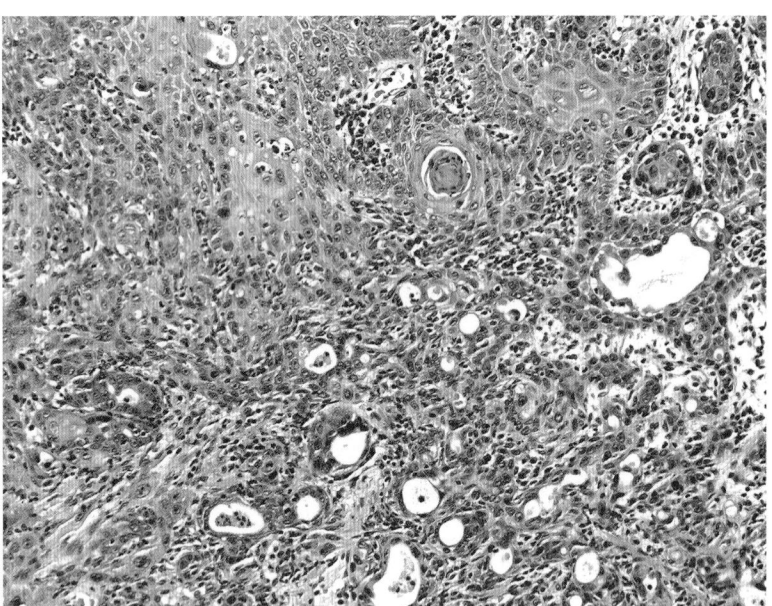

Fig. 11.237
Adenosquamous carcinoma: there is a keratinizing squamous cell carcinoma and an adenocarcinoma forming ducts.

Verrucous carcinoma and papillary squamous cell carcinoma

Clinical features

Verrucous carcinoma presents in older individuals (usually seventh decade) with a predilection for the buccal mucosa and gingiva/alveolar ridge mucosa (more than 70% of cases) and is strongly associated with the use of smokeless tobacco or cigarettes.[1–5] The tumors are white, fungating, cauliflower-like masses, generally several centimeters in size, and have usually been present for several years before patients are finally diagnosed (*Fig. 11.239*). There may be destruction of underlying bone and other structures on a broad advancing front. Reactive lymphadenopathy is often present and nodal metastases are distinctly unusual.[1,4] Between 17% and 20% of patients may have associated leukoplakia (most likely verrucous leukoplakia or proliferative verrucous leukoplakia).[1,4] One study showed 8–12% of verrucous carcinoma exhibited p16 positivity, but none harbored transcriptionally active HPV.[6]

Histologic features

Verrucous carcinoma is characterized by marked parakeratosis with keratin plugs between papillary projections of minimally atypical epithelium. The epithelium forms large, bulbous, frondlike rete ridges that are endophytic and bluntly invasive on a broad advancing front (*Fig. 11.240*). Although there may be slight epithelial atypia, pleomorphism or anaplasia is lacking (*Fig. 11.241*). Lymph node dissection does not usually reveal metastatic disease.[7]

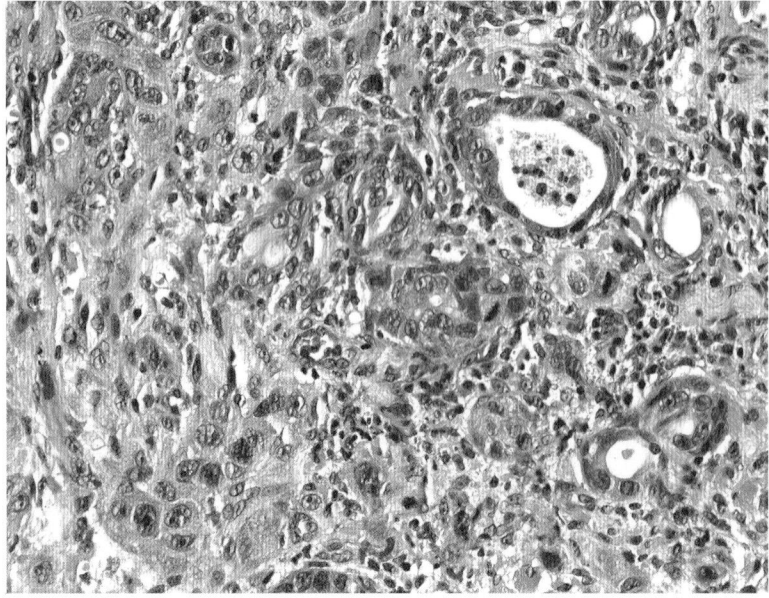

Fig. 11.238
Adenosquamous carcinoma: conventional squamous cell carcinoma is present on the left and adenocarcinoma on the right.

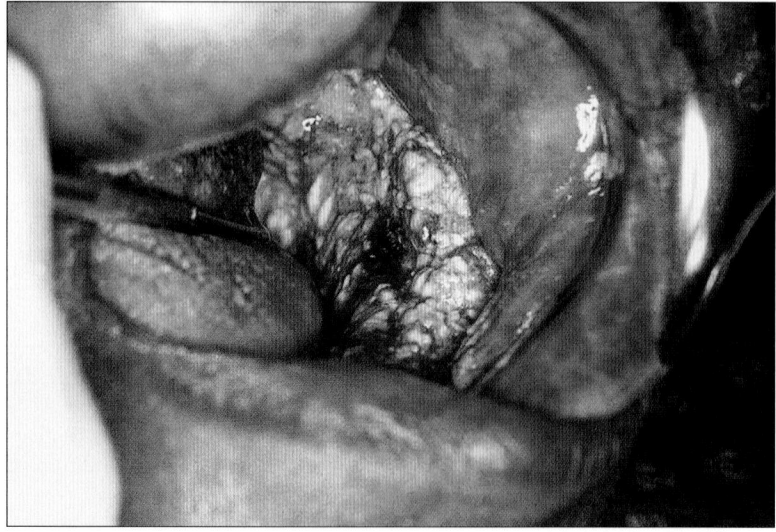

Fig. 11.239
Verrucous carcinoma: there is a warty mass in the mandibular buccal mucosa and sulcus.

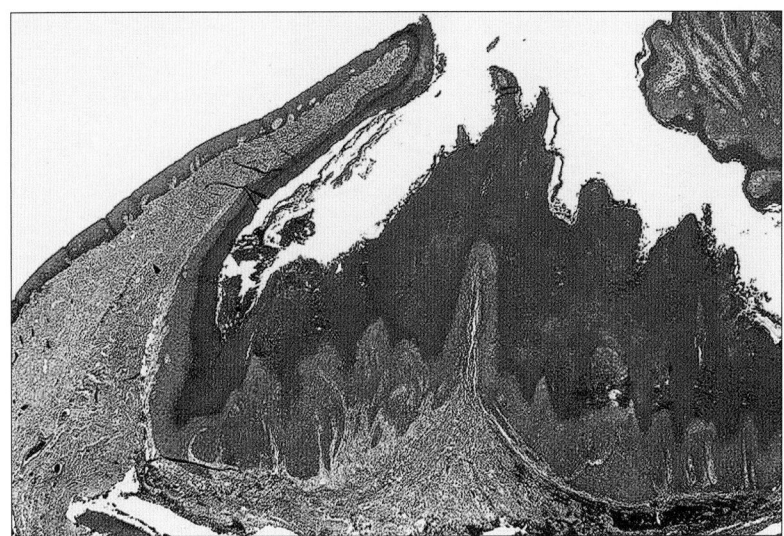

Fig. 11.240
Verrucous carcinoma: there is an endophytic proliferation of squamous epithelium with a verrucous morphology and a broadly invasive front; note the normal gingival epithelium at the periphery.

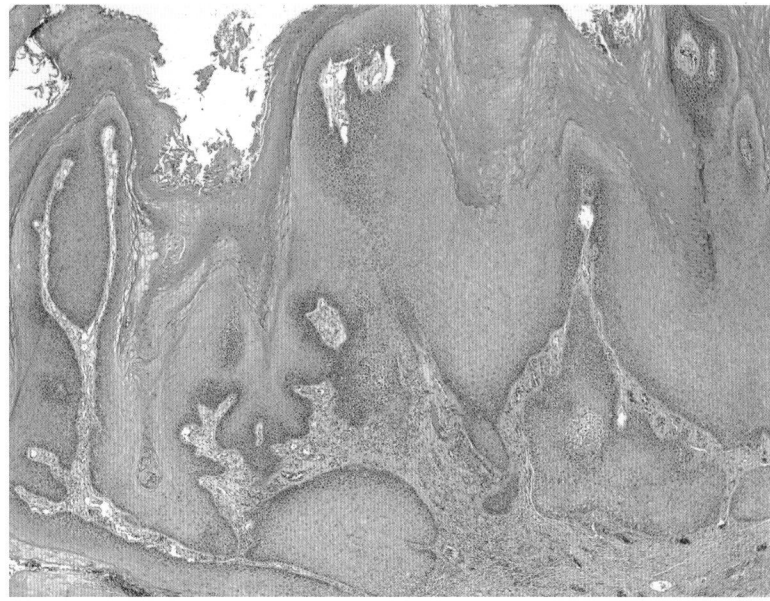

Fig. 11.242
Bluntly invasive squamous cell carcinoma: there is a papillary proliferation of squamous epithelium with parakeratosis and substantial cytological atypia even at this power.

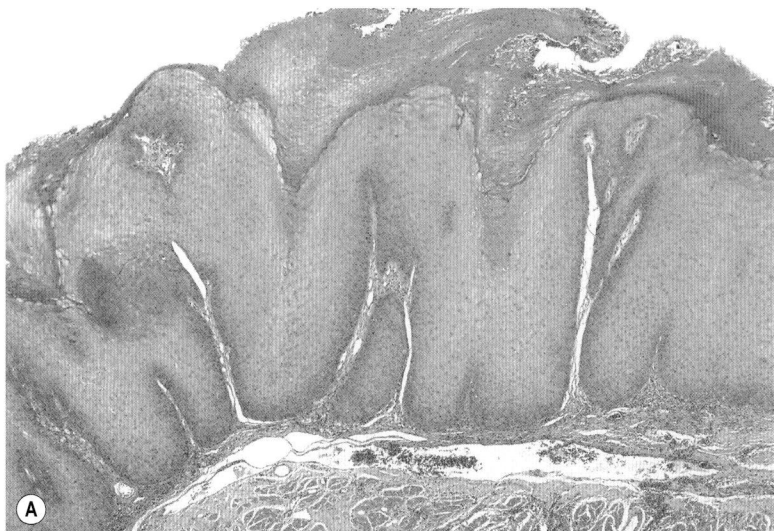

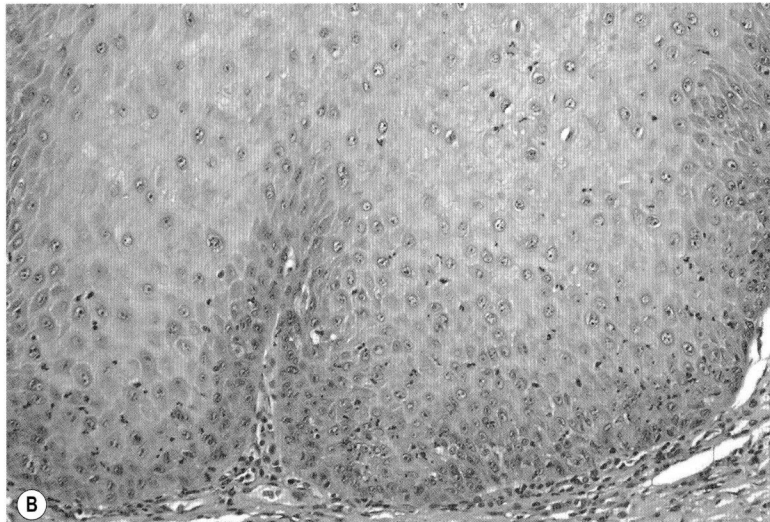

Fig. 11.241
Verrucous carcinoma: (**A**) there is a papillary proliferation of squamous epithelium with parakeratosis, forming frondlike rete ridges; (**B**) there is minimal cytological atypia and no single cell infiltration of the stroma.

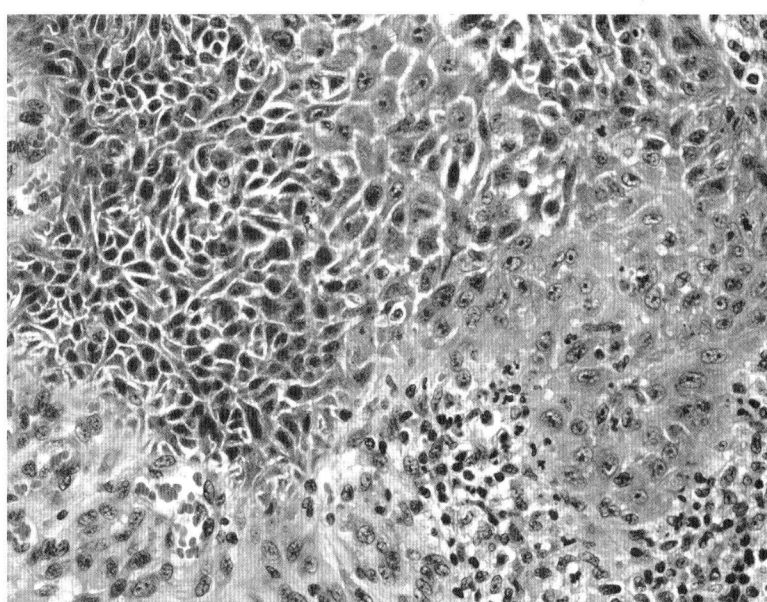

Fig. 11.243
Bluntly invasive squamous cell carcinoma: the tumor exhibits substantial cytological atypia namely pleomorphism and large nuclei with coarse chromatin and hyperchromatic nuclei.

A variant has been described where there is obvious dysplasia within epithelial cells but still without single cell infiltration of the stroma (*Figs 11.242* and *11.243*). There is lack of consensus regarding terminology for such lesions, which have been referred to as bluntly invasive well-differentiated papillary squamous cell carcinoma (see below) or atypical endophytic squamous proliferation.[8] Such tumors are likely to have similar minimal metastatic potential as conventional verrucous carcinoma.

Foci of more typical infiltrative squamous cell carcinoma may be seen in 20% of tumors, the so-called 'hybrid tumor'. These foci may be responsible for a higher recurrence rate (approximately 30%).[8] Strictly, such tumors probably should be diagnosed as papillary well-differentiated squamous cell carcinoma rather than verrucous carcinoma.

An important variant is the papillary squamous cell carcinoma, which is much more common within the oropharynx (including the palatine tonsil and base of tongue) and larynx, compared with the anterior oral cavity

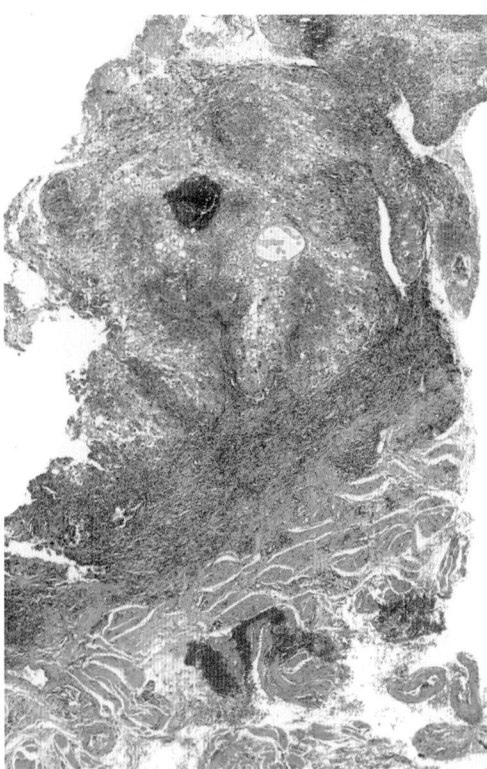

Fig. 11.244
Papillary squamous cell carcinoma: the papillary projections of malignant epithelial cells are nonkeratinized and there is stromal invasion.

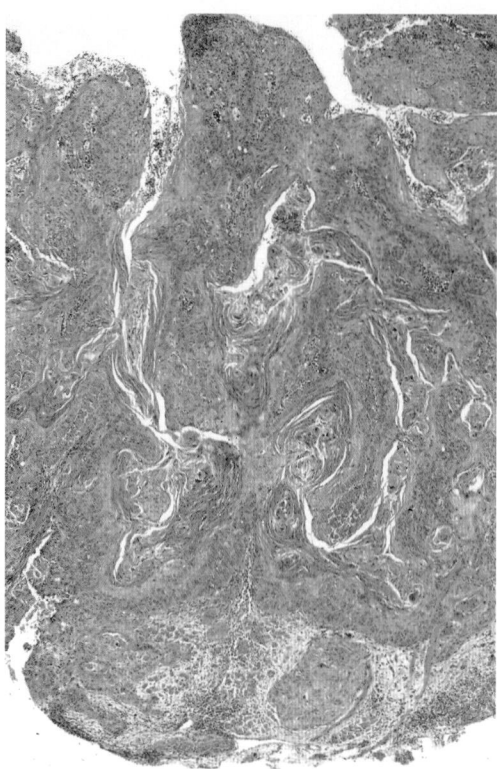

Fig. 11.246
Papillary squamous cell carcinoma: there is a papillary proliferation of squamous epithelium that forms infiltrative islands of tumor cells.

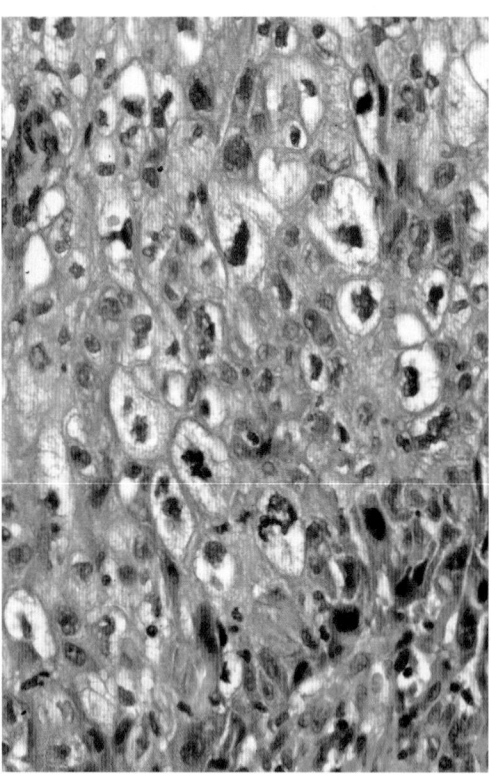

Fig. 11.245
Papillary squamous cell carcinoma: there is marked pleomorphism and koilocyte-like cells.

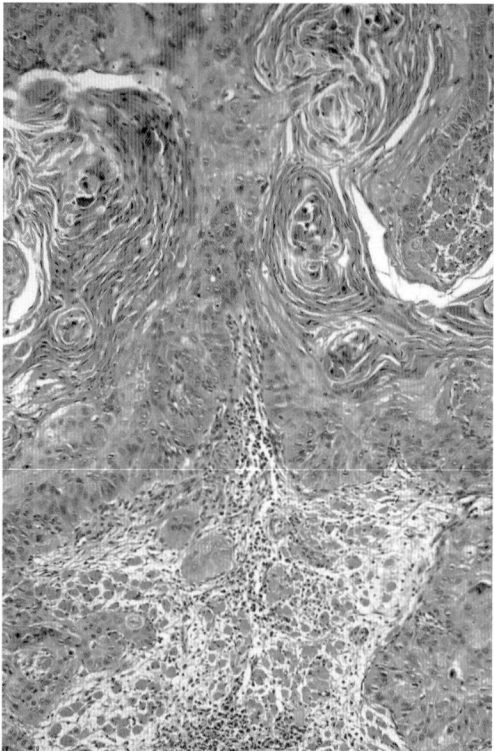

Fig. 11.247
Papillary squamous cell carcinoma: the tumor islands form keratin pearls and are hyperchromatic and pleomorphic.

where it occurs on the gingiva, palatal mucosa, and buccal mucosa.[9] There are two subtypes, both characterized by a papillary growth pattern:

- The laryngeal and oropharyngeal tumors occur mostly in men and consist of an invasive papillary proliferation of minimally to nonkeratinizing epithelium with highly atypical, hyperchromatic epithelial cells with high nuclear:cytoplasmic ratio, and numerous mitoses overlying fibrovascular cores (Figs 11.244 and 11.245).[10–12] The in situ portion of the tumor resembles a squamous papilloma with carcinoma in situ. Many are p16 positive, and up to 68% are associated with high-risk HPV.[13]

- In contrast, oral papillary squamous cell carcinomas are slightly more frequent in women and generally well differentiated, although

they usually show varying degrees of dysplasia in contrast to the bland histology typical of verrucous carcinoma (see above), and are conventionally invasive (Figs 11.246 and 11.247).[14] p16 expression is generally weak and focal, and they do not harbor high-risk HPV.[9]

Differential diagnosis

Although the term 'carcinoma cuniculatum' is sometimes used interchangeably with verrucous carcinoma, it should be considered a separate entity. The overlying mucosa is generally not as overtly exophytic warty, but may have a multinodular appearance, and characteristically exhibits many sinus tracts that connect with underlying burrows and cystic spaces within the tumor mass (Fig. 11.248).[15–17]

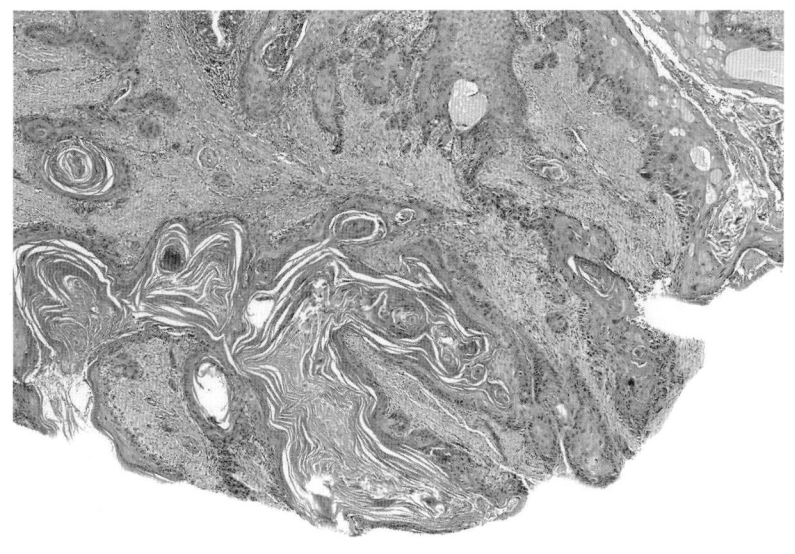

Fig. 11.248
Carcinoma cuniculatum: the tumor forms interconnected burrows filled with keratin surrounded by carcinomatous cells.

ORAL LYMPHOMA

Non-Hodgkin lymphoma is the second most common malignancy in the oral cavity and accounts for 3–4% of all oral malignancies.[1] The most frequently affected sites are palatal mucosa, gingiva, and tongue, and some cases occur as primary intraosseous malignancies.[2,3] Patients present with diffuse swelling and masses at affected sites, and teeth become mobile if bone is involved. The most common lymphoma is diffuse large B-cell lymphoma, which accounts for up to 68% of oral lymphomas; follicular and marginal zone lymphomas are two other lymphomas seen with some frequency (21% combined).[4] Plasmablastic lymphoma is primarily encountered in the oral cavity in patients with HIV/AIDS, and is associated with Epstein-Barr virus.[5–7] Finally, involvement of the jawbones and oral soft tissues is noted in 14% of patients with multiple myeloma, and the head and neck is the most common site of extramedullary plasmacytomas.[8–10]

PIGMENTED LESIONS

Amalgam tattoo

Clinical features

These occur in adults as asymptomatic gray, bluish, black or slate-colored macules on the gingiva/alveolar ridge mucosa (approximately 50%), the buccal mucosa (approximately 25%), or the floor of mouth (approximately 10%), although any site may be affected (Figs 11.249 and 11.250).[1,2]

Pathogenesis and histologic features

Particles of amalgam restorations may leach from contacting restorations or amalgam retrograde restorations after root canal therapy, dislodge during tooth extractions and lodge in the extraction socket, or be traumatically implanted into the mucosa during placement or removal of a restoration. Dental amalgam is a mixture of mostly silver and tin and other metals in smaller amounts, and mercury. The silver stains agryrophillic fibers (type III collagen/reticular fibers) within the connective tissue. It is believed that metallothioneins (low molecular weight proteins that bind metals) are also present within tattoos and bind metals, preventing local and systemic toxicity.[3]

Amalgam deposits in the tissue in several ways. It is most often present as fine, golden-brown dusty granules dispersed in a beaded fashion along connective tissue fibers and the basement membrane of blood vessels and

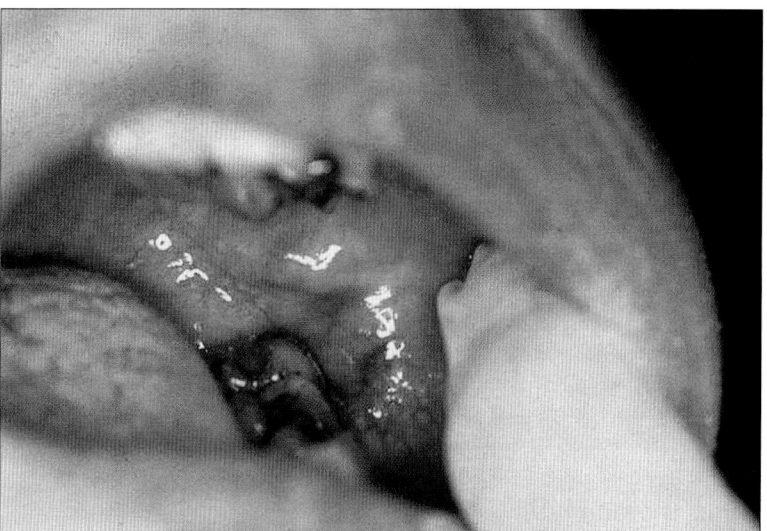

Fig. 11.249
Amalgam tattoo: there are slate-gray macules on the left buccal mucosa corresponding to some large amalgam restorations.

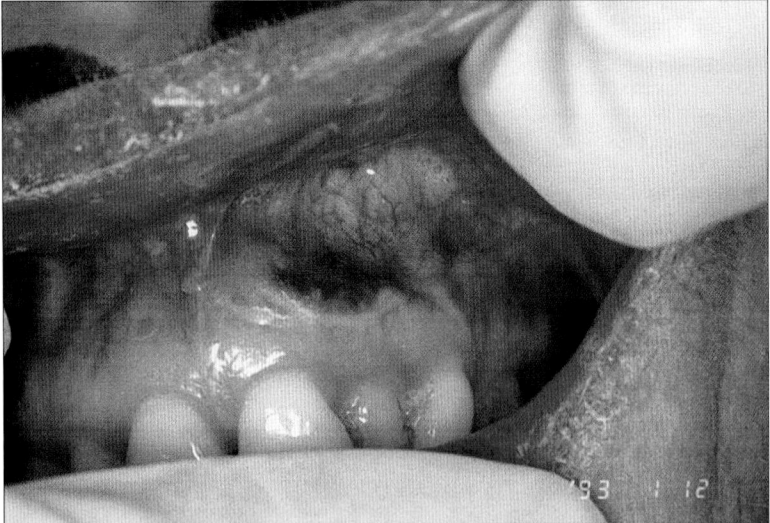

Fig. 11.250
Amalgam tattoo: there is a blue-black macule on the attached gingiva superior to a semilunar scar; this tattoo is caused by a root canal-related surgical procedure.

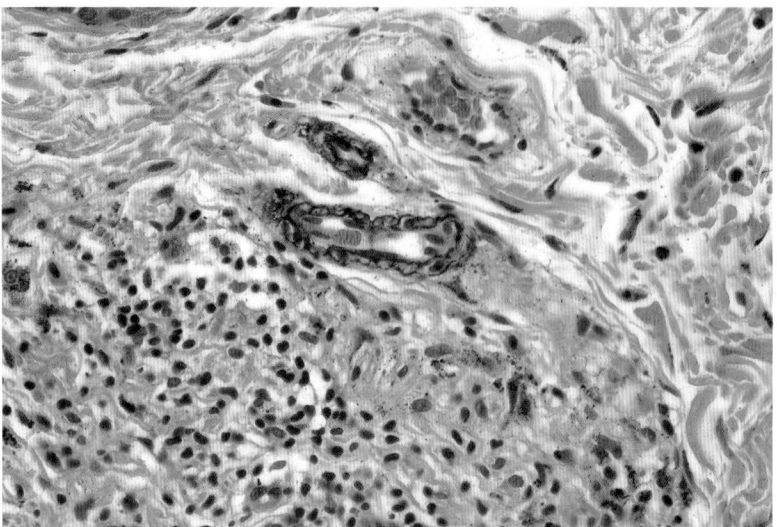

Fig. 11.252
Amalgam tattoo: note the typical staining of the vascular basement membrane.

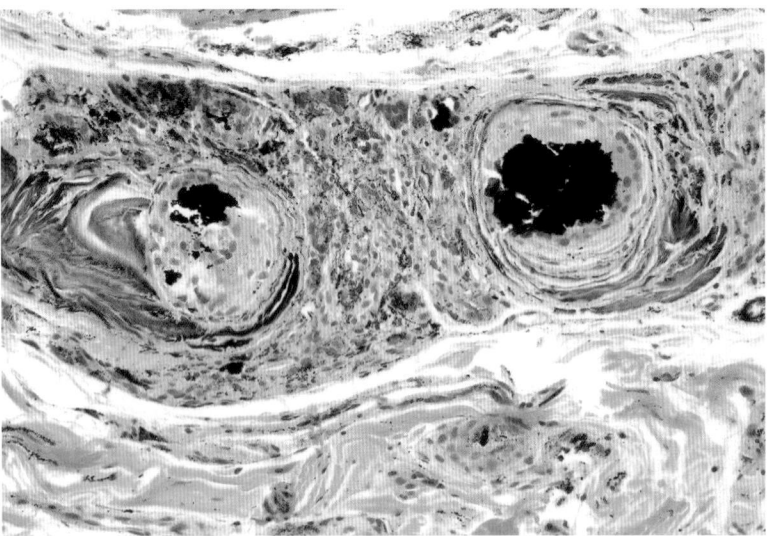

Fig. 11.251
Amalgam tattoo: there are coarse and fine granules of amalgam associated with foreign body granulomata; the connective tissue fibers are stained brown by the amalgam.

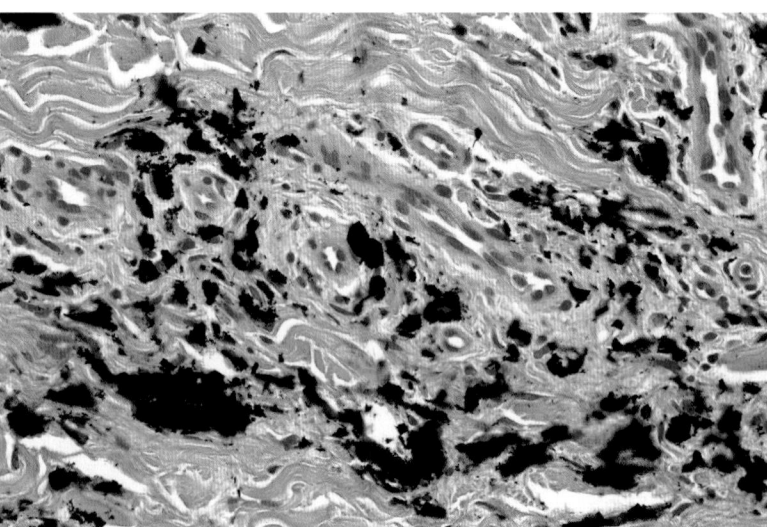

Fig. 11.253
Graphite tattoo: there are large deposits of black granular material that do not stain the connective tissue fibers or dispose along them.

the epithelium, endomysium and perineurium (*Figs 11.251* and *11.252*).[1] The collagen itself may sometimes be stained a golden color. Larger black fragments are usually associated with a foreign body reaction with particles within multinucleated giant cells.[1,2,4] Scarring is almost always present, confirming its traumatic etiology. The particles contain silver, copper, and other metals typical for amalgam.[5]

Differential diagnosis

Graphite (pencil lead) are larger and coarser and do not stain or dispose along the connective tissue fibers (*Fig. 11.253*). It maintains yellow birefringence (especially at the edges of the particles) after treatment with 10% ammonium sulfide, unlike amalgam.[6] Aluminum and silicon (hardeners for graphite) are identified using dispersive X-ray microanalysis.[7]

Silver tattoos of nonamalgam derivation have been reported in patients following silver nitrate cautery.[8]

Oral melanocytic lesions

Five conditions are of particular importance: melanotic macule, medication-induced hypermelanosis, melanoacanthosis, melanocytic nevus, and melanoma.

Oral melanotic macule

Clinical features

These are the most common melanocytic lesions in the oral cavity.[1-3]

These are two to three times more frequently encountered in adult females, and most are solitary (two-thirds solitary, one-third multiple). They appear as well-demarcated, tan-to-brown, evenly pigmented macules measuring less than 1.0 cm often occurring on the lips (usually lower, and referred to as labial melanotic macule), palatal mucosa, gingiva, or buccal mucosa; lesions have usually been present for months (*Fig. 11.254*).[1,4-6] The intensity of pigmentation is usually constant unlike in ephelides, which tend to darken with sun exposure. Biopsy is usually performed to exclude a melanoma.

Pathogenesis and histologic features

Solitary melanotic macules are likely to represent postinflammatory hypermelanosis, a condition poorly recognized in the dental community. Patients are generally not followed up after biopsy to document resolution which, as on the skin, may take months to years. Some patients report a strong family history of this condition.

Multifocal melanotic macules may be idiopathic or may be syndromic. These include the Laugier-Hunziker syndrome (melanotic macules on the

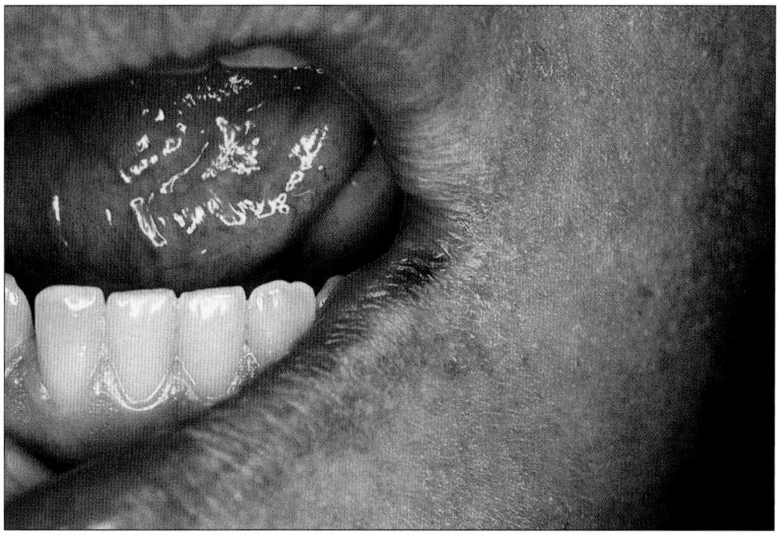

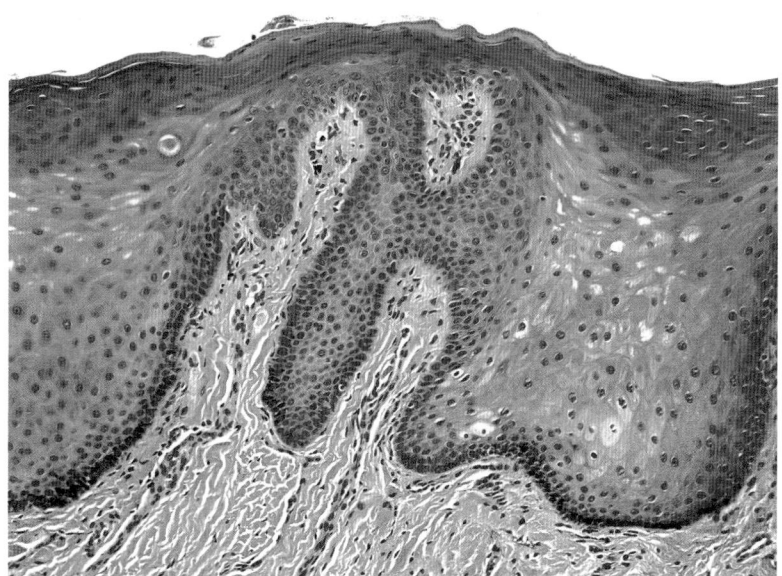

Fig. 11.254
Oral melanotic macule: note the typical dark brown-to-black macule on the vermilion.

Fig. 11.255
Oral melanotic macule: there is increased melanization of the basal cells in the absence of melanocytic hyperplasia; melanophages are present in the papillary lamina propria.

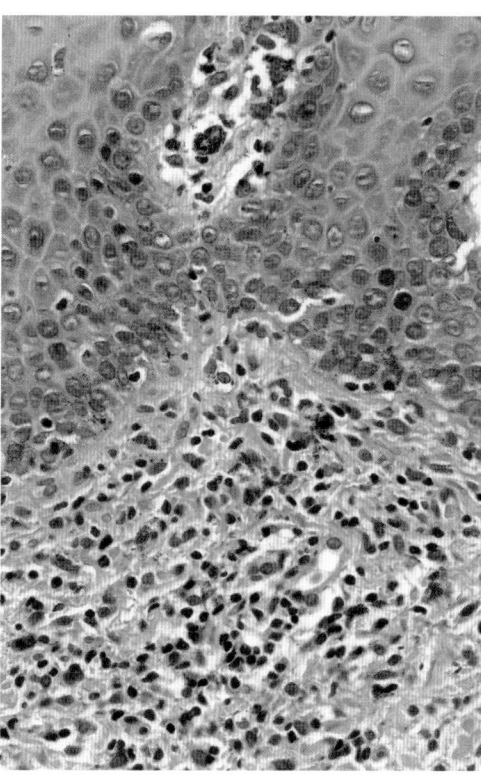

Fig. 11.256
Post-inflammatory hypermelanosis: there is increased melanization of the basal cells, vascular ectasia, chronic inflammation, and many melanophages in the lamina propria.

oral and genital mucosa with melanonychia striata),[7,8] neurofibromatosis, Addison disease, Peutz-Jegher syndrome (associated with intestinal polyposis), and McCune-Albright syndrome (associated with endocrinopathy and bone lesions).

The oral melanotic macule is characterized by increased melanin pigmentation in the basal cell layer of the epithelium, usually localized to the tips of the rete ridges with no or only minimal melanocytic hyperplasia (Fig. 11.255).[1,3,9,10] There are increased numbers of melanophages in the lamina propria, melanin incontinence, variable lymphocytic infiltrate, and ectatic capillaries. There may be associated mild hyperkeratosis, parakeratosis, and acanthosis, all suggestive of a reactive, inflammatory lesion. Such findings are also seen in postinflammatory hypermelanosis associated with interface stomatitides such as lichen planus (Fig. 11.256).

Ultrastructurally, stage III and stage IV heavily melanized melanosomes are clustered in complexes within melanocytes, keratinocytes, and melanophages.[9]

Differential diagnosis

Smoker's melanosis exhibit the same features and is also likely to represent postinflammatory hypermelanosis.[11] Cases of melanotic macules associated

with syndromes as described above have similar histopathology but generally without significant inflammation.

The pigment in medication-induced hyperpigmentation is present as regular, brown spherical granules within the lamina propria often in linear array likely because they are present within cytoplasmic processes of macrophages or dendritic cells; there is no pigment within basal cells (see later).

Ephelides occur on sun-exposed areas and the darkness of pigmentation increases with sun exposure. Lentigo shows epithelial and melanocytic hyperplasia in addition to increased melanin pigmentation, and rare intraoral cases have been identified.[12]

Melanoacanthosis

Clinical features

Melanoacanthosis (oral melanoacanthoma) should not be confused with cutaneous melanoacanthoma. More than 70% of cases occur in young black females, and it typically presents in areas that are susceptible to trauma such as the buccal mucosa, lower lip, palatal mucosa, and gingiva.[1-5] The macules have a slightly rough surface and are brown, black, or bluish (Fig. 11.257). The lesion may be well or poorly demarcated. Most lesions are solitary although rare cases are multifocal.[6] A history of trauma is present in only 50% of cases. Lesions may grow rapidly to several centimeters in size over a few weeks, and complete resolution occurs within months.

Pathogenesis and histologic features

It is likely that oral melanoacanthosis is a form of postinflammatory hypermelanosis, precipitated by trauma with subsequent inflammation resulting in reactive hyperplasia of dendritic melanocytes.

There is slight parakeratosis and acanthosis and, usually, spongiosis (Fig. 11.258). Numerous dendritic melanocytes and their melanin-laden processes are found insinuating between keratinocytes throughout the full thickness of the epithelium (Fig. 11.259).[1-7] Such transmigration of melanocytes should not be overdiagnosed as melanoma since there is no cytological atypia. Melanophages, a mild lymphocytic infiltrate, and vascular ectasia may also be seen in the lamina propria. Sometimes, the spongiosis may be so severe as to form spongiform vesicles.[8] Studies for S100 and Melan-A are positive.[3,9]

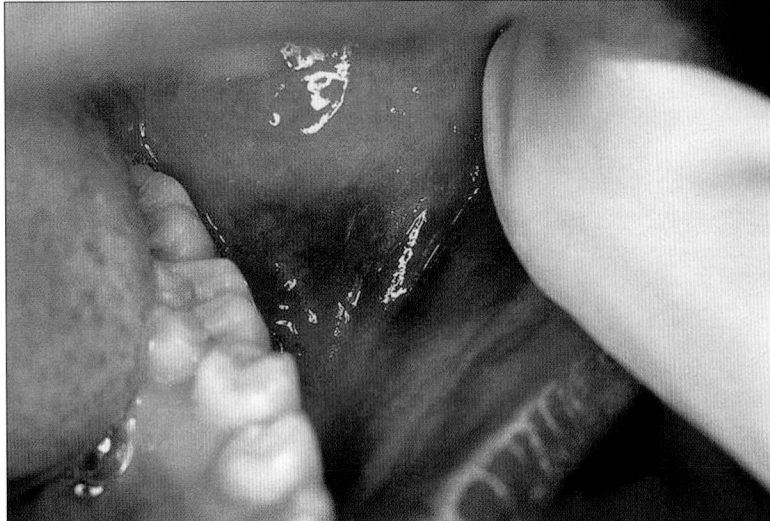

Fig. 11.257
Melanoacanthosis: there is a blue-black macule on the buccal mucosa that
enlarged rapidly over a few weeks.

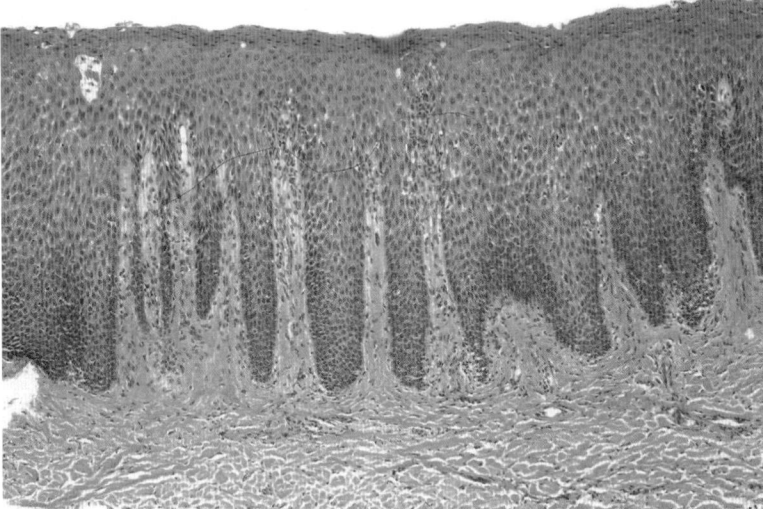

Fig. 11.258
Melanoacanthosis: there is parakeratosis, acanthosis, spongiosis, and melanocytic
hyperplasia involving the full thickness of the epithelium.

Differential diagnosis

Melanoacanthosis differs from a junctional melanocytic nevus by the
absence of nesting of melanocytes at the interface. The benign cytology of
the melanocytes readily distinguishes this lesion from oral melanoma, even
though there is epithelial transmigration.

Medication-induced oral pigmentation

Clinical features

These present as slate-blue macular pigmentation usually of the hard palatal
and gingiva. The cutaneous tissues may or may not be involved. The medications involved include minocycline, antimalarial agents, clofazamine, birth
control medications, amiodarone, tyrosine kinase inhibitors such as imatinib, and drugs that contain heavy metals.[1-7] Tetracycline becomes incorporated into hydroxyapatite crystals of bone and teeth, and it is common for
the pigmented bone to show through the mucosa as gray macular areas.[8]
Extracted teeth also have a grayish-green cast.

Pathogenesis and histopathological features

The metabolites of these medications are either themselves pigmented or
chelate to hemosiderin and melanin to form these pigment granules.

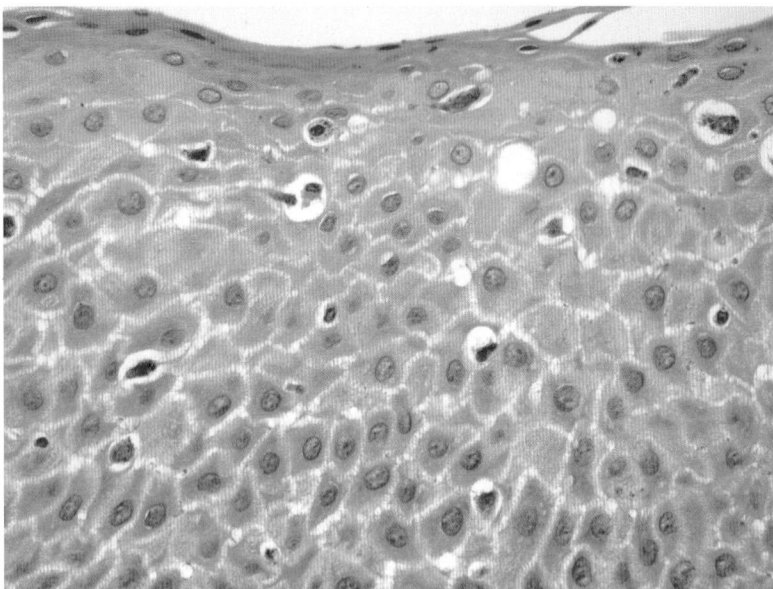

Fig. 11.259
Melanoacanthosis: benign dendritic melanocytes are present throughout the full
thickness of the epithelium.

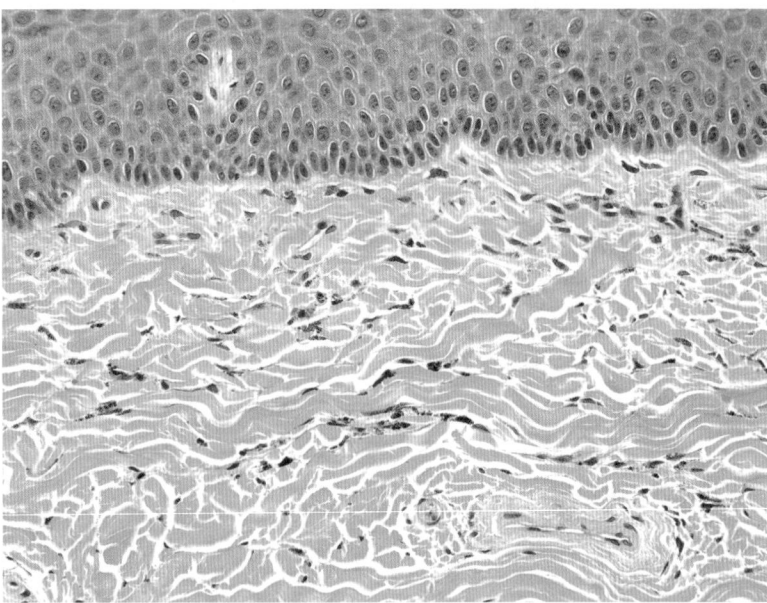

Fig. 11.260
Imatinib-induced pigmentation: there are small, spherical, brown pigment granules
disposed along connective tissue fibers.

There is deposition of small, 1–5 micron, brown spherical granules in
the superficial lamina propria that are disposed, often in a linear fashion,
along connective tissue fibers likely within cytoplasmic processes of macrophages or dendritic cells (*Fig. 11.260*). Importantly, there is no increased
melanin deposition within the basal keratinocytes. The granules often stain
for melanin (Fontana Masson) and iron (Prussian blue) (*Fig. 11.261*).[5-7]

Differential diagnosis

Many medication-induced hyperpigmentary states are not caused by metabolites of the medication, but rather represent postinflammatory hypermelanosis. This is particularly common if the medications cause a lichenoid or
interface stomatitis. In such cases, the lesions almost always show increased
melanin pigment within the basal keratinocytes (even if a lymphocytic band
at the interface is not present), and the stain for iron will be negative. They
also tend to be located at sites other than the palatal mucosa.

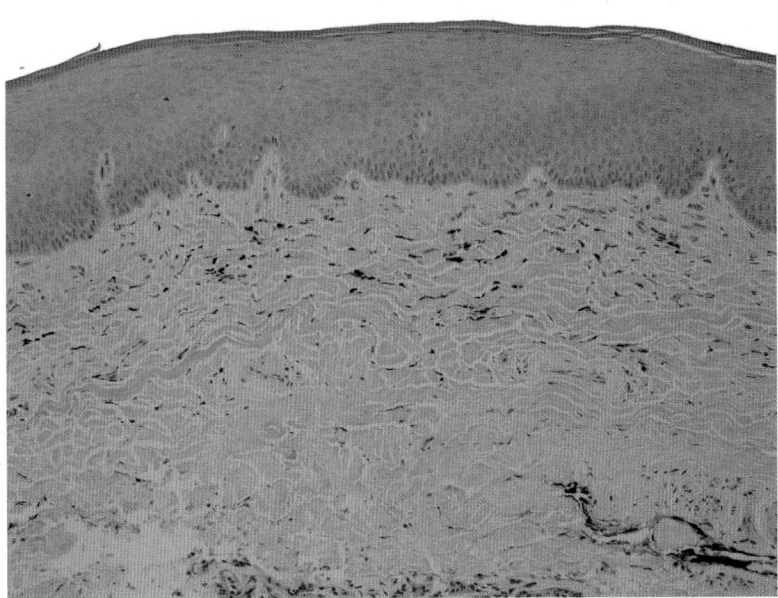

Fig. 11.261
Imatinib-induced pigmentation: the Prussian blue stain is positive for the presence of iron.

Oral melanocytic nevus

Clinical features

Oral melanocytic nevi are generally diagnosed and biopsied in the second to fourth decades of life, with a female predilection (2:1). Approximately 85% are clinically pigmented (gray, brown, blue or black, or a combination thereof), and almost all are raised, being nodular or papular lesions.[1-3] The hard palatal mucosa and buccal mucosa are the favored sites, followed by the lip mucosa, gingiva, and vermilion. Seventy-five percent of all intraoral blue nevi occur as macules on the palatal mucosa, with the lip mucosa being the second most frequently affected site, whereas banal intramucosal melanocytic nevi occur on the palatal and buccal mucosa equally.[4]

Histologic features

Melanocytic nevi in the oral cavity are histologically identical to those found on the skin. The intramucosal nevus (counterpart of the dermal nevus) is the most common (63–80%), followed by the blue nevus (8–17%) and compound nevus (6–17%).[1,4-7] The intramucosal nevus consists of nests of epithelioid melanocytes superficially with downward maturation. Epithelial hyperplasia is seen in association with intramucosal nevi in approximately 50% of cases, sometimes associated with benign lentiginous melanocytic hyperplasia. Approximately 15% are nonpigmented. Nevus cells are also sometimes seen within the underlying adipose tissue and muscle.[1] The spindled cells of blue nevi are variably pigmented and dispersed within the lamina propria. Oral melanocytic nevi are immunopositive for S100 protein and MART-1, and blue nevi also exhibit positivity for HMB-45.[8] Combined nevus, Spitz, congenital, and balloon cell nevi have also been described, albeit rarely[4,9-12] Mutation of *BRAF V600E* have been identified in oral melanocytic nevi, as has *GNAQ209* mutation in a blue nevus.[13] There is no risk of malignant transformation to melanoma.[14]

Oral melanoma

Clinical features

Primary oral melanomas comprise 20–40% of mucosal head and neck melanomas, which, in turn, comprise 1–3% of all melanomas. It is more common in the Japanese and in blacks.[1-5] Tumors are most often seen in the seventh decade of life, with a male predilection. The hard palatal mucosa and maxillary gingiva are affected in more than 70% of cases.[6] Early lesions that are in situ, appear as large (usually greater than 1 cm), macular melanotic lesions that progressively spread over the mucosa, and have uneven borders and uneven pigmentation. As this progresses, plaques, nodules, or mass lesions become apparent, sometimes with pain and bleeding.[2,4,7,8] Oral lesions behave similarly to acral melanoma, and between 20% and 40% of patients present with lymph node metastases.[1-3] Most mucosal melanomas are negative for *BRAF* mutation, but may express *KIT* and *NRAS* mutations.[9,10] Prognostic stage groups based on the TNM system are no longer used in the 2017 American Joint Committee on Cancer guidelines issued in 2016.[10]

Overall, the prognosis for oral tumors is much worse than that for cutaneous melanoma and the 5-year survival rate is generally <30%.[1-3,5,11] A high rate of nodal metastasis, thick tumor at presentation, extensive lateral spread of tumor, and the complicated anatomy of the maxillary complex make it difficult to completely excise the majority of these lesions.

Histologic features

Most oral melanomas arise from pre-existing intraepithelial melanocytic dysplasia or atypical melanocytic hyperplasia that is either lentiginous or pagetoid, similar to cases of acral lentiginous melanoma.[12] Common patterns are spindled or fasciculated, solid, and peritheliomatous, with storiform, pseudopapillary, and pseudoalveorlar forms being less common.[10] Tumor cells are often spindled, epithelioid, plasmacytoid, rhabdoid, or clear. Tumors are amelanotic in 15–50% of cases.[5,13] Tumor thickness greater than 5 mm, presence of vascular invasion, presence of bcl2 in the initial tumor, and the development of nodal and distant metastases predict a worse prognosis.[3,14,15] Desmoplastic melanoma has been reported in the oral cavity as has cartilaginous metaplasia.[16-18] Results of immunohistochemical studies are identical to those for cutaneous melanomas, namely, positivity for S100 protein, SOX10, MART-1, HMB-45, and MITF.

One other intraoral tumor that presents with melanotic pigmentation is the melanotic neuroectodermal tumor of infancy. This occurs as an intraosseous lesion that usually erodes through the cortical bone into the soft tissues, and has an epithelioid cell population that contains melanin and is positive for melanocytic markers, and a neuroblast-like cell population positive for neuroendocrine markers.[19-21]

OTHER TUMORS

Granular cell tumor

Clinical features

The granular cell tumor occurs in females twice as often as in males, and the mean age at presentation is in the fourth decade, although cases have been reported in the first two decades of life.[1] It presents at a variety of sites, most commonly the skin (38% of cases), the tongue (23–28%), the breast (16%), and the larynx, especially the true cord (8%).[2-4] In the mouth, more than 80% of cases occur in the tongue, with the lips, buccal mucosa, and floor of mouth being other sites of involvement.[5] Approximately 8% of cases are multiple.[2] The lesions are yellowish-white, firm and indurated, painless masses or plaques generally measuring less than 2 cm in greatest dimension (*Fig. 11.262*). There is little tendency to recur even after incomplete excision.

Pathogenesis and histologic features

This tumor is immunopositive for neural markers.[6,7]

The overlying epithelium exhibits pseudoepitheliomatous hyperplasia in one-third to two-thirds of cases, which in some tumors is so marked as to result in a misdiagnosis of invasive squamous cell carcinoma.[1,4,6,7] The tumor is unencapsulated and presents as nests, cords, and sheets of granular

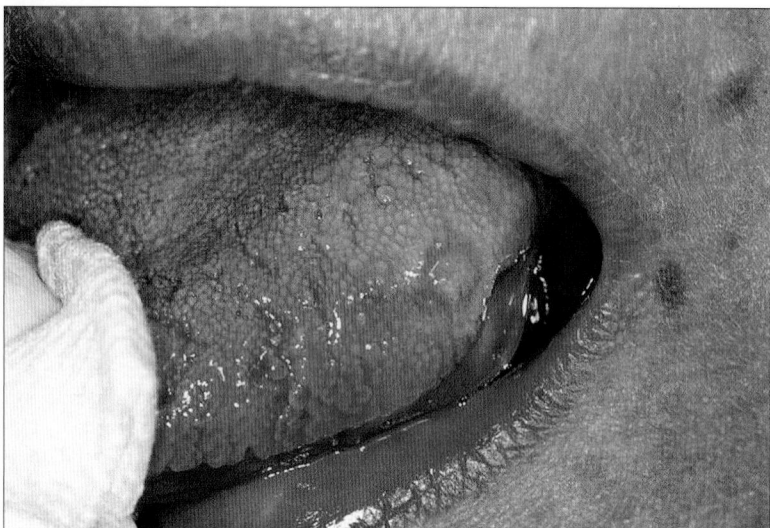

Fig. 11.262
Granular cell tumor: note the small plaque on the left in the tongue.

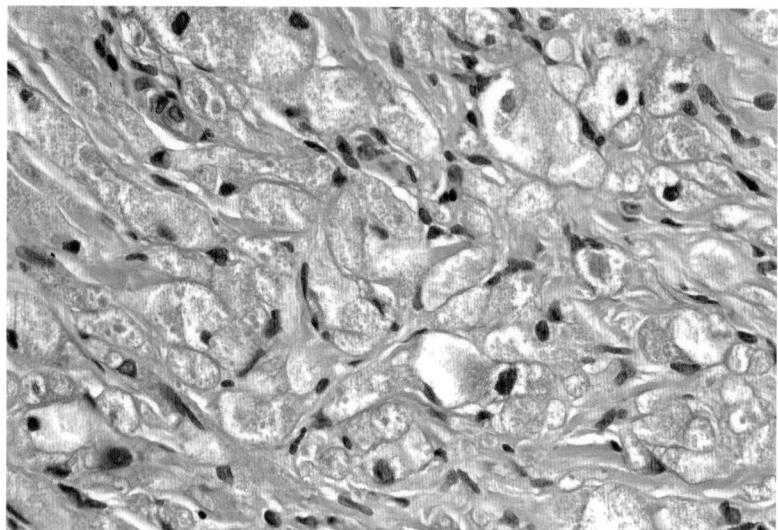

Fig. 11.264
Granular cell tumor: the cells are polyhedral with pale granular cytoplasm and small nuclei; intracytoplasmic eosinophilic globules (pustule ovoid bodies) are present.

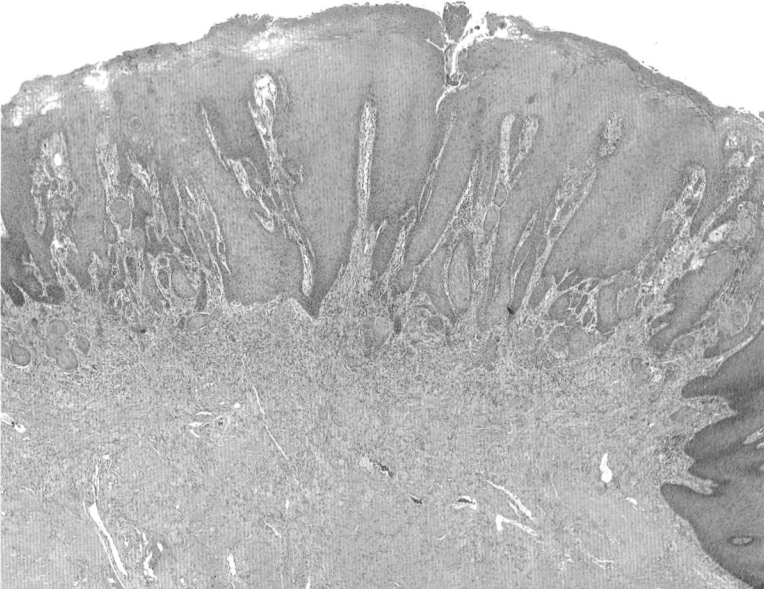

Fig. 11.263
Granular cell tumor: granular cells fill the lamina propria and insinuate between the muscle fibers of the tongue, and there is pseudoepitheliomatous hyperplasia.

cells that often abut the epithelium, filling the lamina propria and infiltrating the underlying muscle (*Fig. 11.263*).[1] There is usually close association between the tumor cells and skeletal muscle, nerves, and blood vessels.[1,7,8] Cells are large and polygonal with either distinct or indistinct cell borders and a small nucleus (*Fig. 11.264*).[1] The abundant cytoplasm contains granules that are PAS positive and diastase resistant. Tumor cells are positive for S100 protein, CD68, and PGP9.5, while studies for muscle and histiocytic markers are negative.[7-13]

Ultrastructurally, the granular cells contain autophagic granules and vesicular bodies.[14] Membrane-bound angulate bodies represent angular lysosomes. A basal lamina is sometimes seen around the cells, suggesting schwannian derivation.

Malignant granular cell tumors are rare and exhibit pleomorphism, mitoses, necrosis, and spindling of cells with a similar staining pattern. They may metastasize.[15,16]

Differential diagnosis

There is a variant of the granular cell tumor that is not immunopositive for S100 protein – the primitive non-neural granular cell tumor. This lesion is polypoid with an epithelial collarette, and the granular cells exhibit slight nuclear atypia.[17-19] The congenital granular cell tumor is also S100 negative and has a delicate arborizing vasculature and does not exhibit pseudoepitheliomatous hyperplasia. Granular cell change may also be observed focally in many other tumors likely as a degenerative phenomenon.[18]

Ectomesenchymal chondromyxoid tumor

Clinical features

This unusual nodular tumor of the anterior tongue dorsum occurs in the third to fourth decades of life.[1,2]

Histologic features

Some authorities consider this a soft tissue myoepithelioma, and a subset of these tumors exhibits *EWSR1* rearrangement, similar to soft tissue myoepithelioma.[3] The tumor is a well-circumscribed but unencapsulated, lobular proliferation of tumor cells in the superficial tongue musculature, arranged in sheets, strands, and cords in a chondromyxoid stroma with cleftlike spaces (*Fig. 11.265*).[1,2,4-6] Cells are polygonal, ovoid, and fusiform with small nuclei and faintly basophilic cytoplasm. There may be focal nuclear hyperchromatism and bi- or multinucleation. The myxoid nature of the stroma often gives the tumor a reticular appearance, and pseudocyst formation is seen in 50% of cases (*Fig. 11.266*). Muscle fibers are often trapped at the periphery of the tumor.[7]

The tumor cells are immunopositive for vimentin, GFAP, S100 protein, CD57, SMA, and smooth muscle myosin heavy chain.[1,2,4,5] There is variable positivity for AE1/AE3, CAM 5.2, EMA and p63. Tumors are negative for desmin but may be positive for CD56.[1,2,8]

Ultrastructurally, basal lamina is focally present, but desmosomes and dense bodies are absent.[1]

Access **ExpertConsult.com** for the complete list of references

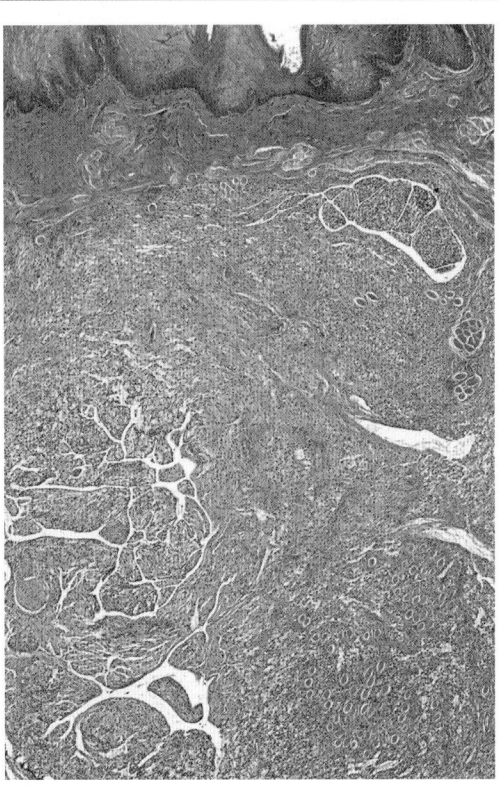

Fig. 11.265
Ectomesenchymal
chondromyxoid tumor of
the tongue: the tumor is
discrete and myxoid, with
many cleftlike spaces.

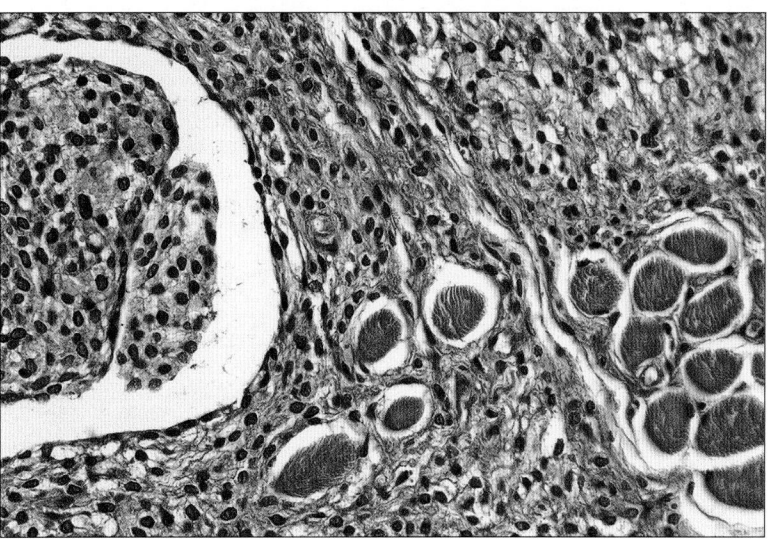

Fig. 11.266
Ectomesenchymal chondromyxoid tumor of the tongue: the tumor cells are
epithelioid and spindled and there is entrapment of muscle fibers.

Diseases of the anogenital skin

Eduardo Calonje, Fiona Lewis, Chris Bunker, Diego Fernando Sánchez Martínez and Antonio L. Cubilla

See
www.expertconsult.com
for references and additional material

Introduction

This section concerns itself principally with dermatological disorders specific to the anogenital skin. Many of the dermatological conditions that present in the skin elsewhere sometimes affect the anogenital area although this site may be one of predilection. Clinical and histologic features can be modified by the chronicity of the problem, treatments applied, and the occlusive effect of this natural flexural site.

Over the years, various classifications have been devised for vulval disorders.[1] Terms such as squamous cell hyperplasia are clinically meaningless and at best histologically descriptive. There has been an attempt to link the clinical and histologic features of vulval disease,[2] and the classification and terminology for squamous vulval intraepithelial neoplasia (VIN) and penile intraepithelial neoplasia (PeIN) are discussed later.

The anogenital area is covered by both skin and mucous membrane, i.e., keratinized and nonkeratinized stratified squamous epithelium. The transition from skin to mucosa is characterized by a subtle modification in the properties of the epithelia at their junctions. It is, therefore, critically important that the site sampled for histologic analysis is always specified so as to avoid confusion and misinterpretation, and there must be careful clinicopathological correlation with an open dialogue between the clinician and the pathologist. The method of biopsy must also be made to the pathologist as the use of topical anesthesia can cause epidermal changes, which can be important diagnostic pitfalls.[3]

Normal female anatomy

The vulva comprises the mons pubis, the labia majora and minora, the vestibule, the clitoris (including the prepuce and frenulum), the glands of Bartholin and Skene, the hymen, posterior commissure, fossa navicularis, introitus, and the external urethral orifice (*Fig. 12.1*).

Histologic features

The anogenital region, as with other mucocutaneous sites, is characterized by a gradual transition from skin to a mucosal surface.

Labia majora and perianal skin

Histologic features

These sites most closely resemble skin from other regions of the body since the epithelium is keratinized and stratified and adnexal structures are represented. The epithelium of the labia majora normally contains occasional lymphocytes, which are found in very small numbers around the superficial dermal vasculature. In the labia majora, sebaceous glands are present in association with hair follicles and both anogenital mammary-like glands are typically present. On the medial aspect of the labia majora, the hair

follicles become modified and there is often no hair seen although sebaceous glands are still present (*Fig. 12.2*). Some may open directly onto the epithelium (Fordyce spots, see below). In the deep dermis, a layer of smooth muscle known as the tunica dartos labialis is seen. The subcutaneous tissue of the labia majora tends to be prominent in women of reproductive age but decreases in amount after the menopause. The labium majus contains a long smooth muscle called the cremaster. The skin of the perianal area shows numerous terminal hairs with sebaceous glands.

Labia minora and clitoral prepuce

Histologic features

The labia minora represent the female equivalent of the penile corpus spongiosum. They are located lateral to the vaginal vestibule, medial to the labia majora, and are covered by stratified, often pigmented, squamous epithelium. In most females, adnexal structures are absent, as is subcutaneous tissue. The stroma is richly vascular and contains abundant erectile tissue and elastic fibers.

The pilosebaceous unit is incomplete, as the sebaceous gland is not usually associated with a hair follicle and opens directly onto the surface. Anogenital mammary-like glands are sparse and subcutaneous fat is not seen.

Glans clitoris

Histologic features

The epithelium is stratified and keratinized. No adnexal structures are present. The glans clitoris, unlike its male counterpart, does not contain a corpus spongiosum. The frenulum and the prepuce originate from the labia minora and contain abundant sebaceous and mucus-secreting glands.

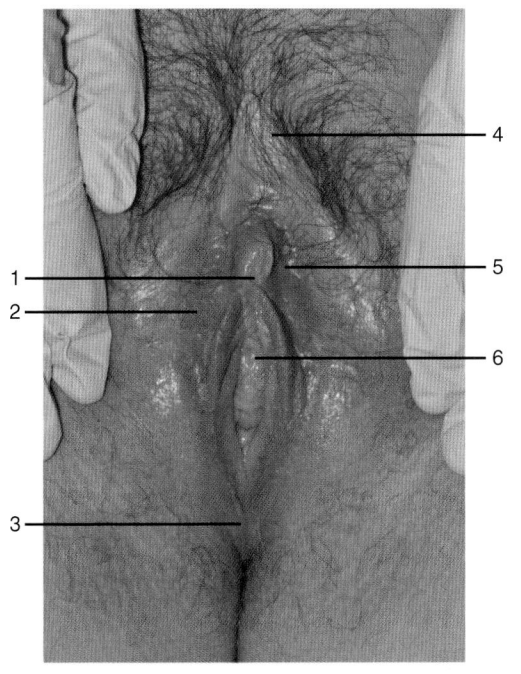

1. Glans clitoris
2. Labium majus
3. Posterior labial commissure
4. Prepuce of clitoris
5. Labium minus
6. External orifice of urethra

Fig. 12.1
Normal vulva showing the major anatomical landmarks.

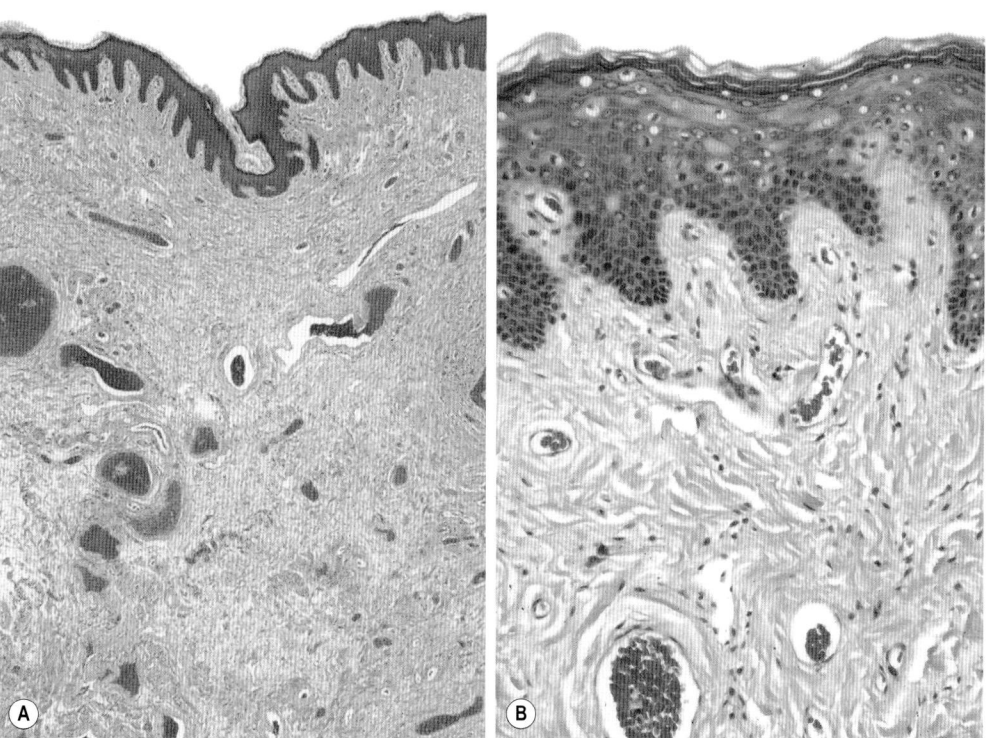

Fig. 12.2
(**A**, **B**) Normal vulva: medial aspect of labium majus. The epidermis is keratinized. The dermis is richly vascular. Hair follicles are absent.

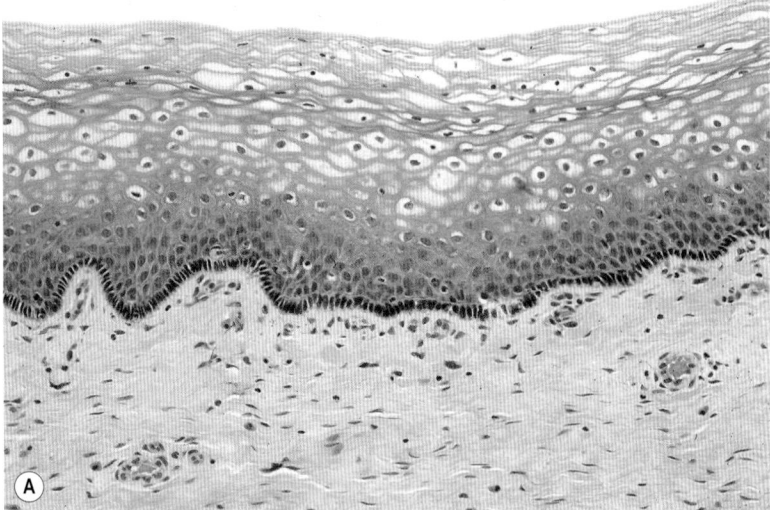

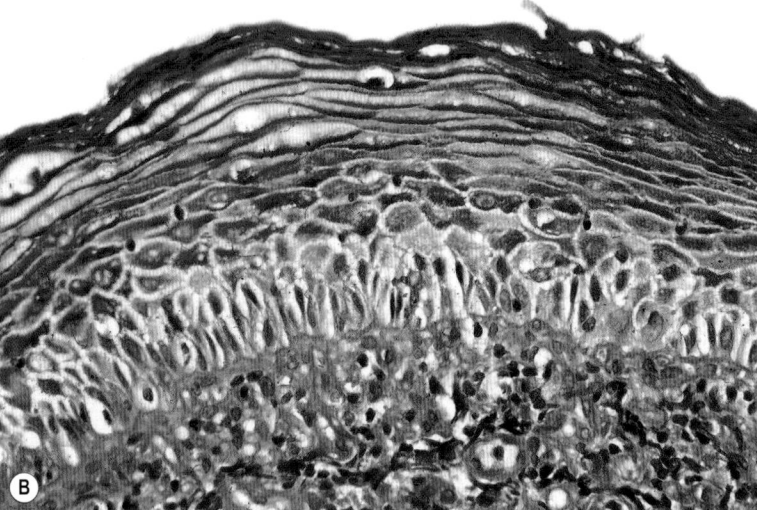

Fig. 12.3
Vestibule: (**A**) the epithelium is nonkeratinizing and rich in glycogen. Cutaneous appendages are absent at this site; (**B**) the epithelium is strongly PAS positive.

Vestibule

Histologic features

The epithelium is stratified and nonkeratinized, i.e., it is a mucosa (*Fig. 12.3*). Both the vagina and the urethra open into the vestibule. Bartholin glands are located deep to the posterior third of the labia majora. They represent the equivalent of Cowper glands or the bulbourethral glands in the male. The ducts of Bartholin and Skene glands and the minor vestibular glands open into the vestibule.

Normal male anatomy

The penis, as well as being essential for sexual intercourse, is also the conduit for urinary excretion. The scrotum is an extracorporeal sac, which contains the testes at an ideal ambient temperature for spermatogenesis. The natal cleft and the inguinal (crural) folds are special sites of importance because they are areas where two layers of skin come into close apposition. They constitute the flexural junctions between the lower limbs and the trunk and also surround the mucocutaneous junctions of the anus and genitalia. The perineum lies between the anus and the scrotum, and the skin at this site is tightly tethered to the underlying tissues.

The prepuce has been present in primates for at least 65 million years and indeed this may be an underestimate, 100 million years having been suggested. The female counterpart is the clitoral hood. Only 4% of boys have a retractable foreskin at birth, 15% at 6 months, 50% at 1 year, and 80–90% at 3 years.[1] The separation of the mucosa of the prepuce and glans is usually complete by 17 years.[2–4] The prepuce is composed of specialized protective and erogenous tissue. The protection it affords is both physical and immunological.[4] Its structures (e.g., the penile dartos muscle and the corpuscular receptor-rich ridged band) and secretions are held to be important for normal function. The foreskin is of variable length and retractability in uncircumcised men.

The anatomical position, when one considers the features of the normal penis, is that of full penile erection. Thus the dorsal aspect of the penis is the surface that is in direct contiguity with the abdomen, being the ventral surface of the body.

Histologic features

The pattern of keratinization of the epithelium varies throughout the anogenital area, most markedly in the transition from true urothelium to true skin. There is controversy over the definition of 'mucosa' but there is no doubt that the penile urethra does possess a true mucosa, whereas the glans of the circumcised male does not; the glans and inner prepuce of the uncircumcised male probably does not display mucosa but the outer prepuce does. There are several epithelial transition zones. The proximal (pre-prostatic and prostatic) urethra is lined by transitional epithelium, the membranous spongy penile urethra by pseudostratified columnar epithelium. The distal penile urethra is lined by stratified or pseudo-stratified squamous epithelium incorporating a single layer of columnar cells at the surface and contains Littre glands, the distal 5–6 mm of penile urethra, which includes the navicular fossa, manifests a 6–10 cell layer of nonkeratinizing squamous epithelium, contains no adnexae, and is continuous with the epithelium of the uncircumcised glans (which may show some thin keratinization, although some accounts state that the glans is not keratinized in the uncircumcised) and inner preputial epithelium; the outer preputial epithelium is identical to skin. Just as there is wide variability in the size and shape of the navicular fossa, the site of the epithelial transition zones and probably the degree of keratinization of the glans and the disposition of adnexa may vary. Presumed multipotential, mucous secreting cells have been described in the perimeatal epithelium, and mucinous metaplasia of glans and foreskin have also been observed.[5] Also, the final transition will depend on the length of the foreskin: it is our experience that male genital lichen sclerosus (LS) has a greater predilection for the male with a longer foreskin (as does penile cancer). The wide spectrum of differentiation of the male urogenital tract is accompanied by changes in the expression of epithelial cytokeratins, but this is relatively unexplored territory.[6] Normal regional histology is illustrated in *Figs 12.4–12.9*.

Embryology

The anatomical position, the arrangement of all of the structures in the area, the normal histology, and some of the histopathology are explained by the embryology (*Figs 12.10* and *12.11*).[1,2] Around the third week of fetal development, mesenchymal cells derived from the primitive streak form ridges of tissue around the cloacal membrane. These cloacal folds are joined anteriorly and cranially and form the genital tubercle. Posteriorly and caudally, they are partially joined to form an annulus. The underlying cloacal membrane is now subdivided into urogenital and anal membranes craniocaudally by about 6 weeks. During the same period, lateral genital swellings develop that will form either the scrotum or labia majora.

From this point, differentiation of the external genitalia occurs in a gender-specific manner, driven in the male by fetal testicular androgens. The genital tubercle lengthens, creating a urethral groove. This eventually becomes the urethral canal when the folds fuse at about 12 weeks. The penile urethra has an epithelium derived therefore from endoderm. It is incomplete cranially where the glans has developed from the genital tubercle. The glanular urethra, the navicular fossa, and the meatus are derived from an invading cord of ectoderm that eventually becomes canalized. There is wide variability in the size and shape of the navicular fossa in men, testifying to the variable consequences of this embryological process. The scrotal swellings fuse posteriorly at about 14 weeks. They are not occupied

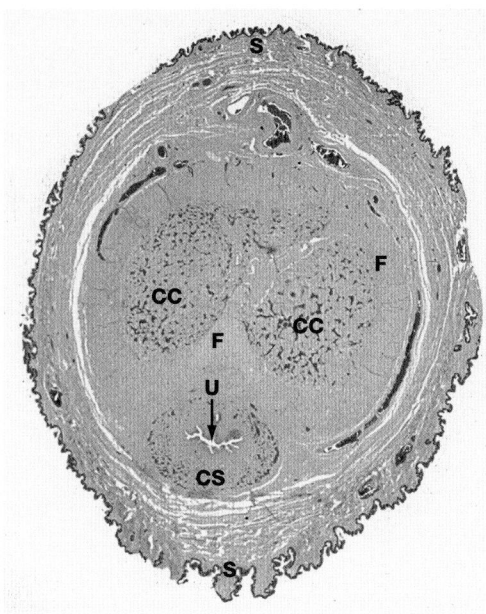

Fig. 12.4
Penis: this transverse section of the human penis shows the arrangement of the erectile tissues, which exist in the form of three columns. The two dorsal columns are called the *corpora cavernosa (CC)* and the single ventral column is the *corpus spongiosum (CS)*, through which runs the *penile urethra (U)*. At its distal end, the corpus spongiosum expands to form the *glans penis*. The erectile corpora are enclosed within, and separated by, a fibrocollagenous capsule *(F)*. The erectile centre of the penis is enclosed in a sheath of skin *S* to which it is connected by a loose subcutis containing prominent blood vessels. Reproduced with permission from Young B. et al., Wheater's Functional Histology, 5th edition. © Churchill Livingstone, 2006.

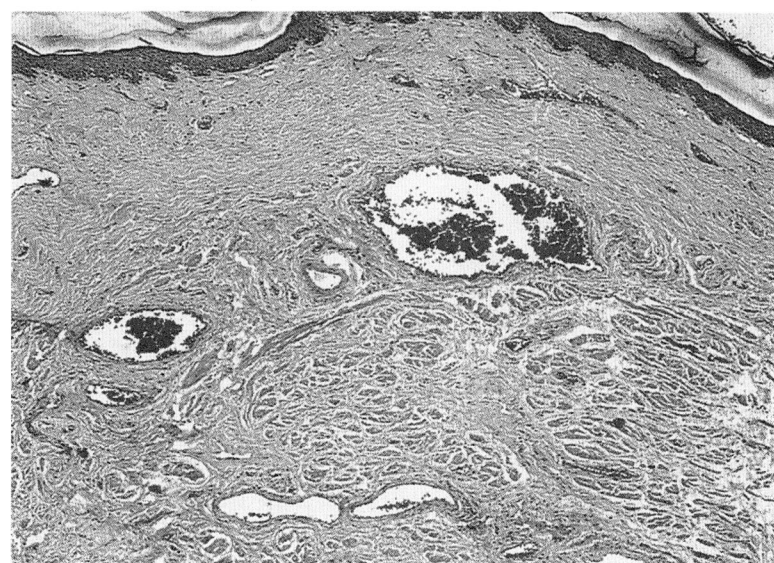

Fig. 12.6
Normal histology of the penis, balanopreputial sulcus. Histologic components of both glans and penile body are present. This specimen from a circumcised person shows the mucosa at top, lamina propria below, then dartos, or smooth muscle layer and Buck fascia. H&E. Courtesy of and reproduced with permission from Sternberg, S.S., ed. Histology for Pathologists, 2nd edition. Philadelphia: Lippincott, Williams and Wilkins, 1997.

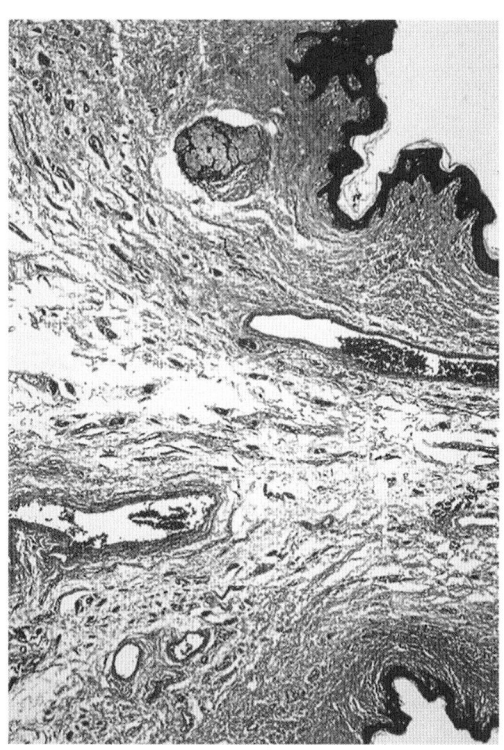

Fig. 12.5
Normal histology of the penis. Foreskin. Full thickness of prepuce shows all five layers: keratinized stratified squamous epithelium, dermis with sebaceous glands, dartos, submucosa, and squamous mucosa. H&E. Courtesy of and reproduced with permission from Sternberg, S.S., ed. Histology for Pathologists, 2nd edition. Philadelphia: Lippincott, Williams and Wilkins, 1997.

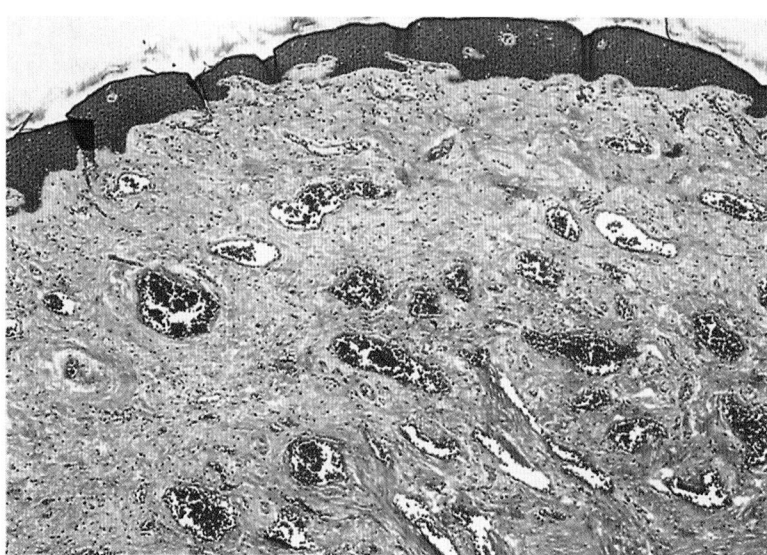

Fig. 12.7
Normal histology of the penis. Glans penis. The three layers of glans are noted: nonkeratinized stratified mucosa, lamina propria, and corpus spongiosum. H&E. Reproduced with permission from Sternberg, S.S., ed. Histology for Pathologists, 2nd edition. Philadelphia: Lippincott, Williams and Wilkins, 1997.

the urogenital sinus anteriorly and the anorectal canal posteriorly. The anal membrane disintegrates at about 9 weeks to open into an ectodermal anal pit formed in the posterior cloacal (anal) folds. The prepuce[3,4] is formed by a midline collision of ectoderm, neuroectoderm, and mesenchyme, resulting in a pentalaminar structure consisting of (inner) squamous mucosal epithelium, lamina propria, dartos muscle, dermis, and glabrous skin (outer). The preputial fold progressively extends, but there is also an ingrowth of a cellular lamella. It then fuses with the mucosa of the glans. At birth, the prepuce is still developing histologically and it is usually incompletely separated from the glans.

In the female, the genital tubercle lengthens and then bends to form the clitoris and is incorporated into the fused anterior genital folds which form the labia minora. The genital swellings which are lateral form the labia majora and become continuous with the mons pubis.

by the testes until about the time of birth. The cloacal membrane is where ectodermal and endodermal tissues are in direct apposition caudally. The separation into urogenital membrane and anal membrane with the formation of the perineum at about 7 weeks is due to the separation of the cloacal portion of the hindgut by the urorectal septum growing caudally between the allantois anteriorly and the hindgut and partitioning the cloaca into

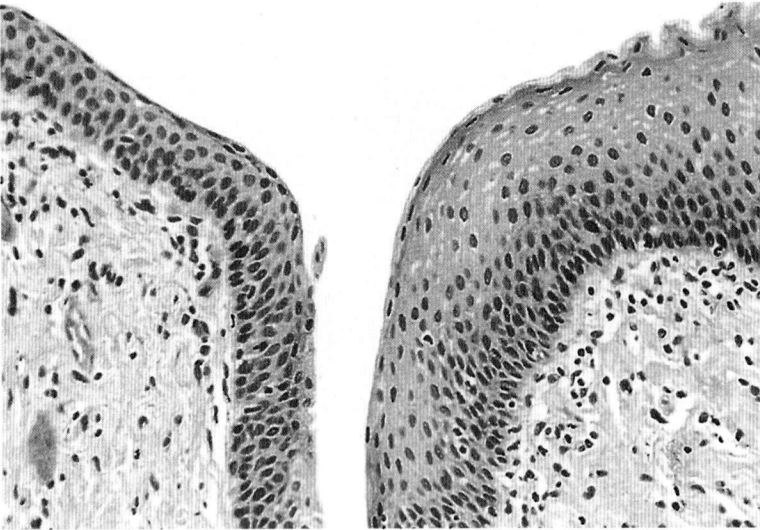

Fig. 12.8
Anal transitional zone (ATZ). Transition from ATZ epithelium *(left)* to squamous zone *(right)*. H&E. Reproduced with permission from Sternberg, S.S., ed. Histology for Pathologists, 2nd edition. Philadelphia: Lippincott, Williams and Wilkins, 1997.

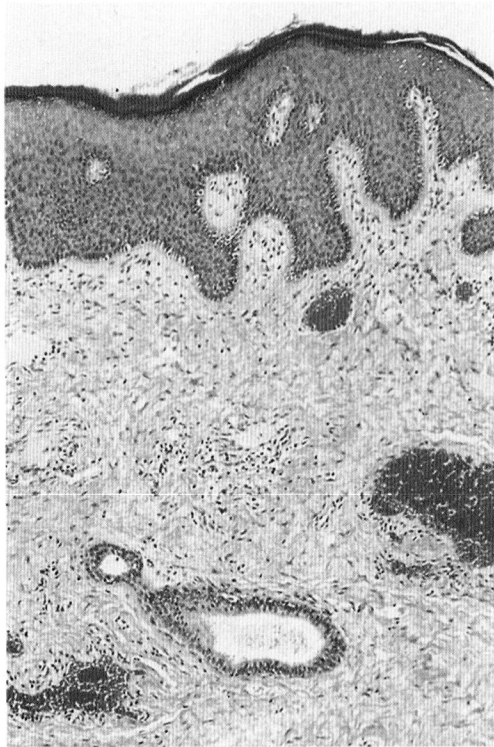

Fig. 12.9
Perianal skin. Keratinized squamous epithelium and an underlying apocrine gland. H&E. Reproduced with permission from Sternberg, S.S., ed. Histology for Pathologists, 2nd edition. Philadelphia: Lippincott, Williams and Wilkins, 1997.

Pubic hair

Pubic hair appears during puberty as vellus hair that is focally replaced by terminal hair. Men have a different pattern of pubic hair than women, but in practice it is one of degree. The distribution of hair and pubic hair varies widely between men.[1] Generally, the abdominal wall, pubic mound, groins, scrotum and perineum are hairy, but the natal cleft, perianal skin, distal penile shaft, prepuce, and glans are hairless.

In females, pubic hair development starts at puberty on the mons pubis and labia majora. The adult distribution with triangular pattern on the mons, with extension to the labia majora and on to the thighs is usually complete by the age of 16–17 years.

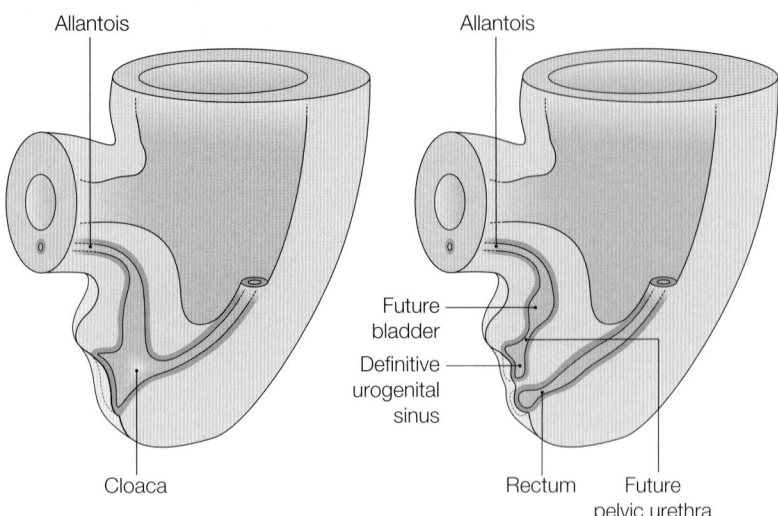

Fig. 12.10
Development of the primitive urogenital sinus. Between 4 and 6 weeks, the urorectal septum splits the cloaca into an anterior primitive urogenital sinus and a posterior rectum. The superior part of the primitive urogenital sinus, continuous with the allantois, forms the bladder. The constricted pelvic urethra at the base of the future bladder forms the membranous urethra in females and the membranous and prostatic urethra in males. The distal expansion of the primitive urogenital sinus, the definitive urogenital sinus, forms the vestibule of the vagina in females and the penile urethra in males. From Bunker C. Male Genital Skin Disease. Saunders Ltd./Elsevier 2004.

Anogenital mammary-like glands

The anogenital area possesses numerous glands (some functionless) regarded in the past as apocrine and eccrine sweat glands. It is now thought that most of these glands represent distinctive structures with close similarities to breast glands and referred to anogenital mammary-like glands (see below). Also, holocrine sebaceous glands are plentiful, usually in association with hair follicles (pilosebaceous units), but also occurring as free glands at some sites such as the anal rim or around the coronal sulcus (Tyson glands). Their secretions lubricate the areas between limb and torso, hair, and mucocutaneous junctions to assist in the voiding of excreta and protect the epithelia from irritation and the penis for sexual activity (the retraction of the foreskin).

Anogenital mammary-like glands, which were first described by van der Putte, are found in anogenital skin, mainly in the interlabial sulci.[1,2] They share morphological, histologic, and immunohistochemical features of mammary glands (*Fig. 12.12*). Superficially, an excretory duct opens directly onto the skin. Excretory ducts are lined by a single layer of epithelial cells and display an external layer of myoepithelial cells. Before entering the epidermis, the ductal epithelial cells become squamous and the myoepithelial cell layer is lost.[3] Occasionally, the opening of the duct into the epidermis is surrounded by clear cells, with features of Toker cells.[3] A deeper coiled or a long straight duct gives rise to several sac-like invaginations forming glands, which typically extend deeper than the apocrine or eccrine glands. The anogenital mammary-like glands are lined by simple columnar epithelium surrounded by a layer of myoepithelial cells. Glands are either simple and round or more complex and composed of lobular structures.[3] A loose or fibrotic stroma surrounds the glandular structures. The immunohistochemical profile of the glandular structures in anogenital glands is very similar to that seen in breast glands. Interestingly, however, the cytokeratin profile of the secretory ducts in anogenital glands is very similar to that seen in eccrine and apocrine glands with the additional finding of expression of CK8 and CK18 in the former.[4] It is thought that tumors arising in the genital skin derive from or show differentiation toward the anogenital glands and these lesions are very similar to tumors occurring in the breast.[5,6] This hypothesis is given further support by a few studies showing similar molecular abnormalities between breast tumors and their genital counterparts.[7,8]

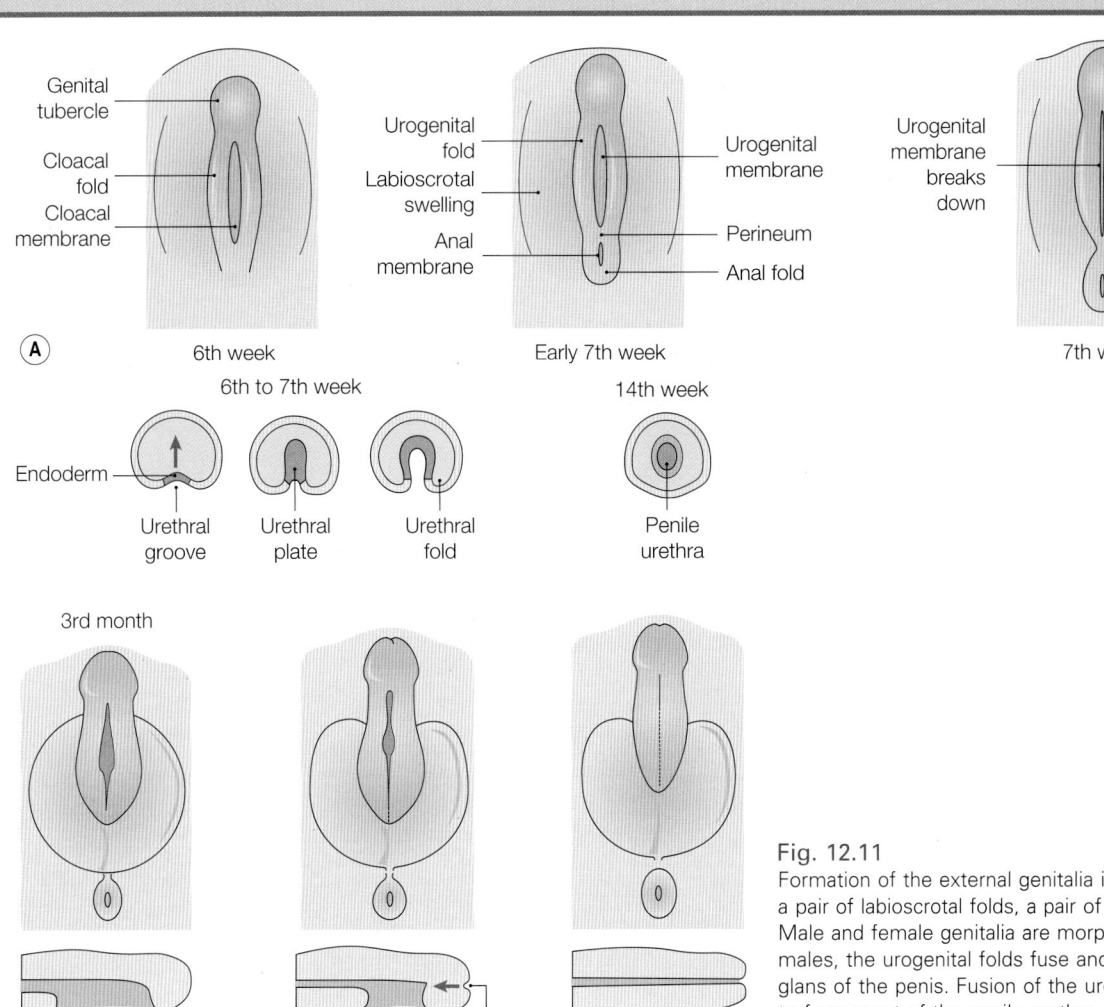

Fig. 12.11
Formation of the external genitalia in males and females. (**A**) The external genitalia form a pair of labioscrotal folds, a pair of urogenital folds and an anterior genital tubercle. Male and female genitalia are morphologically indistinguishable at this stage. (**B**) In males, the urogenital folds fuse and the genital tubercle elongates to form the shaft and glans of the penis. Fusion of the urogenital folds encloses the definite urogenital sinus to form most of the penile urethra. A small region of the distal urethra is formed by the invagination of ectoderms covering the glans. The labioscrotal folds give rise to the scrotum. From Bunker C. Male Genital Skin Disease. Saunders Ltd./Elsevier 2004.

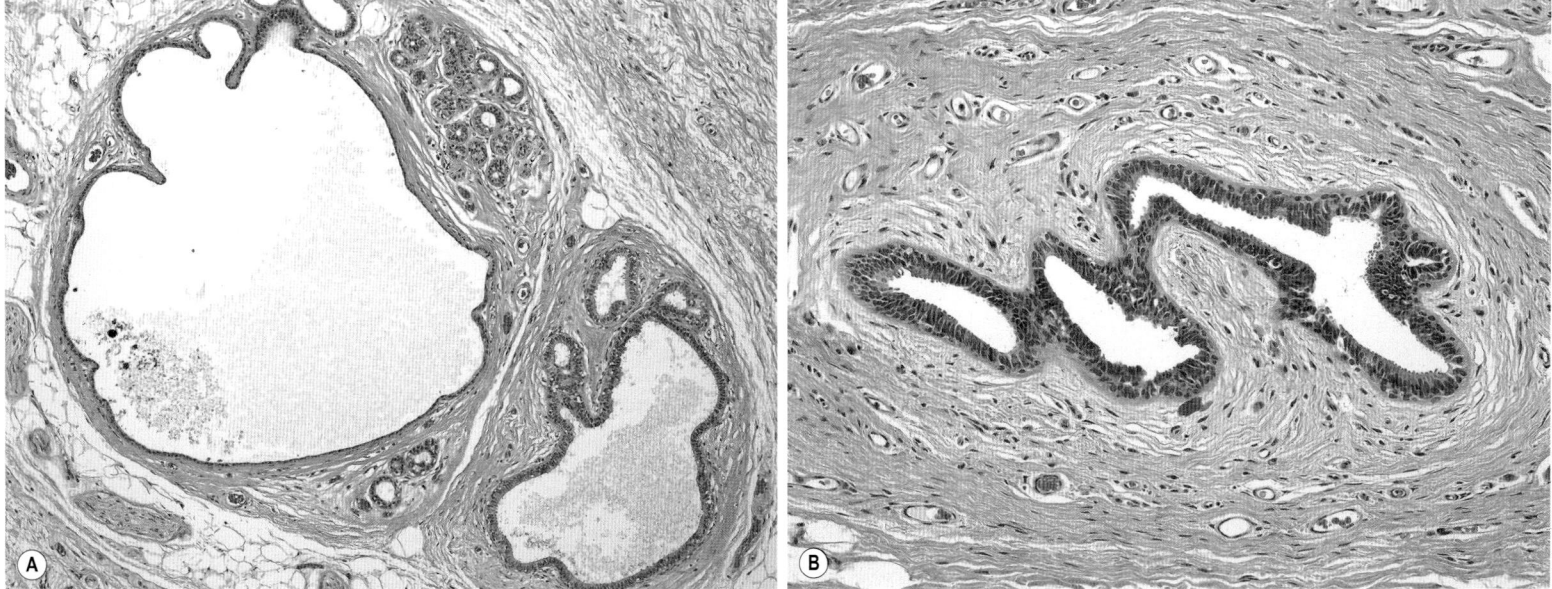

Fig. 12.12
Anogenital mammary-like glands. (**A**) Medium-power view showing glands with focal cystic dilatation; (**B**) high-power view showing a double layered cell wall. Focally, there is a suggestion of apocrine differentiation. By courtesy of D. Kazakov, Charles University Medical Faculty Hospital, Pilsen, Czech Republic.

Normal variants

Pigmentation

The most common variation is constitutive pigmentation due to race. There is often hyperpigmentation of the labia minora in pregnancy. Postinflammatory hyperpigmentation is also common. Linear hyperpigmentation of the ventral penile shaft, along the median raphe, is often seen.

Circumcision

The most common variation is the presence or absence of the foreskin. Circumcision is the oldest elective operation, with evidence of its practice in Ancient Egypt between 2400 and 3000 BC.[1] The operation has been performed for religious, cultural, or medical reasons throughout history.[2] It has been estimated that globally 25% of men have been circumcised.[3] The prevalence of circumcision in any population reflects racial, religious, cultural, and medical differences. The risks and benefits of neonatal circumcision have been the focus of much debate.[4–6] Importantly, circumcision protects men from cancer of the penis, urinary tract, and sexually transmitted infections including human immunodeficiency virus (HIV) and genital dermatoses.[7] However, the incidence of penile cancer is low in Japan and Denmark where circumcision is rare,[8] and therefore other factors are important in its pathogenesis.

Circumcision is indispensible in the management of diseases of the penis and foreskin, including dermatological conditions, and is being investigated for the control of HIV infection. Although the long-held consensus is that there is little evidence of significant adverse effects on health, including psychosexual function, circumcision does have side effects and complications including bleeding, postoperative and other infections, adhesions, fistulae, and keloid.[5]

Acrochordons

Clinical features

Skin tags (acrochordons) are common in the groins, especially in the obese. They may catch on clothing, bleed, and get infected. Fibrosed hemorrhoids can result in perianal skin tags, but larger, fleshier, more edematous skin tags should arouse the suspicion of Crohn disease: they can predate gastrointestinal disease by several years.[1] These lesions are particularly relevant in young patients with diarrhea, abdominal pain, and/or growth retardation.[1]

Histologic features

The histology of a skin tag at this site is identical to that of those occurring elsewhere. The presence of granulomata in anal skin tags is often a clue to the diagnosis of Crohn disease.[2]

Pearly penile papules

Clinical features

Pearly/pink penile papules[1] may be found in 15–50% of men.[2–5] They manifest as flesh-colored, smooth, rounded papules (1–3 mm) occurring predominantly around the coronal margin of the glans, and rarely on the glans. Often, there are rows or rings of papules (*Fig. 12.13*). Ectopic lesions, for example, on the penile shaft, have been reported,[6] including in children.[7] They are frequently mistaken for warts and Tyson or ectopic sebaceous glands. The lesion is analogous to other acral angiofibromas such as adenoma sebaceum, subungual and periungual fibromas, fibrous papule of the nose, acquired acral angiofibroma, and oral fibroma. These lesions may regress with circumcision and old age.[8]

Histologic features

The histology is that of angiofibroma.[9] Human papillomavirus (HPV) DNA is absent.[10,11]

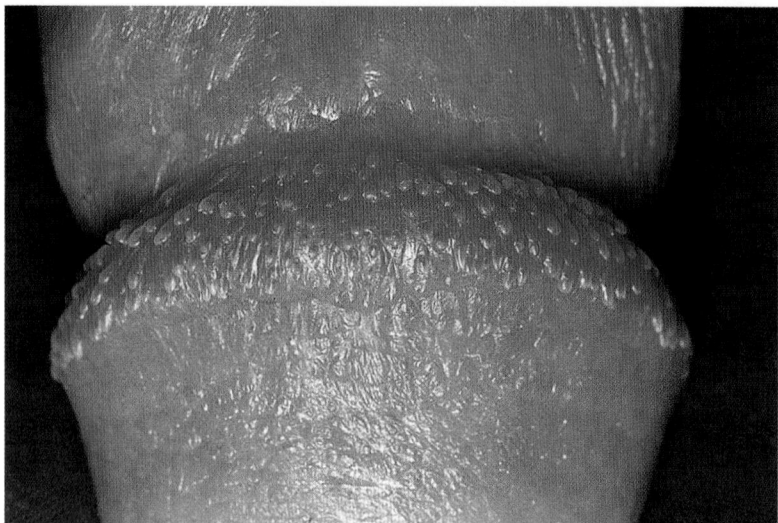

Fig. 12.13
Pearly penile papules. Glans penis, coronal rim. From Bunker C. Male Genital Skin Disease. Saunders Ltd./Elsevier 2004.

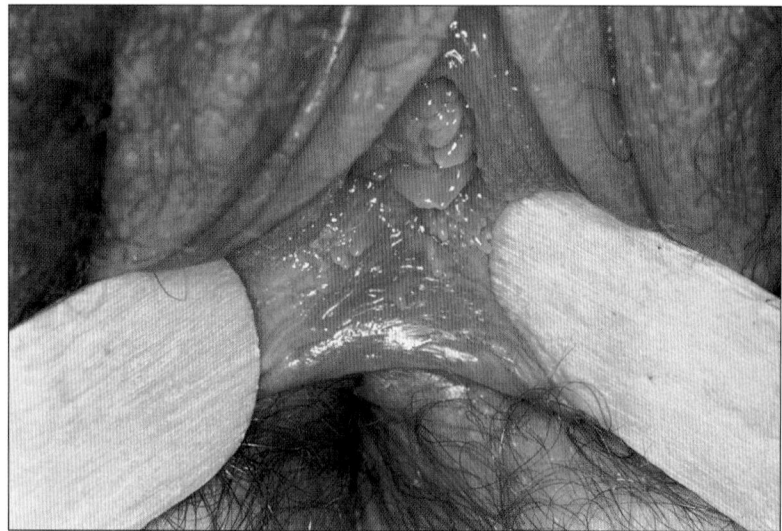

Fig. 12.14
Vestibular papillomatosis: numerous pale papillomata are present in the vestibule and on the labia minora. These are a normal finding and are particularly common in pregnancy. By courtesy of the Institute of Dermatology, London, UK.

Vestibular papillomatosis

Clinical features

Vestibular papillomatosis is not due to HPV infection and is a common finding of no significance.[1,2] It is asymptomatic and is the female equivalent of penile pearly papules. Individual lesions are dome shaped or filiform and arise on a solitary base. They are found on the inner aspect of the labia minora and vestibule[3] (*Fig. 12.14*).

Histologic features

There is a normal or thickened epidermis overlying a central fibrovascular core.

Sebaceous gland hyperplasia

Clinical features

The sebaceous glands of the inner labia majora, the labia minora, and clitoral prepuce do not usually have an associated hair follicle. The glands open

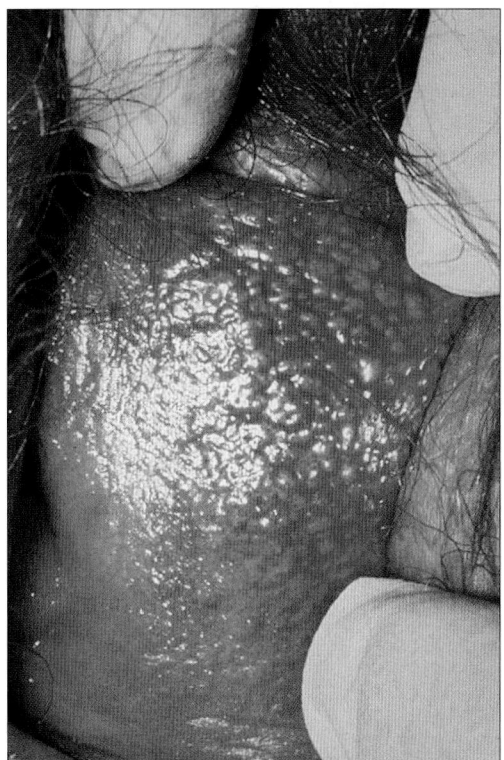

Fig. 12.15
Fordyce spots: hyperplastic sebaceous glands presenting as conspicuous yellow papules. Similar lesions may be seen on the inner lip and oral mucosa. By courtesy of the Institute of Dermatology, London, UK.

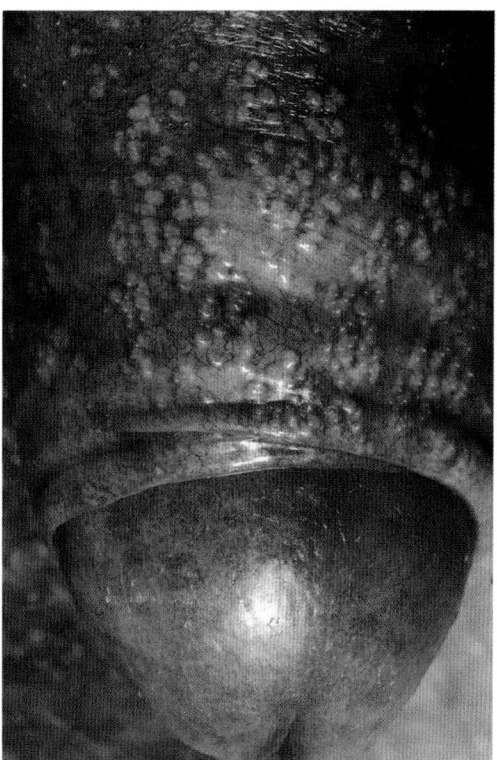

Fig. 12.16
Sebaceous hyperplasia (Fordyce condition). Penis, prepuce. From Bunker C. Male Genital Skin Disease. Saunders Ltd./Elsevier 2004.

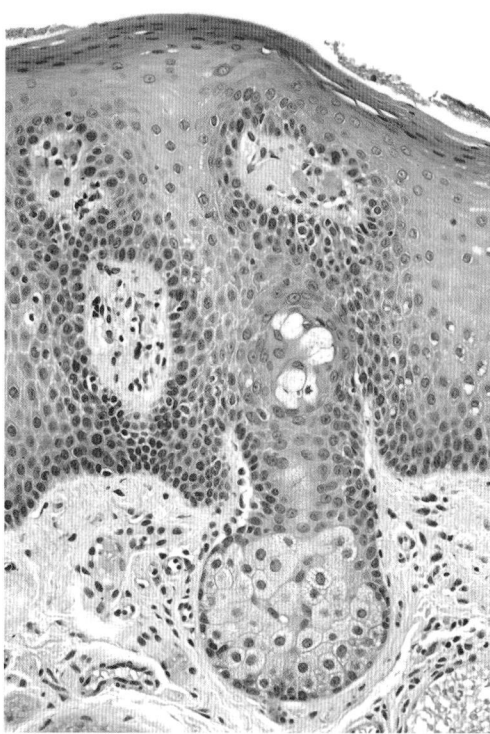

Fig. 12.17
Fordyce spot: this small sebaceous gland can be seen communicating directly with the epidermis.

directly onto the surface and may be very prominent and numerous at these sites. The yellow uniform papules (Fordyce spots) are often seen best if the skin is stretched (*Fig. 12.15*). Sebaceous gland hyperplasia may sometime be associated with pruritus and pain if they enlarge and the contents rupture into the dermis.

In the male, sebaceous gland prominence, Tyson glands, sebaceous hyperplasia, and ectopic sebaceous glands (Fordyce condition) are all virtually synonymous and are common, normal variants of the skin of the scrotal sac and penile shaft (very rarely the glans) but may cause concern to patients, even amounting to dysmorphophobia (*Fig. 12.16*).[1,2]

Histologic features

One or more enlarged sebaceous glands, each composed of numerous lobules, surround a central duct that opens directly into the epidermis (*Fig. 12.17*).

Inflammatory dermatoses

Intertrigo and balanoposthitis

Clinical features

These are non-specific terms.[1] Intertrigo is the name given to any dermatosis occurring in skin folds: any scale is usually rapidly removed by frictional abrasion, and a degree of epithelial loss may result in erosion that renders the site especially susceptible to secondary infection, e.g., with *Candida* (see below).

Balanitis denotes inflammation of the glans penis, while posthitis is inflammation of the prepuce. Balanoposthitis means inflammation of the glans and prepuce and is regarded as a special form of intertrigo. By definition, therefore, balanoposthitis cannot occur in the circumcised male, but balanitis might.

Pathogenesis and histologic features

Generally, dermatologists feel that balanitis, posthitis, and balanoposthitis are probably more common due to inflammatory and precancerous dermatoses, whereas genitourinary physicians teach that most cases are due to infection, usually with *Candida*.[1] However, *Candida* is a ready opportunist so its presence may not always indicate primary infection as the cause of the genital inflammation. Bacteria have increasingly been implicated in the etiology of the disease, particularly *Staphylococcus aureus*.[2] In cases in which *Streptococcus pyogenes* is isolated, it has been suggested that the disease may be sexually transmitted by penile–oral intercourse.[3] Diabetes may be an important predisposing factor to *Candida* and other infective causes or complications of balanoposthitis.[1]

The histologic features are non-specific.

Non-specific balanoposthitis

Clinical experience and histologic evidence indicate that non-specific balanoposthitis is a real entity.[1,2] However, in practice it is a diagnosis of exclusion, because sexually transmitted diseases, eczematous dermatoses, psoriasis, Zoon balanitis (ZB), lichen planus (LP), LS, mucous membrane pemphigoid, and penile carcinoma in situ must be excluded. Non-specific balanoposthitis is a manifestation of a dysfunctional foreskin. Patients generally complain of pain during intercourse and may have variable signs, including eczematous, lichenoid, and Zoonoid inflammation, and even scarring. *Candida* and other organisms can be identified, but they probably represent opportunistic infection. Diabetes should be excluded. In severe cases, medical treatments fail and the only cure is by circumcision. A prior clinical diagnosis may be reversed at this stage by foreskin histology showing LS, LP, or carcinoma in situ. However, experience shows that even where the most thorough histologic examination of the excised prepuce is undertaken, nothing more than non-specific chronic inflammation is found.

Eczema

Clinical features

Seborrheic dermatitis is the most common form of eczema affecting ano-genital skin, followed by irritant contact eczema. Eczema, particularly seborrheic dermatitis, is more common than many other inflammatory dermatoses in uncircumcised males.[1] Allergic contact eczema is rare at genital sites and occurs more typically in a perianal distribution. Involvement of genital skin with atopic eczema is rare.

In infants, eczematous reactions are often seen in the napkin area. Most of these represent a primary irritant dermatitis. Seborrheic dermatitis and a psoriasiform napkin rash can also occur. Some, but not all, patients with the latter condition develop psoriasis later in life.[2]

Histologic features

The histologic features are identical to those seen in eczema affecting other areas of the skin. Psoriasiform napkin rashes show histologic features that overlap with psoriasis.

Seborrheic dermatitis

Clinical features

Seborrheic dermatitis is a common pattern of eczematous disease associated with an abnormal hypersensitivity to the normal commensal cutaneous yeast, *Pityrosporum ovale*. It is discussed in detail elsewhere (Chapter 6). In addition to the classical sites, e.g., scalp (pityriasis capitis, dandruff), ears, glabella and brows, nasolabial folds, axillae, chest and back, the groin, and penis can be involved. Indeed, this may be the sole site, leading to the patient presenting, with pruritus and or bala-noposthitis, to a dermatologist. Some patients may also have a tendency to psoriasis ('sebopsoriasis', 'seboriasis'). On the scalp, on the face, in the flexures, and at anogenital sites, seborrheic dermatitis and psoriasis may be indistinguishable. Seborrheic dermatitis is very common in HIV infection. Diagnosis is achieved on clinical grounds, and it is not usually necessary to do a biopsy. *Pityrosporum* spp. will be seen in large numbers.

In females, seborrheic dermatitis may present as non-specific erythema over the outer labia majora, and there may be some scaling and keratin debris seen in the interlabial sulci (*Fig. 12.18*).

Histology is identical to that of seborrheic dermatitis occurring elsewhere. However, spongiosis can be more prominent.

Infantile gluteal granuloma

Clinical features

Infantile gluteal granuloma (papuloerosive dermatitis of Jacquet and Seves-tre) is a rare condition that has been described mainly in the newborn and infants in the napkin area. It frequently develops in a background of an irritant napkin rash.[1–4] A similar condition has been described in incontinent elderly women with lesions developing on the labia majora (*Fig. 12.19*).[5–8] Oval or round papulonodular lesions present on the convex areas of the perineum, which are in direct contact with the napkin or incontinence pad. They tend to regress spontaneously over a few weeks and occasionally leave scars.

Pathogenesis and histologic features

The etiology of the process is unclear, but occlusion, *Candida* infection, and the application of fluorinated corticosteroids have been implicated. The latter, however, does not seem to be of importance in the incontinent elderly patient.

The histology is fairly non-specific and includes superficial ulceration, focal necrosis, and a prominent mixed inflammatory cell infiltrate with granulomata and numerous lymphocytes and plasma cells. Hemorrhage and hemosiderin deposition can sometimes be present.

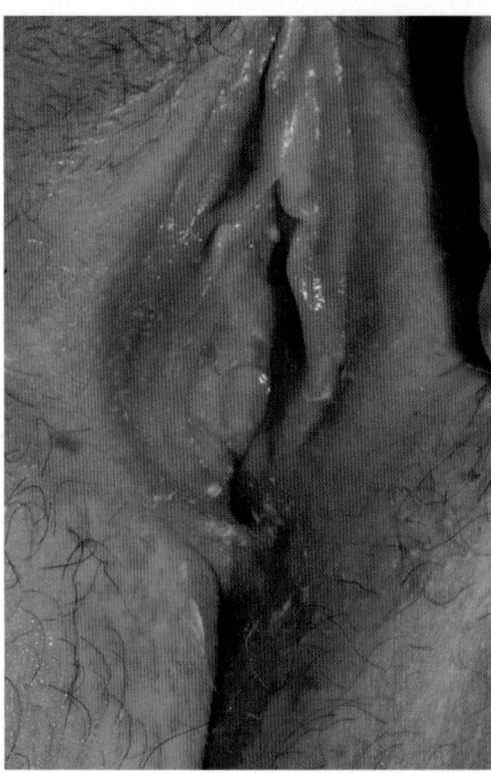

Fig. 12.18
Seborrheic eczema of the vulva – keratin debris in the interlabial sulci. This can mimic candidiasis.

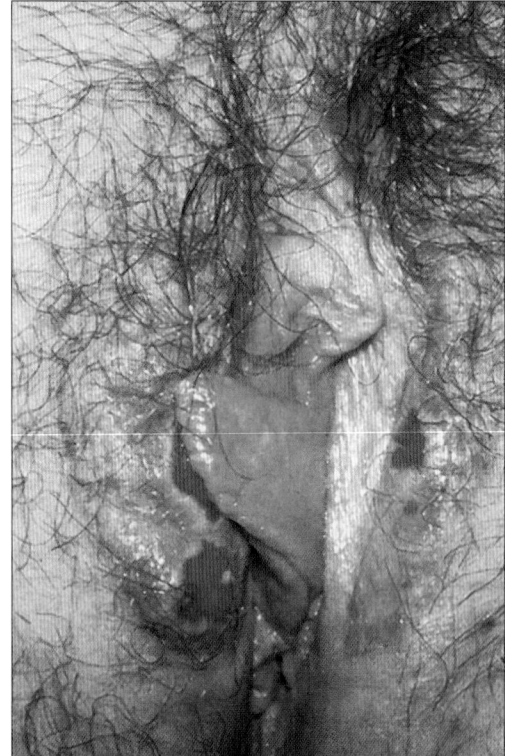

Fig. 12.19
Papuloerosive dermatitis: there are multiple ulcerated papules and nodules predominantly affecting the labia majora. By courtesy of the Institute of Dermatology, London, UK.

Differential diagnosis

Crohn disease and infective granulomatous conditions may need to be excluded but the clinical features of these are usually obvious.

Lichen simplex chronicus

Clinical features

The clinical features of lichen simplex chronicus presenting on genital and anal skin are identical to those seen at other sites of the body. The mons

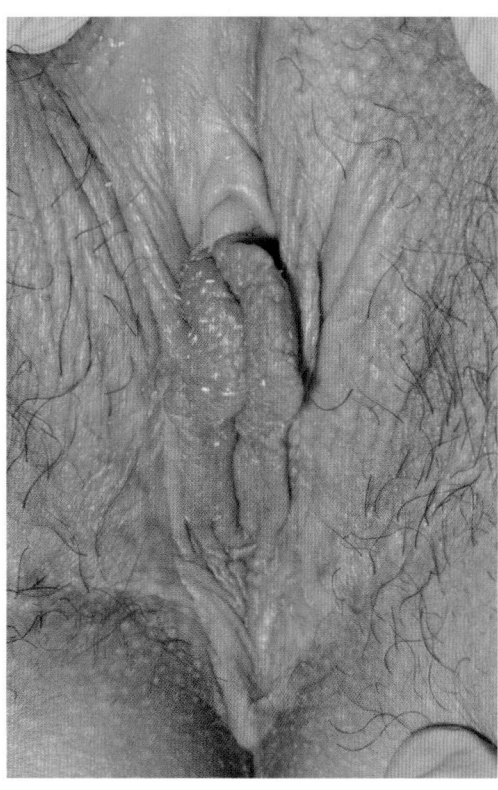

Fig. 12.20
Lichen simplex of
the vulva – marked
lichenification of the labia
majora.

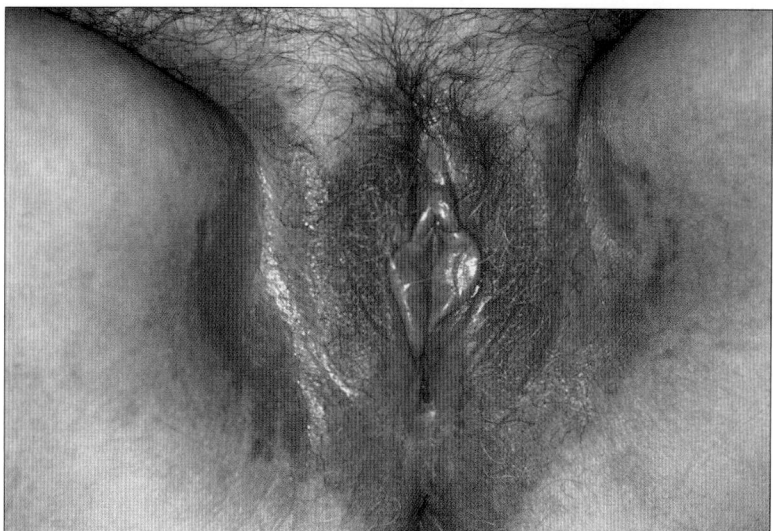

Fig. 12.22
Psoriasis: note the symmetrical, intensely erythematous eruption involving the
groins, vulva and perineum. Scaling is typically absent in flexural disease. The
sharply demarcated border is characteristic. By courtesy of the Institute of
Dermatology, London, UK.

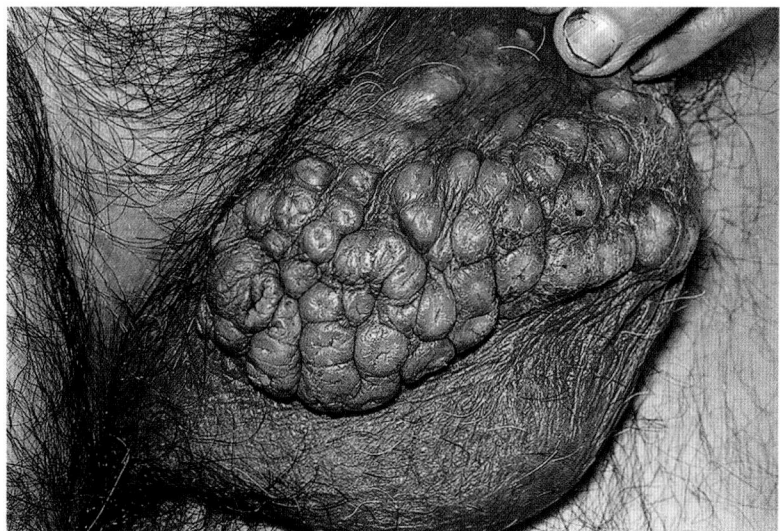

Fig. 12.21
Lichen simplex chronicus. Scrotum. Giant 'pineapple' lesion. From Bunker C. Male
Genital Skin Disease. Saunders Ltd./Elsevier 2004.

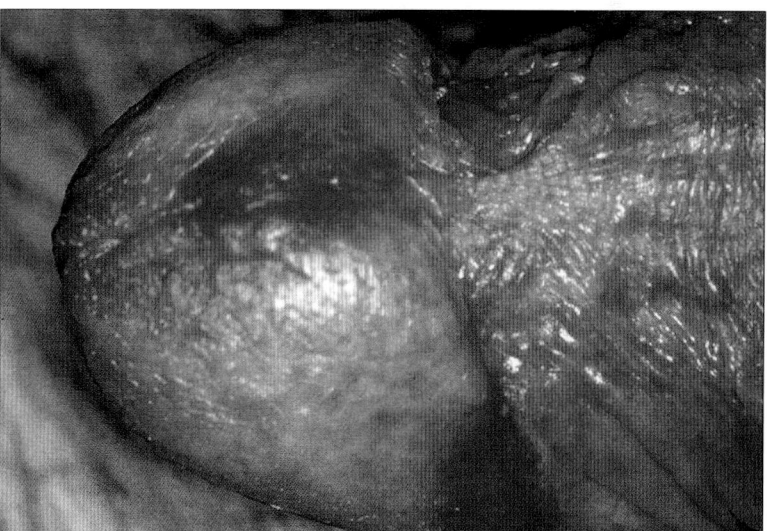

Fig. 12.23
Psoriasis: there are erythematous plaques on the glans penis. By courtesy of the
Institute of Dermatology, London, UK.

pubis or labia majora (*Fig. 12.20*), scrotum and perianal skin are the most
common sites affected. Giant forms (of Pautrier) occur, e.g., on the scrotum,
giving a pineapple appearance (*Fig. 12.21*).

Histologic features

The histologic features are discussed in detail elsewhere, but lichenification
is characterized by hyperkeratosis, hypergranulosis, uniform acanthosis,
fibrosis of the papillary dermis, and an unremarkable low-grade perivascular
infiltrate of mononuclear leukocytes in the superficial dermis. The papillary
dermal fibrosis is streaky and perpendicular to the epidermis. Eosinophils
are often present, in some cases reflecting an element of irritant contact dermatitis. At mucosal sites hyper- and orthokeratosis creates a cornified layer,
resulting in the clinical appearances of white thickened plaques.

Psoriasis

Clinical features

Flexural psoriasis is the most common pattern seen in the anogenital region,
with extension into the genitocrural folds and natal cleft (*Figs 12.22–12.25*).
There are often difficulties clinically in distinguishing between psoriasis and
seborrheic dermatitis. Genital and flexural disease may reflect koebnerization and is relatively common.[1] In the circumcised male, the signs on the
glans and distal penile shaft are similar to those of psoriasis at extragenital
sites, whereas the appearances in the uncircumcised male are of balanoposthitis similar to flexural psoriasis.[2] In females, well-demarcated plaques
generally affect the labia majora with extension on to the mons pubis and
perianal skin. Fissuring is common.[3]

Histologic features

Histology is often unhelpful, as the changes can be non-specific. The typical
features of psoriasis are rarely evident, and the presence of secondary spongiosis is common and may be misleading.

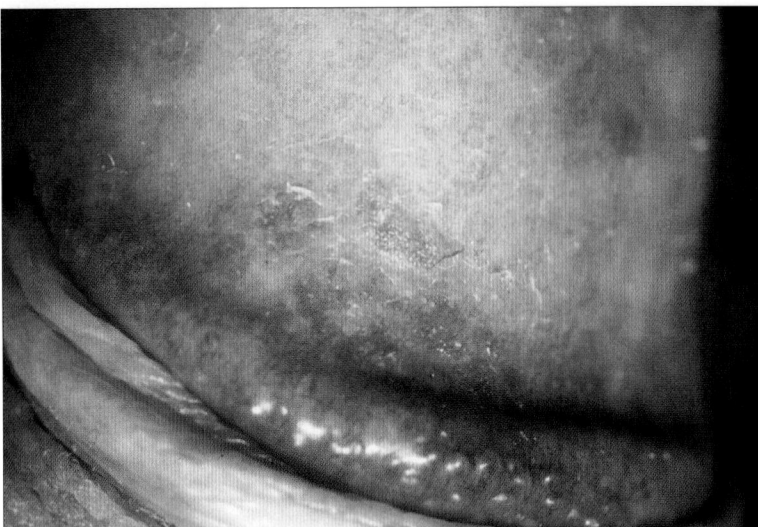

Fig. 12.24
Psoriasis: in this example a slight scale is apparent. By courtesy of the Institute of Dermatology, London, UK.

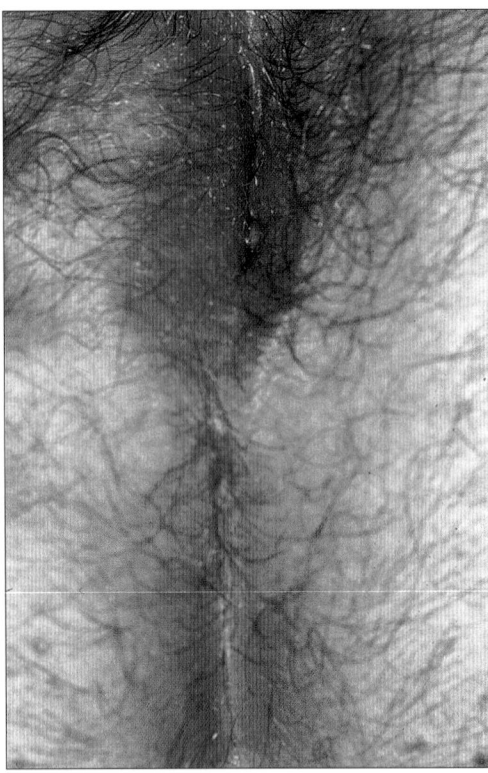

Fig. 12.25
Psoriasis: note the erythematous and slightly scaly plaque affecting the perineum. By courtesy of the Institute of Dermatology, London, UK.

Reactive arthritis

Clinical features

Reactive arthritis (previously known as Reiter syndrome) is part of the same continuum as psoriasis in genetically predisposed individuals.[1] Reactive arthritis is defined by the triad of arthritis, urethritis, and conjunctivitis. It is precipitated by non-specific urethritis, bacillary or amebic dysentery, and associated with HIV infection and the immunogenotype human leukocyte antigen (HLA) B27.[2–6] The classical triad may occur together or develop in sequence, and a range of other symptoms may also be present. It has a worldwide distribution. Reactive arthritis most commonly affects men 20–30 years of age; the male/female sex ratio is approximately 10:1.[1] The syndrome is characterized by a relapsing course.[4]

The condition may follow an enteric or a urogenital infection.[7,8] Shigella dysentery was the first associated enteric infection to be recognized and the causative organisms were either *Shigella flexneri* or *Shigella dysenteriae*.[9]

Salmonella, *Yersinia*, and *Campylobacter* have also been reported preceding reactive arthritis.[10–14]

Sexually transmitted reactive arthritis may occur with a nongonococcal or 'non-specific' urethritis.[7] *Chlamydia trachomatis* is isolated from the genitourinary tract in 40–60% of male cases; isolation is variable, however, and an indirect immunofluorescence test detects chlamydial infection in 90% of patients.[15,16] *Mycoplasma* infection and *Streptococcus viridans* have also been implicated.[17–19] The condition has also been linked to the acquired immunodeficiency syndrome (AIDS).[20–22] Rare associations include *Cyclospora*, *Cryptosporidium*, intravesical bacillus Calmette–Guérin (BCG) immunotherapy, *Gardnerella vaginalis*, hepatitis B immunization, and systemic interferon-alpha (IFN-α) treatment.[23–28]

Reactive arthritis is more likely to occur in predisposed individuals. HLA-B27, which is thought to occur in up to 90% of patients, increases the risk of developing reactive arthritis by 25 times; the disease is also more severe in HLA-B27-positive individuals.[4,29] HLA-B27 in patients with reactive arthritis correlates with ankylosing spondylitis.[4] Reactive arthritis develops in 20% of HLA-B27-positive individuals after a specific infective episode.[30] An association with HLA-B51 has been reported.[31] Rarely, familial instances have been documented.[30] Therefore, it appears that the disease is triggered in genetically predisposed individuals by an unknown mechanism precipitated by infection.

The genitourinary tract is virtually always involved in the form of urethritis, prostatitis, seminal vesiculitis, and hemorrhagic cystitis. Urethral strictures also sometimes occur and females may develop cervicitis.

Bilateral mucopurulent conjunctivitis is the usual form of eye involvement occurring in up to 35% of patients, but occasionally iritis, iridocyclitis, keratitis, or blindness occurs.[32]

Weight-bearing joints and the larger ones (knees, ankles, feet, and wrists) are involved by the arthritis, often together with sacroiliitis. Radiological changes include osteoporosis, erosions and loss of joint space, with multiple joints usually affected.[4,30] Periostitis often affects the metatarsals, the phalanges of the feet, and the tarsal bones; occasionally, ankylosis develops in the small bones of the hands and feet. Ankylosing spondylitis, which is an important manifestation, correlates with a high erythrocyte sedimentation rate (ESR).[30]

In the initial stages of the arthritis the clinical picture resembles that of an acute joint infection, settling to subacute involvement. Although the arthritis in reactive arthritis usually recovers completely, chronic manifestations can sometimes occur; it is important to remember that arthritis may be the only symptom in recurrent episodes.

Skin lesions in reactive arthritis may be similar to those of psoriasis. Cutaneous manifestations include hyperkeratotic cobblestone lesions on the palms and soles and occasionally affecting the trunk and extremities (*Fig. 12.26*). The lesions initially present as erythematous macules; over the course of several days these become hyperkeratotic waxy papules, with an erythematous halo covered by dry hyperkeratotic material. The papules are numerous and eventually coalesce to form thickened horny plaques. Pustular lesions of the palms and soles may also be evident (keratoderma blenorrhagicum) (*Fig. 12.27*).

Circinate balanitis, presenting as a moist superficial erosion, 2–4 mm across, may affect the glans penis and meatus (*Figs 12.28–12.30*). Superficial ulceration of the oral mucosa may also occur, together with reddening and a granular appearance of the surrounding mucous membrane.[4,5]

Stomatitis and nail dystrophy (indistinguishable from that of psoriasis) may be additional features.[4] Weight loss is common.[20] Aortic incompetence is an important late complication, and immunoglobulin A (IgA) nephropathy has been described in a number of patients.[4,33]

Reactive arthritis is rarely reported in females. Vulvitis has been described in a small number of case reports,[34–38] and in one case cervical lesions, presenting as white papules, were seen.[37] The vulval lesions are erythematous and may be ulcerative, eroded, or scaly, and often resemble mucocutaneous candidiasis.

Reactive arthritis may resolve spontaneously, but more often it is characterized by chronicity and recurrences.[4] Rarely, it may prove fatal.[4] Causes of death include aortic incompetence, atrioventricular block, terminal cachexia, systemic amyloidosis, and iatrogenic effects.[39]

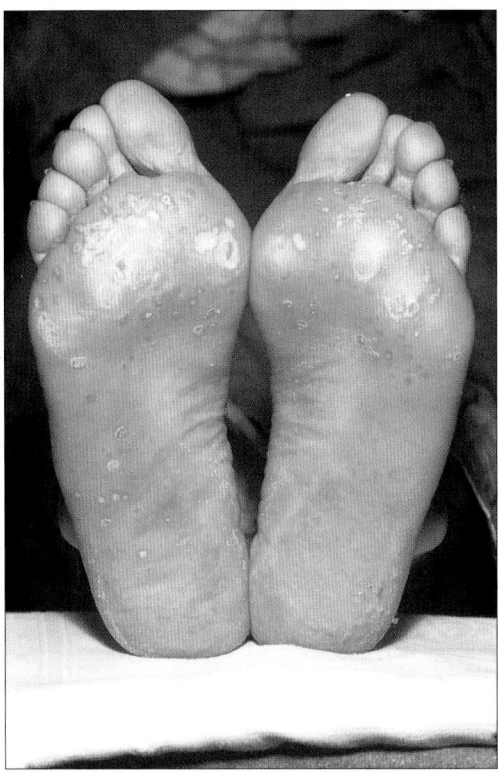

Fig. 12.26
Reactive arthritis: there are bilateral keratotic papules and plaques affecting the soles of the feet. By courtesy of R.A. Marsden, MD, St George's Hospital, London, UK.

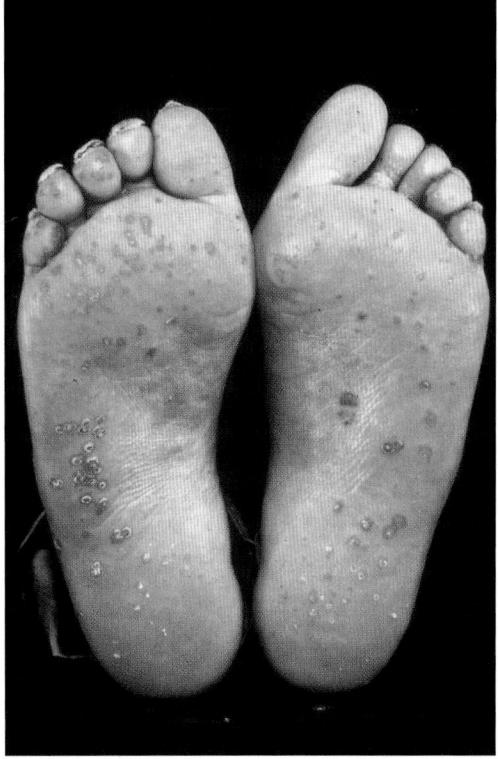

Fig. 12.27
Reactive arthritis: in addition to keratotic papules there are pustular lesions, many of which have ruptured – keratoderma blenorrhagicum. By courtesy of the Institute of Dermatology, London, UK.

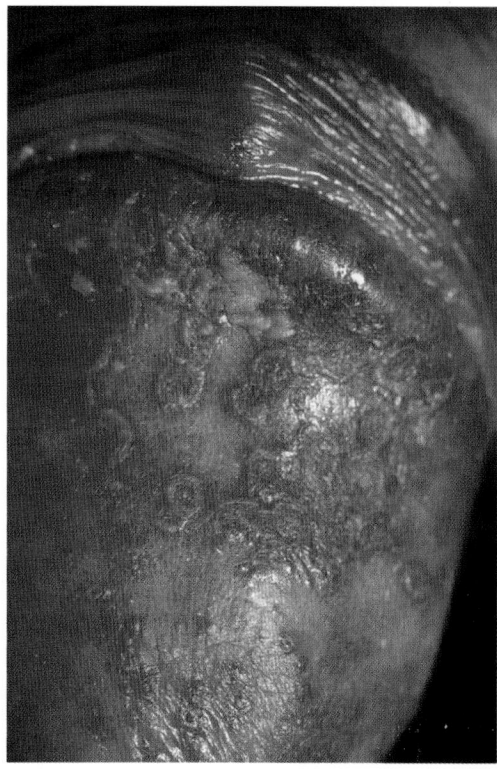

Fig. 12.28
Circinate balanitis. Glans penis. Psoriasiform lesions. From Bunker C. Male Genital Skin Disease. Saunders Ltd./Elsevier 2004.

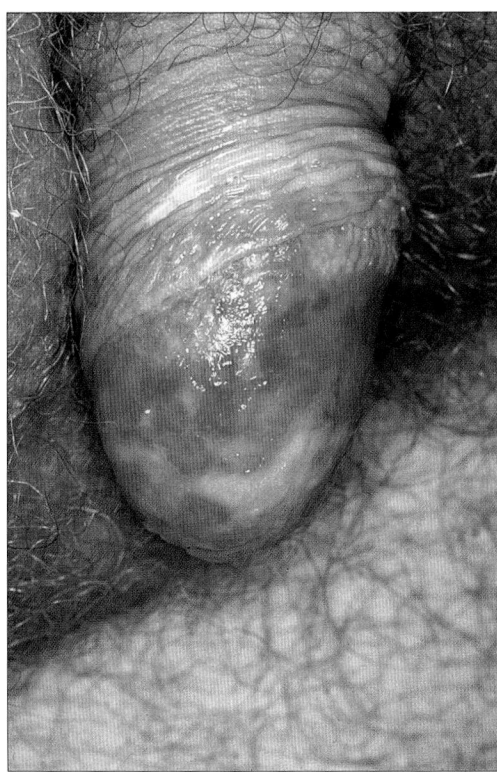

Fig. 12.29
Reactive arthritis: there are multiple erosions on the glans penis. By courtesy of the Institute of Dermatology, London, UK.

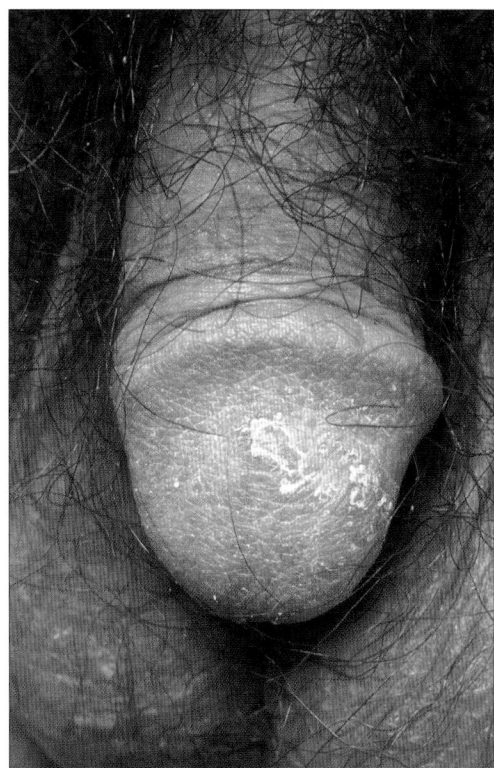

Fig. 12.30
Reactive arthritis: in this patient, there are scaly lesions on the glans penis. By courtesy of the Institute of Dermatology, London, UK.

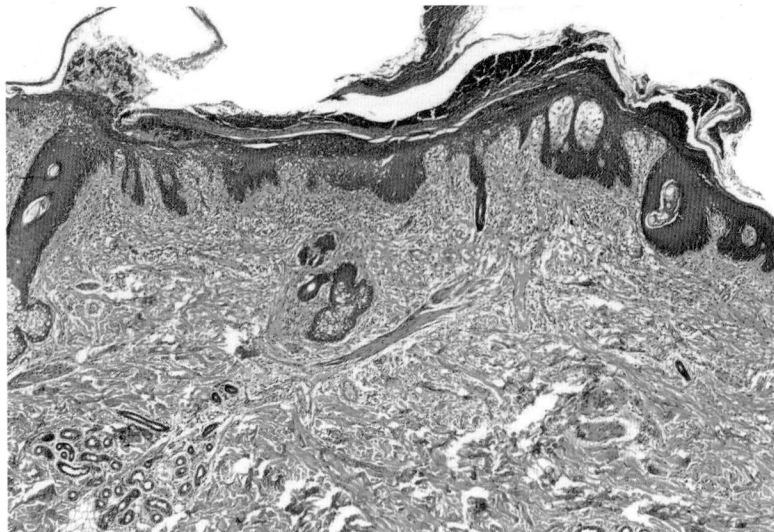

Fig. 12.31
Reactive arthritis: there is parakeratosis overlying a macropustule. The squamous epithelium shows psoriasiform hyperplasia. These features are indistinguishable from pustular psoriasis.

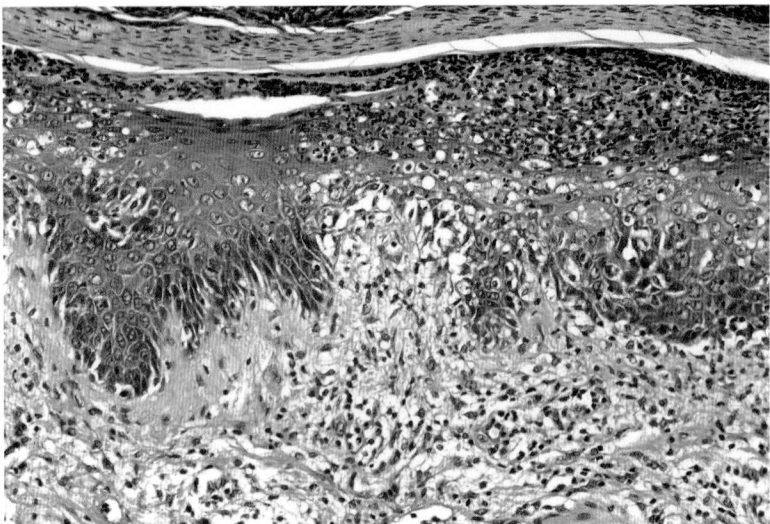

Fig. 12.32
Reactive arthritis: high-power view showing parakeratosis and a pustule.

Histologic features

Essentially, just as the skin lesions of reactive arthritis have psoriasiform morphology (*Fig. 12.31*), they have the same histopathology and ultrastructure as pustular psoriasis.[40]

The epidermis is acanthotic with elongation and hypertrophy of the epidermal ridges and parakeratosis. The suprapapillary plates are thinned and there is infiltration of the epidermis by neutrophils, associated with vacuolation of superficial keratinocytes, together with the formation of spongiform pustules and microabscesses (*Fig. 12.32*). The inflammation extends into the adjacent underlying dermis, where it is predominantly mononuclear. The histology is essentially identical to that seen in pustular psoriasis.[2] Therefore, close clinicopathological correlation is critical to establish a diagnosis. Occasional biopsies from typical lesions of patients with reactive arthritis may disclose an underlying leukocytoclastic vasculitis.[41]

A small number of patients presenting with skin lesions that histologically showed sterile neutrophilic folliculitis with perifollicular vasculopathy have been documented.[42] The authors suggested that this histologic pattern may be a marker of systemic disease. Associations may include reactive arthritis, inflammatory bowel disease, Behçet disease, hepatitis B infection, scrofuloderma, connective tissue diseases, and hematological dyscrasias.

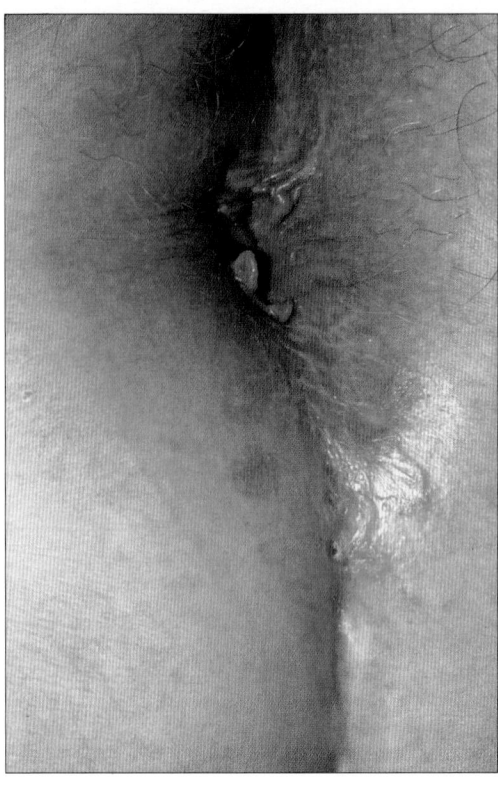

Fig. 12.33
Lichen planus: perineal lesions showing conspicuous striae. By courtesy of the Institute of Dermatology, London, UK.

Patients present with systemic symptoms and variable skin lesions including folliculitis, vasculitis, acneiform eruptions, vesiculopustules, and erythema nodosum-like features.

Early joint lesions are characterized by a neutrophil polymorph inflammatory cell infiltrate with little, if any, synovial changes. Older lesions show features suggestive of rheumatoid arthritis, including lymphoid aggregates, a perivascular chronic inflammatory cell infiltrate, and synovial hyperplasia.[30]

Differential diagnosis

Periodic acid–Schiff (PAS) and/or silver stains should always be performed to exclude a fungal infection which can show similar histologic features.

Lichen planus

Clinical features

Anogenital lesions may be found in up to 40% of patients with generalized disease. In some, however, the disease is restricted to the lower genital tract and/or the perianal region. LP manifests the Koebner phenomenon which may partly explain the orogenital predilection. Genital LP in children is exceptional.[1] Women with oral LP often have genital disease which may be asymptomatic.[2,3]

The lesions are typical, violaceous or white patches, or areas of erythema and erosions. Wickham striae (frequently seen in oral involvement), although sometimes visible, are less often found on anogenital skin (*Fig. 12.33*). The clinical variants of LP affecting the anogenital skin include squamo-papular, erosive, hypertrophic, and hyperpigmented flexural disease (*Figs 12.34–12.41*). Lichen planopilaris has also been described on the vulva.[4]

The erosive form of LP is more common at anogenital sites and can lead to scarring and distortion of the architecture.[5] The vulval vestibule and vagina and cervix may also be involved, and sometimes the vagina and/or the cervix are affected alone.[6,7] There is also an unusual variant of erosive LP in women that involves the oral gingivae, vulval vestibule, and vagina, known as the vulvovaginal-gingival syndrome (*Figs 12.42–12.44*).[8,9] This can lead to severe vulval and vaginal scarring with vaginal adhesions, constriction bands, and, in some cases, complete stenosis.[10] A male equivalent to the vulvovaginal syndrome of Hewitt with chronic erosive gingival and

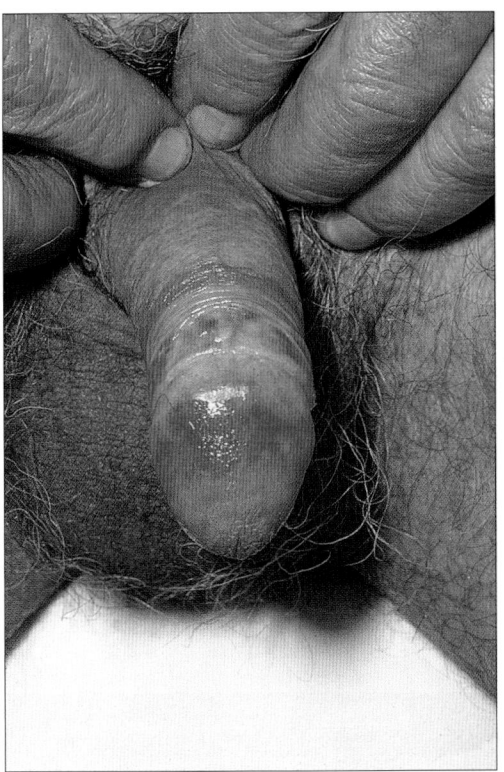

Fig. 12.34
Erosive lichen planus: there is extensive erosion of the glans penis. By courtesy of the Institute of Dermatology, London, UK.

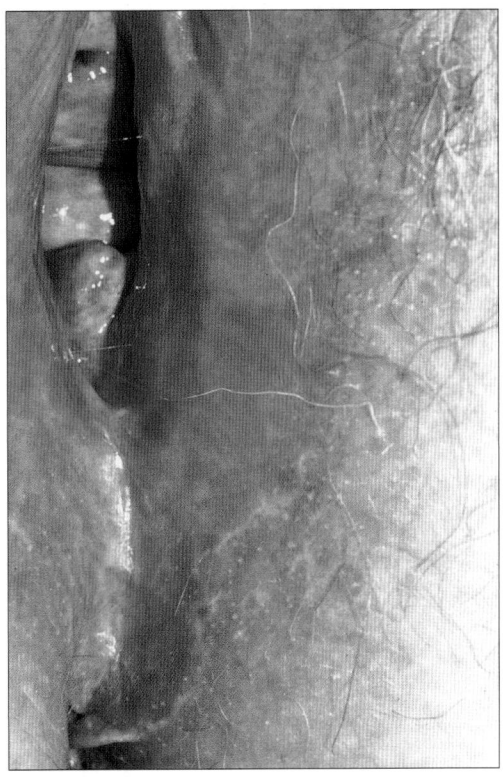

Fig. 12.35
Vulval lichen planus: reticulated lesions of lichen planus extending into the perineum. By courtesy of the Institute of Dermatology, London, UK.

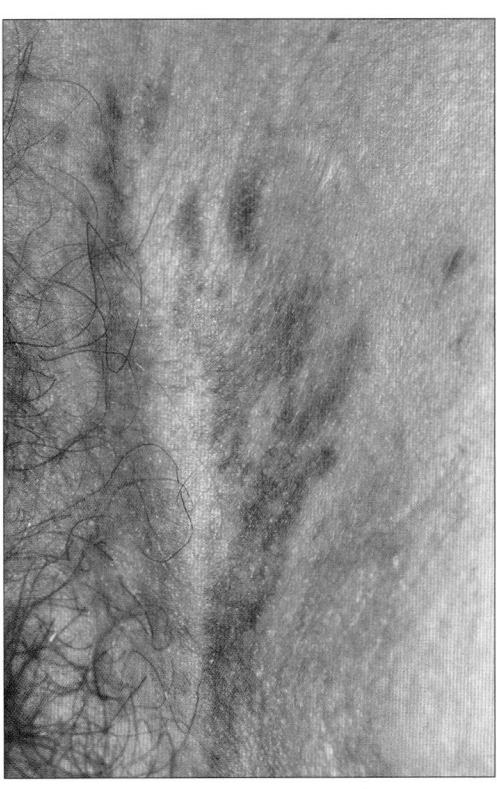

Fig. 12.36
Vulval lichen planus: in this example of resolving disease, there are linear hyperpigmented lesions. By courtesy of the Institute of Dermatology, London, UK.

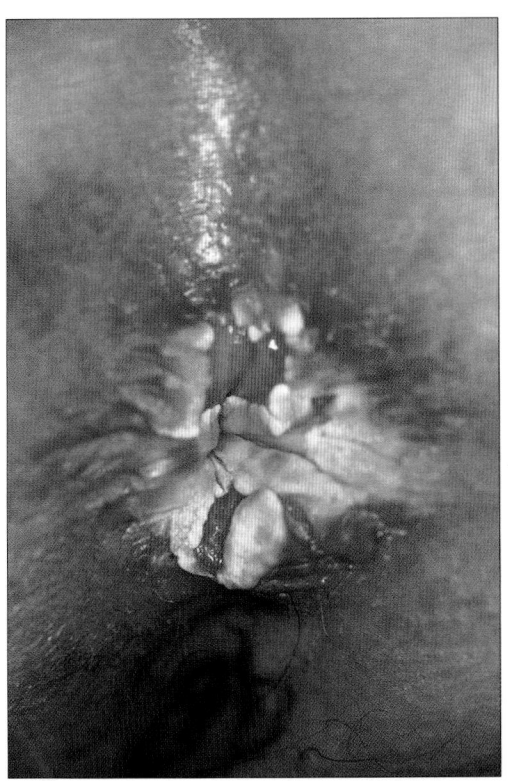

Fig. 12.37
Perineal lichen planus: typical papules with Wickham striae are present. By courtesy of the Institute of Dermatology, London, UK.

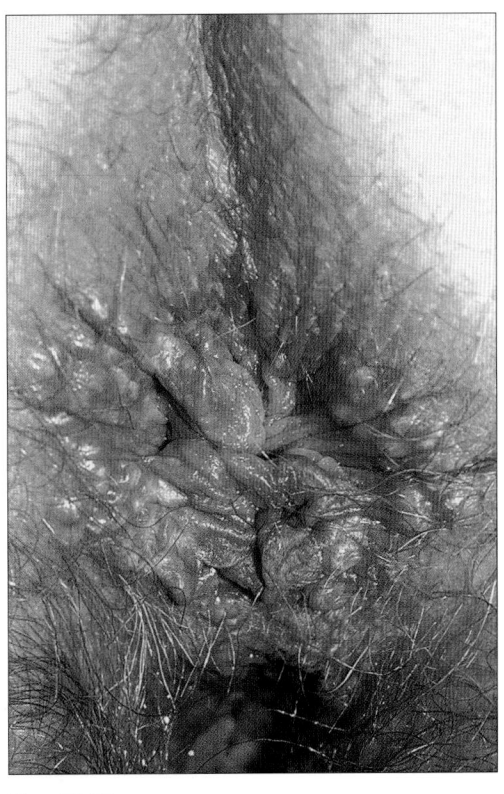

Fig. 12.38
Hypertrophic perianal lichen planus: chronic scratching has resulted in superimposed lichenification. By courtesy of the Institute of Dermatology, London, UK.

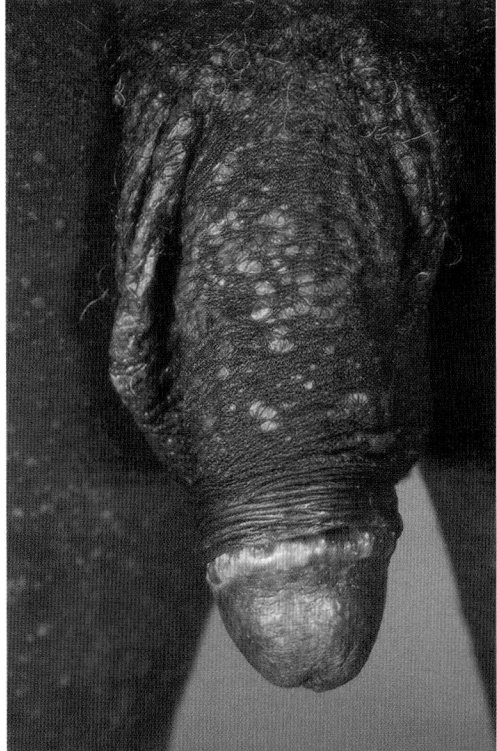

Fig. 12.39
Penile lichen planus: there is involvement of the shaft and glans. From Bunker C. Male Genital Skin Disease. Saunders Ltd./Elsevier 2004.

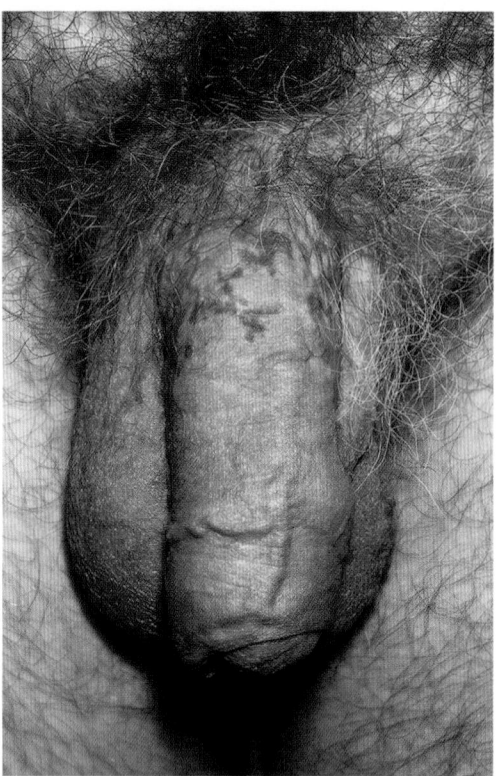

Fig. 12.40
Penile lichen planus: the proximal shaft shows post inflammatory hyperpigmentation. From Bunker C. Male Genital Skin Disease. Saunders Ltd./Elsevier 2004.

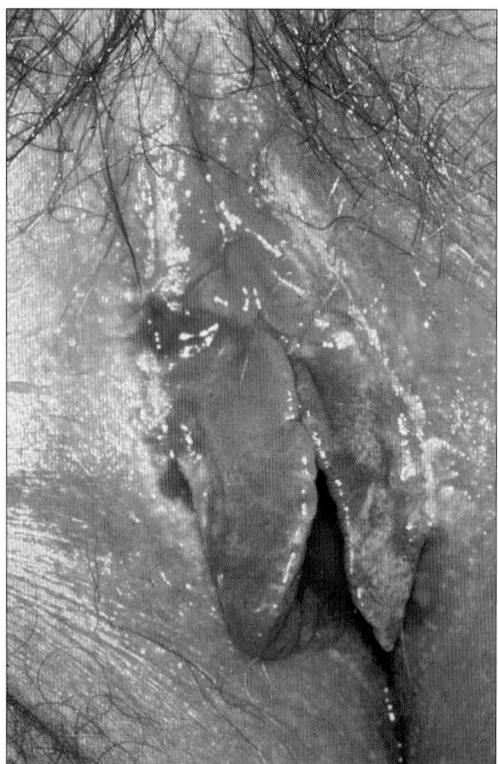

Fig. 12.41
Erosive lichen planus: bilateral erosions are present. By courtesy of the Institute of Dermatology, London, UK.

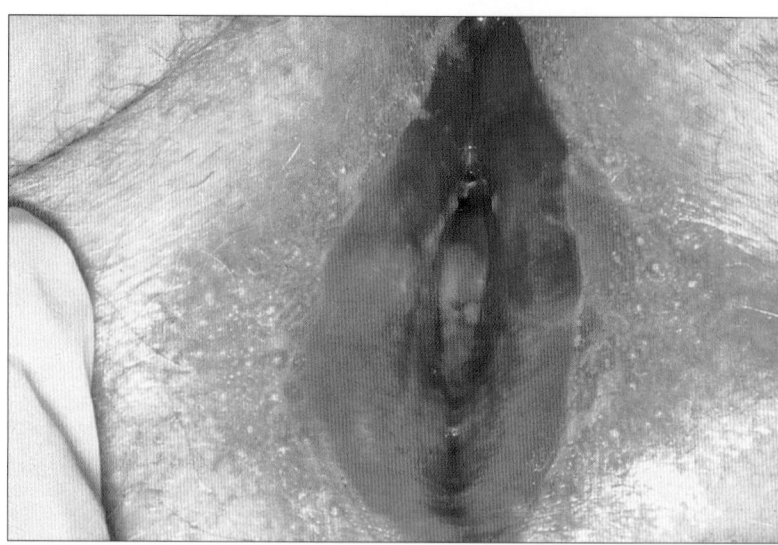

Fig. 12.42
Vulvovaginal-gingival syndrome: there is extensive vestibular erythema and erosion with a surrounding delicate white scale. By courtesy of the Institute of Dermatology, London, UK.

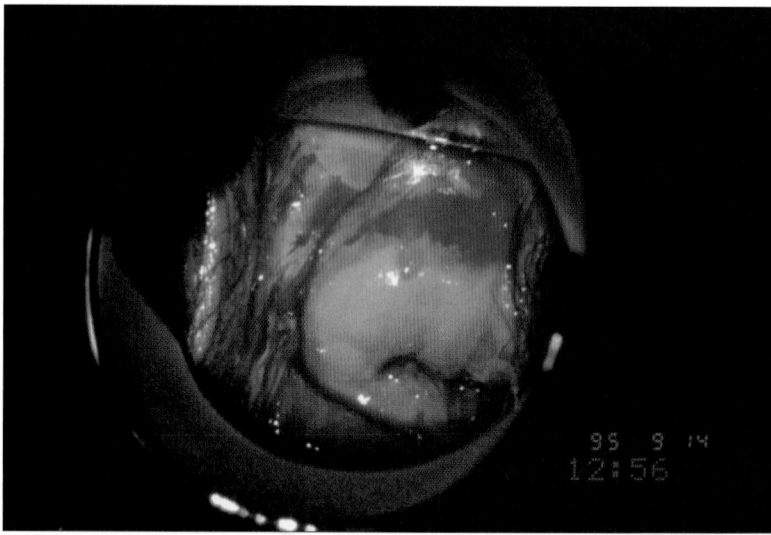

Fig. 12.43
Vulvovaginal-gingival syndrome: there is ulceration of the vagina and cervix. By courtesy of the Institute of Dermatology, London, UK.

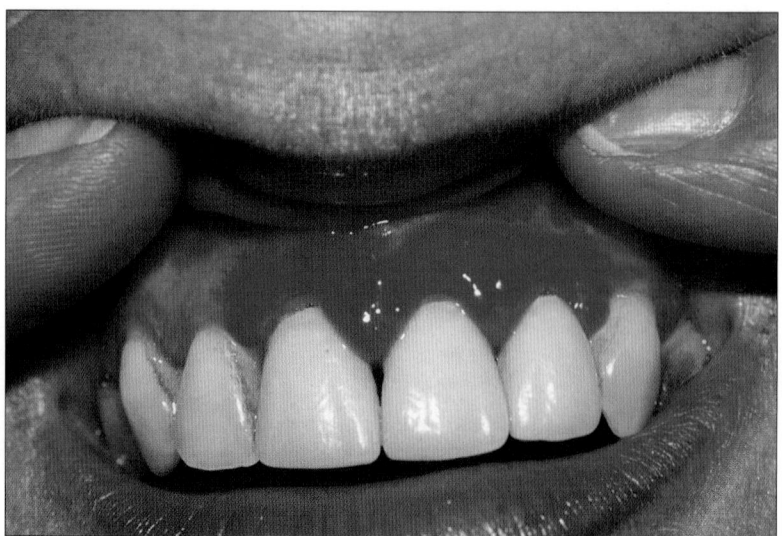

Fig. 12.44
Vulvovaginal-gingival syndrome: note the intense erythema with erosion of the gum. By courtesy of the Institute of Dermatology, London, UK.

genital lesions (genito-gingival syndrome) has been described.[11,12] Patients with genital lesions may have oral, aural, conjunctival, and esophageal involvement.[13–17]

Perianal disease can cause deep, painful fissuring, and it is often the hypertrophic variant that involves this site.

In the male genital, LP can present as phimosis.[18,19] Adhesions are seen in the uncircumcised male, both transcoronal and subcoronal.

Anogenital LP carries a small increased risk of malignancy, usually squamous cell carcinoma (SCC) (*Fig. 12.45*).[20–23] Hypertrophic LP of the glans penis should be regarded as having potential sinister biological behavior.[24]

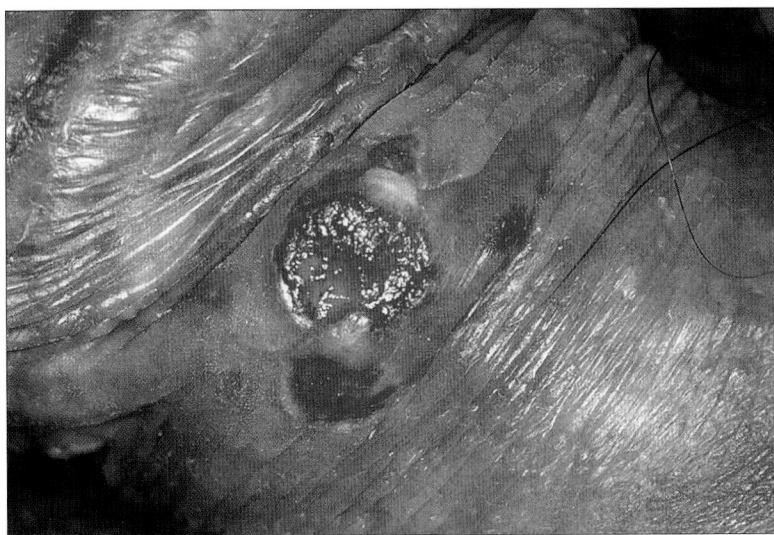

Fig. 12.45
Lichen planus: chronic penile lesion complicated by an ulcerated squamous cell carcinoma. By courtesy of the Institute of Dermatology, London, UK.

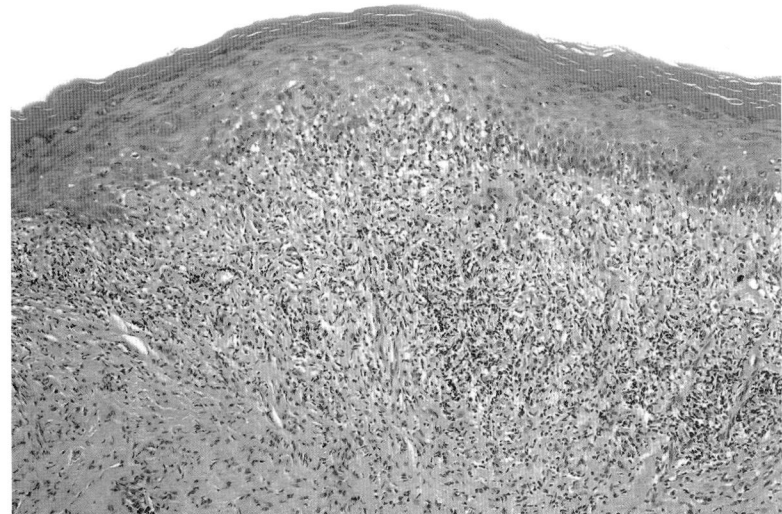

Fig. 12.46
Lichen planus: there is hyperkeratosis, acanthosis, and a bandlike inflammatory cell infiltrate.

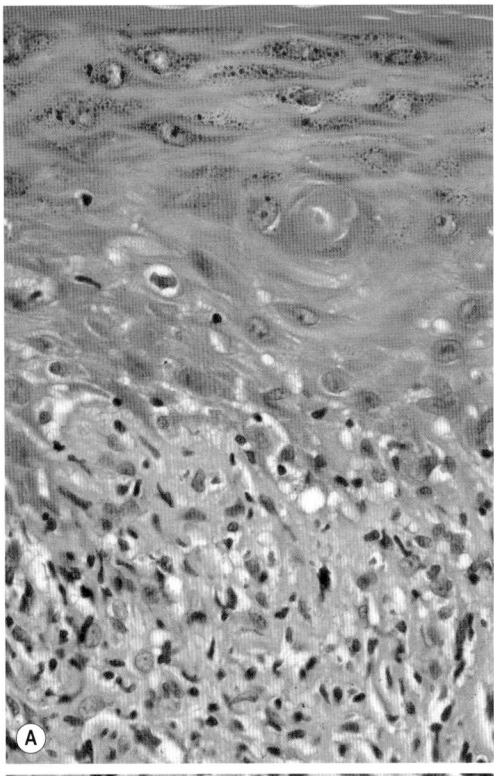

Fig. 12.47
Lichen planus: (**A**) note the hyperkeratosis, hypergranulosis and basal cell hydropic degeneration; (**B**) in contrast to cutaneous disease, plasma cells as shown in this field are often present in genital lesions.

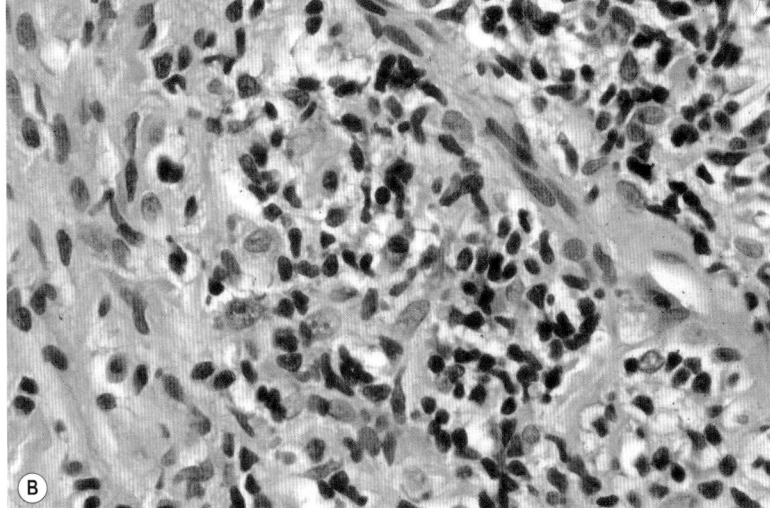

Pathogenesis and histologic features

Studies of oral LP have supported an immunological basis with activated T cell to an unidentified antigenic stimulus.[25] The histologic features of ano-genital LP are often more difficult to recognize than those of LP presenting on nonmucosal surfaces. The epidermis may be effaced or thickened, and there is a dense, band-like infiltrate hugging the dermal–epidermal junction (*Fig. 12.46*). Many genital lesions are mucosal and the inflammatory cell infiltrate is often rich in plasma cells, in contrast with lesions of LP at other sites where lymphocytes and histiocytes predominate (*Fig. 12.47*). The basal layer is often disrupted with some cytological atypia as regeneration takes place. Cytoid bodies may be seen but tend not to be prominent. This is accompanied by parakeratosis. Focal secondary spongiotic changes are not uncommon, particularly in mucosal surfaces. In long-standing disease, the dense, bandlike infiltrate may be replaced by a patchy, scant infiltrate with small foci of lichenoid inflammation. Many cases of male genital LP are misdiagnosed as ZB or LS.

Immunofluorescence studies may show fibrinogen and IgM along the basement membrane zone and, more rarely, IgG or IgA.[26] Cytoid bodies may also be labeled.[26]

Differential diagnosis

The clinical differential diagnosis includes psoriasis, ZB in the male, LS, viral warts, bowenoid papulosis, and porokeratosis. LP is one of the causes of pruritus ani. A biopsy is frequently necessary for diagnostic purposes but is more importantly done in the follow-up of the rare cases of chronic anogenital disease where the development of ulcero-erosive or verrucous features leads to concern about the development of SCC. LP often overlaps with the features of LS, and in some patients the two disorders may coexist. Hyalinization of the papillary dermis or the superficial lamina propria is indicative of the latter condition. In patients suffering from such a chronic overlap syndrome, particular care should be taken to recognize dysplastic areas or SCC. Those patients with predominantly mucosal disease clinically mimic mucous membrane pemphigoid, but immunofluorescence studies are invariably negative. A case of paraneoplastic LP with orogenital involvement and cicatrizing conjunctivitis in association with thymoma has been described.[27]

Sometimes drugs can precipitate a generalized lichenoid eruption. A case of a lichenoid drug eruption confined to the penis due to propranolol has been reported.[28]

Lichen nitidus

Clinical features

This disease has an affinity for the penis.[1] It can be difficult to diagnose because the signs may be subtle even when the lesions are widespread, and when itchy the signs due to excoriation and eczematization may eclipse those due to the lichen nitidus.

Histologic features

Histologically, the appearances are the same as those of lichen nitidus occurring elsewhere.

Porokeratosis

Clinical features

Typical annular lesions with a raised hyperkeratotic margin (see Chapter 3) are classically generalized in distribution but the anogenital skin may be involved. Rarely, the genital skin is affected alone (genital porokeratosis) or, even more rarely, pruritic, occasionally verrucous involvement limited to the perianal and gluteal folds is seen (porokeratosis ptychotropica).[1–3] The differential diagnosis includes LP and amyloid (and the latter has been reported in porokeratosis ptychotropica).[4] An association with bone marrow transplantation has been described.[3]

The condition is exceptionally rare in females.[5]

Histologic features

The histology is distinctive and the same as porokeratosis at other sites. In porokeratosis ptychotropica, most cases have superimposed changes of lichenification which obscures the cornoid lamella. The latter and oblique sectioning means that the condition may be missed unless there is a high index of suspicion and further sections are performed.

Lichen sclerosus

Clinical features

LS is a lymphocyte-mediated dermatosis of unknown etiology.[1] It has a predilection for the anogenital skin in women and genital skin in men. Women are more frequently affected than men (10:1), and it is more common in white than nonwhite patients. It almost never affects men circumcised at birth.[2]

There are two peaks of incidence; in females these occur in the prepubertal years and then post-menopause, and in males in prepubertal and young to middle-aged adult males. When the disease arises in childhood it tends to persist, regression being uncommon.[3] In girls, the condition can present at a very early age with hemorrhagic perianal lesions (*Figs 12.48* and *12.49*). Constipation can occur as a complication of the painful fissuring of the anal canal. If there is marked anogenital involvement, the condition may be mistaken for sexual abuse.[4] Perianal disease does not occur in males, but in boys, genital LS is the most common cause of phimosis. Extragenital lesions occur in 11% of women with genital LS.[5] Such involvement occurs on the upper trunk, groins, upper extremities, neck, lower trunk, and lower extremities in decreasing order of frequency, often at sites of friction (*Figs 12.50* and *12.51*). Involvement of the scalp and face is rare and can be associated with alopecia.[6–8] An exceptional case with plantar involvement has been documented.[9] It is very rare to see extragenital lesions in the absence of genital lesions. The Koebner phenomenon is frequent and LS has been described in association with scars, at the sites of radiotherapy, and insulin injection and in association with a tattoo.[10–13] Lesions can also develop or recur in skin or myocutaneous grafts.[14] Oral involvement including lip lesions as an isolated phenomenon or in association with genital lesions has been described.[15–17] The exact incidence of the latter is unknown, as suspected cases are not often confirmed by histologic examination.[18] LP can coexist with LS, and this may account for some of the oral lesions.[19] Coexistence of LS with morphea has also been documented.[20] A single case

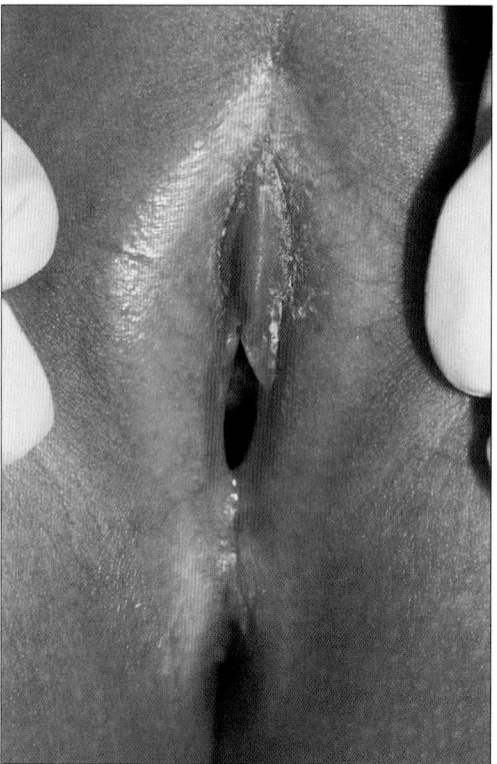

Fig. 12.48
Lichen sclerosus: prepubertal disease showing pallor on upper labia majora and perianal lesions. By courtesy of the Institute of Dermatology, London, UK.

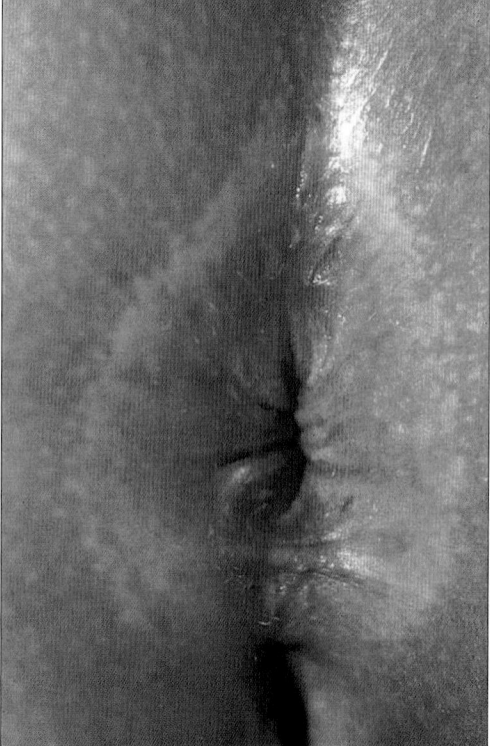

Fig. 12.49
Lichen sclerosus: perianal disease is often present in addition to vulval involvement, giving rise to the so-called hourglass distribution. By courtesy of the Institute of Dermatology, London, UK.

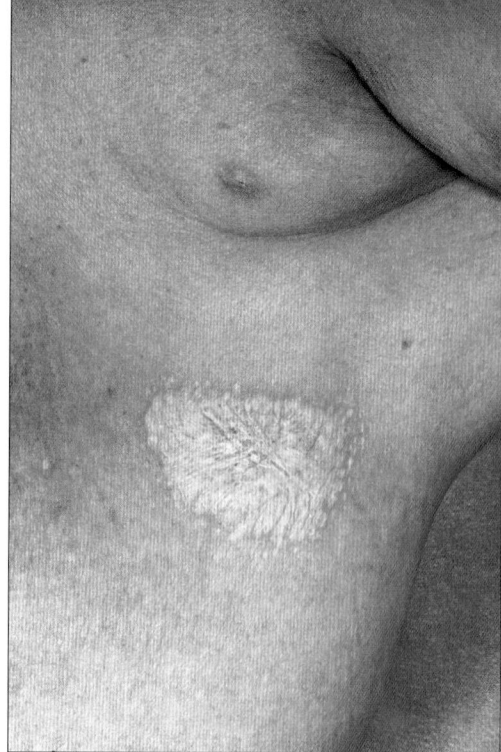

Fig. 12.50
Lichen sclerosus: irregular white plaque. It should be noted that extragenital lesions sometimes occur in the absence of genital lesions. By courtesy of R.A. Marsden, MD, St George's Hospital, London, UK.

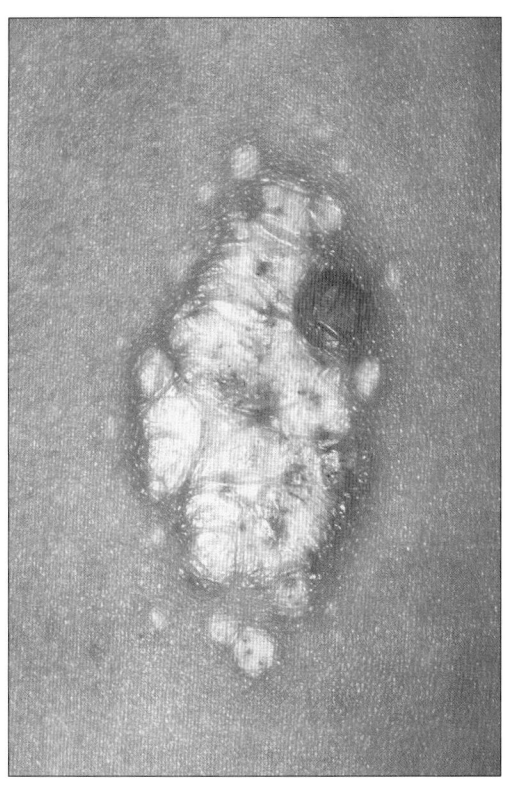

Fig. 12.51
Lichen sclerosus: healing lesion with a typical 'wrinkled tissue paper' appearance. By courtesy of R.A. Marsden, MD, St George's Hospital, London, UK.

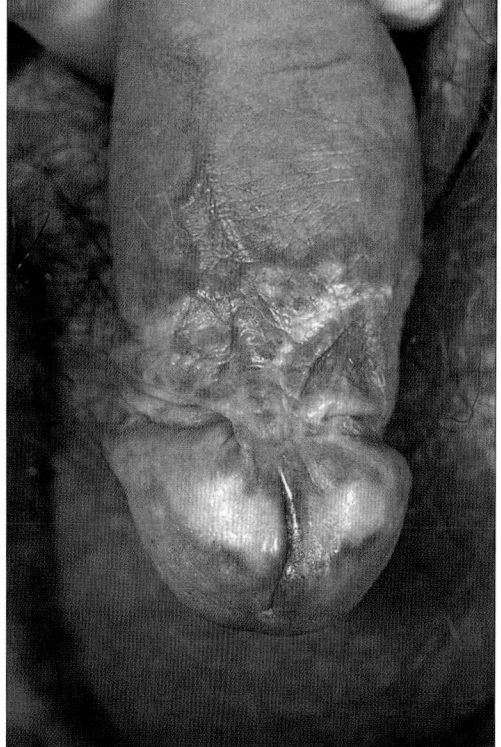

Fig. 12.52
Lichen sclerosus: in males, lesions of the foreskin and glans may be complicated by urethral stricture (so-called balanitis xerotica obliterans). By courtesy of the Institute of Dermatology, London, UK.

of multiple genital and extragenital lesions in a patient receiving imatinib mesylate has been reported.[21] A further case in association with allogeneic stem cell transplantation and another of genital disease developing in scrotal skin used in a case of male-to-female gender reassignment have been documented.[22,23]

The typical lesions of LS are porcelain-white papules and plaques with a crinkled surface. They can coalesce to form plaques. There are often associated ecchymoses and areas of hyperkeratosis. The latter occurs in relation to the appendage ostia, which are dilated, giving rise to the physical sign of delling. Bullae only rarely occur. Common symptoms in women include pruritus, burning, and dyspareunia, and in men coital and urinary difficulties. Although anogenital LS is intensely pruritic, lichenification is often not conspicuous. Female anogenital involvement is typically symmetrical and bilateral, and is described as having a figure-of-eight (hourglass) distribution when it affects the perianal as well as vulval skin. In men the involvement is 'tulip-like' symmetrically affecting the distal penile shaft, glans, and foreskin (not the perianal skin) (*Fig. 12.52*). On the other hand, the presentation may be with complete phimosis (*Fig. 12.53*). Lesions on the vulva predominantly affect the inner aspect of the labia majora, the labia minora, the prepuce of the clitoris, the fossa navicularis, and the posterior commissure (*Figs 12.54* and *12.55*). Penile disease can affect the glans, and distal foreskin, the frenulum, and ventral subcoronal sulcus is a particular target. Inflammation can be lichenoid and Zoonoid. LS is a scarring disorder, and in women there may be marked anatomical changes with resorption of the labia minora, burying of the clitoris, and introital narrowing. The vagina is unaffected. Urethral involvement is very rare.[24] In men there may be complete phimosis, constrictive posthitis due to a sclerotic band ('waisting'), transcoronal and subcoronal adhesions, erosion, ulceration and destruction or obliteration of the frenulum, effacement of the coronal sulcal architecture and definition (e.g., loss of pearly penile papules), and meatal 'pin hole' narrowing. The involvement of the anterior urethra can be serious: 29% of patients undergoing urethroplasty for urethral stricture had pathological evidence of LS.

An important complication of genital LS is the development of dysplasia and SCC. The latter only very exceptionally has been reported in association with extragenital lesions.[25] In the vulva (*Figs 12.56* and *12.57*), dysplastic foci may appear as hyperkeratotic adherent, gray-white areas, ice pick erosions, or fixed areas of erythema. Such changes must be examined histologically. Less than 4% of patients with vulval LS will develop an SCC.[26] It has recently been shown that an important number of cases diagnosed as LS

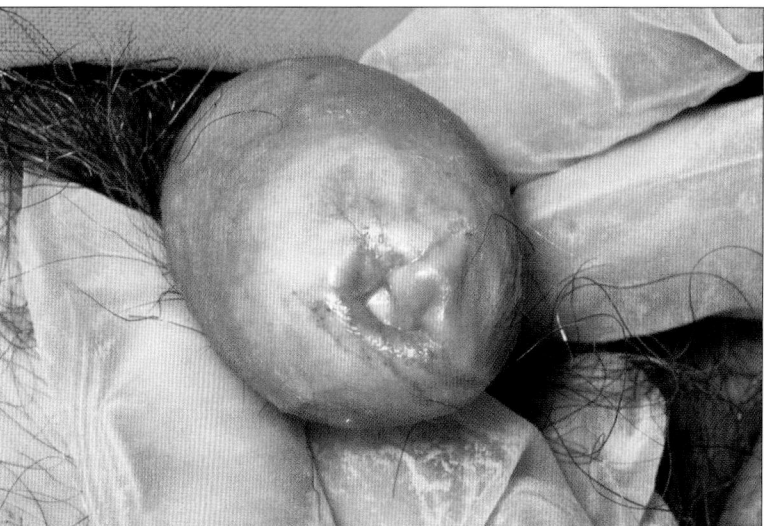

Fig. 12.53
Lichen sclerosus: a more advanced case showing severe phimosis. By courtesy of the Institute of Dermatology, London, UK.

with progression to SCC actually represent differentiated vulvar intraepithelial neoplasia and not LS.[27] The main reason for the high number of misdiagnosed cases is probably the difficulty in diagnosing differentiated vulval neoplasia on histologic grounds. These patients tend to have a more rapid progression to invasive SCC. In the group of patients with true LS and progression, a number of histologic features are seen which are absent in cases without progression. It has been suggested that these criteria can be used to identify patients at risk. They include parakeratosis, dyskeratosis, hyperplasia, and basal cell atypia.[27] In males, the published risk of SCC complicating LS is between 4% and 8%.[28–31] When excision specimens of penile SCC are examined, LS has been found in between 32% and 50% of cases.[31–33] The type of penile SCC associated with LS is not usually associated with HPV.[34] Chronicity, asymmetry, erythema, zoonoid or erythroplasia, erosions, ulcers, and verrucous change must be regarded with a very high index of suspicion and a low threshold for biopsy.

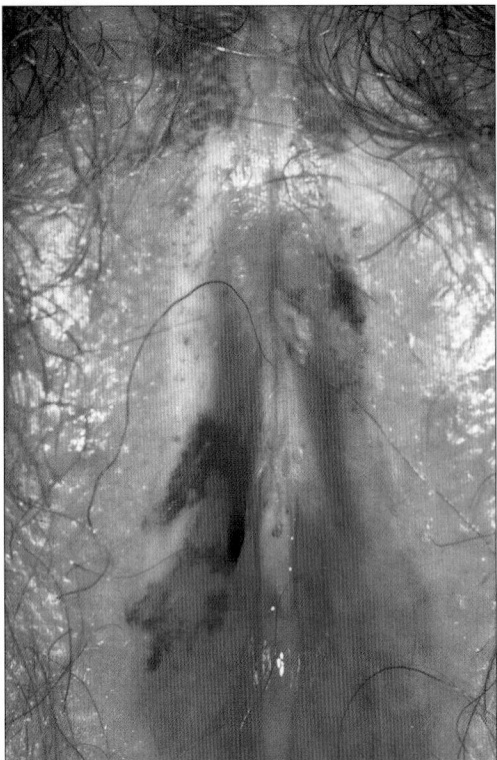

Fig. 12.54
Lichen sclerosus: symmetrical white lesions with
gross atrophy and hemorrhage. By courtesy of the
Institute of Dermatology, London, UK.

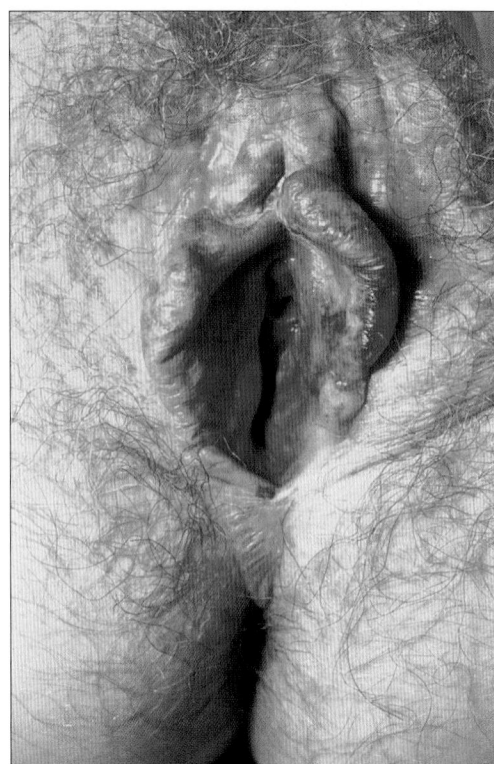

Fig. 12.55
Lichen sclerosus: there is extensive vulval disease
with involvement of the perineum and atrophy. By
courtesy of the Institute of Dermatology, London,
UK.

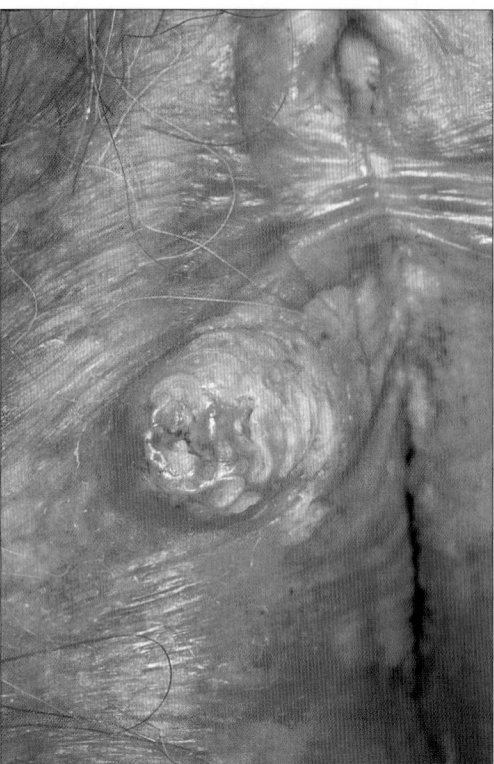

Fig. 12.56
Lichen sclerosus: long-standing disease with
complete loss of the vulval architecture complicated
by the development of an ulcerated squamous
cell carcinoma. By courtesy of the Institute of
Dermatology, London, UK.

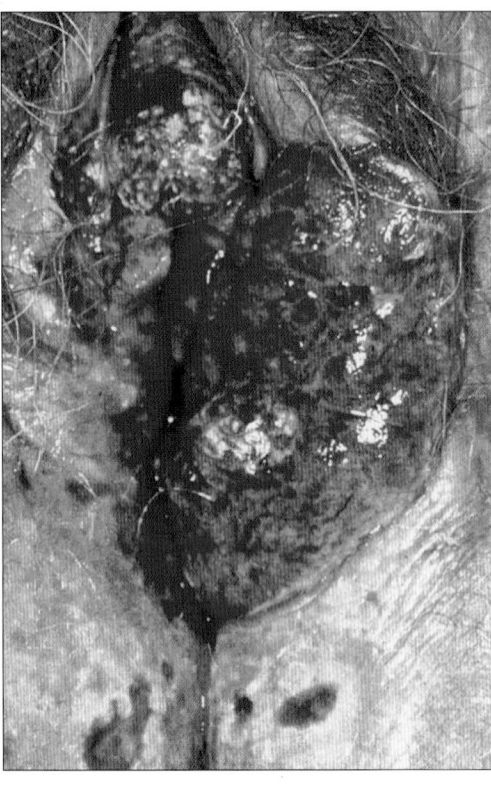

Fig. 12.57
Lichen sclerosus: an
ulcerated squamous cell
carcinoma has destroyed
much of the left side
of the vulva. Note the
background of ulcerated
lichen sclerosus. By
courtesy of the Institute
of Dermatology, London,
UK.

There are reports of atypical melanocytic lesions in association with
LS,[35,36] and careful clinicopathological correlation is needed. Cases of melanoma developing in LS are also reported.[37,38]

Pathogenesis and histologic features

The etiology of LS is not consensually agreed. It has been suggested that
genetic, hormonal, and autoimmune factors may be of importance. Familial
cases are well recognized and have been described in both sexes and in identical and nonidentical twins.[39–42] A recent study found a family history in up
to 12% of patients, suggesting that a number of cases have a genetic component.[43] About 21% of patients with LS have an associated autoimmune
disease including alopecia areata, vitiligo, hyperthyroidism, hypothyroidism,
pernicious anemia, and diabetes mellitus.[44,45] Patients and first-degree relatives may have circulating autoantibodies including those to thyroid, gastric
parietal cell, and smooth muscle in addition to antinuclear factor.[46] A significant association between LS and the presence of class II antigens including
HLA-DQ7, -DR7, -DQ8, and -DQ9 (alone or in combination) has been
reported.[47] It has also been suggested that HLA-A2 possibly exerts a protective role, as it tends to be absent in patients with extensive extragenital
lesions. Also, linkage of HLA-DR4 with -DQ8 is more common in patients
with marked structural damage to the anogenital area. Circulating IgG antibodies to the glycoprotein extracellular matrix protein 1 have been found in
the sera of men and women with genital LS.[48,49] In a few otherwise healthy
children with vulval LS, IgG autoantibodies against the BP180 antigen have
been detected.[50]

Intriguingly, genital LS has been reported in bone marrow transplant
recipients and graft-versus-host disease.[51,52]

Women with genital LS have been found to have a higher incidence
of psoriasis (predominantly extragenital) compared with the general
population.[53,54]

LS developing in premenopausal women has been linked to the use of
oral contraceptives, particularly those with antiandrogenic properties.[55]

Additional proposed etiological factors include absence of collagenase,
an increase in collagen inhibitor enzyme, and decreased elastase activity.
Reduced dihydrotestosterone levels have been described in some patients
and there is one report documenting the histologic presence of variably
acid-fast bacilli.[56,57] As with morphea and atrophoderma, a causal relationship to *Borrelia burgdorferi* has been proposed, but this putative connection derives from cases in Europe and not the United States.[58] There is no
serological evidence in British men with genital LS for an association with

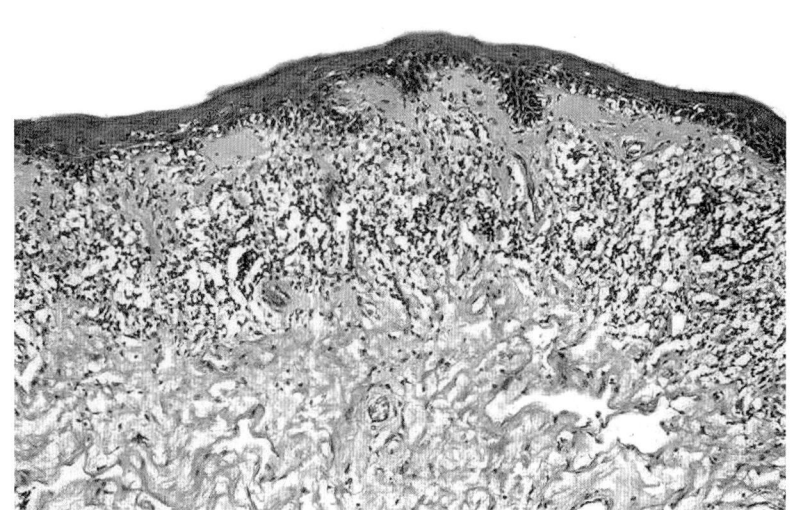

Fig. 12.58
Lichen sclerosus: early lesion showing epidermal atrophy and marked basal cell hydropic degeneration. There is a narrow zone of papillary dermal hyalinization and a bandlike infiltrate is present.

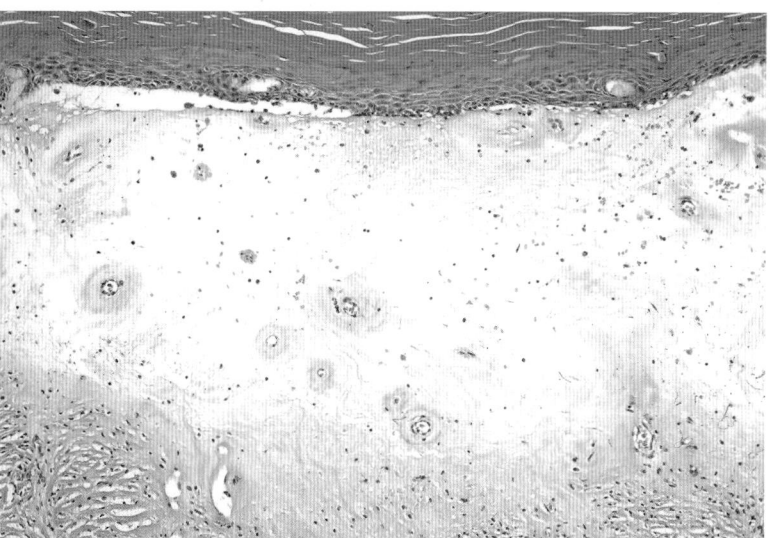

Fig. 12.59
Lichen sclerosus: this example shows the characteristic features of lichen sclerosus. Note the hyperkeratosis, epidermal atrophy, and a broad band of dermal hyalinization. Telangiectatic vessels are prominent.

Borrelia.[59] *Borrelia* has only exceptionally been demonstrated by nested polymerase chain reaction (PCR) in LS.[60] The variable results may be due to techniques used to detect *Borrelia*, and it has been suggested that focus floating microscopy should be the gold standard for detection.[61] HPV (types 6, 16, and 18) has been reported in 70% of cases of childhood penile LS and in 17.4% of adult cases (types 16, 18, 45) compared with 8.7% of normal males in one study and in 33% of adult cases (types 16, 18, 33, 51) in another.[52-64] Topical steroid treatment of LS may lead to HPV reactivation.[65] HPV, however, has not been found in other studies of vulval LS.[66] Epstein–Barr virus (EBV) was reported in 26.5% of samples in the same study. However, the epidemiology and clinical tenor of LS is not that of an infectious or sexually transmitted disease.

In males, obesity, anatomical abnormality, and trauma seem to be contributing factors.[2,24,67] LS has been specifically related to hypospadias and its repair.[24,68] It is often found around urostomies and urethrostomies.[69] The presence of histopathological features of LS in a percentage of acrochordons (skin tags) has led to the suggestion that occlusion of flaccid skin is a pathogenic factor.[70] In men, at least, all the evidence points to LS being due to chronic intermittent occluded contact with urine consequent upon contact with urinary microincontinence.[71]

The histologic changes are identical irrespective of the site involved (*Figs 12.58–12.61*).[72-74] However, genital lesions, as opposed to those occurring at extragenital sites, often show absence of atrophy, lichen simplex chronicus-like changes, spongiosis, more prevalent vascular ectasia, and dermal eosinophils.[75,76] Extragenital LS, on the other hand, seems to be associated in a number of cases with elastophagocytosis, a feature not reported in genital LS.[77] Occasionally, pseudoxanthoma elasticum-like fibers may be seen in patients without pseudoxanthoma elasticum.[78] Fully developed lesions of LS show a thinned, effaced epidermis with interface change and a wide band of hyalinization in the upper dermis and a lymphohistiocytic infiltrate below the hyalinized area. Zoonoid inflammation may be prominent. Marked hyperkeratosis, often associated with follicular plugging on hair-bearing skin, is frequently seen. Subepidermal edema is sometimes present and may be sufficient to cause subepithelial vesiculation (*Fig. 12.62*). Telangiectasia is common and purpura may be an additional feature. Angiokeratoma-like lesions can also develop.[79] A similar phenomenon is that of lymphangiectasia.[80] Early lesions and the periphery of fully developed lesions display lichenoid changes similar to LP (see differential diagnosis). Some cases may be associated with foci of marked and highly irregular acanthosis, often with a very jagged lower border (so-called squamous cell hyperplasia). Such cases should be carefully scrutinized for evidence of epithelial dysplasia (differentiated intraepithelial neoplasia) or adjacent carcinoma. Differentiated intraepithelial neoplasia is by far the most common

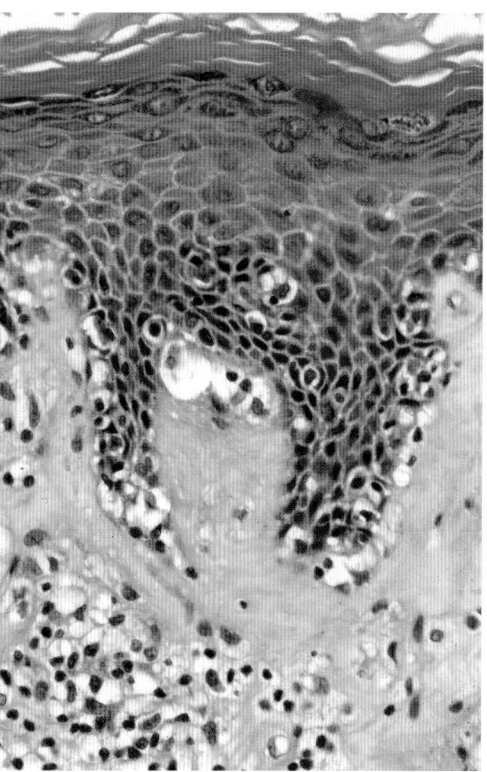

Fig. 12.60
Lichen sclerosus: close-up view of basal cell hydropic degeneration.

type of dysplasia found in SCC associated with LS.[81] Currently, there is no evidence to suggest that oncogenic HPV is associated with LS-related SCC.

The occasional observation of endarteritis in LS led originally to the usage of the term 'obliterans'. In two cases in boys, a dermal lymphohistiocytic and granulomatous phlebitis was found, and one also had evidence of HPV.[82] An exceptional case of LS with associated eosinophilic spongiosis representing superimposed bullous pemphigoid has been reported.[83]

Ultrastructural studies of LS show fragmentation, reduplication, and formation of gaps in the basal lamina.[75,84] Langerhans cells appear to pass through these gaps. The mononuclear infiltrate in LS is composed of an admixture of T-helper and suppressor lymphocytes. Expression of p53 by epidermal cells has been reported in LS.[76,85] The latter is more often seen in cases associated with SCC.[86]

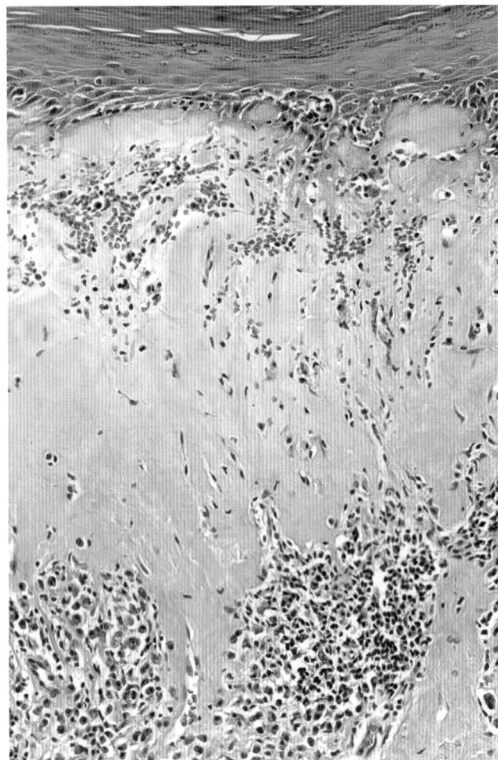

Fig. 12.61
Lichen sclerosus: in this view, the lymphohistiocytic infiltrate is present deep to the zone of hyalinization. There is telangiectasia with hemorrhage.

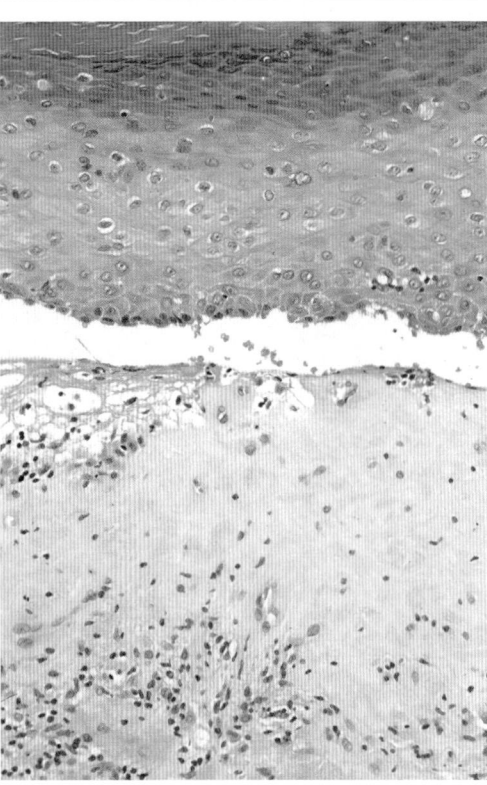

Fig. 12.62
Lichen sclerosus: occasionally, intense edema may result in subepidermal vesiculation.

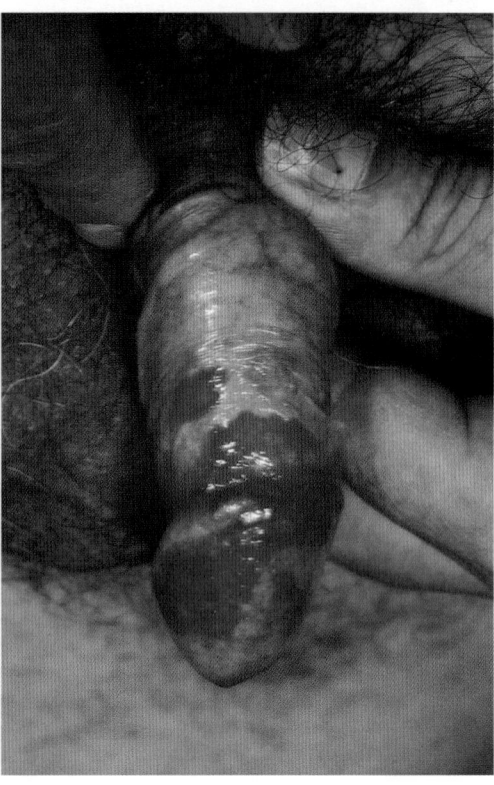

Fig. 12.63
Zoon balanitis: there is involvement of the glans, prepuce, and shaft of the penis. From Bunker C. Male Genital Skin Disease. Saunders Ltd./Elsevier 2004.

Differential diagnosis

Most cases of genital LS can be diagnosed clinically. LP and the much rarer mucous membrane pemphigoid are in the differential diagnosis. A biopsy should be performed if there is any clinical doubt or if the lesions are atypical, eroded, or verrucous. Anogenital LS, particularly early lesions, may be difficult to distinguish from LP. Changes present in the early stages of LS, and absent in LP, include a psoriasiform lichenoid pattern, exocytosis of lymphocytes affecting the basal cell layer, basement membrane thickening, foci of epidermal atrophy, and loss of papillary dermal elastic fibers.[74] Prominent Zoonoid inflammation may conceal subtler underlying LS. The histologic features may simulate mycosis fungoides.[87]

Zoon balanitis

Clinical features

Zoon plasma cell balanitis (ZB) is a disorder of middle-aged and older uncircumcised males, although an analogous condition has been reported to afflict the vulva, mouth, lips, and epiglottis.[1-7] Exceptionally, the disease may present in a circumcised male.[5] True ZB is probably rare with many cases of LS being misdiagnosed as ZB. The presentation is classically indolent and asymptomatic. Well-demarcated, glistening, moist, bright red or brown patches involve the glans and visceral prepuce with sparing of the keratinized penile shaft and foreskin (*Fig. 12.63*). The navicular fossa may be involved. Other signs include dark red stippling – 'cayenne pepper spots' – and purpura with hemosiderin deposition, solitary or multiple lesions of differing sizes (guttate or nummular), characteristically symmetrical about the axis of the coronal sulcus, and 'kissing'. Although vegetative and nodular presentations have been recorded, atypical or unusual morphology should be viewed with great suspicion and biopsied.[8,9] The clinical differential diagnosis includes LS, erosive LP, psoriasis, seborrheic dermatitis, contact dermatitis, fixed drug eruption, secondary syphilis, histoplasmosis, erythroplasia of Queyrat, and Kaposi sarcoma.[10,11] A confident clinical diagnosis is not always possible or safe.[12,13] Therefore, a biopsy is advisable, and the pathologist should actively seek concomitant disease. Overt cases of LS, LP, bowenoid papulosis, and penile cancer often appear to have ZB-like changes both on clinical examination and on histology[9,13-16]: the signs of ZB may be secondary to underlying preputial disease.[8] Probably some of the clinical and histologic variants that have been reported, and the idea that ZB might be a premalignant condition, reflect this phenomenon. ZB indicates a dysfunctional foreskin, potentially concealing a more sinister dermatosis.[10,17,18]

Pathogenesis and histologic features

Since Zoon's original reports, there have been many accounts in the literature, but the etiology remains uncertain. The evidence suggests that ZB is a chronic, reactive, principally irritant dermatosis brought about by a dysfunctional prepuce. Retention of urine and squames and excessive frictional trauma (ZB is often located on the dorsal aspect of the glans and/or the adjacent prepuce, sites of maximal friction on foreskin retraction) create the irritation. There is no evidence of an infectious cause, and immunohistochemical findings suggest that ZB represents a non-specific polyclonal tissue reaction, consistent with an irritant dermatosis.[6,7]

Classically, the epidermis shows attenuation with absent granular and horny layers, and diamond- or lozenge-shaped basal cell keratinocytes with sparse dyskeratosis and spongiosis (*Figs 12.64* and *12.65*). In the dermis, there is a dense band of infiltration with plasma cells of variable density.[13] Other signs include extravasated erythrocytes, hemosiderin, and vascular proliferation. Zoon stressed the presence of the plasma cell infiltrate in this condition, but in practice the plasma cell density can be very variable.[9,13,19]

Zoon vulvitis (plasma cell vulvitis)

This variant of Zoon is the female counterpart of the more common Zoon balanitis and was also described by Zoon after it had been noted by Garnier.[1]

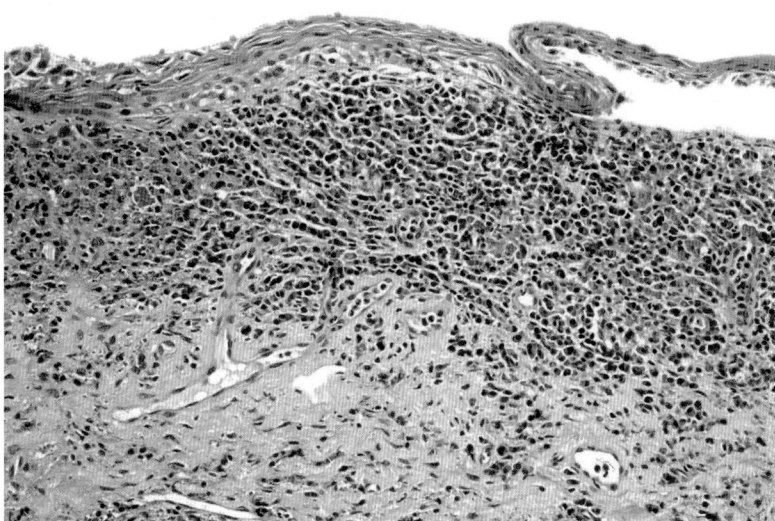

Fig. 12.64
Zoon balanitis: note the epidermal thinning, spongiosis, and a dense superficial inflammatory cell infiltrate.

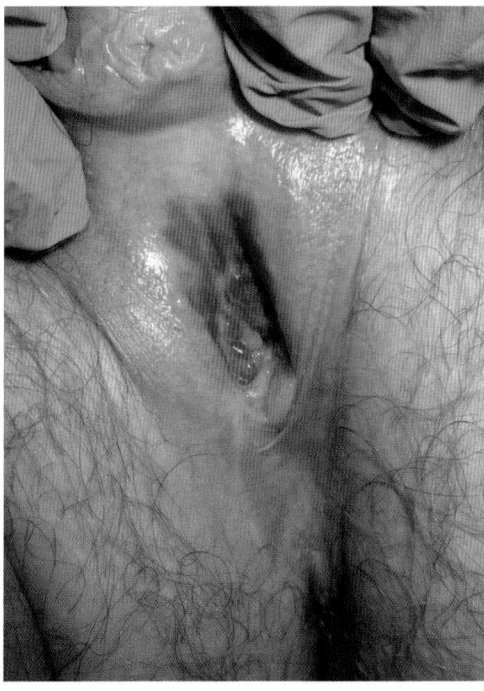

Fig. 12.66
Zoon vulvitis (plasma cell vulvitis): purpuric change at vestibule.

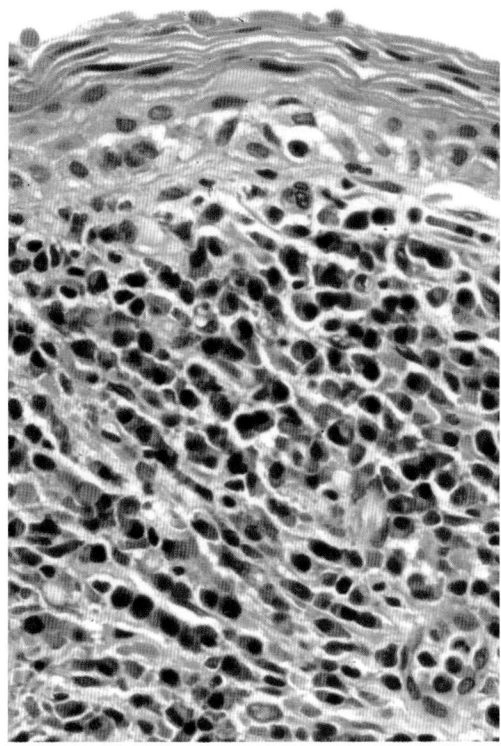

Fig. 12.65
Zoon balanitis: there is 'lozenge-shaped' spongiosis and an intense plasma cell infiltrate.

Clinical features

Lesions in females are rare and affect the vestibule and the labia minora.[2,3] Few lesions have been described on the clitoris. The condition probably is not a single entity but a pattern of inflammation that is seen on a mucosal surface in other chronic dermatoses, particularly LP.[4] The lesions are bright red with a varnished appearance, and sometimes there is cayenne pepper-like speckling. There may also be areas of purpura and hemosiderin pigmentation (Fig. 12.66).

Alternative names proposed for these inflammatory changes include chronic vulval purpura[5] and persistent purpuric dermatitis.[6] Similar lesions have been described in the oral cavity and other mucosal surfaces, including the epiglottis, under names such as plasma cell orificial mucositis and atypical gingivostomatitis.[7]

Histologic features

The histology is the same as that described for ZB. In one histologic study, the percentage of plasma cells seen was felt to be the most important parameter in making the diagnosis.[8] However, the site of the biopsy is important as there are increased numbers of plasma cells seen in the vestibule normally, and this should not be misinterpreted. An exceptional case of Zoon vulvitis with prominent mucinous metaplasia has been described.[9]

Granuloma annulare

A few cases of granuloma annulare affecting the penis have been reported, mainly in children and adolescents.[1–5] An association with LS has been mooted.[6] Erythematous smooth, round, and linear nodules are described. The histology is identical to that seen elsewhere, and often lesions tend to represent deep granuloma annulare.

Vesiculobullous conditions

Subepidermal (bullous pemphigoid and mucous membrane pemphigoid) and intra-epidermal (pemphigus vulgaris) autoimmune blistering diseases are discussed elsewhere. Pemphigus can involve the penis (the glans is the usual site) but very rarely in isolation. Pemphigus vegetans presenting with a 4-year history of indolent tender balanitis, where the glans penis was involved with a moist vegetative plaque with beefy red erosions separating irregular hyperkeratotic mounds, has been reported.[1] Involvement of the penis in mucous membrane pemphigoid is very uncommon and may cause blisters, erosions, ulcers, transcoronal adhesions, scarring, and phimosis.[2]

In the female, mucous membrane pemphigoid can lead to architectural change and is the main differential diagnosis for erosive LP. Vulval involvement in linear IgA disease in children (bullous dermatosis of childhood) can be seen in 80% patients and may present with genital lesions.[3]

The histology of bullous disorders in genital skin is the same as that seen in lesions presenting elsewhere.

Genital papular acantholytic dyskeratosis

This term has been used to describe a condition where papules and nodules develop on the genital skin and may be mistaken for warts.[1] Histologically, lesions demonstrate changes similar to Darier disease and Hailey-Hailey disease.[2,3] It has been proposed that some cases may be a forme fruste of the latter,[4] and there has been a suggestion that it can be considered allelic to

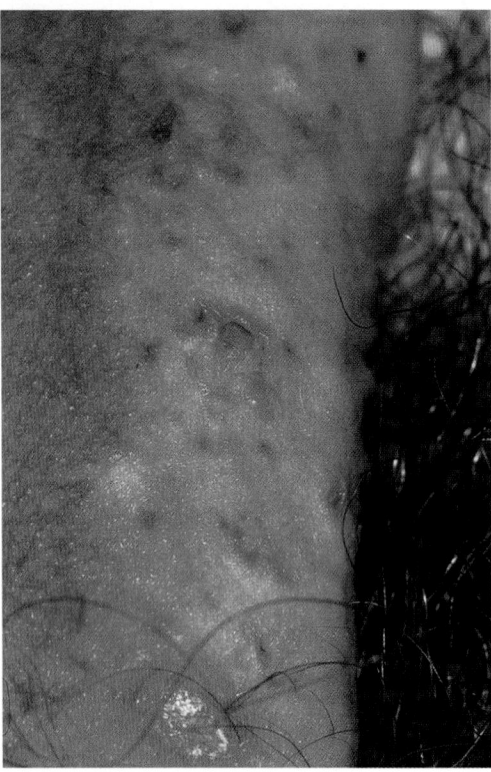

Fig. 12.67
Penile acne: comedones, cysts, and healing inflamed lesions are present on the proximal shaft of the penis. From Bunker C. Male Genital Skin Disease. Saunders Ltd./Elsevier 2004.

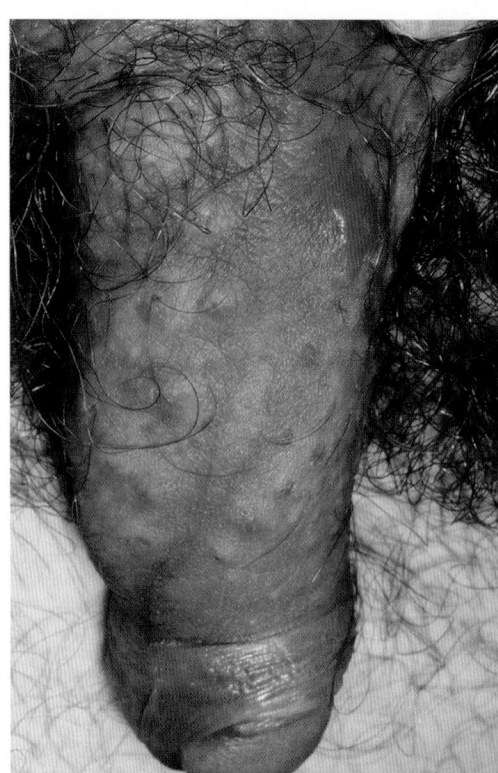

Fig. 12.68
Penile acne: comedones, papules, and nodules are evident. From Bunker C. Male Genital Skin Disease. Saunders Ltd./Elsevier 2004.

Hailey-Hailey disease.[5] Immunofluorescence studies are negative, although one case with positive immunofluorescence consisting of intercellular IgG and C3 has been reported.[6]

Penile acne

Clinical features

This is not an entity that is well recognized in the literature, but it is occasionally encountered in clinical practice. Young men complain of spots, boils, or blackheads, and on examination have comedones, papules, pustules, inflammatory nodules, and scars of the proximal penile shaft (*Figs 12.67* and *12.68*). An important differential diagnosis of acneform disease presenting at any site is chloracne, due to occlusion of the skin with machine oil.

Histologic features

The histology is identical to that of acne at classical sites.

Hidradenitis suppurativa

Clinical features

Hidradenitis suppurativa (acne inversa; chronic perianal pyoderma in Japan and Verneuil disease in France)[1,2] is a chronic inflammatory dermatosis that affects areas rich in apocrine glands. Bridged comedones, folliculitis and furunculosis, deep discharging sinuses, nodules, cysts, and scars may all be present in the groins (*Fig. 12.69*), the natal cleft and buttocks, and in the axillae and under the breasts.[1] The patient may have conglobate acne. Pili incarnati (ingrowing hairs) and secondary folliculitis is a common problem in the bikini area in women but rarely encountered in men (*Fig. 12.70*). It is more common in black individuals and affects the axillae preferentially in women and the perineum in men. A urethral cutaneous fistula and phimosis has been reported.[3] It is a cause of dorsal perforation of the penis.[4,5] Scarring from the disease and its treatment can be extensive (*Fig. 12.71*). The morbidity of hidradenitis may be appalling, interfering with sitting, sleeping, walking, defecation, and sexual activity. Depression is common.

Hidradenitis suppurativa has been considered to be a form of 'apocrine acne'. However, the primary pathological process seems to be associated

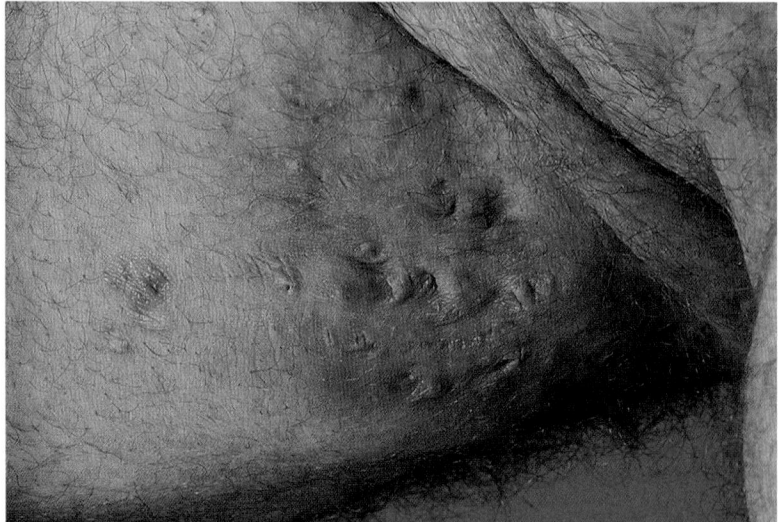

Fig. 12.69
Hidradenitis suppurativa: there is extensive involvement of the groin. From Bunker C. Male Genital Skin Disease. Saunders Ltd./Elsevier 2004.

eminently with the hair follicle. The role of endocrine factors is uncertain as is the *primary* part played by bacteria. Chronicity and tissue destruction lead to the classical physical signs. Disease that has persisted for more than 20 years carries a significant risk of progression to SCC and rarely verrucous carcinoma[6–9]

Hidradenitis is usually a clinical diagnosis. Swabs should be taken for bacteriological analysis. Rarely, a biopsy may be necessary to exclude carcinoma or Crohn disease. Perineal Crohn disease mimics hidradenitis with its granulomatous inflammation, ulceration, and fistula formation, but it is less painful. Also, the disease is absent from the axillae and it is rare for patients to be free of overt gastrointestinal symptoms. Very florid perianal disease can be seen in myeloma and leukemia in homosexual men and AIDS.[10–12]

Histologic features

The histology is identical to that of hidradenitis suppurativa occurring elsewhere.

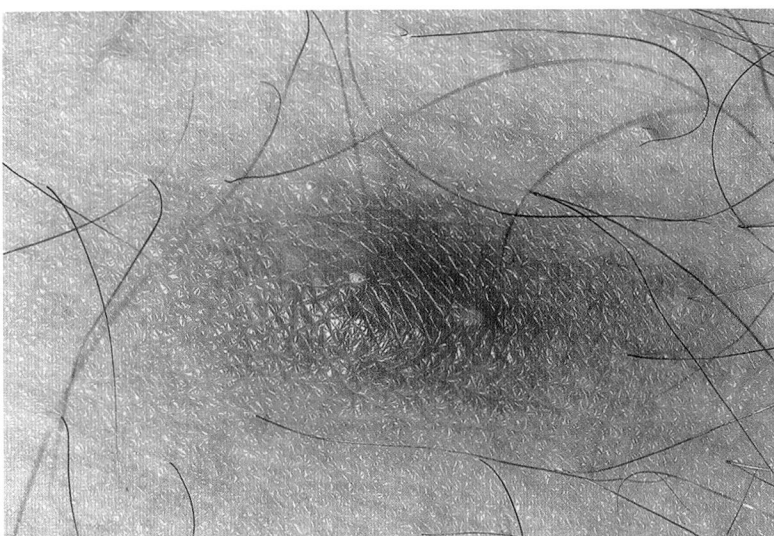

Fig. 12.70
Pili incarnati: lesion from the groin showing and inflamed follicular lesion. From Bunker C. Male Genital Skin Disease. Saunders Ltd./Elsevier 2004.

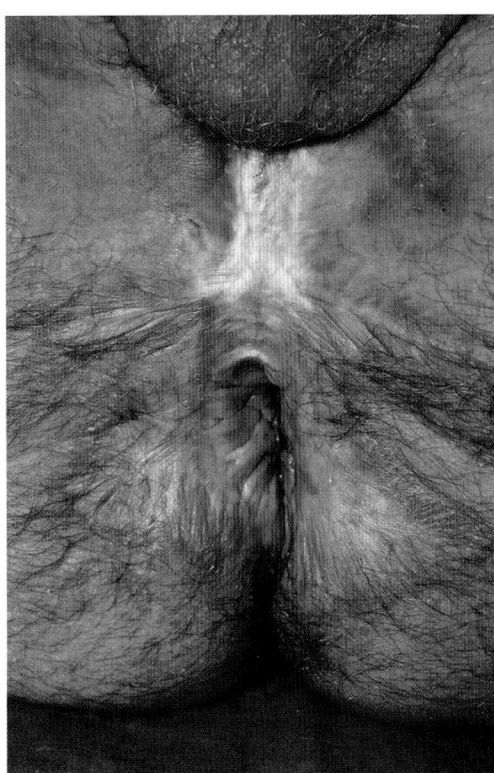

Fig. 12.71
Hidradenitis suppurativa: there is extensive scarring as a result of the disease and also from surgery. Courtesy of Prof. Tim Allen-Mersh, London, UK. From Bunker C. Male Genital Skin Disease. Saunders Ltd./Elsevier 2004.

Aphthous ulceration

Clinical features

The cause of aphthous ulcers is not known. Aphthous ulceration of the penis and scrotum does occur, but this is not an acceptable diagnosis in the perianal skin or genitalia without overt exclusion of sexually transmitted diseases, and culture is reasonable practice.[1] When aphthae occur on the vulva, the usual site involved are the labia majora and minora. They can occur with or without oral aphthae and may be a reactive phenomenon.[2]

The impression is that aphthae and idiopathic orogenital ulceration are more common in HIV infection and worse, symptomatically and morphologically. Giant lesions may occur. In HIV, all mucocutaneous ulcers must be biopsied and cultured; several pathologies may coexist.[1]

Histologic features

The histology of idiopathic aphthous ulceration is entirely non-specific. The main reason why a biopsy is performed is to rule out other pathologies.

Lipschutz ulcer

Clinical features

This condition is seen in teenage girls who present with vulval ulceration of sudden onset. Lesions may be solitary or multiple.[1] The initial lesion is a tender purpuric or hemorrhagic papule that rapidly enlarges and ulcerates. The ulcers are deep and painful, and have sharply delineated erythematous margins. There may be an accompanying fever, malaise, and cervical lymphadenopathy. A similar condition does not occur in males.

Pathogenesis and histologic features

The condition is a toxic reaction to a systemic infection. The most commonly associated infection is EBV infection (infectious mononucleosis).[1] Other associated infections have included typhoid and paratyphoid, mycoplasma, mumps, and cytomegalovirus.[2-5] The microscopic appearance shows non-specific superficial ulceration with granulation tissue, fibrin deposition, and a mixed inflammatory cell infiltrate. It is suggested that a localized lymphocytic arteritis is a common feature[6] The presence of the EBV can be demonstrated by in situ hybridization.

Sclerosing lymphangitis of the penis

Clinical features

Sclerosing lymphangitis of the penis (Mondor disease) is a rare condition which presents as a serpiginous cordlike thickening of the skin near the coronal sulcus.[1-4] Rarely, there is involvement of the dorsal aspect of the shaft. There may be some inflammation and local tenderness. The condition is usually self-limiting and resolves spontaneously after a few weeks. Only occasional cases are persistent and may require surgery.[5] There does not appear to be a female equivalent to this disorder, but there has been a report of the disease involving the upper lip and the labium minus.[6]

Pathogenesis and histologic features

The etiology is unknown but vigorous or traumatic sexual activity is an important precipitant.[7,8] In general, there does not seem to be any relationship to venereal disease although cases have been reported following genital herpes and Chlamydia infection.[9,10] A case developing after coadministration of tadalafil and fluconazole has been documented.[11]

The histologic features are characterized by a thrombosed vascular channel, thought to be of either lymphatic or venous derivation. Some authors separate sclerosing lymphangitis from Mondor disease based on the involvement of lymphatics in the former and veins in the latter.[12] Focal Masson-like (intravascular papillary endothelial hyperplasia) changes may be seen. Later, in the course of the disease, the thrombus is replaced by fibrous tissue and a few scattered mononuclear inflammatory cells are also seen. The wall of the affected vessel later becomes thickened and sclerotic.

Pyoderma gangrenosum

This is a rare genital affliction, including the variant superficial granulomatous pyoderma[1] that can affect the penis and scrotum in adults and children. In children the anogenital area is a site of predilection in addition to the head and neck. Genital pyoderma gangrenosum may occur following local trauma such as urological surgery[1,2] or treatment for cancer.[3] A case has been reported in association with the oncological use of pazopanib (a selective multi-tyrosine kinase inhibitor that blocks tumor growth and inhibits angiogenesis).[4] It may complicate ulcerative colitis[5] or chronic lymphocytic leukemia, or may be idiopathic.[6-9] In idiopathic cases, the diagnosis is frequently delayed because it is not included in the differential by the clinician in pursuit of a diagnosis of cancer or infection. Pathologists may receive biopsies without this possibility being mentioned to them.[10]

Pyoderma gangrenosum of the vulva has been reported after an obstetric laceration.[11]

Histologic features

The histologic features are non-specific identical to those seen in lesions elsewhere.

Penile necrosis

Clinical features

This serious situation has a number of causes and a wide clinical differential diagnoses. Many of the causes are discussed in this and other chapters; for example, decubitus ulcer, the strangulation and tourniquet syndromes and other autoerotic misadventures and causes of artifact (priapism), pyoderma gangrenosum, infections such as herpes simplex, ecthyma gangrenosum and Fournier gangrene, and as a complication of serious illness (e.g., mucormycosis in acute myeloblastic leukemia).[1] Necrosis can be the result of diabetic small vessel and end-stage renal disease[2,3] and chronic renal failure with secondary hyperparathyroidism and calciphylaxis,[4] and can complicate polycythemia, thrombocytopenia and leukemia, cryoglobulinemia, and vasculitis. Inferior vena caval thrombosis as part of disseminated intravascular coagulation can lead to necrosis and gangrene of the penis.[5] Heparin necrosis is a coagulopathy due to heparin-induced thrombocytopenia. Warfarin necrosis is a state of acquired protein C dysfunction.[6,7]

Histologic features

The histologic features consist of extensive necrosis of the skin and deeper tissues, and more specific changes may be found depending on the etiology of the process.

Spontaneous scrotal ulceration

Five cases of spontaneous scrotal ulceration in young, previously fit men have been described by Piñol Aguade.[1] Histology showed non-specific vasculitis, and spontaneous resolution occurred. This entity may be related to idiopathic scrotal panniculitis and fat necrosis. Idiopathic scrotal necrosis in a 2-month-old boy has been documented by Sarihan[2]; trauma, extreme cold, and Fournier gangrene were excluded.

Scrotal fat necrosis

This condition is distinct from other causes of acute scrotum in prepubertal boys.[1] It presents as acute tender, sometimes painful, swelling (classically, but not always, after swimming in cold water). Masses may be palpable in the scrotal wall. The patient is otherwise well, with no fever or leukocytosis.[2,3] In adults, one case of idiopathic scrotal panniculitis has been reported and another associated with pancreatitis.[4,5]

Associations with systemic disease

Crohn disease

Clinical features

Anogenital lesions occur in about 30% of patients with intestinal Crohn disease, either by direct extension of active intestinal disease or occurring at sites distant from any gastrointestinal lesions[1] (so-called 'metastatic disease') such as the face and limbs (*Figs 12.72–12.75*). Skin involvement is more common in patients with colonic disease (up to 80%), and anogenital disease may present years before there is evidence of gastrointestinal disease.[2] Vulval edema can be the only manifestation, and occasionally it is unilateral[3,4] Crohn disease may involve the penis and scrotum, presenting as

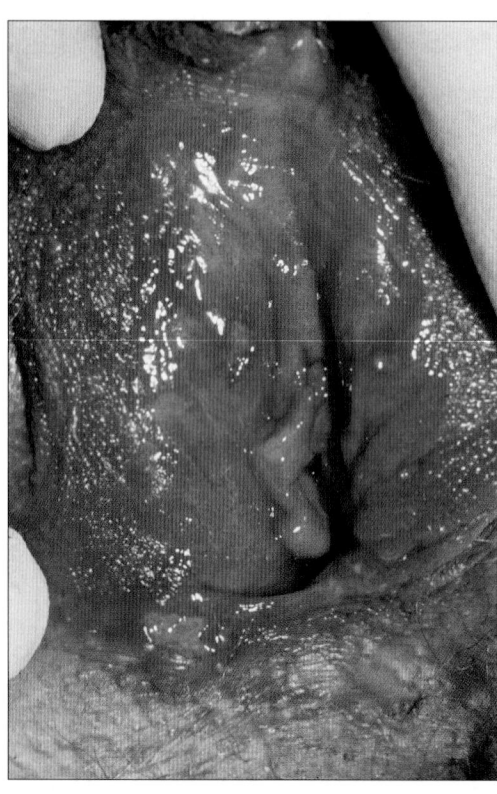

Fig. 12.72
Vulval Crohn disease: there is intense erythema and multiple vestibular erosions are present. By courtesy of the Institute of Dermatology, London, UK.

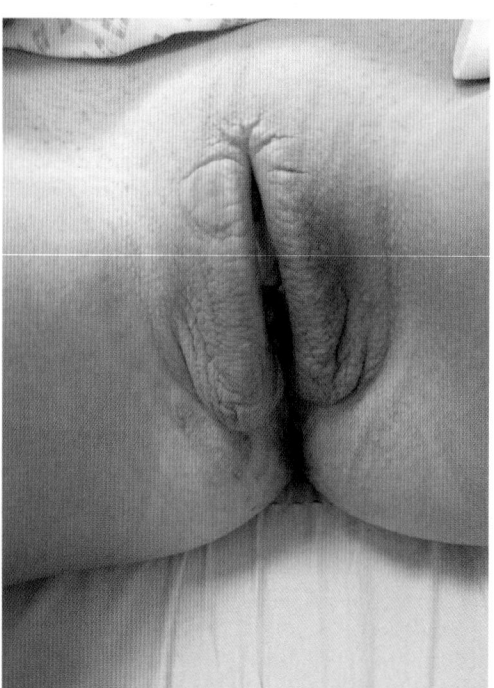

Fig. 12.73
Vulval Crohn disease: in this patient, there is marked edema which is the presenting feature.

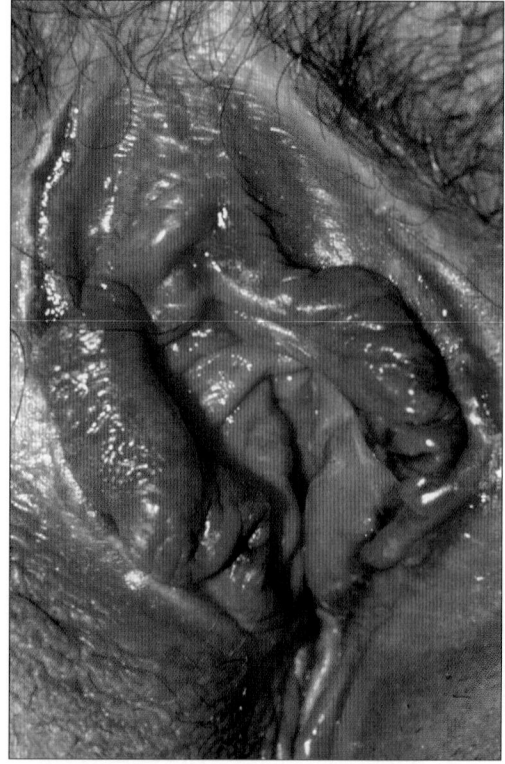

Fig. 12.74
Vulval Crohn disease: note the erythema, edema, and erosions. By courtesy of the Institute of Dermatology, London, UK.

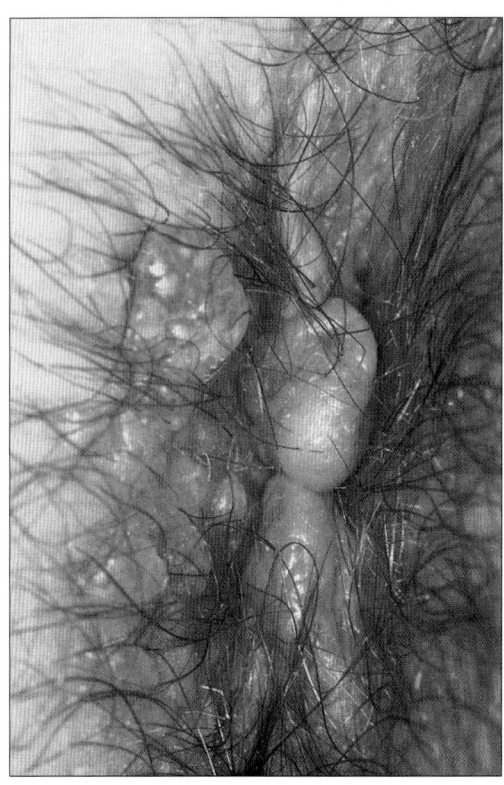

Fig. 12.75
Perianal Crohn disease: multiple skin tags showing massive edema are present. By courtesy of the Institute of Dermatology, London, UK.

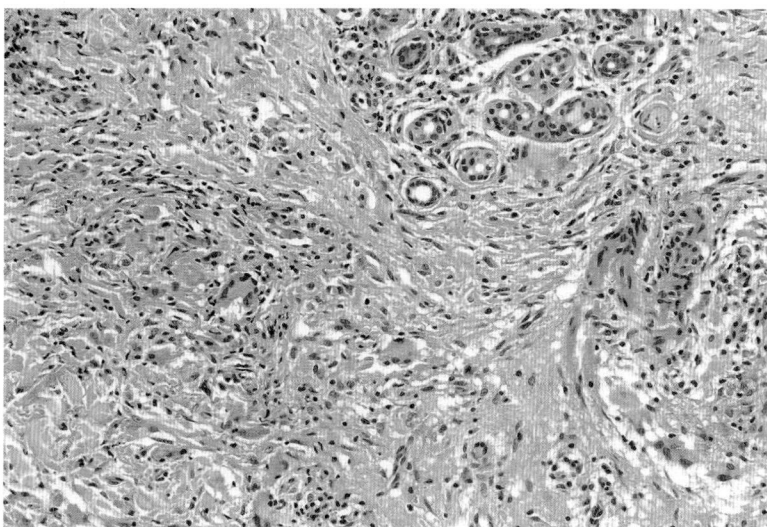

Fig. 12.76
Vulval Crohn disease: there is an ill-defined granulomatous infiltrate with conspicuous giant cells in the deep reticular dermis.

penoscrotal lymphedema.[5,6] More usually, however, the disease is associated with erosions, ulceration, abscesses, skin tags, sinus, and fistula formation.[7] Lesions can exceptionally mimic hidradenitis suppurativa and pyoderma gangrenosum.[8] Deep fissures ('knife-cut' sign) along the skin creases are a characteristic feature. Patients of any age with Crohn disease including children may present with anogenital involvement.[9] Oral involvement includes edema, fissuring, and mucosal 'cobblestoning'. One patient presented with 'metastatic' Crohn disease and oral intraepithelial IgA pustulosis.[10]

Crohn disease is not uncommonly associated with pyoderma gangrenosum and erythema nodosum. Other links include leukocytoclastic vasculitis, erythema elevatum diutinum, granulomatous vasculitis, Sweet syndrome, epidermolysis bullosa acquisita, polyarteritis nodosa, pyostomatitis vegetans, vitiligo, psoriasis, erythema multiforme, lichen nitidus, hidradenitis suppurativa, and acne fulminans.[11–22]

The condition runs a chronic course. Development of Bowen disease in a case of vulvovaginal Crohn disease has been reported.[23] Rarely, SCC may develop in long-standing disease.[24]

Histologic features

The histology may show only edema, dilated lymphatics, or lymphangiectasia. More commonly, there are dermal or rarely subcutaneous noncaseating granulomata mainly of the sarcoidal type (Fig. 12.76). The latter may have a perivascular distribution.[25] Granulomas are usually sparse and may be missed unless multiple sections are examined. The histologic diagnosis can only be made after careful clinicopathological correlation.

Acute hemorrhagic edema of childhood

Clinical features

This is an unusual variant of leukocytoclastic vasculitis of infants and young children that may present as tenderness, redness, and swelling of the penis and scrotum with the development of more widespread hemorrhagic lesions.[1,2]

Pathogenesis and histologic features

Streptococci, staphylococci, and adenoviruses have been implicated. The histology shows typical features of a leukocytoclastic vasculitis.

Behcet disease

Behcet disease is a rare systemic vasculitic disorder characterized by attacks of acute inflammation causing painful orogenital ulceration and ocular involvement. Other skin lesions include erythema nodosum, pseudofolliculitis or acneiform folliculitis, and pathergy. The central nervous system, cardiovascular system, and gastrointestinal system can be severely affected. The pathogenesis is unknown. There is no diagnositic test so the diagnosis is made on the basis of ranked criteria. Histology is usually non-specific and does not distinguish idiopathic aphthae but sometimes necrotising vasculitis is evident.[1–3]

The vulval ulcers are typically larger and deeper than aphthae and can heal with scarring.

Necrotizing vasculitis

Peniloscrotal ulceration due to necrotizing vasculitis in association with Wegener granulomatosis, systemic lupus erythematosus, systemic vasculitis, polyarteritis nodosa, and hereditary spherocytosis with recurrent vascular necrosis has been reported.[1] Rubio et al.[2] describe a case of isolated penile ulceration due to a necrotizing vasculitis, with no evidence of systemic vasculitis that responded to systemic steroids. Fournier gangrene may show histologic evidence of necrotizing vasculitis,[3] and priapism has been documented as a manifestation of isolated genital vasculitis.[4]

Infectious diseases

Erythrasma

Clinical features

Erythrasma is a superficial infection of the skin at flexural sites, particularly in the inguinal and genitocrural folds (Fig. 12.77).[1] The skin between the toes and natal cleft may also be involved. The affected areas are covered in red-brown scaly plaques with well-demarcated edges. The rash is usually asymptomatic or mildly itchy. The affected areas fluoresce coral pink under Wood light. This feature is due to the presence of porphyrin and may be absent in some cases.[2] Very rare cases present with generalized involvement.[3] The disease may appear concomitantly with a dermatophytosis and this often makes the diagnosis difficult.[4]

Pathogenesis and histologic features

The organism involved is an aerobic, Gram-positive corynebacterium, *Corynebacterium minutissimum*,[5] which is a normal skin commensal.

Overgrowth and dermatitis are encouraged by the damp and warm conditions of a flexural zone. Obesity, friction, diabetes, and immunosuppression are all contributory factors.

The characteristic clinical picture and the presence of fluorescence under Wood light obviate the need for biopsies in most cases. A biopsy shows the presence of rods and filamentous organisms in the stratum corneum (*Figs 12.78* and *12.79*). Inflammation is minimal.

Tinea

Tinea (or 'ringworm') refers to superficial dermatophytosis. Tinea is a common disease of the pelvic girdle, especially of the groins (*Figs*

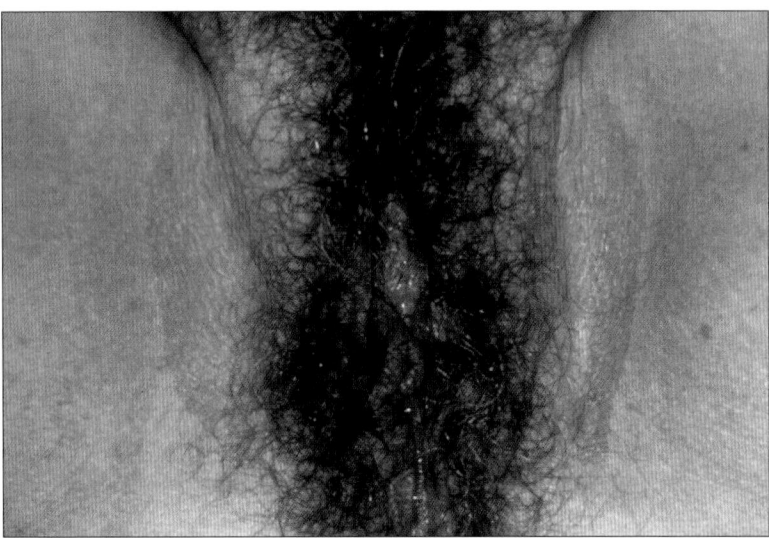

Fig. 12.77
Erythrasma: the flexural distribution and sharply demarcated border are characteristic features. By courtesy of the Institute of Dermatology, London, UK.

12.80–12.82) and is usually due to *Trichophyton rubrum*. It is not always a result of spread from the nails or feet although people with tinea manuum or unguium *can* spread it to the groins or perianal skin. Tinea cruris is itchy, and diagnosed by the presence of red-brown, scaly patches with raised, deeper red edges extending from the groins onto the abdomen (*Fig. 12.83*), buttocks (*Fig. 12.84*), and thighs. Annular lesions are not always obvious. Diagnosis is not always easy, because many patients have been previously misdiagnosed and/or partially treated with topical corticosteroids or topical antifungal agents. This presentation is called tinea incognito (*Fig. 12.85*), where the symptom of itch and the signs of inflammation, including redness, the scale, and the well-demarcated, often scalloped, elevated active margins, have been suppressed, although there is often subtle postinflammatory hyperpigmentation. Folliculitic lesions may be seen.

Tinea of the penis or scrotum[6] is not common, and when it occurs it is usually associated with crural disease. Rarely encountered is tinea on the glans penis with an itch or pain and producing an erythematous patch or a crop of scaly papules. Pandey et al.[7] associated penile tinea (in India) with occlusion due to the wearing of a langota – described as a T-shaped bandage tied over the genitalia.

Trichosporosis

Clinical features

Trichosporosis due to *Trichosporon beigelii* is a common form of genitocrural and perianal intertrigo in India.[1] Predominant symptoms are itching and/or burning. Scaly papules can accompany the intertrigo. Coexisting dermatophyte, *Candida*, trichomycosis, and erythrasma infection may be found. Infection rarely occurs elsewhere, including the scalp.[2,3]

Histologic features

The infection involves the hairs but not the surrounding skin. Microscopic examination of hair shafts shows white or brown soft nodules of varying size that can easily be removed.[2] The diagnosis is suspected by a KOH preparation to identify variable-sized arthrospores and is confirmed by culture.

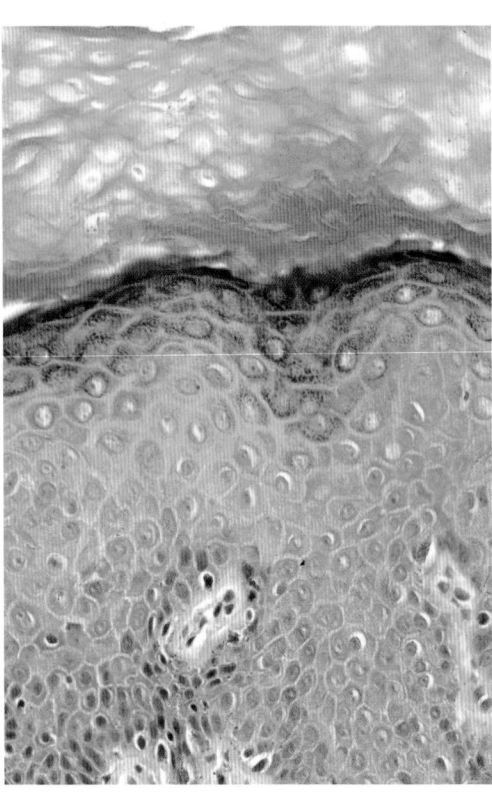

Fig. 12.78
Erythrasma: bacilli are just visible in the upper stratum corneum.

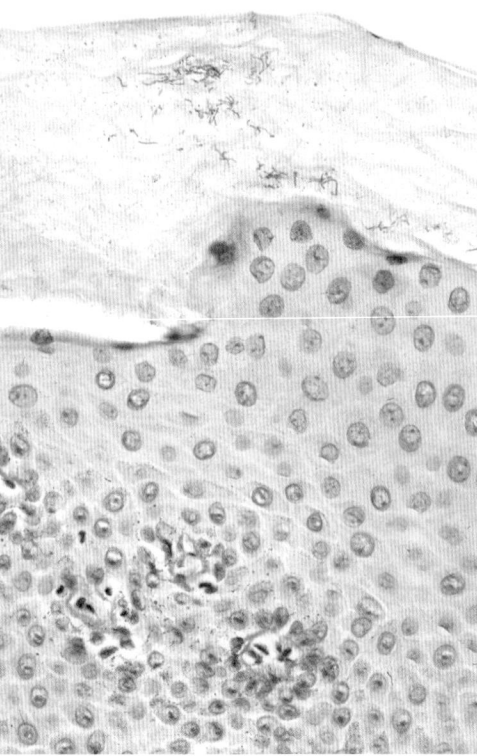

Fig. 12.79
Erythrasma: PAS stain showing elongated bacilli.

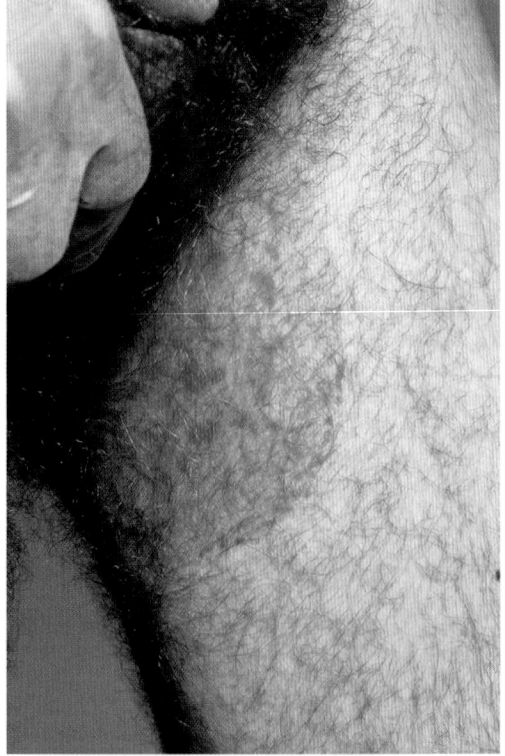

Fig. 12.80
Tinea cruris: there is a large erythematous lesion involving the inner thigh. From Bunker C. Male Genital Skin Disease. Saunders Ltd./Elsevier 2004.

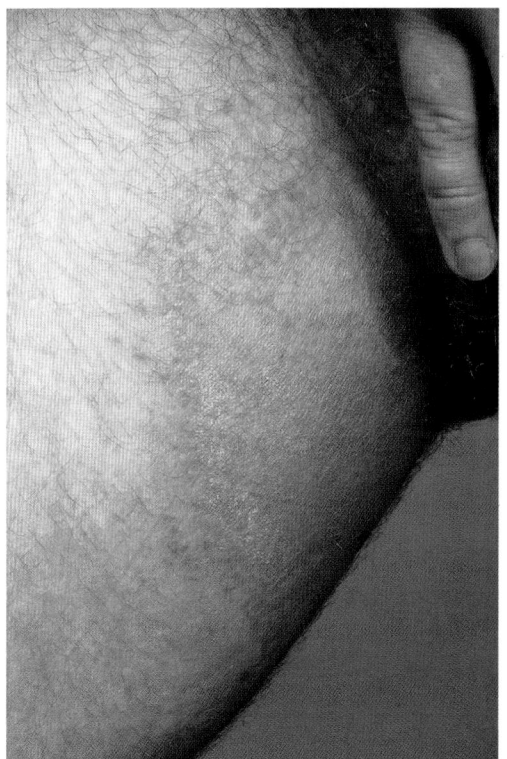

Fig. 12.81
Tinea cruris: note the acute margin. From Bunker C. Male Genital Skin Disease. Saunders Ltd./Elsevier 2004.

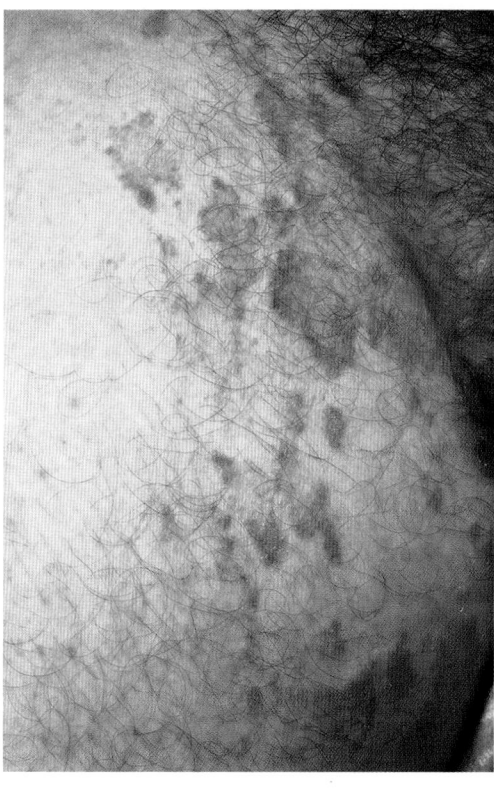

Fig. 12.82
Tinea cruris: close up view. From Bunker C. Male Genital Skin Disease. Saunders Ltd./Elsevier 2004.

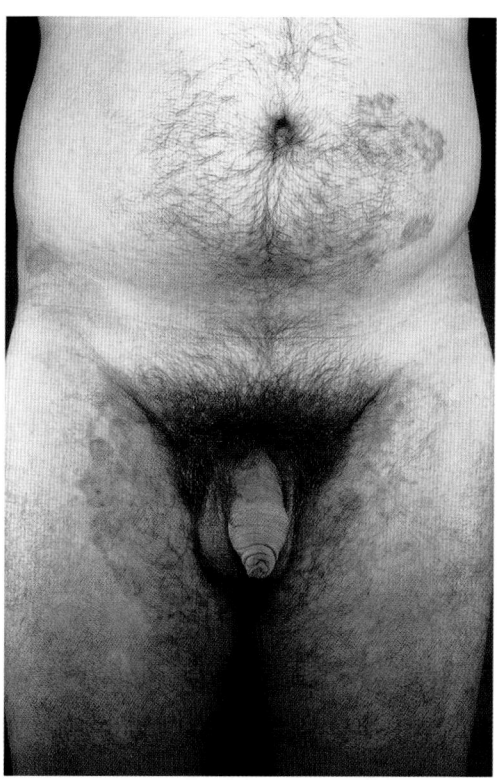

Fig. 12.83
Tinea cruris: in this patient, there is extensive involvement. From Bunker C. Male Genital Skin Disease. Saunders Ltd./Elsevier 2004.

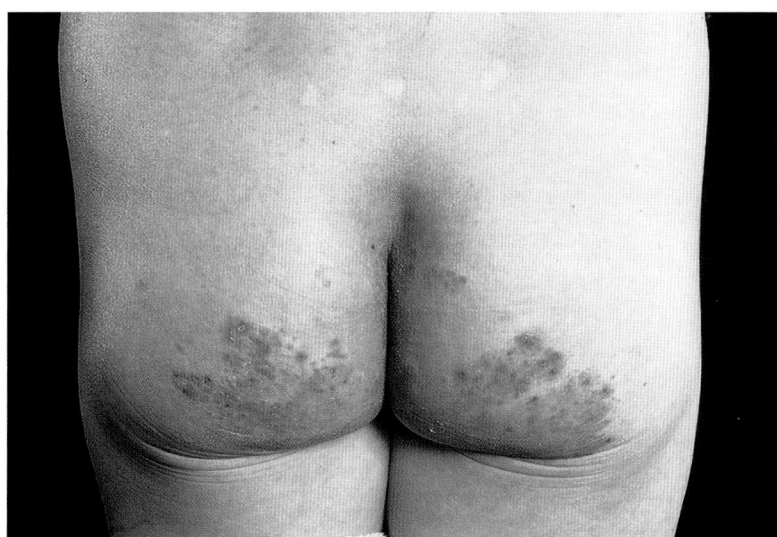

Fig. 12.84
Tinea cruris: note the bilateral involvement of the buttocks.

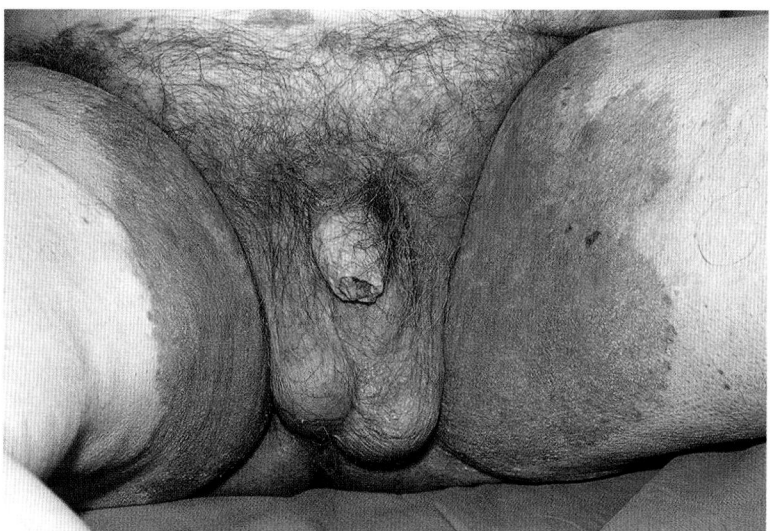

Fig. 12.85
Tinea incognito: there is extensive involvement of the abdomen, groins, thighs and scrotum. This followed injudicious use of topical steroids. From Bunker C. Male Genital Skin Disease. Saunders Ltd./Elsevier 2004.

Condyloma acuminatum (genital warts, HPV infection)

Clinical features

Genital warts (condyloma acuminatum) are usually caused by HPV types 6, 11, 16, 18, 30–32, 42–44, and 51–55.[1] HPV-7, usually associated with warts in butchers, can exceptionally be the cause of condylomas.[2] HPV-6 and 11 account for approximately 90% of these lesions.[3] However, more than one HPV type can be isolated from a single lesion.[4] They occur on the glans penis and prepuce or shaft as soft, fleshy (sometimes filiform) plaques and may extend into the meatus (Figs 12.86 and 12.87). On the shaft, they are less exophytic. Vulval lesions may be bulky and macerated, and can extend into the introitus (Figs 12.88–12.90). Lesions may be difficult to detect on clinical examination.[1] Vulval condylomata usually involve the labia minora, interlabial sulcus, or the area around the introitus. Similar fleshy and filiform soft masses may occur perianally and in the anus, more often in males (Fig. 12.91). Genital warts in children always raise the possibility of sexual abuse but can occur with close nonsexual contact.[5] However, nonvenereal viral warts (verruca vulgaris) mainly caused by HPV type 2 can occur in both young girls and less frequently in adult women, so HPV typing can be very important.[6] Young sexually active adults are the most frequently affected (second and third decades), and often in association with other sexually acquired infections.

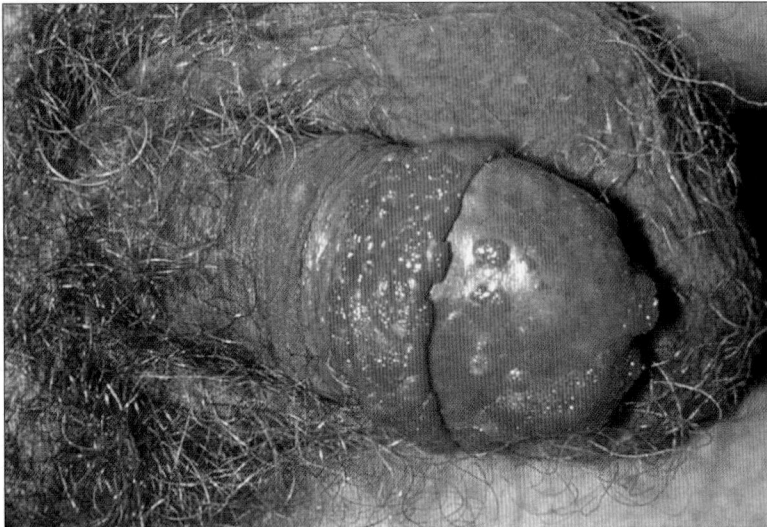

Fig. 12.86
Condyloma acuminatum: multiple erythematous, velvety plaques are present on the glans penis. By courtesy of the Institute of Dermatology, London, UK.

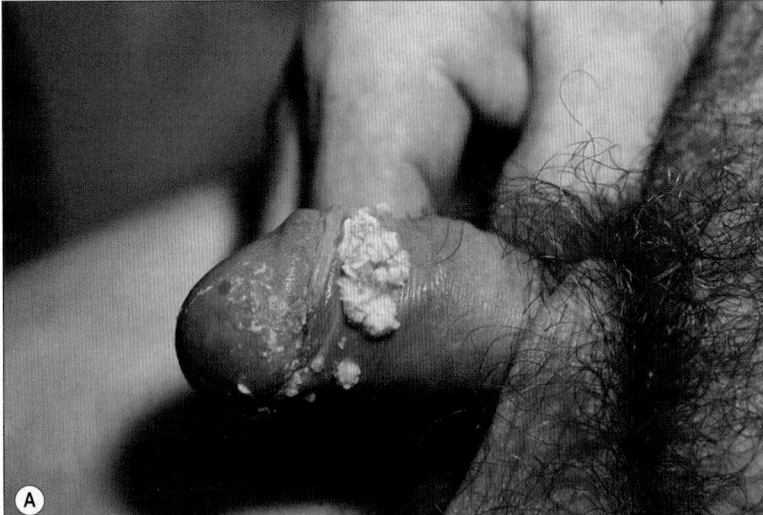

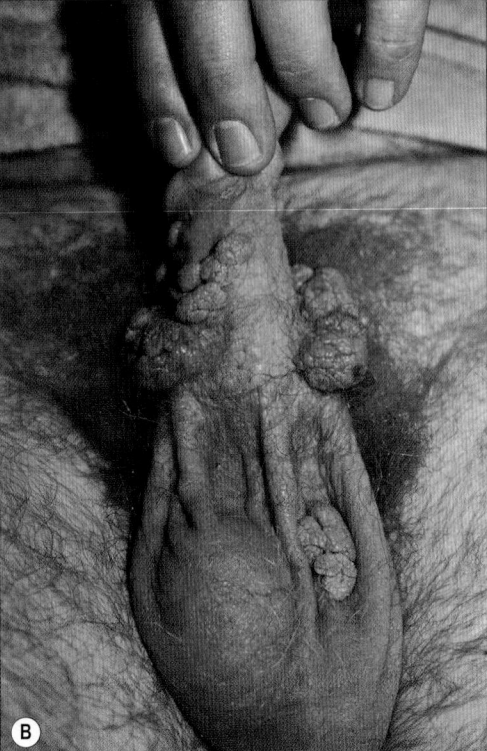

Fig. 12.87
Condyloma acuminatum: (**A**) in this patient, the lesions have a typical filiform appearance; (**B**) multiple condylomata are present on penis and scrotum. By courtesy of the Department of Genitourinary Medicine, St Thomas' Hospital, London, UK.

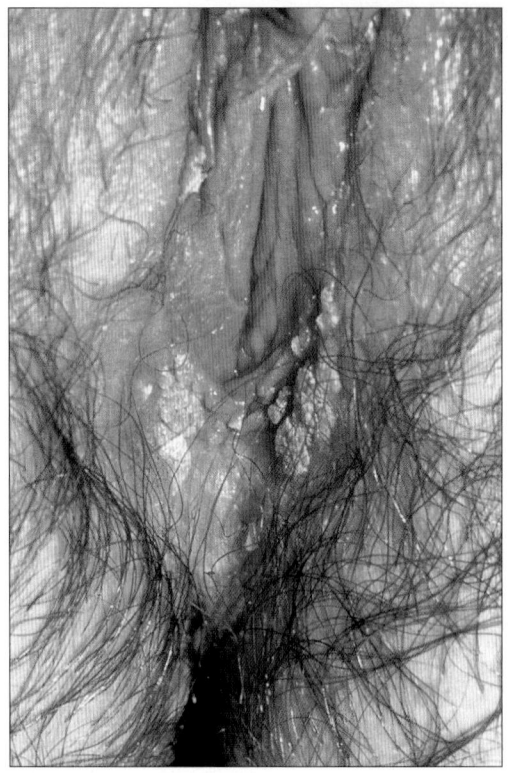

Fig. 12.88
Condyloma acuminatum: multiple gray lesions are evident on the labia minora and around the vestibule. By courtesy of the Institute of Dermatology, London, UK.

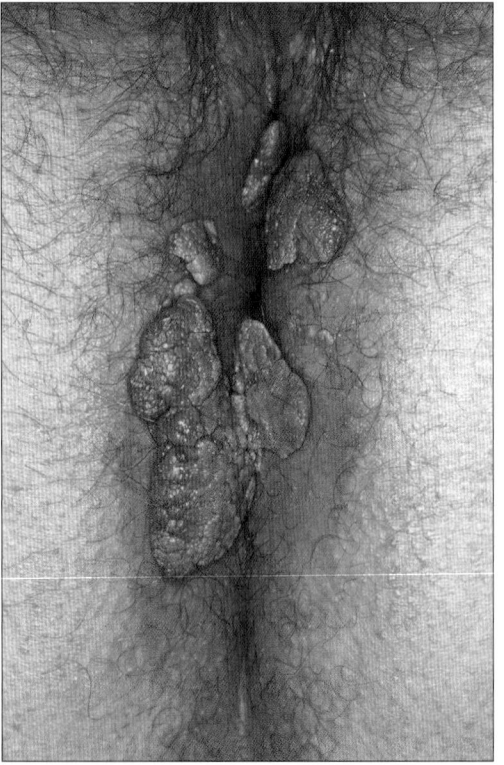

Fig. 12.89
Condyloma acuminatum: in this patient, the condylomata are pedunculated and have extended onto the thighs. By courtesy of the Institute of Dermatology, London, UK.

Rarely, condyloma acuminatum presents in the oral cavity.[7] Condylomata have also been reported in the abdominal pannus fold of a few obese patients.[8]

It is important to recognize that a significant proportion of genital HPV infections are asymptomatic.[1] The female partners of male patients with genital warts have been shown to have an increased risk of cervical HPV infection and intraepithelial neoplasia.[9] Cervical neoplasia associated with preexistent vulval warts has also been related to immunosuppression, at least in some patients.[10] Up to 80% of invasive cervical squamous carcinomas have been shown to contain HPV DNA. Types 16, 18, 31–33, 35, 39, 42, and 51–54 are most commonly associated with cancer of the cervix,

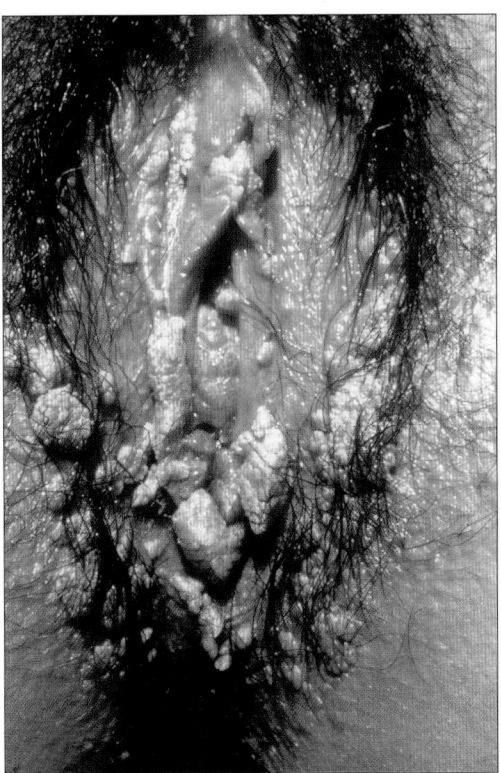

Fig. 12.90
Condyloma acuminatum: there is very extensive disease. The patient is at considerable risk of developing cervical disease. By courtesy of R.A. Marsden, MD, St George's Hospital, London, UK.

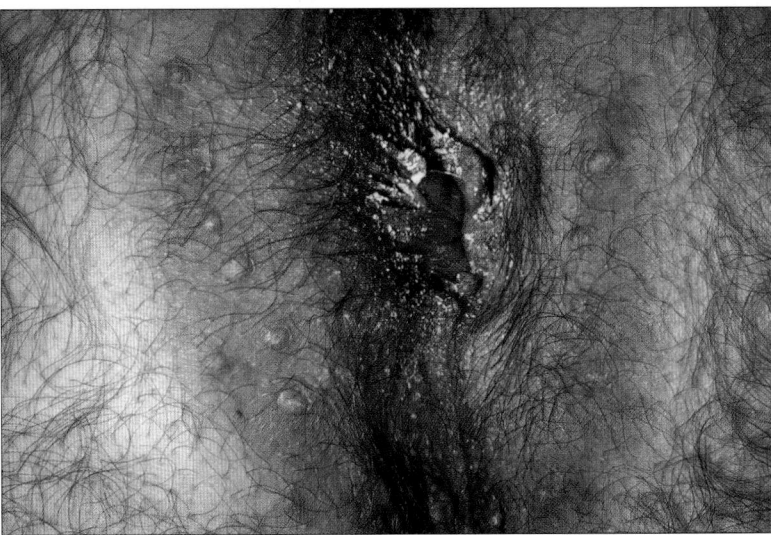

Fig. 12.91
Condyloma acuminatum: perianal involvement is likely to be associated with homosexual activity. By courtesy of R.A. Marsden, MD, St George's Hospital, London, UK.

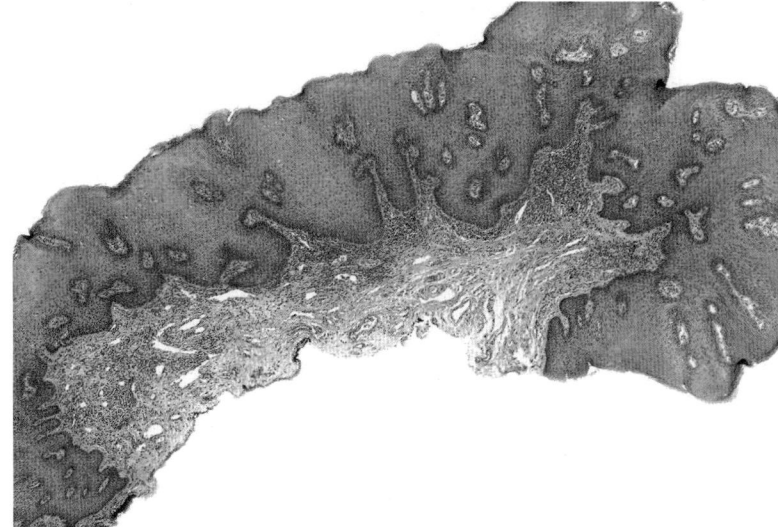

Fig. 12.92
Condyloma acuminatum: there is focal parakeratosis, slight papillomatosis and very marked acanthosis. The lower border is sharply demarcated.

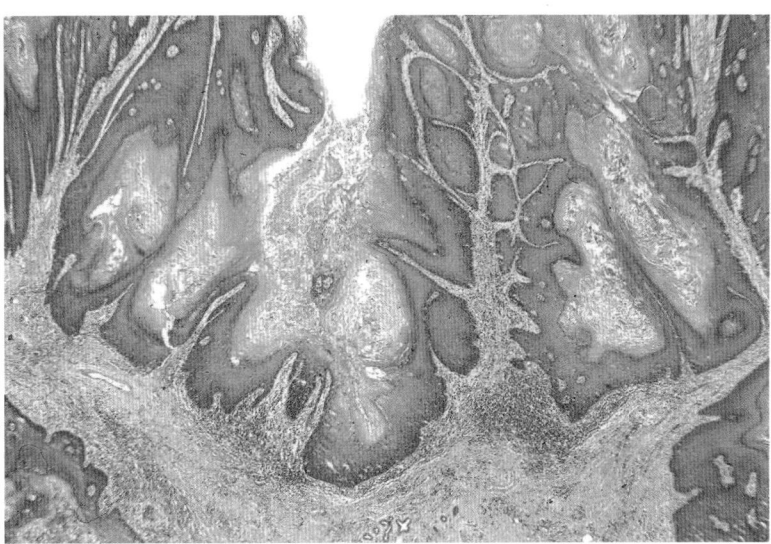

Fig. 12.93
Condyloma acuminatum: this is a much more florid example. Note the gross papillomatosis and very marked acanthosis.

Histologic features

Condylomata acuminata are characterized by marked acanthosis with a solid or trabecular pattern and a broad, rounded, exophytic growth (*Figs 12.92* and *12.93*). There is a sharp, fairly regular, deep margin. The surface of the lesion is hyperkeratotic and parakeratotic. Superficial vacuolated keratinocytes (koilocytes) are characteristic (*Fig. 12.94*). The vacuolated epithelium is often most marked in the declivities. Care must be taken not to confuse koilocytes with the vacuolated, glycogenated keratinocytes of mucosal epithelia or with artifactually vacuolated keratinocytes. Distinction can be made fairly readily as koilocytes have an enlarged, wrinkled, hyperchromatic nucleus.

Care should be taken in the histologic interpretation of lesions that have previously been treated with podophyllin (although this treatment is seldom used nowadays since the advent of imiquimod). These can display prominent degenerative changes with cytoplasmic vacuolation, nuclear enlargement, and metaphase arrest. The changes, however, tend to be more focal, and abnormal mitotic figures are not seen.[17,18] Immunohistochemical stains for papillomavirus common antigen have been used to confirm the diagnosis, but this is only positive in about 60% of cases.[19] More recently, broad-spectrum in situ hybridization in paraffin-embedded tissue has become available.[20]

vulva, and penis[11,12] Malignant transformation of genital warts is rare but may be found in association with penile bowenoid papulosis and VIN usual type (undifferentiated).[11,13] In the most recent classification of VIN,[14] condylomata acuminata are classified as low-grade squamous intraepithelial lesions.[14]

A large, exuberant, and locally destructive variant of condyloma (Buschke-Löwenstein tumor) may rarely be encountered.[15] This is associated with HPV-6, 11, or 16. It is considered by many to be a variant of verrucous carcinoma, a subtype of well-differentiated squamous carcinoma (see below). However, the issue remains controversial and other authors regard it as a distinctive entity. They may show malignant progression if irradiated. The condition has been described in an HIV-positive patient.[16]

Juvenile laryngeal papillomata containing HPV-6 and 11 can be seen in children born to mothers with condylomata acuminata.[1]

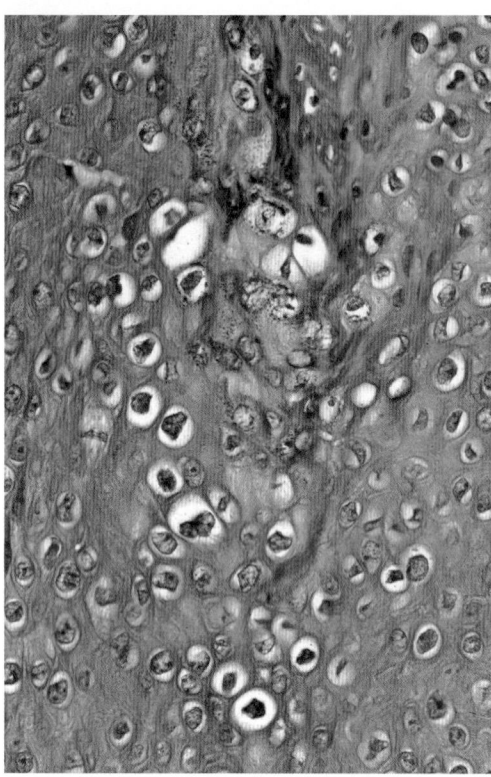

Fig. 12.94
Condyloma acuminatum: there are conspicuous koilocytes with irregular nuclei and vacuolated cytoplasm.

Giant condyloma acuminatum (Buschke-Löwenstein tumor) occurs most frequently on the genitalia, and is larger and more cauliflower-like.[21] It shows some tendency to endophytic growth, but without any suggestion of frank infiltration. It can recur locally. Anal condylomata may develop bowenoid features, and occasionally invasive tumors supervene.[22]

Syphilis

Clinical features

The incidence of syphilis fell dramatically after the introduction of penicillin in the 1940s. In recent years the incidence has been rising annually largely due to the increased number of cases of HIV infection. Drug abuse and high-risk sexual behavior are also contributory factors.[1] The increase in the incidence of syphilis continues, especially in HIV-infected patients with predilection for young homosexual black males.[2]

In the sixteenth century, syphilis carried a high mortality associated with a chronic disfiguring and disabling disease. The disease currently appears less aggressive, even in untreated cases. It is highly infectious, with the risk of transmission from an infected partner estimated at up to 60%.[3] The chance of acquiring the disease depends on the number of exposures, type of sexual practice, and the location and number of the partner's lesions. There is a close relationship between syphilis and HIV infection, and both diseases can be acquired together.[4] It is recognized that diseases such as syphilis that induce genital ulceration increase the risk of acquiring HIV infection.[4]

The causative organism is *Treponema pallidum*, a spirochete with fastidious growth requirements. Transmission is primarily sexual. An endemic form known as bejel, caused by an identical organism, occurs in children living in conditions of poor hygiene and is transmitted by cutaneous inoculation.[5] Other endemic forms have been associated with shared drinking vessels when some members of the community have oral or labial syphilitic lesions.

The typical initial lesion, a chancre, develops 20–30 days after exposure to the organism at the site of inoculation. This can be anywhere on the anogenital skin, more often on the glans penis (especially the coronal sulcus), the shaft, or prepuce, or on the labia majora or minora (*Figs 12.95–12.99*). At least 5% of primary chancres arise at extragenital locations, most commonly oral, but virtually every other part of the skin surface may be affected

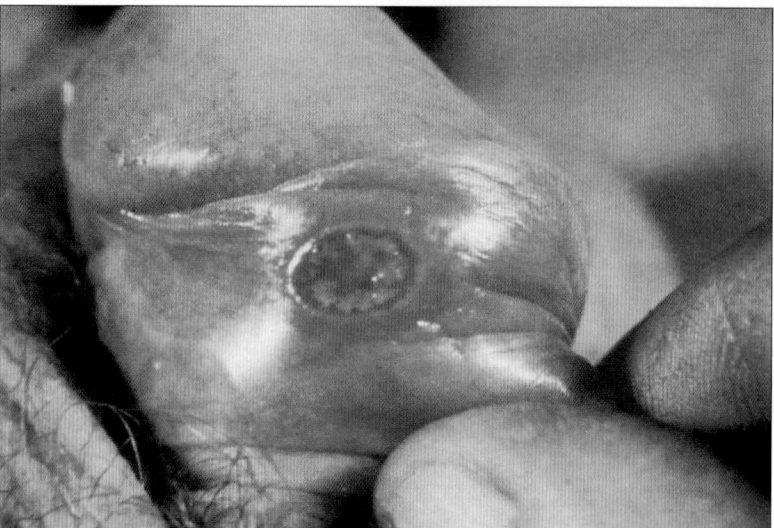

Fig. 12.95
Primary chancre: the chancre is a painless ulcer with an indurated edge. The base is yellow and harbors large numbers of spirochetes. By courtesy of F. Lim, MD, King's College Hospital, London, UK.

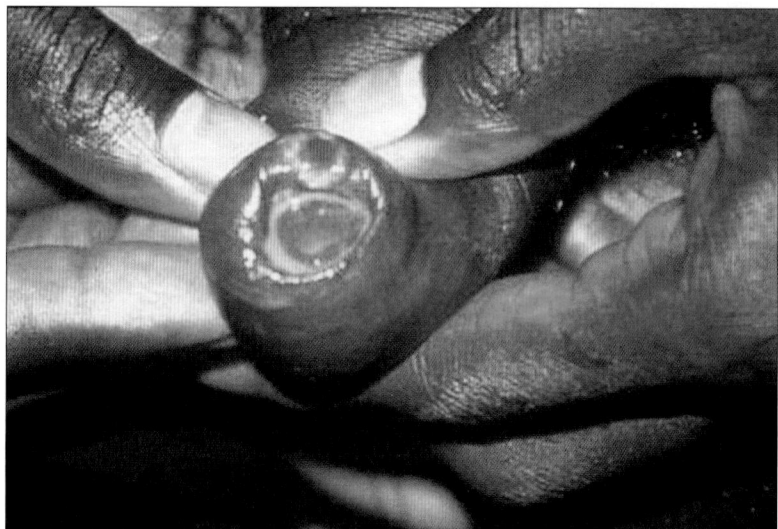

Fig. 12.96
Primary syphilis: painless lymphadenopathy is often present. By courtesy of C. Furlonge, MD, Port of Spain, Trinidad.

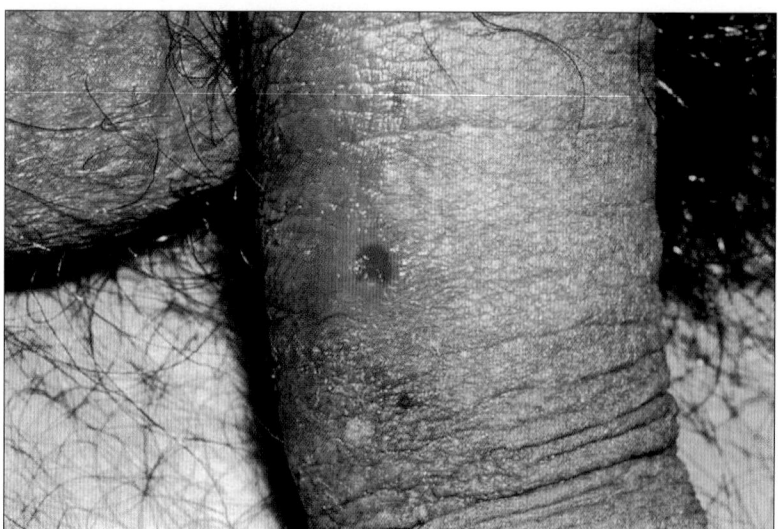

Fig. 12.97
Primary syphilis: in this patient, the chancre has a punched-out appearance. By courtesy of the Institute of Dermatology, London, UK.

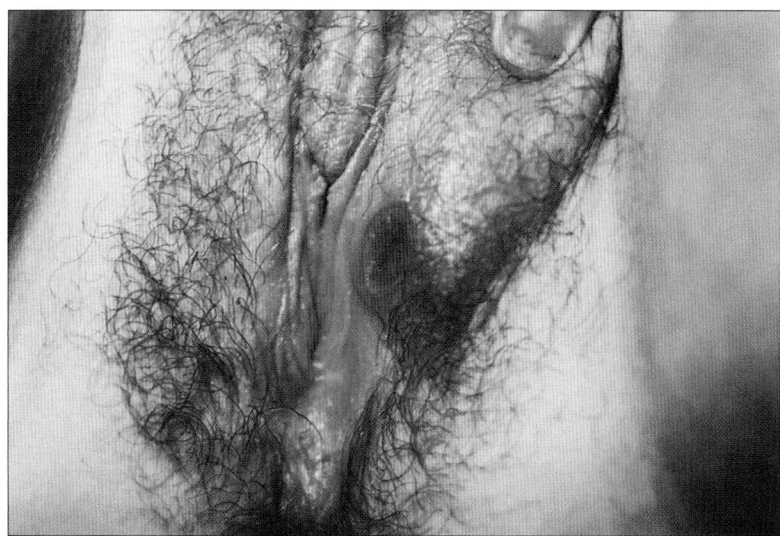

Fig. 12.98
Primary syphilis: a typical chancre is present on the left labium majus. By courtesy of R.N. Thin, MD, St Thomas' Hospital, London, UK.

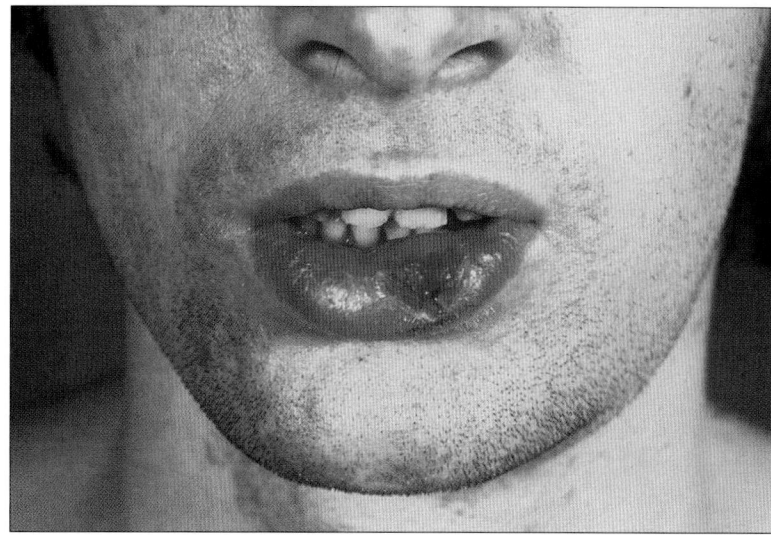

Fig. 12.100
Primary syphilis: oral chancres are most often located on the lip. By courtesy of R.N. Thin, MD, St Thomas' Hospital, London, UK.

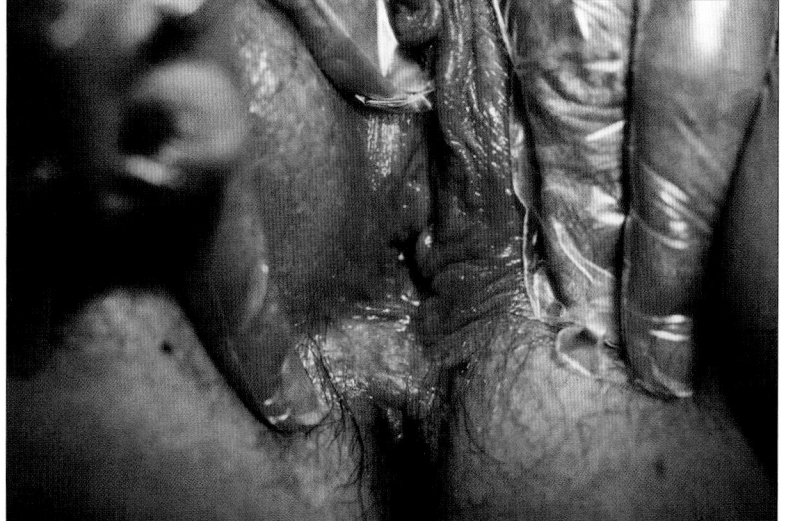

Fig. 12.99
Primary syphilis: typical 'kissing ulcers' are present within the vestibule. By courtesy of D. Barlowe, MD, St Thomas' Hospital, London, UK.

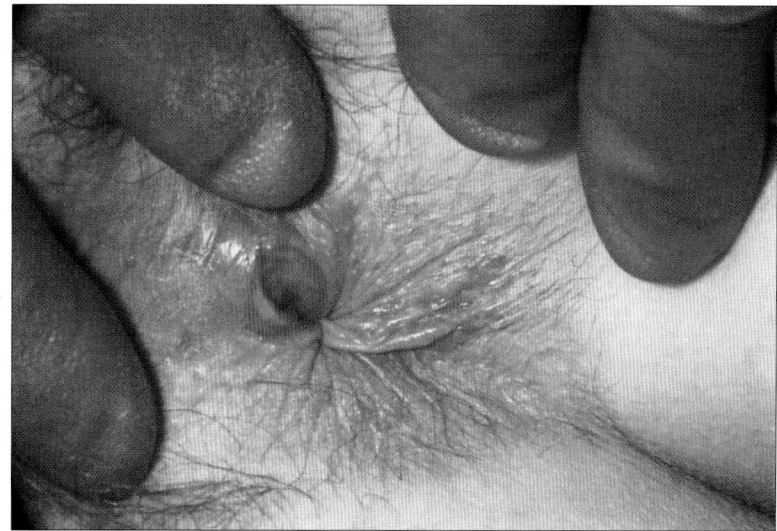

Fig. 12.101
Primary syphilis: a chancre is present at the edge of the anal ostium. By courtesy of R.N. Thin, MD, St Thomas' Hospital, London, UK.

including the tonsils, fingers, eyelids, and nipples (*Figs 12.100* and *12.101*).[6] Lesions in the vagina or cervix may go undetected. The chancre appears as an indurated, punched-out, painless ulcer. It is usually accompanied by painless lymphadenopathy. This resolves without scarring after 1–5 weeks.

The secondary cutaneous lesions (syphilids) are highly infectious and may mimic virtually any skin disorder. They present 6–8 weeks after the appearance of the chancre. They develop insidiously (in up to 80% of patients), with a roseolar, macular–erythematous rash, on the head, face, and neck followed by a polymorphic papular eruption. The macules measure 5–10 mm in diameter, are not pruritic, and particularly occur on the trunk, abdomen, and limbs, especially the palms and soles (*Figs 12.102–12.107*).[7] The papular lesions are characteristically coppery red in color and 3–10 mm in diameter. Hypopigmentation of the neck is known as the 'collar of venus'.

Other manifestations described include condylomata (in intertriginous areas), annular, lichenoid, papulosquamous lesions (psoriasiform), arcuate lesions, corymbose brownish-red papules (Gr. *korymbos*, clusters of ivy flowers), bullous, erythema multiforme-like follicular and pustular variants on the skin, with erosive ulcers (mucous patches), often of 'snail track' type, and the (highly infectious) condylomata lata affecting the mucosae (*Figs 12.108–12.111*).[8–15] Keratoderma can also be seen.[16] Large hypertrophic condylomata are known as framboiseform syphilids.[6] Other variants described

are acneiform, varioliform, and rarely, necrotic (*Fig. 12.112*). Lesions tend to be widely disseminated and often symmetrical in distribution. Papular involvement of the scalp may result in nonscarring, patchy alopecia (*Fig. 12.113*).[17] The alopecia induced by secondary syphilis is known as alopecia syphilitica and has a characteristic, moth-eaten appearance. The beard, eyebrows, and eyelashes may also be affected. Telogen effluvium has also been described.

Rare 'malignant' forms of syphilis (lues maligna) present with rapid progression, papulopustular lesions, much ulceration, and rupial lesions (Gr. *rhypos*, filth; necrotic lesions covered by dirty, lamellated encrustation resembling oyster shells) mainly affecting the face and limbs.[18] Patients can also present with fever, eye involvement, myalgia, lymphadenitis, and hepatosplenomegaly.[19] This form of syphilis has been described in association with HIV infection and is characterized by necrotic and ulcerative lesions.[20]

Secondary syphilis manifestations have typically been described as non-pruritic, but this is not always the case.[21] Indeed, in the series of 105 patients with secondary syphilis published by Chapel, 42% complained of pruritus.[22] Resolution may be accompanied by hypo- or hyperpigmentation. Lymphadenopathy, which may be widespread and is painless and rubbery, occurs in 50–85% of patients. The cutaneous manifestations are often accompanied by pyrexia, headache, weight loss, and non-specific muscle and joint

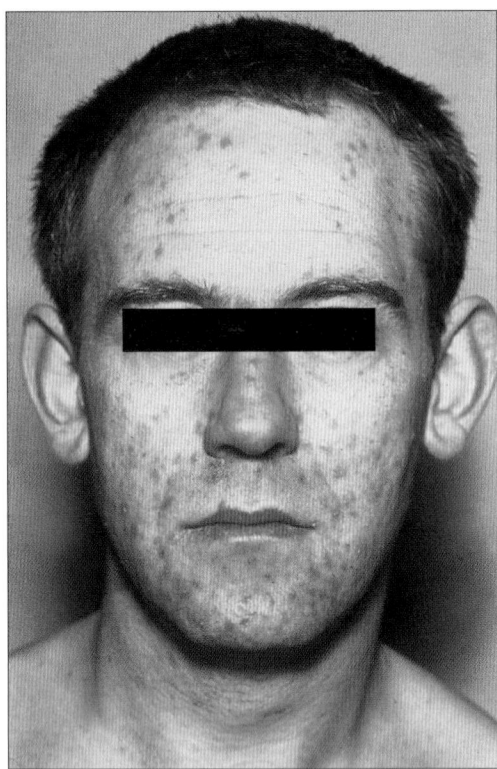

Fig. 12.102
Secondary syphilis:
the face is commonly
affected. Note the
numerous papules. By
courtesy of R.N. Thin,
MD, St Thomas' Hospital,
London, UK.

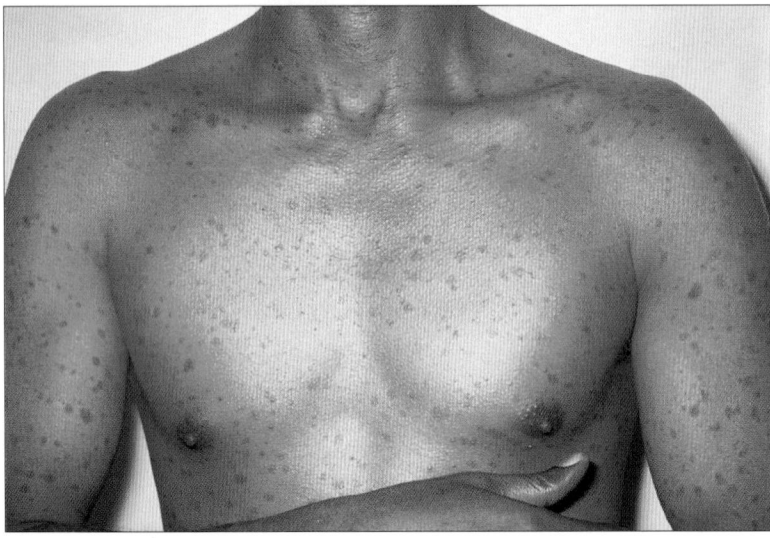

Fig. 12.103
Secondary syphilis: this patient shows a widespread hyperpigmented
maculopapular eruption. By courtesy of C. Furlonge, MD, Port of Spain, Trinidad.

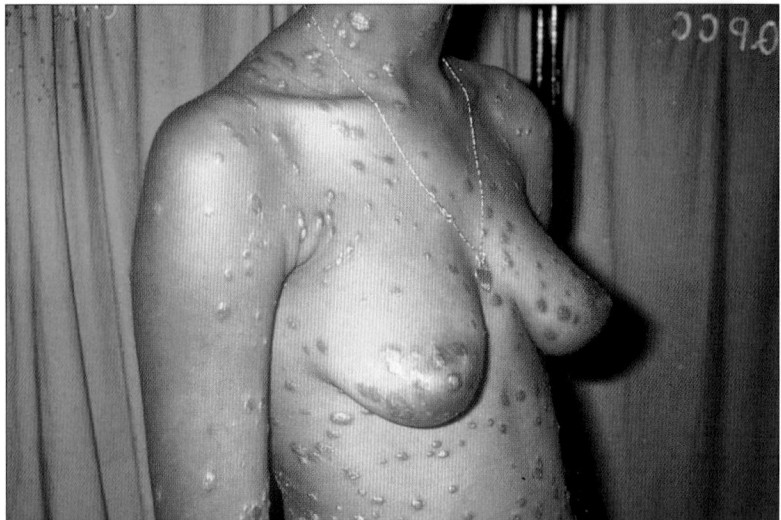

Fig. 12.104
Secondary syphilis: note the widespread papules and nodules many of which
have a hypertrophic appearance. By courtesy of C. Furlonge, MD, Port of Spain,
Trinidad.

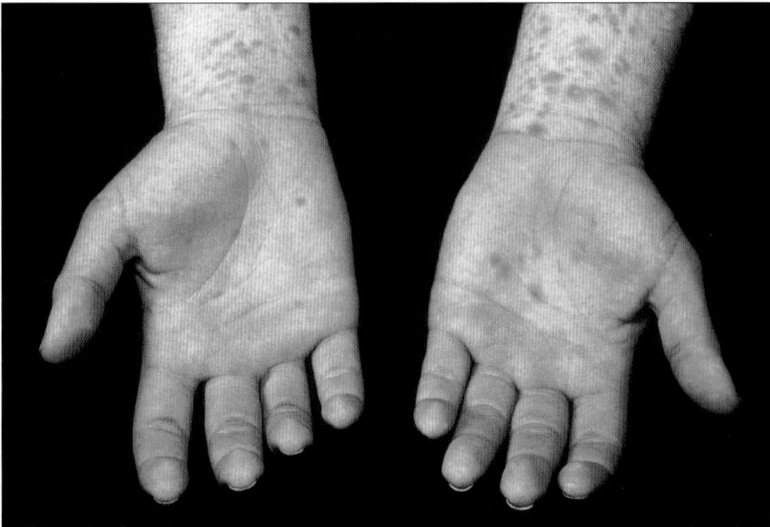

Fig. 12.105
Secondary syphilis: the palms are almost invariably affected. By courtesy of the
Institute of Dermatology, London, UK.

aches. Periostitis can rarely occur.[23] Ocular involvement including uveitis and retinitis can occur at any stage of the disease.[24] Untreated lesions of syphilis resolve in 2–10 weeks, but if treated., there may be a self-limited febrile reaction known as the Jarisch–Herxheimer reaction associated with systemic symptoms.

Atypical clinical forms of syphilis have been reported in HIV-positive patients,[25,26] and multiple genital ulcers may occur in primary syphilis as well as concomitant ulcer with secondary syphilis.[27]

Secondary syphilis is followed by a latent phase, which may precede a change to:
- seronegativity and cure,
- persistent seropositivity without further lesions,
- development of tertiary lesions.

These late lesions involve mainly the cardiovascular (aortic incompetence) and central nervous system (tabes dorsalis and general paresis of the insane), but cutaneous lesions are seen as noduloulcerative lesions and gummata that tend to break down with central necrosis and suppuration. Gummata may

occur up to 15 years after the initial infection. They are painless, frequently ulcerated, firm subcutaneous nodules that show a predilection for the scalp, face, chest, and legs (*Fig. 12.114*).[28] Noduloulcerative late syphilitic lesions present as superficial nodules that extend peripherally and heal centrally to form ulcerated serpiginous plaques. Lesions of tertiary syphilis can be seen in internal organs and may clinically mimic cancer.[29]

Infants born to infected mothers may have widespread lesions reflecting a systemic infection (congenital syphilis). Development of the disease is mainly associated with lack of antenatal screening. These include fibrosis in many organs, with inflammatory changes seen particularly in bones and lungs. Vesicular skin lesions and maldevelopment of teeth and bone are also sometimes evident. Later changes of congenital syphilis are classically frontal bossing, a short maxilla, a high arched palate, chronic interstitial keratitis, notched (Hutchinson) incisors, Mulberry molars, VIII cranial nerve deafness, and saddle nose.[30] Other manifestations include painless hydroarthrosis, perforation of the nasal septum and palate, and cardiovascular and neurological changes, as seen in late-stage adult disease.

Pathogenesis and histologic features

T. pallidum is a slender, coiled organism, 6–16 μm long, capable of an undulating, corkscrew-like motion. The organisms are readily visualized in

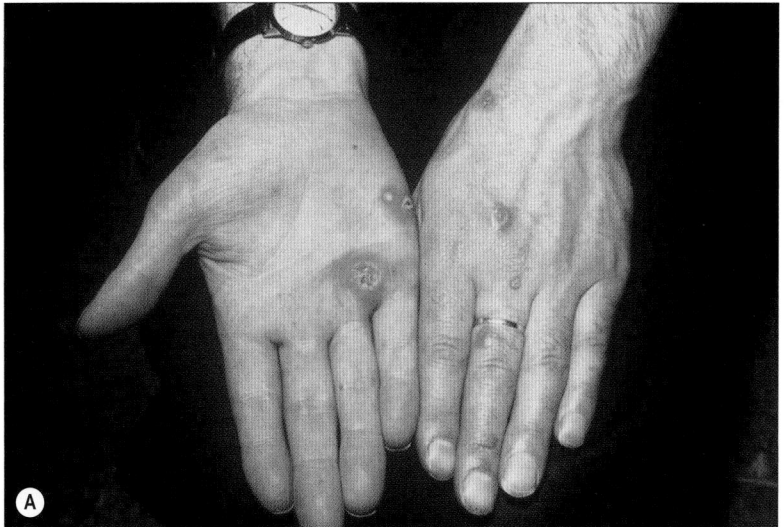

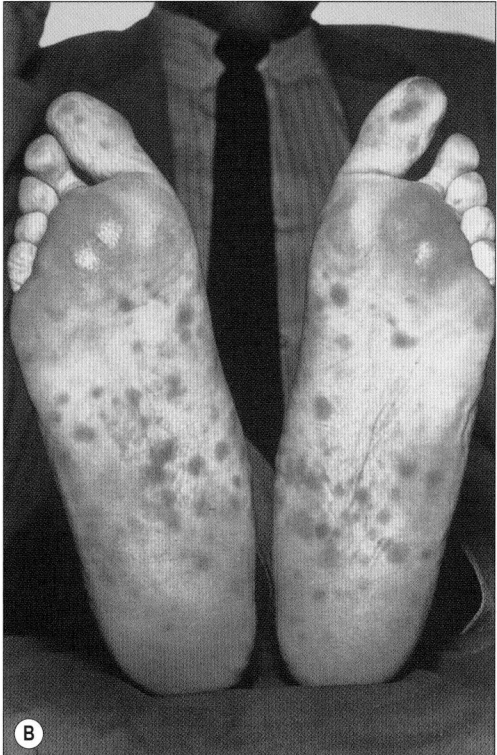

Fig. 12.106
(**A**, **B**) Secondary syphilis: erythematous and scaly papules involving the palms and soles are present in this patient with secondary syphilis. (**A**) By courtesy of R.A. Marsden, MD, St George's Hospital, London, UK; (**B**) by courtesy of R.N. Thin, MD, St Thomas' Hospital, London, UK.

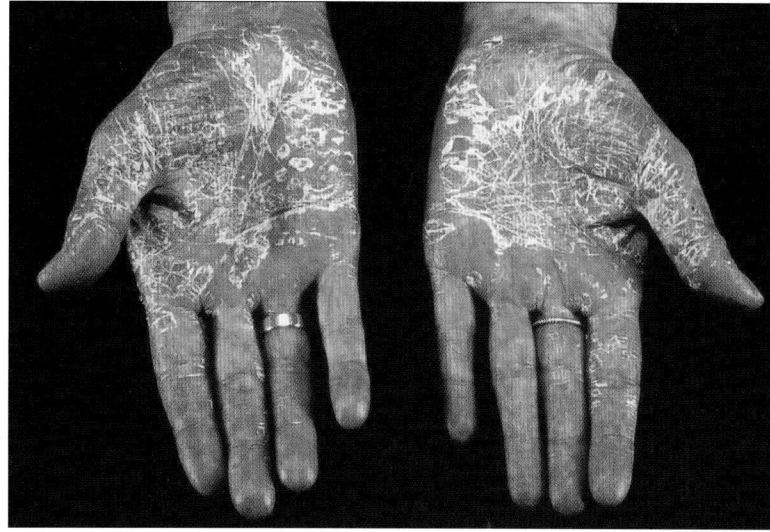

Fig. 12.107
Secondary syphilis: in this patient, typical copper penny macules with surrounding annular scale (Biette collarette) contrast with confluent exfoliation on the palms. By courtesy of the Institute of Dermatology, London, UK.

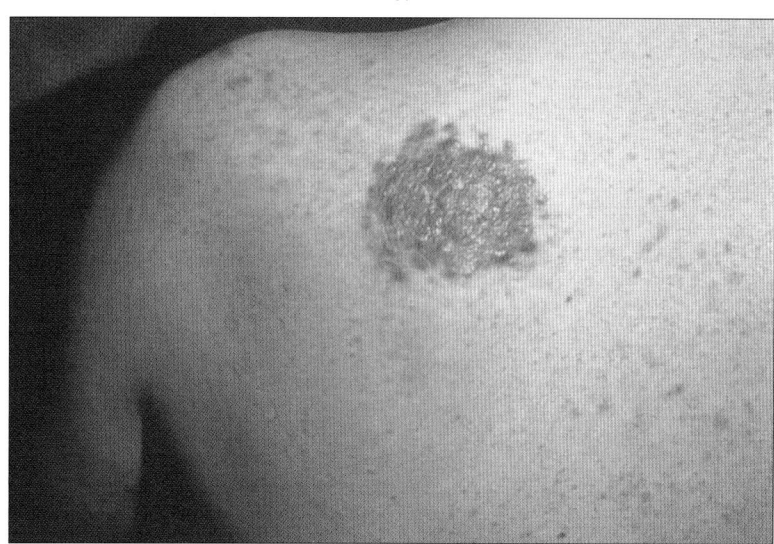

Fig. 12.108
Secondary syphilis: this is a typical corymbose eruption. Note the circumscribed, confluent, erythematous scaly papules. By courtesy of the Institute of Dermatology, London, UK.

material from a primary chancre with dark-field illumination, but can also be grown in culture. The usually nonpathogenic spirochetes, which live as commensals around the gingiva, although still termed *Treponema*, are quite different, not least in that they have a right-handed spiral in contrast to the left-handed spiral of *T. pallidum* and other pathogenic spirochetes.

T. pallidum produces a nonantigenic mucin coat, which may be protective in early infections. This mucoid element may be increased by a component produced by host inflammatory cells. A hyaluronidase is associated with the surface of *T. pallidum* and may facilitate dissemination in tissues.[31]

After the first inoculation of the spirochete through mucosa or abraded skin, the organism becomes systemically distributed before the primary chancre develops at the site of inoculation and numerous spirochetes can again be identified.

The chancre is characterized histologically by initial epidermal hyperplasia with an intense lymphohistiocytic and neutrophil infiltrate in the dermis (*Figs 12.115–12.117*). Plasma cells are present, but may be more numerous in papular and papulosquamous secondary lesions (see below). The overlying epithelium becomes ulcerated, and the adjacent epidermis often shows pseudoepitheliomatous hyperplasia and infiltration by neutrophils. The induration of the primary lesion is due to a large amount of mucoid

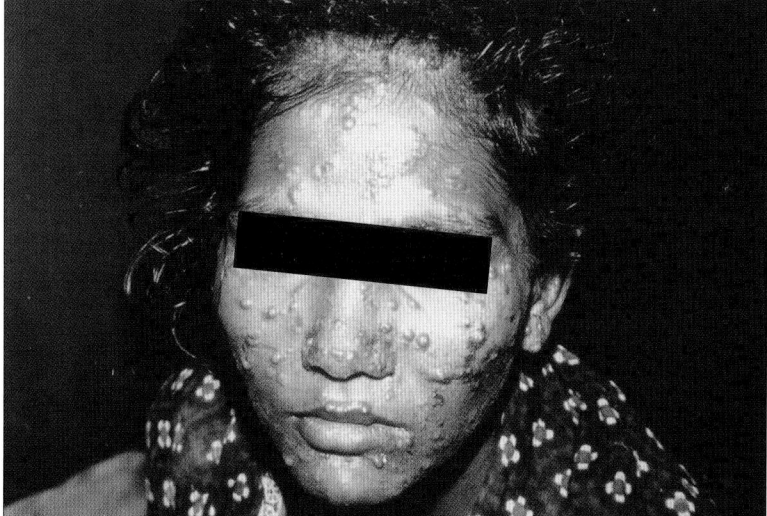

Fig. 12.109
Secondary syphilis: pustular lesions, as seen on this patient's face, are a rare manifestation. By courtesy of R.N. Thin, MD, St Thomas' Hospital, London, UK.

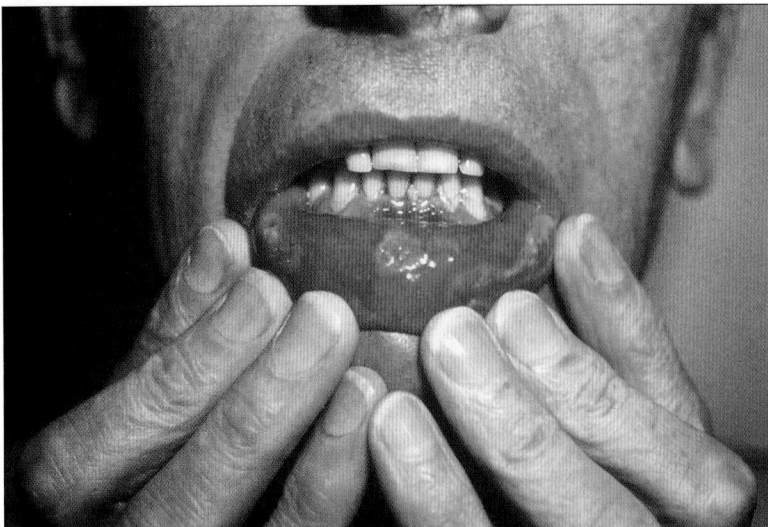

Fig. 12.110
Secondary syphilis: note the symmetrically distributed 'snail track' ulcers. By courtesy of R.N. Thin, MD, St Thomas' Hospital, London, UK.

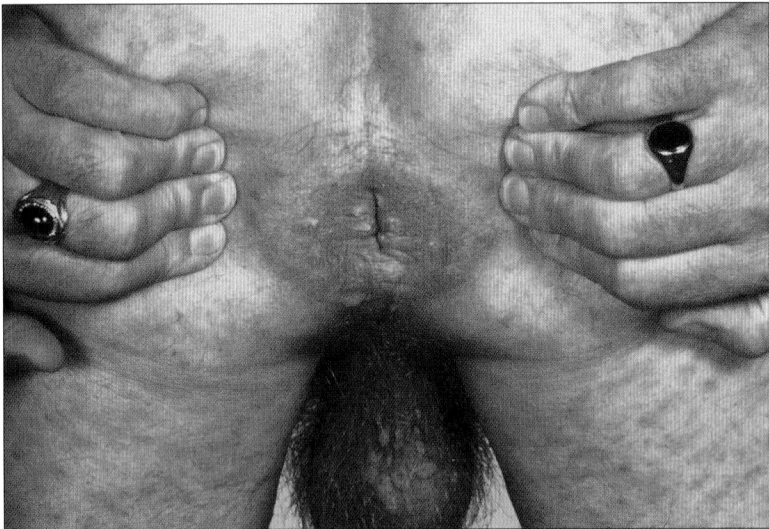

Fig. 12.111
Secondary syphilis: early perianal condylomata lata. By courtesy of R.N. Thin, MD, St Thomas' Hospital, London, UK.

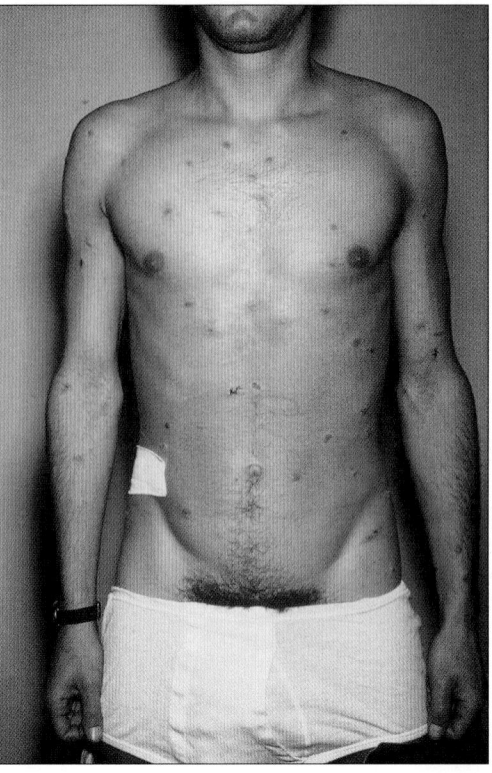

Fig. 12.112
Secondary syphilis: in this patient, the lesions greatly resemble pityriasis lichenoides. By courtesy of R.A. Marsden, MD, St George's Hospital, London, UK.

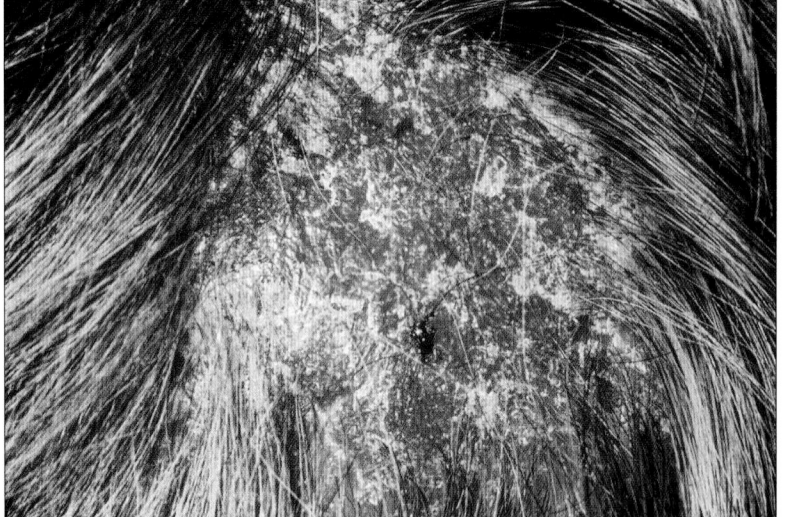

Fig. 12.113
Secondary syphilis: scalp involvement is not uncommon. Note the scaling and hair loss. By courtesy of M.M. Black, MD, Institute of Dermatology, London, UK.

substance. Vascular endothelial cell swelling is often prominent. The organisms can be demonstrated by dark-field examination of a smear taken from the primary lesion. A silver stain such as Warthin-Starry and particularly immunohistochemistry are also useful in demonstrating the organisms in tissue sections. By electron microscopy, the spirochetes are often found in macrophages, endothelial cells, plasma cells, and in the intercellular space close to small blood vessels.[32] Resolution of the chancre, while appearing to coincide with immunity to further infection and demonstration of antibodies, nevertheless does not impede the widespread dissemination and proliferation of the treponeme. This leads to its recrudescence in the secondary phase, a paradox that is not understood.

Secondary lesions show variable appearances depending to some extent on the clinical morphology (*Figs 12.118–12.124*).[33–36] Purely macular lesions are not distinctive and show a rather sparse perivascular lymphohistiocytic infiltrate with few, if any, plasma cells. The epidermis is normal. As the lesions develop a papular morphology, superficial and deep perivascular infiltrates develop, which may also adopt a bandlike distribution. Involvement of the subcutis is rare. Plasma cells become more numerous, and parakeratosis, acanthosis, spongiosis, and exocytosis may be evident. Thick-walled blood vessels with swollen endothelial cells are characteristic. A prominent infiltrate is often present around hair follicles and sweat glands. Early

lesions showing perivascular neutrophils and a heavy neutrophilic infiltrate mimicking Sweet syndrome has been reported.[37] Psoriasiform syphilids show parakeratosis and acanthosis with extended (psoriasiform) epidermal ridges. The inflammatory cell infiltrate is both perivascular and superficial, and bandlike in distribution. Spongiform pustulation and neutrophil exocytosis may be evident, and focal cell hydropic degeneration can sometimes be present.[8,36] Keratinocyte necrosis may occasionally be seen. Leukocytoclastic vasculitis is very rare.[38] A recent study reported the most frequent histologic features to be psoriasiform hyperplasia with slender elongated rete ridges, plasma cells, and endothelial cell swelling.[39]

Erythrocyte extravasation may be a feature of both papular and papulosquamous variants. A granulomatous element has been described in both papular and papulosquamous eruptions, but this is not a constant feature.[36] In addition to a dense dermal infiltrate, large numbers of plasma cells and occasional giant cells are seen in corymbose syphilis. The number of organisms in secondary syphilis varies. Traditionally, they have been identified by

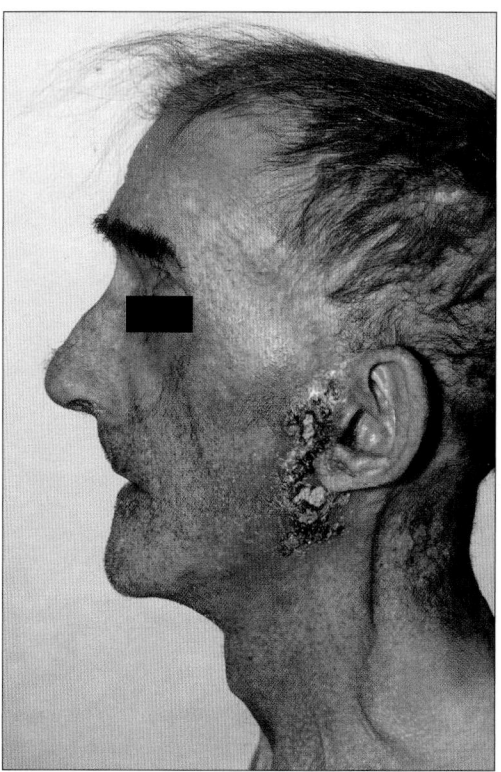

Fig. 12.114
Syphilis: the presence of gummatous cutaneous lesions as seen in this elderly male is now a very rare manifestation. By courtesy of M.M. Black, MD, Institute of Dermatology, London, UK.

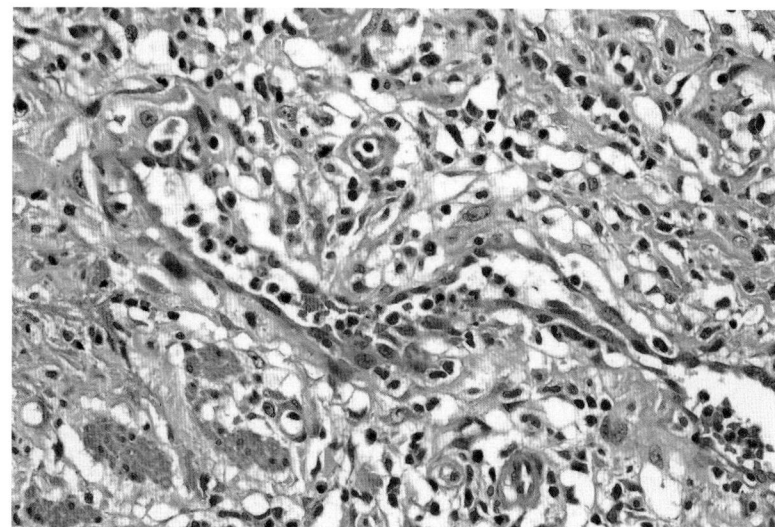

Fig. 12.116
Primary syphilis: note the marked endothelial swelling.

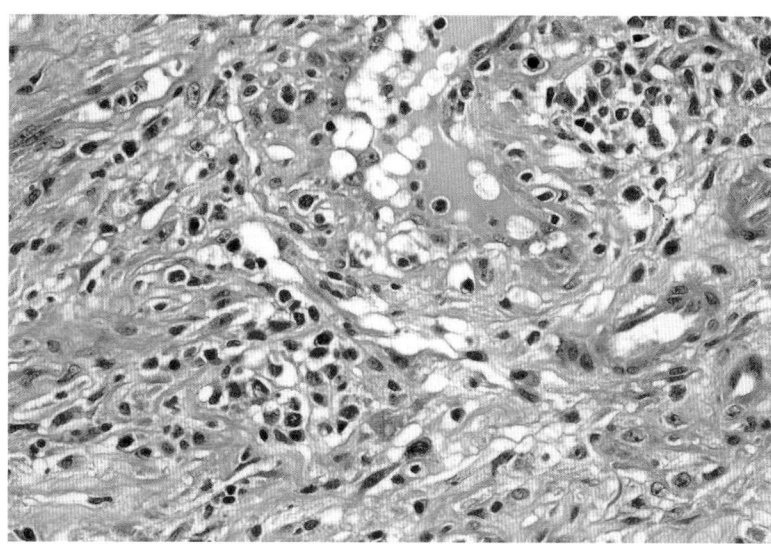

Fig. 12.117
Primary syphilis: the infiltrate consists of lymphocytes, histiocytes, and conspicuous plasma cells.

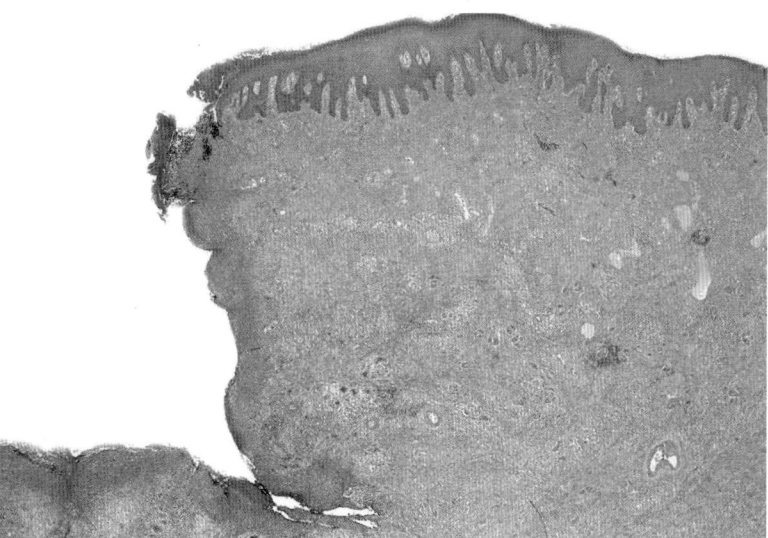

Fig. 12.115
Primary syphilis: biopsy from a chancre on the penis. Note the typical punched-out appearance.

the use of silver stains, mainly Warthin-Starry. However, the latter method is time consuming and difficult to interpret. The organisms can also be identified by PCR, and a polyclonal antibody against *T. pallidum* is available for immunohistochemistry (*Fig. 12.125*).[40–43] Both PCR and immunohistochemistry are much more specific than histochemistry in the diagnosis of syphilis.[42–44] In primary syphilis, the organisms are found both within the epidermis and around blood vessels, whereas in secondary syphilis organisms are mainly found within the epidermis, suggesting that these patterns can be used as an aid in distinction between the two stages of syphilis.[43] The bacteria have also been identified in vivo in the epidermis by the use of reflectance confocal microscopy.[45] In a case of malignant syphilis, a surprisingly very low number of organisms was found in the lesions.[46] Spirochetes have been demonstrated within hair follicles in a case of alopecia syphilitica.[47]

The nodular variants of secondary syphilis may be associated with granulomatous or pseudolymphomatous histology.[48–50] Some lesions can contain

an impressive number of CD30-positive atypical T cells.[51] The granulomata can mimic those of sarcoid and may rarely have a palisaded distribution resembling granuloma annulare.[48,52] The rupial and condylomatous forms are characterized by marked epidermal hyperplasia, spongiosis, and a neutrophil infiltrate. The dermis contains a very heavy inflammatory cell infiltrate including numerous plasma cells. Vascular changes are marked.

Late secondary lesions are typified by histiocytic granulomata. These are not well circumscribed and do not usually include multinucleated giant cells. They can be distinguished from tuberculosis by the presence of numerous plasma cells peripherally and the swollen endothelia of small blood vessels. A case of late latent syphilis with prominent dermal mucin mimicking a connective tissue disease has been reported.[53]

Gummata are characterized by central necrosis similar to caseation, but with a visible suggestion of residual cell outlines (*Fig. 12.126*). The necrosis is surrounded by a lymphohistiocytic and plasma cell infiltrate with fibrosis. Spirochetes are very scanty and very difficult to find with the use of silver stains. Endarteritis is often evident.

Noduloulcerative lesions are granulomatous, and typically there is no significant necrosis. Plasma cells are said to be inconspicuous, which may therefore cause considerable diagnostic difficulty.[54]

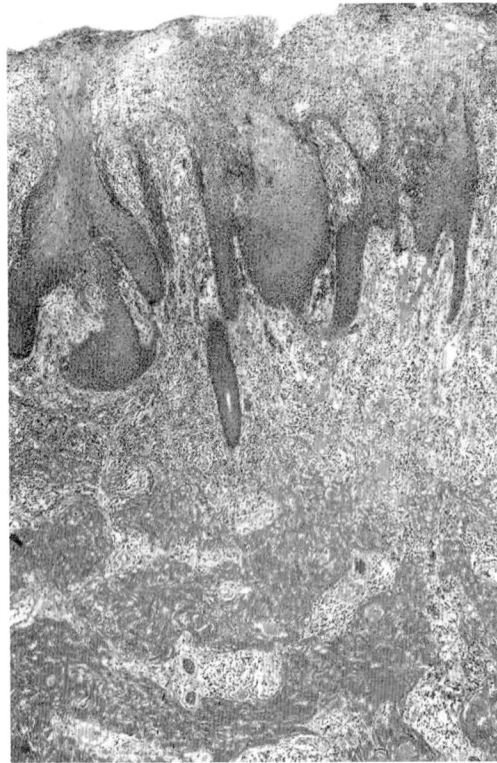

Fig. 12.118
Secondary syphilis: there is very marked hyperkeratosis and parakeratosis. The epidermis shows psoriasiform hyperplasia. A dense inflammatory cell infiltrate is present in the lamina propria. This specimen comes from a condyloma lata.

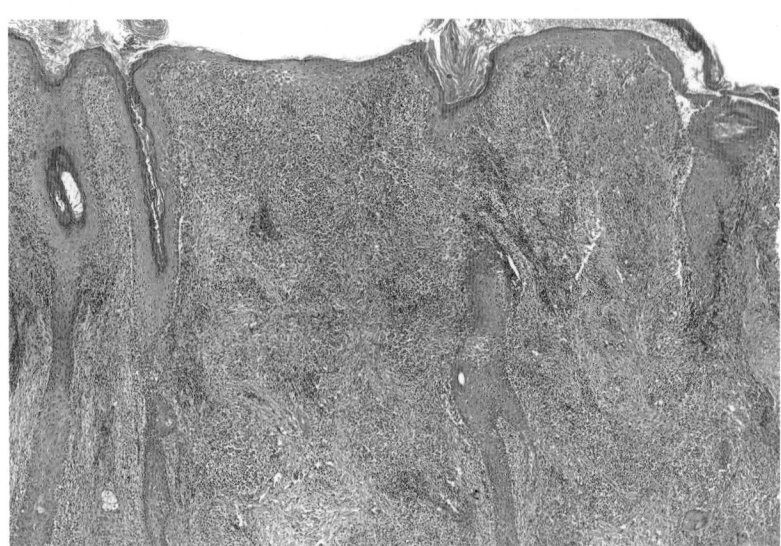

Fig. 12.120
Secondary syphilis: in this example, there is hyperkeratosis, irregular acanthosis and a very dense dermal infiltrate.

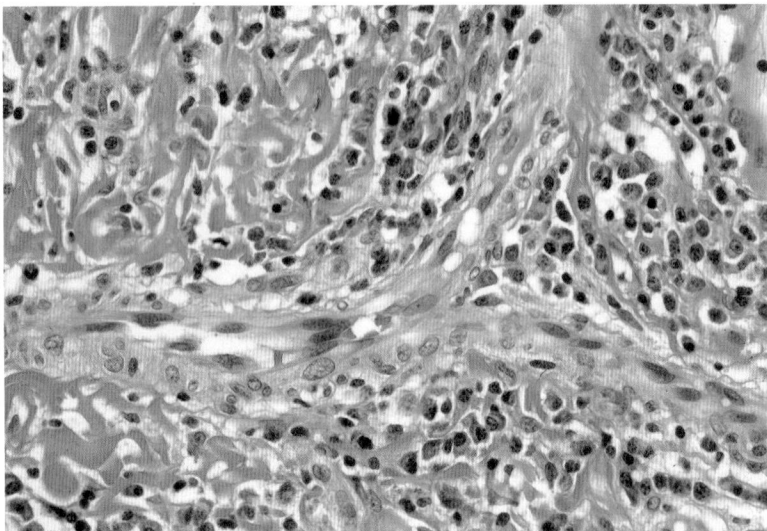

Fig. 12.119
Secondary syphilis: the infiltrate contains large numbers of plasma cells. This specimen comes from a condyloma lata.

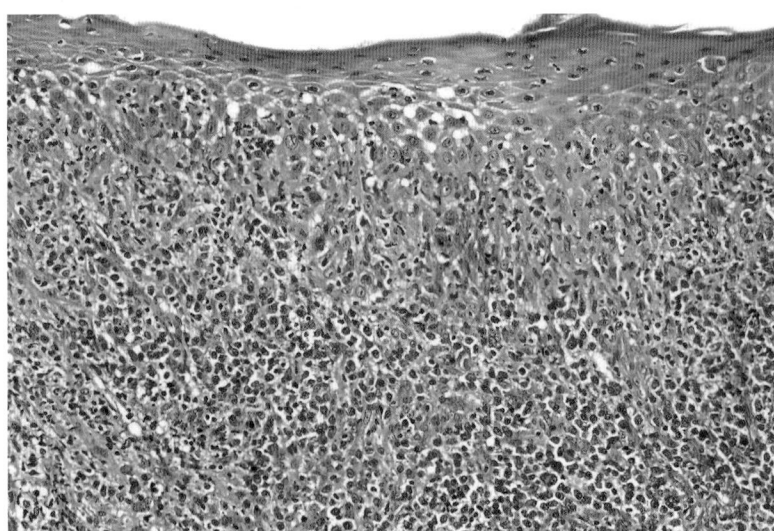

Fig. 12.121
Secondary syphilis: spongiosis is evident.

Granuloma inguinale

Clinical features

Granuloma inguinale (donovanosis) occurs in people with poor hygiene in tropical regions, mainly in India, Brazil, the West Indies, China and West Africa; it was formerly seen in southern United States, but is now rare.[1] The disease is still seen in Australia in the Aboriginal population.[2] The organism is of low infectivity and is presumed to be spread by sexual contact, probably through abraded skin. It occurs most often in the third to fifth decades. The incubation period is uncertain and may range from 2 to 3 weeks to several months.

The initial presentation in females is usually of one or more indurated papules or nodules on the inner aspect of the labia, the fourchette, or around the clitoris (*Fig. 12.127*).[3] In males, the glans, prepuce, coronal sulcus, or shaft is affected (*Fig. 12.128*). Dorsal perforation of the prepuce can occur

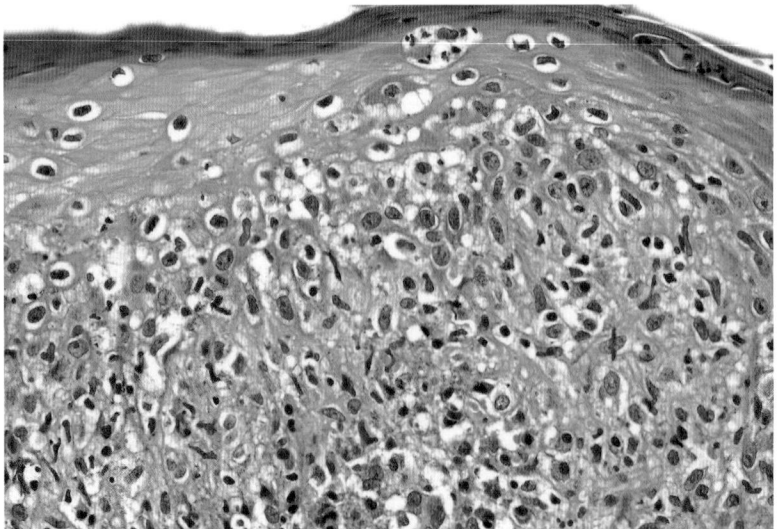

Fig. 12.122
Secondary syphilis: in this field, there is marked interface change.

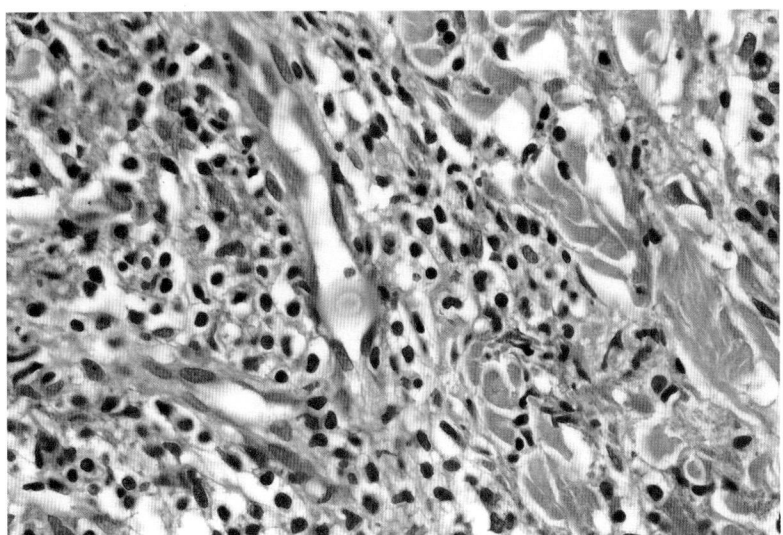

Fig. 12.123
Secondary syphilis: note the marked endothelial cell swelling.

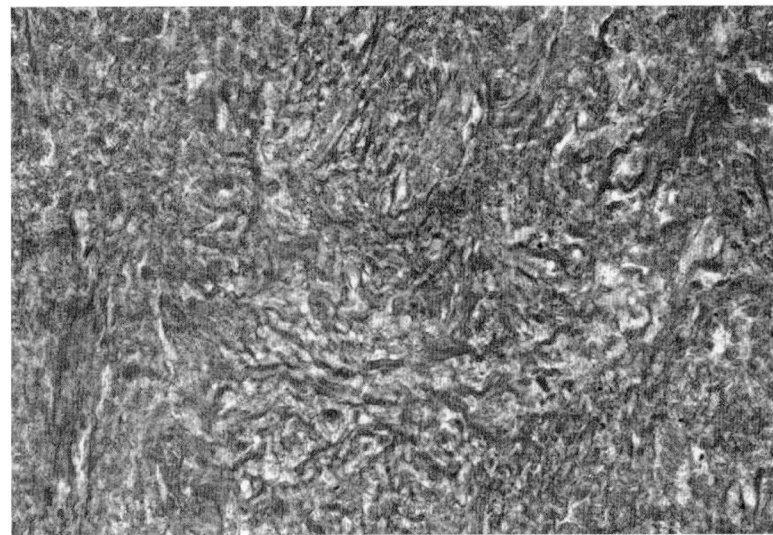

Fig. 12.126
Gumma: high-power view reveals ghost outlines of cells and connective tissue.

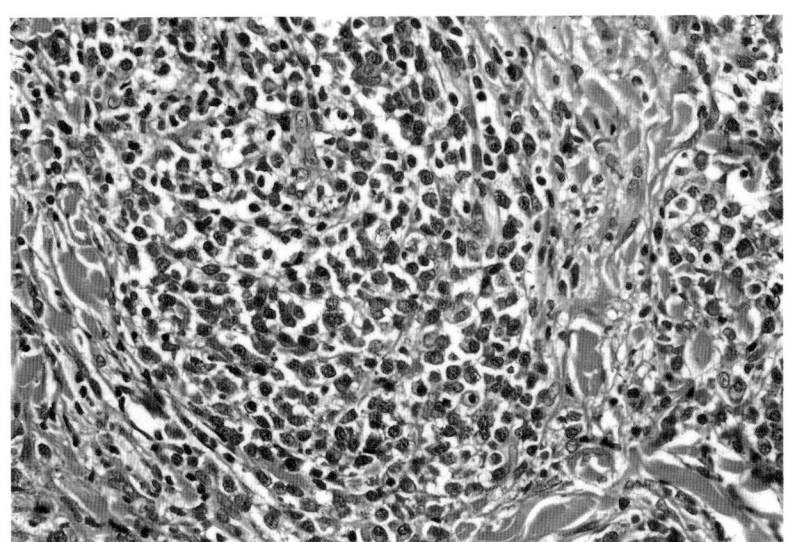

Fig. 12.124
Secondary syphilis: innumerable plasma cells are present.

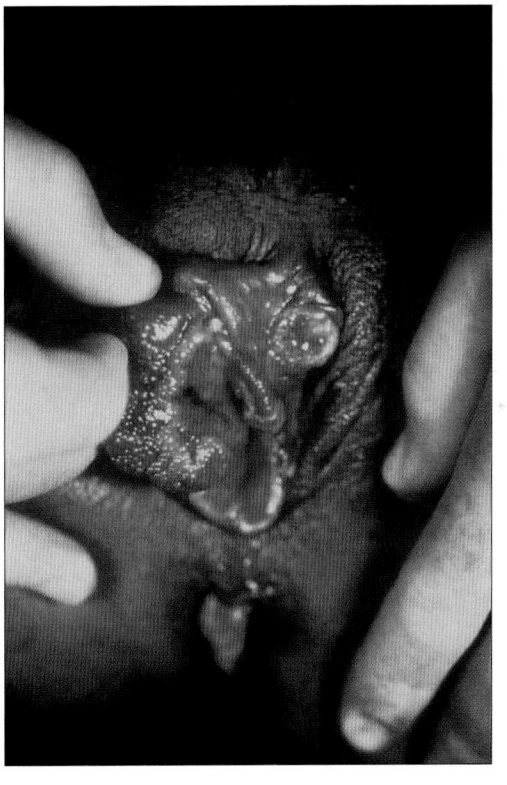

Fig. 12.127
Granuloma inguinale: early lesion showing an ulcerated papule adjacent to the clitoris. By courtesy of J. Lawson, MD, University of Newcastle-upon-Tyne, UK.

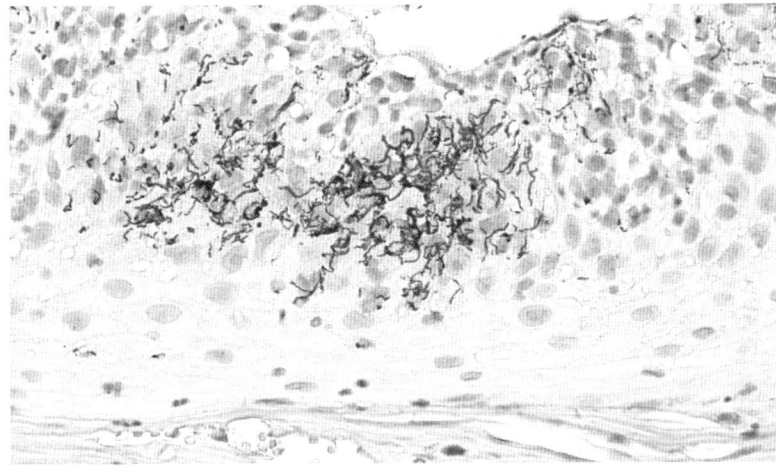

Fig. 12.125
Secondary syphilis: numerous spirochetes are seen by immunohistochemistry within the epidermis in a patient with secondary syphilis.

as a late complication.[4] The perianal and inguinal regions and the cervix may also be involved.[5-7] In one case involving the cervix, there was associated malacoplakia.[7] The papules ulcerate irregularly and extend widely if untreated. The base of the ulcer is 'beefy', and the margins are undermined and indurated. Spread to contiguous 'kissing' areas may sometimes occur. Variants include verrucous, necrotic, and scarring lesions. Primary infection of the lymph nodes does not occur, but painful lymphadenopathy is common due to secondary infection. Rarely, primary extragenital lesions may be seen (mainly mouth or lips but also at unusual sites such as the foot).[8,9] Exceptionally, presentation as a psoas abscess and as a pelvic mass mimicking ovarian cancer has been described.[10,11]

Very occasionally, there is a systemic infection with involvement of many organs including the liver, and osteolytic lesions in bone.[12] The latter may particularly relate to a primary cervical lesion.[1] Spinal compression has also been reported.[13] Later complications include strictures of the urethra, vagina, or anus, destruction of the penile shaft with autoamputation, and pseudoelephantiasis.[14-17] As with other sexually transmitted diseases, patients

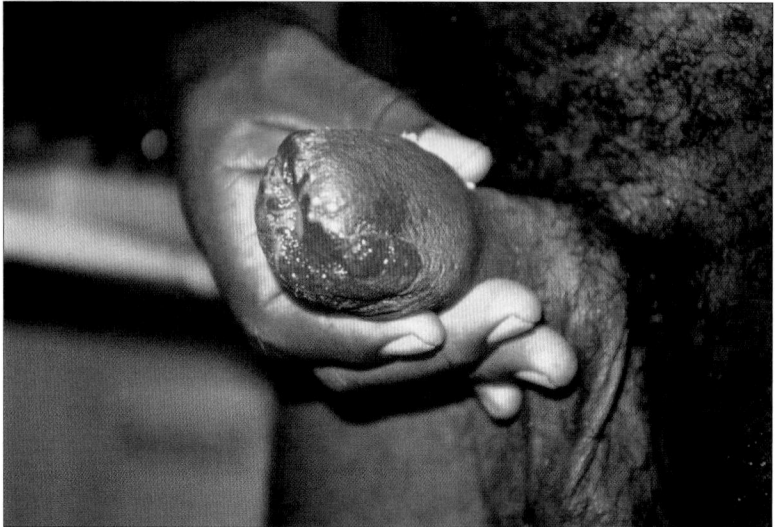

Fig. 12.128
Granuloma inguinale: in this patient, there is extensive ulceration of the glans penis. Note the typical 'beefy' appearance. By courtesy of C. Furlonge, MD, Port of Spain, Trinidad.

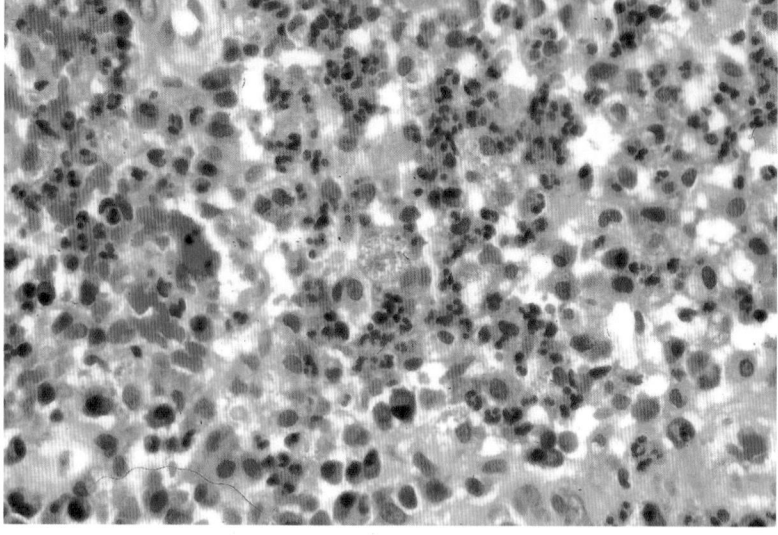

Fig. 12.130
Granuloma inguinale: the infiltrate consists of lymphocytes, neutrophils, plasma cells, and conspicuous pale-staining histiocytes.

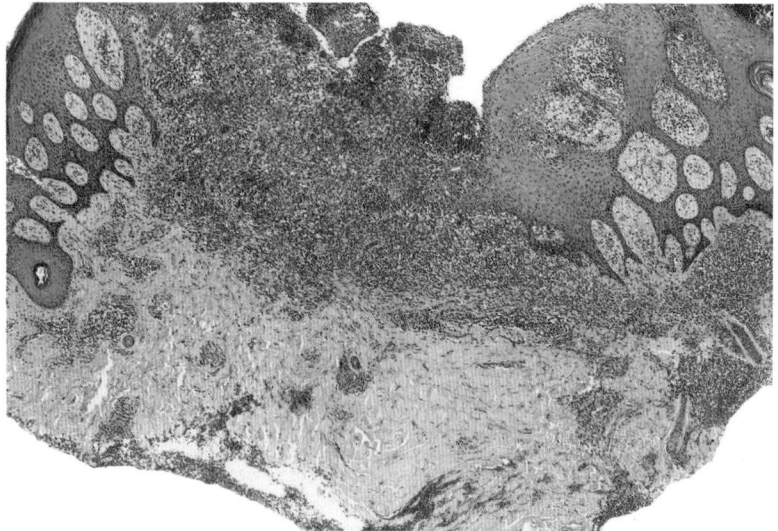

Fig. 12.129
Granuloma inguinale: biopsy from the penis. Note the pseudoepitheliomatous hyperplasia. There are intense inflammatory changes.

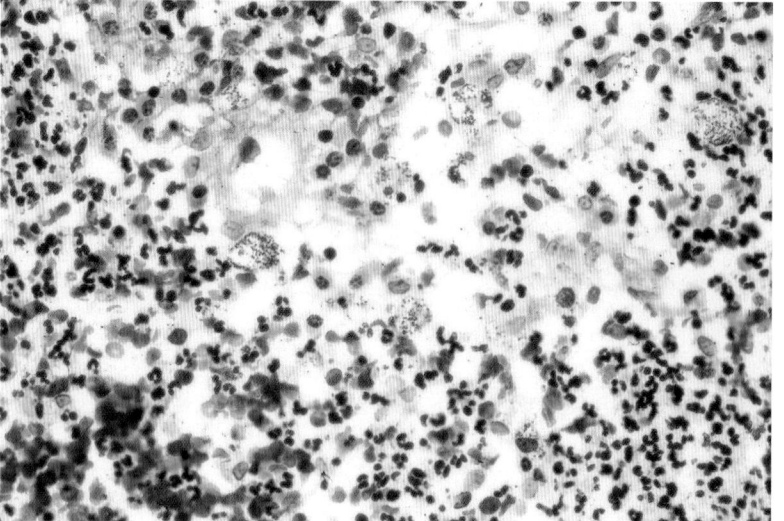

Fig. 12.131
Granuloma inguinale: the histiocytes contain characteristic Donovan bodies (Warthin-Starry stain).

with granuloma inguinale are often HIV positive and may also have syphilis.[18] Genital SCC is an uncommon but important complication.[19,20] Infection in children has rarely been reported and occurs as a result of transmission from an infected mother at birth.[21] Rare manifestations of the disease in children include a mass in the neck, otitis media, and mastoiditis.[22,23]

Pathogenesis and histologic features

Granuloma inguinale is caused by *Calymmatobacterium granulomatis* (formerly *Donovania granulomatis*), an encapsulated short (1–2 μm) Gram-negative rod with characteristic bipolar staining. It is transmitted by sexual contact, but it is of low infectivity.[1] The organism is found in feces, and this may act as a reservoir of infectivity or, in occasional cases, be the source of genital infection. The higher incidence of infection in homosexuals may support this concept.

The lesion is characterized by a very intense inflammatory infiltrate in which plasma cells are predominant (*Fig. 12.129*). Focal formation of neutrophilic microabscesses is frequent. Pathognomonic macrophages contain cytoplasmic cyst-like vacuoles in which bacteria can be demonstrated by staining with Giemsa or the Warthin-Starry reaction (*Figs 12.130* and *12.131*).[24] The bacteria can also be seen extracellularly. In most cases there

is associated acanthosis, which sometimes amounts to pseudoepitheliomatous hyperplasia. Ulceration is common. A large study has demonstrated frequent transepidermal elimination of organisms.[25] It is likely that this phenomenon may be an important mechanism in the spread of the disease.

Diagnosis is confirmed by the identification of typical organisms (Donovan bodies) on a scraping from an ulcer or in a biopsy stained with Giemsa or Warthin-Starry. PCR has also been used successfully to confirm the diagnosis.[26] Dark-field illumination microscopy should be performed to exclude syphilis. By electron microscopy, the encapsulated microorganisms can be demonstrated within the phagosomes of macrophages.[27]

Chancroid

Clinical features

Chancroid (soft chancre, genital ulcer disease) is very common in some tropical areas of Africa, Southeast Asia, Central America, and the Pacific.[1] Poor hygiene is a feature of communities where the disease is endemic. It is associated with an increased risk of transmission or acquisition of HIV.[2] Genital ulcers including chancroid appear to develop more commonly in

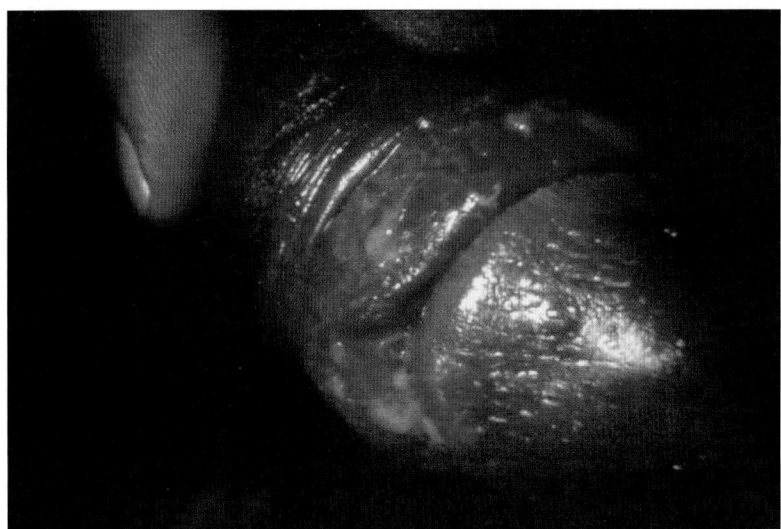

Fig. 12.132
Chancroid: irregular ulcer extending along the coronal sulcus of the penis. By courtesy of R.A. Marsden, MD, St George's Hospital, London, UK.

HIV-positive women during the first month of antiretroviral therapy.[3] It has also been diagnosed more frequently in Western Europe and North America in association with increased travel, immigration and prostitution. Chancroid was endemic in New York City and southern Florida in the 1980s. It represented 3% of genital ulcers in a sexually transmitted disease clinic in Paris.[4] The disease is acquired almost always by sexual contact and has a short incubation period of 3 days to 2 weeks (median, 7 days). Exceptionally, nonsexually transmitted lower limb chancroid ulcers have been reported in patients from Papua New Guinea and Samoa, in both adults and children.[5,6] Concurrence with other sexually transmitted disease including gonorrhea can be seen.[7]

The initial lesion is usually a transient vesicular tender papule, which rapidly ulcerates with copious suppuration. The ulcer is sharply circumscribed with an undermined edge and is typically not indurated. These lesions appear much more commonly in the male, usually on the penis (*Fig. 12.132*). The prepuce, coronal sulcus, frenulum, and glans are the most favored sites. Circumcised males are at lower risk of developing the disease.[8] Lesions in the female are seen on the fourchette, labia majora and minora, and around the clitoris. The perineum and perianal area may also be affected. Multiple ulcers can be present, which have an irregular ragged edge and slough-covered bases. Cervical and vaginal involvement is uncommon. Variants of primary chancroid ulcers include giant and serpiginous forms, follicular, transient, and dwarf lesions; occasionally, a condyloma lata-like presentation may occur.

The ulcers are tender and especially painful when in contact with urine. Lymphadenitis occurs in about 50% of cases approximately 1 week after the genital lesion, and in 50% of these, suppuration (bubo formation) usually follows. Sometimes rupture may occur, resulting in inguinal ulceration. In other cases, the course is variable, some resolving without treatment in a few days while others go on for several weeks, developing phimosis or even gangrene. Systemic infections do not occur.

Pathogenesis and histologic features

Chancroid is caused by *Haemophilus ducreyi*, a Gram-negative coccobacillus, which grows in chains sometimes arranged in parallel. It is transmitted through minor abrasions during sexual intercourse. The subsequent lesion comprises:

- a superficial zone of neutrophils, red cells, bacteria, and cell debris,
- a middle zone of edematous granulation tissue,
- an underlying infiltrate of histiocytes, lymphocytes, and plasma cells (*Figs 12.133* and *12.134*).

The enlarged lymph nodes show central necrosis with a surrounding mixed inflammatory response of neutrophils and macrophages.

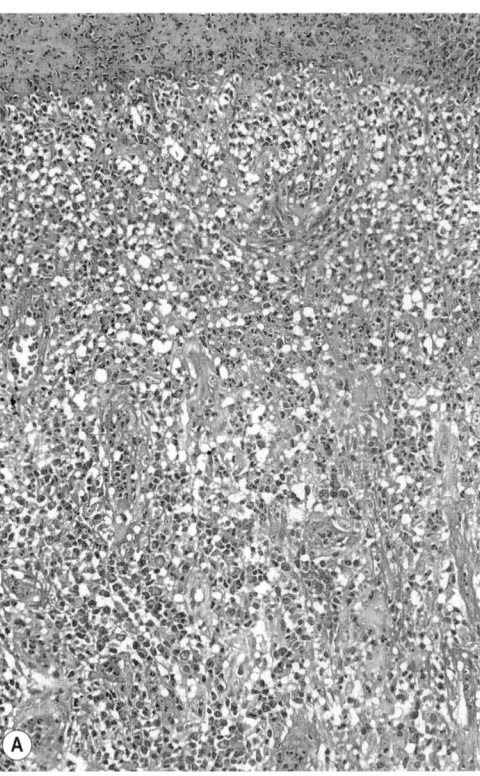
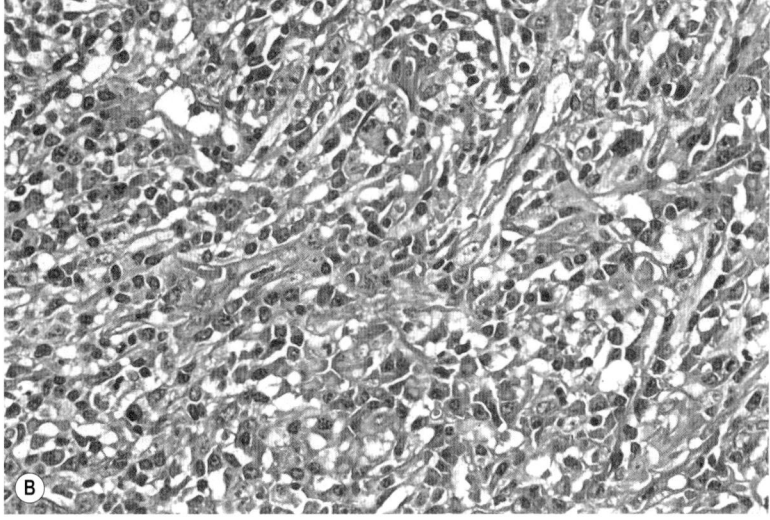

Fig. 12.133
Chancroid: (**A**) biopsy through an ulcer on the glans penis; (**B**) note the conspicuous plasma cells. By courtesy of S. Lucas, MD, St Thomas' Hospital, London, UK.

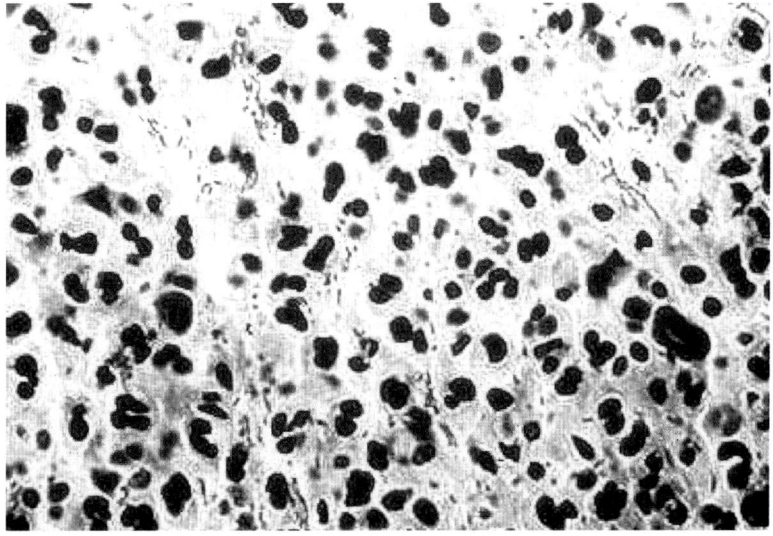

Fig. 12.134
Chancroid: note the coccobacilli growing in chains.

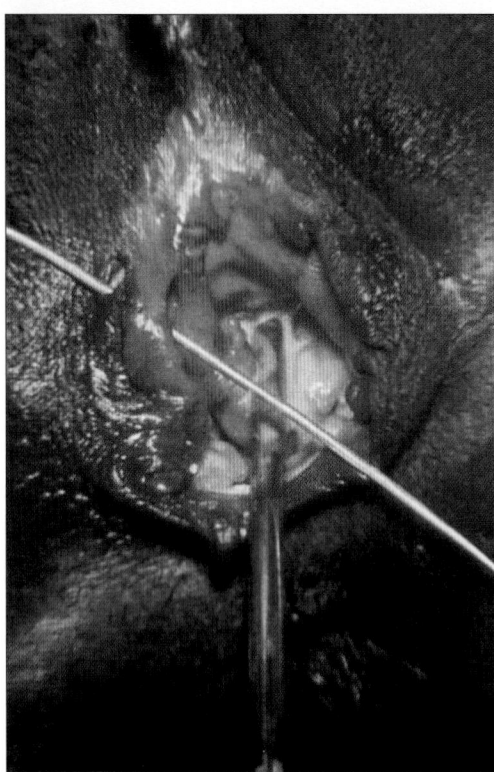

Fig. 12.135
Lymphogranuloma venereum: note the ulcer on the right labium majus. By courtesy of S. Lucas, MD, St. Thomas' Hospital, London, UK.

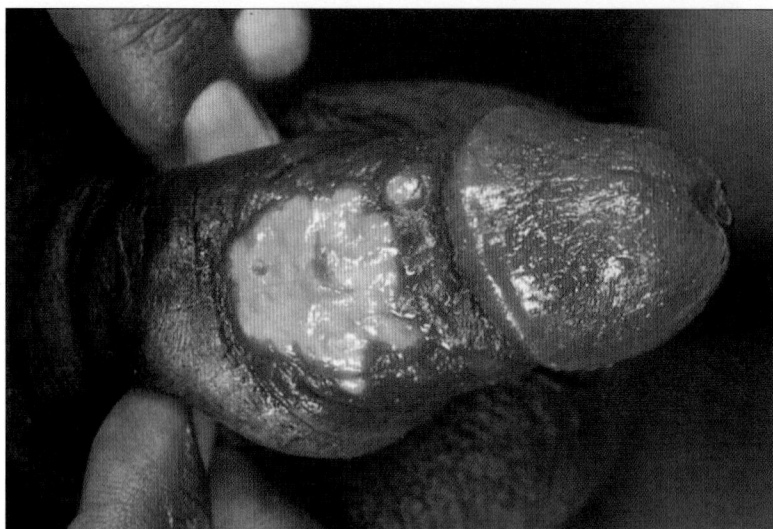

Fig. 12.136
Lymphogranuloma venereum: there is an ulcer on the penile shaft covered with necrotic debris. By courtesy of the Institute of Dermatology, London, UK.

Diagnosis is confirmed by isolation of the organism by culture in a blood-enriched medium containing vancomycin at 33°C. The bacterium may be identified by its chain-like growth in scrapings from the margin of the ulcer, but secondary organisms are often present and it is more helpful to identify the organism in an aspirate from a necrotic lymph node. DNA in situ hybridization and PCR for *H. ducreyi* has been developed.[9,10] DNA from the organism has been detected by PCR in esophageal lesions of HIV-positive patients.[11]

Lymphogranuloma venereum

Clinical features

Lymphogranuloma venereum is endemic in Asia, Africa, and South America and was considered to be rare in developed countries until several outbreaks were reported in a number of European countries and the United States, mainly in homosexuals and in the context of HIV infection.[1,2] It is less common in women.[3]

The disease evolves in three stages:
- In stage 1 disease, the primary lesion develops 3–30 days after contact and is a small, transient, frequently asymptomatic papulovesicle or ulcer on the penis, scrotum, rectum, vulva (most commonly at the fourchette), vagina, and/or cervix (*Figs 12.135* and *12.136*).[4] Primary lesions have been described on the fingers and tongue. Rarely, lymphogranuloma venereum has been reported presenting with a psoas abscess.[5] Cat scratch disease may clinically simulate this disease.[6]
- Stage 2 develops within a few weeks of the primary lesion and consists of enlargement of the inguinal nodes. The pelvic lymph nodes may be enlarged in females. The lymphadenopathy is severe and initially painless and hard; later, the nodes (buboes) soften and discharge viscous pus. The tissue around the nodes becomes involved in the inflammatory process so that they become matted together. Along with lymphadenopathy, the patient may also experience malaise, joint pains, and hepatosplenomegaly. Erythema nodosum, light-sensitive eruptions, and erythema multiforme may complicate this phase and are more common in women.
- Stage 3 disease consists of complications of the early inflammatory changes. Involvement of the deep iliac and perirectal lymph nodes resulting from drainage from a high vaginal, posterior urethral, cervical,

or rectal primary lesion may be complicated by a stricture of the rectum 5–10 cm from the anus.[7] This is associated with periproctitis and proctocolitis, which sometimes fistulates.[8] Rectal carcinoma is an occasional late complication.[9] In both sexes, genital lymphedema and even elephantiasis can develop after the lymphadenopathy. This may be a continuing problem and can be associated with secondary cutaneous erosions and ulceration.

Systemic lesions are rare, and include cardiac and pulmonary involvement, keratoconjunctivitis, episcleritis, uveitis, papilledema and retinal hemorrhages, meningitis, hepatitis, and cutaneous manifestations such as erythema nodosum and erythema multiforme.[10]

Pathogenesis and histologic features

Lymphogranuloma venereum is caused by strains L1, L2, and L3 of the bacterium *C. trachomatis*. The *C. trachomatis* species is divided into 15 prototypic serovars according to analysis of their outer membrane protein.[11] Only serovars L1 to L3 are associated with lymphogranuloma venereum, with the L2 serovar causing most cases. Chlamydiae are nonmobile, coccoid, obligate intracellular parasites. They depend on their host cells for ATP metabolites and multiply within membrane-bound vacuoles in the host macrophage cytoplasm. They stain faintly blue with hematoxylin and eosin (H&E), Gram-negative with the Brown-Hopps tissue Gram stain, and black with the Warthin-Starry silver impregnation technique.[12] On the rare occasions that the primary lesion is viewed histologically, the base of the ulcer is lined by intensely inflamed fibrous granulation tissue. Plasma cells and microabscesses are present. The lymphadenitis has a characteristic picture of stellate central necrosis with neutrophils and a surrounding palisaded granulomatous reaction with occasional giant cells.

The central necrosis is slowly absorbed and replaced by fibrosis. As a consequence, lymphedema develops distally. The lymphatics are typically inflamed and granulomata may be seen.

The diagnostic standard is now nucleic acid amplification testing.[13] PCR may also be used to confirm the diagnosis.[14]

Schistosomiasis

Clinical features

Schistosoma hematobium and *Schistosoma mansoni* are both found extensively in Africa. *S. mansoni* also occurs in the West Indies and in parts of South America. *Schistosoma japonicum* is present in China, Japan, and Southeast Asia. These trematodes (blood flukes) do not often cause major disease of the skin, but skin lesions do occur at various stages of infestation.[1]

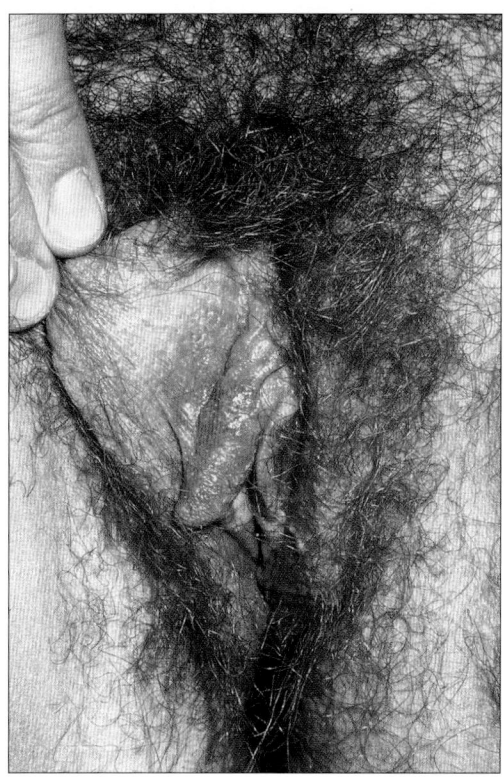

Fig. 12.137
Schistosomiasis: early lesion showing labial erythema and swelling. These features are a response to ova deposition. By courtesy of P. Dowd, MD, Middlesex Hospital, London, UK.

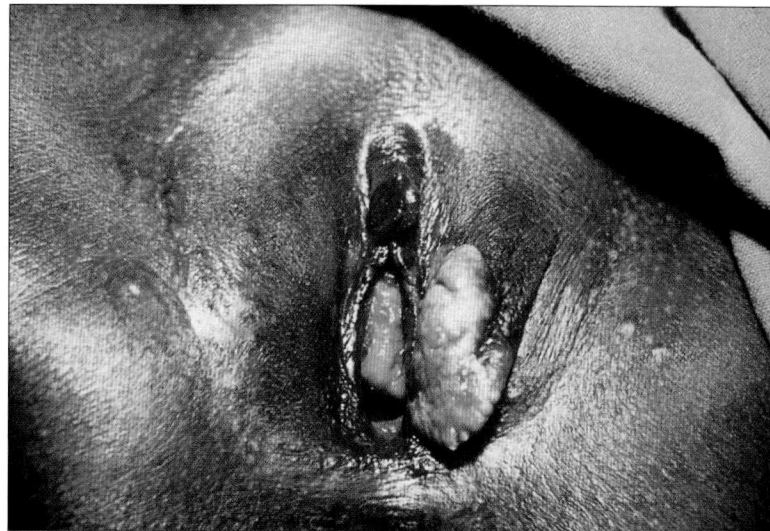

Fig. 12.138
Schistosomiasis: this warty pale nodule has almost completely replaced the left labium majus; other vulval manifestations include schistosomal condylomata, ulcers, and rarely, vitiligo. By courtesy of the late M.S.R. Hutt, MD, St Thomas' Hospital, London, UK.

Invasion of the human host by the aquate cercarial stage may be associated with dermatitis (swimmer's itch). This rash is erythematous, pruritic, and urticarial, but eventually resolves to leave a pigmented spot. It is more often encountered with invasion of avian species.

In schistosomiasis (bilharziasis), the mature worms may be associated non-specifically with erythematous itching macules at the time of release of large numbers of eggs. This probably represents a systemic reaction to antigen liberation. A more severe reaction seen particularly with *S. japonicum* is Katayama disease or Yellow River fever. In addition to erythema, macules, and pruriginous lesions, patients may also have fever, malaise, chills, sweats, arthralgias, headache, lymphadenopathy, hepatosplenomegaly, and peripheral blood eosinophilia.[2]

Specific skin lesions are seen, usually around the genitalia and most often in prepubertal females, when ova are deposited there (*Fig. 12.137*). They appear as grouped solid papules, which subsequently become warty and vegetative, resembling condyloma acuminatum (*Fig. 12.138*). The labia majora are often involved initially. Occasionally, progression to SCC occurs. Periurethral granulomata due to schistosomes may be associated with thrombosis and necrosis, sometimes resulting in fistula formation in the perineum ('watering can perineum'). In late lesions prominent scarring may occur. More rarely, entrapped ova are seen in other areas of skin, but the means of their migration to those sites is not understood. Extragenital lesions of schistosomiasis have been described in the trunk (mainly periumbilical but also in the axilla, back and inframammary area), face, and proximal lower limbs.[3] Facial lesions may be associated with ocular involvement.[4] Extragenital schistosomiasis, also known as extragenital bilharziasis cutanea tarda, is very rare and its recognition is extremely important as it is usually a sentinel as well as a potential external marker of recurrent visceral disease. Interestingly, it has been noted that this type of disease often occurs in pre-existing cutaneous pathology such as squamous papilloma, SCC, scarring, and hidradenitis suppurativa.[3]

Pathogenesis and histologic features

Part of the life cycle of schistosomes takes place in water snails. After their release from the snails, the cercaria penetrates the skin of humans and migrate as schistosomes to the portal veins where they mature into adult male and female worms. Adult females then migrate to the mesenteric plexus (*S. mansoni* and *S. japonicum*) or vesical plexus (*Schistosoma haematobium*). Ova are deposited in the venules, and the clinical and pathological

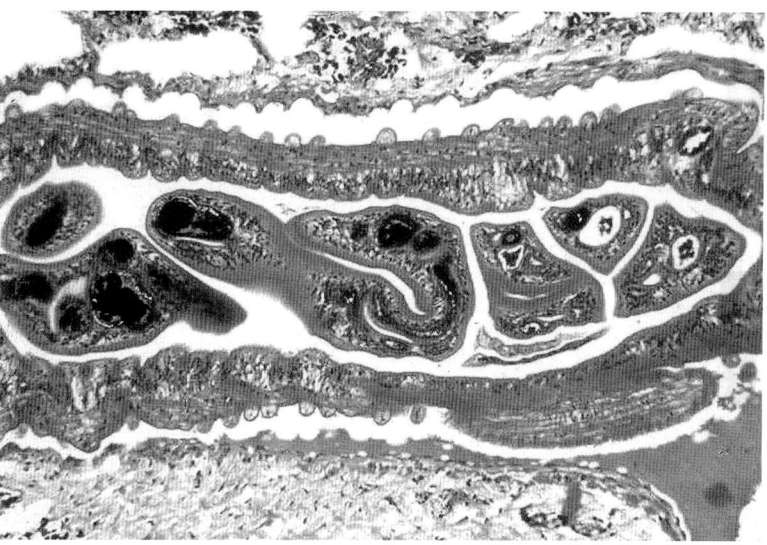

Fig. 12.139
Vulval schistosomiasis: adult worms within a dilated lymphatic; the male characteristically embraces the female in the gynecophoric canal.

sequelae are a direct consequence of the immunological response to their presence.

Eggs are released into the urine or feces where they hatch, releasing miracidia, which enter the snail host. Involvement of the female genital tract is usually due to *S. hematobium* and occurs as a consequence of worms being transported via anastomoses between the vesical and uterovaginal venous plexuses.

Histologically, adult worms are occasionally seen within the lumina of dilated deep dermal veins and lymphatics (*Fig. 12.139*). Viable ova may be present with a recognizable miracidial structure (*Fig. 12.140*). These are usually located within abscesses containing numerous neutrophils and variable numbers of eosinophils. Poorly formed granulomata with Langhans giant cells are also sometimes a feature. *S. hematobium* is recognized by its terminal spine (*Fig. 12.141*). *S. mansoni* has a lateral spine and *S. japonicum* has no spine. The dead ova typically calcify and provoke a chronic, frequently granulomatous, inflammatory response. The overlying epidermis is usually acanthotic, sometimes to the point of pseudoepitheliomatous hyperplasia and may occasionally contain intraepidermal ova undergoing transepidermal elimination (*Fig. 12.142*).[5,6] Smearing crushed biopsies between two

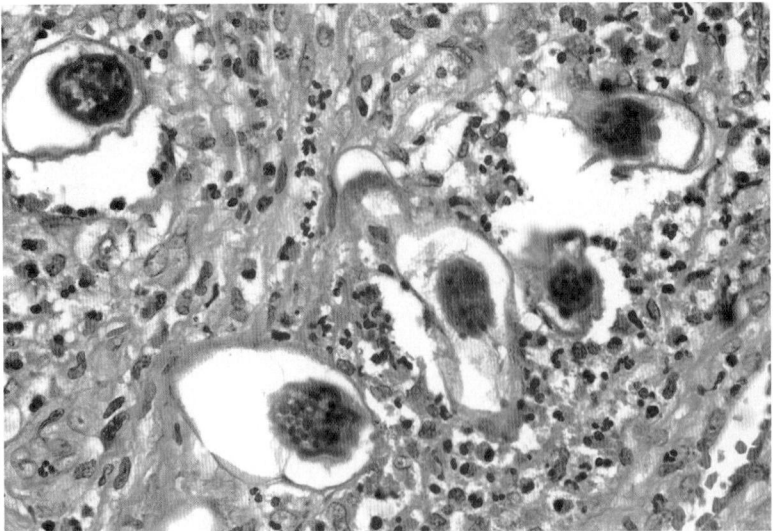

Fig. 12.140
Schistosomiasis: these ova are surrounded by a heavy infiltrate with conspicuous eosinophils.

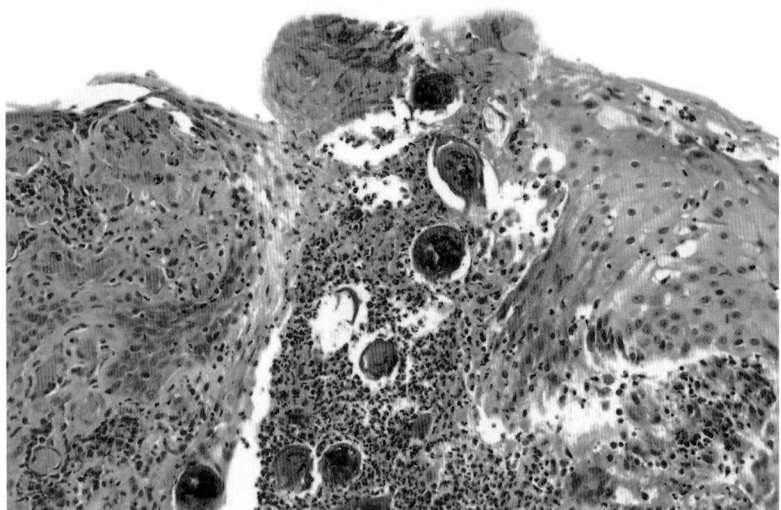

Fig. 12.142
Schistosomiasis: there is marked acanthosis. Ova are present within a breach in the epidermis.

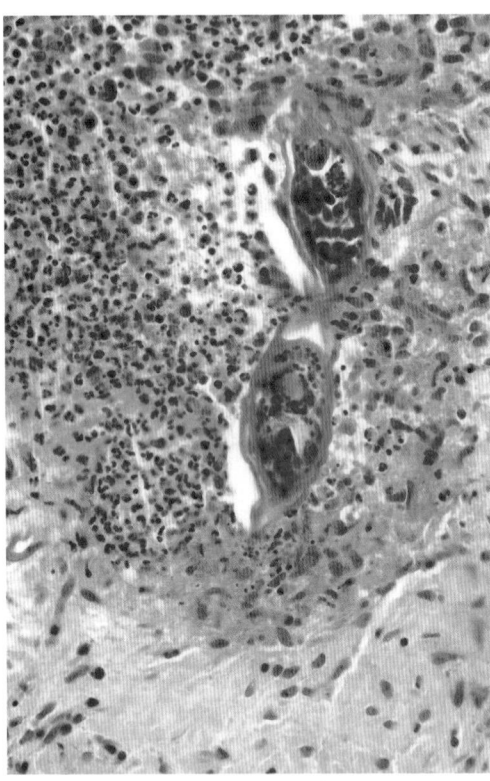

Fig. 12.141
Schistosoma hematobium: the terminal spine is characteristic of this species.

glass slides with 0.5% trypan blue in saline helps to highlight the ova.[7] Adult parasites can sometimes be identified in anogenital and extragenital lesions.[3]

Identification of the type of schistosoma can be made by molecular methods.[8]

Amebiasis cutis

Clinical features

Cutaneous lesions of *Entamoeba histolytica* are rare and more likely to occur in adults,[1] although cases in children have been described.[2] These are most commonly seen after surgical treatment of intestinal or hepatic amebiasis, but may also occur by direct extension, perianally from the bowel or from hepatic involvement, and by direct inoculation of the skin from other infected lesions. Penile amebiasis may follow anal intercourse or vaginal intercourse if the female has amebic vaginitis. HIV infection should be

suspected.[3] Cutaneous lesions have been recorded on the trunk, buttocks, face (including the eyelid and the orbit), genitalia, perineum, and on the legs.[4,5] The cervix is often affected in genital lesions. Subcutaneous swellings called amebomas have been described. Patients with deep tissue involvement tend to have associated contiguous disease, and the prognosis tends to be worse. In HIV/AIDS the outcome is associated with coexisting systemic diseases, and death may ensue in patients with extensive internal involvement.[6]

Lesions present as cutaneous ulcers with a central necrotic zone covered by a purulent exudate, an undermined margin and an erythematous halo. The ulcers are irregular, but sharply defined. They spread and do not heal spontaneously. They are extremely painful and may be destructive. Presentation can also be with fistulae, fissures, abscesses, and polypoid or warty lesions. Occasionally, the latter are large and resemble ulcerating tumors. Sometimes they mimic SCC.[7] Cases of amebiasis presenting as balanitis have been described.[8] Although painful swelling and ulceration are the principal clinical features, frequency, dysuria, and retention may be complications

Histologic features

Lesions are characterized by prominent ulceration, necrosis, and a mixed inflammatory cell infiltrate composed of lymphocytes, histiocytes, plasma cells, and neutrophils. The trophozoites of *E. histolytica* are found within the purulent ulcer exudate and are best identified with PAS staining (*Figs 12.143–12.145*).[9] They are distinguished by their tendency to phagocytose red blood cells. Trophozoites and cysts are usually found in the patient's feces. The organisms are surrounded by neutrophils, with some lymphocytes and plasma cells. The adjacent epidermis appears acanthotic, and this may be marked or pseudoepitheliomatous in verrucous forms. In some cases there is thrombosis or vasculitis with intravascular amebic trophozoites.

Demodecidosis

The pathological role of the mite *Demodex folliculorum* in human cutaneous diseases such as rosacea is controversial. However, Hwang et al.[1] have described a man with a long-standing pruritic eruption of multiple, monomorphic, match-head sized, flesh-colored papules on the penis and scrotum. Histology demonstrated intrafollicular mites and the patient was cured with topical crotamiton.

Malacoplakia

Clinical features

Malacoplakia (soft plaque) is a result of impaired macrophage function in the inflammatory response to bacterial pathogens, most notably *Escherichia*

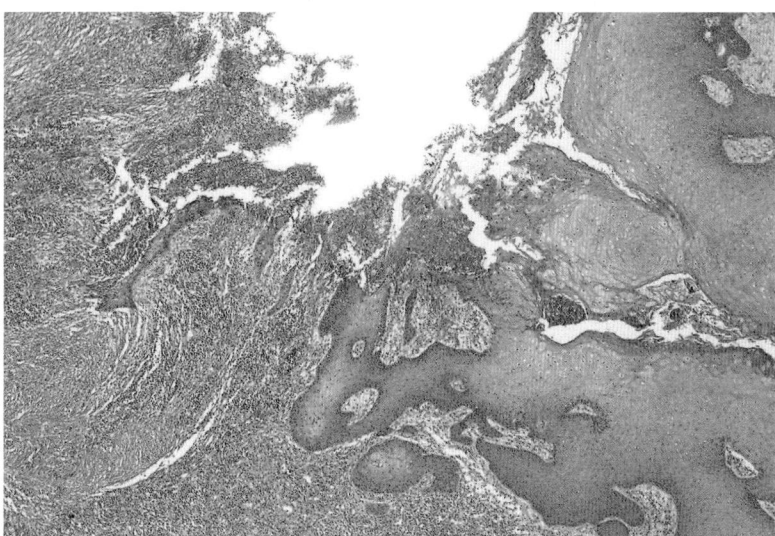

Fig. 12.143
Amebiasis: biopsy from a vulval ulcer, which developed as a result of direct spread from the anus.

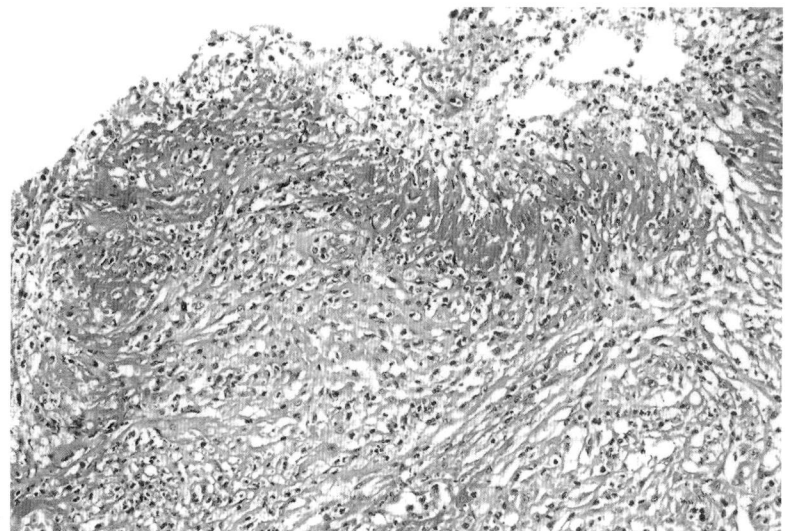

Fig. 12.144
Amebiasis: the floor of the ulcer is covered by a dense fibrinous exudate.

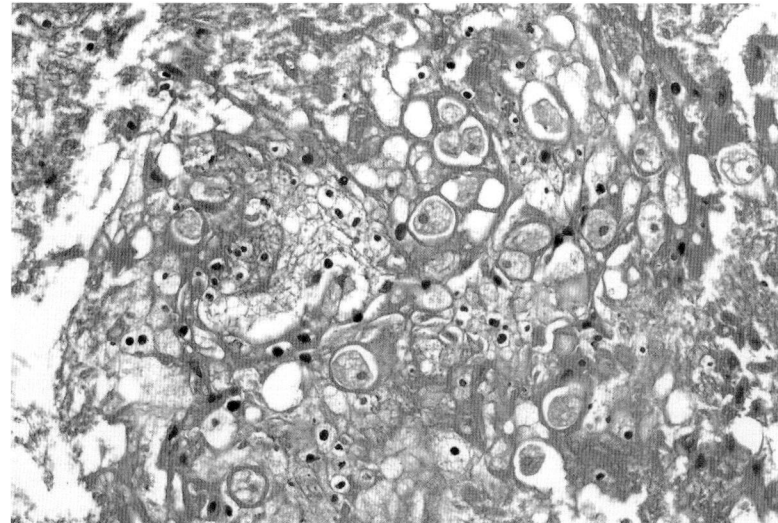

Fig. 12.145
Amebiasis: there are numerous trophozoites present. Note the ingested red blood cells.

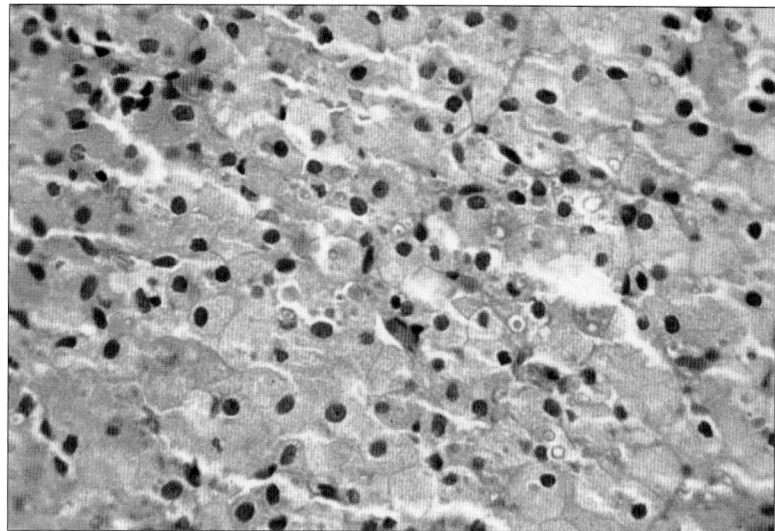

Fig. 12.146
Malacoplakia: the infiltrate consists of histiocytes with eosinophilic cytoplasm. Note the pale blue, laminated Michaelis-Gutmann bodies.

coli, but other organisms, including *S. aureus*, *Proteus*, *Pseudomonas*, *Klebsiella*, and mycobacteria, can be involved. Primary or acquired immunodeficiency has been found in 40% patients.[1] The latter include HIV and solid organ transplantation, mainly renal, and very rarely, heart transplant.[2,3]

It is most frequently described affecting the urinary tract, but it can involve many other organs including the gastrointestinal system, lymph nodes, lower genital tract, brain, bone, lungs, adrenals, and skin.[4,5] Cutaneous lesions may be dermal and/or subcutaneous and are most common around the genitalia (particularly the vulva) or perineum in about 41% of cases, but can be seen at other sites including the trunk in 20% of patients, head and neck in 20%, limbs in 10%, and axilla in 10%.[5] Involvement of Bartholin gland has also rarely been reported.[6] Vaginal bleeding may occur. Concomitant infection with granuloma inguinale of the cervix is described in one patient.[7] Multiple cutaneous sites can be involved, and in an exceptional case there was involvement of the skin with extension into the calvarium and the brain parenchyma.[5] Cutaneous manifestations are variable and include papules, plaques, polyps, ulcers, and sinuses.

Underlying or related conditions, which are usually associated with immunosuppression, include carcinoma, rheumatoid arthritis, systemic lupus erythematosus, hepatitis C, sarcoidosis, leukemia, lymphoma, and transplantation. The skin lesions are nonprogressive, but are typically persistent.

Pathogenesis and histologic features

Malacoplakia is characterized by confluent sheets of histiocytes with eosinophilic granular cytoplasm and small, usually eccentric, nuclei. There are characteristic cytoplasmic, calcified, von Kossa-positive inclusions known as Michaelis-Gutmann bodies (*Figs 12.146* and *12.147*). These are sometimes laminated, and this can be accentuated with PAS staining. They may also be positive on staining with Perl's reaction for iron. The Michaelis-Gutmann body is sufficiently distinctive to allow cytological distinction of malacoplakia in a preparation from a skin scraping.[8,9] The histiocytic infiltrate may be mixed with neutrophils, lymphocytes, and plasma cells, with associated granulation tissue. Electron microscopy of malacoplakia shows the histiocytes to contain numerous phagolysosomes, sometimes with intact and/or partly digested bacteria. It appears that the phagolysosomes accumulate in response to chronic bacterial infections.

Fournier gangrene

Fournier gangrene is analogous to necrotizing fasciitis and Meleney gangrene. The disease begins with urethral or appendageal polybacterial infection. Most of the organisms isolated are resident urethral or lower gastrointestinal flora, and most patients have mixed infections. In children, staphylococci and streptococci are most commonly isolated.[1] A necrotizing

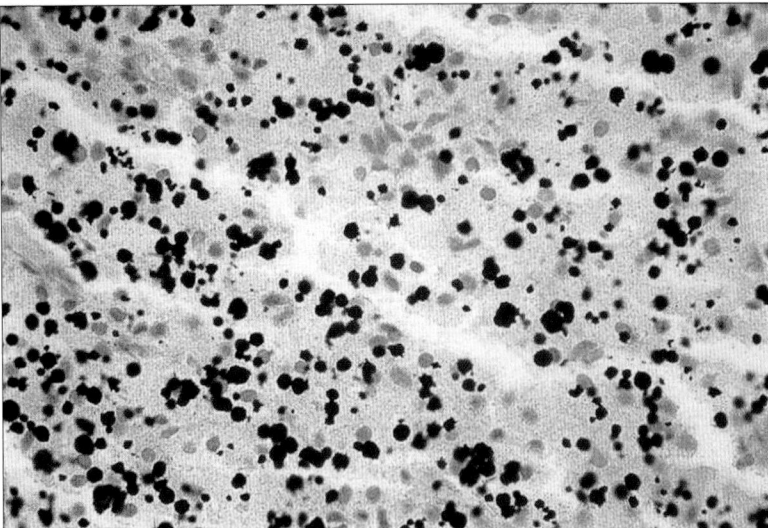

Fig. 12.147
Malacoplakia: the Michaelis-Gutmann bodies can be highlighted with the von Kossa reaction.

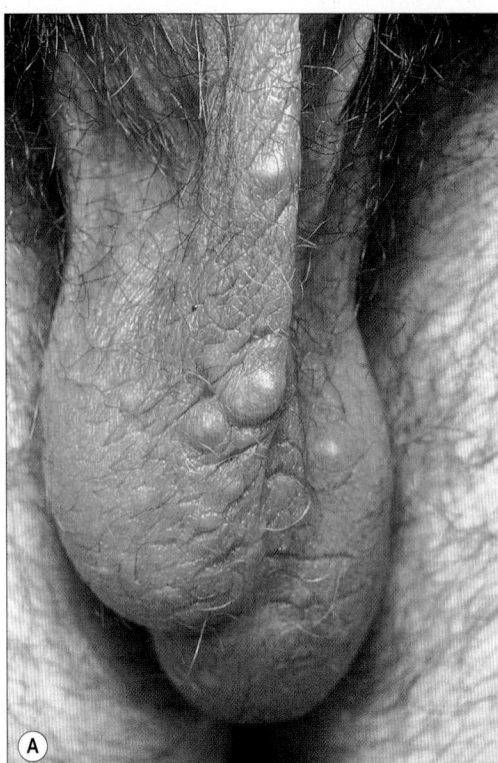

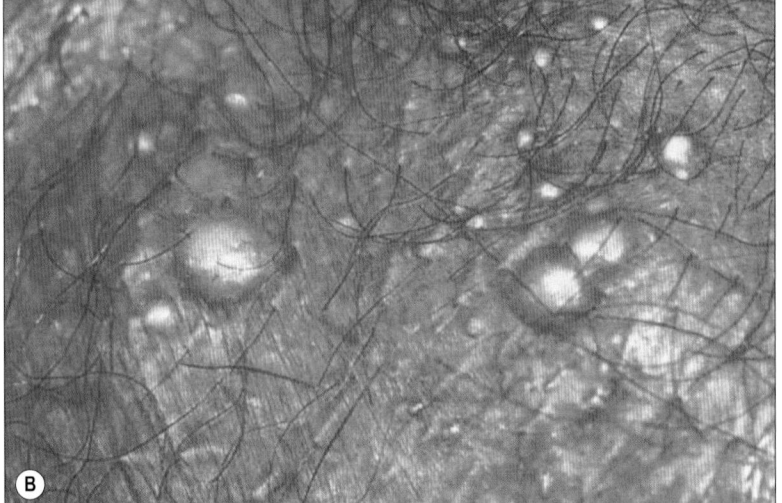

Fig. 12.148
Scrotal calcinosis:
(**A**) characteristic yellow papules and nodules are present; (**B**) close-up view of the lesions. By courtesy of the Institute of Dermatology, London, UK.

vasculitis is initiated that involves skin, subcutis, fascia, and muscle. Classically painful erythematous swelling of the genitals occurs (particularly the scrotum,[2] where a dark red or a black spot may appear) that spreads to perianal or lower abdominal skin, and there may be urinary retention.[3] There is crepitus but no suppuration.[4] In adults there is systemic toxicity, but this may be absent in children.[3] Necrosis of skin and deeper tissues can occur rapidly, and there is a very high mortality unless the diagnosis is made promptly and radical management undertaken. Preceding surgery and instrumentation in patients with the listed risk factors is particularly important.

In adults the mortality is approximately 25%, but it is lower in children.[3,5]

The clinical differential diagnosis of Fournier gangrene includes trauma, herpes simplex, cellulitis (streptococcal, staphylococcal), streptococcal necrotizing fasciitis, gonococcal balanitis and edema, ecthyma gangrenosum, allergic vasculitis, polyarteritis nodosa, necrolytic migratory erythema, vascular occlusion syndromes, and warfarin necrosis.

Miscellaneous conditions

Vulvodynia

Vulvodynia is a clinical, and not a histologic, diagnosis. Biopsy is unhelpful. It is defined as 'vulval pain in the absence of relevant, visible physical findings, or a specific clinically identifiable neurological disorder'.[1] It is a sensory, neuropathic disorder and can be localized and provoked or generalized and spontaneous. Some patients may have an overlap of both types.

Idiopathic calcinosis

Clinical features

Genital calcinosis is uncommon. It occurs much more frequently in the scrotum than in the vulva, where it has only seldom been reported.[1-7] Very rarely, idiopathic calcinosis may develop in the penis or areola of the nipple.[8,9] Lesions present as single or multiple hard nodules in children and young adults (*Fig. 12.148*). Occasionally, nodules break down and discharge chalky material. Some lesions are polypoid and in this setting the clinical diagnosis is difficult if only a single lesion is present.[10-12] Very young children can exceptionally present with single or multiple calcified scrotal lesions secondary to meconium periorchitis.[13,14]

Pathogenesis and histologic features

Although originally thought to represent an idiopathic condition, it more likely that this disorder develops from dystrophic calcification of epidermoid cysts or the contents of cystically dilated eccrine ducts.[15-21] It has also been suggested that the condition can result from dartos muscle degeneration, or cyst wall apoptosis.[22,23] Scrotal calcinosis is characterized by single or multiple dermal nodules of dystrophic calcification (*Fig. 12.149*). In some cases, there is histologic evidence of a preexisting and partially destroyed cyst.

Dermatitis artefacta

Dermatitis artefacta localized to the anogenital area is sometimes encountered (*Figs 12.150–12.152*). At this site the injuries may be sustained in the course of sadomasochistic sexual gratification[1] due to algolagnia (love of pain). A biopsy is usually obtained to exclude genital cancer, but it is important also to consider pyoderma gangrenosum. It should be included in the differential diagnosis of any non-healing or atypical lesion.

Sclerosing lipogranuloma

Clinical features

Sclerosing lipogranuloma (paraffinoma) may involve the scrotum, penis, and exceptionally the epididymus.[1-3] It usually represents a tissue response

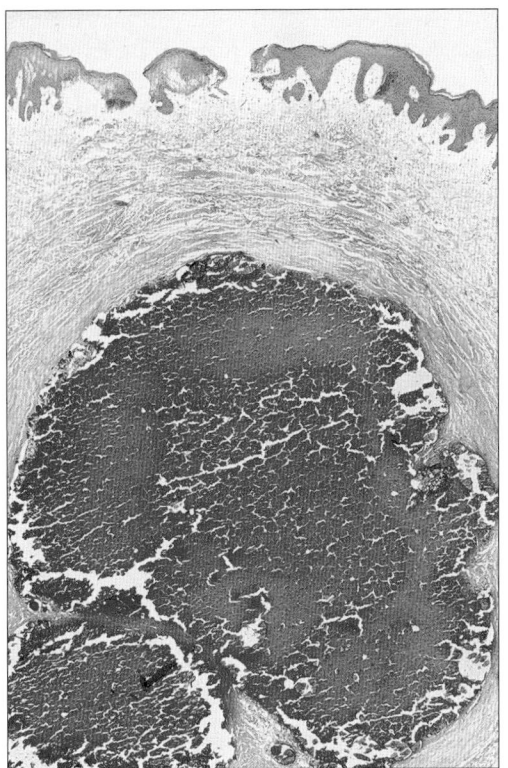

Fig. 12.149
Scrotal calcinosis: the calcium deposits stain purple with hematoxylin and eosin. Sometimes a preexistent epidermoid cyst can be identified.

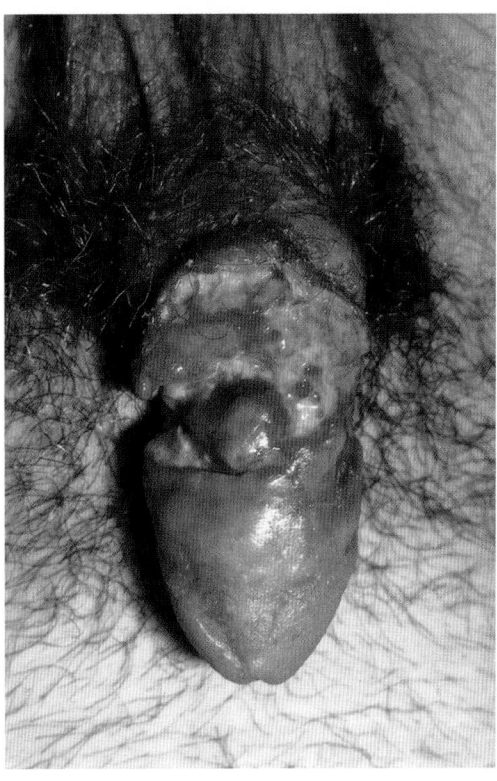

Fig. 12.150
Dermatitis artifacta: there is gross destruction of the penile shaft. From Bunker C. Male Genital Skin Disease. Saunders Ltd./Elsevier 2004.

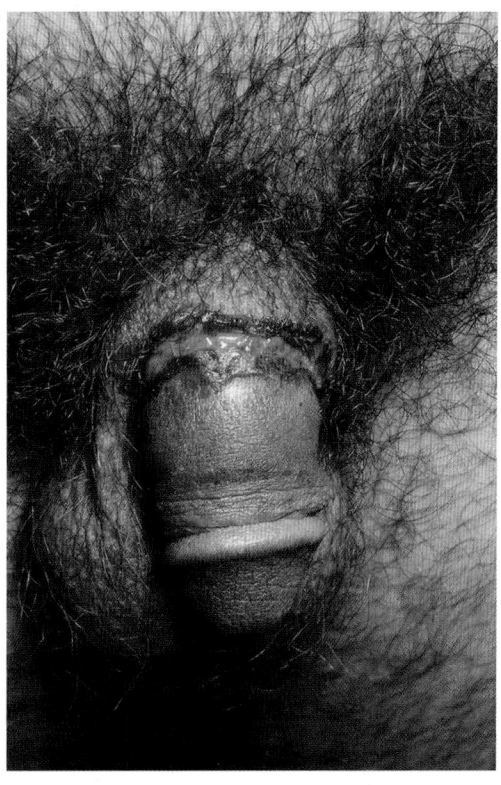

Fig. 12.151
Dermatitis artifacta: note the circumferential ulceration. Reproduced with permission from Bunker C.B. and Mallon E., Management of penile erosions and ulcers, Postgraduate Doctor Middle East, 1998;21:163–168. Copyright © Professional Managerial and Healthcare Publications Limited. From Bunker C. Male Genital Skin Disease. Saunders Ltd./Elsevier 2004.

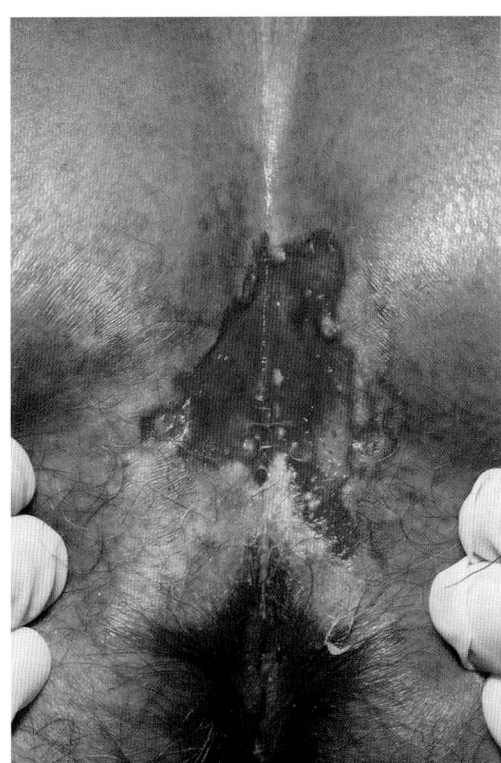

Fig. 12.152
Dermatitis artifacta: this is a view of the natal cleft. Note the central ulceration and surrounding lichenification. From Bunker C. Male Genital Skin Disease. Saunders Ltd./Elsevier 2004.

to exogenous material (usually paraffin, silicone and even mineral oil and Vaseline) and is seen most commonly in the paratesticular area secondary to the injection of size-enhancing materials.[4,5] A very small number of cases of sclerosing lipogranuloma appear to be primary, are more common in Japan, and have predilection for the genitourinary system but can occur elsewhere including the rectum.[6–8] Granulomatous penile nodules (Tanko nodules) have been described due to the insertion of glass spheres under the penile skin.[9]

Histologic features

There is a foreign body-type granulomatous reaction in the dermis. 'Lipid' vacuoles are surrounded by dense fibrous tissue. Rare extensive necrosis in a case of primary sclerosing lipogranuloma has been documented.[8]

Pilonidal sinus

Clinical features

This condition mainly occurs in the sacrococcygeal region and has only rarely been reported as occurring in the penis.[1–8] Only about 20 cases have been reported in the literature. Lesions present in uncircumcised adults with a predilection for the dorsal aspect of the coronal sulcus. It has been postulated that penile pilonidal sinus develops because the coronal sulcus acts as a cleft where hairs can accumulate and eventually penetrate the shaft and the foreskin as a result of friction between these two surfaces. The symptoms are those of chronic inflammation and abscess formation. Pilonidal sinus has been associated with actinomycosis, SCC, and verrucous carcinoma.[1,8–10]

Histologic features

The histopathology is identical to that of pilonidal sinus occurring at the usual site.

Cyclist's vulva

An unusual cause of vulval edema has recently been described that occurs in cyclists.[1] This is usually unilateral and mainly affects the labia majora. It presents as a diffuse unilateral swelling of the vulva that may mimic a soft tissue tumor. The histology shows dilated lymphatics with minor inflammatory change only.

Genital pigmentation

Postinflammatory hyperpigmentation, of non-melanocytic etiology, following an inflammatory dermatosis such as LP is the most common cause of genital pigmentation. However, only melanocytic causes of genital pigmentation are discussed here. They may be difficult to differentiate clinically and, although dermoscopy is of emerging utility, histology is usually needed.[1]

Genital melanosis

Clinical features

Genital melanosis is characterized by pigmentation with no overt evidence of a preceding inflammatory dermatosis.[1-5] However, in men the clinical suspicion is usually raised of past or chronic low-grade LS, LP, ZB, or non-specific balanoposthitis. The pigmentation may vary in its intensity and is typically irregular. The problem usually affects several sites including cutaneous and mucosal surfaces. The pigmentation develops slowly and can be very extensive. In most cases of genital melanosis, lesions become stable and may regress.[6]

Unifocal lesions can also sometimes occur. Small discrete single or multiple lesions are usually described as genital melanotic macules.[4] The most common sites are the glans and shaft of the penis and the inner aspects of the vulva including the vestibule (*Figs 12.153* and *12.154*). Lesions may also affect the vagina and cervix.[7,8]

The condition is considered benign, but there are rare anecdotal reports of melanoma ensuing in areas of melanosis.[9,10] Melanoma rarely occurs in the context of vulval melanosis, and this is likely because in the latter condition there is no increase in the number of melanocytes but only basal cell layer hyperpigmentation. Penile lesions, on the other hand, often display an increase in the number of basal melanocytes. Single lesions are very difficult to distinguish on clinical grounds from either a lentigo or an early junctional nevus.

Cases of multiple genital lesions associated with oral pigmentation have been described as Laugier-Hunziker disease (idiopathic lenticular mucocutaneous pigmentation) (see Chapter 20).[11,12] It is worth remembering that rare cases of Carney complex may present with lentigines in genital skin, and the correct diagnosis will only be possible if close attention is paid to the presence of other markers of this disease.[13,14] Dowling-Degos may also present with genital melanosis.[15]

Histologic features

Genital melanosis is characterized by increased pigmentation of basal keratinocytes and melanocytes (*Fig. 12.155*). By definition, there is no increase in melanocyte number. If, however, melanocytes are present in increased numbers, the term 'genital lentiginosis' may be more appropriate.[16] In real terms, the difference is academic. There is no evidence of junctional activity

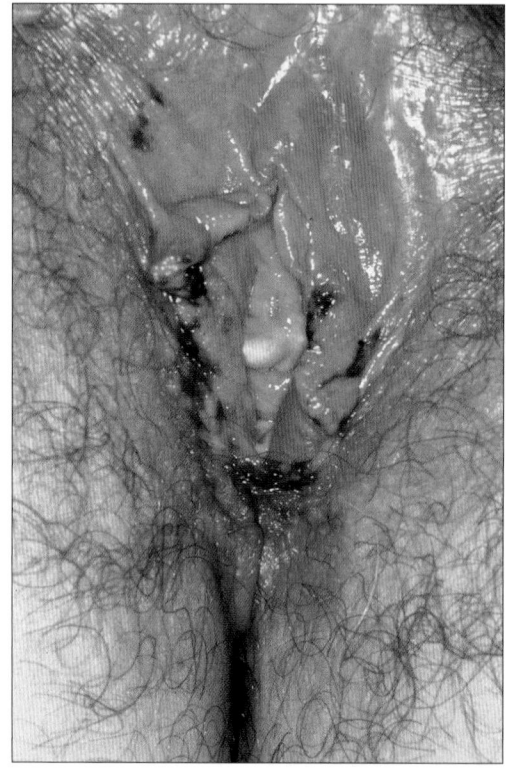

Fig. 12.154
Vulval melanosis: there are multiple irregular pigmented macules on the vulva and adjacent skin. By courtesy of the Institute of Dermatology, London, UK.

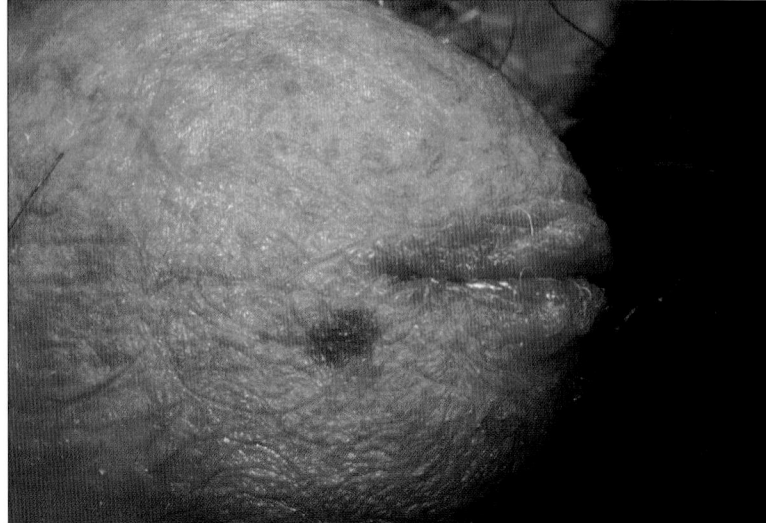

Fig. 12.153
Penile melanotic macule: there is a small irregular pigmented macule on the glans penis. By courtesy of the Institute of Dermatology, London, UK.

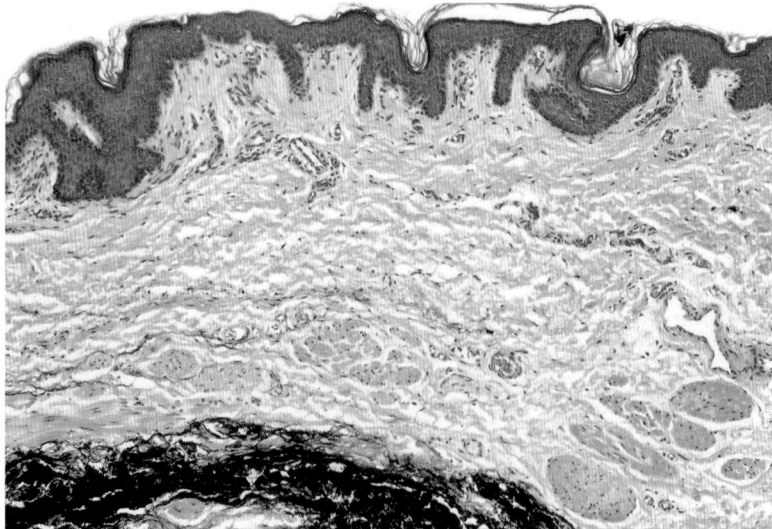

Fig. 12.155
Vulval melanosis: there is marked basal cell pigmentation.

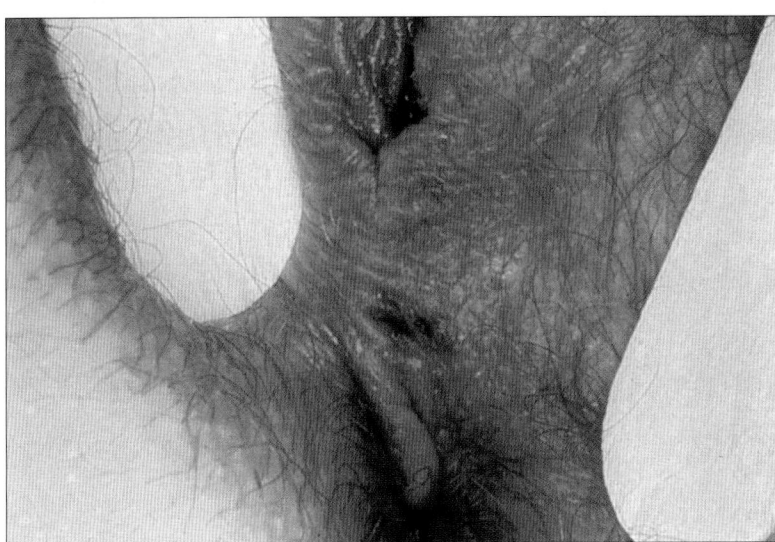

Fig. 12.156
Atypical vulval nevus: there is an irregular darkly pigmented lesion on the perineum. By courtesy of the Institute of Dermatology, London, UK.

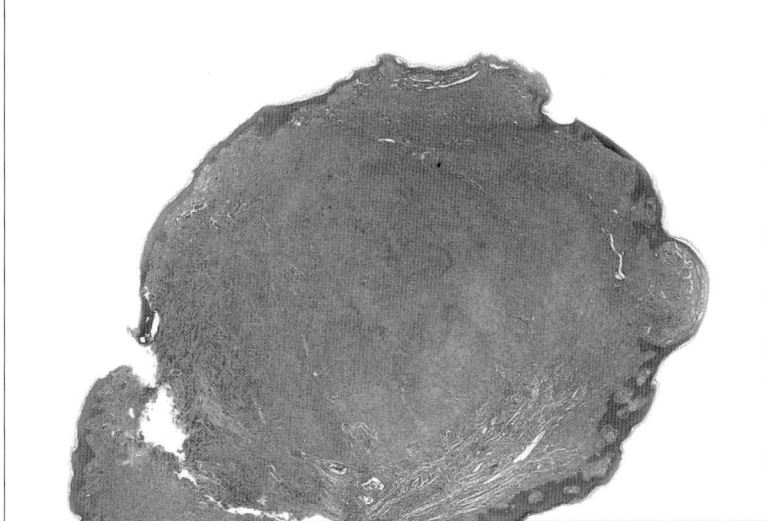

Fig. 12.157
Atypical vulval nevus: scanning view of a polypoid lesion from a 17-year-old female. Note the heavily pigmented nests at the top of the field. By courtesy of the Institute of Dermatology, London, UK.

and, in most cases, cytological atypia is absent. However, it has been suggested that in lesions with increased number of melanocytes and any degree of cytological atypia, there may be an association with melanomas elsewhere in the skin.[6] Pigment-laden macrophages may be conspicuous in the underlying dermis. An important pitfall is the presence of coexistent LS, as the dermal changes may mimic a completely regressed melanoma.[17]

The histologic features of Dowling-Degos disease are specific: moderate orthokeratosis or hyperkeratosis, thinning of the suprapapillary epithelium, 'antler-like' branching of the rete ridges, basal pigmentation with no increase in melanocytic number (S100 normal).[18]

Genital melanocytic nevi

Clinical features

Acquired melanocytic nevi of the genitalia have been estimated to affect 3.5% of children[1] with a male/female ratio of 1.3:1. The prevalence of vulval melanocytic nevi has been reported as 2.3% in one series.[2] Junctional, compound, and dermal nevi can all occur and may demonstrate worrisome histologic features, often raising the possibility of malignancy.[3] Melanocytic lesions presenting in flexural areas (atypical genital nevi, atypical flexural nevi, milk-line nevi, atypical melanocytic nevi of genital type), including the axillae, umbilicus, inguinal creases, pubis, scrotum, and perianal area, similarly may show identical disturbing histologic features.[4]

In women, the presentation is in young girls or adults, and lesions vary in size from a few millimeters to up to 1 cm (Fig. 12.156). Lesions are typically located on the labia minora, mucosal surface of the clitoris, or labia majora.

Pathogenesis and histologic features

Both ordinary and atypical genital nevi can show BRAF V600E mutations as do nevi and melanomas occurring elsewhere.[5] In cases with BRAF mutations, expression of IGFBP7 is maintained, offering a possible explanation as to why these lesions do not have aggressive behavior even harboring BRAF mutations. However, the mutational patterns are different with genital melanomas showing somatic mutations in KIT and TP53.[6]

Banal (ordinary type) and dysplastic nevi are identical to their nongenital counterparts and are discussed elsewhere.

Atypical genital nevi can be a source of considerable diagnostic difficulty and sometimes alarm, which is unfounded as lesions there do not usually progress to melanoma.[3,7,8] Flexural nevi at other sites are often similar although the changes are usually less marked. They may be junctional or compound, symmetrical or asymmetrical, and are typically fairly small, measuring only a few millimeters to 1.0 cm in diameter. The associated

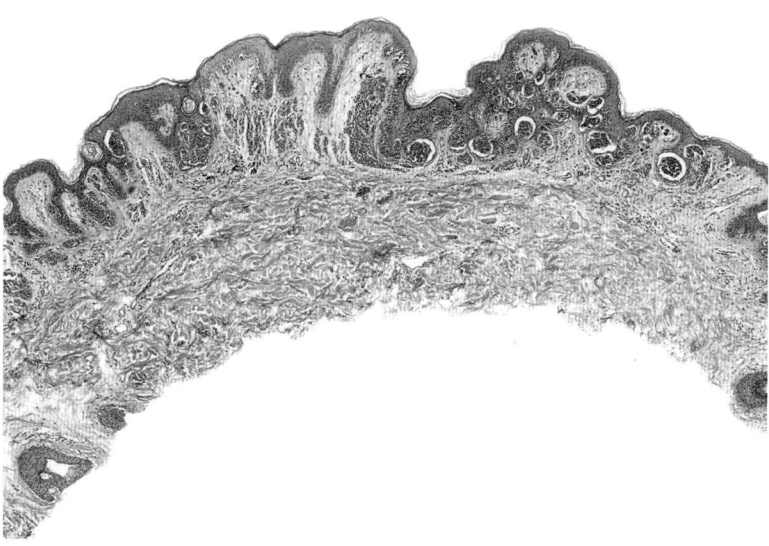

Fig. 12.158
Atypical genital-type nevus: this is a shave biopsy from the labium majus showing a compound melanocytic nevus. The papillomatosis and obvious retraction artifact around the junctional nests are typical features.

epidermis is typically hyperplastic, and papillomatosis can be marked (Figs 12.157 and 12.158). The junctional component is usually lentiginous and nested and commonly involves the adnexae in addition to the epidermis. The nests are often large, surrounded by a retraction artifact and, unlike banal nevi, are situated along the sides in addition to the tips of the rete; they may also be located overlying the dermal papillae (Fig. 12.159). Transepidermal elimination of nests is commonly present, and some degree of pagetoid spread may be a feature.[9] The nevus cells are epithelioid in type and often atypical (Figs 12.160–12.162). The dermal component is composed of morphologically similar nevus cells, which mature with depth. The cytological atypia can affect both junctional and dermal components and in some cases is severe. These features, in addition to dermal mitoses, which are commonly present, may be extreme and raise the possibility of melanoma. Genital melanoma is, however, generally a condition of elderly women. The biological potential of these lesions is benign. Nevertheless, incompletely excised nevi or lesions which extend very close to the radial margin would be best re-excised.

Although there may be some overlap with genital dysplastic nevus, the latter can be distinguished by the presence of elongation of the rete ridges,

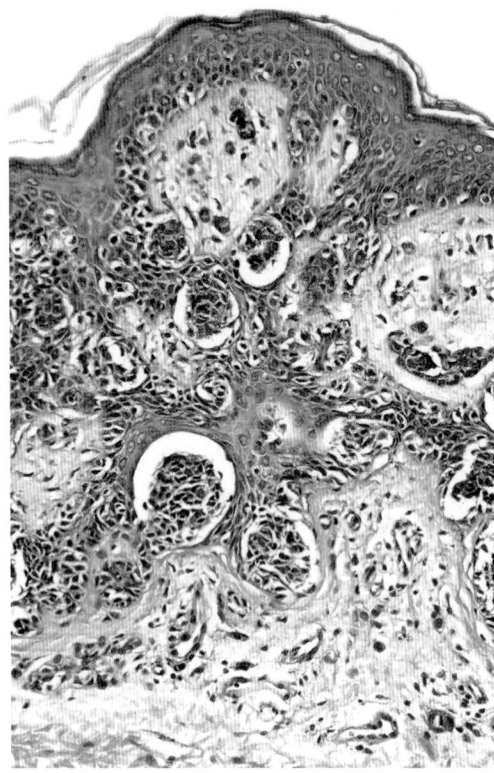

Fig. 12.159
Atypical genital-type nevus: high-power view highlighting the retraction artifact.

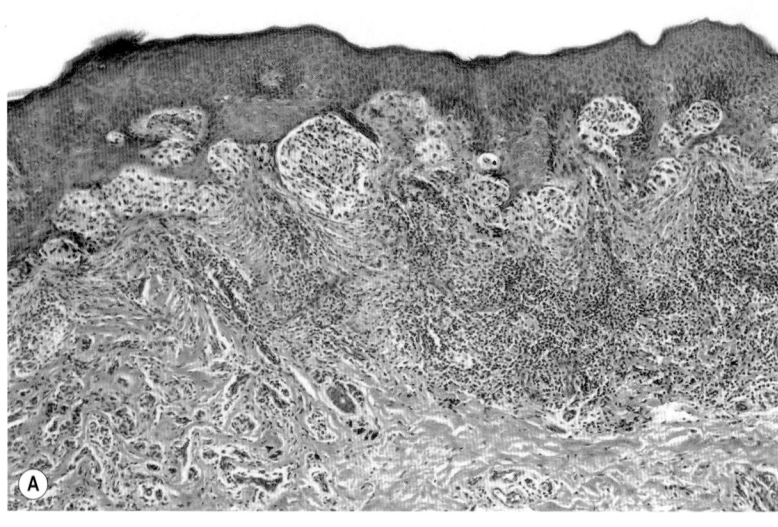

(A)

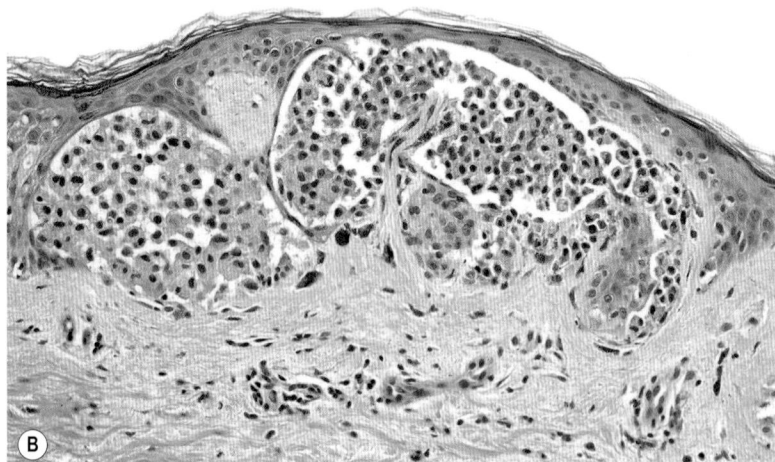

(B)

Fig. 12.160
(**A**, **B**) Atypical genital-type nevus: in this example, the junctional nests are large and due to fine melanin pigmentation; the cytoplasm has a grayish hue. Note the nuclear hyperchromatism.

a more lentiginous distribution of the melanocytes, and the induction of lamellar and eosinophilic fibrosis in the papillary dermis in association with a variable mononuclear inflammatory cell infiltrate and pigmentary incontinence.

Any other type of nevus may occur on genital skin including Spitz nevus, Reed nevus, deep penetrating nevus, and blue nevus. Recently, a small series of epithelioid blue nevi of genital skin in patients with no evidence of Carney complex was reported.[10] These lesions were described on the foreskin and labium minus. Cases of divided or 'kissing' nevus (*Fig. 12.163*) have been reported affecting the penis, analogous to the situation in the eyelid.[11–13]

Congenital 'bathing trunk' nevi may involve the anogenital area and pose significant management problems as they carry a very high risk of multifocal malignant transformation.

Melanoma

Clinical features

Genitourinary melanoma is rare but 10 times more common in women than men in the United States.[1,2] Female genital melanoma accounts for around 3% of all female melanomas and 2–10% of female genital tract malignancies.[3,4] Mucosal female tract melanomas account for 18% of all mucosal melanomas. The vulva is the most frequently involved site followed by the vagina and much less often the cervix (*Fig. 12.164*).[5] The labia majora and the clitoris are the most commonly affected sites. Most patients present in the sixth and seventh decades of life. Less than one-third of cases occur in patients younger than 50 years of age. Melanoma of the vulva in children is exceptional and in some cases reported in association with LS.[6] An association with melanosis is very rare,[7] and a tumor in a young woman, a frequent user of tanning parlors, has been documented.[8]

Clinical presentation varies from flat to raised polypoid brown to black lesions. Ulceration may be present. Less commonly, patients complain of pruritus and/or bleeding. Amelanotic melanomas are reported to be rare, but they represented 27% of all cases in a large Swedish series.[4–9] They may clinically mimic SCC or extramammary Paget disease.

Some tumors arise within a preexisting nevus. A recent study found the latter to occur in around 5% of cases.[4] Most of these are of the superficial spreading type.

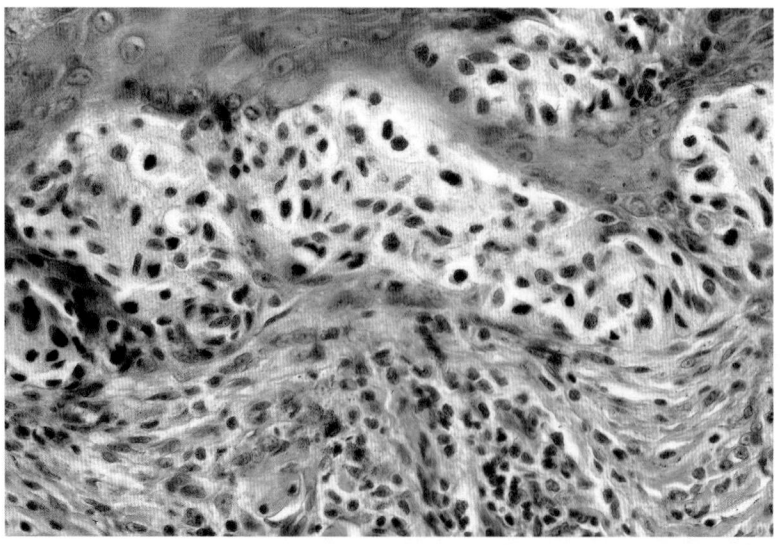

Fig. 12.161
Atypical genital-type nevus: in this field, there is nuclear hyperchromatism and mild pleomorphism.

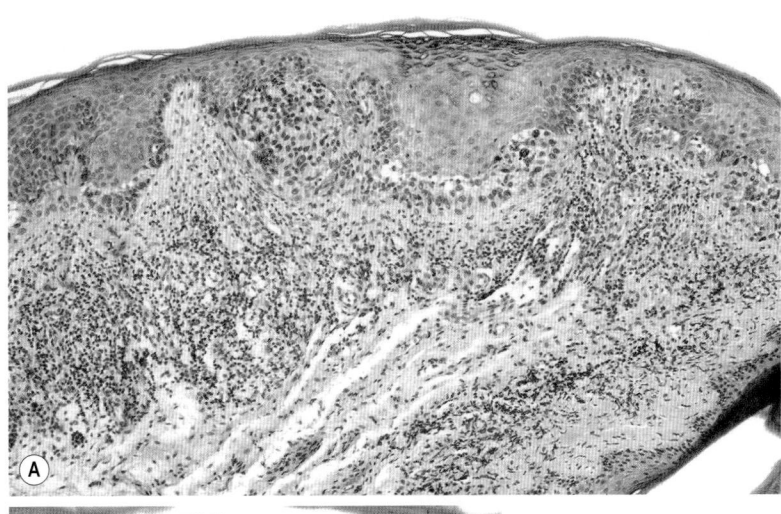

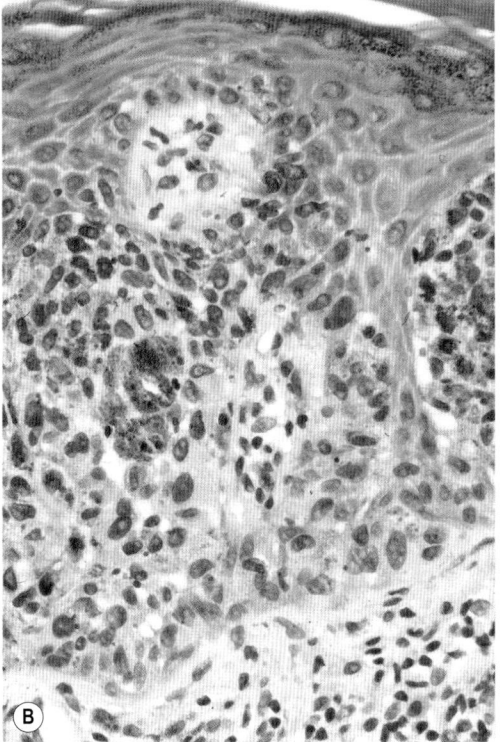

Fig. 12.162
(A, B) Atypical genital-type nevus: this example from the vulva of a 20-year-old female shows severe cytological atypia. The biological behavior of this nevus variant is uncertain although the likelihood of malignancy is very low. It should, however, be completely excised.

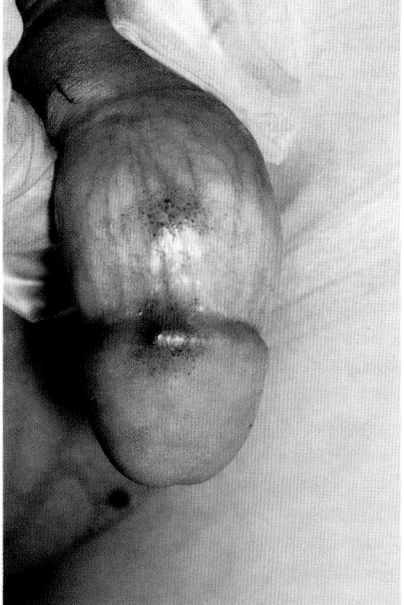

Fig. 12.163
Divided or 'kissing' nevus: note the pigmented lesions on the shaft and the glans penis. From Bunker C. Male Genital Skin Disease. Saunders Ltd./Elsevier 2004.

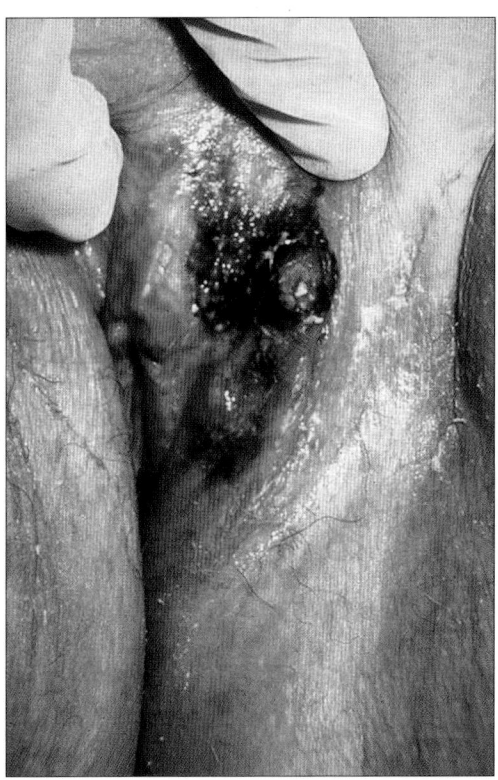

Fig. 12.164
Vulval melanoma: tumors at this site are very rare. They are commonly thick at presentation and therefore generally associated with a poor prognosis. By courtesy of M. Ridley, MD, Institute of Dermatology, London, UK.

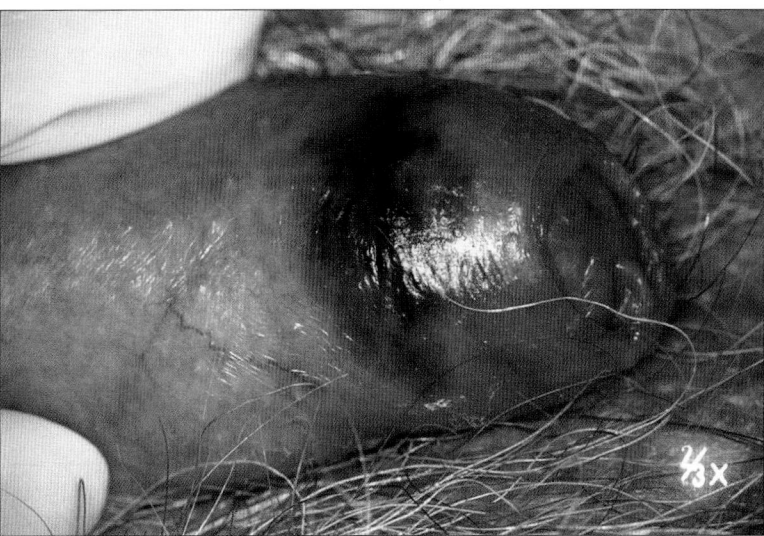

Fig. 12.165
Penile melanoma: note the large size, irregular border, and variable pigmentation. By courtesy of the Institute of Dermatology, London, UK.

A recent study reports a 45% 5-year survival rate for patients with vulval melanoma, which is 15% lower than matched controls with cutaneous melanoma.[10] As with melanomas presenting elsewhere, tumor thickness is the best predictor of survival.[3,11] Staging has also been found to be an independent predictor of survival. In addition, in stage I disease only, ulceration and the presence of clinical amelanosis were found to be independent predictors of survival.[12] Radical surgery for vulval melanoma does not seem to influence outcome. A multivariate analysis of 644 patients with vulval melanoma found that young age, localized disease, and negative lymph nodes were independent prognostic factors.[10] The 5-year disease-specific survival was 75.5%, 38.7%, and 22.1% for patients with localized, regional, and distant disease, respectively.

Melanoma of the male genital skin is very rare, as are those arising around or on the anus (Fig. 12.165).[13–16] Penile metastasis of cutaneous melanoma elsewhere is exceptional.[17] The most common site in men is the glans, but rare cases may present elsewhere, including the shaft and the scrotum.[18–20] The diagnosis can be delayed because of the patient's reluctance to seek medical help.[21] Exceptional cases complicating penile melanosis, penile nevi, have been reported, also a penile melanoma which developed simultaneously with SCC.[22–24] Because of the rarity of the disease, estimation of prognosis is difficult. In the few cases reported, the prognosis appears poor but this seems to be related to late presentation, delay in diagnosis, and problems in achieving complete clearance because of the site. A study of a series of 19 primary mucosal penile melanomas and a review of 47 cases reported in the literature found 2- and 5-year survival rates of 63% and 31%, respectively[25] All patients presenting with nodal and/or distant metastasis died of disease within 2 years.[26] The prognosis is similar in patients who present with metastatic disease on the penis from a primary tumor elsewhere.[25] Poor prognosis was associated with ulceration, Breslow thickness of more than 3.5 mm, and a tumor diameter of more than 15 mm. The behavior of mucosal penile melanoma appears to be the same as cutaneous melanoma elsewhere of similar thickness.

Pathogenesis and histologic features

Unlike cutaneous melanoma, it is difficult to postulate a major role for ultraviolet radiation in genital melanomagenesis. However, a case of melanoma in situ of the glans has been reported in a naturist with a short prepuce.[27] A significant number of mucosal melanomas have shown mutations in c-kit as opposed to melanomas arising in skin exposed intermittently to the sun, in which *BRAF* mutations are frequently found.[28–30] Somatic mutations in P53 are also often seen in genital melanomas.[30] The presence of c-kit mutations offers the possibility of targeted therapy to those melanomas harboring the mutation. A study of vulvar and vaginal melanomas detected HPV-3 and epidermodysplasia verruciformis-associated types of HPV in a number of lesions.[31] Since these HPV types are not usually found in the vulva or vagina, it has been suggested that they may play a role in the pathogenesis of melanomas at these sites.

Histologic features of genital melanoma are identical to melanomas elsewhere. Until recently, there was no consensus as to the most common type of genital melanoma. Recently, however, a large study found that 57% of vulval melanomas were mucosal lentiginous, 22% nodular, 12% unclassified, and 4% superficial spreading.[32] Desmoplastic and neurotropic variants may also occasionally be encountered. Multiple in situ penile melanomas have been documented.[33]

Benign epithelial lesions

Localized epidermolytic hyperkeratosis/epidermolytic acanthoma

Infrequently, epidermal hyperkeratosis can affect the genitalia as a solitary asymptomatic acquired lesion. The vulva, vaginal wall, scrotum, and rarely the prepuce are the genital sites of predilection. Clinically the disorder presents as leukoplakia. Well reviewed by Velazquez et al, the histology as described by Ackerman is of compact hyperkeratosis; clear, differently sized spaces around the nuclei in the strata spinosum and granulosum; reticulate, lightly staining, amphophilic material that forms indistinct cellular boundaries; marked thickening of the granular zone, containing increased variously sized, irregularly shaped keratohyaline bodies. Decrease amounts of keratins 1 and 10 are seen immunohistochemically.[1,2]

Verruciform xanthoma

Verruciform xanthoma is a rare entity that principally affects the mouth. Genitalia are the next most frequently affected, where it presents as a painless, yellow-brown or red, verrucous, sessile, or papillary plaque (*Fig. 12.166*).[1] Histologically, there is hyperkeratosis, focal parakeratosis, and irregular epidermal acanthosis; acantholysis has been reported.[1,2] Rete ridges are lengthened and extend into the dermis, forming areas called dermal papillae and enclosing capillary vessels surrounded by foam cells. These stain with CD 68 but not S100.[1,3] It is thought that the lesion results from apoptotic (probably post-traumatic) epidermal degeneration and that keratinocytic lipid is taken up by dermal macrophages or fibroblasts to form the

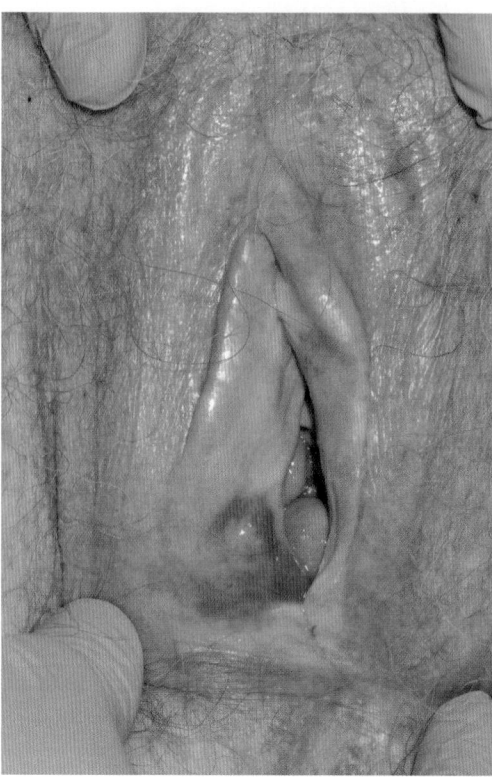

Fig. 12.166
Verruciform xanthoma of the vulva: warty plaque on right labium majus with lichen sclerosus

foam cells.[3,4] An association with squamous carcinoma[5] has been reported, but HPV is not implicated in the pathogenesis of verruciform xanthoma.[6]

In females, an association with LS and other inflammatory conditions has been suggested.[7]

Benign mucinous metaplasia and mucinous syringometaplasia

Benign mucinous metaplasia of the genitalia is exceptionally rare.[1,2] It has been reported on the labia and foreskin. The clinical features are nondistinctive, and histologically benign mucus-containing cells are found within the epidermis with a predilection for the upper layers. It has been reported in ZB and vulvitis and LS.[3] The differential diagnoses are extramammary Paget disease and, in women, VIN with mucinous differentiation. Distinction from extramammary Paget disease is difficult, but the cells in benign mucinous metaplasia lack cytological atypia and contain nuclei with basal orientation.[1] A bandlike inflammatory infiltrate has also been shown to be a common feature in benign mucinous metaplasia.[4]

Mucinous syringometaplasia is very rare in genital skin and can be distinguished from benign mucinous metaplasia because the cells in the former are not confined to the epidermis but extend into adnexal structures.[5]

Endometriosis and endosalpingiosis

Clinical features

Cutaneous endometriosis is uncommon, is predominantly seen in young females, and usually develops in a scar following an abdominal operation such as a cesarean section.[1,2] On occasions, it appears to develop spontaneously in the integument (e.g., in the umbilicus, the inguinal region and the perineum).[3] Endometriosis of the vulva is rare and may occur in an episiotomy scar or after curettage.[4,5] Clinically, it presents as a bluish nodule, which is often painful, and sometimes shows cyclical variation in size and symptoms, occasionally with bleeding during menstruation. Malignant transformation in cutaneous endometriosis is extremely rare.[6]

Cutaneous endosalpingiosis is a similar condition in which cysts lined by tubal epithelium develop as a consequence of salpingectomy.[3] It is exceedingly rare in the skin, and most cases have presented in an abdominal scar

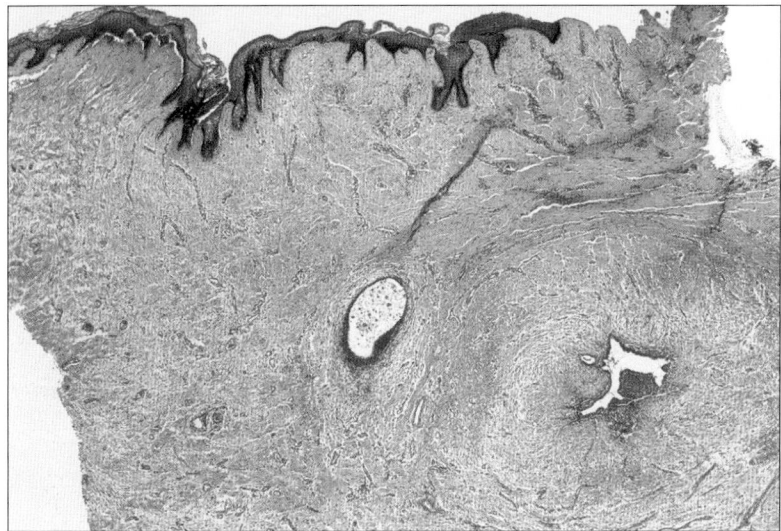

Fig. 12.167
Vulval endometriosis: endometrial glands with edematous stroma are present in the reticular dermis.

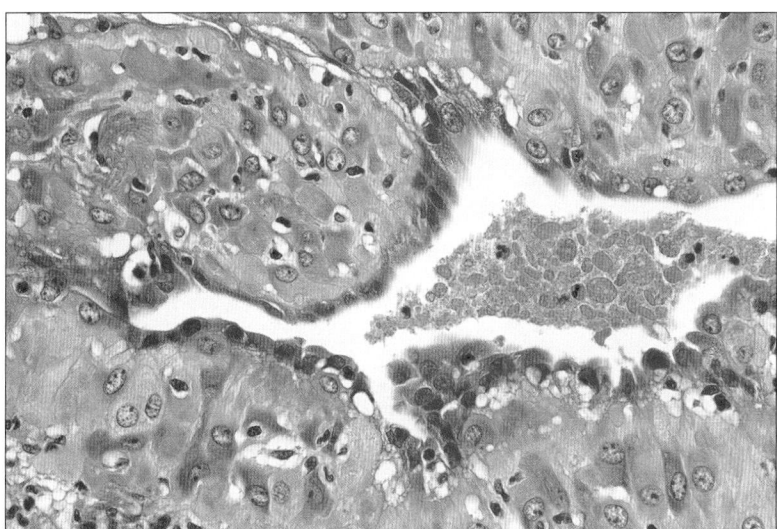

Fig. 12.168
Vulval endometriosis: in this example, there is stromal decidualization.

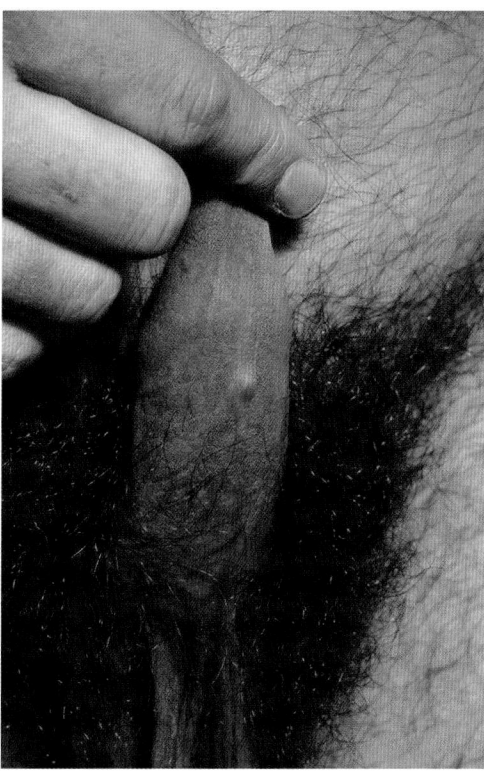

Fig. 12.169
Median raphe cyst: there is a translucent cystic swelling on the glans penis. From Bunker C. Male Genital Skin Disease. Saunders Ltd./ Elsevier 2004.

and occasionally in the umbilicus.[7] One case was associated with severe abdominal pain.[8]

Histologic features

The diagnosis of cutaneous endometriosis depends on the detection of both endometrial glands and stroma (Figs 12.167 and 12.168).[1] Endometrial glands are lined by tall columnar epithelium with basophilic cytoplasm and basally located oval vesicular nuclei. All types of metaplastic changes of the müllerian epithelium can be seen including tubal, oxyphilic, hobnail, mucinous, and papillary syncytial.[9] Mitotic activity may sometimes be marked, and rarely atypical mitotic figures are identified. The stroma is composed of small spindle cells and is usually edematous. Occasionally, decidualization is evident. When the latter is seen, decidual cells are positive for CD30, the latter being a potential pitfall in diagnosis.[10] Other stromal changes include smooth muscle metaplasia, lipoblast-like cells some with intranuclear inclusions, myocytes with degenerative changes, and exceptionally elastosis and perineural invasion. Menstrual bleeding into the deposits often leads to hemosiderin deposition, scarring, and chronic inflammation.

Histologically, in endosalpingiosis, the cyst (which is unilocular) is lined by an admixture of ciliated columnar, nonciliated mucus-secreting columnar, and intercalated dark cells. In contrast to endometriosis, there is no associated stroma and foci of hemorrhage and/or hemosiderin are not seen.

Median raphe cyst

Clinical features

Median raphe cyst (urethroid cyst) is a rare lesion that usually presents on the ventral aspect of the penis of young adults, with a predilection for the glans (Fig. 12.169).[1-4] Perineal and scrotal lesions may occasionally be seen and are rarely polypoid.[5-7] Some lesions present as a cordlike induration.[8] The cyst is usually congenital but tends to become visible only in adult life, often after trauma or infection. Exceptional development after orchiopexy has been documented.[9] Lesions are most commonly solitary, asymptomatic, and measure only a few millimeters in diameter. Large lesions are very rare.[10] Exceptional cases present with multiple cysts and spontaneous regression has also been reported.[11] Pigmented cysts are due to the presence of melanocytes in the lining.[10,12,13] Simple excision is curative.

Pathogenesis and histologic features

It is likely that the cyst originates not as a result of defective closure of the median raphe but secondary to anomalous budding and separation of the urethral columnar epithelium from the urethra.[3]

The cyst is lined by pseudostratified columnar epithelium (Figs 12.170 and 12.171). Rarely, mucin-containing cells or ciliated cells are seen.[14,15] Immunohistochemical stains show that the cells lining the cyst are positive for cytokeratin 7, cytokeratin 13, and CAM 5.2, and negative for cytokeratin 20. It has been suggested that this pattern of keratin expression supports the theory that the cells lining the cyst represent a columnar mucinous epithelium that has undergone immature urothelial metaplasia.[16] Scattered melanocytes and neuroendocrine cells (positive for chromogranin and synaptophysin) may also be identified.[16] Although this lesion may mimic an apocrine cystadenoma, this line of differentiation is unlikely, as the cells in the cyst are negative for human milk fat globulin 1.[17]

Bartholin duct cyst

Clinical features

These lesions present in women of reproductive age as a result of obstruction of the main duct of Bartholin gland.[1] They are relatively uncommon and occur in the posterior aspect of the labium majus, ranging in size from

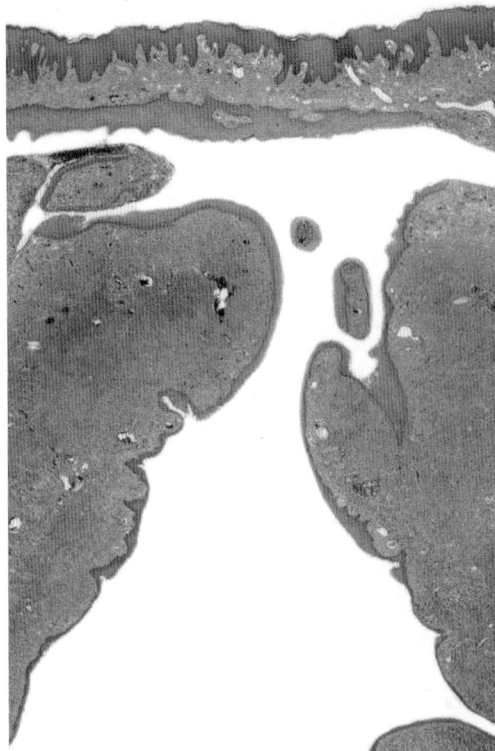

Fig. 12.170
Median raphe cyst: low-power view of cyst. By courtesy of C. Gulmann, MD, Beaumont Hospital, Dublin, Republic of Ireland.

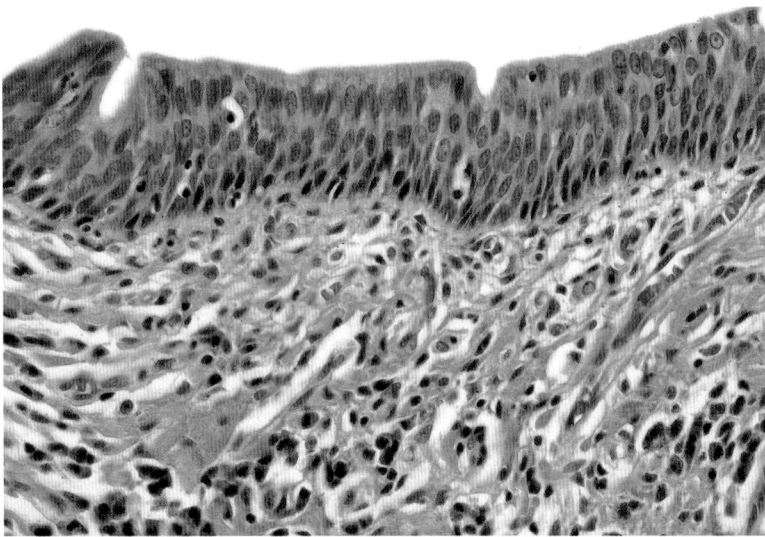

Fig. 12.171
Median raphe cyst: the cyst is lined by pseudostratified epithelium. By courtesy of C. Gulmann, MD, Beaumont Hospital, Dublin, Republic of Ireland.

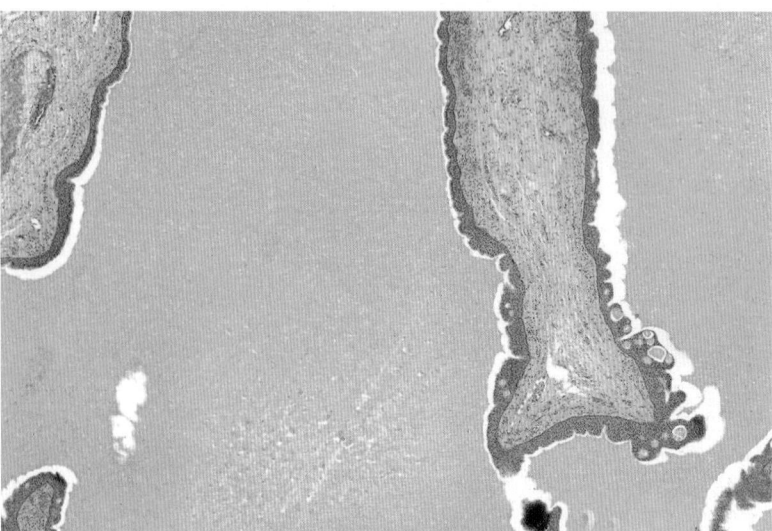

Fig. 12.172
Bartholin duct cyst: low-power view of the cyst. By courtesy of C. Crum, MD, Brigham and Women's Hospital and Harvard Medical School, Boston, USA.

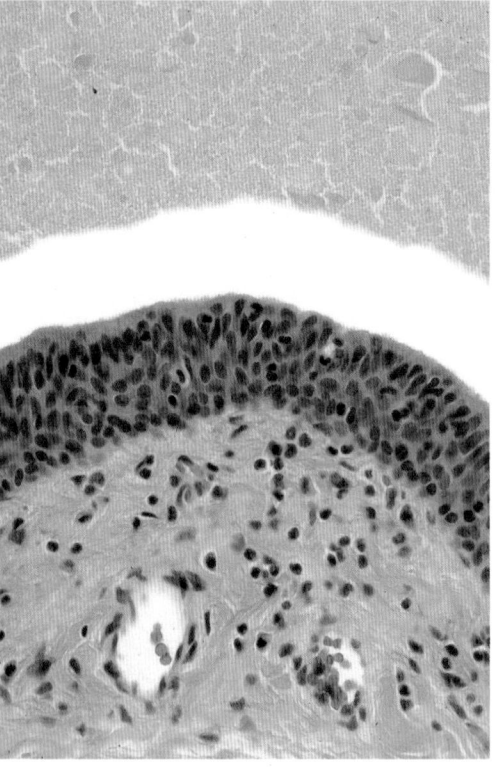

Fig. 12.173
Bartholin duct cyst: the cyst is lined by transitional epithelium. By courtesy of C. Crum, MD, Brigham and Women's Hospital and Harvard Medical School, Boston, USA.

1 cm to several centimeters in diameter. Cysts are usually asymptomatic, but the development of a Bartholin gland abscess is a relatively common complication as the retained glandular secretions become infected.

Histologic features

The cyst is lined by transitional epithelium, which frequently undergoes squamous metaplasia (*Figs 12.172* and *12.173*).[2] Very rarely, a papilloma has been reported developing within a cyst.[3] The exceptional development of a high-grade SCC associated with HPV 16 within a cyst has also been described.[4]

Mucinous cyst

Clinical features

These are rare lesions in men that present as small flesh-colored, midline, translucent, mobile, papules (2 mm) to nodules (25 mm), usually easily

determined to be cystic on clinical grounds.[1,2] They do not have a punctum. Either they are asymptomatic or they become infected or interfere with sex. They have usually been present from birth or childhood and are common near the glans penis or on the foreskin, but may occur anywhere from the urethral meatus to the anus and present at any age in life. The assessment of such cysts should involve the exclusion of secondary infection, for example, gonorrhea.

Vulval lesions are mainly seen in adult women and present as a solitary or, less often, multiple lesions in the vestibule.[3,4] Rare cases are found in adolescents. This cyst arises as a result of obstruction of the duct of a minor vestibular gland. Simple excision is curative.

Pathogenesis and histologic features

Lesions in women were thought to be derived from müllerian epithelium. It is more likely, however, that lesions in both men and women derive from ectopic urogenital sinus epithelium.[2,4] The cyst is lined by a layer

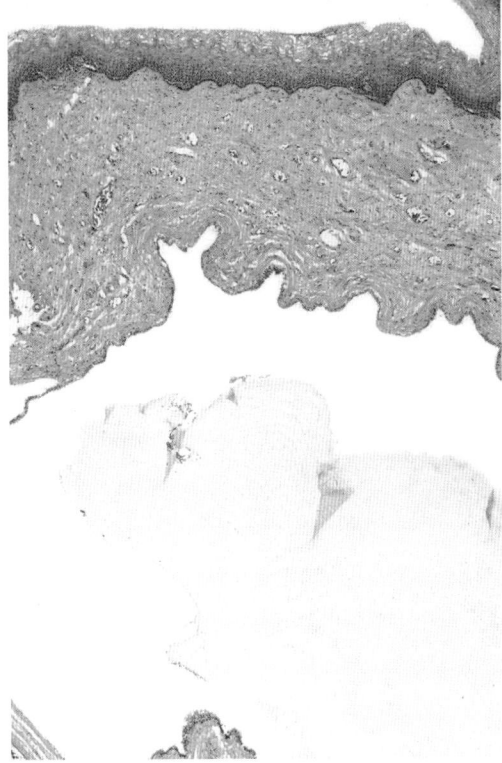

Fig. 12.174
Mucinous cyst: low-power view of mucin-containing cyst. Note the nonkeratinizing surface epithelium. By courtesy of C. Crum, MD, Brigham and Women's Hospital and Harvard Medical School, Boston, USA.

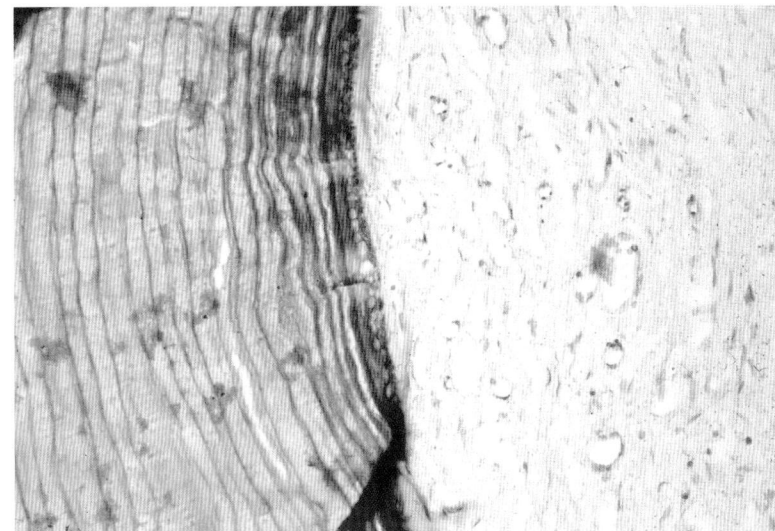

Fig. 12.176
Mucinous cyst: the mucin stains bright red with mucicarmine. By courtesy of C. Crum, MD, Brigham and Women's Hospital and Harvard Medical School, Boston, USA.

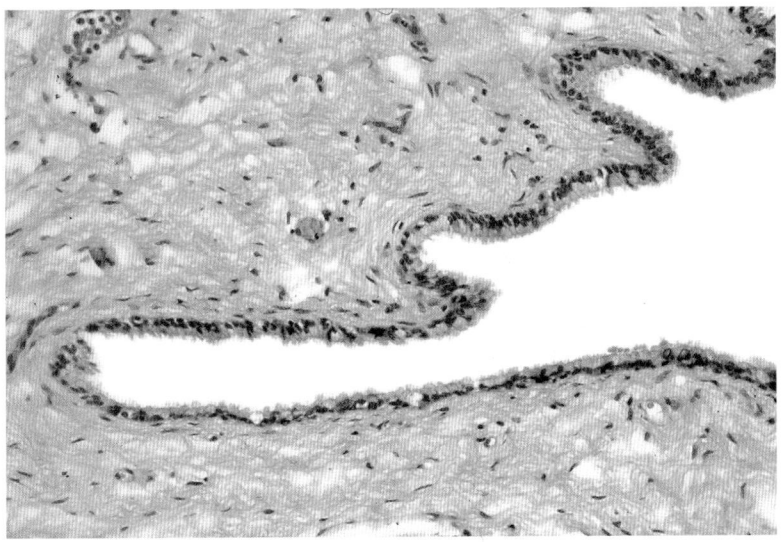

Fig. 12.175
Mucinous cyst: the cyst is lined by mucin-secreting epithelium. By courtesy of C. Crum, MD, Brigham and Women's Hospital and Harvard Medical School, Boston, USA.

of mucinous epithelium with occasional focal squamous metaplasia (*Figs 12.174–12.176*). Myoepithelial cells are not identified.

Mesonephric cyst

Clinical features

This lesion presents in the lateral part of the vulva as a small, asymptomatic, blue-red cystic lesion containing clear fluid. It is thought to be derived from remnants of the mesonephric duct. Simple excision is curative.

Histologic features

The cyst is lined by a single layer of cuboidal or columnar nonciliated cells surrounded by a layer of smooth muscle.[1]

Mesothelial cyst

Clinical features

Mesothelial cyst (cyst of the canal of Nuck) presents as a lesion varying in size from less than 1 cm to 5 cm or more. It arises on the upper and lateral aspect of the labium majus at the level of the insertion of the round ligament. Some cases are associated with an inguinal hernia. Simple excision is curative.

Histologic features

Microscopic examination reveals a unilocular cavity lined by a single layer of flattened mesothelial cells.[1]

Periurethral cyst

Clinical features

This cyst presents as a small or, exceptionally, large swelling lateral to the urethral meatus.[1,2]

Histologic features

Histologic examination shows a cavity lined by transitional epithelium (*Figs 12.177* and *12.178*).

Penile horn

Cutaneous horn (*Fig. 12.179*) is a type of verrucous lesion marked by excessive and increasing keratosis, and a penile horn is a rare lesion with only a handful of reported cases.[1-6] The hyperkeratosis of the cutaneous horn may derive from numerous dermatological lesions including burns, nevi, angiomas, Bowen disease, condylomata, seborrheic keratoses/basal cell papillomas, basal cell carcinoma, pseudoepitheliomatous hyperkeratotic and micaceous balanitis, verrucous carcinoma, and squamous carcinoma.[1,7-10] Chronic inflammation and recent circumcision for long-standing phimosis are important predisposing factors. The lesion is premalignant or, in one-third of cases, malignant at presentation with SCC as the underlying pathology. Precise diagnosis is achieved by adequate excision and histology of the whole lesion, with follow-up because recurrence may occur.[11]

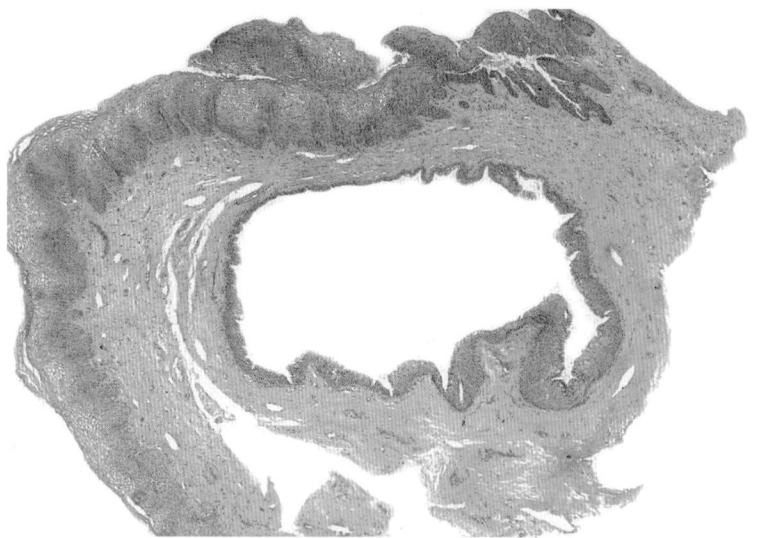

Fig. 12.177
Periurethral cyst: low-power view of unilocular cyst. By courtesy of C. Crum, MD, Brigham and Women's Hospital and Harvard Medical School, Boston, USA.

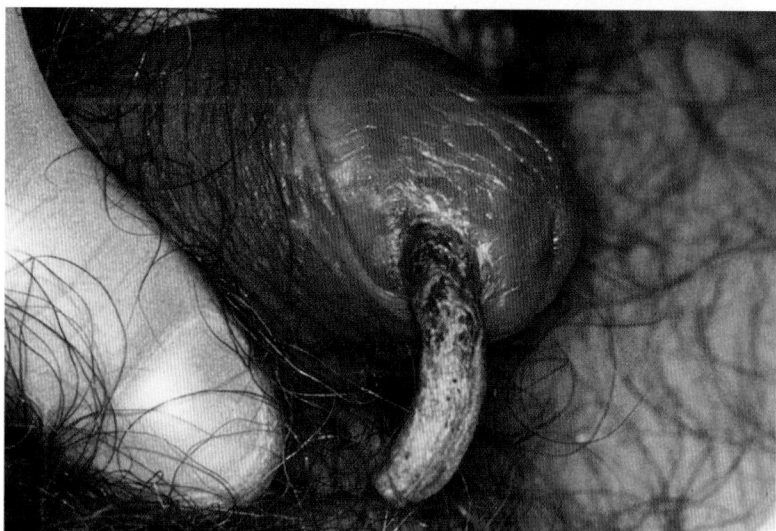

Fig. 12.179
Penile horn: this lesion arose from an underlying squamous cell carcinoma. Courtesy of Dr. J. Ponce de Leon, Barcelona, Spain. Reproduced by kind permission of Blackwell Science from Ponce de Leon J. et al. Cutaneous horn of glans penis. Br J Urol 1994;74:257–8. From Bunker C. Male Genital Skin Disease. Saunders Ltd./Elsevier 2004.

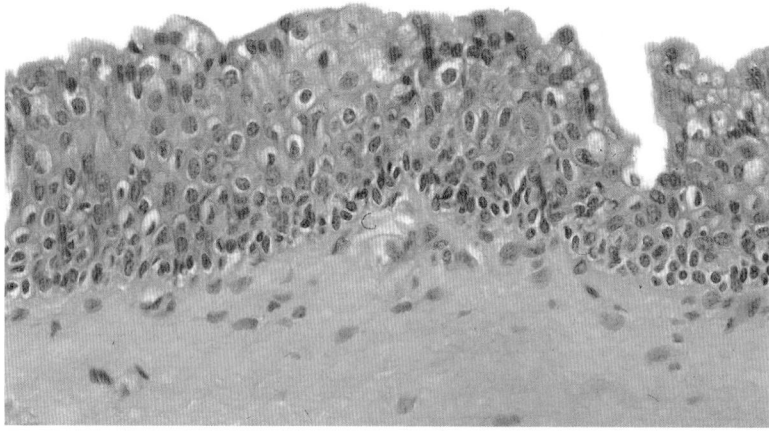

Fig. 12.178
Periurethral cyst: the cyst is lined by transitional epithelium. By courtesy of C. Crum, MD, Brigham and Women's Hospital and Harvard Medical School, Boston, USA.

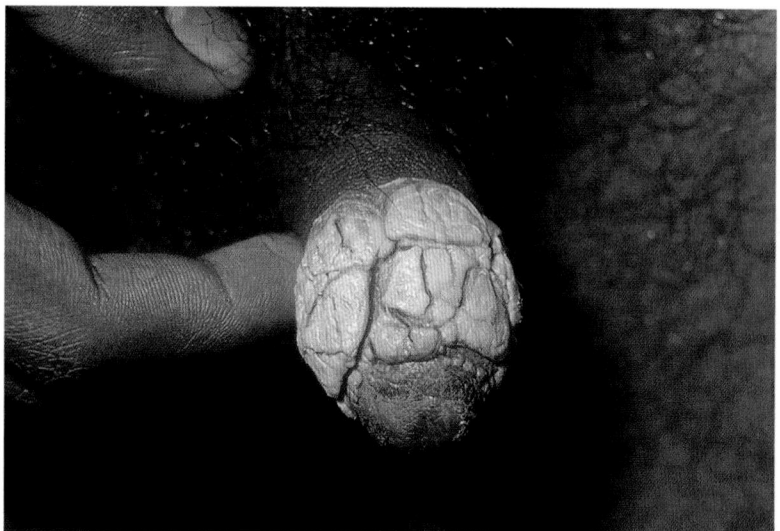

Fig. 12.180
Pseudoepitheliomatous micaceous and keratotic balanitis: verrucous plaques are present on the glans penis. Courtesy of B. Kumar, MD, Chandigarh, India. From Bunker C. Male Genital Skin Disease. Saunders Ltd./Elsevier 2004.

Pseudoepitheliomatous, keratotic, and micaceous balanitis

Clinical features

Pseudoepitheliomatous micaceous and keratotic balanitis (PEMKB) is a rare penile condition that was first described by Lortat-Jacob and Civatte.[1,2] It presents as thick, scaly, micaceous patches[3–6] on the glans penis of older uncircumcised men. Clinically, white, hyperkeratotic, and crusted 'micaceous' plaques develop on the glans penis. These lesions are resistant to treatment, and a verrucous (penile horn) or erosive tumor may emerge from them (*Figs 12.180* and *12.181*). It has been misdiagnosed as reactive arthritis. It is most likely a rare variant of chronic LS with a strong association with verrucous carcinoma and no association with HPV.[7,8] Metastatic spread has not occurred except where there was a penile horn[9] and in one patient who developed an aggressive soft tissue sarcoma of the penis.[10]

Histologic features

Biopsies from early lesions show mild to moderate epidermal hyperplasia with no cytological atypia and a variable focal lichenoid mononuclear inflammatory cell infiltrate. Larger lesions display pseudoepitheliomatous hyperplasia, and often there is transition to verrucous carcinoma.

Genital intraepithelial neoplasia and squamous cell carcinoma

In this text, the term intraepithelial neoplasia is restricted to squamous intraepithelial neoplasia and does not include extramammary Paget disease or melanoma in situ. The terminology used for premalignant vulval epithelial lesions has been confusing and unsatisfactory for many years. In 1986, older terms such as Bowen disease, erythroplasia of Queyrat, bowenoid papulosis, multifocal pigmented Bowen disease, severe dysplasia, and carcinoma in situ, which represented full-thickness atypia, were abandoned in favor of a grading system into three categories similar to that used for cervical intraepithelial neoplasia.[1–3] VIN grades 1, 2, and 3 represent the degree, in thirds, that the epithelium is atypical. This terminology has been extended to include other perineal sites, for example, perianal intraepithelial neoplasia (PaIN 3) and the penis (discussed elsewhere).

Furthermore, unique to the vulval skin, 'VIN 3 differentiated' was introduced to describe a variant where the neoplastic cells do not extend

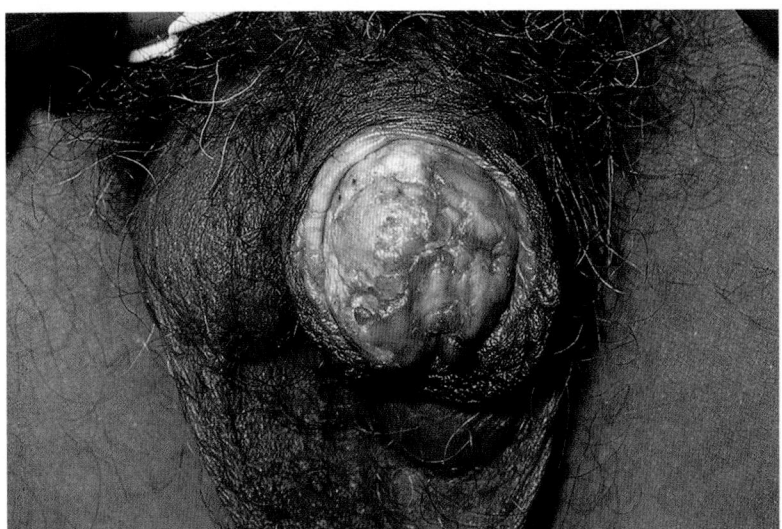

Fig. 12.181
Pseudoepitheliomatous micaceous and keratotic balanitis: note the verrucous plaque. There is underlying lichen sclerosus. Courtesy of B. Kumar, MD, Chandigarh, India. From Bunker C. Male Genital Skin Disease. Saunders Ltd./ Elsevier 2004.

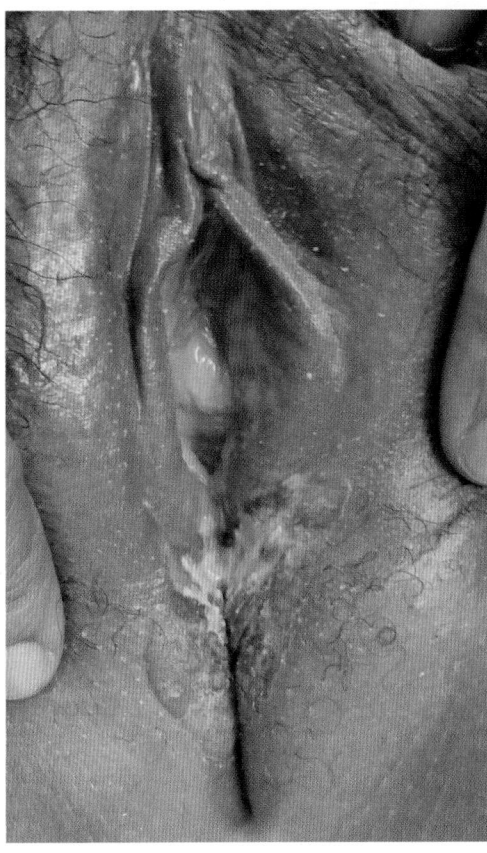

Fig. 12.182
Intraepithelial neoplasia: pigmented VIN. By courtesy of the Institute of Dermatology, London, UK.

throughout the full thickness of the epidermis, which remains well differentiated. However, this terminology does not compare like with like, since the cervix is covered by mucosa and most of the epithelium covering the vulva is skin, the only area that is a mucosa being the vestibule. This newer terminology did not take into account the clinical and biological differences between the cervix and the vulva, and there was also a misconception that there was a natural progression through grades 1–3 to invasive squamous cell carcinoma (SCC). In addition, there were problems with interobserver variation, particularly with VIN 2 and 3, and also poor correlation clinically with some lesions that were histologically VIN 1 and 2.[4] Changes similar to VIN 1 are often found in states where abnormal basal cytology is a result of epithelial reparation (e.g., LP or basal hyperplasia arising from HPV infection). A newer classification was therefore proposed to remove this grading system and replace it with two types of VIN: VIN undifferentiated (usual type) and VIN differentiated.[5]

Undifferentiated usual type VIN. This is atypia involving two-thirds to full thickness of the epidermis of the vulva, previously known as VIN 2 or VIN 3, respectively. This type of VIN is usually associated with the oncogenic type HPV infection. Changes previously described as VIN 1 are now regarded as flat condyloma (HPV-associated).

Differentiated VIN (or carcinoma in situ). This is atypia confined to the basal area of the epidermis, previously termed VIN3 differentiated. This often occurs on a background of LS either surrounding an SCC or just prior to the development of malignant change. This type of VIN does not appear to be associated with HPV infection. Differentiated VIN has a higher risk of progression to invasive SCC.[6]

This terminology is still far from perfect, particularly as differentiated VIN may mistakenly be thought of as having a better prognosis than undifferentiated VIN. Contrariwise, differentiated VIN developing against a background of LS is much more likely to be associated with progression to invasive tumor and aggressive behavior than HPV-associated undifferentiated lesions. Most often, it is seen in vulvectomy specimens from women with SCC arising in a background of lichen simplex or LP. There has been a further reclassification which now includes low- and high-grade squamous intraepithelial lesions (previously undifferentiated VIN usual type), and differentiated VIN remains as a separate category.[7]

Clinical features

Clinical lesions of undifferentiated VIN (usual type) may be unifocal and discrete or multifocal and diffusely distributed about the external genitalia and perineum, where the anus may also be affected. The majority of young

healthy patients have only a small risk of progression to invasive disease but the immunocompromised are at a much greater risk, particularly in the setting of perianal disease.[8] Pigmented multifocal Bowen disease is now classified within the spectrum of VIN.

The morphology of the lesions ranges from papules to plaques, which may be skin-colored, white, erythematous, or pigmented (*Figs 12.182–12.184*). The surface often has a warty texture; less commonly, lesions are papillomatous, particularly around the anus where they may become polypoid (*Fig. 12.185*). The main presenting symptom is pruritus.

Multifocal vulval and perianal lesions are strongly associated with the oncogenic papilloma viruses, particularly HPV-16 and -18, and almost exclusively occurs in smokers.[9] HPV-16 is found more frequently than HPV-18.[10] It is believed that there is a failure of the host to mount an immune response to HPV and that patients who are immunocompromised are at particular risk. However, many of the patients do not have an identifiable immune deficiency. Anogenital intraepithelial neoplasia, in addition to being multifocal, can be multicentric and there is a history in two-thirds of female patients of current or past cervical intraepithelial neoplasia.[11]

Vaginal involvement can occur. The morphology of the lesions is quite variable, some resembling typical warts, others islands of erythema, erosion, or white patches.

Clinical lesions of differentiated VIN (simplex) are not often recognized and are poorly described. Since invasion can develop rapidly, any suspicious areas should be biopsied. It is usually a small hyperkeratotic white papule or plaque or a punched-out ulcer or erosion with a firm border. The lesion invariably arises in a background of a chronic inflammatory dermatosis such as LS, especially if there is associated epidermal acanthosis.

Histologic features
Undifferentiated VIN (usual or classic type)

There is complete loss of cellular stratification throughout the epidermis with large hyperchromatic cells, dyskeratosis, multinucleated cells, and numerous typical and atypical mitoses.[12]

Two distinct types of undifferentiated VIN have been described but are clinically and biologically the same:

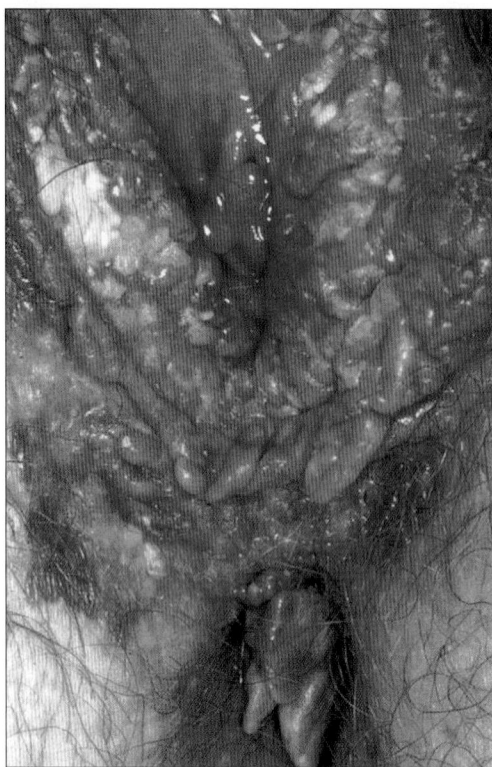

Fig. 12.183
Intraepithelial neoplasia: there are numerous scaly papules accompanied by condylomata. By courtesy of the Institute of Dermatology, London, UK.

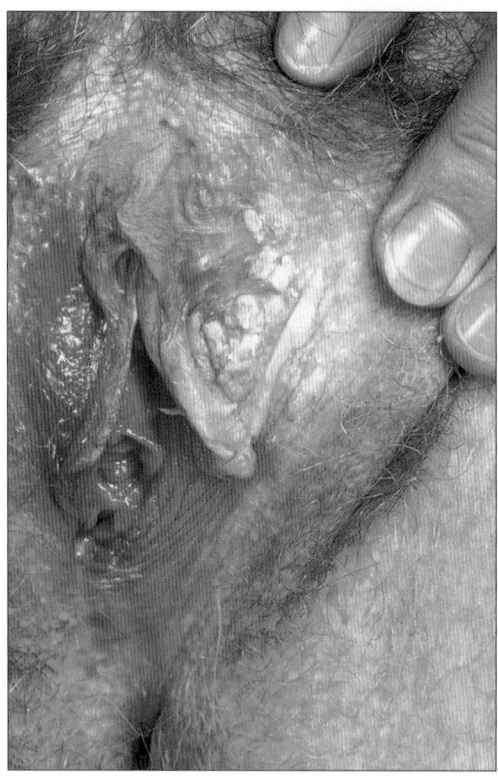

Fig. 12.184
Intraepithelial neoplasia: there is an erythematous plaque with focal scaling. By courtesy of the Institute of Dermatology, London, UK.

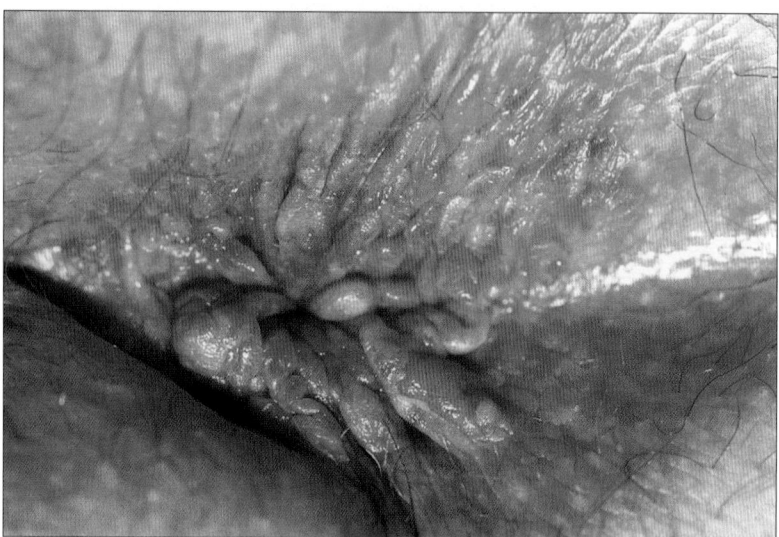

Fig. 12.185
Intraepithelial neoplasia: perianal lesions presenting as multiple small papules. By courtesy of the Institute of Dermatology, London, UK.

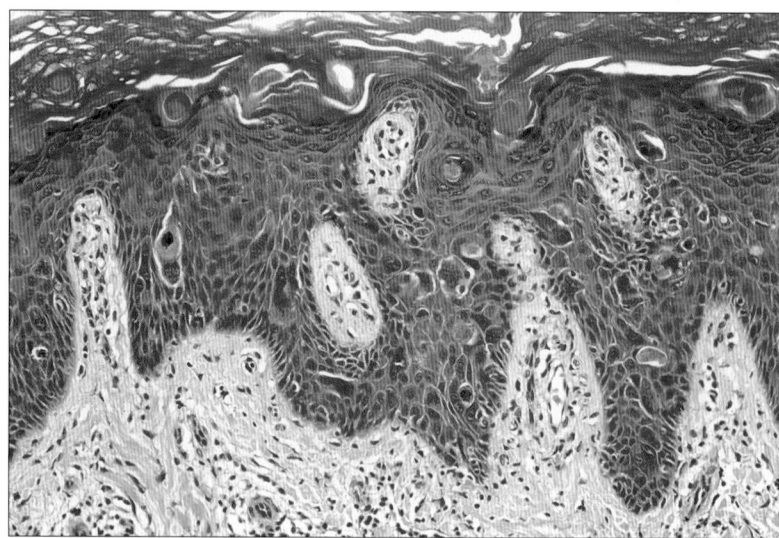

Fig. 12.186
Undifferentiated VIN: there is full-thickness dysplasia with very marked nuclear pleomorphism. Note the abnormal mitosis.

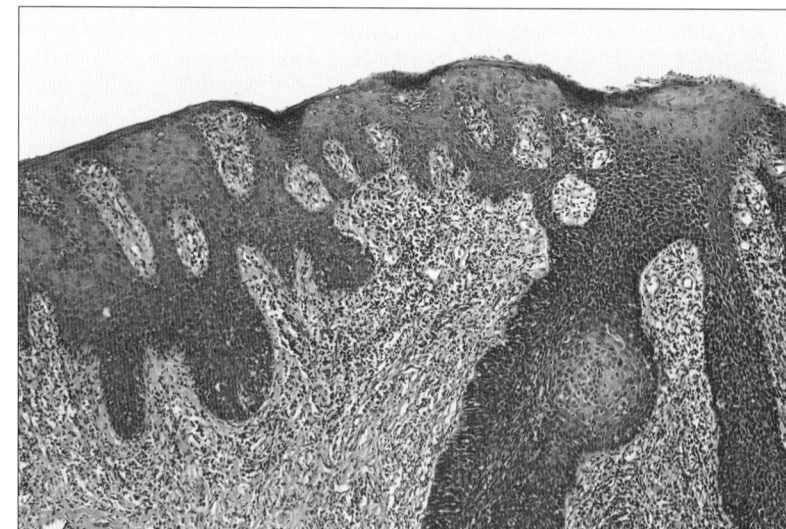

Fig. 12.187
Basaloid VIN: there is full-thickness replacement of the epidermis by a fairly uniform population of small cells with densely basophilic nuclei and imperceptible cytoplasm.

- warty, characterized by individual cell keratinization and premature cellular differentiation; pleomorphism may be marked and abnormal mitoses are often conspicuous (*Fig. 12.186*),
- basaloid, with atypical parabasal cells extending throughout the full thickness of the epithelium (*Fig. 12.187*).

The two variants often overlap histologically and are part of the same spectrum.

Two cases of VIN associated with HPV16 and with prominent mucinous differentiation have been reported.[13]

Undifferentiated VIN tends to be diffusely positive for p16 and negative for p53. In situ hybridization for high risk HPV is usually positive (*Fig. 12.188A and B*).

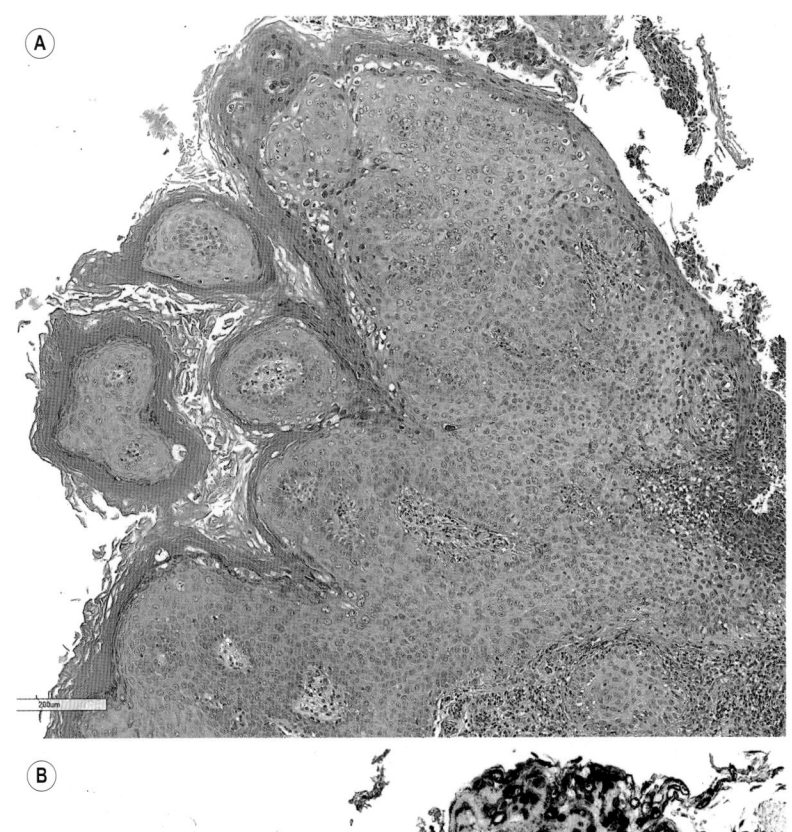

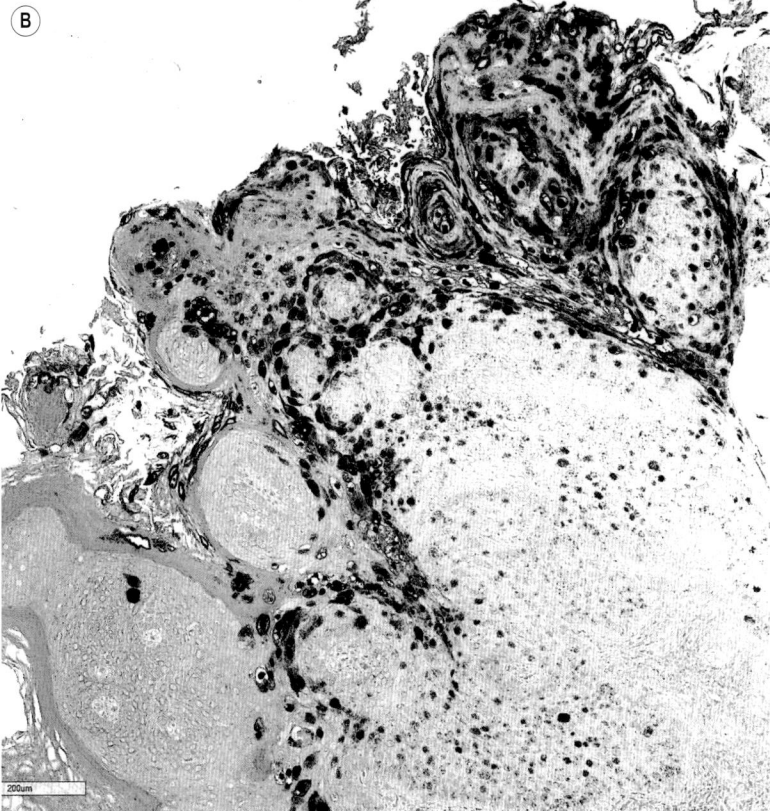

Fig. 12.188
Undifferentiated VIN: (**A**) full-thickness dysplasia; (**B**) nuclear positivity for broad spectrum in situ hybridization for HPV.

Differentiated VIN (simplex)

In some cases of vulval LS there is an associated basal keratinocyte cytological atypia with dyskeratosis and normal differentiation throughout the overlying epithelium (*Fig. 12.189*).[14] The rete ridges may be long and forked with keratin pearls. This change may reflect invasive disease or herald its imminent onset. This change is poorly recognized by many pathologists, and there is a significant risk of a report of VIN 1 being issued, with potentially disastrous consequences.

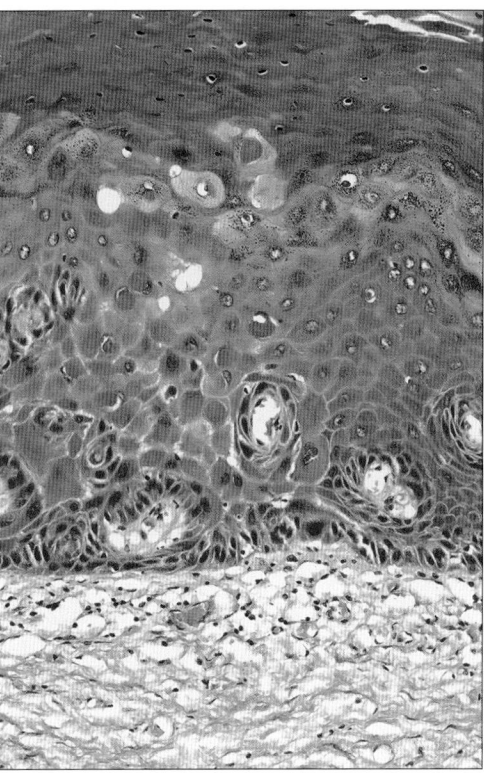

Fig. 12.189
Differentiated VIN: there is basal dysplasia associated with dyskeratosis and normal differentiation. By courtesy of C. Crum, MD, Brigham and Women's Hospital and Harvard Medical School, Boston, USA.

It is important to note that occasional cases of differentiated VIN negative for HPV display complete replacement of the epidermis by basaloid, homogeneous undifferentiated keratinocytes.[15]

Differentiated VIN can be associated with p53 mutations, and p53 is often positive not only in the basal cell layer but also in upper layers of the epidermis. A similar staining pattern can be seen in inflammatory conditions including LS.[16] It has recently been shown that high levels of p53 expression in differentiated VIN correlate with DNA aneuploidy.[17] p16 is usually negative in cases of differentiated VIN.

Squamous cell carcinoma of the genital epithelia

Vulval squamous cell carcinoma

There are two main etiologies for vulval SCC[1,2]:

- The majority (>60% of cases) arise in elderly women against a background of a chronic scarring dermatosis, usually LS but less often LP. In these patients, the tumors develop directly within the background dermatosis and may be preceded by differentiated VIN. They are not usually associated with HPV. SCC arising in the background of differentiated VIN appears to have a higher tendency for local recurrence.[3]
- The second group consists of younger women with a background of undifferentiated VIN (usual type), which is associated with HPV-16 and -18, smoking, and a previous or current history of squamous intraepithelial lesion (SIL/CIN). HPV-16 is the most common type of HPV found in association with vulval SCC.

Interestingly, a recent study of HPV genotypes in invasive vulval SCC found HPV in 70% of cases (mainly HPV-16), and the average age of the patients was 65. Patients with no evidence of HPV were older than those with proven HPV but these differences were not statistically significant.[4]

In addition, much more rarely, vulval carcinoma has been described in association with chronic granulomatous disease, hidradenitis suppurativa, Fanconi anemia, and the genodermatosis Netherton syndrome.[5–9] A tumor in a young woman with Crohn disease and one developing within a localized vulval lesion of Hailey-Hailey disease after tacrolimus therapy have been documented.[10,11]

Patients with the warty and basaloid histologic subtypes of vulval SCC tend to be younger than those with conventional keratinizing SCC, and in one series there seems to be a predominance of black patients with this

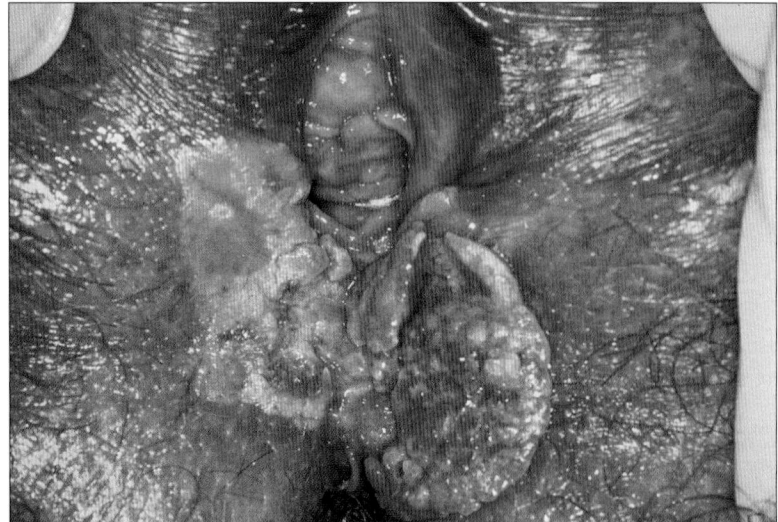

Fig. 12.190
Vulval squamous cell carcinoma: this tumor arose against a background of long-standing carcinoma in situ (Bowen disease). By courtesy of the Institute of Dermatology, London, UK.

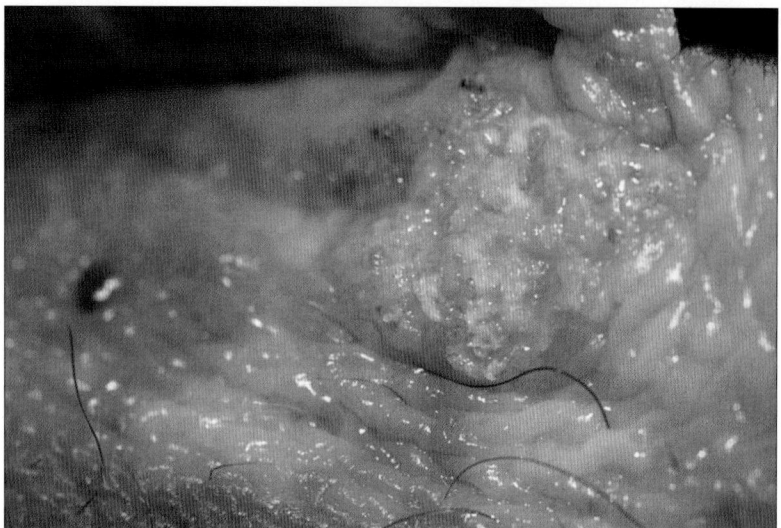

Fig. 12.191
Verrucous carcinoma: note the keratotic warty tumor mass. By courtesy of the Institute of Dermatology, London, UK.

histologic subtype.[12] The majority of vulval SCCs develop on the inner aspect of the labia majora and periclitorally. Patients present with a mass that is sometimes associated with pruritus, ulceration, bleeding, discharge, or pain (*Fig. 12.190*). Multifocal tumors are very rare.[13] Vulval SCC usually spreads via lymphatics to inguinal, femoral, and pelvic lymph nodes. Midline tumors are often associated with bilateral lymph node spread.[14]

The overall 5-year survival for patients with vulval SCC depends on the depth of stromal invasion and the presence or absence of lymph node metastasis.[15] A study has found that patients with stromal invasion of more than 9 mm had higher risk of local recurrence.[16] The presence or absence of lymph node metastasis is the single most important factor determining prognosis.[17] Other factors that have been found to be independently associated with prognosis include older age, advanced stage, size of the tumor, positive margins, and degree of differentiation. It has been suggested that HPV-positive tumors have a worse prognosis than those that are HPV negative.[18] Warty and basaloid SCCs of the vulva are often associated with HPV infection, and there is some suggestion that the prognosis of the basaloid subtype may be worse.[12] Warty SCC of the vulva is more often associated with high risk HPV other than HPV-16.

Tumors with less than 1-mm stromal invasion do not require lymph node dissection and the appropriate surgery is curative.

Verrucous carcinoma

Clinical features

Verrucous carcinoma is a low-grade, slow-growing SCC first described in 1948.[1] The precise incidence of verrucous carcinoma is difficult to assess accurately because of the confusing number of different terms that have been applied to this tumor in the past. There has been some debate as to whether verrucous carcinoma, well-differentiated epidermoid SCC, epithelium cuniculatum, and giant condyloma of Buschke-Löwenstein are all one and the same or separate entities. It is now generally accepted that they are identical lesions.[2,3]

The tumor presents as a warty exophytic plaque and usually occurs at three anatomical sites: the oropharynx, sole of the foot, and the anogenital skin (*Figs 12.191* and *12.192*).[2,4–6] Verrucous carcinoma of the vulva may arise on a background of LS or LP.[7–10] Oral and lower limb neoplasms may be associated with various types of HPV.[11–14] Similarly, genital verrucous carcinoma may be associated with HPV albeit in a minority of cases.[15] The benign histologic appearances of this tumor often lead to an incorrect histologic report of condyloma or squamous papilloma, with resulting under-treatment. Vulval verrucous carcinoma can coexist with ordinary SCC.[16]

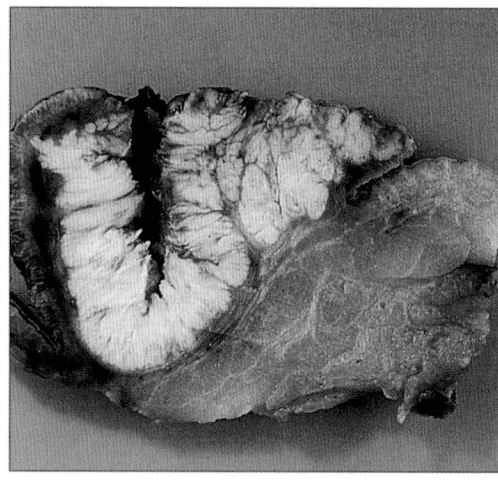

Fig. 12.192
Verrucous carcinoma: this tumor arose in the gluteal cleft of an elderly female. Note the characteristic sharply demarcated lower border.

A case of vulval verrucous carcinoma in an HIV-positive patient has been documented.[17]

Histologic features

Verrucous carcinoma is characterized by an exophytic and endophytic growth pattern.[18,19] The latter, which may extend deeply into subcutaneous tissues or beyond, has a bulbous and sharply delineated lower border, lacking the infiltrative characteristics of conventional SCC (*Figs 12.193–12.195*). The epithelium is well differentiated, showing no appreciable cytological atypia; mitoses, which are generally sparse, are confined to the lower layer. Intraepithelial neutrophil abscesses are commonly present. In some tumors, koilocytes may be seen, supporting an HPV-associated etiology. One study describes a distinctive triad of marked epithelial acanthosis, loss of the granular cell layer with superficial epithelial cell pallor, and multilayered parakeratosis.[20] It has been suggested that this could be a precursor to verrucous carcinoma and is designated vulvar acanthosis with altered differentiation.

Penile intraepithelial neoplasia

In this text, PeIN refers to purely squamous lesions and excludes Paget disease and melanoma in situ. There is a wide spectrum of morphological lesions reflecting the diverse pathogenesis of penile SCC. Historically, the nomenclature used has varied and multiple classification schemes of penile precursor lesions have been proposed[1–6]:

- Bowen disease,
- erythroplasia of Queyrat,

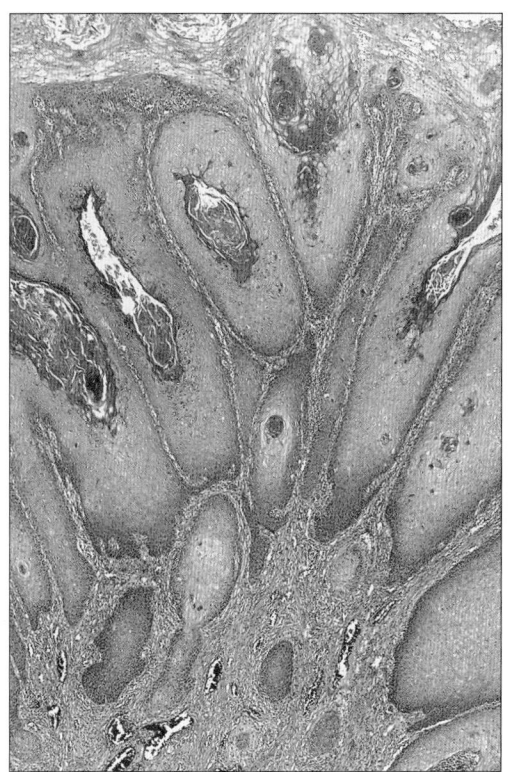

Fig. 12.193
Verrucous carcinoma: low-power view showing the characteristic growth pattern comprising deeply penetrating, blunt, finger-like processes.

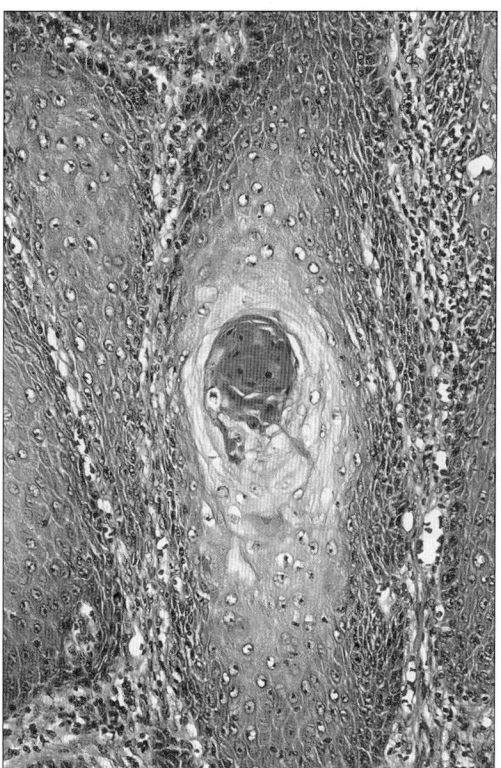

Fig. 12.194
Verrucous carcinoma: the epithelium is uniformly well differentiated and often displays a ground-glass cytoplasmic pallor.

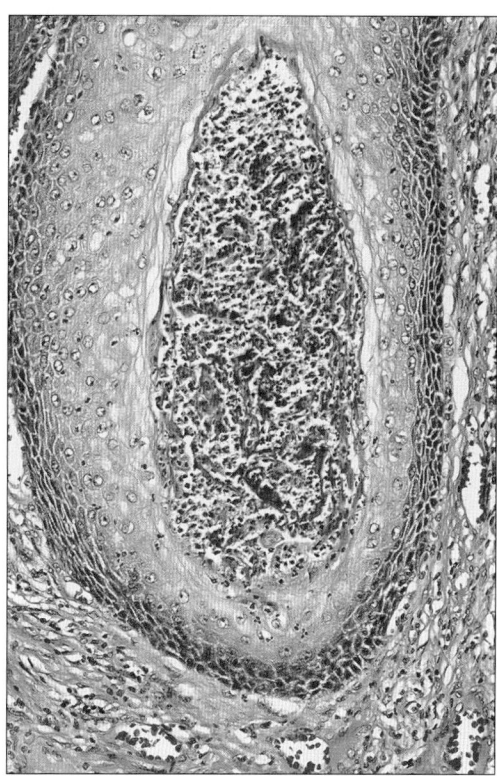

Fig. 12.195
Verrucous carcinoma: intraepithelial neutrophil abscesses are often present.

Table 12.1
Penile intraepithelial neoplasia (PeIN) classification (WHO, 2016)

Non-HPV-related	HPV-related	Other patterns
Differentiated PeIN	Basaloid PeIN Warty PeIN Warty–basaloid PeIN	Pleomorphic Spindle Clear cell Pagetoid

- carcinoma in situ,
- squamous intraepithelial lesion of low and high grade,
- dysplasia,
- penile intrepithelial neoplasia grade 3.

Taking into account similarities in morphology and pathogenesis between vulval and penile carcinoma, we have recently proposed a new nomenclature for penile preinvasive lesions which resulted, with minor changes, in the new WHO classification (*Table 12.1*).[2,7,8] In this section, we present a simplified version taking into account the etiopathogenetic correlation of precursor HPV and non-HPV-related lesions with their invasive counterparts.[9] The term penile intraepithelial neoplasia (PeIN) is preferred over older terminology.[10–13] PeIN is classified into differentiated (non-HPV-related), warty, basaloid, warty–basaloid (HPV-related), and others.

PeIN may be solitary or multifocal, and may or may not be associated with infiltrative SCC. PeIN unassociated with invasive cancer occurs in younger patients and tends to be of basaloid or warty type and positive for HPV. Patients with HIV may also develop warty or basaloid PeIN. Conversely, when PeIN is associated with invasive SCC, the predominant histologic subtype is the differentiated variant, presenting in 65% of the cases and usually negative for HPV. The explanation for this apparent paradox may be the clinical and pathological underrecognition or underdiagnosis of differentitated PeIN. Differentiated PeIN tends to affect the foreskin of older patients whereas basaloid/warty PeIN generally affects the glans of younger patients.

The gross appearance of PeIN is heterogeneous and does not allow a clear distinction between the two main types. Differentiated PeIN tends to be

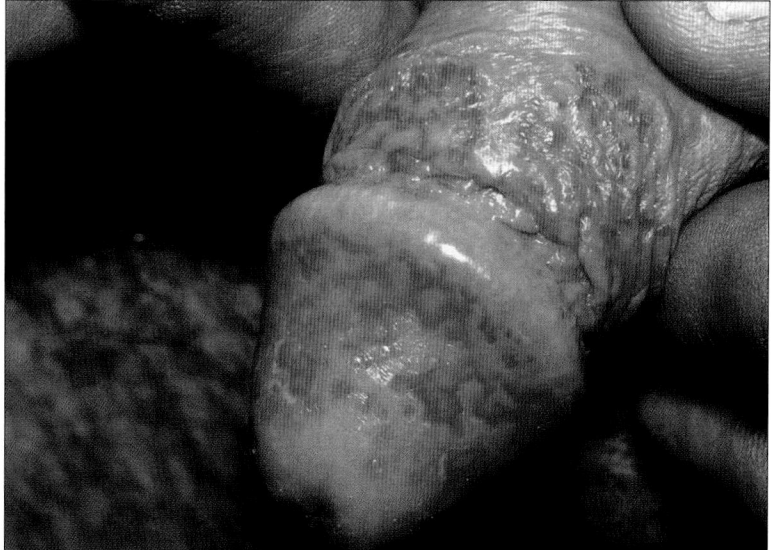

Fig. 12.196
Intraepithelial neoplasia: multiple eroded lesions are present. By courtesy of the Institute of Dermatology, London, UK.

white, whereas HPV-related PeIN is typically reddish or darkly pigmented. Lesions vary from flat to slightly elevated, and can be pearly white or moist erythematous, dark brown or black, and present as macules, papules, or plaques. They may be warty, granular, or villous (*Figs 12.196–12.199*). The contours are sharply delineated or subtle and irregular.

Histologic features

Microscopically, differentiated PeIN is characterized by hyperkeratosis, parakeratosis, variable hypergranulosis, and acanthosis with elongated and anastomosing rete ridges. There is subtle abnormal maturation (enlarged keratinocytes with abundant eosinophilic cytoplasm) (*Fig. 12.200*), whorling

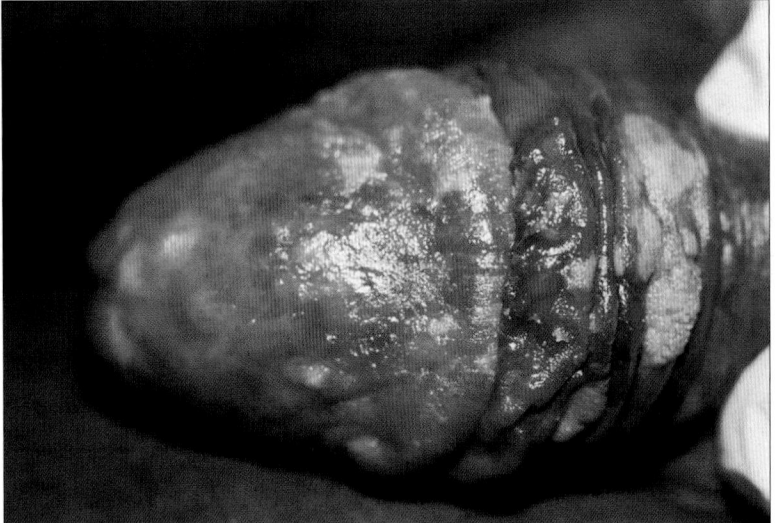

Fig. 12.197
Intraepithelial neoplasia: in this example, viral warts are present in addition to multiple small papules on the glans (bowenoid papulosis). By courtesy of the Institute of Dermatology, London, UK.

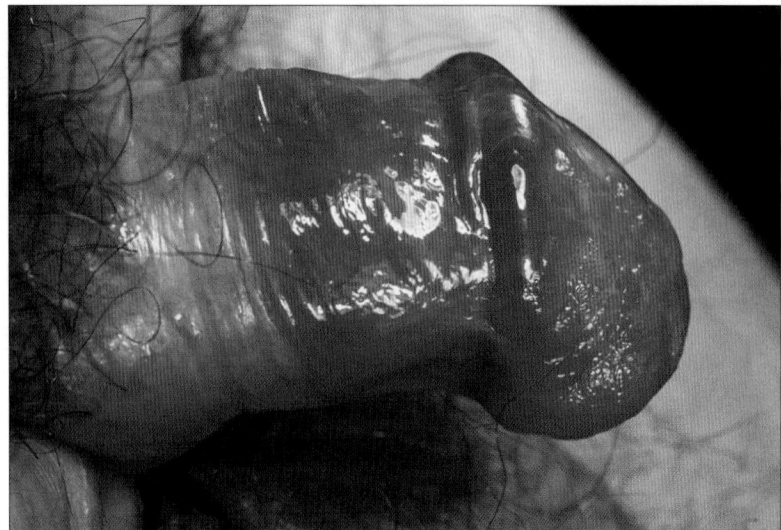

Fig. 12.199
Intraepithelial neoplasia: there is intense erythema of the glans penis and the distal shaft. This lesion is also referred to as Bowen disease and in the older literature as erythroplasia of Queyrat. By courtesy of the Institute of Dermatology, London, UK.

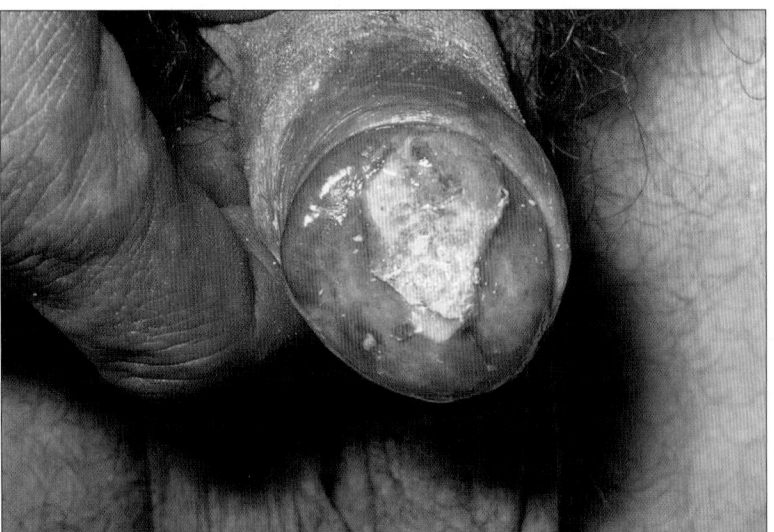

Fig. 12.198
Intraepithelial neoplasia: this patient presented with multiple ulcerated lesions and a thick, scaly plaque. By courtesy of the Institute of Dermatology, London, UK.

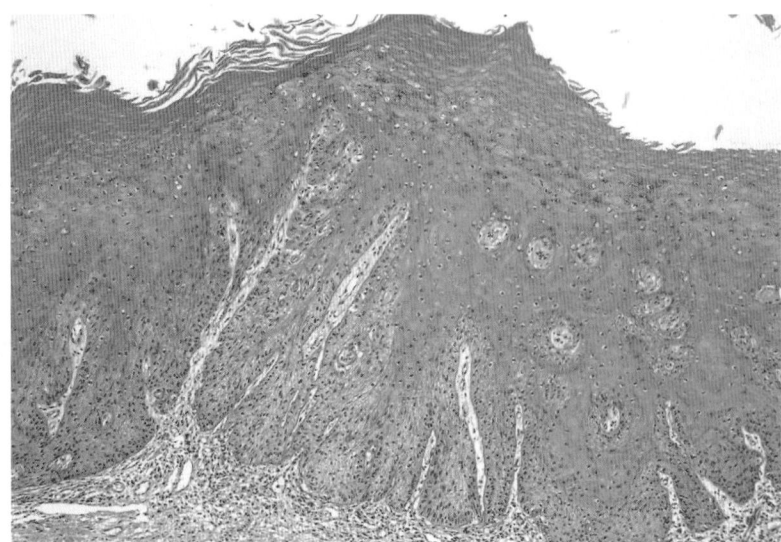

Fig. 12.200
Differentiated PeIN: with acanthosis, hyperkeratosis, retained squamous maturation, and minimal atypia.

and keratin pearl formation (usually in deep rete ridges), prominent intercellular bridges (spongiosis), and sometimes acantholysis. Atypical basal or prickle layer cells are present and a prominent nucleolus may be seen (*Fig. 12.201*). At low power, the atypia may seem to be present only in lower levels of the epidermis; however, at higher magnification, there is subtle but abnormal maturation in all levels of the epithelium (*Figs 12.202–12.204*).

The differential diagnosis is squamous hyperplasia which, by definition, shows no atypia. In the absence of specific penile dermatological conditions which may be associated with hyperplasia, it is likely that most acanthotic squamous lesions represent differentiated PeIN.

It is not surprising that the precursor lesions of well-differentiated invasive tumors show such a high degree of differentiation. It is important to recognize this lesion because it appears to be the most frequent precursor lesion of penile carcinoma, especially of the keratinizing and well-differentiated variants. Unfortunately, most studies on differentiated PeIN are retrospective and have been based on penectomies performed for invasive carcinoma.

There is a preferential association for differentiated PeIN and LS (*Fig. 12.205*).[14] It is therefore important to maintain a high index of suspicion when dealing with hyperkeratotic/hyperplastic epidermal lesions with subtle keratinocytic atypia arising in the setting of long-standing LS.

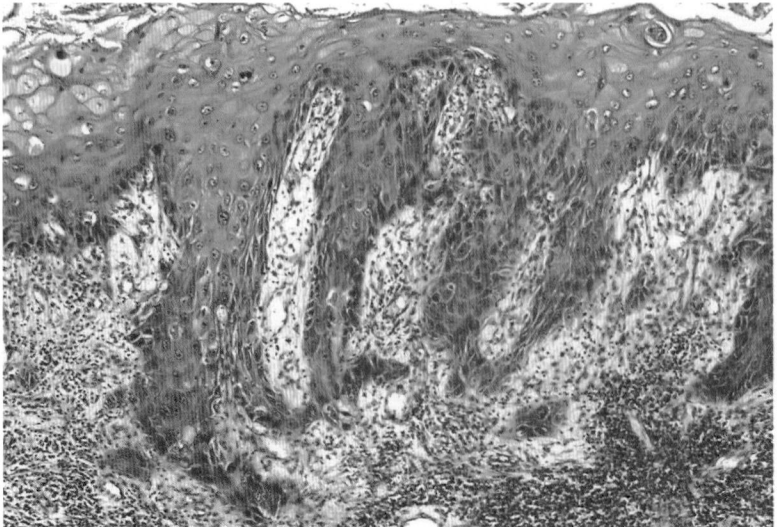

Fig. 12.201
Differentiated PeIN: with marked atypia, more prominent at the bottom layers.

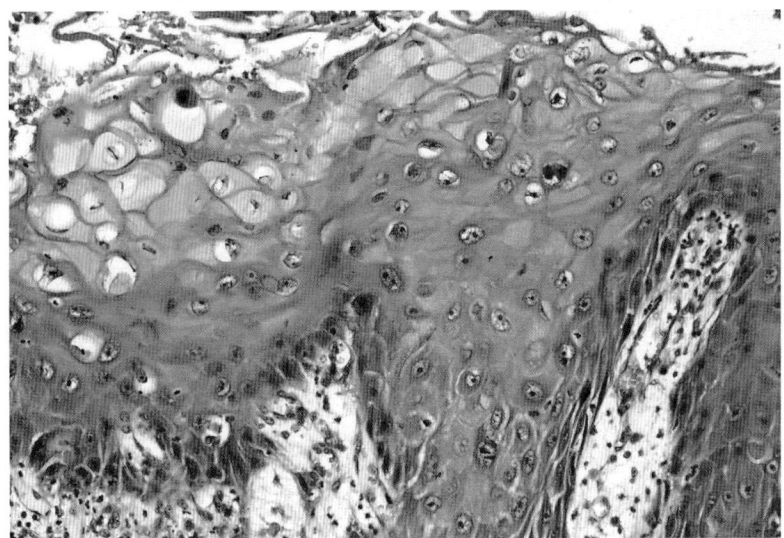

Fig. 12.202
Differentiated PeIN: atypia are seen throughout the epithelium; note the presence of dyskeratosis.

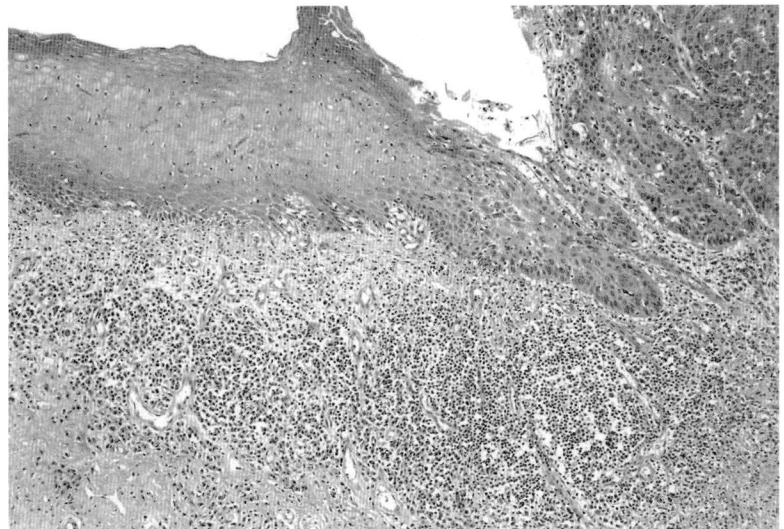

Fig. 12.203
Differentiated PeIN: squamous hyperplasia *(left field)* merging into differentiated PeIN *(center field)*, the latter in continuity with invasive squamous cell carcinoma *(right field)*.

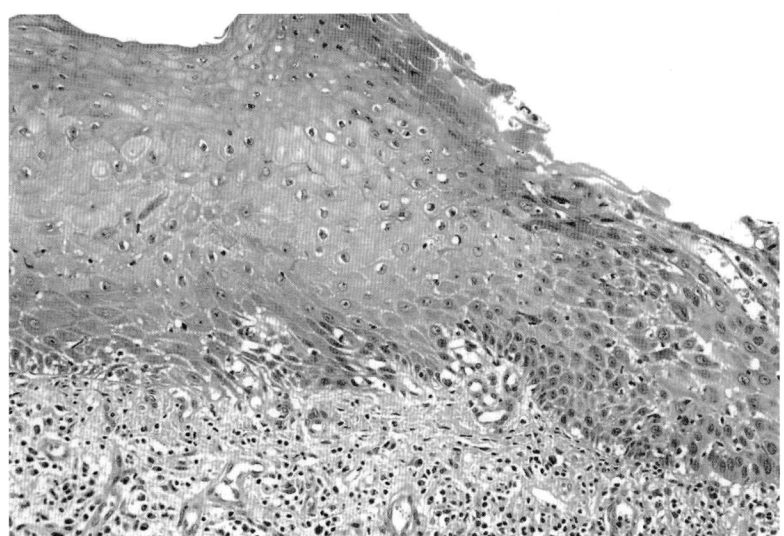

Fig. 12.204
Differentiated PeIN: the presence of nuclear atypia *(right field)* allows the distinction of differentiated PeIN from squamous hyperplasia *(left field)*.

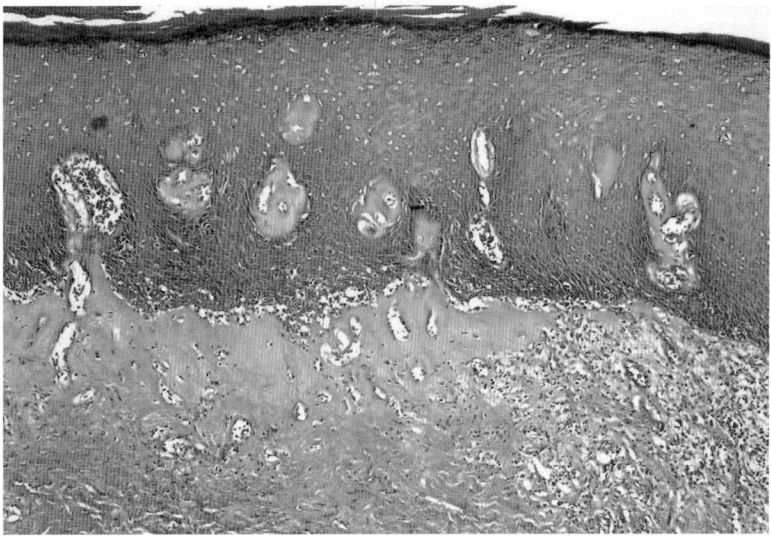

Fig. 12.205
Differentiated PeIN: with underlying lichen sclerosus characterized by dense hyalinized subepithelial tissue.

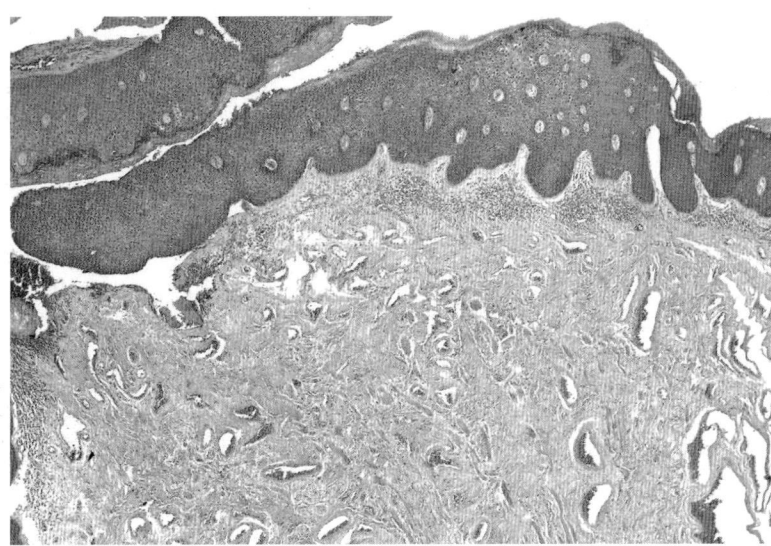

Fig. 12.206
Basaloid PeIN: with acanthosis, parakeratosis, and slightly irregular surface.

Warty/basaloid PeIN (the HPV-related type) shows distinctive morphological features. In accordance with their common pathogenesis, one can frequently find mixtures of warty and basaloid patterns in the same specimen. We classify a lesion as either warty or basaloid when there is more than 90% predominance of one type over the other.

In basaloid PeIN, the epithelium is replaced by a monotonous population of small or intermediate-sized immature cells with high nuclear/cytoplasmic ratio *(Figs 12.206–12.209)*. Short spikes or spindle-shaped cells may be noted. Apoptosis and mitotic figures are numerous. Basaloid PeIN should be distinguished from transitional cell urethral carcinoma in situ, which may secondarily involve the penile meatal region.[15]

In the warty variant, the epithelium has an undulating/spiky surface with atypical parakeratosis. There is cellular pleomorphism and koilocytosis (multinucleation, nuclei with irregular contours, perinuclear halos, and dyskeratosis) *(Figs 12.210–12.212)*. Mitoses may be numerous.

Basaloid lesions are monotonous and flat, whereas warty lesions are spiky and pleomorphic with prominent koilocytosis. Frequently, lesions show overlapping features of both, namely, warty–basaloid PeIN. These mixed lesions have an irregular surface with koilocytic changes while the lower half of the epithelium is predominantly composed of small basaloid cells. This is not a surprising finding, taking into consideration that warty and basaloid carcinomas are both HPV-related tumors. Warty PeIN should

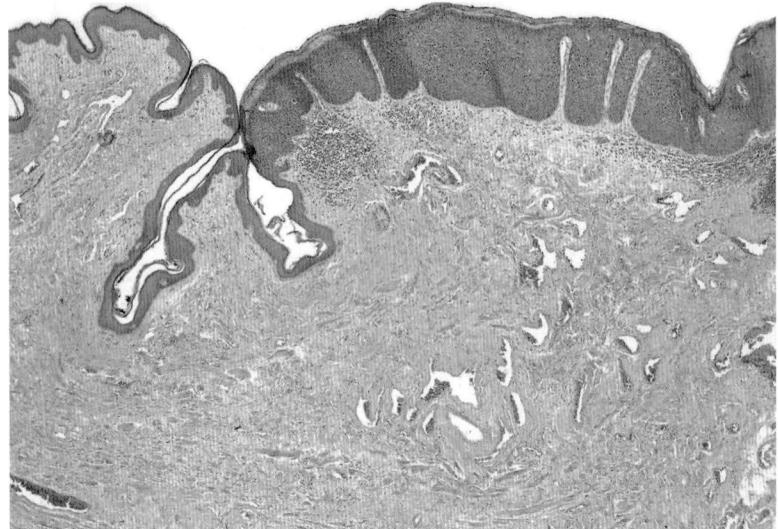

Fig. 12.207
Basaloid PeIN: with epithelial thickening, parakeratosis, and an overall 'blue' appearance due to altered squamous maturation.

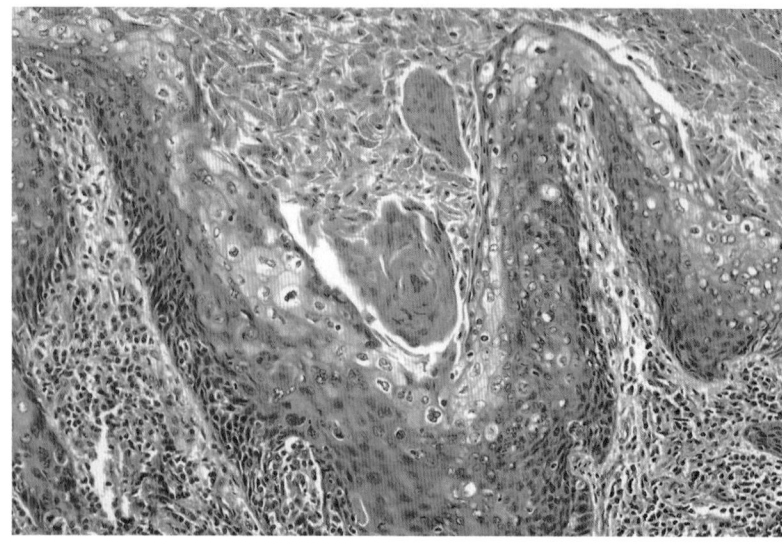

Fig. 12.210
Warty PeIN: with prominent parakeratosis and abundant koilocytes, more prominent at upper layers.

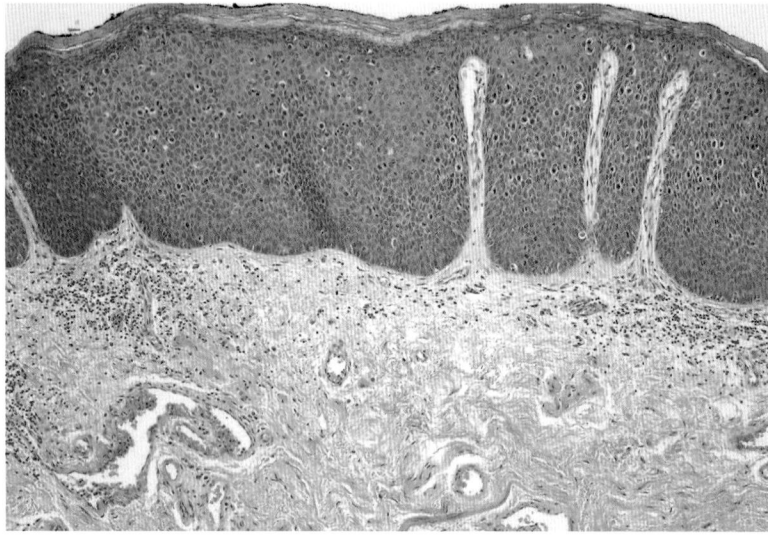

Fig. 12.208
Basaloid PeIN: the epithelium is replaced by a monotonous proliferation of small to medium-sized cells with basal-like features

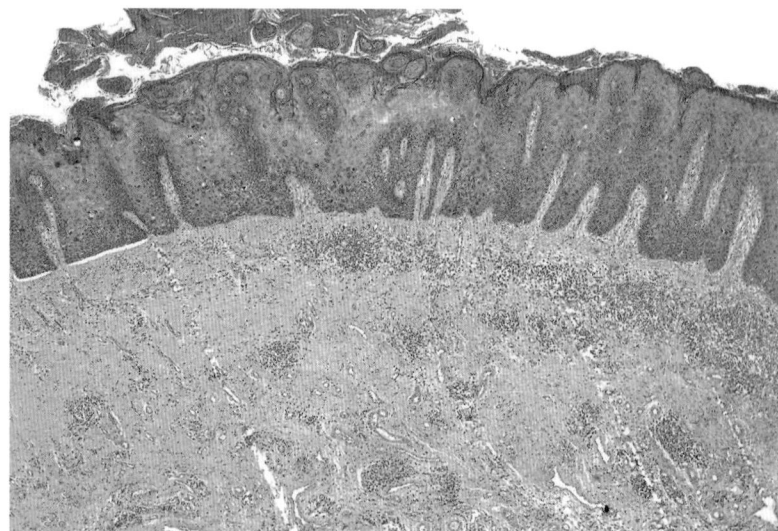

Fig. 12.211
Warty PeIN: showing its characteristic spiky, parakeratotic surface.

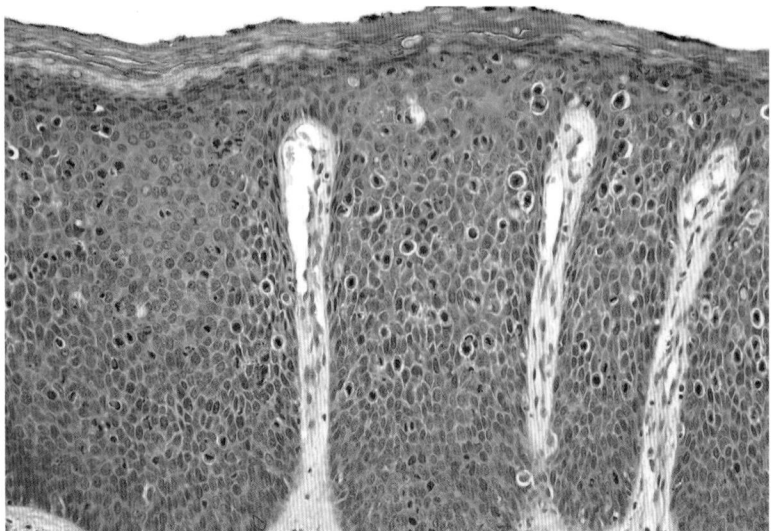

Fig. 12.209
Basaloid PeIN: with abundant mitoses and apoptotic figures throughout the epithelium.

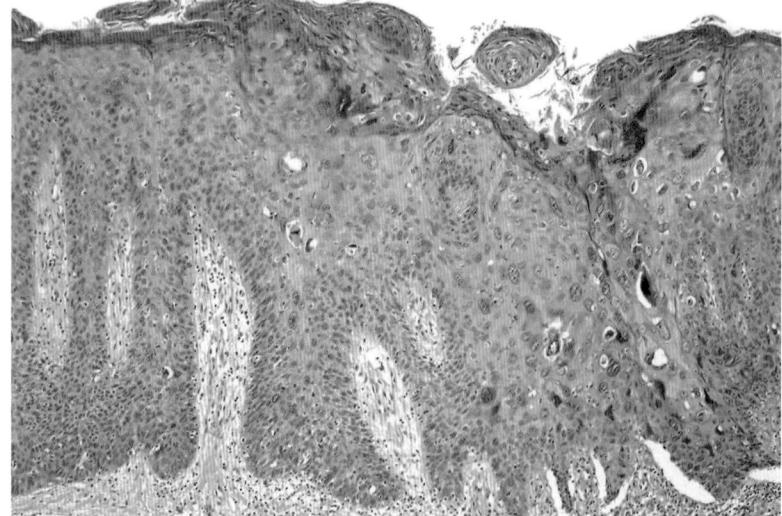

Fig. 12.212
Warty PeIN: nuclear atypia is discernible throughout the epithelium, with conspicuous, sometimes pleomorphic koilocytosis (right field) and marked parakeratosis.

be distinguished from the common condyloma, which does not display atypia except at the level of the upper koilocytotic layer.

Rarely, a mixed lesion composed of differentiated and undifferentiated PeIN is encountered. If an associated invasive cancer is present, it also shows mixed morphology of more than one subtype of invasive SCC.

There are other rare patterns of PeIN. They are less well studied and include pleomorphic, spindle cell, clear cell, pagetoid, and small cell. All of these are likely to represent variants of the HPV-related group.

With few exceptions there is good correlation between the microscopic appearance of the preinvasive lesion and the associated invasive carcinoma. Usual and differentiated subtypes of SCC are associated with differentiated PeIN, while warty and basaloid invasive carcinomas are associated with warty or basaloid PeIN. These observations further support the concept of a bimodal pathway of penile tumorigenesis.[9]

Bowenoid papulosis is a clinical entity. Patients with bowenoid papulosis are younger (mean age, 30 years) than those with penile cancer and present with multiple papules affecting the skin of the shaft, glans, sulcus, or foreskin. Some lesions regress spontaneously.[16–22] The histologic appearance of bowenoid papulosis is undistinguishable from that of basaloid or mixed warty–basaloid PeIN, and the diagnosis should be suggested only when there is a clinical presentation of multiple papular lesions in younger patients.

Penile invasive squamous cell carcinoma

General features

SCC arises on the mucosal surface of the penis extending from the preputial orifice to the urethral meatus, comprising the inner surface of the foreskin, coronal sulcus and glans.[23] SCC presenting on the outer skin of the penis is very unusual.

Penile cancer incidence rates in the West are in the range of 0.3–1.0/100 000 of the population although there is considerable variation among the different countries. The incidence of penile SCC varies from a high incidence in Uganda, Kenya, and some regions of South America, to a lower incidence in Northern Europe and the United States, Japan, and Israel.[2] Comparing cases from the United States and Paraguay, we have found no geographical differences in the morphology, relative incidence of histologic subtypes, or in the presence or absence of HPV according to histologic subtype.[9,24] Several epidemiological studies have indicated the following risk factors: socioeconomic deprivation, poor hygiene, lack of access to running water, phimosis, smegma retention, lack of circumcision, chronic inflammation, history of tear or injury to the penis, physical inactivity, history of warts, ultraviolet irradiation, partner with cervical cancer, immunosuppression, smoking, HPV, and LS.[25–28]

Penile carcinoma in circumcised men is very rare; it has been reported in association with irregular scarring in patients undergoing ritual circumcision. Postcircumcision penile cancer appears to be biologically aggressive.[29]

The overall prevalence of HPV DNA in penile carcinoma (42%) is lower than that seen in cervical carcinoma (nearly 100%) and is similar to vulval carcinoma.[7] Subtypes of penile cancer such as basaloid and condylomatous are consistently associated with HPV, whereas the virus is infrequent in the usual, verrucous, papillary, and sarcomatoid SCC.[9,24] These two groups of tumors appear to develop along different pathogenetic pathways. The new WHO classification of invasive penile SCC takes into account this hypothesis.[2] HPV-16 is the most common type of HPV associated with penile cancer. HPV-related anogenital cancers, including penile carcinoma, are significantly more frequent in HIV-infected patients when compared with the general population.[30,31]

Subtypes of penile squamous cell carcinoma (WHO classification, 2016, *Table 12.2*)

Non-HPV-related
Usual squamous cell carcinoma

Clinical features

The mean age is in the 60s. An exophytic or non-ulcerated lesion is the usual presenting sign. In non-Western countries, up to 40% of patients

Table 12.2

Subtypes of squamous cell carcinoma (WHO, 2016)

Non-HPV-related	HPV-related	Other (rare)
Usual	Basaloid	Solid (medullary)
Pseudohyperplastic	Papillary basaloid	Desmoplastic
Pseudoglandular	Warty	Small cell
Verrucous	Warty–basaloid	
Cuniculatum	Clear cell	
Papillary NOS	Lymphoepithelioma-like	
Adenosquamous		
Sarcomatoid		
Mixed		

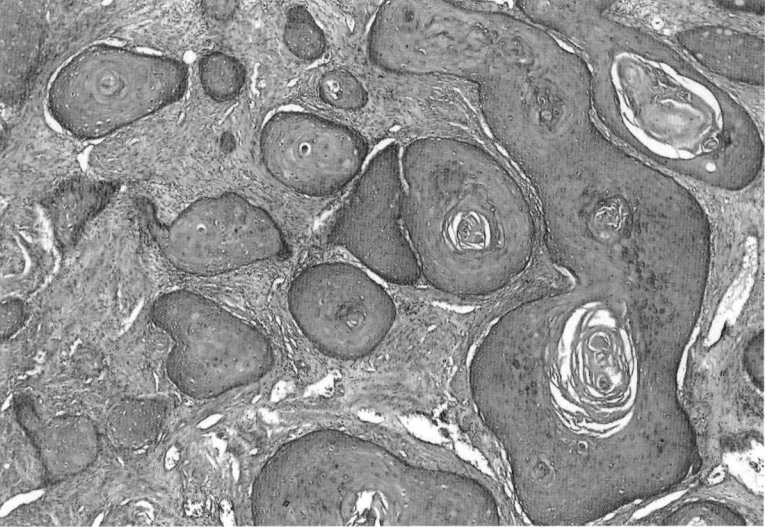

Fig. 12.213

Usual squamous cell carcinoma: well-differentiated (grade 1) usual SCC with keratinizing tumor nests composed of neoplastic cells showing minimal atypia limited to the basal/parabasal layers.

present with inguinal lymph node metastasis and 10% with disseminated disease. This high figure contrasts with a significantly lower incidence of regional and systemic metastasis in North American patients (13% and 2.3%, respectively).[32]

Grossly, the usual type displays wide morphological appearances varying from white-gray exophytic to flat or reddish, ulcerated endophytic masses. The cut surface shows white-gray neoplastic tissues invading variable penile anatomical levels.

Histologic features

Microscopically, tumors vary from well-differentiated keratinizing to solid anaplastic carcinomas with scant keratinization (*Figs 12.213–12.215*). Most tumors are highly keratinized and of moderate differentiation. Poorly differentiated carcinomas may have variable and usually focal amounts of spindled cell, giant cell, solid, acantholytic, clear cell, small cell, warty, basaloid, or glandular components. When these features predominate, there is a morphological justification for separation of the neoplasm as a special subtype of SCC.

Pseudohyperplastic carcinoma

Clinical features

Pseudohyperplastic carcinoma is a low-grade squamous carcinoma preferentially affecting the foreskin of older patients (eighth decade) in association with LS.[33] The tumor is well differentiated, and in small biopsy specimens it may mimic pseudoepitheliomatous hyperplasia. It is often multicentric, and the second or third independent lesion is sometimes verrucous. Grossly, it is a flat or slightly elevated lesion measuring about 2 cm. In a series of 10 cases, recurrence was noted in the glans of one patient who was circumcised

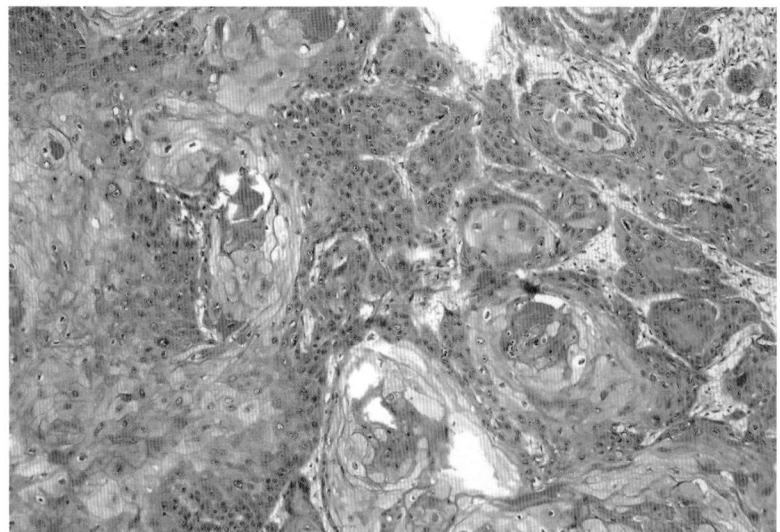

Fig. 12.214
Usual squamous cell carcinoma: moderately differentiated (grade 2) usual SCC with more evident atypia *(upper right field)* but retained squamous maturation.

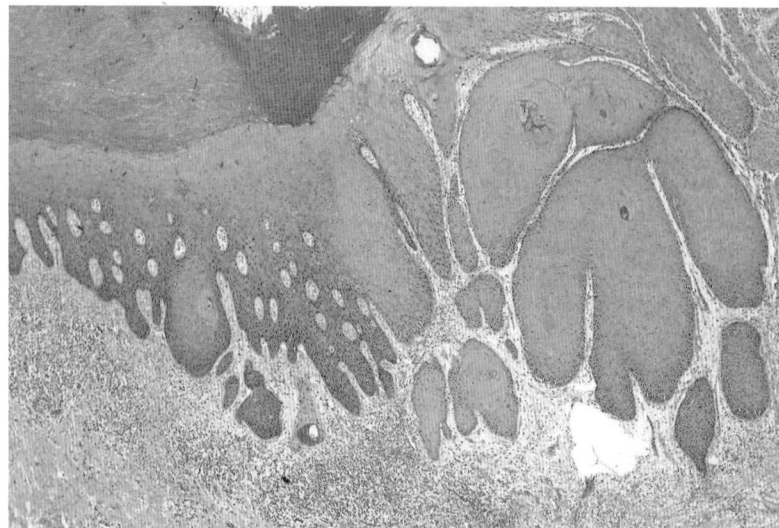

Fig. 12.216
Pseudohyperplastic carcinoma: showing a downward proliferation of irregular tumor nests composed of extremely well-differentiated neoplastic cells.

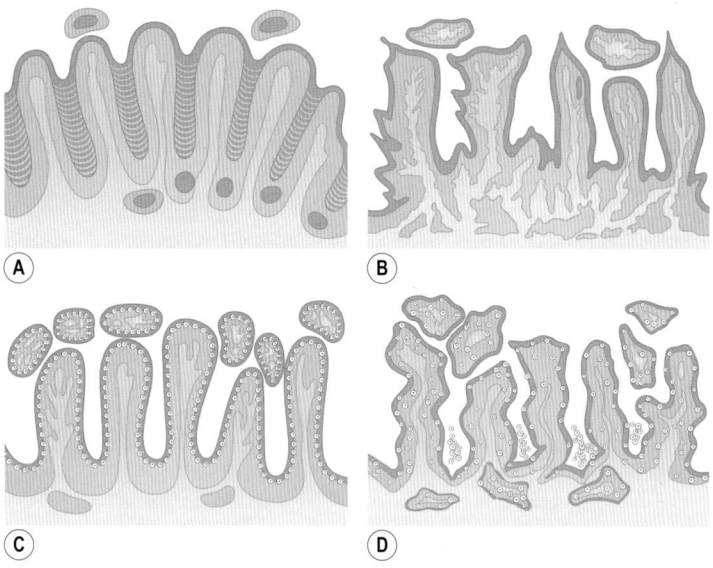

Fig. 12.215
Usual squamous cell carcinoma: poorly differentiated (grade 3) usual SCC with prominent atypia but evidence of squamous differentiation. (**A**) Verrucous carcinoma: tight papillae separated by keratin *(in red)*. Broadly based boundaries between tumor and stroma. (**B**) Papillary carcinoma: irregular papillae without koilocytosis. Jagged tumor–stroma limits. (**C**) Giant condyloma: condylomatous papillae, surface koilocytosis *(white dots)* and broad noninvasive base. (**D**) Warty (condylomatous) carcinoma: irregular condylomatous papillae, diffuse koilocytosis and jagged boundary between tumor and stroma.

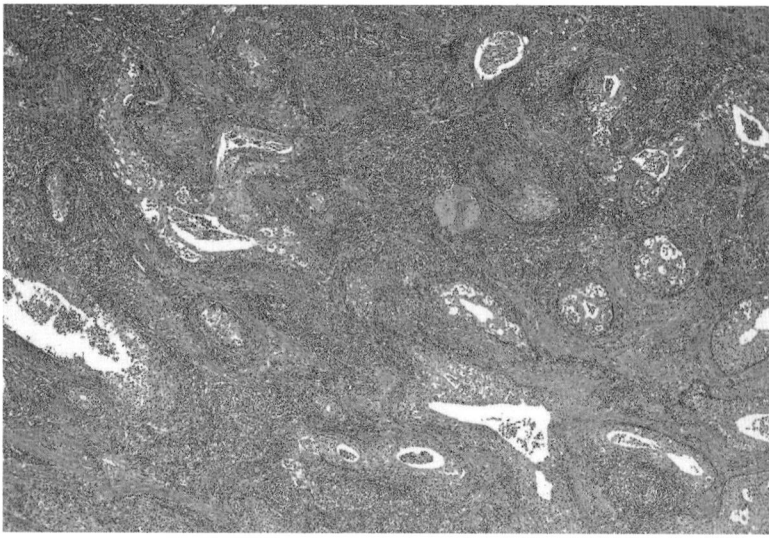

Fig. 12.217
Acantholytic carcinoma: deeply infiltrative tumor nests with extensive areas of central acantholysis, giving the lesion a glandular appearance.

large, involve multiple penile anatomical compartments, and deeply invade into erectile corpora.

Histologic features

The pseudoglandular spaces contain keratin, acantholytic cells, and necrotic debris *(Figs 12.217 and 12.218)*. Carcinoembryonic antigen (CEA) and mucin stains are negative. Compared with usual SCC, pseudoglandular SCC shows higher-grade foci, invades deeper anatomical structures, and is associated with a higher incidence of regional metastasis and mortality. The differential diagnosis includes gland-forming penile tumors (surface adenosquamous, mucoepidermoid, and urethral adenocarcinomas) and the angiosarcomatous variant of sarcomatoid carcinoma.

Verrucous carcinoma

Clinical features

Verrucous carcinoma is a slow-growing, well-differentiated tumor, with a papillomatous appearance and a broad bulbous invasive border. Condyloma, papillary, and condylomatous carcinoma have all been published under the designation of verrucous carcinoma or Buscke-Löwenstein tumor. We have proposed a classification of verruciform neoplasms that helps to

for a multicentric carcinoma of the foreskin 2 years after diagnosis. No metastases developed in any of these cases.

Histologic features

Characteristic microscopic features are keratinizing nests of squamous cells with minimal atypia surrounded by a reactive stroma *(Fig. 12.216)*. The consistent association with LS suggests that this inflammatory condition may play a pathogenetic role.

Pseudoglandular (acantholytic, adenoid) carcinoma

Clinical features

There is prominent acantholysis and the formation of pseudoglandular spaces.[34] The median age of the patient is 54 years. Tumors are generally

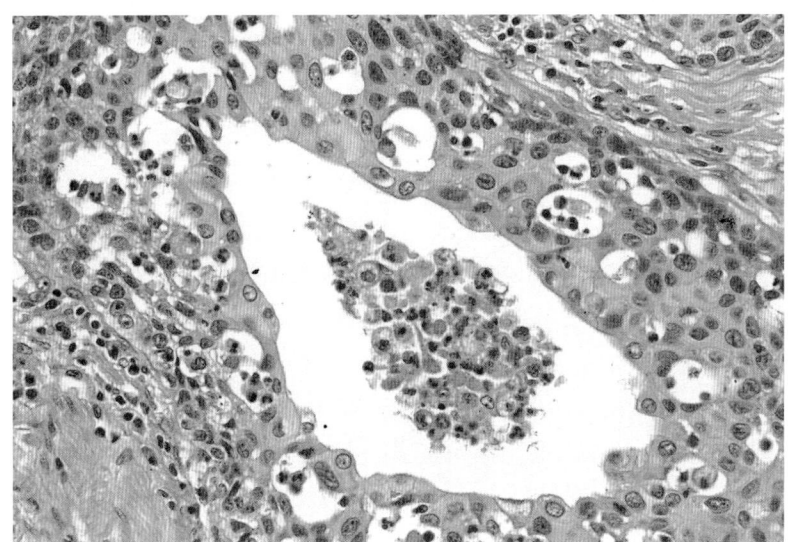

Fig. 12.218
Acantholytic carcinoma: tumor nest with central acantholysis showing an admixture of neutrophils, necrotic debris, and desquamated cells.

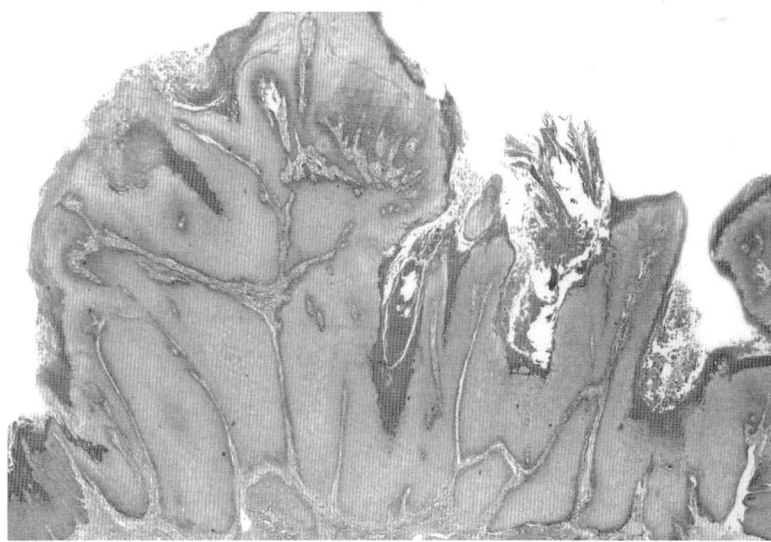

Fig. 12.219
Verrucous carcinoma: exophytic, verruciform proliferation with papillae showing inconspicuous fibrovascular cores.

differentiate verrucous carcinoma from other similar lesions.[35] It is important to follow strict diagnostic criteria since classic penile verrucous carcinoma is associated with virtually no metastatic potential.[36,37] There is a spectrum of combined tumors with focal or significant verrucous features, which need to be distinguished from typical verrucous carcinoma. The most frequent combination is that of a verrucous carcinoma with usual invasive SCC. These mixed or hybrid verrucous carcinomas have a metastatic rate of about 25%.[38–40] Verrucous carcinoma may also be associated with sarcomatoid carcinoma sporadically or after radiation therapy.[41] HPV has been consistently rare or absent in various studies.[9,24,42]

Verrucous carcinoma is rare, accounting for 7% of all penile SCCs.[2] It presents during the sixth to seventh decades and the average duration of the disease is 56 months, the longest among all penile malignant tumors. Any penile epithelial compartment may be affected and it is equally frequent in the foreskin or glans penis. Most tumors are unicentric, but multicentric cases or association with other subtypes such as the pseudohyperplastic variant has been observed.

Grossly, it is an exophytic papillomatous tumor with some variation in the configuration of the papillae, from multinodular with cobblestone morphology to filiform with a spiky appearance. The cut surface reveals a white serrated tumor and a broad demarcation between the lesion and stroma. Verrucous carcinoma is superficial, rarely penetrating beyond lamina propria or superficial dartos or corpus spongiosum.

Histologic features

Microscopically, the tumor is diffusely well differentiated, resembling normal squamous epithelium except for the presence of occasional atypical nuclei in the basal or parabasal layers. Features include papillomatosis, hyper- to orthokeratosis, acanthosis, and a broad-based interface between the tumor and stroma, the latter considered pathognomonic for this tumor. Koilocytosis is not present. Although some papillae may harbor fibrovascular cores, this is not a characteristic feature. The space between papillae is occupied by a keratin-filled crater that on a tangential cut appears as keratin-filled pseudocysts. The stroma may show a dense lymphocytic infiltrate, sometimes blurring the interface between the tumor and the underlying connective tissue (Figs 12.219–12.223). Microscopic small nests of well-differentiated invasive keratinized SCC in the lamina propria (1–3 mm in depth) may rarely be observed. We have not observed metastasis in these cases. A designation for such a lesion could be microinvasive verrucous carcinoma. This entity differs from hybrid verrucous carcinoma where large areas of the tumor show features of a moderately to poorly differentiated invasive typical SCC (Figs 12.224–12.226). Associated lesions which may be seen in the adjacent epithelium include squamous hyperplasia and

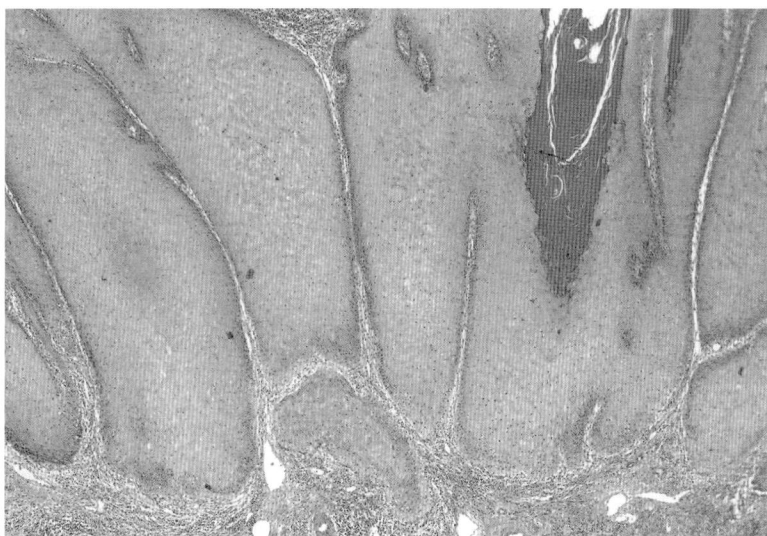

Fig. 12.220
Verrucous carcinoma: showing acanthosis, parakeratosis, papillomatosis, and a broad-based tumor–stroma interface.

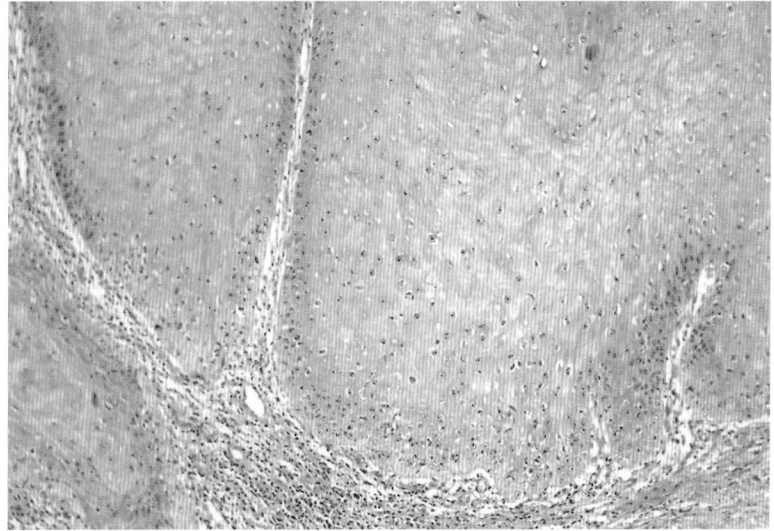

Fig. 12.221
Verrucous carcinoma: neoplastic cells are extremely well-differentiated with minimal atypia limited to the basal/parabasal layers.

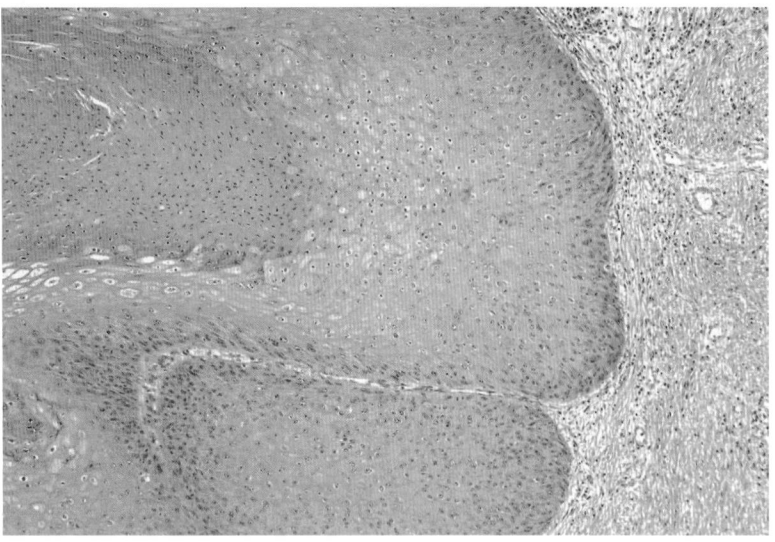

Fig. 12.222
Verrucous carcinoma: with epithelial thickening, minimal atypia, parakeratosis, and a well-defined, rounded tumor front.

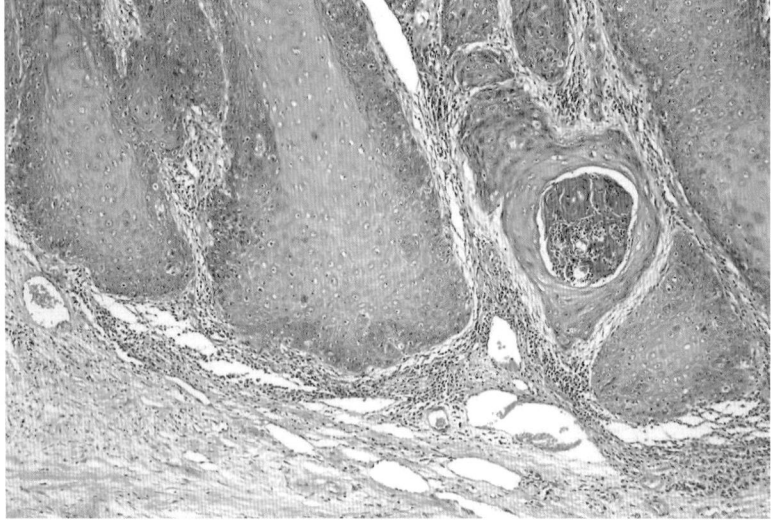

Fig. 12.223
Verrucous carcinoma: with slightly irregular tumor front and foci suspicious for microinvasive verrucous carcinoma *(upper right field)*.

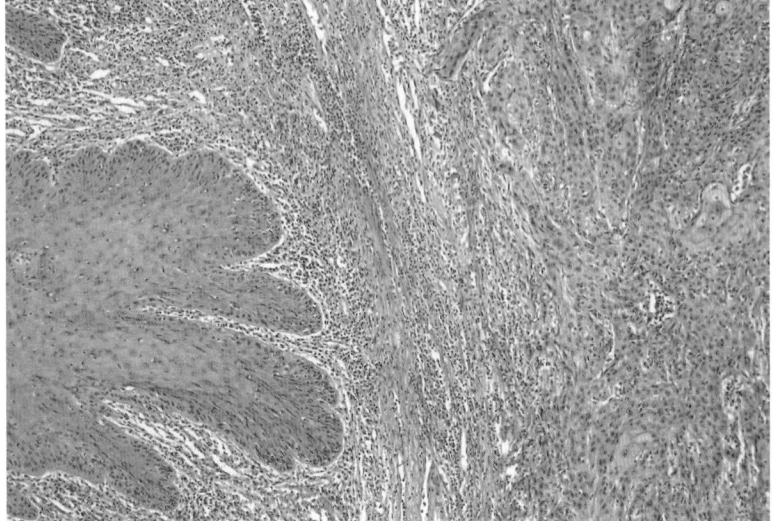

Fig. 12.224
Hybrid verrucous carcinoma: composed of a typical verrucous carcinoma *(left field)* and a usual SCC *(right field)*.

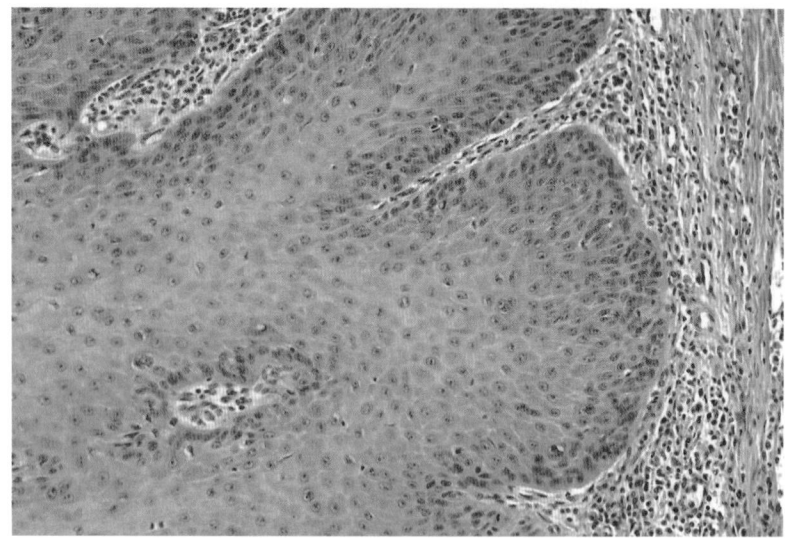

Fig. 12.225
Hybrid verrucous carcinoma: verrucous component with pushing tumor borders and well-differentiated neoplastic cells; note the underlying stromal reaction.

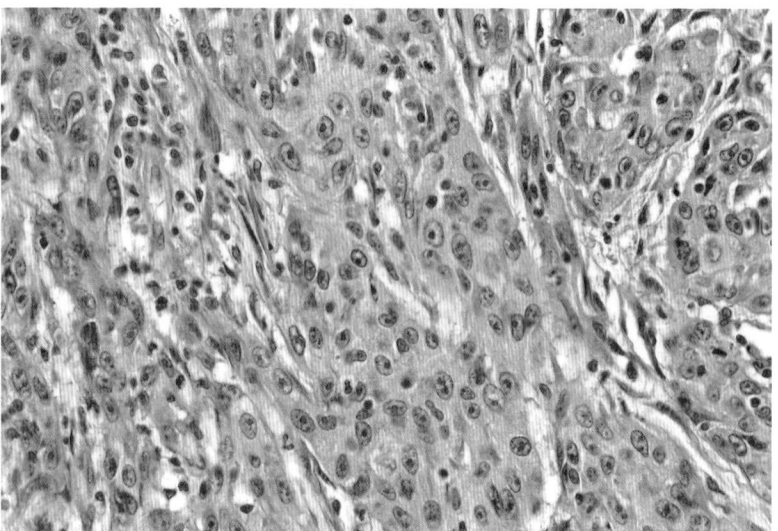

Fig. 12.226
Hybrid verrucous carcinoma: usual SCC component composed of poorly differentiated neoplastic cells.

differentiated PeIN. The hyperplasia often adopts the features of verrucous hyperplasia. LS is a further frequently found associated condition and may be pathogenetically related to verrucous carcinoma.[43] Verrucous carcinoma, if insufficiently resected, is prone to local recurrence. Regional metastases are not seen in typical (pure) lesions.

Carcinoma cuniculatum

Clinical features

This tumor was originally documented on the sole of the foot. It is a deeply penetrating, albeit low-grade SCC which, because of its burrowing growth pattern, was designated epithelioma cuniculatum by Aird in 1954.[44] Seven cases of this unusual variant of SCC have been reported in the penis.[45] The mean age of presentation was 77 years. Grossly, the tumor is white-gray, exo–endophytic and papillomatous with a cobblestone or spiky appearance. It affects the glans and often extends to the coronal sulcus and foreskin (average size, 6 cm). The hallmark of the lesion is visible on the cut surface where deep invaginations of the tumor form irregular, narrow, and elongated neoplastic sinus tracts that connect the surface of the tumor to deep anatomical structures.

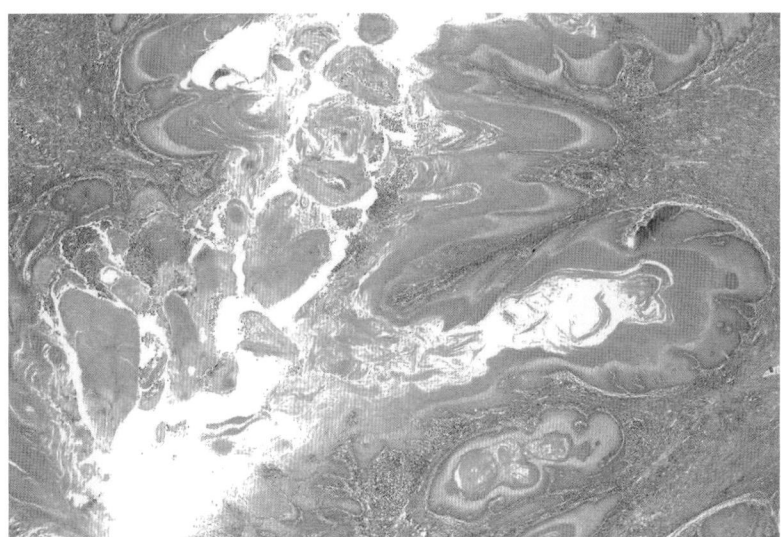

Fig. 12.227
Carcinoma cuniculatum: at low-power view showing its verruciform pattern of growth extending deep into penile erectile tissues.

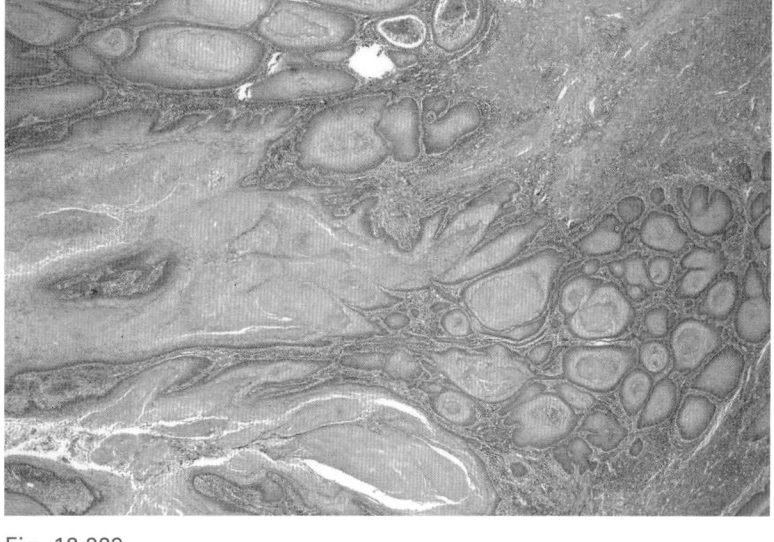

Fig. 12.229
Carcinoma cuniculatum: with its characteristic verruciform pattern of growth *(left field)* associated with an invasive usual SCC *(right field)*.

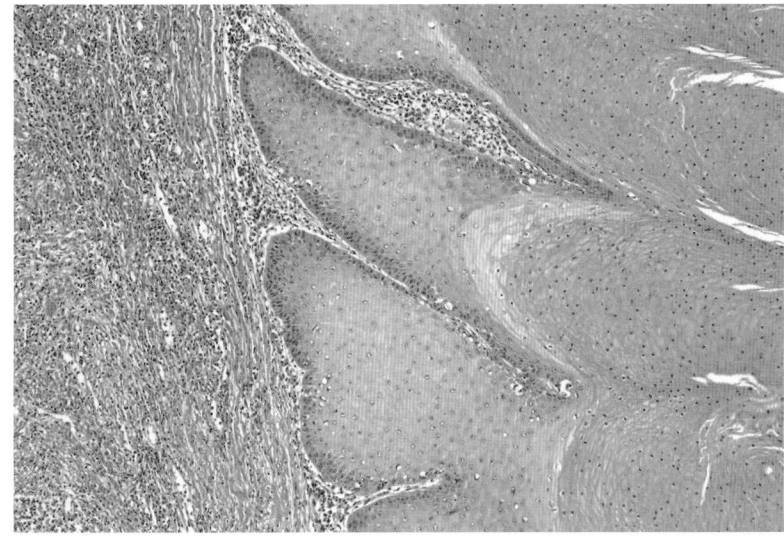

Fig. 12.228
Carcinoma cuniculatum: with a broad-based tumor front, intense stromal reaction, neoplastic cells with minimal atypia, and prominent parakeratosis.

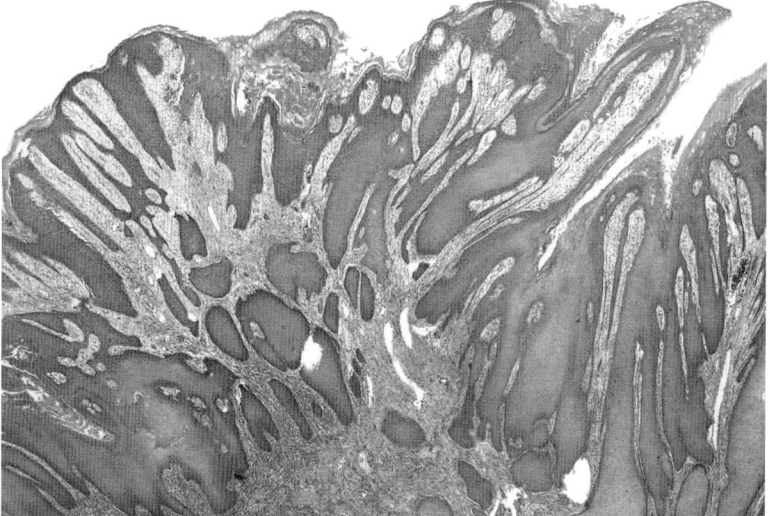

Fig. 12.230
Papillary carcinoma, NOS: with rounded and tipped papillae, hyperkeratosis, and irregular fibrovascular cores.

Despite the deep penetration, none of the reported cases of carcinoma cuniculatum has shown nodal or systemic disease at time of diagnosis.

Histologic features

Microscopically, the tumor partially resembles verrucous carcinoma with a bulbous front of invasion. There may, however, be irregular foci of invasive SCC of the usual type (*Figs 12.227–12.229*). Carcinoma cuniculatum should be distinguished from classical verrucous carcinoma, which is also well differentiated, but rarely invades beyond the lamina propria and has a sharply delineated front.

Papillary carcinoma, not otherwise specified

Clinical features

Papillary carcinoma, not otherwise specified (NOS) is a non-HPV-related verruciform tumor.[2,3,46] Patients are on average around 60 years old. The tumor is grossly exophytic, large, and irregular and involves the glans, coronal sulcus, and foreskin. The cut surface shows a papillary neoplasm involving corpus spongiosum or dartos. Papillary carcinoma is a slow-growing tumor with a low but definite incidence of inguinal nodal metastasis.

Histologic features

Microscopically, the appearance is that of a well-differentiated papillary squamous neoplasm. There is hyperkeratosis and papillomatosis. Papillae are variable and complex, short or long, with or without a fibrovascular core (*Figs 12.230–12.232*). The tips may be straight, undulated, spiky, or blunt. Hyperkeratosis and acanthosis are prominent. Keratin cysts or intraepithelial abscesses are sometimes present. The base of the lesion is irregular and infiltrative. The interface between tumor and stroma is characteristically jagged (*Fig. 12.233*). Koilocytotic-like changes are usually absent. Differentiating features from verrucous and condylomatous carcinoma are based on the heterogeneity of the papillae, the lack of koilocytosis, and the jagged irregular interface between tumor and stroma. The latter feature is crucial to distinguish papillary from verrucous carcinoma. HPV studies may be necessary to differentiate papillary neoplasms, usually negative for HPV, from low-grade condylomatous carcinoma. Another tumor to be distinguished from papillary carcinoma NOS is the infrequent papillary basaloid SCC.[2,47] In this tumor, papillae harbor a thin fibrovascular core and the cells are small and anaplastic, resembling basaloid or transitional carcinoma. This unusual penile neoplasm is often deeply invasive. Low-grade

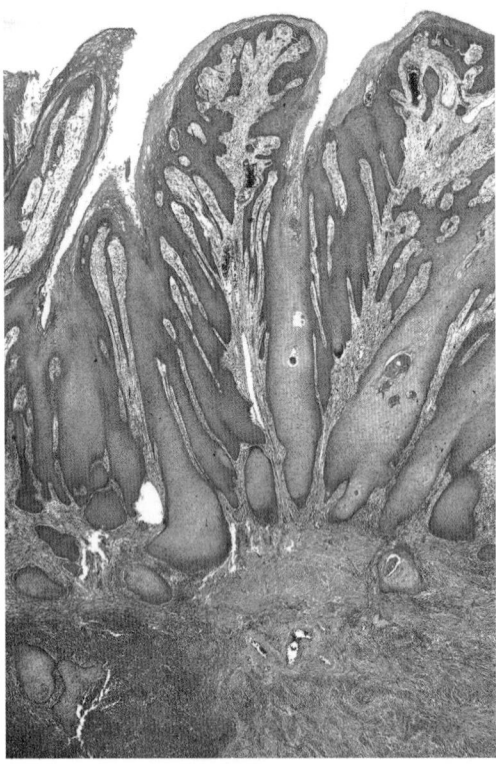

Fig. 12.231
Papillary carcinoma, NOS: with rounded and tipped papillae, hyperkeratosis, and irregular fibrovascular cores.

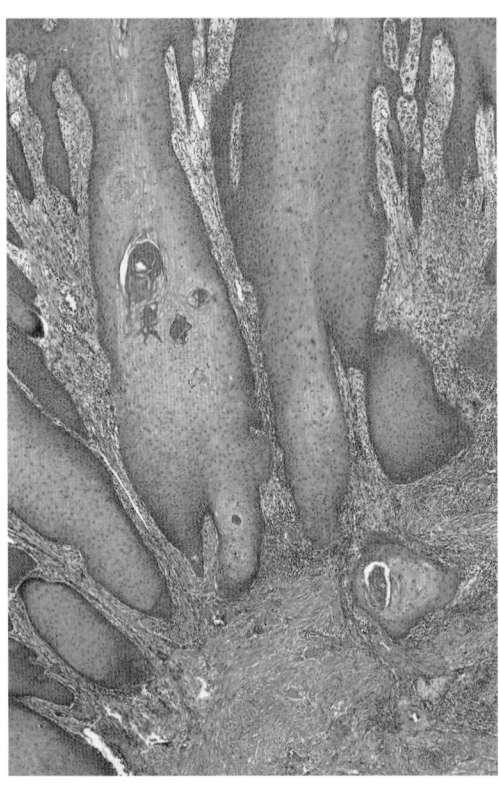

Fig. 12.232
Papillary carcinoma, NOS: showing an irregular, jagged tumor front of invasion and prominent stromal reaction.

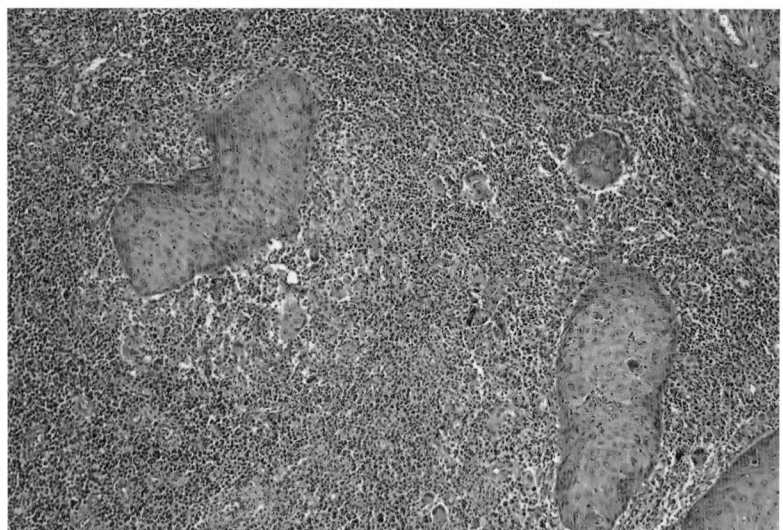

Fig. 12.233
Papillary carcinoma, NOS: irregular tumor nests at the tumor base surrounded by intense chronic inflammation.

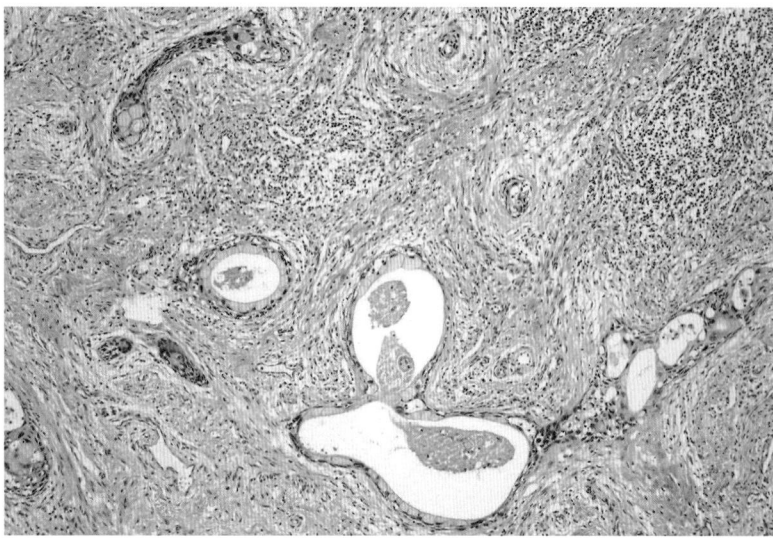

Fig. 12.234
Adenosquamous carcinoma: showing neoplastic nests composed of cells with glandular and squamous differentiation.

squamous intraepithelial lesion and LS are frequently associated with papillary carcinoma.

Adenosquamous carcinoma

Clinical features

Adenosquamous carcinoma is an exceedingly rare variant thought to arise within misplaced glandular cells within the perimeatal region of the penis. It consists of SCC with foci of mucinous glandular differentiation. It is believed to arise from the epithelial surface of the glans, where foci of SCC in situ may be noted. Clinicopathological features and outcome are similar to usual SCC. Grossly, a large firm granular neoplasm deeply invading penile corpora is present. The few reported cases of adenosquamous carcinomas have behaved aggressively with frequent nodal metastasis.

Histologic features

Microscopically, there is an admixture of SCC and mucin secreting adenocarcinoma (*Figs 12.234* and *12.235*). The squamous component generally predominates.[48] The glandular epithelium expresses CEA. Differentiated PeIN is usually present in the adjacent glans mucosa. Adenosquamous carcinomas should be distinguished from mucoepidermoid, adeno-basaloid, and pseudoglandular SCCs. In mucoepidermoid carcinomas, there are isolated cells or group of squamous cells containing mucin without forming glandular structures.[49] In adeno-basaloid tumors, there are well-formed mucin secreting glands but the solid component is a basaloid carcinoma. Pseudoglandular (adenoid or acantholytic) SCC most frequently represents SCC of the usual type in which there is considerable dyskeratosis and acantholysis with secondary pseudolumen formation simulating glandular structures. The lack of mucin production aids in their distinction. Another important differential diagnosis is adenocarcinoma arising in Littre glands. This tumor is ventrally located around the penile urethra.

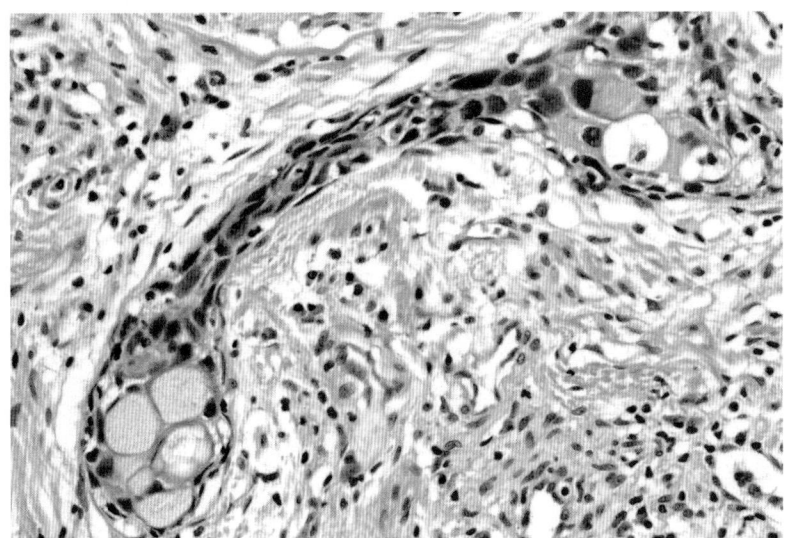

Fig. 12.235
Adenosquamous carcinoma: tumor nest with a high-grade squamous component associated with areas of glandular differentiation.

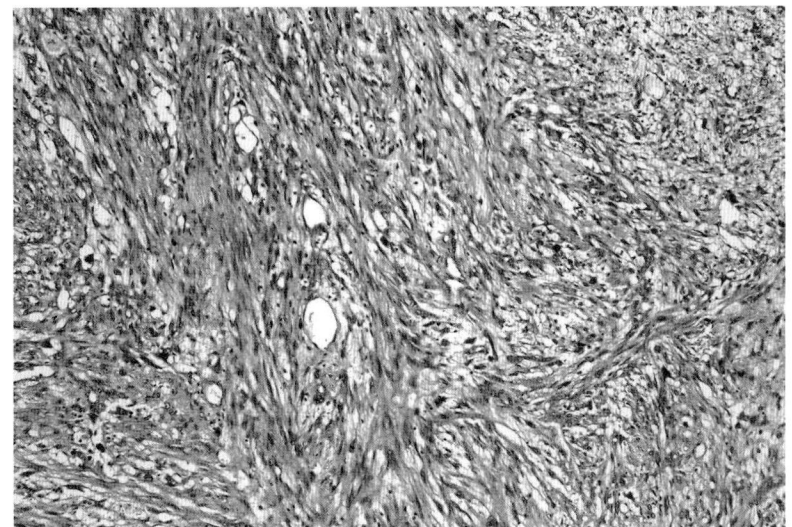

Fig. 12.236
Sarcomatoid carcinoma: composed of neoplastic spindle cells simulating a high-grade sarcoma.

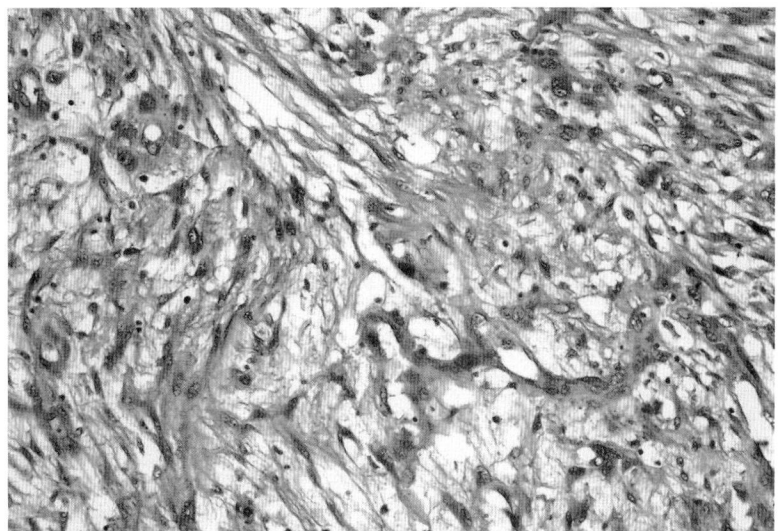

Fig. 12.237
Sarcomatoid carcinoma: high-grade pleomorphic cells intermingled with spindled cells.

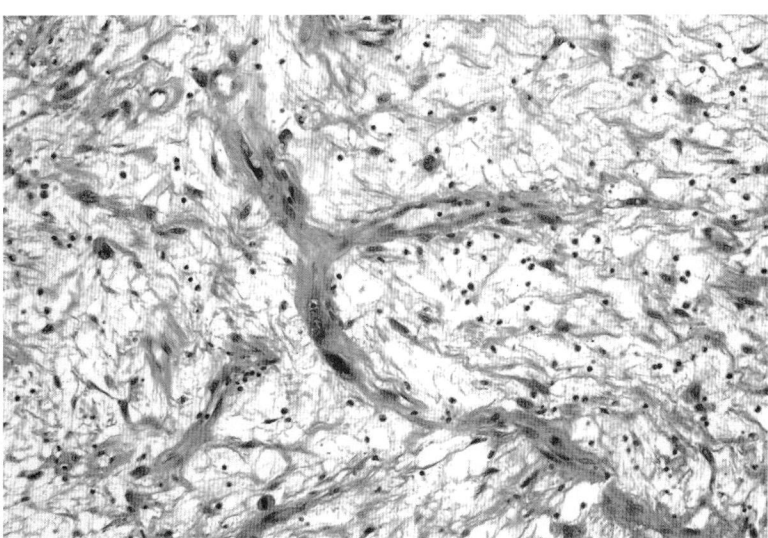

Fig. 12.238
Sarcomatoid carcinoma: pleomorphic and spindled malignant cells in a myxoid background.

Sarcomatoid carcinoma (carcinoma with heterologous differentiation, metaplastic carcinoma)

Clinical features

Sarcomatoid carcinoma is an aggressive penile neoplasm composed predominantly of spindled cells. It may arise de novo, follow a recurrence of usual SCC, or develop after irradiation therapy of a verrucous carcinoma. It accounts for about 1–4% of all penile carcinomas and preferentially involves the glans penis although the foreskin may also be affected.[50] As with usual SCCs, the mean age is around 60 years. Grossly, it presents as a bulky 5–10 cm ulcerated or rounded polypoid mass, which on sectioning shows almost invariably deep invasion into the corpus cavernosum. Regional metastases occur in 85% of sarcomatoid carcinomas, and mortality is high.

Histologic features

Microscopically, there are variable proportions of squamous and spindle cell carcinoma but the latter usually predominates. The sarcomatoid component includes leiomyosarcoma, fibrosarcoma, myxosarcoma, epithelioid angiosarcoma, classic angiosarcoma, and the so-called 'pleomorphic malignant fibrous histiocytoma' (*Figs 12.236–12.240*). Heterologous bone and cartilage formation is sometimes focally present. Rarely, the tumor shows pseudoglandular and/or pseudovascular differentiation (*Figs 12.241* and

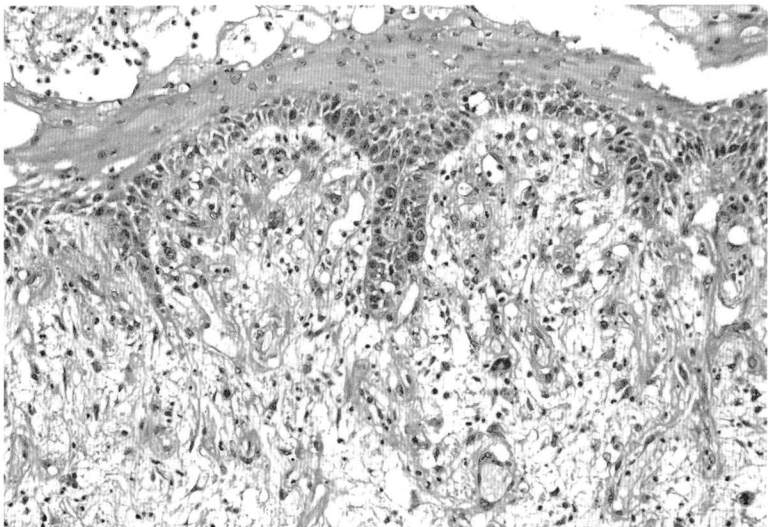

Fig. 12.239
Sarcomatoid carcinoma: differentiated PeIN with underlying sarcomatoid carcinoma.

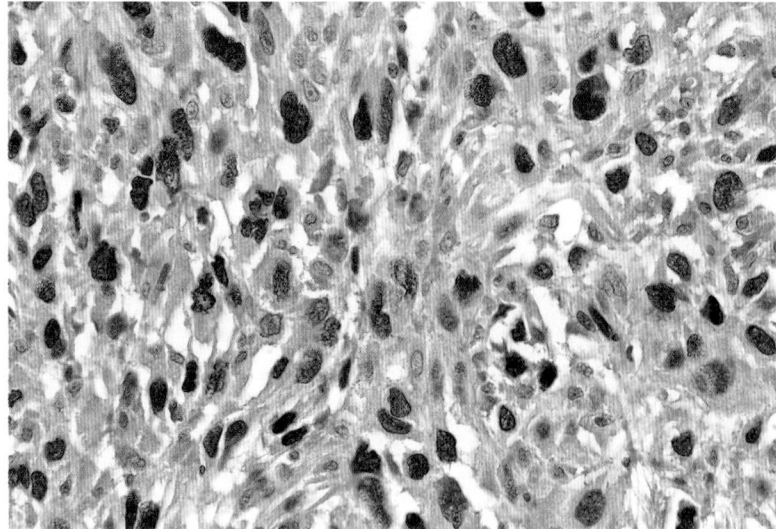

Fig. 12.240
Sarcomatoid carcinoma: neoplastic cells in a sarcomatoid carcinoma showing nuclear positivity for p63 immunohistochemistry.

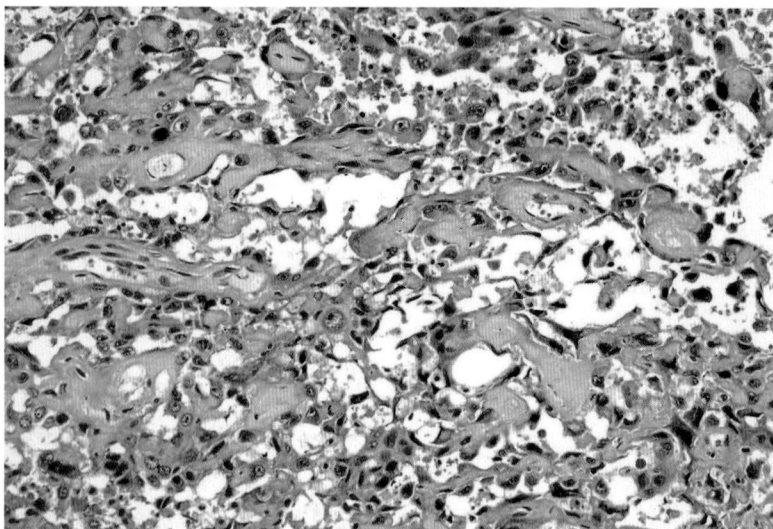

Fig. 12.242
Sarcomatoid carcinoma: high-grade pleomorphic cells mimicking the pattern of growth of angiosarcomas ('pseudoangiosarcomatoid carcinoma').

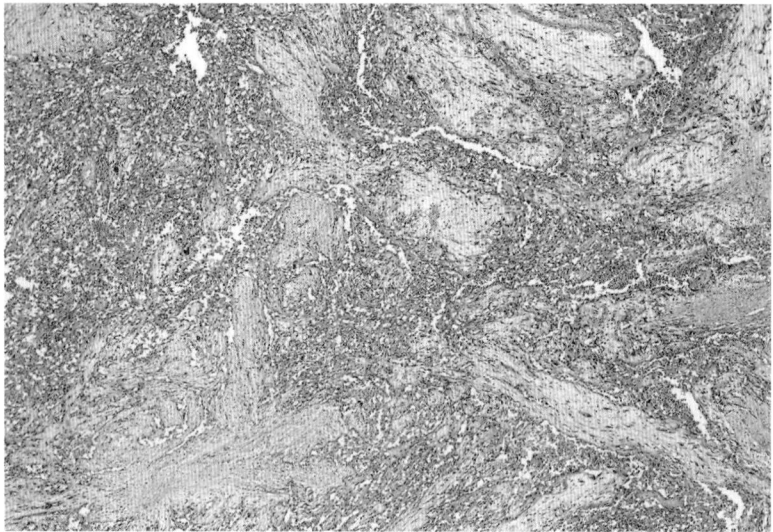

Fig. 12.241
Sarcomatoid carcinoma: low-power view of a sarcomatoid carcinoma with irregular spaces simulating vascular lumina.

12.242). The squamous component typically shows the morphology of usual SCC but areas of verrucous, papillary, or basaloid carcinoma may also be observed, indicating that sarcomatoid transformation may occur in practically any tumor type. HPV is usually absent. Differential diagnosis includes sarcoma and melanoma. Immunohistochemistry is essential for tumors with little or no epithelial component and for small biopsy specimens. The spindle cells are usually positive for vimentin, various cytokeratins, and p63. In our experience, cytokeratin 34betaE12 and p63 appear to be the more specific and sensitive markers to categorize these tumors as epithelial. AE1/AE3 and Cam 5.2 tend to be more variable and often only focally positive, sometimes highlighting scattered single cells. Smooth muscle actin can be focally positive; however, desmin, muscle-specific actin, myogenin, and S100 are negative. Tumors which display specific sarcomatous components such as leiomyosarcoma or angiosarcoma display the expected immunohistochemistry.

Mixed carcinoma

Clinical features

In mixed carcinoma, there are morphological features characteristic of two or more subtypes of SCC. Warty–basaloid and adenosquamous carcinomas are mixed neoplasms but are discussed as separate entities. They represent about 25% of all carcinomas and affect the glans of males in their seventies. Gross features are non-specific with an irregular white-gray mass replacing the distal penis.[51]

Histologic features

There is a variety of mixed tumors, and any subtype in this classification scheme may be found mixed with other subtypes. Usually non-HPV tumors are found mixed with other non-HPV-related subtypes, and the same is true for HPV-related neoplasms. What is important to recognize is the verrucous mixed with usual SCC (hybrid verrucous carcinoma). Typical verrucous carcinomas do not metastasize, whereas regional and systemic spread may occur in mixed verrucous carcinomas. Long-standing benign and or giant condilomas may develop malignant transformation showing areas of usual SCC. HPV-related and non-HPV-related carcinomas may rarely mix. There are rare large complex exophytic verruciform tumors that are difficult to classify, with verrucous, papillary, and condylomatous features.[2]

HPV-related carcinomas
Basaloid carcinoma

Clinical features

Basaloid carcinoma is an aggressive, HPV-related variant of SCC occurring in the fifth decade and preferentially affecting the glans.[52] It has been proposed that it originates within the squamous–transitional junction of the meatal region. Rarely, basaloid carcinoma may develop in the foreskin. It accounts for 4–10% of penile SCCs. The median age is 53 years. More than half of patients show inguinal metastasis at clinical diagnosis. Grossly, there is an ulcerated irregular mass. The cut surface reveals a tan, solid tumor, deeply invasive into the corpus spongiosum or cavernosum.

Histologic features

Microscopically, there are separate or confluent solid nests composed of small basaloid cells, usually with central necrosis (comedonecrosis) or central abrupt keratinization (Figs 12.243–12.246). Nuclei are anaplastic and nucleoli inconspicuous. There are numerous mitotic figures. Occasional palisading at the nest periphery may be noted, but it is usually not as prominent as is seen in basal cell carcinoma of the skin. Basophilic intermediate or large cell nuclei may be noted in some cases. Pseudoglandular features are sometimes present (Figs 12.247 and 12.248) (adenoid–basaloid carcinomas). A papillary variant of basaloid carcinoma, also denominated papillary basaloid carcinoma, has been reported (Fig. 12.249).[47] PeIN of the warty–basaloid type is often found in the epithelium adjacent to the invasive cancer.

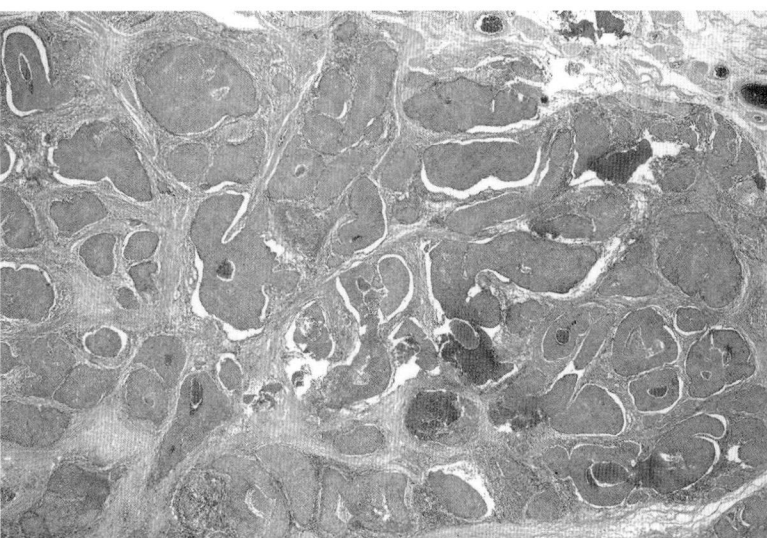

Fig. 12.243
Basaloid carcinoma: at low-power view showing deeply infiltrative tumor nests.

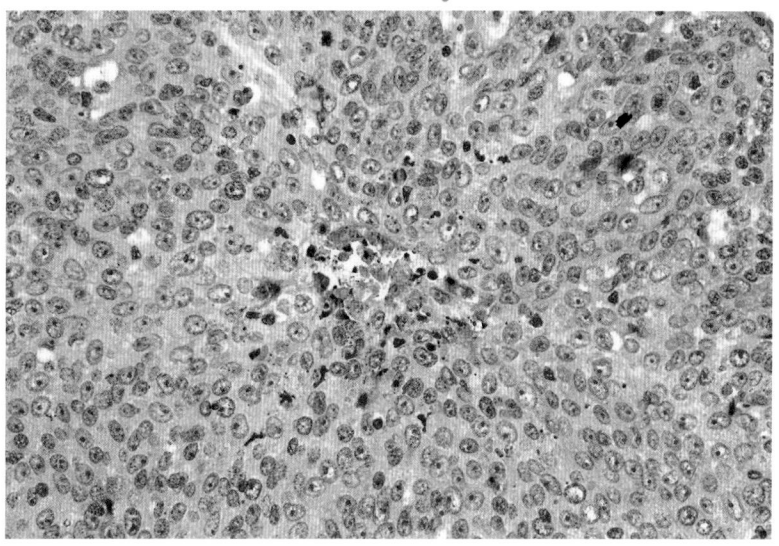

Fig. 12.246
Basaloid carcinoma: composed of neoplastic cells with indistinctive cellular borders, high mitotic/apoptotic rate, and central (comedo-like) necrosis.

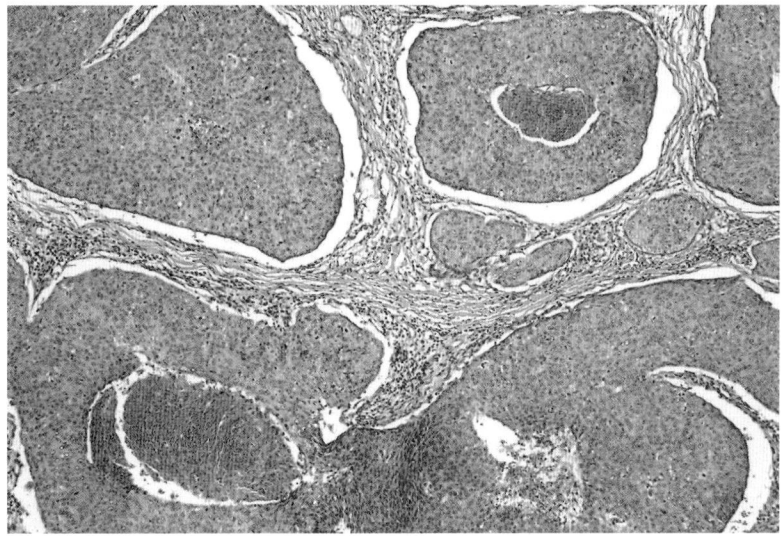

Fig. 12.244
Basaloid carcinoma: with tumor nests showing central, abrupt parakeratosis, and retraction artifact.

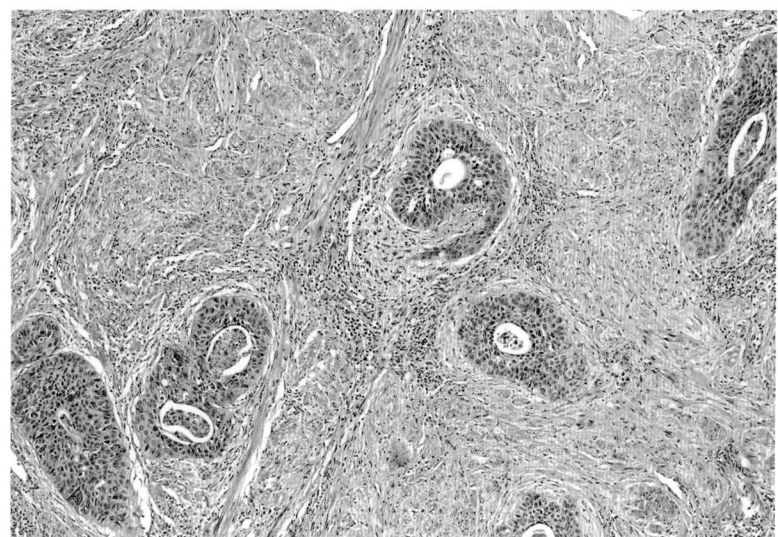

Fig. 12.247
Basaloid carcinoma: with tumor nests exhibiting open central areas due to central necrosis, simulating glandular spaces.

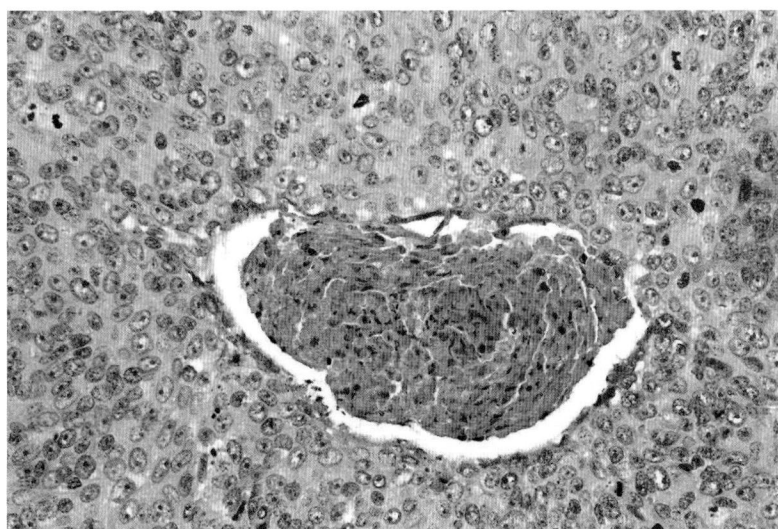

Fig. 12.245
Basaloid carcinoma: tumor nest composed of a monomorphic population of cells with evident atypia and central parakeratotic debris.

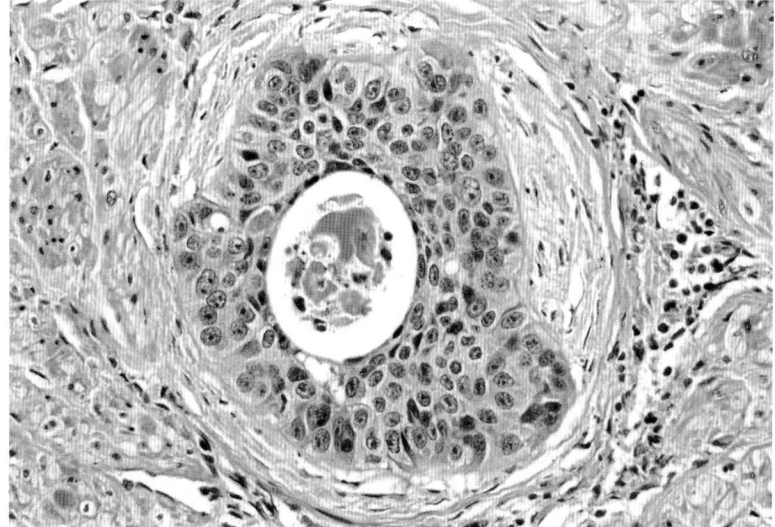

Fig. 12.248
Basaloid carcinoma: with central, necrotic debris and a pseudoglandular appearance.

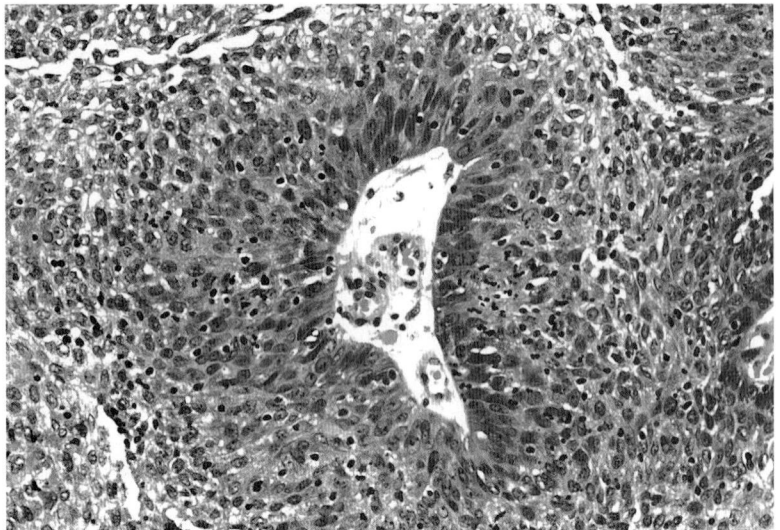

Fig. 12.249
Papillary basaloid variant: papillomatous tumor with a central fibrovascular core. Cells are small and basophilic.

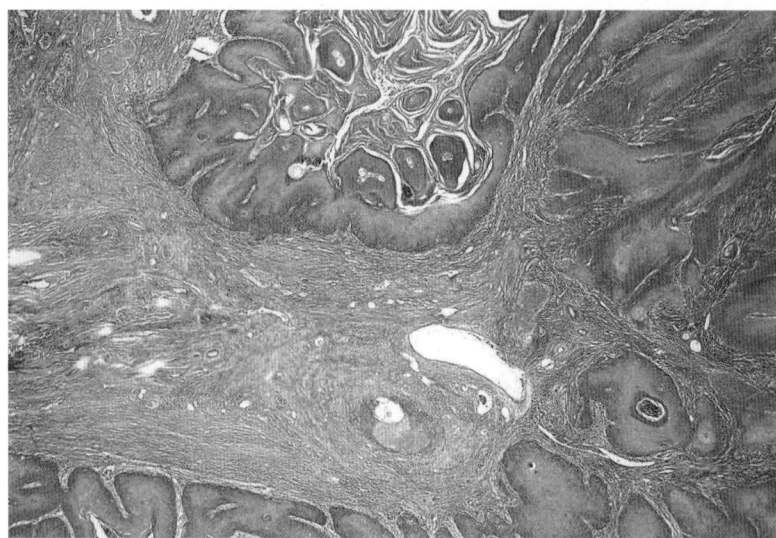

Fig. 12.251
Condylomatous carcinoma: showing an irregular, jagged infiltrative tumor front *(right field)*.

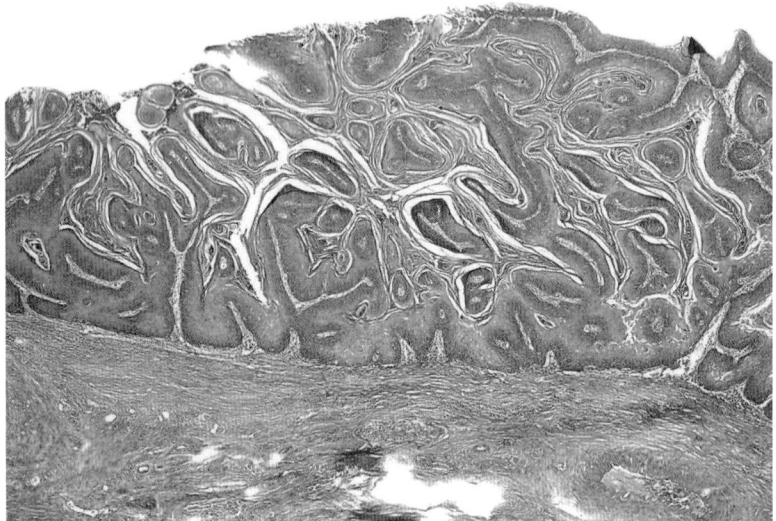

Fig. 12.250
Condylomatous carcinoma: exhibiting an exophytic, papillomatous pattern of growth with conspicuous fibrovascular cores.

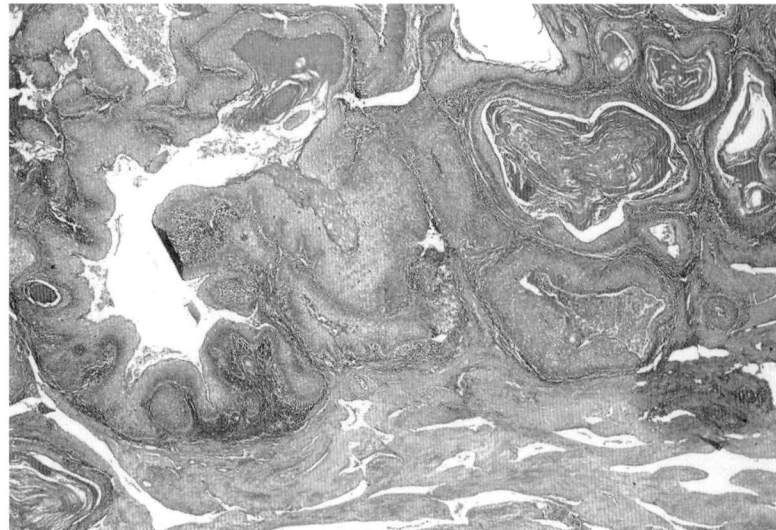

Fig. 12.252
Condylomatous carcinoma: with papillomatosis, evident fibrovascular cores, and irregular tumor–stroma interface.

Condylomatous (warty) carcinoma

Clinical features

Condylomatous carcinoma is a slow-growing, verruciform low- to intermediate-grade HPV-related tumor, grossly similar to giant condyloma but with malignant histology and potential for nodal metastasis.[35] It accounts for 7% of all penile SCCs affecting patients younger than those with the usual SCC. A history of previous viral warts is frequently obtained. The foreskin, coronal sulcus, and glans are usually involved. Macroscopically, the cut surface shows a papillomatous growth generally penetrating into the corpora spongiosa and cavernosa. The interface of tumor and stroma varies from broadly based to jagged and irregular.

Histologic features

Microscopically, the tumor papillae are condylomatous and of various shapes (round, ovoid or spiky, long or short) but always with a prominent central fibrovascular core and koilocytotic changes (*Figs 12.250–12.254*). Unlike benign condyloma, koilocytosis is not restricted to the surface epithelial cells but is also present in deep invasive portions of the tumor (*Fig. 12.255*). Hyper- and parakeratosis, cellular pleomorphism, and clear cell change may be prominent. p16 is positive in nonkeratinized areas. The biological behavior of condylomatous carcinoma is intermediate between that

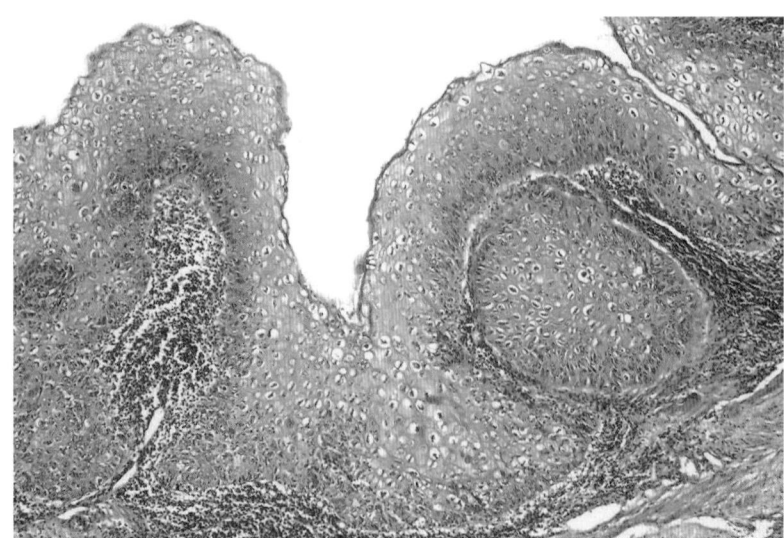

Fig. 12.253
Condylomatous carcinoma: papillae with conspicuous koilocytosis, slight parakeratosis, and underlying chronic stromal reaction.

of other types of low-grade verruciform tumors (verrucous and papillary) and SCC of the usual type. Deeply invasive, high-grade condylomatous carcinoma may be associated with inguinal nodal metastasis.

The differential diagnosis is with other verruciform tumors, verrucous and papillary carcinoma and giant condyloma. The histologic evaluation of type of papillae, presence of koilocytosis, interface of tumor and stroma, and presence of HPV helps in the differentiation of these neoplasms (see Table 12.3).

Koilocytosis, condylomatous papillae, and jagged irregular boundaries between tumor and stroma are present in warty but not in verrucous carcinomas. In papillary carcinomas, papillae are complex and show no koilocytosis. Giant condylomas are broadly based noninvasive tumors with surface koilocytosis (see Table 12.3).[35,53] Associated precursor lesions of condylomatous carcinoma include PeIN of the warty or basaloid types.

Warty–basaloid carcinoma

Clinical features

Mixed tumors composed of warty and basaloid features.[54] They are large neoplasms preferentially affecting the glans, but other compartments may be involved. Patients are usually in the seventh decade of life. Grossly they are exophytic or exo-endophytic. The cut surface may be white-gray serrated at the surface and solid in deeper tissues.

Histologic features

Warty and basaloid features intermixed in various proportions and modalities. Typically, there is a warty carcinoma on the surface and a basaloid carcinoma in the invasive component. Features of warty and basaloid carcinoma may be present in the same tumor nest, with clear cell pleomorphic koilocytotic pattern in the center and a small cell homogenous pattern at the periphery. p16 is positive in both cell type components (Fig. 12.256). The differential diagnosis is with pure warty and basaloid carcinomas and with the papillary variant of basaloid carcinomas. Pure warty carcinomas have no basaloid features, and in pure basaloid carcinomas there are no warty features. The papillary variant of basaloid carcinomas should be distinguished from the papillomatous warty–basaloid carcinomas. In the former the cell pattern is of small uniform basaloid, and in the latter the cell pattern is biphasic with both warty and basaloid cells present in the papillae.

Clear cell carcinoma

Clinical features

Aggressive HPV-related solid tumors arising in penile mucosae predominantly composed of clear cells.[55,56] Grossly they are large, white-gray irregular masses on the foreskin or glans.

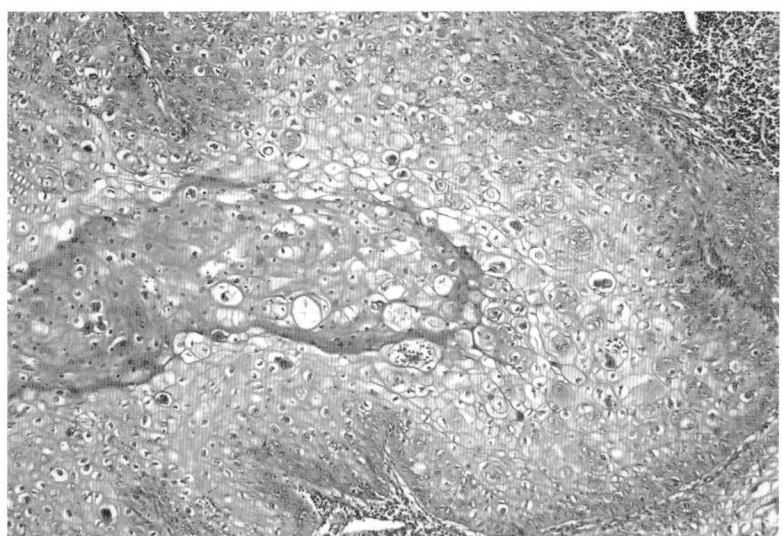

Fig. 12.254
Condylomatous carcinoma: showing abundant koilocytes, more prominent at the upper layers, and marked parakeratosis.

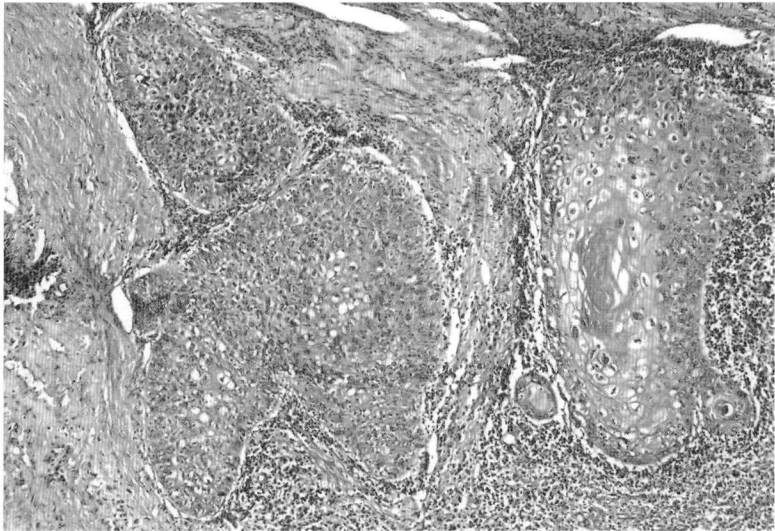

Fig. 12.255
Condylomatous carcinoma: deep infiltrative nests with koilocytes and surrounding stromal reaction.

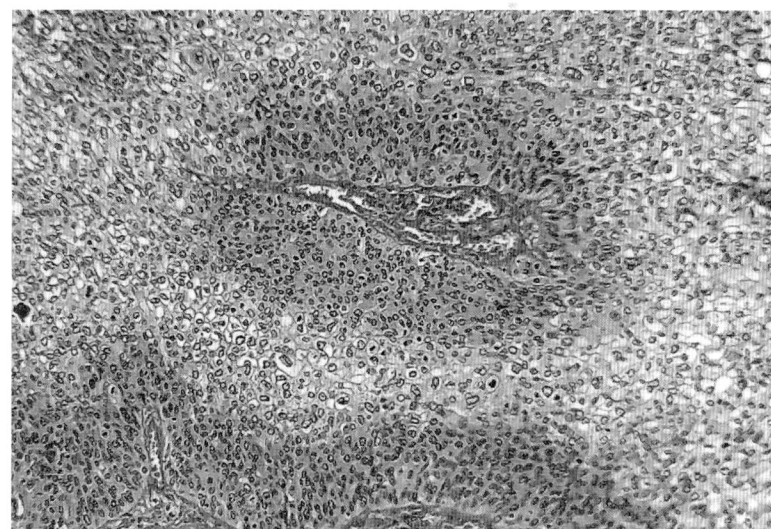

Fig. 12.256
Warty–basaloid carcinoma: a tumor composed of central clear cells and peripheral basaloid cells.

Table 12.3
Differential diagnosis of verruciform tumors

	Papillae	Koilocytosis	Interface	HPV
Warty	Condylomatous	Present phloem	Jagged	+ High risk
Verrucous	Noncondylomatous	Absent	Broad	Absent
Papillary	Complex	Absent	Jagged	Absent
Giant condyloma	Condylomatous	Superficial	Broad	+ Low risk

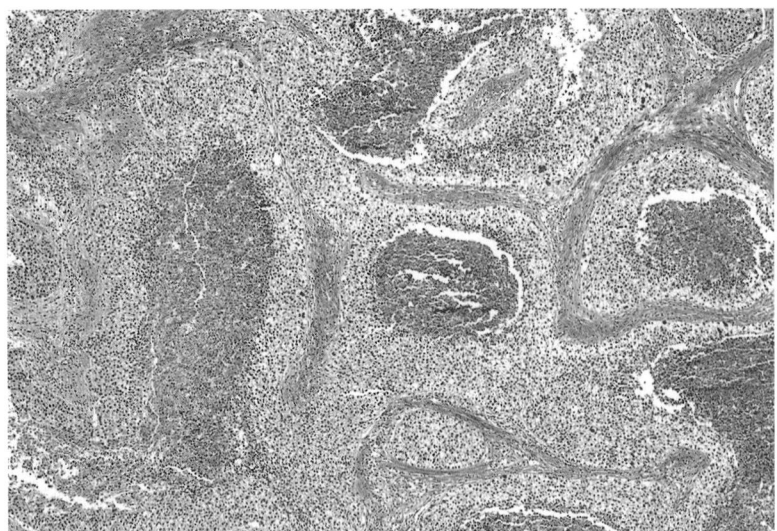

Fig. 12.257
Clear cell carcinoma: there is a confluent nesting pattern with central comedonecrosis.

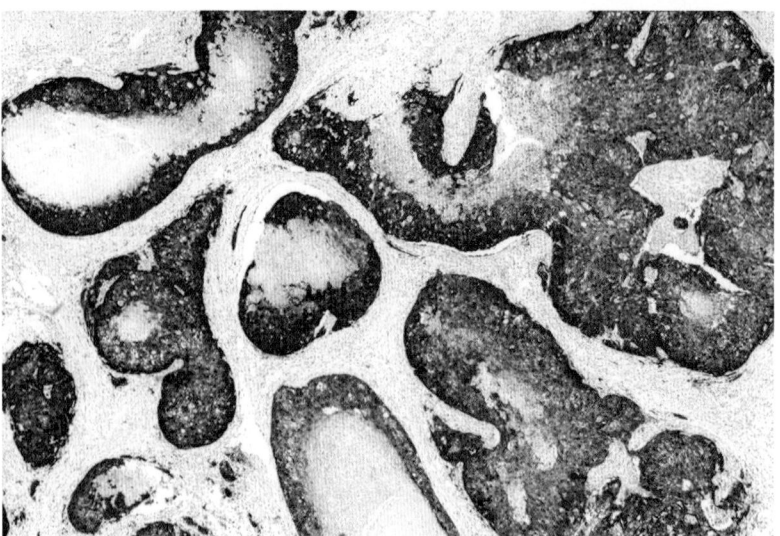

Fig. 12.259
Clear cell carcinoma: p16 immunostain is positive in tumor cells.

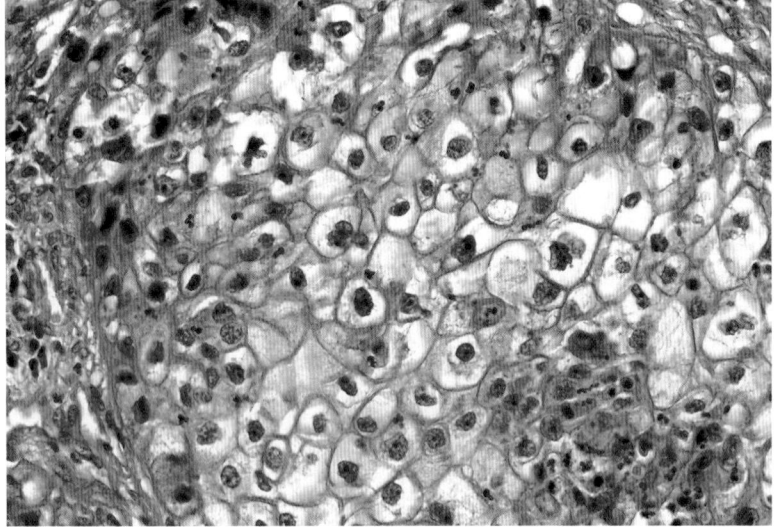

Fig. 12.258
Clear cell carcinoma: composed of polygonal cells with evident atypia and a clear, faintly eosinophilic cytoplasm.

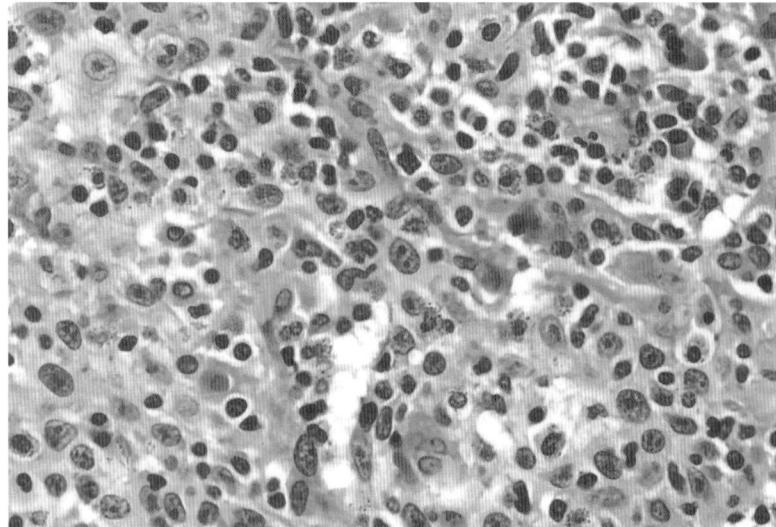

Fig. 12.260
Lymphoepithelioma-like carcinoma: poorly cohesive tumor cells are associated with prominent inflammation.

Histologic features

The growth pattern is nested with clear cell features (*Fig. 12.257*). Comedo-like and geographic necrosis are prominent. The clear cell cytoplasmic feature is uniform throughout the tumor (*Fig. 12.258*). Nuclei are irregular and centrally located. There is PAS-positive intracytoplasmic material. p16 is strongly positive (*Fig. 12.259*). The differential diagnosis is with warty penile carcinoma, skin adnexa sweat gland tumors, and metastatic renal cell carcinoma. Clear cell carcinomas are non-verruciform and solid without the papillary configuration of warty carcinomas. Immunostains may be used to rule out sweat gland and renal cell carcinoma. Positivity for p16, negative in skin and renal tumors, should allow the difference to be made.

Lymphoepithelioma-like carcinoma

Clinical features

This is an extremely rare and poorly differentiated carcinoma. Its name derives from lymphotepithelioma or undifferentiated nasopharyngeal carcinoma. Few cases have been reported.[57,58] EBV stain is negative. Patients are uncircumcised, and the age range is between the sixth and eighth decades of life. Grossly, they present with large tumors in the glans with extension to foreskin.

Histologic features

Poorly differentiated loosely cohesive squamous cells within a dense inflammatory cell stroma, which obscures tumor cell boundaries, with occasional tumor-isolated cells simulating malignant lymphoma (*Fig. 12.260*). The differential diagnosis is with lymphomas and poorly differentiated usual SCCs.

Other rare carcinomas

Tumor arising in the skin appendages of the penile shaft are described elsewhere. Within the penile mucosal compartments, there are rare, poorly differentiated tumors difficult to classify. One of them, still not included in the WHO classification, is the poorly differentiated solid and syncytial medullary carcinoma of the penis.[59] This is an unusual aggressive HPV-related penile neoplasm characterized by a solid or syncytial growth pattern and a prominent tumor or stromal associated inflammatory cell infiltrate (*Figs 12.261* and *12.262*). Neuroendocrine carcinoma Merkel type has been reported.[60] Paget disease may rarely affect the penis.

    Giant condyloma. Described by Buschke and Löwenstein, this is an exophytic tumor which reaches a very large size after many years of evolution.[55] There has been much confusion in the correct classification of this lesion, which has been confused with verrucous carcinoma. In our opinion,

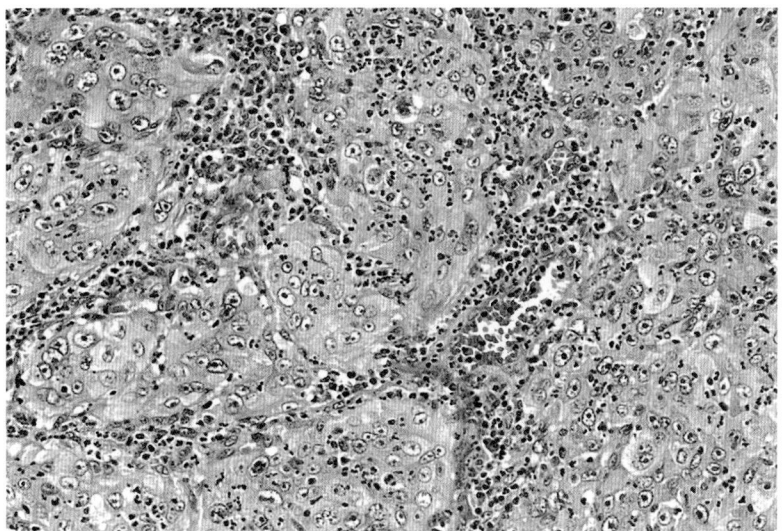

Fig. 12.261
Medullary carcinoma: poorly differentiated nonkeratinizing solid neoplasm with cellular pleomorphism.

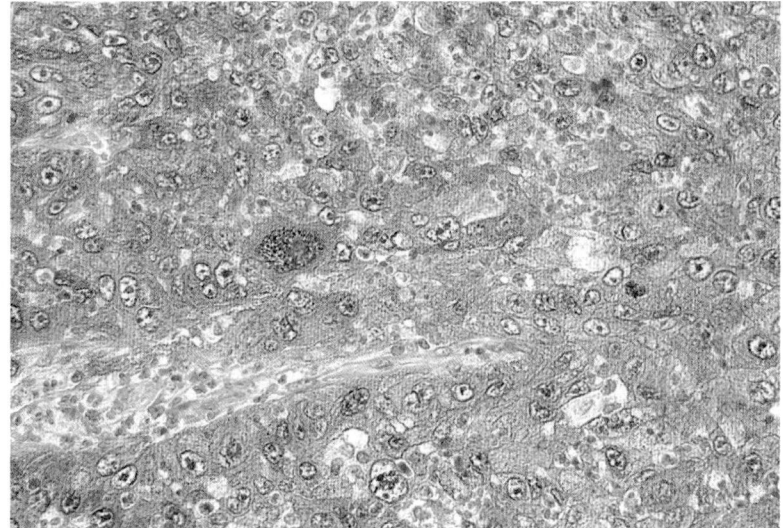

Fig. 12.262
Medullary carcinoma: p16 positive cells in a diffuse pattern.

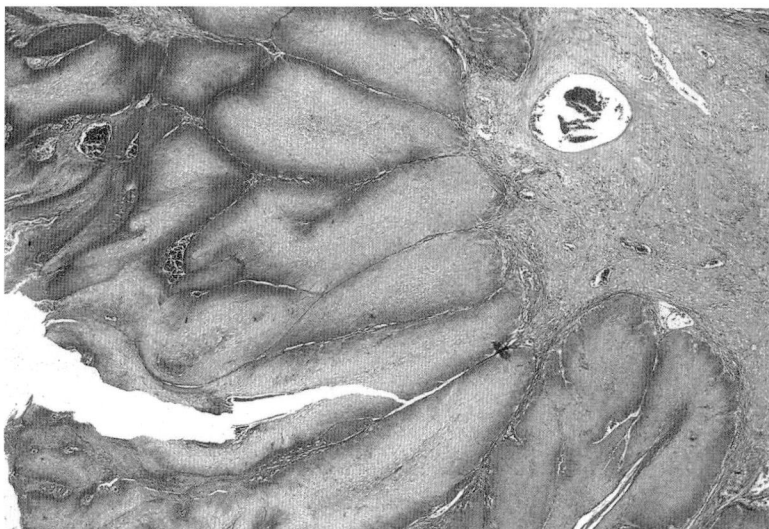

Fig. 12.263
Giant condyloma: showing a papillomatous, exophytic pattern of growth, conspicuous fibrovascular cores, and a broad tumor base.

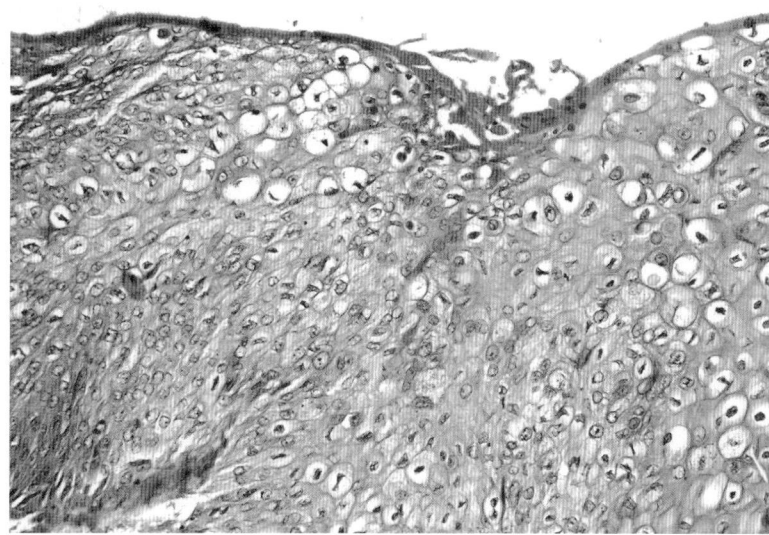

Fig. 12.264
Giant condyloma: with overt koilocytosis, slight parakeratosis, and no cellular atypia.

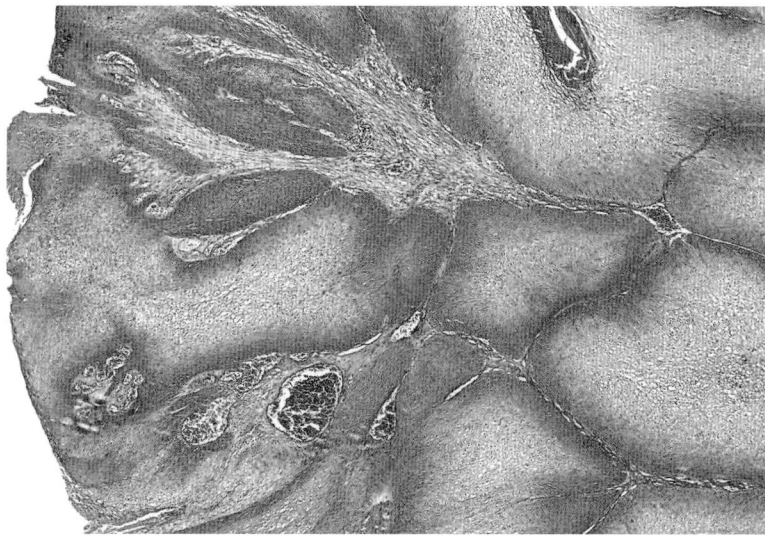

Fig. 12.265
Giant condyloma: with a pushing, downward proliferation extending into penile erectile tissues.

verrucous carcinoma is a different tumor (see above). In giant condylomas, patients are older than those with condyloma acuminatum and younger than those with condylomatous (warty) carcinoma. Grossly, it presents as a cauliflower-like tumor showing a papillomatous growth with a sharp demarcation between the lesion and stroma on the cut surface. The deep border may affect lamina propria, dartos, or corpus spongiosum. Histologically, it may have an exo- add/or endophytic growth pattern with morphology identical to condyloma acuminatum. However, in our recent experience, there is a morphological spectrum:

- entirely benign, composed of differentiated squamous cells, and indistinguishable from condyloma acuminatum,
- focally atypical,
- entirely atypical but without invasion,
- associated with superficial microinvasive SCC,
- associated with overtly invasive SCC (see diagram).

The condylomatous papillae show a central fibrovascular core and superficial koilocytotic changes (*Figs 12.263–12.266*). The differential diagnosis includes condyloma acuminatum and noninvasive condylomatous carcinoma (see *Table 12.3*). Condyloma acuminatum is smaller and affects younger patients, and lesions are usually multiple, affecting not only the squamous epithelium of penile mucosal epithelial compartments but also the outer skin of the foreskin and shaft. Giant condyloma affects older

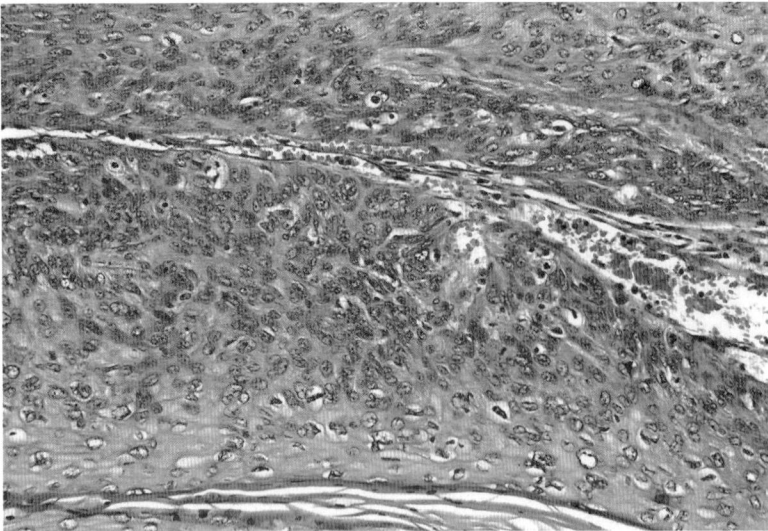

Fig. 12.266
Giant condyloma: with koilocytosis, easily recognized in the upper layers, and mild atypia at the base of the papillae ('atypical condyloma').

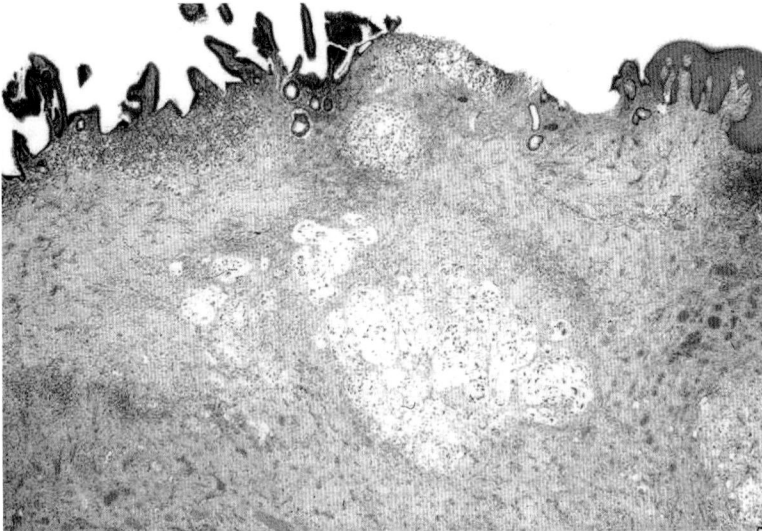

Fig. 12.267
Cloacogenic vulval adenocarcinoma: scanning view showing vulval squamous epithelium on the far right. Colonic epithelium is present on the left. Mucus-secreting carcinoma extends throughout the underlying connective tissue.

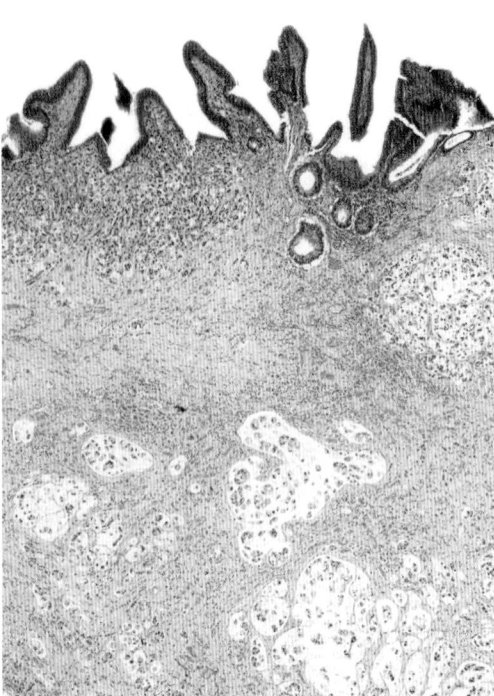

Fig. 12.268
Cloacogenic vulval adenocarcinoma: the tumor is associated with abundant mucin secretion forming large lakes.

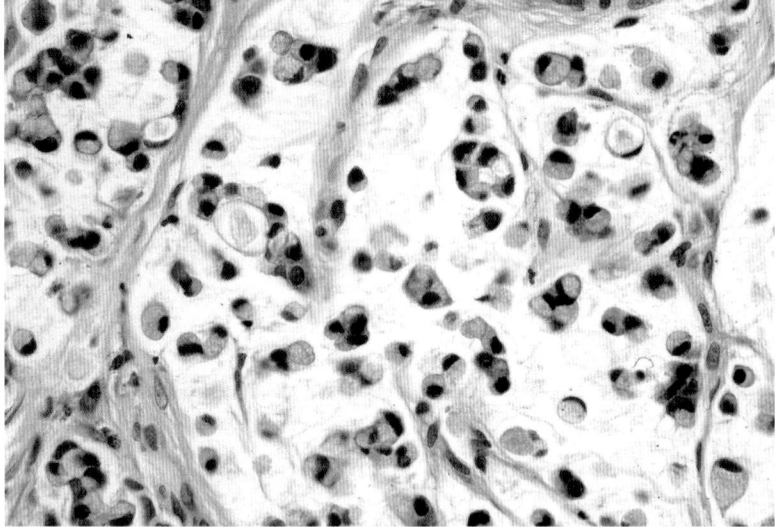

Fig. 12.269
Cloacogenic vulval adenocarcinoma: close-up view showing the tumor cells distended by intracytoplasmic mucin.

patients, is usually bulky and unicentric. The distinction of giant condyloma from well-differentiated condylomatous carcinoma may be difficult. Identification of low-risk HPV in giant condyloma and HPV-16 in condylomatous carcinomas may aid in the differential diagnosis.

Cloacogenic carcinoma

This rare tumor presents in middle-aged women as a superficial ulcerated adenocarcinoma composed of colonic-type glands arising in direct continuity with vulval surface epithelium (Figs 12.267–12.269).[1-4] It is independent of the perivulval glands and, by definition, direct extension or metastasis from an underlying large intestinal or visceral adenocarcinoma has been excluded. The clinical features are not distinctive but tumors may present as lesions simulating Bartholin gland infection.[5] In a single case, the neoplastic glands also contained Paneth cells.[6] The origin of this tumor is not known, but it is thought most probably to arise from an area of gastrointestinal metaplasia or from heterotopic intestinal tissue (Fig. 12.270). Vulval cloacogenic carcinoma should not be confused with the similarly named tumor of the anal canal. Tumor cells are positive for CK7 and CK20 and negative for estrogen and progesterone receptors.[7]

Tumors of anogenital mammary-like glands

The anogenital glands seen in the vulva and scrotum were first described by van der Putte, having previously been thought to be ectopic mammary tissue.[1,2] They are most commonly found in the interlabial sulci and perineum. Histologically, they have features similar to mammary ducts and often show apocrine change. Their immunohistochemical profile is similar to that of normal breast tissue.[3] Furthermore some molecular alterations in benign and malignant anogenital mammary-like glands are similar to the counterparts presenting on breast tissue.[4-6]

Anogenital mammary-like glands can undergo neoplastic change identical to those seen in many breast tumors both benign (including hamartomas) and malignant. So far, a wide range of tumors have been described including hidradenoma papilliferum (equivalent to breast intraductal papilloma), lactating adenoma, tubular adenoma, fibroadenoma, juvenile-type

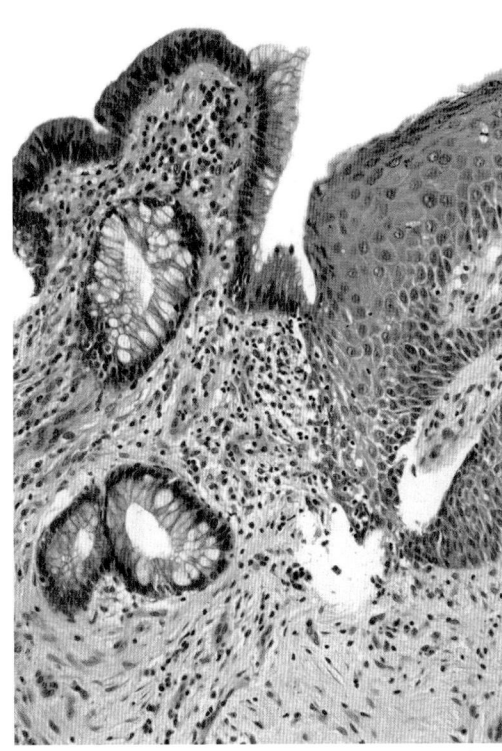

Fig. 12.270
Cloacogenic vulval
adenocarcinoma:
high-power view of
the junction between
squamous and colonic
epithelium.

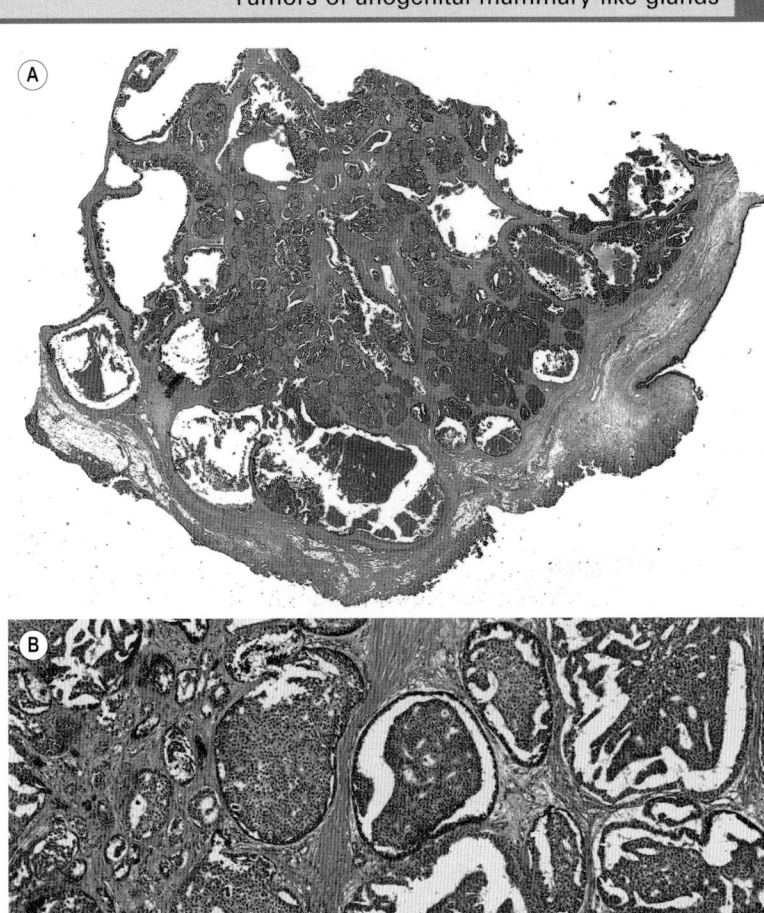

Fig. 12.271
(**A**, **B**). Adenocarcinoma of anogenital mammary-type glands: low- and high-power views highlighting the similarities to breast adenocarcinoma. By courtesy of Dr Catherine Stefanato, St John's Institute of Dermatology, London, UK.

fibroadenoma, benign and low-grade (but not malignant) phyllodes tumor, mammary type in situ and invasive carcinoma (*Fig. 12.271A* and *B*), mammary type mixed ductal and lobular invasive carcinoma, mammary type tubulolobular carcinoma, and mucinous (colloidal) carcinoma and adenoid cystic carcinoma.[7–13] Most of these neoplasms except hidradenoma papilliferum are very rare. Hyperplastic changes identical to those seen in breast lesions may also be identified. An unusual proliferative lesion of anogenital glands in a single patient with Cowden syndrome has been described.[14] Pseudoangiomatous stromal hyperplasia has also been described in the setting of other lesions.[15]

Papillary hidradenoma (hidradenoma papilliferum)

Clinical features

Papillary hidradenoma (hidradenoma papilliferum) occurs almost exclusively in females.[1,2] A single example of a perianal variant has been described in a male.[3] The age range is wide, with tumors presenting in adult females with a predilection for the fifth and sixth decades of life.

Papillary hidradenoma typically presents as a small (1–2 cm diameter) solitary asymptomatic nodule in a vulval, perineal, or perianal location.[4,5] Rare lesions attain a large size.[6] Lesions may present with bleeding or pruritus and rarely ulcerated. Most often it affects the labium majus, but on occasion it arises on the lateral aspect of the labium minus, fourchette, or clitoris (*Fig. 12.272*), and is seen at the sites of anogenital mammary-like glands.[5,7] Perianal lesions are very uncommon.[8] Rarely, tumors are multiple and such cases tend to be located on the same side of the vulva.[1] Very rarely, lesions have been described on the nipple, eyelid, and external auditory canal.[9,10]

Pathogenesis and histologic features

This tumor is likely to be derived from anogenital mammary-like glands, and although the name mammary-like gland adenoma of the vulva has been proposed this has not been universally accepted.[4] The lesion is the equivalent of mammary intraductal papilloma.[11,12] The close relationship between tumors is further given support by a similar immunohistochemical profile and mutations in both neoplasms.[11,13,14] The latter include PIK3CA and AKT1 mutations.[13,14]

The epidermis may be normal, acanthotic, or ulcerated. A connection to the epidermis, and less commonly to the infundibulae of hair follicles, may be seen. In such cases, tumors resemble syringocystadenoma papilliferum, even displaying prominent plasma cells in the stroma.[11,15] The tumor forms a fairly well-demarcated nodule in the dermis or lamina propria and sometimes shows foci of continuity with the overlying epithelium. The growth pattern consists of a mixture of tubular, papillary, and solid areas.[4] It is composed of epithelium-covered papillary processes projecting into cystic spaces (*Fig. 12.273*). Cystic change, sometimes prominent, is seen in a small percentage of cases The epithelial lining is typically double layered, comprising outer small myoepithelial cells with oval hyperchromatic nuclei and inner tall columnar cells with eosinophilic cytoplasm, often manifesting decapitation secretion, indicating apocrine lineage (*Figs 12.274* and *12.275*). Cytological atypia is mild or absent. Squamous and mucinous metaplasia are very rarely identified.[11] Oxyphilic metaplasia of tumor cells is common, and tumor cells display more cytological atypia and a single prominent nucleolus.[16] Tumor cells are epithelial and myoepithelial, and the latter can display clear cell change.[4] Clear cell change in epithelial cells (lamprocytes) is very rare.[11] Occasionally, the lining is only one cell thick (columnar). Diastase-resistant, PAS-positive intracytoplasmic granules are usually present. The occasional finding of a normal mitotic figure has no sinister implication. The larger villi have a fibrous core in which occasional ductal structures may be identified. Often, the fibrous tissue surrounding the tumor is compressed to form a pseudocapsule. Some tumors have a pattern

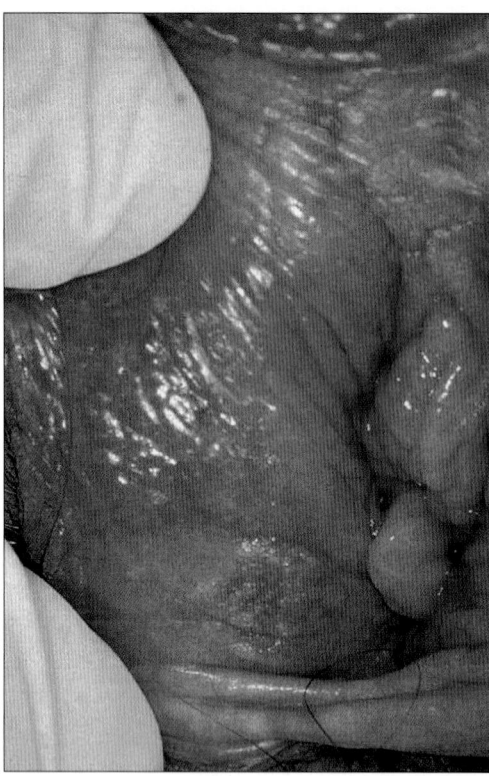

Fig. 12.272
Papillary hidradenoma: the lesion presents as a warty nodule. By courtesy of the Institute of Dermatology, London, UK.

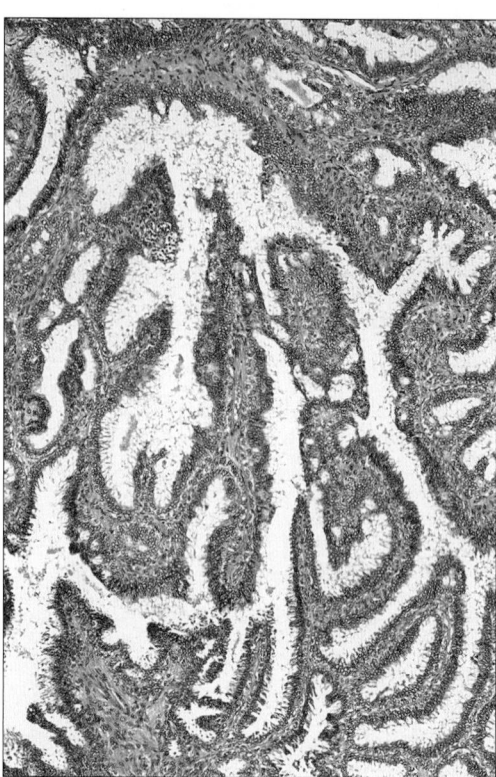

Fig. 12.274
Papillary hidradenoma: the papillae have a fibrovascular core.

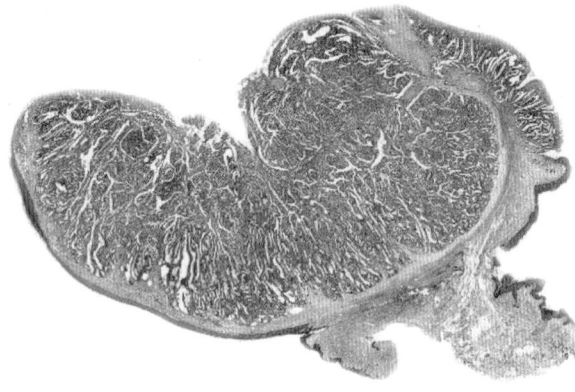

Fig. 12.273
Papillary hidradenoma: whole mount preparation showing sharply circumscribed papillary tumor.

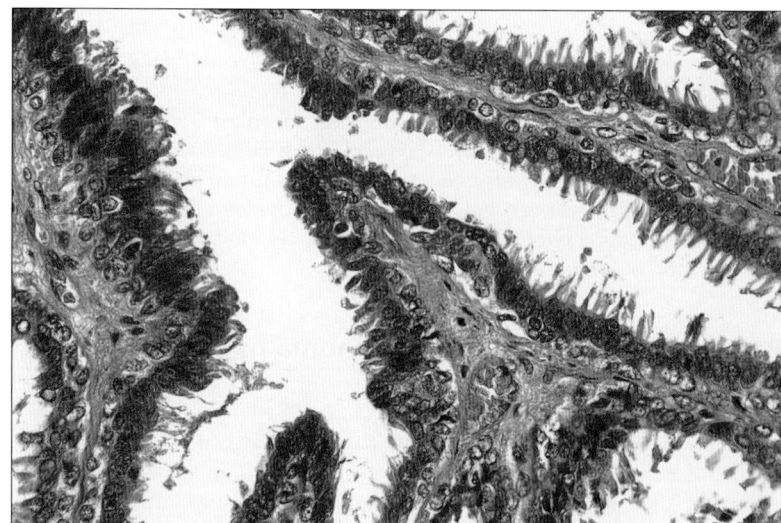

Fig. 12.275
Papillary hidradenoma: the papillae are covered by a double layer of epithelial cells, the inner showing typical decapitation secretion.

identical to those of breast tumors including erosive adenomatosis, sclerosing adenosis, and ductal hyperplasia.[4] An inflammatory cell component is not a significant feature except in ulcerated lesions and those connected to the overlying epithelium, but foamy histiocytes can be seen. In the surrounding stroma, residual anogenital mammary-like glands are found and may display hyperplasia.[11]

Very rarely, coexistence with extramammary Paget is noted.[11] Exceptionally rarely, a malignant variant has been reported.[16–18] The diagnosis of a handful of invasive cases reported in the literature including one described as an adenosquamous carcinoma, has been challenged and so far only cases of carcinoma in situ developing within the tumors have been accepted as genuine. In these cases, involved glands are associated with an intact layer of pericytes. In a single case, association with HPV16 was reported.

HPV has only occasionally been detected in this tumor, but this is not likely to have an etiological link.[19]

Fibroadenoma and phyllodes tumor

Clinical features

Genital fibroadenoma and phyllodes tumor are identical to those tumors occurring in breast tissue but in contrast to the latter, their incidence is very low.[1–6] The vast majority present in females, with only one case reported in the perianal skin of a male.[7] Most tumors are solitary and present as an asymptomatic, slowly growing nodular lesion with variable size, usually several centimeters. The vulva is the most common site with rare lesions developing in the perineum, perianal skin, or pubis. Multiple and bilateral lesions are vanishingly rare as is the occurrence of simultaneous lesions involving the breast and genital skin. Local recurrence may be seen in phyllodes tumor.

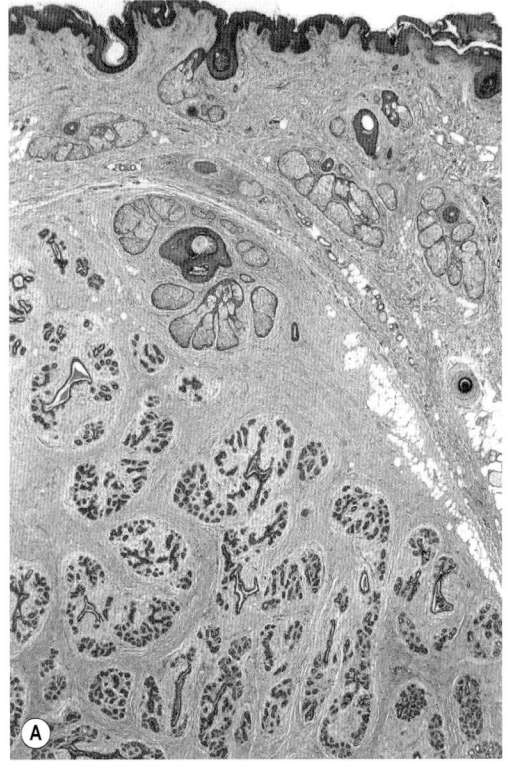

Fig. 12.276
(**A**, **B**) Fibroadenoma of anogenital mammary-type glands: prominent glandular and stromal elements identical to lesions seen in the breast.

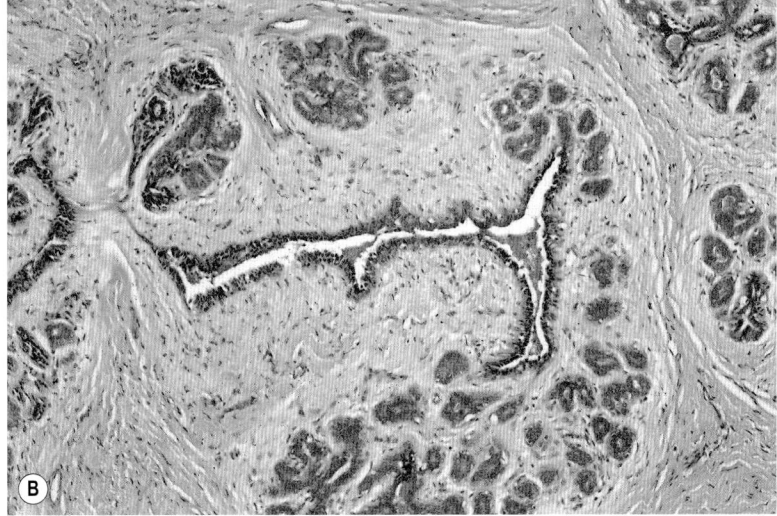

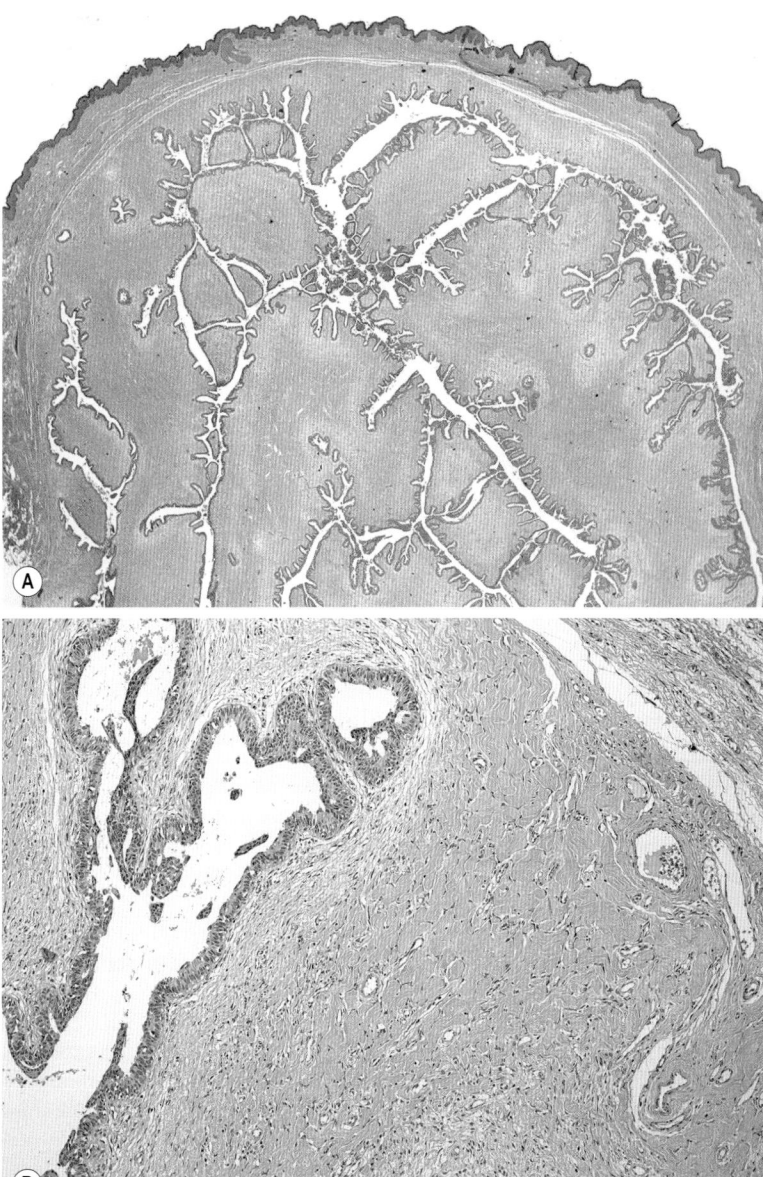

Fig. 12.277
(**A**, **B**) Pseudoangiomatous stromal hyperplasia in the setting of a phyllodes tumor. (**A**) Low magnification of a phyllodes tumor arising from the anogenital mammary-type glands. (**B**) Stromal changes with slit-like spaces lined by spindle-shaped cells and closely mimicking vascular spaces. Courtesy of Dr Dmitry Kazakov, Pilsen, Czech Republic.

Pathogenesis and histologic features

Mutations in *MEK* have been found in one vulvar fibroadenoma, and alterations in *ABL1* and *TP53* have been described in one case of low-grade phyllodes tumor.[8]

Histologically, tumors are fibroepithelial lesions identical to those described in the breast. Fibroadenomas are well-circumscribed and consist of varying proportions of epithelial and stromal elements (*Fig. 12.276A* and *B*). The stroma is hypocellular and loose, and consists of bland spindle-shaped cells with very low or no mitotic activity. In cases with prominent stroma, there is narrowing of the glandular spaces with a slit-like appearance (intra-canalicular pattern). In areas where the stroma surrounds round ducts, the pattern is known as pericanalicular. Fibrocystic changes may be seen. The epithelial glandular cells may show decapitation secretion and squamous metaplasia is exceptional.[1,2] Fatty and myoid metaplasia may be rarely observed. Epithelial cells are positive for keratins and estrogen and progesterone receptors, myoepithelial cells are focally positive for S100 and positive for SMA and calponin, and stromal cells are positive for

CD34 and focally positive for SMA.[1,2] In very rare cases, features may be those of a mammary-type juvenile fibroadenoma or a lactating adenoma.[1,2] Pseudoangiomatous stromal hyperplasia and exceptionally giant cells may also be seen.[1,2,9] In pseudoangiomatous hyperplasia, there is a proliferation of bland spindle-shaped cells that appear to be lining slit-like spaces mimicking vascular channels (*Fig. 12.277A* and *B*). Distinction from a low-grade angiosarcoma may be difficult, but in the former, there is cytological atypia, mitotic activity, and multilayering, and cells are positive for vascular markers. A single case of a tumor combining features of fibroadenoma, hidradenoma papilliferum, and pseudoangiomatous stromal hyperplasia has been reported.[10] Phyllodes tumors are circumscribed with a hypercellular stroma that tends to be more pronounced around glandular structures (*Fig. 12.278*). The stroma displays leaf-like projections into the glandular structures. The stroma in reported cases of genital phyllodes tumor has been benign or low grade.[1,2] Mitotic activity is low. Pseudoangiomatous stromal hyperplasia may be seen.[9]

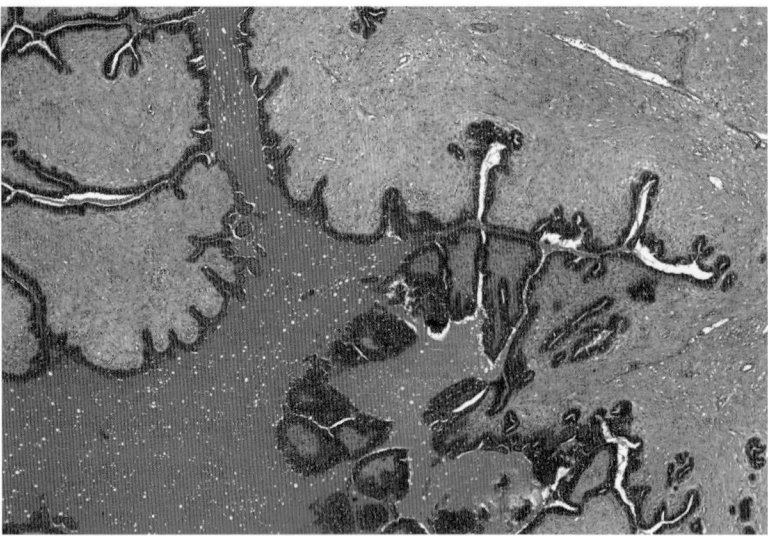

Fig. 12.278
Phyllodes tumor: fibroepithelial tumor with a more cellular stroma protruding with a leaf-like pattern into the glandular spaces.

Benign tumors of Bartholin gland

Clinical features

Benign tumors of the Bartholin gland are very rare and the vast majority are nodular hyperplasias.[1] They occur mainly in young women, with an average age of 36 years.[2] Adenomas and adenomyomas are very rare.[1,3,4] They all present as a small asymptomatic mass on the posterolateral aspect of the vulva and are usually diagnosed clinically as a cyst. Bilateral lesions are very rare.[5] Both hyperplasia and adenomas may be associated with pain.[5,6]

Histologic features

Nodular hyperplasia is well circumscribed and lobular with preservation of the normal duct–acinar relationship.[1] Focal inflammation and squamous metaplasia of the ducts is commonly seen. Dilated ducts and sometimes ruptured ducts with extravasated mucin can be noted.[7] Adenomas are well circumscribed and composed of small- to medium-sized glands with focal papillary projections and lined by columnar, mucin-producing cells with no cytological atypia and very rare mitotic figures. Tubules and acini proliferate in a haphazard way in contrast to the hyperplasias, where the normal architecture is preserved.[1] In one case of hyperplasia, clonality was demonstrated, suggesting that the process may be neoplastic rather than reactive.[7]

A single case of a papilloma arising from the duct of a Bartholin cyst has been reported.[8]

Adenoma of minor vestibular glands

Clinical features

Adenoma of minor vestibular glands (paravestibular tumor) is exceedingly rare and occurs in the vulvar vestibule.[1–3] It is likely that it represents a hyperplasia rather than a true neoplasm. The lesion is very small and usually represents an incidental finding in a biopsy taken for another reason.

Histologic features

Histologically, it consists of a small nodular aggregate of mucin-secreting glands lined by columnar cells.

Bartholin gland carcinoma

Clinical features

This rare tumor accounts for approximately 5% of vulval neoplasms.[1,2] It presents as a painless, hard, deep subcutaneous nodule, which, as it expands, becomes fixed and painful. The lesion measures from 1 cm to several centimeters and is located in the posterior aspect of the labium majus. It often invades deeply into fat, muscle, or bone and may be associated with a Bartholin gland abscess. The diagnosis is often delayed because of the latter association. Adult and elderly women are usually affected. Exceptional cases have been described during pregnancy.[3]

It is often difficult to decide when a tumor has originated from Bartholin gland, and particular attention should be paid to exclude a metastasis from elsewhere. Distinction from a sweat gland carcinoma can also be a diagnostic problem. Rarely, the tumor is associated with extramammary Paget disease.[4] In recent years, a consistent association has been found between these tumors and HPV-16.[5,6] Recurrence rates vary and have been reported to be as high as 54%.[7] Up to 40% of patients present with inguinofemoral metastases. The survival rates are similar to those with other types of vulval carcinoma.[1] Adenoid cystic carcinoma of Bartholin gland has a high local recurrence rate and occasionally presents with metastatic disease.[8]

Histologic features

About 40% of Bartholin gland carcinomas are adenocarcinomas.[3] A further 40% are SCCs and 15% are adenoid cystic carcinomas. The remainder are transitional, adenosquamous, or anaplastic carcinomas.[9] A case of lymphoepithelioma-like carcinoma and two low-grade epithelial–myoepithelial carcinoma of the Bartholin gland have been documented.[10,11] A case of high-grade squamous intraepithelial neoplasia in a Bartholin cyst has also been reported.[12]

Exceptional cases of neuroendocrine carcinoma have also been described.[13] Malignant mixed tumor very rarely originates from Bartholin glands.[14] A neoplasm can only be accepted as originating from the gland if there is continuity with it. Adenocarcinomas may be mucinous or papillary. Cytogenetic analysis of a single case of adenoid cystic carcinoma of Bartholin gland revealed complex chromosomal abnormalities involving chromosomes 1, 4, 6, 11, 14 and 22.[15]

Other vulval adnexal neoplasms

Adnexal neoplasms both benign and malignant that occur elsewhere in the skin may rarely present in vulval skin. They are identical to the lesions presenting elsewhere and will not be described in detail. These tumors include syringoma (usually of the eruptive type), poroma, spiradenoma, cylindroma, pilomatricoma, trichoepithelioma, sebaceoma, spiradenocarcinoma, apocrine carcinoma, and sebaceous carcinoma.[1]

Basal cell carcinoma

Clinical features

Basal cell carcinoma can arise on the anogenital skin (*Figs 12.279* and *12.280*). Prior genital irradiation for cancer or ringworm is a theoretical risk factor that appertains to basal cell carcinoma at other sites. Vulval and penile tumors are seen mainly in elderly patients.[1,2] They usually present as an eroded papule or plaque, which may be pigmented. Less commonly, the tumor forms a nodule or an ulcer. Symptoms vary from discomfort to pruritus.[3,4] Neoplasms occur most frequently on the labia majora, but can occur on the perianal skin in both sexes.[1] They are sometimes multiple.[5] Tumors can rarely occur in the context of Gorlin syndrome.[6] Inadequate excision accounts for a high recurrence rate and exceptional metastases to regional lymph nodes.[7,8] Mohs surgery is often recommended to ensure adequate local excision and acceptable cosmetic results.[9]

Histologic features

Histologically, the appearances are identical to basal cell carcinomas occurring elsewhere. There has been one case report of the variant fibroepithelioma of Pinkus affecting the base of the penis.[10] The patchy expression of p16 in vulval basal cell carcinomas can help to distinguish them from a basaloid SCC, which shows diffuse staining.[11]

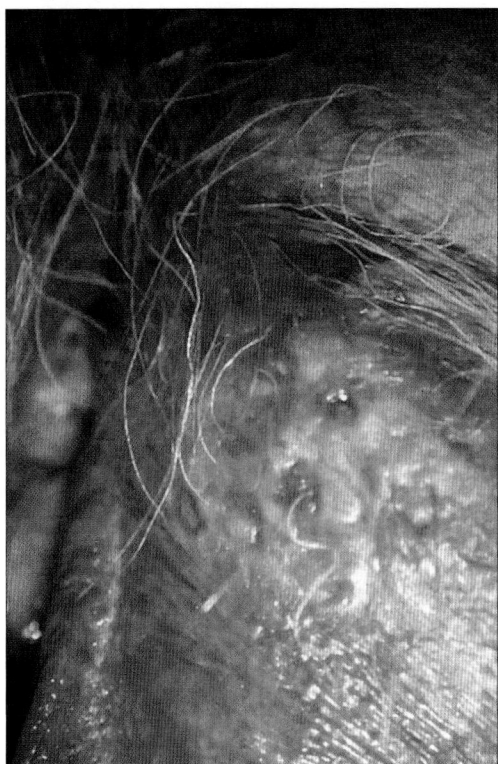

Fig. 12.279
Vulval basal cell carcinoma: erythematous, keratotic plaque on left labium majus. By courtesy of the Institute of Dermatology, London, UK.

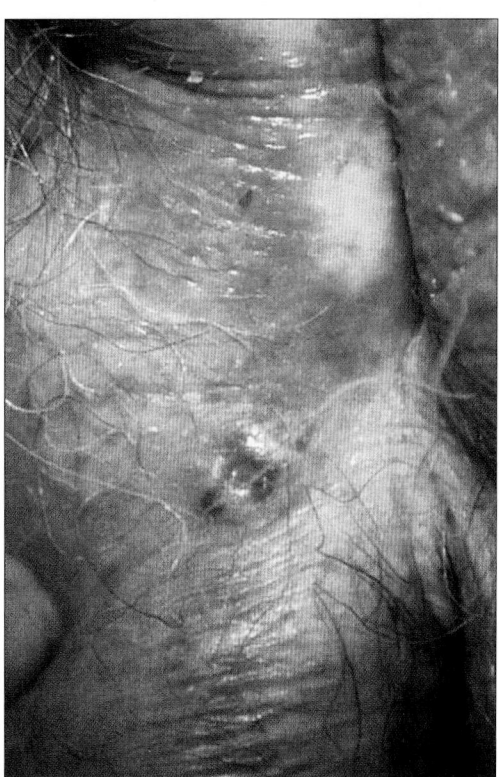

Fig. 12.280
Perianal basal cell carcinoma: ulcerated perianal nodule with a pearly white rolled border. By courtesy of the Institute of Dermatology, London, UK.

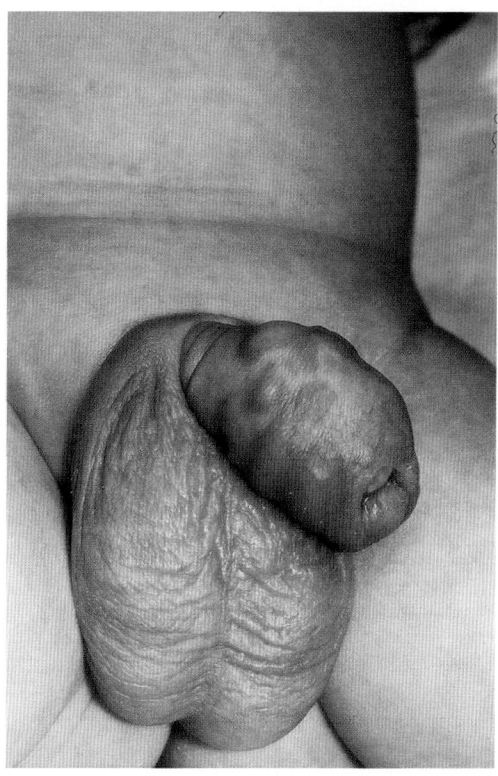

Fig. 12.281
Juvenile xanthogranuloma: lesions are present on the lateral shaft of the penis. Courtesy of R. Haufmann, Ulm, Germany. Reproduced with permission from Haufmann R.E., Bachor, R. Juvenile xanthogranuloma of the penis. J Urol. 1993:150:456–457. From Bunker C. Male Genital Skin Disease. Saunders Ltd./Elsevier 2004.

Metastatic tumors

The anogenital skin is a rare site for metastatic tumors.[1-4] Those that are described are usually from a nearby primary site; for example, vulval metastases may be derived from vaginal, cervical, endometrial, ovarian, renal cell carcinoma, and choriocarcinoma. A large study of metastatic vulval tumors found that about 46.9% arise from gynecological and 43.9% from nongynecological primary tumors. The rest of the tumors were metastases from an unknown primary.[4] Vulval metastases usually present as a mass or, less commonly, with pain or ulceration.[4] Penile metastases most often arise from the prostate, colon, bladder, and kidney. Rarely, they derive from elsewhere including pulmonary carcinoma, SCC of the tongue and cutaneous melanoma.[5] The metastases are most commonly sited on the labia majora or periclitorally and in the corpus cavernosum of the penis. Tumor thrombi are often found in the erectile tissue of the penis, predominantly in the corpora cavernosa.[5] Penile metastasis may result in priapism.[6] They usually represent an ominous sign.[5] Metastases may also arise in an episiotomy scar. An exceptional metastasis to a Bartholin gland has been reported.[7,8]

Lymphoma and leukemia

Although lymphoma is the most frequent secondary tumor of the testis, it is rare in other parts of the urogenital tract, and few case reports exist.[1,2] Primary anal lymphomas are also extremely rare and the cases described have been anorectal, mainly of the plasmablastic variant, associated with EBV and AIDS.[3]

Dehner and Smith included two cases of primary lymphoma in their series of soft tissue tumors of the penis, both presenting as painless subcutaneous nodules without evidence of systemic lymphoma.[4] One case presented with painless priapism and erythematous nodular ulceration of the shaft of the penis, another case with progressive swelling of the glans penis, and another with chronic penile ulceration.[5,6]

Doll and Diaz-Arias described a fungating nodular tumor of the scrotum in an HIV-negative homosexual that was shown to be immunoblastic T-cell lymphoma.[7]

Ulceration of the penis due to leukemic infiltration secondary to chronic lymphocytic leukemia has been reported.[8,9] Scrotal ulceration due to leukemia cutis in acute myelogenous leukemia has also occurred.[10,11] Lymphoma may present with perianal ulceration abscess and suppuration.[12] Perianal infiltration, ulceration, or abscess occurs in 5% of hematological malignancies.[13]

The histopathology of genital lymphomas is identical to that occurring elsewhere in the skin. The most commonly reported anogenital B-cell lymphoma is of the diffuse large cell type.

Non-Hodgkin and Hodgkin lymphomas may rarely involve the vulva.[14,15] A myeloid sarcoma of the vulva has been reported as the presenting feature of acute myeloid leukemia.[16]

Juvenile xanthogranuloma

This lesion usually affects the head and trunk but can also involve the genitalia (*Fig. 12.281*).[1] Multifocal penile presentation has been documented,[2] as well as a solitary perineal papule[3] and a scrotal swelling.[4] Clinicopathologically identical solitary lesions may be seen in adults.[5] The histology is of lipid-laden histiocytes and giant cells, negative for CD1 and langerin, which are found in Langerhans cell histiocytosis. S100 may be positive in about 25% of cases. Juvenile xanthogranuloma is not associated with abnormal lipids but there may be a relationship with urticaria pigmentosa, diabetes mellitus, neurofibromatosis, cytomegalovirus infection, and leukemia.

A case of an isolated clitoral lesion is described.[6]

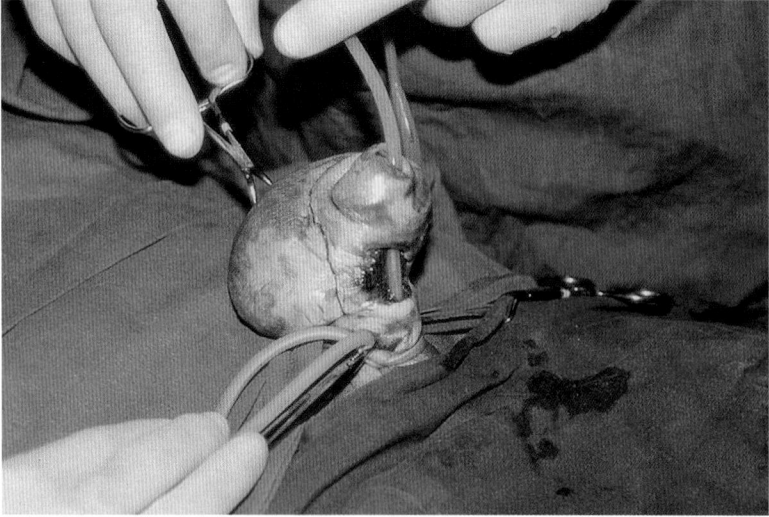

Fig. 12.282
Chronic edema simulating a keloid: note the dorsal proximal swelling and ventral urethral fistula. Courtesy of Dr Rameshwar Bang, Safat, Kuwait. Reproduced from Bang R.L. Penile edema induced by continuous condom catheter use and mimicking keloid scar. Scand J Urol Nephrol 1994;28:333–5. From Bunker C. Male Genital Skin Disease. Saunders Ltd./Elsevier 2004.

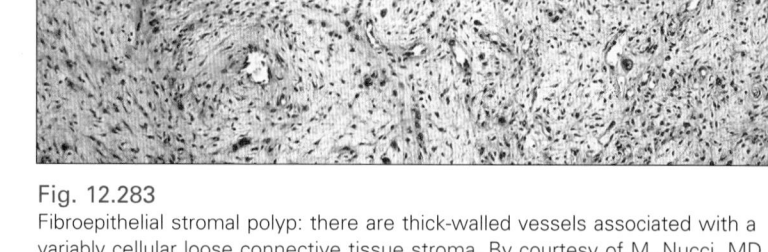

Fig. 12.283
Fibroepithelial stromal polyp: there are thick-walled vessels associated with a variably cellular loose connective tissue stroma. By courtesy of M. Nucci, MD, Brigham and Women's Hospital and Harvard Medical School, Boston, USA.

Langerhans cell histiocytosis

This condition is regarded as an abnormality of immune function. It usually affects the genital area as part of disseminated disease but can rarely appear at this site alone.[1–3] Females are affected much more often than males, and presentation can occur at any age from infancy to old age. Anogenital lesions may present as ulcers, erosions, papules, nodules, or plaques. Involvement of the penis is very rare.[4] Presentation as a fleshy papule on the dorsal penis[5] and primary penile ulceration[6] have been reported.

In infants, the diaper area may be affected, typically with a seborrheic-like dermatitis or purpuric papules. There are isolated reports of Langerhans cell histiocytosis occurring with LS.[7,8]

Soft tissue tumors

Keloid

It has been asserted that the skin of the penis never forms keloid,[1,2] but it has been reported after circumcision[3] and other forms of trauma[4,5] and may be more common than suspected.[6] Keloid has been simulated on the dorsum of the penis (Fig. 12.282) by chronic edema caused by a condom catheter.[7]

Fibroepithelial stromal polyp

Clinical features

Fibroepithelial stromal polyp (mesodermal stromal polyp, pseudosarcoma botryoides), which presents in women of reproductive age, predominantly affects the vagina (usually the lower third) and, less commonly, the vulva.[1–9] Involvement of the cervix is rare.[2] Presentation in the very young (including a congenital lesion) or the elderly is uncommon.[10,11] Interestingly, about one-third of patients are pregnant, suggesting that hormonal influences play a significant role in the pathogenesis of these tumors.[5] Lesions can be single or, more rarely, multiple and bilateral,[12] the latter occurrence being most frequently seen in pregnancy. Tumors are usually less than 5 cm in diameter and are often pedunculated. Giant lesions are exceptional,[13,14] but lesions up to 18 cm have been reported.[15] Local recurrence may occur following incomplete excision but the behavior is benign.

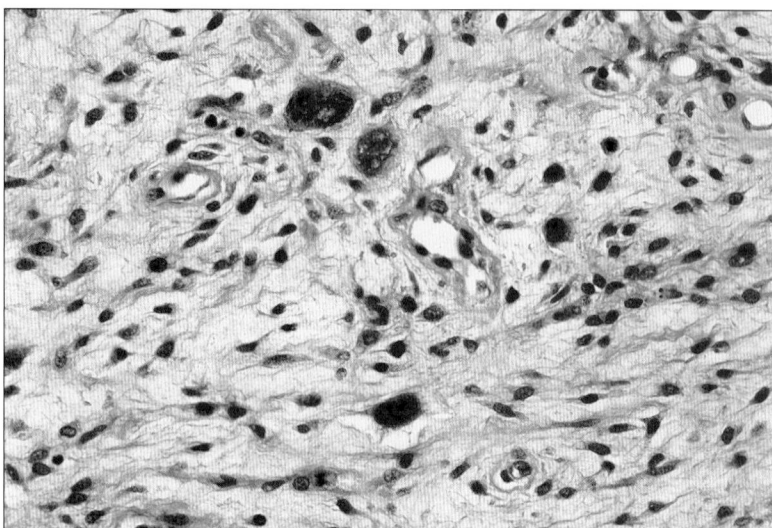

Fig. 12.284
Fibroepithelial stromal polyp: in this field, there is striking nuclear atypia. By courtesy of M. Nucci, MD, Brigham and Women's Hospital and Harvard Medical School, Boston, USA.

Histologic features

Low-power examination reveals a polypoid and often pedunculated lesion with fibrovascular stroma and showing variable cellularity. Small to medium-sized blood vessels with thick walls are conspicuous (Fig. 12.283). Hypocellular tumors contain abundant collagen and only scattered spindle-shaped or stellate cells displaying mild focal or no cytological atypia and occasional to frequent multinucleated cells. With increasingly cellular tumors, there is more prominent cytological atypia and mitotic figures may be conspicuous (Figs 12.284 and 12.285).[8,9,16]

Occasional atypical forms may be seen. Such variants are more frequent in pregnant patients. Multinucleated tumor cells become more prominent with a tendency to concentrate in the stroma adjacent to the epithelium. The cellularity is more prominent toward the center of the lesion.[8] Small collections of mononuclear inflammatory cells are also commonly present.

Tumor cells are positive for desmin, vimentin, and estrogen and progesterone receptors.[9,17,18] Positivity for actin is rare and macrophage markers are negative.[12]

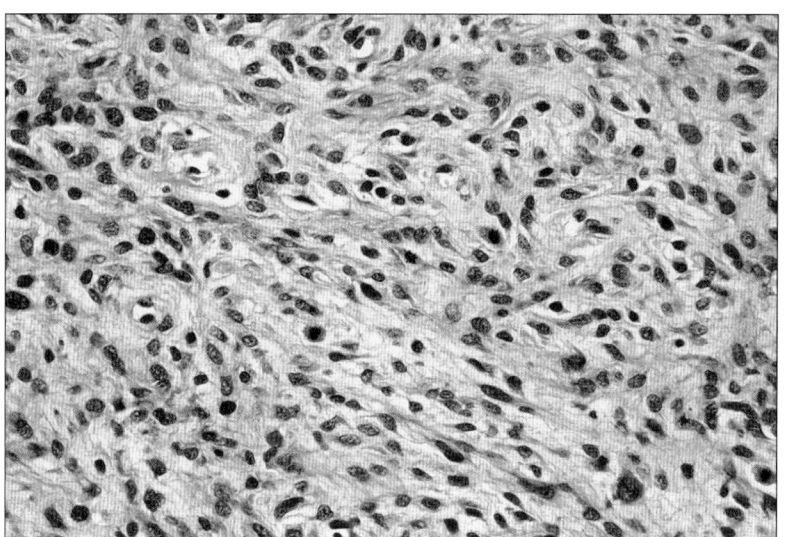

Fig. 12.285
Fibroepithelial stromal polyp: the presence of multiple mitoses as shown in this field can be a source of concern to the unwary. By courtesy of M. Nucci, MD, Brigham and Women's Hospital and Harvard Medical School, Boston, USA.

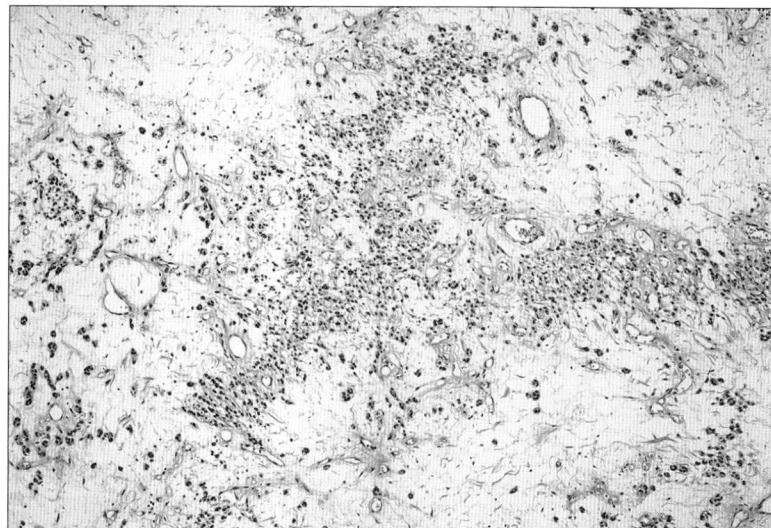

Fig. 12.286
Angiomyofibroblastoma: low-power view showing a richly vascular tumor. In this example, there is a strikingly myxoid stroma. By courtesy of M. Nucci, MD, and C.D.M. Fletcher, MD, Brigham and Women's Hospital and Harvard Medical School, Boston, USA.

Ultrastructural studies show cells with features of fibroblasts and myofibroblasts.[18,19]

Differential diagnosis

The main differential diagnosis, particularly for lesions presenting in the vagina, is sarcoma botryoides. The latter lesion, by contrast, tends to occur at a much younger age, lacks a cambium layer, displays invasion of the epithelium by tumor cells, and is composed of small, undifferentiated tumor cells.[20] Focal myogenin expression occurs uncommonly in fibroepithelial polyps and may result in misdiagnosis such as sarcoma botryoides.[21]

Lymphedematous fibroepithelial polyp of the glans penis and prepuce

Clinical features

Only a handful of cases of this distinctive entity have been reported.[1] Patients developed polypoid or cauliflower-like, usually long-standing, lesions on the glans penis or prepuce associated with chronic catheter use and phimosis. All reported cases are in adults with a median age of 40 years. There may be local recurrences.

Histologic features

Lesions are polypoid with a hyperplastic epidermis and an edematous stroma with telangiectasia and sometimes focal proliferation of vascular channels. In the background, there are mono- or multinucleated stromal cells and scattered mononuclear inflammatory cells, mainly lymphocytes. The stromal cells are focally positive for actin and desmin.

Prepubertal vulval fibroma

Clinical features

This distinctive vulval lesion has been also described as 'childhood asymmetric labium majus enlargement'.[1,2] Lesions involve the labium majus and present as a unilateral and exceptionally bilateral swelling in girls between the ages of 3 and 13 years. A similar case in a postmenopausal patient has been documented.[3]

Histologic features

The lesion is poorly circumscribed, lies within the dermis and subcutis, and consists of a poorly cellular mass with abundant collagen, edema, and focal myxoid change. The cells within the tumor are positive for CD34.

Angiomyofibroblastoma

Clinical features

This is a distinctive benign soft tissue tumor of the external genitalia and perineum that must be distinguished from aggressive angiomyxoma (see below).[1–5] Rare cases have been documented in the vagina, fallopian tube, urethra, and retroperitoneum.[6–9] It most commonly affects females of reproductive age but has also been described in the elderly.[4] Cases in males are exceptional.[10] A tumor sharing many clinical and histologic features with angiomyofibroblastoma has been reported in the male genital tract as angiomyofibroblastoma-like tumor. These are described in the scrotum and groin, and histologically show hybrid features between angiomyofibroblastoma and spindle cell lipoma.[11,12]

Angiomyofibroblastoma presents as a slowly growing, small (usually less than 5 cm diameter), asymptomatic subcutaneous mass in the vulva or, less commonly, in the vagina. They are frequently confused with a Bartholin gland cyst. Polypoid morphology is rare.[13] but a pedunculated variant is recognized.[14] In males, tumors occur on the scrotum and rarely in the perineum, groin, and spermatic cord.[15–17] Their behavior is generally benign with little or no tendency for recurrence although a single malignant case has been reported.[18,19] This tumor consisted of typical areas of angiomyofibroblastoma with areas of high-grade myxoid sarcoma.

Histologic features

Angiomyofibroblastoma is well circumscribed and surrounded by a fibrous pseudocapsule. Scanning magnification reveals a tumor with hypo- and hypercellular areas and a prominent vascular network composed of thin-walled dilated vascular channels (*Figs 12.286* and *12.287*). The hypocellular areas display prominent myxoid change. Tumor cells are plump, epithelioid, or spindle-shaped with imperceptible to abundant pink cytoplasm, finely dispersed chromatin, and inconspicuous nucleoli. They tend to concentrate around the vascular channels. Multinucleated forms are frequent. Epithelioid cells with hyaline cytoplasm often have a plasmacytoid appearance. Cytological atypia is absent and mitotic figures are usually rare or exceptionally more prominent.[20] Scattered lymphocytes and mast cells are often present. Intratumoral mature adipocytes are present in a number of cases and may represent most of the tumor (lipomatous variant of angiomyofibroblastoma).[5,21,22] Degenerative nuclear hyperchromatism may sometimes be present.

The tumor cells are diffusely and strongly positive for desmin, but in only occasional cases are they positive for either smooth-muscle actin or

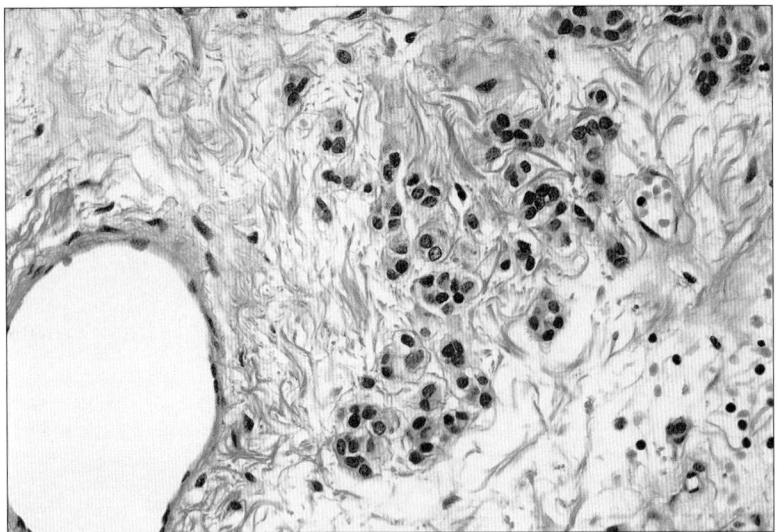

Fig. 12.287
Angiomyofibroblastoma: the tumor cells have eosinophilic cytoplasm and small nuclei. Nucleoli are not apparent. By courtesy of M. Nucci, MD, and C.D.M. Fletcher, MD, Brigham and Women's Hospital and Harvard Medical School, Boston, USA.

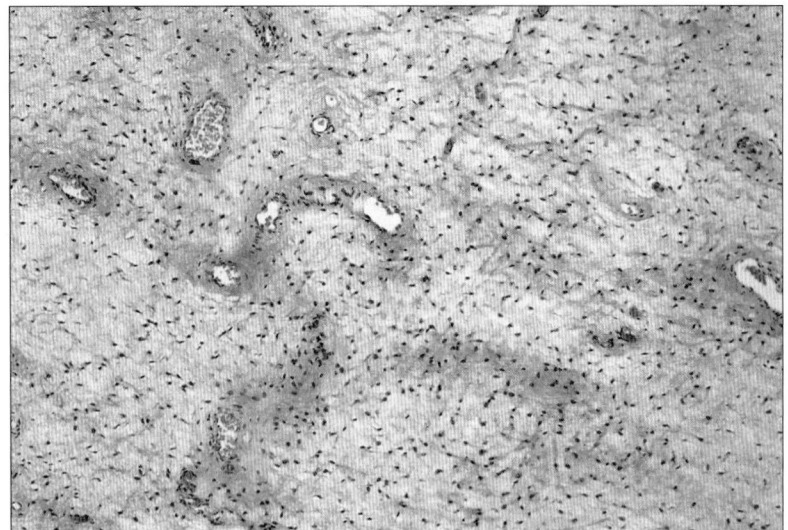

Fig. 12.288
Aggressive angiomyxoma: there are conspicuous blood vessels dispersed in a myxoid stroma. By courtesy of M. Nucci, MD, Brigham and Women's Hospital and Harvard Medical School, Boston, USA.

pan-muscle actin. Estrogen and progesterone receptor can be positive.[5] CD34 is only exceptionally positive. Epithelial markers, S100, and myoglobin are negative.

Ultrastructural studies suggest myofibroblastic differentiation.[1,3,4]

Differential diagnosis

Distinction from aggressive angiomyxoma is not usually difficult as the latter is larger (usually more than 5 cm), infiltrative, less cellular and vascular, and contains vessels with thicker walls. However, tumors with hybrid features of angiomyofibroblastoma and aggressive angiomyxoma have been reported.[23] Despite this, it is controversial whether both entities are related. Aggressive angiomyxoma has rearrangements of HMGA2, a member of the high-mobility-group protein family involved in alteration of chromatin structure and in the transcription of many genes. The latter feature has not been found in angiomyofibroblastoma.[24] The rare cases of hybrid tumors are best classified and treated as aggressive angiomyxoma, and, if possible, cytogenetic analysis or immunohistochemistry for HMGA2 should be performed. By immunohistochemistry, nuclear staining for this protein is seen in the majority of (but not all) aggressive angiomyxomas, and it tends to be negative in angiomyofibroblastoma.[25,26] However, it is important to take into consideration that there is not always correlation between the translocation and protein expression.

Aggressive angiomyxoma

Clinical features

This tumor presents as a slowly growing asymptomatic mass involving the pelvis and perineum.[1-6] Exceptionally, the lesion can present in the retroperitoneum.[7] It mainly affects females in the third or fourth decade of life, and it is exceptionally rare in children.[8,9] Less than 5% of cases occur in males, with predilection for the scrotum, perineum, or groin.[10-12] In males, lesions may mimic a hydrocele or an inguinal hernia.[13,14] Tumors are often 10 cm or more in diameter and can sometimes attain a very large size. Genitourinary and anorectal symptoms usually ensue due to external compression by the tumor. In females, lesions present mainly in the vulva or perineum followed by the vagina and the pelvis. Because of its extensive infiltrative growth, complete surgical excision is often difficult; local recurrences are therefore frequent and occur in up to 30% of cases. Metastasis are exceptional.[15,16]

Rare case reports have been published of tumors displaying prominent reduction in size after treatment with gonadotrophin releasing hormone agonists.[17,18]

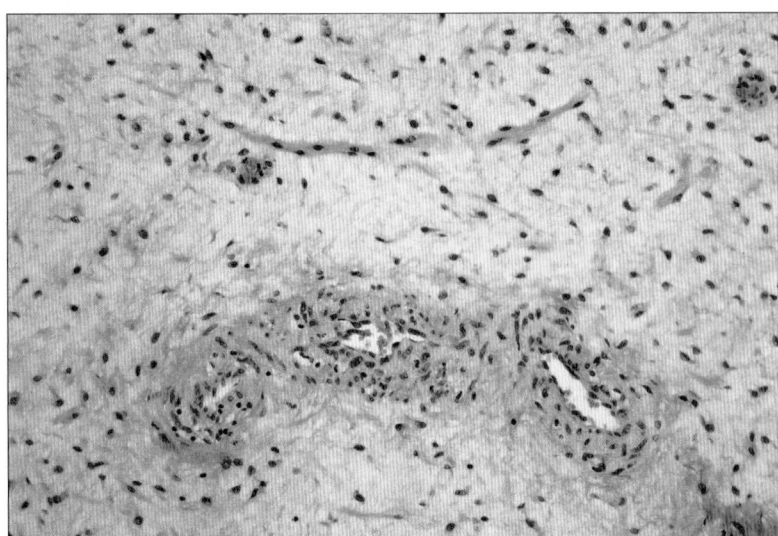

Fig. 12.289
Aggressive angiomyxoma: in this view, a smooth muscle bundle is evident in the upper field. By courtesy of M. Nucci, MD, Brigham and Women's Hospital and Harvard Medical School, Boston, USA.

Histologic features

Macroscopic examination reveals a soft, ill-defined, lobulated tumor with myxoid change. Microscopically, the lesion is infiltrative, with numerous small- and medium-sized blood vessels and a small number of tumor cells in a myxoid stroma (*Figs 12.288–12.290*). The blood vessels have thick walls, which are often hyalinized. Tumor cells are small, spindle-shaped, or stellate with ill-defined pale pink cytoplasm and vesicular nuclei. Cytological atypia is absent and mitotic figures are rare. Bundles of smooth muscle are frequently seen adjacent to blood vessels, a finding that can be highlighted by a desmin stain.[10] Residual normal structures including glands and smooth muscle are often entrapped by the tumor. Scattered mast cells are often present. Multinucleated giant cells similar to those found in stromal polyps are occasionally found. Some cases overlap histologically with angiomyofibroblastoma (see above).

Immunohistochemically, tumor cells are positive for smooth-muscle actin and desmin. Positivity for estrogen and progesterone receptors is also seen, and in men androgen receptors are positive.[5,7,19] Cytogenetic analysis of a number of aggressive angiomyxomas has often shown rearrangements of

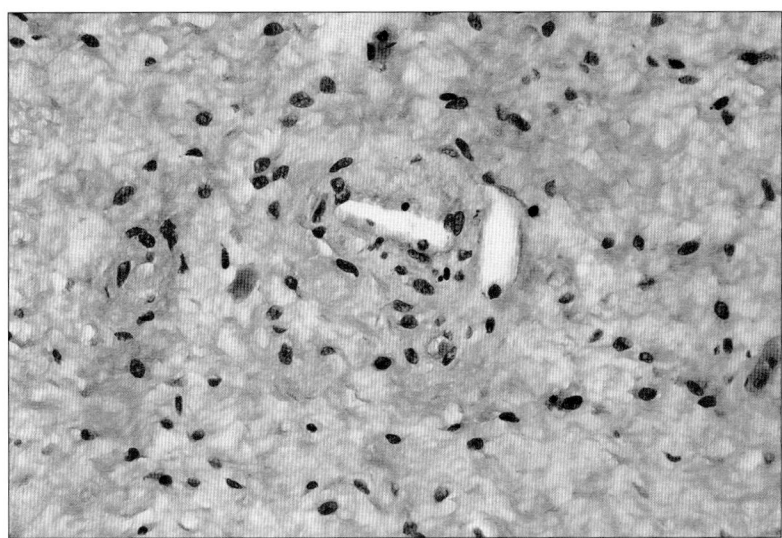

Fig. 12.290
Aggressive angiomyxoma: high-power view showing a uniform cellular population. There is no pleomorphism. By courtesy of M. Nucci, MD, Brigham and Women's Hospital and Harvard Medical School, Boston, USA.

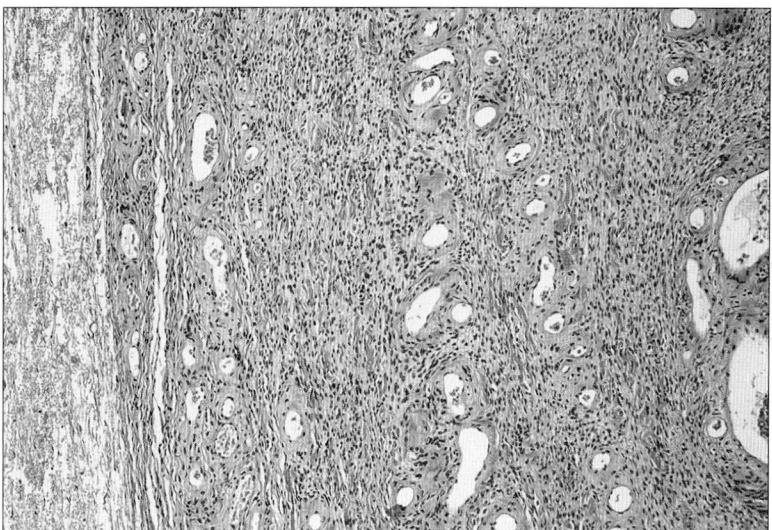

Fig. 12.291
Cellular angiofibroma: the tumor is characterized by thick-walled, hyalinized blood vessels associated with a densely cellular stroma. By courtesy of M. Nucci, MD, Brigham and Women's Hospital and Harvard Medical School, Boston, USA.

chromosome 12q13–15. The latter results in an aberrant expression of HMGA2 (a member of the high-mobility-group protein family previously known as HMGIC).[20–24] Interestingly, the area involved (12q14–15) is the same as that reported in a number of other tumors including leiomyoma and lipomatous neoplasms. Staining for HMGA2 may be useful to distinguish aggressive angiomyxoma from potential mimics, mainly angiomyofibroblastoma (see under the latter), but this marker, although sensitive, is not very specific.[25,26]

Electron microscopy shows cells with features of fibroblasts and myofibroblasts.[5]

Differential diagnosis

See angiomyofibroblastoma.

Chronic lymphedema of the vulva may give rise to a lymphedematous pseudotumor that can mimic aggressive angiomyxoma.[27] In the former, however, there is massive edema rather than myxoid change, and telangiectatic lymphatics focally surrounded by lymphocytes. Identical changes may be seen in massive localized lymphedema secondary to morbid obesity.

Cellular angiofibroma

Clinical features

Cellular angiofibroma is a distinctive tumor that occurs mainly on the vulva of middle-aged women,[1–7] and very rarely in the vagina.[6,7] Presentation in males is less common, with lesions occurring in the inguinoscrotal region or rarely in the perianal region.[1,2,6,7] Exceptional cases have been reported in the retroperitoneum and in the subcutaneous tissue of the chest, abdomen, knee, retroperitoneum, urethra, anus, prostate, upper eyelid, oral mucosa, and elbow.[2,7–12] Tumors tend to be small and behavior is benign, with almost no tendency for local recurrence.[1,7,13] Very large lesions are exceptional.[14,15] Two testicular lesions presenting simultaneously have been described.[16] Sarcomatous change has been reported, but so far this has not been associated with aggressive behavior.[7,17–19]

Pathogenesis and histologic features

Cytogenetic analysis of cellular angiofibroma has shown loss of chromosome 13q14, a feature also seen in spindle cell lipoma and mammary-type myofibroblastoma.[7,20–22] In conjunction with histologic similarities, this gives further support to a link between these neoplasms. The cytogenetic abnormality described results in loss of nuclear expression of the Rb protein, a feature that is useful in distinction from histologic mimics.[23]

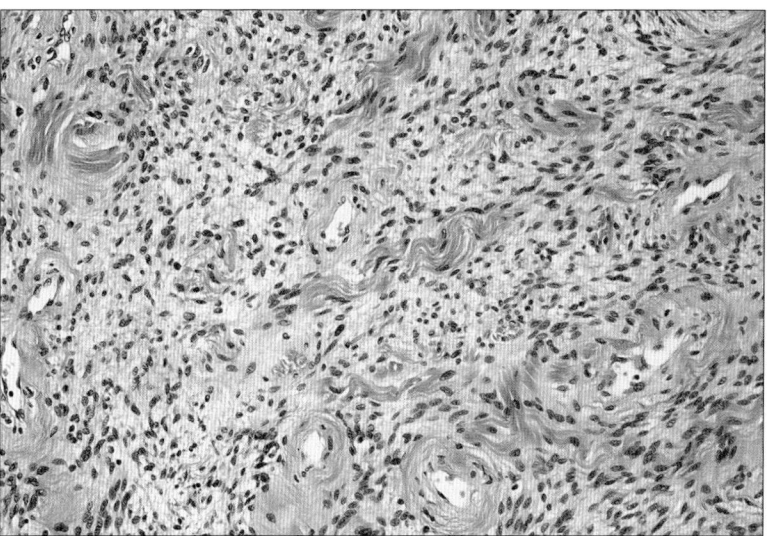

Fig. 12.292
Cellular angiofibroma: note the associated collagen fibers. By courtesy of M. Nucci, MD, Brigham and Women's Hospital and Harvard Medical School, Boston, USA.

Tumors are well circumscribed but unencapsulated, with only occasional extension into the surrounding soft tissues (Figs 12.291–12.293).[1] An infiltrative pattern is rare.[7] Most lesions are fairly cellular and composed of short, bland, spindle-shaped cells with poorly defined pale eosinophilic cytoplasm and vesicular nuclei. Nuclear grooves and intranuclear inclusions are common. The number of mitotic figures varies, but sometimes they may be prominent. Thick-walled, medium-sized hyalinized blood vessels are frequent in addition to slender collagen bundles and mast cells. Pseudovascular spaces are sometimes seen. Mature adipocytes are frequently present (in up to 30% of cases). Focal cytological atypia resembling symplastic changes seen in other tumors are described, and sarcomatous transformation can be identified.[7,17–19,24,25] Malignant areas usually show high cellularity, cytologic atypia, and multinucleated cells.[7] Tumors may rarely show features of a pleomorphic liposarcoma or of an atypical lipomatous tumor.[6,18,19]

Tumor cells are positive for vimentin and are positive for CD34 in up to 50% of cases. Staining for actin, desmin, caldesmon, S100 protein, and epithelial markers is negative.[1,2]

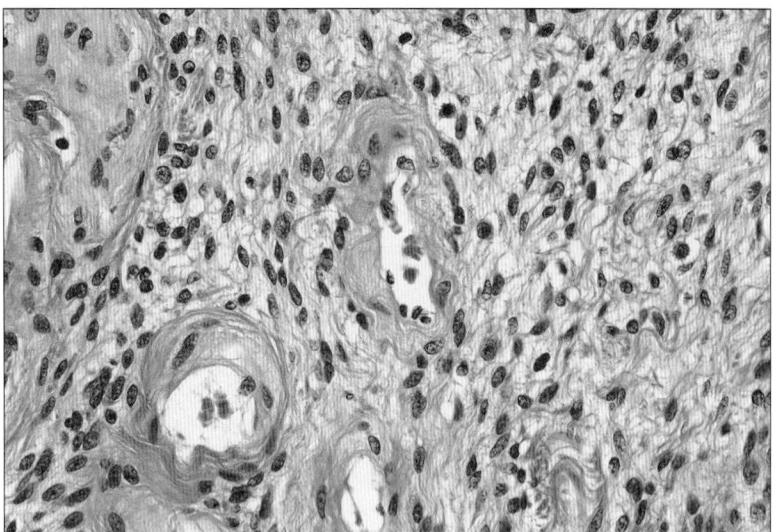

Fig. 12.293
Cellular angiofibroma: the tumor cells are small, uniform and have round to oval vesicular nuclei. By courtesy of M. Nucci, MD, Brigham and Women's Hospital and Harvard Medical School, Boston, USA.

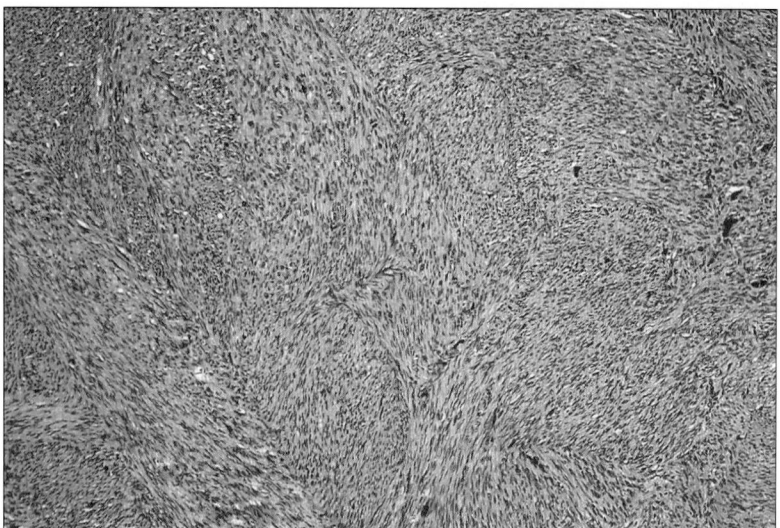

Fig. 12.294
Vulval leiomyosarcoma: this low-power view shows fascicles of tumor cells with eosinophilic cytoplasm. By courtesy of C. Crum, MD, Brigham and Women's Hospital and Harvard Medical School, Boston, USA.

Differential diagnosis

Distinction is mainly with angiomyofibroblastoma. The latter consists of more epithelioid desmin-positive cells with a nested pattern and a tendency for perivascular distribution. Cellular angiofibroma is negative for desmin and is often positive for CD34.

Genital leiomyoma

Clinical features

Genital leiomyoma comprises those lesions arising from the vulva, scrotum, and nipple. Tumors arising in the vulva and scrotum are distinctive from other cutaneous leiomyomas including pilar leiomyoma and angioleiomyoma.[1] Leiomyomas arising in the nipple are similar to pilar leiomyoma.

Vulval leiomyomas are relatively rare and present mainly in women of reproductive age as an asymptomatic swelling.[1–5] Clinical features are not distinctive. Tumors are subcutaneous, well circumscribed, and are often clinically diagnosed as a cyst. The majority of benign lesions are less than 5 cm in diameter and present in the labia. Rare cases arise in the clitoris.[6] Tumors may increase in size during pregnancy and also in association with estrogen/progesterone replacement therapy.[7] Benign tumors are typically well-circumscribed and small, but only histologic examination allows for distinction between benign, low-grade malignant and malignant tumors.

In males,[8] it presents as a painless, slow-growing, palpable mass (papule or nodule), and/or difficulty with micturition[9] if it affects the penis; or swelling of the scrotum where it arises from the tunica dartos scroti.[1,10–12] Scrotal tumors are less common and tend to be larger than their vulval counterparts.[13,14] They present as an asymptomatic mass that may occasionally be polypoid.[14] Rare cases are associated with prominent warty epidermal hyperplasia and resemble condyloma acuminatum.[15] Other benign smooth muscle lesions of the scrotum such as hamartoma of the dartos muscle are exceedingly rare.[16]

Histologic features

Cytogenetic analysis of a single vulval leiomyoma showed pericentric inversion of (12)(p12q13–14).[17] Although the HMGA2 gene is not involved in the breakpoint, the proximity of the gene to the breakpoint resulted in activation of the gene and tumor cells expressed HMGA2, a feature that is seen in genital leiomyomas.[17]

Tumors are well circumscribed and noninfiltrative with variable cellularity.[1–3] They are composed of admixed spindled and epithelioid cells, often with a single cell type predominating.[4,18,19] Lesions with a spindled cell component are very similar to those found in the uterus and consist of bundles of cells with well-defined eosinophilic cytoplasm, vesicular cigar-shaped nuclei, and an inconspicuous nucleolus. Focal myxoid change and hyalinization are commonly seen and sometimes this results in a plexiform appearance. Epithelioid tumor cells have abundant eosinophilic or pale-staining cytoplasm.

Because of the rarity of vulval smooth muscle tumors, it is often difficult to separate benign lesions from those with potential for local recurrence or metastasis (see below). It has been suggested that a tumor with any evidence of mitotic activity, nuclear pleomorphism, or an infiltrative margin should be regarded as having at least the potential for local recurrence.[4] In such cases, excision with a margin of at least 1 cm should be recommended.[4]

Since scrotal leiomyomas are so rare, there is even less information relating to their histologic evaluation. Symplastic scrotal leiomyomas may have an ill-defined infiltrative margin and can display cytological atypia ranging from moderate to severe.[20,21] The latter, however, is degenerative in nature with frequent multinucleated cells, low nuclear/cytoplasmic ratio, and smudged chromatin.[21] Lesions are also smaller and less cellular than leiomyosarcomas and lack mitotic activity.

Leiomyosarcoma

Clinical features

Vulval leiomyosarcoma is rare and presents in middle-aged to elderly patients as an asymptomatic mass mainly affecting the labia.[1–6] Malignancy is not usually suspected on clinical examination unless the mass is large and poorly circumscribed. Lesions may be confused with a Bartholin gland cyst.[6,7]

Scrotal leiomyosarcomas are exceptional and present as an asymptomatic, rapidly growing mass in elderly patients.[8,9]

Wide local excision is the treatment of choice. It is difficult to predict the outcome because of their rarity and the lack of large studies with adequate follow-up information.

Histologic features

It has recently been proposed that vulval leiomyosarcomas should be evaluated and classified according to the criteria and nomenclature proposed for uterine smooth muscle tumors.[10] Accepted criteria for the histologic diagnosis of leiomyosarcoma include (*Figs 12.294–12.296*)[1,2,11]:

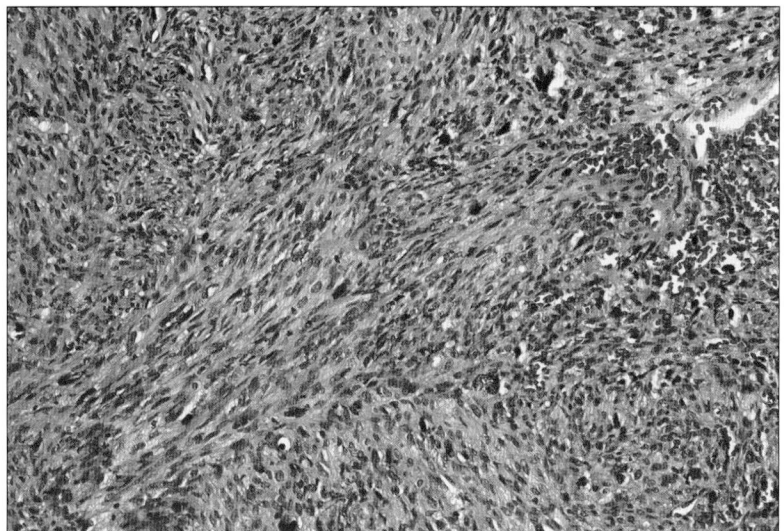

Fig. 12.295
Vulval leiomyosarcoma: note the nuclear pleomorphism. By courtesy of C. Crum, MD, Brigham and Women's Hospital and Harvard Medical School, Boston, USA.

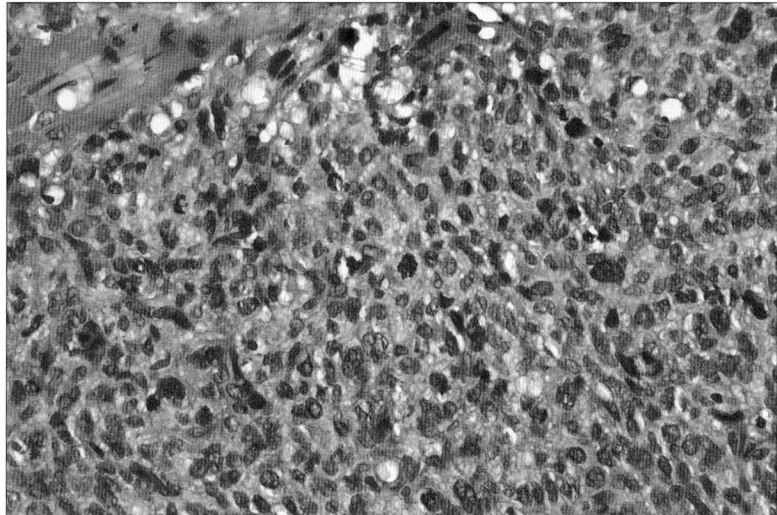

Fig. 12.296
Vulval leiomyosarcoma: high-power view showing a mitotic figure in the center of the field. By courtesy of C. Crum, MD, Brigham and Women's Hospital and Harvard Medical School, Boston, USA.

- size larger than 5 cm in diameter,
- infiltrative margins,
- more than 5 mitoses/10 high-power fields (HPF),
- moderate to severe cytological atypia.

Tumor necrosis should also be regarded as evidence of malignancy.[11]

Vulval leiomyomatosis

Clinical features

This rare condition is characterized by multiple leiomyomas in the vulva associated with esophageal leiomyomas.[1–8] The vulval tumors may appear before, concomitantly, or after the development of esophageal lesions. Involvement of the clitoris is sometimes noted. Patients can also present with Alport syndrome, characterized by inherited glomerulonephritis, ocular abnormalities, and deafness.[5]

Pathogenesis and histologic features

The pathogenesis of the disease is unknown, but deletions and mutations in the COL4A6 and COL4A5 genes have been described.[5,7] These

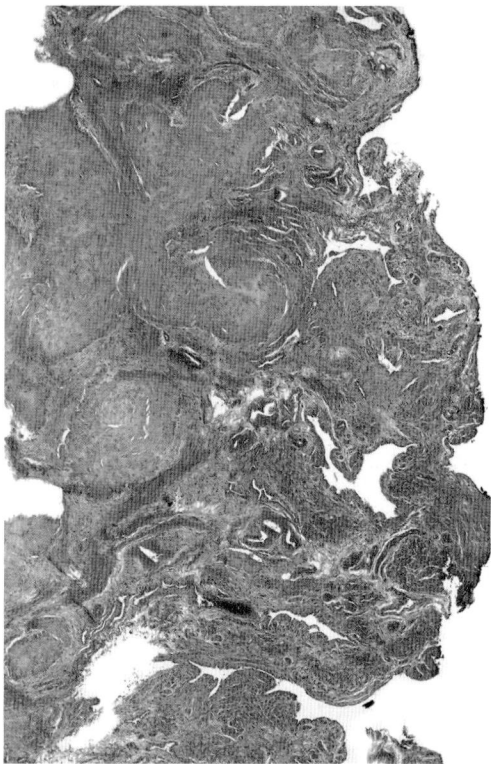

Fig. 12.297
Myointimoma: note the multinodular and plexiform growth pattern.

genetic alterations are associated with defects in type IV collagen in Alport syndrome.

Vulval and esophageal leiomyomas are identical to those occurring sporadically.

Myointimoma

Clinical features

This is a rare, recently described tumor involving the corpus spongiosum of the glans penis.[1] The original series consisted of adult patients, but a recent small series in children and adolescents has been reported.[1,2] Few single case reports have been presented.[3–5] Lesions are small (usually less than 1 cm) and asymptomatic. It does not seem to be related to trauma. The behavior is benign with no tendency for local recurrence.[1,2]

Histologic features

Low-power examination reveals a diffuse myointimal proliferation of the blood vessels of the corpus spongiosum of the glans penis in a plexiform growth pattern (Figs 12.297–12.299). The proliferating cells are bland and spindled with abundant pink cytoplasm and vesicular nuclei. A minority of the cells display features more reminiscent of fibroblasts. The background stroma is sclerotic and myxoid. Focal degenerative changes may be seen and mitotic figures are absent.

The spindled cells are positive for smooth-muscle actin, muscle-specific actin, and calponin but negative for desmin.

Differential diagnosis

This tumor must be distinguished from myofibroma, intravascular nodular fasciitis, and vascular leiomyoma.

Postoperative spindle-cell nodule

Clinical features

This rare reactive lesion presents as a small nodule at the site of a previous surgical procedure on the genitourinary tract including the bladder, vulva, and vagina.[1–4] It grows rapidly and is usually asymptomatic.[1–3] Local recurrence is not common.

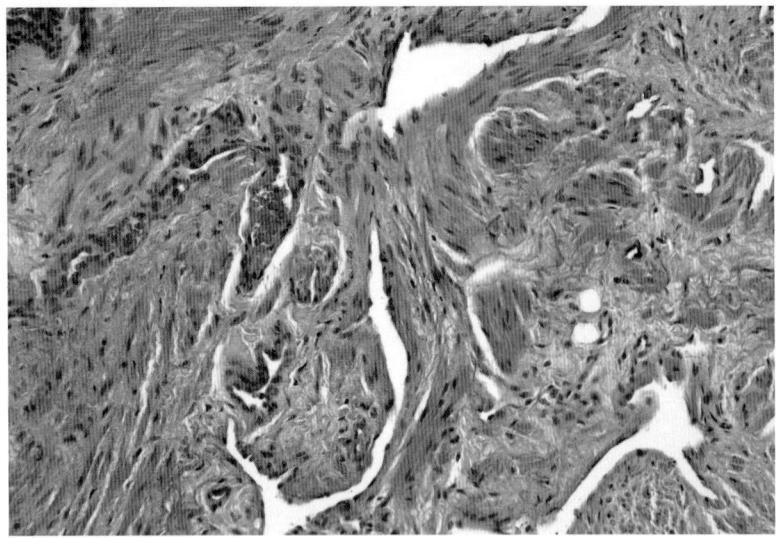

Fig. 12.298
Myointimoma: the vascular lumina are compressed by the proliferation of spindle-shaped cells.

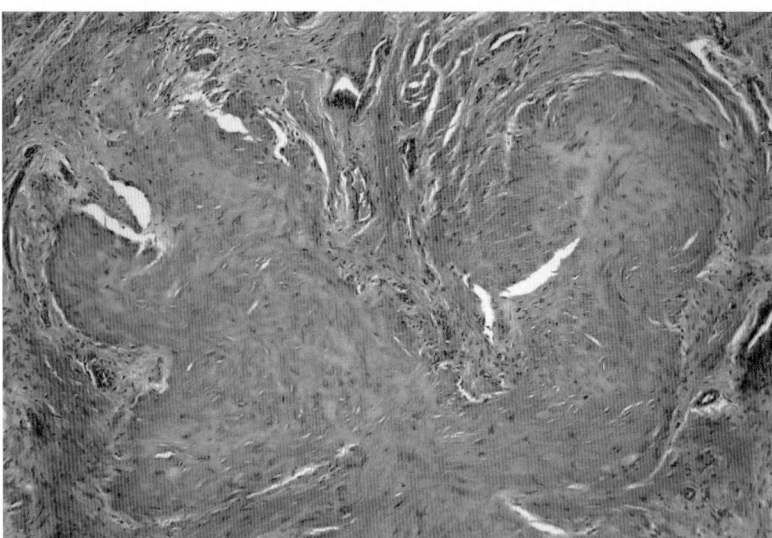

Fig. 12.299
Myointimoma: areas of hyalinization may be seen.

Pathogenesis and histologic features

The lesion is regarded as a non-neoplastic reparative phenomenon. Interestingly, trisomy 7 has been reported in two cases.[5] The nodule is poorly circumscribed and resembles nodular fasciitis.[1-3] It is composed of bundles of plump myofibroblast-like cells dispersed in a myxoid or edematous background. Nuclei may be bland or hyperchromatic. Small blood vessels, foci of hemorrhage, lymphocytes, and neutrophils are additional features. Mitotic figures are common.

Access **ExpertConsult.com** for the complete list of references

Degenerative and metabolic diseases

See
www.expertconsult.com
for references and
additional material

The hyperlipidemias

The hyperlipidemias may present as cutaneous xanthomata, which are localized aggregates of histiocytes containing accumulated lipid (primarily free and esterified cholesterol), in the form of five main clinical types:
- eruptive,
- tendinous,
- tuberous,
- planar,
- disseminated.[1]

The last, xanthoma disseminatum, in which serum lipid levels are normal, is discussed in Chapter 29 (see xanthogranuloma). Xanthoma cells are histiocytes and express CD4, CD11c, CD14b, CD68 and CD163 in addition to human leukocyte antigen (HLA) class II antigens.[2,3]

Hyperlipidemias may be primary, or secondary to conditions such as diabetes mellitus, obesity, pancreatitis, renal disease (the nephrotic syndrome or chronic renal failure), hypothyroidism, alcohol consumption, pregnancy, cholestatic liver disease (e.g., primary biliary cirrhosis), and paraproteinemias. Drug-induced hyperlipidemia also occurs as a result of administration of estrogens, corticosteroids, or 13-cis-retinoic acid. It is often associated with serious, potentially life-threatening disorders, such as atherosclerosis (low-density lipoproteins) and pancreatitis (hypertriglyceridemia).[4]

The presence of xanthomata commonly represents a cutaneous manifestation of systemic disease, and their recognition should therefore be followed by exhaustive investigations to exclude the latter (Table 13.1).[2,5] Although not a hard and fast rule, xanthoma morphology and distribution can sometimes point toward specific hyperlipidemia variants.

The plasma lipids are composed of triglycerides and cholesterol; these are insoluble and their transport is facilitated by their aggregation into lipoproteins. The latter are macromolecular complexes composed of an outer shell of hydrophilic phospholipids, nonesterified cholesterol, and apo(lipo) proteins, which emulsify the associated hydrophobic core of triglycerides and cholesterol ester.[5] There are a large number of apoproteins, with variable structure and function (e.g., ApoB-48, which is required for the secretion of chylomicrons into the thoracic duct).[4] In addition to giving structure to the lipoprotein, apoproteins also represent ligands for specific receptors (e.g., ApoE is a ligand for liver chylomicron receptors). They also act as cofactors for a number of lipid-modifying enzymes (e.g., ApoCII activates lipoprotein lipase).[6] Lipoprotein metabolism, which is summarized in Fig. 13.1, involves both exogenous (dietary) and endogenous pathways.[7] For more detailed information the reader is particularly referred to references 1 and 7.

The classification of hyperlipidemias is based upon the electrophoretic separation, on paper or agarose gel, of abnormal quantities of lipoprotein in the plasma (Fig. 13.2). There are seven main classes of lipoprotein, with differing electrophoretic mobilities:
- chylomicrons, which are composed predominantly of exogenous triglycerides produced by small intestinal mucosal epithelium in response to dietary lipid,
- very low density (pre-beta) lipoproteins (VLDL) of hepatic derivation, which are particularly involved in the transportation of endogenous triglyceride,
- intermediate density lipoproteins (IDL), which are thought to be VLDL remnants,

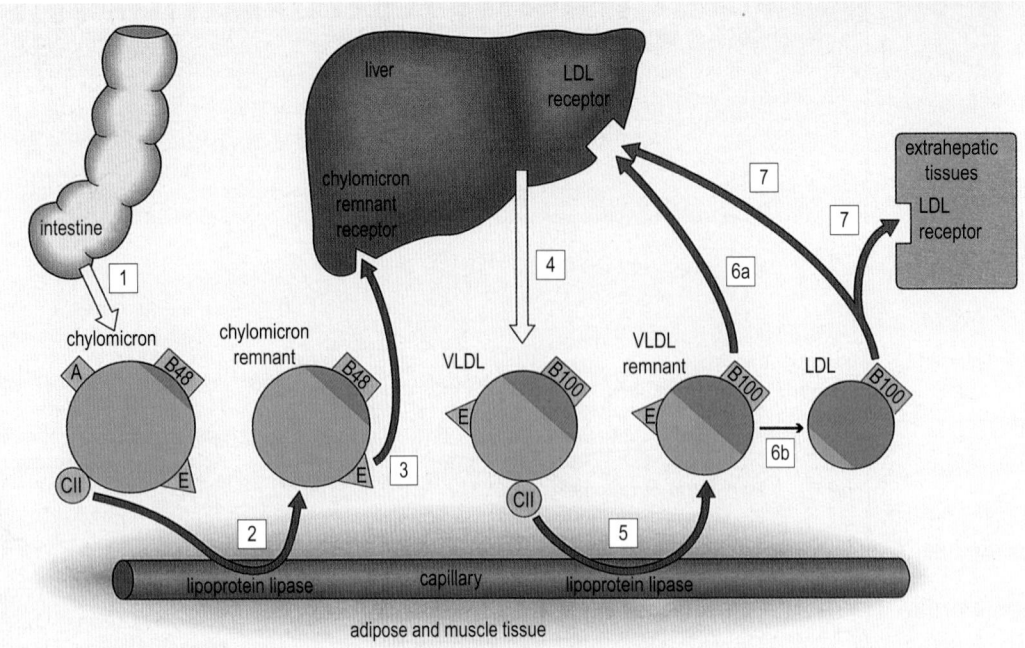

Fig. 13.1

Lipoprotein metabolism. (LDL, low density lipoprotein; VLDL, very low density lipoprotein.) Reproduced with permission from Cruz, P.D., East, C., Bergstresser, P.R. (1988) Journal of the American Academy of Dermatology, 19, 95–111.

Table 13.1
Classification of xanthomatous disorders

Hyperlipidemic xanthomatoses: disorders characterized by elevated plasma triglycerides or cholesterol		Normolipidemic xanthomatoses: disorders characterized by normal plasma triglycerides and cholesterol	
Primary hyperlipoproteinemias	Elevated plasma triglycerides lipoprotein lipase deficiency familial hyperlipoproteinemia, type V familial hypertriglyceridemia Elevated plasma triglycerides and cholesterol familial dysbetalipoproteinemia, type III Elevated plasma cholesterol familial hypercholesterolemia	Disorders characterized by altered lipoprotein content or structure	Accumulation of unusual sterols in LDL cerebrotendinous xanthomatosis (cholestanol) sitosterolemia (sitosterol, campesterol, stigmasterol, etc.) Deficiency of HDL plantar and buccal mucosal xanthomas diffuse plane xanthomas Normocholesterolemic dysbetalipoproteinemia tuberous xanthelasmas Hyperapobetalipoproteinemia tendon xanthomas xanthelasmas
Secondary hyperlipoproteinemias	Elevated plasma triglycerides diabetes mellitus drug-induced chylomicronemia alcohol estrogens retinoids hypothyroidism nephrotic syndrome type I glycogen storage disease (von Gierke disease) Elevated plasma cholesterol hepatic cholestasis primary biliary cirrhosis biliary atresia hypothyroidism dysglobulinemias or paraproteinemias multiple myeloma	Disorders associated with antibodies directed against lipoprotein components	Multiple myeloma Other paraproteinemias
		States with no demonstrated lipoprotein abnormalities	Underlying lymphoproliferative disease multiple myeloma cryoglobulinemia Waldenström macroglobulinemia leukemia lymphoma other Xanthomatosis antedated by local tissue alterations normolipemic eruptive xanthomas (after erythema) xanthelasmas and planar xanthomas (after erythroderma) Verruciform xanthomas (in areas of dystrophic epidermolysis bullosa) Other hereditary tendinous and tuberous xanthomas normolipemic tendon and tuberous xanthomas normolipemic subcutaneous xanthomatosis

HDL, high density lipoprotein; LDL, low density lipoprotein.
Reprinted from Cruz, P.D., East, C., Bergstresser, P.R. (1988) Journal of the American Academy of Dermatology, 19, 95–111 with permission from the American Academy of Dermatology, Inc.

- low density (beta) lipoproteins (LDL), which are mainly involved in cholesterol transport and derived from IDL or else produced by the liver,
- high density (alpha) lipoproteins (HDL) composed predominantly of lipoprotein and equal quantities of cholesterol and phospholipid,
- high density lipoprotein variant HDL2,[1,6]
- high density lipoprotein variant HDL3.[1,6]

The hyperlipidemias are classified into six types according to the lipoprotein anomaly present (*Table 13.2*). However, it should be noted that each of these six types may result from a variety of pathogeneses, including those of a known or presumed genetic basis and others that complicate a diverse group of disease processes (secondary hyperlipidemia).[8–10] HDLs are not atherogenic.[4] Indeed, their function is to remove cholesterol from the tissues and high levels serve to protect against vascular disease.[6] Conversely, HDL deficiency (e.g., Tangier disease) is associated with cholesterol accumulation.[11]

The lipid content of xanthomata is probably mostly derived from the plasma, presumably by lipoprotein (particularly LDL and VLDL) permeation of blood vessel walls with the release of lipid and its subsequent phagocytosis by histiocytes, although localized lipogenesis may also be of importance.[11–14] The subgroups and proportions of lipid deposited within xanthomata are similar to those found in atheromatous plaques, raising the possibility of a shared pathogenesis.[1]

Xanthomata are, however, not always associated with hypercholesterolemia or hyperlipoproteinemia.[15] Under such circumstances, they may evolve as a consequence of altered lipoprotein content or structure, represent local tissue changes or develop as a consequence of systemic disease including lymphoma, multiple myeloma, and Waldenström macroglobulinemia.[16] Normocholesterolemic xanthomata can therefore arise as a consequence of the accumulation of cholesterol-like substances within histiocytes (e.g., cerebrotendinous xanthomatosis and β-sitosterolemia).

Cerebrotendinous xanthomatosis represents an abnormality of bile acid metabolism inherited in an autosomal recessive pattern.[17–19] As a consequence of mitochondrial enzyme sterol 27-hydroxylase deficiency and resultant impaired oxidation of the cholesterol side chain during the production of cholic acid, cholestanol (and cholesterol) accumulates in the tissues, especially the tendons, lungs, and brain. The xanthomata particularly affect the Achilles tendons and the tendons of the knees, elbows, and the interphalangeal joints.[20] In addition to tendinous xanthomata, patients develop juvenile cataracts and progressive neurological dysfunction including mental retardation, dementia, pyramidal signs, cerebellar ataxia, spinal cord paresis, and sensory changes due to dysmyelination.[19,21,22] Coronary atherosclerosis,

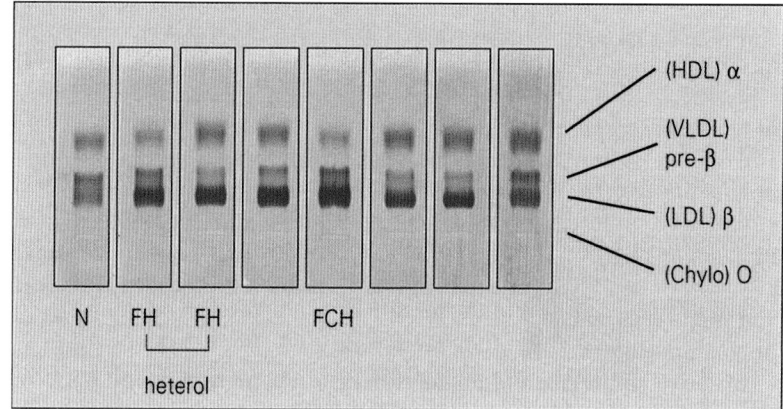

Fig. 13.2
Hyperlipidemia: electrophoretic separation of serum lipids. (Chylo, chylomicron; HDL, high density lipoprotein; LDL, low density lipoprotein; VLDL, very low density lipoprotein.) By courtesy of B. Lewis, MD, St Thomas' Hospital, London, UK.

Table 13.2
Classification of hyperlipidemias

Type	Anomaly	Primary cause	Secondary cause	Atherogenesis	Xanthoma	Associations
I	Raised chylomicrons	Familial lipoprotein lipase deficiency Apoprotein CII deficiency	–	–	Eruptive	Hepatomegaly Pancreatitis Lipemia retinalis Abdominal pain
IIA	Raised LDL	Familial hypercholesterolemia Familial multiple type hyper lipoproteinemia Common hypercholesterolemia	Hepatoma Porphyria Myxedema Anorexia nervosa Nephrotic syndrome Cushing syndrome	+	Tendinous Xanthelasma Arcus Tuberous (rare)	–
IIB	Raised LDL and VLDL	Familial hypercholesterolemia Familial multiple type hyperlipidemia	Nephrotic syndrome Cushing syndrome	+	Tendinous Xanthelasma Arcus Tuberous	–
III	Raised IDL	Familial dysbetalipoproteinemia	Paraproteinemia	+	Palmar Tendinous Tuberous	Diabetes Gout Obesity
IV	Raised VLDL	Familial multiple type hyperlipidemia Familial hypertriglyceridemia Sporadic hypertriglyceridemia	Diabetes Uremia Paraproteinemia Alcoholism Lipodystrophy Obesity	+	Eruptive Tendinous Tuberous	–
V	Raised chylomicrons and VLDL	Familial multiple type hyperlipoproteinemia Familial lipoprotein lipase deficiency Apoprotein CII deficiency Familial hypertriglyceridemia Familial type V hyperlipoproteinemia	Diabetes Obesity Pancreatitis	+	Eruptive	Hepatomegaly Pancreatitis Lipemia retinalis

IDL, intermediate density lipoprotein; LDL, low density lipoprotein; VLDL, very low density lipoprotein.

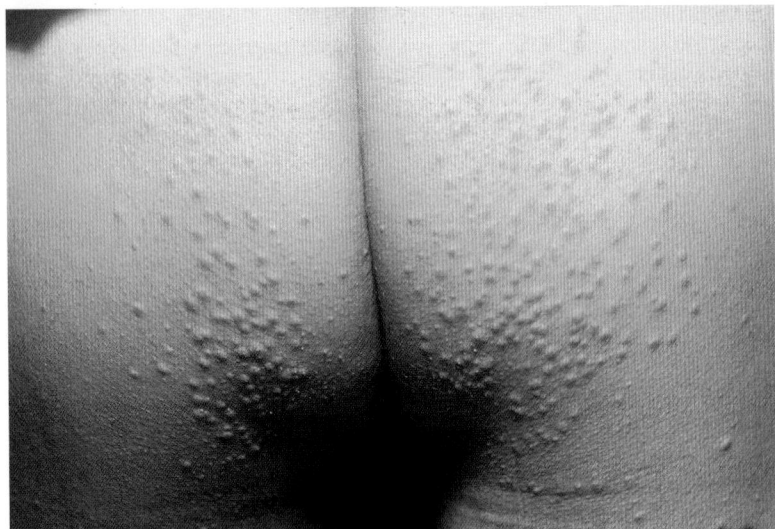

Fig. 13.3
Eruptive xanthoma: numerous small yellow papules are present on the buttocks.
By courtesy of R.A. Marsden, MD, St George's Hospital, London, UK.

endocrine abnormalities, and diarrhea may also be present. In addition to cholestanol accumulation, cerebrotendinous xanthomatosis has been shown to be characterized by abnormal HDLs, which result in impaired cholesterol (and cholestanol) transport and contribute to the consequent xanthomatization.[17] The mortality is high, patients usually dying in the fourth to sixth decades, most often from progressive neurological dysfunction, pseudobulbar paralysis or myocardial infarction.[22]

Tendinous and tuberous xanthomata may also represent a manifestation of β-sitosterolemia. This is an autosomal recessive condition in which increased intestinal absorption of the plant sterols β-sitosterol, campesterol, and stigmasterol results in tissue deposition along with cholesterol and subsequent xanthoma formation.[23–25] Normally these sterols are almost completely unabsorbed from the gastrointestinal tract. β-Sitosterolemia is associated with an increased risk of atherosclerosis.[4]

Xanthomata may occur in extracutaneous locations mimicking tumors in patients with hyperlipidemia. Sites include deep soft tissues and mediastinum.[26]

Eruptive xanthomata

Clinical features

Eruptive xanthomata are small (1–4 mm) yellowish papules with a red halo that have a predilection for the buttocks, shoulders, and extensor surfaces of the limbs (Fig. 13.3).[1] They may also present in the antecubital and popliteal fossae, axillae, lips, eyelids, and ears.[2] They often appear in crops and may wax and wane with plasma lipoprotein levels.[3] Lesions usually resolve spontaneously over a period of weeks. Pruritus is frequently present and the papules are sometimes tender.[2] Eruptive xanthomata may rarely display a Koebner phenomenon.[4,5] Healing is occasionally associated with the development of hyperpigmented scars.[2] Cutaneous lesions of Langerhans cell histiocytosis and cutaneous involvement by adenocarcinoma may mimic eruptive xanthoma.[6,7]

Eruptive xanthomata are associated with hypertriglyceridemia and most often occur in hyperchylomicronemic states. Sometimes their presence correlates with increased levels of VLDL. The most common cause, however, is secondary hyperlipoproteinemia (HPL), especially in those cases associated with diabetes mellitus and alcohol ingestion, or in those that are drug induced (e.g., due to exogenous estrogens, corticosteroids or retinoids).[2,8] They may also develop as a consequence of decreased lipoprotein lipase activity, ApoCII deficiency or increased synthesis of VLDL, which effectively blocks chylomicron access to lipoprotein lipase.[2,9] Eruptive xanthomata are therefore often accompanied by other features of hyperlipidemia, including lipemia retinalis, hepatosplenomegaly, abdominal pain, and pancreatitis.

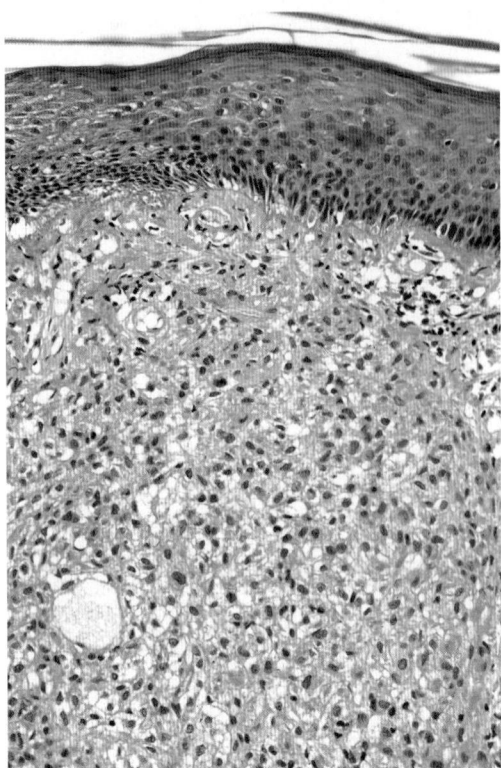

Fig. 13.4
Eruptive xanthoma: biopsy of an established lesion. The histiocytes have abundant vacuolated cytoplasm.

They may also rarely develop as a manifestation of primary hyperlipoproteinemia (HPL), particularly autosomal recessive lipoprotein lipase deficiency (HPL type I) in children and familial HPL type V in adults.[10,11] An exceptional association with β-sitosterolemia, a condition usually presenting with tuberous or tendinous xanthomata, has been documented.[12] Much rarer associations include familial hypertriglyceridemia, the nephrotic syndrome, chronic pancreatitis, von Gierke disease, and hypothyroidism.[8,13,14] An association with acanthosis nigricans (AN) has also been reported.[15] Dystrophic xanthomatization resulting in eruptive xanthomas at the site of prior herpes zoster as a manifestation of Wolf isotopic response has also been reported.[16] There are also reports of eruptive xanthomas developing in tattoos.[17,18]

Histologic features

The histologic features are seen predominantly within the superficial reticular dermis. In early lesions histiocytes are numerous and the fully developed 'foam cells', which characterize xanthomata, are sometimes few in number. The infiltrate may also contain an admixture of lymphocytes and neutrophils.[19,20] In an established papule, xanthoma cells with characteristic clear or foamy cytoplasm form the predominant cell type (Figs 13.4–13.6). Occasional cases show a palisading appearance at low magnification and urate-like crystals.[13,21,22]

Eruptive xanthomata often develop rapidly over the course of several days and occasionally are associated with spontaneous resolution. The quantity of intracytoplasmic lipid (predominantly triglyceride in contrast to other xanthomata, which contain mostly cholesterol) is in a state of flux and may be associated with extracellular deposition, a phenomenon that is rare or absent in the other types of xanthomata. In all xanthomata the lipid within the macrophage stains positively with fat stains such as oil red O, scarlet or Sudan red (Fig. 13.7).

Differential diagnosis

There can be confusion with granuloma annulare histologically as both conditions have certain features in common, namely a dermal interstitial histiocytic infiltrate with variably increased mucin.[13,19,20] Although extracellular lipid may disrupt dermal collagen, necrobiosis is not characteristic of

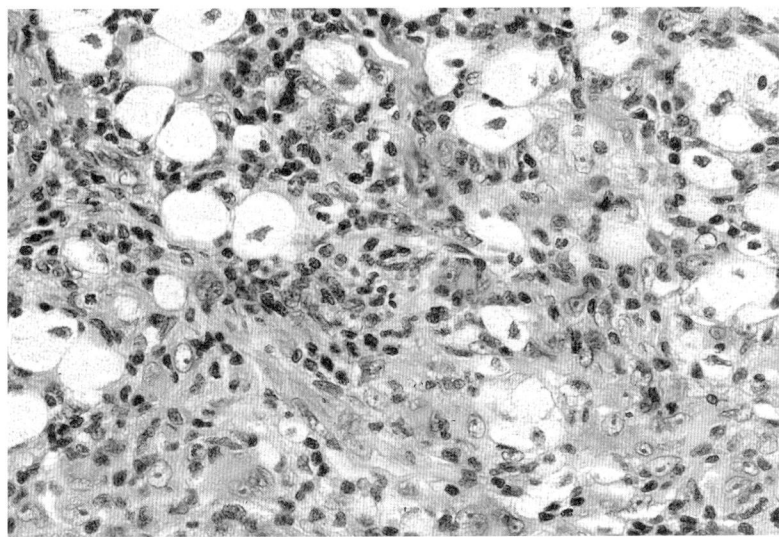

Fig. 13.5
Eruptive xanthoma: high-power view showing an admixture of vacuolated xanthoma cells and nonlipidized variants with abundant eosinophilic cytoplasm.

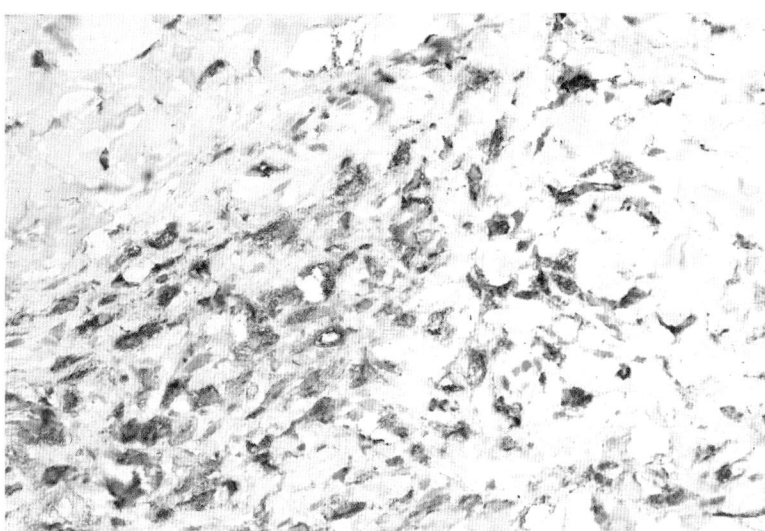

Fig. 13.6
Eruptive xanthoma: the histiocytes express CD68.

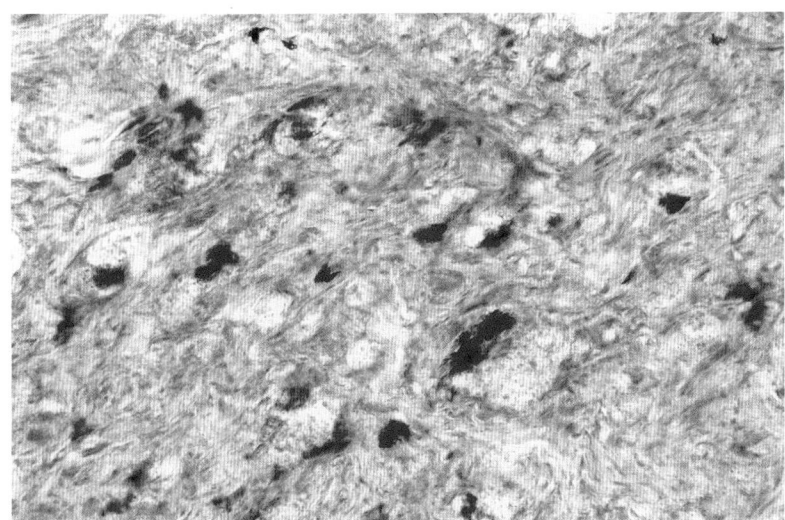

Fig. 13.7
Eruptive xanthoma: the lipid within the macrophages stains positively with oil red O.

eruptive xanthoma and palisading is not a feature of the latter. Additionally, it contains few giant cells and the perivascular infiltrate is histiocytic, in contrast to the perivascular lymphocytes seen in granuloma annulare.[13] Cases of eruptive xanthoma with urate-like crystals have been misdiagnosed as gout.[22] Immunohistochemical studies of these urate-like crystals suggest that they are, not surprisingly, composed of chylomicrons.[23]

Tendinous xanthomata

Clinical features

Tendinous xanthomata, which are associated with raised LDL levels, are slowly enlarging subcutaneous tumors that occur in tendons (especially those of the hands, knees, elbows, and the Achilles tendon), ligaments, fascia, and periosteum (*Figs 13.8* and *13.9*).[1] The overlying skin, which appears normal, is freely moveable over the surface and small tendon xanthomata may be difficult to palpate.[1] The lesions characteristically 'move with the tendons' and are thought to be trauma related.[2] The presence of these xanthomata is most frequently a feature of heterozygous familial (LDL receptor deficiency) hypercholesterolemia.[2-4] There is a high risk of

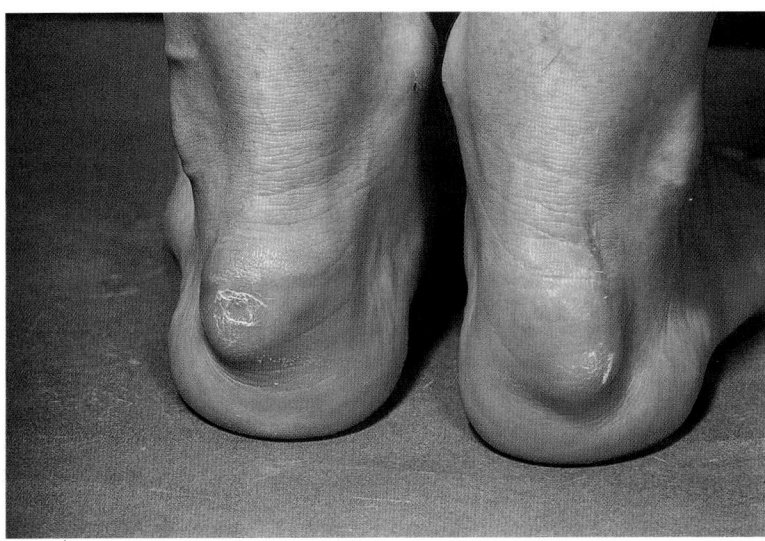

Fig. 13.8
Tendinous xanthoma: typical nodules on the heels. These lesions are often related to trauma; the Achilles tendon is a classical site. By courtesy of A.F. Lant, MD, and J. Dequeker, MD, London, UK.

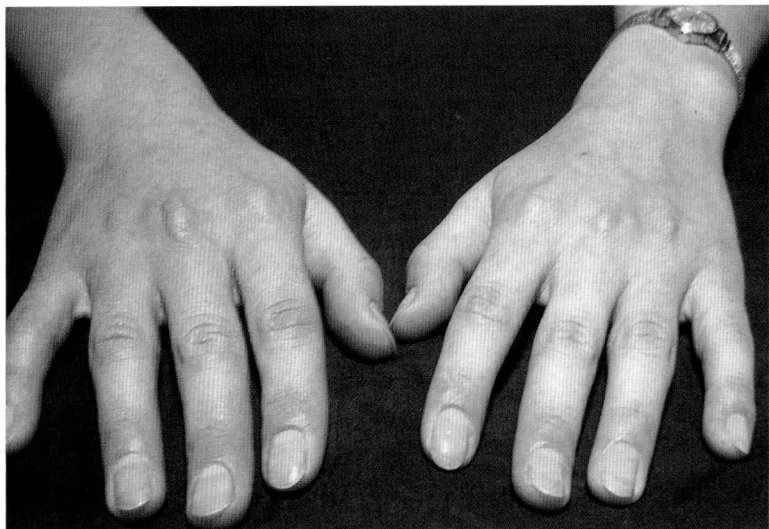

Fig. 13.9
Tendinous xanthoma: xanthomata are present overlying the knuckles. By courtesy of the Institute of Dermatology, London, UK.

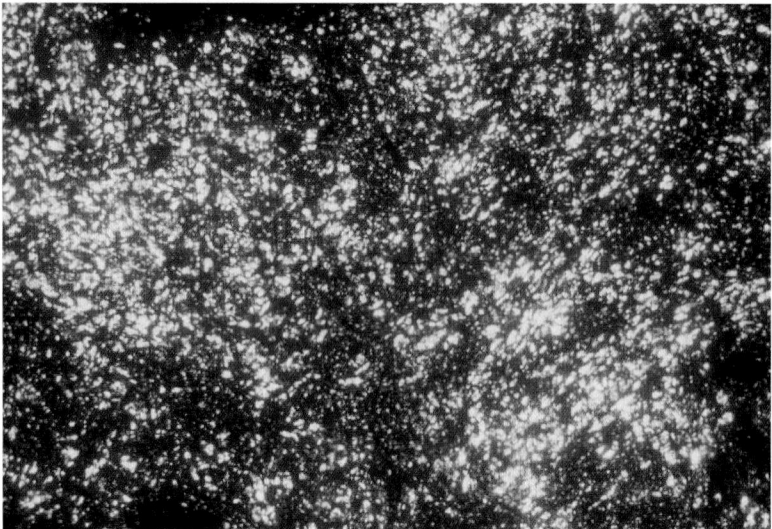

Fig. 13.10
Tendinous xanthoma: intense birefringence of deposits in polarized light (oil red O).

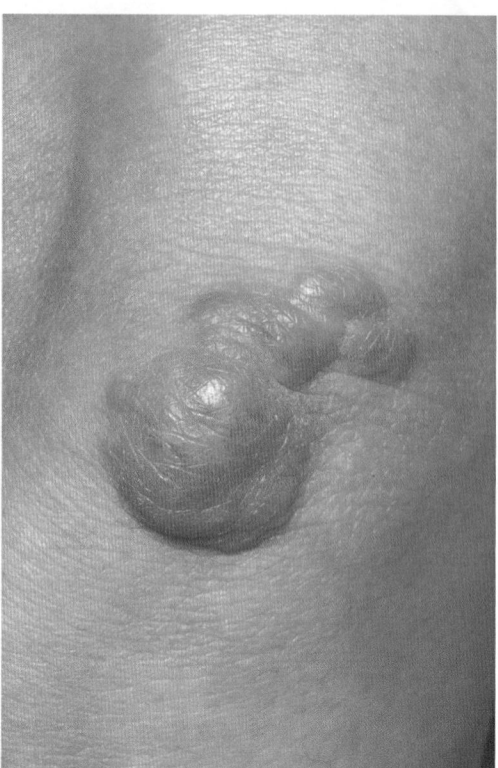

Fig. 13.11
Tuberous xanthoma: firm erythematous nodules over the elbow. By courtesy of R.A. Marsden, MD, St George's Hospital, London, UK.

associated coronary atherosclerosis. A meta-analysis demonstrated a three-fold increased risk of cardiovascular disease in patients with familial hypercholesterolemia and tendinous xanthomata compared to those without cutaneous lesions.[5] Tendinous xanthomata are also seen in familial combined hyperlipidemia, normocholesterolemic states such as cerebrotendinous xanthomatosis (cholestanolosis) and β-sitosterolemia, and the nephrotic syndrome.[2,6–10] Cerebrotendinous xanthomatosis is an autosomal recessive disease caused by a mutation in *CYP27A1*, the sterol 27-hydroxylase gene that is an important regulator of brain cholesterol homoestasis.[11] This results in xanthoma in the brain as well as tendons.

Clinically, the lesions, which may be mistaken for gouty tophi and rheumatoid nodules, are sometimes found in association with tuberous xanthomata and xanthelasmata.

Histologic features

Tendinous xanthomata are composed of multiple nodules containing xanthoma cells, accompanied in early lesions by an admixture of inflammatory cells including non-lipidized histiocytes, lymphocytes, and neutrophil polymorphs. The deposits in tendinous xanthoma are doubly refractile to polarized light (*Fig. 13.10*). Older lesions are characteristically associated with fibrosis.

Tuberous xanthomata

Clinical features

Tuberous xanthomata are firm yellow–red papules and nodules, which are found most frequently on the extensor aspect of the knees, elbows, and buttocks (*Figs 13.11–13.13*).[1] Lesions sometimes also occur on the hands and palms.[2] Rare cases involve cheeks and nose.[3] They are most characteristically seen in familial dysbetalipoproteinemia type III, and there is a particular risk of peripheral vascular disease.[4] Four other conditions may also be characterized by tuberous xanthomatosis:

- homozygous familial hypercholesterolemia,
- cerebrotendinous xanthomatosis,
- β-sitosterolemia,[1]
- type IV HPL.[5]

Tuberous xanthomata also occur in secondary hyperlipidemia (e.g., due to the nephrotic syndrome or hypothyroidism). Protease inhibitors may cause hyperlipidemia, and ritonavir has been reported to induce tuberous and tendinous xanthoma lesions.[6] Clinically, tuberous xanthomata occasionally resemble the lesions of erythema elevatum diutinum. Tuberous and tendinous normolipemic xanthomata have been described but it seems that, with adequate follow-up, patients usually develop some form of hyperlipidemia.[7]

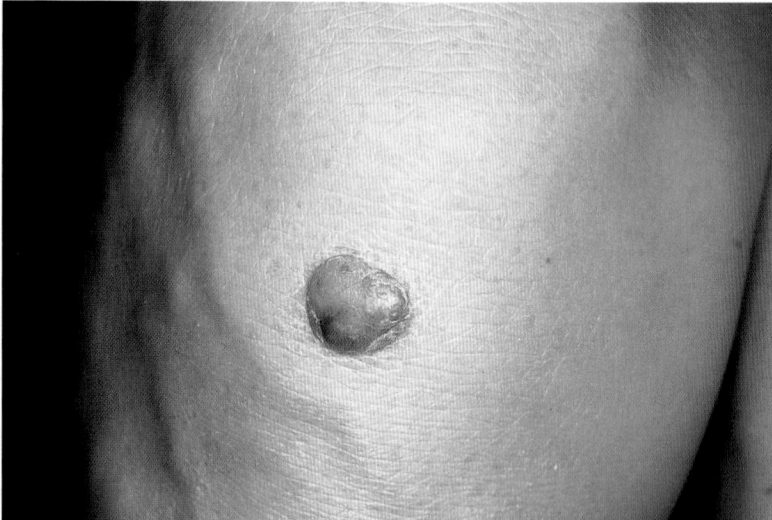

Fig. 13.12
Tuberous xanthoma: erythematous nodule on the back of the arm. By courtesy of the Institute of Dermatology, London, UK.

Cholesterotic fibrous histiocytomas may be associated with hyperlipidemia and often simulate a tuberous xanthoma clinically and histologically.[8] A rare case of undifferentiated pleomorphic sarcoma (malignant fibrous histiocytoma) clinically presenting as a tuberous xanthoma in a patient with type IIA HPL has been documented.[9]

Histologic features

Tuberous xanthomata consist of multiple nodules in the reticular dermis and sometimes the subcutaneous fat (*Fig. 13.14*). Their appearance varies, depending upon their stage of evolution (*Fig. 13.15*). Xanthoma cells predominate in early lesions, but with maturity fibrosis supervenes (*Fig. 13.16*). On occasion, foreign body giant cell granulomata containing cholesterol

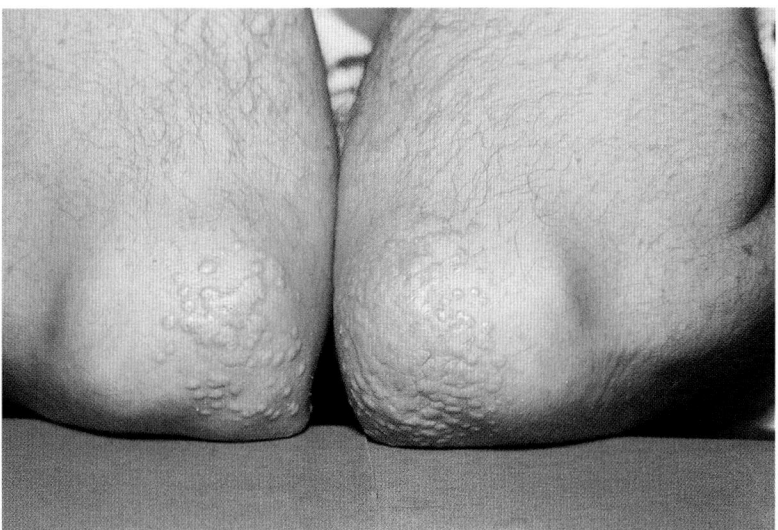

Fig. 13.13
Tuberous xanthoma: in this example, eruptive lesions are present on the elbows. By courtesy of the Institute of Dermatology, London, UK.

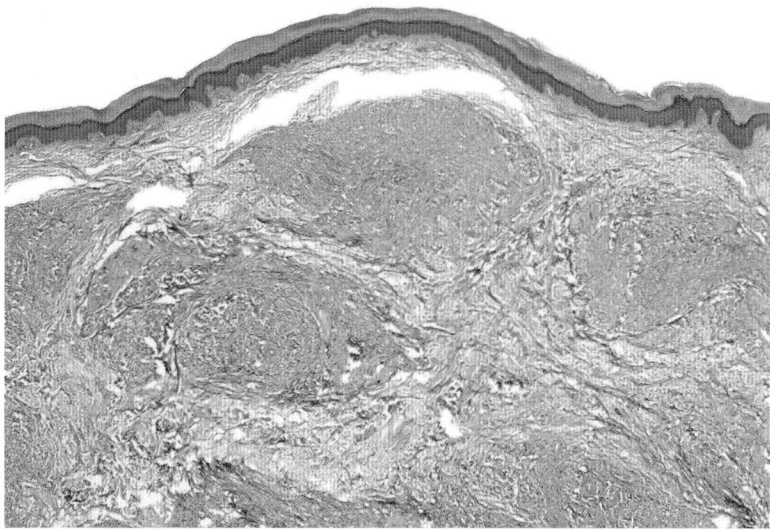

Fig. 13.14
Tuberous xanthoma: several nodules are present in the reticular dermis.

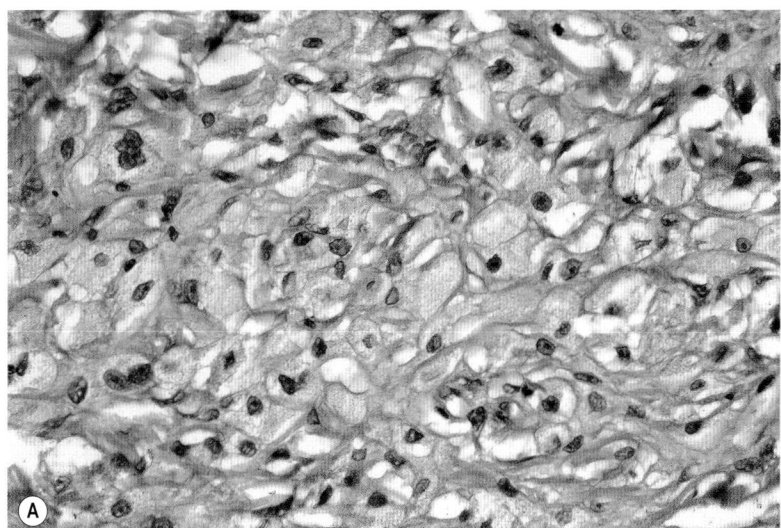

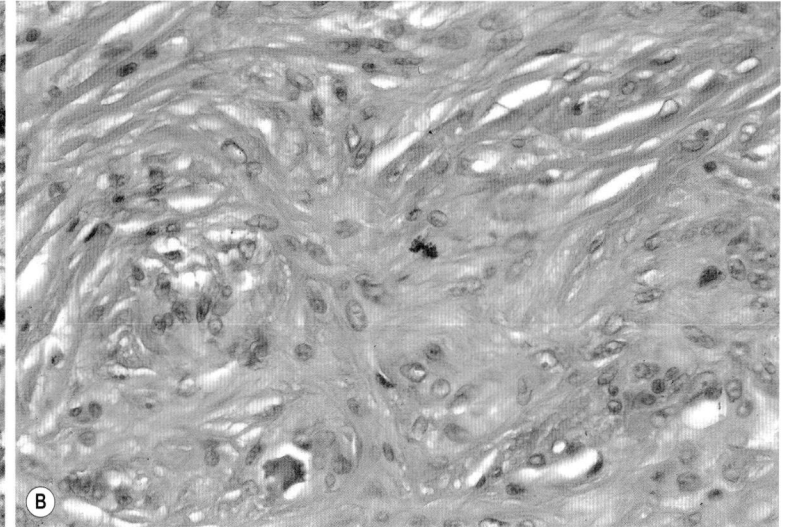

Fig. 13.15
Tuberous xanthoma: (**A**) the infiltrate is composed of uniform xanthoma cells characterized by pale, foamy cytoplasm and small central vesicular nuclei; (**B**) occasional normal mitoses are commonly present.

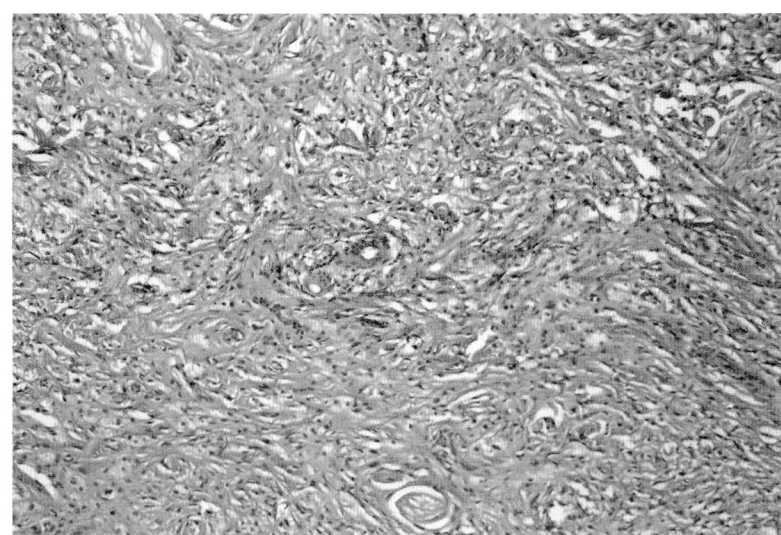

Fig. 13.16
Tuberous xanthoma: there is marked scarring.

clefts are seen and a perivascular chronic inflammatory cell infiltrate is sometimes evident (*Fig. 13.17*).

Differential diagnosis

Heavily lipidized fibrous histiocytomas that tend to occur mainly around the ankle may histologically mimic tuberous xanthoma.[10] The latter lesions lack the architecture of fibrous histiocytomas, have a nodular/multinodular growth pattern with variable fibrosis and lack epidermal hyperplasia and the hyalinization of collagen pattern seen at the periphery of fibrous histiocytomas.

Planar xanthomata

Clinical features

Planar xanthomata are typically soft yellow dermal macules or plaques that occur most frequently around the eyes, where they are known as xanthelasmata (*Fig. 13.18*).[1,2] About 50% of patients with xanthelasmata have associated hyperlipidemia (hypercholesterolemia or HPL type III) which is often accompanied by a cholesterol corneal arcus.[3-5] Many of those who

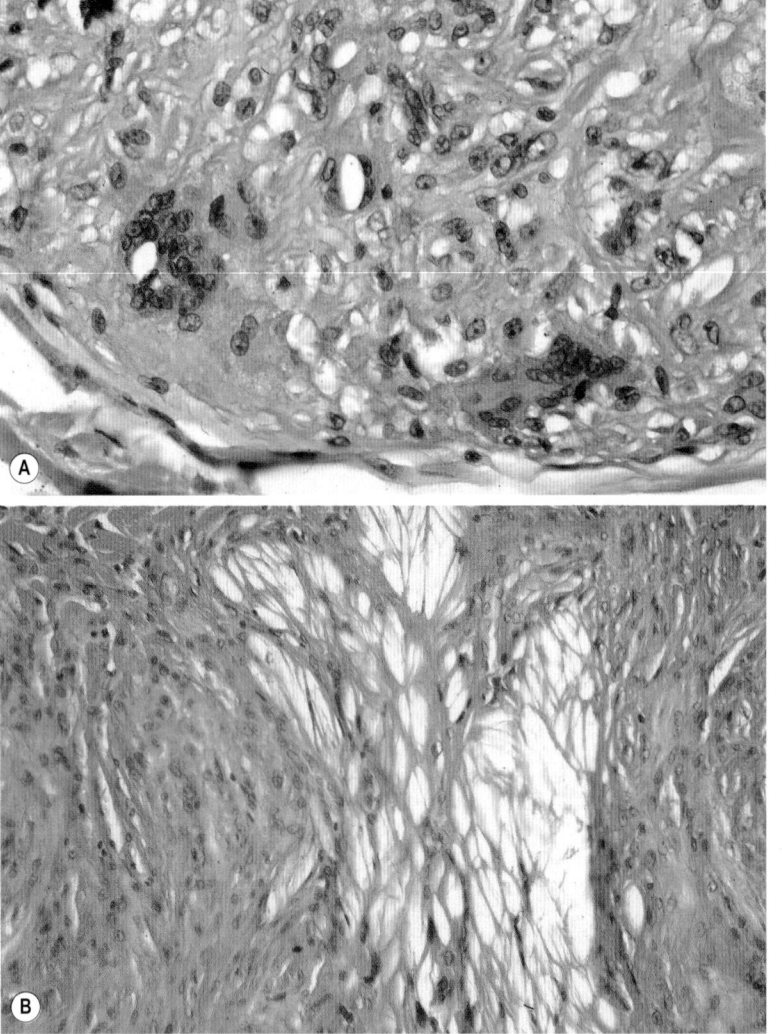

Fig. 13.17
(A, B) Tuberous xanthoma: in addition to xanthoma cells, occasionally there are foreign body giant cells containing cholesterol clefts. The lipid has been dissolved out during processing.

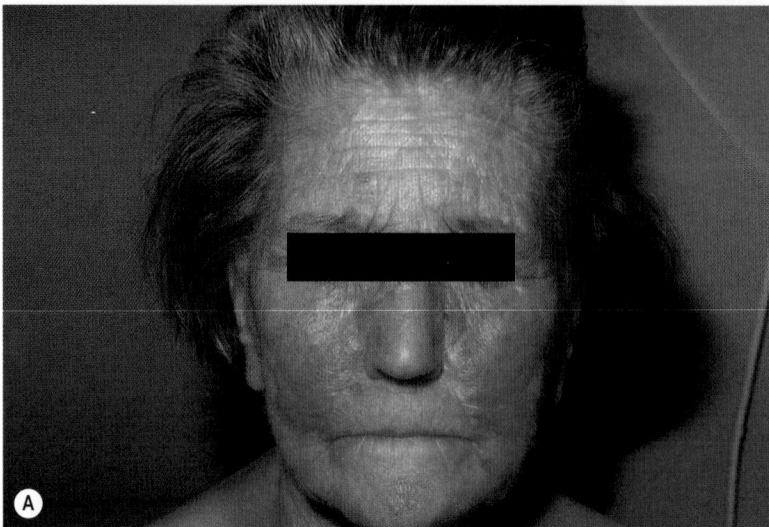

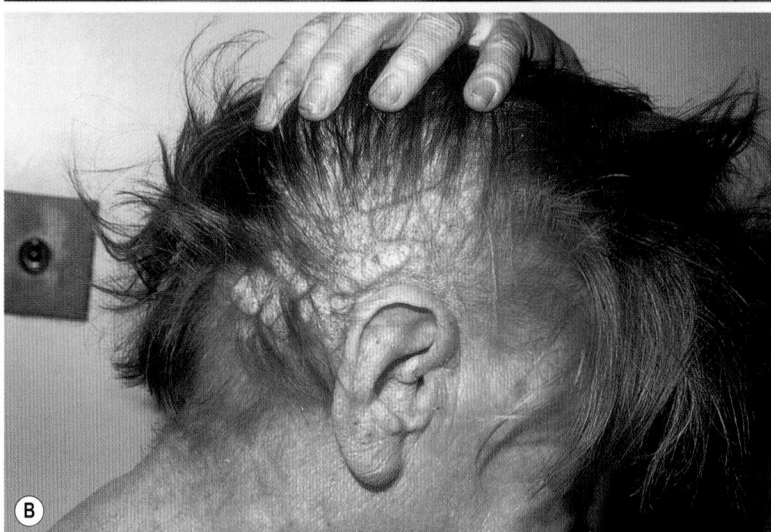

Fig. 13.19
Planar xanthoma: (A) widely distributed lesions over the forehead, eyelids, and cheeks; (B) extensive yellow plaques on the scalp. This appearance should prompt a search for an associated paraproteinemia. By courtesy of R.A. Marsden, MD, St George's Hospital, London, UK.

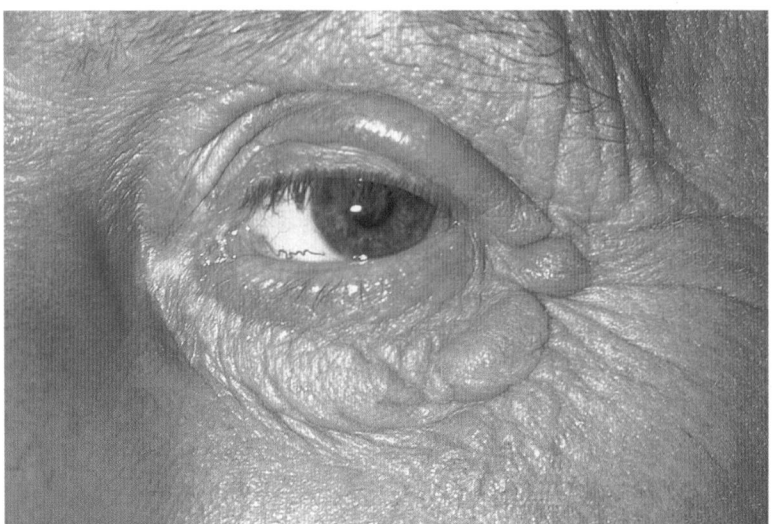

Fig. 13.18
Xanthelasmata: note the yellow, periorbital plaques. These are a common manifestation of hypercholesterolemia. By courtesy of the Institute of Dermatology, London, UK.

appear biochemically normal on routine testing, however, are shown to have subtle abnormalities of lipid metabolism on more detailed analysis.[6] There is a particularly increased risk of coronary artery atherosclerosis in younger patients.[1] When very extensive (diffuse or generalized plane xanthomatosis) and associated with orange–yellow planar xanthomata around the head and neck, and occasionally the upper trunk and arms, there may be an associated systemic disorder such as multiple myeloma with paraproteinemia, cryoglobulinemia, benign paraproteinemia or, less commonly, leukemia and rheumatoid arthritis (necrobiotic xanthogranuloma) (Fig. 13.19).[1,3,7–14] More exceptional associations include idiopathic Bence Jones proteinuria, Sézary syndrome, Castleman disease, relapsing polychondritis, acquired palmoplantar keratoderma, adult T-cell leukemia/lymphoma, and Takayasu disease.[15–21] A patient with monoclonal gammopathy and cutaneous lesions with features of both plane xanthoma and amyloidosis has been documented.[22] The latter case was also associated with myeloma.

In cases of myeloma and plane xanthoma, it has been demonstrated that complexes form between serum lipoproteins and paraprotein, suggesting that this interaction may induce a hyperlipidemia and xanthoma formation.[23,24] The serum lipid levels of patients with diffuse plane xanthomata are normal or raised. Plane xanthomata may present in the gingiva and, in this location, are usually associated with hyperlipidemia.[25] An exceptional case has been described in an infant presenting with normolipemic papular and nodular lesions progressing to plane xanthomata and resulting

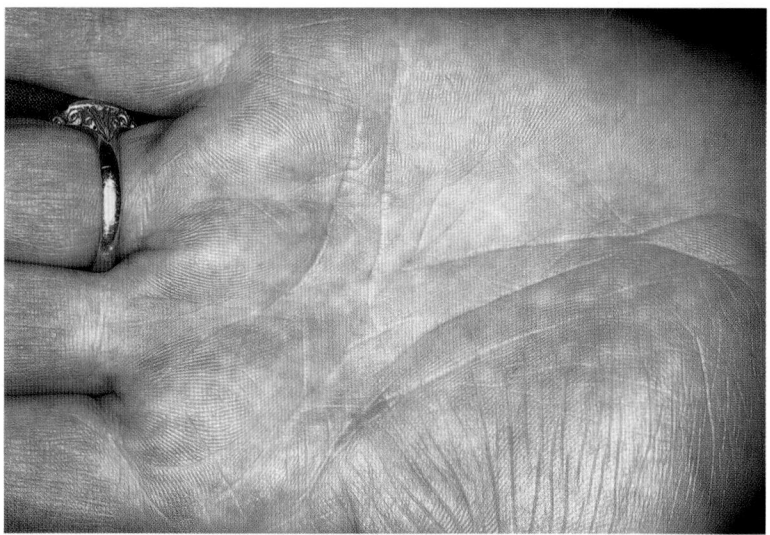

Fig. 13.20
Planar xanthoma: palmar lesions presenting as discrete macules with accentuation in the skin creases. By courtesy of R.A. Marsden, MD, St George's Hospital, London, UK.

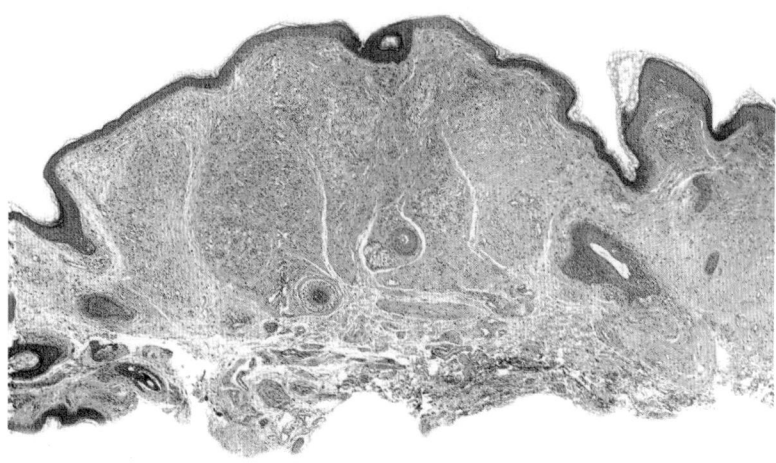

Fig. 13.21
Planar xanthoma: a dense infiltrate is present in the upper dermis.

in spontaneous resolution.[26] Diffuse plane normolipemic xanthomata with mucosal and conjunctival involvement and aortic valve xanthomatosis may occur exceptionally.[27] Lesions have been reported that clinically resembled plane xanthomata in a patient with systemic lupus erythematosus but histologically showed degeneration of collagen bundles with secondary fat deposition.[28]

Intertriginous xanthomata seen in patients with raised LDLs and pathognomonic of homozygous familial hypercholesterolemia present as yellow papules and plaques, often with a cobblestone appearance. These occur in the finger webspaces and to a lesser extent in the axillae and antecubital and popliteal fossae.[29] They have a particularly high association with early and severe atherosclerosis. Intertriginous xanthomata may also rarely be seen in heterozygous familial hypercholesterolemia.[30]

Planar xanthomata presenting as yellow-orange macules in the skin creases of the palm and fingers (xanthoma striatum palmare) are diagnostic of familial dysbetalipoproteinemia (HPL type III, broad beta disease) (*Fig. 13.20*), which is due to an abnormality of the apoprotein ApoE (homozygous ApoE2/E2).[1,2,31] This results in impaired uptake of lipoprotein remnant particles by the liver and macrophages with resultant HPL and increased atherogenesis.[30] Interestingly, the tendency to familial dysbetalipoproteinemia is present in 1% of the population, but a second lipid abnormality appears to be necessary to induce symptoms.[30]

Plane xanthomata of cholestasis, for example due to primary biliary cirrhosis and biliary atresia, present as well-demarcated, beige–orange plaques that are particularly found on the hands and feet, but may occur elsewhere.[2] They can also develop in patients with diabetes mellitus and have been described in the setting of cholestasis resulting from chronic graft-versus-host disease.[32]

Planar xanthomata have also been described as a feature of HDL deficiency.[33]

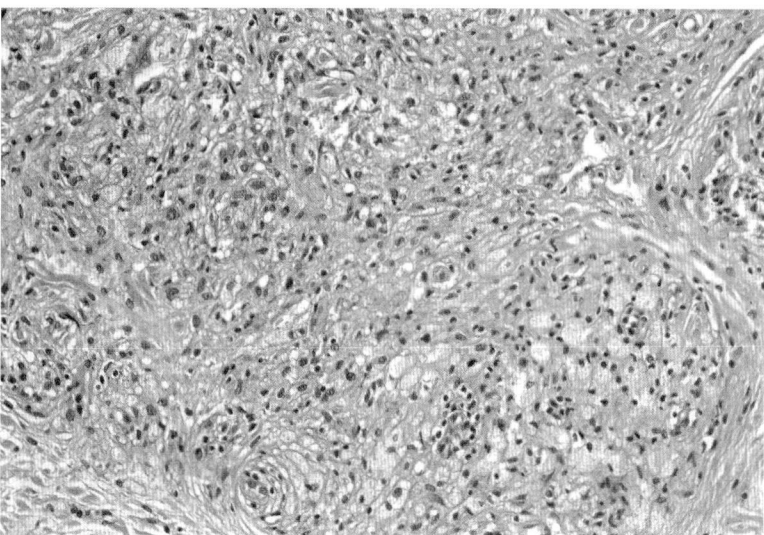

Fig. 13.22
Planar xanthoma: there is an admixture on nonlipidized and lipidized histiocytes.

Histologic features

In planar xanthomata, the characteristic lipid-laden foam cells are situated within the superficial dermis (*Figs 13.21–13.23*). There is minimal fibrosis. In rare cases, the histology may overlap with that of necrobiotic xanthogranuloma.[34.]

Verruciform xanthoma

Clinical features

The verruciform xanthoma is an uncommon, asymptomatic lesion, which occurs predominantly in the oral cavity of adults in their fifth or sixth decade

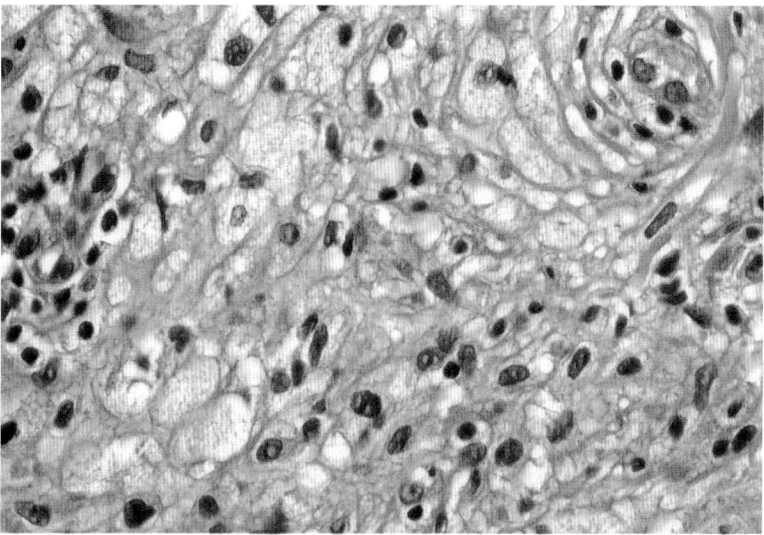

Fig. 13.23
Planar xanthoma: in addition to xanthoma cells, there are scattered lymphocytes.

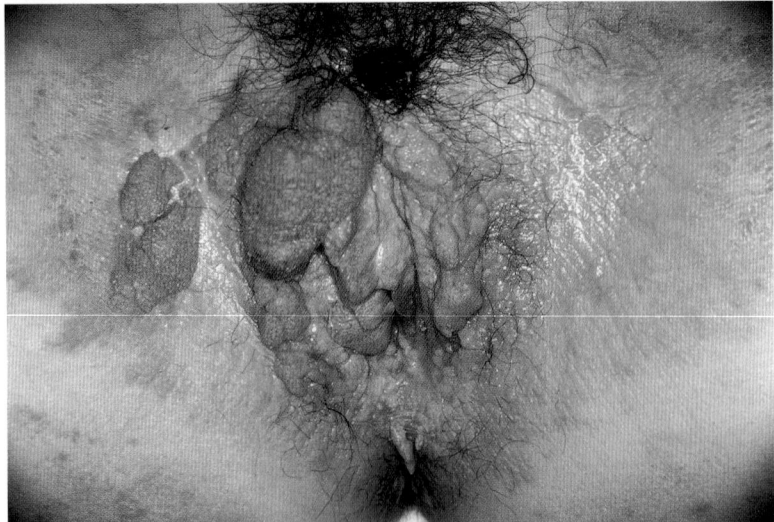

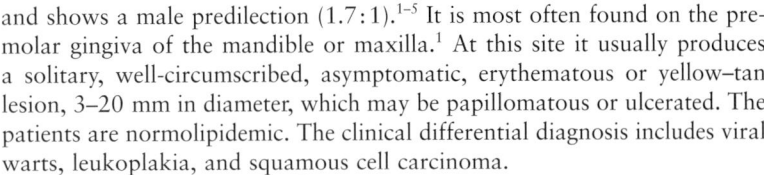

Fig. 13.24
Verruciform xanthoma: in this unusual gross example, there are numerous warty and polypoid lesions showing extensive involvement of the vulva, perineum, and thighs. A viral etiology was initially suspected clinically.

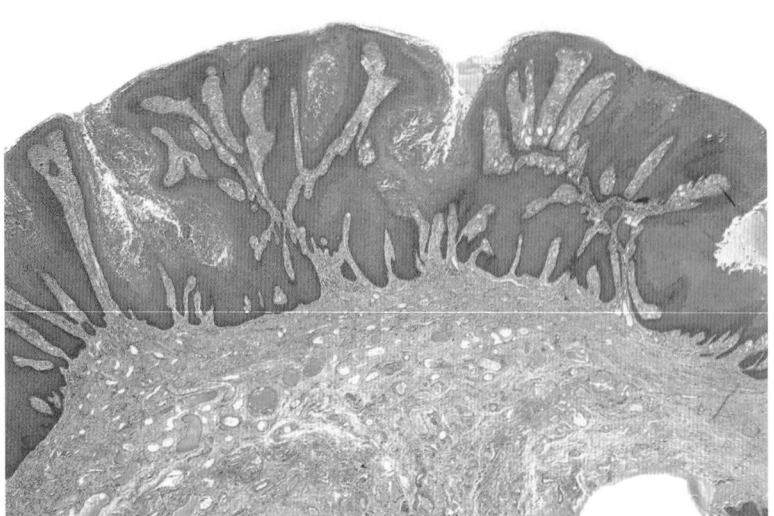

Fig. 13.25
Verruciform xanthoma: there is marked acanthosis, hyperkeratosis, and a level lower border.

and shows a male predilection (1.7:1).[1-5] It is most often found on the premolar gingiva of the mandible or maxilla.[1] At this site it usually produces a solitary, well-circumscribed, asymptomatic, erythematous or yellow–tan lesion, 3–20 mm in diameter, which may be papillomatous or ulcerated. The patients are normolipidemic. The clinical differential diagnosis includes viral warts, leukoplakia, and squamous cell carcinoma.

Verruciform xanthomata of the skin, which are extremely rare, have been described at a variety of sites including the ear, nose, lip, digits, and arm.[6-13] Most cases described, however, have arisen on anogenital skin (*Fig. 13.24*).[14-22] It may also develop as a reactive phenomenon within epidermolytic acanthoma, seborrheic keratoses, epidermal nevi (including patients with inflammatory linear verrucous epidermal nevus or with the epidermal nevus syndrome), lymphangioma circumscriptum, and has been recorded as a complication of lymphedema.[9,23-32] It has been described in association with longstanding discoid lupus erythematosus, lichen sclerosus, lichen planus, complicating ulceration in epidermolysis bullosa, congenital hemidysplasia with ichthyosiform erythroderma and limb defects syndrome (CHILD syndrome) and in association with squamous cell carcinoma of the penis.[33-43] Occasionally, verruciform xanthomata are multifocal.[6] Such a case has been described as multiple lesions in the upper aerodigestive tract of a child with a systemic lipid storage disease.[38] Multiple verruciform xanthomata have also been reported in the anogenital region several years following necrotizing fasciitis of the perineum and in the oral mucosa in a patient with chronic graft-versus-host disease.[39,44] A rare case of disseminated lesions has been described on the hands, feet, and anogenital region and another with similar widespread disease that also included the oral cavity.[45,46]

In the skin, verruciform xanthoma usually presents as a gray or pink nodule or as a plaque with a variably warty surface. Untreated, the lesions have a long duration and behave in a benign fashion, recurrence being very uncommon after local excision.

Pathogenesis and histologic features

The etiology and pathogenesis of the verruciform xanthoma are unknown. Originally, a viral infection by human papillomavirus (HPV) was suspected. Although most studies have not demonstrated definitive evidence to support this hypothesis, there are isolated reports demonstrating HPV DNA by polymerase chain reaction (PCR) in the lesions.[47-50] Additionally, it has been suggested that keratinocyte necrosis may lead to the release of intracellular lipids, with resultant macrophage influx and xanthomatization.[3,49,51] The inciting event leading to keratinocyte necrosis has not been identified. Immunohistochemical and electron microscopic studies give some credence to support to this latter hypothesis (see below). More recently, it has been proposed that localized lymphedema is a critical factor in some cases, as the

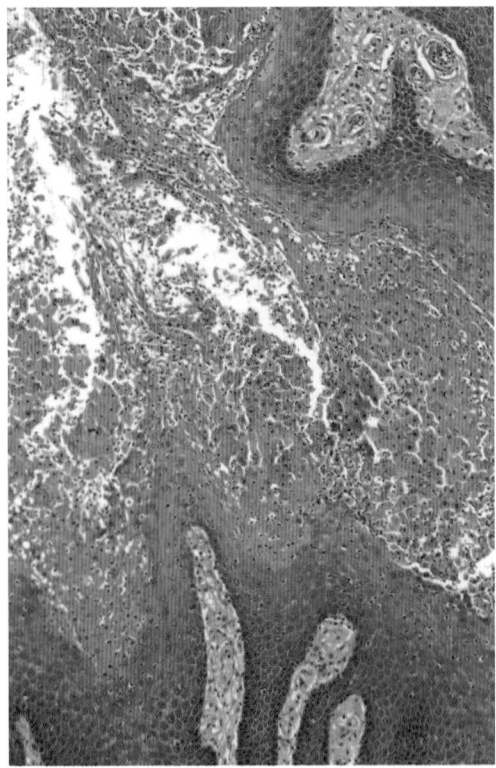

Fig. 13.26
Verruciform xanthoma: there is extensive keratinocyte necrosis associated with a polymorph infiltrate.

same types of lipid-laden macrophages are seen in other conditions associated with chronic lymphedema.[31,32]

Verruciform xanthoma is an exophytic lesion characterized by massive but regular acanthosis, variable papillomatosis, parakeratosis, and hyperkeratosis (*Fig. 13.25*).[47] Neutrophils, and neutrophilic debris are frequently observed at the level of the stratum corneum. Bacterial colonies may also be evident in the parakeratotic stratum corneum. The acanthosis is associated with uniform, bulbous epidermal ridges, all of which penetrate to the same depth, giving a characteristically level lower border. The expanded ridges are associated with marked central keratinocyte necrosis and a heavy neutrophil polymorph inflammatory cell infiltrate (*Fig. 13.26*). There is no epithelial atypia and viral inclusions are invariably absent. The accentuated papillary dermis between the elongated epidermal ridges contains

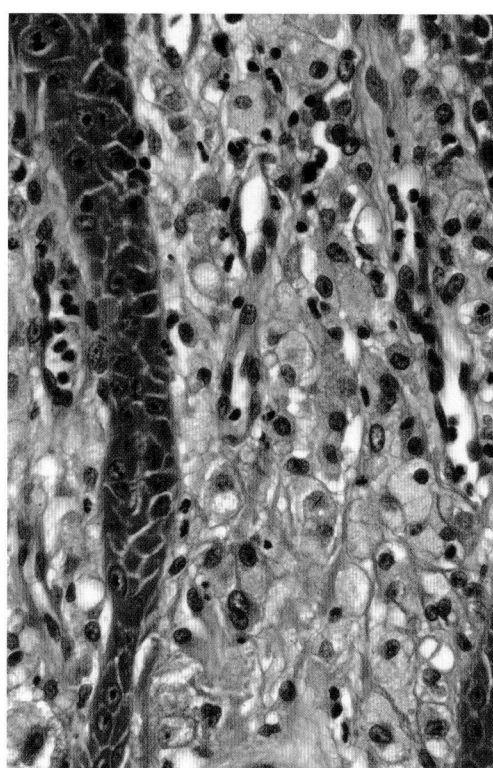

Fig. 13.27
Verruciform xanthoma: in the papillary dermis there is an infiltrate of uniform xanthoma cells.

large numbers of eosinophilic foamy to granular xanthoma cells, which stain positively with lipid stains, but not usually with the diastase–periodic acid-Schiff (PAS) technique (Fig. 13.27). No foreign body or Touton giant cells are present. At the base of the lesion the epidermis may show focal basal cell hydropic degeneration associated with patchy loss of basement membrane. The reticular dermis deep to the lesion often contains a moderately dense lymphocyte–plasma cell infiltrate, which at the edge of the lesion sometimes adopts a lichenoid distribution. Typically, vascular ectasia is seen beneath the lesion, possibly giving support to the lymphedema hypothesis. Oral examples are similar to their cutaneous counterparts, but they lack compact hyperkeratosis.[48]

Older studies showed that the fully formed foamy cells are negative for histiocytic markers including factor XIIIa, Mac 387, Ham-56, and KP1 (CD68) while the incompletely lipidized cells are diffusely positive for KP1 and weakly positive for FXIIIa and keratin.[49,52] Nonlipidized cells located in the periphery of the infiltrate are diffusely positive for FXIIIa only. This staining pattern has led to the suggestion that FXIIIa-positive dermal dendritic cells in the setting of damaged keratinocytes play an active role in the formation of the lipid cells seen in this condition.[49] The mechanism of keratinocyte damage is not fully elucidated. One theory proposes that the macrophages play an active role in keratinocyte cleavage and keratinolysis with secondary release of epithelial lipid. Macrophage recruitment is postulated to occur as a consequence of CD8-positive T cells present in the submucosa.[52,53] A more recent study of oral verruciform xanthomas showed diffuse, strong immunoreactivity for CD68 in all of the xanthoma cells and moderate immunoreactivity for CD163 and CD63 regardless of the degree of lipidization.[54]

Ultrastructural studies have revealed histiocytes containing numerous nonmembrane-bound lipid droplets, lysosomes, and myelin figures.[15,55] Smaller numbers of these lipid inclusions may be found in the overlying keratinocytes and in the intercellular space. In one report, basal melanocytes were found to contain conspicuous lipid droplets.[56] This was accompanied by evidence that the latter had been released into the basal intercellular space in association with disruption of the basal lamina, thereby providing a source for the lipid within the dermal macrophages.

Differential diagnosis

Verruciform xanthoma must be distinguished from viral warts, granular cell tumor, and verrucous carcinoma:

- *Viral warts*: verruciform xanthoma lacks the vacuolation, clumped keratohyalin granules and tiers of parakeratosis seen in a viral wart. Inclusions are not a feature.
- In *granular cell tumor* the hyperplastic overlying squamous epithelium often shows an infiltrative growth pattern, in contrast to the exophytic nature of verruciform xanthoma. The granular cells are larger, often have a syncytial appearance, and typically stain positively with the PAS reaction.
- *Verrucous carcinoma* has both exophytic and endophytic components, the latter appearing as deeply penetrating bulbous epithelial processes. The epithelium often has a 'watery' appearance and xanthoma cells are not a feature.

Angiokeratoma corporis diffusum

Clinical features

Angiokeratoma corporis diffusum (Anderson-Fabry disease) is a sex-linked recessive disorder of glycosphingolipid metabolism with a high mortality. It is very rare with an approximate incidence of 1 in 200 000.[1] Deficiency of the lysosomal enzyme α-galactosidase A leads to the widespread accumulation of neutral glycolipids, mainly globotriaosylceramide (GB3, ceramide trihexoside), and elevated urinary trihexoxylceramide levels.[1–6]

Globotriaosylceramide is normally broken down by α-galactosidase A to produce galactose and lactosylceramide. The full-blown syndrome is normally seen only in men, since female carriers have 15% to 40% greater enzyme activity than their male siblings or offspring. Heterozygotes, however, usually display abnormal ophthalmological and ultrastructural features.[7] Occasionally, heterozygous females may manifest signs and symptoms due to extreme X inactivation (lyonization) of the healthy X-chromosome.[7,8] Cutaneous lesions are believed to occur in about 20% of heterozygous females.[9]

In males, the disease normally presents in childhood as episodes of excruciating intermittent pain, frequently in the fingers and toes.[10] The attacks may be accompanied by fever, edema, and malaise. Patients may also have hypohidrosis, lymphedema, acroparesthesia, and peripheral vasomotor disturbance affecting the heart, kidney, and central nervous system (CNS). Heat intolerance and telangiectases of the ears are often present early in the course of the disease.[11,12]

The characteristic angiokeratomata develop after puberty and present as tiny red–black bilaterally symmetrical papules, 0.5–2 mm in diameter, with slight hyperkeratosis.[10] Lesions are typically seen in the bathing trunk distribution including the thighs, buttocks, lower back, penis, and scrotum, although occasional lesions may also be seen on the trunk or buccal mucosa (Figs 13.28 and 13.29). The number of angiokeratomata is highly variable. Atypical cases can present with an oligosymptomatic phenotype which includes only very few cutaneous angiokeratomata and asymptomatic involvement of organs such as the kidney and the heart.[13] A female heterozygote with multiple nonkeratotic cutaneous angiomas has also been described.[14] Nonvascular proliferations have been reported in patients with Fabry disease, including polyarteritis nodosa and leg ulcers.[15,16] Telangiectasias develop in up to one-fourth of affected males.[12,17,18] The presence of angiokeratomas and telangiectasias has been correlated with disease severity.[17]

In a patient in whom the diagnosis is suspected, confirmation can usually be obtained by an ophthalmic examination. The conjunctival vessels may be tortuous or aneurysmal, as may the retinal vessels, and slit-lamp examination of the eyes reveals characteristic whorled, corneal linear opacities (verticillate cornea) (Fig. 13.30). Enzyme assay of α-galactosidase A can be performed using peripheral leukocytes or cutaneous fibroblasts. Hair root analysis has been recommended for the detection of heterozygotes.[19]

Affected males can develop transient cerebrovascular accidents, but one of the most common causes of death is renal failure.[20–22] In the early stages, proteinuria is seen and microscopy of the urinary sediment sometimes

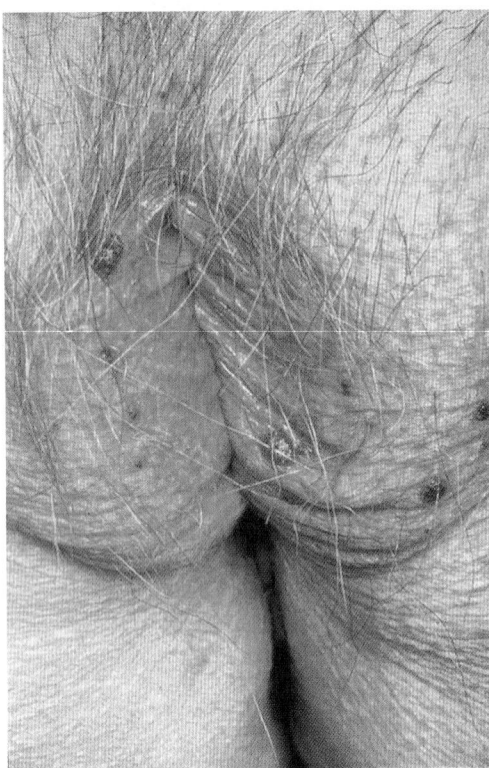

Fig. 13.28
Angiokeratoma corporis diffusum: tiny grouped red papules are present on the buttocks, a characteristic site. By courtesy of the Institute of Dermatology, London, UK.

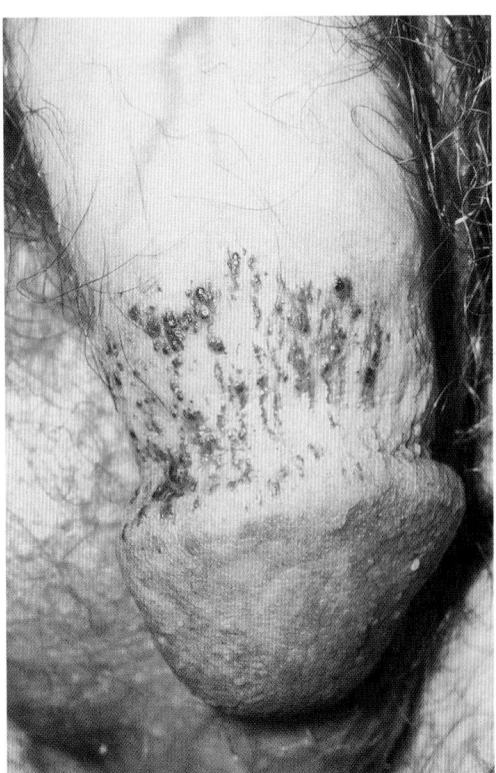

Fig. 13.29
Angiokeratoma corporis diffusum: conspicuous angiokeratomata on the penis, a commonly affected site. By courtesy of R.A. Marsden, MD, St George's Hospital, London, UK.

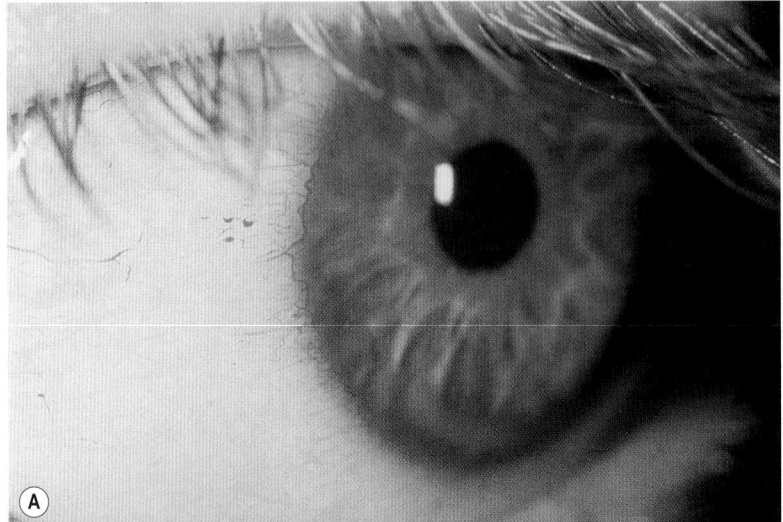

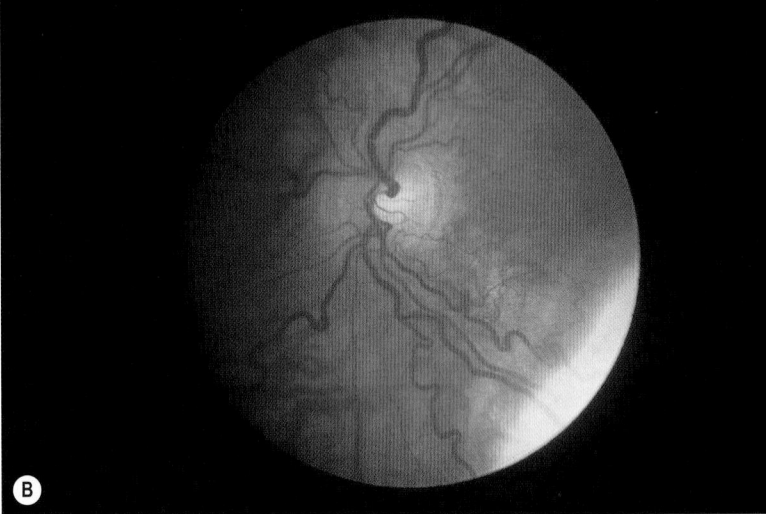

Fig. 13.30
Angiokeratoma corporis diffusum: (**A**) tortuous conjunctival vessels; (**B**) tortuous retinal vessels. By courtesy of S. Parker, MD, St Thomas' Hospital, London, UK.

reveals characteristic lipid-laden cells even before proteinuria develops (*Fig. 13.31*). Electron microscopy may reveal the typical inclusions (*Fig. 13.32*).

Cardiac involvement is found in approximately 20% of patients.[22,23] Glycosphingolipid deposits in the conducting system, myocardium, endocardium, and valves may give rise to angina, electrocardiographic abnormalities, hypertrophic cardiomyopathy, hypertension, mitral valve incompetence, and aortic medial degeneration.[24–30] Cardiovascular disease was found to be the most common cause of death in patients in a study of the Fabry registry, but cardiovascular outcomes are linked to coexisting severe chronic renal disease.[31,32]

Oral and dental abnormalities are more common than previously realized and include the presence of cysts/pseudocysts of the maxillary sinuses and maxillary prognathism.[33]

Pathogenesis and histologic features

A variety of genetic defects has been identified including point mutations, gene rearrangements, and deletions resulting in defects of α-galactosidase A.[34–37] However, rare patients with angiokeratoma corporis diffusum but without detectable mutation in the α-galactosidase gene have been described.[38–40] Patients with Fabry disease have elevated serum levels of vascular endothelial growth factor (VEGF-a), which could account for the vascular proliferation seen in this disease.[41]

The skin lesions are composed of ectatic blood-filled vessels in the papillary dermis, associated with slight hyperkeratosis (*Figs 13.33* and *13.34*). A characteristic feature is vacuolation of endothelial cells due to lipid deposits.

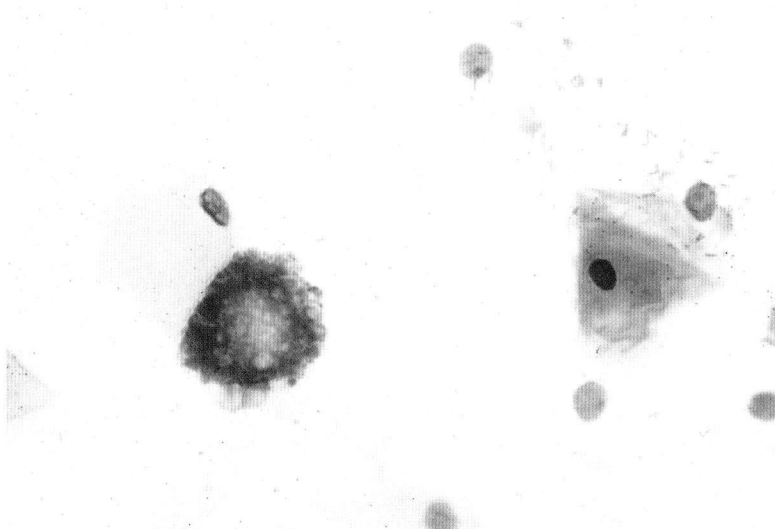

Fig. 13.31
Angiokeratoma corporis diffusum: urinary sediment stained with toluidine blue. The metachromasia (purple coloration) is due to the presence of intracytoplasmic sulfatides.

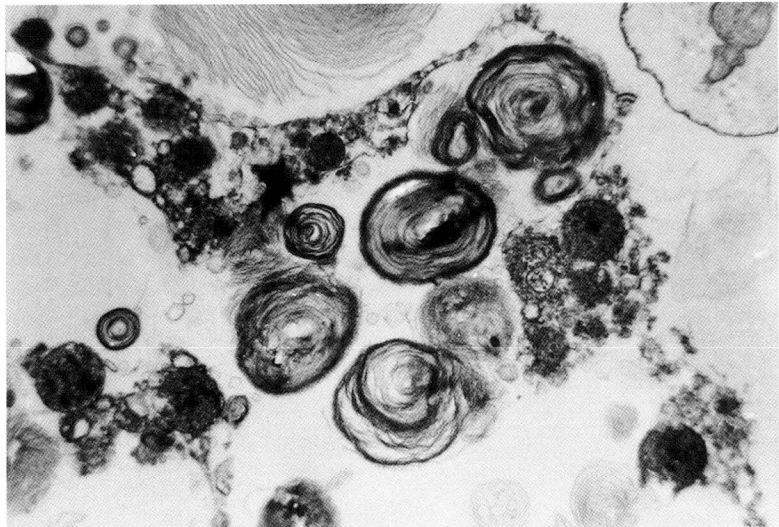

Fig. 13.32
Angiokeratoma corporis diffusum: electron micrograph of urine sediment, showing typical concentrically lamellated inclusions.

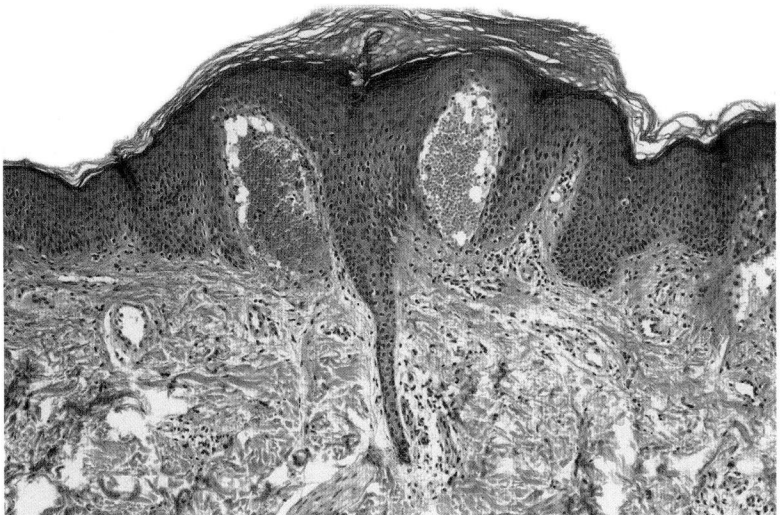

Fig. 13.33
Angiokeratoma corporis diffusum: ectatic blood-filled vascular channels expand the papillary dermis. Note the hyperkeratosis.

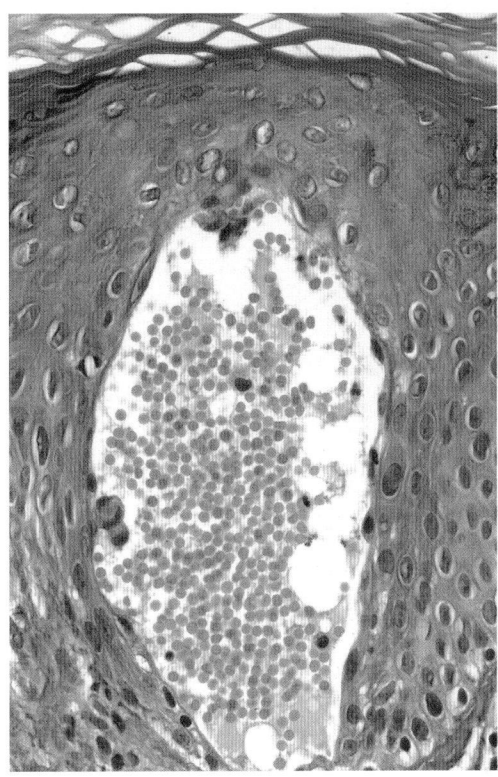

Fig. 13.34
Angiokeratoma corporis diffusum: close-up view.

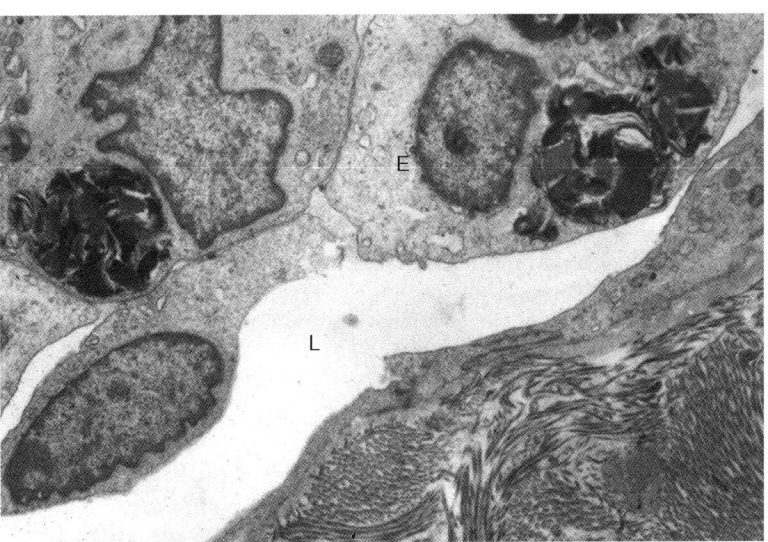

Fig. 13.35
Angiokeratoma corporis diffusum: the endothelial cells of this small blood vessel contain typical inclusions (L, lumen; E, endothelial cell).

The latter are doubly refractile and can usually be demonstrated in frozen material tissue sections. They may also be identified in toluidine blue-stained material. On electron microscopy, lamellar electron-dense inclusion bodies are present within endothelial cells, pericytes, smooth muscle cells, fibroblasts, sweat gland epithelium, and macrophages. It is believed that these are due to lipid deposition within lysosomes (*Fig. 13.35*). Lamellar bodies have also been identified in the endothelial cells of affected vessels with polyarteritis nodosa in a patient with Fabry disease.[15]

Differential diagnosis

Other forms of angiokeratomata, for example those of Mibelli or Fordyce, should be clinically distinguishable by their site and distribution although their histopathological appearances are identical. It should be noted, however, that diffuse angiokeratomata may also be seen in fucosidosis, α-galactosidosis,

Table 13.3
Classification of the amyloidoses

Systemic amyloidosis	Localized amyloidosis
Primary (due to an occult plasma cell dyscrasia)	Organs other than the skin*
Myeloma associated	Primary cutaneous
Secondary	Lichen, macular, and biphasic
Hemodialysis associated	Secondary cutaneous
Heredofamilial[†]	Associated with neoplasms, porokeratosis, and PUVA therapy
Amyloid elastosis	Familial cutaneous, nodular

*Not discussed further in this chapter.
[†]Including familial Mediterranean fever, Muckle-Wells syndrome, familial amyloidotic polyneuropathy.

sialidosis, aspartylglycosaminuria, α-N-acetylgalactosaminidase deficiency (Kanzaki disease), human beta-mannosidosis, adult-onset GM1 gangliosidosis, and indeed, diffuse angiokeratomata of a benign type may occur in patients with normal enzyme activities.[42–47] Widespread angiokeratomata have also been described as an exceptional finding in tuberous sclerosis and in a patient with Hodgkin lymphoma as a possible paraneoplastic syndrome.[48,49]

The amyloidoses

Amyloidosis is characterized by the extracellular deposition of a protein associated with particular tinctorial and ultrastructural properties. The amyloidoses are classified according to whether the amyloid deposition is systemic or localized (*Table 13.3*).

The most characteristic staining patterns of amyloid are seen with Congo red or Dylon (cotton dye pagoda red No. 9), which show apple-green birefringence under polarized light (*Fig. 13.36*).[1] Unfortunately, this is not specific, and green birefringence may also be seen with collagen and in colloid milium, porphyria, and lipoid proteinosis. Amyloid deposits, which are PAS positive, may also be identified by the cotton dye Sirius red, or metachromatically using methyl or cresyl violet.[2] Further confirmatory evidence can be obtained by staining with thioflavine-T and examination using fluorescence microscopy or by immunocytochemistry (see below) (*Fig. 13.37*).

Amyloid shows characteristic and specific electron microscopic features of rigid, straight, nonbranching amyloid filaments with a diameter of 6–10 nm showing a hollow core on cross-section (*Fig. 13.38*).[3] They are haphazardly distributed, lack the cross-banding of collagen, and are embedded in an electron-dense amorphous ground substance, which is probably composed of polysaccharides.

X-ray diffraction and infrared spectroscopy reveal a beta-pleated antiparallel configuration.[4,5] Fibrils with a beta-pleated configuration are insoluble and highly resistant to proteolysis. This, combined with a lack of immunogenicity, results in their persistence at the site of deposition and subsequent tissue-damaging effects.

All forms of amyloid contain up to 14% by dry weight of a nonfibrillary protein, the serum amyloid P (SAP) component.[2,6] The function of SAP is unknown, but it has been suggested that it may be primarily involved in the deposition and maintenance of the fibrillary components.[2] Its presence, identified immunohistochemically, is a useful adjunct to the diagnosis of amyloidosis.[7] However, it should be appreciated that the antibody also labels degenerate elastic fibers. The fibrillary component, however, may be derived in very different ways in each of the recognized types of amyloidosis:[8]

- In primary and myeloma-associated amyloidoses it consists of immunoglobulin light chains (most often of lambda type, or a part thereof).
- In the secondary form the fibrillary component is composed of amyloid A protein, which is derived from a normal serum constituent known as serum amyloid A protein. This serum protein, which is an HDL3-associated apolipoprotein, is an acute phase reactant.[2,8]

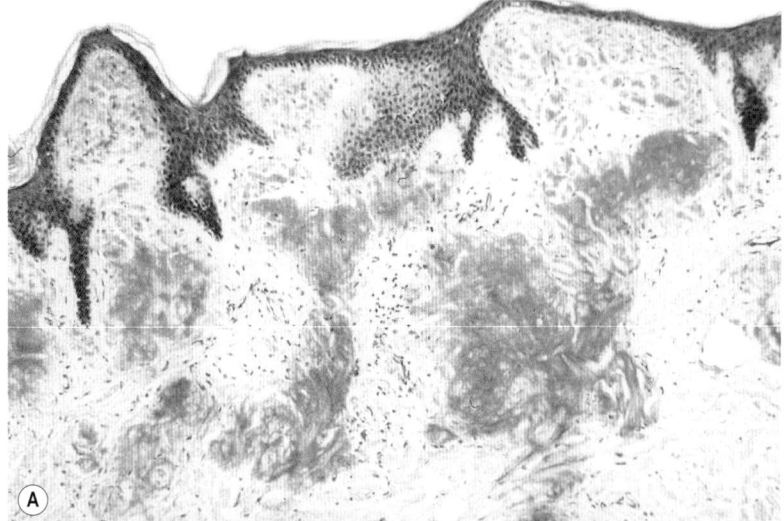
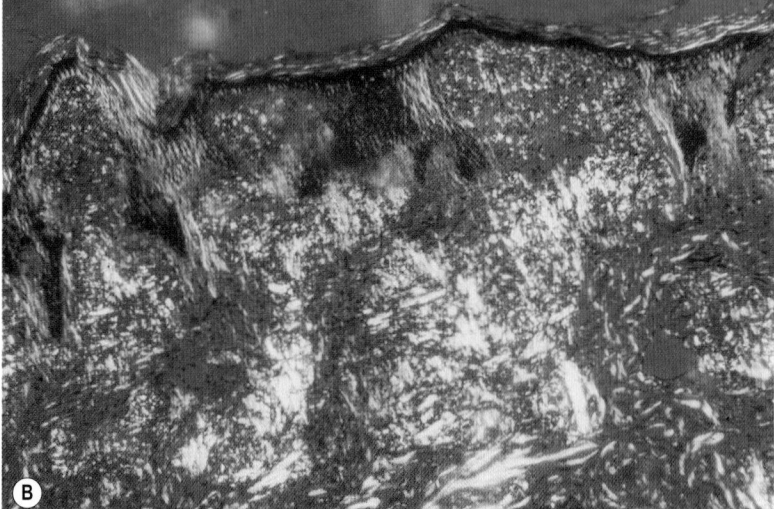

Fig. 13.36
Cutaneous amyloidosis: (**A**) positive staining with Congo red; (**B**) there is intense apple-green birefringence when viewed with polarized light.

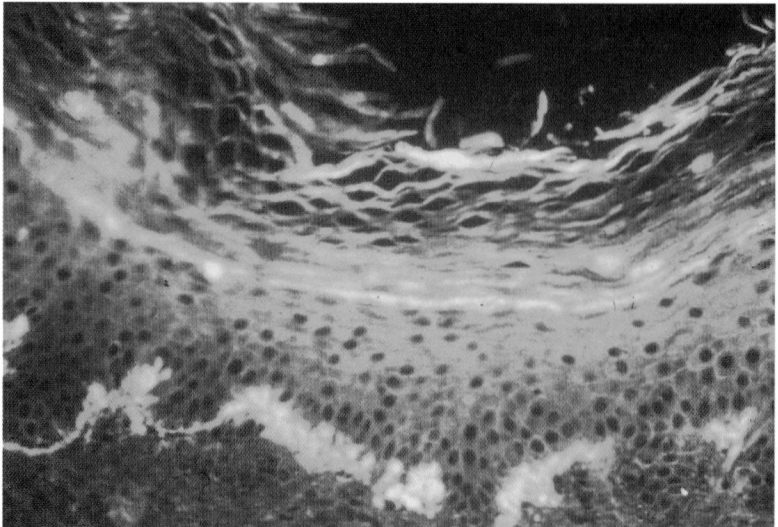

Fig. 13.37
Cutaneous amyloidosis: positive immunofluorescence just beneath the epidermis in a case of macular amyloid (thioflavine-T).

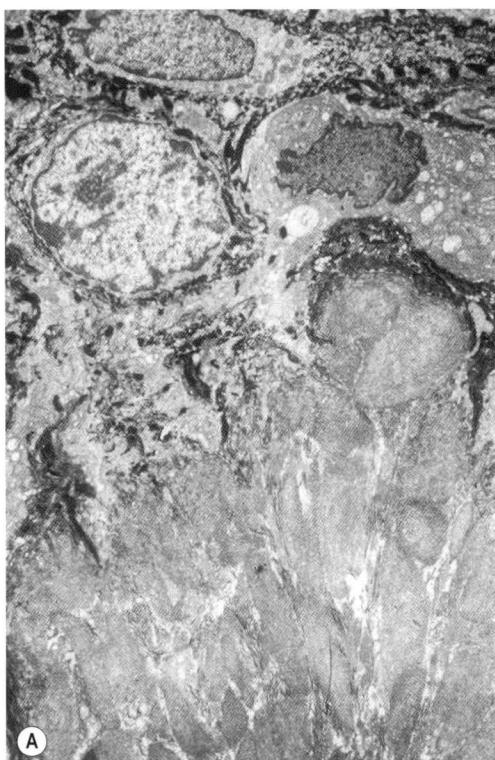

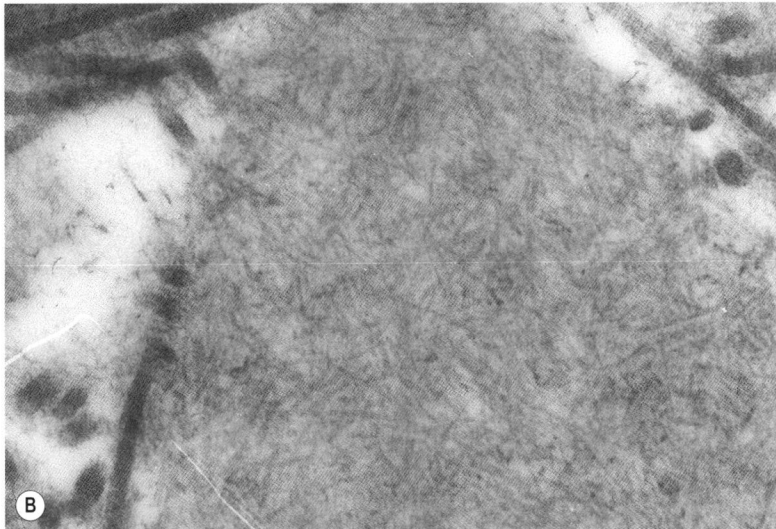

Fig. 13.38
Cutaneous amyloidosis: (**A**) electron micrograph of macular amyloidosis showing nodular deposits in the superficial dermis; (**B**) the characteristic randomly orientated, straight, nonbranching appearance of amyloid filaments.

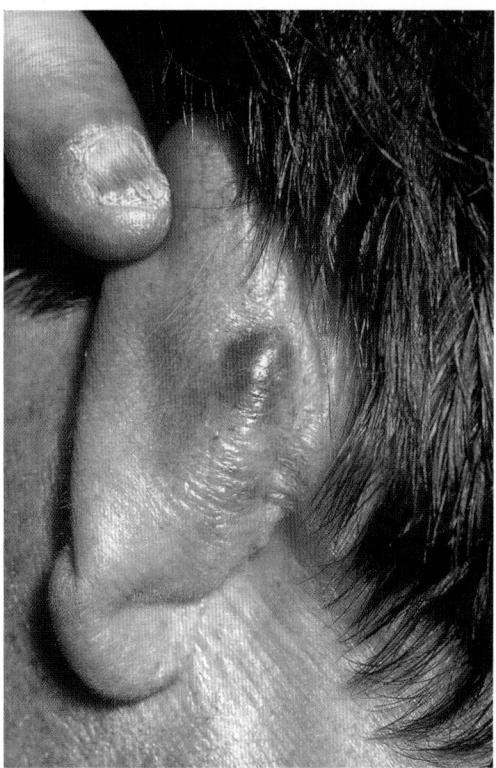

Fig. 13.39
Primary systemic amyloidosis: a waxy nodule is present behind the ear. Note the purpura. By courtesy of R.A. Marsden, MD, St George's Hospital, London, UK.

- Primary cutaneous amyloidosis is derived from filamentous degeneration of keratin filaments (amyloid-K) (see below).[9,10]

The capacity to form amyloid in the primary and myeloma-associated variants appears to be dependent upon the inherent ability of a segment of the variable region of the light chain to adopt a beta-pleated configuration.[3] This capability is only evident in a proportion of (so-called amyloidogenic) Bence Jones proteins, which explains why not all patients with multiple myeloma develop amyloidosis. Primary and myeloma-associated amyloidoses can be distinguished histochemically from secondary amyloidosis using the potassium permanganate reaction.[11] The former are potassium permanganate resistant whereas the latter is sensitive and loses its affinity for Congo red following exposure. 'Endocrine' amyloid is also resistant to the effects of potassium permanganate solution, as is senile cardiac amyloid. Therefore, although the amyloidoses all include, by definition, amyloid deposition, they in fact represent a very diverse group of conditions.

Primary and myeloma-associated systemic amyloidoses

Cutaneous disease occurs in up to 40% of patients with primary (due to occult plasma cell dyscrasia) and myeloma-associated systemic amyloidosis.[1-5]

Clinical features

Primary and myeloma-associated systemic amyloidoses predominantly affect the elderly (mean onset at 65 years of age) and show a slight predilection for males.[2] Up to 15% of patients with myeloma have coexisting primary amyloidosis. Occasional patients present with primary systemic amyloidosis and only develop multiple myeloma later.[6]

The early clinical changes, which are often mild, non-specific, and very difficult to diagnose, include weight loss, hoarseness, dyspnea, fatigue, paresthesia, and lightheadedness.[7] Subsequently, the most frequent features are development of the carpal tunnel syndrome and edema due to renal and cardiac involvement. Bilateral carpal tunnel syndrome may be the first symptom of the disease.[8]

The commonest cutaneous manifestation is hemorrhage (purpura, petechiae, and frank ecchymoses) due to deposition of amyloid within blood vessel walls, with resultant fragility (*Figs 13.39–13.42*).[9] It occurs most typically on the hands (often posttraumatic) and around the eyes, when the purpura may follow proctoscopy or vomiting (*Fig. 13.43*). Lesions are sometimes also evident in the nasolabial folds, the neck, axillae, umbilicus, anogenital region, and within the oral cavity.[4,10-12] Prominent hemorrhagic bullae may be present.[12,13] Rarely, systemic amyloidosis presents with solitary vulval lesions which may mimic a condyloma acuminatum.[14,15]

Blistering is sometimes an additional feature, which occurs due to cleavage developing within the amyloid deposits as a consequence of shearing stresses.[12,16-29] The blisters are often hemorrhagic, and occur most often on the tongue, buccal or labial mucosa although they may be more widespread and thus mimic those of bullous pemphigoid.[16,27] Blisters can sometimes arise on the dorsal surfaces of the hands and fingers and the extensor aspect of the forearms and epidermolysis bullosa acquisita then enters the differential diagnosis (*Fig. 13.44*). Healed lesions are sometimes associated with the development of milia.[21] Bullous amyloidosis most often develops in patients with systemic disease, particularly myeloma associated.[18] Rarely, however, it

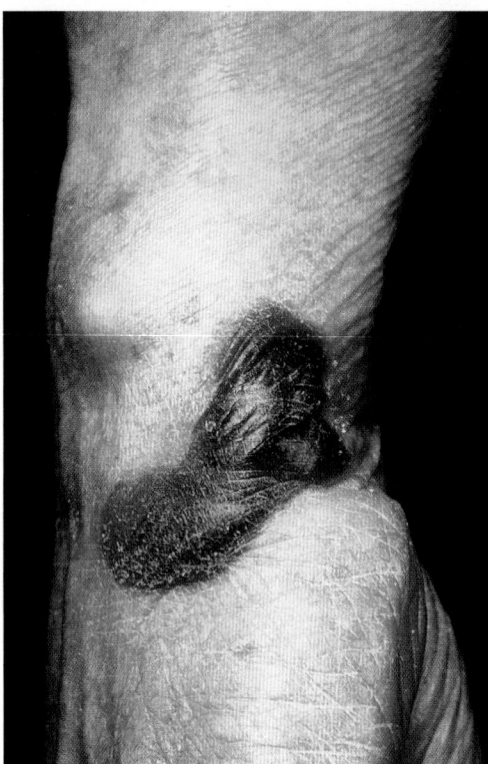

Fig. 13.40
Primary systemic amyloidosis: hemorrhagic bullous lesion on wrist. By courtesy of the Institute of Dermatology, London, UK.

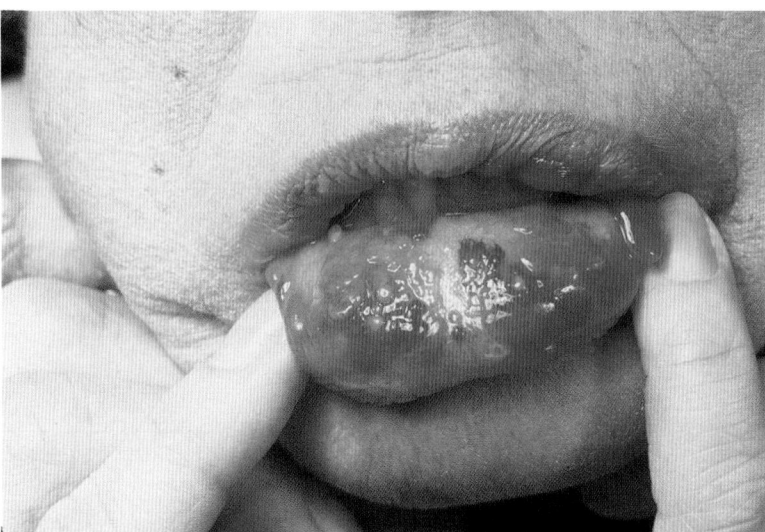

Fig. 13.41
Primary systemic amyloidosis: papular mucosal lesions with hemorrhage on the inner aspect of the lower lip. By courtesy of R.A. Marsden, MD, St George's Hospital, London, UK.

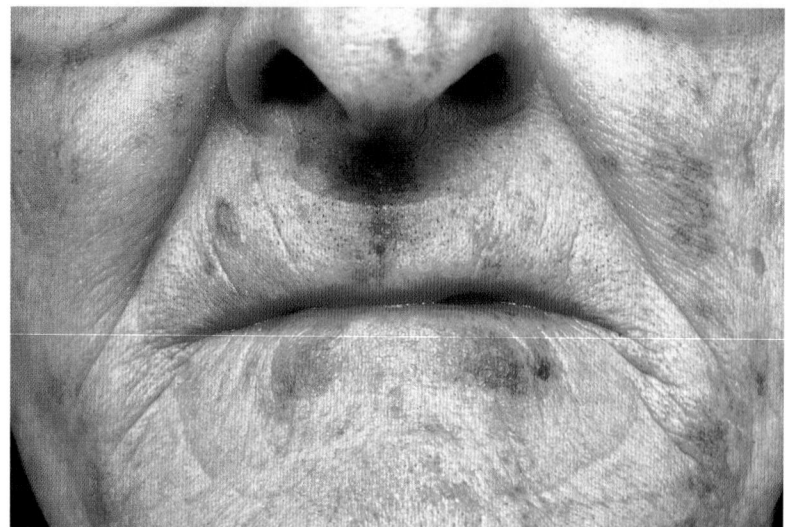

Fig. 13.42
Primary systemic amyloidosis: erythematous and purpuric lesions on the face of an elderly male. By courtesy of the Institute of Dermatology, London, UK.

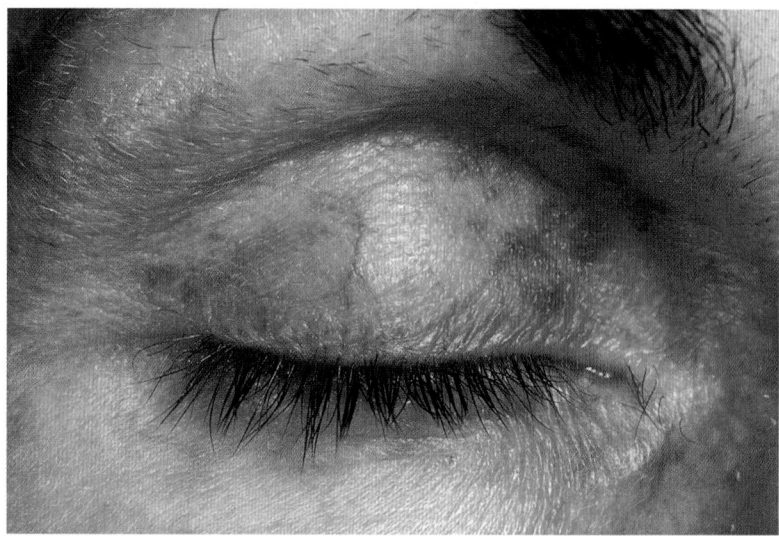

Fig. 13.43
Primary systemic amyloidosis: small macular purpuric lesions at a classical site. By courtesy of R.A. Marsden, MD, St George's Hospital, London, UK.

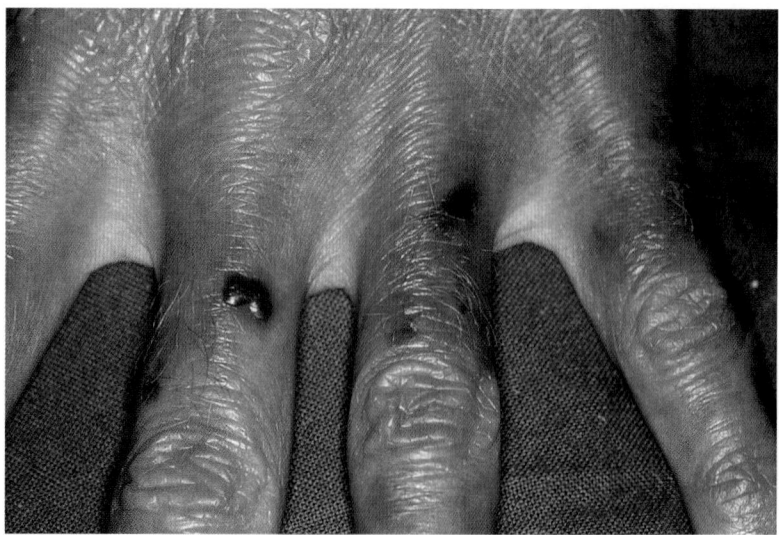

Fig. 13.44
Primary systemic amyloidosis: blood-filled blisters on the dorsal aspect of the fingers. By courtesy of R.A. Marsden, MD, St George's Hospital, London, UK.

may complicate primary cutaneous amyloidosis.[16,26,28,29] Rare cases present an elastolytic appearance and development of cordlike indurations associated with intermittent claudication. Prominent perivascular deposition of amyloid has been documented in these patients.[30,31]

In more advanced cases, waxy, smooth, shiny papules, plaques, and even nodules develop. Cystic nodular lesions have also been reported.[32] The papules are skin-colored or yellow and have a dome-shaped appearance.[10,33] They are found predominantly on the face (especially the eyelids), head and neck, axillae, umbilicus, inguinal region, and the perineum.[4,10] In severely affected patients the clinical appearances with taut skin, particularly affecting the face, hands, and digits, may mimic scleroderma.[10,33] Alopecia and nail dystrophy are sometimes evident (Fig. 13.45).[34–36] Chronic paronychia,

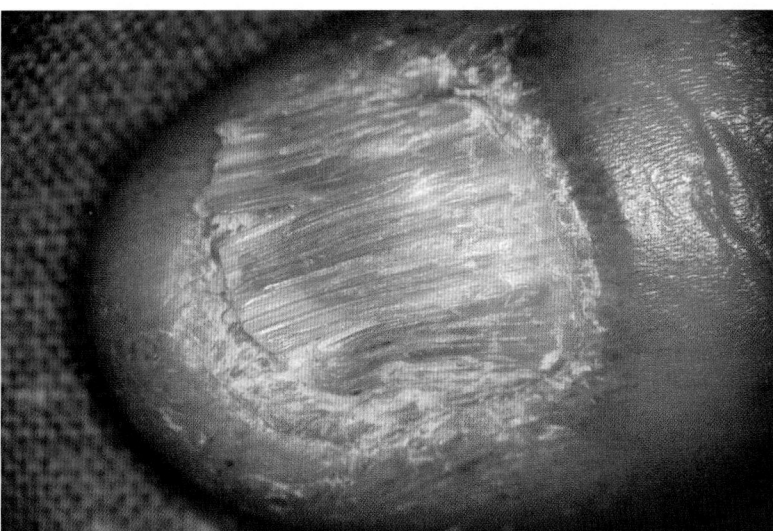

Fig. 13.45
Primary systemic amyloidosis: nail dystrophy as seen in this example is a very rare manifestation. By courtesy of R.A. Marsden, MD, St George's Hospital, London, UK.

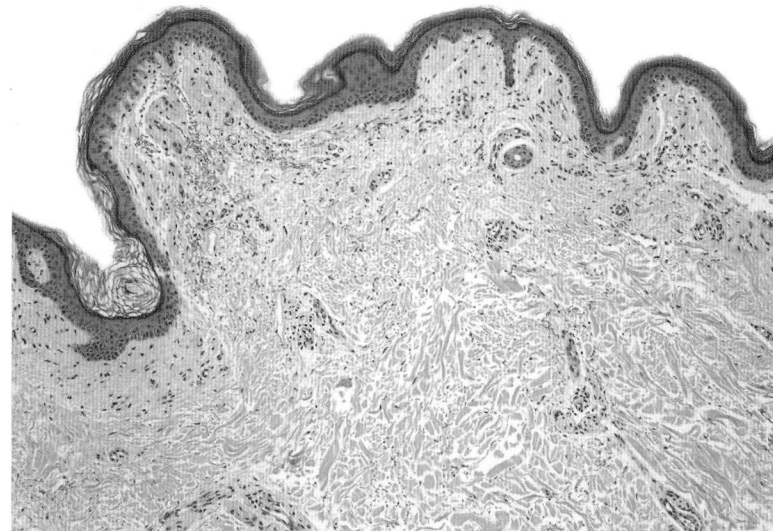

Fig. 13.47
Primary systemic amyloidosis: the superficial blood vessels are thickened due to amyloid deposition.

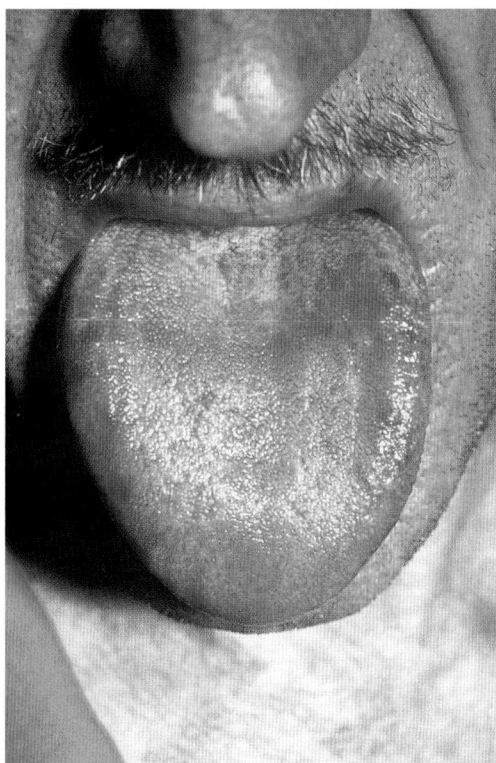

Fig. 13.46
Primary systemic amyloidosis: macroglossia. By courtesy of R.A. Marsden, MD, St George's Hospital, London, UK.

neuropathy, and renal failure or the nephrotic syndrome. Splenomegaly is a feature in less than 10% of cases.[5] Intestinal involvement can lead to malabsorption or an ulcerative colitis-like picture, sometimes with hemorrhage.[4] Pseudo-obstruction, diarrhea, and constipation can also occur.[7] There is no effective treatment for systemic primary amyloidosis and the prognosis is therefore grave. Mortality relates primarily to cardiac and renal involvement.[2,3]

Histologic features

Masses of eosinophilic, amorphous, fissured material are present in the dermis and subcutaneous tissues.[10,43] The overlying epidermis is often stretched and flattened, but – in contrast to the macular and lichenoid variants – shows no evidence of amyloid deposition. In mild cases the changes may be limited to the perivascular tissues, but in more extensive disease large aggregates are usually evident. Involvement of blood vessel walls, arrector pili muscles, skin adnexa, and subcutaneous fat (amyloid rings) is frequently present (Figs 13.47 and 13.48).[4,10,33] Amyloid deposits around the pilosebaceous units may be accompanied by follicular atrophy with resultant hair loss.[10] There is usually little secondary inflammatory cell infiltration.

In those cases associated with blistering, the vesicle appears in an intradermal or less commonly subepidermal location. The dermis, in addition to showing amyloid deposits, often in association with blood vessel walls, also shows a fragmented appearance due to the presence of cleft like spaces.[15] Purpura is frequently marked.

Clinically normal skin shows histologic evidence of amyloid deposition in up to 50% of patients.[33]

An exceptional case of reactive eccrine syringofibroadenomatosis secondary to primary cutaneous amyloidosis has been reported.[44]

Secondary amyloidosis

Secondary amyloidosis develops as a consequence of chronic inflammatory conditions or infections. Cutaneous involvement has not been recognized as a clinical feature of secondary systemic amyloidosis. Yet in one publication it was described in eight out of nine patients with amyloidosis complicating rheumatoid arthritis.[1] It is of interest to note that a considerable number of chronic dermatoses may be associated with the development of secondary amyloidosis including psoriasis, lepromatous leprosy, hidradenitis suppurativa, chronically infected burns, and dystrophic epidermolysis bullosa.[2–4] In patients with no cutaneous lesions and symptoms suggestive of systemic amyloidosis, the diagnosis can be confirmed by Congo red staining of abdominal fat fine-needle aspirates or biopsies.[5–10] Most studies have shown

palmodigital erythematous swelling, and induration of the hands have been described.[37] The presence of these features in conjunction with macroglossia and the carpal tunnel syndrome is highly suggestive of primary or myeloma-associated systemic amyloidosis (Fig. 13.46). In addition to macroglossia, the tongue may be covered with waxy papules, nodules, and plaques and occasionally it is ulcerated or fissured.[4] As a consequence, speaking and swallowing difficulties are not infrequently encountered. The sicca syndrome may also be a manifestation of primary systemic amyloidosis.[36,38,39] Exceptionally, association with normolipemic xanthoma has also been documented.[40–42]

Hepatomegaly is found in about 50% of cases and there may also be evidence of cardiomyopathy with arrhythmia or heart failure, peripheral

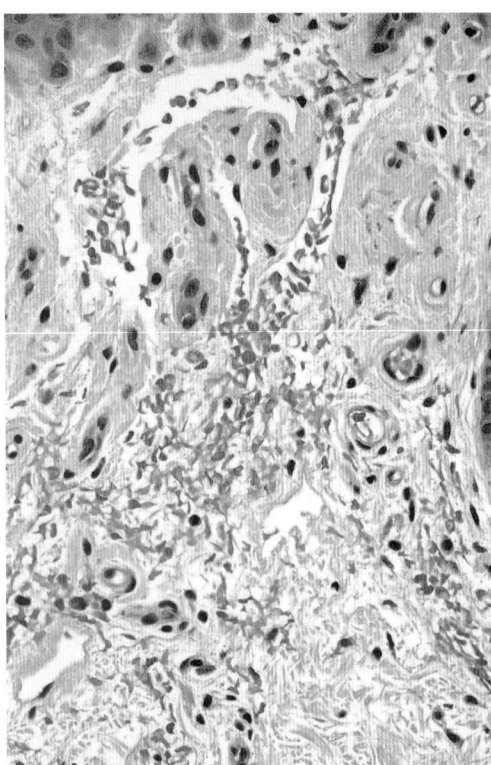

Fig. 13.48
Primary systemic amyloidosis: high-power view of *Fig. 13.47*. Note the red cell extravasation.

good sensitivity and specificity (~70–90%), but others have demonstrated poor sensitivity in abdominal fat pad biopsies.[10]

Although frank clinical lesions are not commonly a feature of secondary amyloidosis, sometimes small deposits are found in specimens of normal skin.[11] Usually these are present in a perivascular location, but may occasionally be present elsewhere in the dermis or even in subcutaneous fat.[12] Deposition of amyloid around sweat glands may also be seen. Deposits are said to be focal and abdominal subcutaneous fat has been recommended as the site that is most likely to be positive.[1,5,13] Hemodialysis-associated amyloidosis is a distinctive form of secondary amyloidosis and is described below.

Hemodialysis-associated amyloidosis

Clinical features

This variant of amyloidosis, induced by beta-2-microglobulin, occurs in patients on long-term hemodialysis.[1–5] Exceptionally, cases may present after short-term hemodialysis.[6] The most commonly involved organs are the heart, gastrointestinal tract, and lungs.[1] Interestingly, the disease does not seem to involve the spleen.[1] Carpal tunnel syndrome, polyarthralgia, and destructive spondyloarthropathy have also been documented.[4,7–9] The walls of blood vessels are often involved, whereas bone lesions are relatively rare, although pathological fractures may occur.[7,9,10] Cutaneous involvement, which is very uncommon, has been reported to present as subcutaneous masses in the buttocks and shoulder, lichenoid papules and a wrinkled appearance of the skin of the palmar aspect of the fingers.[6,7,10–13] Rare cases of amyloidoma of the tongue and external auditory canal have been reported.[14–16]

Histologic features

In cases with skin involvement, the amyloid deposits have been found either in the subcutaneous tissue or in the papillary and reticular dermis, around sweat glands and hair follicles.[6,7,10–13] Occasionally, special stains are unhelpful in demonstrating amyloid and confirmation of the diagnosis by electron microscopy or, mass spectroscopy can confirm the diagnosis.[17]

12-Heredofamilial amyloidoses

Familial Mediterranean fever

Clinical features

This is an autosomal recessive inherited autoinflammatory disease. It is divided into two phenotypes: types 1 and 2. Type 1 is associated characterized by episodes of fever, serositis, peritonitis, synovitis, and in rare instances pericarditis and meningitis. Amyloidosis can result from the recurrent inflammatory episodes. In type 2, patients present initially with amyloidosis and are otherwise asymptomatic.[1–5] Cutaneous lesions are rare and consist of Henoch-Schönlein purpura and erythema of the lower limbs mimicking erysipelas.[1,6] Panniculitis, recurrent urticaria, polyarteritis nodosa, psoriasis-like lesions, bullous skin lesions, perivascular lymphocytic dermatitis, and sarcoidosis may also occur.[7–14] Nail fold capillary abnormalities consisting of increased tortuosity and enlargement of capillary loops have also been documented.[15,16] Cutaneous amyloid deposition has not been described.

Pathogenesis and histologic features

Familial Mediterranean fever is cause by mutations in *MEFV* on chromosome 16p13, a gene that encodes pyrin, a protein involved in deactivating the immune response.[5] Defects in pyrin lead to over production of interleukin-1, resulting in a proinflammatory state contributing to the formation of amyloid.[17] In familial Mediterranean fever, a serum precursor protein forms the amyloid in this condition. This precursor is a HDL known as serum amyloid A.

The erysipelas-like lesions are characterized by a perivascular mixed infiltrate of lymphocytes, histiocytes, and neutrophils with leukocytoclasia.[6] Vasculitis is not seen, although on direct immunofluorescence perivascular C3 and, less consistently IgM and fibrinogen, have been reported.[6] However, as noted above, leukocytoclastic vasculitis may be seen in this disease.

Cryopin-associated periodic syndrome (Muckle-Wells syndrome, familial cold autoinflammatory syndrome and neonatal-onset multisystem inflammatory disorder)

Cryopin-associated periodic syndrome is an autosomal inherited disease with variable penetrance that encompasses a spectrum of diseases that includes Muckle-Wells syndrome, familial cold autoinflammatory syndrome, and neonatal-onset multisystem inflammatory disorder.[1,2] All of the conditions have in common recurrent fevers, joint pain, and urticaria. They variably may have systemic amyloidosis, deafness, conjunctivitis, and severe neurological manifestations.[3,4] In the spectrum of disease, familial cold autoinflammatory syndrome represents the mild end of the spectrum and neonatal-onset multisystem inflammatory disorder the severe end.[1] In familial cold autoinflammatory syndrome, there is no deafness and the episodes of urticaria are precipitated by cold. Amyloidosis is more common in Muckle-Wells syndrome and severe neurologic manifestations are more common in neonatal-onset multisystem inflammatory disorder.[1,2] The same serum precursor protein (serum amyloid A) produces the amyloid. Cutaneous amyloidosis is not typically seen in Muckle-Wells syndrome. The disease is related to a gain in function mutation of *NLRP3* (also called *CIAS1*) that encodes cryopyrin, a protein that plays a role in the regulation of inflammation, and apoptosis via caspase-1-interleukin-1 axis.[1,2,5,6] Six patients with Muckle-Wells syndrome were described as having sclerotic, hyperpigmented plaques with hypertrichosis on the extremities and abdomen.[7]

The urticarial lesions are characterized by an upper to mid-dermal infiltrate of neutrophils with a few eosinophils and dermal edema.[8,9] Neutrophils are seen intravascularly and in vessel walls as well as around eccrine glands.[8,9] Although vasculitis has not been described, some vessels may contain fibrinoid deposits. Histologic features of the sclerotic lesions include dermal thickening with sclerosis of collagen bundles, fragmentation and thickening of elastic fibers, focal calcification of degenerated elastic fibers, superficial and deep perivascular and interstitial infiltrate of lymphocytes and histiocytes, numerous plasma cells and admixed eosinophils and mast cells.[7]

Familial amyloidotic polyneuropathy

Clinical features

Familial amyloidotic polyneuropathy is an autosomal dominant disease in which the deposition of amyloid occurs predominantly in peripheral nerves. The amyloid deposits in this disease consist in most cases of variant transthyretin with single amino acid substitutions.[1-3] Clinical manifestations include sensory then motor peripheral neuropathy predominantly affecting the limbs and autonomic dysfunction manifesting as alternating diarrhea and constipation, urinary incontinence, orthostatic hypotension, and sexual dysfunction.[3] The cutaneous manifestations comprise nonhealing ulcers, multiple atrophic scars, and anhidrosis of the lower limbs.[4,5] Patients may also have seborrheic dermatitis, acne, and onychomycosis, though some of these may be coincidental.[6] In some patients petechiae can be induced by gentle stroking of the skin.

Histologic features

Histologically, biopsies from clinically normal skin reveal the presence of amyloid in blood vessel walls, sweat glands, and arrector pili muscle.[4]

Amyloid elastosis

Clinical features

Amyloid elastosis is a very rare disease, characterized by cutaneous deposits of amyloid in association with elastic fibers of the skin. Only a handful of cases have been reported to date, all in the setting of systemic amyloidosis, except for one in the setting of primary cutaneous amyloidosis.[1-7] The clinical manifestations are variable. Most have skin-colored to yellow cobblestoned papules and plaques. Some patients had a pseudoxanthoma-like lesions on the neck and/or intertriginous areas.[1,2,3,6] One patient had widespread skin-colored papules and a whitish cobblestone plaque around the urethral meatus.[4] Some patients had cordlike thickening of superficial blood vessels, livedo reticularis-like changes on the trunk, Raynaud phenomenon, venous and arterial thrombosis, and the nephrotic syndrome.[1,2] The patient with primary cutaneous amyloidosis presented a plaque with prominent skin folds and peripheral erythema involving his left axilla.[7] The causes of the systemic amyloidosis included lambda light chain paraprotein and myeloma.[2-6]

Histologic features

Amyloid is seen in the dermis, around adnexal structures, surrounding elastic fibers, sometimes forming small globules, and in blood vessel walls, together with striking deposits in the dermal, subcutaneous, and serosal elastic tissue.[1-3,7]

Primary localized cutaneous amyloidosis, lichen and macular types

Clinical features

Lichen and macular amyloidoses (skin-limited amyloidoses) represent different manifestations of the same process and both entities may coexist (biphasic amyloidosis) or one may transform into the other.[1-4] A large study of primary localized cutaneous amyloidosis found that 67% of cases represented lichen amyloidosis, 8% macular amyloidosis, and 25% biphasic variants.[5] Although most cases are sporadic, up to 10% of patients demonstrate an autosomal dominant inheritance pattern (see familial primary cutaneous amyloidosis).[6,7]

Macular primary cutaneous amyloidosis. This is most commonly seen in patients from the Middle East, Asia, and Central and South America.[1,8] It affects females more often than males (3:1), is seen in younger age groups, and is usually a chronic condition.[9,10] Patients present with a macular, dark brown or grayish, symmetrical pigmentation, which occurs most frequently on the upper chest and back, although the extremities and face may also be affected (Fig. 13.49).[1,9] The lesions sometimes have a very characteristic reticulated or rippled appearance, which can be quite subtle, and they are

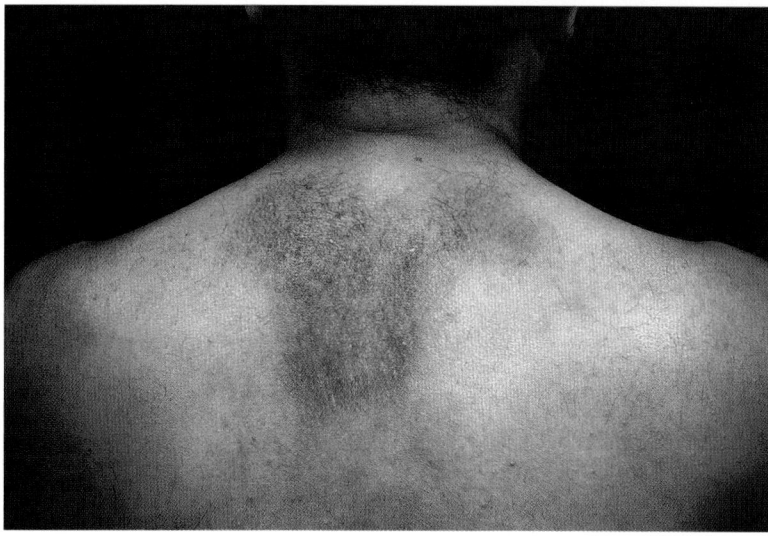

Fig. 13.49
Macular amyloid: hyperpigmented lesion in a characteristic site. By courtesy of R.A. Marsden, MD, St George's Hospital, London, UK.

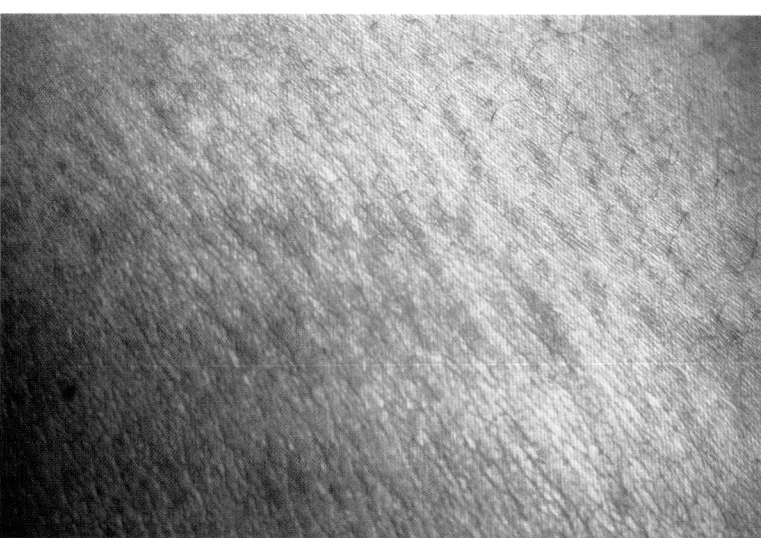

Fig. 13.50
Macular amyloid: close-up view of a lesion showing the typically rippled appearance. By courtesy of R.A. Marsden, MD, St George's Hospital, London, UK.

usually moderately pruritic (Fig. 13.50). More commonly, however, macular amyloid appears as small, 2–3 mm diameter lesions or else as confluent macular foci, which sometimes have superimposed micropapules.[8] Lesions sometimes follow Blaschko lines, resembling incontinentia pigmenti.[11,12] Exceptionally, widespread diffuse pigmentation occurs.[13] Predominantly hypopigmented macules have been described, mimicking guttate morphea and vitiligo.[14]

Papular or lichen amyloidosis. In papular or lichen amyloidosis, discrete papules and/or plaques occur, which are often scaly, persistent, and pigmented (Fig. 13.51). They are usually severely pruritic. Excoriations, lichenification, and nodular prurigo-like lesions due to chronic scratching are sometimes evident.[10] Lesions are especially common on the front of the shins and extensor aspect of the forearms (Figs 13.52 and 13.53).[15,16] The calves, ankles, dorsa of the feet, thighs, and trunk may also be affected.[17-19] Presentation is most often in young adults. The sex incidence is equal.[1,20] Lichen amyloidosis shows a predilection for the Chinese race and familial cases have been recorded.[18,19] An association with Epstein-Barr virus infection has been reported in a single case, but this was not confirmed in a larger study.[21]

Association with systemic disease is probably coincidental but there have been a number of cases described with progressive systemic sclerosis.[22,23]

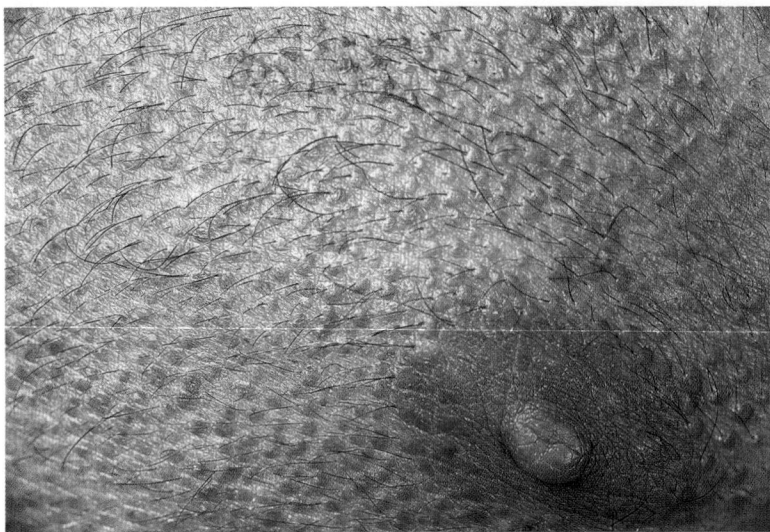

Fig. 13.51
Lichen amyloidosis: pigmented papules on the chest. By courtesy of R.A. Marsden, MD, St George's Hospital, London, UK.

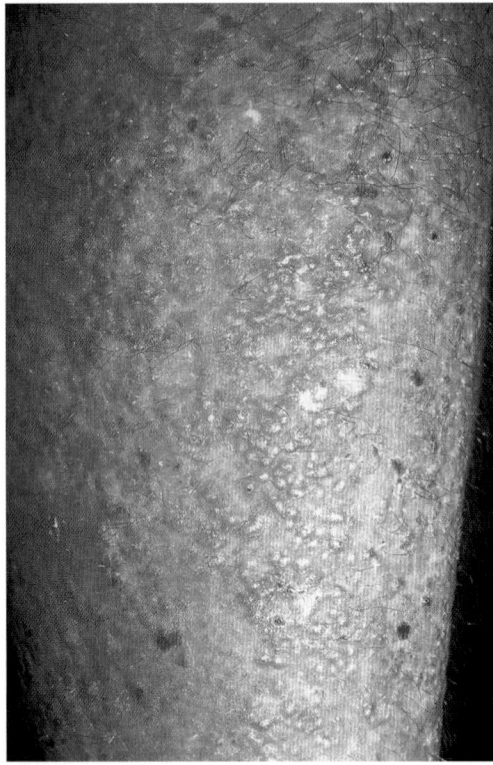

Fig. 13.52
Lichen amyloidosis: scaly lichenoid papules on the shin. By courtesy of R.A. Marsden, MD, St George's Hospital, London, UK.

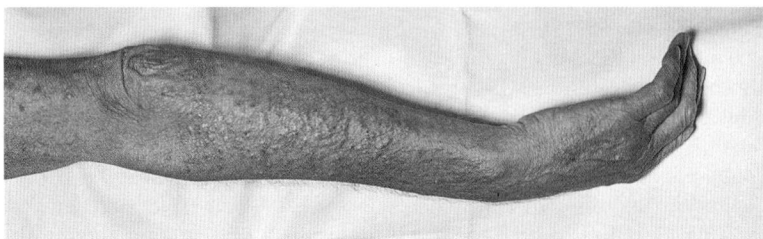

Fig. 13.53
Lichen amyloidosis: grouped, erythematoviolaceous papules, with a lichenoid surface and showing excoriations in some areas. By courtesy of R.A. Marsden, MD, St George's Hospital, London, UK.

Other primary cutaneous amyloidoses. These include anosacral and poikilodermatous variants:

- Anosacral amyloidosis presents as scaly hyperpigmented macules and lichenoid papules spreading out from the perianal skin.[24,25] It is seen in patients from Japan and China and is very rare. The disease may present early in life and its cause has not been established, although a relationship to keratinocyte apoptosis has been suggested.[25] Clinically, lesions can be confused with lichen simplex chronicus, a dermatophyte infection or even postinflammatory hyperpigmentation.
- Poikiloderma-like cutaneous amyloidosis is an extremely rare manifestation of localized cutaneous amyloidosis.[26,27] Patients present with poikilodermatous skin lesions and lichenoid papules. It may be associated with photosensitivity, short stature, and palmoplantar keratoderma.[27] Blisters are rarely seen. The condition presents early in life or in young adults. Confusion with other conditions associated with poikiloderma, including poikiloderma atrophicans vasculare, is possible. A single case of poikiloderma-like amyloidosis associated with lichen, dyschromic, and bullous variants has been described.[28]

Pathogenesis and histologic features

Chronic irritation to the skin has been proposed as the cause of amyloid deposition in the macular and lichenoid variants, although this has never been proven.[29,30] The documentation, however, of friction amyloidosis due to nylon brush skin massage and towels does offer some support to this hypothesis.[31–34] It may be that chronic trauma in a susceptible or 'primed' individual may be associated with an increased risk of developing cutaneous amyloidosis. It has been suggested that amyloid deposition in lichen amyloidosis is a consequence of scratching, as pruritus tends to be the presenting symptom even before amyloid is detected in skin biopsies.[35] The chronic damage to the epidermis induces apoptosis of keratinocytes and this leads to amyloid deposition in the papillary dermis. A similar mechanism has been proposed in notalgia paresthetica. This is a condition characterized by pruritus, a burning sensation, and paresthesia or hyperesthesia in an area of the back between dermatomes D2 and D6.[36,37] The resultant irritation and scratching induce cutaneous hyperpigmentation and amyloid deposition. It has even been suggested that the cutaneous amyloidosis observed in patients with multiple endocrine neoplasia type 2A is secondary to notalgia paresthetica (see below).[38]

In both variants the amyloid is deposited high in the papillary dermis, often immediately adjacent to the epidermis.[8,9,17,39,40]

In the macular type, the amount of amyloid present is often very small and focally distributed. It frequently has a faceted appearance (*Figs 13.54–13.56*).[2,9] Special stains and/or immunocytochemistry are sometimes necessary as the deposits can easily be missed. Intraepidermal cytoid bodies

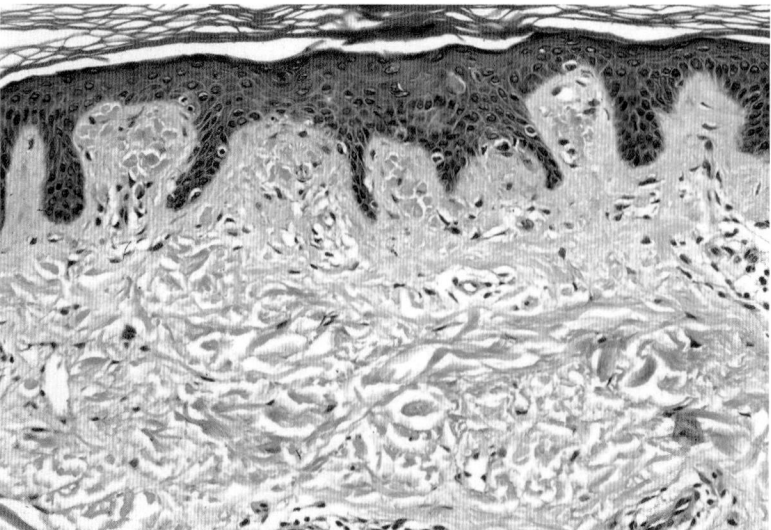

Fig. 13.54
Macular amyloidosis: typical eosinophilic faceted deposits are present in the papillary dermis.

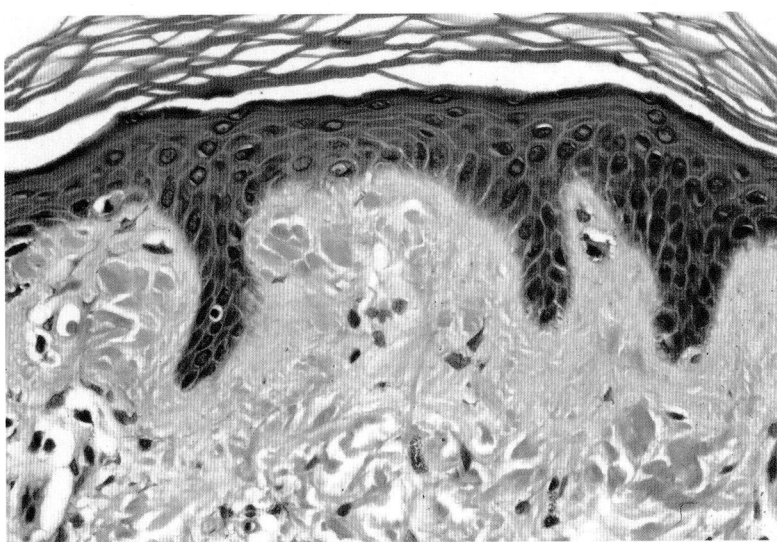

Fig. 13.55
Macular amyloidosis: close-up view of faceted deposits.

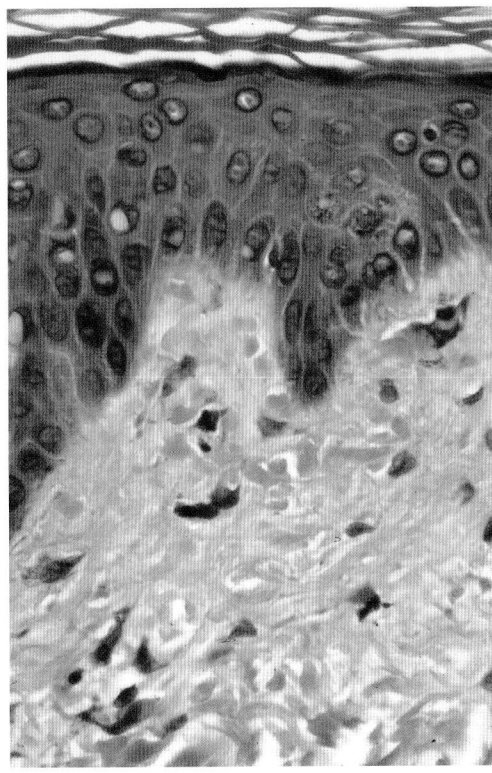

Fig. 13.56
Macular amyloidosis: pigmentary incontinence is typically present.

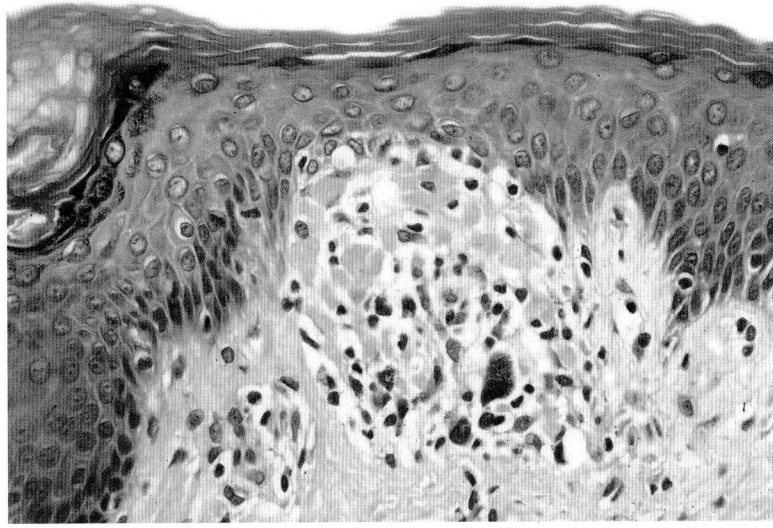

Fig. 13.57
Lichen amyloidosis: there is hyperkeratosis, acanthosis, and basal cell hydropic degeneration; small eosinophilic globules are present in the papillary dermis. A mild chronic inflammatory cell infiltrate is present. Note the pigmentary incontinence.

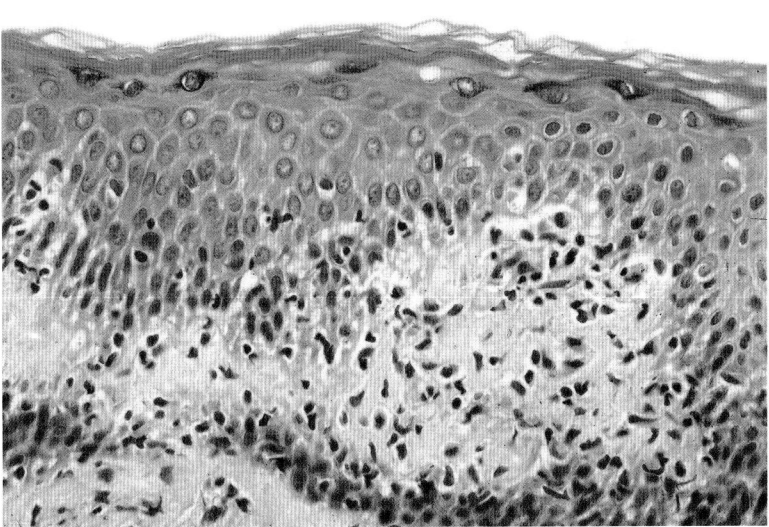

Fig. 13.58
Lichen amyloidosis: in this view, there is interface change and a lymphocytic infiltrate.

are present in about 33% of cases.[8] Typically, there is associated pigmentary incontinence, but only minor epidermal changes of hyperkeratosis and acanthosis are generally evident. Melanin pigment may be present in the stratum corneum. A slight perivascular chronic inflammatory cell infiltrate is often found in the superficial dermis.[9] Mild vacuolar interface alteration can be present.[14]

In papular or lichen amyloidosis, the histopathological changes are similar and cannot be reliably distinguished from those of the macular variant, except that the quantities deposited are greater and there is often more marked epidermal acanthosis, hypergranulosis, and hyperkeratosis. Basal cell hydropic degeneration may be evident and colloid bodies are usually visible (*Figs 13.57* and *13.58*).[1] Satellite cell necrosis is sometimes a feature.[1] A superficial perivascular chronic inflammatory cell infiltrate is typically present.

When special stains fail to demonstrate the presence of amyloid, ultrastructural studies are usually successful in detecting the presence of the protein.[41]

In contrast to skin involvement in systemic disease, blood vessel deposits are not a feature of primary cutaneous localized lesions.

In earlier literature it was postulated that the amyloid might have been derived from mast cells or fibroblasts. The application of newer technology, however, has shown that it is indisputably of keratinocyte derivation, and amyloid deposits have been shown to contain disulfide bonds and bullous pemphigoid antigen.[8] Numerous recent publications confirm the presence of epidermal keratin in the deposits in both macular and lichenoid forms using monoclonal immunocytochemistry.[3,42–50] The amyloid of the skin-limited variants, so-called amyloid-K, has been shown to contain 50 and 67 kD keratin filaments.[29,49] Apolipoprotein E, one of the proteins found in the amyloid plaque of Alzheimer disease and in systemic amyloidosis, has also been demonstrated in the amyloid present in localized cutaneous amyloidosis.[51,52] Electron microscopic studies have provided further evidence that amyloid-K is of keratinocyte origin by showing tonofilament filamentous (apoptotic) degeneration into amyloid filaments both within the epidermis

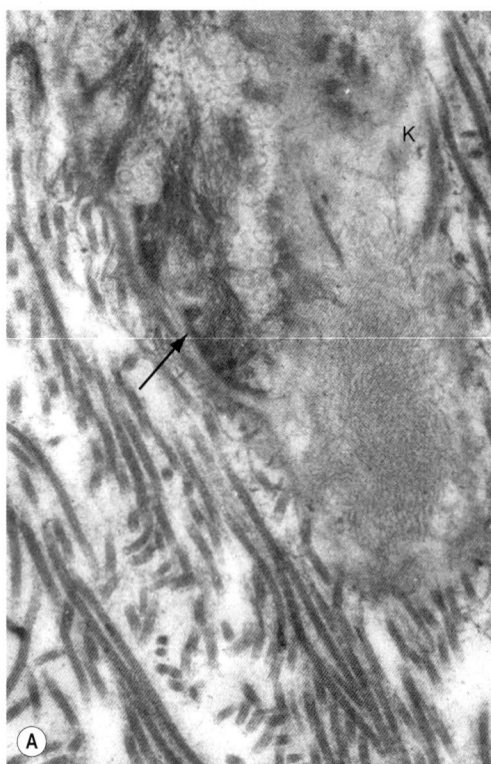

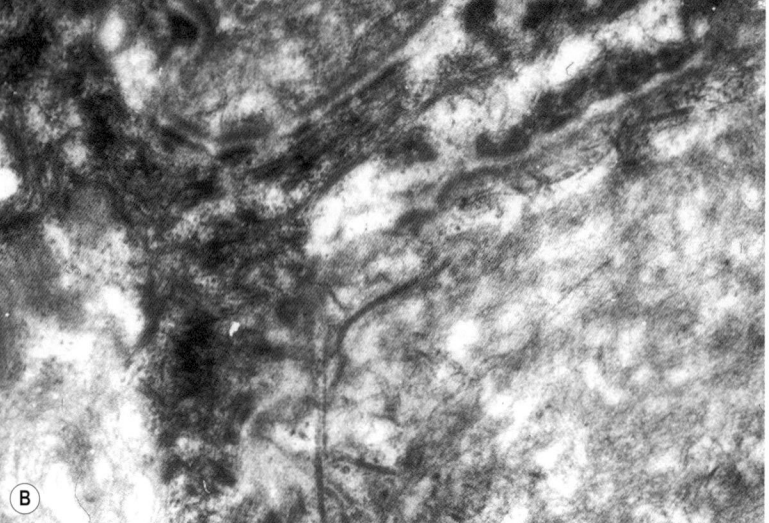

Fig. 13.59
Lichen amyloidosis: (**A**) early filamentous degeneration is seen in this basal keratinocyte (**K**), lamina densa is arrowed; (**B**) compare the organized appearance of the tonofilaments with the haphazardly orientated amyloid immediately adjacent to the lamina densa.

and in the immediately adjacent dermis.[53] Under normal circumstances, apoptotic keratinocytes (cytoid bodies) are either shed as a consequence of epidermal upward migration or are released into the dermis where they are removed by an inflammatory response as is seen, for example, in lichen planus. In macular and lichenoid cutaneous amyloidosis it appears that the above disposal mechanism is either overwhelmed or nonfunctioning.

Early ultrastructural changes consist of loss of tonofilament electron density and development of a wavy morphology accompanied by internalization of desmosomes, thickening of the keratinocyte cell membrane, and the acquisition of hemidesmosome-like attachments to neighboring cells.[29] Cytoplasmic and nuclear remnants are frequently present in the more superficial deposits. It is thought that on entering the dermis, fibroblasts and macrophages convert the degenerate keratin into amyloid filaments (*Fig. 13.59*).[53] The precise mechanism is unknown, but it must involve the conversion of the normal alpha tertiary structure of tonofilaments into the beta-pleated configuration of amyloid. The filaments of amyloid and cytoid

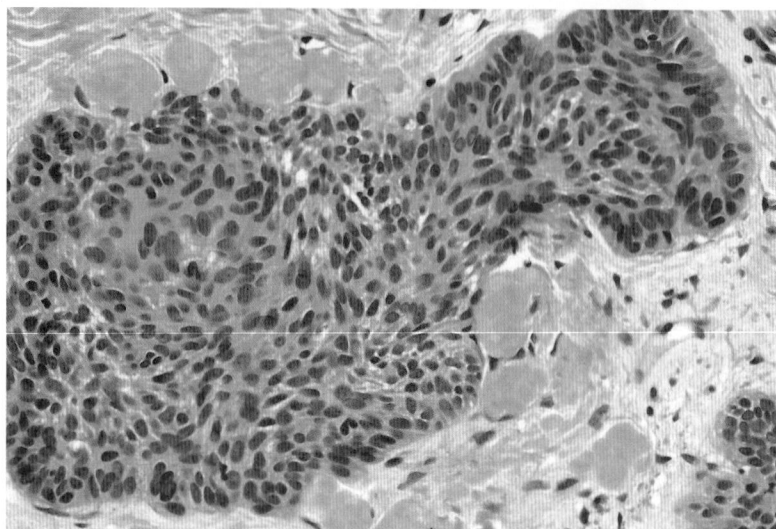

Fig. 13.60
Tumor-associated amyloid: amyloid deposits in a basal cell carcinoma.

bodies show ultrastructural differences. Amyloid fibrils are irregularly distributed whereas the filaments in cytoid bodies are arranged in bundles or whorls.[54]

It is postulated that the development of localized cutaneous amyloidosis is dependent upon mild chronic trauma resulting in excessive production of cytoid bodies and their subsequent conversion into amyloid deposits. It would seem that despite a normal humoral response as shown by the presence of IgM and IgG in association with complement fixation, the normal cellular response whereby apoptotic keratinocytes are removed is lacking.[29,55-57]

Amyloid deposits are frequently found in intimate association with dermal elastic fibers and the deposits in macular amyloidosis have been shown to contain fibrillin.[58] Whether this is of pathogenetic significance or is merely a secondary phenomenon is uncertain.

The apoptotic theory of amyloidogenesis in the cutaneous variants has, however, been challenged. On the basis of finding amyloid deposits immediately below the basal keratinocyte, separating its cell membrane from the lamina densa in the absence of any evidence of filamentous degeneration, it has been suggested that cutaneous amyloid deposits may also be a direct secretory product of keratinocytes.[59,60] It could be that both mechanisms are in operation.

Secondary localized cutaneous amyloidosis

Microscopic foci of amyloid have been described in a number of cutaneous neoplasms including basal cell carcinoma, sweat gland tumors, syringocystadenoma papilliferum, pilomatrixoma, trichoepithelioma, trichoblastoma, intradermal nevus, dermatofibroma, seborrheic keratosis, solar keratosis, and Bowen disease (*Fig. 13.60*).[1-7] The amyloid in most cases appears to be derived from tumor cells. Porokeratosis has also been reported in association with dermal amyloid deposition as a result of apoptosis of keratinocytes.[8,9] Mycosis fungoides and discoid lupus erythematosus may exceptionally be seen associated with localized cutaneous amyloidosis.[10,11]

Cutaneous amyloid deposition may also rarely be seen as a consequence of chronic epidermal damage following PUVA therapy.[12,13] So-called concha amyloidosis due to chronic actinic damage to the ear has also been documented.[14,15]

Repeated insulin injections at the same site have been reported as inducing amyloid in the skin, rarely with coexisting acanthosis nigricans overlying the amyloid.[16-20]

Familial primary cutaneous amyloidosis

Familial primary cutaneous amyloidosis is a very rare autosomal dominant variant of amyloidosis that presents with manifestations of either macular and/or lichenoid amyloidosis.[1-5] Lichen amyloidosis is also seen in patients with multiple endocrine neoplasia type 2A (Sipple syndrome).[6-8] Germline mutations of the *RET* proto-oncogene on chromosome 10 involving cysteine residues have been consistently described in Sipple syndrome. However, familial primary cutaneous amyloidosis without Sipple syndrome does not show *RET* mutations, clearly indicating that they are different conditions.[6,9]

Genetic studies in patients with familial primary cutaneous amyloidosis have identified mutations in *OSMR*, which encodes oncostatin M receptor beta, which is expressed in various tissues including keratinocytes, cutaneous nerves, and in the dorsal root ganglion.[10-17] This is an interleukin-6 family cytokine receptor, and it is speculated that mutations in it lead to dysfunctional cell signaling resulting in apoptosis of keratinocytes, amyloid deposition, and reduction of nerve fibers, which causes pruritus.[10,18] Not all patients with familial primary cutaneous amyloidosis have been shown to have the same mutation in chromosome 5, indicating genetic heterogeneity in this disease.[19] The histopathological findings are identical to those described in the primary nonfamilial variants of localized cutaneous amyloidosis.

Amyloidosis cutis dyschromica (vitiliginous) is another familial variant of primary cutaneous amyloidosis characterized by reticulate hyper- and hypopigmentation of the trunk and limbs, with onset typically in childhood.[20-28] Papules, atrophy, and telangiectasia are usually not present. One patient with concomitant morphea has been described.[24] It has been suggested that the disease is caused by hypersensitivity to ultraviolet B light with possible DNA repair defects.[22] Histologically, the amyloid is present in the papillary dermis. Amyloidosis cutis dyschromica may represent the same disease described as X-linked reticulate pigmentary disorder in which cutaneous amyloidosis occurs as a secondary phenomenon in patients with a disease characterized by failure to thrive, chronic respiratory disease, photophobia with corneal dystrophy, and gastrointestinal disease.[29,30]

Nodular amyloidosis

Clinical features

In this rare variant, which is more common in females, pink–brown single or multiple nodules develop on the trunk, extremities, genitalia, face or scalp (*Fig. 13.61*).[1-13] Bilateral nodular amyloidosis of the eyelids in the absence of systemic amyloidosis has rarely been documented.[14] The lesions often have a waxy appearance and the surface may be atrophic or ulcerated. Most cases of nodular amyloidosis are limited to skin and only 7% show progression to systemic amyloidosis.[7,15] Occasional reports have documented monoclonal paraproteinemia, lymphoplasmacytoid lymphoma, marginal zone lymphoma, Sjögren syndrome, proteinuria, bone marrow abnormalities, and a positive rectal biopsy.[16-25] It has also been reported in association with psoriasis, eczema, and cirrhosis.[26-28] Nodular cutaneous amyloidosis has also been described in association with carpal tunnel syndrome induced by the amyloidogenic transthyretin His 114 variant.[29] An unusual variant of nodular amyloidosis with bilateral plantar involvement is very occasionally encountered.[30]

Histologic features

The histologic appearances cannot be distinguished from those of systemic amyloidosis and, indeed, as in primary amyloidosis, the amyloid consists of light chain-derived AL protein.[31-34] It is thought likely that this nodular variant results from local production of light chains by a localized group of plasma cells.[1] PCR studies have demonstrated that the infiltrating plasma cells in cases of nodular amyloidosis are usually monoclonal.[35,36] Polyclonality, however, has also been reported.[17] In all patients with nodular amyloidosis, it is important to exclude systemic disease.[2,7] A rare case of nodular amyloidosis secondary to keratin derived amyloid has been described.[37]

The deposits of amyloid are present in both the papillary and reticular dermis and may involve the subcutaneous fat (*Figs 13.62–13.64*). Sometimes

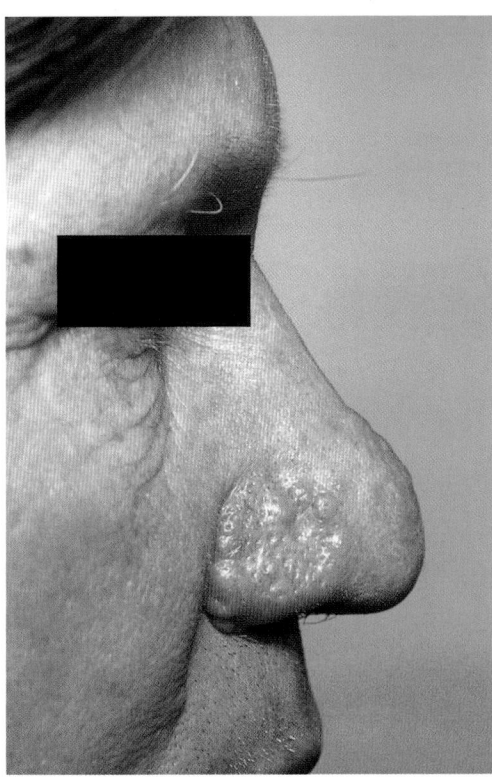

Fig. 13.61
Nodular amyloidosis: an irregular infiltrated plaque limited to the nose.

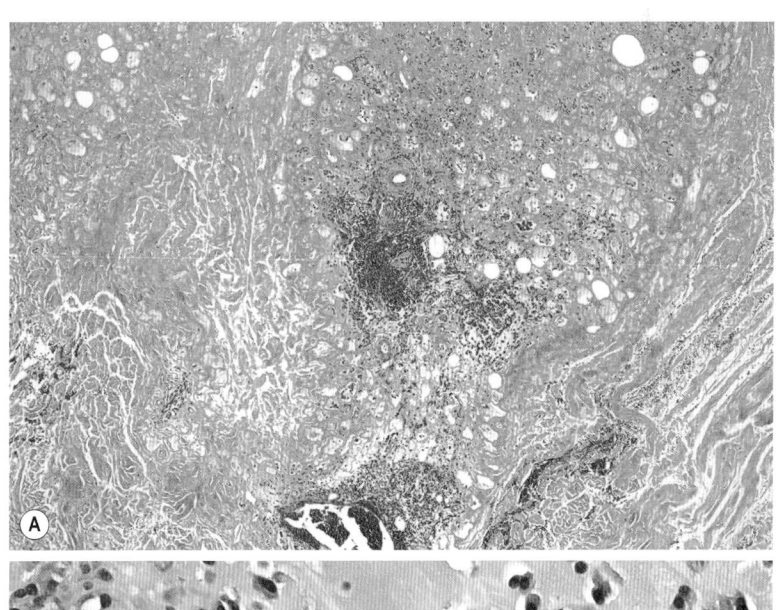

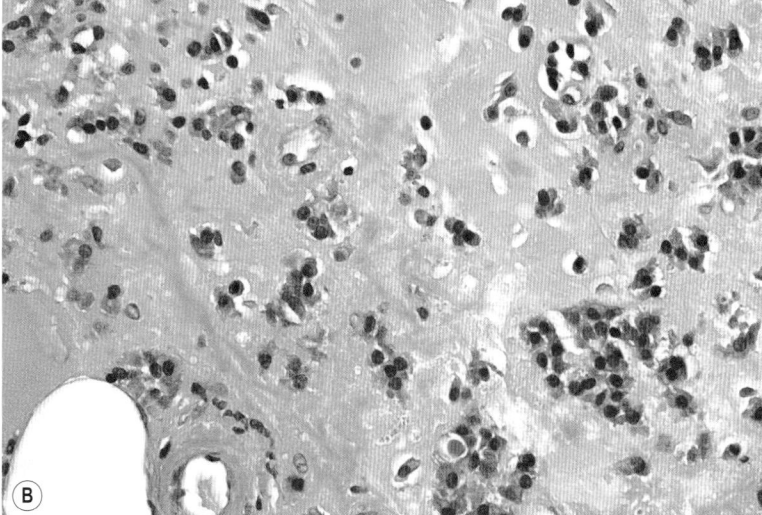

Fig. 13.62
Nodular amyloidosis: (**A**) massive deposits of amyloid are present in the dermis; (**B**) there is a heavy associated plasma cell infiltrate.

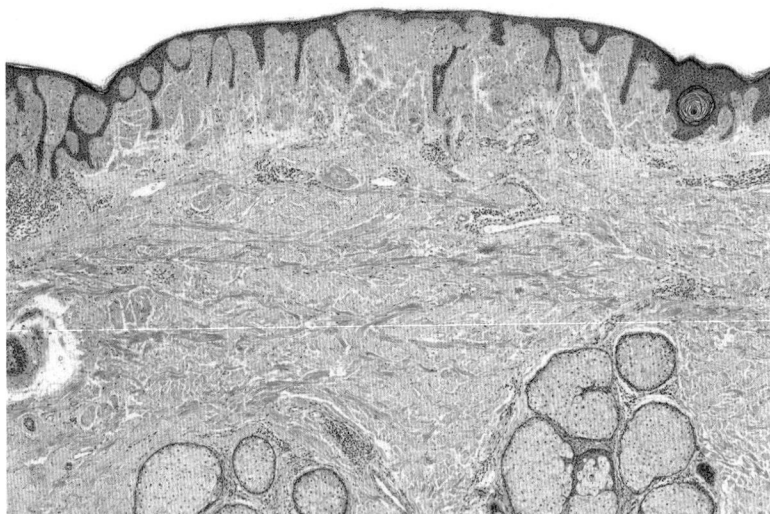

Fig. 13.63
Nodular amyloidosis: in this example there is a broad bandlike deposit in the upper dermis.

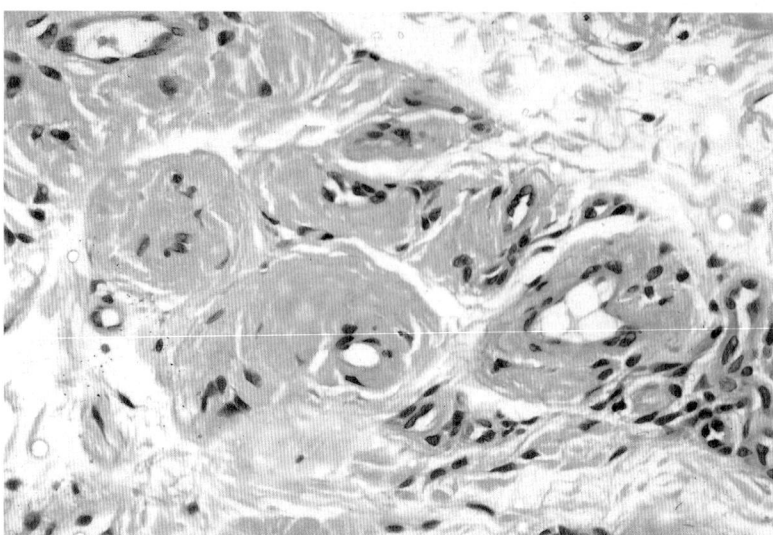

Fig. 13.65
Nodular amyloidosis: amyloid deposits have thickened the blood vessel walls.

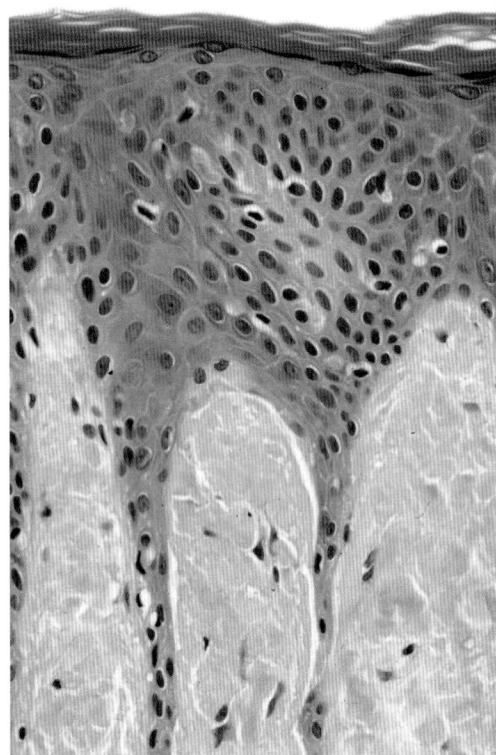

Fig. 13.64
Nodular amyloid: the amyloid deposits fill the papillary dermis.

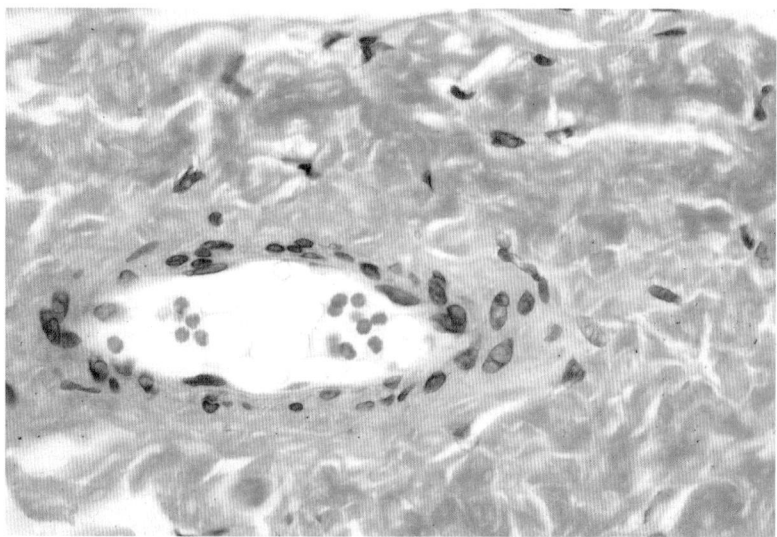

Fig. 13.66
Nodular amyloid: the deposits are strongly Congo red positive.

the vasculature and nerve sheaths are affected (*Figs 13.65–13.67*).[2] Characteristically, plasma cells are seen around blood vessels and at the margin of the amyloid deposits (*Fig. 13.68*).[4,38] Rarely, an associated foreign body giant cell reaction with phagocytosis of amyloid and/or calcification are evident.[4,6]

Colloid milium

Colloid milium, which is characterized by the deposition of amorphous, eosinophilic granular deposits in the superficial dermis, has a number of subtypes including the juvenile and adult variants. It may also develop as a manifestation of ochronosis due to use of the skin bleaching agent hydroquinone or exposure to fertilizers.[1,2] Two other variants – nodular colloid degeneration and paracolloid of the skin – are probably variants of nodular

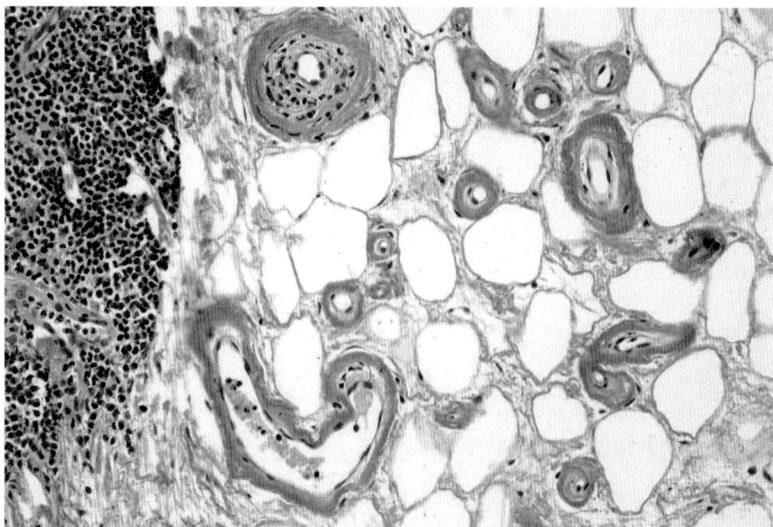

Fig. 13.67
Nodular amyloid: in this example, vessels in the subcutaneous fat showing striking involvement.

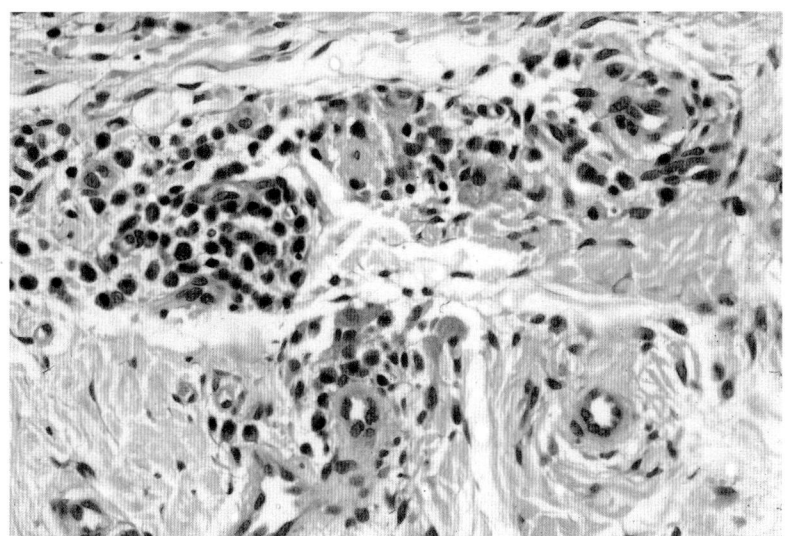

Fig. 13.68
Nodular amyloidosis: there is a conspicuous plasma cell infiltrate.

amyloidosis.[3-5] An alternative name proposed for adult colloid milium is papular elastosis.[6]

Juvenile colloid milium

Clinical features

The juvenile variant, which is exceedingly rare, develops in children before puberty and sometimes has a familial incidence.[7-9] Patients present with discrete, or sometimes confluent, papules measuring 0.2–1.5 cm in diameter.[8-10] An unusual periocular and perioral linear pattern has been reported.[9] Lesions, which are yellow–brown in color, appear translucent and when punctured characteristically express gelatinous material. The underlying tissues often feel indurated. Juvenile colloid milium predominantly affects the face, in particular the cheeks, nose, and around the mouth (Figs 13.69–13.71). Induction of purpura after stroking has been described in both juvenile and adult colloid milium.[11] This phenomenon has been attributed to vascular fragility due to infiltration of the blood vessel walls by colloid material. Exceptionally, juvenile colloid milia may present with gingival deposits and ligneous conjunctivitis as a result of infiltration of these tissues by colloid-like material.[12-14]

Pathogenesis and histologic features

Although the etiology remains unknown, in some cases at least, sunlight plays an important role. The pathogenesis, however, shows considerable overlap with macular and lichenoid amyloidosis. Juvenile colloid milium represents a primary degenerative disorder of epidermal keratinocytes, which through the process of apoptosis are transformed into colloid bodies within the superficial dermis.

The initial change is one of filamentous transformation whereby the relatively straight electron-dense keratin filaments are converted into shortened, curved 8–10 nm filaments arranged in weaved or whorled fascicles (Fig. 13.72).[10] Occasionally, both types of filament may be identified simultaneously within the cytoplasm of basal keratinocytes. With progression, filamentous transformation comes to affect the entire cell, and nuclear, cytoplasmic, and desmosomal remnants may be identified within the filamentous mass (Fig. 13.73). Residual desmosomes are sometimes present around the border of the colloid deposit. Finally, the apoptotic cell is extruded into the adjacent dermis. In addition to the transformed filaments characteristic of all cytoid bodies, amyloid filaments have also been identified in juvenile colloid milium, thereby prompting the authors to classify this entity along with other amyloid-K dermatoses.[3] Positive labeling of the deposits for epidermal keratin gives support to this hypothesis.[3,15]

Juvenile colloid milium has also been shown by direct immunofluorescence to be accompanied by immunoglobulin, complement, and fibrin

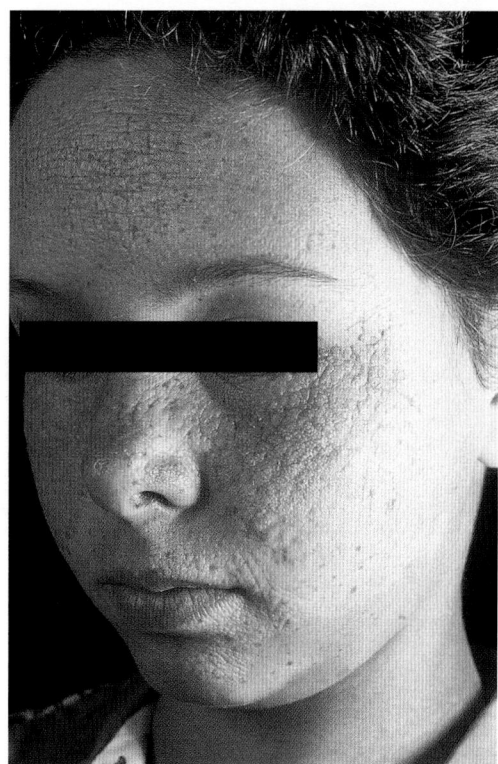

Fig. 13.69
Juvenile colloid milium: there is papular thickening of the skin, particularly involving the cheeks, nose, and forehead. By courtesy of S. Handfield-Jones, MD, Institute of Dermatology, London, UK.

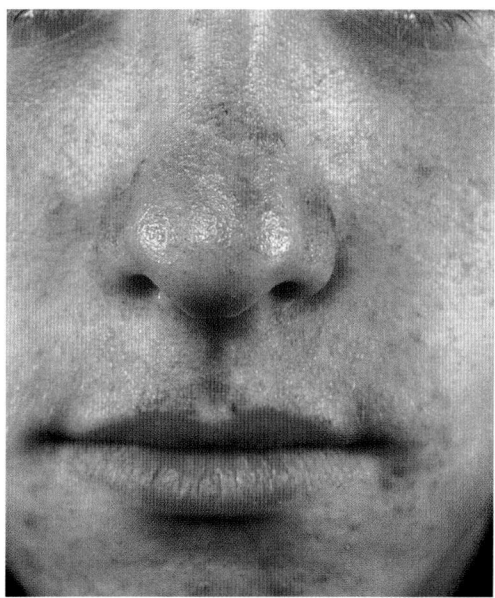

Fig. 13.70
Juvenile colloid milium: this less severely affected child shows typical yellow–brown translucent papules on the nose and upper lip. By courtesy of S. Handfield-Jones, MD, Institute of Dermatology, London, UK.

deposits.[8] Whether this represents an autoimmune-mediated reaction as is seen in macular-lichenoid amyloidosis or a secondary non-specific reactive phenomenon has yet to be determined.

Histologically, the deposits are present in the superficial dermis where they impinge on the overlying and often somewhat frayed epidermis (Figs 13.74–13.77). The colloid is composed of eosinophilic amorphous aggregates, often showing a fractured appearance. The overlying epithelium shows prominent cytoid bodies, while laterally, acanthosis associated with downward and inward growth results in cuffing or even encirclement of

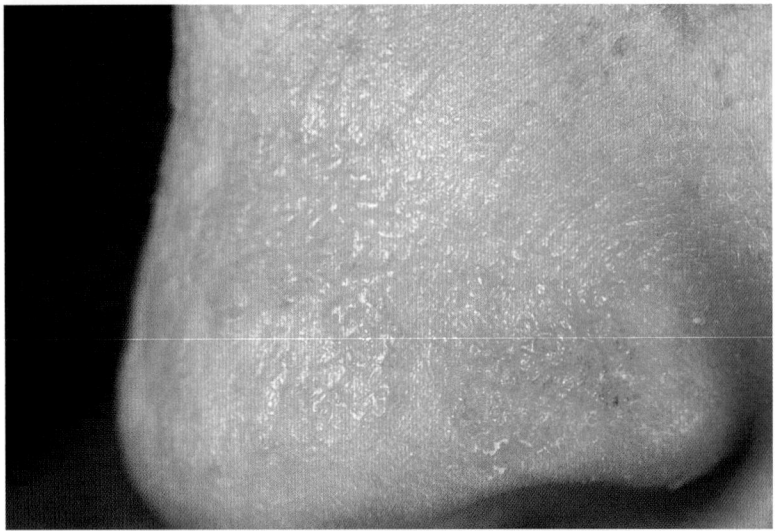

Fig. 13.71
Juvenile colloid milium: close-up view from the brother of the patient shown in
Fig. 13.70. By courtesy of S. Handfield-Jones, MD, Institute of Dermatology,
London, UK.

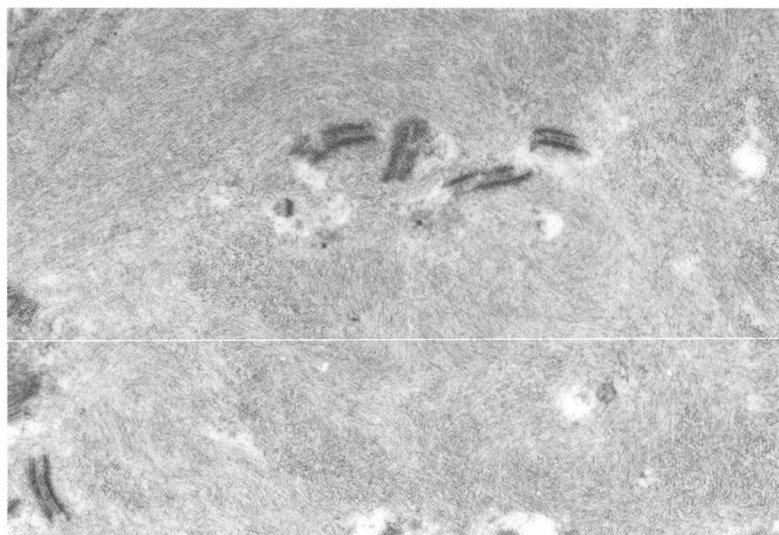

Fig. 13.73
Juvenile colloid milium: internalized desmosomes are evident within this
degenerate keratinocyte.

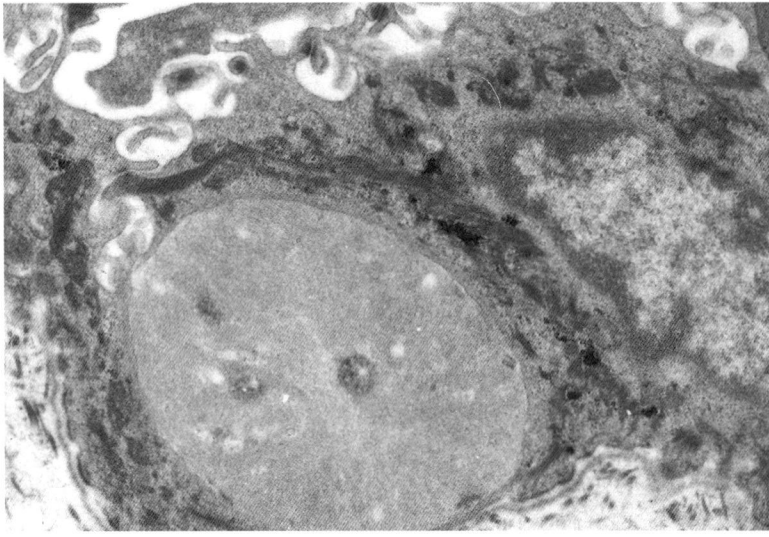

Fig. 13.72
Juvenile colloid milium: this shows an apoptotic keratinocyte, the cytoplasm of
which is filled with fascicles of pale-staining filaments that contrast strikingly with
adjacent tonofilaments.

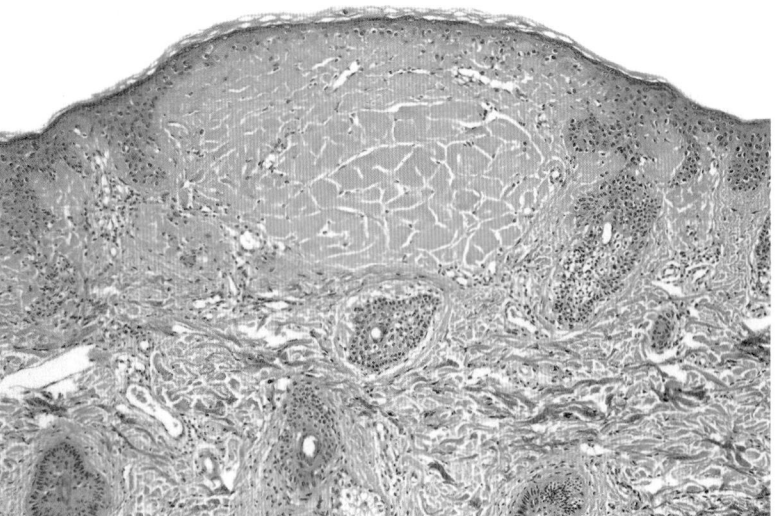

Fig. 13.74
Juvenile colloid milium: the papule consists of an intradermal deposit of
eosinophilic material. There is no inflammatory response.

the colloid islands by an epidermal collarette.[3] An admixture of fibroblasts
and mast cells may be evident and pigmentary incontinence is sometimes
present. Juvenile colloid milium is histochemically indistinguishable from
amyloid: it is diastase-resistant, PAS positive, thioflavine-T positive, and
shows positive staining with Congo red with apple-green birefringence.

Adult colloid milium

Clinical features

This variant, which is much commoner than the childhood form, affects
middle-aged patients and shows a predilection for males. Outdoor workers
are most often affected and lesions seen on sun-exposed skin are often
accompanied by the features of solar elastosis, giving rise to the synonym
of papular elastosis.

Adult colloid milium presents as dome-shaped yellowish translucent
papules measuring 0.1–0.5 cm in diameter and, in common with juvenile
colloid milium, they contain gelatinous material. Lesions are most often
seen on the face, ears, neck, and the dorsum of the hands (*Fig. 13.78*) and

may be skin-colored to brown.[3,16] Adult colloid milium affects fair-skinned
patients and follows excessive sun exposure. This has been dramatically
illustrated in patients whose lesions are limited to sun-exposed areas of the
body.[17,18] Adult colloid milium has also been reported following the excessive use of cosmetic ultraviolet A (UVA) sunbed exposure.[19] A rare association with multiple myeloma has been described.[20] A further report described
a patient who developed lesions of adult colloid milia in areas exposed to
mineral oils.[21] A single case has also been described in a patient with beta
thalassemia major.[22] Rare cases of pigmented colloid milium have been documented as a consequence of exogenous ochronosis due to bleaching creams
and fertilizers.[1,16]

Pathogenesis and histologic features

In contrast to the keratinocyte changes seen in the juvenile variant, adult
colloid milium represents an extreme degree of actinic damage centered
upon the upper dermal elastic fibers. Although earlier studies suggested
that the colloid might have represented abnormal collagen or a fibroblast
secretory product, more recent studies suggest that it derives from actinic
elastoid.[17,23–25]

Ultrastructural studies have shown that there is direct continuity between
actinic elastoid and the colloid deposits and that, within the electron-dense

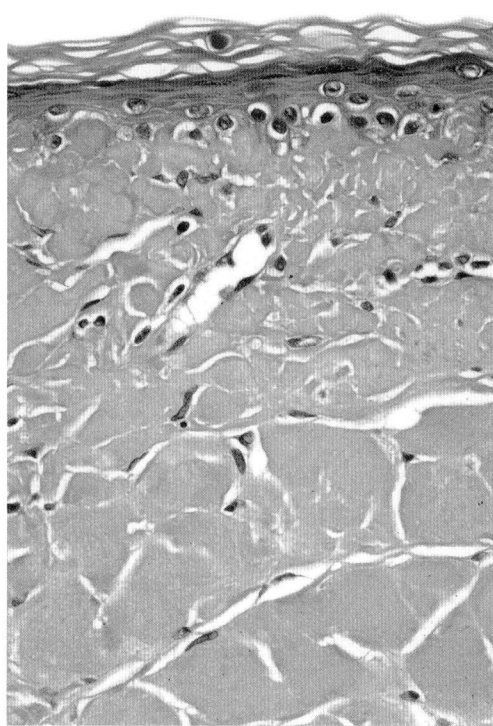

Fig. 13.75
Juvenile colloid milium: this high-power view shows the faceted nature of the deposit.

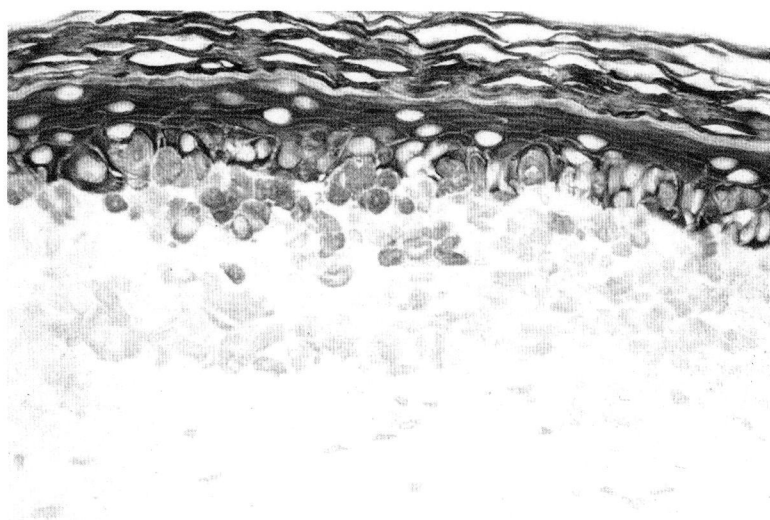

Fig. 13.77
Juvenile colloid milium: the amorphous material that characterizes this condition is of epidermal derivation. Tonofilaments undergo filamentous degeneration (apoptosis). Note the keratin positivity of the colloid aggregates (pankeratin).

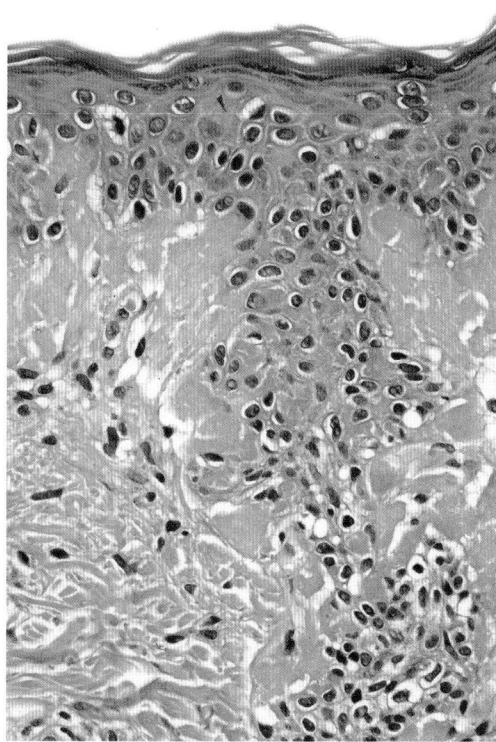

Fig. 13.76
Juvenile colloid milium: the adjacent epidermis shows massive apoptosis.

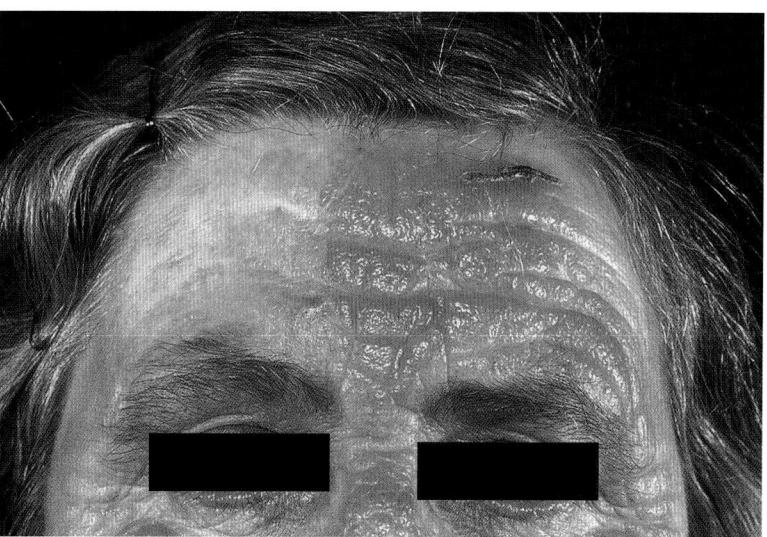

Fig. 13.78
Adult colloid milium: predominantly unilateral, streaked, orange plaque involving the forehead and nose. By courtesy of the Institute of Dermatology, London, UK.

label with antikeratin antibodies, and immunoglobulins and complement are absent.

Histologically, the eosinophilic amorphous, autofluorescent clefted deposits are typically separated from the epidermis by a grenz zone containing normal collagen (Figs 13.79 and 13.80).[24] Fibroblasts often occupy the fissures between the fragmented deposits.[24]

Histochemically, adult colloid milium is diastase-resistant, PAS positive, thioflavine-T positive, and demonstrates apple-green birefringence with Congo red.[17] It is also Dylon positive.[2] Colloid milium can be difficult to distinguish from amyloidosis, and electron microscopy may be necessary.[29,30]

Hyalinosis cutis et mucosae

Clinical features

Hyalinosis cutis et mucosae (Urbach-Wiethe disease, lipoid proteinosis), is a very rare, autosomal recessive condition first described in 1929 in which hyaline material is deposited in virtually any organ in the body, but particularly the skin, the pharyngeal mucosa, and the larynx.[1-10] It has been reported most frequently in South Africa (descendants of German and

colloid, remnants of both normal and elastotic fibers may sometimes be identified.[24,26] Amyloid filaments are not present. Further support for this hypothesis is given by the identification of SAP component within the colloid deposits.[24] Although this protein is characteristically present within amyloid, it is also a constant component of normal elastic tissue and has also been identified in actinic elastoid.[27,28] Adult colloid milium does not

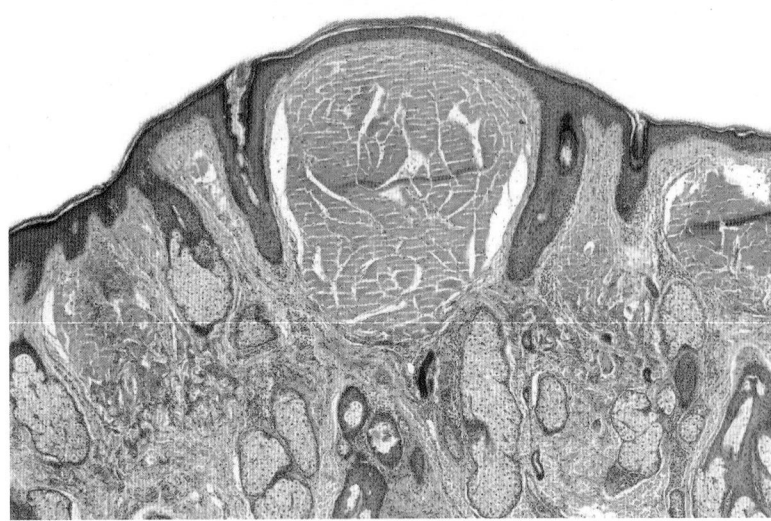

Fig. 13.79
Adult colloid milium: deposits of eosinophilic material are present in the superficial dermis. There is adjacent solar elastosis.

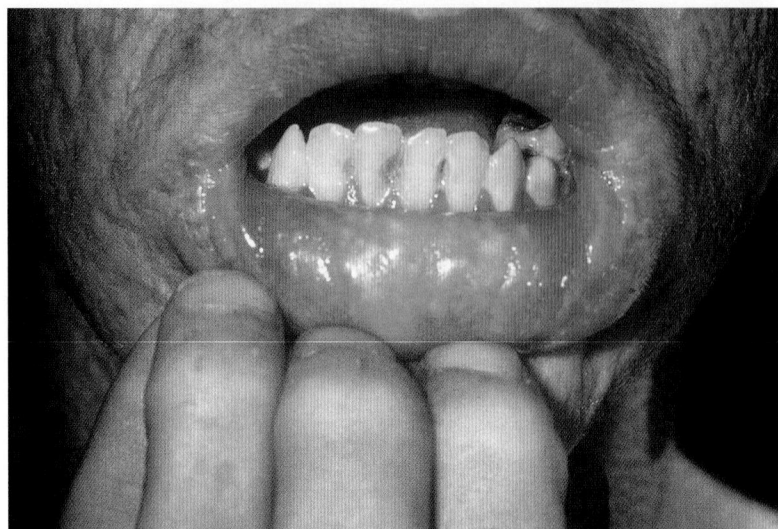

Fig. 13.81
Lipoid proteinosis: small pale papules are present on the mucosal aspect of the lower lip. By courtesy of the Institute of Dermatology, London, UK.

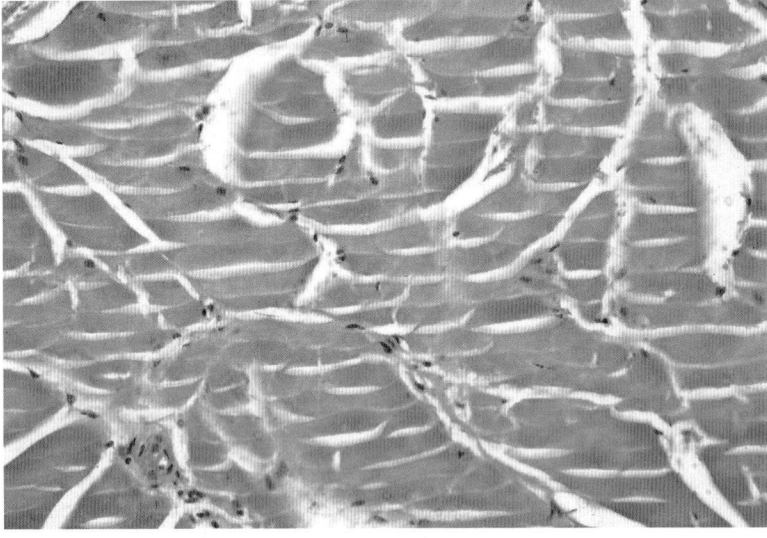

Fig. 13.80
Adult colloid milium: the typical faceted appearance.

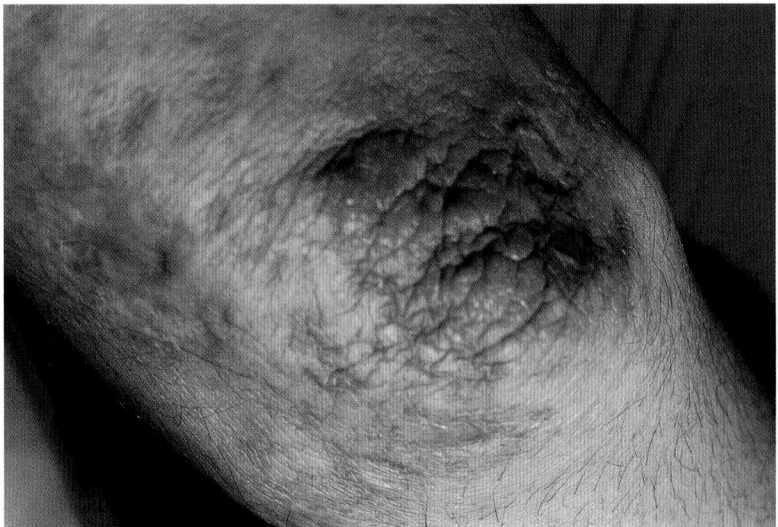

Fig. 13.82
Lipoid proteinosis: marked thickening of the skin is present with conspicuous scarring. By courtesy of R.A. Marsden, MD, St George's Hospital, London, UK.

Dutch immigrants) and Sweden, and it has been suggested that up to 35% of documented cases have had South African lineage.[11–14]

The gene for lipoid proteinosis has been mapped to chromosome 1q21 and the disease is caused by mutations in the extracellular matrix protein 1 gene (ECM1) which lead to partial or complete loss of function of the protein.[15–21] ECM1 is thought to play a critical role in dermal structure and organization by binding to dermal ground substance (molecules such as perlecan and matrix metalloproteinases), in the formation and maintenance of the basement membrane, and in stromal signaling.[20] It has been called 'biological super-glue'.[20,21] It is also overexpressed in cancers, influencing tumor growth and metastasis.[20] Over 40 different mutations in this gene have been reported in association with lipoid proteinosis, and studies thus far have not demonstrated a relationship between the specific type of mutation and clinical phenotype.[20,21] Interestingly, patients with lichen sclerosus have autoantibodies to ECM1.[22]

The initial symptom, a hoarse cry, develops in infancy and results from incomplete closure of the vocal cords, which are thickened and irregular due to the hyaline deposits. Induration of the oral mucosa (including the inner aspect of the lips, the gingivae, uvula, palate, and floor of the mouth) begins in childhood and is progressive, so that adults have extensive yellow infiltration (Fig. 13.81).[4,10,23] The lower lip often assumes a cobblestone

appearance. The tongue also tends to be thick and immobile with sublingual frenulum thickening and ankyloglossia. Recurrent ulcers on the tongue have been described.[5] Nail growth is frequently abnormal and the upper incisors, premolars or molars can be hypoplastic or aplastic.[6]

Early inflammatory skin lesions (bullae, pustules, and crusts) are followed by acneiform infiltrated scars on the face and limbs (Fig. 13.82).[13] Papulonodular lesions develop on the face, fingers, and around the eyelashes, where they produce the pathognomonic 'string of beads' appearance (moniliform blepharosis) (Fig. 13.83). Thicker xanthoma-like plaques, which sometimes become verrucous, later develop on the areas of trauma including the knees, elbows, feet, and hands.[24] With chronicity in severely affected patients the entire skin becomes yellow, waxy, and thickened, particularly the flexures.[25] Similar lesions in the scalp may produce alopecia, which can be patchy or diffuse.[6,11]

Intracranial disease sometimes occurs, associated with calcification, which is thought to complicate deposition of hyaline material around cerebral blood vessels and basal ganglia.[4] Epilepsy is a not uncommon result.[24,26–29] Other neurological manifestations include memory loss, rage attacks, and mild mental retardation.[17,30–32]

Involvement of the small bowel by the disease may lead to intestinal bleeding.[33]

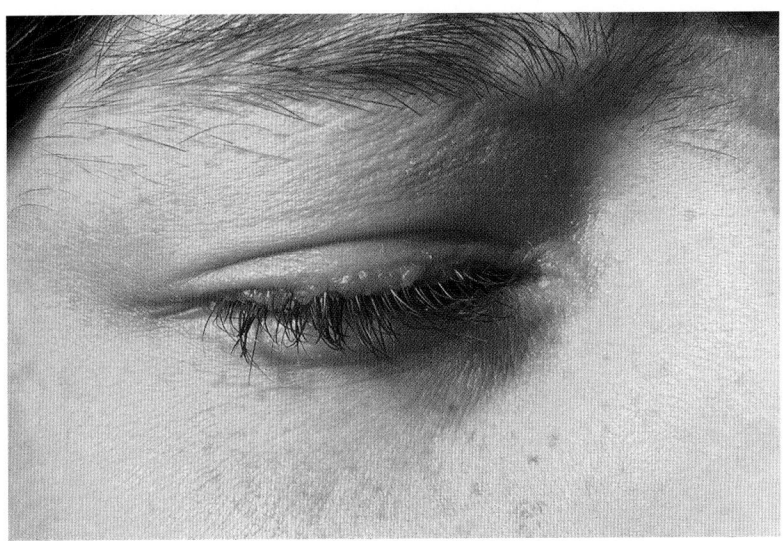

Fig. 13.83
Lipoid proteinosis: note the waxy nodules on the upper eyelid, producing the typical 'string of beads' appearance. By courtesy of the Institute of Dermatology, London, UK.

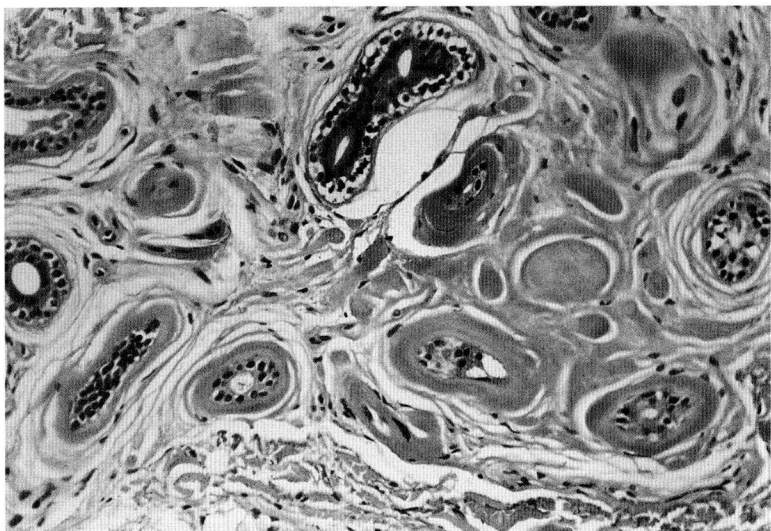

Fig. 13.85
Lipoid proteinosis: in this advanced example, there is considerable involvement of eccrine sweat glands which, as a result, are atrophic.

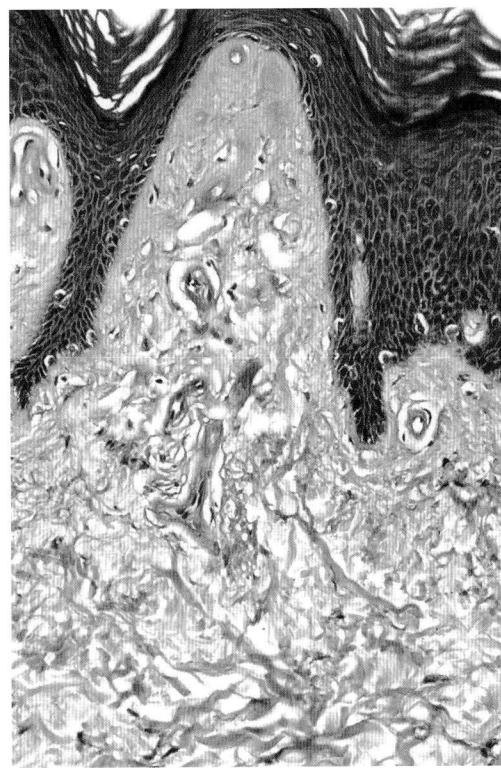

Fig. 13.84
Lipid proteinosis: the blood vessel walls are thickened by pale-staining, eosinophilic homogeneous material.

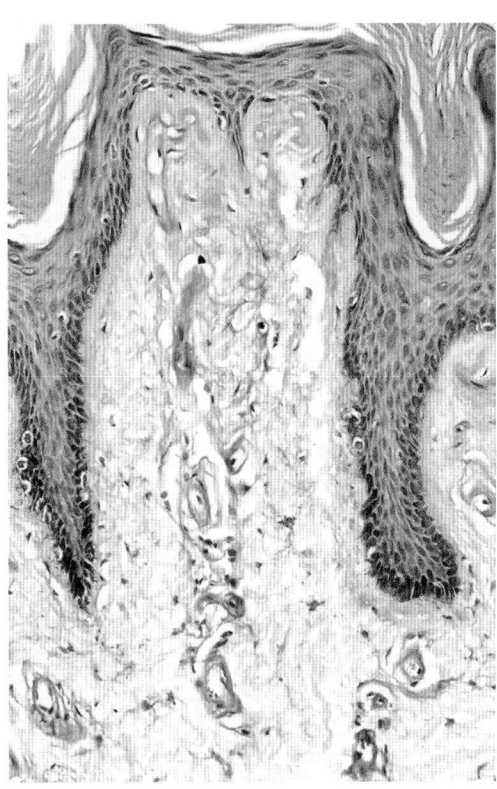

Fig. 13.86
Lipoid proteinosis: the deposit is strongly periodic acid–Schiff positive (diastase-resistant).

The disease is usually associated with normal life expectancy although there might be some increase in the mortality rate during childhood due to respiratory insufficiency.[2]

Pathogenesis and histologic features

The epidermis is acanthotic and occasionally papillomatous, with overlying hyperkeratosis. Homogeneous eosinophilic material is distributed in a very characteristic pattern in the dermis.[11] Initially, it is found around capillaries and concentrically around sweat coils (Figs 13.84 and 13.85); later, more extensive deposits are seen, which tend to be vertically orientated within the dermis.[34] The hair follicles and arrector pili muscles are often surrounded by a hyaline mantle.[35] In advanced cases, the perineurium of nerves can also be affected.[36] This material stains very strongly with PAS

(diastase-resistant) and only very weakly with Congo red and thioflavine-T (Fig. 13.86). The name lipoid is used because the hyaline material usually has a lipid component.[37]

Ultrastructurally, the deposit is amorphous, electron-dense, and may contain ill-defined, anastomosing amyloid-like (5–10 nm) filaments and delicate collagen fibers (Figs 13.87 and 13.88).[35] Reduplication of basal lamina is evident around blood vessels, hair follicles, and sweat glands, and excess type IV collagen has been demonstrated immunohistochemically.[11,24,25,38] The fibroblasts contain abundant rough endoplasmic reticulum and numerous mitochondria. Intracytoplasmic inclusions, probably lysosomal in nature, have also been described.

The etiology of bullous lesions in lipoid proteinosis is unclear. A recent report sheds light on a possible pathogenesis. It describes subcorneal and

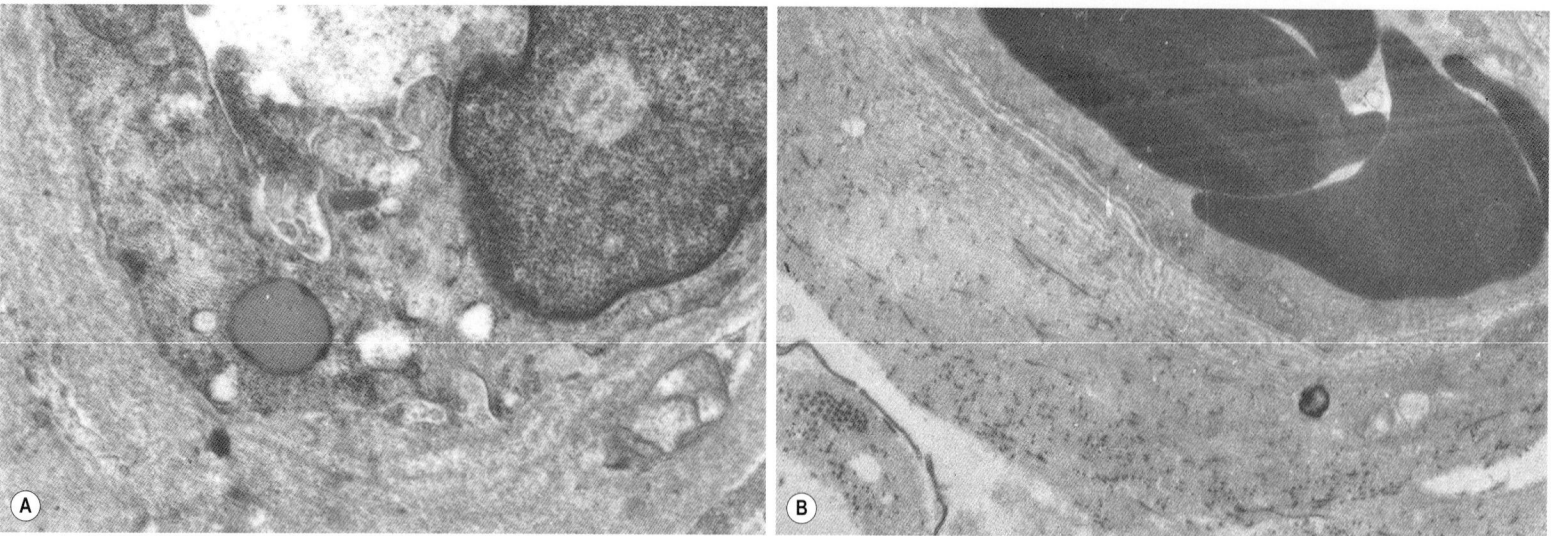

Fig. 13.87
(**A, B**) Lipoid proteinosis: transverse section through blood vessel showing reduplication of the basement membrane.

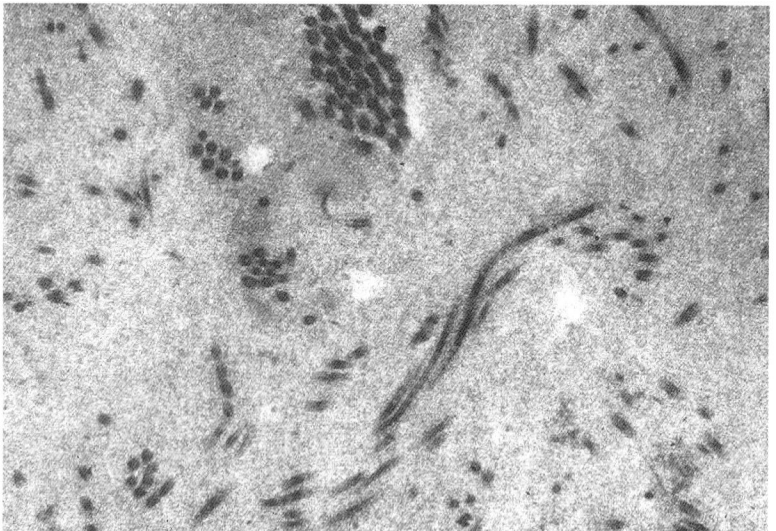

Fig. 13.88
Lipoid proteinosis: high-power view of amorphous electron-dense material containing occasional collagen fibers.

intraepidermal acantholysis without dyskeratosis in a child with lipoid proteinosis.[39] Subepidermal clefting was also noted but thought to be artifactual. Direct immunofluorescence studies were negative.

Despite considerable research, the precise pathogenesis of lipoid proteinosis remains an enigma. Quantitative abnormalities of dermal collagen have been clearly demonstrated, but little is known about the nature of the hyaline deposits other than that they are probably composed of an admixture of glycoproteins, glycosaminoglycans, and lipids, as may be determined by special staining techniques.[11]

Numerous mechanisms have been hypothesized, but none has satisfactorily unraveled the nature of the primary disturbance in this disease. The identification of lipid droplets within the hyaline deposits therefore led to the suggestion that lipoid proteinosis might represent a systemic lipoidosis.[11] However, the lipid deposition is very variable and lesional chemical analyses have not demonstrated any consistent abnormalities. Fibroblast tissue culture experiments have not supported this concept.[37] It probably denotes a secondary phenomenon. The ultrastructural finding of intracytoplasmic inclusions – including myelin figures and lysosomes accompanied by an increased fibroblast hexuronic acid content – has raised the possibility of a lysosomal storage disorder.[40] This has recently been given further support by the demonstration of abnormal lysosomes in eccrine cells and histiocytes in two patients with this disease.[41] These lysosomes were found to contain amorphous granular material, zebra bodies, and curved tubular profiles. The curved tubular profiles are similar to those found in Farber disease and it has been suggested that lipoid proteinosis represents a disease with not only impaired production of collagen but also with alterations in ceramide metabolism.

A number of publications have described a variety of changes in the dermal collagen content.[42] The reduplicated basement membrane laminae noted ultrastructurally have been shown to be composed of laminin accompanied by collagen types III and IV.[43] This feature, however, is of doubtful significance as similar appearances have been described in a wide variety of conditions including psoriasis, systemic lupus erythematosus, and diabetes mellitus.[11] Basement membrane replication most likely represents a non-specific secondary response to a range of stimuli.

Dry weight studies of lipoid proteinosis dermis have shown an apparent decrease in collagen content, although there appears to be a relative increase in collagen types III and V compared with collagen type I.[44] Immunofluorescence data, however, suggest that there are reduced absolute levels of both type I and type III collagen.[11] In vitro studies of fibroblast collagen synthesis, as determined by radioactive hydroxyproline synthesis, have revealed no significant abnormality.[24] Fibroblasts, however, have reduced replicative capacity. Investigations have disclosed reduced fibroblast type I procollagen mRNA and a diminished type I:III procollagen mRNA ratio.[24] Type IV procollagen mRNA levels have been shown to be raised.[45] No DNA abnormalities or chromosomal alternations have yet been identified in lipoid proteinosis.

It is likely that the collagen changes are not directly responsible for the accumulation of the granular hyaline material so characteristic of this disorder. It is, however, most probably of fibroblast derivation.[46]

Cutaneous macroglobulinosis

Clinical features

Cutaneous macroglobulinosis (IgM storage papules) is a rarely documented manifestation of Waldenström macroglobulinemia.[1–16] The latter is a chronic lymphoproliferative condition that typically presents in the fifth and sixth decades and shows a slight predilection for males.[5] It is characterized by proliferation of lymphoplasmacytoid cells in the bone marrow, lymph node, and spleen and IgM paraproteinemia.[5] Patients present with weakness, fatigue, weight loss, anemia, mucous membrane bleeding, retinal hemorrhages, lymphadenopathy, hepatosplenomegaly, peripheral neuropathy, and the hyperviscosity syndrome.[7,8] Skin involvement is very uncommon and includes papules, nodules, tumors, plaques, and macroglobulinosis cutis. Additional features that are sometimes encountered include purpura, xanthomata, cryoglobulinemia, and Raynaud phenomenon.[7]

Clinically, macroglobulinosis presents as sometimes pruritic, skin-colored, erythematous or translucent papules measuring up to 1.0 cm in diameter distributed predominantly on extensor sites including knees, elbows, buttocks, and the arms and legs.[7] Umbilication, erosion, and crusting and hyperkeratosis are commonly seen.[5,9,10,11,15] Cutaneous tumor deposits present as violaceous nodules and plaques.

Histologic features

The papules are characterized by homogeneous eosinophilic material in the papillary and reticular dermis (Fig. 13.89).[2,11] Hair follicles and eccrine glands may be encased.[2,11] The deposits are PAS positive but are Congo red negative (Fig. 13.90). Vessels may also show occlusion by the same

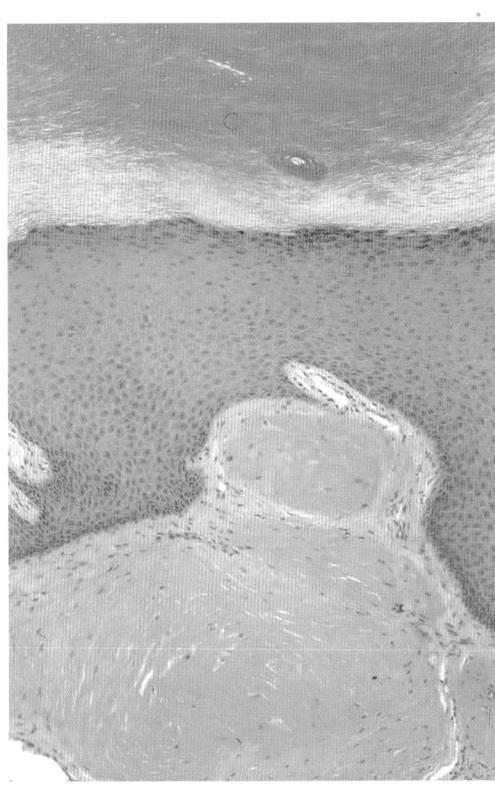

Fig. 13.89
Macroglobulinosis cutis: these are nodular deposits of eosinophilic material in the superficial dermis. By courtesy of A. Wang, MD, Brigham and Women's Hospital, Boston, USA.

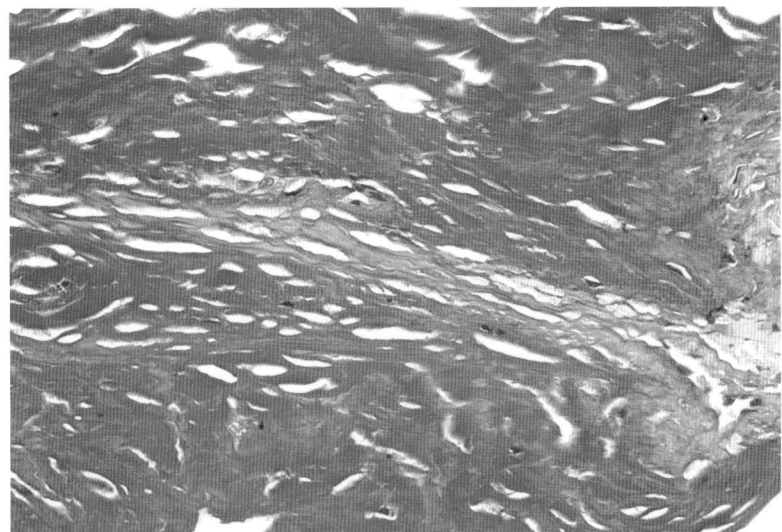

Fig. 13.90
Macroglobulinosis cutis: the material is strongly periodic acid–Schiff positive. By courtesy of A. Wang, MD, Brigham and Women's Hospital, Boston, USA.

material.[11] A lymphoplasmacytoid infiltrate is variably present.[7] The plasma cells may contain intracytoplasmic IgM-rich vacuoles.[4]

Direct immunofluorescence and immunohistochemistry show that the deposits stain strongly for IgM.[2,5,7,11]

Ultrastructurally, the deposits are composed of amorphous or granular and sometimes filamentous material which by immunoelectron microscopy consists of IgM.[1–3,7] The periodicity of amyloid is absent in the filamentous component.[7]

The plaques and tumor nodules are composed of lymphoplasmacytoid infiltrates.

Porphyria

The porphyrias constitute a heterogeneous group of conditions characterized by the excessive production of porphyrins or their precursors resulting from defects in the activity of the enzymes regulating heme synthesis (Fig. 13.91).[1–12] Porphyrin synthesis occurs mainly in the erythropoietic

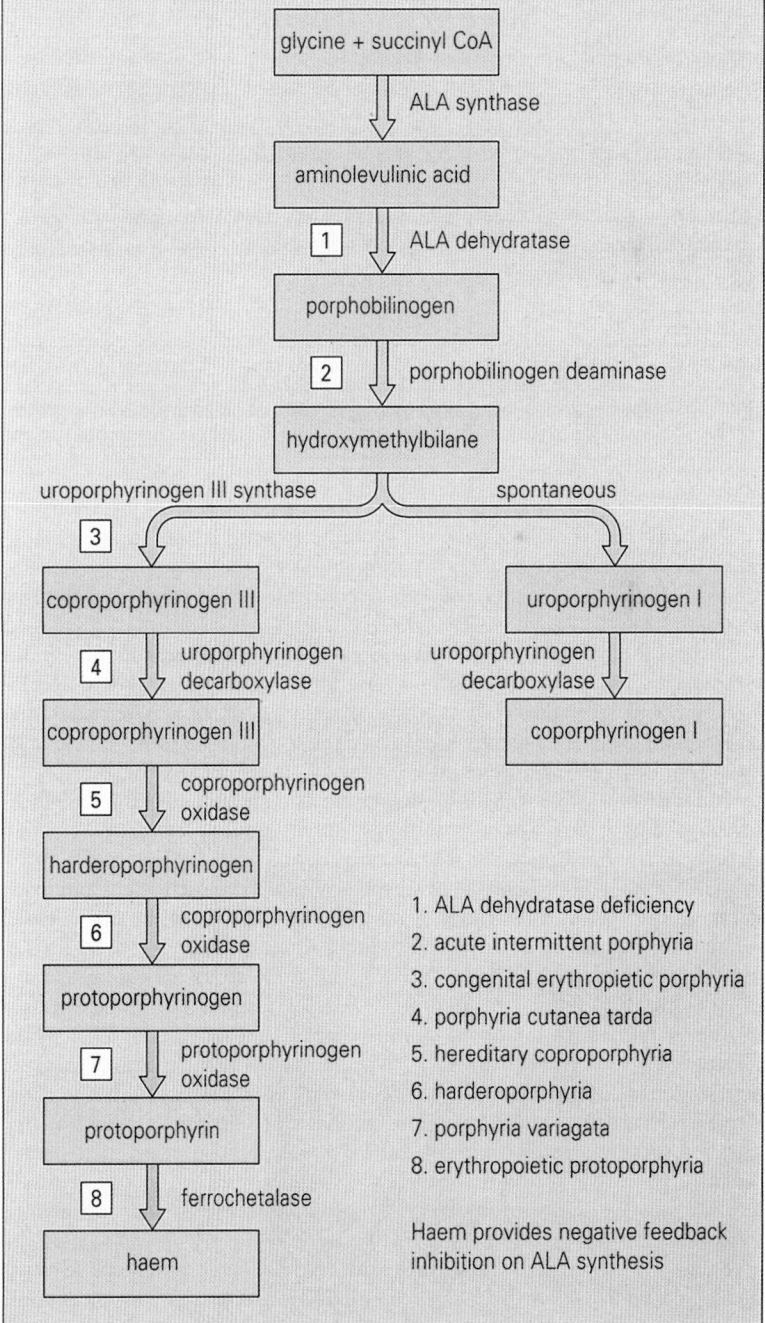

Fig. 13.91
Biochemistry of porphyria. Reproduced with permission from Young, J.W., and Conte, E.T. (1991) International Journal of Dermatology, 30, 399–406.

Table 13.4
Classification of porphyria

Condition	Mode of inheritance	Enzyme defect	Site of metabolic expression	Laboratory abnormality
Non-acute porphyrias producing cutaneous lesions				
Congenital erythropoietic porphyria	Autosomal recessive		Erythroid cells	Elevated uroporphyrin Coproporphyrin in urine and feces
Porphyria cutanea tarda				Urinary uroporphyrin: coproporphyrin = 3:1
inherited	Autosomal dominant	URO-D	Hepatocytes	Elevated urinary uroporphyrin
sporadic toxic	Acquired/sporadic Acquired	URO-D		Urinary and stool isocoporphyrins
Erythropoietic protoporphyria	Autosomal dominant	Ferrochelatase	Erythroid cells and hepatocyte	Normal urine Elevated plasma, RBC and stool protoporphyrin Elevated fecal and RBC coproporphyrin
Hepatoerythropoietic porphyria	Autosomal recessive	URO-D (severe)	Erythroid cells and hepatocyte	Increased urine and stool URO Elevated stool coproporphyrin and isocoproporphyrin Elevated RBC protoporphyrin
Acute porphyrias (porphyrias producing abdominal, neurological, and psychiatric symptoms)				
Acute intermittent porphyria	Autosomal dominant	Porphobilinogen deaminase	Hepatocyte	Stool and blood usually normal Elevated urinary ALA and PBG
ALA dehydratase deficiency	Autosomal recessive	ALA dehydratase (porphobilinogen synthase)	?	ALA alone elevated
Porphyrias producing abdominal, neurological, psychiatric, and cutaneous manifestations				
Variegate porphyria	Autosomal dominant	Protoporphyrinogen oxidase	Hepatocyte	Urine normal between attacks Increased stool protoporphyrins and coproporphyrin Increased urinary ALA and PBG during attacks
Hereditary coproporphyria	Autosomal dominant	Coproporphyrinogen oxidase	Hepatocyte	Increased stool and urine coproporphyrins

ALA, aminolevulinic acid; PBG, porphobilinogen; RBC, red blood cell; URO, uroporphyrinogen.
Reproduced with permission from Young, J.W., Conte, E.T. (1991) International Journal of Dermatology, 30, 399–406.

system and the liver. Deficiency of a specific enzyme results in an accumulation of heme precursors due to stimulation of the rate-limiting enzyme aminolevulinic acid synthetase as a consequence of diminished heme concentration.[10,13]

Genetic mutations account for the enzyme deficiencies seen in the various types of porphyria. These mutations have all been delineated at a molecular level, are very heterogeneous, and often result in enzyme deficiencies that may remain silent throughout life.[13] If a patient is homozygous for a specific mutation, however, symptoms usually develop even in early life.

Patients may present with acute porphyria (abdominal pain with neurological and/or psychiatric symptoms) often induced by drugs, fasting, alcohol or sex hormones.[14–17] The enzyme defect leads to the accumulation in the skin of a photosensitizing porphyrin, which absorbs light predominantly in the 400–410 nm range. The energy absorbed may then be released to adjacent nucleic acids or proteins, either directly or indirectly by involving acceptor molecules, such as oxygen, and toxic changes causing damage to lysosomal and cellular membranes result.[16,17] There is also some evidence to suggest that activation of the complement cascade may be involved in the phototoxic reaction mechanism.[16,17] The cutaneous manifestations in acute attacks consist of prominent erythema in sun-exposed areas with a burning sensation. Subacute or chronic skin involvement consists of skin fragility, blister formation, and progressive scarring. Exceptional cases of a photosensitive bullous eruption associated with transient elevation of porphyrin levels have been described in neonates during phototherapy for treatment of hyperbilirubinemia due to hemolytic disease.[18,19]

Porphyria is primarily classified into erythropoietic and hepatic types depending upon which tissue is predominantly affected. The erythropoietic porphyrias (congenital erythropoietic porphyria and erythropoietic protoporphyria) are characterized by altered heme synthesis mainly in the bone marrow. In the hepatic porphyrias the altered synthesis mainly occurs in the liver (porphyria cutanea tarda, hepatoerythropoietic porphyria, acute

intermittent porphyria, aminolevulinic acid (ALA) dehydratase deficiency, variegate porphyria, and hereditary coproporphyria). Of the eight major types of porphyria, six are associated with cutaneous disease (*Table 13.4*). The clinical and biochemical findings are very different in these six types of porphyria, although the cutaneous histology is similar in all.[20–23] Type II porphyria cutanea tarda, hereditary coproporphyria, variegate porphyria, and erythropoietic protoporphyria are all inherited as autosomal dominants with incomplete penetrance. Fewer than 20% of affected individuals display symptoms and patients often deny a family history.[2]

Congenital erythropoietic porphyria

Clinical features

Congenital erythropoietic porphyria (Gunther disease) is the most severe and mutilating of the erythropoietic porphyrias. It is inherited as an autosomal recessive and develops as a consequence of deficiency of the fourth enzyme of the heme pathway (uroporphyrinogen III synthase) resulting in excessive production of uroporphyrin I and coproporphyrin I, which give the urine a pink–burgundy color.[1–4] Patients with the more severe form of the disease may present with fetal hydrops.[4,5] The diapers of affected children usually show a characteristic pink stain. Uroporphyrin I accumulates in the bone marrow, peripheral blood, and other organs. It has been demonstrated that there is a clear correlation between the degree of porphyrin excess and disease severity.[6] There is increased production of uroporphyrins and coproporphyrins in the urine and coproporphyrins in the feces.

Affected patients develop intense photosensitivity to sunlight as well as to fluorescent light, typically in infancy (*Fig. 13.92*). Symptoms include painful and pruritic erythema and swelling, which occurs within minutes of sun exposure. Vesicles and bullae are supervened by a mutilating scarring process on the face and hands, where autoamputation may occur (*Figs 13.93*

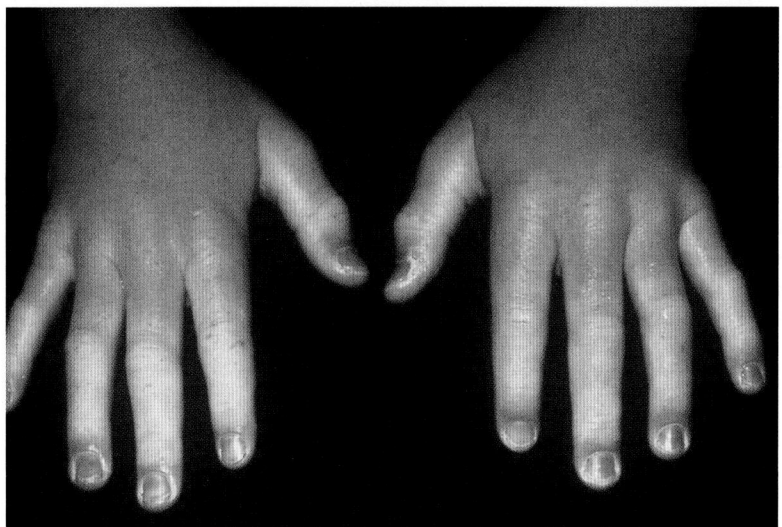

Fig. 13.92
Congenital erythropoietic porphyria (Gunther disease): this variant is associated with severe photosensitivity. There is marked erythema and edema of the backs of the hands and fingers. Scarring frequently supervenes. By courtesy of G. Murphy, MD, Beaumont Hospital, Dublin, Eire.

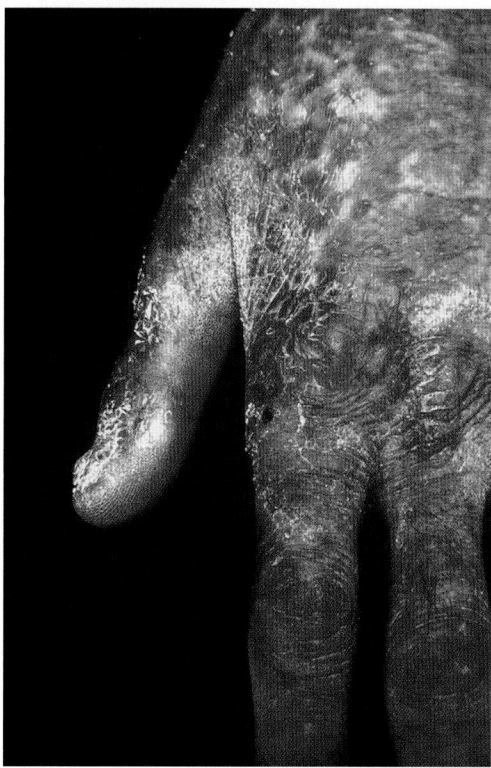

Fig. 13.94
Congenital erythropoietic porphyria (Gunther disease): adult patient showing very severe photodamage. By courtesy of the Institute of Dermatology, London, UK.

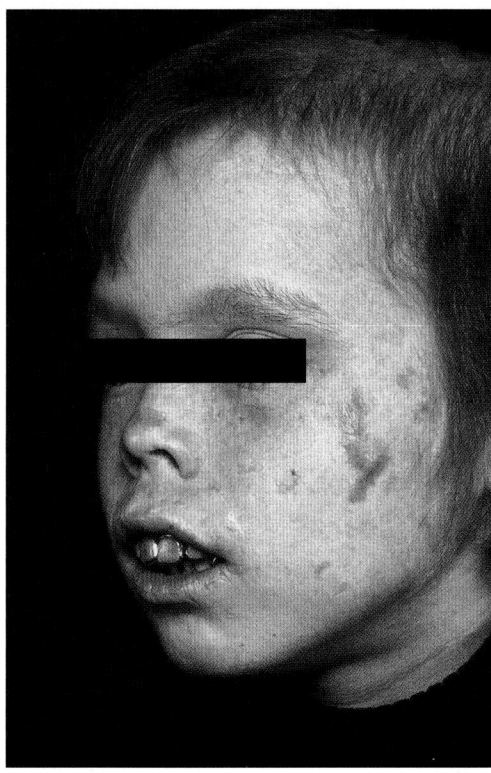

Fig. 13.93
Congenital erythropoietic porphyria (Gunther disease): in this severely affected patient, there is marked hyperpigmented scarring on the cheeks, nose, and around the mouth. The brownish discoloration of the teeth is characteristic. By courtesy of G. Murphy, MD, Beaumont Hospital, Dublin, Eire.

and 13.94). A rare case of metastatic squamous cell carcinoma has been reported in an amputation stump.[7] Sclerodermoid change is sometimes seen.[8] A case resembling pseudoxanthoma elasticum (PXE) has also been reported.[9] Coarse hair may be found on the face, and lanugo hair develops on the limbs. Pigmentary changes are sometimes evident. In addition, patients develop cicatricial alopecia of the scalp, nail changes, conjunctivitis, ectropion, keratoconjunctivitis, symblepharon, blepharitis, necrotizing scleritis, or brown staining of the teeth (erythrodontia).[4,10–14] The teeth characteristically fluoresce intense orange–red with Wood light (400 nm).[14] The sclera also demonstrates pink fluorescence under Wood light.[15]

Hemolytic anemia and splenomegaly occur in a large proportion of the patients and hypersplenism is sometimes a feature. Patients with congenital erythropoietic porphyria have an increased risk of bone fragility with resultant fractures and developmental defects.[2] Acro-osteolysis, soft tissue calcifications, and widening of the diploic space have also been documented.[16,17] Early death may result, often in the third decade. Rare cases are associated with the nephrotic syndrome, probably secondary to renal siderosis.[18] A delayed late-onset variant has rarely been described.[19–22] Some of these patients present with thrombocytopenia and others with myelodysplasia.[21–25]

The URO-synthase gene has been mapped to chromosome 10q25.3-q26.[3,4,21] The molecular defects in this disease are very heterogeneous and greater than 38 mutations in the URO-synthase gene have already been described.[25–34] These include single base substitutions, insertions and deletions, and splicing defects. By far the most common mutation is C73R, which has been found in up to 40% of patients with the disease. Two other relatively common mutations include L4F and T228M, seen in 8% and 7% of patients, respectively.[26] Prenatal diagnosis of the disease is possible not only by measurement of uroporphyrin I levels in amniotic fluid, but also by DNA mutation analysis.[35]

Erythropoietic protoporphyria

Clinical features

Although this condition was not recognized until 1961, it is now known to be the second commonest type of porphyria. It results from increased production of protoporphyrin due to diminished ferrochelatase (heme synthase) activity.[1–3] Ferrochelatase is the enzyme responsible for the combination between protoporphyrin IX and iron to form heme. Urinary porphyrins are normal because protoporphyrins are insoluble in water. Protoporphyrin is elevated in plasma, erythrocytes, and occasionally in the feces.[1] Coproporphyrins may be found in erythrocytes and feces. The mode of inheritance is predominantly autosomal dominant with incomplete penetrance although an autosomal recessive inheritance has also rarely been reported.[4–6] The gene for ferrochelatase has been mapped to the long arm of chromosome 18 (18q21.3).[7] A less common genetic variant is the X-linked dominant form

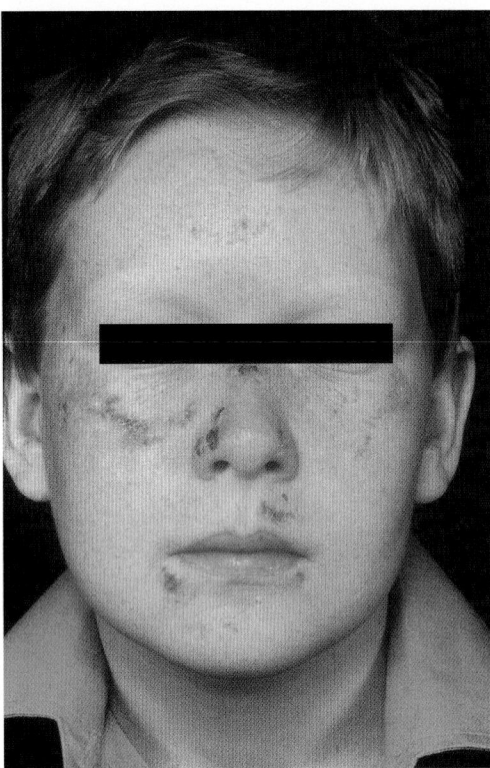

Fig. 13.95
Erythropoietic protoporphyria: crusted lesions are present on the cheeks, nose, and around the mouth. By courtesy of G. Murphy, MD, Beaumont Hospital, Dublin, Eire.

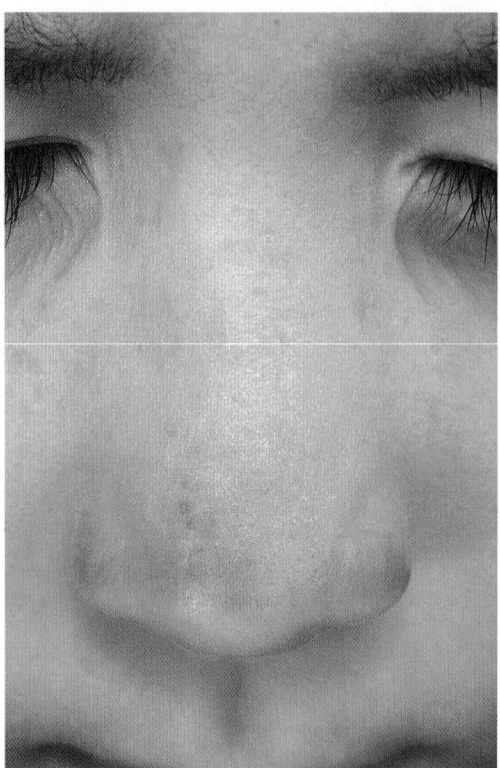

Fig. 13.97
Erythropoietic protoporphyria: there are characteristic, depressed, small linear scars on the bridge and sides of this patient's nose. By courtesy of the Institute of Dermatology, London, UK.

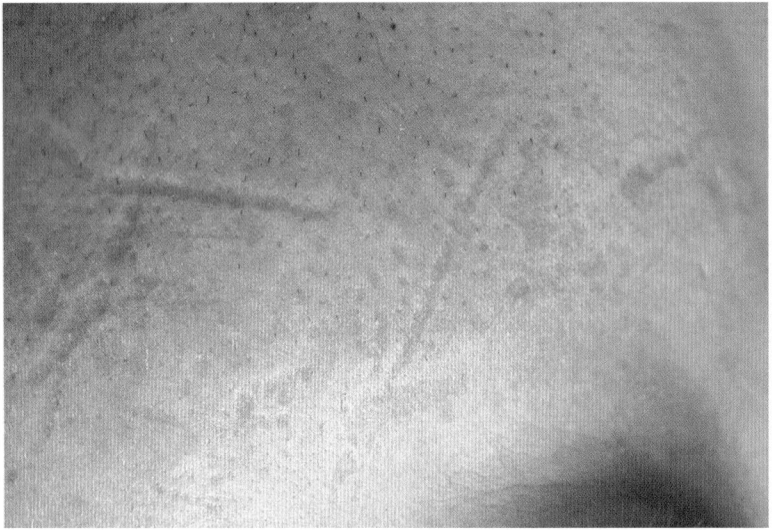

Fig. 13.96
Erythropoietic protoporphyria: there is marked scarring. Note the depressed linear lesions. By courtesy of G. Murphy, MD, Beaumont Hospital, Dublin, Eire.

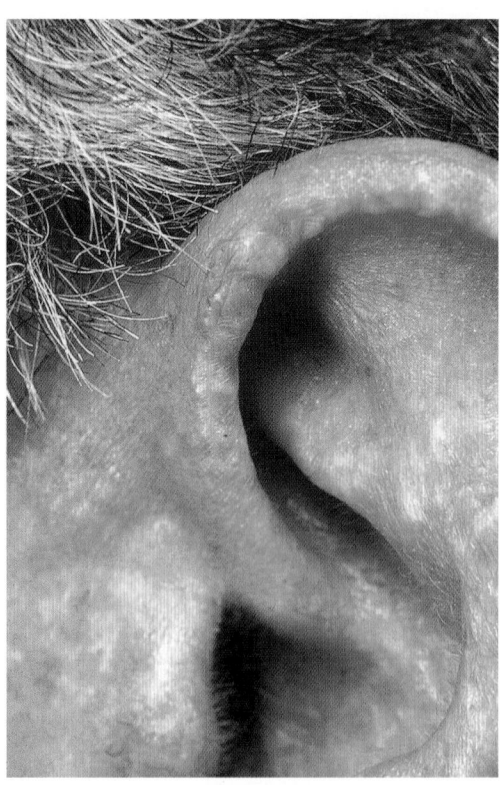

Fig. 13.98
Erythropoietic protoporphyria: there is very severe actinic damage. By courtesy of the Institute of Dermatology, London, UK.

caused by a gain of function mutation in erythroid-specific 5-aminolevulinate synthase on the X-chromosome.[8–12] This form appears to be more common in North Africa.[11]

The variable clinical manifestations of this disease are probably the result of heterogeneity of the ferrochelatase gene defects.[4,13,14] Acute photosensitivity usually presents in early childhood.[15] A painful burning erythema with edema occurs immediately after exposure to sunlight.[16] Petechiae can occur, particularly with prolonged exposure. Vesicles are uncommon, but a scaly, erythematous reaction may be seen, leading to circular or linear depressed scars on the face (particularly on the bridge of the nose and around the mouth) and over the knuckles (Figs 13.95–13.99).[1] Purpura and urticaria are sometimes seen. There may also be a waxlike thickening of the skin, particularly of the dorsum of the hands and, more rarely, the face (Fig. 13.100).[1] Bullae and milia have been documented exceptionally.[3] A further case presented with pseudoainhum.[17] An association with lupus erythematosus is very rare.[18] Hypertrichosis and hyperpigmentation are not typically seen.[2]

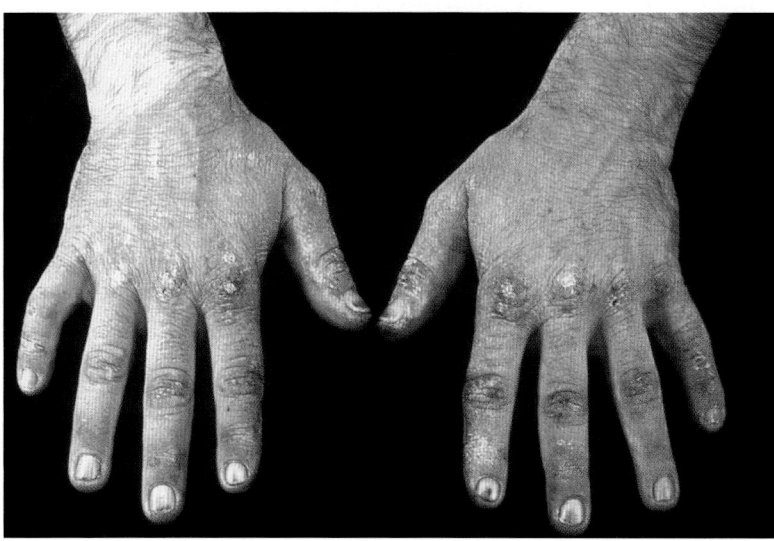

Fig. 13.99
Erythropoietic protoporphyria: note the characteristic scaly scars over the knuckles. By courtesy of the Institute of Dermatology, London, UK.

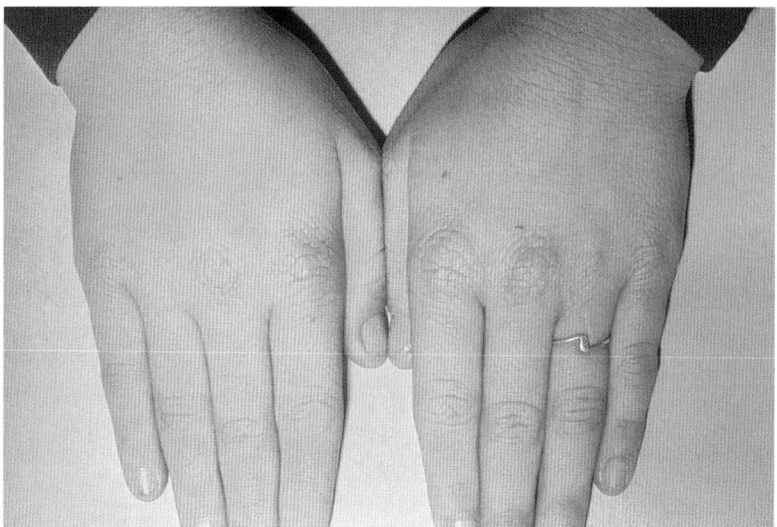

Fig. 13.100
Erythropoietic protoporphyria: there is characteristic waxy thickening of the skin of the hands. By courtesy of G. Murphy, MD, Beaumont Hospital, Dublin, Eire.

In the majority of cases the disease is limited to the skin, but some affected patients develop protoporphyrin-rich gallstones, and 5% to 10% of patients develop liver disease, which may progress to liver failure in fewer than 5% of patients and rarely to cirrhosis.[7,19-21] Patients who develop liver failure typically have the autosomal recessive or X-linked dominant forms of transmission.[11,22] Neurological manifestations are not common. Anemia is rare and if present is very mild.

Recently, a late-onset variant has been described, which is more commonly associated with hematological malignancy, where the disease occurs secondary to an acquired somatic mutation in the malignant clone within the bone marrow.[23-26] Exacerbation of the disease by blood transfusion and by iron ingestion has been described.[27,28]

Hereditary coproporphyria

Clinical features

This very rare autosomal dominant form of porphyria develops as a result of a deficiency of coproporphyrinogen oxidase.[1,2] This enzyme catalyzes the sixth step in the heme biosynthetic pathway. It has been mapped to the long arm of chromosome 3 (3q11.2).[3] A number of different mutations have been documented.[4,5] Heterozygous patients often do not manifest symptoms of the disease.[6] In those who develop symptoms, these usually appear after puberty. Affected patients develop intermittent attacks of abdominal pain in association with neurological and psychiatric manifestations. About 30% of cases develop photosensitivity, usually at the time of the acute attacks. The cutaneous changes are similar to those described for porphyria cutanea tarda. The disease may be precipitated by pregnancy, the contraceptive pill, fasting, infections, and the anabolic steroid methandrostenolone.[3,7-9] Diagnosis is confirmed by the presence of increased excretion of coproporphyrinogen III in urine and feces. Porphobilinogen and aminolevulinic acid are increased during the episodic attacks.

Harderoporphyria is regarded as a variant form of hereditary coproporphyria in which hematological alterations predominate.[2,10] Patients present with jaundice, severe chronic hemolytic anemia starting in the neonatal period, hepatosplenomegaly, and photosensitivity. Neuropsychiatric symptoms or abdominal pain are not seen. These patients usually have a specific mutation (K404E) on one or both alleles of the coproporphyrinogen gene.[11]

Porphyria cutanea tarda

Clinical features

This is the commonest type of porphyria and usually manifests in middle age.[1-3] It shows a marked male predominance.[4] The highest incidence is found in the South African Bantu.[4] Cases are also often seen in Europe and North America.

There are two main forms of porphyria cutanea tarda: familial and sporadic.[1] Both variants have in common a reduced activity of uroporphyrinogen decarboxylase (URO-D), which catalyzes the decarboxylation of uroporphyrinogen to coproporphyrinogen. In the familial variant there is decreased URO-D activity in erythrocytes and most other tissues while in the sporadic form there is decreased URO-D activity restricted to the liver.[5,6] In rare familial cases, normal URO-D activity has been reported in erythrocytes.[7]

The rare familial form exhibits an autosomal dominant inheritance. The onset tends to be earlier than that of the sporadic form and the exceptional cases occurring in childhood are usually familial. The disease is related to many different mutations in the *UROD* gene.[8,9] There is no clear correlation between disease severity and the type of mutation.[10] Porphyria cutanea tarda may be precipitated by many exogenous factors, including alcohol abuse, iron overload, childbirth, and sun exposure.[11] Pregnancy may exacerbate the symptoms of the disease during the first trimester.[12] Multiple factors often contribute to precipitate the disease in a given patient.[13] Rare cases of familial porphyria cutanea tarda present with constrictive pericarditis.[14]

The second much more common form is sporadic or acquired. Up to 80% of patients with porphyria cutanea tarda have the sporadic form of the disease. It has been demonstrated that sporadic porphyria cutanea tarda is a multifactorial disorder involving a combination of genetic and environmental factors. Recent studies have demonstrated that the hemochromatosis gene mutations C282Y and H63D represent a susceptibility factor in Western European and Australian patients affected by this form of the disease.[15-20] These mutations probably induce the disease through iron overload. It has also been suggested that the IVS4+198 T allele in the human transferrin receptor-1 may play an independent role in the development of the disease.[15] However, this has not been substantiated in other studies.[18] Coinheritance of mutations in the uroporphyrinogen decarboxylase and in the hemochromatosis genes appears to accelerate the onset of porphyria cutanea tarda.[21] Sporadic cases mainly occur in patients exposed to a variety of hepatotoxic chemicals, such as ethanol, estrogens, griseofulvin, vitamin B_{12}, sulfonamides, tamoxifen, pravastatin, barbiturates, hydantoins, and chlorinated hydrocarbons: for example, an epidemic form occurred in Turkey due to exposure to the fungicide hexachlorobenzene.[22-26] Rare associations include diabetes mellitus, Wilson disease, myelofibrosis, the CREST syndrome, and hepatocellular carcinoma.[27-30]

Increased hepatic iron stores are a major predisposing factor.[6,20,31,32] The mechanism by which this happens is not well understood. Iron catalyzes the formation of reactive oxygen species and this may enhance uroporphyrin

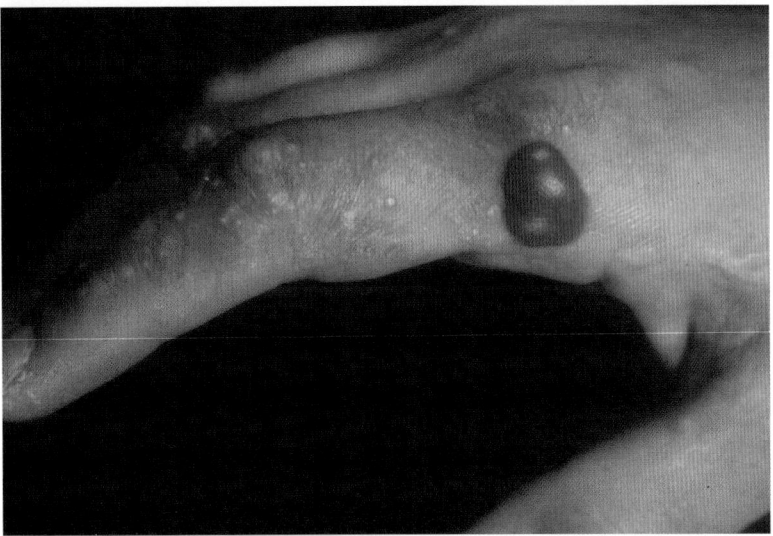

Fig. 13.101
Porphyria cutanea tarda: in addition to a blood-filled vesicle there are numerous milia. By courtesy of G. Murphy, MD, Beaumont Hospital, Dublin, Eire.

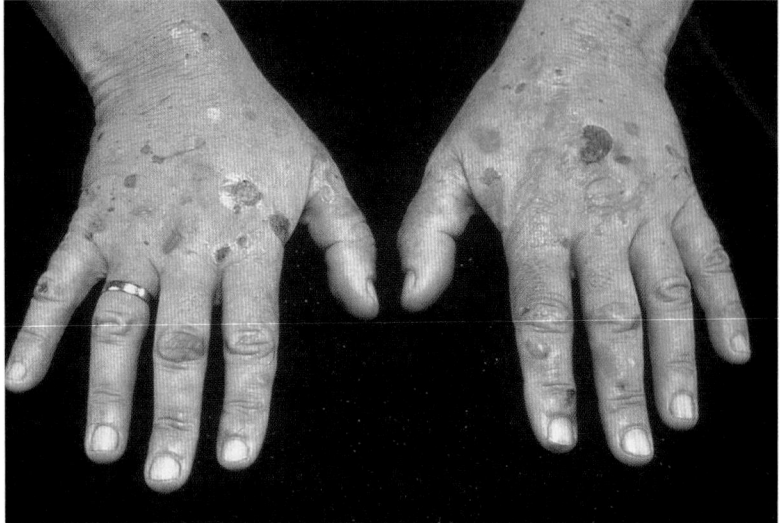

Fig. 13.102
Porphyria cutanea tarda: there are numerous ruptured blisters. Milia are also evident. By courtesy of the Institute of Dermatology, London, UK.

formation by increasing the rate at which uroporphyrinogen is oxidized to uroporphyrin, leading to the manifestations of the disease. A second possible proposed mechanism considers the indirect inhibition of uroporphyrinogen decarboxylase by iron. Whatever the mechanism, the iron overload has important therapeutic implications as venesection can induce a remission.

Hepatitis C virus infection is often associated with porphyria cutanea tarda.[32-35] A frequent association is also the acquired immunodeficiency syndrome (AIDS).[36-43] AIDS patients with porphyria cutanea tarda are often hepatitis C virus-positive.[43,44] Patients who have had both acquired and familial variants have developed the typical features of increased skin fragility, blistering, hyperpigmentation, and hypertrichosis, but scarring and milia have rarely been evident.[45] Often, the development of porphyria has preceded the diagnosis of HIV infection.[41] In many instances this has been related to excessive alcohol consumption and/or infectious hepatitis, particularly hepatitis C.[40,46] The association has been reported too often to be merely fortuitous and liver damage seems to be the common denominator. The causal agent (be it hepatitis C virus or HIV) seems to have a direct effect upon hepatocyte porphyrin metabolism. It has been demonstrated that elevated serum porphyrin levels occur in early-stage HIV infection and hepatitis C infection.[47] Porphyria cutanea tarda has also been described in association with nonalcoholic liver disease, chronic hemodialysis, noninsulin dependent diabetes mellitus and lupus erythematosus.[1,48,49] An autoantibody study in a large series of patients with lupus erythematosus suggests that the association is fortuitous.[50] The association with hematological malignancies, including leukemia and lymphoma, is usually related to the treatment, particularly repeated blood transfusions.[51,52]

Typically, blisters occur on light-exposed skin and are traumatic or actinically induced (Figs 13.101–13.103).[4] Cutaneous fragility is usually marked. The blisters are slow to heal and leave superficial atrophic scars with milia. Although they are most often seen on the backs of the hands, they may also be found on the palms, face, scalp, forearms, trunk, and under the finger nails.[4] Hypertrichosis and premature aging with chronic actinic damage are usual and sclerodermatous changes may be marked (Fig. 13.104). The hypertrichosis is characterized by long dark lanugo hair developing about the cheeks and temples, the eyebrows, ears, and arms (Fig. 13.105).[4] The sclerodermatous features, which are more common in females, are found on both light-exposed and unexposed skin. Sites that are particularly affected include the face, neck, scalp, chest, and backs of hands, and often there is hyper- or hypopigmentation or both.[4,53-55] In rare cases, patients may clinically present as scleroderma without other manifestations of porphyria cutanea tarda.[55] Hyperpigmentation, if present, may be diffuse, reticulate or spotty. Preauricular calcification is a common complication. The dermal fibrosis appears to be related particularly to high uroporphyrin

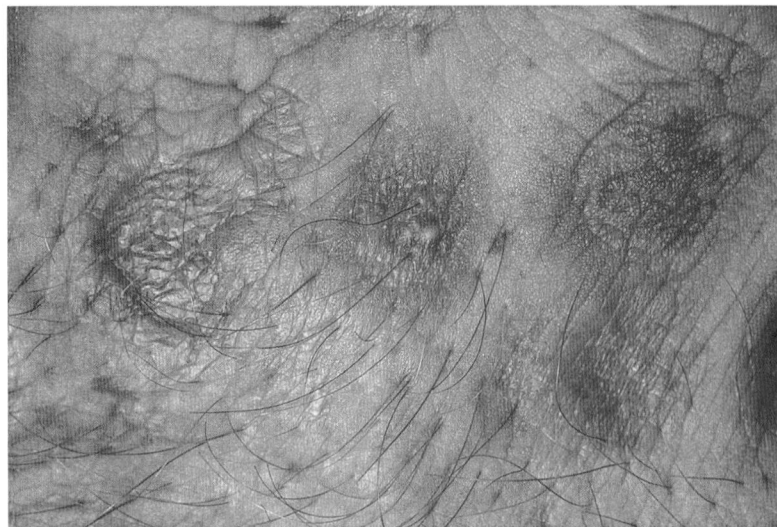

Fig. 13.103
Porphyria cutanea tarda: note the scarring and milia. By courtesy of the Institute of Dermatology, London, UK.

levels.[53] Uroporphyrin has been shown to stimulate fibroblast collagen synthesis independent of ultraviolet light.[56]

Uncommon cutaneous manifestations of porphyria cutanea tarda include alopecia affecting the frontoparietal, temporal, and occipital regions of the scalp, and centrofacial papular lymphangiectasis.[57-59] Hair darkening has also been reported.[60] Very rare cases have been documented presenting with plaques or simulating solar urticaria.[61,62]

Acute attacks are not a feature of this variant. Biochemical evidence of liver involvement is common, but clinical manifestations are unusual.[1] Urinary porphyrin levels are increased and result in pink–red fluorescence with a Wood lamp.[63]

The diagnosis is confirmed by the presence of uroporphyrin and heptacarboxylic porphyrins in urine and plasma and by the presence of isocoproporphyrin in feces.

Hepatoerythropoietic porphyria

Clinical features

Hepatoerythropoietic porphyria is very rare and, in fact, represents the homozygous form of familial porphyria cutanea tarda.[1] Both diseases share

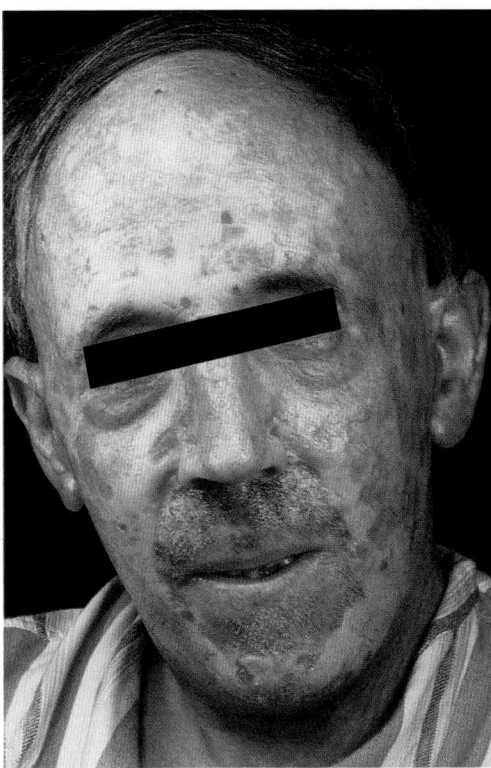

Fig. 13.104
Porphyria cutanea tarda: there is marked facial scarring with sclerodermiform features. By courtesy of G. Murphy, MD, Beaumont Hospital, Dublin, Eire.

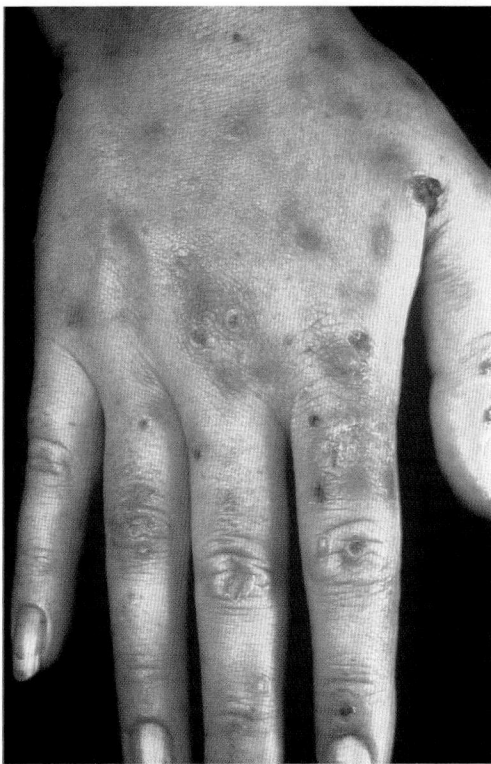

Fig. 13.106
Variegate porphyria: numerous ruptured vesicles are present on the back of the hand and fingers. By courtesy of G. Murphy, MD, Beaumont Hospital, Dublin, Eire.

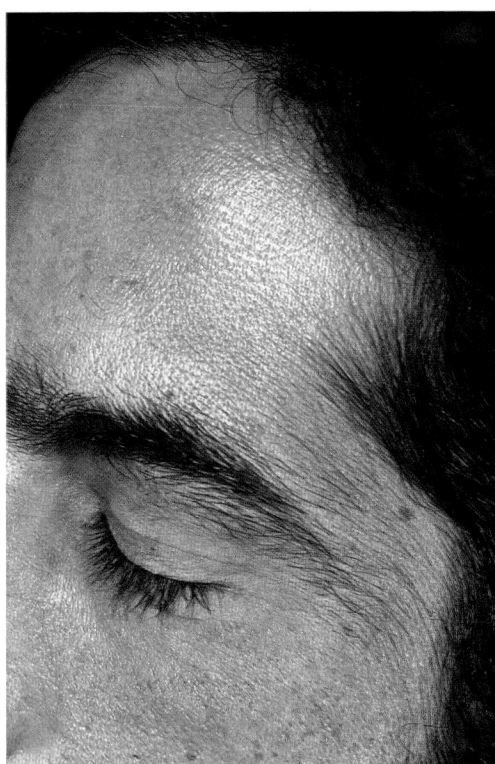

Fig. 13.105
Porphyria cutanea tarda: hypertrichosis as seen in this patient is a very typical feature. By courtesy of the Institute of Dermatology, London, UK.

mutations.[8,9] Extreme immediate photosensitivity occurs in infancy.[10–12] Erythema, edema, and vesicles lead to severe scarring, with hypertrichosis and sclerodermatous changes in exposed areas.[13] Ocular features include photophobia, conjunctivitis, and scleromalacia perforans.[14] Hepatitis, cirrhosis, and normochromic anemia may also occur.

Variegate porphyria

Clinical features

This familial type of porphyria manifests the cutaneous features of porphyria cutanea tarda and the acute abdominal and neurological attacks of acute intermittent porphyria, both of which usually become apparent in the second or third decade (*Figs 13.106–13.109*).[1,2] It is particularly common in South Africa where it can be traced to the descendants of a single Dutch family.[2,3] It is an autosomal dominantly inherited condition and more severely affected homozygotes have been recognized (*Figs 13.110 and 13.111*). Variegate porphyria is associated with diminished activity of protoporphyrinogen oxidase, the penultimate enzyme in the heme biosynthetic pathway.[4] Several different mutations have been demonstrated in the protoporphyrin oxidase gene on chromosome 1q22-23.[5–7] The genotype is not a significant determinant of the clinical manifestations.[8–10] Usually, there is approximately a 50% reduction in the activity of the enzyme.[10]

Acute attacks may be precipitated by a wide range of drugs that induce hepatic microsomal activity, including barbiturates, alcohol, oral contraceptives, pregnancy, anticonvulsants, and sulfonamides.[11–14] Acute variegate porphyria has also presented during an episode of viral hepatitis.[11] The cutaneous manifestations are sometimes mild or absent during the acute attack and the condition may therefore be misdiagnosed as acute intermittent porphyria.[2]

Histologic features of the porphyrias

Direct immunofluorescence reveals immunoglobulin (particularly IgG and to a lesser extent IgM), fibrinogen, and C3 outlining characteristic donut-shaped blood vessels in the papillary dermis (*Fig. 13.112*). Although

some of the mutations that have been described.[2] This form of porphyria is also heterogeneous and different mutations in the *UROD* gene may occur.[3–7] The activity of uroporphyrinogen decarboxylase is much lower than in porphyria cutanea tarda. As a consequence, disease manifestations are typically severe. Mild variants have been reported in association with certain genetic

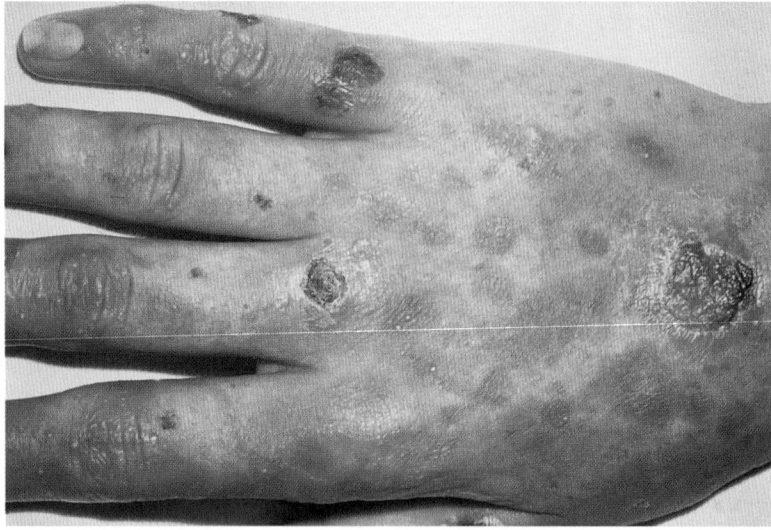

Fig. 13.107
Variegate porphyria: there are ruptured blisters with scarring and milia. By courtesy of the Institute of Dermatology, London, UK.

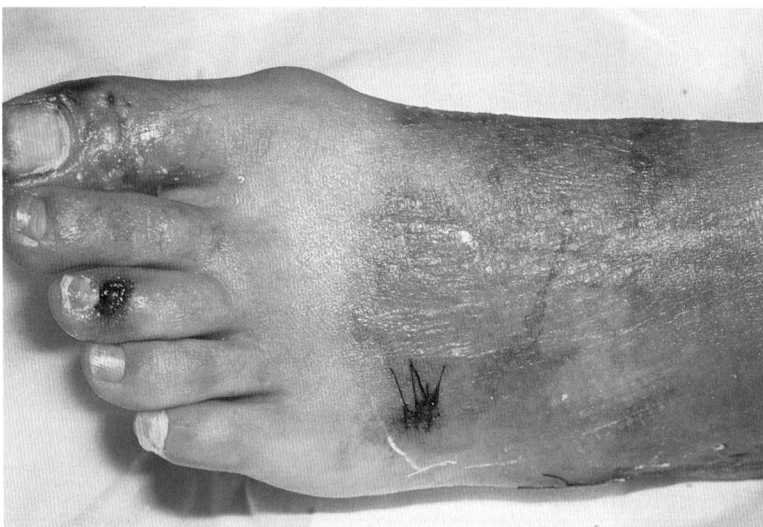

Fig. 13.108
Variegate porphyria: note the blistering over the toes and dorsum of the foot. By courtesy of the Institute of Dermatology, London, UK.

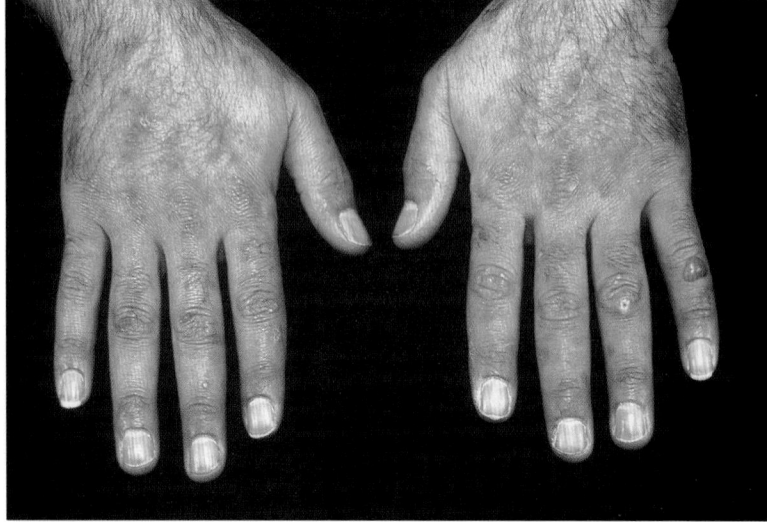

Fig. 13.109
Variegate porphyria: an intact blister is present on the left little finger. Elsewhere, there is marked scarring and milia are present. By courtesy of the Institute of Dermatology, London, UK.

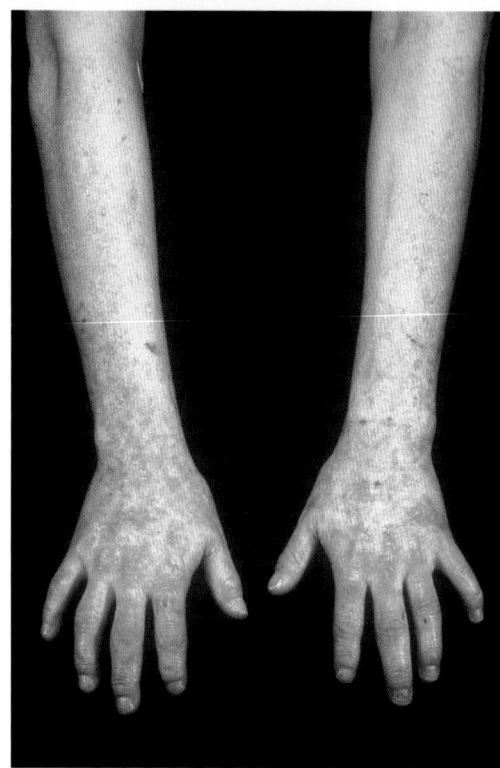

Fig. 13.110
Homozygous variegate porphyria: there is marked scarring of the dorsal surface of the forearms, hands, and fingers. By courtesy of the Institute of Dermatology, London, UK.

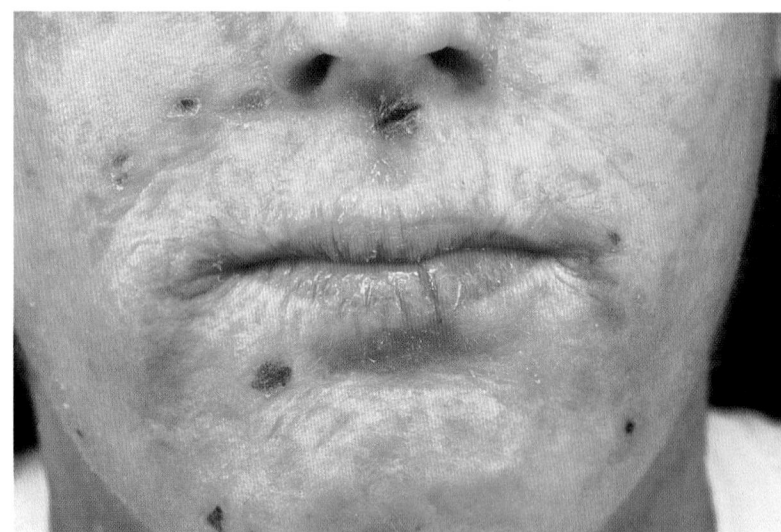

Fig. 13.111
Homozygous variegate porphyria: note the perioral erosions and scarring. By courtesy of the Institute of Dermatology, London, UK.

this is particularly evident in erythropoietic protoporphyria, it is also a feature of the other 'cutaneous' variants.[1-3] Immunoreactants are also frequently present at the dermal–epidermal junction and have been identified within the basement membrane region of eccrine sweat glands and ducts.[1-5] This finding is believed to be due to the non-specific binding of serum components rather than an immunologically mediated reaction.[4] In addition, both type IV collagen and laminin are present in increased amounts, thereby contributing to the vessel wall thickening.[6] Cytoid bodies are also commonly evident.[4] Direct immunofluorescence studies have demonstrated granular and homogenous deposition of the membrane attack complex C5b-9 in vessel walls of the superficial and mid dermis in patients with porphyria cutanea tarda. It is proposed that UV light activated uroporphyrins

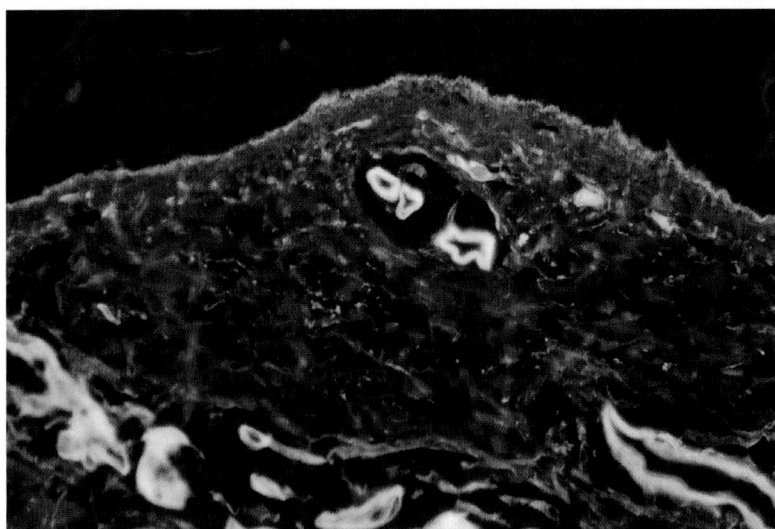

Fig. 13.112
Porphyria cutanea tarda: the superficial blood vessels show striking IgG circumferential deposition.

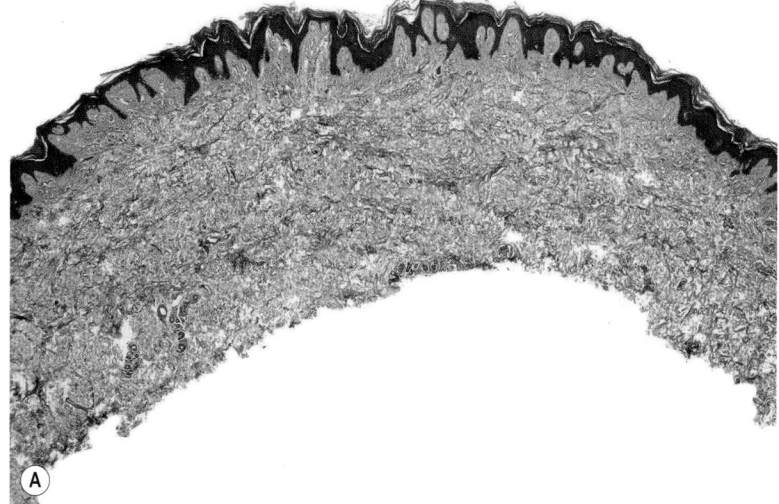

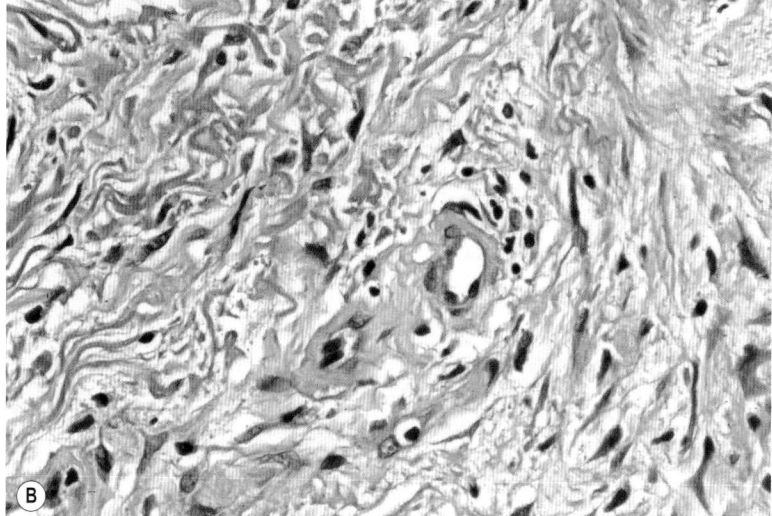

Fig. 13.113
(**A**, **B**) Porphyria cutanea tarda: the superficial vessels are thickened and appear hyalinized.

in turn activate complement, possibly playing a pathological role.[7] Indirect immunofluorescence is invariably negative for basement membrane zone autoantibodies.

The histologic changes for all types of porphyria are very similar. The characteristic feature is the presence of a PAS-positive, diastase-resistant, hyaline material around the blood vessels of affected skin (*Figs 13.113* and *13.114*). In mild disease the deposits are delicate and are usually limited to the papillary dermal blood vessels, but in more severe cases the deposits are widespread, occur more deeply in the dermis, and give the vessel walls a characteristic lamellated appearance. These appearances are particularly conspicuous in erythropoietic protoporphyria.[1,8] Alcian blue-positive mucin is sometimes evident around the blood vessels and to a lesser extent at the dermal–epidermal junction in both porphyria cutanea tarda and erythropoietic protoporphyria.[1] Lipid droplets are sometimes also demonstrable. A false-positive Congo red stain for amyloid may be evident in the lower dermis.[1]

Electron microscopic observations include considerable basement membrane reduplication around the dermal vasculature and to a lesser extent at the dermal–epidermal junction (*Fig. 13.115*).[1,8] This is consistent with the effects of repetitive endothelial cell injury and regeneration with subsequent new basement membrane formation. In addition, finely fibrillar material is typically present both around the vessels and at the epidermal basement membrane region. Irregular electron-dense amorphous deposits may also be evident.[1]

There may be subepidermal blisters, characteristically associated with slight mononuclear inflammatory cell infiltration (*Figs 13.116* and *13.117*). Neutrophil polymorphs showing leukocytoclasis have been described in acute lesions of erythropoietic protoporphyria and red cell extravasation is sometimes evident.[9] Festooning of the dermal papillae is often, though not invariably, present. The plane of cleavage appears to be variable.[3,10] Some blisters arise beneath the lamina densa in the superficial dermis similar to epidermolysis bullosa acquisita. In others, they develop within the reduplicated basement membrane constituents. Most often, however, as shown by antigen mapping experiments, blistering commences in the lamina lucida.[10,11] Type IV collagen and laminin are therefore usually present along the floor of the blister while bullous pemphigoid antigen is evident in the roof. Linear segmented structures composed of type IV collagen and laminin have been identified in the roof of blisters from patients with porphyria cutanea tarda.[3,12] These so-called caterpillar bodies may also be seen in specimens from patients with erythropoietic protoporphyria and drug-induced pseudoporphyria (*Fig. 13.117b*).[13] They are PAS positive and appear as globules arranged in a linear fashion in the epidermis overlying the subepidermal blisters. Ultrastructural studies suggest that these bodies represent a combination of degenerating keratinocytes, colloid bodies, and basement

membrane fragments formed by repeated blistering and re-epithelialization.[14] Caterpillar bodies are present in up to 43% of porphyria cutanea tarda specimens.[15] 'Caterpillar body-like clusters' have also been identified in patients with porphyria cutanea tarda, erythropoietic protoporphyria, bullous pemphigoid, and junctional and dystrophic epidermolysis bullosa. These clusters were histologically identical to classical caterpillar bodies, but did not stain for type IV collagen or PAS stains.[15]

Rarely, a lichenoid tissue reaction has been documented in porphyria cutanea tarda.[16]

The histologic features of the blisters seen in variegate porphyria are identical to those described for porphyria cutanea tarda.[17]

A secondary sclerodermatous change is frequently present in more chronic lesions, characterized by thickened collagen bundles and reduced numbers of cutaneous adnexae (*Fig. 13.118*).[4,8,18] Diastase-resistant, PAS-positive material may be identified throughout the involved dermis.[1] This is particularly marked in porphyria cutanea tarda. Its distinction from the dermal changes of scleroderma may be very difficult, but it has been said that the texture of the collagen bundles is somewhat looser in porphyria.[1] The clinical distribution of sclerodermoid changes in porphyrias in sun-exposed skin aids in the distinction.[19] Basement membrane thickening due to diastase-resistant, PAS-positive material is usually present, particularly in porphyria cutanea tarda.[1,8] Solar elastosis is often evident in the latter condition, but this is probably largely a consequence of the age of the patient and is unlikely to be a fundamental process (*Fig. 13.119*). It is not a feature of erythropoietic protoporphyria.[1,8]

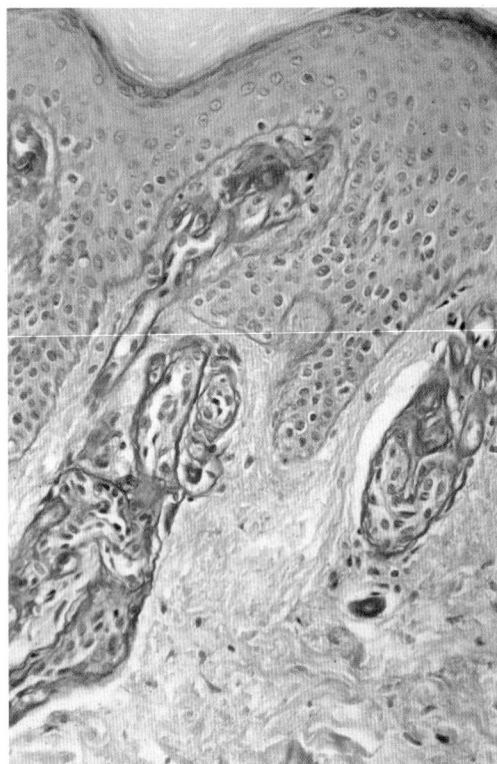

Fig. 13.114
Erythropoietic protoporphyria: the appearances are much more dramatic in this periodic acid–Schiff-stained section.

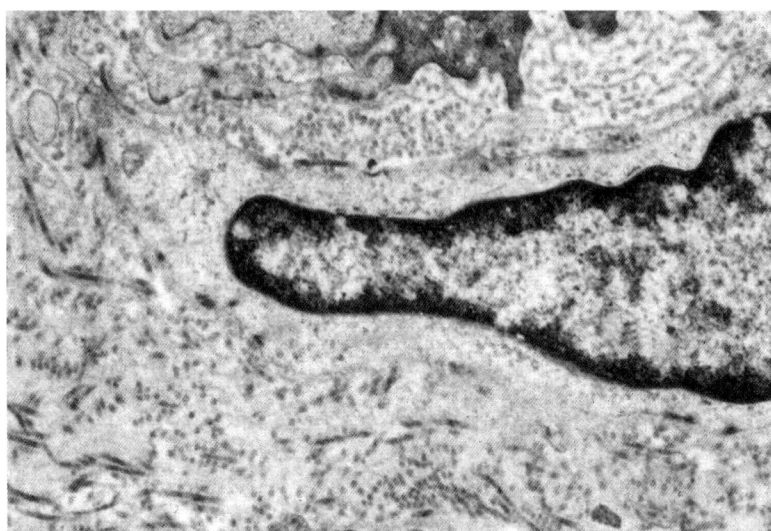

Fig. 13.115
Porphyria cutanea tarda: there is striking basement membrane reduplication surrounding this small dermal vessel.

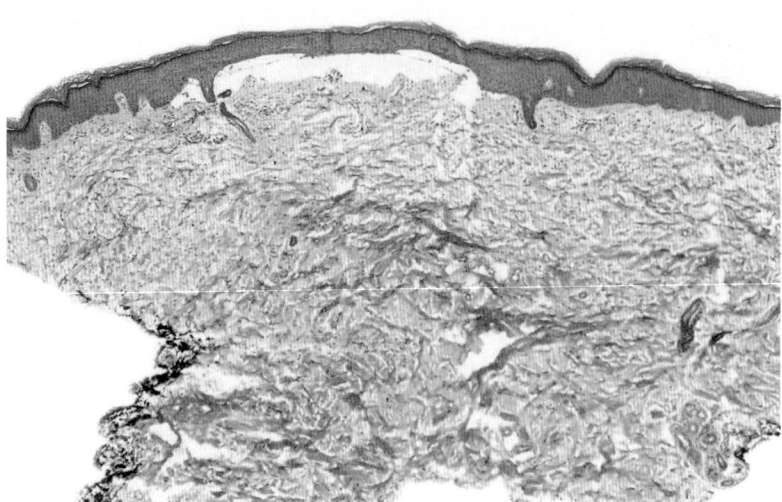

Fig. 13.116
Porphyria cutanea tarda: a bland subepidermal blister is present.

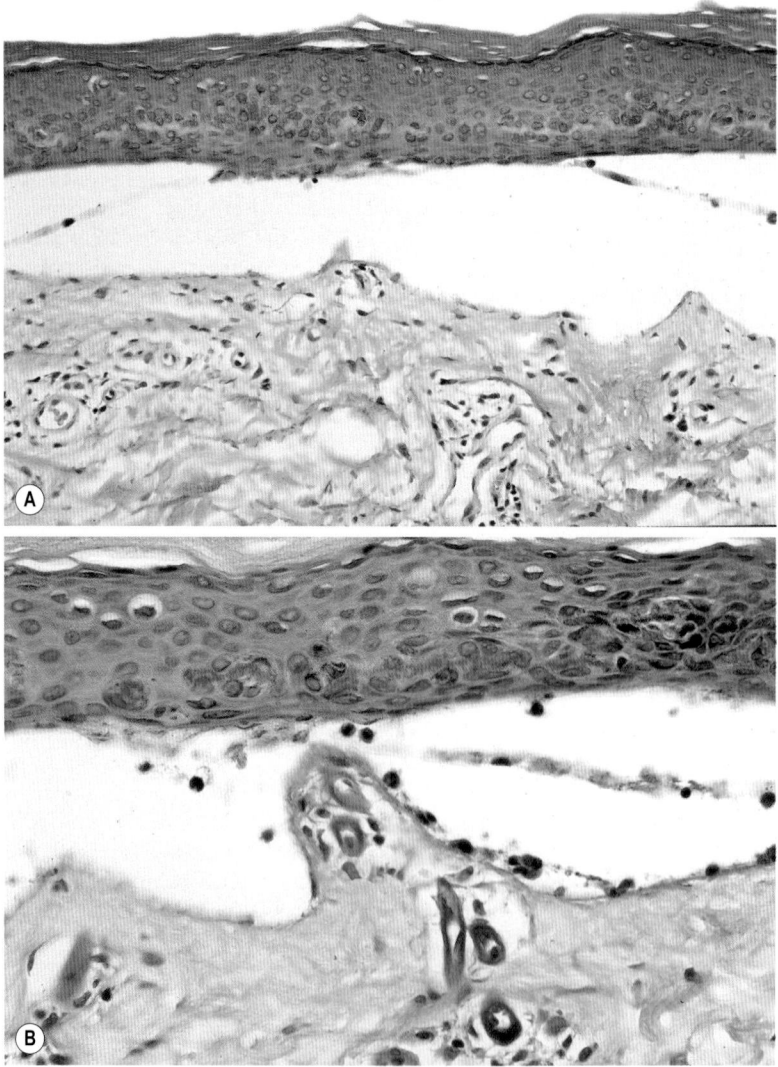

Fig. 13.117
Porphyria cutanea tarda: (**A**) the blister is cell free; (**B**) the superficial vessels are thickened (periodic acid–Schiff). Note the caterpillar bodies in the overlying epidermis.

In the alopecia associated with porphyria cutanea tarda, the initial changes are those of swelling and homogenization of the perifollicular connective tissue sheath.[20] Later, the features of sclerodermatous transformation of the reticular dermis supervene. Centrofacial papular lymphangiectasis is characterized by the presence of dilated lymphatics in the superficial dermis.[21]

The hepatic changes of porphyria cutanea tarda are variable and include needle-shaped uroporphyrin crystals, hepatitis, liver cell degeneration and regeneration, fatty change, hemosiderosis, and scarring, sometimes amounting to cirrhosis (*Fig. 13.120*).[20,22,23] There is an increased risk of hepatocellular carcinoma.[23–27] Hepatic changes of erythropoietic protoporphyria include birefringent, dark brown, protoporphyrin crystal deposition in the

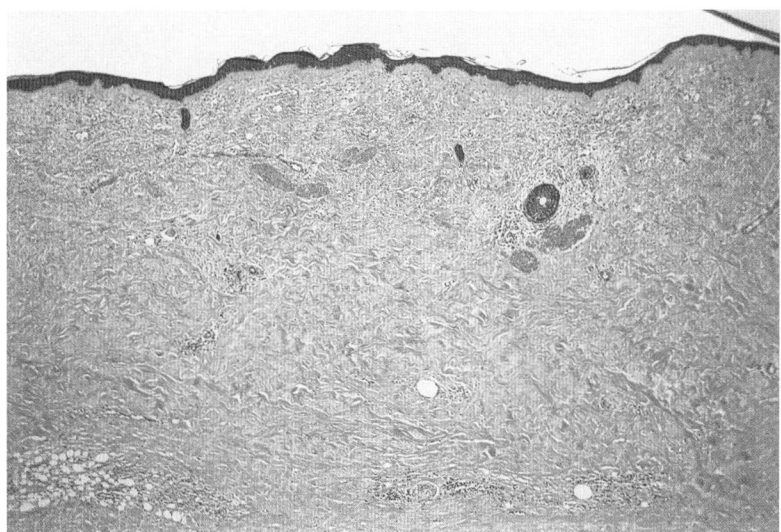

Fig. 13.118
Porphyria cutanea tarda: there is intense scarring of the entire dermis. The fat entrapment is reminiscent of scleroderma.

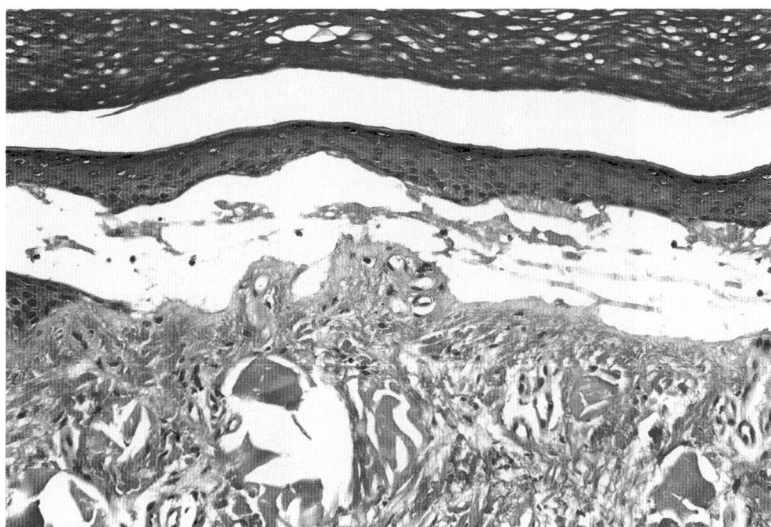

Fig. 13.119
Porphyria cutanea tarda: there is colloid milium-like solar elastosis deep to this blister.

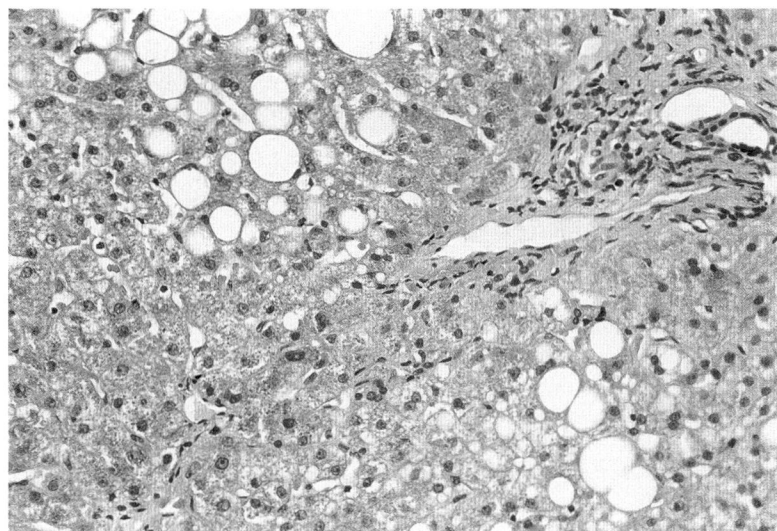

Fig. 13.120
Porphyria cutanea tarda: in addition to fatty change and mild chronic inflammation, brown uroporphyrin crystals are evident.

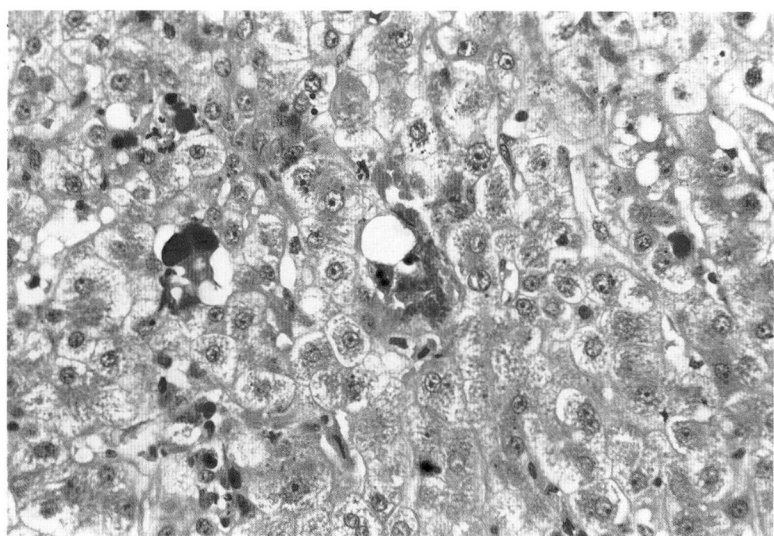

Fig. 13.121
Erythropoietic protoporphyria: the Kupffer cells contain abundant brown pigment. By courtesy of D.R. Davies, MD, St Thomas' Hospital, London, UK.

hepatocytes and Kupffer cells, hepatocyte necrosis, portal and periportal fibrosis, cholestasis and, less commonly, cirrhosis (*Fig. 13.121*).[28]

Differential diagnosis

The major differential diagnosis histologically is between porphyria, pseudoporphyria, epidermolysis bullosa acquisita and congenita, and bullous amyloidosis. All produce cell-poor or cell-free subepidermal blisters. Their distinction is readily made in the majority of cases with clinical information, immunofluorescence studies, and Congo red staining.

Pseudoporphyria

Clinical features

Pseudoporphyria (drug-induced pseudoporphyria, drug-induced pseudoporphyria cutanea tarda, pseudoporphyria cutanea tarda, bullous dermatosis in end-stage renal failure, bullous dermatosis of hemodialysis) refers to a photodistributed blistering dermatosis resembling porphyria cutanea tarda but in the absence of any serum, urine, or stool porphyrin abnormality (*Figs 13.122–13.125*).[1] It is now recognized as having many causes including drugs, excessive UVA (including the use of sunbeds), and sunlight exposure and may develop in patients undergoing hemodialysis for chronic renal failure.[1–24] Pseudoporphyria occurs in up to 6% of patients receiving hemodialysis.[25] It has also been described in patients self-medicating with chlorophyll.[26]

Small tense blisters develop on the backs of the hands and fingers, and occasionally involve the face, upper chest, and legs.[1,2] Milia, skin fragility, photosensitivity, and scarring are often present. Hypertrichosis, hyperpigmentation, sclerodermoid changes, and dystrophic calcification as seen in porphyria cutanea tarda are not features of pseudoporphyria.[1] In children affected with this condition (usually receiving naproxen for juvenile arthritis), facial scarring reminiscent of erythropoietic protoporphyria has been documented.[7,27] In general, hepatic abnormalities appear to be absent.[1]

Pathogenesis and histologic features

Pseudoporphyria is a UVA-related phototoxic dermatosis.[1] It may develop following both hemodialysis and peritoneal dialysis and also in patients with chronic renal failure in the absence of dialysis. Suggested risk factors in such patients include iron overload, aluminum intoxication, PVC-induced photosensitivity, drugs, and ethanol.[1,2] The condition has also been documented following use of nonsteroidal anti-inflammatory medications, including naproxen and cyclooxygenase inhibitors.[7–10,19] A wide variety of other drugs, including various antibiotics (e.g., nalidixic acid, tetracyclines, and ciprofloxacin), antifungals (e.g., voriconazole), diuretics (e.g., furosemide

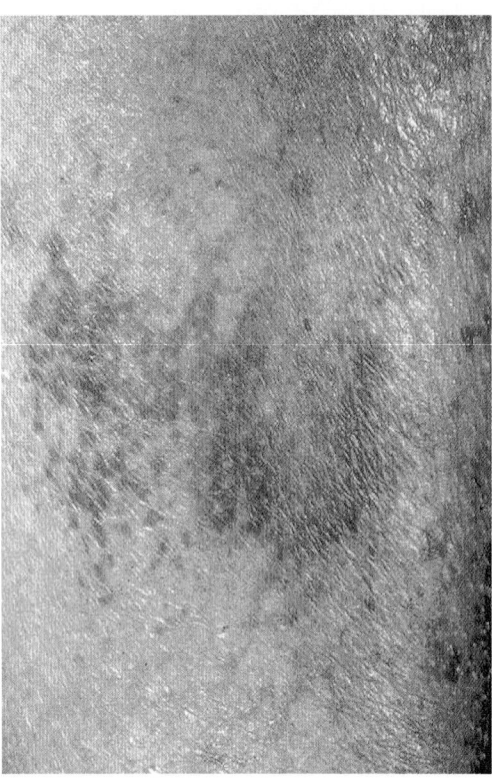

Fig. 13.122
Pseudoporphyria: there is extensive purpura with freckling and conspicuous excoriations. The patient had used a sunbed for a number of years. By courtesy of G.M. Murphy, MD, Beaumont Hospital, Dublin, Eire.

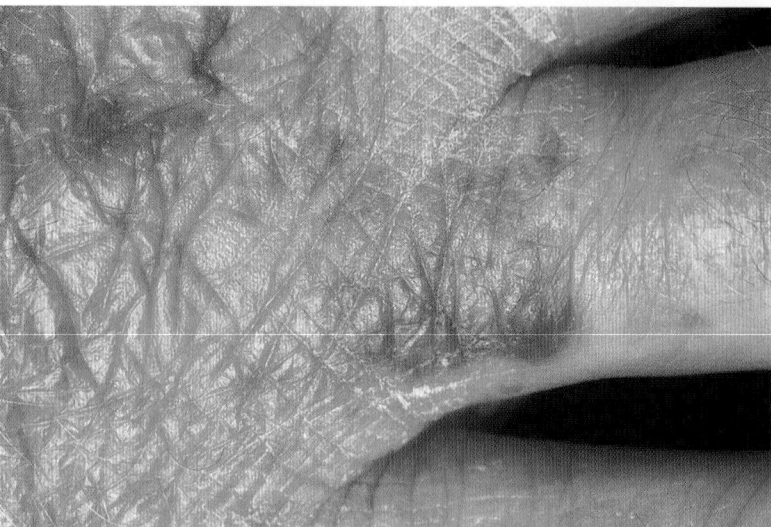

Fig. 13.124
Pseudoporphyria: note the hemorrhagic blister overlying the knuckle. By courtesy of G.M. Murphy, MD, Beaumont Hospital, Dublin, Eire.

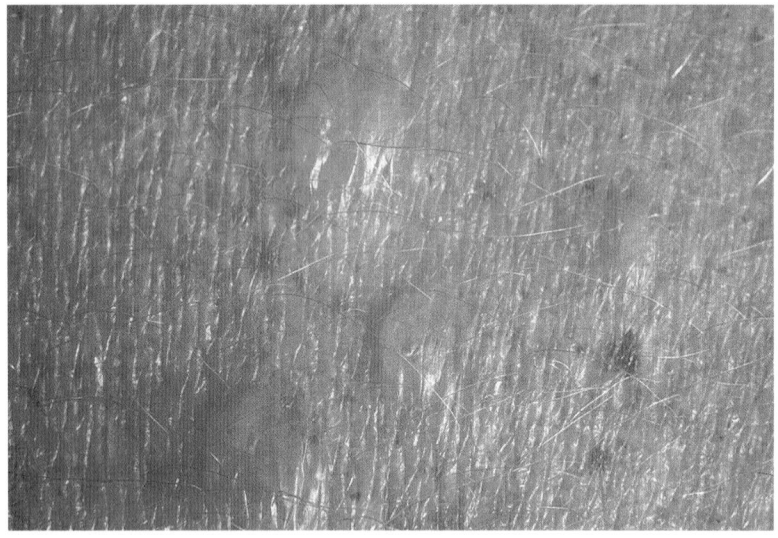

Fig. 13.123
Pseudoporphyria: small tense grouped vesicles are present on the arm. By courtesy of G.M. Murphy, MD, Beaumont Hospital, Dublin, Eire.

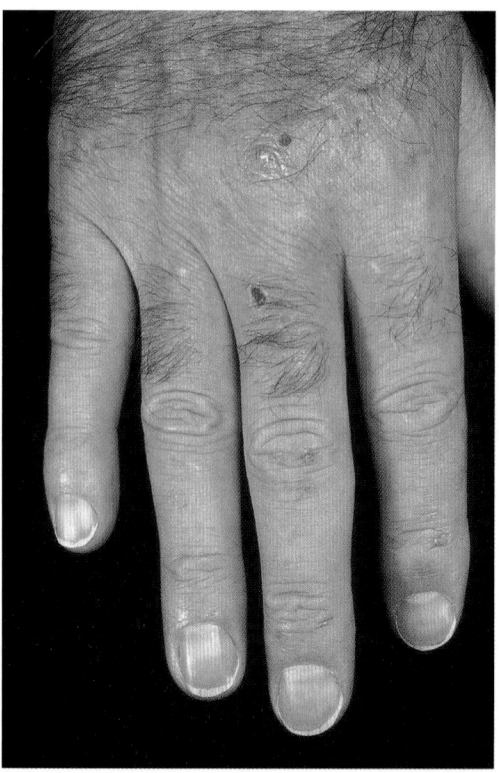

Fig. 13.125
Pseudoporphyria: there are multiple erosions and milia. By courtesy of the Institute of Dermatology, London, UK.

(frusemide), torsemide), metformin, finasteride, tyrosine kinase inhibitors, ciclosporin, and oral contraceptives have also been incriminated. [13–24,27–34] The use of UVA suntanning beds is also a well-recognized cause of pseudoporphyria.[12,35] Young females are almost exclusively affected and PUVA therapy has also rarely been incriminated.[1] A rare case of narrow-band UVB-induced pseudoporphyria has been reported in a patient being treated for psoriasis. [24]

The blisters are subepidermal and rather bland, containing perhaps a little fibrin and, occasionally, red blood cells (Fig. 13.126).[7,11,34,36] The floor of the blister is typically lined by well-preserved dermal papillae (festooning). There is usually no significant inflammatory component although occasionally, a light perivascular lymphocytic infiltrate may be seen in the superficial dermis. Thickening of the superficial vessels (highlighted by a PAS stain) and dermal sclerosis with elastosis may be apparent.

Direct immunofluorescence reveals Ig (usually IgG, IgM, and sometimes IgA) with C3 around the superficial vasculature in a donut distribution and as a fine granular deposit at the epidermal basement membrane region (Fig. 13.127).[2,7,27,28,35–37] Indirect immunofluorescence is invariably negative.[2]

On electron microscopic examination, the plane of cleavage is variable: in some it has been shown to be within the lamina lucida, whereas in others it has been deep to the lamina densa (Fig. 13.128).[7,38,39] As in porphyria cutanea tarda, basement membrane reduplication is typically present both at the dermal–epidermal junction and also around the superficial vasculature (Fig. 13.129).[7]

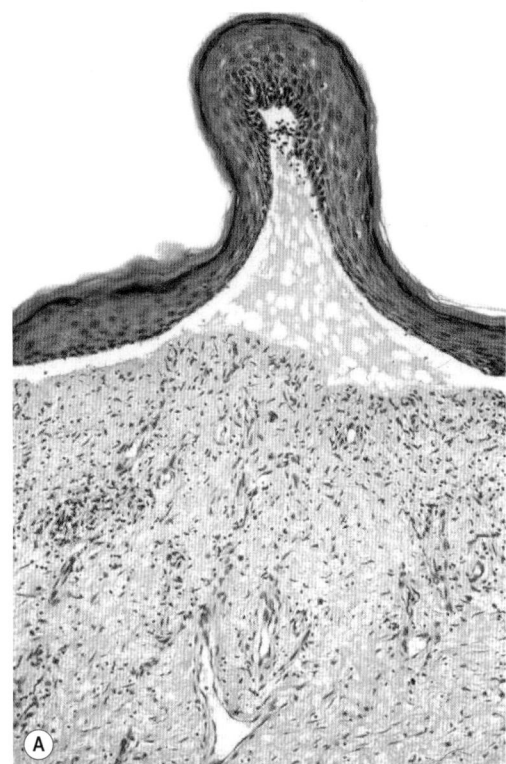

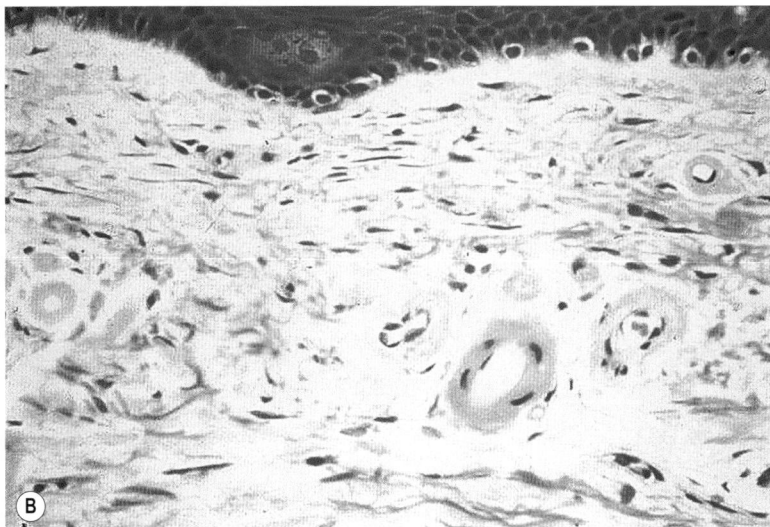

Fig. 13.126
Pseudoporphyria: (**A**) there is a subepidermal blister; (**B**) the superficial dermal vessels are thickened with a hyaline deposit. (**B**) By courtesy of G.M. Murphy, MD, Beaumont Hospital, Dublin, Eire.

Differential diagnosis

The invariably negative indirect immunofluorescence and absence of porphyrin abnormalities distinguish this disease from autoimmune bullous dermatoses and porphyria cutanea tarda.[40,41]

Gout

Clinical features

Gout represents a group of disorders of purine metabolism in which elevated levels of uric acid occurs.[1–4] The majority of affected patients have reduced excretion of purines which may be caused by diuretic therapy or renal disease. Hyperuricemia may also complicate diabetic ketoacidosis and starvation, and can develop in patients with sarcoidosis and psoriasis.[5,6] Some have increased purine synthesis and this type of disturbance can occur dramatically in the myeloproliferative diseases, particularly following

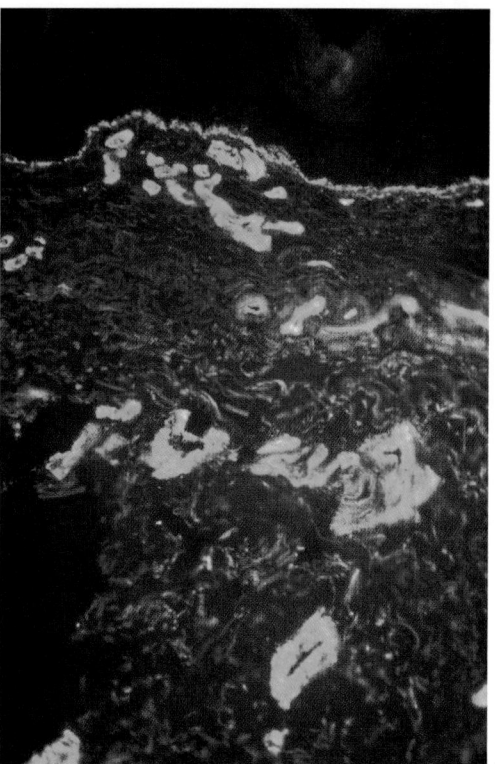

Fig. 13.127
Pseudoporphyria: the vessel wall thickening is in part due to excess type IV collagen, as shown in this field. By courtesy of G.M. Murphy, MD, Beaumont Hospital, Dublin, Eire.

therapy with cytotoxic drugs. Less commonly, gout represents a primary inherited disorder of purine metabolism. A number of enzymatic defects are recognized, including hypoxanthine guanine phosphoribosyltransferase activity (X-linked recessive), abnormal phosphoribosylpyrophosphate synthetase variants (X-linked dominant) and glucose-6-phosphatase deficiency.[4] These defects represent a small proportion of patients with gout. More recent genome-wide association studies have rapidly expanded the knowledge of other genetic defects responsible for the disease.[7–10] Many of the implicated genes are believed to function as urate transporters in the renal tubules.[8–10]

Males are affected more often than females and presentation is usually in the fourth to sixth decades. However, the incidence in females is rising, particularly in those on diuretics and those with altered renal function.[11] The prevalence of the disease is higher in black patients.[12]

Gout produces recurrent, acute, exceedingly painful monoarticular arthritis, classically of the great toe, but also of the large joints of the legs. Many patients present initially with acute inflammation of the first metatarsophalangeal joint (podagra).[13] The affected joint is characteristically exceedingly tender, hot, and erythematous, and cellulitis may therefore enter the differential diagnosis. Precipitating factors include trauma, excessive alcohol consumption, dietary excess (particularly red meat consumption), lead exposure, hypertension, renal insufficiency, surgery, and infections.[4,13–16] Alcohol and obesity are associated with increased nucleotide catabolism and decreased urate excretion.[17–19] Not surprisingly, more recent studies indicate a close relationship with the metabolic syndrome, and as a consequence patients with gout also have an increased risk of diabetes, myocardial infarction, and premature death.[8,20] Certain medications, including diuretics (loop and thiazide), low-dose aspirin, and ciclosporin increase the risk of gout.[15,21] With chronicity, a disabling and often crippling arthritis may develop, particularly affecting the hands and feet.[3] Subsequently, uric acid crystal deposition in skin and soft tissues produces gouty tophi; these nodules are seen most commonly on the external ear, but also over the elbows and on the digits (*Fig. 13.130*). When large, they often discharge a chalky material. Rare clinical presentations include bullous lesions, a fungating mass, and sparing of hemiplegic limbs by the tophi.[22–24] Nowadays, only a minority of patients

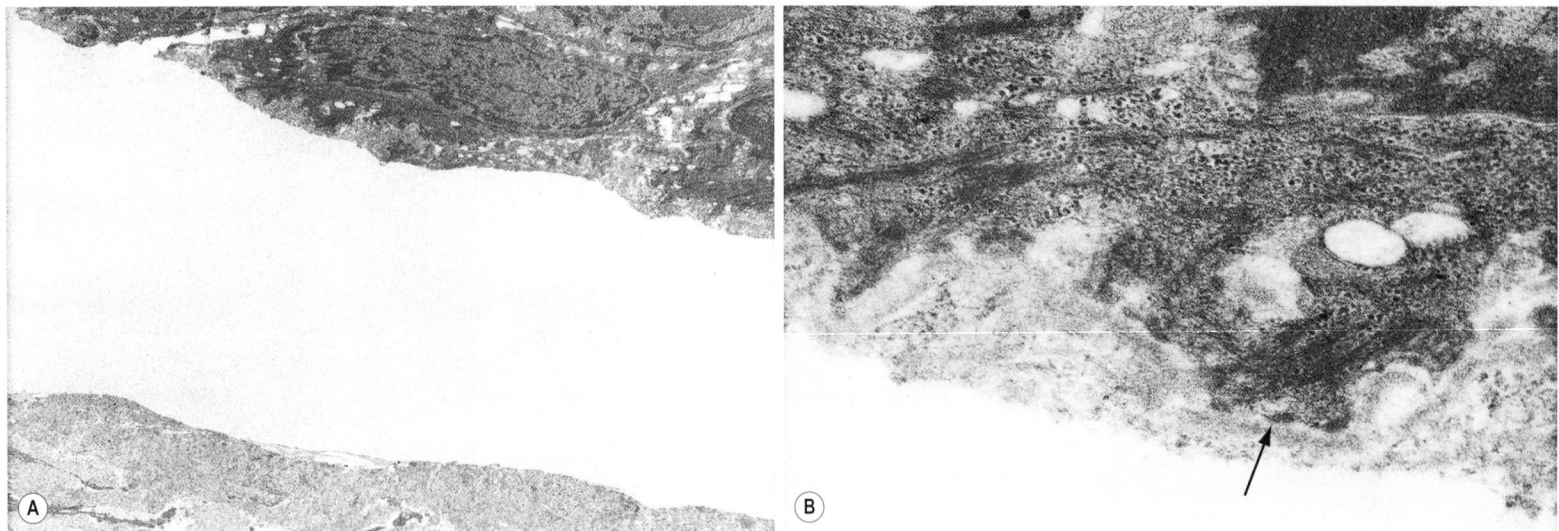

Fig. 13.128
(**A**, **B**) Pseudoporphyria: in this example, the blister is located in the superficial papillary dermis deep to the lamina densa (*arrowed*).

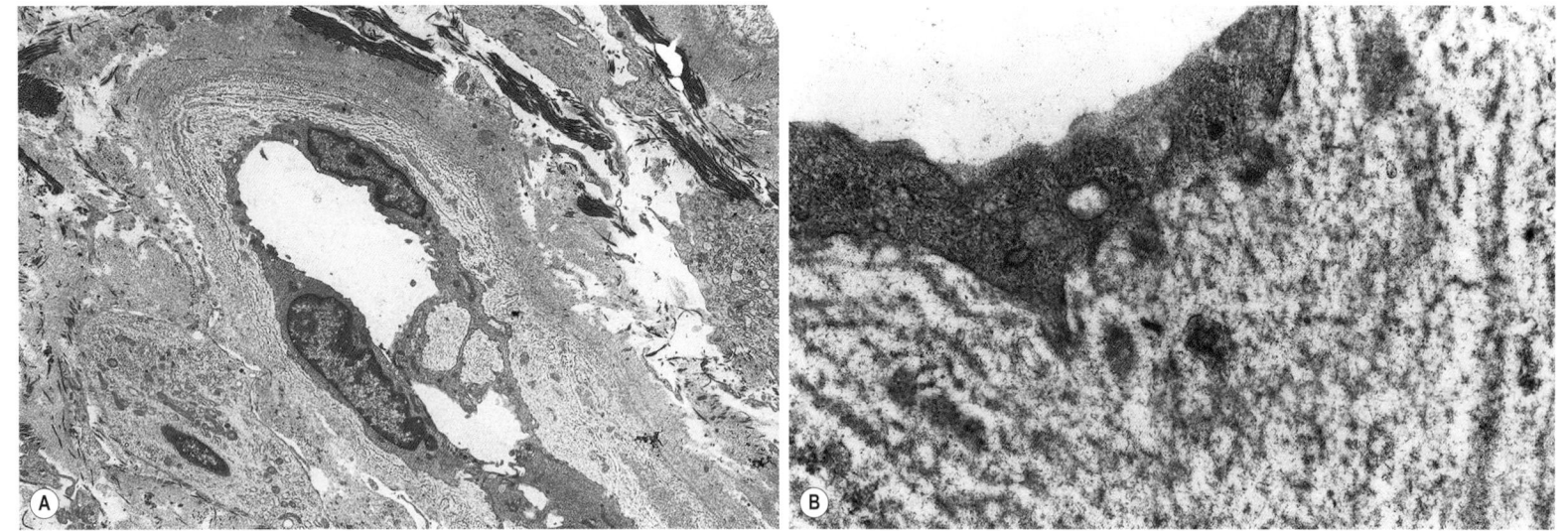

Fig. 13.129
(**A**, **B**) Pseudoporphyria: note the striking basement membrane duplication.

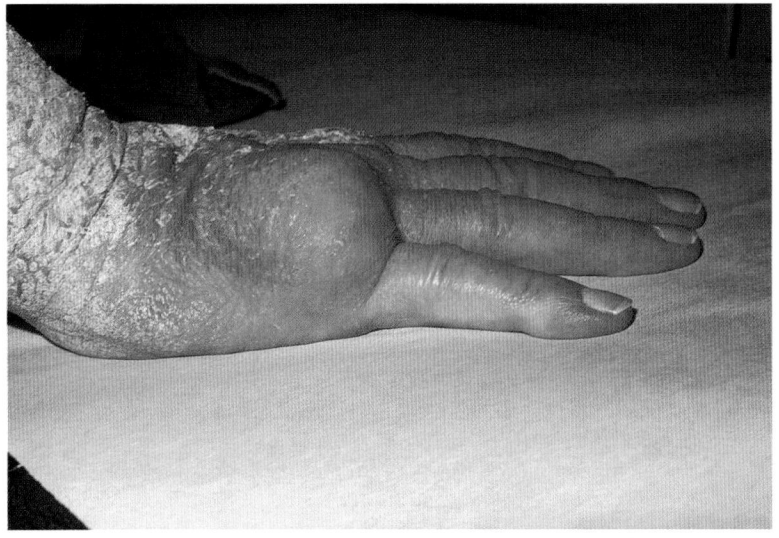

Fig. 13.130
Gout: massive deposit on the dorsal aspect of the hand.

present with tophi because of improvement in the diagnosis and treatment of the disease.[25] Tophi are rarely the first manifestation of the disease.[26,27] They have exceptionally been described in the mitral valve, breast, nose, cervical spine, sacroiliac joint, larynx, and eyes.[28–34] Bone involvement gives rise to characteristic lytic lesions in the distal subchondral region of the digits.[4] Fracture due to bone erosion has been reported.[35]

Renal disease, which is an important complication, presents as urate nephropathy and/or uric acid nephrolithiasis.[20,36,37] In secondary types associated with increased cell turnover, including myeloproliferative disease and multiple myeloma, acute precipitation of uric acid crystals sometimes occurs in the collecting ducts of the kidney during chemotherapy. Uric acid nephropathy may also develop in patients with the inherited variants. Patients present with acute renal failure. More commonly, in primary gout, renal stones are a feature, and chronic urate nephropathy (due to deposition of monosodium urate monohydrate salt crystals in the interstitial tissues of the kidney), presenting as mild proteinuria and hypertension, occasionally develops.[4] Uric acid stones develop in about 40% of patients with gout secondary to myeloproliferative diseases and in 10–25% of patients with the primary variants.[4]

The diagnosis of gout rests primarily on the identification of uric acid crystals within joint fluid or tophi rather than on serum uric acid levels,

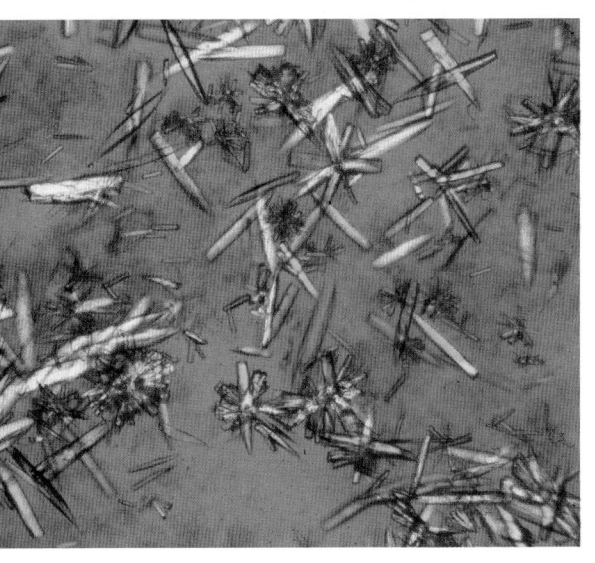

Fig. 13.131
Gout: characteristic needle-shaped crystals. By courtesy of G.T. McKee, MD, Massachusetts General Hospital, Boston, USA.

which can be unreliable. Acute attacks of gout can be associated with normal uric acid levels.[13]

Histologic features

The demonstration of uric acid crystals in tophi requires alcohol fixation and anhydrous processing because monosodium urate is water soluble (Fig. 13.131).[38] In formalin-fixed sections, uric acid crystals appear as amorphous material in the dermis or subcutaneous tissues, surrounded by a marked granulomatous response in which many giant cells are usually evident (Figs 13.132 and 13.133). Urate crystals can sometimes be detected in formalin-fixed tissue by polariscopy of 10-micron-thick, unstained sections from the paraffin block.[39] Calcification may be a late complication. In secondarily infected lesions, a neutrophil polymorph infiltrate is sometimes present.[40] In alcohol-fixed sections, the deposits are seen to be composed of needle-shaped brown crystals, which lie in bundles and show negative birefringence with polarized light and a first-order red compensator filter (Figs 13.134 and 13.135).[41]

Ochronosis

The term 'ochronosis' was first used by Virchow in 1866 to describe a clinical condition in which blue–black cutaneous pigmentation in the skin was associated with the microscopic deposition of an ochre-colored pigment. There are two main types: alkaptonuria and exogenous ochronosis.

Alkaptonuria

Clinical features

This is an autosomal recessively inherited condition (with an approximate incidence of $1:10^6$) in which deficiency of homogentisate 1,2-dioxygenase (HGD) in the liver and kidneys (necessary for the catabolism of phenylalanine and tyrosine) leads to the accumulation of homogentisic acid (2,5-hydroquinone acetic acid) in cartilage, tendon, skin, and fibrous tissue.[1–5] The condition is particularly seen in patients of Eastern European origin, mainly those from Slovakia where the incidence is as high as $1:19\,000$.[6] Clinical features relate particularly to joint and cardiovascular involvement, renal and prostatic stones, and ocular and cutaneous lesions. Alkaptonuria, or blackening of the urine after standing or alkalinization due to oxidation of homogentisic acid, usually becomes obvious in childhood. Most patients present with either dark urine or early-onset arthritis. The blue–black discoloration of the tissues (known as ochronosis) is due in part to the Tyndall effect.

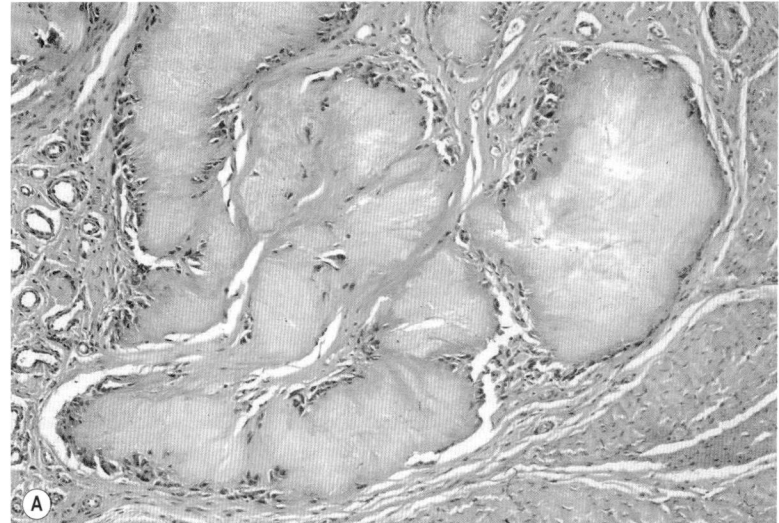

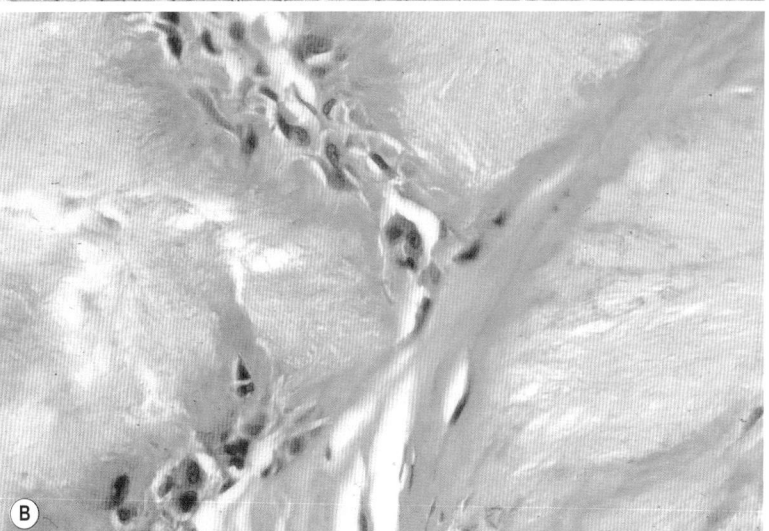

Fig. 13.132
Gout: (A) circumscribed deposits of uric acid are scattered within the dermis, note the accompanying fibrosis; (B) formalin fixation has destroyed the uric acid crystals to leave amorphous eosinophilic material.

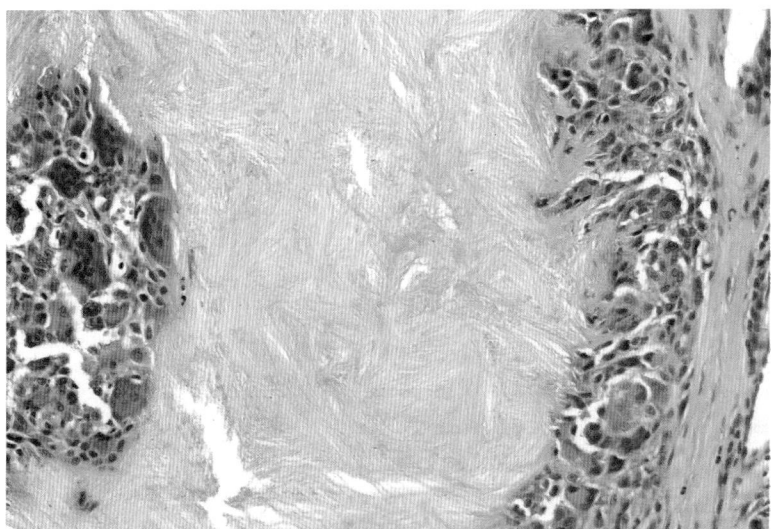

Fig. 13.133
Gout: multinucleate giant cells are present.

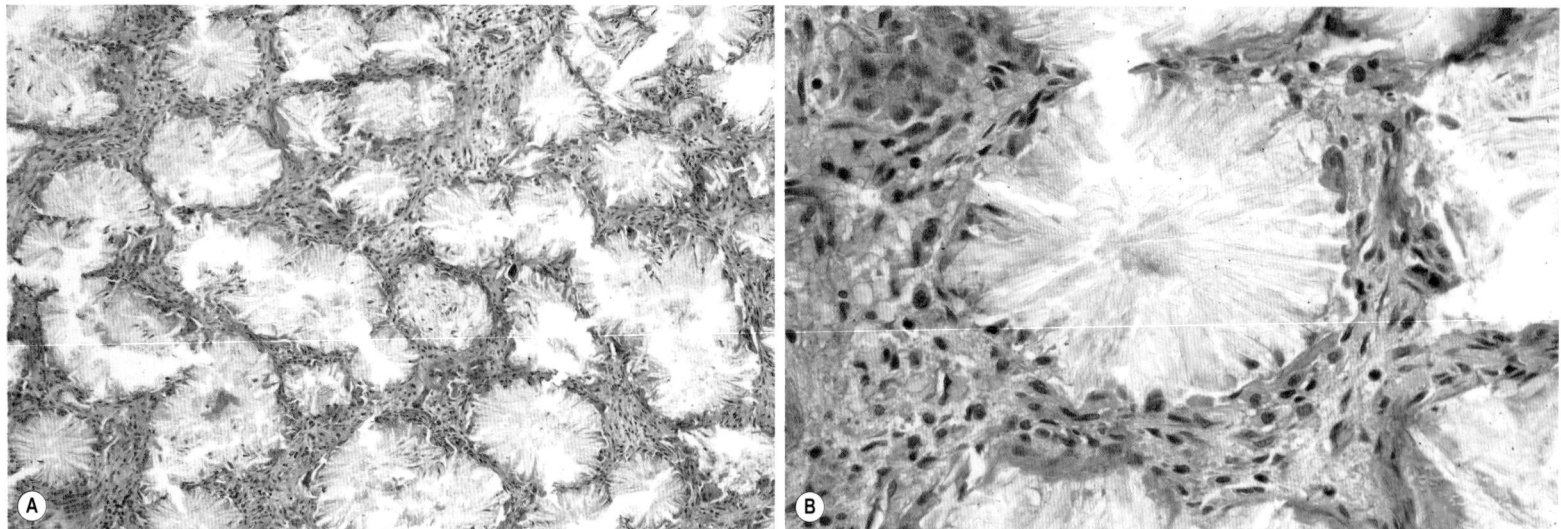

Fig. 13.134
(**A**, **B**) Gout: characteristic needle-shaped uric acid crystals are seen in alcohol-fixed and anhydrous processed material.

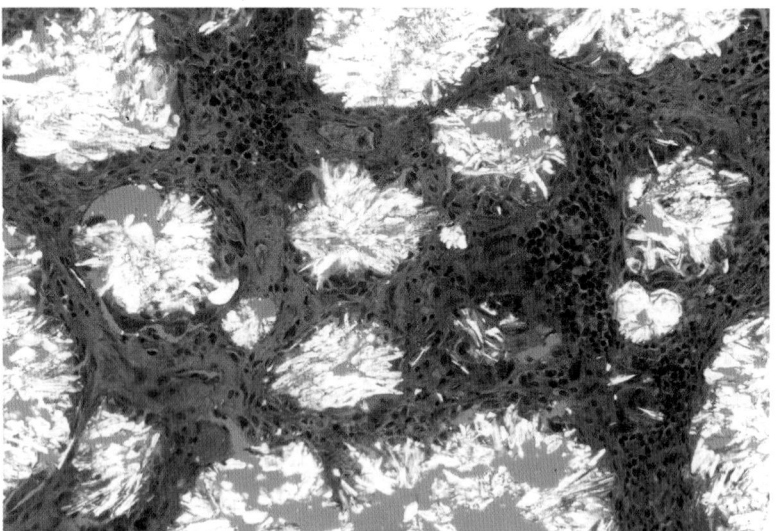

Fig. 13.135
Gout: the crystals display striking birefringence when viewed with polarized light.

The cutaneous changes develop later, at about 30–40 years of age. They are seen particularly on sun-exposed skin and areas with maximum numbers of sweat glands.[1-4] Deposition of polymerized oxidase pigment in the ear cartilage produces painful thickening and blue–black speckled discoloration. Involvement of the eardrum and ossicles may result in tinnitus and deafness.[4] Subsequently, discoloration of the sclera, conjunctiva, tendons, and skin of the face, hands, and flexures occurs.[7] A rare case of vaginal hyperpigmentation has been reported.[8] The skin pigmentation may be more prominent on the palms and soles.[9,10] Finally, a characteristic arthritis, which is often severe, develops in almost all patients.[4,11] Low back pain is followed by involvement of the large joints of the limbs. Spinal involvement leads to disc herniation, spondylosis, and osteophytosis with resultant limitation of movement and loss of height.[1,12] Musculoskeletal disease caused by alkaptonuria can be severe and result in significant disability.[13,14] Despite widespread morbidity, alkaptonuria is not associated with significant mortality, and life expectancy is typically normal, though mortality related to renal disease or cardiac complications has been reported.[1,15,16]

Osteoarticular involvement – which is particularly evident in the knees, shoulders, and hips, and in advanced cases the vertebral column – is characterized by pigmentation of the articular cartilage, synovium, and capsule associated with fibrillation, fragmentation, calcification, and erosion.[13,14] Osteoarthritis may also be evident and chronic non-specific synovitis is commonly present. Cardiovascular involvement occurs in up to 50% of

patients and mainly consists of pigmentation and calcification of the aortic valve, which may lead to stenosis.[17-20] The cardiac manifestations appear to be independent from other cardiac risk factors.[20] Cardiovascular pigmentation, which is especially seen on the endocardium and valves (aortic and mitral), also affects the intima and media of arteries. Surprisingly, even with heavy pigment deposition and smooth muscle cell degeneration, aneurysm formation is not a feature of vascular involvement.[21]

In up to 60% of patients the kidneys typically show very marked pigmentation, especially involving the pyramids and calculi.[22] Ochronotic prostatic stones are a nearly invariable feature, but bladder calculi are much less frequent.[4,21] In addition to stones, patients may develop chronic renal disease.[15,16] A case with a rapidly fatal course in a patient with chronic renal disease has been reported. This patient had intravascular hemolysis related to toxic effects from elevated plasma soluble melanins due to accumulation of homogentisic acid that precipitated acute renal failure.[23] Asymptomatic ocular involvement is seen in up to 70% of patients.[24] Pigmentation particularly affects the sclera and to a lesser extent the conjunctiva and cornea.[7,21] The lesions are typically noninflammatory.

Ochronotic pigmentation is frequently seen in the hyaline cartilage of the larynx, trachea, and bronchi.[21,25] Involvement of endocrine organs, CNS, and teeth is rare.[26-28]

Exogenous ochronosis

Clinical features

Deposition in the skin of an identical pigment to that seen in alkaptonuria may occur as a result of the application of phenol (carbolic acid) to leg ulcers, therapy with resorcinol and picric acid, the oral and intramuscular administration of antimalarials such as chloroquine, and the application to dark skin of bleaching creams containing hydroquinone, most often in black women.[29-42] Antimalarials result in slate-gray pigmentation affecting the knees, face, palate, and subungual regions.[43] In hydroquinone-induced ochronosis, lesions occur particularly over bony prominences such as the forehead, temples, nose, and lower jaws and also on the sides of the neck (*Fig. 13.136*).[33] Time to onset of lesions is approximately 6 months. The first stage is characterized by erythema and mild hyperpigmentation.[30] Subsequently, the hyperpigmentation intensifies and patients develop widespread 'caviar-like' black papules; cutaneous atrophy and colloid milia may also occur.[44] In longstanding disease, nodules develop.[30,45-47] Hydroquinone-induced ochronosis is a major problem in the black population of South Africa. In one series the prevalence among users of skin lighteners was almost 70%.[34] The reason for the high incidence of ochronosis in this population is not entirely clear but is thought to be due in part to high concentrations of hydroquinone used in their products and the synergistic

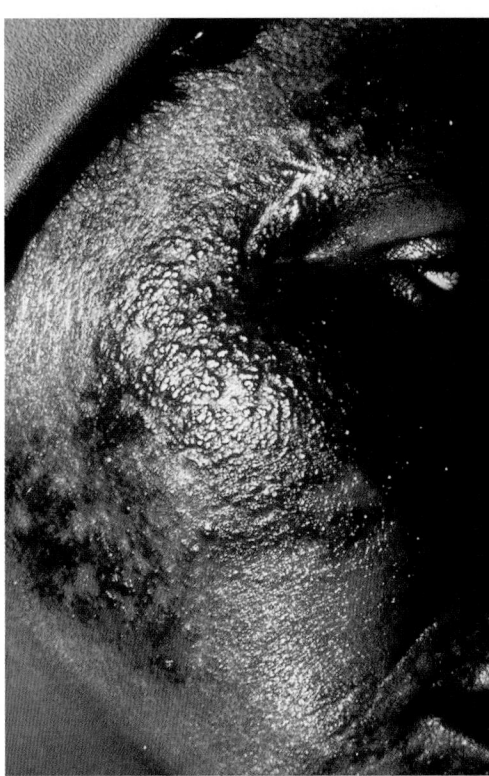

Fig. 13.136
Exogenous ochronosis: hyperpigmented plaque with numerous colloid milia in a Bantu female. The lesions developed as a consequence of the application of hydroquinone bleaching cream.

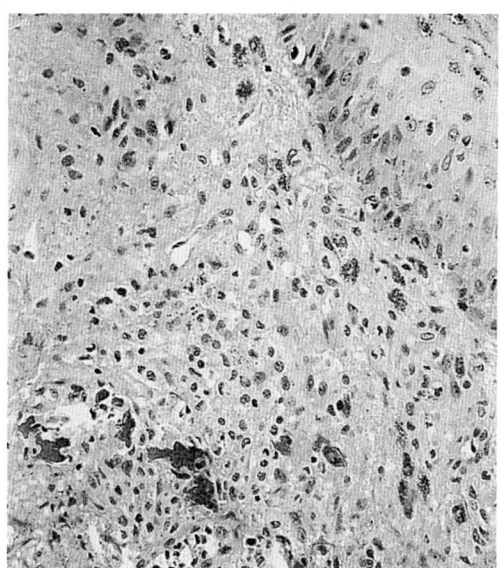

Fig. 13.137
Ochronosis: typical swollen, irregular, golden-brown fibers are seen (bottom left).

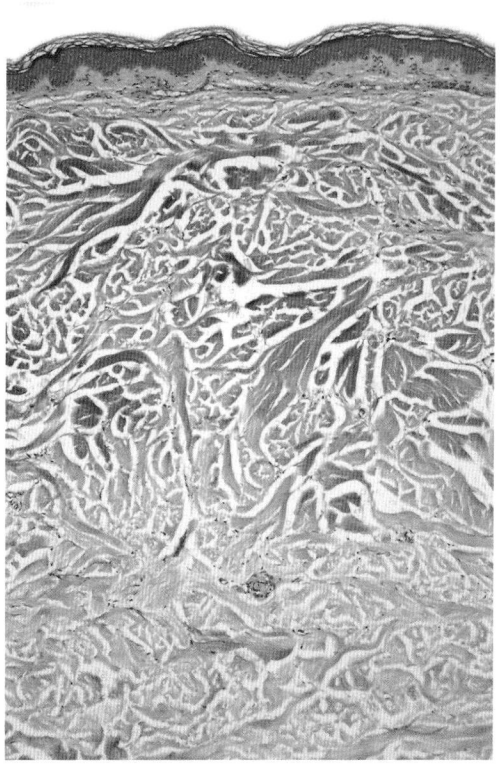

Fig. 13.138
Exogenous ochronosis: early lesion showing markedly swollen collagen fibers.

effect of multiple compounds used in combination with hydroquinone such as mercury and resorcinol, which can also cause ochronosis.[30] Exogenous ochronosis due to hydroquinone is thought to be photoactivated. Exogenous ochronosis tends to chronicity. In addition to causing ochronosis, hydroquinones containing bleaching creams have been shown to be carcinogenic in rodents. As a result, in 2006, the US Food and Drug Administration proposed a ban on all over-the-counter bleaching creams containing hydroquinone, although this proposal has not gone into effect.[35]

Pathogenesis and histologic features

In alkaptonuria, as a result of the deficiency of HGD, homogentisic acid is oxidized and polymerized by polyphenol oxidase to form benzoquinone acetic acid. This results in a black pigment that binds irreversibly to collagen. Polyphenol oxidase is particularly common in cartilage and skin and this reflects in their preferential involvement. The pigment formed has not been characterized but there are some similarities to melanin.[48] It appears that the pigment deposition occurs in both previously damaged collagen and normal collagen. The gene responsible for alkaptonuria has been localized to chromosome 3q.23-21.[49–51] The human HGD gene has been cloned and it has been shown that patients with alkaptonuria carry two copies of a loss-of-function HGD allele.[52] Over 100 different genetic mutations have been identified thus far in the HGD gene.[51,53] A study of patients with alkaptonuria has demonstrated that they have a significantly higher prevalence of HLA-DR7 than those without the disease.[54]

The exact pathogenesis of exogenous ochronosis is not known. Proposed mechanisms include:
- the inhibition in the skin of HGD by hydroquinone with formation of pigment,[55]
- increased tyrosinase activity induced by hydroquinone.[29]

Ochronosis presents as yellow–brown, sharply defined, irregularly shaped and frequently fragmented fibers in the superficial dermis (Fig. 13.137).[1,32] The ochronotic pigment is autofluorescent, appears black with methylene blue, but does not stain with van Gieson, Perl stains or the Masson-Fontana reaction.[1] Pigment granules are often present in the epithelium and basement membrane of sweat glands, in endothelial cells, and within dermal macrophages.[21,25] In ochronosis, due to hydroquinones, the skin may, in addition, show melanophages in the upper dermis associated with depigmentation of the epidermal melanocytes.[45]

In early lesions the collagen fibers appear basophilic and swollen before developing the characteristic yellow ochronotic morphology (Fig. 13.138).[56] With chronicity, large amorphous eosinophilic granules may develop, resembling colloid milium.[45] Solar elastosis and foreign body granulomata (sometimes indistinguishable from sarcoidosis) are less common features.[32,33,47,57] An actinic granuloma-like variant has been described.[58] Transepidermal and transfollicular elimination of ochronotic fibers has occasionally been documented.[47,58]

Antimalarial pigmentation is due to melanin and hemosiderin deposition in addition to the classical ochronotic fibers.[1]

Electron microscopic studies have shown that initially electron-dense ochronotic pigment is deposited around swollen collagen fibrils that characteristically lose their banding pattern.[45] These fibrils subsequently degenerate until the whole collagen fiber is replaced by amorphous ochronotic pigment. Rupture of the fibrils also occurs, so that the pigment comes to lie scattered free in the dermis. Phagocytosis of the latter by macrophages and giant cells may be seen.[21,32] The colloid milium-like deposits in hydroquinone-associated ochronosis consist of electron-dense granular material lacking a significant fibrillar component.[45]

Hartnup disease

Clinical features

Hartnup disease is an autosomal recessive disorder characterized by defective gastrointestinal absorption and renal reabsorption of monoamine and monocarboxylic amino acids due to a defect in the neutral brush border system.[1] One of the effects is tryptophan deficiency.[2] The disease typically presents in childhood. In addition to a pellagra eruption (see below), patients also have a characteristic aminoaciduria and cerebellar ataxia.[3,4] An uncommon cutaneous manifestation is an acrodermatitis-like eruption involving the perioral region, perineum and acral skin.[5-7] The disease may, however, sometimes be so mild as to remain asymptomatic.[8] Additional symptoms include diarrhea and CNS dysfunction ranging from mild apathy to psychosis and frank dementia.[7,9] An exceptional case of a patient with identical symptoms and signs of Hartnup disease in the absence of a recognized metabolic abnormality or aminoaciduria has been described.[10] The disease has been mapped to chromosome 5p15 and the defective gene is *SLC6A19*, a sodium dependent neutral amino acid transporter.[11-13]

Histologic features

The cutaneous histology is identical to that of pellagra (see below).

Pellagra

Clinical features

Pellagra develops as a consequence of deficiency of nicotinic acid (niacin, vitamin B₃) or its precursor tryptophan.[1-3] The cause may be dietary. It has traditionally been associated with high consumption of corn.[3] In developed countries it is most frequently observed in alcoholics, in those living in conditions of socioeconomic deprivation, and in patients with anorexia nervosa or malabsorption due to extensive gastrointestinal disease (e.g., partial gastrectomy, gastroenterostomy, and Crohn disease).[1,4] A severe case of cytomegalovirus colitis in an immunocompetent patient has also been associated with pellagra.[5] It is sometimes also a feature of the carcinoid syndrome because the tumor cells consume available tryptophan to produce serotonin.[5,6] Pellagra occasionally develops after therapy with a number of drugs, including isoniazid, 6-mercaptopurine, 5-fluorouracil, ethionamide, and phenobarbital.[6-13] It can occur in Hartnup disease and in association with defects in the metabolism of tryptophan.[14] Rare cases have also been associated with megaduodenum, congenital duodenal diaphragm, and Sjögren syndrome.[15-17] Pellagra is particularly prominent in parts of Africa and Asia where nutritional deficiencies are prevalent.[1] A rare case has been described in association with the intake of alternative medicines.[18] A further report describes an association with amyloidosis secondary to multiple myeloma.[19] A pellagra-like eruption partially responsive to niacin associated with xeroderma pigmentosum/Cockayne syndrome complex has been reported.[20]

The classic triad of pellagra is 'dermatitis, diarrhea, and dementia'. The skin eruption of pellagra is photosensitive in nature. An initial painful sunburn-like erythema subsides to leave a dusky brownish discoloration with a dry scaly appearance (*Figs 13.139* and *13.140*). Blisters may sometimes be evident. The eruption is typically sharply demarcated, symmetrical, and occurs on the backs of the hands (most commonly), the forearms, the knees, central chest, neck, and face.[7] The thickened skin around the photo-exposed skin of the neck typically resembles a necklace (Casal necklace). Other

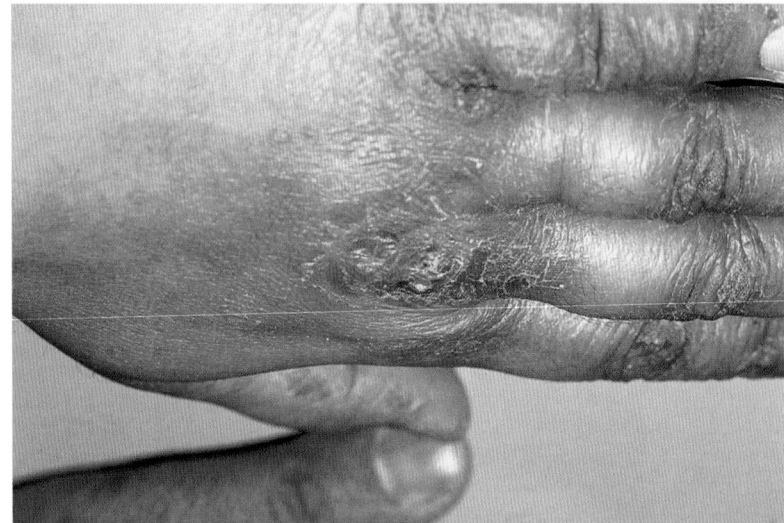

Fig. 13.139
Pellagra: scaling and hyperpigmentation are present on the dorsal aspect of the knuckles and fingers. By courtesy of the Institute of Dermatology, London, UK.

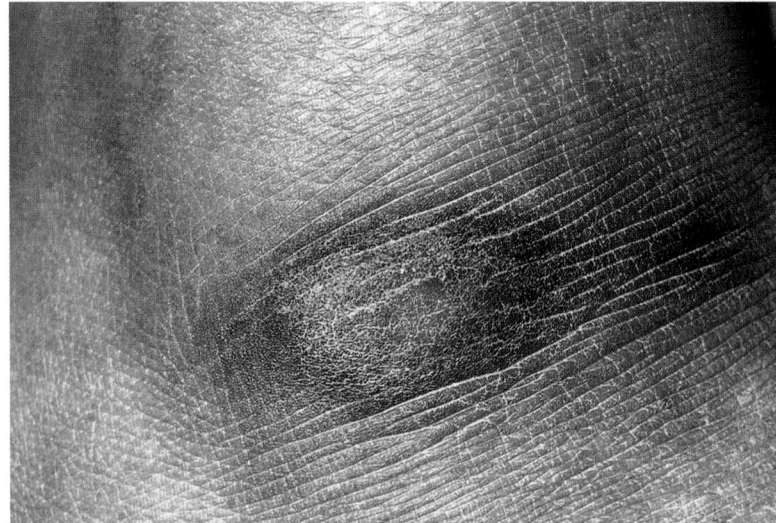

Fig. 13.140
Pellagra: close-up view of hyperpigmentation and scaling. By courtesy of the Institute of Dermatology, London, UK.

features sometimes present include cheilosis, glossitis, angular stomatitis, and oral or perianal sores.[3,7]

Gastrointestinal disease in pellagra manifests as nausea, vomiting, abdominal pain, gastritis, and diarrhea. Neurological involvement evolves with headache, depression, and ataxia initially then more severe symptoms of disorientation, delirium, coma and eventually death.[3]

Histologic features

The appearances in pellagra are usually non-specific. There is hyperkeratosis, parakeratosis, and acanthosis associated with increased melanin pigmentation and, in early lesions, keratinocyte vacuolation in the upper reaches of the epidermis.[7,8] Telangiectasia and a perivascular chronic inflammatory cell infiltrate in the upper dermis may also be evident. Older lesions sometimes show epidermal psoriasiform hyperplasia.[21] In some instances the histology can resemble that of necrolytic migratory erythema and acrodermatitis enteropathica.

Differential diagnosis

The diagnosis is very much dependent upon clinicopathological correlation, particularly in those cases that resemble necrolytic migratory erythema and acrodermatitis enteropathica.

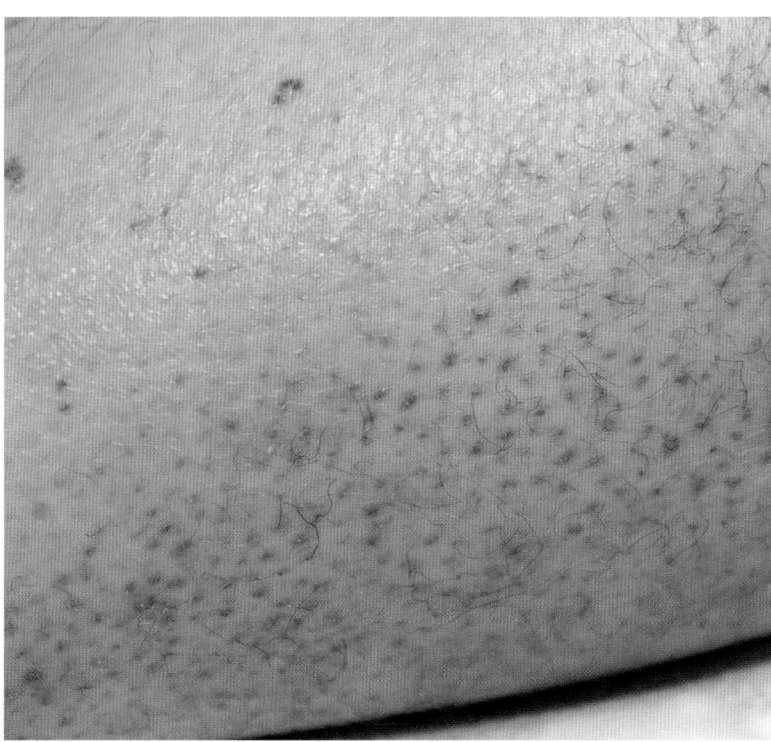

Fig. 13.141
Scurvy: the hairs have a coiled, corkscrew shape and there is perifollicular hemorrhage. By courtesy of Melissa Piliang, MD, Cleveland Clinic, Cleveland, USA.

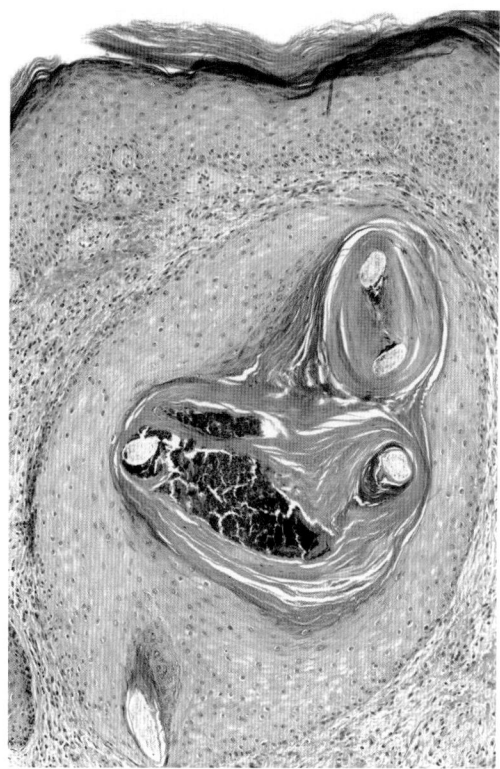

Fig. 13.142
Scurvy: the hair follicle is dilated and there is a typical corkscrew hair cut in multiple planes. Note the surrounding chronic inflammation and red cell extravasation. By courtesy of S. Tahan, MD, Beth Israel and Deaconess Medical Center, Boston, USA.

Scurvy

Clinical features

Scurvy, due to vitamin C deficiency, results from a diet inadequate in fresh fruit and vegetables and is nowadays most often encountered following inappropriate dieting and food fads, in alcoholics and socially isolated individuals, and in patients with malabsorption secondary to underlying bowel diseases, including Crohn disease, Whipple disease, and gastro-intestinal chronic graft-versus-host disease.[1-4] Scurvy is rare in children but does occur in those with developmental and psychiatric disorders. It may also be secondary to drinking boiled or evaporated milk that is deficient in vitamin C.[5]

Cutaneous manifestations include dry skin, follicular hyperkeratoses (particularly affecting the forearms, legs, and abdomen), perifollicular hemorrhages with coiled hair (especially affecting the legs), petechiae and subungual splinter hemorrhages, leg edema, alopecia, erythematous swollen and bleeding gums with tooth loss, and clinical evidence of poor wound healing (*Fig. 13.141*).[1-8] Painful subperiosteal hemorrhage, 'Barlow disease', is characteristically seen in infants.[5] Less specific manifestations, which may cause a delay in diagnosis, include fatigue, arthralgia, myalgias, and in children a refusal to walk.[6,9]

Pathogenesis and histologic features

Vitamin C is necessary for hydroxylation of proline and lysine residues during the conversion of procollagen into collagen fibers. As a result of impaired collagen synthesis, basement membrane synthesis is defective, with consequent loss of blood vessel wall integrity. This, combined with impaired dermal connective tissue constituents, results in a bleeding tendency.

The cutaneous features include follicular dilatation and keratin plugging, perifollicular hemorrhages with chronic inflammation, and hemosiderin deposition.[7,10-12] The alopecia is characterized by hair shaft fracture and corkscrew hairs within a dilated and plugged follicle (*Fig. 13.142*).[1,7,13] In some cases, the corkscrew hairs may be less apparent, but perifollicular hemorrhage is a clue to the diagnosis (*Fig. 13.143*).

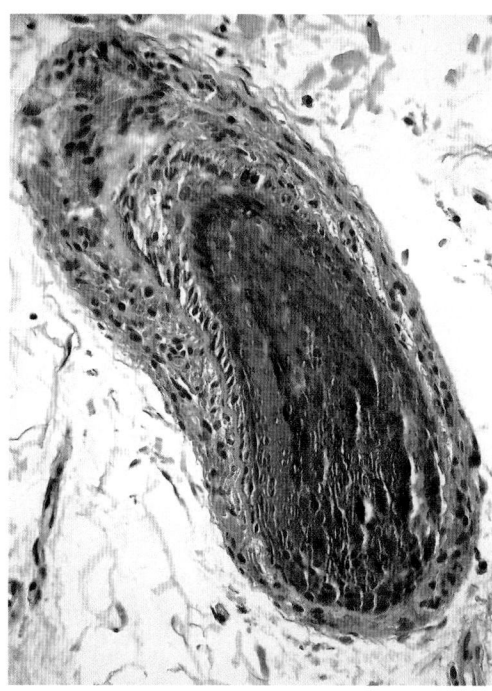

Fig. 13.143
Scurvy: In cases where the corkscrew hairs are less evident, perifollicular hemorrhage is a helpful clue. By courtesy of Melissa Piliang, MD, Cleveland Clinic, Cleveland, USA.

Calcinosis cutis

Calcinosis cutis may occur when connective tissue is abnormal (dystrophic) or where calcium or phosphate levels in the blood are high (metastatic); alternatively, there may be no obvious underlying cause (idiopathic) (*Table 13.5*).[1-3]

Table 13.5
Classification of calcinosis cutis

Type	Distribution	Clinical features
Dystrophic	Localized Widespread	Acne scars; fat cell necrosis; epidermoid cysts; pilomatrixoma; infantile calcinosis of the heel Dermatomyositis; systemic lupus erythematosus; Ehlers-Danlos syndrome; pseudoxanthoma elasticum
Metastatic	Hypercalcemic	Hyperparathyroidism; sarcoidosis; vitamin D excess; milk alkali syndrome; destructive bone disease
	Normocalcemic	Chronic renal failure; pseudohypoparathyroidism
Idiopathic	Generalized Localized	Calcinosis universalis Subepidermal calcified nodule; localized idiopathic dermal calcinosis; tumoral; scrotal

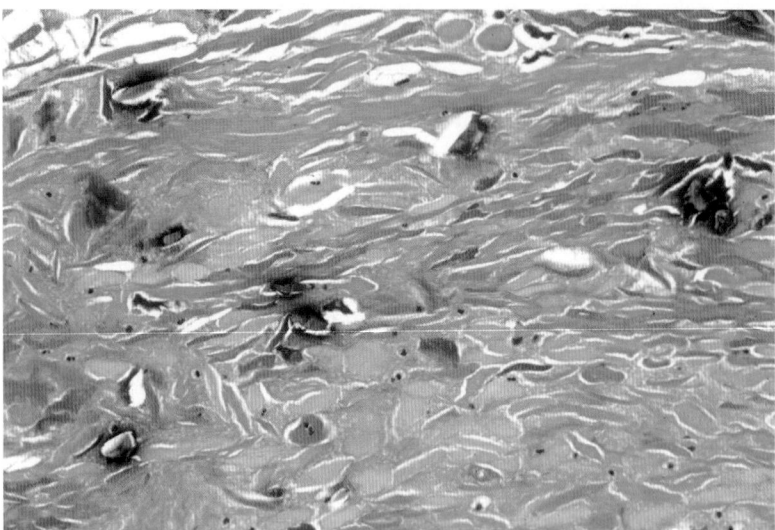

Fig. 13.144
Dystrophic calcinosis cutis: calcification has developed in this ruptured cyst.

Dystrophic calcinosis cutis

Clinical features

In this, the most common variant of calcinosis, the changes are limited to the dermis and subcutaneous tissues and there is no involvement of internal organs. This form of calcinosis always occurs in tissue that has been previously damaged either by external agents or as the result of a disease. Under this variant, iatrogenic calcinosis cutis induced by local application of chemicals or medications is also included. In the localized form of dystrophic calcinosis cutis, the underlying anomaly may be inflammatory or traumatic in nature, for example acne scars, burns, fat necrosis or subcutaneous and intramuscular injections.[4–7] Calcification and necrosis have been reported following electroencephalography and electromyography.[8,9] Calcification is a characteristic feature of pancreatic disease-associated panniculitis and in older lesions of subcutaneous fat necrosis of the newborn. Auricular calcification (also known as 'petrified ear') may occur as a result of chondritis, trauma or frostbite.[1,10,11] Less commonly, it is associated with hypercalcemia associated with systemic disorders and endocrinopathies.[10,11] A distinct example of dystrophic calcification is infantile calcinosis cutis of the heel, in which calcific dermal nodules develop approximately 1 year after birth in infants who have had multiple heel punctures for venesection.[12,13] A rare case as a complication of radiation therapy for breast cancer has been described.[14] An exceptional case following cutaneous exposure to a calcium chloride solution has been reported.[15]

Localized dystrophic calcinosis may also complicate epithelial cysts or neoplasms (*Fig. 13.144*).[16] It is particularly seen within the keratin of trichilemmal cysts. Calcification may occur in many adnexal tumors, for example pilomatrixoma, desmoplastic trichoepithelioma, and microcystic adnexal carcinoma. It is much more common in basal cell carcinoma than in squamous cell carcinoma.[17,18] Subungual epidermoid inclusions are rare tumors of the nail bed in which calcification may occur.[19]

Calcinosis cutis has also been documented following the intravenous administration of calcium chloride, phosphate, and gluconate (iatrogenic calcinosis cutis) (*Fig. 13.145*).[20–23] Lesions consist of multiple, erythematous nodules, which can ulcerate. They usually develop within a few weeks of exposure.[22] Deep soft tissue calcification has been described in association with pentazocine and pitressin.[23,24] Similar reactions following calcium-containing heparin in patients with renal insufficiency have also been reported.[25,26]

Widespread dystrophic calcification occurs most commonly as a sequel to connective tissue disease (*Figs 13.146* and *13.147*). Localized dystrophic calcification with bone formation has also been described in mixed connective tissue disease.[27,28] Dermatomyositis, especially in children, may be complicated by extensive deposits of calcium in the skin and subcutaneous tissues, muscles, and tendons and the dystrophic calcification may be

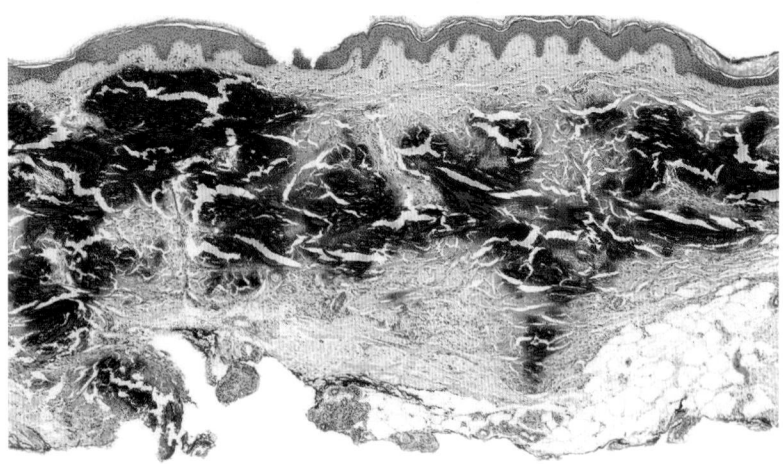

Fig. 13.145
Iatrogenic calcinosis cutis: this widespread dermal calcification followed calcium gluconate infusion.

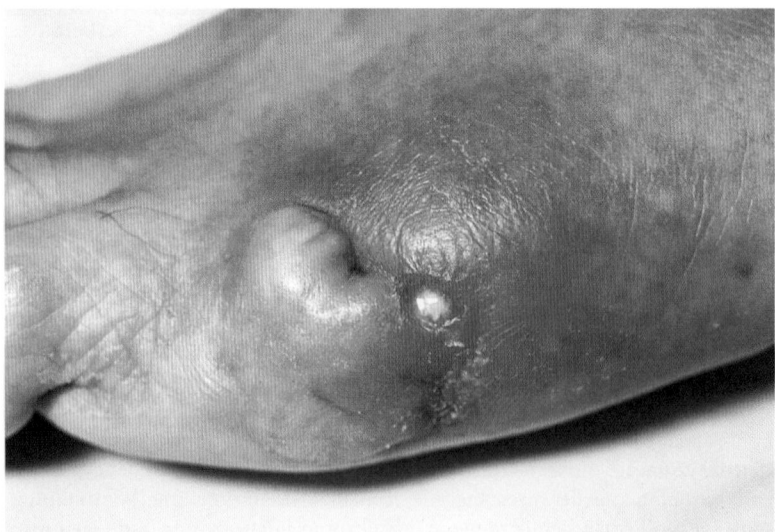

Fig. 13.146
Dystrophic calcinosis cutis: this large deposit is associated with focal ulceration and transepidermal elimination. By courtesy of the Institute of Dermatology, London, UK.

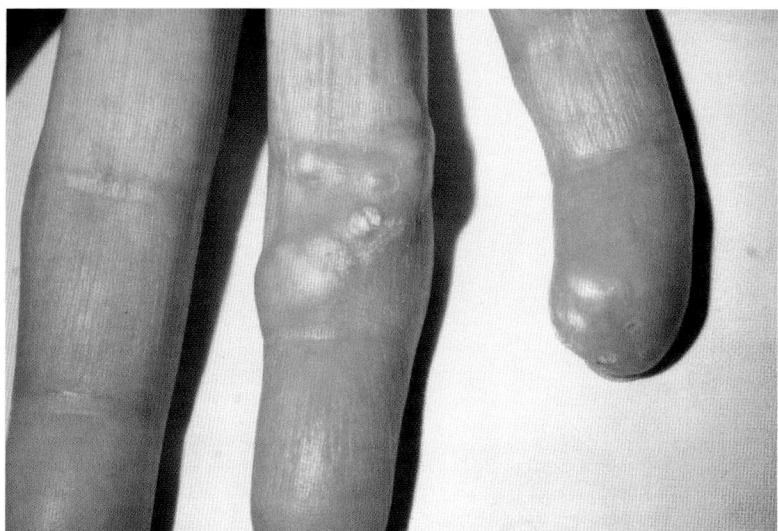

Fig. 13.147
Dystrophic calcinosis cutis: multiple digital deposits are present. By courtesy of the Institute of Dermatology, London, UK.

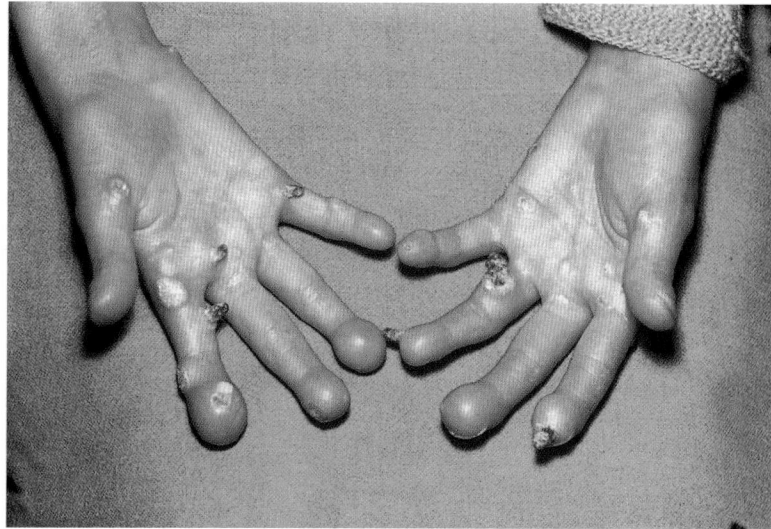

Fig. 13.148
Metastatic calcinosis cutis: there are gross deposits, many ulcerated. By courtesy of R.A. Marsden, MD, St George's Hospital, London, UK.

the presenting sign.[29,30] Scleroderma, especially the CREST variant, tends to show localized deposition of calcium, particularly on the digits and over bony prominences. Fingertip lesions are a common presentation in patients with Raynaud phenomenon (with or without underlying connective tissue disease) and have also been reported in a patient with Sjögren syndrome who did not have Raynaud syndrome.[31,32] Systemic lupus erythematosus is infrequently associated with calcinosis.[33,34] It is usually an incidental radiological observation, most commonly seen in the buttocks and extremities and unassociated with panniculitis. Mostly it develops in patients with severe acute disease, including cardiac, renal, or CNS manifestations.[2] It also appears to correlate with high doses of corticosteroids and myositis.[35,36] Calcification complicating discoid lupus erythematosus and subacute lupus erythematosus is limited to isolated case reports.[37-39] Lupus panniculitis and other types of panniculitis (including pancreatic fat necrosis) may also be associated with calcification.[40] Patients with porphyria cutanea tarda rarely develop calcinosis cutis. Lesions are most common on the scalp, neck, preauricular area, and hands, and are more likely to develop in patients with sclerodermoid disease.[41] Calcium is also deposited in inherited connective tissue disorders, especially Werner syndrome, pseudoxanthoma elasticum (PXE), and Ehlers-Danlos syndrome, in which small calcific nodules typically develop within atrophic scars over bony prominences. Alternatively, dystrophic calcification in PXE may occur as large, painful, pruritic nodules in areas involved by the underlying disease.[42]

Calcification has been described in patients with nephrogenic systemic fibrosis, associated with the cutaneous lesions as well as in fascia and muscle.[43,44] The etiology of calcification in this disease is debated. Some believe it occurs secondarily as part of a dystrophic process while others contend that calcification is intrinsic to the pathological process, particularly as it is also seen in vessels, in patterns resembling calciphylaxis.[45]

Metastatic calcinosis cutis

Clinical features

Metastatic calcification occurs as a result of hypercalcemia or hyperphosphatemia as may be seen in chronic renal failure, hyperparathyroidism, and sarcoidosis.[46-49] It has also been reported secondary to leukemia.[50-52] Calcium deposits occur in the skin, subcutaneous tissues, muscle, tendon, and internal organs. In the skin, the clinical appearances are of hard nodules and plaques, which may ulcerate to liberate chalky material and ultimately leave a scar (*Fig. 13.148*). This may be particularly frequently seen over large joints, the iliac crest or in the flexures. Fingertip lesions are usually very painful. A case report describes a patient with vulvar cystic nodules and hyperphosphatemia.[53]

Albright hereditary osteodystrophy is a genetic disorder associated with end-organ resistance to parathyroid hormone. Patients present in infancy or childhood with obesity, short stature, mild mental retardation, shortened fourth and fifth metacarpals, cutaneous calcification, osteoma cutis, and calcifying aponeurotic fibroma-like lesions.[54-56] The skin lesions are typically multiple erythematous to purpuric papules, plaques, and nodules on the trunk and extremities.

Vascular calcification with thrombosis may lead to livedo reticularis, ulceration, and gangrene, particularly affecting the hands, fingers, toes, and lower legs (so-called clinical calciphylaxis).[49,57,58] A frequent complication is sepsis and this often results in death. Patients usually have chronic renal failure in association with hyperphosphatemia and hyperparathyroidism.[59-61] Other conditions associated with calciphylaxis include hypervitaminosis D and A, hypercalcemia, primary or secondary hyperparathyroidism, AIDS, and protein C deficiency.[62,63] The exact mechanism of calciphylaxis is not clear, but it seems to be related to an imbalance in calcium and/or phosphorus metabolism.[64,65] Rarely, the condition occurs in patients with normal levels of calcium and phosphorus.[64-68]

Idiopathic calcinosis cutis

Clinical features

There are six main clinical types of calcinosis in which there is usually no known predisposing condition:
- In *calcinosis universalis*, there is progressive deposition of calcium in the skin and subcutaneous tissue, producing discharging hard nodules and plaques very similar clinically to those seen in metastatic calcification.[69-72] This condition has been associated with dermatomyositis, lupus erythematosus, scleroderma, and chronic graft-versus-host disease.[73-77] Therefore some cases may represent manifestations of other diseases in which the acute phase was not diagnosed.
- In contrast, *idiopathic calcinosis* may occur as a solitary nodule on the extremities and face, particularly the eyelids (subepidermal calcified nodule, cutaneous calculus).[78,79] It usually presents in early childhood and is more common in males; the majority of the nodules are hyperkeratotic and tender on palpation. Rarely, it may be present at birth and occasionally multiple lesions are present.[80]
- *Localized idiopathic dermal calcinosis* may also occur as a solitary nodule on the limbs.[81,82] The fingers and elbows are particularly affected.[1] An equivalent lesion, designated oral mucosal calcified nodule, which affects the gingiva, tongue, and palate has been documented.[83-86]

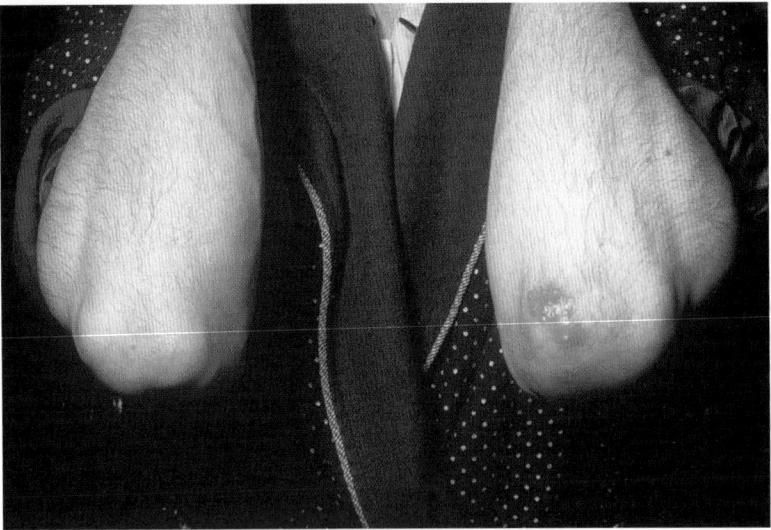

Fig. 13.149
Tumoral calcinosis: bilateral nodules over the elbows, with perforation on the patient's left. By courtesy of R.A. Marsden, MD, St George's Hospital, London, UK.

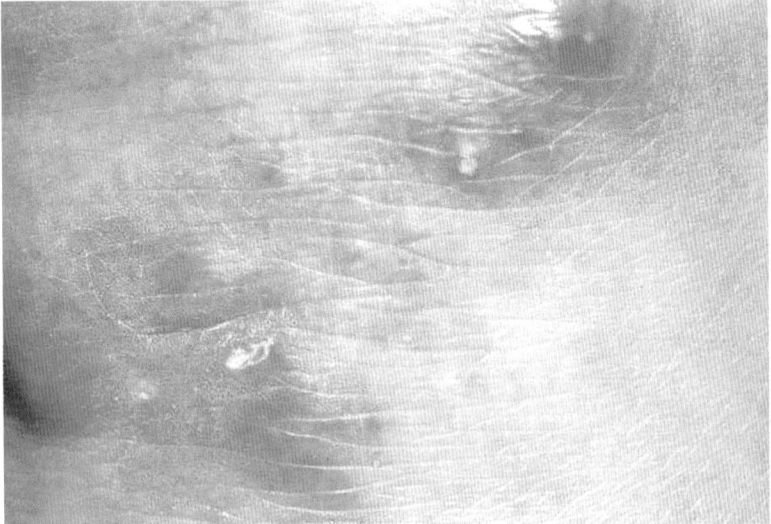

Fig. 13.150
Tumoral calcinosis: these small deposits are undergoing transepidermal elimination. By courtesy of R.A. Marsden, MD, St George's Hospital, London, UK.

- In *tumoral calcinosis*, large deposits of calcium are present in the skin and subcutaneous tissues, typically over bony prominences (hip, elbow, and scapula) (*Figs 13.149* and *13.150*). It is rare in Europe and North America, but is not uncommon in South, Central and East Africa and Papua New Guinea, where it is known as hip stone. It shows a female preponderance (2:1) and affects younger age groups. These deep deposits may be visualized radiologically (*Fig. 13.151*). Although most cases are idiopathic, there is a genetic defect is a small percentage, discussed below.
- *Scrotal calcinosis* may occur spontaneously. Patients present in childhood or early adulthood with multiple, asymptomatic, flesh-colored or yellow nodules of varying sizes, which often release granular chalky material.[87] A similar finding on the penis has also been reported in young men with no prior history of trauma and without a known underlying adnexal lesion.[88]
- Finally, *milia-like idiopathic calcinosis cutis* is a rare condition seen in children (usually under the age of 21 years).[89–93] Lesions are multiple, skin colored to whitish papules with a generalized distribution. Perforation may occur. Most cases are idiopathic. Two-thirds of cases have been associated with Down syndrome and up to one-third of

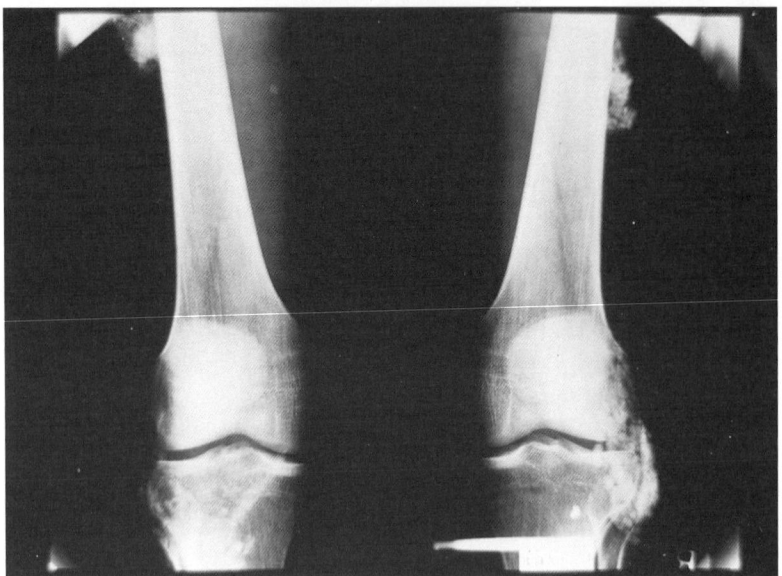

Fig. 13.151
Tumoral calcinosis: subcutaneous deposits are present overlying the thigh and lateral border of the knee. By courtesy of R.A. Marsden, MD, St George's Hospital, London, UK.

patients have coexisting syringomata. An association with acne is rarely seen. Lesions resolve spontaneously without scarring.

Pathogenesis and histologic features

Calcium stains blue with hematoxylin and eosin. In calcinosis cutis a rather homogeneous deep blue material is seen, either as small superficial deposits or as deeper globular ones (*Fig. 13.152*). Owing to the concomitant presence of phosphate and carbonate, the deposit stains black with the Von Kossa stain (*Fig. 13.153*).

The presence of calcium in the skin variably excites a foreign body reaction, so giant cells are sometimes seen at the edge of the deposit. On other occasions a chronic inflammatory cell infiltrate is present. Transepidermal elimination of calcified debris is sometimes a feature.[4]

Dystrophic calcification due to extravasation of intravenous solutions containing calcium is characterized by dermal calcium surrounding degenerated collagen bundles.[22] Lesions caused by calcium-containing heparin also demonstrate calcium in fat lobules, surrounding adipocytes, in septa as well as within the media of small vessels in the subcutaneous fat and dermis.[22] There may be fibrosis of vessel walls; however, thrombosis is not a usual feature.[24,26]

In calciphylaxis, there is prominent calcification of walls of dermal and subcutaneous small blood vessels (*Fig. 13.154*).[64] Often, the findings also include some degree of intimal proliferation and thrombosis. These changes result in prominent ischemic necrosis with extensive fat necrosis. Calcification of the surrounding fat may also be seen.

The pathogenesis of calciphylaxis is not completely understood. Recent studies point to osteopontin as a possible factor.[65,94] Osteopontin is a phosphoprotein adhesion molecule with a high affinity for calcium. It is normally expressed by various cell types, including osteoblasts, osteocytes, fibroblasts, macrophages, and smooth muscle cells. It plays an important role in bone remodeling. Previous studies have suggested a role for osteopontin in calcification of heart valves and pilomatrixoma.[95,96] Osteopontin expression in the media and, less often, the intima of vessel walls and surrounding adipocytes in the subcutaneous fat in areas involved by calcification in calciphylaxis has been demonstrated.[94] Calciphylaxis may in part be caused by osteogenic differentiation of vascular smooth muscle cells.

Calcification deposits in nephrogenic systemic fibrosis occur in the dermis, associated with CD34-positive spindle-shaped cells and in the media of small arteries in the deep dermis and subcutaneous fat, similar to that seen in calciphylaxis.[45]

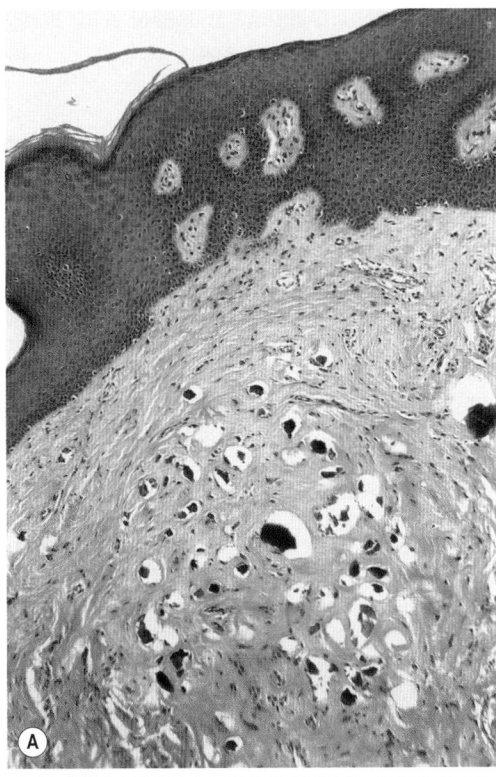

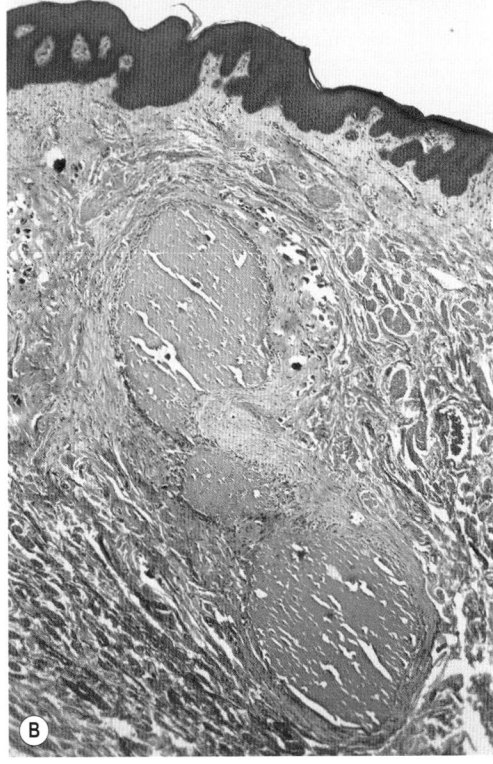

Fig. 13.152
Calcinosis cutis: (**A**) small deposits of intensely basophilic material are present in the superficial dermis; (**B**) these calcium deposits are associated with scarring.

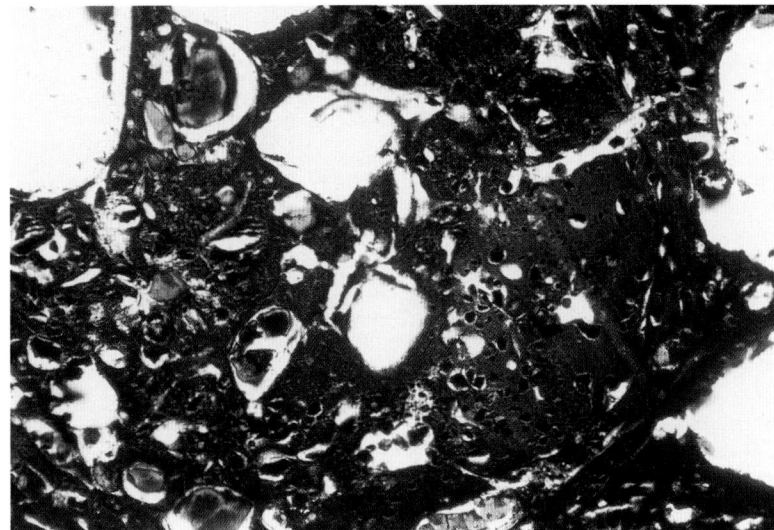

Fig. 13.153
Calcinosis cutis: the calcified deposit stains positively with the Von Kossa reaction.

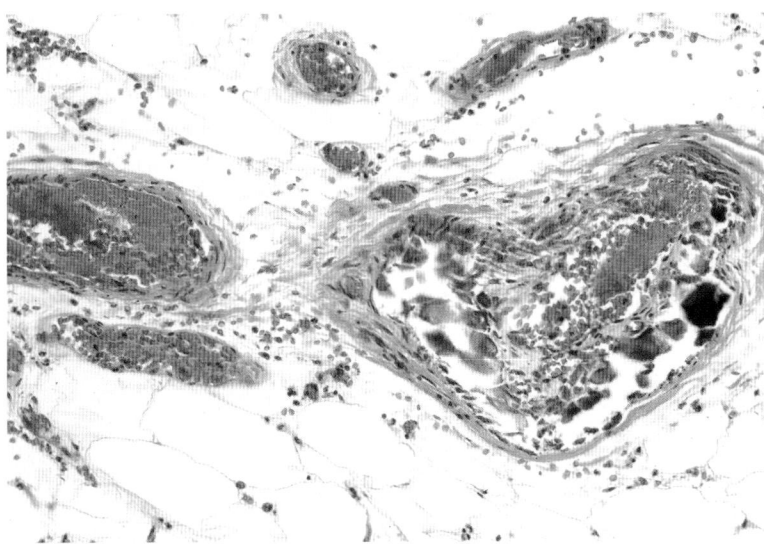

Fig. 13.154
Calciphylaxis: note the subendothelial calcification and thrombosis.

A report of an exceptional case of metastatic calcification showed calcification only of sweat ducts.[97]

There may be histologic evidence of the underlying disease process. In localized dystrophic calcinosis, for example, there is sometimes evidence of a preceding cyst particularly of the trichilemmal variant. In widespread dystrophic calcinosis cutis secondary to connective tissue disease, there is occasionally evidence of preceding collagen degeneration.

In a subepidermal calcified nodule, there is sometimes pseudoepitheliomatous hyperplasia, associated with transepidermal elimination of calcium.

In tumoral calcinosis the histologic features depend upon the stage of evolution of the lesion (*Figs 13.155–13.157*).[98] In early examples, multiple cystic spaces lined by epithelioid and giant cells are seen. The cyst lumina contain eosinophilic debris undergoing calcification. In advanced lesions, densely calcified material is seen embedded in hyalinized connective tissue. The occasional finding of necrobiosis and vasculitis may have pathogenetic significance. In the familial form of tumoral calcinosis, mutations in *FGF23*, *GALNT3*, or *KLOTHO* may be seen.[99–102] These mutations result in hyperphosphatemia with increased phosphate reabsorption, elevated 1,25-dihydroxyvitamin D(3), and deposition of large calcific masses.

The pathogenesis of the scrotal variant is most probably calcification of the contents of pre-existent dermal cysts, mostly epidermoid, but occasionally pilar.[90,103–108] Some authors have failed to detect an epithelial component;[54] however, this may be a reflection of the age of the lesion. In two different studies, residual epidermal cysts were present in over 50% of cases.[106,108] In many examples, typical epidermoid lining epithelium surrounds the calcified deposit and sometimes residual keratinous contents are visible. A foreign body giant cell reaction is not uncommon.

The etiology of milia-like calcinosis cutis is unclear. Theories include increased calcium content of excreted sweat and calcification of a pre-existing cyst.[89] Histologically, there is a focus of calcium in the papillary dermis

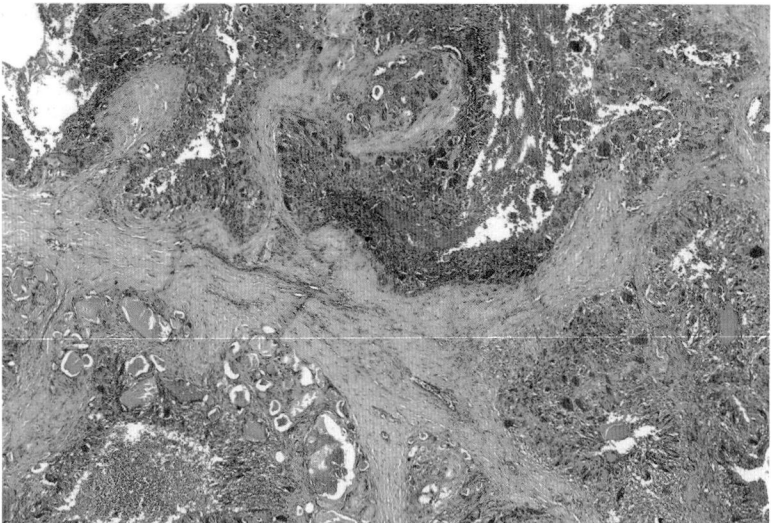

Fig. 13.155
Tumoral calcinosis: this low-power view shows a dense hyalinized stroma with numerous cystic cavities containing necrotic and calcified debris.

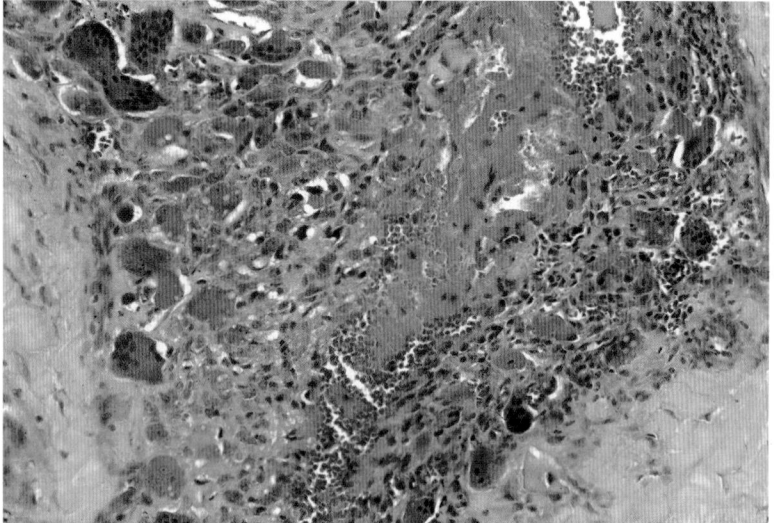

Fig. 13.156
Tumoral calcinosis: early lesions characteristically show a histiocytic and giant cell palisade around eosinophilic, degenerate connective tissue.

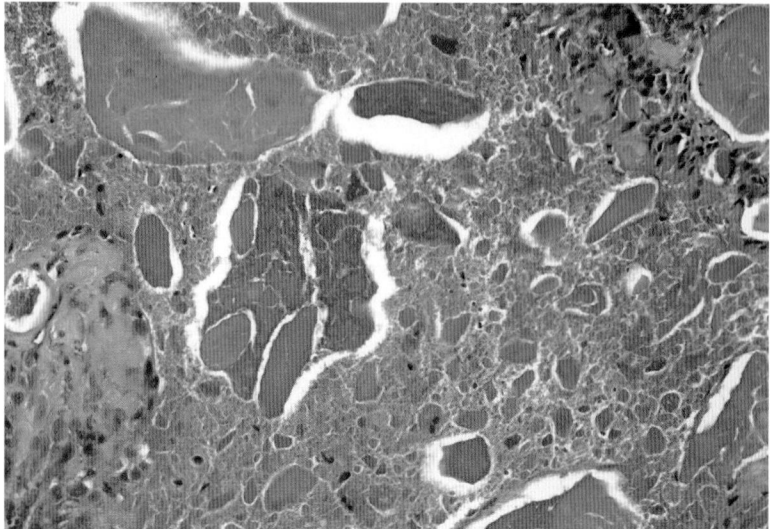

Fig. 13.157
Tumoral calcinosis: in older lesions, calcified deposits lie within lacunae.

surrounded by a lymphocytic infiltrate and giant cells. Perforation may be present.[89–93] Cyst epithelium is not present.

The mucinoses

The mucinoses are a group of conditions in which accumulation of acid glycosaminoglycans (mucin), particularly hyaluronic acid and to a lesser extent chondroitin (-4 and -6) sulfate and heparin, occurs either diffusely or focally in the dermis (*Table 13.6*).[1–6] Mucinosis also may occur as a secondary phenomenon in dermatoses such as lupus erythematosus, scleroderma, dermatomyositis, Degos disease, granuloma annulare, and chronic graft-versus-host disease.[5,7,8] In this chapter, however, only primary cutaneous mucinoses are the focus.

The glycosaminoglycans, which are secreted by fibroblasts, are constituents of normal cell membranes and connective tissue. This substance is usually secreted in only small amounts by fibroblasts. It is not clear why mucin production is increased in pathological states. Although the cause is probably multifactorial, it has been suggested that cytokines and/or immunoglobulins and unidentified factors in the serum of affected patients can induce synthesis of glycosaminoglycans.[5,9–11] Cytokines that play an important role in this process include tumor necrosis factor, interleukin-1, and transforming growth factor beta (TGF-β).[5,12,13] Actively secreting fibroblasts have a characteristic stellate shape and contain intracytoplasmic secretory vesicles; their presence in sections should therefore prompt a careful search for mucin deposition (*Figs 13.158–13.160*).

Table 13.6
Classification of the dermal mucinoses

Diffuse
lichen myxedematosus – generalized form (scleromyxedema)
scleredema
reticular erythematous mucinosis
generalized myxedema
pretibial myxedema
hereditary progressive mucinous histiocytosis
Focal
lichen myxedematosus – discrete papular form
acral persistent papular mucinosis
papular and nodular mucinosis associated with lupus erythematosus
self-healing juvenile cutaneous mucinosis
cutaneous mucinosis of infancy
cutaneous focal mucinosis
myxoid cyst
Follicular
follicular mucinosis

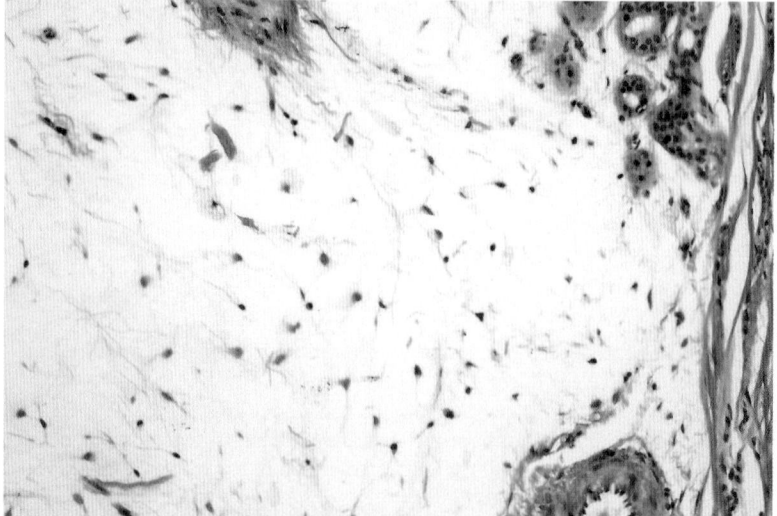

Fig. 13.158
Myxoma: Note abundant stromal mucin.

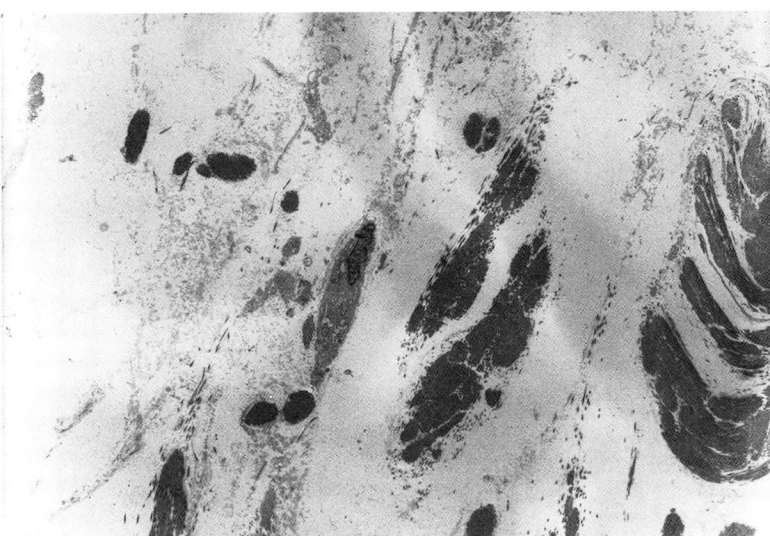

Fig. 13.159
Mucinosis: this electron micrograph from a patient with acral persistent papular mucinosis shows collagen bundles widely separated by a faintly electron-dense granular deposit.

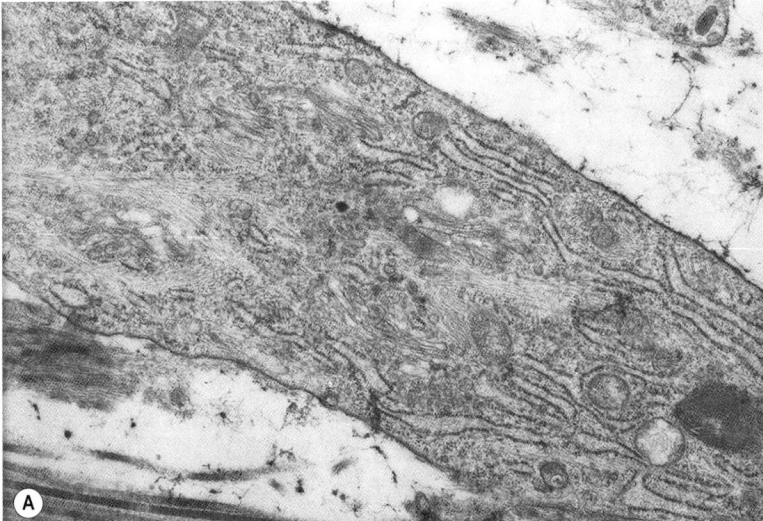

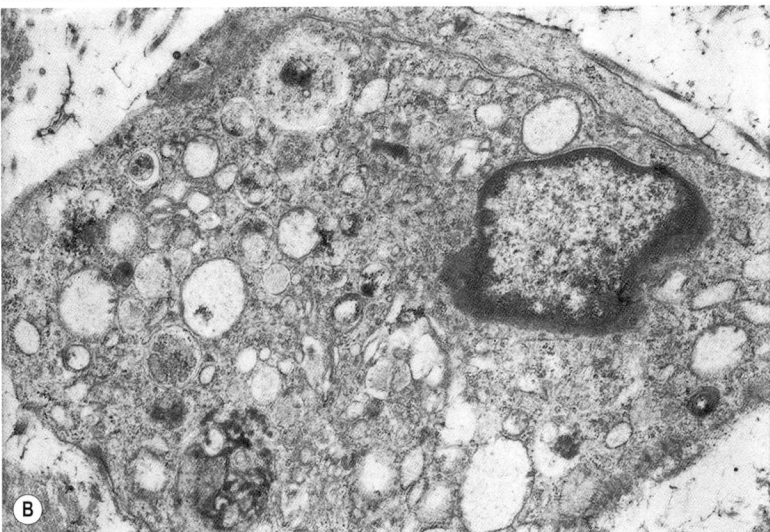

Fig. 13.160
Mucinosis: (**A**) actively secreting fibroblasts contain abundant rough endoplasmic reticulum; (**B**) numerous intracytoplasmic vesicles containing amorphous material are commonly present.

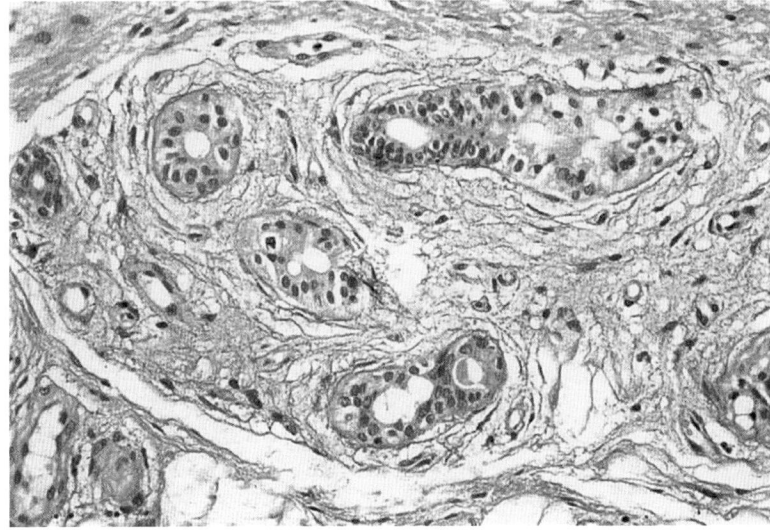

Fig. 13.161
Eccrine sweat gland: this section of normal skin from the sole of the foot shows abundant dermal mucin when stained with Ehrlich hematoxylin.

Hyaluronic acid stains with colloidal iron (blue–green), Alcian blue at pH 2.5 (blue) (but not at pH 0.4), and mucicarmine (red) but it is negative for PAS. It also stains metachromatically with toluidine blue, methylene blue, and thionine.[14] Sulfated acid mucins stain with Alcian blue at pH 0.5 and aldehyde-fuschin.[2] Hyaluronic acid absorbs enormous amounts of water, which accounts for the induration and thickening common to this group of conditions.[15]

Routine fixation and processing results in an anhydrous state so that mucin presents as basophilic strands and granules in hematoxylin and eosin stained sections.[3] In normal skin it is found particularly around appendages and the vasculature (*Fig. 13.161*). In the cutaneous mucinoses the deposits are hyaluronidase sensitive because most of the mucin present is hyaluronic acid. The excessive mucin disrupts the collagen fibers, giving them a frayed appearance. In general, with the exception of scleromyxedema, there is considerable histologic overlap within this group of conditions. Diagnosis depends considerably upon clinical features and the results of biochemical investigations.[15]

There are five major mucinoses:
- generalized myxedema,
- pretibial myxedema,
- lichen myxedematosus,
- reticular erythematous mucinosis,
- scleredema.

Follicular mucinosis is considered in Chapter 29.

Generalized myxedema

Clinical features

Generalized myxedema occurs as a consequence of severe hypothyroidism. Patients with myxedema may appear pale yellow due to the combined effects of edema, anemia, and carotenemia.[1,2] The last, which is due to defective conversion of beta-carotene to vitamin A in the liver, is seen particularly on the palms, soles, and in the nasolabial folds.[3] Rarely, the color change is generalized.[4] The skin is cool, dry, coarse, waxy, and puffy, especially around the eyes and cheeks, and the hands and feet may show nonpitting edema (*Fig. 13.162*).[3,5–7] The face is often expressionless. Eccrine and sebaceous gland secretions are reduced and this may result in xerosis, an ichthyotic appearance, or asteatotic eczema.[4] Hyperkeratosis over bony prominences resembling avitaminosis A is also sometimes evident.[8] Alopecia is a common finding and the outer third of the eyebrows is typically affected. There is usually thinning of the beard and sexual hair in addition to loss of the scalp hair. Myxedema is associated with a greatly increased percentage of hair follicles in the telogen phase.[9] The rate of hair growth is

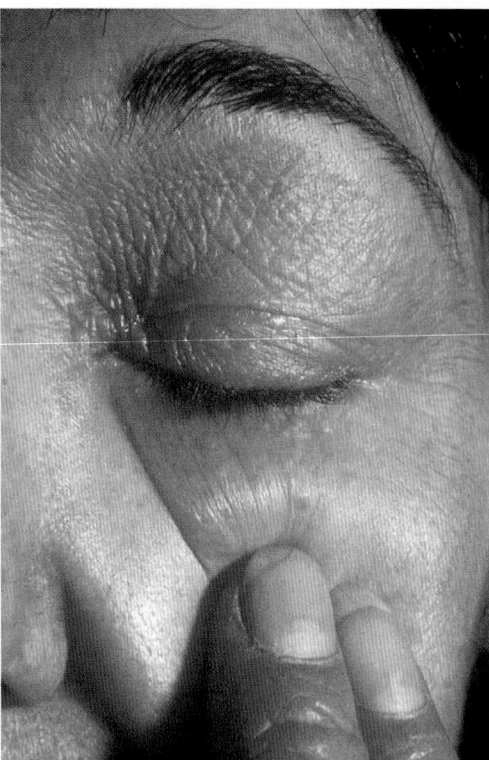

Fig. 13.162
Generalized myxedema: note the waxy infiltrated plaques on the eyelid. By courtesy of R.A. Marsden, MD, St George's Hospital, London, UK.

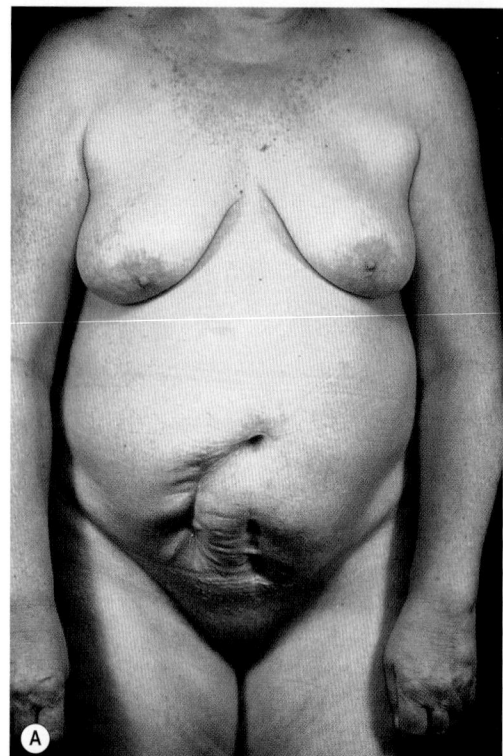

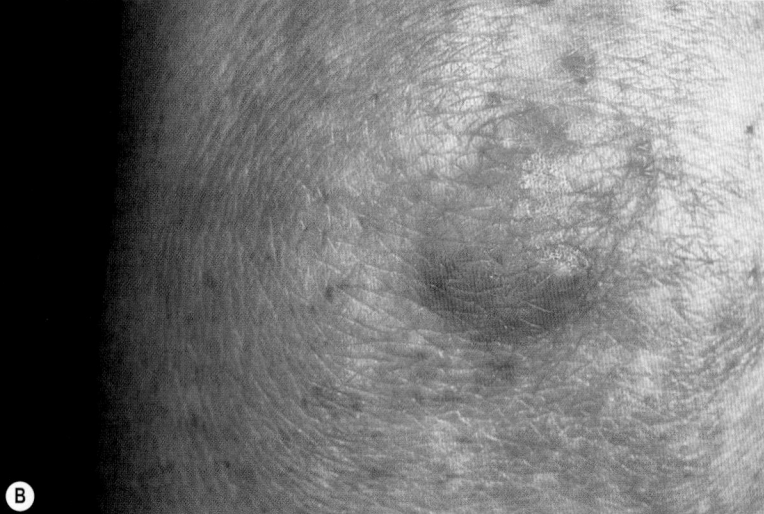

Fig. 13.163
(**A**, **B**) Generalized myxedema: this patient has widespread xanthomata. By courtesy of the Institute of Dermatology, London, UK.

also diminished. Residual hair is dry, coarse, and brittle.[3] The nails often become thin, brittle, and striated.[1] Additional cutaneous manifestations have included pruritic papular lesions, purpura and ecchymoses, impaired healing, generalized follicular mucinosis, and multiple focal cutaneous mucinoses.[1,5,9–11] Oropharyngeal and laryngeal involvement is common and many patients are hoarse. Patients with myxedema have an increased risk of developing hyperlipidemia with resultant eruptive and tuberous xanthomata (*Fig. 13.163*).

Histologic features

The epidermis may show mild hyperkeratosis with occasional follicular plugging.[3] Most frequently, the dermal changes are subtle and nondiagnostic. However, in cases of greater severity, there is slight swelling and separation of the collagen bundles with edema, and special stains show that small quantities of mucin are present within the dermis and occasionally in the subcutaneous fat.[12] Fibroblastic proliferation is not a feature of generalized myxedema.[13]

Localized (pretibial) myxedema

Clinical features

Localized (pretibial) myxedema is most often associated with hyperthyroidism.[1] It occurs in 3–5% of cases.[2] It is one of three processes classically seen in autoimmune thyroid (Graves) disease, the other two being exophthalmos and thyroid acropachy (clubbing of the digits associated with subperiosteal new bone formation). Pretibial myxedema, also known as 'Graves or thyroid dermopathy', is usually a late manifestation of Graves disease and follows the development of Graves ophthalmopathy.[3] It has only been reported exceptionally preceding the diagnosis of Graves disease and in the absence of ophthalmopathy.[4] In 10% of cases of Graves disease, patients are not clinically hyperthyroid.[5] They may be hypothyroid or euthyroid.[5] Pretibial myxedema can rarely be associated with Hashimoto thyroiditis.[6–8] Pink or yellow waxy plaques, nodules, and sometimes 'tumors' develop, most frequently first on the anterolateral aspects of the lower legs (*Fig. 13.164*). Lesions are classically nonpitting. In some patients there is induration with prominence of the follicles, giving rise to a peau d'orange appearance, and secondary hypertrichosis is occasionally marked. Localized hyperhidrosis at the site of the myxedema may also rarely occur.[9] The disease may progress to involve much of the lower leg, which rarely becomes grossly elephantiasiform (*Fig. 13.165*).[2,10–13] The feet and toes sometimes can be involved.[12,14] Small lesions are usually asymptomatic or mildly pruritic; the larger plaques are often painful.[15] Infrequently, localized myxedema occurs on other sites, such as the arms, shoulders, abdomen, neck, face, and even the ears (*Fig. 13.166*).[16] Nodular lesions rarely occur on the hands.[17] Deposition on the forearm has been described as 'preradial myxedema'.[17,18] Occurrence at atypical sites is most likely related to trauma.[19–21] For example, it has been described localized to scar tissue.[20,22–24] The latter includes the site of a smallpox vaccination scar.[25] Presentation at the site of a thigh donor graft site has also been reported.[26]

Rare patients with pretibial myxedema have no evidence of thyroid disease. Biopsies from these patients tend to show changes associated with stasis and this feature is useful in the histologic differential diagnosis.[27] One

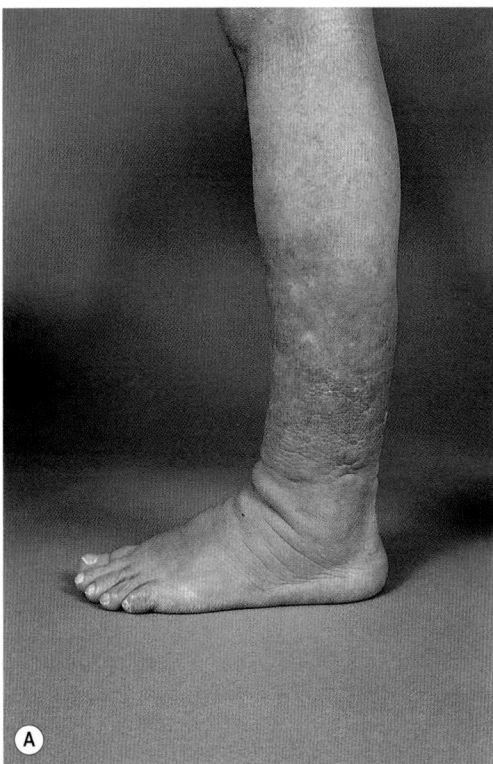

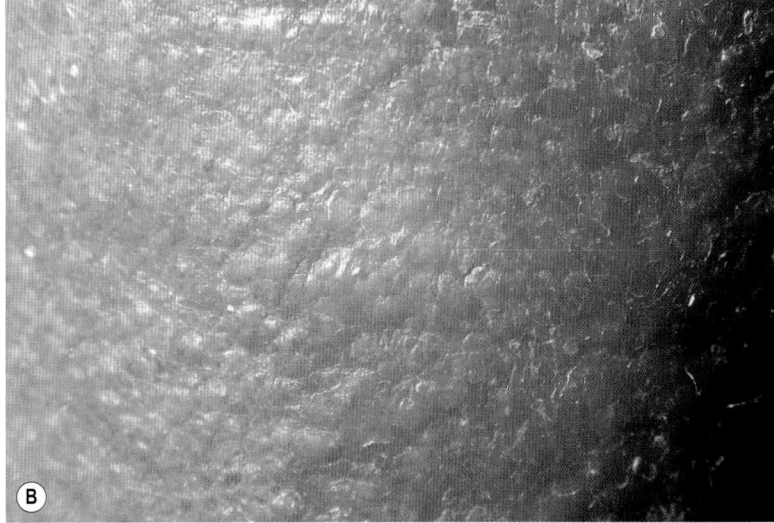

Fig. 13.164
Pretibial myxedema: (**A**) erythematous, somewhat translucent plaques are present over the shin; (**B**) close-up view. By courtesy of R.A. Marsden, MD, St George's Hospital, London, UK.

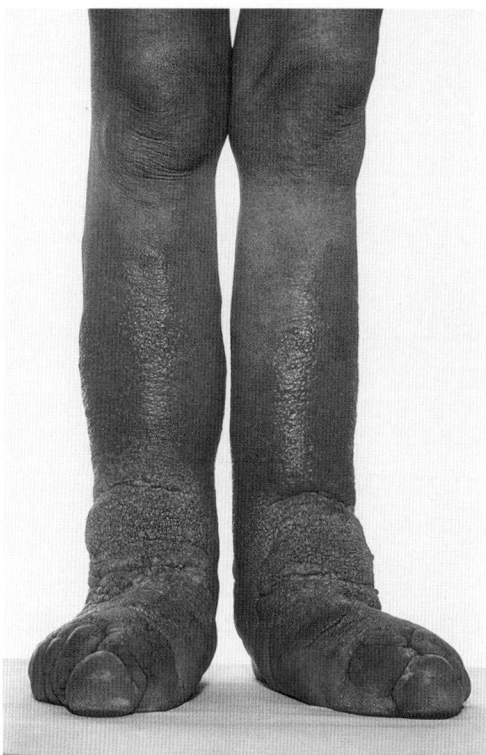

Fig. 13.165
Pretibial myxedema: in this extreme example, the features resemble elephantiasis. By courtesy of R.A. Marsden, MD, St George's Hospital, London, UK.

such variant has been described in morbidly obese patients with lymph-edema.[28,29] Lesions occur as papules, vesicles, and nodules on the pretibial surfaces.

Pretibial myxedema is sometimes self-limiting, involution occurring after a number of years. Complete remission occurs in up to 26% of cases but this depends on the severity of the disease.[5,30]

An exceptional form of pretibial mucin deposition that may be confused with pretibial myxedema associated with Graves disease has been documented in association with Sjögren syndrome under the name acral ichthyosiform mucinosis.[31] In the cases described, the patients had normal thyroid function tests and the mucin deposition was predominantly in the papillary dermis.

Pathogenesis and histologic features

The etiology is uncertain; the presence of pretibial myxedema is usually associated with detection of long-acting thyroid stimulator (LATS) in the serum, but LATS is not believed to be causal.[32] It was suggested in 1978 that a fibroblast stimulating factor associated with mucigenic properties isolated from the serum of patients with pretibial myxedema might play a role in the pathogenesis of the disease.[33] Subsequent studies have shown that fibroblasts in pretibial skin and in the orbit of affected patients contain sequences identical to those of the thyroid stimulating hormone receptor.[34,35] It has also been proposed that the fibroblasts might contain a cross-reacting protein rather than the true receptor, which binds with the autoantibodies against thyroid stimulating factor receptor.[36,37] Based on these observations, it has been proposed that autoantibodies against thyroid-stimulating hormone receptor react with fibroblasts containing these sequences, resulting in production of cytokines and induction of increased glycosaminoglycan secretion.[36,37]

Localization to the legs most typically is thought to be due to dependency and mechanical factors.[3] Additionally, tobacco is a known risk factor for the development of pretibial myxedema and Graves ophthalmopathy; however, the precise mechanism for this is presently unknown.[3]

The epidermis is often hyperkeratotic with follicular plugging; in gross cases, it may be papillomatous and acanthotic. The reticular dermis shows separation of collagen bundles by large quantities of mucin (*Figs 13.167* and *13.168*).[1] Fragmentation of collagen fibers can be seen.[3] Stellate fibroblasts are evident, but there is usually no increase in their number except perhaps in the more elephantiasiform examples. Lesions seen in the setting of lymphedema and obesity are also characterized by small vessel angiogenesis, vessel wall thickening, edema, and hemosiderin deposition.[28,29]

Immunofluorescent studies are usually negative, although granular deposits of IgM have been identified within the superficial papillary dermis.[15]

Electron microscopic studies show amorphous granular material both within fibroblast endoplasmic reticulum, coating the surface of the fibroblast, and in the interstitium surrounding the widely separated collagen and elastic fibers.[11] Tubuloreticular structures have been identified in the cytoplasm of endothelial cells in one case and in the dermis of another.[15,22]

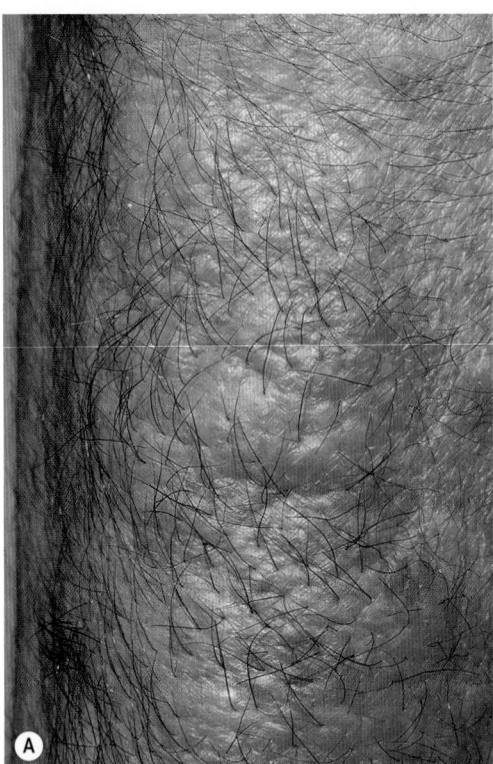

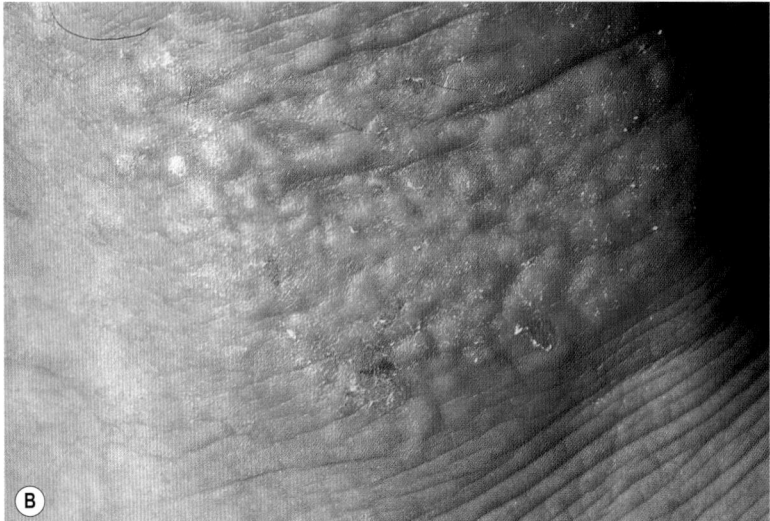

Fig. 13.166
(**A**, **B**) Localized myxedema: these pictures came from same patient shown in *Fig. 13.162*. Following a road traffic accident, the patient developed additional mucinous deposits on her arm close to the site of a fracture. By courtesy of P.G. Goodwin, MD, The Royal Bournemouth Hospital, UK.

Lichen myxedematosus/scleromyxedema

Clinical features

As originally classified, there were four variants of this rare disease of adults.[1] These were:

- generalized lichenoid papular eruption (*Figs 13.169* and *13.170*),
- discrete papular variant presenting as much smaller numbers of flesh-colored papules on the trunk and extremities (*Fig. 13.171*),
- localized and generalized lichenoid plaques mimicking lichen planus,
- urticarial or nodular lesions, which often evolved into the generalized papular form.[2,3]

With the subsequent delineation of new entities, the validity of this classification was called into question.[4] Lichen myxedematosus is now divided into three forms:[5–8]

- a localized form, which includes several variants: discrete papular lesions occurring at any site, acral persistent papular mucinosis (see

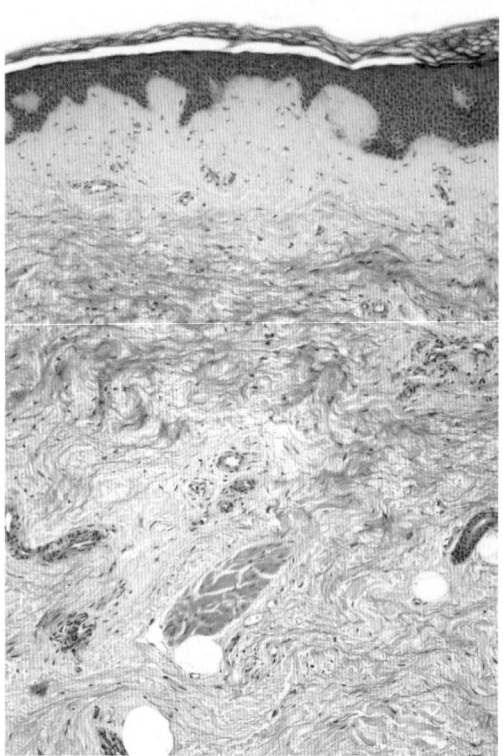

Fig. 13.167
Pretibial myxedema: there is loss of collagen fibers associated with mucin deposition.

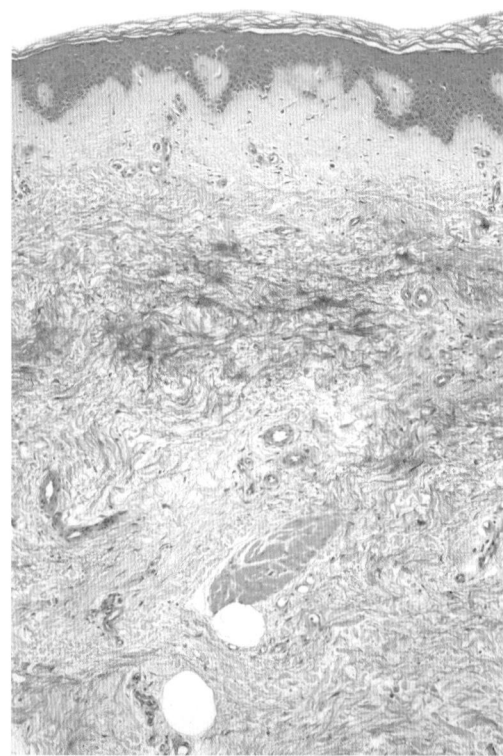

Fig. 13.168
Pretibial myxedema: the mucin (hyaluronic acid) stains positively with Alcian blue.

below), self-healing papular mucinosis (see below), papular mucinosis of infancy (see below), and nodular mucinosis,

- a generalized form (scleromyxedema) characterized by lichenoid papules, indurated and thickened skin, and a monoclonal gammopathy; by definition, thyroid function is invariably normal,

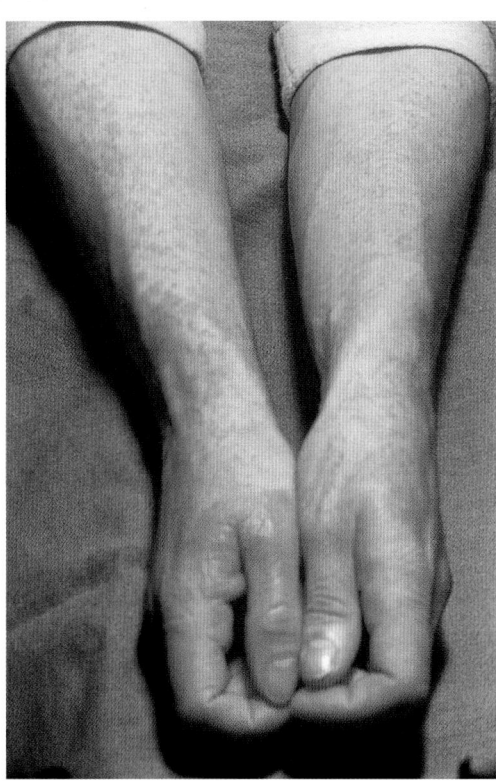

Fig. 13.169
Lichen myxedematosus: erythematous papules are widely distributed over the forearms. A more diffuse plaque is present over the dorsum of the left hand.

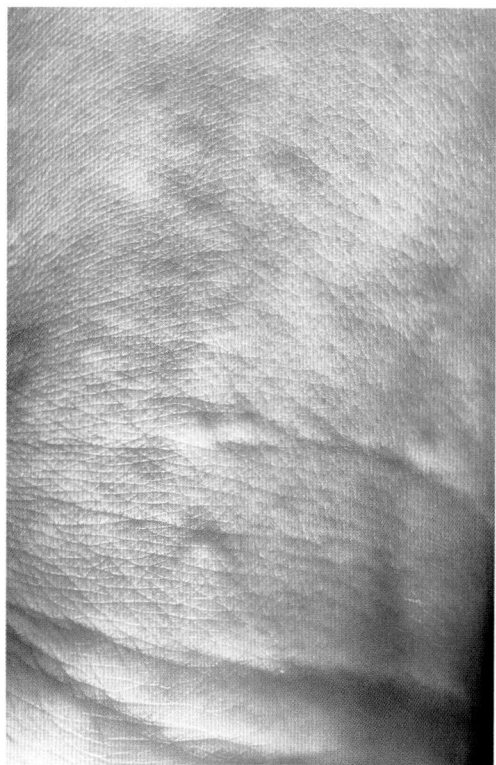

Fig. 13.171
Lichen myxedematosus: this is an example of the discrete papular form showing small numbers of papules on the anterior wrist. By courtesy of R.A. Marsden, MD, St George's Hospital, London, UK.

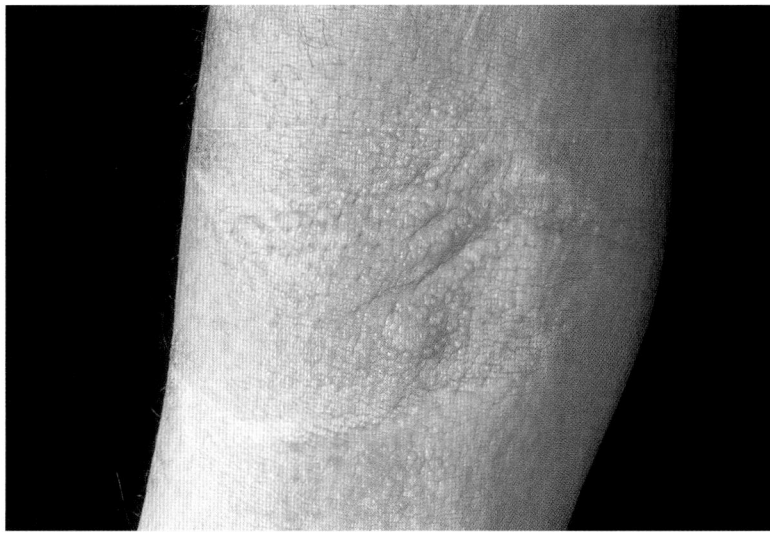

Fig. 13.170
Lichen myxedematosus: numerous papules are present in the antecubital fossa. By courtesy of R.A. Marsden, MD, St George's Hospital, London, UK.

- an atypical or intermediate form where patients may have generalized lesions without systemic symptoms/gammopathy, localized lesions with systemic symptoms/gammopathy or other manifestations that do not strictly fulfill criteria for either the localized or generalized variants.

The generalized form of lichen myxedematosus (scleromyxedema) occurs equally in males and females and is seen most often in the fourth and fifth decades.[3] It often presents on the hands and wrists, but soon becomes generalized although lesions are particularly seen on the hands, elbows, neck, face, and upper trunk.[9-11] Prominent linear papules may be evident on the forehead, neck, axillae, and behind the ears.[12] The papules are small, 2–3 mm in diameter, white or erythematous, and often have a waxy consistency. They tend to coalesce to form infiltrated plaques and, when associated with hardening and thickening of the underlying skin (scleromyxedema), result

in tethering and limitation of movement, so that sclerodactyly, microstomia, and a mask-like facies may result (*Fig. 13.172*).[4,11] Gross involvement of the glabellar skin sometimes causes a leonine appearance.[11,13] A rare patient with leonine facies and tumor-like nodules mimicking lymphoma has been reported.[14] The lack of acral calcification and absence of Raynaud phenomenon help to distinguish this condition from scleroderma. The mucous membranes are not usually affected.[3] The lesions are variably pruritic.

There are occasional reports of systemic symptoms. Esophageal aperistalsis, peripheral neuropathy, proximal myopathy, and cardiac and cerebrovascular diseases have all been described.[4,11,15,16] There has been little postmortem confirmation of visceral involvement and therefore it is likely that many of these associations are no more than coincidental. Neurological manifestations have, however, been reported most often and are probably of significance. They have included acute psychoses, encephalopathy and coma, epileptiform seizures, aphasia, memory loss, depression, and motor dysfunction.[9,15-18] Dermatoneuro syndrome describes a rare manifestation of CNS disease where patients develop high fever, flulike symptoms followed by seizures, and coma.[16,19,20] Carpal tunnel syndrome has also been reported fairly frequently.[21-23] Pulmonary involvement is not uncommon and consists of restrictive or obstructive disease and pulmonary hypertension.[16,24] Renal disease similar to that seen in scleroderma is rare.[25,26] There is usually no relationship between lichen myxedematosus and neoplasia, but patients with underlying Hodgkin lymphoma, myeloid leukemia, hepatocellular carcinoma, thymic carcinoma, and seminoma has been reported.[16,27-29] Rare cases associated with HIV infection have also been documented.[30,31] Further associations include chronic hepatitis C and dermatomyositis.[32-34] The latter finding is interesting because in the past, inflammatory myopathy not dermatomyositis has been described in association with scleromyxedema.[35] It has been suggested that the development of myopathy is associated with a poor prognosis.[35] A case associated with immune thrombocytopenia and atypical nodular lesions has been reported.[36]

Scleromyxedema is usually (but not invariably) associated with a paraproteinemia; most often this is IgG with lambda light chains.[11,17,37-40] Occasionally it has been of the IgM or IgA class.[3] An occasional association

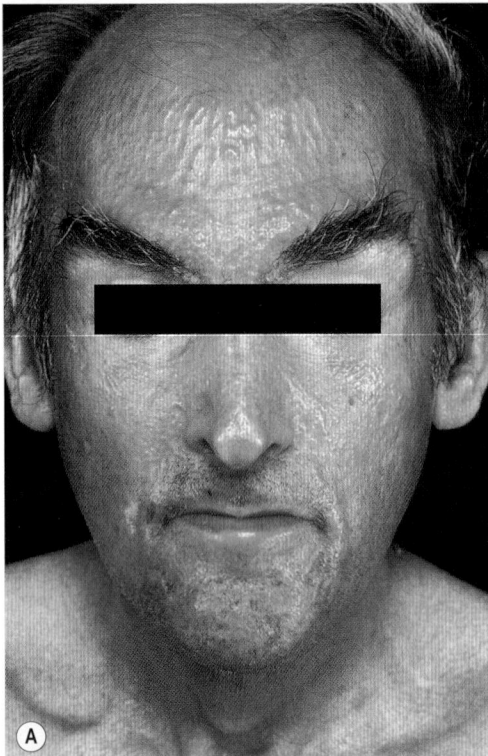

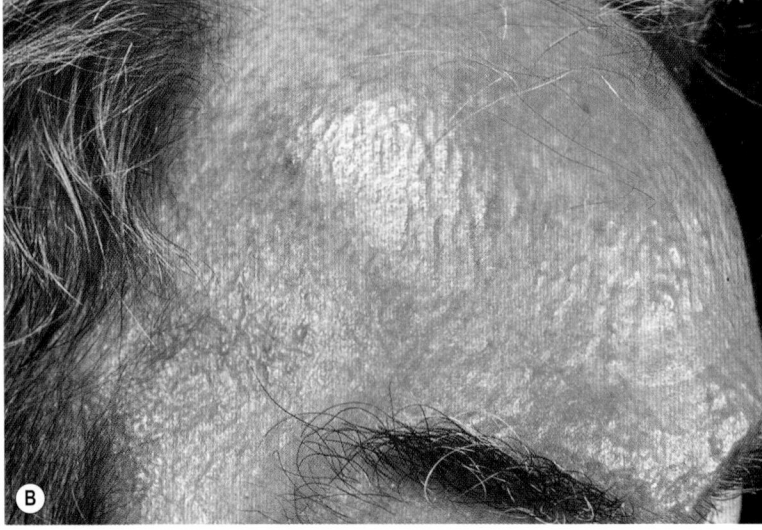

Fig. 13.172
(**A**, **B**) Scleromyxedema: this severely affected patient shows sclerosis and linear papules on the forehead. Note the pinched, mask-like facies. By courtesy of R.A. Marsden, MD, St George's Hospital, London, UK.

with multiple myeloma has also been noted but occurs in less than 10% of patients.[5,9]

Pathogenesis and histologic features

The pathogenesis of lichen myxedematosus is unknown. There is no evidence to suggest that the paraprotein is responsible for the fibroblastic proliferation. However, serum from scleromyxedema patients has been shown to contain a nonparaprotein-associated fibroblast growth factor. This requires further characterization.[8,41] There is some evidence to suggest that the paraprotein may, however, have mucinogenic properties.[42,43] Fibroblasts grown in tissue culture produce greater quantities of hyaluronic acid and sulfated glycosaminoglycans than normal controls.[44] Collagen synthesis, as determined by H3-hydroxyproline estimations, is diminished.

Immunofluorescent studies have revealed immunoglobulin (IgG and to a lesser extent IgM) in the reticular dermis or just below the epidermis in 35% of cases.[13] Indirect immunofluorescence is invariably negative.

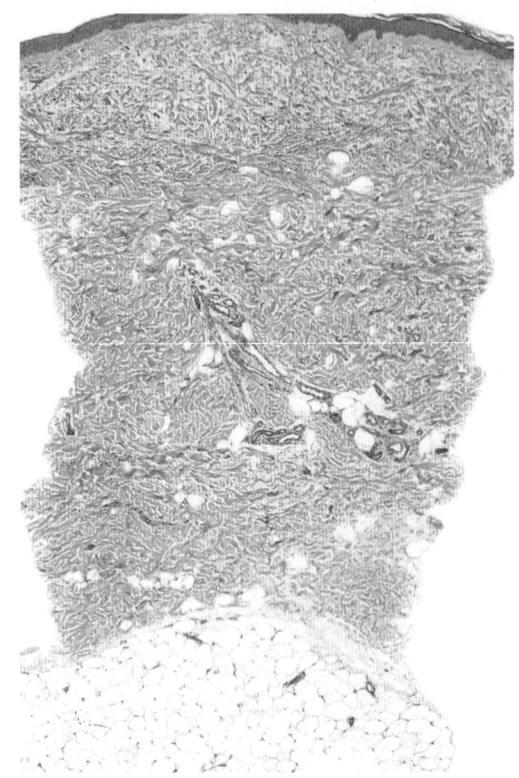

Fig. 13.173
Lichen myxedematosus: increased mucin is evident in the superficial dermis.

The epidermis may be normal, acanthotic, or atrophic, and sometimes hyperkeratosis with parakeratosis is evident. In early lesions stellate fibroblasts are seen between disorganized collagen fibers in the reticular dermis (*Figs 13.173* and *13.174*).[3,7] The papillary dermis is not affected. Increased numbers of mast cells are sometimes present.[29] Focal deposits of mucin are readily identifiable (*Fig. 13.175*).[2] A slight perivascular chronic inflammatory cell infiltrate is often seen in the superficial dermis.

In the more severe scleromyxedema variant, fibroblasts are numerous and there is consequent fibrosis and thickening of the dermis (*Figs 13.176–13.178*).[4,45] Mucin deposits may be less evident or even absent.[12] Decreased elastic fibers have occasionally been reported.[3] A chronic inflammatory cell infiltrate is frequently present surrounding the superficial vasculature.

A less common granulomatous variant of scleromyxedema has been described in which there is an interstitial histiocytic infiltrate with giant cells, similar to granuloma annulare or interstitial granulomatous dermatitis.[45–49] Although there is increased mucin, prominent stellate fibroblasts and dense bundles of collagen are not a feature. This variant may be more common than previously realized, representing close to 30% of cases in one series.[45]

Ultrastructural studies show active fibroblasts characterized by abundant rough endoplasmic reticulum and Golgi apparatus, increased numbers of mitochondria, and cytoplasmic inclusions accompanied by collagen deposition.[50]

Systemic involvement has only rarely been documented. Mucin deposition has been described in the adventitia of visceral blood vessels and in the renal papillae in single case reports.[9,50] It has also been described within rectal mucosa and in muscle in one patient with scleromyxedema. Whether this represents true primary involvement or a secondary unrelated phenomenon is uncertain. In a particularly unusual case the features of systemic sclerosis were found in the kidney.[9] In the absence of any autopsy evidence of further sclerodermatous lesions, it may be that the renal vascular and glomerular changes reflected unrecognized scleromyxedematous pathology. Demyelination and focal gliosis have also been reported.[13,51] Nevertheless, autopsy studies have usually shown no evidence of widespread mucinosis, and it is likely that in the great majority of cases the pathological changes are limited to the skin.

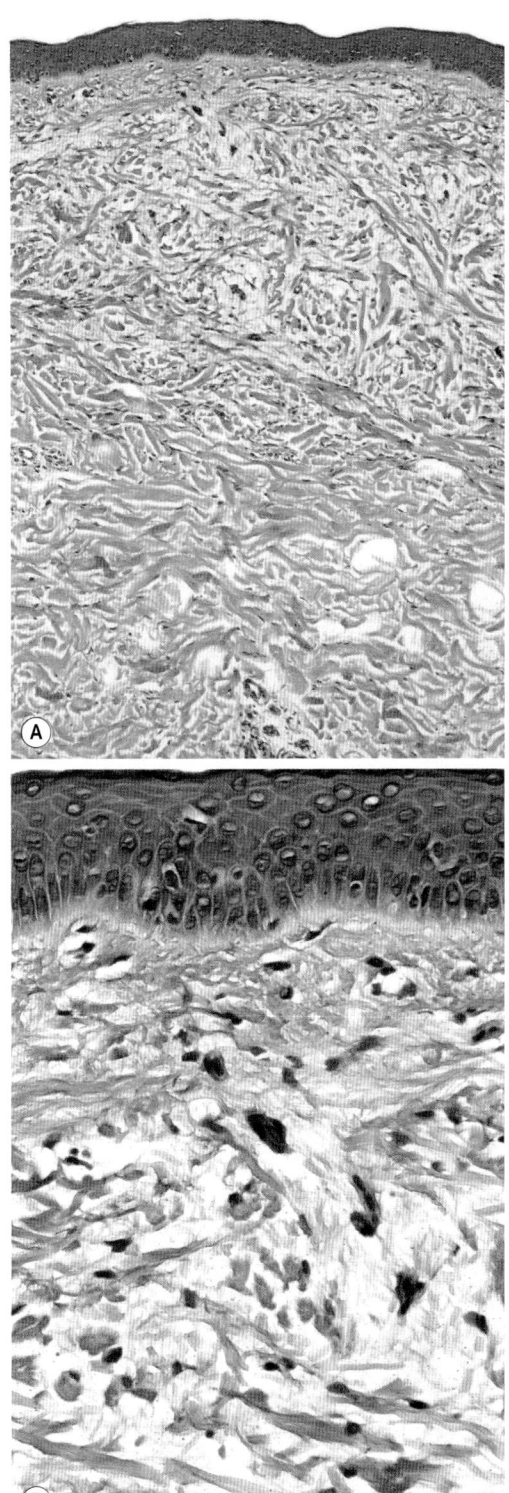

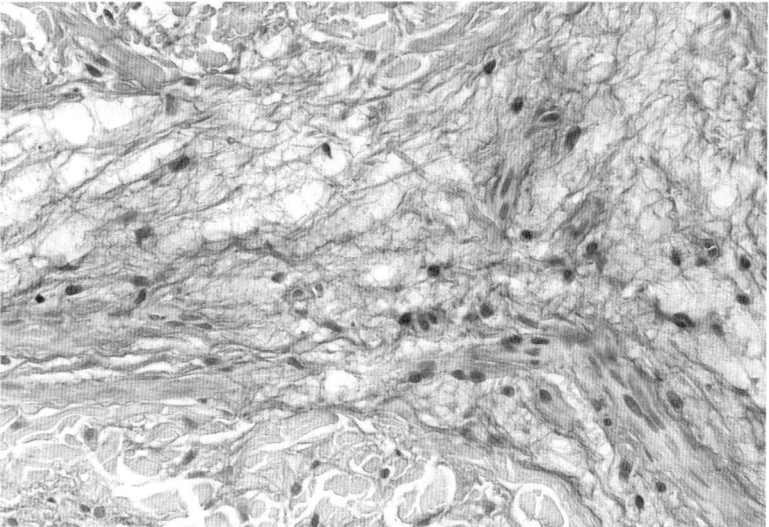

Fig. 13.175
Lichen myxedematosus: staining with colloidal iron emphasizes the mucin deposits.

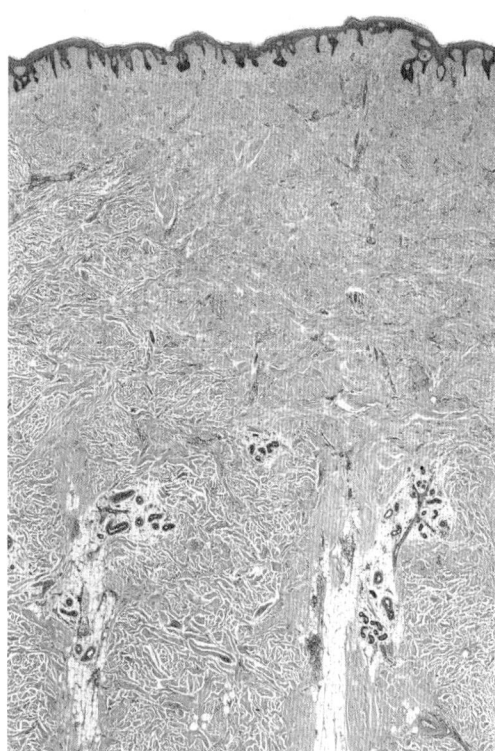

Fig. 13.176
Scleromyxedema: the dermis is markedly thickened. There is fibrosis and increased numbers of fibroblasts are evident.

Fig. 13.174
(**A**, **B**) Lichen myxedematosus: the collagen fibers are widely separated by mucin deposits. Fibroblasts are increased in number.

Differential diagnosis

It may be impossible to distinguish scleromyxedema from nephrogenic systemic fibrosis based solely on histopathological features.[52] Both conditions demonstrate an intradermal proliferation of spindled cells associated with increased mucin. The spindled cells stain for CD34, factor XIIIa, and procollagen I in both disorders. Although correlation with clinical parameters is critical for ultimate distinction between the two disorders, the depth of the infiltrate may be a helpful differentiating feature.[53,54] In scleromyxedema the infiltrate is confined to the mid to deep dermis, whereas in nephrogenic

systemic fibrosis the process begins in the dermis but also extends into the septa of the subcutaneous fat. In the absence of adequate clinical information, the changes seen in established lesions of lichen myxedematosus may be confused with those seen in a dermatofibroma. Epidermal changes, polymorphism and hyalinization of collagen bundles at the periphery of the proliferation are absent in the former.

Acral persistent papular mucinosis

Clinical features

This rare condition, which predominantly affects females, is characterized by the development of persistent multiple discrete and often symmetrical

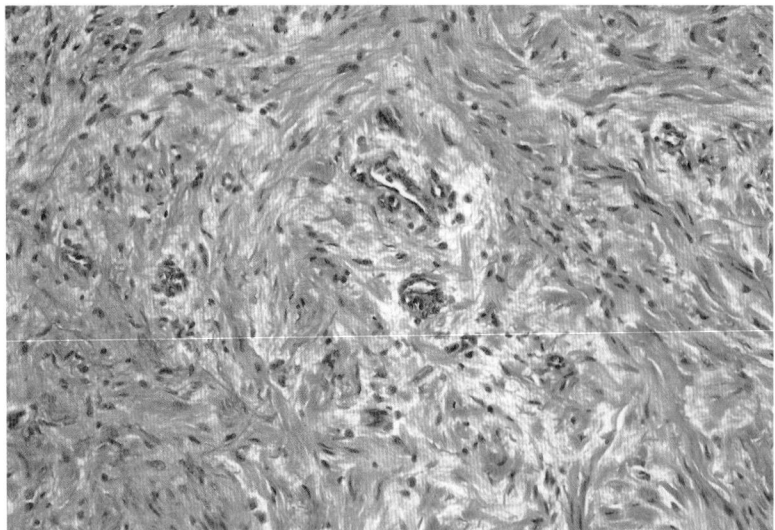

Fig. 13.177
Scleromyxedema: delicate strands of mucin separate the collagen fibers.

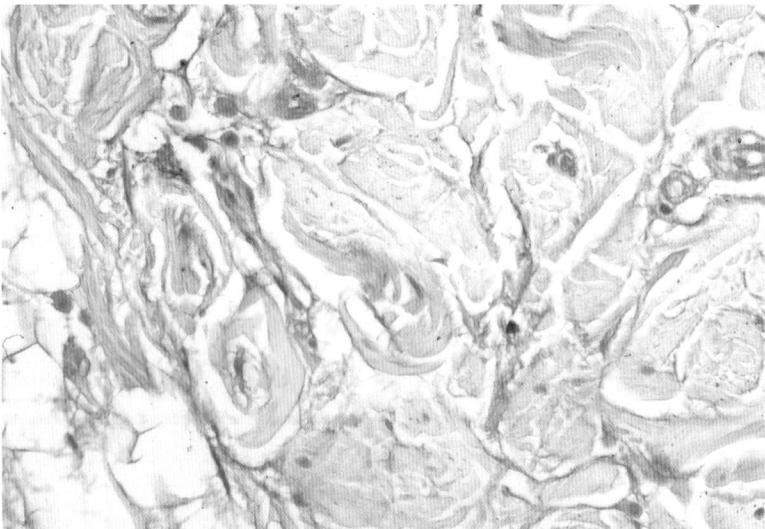

Fig. 13.178
Scleromyxedema: Alcian blue.

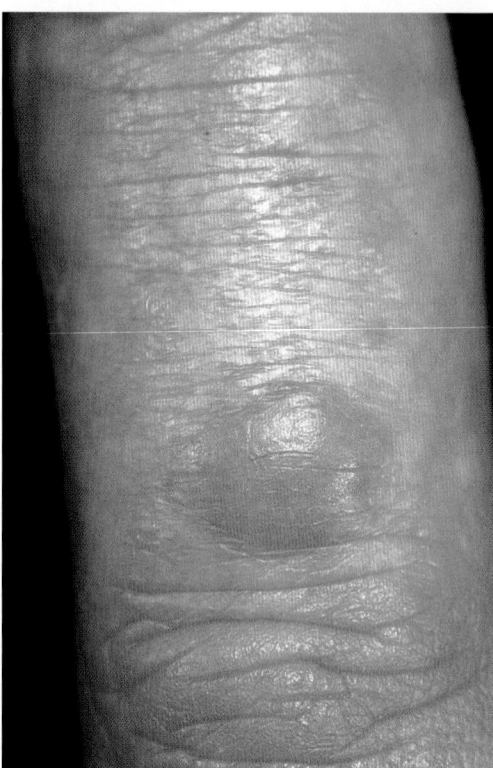

Fig. 13.179
Acral persistent papular mucinosis: discrete papule on the dorsal surface of a forefinger. This patient had similar lesions on the arms. By courtesy of R.A. Marsden, MD, St George's Hospital, London, UK.

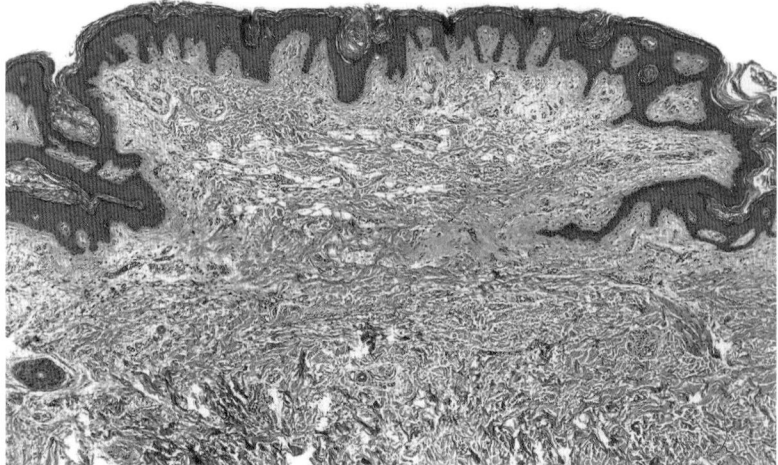

Fig. 13.180
Acral persistent papular mucinosis: note the presence of a discrete superficial papule with a well-developed collarette.

smooth-surfaced small papules (2–7 mm) on the dorsal aspects of the hands and wrists, sometimes extending on to the forearms (Fig. 13.179).[1–4] The condition is generally regarded as a localized variant of lichen myxedematosus.[5–11] The papules are ivory or flesh-colored and translucent, and on puncture characteristically contain clear viscous fluid.[2] Lesions do not occur on the face or trunk and there is no thickening or induration of the skin.[12] Pruritus is exceptional.[13] Occurrence in two sisters has been reported, raising the possibility of a familial form of the disease.[14] Acral persistent papular mucinosis is not usually known to be associated with any systemic abnormalities, such as thyroid disease or paraproteinemia.[15,16] An exceptional case associated with IgA monoclonal gammopathy has been reported.[17]

Histologic features

The papules show extensive mucin deposition in the upper reticular dermis separated by a grenz zone from the overlying epidermis (Figs 13.180 and 13.181).[10,12,18,19] Increased numbers of spindled or stellate-shaped fibroblasts may occasionally be evident.[20] Fibrosis, however, as seen in lichen myxedematosus, is not a feature of this condition. Direct immunofluorescence has revealed granular IgM at the dermal–epidermal junction and linear IgG around the eccrine glands in one case.[2] Ultrastructural studies reveal active fibroblasts with prominent dilated rough endoplasmic reticulum. The collagen bundles are widely separated and focal deposits of electron-dense amorphous material are evident.[5] Conspicuous lamellated electron-dense lysosomes have been described in one case.[20] This probably represents a non-specific secondary change.

Cutaneous mucinosis of infancy

Clinical features

This variant of papular mucinosis is very rare.[1–4] It has been suggested that the condition might represent a pediatric localized form of lichen myxedematosus.[5,6] Familial cases have been documented.[5]

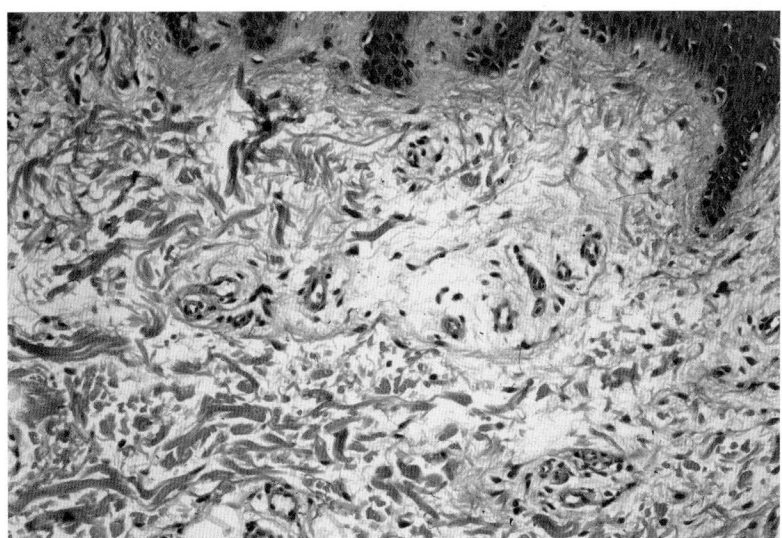

Fig. 13.181
Acral persistent papular mucinosis: close-up view showing mucin deposits.

The eruption consists of densely grouped, firm, 1–2 mm papules on the elbows and smaller numbers of more dispersed lesions about the forearms and dorsa of the hands.[1] Congenital linear papules on the backs of two fingers have been reported in one infant and another was born with clustered papules on the lower back.[2,3] Another patient presented with a cobblestoned plaque on the thigh.[4] Congenital cases presenting with papules on the fingers and toes or widespread eruption involving the trunk, neck, and extremities have been described.[7,8] Owing to the paucity of cases, the natural history and prognosis of this condition are unknown, though some lesions spontaneously regress.[7,8]

Histologic features

Excessive mucin (hyaluronic acid) is present in the papillary and/or reticular dermis under a variably acanthotic epidermis.[1,7,8] Sectioning artifact may make the deposits appear to have an intraepidermal location.[1] Biopsies from late lesions show features identical to those of lichen myxedematosus with fibrosis and proliferation of dermal fibroblasts.[4] A perivascular chronic inflammatory cell infiltrate is evident in the superficial dermis.

Self-healing juvenile cutaneous mucinosis

Clinical features

This is an extremely rare condition, only a few cases having been documented.[1–20] It most commonly presents in children, with a rapid onset of asymptomatic erythematous papules, nodules, and plaques, which show a predilection for the face, neck, scalp, abdomen, and extremities, accompanied by deep nodules on the face and periarticular regions.[1,12,18] The plaques have a characteristic appearance as linear groups of papules, giving the skin a corrugated appearance.[3] The deep nodules can mimic fasciitis.[11,18] The eruption resolves within a period of weeks to months. Mild arthritis involving the elbows, knees, and interphalangeal joints has been documented as has possible polychondritis.[1,3] These latter manifestations may be persistent.[1] In one patient, bilateral carpal tunnel syndrome was present. Non-specific features of fatigue, weight loss, and myalgia may also be evident. The age of those who are typically affected ranges from infancy to teenagers. Exceptionally, the disease presents in adults.[14–17] There is no evidence of thyroid dysfunction or paraproteinemia.

Pathogenesis and histologic features

The etiology is unknown although it has been suggested that the fibroblast activity may have been stimulated by a preceding viral infection.[3]

Histologically, the epidermis is normal or may show mild hyperkeratosis. Mucin deposition is seen in the papillary and upper reticular dermis

separating and splitting the collagen bundles. In one case the mucin was PAS positive and identified as a sialomucin, whereas in others it was found to consist of hyaluronic acid.[1,3,9,10,12,14,16] Fibroblasts are slightly increased in number and a mild chronic inflammatory cell infiltrate surrounds the superficial vasculature. Deeper nodules demonstrate similar involvement of the septa and lobules of the subcutaneous fat, which can also extend into the fascia.[11,18] Epithelioid, ganglion-like histiocytes/myofibroblasts can be seen and may cause confusion with proliferative or nodular fasciitis.[11,12,18,19]

Reticular erythematous mucinosis

This condition is described in Chapter 8.

Scleredema

Clinical features

Scleredema (Buschke) is a rare primary mucinosis that presents with non-pitting indurated edema and associated dermal hardening in the absence of any significant clinical abnormality of the overlying skin.[1,2] Three distinct subtypes are recognized:[2–5]

- Most commonly seen is an acute variant predominantly affecting children and characterized by a rapid onset arising a few weeks after an infection, most often of the upper respiratory tract. Streptococcal infections are particularly implicated, but cases have followed a variety of viral illnesses including measles, mumps, influenza, cytomegalovirus infection, chickenpox, and *Mycoplasma pneumoniae* infection.[6–9] Scleredema has also occurred in the setting of chronic scabies and secondary streptococcal infection.[10] Although many of these cases resolve spontaneously within a period of months and years, a significant number are persistent and exacerbations are not uncommon.[11] Females are affected more often than males and the disease is more common in the winter months.[12] Sometimes there is a prodromal illness of malaise, myalgia, generalized myasthenia, and arthralgia.[11] Some patients develop a variety of cutaneous manifestations including transient erythema, urticarial or annular eruptions, and dermographism before the onset of the more typical features.[4] Scleredema in children may exceptionally present overlapping features with eosinophilic fasciitis.[13]
- Secondly, scleredema may have an insidious onset unaccompanied by any previous acute illness.[2]
- Lastly, scleredema sometimes develops in association with late-onset diabetes mellitus. Patients, more often males, are often obese and there are usually other manifestations of diabetes, including nephropathy, hypertension, coronary and peripheral vascular insufficiency, retinopathy, and peripheral neuropathy.[2,14,15] The diabetes commonly precedes the development of scleredema, which is usually widespread and associated with a chronic course.[1,16,17] This variant of scleredema does not tend to resolve spontaneously or with treatment, though there have been reports with improvement with combinations of PUVA and colchicine or UVA with or without colchicine.[18–20]

Scleredema is occasionally associated with a paraproteinemia (usually IgG, but sometimes IgA) and rarely multiple myeloma.[21–24] There is no evidence that the paraprotein results in the skin lesions; hence it is probably a secondary phenomenon. Evolution to systemic amyloidosis has been reported in one patient.[24]

It should be noted that despite the original nomenclature of scleredema adultorum, many of the patients are, in fact, children.[11,12,25] Only very rarely are childhood cases associated with diabetes.[25] An exceptional case of congenital scleredema has been reported.[26]

Rare cases have had associated primary and secondary hyperparathyroidism, rheumatoid arthritis, Sjögren syndrome, and sarcoidosis.[27–31] Scleredema has also been described in HIV infection, in association with a nuchal fibroma, following exposure to organic solvent, in the setting of a malignant insulinoma and carcinoid, with acanthosis nigricans, with generalized hyperpigmentation, and as an adverse consequence of infliximab.[14,22,32–37] The cutaneous manifestations are similar for all three subtypes, differences being merely a matter of degree.

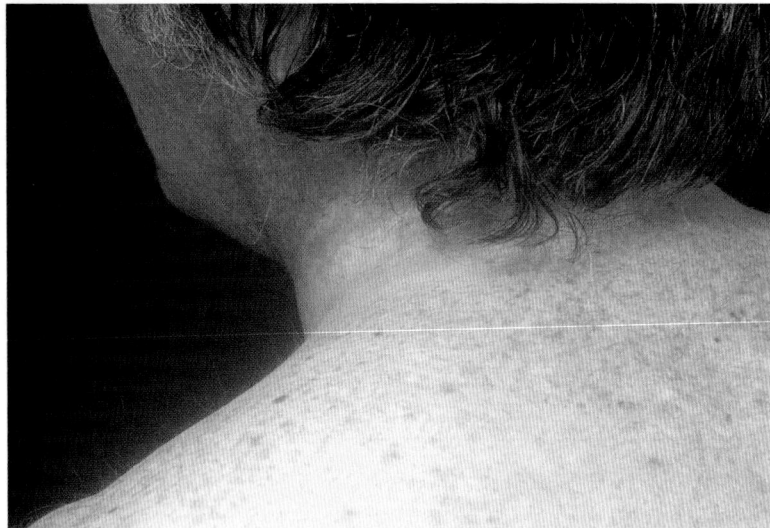

Fig. 13.182
Scleredema: a diffuse, firm thickening of the tissues is present over the neck and shoulders. By courtesy of G. Murphy, MD, Institute of Dermatology, London, UK.

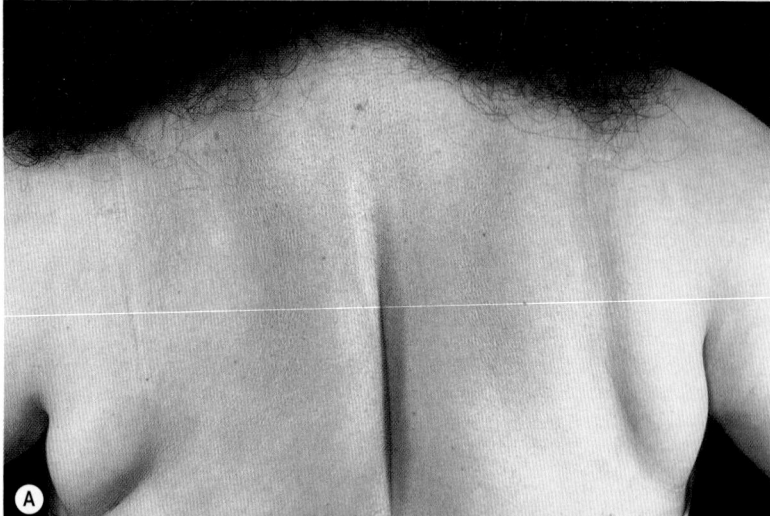

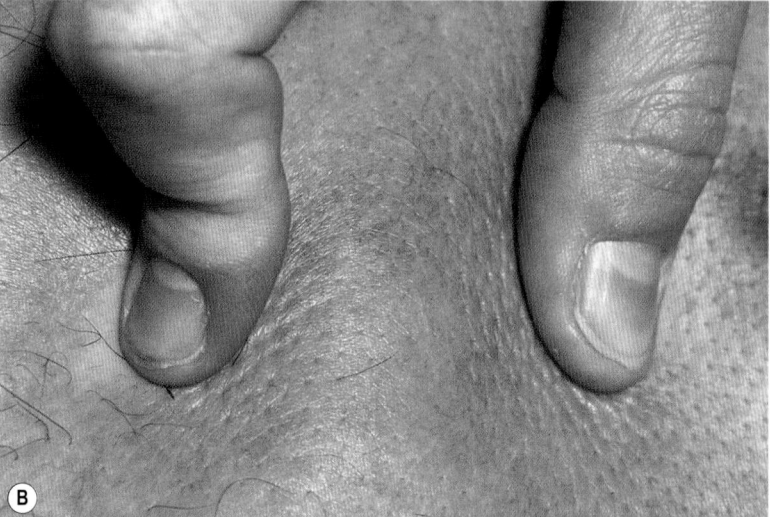

Fig. 13.183
(**A**, **B**) Scleredema: there is marked thickening and induration of the skin of the upper back. By courtesy of G. Murphy, MD, Beaumont Hospital, Dublin, Eire.

Patients present with symmetrical nonpitting edema and dermal hardening, which particularly affects the posterior and lateral aspects of the neck (*Fig. 13.182*).[2] The face, anterior neck, upper trunk, and upper limbs are also frequently affected.[1] Rarely, the disease may spread to the lower abdomen and legs. Confinement of the changes to the thighs has been described.[38] The hands and feet are rarely affected and genital involvement is uncommon.[10,39] Lesional skin is shiny and feels hard, and wrinkling is impossible due to involvement of the papillary dermis (*Fig. 13.183*). In severely affected patients reduced mobility is often a problem. The face may be expressionless, the lines of cleavage lost, and smiling and mouth opening may be difficult.[1] The overlying skin may demonstrate erythema, hyperpigmentation, and/or a peau d'orange appearance. An unusual case with hyperkeratosis has been described.[8]

In some patients systemic disease may be evident, including pericardial, pleural, and peritoneal effusions, dysarthria and dysphagia due to tongue and pharyngeal lesions, hepatosplenomegaly, cardiac and skeletal muscle manifestations, parotid gland involvement, and ocular changes presenting as induration of the eyelids and conjunctivae.[11,12,40] Periorbital edema can be the sole presentation.[41,42] In cases with systemic involvement, mucin deposition has been demonstrated in the bone marrow, liver, nerve, salivary gland, and heart.[43–45] Cardiac and pulmonary disease may exceptionally lead to death.[46]

Pathogenesis and histologic features

The pathogenesis of scleredema is unknown. The serum from one patient with scleredema and a paraprotein markedly stimulated collagen production in normal skin fibroblast cultures, suggesting that a circulating factor(s) probably related to the paraprotein might induce the dermal fibrosis.[47] The involved skin shows increased synthesis of type I collagen, which appears to be responsible, at least in part, for the dermal fibrosis.[48,49] The fibroblasts in involved skin from individuals with scleredema show increased protein production, collagen synthesis, and glucosamine incorporation. This correlation is associated with increased levels of type I and type III collagen.[50] Biochemical analysis of involved skin in scleredema has confirmed an increase in glycosaminoglycans, the main component being hyaluronic acid.[51]

The histologic features are often subtle and the diagnosis is difficult. The epidermis may be slightly thinned or appear normal. The reticular dermis is greatly thickened, often at the expense of the subcutaneous fat, and the eccrine glands therefore become abnormally situated within the upper third or mid dermis (*Figs 13.184* and *13.185*).[1] In some cases eccrine glands may be markedly reduced in number.[52] The collagen fibers are broadened and, particularly in the earlier stages, are abnormally separated by clear spaces (dermal fenestration).[2] The latter may contain small quantities of mucin, but often special stains (Alcian blue, colloidal iron) and multiple biopsies are

necessary for their demonstration (*Fig. 13.186*).[17,53] Up to one-third of cases may not demonstrate mucin even with the aid of special stains.[54] Fibroblasts are present in normal numbers. A mild chronic inflammatory cell infiltrate is sometimes evident in the superficial dermis and mast cells may be increased in number (*Fig. 13.187*).[1] Direct immunofluorescence studies are negative.[2,21]

Differential diagnosis

Scleredema may be distinguished clinically from scleroderma by the absence of Raynaud phenomenon, acral sclerosis with calcification, pigmentary changes, and telangiectasia.[2] Histologically, the appendages are atrophic and compressed or absent in scleroderma, inflammation usually with the presence of plasma cells is identified and there is diffuse dermal sclerosis rather than the fenestrated appearance seen in scleredema.

Papular and nodular cutaneous mucinosis of systemic lupus erythematosus

Clinical features

Mucin deposition as a specific clinical manifestation of lupus erythematosus has been recorded only rarely in the literature yet is said to occur in up to 1.5% of dermatological patients with this disease.[1–3] The condition presents as asymptomatic, flesh-colored, occasionally umbilicated papules and nodules on the neck, trunk, and upper limbs.[4–17] Presentation with

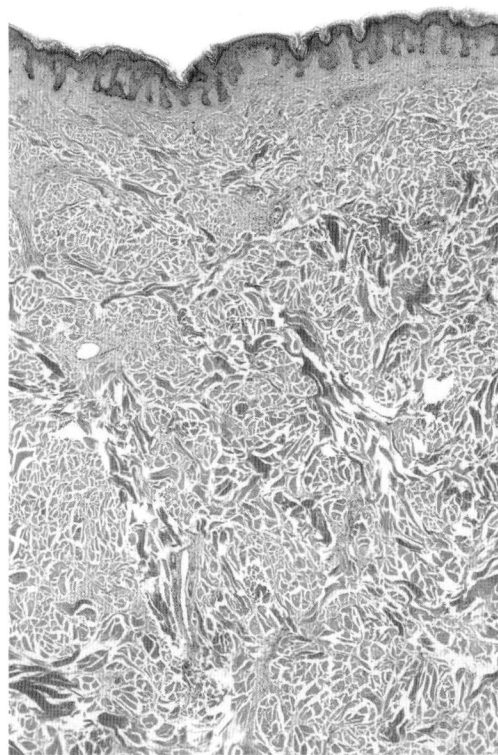

Fig. 13.184
Scleredema: early lesion showing collagen bundle separation.

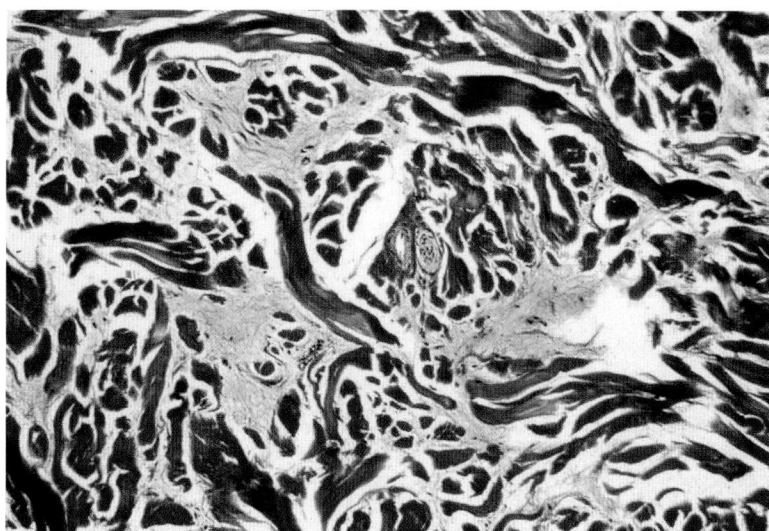

Fig. 13.186
Scleredema: the abundant mucin is highlighted by Alcian blue/chromotrophe 2R staining.

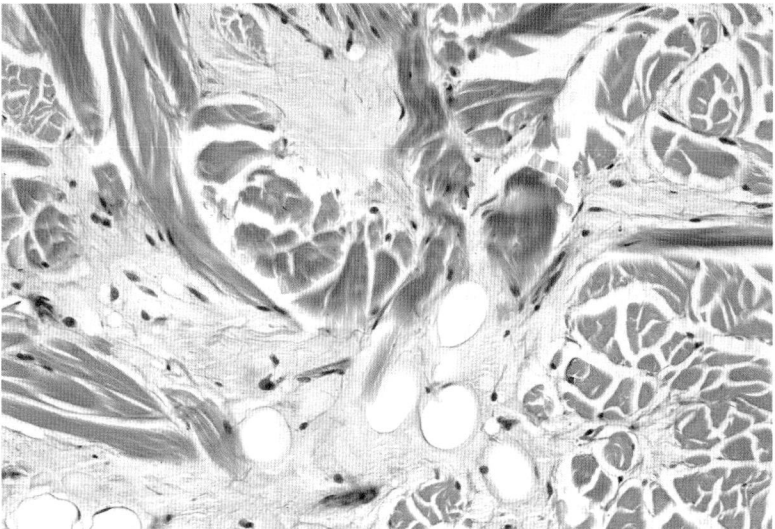

Fig. 13.185
Scleredema: the collagen fibers appear swollen. There is excess mucin.

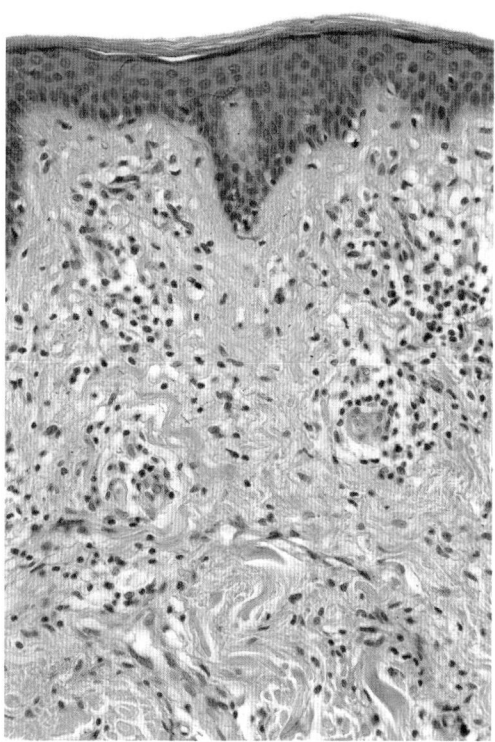

Fig. 13.187
Scleredema: superficial dermal lymphohistiocytic infiltrate.

massive cutaneous mucinosis has also rarely been reported.[18] The papules may rarely be hyperpigmented.[19] Lesions are best appreciated using tangential light, which gives the skin a lumpy appearance.[5] Mucin deposition occurs most often in patients with the systemic variant, usually with diffuse antinuclear factor and anti-DNA antibodies, and is particularly associated with joint and kidney lesions.[4,11,13-20] There are, however, occasional reports of its occurrence in patients with discoid and subacute cutaneous lupus erythematosus.[4,7-9] An inconstant relationship to sunlight has been recorded.[4,21] Exceptionally, systemic sclerosis may present with similar papular and nodular mucinous lesions.[22]

Histologic features

The epidermis shows no significant features; in particular, the changes of lupus erythematosus are usually absent. However, an interface change has been described in a single case.[23] The mucin is present in the papillary and upper reticular dermis associated with a slight perivascular chronic inflammatory cell infiltrate.[4,24] Fragmentation of collagen bundles has been noted in one case in association with mucin accumulation.[11] A case with features of interstitial granulomatous dermatitis has also been described.[25]

Direct immunofluorescence may show linear or granular immunoglobulin (IgG, IgM) deposits and complement at the dermal–epidermal junction.

Myxoid cyst

Clinical features

Cutaneous myxoid cyst, sometimes inappropriately referred to as synovial cyst, presents as a soft or fluctuant cystic nodule on the dorsal aspect of the distal interphalangeal, the metacarpophalangeal and, less frequently, the metatarsophalangeal joints (Figs 13.188 and 13.189).[1,2] An exceptional

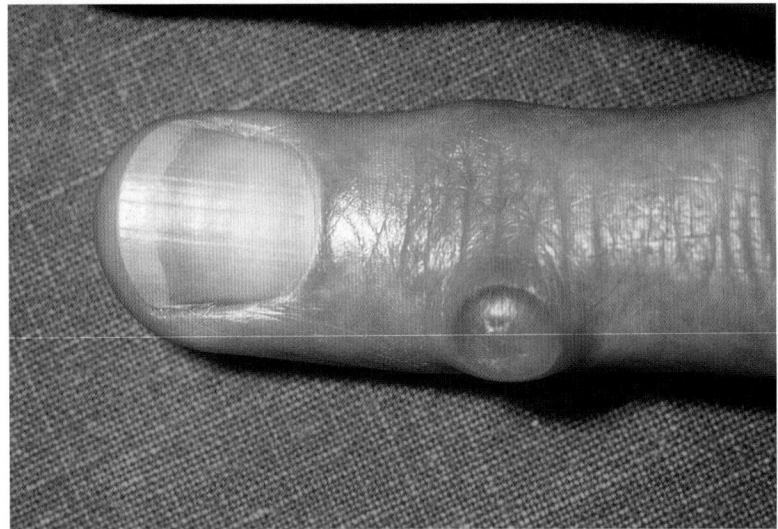

Fig. 13.188
Myxoid cyst: the translucency is typical. By courtesy of R.A. Marsden, MD, St George's Hospital, London, UK.

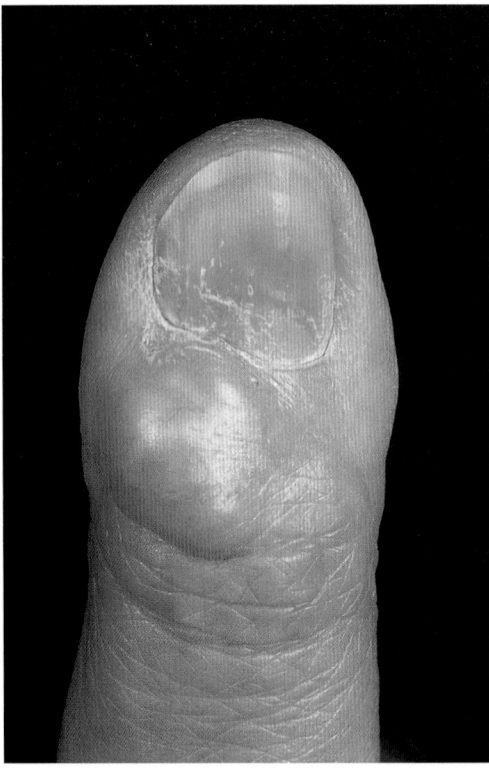

Fig. 13.189
Myxoid cyst: localization over the distal interphalangeal joint is characteristic. By courtesy of the Institute of Dermatology, London, UK.

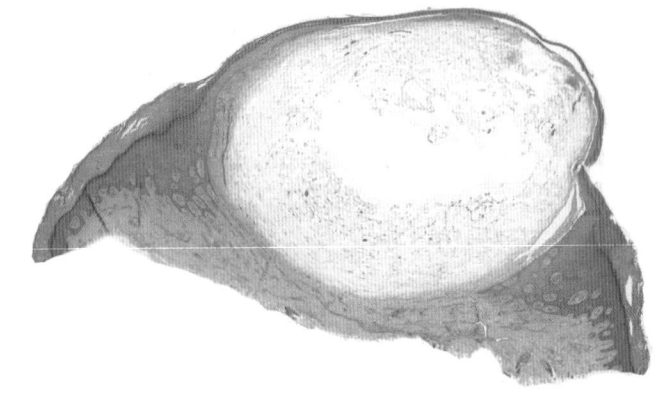

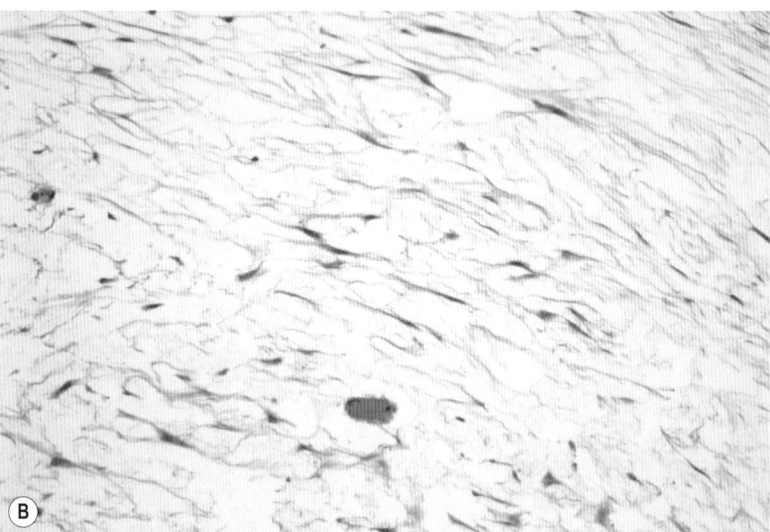

Fig. 13.190
(**A**, **B**) Myxoid cyst: excessive mucin deposition has resulted in this fluid-filled cyst. The overlying epithelium may appear attenuated or verrucous and occasionally the cyst is, in part, intraepidermal in location.

case occurring on the lateral aspect of the knee has been described.[3] Occasionally, lesions are multiple.[4,5] Cutaneous myxoid cysts may present at any age and are more common in females. The surface is usually smooth, although verrucous variants are occasionally encountered. The cyst contains clear, yellow, viscous fluid. Lesions are often painful or tender. Myxoid cyst involving the proximal nail fold can be associated with longitudinal grooving of the nail.[6] Although the precise cause is not well elucidated, underlying osteoarthrosis is sometimes evident, and repetitive trauma is proposed to be one possible mechanism.[1,4]

Histologic features

The cyst is devoid of any lining and consists of a large pool of mucin containing spindled/stellate fibroblasts with prominent cytoplasmic processes

(*Fig. 13.190*). The overlying epidermis is often atrophic and hyperkeratotic, and acanthosis may be seen at the edges. Early lesions are sometimes indistinguishable from cutaneous focal mucinosis. There is no evidence of any connection with an underlying joint.

Cutaneous focal mucinosis

Clinical features

Cutaneous focal mucinosis presents as an asymptomatic, usually solitary, dermal papule or nodule most commonly on the face, neck, trunk, or extremities of adults.[1-6] A case involving the areola has been recently reported.[7] It is not seen in relation to the joints of the hands, feet, or wrists. The lesion is usually dome-shaped, white or flesh-colored and sometimes has an erythematous halo.[2] Occasional verrucous variants have been documented.[1] There is usually no evidence of an associated thyroid abnormality. Exceptional cases, however, are associated with reticular erythematous mucinosis or scleromyxedema.[8] Multiple lesions are rare.[9]

Histologic features

The lesion is usually located in the mid and upper dermis, often separated from the epidermis by a grenz zone of dermal sparing.[2] It consists of a localized, but usually poorly delineated, focus of mucin deposition containing increased numbers of spindle-shaped cells and stellate fibroblasts

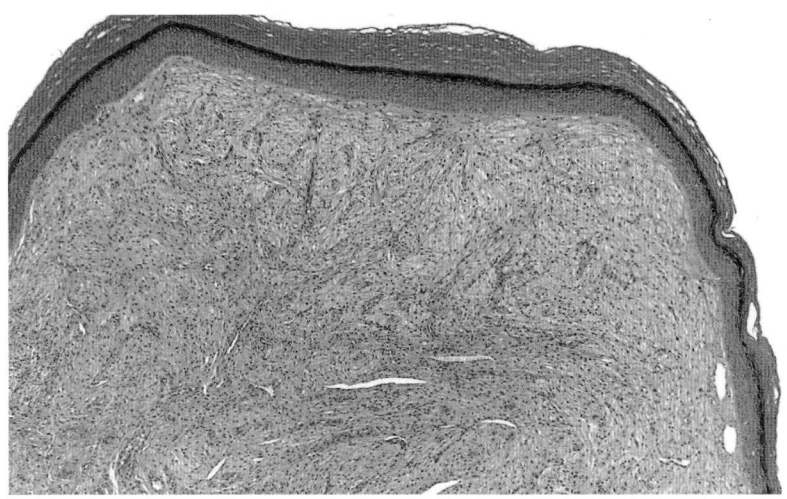

Fig. 13.191
Focal dermal mucinosis: mucin deposition in upper dermis with scattered widely spaced collagen bundles.

with elongated cytoplasmic processes.[2] Sometimes these contain conspicuous intracytoplasmic vacuoles.[3] Collagen fibers are usually diminished in number, but some collagen fibers are often present within the collection of dermal mucin (*Fig. 13.191*).[4,10] A mild perivascular chronic inflammatory cell infiltrate is often present in the adjacent dermis. There may be an increase in the number of small-caliber blood vessels. The overlying epidermis is typically uninvolved; however, immature follicular germ-like induction can occur.[11]

Ultrastructurally, the fibroblasts contain prominent rough endoplasmic reticulum and membrane-bound intracytoplasmic vesicles containing abundant granular electron-dense material.[3]

Differential diagnosis

Cutaneous focal mucinosis must be distinguished from superficial angiomyxoma, a benign myxoid cutaneous and subcutaneous lesion with a tendency for local recurrence, associated with Carney complex. Superficial angiomyxoma has a distinctly lobular growth pattern, typically without entrapped/retained collagen fibers and a more developed thin-walled vasculature. Admixed stromal neutrophils are often present in superficial angiomyxoma, and secondary proliferation of adnexal structures may be seen.[10,11]

Mucinous nevus

Clinical features

Mucinous nevus (nevus mucinosis) is a rare lesion that may be congenital or acquired.[1–8] The most common sites affected are either the trunk or lower limbs. Patients present with papules, nodules and/or plaquelike lesions, usually with a linear or dermatomal distribution.[4] Large pedunculated lesions are rare.[8,9] A familial case has been described in two young brothers.[10]

Histologic features

Histologically, the mucin is located in the superficial dermis where it replaces the collagen and elastic fibers.[5] Some cases are associated with epidermal hyperplasia and these may represent a combined epidermal and mucinous nevus.[3,11] A case with dilated pores, termed follicular mucinous nevus, has been reported.[12] A recent immunohistochemical evaluation demonstrated that the stromal cells are CD34 positive, with rare cells staining for factor XIIIA.[13]

Differential diagnosis

These lesions must be distinguished from the mucinous eccrine nevus, which comprises abundant mucin surrounding eccrine glands and ducts.[14]

Neuropathia mucinosa cutanea

There is only one case report of this condition, which presented in a young male with hyperesthesia and livedoid lesions on the lower limbs. A biopsy of these lesions revealed hypertrophic nerves surrounded by mucin.[1]

Self-healing infantile familial cutaneous mucinosis

This very rare entity has been reported only once, in two brothers. Multiple lesions developed during the first few months of life and in one patient regressed spontaneously over a few years.[1]

Localized mucinosis secondary to venous insufficiency

A form of localized mucinosis related to stasis change has been described.[1–3] Patients developed violaceous plaques and coalescing papules on the lower extremities.[1,2] The lesions were painful and occurred in the setting of venous stasis. There was no history of thyroid disease, connective tissue disease or antecedent treatment with ultraviolet light. The histologic features consisted of large amounts of mucin deposition in the papillary and reticular dermis with characteristic extension around the eccrine glands. There was a slight increase in the number of blood vessels that demonstrated thickened walls. However, an inflammatory infiltrate was not present. The pathogenesis of this condition is unknown.

Hereditary progressive mucinous histiocytosis

Clinical features

Hereditary progressive mucinous histiocytosis was originally described as a familial histiocytosis presenting in women.[1] Since the original description, a number of additional cases have been reported.[2–13] Most cases are familial, but sporadic cases have been described.[6,8] It is a rare non-Langerhans cell histiocytosis that typically presents in the second decade of life. Rarely it can present congenitally or in the first few months of life.[4,12] Females are much more commonly affected than males, but a few cases in males have been described.[9,12] The lesions present as skin-colored to red–brown 1–10 mm papules, most commonly on the dorsal hands, forearms, face, and legs.[1–13] Less commonly it may involve the trunk. Mucosal membranes are not involved. Usually the papules are asymptomatic, but pruritus has been occasionally reported.[9,12] The lesions persist without spontaneous regression.

Pathogenesis and histologic features

The pathogenesis is uncertain. Though no specific gene defect has been described, the familial clustering suggests either an autosomal dominant pattern of inheritance influenced by female hormones or, less likely, X-linked dominant inheritance that is lethal in utero to males. The fact that the eruption usually begins in the second decade and the occasional cases in males supports the former hypothesis.

Histologically, the lesion is characterized by a well-circumscribed proliferation of epithelioid histiocytes to spindled cells in the upper to mid dermis associated with increased dermal mucin (*Figs 13.192* and *13.193*).[1–13] Dilated vessels may be present and occasional cases have increased mast cells.[1,6] The cellular constituents may vary somewhat depending on the age of the individual lesion. In early lesions, the epithelioid cells may predominate while the spindled cells tend to be more numerous in older lesions.[1,6] It has been hypothesized that cytokine production by the histiocytes results in fibroblast proliferation and angiogenesis, leading to the proliferation of spindled cells in older lesions.[3]

The immunophenotype is somewhat variable. The lesional cells are usually positive for lysozyme, but inconsistently positive for CD68.[3,5,6,8–10] Generally, the histiocytic cells are positive for CD68, while the spindled cells are often negative. The histiocytic cells are also positive for alpha-1 antitrypsin, alpha-1antichymotrypsin, and CD31.[1,6,9] The spindled cells may be positive for CD34.[3] Variable positivity for factor XIIIa has been reported.[6,8,10] Importantly, both the histiocytic and spindled cells are consistently negative

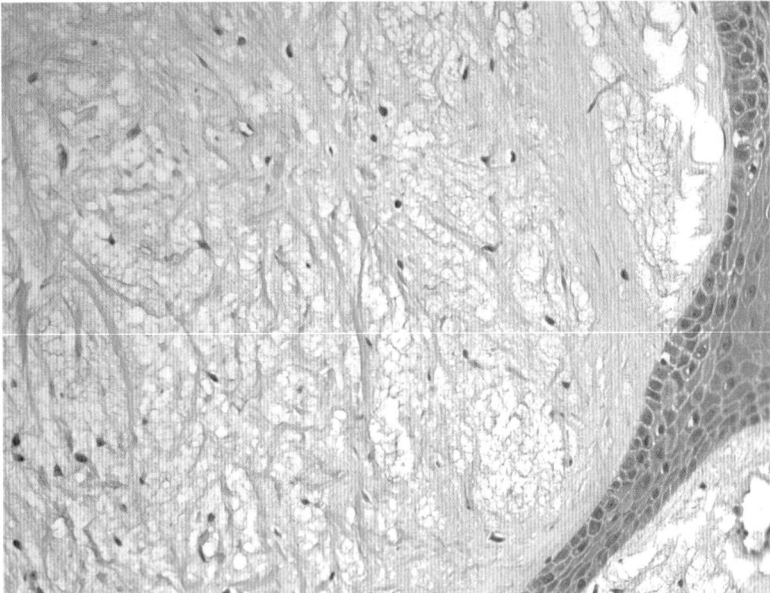

Fig. 13.192
Hereditary progressive mucinous histiocytosis. Nodular dermal infiltrate of histiocytes in a mucinous/myxoid background. By courtesy of C-K Sui, S-C Chao and J. Y-Y Lee, Tainan, Taiwan.

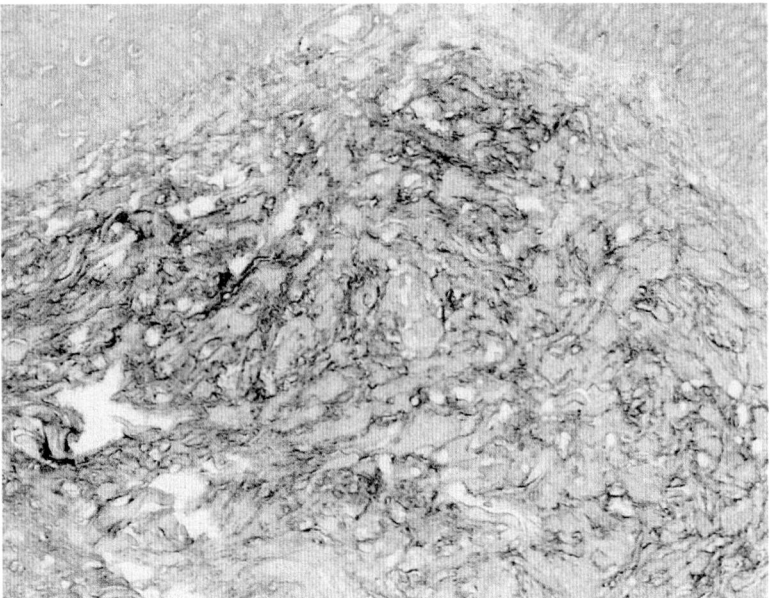

Fig. 13.193
Hereditary progressive mucinous histiocytosis. Colloidal iron highlighting prominent dermal mucin. By courtesy of C-K Sui, S-C Chao and J. Y-Y Lee, Tainan, Taiwan.

for S100 protein and CD1a. The dermal mucin can be highlighted with Alcian blue at pH 2.5 or toluidine blue cytochemical stains.[1,8,10]

Ultrastructural examination reveals intracellular structures reminiscent of lysosomal storage diseases. Within the cytoplasm of the histiocytes, there are circular osmophilic myelin bodies and zebra bodies.[1–11]

Differential diagnosis

Clinically the differential diagnosis includes generalized eruptive histiocytoma, xanthoma disseminatum, and progressive nodular histiocytosis. None of these entities is associated with increased dermal mucin. Histologically, the differential diagnosis includes acral persistent mucinosis, focal dermal mucinosis, superficial angiomyxoma, scleromyxedema, granuloma annulare and myxoid dermatofibroma. Acral persistent mucinosis is not familial and lacks a histiocytic proliferation. Focal dermal mucinosis and superficial angiomyxoma are typically solitary lesions and do not have a histiocytic

proliferation. Scleromyxedema is more widespread, less well circumscribed, has plasma cells, and is associated with a paraproteinemia. Although palisading has been reported in hereditary progressive mucinosis potentially causing confusion with granuloma annulare, necrobiotic collagen is not a feature of hereditary progressive mucinosis. Myxoid dermatofibromas are actually quite rare and would not present as multiple lesions.

Secondary cutaneous mucinoses

Clinical features

Mucinous lesions on the skin have been described as part of a reactive process associated with various triggers. A patient recently developed multiple erythematous to skin-colored papules following infection with varicella-zoster virus.[1,2] The lesions occurred in the same dermatome affected by postherpetic neuralgia and resolved as the pain improved. Mucinosis complicated by cutaneous necrosis can occur following injection with interferon. Recombinant interferon-beta-1b and interferon alfacon-1 have been implicated in the setting of treatment for multiple sclerosis and hepatitis C, respectively.[3,4] Erythematous ulcerative plaques develop at injection sites. Additionally, mucinosis papules and plaques have been described in the vicinity of a recently replaced joint.[5]

Histologic features

These mucinous disorders are characterized by intradermal mucin without a significant increase in dermal fibroblasts.[1–5] Ulcerative lesions associated with interferon injections can also demonstrate intravascular thrombi.[4]

Acanthosis nigricans

Clinical features

Acanthosis nigricans develops under a variety of circumstances.[1–3] In addition to the well-recognized tumor-associated variant, acanthosis nigricans may present with benign familial forms, endocrinopathy and drug-related variants, and the condition can be seen in association with a range of congenital conditions including lipoatrophy, leprechaunism, and the type A and type B syndromes described below. Genetic conditions associated with acanthosis nigricans include:

- Alstrom syndrome (retinopathy, progressive sensorineural hearing loss, and truncal obesity),
- Crouzon syndrome (facial palsy, sensorineural hearing loss with skeletal and mental retardation),
- Seip-Lawrence syndrome (congenital lipodystrophic diabetes),
- Costello syndrome (postnatal growth deficiency, coarse facies, redundant skin of the neck, palms, soles, and fingers, dark skin, and papillomas),
- Bannayan-Riley-Ruvalcaba syndrome (subcutaneous lipomas, vascular malformations, lentigines of the penis and vulva, warty lesions, macrocephaly, mental retardation, intestinal polyposis, skeletal abnormalities, vascular malformations of the central nervous system, and thyroid tumors),[4–8]
- Lelis syndrome (ectodermal dysplasia with hypotrichosis, hypohidrosis, hypodontia, palmoplantar hyperkeratosis, and perioral furrows).[9]

Acanthosis nigricans has been described in association with a missense mutation of the fibroblast growth factor receptor.[4] This disease is also associated with severe neurological impairment and severe achondroplasia.[10] Additional rare associations include Wilson disease (hepatolenticular degeneration) and primary biliary cirrhosis.[11,12] In the latter case, the acanthosis nigricans resolved after liver transplantation. In an exceptional family with several members affected by acanthosis nigricans, absence of the eyebrows and eyelashes and sparse hair elsewhere has been reported.[13]

Development of acanthosis nigricans may also antedate or present concomitantly with a variety of connective tissue diseases including systemic lupus erythematosus, systemic sclerosis, and dermatomyositis.[14–17] The condition is characterized by the presence of symmetrical brown velvety or verrucous plaques with a predilection for intertriginous sites, such as the back

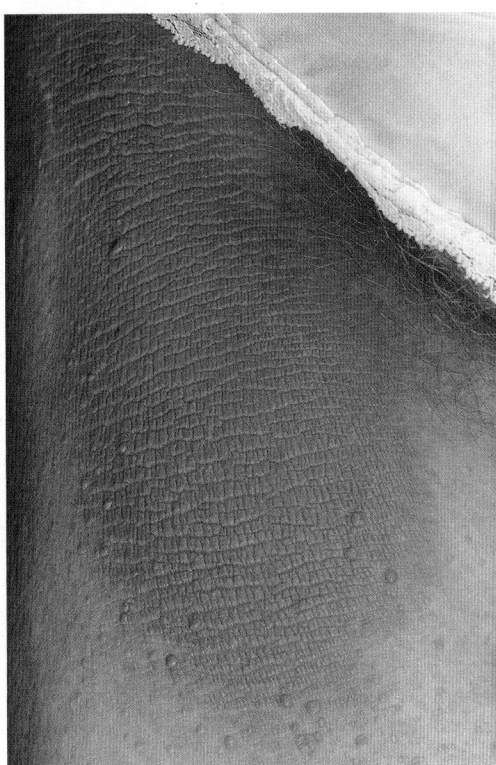

Fig. 13.194
Acanthosis nigricans: thickening of the skin of the groin. By courtesy of R.A. Marsden, MD, St George's Hospital, London, UK.

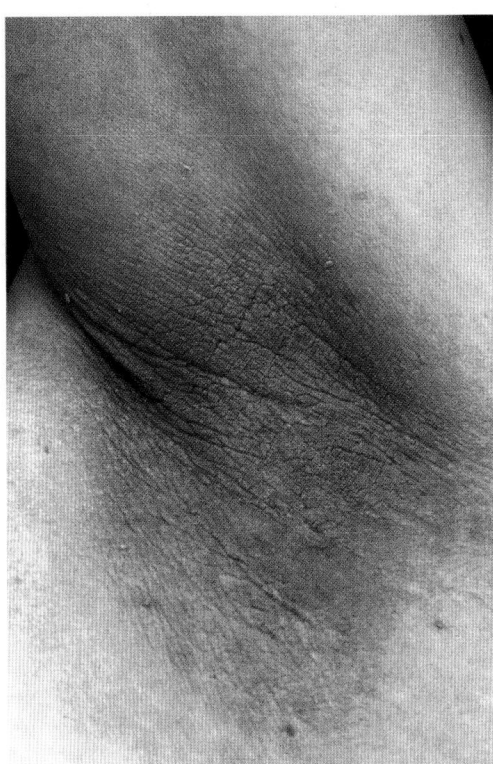

Fig. 13.195
Acanthosis nigricans: there is velvety thickening of the axillary skin. By courtesy of the Institute of Dermatology, London, UK.

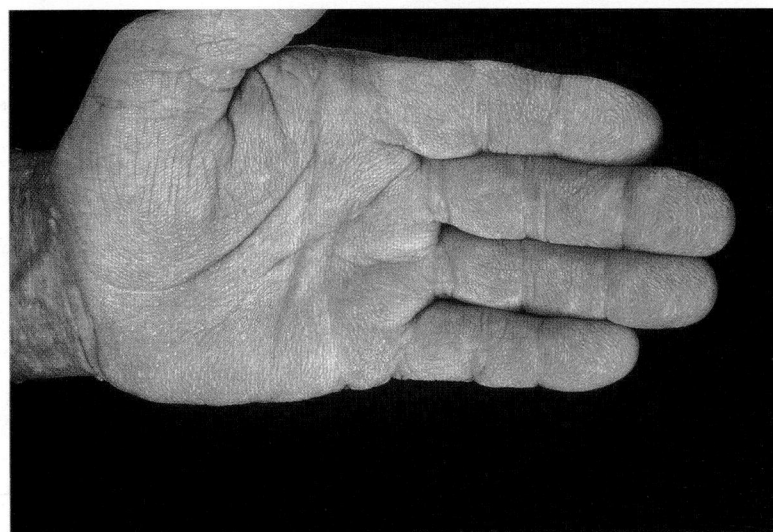

Fig. 13.196
Acanthosis nigricans: tripe palms. The palmar skin is thickened and the creases are accentuated. By courtesy of the Institute of Dermatology, London, UK.

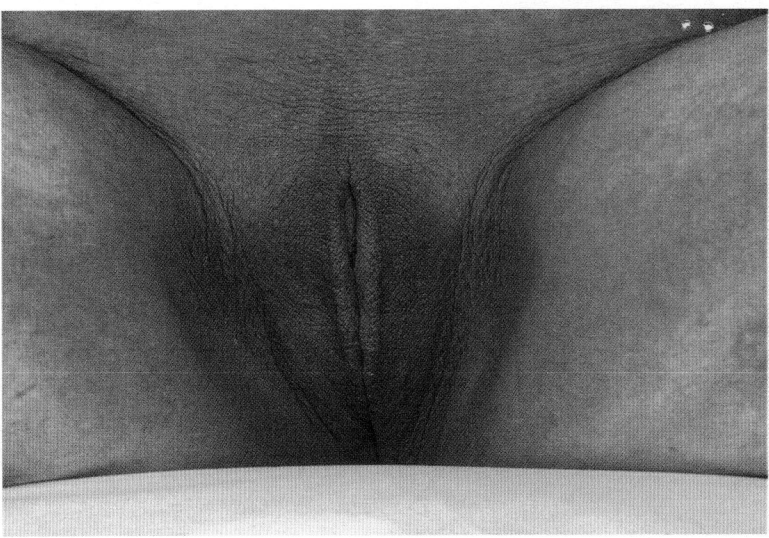

Fig. 13.197
Acanthosis nigricans: the skin of the groins and vulva is thickened and hyperpigmented. By courtesy of R.A. Marsden, MD, St George's Hospital, London, UK.

of the neck, groin, and axillae (*Figs 13.194* and *13.195*). In more extreme forms the changes may be generalized.[18] Involvement of the eyelids also rarely occurs.[19–21] In addition, there is sometimes brown thickening of the skin over the dorsum of the fingers or, rarely, the palms of the hands (tripe palms) (*Fig. 13.196*). The latter is a distinctive appearance due to broadened epidermal ridges and deep sulci giving the skin a velvety rugose texture.[22] Tripe palms are frequently associated with a variety of internal malignancies and often (but not invariably) accompany acanthosis nigricans.[23–29] However, the lesion may also represent a benign reversible phenomenon unassociated with neoplasia. Less frequently, there are similar changes on mucosal surfaces, such as the mouth (particularly the tongue and upper lip) or genitalia (*Fig. 13.197*).[30,31] The latter changes are more common in cases related to malignancy.

Oral lesions have been reported in 25% to 50% of all cases of acanthosis nigricans and this presentation is a marker for potential underlying malignancy.[29,30,32–34] At least 35% of patients with oral acanthosis nigricans have an associated malignancy.[30,32,35] The tongue lesions consist of hypertrophied filiform papillae producing a deeply fissured papillomatous surface and the lips develop papillary and verrucous lesions.[30] The palate and buccal mucosa may also be involved.[35] Oral lesions are usually nonpigmented. Involvement of the esophagus is rare and is almost invariably associated with malignancy, particularly in the gastrointestinal tract.[36]

A drug-induced variant has been documented, and glucocorticoids, nicotinic acid, oral contraceptives, and diethylstilbestrol have been implicated.[37] Acanthosis nigricans has also been reported in association with somatotrophin therapy.[38] It has also been seen as a complication of testosterone injections and at insulin injection sites.[39,40]

Rarely, the disease presents as an autosomal dominant nevoid lesion, which may present at birth, in childhood, or at puberty.[41,42] The condition has also been reported in association with Cohen syndrome (truncal obesity, hypotonia, mental retardation, microcephaly, and ocular abnormalities).[43]

So-called benign familial acanthosis nigricans occurs more commonly in females. This autosomal dominantly inherited condition usually presents in early childhood with lesions that particularly affect the face, dorsal surfaces of the fingers, and the flexures.[44] There are usually no associated endocrinopathies or congenital abnormalities.

Acanthosis nigricans presents in up to 51% of patients with Down syndrome and is probably due to insulin resistance.[45] It has also been described in up to 5% of patients with severe atopic dermatitis, but the pathogenesis in this setting is unknown.[45]

It may occur in the setting of malignancy, as discussed above, and may be the presenting sign of occult neoplasms. The sex incidence is equal. Malignant acanthosis nigricans is often severe, widely disseminated, and has a rapid course. Lesions may also be pruritic and are more difficult to treat. Tumors that are particularly associated include gastric adenocarcinoma and, less often, malignancies of the extrahepatic biliary tree, breast, pancreas, bladder, and colon.[23,25,27,29,34,36,46,47] Ovarian and uterine tumors, bronchial squamous and adenocarcinoma, and lymphoma have also been implicated.[26,33,48]

Acanthosis nigricans as an indicator of insulin resistance has been reported in HIV-positive patients receiving treatment with protease inhibitors.[49]

The malignant form sometimes develops in association with other cutaneous markers of internal malignancy, including palmoplantar hyperkeratosis, eruptive seborrheic keratoses (Leser-Trélat sign), and florid cutaneous papillomatosis.[26,50] The last condition presents as numerous viral wartlike itchy papillomata, which show a predilection for the trunk and extremities and invariably accompany an internal malignancy, most often gastric adenocarcinoma. The course of malignant acanthosis nigricans usually parallels that of the underlying neoplasm, which is generally aggressive and associated with a high mortality. Lesions may sometimes abate following surgical removal of the tumor, only to return with its recurrence.

Acanthosis nigricans is also associated with a wide range of endocrine diseases, including Cushing disease, acromegaly, gigantism, Addison disease, polycystic ovary syndrome, diabetes mellitus, and thyroid disorders. The association between hyperandrogenism (HA), insulin resistance (IR), and acanthosis nigricans (AN) is known as HAIR-AN syndrome. There appears to be an association between acanthosis nigricans, obesity, hypertension, ischemic heart disease, and type 2 diabetes, the inheritance of which is autosomal dominant.[51] Acanthosis nigricans may also occur in nonobese patients in association with diabetes mellitus and insulin resistance due to diminished receptor binding.[52–57] Patients with this sporadic syndrome are divided into two groups:

- In type A, the patients are young (particularly black) women with acanthosis nigricans, primary amenorrhea with hypertestosteronemia, virilization, increased somatic growth, hyperglycemia and hyperinsulinemia, with insulin resistance due to a congenital defect of insulin receptors.
- In type B, the patients are older and have features suggesting other autoimmune diseases, including raised erythrocyte sedimentation rate (ESR), proteinuria, and hypocomplementemia with antinuclear and anti-DNA antibodies. Antibodies directed against the insulin receptor may be detected.
- A third type, type C, has recently been proposed, in which acanthosis nigricans and insulin resistance are associated with a postinsulin receptor defect.

Studies have found that the presence of acanthosis nigricans in African-Americans and Native Americans is a cutaneous marker of hyperinsulinemia and insulin resistance.[58,59]

Obesity-associated acanthosis nigricans, previously called pseudoacanthosis nigricans, develops in the flexures of obese patients. This is the most common type of acanthosis nigricans in children and adults and is associated with insulin resistance.[60–63]

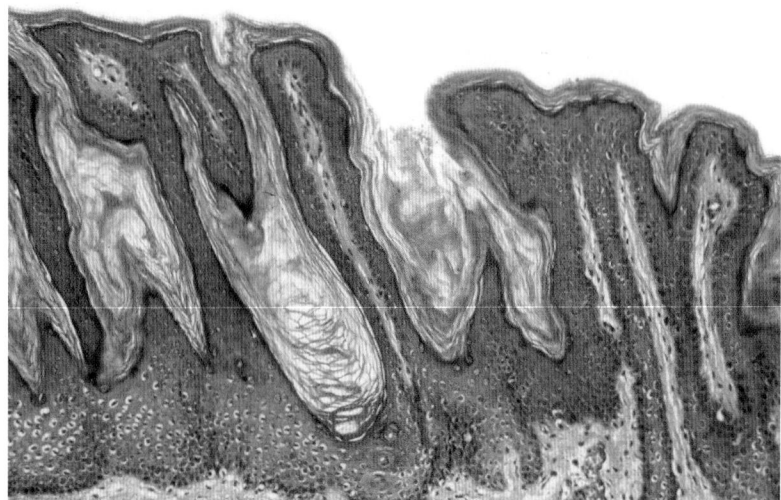

Fig. 13.198
Acanthosis nigricans: there is hyperkeratosis, papillomatosis, and slight acanthosis.

Transient acanthosis nigricans-like lesions have been described at the sites of healing lesions of pemphigus vulgaris and pemphigus foliaceous.[64,65]

Acanthosis nigricans-like lesions have been described after local application of fusidic acid.[66]

Pathogenesis and histologic features

The pathogenesis is uncertain, although in the diabetes-associated patients hyperinsulinemia is likely to be of importance.[55] In malignancy-related acanthosis nigricans, peptide or hormonal secretion appears to be of significance in at least a proportion of cases.[46] It has been demonstrated that some malignant tumors secrete transforming growth factor alpha (TGF-α) in large quantities and this stimulates proliferation of keratinocytes.[67]

The histopathological findings are subtle, comprising delicate, elongate papillomatosis, hyperkeratosis and slight acanthosis, sometimes alternating with foci of atrophy (Fig. 13.198). The occasional presence of keratin-filled cysts may result in a seborrheic keratosis-like appearance.[30] Despite the clinically obvious brown appearance of the lesions, there is normally little increase in the amount of melanin present. A non-specific perivascular chronic inflammatory cell infiltrate is sometimes evident in the superficial dermis. Distinguishing this type of benign acanthosis from others, such as epidermal nevi may be difficult.

Oral lesions show hyperkeratosis and patchy parakeratosis associated with marked acanthosis and epithelial papillary hyperplasia.[30]

Tripe palms are characterized by hyperkeratosis, acanthosis, and papillary dermal hypertrophy.[22]

Florid cutaneous papillomatosis is also characterized by hyperkeratosis, papillomatosis, and acanthosis.[50]

Acrodermatitis enteropathica

Clinical features

Acrodermatitis enteropathica is a rare autosomal recessive inherited disorder of zinc malabsorption, which predominantly affects infants and responds dramatically to dietary zinc supplements.[1–4] It presents with diarrhea, stomatitis, irritability, and failure to thrive, accompanied by erythematous scaly and crusted lesions with vesicles, pustules, and erosions, predominantly affecting the extremities, perineal, and periorificial region (Figs 13.199 and 13.200). Frankly bullous lesions have been described.[5] Nonscarring alopecia may also be present. Additional features include nail dystrophy, prolonged wound healing, impetiginization, short stature, psychiatric symptoms, and photophobia.[1–7] Corneal lesions and decreased visual acuity have also exceptionally been reported.[8,9] Patients are also prone to developing infections, particularly by bacteria and fungi, illustrating the importance of

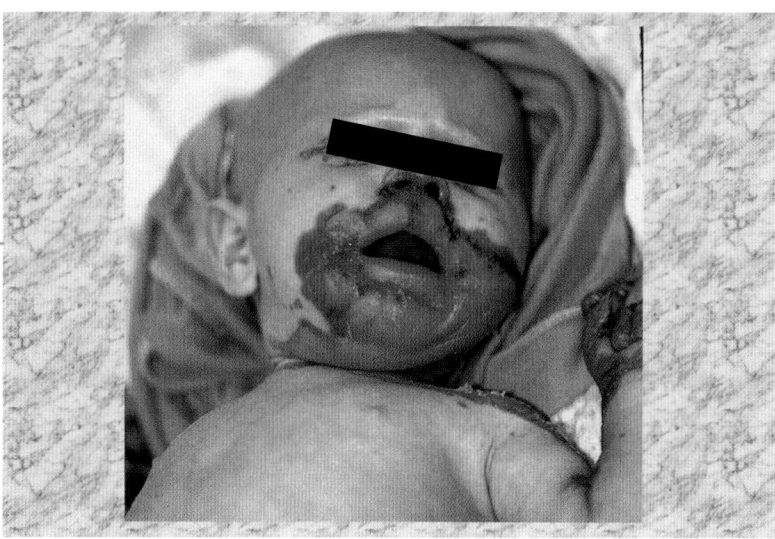

Fig. 13.199
Acrodermatitis enteropathica: extensive crusted erosions in a characteristic distribution. By courtesy of Z.S. Tannous, MD, Harvard Medical School, Boston, USA.

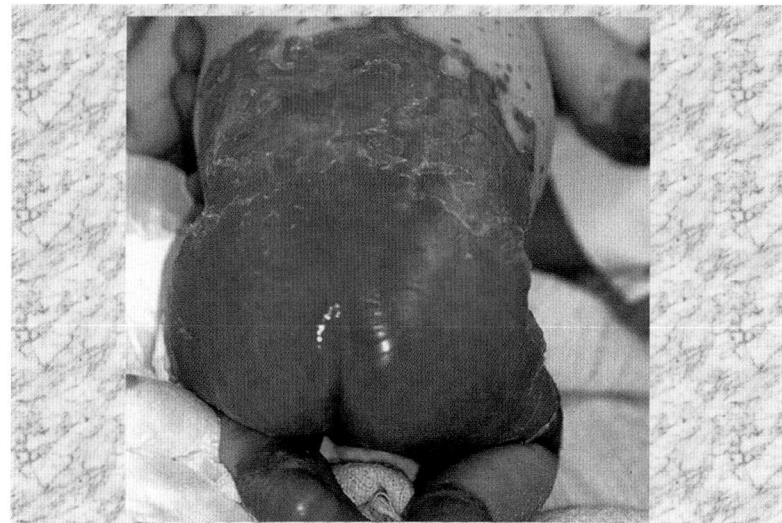

Fig. 13.200
Acrodermatitis enteropathica: in this infant, there is very extensive involvement with widespread erosion. By courtesy of Z.S. Tannous, MD, Harvard Medical School, Boston, USA.

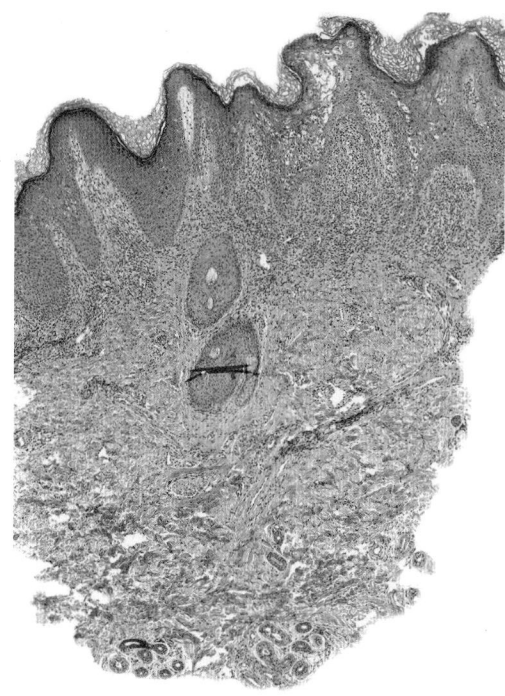

Fig. 13.201
Acrodermatitis enteropathica: low-power view showing hyperkeratosis and marked epidermal eosinophilia on the right side.

The changes are due not only to zinc deficiency, but also to a deficiency in branched chain amino acids including isoleucine.[63,64] This is induced by the low protein diet that these patients receive. Acrodermatitis enteropathica has also been described in relation to HIV infection.[65]

Pathogenesis and histologic features

The manifestations of acrodermatitis enteropathica result from insufficient absorption of zinc by the intestine. The mechanism of the disease involves a defect in a zinc transporting protein. Initial studies of genes that encode for proteins important in the transport of zinc including SLC30A4 and ZNT4 did not show association with the disease.[66–68] More recently, the gene for acrodermatitis enteropathica has been identified on chromosome 8q24.3.[69] This gene, designated SLC39A4, encodes a histidine-rich transmembrane protein known as hZIP4 which is involved in zinc uptake.[70–76] The mutation in acrodermatitis enteropathica also affects zinc metabolism in fibroblasts and reduces the activity of 5'-nucleotidase.[78,79] Over 30 different mutations in this gene have been described thus far in association with acrodermatitis enteropathica.[75–77,80–84] The vast majority of patients carry a homozygous or compound heterozygous mutation in SLC39A4. However, there are some without such an identifiable genetic mutation, indicating that other genetic factors may possibly play a causative role in the disease.[75]

The mechanism of infections in acrodermatitis enteropathica is related to alterations in the immune system due to zinc deficiency.[12,13] Zinc is critical to the development and function of lymphocytes, neutrophils, macrophages, NK cells, and cytokine production. It also functions as an antioxidant and prevents cellular damage by free radicals.[13] Lymphopenia and thymic atrophy are frequent findings in acrodermatitis enteropathica and are due to the loss of B- and T-cell precursors in the bone marrow. The zinc deficiency induces apoptosis mediated by glucocorticoids with resultant decrease in lymphopoiesis.

The histopathology varies according to the stage of evolution.[85] Very early lesions show subtle changes consisting of focal parakeratosis alternating with orthokeratosis. As lesions advance, the parakeratosis becomes more prominent and confluent and the stratum granulosum is decreased or absent. The keratinocytes in the upper layers of the epidermis display marked cytoplasmic pallor (Figs 13.201 and 13.202). In addition there is focal spongiosis. Dyskeratotic cells are rarely seen.

normal zinc levels in maintaining the integrity of the immune system.[10–13] The disease can persist into adulthood or rarely be diagnosed for the first time in adult life.[14–16] An acquired variant may complicate artificially fed or, rarely, breast-fed infants either full term or premature.[17–28] This is due to the low concentration of zinc in breast milk secondary to a defect in zinc uptake from maternal serum into the breast.[28] In premature infants, the problem is aggravated by the low gastrointestinal absorption of zinc and low body stores of zinc that were transferred from mother to fetus in the last 10 weeks of pregnancy.[28,29]

Many other conditions with acquired zinc deficiency have been associated with signs and symptoms of acrodermatitis enteropathica including Crohn disease, alcoholic cirrhosis, alcoholic pancreatitis, intestinal bypass operation, chemotherapy for hematological malignancies, anorexia nervosa, lymphoma, biotin deficiency, dialysis, cystic fibrosis, Hartnup disease, essential fatty acid deficiency, citrullinemia, deficiency of ornithine transcarbamylase, following total intravenous hyperalimentation, and celiac disease.[9,30–55] A similar picture has also been described in a number of aminoacidopathies and organic acidemias. The latter include methylmalonic acidemia, propionic acidemia, glutaric aciduria type I, and nonketotic hyperglycinemia.[56–62]

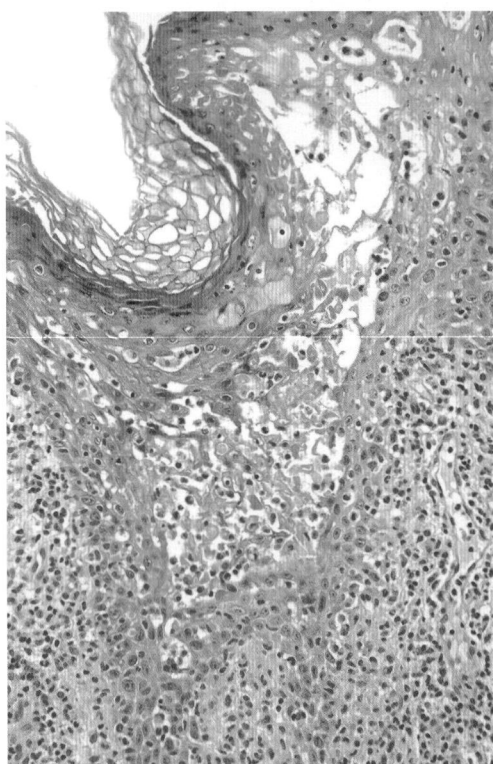

Fig. 13.202
Acrodermatitis enteropathica: keratinocyte necrosis is seen in this high-power view.

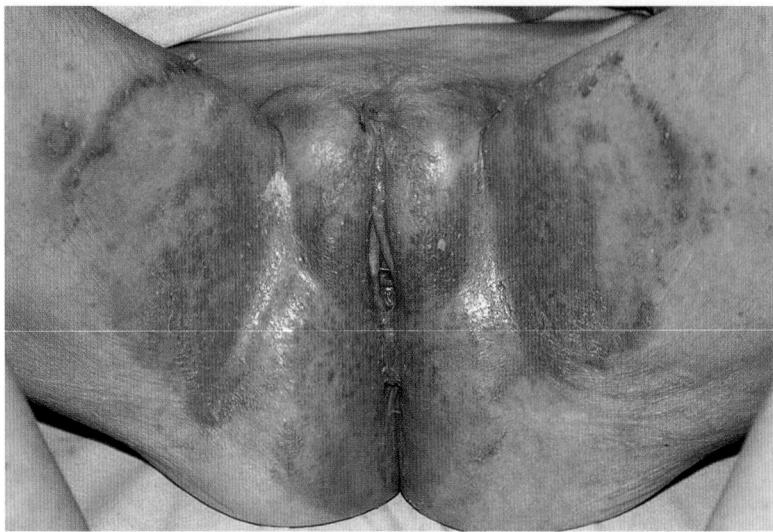

Fig. 13.203
Necrolytic migratory erythema: note the intense erythema in a characteristic distribution. By courtesy of the Institute of Dermatology, London, UK.

In late stages there is cytoplasmic vacuolation and necrosis which may result in intraepidermal vesicles or occasionally progress to blister formation.[86,87] Subcorneal pustules may be seen and usually indicate secondary infection. An atypical case of bullous acrodermatitis enteropathica with a lichenoid infiltrate has been reported.[88]

Differential diagnosis

Histologically, acrodermatitis enteropathica is indistinguishable from necrolytic migratory erythema and pellagra. Very similar histologic features are also seen in necrolytic acral erythema, a condition that occurs on the dorsum of the feet and legs of patients with hepatitis C infection.[89–91] Lesions are erythematous and psoriasiform plaques and decreased serum and lesional zinc levels have been associated with this condition.[91,92] Prominent pallor of keratinocytes in the upper layers of the epidermis is also seen in deficiency of the M subunit of lactate dehydrogenase.[93,94] The cutaneous manifestation of the latter condition has been described as annually recurring acroerythema.[95]

Necrolytic migratory erythema

Clinical features

Necrolytic migratory erythema is a distinctive dermatosis that is classically seen in patients with the glucagonoma syndrome.[1–9] The latter, due to a slowly progressive malignant tumor of the pancreatic islets, consists of hyperglucagonemia, diabetes mellitus, glossitis, normochromic normocytic anemia, nausea, diarrhea, abdominal pain, neurological symptoms (ataxia and fecal and urinary incontinence), thromboembolic pathology (deep vein thrombosis and pulmonary thromboembolism), and weight loss in addition to the cutaneous manifestations.[10] About 57% of patients present with the typical visceral, cutaneous, and laboratory abnormalities.[11] Exceptional cases of glucagonoma arise from the duodenum, kidney, and lung.[12–14]

Necrolytic migratory erythema, so-called because of its superficial resemblance to toxic epidermal necrolysis and the waxing and waning nature of the eruption, is seen most frequently on the central face, particularly around the mouth, on the perineum and other intertriginous sites, the thighs,

buttocks, and distal limbs (*Fig. 13.203*).[3] Patients most often present in their sixth decade (median 52 years) with intense erythema, which progresses to flaccid bullae that rupture readily and develop crusting.[11,15] A rare pediatric case has been described.[16] Pressure, friction, and trauma have occasionally been noted to precipitate the eruption.[8] Central healing with active borders gives rise to annular and serpiginous lesions. Lesions are often painful and pruritic.

Postinflammatory hyperpigmentation follows resolution. Individual lesions usually last 1–2 weeks and, characteristically, lesions in varying stages of evolution are evident at any one time.[8,15]

Additional features may include stomatitis, angular cheilitis, blepharitis, conjunctivitis, hair loss, and nail changes.[9–11] Laboratory investigations commonly reveal an abnormal glucose tolerance test, normochromic normocytic anemia, hypoproteinemia, hypoalbuminemia, and hypoaminoacidemia.[9,17] Low amino acid levels were detected in 96% of patients in one reported series.[18] However, in larger series, the percentage of patients with low amino acid levels has been lower, ranging between 41% and 78%.[10,11] Patients with low amino acid levels may respond to intravenous replacement.[19]

Glucagonoma syndrome may constitute part of the multiple endocrine neoplasia syndrome.[18]

Rarely, necrolytic migratory erythema has been described in the absence of a glucagonoma, so-called 'pseudo-glucagonoma syndrome'.[20–33] Abnormal liver function tests have usually been present and it has been suggested that this may have resulted in impaired glucagon catabolism with resultant hyperglucagonemia or raised levels of one of the glucagon immunofractions.[22] Patients have had associated gastrointestinal malabsorption disorders, such as celiac disease, ulcerative colitis, Crohn disease, short bowel syndrome, and liver diseases, including cirrhosis and hepatitis, as well as chronic pancreatitis, cystic fibrosis, and other malignancies.[25,28–33] A study of 24 patients with nonglucagonoma-associated necrolytic migratory erythema found increased glucagon in 52% of patients and low zinc levels in 37% of patients.[25]

Despite its relatively indolent growth characteristics, a large majority of tumors have metastasized by the time of diagnosis.

Pathogenesis and histologic features

The precise etiology of necrolytic migratory erythema is unknown. Although it is certainly related to hyperglucagonemia, this is not necessarily causal. Therefore, although the signs and symptoms rapidly abate following surgery or the use of glucagon secretion inhibitors such as somatostatin, hyperglucagonemia does not readily explain the intermittent nature of the eruption.[22] The topical or intradermal application of glucagon does not produce the dermatoses.[8] Similarly, there are alternative causes of hyperglucagonemia, including burns and acute trauma, diabetes mellitus, septicemia, cirrhosis,

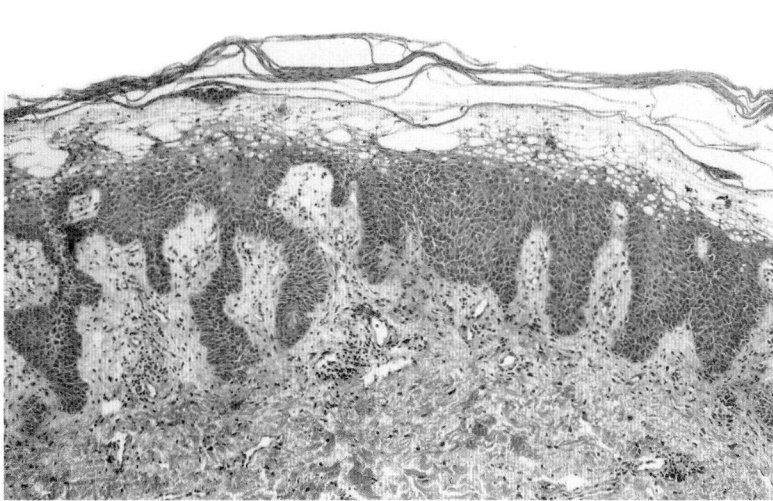

Fig. 13.204
Necrolytic migratory erythema: low-power view showing extensive vacuolation with vesiculation.

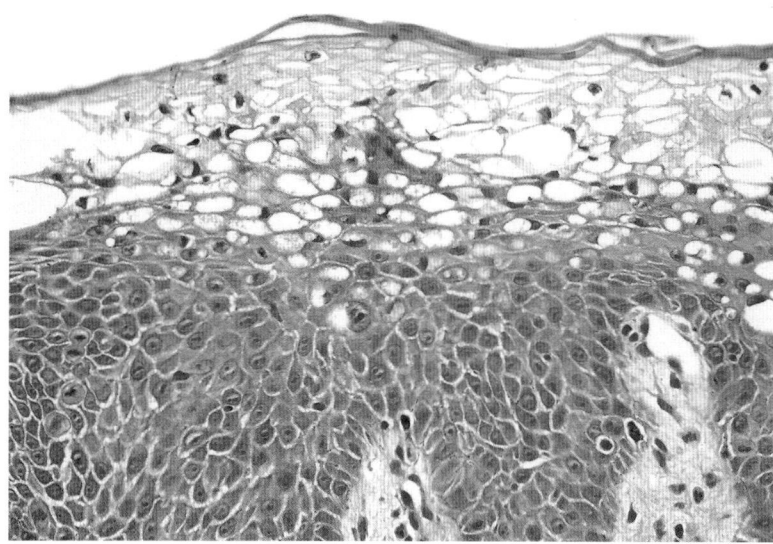

Fig. 13.205
Necrolytic migratory erythema: close-up view of *Fig. 13.199.*

renal failure, Cushing syndrome, and primary hyperglucagonemia, in which necrolytic migratory erythema is not a feature.[17]

Hypoaminoacidemia is an extremely common manifestation and it may have pathogenetic significance for the cutaneous lesions, as evidenced by the fact that the condition may respond to amino acid replacement.[19] It has been proposed that the diminished amino acid availability may result in epidermal protein depletion and eventual necrosis.[15] Certainly, treatment with intravenous amino acids has been shown to control the eruption, but it is possible that this is coincidental, considering the characteristic fluctuating course of the dermatoses.[22] Fatty acid and zinc deficiency and abnormal arachidonic acid distribution have also been proposed as pathogenetic mechanisms.[9,33] It has been suggested that diminished tryptophan levels may be the cause of the dermatoses.[9] A further hypothesis points to hepatic dysfunction as having a role in the pathogenesis of the disease.[22,23,25,27,34] This is mainly based on the fact that patients with necrolytic migratory erythema and absence of glucagonoma often have liver dysfunction. The model of 'multifactorial malnutrition' has been suggested as an explanation for the several disorders associated with this disease.[27] It is proposed that deficiencies in zinc, amino acids, fatty acids, and protein result in a metabolic alteration which affects a final common pathway that manifests clinically with epidermal inflammation and necrosis in areas of trauma. The precise pathways involved remain unknown.

Histologic examination reveals parakeratosis accompanied by vacuolation and pallor of the mid and upper keratinocytes (*Figs 13.204–13.206*).[35] Dyskeratosis has been described as a clue to early diagnosis.[36] This is accompanied by necrosis and separation of the upper layers of the epidermis, giving rise to intraepidermal clefting or vesiculation.[35] A neutrophilic infiltrate may be evident, particularly in well-established lesions.[37] Subcorneal pustulation has also been described.[17] This may develop in a background of epidermal necrosis or, less often, represents an isolated phenomenon.[37] Suprabasal acantholysis has exceptionally been described.[38] The dermis shows a lymphohistiocytic chronic inflammatory cell infiltrate surrounding dilated blood vessels. In lesions associated with pustulation, neutrophils may also be present. In some biopsies the changes may be predominantly spongiotic. Older lesions may show parakeratosis, marked acanthosis, and papillary dermal angiogenesis, and psoriasis may therefore enter the differential diagnosis.[7,35,37] Pustular folliculitis in association with more typical features has also been described.[37]

Immunofluorescence studies are invariably negative.[13,15,33,37,39]

An ultrastructural study revealed widening of the intercellular space with reduced numbers of desmosomes in the absence of acantholysis.[40] Cytoplasmic vacuolation with lysed organelles and dyskeratotic cells was also present. These changes are largely degenerative and non-specific.

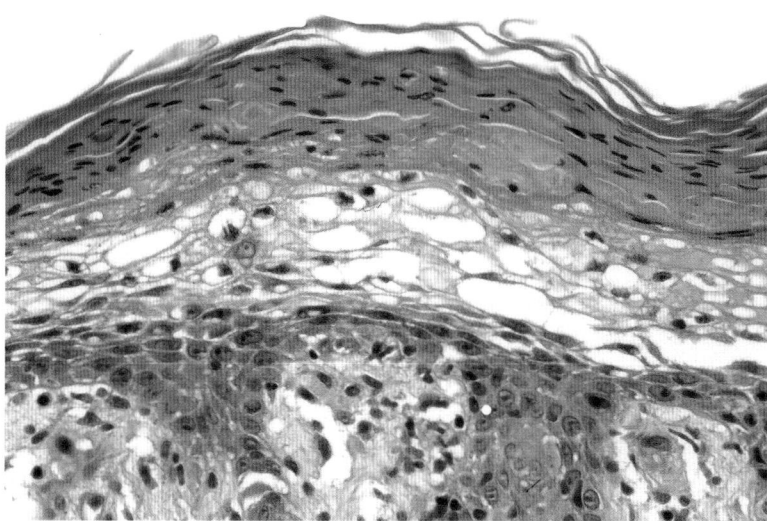

Fig. 13.206
Necrolytic migratory erythema: high-power view showing marked overlying parakeratosis.

Differential diagnosis

Necrolytic migratory erythema shows considerable clinicopathological overlap with acrodermatitis enteropathica, and niacin and zinc deficiencies, suggesting a possible shared pathogenesis.[9] Pellagra can also show similar histologic features. The histology of necrolytic acral erythema is that of necrolytic migratory erythema. This condition is, however, associated with hepatitis C infection and clinically tends to be restricted to the dorsum of the feet, with less common involvement of the lower legs and dorsal hands.[41]

If subcorneal pustules are evident, impetigo, dermatophyte infection, pustular psoriasis, subcorneal pustular dermatosis, IgA pemphigus, and pemphigus foliaceus enter the differential diagnosis. Multiple biopsies are sometimes necessary before the correct diagnosis can be established.

Bullosis diabeticorum

Clinical features

There are numerous cutaneous manifestations of diabetes mellitus. These include vascular complications, such as peripheral gangrene, especially affecting the foot, and infective lesions including candidiasis and dermatophytosis. Other dermatological features include necrobiosis lipoidica diabeticorum, disseminated granuloma annulare, acanthosis nigricans, eruptive xanthomata, scleredema, diabetic dermopathy (shin spots), waxy skin, and bullous lesions.[1–4]

Bullosis diabeticorum (bullous eruption of diabetes mellitus) is rare, affecting approximately 0.16% of diabetics, and affects men more commonly (male:female ratio 2:1).[5] It usually presents as spontaneous blisters, typically without underlying inflammation, affecting the periphery. Lesions, which are sometimes mildly painful or associated with a burning sensation, are found most often on the feet and lower legs, although the hands may also be affected.[6–11] Blisters range in size from a few millimeters to a few centimeters and can evolve rapidly and become hemorrhagic.[4] The lesions, which are often recurrent, commonly heal in a few weeks and are not associated with scarring. Rarely, secondary ulceration and infection can occur.[5] Associated osteomyelitis has been reported.[12]

Pathogenesis and histologic features

The cause of blistering in diabetic patients is unknown, but theories implicating a vascular or neurological mechanism have been favored in the literature. The occasional finding of epidermal infarction overlying the blister cavity favors the former in at least some patients.[6] The discovery that diabetic patients have a diminished threshold for suction-induced blisters may have pathogenetic significance.[13] Others have suggested an abnormality of calcium and magnesium metabolism as a consequence of diabetic nephropathy.[14] There is evidence that the lesions are more likely to occur during episodes of hyperglycemia.[15] Despite lesions being predominantly acral in distribution, trauma does not seem to be generally implicated. In all likelihood, the cause is probably multifactorial.

The reported histopathological features have been variable and include subcorneal, suprabasal, and subepidermal vesiculation, sometimes associated with spongiosis (*Figs 13.207* and *13.208*).[11,14,16,17] Some of the discrepancies may be due, at least in part, to variable ages of the lesions, biopsies with re-epithelialization resulting in an apparent intraepidermal location. Electron microscopic studies in two cases have shown that the plane of separation is through the lamina lucida in the subepidermal lesions.[6,14] Absence of hemidesmosomes and anchoring filaments has also been described.[14]

Immunofluorescence studies are almost invariably negative, although one report described IgM and C3 around the superficial vasculature in uninvolved skin.[18]

Differential diagnosis

The differential diagnosis is dependent on the histologic features of a given lesion. In cases with subepidermal blister formation, the differential diagnosis includes epidermolysis bullosa acquisita and porphyria cutanea tarda. Epidermolysis bullosa acquisita is associated with skin fragility, and immunofluorescence studies reveal IgG along the basement membrane zone. Porphyria cutanea tarda, as previously discussed, has PAS-positive, diastase-resistant, hyaline material around the blood vessels of affected skin and the blisters may have so-called caterpillar bodies. For lesions with intraepidermal vesicles, dyshidrotic eczema could be considered, but bullous diabeticorum lacks a significant inflammatory infiltrate.

The authors would like to acknowledge the work of Nooshin Brinster on the previous edition of this chapter.

Access **ExpertConsult.com** for the complete list of references

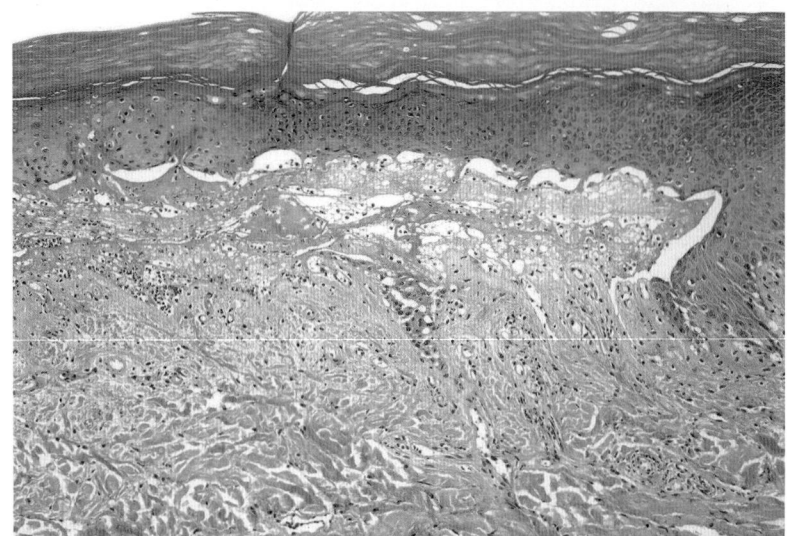

Fig. 13.207
Bullous eruption of diabetes: this example from the fingertip shows a subepidermal vesicle.

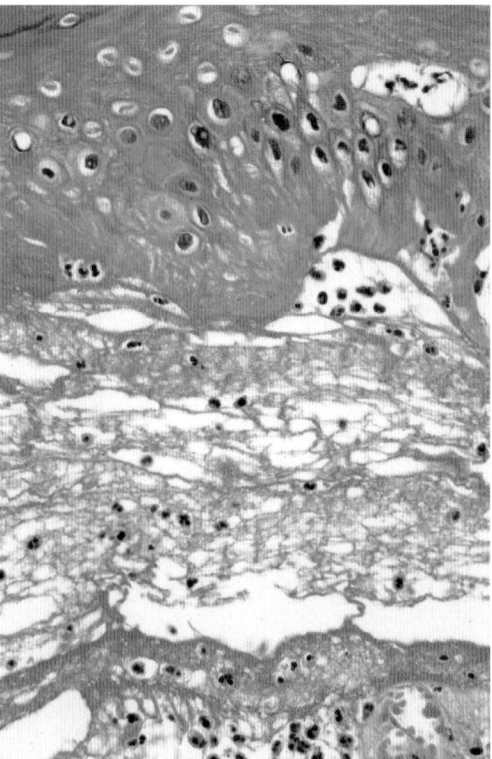

Fig. 13.208
Bullous eruption of diabetes: in this field, the epidermis shows the changes of infarction. Note the intense cytoplasmic eosinophilia and absence of nuclei.

See
www.expertconsult.com
for references and
additional material

Cutaneous adverse reactions to drugs

CHAPTER 14

ADVERSE DRUG REACTIONS – INTRODUCTION

Adverse drug reactions are unintended and undesired effects of drugs used for prevention, diagnosis, or treatment of disease.[1,2] In light of the ever-increasing number of medications available, it should come as no surprise that such reactions are extremely common. The incidence statistics vary considerably depending upon the method by which the data are derived and the nature of the population under study.[3] Estimates, however, range from 2% to 7% of hospital inpatients.[4–9] Although most reactions are mild, they are sometimes severe and a source of considerable morbidity and occasional mortality.[6,7]

The diagnosis of an adverse drug reaction is frequently problematical, the clinical appearances often being similar, if not identical, to a number of primary dermatoses and infectious conditions (particularly viral exanthems) and, in the context of transplantation patients, graft-versus-host disease (GVHD). The histologic diagnosis can also be extremely difficult, as drug reactions can demonstrate several inflammatory histologic patterns that mimic other dermatoses (i.e., spongiotic, psoriasiform, lichenoid, pityriasiform).[10] The problem is exacerbated in the immunologically compromised patient. Frequently, the diagnostic difficulties are worsened by the multitude of drugs prescribed. The problem is further compounded by the multiplicity of different eruptions that any one particular drug may induce.

Contrariwise, a given clinical appearance may be caused by a large number of unrelated drugs.[11]

The prevalence of agents responsible for adverse drug reactions reflects the prescribing tendencies for any given population as much as the relative risks ascribed to any particular drug.[12] It should come as no surprise, therefore, that – in a hospital environment – antibiotics, nonsteroidal anti-inflammatory drugs (NSAIDs), and psychotropic drugs are commonly reported as being the most frequently incriminated.[8,13] Oral anticoagulants, low-dose aspirin, and digoxin are also frequent causes.[13] In a large hospital survey, penicillin and sulfonamides accounted for over 80% of all adverse drug reactions.[8] Experience in general practice has been much less often documented. In a survey from the Netherlands, sulfonamide-trimethoprim combinations, fluoroquinolones, and penicillin were the most common antibacterials causing drug-related eruptions.[3] In the series of approximately 150 000 patients, 1% developed a reaction.

Adverse drug reactions are mostly nonimmunologically mediated. They develop either as a result of an unwanted but known property of the drug (and hence are entirely predictable) or as a consequence of drug intolerance/idiosyncrasy (and are completely unpredictable).[5,14–17] The former are by far the more common, accounting for approximately 80% of all adverse drug reactions. Less often, adverse drug reactions represent a manifestation of an immunological phenomenon, so-called allergic drug reactions.[5,17] Although in theory the above subdivisions are sharply defined, in many patients the underlying pathogenetic mechanisms are far from clear.[15]

Adverse drug reactions are particularly encountered in certain population groups, for example, the elderly, females, patients with Sjögren syndrome, and those suffering from the effects of immune deficiency including patients receiving immunosuppressive therapy and those suffering from the acquired immunodeficiency syndrome (AIDS).[5,18]

Adverse drug reactions can be divided into three categories: type A, type B, and type C.[1,12,19]

Type A drug reactions

Type A reactions, which are predictable and are related to the pharmacological actions or metabolism of the drug, include[1]:
- side effects,
- drug toxicity,
- drug interactions.

Side effects

Side effects, which occur with almost all drugs, represent unwanted pharmacological actions. For example, methotrexate, cyclophosphamide, and nitrosourea commonly result in anagen alopecia by inducing Bax protein-mediated apoptosis.[20–24] Gold may be associated with cutaneous pigmentation (chrysiasis) and penicillamine can be associated with the development of skin laxity and fragility.[25–28]

Drug toxicity

Drug toxicity develops as a consequence of the gradual accumulation of a drug or its metabolite (e.g., minocycline or amiodarone deposition with resultant abnormal pigmentation).[17,29–32] Delayed toxicity may take months to many years before expression (e.g., arsenical keratoses).[33–37]

Drug interactions

Drug interactions develop when one drug alters the pharmacological efficacy of another that is given concurrently.[12,13,38,39] The effect may enhance or diminish the effect of the drug with resultant toxicity or loss of therapeutic value.[15,16] Drug interactions are thought to arise when one drug affects clearance of the other as a consequence of several mechanisms including[3,4]:
- alteration in the rate of absorption resulting in diminished drug levels,
- alteration in the renal excretion resulting in inappropriately high drug levels,
- plasma protein or tissue drug binding site competition resulting in displacement and inappropriately high drug levels,
- alterations in hepatic cytochrome P-450-mediated drug metabolism.

The last is believed to be of particular importance and includes increased enzyme synthesis with excessive drug degradation and diminished circulating or tissue levels and inhibition of drug breakdown with increased circulating and tissue levels.[37,39]

Drug interactions are of particular importance in the elderly, the immunosuppressed, and in those patients receiving multiple medications.[3,4]

Type B drug reactions

Type B reactions are uncommon and unpredictable. They do not have an allergic pathogenesis and include[1]:
- idiosyncratic drug reactions,
- exacerbation of a pre-existing condition,
- pseudoallergic drug reactions.

Idiosyncratic drug reactions

Idiosyncratic reactions (drug intolerance) develop as a result of genetic or metabolic influences. They may represent the effects of abnormal or altered hepatic drug metabolism. For example, a lupus erythematosus-like condition is a rare complication of hydralazine therapy in the average population, but the risk is greatly increased in patients who metabolize the drug slowly.[3,7]

Drug-induced lupus erythematosus may also be caused by procainamide, chlorpromazine, isoniazid, methyldopa, penicillamine, minocycline, quinidine, and sulfasalazine.[39–41] Cefaclor-induced serum sickness-like eruptions and the antiepileptic hypersensitivity syndrome are also believed to result from reactive intermediate metabolic products.[42,43]

Exacerbation of a pre-existing condition

This is a not uncommon problem; for example, lithium, beta blockers, antimalarial drugs, NSAIDs, and tetracycline may precipitate, aggravate, or induce a psoriatic eruption.[4,44–48]

Pseudoallergic drug reactions

Pseudoallergic reactions result from the nonimmunologically mediated release of effector substances such as histamine from tissue-bound mast cells or circulating basophils with resultant urticarial reactions, angioneurotic edema, and anaphylaxis.[1,4] The complement system can also be activated by similar nonimmune mechanisms, and there is evidence that perturbation of arachidonic acid metabolism may be involved in some cases.[1,3,20] Drugs that have been incriminated in such pseudoallergic reactions include radiocontrast media, NSAIDs, acetyl salicylic acid, opium derivatives, codeine, curare, d-tubocurare, polymyxin B, and angiotensin-converting enzyme (ACE) inhibitors.[49–53]

Type C drug reactions

Type C reactions are rare, immunologically mediated, and develop as a consequence of previous exposure to the drug with resultant allergy.[1] The majority of drugs are of low molecular weight (less than 1000 Daltons) and therefore on their own are incapable of eliciting an immune response. By functioning as haptens and forming conjugates with carrier plasma proteins or cell membrane constituents, they develop immunogenic potential.[1,2,20] The ability of the majority of drugs to cause an immune response is therefore dependent on whether it is able to bind to circulating or tissue protein.[54] A number of drugs are likely to induce allergic reactions, including antibiotics, anticonvulsants, chemotherapeutic agents, heparin, insulin, protamine, and biological response modifiers such as interferons (IFNs) and growth factors.[1] A variety of mechanisms may be involved in cutaneous drug-induced hypersensitivity reactions including[14]:
- IgE-mediated type 1 reactions,
- immune complex-associated type 3 reactions,
- type 4 delayed hypersensitivity reactions.

IgE-mediated type 1 cutaneous reactions

In type 1 reactions, the release of histamine and other chemical mediators from tissue-fixed mast cells results in increased vascular permeability with development of edema in the dermis or deeper tissues.[5,20] Immediate reactions which develop within an hour or less of drug exposure present as urticaria, angioedema, or anaphylaxis, whereas accelerated reactions which develop from 1 to 72 hours following the administration of the drug are usually urticarial.[20] Urticaria following treatment with penicillin is a typical type 1 reaction. Certain other antibiotics, antisera, and gammaglobulin are also common offenders.[14]

The most common cause of anaphylaxis is penicillin.[55] Other causes include foods, stings, anesthetics, muscle relaxants, latex, contrast material, antibiotics, and allergenic extracts.[55–57] In addition to histamine, anaphylaxis is mediated through a number of substances including prostaglandin D2, leukotriene C4, interleukin (IL)-4 and IL-13, and tumor necrosis factor alpha (TNF-α).[54]

Immune complex-associated type 3 reactions

Type 3 reactions are expressed as urticaria, the Arthus reaction, serum sickness, and leukocytoclastic (allergic) vasculitis.[14] The disease manifests a week or more after exposure to the drug, by which time sufficient circulating antibody has been generated to result in immune complexes of an appropriate size to avoid phagocytosis. Their deposition in the tissues or within blood vessel walls is accompanied by complement fixation and resultant acute inflammatory reaction.

Delayed hypersensitivity type 4 reactions

Delayed hypersensitivity reactions are T-lymphocyte mediated and exemplified in acute allergic contact dermatitis.[14,20] Cytotoxic T-cell-mediated reactions are of importance in many other adverse allergic drug reactions including exanthematous/morbilliform, bullous, and interface variants.[58-61] Although most delayed hypersensitivity reactions are immune responses to the hapten-carrier complex, recent studies indicate that some drugs may be capable of directly activating the immune system, independent of a covalent drug-peptide complex.[62] Certain medications may directly bind T-cell receptors (TCRs) and major histocompatibility complex (MHC) molecules and trigger the release of cytokines which recruit specific leukocytes. The delayed hypersensitivity reactions may be subclassified based on the cell type recruited: monocytes (type 4a), eosinophils (type 4b), T cells (type 4c), and neutrophils (type IVd). The resultant clinical phenotype may be determined by which cells are involved.[62]

ADVERSE DRUG REACTIONS – CLINICAL MANIFESTATIONS

Although the range of drugs that may result in adverse drug reactions is extensive, the variety of clinical responses encountered is fairly limited. Many drugs may cause more than one clinical response, and any given reaction pattern may result from a wide range of drugs. There are, however, a number of clinicopathological responses that are fairly unique to a particular drug and these are dealt with individually, later in this chapter.[1-8]

Adverse drug reactions may therefore present with a considerable number of clinical manifestations as outlined in *Box 14.1*.[1,2]

Exanthematous reactions

Clinical features

Exanthematous (morbilliform, maculopapular) reactions are the most frequently encountered adverse drug reaction, accounting for 51% to 95% of skin reactions, and mimic a variety of infective conditions including scarlet fever, measles, and rubella (*Figs 14.1* and *14.2*).[1-5] Patients present with erythematous macules and papules that may become confluent or gyrate/polycyclic. Pruritus, low-grade fever, and eosinophilia are sometimes present.[2] The eruption is often symmetrical and usually presents on the trunk and extremities or sites of pressure and trauma.[1] The palms and soles are sometimes affected but the mucous membranes are not usually involved.

Exanthematous eruptions typically develop within 1–2 weeks of starting the drug.[1] Occasionally, the eruption is delayed and may even present after the treatment has ceased.[1,6] In more seriously affected patients the eruption can progress to erythroderma (exfoliative dermatitis), in which the erythema becomes generalized and is often accompanied by scaling.[7] Resolution of exanthematous drug reactions is characterized by exfoliation and sometimes

Box 14.1
Clinical manifestations of adverse drug reactions

- Exanthematous reactions
- Urticaria, angioedema and anaphylaxis
- Serum sickness
- Phototoxic/photoallergic eruptions
- Hypersensitivity syndrome
- Lichenoid drug reactions
- Fixed drug eruptions
- Erythema multiforme
- Stevens-Johnson syndrome/toxic epidermal necrolysis
- Pigmentary abnormalities
- Vasculitis
- Purpura
- Granulomatous drug reactions
- Erythema nodosum
- Drug-induced alopecia
- Lupus erythematosus-like drug reactions
- Bullous drug reactions
- Psoriasiform drug reactions
- Pityriasis rosea-like eruptions
- Pustular drug reactions
- Ichthyosiform drug reactions
- Pseudolymphomatous drug reactions
- Eczematous drug reactions

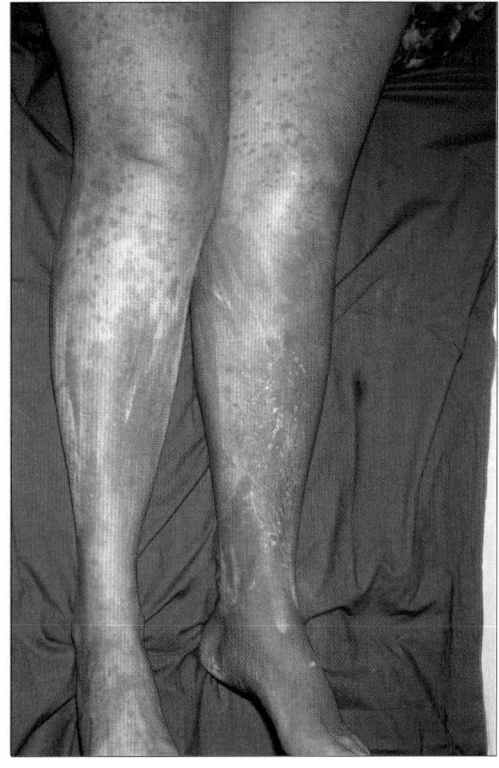

Fig. 14.1
Exanthematous drug reaction: typical erythematous maculopapular eruption on the lower extremities due to ampicillin. By courtesy of the Institute of Dermatology, London, UK.

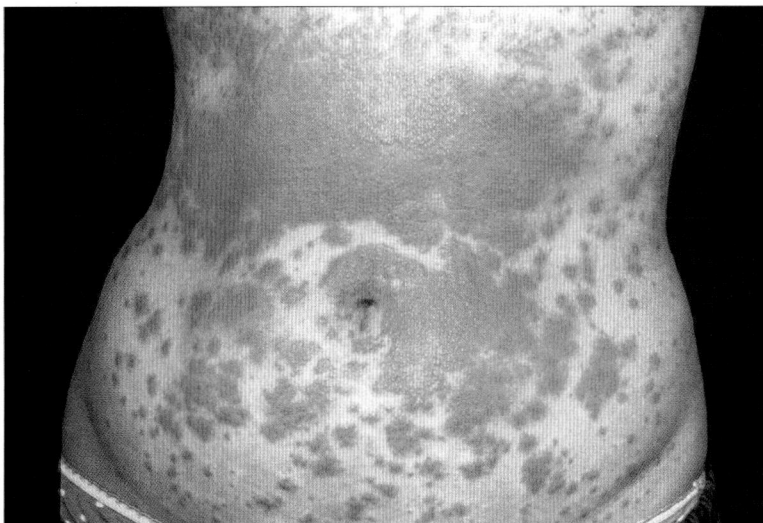

Fig. 14.2
Exanthematous drug reaction: more extensive lesions on the abdomen associated with amoxicillin therapy. By courtesy of the Institute of Dermatology, London, UK.

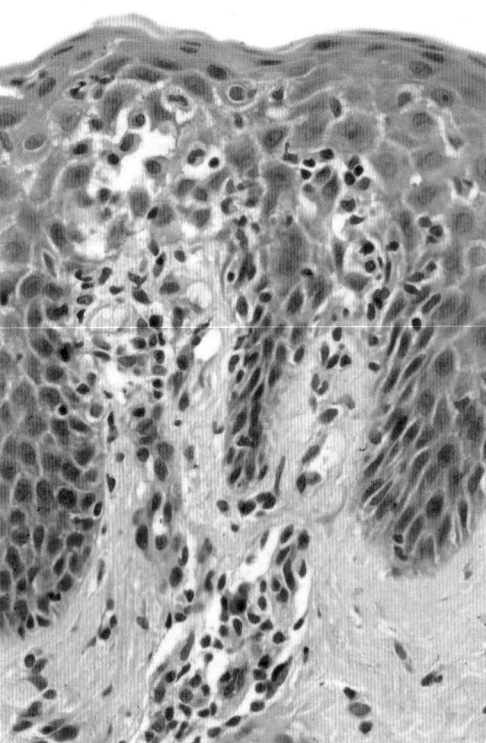

Fig. 14.3
Exanthematous drug reaction: early lesion due to penicillin showing slight interface change, spongiosis, and lymphocytic exocytosis. There is a superficial perivascular lymphocytic infiltrate, and one or two plasma cells are present.

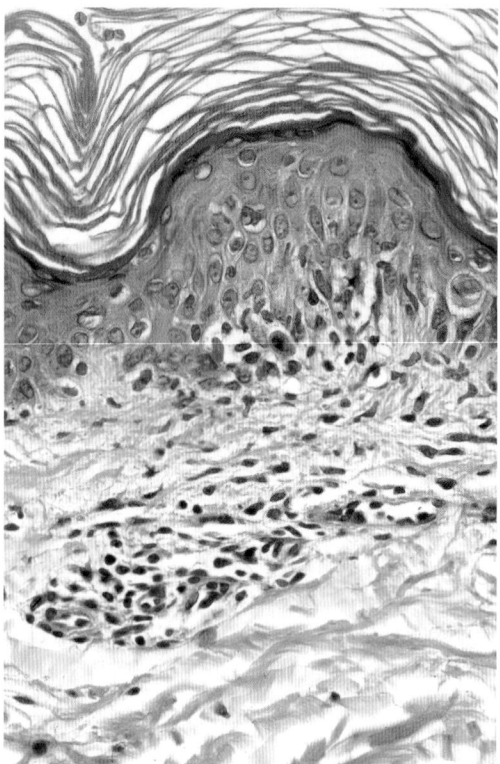

Fig. 14.4
Exanthematous drug reaction: in this example, due to carbamazepine therapy, there is spongiosis, dyskeratosis, and interface change associated with lymphocytic exocytosis.

is followed by postinflammatory hyper- or hypopigmentation.[1] Penicillin, sulfonamides, ampicillin, amoxicillin, phenylbutazone, isoniazid, barbiturates, phenytoin, carbamazepine, benzodiazepines, gold, and trimethoprim are especially incriminated, but a wide range of medications can induce exanthematous drug eruptions.[1,8–11] Patients who suffer from infectious mononucleosis are at risk of developing an exanthematous reaction following therapy with ampicillin or amoxicillin.[12] Dietary supplements can also induce a similar cutaneous eruption.[13]

Pathogenesis and histologic features

The pathogenesis of exanthematous drug reactions is not fully understood, although a cytotoxic T-cell-mediated reaction is likely in most cases (see below).

The histologic features are often subtle. Although the epidermis may appear normal, focal parakeratosis is commonly present. The characteristic changes include lymphocytic exocytosis with mild spongiosis, typically accompanied by basal cell liquefactive degeneration and a few dyskeratotic keratinocytes (*Figs 14.3–14.7*).[14,15] In some cases, no interface change is histologically apparent. The dermis shows a perivascular infiltrate of lymphocytes and histiocytes with variable numbers of eosinophils. Eosinophils – although often emphasized in the literature as an important feature of drug reactions – can, in our experience, be very scanty or even absent. Sometimes marked edema is seen, particularly if an urticarial element is clinically evident. Red cell extravasation may also be a feature in those lesions that include a purpuric component.

By immunohistochemistry, the lymphocytes are largely CD3+ T-cells with a predominance of CD4+ cells in the superficial perivascular infiltrate.[16] Lymphocytes at the dermal–epidermal junction and within the epidermis consist of approximately equal numbers of CD4+ and CD8+ forms.[16–21] These latter cells regularly express human leukocyte antigen (HLA)-DR and a subpopulation also expresses CD25.[21] There is an admixture of T-helper Th1 and Th2 cells.[20] Occasionally, the infiltrate is almost entirely composed of the CD4+ lymphocytes and, contrariwise in human immunodeficiency virus (HIV)-positive patients, the infiltrate may consist of CD8+ cells alone.[16,19] CD1a+ dendritic cells and CD68+ histiocytes are also present.[20]

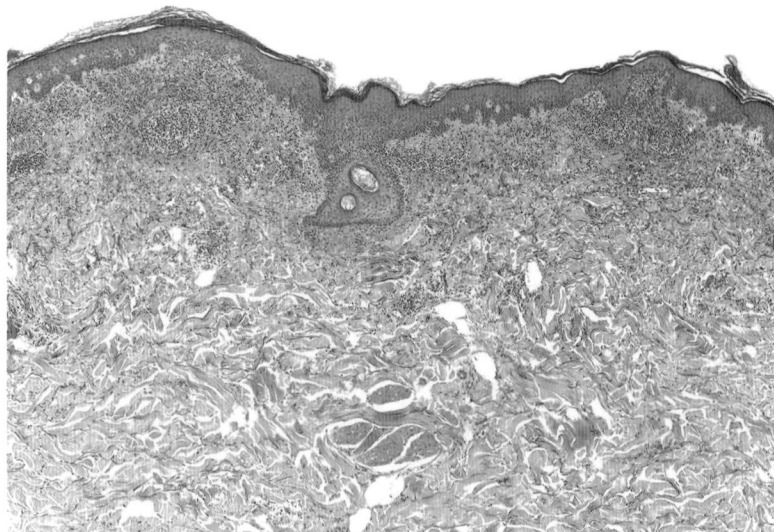

Fig. 14.5
Exanthematous drug reaction: low-power view showing focal parakeratosis, mild acanthosis, and a heavy upper dermal inflammatory cell infiltrate.

CD56+ natural killer (NK) cells may be identified.[19] Cytotoxic pathways mediated by perforin and granzyme B have been shown to be of particular importance in exanthematous drug reactions.[18,20,21] Fas/Fas-L cytotoxic mechanisms are not thought to be of relevance.[16]

The features of drug-induced erythroderma are rather non-specific and include parakeratosis and psoriasiform hyperplasia, sometimes accompanied by mild spongiosis. Eosinophils may be identified within the dermal chronic inflammatory cell infiltrate.

Differential diagnosis

Exanthematous adverse drug reactions are a frequent feature in transplantation patients who are usually taking multiple medications and, therefore, must be distinguished from acute GVHD. In reality, it is difficult, if not

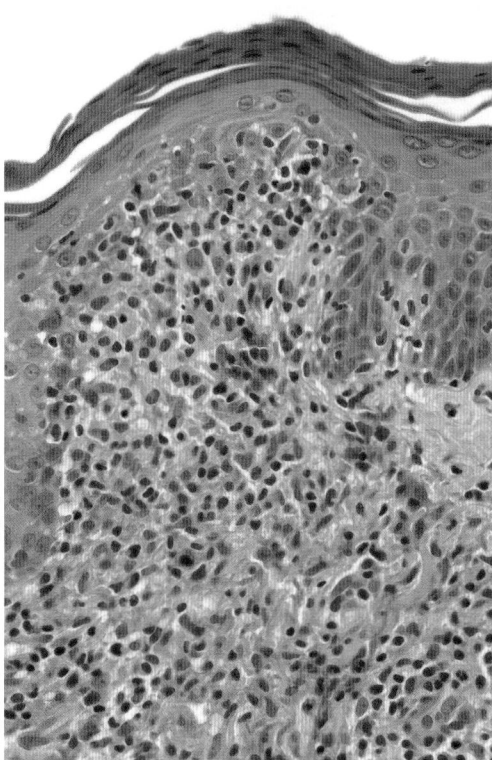

Fig. 14.6
Exanthematous drug reaction: in this high-power view, there is parakeratosis, focal spongiosis and lymphocytic exocytosis. A heavy dermal infiltrate is present with one or two eosinophils.

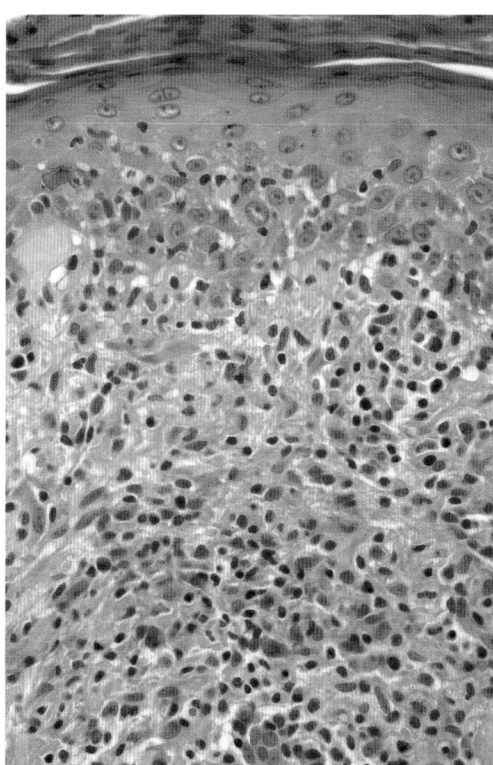

Fig. 14.7
Exanthematous drug reaction: note the interface change and cytoid bodies.

impossible, to make this distinction histologically. Previously, the presence of eosinophils was thought to support a drug reaction. However, tissue eosinophils can be seen in both GVHD and drug reactions.[22] It is only when eosinophils are relatively numerous (≥ 16 per 10 high-power fields [HPFs]) can a drug reaction be strongly favored over GVHD.[23] A viral exanthem also commonly enters the differential diagnosis – the histologic findings are

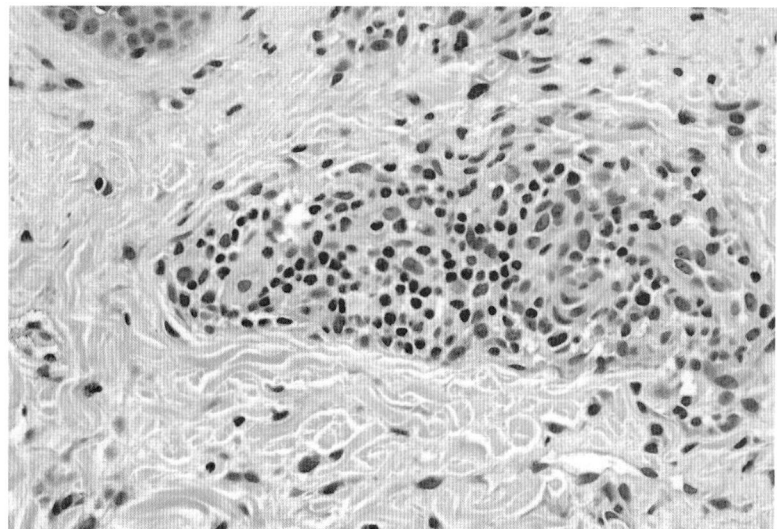

Fig. 14.8
Urticarial drug reaction: high-power view showing a predominately perivascular lymphohistiocytic infiltrate with one or two eosinophils.

often indistinguishable although the presence of eosinophils may favor a drug reaction.

Urticarial reactions, angioedema and anaphylaxis

Clinical features

Urticaria is the second most common adverse drug reaction.[1] It is characterized by pruritic, erythematous, and edematous wheals. If accompanied by marked edema involving the deeper dermis and subcutaneous fat, or if the submucosal layers are affected, angioedema results.[2–4] Urticaria can also be a manifestation of serum sickness and anaphylaxis.

Urticarial reactions may be caused by a large number of drugs. In a large retrospective study from Thailand, 147 different drugs were presumed etiological agents of drug-induced urticaria.[5] Antibiotics, especially cephalosporins, and NSAIDs were most commonly implicated.[5] Other common causes include aspirin, penicillin, ACE inhibitors, and blood products.[6–8] Drugs that directly stimulate mast cell release of vasoactive substances such as histamine can cause urticaria, and include opiates, curare, vancomycin, and polymyxin B.[3,9,10] Radiocontrast media may have a similar effect.[3] Urticarial reactions due to aspirin and NSAIDs are thought to sometimes be a result of abnormal arachidonic acid metabolism.[3,11]

Pathogenesis and histologic features

The pathogenesis of urticarial drug reactions includes IgE-mediated type 1 reactions, immune complex mechanisms, and pseudoallergic phenomena (non-IgE-mediated).[6,12,13] Ultrastructural studies have found mast cell tryptase and FXIII in the superficial nerves of patients with drug-induced urticaria, possibly contributing to the symptomotology.[14] There is evidence that chemokines may also play a role.

Histologically, urticaria is characterized by dermal edema and vascular dilatation accompanied by a perivascular infiltrate consisting of lymphocytes and eosinophils (*Fig. 14.8*). Edema is often difficult to appreciate histologically but may be inferred by separation of collagen bundles. Mast cell degranulation may be present.[3] Vasculitis is not a feature.

Angioedema is characterized by edema extending into the deeper dermis and subcutaneous fat.

Serum sickness/serum sickness-like drug reactions

Clinical features

Serum sickness develops within 1–3 weeks after taking the serum or vaccine.[1–11] It presents with an erythematous maculopapular or urticarial response or with palpable purpura variably accompanied by fever, arthralgia, myalgia, arthritis, lymphadenopathy, glomerulonephritis, myocarditis, and neuritis (*Fig. 14.9*).[1-4] The cutaneous manifestations often commence on the sides of the fingers, toes, and hands before becoming more generalized.[2] A wide range of drugs has been implicated in the development of serum sickness-like drug reactions including phenytoin, phenylbutazone, and carbamazepine. Antibiotics are also a common offender, with cefaclor featured most prominently along with other antibiotics such as cefprozil, ciprofloxacin, minocycline, penicillin V, amoxicillin, flucloxacillin, and co-trimoxazole.[6,12-22] More recently, therapy with monoclonal antibodies such as rituximab, infliximab, natalizumab, and omalizumab has been associated with serum sickness-like reactions.[23-29] It has also been seen in transplant patients receiving rabbit antithymocyte globulin treatment.[30-32]

Pathogenesis and histologic features

Serum sickness is thought to represent an immune complex-mediated type 3 reaction although the possibility of direct toxicity against vessel wall, autoimmunity, and cell-mediated cytotoxicity have been proposed as alternative pathogenetic mechanisms.[2] Direct immunofluorescence reveals immunoglobulin and C3 in relation to blood vessel walls.[6]

The histologic features are those of leukocytoclastic vasculitis (*Fig. 14.10*).[33] Patients with a serum sickness-like drug reaction with histologic findings reminiscent of neutrophilic urticaria have been described.[27,34]

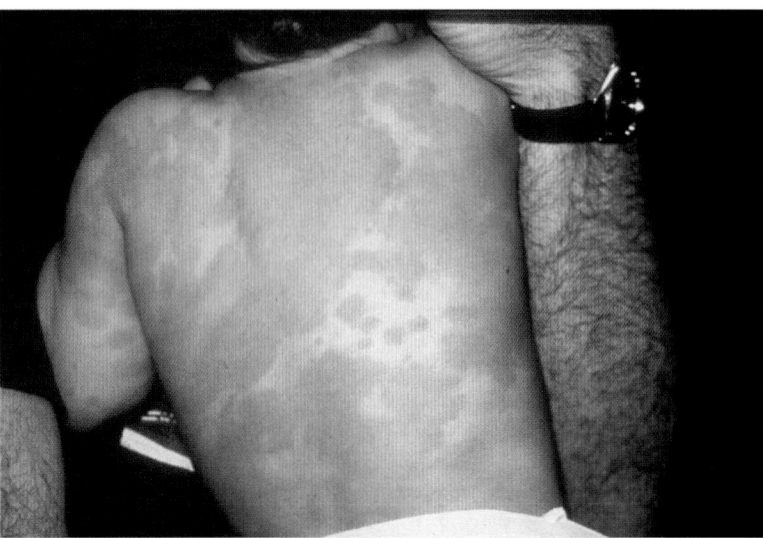

Fig. 14.9
Serum sickness: there is a widespread erythematous and urticarial eruption.

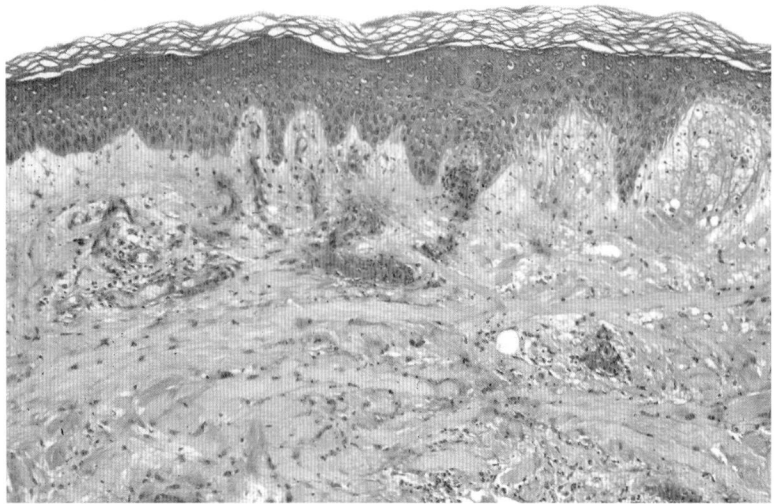

Fig. 14.10
Serum sickness: there is a florid leukocytoclastic vasculitis.

Phototoxic and photoallergic reactions

Clinical features

There are two types of photosensitive drug reactions: phototoxic and photoallergic. Phototoxic reactions are more common; however, they are not necessarily mutually exclusive and are not always clinically distinguishable.[1-30] They are relatively common, representing up to 8% of adverse drug reactions.[31] The clinical appearances of acute phototoxic reactions mimic severe sunburn and include erythema, edema, and blistering with subsequent desquamation and postinflammatory hyperpigmentation (*Figs 14.11* and *14.12*).[6,7] Typically, only exposed skin is affected, and it occurs minutes

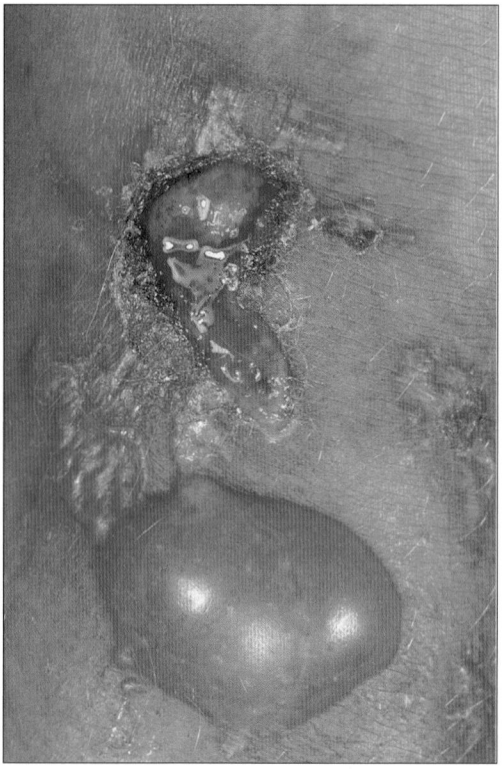

Fig. 14.11
Phototoxic drug reaction: in this example, there are well-developed blisters arising on an erythematous base.

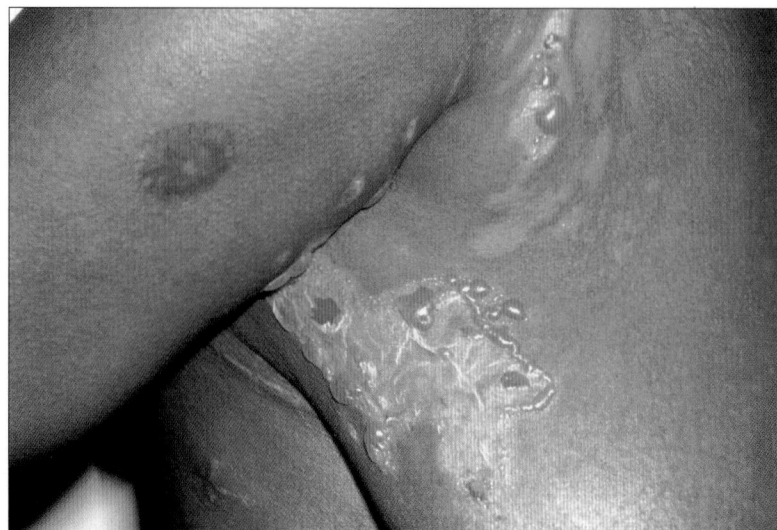

Fig. 14.12
Phototoxic drug reaction: the lesions in this patient followed PUVA therapy. By courtesy of the Institute of Dermatology, London, UK.

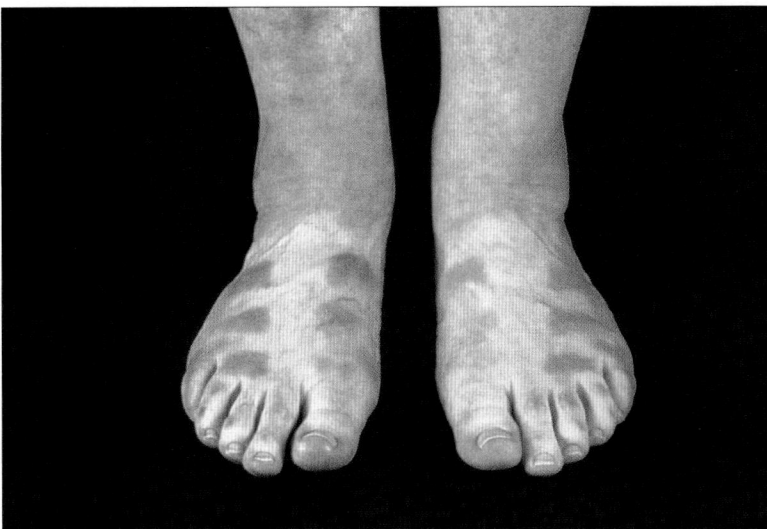

Fig. 14.13
Photoallergic drug reaction: note the obvious sparing of covered skin. By courtesy of the Institute of Dermatology, London, UK.

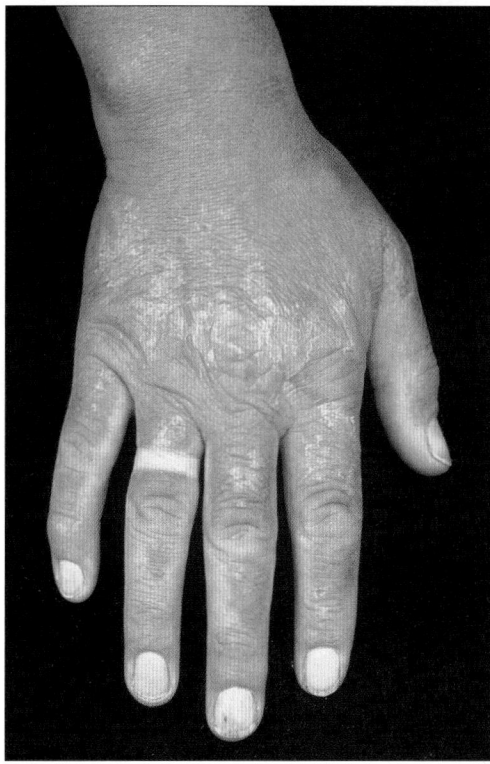

Fig. 14.14
Photoallergic drug reaction: this example resulted from treatment with tetracycline. By courtesy of the Institute of Dermatology, London, UK.

to hours after sun exposure. Phototoxicity has also been associated with onycholysis.[21,25]

Chronic phototoxicity presents with poikilodermatous features including hyper- and hypopigmentation, epidermal atrophy, and telangiectasia. It is an important feature of the porphyrias and the inherited photodermatoses such as xeroderma pigmentosum, Rothmund-Thomson syndrome, and Bloom syndrome. It rarely results from drug treatment but may follow long-term therapy with psoralen and UVA (PUVA therapy), where there is also an increased incidence of actinic keratosis, basal cell carcinoma, squamous cell carcinoma, and, more rarely, melanoma.[6,32–35]

Drugs that are incriminated in acute phototoxic reactions include thiazide diuretics, sulfonamides, tetracycline antibiotics, NSAIDs (including naproxen, diclofenac, and ketoprofen), phenothiazines (particularly chlorpromazine), amiodarone, tars, psoralens, antidepressants, chemotherapeutics, calcium channel blockers, and atovastatin.[6–13,19,20,23,24,29,36] Phototoxicity has also been described with use of St. John's wort and following photodynamic therapy.[22,26] Porphyrins are potent phototoxic sensitizers.[6] In this instance, the damage affects the dermal constituents including the vasculature, leaving the epidermis relatively unaffected.

The clinical appearances of photoallergic drug reactions are variable and include eczematous and lichenoid dermatitides (*Figs 14.13* and *14.14*).[14] Patients may also have erythema multiforme (EM), telangiectasia, hyperpigmentation, and pseudoporphyria.[36] The rash usually develops 24 hours or more after sun exposure. Unlike phototoxic reactions, unexposed skin may also be affected in addition to exposed skin.[7] Typically, the dermatitis resolves after withdrawal of the offending agent. Rarely, a persistent light reaction may occur in which the photodermatitis persists despite removal of the photosensitizing chemical. This usually occurs in the setting of photoallergic contact dermatitis.

The majority of photoallergic reactions are induced by the application of topical medicaments and chemicals (contact photoallergy) including antihistamines, local anesthetics, chlorpromazine, hydrocortisone sunscreens containing *p*-aminobenzoic acid, and halogenated phenolic compounds in soaps and fragrances (e.g., 6-methylcoumarin and musk ambrette).[2,7,15,17] Photoallergy can also follow systemic administration of drugs including sulfonamides, griseofulvin, phenothiazines, tetracyclines, NSAIDs, chloroquine, thiazides, ACE inhibitors, antidepressants, cholesterol lowering drugs, amiodarone, and some chemotherapeutic drugs.[8,18,36] Diagnosis is best confirmed by a photopatch test.

Phytophotodermatitis represents a phototoxic drug reaction due to contact with plants containing furanocoumarins.[37–39] Patients develop erythema followed by postinflammatory hyperpigmentation. Rarely, blisters may develop (*Fig. 14.15*).[37] Members of the Umbelliferae, Rutaceae, and Moraceae families are implicated.[38,39]

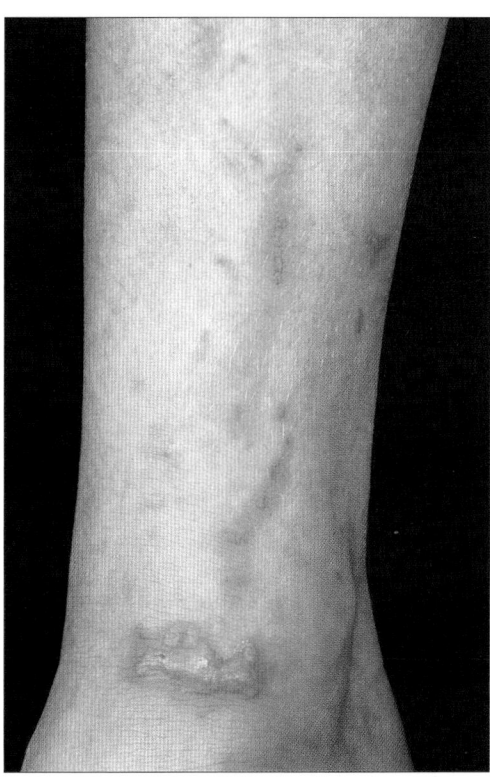

Fig. 14.15
Phytophotodermatitis: this variant represents an allergic reaction to a plant chemical. Linear lesions on the limbs are characteristic and usually follow gardening. By courtesy of the Institute of Dermatology, London, UK.

Pathogenesis and histologic features

Photosensitization has been described as a process whereby 'a reaction to nonionizing radiation occurs as a consequence of the introduction of a radiation-absorbing reagent (the sensitizer), which induces another substance (the substrate) to undergo chemical change'.[1–6] There are two basic

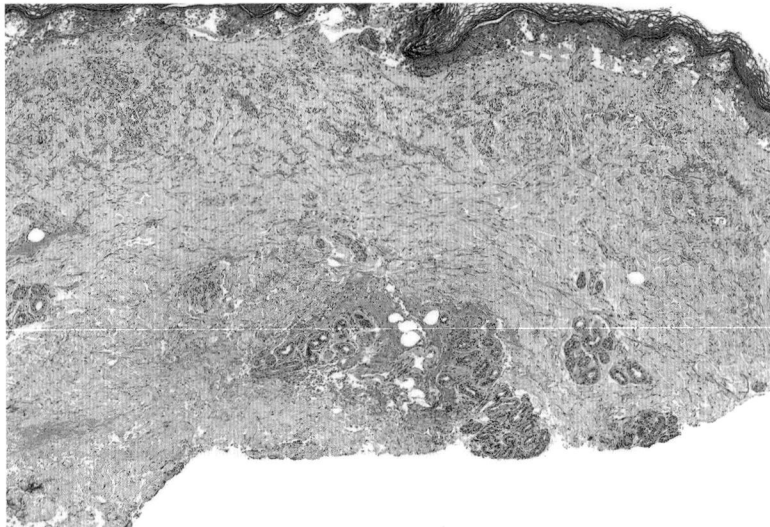

Fig. 14.16
Phototoxic drug reaction: this is a very severe reaction. Dermal edema has resulted in subepidermal vesiculation.

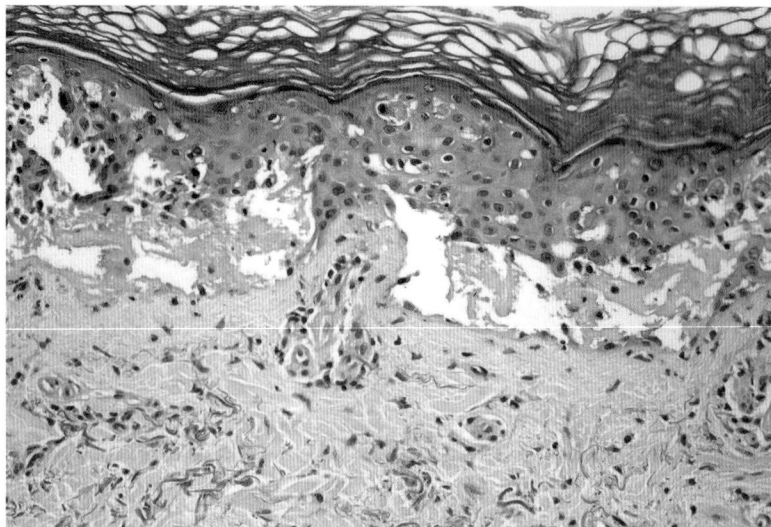

Fig. 14.17
Phototoxic drug reaction: note the multiple necrotic keratinocytes (sunburn cells). The blister cavity is cell-free and the dermal papillae are preserved (festooning).

mechanisms: phototoxic and photoallergic. While an enormous range of drugs has been implicated in photosensitivity reactions, NSAIDs, phenothiazines, amiodarone, antibiotics, and antifungal agents such as griseofulvin appear to be of particular importance.[30]

Two types of phototoxic reactions are recognized: photodynamic and nonphotodynamic.[6,40]

- Photodynamic reactions are oxygen-dependent and result in singlet oxygen or superoxide anions which cause injury to cellular constituents such as cell membranes, cytoplasmic proteins, and nucleic acids.
- Nonphotodynamic reactions are oxygen independent and damage DNA or RNA directly.

Many drug reactions are photodynamic, whereas psoralen represents a nonphotodynamic reaction. Phototoxic reactions do not depend on prior exposure to the drug and will affect all patients of the same skin type provided that sufficient bound drug is available for reaction with the appropriate radiation.[1] The action spectrum for phototoxicity is UVA, and less often UVB and visible light.[40]

Photoallergic drug-induced photosensitivity is immunologically mediated and represents a delayed papular, vesicular, or eczematous response.[6,40] It is a lymphocyte-mediated delayed hypersensitivity type IV reaction. It typically requires previous exposure to the drug or chemical.[1,5,40] Only a proportion of patients taking the drug will develop a reaction. Photoallergic reactions are usually induced by UVA.[1,2,40]

The histologic appearances of acute phototoxic reactions include conspicuous apoptotic keratinocytes (sunburn cells), which in severe cases may affect the entire epidermis, with variable neutrophil exocytosis, dermal edema, and a perivascular lymphohistiocytic infiltrate with small numbers of neutrophils and eosinophils (Figs 14.16 and 14.17).[40,41]

Chronic lesions are characterized by hyperkeratosis, hypergranulosis, variable acanthosis and epidermal atrophy, increased melanin pigmentation, melanocyte hyperplasia, and pigmentary incontinence.[41] Elastosis and telangiectatic vessels may be conspicuous, and in severely affected patients stellate atypical myofibroblasts can be a feature. Epidermal disorganization and dyskeratosis may also be present.[6]

The histologic appearances of drug-induced photoallergic reactions include spongiosis (often with vesiculation, lymphocytic, and eosinophil exocytosis), accompanied by papillary dermal edema and an upper dermal lymphohistiocytic infiltrate with variable numbers of eosinophils.[40,41]

Drug reaction with eosinophilia and systemic symptoms

Drug reaction with eosinophilia and systemic symptoms (DRESS) was previously known as anticonvulsant hypersensitivity syndrome because of its

Table 14.1

Common drugs associated with drug reaction with eosinophilia and systemic symptoms

Drug category	Drug name
Anticonvulsant	Carbamazepine, lamotrigine, phenobarbital, phenytoin, valproic acid, and zonisamide
Antimicrobial	Ampicillin, cefotaxime, dapsone, ethambutol, isoniazid, linezolid, metronidazole, minocycline, pyrazinamide, quinine, rifampin, sulfasalazine, streptomycin, trimethoprim-sulfamethoxazole, and vancomycin
Antiviral	Abacavir, nevirapine, and zalcitabine
Antidepressant	Bupropion and fluoxetine
Antihypertensive	Amlodipine and captopril
Biologic	Efalizumab and imatinib
NSAID	Celecoxib and ibuprofen
Miscellaneous	Allopurinol, epoetin alfa, mexiletine, and ranitidine

NSAID, Nonsteroidal anti-inflammatory drug.
Reproduced with permission from Husain Z., Reddy B.Y., Schwartz R.A. DRESS syndrome: Part I. Clinical perspectives. *J Am Acad Dermatol.* **68**, 2013;693.e1-14; quiz 706-8.

close link with anticonvulsants.[1–10] Cutaneous eruptions associated with anticonvulsants include erythematous maculopapular lesions, erythroderma, acneiform lesions, hypo- and hyperpigmentation, vasculitis, EM, and toxic epidermal necrolysis (TEN), and can affect up to 19% of patients on anticonvulsants, especially phenytoin.[1–8] However, in addition to anticonvulsants, DRESS may be triggered by numerous types of medications including allopurinol, azathioprine, numerous antibiotics (especially dapsone, minocycline and sulfonamides), terbinafine, antivirals, antidepressants, antihypertensives, biologics, NSAIDs, and miscellaneous other drugs (*Table 14.1*).[11–17] DRESS is now the preferred terminology.[17] Pseudolymphomatous drug reactions may also occur, and these are discussed later in the chapter.

DRESS is typically defined by a triad of pyrexia, exanthematous skin rash, and evidence of systemic involvement.[7] Three different systems for diagnostic criteria have been proposed.[17–20] In clinical practice, the criteria proposed by Bocquet et al may be the simplest to apply to ensure that the diagnosis is not missed.[21] In this system, the diagnosis requires three criteria: cutaneous drug eruption, hematological abnormalities, and systemic involvement.[18] The hematological abnormalities include eosinophilia $\geq 1.5 \times 10^9$/L and atypical lymphocytes. Systemic involvement includes any

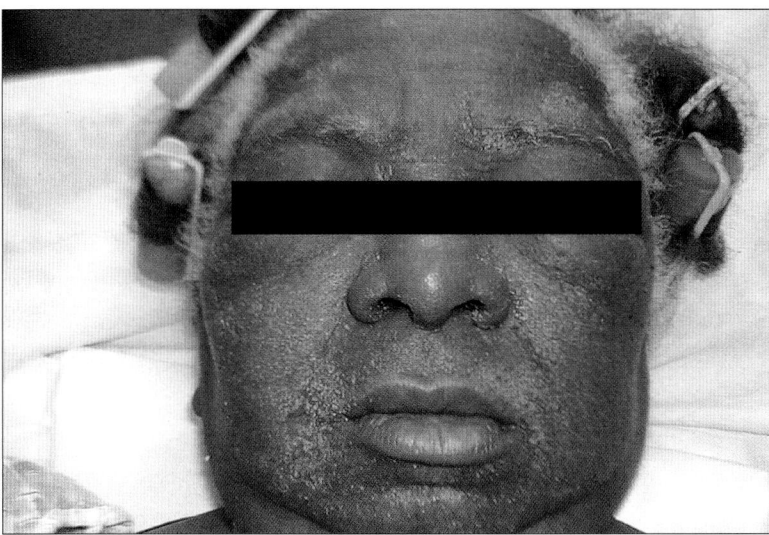

Fig. 14.18
Anticonvulsant hypersensitivity syndrome: there is striking facial edema with periorbital accentuation. By courtesy of C.C. Kim, MD, Department of Dermatology, Harvard Medical School, Boston, USA.

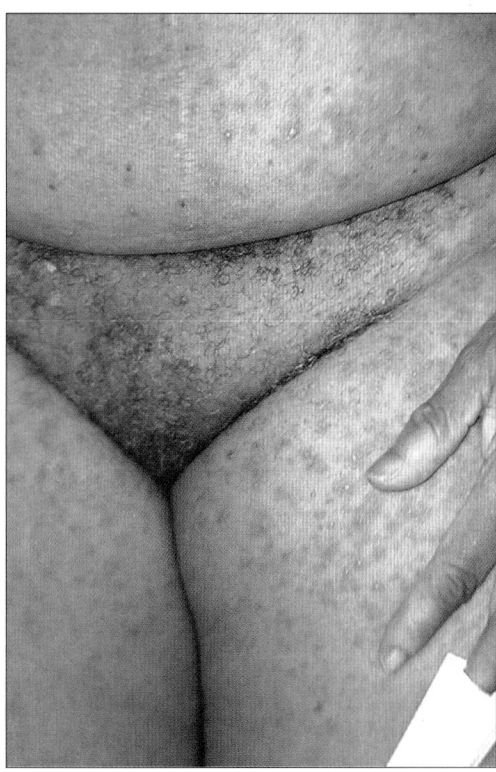

Fig. 14.19
Anticonvulsant hypersensitivity syndrome: there is a maculopapular eruption and pustules are present. By courtesy of C.C. Kim, MD, Department of Dermatology, Harvard Medical School, Boston, USA.

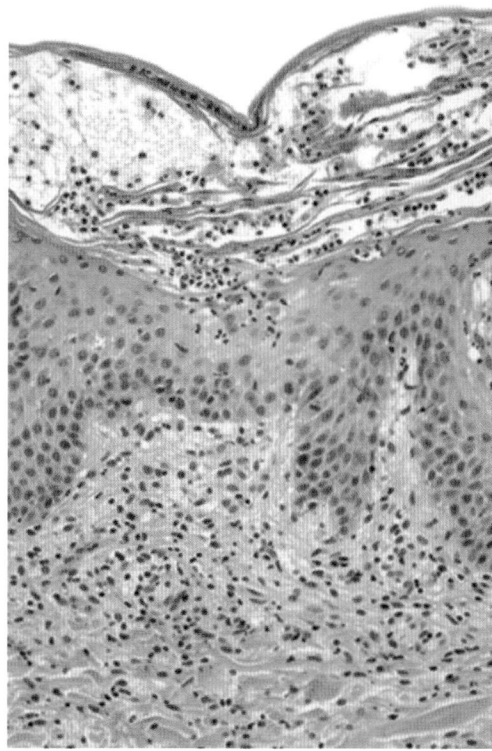

Fig. 14.20
Anticonvulsant hypersensitivity syndrome: this example shows a subcorneal pustule.

of the following: lymphadenopathy, hepatitis with liver transaminases ≥2× normal, interstitial nephritis, interstitial pneumonitis, or carditis. Lymphadenopathy and hepatitis are, by far, the most common systemic manifestation.[17] Liver involvement is seen in 70–95% of patients.[22,23] DRESS typically starts 1–8 weeks after initiation of the drug. The syndrome is more common in black patients. There is no sex predilection.[4] Children may be affected.[24–28] Clinical features include pyrexia, a maculopapular or erythrodermatous eruption, facial or periorbital edema, strawberry tongue, tender lymphadenopathy, myositis, and hepatitis associated with leukocytosis and eosinophilia (Figs 14.18 and 14.19).[5,6] Less often, the cutaneous manifestations include localized or generalized follicular pustules, EM,

and TEN.[4,6,28–31] In patients with the pustular variant, lesions present on the scalp before becoming generalized.[32,33] Conjunctivitis and/or pharyngitis may also be present.[2] Renal, pulmonary (interstitial pneumonitis), and hematological (atypical lymphocytosis) involvement sometimes occur.[5,17] Certain drugs are more commonly implicated in specific organ systems.[17] Liver involvement is strongly associated with phenytoin, minocycline, and dapsone. Renal involvement is most commonly associated with allopurinol, carbamazepine, and dapsone. Minocycline is the most common triggering agent for pulmonary involvement, whereas ampicillin and minocycline are the most common drugs linked to cardiac involvement. The prognosis of this syndrome is variable, with most fatalities secondary to hepatic involvement.[17,34,35] In patients with hepatitis, the mortality is approximately 10–20%.[5,17,36]

Pathogenesis and histologic features

The precise etiology of this syndrome is uncertain but appears to be multifactorial. Patients with mutations in drug detoxification enzymes have an increased risk of DRESS.[17] It is thought to result from an inability to detoxify arene oxide anticonvulsant metabolites due to absence, possibly genetically determined, of specific hydrolases. These genetic differences may help explain familial cases and the increased risk of DRESS in black patients.[17] Immunology may also play a role. Immunosuppressed patients are at increased risk, possibly secondary to reactivation of herpesvirus infections, including reactivation of human herpes virus 6 and 7, Epstein-Barr virus (EBV), and cytomegalovirus.[17,37–42] HHV-6 DNA and mRNA has been detected in the skin of patients with DRESS.[17] Clinical manifestations of primary HHV-6 can closely mimic DRESS, suggesting that viral reactivation may play a significant role.[17] Patients with DRESS have increased plasmacytoid dendritic cells (PDC) in the skin and decreased amounts in the circulation, possibly contributing to viral reactivation.[43] Patients have increased levels of IL-5, contributing to eosinophilia.[44–46] Therefore, it appears to be a complex interactions with biochemical, genetic, and immunological factors that contribute to DRESS.

The histologic features vary from spongiotic dermatitis to those of EM or TEN. Pustular lesions are characterized by a subcorneal pustule associated with follicular infundibular dilatation (Figs 14.20 and 14.21).[8,17]

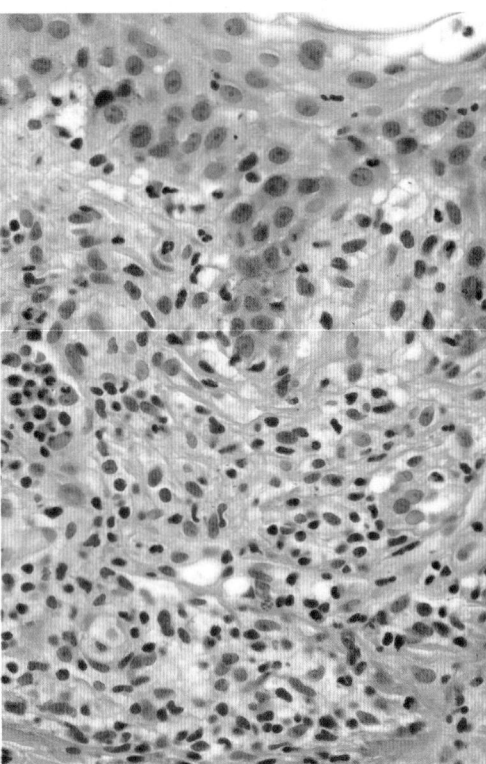

Fig. 14.21
Anticonvulsant hypersensitivity syndrome: the underlying dermis shows a superficial dermal perivascular lymphohistiocytic infiltrate with scattered eosinophils.

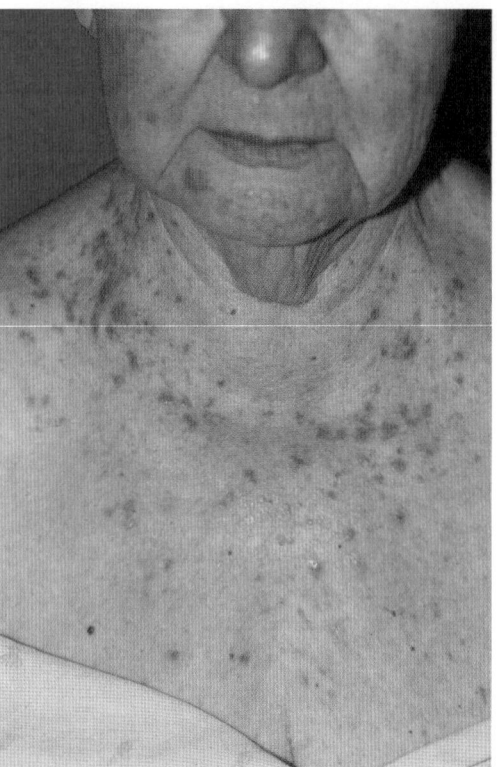

Fig. 14.22
Lichenoid drug reaction: lichenoid papules are widely distributed about the patient's face and upper chest.

Lichenoid and interface drug reactions

Clinical features

Lichenoid drug reactions account for approximately 5% of adverse drug reactions.[1] Lichenoid drug reactions are clinically similar to lichen planus, although lesions are often larger. Wickham striae are usually not apparent.[2–5] Mucosal involvement is rare and clinically and histologically resembles oral lichen planus.[6–8] In contrast to lichen planus, where lesions are characteristically on the flexural surfaces of the forearms, the legs, and the genitalia, in lichenoid drug reactions the trunk and extremities are more often affected (*Figs 14.22* and *14.23*).[9,10] The eruption may sometimes be photodistributed and predominantly affect the hands and forearms, although other sun-exposed sites can be involved.[5,10,11] The latent period between starting the drug and the onset of the eruption is often long, which can take months or even years.[5] Atypical features including eczematous and psoriasiform lesions are sometimes seen, and bullous or ulcerative variants are occasionally encountered.[4,5,12] Postinflammatory hyperpigmentation may be very marked and is often persistent. Scarring alopecia is sometimes present, and some patients may develop anhidrosis.[5]

Although many drugs can cause a lichenoid reaction, those of particular importance include gold, antimalarials such as quinine and quinidine, penicillamine, captopril, various beta blockers (e.g., propranolol), lithium, thiazide diuretics, furosemide (frusemide), spironolactone, and ethambutol.[5,11–23] More recently, the TNF-α inhibitors (infliximab, adalimumab, and etanercept), imatinib mesylate, and PD-1 and PD-L1 inhibitors have been associated with lichenoid eruptions.[24–34] Lichenoid drug reactions have also been associated with hepatitis B, influenza, and human papilloma virus vaccinations.[34–38]

Contact with *p*-phenylenediamine by workers engaged in the photographic color developing process and hairdressers may also result in a cutaneous lichenoid reaction. This is of two types:

- Continuous exposure to small amounts results in the appearance of typical lichen planus.

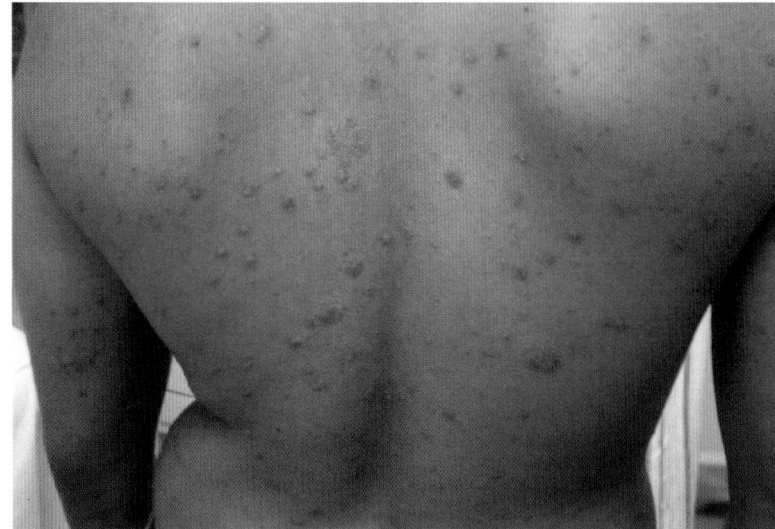

Fig. 14.23
Lichenoid drug reaction: lichenoid papules on the back. By courtesy of B. Al-Mahmoud, MD, Doha, Qatar.

- If exposed to a single large dose, the features are those of a lichenoid contact dermatitis.[5]

Other causes of a contact lichenoid eruption include dental restorative materials, musk ambrette, nickel, and gold.[5]

Captopril and cinnarizine may cause lichen planus pemphigoides-like eruptions (see bullous drug reactions below).[39,40]

Histologic features

The histologic features are frequently indistinguishable from typical lichen planus, although focal parakeratosis and spongiosis are sometimes present and interface change may be patchy (*Figs 14.24–14.26*). The epidermis is often thinner and hypergranulosis less marked.[19] Cytoid bodies may be found in the upper granular cell layer or even in the stratum corneum.[9,11]

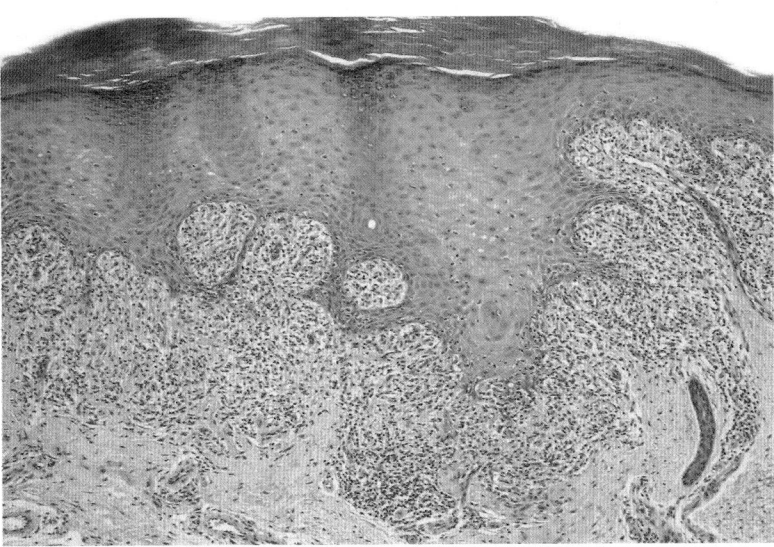

Fig. 14.24
Lichenoid drug reaction: there is hyperkeratosis, hypergranulosis with interface change. Note the superficial bandlike infiltrate. The appearances are indistinguishable from idiopathic lichen planus.

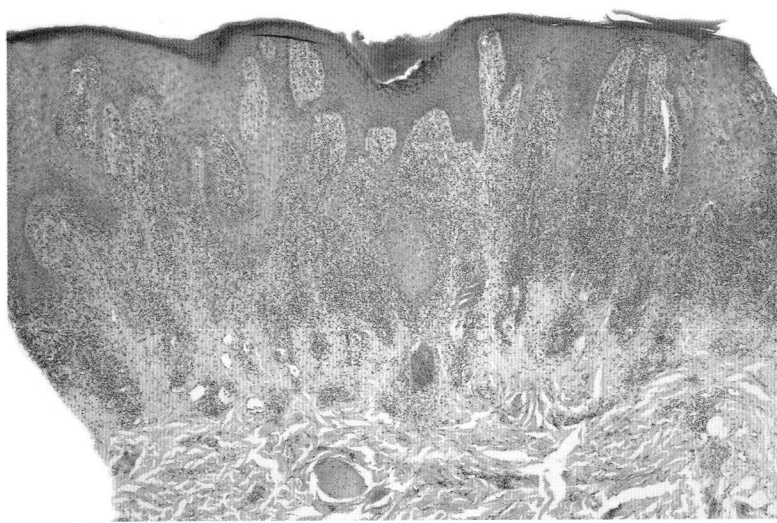

Fig. 14.25
Lichenoid drug reaction: In this example, the changes of hypertrophic lichen planus-like lesions are evident. There is pseudoepitheliomatous hyperplasia and a dense upper dermal lymphohistiocytic infiltrate.

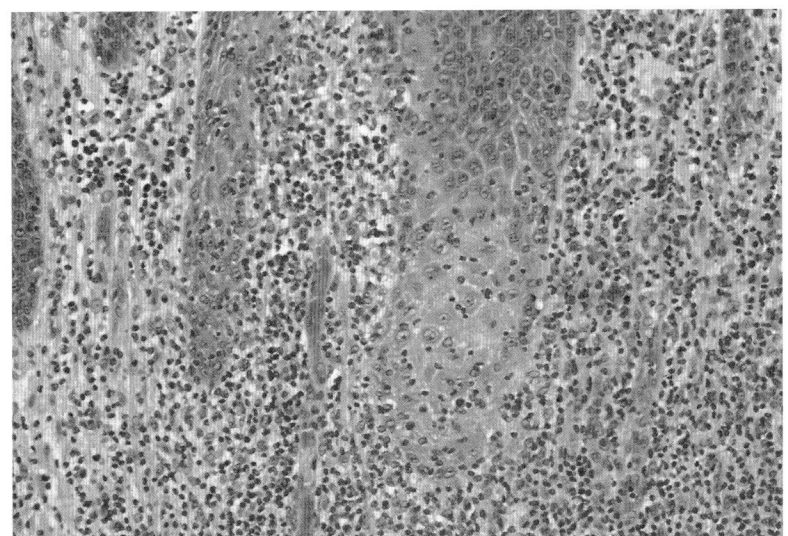

Fig. 14.26
Lichenoid drug reaction: focal interface change is present. Eosinophils are conspicuous.

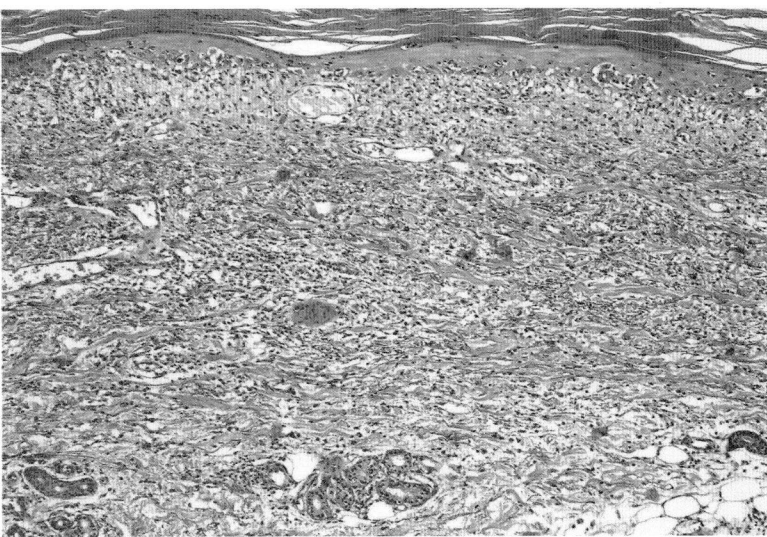

Fig. 14.27
Interface drug reaction: more extensive lesion due to propranolol showing hyperkeratosis, widespread apoptosis, upper dermal edema, and a superficial chronic inflammatory cell infiltrate.

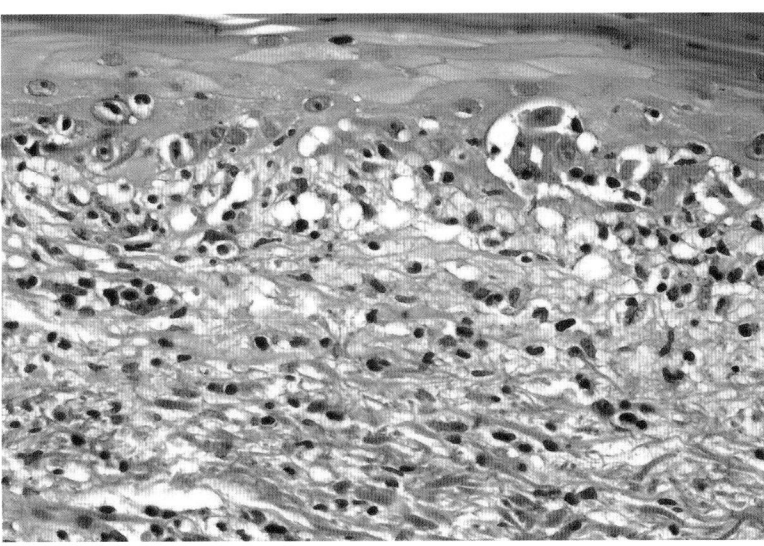

Fig. 14.28
Interface drug reaction: there are numerous apoptotic keratinocytes and severe interface change is evident.

Sometimes, eosinophils and occasionally plasma cells are found in the dermal infiltrate.[9] Focal interruption of the granular cell layer, exocytosis of lymphoid cells into the upper epidermis, and a perivascular infiltrate in the deeper dermis are said to be additional helpful diagnostic pointers.[11] Photodistributed lichenoid drug reactions are said to more closely resemble idiopathic lichen planus than nonphotodistributed variants.[9] The changes that allow distinction from lichen planus are often seen in hypertrophic lichen planus. However, in lichenoid drug eruptions, prominent hyperplasia is hardly ever present. With some drug reactions, interface changes are present in the absence of a background of epidermal lichenoid features (*Figs 14.27* and *14.28*). In lichenoid drug reactions secondary to anti-PD1 and anti-PD-L1 medications, spongiosis and epidermal necrosis are more prominent, and there are an increased number of histiocytes in the infiltrate.[30]

Fixed drug eruptions

Clinical features

Fixed drug eruptions present as one or more circumscribed erythematous to violaceous or brown plaques that show a predilection for the extremities

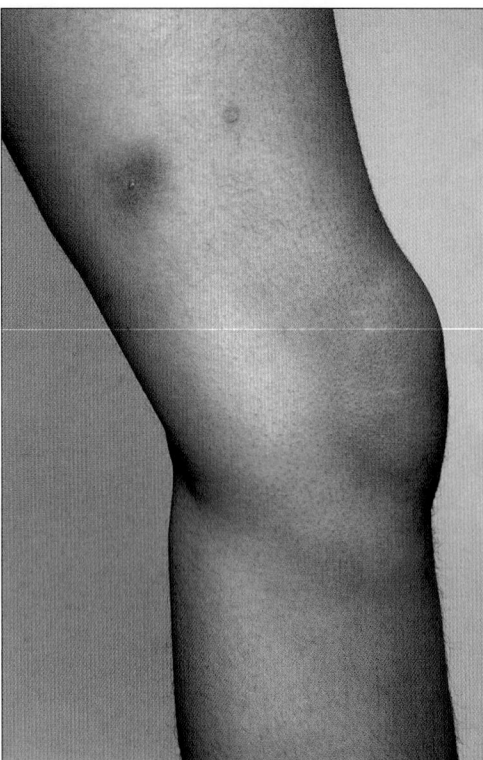

Fig. 14.29
Fixed drug eruption: typical localized brown plaque with a small central blister. By courtesy of the Institute of Dermatology, London, UK.

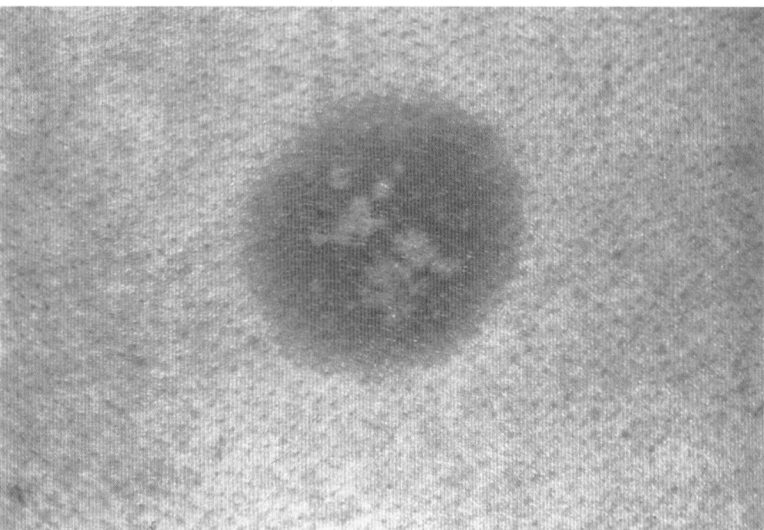

Fig. 14.30
Fixed drug eruption: early, sharply delineated erythematous lesion. By courtesy of the Institute of Dermatology, London, UK.

including the hands, feet, and external genitalia (*Figs 14.29* and *14.30*).[1–8] The mucous membranes may be affected, either alone or in association with cutaneous manifestations.[3] Lesions – which may be pruritic or present with a burning sensation – typically recur at the same site on rechallenge with the offending drug. They usually develop within 30 minutes to 8 hours after taking the drug.[3] Vesiculation and blistering are common. Resolution is typically marked by postinflammatory hyperpigmentation varying from brown to brown-violet or even black.[6] In cases with multiple lesions, the multiple pigmented patches result in an appearance described as 'Dalmatian dog'. Occasionally, the eruption is generalized and resembles TEN.[9,10] Although the number of drugs that are capable of eliciting a fixed reaction is very large, those that are said to be more commonly incriminated include barbiturates, phenylbutazone, ibuprofen, acetyl salicylic acid, sulfonamides, trimethoprim-sulfamethoxazole, tetracyclines, dapsone, phenolphthalein, and quinine.[2,3,6] In a large retrospective study from Singapore, the NSAID drug etoricoxib was responsible for close to 40% of fixed drug eruptions.[11]

Pathogenesis and histologic features

Fixed drug eruption is unique owing to the precise localization of the eruption and its recurrence at the same site on rechallenge. To understand this process, initial research was directed toward identifying the site of cutaneous memory. Autotransplantation experiments in which normal skin was grafted to a previously affected site and vice versa, followed by rechallenge with the causative drug, produced conflicting results. Some workers found that following challenge, grafted normal skin was unaffected, whereas transplanted previously affected skin developed erythema and became symptomatic.[12] Others experienced quite the opposite results.[13]

Immunofluorescence studies have been equally conflicting. While some authors have documented in vivo bound immunoglobulin and complement in the intercellular region of the epidermis or at its basement membrane, the majority of investigations have been negative.[14,15]

It seems unlikely, therefore, that humoral immunity has a significant part to play in the pathogenesis of fixed drug eruption. Current research is directed toward understanding the role of cellular immunity. On initial exposure, the drug appears to bind to the epidermal keratinocytes (thereby functioning as a hapten) and is presented by Langerhans cells to lymphocytes within the dermis or in local lymph nodes. This stimulates an effector CD8+ lymphocyte population which, on returning to the epidermis, produces various cytokines including IFN-gamma (IFN-γ) and TNF-α, which result in epidermal necrosis.[16,17] Keratinocyte death is believed to be mediated by both cytolytic pathways (e.g., perforin, granzyme A, and granzyme B) and FAS-mediated apoptosis.[16–18] Resolution of the disease is thought to be due to recruitment of CD4+ T cells into the epidermis which suppress CD8+ T-cell activation and limit cell destruction, possibly via production of IL-10.[19]

Although the precise mechanism by which memory in fixed drug eruption is achieved is incompletely understood, there is now considerable evidence to suggest that an intraepidermal effector-memory CD8+ T-cell population residing in the epidermis after the initial drug reaction is of particular importance.[15–22] Such cells are defined immunohistochemically by expression of CD3, CD45RA, TCR-alpha beta, CD11a, and CD11b, and absence of CD27, CD28, and CD62L.[21,23] It has been demonstrated that they remain in a state of activation (CD69+) in the unchallenged state and, following exposure to the drug, rapidly up-regulate IFN-γ expression and induce FAS and FAS-ligand expression, soon followed by epidermal necrosis.[18,22] The localization may be related to site-specific, tissue resident T cells that remain after the eruption resolves and subsequently reactivate on re-exposure to the offending agent.[24]

Histologically, the acute fixed drug eruption is characterized by marked basal cell hydropic degeneration, with lymphocyte tagging along the dermal–epidermal junction and individual keratinocyte necrosis (*Figs 14.31–14.33*).[25] Marked pigmentary incontinence is typical. Subepidermal vesiculation may be a feature of advanced lesions. Lymphocytes, histiocytes, and neutrophils are evident in the upper dermis. Eosinophils may sometimes be prominent. In late lesions, pigmentary incontinence may be the sole histologic finding.

Erythema multiforme

Although infectious agents (herpes simplex virus, *Mycoplasma* species) are the most common cause of EM, medications, or a combination of medications and viral infections, are implicated in a subset of patients. Drugs with the strongest association include antibiotics, anticonvulsants, and NSAIDs.[1] Sulfonamides, specifically trimethoprim-sulfamethoxazole, carry the highest relative risk. Other causative antibiotics include aminopenicillins, quinolones, cephalosporins, and tetracyclines. The anticonvulsants associated with EM most often are phenobarbital, carbamazepine, phenytoin, and valproic acid. EM due to a combined viral infections and drug exposure has been described with cytomegalovirus and EBV.[2,3] Despite the known associations,

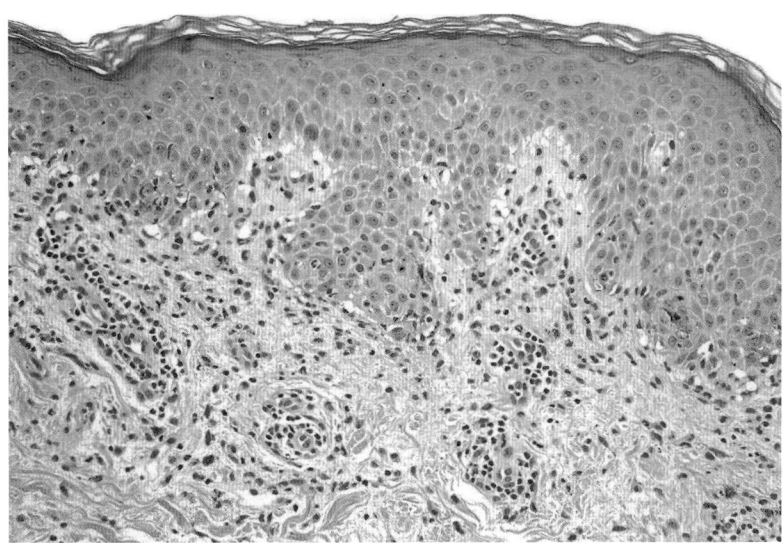

Fig. 14.31
Fixed drug eruption: there is epidermal hyperplasia, interface change, and a superficial dermal chronic inflammatory cell infiltrate.

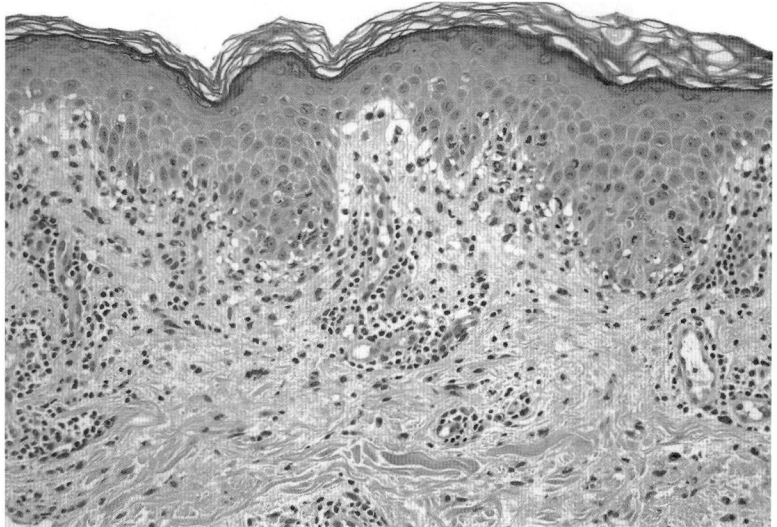

Fig. 14.33
Fixed drug eruption: in this example, the infiltrate has a predominantly perivascular distribution.

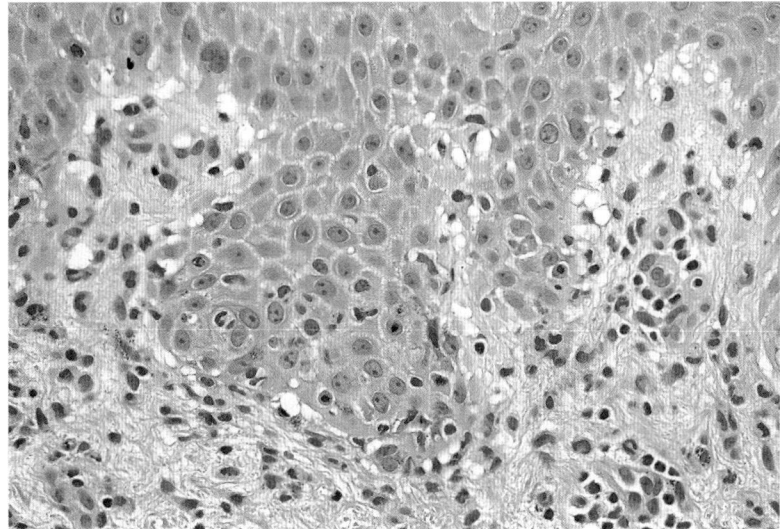

Fig. 14.32
Fixed drug eruption: high-power view showing apoptosis and interface change.

the underlying trigger may be unknown in more than half of patients affected.[4]

Stevens-Johnson syndrome and toxic epidermal necrolysis

In contrast to EM, Stevens-Johnson syndrome (SJS) and TEN are much more strongly associated with medication use.[1,2] The profile of implicated drugs is similar to that seen in EM (see above).[3,4] Studies on newer medications cite strong associations for nevirapine and lamotrigine, and weaker but significant associations for sertraline, pantoprazole, and tramadol.[5] In a recent study, allopurinol was the most common trigger, accounting for 20% of cases over a 10-year period.[6]

Drug-induced hyperpigmentation

Clinical features

Cutaneous hyperpigmentation is a frequent complication of drug therapy. It may result from increased melanin synthesis or deposition of the drug or its metabolite within the skin.[1–5] Heavy metals can also result in skin

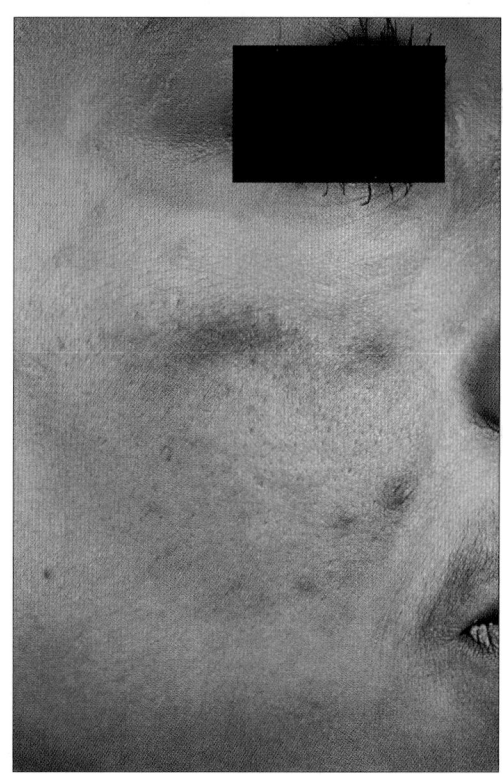

Fig. 14.34
Minocycline pigmentation: extensive lesions involving the cheek and periorbital region. By courtesy of the Institute of Dermatology, London, UK.

pigmentation.[4] Most often, however, it results from postinflammatory hyperpigmentation.[3]

Long-term treatment with minocycline might result in usually reversible (types I and II) cutaneous pigmentation.[6–13] Three clinical variants of cutaneous minocycline pigmentation are generally recognized (*Figs 14.34–14.36*):
- Type I: blue-black macules localized to areas of scarring and inflammation (e.g., facial acne scars),
- Type II (most common): blue-black, brown or slate-gray pigmentation on the shins, ankles, and arms,
- Type III: generalized muddy-brown pigmentation which may be exacerbated on sunlight-exposed regions.

A fourth variant affecting the lips and possibly representing a fixed drug eruption has been described.[14]

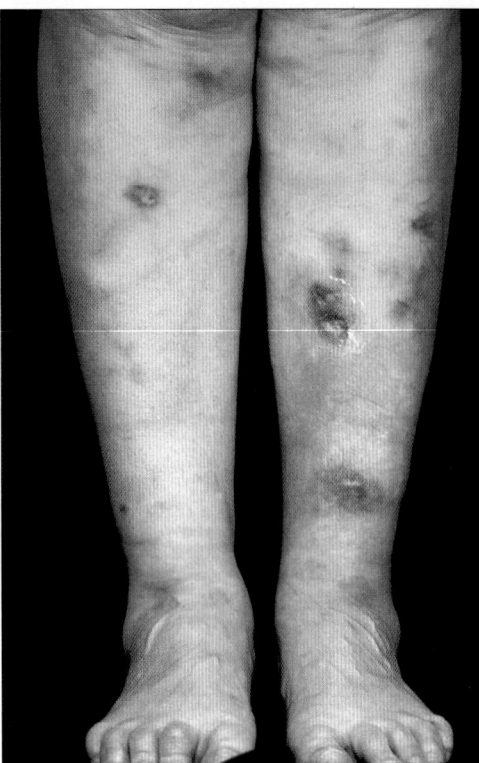

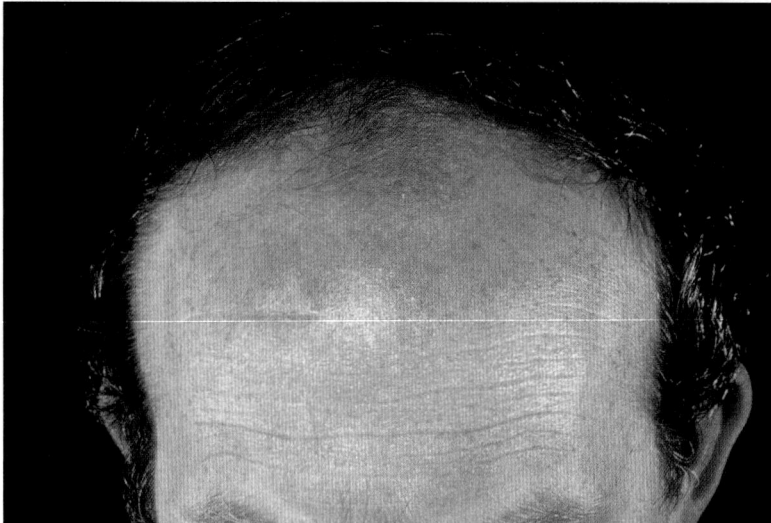

Fig. 14.37
Amiodarone pigmentation: note the slate-gray discoloration on the forehead, a characteristic site. By courtesy of the Institute of Dermatology, London, UK.

Fig. 14.35
Minocycline pigmentation: these blue-black lesions have developed in a patient with pyoderma gangrenosum. By courtesy of the Institute of Dermatology, London, UK.

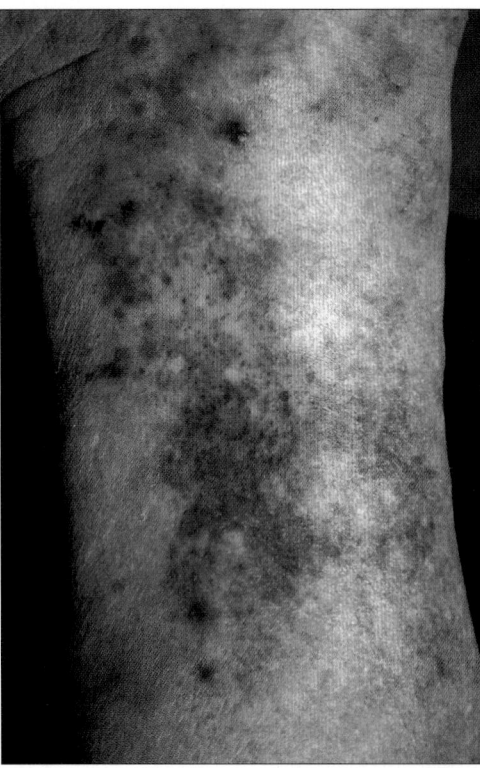

Fig. 14.36
Minocycline pigmentation; typical pigmentation affecting the shin. By courtesy of the Institute of Dermatology, London, UK.

Localized minocycline pigmentation as a complication of cosmetic laser procedures have also been reported.[15,16]

Nail pigmentation most often presents as a persistent slate-gray coloration of the proximal nail bed.[17] Additional features include longitudinal melanonychia, diffuse nail pigmentation, and photo-onycholysis.[17]

Minocycline may involve the teeth (causing a green-gray or blue-gray discoloration), predominantly affecting the middle and occasionally the incisal thirds of the crown.[18] Lesions of the oral mucosa are rare although pigmentation has been described on the buccal mucosa, gingiva, tongue, and lips.[19-23] The bones underlying the oral cavity (black bone disease) represent the single site most commonly affected by minocycline pigmentation.[24] This is best visualized by inspecting the maxillary and mandibular anterior alveolar mucosa.[14] The hard palate and lingual alveolar bone are also commonly affected.[14]

The conjunctiva, sclera, thyroid (black thyroid), aorta, endocardium, and atherosclerotic plaques may also be involved in minocycline pigmentation.[25-34] Minocycline pigmentation may also affect the vulvar/vaginal mucosa and may clinically mimic a melanocytic lesion.[35]

Many other tetracyclines including methacycline and tetracycline hydrochloride have also been associated with cutaneous pigmentation.[36,37]

Amiodarone, which is used primarily in the treatment of cardiac arrhythmias, is associated with a phototoxic/photosensitivity reaction in up to 50% of patients.[38-44] In addition, cutaneous golden-brown to slate-gray or blue/violaceous pigmentation predominantly affecting the exposed surfaces including the face and the backs of the hands may develop, especially in those receiving high doses over a protracted period of time (Fig. 14.37).[38] Pigmentation is also sometimes seen in the sclera and cornea.[41]

Antimalarials also result in abnormal skin pigmentation.[45-48] Mepacrine (quinacrine) typically produces a yellow coloration although localized blue-black mucocutaneous lesions have been described (Figs 14.38 and 14.39).[48] Chloroquine and hydroxychloroquine cause yellow-brown to gray pigmentation.[2,45-47] Sun-exposed skin is predominantly affected, although mucosal pigmentation may also occur.[49]

In addition to causing photosensitivity and contact dermatitis, chlorpromazine therapy (particularly when protracted and in high doses) can result in cutaneous pigmentation, especially on sun-exposed skin such as the face, dorsum of the hands, and the neck.[2,50-53] Patients may present with a golden brown, tanned appearance while others develop a slate-gray, bluish, or purple appearance. The cornea and lens of the eye can also be involved.[2]

Long-term treatment with imipramine may result in photodistributed hyperpigmentation affecting the face, neck, 'V' of chest, arms, and hands (Fig. 14.40).[54-56] The coloration varies from golden brown to blue-gray or slate-gray. The irises may also darken.

Photodistributed blue-gray pigmentation has been documented following treatment with desipramine.[57]

Heavy metals including gold, silver, and mercury can all result in cutaneous pigmentation (see below).

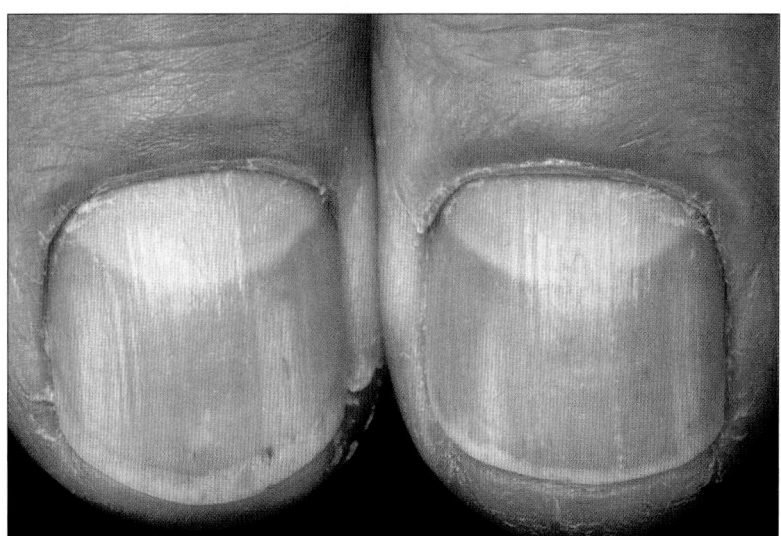

Fig. 14.38
Mepacrine pigmentation: a yellow discoloration is characteristic. By courtesy of the Institute of Dermatology, London, UK.

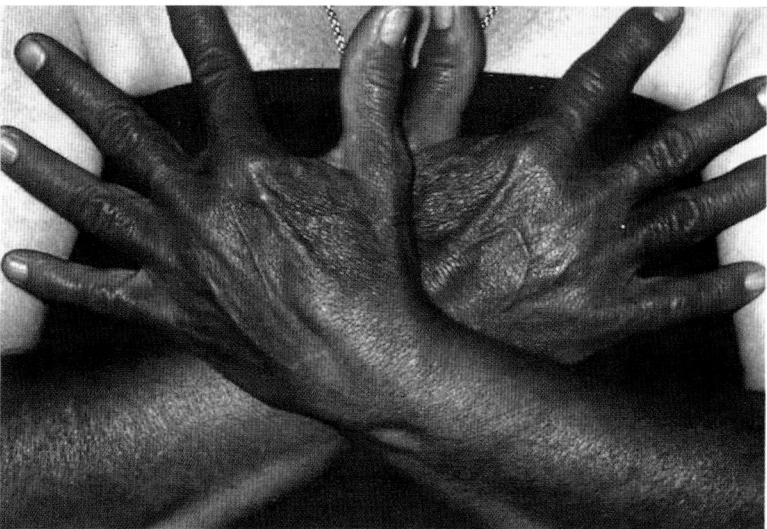

Fig. 14.40
Imipramine pigmentation: note the intense brown pigment of the hands and forearms in comparison with the chest. By courtesy of L. Cohen, MD, Cohen Dermatopathology, Massachusetts, USA.

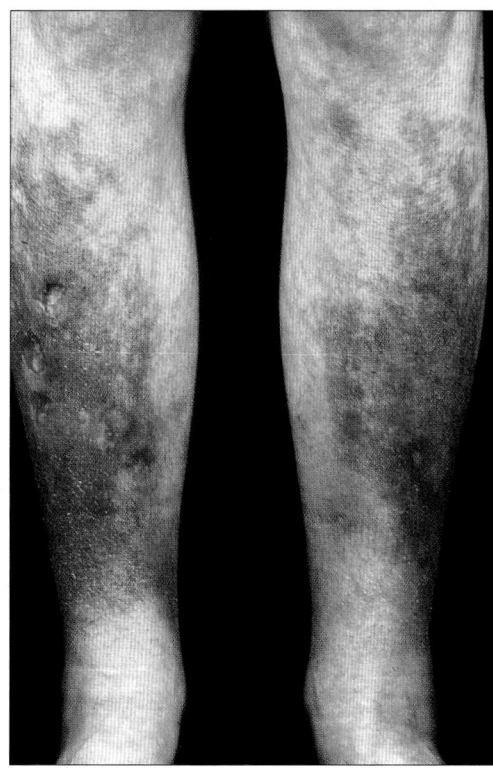

Fig. 14.39
Mepacrine pigmentation: in this patient, the drug resulted in black lesions. By courtesy of the Institute of Dermatology, London, UK.

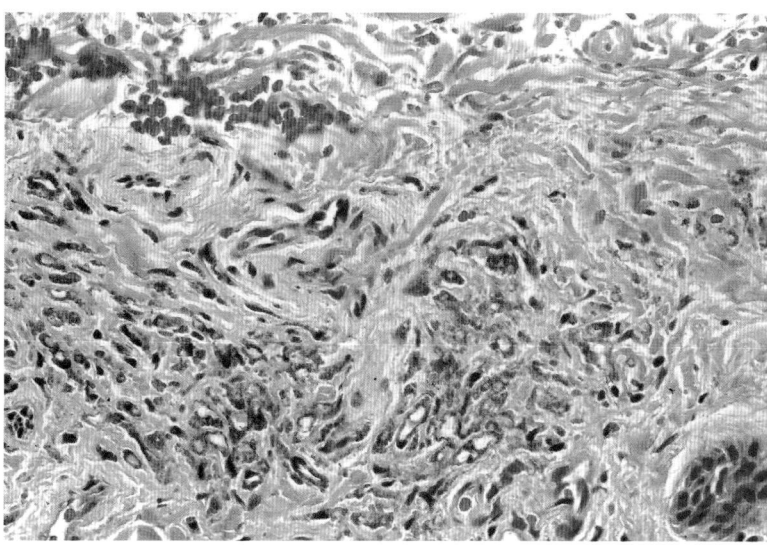

Fig. 14.41
Minocycline pigmentation: note the presence of perivascular granular brown pigment.

Pathogenesis and histologic features

The histologic features of minocycline pigmentation are variable.[7,10,11,14] In types I and II variants, golden brown to brown-black granules are found predominantly within macrophages distributed mainly around the vasculature and sweat gland coils (*Fig. 14.41*). The pigment, which fluoresces yellow under ultraviolet light, stains positively with both Masson-Fontana and Perls Prussian blue reactions in type II variants (*Figs 14.42* and *14.43*).[11] The pigment is periodic acid-Schiff (PAS) negative. In contrast, in type I, the pigment only stains with Perls reaction. It is believed to represent minocycline or its breakdown product chelated with hemosiderin, ferritin, or iron.[7] Calcium, sulfur, and chlorine are also present, but melanin is absent.[11] Melanocytes and the epidermis show no increase in melanin pigmentation in types I and II variants. Type III hyperpigmentation is characterized by

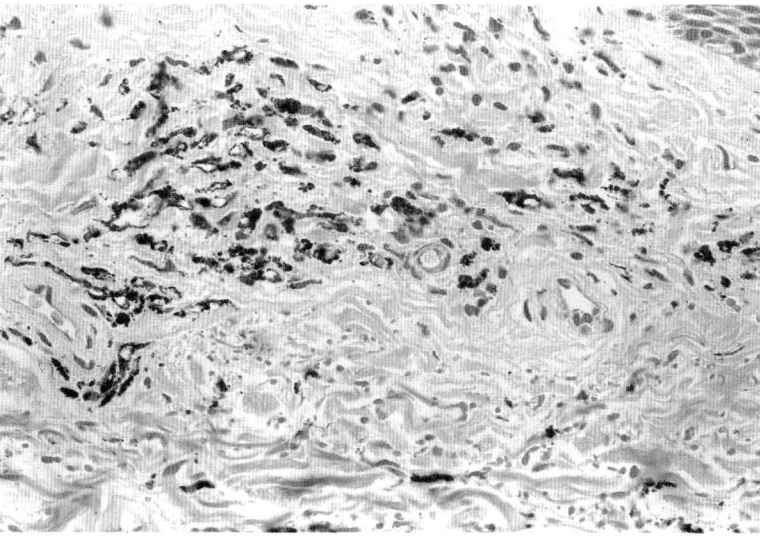

Fig. 14.42
Minocycline pigmentation: the pigment stains positively with Masson-Fontana.

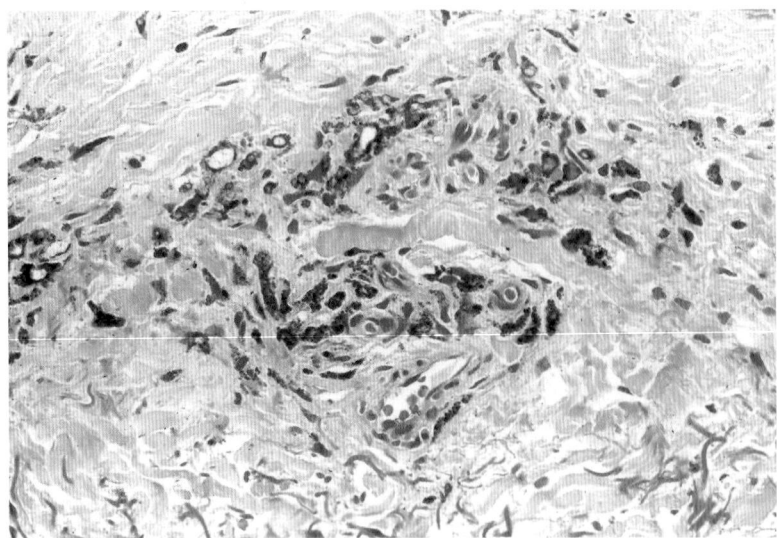

Fig. 14.43
Minocycline pigmentation: the pigment also stains with Prussian blue.

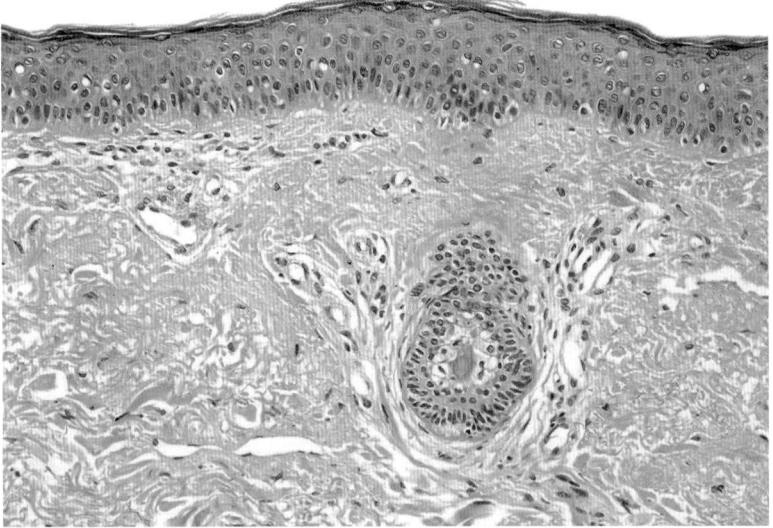

Fig. 14.44
Amiodarone pigmentation: pigmented macrophages are present in a perivascular distribution.

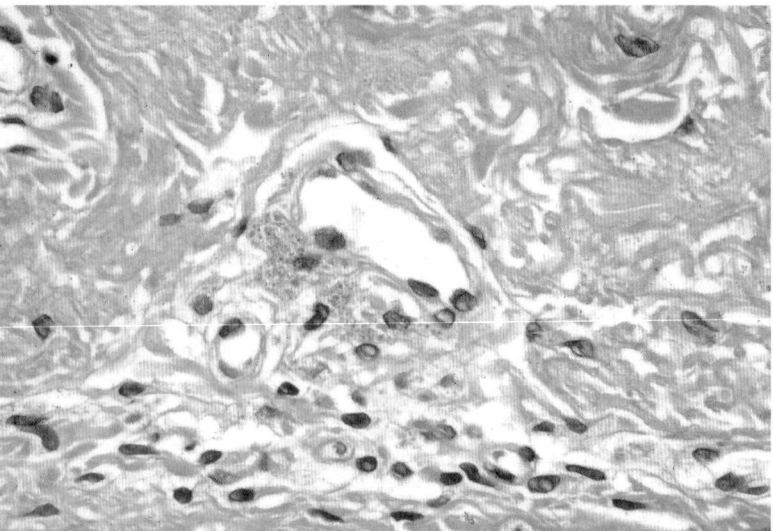

Fig. 14.45
Amiodarone pigmentation: high-power view.

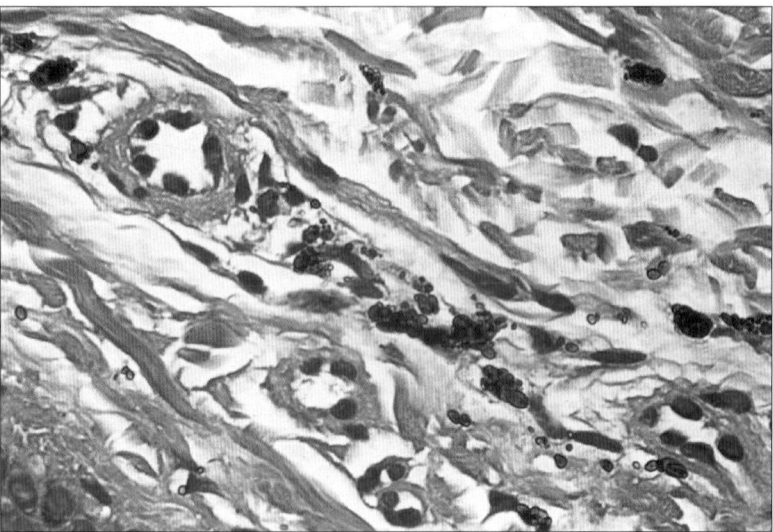

Fig. 14.46
Imipramine pigmentation: typical golden-brown granules. Note that the Prussian blue reaction is negative. By courtesy of L. Cohen, MD, Cohen Dermatopathology, Massachusetts, USA.

an increase in epidermal basal cell melanin pigmentation.[6] The Perls stain is negative. Minocycline pigmentation of the subcutaneous fat has been described in the clinical setting of type II disease.[58,59] Histologically, there is pigment within macrophages and giant cells in the subcutaneous fat, with positive staining for Masson-Fontana and variable staining with Perls reaction. One study also described green-gray nonrefractile globules within macrophages in the fat.[59]

Histologically, amiodarone pigmentation is characterized by macrophages containing PAS-positive, yellow-brown lipofuscin-like granules located in a perivascular distribution (Figs 14.44 and 14.45).[38] Melanin pigmentation of the epidermis is not increased; indeed, its absence in involved skin has recently been documented.[44] By electron microscopy, the granules are located within lysosomes.[39,43] Lamellar myelin bodies may also be identified.[25] Similar inclusions may be found in the hepatocytes, Kupffer cells, pulmonary macrophages, and neutrophils.

In mepacrine (quinacrine) pigmentation, yellow-brown pigment is found within the cytoplasm of histiocytes throughout the dermis.[48] The pigment is weakly positive with the Perls Prussian blue reaction for iron and is Masson-Fontana negative.[44,49] The histologic findings in hydroxychloroquine-related pigmentation have been described as yellow-brown granular deposits within macrophages and extracellularly.[60]

These granules are nonrefractile and stain positively with Masson-Fontana and are negative for iron.[60]

Histologically, chlorpromazine hyperpigmentation is characterized by golden brown macrophage-bound granules surrounding the superficial vasculature. The granules are positive with the Masson-Fontana reaction but do not stain with Perls Prussian blue.[53] Ultrastructurally, the pigment is lysosome bound and present in endothelial cells, fibroblasts, Schwann, and smooth muscle cells, in addition to macrophages.[50,51] Increased melanin also contributes to the cutaneous pigmentation.[50]

Histologically, imipramine and desipramine hyperpigmentation contain Masson-Fontana positive golden brown granules within the upper dermis, lying both free and within macrophages (Fig. 14.46).[54,55,57] Perls Prussian blue is negative. Ultrastructurally, histiocytes contain melanosomes in addition to lysosomal-bound electron-dense granules.[54]

Vasculitic drug reactions

Adverse drug reactions are a common cause of vasculitis, accounting for up to 30% of vasculitides.[1–3] In a study of hospitalized patients with adverse medication reactions, approximately 3% were vasculitis in nature.[4] An immune complex mechanism mostly represents the pathogenesis in the

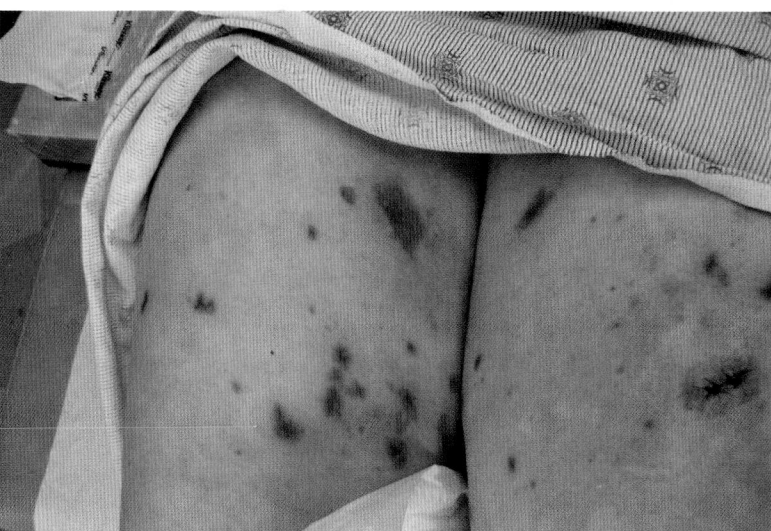

Fig. 14.47
Vasculitic drug reaction: hemorrhagic papules and plaques with central necrosis complicating treatment with propylthiouracil. By courtesy of M. Mailberger, MD, Virginia Commonwealth University, Richmond, Virginia, USA.

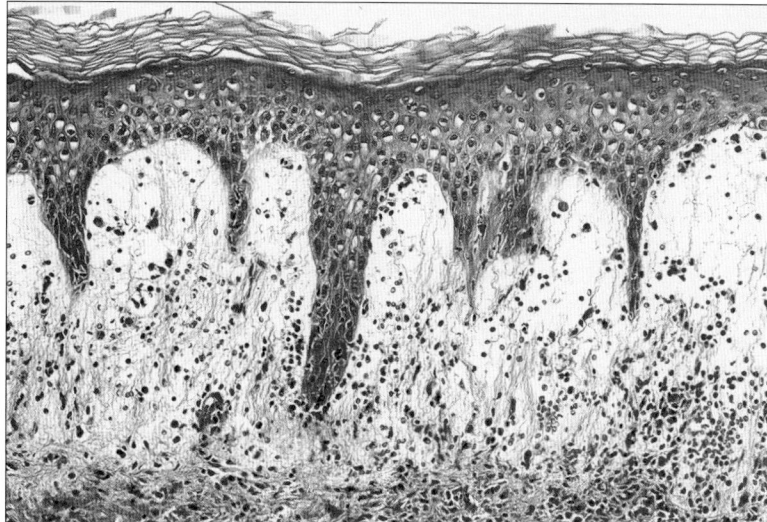

Fig. 14.49
Purpuric drug reaction: there is massive subepidermal edema with red cell extravasation.

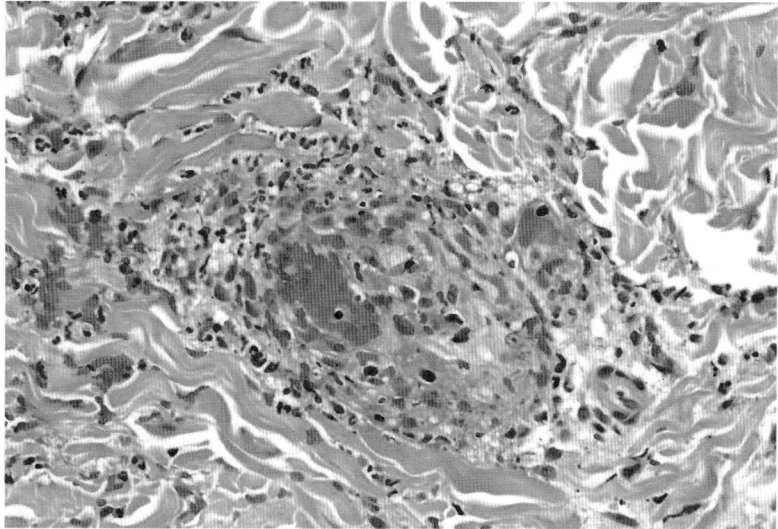

Fig. 14.48
Vasculitic drug reaction: there is acute vasculitis with thrombosis.

majority of cases. A wide range of drugs has been implicated, including anti-infective agents, cancer chemotherapeutic agents and adjuvants, psychoactive and cardiovascular drugs, diuretics, anticoagulants, beta-adrenergic receptor agonists, and anticonvulsants.[2] The more important agents include trimethoprim, penicillin, sulfonamides, NSAIDs, and aspirin.[5] Other implicated drugs include cimetidine, clarithromycin, coumadin, furosemide (frusemide), hydralazine, ibuprofen, iodides, phenacetin, phenothiazines, procainamide, rifampin, propylthiouracil, and streptokinase (*Figs 14.47* and *14.48*).[6–15] Anti-TNF-α therapies have been linked to vasculitic reactions.[16,17] Vasculitis has also been associated with ustekinumab.[18] As discussed in the chapter on vasculitis, levamisole tainted cocaine is another cause of drug-induced vasculitis.[19]

Granulomatous vasculitis has been described following treatment with chlorothiazide, allopurinol, phenytoin, and carbamazepine.[6,20–22]

Purpuric drug reactions

Clinical features

Purpura may be a manifestation of an adverse drug reaction. Causes include NSAIDs, diuretics, meprobamate, zomepirac sodium, ampicillin,

pseudoephedrine, linezolid, and lidocaine/prilocaine cream.[1–4] Purpuric eruptions at friction sites have been associated with angiotensin II receptor inhibitors.[5]

Histologic features

The histologic features are those of red cell extravasation in the absence of changes of vasculitis (*Fig. 14.49*).

Granulomatous drug reactions

Clinical features

Interstitial granulomatous drug reactions are rare and have been associated with a number of drugs including calcium channel blockers, ACE inhibitors, beta blockers, lipid-lowering agents, diuretics, NSAIDs, antihistamines, anticonvulsants, and antidepressants.[1] IL-1 inhibitor (anakinra), adalimumab, sorafenib, ganciclovir, thalidomide, desmopressin, allopurinol, febuxostat, and quetiapine have also been associated with an interstitial granulomatous reaction.[2–9] This reaction pattern may also be related to a variety of systemic illnesses including rheumatoid arthritis, hepatobiliary disease, diabetes mellitus, Crohn disease, and chronic infections such as hepatitis C, herpes simplex/varicella-zoster, EBV, and HIV.[2] Patients present with erythematous to violaceous, nonpruritic, irregular and sometimes annular papules or plaques predominantly affecting the inner arms, inner thighs, and the groins (*Fig. 14.50*).[1] Erythroderma in a case of anticonvulsant-induced hypersensitivity syndrome has also been described.[4] A patient with an allopurinol triggered granulomatous drug eruption also had coexisting DRESS syndrome.[7]

Histologic features

Histologically, the eruption is characterized by an interstitial infiltrate of lymphocytes, histiocytes, eosinophils, plasma cells, and multinucleate giant cells, sometimes associated with increased dermal mucin and showing more than a superficial resemblance to interstitial granuloma annulare (*Figs 14.51* and *14.52*). Fragmentation of collagen fibers and elastic tissue is commonly evident and phagocytosis of connective tissue debris by giant cells is typically seen (*Figs 14.53* and *14.54*). Discrete granulomata may also be identified and granulomatous vasculitis has been documented.[10,11] Flame figures and Churg-Strauss-like granulomata have also been described.[12,13] Atypical lymphocytes with hyperchromatic, irregular, and variably enlarged nuclei showing epidermotropism are present in up to 50% of cases.[1] In rare cases, the granulomatous drug eruption can have epidermotropism and positive clonality mimicking granulomatous mycosis fungoides.[14] The changes of interface dermatitis, sometimes with an associated lichenoid infiltrate, are found in the majority of cases.[1,11]

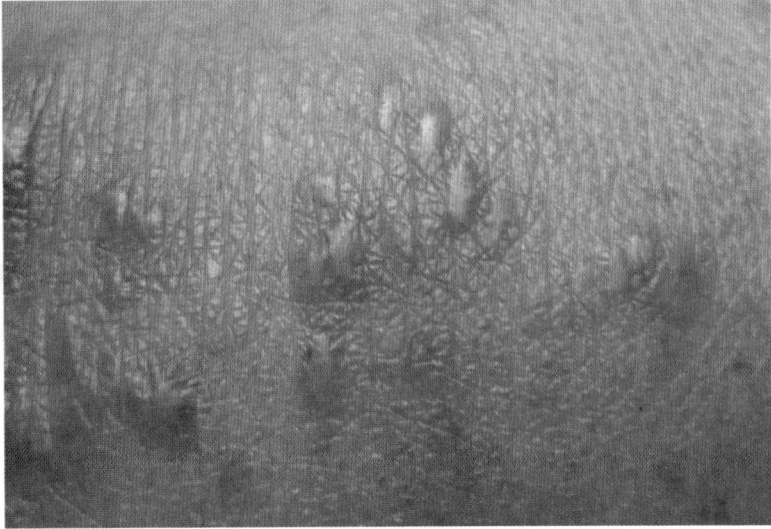

Fig. 14.50
Lichenoid and granulomatous dermatitis: note the flat-topped lichenoid papules. This reaction developed during rituximab therapy. By courtesy of J. Francis, MD, Virginia Commonwealth University, Richmond, Virginia, USA.

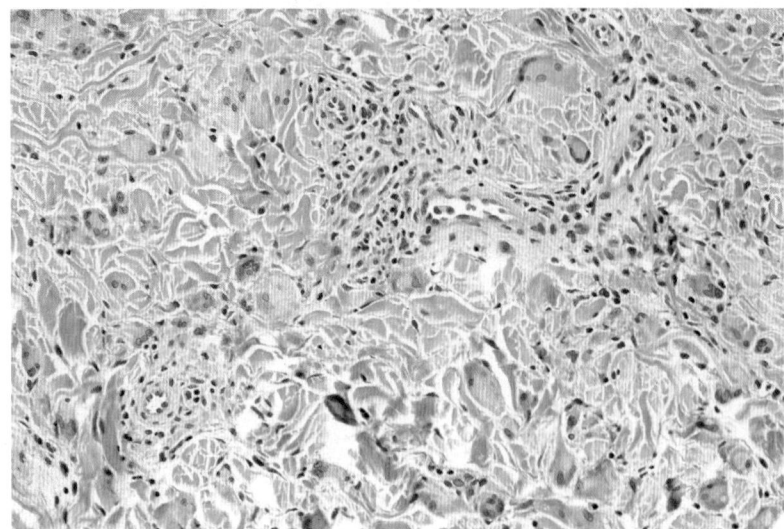

Fig. 14.52
Granulomatous drug reaction: in this example, there is an obvious interstitial distribution reminiscent of granuloma annulare.

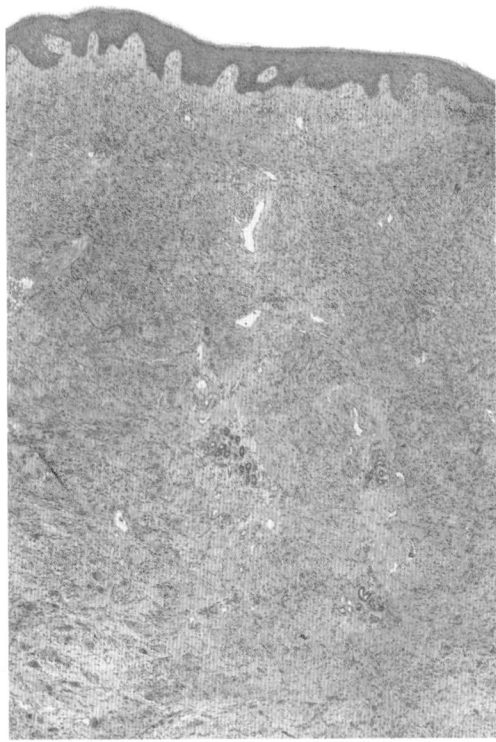

Fig. 14.51
Granulomatous drug reaction: there is a marked infiltrate involving the full thickness of the dermis.

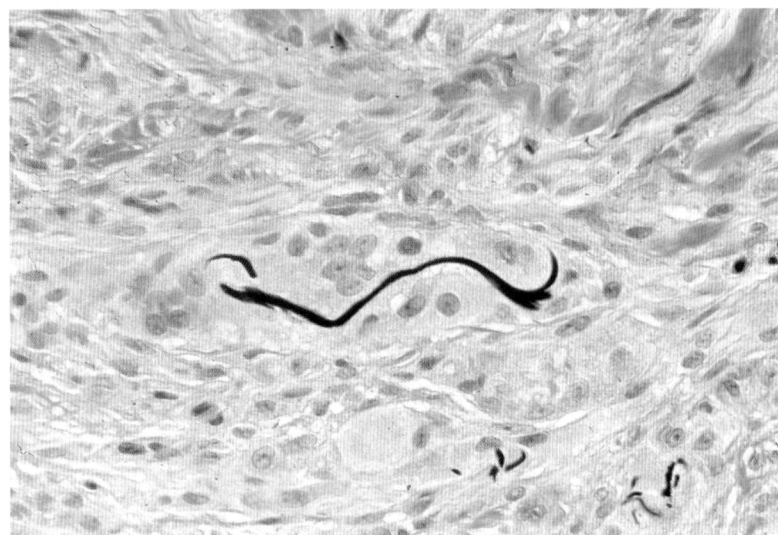

Fig. 14.53
Granulomatous drug reaction: there is extensive elastophagocytosis (elastic van Gieson).

Differential diagnosis

Interstitial granulomatous drug reactions must be distinguished from granuloma annulare and systemic disease-associated lesions as described above. Granuloma annulare is not usually associated with interface dermatitis, and necrobiosis and mucin deposition are not typical features of granulomatous drug reactions. Systemic disease-associated granulomatous dermatitis is usually associated with vasculitic and/or thrombotic phenomena.[13] In cases where significant lymphoid atypia is present, cutaneous T-cell lymphoma enters the differential diagnosis.[14] When elastophagocytosis is marked, granulomatous slack skin or an elastolytic granuloma may be important diagnostic considerations. Correlation with clinical history and resolution with withdrawal of the triggering agent is critical in confirming the diagnosis.

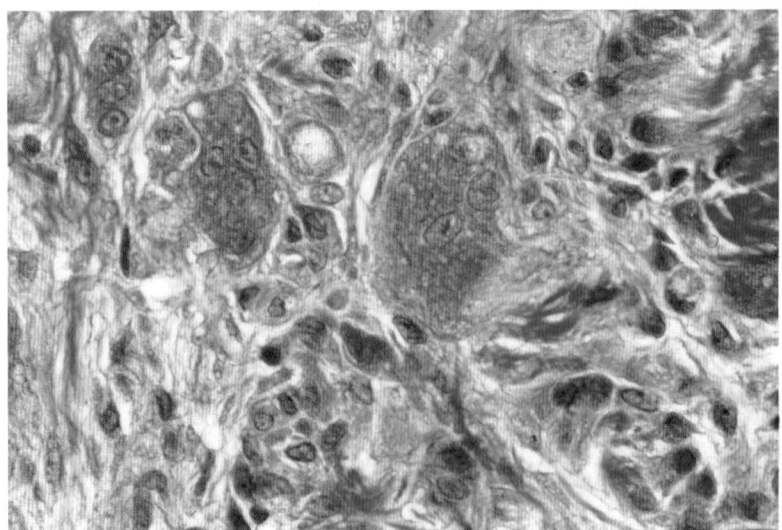

Fig. 14.54
Granulomatous drug reaction: phagocytosis of collagen may also be seen (Masson trichrome).

Drug-induced erythema nodosum

This topic is discussed in the chapter on panniculitis.

Drug-induced alopecia

Drug-induced alopecia is usually reversible, predominantly nonscarring, and affects females more often than males.[1–4]

Anagen effluvium, in which hair growth stops due to cessation of mitotic activity, is a common feature of anticancer therapy and often develops days or a few weeks after starting the drug.[1,2] The scalp and beard areas, which contain a high percentage of anagen follicles, are particularly affected. It especially complicates combination chemotherapy and is likely to be severe.[5] Although all anticancer drugs may be associated with some degree of alopecia, particular offenders include bleomycin, cyclophosphamide, dactinomycin, daunorubicin, doxorubicin, 5-fluorouracil, ifosfamide, and vindesine.[1,2] There is some variation in drug effect. Some cause alopecia in all individuals whereas others affect only a minority of patients.[5] In addition to traditional chemotherapeutics, targeted chemotherapeutics, especially vismodegib, sorafenib, and vemurafenib, are associated with alopecia.[6] TNF-α antagonists and endocrine-based chemotherapies are also associated with alopecia.[7,8]

Telogen effluvium, in which hairs are transformed into the telogen phase, develops several months after commencing therapy.[1] Anticoagulants, including heparin and warfarin and dextran sulfate, cause telogen effluvium in up to 50% of patients.[3,5,9–14] Other causes include antithyroid drugs such as iodine, thiouracil and carbimazole, oral contraceptives, lithium, IFNs, retinoids, and pramipexole.[5,15–17]

Alopecia areata may develop as a consequence of TNF-α inhibitors such as adalimumab, etanercept, and infliximab.[18–21] Case reports of alopecia areata have also been reported secondary to acitretin, vandetanib, and ustekinumab.[22–24]

Drug-induced lupus erythematosus

Clinical features

Drug-induced systemic lupus erythematosus was first described as a complication of hydralazine.[1–8] It has also been reported in association with procainamide, quinidine, sulfasalazine, chlorpromazine, penicillamine, methyldopa, carbamazepine, acebutalol, isoniazid, captopril, propylthiouracil, and minocycline.[2,3] Therapy with TNF-α inhibitors has been associated with a lupus-like syndrome.[9,10] Imiquimod can also induce a lupus-like reaction that histologically and clinically resemble subacute cutaneous lupus erythematosus.[11–14] With the exception of hydralazine and procainamide (high risk) and quinidine (medium risk), the other associations are low risk.[2] Laboratory investigations reveal anti-Ro, anti-La, and antinuclear antibodies (ANAs) in the majority of cases.[1] Subacute cutaneous lupus erythematosus-like features have been described following treatment with terbinafine.[15–17] Localized cutaneous lupus lesions occurring at the site of IFN injection have been reported.[18] Cutaneous lesions including malar erythema, discoid lesions, photosensitivity, oral ulceration, and alopecia are rare.[2] Anti-TNF-α therapy-induced lupus may result in a higher incidence of cutaneous lesions, hypocomplementemia, and positive serology for double-stranded DNA as compared to other medications.[17] Symptoms typically develop months to years after initiating therapy.[19] Diagnostic criteria have been defined as follows[2]:

- continuous treatment with the suspected drug for 1 month or longer,
- common presenting symptoms include arthralgias/arthritis, myositis, serositis, malaise and fever,
- antihistone antibodies frequent, particularly IgG anti-([H2A-H2B]-DNA),
- most importantly, clinical improvement within days or weeks after stopping the suspected drug.

Histologic features

The histologic features of cutaneous lesions are indistinguishable from those seen in the idiopathic forms.[14,20]

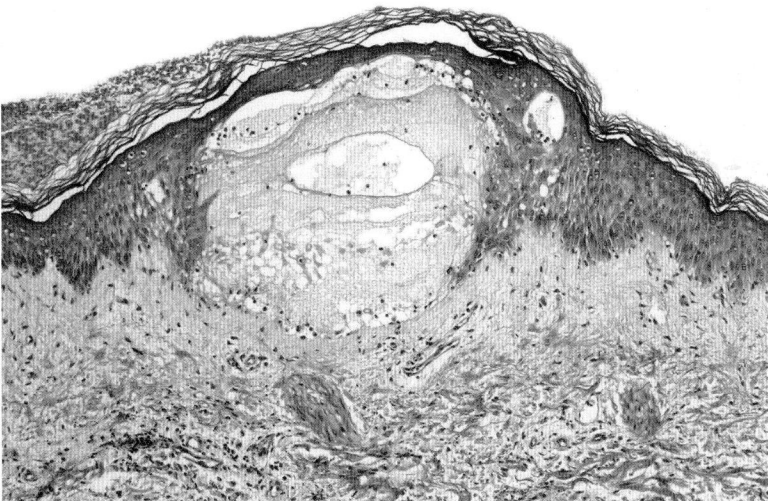

Fig. 14.55
Bullous drug reaction: this subepidermal blister arose against a background of an exanthematous drug reaction.

Bullous drug reactions

Blisters may develop within the setting of an adverse drug reaction either as a consequence of severe spongiosis or marked interface change or they may reflect drug-related autoimmune bullous disorders (*Fig. 14.55*). In this section, only the last are discussed. These include drug-induced linear IgA disease, bullous pemphigoid, epidermolysis bullosa acquisita, pemphigus variants, and drug-induced pseudoporphyria. Many alleged drug reactions are single case reports, particularly in patients taking multiple medications. It is often difficult to determine which associations are therefore coincidental and which are genuine. In occasional reports, recrudescence following re-exposure to the offending agent has been documented.

The precise mechanism of drug-induced blistering is unknown, although multiple factors have been suggested[1]:

- Direct toxicity to basement membrane constituents or intercellular junctions with resultant autoantibody production.
- The drug may function as a hapten.
- The drug may be antigenically similar to a basement membrane or intercellular junction constituent.
- Perturbation of the immune system with inappropriate production of antibasement membrane antibodies.
- Drug-induced abnormality of cell membrane calcium metabolism.

Drug-induced linear IgA disease

Drug-induced linear IgA disease is most often associated with intravenous therapy with vancomycin.[1–10] Similar eruptions, however, have also been described following treatment with trimethoprim-sulfamethoxazole, penicillin, phenytoin, somatostatin, lithium, amiodarone, captopril, cefamandole, ceftriaxone, ciclosporine, IL-2, IFN-alpha, penicillin, amoxicillin, vigabatrin, diclophenac, ketoprofen, buprenorphine, infliximab, piperacillin-tazobactam, ustekinumab, and following vaccination for human papilloma virus.[2,11–27] Cutaneous manifestations of vancomycin-induced linear IgA disease include pruritic, erythematous, urticarial, targetoid, and bullous lesions with a predilection for the trunk, extremities, palms, and soles (*Figs 14.56* and *14.57*).[1] Morbilliform lesions have also been described.[8] Mucosal involvement is present in up to 40% of cases. As such, there can be considerable clinical overlap with EM and TEN.[2,9,10] Laryngeal involvement has been documented.[20] Drug-induced linear IgA disease tends to be more severe than spontaneous forms.[28]

Pathogenesis and histologic features

By definition, linear IgA deposition along the basement membrane region is present in all cases (*Fig. 14.58*). C3 is seen in approximately 20% of cases.[7]

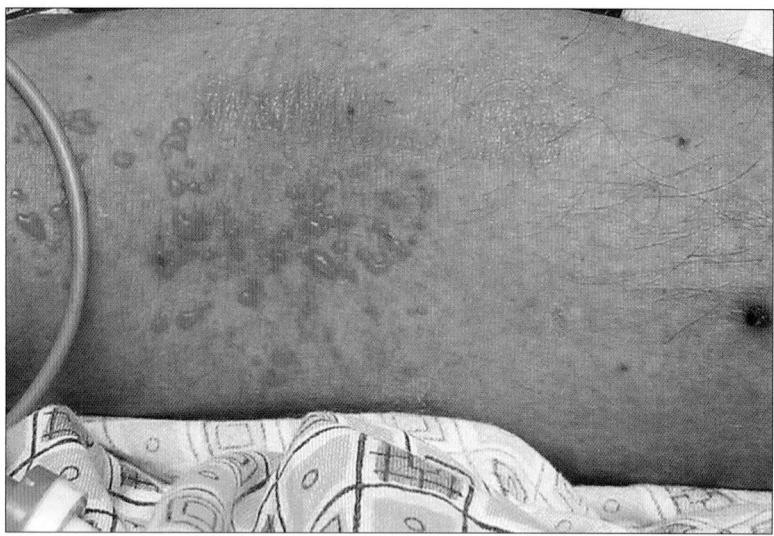

Fig. 14.56
Drug-induced linear IgA disease: these blisters developed following treatment with vancomycin. By courtesy of B.A. Solky, MD, Department of Dermatology, Harvard Medical School, Boston, USA.

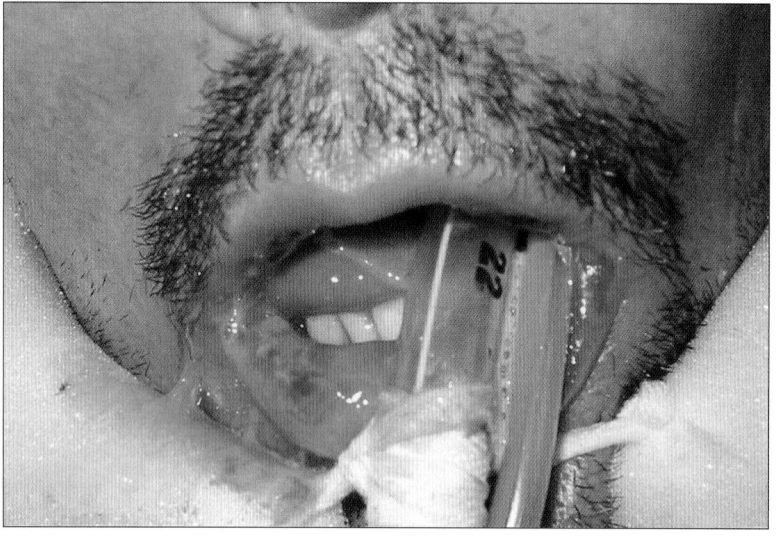

Fig. 14.57
Drug-induced linear IgA disease: oral lesions were also present. By courtesy of B.A. Solky, MD, Department of Dermatology, Harvard Medical School, Boston, USA.

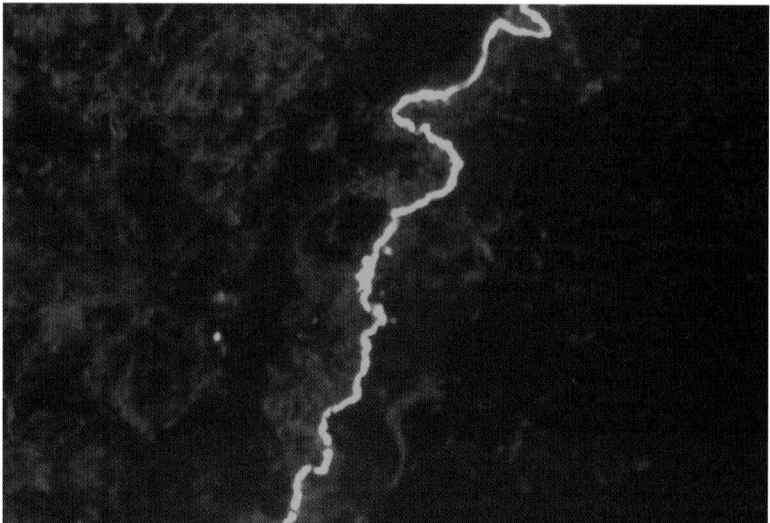

Fig. 14.58
Vancomycin-induced linear IgA disease: immunofluorescence showed strong basement membrane deposition of IgA.

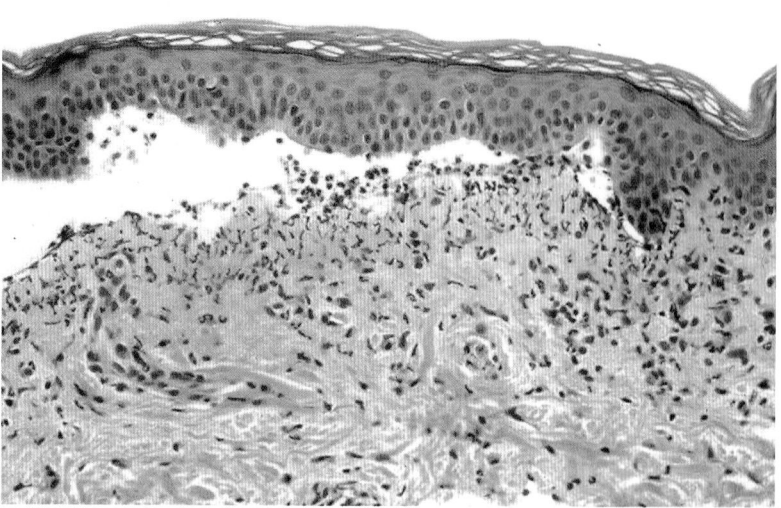

Fig. 14.59
Vancomycin-induced linear IgA disease: this case showed a neutrophil-rich subepidermal blister.

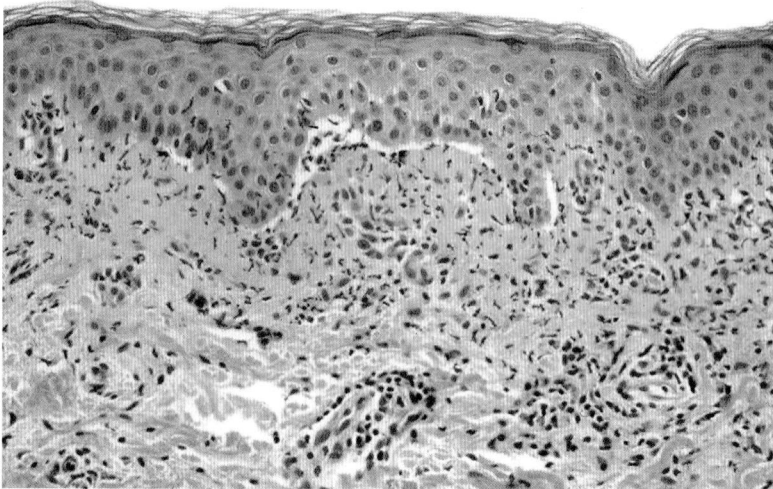

Fig. 14.60
Vancomycin-induced linear IgA disease: the adjacent skin showed neutrophil dermal papillary microabscesses.

Linear IgG may also very exceptionally be present, although distinction from drug-induced bullous pemphigoid can then be problematical.[3,17] Such cases may, in fact, represent examples of drug-induced IgA-mediated bullous pemphigoid.[21] Circulating IgA antibasement membrane zone antibodies are found in 25% of cases.[1] Split skin studies predominantly localize to the floor of the blister cavity.[1,2] By immunoelectron microscopy, the results are heterogeneous, IgA having been detected within the lamina lucida, lamina densa, and in the sublamina densa.[18-20] Western immunoblotting has detected a number of antigens including a 230-kD antigen (bullous pemphigoid antigen 1), a 97-kD antigen (an anchoring filament protein), and also a 250-kD antigen corresponding to type VII collagen.[19,20]

Histologically, a neutrophil-rich subepidermal blister is seen in the majority of cases, but sometimes eosinophils are conspicuous (Figs 14.59–14.61).[2]

Drug-induced bullous pemphigoid

Clinical features

A variety of drugs including captopril, ciprofloxacin, chloroquine, furosemide (frusemide), ibuprofen, mefenamic acid, nifedipine, penicillamine,

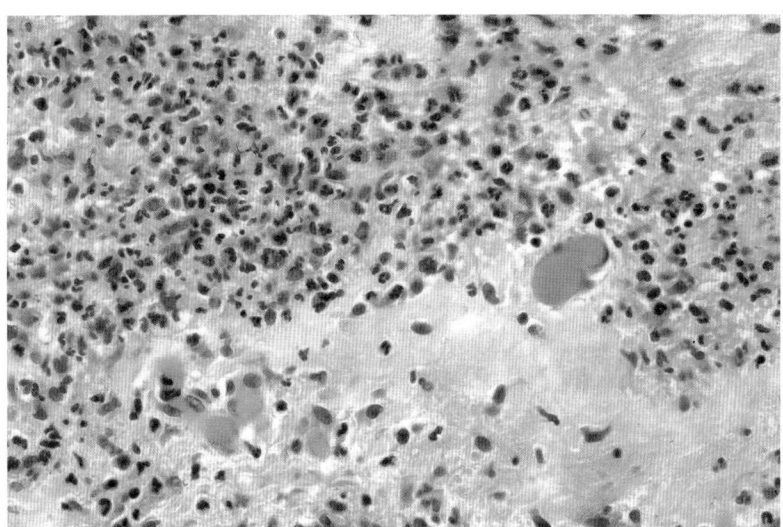

Fig. 14.61
Vancomycin-induced linear IgA disease: conspicuous eosinophils may raise suspicion for bullous pemphigoid if the clinical information is unavailable.

penicillins, phenacetin, sulfasalazine, spironolactone, enoxaparin, dipeptidyl peptidase IV inhibitors, metronidazole, mammalian target of rapamycin (mTOR) inhibitors, and levofloxacin have been incriminated in alleged drug-induced bullous and mucosal pemphigoid.[1–19] Of these, antirheumatics, cardiovascular drugs, and antimicrobial drugs are the most important.[6] Penicillamine is among the most commonly incriminated (mucosal more than bullous), usually in rheumatoid arthritis patients.[6,20–21] Furosemide (frusemide) is believed to be an important cause of drug-induced bullous pemphigoid, although recently this has been challenged, with the author suggesting that diagnoses of pseudoporphyria or epidermolysis bullosa acquisita may be more appropriate.[6,22,23] The ACE inhibitors, captopril and enalapril, have both been associated with immunologically proven bullous pemphigoid.[2,8] The penicillins including amoxicillin and procaine penicillin G are the most frequently implicated antibiotics.[6]

Clinically, drug-induced bullous pemphigoid is similar to idiopathic disease although the lesions are often polymorphic, mimicking other drug-induced bullous dermatoses such as EM, eczematous dermatitis, and porphyria cutanea tarda.[6] In drug-induced disease, mucous membranes are often involved, thereby blurring the distinction between bullous and mucosal variants of pemphigoid. In some patients, there appears to be overlap between bullous pemphigoid and pemphigus vulgaris.[6]

Histologic features

Drug-induced variants are characterized by linear IgG and C3 along the basement membrane region on direct immunofluorescence.[7,8] By indirect immunofluorescence, the antibodies bind to the epidermal side (roof) of split skin.[2,5,6] Western immunoblotting has demonstrated that the antibodies react with both the 230- and 180-kD bullous pemphigoid antigens.[2,3]

Histologically, drug-induced variants are similar to typical bullous pemphigoid, being characterized by an eosinophil-rich subepidermal blister.

Drug-induced epidermolysis bullosa acquisita

Drug-induced epidermolysis bullosa acquisita has been described following treatment with granulocyte-macrophage colony-stimulating factor (GM-CSF) and in a patient receiving vancomycin and gentamicin therapy.[1,2] In both patients, the blisters were subepidermal and eosinophil rich; direct immunofluorescence disclosed linear IgA and IgG deposits at the basement membrane region. Split skin indirect immunofluorescence in the former patient labeled the floor of the blister cavity and by immunoelectron microscopy the deposits were localized to the lamina densa and the sublamina densa region.[1] In the latter patient, IgG antibodies against type VII collagen were recognized by an enzyme-linked immunosorbent assay

(ELISA).[2] An epidermolysis bullosa acquisita-like reaction has also been described after treatment with penicillamine. Histologic features included a pauci-inflammatory subepidermal blister. Linear deposition of C3, IgG, and IgM are seen on direct immunofluorescence, and IgG labels to the base of the blister on salt-spilt direct immunofluorescence.[3]

A significant number of cases of vancomycin-induced linear IgA disease are characterized by antibodies which label the floor of split skin on indirect immunofluorescence. Many of these might represent examples of drug-induced epidermolysis bullosa acquisita.[2] An epidermolysis bullosa acquisita-like blistering dermatosis has been described with penicillamine therapy, but this has not been confirmed with immunofluorescent or molecular data.[3]

Drug-induced pemphigus

Clinical features

Pemphigus may be related to a wide range of drugs, either directly as a causative factor or indirectly as a precipitating or triggering factor.[1–15] The range of drugs is quite wide but many belong to the thiol group of compounds (characterized by the presence of an -SH group) including penicillamine, captopril, bucillamine, and thiopronine.[1,4,15] Thiol-induced acantholysis is mediated by both immune and direct biochemical mechanisms.[5] Penicillamine most often induces pemphigus in the setting of rheumatoid arthritis.[6] Although foliaceus is most commonly encountered, vulgaris, erythematosus, and herpetiform variants may occur.[2,6–8,15] Other drugs that contain sulfur, which can also form -SH groups, include gold compounds, penicillins, rifampicin, and cephalosporins.[4] Topical application of imiquimod has been reported to cause pemphigus foliaceus and vegetans.[16–18] Additionally, both pemphigus foliaceus and vulgaris lesions have been described as a consequence of radiotherapy.[19–22] Clinically, drug-induced pemphigus can resemble vulgaris, foliaceus, erythematosus, and vegetans variants, the first being most often encountered.[4] In the older literature, foliaceus variants were typical but with a change in prescribing habits to non-thiol-related drugs, vulgaris-type cases are more frequently seen.[4] In most cases of imiquimod-induced pemphigus foliaceus, disease is localized to the sites of application, although there is one report of both localized and distant lesions.[17] In the setting of radiotherapy, all patients developed pemphigus at the site of radiation.[19–24] One patient also had distant lesions.[25]

Pathogenesis and histologic features

Histologically, drug-induced and idiopathic variants are indistinguishable.[26] Intercellular IgG and circulating antibodies are variable in drug-induced pemphigus, although in a series of 10 patients all had positive direct immunofluorescence and 80% had circulating antibodies.[4] Such antibodies may recognize desmoglein 3 and/or 1.[1,25]

Drug-induced pseudoporphyria

Clinical features

Pseudoporphyria is a rare blistering disease that clinically and histologically mimics porphyria but which develops in the setting of normal porphyrin metabolism (*Fig. 14.62*). There are many causes including drugs, chronic renal failure usually in the setting of dialysis, excessive sun exposure, and UVA. It has also been described following excessive use of sunbeds.[1–15] The most common medications include diuretics such as furosemide (frusemide) and NSAIDs, particularly naproxen. Other drugs include isotretinoin and the oral contraceptive. More recently imatinib, sunitinib, voriconazole, and diclofenac have been implicated.[14–19]

Pathogenesis and histologic features

The pathogenesis of pseudoporphyria is unknown, but it may (at least in some patients) represent a phototoxic photosensitivity reaction.[12]

Histologically, pseudoporphyria is identical to porphyria cutanea tarda. Typical lesions are characterized by a subepidermal cell-free blister, typically with preservation of the dermal papillae (festooning) and thickening of the vessel walls in the superficial dermis.

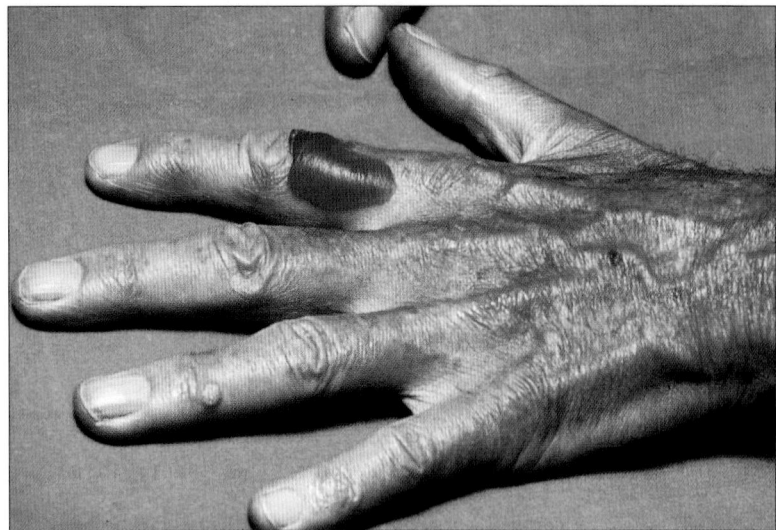

Fig. 14.62
Pseudoporphyria: trauma-induced blisters on the backs of the hands and fingers are characteristic. By courtesy of the Institute of Dermatology, London, UK.

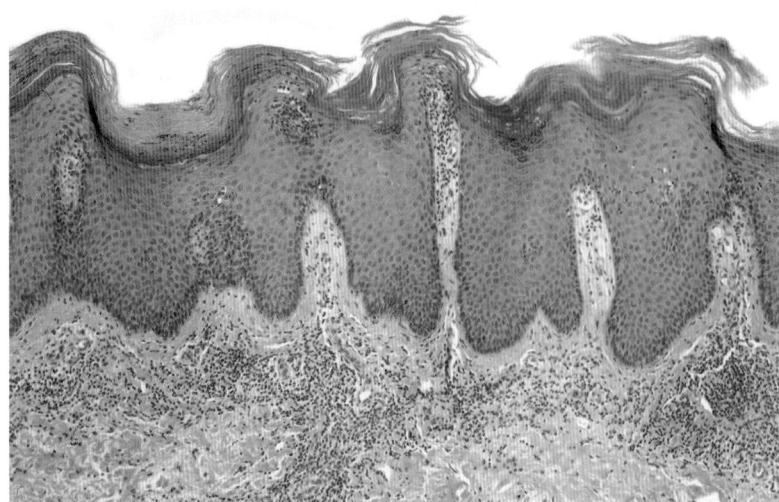

Fig. 14.63
Psoriasiform drug eruption: there is confluent parakeratosis with elongated, broadened, and partially fused rete ridges.

By immunofluorescence, immunoglobulin (most commonly IgG) is present at the dermal–epidermal junction and also outlining the superficial dermal vasculature.

Psoriasiform drug reactions

Clinical features

Psoriasis and psoriasiform dermatoses can be caused by a number of drugs including lithium, beta blockers, NSAIDs, synthetic antimalarials, and tetracycline.[1-5] Drug-induced disease may have variable presentations including[1,2]:

- exacerbation of pre-existing psoriasis,
- induction of new lesions in uninvolved psoriatic skin,
- precipitation of psoriasis de novo,
- resistance to treatment.

Lithium-induced psoriasis varies from exacerbation of pre-existing psoriasis to development of new disease.[2] Manifestations vary from plaque disease to generalized pustular psoriasis, palmoplantar pustulosis, scalp psoriasis, and psoriatic erythroderma.[2,6-8] Latency varies from 1 week to years or more.[2]

Beta blockers (e.g., propranolol, oxprenolol, pindolol, alprenolol, and the now discontinued practolol), antimalarials (e.g., chloroquine and hydroxychloroquine) and NSAIDs (e.g., indomethacin, phenylbutazone, oxyphenylbutazone, and ibuprofen) can also induce psoriasiform eruptions or result in exacerbations and flares.[1,2,9-15]

The increasing use of TNF-α inhibitors is associated with new-onset or exacerbated psoriasiform eruptions.[16-21] TNF-α inhibitors-induced psoriasis may be seen in approximately 1% of patients on the medication.[22] Most patients develop palmoplantar pustulosis or plaque-type psoriasis.[18-20] The average time to onset of lesions is 6–10 months, although the range is variable.[16-21] It is speculated that inhibition of TNF-α increases levels of type 1 IFNs which result in psoriasiform lesions.[21]

A large number of other drugs have been linked with exacerbation of psoriasis or development of new disease. These include the antifungal agent terbinafine, antibiotics such as penicillin and tetracycline, digoxin, amiodarone, IFN-α, recombinant IFN-α, erlotinib, and imiquimod.[2,23-34]

Histologic features

The histologic features overlap lichen simplex chronicus and psoriasis. Occasionally, they are indistinguishable from psoriasis vulgaris (Figs 14.63–14.65) or pustular psoriasis. Psoriasis secondary to TNF-α inhibitors may also demonstrate lichenoid inflammation and spongiosis.[21,35]

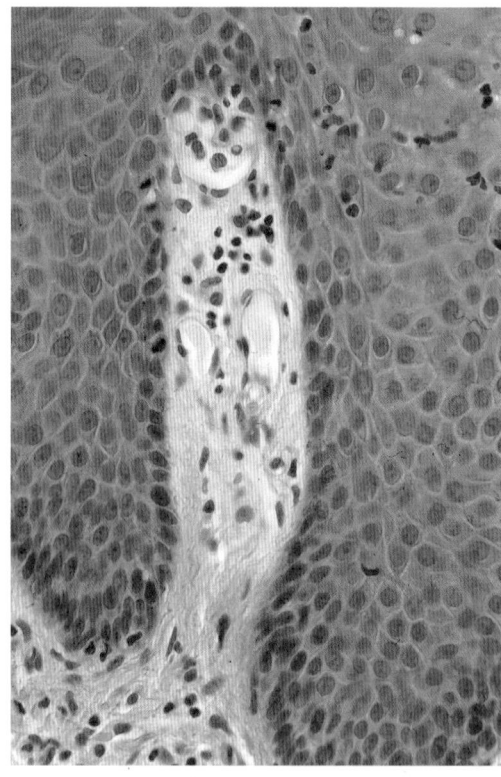

Fig. 14.64
Psoriasiform drug reaction: the capillaries in the dermal papillae are tortuous and dilated.

Pityriasiform drug reactions

Clinical features

Pityriasiform drug reactions may be particularly caused by ACE inhibitors and gold.[1-4] Less often, terbinafine, omeprazole, benfluorex, arsenicals, bismuth compounds, isotretinoin, naproxen, acetaminophen, barbiturates, and bacille Calmette-Guérin (BCG) therapy have been implicated.[5-13] The tyrosine kinase inhibitors imatinib and ponatinib have been associated with pityriasiform dermatitis.[12-16] Patients present with small erythematous lesions accompanied by a peripheral scale, which may follow Langer lines (cleavage lines), giving rise to the typical 'fir tree' appearance. The trunk and extremities are predominantly affected.

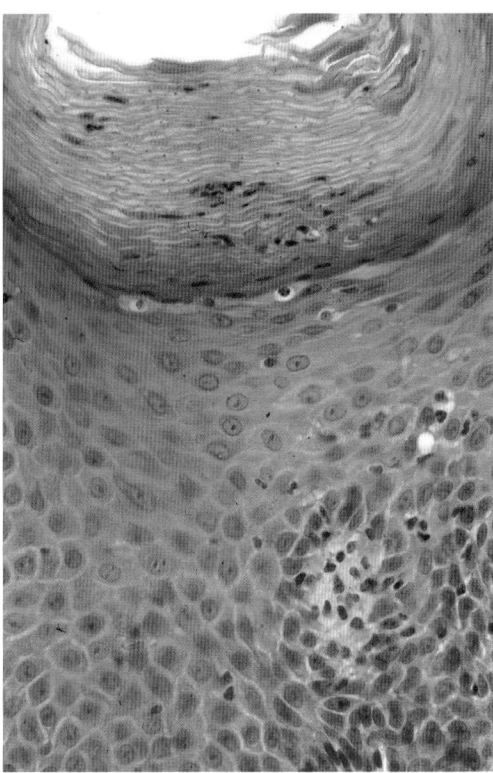

Fig. 14.65
Psoriasiform drug reaction: neutrophils are present in the stratum corneum.

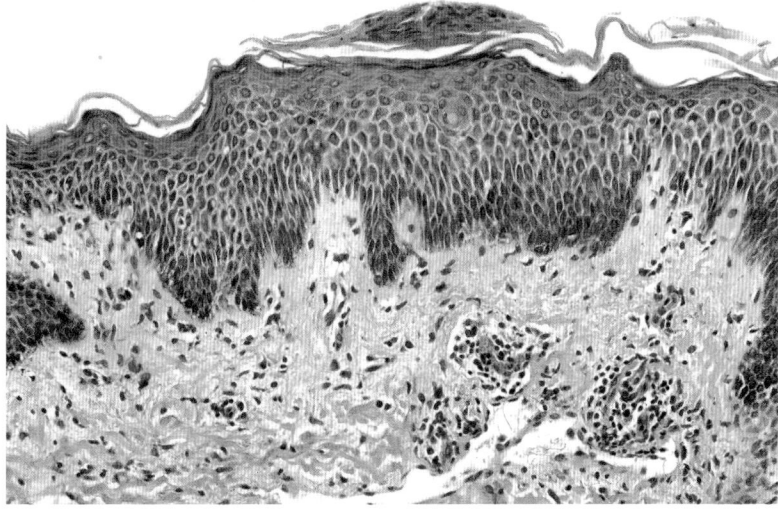

Fig. 14.66
Pityriasiform drug reaction: there is a focal parakeratotic scale associated with acanthosis and spongiosis. A perivascular chronic inflammatory cell infiltrate surrounds the superficial vasculature.

Histologic features

Histologically, pityriasiform drug reactions are typically characterized by patchy parakeratosis, focal spongiosis with lymphocytic exocytosis, and a superficial perivascular lymphocytic infiltrate, sometimes associated with red cell extravasation (*Fig. 14.66*)[3,6] On occasions, clinically typical pityriasiform drug eruptions may demonstrate a more psoriasiform histology.[9]

Pustular drug reactions

Clinical features

Drug-induced pustules are a manifestation of reactions to corticosteroids, anabolic steroids, oral contraceptives, isoniazid, haloperidol, and lithium

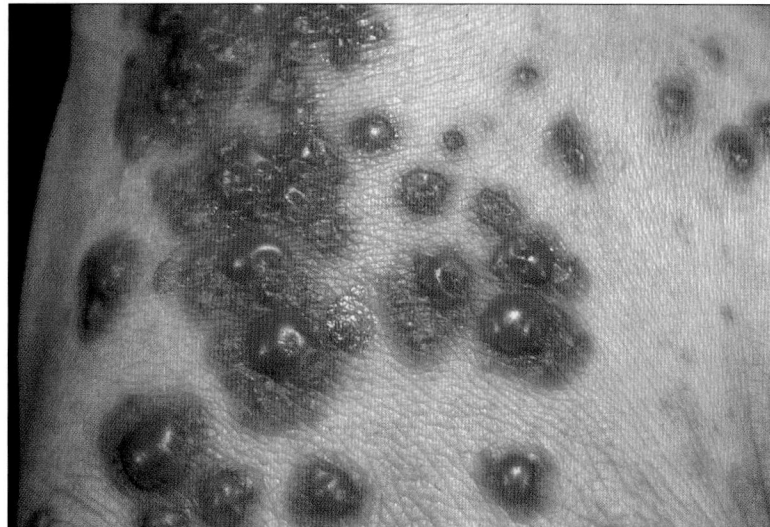

Fig. 14.67
Pustular drug reaction: numerous pustules are present on an erythematous background. By courtesy of the Institute of Dermatology, London, UK.

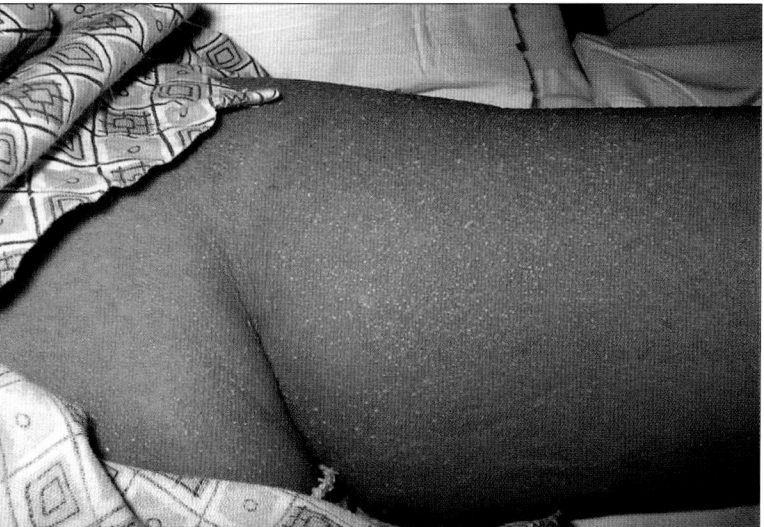

Fig. 14.68
Acute generalized exanthematous pustulosis: tiny pustules are evident. There is intense erythema. By courtesy of B.A. Solky, MD, Department of Dermatology, Harvard Medical School, Boston, USA.

therapy (*Fig. 14.67*).[1] In addition, they are a feature of the halogenodermas (see below).

Pustules are also the main feature of acute generalized exanthematous pustulosis (AGEP, toxic pustuloderma) (*Fig. 14.68*). This rare condition is characterized by the sudden onset of numerous small, nonfollicular pustules arising against a background of pruritic or burning edematous erythroderma.[2–12] The eruption often starts on the face or in the intertriginous regions but soon becomes generalized.[3] The mucous membranes are affected in a minority of patients.[3] Facial edema, purpura, vesicles, blisters, and EM-like lesions have also been described.[3,6] Pyrexia is usually present. Although in the majority of patients there is no history of significant previous skin disease, in some there is a background of psoriasis.[3] The eruption usually resolves rapidly and is followed by widespread desquamation.[9] Peripheral leukocytosis with high neutrophil levels and sometimes eosinophilia can be present.[3,9]

While this disorder may occur as a feature of mercury toxicity or follow a viral infection (particularly enteroviruses) or spider bite, in the majority of cases it represents an adverse drug reaction.[3,13,14] In most patients, the eruption has followed antibiotic therapy including penicillin, amoxicillin, ampicillin, metronidazole, trimethoprim, erythromycin, and clindamycin.[3,9,15]

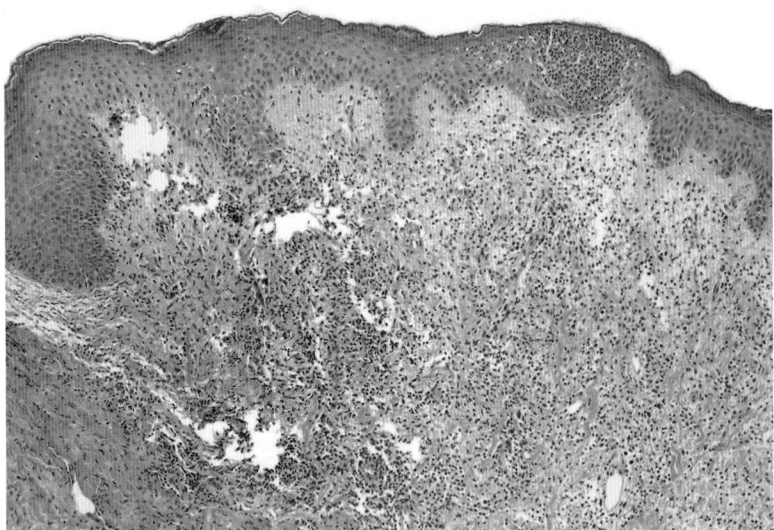

Fig. 14.69
Acute generalized exanthematous pustulosis: there is a subcorneal pustule. The dermis is intensely inflamed.

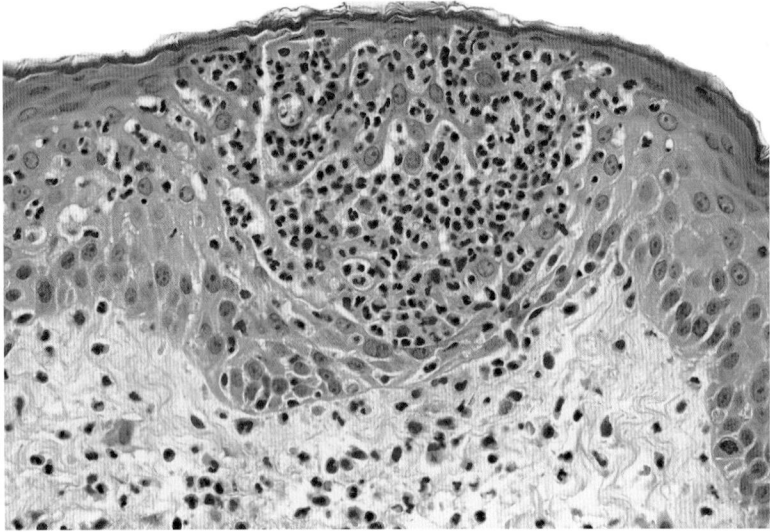

Fig. 14.70
Acute generalized exanthematous pustulosis: high-power view of pustule. Note the acantholysis.

Analgesics (e.g., acetaminophen), antiepileptics (e.g., carbamazepine), antidiabetics (e.g., carbutamide), antifungals (e.g., terbinafine), antimalarials (e.g., hydroxychloroquine), proton pump inhibitors, herbal medicines, and many other drugs have also been implicated.[3,11,12,16–26] The condition often develops rapidly following the administration of the drug, typically within 24–48 hours and sometimes more rapidly.[3,7,15–26]

Histologic features

The pustules are present in a subcorneal and/or intraepidermal location and sometimes contain a few acantholytic keratinocytes in addition to large numbers of neutrophils (*Figs 14.69* and *14.70*).[3,9] A background of spongiosis is usually evident. The dermal papillae are often edematous, and occasionally subepidermal vesiculation is a feature. A perivascular infiltrate of lymphocytes and histiocytes with conspicuous neutrophils and variable numbers of eosinophils is generally present in the superficial dermis. Leukocytoclastic vasculitis may be a feature in a significant proportion of cases.[3,9,11]

Differential diagnosis

The differential diagnosis includes pustular psoriasis, subcorneal pustular dermatosis, IgA pemphigus, pustular necrotizing angiitis, and acute

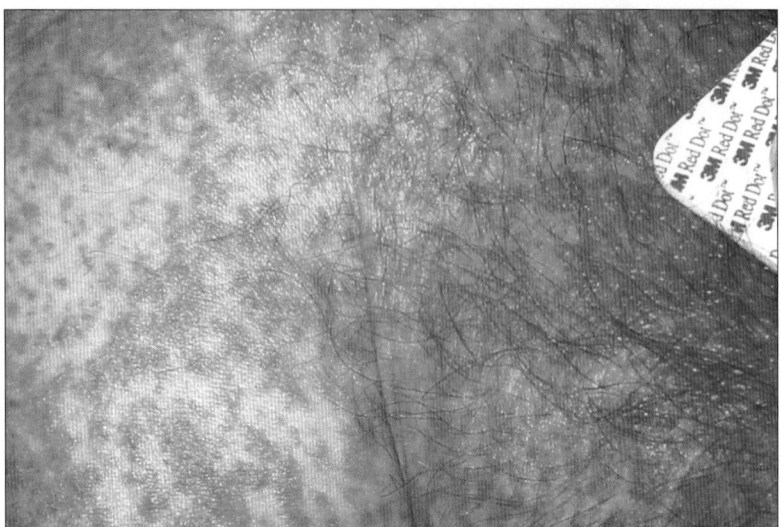

Fig. 14.71
Drug-induced pseudolymphoma: this patient developed a maculopapular eruption following treatment with phenytoin.

generalized pustular bacterid.[22,23] The rapid onset after introduction of a new medication is an important clue to the diagnosis.

Ichthyosiform drug reactions

Clinical features

Exceptionally, acquired ichthyosis following lipid-lowering agents (including triparanol and diazacholesterol) and kava consumption has been documented.[1–3] The clinical features may resemble ichthyosis vulgaris or lamellar ichthyosis.

Histologic features

In ichthyosis vulgaris-like drug-induced variants, there is mild hyperkeratosis associated with a diminished to absent granular cell layer. A mild superficial perivascular lymphohistiocytic infiltrate with occasional eosinophils may be present.

In the lamellar ichthyosis-like variant, there is marked hyperkeratosis, mild acanthosis, and a normal or thickened granular cell layer.

Drug-induced pseudolymphoma

Clinical features

Drug-induced pseudolymphoma includes pseudolymphomatous reactions to systemically administered medications (lymphomatoid drug eruption) and the much less frequent contact variant associated with locally administered agents (lymphomatoid contact dermatitis).[1–3]

Lymphomatoid drug eruptions are commonly a T-cell type, although B-cell lymphomatoid drug eruptions are also recognized. T-cell variants are divided into anticonvulsant-related and nonanticonvulsant-related variants.[2]

Anticonvulsant-related T-cell lymphomatoid drug eruption typically develops within weeks or months of commencing treatment. Patients present with pyrexia, lymphadenopathy, and an eruption of single or generalized lesions comprising erythematous, morbilliform maculopapules, plaques, nodules or tumors often associated with leukocytosis, circulating Sézary cells, eosinophilia, hepatosplenomegaly, and variable liver dysfunction (*Fig. 14.71*).[2,4–16] Vesicles and purpuric lesions have also been described.[14] Sézary syndrome-like features may rarely be seen.[17] A number of anticonvulsants have been implicated including phenytoin, primidone, mephenytoin, carbamazepine, phenobarbital, and trimethadione.[2]

Nonanticonvulsant-related pseudolymphomatous reactions present similarly with single lesions or multiple papules, plaques, and nodules.

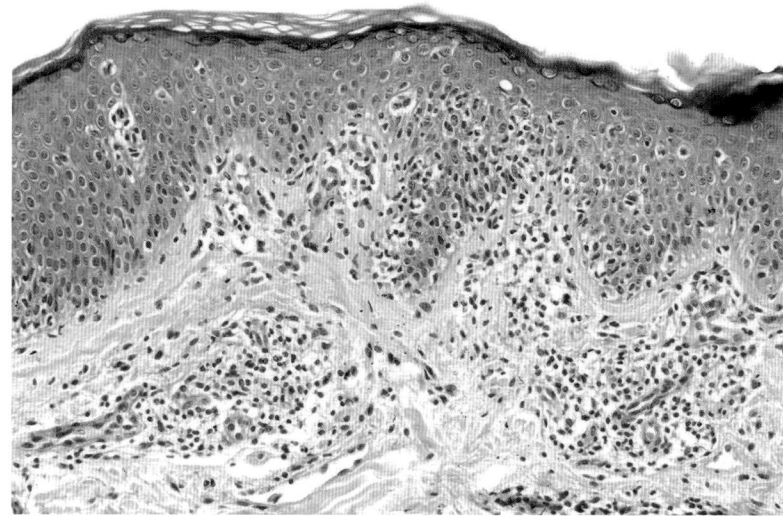

Fig. 14.72
Drug-induced pseudolymphoma: there is an atypical superficial perivascular lymphocytic infiltrate. Note the marked epidermotropism. The histological features are suggestive of mycosis fungoides.

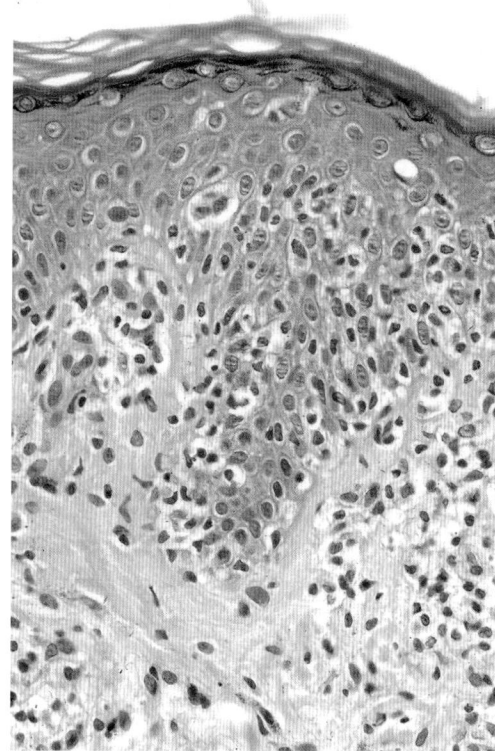

Fig. 14.73
Drug-induced pseudolymphoma: the lymphocytes are surrounded by a well-developed retraction artifact and there is a small Pautrier microabscess.

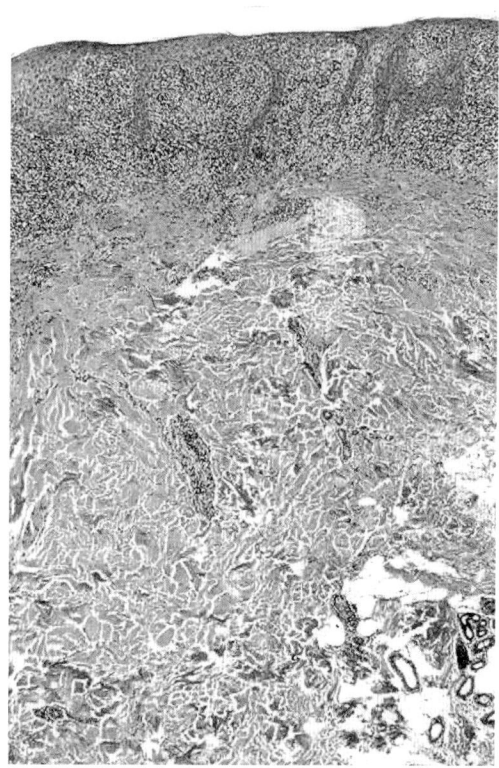

Fig. 14.74
Carbamazepine-induced pseudolymphoma: in this example, there is a dense bandlike upper dermal lymphocytic infiltrate.

Associated drugs include antihypertensives, antidepressants, tranquilizers, beta blockers, calcium channel blockers, diuretics, NSAIDs, antibiotics, tyrosine kinase inhibitors, and ciclosporine.[2,18–27] Sézary syndrome-like features have also been documented.[28]

Lymphomatoid contact dermatitis is much less common and usually represents a T-cell reaction to a contact allergen that histologically shows features reminiscent of mycosis fungoides.[2,29–41] Patients present with pruritic, localized to generalized scaly papules and plaques.[2] A number of antigens have been incriminated including matchbox striking surface antigens, ethylenediamine dihydrochloride, isopropyl-diphenylenediamine, phosphorus, nickel, gold, cobalt naphthenate, *para*-phenylenediamine, methylisothiazolinone, methylchoroisothiazolinone/methylisothiazolinone and paraben mix, textile dyes, and exotic wood on a toilet seat.

B-cell lymphomatoid drug reaction is rare but has been described in association with fluoxetine hydrochloride, amitriptyline hydrochloride, and levofloxacin.[2,21,22,42] Patients present with solitary nodules, multiple infiltrative plaques, or multiple papules.

B-cell lymphomatoid contact reactions may be seen with gold and nickel earrings. Patients present with one or more firm, erythematous nodules at the site of piercing.[43–45]

B-cell and, less commonly, T-cell pseudolymphomatous reactions may develop within tattoos.[46–52] Papules and nodules localized to the tattoo occur months to years after tattoo placement. The most common culprit is red pigment, although reactions to blue, green, and black dyes have been reported.[49,50,52] Both metals and organic synthetic pigments are implicated as antigens in such reactions.

Pathogenesis and histologic features

The pathogenesis of lymphomatoid drug reactions is not completely understood, but is thought to be secondary to immune dysregulation.[27,53] Studies show that medications implicated in drug-induced pseudolymphoma can induce proliferation of T cells and inhibit suppressor T cells, both in vivo and in vitro.[53,54] This may lead to an increase in helper T cells as well as B cells, resulting in T-cell and B-cell pseudolymphoma, respectively.

Drug-induced T-cell pseudolymphoma most often presents as a dense superficial perivascular or bandlike infiltrate composed of lymphocytes, histiocytes, and atypical lymphoid cells with irregular, enlarged, and hyperchromatic nuclei (*Figs 14.72–14.76*).[55] Cerebriform variants may be seen, and there is often associated epidermotropism. Pautrier-like microabscesses reminiscent of mycosis fungoides, however, are only occasionally identified. Eosinophils are frequently evident and often the epidermis shows significant spongiosis. Giant cells, collections of histiocytes, and epithelioid granulomata may also be evident. Dense nodular and tumorlike variants more suggestive of anaplastic T-cell lymphoma may also be encountered (*Figs 14.77–14.79*). A follicular mucinosis-like variant has rarely been described.[22] The infiltrate may also have a prominent angiocentric pattern with numerous immunoblasts.[56] A clinical case of AGEP secondary to clindamycin that histologically mimicked a lymphomatoid drug reaction has also been reported.[57]

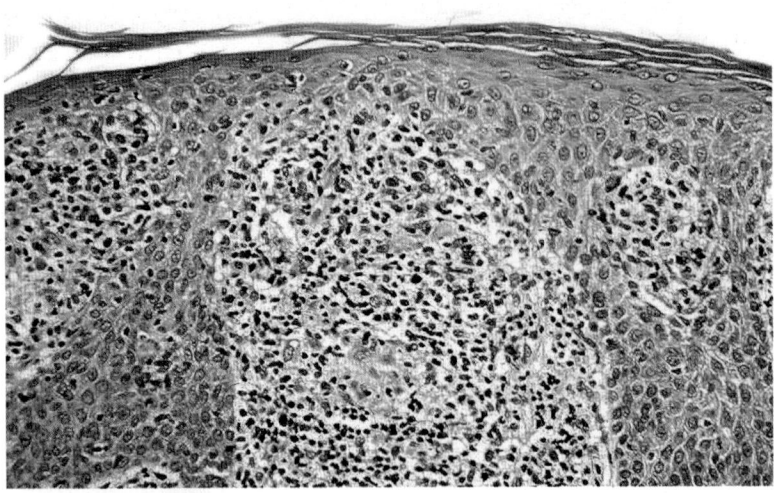

Fig. 14.75
Carbamazepine-induced pseudolymphoma: there is marked lymphocytic atypia. Cerebriform cells are present. The features are very suggestive of plaque stage mycosis fungoides.

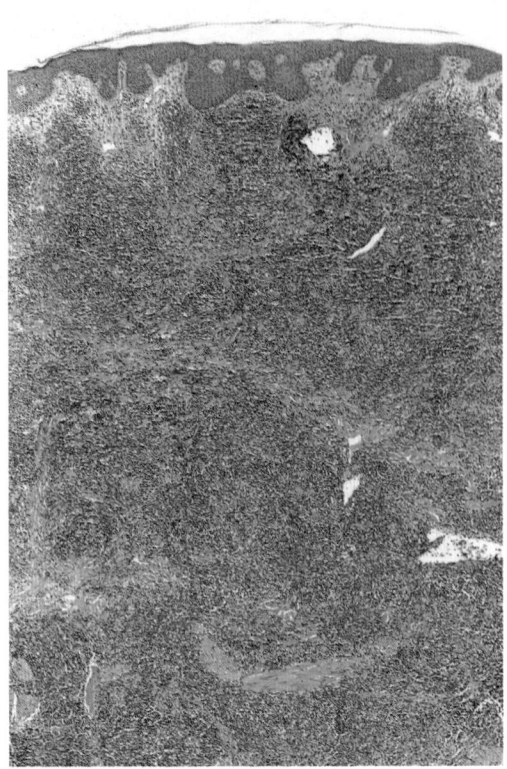

Fig. 14.77
Drug-induced pseudolymphoma: this very dense dermal infiltrate developed following treatment with an antidepressant. Multiple cutaneous nodules were present.

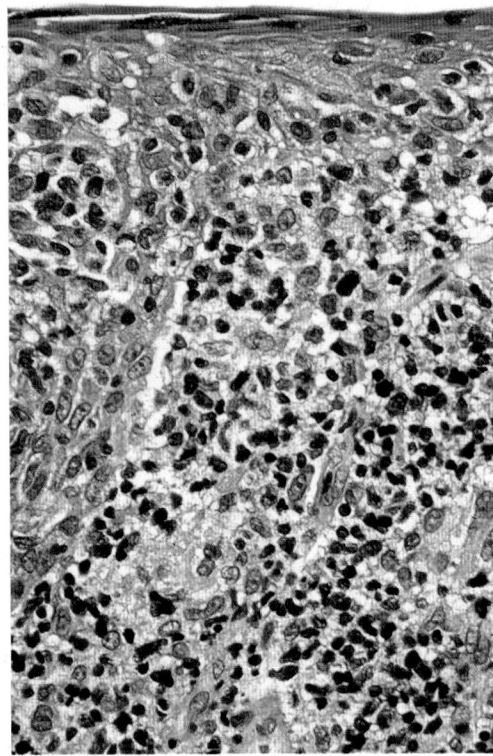

Fig. 14.76
Carbamazepine-induced pseudolymphoma: diagnosis depends on careful clinicopathological correlation.

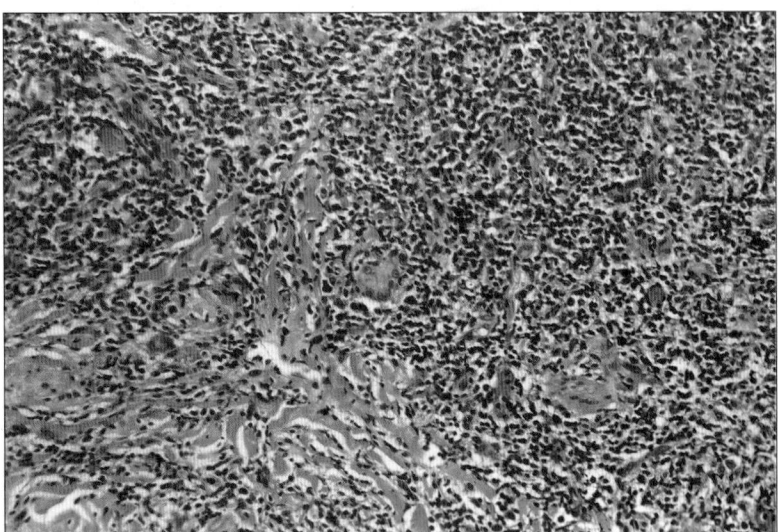

Fig. 14.78
Drug-induced pseudolymphoma: scattered multinucleated giant cells are evident.

By immunohistochemistry, the infiltrate consists of CD3+ T cells. CD4+ cells most often outnumber CD8+ forms, and CD20+ B cells are either extremely sparse or absent. A CD8+ variant has, however, been described following treatment with gemcitabine and infliximab.[58,59] CD30 expression with resultant confusion with an anaplastic large cell lymphoma or lymphomatoid papulosis has also been described.[11,24,27,56,59,60]

Reported TCR gene rearrangement studies have disclosed a clonal population in only a small minority of patients.[5,6,12,14]

Lymphomatoid contact dermatitis most often is reminiscent of mycosis fungoides and is characterized by a superficial dermal bandlike infiltrate composed of atypical lymphocytes and histiocytes with variable lymphocyte epidermotropism. The epidermis is typically acanthotic, and spongiosis may sometimes be present.

Immunohistochemical analysis has been reported in a small number of cases. The atypical lymphocytes usually express CD3 and CD4 with no loss of CD5 and CD7. A CD8 predominant variant has been documented.[34]

In the limited number of cases in which TCR gene rearrangements have been documented, most disclosed a polyclonal pattern while true monoclonal bands are rare.[31,34,36,61]

B-cell lymphomatoid drug reactions are characterized by a nodular or diffuse pandermal infiltrate, often accompanied by extension into the subcutaneous fat. The infiltrate consists of lymphocytes and histiocytes with

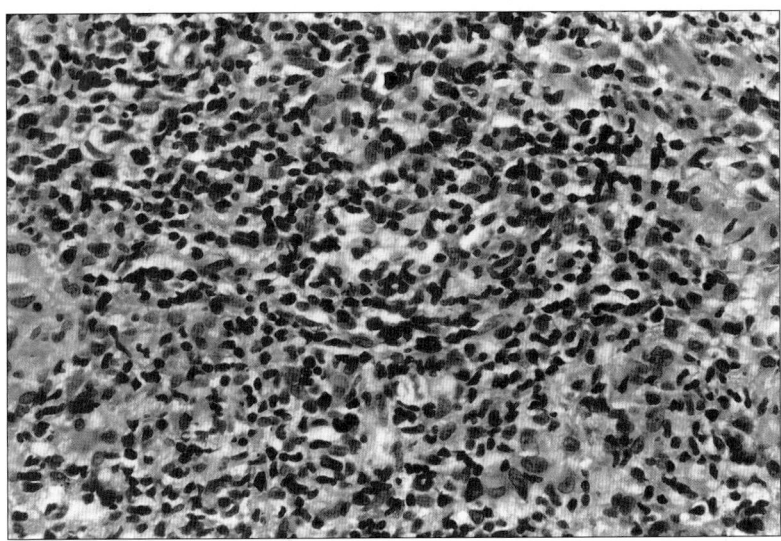

Fig. 14.79
Drug-induced pseudolymphoma: there is marked lymphocytic atypia. The nodules melted away following withdrawal of drug.

variable numbers of plasma cells and eosinophils. Mitoses are sometimes numerous. Blasts are often present and lymphoid follicles with germinal centers may be evident.

By immunohistochemistry, the majority of the lymphocytes are CD20+ B cells although a subpopulation of CD3+ T-cells is also present. Identification of CD21+ follicular dendritic cells may be helpful in confirming the presence of poorly developed follicles. Kappa and lambda immunohistochemistry invariably show no evidence of light chain restriction.

Tattoo-associated pseudolymphomas may be of the B- or T-cell type, with a B-cell pattern being more common. In addition to the features described above, there is tattoo pigment extracellularly and within macrophages. Rarely, a lichenoid infiltrate is present.[50]

Differential diagnosis

Distinction between cutaneous lymphoma and a drug-induced pseudolymphoma can be exceedingly difficult. Features that favor a drug-induced process over mycosis fungoides include vacuolar alteration, keratinocyte necrosis, spongiosis, and papillary dermal edema.[53] However, there can be considerable histologic overlap, and rare instances of a TCR gene rearrangement necessitate close clinicopathological correlation. If cutaneous pseudolymphoma is suspected, the most effective way to make the distinction is withdrawal of the suspected drug. It is important that correlation always be undertaken in any case of an unanticipated lymphoma in order that reactive conditions do not receive inappropriate lymphoma treatment. True cutaneous lymphomas may be drug-induced like in the case of CD30(+) anaplastic large cell lymphoma associated with fingolimod used in the treatment of multiple sclerosis.[51a]

Specific drug reactions

Arsenic

Clinical features

Arsenic exposure can be encountered under a variety of circumstances.[1-7] It may be a constituent of proprietary medicines and is an active component of pesticides and herbicides.[3] Fowler's solution – once used in the treatment of psoriasis and other dermatological disorders – contained 1% potassium arsenate.[1,3] The most common source of arsenic exposure now is through contaminated groundwater. For many years (as a consequence of its use as an insecticide), it was an ingredient in cigarette tobacco.[2,4] High levels of arsenic occur in the mining and smelting industries.[3]

Exposure to arsenic may cause acute arsenical dermatitis, although more commonly patients are seen with long-term sequelae.[2-7] The former presents with a diffuse erythematous papular or pustular/bullous dermatosis that can progress to exfoliative dermatitis.[5] Transverse white nail striations may be a feature.[5] Rarely, TEN can develop.[8] Irritant nail dermatitis has also been reported.[9] Chronic complications of arsenic exposure include pigmentary disturbances and cutaneous tumors. Patients are also at increased risk of internal malignancies.[1,7] Other systemic manifestations include atherosclerosis, hepatic fibrosis, peripheral neuropathy, respiratory disease, and diabetes mellitus.[7]

Characteristic of arsenicism is the 'rain drops on a dusty road' appearance in which patients develop hyperpigmented macules containing foci of hypopigmentation and areas of darker pigmentation.[7,10-12] Lesions are often seen on the trunk and in heavily pigmented regions such as the areola and flexural creases.[3] The cutaneous pigmentary changes are especially seen in Asian populations.[3]

Palmar and plantar keratoses are common and present 2 years or more after exposure.[5] After many years, they may be associated with malignant transformation.[7]

Skin tumors are a late manifestation, are often multiple, and are particularly found on non-sun-exposed sites. Bowen disease, squamous cell carcinoma, and superficial basal cell carcinoma may develop.[1,2]

Patients with evidence of arsenic exposure should be investigated for visceral malignancies, particularly carcinoma of the lung, bladder, and kidney.[7,13,14] There are occasional reports documenting an association between arsenic and hepatic angiosarcoma.[15,16]

Pathogenesis and histologic features

The mechanism of arsenic carcinogenesis is multifactorial. Arsenic is methylated as part of the metabolization process.[6] This results in free radicals which damage DNA, contribute to chromosomal aberrations, and increase sister chromatid exchange.[7] Arsenic also impairs the DNA repair process and diminishes p53 activity.[17] Transcription factors, cytokines, and cell signaling pathways critical to regulation of cellular proliferation and differentiation are also affected by arsenic and lead to uncontrolled cell growth and de-differentiation.[7,17,18] Decreased methylation capacities and a specific NALP2 polymorphism are associated with an increased risk of developing arsenic-related skin lesions.[19,20]

Histologically, cutaneous hyperpigmentation demonstrates increased melanin synthesis, with excess pigment being present at all levels of the epidermis.[3] There is no evidence of melanocytic proliferation. Skin cancers arising as a result of arsenic exposure show no distinguishing features histologically and are described elsewhere.

Iododerma

Clinical features

Potassium iodide is encountered in various settings. It is often included in expectorants/bronchodilators and is used for treatment of thyroid disease and as a radiocontrast medium.

Adverse reactions are rare.[1-9] Acneiform papulo/pustular lesions are most common and affect the face, neck, and back.[3,4] Erythematous, urticarial, vesiculobullous, and pustular psoriasis-like lesions have been described.[1,7,10,11] Rarely, chemical burnlike changes develop in patients, often postsurgical, when there is concomitant occlusion and maceration.[9] Lesions affecting the lower limbs may be petechial, hemorrhagic, or resemble erythema nodosum.[1,2] Nodular and ulcerated vegetative plaques constitute more extreme forms. This latter variant affects the face, shoulders, trunk, and extremities and presents as 1–7 cm disfiguring, crusted, erythematous lesions, sometimes with central umbilication (Figs 14.80 and 14.81).[3] Healing may be complicated with scarring.

Iododerma is associated with multiple myeloma, polyarteritis nodosa, lymphoma, and glomerulonephritis.[3,7,12] Renal insufficiency may be a predisposing factor.

Pathogenesis and histologic features

Although delayed hypersensitivity is believed to represent the underlying pathogenesis, the precise mechanism is unknown. Acute lesions are

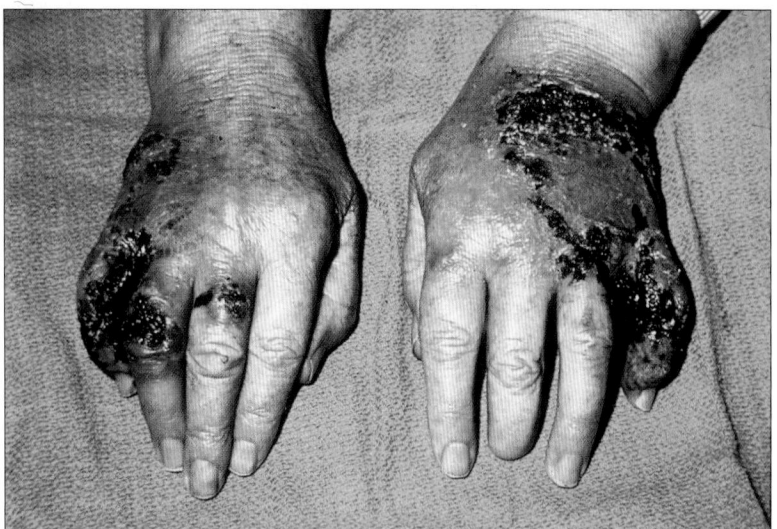

Fig. 14.80
Iododerma: ulcerated vegetative plaques are present on the backs of the hands and fingers. By courtesy of the Institute of Dermatology, London, UK.

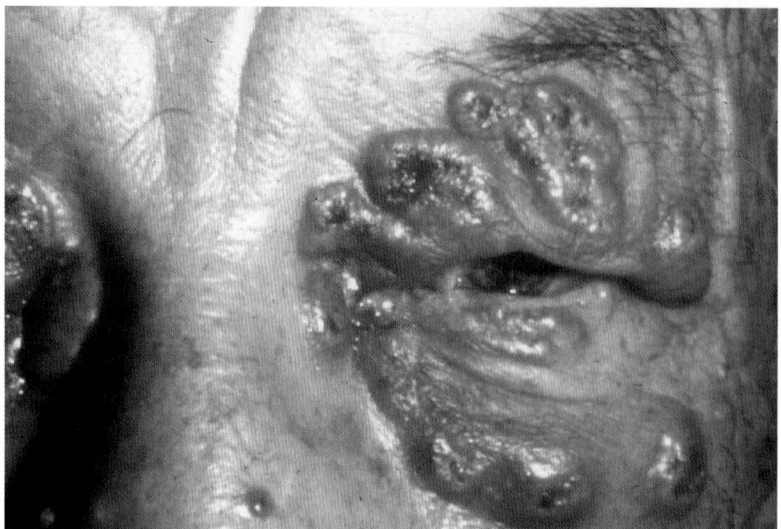

Fig. 14.82
Bromoderma: vegetant plaques and nodules are seen around the eye. Ulceration is present. By courtesy of the late M. Beare, MD, Royal Victoria Hospital, Belfast, N. Ireland.

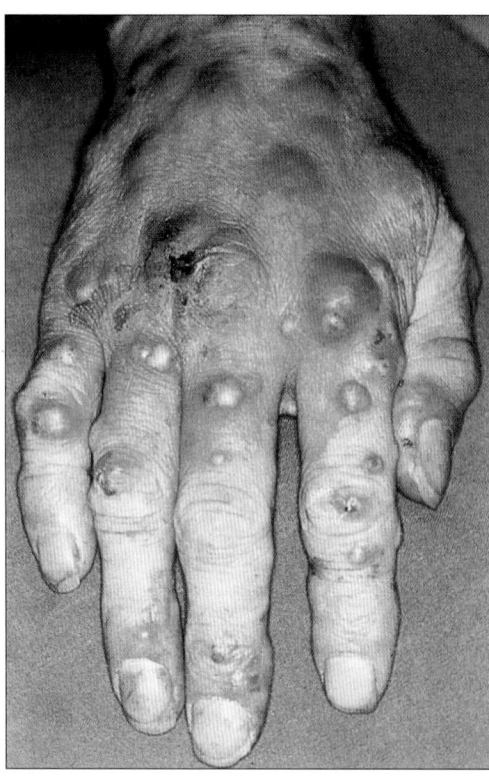

Fig. 14.81
Iododerma: in this patient, nodules are conspicuous. Superimposed pustules are evident. By courtesy of the Institute of Dermatology, London, UK.

characterized by an intense dermal neutrophil-rich infiltrate. With chronicity, pseudoepitheliomatous hyperplasia and ulceration are common. Neutrophil microabscesses may be seen in the epidermis and the dermis; in some cases, there is focal leukocytoclastic vasculitis.[3,5]

Differential diagnosis

Histologically, the nodular lesions of iododerma resemble an infective process such as blastomycosis or an atypical mycobacterial condition. The presence of occasional eosinophils within the infiltrate and epidermal degeneration in association with the abscesses may result in confusion with pemphigus vegetans. In early lesions, when the epidermis is normal thickness, the features can be mistaken for Sweet syndrome and pyoderma gangrenosum.

Bromoderma

Clinical features

Methyl bromide has been used as a pesticide and disinfectant and in the pharmaceutical, film, and dye industries.[1–5] It may be found in sedative syrups and expectorants. Although occupational exposure is associated with severe respiratory effects including pulmonary edema, occasional reports of skin contact have also been documented.[3,4] Potassium bromide is used as an anticonvulsant in many parts of the world. Other sources of exposure include brominated pool disinfectants and brominated vegetable oil, a product used in citrus-flavored drinks.[6] In Japan and other countries, over-the-counter bromide-containing sedatives can be a source of exposure.[7] Bromoderma has also been reported in a patient with a pituitary adenoma treated with bromocriptine.[8]

Patients present with sharply circumscribed erythematous lesions containing vesicles and bullae.[4] Intertriginous regions and sites of mechanical pressure are predominantly affected. Ingested bromide may give rise to hyperpigmentation, urticaria, acneiform/pustular lesions (acne bromica), vegetative and ulcerated plaques (vegetant bromoderma, tuberous bromoderma), necrotizing panniculitis, and pyoderma gangrenosum-like ulcers (Fig. 14.82).[7,9–14] Lesions may be multiple or solitary. Vegetant bromoderma most often presents on the face, scalp, and legs and predominantly affects infants.[8] It is commonly mistaken for an infection. A case which complicated bromine secretion in breast milk has been documented.[15]

Histologic features

Cutaneous lesions that develop following acute exposure to methyl bromide are characterized by spongiosis, keratinocyte necrosis, papillary dermal edema, and subepidermal blister formation.[4] A perivascular inflammatory cell infiltrate containing neutrophils, eosinophils, and smaller numbers of lymphocytes and histiocytes is present in the superficial dermis.

In vegetating lesions, there is striking pseudoepitheliomatous hyperplasia with intraepidermal and dermal abscesses accompanied by an intense neutrophil, eosinophil, and lymphohistiocytic infiltrate in the underlying dermis. Ulceration resembling pyoderma gangrenosum may be present.[7]

Urticarial lesions show papillary dermal edema accompanied by a neutrophil and eosinophil-rich infiltrate.[4]

Differential diagnosis

Vegetating lesions may be easily confused with deep fungal and atypical mycobacterial infections. Pemphigus vegetans also enters the differential diagnosis. Sweet syndrome and pyoderma gangrenosum also have some similarities. The diagnosis may be most easily reached by careful clinico-pathological correlation.[13]

Warfarin

Warfarin (coumadin) may be associated with a number of adverse reactions including hemorrhage, alopecia, urticaria, maculopapular eruptions, dermatitis, purple toe syndrome, and leukocytoclastic vasculitis.[1-8] Cutaneous necrosis develops in 0.01–0.1% of patients and may cause severe morbidity and significant mortality.[5]

Clinical features

Warfarin necrosis typically develops 3 to 6 days after starting anticoagulation therapy. Paresthesia is present initially and is followed by a painful, well-circumscribed, edematous, and erythematous plaque resembling peau d'orange with purpura.[1,5] Large blood-filled blisters that rapidly break down, accompanied by progressive necrosis of the underlying dermis and subcutaneous fat, are later sequelae. Tissue destruction is often considerable and the resultant scarring is very disfiguring. Occasionally, the onset of this condition is delayed for weeks or months, although in most instances this reflects an interrupted therapeutic regimen.[9-11]

The condition shows a predilection for obese females (85%) and predominantly affects the breasts, buttocks, and thighs.[2] The reason for the female predominance is unknown. In males, the thighs and buttocks are also affected and sometimes the penis is involved. Occasionally, lesions are seen on the hands. Deeper soft tissues and internal viscera are not affected.

Patients almost invariably have received anticoagulation for thrombophlebitis (deep venous thrombosis) and/or pulmonary embolism. Patients who receive warfarin for treatment of cardiovascular disorders such as atrial fibrillation only very exceptionally develop this condition.[5]

Pathogenesis and histologic features

Cutaneous necrosis rarely complicates therapy with warfarin. Although hypersensitivity reactions and direct toxicity have been postulated as etiological factors, an imbalance in the ratio of procoagulative and anticoagulative factors is currently thought to be most important.[5] In addition to depressing the vitamin K-dependent clotting factors II, VII, IX, and X, warfarin reduces the levels of naturally occurring anticoagulants including protein C, protein S, and antithrombin III. It first affects protein C, which has an extremely short half-life, and until the anticoagulative effect comes into play with depressed levels of coagulating factors, the patient is paradoxically at increased risk of thrombosis. Why this should so rarely result in skin necrosis is uncertain.

Congenital protein C deficiency is an important predisposing factor in some patients. This is a relatively common autosomal dominant condition that affects between 1:200 and 1:300 of the population. Protein C is activated by thrombin under the influence of the cofactor thrombomodulin.[5] The activated form inactivates factors VIIIa and Va, which inhibit conversion of factor X to factor Xa and prothrombin to thrombin with resultant inhibition of coagulation.[5] Protein C deficiency is, therefore, associated with a thrombotic tendency.[12] Approximately 30% of patients who develop warfarin necrosis have an underlying protein C deficiency.[2] Warfarin therapy, therefore, tips the balance in an already protein C-deficient patient. The proposed mechanism, however, by no means offers an explanation in the majority of cases.

Acquired or congenital deficiency of protein S may also be of importance in a small number of cases.[13-16] Protein S is a vitamin K-dependent cofactor for activated protein C.[5] Acquired protein S deficiency may be encountered in patients with renal failure or antiphospholipid syndrome, or who are undergoing hemodialysis.[17,18]

An episode of thrombophlebitis and/or pulmonary embolism leading to the warfarin therapy seems to be of major etiological importance.[1,2] It is proposed that the vascular inflammatory changes play a role in precipitating the thrombotic tendency by reducing endothelial cell thrombomodulin levels, inactivating protein S and decreasing fibrinolytic activity.[1-4] Protein C or protein S deficiency (inherited or developing as a consequence of warfarin therapy) may then represent an additional predisposing factor. Other

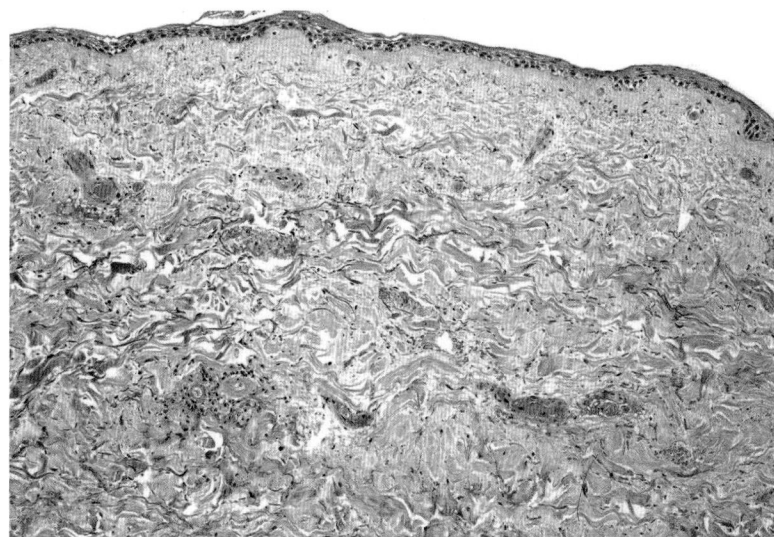

Fig. 14.83
Warfarin necrosis: there are thrombosed vessels throughout the superficial dermis associated with epidermal regeneration.

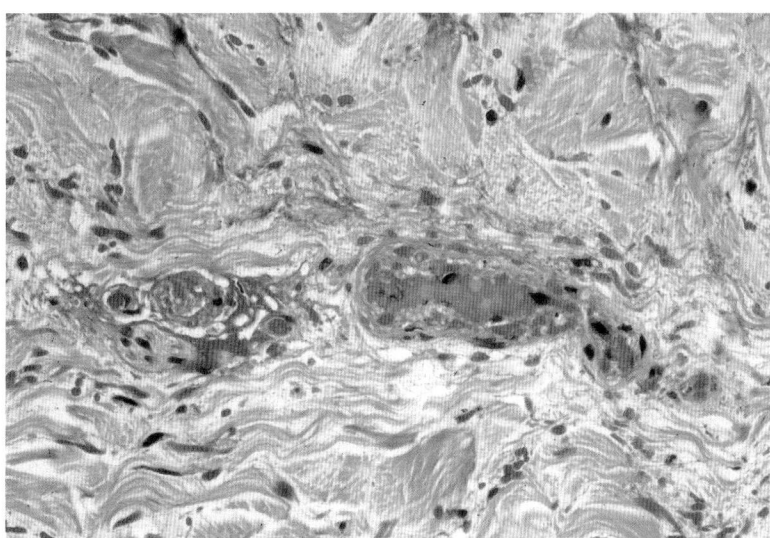

Fig. 14.84
Warfarin necrosis: high-power view of Fig. 14.83.

conditions that predispose to the development of warfarin necrosis include reduced antithrombin III levels, lupus anticoagulant syndrome, factor V Leiden, and prothrombin gene mutation.[19-21]

Histologically, warfarin-associated skin necrosis is characterized by fibrin thrombi in the small veins and venules of the dermis and subcutaneous fat, with widespread erythrocyte extravasation (Figs 14.83 and 14.84). In advanced lesions, subepidermal blood-filled blisters are seen. In older lesions, the changes of infarction are superimposed; however, vasculitis is not typically a feature. However, warfarin-induced leukocytoclastic vasculitis has been reported.[22,23] Arteries are not affected.

Differential diagnosis

Identical histologic features may be seen in a number of conditions including antiphospholipid antibodies, hereditary hypercoagulation disorders (factor V Leiden mutations, protein C or S, and antithrombin III deficiencies) in the absence of warfarin therapy, heparin-induced thrombocytopenia (HIT) syndrome, and disseminated intravascular coagulation (DIC). Cryoglobulinemia and cryofibrinogenemia may also have to be excluded. Calciphylaxis can be excluded by the absence of vascular calcification. The diagnosis ultimately depends upon adequate clinicopathological correlation.

Heparin

Adverse side effects of heparin include hemorrhage, urticaria, anaphylaxis, macular erythema, and alopecia.[1-3] Of greater significance, patients may develop thrombocytopenia, paradoxical thrombosis, and skin necrosis – HIT syndrome.[1-6]

Clinical features

Urticarial reactions are exceptionally rare.[7-9] Delayed hypersensitivity reactions are the most common of the adverse cutaneous responses to heparin, occurring in 7.5% of patients.[9,10] Macular erythema and eczematous lesions occur at the injection site. There is a striking female predominance.[2,11] Rarely, blisters may develop, and exceptionally the erythema becomes generalized.[10]

Hemorrhagic vesicles have also been described in patients given low molecular weight heparin.[12,13] Reported patients have been elderly and received the medication while hospitalized. Lesions develop distant from injection sites and occur on the extremities.

HIT syndrome – in addition to definitional thrombocytopenia – is characterized by thrombosis (venous more often than arterial), which accounts for the high morbidity and potential mortality.[4,6] Venous thrombosis results in deep venous lesions in the lower legs in up to 50% of patients, and of these 25% may develop pulmonary embolism.[6] Additional complications include warfarin-induced limb gangrene, adrenal hemorrhage, and DIC.[6] Arterial thrombosis is more likely in catheterized or traumatized arteries and may affect the aorta and ileofemoral arteries, resulting in peripheral gangrene, myocardial infarction, or stroke.[4,6,14]

Cutaneous necrosis develops in 10–20% of patients with the HIT syndrome.[6,15] The injection site is predominantly involved, but more distant areas (thighs, abdomen, and buttocks) may also be affected in a minority of patients.[1,2,16-25] Initial lesions are painful or burning erythematous plaques followed by ulceration and tissue necrosis.[2] The condition shows a predilection for middle-aged females and the obese.[2,16]

Thrombocytopenia and thromboembolism are potentially life-threatening complications.

Pathogenesis and histologic features

The HIT syndrome results from platelet activating HIT/PF4 antibodies induced in response to a platelet factor 4-heparin complex.[1,23,24] The resulting immune complexes bind to platelet Fc receptors and activate platelets. In addition, the antibody reacts with surface endothelial cell platelet factor 4-inducing endothelial cell injury and thrombosis.[4,24] Only a minority of patients with HIT antibodies develop skin necrosis, and it is postulated that additional prothrombotic factors such as protein C or S deficiency are necessary for the development of thrombosis and its sequelae.[1] Adverse side effects are more common and more severe in patients receiving unfractionated as opposed to low molecular weight heparin.[25] Extensive necrosis has been triggered by low molecular weight heparin in a patient with underlying lupus erythematosus and antiphospholipid syndrome.[26]

The histologic features of the macular erythema are those of spongiotic dermatitis. Within the superficial dermis is a perivascular lymphohistiocytic infiltrate with variable numbers of eosinophils. The lymphocytes are predominantly of the T-helper subclass.[27]

Heparin-induced cutaneous necrosis is characterized by widespread superficial small vessel (capillary and venule) thrombi accompanied by hemorrhage and necrosis.[17,18] The presence of leukocytoclastic vasculitis is variable.[2]

Bullous hemorrhagic lesions are intraepidermal blisters filled with extravasated red blood cells.[12,13] Perivascular lymphocytes, histiocytes, and eosinophils are variably present. Leukocytoclastic vasculitis is absent. Direct immunofluorescence studies are negative.

Penicillamine

Clinical features

Penicillamine therapy is associated with various adverse reactions including exanthematous eruptions, urticaria, lichenoid reactions, papulosquamous

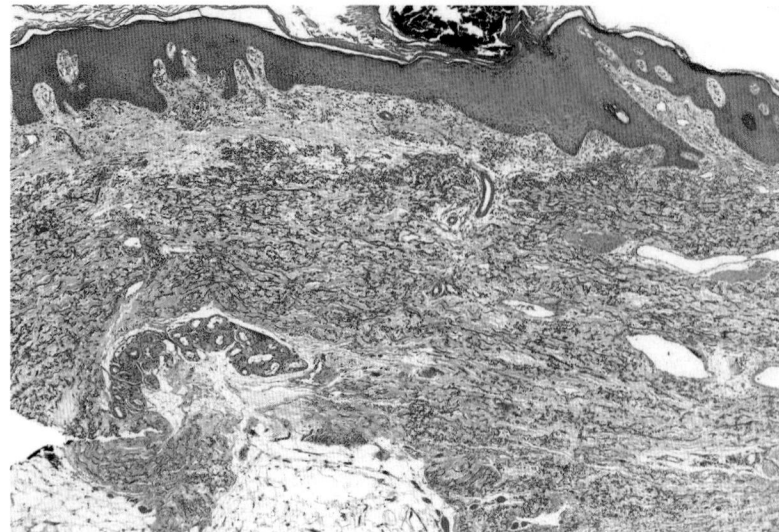

Fig. 14.85
Penicillamine dermopathy: there are thickened, intensely eosinophilic elastic fibers throughout the reticular dermis.

dermatoses, alopecia, hypertrichosis, nail changes, dermatomyositis, systemic lupus erythematosus, pemphigus vulgaris, pemphigus foliaceus, pemphigus erythema, and bullous and mucosal pemphigoid.[1-13] The autoimmune blistering dermatoses complicating penicillamine therapy are not dose dependent and are seen particularly in patients with other immunologically mediated diseases including rheumatoid arthritis and systemic sclerosis.[9] Pemphigus is by far the most common bullous disorder associated with penicillamine, pemphigus foliaceus being the most frequent variant encountered.[4,9] Herpetiform pemphigus has also rarely been described as complicating the use of penicillamine.[10,11] Additional manifestations – particularly seen in patients taking high doses in the treatment of Wilson disease and cystinuria – include penicillamine dermopathy, elastosis perforans serpiginosa, skin fragility with hemorrhages and milia formation on the extensor surfaces, wrinkling and anetoderma-like changes, cutis laxa, and pseudoxanthoma elasticum-like appearances.[13-20] Patients on long-term therapy may present with small yellow papules resembling a plucked-chicken appearance or disfiguring loose folds of skin particularly affecting the flexures.[17,18]

Pathogenesis and histologic features

Penicillamine acts by impairing cross-linking in newly formed collagen and elastic fibers.[14] It also binds aldehydes to the surfaces of macrophages and amine groups on T cells, and this could represent a mechanism for triggering autoimmune reactions. contributing to an autoimmune reaction.[21,22] The histologic features include increased numbers of abnormally formed elastic fibers in the reticular dermis (Fig. 14.85). These are thickened with irregular serrated appearance on cross section. When viewed in a longitudinal plane, the fibers show conspicuous lateral projections (Figs 14.86 and 14.87).

Evidence of similar elastic tissue damage has been documented in the joint capsules, lungs, intestine, and large elastic arteries.[14]

Gold

Clinical features

Gold therapy may result in eczematous, lichenoid, pityriasiform, and psoriasiform dermatoses and stomatitis.

Cutaneous pigmentation that results from parenteral treatment with gold salts is known as chrysiasis (auriasis, chrysoderma, hautaurosis).[1-5] It is a photodependent, irreversible condition most often documented in patients with rheumatoid arthritis.[2,3] Patients are at risk once a threshold of 50 mg/kg of gold is reached.[1] Disease severity correlates with the cumulative dose of gold.[6] Coloration varies from mauve/blue to blue to slate-gray.[2] The sun-exposed skin of the face is particularly affected. In severe cases, lesions may be seen on the neck, front of chest, and backs of the forearms

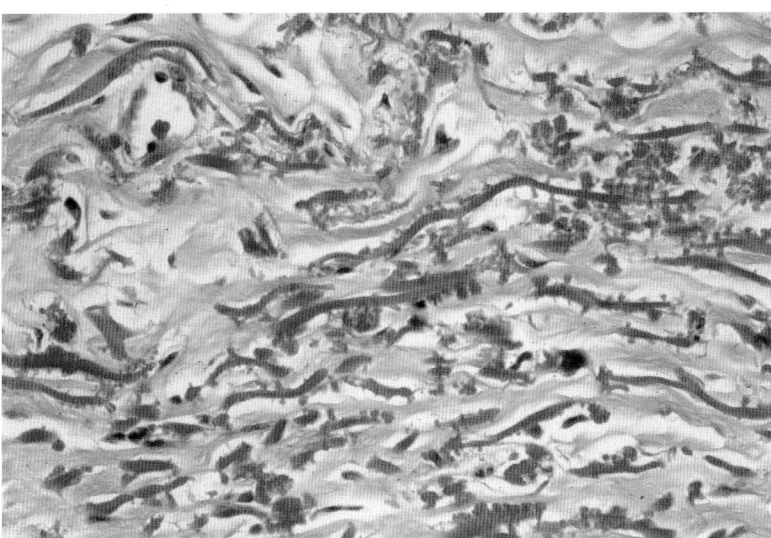

Fig. 14.86
Penicillamine dermopathy: the serrated appearance is characteristic.

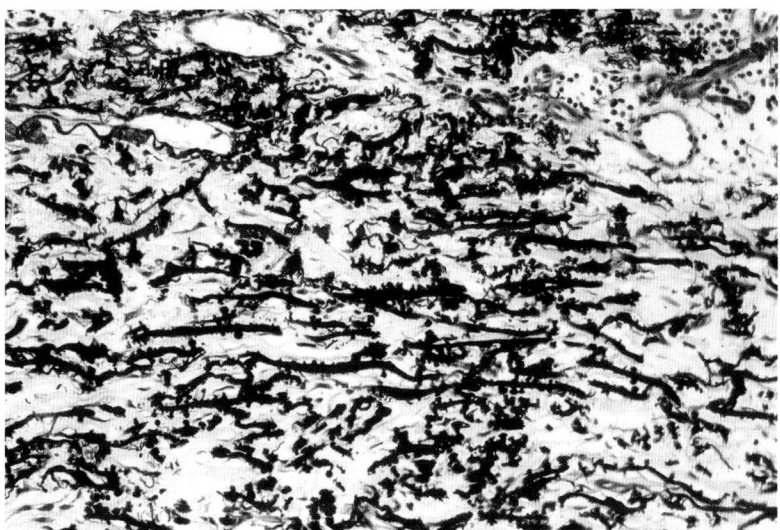

Fig. 14.87
Penicillamine dermopathy: the changes can be highlighted by an elastic tissue stain.

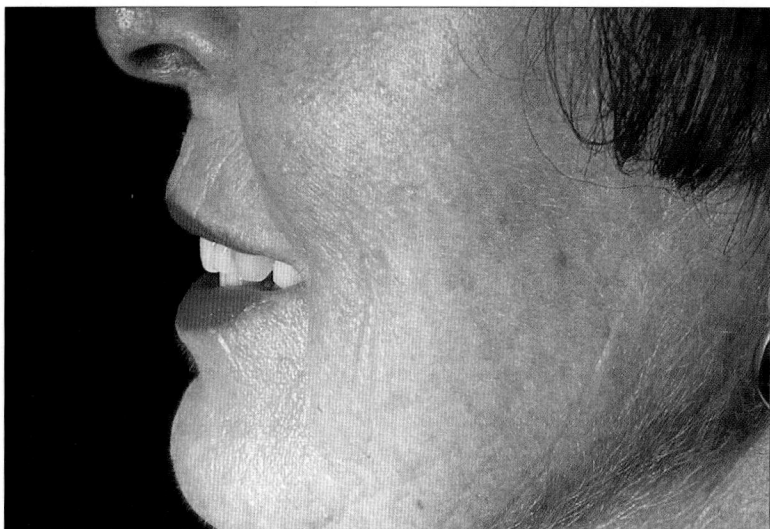

Fig. 14.88
Chrysiasis: multiple foci of blue discoloration are present on the cheek. By courtesy of J. Kerner, MD, Department of Dermatology, Harvard Medical School, Boston, USA.

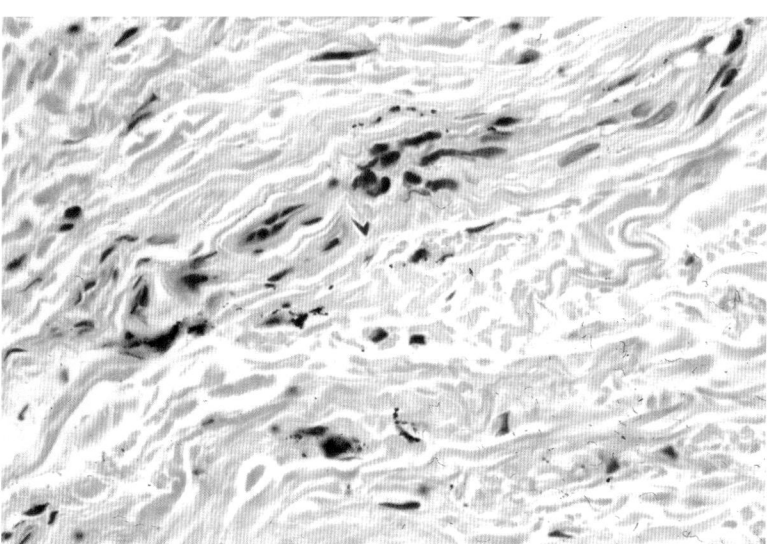

Fig. 14.89
Chrysiasis: there are fine black granules both within macrophages and lying free around the superficial vasculature. By courtesy of S. Lyle, MD, Beth Israel Deaconess Medical Center, Boston, USA.

and hands (*Fig. 14.88*).[2] In bald patients, scalp involvement is sometimes apparent. Pigmentation has also been described in the sclera and buccal mucosa.[2]

Pathogenesis and histologic features

The pathogenesis of chrysiasis is uncertain. It is probably related to an effect of UV radiation on tissue-bound gold particles. Support for this hypothesis is the observation that skin lesions can be induced by UVB irradiation of sunlight-protected skin.[7] Similarly, typical skin lesions have been described following Q-switched ruby laser treatment in patients treated with gold.[8-11]

Chrysiasis is characterized by deposits of small black macrophage-bound particles surrounding the vessels in the deeper reticular dermis and around the sweat gland coils (*Fig. 14.89*).[2] Perls Prussian blue (hemosiderin) and Masson-Fontana staining for melanin are negative. The gold particles show orange-red birefringence with cross-polarized light.[12] There is no inflammatory response. Epidermal melanin pigmentation usually appears normal.[2] A localized form of chrysiasis with sclerosing lipogranulomas at injection sites has also been reported.[13]

By electron microscopy, the gold appears as granular, particulate, and filamentous material, sometimes showing a starlike morphology within phagolysosomes (aurosomes). The diagnosis can be confirmed by electron/X-ray probe microanalysis.[2,4,13-16]

Differential diagnosis

Gold pigment must be distinguished from silver deposits (argyria), mercury, and tattoo pigment.[5,10] Silver pigment is predominantly deposited in relation to basement membranes, particularly of the sweat glands. It does not show orange-red birefringence with cross-polarized light.[10] Mercury particles are large (up to 340 μm in diameter) and brown-black in color. Tattoo usually consists of a variety of different pigments of varying colors. Clinical history should readily establish the diagnosis in the majority of cases.

Silver

Clinical features

Generalized tissue accumulation of silver (argyria) follows dietary, medicinal, and industrial exposure to silver compounds.[1-9] Occupational exposure may be encountered in silver mining and smelting, electroplating, and in the photographic industries.[3] Silver deposits are found in the skin and mucous membranes in addition to internal viscera, particularly liver, spleen,

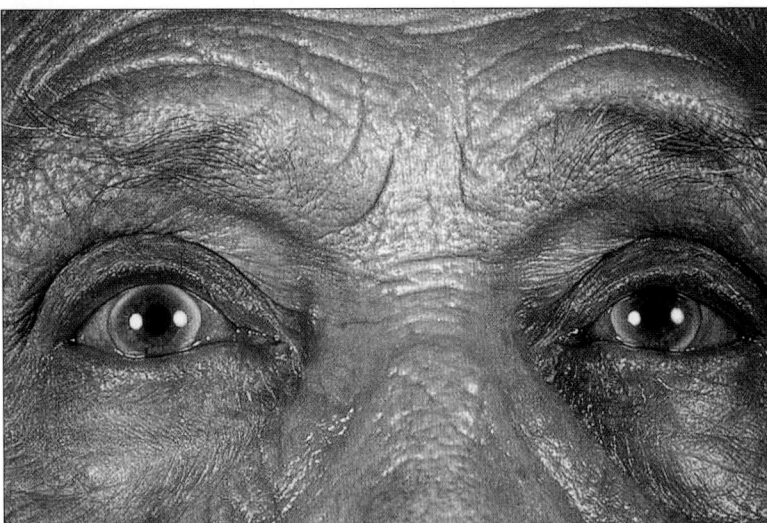

Fig. 14.90
Argyria: there is striking slate-blue pigmentation; the eyes are also affected. By courtesy of the Institute of Dermatology, London, UK.

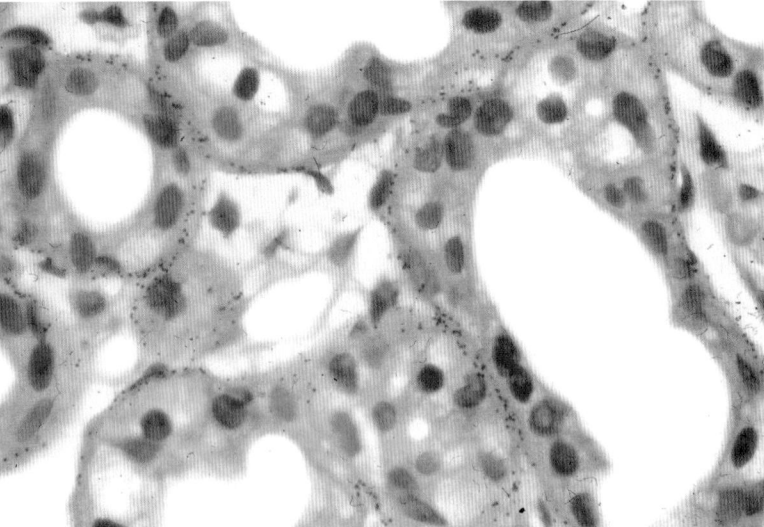

Fig. 14.91
Argyria: note the fine silver granules outlining the basement membrane of the sweat gland epithelium.

adrenals, muscle, and brain (*Fig. 14.90*).[1] Argyria initially presents in the gingivae as a slate-blue line due to deposition of metallic silver and silver sulfide.[1–3] Cutaneous manifestations affect the sun-exposed sites of the face, neck, and backs of hands.[6] The nails may also be involved. Ocular involvement presents as a bluish-gray to brownish-black coloration.

Localized argyria has been documented due to silver earrings, orthodontic surgery, acupuncture, silver polishing, and the application of topical silver sulfadiazine.[10–19] In the absence of clinical information, a diagnosis of blue nevus may mistakenly be made.[11,20]

Histologic features

Argyria results from deposition of metallic silver and silver sulfide. Pigmentation is intensified by sunlight due to silver reduction analogous to photographic processing.[6] There is also increased epidermal melanin synthesis.

Silver granules are found in association with the vascular and adnexal basement membranes and adjacent to dermal elastic fibers (*Fig. 14.91*).[2,21] They measure less than 1.0 μm in diameter and appear brown-black in hematoxylin and eosin stained sections.[6] Rarely, argyria can have some overlap with ochronosis.[22] Ultrastructurally, the silver granules may be membrane bound within macrophage lysosomes or lie freely in the dermis.[8] The diagnosis can be confirmed by X-ray microanalysis.[6,9,21]

Mercury

Clinical features

Mercury exposure is encountered under a variety of circumstances.[1–3] It occurs in three different forms: metallic, inorganic, and organic mercury.[1]

- Metallic mercury, which is a liquid at room temperature, is present in vapor from heating amalgam and paints and in mercury thermometers.[4]
- Inorganic mercurial salts may be present in laxatives, pesticides, antiseptics, and germicides.[1,5]
- Organomercurials are used as industrial antifungal agents.[4]

Dermatological reactions to metallic mercury include mercury granuloma and mercury exanthem (mercury-induced AGEP). Mercury granuloma follows penetrating skin wounds as might result from a broken thermometer, attempted homicide, or suicide. Patients present with a flesh-colored to red or hyperpigmented nodule at the site of implantation.[6–10] Membranous fat necrosis following subcutaneous mercury injection has also been documented.[11] Mercury exanthem follows exposure to metallic mercury (as may follow breaking a thermometer) in a previously sensitized patient.[12–22] The eruption presents as a vivid erythema, which particularly affects the flexural sites of the body (so-called 'Baboon syndrome').[17] An inverted V-shaped erythema affecting the upper anteromedial aspects of both thighs is characteristic.[12,16] Sterile pustules commonly develop and a purpuric element may develop. Pyrexia and peripheral leukocytosis are typically present. The dermatosis resolves by desquamation.

Topical mercury cream has been (and is still in some countries) used as a skin-bleaching agent.[6,23–26] Continuous and protracted use results in slate-gray pigmentation affecting the flexures. The eyelids, nasolabial folds, and neck creases are sites of predilection.[27,28]

Parenteral use of mercury results in pigmentation of the gingivae.[28] A lichenoid drug reaction has been documented following acute mercury poisoning.[29]

Dental workers are at risk of allergic contact dermatitis from exposure to mercury or mercury salts.[30]

Mercury may also be associated with palmar/plantar peeling in children (pink disease, acrodynia, erythredema), palmar/plantar hyperkeratosis, and acanthosis nigricans-like skin lesions.[31] Pink disease is rarely encountered nowadays due to control of mercury in medications and in the environment.[32–34] The condition is still occasionally seen and may be a problem in developing countries. It presents in infants and young children following chronic mercury exposure, for example, in diaper powders, laxatives, paint, fluorescent light bulbs, or other household sources.[1] It is characterized by the development of characteristic painful swelling and pink coloration of the tip of the nose, fingers, and toes.[1,11] As the condition resolves, the palms and soles show intense sweating and desquamation.[1] Sterility in males is a potential long-term sequel.[33]

Lichenoid and granulomatous inflammatory reactions may complicate use of mercuric sulfide (cinnabar) to provide the red color in tattoos.[35–37] Pseudolymphomatous reactions to mercury have also been documented.[38,39]

Amalgam tattoo reactions are discussed elsewhere.

Histologic features

Mercury pigment is brown-black, round, and opaque, and measures up to 340 μm in diameter (*Fig. 14.92*).[5–7,40] The granules are found within macrophages in addition to extracellular dermal deposition. They are localized around the superficial vasculature and in association with the connective tissue elements.[40]

Mercury granulomata are characterized by local necrosis associated with free mercury globules surrounded by an intense foreign body granulomatous reaction with lymphocytes, histiocytes, plasma cells, neutrophils, and varying numbers of eosinophils.[6,7,9] Ulceration is common, and the epidermis may show pseudoepitheliomatous hyperplasia.

Mercury exanthem is characterized by subcorneal and/or intraepidermal pustules which may contain acantholytic keratinocytes in addition to large numbers of neutrophils.[13] Background spongiosis is usually evident. The dermal papillae are often edematous, and occasionally subepidermal vesiculation is a feature. A perivascular infiltrate of lymphocytes and histiocytes

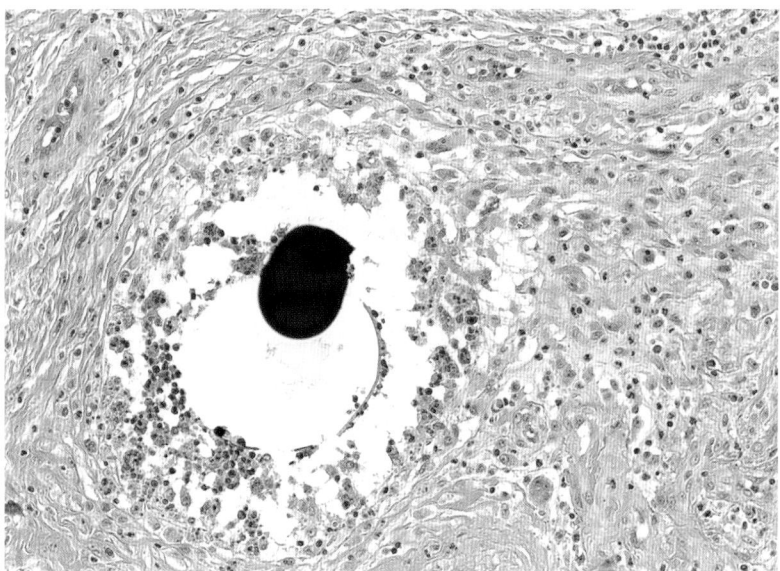

Fig. 14.92
Mercury pigmentation: the round black deposit of mercury is surrounded by a suppurative granuloma.

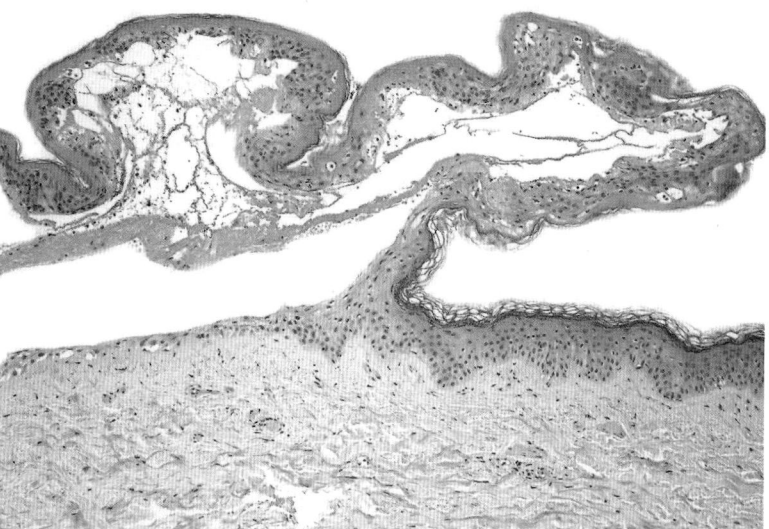

Fig. 14.93
Coma blister: there is a subepidermal blister. Re-epithelialization along the floor is present.

with conspicuous neutrophils and variable numbers of eosinophils is present in the superficial dermis. Leukocytoclastic vasculitis may be a feature in a significant proportion of cases.[13]

Cutaneous pigmentation following chronic local exposure to mercury is characterized by increased melanin pigment in the epidermis accompanied by mercury granules in the papillary dermis.[26] Iron stains are negative.[1]

Pink disease is characterized by sweat gland hyperplasia and a non-specific dermal inflammatory cell infiltrate.[1]

Bismuth

Clinical features

Bismuth may be used for gastrointestinal complaints including gastritis and peptic ulceration.[1-3] Adverse cutaneous reactions include erythroderma, exanthemata, purpuric eruptions, stomatitis, urticaria, livedo-like dermatitis, pityriasis rosea-like dermatitis, allergic contact dermatitis to topical therapy containing bismuth.[2-6] Generalized pigmentation may follow prolonged parenteral and oral use. Patients develop a generalized blue-gray pigmentation, which also affects the conjunctivae and oral mucosa.[1] A blue-black line at the gingival margin is pathognomonic.[1] Transient black lingual pigmentation has also been reported.[7]

Histologic features

Bismuth appears as small dark granules in the dermis and within sweat gland basement membranes.[3] Transfollicular elimination has been documented.[2]

Voriconazole

Clinical features

Voriconazole is a second-generation broad-spectrum triazole antifungal that acts by inhibiting fungal cytochrome 450 enzymes. It is well tolerated, and it is commonly used to treat fungal infections, particularly in immunocompromised patients. It may be associated with a number of side effects including nausea, vomiting, diarrhea, visual disturbances, cheilitis, EM, SJS, TEN, pseudoporphyria, blistering, facial erythema, and mucocutaneous retinoid-like effects.[1-4] One of the most important side effects is photosensitivity, initially reported to occur in about 1–2% of patients and after long-term therapy.[5-7] Photosensitivity may be more common in pediatric patients, affecting up to 20% of patients on the drug.[8] Although the photosensitivity subsides when the treatment is stopped, photoaging also occurs

and it persists. The latter is associated with multiple lentigines and premature dermatoheliosis.[5-7] Furthermore, some patients, even children, have developed aggressive squamous cell carcinomas and melanomas in situ have also been reported in adults.[9-16]

Histologic features

All the cutaneous manifestations of voriconazole therapy show the same histologic features of their counterparts not induced by drugs.

Lithium

Clinical features

Lithium therapy is associated with cutaneous side effects in up to 45% of patients.[1,2] It is known to precipitate or aggravate psoriasis, in particular, pustular lesions.[3-7] Other cutaneous adverse effects include maculopapular eruptions, seborrheic dermatitis, exfoliative dermatitis, atypical acneiform lesions (predominantly affecting the forearms and legs), pustular eruptions, hidradenitis suppurativa, keratosis pilaris-like lesions, palmoplantar hyperkeratosis, bullous disorders, and hair, nail, and mucosal changes.[8-13] Exacerbation and the development of Darier disease has rarely been documented.[14]

Barbiturates and coma blisters

Clinical features

Barbiturates may be associated with a wide range of adverse drug reactions including EM, TEN, hypersensitivity syndrome, and pseudolymphoma.[1,2]

In company with many other sedative drugs, including chlorpromazine, imipramine, and meprobamate, barbiturates, particularly when taken in overdose, may result in blisters (coma blisters), related especially to sites of trauma.[3-8]

Pathogenesis and histologic features

These lesions probably develop as a result of focal persistent hypoxia and ischemia due to chronic localized pressure. They may develop in a comatose patient whatever the cause. Direct toxic effect may be of importance in some patients, as similar blisters have complicated localized barbiturate extravasation.

Histologically, the blisters are subepidermal in location and are often accompanied by infarction of the overlying epidermis (Fig. 14.93). Sweat gland necrosis is characteristic.

Chemotherapeutic agents

Clinical features

The rapid rate of epidermal and mucosal turnover results in a high degree of susceptibility to the effects of chemotherapeutic agents. Among the most commonly encountered adverse responses are stomatitis, alopecia, and pigmentary changes.[1–8]

Stomatitis is very common and presents as burning erythema, followed by the development of extremely painful erosions and ulcers.[2] Commonly implicated drugs include cyclophosphamide, methotrexate, bleomycin, cytarabine, doxorubicin, daunorubicin, dactinomycin, 5-fluorouracil, IL-2, hydroxyurea, and mercaptopurine.[5,7] Secondary infection, such as with herpes simplex virus or *Candida albicans*, is an important complication.

Proliferating hair follicles are highly susceptible to chemotherapeutic agents and as a consequence anagen effluvium (in which there is loss of much of the body hair) is a common and distressing complication.[7,8] This is reversible once treatment is completed, although subsequent regrowth of hair may be accompanied by a change in color or texture.[1] Concomitant premature catagen and telogen effluvium can result in total baldness.[2] Drugs most often implicated include bleomycin, cyclophosphamide, daunorubicin, docetaxel, doxorubicin, etoposide, ifosfamide, mechlorethamine, methotrexate, mitoxantrone, and paclitaxel.[1] Nail changes, including pale transverse ridges (Beau lines), develop as a result of mitosis inhibition with consequent temporary growth arrest and may be due to bleomycin, cyclophosphamide, and doxorubicin.[5] Onycholysis can follow treatment with docetaxel, fluorouracil, and mitoxantrone.[7] Transverse striate leukonychia (Mees lines), which result from periodic disruption of nail plate keratinization, classically have been described in association with arsenic poisoning.[9] Similar lesions have been documented with a number of agents including ciclosporine and daunorubicin.[10,11]

Maculopapular eruptions may be caused by several chemotherapeutic drugs including azathioprine, 5-fluorouracil, chlorambucil, melphalan, hydroxyurea, fludarabine, cladribine, gemcitabine, and pemetrexed.[6,12] These are frequently a source of clinical diagnostic difficulty, as infectious diseases – including viral exanthemas and, in patients who have undergone transplantation, acute GVHD – are often within the differential diagnosis.

Cutaneous hyperpigmentation is a common complication of chemotherapeutic agents and often affects the hair, nails, and mucosae in addition to the skin.[1–8,12–15] Hypopigmentation is less commonly seen.[5] The mechanism for increased melanin synthesis by melanocytes is unknown. Alkylating agents including busulfan, cyclophosphamide, ifosfamide, hydroxyurea, 5-fluorouracil, methotrexate, and thiotepa are among the most often implicated agents.[5,12,16,17] Nail changes (including diffuse pigmentation, longitudinal and transverse banding or streaks) are particularly seen with cyclophosphamide, daunorubicin, doxorubicin, 5-fluorouracil, and hydroxyurea.[2,9] Cyclophosphamide also causes hyperpigmentation of the palms and fingers.[12,15] Immediate or delayed tanning following sun exposure is a frequent complication of 5-fluorouracil. Rarely, patients may develop linear erythema, complicated by pigmentation around an injection site, so-called serpentine supravenous hyperpigmentation.[7,17–20] Similar lesions have followed treatment with actinomycin and nitrosourea.[21,22] Hair pigmentation can result from tamoxifen therapy.[1,23] Bleomycin therapy is associated with cutaneous pigmentation affecting between 30% and 60% of patients.[2,24] Pathognomonic linear flagellate streaks may develop on the skin of the trunk and proximal extremities.[25–32] This flagellate pattern has also been reported in a patient receiving bendamustine.[33] It is suggested that lesions develop as a consequence of trauma-induced vasodilatation with resultant local increased concentration of bleomycin. An early inflammatory phase, due to scratching, has occasionally been documented, suggesting that the pigmentation occurs as a consequence of postinflammatory changes. A similar problem of patterned hyperpigmentation has been documented following treatment with thiotepa (triethylene thiophosphoramide). Localized occlusion during treatment (e.g., with adhesive bandages) may cause retention of thio-TEPA-rich sweat and subsequent reversible hyperpigmentation confined to the occluded surfaces.[12,34,35] Transverse banding of hair shafts

following therapy with methotrexate – the so-called 'flag sign' – has also been documented.[36]

Hand-foot syndrome, also called chemotherapy-induced acral erythema acral erythrodysthesia or palmar-plantar erythrodysthesia, is commonly seen in patients receiving chemotherapy.[37–41] The most commonly implicated agents include pegylated liposomal doxorubicin, capecitabine, docetaxel, and doxorubicin.[41] Patients develop symmetric erythema, edema, and neuropathic pain involving the hands and feet that can progress to blistering with desquamation and ulceration.[41] Hand-foot syndrome can also be accompanied by hyperpigmentation in patients treated with capecitabine. This is discussed in more detail below.

Chemotherapeutic agents may interact with radiation therapy to result in various unusual manifestations including photosensitivity, radiation enhancement, radiation recall, and reactivation.

Photosensitivity may be induced by dacarbazine, 5-fluorouracil, hydroxyurea, and vinblastine.[7]

Radiation enhancement, which may be a feature of both dactinomycin and doxorubicin therapy, is due to impaired repair of radiation-induced sublethal cellular damage.[2,5] As a consequence, the effects of radiation therapy are amplified. Clinical manifestations include increased erythema, hyperpigmentation, erosions, blistering, and necrosis at the site of radiation therapy.[32] Radiation enhancement has also been encountered following therapy with adriamycin, bleomycin, cisplatin, 5-fluorouracil, hydroxyurea, and methotrexate.[5,7]

Radiation recall presents as erythema, vesiculation, and desquamation at the site of previous irradiation and may develop months or years after completion of treatment.[2] The mechanism is unknown. Dactinomycin is particularly incriminated.[2] A similar response has also been reported following therapy with adriamycin, bleomycin, cytarabine, doxorubicin, etoposide, 5-fluorouracil, hydroxyurea, melphalan, methotrexate, tamoxifen, and vinblastine.[7,42,43] Radiation recall reactions have been described following treatment with paclitaxel, gemcitabine, docetaxel, IFN-α2b, dacarbazine, acyclovir, capecitabine, chlorambucil, and sorafenib.[12,44–54]

Reactivation of ultraviolet light-induced erythema has been described as a complication of methotrexate and suramin therapy.[7,55] Manifestations include vesiculation and erythema.

Inflammatory changes affecting pre-existing actinic keratoses and seborrheic keratoses have been described following treatment with cisplatin, cytarabine, dacarbazine, dactinomycin, doxorubicin, 5-fluorouracil, 6-thioguanine, and vincristine.[4,5] The affected keratoses become pruritic and erythematous. It is suggested that such changes are analogous to radiation recall phenomena.[4]

Hypersensitivity reactions (including urticaria, angioedema, serum sickness, anaphylaxis, generalized dermatitis, and fixed drug eruption) are uncommon complications of chemotherapy. Although a wide range of agents may result in these responses, L-asparaginase, intravenous melphalan, and cisplatin have been particularly incriminated.[2,56,57] Cyclophosphamide, daunorubicin, doxorubicin, methotrexate, and procarbazine have also been implicated.[57] Dacarbazine and procarbazine may cause fixed drug reactions.[1] Immune complex-mediated reactions including vasculitis and some cases of EM or TEN may rarely be a result of treatment with hydroxyurea and mechlorethamine.[5] Contact dermatitis is an uncommon but important complication of topical mechlorethamine (mustard) therapy.[58]

An interstitial granulomatous maculopapular eruption following low-dose methotrexate in the treatment of collagen vascular diseases including lupus erythematosus and rheumatoid arthritis has been described.[59] The buttocks and limbs are commonly affected.

Newer chemotherapeutic agents have emerged that selectively target specific cellular pathways. Their increasing use has also resulted in diverse cutaneous side effects.[60,61] One class of such drugs is the epidermal growth factor receptor (EGFR) inhibitors which are used to treat non-small cell lung cancer, breast, colon, pancreatic, and squamous cell carcinoma of the head and neck.[62] Examples include cetuximab, gefitinib, erlotinib, and panitumab. Since EGFR is expressed in keratinocytes, follicular epithelium, eccrine glands, and sebaceous cells, adverse effects on the skin and appendages are common.[63] Acute folliculitis on the face and trunk is most common (*Fig. 14.94*).[60–62,64,65] Other potential side effects include dry skin (eczema

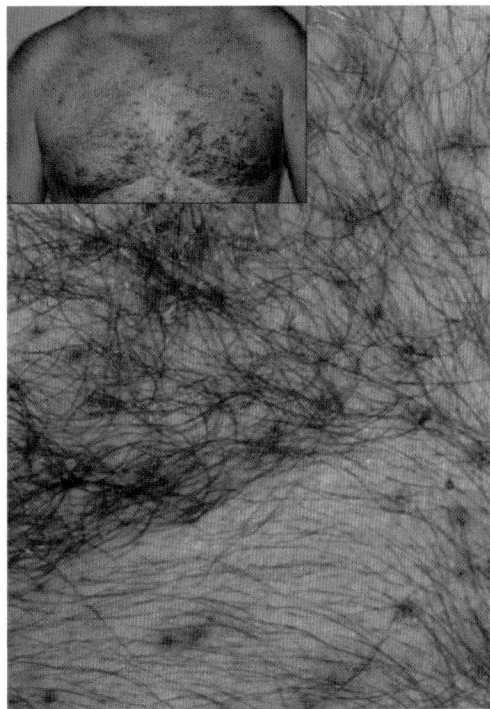

Fig. 14.94
Acneiform eruption in patient on EGFR inhibitor cetuximab. By courtesy of Klaus Busam, MD, Memorial Sloan Kettering Cancer Center, New York, New York, USA.

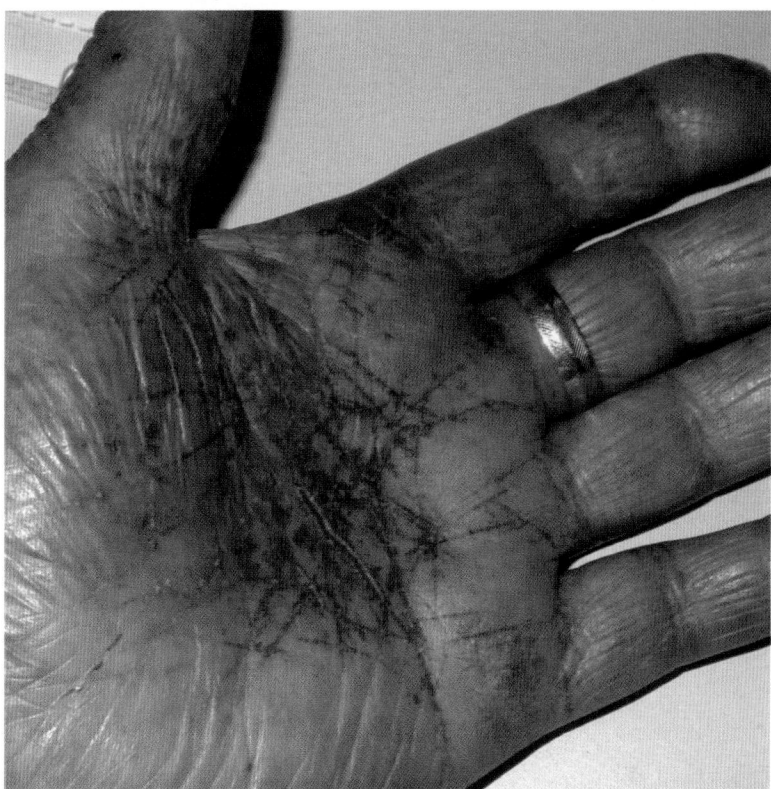

Fig. 14.96
Painful palmar fissures in patient on EGFR inhibitor cetuximab.

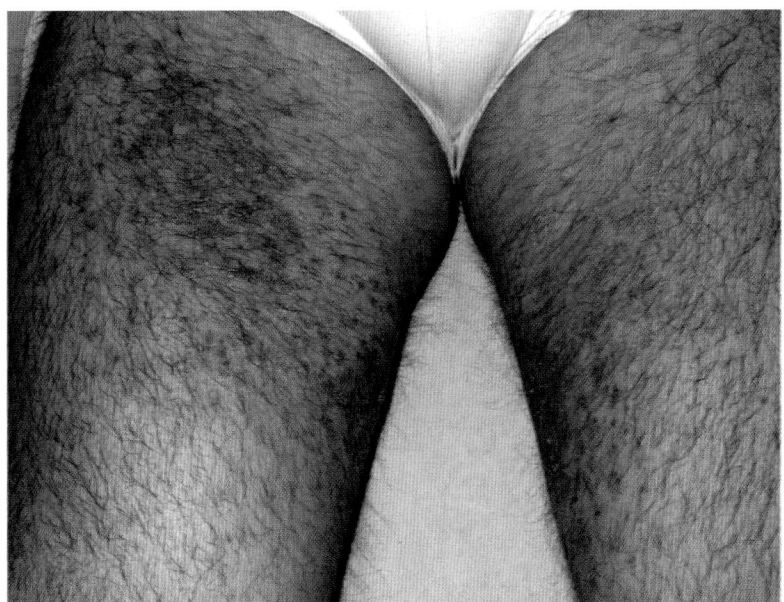

Fig. 14.95
Severe asteatotic eczema in patient on EGFR inhibitor panitumab.

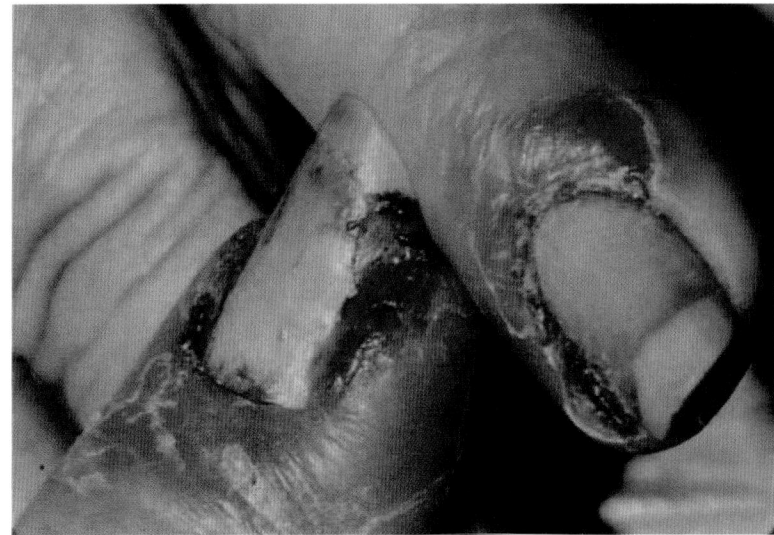

Fig. 14.97
Severe paronychia in patient on EGFR inhibitor cetuximab. By courtesy of Klaus Busam, MD, Memorial Sloan Kettering Cancer Center, New York, New York, USA.

craquelé) (*Fig. 14.95*) with painful fissures (*Fig. 14.96*), pruritus, nail alterations (paronychia, ingrown nails, nail fold fissures, onycholysis, splinter hemorrhages, pyogenic granulomas) (*Fig. 14.97*), hair changes (frontal alopecia, trichomegaly of eyelashes (*Fig. 14.98*), altered hair texture), and mucositis (*Fig. 14.99*).[60–69] Rare cases of vasculitis have also been reported (*Fig. 14.100*).[70]

Tyrosine kinase inhibitors imatinib, dasatinib, and nilotinib are used to treat chronic myeloid leukemia (CML).[60] Imatinib is also approved for treatment of gastrointestinal stromal tumor (GIST) and rare cases of inoperable or metastatic dermatofibrosarcoma protuberans. A wide range of cutaneous effects have been reported with these medications, the more common being hyper-, hypo- and de-pigmentation and macular-papular exanthems.[60,61,71,72] Patients may also develop edema and, less commonly, urticarial, lichenoid,

pityriasiform, and psoriasiform eruptions.[61] SJS, AGEP, Sweet syndrome, neutrophilic eccrine hidradenitis, neutrophilic panniculitis, and lymphomatoid drug reactions have also been reported.[61]

Sorafenib and sunitinib are multikinase inhibitors currently approved for treatment of a variety of malignancies, including, renal cell carcinoma, hepatocellular carcinoma melanoma, non-small cell lung carcinoma, pancreatic carcinoma, colon cancer, breast cancer, melanoma, and GIST.[60,61,73] The hand–foot skin reaction is seen in up to up to two-thirds of patients, typically 2 to 4 weeks after initiating treatment, and characterized by painful erythema and edema of the palms and soles (*Fig. 14.101*).[60,61,63,74–76] There may be associated paresthesia and desquamation. The lesions are discrete

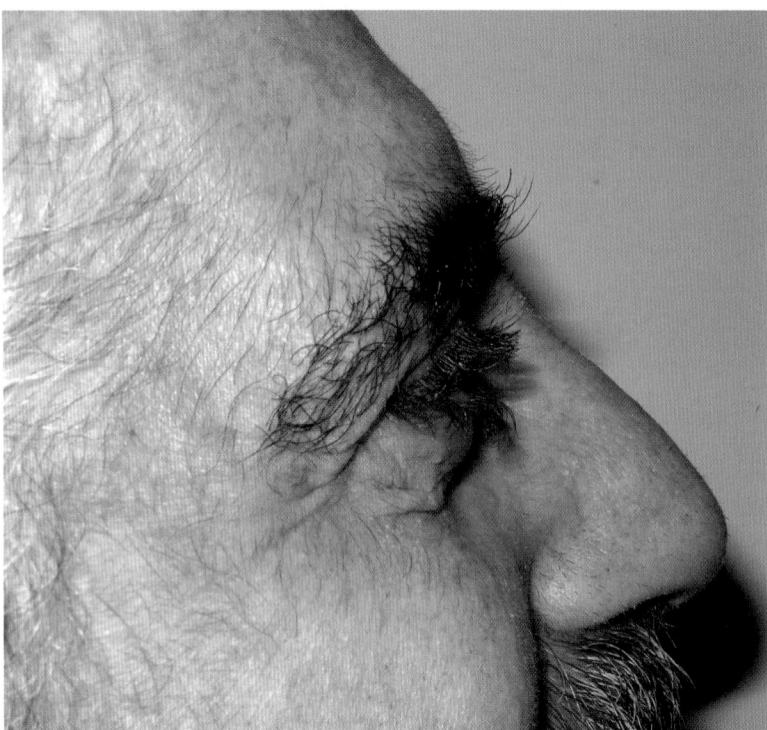

Fig. 14.98
Trichomegalia in patient on EGFR inhibitor panitumab.

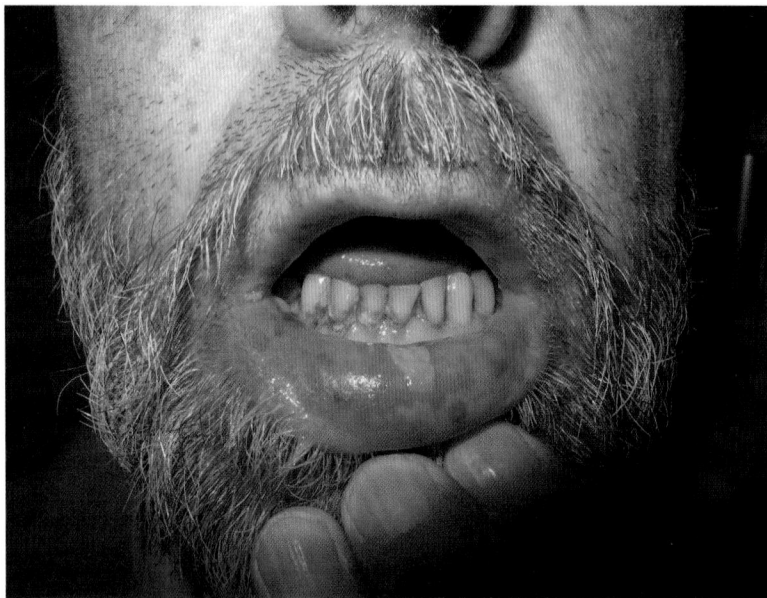

Fig. 14.99
Mucositis in patient on EGFR inhibitor panitumab.

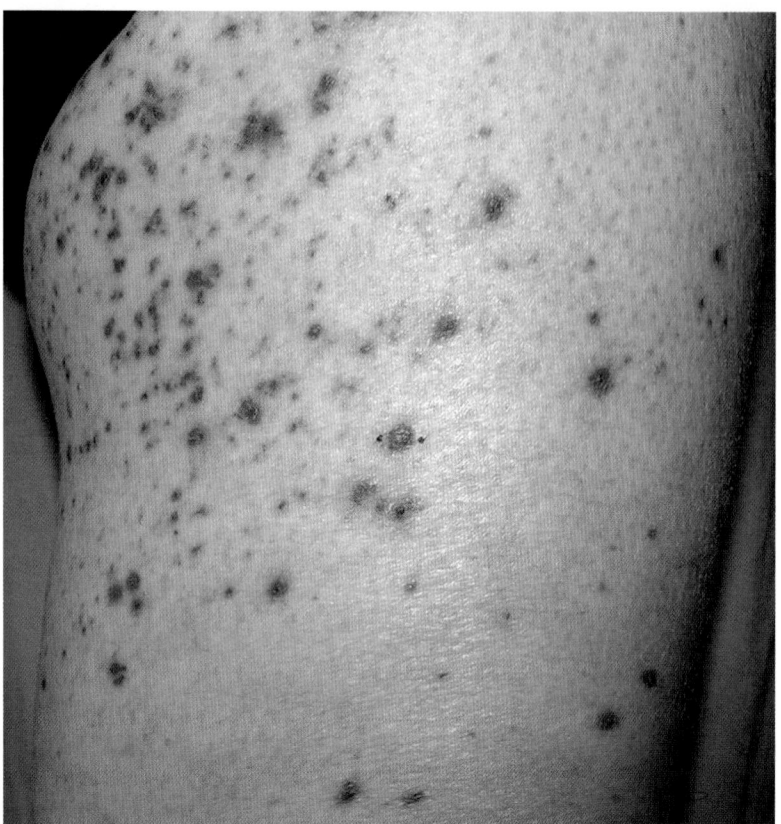

Fig. 14.100
Vasculitic drug reaction in patient on EGFR inhibitor. By courtesy of Chao-Kai Hsu, MD, Sheau-Chiou Chao and Julia Yu-Yun, National Cheng Kung University Hospital, Tainan, Taiwan.

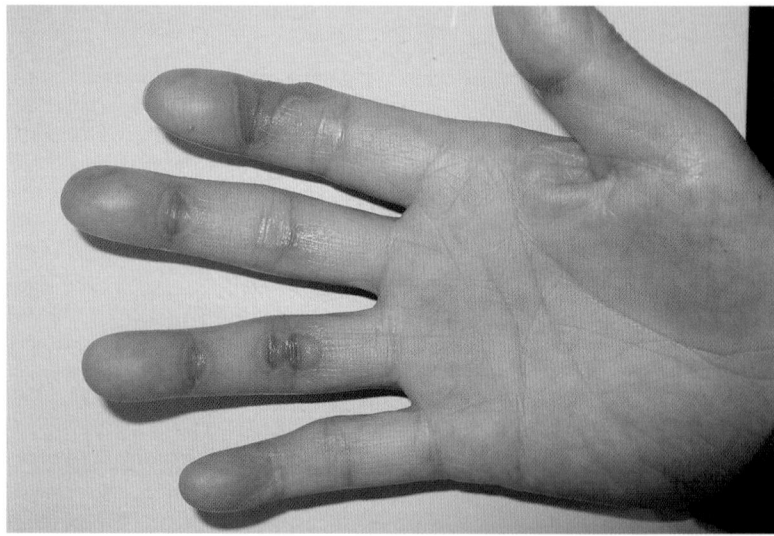

Fig. 14. 101
Chemotherapy-related drug reaction: there are discrete palmar bullae with a rim of erythema. The patient had been taking sorafenib. By courtesy of R. Lee, MD, Virginia Commonwealth University, Richmond, Virginia, USA.

and accompanied by hyperkeratosis, a feature not usually seen in acral erythema associated with traditional chemotherapeutic agents.[41,63] In contrast to hand-foot syndrome discussed above, hand–foot skin reaction also affects the soles more than the palms, although there is significant clinical overlap.[41] Other cutaneous reactions linked to sorafenib include pruritus, alopecia, actinic keratoses, and squamous cell carcinoma.[60,61,77,78]

Vismodegib is an inhibitor of the smoothened receptor in the hedgehog pathway that is used for the treatment of metastatic and advanced basal cell carcinoma. The most common cutaneous side effect is alopecia, seen in over 60% of patients.[61] Patients also may experience muscle spasms, dysgeusia, fatigue, nausea, and diarrhea.

Bortezomib, a proteasome inhibitor used to treat hematopoietic malignances, has been associated with morbilliform eruptions, ulcerations,

CD30-positive lymphomatoid drug reaction, edematous plaques, vasculitis, and interface dermatitis.[61,79–82]

Vemurafenib and dabrafenib are BRAF inhibitors of the mitogen-activated protein kinase (MAPK) pathway used in the treatment of metastatic melanoma. The most common cutaneous side effects are an exanthematous rash and photsensitivity.[61] SJS/TEN, DRESS, seborrheic dermatitis, and acneiform eruptions have also been reported.[83–86] Development of verrucal keratoses, keratoacanthomas, squamous cell carcinoma in situ, and invasive squamous cell carcinoma are seen in approximately 10% of

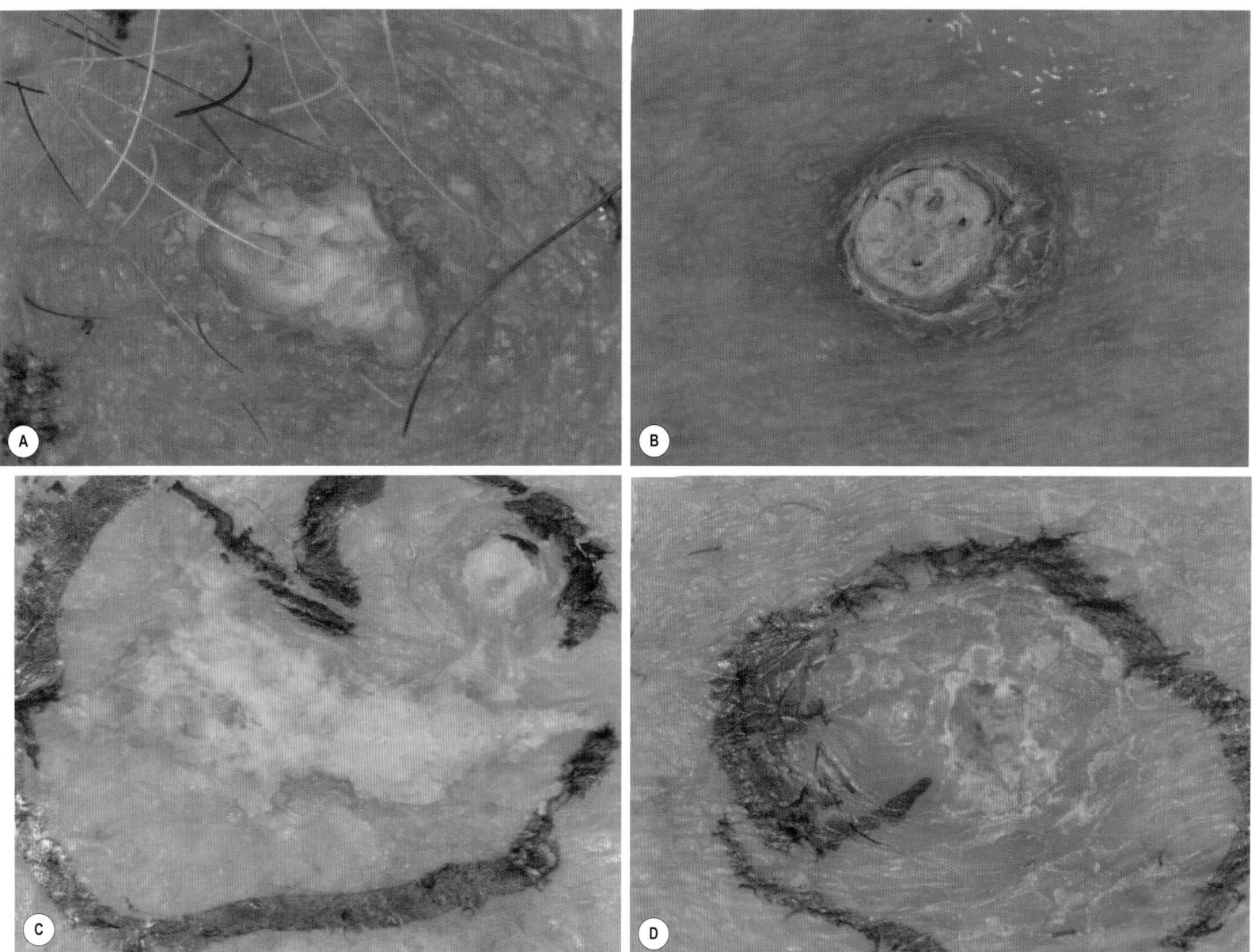

Fig. 14.102
Keratotic lesions seen in patients on vemurafenib including: (**A**) verrucal keratosis; (**B**) keratoacanthoma; (**C**) squamous cell carcinoma in situ; (**D**) invasive squamous cell carcinoma. By courtesy of Klaus Busam, MD, Memorial Sloan Kettering Cancer Center, New York, New York, USA.

patients (*Fig. 14.102*).[61] Trametinib, an inhibitor of MEK1 and MEK2 of the MAPK pathway, is associated with exanthematous rashes and acneiform eruptions, but not cutaneous squamous cell carcinoma.[61,87] Erythema nodosum-like lesions have also been associated with this group of drugs.[88]

Immunotherapy checkpoint inhibitors are a new chemotherapeutic option for treatment of melanoma. Ipilumimab, an anti-CTLA-4 immunotherapy, may be complicated by pruritus, a morbilliform rash, vitiligo, and, less commonly, prurigo nodularis, lichenoid dermatitis, pyoderma-gangrenosum-like ulcerations, photosensitivity, radiation recall, TEN, alopecia, and DRESS.[89] Nivolumab and pembrolizumab are anti-PD-1 antibody immunotherapies. Morbilliform drug eruptions, lichenoid dermatitis, and vitiligo are the most common adverse cutaneous reactions.[90] Psoriasiform dermatitis, lupus erythematosus, and pemphigoid-like reactions have also been reported as side effects.[89,90]

Histologic features

The histologic features largely depend on the type of drug reaction seen in the patient. Interface dermatitis represents the most frequently encountered histologic appearance in chemotherapy adverse drug reactions (*Figs 14.103–14.105*).[90–93] In addition to the epidermis, both follicular and sweat gland/duct epithelium may be affected. Appearances are variable, ranging from lichen planus-like changes (including hyperkeratosis, hypergranulosis, acanthosis, basal cell hydropic degeneration, and apoptosis) to lupus erythematosus-like reactions in which the epidermis is markedly atrophic. The combination of interface changes with severe maturation arrest (dysmaturation) is pathognomonic of chemotherapy-related reactions. It is particularly a feature of patients receiving long-term chemotherapy, high-dose chemotherapy, and multiagent chemotherapy. In addition to impaired maturation, the epidermis appears disorganized and individual keratinocytes are enlarged with pleomorphic nuclei containing conspicuous nucleoli (*Fig. 14.106*). These changes are particularly associated with bleomycin, busulfan, and hydroxyurea. Eccrine squamous syringometaplasia (squamous metaplasia of the dermal sweat ducts) may be seen with a variety of chemotherapeutic agents including methotrexate, bleomycin, pegylated liposomal doxorubicin, vincristine, dabrafenib, vemurafenib, tamoxifen, and docetaxel.[94–102] Checkpoint inhibitor reactions most frequently result in a lichenoid interface dermatitis that shows significant histologic overlap with lichen planus (*Fig. 14.107*).[103] The epidermis also exhibits acanthosis but lacks the dysmaturation of traditional chemotherapeutic agents.

Etoposide, a podophyllin derivative, in addition to causing maturation abnormalities, can cause metaphase arrest with characteristic fragmented nuclear chromatin resulting in so-called 'starburst cells'.[104]

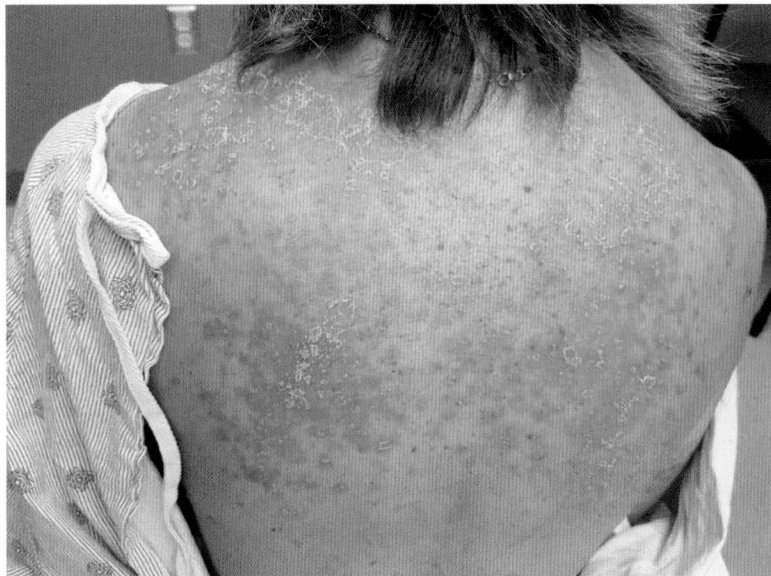

Fig. 14.103
Lichenoid dermatitis secondary to Nivolumab. By courtesy of Adrienne Choksi, MD, MD Anderson Cancer Center, Houston, Texas, USA.

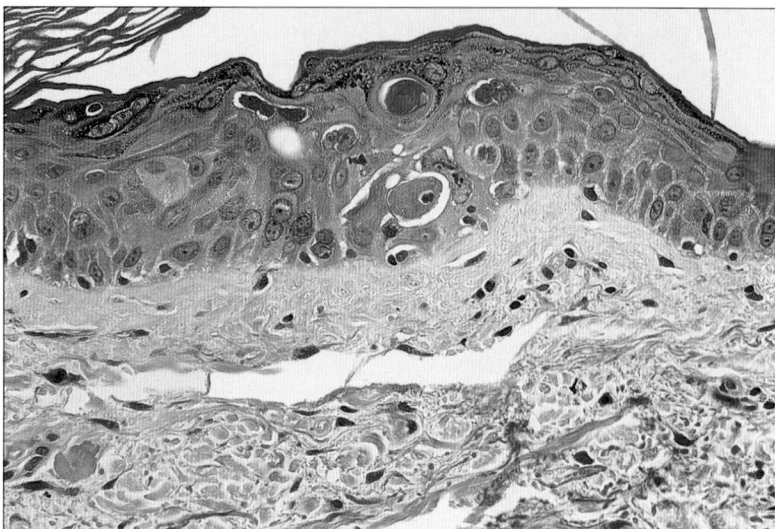

Fig. 14.105
Chemotherapy-related drug reaction: there is striking dyskeratosis and abnormal maturation. The latter is a common feature of chemotherapy reactions.

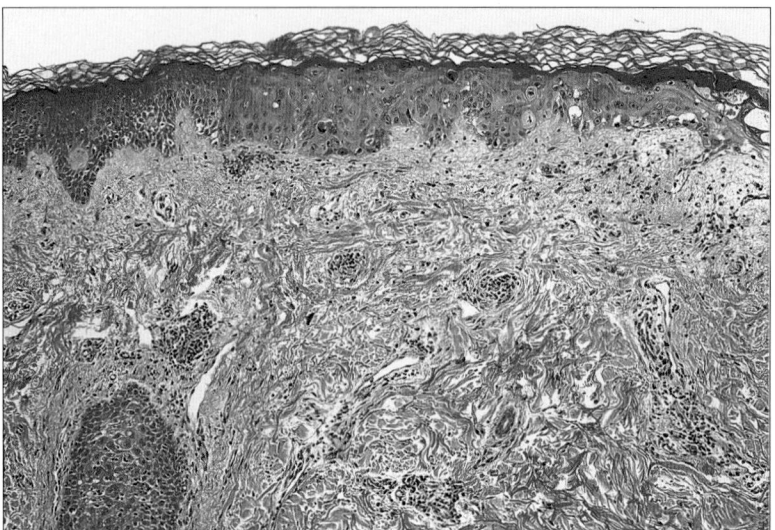

Fig. 14.104
Chemotherapy-related drug reaction: there are interface changes with basal cell hydropic degeneration and apoptosis.

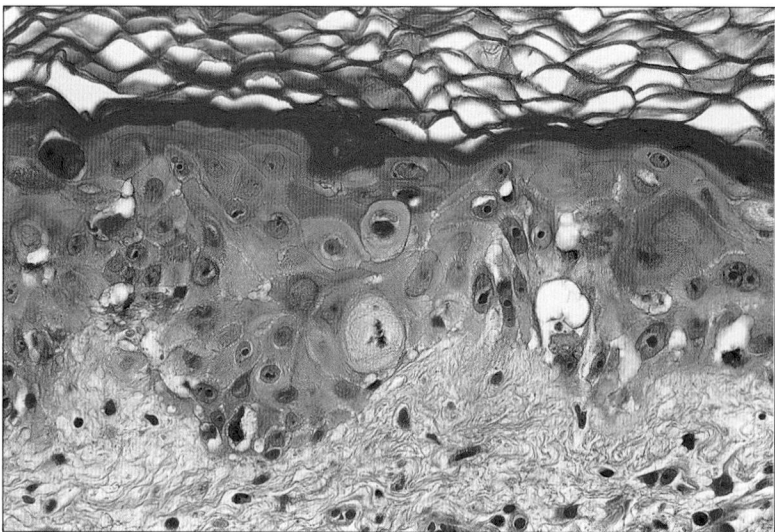

Fig. 14.106
Chemotherapy-related drug reaction: close-up view.

Hyperpigmentation complicating busulfan therapy predominantly affects the basal layer of the epidermis but may also extend throughout the full thickness and is often accompanied by pigmentary incontinence due to melanocyte toxicity.[105] Similarly, bleomycin-induced hyperpigmentation is characterized by epidermal hyperpigmentation and pigmentary incontinence.[106] Melanocytes are present in normal numbers. The early inflammatory phase is characterized by a superficial perivascular infiltrate of lymphocytes, histiocytes, occasional neutrophils, plasma cells, and eosinophils. Some authors, however, have described basal cell pigmentation in the absence of pigmentary incontinence.[28,107] Lymphocytic vasculitis has also been reported.[29]

Thio-TEPA-induced pigmentation is similarly characterized by melanin pigment within all layers of the epidermis including the stratum corneum, accompanied by basal cell hydropic degeneration and pigmentary incontinence.[34] A mild perivascular lymphohistiocytic infiltrate is present in the superficial dermis. The melanocyte concentration is normal.

Radiation recall is characterized by epidermal atrophy, basal cell hydropic degeneration, and superficial dermal vascular ectasia.

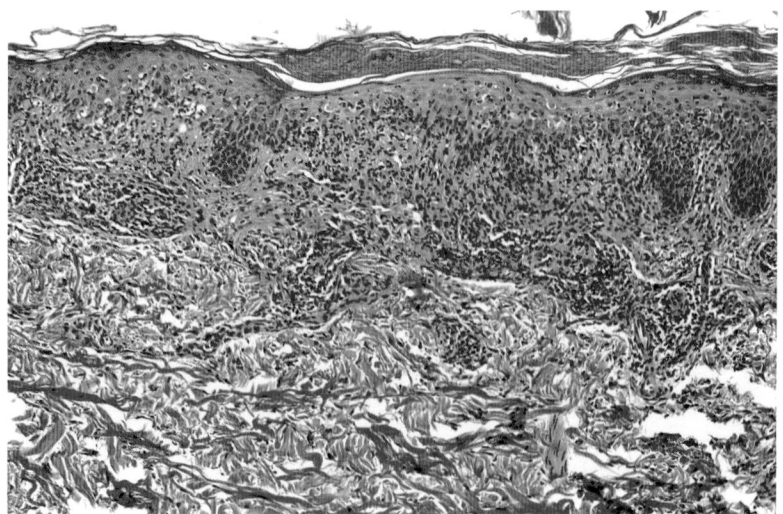

Fig. 14.107
Lichenoid interface drug reaction secondary to PD1 inhibitor. By courtesy of Michael T. Tetzlaff, MD, PhD, The University of MD Anderson Cancer Center, Houston, Texas, USA.

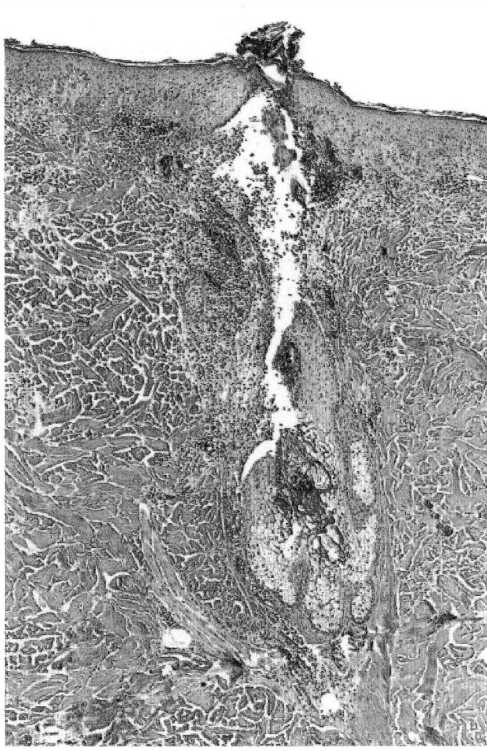

Fig. 14.108
Pustular folliculitis secondary to EGFR inhibitor. By courtesy of Klaus Busam, MD, Memorial Sloan Kettering Cancer Center, New York, New York, USA.

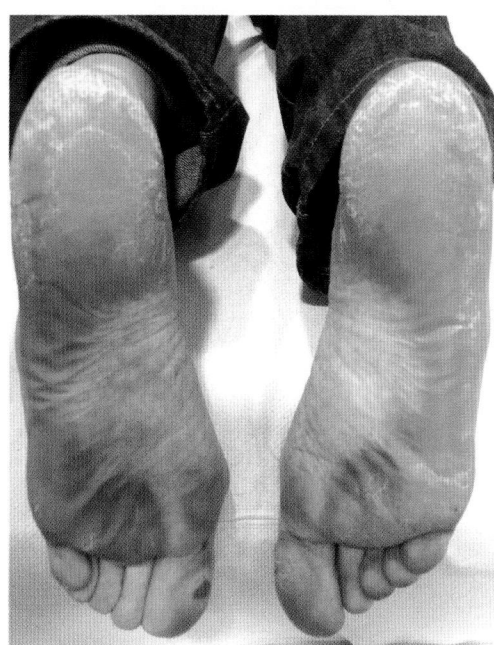

Fig. 14.109
Chemotherapy induced acral erythema characterized by circumscribed erythematous macules on soles. By courtesy of Eduardo Rozas Munoz, MD, Hospital de la Santa Creu I Sant Pau, Barcelona, Spain.

In addition to anagen alopecia and interface changes, pustular folliculitis and allergic contact dermatitis (5-fluorouracil) may be a feature of chemotherapy-associated adverse reactions, particularly with dactinomycin and 5-fluorouracil.[108,109]

Hypersensitivity reactions including urticaria, angioedema, and maculopapular eruptions are histologically no different from other drug-induced lesions (see above).

Dermal sclerosis may be a feature of bleomycin and docetaxel therapy.[110]

Extravasation of chemotherapeutic agents including cisplatin, dactinomycin, daunorubicin, doxorubicin, etoposide, idarubicin, mechlorethamine, mithramycin, paclitaxel, vinblastine, and vincristine may result in chemical cellulitis and tissue necrosis.[1]

Spongiotic dermatitis is rarely seen as a complication of systemic chemotherapy but has been described following treatment with methotrexate, 5-fluorouracil, and dacarbazine.[92,93] It is much more commonly encountered following topical chemotherapeutic agents including 5-fluorouracil and mechlorethamine.

The interstitial granulomatous reaction associated with low-dose methotrexate therapy is characterized by a largely histiocytic interstitial infiltrate with small numbers of neutrophils.[55] Vasculitis is not a feature. The histiocytes may surround neutrophil aggregates, and a characteristic feature is histiocytes forming a palisade around collagen fibers.[78]

Pustular folliculitis secondary to EGFR inhibitors demonstrates a dilated, hyperkeratotic follicular infundibulum.[76] The perifollicular infiltrate initially contains lymphocytes and later becomes neutrophilic (*Fig. 14.108*). Epidermal dysmaturation and extravasation of red blood cells are also seen.[111] Vasculitis secondary to EGFR inhibitors is rare, showing features of typical leukocytoclastic vasculitis.

The histologic features of hand-foot eruption seen with multikinase inhibitors sorafenib and sunitinib include vacuolar interface alteration along the dermal–epidermal junction, dyskeratotic keratinocytes, and a thin to absent granular cell layer with variable parakeratosis.[63,73] Mitotic figures may also be seen predominantly in the spinous layer. Intraepidermal cleavage occurs as a consequence of epidermal cell necrosis. Intradermal perivascular inflammation is sparse and contains mononuclear cells with inconspicuous eosinophils. Vasculitis is not seen.

Chemotherapy-induced acral erythema

Clinical features

Chemotherapy-induced acral erythema (acral erythema, hand-foot syndrome, palmoplantar erythrodysesthesia syndrome, toxic erythema of the palms and soles) in which the patient presents with circumscribed, extremely painful, and tender erythematous macules on the palms, fingertips, and soles has been described following treatment with 5-fluorouracil, cyclophosphamide, cytarabine, daunorubicin, doxorubicin, and vincristine (*Fig. 14.109*).[1–12] Pegylated liposomal doxorubicin, capecitabine, docetaxel, and doxorubicin are now the most commonly implicated drugs.[13] Etoposide, mercaptopurine, methotrexate, and vinblastine have also been incriminated. Patients subsequently develop blisters followed by desquamation.

Histologic features

The histologic features include basal cell liquefactive degeneration, keratinocyte necrosis, and mild spongiosis.[1–3,14] There is papillary dermal edema, vascular dilatation, and a mild superficial perivascular lymphohistiocytic infiltrate. Features of syringosquamous metaplasia and eccrine neutrophilic hidradenitis are rarely seen.[15,16]

In one case, immunohistochemistry of the dermal lymphocytes disclosed a CD3+, CD16+, CD56+, leukocyte function antigen-1 positive phenotype suggestive of NK T-cells.[17] The eccrine ducts expressed HLA-DR and intercellular adhesion molecule-1 (ICAM-1).[18]

Differential diagnosis

The features are indistinguishable from those of GVHD. Distinction is dependent upon clinicopathological correlation. Compared to hand-foot reaction associated with multikinase inhibitors, there is no diminution of the granular cell layer, parakeratosis, or intraepidermal mitoses.[17]

Chemotherapy-associated eccrine gland reactions

Although there is some histologic overlap between neutrophil eccrine hidradenitis and eccrine syringosquamous metaplasia, more often they present independently of one another and, as such, they are considered separately.

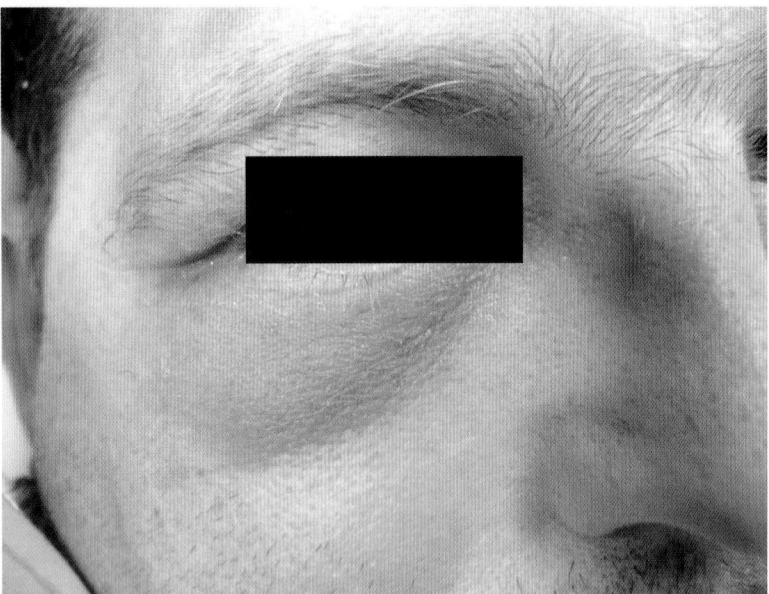

Fig. 14.110
Neutrophilic eccrine hidradenitis secondary to cytarabine manifesting as cellulitis-like plaques on the face. By courtesy of Scott Guenthner, MD, Plainfield, Indiana, USA.

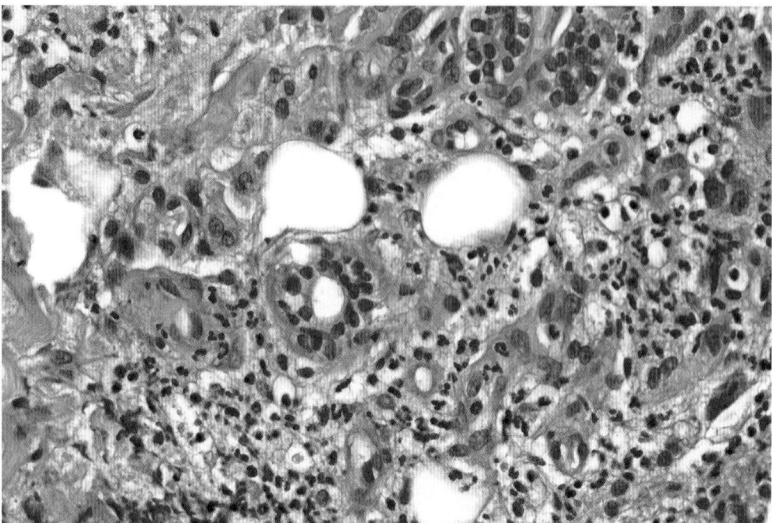

Fig. 14.111
Neutrophilic eccrine hidradenitis: there is a neutrophil infiltrate involving the eccrine gland. Note the sparing of the duct in the center of the field.

Neutrophilic eccrine hidradenitis

Clinical features

This rare eccrine gland reaction was initially reported in a patient receiving induction chemotherapy including doxorubicin and cytarabine in the treatment of acute myelogenous leukemia.[1] Subsequently, a similar eruption was described in patients with a number of other malignancies such as Hodgkin lymphoma, non-Hodgkin lymphoma, breast carcinoma, Wilms tumor, osteosarcoma, and testicular tumors including embryonal carcinoma and teratoma.[2–7] Further cases developing in association with acute myelogenous leukemia have also been documented.[8,9] Additional chemotherapeutic agents including bleomycin, chlorambucil, daunorubicin, dactinomycin, vincristine, lomustine, mitoxantrone, thioguanine, cis-platinum, vinblastine, topotecan, cyclophosphamide, 5-fluorouracil, carbamazepine, cetuximab, and BRAF inhibitors may also be causative, although cytarabine has been most commonly implicated.[10–13] A case following the use of GM-CSF has been reported.[14] It should be noted, however, that neutrophilic eccrine hidradenitis has also been described as a prodromal manifestation of acute myelogenous leukemia in the absence of chemotherapy.[15] The condition has been described in HIV-positive patients receiving zidovudine and as a complication of treatment with acetaminophen.[16–19]

Clinically, patients (who are commonly febrile) develop a polymorphous eruption consisting of variably asymptomatic or tender erythematous to violaceous macules, papules, plaques, nodules, and pustules, which most often presents within 1 or 2 weeks of starting chemotherapy.[4] Lesions may be very numerous and, although there does not appear to be a site predilection, the trunk and upper limbs are most often affected.[5] Facial involvement may also occur, manifesting as periorbital edema, violaceous plaques, and lesions that mimic cellulitis (Fig. 14.110).[20–22] Ear involvement seen as bilateral tender erythema has been documented.[23] An atypical presentation with symmetrical, erythematous plaques isolated to the breasts has also been reported.[24] The lesions desquamate and usually heal spontaneously within 1–3 weeks.[4] Postinflammatory hyperpigmentation and scarring are not usually features. Recurrence following the reintroduction of chemotherapy has been documented.[1,8] Clinically, an infectious condition, leukemia cutis, bullous pyoderma, atypical pyoderma gangrenosum, or Sweet disease is most often suspected.[8]

Pathogenesis and histologic features

The pathogenesis of this condition is unknown, but it has been proposed that the drug may be concentrated in the sweat glands, thereby exerting a direct toxic effect on the secretory epithelial cells.[1,2] This view is supported by the report of a patient with clinical lesions identical to neutrophilic eccrine hidradenitis without histologic evidence of neutrophilic infiltration in a neutropenic patient.[25] Alternatively, it has been suggested that the condition may represent part of the spectrum of acute neutrophilic dermatoses which also includes Sweet syndrome and pyoderma gangrenosum.[4] Presentation as a prodromal manifestation of leukemia before the introduction of chemotherapy and its development in an otherwise healthy person as a probable complication of prolonged pressure suggests that the etiology is likely to be multifactorial.[15,19]

The most significant histologic features are seen in the deeper reticular dermis and subcutaneous fat where a dense neutrophil polymorph infiltrate surrounds the eccrine secretory coils (Fig. 14.111). The coiled and straight dermal ducts are typically unaffected. Leukocytoclasis is sometimes evident.[4,26] The glandular epithelium shows neutrophil infiltration, nuclear pyknosis, cytoplasmic eosinophilia, or vacuolation and often appears sloughed off into the lumen of the gland.[7] Syringosquamous metaplasia may additionally be present; rarely, necrosis of the eccrine gland is seen in the absence of significant inflammation.[8,20,27,28] The periadnexal fibroadipose tissue stroma typically shows mucinous degeneration and a variable infiltrate of neutrophils, lymphocytes, histiocytes, and eosinophils.[8] Recently, it has been shown that the apocrine glands may be affected in addition to the eccrine glands.[29] There is no evidence of vasculitis.

Differential diagnosis

Idiopathic plantar hidradenitis (idiopathic recurrent palmoplantar hidradenitis in children, neutrophilic eccrine hidradenitis in children) is a rare dermatosis in which tender, painful, erythematous papules, plaques, and nodules, 0.5–3.0 cm in diameter, develop on the soles of the feet of children.[30–34] Pustular lesions have been reported.[35] Less often, concomitant palmar involvement has been documented.[31] Recurrences are not uncommon. The condition shows a predilection for females (2:1).[30] Incidence shows seasonal variation, with lesions developing most often in spring and autumn. Adults may also rarely be affected.[36] Although trauma does not appear to be an etiological factor, chronic pressure is probably of importance. Prolonged immersion in hot bath water preceded the development of lesions in a number of cases. Pyrexia is not usually present, and the patients are otherwise well. The condition generally clears spontaneously.

In contrast to eccrine neutrophilic hidradenitis, the changes are centered on the coiled duct and proximal straight duct, the secretory apparatus usually being spared or only minimally affected.[30] There is an intense neutrophil infiltrate surrounding and involving the ductal epithelium associated with epithelial degenerative changes and necrosis. Abscess formation may also be a feature. Eccrine syringosquamous metaplasia is not seen.

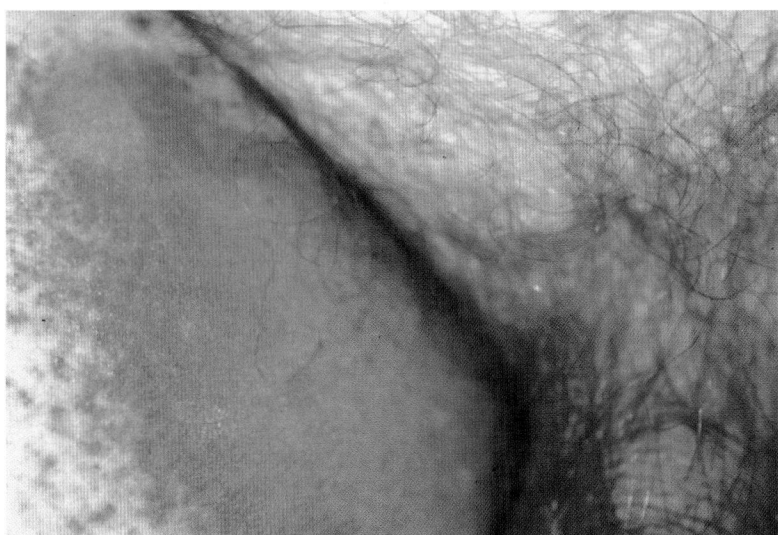

Fig. 14.112
Eccrine squamous syringometaplasia: there is an erythematous patch with a dusky center on the thigh and in the inguinal fold.

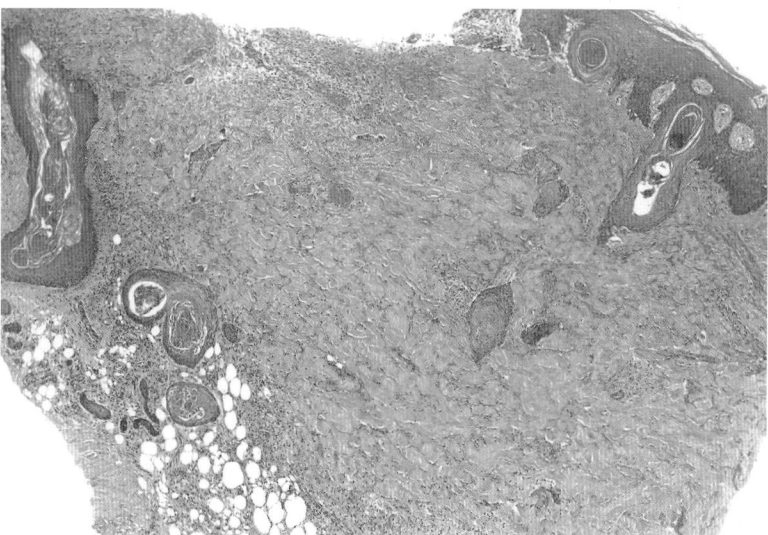

Fig. 14.113
Eccrine squamous syringometaplasia: the eccrine ductal wall is replaced with squamous epithelium.

Rarely, neutrophilic eccrine hidradenitis may represent a primary infectious process, for example, *Serratio* spp., *Enterobacter cloacae*, *Staphylococcus aureus*, and *Nocardia asteroides*.[37-39]

Eccrine squamous syringometaplasia

Clinical features

Eccrine squamous syringometaplasia (syringosquamous metaplasia) is a histologically distinctive eruption that may rarely develop following chemotherapy.[1-3] Patients present with erythematous papules often in a generalized distribution following the administration of a number of chemotherapeutic agents including bleomycin, cytarabine, daunorubicin, doxorubicin, and *cis*-platinum (*Fig. 14.112*). A similar response has been seen with the kinase inhibitors sunitinib, imatinib, vemurafenib, and dabrafenib.[4-8] Pustules and vesicles are sometimes seen. Presentation as acral erythema has also been documented.[9,10]

Histologic features

The changes primarily affect the upper portion of the eccrine duct and consist of squamous metaplasia associated with apoptosis of the lining epithelium (*Figs 14.113* and *14.114*).[1] Periductal edema and fibrosis may also be seen. A perivascular infiltrate consisting of lymphocytes and occasionally neutrophils is present in the surrounding dermis.

Differential diagnosis

Eccrine squamous syringometaplasia may occur in a wide variety of settings. It may be found adjacent to cutaneous ulcers, following severe burns, at radiation sites, as a feature in panniculitis, linear scleroderma, morphea, pyoderma gangrenosum, in fibrous hamartoma of infancy, in recall phenomenon, in association with tumors including squamous cell carcinoma and keratoacanthoma, and in infections including herpes virus, cytomegalovirus, and HIV.[11-20] It has also been described as a complication of benoxaprofen therapy.[21] In these settings, it is critical to recognize the underlying primary process. Differentiating the process from squamous cell carcinoma is also critical. The absence of overlying dysplasia in the epidermis and the continuity of the process with eccrine ducts allows distinction.

Adverse reactions to cytokine therapy

Clinical features

A very wide range of adverse reactions to the large number of recombinant cytokines available as therapeutic agents has been described.[1] These

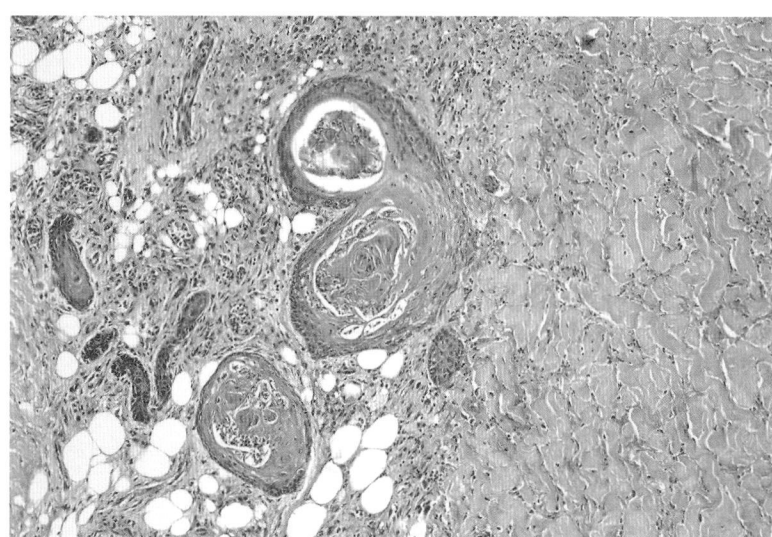

Fig. 14. 114
Eccrine squamous syringometaplasia: high-power view.

are very comprehensively documented in the review article of Asnis and Gaspari.[2] The majority of these agents have, to a greater or lesser extent, been associated with local injection site reactions (painful or pruritic erythematous wheals).[2] Only a limited number of cytokines, which may be associated with more specific dermatological manifestations, are included in this section.

Granulocyte colony-stimulating factor (G-CSF, filgrastim; a glycoprotein that stimulates proliferation and differentiation of neutrophils) therapy has been associated with a number of dermatological conditions including bullous pyoderma gangrenosum, folliculitis, leukocytoclastic vasculitis, and Sweet syndrome.[2-9] G-CSF and GM-CSF have also been incriminated in exacerbation of pre-existent leukocytoclastic vasculitis, psoriasis, a generalized erythematous eruption, erythematous plaques, and a localized lichenoid reaction.[10-15]

A number of adverse reactions have been described following treatment with GM-CSF (a growth factor which stimulates proliferation and differentiation of neutrophils, monocytes, and eosinophils) including localized angioedema, facial flushing, and generalized erythematous, maculopapular, exfoliative, urticarial, pruritic, and pustular cutaneous reactions.[2,16-19] Localized pustular and vasculitic reactions, generalized folliculitis, epidermolysis bullosa acquisita, and alopecia have also followed treatment with GM-CSF.[2,7,18-21]

The use of IFN-α may be followed by localized erythema and, less often, skin necrosis. It is followed by the development of alopecia in up to 10% of patients.[22] Psoriasis, pyoderma gangrenosum, localized granulomatous and suppurative lesions, ulcers, vasculitis, systemic lupus erythematosus, eosinophilic fasciitis, eczematous lesions, photosensitivity, paraneoplastic pemphigus, and a localized lupus-like reaction have also complicated its use.[2,23–30] Sarcoidosis induced by IFN-α is also well documented.[31–33] Cutaneous and systemic disease may occur as a consequence of enhanced helper T-cell type 1 (Th1) immune response, resulting in granulomatous inflammation.

Pegylated IFN-α, used increasingly for its improved bioavailability compared to traditional IFN, has been linked to hyperpigmentation.[34–36] Expression of α-melanocyte stimulating hormone receptors is increased by IFN, and is thought to be the cause of lingual and cutaneous darkening. Cutaneous lesions are reported to occur at sites of injection and elsewhere, including the face, trunk, extremities, and nails. Lesions develop weeks to months after starting therapy.

Single case reports have documented instances of fatal pemphigus vulgaris and allergic facial contact dermatitis following treatment with IFN-β.[37,38] Erythematous plaques, cutaneous ulceration, necrosis, vasculitis, sclerodermiform lesions, and lobular panniculitis have also been documented.[39–45]

IFN-γ may induce psoriatic plaques at the injection site, and its use has been shown to induce erythema nodosum leprosum in patients with leprosy.[46,47]

IL-2, which is produced by activated T lymphocytes, stimulates the production of a number of cytokines including IFN-γ, TNF, and GM-CSF in addition to inducing differentiation of an activated killer cell population which has a cytotoxic effect on tumor cells.[48,49] Dermatological complications of recombinant IL-2 (r IL-2) therapy include a desquamating, diffuse erythematous macular eruption, pruritus, purpura, telogen effluvium, mucositis with aphthous ulcers, and glossitis.[2,48] TEN-like blistering dermatoses, pemphigus vulgaris, linear IgA disease, vitiligo, and erythema nodosum have also been reported.[2,29,50–54] IL-2 therapy may be associated with exacerbation of psoriasis.[55,56]

Pruritus, facial edema, and a transient acantholytic dermatosis-like eruption affecting the chest, back, and proximal extremities have been described following treatment with IL-4, and there is a case report describing the development of vitiligo in association with recombinant IL-4 therapy.[57,58]

Histologic features

Histologically, the erythematous lesions associated with G-CSF show epidermal acanthosis, parakeratosis, eosinophilic spongiosis with abscess formation, and interface changes.[14] The lichenoid eruption is characterized by hyperkeratosis, dyskeratosis, and interface change accompanied by a lymphocytic infiltrate.[15] An atypical dermal monocytic infiltrate characterized by nuclear pleomorphism and mitotic activity has been documented.[59]

The erythematous maculopapular eruption associated with GM-CSF is characterized by edema and a superficial perivascular and interstitial inflammatory cell infiltrate composed of T-helper lymphocytes, histiocytes, eosinophils, and conspicuous neutrophils accompanied by epidermal spongiosis and lymphocyte/neutrophil exocytosis.[16–18] Focal dyskeratosis may also be a feature.[16]

The histologic features of hyperpigmentation from pegylated IFN-α include increased melanin along the basal layer of the epidermis and papillary dermal melanophages.[35] There is no associated iron deposition.

Lobular panniculitis associated with IFN-β demonstrates a spectrum of changes.[45] Early on, there is a neutrophil-rich lobular panniculitis with sterile microabscess formation. Intravascular thrombi without vasculitis, increased interstitial mucin, and microcalcification may be seen. Areas of fat saponification with microcalcification are typical and must be distinguished from pancreatitis-associated panniculitis. As lesions become longstanding, there is less inflammation, predominantly composed of mononuclear cells with septal fibrosis and calcification surrounding adipocytes.

IL-2 skin reactions are characterized by interface vacuolar degeneration with rare necrotic keratinocytes accompanied by lymphocyte exocytosis and focal spongiosis.[3,48,56] Papillary dermal edema is present with a superficial perivascular lymphohistiocytic infiltrate. Rarely, epidermal necrosis may be extensive.[48]

The infiltrate consists predominantly of CD3+/CD4+/CD25-/HLA-DR+ T-helper cells with a small subpopulation of CD8+ lymphocytes. Endothelial cells and keratinocytes express ICAM-1.[48]

Histologically, the transient acantholytic dermatosis-like eruption associated with IL-4 therapy is characterized by acantholysis and suprabasal cleft formation with dyskeratosis, spongiosis, and a superficial perivascular lymphohistiocytic infiltrate with rare eosinophils.[55] Immunofluorescence studies have not been performed.

Cutaneous reaction of lymphocyte recovery

Clinical features

This unusual condition follows return of lymphocytes to the general circulation and skin after induction or augmentation chemotherapy.[1,2] It has been described most often following combined cytarabine and daunorubicin treatment and also following treatment with amsacrine, etoposide, IFN, cyclophosphamide, and vincristine.[3] Patients present with a pruritic, erythematous maculopapular eruption associated with pyrexia.[1] The eruption resolves with desquamation.[2]

Histologic features

The histologic features include mild spongiosis with lymphocyte exocytosis associated with interface change, keratinocyte atypia with impaired maturation (chemotherapy effect), and minimal dyskeratosis.[1,2] There is vascular dilatation, and a perivascular lymphocytic infiltrate is present in the superficial dermis. Eosinophils are absent.[2] Exceptionally, epidermal lymphocyte infiltration may be very marked so as to mimic mycosis fungoides.[4]

The infiltrate is composed of CD3+/CD4+ T-helper cells with a smaller subpopulation of CD8+ cells.[2] The lymphocytes may also express CD25.[4] Epidermal Langerhans cells are reduced in number, and there is minimal to absent keratinocyte HLA-DR and ICAM-1 expression.[2,4]

Nuclear pleomorphism with hyperchromatism and expression of CD30, CD25, and HLA-DR has been described in the eruption of lymphocyte recovery in patients who have also received human recombinant cytokines including GM-CSF and IL-3.[5]

Differential diagnosis

The features are indistinguishable from exanthematous drug reactions, viral infections, and acute GVHD.[6]

Dental amalgam tattoos

Clinical features

Dental amalgam tattoos develop following the accidental implantation of dental amalgam into the soft tissue of the mouth following a dental procedure. Lesions, which are most commonly found on the buccal, gingival, and alveolar mucosa, measure from 0.10 to 1.5 cm and present as flat gray to blue-gray or slate-colored lesions.[1]

Histologic features

Amalgam tattoos, which consist of mercury and silver, sometimes accompanied by tin, present as fine to globular, brown to black deposits lying free or within macrophages and also deposited on the elastic tissue fibers and blood vessels within the lamina propria (*Fig. 14.115*).[2–4]

Tumor necrosis factor-α inhibitors

The use of TNF-α inhibitors has rapidly expanded over the past decade. Etanercept, infliximab, and adalimumab are Food and Drug Administration approved for treatment of plaque-type psoriasis, rheumatoid arthritis, and ankylosing spondylitis. Other indications for its use include Crohn disease, ulcerative colitis, and juvenile idiopathic arthritis. As use of these medications has increased, so too has the side effect profile.

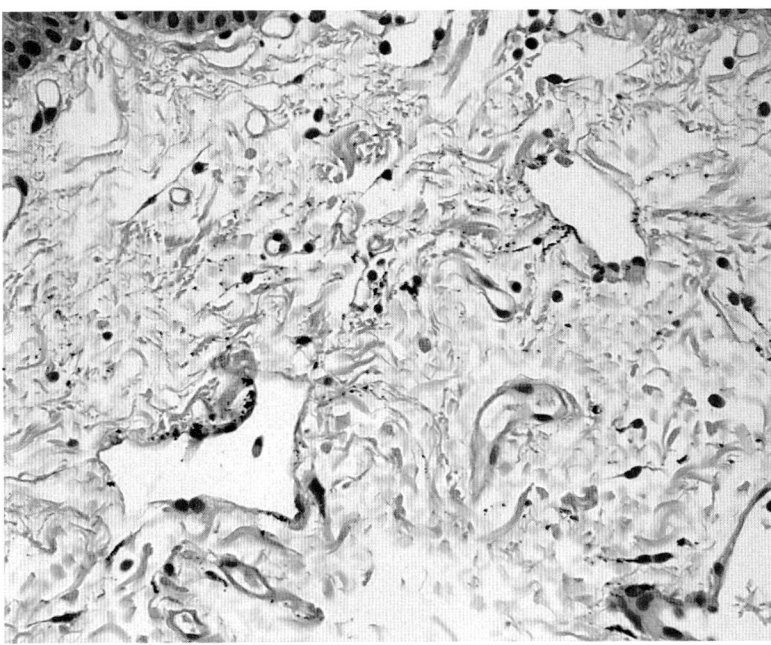

Fig. 14.115
Dental amalgam tattoo consisting of black exogenous pigment deposited on elastic fibers and blood vessel walls.

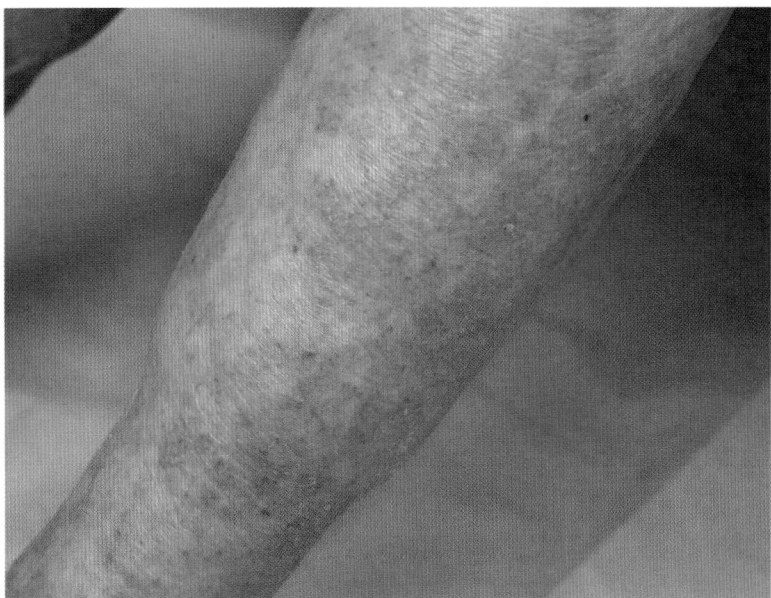

Fig. 14.117
Tumor necrosis factor-α inhibitor reaction: erythematous, psoriasiform plaques are present on the lower leg. By courtesy of J. Nunley, MD, Virginia Commonwealth University, Richmond, Virginia, USA.

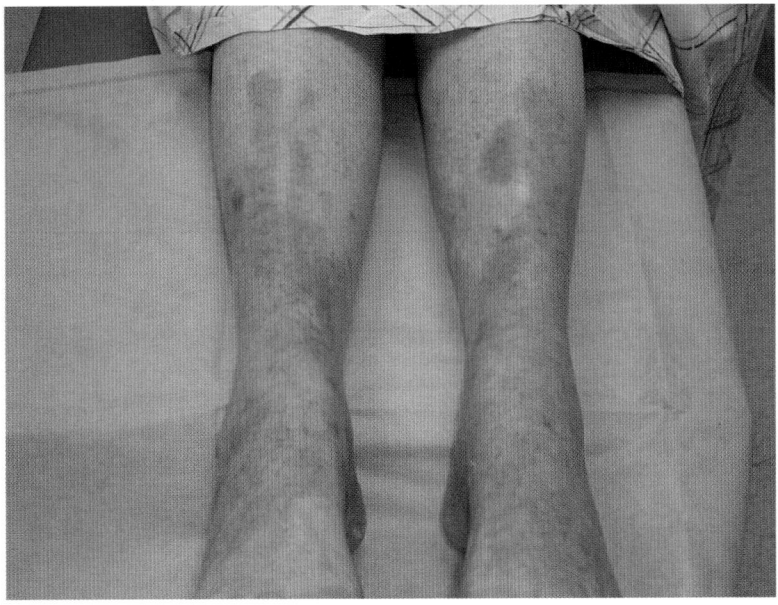

Fig. 14.116
Tumor necrosis factor-α inhibitor reaction: there are thin psoriasiform plaques on the lower legs.

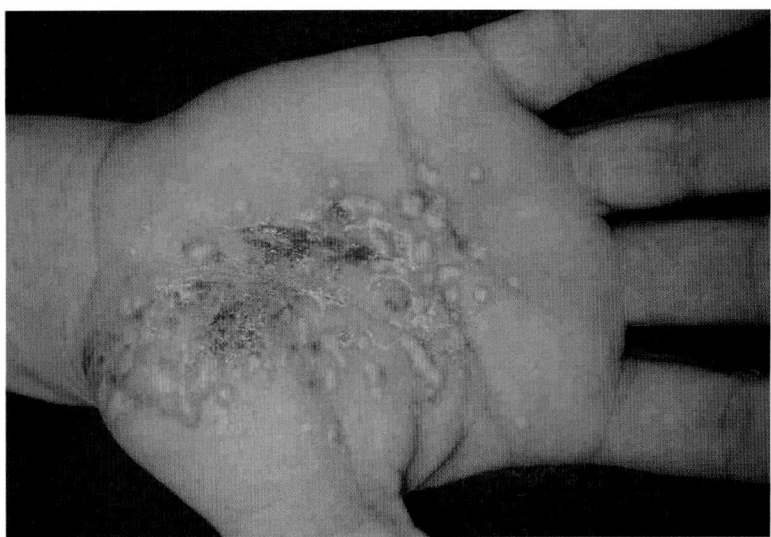

Fig. 14.118
Tumor necrosis factor-α inhibitor reaction: there are tense palmar pustules identical to those seen in palmar-plantar psoriasis.

The most common adverse dermatological effect is injection site reaction, occurring in up to one-third of patients.[1–3] Erythematous, edematous, eczematous lesions are described most commonly, although discoid lupus erythematosus and localized vasculitis have been reported.[1–4] Generalized vasculitis may also occur, either following localized lesions or de novo, involving the skin and other organ systems (kidneys, central and peripheral nervous systems, serosa, myocardium, lung, gall bladder).[5–7]

Paradoxically, a common cutaneous side effect seen distant from the injection site is psoriasis.[8–10] Both psoriasis vulgaris and palmar–plantar pustular psoriasis have been described, predominantly in patients treated for rheumatoid arthritis, ankylosing spondylitis, and Crohn disease (*Figs 14.116–14.118*).[10] Most psoriasiform reactions occur 6 to 10 months after starting therapy.[10,11] The proposed mechanism is increased IFN-α production by PDC as a consequence of TNF-α inhibition, which has been shown to induce psoriasis lesions.[12–14]

There is clinical overlap between the psoriasiform and lichenoid dermatitides associated with the TNF-α inhibitors. The clinical appearance of the lichenoid eruptions may resemble lichen planus, psoriasis, or be non-specific erythematous macules and papules.[15,16] The mechanism for development of these lesions is not well understood but is thought to be a consequence of cytokine imbalance.[17] The eruption begins weeks to months after starting TNF-α inhibition therapy.

Cutaneous infections are a well-known risk with TNF-α inhibitor therapy and include folliculitis, herpes simplex, tinea corporis, tinea versicolor, and rare cases of aspergillosis.[18–21]

An emerging reaction seen in the setting of TNF-α inhibition is granulomatous inflammation. Case reports describe cutaneous, pulmonary, and nodal sarcoidosis which improves upon discontinuation of therapy.[22–24] Additional reports include interstitial granulomatous dermatitis and granuloma annulare.[25,26]

Lupus-like syndromes may also occur as a consequence of therapy with TNF-α inhibitors.[27,28] Neutrophilic eccrine hidradenitis and Sweet syndrome-like reactions have also been reported.[29]

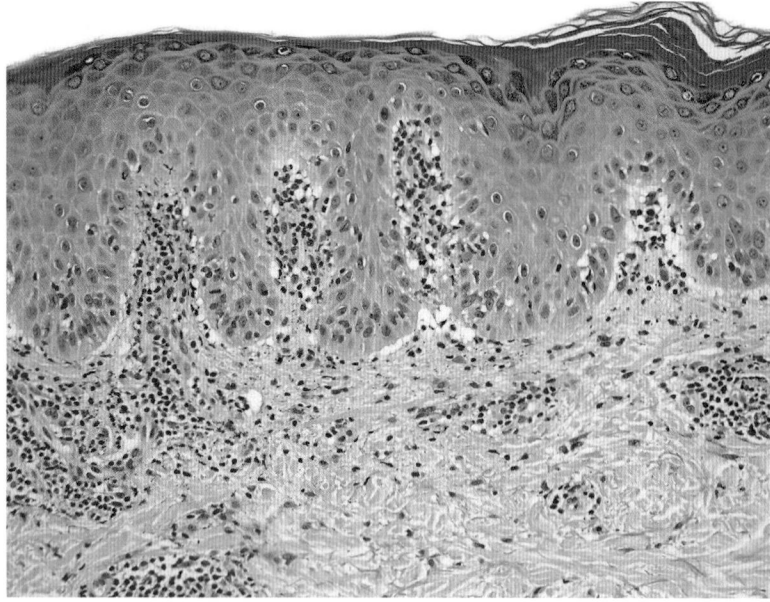

Fig. 14.119
Tumor necrosis factor-α inhibitor reaction: there is hyperkeratosis, hypergranulosis, psoriasiform hyperplasia, and interface change with a superficial perivascular lymphohistiocytic infiltrate.

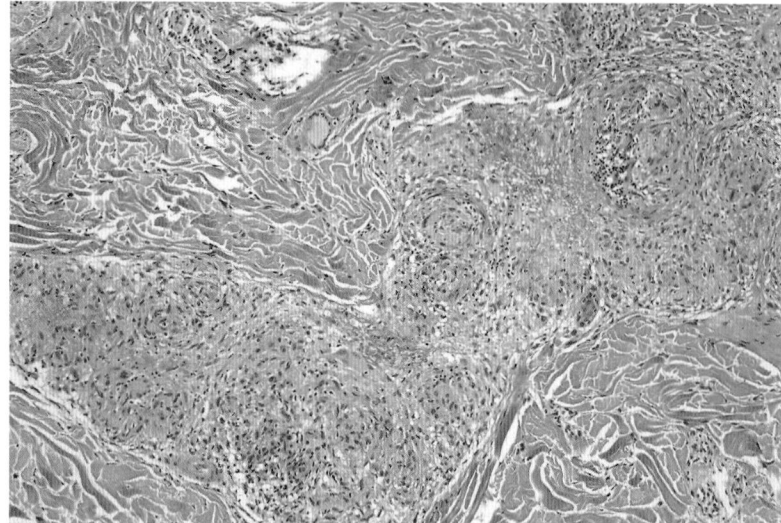

Fig. 14.120
Tumor necrosis factor-α inhibitor reaction: in this example, the features are indistinguishable from sarcoidosis.

Histologic features

Injection site reactions are characterized by dermal edema, a perivascular lymphocytic infiltrate with eosinophils.[1,2,4] Immunohistochemical studies demonstrate CD8-predominant T cells.[1]

Vasculitis in the setting of TNF-α inhibitor therapy may involve small- or medium-sized vessels with leukocytoclastic changes.[10] Necrotizing features and extravascular granulomatous inflammation have been described.

Psoriasis induced by TNF-α inhibitors resembles pustular psoriasis or psoriasis vulgaris, with variable presence of spongiosis and lichenoid inflammation.[13] The dermal infiltrate contains mononuclear cells, although eosinophils may be present.[13]

The few histologic descriptions of TNF-α inhibitor-associated lichenoid dermatitis available closely resemble lichen planus, with a lichenoid infiltrate of mononuclear cells, melanophages involving a hyperplastic epidermis, hyperkeratosis, and hypergranulosis.[15,16] Psoriasiform hyperplasia may be superimposed (*Fig. 14.119*). Vacuolar interface dermatitis may also be seen.[29]

TNF-α inhibitor associated sarcoidosis is characterized by noncaseating granulomata in the dermis and/or subcutis (*Figs 14.120* and *14.121*).[22] Necrotizing foci are rarely described. Interstitial granulomatous dermatitis demonstrates a diffuse intradermal infiltrate of histiocytes and lymphocytes with a variable number of eosinophils and occasional neutrophils.[25] There is no increased dermal mucin or vasculitis. Interface changes occur but are not common.

Other patterns that have been reported include pustular folliculitis, Sweet syndrome-like eruptions, and neutrophilic eccrine hidradenitis.[29]

Esthetic microimplants

Cosmetic dermatology is a rapidly evolving industry. The demand for 'non-surgical' rejuvenation has seen a rise in the number of implants and injectable materials available to patients. Unfortunately, inflammatory reactions to these agents occur.

There are several categories of fillers which may be permanent or resorbable (*Table 14.2*). Fillers are either polymers, which function as volumizers, creating effect by taking up space, or a combination of degradable polymer and microparticles.[1] The microparticles serve as a lattice upon which the host's response (often collagen induction) contributes partially or completely to the filler's effect. The microparticles may or may not be degraded over time.

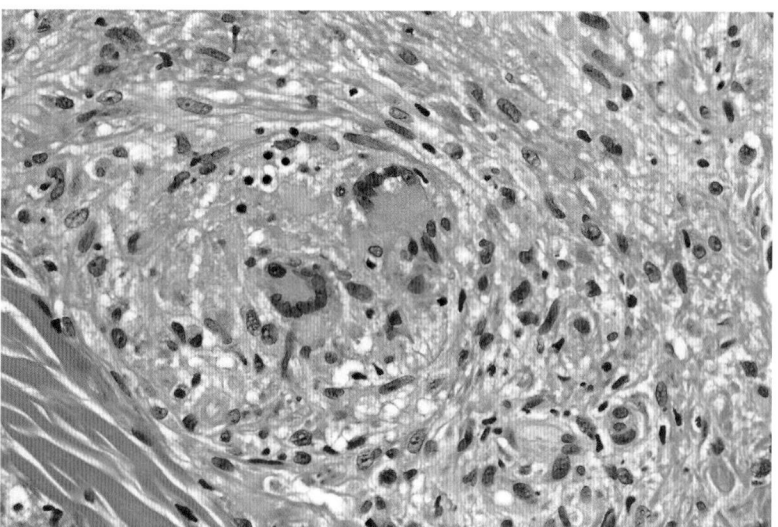

Fig. 14.121
Tumor necrosis factor-α inhibitor reaction: high-power view.

Silicone was one of the first agents used for soft tissue augmentation, in the 1950s. It was banned in the United States in 1982 due to concerns over adverse effects such as migration to distant locations.[2,3] Inflammatory nodules ('siliconomas') may also develop, sometimes years later. At present, two new forms of liquid silicone are available, Silikon 1000 and Adatosil 5000, for treatment of retinal detachment.[1] The former is more easily injected and is used off-label for cosmetic purposes. Polydimethylsiloxane/polyvinyl pyrrolidone (Bioplastique) contains particles of solid silicone and is available for injection into the subcutaneous fat (*Fig. 14.122*).[4]

As a consequence of the ban on silicone, bovine collagen was developed. There is a 1–3% rate of allergic reactions, despite double skin testing.[4] Many such reactions are localized erythema and edema which occur in the first weeks to months after injection, although recurrent inflammation, years later, has been described. Other potential complications include localized glabellar necrosis, granulomata, and abscess formation.[5] Granulomata present as erythematous nodules at the site of treatment and are seen within a few months following injection. Sometimes, lesions are seen years later. Abscesses typically occur weeks to months after injection.[4,5] Polymethyl-methacrylate microspheres and bovine collagen (Artecoll, Arteplast, and Artefill) is a temporary filler that uses a solution of bovine collagen as a carrier. Patients may rarely develop telangiectasias, hypertrophic scarring, allergic reactions, and granuloma formation.[5]

Table 14.2
Esthetic microimplants

Chemical ingredient	Product name(s)
Resorbable	
Bovine collagen	Zyderm, Zyplast
Human collagen	Cosmoderm, Cosmoplast, Cymetra
Porcine collagen	Evolence
Hyaluronic acid (nonanimal)	Restylane, Captique, Perlane, Juvederm
Hyaluronic acid (animal)	Hylaform, Hylaform plus
Poly-L-lactic acid	Newfill, Sculptra
Hydroxy-polyethylene/ hydroxyl-polypropylene	Profill
Calcium hydroxylapatite	Radiesse, Radiance
Permanent	
Bovine collagen/polymethyl methacrylate microspheres (PMAA)	Artecoll, Arteplast, Artefill, Metacril
Hyaluronic acid/ polyhydroxyethylmethacrylate (HEMA)/ethylmethacrylate (EEMA)	DermaLive, DermaDeep
Silicone (dimethyl polysiloxane)	Silikon 1000, Silskin, Adatosil 5000
Polydimethylsiloxane/polyvinyl pyrrolidone	Bioplastique
Polyacrylamide gel (PAAG)	Aquamid
Polyacrylamide and polyvinyl acid	Evolution
Polyalkylimide gel	Bio-Alcamid
Polytetrafluoroethylene	Gore-Tex

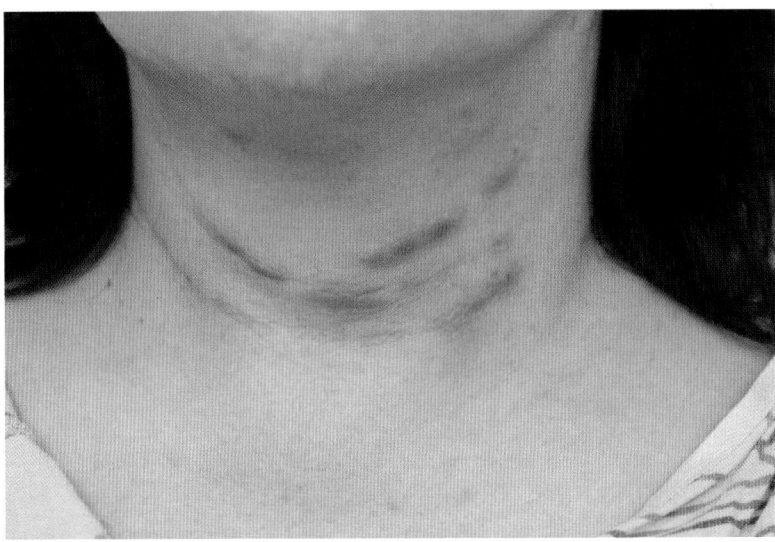

Fig. 14.122
Restylane nodules: linear arrangement of nodules along the neck creases.

Human-derived bioengineered collagen was developed as an alternative to bovine collagen. Most reactions consist of localized bruising at sites of injection, but rare granulomatous reactions have been reported.[5]

Hyaluronic acid is a temporary filler commonly used to correct facial creases and wrinkles. There are two types of hyaluronic acid fillers: non-animal, derived from fermentation of bacteria (*Streptococcus equi*), and animal, derived from chicken combs.[5–7] Hypersensitivity reactions, although rare, have been reported in up to 0.8% of patients.[4,8] Injection site reactions are most common, with temporary erythema, edema, and bruising within the first 14 days following injection.[9] Delayed reactions are less common and present as erythematous, firm nodules along the sites of injection weeks to months later.[6–12] There are two types of nodules: granulomatous and nongranulomatous. The etiology of the granulomatous response is unclear. There is speculation that it could be secondary to impurities related to the fermentation process in the nonanimal-derived form.[13] Additional side effects to hyaluronic acid include sterile abscesses, hyperpigmentation, and a livedoid, reticular pattern in the area of injection.[8]

Hydroxyethylmethacrylate/ethylmethacrylate fragments and hyaluronic acid (DermaLive and DermaDeep) is a permanent filler. It can result in edema, induration, and granulomatous inflammation.[5]

Foreign-body granulomata have also been seen following injection with poly-L-lactic acid (Newfill, Sculptra) and polyacrylamide gel (PAAG; Aquamid).[4–6] Hydroxy-polyethylene/hydroxyl-polypropylene (Profill) is also associated with lipoatrophy.[4]

Calcium hydroxylapatite is a resorbable filler of calcium hydroxylapatite microspheres that stimulate the endogenous production of collagen. Occasional granulomatous reactions occur.[5]

Polytetrafluoroethylene (Gore-Tex) has been used for lip augmentation and has resulted in ulcerated nodules with pustules.[14]

Immediate-type reactions such as erythema, edema, and bruising have also been described with other fillers, including hydroxy-polyethylene/ hydroxyl-polypropylene (Profill), polyacrylamide-containing products, and poly-L-lactic acid.[4,14]

Infection is a potential complication following any cosmetic procedure.[14] Early infections, occurring within 2 weeks, are typically secondary to bacteria such as *S. aureus* or *Streptococcus*.[3,14] Later infections may be due to atypical mycobacteria such as *Mycobacterium chelonae*, *Mycobacterium fortuitum*, and abscesses.[14]

Histologic features

Silicone nodules contain multiple vacuoles in the dermis, subcutis, and skeletal muscle.[3,4,13] Vacuoles are variable in size and shape and resemble Swiss cheese. These are actually empty spaces where silicone was lost during processing. They are surrounded by giant cells and histiocytes which contain intracytoplasmic vacuoles.[15] The latter may mimic lipoblasts. Additionally, impurities in the silicone result in birefringent foreign material within giant cells.[3–5] Surrounding fibrosis may also be noted.[3] The silicone particles in polydimethylsiloxane/polyvinyl pyrrolidone are too large to be phagocytosed by histiocytes.[1] The material induces a foreign-body giant cell reaction and fibrosis. The particles are identified as translucent, jagged structures within cystic spaces.[4,5]

Bovine collagen is distinguished from human collagen by its lighter eosinophilic color, thicker bundles, and more amorphous, acellular appearance.[4,5] When recurrent inflammatory reactions develop in hypersensitive patients, there is a perivascular mononuclear cell infiltrate with a mixture of neutrophils, mononuclear cells, and eosinophils within implanted collagen.[4,15]

Early granulomatous nodules are composed of a mixture of mononuclear cells, giant cells, eosinophils, neutrophils, and plasma cells surrounding, but not infiltrating, the collagen implant.[4] Later lesions have a denser and deeper infiltrate. Birefringent material is not seen. In contrast, nodules due to polymethyl-methacrylate microspheres and bovine collagen (PMAA) (Artecoll) contain a diffuse and nodular granulomatous infiltrate which surrounds cystic spaces, mimicking fat cells and with a Swiss cheese appearance.[3,5,15] Located in the center of the spaces are nonbirefringent, round, translucent, well-circumscribed foreign bodies (*Fig. 14.123*). This foreign material is the PMMA microsphere, which also induces surrounding fibrosis. The fibrosis contributes to the filling effect. Hyaluronic acid with polyhydroxyethylmethacrylate (HEMA)/ethylmethacrylate (EEMA) (DermaLive, DermaDeep) reactions are very similar histologically to Artecoll, as they also contain methacrylate microspheres, but the foreign material has a more polygonal appearance.[3,5,15] Calcification of the foreign material has been described with DermaLive.[1] Asteroid bodies may be present in both reactions.[15]

Abscesses seen as a consequence of collagen implants show a dense neutrophilic infiltrate with admixed plasma cells, histiocytes, and mononuclear cells.[4] Giant cells surround implanted collagen, and granulomata may be present.

Nongranulomatous inflammatory nodules related to hyaluronic acid injection are characterized by a superficial and deep perivascular and

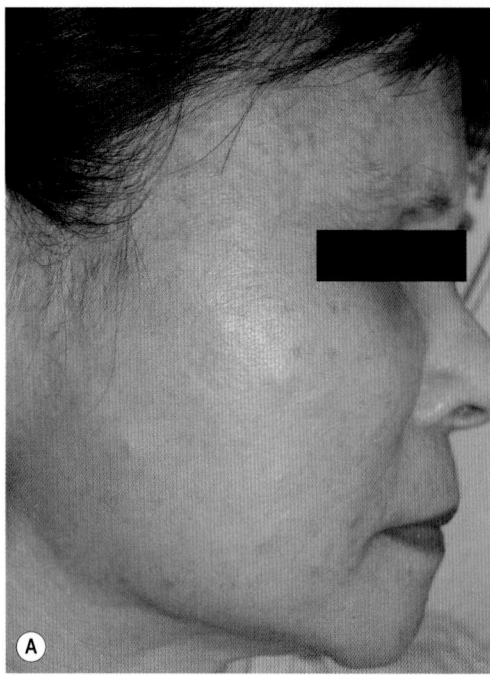

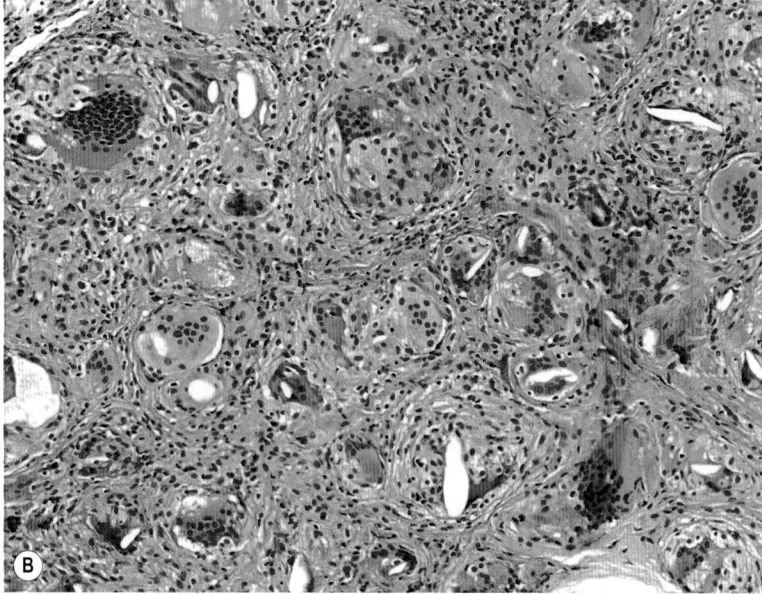

Fig. 14.123
(**A**) Clinical reaction to poly-L-lactic acid filler. (**B**) Reaction to a poly-L-lactic acid with granulomas containing spiky translucent material. By courtesy of Chao-Kai Hsu, MD, Sheau-Chiou Chao, and Julia Yu-Yun, National Cheng Kung University Hospital, Tainan, Taiwan.

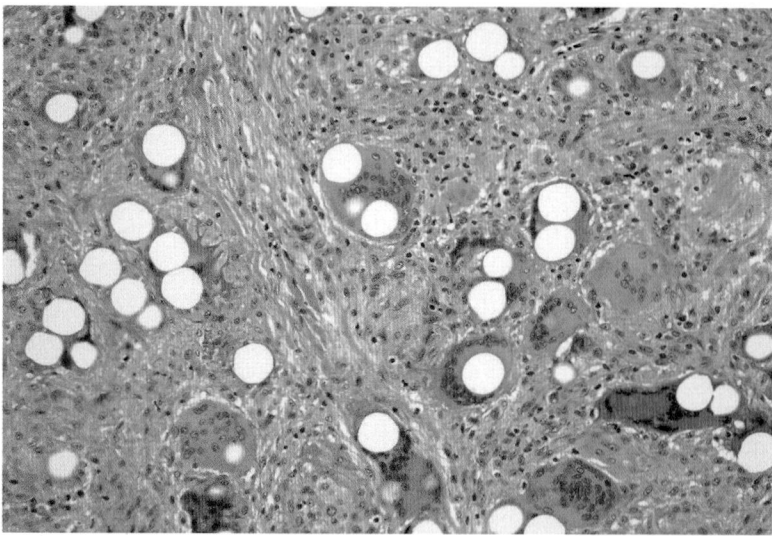

Fig. 14.124
Reaction to Artecoll: note the foreign body granulomatous reaction and the typical Swiss cheese appearance.

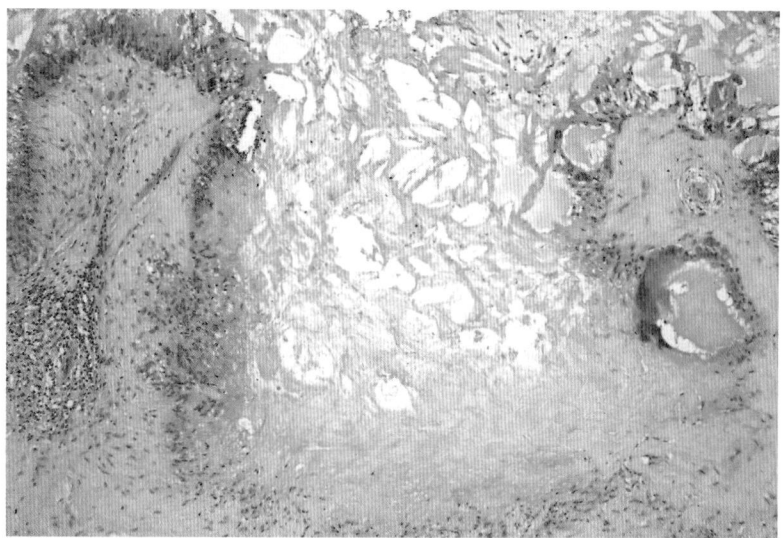

Fig. 14. 125
Reaction to Bio-Alcamid: the central necrobiosis with a surrounding rim of histiocytes shows a striking resemblance to granuloma annulare.

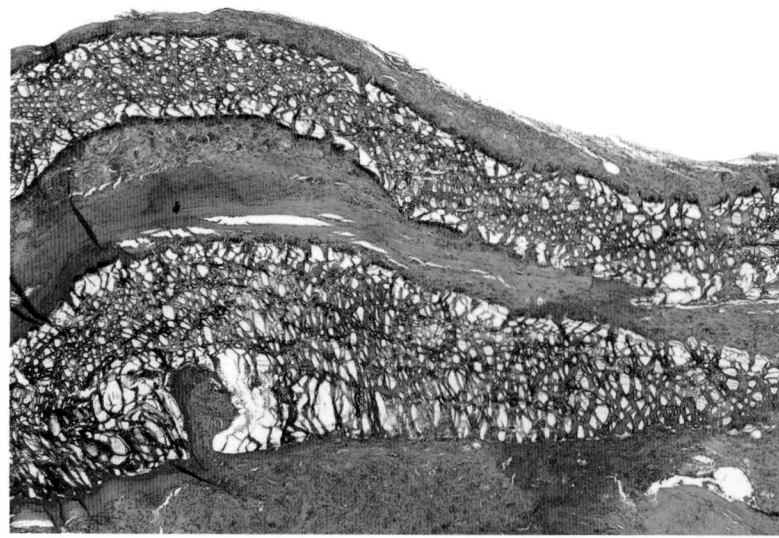

Fig. 14.126
Reaction to Gore-Tex: the mesh is surrounded by dense fibrous tissue.

periadnexal infiltrate of mononuclear cells with several eosinophils.[13] Implanted hyaluronic acid is not seen. In contrast, the granulomatous nodules contain a striking nodular infiltrate of foreign body giant cells, histiocytes, and eosinophils surrounding pools of basophilic foreign material which stain with Alcian blue (pH 2.7).[4,14] Polyacrylamide gel (Aquamid) has similar features, but is distinguished from injected hyaluronic acid by the presence of necrotic tissue admixed with the basophilic foreign material.[5,14]

Poly-L-lactic acid (Newfill, Sculptra) nodules are granulomatous and are distinguished by spiky, long translucent bodies within giant cells (*Fig. 14.124*).[4,14] They are irregular in shape and birefringent.

Reactions to Bio-Alcamid (polyalkylimide gel) display palisading granulomas with scattered giant cells and a central area of amorphous material that may mimic deep granuloma annulare or rheumatoid nodule (*Fig. 14.125*).[5,15]

Ulcers caused by polytetrafluoroethylene (Gore-Tex) demonstrate variably sized threads of material surrounded by neutrophils and granulation tissue (*Fig. 14.126*).[14]

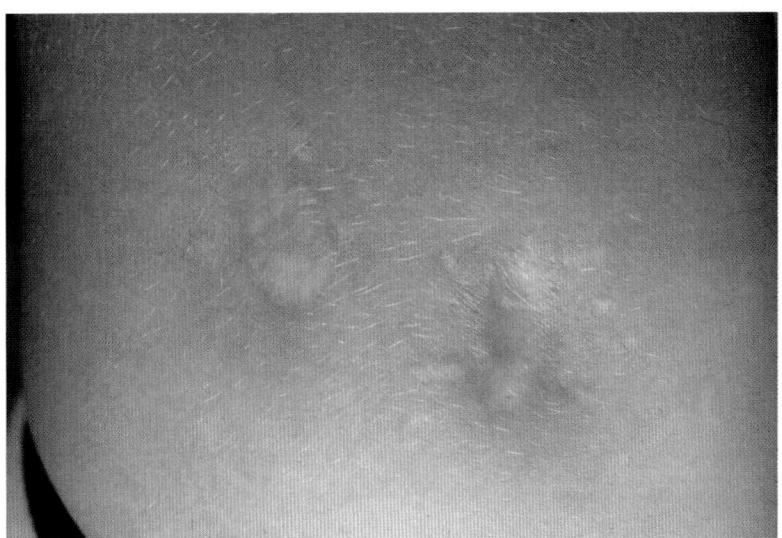

Fig. 14.127
Aluminum granuloma: multiple depressed nodules with scarring are evident. From the collection of the late N.P. Smith, MD, Institute of Dermatology, London, UK.

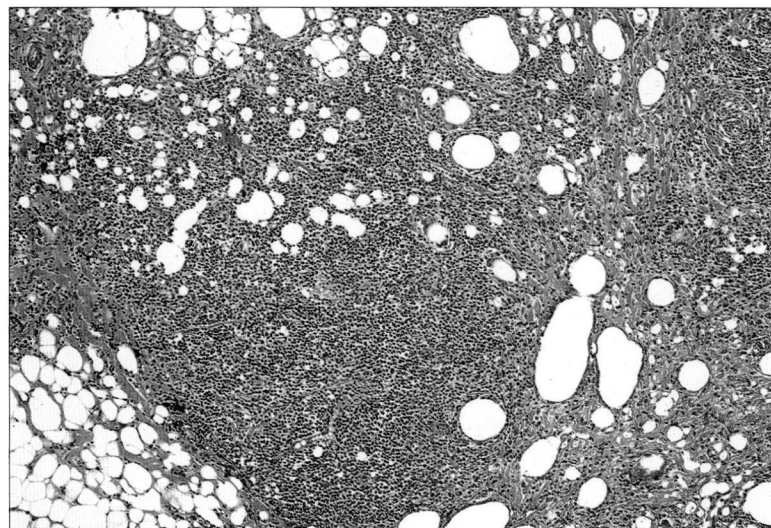

Fig. 14.128
Aluminum granuloma: there is a dense inflammatory cell infiltrate within the subcutaneous fat.

Infectious lesions demonstrate variable findings depending on the causative organism. Mycobacterial infections may present as granulomatous nodules, and appropriate tissue stains and culture are necessary.

Aluminum granuloma

Clinical features

Aluminum granuloma refers to the persistent, sometimes painful, subcutaneous nodules that develop at the sites of vaccination or hyposensitization with agents containing aluminum hydroxide as an absorbing agent (Fig. 14.127).[1-5] If a vaccine is erroneously applied intradermally, lesions may occur within the dermis.[6] The term granuloma is a misnomer as lesions do not usually consist of granulomatous inflammation. The lesions develop after a few weeks or years after the injections and are thought to be secondary to a hypersensitivity reaction to aluminum hydroxide. Often, patients have a contact allergy to aluminum as demonstrated by positive patch tests to aluminum hydroxide.[7] The most common vaccine associated with this reaction is tetanus toxoid, but any vaccine containing aluminum hydroxide as an absorbent may induce the reaction, including hepatitis A and C and human papillomavirus vaccines.[8]

Intramuscular vaccines induce a condition described as macrophagic myofasciitis. This condition has been described both in children and adults.[9,10]

Pathogenesis and histologic features

The occurrence of the nodules appears to be the result of a delayed hypersensitivity reaction to aluminum.

Four histologic patterns, which can overlap, may be found[11]:

- A predominantly lobular panniculitis with fairly non-specific findings including focal inflammation consisting of lymphocytes, histiocytes, and plasma cells with fat necrosis. Loose subcutaneous collections of histiocytes with a slightly granular, bluish cytoplasm are always found, but their number varies and the change may be subtle.
- A prominent subcutaneous, predominantly mononuclear, inflammatory cell infiltrate with eosinophils and focal formation of germinal centers often mimicking a marginal zone lymphoma (Figs 14.128–14.130). Plasma cells are often prominent. Careful examination reveals scattered grouped histiocytes with bluish granular cytoplasm.
- A deep granuloma annulare-like infiltrate with numerous histiocytes surrounding an area of necrobiosis (Figs 14.131 and 14.132). All the histiocytes show a characteristic bluish granular cytoplasm.
- A pattern with hyaline necrosis of the subcutaneous lobule mimicking lupus profundus. This is associated with lymphocytes, and plasma cells

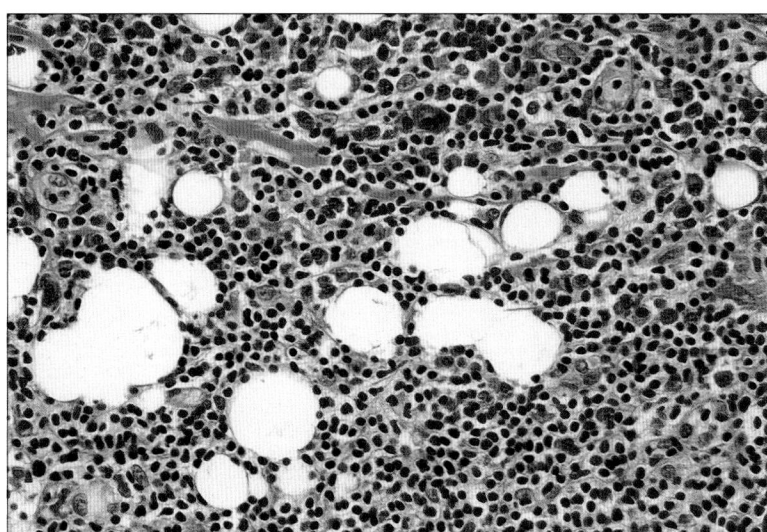

Fig. 14.129
Aluminum granuloma: the infiltrate consists of lymphocytes, histiocytes, and plasma cells.

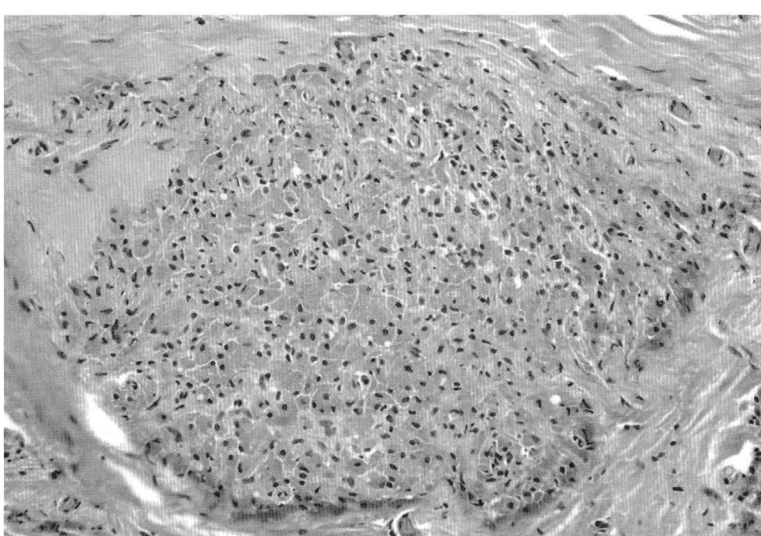

Fig. 14.130
Aluminum granuloma: the histiocytes have markedly granular cytoplasm due to the presence of aluminum.

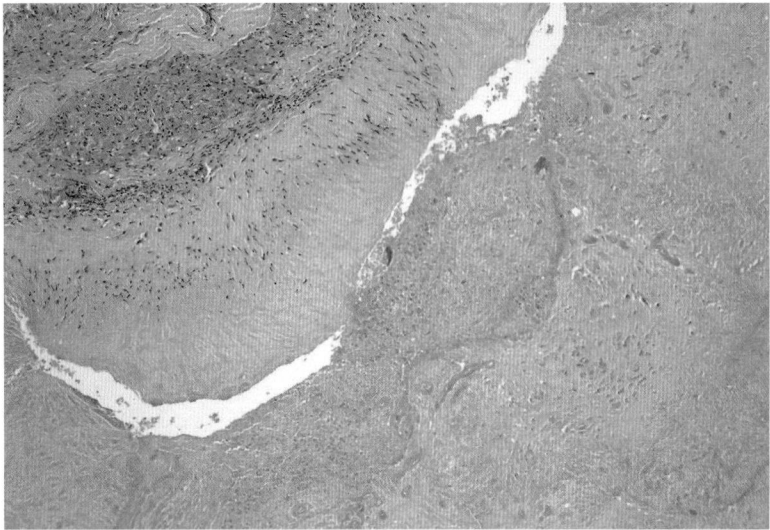

Fig. 14.131
Aluminum granuloma: in this example, there is a palisading granuloma surrounding a necrobiotic nodule.

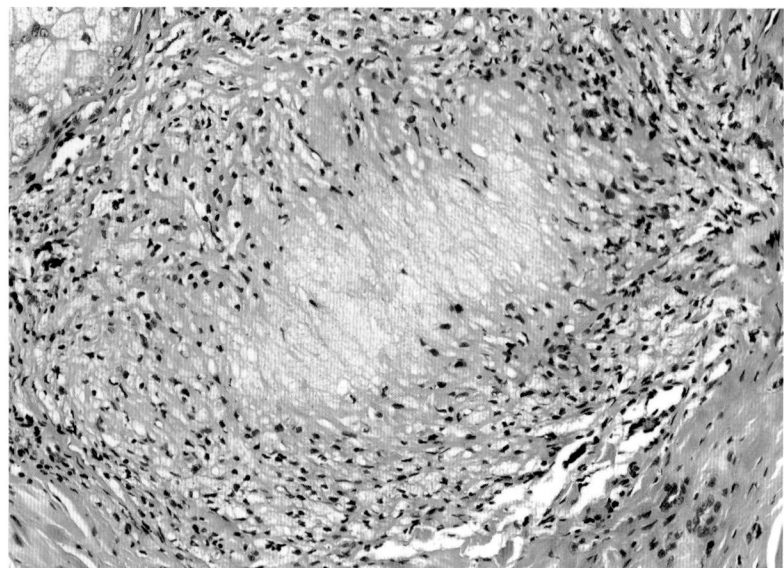

Fig. 14.133
Reaction to steroid injection: mucinous material surrounded by palisaded histiocytes and mimicking granuloma annulare. Courtesy of Dr Isabel Viana, Centro Hospitalar de Lisboa Ocidental, Lisboa, Portugal.

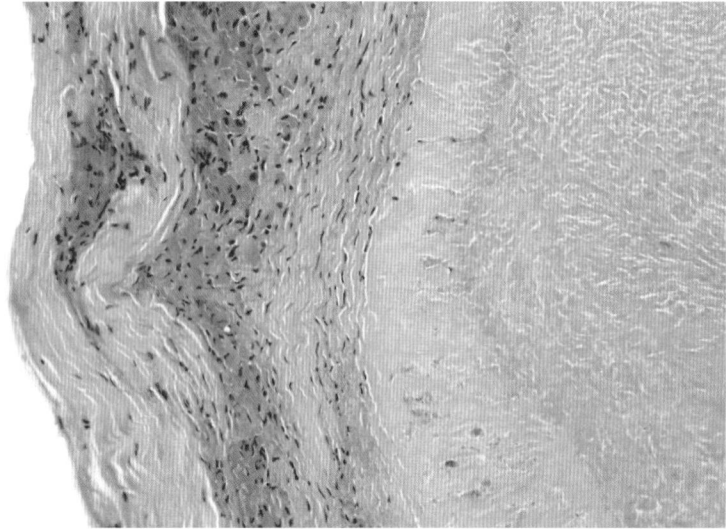

Fig. 14.132
Aluminum granuloma: the histiocytes have finely granular cytoplasm.

and germinal centers may also be seen. Careful examination reveals the presence of typical histiocytes with bluish granular cytoplasm.

A case with numerous mast cells and associated with urticaria has been described.[12]

The material within the histiocytes represents aluminum. Confirmation of the presence of aluminum can be done histochemically with the use of azurin stain or by energy dispersive X-ray microanalysis.

Adverse reactions to corticosteroid injections

Clinical features

Localized injections of corticosteroids is a ubiquitous practice in dermatology. One of the most common adverse reactions is localized atrophy and localized hypopigmentation.[1–3] The atrophy can sometimes clinically resemble morphea.[3] The atrophic changes can develop a linear pattern, following lymphatic drainage.[4,5] Patients may also develop localized alopecia.[6]

Histologic features

Atrophic changes include loss and thinning of rete ridges with vascular ectasia.[1,3] less commonly, foreign body-type granulomas and rheumatoid nodule/granuloma annulare-like granulomas may develop at injection sites.[7–9] Small, elongated spaces are typical, and occasionally birefringment crystals are seen.[9] The granulomatous reaction can surround amorphous mucinous material (*Fig. 14.133*).[10,11] This material is not hyaluronic acid and should not be confused with primary dermal mucinosis.[10] Titanium dioxide added to topical and injectable steroids like triamcinolone may exceptionally induce blue discoloration at the site of application.[12] Titanium dioxide can only be demonstrated by scanning electron microscopy with energy dispersive X-ray spectroscopy analysis.

Alpha-melanocyte stimulating hormone analogues (melanotan I and II)

Melanotan I and II are superpotent analogues of alpha-melanocyte stimulating hormone that have photoprotective effects. They appear to be increasingly used by patients who want to develop a prominent tan. Although they are not licensed for this purpose, they can be obtained through the Internet. Their administration not only induces prominent tanning but also induces enlargement and darkening of pre-existing nevi. Histology of these nevi has not been described in detail, but the few removed lesions in two patients did not show evidence of malignancy.[1]

EMLA cream (prilocaine-lidocaine emulsion)

Clinical features

EMLA is a eutectic mixture of prilocaine and lidocaine that is used widely as a cream to provide local anesthesia, particularly in children and in adults in genital areas. Very few side effects occur with its application, among them a petechial eruption, contact urticaria, allergic contact dermatitis, and irritant contact dermatitis.[1–4] For dermatopathologists, however, what is more important about EMLA are the subtle changes that it can cause at a microscopic level, leading to difficulties in interpretation.[5] These changes appear to be related to the time that the cream is applied to the patient and they may be more common in skin in which the biopsy is performed as a result of an inflammatory process.

Histologic features

In cases of irritant contact dermatitis, the features consist of confluent necrosis of the upper layers of the epidermis, focal interface change with hydropic degeneration of basal cells and clefting at the dermal–epidermal junction and an upper dermal mixed inflammatory cell infiltrate with neutrophils.[4] The changes mimic a necrolytic erythema or GVHD. In cases with no clinical evidence of a side effect, there is vacuolization of the granular cell layer and upper stratum spinosum and focal areas with hydropic degeneration of basal cells and clefting at the dermal–epidermal junction.[5] The latter changes may mimic epidermolysis bullosa (*Fig. 14.134*). By electron microscopy, the appearances mimic a lysosomal storage disorder with empty lysosomal inclusions.[6] The latter change has been attributed to the castor oil contained in EMLA cream.

Access **ExpertConsult.com** for the complete list for references

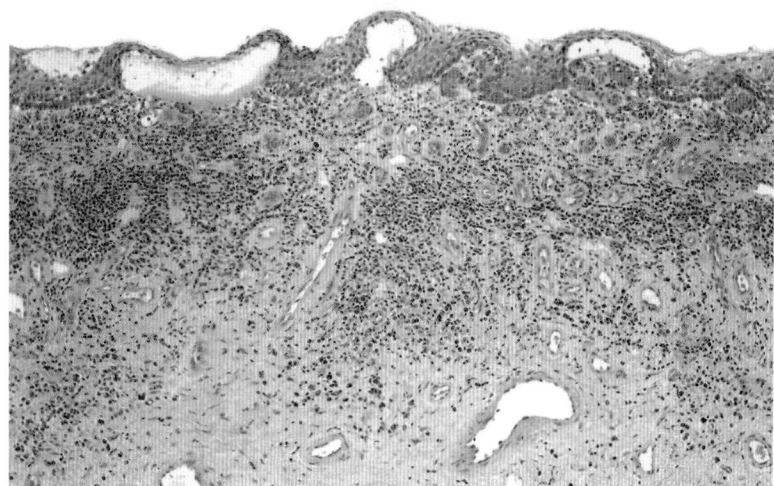

Fig. 14.134
Reaction to EMLA cream: in this example, there are multiple small foci of subepidermal vesiculation.

CHAPTER

15

Neutrophilic and
eosinophilic dermatoses

See
www.expertconsult.com
for references and
additional material

Pyoderma gangrenosum

Clinical features

Pyoderma gangrenosum is an uncommon disease of obscure etiology.[1–12] It appears to be somewhat more common in women and, although it may occur at any age, most patients are in their fourth or fifth decade.[4] Presentation in children is uncommon, but it has been seen even in infants,[13–25] and rare familial cases have been documented.[26–29] The disease may also present in pregnancy, and in this setting it is associated with an underlying disease process in about 30–50% of the cases.[30–34] Large, necrotic ulcers, often 10 cm or more in diameter, characterize the disease (Fig. 15.1). Lesions may arise from acneiform pustules or on a background of erythematous nodules. Typically, the ulcers have undermined edges and red–purple borders (Fig. 15.2). They may be solitary or multiple, and occur most often on the lower limbs, although other sites such as the trunk, face, arms, hands, and buttocks are sometimes affected (Fig. 15.3).[4,5,35–37] Rare sites of involvement include the oropharyngeal region, hand, eyelid, eye, vulva, penis, scrotum, and the cervix.[38–55] The ulcers are painful and tender, and may persist for months or years. Complications usually result from the site of the lesion and can include cranial osteolysis, nasal perforation, and tendon rupture.[18,56,57] Recurrent attacks are not uncommon.[2] Cribriform scarring often follows healing. Systemic involvement has rarely been documented, affecting the lungs, liver, bone, joints, pancreas, heart, and spleen.[58–66]

Occasionally, bullous or pustular variants are encountered.[4,67–83] One large study found that bullous lesions are more common on the upper extremities, and they appear to be more frequently associated with hematological malignancy.[4] Such lesions are sometimes designated atypical pyoderma gangrenosum.[4,68] A vegetative form has also been described.[84–89] Some patients have more than one clinical type concurrently.[80,82,86]

A particularly interesting feature seen in 20–50% of cases is development of lesions in traumatized areas (pathergy).[4,10,90,91] Lesions may occur at sites of surgery and have been reported after cholecystectomy, breast reduction or augmentation, splenectomy, hysterectomy, cesarean section, appendectomy, cardiac surgery, orthopedic surgery, herniorrhaphy, bowel bypass procedure, excision of anal condyloma, at the site of a fasciocutaneous flap, a laparoscopic port insertion site, and in an amputation stump (Fig. 15.4).[92–119] In the postoperative setting, women appear to be disproportionately affected, with breast reconstruction surgery being the most common inciting incident.[119] They also occur following rather trivial trauma such as injection or intravenous access site, arteriovenous dialysis shunt, blood-drawing, acupuncture, or a tattoo.[4,120–125] Pressure from use of seat belts in automobiles has been associated with subsequent lesion development.[126] Presentation has even been documented at the location of a spider bite.[127] One case reports involvement of the scalp after receiving hair highlights at a salon, which could be due to physical and/or chemical trauma.[128]

A variety of drugs have been implicated as potential triggers, including, alpha-2b interferon (IFN-α2b), isotretinoin, sulpiride, propylthiouracil, lenalidomide, rituximab, sunitinib, imatinib, gefitinib, pazopanib, ipilimumab, and adalimumab.[128–147] Paradoxically, some of these medications (e.g., rituximab, ipilimumab, and adalimumab) have been used to treat pyoderma gangrenosum.

Pyoderma gangrenosum after combination therapy with cytosine arabinoside, aclarubicin, and granulocyte colony-stimulating factor for myelodysplastic syndrome has been reported.[148] Pyoderma gangrenosum has also been linked to levamisole-adulterated cocaine abuse.[149–151] A granulomatous and suppurative dermatitis that may mimic pyoderma gangrenosum has been documented at the site of interferon-alpha (IFN-α) injections.[152] Sclerotherapy has also been complicated by pyoderma gangrenosum on rare occasions.[153] Of particular importance is the known association of pyoderma gangrenosum with a variety of conditions[4,11,12,154] (in up to 50% of patients[2]) as outlined in Table 15.1. Of these, inflammatory bowel disease (both Crohn disease and ulcerative colitis) and arthritis show the most well-established links.[155–158] Pyoderma gangrenosum is reported to complicate around 1–2% of inflammatory bowel disease patients.[158–161] In one study, 27% of patients had associated inflammatory bowel disease and 20% of patients had arthritis.[4] In this same study, 27% of patients with superficial 'atypical' pyoderma gangrenosum had an associated hematological disorder.[4] In another large study, idiopathic pyoderma gangrenosum and that associated with chronic inflammatory bowel disease were found to be more common in females, whereas pyoderma gangrenosum associated with hematological malignancy was more common in males.[5] While pyoderma gangrenosum can fluctuate with inflammatory bowel disease activity, it may also be a presenting or heralding feature. The presence of pyoderma gangrenosum as a complication of inflammatory bowel disease does not appear to be an independent predictor of severity of the bowel disease.[162,163] Although pyoderma gangrenosum lesions may improve as inflammatory bowel disease is brought under control, specific treatment is usually required.[163] Most of the other numerous, rare associations mentioned in Table 15.1 are likely to be fortuitous, as a report of simple coexistence does not strictly imply

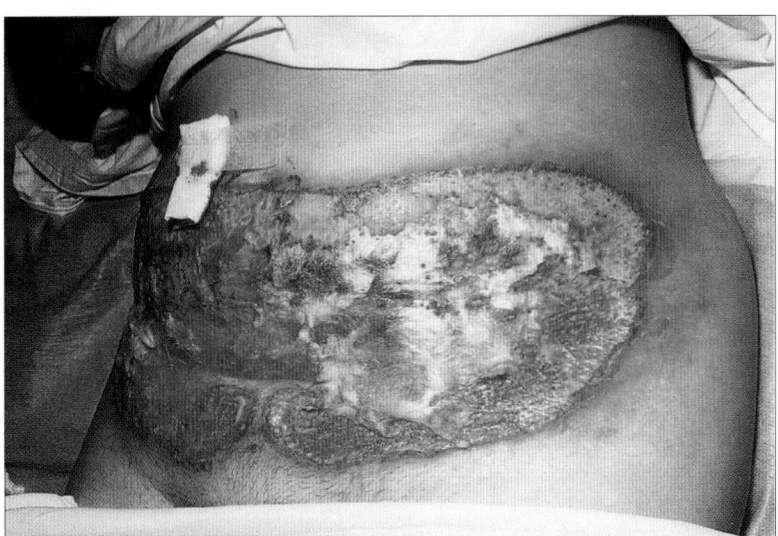

Fig. 15.1
Pyoderma gangrenosum: this unusually severe example is associated with very extensive tissue destruction resembling necrotizing fasciitis. By courtesy of R.A. Marsden, MD, St George's Hospital, London, UK.

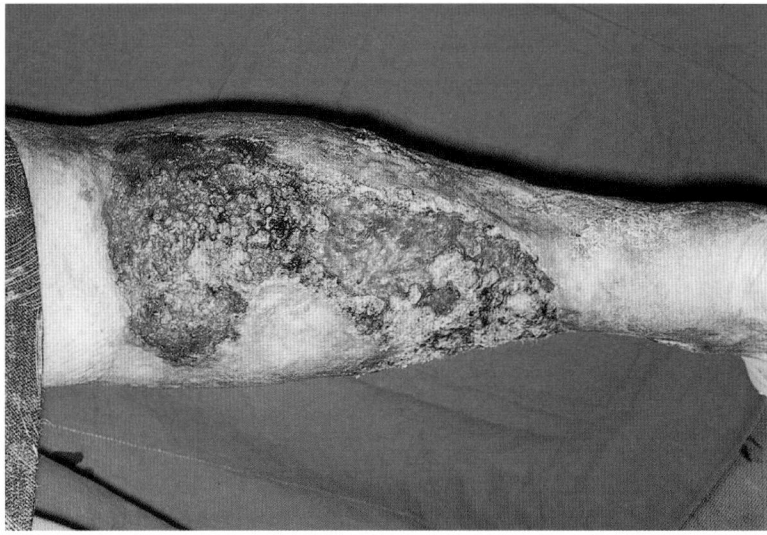

Fig. 15.3
Pyoderma gangrenosum: an extensive lesion with marked crusting and undermining in the proximal and medial margins. By courtesy of R.A. Marsden, MD, St George's Hospital, London, UK.

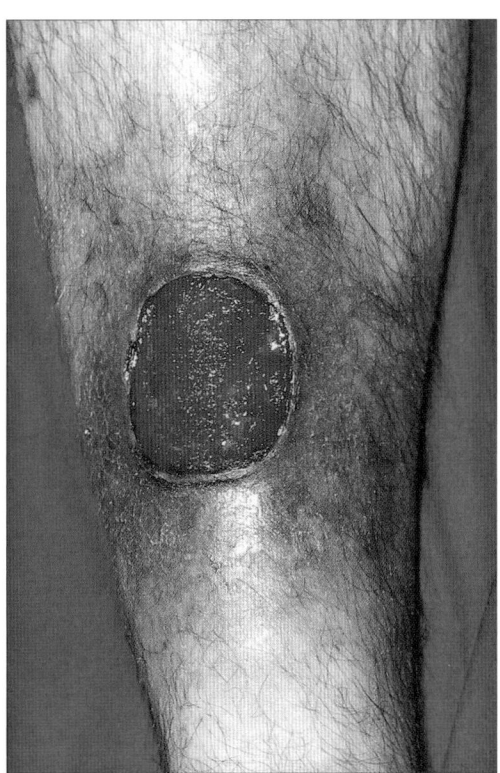

Fig. 15.2
Pyoderma gangrenosum: this shows an area of ulceration with a typical undermined purplish border. By courtesy of R.A. Marsden, MD, St George's Hospital, London, UK.

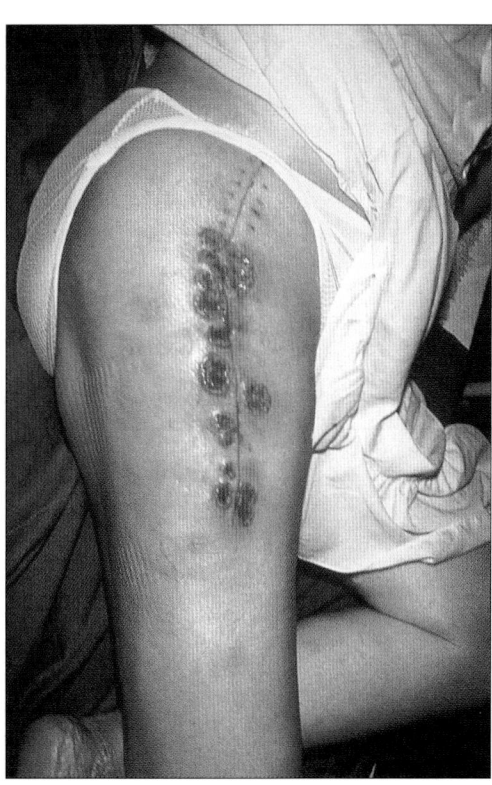

Fig. 15.4
Pyoderma gangrenosum: multiple early lesions at the site of previous surgery. By courtesy of R.A. Marsden, MD, St George's Hospital, London, UK.

a meaningful association.[164] In any event, a diagnosis of pyoderma gangrenosum should always prompt an evaluation for an underlying disease association. Pyoderma gangrenosum-like lesions have been reported as the presenting feature of antiphospholipid antibody syndrome.[165] Other underlying conditions causing lesions that mimic pyoderma gangrenosum are also well described including inflammatory and infectious processes, vasculopathies, and malignancies, stressing the importance of careful clinical investigation.[166–176]

The disease may also occur in association with other neutrophilic dermatoses including Sweet syndrome and other dermatological diseases, such as lupus erythematosus and erythema nodosum, the latter typically in the background of concomitant inflammatory bowel disease.[177–182] Pyoderma

gangrenosum is one of the components of an autosomal dominant syndrome known as PAPA (pyogenic sterile arthritis, pyoderma gangrenosum and acne).[183] This syndrome has been mapped to chromosome 15q and is associated with mutations in the gene *CD2BP1/PSTPIP1*.[184–194] These mutations increase the binding affinity of this gene product to pyrin, overcoming the autoinhibition of this homotrimer and allowing activation of the downstream innate immune response.[189–191] Ultimately, this mutation leads to an increase in caspase-1 activation, an underlying feature of multiple inherited autoinflammatory syndromes.[195] These findings indicate that pyoderma gangrenosum may be best regarded as an autoinflammatory or autoimmune disease, and the pathways being studied in PAPA syndrome may also eventually shed light onto the pathogenic mechanisms of sporadic

Table 15.1

Conditions associated with pyoderma gangrenosum (alphabetical order)

- Acne fulminans, acne conglobata and hidradenitis suppurativa[265-269]
- Acquired ichthyosis[270]
- Acute myeloid leukemia[271]
- Allergic contact dermatitis from rubber[272]
- Anaplastic large cell lymphoma[273]
- Antineutrophil cytoplasmic antibodies[274-276]
- Arthritis (either seronegative or rheumatoid arthritis), ankylosing spondylitis, and osteoarthrosis[4,277-279]
- Autoimmune neutropenia of infancy[280]
- Behçet disease[281]
- Bullous systemic lupus erythematosus[282]
- Burns/scalding[283,284]
- C7 deficiency[285]
- Chronic idiopathic myelofibrosis[286]
- Chronic myelomonocytic leukemia[287]
- Chronic renal failure[288]
- *Chlamydia pneumoniae*[289]
- Cogan syndrome (interstitial keratitis and vestibuloauditory dysfunction)[290]
- Collagenous colitis[291,292]
- Colorectal carcinoma[293]
- Cutaneous T-cell lymphoma[294]
- Cryofibrinogenemia[295]
- Cryoglobulinemia[6]
- Diverticular disease[296]
- Essential thrombocythemia[297]
- Fanconi anemia[298]
- Factor V Leiden deficiency[295]
- Gastric carcinoma[227,299]
- Graves disease[300]
- Glomerulonephritis[301]
- Hepatitis, autoimmune and viral[229,302-306]
- Human immunodeficiency virus (HIV) infection[307-309]
- Hypertrophic osteoarthropathy[310]
- Hypogammaglobulinemia[311,312]
- Inflammatory bowel disease: both ulcerative colitis and Crohn disease[2,4,159]
- Juvenile idiopathic arthritis[313]
- Kartagener syndrome[314]
- Klinefelter syndrome[315]
- Lupus anticoagulant[316]
- Monoclonal gammopathy (most often IgA); usually benign but may lead to multiple myeloma[2,69,279,317]
- Multiple sclerosis[318]
- Myelodysplastic syndrome[319,320]
- Myelofibrosis[321]
- Myeloid leukemia[70,72,228,322]
- Osteomyelitis[12,323]
- Paroxysmal nocturnal hemoglobulinuria[324]
- Polycythemia rubra vera[279]
- Psoriasis[325]
- Renal transplant[328,326]
- SAPHO syndrome (synovitis, acne, pustulosis, hyperostosis, osteitis)[327,328]
- Sarcoidosis[329]
- Sjogren syndrome[330]
- Subcorneal pustular dermatosis[331,332]
- Systemic lupus erythematosus[333]
- Systemic sclerosis[334]
- Tuberculosis[335]
- Varicella (chickenpox)[336]
- Vasculitis, including Takayasu disease, erythema elevatum diutinum, and cutaneous granulomatosis[337-343]

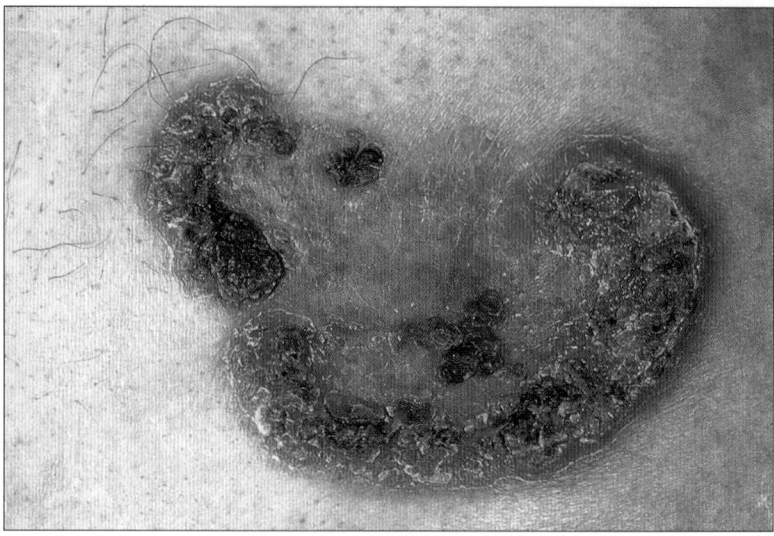

Fig. 15.5

Superficial granulomatous pyoderma: crusted superficial lesion with a cribriform appearance. By courtesy of the Institute of Dermatology, London, UK.

described, and a patient with a mutation in *NCSTN*, a gene implicated in hidradenitis suppurativa, has been reported.[200,201] Pyoderma gangrenosum has also been associated with LAD-1 (leukocyte adhesion deficiency-1) secondary to mutation of *ITGB2*.[202-204]

Para- and peristomal involvement in patients with ileostomy or colostomy for inflammatory bowel disease is a well-recognized phenomenon.[4,205-211] In a large series, 13% of patients had peristomal pyoderma.[4] Both Crohn disease and ulcerative colitis are associated with this complication.[4,208-212] It should be noted that peristomal pyoderma gangrenosum has been seen in the absence of inflammatory bowel disease.[205,206] It has been documented in patients with ostomy for gastrointestinal carcinoma and diverticular disease.[205,206] Pyoderma gangrenosum may also occur at urostomy sites following cystectomy for bladder carcinoma.[206]

Superficial granulomatous pyoderma is believed to represent a superficial and rare variant of pyoderma gangrenosum.[3,212-218] However, the latter is controversial as patients with this condition usually do not have associated systemic disease and the histologic features are different with predominance of suppurative granulomas (see below). Patients develop single or sometimes multiple superficial ulcerated lesions with vegetative borders (for this reason, this variant is sometimes referred to as 'vegetative variant of pyoderma gangrenosum') as a consequence of trauma, frequently surgical (*Fig. 15.5*). Pain is an occasional feature. The ulcers have a cleaner base than those seen in classic pyoderma. Lesions are most commonly found on the trunk and upper extremities, and heal with cribriform scarring (*Fig. 15.6*). Draining sinuses are occasionally evident. Often there is no evidence of underlying systemic disease. Superficial granulomatous pyoderma is more likely to follow a chronic course compared with classic pyoderma gangrenosum.[218] Rare cases involving the face, eye, and vulva have been reported.[219-222]

So-called 'malignant pyoderma' is a controversial designation which we believe should be avoided. Some authors have used the term to describe a variant of pyoderma gangrenosum predominantly affecting the head and neck.[223-226] It has been postulated that at least some cases of so-called malignant pyoderma more likely represent cutaneous granulomatosis with polyangiitis (cutaneous granulomatosis).[226]

One study found that over 50% of patients with pyoderma gangrenosum required long-term therapy to control their disease.[5] The disease may be fatal in some cases, particularly if diagnosis is delayed.[6,227] In another study, 2 of the 21 patients reported died of pyoderma gangrenosum secondary to pulmonary involvement.[6]

Pathogenesis and histologic features

The precise pathogenesis of pyoderma gangrenosum is uncertain. The current state of knowledge suggests that it is due to immune dysfunction,

pyoderma gangrenosum.[196] A related syndrome with hidradenitis instead of pyogenic arthritis (PASH) associated with mutations in *PSTPIP1* has been described.[197-199] Some patients have hidradenitis with arthritis (PAPASH).[200] The genetics of pyoderma gangrenosum and these related syndromes is more complex than is appreciated. Cases lacking mutations in *PSTPIP1* have been

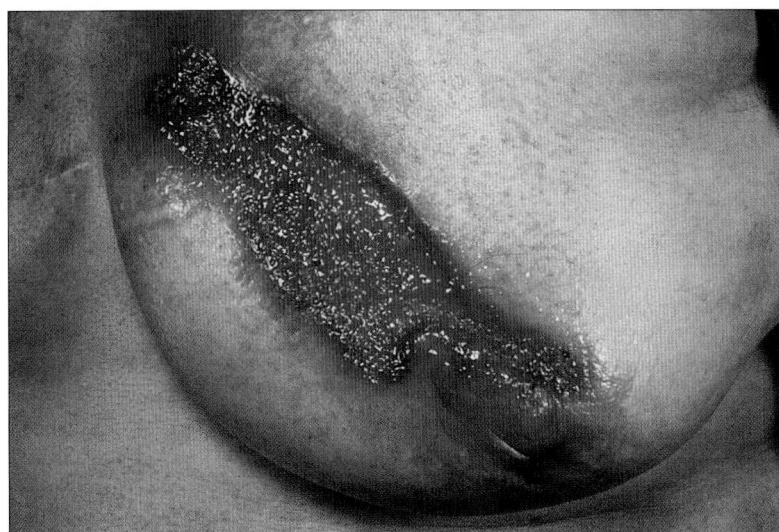

Fig. 15.6
Superficial granulomatous pyoderma: this field shows extensive ulceration of the breast. By courtesy of R.K. Winkelmann, MD, Mayo Clinic, Scottsdale, Arizona, USA.

perhaps innate, and/or that it develops on a vasculitic basis.[10,12,186,228-233] A variety of immunological abnormalities have been described including:

- absent delayed hypersensitivity reactions to common antigens such as mycobacteria and *Candida albicans*
- defective neutrophil chemotaxis and irregular neutrophil trafficking
- impaired neutrophil phagocytosis
- diminished lymphokine (migration inhibition factor) production[12,228,229,231]
- overexpression of interleukin (IL)-8, a potent chemotactic polypeptide for neutrophils, has been reported in lesional tissue and may be an important pathogenetic factor[234,235]
- reduction in IL-8 and related molecules has been noted following successful therapy[236]
- overexpression of IL-17 and 23[237-239]
- aberrant neutrophil trafficking and metabolic integrin β2-CR3 and -CR4 oscillations in lesional tissue[240,241]
- elevated levels of HIF2a and downstream effectors vascular endothelial growth factor (VEGF) and Ang-2 have been noted in disseminated disease, suggesting that angiogenesis in improper control of the neutrophil oxidative burst may be involved[242]
- elevated tumor necrosis factor-alpha (TNF-α), MMP-9, and MMP-10 have also been noted[237,243]
- TNF-α may have some of its effects mediated by keratinocyte secretion of elafin, an elastase inhibitor.[244] Indeed, anti-TNF-α therapy has been described to show some efficacy[245-251]; however, a case has also been described in association with TNF-α antagonists used to treat rheumatoid arthritis and the relationship may be complex.[252]

The results of immunofluorescence studies in large series of patients have revealed both immunoglobulins (usually IgM) and complement in blood vessel walls in the dermis of the leading edge of the ulcer.[253,254] Another study, however, failed to substantiate this finding, and immunofluorescence should not be considered and ancillary diagnostic test.[2] There is no evidence to support an infective pathogenesis.[255]

Expanding T-cell clones in both the skin and circulation have been described in a small series of patients, indicating that T-cell response plays a role in the disease and may be triggered by a local stimulus in the skin.[256] T-cell clonality has been described in pyoderma gangrenosum in the absence of an underlying myeloproliferative disease.[257]

In general, the histopathology is that of non-specific ulceration with abscess formation (*Fig. 15.7*). The adjacent dermis shows acute and chronic inflammation. A pseudo-Pelger-Huet phenomenon with hyposegmented neutrophils making recognition difficult has been described in one patient.[258] Early lesions may present with subcorneal pustulation (*Fig. 15.8*). Although the histologic features of both leukocytoclastic and lymphocyte-mediated

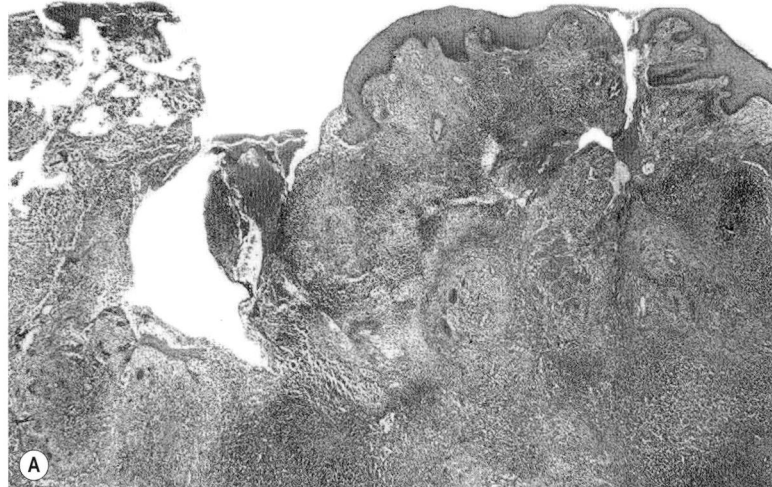

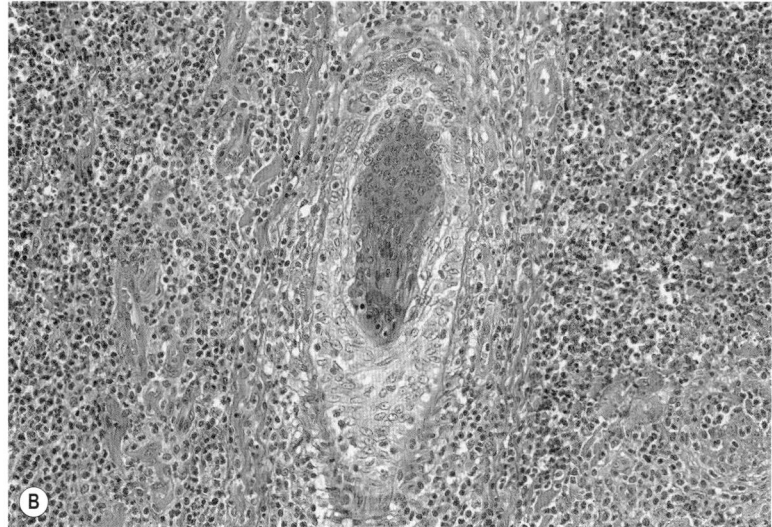

Fig. 15.7
(**A**, **B**) Pyoderma gangrenosum: in this biopsy from the edge of an ulcer, there are massive intradermal inflammatory changes, with abscess formation.

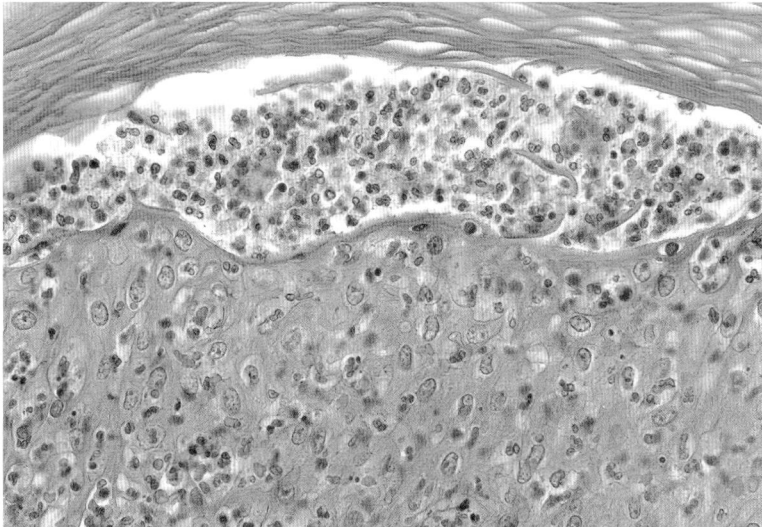

Fig. 15.8
Pyoderma gangrenosum: early acneiform lesion showing a subcorneal pustule.

vasculitis have been described, it is our experience that any vasculitis present is usually located within the floor of the ulcer or in the immediate adjacent tissues and is, therefore, more likely to be a consequence, rather than a cause, of the lesion (*Fig. 15.9*).[1,259] It has been suggested by some that some lesions of pyoderma gangrenosum may be initiated by acute folliculitis.[260]

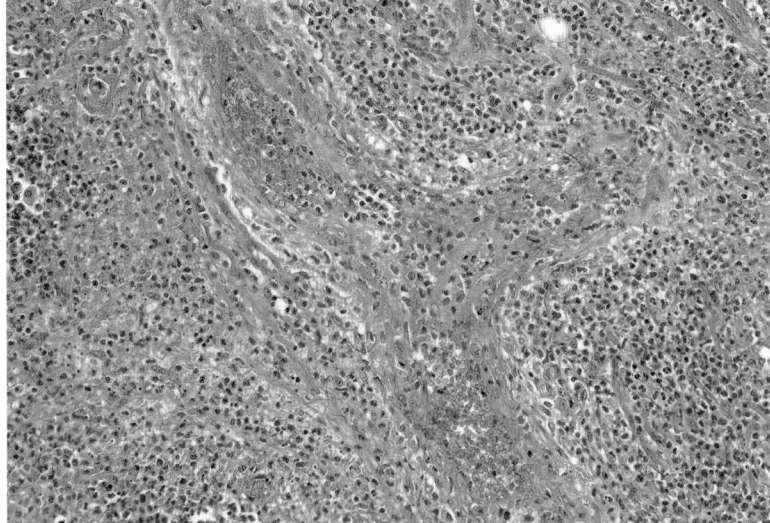

Fig. 15.9
Pyoderma gangrenosum: acute necrotizing vasculitis. It is likely that any active inflammation of the blood vessel walls is a result of the surrounding inflammation rather than its cause.

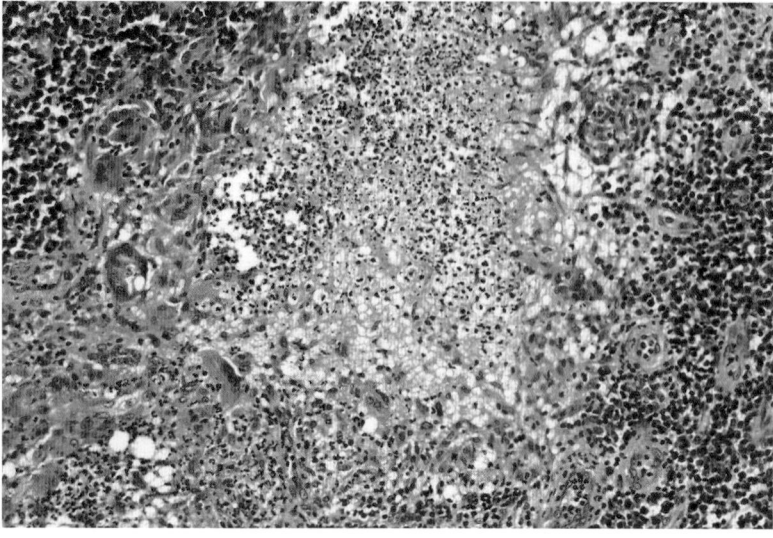

Fig. 15.11
Superficial granulomatous pyoderma: the zoned inflammatory reaction is clearly seen. Note the central abscess and surrounding granulomatous inflammation.

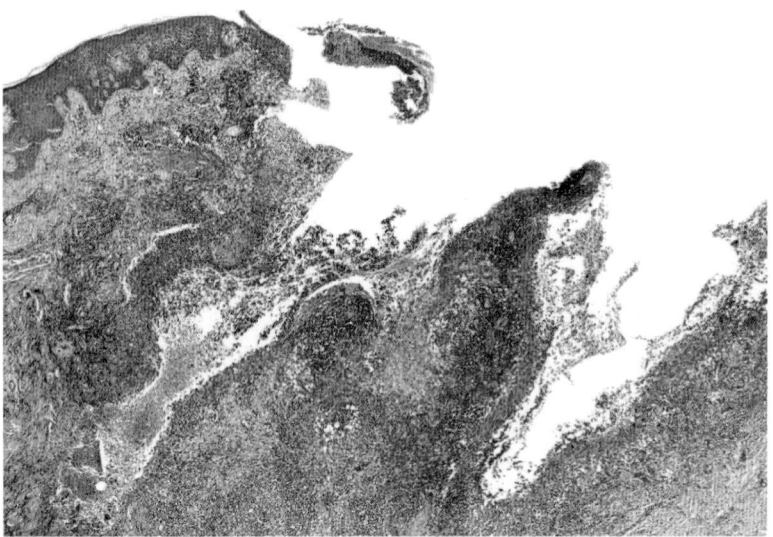

Fig. 15.10
Superficial granulomatous pyoderma: low-power view showing an undermining ulcer.

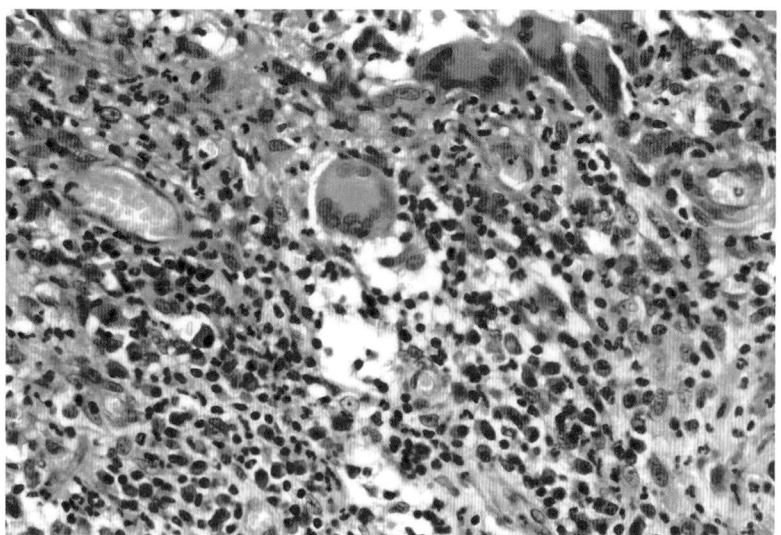

Fig. 15.12
Superficial granulomatous pyoderma: high-power view showing multinucleate giant cells. There are also conspicuous plasma cells.

Giant cells appear to be a common feature of pyoderma gangrenosum in patients with Crohn disease.[7] In one study, they were present in 6 of 13 patients with associated inflammatory bowel disease; of these, 5 had Crohn disease and 1 had ulcerative colitis.[7] Giant cells were not found in any biopsies from 22 patients without associated inflammatory bowel disease.

Superficial granulomatous pyoderma is characterized by a zoned inflammatory infiltrate in the superficial dermis.[3] Focal and sterile abscesses are surrounded by a zone of granulomatous inflammation, mainly suppurative granulomas, bordered by a rim of lymphocytes and plasma cells (Figs 15.10–15.12).[3] Hemorrhage is often present and eosinophils may be evident. Any vasculitic change is thought to be secondary. The adjacent tissues may show scarring. Acanthosis and pseudoepitheliomatous hyperplasia predominantly, but not exclusively of the infundibular portion of hair follicles are frequently noted. Foreign material including starch, sutures, vegetable matter, wood, and hair has been identified in a large proportion of these cases.[3] It should be noted that not all cases of pyoderma gangrenosum with granulomatous inflammation are limited to the superficial dermis. Some cases show involvement of the deep dermis and even subcutaneous tissue.

Differential diagnosis

The histopathological findings in pyoderma gangrenosum are non-specific, and the diagnosis is primarily one of exclusion.[261] Since surgery is used to manage some of the disorders considered in the histologic and clinical differential diagnosis – but is contraindicated in the treatment of pyoderma gangrenosum – early and accurate diagnosis is critical. Surgery, which tends to exacerbate the disease, is generally contraindicated in pyoderma cases because of the pathergic response. The mainstay of therapy is medical management, such as corticosteroids and more recently targeted therapies. Unfortunately, patients with pyoderma are often misdiagnosed early in the course of their disease, and the diagnosis is sometimes made only after multiple unsuccessful (and damaging) surgeries have been performed. In one study, an average of five physicians had examined the patient before a correct diagnosis was rendered.[35] To avoid this error, obtaining accurate clinical information on wounds and debridement specimens is essential.

Culture is required to exclude infection (bacterial, mycobacterial, fungal). Necrotizing fasciitis tends to affect deeper fascial and subcutaneous tissue, while pyoderma is centered in the dermis (albeit some spillover into the subcutis may be seen). Usually, sheets of bacteria are evident in untreated necrotizing fasciitis. Distinguishing these two conditions is critical since the treatments are diametrical opposites with surgery and antibiotics for necrotizing fasciitis and avoidance of surgery with systemic anti-immune treatment and supportive wound care for pyoderma gangrenosum.[262–264]

Sweet syndrome is generally not associated with ulceration and shows more prominent karyorrhexis relative to the number of neutrophils, and the inflammatory cell infiltrate tends to be restricted to the dermis. Bite reactions, particularly resulting from the brown recluse or other spiders, may show similar histologic features, and eosinophils may not be a prominent feature in early lesions of bites. Clinical information is necessary to distinguish pyoderma from many other forms of ulcer such as those due to trauma.

Although some authors have noted lymphocytic or neutrophilic vasculitis in lesions of pyoderma gangrenosum, this finding, in our experience, is limited to areas adjacent to the ulcer and likely represents a secondary finding.[5] Indeed, it has been our experience that 'secondary' vasculitis is frequently present at the border of ulcers of many different etiologies in patients without any genuine underlying 'primary' vasculitic process. Evaluation for vasculitis as a cause of ulceration, therefore, depends upon examination of blood vessels in areas of dermis and subcutaneous tissue away from the ulcer.

It cannot be overemphasized how important accurate clinical information is in establishing the correct diagnosis. Failing to recognize this disease early in its course can be disastrous for the patient.

Acute febrile neutrophilic dermatosis (Sweet syndrome)

Clinical features

Acute febrile neutrophilic dermatosis (Sweet syndrome) is an uncommon disease of unknown etiology and pathogenesis.[1–11] It is associated with a marked female predilection (5:1), and most patients affected are in their third through sixth decades. It may, however, occasionally be seen in children, and a few cases presenting in infancy have been documented.[12–28] Infant brothers who both had Sweet syndrome have been reported.[26] Patients present with variable numbers of asymmetrically distributed, frequently bilateral, circumscribed, tender, and painful red plaques or nodules, particularly on the face, neck, and upper and lower limbs (Figs 15.13–15.15). An acral form of this condition is now termed neurophilic (or pustular) dermatosis of the dorsal hands (Fig. 15.16).[29–38] Whether this represents a distinct disease or a peculiarly localized variant of Sweet syndrome is uncertain.

Occasionally, the lesions may become bullous or pustular.[39–46] The plaques vary from about 1 to 4 cm in diameter and typically heal without

scarring. Recurrences develop in approximately one-third of patients and postinflammatory hyperpigmentation is sometimes seen.[47,48] Pathergy and koebnerization are occasional features, and necrosis with ulceration may rarely be encountered.[7,49–51] Sweet syndrome may present with lesions mimicking palmoplantar pustulosis and sometimes erythema nodosum-like lesions are present.[39,52,53] A Sweet syndrome-like eruption has been described in association with exposure to light.[54]

Sweet syndrome often follows an upper respiratory tract infection. In some cases, it is a complication of drug treatment, for example, carbamazepine, furosemide, hydralazine, co-trimoxazole, abacavir, azathioprine, ofloxacin, doxycycline, clindamycin, minocycline, trimethoprim–sulfamethoxazole, bortezomib, lenalidomide, imatinib mesylate, nilotinib, etanercept, granulocyte

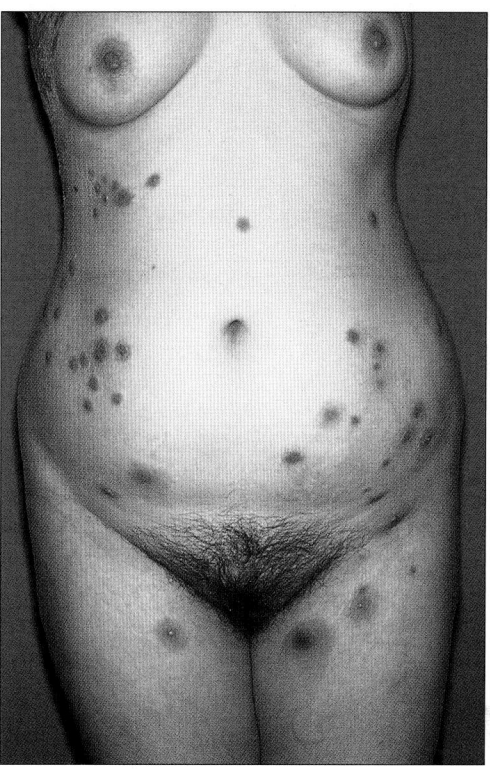

Fig. 15.14
Sweet syndrome: characteristic edematous red plaques (some showing ulceration and pustulation) are widely distributed on the trunk and proximal limbs. By courtesy of R.A. Marsden, MD, St George's Hospital, London, UK.

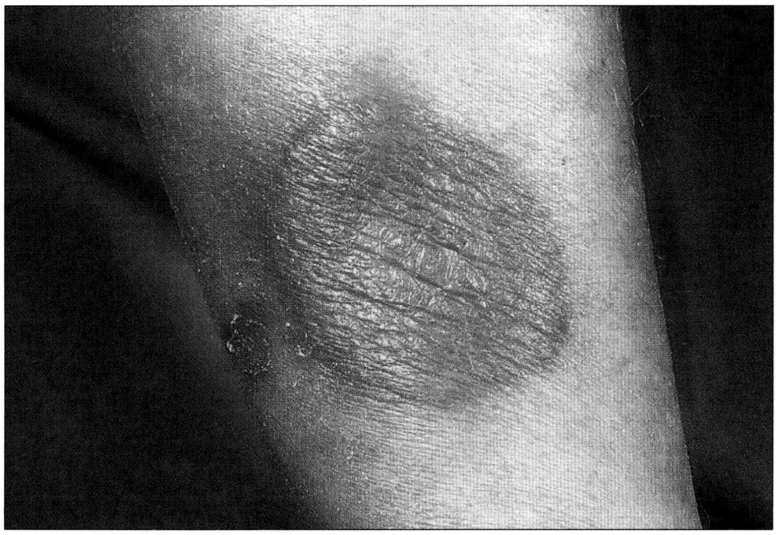

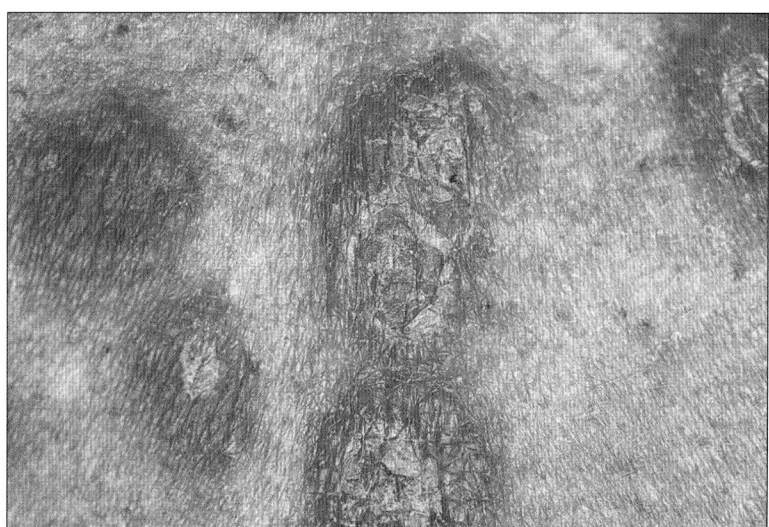

Fig. 15.13
Sweet syndrome: an erythematous plaque on the forearm. By courtesy of R.A. Marsden, MD, St George's Hospital, London, UK.

Fig. 15.15
Sweet syndrome: close-up view of typical plaques. By courtesy of the Institute of Dermatology, London, UK.

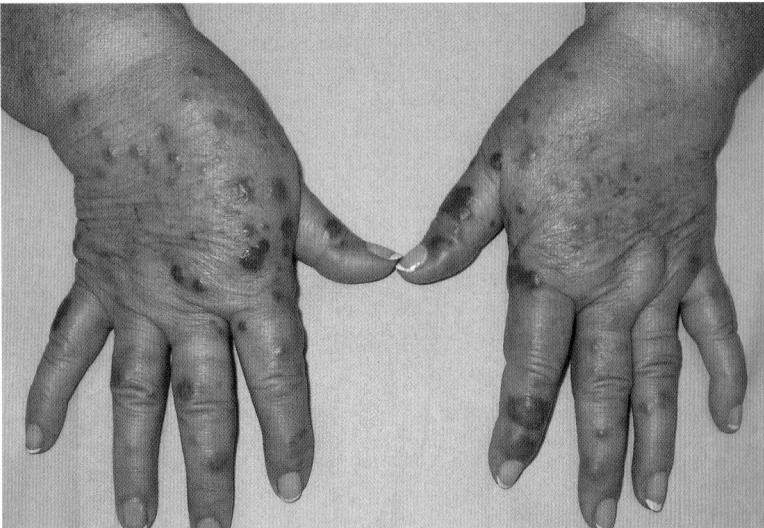

Fig. 15.16
Sweet syndrome: acral lesions on the dorsal surface of the hands and fingers, some with a hemorrhagic appearance. By courtesy of J.C. Pascual, MD, Alicante, Spain.

Table 15.2
Conditions associated with Sweet syndrome

Bacille Calmette-Guérin (BCG) vaccination[200]
Behçet disease[201,202]
Bronchiolitis obliterans[203]
Celiac disease[204]
Chronic granulomatous disease[205]
Dermatomyositis[206,207]
Drugs[71]
Encephalitis[208]
Erythema nodosum[103]
Generalized granuloma annulare[209]
Hematological malignancies (and myelodysplastic syndrome)[116]
Hepatitis B[210]
Infection with *Apnocytophaga canimorsus, Chlamydia pneumoniae, Coccidiodes immitis*, Cytomegalovirus, *Francisella tularensis, Helicobacter pylori*, Hepatitis C, human immunodeficiency virus (HIV), *Pasteurella multocida, Salmonella enteritidis*, and *Staphylococcus epidermidis* and *Staphylococcus aureus*[211–224]
Inflammatory bowel disease (including ulcerative colitis and Crohn disease)[225,226]
Nontuberculous mycobacterial infection[227,228]
Pigmented villonodular synovitis[229]
Polycythemia rubra vera[230,231]
Pregnancy[232]
Prothrombin gene (G20210A) mutation[233]
Relapsing polychondritis[234,235]
Sarcoidosis[236–238]
Scrofuloderma[239]
Sjögren syndrome[240]
Solid tumor malignancy[112,130]
Still disease[241]
Subacute and systemic cutaneous lupus erythematosus[242–244]
Surgery[245]
Thyroid disease (Graves disease and Hashimoto thyroiditis)[246,247]
Tuberculosis[248]
Upper respiratory tract infection[10]
Urticaria pigmentosa[7]

colony-stimulating factor (G-CSF), radiocontrast agent, some vaccines, oral contraceptives, all-*trans*-retinoic acid, isotretinoin, nitrofurantoin, diazepam, clozapine, celecoxib, ketoconazole, azacitidine, omeprazole, mitoxantrone, vemurafenib, azathioprine, ipilimumab, and interferon (IFN).[39,40,55–91] The temporal relationship with administration, development of symptoms, and resolution with withdrawal of the offending drug establishes the cause in drug-induced cases.[55,78,91] The disease has also been reported after chemotherapy in patients with acute myeloid leukemia.[92,93] Sweet syndrome can be broadly reviewed as falling into three general categories:

- classic (and often idiopathic),
- malignancy-associated (paraneoplastic),
- drug-induced.[10]

Patients may also have conjunctivitis, episcleritis, iritis, polyneuropathy, oral involvement (superficial ulcers), and arthralgias.[39,94–98] The larger joints are usually affected, and involvement tends to be migratory.[5] Patients with concurrent Sweet syndrome and erythema nodosum have been described, and it is possible that these two disorders share common pathogenetic mechanisms.[99,100] Dyssynchronous and synchronous Sweet syndrome and erythema nodosum may occur.[101–106]

Sweet syndrome is of particular importance since 10% to 40% of cases are associated with hematological malignancy such as leukemia (monocytic or myelomonocytic, including leukemia cutis), myelodysplasia, lymphoma, and multiple myeloma.[107–122] Development of the disease may herald a relapse of the leukemia or precede it.[123–125] Sweet syndrome has also been reported in patients with monoclonal gammopathy and myelodysplasia in the absence of frank leukemia or lymphoma.[124,126,127] Hemophagocytic syndrome is also a reported association.[128,129] The clinical lesions of Sweet syndrome are said to be more severe in patients with underlying hematological disease.[113] An association with urticaria pigmentosa has also been documented.[7]

Solid tumors may also be associated with Sweet syndrome in up to 7% of patients, including:

- testicular,
- bladder,
- gastrointestinal,
- breast,
- lung,
- ovary,
- prostate,
- gallbladder,
- thyroid,
- oral squamous cell carcinoma.[7,39,48,49,102,107–110,113,126,130–136]

A rare case following treatment of herpes simplex in a patient with metastatic breast carcinoma and another associated with post-mastectomy

lymphedema have been reported.[137,138] Sweet syndrome has been described in conjunction with numerous conditions, some of which are listed in *Table 15.2*. While its association with hematological and internal malignancies, upper respiratory tract infections, drugs, and certain inflammatory disorders such as erythema nodosum, rheumatoid arthritis, and sarcoidosis appears repeatedly, many of the others listed in the literature could be coincidental.

Systemic involvement may be a feature of Sweet syndrome with lesions described in the eye, lung, kidney, central nervous system, vagina, liver, gastrointestinal tract, and skeletal muscle.[7,111,139–150] Neural involvement appears to be strongly associated with human leukocyte antigen (HLA-Cw1).[147] An exceptional case with gingival hyperplasia and myositis in the absence of cutaneous involvement has been documented.[151]

Associated features include pyrexia, neutrophilia, and a raised erythrocyte sedimentation rate (ESR). Patients with antineutrophil cytoplasmic antibodies (ANCA) have been reported, and this finding may be more common with Sweet syndrome localized to the dorsal hands.[152–154] The presence of ANCA, however, is not a consistent finding.[7]

Pathogenesis and histologic features

The etiology of Sweet syndrome is unknown; however, the disease most probably represents an unusual hypersensitivity reaction secondary to cytokine production.[155] It is likely that neutrophils are activated by IL-1 and that Sweet syndrome represents a cytokine-mediated inflammatory reaction to a wide variety of different antigens including bacteria, viruses, drugs, and malignancies.[156–159] Demonstration of elevated serum IL-1α, IL-1β, IL-2, and interferon-gamma (IFN-γ), but not IL-4, suggests that type 1 (but not type 2) helper T cells (Th) play a role in the pathogenesis.[160,161] Not surprisingly, since exogenous treatment with G-CSF is associated with Sweet syndrome, endogenous G-CSF has been shown to be elevated in some cases.[162]

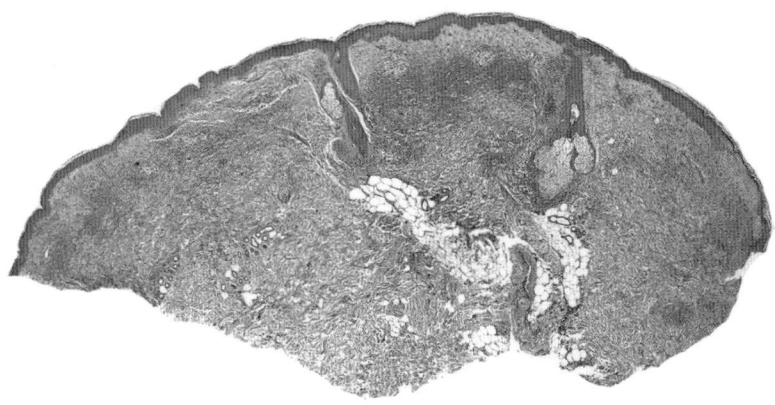

Fig. 15.17
Sweet syndrome: an intense inflammatory cell infiltrate is present in the dermis.

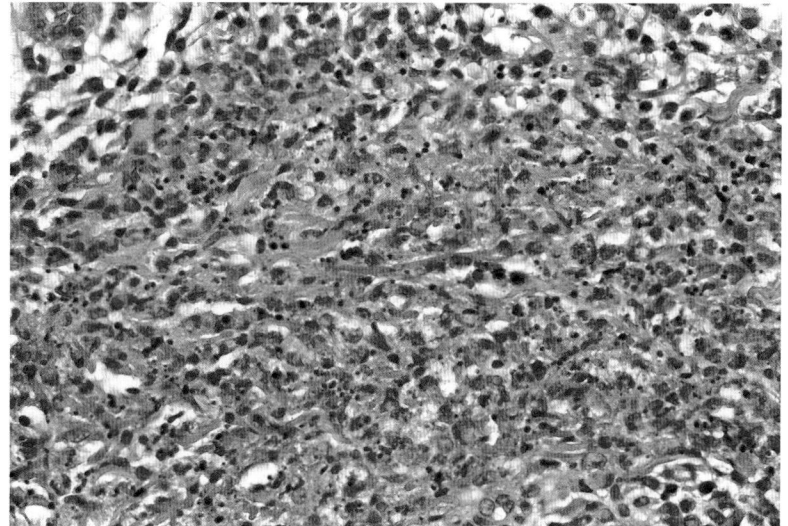

Fig. 15.18
Sweet syndrome: the infiltrate consists largely of neutrophils. There is edema and marked leukocytoclasis.

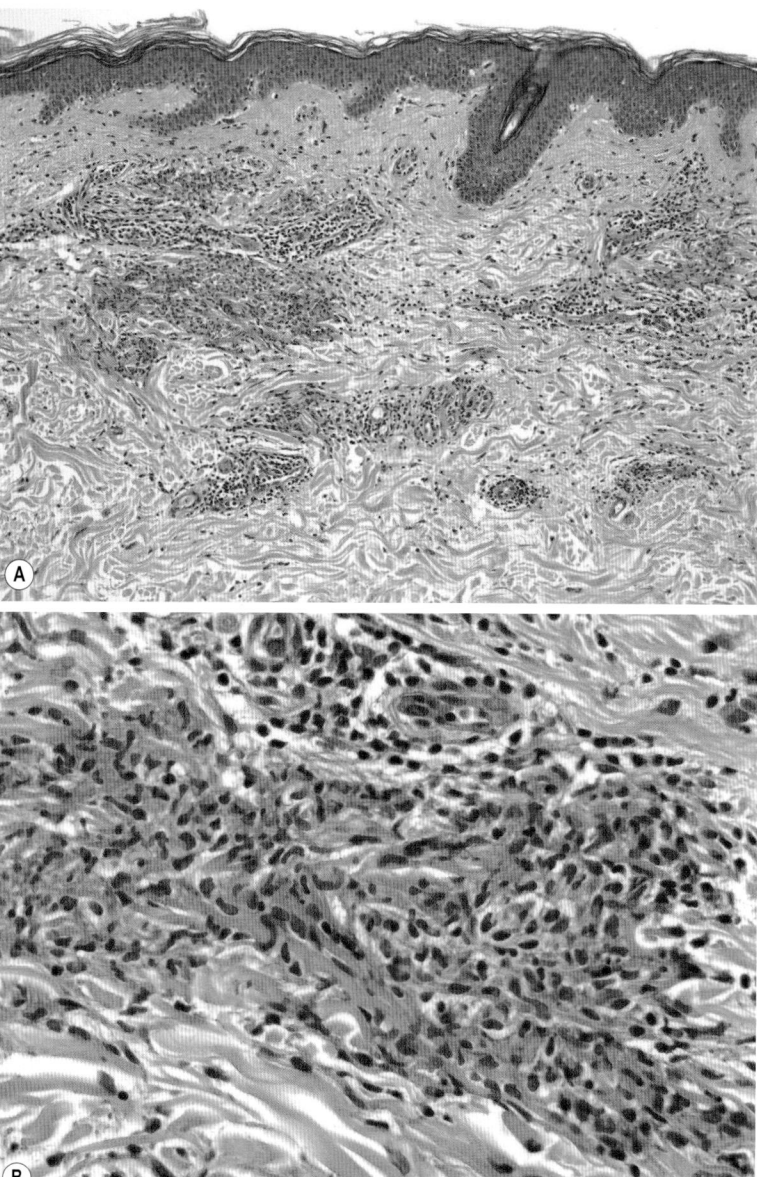

Fig. 15.19
(A, B) Histiocytoid Sweet syndrome: the proliferation is characterized by immature myeloid cells that resemble histiocytes. By courtesy of B. Luzar, MD, University of Ljubljana, Ljubljana.

In patients with G-CSF-associated Sweet syndrome, it has been suggested that the condition represents a form of neutrophilic recovery syndrome.[163] The occasional presence of immune complexes in blood vessel walls may have pathogenetic significance.[39]

Clonality in the skin infiltrate of a patient with Sweet syndrome and acute myelogenous leukemia undergoing treatment with G-CSF has been demonstrated, suggesting that the infiltrate may be the result of therapy-induced differentiation of neoplastic cells.[164] However, a further demonstrating clonality in four patients in the absence of myeloproliferative disease argues against that theory.[165]

Histologically, the epidermis in Sweet syndrome is usually unaffected although occasionally slight spongiosis is present; rarely, vesiculation, spongiform pustules, and necrotic keratinocytes have been described.[39] The cardinal feature, however, is an intense neutrophil polymorph infiltrate within the reticular dermis (Fig. 15.17).[3,166] This may be diffuse or perivascular in distribution and often surrounds the sweat ducts. Typically, leukocytoclasis is marked (Fig. 15.18). Admixed with the neutrophil polymorphs are variable numbers of lymphocytes, and histiocytes. Eosinophils are exceptional and when seen tend to be sparse. Ingestion of nuclear debris by histiocytes is sometimes a conspicuous feature. Rarely, degenerating neutrophils can resemble Cryptococcus.[167,168] A histiocytic/histiocytoid form of the disease has increasingly been recognized.[39,169–180] In this variant, the infiltrate is composed of mononuclear cells with lightly eosinophilic cytoplasm resembling histiocytes (Fig. 15.19). This is more likely to represent a stage in the evolution of the disease rather than a specific variant of Sweet syndrome. It has been postulated that the histiocyte-like cells seen represent immature

granulocytes based on immunoreactivity for myeloperoxidase in addition to histiocytic markers in most of the cells.[177] Cells are positive for CD15, CD45, CD43, CD68, MAC-386, HAM56, lysozyme, and myeloperoxidase CD33. Awareness of this form of presentation is important to avoid a misdiagnosis. Exceptionally, cells in histiocytoid Sweet appear haloed mimicking a cryptococcal infection.[181] Given the presence of a mononuclear cell infiltrate in these cases, it is extremely important to exclude leukemia cutis. Special stains and clinicopathological correlation are therefore paramount.

Often, the papillary dermis shows very marked edema, which sometimes results in subepidermal vesiculation (Fig. 15.20). Rarely, the presence of dermal papillary neutrophil microabscesses may cause diagnostic confusion with dermatitis herpetiformis (Fig. 15.21).[166] In Sweet syndrome, the blood vessels are dilated and may show endothelial swelling but changes of frank vasculitis are generally absent in our experience (and certainly not prominent). However, others have reported features of vasculitis such as nuclear dust, extravasation of erythrocytes, and fibrin deposition in and around vessels walls, and thus argue that the presence of vasculitis should not exclude this diagnosis.[182–184] Purpura is sometimes evident.[185,186] Immunofluorescence examination of skin biopsies in Sweet syndrome is usually negative for immunoreactants in the walls of the vasculature.

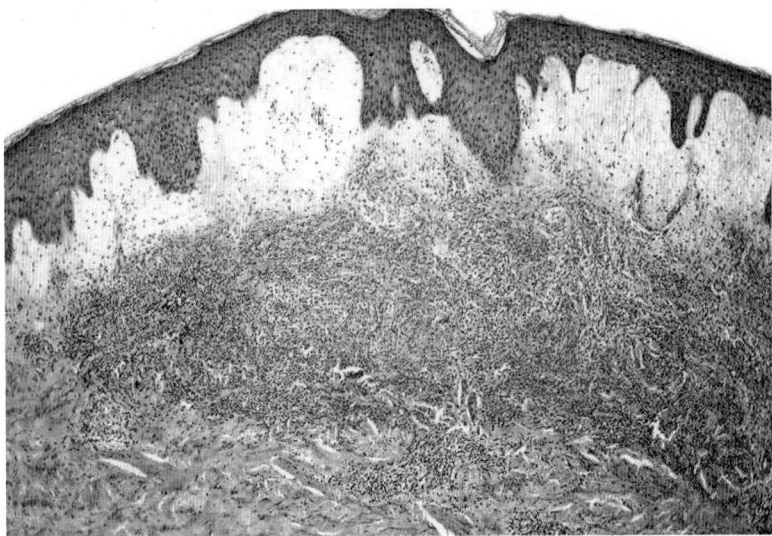

Fig. 15.20
Sweet syndrome: marked papillary dermal edema is commonly present and sometimes this is associated with subepidermal vesiculation.

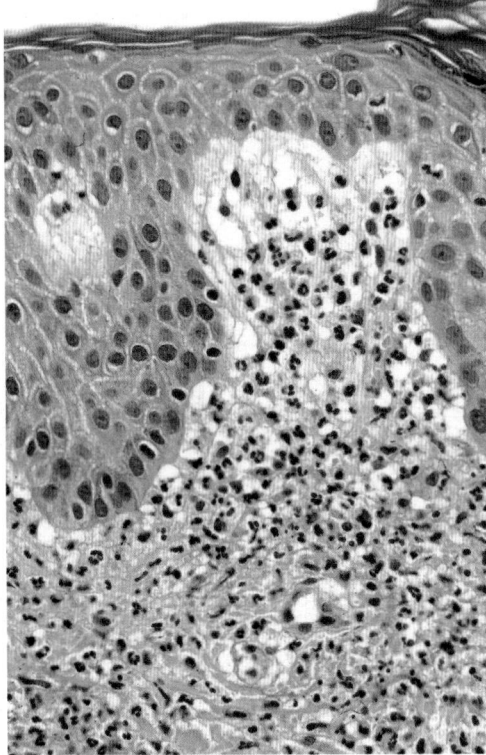

Fig. 15.21
Sweet syndrome: the occasional presence of dermal papillary neutrophil microabscesses can result in confusion with dermatitis herpetiformis.

Cases associated with leukocytoclastic neutrophilic lobular panniculitis, have been reported, and this may represent subcutaneous Sweet syndrome.[187–189] In other cases, the infiltrate may be predominantly composed of lymphocytes and histiocytes and, less commonly, neutrophils.[166,176,190,191] Sweet syndrome has also been associated with an erythema nodosum-like panniculitis.[192] Recently, cases with widespread cellulitis-like erythematous plaques have been described, termed giant cellulitis-like Sweet syndrome.[193,194] This form can be either neutrophilic or histiocytoid. Elastophagocytosis and cutis laxa have been reported with resolution of Sweet syndrome lesions.[195–197]

Differential diagnosis

The presence of prominent fibrinoid vascular change can distinguish necrotizing vasculidities such as leukocytoclastic vasculitis, erythema elevatum

diutinum, and granuloma faciale from Sweet syndrome; the clinical presentation and distribution of disease are also extremely helpful. In granuloma faciale, fibrinoid necrosis is often minimal and eosinophils tend to be prominent. Late lesions of erythema elevatum diutinum and granuloma faciale show fibrosis, a feature not seen in Sweet syndrome. Clinically, the presence of characteristic large ulcers helps distinguish pyoderma gangrenosum from Sweet syndrome. Also, pyoderma gangrenosum does not usually show the extent of karyorrhexis that is a typical feature of Sweet syndrome. A Gram stain and periodic acid-Schiff (PAS) or culture may be necessary to exclude infection. Distinction from some other forms of neutrophilic dermatosis including bowel bypass syndrome may be a definitional issue since the clinical setting determines the terminology applied.[7] Behçet disease may also be associated with lesions similar to those seen in Sweet syndrome. Clinical correlation should ensure the correct diagnosis. CD30-positive forms can sometimes be found in Sweet syndrome, raising the possibility of lymphomatoid papulosis. However, neutrophils are usually rare in the latter condition and the number of CD30-positive cells in Sweet syndrome is not prominent.[198] Knowledge of coexisting rheumatoid arthritis or systemic lupus eyrthematosus helps distinguish Sweet syndrome from rheumatoid neutrophilic dermatosis and systemic lupus erythematosus (SLE)-associated neutrophilic dermatosis, respectively. Although it has been suggested that in the later the dermal infiltrate tends to be paucicellular in contrast with the heavier infiltrate seen in Sweet syndrome, in fact moderate to prominent dermal neutrophilic infiltrates are more commonly seen in lupus.[199] Therefore, distinction from Sweet syndrome is impossible without clinicopathological correlation.

Neutrophilic dermatoses associated with gastrointestinal and hepatobiliary disease

Clinical features

Pyoderma gangrenosum, the most common neutrophilic dermatosis affecting patients with gastrointestinal disease (particularly ulcerative colitis), is discussed above. The spectrum of lesions described in this section shares many histologic (and likely pathogenetic) features with pyoderma gangrenosum but lack the characteristic progressive ulceration. Neutrophilic dermatoses associated with gastrointestinal disease may best be regarded as a continuum, with pyoderma gangrenosum representing an extreme end of the spectrum.

A syndrome of arthritis and pustular skin lesions was initially described in patients with inflammatory bowel and liver disease, and also in patients who have undergone jejunoileal bypass, gastric bypass, or Billroth II surgery for morbid obesity, but now has been described in other gastrointestinal disorders including Crohn disease and ulcerative colitis.[1–11] Up to 20% of patients with jejunoileal bypass develop this condition.[4,12] It has also been noted in association with peptic ulceration, appendicitis, and diverticular disease.[13,14] An increasing number of papers call this process bowel-associated dermatosis-arthritis syndrome (BADAS); this terminology currently appears to be that preferred by the majority of authors.

The skin lesions may be papular or vesicular, or form large necrotic lesions resembling pyoderma gangrenosum. They are usually found on the trunk or extremities. Oral involvement has also been described.[2] Associated panniculitis, which may resemble erythema nodosum, is a feature in some patients. Cutaneous manifestations often recur with exacerbation of the associated gastrointestinal disease.[4] Some patients have an elevated ESR.[4] The disease occasionally responds to antibiotic or steroid therapy.

A recurring vesiculopustular eruption may be seen in patients with hepatobiliary disease.[15] The lesions – which can be pruritic and sometimes heal with an atrophic scar – often present on the extremities. In some patients, the eruption represents a necrotizing folliculitis.[15] Occasionally, the cutaneous lesions precede the features of the hepatobiliary disease. A similar eruption may rarely be seen in Crohn disease.[16]

Patients with Crohn disease can also be complicated by disseminated abscesses involving the spleen, lymph nodes, liver, pancreas, and brain.[16,17] In some of these, the abscesses occurred before the diagnosis of Crohn disease. Histologically, a granulomatous element was commonly present. Successful treatment with immunosuppressive therapy suggests that such lesions may represent an unusual extraintestinal manifestation of Crohn disease.[16]

An unusual presentation of aseptic pustulosis largely restricted to skin folds has been described in patients with inflammatory bowel disease. This seems to be a paradoxical reaction to TNF-α blockers.[18,19]

The description of these entities suggests that they are overlapping or perhaps represent a disease continuum. BADAS is the most rigorously defined among these, and this terminology can probably be employed for all of the conditions mentioned above.

Pathogenesis and histologic features

The presence of circulating immune complexes in occasional patients has led some authors to postulate a pathogenic role.[20,21] It is postulated that bacterial overgrowth may play a role in the development of such circulating immune complexes.[4] In patients with the paradoxical reaction to TNF-α blockers, the lesions had increased expression of IL-1, TNF-α, IL-17, IL-8 and matrix metalloproteinases.[19] These observations are consistent with the concept that BADAS is an autoinflammatory disease similar to other neutrophilic dermatoses.[20]

The histopathological findings, which are non-specific, are those of a neutrophilic dermatosis. The lesions show variable dermal edema and necrosis associated with a perivascular and interstitial neutrophilic infiltrate. Variable numbers of lymphocytes and histiocytes may also be present. Abundant karyorrhexis gives rise to a histologic pattern similar to acute febrile neutrophilic dermatosis (Sweet syndrome) (*Fig. 15.22*). Leukocytoclastic vasculitis and pustular vasculitis have also been documented.[22–24] The inflammation is often limited to the dermis, but in some patients it may be seen to involve the subcutaneous fat, resulting in erythema nodosum or an erythema nodosum-like panniculitis.

The small number of cases described in patients with hepatobiliary disease has shown bullae associated with a dermal neutrophilic infiltrate, sometimes accompanied by eccrine hidradenitis or folliculitis.[15]

Differential diagnosis

The main differential diagnoses include infection, Sweet syndrome, pyoderma gangrenosum, and rheumatoid neutrophilic dermatitis. Clinical history is essential to distinguish these conditions.

The literature relating to BADAS and Sweet syndrome is often confusing, and it seems likely that some patients who have been reported as the former would actually have been better classified as the latter. Contrariwise, occasional patients who presented with features more typical of BADAS have, in fact, been reported as Sweet syndrome.[25,26] In many patients, such a distinction is semantic. In others, however, the clinical lesions are quite inconsistent with Sweet syndrome and in these patients a designation of BADAS is probably more appropriate.

Pyoderma gangrenosum is another neutrophilic dermatosis which patients with gastrointestinal disease are at risk of developing. Clinically, it may be distinguished by the progressive expansile nature of the cutaneous ulcers.[4] Since the biopsy findings may be similar, clinical correlation is essential to distinguish this condition from BADAS.

It is likely, given the histologic and clinical spectrum encountered in the neutrophilic dermatoses associated with gastrointestinal and hepatobiliary disease, that they result from similar or shared pathogenetic mechanisms. Clearly, more research may clarify their precise pathogenesis and contribute to a more satisfactory classification system.

Rheumatoid neutrophilic dermatitis

Clinical features

Rheumatoid neutrophilic dermatitis is an uncommon eruption seen in patients with rheumatoid arthritis.[1] It presents most often as papules, nodules, and plaques on the extensor surfaces of the extremities, neck, and trunk. In some patients, it may clinically resemble urticaria.[2–7] Bullous and pustular lesions have also been described.[8–11] The lesions, which can ulcerate, are often pruritic or painful, and sometimes show an annular configuration.[3,12,13] The disease is uncommon, as evidenced by documentation in

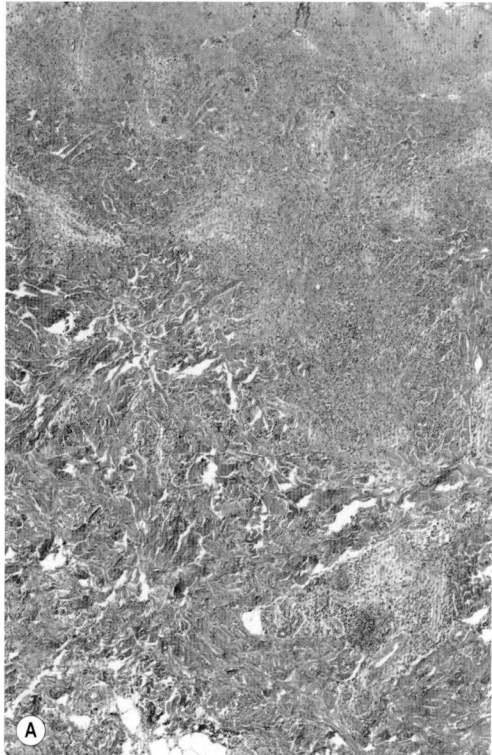

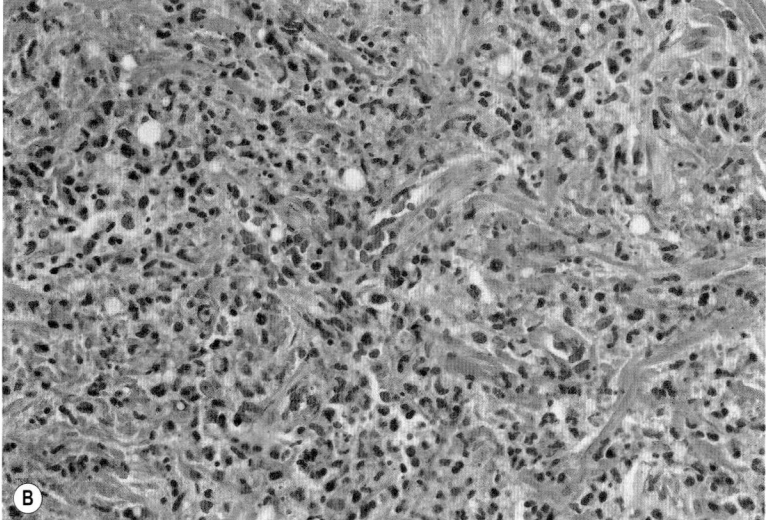

Fig. 15.22
(**A**, **B**) Neutrophilic dermatosis associated with gastrointestinal disease: there is an intense dermal neutrophilic infiltrate indistinguishable from Sweet syndrome.

just two of 142 and two of 215 patients with rheumatoid arthritis seeking medical attention for skin disorders in academic clinics in Japan and Turkey, respectively.[4,14] The presence of rheumatoid neutrophilic dermatitis correlates with the severity of the patient's joint disease.[4]

Typically, lesions last for up to several weeks.[2] In some patients, the condition resolves spontaneously; in others, it responds to steroid, dapsone, or sulfamethoxypyridamine therapy.[2,5,12]

Patients with seronegative arthritis but with cutaneous findings similar to rheumatoid neutrophilic dermatitis have recently been reported.[15–18]

Magro and Crowson have described sterile neutrophilic folliculitis associated with a Sweet syndrome-like histology in a setting of systemic disease including rheumatoid arthritis, Crohn disease, connective tissue disease, hepatitis, Behçet disease, atopy, hematological dyscrasia, and mycobacterial infection.[19] A similar folliculocentric acute inflammatory process has also been documented in patients with ulcerative colitis.[20,21] It would seem probable that these reports reflect a similar condition or spectrum of disease that likely shares common histopathogenetic mechanisms.

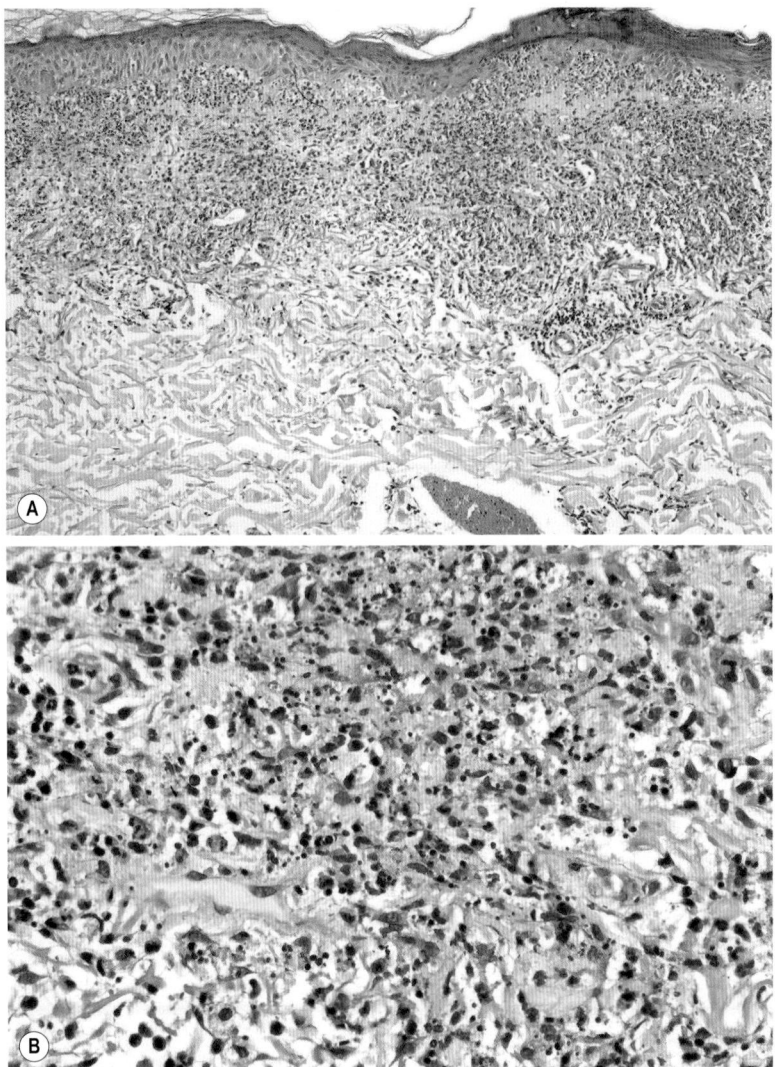

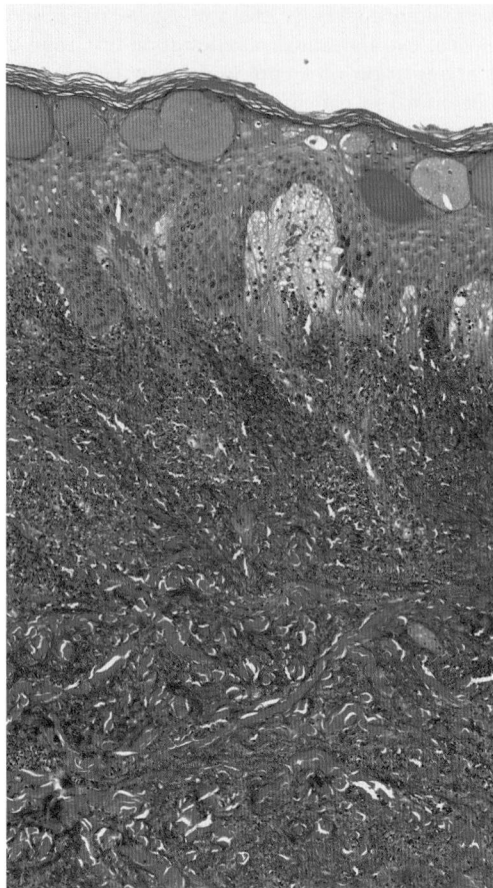

Fig. 15.24
Rheumatoid neutrophilic dermatosis: in some cases, there is prominent spongiosis of the epidermis with microvesicale formation. By courtesy of Dr. Jennifer S. Ko, MD, PhD, Cleveland Clinic, Cleveland, USA.

Fig. 15.23
(**A**, **B**) Rheumatoid neutrophilic dermatitis: there is an intense upper dermal neutrophilic infiltrate with conspicuous karyorrhexis. By courtesy of J. Cohen, MD, Dermatopathology Laboratory, Tucson, USA.

Pathogenesis and histologic features

The pathogenesis of rheumatoid neutrophilic dermatitis is not well understood, but some authors have suggested that it may represent an immune complex-mediated disease.[3,5] Likely, it is related to autoinflammatory disease related to a combination of IL-1, TNF-α and other cytokines similar to other neutrophilic dermatoses.[22]

Histologically, it is characterized by a dermal neutrophilic infiltrate with variable karyorrhexis (*Fig. 15.23*). In some cases, however, karyorrhexis is minimal or absent. Variable numbers of histiocytes, plasma cells, and eosinophils may be present; abscess formation is sometimes a feature.[2,3,5] Occasionally, the inflammatory infiltrate extends into the subcutaneous fat.[3,7] The overlying epidermis may show spongiosis and intraepidermal vesiculation (*Fig. 15.24*).[5]

Differential diagnosis

Infection must be considered in the differential diagnosis, particularly as patients are often at risk of infection as a result of immunosuppressive therapy. Furthermore, the cutaneous eruption may be treated with steroids, and failure to diagnose an underlying infective process could have disastrous consequences. Gram, AFB/acid fast, and silver stains for microorganisms should be routinely performed and the diagnosis made only after infection has been excluded. We have encountered several patients with rheumatoid arthritis on steroid therapy who developed pustular infiltrates associated with *Mycobacterium chelonae* infection.

Pyoderma gangrenosum may show similar, if not identical, features but differs by progressive ulceration. It should be remembered that patients with rheumatoid arthritis may also develop pyoderma gangrenosum.[4] Clinical correlation is necessary to distinguish these entities. Pyoderma gangrenosum may form part of a continuum that may eventually prove to share similar pathogenetic mechanisms. To those who hold this view, documentation of a patient with concurrent typical features of both pyoderma gangrenosum and rheumatoid neutrophilic dermatitis should not be surprising.[23]

Some authors have pointed out that rheumatoid neutrophilic dermatitis might be classified as a variant of Sweet syndrome.[2] Certainly, the biopsy findings may be very similar. The lack of fever and the general malaise that accompany Sweet syndrome are distinguishing clinical findings. The presence of gastrointestinal disease distinguishes rheumatoid neutrophilic dermatitis from BADAS. As with pyoderma gangrenosum, one might consider Sweet syndrome and rheumatoid neutrophilic dermatitis to form a spectrum of disease.[2] It is the characteristic clinical settings that allow these disorders to be distinguished.

Patients with rheumatoid arthritis may sometimes develop lesions which show histologic overlap with rheumatoid neutrophilic dermatitis but which can be distinguished by the presence of a palisading necrobiotic and granulomatous component (termed palisaded neutrophilic granulomatous dermatitis).[24] This spectrum also includes interstitial granulomatous dermatitis encountered in a setting of systemic disease (including rheumatoid arthritis). Patients, predominantly adults, present with papules and nodules which particularly affect the extremities or trunk; these are often distributed in a linear pattern.[25,26] The presence of necrobiosis associated with a histiocytic response reminiscent of granuloma annulare or necrobiosis lipoidica in addition to acute inflammation and variable karyorrhexis helps distinguish these lesions from typical rheumatoid neutrophilic dermatitis. A case has been described in a patient with rheumatoid arthritis treated with adalimumab.[27]

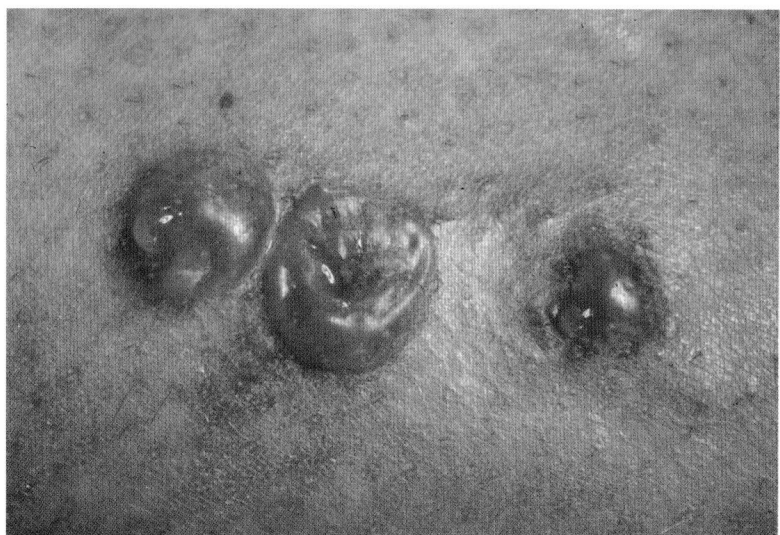

Fig. 15.25
Bullous insect bite reaction: there are large fluid-filled bullae in this close-up view from the lower leg. From the collection of the late N.P. Smith, MD, the Institute of Dermatology, London, UK.

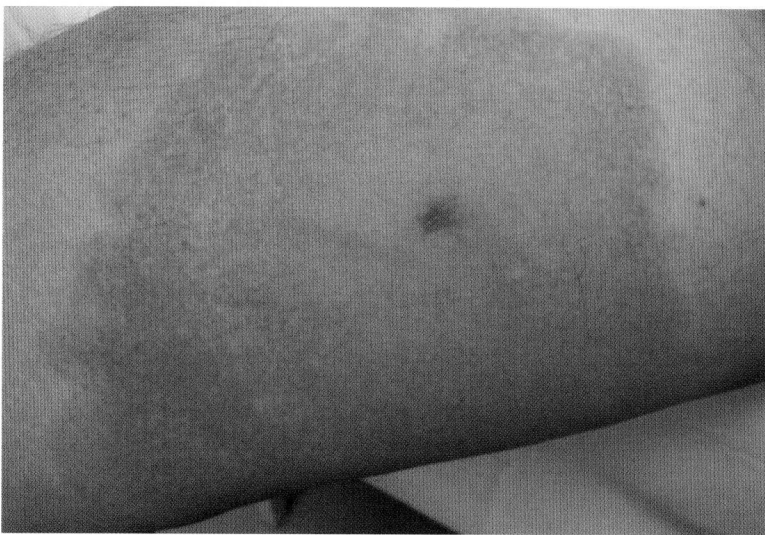

Fig. 15.26
Spider bite: note the central eschar and surrounding erythema. Courtesy of Al Mahmoud, MD, Doha, Qatar.

Lesions in which the neutrophilic infiltrate is associated with dermal papillary abscess formation may be mistaken for dermatitis herpetiformis, linear IgA disease, and bullous SLE. IMF staining may be necessary in problematic cases.

The presence of vascular necrosis and fibrinoid change distinguishes rheumatoid neutrophilic dermatitis from vasculitis.[28] It must be emphasized that a careful search for evidence of vasculitis is not simply an academic exercise, since patients with rheumatoid arthritis are also at risk of developing vasculitis. In fact, patients with rheumatoid arthritis may present with lesions histologically showing extravascular palisading granulomas, diffuse neutrophilic infiltrates, or vasculitis (neutrophilic, lymphocytic, or granulomatous). The different patterns may overlap, and classification should be based on the dominant histologic pattern.

Arthropod and arachnid bite reactions

Clinical features

The vast majority of insect bites pose little more than a minor annoyance. The reaction that results from a given bite depends on the nature of the offending insect and the patient's immune response. The clinical response to a bite may vary from a trivial erythematous papule to a large nodule associated with marked pruritus and ulceration. Vesicles are sometimes seen in severe reactions (*Fig. 15.25*). Careful inspection will often reveal a punctum at the site where insect mouth parts entered skin.

While arthropod bites are rarely of clinical importance, reactions following the bite of certain arachnids can lead to a more serious clinical lesion (*Fig. 15.26*). Many different species of spiders may bite humans, and reactions to the most significant and well described – the brown recluse and the black widow – are detailed below.[1-4]

Brown recluse spider

The brown recluse spider (*Loxosceles reclusa*) bite begins as a painful bluish macule, papule, or nodule, often with a bruise-like appearance. A central punctum is commonly observed. The thigh was the involved site in almost 50% of cases, with the arm and abdomen accounting for most of the remainder in a large series from a single center of more than 50 patients with presumed bites.[5] However, in some patients, blistering and ulceration, often progressing to a large necrotic lesion, is a feature.[6] The lesion is often trivial. Chronic ulceration mimicking pyoderma gangrenosum may rarely ensue.[7] The brown recluse is most commonly encountered in rural areas of the Midwest, south-central, and southeastern United States and is easily identified by a violin-shaped marking on the cephalothorax that gives it its

vernacular name of 'fiddleback' spider.[8] Most bites are seasonal, occurring between the months of April and October.[9] However, other spiders are often misidentified as brown recluse, and the diagnosis may be overused as the spider is often not identified at the time of the bite.[10-14] This makes much of the existing literature suspect.[15]

Phospholipase D/sphingomyelinase-D in the venom of the brown recluse spider is thought to be responsible for the extensive necrosis that results in some patients.[16,17] Spider bites may be associated with morbilliform rash, malaise, fever, nausea, hemoglobinuria, arthralgias, and vomiting.[6,18-20] More serious complications (e.g., renal failure, shock, disseminated intravascular coagulation, acute hemolytic anemia, intravascular hemolysis, and a single case of bilateral optic neuropathy) have also been described.[18,21-26] Many of the effects of the venom appear to be dose-dependent rather than idiosyncratic.[27,28] ELISA-based assays to detect the *Loxosceles* venom at the site of the bite are available and can be helpful to confirm the diagnosis, as detectable toxin may persist for more than 2 weeks.[29-33] Anti-loxoscelic sera are available for use in severe cases.[34,35]

Widow spiders

The five species of widow spiders found in the United States, including the notorious black widow (*Latrodectus mactans*), are most commonly encountered in the southern states. Compared with the brown recluse, bites by widow spiders are much less commonly encountered by healthcare providers. Many presumed or self-reported arachnid bites are ultimately discovered to be skin and soft tissue infections.[36] The bite often shows a targetoid appearance with a pale center surrounded by an outer erythematous rim.[37] A bite from a black widow spider is commonly associated with severe pain in the vicinity of the bite as well as systemic symptoms such as general malaise, abdominal pain, nausea, headache, and muscle spasms.[6,18,37] Priapism has been noted as a rare complication.[38] Occasionally, patients die as a result of the bite.[21,39]

Alpha-latrotoxin is an active component of the venom that binds to presynaptic nerve terminals and stimulates massive neurotransmitter release. The neurological symptoms are termed latrodectism and consist of pain, diaphoresis, and non-specific systemic symptoms sometimes combined with additional autonomic or neurological dysfunction.[40] Equine-derived antisera is available and effective as a treatment.[41,42] Recombinant antisera are under development.[43]

Hobo spider

Recently, the Hobo spider (*Tegenaria agrestis*) has been implicated as a cause of significant bite reactions in the Pacific Northwest with migration to Montana and Colorado and evidence of continuing eastward expansion.[44,45]

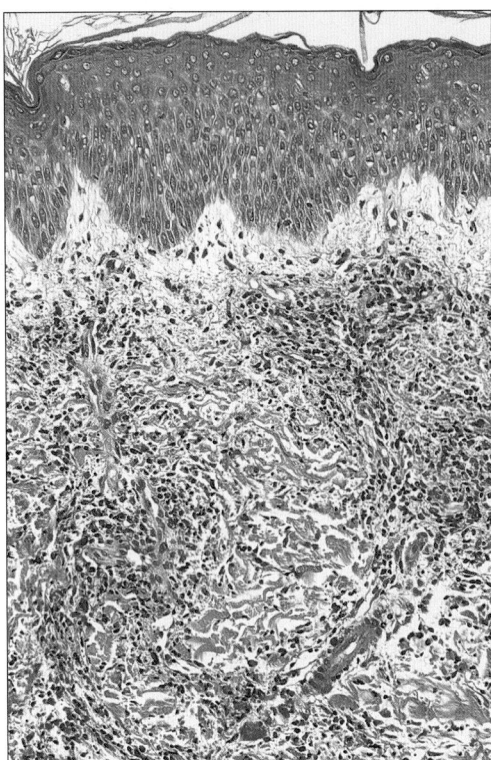

Fig. 15.27
Arthropod bite reaction: there is a heavy perivascular and interstitial infiltrate.

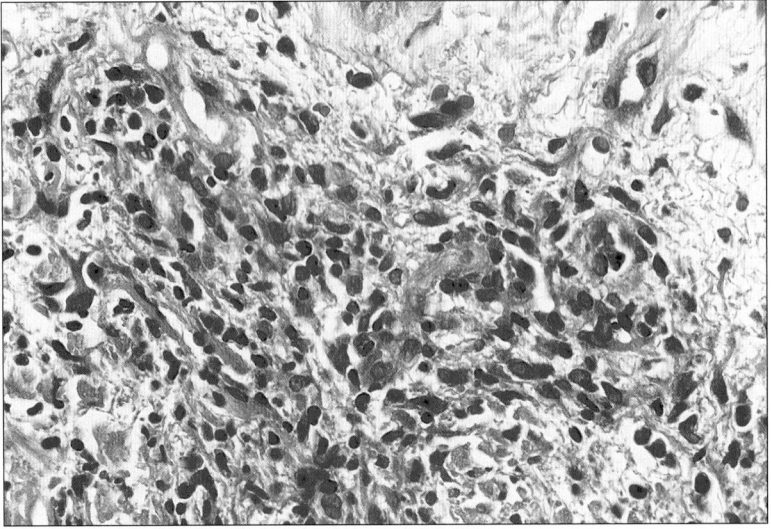

Fig. 15.28
Arthropod bite reaction: note the conspicuous eosinophils.

While bites from this spider are believed to cause dermonecrotic injuries, additional studies are necessary to confirm this impression, as not all confirmed bites from this spider result in significant tissue necrosis.[46–48]

Histologic features

Just as there is a spectrum of clinical response to an insect bite, the histopathological features also vary.

The typical arthropod bite reaction, such as follows a mosquito bite, is characterized by a wedge-shaped polymorphic inflammatory cell infiltrate composed of lymphocytes, histiocytes, eosinophils, and sometimes neutrophils (*Figs 15.27* and *15.28*). Spongiosis (occasionally with vesicle formation) and dermal edema are variably seen (*Figs 15.29–15.32*), but in many cases the epidermis can appear relatively unremarkable. Ulceration with scale-crust commonly forms in excoriated lesions. In some cases, insect mouth parts are identified in the center of the lesion. In our experience,

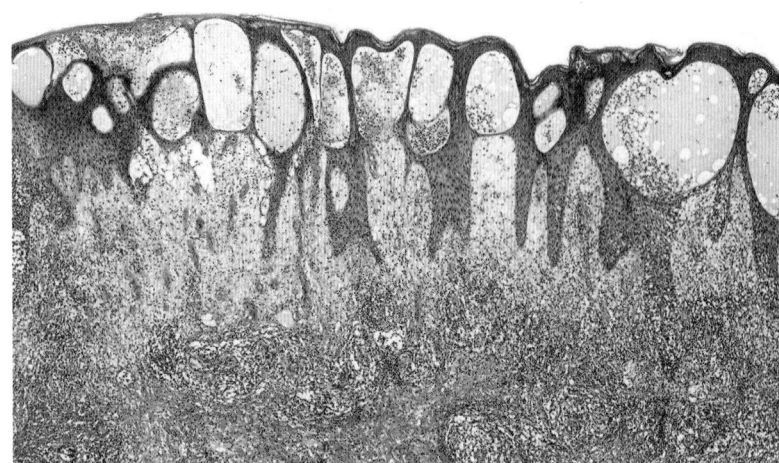

Fig. 15.29
Bullous arthropod bite reaction: massive subepidermal edema has resulted in a multiloculated subepidermal blister.

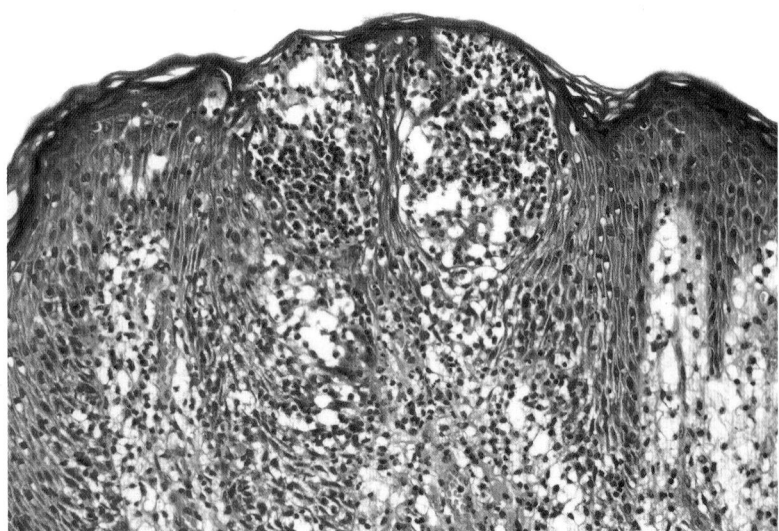

Fig. 15.30
Bullous arthropod bite reaction: eosinophilic spongiosis is present at the edge of the lesion.

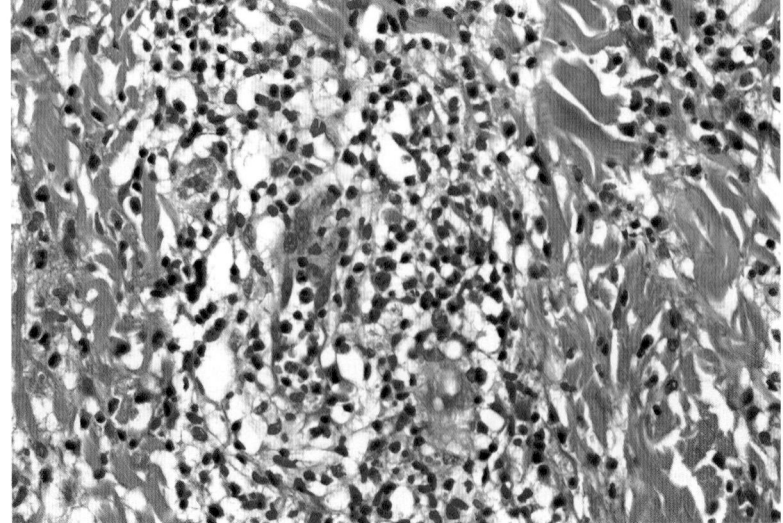

Fig. 15.31
Bullous arthropod bite reaction: there is a lymphocytic and eosinophilic perivascular and interstitial infiltrate.

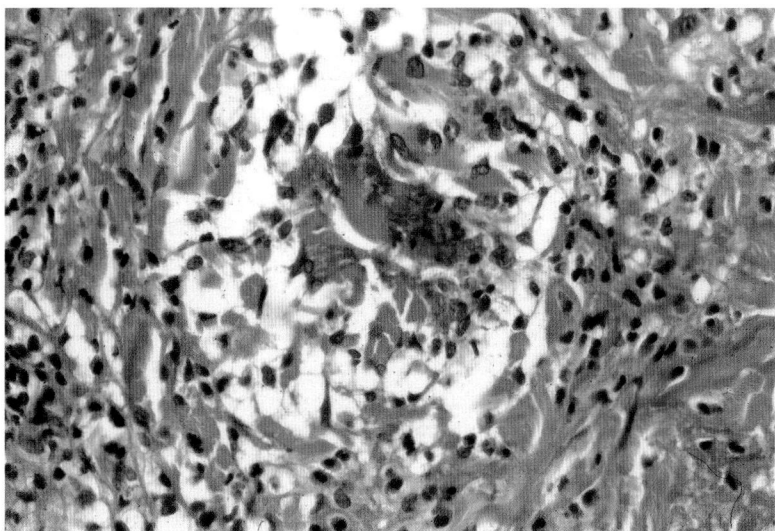

Fig. 15.32
Bullous arthropod bite reaction: high-power view showing a flame figure.

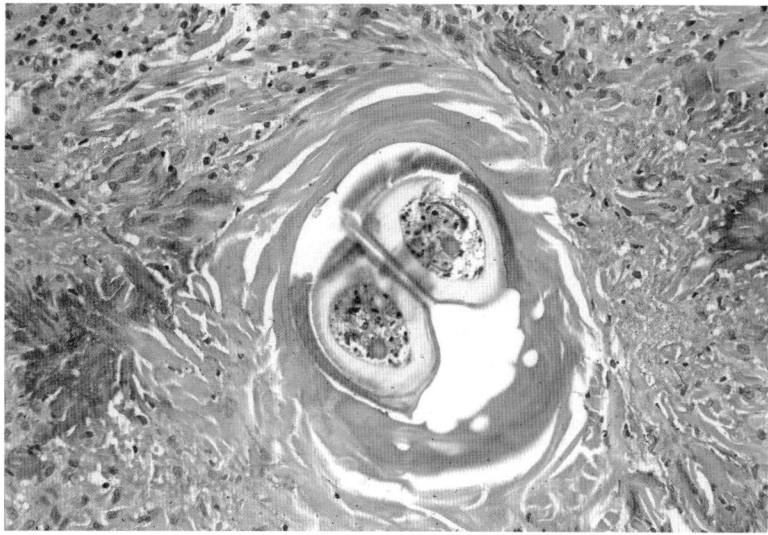

Fig. 15.34
Tick bite reaction: high-power view showing tick parts and multiple flame figures.

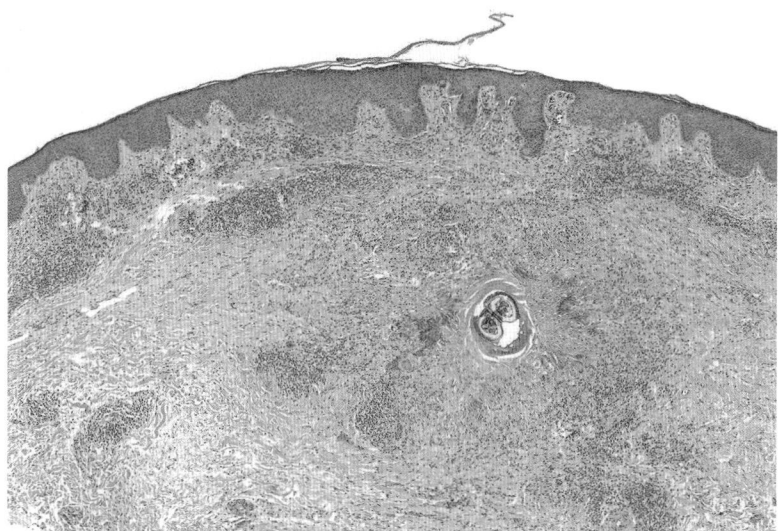

Fig. 15.33
Tick bite reaction: low-power view showing a heavy dermal inflammatory cell infiltrate. Tick parts are seen in the center of the field.

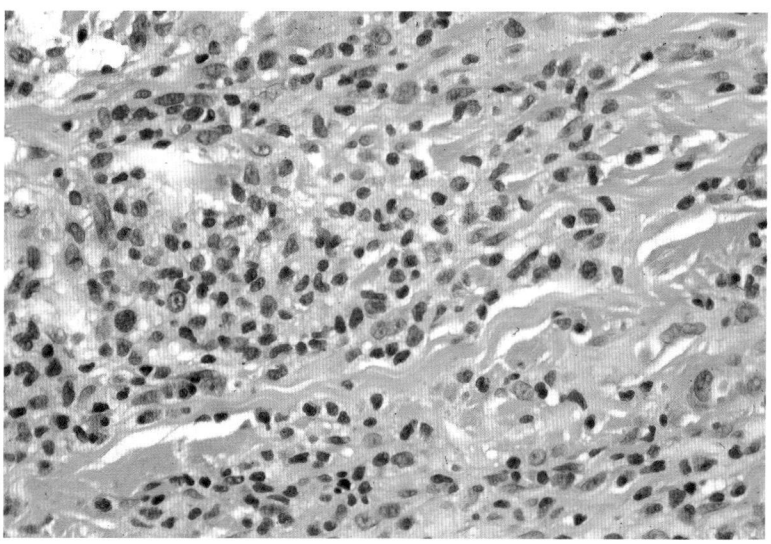

Fig. 15.35
Tick bite reaction: there is a dense infiltrate of lymphocytes, histiocytes, and conspicuous eosinophils.

this is more common in biopsies from tick bites than arachnid bites (*Figs 15.33–15.35*).

As with arthropod bite reactions, the histologic sequelae from arachnid bite are variable. Compared with the former, arachnid bite reactions are typically associated with more extensive necrosis and suppurative inflammation. Necrosis may extend to involve the subcutaneous fat and muscle.[6] Variable numbers of eosinophils and lymphocytes are present, and marked dermal edema is often a feature.[6] Secondary vasculitis, involving vessels within the lesion or in the immediate surrounding tissue, may be a feature in some cases. Injection of brown recluse spider venom into rabbits results in 'mummified' coagulation necrosis, a mixed inflammatory cell infiltrate, and vasculitis.[49]

Differential diagnosis

The histologic findings in biopsies of insect bites, short of identifying mouth parts in the specimen, are non-specific. The main differential diagnosis includes hypersensitivity reactions. The characteristic wedge shape of the infiltrate is an important clue to the diagnosis. Although scattered large atypical lymphocytes may be seen in bite reactions, these cells are more numerous and often arranged in aggregates in lymphomatoid papulosis. Bite reactions with a dense eosinophil-rich infiltrate may be indistinguishable

from Wells syndrome. The occasional presence of flame figures heightens the similarity. Clinical correlation may be necessary to distinguish these two conditions.

The histologic findings associated with arachnid bite are also non-specific. Arachnid bites must be distinguished from pyoderma gangrenosum, factitial disease, primary vasculitis, and infections including cellulitis and necrotizing fasciitis. Arachnid envenomation appears to be overreported; thus, some cases have been reported in regions where the spiders have never been documented to exist. ELISA-based assays may be helpful to confirm the diagnosis. Without definitive evidence of involvement of an arachnid, the diagnosis must be considered one of exclusion so as not to overlook important clinical alternatives with a different treatment approach.

Seabather's eruption and coelenterate stings

Clinical features

Seabather's eruption, sometimes referred to as 'sea lice', is attributed to stings from larval forms of coelenterates, often the thimble jellyfish (*Linuche unguiculata scyphomedusae*).[1–4] Typically, patients develop a papular eruption in areas covered by the bathing suit, often accentuated where the suit is tight fitting, such as the waistline.[5,6] The eruption is usually pruritic and may cause a burning sensation. Patients sometimes experience systemic symptoms such as malaise, fever, nausea, diarrhea, and vomiting.

Reactions to coelenterates such as jellyfish vary from minor irritation to fatal reactions following stings by highly venomous species such as the 'box jellyfish' (*Chironex fleckeri* and *Chiropsalmus quadrigatus*).[7] Jellyfish stings are often erythematous and show a 'whiplash-like' appearance.[7,8] Certain species may have more serious consequences, such as the Portuguese man-of-war (*Physalia physalis*), where systemic effects from neurotoxins can be seen, including cramping of muscles, respiratory distress, profound hypotension, and even death in extreme cases.[9–12] It appears that the length of the nematocyst tube may correlate whether a jellyfish has the ability to sting; jellyfish with longer nematocysts can result in stings while those with shorter ones do not.[13]

A topically applied envenomation inhibitor based on the mucous coat of clown fish is effective in dramatically reducing both some coelenterate stings and seabather's eruption, although it may lack efficacy against certain coelenterate species.[14,15]

Histologic features

Biopsy of papules of seabather's eruption shows a non-specific perivascular inflammatory cell infiltrate composed of variable numbers of lymphocytes, eosinophils, and neutrophils.[2] Epidermal changes are apparently not usually a feature.[2]

Only few authors have reported the histologic findings following reaction to coelenterate stings. Non-specific perivascular inflammation with lymphocytes and variable numbers of eosinophils appear to be characteristic. Some cases show dense, sheetlike aggregates of lymphocytes, and histiocytes.[16] Variable dermal edema may be an additional feature. Spongiosis and vesicle formation are also sometimes described.[16–18] One fatal case showed only vascular congestion without significant inflammation, a histologic picture that likely reflects the fact that the patient died only 40 minutes after being stung.[6] Only occasionally are nematocyst capsules and tubes identified.[6,18]

Differential diagnosis

The histologic differential diagnosis of reactions to coelenterates includes other hypersensitivity reactions. Short of finding nematocysts, the diagnosis depends entirely on clinical correlation.

Erythema marginatum rheumaticum

Clinical features

Once a common disease, it was thought that, with the effective antibiotic treatment of the causative infection, rheumatic fever would become of historical interest only. However, there has been a resurgence of the condition over the past few decades, particularly in developing countries.[1–5]

Rheumatic fever is an immunologically mediated disease that follows an infection with Lancefield group A beta-hemolytic streptococcus. The infection causes pharyngitis and carditis. Additional features include polyarthritis, a neurological movement disorder known as Sydenham chorea, and subcutaneous nodules.[6] Carditis, characterized by a valvular disease, is a major cause of morbidity and mortality.

Erythema marginatum rheumaticum is the designation given to the distinctive annular or polycyclic eruption of rheumatic fever. The lesions are nonpruritic, multiple, flat, erythematous maculopapules which change and spread over hours, and are often recurrent. The trunk and proximal extremities are most frequently affected.[2,7] The hands and face may also be involved.[4] By definition, erythema marginatum rheumaticum is associated with rheumatic fever, but occurs in only 1–18% of patients.[1] Some studies have failed to identify significant HLA associations.[3,8] However, there are conflicting reports of certain HLA subtypes and the disease.[9]

Pathogenesis and histologic features

The pathogenesis of rheumatic fever is incompletely understood. It appears likely that it results from a hypersensitivity reaction triggered by streptococcal infection. Specifically, patients develop autoantibodies that cross-react

with streptococcal antigens due to molecular mimicry.[10] For example, autoantibodies cross-react with cardiac muscle, causing carditis. Mice immunized with the streptococcal M protein develop myocarditis.[10] Bradykinin in dense deposits can be seen in stromal and endothelial tissues, suggesting it may mediate some facets of this condition.[11]

Variable numbers of neutrophils (sometimes associated with leukocytoclasis) and mononuclear cells are present in the infiltrate.[8,12] Importantly, however, there is no evidence of vasculitis. Dermal papillary neutrophil microabscesses have occasionally been described.[8]

It has been reported that rare cases are devoid of neutrophils and the infiltrate is instead composed of lymphocytes and histiocytes.[13]

Differential diagnosis

The biopsy findings in erythema marginatum are non-specific. Similar histologic features may be seen in patients with Still disease and acute lupus erythematosus. Careful search for vascular damage is necessary to exclude leukocytoclastic vasculitis. Special stains and culture to rule out an infectious etiology are sometimes required. Urticaria can demonstrate perivascular neutrophils, but additionally it shows significant dermal edema, and an interstitial inflammatory cell infiltrate, including neutrophils, eosinophils, and lymphocytes

Still disease

Clinical features

Juvenile rheumatoid arthritis or systemic juvenile idiopathic arthritis (Still disease) is a heterogeneous group of disorders which share in common an inflammatory arthritis with many features similar to rheumatoid arthritis in adults. Juvenile rheumatoid arthritis patients, however, are seronegative for rheumatoid factor.[1] There are marked differences in prevalence from region to region. Whites in Europe, the United States, and Australia (4 per 1000) have the highest prevalence.[2,3] One study has suggested that the incidence of the disease is decreasing.[4] This same study also documented incidence peaks indicating a possible cyclical pattern.[4] Other studies have found seasonal variation in certain regions such as the Canadian prairies.[5] However, such seasonal onset has not been apparent in other areas of Canada, in Denmark, or in Japan.[5–8]

Juvenile rheumatoid arthritis is classified into three variants: pauciarticular, polyarticular, and systemic onset.
- The pauciarticular (oligoarticular) form is characterized by arthritis involving up to a maximum of four joints. Systemic manifestations are uncommon. Uveitis, however, is frequently present.
- The polyarticular form is manifest by symmetrical arthritis typically involving the knees, wrists, and ankles. Fever and hepatosplenomegaly are sometimes present.
- The systemic-onset form is a severe variant in which lymphadenopathy, fever, and rash precede development of polyarteritis, which most often affects the knees, ankles, and wrists.[9] Additional features may include hepatosplenomegaly and effusions. In general, the term Still disease is restricted to this form of juvenile rheumatoid arthritis; however, some authors use it for any of the variants. The majority of patients with the systemic form have the characteristic rash in contrast to the pauci- and polyarticular variants in which only 20–40% are affected.[9]

The rash of Still disease is typically evanescent, and is characterized by a faint erythematous (salmon-colored), sometimes pruritic, macular eruption involving the trunk, extremities, head, and neck.[9–12] Often, there is an association between onset of rash and febrile episodes, particularly in the late afternoon or evening.[9,11] The rash is typically present for only a short period, usually a matter of a few hours; however, some lesions persist for more than 24 hours.[9,11,12] It characteristically reappears without regard for its former distribution.[11] Macules are often only a few millimeters in size but frequently become confluent to form larger lesions. Central pallor is sometimes a feature of the latter.[10] The eruption – which may persist for weeks to years – tends to localize to areas of mild trauma and pressure.[9,11]

Laboratory abnormalities include elevated ESR and C-reactive protein. Serum immunoglobulins may also be raised. Patients often have leukocytosis

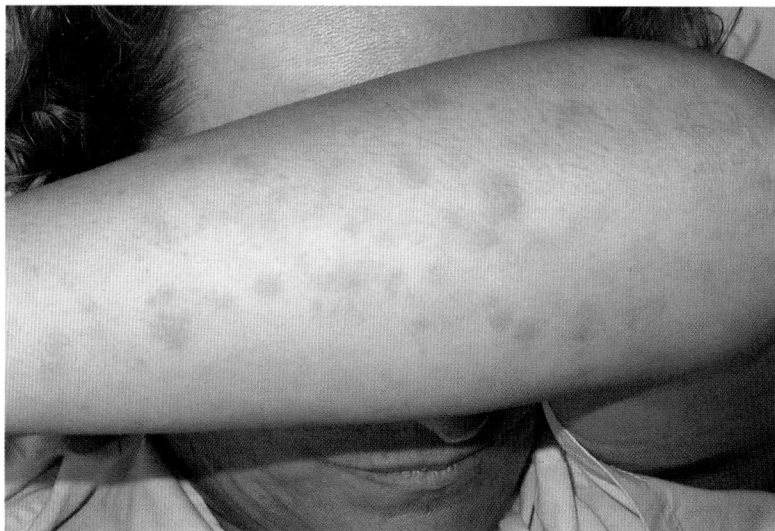

Fig. 15.36
Still disease in an adult: there are multiple erythematous macules. By courtesy of J.C. Pascual, MD, Alicante, Spain.

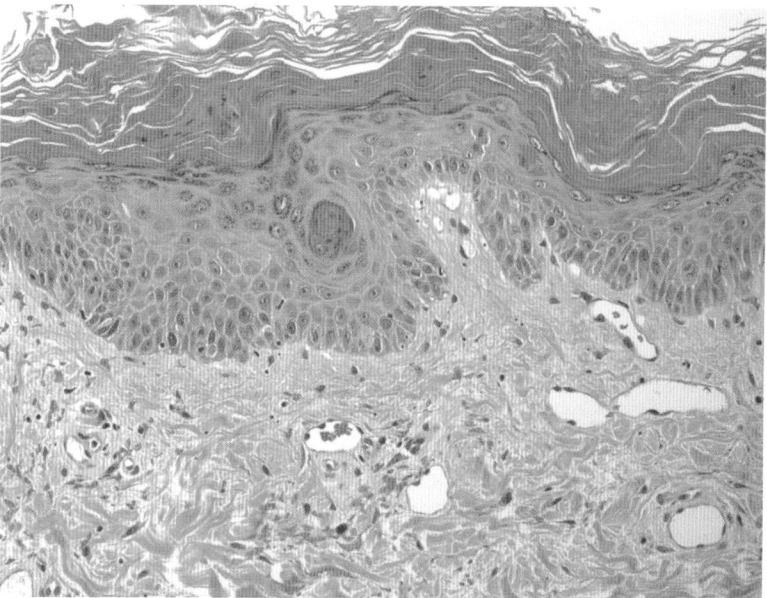

Fig. 15.37
Adult onset Still disease: there are numerous dyskeratotic cells in stratum corneum and upper epidermis.

and increased ferritin levels and may have anemia, and thrombocytosis.[12] Occasional patients have rheumatoid factor, and some authors consider this to represent bona fide juvenile rheumatoid arthritis. Antinuclear antibodies are commonly found in patients with pauci- and polyarticular variants of the disease.[8] In contrast, antinuclear antibody is usually not present in the systemic-onset form.

It is very difficult to predict the outcome of this disease in the individual patient. Approximately 50% of patients experience symptoms into adulthood. Progression of juvenile rheumatoid arthritis to SLE has been documented.[13] Serious complications including uveitis, cardiac tamponade, portal vein thrombosis, liver failure, disseminated intravascular coagulation, parenchymal lung disease, and hemophagocytic syndrome have been documented.[14–22]

Despite the name juvenile rheumatoid arthritis, Still disease is not limited to the pediatric population. Adult onset is well described in the literature (Fig. 15.36).[12,23–29] Patients with the adult form of the disease may develop persistent papules and plaques and hyperpigmentation.[30] Lesions are mainly seen on the face, neck, trunk, and extensor surfaces of the extremities.

Pathogenesis and histologic features

The pathogenesis of juvenile rheumatoid arthritis is poorly understood. It would seem likely, however, that the various subtypes have different etiologies. Thus:

- IL-2 mRNA is detected more often in pauciarticular juvenile rheumatoid arthritis than in the polyarticular form.[31]
- A shift toward a Th1 type cytokine profile is seen with increased serum levels of IFN-γ, IL-6, IL-18, and TNF-α.[28,31,32]
- IL-18 may play a particularly crucial role in activating macrophages and inducing the TH1 cytokine profile in Still disease.[28]

It has been suggested that nucleotide-binding and oligomerization domain (NOD)-like receptors (NLR) that detect microbes and help constitute the inflammasome (a complex of proteins which initiates an inflammatory reaction) may be involved in autoimmune disease generally and in Still disease in particular.[33,34]

Data suggesting that the incidence of the disease is decreasing with cyclical peaks raise the possibility that environmental factors could play a role in the pathogenesis.[4] Demonstration of T-cell oligoclonal expansions within synovial tissue suggests that an antigen or group of antigens may trigger the disease.[35] The nature of such triggering factors, however, has not yet been identified.

The prevalence of autoimmune disease is increased in relatives of patients with juvenile rheumatoid arthritis compared with control subjects, suggesting that shared susceptibility genes may be of importance in the pathogenesis of juvenile rheumatoid arthritis and other autoimmune diseases.[36]

The influence of various HLA alleles and their association with juvenile rheumatoid arthritis has been an area of considerable interest and has yielded a complex picture of the relationship between certain HLA alleles and risk of disease.[37] HLA-A2, DR8, DR5, and DPB1*0201 are associated with increased risk of pauciarticular disease early in life.[37] While B27 and DR4 may be protective in the early years, these alleles seem to confer increased risk of disease later in life.[38]

CD4-reactive T lymphocytes are the predominant cell type in the inflamed synovium.[39] As with other autoimmune disorders, production of predominantly Th1 cytokines (IFN-γ and IFN-β) has been observed in the synovium of juvenile rheumatoid arthritis patients.[39,40]

The biopsy findings are non-specific and variable. There is often a perivascular neutrophilic infiltrate.[10,12] In some cases, mononuclear cells are the predominant cell type, and in others there is a mixed infiltrate of neutrophils and mononuclear cells.[9,11,12] A neutrophilic panniculitis may be associated with the disease.[41] In adult-onset Still disease, distinctive histologic features have been described particularly in the persistent papules and plaques sometimes seen in the disease. The epidermis displays dyskeratotic keratinocytes in single units or aggregates (Fig. 15.37).[12,30] They tend to be present mainly in the upper layers of the epidermis and even in the stratum corneum.[12,30,42] Other changes include subcorneal pustules, upper dermal lymphocytes and neutrophils, interface change, neutrophilic eccrine hidradenitis, and increased dermal mucin.[12,30,42]

Differential diagnosis

The histologic findings, as indicated above, are variable and non-specific. Clinical correlation is necessary to establish the diagnosis. The differential diagnosis includes infection, and culture and stains for microorganisms should be performed when necessary. The absence of fibrinoid change and necrosis of blood vessel walls distinguishes the lesions from leukocytoclastic vasculitis. The presence of dyskeratotic cells could suggest an irritant contact dermatitis, but that entity has less inflammation and a different clinical presentation.

Urticaria

Clinical features

Urticaria is an extremely common group of disorders that share common clinical and histologic features (Table 15.3).[1] The lifetime incidence approaches one in five people.[2] As will be seen later, urticaria has many

Table 15.3
Classification of urticaria subtypes (presenting with wheals and/or angioedema)

Types	Subtypes	Definition
Spontaneous urticaria	Acute spontaneous urticaria	Spontaneous wheals and/or angioedema <6 weeks
	Chronic spontaneous urticaria	Spontaneous wheals and/or angioedema >6 weeks
Physical urticaria	Cold contact urticaria	Eliciting factor: cold objects/air/fluids/wind
	Delayed pressure urticaria	Eliciting factor: vertical pressure (wheals arising with a 3–12 h latency)
	Heat contact urticaria	Eliciting factor: localized heat
	Solar urticaria	Eliciting factor: UV and/or visible light
	Urticaria factitia/dermographic urticaria	Eliciting factor: mechanical shearing forces (wheals arising after 1–5 min)
	Vibratory urticaria/angioedema	Eliciting factor: vibratory forces, e.g., pneumatic hammer
Other urticaria types	Aquagenic urticaria	Eliciting factor: water
	Cholinergic urticaria	Elicitation by increase of body core temperature due to physical exercises, spicy food
	Contact urticaria	Elicitation by contact with urticariogenic substance
	Exercise induced anaphylaxis/urticaria	Eliciting factor: physical exercise

Table 2 from Zuberbier T, Asero R, Bindslev-Jensen C, et al. EAACI/GA2LEN/EDF/WAO guideline: definition, classification and diagnosis of urticaria. Allergy 2009; 64:1417–1426.

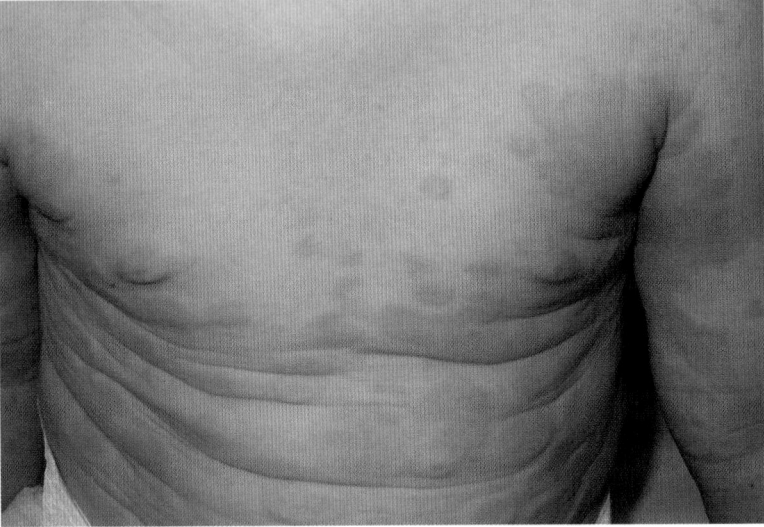

Fig. 15.38
Urticaria: erythematous, edematous, coalescing plaques on the trunk and proximal extremities of an infant. By courtesy of J.C. Pascual, MD, Alicante, Spain.

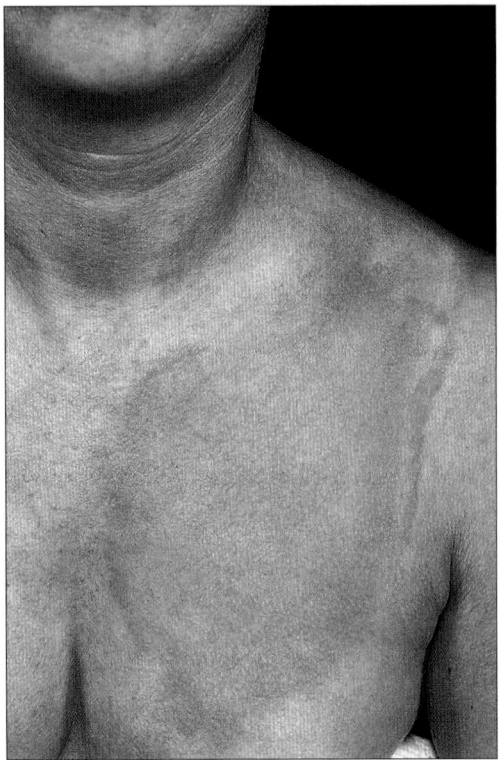

Fig. 15.39
Urticaria: in this patient, the erythematous border is well demonstrated. By courtesy of the Institute of Dermatology, London, UK.

different etiologies but, more often than not, the cause remains unknown and the disease is then classified as idiopathic. In some patients, more than one stimulus may elicit symptoms.[3] The clinical common denominator in urticaria is the development of 'hives' or 'wheals' – raised edematous lesions – which are often surrounded by a zone of erythema and are commonly pruritic (*Figs 15.37–15.40*).[4,5] Dermatographism – pressure or light scratching resulting in linear urticarial lesions – is a common symptom. Urticaria may develop in only seconds. Lesions usually resolve in less than a few hours. By definition, lesions in patients with chronic urticaria, however, persist over a period in excess of 6 weeks.[5,6] In addition, individual lesions in patients with chronic urticaria often last longer – up to 36 hours.[4]

Given that urticaria is best viewed not as a single disease but as a group of related disorders, it comes as no surprise that the natural history of urticaria is highly variable.[2] Resolution is seen in 50% of patients within a few years of onset; however, in some patients the disease persists for decades.[2,5] The severity of symptoms is also variable. For many patients, the disease is a minor annoyance; for others, however, it can result in significant impacts in quality of life and severe reactions may be associated with life-threatening anaphylaxis.[7]

Physical causes of urticaria include sunlight, cold, heat, pressure, and vibration.

Solar urticaria

Solar urticaria is characterized by development of wheals and pruritus that usually develop within minutes at sites exposed to light (*Fig. 15.41*).[8,9] A sensitizing agent, such as a drug, may be necessary.[10–12] In some patients, lesions even arise in areas covered by light clothing.[13] 'Fixed solar urticaria' is a designation given to a rare form of urticaria seen in patients who develop lesions at the same sites with repeated light exposure.[14,15] Solar urticaria has also been described following exposure to infrared and ultraviolet radiation.[16,17]

Aquagenic urticaria

'Aquagenic urticaria' is a bizarre variant of physical urticaria in which patients develop lesions following exposure to water (regardless of temperature).[18,19] Extracutaneous manifestations such as migraine headache and familial occurrence has been described on rare occasion.[20–22] Thankfully, patients do not develop symptoms from drinking water.[5,23] Application of petrolatum ointment or other barrier cream prior to water exposure helps to prevent lesion development.[18,24,25] It has been postulated that a water-soluble epidermal antigen may be responsible for such symptoms, since aqueous extracts of callus cause symptoms in patients' skin but not in that of controls.[26] Increased water salinity has also been implicated.[27]

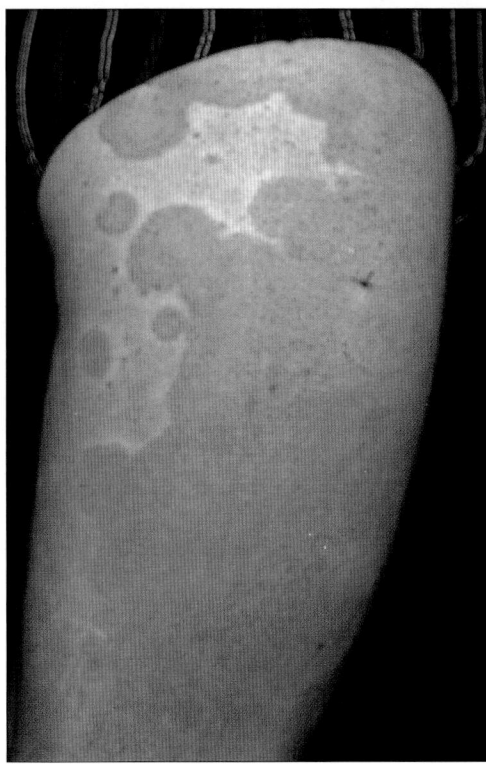

Fig. 15.40
Urticaria: in this extreme example, there is intense erythema. By courtesy of the Institute of Dermatology, London, UK.

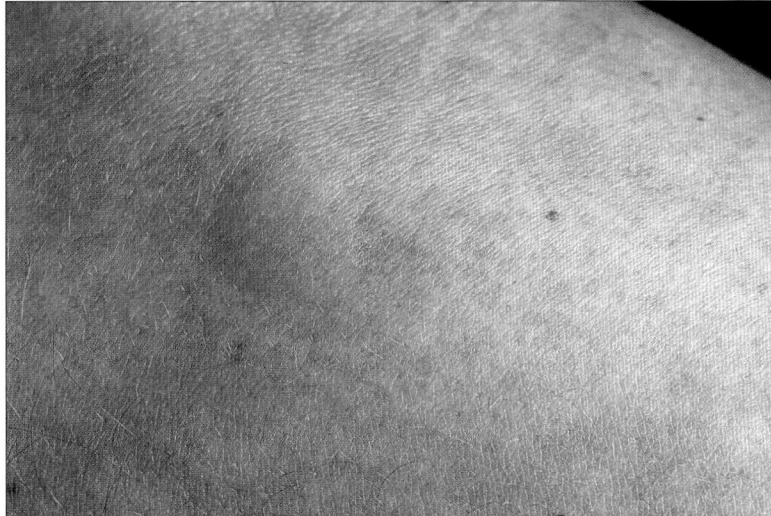

Fig. 15.41
Solar urticaria: in this patient, urticaria developed after exposure to sunlight. By courtesy of the Institute of Dermatology, London, UK.

Cold urticaria

Placing an ice cube on the skin of patients may elicit a wheal – a condition designated 'cold urticaria'.[5,28] Some patients, however, develop symptoms only after generalized cooling of the body.[5,29] Occasionally, drinking cold liquids, bathing in cold water, or exposure to cold air elicits symptoms.[5,30] Prolonged exposure to cold can result in generalized symptoms, including headache, dyspnea, hypotension, anaphylaxis, and loss of consciousness.[30,31] The condition can be associated with other types of physical urticaria. Very rarely, there is associated cryoglobulinemia and in some cases the condition follows a viral infection or drug ingestion.[28,32,33]

Familial cold urticaria (familial cold autoinflammatory syndrome) which follows exposure to cold is an autosomal dominant condition characterized by[34–37]:

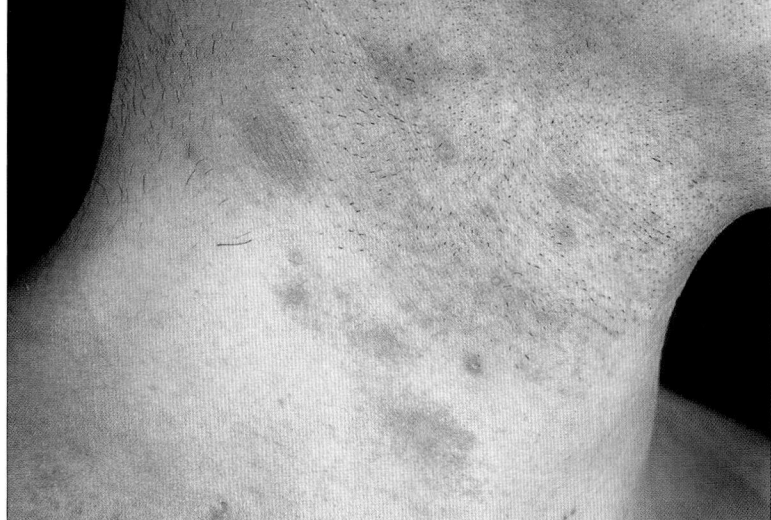

Fig. 15.42
Cholinergic urticaria: in this variant, urticaria follows heat, emotional stress, or a spicy meal. By courtesy of the Institute of Dermatology, London, UK.

- urticaria,
- fever,
- arthralgias,
- arthritis,
- conjunctivitis,
- leukocytosis.

Patients with this syndrome develop symptoms with a decrease in body temperature but do not develop wheals at the site of an ice cube applied to skin. Patients have been shown to have gain of function mutations in the *NLRP3* gene (also known as *CIAS1*) on chromosome 1q44 encoding the protein cryopryin. This protein is part of the cytosolic inflammasome protein complex and involved in its activation.[38–46] Most patients have missense mutations resulting in increased production of IL-1.[46] Interestingly, Muckle-Wells syndrome is associated with the same gene and consists of periodic fever, frequent sensorineural hearing loss, amyloidosis, and recurrent urticaria not linked to cold exposure.[39,47] In addition, neonatal-onset multisystem inflammatory disease also maps to this gene.[48] The spectrum of autoinflammatory disorders is now referred to as the cryopinopathies.[49,50]

Urticaria induced by heat has rarely been documented.[51–53]

Delayed pressure urticaria

Patients with 'delayed pressure urticaria' develop lesions at sites of pressure, such as areas of tight clothing.[5,54] This form of urticaria is seen in 40% of patients with chronic urticaria (see below).[5,55,56]

Cholinergic urticaria

Cholinergic urticaria – one of the most common subtypes of urticaria – is thought to result from release of cholinergic substances by nerves.[57–59] Evidence in support of this theory includes the observation that wheals may be elicited by the injection of cholinergic compounds, and injection of anticholinergic agents blocks wheal formation.[57] Furthermore, wheals do not develop in skin innervated by nerves injected with local anesthetic, and application of scopolamine to skin prevents aquagenic urticaria.[23,57] Common causes of cholinergic urticaria include increase in body temperature (e.g., following a hot bath or shower), emotional stress, exercise, or consumption of spicy food (*Fig. 15.42*).[5,57,60] A significant proportion may be from autologous sweat hypersesnsitivity.[61] Familial cases of cholinergic urticaria have been reported.[62]

Contact urticaria

Contact urticaria may be divided into two main subtypes: allergic and irritant.[5]

- Allergic contact urticaria is a hypersensitivity reaction following exposure to an allergen such as chemicals, foods, latex, plants, fruits and vegetables, and animal-derived antigens.[63–66] Not surprisingly, this form of urticaria often occurs in patients with a history of atopy.[63,67]

- Irritant contact urticaria is a nonimmunologically mediated form of urticaria secondary to a wide variety of substances found in cosmetics, food, and medications.[63]

Urticarial angioedema

Patients with urticaria often develop angioedema characterized by edematous swelling of the lips, eyelids, and tissues of the oropharynx.[5,68,69] Two main subtypes of angioedema are recognized: hereditary and nonhereditary (acquired).

- Hereditary angioedema is rare, autosomal dominantly inherited, and due to C1-esterase inhibitor deficiency.[70]
- Acquired angioedema is caused by drug reactions, allergic reactions, reaction to physical agents, hypereosinophilia, and acquired (nonhereditary) C1-esterase deficiency.[69]

An idiopathic variant is also recognized.

Physical urticaria, secondary to vibration, cold, and sunlight, as well as contact (type I) hypersensitivity reaction and cholinergic urticaria may be associated with angioedema.[69]

Urticarial vasculitis

Urticarial vasculitis is an uncommon condition which combines clinical features of chronic urticaria and histologic findings of leukocytoclastic or lymphocytic venulitis.[71–75] A type III hypersensitivity reaction (caused by antibody–antigen complexes) appears to be the underlying etiology in a subset of patients.[75,76] In many patients, however, no underlying cause is discovered.

Urticarial vasculitis is associated with a female predominance (2:1) and is most often seen in young to middle-aged adults. Urticarial lesions tend to last 24–72 hours and may be associated with pruritus, a burning sensation or pain.[75,78–80] The frequency of attacks varies from daily to monthly. Hyperpigmentation can be present at resolution.

The spectrum of illness ranges from mild symptoms to a serious systemic illness.[81] In addition to urticarial skin lesions, patients can also have angioedema, gastrointestinal symptoms, and evidence of renal involvement. Necrotic skin lesions are not usually seen. Other systemic manifestations/associations include joint pain, stiffness, and swelling; however, frank arthritis is extremely rare. Some patients have proteinuria and hematuria. Rarely, renal biopsy reveals the features of focal or diffuse proliferative glomerulonephritis. Crescentic glomerulonephritis and mesangial and membranous nephropathy have been described in some patients.[81–83] The ESR is frequently raised.

Rarely, urticarial vasculitis has been documented in association with malignancy, a relationship which may be coincidental.[75,81,84–89]

Hypocomplementemia is seen in many patients, and the presence of this sign correlates with systemic involvement and a high prevalence of autoantibodies to endothelial cells.[76,81,90–92] Patients with Schnitzler syndrome have urticarial vasculitis and monoclonal IgM gammopathy.[90–100] Hepatosplenomegaly, elevated ESR, raised white blood cell count, fever, and joint pain are frequent features.[94–96] Occasional patients have an associated lymphoproliferative disorder.[79] This disease is associated with anti-C1q autoantibodies in over half of the patients and likely mediate the disease in this subgroup.[101,102]

Urticarial vasculitis (especially the hypocomplementemic variant) is often associated with or precedes development of a variety of systemic diseases, including myeloma, hepatitis B and C, SLE, arthritis, interstitial lung disease, pericarditis, mixed connective tissue disease, inflammatory bowel disease, serum sickness, polyarteritis nodosa, granulomatosis with polyangiitis, viral infections, Sjögren syndrome, cryoglobulinemia, polycythemia rubra vera, reaction to drugs, and as a response to sunlight.[75,81,89,90,101–113] Urticarial vasculitis has also been documented in association with pregnancy, exercise, and cocaine use.[114–116] Ocular disease (including uveitis, scleritis, conjunctivitis, or episcleritis) is a very common feature.[81,117] Patients with hypocomplementemia appear to be at risk of developing more severe disease.[103] Obviously, a diagnosis of urticarial vasculitis in any patient should initiate an evaluation for underlying disease.[118]

Drug-induced urticaria

Drug-induced urticaria is fairly common. It is present in 0.16% of medical inpatients and in 9% of cases of chronic urticaria or angioedema seen in dermatology outpatient departments.[119,120] The drugs most commonly implicated are sulfonamides, penicillins, and non-steroidal anti-inflammatory medications.[119] Aspirin may induce acute urticaria, worsen chronic urticaria, or act as a cofactor to induce anaphylaxis.[121] Other less common drug associations include antipsychotics, alendronate, recombinant IFN-β, cetirizine, bleomycin, and IL-3.[121–127] Many of these reactions are mediated by IgE antibodies, but some result from direct activation of mast cells or interact with another pathway that augments the urticaria reaction.[128] In this last category, modulation of arachidonic acid metabolites by aspirin and other agents can help initiate or exacerbate urticaria.[129] A variety of genetic polymorphisms in different components of the inflammatory cascade have been linked to aspirin-induced urticaria, including the leukotriene C4 synthase, the prostaglandin E2 receptor subtype EP4, IL18 promoter, thromboxane A2 receptor, and adenosine A3 receptor.[130–138]

Other urticarial associations

Urticaria has also been documented in association with autoimmune progesterone dermatitis, dermatophytosis, candidiasis, parasites (anisakiasis), consumption of tonic water, nicotine, alcohol consumption, and hepatitis B vaccination.[139–145]

Pathogenesis and histologic features

As has been stated above, urticaria is probably best viewed as a group of disorders sharing common clinical and histologic features. The pathogenesis of some forms of urticaria (e.g., allergic contact urticaria) is well understood; however, the precise pathogenesis of many cases of urticaria is obscure.[146] Mast cell degranulation with perhaps some involvement of basophils appears to be a common denominator in the pathway of most types of urticaria.[147,148]

Release of histamine following a hypersensitivity reaction after exposure to an allergen is the basis for allergic contact urticaria.[68] In sensitized patients, an allergen binds to IgE on mast cells causing degranulation and the release of histamine, eosinophil chemotactic factor, prostaglandin, leukotrienes, platelet activating factor, and enzymes.[63,146,147,149,150] Similarly, IgE-mediated mast cell degranulation also underlies the pathogenesis of allergic contact urticaria in which direct contact with allergens on skin bind to the surface IgE on mast cells causing release of histamine and other inflammatory mediators. Autoantibodies against the IgE high-affinity receptor (FcεRI) or to IgE itself are present in about 30% of patients with chronic urticaria, designated autoimmune urticaria, a type II hypersensitivity reaction.[146,151–155] Patients with physical urticaria or with connective tissue or autoimmune bullous disease may also have anti-FcεRI. However, in the last group of patients, the autoantibodies are nonfunctional (non-histamine releasing), whereas in chronic urticaria, the antibodies are functional (histamine releasing).[154–156] A type III hypersensitivity reaction, caused by circulating antigen–antibody immune complexes, underlies a form of urticaria associated with serum sickness.

There is growing evidence that infection with *Helicobacter pylori* may play a causative role in chronic urticaria in a subset of patients, including cases where the urticaria resolved after treatment and returned on reinfection.[157–165]

The pathogenesis of irritant contact urticaria is not well understood, but evidence suggests that degranulation of mast cells due to direct, nonimmunologically mediated contact causes release of vasogenic mediators.[63,147] Similarly, it is thought that the physical urticarias (heat, cold, pressure, vibration, water) also result from a direct effect on mast cells in susceptible individuals.[150]

Some investigators have suggested that solar urticaria results from a type I hypersensitivity reaction to a photo-induced antigen eliciting IgE-mediated mast cell degranulation.[13] An intriguing study has shown that most patients (77%) develop an urticarial reaction when challenged with autologous serum that has been irradiated using the same spectrum of light that induces lesions in each particular patient.[166] Furthermore, patients with 'fixed'

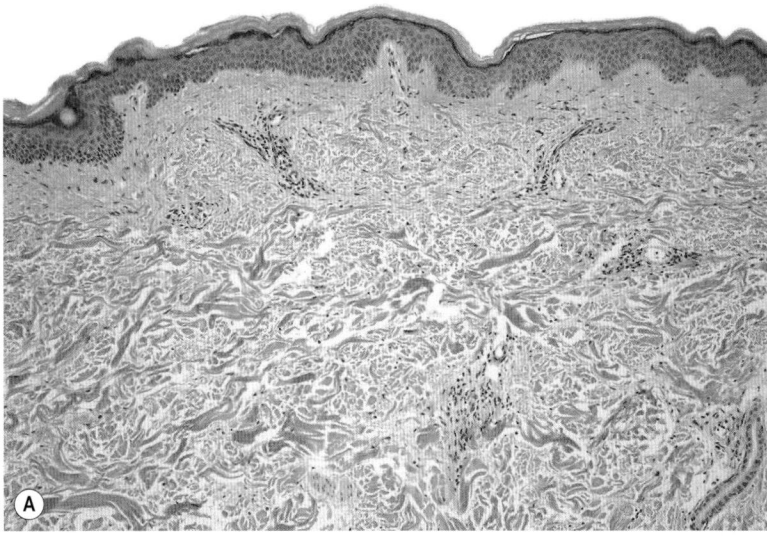

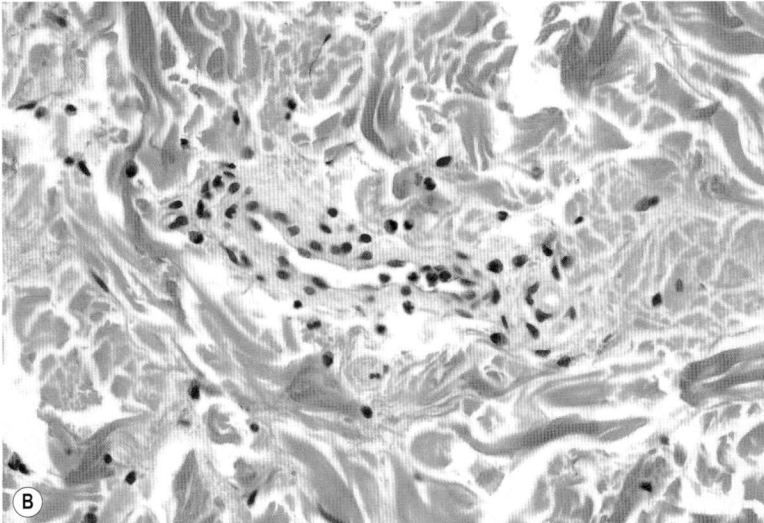

Fig. 15.43
Urticaria: (**A**) at low-power examination, the features are easily overlooked. There is a light perivascular infiltrate and the collagen fibers appear separated; (**B**) at high power, there is edema and a light perivascular infiltrate of lymphocytes with scattered eosinophils.

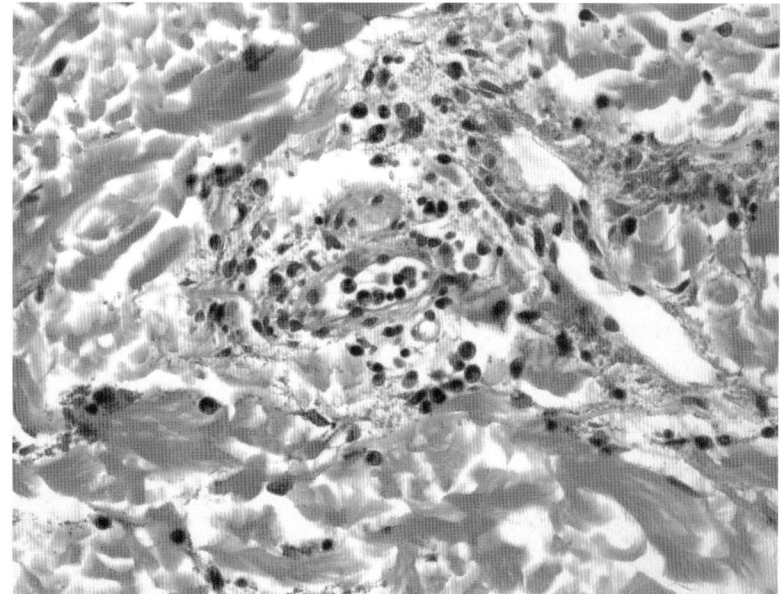

Fig. 15.44
Urticaria: in some cases intravascular neutrophils are prominent, and their presence can be a clue to the diagnosis.

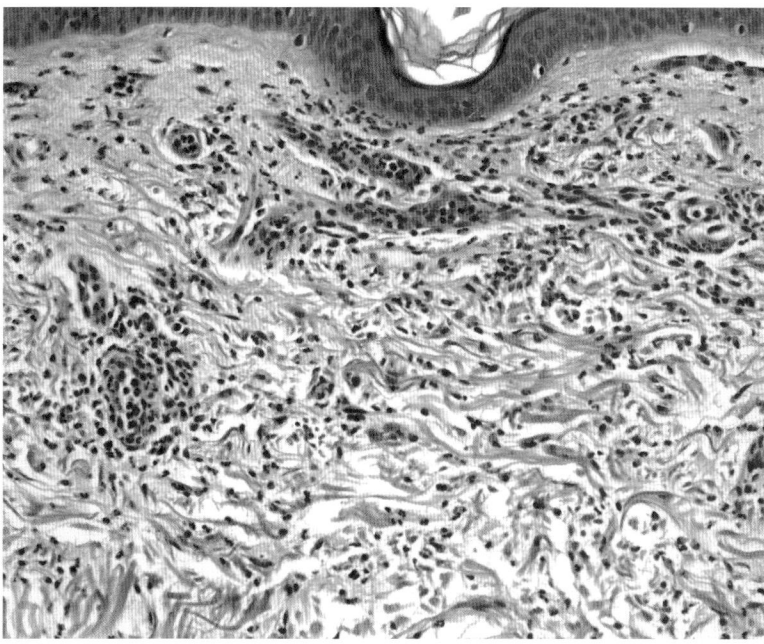

Fig. 15.45
Urticarial vasculitis: in this case there is a perivascular infiltrate of neutrophils and eosinophils with leukocytoclasia, subtle extravasation of erythrocytes but no fibrinoid necrosis of blood vessels.

urticaria develop lesions at the same specific sites that are affected by light exposure following injection with irradiated plasma.[18] Consistent with these observations, some patients with severe solar urticaria may be effectively treated by plasma exchange.[167,168]

A type III hypersensitivity reaction (caused by antibody–antigen complexes) appears to be the underlying etiology in some patients with urticarial vasculitis; however, no underlying cause is discovered in many patients.[77,81] More recently, urticarial vasculitis has been excluded from the formal urticaria group of disorders by some authors due to its variant pathogenic mechanism, but is still considered in this section for historical purposes.[2]

The biopsy findings in urticaria are non-specific. Dermal edema may be mild or severe, and its presence is confirmed by separation of dermal reticular collagen fibers. An often sparse dermal perivascular and interstitial mixed inflammatory infiltrate composed of variable numbers of lymphocytes, neutrophils, and eosinophils is present (*Fig. 15.43*). An increased number of intravascular neutrophils are a frequent finding, although this is not invariable (*Fig. 15.44*). Of interest, mast cells – which play such an important role in the pathogenesis of urticaria – do not appear to be increased in number except in chronic urticaria.[153,169] Usually, more inflammatory cells are seen in lesions of chronic urticaria compared to those of acute urticaria.[169]

Urticarial vasculitis combines histologic features of urticaria with superimposed vascular damage. The vasculitis affects the superficial vascular plexus and shows features of a leukocytoclastic subtype; however, compared with typical leukocytoclastic vasculitis, the histologic findings tend to be subtle and are easily overlooked (*Fig. 15.45*). Mild or focal fibrinoid change apparent on only a few sections associated with few neutrophils and sparse karyorrhexis is typical. Some authors have shown that endothelial necrosis is unusual.[77] Occasionally, impressive necrotizing vasculitis (features of typical leukocytoclastic vasculitis) may be seen. In some cases, the infiltrate is predominantly lymphocytic and the lesion has the appearance of a lymphocytic vasculitis.[75] In summary, urticarial vasculitis appears as a continuum, ranging from urticaria with very mild vascular injury (most cases) to frank necrotizing vasculitis.[170]

Differential diagnosis

The diagnosis requires careful clinical correlation. The biopsy findings are often very subtle: the dermal edema and sparse inflammatory infiltrate may be easily overlooked. A definitive diagnosis sometimes requires testing for response to particular antigens. Other forms of hypersensitivity reaction such as arthropod bite and drug eruption can show similar features and require clinical correlation to distinguish them from urticaria. Clinical correlation is necessary to distinguish urticarial vasculitis from other forms of leukocytoclastic vasculitis. Although urticarial vasculitis is often associated with subtle low-grade vascular injury, this pattern should not be relied on in the distinction from other forms of vasculitis. In short, the pathologist's role in diagnosis is to confirm the presence of vasculitis.

Papular urticaria

Clinical features

Although papular urticaria (prurigo mitis) is often described as a variant of urticaria, and the histologic picture is that of an urticarial dermatitis, the lesions are persistent and patients do not fulfill the criteria for the diagnosis of urticaria. In the latter, lesions are self-limited even in cases of chronic urticaria. The condition is generally regarded as a variant of an insect bite reaction.[1-4] Papular urticaria has no sex predilection, and although the age range is wide, it tends to be more frequent in children. It presents as small, itchy, red papules that tend to appear in crops. Most lesions are no more than a few millimeters in diameter but larger lesions may be seen. They are more usually seen on exposed areas of the body and tend to be more prevalent during the summer months. Changes secondary to scratching including excoriations are frequent. There are no associations with systemic disease.

Pathogenesis and histologic features

The pathogenesis is not entirely clear, but it is generally believed that the condition is triggered by a hypersensitivity reaction to insect or arthropod bites.[5,6] Many insects and arthropods have been implicated in the disease including fleas, carpet beetles, lice, bedbugs, mosquitoes, and even caterpillars. This is further supported by the rash clearing after the patient returns from holidays or after moving to a new house. A study found evidence of IgG against bedbugs (*Cimex lectularius*) in affected patients, suggesting a role in the pathogenesis of the disease.[6] In papular urticaria related to flea bites, patients appear to react to a variety of low molecular weight antigens derived from fleas.[7,8] Patients with papular urticaria secondary to fleas may be related to an aberrant T-helper (Th17) response and increased production IL-10. This may be related to an impaired dendritic cell response in these patients.[9]

The histologic features are fairly non-specific. In intact lesions, the epidermis is unremarkable or slightly acanthotic. Changes of excoriation may be evident. In the dermis there is a mild to moderate, superficial, and deep, often wedge-shaped, mainly perivascular inflammatory cell infiltrate composed of lymphocytes, histiocytes, and eosinophils.[7] Neutrophils can be seen in some cases.[10] A few CD30-positive lymphocytes are sometimes present.

Neutrophilic urticarial dermatosis

Clinical features

Neutrophilic urticarial dermatosis represents a particular cutaneous manifestation that may be seen in a variety of autoinflammatory disorders, including Schnitzler syndrome, Still disease, cryopyrin-associated periodic syndrome, SLE, rheumatoid arthritis, Sjögren syndrome, and other autoimmune diseases, as well as IgA monoclonal gammopathy and IgA myeloma.[1-14] Clinically, patients present with present with variably pruritic, pale erythematous macules, papules, or plaques that resolve within 24–72 hours (*Fig. 15.46*).[1,4]

Pathogenesis and histologic features

The pathogenesis is incompletely understood and, given the multiple different disease associations, likely multifactorial. The pathogenesis, while incompletely understood, involves the proinflammatory effects of IL-β and IL-17. In cryopyrin-associated periodic syndrome, there is a mutation in *NLRP3* (NOD-like receptor 3) that results in increased IL-β production and recruitment of neutrophils.[10,12] A defined gene mutation is not known in Schnitzler syndrome, but cutaneous mast cells express IL-β and neutrophils in the dermis express IL-17.[15] Interestingly, IL-β positive mast cells are less

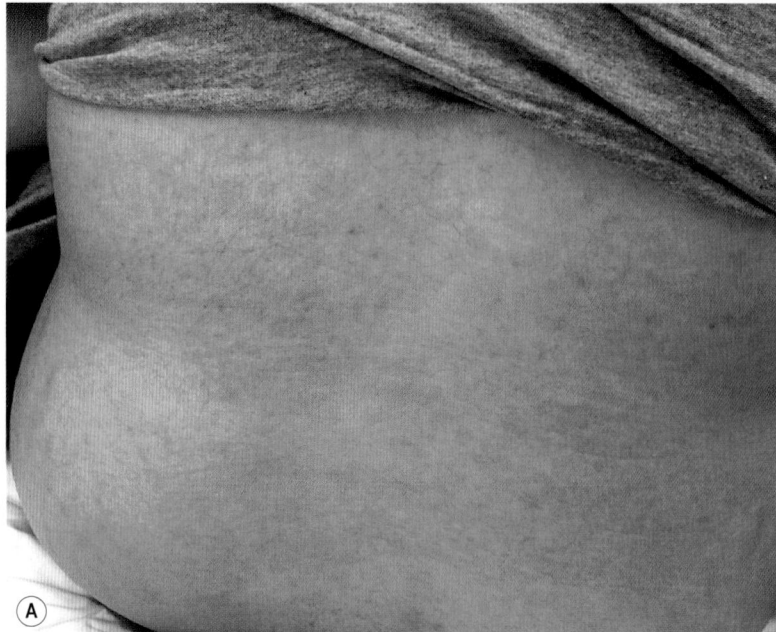

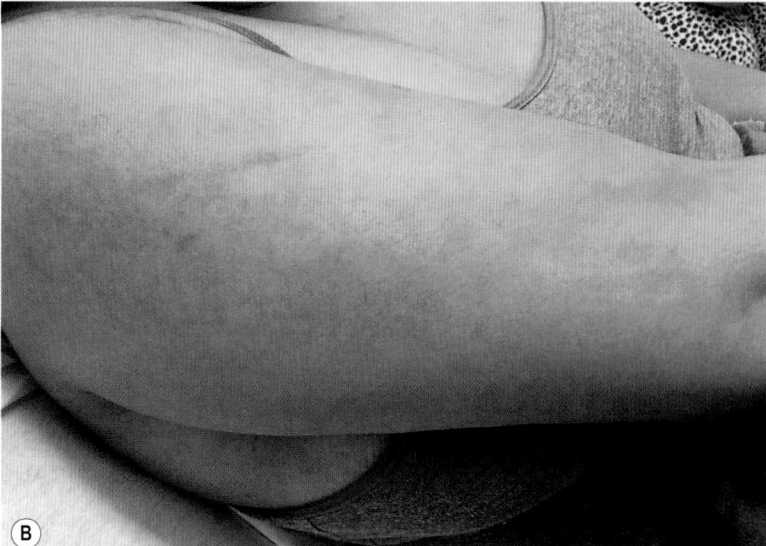

Fig. 15.46
Urticarial eruption in patient with Schnitzler syndrome involving the back (A) and arms (B). By courtesy of Dr. Anthony P. Fernandez, Cleveland Clinic, Cleveland, USA.

common in cryopyrin-associated periodic syndrome and IL-17-positve neutrophils are not seen in cryopyrin-associated periodic syndrome, indicative of multiple pathways to a common cutaneous and histologic presentation.[15]

Microscopically, neutrophilic urticarial dermatosis is associated with a dermal infiltrate of neutrophils. The infiltrate has both a perivascular and interstitial pattern and can be relatively mild to dense, mimicking Sweet syndrome (*Fig. 15.47*).[1,4,16] Similar to Sweet syndrome, leukocytoclasis in the absence of vasculitis is common. Necrobiotic collagen bundles are sometimes present and the neutrophils can intercalate between collagen bundles in a manner similar to metastatic breast carcinoma (*Fig. 15.48*). The neutrophils may extend into the epithelium of the epidermis or adnexal structures, and this neutrophilic epitheliotropism is relatively sensitive and specific for neutrophilic urticarial dermatosis.[16]

Differential diagnosis

The differential diagnosis includes Sweet syndrome, urticaria, leukocytoclastic vasculitis, and cellulitis. Sweet syndrome is clinically different with more indurated plaques and nodules and prominent dermal edema. Conventional urticaria usually has eosinophils associated with the infiltrate. Leukocytoclastic vasculitis has damage to the vascular walls, a feature not seen in

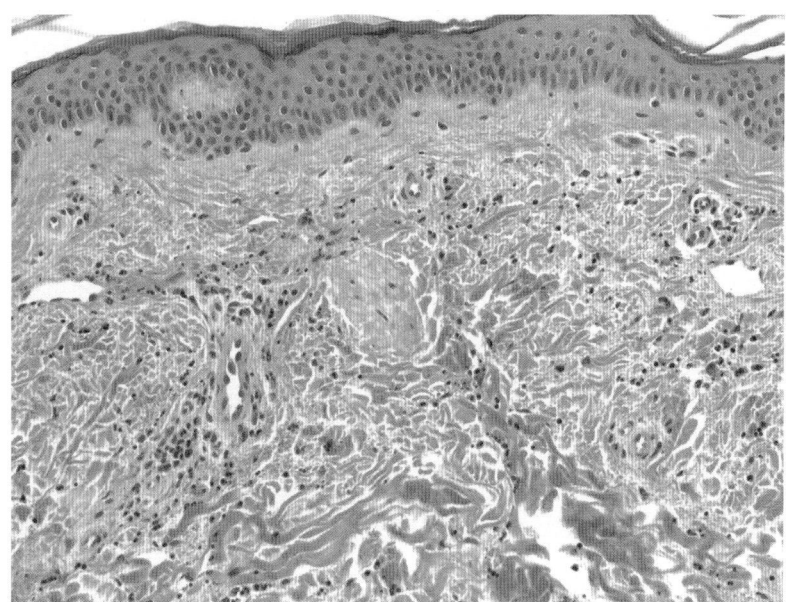

Fig. 15.47
Mild perivascular neutrophilic infiltrate in patient with Schnitzler syndrome. By courtesy of Dr. Anthony P. Fernandez, Cleveland Clinic, Cleveland, USA.

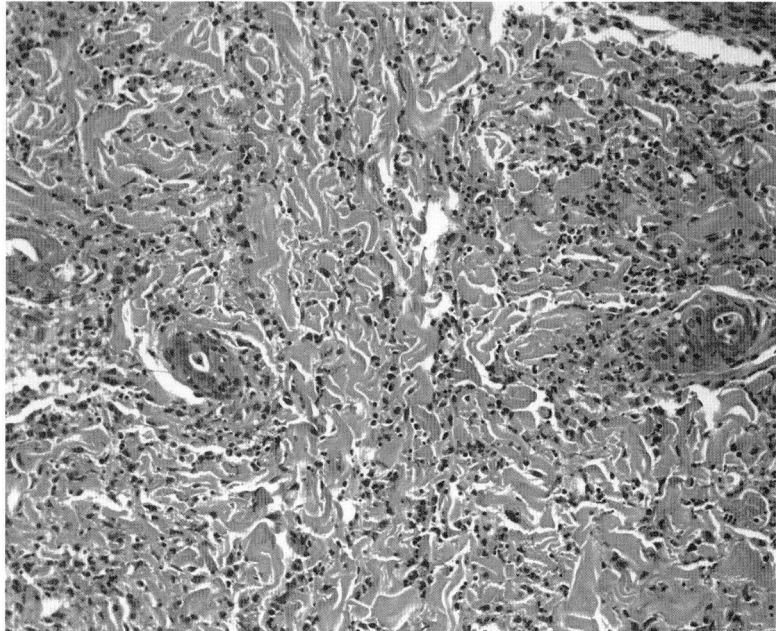

Fig. 15.48
Biopsy from patient with neutrophilic urticarial dermatitis with interstitial infiltrate with cordlike pattern intercalating between collagen bundles.

neutrophilic urticarial dermatosis. Although cellulitis could be histologically indistinguishable, it is clinically different.

Cutaneous atypical neutrophilic dermatosis with lipodystrophy and elevated temperature

Cutaneous atypical neutrophilic dermatosis with lipodystrophy and elevated temperature (CANDLE) is a distinctive, rare, autoinflammatory disease previously described as Nakajo-Nishimura disease, joint contractures, muscle atrophy, microcytic anemia and panniculitis induced lipodystrophy (JMP), or Japanese autoinflammatory syndrome with lipodystrophy.[1–3]

The condition presents early in life with recurrent, almost daily episodes of fever poorly responsive to non-steroidal anti-inflammatory drugs, purpuric, annular, violaceous skin plaques, low height and weight, eyelid swelling, lipodystrophy, increased ESR and CRP, hypochromic anemia, and elevated liver enzymes. Other less common manifestations include perioral swelling, arthralgia, hepatosplenomegaly, basal ganglia calcifications, chondritis of the ear and nose, aseptic meningitis, and conjunctivitis and episcleritis.[1–3]

Pathogenesis and histologic features

The pattern of transmission of the disease suggests that it is an autosomal recessive condition. Mutations in *PSMB8* have been documented in most patients. This gene encodes many of the components of proteasomes, and alterations in these components lead to malfunction of proteasomes with accumulation of protein waste products in the cells.[4–6] It appears that these patients also have a unique dysregulation of the IFN signaling pathway that contributes to many manifestations of the disease.[7]

Histologically, a prominent perivascular and interstitial cell infiltrate that may extend into the subcutaneous tissue, is seen. The infiltrate consists mainly of large mononuclear cells with pale cytoplasm, vesicular bean-shaped or oval vesicular nuclei, and a small nucleolus. These cells resemble those seen in leukemia and cutaneous infiltrates of myelodysplastic syndrome. Mitotic activity is present, and in the background there are neutrophils sometimes with nuclear dust, eosinophils, and lymphocytes.[1,8] By immunohistochemistry, the large cells are positive for KP1 (CD68), lysozyme, CD45, and myeloperoxidase.[1,8]

Differential diagnosis

In view of the presence of immature myelo-monocytic cells, distinction from leukemia cutis, the cutaneous infiltrates of myelodysplastic syndrome, and histiocytic Sweet syndrome may be difficult. Close clinicopathological correlation is critical as patients with CANDLE do not develop or have leukemia or myeolodysplastic syndrome, and histiocytic Sweet syndrome does not tend to occur early in life.

Hypereosinophilic syndrome

Clinical features

The hypereosinophilic syndrome was previously defined as an idiopathic condition characterized by persistent eosinophilia (more than 1.5×10^9/L) for at least 6 months and with involvement of one or more organs.[1–4] This definition has undergone revisions to include other diseases associated with eosinophilia such as eosinophilic pneumonia, eosinophilic gastrointestinal disorders, and eosinophilic granulomatosis with polyangiitis (formerly Churg-Strauss syndrome and discussed in the chapter on vasculitis). The definition has also been modified to include patients with peripheral eosinophils with substantial tissue eosinophilia, removing the requirement of an absolute eosinophil count $>1.5 \times 10^9$/L.[5] Similarly, the time requirement of 6 months has been shortened to 1 month since some patients developed end-organ damage with less peripheral eosinophilia in a shorter period.[6] The diagnosis should be made only after other causes of eosinophilia, particularly parasitic infections, have been excluded. The heart, lungs, central and peripheral nervous system, liver, and skin are commonly affected. The disease, which may sometimes prove fatal, generally presents in adults.

Cutaneous lesions are seen in over 50% of patients and usually consist of either pruritic papules and nodules or urticaria and angioedema.[5,7] Rarely, skin lesions represent an initial manifestation, and in this setting, annular erythema and erythroderma have been reported.[8–12] Oral and genital erosions/ulcerations are quite characteristic and can be the first manifestation of the disease.[5,13,14] Other cutaneous features include livedo reticularis, cutaneous infarction, deep vein thrombosis, blisters, aquagenic pruritus, erythema gyratum repens, and Wells syndrome.[5,15–21] Hypereosinophilic syndrome has been reported in association with lymphomatoid papulosis, T-cell lymphoma, myeloid neoplasms, systemic mast cell disease, SLE, and HIV infection.[5,6,22–27]

Pathogenesis and histologic features

The etiology is unknown. It has sometimes been categorized into:
- idiopathic,
- clonal (primary clonal expansion of eosinophils),
- familial (autosomal dominant),
- secondary types.[5,6,22,28]

Some forms of clonal eosinophilia best regarded as variants of eosinophilic leukemia, (malignancy-associated) harbor a distinctive *FIP1L1-PDGFRA* fusion (FIP1L1: Fip1-like; PDGFRA: platelet-derived growth factor receptor A) and are amenable to targeted therapies.[29–31] Secondary cases result from other causes such as an underlying malignancy particularly lymphoid neoplasms. The lymphoid or lymphocytic variant of hypereosinophilic syndrome results from circulating T lymphocytes that are usually CD3-CD4+, are frequently clonal and drive a polyclonal proliferation of eosinophils.[32] The latter is the result of production of IL-5 by the clonal T cells. This variant of the disease may be very rarely complicated by the development of T-cell lymphoma, cutaneous or systemic. Idiopathic is what remains when these first two categories are excluded. Besides elevated serum levels of IL-5, elevated serum levels of IL-10 and soluble IL-2 receptor have also been documented.[33] IL-2 stimulates release of eosinophilic cationic protein from eosinophils which contain IL-2 receptor (CD25), and this results in tissue damage.

The histologic findings vary according to the type of lesion biopsied. Urticarial and papular lesions show a superficial and deep perivascular and interstitial mixed inflammatory cell infiltrate with variable numbers of eosinophils and scattered lymphocytes, histiocytes, and occasional plasma cells. Rare flame figures may be present and may occasionally be prominent. Dermal edema is seen particularly in urticarial lesions. Eosinophils are not always prominent, and the findings can be entirely non-specific. Microthrombi are present in some cases and sometimes correlate with the severity of the disease.[15,34] In the lymphocytic variant of the disease an exceptional case of cutaneous lesions with a CD30 positive clonal T-cell lymphoid proliferation has been described.[35]

Eosinophilic cellulitis

Clinical features

Eosinophilic cellulitis (Wells syndrome) is an uncommon disorder, characterized by recurrent erythematous and edematous plaques.[1–6] It occurs with an equal sex ratio, and there is a large age range, with a mean age of 37 years.[7] It is sometimes also encountered in children and rare cases have been documented in neonates.[7–11] It appears that cases occurring in childhood may be particularly severe. Scalp involvement, with alopecia and scarring, is a feature in some patients.[7,8]

The disease particularly affects the extremities and trunk. Although it presents most commonly as well-defined (cellulitis-like) annular erythematous plaques, which are edematous and firm, a wide variety of clinical appearances have been described including blistering, nodular, papulovesicular eruptions, and itchy excoriated inflammatory papules (*Figs 15.49–15.51*).[7,12–14] The plaques, which cause pain and pruritus in some patients, typically heal without scarring.[7] Eosinophilic cellulitis has been associated with urticaria.[15] Dermatographism can be a feature.[16] With progression, the lesions sometimes adopt a greenish hue. Clinically, the lesion may occasionally be mistaken for an infective process.[17] The disease tends to be episodic, with remissions and relapses, which can last from months to years.

Large bullae are seen in rare patients.[18] An unusual pattern of involvement following Blaschko lines has been reported, and it has been proposed that this form represents cutaneous mosaicism.[19]

Rarely, eosinophilic cellulitis is associated with a malignant neoplasm. Cases accompanied by eosinophilic leukemia, colonic carcinoma, squamous cell carcinoma of the lung, and non-Hodgkin lymphoma have been described.[20–23] Associations with HIV, hypereosinophilic syndrome, ulcerative colitis, tetanus or thiomersal-containing vaccine, varicella infection, Churg Strauss syndrome, and IgG4-related disease have occasionally been documented.[24–33] Some cases of eosinophilic cellulitis appear to be triggered by medications, including antibiotics, anticholinergic agents, anesthetics, non-steroidal anti-inflammatory drugs, thyroid medications, and thiazide diuretics.[34] A case associated with a henna tattoo has also been reported.[35]

Exceptional familial cases have been reported.[36,37] In one family, the disease showed an autosomal dominant pattern of inheritance and was

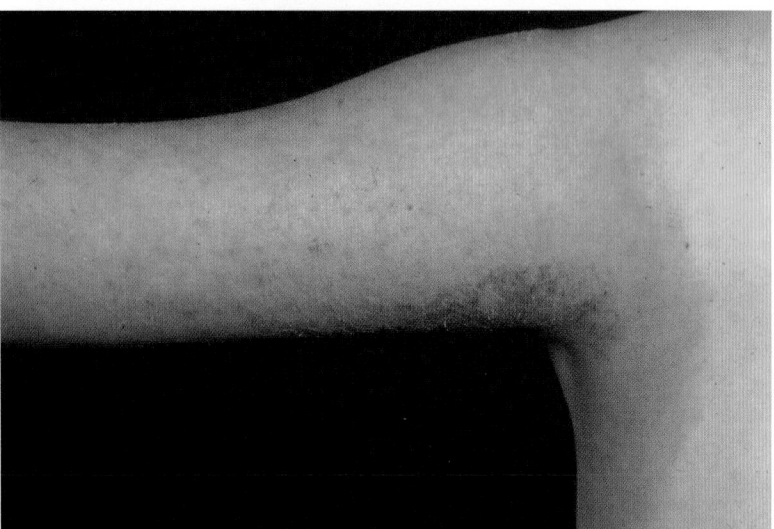

Fig. 15.49
Eosinophilic cellulitis: there is a large erythematous swollen plaque. The limbs are commonly affected. From the collection of the late N.P. Smith, MD, the Institute of Dermatology, London, UK.

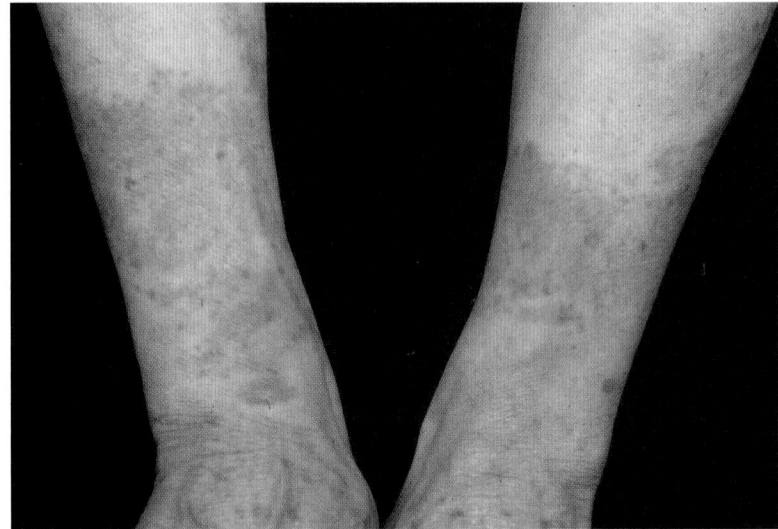

Fig. 15.50
Eosinophilic cellulitis: in this patient, there is striking symmetry. From the collection of the late N.P. Smith, MD, the Institute of Dermatology, London, UK.

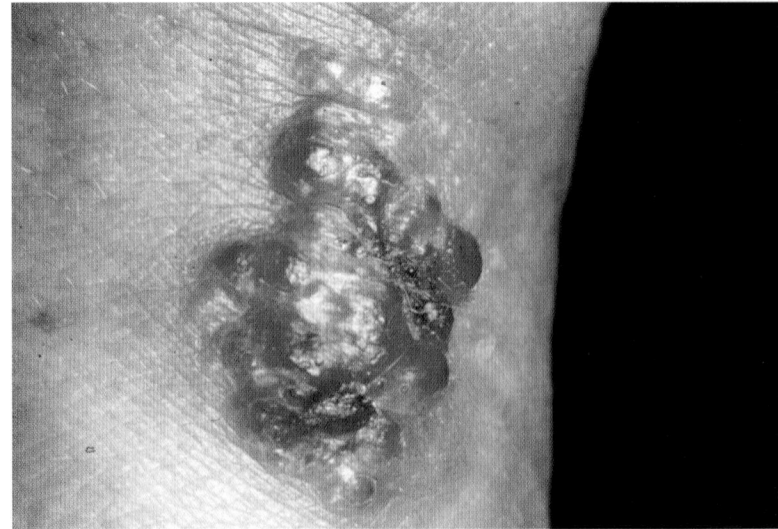

Fig. 15.51
Eosinophilic cellulitis: bullous lesion with a hint of greenish discoloration in the adjacent skin. From the collection of the late N.P. Smith, MD, Institute of Dermatology, London, UK.

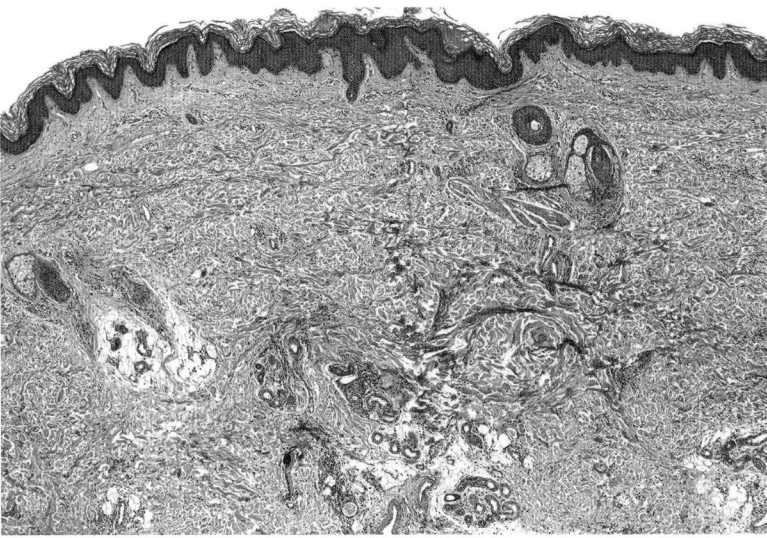

Fig. 15.52
Eosinophilic cellulitis: there is a light, deep dermal chronic inflammatory cell infiltrate. A flame figure is present.

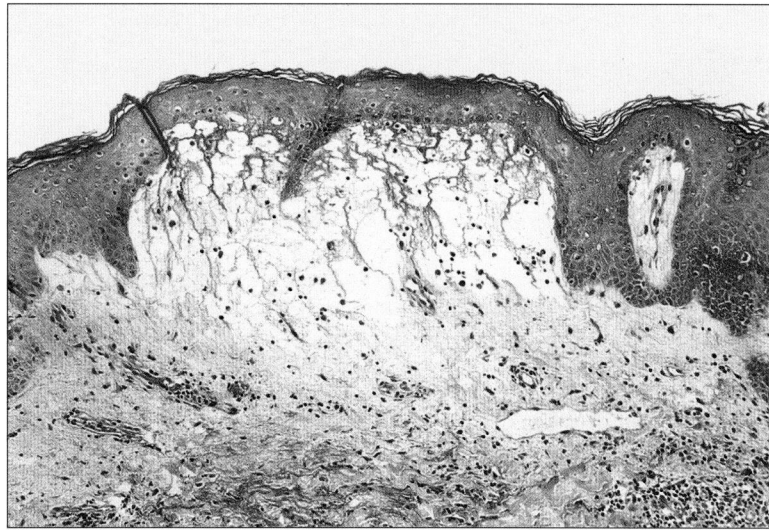

Fig. 15.54
Eosinophilic cellulitis: subepidermal vesiculation as seen here is not uncommon. The blister cavity may contain numerous eosinophils reminiscent of bullous pemphigoid.

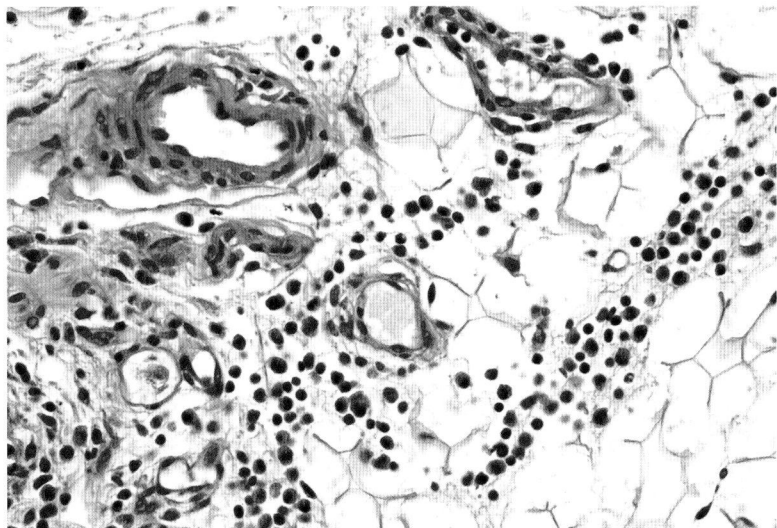

Fig. 15.53
Eosinophilic cellulitis: the infiltrate is composed of lymphocytes and histiocytes with conspicuous eosinophils and extends into the subcutaneous fat.

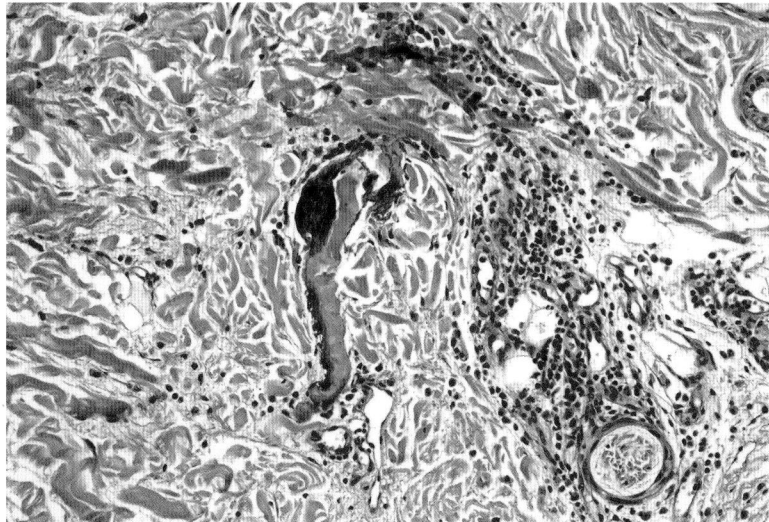

Fig. 15.55
Eosinophilic cellulitis: flame figures are typically present.

associated with developmental delay and dysmorphic body habitus.[36] In another family, the lesions were first noted during infancy.[37]

Pathogenesis and histologic features

The pathogenesis is unknown and may simply represent an eosinophil-rich inflammatory reaction to a variety of insults. The only consistent association appears to be a peripheral eosinophilia, manifested either as an elevated total eosinophil count or as an increased percentage of eosinophils. Clinical activity appears to correlate with increased eosinophil cation protein and IL-5 levels in the peripheral blood in addition to blood and bone marrow eosinophilia.[38]

An elevated ESR is occasionally present. It is possible that some patients represent the benign end of the spectrum of the hypereosinophilic syndrome discussed in the previous section.

Histologically, early lesions of eosinophilic cellulitis are characterized by a diffuse and heavy dermal infiltrate of eosinophils: this occurs either in the superficial dermis, as a bandlike infiltrate, or in the deep dermis with extension into the underlying subcutaneous tissue, fascia, and muscle (Figs 15.52 and 15.53).[2,39,40] In addition, lymphocytes and plasma cells may be present. There is sometimes edema of the papillary dermis to such an extent that subepidermal bullae develop (Fig. 15.54).[39] The epidermis can be spongiotic

and occasionally intraepidermal vesicles are present.[39] Early lesions may be indistinguishable from an arthropod bite reaction.[41] Over a period of 1–3 weeks, the eosinophils degranulate and degenerate, and eosinophilic material and nuclear debris are deposited on collagen fibers to produce 'flame figures' (Fig. 15.55).[39–42] Sometimes these are surrounded by histiocytes and multinucleated giant cells (Fig. 15.56). There is no evidence of primary collagen degeneration. It is likely that flame figures represent a non-specific eosinophil reaction pattern to a variety of different provoking stimuli.[42] Later, the lesion becomes more granulomatous and giant cells are occasionally prominent.[43] Extravasation of red blood cells is sometimes evident, but vasculitis is not usually a feature, except for rare cases reported to evolve into Churg-Strauss syndrome.[31,32,40]

Indirect immunofluorescence studies have shown that flame figures contain extracellular eosinophil granule major basic protein.[44] Ultrastructural investigation confirms that the eosinophil granules invest the associated collagen fibers.[45] Direct immunofluorescence has demonstrated immunoglobulins and/or complement in blood vessel walls in a minority of cases.[2,7,17,42]

Differential diagnosis

The histologic features of eosinophilic infiltration with 'flame figures', although characteristic of Wells syndrome, are not pathognomonic.[46] Similar

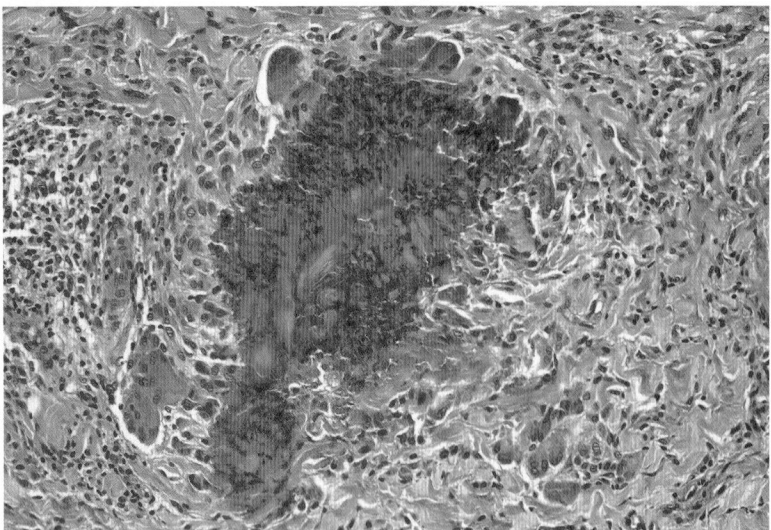

Fig. 15.56
Eosinophilic cellulitis: in this example, a flame figure is surrounded by an intense granulomatous infiltrate.

features may be seen in arthropod bite reactions, spider bites, onchocerciasis, drug hypersensitivity reactions, diffuse erythema, tinea infection, atopic eczema, allergic contact dermatitis, urticarial vasculitis, eosinophilic pustular folliculitis, bullous pemphigoid, herpes gestationis, the hypereosinophilic syndrome, and cutaneous mastocytoma.[2,42,47-53] Prominent flame figures are also seen in eosinophilic ulcer of the oral mucosa.[54-56] It should be emphasized that in regions where parasitic infections are endemic, lesions with the histologic appearance of eosinophilic cellulitis have a high likelihood of representing parasitic infection such as giardiasis, toxocariasis, and onchocerciasis.[57-59] In eosinophilic fasciitis, diffuse fibrosis of the deep dermis with extension into the fibrous septa of the subcutaneous fat and involvement of the fascia allow for easy distinction from Wells syndrome.

Eosinophilic pustular folliculitis

Clinical features

Eosinophilic pustular folliculitis (Ofuji disease) is a rare dermatosis seen primarily in Japanese and Chinese patients, although occasional reports from Europe and the USA are encountered.[1-5] It is a disease which particularly affects the seborrheic regions and, therefore, lesions are predominantly present on the face and back.[6,7] The extensor surfaces of the upper limbs are also frequently affected. Acral involvement is uncommon.[7-10] Patients present with crops of occasionally pruritic, sterile follicular papulopustules measuring 1–2 mm in diameter, grouped to form small plaques, which characteristically spread centrifugally to produce an annular or serpiginous lesion.[1,6] The disease is typically recurrent, and spontaneous resolution within months to several years is characteristic.[11,12] Healing is often associated with residual postinflammatory hyperpigmentation.[1] The peak incidence is in the third and fourth decades, although children and infants can be affected.[7,14-17] Males have been thought to be predominantly affected (5:1), but recent studies have shown an equal sex incidence.[7,13,18] Sometimes there is a past or present history of acne vulgaris.

Extensive laboratory investigations reveal leukocytosis with hypereosinophilia.[18] Serum IgE levels may be increased.[5,19,20]

Similar cases have been reported in Caucasians in association with HIV infection.[3,4,21-28] However, based on the clinical and histologic findings, many authors regard HIV-associated eosinophilic folliculitis as a separate entity.[25,27] Pruritus, which is always present in patients with HIV-associated eosinophilic folliculitis, is seen only on occasional patients with Ofuji disease.[29]

A small number of childhood cases of eosinophilic pustular folliculitis, including several in neonates, have also been reported.[16,17,30-36] Some authors prefer to categorize these as a separate entity, whereas others feel that this category does not form a distinct condition.[5,13,33,37] In children, the scalp is particularly involved. There is less of a tendency to affect the seborrheic regions and polycyclic patterns are not evident.[30]

Eosinophilic pustular folliculitis has been described in association with non-Hodgkin lymphoma, Hodgkin lymphoma, polycythemia rubra vera, myelodysplastic syndrome, bone marrow transplant for aplastic anemia, eosinophilic cellulitis, hepatitis C viral infection, and the nevoid basal cell carcinoma syndrome.[13,38-46] A few cases induced by allopurinol, timepidium bromide, carbamazepine, and chemotherapy for breast carcinoma have also been documented.[47-50]

Pathogenesis and histologic features

The etiology and pathogenesis of eosinophil pustular folliculitis are unknown. The possibility of an inherited or contagious cause for the disease has been raised by the observation of the disease in siblings.[51] However, there is no firm evidence of an infective cause. A variety of immunological abnormalities have been described including:

- raised IgE levels,
- low immunoglobulin levels,
- defects of neutrophil motility.[6,20,33]

A pemphigus-like antibody and an antibasal keratinocyte antibody have also been recorded in patients with this disease.[52,53]

The seborrheic distribution raises a possible role for sebaceous glands in the pathogenesis.[10] A lipid-soluble eosinophil chemotactic factor has been identified from epidermal surface lipids.[54] The association of eosinophil pustular folliculitis with AIDS (if indeed this is the same disease) raises the interesting possibility of a diminished T-helper lymphocyte-mediated pathogenesis. An increased number of mast cells have been described around hair follicles and sebaceous glands, suggesting a role for these cells in the development of the disease.[55] A more recent study demonstrated that prostaglandin synthase may result in sebocyte production of eotaxin, a chemoattractant for eosinophils.[56]

In early lesions, spongiosis of the outer root sheath of the infundibulum with an accompanying eosinophil and mononuclear cell infiltrate is characteristic.[6,57] As the disease progresses, vesiculation and pustulation are seen deep to the stratum corneum, often extending into the sebaceous gland (Fig. 15.56). The epithelium is infiltrated by large numbers of eosinophils with an admixture of neutrophils and mononuclear cells. In the superficial dermis, there is a perivascular mononuclear and eosinophil infiltrate. Follicular mucinosis has been described.[57-62]

Differential diagnosis

As mentioned above, there is considerable overlap between eosinophilic folliculitis associated with HIV infection and Ofuji disease. The latter condition tends to form arcuate plaques. Histologically, well-developed large eosinophilic pustules in the pilar canals are characteristic of Ofuji disease but are less common in HIV-associated eosinophilic folliculitis.[63]

Identical histology may be seen in epidermal fungal infections, and special stains are essential to exclude this possibility.[55,57,64-67]

It can also be difficult to differentiate eosinophilic folliculitis from mycosis fungoides. Initial lesions of mycosis fungoides can sometimes resemble eosinophilic folliculitis. Similarly, anaplastic large cell lymphoma can have lesions mimicking eosinophilic folliculitis.[57] The presence of atypical lymphocytes, clonality studies, and multiple biopsies over time may help clarify the differential diagnosis.

Incontinentia pigmenti

Clinical features

Incontinentia pigmenti (Bloch-Sulzberger syndrome) is a rare systemic illness with a striking female bias (in excess of 37:1), as affected males usually die in utero.[1-3] It has an X-linked dominant mode of inheritance.[4] Cutaneous manifestations usually present at birth or during the first few weeks of life.[1] There may also be lesions affecting the hair, teeth, nails, eyes, skeleton, and the central nervous system in up to 80% of patients.[1,4] The phenotype in females is variable, manifestations being dependent on the effects of

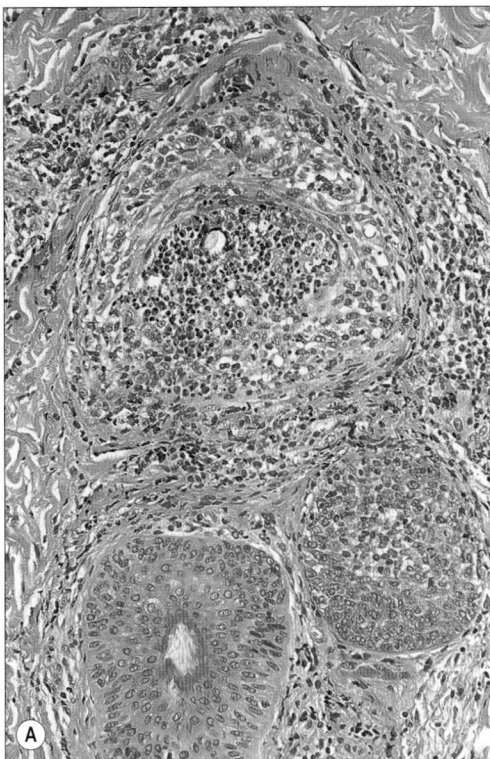

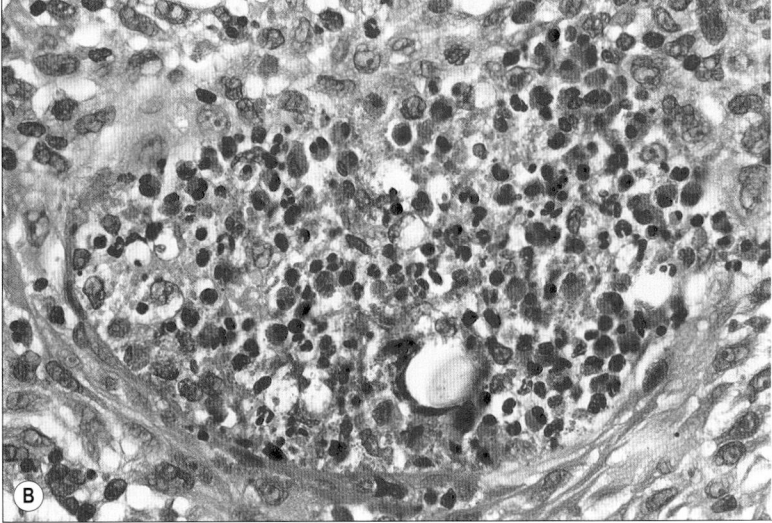

Fig. 15.57
(**A**, **B**) Eosinophilic pustular folliculitis: there is spongiosis associated with an eosinophil-rich abscess.

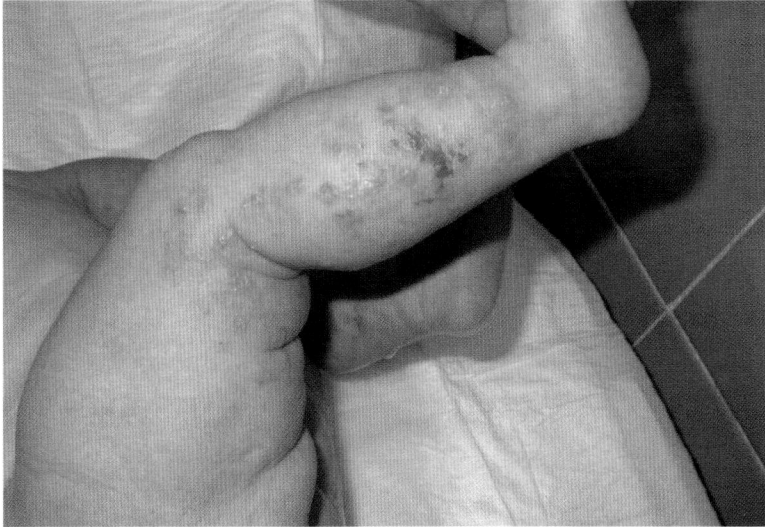

Fig. 15.58
Incontinentia pigmenti: the inflammatory stage is characterized by erythema, linear clusters of intact vesicles, crusts, and scaling. By courtesy of J.C. Pascual, MD, Alicante, Spain.

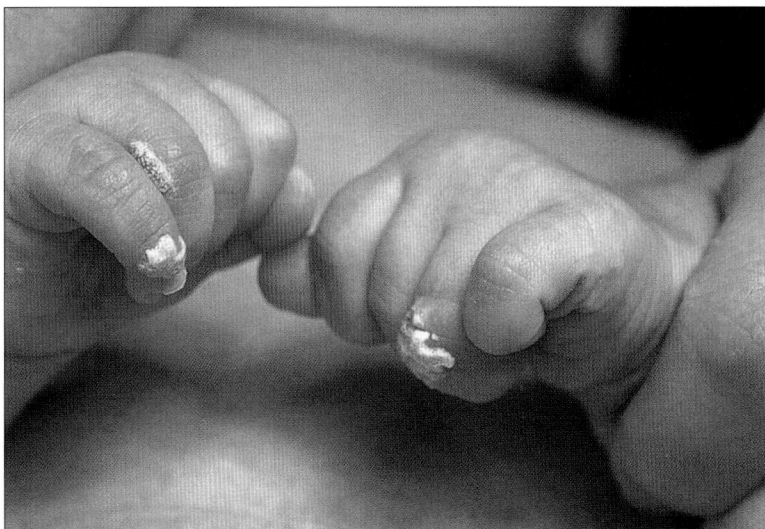

Fig. 15.59
Incontinentia pigmenti: verrucous lesions, seen in the second stage, predominantly affect the extremities. By courtesy of the Institute of Dermatology, London, UK.

mosaicism resulting from X-chromosome lyonization.[5] It has occasionally been described in identical twins.[6] The disease is rarely transmitted from father to daughter.[7]

Most males with incontinentia pigmenti die in utero, and only very rare patients survive. As with females, it is associated with the same phenotypic mosaicism.[8] In the majority of cases of male involvement, it develops in association with Klinefelter syndrome.[9–12] Half chromatid mutation, or more recently an unstable pre-mutation, has been offered as explanation for affected males with a normal karyotype.[11,12] Only extraordinary cases have been reported in normal XY males, secondary to somatic mosaicism.[13]

Typically, the condition has four stages:[14–16]

- Stage 1, comprising erythema and linear vesiculation on the trunk and extremities, is apparent at birth or during the first 2 weeks of life (*Fig. 15.57*).[16,17] Characteristically, the face is unaffected. Patients usually show associated leukocytosis and eosinophilia. On average, the blistering stage completely resolves within 4 months.[5]
- Stage 2, which is uncommon and usually transitory, consists of hyperkeratotic verrucous papules and plaques most frequently found on the extremities (*Fig. 15.58*). The verrucous lesions develop at sites of previous blistering.[16,17] They may resemble linear epidermal nevi.[16,18] This stage (when present) appears during the second to sixth weeks of life and usually resolves completely by 6 months.[5]
- Stage 3, which is pathognomonic of incontinentia pigmenti, presents as bizarre reticulated pigmentation, generally between the 12th and 26th weeks after birth. It sometimes occurs de novo. The brown to slate-gray pigmentation appears as splashes, streaks, and whorls (sometimes referred to as 'Chinese lettering') on the torso and extremities (*Fig. 15.59*). The nipples are typically hyperpigmented and involvement of the groin and axillae is characteristic.[5] The pigmentation appears to develop independently of the bullous lesions or verrucous plaques and follows Blaschko lines.[16,17] Resolution of lesions is associated with atrophy and the pigmentation is usually imperceptible by adulthood.
- Stage 4, usually presenting in adulthood, shows only residual changes that may be visible as occasional atrophic, hypopigmented, hairless, reticulated patches and streaks best seen on the lower legs.[1,5,18]

Additional cutaneous lesions include mild nail dystrophy (40%), scalp alopecia at the vertex, and the woolly hair nevus.[4,5,16] A whorled scarring alopecia following the lines of Blaschko has been documented.[2,19] At this point,

Table 15.4
General manifestations of incontinentia pigmenti

System	Abnormality
Scalp	Scarring Alopecia of variable severity
Nails	Occasional dystrophy
Teeth	Partial/complete absence Conical (pegged)
Eyes	Strabismus Blindness Cataracts Atrophy of optic nerve
Central nervous system	Spastic paralysis Mental retardation Convulsions

the skin lesions cease to be problematic, and other issues such as ocular involvement are the focus of concern.[20–22]

Painful subungual digital verrucous nodules are occasional late features of incontinentia pigmenti.[16,23–25] They are usually multiple, affect the hands more often than the feet, and, in addition to nail destruction, they can also be associated with scalloped resorption of the underlying phalanx.[25] Spontaneous regression is sometimes seen. Clinically, these nodules may be mistaken for a wart, subungual fibroma, keratoacanthoma, or squamous cell carcinoma.[22]

Dermatoglyphic patterns presenting in patients and also in nonaffected family members have been described.[26]

Some patients develop episodes of late reactivation of the disease in hyperpigmented streaks, and this appears to be related to a preceding infection.[27] It suggests that the mutated cells persist in the epidermis for a long period of time.

There can be widespread systemic involvement (*Table 15.4*). Dental abnormalities include hypodontia, delayed eruption, impaction, and crown malformations such as conical forms and accessory cusps.[5,18,28–31]

The most characteristic ocular changes are strabismus, microphthalmos, cataract, and optic atrophy.[22,32] Retinal detachment with a fibrovascular retrolental membrane is the commonest intraocular abnormality.[22,33–36]

Central nervous system involvement may result in encephalopathy, seizures, mental retardation, microcephaly, cerebellar ataxia, and motor effects including spastic quadriplegia, hemiplegia, slow motor development, and psychomotor retardation.[1,37–41] There is some evidence to suggest that incontinentia pigmenti can be associated with chromosomal instability and a slightly increased susceptibility to cancer; cutaneous squamous cell carcinoma has been described in a 16-year-old.[42,43] A unique case associated with twenty-nail dystrophy has been reported.[44]

Pathogenesis and histologic features

Considerable data have been published which sheds much light on the pathogenesis of this disease:

- Linkage analysis has demonstrated two incontinentia pigmenti loci that reside within the long arm of the X chromosome at Xq11 (*IP1*) and Xq28 (*IP2*).[5,45,46]
- Mutations in the gene for the inhibitor of kappa light polypeptide gene enhancer in B cells, kinase gamma (*IKBKG*) also called nuclear factor (NF)-κB gene modulator (*NEMO*), which plays a role in inhibiting TNF-induced apoptosis, has been shown to be responsible for development of the disease.[47–50]
- A mouse model has been created by disruption of NEMO, which leads to lethality in males and heterozygous females with skin and eye lesions similar to incontinentia pigmenti.[51,52] Biopsy of skin lesions of diseased animals shows increased keratinocyte apoptosis, inflammation, and pigment incontinence.[51]
- A relationship between incontinentia pigmenti and the osteopetrosis, lymphedema, anhidrotic ectodermal dysplasia, immunodeficiency (OL-EDA-ID) syndrome has recently been suggested in a patients who

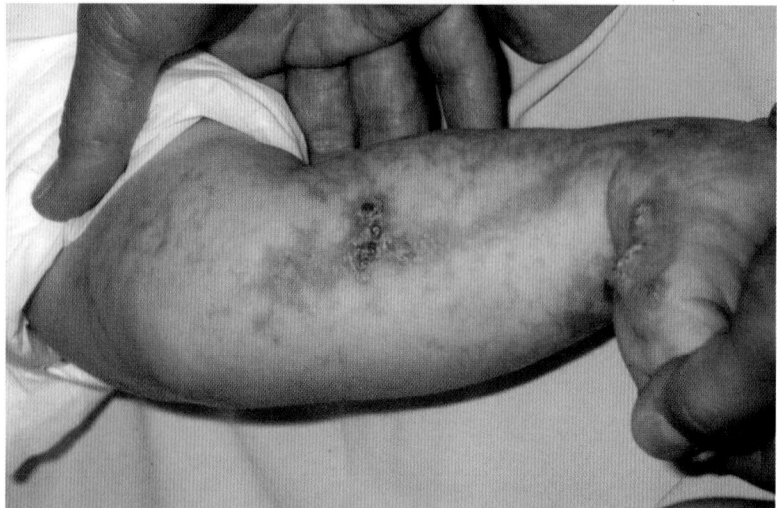

Fig. 15.60
Incontinentia pigmenti: the whorl-like distribution of the pigment is characteristic. From the collection of the late N.P. Smith, MD, the Institute of Dermatology, London, UK.

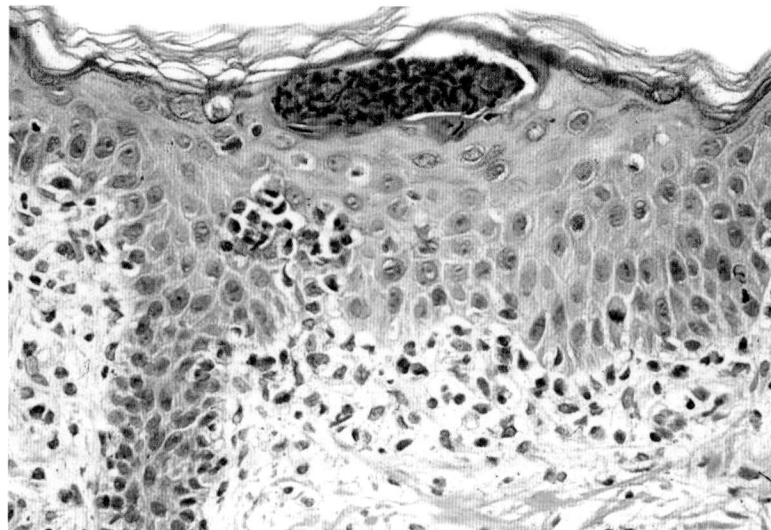

Fig. 15.61
Incontinentia pigmenti: vesicular stage showing a subcorneal eosinophil pustule and intraepidermal eosinophils.

presented with the latter syndrome born to mothers with features of incontinentia pigmenti.[53,54] Both diseases are associated with mutations in *NEMO/IKBKG*.[54–56] Male patients with the disease often have less deleterious mutations and present with ectodermal dysplasia and immunodeficiency.[10]

- Eotaxin (an NF-kappaB-activated chemokine) is strongly expressed in the suprabasal epidermis of involved skin in patients with the disease.[57] This expression is concomitant with the upper epidermal accumulation of eosinophils, suggesting a pathogenetic role for this chemokine.

Histologic examination of lesions in the vesicular stage (stage 1) shows eosinophilic spongiosis (*Fig. 15.60*). Occasionally, aggregates of dyskeratotic cells are evident (*Fig. 15.61*).[4] A chronic inflammatory cell infiltrate with conspicuous eosinophilia may be present within the dermis.

The verrucous lesions (stage 2) are characterized by hyperkeratosis, acanthosis, papillomatosis, and focal dyskeratosis (*Fig. 15.62*).[24] The dyskeratotic cells are typically arranged in a whorled configuration.

Stage 3 lesions manifest marked pigmentary incontinence with numerous melanophages in the dermis associated with epidermal basal cell degeneration.

End-stage lesions display epidermal atrophy, and there may be loss of the adnexae. Melanocytes appear to be present in reduced or normal numbers

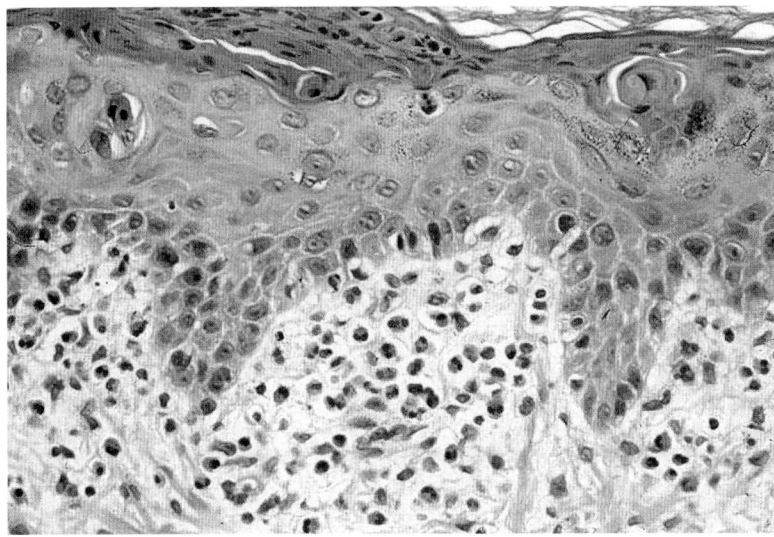

Fig. 15.62
Incontinentia pigmenti: there is dyskeratosis and an upper dermal eosinophil-rich infiltrate.

and ultrastructurally have shown no significant lesion except for one report in which small non-dendritic forms with degenerate melanosomes were described.[6,58] Some authors have recommended biopsy of these late lesions in adulthood as helpful for diagnosis.[59]

Molecular testing is available for confirmation of difficult cases and such techniques can also be applied to prenatal testing.[3,60–62]

The subungual verrucous nodules display features identical to those described in subungual keratoacanthoma with lobules of glassy cells associated with prominent hyperkeratosis, hypergranulosis, and striking dyskeratotic cells throughout the epidermis.[24,25]

Differential diagnosis

Clinically, incontinentia pigmenti may be confused with hypomelanosis of Ito (incontinentia pigmenti achromians), and the central nervous system involvement in both diseases is similar.[63D] The latter condition, however, is characterized by cutaneous pigmentary changes in the absence of either vesicular or verrucous lesions.

Many conditions are associated with eosinophilic spongiosis, but with adequate clinical information none should pose diagnostic problems. Toxic erythema of the neonate can be distinguished histologically from incontinentia pigmenti by the absence of spongiosis in the former condition.

Toxic erythema of the neonate

Clinical features

Toxic erythema of the neonate (erythema toxicum, erythema toxicum neonatorum) is a very common, self-limiting disorder that presents as an asymptomatic erythematous macular rash usually in the first few days of life. Very rarely, the eruption occurs a week or more after birth.[1] It affects up to 50% of neonates. In survey studies from Japan, Australia, China, and India, toxic erythema was found in up to 40.8%, 34.8%, 33.7%, and 20.6% of infants, respectively.[2–5] In a prospective study, the prevalence was 16.7% and more common in Caucasians and newborns with higher birth weights, greater gestational age, and in newborns delivered vaginally.[6]

It may be associated with papules, and occasionally pustule formation is evident. It most often involves the trunk, thighs, and buttocks but may also involve the head and neck and extremities.[6,7] Lesions usually resolve in a few days.

Pathogenesis and histologic features

The etiology of this condition is obscure, but some have suggested an immune reaction to postnatal cutaneous commensal microbial colonization, perhaps partially mediated by mast cells.[8,9]

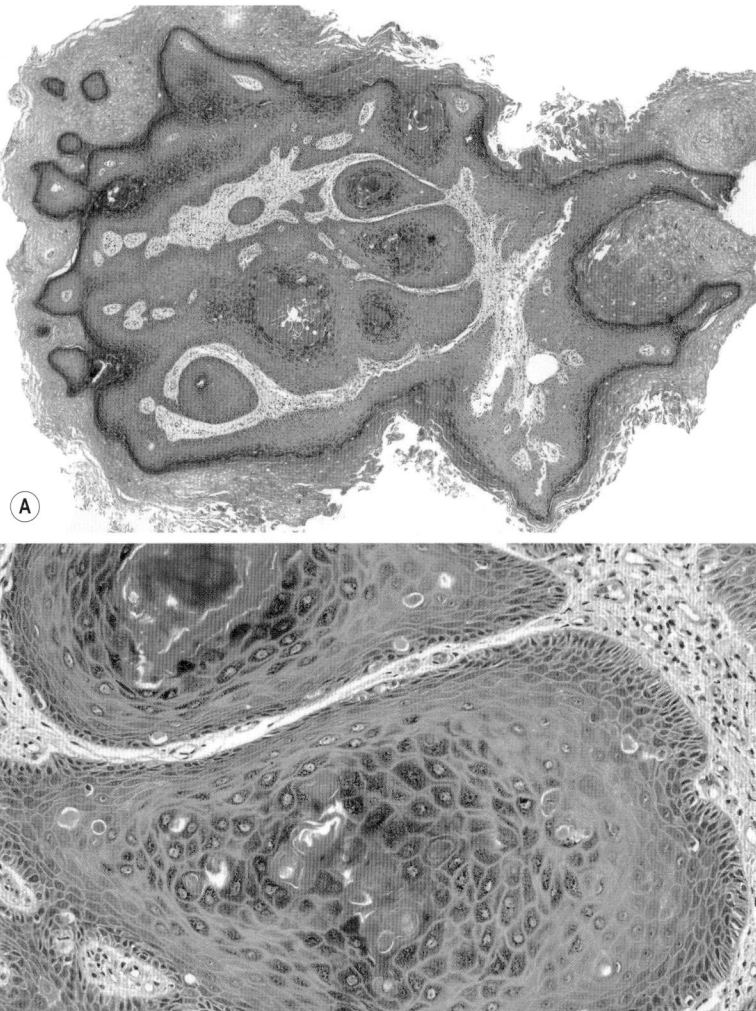

Fig. 15.63
(A, B) Incontinentia pigmenti: verrucous stage showing massive hyperkeratosis, papillomatosis, acanthosis, and numerous dyskeratotic cells.

Early erythematous lesions show a somewhat nondescript perivascular inflammatory cell infiltrate with conspicuous eosinophils, which can be seen penetrating the epidermis in close proximity to hair follicles. The pustules are characteristically intrafollicular, sometimes subcorneal or intraepidermal, and contain large numbers of eosinophils and occasional neutrophils.[10]

Differential diagnosis

Toxic erythema of the neonate must be distinguished from incontinentia pigmenti. The latter, however, is characterized by eosinophilic spongiosis, a feature not seen in toxic erythema. In miliaria rubra, the vesicles are related to sweat ducts rather than hair follicles and typically contain mononuclear cells rather than eosinophils.

Hidradenitis suppurativa

Clinical features

Hidradenitis suppurativa (acne inversa, apocrine acne) is a common disease.[1–3] The prevalence varies from <1.0% to 4%.[4–7]

It is a chronic relapsing suppurative inflammation of regions where apocrine glands occur, i.e., the axilla, inguinal folds, perineum, genitalia, and periareolar region (Fig. 15.63).[7,8] It usually occurs postpubertally in both sexes, more commonly in women.[5] Karl Marx was famously afflicted.[1–12] The disease is seen most frequently in young adults, although its first presentation may be in older individuals and also before puberty.[13–15] In

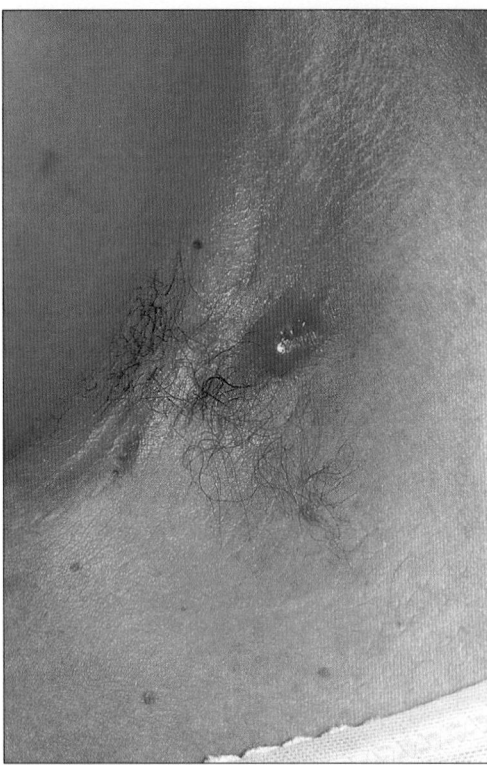

Fig. 15.64
Hidradenitis suppurativa: early lesion presenting as an erythematous nodule discharging clear fluid. The axilla is a commonly affected site. By courtesy of R.A. Marsden, MD, St George's Hospital, London, UK.

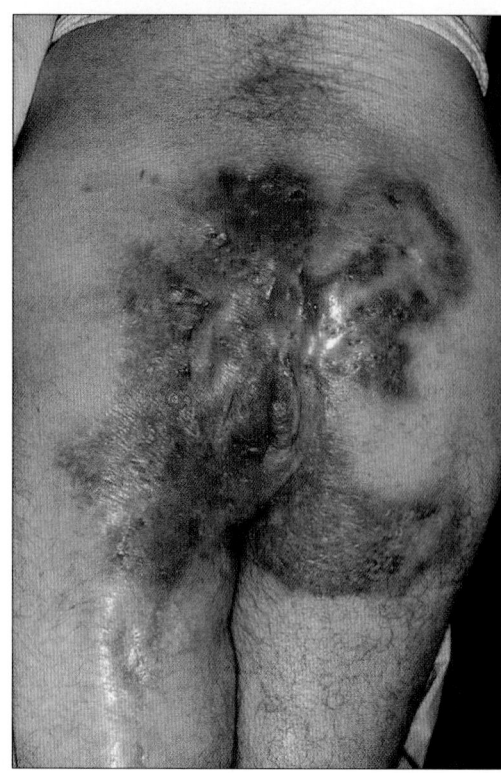

Fig. 15.65
Hidradenitis suppurativa: in this very severe example, there is marked scarring and numerous sinuses are present. By courtesy of R.A. Marsden, MD, St George's Hospital, London, UK.

prepubertal children, there is frequently a family history.[15] Initially, there is a firm painful nodule in the groin or axilla. The nodule can involute slowly or else discharge pus through the skin; the discharge of pus is not copious, but is chronic and often malodorous. In the late stages, a complex interconnecting system of sinuses extends deeply into the dermis and subcutaneous fat with extensive dense fibrosis (*Fig. 15.64*).[16]

Axillary lesions are more common in women and genitoinguinal lesions are more common in men. Changes may be confined to one region or occur in both, but the axillary region is involved in over 70% of cases.[17] Some reports have attached etiological importance to axillary shaving and the use of deodorants, but this is not generally accepted.[17,18] Obesity, metabolic syndrome, diabetes mellitus, inflammatory bowel disease, arthritis, and smoking are associated.[6,19–22] In one study, nearly 90% of German patients were smokers (expected prevalence rate 27%).[13] Whether cessation of smoking improves the course of the disease is unknown.[23] Patients with the hidradenitis suppurativa appear to be at increased risk of developing nonmelanoma skin cancer, but it is usually late onset (~25 years) and may be due to the complications of a chronic inflammatory state.[22,24]

The lesions are clearly maintained by bacterial infection as various organisms are often grown.[25] Symptomatic improvement can be achieved with long-term antibiotics. Perineal lesions are often severe and complicated by abscesses, fistulae, and draining sinus tracts.[17]

Lesions are also rarely seen on the malar region of the face and even on the eyelids (glands of Moll), sites with modified apocrine glands.

Hidradenitis suppurativa can be present in association with conditions which are said to be pathologically similar, namely, acne conglobata and dissecting folliculitis of the scalp. These three conditions have been referred to collectively as the 'follicular occlusion triad'.[26] Any one condition, however, may occur separately. Acne conglobata, an extremely severe nodulocystic variant of acne, occurs extensively on the trunk, buttocks, and limbs with predilection for males.[27] The disease has been described in association with HIV and following pregnancy.[28,29] Dissecting folliculitis (folliculitis capitis abscedens et suffodiens) is centered on the vertex of the scalp and is characterized by boggy tender lesions that tend to become confluent with formation of draining sinuses and suppuration.[30–33] The disease presents more

commonly in black males, and it is very rarely familial.[34] Radical surgery is often the only satisfactory means of terminating the process. All the diseases in the follicular occlusion triad can occasionally be complicated by progression to cellulitis and septicemia. Squamous carcinoma (including the verrucous variant) is a rare and late additional complication.[35–42] As with Marjolin ulcer–cancer, the carcinomas are capable of aggressive invasion and metastasis (50%) and are generally associated with a poor prognosis.[17] Such tumors arise most frequently on the buttocks and are more often seen in males.[38] Hidradenitis has been shown to be associated with systemic granulomatous lesions, in particular, Crohn disease.[19,22,43–45] An association with spondyloarthropathy, Dowling-Degos disease, and lithium therapy has also been documented.[22,46–48]

Treatment of this disease is difficult due to its chronic relapsing nature. Surgery is often used to remove affected areas, but the cure rate in some studies is very low.[49] Nevertheless, occasional patients are satisfied with the relief of symptoms, albeit temporary, afforded by surgery.[49] Other studies have shown a low recurrence rate following wide excision.[50,51] Early surgical treatment appears to increase the chance of success.[52] Recently, new-generation immunosuppressive agents and biological medications have shown some efficacy.[53,54] Hormonal regulation has also been employed with more limited success.[55,56]

Pathogenesis and histologic features

The pathogenesis of hidradenitis suppurativa remains poorly understood.[57–62] It has generally been thought that the earliest lesion is an acute inflammatory process involving the apocrine duct and gland, which extends into the surrounding connective tissue with subsequent abscess and sinus formation (*Fig. 15.65*).[57] Other authors, however, believe that eccrine hidradenitis is more commonly found than apocrine involvement, and yet others think that the primary event is follicular obstruction.[38,59] Some data suggest overactivation of the innate immune system, but a deeper underlying cause remains elusive.[25,63,64]

The provocation for the initial 'apocrinitis' is believed by some to be keratin occlusion of the corresponding hair follicle. Certainly, keratin plugging of follicles and sinuses and inflammation in and around the hair follicle are regularly seen.[58] In one study, follicular occlusion was present in all of 118 specimens examined in patients with disease duration that ranged from as little as 1 month to many years.[60] The anatomic distribution of the lesions also supports the concept of an underlying apocrine gland defect. The condition has some similarity to Fox-Fordyce disease, which is more convincingly associated with an inflammatory process of the apocrine duct. Fox-Fordyce disease has the same sex predilection, age incidence, and anatomic distribution, and it, too, is alleviated by pregnancy. Interestingly, some cases of Fox-Fordyce disease have been reported to progress to hidradenitis suppurativa.

The other members of the follicular occlusion triad – acne conglobata and dissecting folliculitis – are both clearly associated with keratin plugging.

There is no doubt that the main symptoms and chronic disability are related to the sinuses and fibrosis; these are largely due to the chronic secondary infection, since injection of sterile apocrine sweat into tissues does not induce an inflammatory response.

Organisms that may be found include *Staphylococcus aureus*, *Streptococcus viridans*, *Escherichia coli*, *Proteus mirabilis*, *Klebsiella* spp., *Pseudomonas aeruginosa*, *Streptococcus milleri*, and anaerobic organisms. Coagulase-negative *S. aureus* is the most common bacterium isolated from the depth of the lesions.[25,65] Anaerobic organisms are responsible for the offensive smell, which can be a major problem for the patient. Generally, no immune deficiency is detectable, but there have been occasional reports of a functional neutrophil deficiency.

In considering the pathogenesis of this condition, it must also be noted that some cases clearly develop as an autosomal dominantly inherited tendency.[66,67] Others have no suggestion of familial incidence.

The disease has been simulated in 3 of 12 normal volunteers by occlusion of axillary skin with atropine tape following depilation.[68] The latter in itself could be expected to produce some pathology, which is clearly not seen in the normal individual. The absence of lesions in 75% of these volunteers shows at least that there is some variation in susceptibility to developing the disease. This experimental induction of the disease has not been repeated.

In a study of 42 women with hidradenitis suppurativa, the authors noted premenstrual exacerbation of symptoms in two-thirds of patients and over one-third of patients reported menstrual irregularities.[69] In this same study, testosterone and free androgen index were higher compared with control patients.[69] In contrast, another study was not able to correlate hyperandrogenism and development of hidradenitis in women.[9,70] Pregnancy may relieve the symptoms of the disease.

In summary, the precise pathogenesis of hidradenitis suppurativa is not well understood. It seems likely, however, that while many patients have a tendency to follicular occlusion with resultant acne-like lesions, some individuals show an additional, occasionally inherited, tendency for follicular obstruction to cause, or be associated with, inflammation of the apocrine duct. With the additional occlusive effects of obesity and secondary infection, often by mixed organisms, there is a resultant florid destructive folliculitis centered on, or also involving, the apocrine glands. The secondary bacterial infection perpetuates the chronic inflammatory and scarring nature of the process. A defect in the immune system would be expected to exacerbate this vicious circle, but no consistent abnormality has yet been identified.[71,72] The changes with pregnancy and menstrual cycle can be attributed to the hormonal effects on the apocrine gland and do not appear to be of primary importance.

Biopsies of established hidradenitis suppurativa show sinus tracts with marked suppuration and frank abscess formation. The sinus tracts are lined by a mixture of granulation tissue and squamous epithelium (*Figs 15.66* and *15.67*). The latter extends from the associated follicular epithelium. These inflammatory sinus tracts usually contain desquamated keratin and sometimes hair shafts, and are surrounded by dense fibrosis.[60] The suppuration may extend into adjacent connective tissue where there can also be a chronic inflammatory infiltrate frequently including histiocytes and giant cells that are sometimes related to keratin fragments. At this stage, apocrine glands are conspicuously absent in the scarred and inflamed area, although adjacent apocrine glands often appear quite normal. Although some authors have emphasized the presence of acute inflammation of apocrine glands, in our experience, this is an uncommon finding in routine surgical specimens.

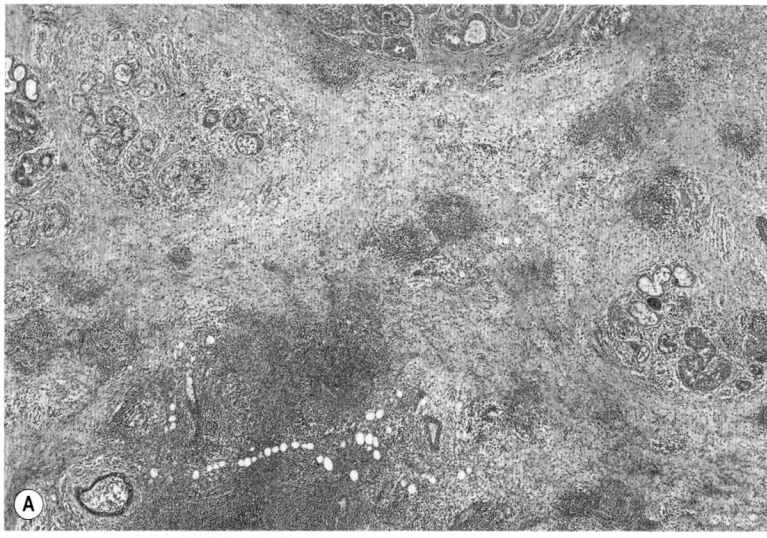
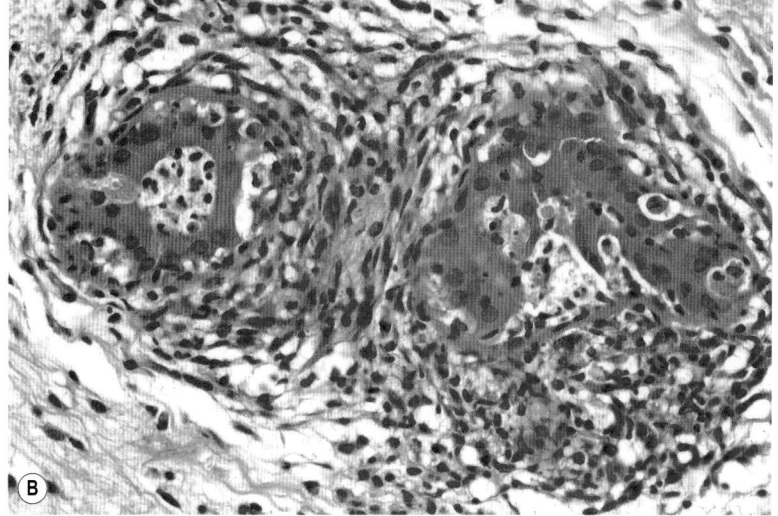

Fig. 15.66
(**A**, **B**) Hidradenitis suppurativa: early lesion showing acute inflammation involving the apocrine gland.

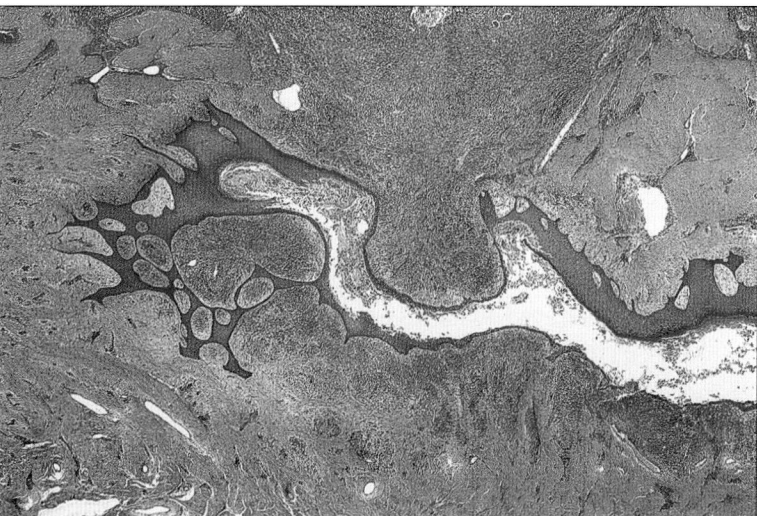

Fig. 15.67
Hidradenitis suppurativa: the sinuses are lined by stratified squamous epithelium and surrounded by fibrosis and inflammation.

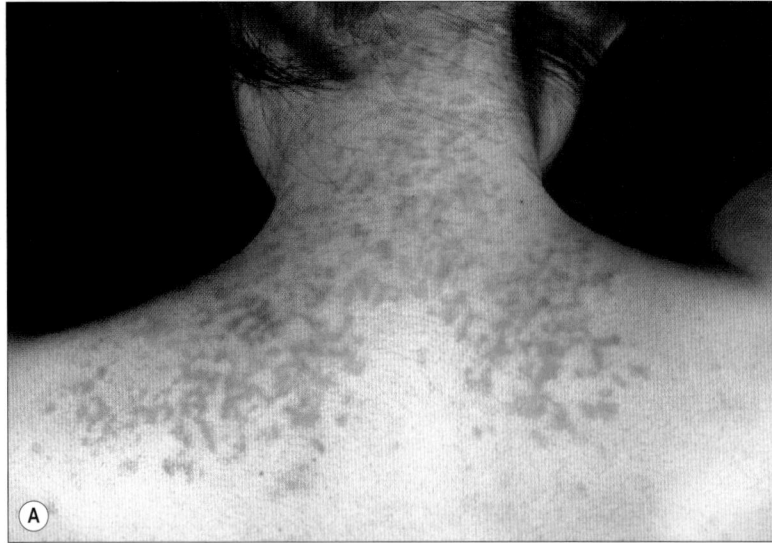

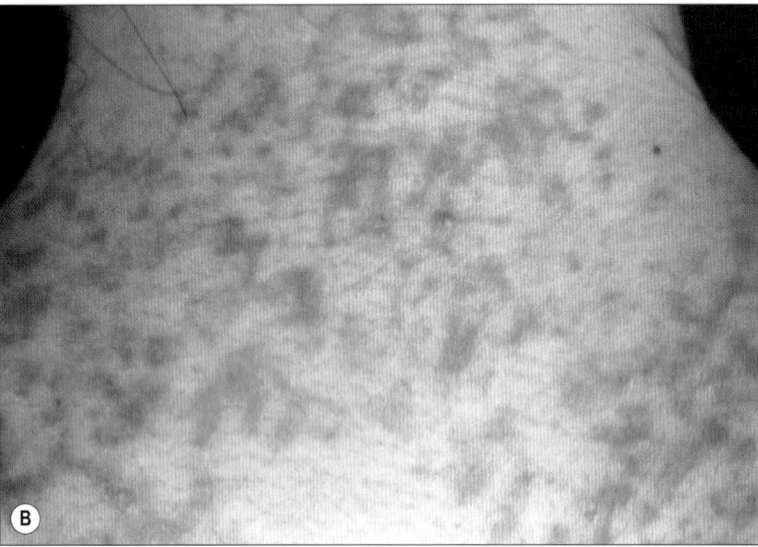

Fig. 15.68
Prurigo pigmentosa: reticulate urticarial papules on (**A**) the upper back and (**B**) the neck. By courtesy of the Institute of Dermatology, London, UK.

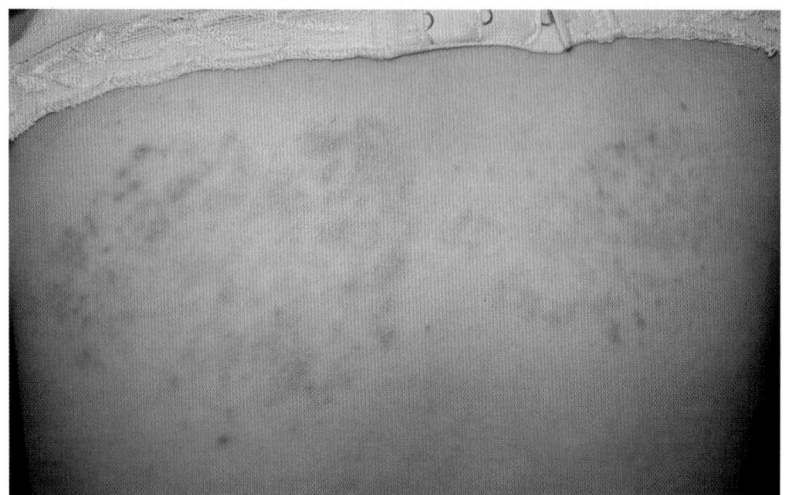

Fig. 15.69
Prurigo pigmentosa: late lesions with typical reticulate hyperpigmentation. By courtesy of Drs. Chao-Kai Hsu and Prof. Julia Yu-Yun Lee, Tainan, Taiwan.

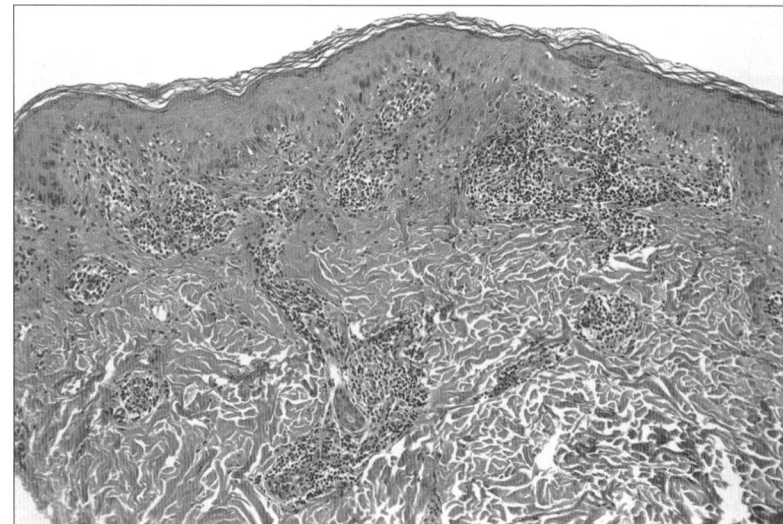

Fig. 15.70
Prurigo pigmentosa: superficial perivascular infiltrate in an established lesion.

Others have also found primary inflammation of apocrine glands in only a minority of specimens.[59,73]

Differential diagnosis

The main differential diagnoses are primary infection, a response to a ruptured epidermal inclusion cyst, or wounds. Clinical correlation and special stains for microorganisms are necessary to establish the correct diagnosis.

Prurigo pigmentosa

Clinical features

Prurigo pigmentosa is a distinctive inflammatory dermatosis first described by Nagashima in 1978.[1-6] Most cases occur in Japanese patients although the disease appears to have a wider distribution and may have been underdiagnosed in the past.[6-12] Most cases present in young adults and there is a predilection for females. Cases in small children are very uncommon. The disease also seems to have a predilection for patients in Sicily, Turkey, and Iran.[13-16] It presents as very pruritic urticarial papules, papulovesicles, and vesicles in a reticular pattern on the back, neck, and chest.[17,18] (*Fig. 15.68*) Pustules are rarely seen.[19] Involvement of the lower trunk may be seen and lesions on the face are exceptional.[20,21] Lesions last for a few days and heal, leaving a reticulate hyperpigmentation (*Fig. 15.69*). Recurrences are frequent. It most commonly occurs in the spring and summer. Unilateral

or segmental cases are exceptional.[22,23] Associations with diabetes mellitus, ketosis, anorexia nervosa, bismuth, and allergic contact dermatitis to chromium and nickel have been documented.[24-34] Rare associations with an atopic diathesis, pregnancy and primary biliary cirrhosis, Sjögren disease, *H. pylori* infection, after bariatric surgery, and in a pregnant woman with hyperemesis gravidarum have also been reported.[35-41] *H. pylori* organisms have been identified in a dilated hair follicle of an affected patient.[42] A prurigo pigmentosa-like rash has been reported in a case of adult-onset Still disease.[43,44] A case in white monozygotic twins has been described.[45]

Pathogenesis and histologic features

The pathogenesis of the disease is as yet unknown although some cases may be induced by ketosis or allergic contact dermatitis to chromium and nickel.[24-29,33,34,46] Antinuclear antibodies have been reported in some patients but it is not clear whether this has pathogenetic importance or represents a coincidence.[47] The detection of *Borrelia garinii* and *Borrelia afzelii* in skin specimens with serological evidence of *Borrelia* infection in three reported cases has raised the possibility that this is an unusual manifestation of the disease.[48] It has also been suggested that the disease is an inflammatory variant of confluent and reticulated papillomatosis.[49]

Early lesions show a superficial perivascular inflammatory cell infiltrate composed of neutrophils (*Fig. 15.70*). In these early lesions, dermatitis

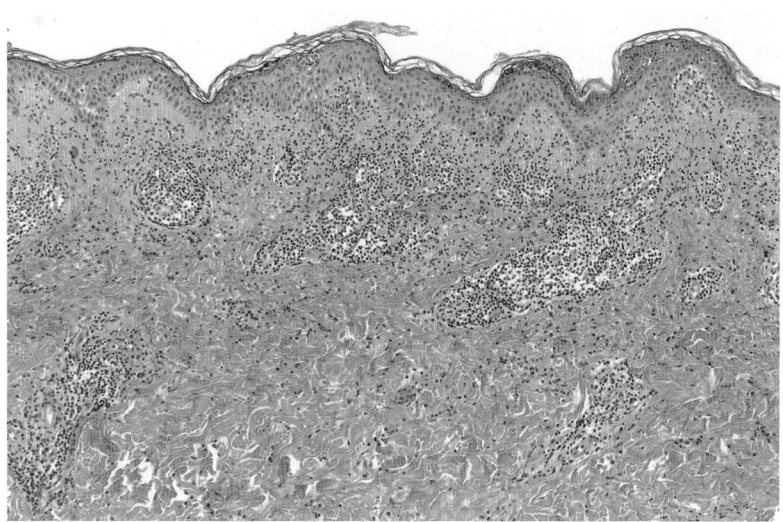

Fig. 15.71
Prurigo Pigmentosa: as the lesion evolves, there is exocytosis of neutrophils into the epidermis, with spongiosis and necrotic keratinocytes.

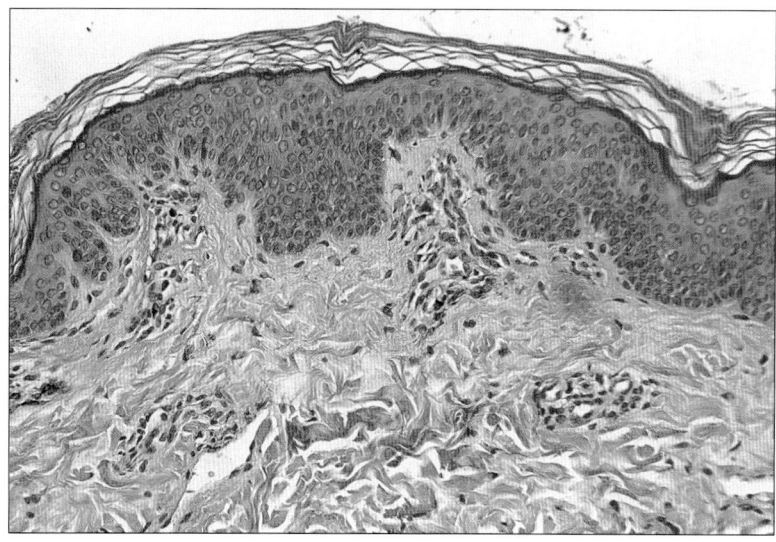

Fig. 15.73
Prurigo pigmentosa, late lesion: mild acanthosis with hyperkeratosis and pigment incontinence.

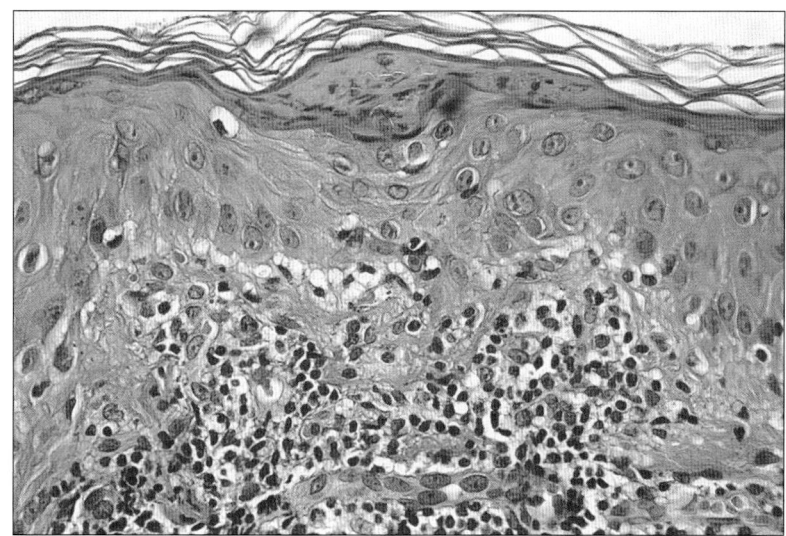

Fig. 15.72
Prurigo pigmentosa: focal lichenoid change combined with spongiosis and some exocytosis of lymphocytes. Neutrophils have been replaced by lymphocytes and histiocytes.

herpetiformis-like changes have been described.[50] As the disease progresses, neutrophils may be seen in the papillary dermis and extending into the epidermis. This is associated with spongiosis, ballooning, and scattered necrotic keratinocytes.[6,51] As the lesions evolve, epidermal neutrophilic microabscesses may be found and dermal eosinophils and lymphocytes are seen (*Fig. 15.71*). A focal lichenoid pattern may be present (*Fig. 15.72*). Hydropic degeneration of basal cells is very focal, and colloid bodies are not usually detected. Microvesicle formation is present in some cases but subepidermal blister formation is rare.[51] Epidermal acanthosis and hyperkeratosis are features in late stages along with pigment incontinence and melanophages (*Fig. 15.73*). Follicular involvement in the form of bacterial colonies in the hair follicle, folliculitis, and perifolliculitis has been reported in 78% in a series of cases.[52]

Access **ExpertConsult.com** for the complete list of references

Vascular diseases

See
www.expertconsult.com
for references and
additional material

Introduction

Vasculitis and other forms of vascular damage are the subjects of this chapter. Although minimal criteria for the diagnosis of vasculitis may differ among experts, the presence of inflammation and some evidence of vascular damage in the form of vessel wall/endothelial cell necrosis or fibrinoid change fulfill most authorities' criteria for a diagnosis of vasculitis. Some, however, apply the term less restrictively to vascular inflammation associated with non-specific histologic features, such as extravasated red cells, endothelial swelling, or karyorrhexis but without fibrinoid change or necrosis. When encountering such cases, we prefer to designate them as 'low-grade vascular damage' and include a comment that, although the findings may represent very early vasculitis, they do not meet strict criteria for necrotizing vasculitis. That inflammatory vascular disease is represented by a broad spectrum of histologic changes cannot be overemphasized.

The histologic features of most forms of vasculitis are not specific for an entity per se. A specific diagnosis requires careful clinical, histologic, and serological (i.e., presence of antineutrophil antibodies) correlation.[1] The role of the pathologist in evaluating a biopsy is to confirm or deny the presence of vasculitis, and to describe the nature of the inflammatory infiltrate and the type(s) and size(s) of the vessel(s) involved. A histologic differential diagnosis is established to guide patient evaluation. Correct biopsy technique and timing are important to allow for adequate assessment for vasculitis. Incisional biopsies to include sufficient subcutis and larger subcutaneous vessels within the first 48 hours after development of the lesion yield the best results.[1]

A pathological diagnosis of vasculitis may indicate a primary or secondary disease (i.e., in the setting of connective tissue disease). Secondary forms of vascular disease may manifest as diverse histologic patterns. For example, connective tissue diseases may be associated with either a small-vessel leukocytoclastic disease or a large-vessel vasculitis. Likewise, different histologic patterns may be seen in association with a given primary vasculitis. As an example, granulomatosis with polyangiitis may be linked with either leukocytoclastic or granulomatous vasculitis.

The myriad schemata for the classification of the vasculitides are a reflection of the complexity of this controversial class of diseases. Over the last decade or so, several new classifications have emerged that attempt to combine both histologic and clinical information (Table 16.1).[2-5] More recently, the revised Chapel Hill consensus has updated the nomenclature of vasculitidies.[3] Undoubtedly, these will continue to be refined as a more complete understanding of the pathogenesis of these diseases is gained.

Leukocytoclastic vasculitis

Clinical features

Leukocytoclastic vasculitis (allergic vasculitis, cutaneous leukocytoclastic angiitis, hypersensitivity vasculitis, leukocytoclastic angiitis) is the commonest form of vasculitis.[1-7] It is not a disease entity but represents a vascular reaction pattern due to circulating immune complexes that may either be idiopathic or caused by a number of underlying disorders. The antigens possibly involved are summarized in Table 16.2.[1-8] The most frequent associations are drugs in addition to infections.[9,10] In over 40% of cases, however, no underlying condition can be identified.[11] Although the condition may be limited to the skin, it is important to recognize that it can also be associated with systemic manifestations involving the joints, kidneys, and gastrointestinal system in between 15% and 50% of patients.[5,11-14] The disease occurs equally in men and women, and may present in any age group.

Skin lesions are typically polymorphic, but palpable purpura (nonblanching erythematous papules) is the commonest manifestation (Fig. 16.1). Urticarial, bullous or vesicular, ulceroinfarctive, nodular, pustular, livedoid, and annular lesions may also be encountered (Figs 16.2–16.8).[15-19] The

Table 16.1

Types and definitions of vasculitis adopted by the 2012 Chapel Hill Consensus Conference on the Nomenclature of Systemic Vasculitis

CHCC2012 name	CHCC2012 definition
Large vessel vasculitis	Vasculitis affecting large arteries more often than other vasculitides. Large arteries are the aorta and its major branches. Any size artery may be affected.
Takayasu arteritis	Arteritis, often granulomatous, predominantly affecting the aorta and/or its major branches. Onset usually in patients younger than 50 years.
Giant cell arteritis	Arteritis, often granulomatous, usually affecting the aorta and/or its major branches, with a predilection for the branches of the carotid and vertebral arteries. Often involves the temporal artery. Onset usually in patients older than 50 years and often associated with polymyalgia rheumatica.
Medium vessel vasculitis	Vasculitis predominantly affecting medium arteries defined as the main visceral arteries and their branches. Any size artery may be affected. Inflammatory aneurysms and stenoses are common.
Polyarteritis nodosa	Necrotizing arteritis of medium or small arteries without glomerulonephritis or vasculitis in arterioles, capillaries, or venules, and not associated with antineutrophil cytoplasmic antibodies (ANCAs).
Kawasaki disease	Arteritis associated with the mucocutaneous lymph node syndrome and predominantly affecting medium and small arteries. Coronary arteries are often involved. Aorta and large arteries may be involved. Usually occurs in infants and young children.
Small-vessel vasculitis	Vasculitis predominantly affecting small vessels, defined as small intraparenchymal arteries, arterioles, capillaries, and venules. Medium arteries and veins may be affected.
ANCA-associated vasculitis	Necrotizing vasculitis, with few or no immune deposits, predominantly affecting small vessels (i.e., capillaries, venules, arterioles, and small arteries), associated with myeloperoxidase (MPO) ANCA or proteinase 3 (PR3) ANCA. Not all patients have ANCA. Add a prefix indicating ANCA reactivity, e.g., MPO-ANCA, PR3-ANCA, ANCA-negative.
Microscopic polyangiitis	Necrotizing vasculitis, with few or no immune deposits, predominantly affecting small vessels (i.e., capillaries, venules, or arterioles). Necrotizing arteritis involving small and medium arteries may be present. Necrotizing glomerulonephritis is very common. Pulmonary capillaritis often occurs. Granulomatous inflammation is absent.
Granulomatosis with polyangiitis (Wegener)	Necrotizing granulomatous inflammation usually involving the upper and lower respiratory tract, and necrotizing vasculitis affecting predominantly small to medium vessels (e.g., capillaries, venules, arterioles, arteries, and veins). Necrotizing glomerulonephritis is common.
Eosinophilic granulomatosis with polyangiitis (Churg-Strauss)	Eosinophil-rich and necrotizing granulomatous inflammation often involving the respiratory tract, and necrotizing vasculitis predominantly affecting small to medium vessels, and associated with asthma and eosinophilia. ANCA is more frequent when glomerulonephritis is present.
Immune complex vasculitis	Vasculitis with moderate to marked vessel wall deposits of immunoglobulin and/or complement components predominantly affecting small vessels (i.e., capillaries, venules, arterioles, and small arteries). Glomerulonephritis is frequent.
Cryoglobulinemic vasculitis	Vasculitis with cryoglobulin immune deposits affecting small vessels (predominantly capillaries, venules, or arterioles) and associated with serum cryoglobulins. Skin, glomeruli, and peripheral nerves are often involved.
IgA vasculitis (Henoch-Schönlein)	Vasculitis, with IgA1-dominant immune deposits, affecting small vessels (predominantly capillaries, venules, or arterioles). Often involves skin and gastrointestinal tract, and frequently causes arthritis. Glomerulonephritis indistinguishable from IgA nephropathy may occur.
Hypocomplementemic urticarial vasculitis	Vasculitis accompanied by urticaria and hypocomplementemia affecting small vessels (i.e., capillaries, venules, or arterioles), and associated with anti-C1q antibodies. Glomerulonephritis, arthritis, obstructive pulmonary disease, and ocular inflammation are common.
Variable vessel vasculitis	Vasculitis with no predominant type of vessel involved that can affect vessels of any size (small, medium, and large) and type (arteries, veins, and capillaries).
Behçet disease	Vasculitis occurring in patients with Behçet disease that can affect arteries or veins. Behçet disease is characterized by recurrent oral and/or genital aphthous ulcers accompanied by cutaneous, ocular, articular, gastrointestinal, and/or central nervous system inflammatory lesions. Small-vessel vasculitis, thromboangiitis, thrombosis, arteritis, and arterial aneurysms may occur.
Cogan syndrome	Vasculitis occurring in patients with Cogan syndrome. Cogan syndrome characterized by ocular inflammatory lesions, including interstitial keratitis, uveitis, and episcleritis, and inner ear disease, including sensorineural hearing loss and vestibular dysfunction. Vasculitic manifestations may include arteritis (affecting small, medium, or large arteries), aortitis, aortic aneurysms, and aortic and mitral valvulitis.
Single-organ vasculitis	Vasculitis in arteries or veins of any size in a single organ that has no features that indicate that it is a limited expression of a systemic vasculitis. The involved organ and vessel type should be included in the name (e.g., cutaneous small-vessel vasculitis, testicular arteritis, central nervous system vasculitis). Vasculitis distribution may be unifocal or multifocal (diffuse) within an organ. Some patients originally diagnosed as having SOV will develop additional disease manifestations that warrant redefining the case as one of the systemic vasculitides (e.g., cutaneous arteritis later becoming systemic polyarteritis nodosa, etc.).
Vasculitis associated with systemic disease	Vasculitis that is associated with and may be secondary to (caused by) a systemic disease. The name (diagnosis) should have a prefix term specifying the systemic disease (e.g., rheumatoid vasculitis, lupus vasculitis, etc.).
Vasculitis associated with probable etiology	Vasculitis that is associated with a probable specific etiology. The name (diagnosis) should have a prefix term specifying the association (e.g., hydralazine-associated microscopic polyangiitis, hepatitis B virus–associated vasculitis, hepatitis C virus–associated cryoglobulinemic vasculitis, etc.).

Reproduced with permission from Jennette, J.C., et al. 2013 *Arthritis & Rheumatism*, 65, 1–11.

Table 16.2
Possible causes of allergic vasculitis

- Infection
  - bacterial: *Streptococcus*
  - mycobacterial: *Mycobacterium tuberculosis*
  - viral: hepatitis, influenza
  - cytomegalovirus
  - HIV infection
  - leprosy
- Drugs
  - aspirin, phenacetin, sulfonamides, penicillin, iodides, phenothiazines
- Chemicals
  - insecticides, weed killers, petroleum products
- Foreign proteins
  - serum sickness
  - hyposensitization antigens
- Associated diseases
  - autoimmune diseases: systemic lupus erythematosus, inflammatory bowel disease
  - hemolytic anemia
  - Hodgkin lymphoma, carcinoma
  - rheumatoid arthritis
  - mixed connective tissue disease
  - dermatomyositis
  - relapsing polychondritis
  - Sjögren syndrome
  - IgA vasculitis
  - cryoglobulinemia
  - polyarteritis nodosa
  - Granulomatosis with polyangiitis
  - Churg-Strauss disease
  - granuloma faciale
  - erythema elevatum diutinum
  - Waldenström hypergammaglobulinemia
  - sarcoidosis

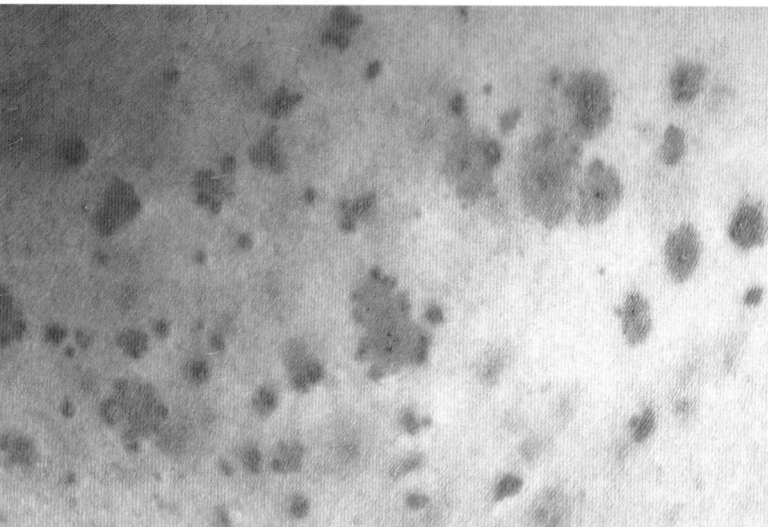

Fig. 16.2
Leukocytoclastic vasculitis: close-up view showing small erythematous lesions. By courtesy of the Institute of Dermatology, London, UK.

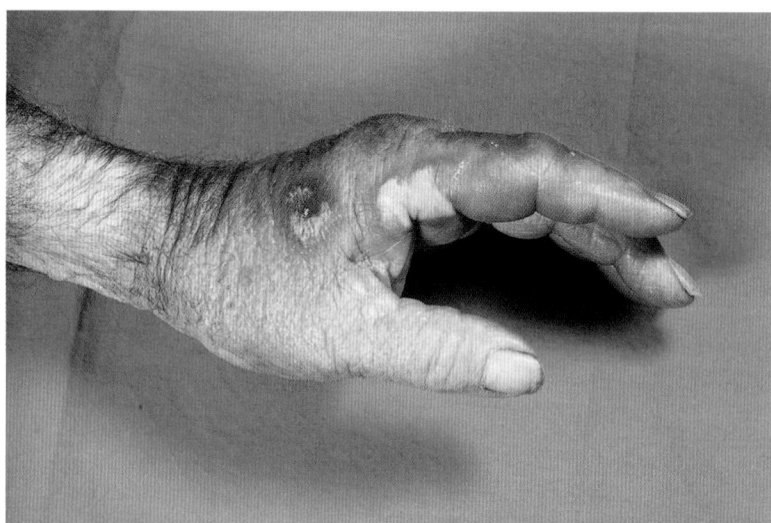

Fig. 16.3
Leukocytoclastic vasculitis: in this patient an extensive purpuric eruption showing central necrosis is evident. By courtesy of R.A. Marsden, MD, St George's Hospital, London, UK.

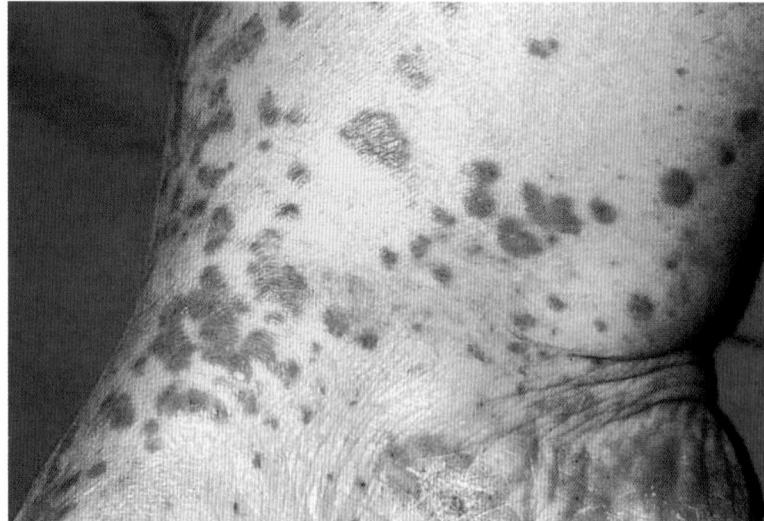

Fig. 16.1
Leukocytoclastic vasculitis: typical erythematous maculopapular lesions are present on the medial aspect of the ankle. By courtesy of R.A. Marsden, MD, St George's Hospital, London, UK.

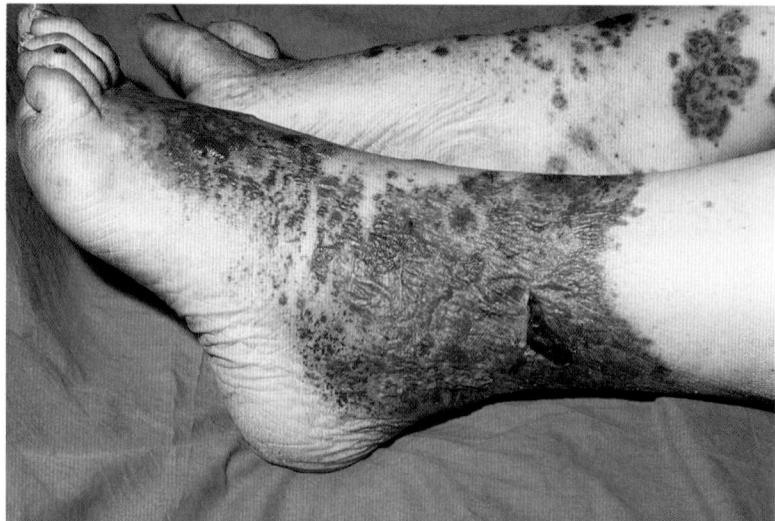

Fig. 16.4
Leukocytoclastic vasculitis: here confluent purpura with ulceration is present. By courtesy of R.A. Marsden, MD, St George's Hospital, London, UK.

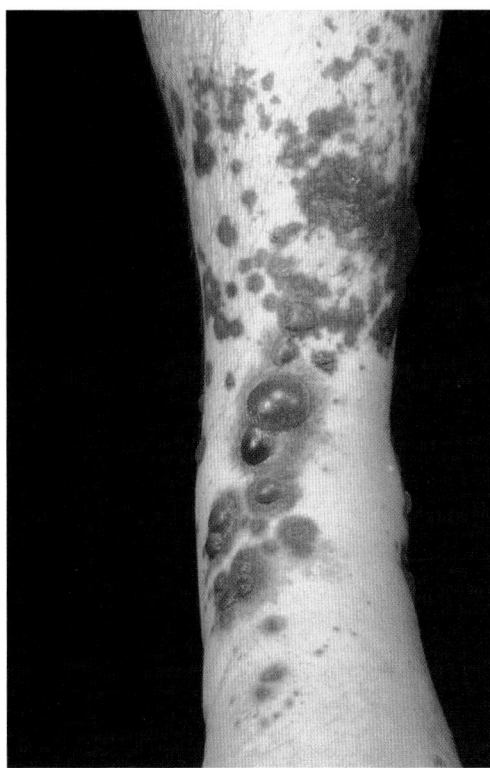

Fig. 16.5
Leukocytoclastic vasculitis: this patient presented with bullous lesions which developed as a consequence of thrombosis with epidermal infarction. By courtesy of the Institute of Dermatology, London, UK.

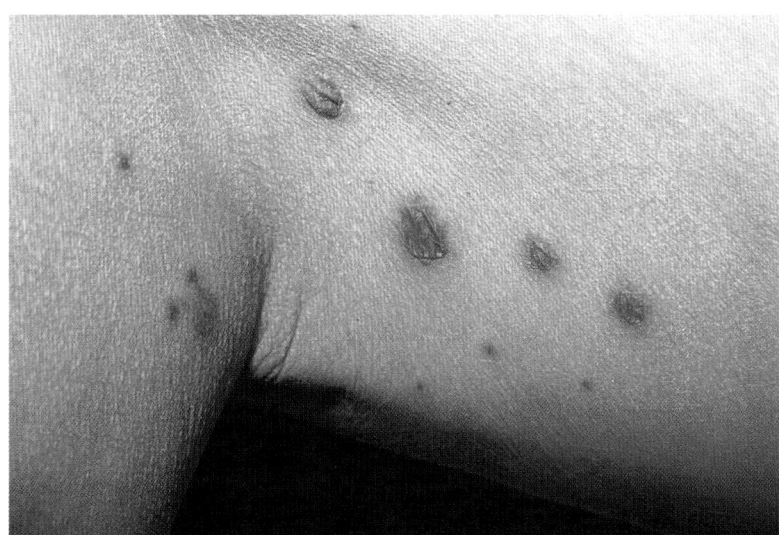

Fig. 16.6
Leukocytoclastic vasculitis: nodular lesions. By courtesy of the Institute of Dermatology, London, UK.

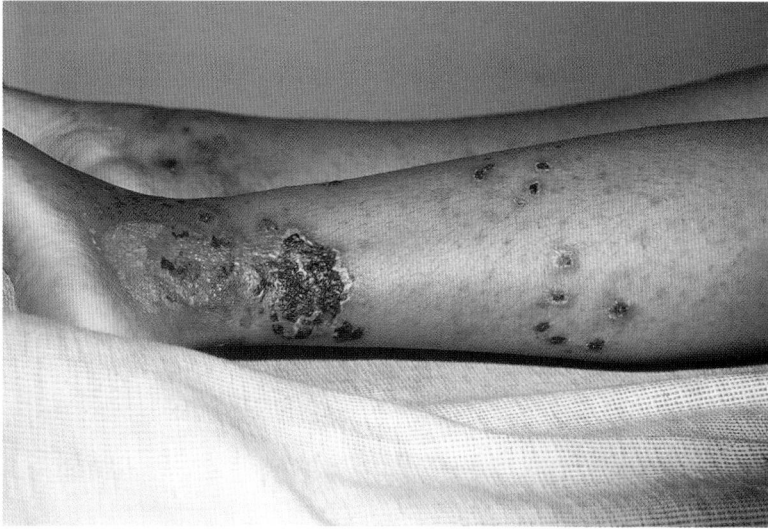

Fig. 16.7
Leukocytoclastic vasculitis: in this patient, there are extensive ulceroinfarctive lesions. By courtesy of the Institute of Dermatology, London, UK.

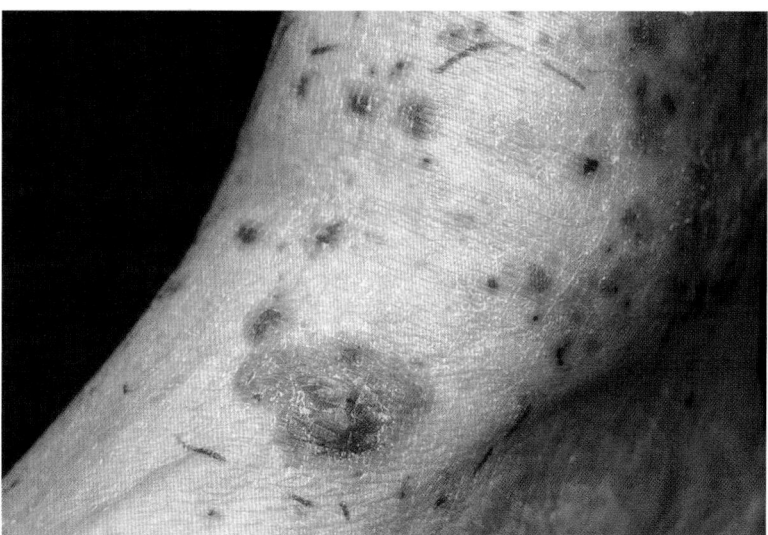

Fig. 16.8
Leukocytoclastic vasculitis: close-up view of a hemorrhagic blister. By courtesy of the Institute of Dermatology, London, UK.

lesions measure from 1 mm to several centimeters in diameter. Occasionally, annular erythema multiforme-like lesions occur (*Fig. 16.9*). The lower legs are affected most often, but lesions can present at a wide variety of sites, including the buttocks, arms, feet, ankles, trunk, and face, particularly in more seriously affected patients (*Figs 16.10* and *16.11*). Lesions may be noted in the skin of dependent areas of bedridden patients, such as the back and buttocks. A frequent accompaniment is edema of the lower legs or ankles (*Fig. 16.12*). Patients either experience a single occurrence or develop frequent recurrences over months or years. The eruption often occurs in episodes at irregular intervals, each lasting 1–4 weeks. Lesions usually heal completely, although on occasions atrophic scars and hyperpigmentation may occur. Rarely, leukocytoclastic vasculitis shows an erythema gyratum repens gross morphology.[20]

Although occasional cases are asymptomatic, patients not uncommonly complain of pruritus or burning; less frequently, pain is a feature. Additional features, which are sometimes present, include abdominal pain and gastrointestinal bleeding, joint pains with associated erythema and swelling, and evidence of renal involvement.[14,21] In severe cases, the features resemble acute glomerulonephritis and the nephrotic syndrome may even supervene. Rarely, patients have respiratory involvement (nodular or diffuse infiltrative lesions on X-ray examination), and very exceptionally the central or peripheral nervous system is affected, causing symptoms such as headache, diplopia, and dysphagia.[14]

In one study, drug therapy, often following an upper respiratory tract infection, was the inciting event in 45% of patients.[22] Numerous drugs have been implicated as a trigger including nonsteroidal anti-inflammatory drugs (aspirin, ibuprofen, naproxen, phenylbutazone), phenytoin, quinidine, amiodarone, potassium iodide, allopurinol, sulfonamides, griseofulvin, penicillin, erythromycin, clindamycin, oxacillin, vancomycin, ofloxacin, clarithromycin, furosemide (frusemide), thiazides, cimetidine, omeprazole, gabapentin, orlistat, zidovudine, indinavir, efavirenz, lisinopril, sotalol, insulin, retinoids, propylthiouracil, thiouracil, mefloquine, methotrexate, azathioprine, sirolimus, granulocyte colony-stimulating factor, haloperidol,

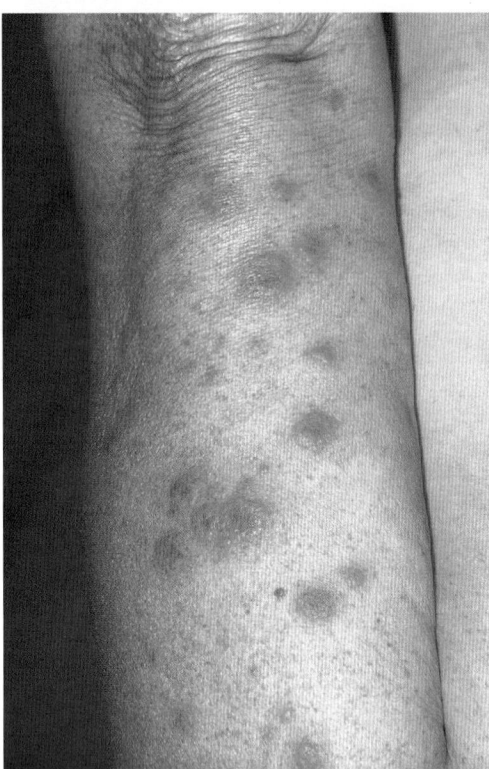

Fig. 16.9
Leukocytoclastic vasculitis: these urticarial lesions on the back of the arm resemble those of erythema multiforme. By courtesy of R.A. Marsden, MD, St George's Hospital, London, UK.

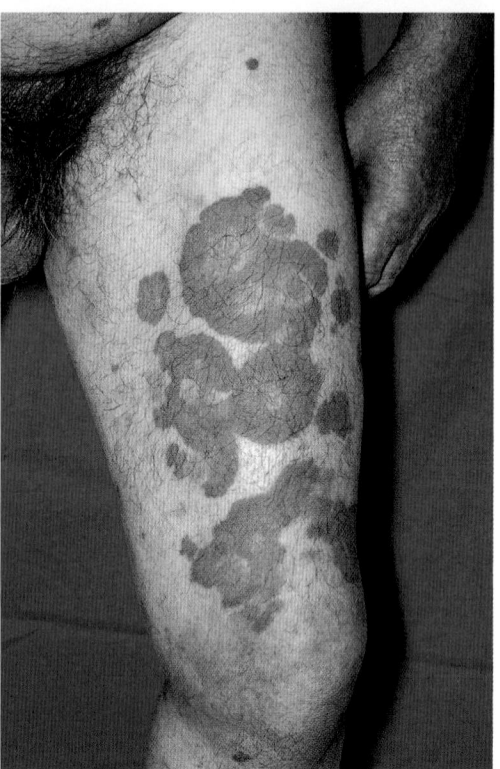

Fig. 16.11
Leukocytoclastic vasculitis: this patient has serological evidence of systemic lupus erythematosus.

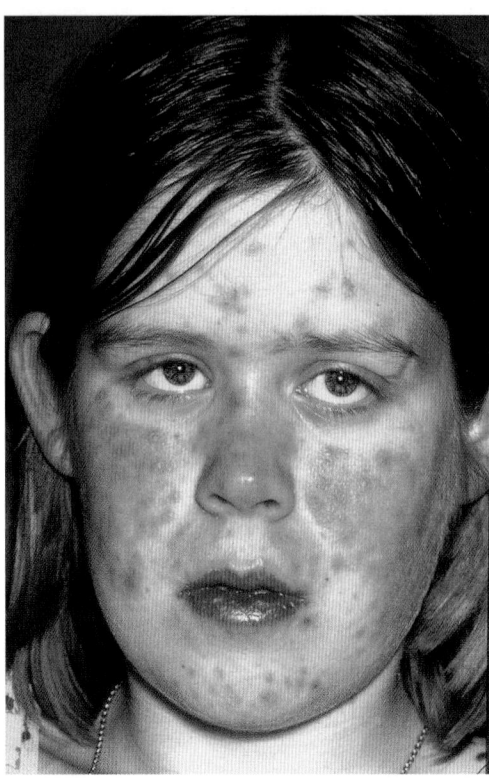

Fig. 16.10
Leukocytoclastic vasculitis: lesions may be widely disseminated in severely affected patients. By courtesy of R.A. Marsden, MD, St George's Hospital, London, UK.

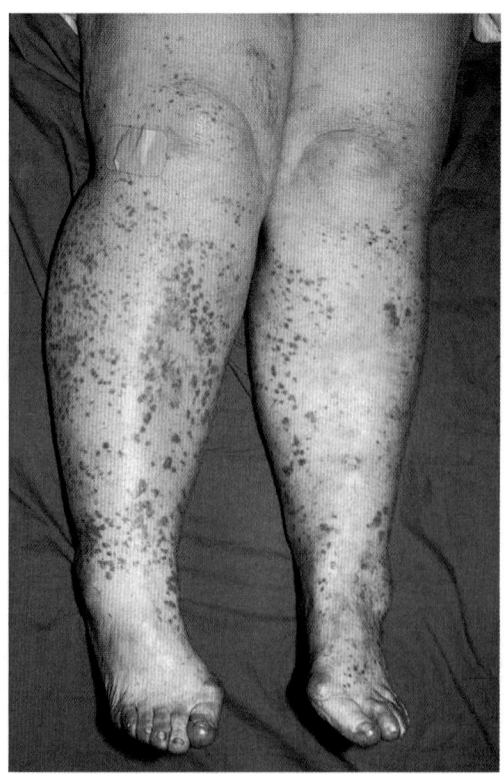

Fig. 16.12
Leukocytoclastic vasculitis: in addition to the typical maculopapular eruption there is marked swelling of the legs. By courtesy of R.A. Marsden, MD, St George's Hospital, London, UK.

cytarabine, erlotinib, rituximab, cinacalcet, famciclovir, rifampin, pyrazinamide, insulin aspart, metformin, gold, and disulfiram.[2,23–65] Levamisole has been described as producing a vasculitis localized to the ears in children.[66,67] More recently, levamisole has been implicated in vasculitis and thrombotic vasculopathy related to cocaine abuse, discussed in more detail below.[68–75] Localized leukocytoclastic vasculitis may occur at the site of interferon alpha injection.[76,77]

Collagen vascular disease (most often rheumatoid arthritis and lupus erythematosus) is commonly associated with leukocytoclastic vasculitis,[2,78] and in one study it was found in 21% of patients.[2] The presence of leukocytoclastic vasculitis in a patient with dermatomyositis raises the possibility of associated malignancy.[79–81]

Infection is also commonly associated with leukocytoclastic vasculitis, with bacterial, fungal, and viral infection all being implicated.[82] Associated bacterial infections include streptococci, *Klebsiella pneumoniae*, *Mycobacterium tuberculosis*, and *Mycoplasma pneumoniae*.[83–85] Systemic cat scratch disease presenting as leukocytoclastic vasculitis has been documented.[86] Hepatitis C infection is a particularly frequent association. It should be noted that hepatitis C is also often associated with cryoglobulins (see section on cryoglobulinemia).[87–91]

Inflammatory bowel disease, both ulcerative colitis and Crohn disease, may be coupled with leukocytoclastic vasculitis.[92–106] One study suggested that vasculitis was more commonly a complication of Crohn disease rather than ulcerative colitis.[106] In some patients with inflammatory bowel disease, there is evidence that implicates treatment with tumor necrosis alpha inhibitors as the inciting factor.[107–109] Further rare associations include sarcoidosis, α_1-antitrypsin deficiency, cystic fibrosis, and the Wiskott-Aldrich syndrome.[17,110,111]

Physical exercise has also been related to the development of leukocytoclastic vasculitis. Outdoor activities in hot weather such as walking, running, golfing (golfer's vasculitis), swimming, and dancing have especially been implicated and middle aged to elderly individuals are more frequently affected.[111–115] In the setting of exercise-induced vasculitis, venous stasis may be a contributing factor.[115] Leukocytoclastic vasculitis rarely represents a paraneoplastic manifestation of an underlying malignancy, especially leukemia and lymphoma.[116] Hairy cell leukemia is particularly often associated with leukocytoclastic vasculitis but other forms of vasculitis may also be seen.[117,118] In one study of 42 patients with hairy cell leukemia and vasculitis, 21 had leukocytoclastic vasculitis and 17 had polyarteritis nodosa.[117] In addition, four patients had direct infiltration of vessel walls by leukemic cells (see also section on paraneoplastic vasculitis). Although uncommon, leukocytoclastic vasculitis may also be seen in patients with a variety of solid tumors including non-small cell carcinoma of lung, adenocarcinoma of breast, colon, prostate, and kidney, papillary thyroid carcinoma, thymoma, and chondrosarcoma.[119–122]

Leukocytoclastic vasculitis can be a manifestation of human immunodeficiency virus (HIV) infection.[123,124] Unusual associations of this condition include the use of a nicotine patch, drug additives, sodium benzoate, protein A column pheresis, interleukin-12 receptor beta-1 deficiency, prolonged exercise, and as a complication of an infected hip prosthesis.[125–131]

Laboratory investigation may reveal an elevated erythrocyte sedimentation rate (ESR), proteinuria, or hematuria. In some idiopathic cases and in those associated with systemic disease (e.g., rheumatoid arthritis, systemic lupus erythematosus (SLE), and Sjögren syndrome), hypocomplementemia is sometimes evident.[5] Urinalysis may reveal proteinuria or hematuria. Cryoglobulins have been found in up to 25% of patients.[2] Perinuclear staining antineutrophil antibodies are present in about 20% of patients.[2,132]

The outcome of leukocytoclastic vasculitis is variable, ranging from a mild, self-limiting illness through to a serious, potentially fatal disorder due particularly to renal involvement.[21] About 1.9% of patients die of systemic disease.[2] Most patients have a benign outcome. An acute clinical course is seen in approximately 50% of patients.[2,11] A chronic course or one characterized by relapses and remissions is seen in some patients.[2] In one study of patients with hypersensitivity vasculitis, 54 did not require therapy, 26 were treated with nonsteroidal anti-inflammatory medications, and 14 required immunosuppressive agents, most often corticosteroids.[22]

Specific syndromes associated with leukocytoclastic vasculitis, such as urticarial vasculitis and Henoch-Schönlein purpura, are discussed under separate headings in this chapter.

Pathogenesis and histologic features

Leukocytoclastic vasculitis is an immune complex-mediated disorder similar to the classic Arthus reaction.[133] Immune complexes are deposited in the walls of small blood vessels.[5] This is associated with activation of the complement cascade and the production of C5a (a neutrophil polymorph chemotactant). The resultant polymorph influx is associated with release of lysosomal enzymes, including elastases and collagenases, resulting in blood vessel wall damage, fibrin deposition, and the release of red blood cells (purpura) into the perivenular connective tissue. Thrombosis may ensue and, in particularly severe examples, epidermal ischemic damage results. Lesions are particularly seen on the lower legs because of hydrostasis and blood vessel flow sludging.[5]

Evidence for an immune complex-mediated pathogenesis is convincing.[1] Patients have been clinically proven to have high levels of circulating immune complexes, and these are shown to correlate with vasculitic lesions. Immunoglobulin and complement can be identified in vitro, by immunofluorescence or immunoperoxidase techniques, and in biopsies from blood vessel wall lesions less than 24 hours old (*Fig. 16.13*).[134] Immune complexes can be identified ultrastructurally as clumps of electron-dense material, usually within the basement membrane between endothelial cells and pericytes of postcapillary venules. Examination of apparently uninvolved skin from patients with leukocytoclastic vasculitis sometimes shows immunoglobulin and complement within the walls of dermal blood vessels. If histamine is injected into uninvolved skin 3–4 hours previously, all the features of leukocytoclastic vasculitis are evident at biopsy, including neutrophil degeneration; this suggests that the immunoreactants are a cause rather than a consequence of the vasculitis.[1]

The findings of immunofluorescence studies vary according to the age of the lesion. Immunoglobulins have been described in up to 81% of patients.[9] In early lesions, C3 and IgM predominate, in fully developed lesions there is predominance of fibrinogen and IgG, and in late lesions fibrinogen and C3 are detected.[9]

Some authors, noting that early lesions may contain abundant CD3+, CD4+, and CD1a+ cells, have suggested that cell-mediated immune mechanisms may also play a role in the pathogenesis of leukocytoclastic vasculitis.[9] Consistent with this hypothesis is the demonstration of Langerhans cells in the late phase of vasculitis.[135] Expression of 72 kD heat shock protein and the presence of gamma/delta T cells in patients with vasculitis

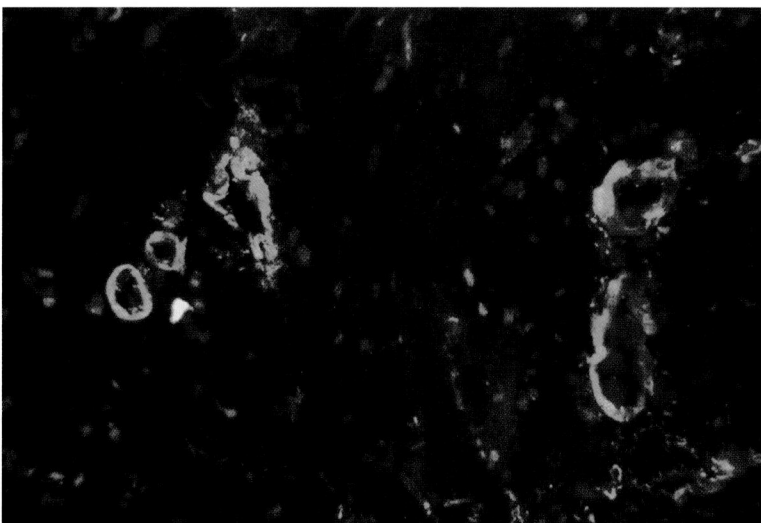

Fig. 16.13
Leukocytoclastic vasculitis: IgM is present in the blood vessel walls (direct immunofluorescence). By courtesy of B. Bhogal, FIMLS, Institute of Dermatology, London, UK.

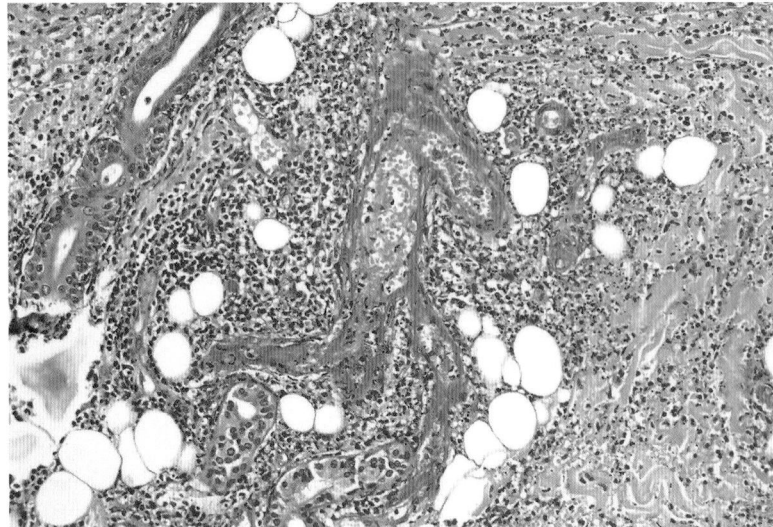

Fig. 16.14
Leukocytoclastic vasculitis: the blood vessels show florid fibrinoid necrosis and intense inflammation.

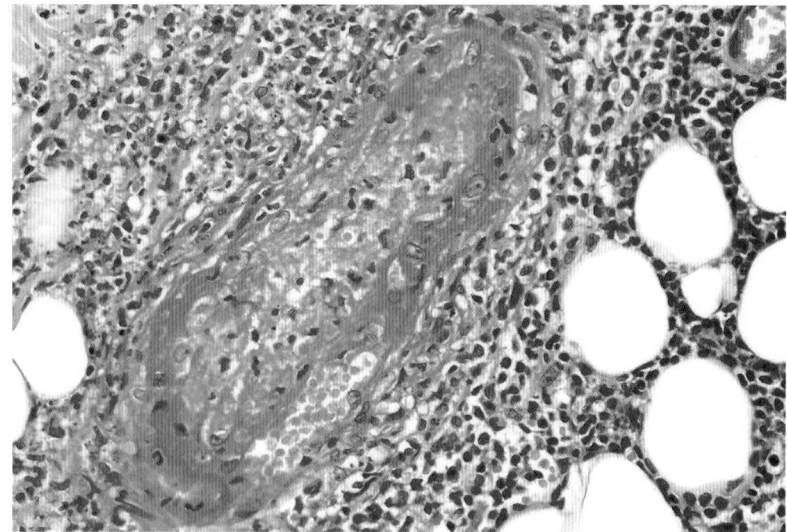

Fig. 16.16
Leukocytoclastic vasculitis: high-power view showing fibrinoid necrosis and a mixed inflammatory cell infiltrate composed of neutrophils, eosinophils, and lymphocytes. There is marked leukocytoclasis (karyorrhexis, nuclear dust).

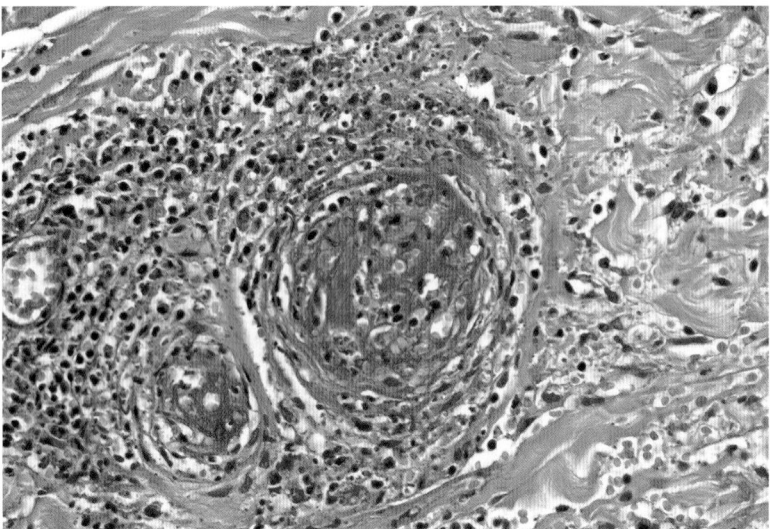

Fig. 16.15
Leukocytoclastic vasculitis: high-power view showing complete vessel wall destruction.

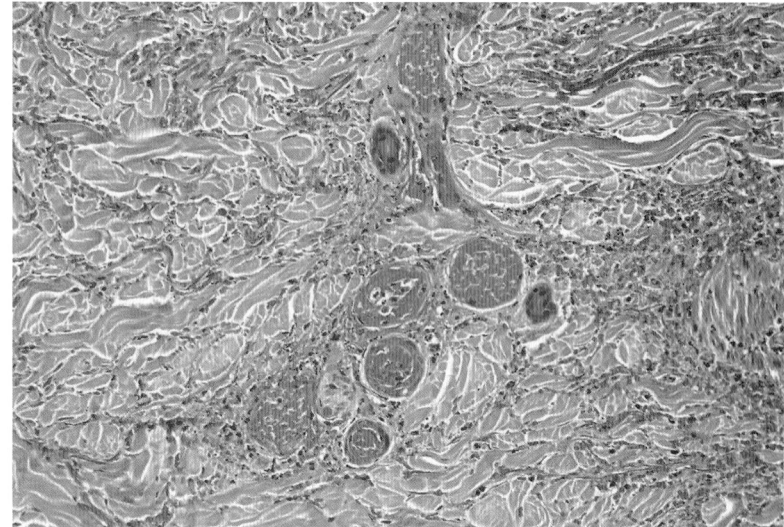

Fig. 16.17
Leukocytoclastic vasculitis: vascular thrombosis as seen in this field is not uncommon.

associated with infection have led one group of authors to postulate that the cell-mediated immune response plays an important role in that subset.[136]

In leukocytoclastic vasculitis, it is the postcapillary venule and the capillary loops (and not the arteriole) which are primarily affected, usually within the superficial dermis (*Figs 16.14* and *16.15*). In severe cases, particularly those associated with malignancy or connective tissue disease, the inflammatory changes extend into the vasculature of the deep reticular dermis or even the subcutaneous fat.[10] The histologic features are similar irrespective of the underlying etiology.

The histologic features of leukocytoclastic vasculitis are those of fibrinoid necrosis associated with endothelial cell swelling and infiltration of the blood vessel walls by neutrophils and conspicuous nuclear dust (*Fig. 16.16*).[2,132,137,138] Variable numbers of mononuclear cells and eosinophils may be seen. In early lesions, nuclear dust is associated with a perivascular neutrophilic infiltrate but multiple tissue sections may be needed to identify fibrinoid vascular changes. The former features, even without unequivocal fibrinoid change, are suggestive of an evolving leukocytoclastic vasculitis. In late lesions lymphocytes may be more prominent than neutrophils.

Intravascular thrombi and ischemic necrosis of the overlying epidermis (often with bullae formation) may sometimes be seen (*Figs 16.17–16.19*). Occasionally, one may encounter intradermal or subepidermal pustules.

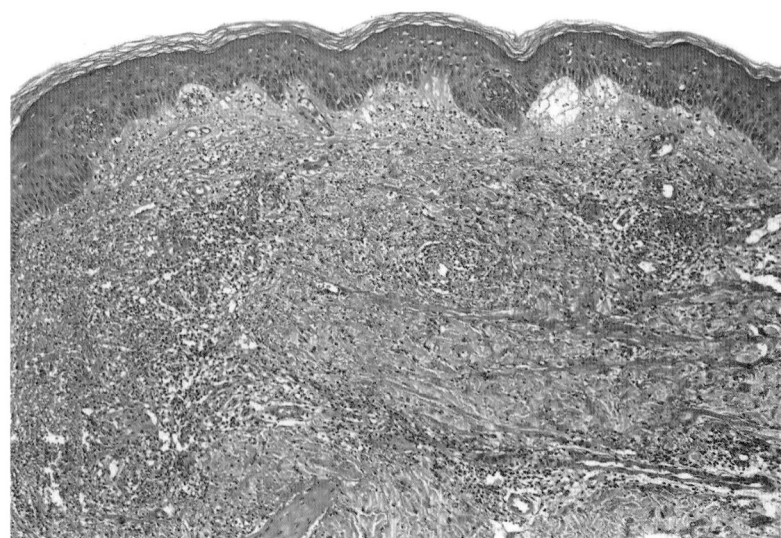

Fig. 16.18
Leukocytoclastic vasculitis: in this example, there is incipient subepidermal vesiculation.

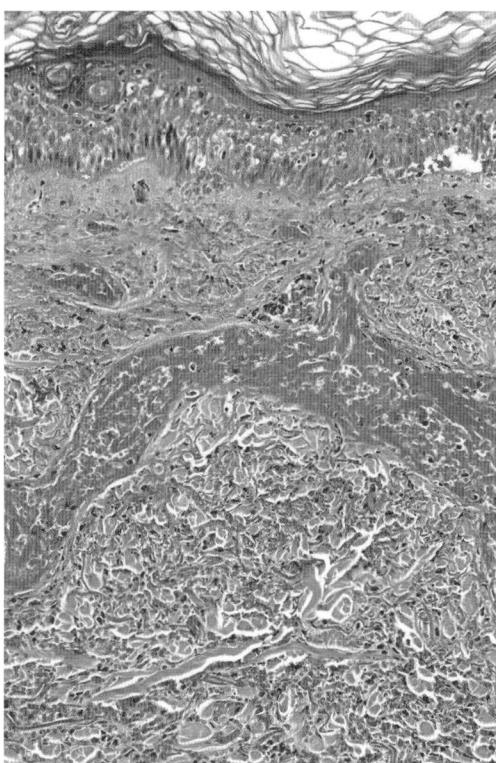

Fig. 16.19
Leukocytoclastic vasculitis: vascular thrombosis is accompanied by epidermal infarction. Note the cytoplasmic eosinophilia and loss of nuclei.

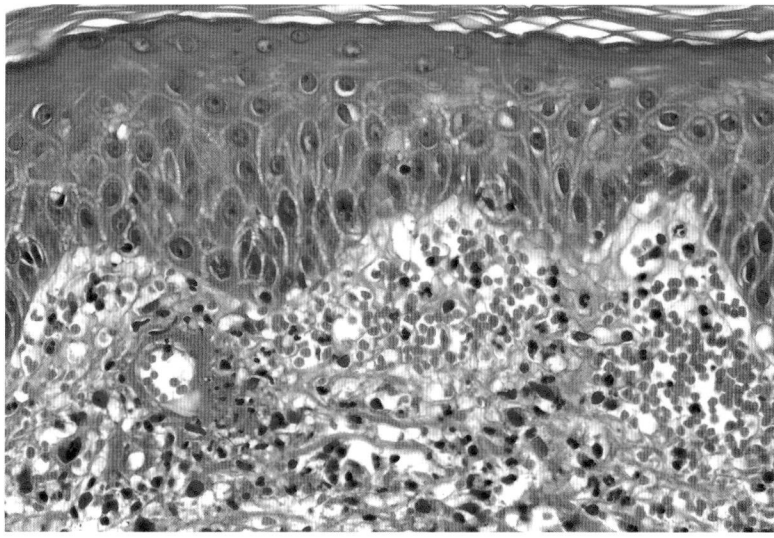

Fig. 16.20
Leukocytoclastic vasculitis: note the marked red cell extravasation.

In patients with associated hypocomplementemia, neutrophils are predominant with far fewer lymphocytes; patients who are normocomplementemic may show lymphocyte predominance. In the surrounding connective tissue, red cell extravasation, edema, and an inflammatory neutrophil infiltrate associated with karyorrhexis (leukocytoclasis) are typically present (*Fig. 16.20*).

The severity of the histopathological changes in the cutaneous lesions of leukocytoclastic vasculitis does not predict extracutaneous involvement.[139]

Differential diagnosis

The diagnosis is relatively straightforward. It is critical to understand that leukocytoclastic vasculitis is not a disease sui generis. Rather, it represents a reaction pattern due to circulating immune complexes that may be caused by myriad underlying disorders. Furthermore, leukocytoclastic vasculitis is frequently encountered in association with other forms of vasculitis. For example, it is much more commonly encountered in patients with granulomatosis with polyangiitis than granulomatous vasculitis. Therefore, a biopsy showing leukocytoclastic vasculitis does not exclude diseases that may be associated with other forms of vasculitis. Sometimes it coexists with a large-vessel vasculitis. An inadequate biopsy that does not include deep dermis and subcutaneous tissue containing large vessels can produce misleading results. The presence of leukocytoclastic vasculitis in a superficial biopsy does not exclude an associated large-vessel vasculitis; therefore the report of a superficial biopsy from a patient suspected of having large-vessel vasculitis should comment on the lack of larger vessels for evaluation.

Sweet syndrome may resemble leukocytoclastic vasculitis; however, the presence of a diffuse (rather than predominantly perivascular) neutrophilic infiltrate without fibrinoid vascular change or necrosis favors the former condition.

IgA vasculitis (Henoch-Schönlein purpura)

Clinical features

IgA vasculitis (Henoch-Schönlein purpura) is a syndrome characterized by abdominal pain, joint symptoms, and palpable purpura secondary to leukocytoclastic vasculitis, and caused by circulating IgA immune complexes. The disease typically involves children (males more often than females), although adults may also be affected.[1-6] Occurrence during pregnancy has only rarely been documented.[7] In a large study of children with Henoch-Schönlein purpura, 92% of patients were less than 10 years of age.[8]

It often complicates an upper respiratory tract infection and is characterized by a seasonal incidence with a peak in winter.[1] Clustering of cases has been described, leading one group of authors to postulate that person-to-person spread of an infectious agent plays a role in the pathogenesis of this syndrome.[9] Although it may follow a streptococcal throat infection, it sometimes develops after a wide variety of other infective conditions including amebiasis, chickenpox, hepatitis, HIV, yersiniosis, and infection by *Toxocara canis*, *Helicobacter pylori*, *Pseudomonas aeruginosa*, *Staphylococcus aureus*, *Escherichia coli*, and erythrovirus (formerly parvovirus) B19.[10-15] In one series >30% had documentation of some sort of an infection prior to the development of vasculitis.[5] Additional causes include adverse reactions to drugs such as ampicillin, penicillin, erythromycin, clarithromycin, glyburide, etanercept, infliximab, and adulmumab.[16-22] An association with cocaine inhalation has also been described.[23] In one study, drug therapy may have been a precipitating cause in 26% of patients.[24]

As noted above, classic IgA vasculitis is characterized by a triad of purpura, abdominal pain, and arthralgia. The cutaneous clinical findings are those of leukocytoclastic vasculitis. Cutaneous lesions are most frequently the presenting symptom and comprise palpable purpura predominantly affecting the lower limbs, thighs, and buttocks (*Fig. 16.21*).[1,5,25-27] Targetoid lesions are often present.[28] Hemorrhagic bullae are uncommon.[5,29-31] Rare pustules and subcutaneous nodules have also been documented.[5,32] A prodrome of itchy urticaria is sometimes described.[2] Children often have edema, particularly of the feet and lower legs, although it may be more widespread.

In one large study, arthritis was seen in 82% of patients and was the presenting feature in 24%.[8] Joint involvement consists of migratory arthralgia predominantly affecting the large joints of the lower limbs. Involvement of the upper extremity occurred in 37%, with the hand and wrist being more often affected than the elbow.[8]

Intestinal involvement with resultant red cell extravasation or hemorrhage leads to abdominal pain and gastrointestinal bleeding. Abdominal pain was noted in 63% of patients in one study of 100 consecutive children presenting with the condition.[8] Gastrointestinal disease develops as a consequence of acute vasculitis. Bleeding may be either occult or in the form of bloody stools.[8] Intussusception is an occasional complication.[33,34] Abdominal pain was the presenting complaint in 19% of patients in one study.[8] Endoscopy may reveal hemorrhage, ulceration, and erosions.[35] IgA is often noted in capillaries of the gastrointestinal tract but frank necrotizing vasculitis was

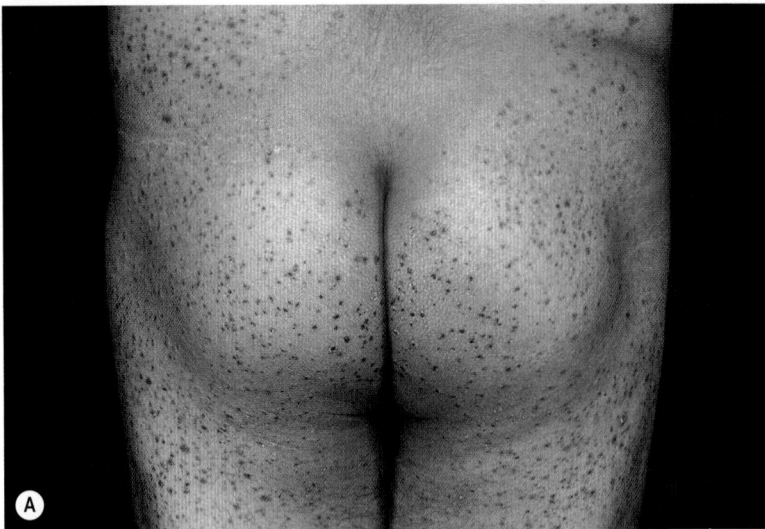

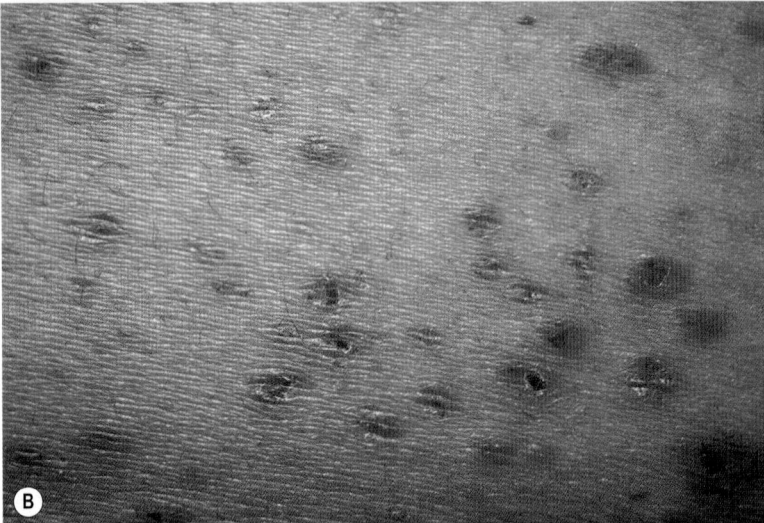

Fig. 16.21

(**A**, **B**) Henoch-Schönlein purpura: palpable purpura in the classical distribution on the buttocks and thighs. From the collection of the late N.P. Smith, MD, the Institute of Dermatology, London, UK.

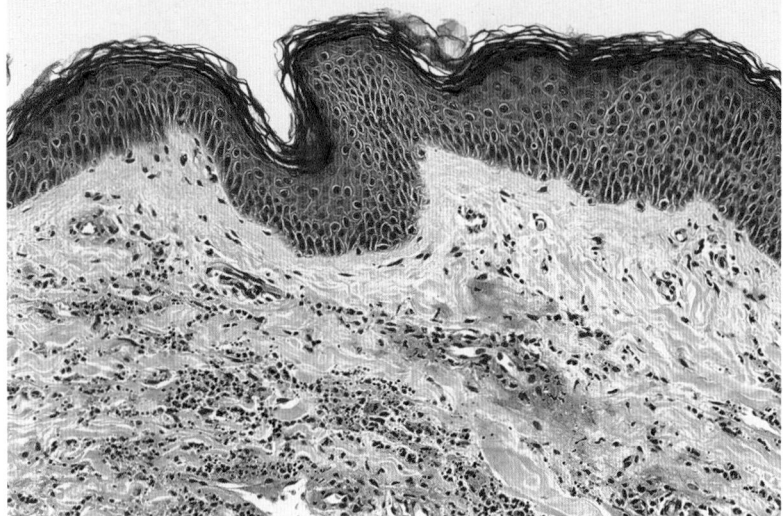

Fig. 16.22

Henoch-Schönlein purpura: this small venule shows striking fibrinoid change. There is considerable red cell extravasation.

not seen in any patients in two series.[35,36] Rarely, gastrointestinal involvement with minimal skin lesions is encountered.[37]

Renal symptoms are variable and include microscopic hematuria, acute nephritic syndrome, nephrotic syndrome, and acute or chronic renal failure. The pathological features seen on renal biopsy range from mild focal glomerulonephritis to necrotizing or proliferative glomerulonephritis.[1,8] In a consecutive series of 100 pediatric patients, a single patient required transplantation.[8] Patients older than 7 years are at increased risk of renal involvement.[38]

Orchitis is a recognized complication of IgA vasculitis, affecting 14% of male patients.[8,25]

Neurological involvement may be manifested by headaches, seizures, mental status changes, and, less frequently, ataxia and peripheral neuropathy.[39–41] Neurological manifestations may be seen in up to one third of patients.[41]

Low serum C3, leukopenia, and thrombocytopenia are rare findings.[42]

IgA vasculitis in children is generally associated with a good prognosis, with less than 2% suffering long-term morbidity.[43,44] However, patients do occasionally die from renal failure, gastrointestinal infarction, or respiratory involvement. In contrast to pediatric patients, adults are thought to have a worse prognosis, with remission of renal disease seen in as low as 21% of patients.[45] In contrast, one study found that although older patients had more severe symptoms, including frequent renal involvement, prognosis was equally good in young and older patients.[46] In another study, complete recovery was seen in 67% of adults after a median follow-up period of 36

months.[12] In a further series, a third of patients suffered at least one recurrence of symptoms, usually within a few months of initial presentation.[8] Recurrences were also found to be more frequent in patients >8 years of age and in those with nephritis.[25]

Solid tumors including lung, prostate, breast and gastrointestinal cancer, and hematological malignancy have been associated with IgA vasculitis.[47–51] One study found that nearly a third of adults with IgA vasculitis purpura had an associated tumor.[47] For this reason, the authors concluded that physicians should suspect an underlying malignancy in older patients (especially males of 40 years or more) with IgA vasculitis.[48]

Pulmonary hemorrhage is a rare complication that may prove fatal.[52,53]

Pathogenesis and histologic features

An incomplete picture of the pathogenesis of IgA vasculitis/Henoch-Schönlein purpura has emerged. As noted above, it seems a wide variety of infective agents may trigger this disease. It is associated with IgA deposition in blood vessel walls, both in the dermis and in the renal glomerulus (mesangium). IgA1 is the major IgA subclass found in the dermal, gastrointestinal, and glomerular blood vessels.[54,55] Fibrinogen and C3 are also usually present. Raised levels of serum IgA and IgE are present in some, but not all, patients.[8] IgA antineutrophil cytoplasmic antibodies (ANCA) and IgA anticardiolipin antibodies have also been documented.[56,57] There is evidence that patients have an increased number of IgA-type B cells.[58] More recently, IgA-binding regions from streptococcal M proteins have been identified in a significant subset of skin and renal biopsies from patients with Henoch-Schönlein purpura.[59]

The finding of IgA deposition by immunofluorescence is not equivalent to a diagnosis of IgA vasculitis and must be correlated with the clinical presentation.[60] A vasculitis with the presence of IgA deposition in patients lacking other typical features of Henoch-Schönlein purpura has been described in association with cancer, granulomatosis with polyangiitis, and inflammatory bowel disease.[61] The observation of an association between DRB1*01 and DRB1*11 and Henoch-Schönlein purpura suggests a genetic susceptibility in some patients.[62,63] Other authors have suggested that DQA1*0301 and C4 deletion may also represent risk factors for IgA nephropathy as well as Henoch-Schönlein nephritis.[64] In a study from Taiwan, children with atopic dermatitis had a 1.75-fold increased risk for IgA vasculitis compared with matched controls.[65]

Biopsies of cutaneous lesions show features of typical leukocytoclastic vasculitis (*Fig. 16.22*).

Differential diagnosis

The histologic differential diagnosis includes other forms of leukocytoclastic vasculitis. Since IgA deposition can be seen in the blood vessel walls of patients with leukocytoclastic vasculitis but without of the clinical manifestations of IgA vasculitis/Henoch-Schönlein purpura, this finding is not diagnostic in isolation.[60,66] In one study, only 24% of patients with vascular IgA deposition had Henoch-Schönlein purpura.[66] Other studies have demonstrated a strong correlation with vascular deposits of IgA and IgA vasculitis.[5,67,68] The sensitivity and specificity has been reported to exceed 80%.[5] Nevertheless, careful clinical correlation is necessary to establish the diagnosis.

Infantile acute hemorrhagic edema

Clinical features

Infantile hemorrhagic edema is a form of leukocytoclastic vasculitis that is mostly seen in newborns but has also been described in the first 3 years of life and occasionally in older children.[1-11] The disease is usually limited to the skin but mucosal involvement may be an additional feature.[10] Transient renal involvement with microscopic hematuria and proteinemia, hypocomplementemia, abdominal pain, and elevated transaminases are exceptional additional findings.[12,13] It frequently follows vaccination or infection including otitis, upper respiratory tract infection, or conjunctivitis.[1,10,11] An association with cytomegalovirus, herpes simplex virus-1, or rotavirus infection has been documented.[14-16] Since many children had received antibiotics for infection prior to development of lesions, a subset of cases may represent reaction to medication.[1] This disease has a peak incidence in the winter months.

Skin lesions are widely distributed, and often involve the head and neck, and limbs. They present as purpuric lesions that often have a rosette or targetoid configuration.[2,3] The cheeks and ears seem to be sites of predilection.[3,11] Resolution within a few weeks is typical and recurrences are not reported.[1,11,17]

An elevated ESR and leukocytosis are usually present.

Pathogenesis and histologic features

The pathogenesis of infantile hemorrhagic edema is unknown; however, it is likely that the disease is immune mediated. Biopsy shows features of leukocytoclastic vasculitis with variable fibrinoid necrosis.[3]

Differential diagnosis

Some authors consider infantile hemorrhagic edema to be a variant of IgA vasculitis. Others do not agree, arguing that the absence of perivascular IgA on immunofluorescence staining, absence of systemic involvement in most patients, and the benign clinical course do not support this view.[3,18] However, a very interesting link between the two diseases has been postulated.[19] Goraya and Kaur note that, since the IgA immune system in infants is immature, if acute hemorrhagic edema were related to IgA vasculitis, the patient would be incapable of mounting an IgA-mediated immune response and this would explain the lack of IgA on immunofluorescence studies in the majority of patients.[19] Clearly, further study of this disorder is necessary to elucidate its pathogenesis and to clarify its nosological position in the classification of leukocytoclastic vasculitis.

Urticarial vasculitis

Clinical features

Urticarial vasculitis is an uncommon condition characterized clinically by urticaria and histologically by leukocytoclastic venulitis.[1-5] In addition to urticarial skin lesions, patients may also experience angioedema, arthralgia, gastrointestinal symptoms, and evidence of renal involvement.[6,7] The term encompasses a spectrum of illness, with some patients experiencing only mild symptoms while others develop serious systemic involvement.[7,8]

Urticarial vasculitis is most often seen in the third to fifth decades and shows a female predominance.[7] The cutaneous lesions are urticarial in appearance, consisting of edematous, raised, erythematous plaques associated with nonblanchable purpura (*Figs 16.23* and *16.24*). However, in contrast to uncomplicated urticaria, cutaneous lesions of urticarial vasculitis

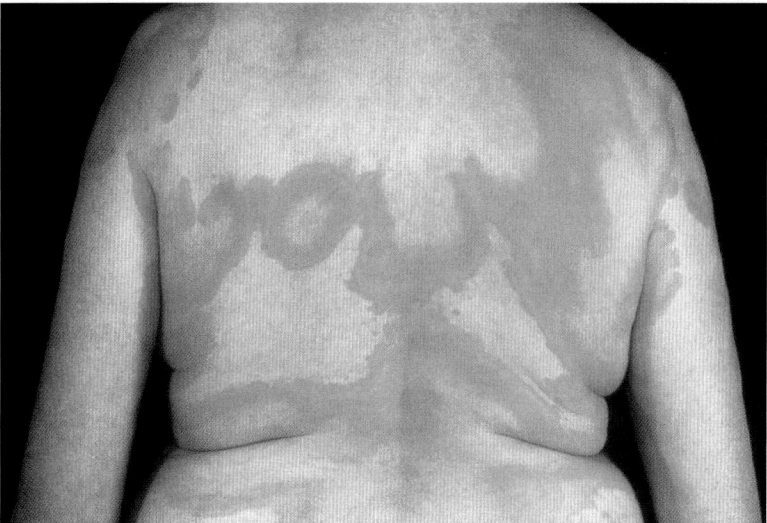

Fig. 16.23
Urticarial vasculitis: this very large lesion has developed a bizarre outline due to central clearing. By courtesy of the Institute of Dermatology, London, UK.

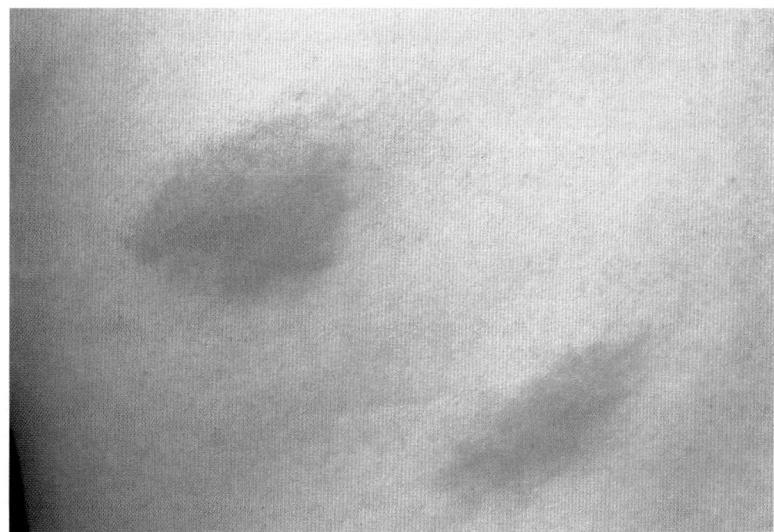

Fig. 16.24
Urticarial vasculitis: close-up view. By courtesy of the Institute of Dermatology, London, UK.

often last 24–72 hours.[9] Patients commonly complain of pruritus, burning, or pain. The frequency of cutaneous symptoms varies considerably, from daily to monthly.

Joint pain, stiffness, and swelling, particularly of the hands, elbows, feet, ankles, and knees, are seen; however, frank arthritis is extremely rare.[10] Hypocomplementemia, which correlates with systemic involvement, is a feature in many patients.[4,7,8,11-13] Patients with hypocomplementemia may have musculoskeletal involvement, ocular involvement, pulmonary involvement, and gastrointestinal involvement in decreasing order of frequency.[13] Proteinuria and hematuria may also be noted. Rarely, patients develop focal or diffuse proliferative glomerulonephritis. Crescentic glomerulonephritis, mesangial glomerulonephritis, and membranous nephropathy have also been documented.[8,14-19] Gastrointestinal symptoms can include abdominal pain, nausea, vomiting, and diarrhea, and an associated peripheral neuropathy has been reported.[13,20]

The ESR is raised in many patients with hypocomplementemia. There may also be depression of the early classic pathway components C1q, C4, and C2. Patients with hypocomplementemic urticarial vasculitis have a high prevalence of autoantibodies to endothelial cells.[21,22] Elevated rheumatoid factor has also been reported.[23]

Schnitzler syndrome is a term that has been applied to patients with urticarial vasculitis and monoclonal IgM gammopathy.[24–29] Hepatospleno-megaly, elevated ESR and white blood cell count, fever, and joint pain are characteristic features.[25–27] An associated monoclonal IgA gammopathy has been reported and an underlying lymphoproliferative disorder is present in some patients.[24,30,31] In one series, 90% had a monoclonal IgM gammopathy, 5% had a monoclonal IgA gammopathy, and 5% had a monoclonal IgG gammopathy. Interestingly, these patients had perivascular and/or interstitial neutrophilic infiltrate or a mononuclear infiltrate with eosinophils, but none had vasculitis.[32] The current Strasbourg criteria in fact do not require vasculitis. Obligate criteria include a chronic urticarial rash and a monoclonal IgM or IgG gammopathy. Minor criteria include recurrent fever, objective findings of abnormal bone remodeling, neutrophilic dermal infiltrate, and leukocytosis and/or elevated CRP. Patients with IgM paraproteinemia require both obligate criteria and two minor criteria, while patients with IgG paraprotein-emia require both obligate criteria and three minor criteria.[33] These criteria have >80% sensitivity and >90% specificity for the diagnosis.[34]

Importantly, urticarial vasculitis (especially the hypocomplementemic variant) is often associated with, or heralds the onset of, a variety of systemic diseases, including SLE, arthritis, interstitial lung disease, pericarditis, mixed connective tissue disease, systemic sclerosis, relapsing polychondritis, hepatitis, inflammatory bowel disease, serum sickness, polyarteritis nodosa and Granulomatosis with polyangiitis, viral infection, Sjögren syndrome, cryoglobulinemia, polycythemia rubra vera, reaction to drugs (including cocaine and diltiazem), and as a response to sunlight.[8,13,14,35–46] The condition may be exacerbated by methotrexate.[47] More than 50% of patients had uveitis, scleritis, conjunctivitis, or episcleritis.[8,13] It appears that patients with hypocomplementemia have more severe disease.[38] Some authors have postulated that hypocomplementemic urticarial vasculitis represents a subset of SLE. Others, however, have failed to confirm this observation.[8,48,49]

Urticarial vasculitis has been documented in association with malignancy.[8,50–58] Given the rarity of this association, this may well be coincidental. Nevertheless, a diagnosis of urticarial vasculitis should always initiate an evaluation for possible underlying disease. Urticarial vasculitis usually has a benign outcome.[8]

Pathogenesis and histologic features

In many patients, no underlying cause is discovered. In others, antibody-antigen complexes (a type III hypersensitivity reaction) is implicated.[4,5] Mutations in *DNASE1L3* have been identified in two families with autosomal recessive hypocomplementemic urticarial vasculitis.[59] Mutations in this same gene have been implicated in SLE.

The vasculitis affects the superficial vascular plexus and is characterized by a leukocytoclastic pattern (*Fig. 16.25*). Extravasation of red blood cells is evidence of vascular damage. A background of dermal edema may be seen. Often, the histologic features are subtle and are easily overlooked, with only focal fibrinoid vascular change, few neutrophils, and sparse karyorrhexis. In our experience, the vasculitis is usually low grade or subtle in nature; however, more impressive necrotizing vasculitis is seen in some patients. Others have shown that endothelial necrosis is unusual.[5]

In summary, urticarial vasculitis may show a spectrum of histologic changes ranging from urticaria with very mild vascular injury to frank necrotizing vasculitis.[60]

Differential diagnosis

Clinical correlation is necessary to distinguish urticarial vasculitis from other forms of leukocytoclastic vasculitis. Although urticarial vasculitis is often associated with subtle low-grade vascular injury, this feature should not be relied upon in its distinction from other forms of vasculitis. In short, the pathologist's role in diagnosis is to confirm the presence of vasculitis.

Granulomatosis with polyangiitis

Clinical features

Granulomatosis with polyangiitis is a multisystem vascular disease associated with high morbidity and mortality.[1–3] Before the introduction of

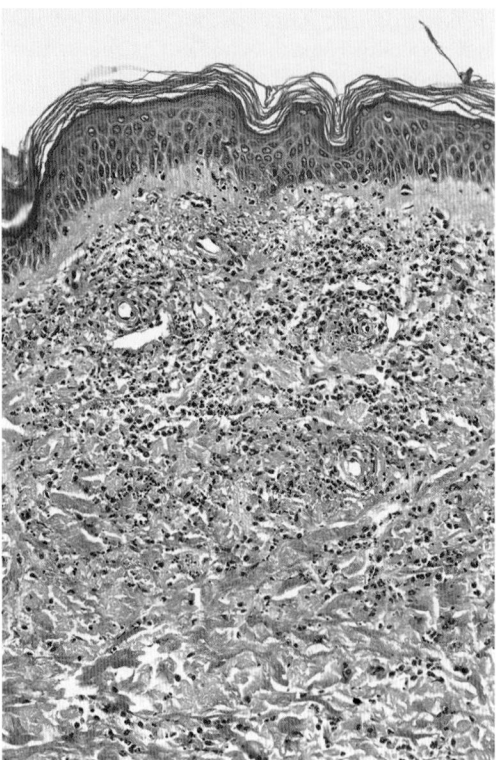

Fig. 16.25
Urticarial vasculitis: the changes are unusually florid in this example.

cyclophosphamide therapy it was associated with a dismal prognosis. Mean survival was of the order of 5 months following diagnosis and approximately 80% of patients died within 1 year, most as a consequence of renal involvement.

Although it may present in a wide variety of age groups, from infancy to the elderly, it is the middle aged that are predominantly affected, with a peak incidence in the fourth decade.[1–5] There is a slight predilection for males (3:2). In one large study, 97% of patients were Caucasians.[6]

Granulomatosis with polyangiitis comprises a triad of characteristics:
- necrotizing, destructive, granulomatous lesions in the upper respiratory tract (nose, nasal sinuses, nasopharynx, and larynx) and/or in the lower respiratory tract (trachea, bronchi or lungs); frequently, both are present. Similar lesions may also be found in virtually any organ in the body,
- a generalized focal vasculitis occurring in a wide variety of sites, but particularly affecting the lungs,
- glomerulonephritis.[3,7,8]

Early in the disease, when patients may not have developed the full clinical triad, definitive diagnosis can be difficult or impossible (see *Table 16.3*). According to the current Chapel Hill criteria, glomerulonephritis is not requisite for the diagnosis.[3] The most common presenting symptoms relate to involvement of the nose and nasal sinuses, and include severe and often purulent nasal discharge or evidence of sinusitis with pain and discharge. Clinical examination may reveal mucosal ulceration, perforated septum, paranasal sinusitis, or a saddle-nose deformity. Serous or purulent otitis media is occasionally a presenting feature. Middle and inner ear involvement is also a common manifestation of disease.[9–12]

Pulmonary lesions are present in up to 90% and patients may have cough, chest pain, or hemoptysis.[12] Radiological examination frequently reveals solitary or more commonly multiple nodular opacities, which are often bilateral, may be diffuse or sharply delineated, and are typically transient. Cavitation is frequently a feature. Lesions may present as large nodules that are clinically and radiologically suspicious for malignancy.

Renal involvement is usually in the form of focal segmental necrotizing glomerulonephritis.[12] Urinalysis typically reveals hematuria (often microscopic), proteinuria, and red cell casts.

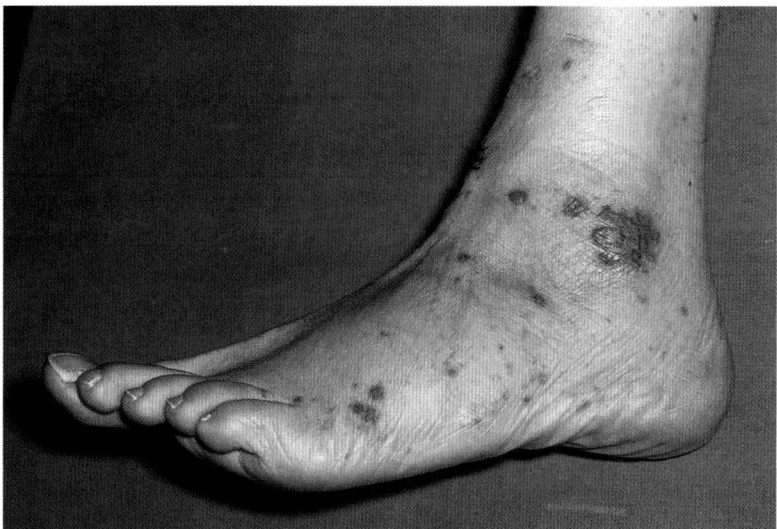

Fig. 16.26
Granulomatosis with polyangiitis: multiple purpuric macules and papules. By courtesy of D. McGibbon, MD, St Thomas' Hospital, London, UK.

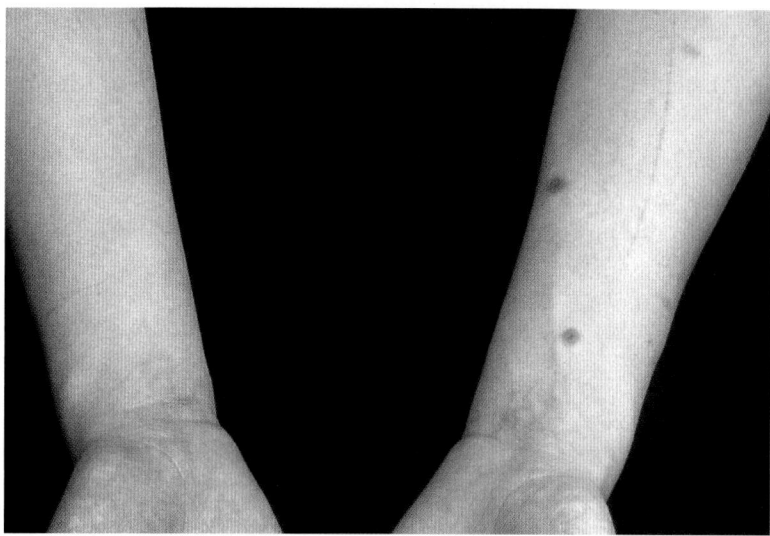

Fig. 16.27
Granulomatosis with polyangiitis: cutaneous nodules as seen in this patient are a not uncommon manifestation. By courtesy of the Institute of Dermatology, London, UK.

Table 16.3
1990 criteria for the classification of granulomatosis with polyangiitis (traditional format)*

Criterion	Definition
Nasal or oral inflammation	Development of painful or painless oral ulcers or purulent or bloody nasal discharge
Abnormal chest radiograph	Chest radiograph showing the presence of nodules, fixed infiltrates or cavities
Urinary sediment	Microhematuria (>5 red blood cells per high-power field) or red cell casts in urine sediment
Granulomatous inflammation on biopsy	Histologic changes showing granulomatous inflammation within the wall of an artery or in the perivascular or extravascular area (artery or arteriole)

*For purposes of classification, a patient shall be said to have Granulomatosis with polyangiitis if at least two of these four criteria are present. The presence of any two or more criteria yields a sensitivity of 88.2% and a specificity of 92.0%
Reproduced with permission from Leavitt, R.Y. (1990) *Arthritis & Rheumatism*, 33, 1101–1107.

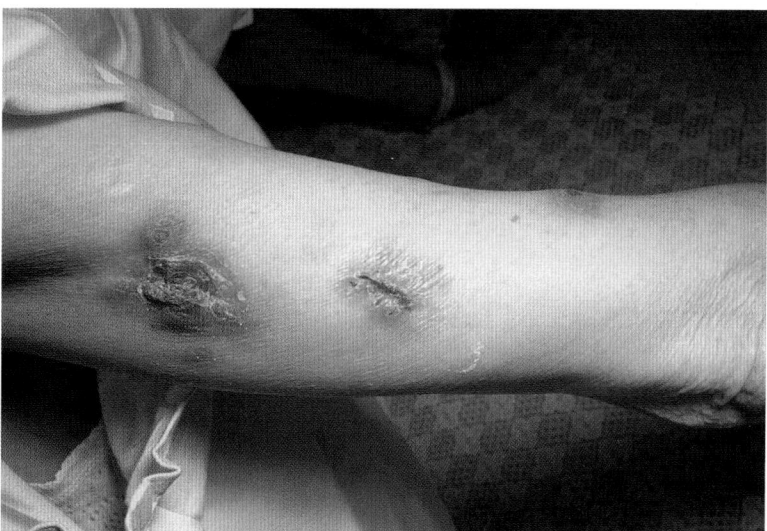

Fig. 16.28
Granulomatosis with polyangiitis: this patient has ulcerating plaques and nodules. By courtesy of the Institute of Dermatology, London, UK.

Joint involvement may present as arthralgia or, less commonly, frank arthritis.

In one large series, 34% of patients developed neurological involvement.[13] Peripheral neuropathy was seen in 16%.[13] Central nervous system (CNS) lesions are not uncommon and occur either as a consequence of direct extension through the base of the skull from sinus involvement or as a result of meningeal or intracerebral necrotizing granulomata. Patients may experience myelopathy or neuropathy.[14] Vasculitis involving intracerebral vessels can also result in cerebral lesions. Patients develop cranioneuropathy, cerebrovascular accidents, or seizures.[13] Involvement of the vasa nervosa may give rise to mononeuritis multiplex.

Ocular lesions result in a variety of complications including conjunctivitis, granulomatous keratitis, sclerouveitis, and orbital pseudotumor. Proptosis is sometimes a feature.[15] Involvement of the temporal artery results in features (i.e., vision loss, jaw claudication) similar to those seen in temporal arteritis.[16]

Cutaneous manifestations are common, occurring in about 10% to 50% of patients.[12,17–20] Several different types of skin lesion may be encountered, including vasculitic lesions with purpura, bruising, and nodule formation (*Figs 16.26–16.28*). Pyoderma gangrenosum-like lesions with necrosis and ulceration that have a predilection for the lower limbs are sometimes encountered. The presence of skin lesions appears to correlate with disease activity. Oral ulceration is common.[20,21]

In addition to the organ-specific features noted above, patients also often have a variety of constitutional symptoms, including anorexia, weight loss, fever, and general malaise.

Two limited forms are recognized: pathergic granulomatosis and limited pulmonary granulomatosis.[22–24]

- Pathergic granulomatosis is of particular importance because mucosal and cutaneous lesions may predominate and persist for very long periods of time before intractable renal failure develops. In the absence of evidence of pulmonary and renal involvement, there may be a delay in establishing the diagnosis and administration of appropriate chemotherapy, with resultant increased morbidity and mortality. Patients with this variant are at particular risk of facial mutilation; sites especially involved include the nose, nasopharynx, sinuses, and middle ears (*Fig. 16.29*).
- In limited pulmonary granulomatosis patients have respiratory symptoms with associated fever and weight loss. Radiologically, multiple bilateral discrete nodular infiltrates and thin-walled cavitating lesions are seen, usually in the lower lobes. No evidence for renal involvement is present. Patients with this variant appear to have a somewhat better prognosis than those with classic (generalized) granulomatosis with polyangiitis.

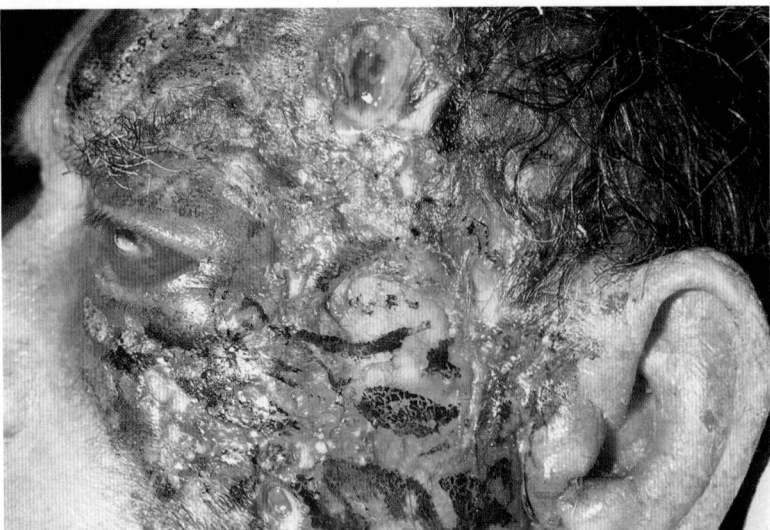

Fig. 16.29
Pathergic granulomatosis: gross necrosis and ulceration have resulted in very disfiguring tissue damage.

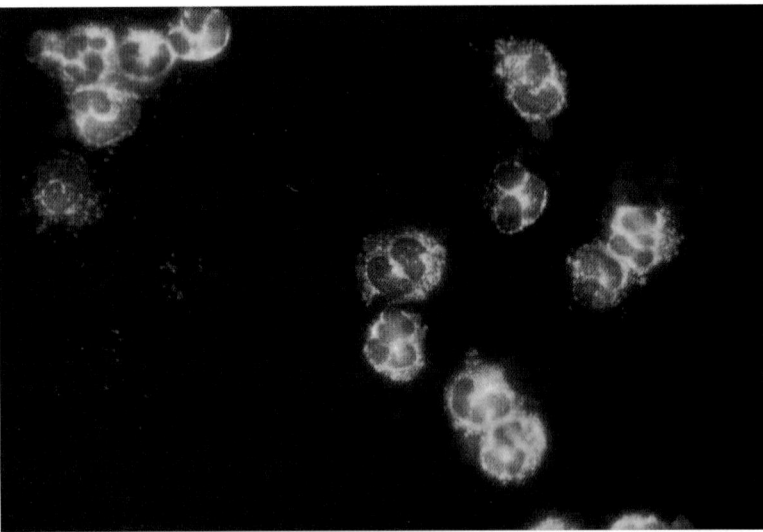

Fig. 16.30
Granulomatosis with polyangiitis: c-ANCA. By courtesy of G. Swana, MD, St Thomas' Hospital, London, UK.

It has been suggested that the presence of extravascular granulomata (particularly affecting the ears, nose, throat, orbit, or lung) in association with a positive serum cytoplasmic-antineutrophil cytoplasmic antibody (c-ANCA) represents the earliest stage in the evolution of granulomatosis with polyangiitis.[25] There are cases in which patients had relatively minor symptoms in which serological testing for c-ANCA helped establish the diagnosis.[26] There are also case reports of patients with smoldering symptoms that fully develop vasculitis after many years.[27] While these cases are exceptional, it does suggest that some cases may be diagnosed at an early stage before the development of more serious multisystem disease and, hence, earlier treatment.

Greater than 90% of patients with granulomatosis and polyangiitis have ANCA detected in their sera; rising titers have been shown to correlate with disease activity and are a valuable method of predicting relapse.[2,28,29] Typically, the indirect immunofluorescence shows a cytoplasmic pattern of staining (c-ANCA) (*Fig. 16.30*).[1] In the majority (70–80%) of patients with active disease ANCAs are directed against proteinase 3 (PR3) while ANCAs against myeloperoxidase (MPO) are detected in approximately 10% of patients.[30,31] Some patients who are negative for ANCAs by conventional methods have antibodies to lysosome-associated membrane glycoprotein 2, while others have antibodies for a MPO peptide not detected by conventional methods.[29] ANCAs have also been detected in patients with Takayasu arteritis, eosinophilic granulomatosis with polyangiitis (Churg-Strauss syndrome), Kawasaki arteritis, microscopic polyangiitis, and idiopathic crescentic glomerulonephritis.[28,32,33]

Pathogenesis and histologic features

This rare disease is thought to represent a hypersensitivity reaction triggered by a variety of stimuli, including infections, environmental factors, and medications in genetically susceptible patients.[34]. Response to immunosuppressive therapy and the increased risk for patients with MHC class II HLA-DP1*0401, MHC class II HLA-DRB1 ' 15, or MHC class II HLADRB '1501 are consistent with this hypothesis.[35] The presence of ANCAs against PR3 and to a lesser amount MPO in most patients with granulomatosis with polyangiitis and the correlation of circulating levels of ANCAs with disease activity supports a role in the pathogenesis of this disease, as do animal models of ANCA-associated vasculitis.[36] Additionally, although immune complexes have not been demonstrated, disease activity is ameliorated with plasma exchange. Thus, there is compelling evidence suggesting ANCAs are central to pathogenesis, most likely through activation of neutrophils, lymphocytes, and macrophages.[37] In particular, abnormal numbers and function in regulatory T cells (T_{reg}) have been demonstrated in patients with granulomatosis and polyangiitis and appear to also correlate with disease activity.[38–40] However, the precise mechanism action of ANCAs is not yet fully understood.[37]

It is postulated that exposure to an antigen (or antigens) may trigger ANCAs that have pathophysiological effects leading to tissue destruction.[34,41] Infectious agents have received some attention as potentially playing a role in the pathogenesis of granulomatosis with polyangiitis. It is interesting to note that relapses of the disease may follow infection.[37] In some patients, a complete or partial remission is achieved with antibiotic treatment combined with immunosuppressive agents.[37,42] Trimethoprim-sulfamethoxazole has also been used to reduce the frequency of relapses in patients with granulomatosis and polyangiitis.[43] Patients who are chronic nasal carriers of *S. aureus* seem to have a higher relapse rate compared with noncarriers.[44] Furthermore, antibodies against hepatitis C virus, Epstein-Barr virus, and *H. pylori* as well as IgG antibodies against *Toxoplasma gondii* and IgM antibodies against cytomegalovirus are significantly more common in patients with granulomatosis with polyangiitis than in unaffected individuals.[45] Gastrointestinal and renal manifestation correlates well with the presence of IgG antibodies to cytomegalovirus while otolaryngeal manifestation is more common in patients with IgG antibodies to the Epstein-Barr virus early antigen.[45] Despite considerable research to establish a possible relationship between granulomatosis with polyangiitis and infection, a categoric role in the disease is elusive.[46]

In addition to that for infectious agents, a search for putative roles for physical agents in the environment has also been undertaken. Perhaps most attention has focused on silicon compounds.[47–49] One case-control study showed that exposure to silicon-containing compounds conferred a sevenfold risk for the development of granulomatosis with polyangiitis.[48] It has been postulated that silica-induced apoptosis of inflammatory cells may release lysosomal enzymes that stimulate ANCAs.[37,47]

Pulmonary lesions are characterized by necrotizing granulomatous inflammation that may bear more than a superficial resemblance to the caseation of pulmonary tuberculosis (*Fig. 16.31*).[50] The similarity is increased by the presence of large numbers of Langhans giant cells at the periphery of the necrotic focus (*Fig. 16.32*). In addition, the features of an active angiitis are present; this may involve both arteries and veins and frequently has a granulomatous component (*Fig. 16.33*). The adjacent parenchyma is chronically inflamed and often shows severe, diffuse, interstitial fibrosis.

Early renal lesions are characterized by focal segmental glomerulonephritis. In more advanced cases the glomerulitis becomes generalized, with fibrinoid necrosis and widespread epithelial crescent formation.[51] The renal interstitial tissue may contain necrotizing granulomata, and vasculitis is sometimes a feature. Immunofluorescence occasionally reveals granular deposits of immunoglobulin and complement along the glomerular capillary walls. This is taken as evidence for possible immune complex involvement. Similar granulomata and evidence of vasculitis have been described in all organ systems of the body, but are particularly often seen in the spleen.

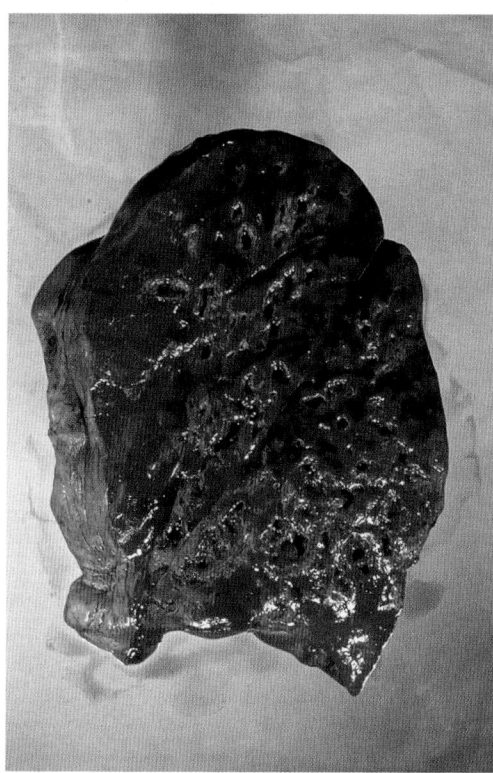

Fig. 16.31
Granulomatosis with polyangiitis: this postmortem lung specimen shows consolidation and numerous abscesses. By courtesy of B. Corrin, MD, Brompton Hospital, London, UK.

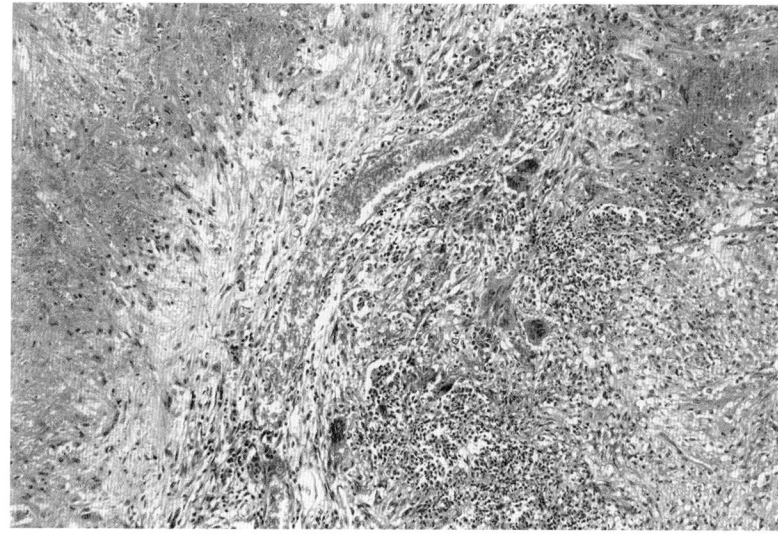

Fig. 16.32
Granulomatosis with polyangiitis: this lung section shows extensive necrosis associated with a granulomatous infiltrate containing Langhans giant cells. These appearances resemble pulmonary tuberculosis.

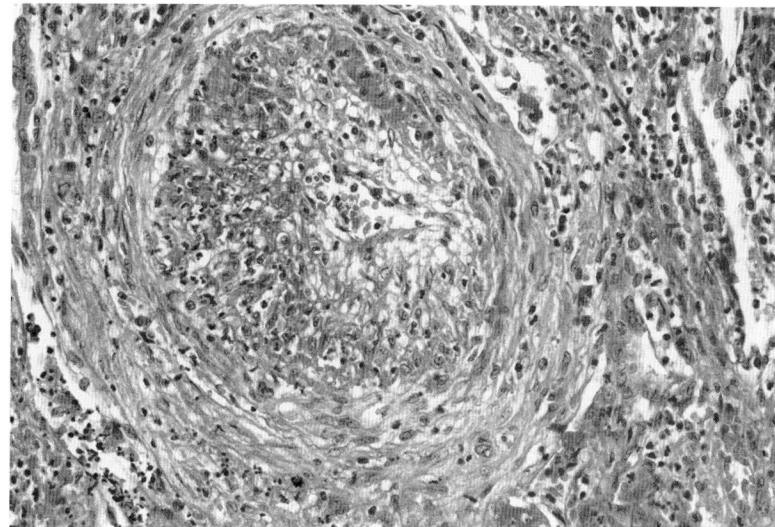

Fig. 16.33
Granulomatosis with polyangiitis: a branch of the pulmonary artery shows necrotizing arteritis with fibrointimal thickening.

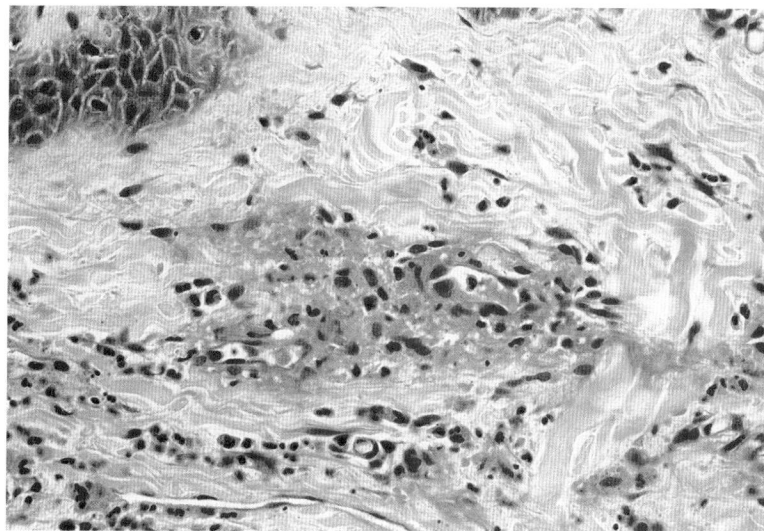

Fig. 16.34
Granulomatosis with polyangiitis: leukocytoclastic vasculitis as shown in this field is the most frequently encountered cutaneous lesion.

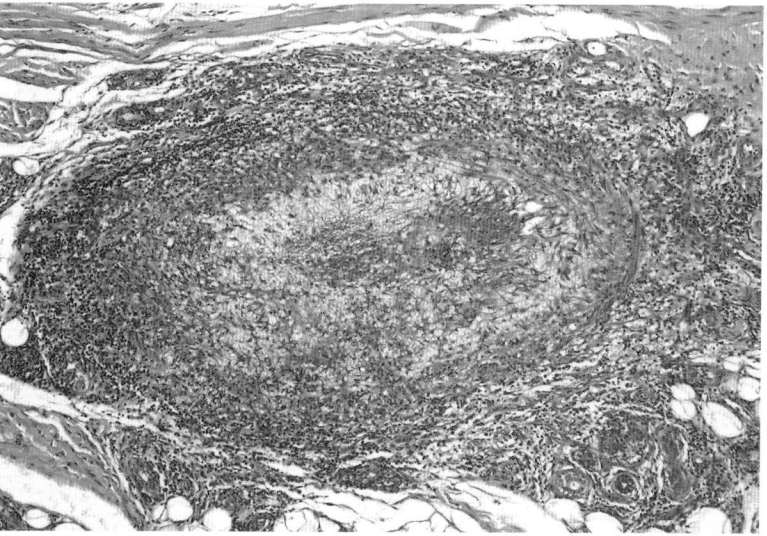

Fig. 16.35
Granulomatosis with polyangiitis: large vessel showing intense chronic inflammation, thrombosis, and intimal fibrosis.

Cutaneous lesions reveal a variety of features, including necrotizing vasculitis, in which small and/or medium-sized dermal vessels display fibrinoid necrosis, a neutrophil polymorphonuclear infiltrate, and leukocytoclasis (*Figs 16.34* and *16.35*). In one series, 80% of biopsies from patients with cutaneous lesions (of 244 patients in this series, 14% had cutaneous lesions) showed leukocytoclastic vasculitis.[19] In another study, nearly a third showed leukocytoclastic vasculitis and another third showed non-specific chronic inflammation.[52] In this study, nearly 50% of patients had entirely non-specific findings. Extravasated red blood cells are invariably present.[17,18] In severe cases, the epidermis may show ischemic necrosis. Bone fide granulomatous vasculitis of skin appears to be a very rare feature.[52,53] In fact,

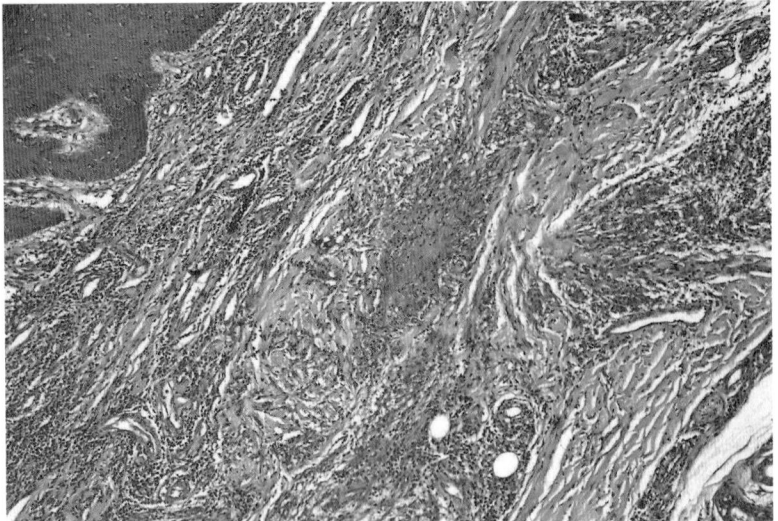

Fig. 16.36
Granulomatosis with polyangiitis: low-power view of a necrotizing dermal granuloma.

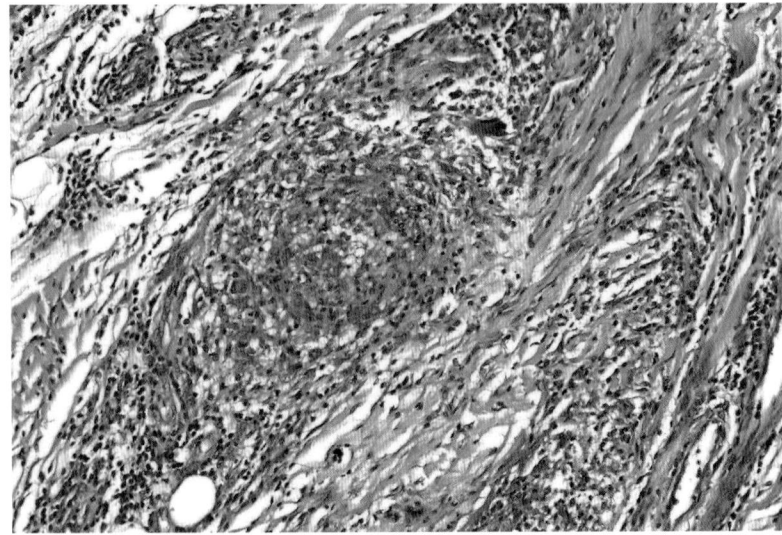

Fig. 16.37
Granulomatosis with polyangiitis: high-power view of an ill-defined granuloma.

Table 16.4
1990 criteria for the classification of Churg-Strauss syndrome (traditional format)*

Criterion	No. of CSS patients (n = 20)	Sensitivity (%)	No. of control patients (n = 787)	Specificity (%)
Asthma	19	100	782	96.3
Eosinophilia >10%	20	95	708	96.6
Neuropathy (mono or poly)	20	75	781	79.8
Pulmonary infiltrates, non-fixed	20	40	736	92.4
Paranasal sinus abnormality	14	85.7	366	79.3
Extravascular eosinophils	16	81.3	385	84.4

*For classification purposes, a patient shall be said to have Churg-Strauss syndrome (CSS) if at least four of these six criteria are positive. The presence of any four or more of the six criteria yields a sensitivity of 85% and a specificity of 99.7%.
Reproduced with permission from Masi, A.T. (1990) *Arthritis & Rheumatism*, 33, 1094–1100.

one study failed to demonstrate granulomatous vasculitis in 75 skin biopsies from 46 patients.[52] In other patients, there may be granulomatous infiltration of the dermis, which may be related to foci of collagen necrosis and sometimes resembles the granulomas seen in eosinophilic granulomatosis with polyangiitis (*Figs 16.36* and *16.37*). In some cases, extensive geographic zones of necrosis are present, associated with a mixed inflammatory cell infiltrate including variable numbers of histiocytes, giant cells, lymphocytes, eosinophils, and plasma cells. Erythema nodosum and granuloma annulare-like lesions may also be encountered.[52]

Differential diagnosis

As mentioned above, early in the course of the disease, when patients may not have developed the full clinical triad, definitive diagnosis is sometimes impossible.

In those instances where a granulomatous dermal infiltrate occurs in the absence of vasculitis, a host of conditions enters the differential diagnosis, including sarcoidosis and infections, particularly mycobacterial and fungal. Granulomatous vasculitis may also be seen in association with lymphoproliferative diseases, including lymphoma, angioimmunoblastic lymphadenopathy, and leukemia.[54]

Microscopic polyangiitis can be confused with granulomatosis with polyangiitis. The presence of granulomatous inflammation in the lung would favor the latter. Microscopic polyangiitis is approached as a diagnosis of exclusion, as mentioned previously. In fact, a diagnosis may be revised as the pattern of clinical involvement changes. For example, patients who appear to fit criteria for microscopic polyangiitis may eventually develop manifestation allowing for classification as granulomatosis with polyangiitis.[55]

When granulomata and/or allergic vasculitis are the only features, it may not be possible to histologically distinguish granulomatosis with polyangiitis from eosinophilic granulomatosis with polyangiitis. A high eosinophil content, however, is somewhat suggestive of the latter condition but certainly not diagnostic, as this finding may sometimes be seen in granulomatosis with polyangiitis.[54] Therefore, distinction of granulomatosis with polyangiitis from other forms of granulomatous inflammation and leukocytoclastic and granulomatous vasculitis requires careful clinicopathological and serological correlation.

Eosinophilic granulomatosis with polyangiitis

Clinical features

Eosinophilic granulomatosis with polyangiitis (Churg-Strauss syndrome) is a very rare disease that combines the features of asthma, fever, multisystem necrotizing vasculitis, extravascular granulomata, and hypereosinophilia.[1,2] Although there is clinical overlap, it can be distinguished from polyarteritis nodosa and granulomatosis with polyangiitis (see *Table 16.4*). The criteria published by the Chapel Hill Consensus conference differ somewhat.[3] In this scheme, eosinophilic granulomatosis with polyangiitis is defined as 'eosinophil-rich and granulomatous inflammation involving the respiratory tract, and necrotizing vasculitis affecting small to medium-sized arteries, and associated with asthma and eosinophilia'.[3] Given differences in classification criteria, it comes as no surprise that inconsistencies between these classification schemes exist.[4,5] One study found good concordance between classification schemes for the diagnosis of granulomatosis with polyangiitis but not eosinophilic granulomatosis with polyangiitis.[4] As we gain further understanding of this disease, refinement of diagnostic criteria is likely.

Eosinophilic granulomatosis with polyangiitis may present in a wide range of age groups, but most patients are adults, those in the third and fourth decades being most commonly affected. The disease has a slight male predominance.[6-9] Presentation in children is very rare, and most commonly involves teenaged patients.[10-14]

Asthma and necrotizing vasculitis are almost invariably present. Asthma often precedes the onset of vasculitis, sometimes by many years, or these features develop simultaneously. In one large study, asthma preceded definitive diagnosis in 94% of patients.[1] Asthma may be associated with transient pulmonary infiltrates (Loeffler syndrome) or there can be full-blown chronic eosinophilic pneumonitis.[6] There is some evidence to suggest that patients in whom vasculitis occurs rapidly after presentation of asthma have a particularly poor prognosis. It has been suggested that, in some cases, treatment for allergic rhinitis with steroids suppresses the full-blown syndrome.[15,16] An association between treatment of asthma with antileukotrienes and development of eosinophilic granulomatosis with polyangiitis has been suggested.[2,17] The association is controversial and what role, if any, antileukotrienes play in development of disease in these patients is unclear. However, it has also been proposed that it is the withdrawal of the steroids and not the administration of antileukotrienes that leads to disease.[2] Further investigation is required to resolve this controversy. Eosinophilic granulomatosis with polyangiitis has also been described following treatment with anti-IgE antibodies (omalizumab) for asthma and may represent unmasking of the disease while reducing steroid treatment.[18,19]

Common manifestations of upper respiratory tract involvement include allergic rhinitis (which is sometimes associated with polyp formation and sinusitis) and hay fever. A family history of atopy and allergic reactions to inhaled antigens and drugs is often present.

Chest radiography frequently confirms the presence of pulmonary involvement, which takes a variety of forms including transient patchy infiltrates, discrete noncavitating nodular masses, or diffuse interstitial disease. On CT scan, pulmonary infiltrates may take the form of opacification, nodules, or bronchial wall and interlobular septal thickening.[20] Bronchoalveolar lavage reveals alveolar eosinophilia.[1] Certain patients develop an eosinophil-rich pleural effusion.[1]

In addition to pulmonary lesions, systemic involvement most commonly affects the heart, nervous system, gut, and kidneys.[6] Cardiac lesions may be a cause of dysrhythmia or sudden death. Cardiac manifestations also include valvulopathy, ventricular insufficiency, global cardiac insufficiency, and endomyocarditis.[1,21-27] Pericardial effusion was seen in 23% of patients in one study.[1] Complications relating to cardiac involvement are the most common cause of death in patients with eosinophilic granulomatosis with polyangiitis. Nearly 40% of deaths are due to cardiac involvement.[1]

Neurological manifestations are frequent, particularly mononeuritis multiplex and symmetric polyneuropathy.[28-31] In one large study, 72% of patients developed mononeuritis multiplex.[1,30] Intracerebral hemorrhage or infarction sometimes develops.[27,28] Ischemic optic and bilateral trigeminal neuropathy are rare complications.[29] Myalgia, epilepsy, hydrocephalus, chorea, and vertigo are further occasional features.[31]

Evidence of gastrointestinal involvement, such as nausea, bleeding, vomiting, and abdominal pain, is often found. In one study, one-third of patients experienced gastrointestinal symptoms, usually abdominal pain.[1] Diffuse bowel ischemia is an uncommon but serious complication.[1,33]

Renal disease in eosinophilic granulomatosis with polyangiitis is usually manifest as glomerulonephritis, most often a focal segmental glomerulonephritis.[1,32] Patients with renal involvement show hematuria, proteinuria, and increased creatinine.[1] Renal infarction appears to be a rare complication.[1]

Rheumatological involvement in the form of polyarthralgia and constitutional symptoms, including fever, anemia, and weight loss, is common.[1]

Amyloidosis is a rare complication.[34-36] Exceptionally, eosinophilic granulomatosis with polyangiitis may present with temporal nongiant cell arteritis.[37] Involvement of the breast occurs exceptionally as eosinophilic mastitis.[38-40] A limited form of the disease has been described.[41,42]

Cutaneous lesions are seen in 40% to 70% of patients and include petechiae, purpura, papules, vesicles, facial erythema, urticaria, and

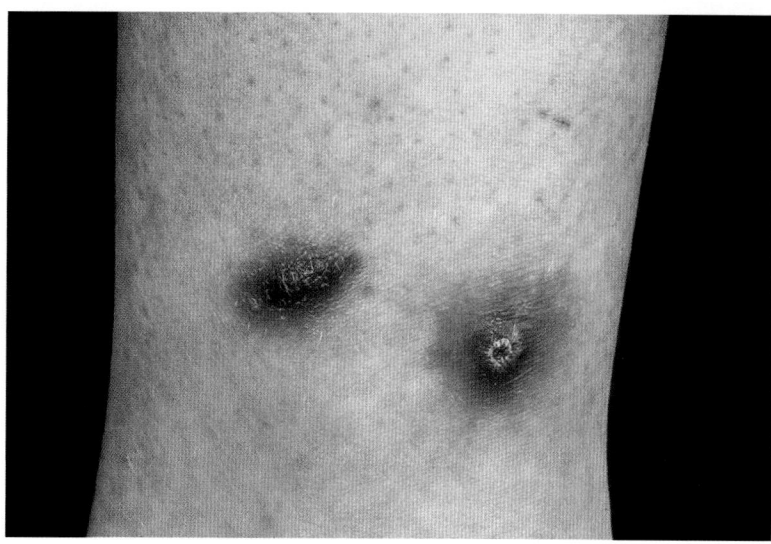

Fig. 16.38
Eosinophilic granulomatosis with polyangiitis: this patient presented with painful nodules on the limbs. By courtesy of the Institute of Dermatology, London, UK.

ulceration.[42-48] Cutaneous infarction and bullae are less common manifestations.[46,49] Livedo reticularis involving the lower limbs is occasionally a feature. Patients may also develop tender nodules, which particularly affect the extensor aspects of the arms, legs, hands, and feet (Fig. 16.38). The sacrum, buttocks, and scalp can also be involved. The cutaneous lesions tend to appear in crops with spontaneous relapses and remissions.

Eosinophilic granulomatosis with polyangiitis has been seen in association with HIV infection, hepatitis B, Wells syndrome, and bronchopulmonary candidiasis.[50-53] The disease has also been described in association with drugs including fluticasone and cocaine.[54,55]

Laboratory investigation usually reveals leukocytosis and a raised ESR in association with peripheral blood eosinophilia.[46] Blood eosinophilia often decreases with treatment but some authors stress that such a response should not be taken as evidence that disease activity is under control.[56] ANCAs are demonstrated in many patients (see below).

Pathogenesis and histologic features

The etiology and pathogenesis of eosinophilic granulomatosis with polyangiitis is poorly understood. The presence of perinuclear-antineutrophil cytoplasmic antibodies (p-ANCA) in many patients is of considerable interest.[57-60] ANCAs are detected in approximately 40% of patients.[61-63] The ANCAs seen in these patients usually target MPO.[63] However, the various types of ANCA are non-specific, being present in a spectrum of disease.[64] Their presence is associated with higher risk of developing glomerulonephritis, peripheral neuropathy, and alveolar hemorrhage while absence of ANCAs is linked to heart disease and fever.[62,63,65,66] ANCAs may activate neutrophils, causing degranulation and vascular injury.[67] T lymphocytes can also be stimulated, leading to endothelial cell injury.[67] As with other ANCA-associated vasculitides, it is suspected that they play a role in the pathogenesis; however, the precise mechanism, particularly triggering factors, is not yet known. Persistence of ANCAs with therapy may be of limited value in making treatment decisions.[68] One group has found that, although there is poor correlation between ANCA titer and disease activity, disappearance of ANCA can reflect absent disease activity.[69]

Pulmonary lesions comprise variably sized (up to 1.5 cm) nodules, ranging from only a few lesions to hundreds which may coalesce. Histologically, they are composed of granulomata with central necrosis and surrounding epithelioid histiocytes with occasional giant cells. Large numbers of eosinophils with an admixture of lymphocytes, neutrophils, plasma cells, and histiocytes infiltrate the adjacent lung parenchyma. Vasculitis involving small arteries and sometimes veins is also present.

Cutaneous lesions are variable. A common feature is the so-called Churg-Strauss (extravascular) granuloma. Early lesions are characterized by focal collagen degeneration in association with a varying and mixed

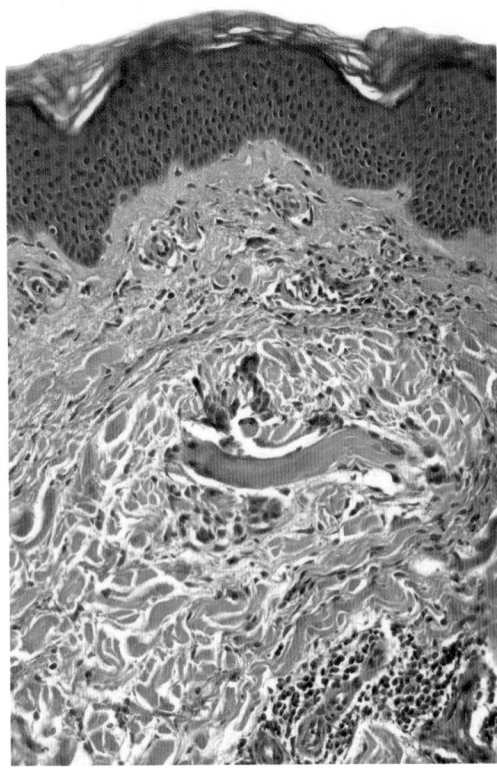

Fig. 16.39
Eosinophilic granulomatosis with polyangiitis: this early lesion shows a swollen collagen fiber in the superficial dermis. Note the surrounding multinucleate giant cells.

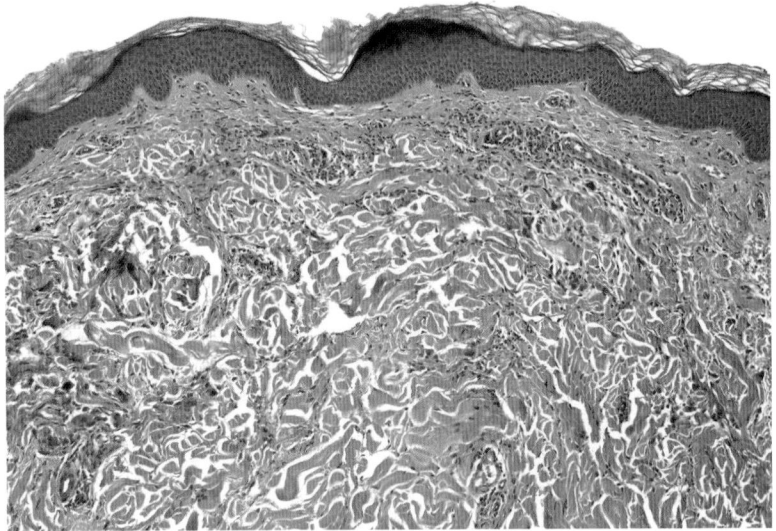

Fig. 16.40
Eosinophilic granulomatosis with polyangiitis: medium-power view showing swelling of the dermal collagen fibers and a perivascular chronic inflammatory cell infiltrate.

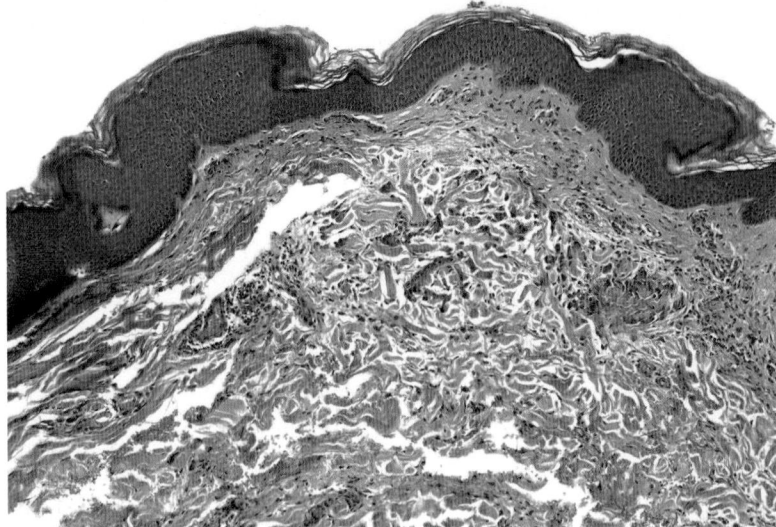

Fig. 16.41
Eosinophilic granulomatosis with polyangiitis: in this field there is a more obvious granulomatous infiltrate.

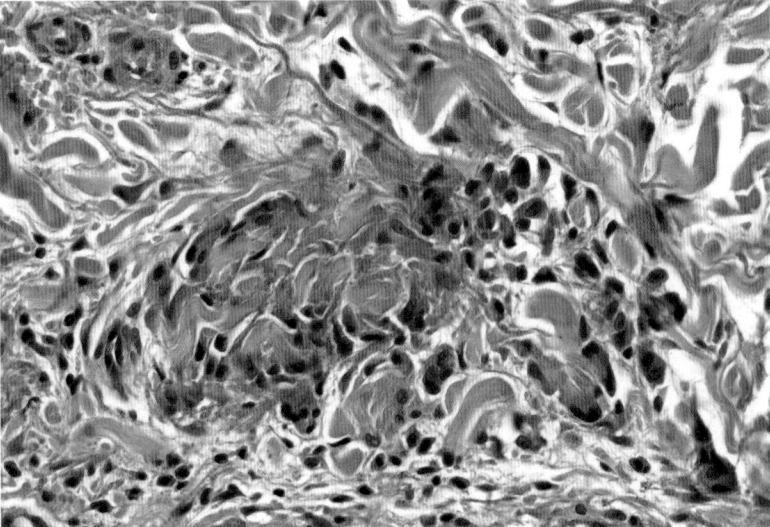

Fig. 16.42
Eosinophilic granulomatosis with polyangiitis: this florid example shows a granulomatous infiltrate containing prominent giant cells. By courtesy of E. Wilson Jones, MD, Institute of Dermatology, London, UK.

inflammatory cell infiltrate comprising neutrophils, lymphocytes, and histiocytes (*Figs 16.39* and *16.40*). Eosinophils may be sparse or numerous. Leukocytoclasis is often a feature. In more advanced examples the granuloma is more mature in appearance, consisting of a central zone of collagen necrosis surrounded by a peripheral palisade of epithelioid and giant cells (*Figs 16.41* and *16.42*). In some examples, the features are those of a rather diffuse and ill-defined granulomatous inflammatory process without obvious collagen degeneration. Commonly, features of necrotizing vasculitis are evident: fibrinoid necrosis accompanied by an eosinophilic and neutrophilic infiltrate with leukocytoclasis involving the more superficial small blood vessels (*Fig. 16.43*). There may be epidermal ischemic necrosis. In one

study, 16 of 37 biopsies (taken from 29 patients) showed leukocytoclastic vasculitis.[45] Occasionally, the arteries in the dermis and subcutaneous fat show changes similar to those seen in polyarteritis nodosa.[46] Additionally, acute and chronic panniculitis with eosinophils has been described.[46]

Differential diagnosis

The histologic features encountered in skin biopsies of patients with eosinophilic granulomatosis with polyangiitis are not diagnostic. Careful clinico-pathological and serological evaluation is necessary to establish a definitive diagnosis. Although eosinophilic granulomatosis with polyangiitis, polyarteritis nodosa, and granulomatosis with polyangiitis show both clinical and histologic overlap, research over the last several decades leaves no doubt that they represent distinctive entities. Nonetheless, they form a spectrum of disease with similar pathogenesis, although there are sufficient differences to justify their separate classification:

- Asthma may be seen in both polyarteritis nodosa and eosinophilic granulomatosis with polyangiitis, but characteristically polyarteritis affects medium-sized and small arteries, while eosinophilic granulomatosis with polyangiitis typically affects small arteries and veins.

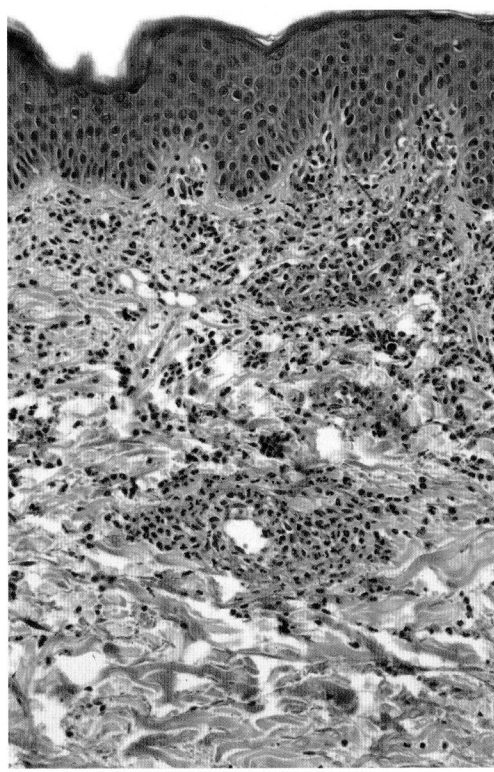

Fig. 16.43
Eosinophilic granulomatosis with polyangiitis: the features of small-vessel leukocytoclastic vasculitis are evident.

- The neutrophil dominates the inflammatory cell infiltrate in polyarteritis nodosa, whereas in eosinophilic granulomatosis with polyangiitis is the eosinophil.
- Necrotizing extravascular granulomata are not a feature of polyarteritis nodosa.
- Patients with granulomatosis with polyangiitis present with ulceroproliferative lesions of the upper respiratory tract, chest pain, and hemoptysis rather than asthma.
- Marked eosinophilia is uncommon in granulomatosis with polyangiitis. Churg-Strauss granulomata may be seen in granulomatosis with polyangiitis; however, the necrosis is more often of the tuberculocoagulative type. Granulomatous vasculitis is not a feature of eosinophilic granulomatosis with polyangiitis, though is not a sensitive feature for discrimination.

It must be stressed that Churg-Straus granulomata should not be taken as pathognomonic for eosinophilic granulomatosis with polyangiitis (Churg-Strauss syndrome). Churg-Strauss granulomata, or nearly identical lesions, has been described in the setting of other systemic diseases including rheumatoid arthritis, lupus erythematosus, other forms of vasculitis (granulomatosis with polyangiitis, polyarteritis nodosa, Takayasu arteritis), lymphoproliferative disorders, Crohn disease and ulcerative colitis, bacterial endocarditis, and hepatitis.[46,70–74]

Microscopic polyangiitis

Clinical features

Microscopic polyangiitis (microscopic polyarteritis) is a necrotizing vasculitis predominantly affecting small vessels with few to no immune complexes.[1] Patients often present with non-specific constitutional symptoms including malaise, fever, and myalgia. There may be a past history of sore throat or a flulike illness, which obviously raises the possibility of an iatrogenic pathogenesis for the subsequent vasculitic process.[2] Renal involvement, consisting of glomerulonephritis, is seen in about 90% of patients, manifesting as microscopic hematuria, proteinuria, or acute renal failure.[2–6] Hypertension is present in a large proportion of patients. Pulmonary lesions present as hemoptysis, pulmonary fibrosis, and intrapulmonary hemorrhage, which

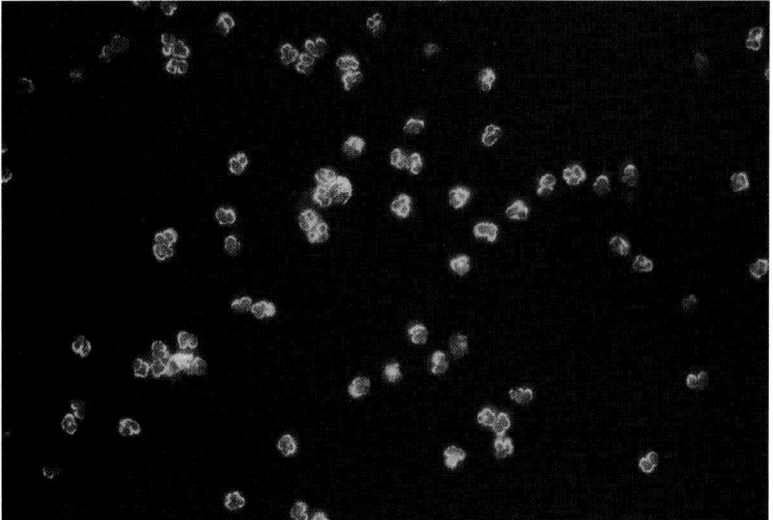

Fig. 16.44
Microscopic polyarteritis: p-ANCA. By courtesy of G. Swana, MD, St Thomas' Hospital, London, UK.

can prove fatal.[7,8] In one large series from a single institution, over 80% of patients had pulmonary symptoms, suggesting pulmonary involvement may be more common than previously recognized.[9]

Cutaneous involvement is seen in in approximately 40% of patients.[2–6] Dermatological signs include purpura, erythema, splinter hemorrhages, and leg ulceration.[6] Bullous presentation and urticaria are occasionally encountered but cutaneous nodules and livedo are rare features of this disease due to absence of involvement of larger vessels.[10–12] Other manifestations such as nervous system lesions, gastrointestinal bleeding with pain, and diarrhea, are sometimes evident.[13–16]

Microscopic polyangiitis is a member of the ANCA-associated vasculitides. Microscopic polyangiitis is usually associated with positive neutrophil cytoplasmic antibodies, typically of the antimyeloperoxidase (perinuclear-antineutrophil cytoplasmic antibody, p-ANCA) subtype (*Fig. 16.44*).[17] In microscopic polyangiitis, about 70% of patients have ANCA directed against MPO (MPO-ANCA), while the remainder have proteinase 3 (PR3)-ANCA.[4]

Other laboratory findings in microscopic polyarteritis include a raised ESR, normochromic normocytic anemia, leukocytosis with neutrophilia and thrombocytosis, raised C-reactive protein, and raised α-1 and α-2 globulins. Rheumatoid factor and immune complexes are present in less than 50% of patients.[5] Anti-DNA antibodies are not a feature. Cutaneous immunofluorescence is usually negative.

This disease is of particular importance due to its high morbidity and mortality, with a 5-year survival of approximately only 65%.[5] As a result of improved medical treatment outcome has significantly improved over the past few decades, with a quoted 5-year survival of 81%.[18] Severe renal disease and disease relapse are the best indicators for poor prognosis.[18]

Pathogenesis and histologic features

The precise pathogenesis is uncertain, but ANCAs are clearly implicated. In vitro and mouse studies implicated MPO-ANCA as a causative agent in microscopic polyangiitis.[4] Glomerulonephritis can be induced by injection of MPO-IgG into recipient mice.[19] There have also been reports suggesting an etiological link related to silica exposure, but this evidence is not conclusive.[20–22]

Microscopic polyangiitis (microscopic polyarteritis) is characterized by small-vessel leukocytoclastic vasculitis, which may predominantly affect the muscular arterioles, capillaries, and venules (*Fig. 16.45*).[2,16,23] Necrotizing vasculitis with fibrinoid necrosis and variable numbers of neutrophils and monocytes is seen. In early lesions, neutrophils associated with karyorrhexis predominate, while lymphocytes and histiocytes dominate the infiltrate in older lesions. Renal lesions include focal segmental necrotizing glomerulonephritis (often with crescents), vasculitis, interstitial inflammation, and

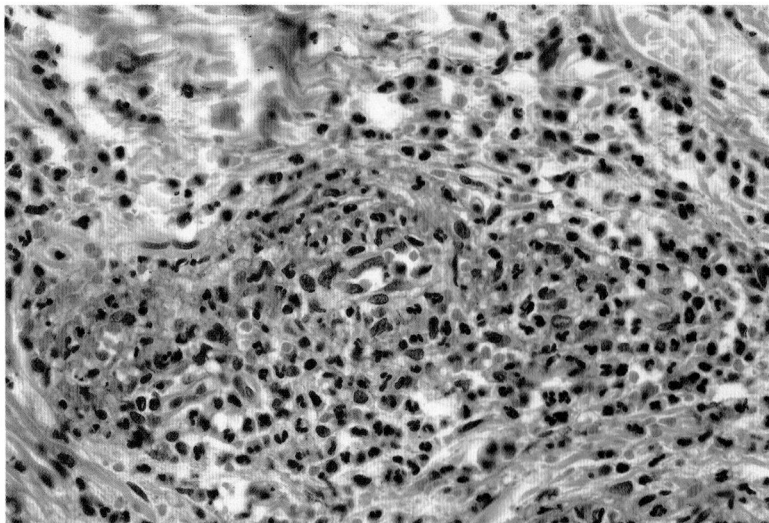

Fig. 16.45
Microscopic polyarteritis nodosa: acute necrotizing vasculitis of a small muscular arteriole is evident. Numerous eosinophils are present.

Table 16.5
1990 criteria for the classification of polyarteritis nodosa (traditional format)*

Criterion	Definition
Weight loss ≥ 4 kg	Loss of 4 kg or more of body weight since illness began not due to dieting or other factors
Livedo reticularis	Mottled reticular pattern over the skin of portions of the extremities or torso
Testicular pain or tenderness	Pain or tenderness of the testicles not due to infection, trauma or other causes
Myalgias, weakness, or leg tenderness	Diffuse myalgias (excluding shoulder and hip girdle) or weakness of muscles or tenderness of leg muscles
Mononeuropathy or polyneuropathy	Development of mononeuropathy, multiple mononeuropathies, or polyneuropathy
Diastolic BP > 9 mmHg	Development of hypertension with the diastolic BP higher than 90 mmHg
Elevated BUN or creatinine	Elevation of BUN >40 mg/dL or creatinine >1.5 mg/dL not due to dehydration or obstruction
Hepatitis B virus	Presence of hepatitis B surface antigen or antibody in serum
Arteriographic abnormality	Arteriogram showing aneurysms or occlusions of the vesical arteries not due to arteriosclerosis, fibromuscular dysplasia, or other noninflammatory causes
Biopsy of small or medium-sized artery	Histologic changes showing the presence of granulocytes or granulocytes and mononuclear leukocytes containing PMN in the artery wall

*For classification purposes, a patient shall be said to have polyarteritis nodosa if at least 3 of these 10 criteria are present.
The presence of any three or more criteria yields a sensitivity of 82.2% and a specificity of 86.6%.
BP, blood pressure; BUN, blood urea nitrogen; PMN, polymorphonuclear neutrophils.
Reproduced with permission from Lightfoot, D.W. (1991) *Current Opinion in Rheumatology*, 3, 3–7.

tubular atrophy. Large-vessel disease, visceral infarction, and granulomatous inflammation are not features.

Differential diagnosis

The absence of involvement of capillaries and venules in classic polyarteritis nodosa is a major point of distinction from microscopic polyangiitis. IgA vasculitis and conventional leukocytoclastic vasculitis tend to affect superficial vessels predominantly, whereas microscopic polyangiitis usually involves superficial and deep vessels. However, this is not sufficiently reliable. Microscopic polyangiitis may also be confused with granulomatosis with polyangiitis and eosinophilic granulomatosis with polyangiitis (Churg-Strauss syndrome). The presence of granulomatous inflammation in the lung favors the first of the last two conditions. The presence of blood eosinophilia and asthma favors a diagnosis of eosinophilic granulomatosis with polyangiitis. Ultimately, microscopic polyangiitis is a diagnosis of exclusion. Therefore, the biopsy findings must never be used in isolation to determine the diagnosis. Only after careful clinical, serological, and histologic correlation should a definitive diagnosis be rendered. Careful clinical investigation is required to evaluate for underlying causes/disease associations.

Polyarteritis nodosa

Classic polyarteritis nodosa (Kussmaul-Maier disease) is a rare systemic vasculitis predominantly involving medium-sized and small arteries.[1,2] Some view the disorder not as a disease sui generis but, less restrictively, as a syndrome with many triggering causes and disease associations. Classic polyarteritis nodosa overlaps both clinically and histologically with microscopic polyangiitis (microscopic polyarteritis nodosa, microscopic polyarteritis), but polyarteritis nodosa is predominantly a medium vessel vasculitis while microscopic polyangiitis is predominantly a small-vessel vasculitis and is discussed elsewhere.[2]

Clinical features
Classical polyarteritis nodosa

Classic polyarteritis nodosa is a multisystem disease with protean clinical manifestations (*Table 16.5*).[1,3–6] It should be noted that the 1990 criteria from the American College of Rheumatology did not distinguish polyarteritis nodosa from microscopic polyarteritis. However, in the more recent Chapel Hill consensus nomenclature, they are divided by the size of vessel involved (see *Table 16.1*).[2,6] Polyarteritis nodosa is associated with significant morbidity and mortality even when treated with corticosteroids. With therapy, survival is in the range of 75% to 80%.[1] Although a wide age group may be affected, patients are most often in their fifth or sixth

decade.[6,7] There is a male predilection (4:1). Patients commonly present with constitutional symptoms including weight loss, pyrexia, and anorexia.[1]

Cutaneous lesions are common and are present in 30% to 60% of patients.[6–12] Palpable purpuric lesions and foci of ulceration, particularly involving the lower limbs, are most often found (*Figs 16.46–16.48*).[11] Livedo reticularis is also a common cutaneous manifestation (*Fig. 16.49*). Cutaneous nodules may also be seen. A maculopapular rash, vesiculation, and pustular lesions are occasional features (*Figs 16.50–16.53*).

Joint involvement (arthralgias and arthritis) is often present; arthritis is usually asymmetrical and particularly affects the lower limbs. Non-specific muscle pain and weakness are additional features. Muscle wasting is commonly found.

Both peripheral and CNS involvement are often encountered. The former presents as sensory neuropathies (numbness or paresthesias), motor neuropathies (wrist or foot drop), and combined sensorimotor lesions (mononeuritis multiplex and polyneuropathy). CNS involvement may present as confusion, disorientation, or delirium. Eye involvement is a rare feature of polyarteritis nodosa.[13,14] Complications include choroidal infarction, ischemic optic neuropathy, retinal artery occlusion, episcleritis, ulcerative keratitis, uveitis, and orbital pseudotumor.[13–16]

Involvement of the kidney is common and is of major importance because its sequelae – renal failure and hypertension – are among the commonest causes of death in this disease.[1,6,12] Patients on occasion have episodes of loin pain due to renal infarction. Hypertension is often present in patients with classical polyarteritis nodosa and in some patients it may enter the malignant phase. Urinalysis for proteinuria, hematuria and red cell casts, and serum creatinine estimations are therefore mandatory early investigations.

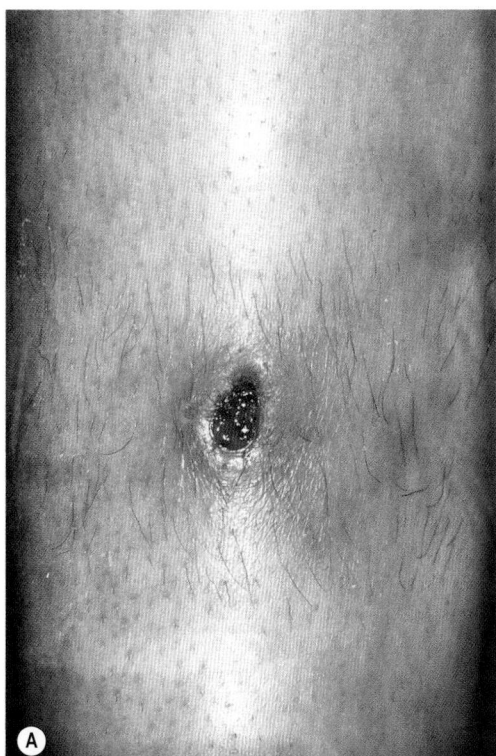

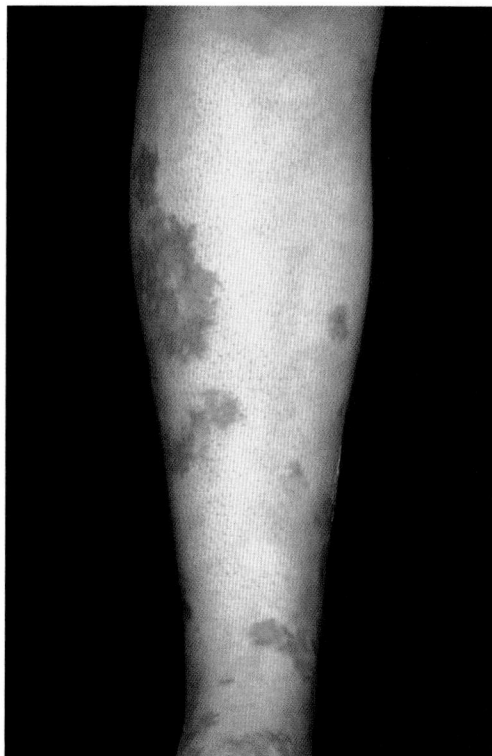

Fig. 16.47
Polyarteritis nodosa: this patient presented with large hemorrhagic lesions on the legs. By courtesy of the Institute of Dermatology, London, UK.

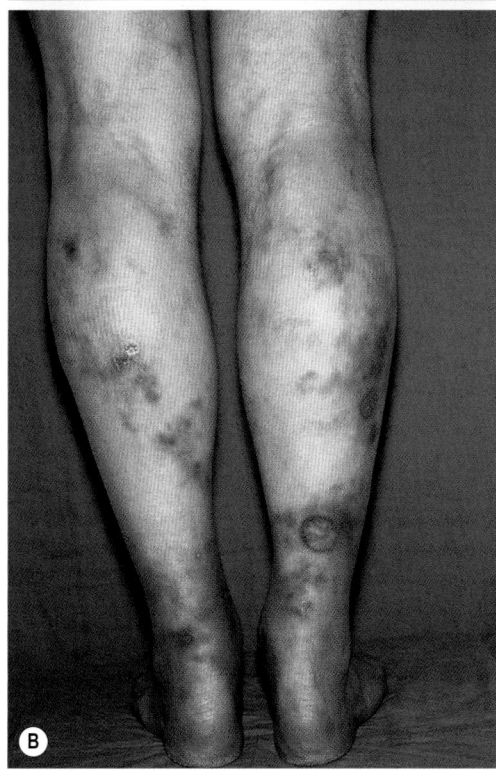

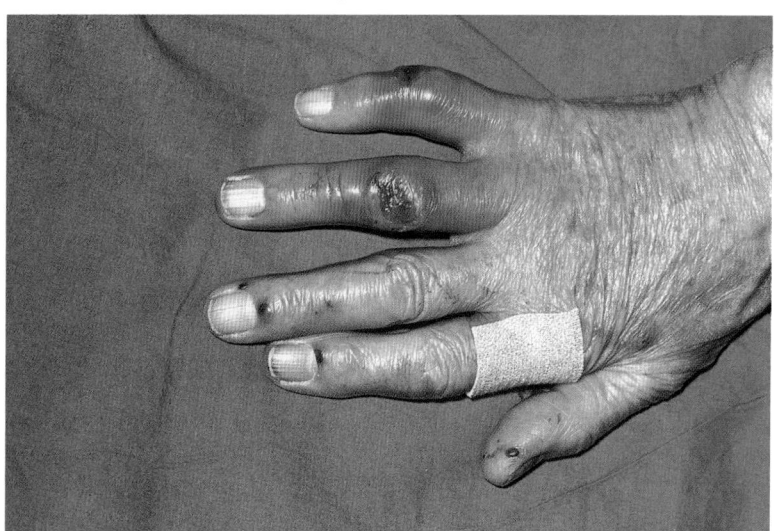

Fig. 16.48
Polyarteritis nodosa: epidermal infarction has resulted in these digital ulcers. By courtesy of R.A. Marsden, MD, St George's Hospital, London, UK.

Fig. 16.46
Polyarteritis nodosa: (A) a sharply defined ulcer with an indurated purplish border on the shin; (B) multiple ulcers, nodules, and foci of livedo reticularis. By courtesy of R.A. Marsden, MD, St George's Hospital, London, UK.

Gastrointestinal involvement is also an important cause of morbidity and mortality.[6,12,17,18] Symptoms include nausea, vomiting, and abdominal pain. Serious complications include gastrointestinal hemorrhage, perforation, and infarction, the last being a not uncommon cause of death. Involvement of the hepatobiliary tract may also be seen.[19,20] Involvement of the gallbladder and pancreas has also been reported and can represent an incidental finding or patients may present with symptoms of acute cholecystitis.[21,22]

Cardiac involvement occurs in less than one third of cases.[6,12] Manifestations include pericarditis, arrhythmias, and myocardial infarction due to coronary artery involvement (Fig. 16.54).[23] Although it is often stated that polyarteritis nodosa does not involve the lung, in exceptional cases pulmonary involvement is seen and patients occasionally complain of asthma, hemoptysis, and effusions. Although clinical involvement of the lungs is rare, autopsy evaluation has shown that arteritis affecting the bronchial arteries is not uncommon, being seen in 70% in one small series.[24]

Orchitis, usually unilateral, is a characteristic feature of polyarteritis nodosa.[25–27] Affected patients present with symptoms of acute orchitis or features that suggest a testicular neoplasm.[25,27]

Laboratory investigations often reveal anemia, leukocytosis, and a raised ESR. Low-titer rheumatoid factor and antinuclear antibody are sometimes features and, in occasional patients, a cryoglobulin is identified. Diminished serum complement levels may also be detected. ANCAs are uncommonly

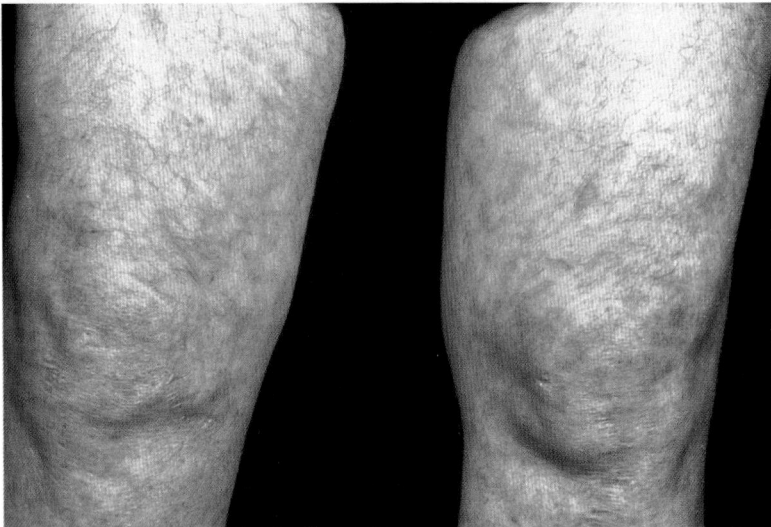

Fig. 16.49
Polyarteritis nodosa: this patient shows florid livedo reticularis. By courtesy of the
Institute of Dermatology, London, UK.

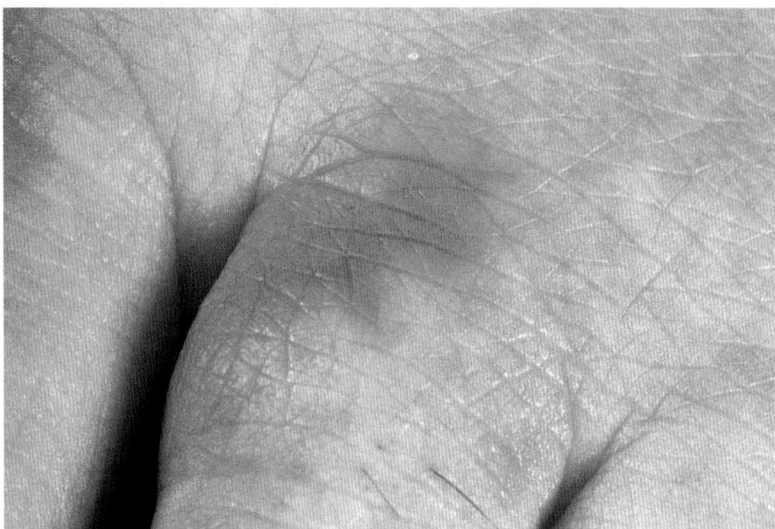

Fig. 16.52
Polyarteritis nodosa: this patient presented with acral erythematous lesions. By
courtesy of the Institute of Dermatology, London, UK.

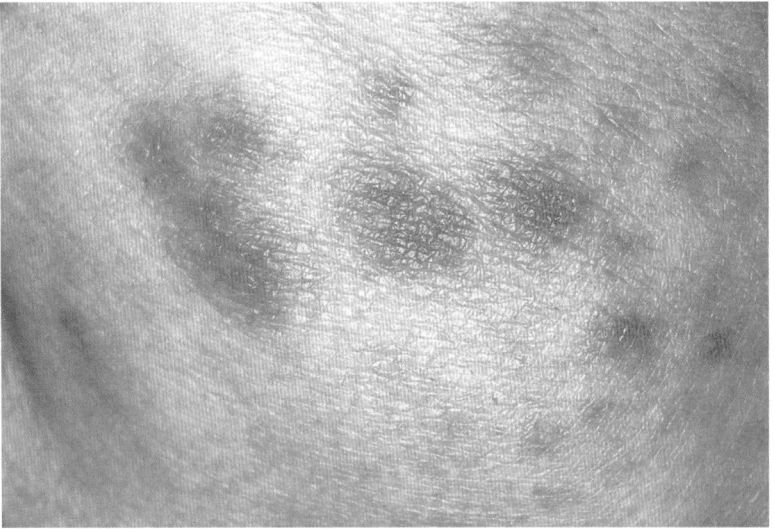

Fig. 16.50
Polyarteritis nodosa: erythematous macules are occasionally seen. By courtesy of
the Institute of Dermatology, London, UK.

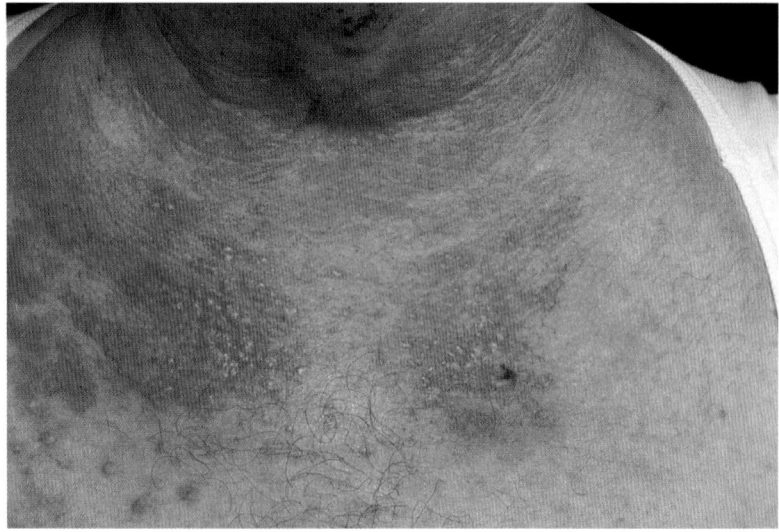

Fig. 16.53
Polyarteritis nodosa: in some patients, an intense neutrophil infiltrate results
in pustular lesions as seen in this patient. By courtesy of the Institute of
Dermatology, London, UK.

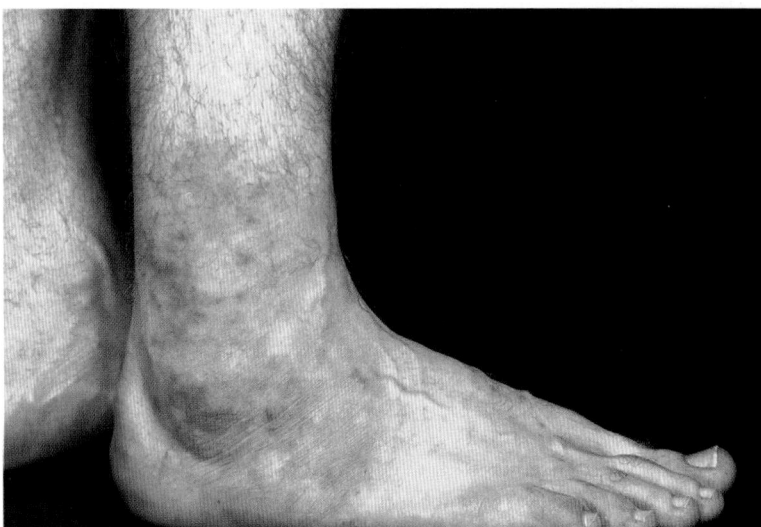

Fig. 16.51
Polyarteritis nodosa: erythematous papules are present around this patient's
ankles. By courtesy of the Institute of Dermatology, London, UK.

seen in patients with classic polyarteritis nodosa. One group with extensive
experience estimates that less than 5% of patients with the classic form of
the disease have ANCAs.[28] However, the presence of ANCAs should prompt
strong consideration of an ANCA-related vasculitis rather than polyarteritis nodosa.[6] Polyarteritis nodosa in children may present in two forms: the
infantile variant, which may be related to Kawasaki disease, and a childhood form, which is similar to adult polyarteritis nodosa (see also section
on Kawasaki disease).[29]

Cutaneous polyarteritis nodosa

In addition to classic polyarteritis nodosa, 'localized (cutaneous) polyarteritis nodosa' has also been described.[30–39] This is a relatively benign variant in
which patients develop cutaneous lesions, often over very prolonged periods,
but serious visceral involvement is, by definition, never a feature. In one
study, none of 79 patients with cutaneous polyarteritis nodosa who were
followed for an average of 6.9 years developed systemic vasculitis.[30] It may
occur at any age, including childhood, and shows no sex predilection. The
disease has occasionally been associated with minocycline treatment.[40–42]

Patients have recurrent episodes during which tender, painful nodules
develop, particularly on the lower legs, although these may sometimes be

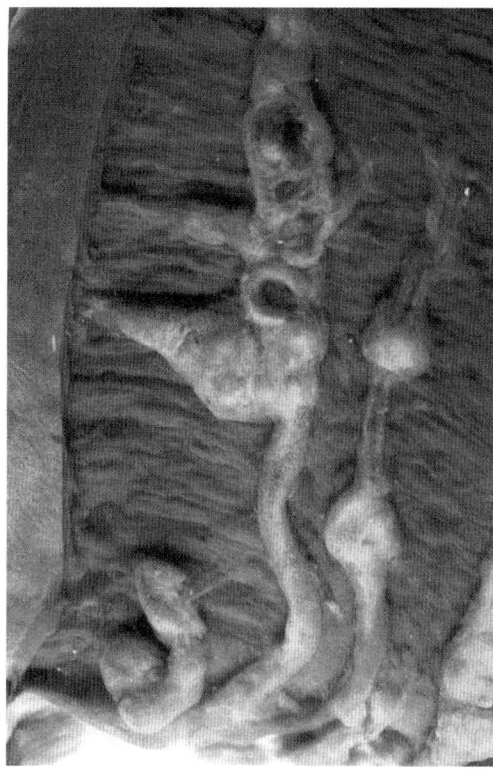

Fig. 16.54
Polyarteritis nodosa: coronary arteries showing conspicuous aneurysmal dilatation are now very rarely seen (museum specimen). By courtesy of the Department of Pathology, St Thomas' Hospital, London, UK.

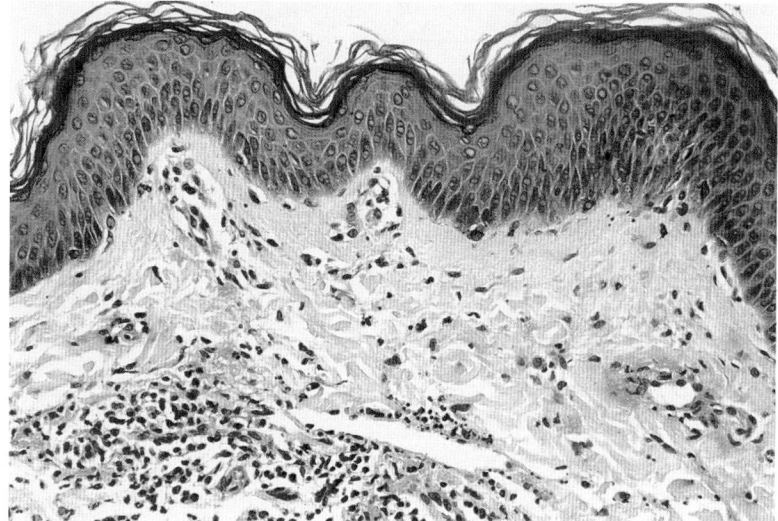

Fig. 16.55
Polyarteritis nodosa: in this case the features are those of a superficial leukocytoclastic vasculitis. It is important to remember that this histologic lesion may represent a serious systemic disease.

quite widespread. Individual lesions vary from 2 mm to 2 cm in diameter. In the early stages they are pink or red, while more established nodules may have a purplish coloration. Patients sometimes also manifest livedo reticularis, usually on the lower legs and often related to groups of nodules. Other complications include ulceration and, rarely, gangrene. Very occasionally, patients develop lesions reminiscent of atrophie blanche.[30]

Other features include fever, malaise, arthralgias, and myalgias, and peripheral nerves may be affected, but there is never any evidence of more widespread visceral involvement.[32,36,37]

Immunofluorescence often reveals IgM and/or complement in the walls of cutaneous arteries, suggesting a possible immune complex pathogenesis.[43] Rare reports of infants of mothers with cutaneous polyarteritis developing the disease and experiencing subsequent resolution are suggestive of a pathogenic circulating factor.[44]

Pathogenesis and histologic features

The pathogenesis of polyarteritis nodosa is poorly understood. Classic polyarteritis nodosa has been suggested to be immune-complex mediated, on the basis of serum immune-complex levels, immunofluorescence investigations, and ultrastructural studies. However, in many patients immune complexes cannot be demonstrated and their role in the development of this disease is controversial. Important suspect antigens include hepatitis B virus (HBV) surface antigens and cryoglobulins.[45–48] It has been shown that a significant number of patients with polyarteritis nodosa have circulating HBV antigen.[10,48] Furthermore, circulating immune complexes containing HBV antigen and immunoglobulin have been characterized in occasional patients.[10] HBV surface antigen has also been identified within affected vessels in a small number of patients.[10] A decrease in HBV-associated cases of polyarteritis nodosa in France has been reported and it has been suggested that this phenomenon is the result of vaccination programs.[49] Rarely, however, polyarteritis nodosa may also develop following hepatitis B vaccination.[50] Human immunodeficiency viral infection has also been reported in cases of polyarteritis nodosa or a polyarteritis nodosa-like syndrome.[51–57]

Evidence of hepatitis C viral infection has been documented in some patients. In one study, 20% of patients had antibodies against hepatitis C

virus.[56,58] Parvovirus infection has been associated with polyarteritis nodosa in occasional cases.[59,60]

In childhood polyarteritis nodosa, there appears to be a striking association with group A streptococci.[61]

Although there is some evidence to suggest a role for immune complexes generated during infection, such a relationship cannot be demonstrated in many cases. Therefore, the pathogenesis of classic polyarteritis nodosa is unclear in many patients.

In a small subset of patients, the disease is related to deficiency of adenosine deaminase 2 (DADA2). This is a recently described autoinflammatory disease secondary to mutations of *CECR1* on chromosome 22q11.1. It is characterized by early childhood onset of livedoid vasculopathy with CNS involvement and mild immunodeficiency. Patients frequently have clinical and histopathological findings indistinguishable from polyarteritis nodosa, reflecting that concept of multiple pathogenetic pathways.[62,63] The early onset is in stark contrast to conventional polyarteritis nodosa. Therefore, investigation for this possible genetic condition should be considered in cases encountered in infants and young children.

The histologic features of the cutaneous lesions in both the classic and localized variants of polyarteritis nodosa are similar and changes are variable.[64–66] In some instances, the changes are indistinguishable from leukocytoclastic vasculitis involving the superficial dermal vessels (*Fig. 16.55*). More characteristic, however, is the finding of necrotizing vasculitis involving the muscular arteries of the deep dermis or subcutaneous fat; these are the changes that are also seen in the internal viscera, often associated with infarction (*Fig. 16.56*). Although the whole circumference and thickness of the vessel wall is often affected, sometimes the changes are focal. Typically in polyarteritis nodosa, the vascular changes are discontinuous, with uninvolved skip lesions between affected segments (*Fig. 16.57*).

The acute changes, those of fibrinoid necrosis, involve the muscle coat and often destroy the internal elastic lamina; this is often best appreciated by the use of a stain for elastic tissue (*Fig. 16.58*). Associated with the necrosis is an inflammatory cell infiltrate of neutrophils, eosinophils, and mononuclear cells. Leukocytoclasis is sometimes an additional feature. Thrombosis is common and may be complicated by ischemic necrosis of the surface epithelium. Healing lesions are associated with fibroblastic proliferation and eventual fibrous scarring. In the healing phase a lymphocytic infiltrate rather than a neutrophilic infiltrate is often present.[68,69] Endarteritis is often evident and any disruption of the internal elastic lamina is permanent. A characteristic feature that often presents in wedge biopsies that contain multiple vessels is the presence of lesions at varying stages of evolution. Deep, surgical incisional biopsies are essential for the diagnosis of cutaneous involvement in polyarteritis nodosa. A punch biopsy will often

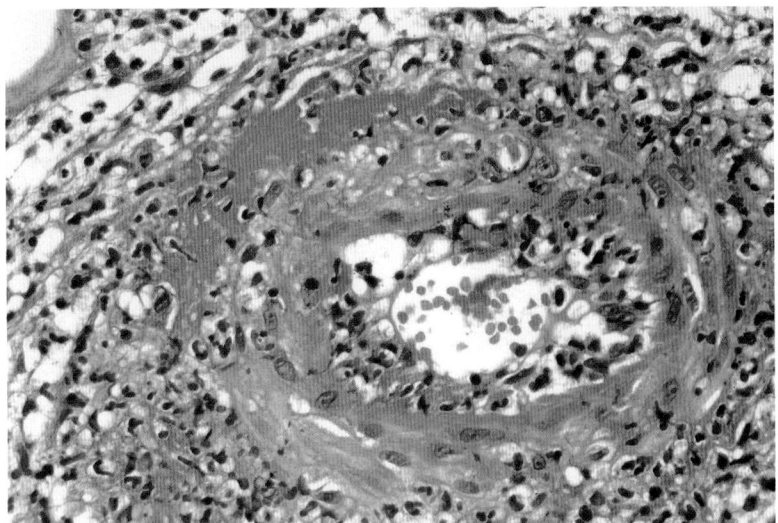

Fig. 16.56
Polyarteritis nodosa: high-power view showing fibrinoid necrosis.

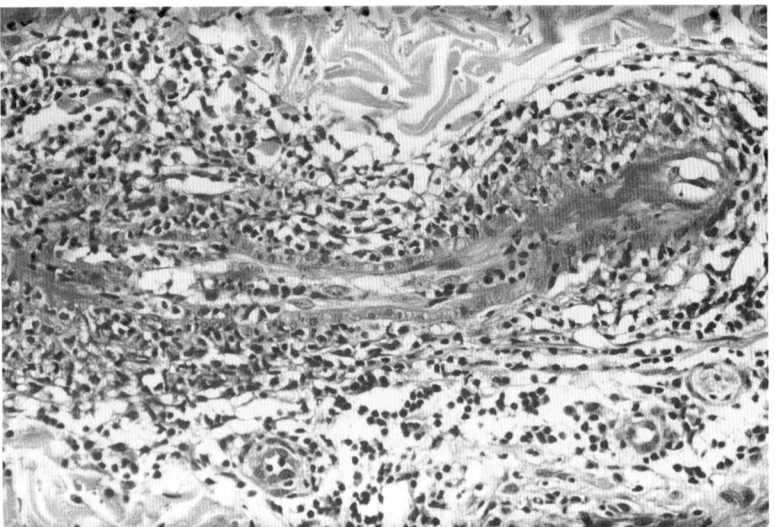

Fig. 16.57
Polyarteritis nodosa: while fibrinoid necrosis involves both lateral extremities of this vascular segment, the middle portion is relatively unaffected.

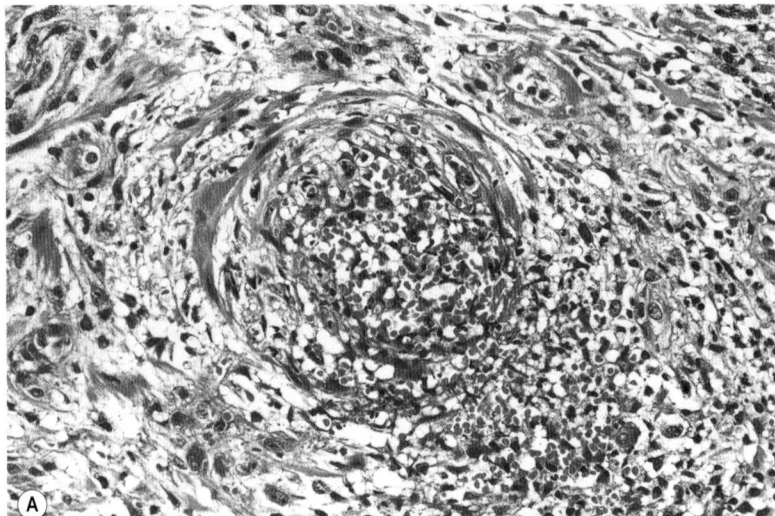

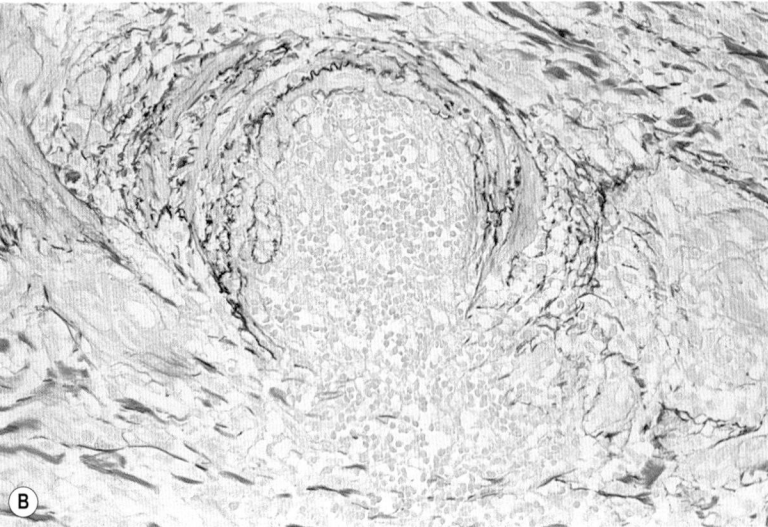

Fig. 16.58
Polyarteritis nodosa: (**A**) there is marked red cell extravasation; (**B**) elastic–van Gieson staining shows disruption of the internal elastic lamina.

not sample larger vessels that are typically affected. Furthermore, the diagnosis is subject to sampling error due to the multifocal nature of the disease. Aneurysm formation may sometimes be appreciated microscopically.[1]

Internal visceral involvement is based upon the effects of necrotizing arteritis. Interestingly, nodular swellings (aneurysms) are much more obvious. The effects depend upon the relative interplay of infarction and hemorrhage. Renal involvement in classical polyarteritis nodosa is predominantly due to large-vessel vasculitis, with resultant thrombosis and infarction, coupled with the effects of hypertension (*Fig. 16.59*).[67] Patients may also manifest focal, segmental proliferative or necrotizing glomerulonephritis similar to that seen in patients with microscopic polyarteritis nodosa (*Fig. 16.60*).

Differential diagnosis

Distinction between classic polyarteritis nodosa and microscopic polyangiitis is based on the size of vessels involved, spectrum and type of organ involvement, and presence of ANCAs. Similar to polyarteritis nodosa, erythema induratum frequently shows vasculitis of medium-sized vessels, but also has an associated lobular panniculitis in contrast to polyarteritis nodosa. Cutaneous lymphocytic thrombophilic/macular lymphocytic arteritis likely represents the healing phase of polyarteritis nodosa rather than a distinct entity.[68–70]

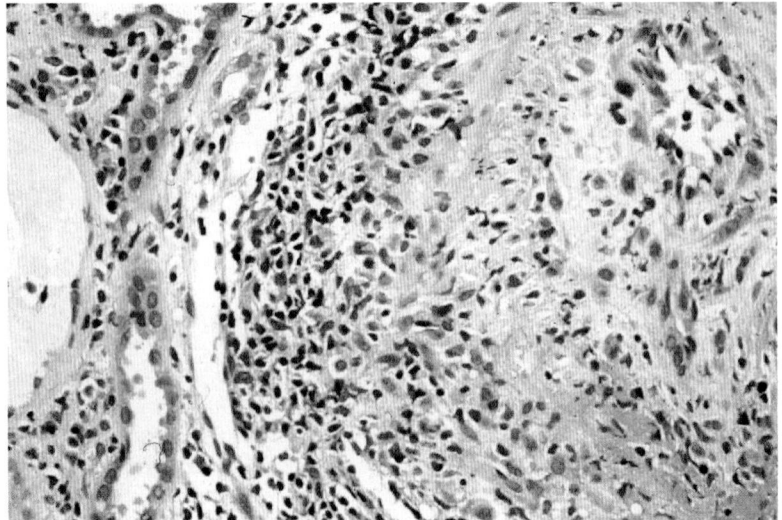

Fig. 16.59
Polyarteritis nodosa: in this kidney section an arcuate artery shows necrotizing vasculitis and fibrointimal thickening. The inflammatory cell infiltrate contains conspicuous eosinophils.

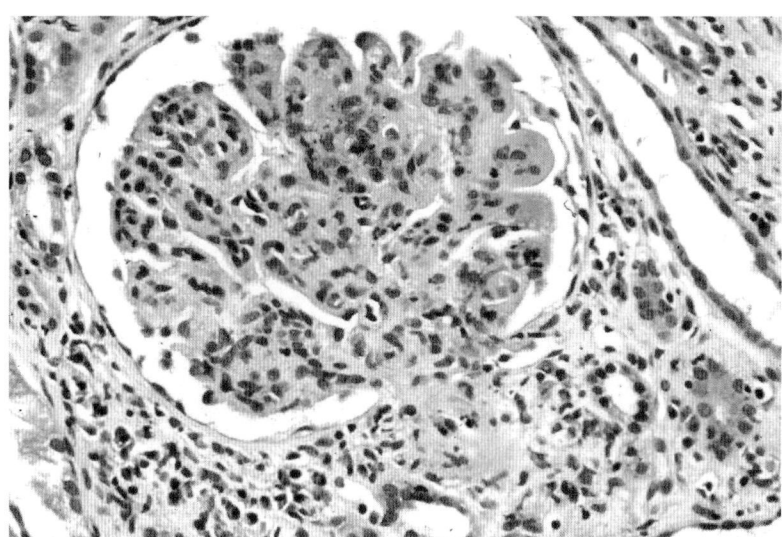

Fig. 16.60
Polyarteritis nodosa: segmental necrotizing glomerulonephritis.

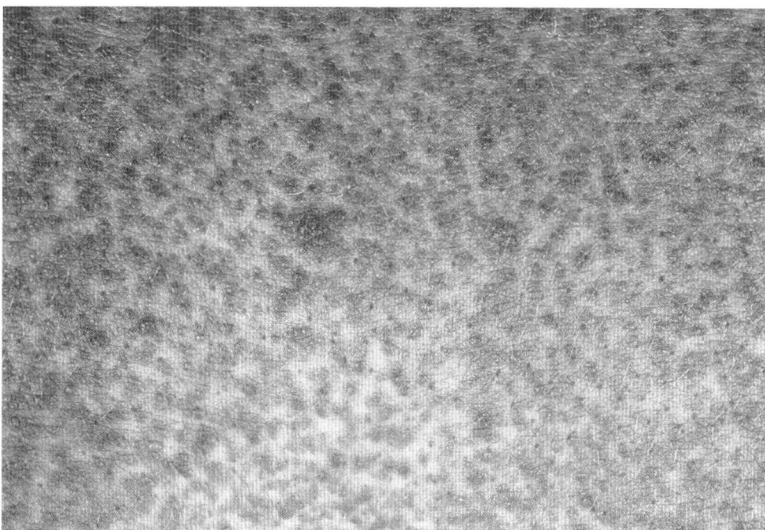

Fig. 16.61
Kawasaki disease: erythematous macular eruption. By courtesy of W.G. Phillips, MD, Institute of Dermatology, London, UK.

Table 16.6
Kawasaki syndrome: diagnostic guidelines

- Fever lasting ≥5 days
- Polymorphous rash
- Bilaterial conjunctival injection
- At least one of the following changes of the mucosal membranes:
  - erythema or fissuring of the lips
  - strawberry tongue
  - diffuse injection of oral and pharyngeal mucosa
- Acute non-purulent cervical lymphadenopathy (at least one node ≥1.5 cm)
- At least one of the following changes of the peripheral extremities:
  - erythema of palms and soles
  - indurative edema of hands and feet
  - membranous desquamation from fingertips

Fever plus four of the above criteria must be present for a secure diagnosis; other illness that can present with similar clinical findings must be excluded.
Reproduced with permission from Wortman, D.W. (1992) *Seminars in Dermatology*, 11, 37–47.

Kawasaki disease (mucocutaneous lymph node syndrome)

Kawasaki disease (mucocutaneous lymph node syndrome) is a multisystem disease that predominantly affects infants and young children.[1–6] Although it was first described, and shows a marked preponderance, in Japan, it has been diagnosed worldwide and in all races. Kawasaki disease is characterized by both endemic and epidemic variants.[4] The incidence among Japanese children is 16–150/100 000/year whereas in white children the incidence is 6–21/100 000/year.[4,6,7] The incidence of reported disease in the United States is rising but has been attributed to increased physician awareness.[8,9] Kawasaki disease shows a male predominance and occurs most frequently in children aged 6–18 months.[10] Adults are only rarely affected.[11–14] Kawasaki syndrome is thought to have an infectious etiology on the basis of symptoms of fever and exanthem, age distribution, seasonality (peaks in winter and spring), and occurrence of community-wide epidemics.[15]

Clinical features

The diagnostic features of Kawasaki syndrome are summarized in *Table 16.6* and include:
- a spiking fever unresponsive to antibiotic therapy,
- an erythematous polymorphic cutaneous eruption (*Fig. 16.61*),
- erythema, edema, and induration of the extremities followed by cutaneous desquamation of the tips of the fingers and toes (*Fig. 16.62*),

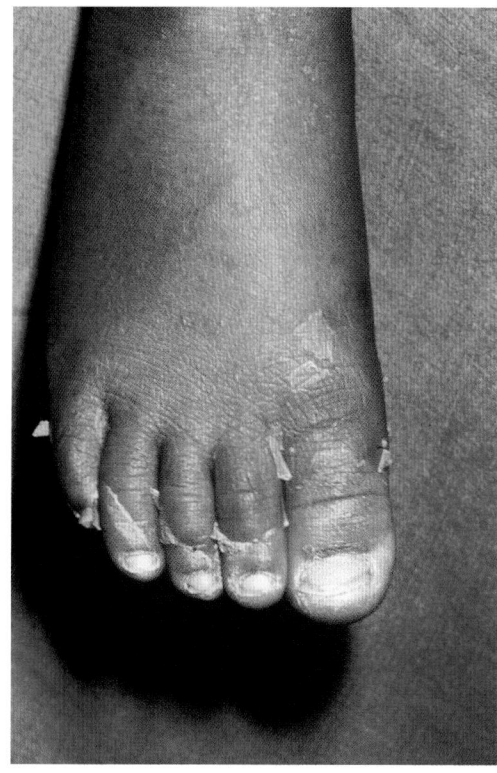

Fig. 16.62
Kawasaki disease: desquamation of the skin of the toes is a characteristic finding. By courtesy of J. Ross, MD, Lewisham Hospital, London, UK.

- oropharyngeal mucosal changes including edema, erythema, and fissuring of the lips, erythema of the cheeks, and a strawberry (scarletiform) tongue (*Figs 16.63* and *16.64*),
- bilateral, nonexudative conjunctivitis,
- nonsuppurative cervical lymphadenopathy.

In an appropriate clinical context, children are judged to have Kawasaki syndrome if they show a high fever plus four of the signs described above.[4,6,16] This has been amended to include coronary artery aneurysm plus three of the above features.[4]

The cutaneous findings are variable and include erythematous, macular, maculopapular (morbilliform), urticarial, pustular, erythema multiforme-like (targetoid), and erythema marginatum-like lesions.[2,6,17] A vesiculopustular eruption has also been reported.[18] The skin lesions show a propensity for

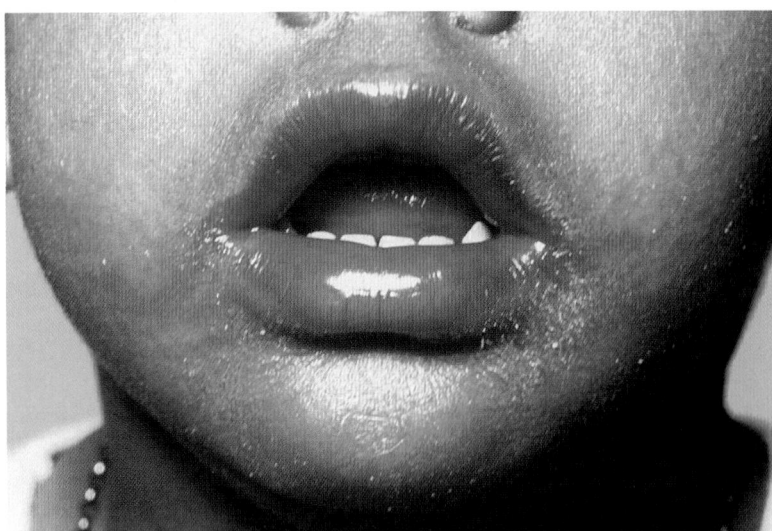

Fig. 16.63
Kawasaki disease: the lips are erythematous and swollen. Angular cheilitis is evident. By courtesy of J. Ross, MD, Lewisham Hospital, London, UK.

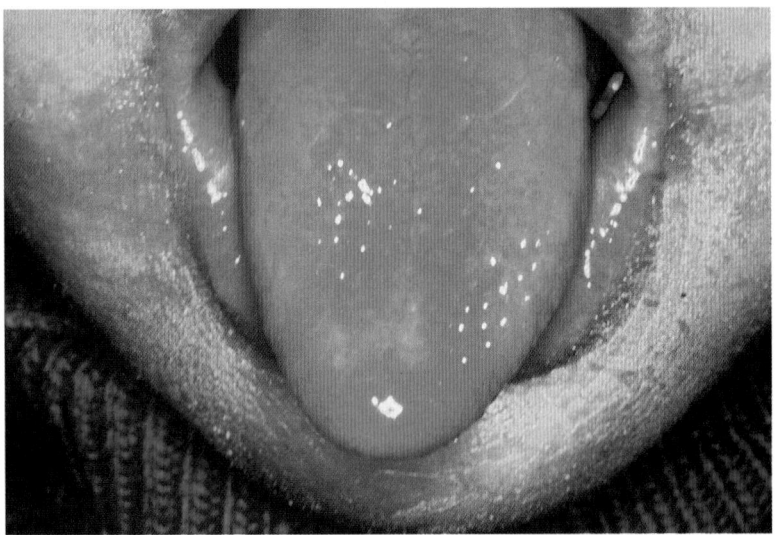

Fig. 16.64
Kawasaki disease: the tongue shows intense erythema. By courtesy of J. Ross, MD, Lewisham Hospital, London, UK.

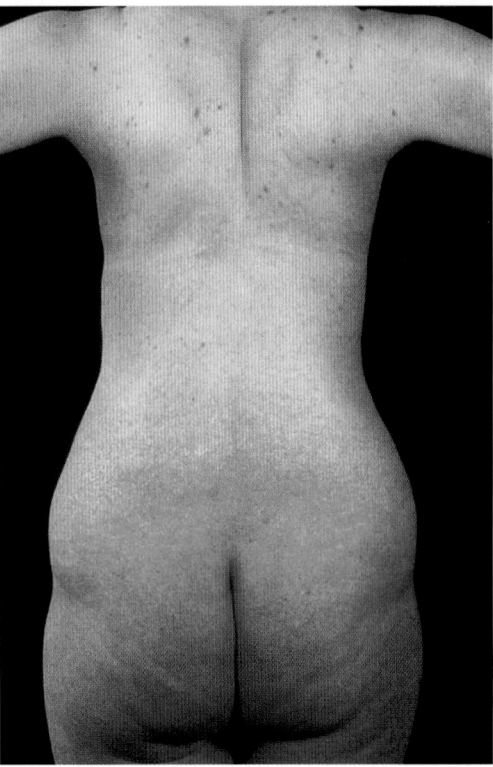

Fig. 16.65
Kawasaki disease: disease in an adult is very rare. In this patient, the erythema particularly affects the buttocks and thighs. By courtesy of W.G. Phillips, MD, Institute of Dermatology, London, UK.

the trunk and extremities, but may be more generalized. A diffuse, erythematous macular or plaquelike eruption involving the perineum is said to be characteristic.[5,6] This can be pruritic or painful and typically desquamates. Transverse orange-brown or white color changes of nails can be seen in up to 75% of cases.[19] Beau lines are another nail finding.[6] Rare cases of alopecia have been described.[20]

Cervical lymphadenopathy affects 50% to 75% of patients and may be unilateral or bilateral and involves one or a group of nodes.

Cardiovascular involvement is characteristic and is the most important cause of morbidity and mortality.[2] Some 50% of patients show evidence of myocarditis, which may progress to congestive cardiac failure. Pericardial effusion (subclinical) is not uncommon. Of particular significance is the development of coronary artery ectasia or aneurysm, a feature that develops in 15% to 25% of patients, which may be complicated by coronary artery ischemia, thrombosis, and infarction. In 2% of patients, it proves fatal.[13] In a very large follow-up study of 594 patients, the incidence of coronary artery aneurysm was 25%.[21] Angiographic evidence of regression was seen in 55% of patients.[21] There is an inverse relationship between the size of the aneurysm and the likelihood of resolution: large aneurysms, especially giant aneurysms (defined as greater than 8.0 mm), tend to persist, or become obstructed or stenotic.[22]

Gastrointestinal involvement presents as abdominal pain, vomiting, and diarrhea. Liver lesions may result in abnormal liver function tests and, less often, jaundice. Pancreatitis and hydrops of the gallbladder are seen in approximately 10% of patients.[2]

Neurological symptoms develop in about 30% of patients and include features of aseptic meningitis, seizures, and transient paralyses.[2] Arthralgias and arthritis are present in up to 30% to 40%, although chronicity is not a feature. Renal involvement manifests as sterile pyuria, hematuria, and infarction.

The features of adult Kawasaki syndrome are essentially those described above and can include erythema of the buttocks, as illustrated in *Fig. 16.65*. Coronary artery aneurysm, however, appears to be a less common complication.[11] It is important to differentiate this condition from staphylococcal toxic shock syndrome.[23]

Occasionally, patients develop a relapse, which may occur years after initial disease and resolution.[24]

Pathogenesis and histologic features

The etiology of this disease is unknown, but an infectious trigger is likely. Some evidence points to an immunoregulatory defect of T cells stimulated by superantigen-producing strains of *Streptococcus pyogenes* and *S. aureus*.[23,25,26] Superantigens are a class of microbial antigens that are thought to be capable of stimulating a large number of naive T cells in a non-specific manner by binding to histocompatibility antigens on antigen-presenting cells leading to T-cell activation. Superantigens have been postulated to play a role in the pathogenesis of a number of skin diseases in addition to Kawasaki disease, such as atopic dermatitis, psoriasis, and toxic shock syndrome. However, in one study, superantigen-producing bacteria were found in 56% of cultures (taken from throat, rectum, and groin) from patients with Kawasaki disease compared with 35% of controls with positive culture.[27] These differences did not achieve statistical significance. Another study found strains of streptococci and staphylococci in the jejunum of patients with Kawasaki disease but not in controls.[28] These same authors, in a follow-up study, found V beta 2+ T cells selectively increased in small bowel mucosa of Kawasaki patients compared with control subjects.[29] Other research has demonstrated IgA plasma cells and oligoclonal IgA response in affected arterial tissue, suggesting that the disease may be triggered from a pathogen at a mucosal site.[30] Clearly, further research is necessary to elucidate the precise pathogenesis of Kawasaki disease.

Other infectious agents that have been implicated, but not proved to be involved in the pathogenesis of Kawasaki disease, include retroviruses, rickettsiae, spirochetes *Propionibacterium acnes*, *M. pneumoniae*, Epstein-Barr virus, and adenoviruses.[5,6,31] Additionally favored hypotheses include exposure to house mites and recently cleaned or shampooed carpet, living in close proximity to open water or complicating a recent respiratory illness.[15] It is likely that Kawasaki disease represents a vasculitic disorder developing as a consequence of multiple infectious agents in a genetically susceptible individual.

Of interest, there is a growing body of literature reporting Kawasaki disease, or a Kawasaki-like syndrome, in patients infected with the HIV.[32–34]

The histopathological features of cutaneous lesions in Kawasaki disease are often non-specific and comprise severe edema of the papillary dermis accompanied by vascular dilatation, endothelial cell swelling, and degeneration associated with a superficial perivascular mononuclear infiltrate.[5] Immunopathological studies have shown the infiltrate is usually composed of CD4+ T lymphocytes and macrophages.[35] Occasionally, however, the features of a leukocytoclastic vasculitis are evident (*Fig. 16.66*). The epidermis may show mild basal cell degeneration.[5] Vesiculopustular lesions develop on the basis of subcorneal spongiform pustulation.[10]

Systemic lesions are characterized by necrotizing vasculitis.[23,36,37] Aneurysm with mural thrombus formation may be evident in advanced lesions.

Lymph node involvement includes vasculitis, focal necrosis, and infarction.

Differential diagnosis

The mucocutaneous manifestations of Kawasaki disease show considerable overlap with those seen in the toxic shock syndrome, which is not surprising, given that they appear to share a similar pathogenesis. Palmoplantar erythema, cutaneous desquamation, conjunctivitis, and pharyngitis are therefore common to both.[38] Toxic shock syndrome (which has been linked to staphylococcal exotoxin complicating constant tampon use in menstruating females) is, however, not associated with systemic vascular involvement. Histologically, it is characterized by a mild, superficial, perivascular lymphocytic infiltrate associated with edema of the papillary dermis and no evidence of vasculitis.[39]

Granuloma faciale

Clinical features

Granuloma faciale is a localized form of leukocytoclastic vasculitis of uncertain pathogenesis. Although children may be affected, most cases occur in people who are middle aged or older, most commonly in men.[1] Lesions occur most commonly on the face and are single or more often multiple, erythematous or brownish red, soft discrete papules, plaques or nodules up to several centimeters in diameter (*Fig. 16.67*).[2–4] The surface often shows dilated follicles and fine telangiectasia (*Fig. 16.68*). Common sites include the nose, malar prominence, forehead, and ear (*Fig. 16.69*). A case simulating rhinophyma has been documented.[5] Extrafacial lesions may occur

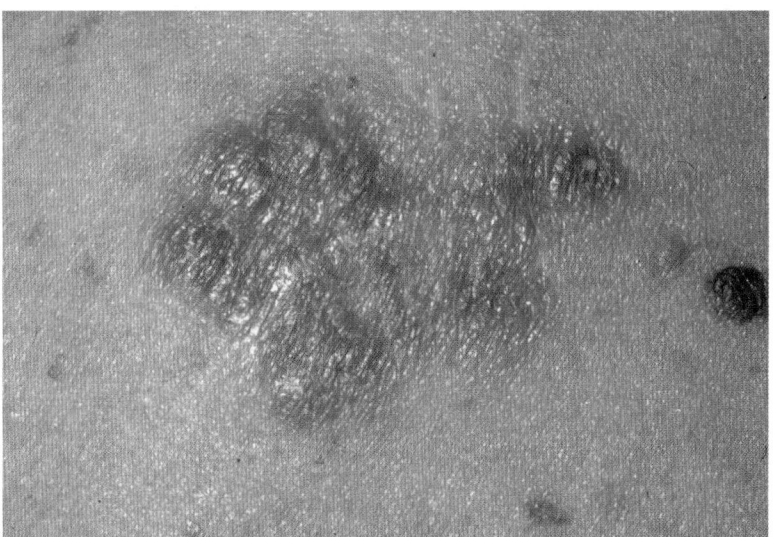

Fig. 16.67
Granuloma faciale: multiple brown nodules. From the collection of the late N.P. Smith, MD, the Institute of Dermatology, London, UK.

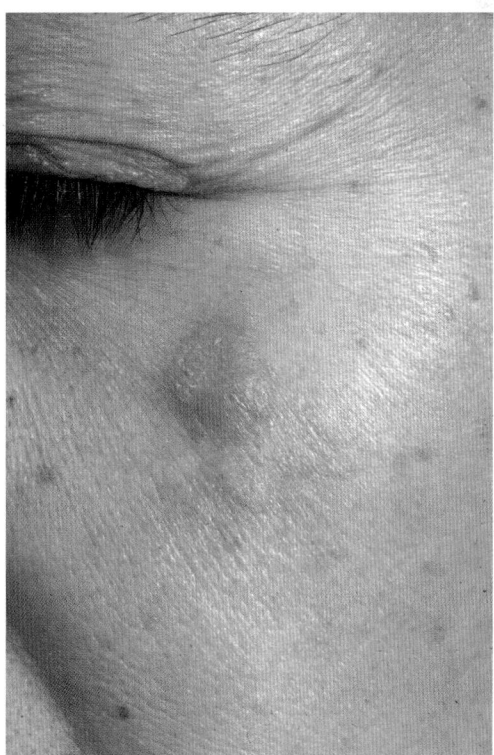

Fig. 16.68
Granuloma faciale: the face is a commonly affected site. From the collection of the late N.P. Smith, MD, the Institute of Dermatology, London, UK.

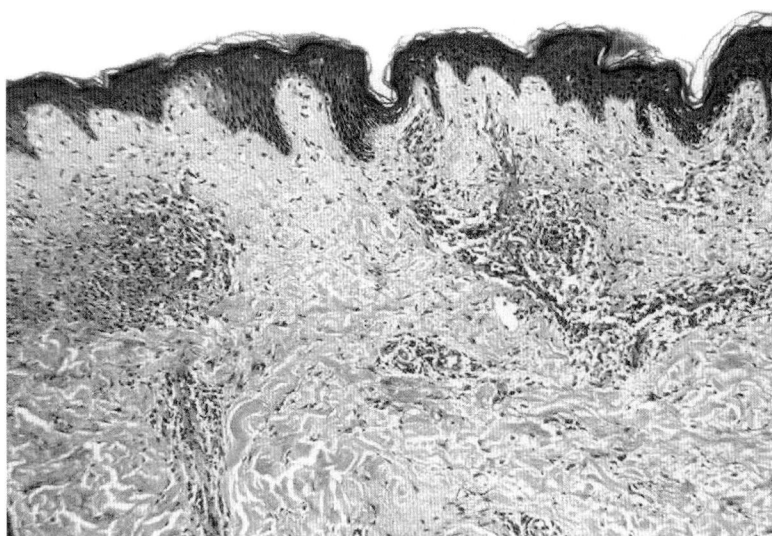

Fig. 16.66
Kawasaki disease: in this example, the features of severe, acute leukocytoclastic vasculitis are present in the superficial dermis. This is an uncommon finding. By courtesy of W.G. Phillips, MD, Institute of Dermatology, London, UK.

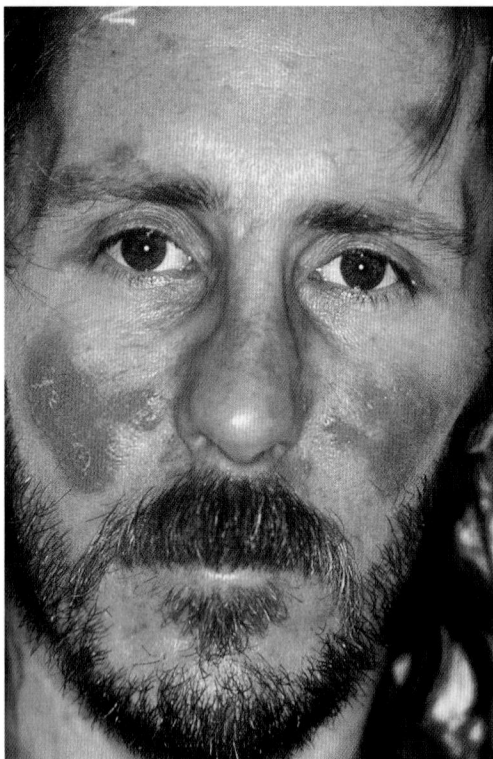

Fig. 16.69
Granuloma faciale: the lesions are frequently multiple. By courtesy of K. Liddell, MD, Eastbourne District Hospital, East Sussex, UK.

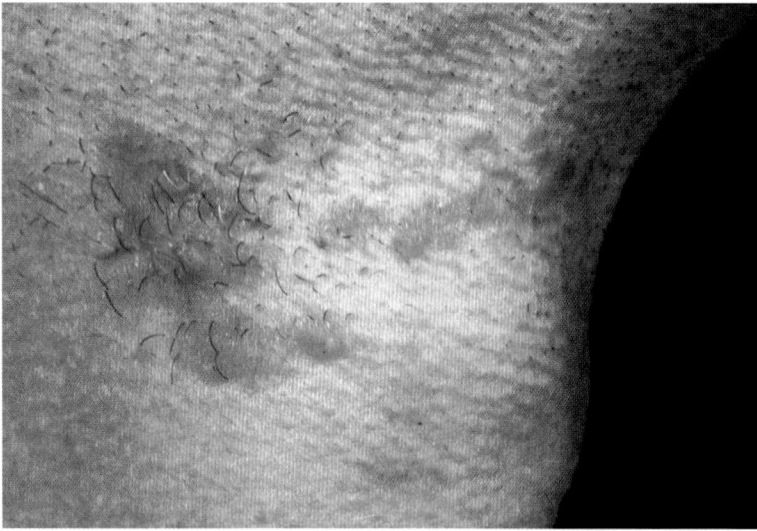

Fig. 16.70
Granuloma faciale: there are multiple lesions on this patient's neck. By courtesy of the Institute of Dermatology, London, UK.

on the extremities, neck, chest, and scalp (*Fig. 16.70*).[1,6–14] Although often asymptomatic, patients sometimes report symptoms of mild pruritus or stinging. There is no evidence of associated systemic involvement. Granuloma faciale tends to chronicity and is typified by periods of relapse and partial remissions. Treatment is very difficult and recurrences manifest after surgical excision, even at the site of full-thickness grafting.[15]

A histologically similar lesion affecting the mucosa of the upper respiratory tract has been designated 'eosinophilic angiocentric fibrosis'. Concurrent cases of granuloma faciale and eosinophilic angiocentric fibrosis have been described.[16–21] This suggests that the two diseases represent part of the same spectrum.

Granuloma faciale has been documented in a patient with prostate carcinoma.[22] Any relationship with tumors is likely to be coincidental.

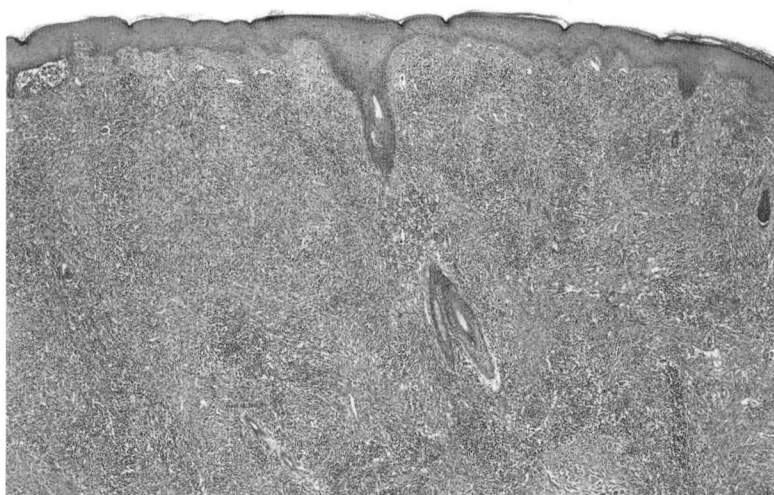

Fig. 16.71
Granuloma faciale: a dense inflammatory cell infiltrate is present in the dermis. Note the conspicuously spared grenz zone.

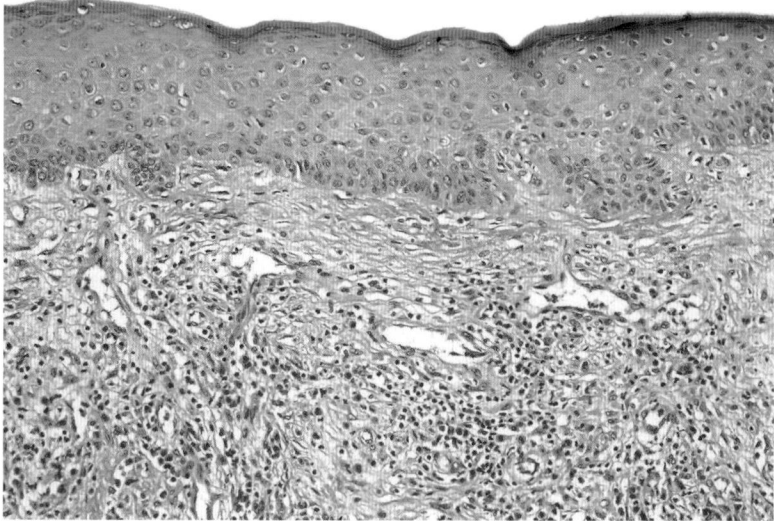

Fig. 16.72
Granuloma faciale: close-up view of grenz zone.

Pathogenesis and histologic features

Examination of lesional biopsies by immunofluorescence reveals granular IgG and complement along the epidermal-dermal junction, outlining the hair follicles, and also within the walls of blood vessels; less often IgA and IgM are present, and there is abundant fibrin.[23–25] Granuloma faciale is, therefore, a chronic vasculitis and may be immune complex mediated. However, some authors consider the above immunofluorescence findings non-specific. Immunohistochemistry shows the presence of abundant eosinophilic cationic protein.[26] T-helper lymphocytes represent the main nonmyelocytic cell in the infiltrate and it has been suggested that they play a role in the pathogenesis of the disease, being attracted to the site by gamma-interferon.[27]

Some cases of granuloma faciale may be related to IgG4-associated sclerosing diseases. In one study, just over 20% of granuloma faciale cases met immunohistochemical criteria for IgG4 sclerosing diseases.[28] In contrast, another large series demonstrated no evidence of IgG4-related disease, suggesting that the association may be less common.[29]

Histologically, granuloma faciale is characterized by a dense cellular infiltrate, which often has a nodular outline (*Fig. 16.71*).[30] This infiltrate usually occupies the mid-dermis, although the deep dermis and the subcutaneous fat may be involved; it typically spares the immediate subepidermis and hair follicles, forming a 'grenz zone' (*Fig. 16.72*). The infiltrate is polymorphic, being composed of large numbers of eosinophils, neutrophils

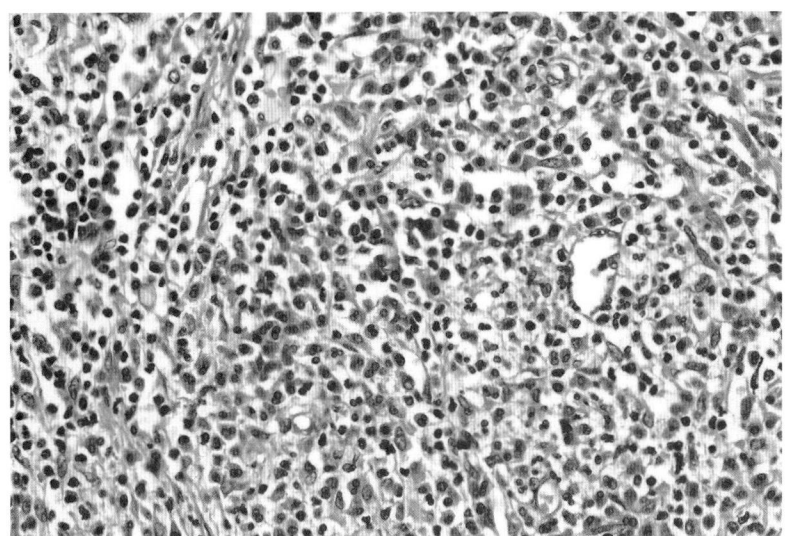

Fig. 16.73
Granuloma faciale: the infiltrate contains large numbers of eosinophils as well as lymphocytes, histiocytes, and occasional polymorphs and plasma cells.

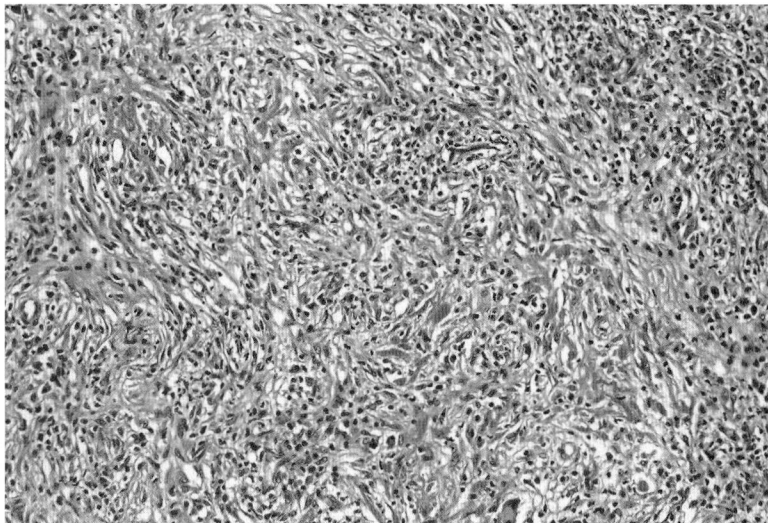

Fig. 16.75
Granuloma faciale: there is a well-developed storiform pattern.

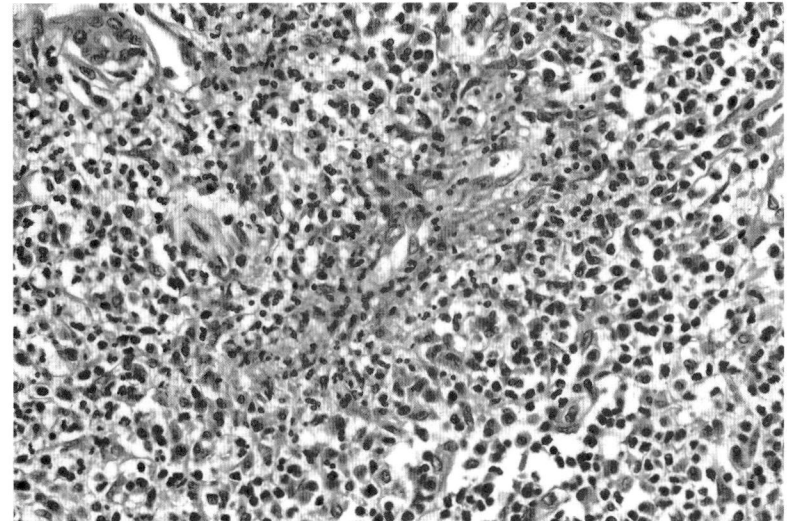

Fig. 16.74
Granuloma faciale: this dilated blood vessel shows marked endothelial swelling, fibrin deposition, and disruption of its wall.

(often displaying leukocytoclasis), and an admixture of plasma cells, mast cells, and lymphocytes (*Fig. 16.73*).[31] Red cell extravasation is often present. Blood vessels, which often appear increased in number, are dilated and may show infiltration of their walls by eosinophils with fibrin deposition (*Fig. 16.74*). Diagnostic features of vasculitis, namely inflammation of vessel walls associated with fibrinoid change, may be difficult to identify or absent in some lesions.[6] In other cases, fibrin is widely distributed in the dermis. Older lesions may show fibrosis and hemosiderin deposition.[1] The microscopic picture in late stages overlaps with that seen in erythema elevatum diutinum (*Fig. 16.75*).[1]

An ultrastructural study of a case of granuloma faciale has shown that the cytoplasmic granules in the eosinophils display alterations and Langerhans cells are absent.[32]

Differential diagnosis

The morphological features of granuloma faciale are distinctive. The presence of a mixed infiltrate with a grenz zone distinguishes it from neutrophilic dermatoses and leukocytoclastic vasculitis. Erythema elevatum diutinum, another form of localized vasculitis, tends to be located on the extensor surfaces of the extremities and shows more sclerosis, more neutrophils, and fewer eosinophils. The presence of large numbers of eosinophils may raise the possibility of a Langerhans cell proliferative disorder; however, the presence of only scattered Langerhans cells and a grenz zone (Langerhans cell proliferative disorders tend to be epidermotropic) with significant numbers of neutrophils favors granuloma faciale. The grenz zone also helps to distinguish granuloma faciale from hypersensitivity reactions, such as to an arthropod bite. Epithelioid hemangioma (angiolymphoid hyperplasia) is distinguished by the presence of a lobular proliferation of vessels lined by epithelioid endothelial cells. An exceptional case of infection by *Trichophyton rubrum* with histology mimicking that of granuloma faciale has been documented.[33]

Histologic features identical to those of granuloma faciale may be seen in patients presenting with a solitary lesion (papule, nodule, or plaque) that does not have the clinical appearance or location typical of the disease. The histologic picture in these cases has been described as chronic fibrosing vasculitis. As there is also histologic overlap with erythema elevatum diutinum, it has been suggested that the microscopic appearances represent a non-specific inflammatory reaction pattern.[34] Therefore, establishing the diagnosis requires close clinicopathological correlation.

Erythema elevatum diutinum

Clinical features

This uncommon disease represents a localized variant of leukocytoclastic vasculitis.[1–3] Although it can occur in any age group, patients are usually in their third to fifth decade.[4] Incidence is equal in men and women. Patients present with papules and nodules measuring up to about 1 cm in diameter; they may also develop round or oval, indurated, elevated plaques 5–6 cm in diameter. Lesions are red or purple, although some have a yellowish tinge, which may be confused with a xanthomatous process. Bullous lesions are occasionally present and an annular distribution has been reported.[1,5,6] The disease is characteristically persistent and the distribution of the lesions often symmetrical. Large nodules resembling keloids or tumors are sometimes found.[7,8]

Lesions are located particularly in relation to the extensor surfaces of the joints and are, therefore, seen on the backs of the hands and fingers, wrists, elbows, knees, ankles, and toes (*Figs 16.76* and *16.77*). The buttocks may also be affected, but the trunk is usually spared.[9] We have observed a case with oral involvement. Although lesions are often asymptomatic, some patients complain of itching and pain, and symptoms are frequently made worse in a cold environment. Patients sometimes also have arthralgia. Eye involvement includes keratolysis and ulcerative keratitis with positive rheumatoid factor.[10–13] Although the disease is chronic and progressive, resolution usually occurs by 5–10 years. The disease characteristically responds to dapsone.

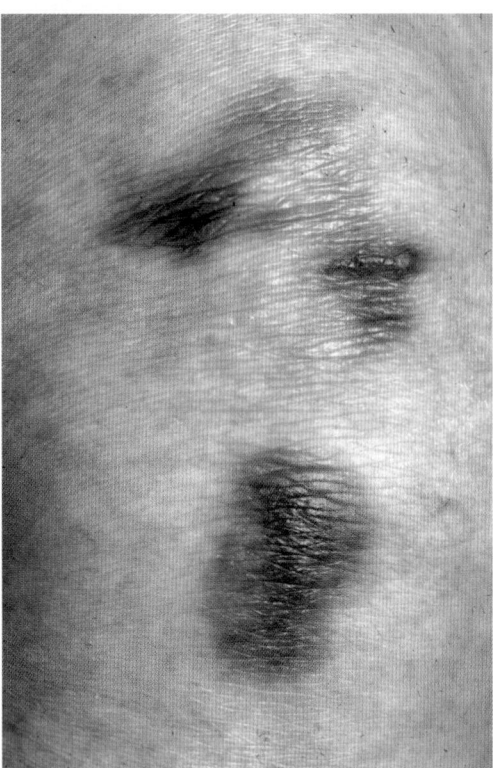

Fig. 16.76
Erythema elevatum diutinum: tuberose nodules present on the elbow. From the collection of the late N.P. Smith, MD, the Institute of Dermatology, London, UK.

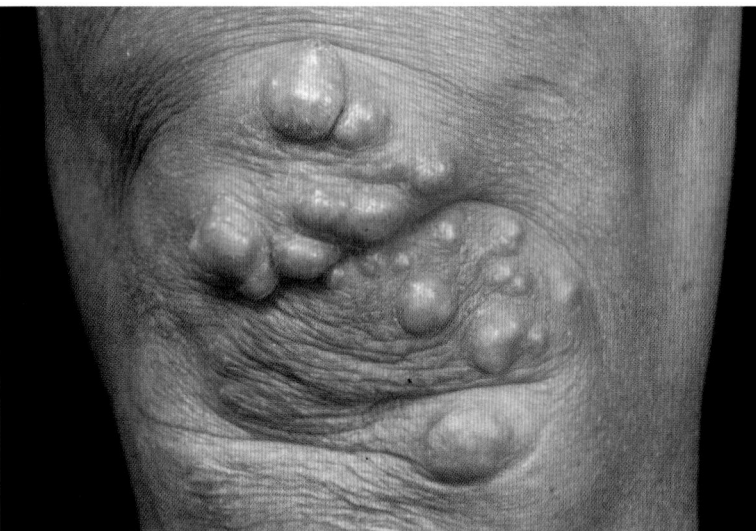

Fig. 16.77
Erythema elevatum diutinum: the extensor surfaces are commonly affected. From the collection of the late N.P. Smith, MD, the Institute of Dermatology, London, UK.

Systemic involvement does not usually occur but pulmonary infiltrates have exceptionally been documented.[14]

An association with paraproteinemia is frequently present, often of the IgA subtype.[1,15–19] Hyperimmunoglobulinemia D syndrome is a further rare association.[20] An underlying myelodysplastic syndrome or a hematological malignancy (e.g., multiple myeloma, B-cell lymphoma, and chronic lymphocytic leukemia) has been found in some patients.[1,21–25] Often, the skin lesions precede development of the hematological disorder.[1] In one study, an average of 7.8 years separated onset of skin lesions and development of a myeloproliferative disorder.[1,26]

Erythema elevatum diutinum has rarely also been associated with other malignancies such as pulmonary lymphoepithelioma-like carcinoma and breast carcinoma.[27,28]

Inflammatory bowel disease – both Crohn disease and ulcerative colitis – has also been associated with erythema elevatum diutinum.[29–31] Interestingly, in one patient with Crohn disease, skin lesions seemed to appear during exacerbation of bowel symptoms.[29] In another patient with ulcerative colitis, onset of erythema elevatum diutinum lesions coincided with presentation of bowel disease, and skin lesions resolved following colectomy.[30] Erythema elevatum diutinum has also been reported in association with celiac disease.[32–34] In one patient with celiac disease, skin lesions resolved with the introduction of a gluten-free diet.[33]

Rheumatoid arthritis has been described in conjunction with erythema elevatum diutinum.[35–37] Other reported associations include granulomatosis with polyangiitis, relapsing polychondritis, pyoderma gangrenosum, Sweet syndrome, cutaneous lupus erythematosus, nodular scleritis and panuveitis, Hashimoto thyroiditis, juvenile idiopathic arthritis, Sjögren syndrome, dermatomyositis, and dermatitis herpetiformis.[38–50] Erythema elevatum diutinum is also seen in patients with HIV infection.[51–56] In HIV-infected patients, lesions may mimic Kaposi sarcoma.[51,57] Extensive acro-osteolysis has been described in a single case.[58] The exceptional association with pityriasis rubra pilaris and mosquito bites is probably coincidental.[59]

Although it has been suggested that a condition described as 'neutrophilic dermatosis of the dorsal hands' may be part of the spectrum of erythema elevatum diutinum, it is more likely to represent a variant of Sweet syndrome.[60]

Pathogenesis and histologic features

Erythema elevatum diutinum is possibly immune complex mediated. Both a streptococcal antigen and *E. coli* have been implicated.[2,61] As mentioned above, the disease has also been recorded in association with cryoglobulin IgA, monoclonal or biclonal gammopathy, multiple myeloma, hairy cell leukemia, and polycythemia rubra vera.[1,62–64] In addition, IgA ANCA and less frequently IgG ANCA have been identified in patient's serum.[65] In early lesions, there is increased expression of the beta (2)-integrins CR3 and LFA-1 and this diminishes in older lesions.[66] Peripheral blood neutrophils show increased migration in response to interleukin-8 (IL-8) and decreased responsiveness to the bacterial peptide analog N-formyl-methionyl-leucyl-phenylalanine. These findings suggest that in erythema elevatum diutinum the recruitment of neutrophils occurs as a result of activation of cytokines such as IL-8.[66] Immune complexes and bacterial peptides sustain the persistent local inflammatory response.[66] There appears to be no association with IgG4-related diseases.[67,68]

Biopsy of early lesions reveals typical features of leukocytoclastic vasculitis (*Fig. 16.78*).[1,69] The epidermis may show acanthosis and parakeratosis. Fibrinoid necrosis and infiltration of the superficial vessels by neutrophil polymorphs are present. The perivenular connective tissue contains abundant fibrin and a dense inflammatory cell infiltrate of neutrophils, histiocytes, lymphocytes, and eosinophils. Leukocytoclasis is usually evident.

Older lesions are characterized by the development of granulation tissue and fibrous scarring, although even then, foci of neutrophilic vasculitis may be found after examination of multiple sections (*Fig. 16.79*). In 'burnt out' lesions, vasculitis may not be present. Granulation tissue and dense scarring mark the site of the previous acute inflammatory process. In older lesions the scarring often shows a storiform pattern (*Fig. 16.80*). Interstitial lipid deposition described in the past as extracellular cholesterolosis is uncommon.

In ocular lesions, leukocytoclastic vasculitis with focal granulomatous inflammation has been described.[11]

Rare histopathological features described include palisaded necrotizing granuloma and pyogenic granuloma-like features.[59]

Differential diagnosis

Erythema elevatum diutinum typically involves the dermis and must, therefore, be distinguished from granuloma faciale. Granuloma faciale usually shows an eosinophil predominance whereas in erythema elevatum diutinum neutrophils are much more numerous. However, the histologic features of late lesions in both entities often overlap and similar appearances are found in chronic fibrosing vasculitis. The latter represents a non-specific reaction pattern that is occasionally seen in solitary lesions from patients who have no clinical features of either granuloma faciale or erythema elevatum

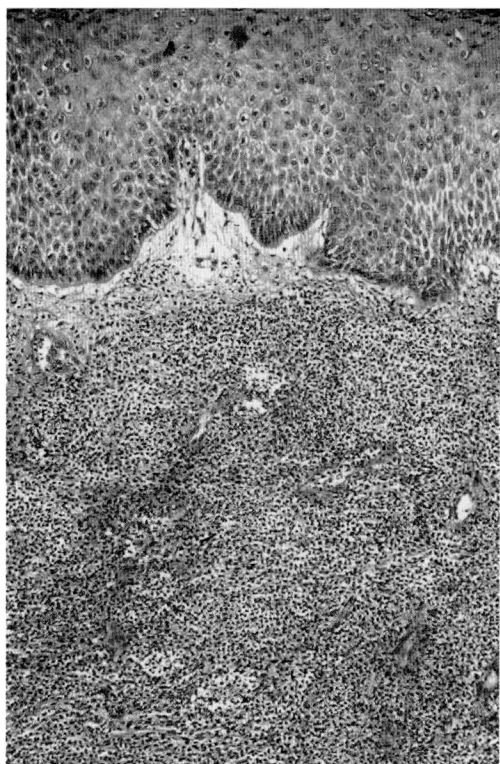

Fig. 16.78
Erythema elevatum diutinum: early lesion showing leukocytoclastic vasculitis in a background of a Sweet syndrome-like neutrophil infiltrate.

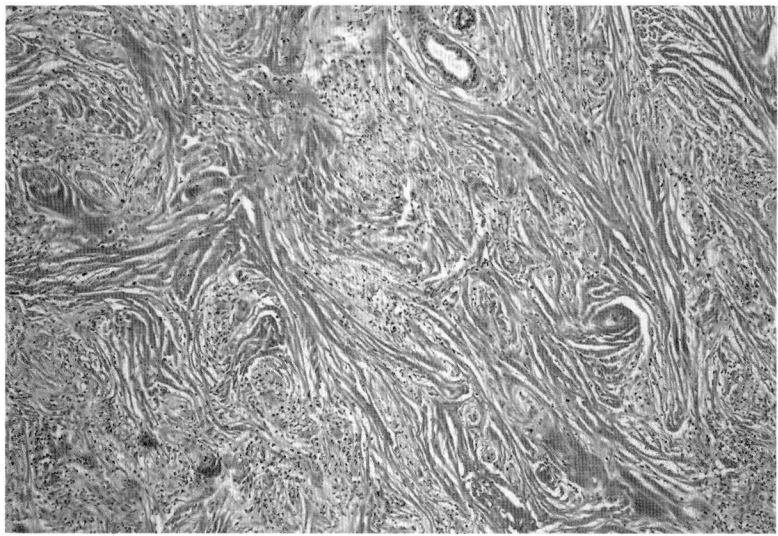

Fig. 16.79
Erythema elevatum diutinum: older lesion showing scar tissue with a vaguely storiform growth pattern.

diutinum.[70] Distinction from Sweet syndrome is afforded by the presence of neutrophilic vasculitis. Older sclerotic lesions, particularly when they present as mass lesions, may be mistaken for a neoplastic process or dermatofibroma.[8] The presence of a leukocytoclastic vasculitis and neutrophilic infiltrate with karyorrhexis favors erythema elevatum diutinum.

Behçet disease

Clinical features

This rare disease was originally described as a combination of recurrent oral and genital ulceration associated with uveitis. However, it is now known to represent a systemic illness with lesions involving the joints and central nervous, vascular, respiratory, gastrointestinal, and urogenital systems, in

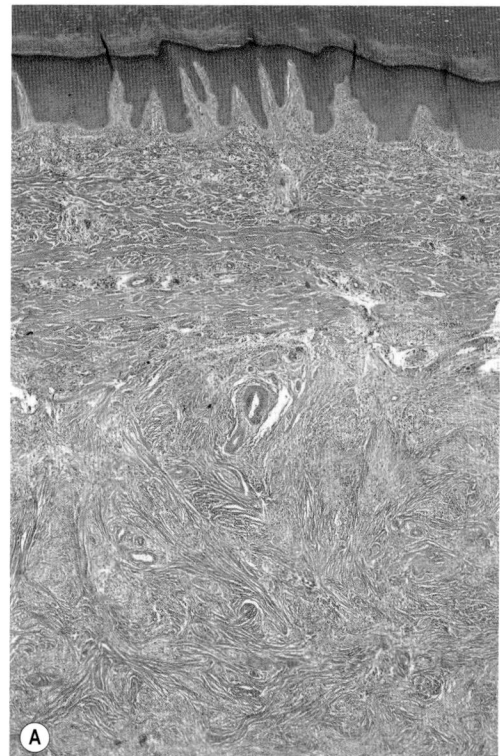

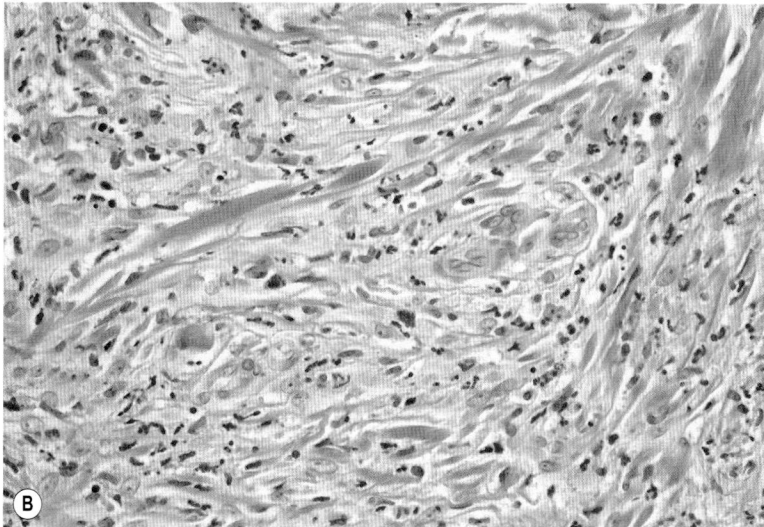

Fig. 16.80
(A, B) Erythema elevatum diutinum: this example was clinically thought to represent a keloid. There is a circumscribed dermal nodule composed of spindle cells in a hyalinized stroma. Focally perivascular nuclear debris is evident and there are scattered eosinophils.

addition to mucous membranes and integument (Table 16.7).[1-13] Although it is seen worldwide, it has a high incidence in Japan, Southeast Asia, the Middle East, Turkey, and some countries bordering the Mediterranean. Behçet disease shows a male predominance and most commonly presents in young adults with a peak incidence of onset in the third decade.[14] Children may also be affected with an approximately equal sex incidence.[15] One study has suggested that the disease is less aggressive in children.[16] Some data appear to indicate that males have a higher mortality rate.[17]

The International Study Group established diagnostic criteria for Behçet disease in 1990 and these are summarized in Table 16.8.[4] It should be kept in mind that these criteria are somewhat controversial.[18] More research is necessary before we can fully understand this complex disease.

Recurrent oral ulceration is an invariable feature. Some patients have a long history of oral ulceration before developing other features that allow for a definitive diagnosis of Behçet disease. Ulcers typically measure up to 1 cm across but may be larger. They develop anywhere in the oral cavity,

Table 16.7
Behçet disease: frequency of organ involvement

Sign or symptom	Incidence (%)
Oral ulcers	90–100
Genital ulcers	64–88
Ocular lesions	27–90
Cutaneous lesions	48–88
Joint manifestations	18–64
Neurological features	10–29
Intestinal manifestations	0–59
Thrombophlebitis	10–37

Reproduced with permission from Arbesfield, S.J. and Kurban, A.K. (1988) *Journal of the American Academy of Dermatology*, 19, 767–779. Copyright © The American Academy of Dermatology, Inc.

Table 16.8
Behçet disease: diagnostic criteria*

Criterion	Definition
Recurrent oral ulceration	Minor aphthous, major aphthous, or herpetiform ulceration observed by physician or patient, and recurrent at least three times in one 12-month period
Plus two of:	
Recurrent genital ulceration	Aphthous ulceration or scarring, observed by physician or patient
Eye lesions	Anterior uveitis, posterior uveitis, or cells in vitreous on slit lamp examination or Retinal vasculitis observed by ophthalmologist
Skin lesions	Erythema nodosum observed by physician or patient, pseudofolliculitis or papulopustular lesions; or acneiform nodules observed by physician, patient not on corticosteroid treatment
Positive pathergy test	Read by physician at 24–48 hours

*Findings applicable only in the absence of other clinical explanations.
Reprinted with permission from Elsevier (International Study Group for Behçet's Disease (1990) *Lancet*, 335, 1078–1080).

in the pharynx, and even in the larynx (*Fig. 16.81*).[19] They are exquisitely painful, and usually regress spontaneously within 14 days although they can persist for much longer. A yellow, necrotic crust covers the ulcer floor. Some patients develop ulcerations in a herpetiform configuration.[20] Patients with larger ulcers tend to have greater severity of oral disease with more frequent relapses.[20]

Cutaneous lesions are common, recurrent, and comprise a wide variety of manifestations including erythema nodosum-like lesions, usually on the lower extremities.[21,22] Patients may also develop acneiform papules and pustules, furuncles, pyoderma, and thrombophlebitis (*Fig. 16.82*). In one very large study, papulopustular lesions (followed by erythema nodosum-like nodules) were the most commonly encountered skin manifestation.[7] Patients have also been described with Sweet syndrome-like features.[23]

Typical of Behçet disease, and an important diagnostic clue, is development of sterile pustules at sites of mild skin trauma such as injection sites (pathergic response) (*Fig. 16.83*).[24,25] Paradoxically, some authors have found that wound healing after 4 mm punch biopsy does not seem to differ compared with control subjects.[26]

Genital lesions, similar in appearance to those of the oral mucosa, occur on the scrotum, penis, vagina, and vulva (*Figs 16.84* and *16.85*).[7]

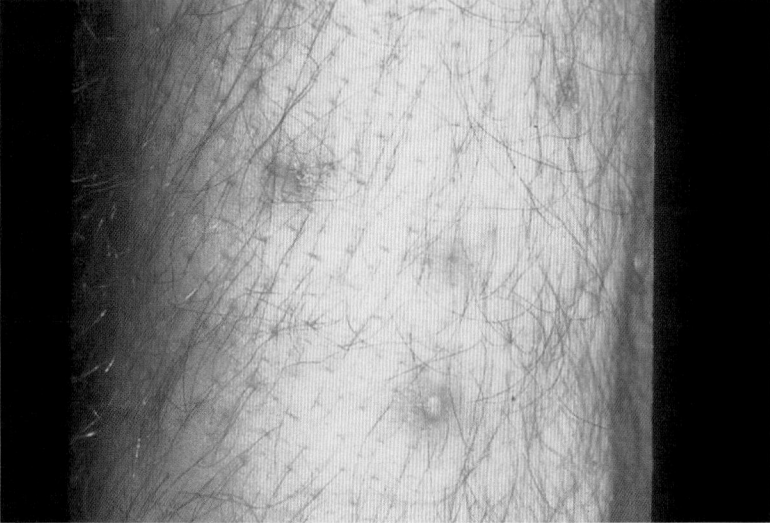

Fig. 16.82
Behçet disease: typical pustules on the lower leg. By courtesy of R.A. Marsden, MD, St George's Hospital, London, UK.

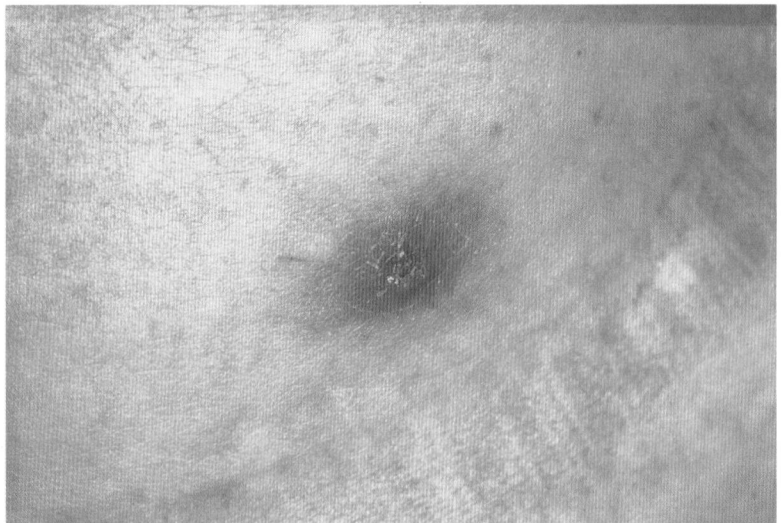

Fig. 16.83
Behçet disease: this ruptured pustule developed at the site of a previous venipuncture. Such a positive provocation test is virtually pathognomonic for Behçet disease. By courtesy of D.A.H. Yates, MD, St Thomas' Hospital, London, UK.

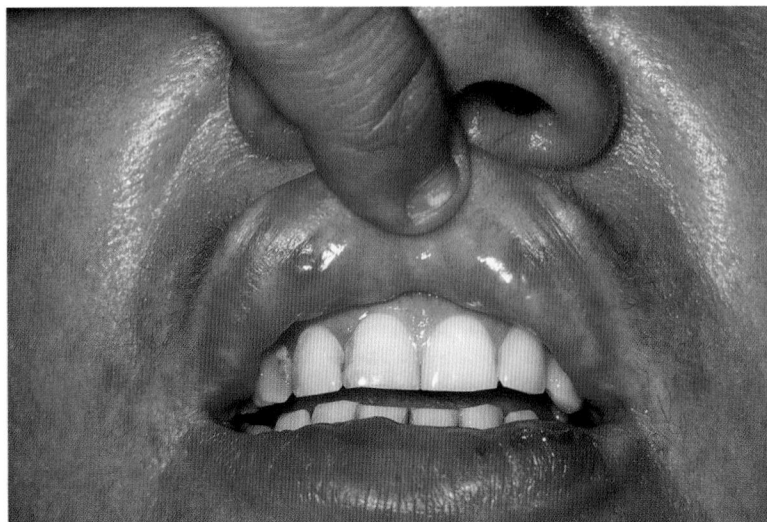

Fig. 16.81
Behçet disease: superficial ulcers are present on the inner aspect of both lips. By courtesy of R.A. Marsden, MD, St George's Hospital, London, UK.

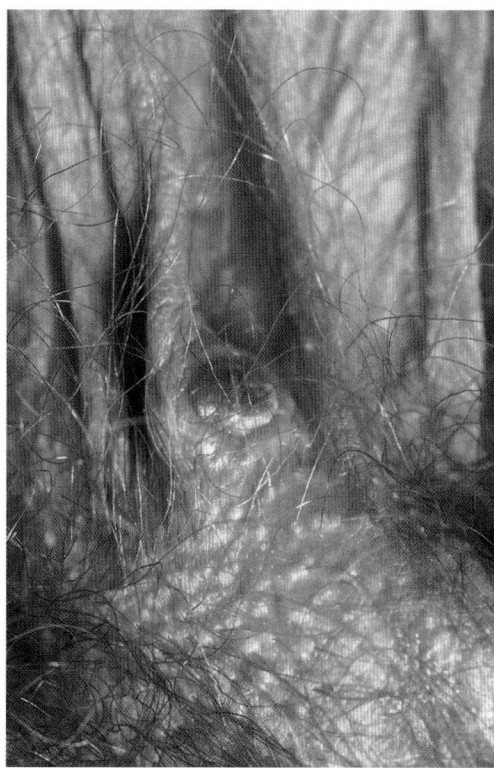

Fig. 16.84
Behçet disease: there is a typical scrotal ulcer with central slough. By courtesy of D.A.H. Yates, MD, St Thomas' Hospital, London, UK.

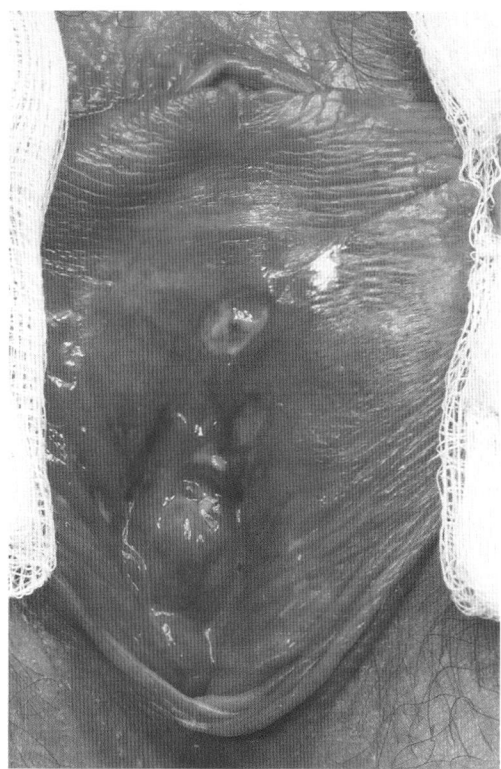

Fig. 16.85
Behçet disease: multiple superficial vulval ulcers are present. By courtesy of R.A. Marsden, MD, St George's Hospital, London, UK.

Ocular involvement is important because, if left untreated, it may progress to cataracts and blindness. Both eyes are affected in the majority of patients. Almost any part of the eye is affected and bilateral inflammation of the anterior segment (anterior uveitis), posterior uveitis with hypopyon, and vitreitis are said to be pathognomonic.[27,28] Uveitis is more common and

is associated with a more severe clinical course in males, potentially leading to loss of vision.[28] Conjunctivitis, corneal ulceration, choroiditis, and retinal vessel involvement (arterial and venous vasculitis) are sometimes additional features.

Joint involvement is not uncommon and usually affects the knees, ankles, elbows, and wrists.[29] A mono- or oligoarticular pattern is typical. The affected joints are swollen, red, tender, and painful. It is of interest that despite many years of arthritic symptoms, joint deformities do not develop.

Vascular disease in Behçet disease takes the form of both thrombo-occlusive disease and frank vasculitis. Vascular involvement is an important cause of both morbidity and mortality and is seen in approximately one-third of patients.[30,31] Males appear to be at an increased risk.[31] Thrombophlebitis is common and can affect both superficial and deep veins of the limbs. Superior and inferior vena caval obstruction are not uncommon complications. A particularly perilous form of vascular involvement is hepatic vein occlusion (Budd-Chiari syndrome), which is associated with a high mortality.[13,32] Pulmonary artery aneurysm occurs in approximately 1% of patients and is associated with a 50% mortality rate.[33,34]

The inflammation may affect virtually any artery and the development of an aneurysm with subsequent rupture is an important cause of death.

Respiratory involvement presents as dyspnea, cough, pleuritic chest pain, and hemoptysis.[36] The last, due to pulmonary artery–bronchial fistula formation, is an important cause of death. Lung involvement occurs in up to 5% of patients.[35]

Intestinal involvement particularly affects the ileocecal region; ulcers may be complicated by perforation, presenting as an intra-abdominal emergency necessitating surgical intervention.[36–38] Interestingly, one group has reported seasonal variation in Behçet disease flares suggesting an exogenous component or trigger.[39] The esophagus is uncommonly affected by ulcers and erosion, stenosis or esophagitis.[40]

Involvement of the nervous system, which is associated with a poor prognosis, occurs in up to 25% of patients.[12,41] Lesions develop anywhere in the central and peripheral components and, therefore, virtually any neurological sign or symptom may be seen, including sensory losses, strokes, and spinal cord, cranial and peripheral nerve lesions. Dural sinus thrombosis is a well-recognized complication.[41]

The kidney is affected in up to 55% of patients and manifestations include amyloidosis, glomerulonephritis, interstitial nephritis, vasculitis, and IgA nephropathy.[42–46]

A study of relative organ system involvement has led to a subclassification of a spectrum of Behçet disease.[47,48] The mortality of Behçet disease is, however, surprisingly low, of the order of 2% to 4%.

Pathogenesis and histologic features

Although the precise etiology and pathogenesis are unknown. It is likely that there is an altered immune response in patients with Behçet disease. It has been suggested that heat shock proteins may play an important role in its pathogenesis.[49,50] They have been found to be elevated in serum together with increased levels of vascular endothelial growth factor (VEGF) and antiphospholipid antibodies independent of disease activity.[51] Heat shock proteins reactive in Behçet patients induce uveitis in rats.[50] Increased VEGF levels correlate significantly with the presence of vascular or ocular disease.[51] Oligoclonal expansion of T cells in some patients with Behçet disease has been documented.[52] In one study, serum IL-12 and peripheral Th1 lymphocyte levels correlated with disease activity.[53]

The increased peripheral Th1 lymphocyte levels would seem to correlate with molecular findings. Genome wide association studies have identified associations with the *IL23R-IL12RB2*, *IL10*, *STAT4*, *CCR1-CCR3*, *KLRC4*, *ERAP1*, *TNFAIP3*, and *FUT2* loci. These genes are associated with polarization toward a Th1 phenotype.[54]

Complement components C3 and C9 have been identified in blood vessel walls in oral biopsies.[48] Increased interleukin levels associated with increased B-cell activity have also been described.[55] Of possible importance in the pathogenesis is the frequent presence of high levels of circulating immune complexes and the common detection of immunoglobulins (particularly IgM) and complement in blood vessel walls.[56–58] Behçet disease is associated with human leukocyte antigen (HLA)-B5, -B12, -B15, -B27,

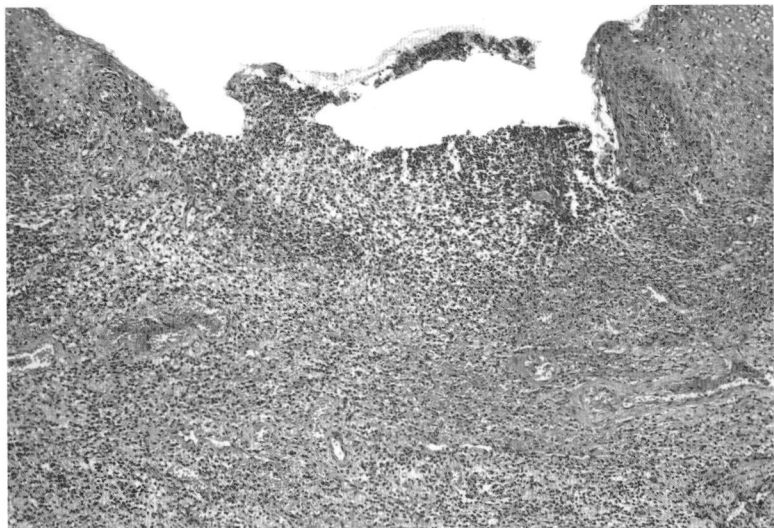

Fig. 16.86
Behçet disease: this field shows a superficial vulval ulcer with an intense neutrophilic infiltrate and changes of acute vasculitis.

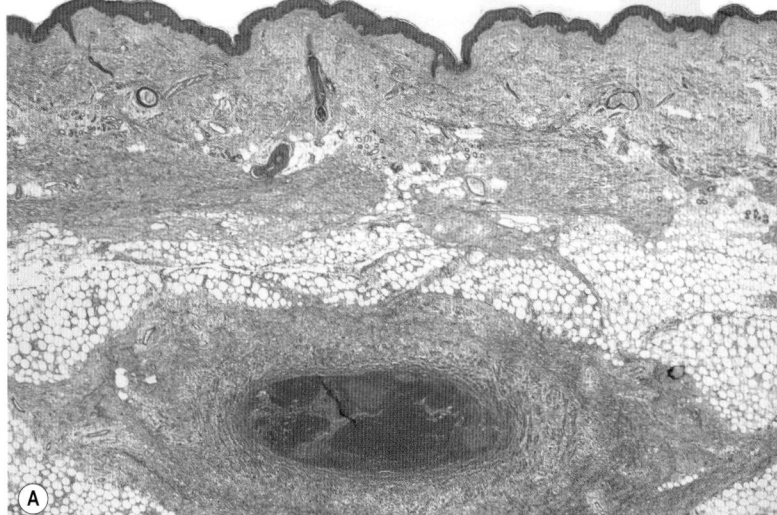

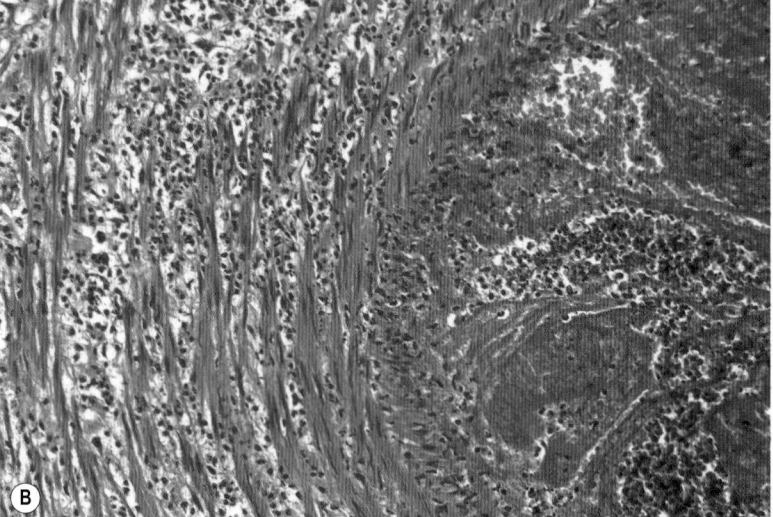

Fig. 16.88
(**A**, **B**) Behçet disease: this section shows thrombophlebitis involving a vein in the subcutaneous fat. The vessel is infiltrated by large numbers of lymphocytes.

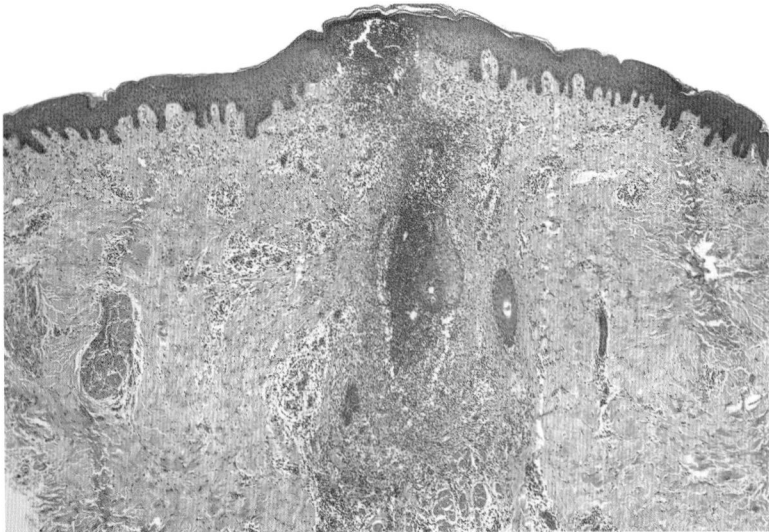

Fig. 16.87
Behçet disease: there is florid suppurative acute folliculitis.

-A26, and particularly with HLA-BW51.[30,54] Anticardiolipin antibodies have been described.[30]

Despite the accumulation of considerable immunological and genetic data, the underlying antigen or other stimulus that drives these changes, and is ultimately responsible for the disease, remains elusive.

The histologic features are in themselves largely non-specific.[48,55,59,60] The diagnosis of Behçet disease is essentially clinical. The pathological features that may be detected include both lymphocytic and necrotizing vasculitis affecting the superficial postcapillary venules with associated fibrinoid necrosis (*Fig. 16.86*).[59] In one study, nearly 50% of patients had evidence of vasculitis.[61] Often, however, such vasculitic changes appear to be a consequence, rather than a cause, of the dermal or mucosal inflammatory changes.[60] Endothelial swelling may be a feature and there is often an associated lymphocytic perivascular infiltrate, although sometimes neutrophils are abundant.[62] Venulitis and phlebitis were the most common forms of vasculitis seen in one series of patients.[18] In this study, phlebitis/venulitis was seen in 48% of patients while leukocytoclastic vasculitis and lymphocytic vasculitis were seen in 17% and 31% of patients, respectively.[61]

Non-specific features include a diffuse neutrophil polymorph dermal infiltrate with or without abscess formation, corresponding clinically to pustular lesions, acute folliculitis, and acneiform folliculocentric pustular changes (*Fig. 16.87*).[18,63,64] Biopsy after needle trauma in one study showed

a neutrophilic infiltrate with intraepidermal pustules. Vasculitis was not seen in pathergic lesions in this study.[65] Other authors have found that the pathergic lesions may show leukocytoclastic vasculitis or Sweet syndrome-like features.[24]

The erythema nodosum-like lesions correspond to necrotizing vasculitis of the subcutaneous vessels, usually associated with thrombosis. Septal and lobular panniculitis have also been described.[19] Superficial thrombophlebitis is present in up to 30% of patients (*Fig. 16.88*).[47] Oral lesions and genital ulcers show non-specific ulceration, accompanied in some instances by leukocytoclastic or lymphocytic vasculitis.

Pulmonary involvement is characterized by pulmonary artery vasculitis, sometimes also affecting the veins and capillaries.[35] Thrombosis, infarction, hemorrhage, and the development of aneurysm are important sequelae. The inflammation is usually transmural and may be associated with damage to the associated elastic tissue. Older destructive vascular lesions are characterized by fibrous scarring.

Cerebral lesions in the early stage are characterized by a perivenular lymphocytic infiltrate. In the more advanced lesions there is extensive demyelination resembling multiple sclerosis.[30]

Differential diagnosis

Given the myriad non-specific histologic manifestations that Behçet disease may produce, it comes as no surprise that the histologic differential diagnosis is usually broad. The authors of one large study stated that clinical data are most important in establishing a diagnosis and suggested that the role of biopsy is to confirm the clinical impression.[7] Others propose that biopsy is critical to evaluate for vessel-based pathology as clinical distinction from pustular (non-vascular) lesions may be important.[18] It is likely that the criteria for diagnosis of Behçet disease will continue to be refined.

The differential diagnosis includes other causes of folliculitis, infection, erythema nodosum, connective tissue disease, neutrophilic and lymphocytic vasculitis, and neutrophilic dermatoses. There are no pathognomonic histologic changes. Both clinical and pathological data must be considered before arriving at a final diagnosis.[7]

Thromboangiitis obliterans

Clinical features

Thromboangiitis obliterans (Buerger disease) is most often seen in young adults and is much more common in males than in females.[1] However, the ratio of men to women is shifting, with the disease becoming more common in women.[2,3] In one large study, 23% of patients were female.[2] In addition, the disease is seen more frequently in older patients.[2] Buerger disease occurs almost exclusively in smokers. Although most patients are considered 'heavy' smokers, some smoke less than a pack of cigarettes a day.[4] In fact, some authors view a history of smoking a necessary criterion for diagnosis. In one study from Japan, nonsmokers with Buerger disease were more likely to be women.[5] In Bangladesh, smoking bidis (a hand-rolled, additive-free, unprocessed form of tobacco) is particularly associated with this disease.[6]

The worldwide incidence of Buerger disease differs dramatically from region to region. For example, the incidence is 50-fold greater in Nepal compared with North America.[7] This disease has its highest prevalence in Eastern Europe, the Middle East, and Asia. Patients most often present with painful cyanotic lesions of the extremities, especially the fingers or toes, which may ulcerate and become gangrenous (Fig. 16.89). Sensitivity to cold is a common complaint.

Resolution of disease usually follows cessation of smoking.[8,9] Patients who continue to smoke suffer autoamputation of digits and distal extremities. In one study, only 2% of patients who quit smoking had amputations. In contrast, 42% of those that continued to smoke required amputation.[2]

In most patients, the disease is limited to the extremities; however, some patients develop visceral involvement,[10–13] and this can prove fatal.[10] The vessels of the brain, intestine, heart, kidney, and lung may therefore be affected.[14–17] Occasional patients have involvement of multiple organs.[18]

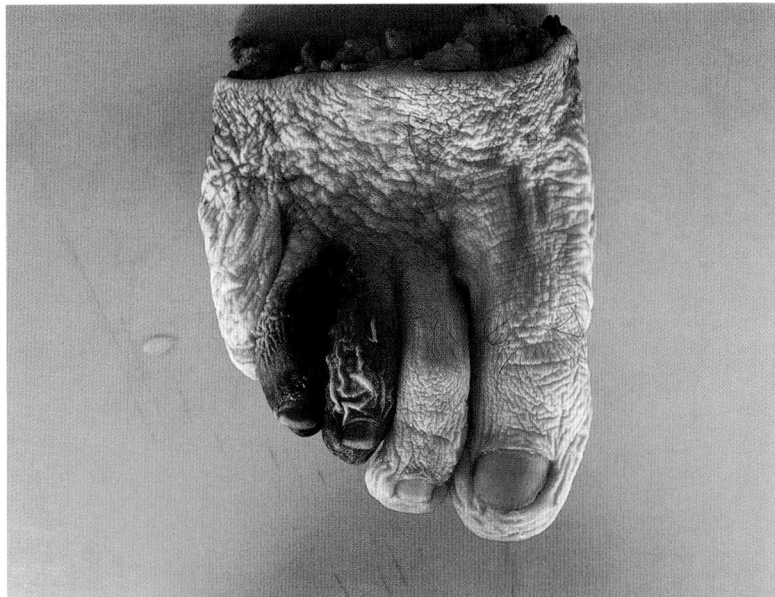

Fig. 16.89
Thromboangiitis obliterans: digital gangrene is present in this amputation specimen.

Pathogenesis and histologic features

The pathogenesis of thromboangiitis obliterans is poorly understood. Clearly, the strong association with smoking suggests that this habit plays an important role in eliciting thrombosis and resultant ischemia.[19] It is unclear if tobacco products are toxic to endothelial cells or elicit immune reactions that damage vessels. Of interest, the disease has been described in patients who use smokeless tobacco.[20] Antiendothelial antibodies are elevated in a subset of patients with Buerger disease.[21] Furthermore, disease activity correlates with antiendothelial cell antibody titers.[21] Response to acetylcholine, an endothelium-dependent vasodilator, is diminished in 'nondiseased' extremities of thromboangiitis obliterans patients compared with control subjects.[22] IgG, IgM, and IgA are present along the internal elastic lamina.[23]

Injury to endothelial cells may play an initiating role. Endothelial cells in lesional tissue have increased expression of adhesion molecules VCAM-1, ICAM-1, and E-selectin, which allows for attachment of inflammatory cells and triggering the inflammatory response.[24]

Thromboangiitis obliterans patients also have higher levels of TNF-α, IL-1β, IL-4, IL-17, and IL-23 compared with matched controls.[24] This could contribute to a proinflammatory and autoimmunity environment.

Lesions are characterized by thrombosis of small or medium-sized arteries and, less commonly, veins associated with a variable inflammatory infiltrate composed of a mixture of neutrophils, lymphocytes, eosinophils, histiocytes, and giant cells.[19,25] Immunohistochemical studies have confirmed the heterogeneous nature of the infiltrate. T cells, B cells, macrophages, and dendritic cells may all be present.[23] CD4-positive T cells outnumber CD8-positive cells and T-cell-mediated inflammation appears to be of significance in the development of the disease.[24,26] A characteristic finding is the presence of a microabscess associated with an intraluminal thrombus. Inflammatory cells may be seen in all layers of the vessel wall (Fig. 16.90). Preservation of the internal elastic lamina is a typical feature.[19]

As lesions age, thrombi become organized and are replaced by fibrosis, and eventually the vessel is recanalized (Fig. 16.91). A definitive diagnosis based on biopsy findings is not possible during the later stages of organization.

Differential diagnosis

The histopathological features are probably not specific for thromboangiitis obliterans (Buerger disease), and differential diagnosis includes other thrombotic vasculopathies. Clinical correlation is advised before rendering a definitive diagnosis. Preservation of the internal elastic lamina is a characteristic feature and is said to help in distinction from other vasculitides.[19,27]

Giant cell arteritis (temporal arteritis)

Clinical features

Giant cell arteritis, formerly also called temporal arteritis, is a disease of the elderly that shows a marked female predominance (3:1).[1,2] It is a generalized vasculitis that predominantly affects large and medium-sized arteries.[3] It is mainly seen in Caucasians and its etiology is unknown.[2,3]

Five of the American College of Rheumatology 1990 criteria are outlined in Table 16.9.[1] Classically, the temporal arteries are primarily affected, but giant cell arteritis may also affect the occipital or facial arteries and, in fact, has the potential to involve virtually any medium-sized or large vessel, including the aorta and its branches.[3] Given that temporal arteries may be uninvolved, giant cell arteritis is the preferred terminology in the current Chapel Hill Consensus conference classification.[4] Patients with giant cell arteritis classically present with severe headache, pyrexia, and throbbing scalp pain. Clinical examination may reveal scalp tenderness and the skin overlying the affected vessel may be erythematous, edematous, or appear bruised.[5,6] Palpation often reveals a cordlike and nodular vessel. Pulsation can be diminished or absent.

Visual disturbance, present in 25% to 50% of patients, due to involvement of the ophthalmic or retinal vessels is an important complication which sometimes results in blindness.[6] Lesions of the CNS may result in

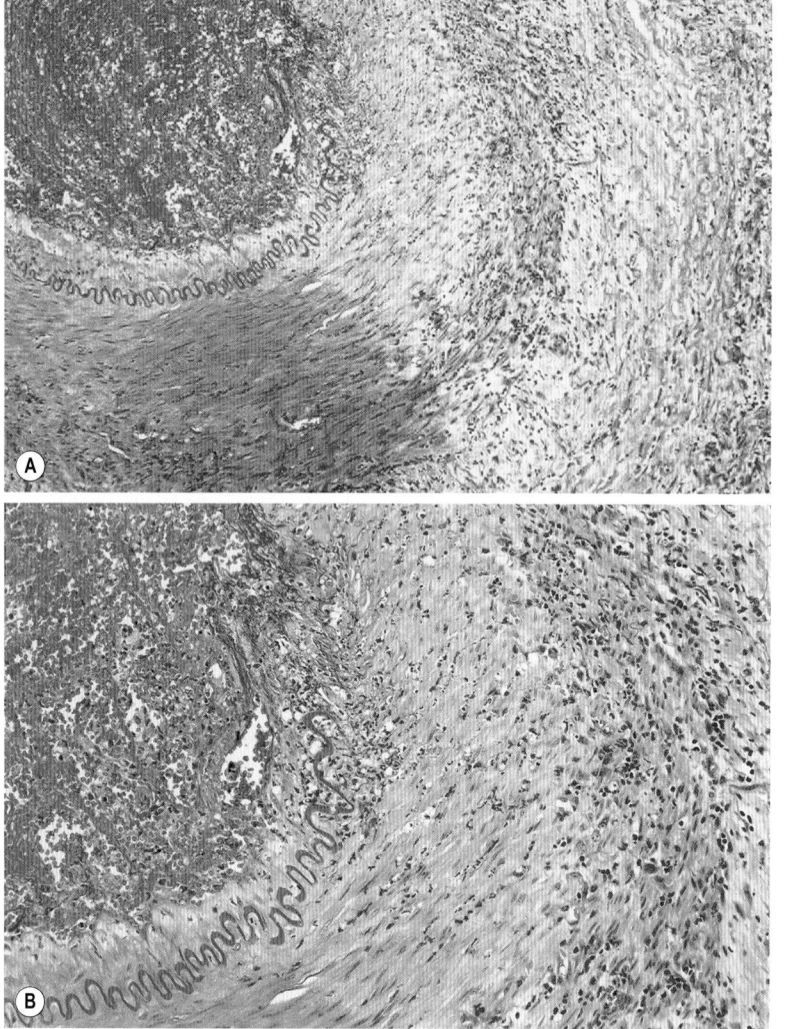

Fig. 16.90
(A, B) Thromboangiitis obliterans: this acute lesion shows pan-mural inflammation with abscess formation and thrombosis.

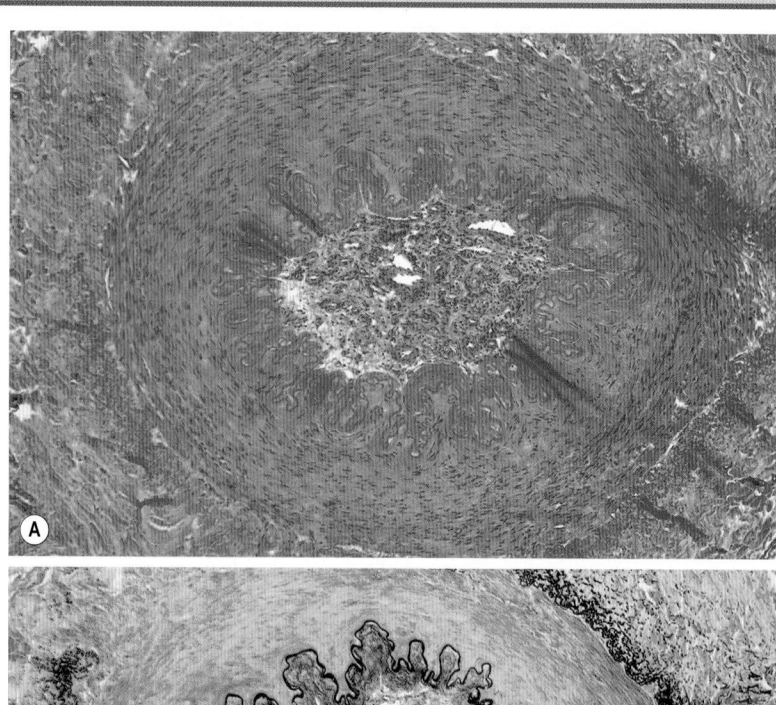

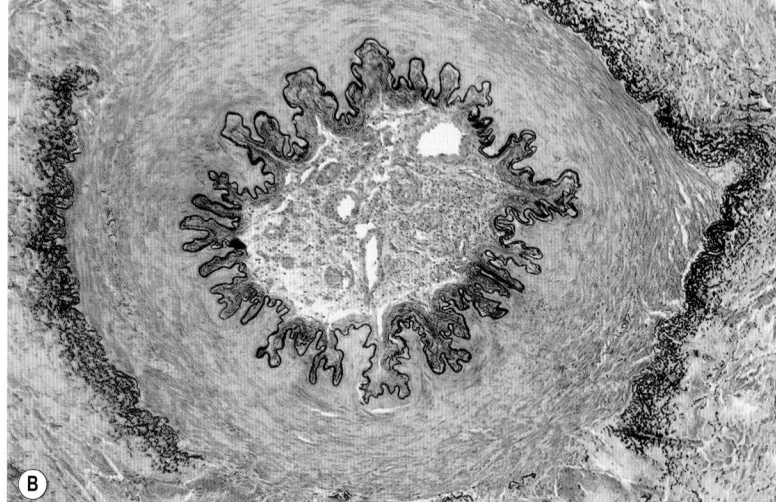

Fig. 16.91
(A, B) Thromboangiitis obliterans: old lesion showing luminal obliteration and recanalization. Note the intact elastic lamina.

stroke, subarachnoid hemorrhage, or mental confusion, and aural involvement can cause deafness. In one large study, neurological problems were present in nearly one-third of patients.[7] Peripheral neuropathic syndromes are evident in 14% of patients.[5] Often the associated lymph nodes are enlarged and tender. Symptoms of polymyalgia rheumatica (i.e., stiffness, weakness, aching and pain in the muscles of the neck, limb girdles, and upper limbs) are extremely common, occurring in 40% to 75% of patients with giant cell arteritis.[8,9] Giant cell arteritis, however, is present in approximately 20% of patients with polymyalgia rheumatica.[9] Laboratory investigations typically reveal mild anemia, neutrophilia, and a very high ESR. Elevated levels of von Willebrand factor are characteristic.[10] Patients may also have hyperthyroidism and abnormal liver function tests with elevated alkaline phosphatase and transaminases.[6]

Cutaneous lesions other than those mentioned above are uncommon, presumably reflecting the vast collateral circulation of the integument.[11–12] Patients may occasionally manifest ulcers (sometimes quite widespread), massive necrosis, bullae, and gangrene (Fig. 16.92).[13,14] Involvement of the lingual artery can cause glossitis or gangrene of the tongue.[15,16] Masticatory claudication is an additional feature.[6]

Rare patients with disseminated visceral arteritis with giant cell arteritis-like histologic features have been described.[17] The heart, lungs, kidneys, stomach, pancreas, and liver may be involved.[17] It is debatable what terminology should be applied to such rare and unusual cases.

Life expectancy does not seem to be adversely affected by having temporal arteritis.[18]

Table 16.9
1990 criteria for the classification of giant cell (temporal) arteritis (traditional format)*

Criterion	Definition
Age at disease onset ≥50 years	Development of symptoms or findings beginning at age 50 or older
New headache	New onset of, or new type of, localized pain in the head
Temporal artery abnormality	Temporal artery tenderness to palpation or decreased pulsation, unrelated to arteriosclerosis of cervical arteries
Elevated ESR	ESR ≥50 mm/h by the Westergren method
Abnormal artery biopsy	Biopsy specimen with artery showing vasculitis characterized by a predominance of mononuclear cell infiltration or granulomatous inflammation, usually with multinucleated giant cells

*For purposes of classification, a patient shall be said to have giant cell (temporal) arteritis if at least three of these five criteria are present. The presence of any three or more criteria yields a sensitivity of 93.5% and a specificity of 91.2%.
Reproduced with permission from Hunder, G.G. (1990) *Arthritis & Rheumatism*, 33, 1122–1128.

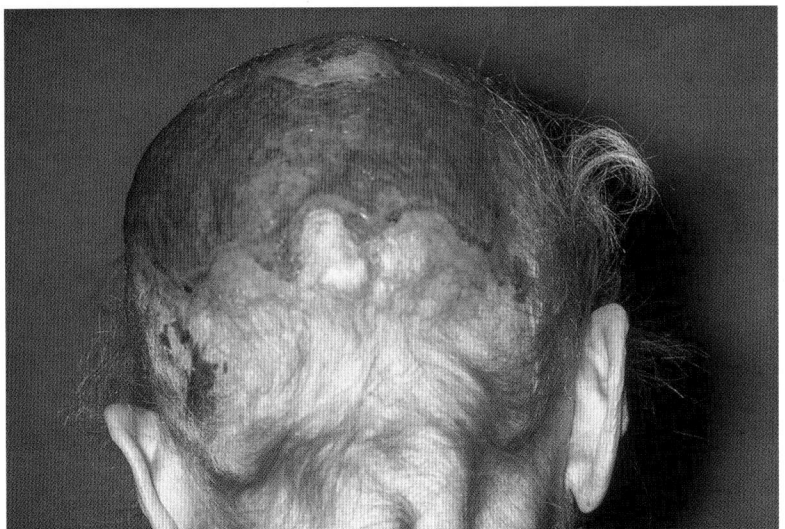

Fig. 16.92
Giant cell arteritis: severe ischemic necrosis with ulceration has destroyed most of this patient's scalp. By courtesy of D. McGibbon, MD, St Thomas' Hospital, London, UK.

The vast majority of patients have an elevated ESR.[19] C-reactive protein is also typically elevated.[19] Elevated levels of anticardiolipin antibodies are frequently present.[20–23] Some studies suggest that the presence of anticardiolipin antibodies correlates with more severe vascular damage.[22,23] In most patients, anticardiolipin antibody titers return to normal range with steroid therapy.[21]

Pathogenesis and histologic features

The pathogenesis of giant cell arteritis is poorly understood. Although an immunological mechanism has been suggested, it has not been proven. Evidence of familial aggregation and an increased incidence of the HLA-DR4 antigen have raised the possibility of a genetic influence.[3] However, consistent reproducible HLA associations have not been demonstrated in all populations.

It has been suggested that giant cell arteritis is an autoimmune disease perhaps directed, at least in part, against the vascular elastic lamina.[3] T cells in the infiltrate are predominantly of the helper subclass and expression of HLA-DR has been recorded, thereby suggesting that they are activated.[3] The lymphocytes have been shown to respond to antibodies against transferrin and IL-2 receptors.[24] Proliferation of mononuclear cells following incubation in cultures containing elastin-derived peptides is increased compared with control subjects.[25] This finding suggests elastin-derived peptides are the targets of T cells in giant cell arteritis.[25] Disease activity has been shown to correlate with plasma concentrations of IL-6.[26] It has also been shown that CD4-positive T-cell expressing CD161 are present in the arterial wall. These cells then polarize into Th1 and Th17 cells, resulting in IFN-γ production that activates macrophages, giant cells, and vascular smooth muscle cells.[27] This could account for the vascular damage and resulting ischemia.

The demonstration by some authors of a fluctuating cyclical pattern of incidence has raised the possibility of an infectious agent or other triggering factor playing a significant pathogenetic role.[28–30] A study from the Mayo Clinic showed a variation in incidence with peak periods occurring approximately every 7 years.[28] Similarly, a study from Denmark demonstrated marked variation in the incidence of temporal arteritis with five peak periods.[30] Of these, there appeared to be association with two epidemics of *M. pneumoniae* infection, two possibly related to erythrovirus (parvovirus) B19 epidemics, and one peak that may have been related to an epidemic of *Chlamydia pneumoniae*.[30] Another study showed a threefold increased likelihood of infection in patients with giant cell arteritis compared with control subjects.[31] An association between giant cell arteritis and antibodies to parainfluenza type 1 has been demonstrated.[32,33] Other large studies have found no seasonal variation, casting some doubt on the infectious hypothesis.[34] A different hypothesis implicated altered endogenous material due to age- or

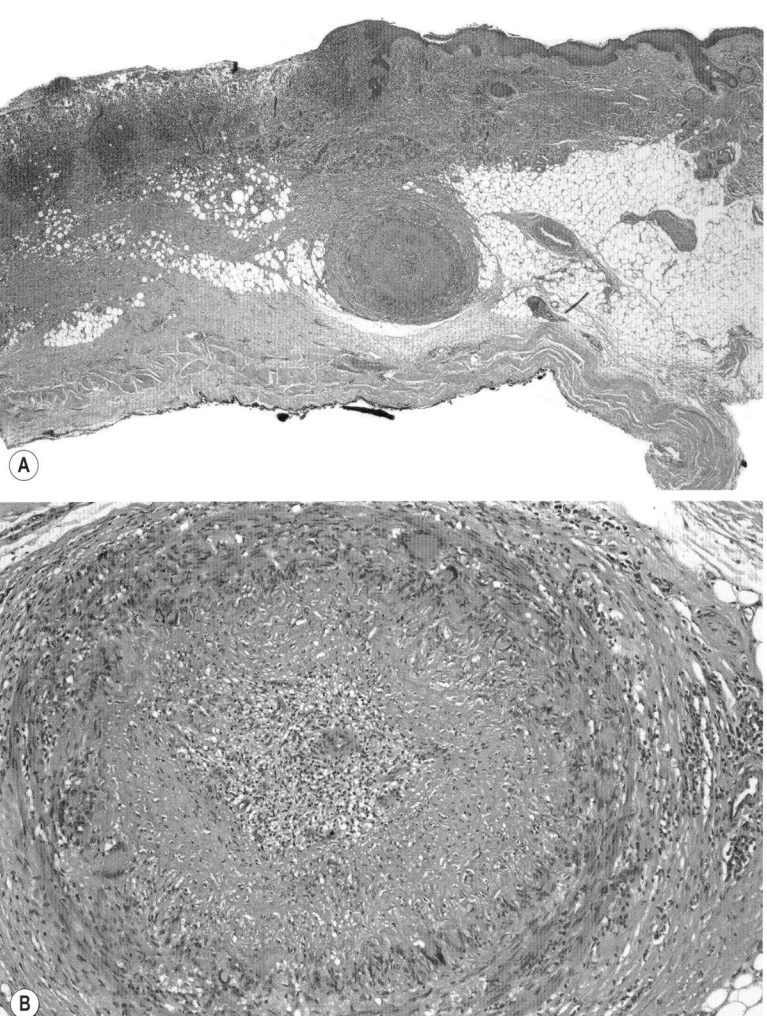

Fig. 16.93
(A, B) Giant cell arteritis: this scalp biopsy showed multiple affected vessels. By courtesy of P.A. Burton, MD, Southmead Hospital, Bristol, UK.

sun damage-related changes.[35–37] Despite these observations, the precise triggering factors and the pathogenesis of giant cell arteritis remain unclear.

The lesions of giant cell arteritis are typically focal in distribution; therefore, the vessel should be carefully palpated to find an obviously affected segment before a biopsy is undertaken. Even then, false negatives are not uncommon (see below). The lesion is granulomatous in nature and may affect only part or the whole circumference of the vessel wall (*Fig. 16.93*).[38] The infiltrate, which particularly affects the intima and media, is composed of lymphocytes, plasma cells, histiocytes, and variable numbers of giant cells of both foreign body and Langhans type (*Fig. 16.94*). Giant cells are sometimes relatively sparse and multiple levels have to be examined before they are identified. On occasion, they are absent. Typical of giant cell arteritis is damage to the internal elastic lamina, which appears swollen and fragmented, and portions may be identified within the cytoplasm of giant cells (*Fig. 16.95*).[5]

A second, less common form consists of a panarteritis composed of lymphocytes, macrophages, neutrophils, and eosinophils but giant cells are absent. Varying degrees of vessel wall necrosis are evident and the vessel is often thrombosed.

In the late stages of the disease, fibrous scarring takes place and a reconstituted, often multilayered, internal elastic lamina may be identified. In cases of doubt, an elastic tissue stain can prove invaluable. The thrombus is on occasions recanalized.

Initiation of corticosteroid treatment before biopsy influences the histologic appearances.[39] Giant cells are rare or entirely absent, there are large

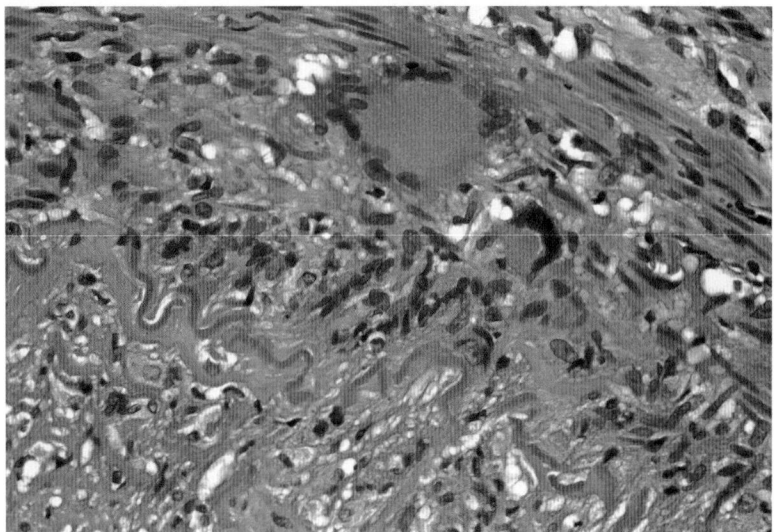

Fig. 16.94
Giant cell arteritis: the intima and media are infiltrated by a dense chronic inflammatory cell infiltrate containing conspicuous Langhans giant cells. By courtesy of P.A. Burton, MD, Southmead Hospital, Bristol, UK.

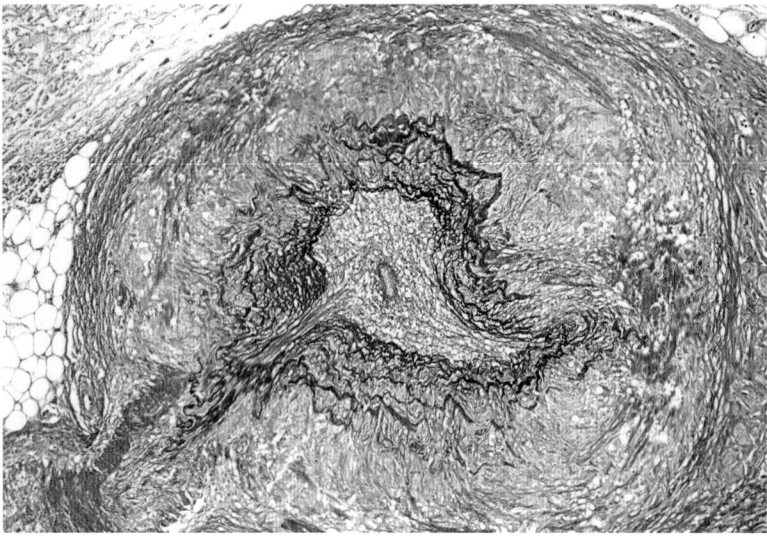

Fig. 16.95
Giant cell arteritis: there is fragmentation of the internal elastic lamina. By courtesy of P.A. Burton, MD, Southmead Hospital, Bristol, UK.

circumferential defects in the elastic lamina, and there is a mantle of lymphocytes and epithelioid histiocytes between the outer muscular layer and the adventitia.[39] These changes can be noted as early as 1 week following steroid treatment.[39]

It is crucial to note that patients with classic symptoms of giant cell arteritis may have a negative biopsy, most likely due to the multifocal nature of the arteritis and sampling bias. Negative biopsies may be seen in 15% to 44% of patients with clinical manifestations of giant cell arteritis.[40,41] Therefore, a negative biopsy does not necessarily exclude this disease. Given the consequences of delayed or no treatment, it is often necessary to treat selected patients even without definitive biopsy diagnosis. One study found that patients with giant cell arteritis who have constitutional symptoms or an abnormal temporal artery detected by physical examination are more likely to have a positive biopsy.[42] Doppler flow studies may be used to improve the sensitivity of biopsy.[43] Magnetic resonance imaging can also be useful in biopsy negative cases, but they need to be done promptly, as corticosteroid therapy can reduce the sensitivity of the test.[44] Given the multifocal nature of giant cell arteritis, the diagnostic yield, not surprisingly, is likely improved with longer artery length biopsied and increased number of sections examined.[45]

Differential diagnosis

The histologic findings are identical to those seen in some patients with Takayasu arteritis, another form of giant cell arteritis. Careful clinical correlation is required to distinguish these conditions and, since overlap exists, many cases are not easily subclassified. Some authors consider these diseases part of a continuum of giant cell vasculitis, with patient age being an important discriminator: patients under age 40 are more likely to have Takayasu arteritis; those over 50 are more likely to have giant cell arteritis.

It should be noted that fragmentation of the internal elastic lamina may result from either age-related changes or atherosclerosis and these conditions may be difficult to distinguish from healed arteritis. The presence of medial scarring is suggestive of giant cell arteritis. The extent of destruction, particularly confluent loss of the internal elastic lamina, is said to correlate with probability of healed arteritis.[8]

Juvenile temporal arteritis

Clinical features

Juvenile temporal arteritis is a rare and poorly defined entity first reported in 1975.[1] Thus far, only approximately 20 cases have been reported in the literature.[2–10] The disease is unrelated to classic temporal arteritis and is not associated with abnormal ESR or signs of systemic involvement. It occurs in patients under the age of 40, most commonly manifesting as a unilateral painless nodule or swelling of a few centimeters in the temporal area.[1–10] Painful presentation and bilateral involvement are rare features.[2–4] The disease may be accompanied by blood eosinophilia and it may be related to or associated with Kimura disease.[4,5,7,9–11]

Histologic features

Juvenile temporal arteritis is characterized by intimal proliferation and disruption of the media of the temporal artery associated with a heavy chronic inflammatory infiltrate composed predominantly of lymphocytes and eosinophils.[10] Endothelial proliferation is an additional finding and formation of lymphoid follicles and germinal centers may be present.[12] Giant cells as seen in classical temporal arteritis are not a feature.

Takayasu arteritis

Clinical features

Takayasu arteritis (pulseless disease, giant cell arteritis) is a rare granulomatous disease that predominantly affects the aorta and its major branches and results in vascular stenoses with bruits and diminished or absent pulses (hence the term 'pulseless disease').[1,2] Aneurysm formation may be an additional feature. It predominantly affects females (7:1), most often involves the upper limbs, and usually presents in the second or third decade. Although most patients are young adults, the disease is also seen in children.[3–7] It is rare in Europe and the United States, occurring more often in Japan, China, Korea, Southeast Asia, India, and Mexico.[2] It appears to have two stages:

- an acute systemic illness characterized by fever, malaise, arthralgias, myalgias, and ocular lesions including uveitis and episcleritis,
- a chronic stage of large-vessel involvement.[8]

Current diagnostic criteria are shown in *Table 16.10*. In addition to the obligatory criterion, the presence of two major criteria, one major plus two or more minor, or four or more minor criteria, is associated with a high probability of Takayasu arteritis.[9]

Cutaneous manifestations have been described in up to 50% of patients and include Raynaud syndrome (due to large-vessel involvement), acute inflammatory nodules and erythema nodosum-like features (particularly in Europe and North America), pyoderma gangrenosum-like lesions (especially in the Japanese), pseudoerythema induratum, superficial phlebitis, tuberculid eruptions, and purpura (*Fig. 16.96*).[8,10,11] Patients may present with cutaneous necrotizing vasculitis.[11] Rare associations with Sweet syndrome, pyoderma gangrenosum, and ulcerative cutaneous sarcoidosis have been reported.[12,13]

Table 16.10
Takayasu arteritis: diagnostic criteria

- Obligatory criterion
  - age <40 years
- Major criteria
  - left mid subclavian artery lesion
  - right mid subclavian artery lesion
  - Minor criteria
  - high ESR
  - carotid artery tenderness
  - hypertension
  - aortic regurgitation or annuloaortic ectasia
  - pulmonary artery lesion
  - left mid common carotid lesion
  - distal brachiocephalic trunk lesion
  - descending thoracic aorta lesion
  - abdominal aorta lesion

Reproduced with permission from Bentsson, B.A. and Anderson, T. (1991) *Current Opinion in Rheumatology*, 3, 15–22.

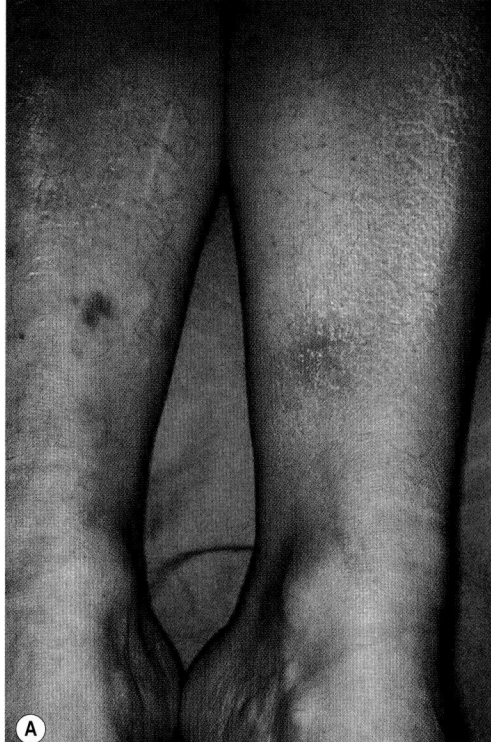

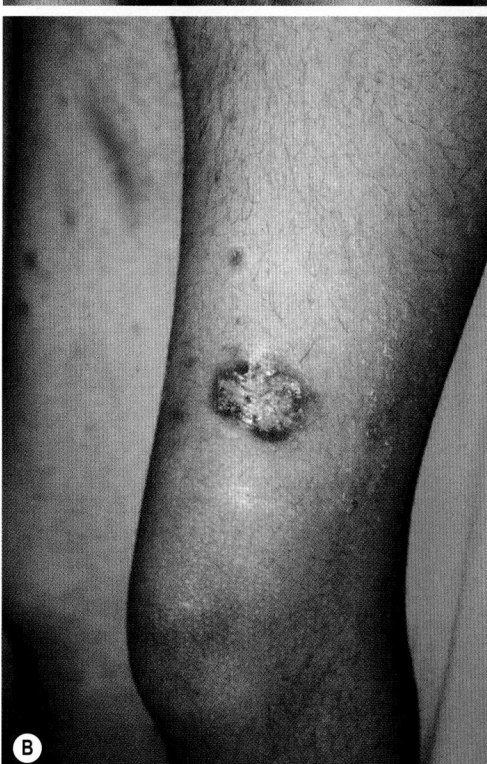

Fig. 16.96
Takayasu arteritis: (**A**) this patient presented with multiple lesions as seen here on the lower legs; (**B**) a large ulcerated inflammatory nodule is present on the left thigh. By courtesy of P. Godeau, MD, and C. Francès, MD, Groupe Hospitalier, Pitié-Salpêtrière, Paris, France.

Cases have been reported describing an overlap between Takayasu arteritis and polyarteritis nodosa.[9] Rare patients with a lupus-like malar flush and an urticarial reaction with livedo reticularis have been documented.[10] Renal artery involvement with stenosis causes severe hypertension secondary to renin secretion. Stroke due to severe hypertension is a serious complication in some patients. Patients with Takayasu arteritis also have an increased incidence of associated Crohn disease.[15]

Pathogenesis and histologic features

The etiology and pathogenesis of Takayasu arteritis is poorly understood. Occasionally, other diseases are seen in association with Takayasu arteritis including tuberculosis, inflammatory bowel disease, polymyositis, sarcoidosis, and rheumatoid arthritis.[1,8,14,16–18] Coexpression with polyarteritis nodosa raises the possibility of an autoimmune phenomenon.[19]

A genetic component may also be present. Takayasu arteritis is associated with HLA-B*52, HLA-B*39, HLA-DRB1*1502, HLA-DRB1*0405, HLA-B/MICA, and HLA-DQB1/HLA-DRB1.[20] There is also an association with genes for FC-gamma receptor IIA and FC-gamma receptor IIIA.[20] The latter two haplotypes have also been associated with giant cell arteritis.[21]

The diagnosis is usually made by clinical and radiological correlation; however, in some cases tissue is sent to the pathologist. The histologic features are variable and include granulomatous vasculitis indistinguishable from giant cell arteritis, leukocytoclastic vasculitis, lymphocytic vasculitis, and polyarteritis nodosa-like features (*Figs 16.97* and *16.98*).[8–10,19,22]

Septal and lobular panniculitis with granulomatous vasculitis may be the underlying histology of erythematous nodules and erythema nodosum-like lesions.[10] Features of Churg-Strauss granulomata have also been reported.[8]

Differential diagnosis

As can be seen from the above discussion, several different patterns of vasculitis may be encountered in Takayasu arteritis. Furthermore, the histologic findings seen in this disease may be identical to other forms of vasculitis. Therefore, careful clinical and radiological correlation is necessary to establish the correct diagnosis.

Infection-related vasculitis

Infection must be considered in the evaluation of many forms of vasculitis, particularly leukocytoclastic vasculitis. Infective vasculitis is caused by a wide variety of agents including bacteria, fungi, protozoa, viruses, spirochetes, and rickettsiae (*Table 16.11*). The relationship between particular microorganisms and vascular lesions is covered under the specific infection in Chapter 18. In general terms, vessel wall damage may occur as a consequence of direct microbial toxic damage or else develop as a complication of an immunologically mediated injury (*Table 16.12*).[1]

Bacterial arteritis can develop as a result of embolization from valvular lesions in patients with infective endocarditis. Although many different organisms are of etiological importance in the latter condition, staphylococcal and streptococcal infections remain the most important.[2] It may also occur by direct spread from an adjacent septic focus, by lymphatic spread, or represent a manifestation of underlying bacteremia or septicemia. There also appears to be a significant relationship between group A streptococci and childhood polyarteritis nodosa, both cutaneous and generalized.[3] In

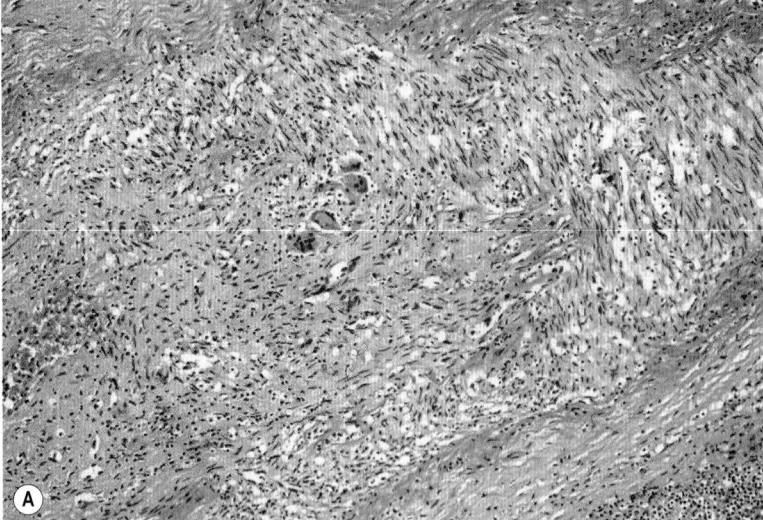

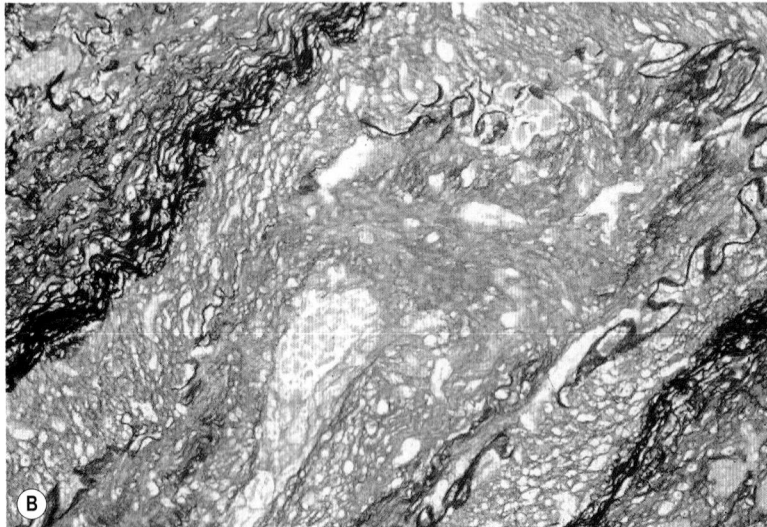

Fig. 16.97
(**A**, **B**) Takayasu arteritis: this occluded artery was present with a thickened septum of the subcutaneous fat from the thigh of a young woman.

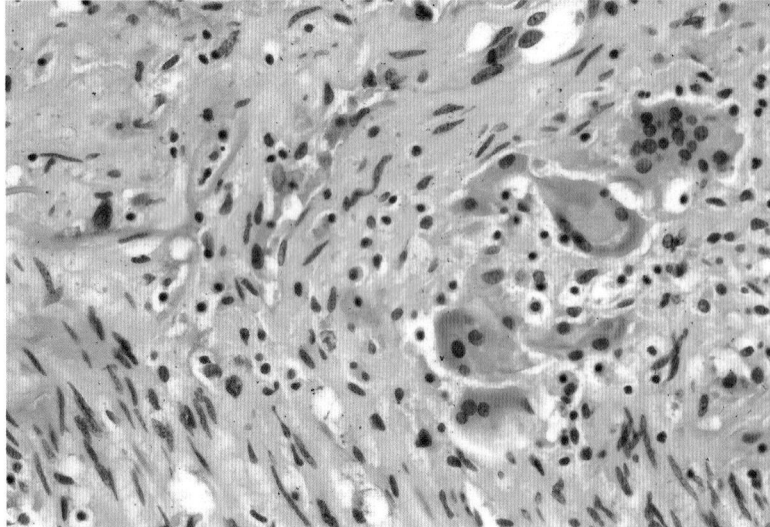

Fig. 16.98
Takayasu arteritis: high-power view showing granulomatous inflammation. The features are indistinguishable from giant cell arteritis.

Table 16.11
Infections known to be associated with clinically defined vasculitis

Vasculitic syndrome	Infective agent

Leukocytoclastic vasculitis (including IgA vasculitis)	Bacterial
	  Streptococcus
	  Staphylococcus
	  Salmonella
	  Yersinia
	  Mycobacterium
	Viral
	  varicella-zoster
	  hepatitis B
	  cytomegalovirus
	  influenza

Polyarteritis nodosa	Bacterial
	  Streptococcus
	Viral
	  hepatitis A, B, C
	  human immunodeficiency virus
	  cytomegalovirus
	  human T-cell leukemia
	  erythrovirus

Isolated granulomatous vasculitis of the central nervous system	*Treponema pallidum*
	Mycobacterium tuberculosis
	Fungal
	  Coccidioides
	  Actinomyces
	  Cryptococcus
	  Histoplasma
	  Nocardia
	  Aspergillus
	Borrelia burgorferi (Lyme)
	Varicella-zoster

Kawasaki disease	Bacterial
	  Streptococcus
	  Salmonella
	  Yersinia
	  Mycoplasma
	Viral
	  parainfluenza
	  rotavirus

Reproduced with permission from Mader, R. and Keystone, E.C. (1992) *Current Opinion in Rheumatology*, 4, 35–38.

Table 16.12
Mechanisms for infection-associated vasculitis

- Direct microbial toxicity
  - direct endothelial infection
  - effect of microbial toxins
- Immune mediated
  - humoral: soluble immune complexes; in situ complex formation
  - cellular: cytotoxic cell reaction (T cell, NK cell, other); polyclonal T- or B-cell response; monoclonal T- or B-cell response

NK, natural killer.
Reproduced with permission from Calabrese, L.H. (1991) *Rheumatic Disease Clinics of North America*, 17, 131–147.

addition, Kawasaki disease has been reported in association with group A streptococci, possibly as a result of superantigen stimulation.[4] Gonococcal bacteremia due to *Neisseria gonorrhea* is another important cause of vasculitis. Neisseria meningitis infection may result in vasculitis associated with considerable morbidity and mortality.

The histologic features of small-vessel involvement are variable and depend to some extent on the nature of the causative organism. Suppurative features are most likely to be due to staphylococcal, streptococcal, *Pseudomonas* or *Klebsiella* infection.[2] A Gram stain is advisable in all suspected cases.

Obviously, in the context of immunosuppressed patients, the range of bacteria and fungi that can be implicated is very broad. In cases of suspected cutaneous infective vasculitis, especially in immunosuppressed patients, a detailed clinical history is essential and the judicious use of special stains is highly advisable.

Candidiasis, aspergillosis, cryptococcosis, and mucormycosis are of special importance. *M. tuberculosis* is also sometimes a cause of vascular damage. It tends to affect veins rather than arteries.[2] The features are usually those of a granulomatous thrombophlebitis, usually in the absence of caseation necrosis, although sometimes this is a feature. Occasionally, however, arteries are primarily affected (*Fig. 16.99*).

Lepra bacilli are very commonly seen in endothelial and vascular smooth muscle cells in lepromatous leprosy. Vasculitis in the setting of leprosy (erythema nodosum leprosum) is a common cause of vasculitis in regions of the world where this disease is endemic.

Vascular lesions in the skin accompany a variety of rickettsial infections including epidemic typhus, scrub typhus, and Rocky Mountain spotted fever.[2,5] The histologic features include endothelial swelling and a mixed inflammatory cell infiltrate of T lymphocytes, macrophages, and occasionally neutrophils.[2] Thrombosis is sometimes present.

Small-vessel vasculitis may be seen in all three stages of syphilis. The features vary from a non-specific lymphocytic inflammation through to necrotizing granulomatous angiitis.[6–8] *Treponema pallidum*, however, is very rarely identified.[2] Cutaneous vasculitis is an occasional feature of Lyme disease.[2]

The best known viral association with vasculitis is hepatitis B, which has been described in association with polyarteritis nodosa, leukocytoclastic vasculitis, and mixed cryoglobulinemia, and hepatitis C associated mixed cryoglobulinemia and leukocytoclastic vasculitis.[1,9–12] Evidence of hepatitis B infection is found in approximately 35% of all patients with polyarteritis nodosa.[1]

HIV may be present in a very wide spectrum of vasculitic lesions including polyarteritis nodosa, eosinophilic granulomatosis with polyangiitis, leukocytoclastic vasculitis, IgA vasculitis, lymphomatoid granulomatosis, and primary angiitis of the central nervous system.[13–15] Whether these represent a direct effect of HIV, or are a consequence of coexisting viral infections known to cause vasculitis (e.g., cytomegalovirus, HBV or Epstein-Barr virus), is unknown.[10] The identification of HIV within endothelial cells adds some support to the former possibility.[16]

Paraneoplastic vasculitis

Clinical features

Occasionally, cutaneous vasculitis is a marker of an underlying systemic malignancy (*Table 16.13*).[1–12] Most commonly the vasculitis is associated with hematological malignancies.[12] There are also reports of an association with solid tumors.[1,4,6,12–17] Vasculitis has nevertheless been reported in patients with carcinoma of the kidney, breast, ovary, lung, nasopharynx, stomach, small bowel, colon, prostate, and thyroid, and chondrosarcoma. Some of these associations may represent coincidence. Leukocytoclastic vasculitis is the most common pattern of vasculitis associated with malignancy but large-vessel vasculitis may also be seen. Of interest, vasculitis can be present at the time of initial diagnosis and also herald the onset of relapse.[4] Solid tumors and hematological malignancy have been associated with IgA vasculitis.[7,10–12] One study found that nearly a third of adults with Henoch-Schönlein purpura had an associated malignancy.[10] For this reason, the authors concluded that physicians should suspect underlying malignancy in older patients (especially men of more than 40 years) with IgA vasculitis.[10]

In contrast to solid tumors, there does appear to be a more definitive relationship between cutaneous vasculitis and hematological and lymphoreticular neoplasms including hairy cell leukemia, acute and chronic myeloid leukemia, multiple myeloma, and non-Hodgkin lymphoma.[1]

In general, patients present with the features of leukocytoclastic vasculitis, and occasionally arthralgia or arthritis is evident. Cutaneous manifestations include maculopapular eruptions, purpura, urticaria, peripheral ulcers, and gangrene.[12,18] Although vasculitis is seen in patients with a spectrum of hematological malignancies, hairy cell leukemia is particularly associated with leukocytoclastic vasculitis and a polyarteritis nodosa-like picture, including systemic lesions.[4–6] In one study of 42 patients with hairy cell leukemia and vasculitis, 21 also had leukocytoclastic vasculitis and 17 had polyarteritis nodosa.[4] In addition, four patients had direct infiltration of vessel walls by leukemic cells. Hodgkin lymphoma has occasionally been linked to

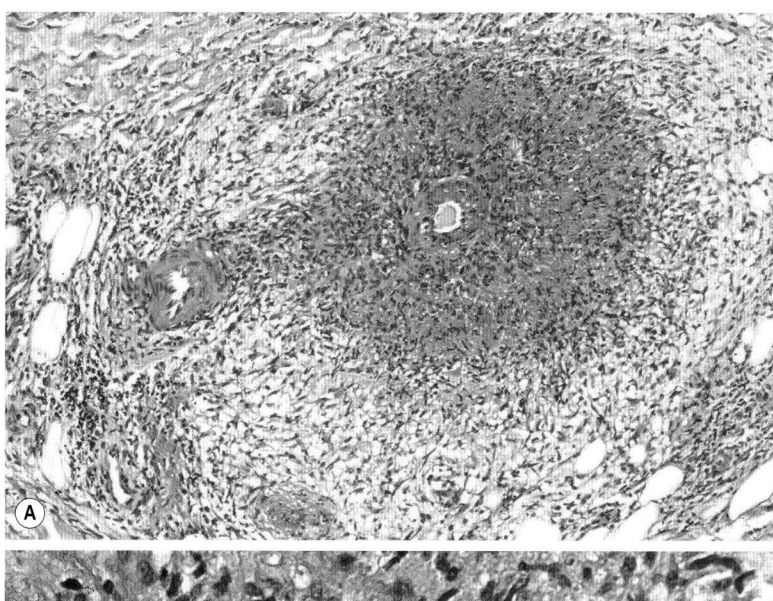

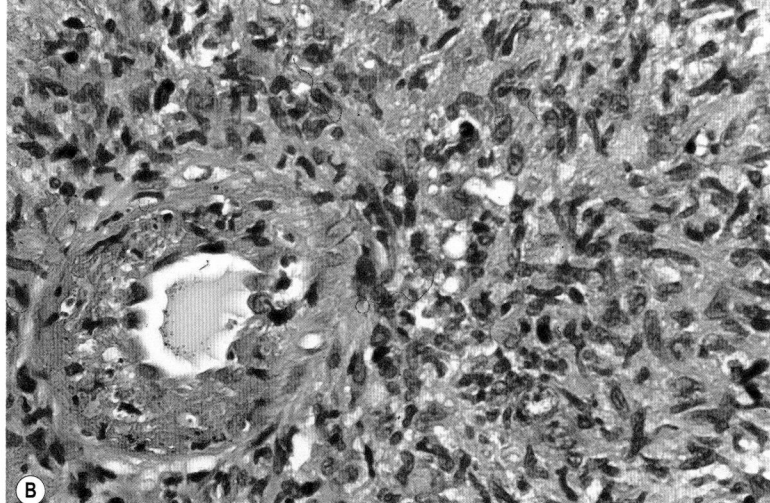

Fig. 16.99
(**A**, **B**) Tuberculous vasculitis: this patient with miliary tuberculosis presented with ischemic cutaneous lesions. Note the granulomatous inflammation.

Table 16.13
Vasculopathic syndromes associated with malignancy

- Migratory superficial thrombophlebitis
- Deep venous thrombosis
- Nonbacterial thrombotic endocarditis
- Anticardiolipin antibody syndrome
- Embolic features associated with atrial myxoma
- Raynaud phenomenon
- Erythema nodosum
- Hyperviscosity syndrome
- Cryoglobulinemia
- Lambda light chain vasculopathy
- Cutaneous vasculitis
- Systemic vasculitis

Reproduced with permission from Mertz, L.E. and Conn, D.L. (1992) *Current Opinion in Rheumatology*, 9, 39–46.

erythema nodosum, and myelodysplasia has been found in conjunction with leukocytoclastic vasculitis.[19,20] Multiple myeloma is particularly associated with nonthrombocytopenic purpura.[21] It has been documented that lymphocytic vasculitis is a relatively common form of paraneoplastic vasculitis associated with lymphoproliferative disorders.[22]

It is important to note that these vasculitic phenomena may antedate the clinical manifestations of the underlying malignancy. In one retrospective study from a single tertiary care institution, the diagnosis of vasculitis in all 16 cases preceded the diagnosis of malignancy.[12] Therefore, patients with an unexplained vasculitic rash should be investigated with this in mind.[2,12] In hairy cell leukemia, vasculitis often follows splenectomy.[5,18]

Pathogenesis and histologic features

The pathogenesis of paraneoplastic vasculitis has not been well studied, but could include immune complexes, cross-reacting antigens, and direct tumor (leukemic blast) infiltration of blood vessel walls.

Leukocytoclastic, polyarteritis nodosa-like, and lymphocytic forms of paraneoplastic vasculitis have all been described and show histologic features similar to their nonparaneoplastic counterparts.[22]

Cases of vasculitis in the setting of myelomonocytic or monocytic leukemia cutis have been described in which the vascular injury was mediated by leukemic blasts.[23,24] The term 'leukemic vasculitis' has been proposed for this form of vasculitis.[23] In these cases, the vasculitis ranged from mild microvascular injury to frank necrotizing vasculitis.[23–25] The former was characterized by low-grade vascular injury with endothelial cell swelling and focal fibrin deposition. Frank necrotizing vasculitis shows infiltration of the vessel wall by neoplastic cells associated with necrosis and fibrin deposition in a pattern that resembles polyarteritis nodosa. Hairy cell leukemia may also show infiltration of vessel walls by leukemic cells.[4,5]

Vasculitis associated with palisaded neutrophilic and granulomatous dermatitis

Clinical features

Occasionally, granuloma annulare, necrobiosis lipoidica, and rheumatoid nodule-like lesions associated with vasculitis are encountered.[1,2] This group of disorders, which is almost always associated with systemic disease, is also discussed in Chapter 9. A number of different terms have been applied, including palisaded neutrophilic and granulomatous dermatitis (of immune complex disease), interstitial granulomatous dermatitis with arthritis, rheumatoid papules, superficial ulcerating rheumatoid necrobiosis, cutaneous extravascular necrotizing granuloma, and Churg-Strauss granuloma.[1–6] Many types of underlying systemic disease have been reported in association with these lesions, including rheumatoid arthritis, lupus erythematosus, Sjögren syndrome, thyroiditis, Raynaud syndrome, hepatitis, inflammatory bowel disease, lymphoproliferative disorders, myelodysplastic syndrome, vasculitis (granulomatosis with polyangiitis, eosinophilic granulomatosis with polyangiitis, Takayasu arteritis, periarteritis nodosa), hemolytic uremic syndrome (HUS), thrombotic thrombocytopenic purpura (TTP), mixed cryoglobulinemia, drug reactions, carcinoma, diabetes mellitus, and infection (streptococcal, HIV, Epstein-Barr virus, erythrovirus).[1–4] Patients without underlying systemic disease have also been reported.[7]

The lesions are usually papules and nodules, or plaques with a predilection for the extremities or trunk in an adult.[2,6,7,8] They are often arranged in a linear pattern, which may be confluent linear bands or cords that are said to have a 'ropelike' quality.

Pathogenesis and histologic features

The pathogenesis of palisaded neutrophilic and granulomatous dermatitis likely depends on the associated/underlying disease. An autoimmune-mediated vasculitis probably plays an important role in at least a subset of cases.

As noted above, this is not a single disease but rather a group of disorders showing a broad spectrum of histology sharing the common denominator of a prominent neutrophilic infiltrate with or without vasculitis in a background of palisading granulomatous inflammation. When present, vasculitis usually shows the features of leukocytoclastic vasculitis.

Differential diagnosis

The precise terminology that is preferred by the dermatopathologist is probably not important. More significant than the nosological nuances is rendering a report that alerts the clinician to the possibility that the patient may have underlying systemic disease, and when such lesions are encountered appropriate clinical evaluation is necessary.

Lymphocytic vasculitis

Lymphocytic vasculitis is sometimes diagnosed in cases in which a perivascular lymphocytic infiltrate is associated with vascular damage (*Fig. 16.100*). In many cases, the vascular changes are subtle and minimal, including only endothelial swelling and extravasated blood cells and sometimes focal fibrin deposition. Not surprisingly, the concept of lymphocytic vasculitis is somewhat controversial.[1–5] This category of vasculitis has been embraced by some authors and rejected by others. To a large extent, the controversy is the result of a lack of precisely defined criteria for diagnosis. Kossard has defined lymphocytic vasculitis as an overlapping spectrum of changes varying from angiodestruction to endovasculitis and including a pattern defined as lichenoid lymphocytic vasculitis.[6]

It is arguable that the term 'vasculitis' should not be applied to lesions with minimal vascular damage. Regardless of terminology, it is important for the pathologist to render a report that distinguishes cases of low-grade vascular injury associated with a lymphocytic infiltrate from frank necrotizing

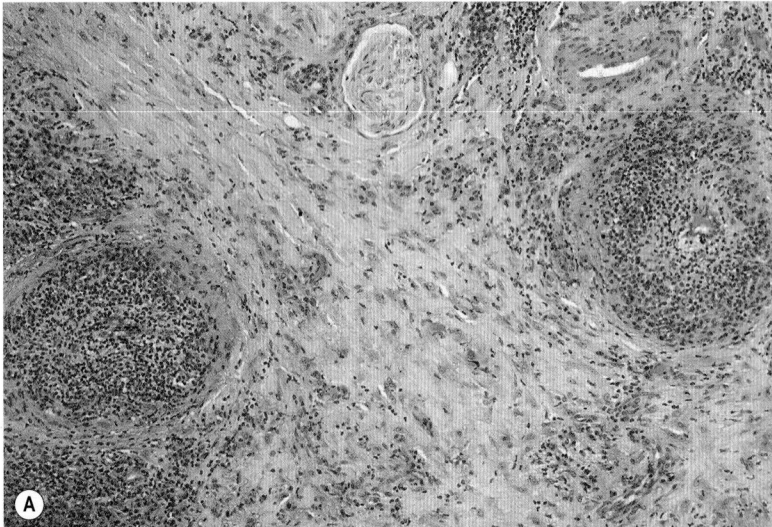

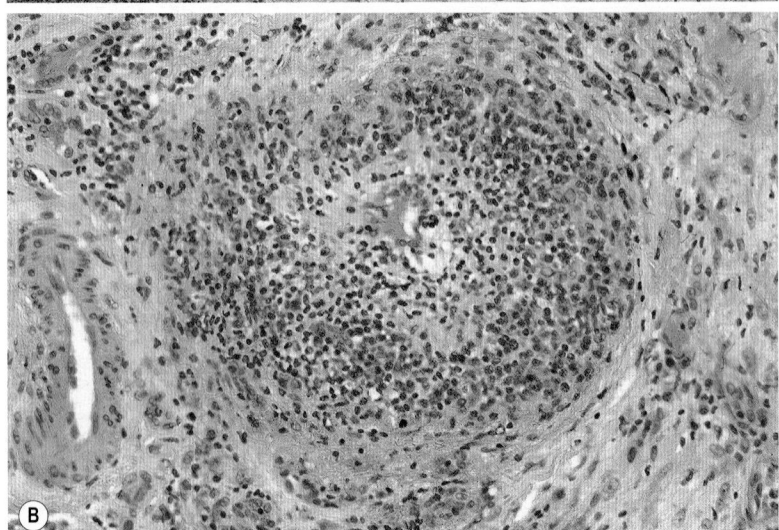

Fig. 16.100
(**A**, **B**) Lymphocytic vasculitis: there is mural fibrinoid necrosis accompanied by a dense lymphocytic infiltrate. These images come from a patient with very severe perniosis.

Table 16.14
Causes of lymphocytic vasculitis

- Behçet disease
- Connective tissue disease
- Malignant atrophic papulosis
- Drug eruptions
- 'Gyrate erythemas' (e.g., erythema annulare centrifugum)
- Infection (especially viral and rickettsial)
- Insect bite reactions
- Kawasaki syndrome
- Livedoid vasculopathy/atrophie blanche
- Lymphomatoid papulosis
- Perniosis (chilblains)
- Pityriasis lichenoides
- Pigmented purpuric dermatoses
- Polymorphic eruption of pregnancy
- Polymorphous light eruption
- Prurigo of pregnancy

vasculitis. Furthermore, it is important to distinguish lymphocytic from neutrophilic vasculitides.

To avoid any ambiguity, in cases with low-grade vascular injury, we often apply the term low-grade lymphocytic vasculitis and mention in our report that frank necrotizing vasculitis is not present. If strict criteria are used – requiring vascular necrosis or significant fibrinoid change for a diagnosis of vasculitis – frank necrotizing lymphocytic vasculitis is an uncommon condition. The differential diagnosis of lymphocytic vasculitis is broad and many entities associated with a perivascular lymphocytic infiltrate may, on occasion, cause vascular changes that warrant a diagnosis of non-necrotizing lymphocytic vasculitis (*Table 16.14*). Entities that exceptionally show features of lymphocytic vasculitis are discussed in their appropriate chapters. Diseases commonly associated with lymphocytic vasculitis include Degos disease, perniosis, Behçet disease, livedo vasculitis, and Kawasaki disease. Other rare associations of lymphocytic vasculitis include leukemia and the tumor necrosis factor receptor-associated periodic syndrome. The latter is a periodic fever syndrome associated with a skin eruption presenting with macules and plaques in early life. It results from mutations in the *TNFRS-FIA*, the gene encoding the tumor necrosis factor receptor.[7,8]

Malignant atrophic papulosis

Clinical features

Malignant atrophic papulosis (Degos disease, Köhlmeier-Degos disease, lethal intestinocutaneous syndrome) is a rare disorder affecting multiple systems and usually associated with a poor prognosis.[1–4] It is of unknown etiology, shows a male predominance (3:1), and usually affects the young and middle aged. The mean age at presentation is 33 years; however, a wide age range at diagnosis (from infancy to 67 years) has been described.[5,6] Occasional instances of familial involvement have been recorded.[7–9] Presentation during pregnancy may rarely occur.[10]

The cutaneous lesions are distinctive, although similar lesions can be a manifestation of other diseases, including SLE, systemic sclerosis, dermatomyositis, rheumatoid arthritis, and Crohn disease.[11–17] It has been proposed that malignant atrophic papulosis represents a reaction pattern mainly seen in lupus erythematosus and not a specific disease per se.[17,18] Lesions, which may be quite numerous, appear in crops, initially as pinkish or yellow-gray papules up to 5 mm in diameter and showing a predilection for the trunk and proximal extremities. Characteristically, the palms, soles, face, and scalp are spared.[19] The papules are usually asymptomatic and do not ulcerate or scar. With progression, they develop a characteristic appearance: discrete small patches composed of a central zone with a depressed white, porcelain-like appearance and a fine scale, surrounded by a narrow red or violaceous rim associated with fine telangiectasia (*Fig. 16.101*).[19] On rare occasions, similar lesions are found on the buccal and genital mucosa. Penile ulceration has rarely been documented.[19,20] Sometimes, avascular conjunctival pale patches are seen.[21]

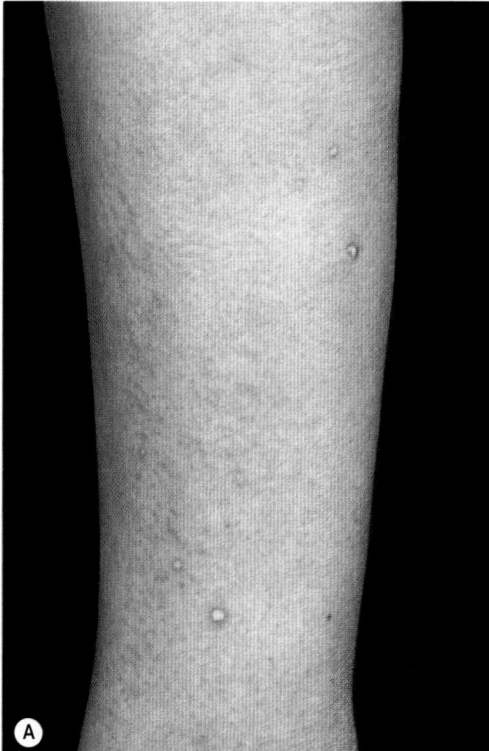
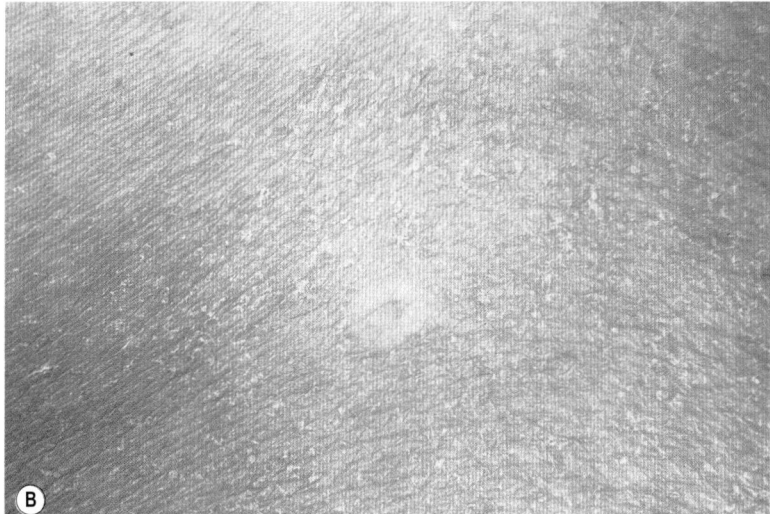

Fig. 16.101
(**A**, **B**) Malignant atrophic papulosis: note the typical small papules with depressed centers and fine white scaling. By courtesy of the Institute of Dermatology, London, UK.

Intestinal manifestations are variable. While any segment of the intestinal system from the oral cavity to the anus may be involved, it is predominantly the small intestine that is affected.[13] Some patients are asymptomatic while others complain of indigestion, diarrhea, constipation or abdominal distension and pain. Laparoscopy usually reveals characteristic subserosal white, yellow, or pinkish plaques, typically slightly depressed and several centimeters in diameter.[22] Of great importance, some patients develop small intestinal perforation with resultant peritonitis. Fistulae involving the small bowel may develop as a complication.[22–24] Omental necrosis may also be seen.[25] Rarely, intestinal involvement precedes the cutaneous features.[26] Acute small bowel perforation can be the first manifestation of the disease.[27] In addition, intestinal lesions sometimes develop many years after an initial cutaneous presentation.

The condition may involve both the peripheral and central nervous systems and occasionally such lesions dominate the clinical features.[27–35] Symptoms are variable and are occasionally multiple due to various sites being affected. For example, hemi- and quadriplegias, sensory losses, and cranial nerve lesions may all be encountered.[35,36]

Malignant atrophic papulosis is a truly systemic illness in most patients. Lesions are found in a variety of sites including the heart, lungs, kidneys, bladder, and liver.[19,22,37–44]

Although this disease is usually associated with a poor prognosis and high mortality, there does appear to be a subset of patients in whom the cutaneous features are the sole manifestation and evolution is benign.[10,45–51] Intestinal involvement appears to correlate particularly with a poor outlook.[52,53] Mortality is especially correlated with intestinal perforation.[53]

Malignant atrophic papulosis has been reported in a patient with acquired immunodeficiency syndrome.[54]

Pathogenesis and histologic features

The precise etiology is unknown, although viral, genetic, autoimmune mechanisms, and fibrinolysis have all been implicated.[55,56] Since lesions are sometimes not associated with significant inflammation, it is debatable whether classification as a true vasculitis is appropriate. The pathogenesis is that of vascular thrombosis, the essential pathology of the lesions being that of infarction.[1] A focal fibrinolytic defect within the center of the infarcted lesions and alterations of fibrinolysis and platelet function have been described, but these are not consistent findings.[1,57,58] It has been proposed that endothelial swelling and proliferation with secondary thrombosis is the primary pathogenesis.[1] Consistent with this hypothesis is the documentation of a patient with malignant atrophic papulosis associated with elevated anticardiolipin antibodies.[59] Others, however, have not been able to corroborate this finding.[60]

In most cases, the cause of the initial endothelial vascular insult is unknown, but a mononuclear vasculitis may play a role in the pathogenesis.[4] Most authors regard the mucin deposition described below as a secondary event developing as a consequence of dermal ischemia.

The established cutaneous lesion has a characteristic appearance.[61,62] The overlying epidermis is hyperkeratotic and atrophic. Immediately beneath this is a wedge-shaped zone of dermal infarction with the base parallel to the surface epithelium: it is typically pale in color, relatively acellular, and associated with mucin deposition (*Figs 16.102* and *16.103*).[63] The latter is metachromatic with toluidine blue and demonstrates hyaluronidase-sensitive Alcian blue staining. Older lesions are frequently ulcerated. Often, the vessels adjacent and deep to the infarct are hyalinized and show a perivascular lymphocytic infiltrate (*Figs 16.104* and *16.105*). Usually, but not invariably, an endovasculitis can be demonstrated in the blood vessels at the apex of the lesion: this consists of endothelial cell hyperplasia, sometimes complicated by thrombosis. The internal elastic lamina, media, and serosa

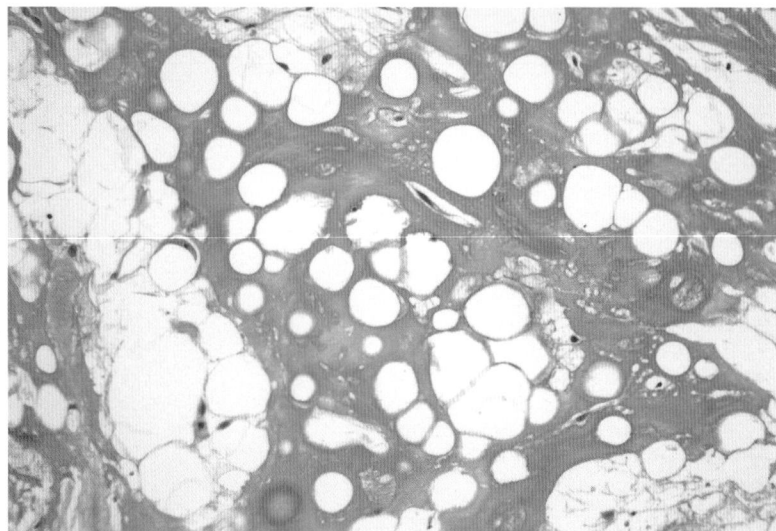

Fig. 16.103
Malignant atrophic papulosis: high-power view showing hyalinized fat necrosis.

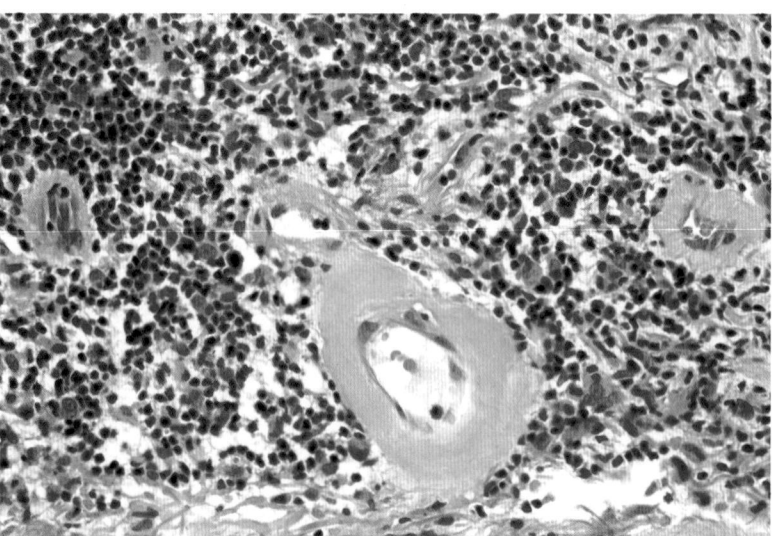

Fig. 16.104
Malignant atrophic papulosis: high-power view showing blood vessel wall hyalinization and a heavy lymphocytic infiltrate.

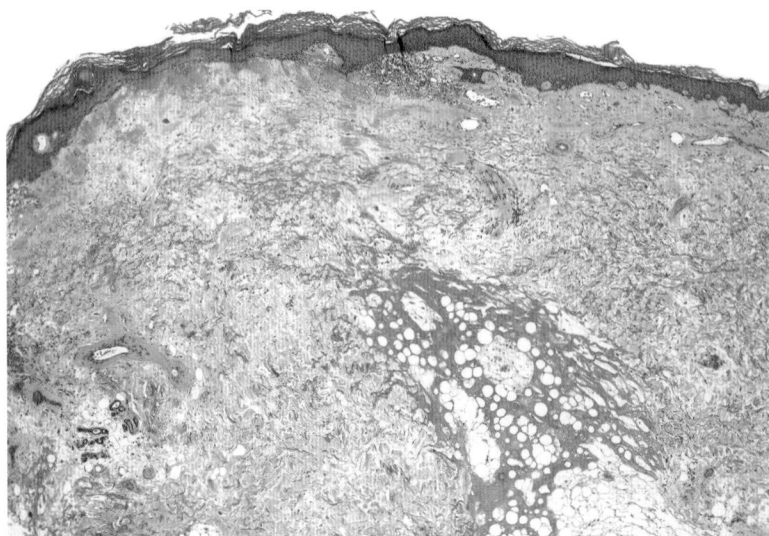

Fig. 16.102
Malignant atrophic papulosis: there is hyperkeratosis and epidermal atrophy associated with a zone of dermal infarction. Note the ectatic vessels.

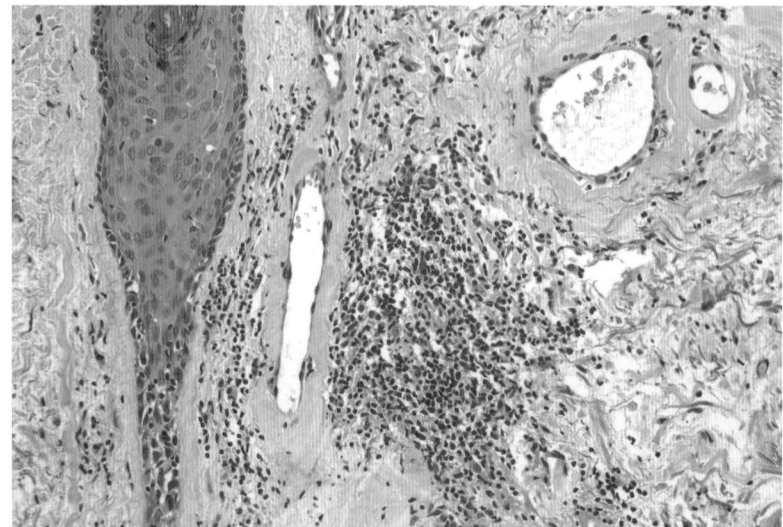

Fig. 16.105
Malignant atrophic papulosis: the superficial blood vessels are thickened and hyalinized.

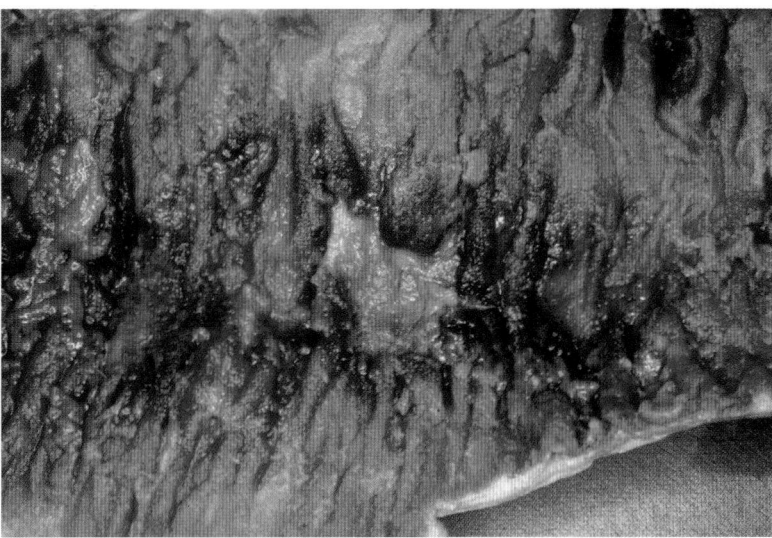

Fig. 16.106
Malignant atrophic papulosis: section of jejunum showing ulceration of the mucosa with surrounding intense congestion. By courtesy of C.J.J. Mulder, MD, Rijnstate Hospital, Arnhem, The Netherlands.

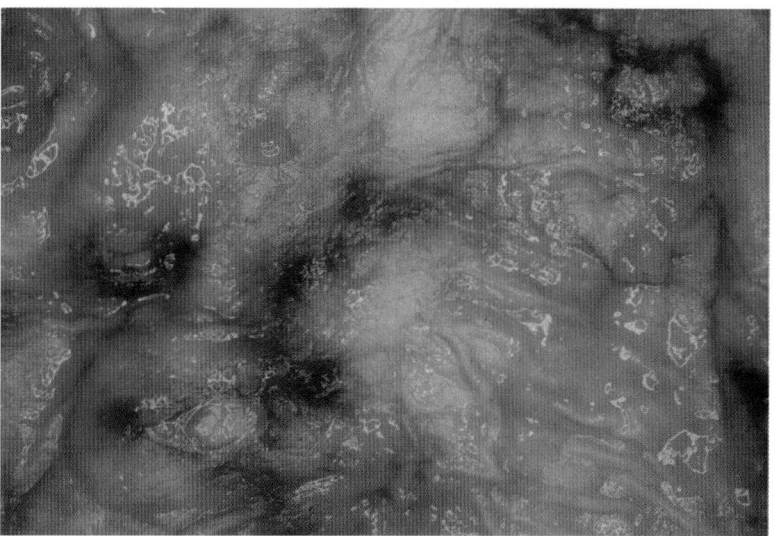

Fig. 16.108
Malignant atrophic papulosis: section of rectum showing focal congestion and ulceration. By courtesy of C.J.J. Mulder, MD, Rijnstate Hospital, Arnhem, The Netherlands.

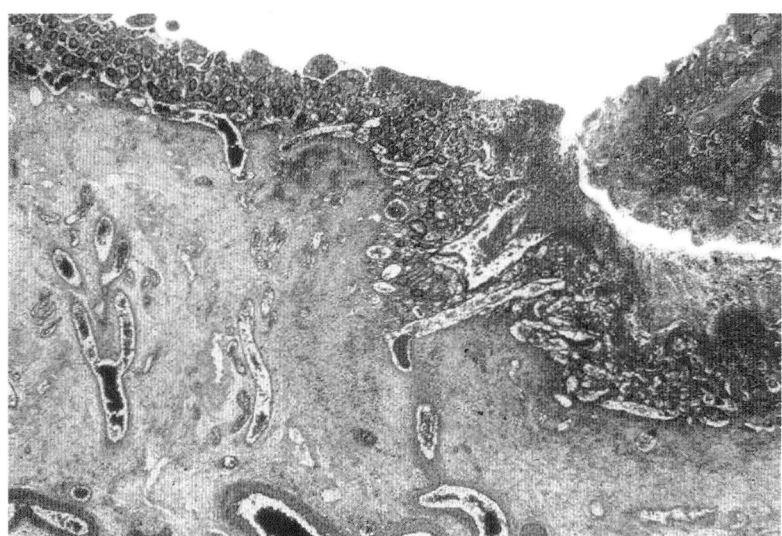

Fig. 16.107
Malignant atrophic papulosis: histologic section of jejunum shown in Fig. 16.106. Note the acute inflammation and ulceration. By courtesy of C.J.J. Mulder, MD, Rijnstate Hospital, Arnhem, The Netherlands.

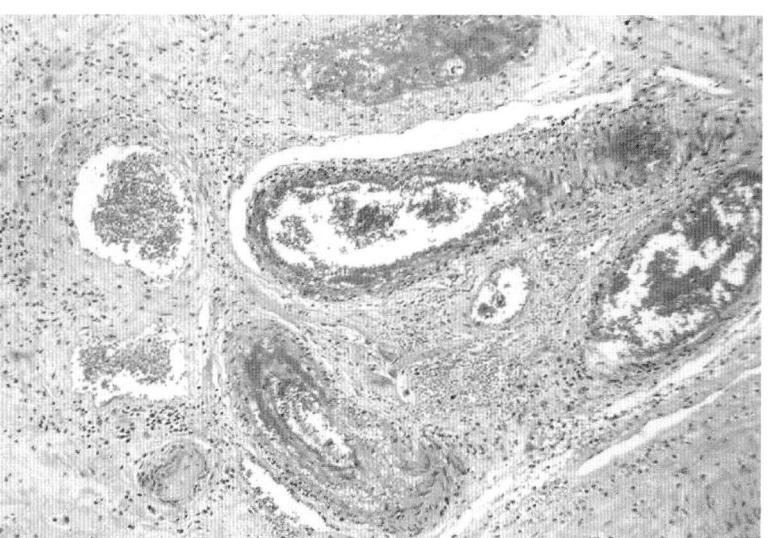

Fig. 16.109
Malignant atrophic papulosis: histologic section of the submucosa of the rectum. There is acute vasculitis with thrombosis. By courtesy of C.J.J. Mulder, MD, Rijnstate Hospital, Arnhem, The Netherlands.

are usually not involved. A panniculitis mimicking lupus erythematosus profundus has been described.[64]

Microscopic examination of the bowel lesions reveals transmural intestinal inflammation with ulceration and hemorrhage. The latter may involve the small and large intestines including the rectum (*Figs 16.106–16.109*). Vascular changes have included gross intimal thickening with consequent severe diminution in the lumen diameter, thrombosis, and acute vasculitis.[65]

Differential diagnosis

As mentioned above, the cutaneous findings are distinctive and diagnosis should be relatively straightforward. However, it should be kept in mind that although the cutaneous lesions of malignant atrophic papulosis are typical, similar lesions have been described in patients with other diseases, such as SLE, systemic sclerosis, rheumatoid arthritis, dermatomyositis, and Crohn disease.[11–16,66] A search for underlying or associated disorders is therefore advised.

Livedoid vasculopathy and atrophie blanche

Clinical features

Livedoid vasculopathy and atrophie blanche (also referred to as livedo vasculitis, livedoid vasculitis, and segmental hyalinizing vasculitis) have traditionally been used interchangeably. It is a common dermatosis that usually occurs in young to middle-aged women.[1–5] However, it has been argued that the term livedoid vasculopathy be used to describe the disease entity, and that atrophie blanche be used as a description of a certain pattern of clinical manifestation that is often, though not invariably, associated with livedoid vasculopathy.[5] In addition to the association with the thrombotic vasculopathy that is livedoid vasculopathy, the changes of atrophie blanche may be seen in chronic venous insufficiency.[5] Early in the course the patients may present with painful purpuric papules and plaques that progress to ulcers.[5] In its fully established state, the lesions may develop into atrophie blanche consisting of one or more irregular, smooth, atrophic plaques surrounded

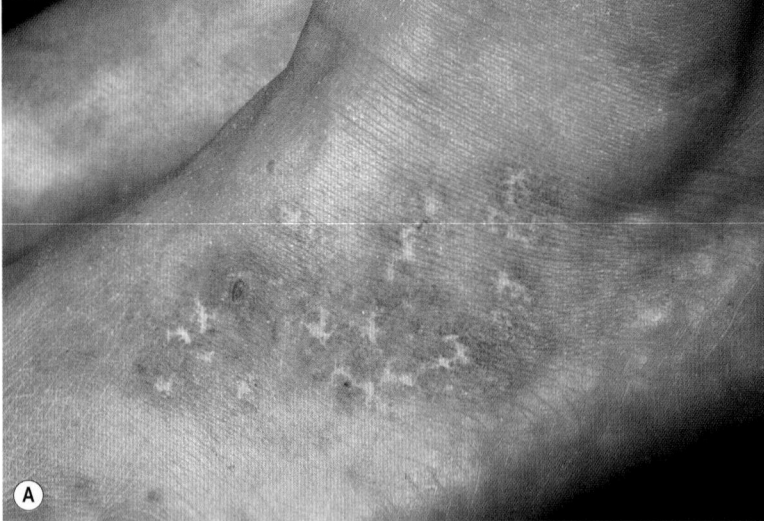

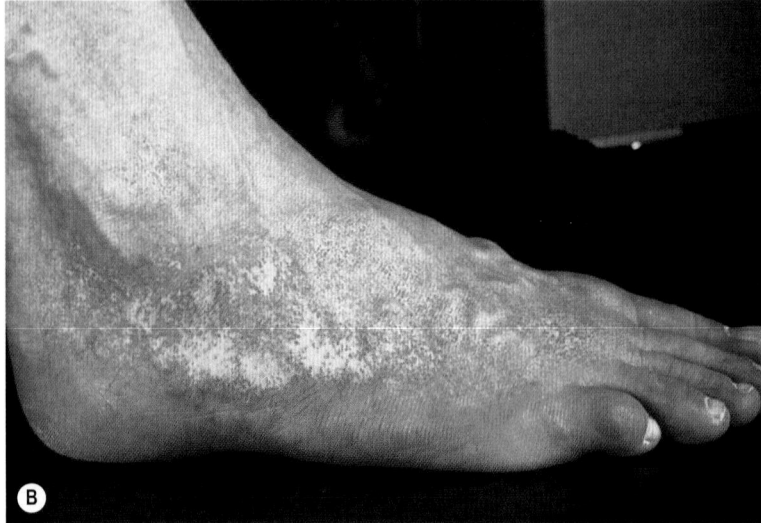

Fig. 16.110
Livedoid vasculopathy: (**A**) there is ulceration with erythema and scaling; (**B**) this example shows marked hyperpigmentation with scarring and atrophy around the ankle and extending onto the dorsum of the foot. By courtesy of the Institute of Dermatology, London, UK.

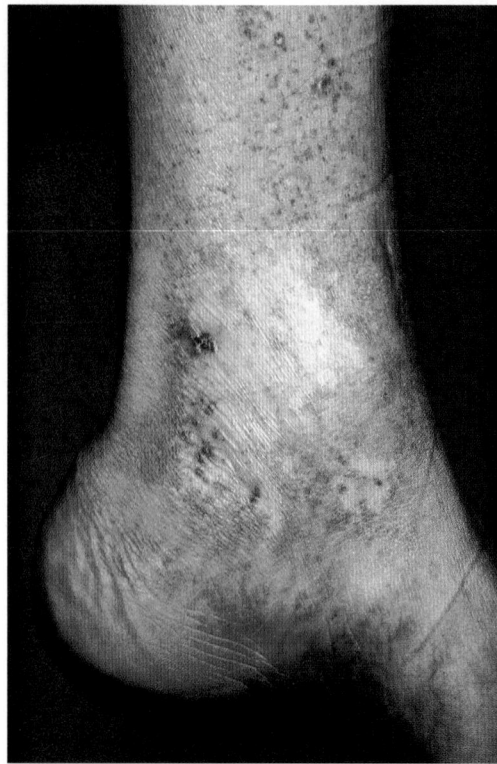

Fig. 16.111
Livedoid vasculopathy/atrophie blanche: an extensive ivory-white area of scarring overlies the medial malleolus. By courtesy of R.A. Marsden, St George's Hospital, London, UK.

by a hyperpigmented border and telangiectases (*Figs 16.110* and *16.111*). Ulcerative lesions of two types may precede it:
- small (1–5 mm diameter), very painful erythematous purpuric areas that ulcerate and heal slowly,
- chronic large areas of ulceration up to 5 cm in diameter, which, after a long period of time, heal to form extensive areas of atrophic plaque.

The condition shows seasonal variation, typically worsening in the summer months. Lesions recur at periodic intervals and are predominantly located on the lower legs, ankles, and the dorsal surfaces of the feet. Occasionally, however, they are found around the forearms, fingers, and hands or even in a more widespread distribution.[3,6,7] The clinical manifestation of atrophie blanche is often associated with signs of venous stasis.[8,9]

Approximately half of patients involved have coagulation abnormalities, including factor V Leiden mutation, decreased protein C or protein S activity, prothrombin G20210A mutation, anticardiolipin antibodies, homocysteinemia, lupus anticoagulant, cryoglobulinemia, and methylenetetrahydrofolate reductase mutation.[4,5,10–18] One study found 17% of lupus patients were affected.[19] This study also noted that the pattern of cutaneous lesions was somewhat unusual, with involvement of the knees, elbows, fingers, soles, and the back.[19] The same study suggested that patients with lupus erythematosus who have atrophie blanche are at an increased risk of developing lupus CNS involvement.[19]

Pathogenesis and histologic features

The pathogenesis of livedoid vasculopathy is not entirely understood but is clearly a thrombotic vasculopathy resulting in ischemia. Hydrostatic pressure certainly contributes to the development, given the predilection for the distal lower extremities and the association with venous insufficiency in some cases. Both immunoglobulin (usually IgM, less often IgG and IgA) and complement within the blood vessel walls raise the possibility of an immunological pathogenesis in some cases.[20] It has been associated with a localized defect of tissue plasminogen activator.[3,21] The location of the lesions suggests that trauma may also play some role in development of some lesions. As previously mentioned, many cases are associated with disorders of coagulation, suggesting an underlying coagulopathy is the basis of disorder.[4,5,10–18] Elevated levels of lipoprotein(a) are associated with livedoid vasculopathy and may also contribute to a prothrombotic state.[22]

Early and ulcerative lesions are characterized by the presence of increased numbers of dermal vessels containing fibrin within their walls in addition to intraluminal fibrinoid plugs (*Figs 16.112–16.114*). The latter are typically diastase resistant and periodic acid-Schiff (PAS) positive, and can also be highlighted by use of the phosphotungstic acid–hematoxylin stain (*Fig. 16.115*). Inflammatory destruction of blood vessels is, however, not a feature and therefore this disorder is not a true vasculitis. Variable degrees of red cell extravasation are evident, and hemosiderin pigment is often present. A perivascular lymphohistiocytic infiltrate of varying intensity is usually found, and dermal mast cells are often increased in number. Ulcerative lesions show infarction of the superficial dermis and epidermis. In the fully established atrophic plaque, in addition to the vascular changes, the epidermis is atrophic and the dermis shows dense scleroderma-like scarring.

Differential diagnosis

The histologic features in the appropriate clinical setting are diagnostic. Coagulopathies are associated with intraluminal fibrinoid plugs but not extensive fibrinoid change of the vessel wall. Lesions with the clinical manifestation of atrophie blanche show some of the features seen in stasis

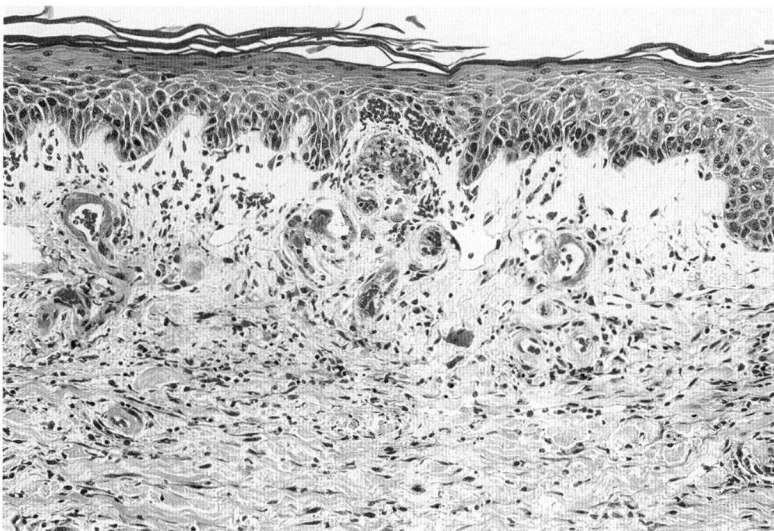

Fig. 16.112
Livedoid vasculopathy: the vessels in the papillary dermis are increased in number and show mural fibrin deposition. There is underlying scarring.

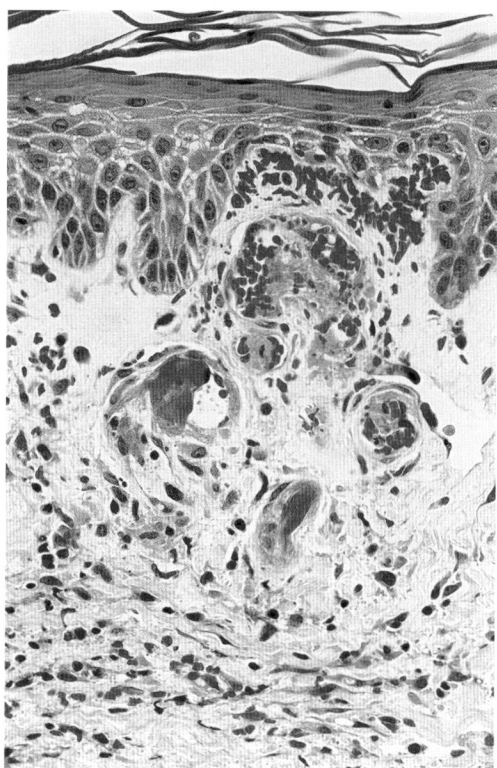

Fig. 16.114
Livedoid vasculopathy: occluded vessels are present. There is marked red blood cell extravasation.

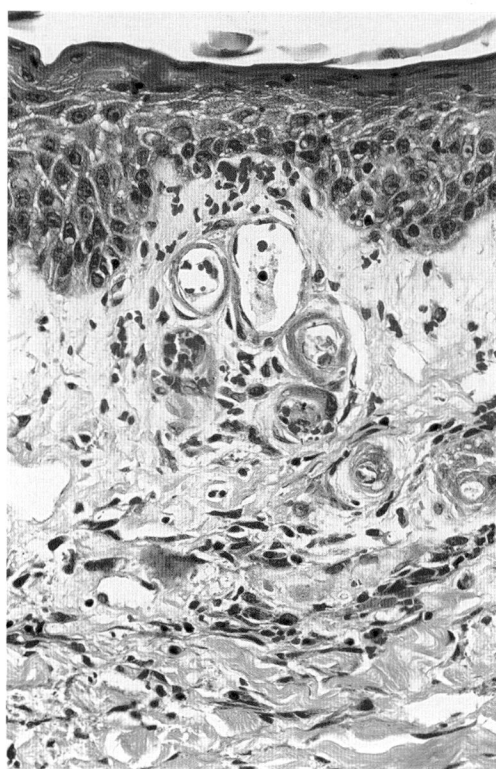

Fig. 16.113
Livedoid vasculopathy: high-power view of vessels.

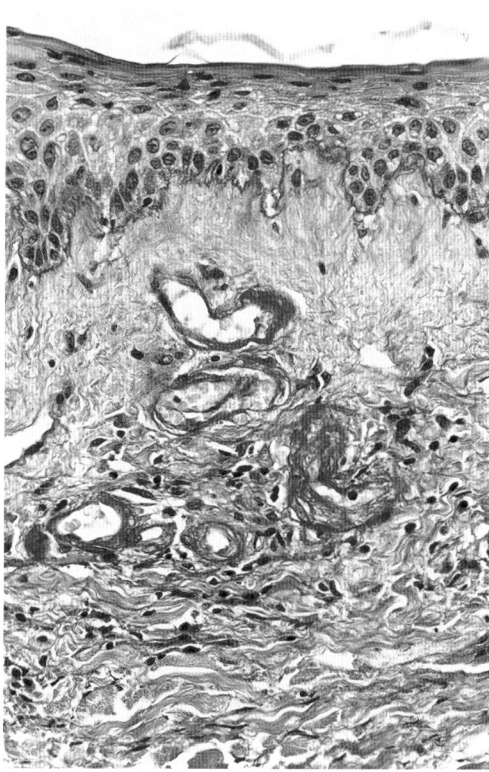

Fig. 16.115
Livedoid vasculopathy: the vessel walls are strongly PAS positive, diastase resistant.

dermatitis, such as clustering of vessels in the superficial dermis; however, uncomplicated stasis does not show fibrinoid change.

Dermatological manifestations of cholesterol crystal embolism and embolism from atrial myxoma

Clinical features

Cholesterol crystal embolism is a disease of the elderly and typically occurs in males (4:1), thereby reflecting the demographics of atherosclerosis.[1,2] Cholesterol embolism may occur spontaneously or complicate trauma to the aorta or other large arteries.[1,3] It can be seen following warfarin therapy.[4] Systemic symptoms due to infarction are variable and depend upon the organ embolized. Necrotizing vasculitis has been described following cholesterol crystal embolization.[5] Multisystem involvement sometimes results in an initial diagnosis of vasculitis.

Patients commonly manifest pyrexia, myalgia, and a sudden onset of systemic hypertension as well as renal failure and cutaneous lesions.[6] An

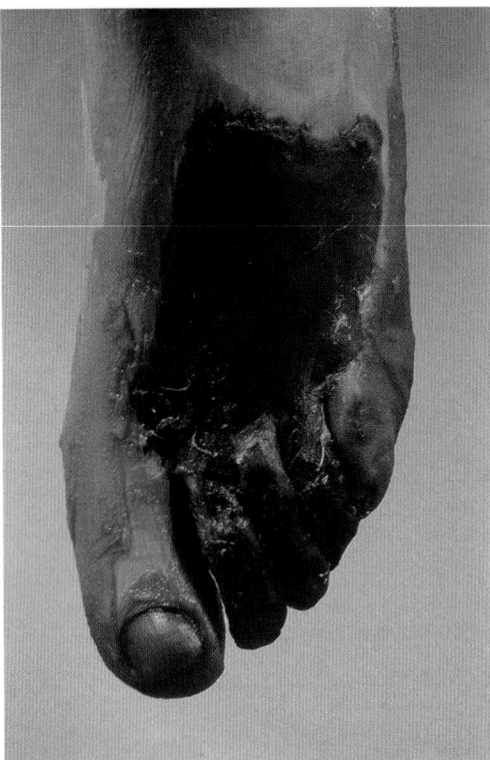

Fig. 16.116
Cholesterol embolism: there is extensive infarction of the toes of this elderly male patient.

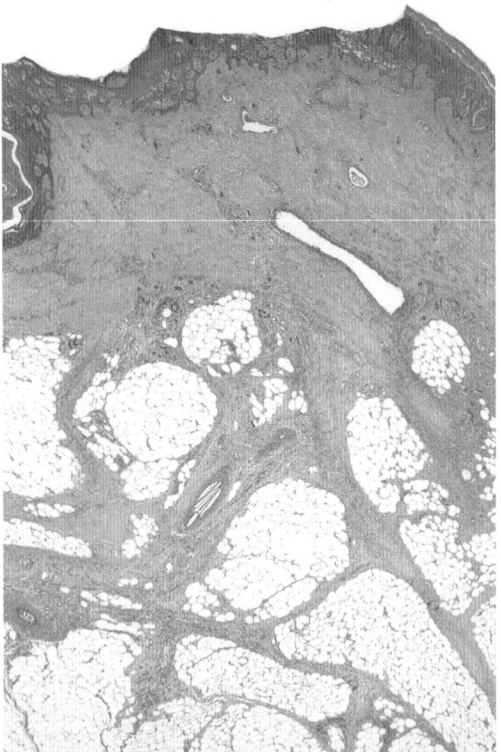

Fig. 16.117
Cholesterol emboli: there is ulceration and dermal scar tissue extending into the septa of the subcutaneous fat. Needle-shaped crystals are present in the lumen of an artery in the middle of the field.

increased ESR, blood eosinophilia, and raised serum creatinine are additional features. Cutaneous manifestations are common and include:

- livedo reticularis, often bilateral, affecting the feet and legs and sometimes extending up to involve the trunk,[7]
- gangrene of the toes (*Fig. 16.116*),
- cyanosis,
- purple discoloration of the toes,
- cutaneous ulceration,
- nodules on the legs, thighs, feet, and toes,
- purpuric lesions on the legs and feet.

The cutaneous lesions of cholesterol crystal embolism therefore mimic many other vascular lesions, and biopsy is essential for diagnosis. Mortality is very high due to cardiac and CNS involvement.

Cardiac myxomas are rare but represent the most frequent primary cardiac tumor. Although benign, they are a marker of Carney complex and early recognition is imperative as distant embolization is an important complication associated with high mortality. Cutaneous symptoms include erythematous macules and papules predominantly of acral sites, digital cyanosis, petechiae, splinter hemorrhages, telangiectasia, and livedo reticularis.[8–16]

Pathogenesis and histologic features

Cholesterol emboli are found in the small to large arteries and arterioles of the deep dermis or subcutaneous fat (*Figs 16.117* and *16.118*). Diagnosis depends upon the identification of typical biconvex cleft- or needle-shaped empty spaces (representing evanescent cholesterol crystals dissolved during tissue processing) often associated with atheromatous debris or luminal thrombosis. It is essential, therefore, that deep biopsies are taken. Multiple levels should also be examined because emboli tend to be patchily distributed and are often difficult to detect. The skin supplied by the occluded vessel may be infarcted.

Emboli from atrial myxomas are characterized by the presence of myxoid material within medium-sized vessels. Due to vascular occlusion, this is accompanied by fibrin deposition and a reactive vascular proliferation. Demonstration of the myxoid substance is often difficult and commonly requires examination of multiple levels.

Disseminated intravascular coagulation

Clinical features

Disseminated intravascular coagulation (DIC) is a consumptive coagulopathy that is associated with a wide variety of underlying disorders, many of them life threatening. It is not uncommonly seen in very ill patients and may be acute, subacute, or chronic. Purpura fulminans is a term that has been applied to infection-associated DIC in children. Some authors have applied the term less restrictively to a severe form of DIC associated with high morbidity and mortality.[1,2] Purpura fulminans is characterized by an acute syndrome of rapidly progressive and extensive hemorrhagic skin necrosis associated with dermal vascular thrombosis and vascular collapse due to DIC.[3,4] A common presentation is symmetrical purpura of the fingers and toes.

DIC is commonly associated with complications of pregnancy and delivery, such as abruptio placentae, sepsis, and amniotic fluid embolism. A wide variety of infections, including bacterial sepsis, meningococcemia, and fungal infections, may also be associated. Massive trauma, heat stroke, shock, snakebite, poisoning, and burns can cause DIC. Malignant neoplasms (including carcinoma of the stomach, breast and colon, small cell carcinoma of the lung, brain, and pancreas) and hematological malignancies have also been associated with this condition.[5–14]

Purpura fulminans occurs predominantly in children and has an equal incidence in males and females. It develops as a complication of a prodromal infectious illness, most commonly meningococcemia, scarlet fever, viral upper respiratory tract infection, chickenpox, rubella, and other exanthemata.[15] The disease shows some seasonal variation, being more common in winter and spring. Children develop large confluent ecchymoses, which particularly affect the buttocks, legs, and feet, and commonly appear on the upper limbs and abdomen (*Fig. 16.119*). The ecchymoses frequently become necrotic, and blood-filled blisters are often found. On occasion the limbs become gangrenous (*Fig. 16.120*). Fever and hypotension accompany the cutaneous lesions.

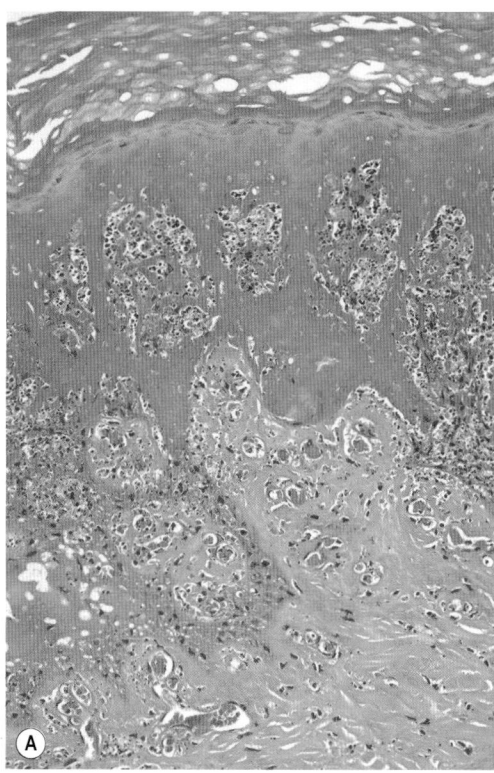

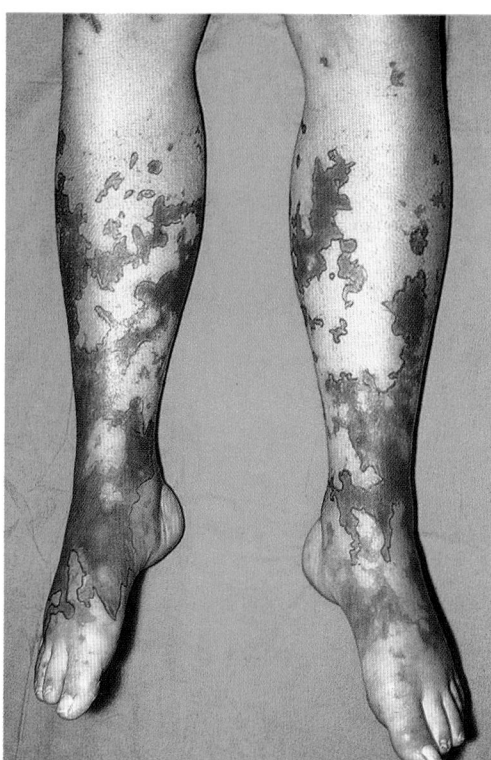

Fig. 16.119
Purpura fulminans: bilateral extensive ecchymoses are present on this child's legs. By courtesy of D. McGibbon, MD, St Thomas' Hospital, London, UK.

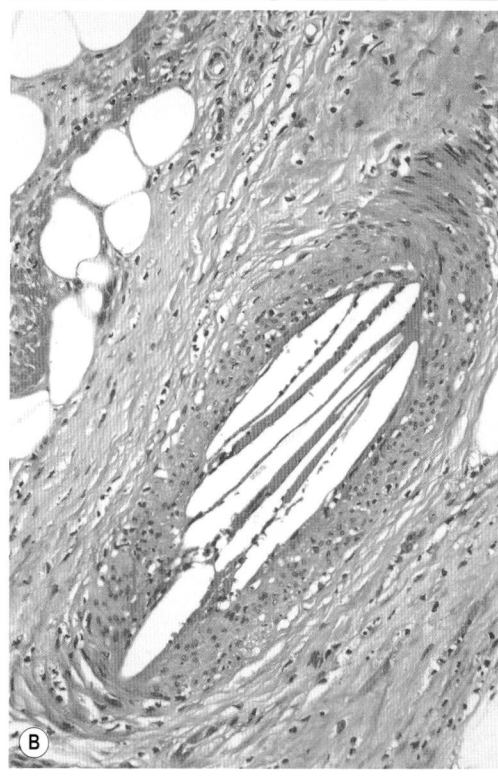

Fig. 16.118
Cholesterol embolism: (**A**) the overlying epidermis shows full-thickness infarction; (**B**) high-power view of cholesterol clefts.

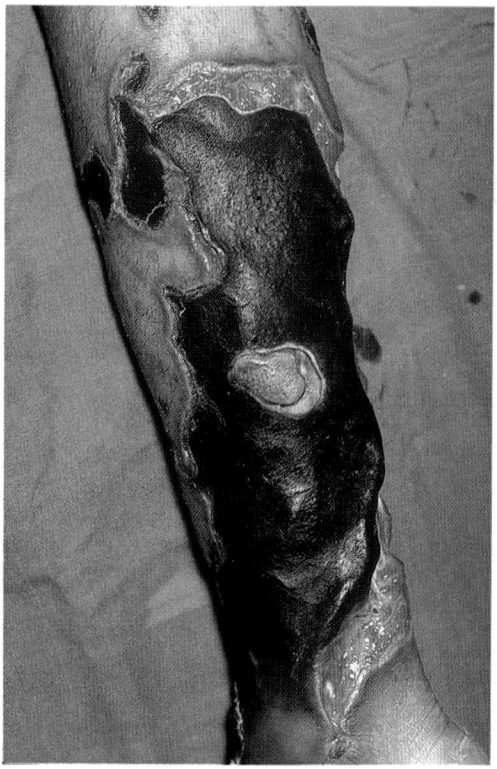

Fig. 16.120
Purpura fulminans: there is complete gangrene of the skin. By courtesy of D. McGibbon, MD, St Thomas' Hospital, London, UK.

Hematological studies reveal thrombocytopenia, anemia, and often a leukocytosis. The prothrombin and bleeding times are prolonged. Fibrinogen levels are low and fibrin-fibrinogen degradation products elevated.

Pathogenesis and histologic features

As stated above, DIC is not a disease sui generis but represents a coagulopathy resulting from a large number of disorders. These conditions trigger DIC either by causing direct injury to endothelial cells, which causes platelet aggregation, or by increasing circulating procoagulant factors, often tissue factor. The consequences are thrombosis, fibrinolysis leading to depletion of fibrin, clotting factors and platelets, vascular occlusion, tissue ischemia, and hemorrhage. Clotting factors may be consumed at a rate that exceeds the ability of the liver for synthesis. The coagulopathy, in turn, causes a hemolytic anemia by damaging red blood cells.

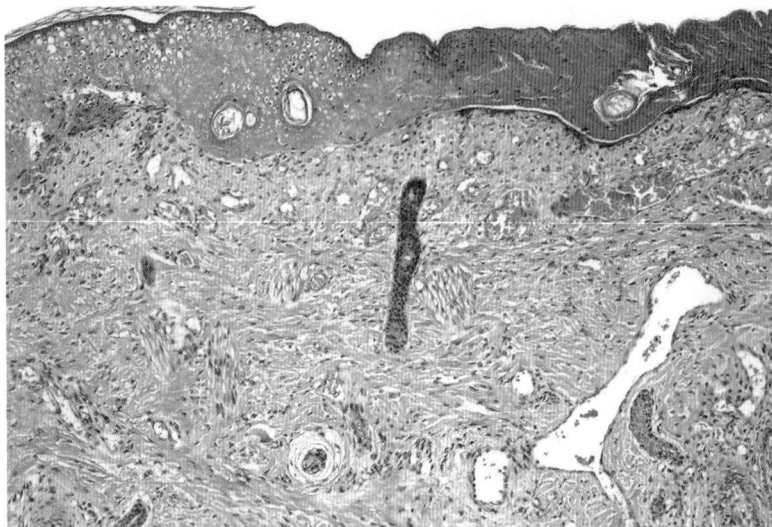

Fig. 16.121
Purpura fulminans: there is epidermal infarction.

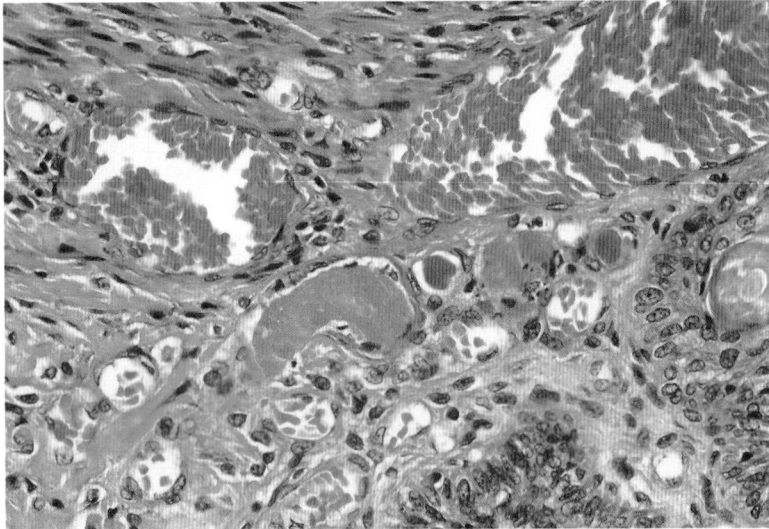

Fig. 16.122
Purpura fulminans: numerous small thrombi are seen in the superficial vessels.

Purpura fulminans is sometimes a manifestation of hereditary protein C deficiency, protein S deficiency, Coumadin therapy, and antiphospholipid antibodies.[3,16]

Biopsy of skin lesions in patients with DIC is characterized by fibrin, platelet, or mixed thrombi in the capillaries and venules, particularly of the skin, but also commonly affecting the internal viscera, including the kidneys, bowel, bladder, and brain (*Figs 16.121* and *16.122*).[3] The number of vessels containing thrombi ranges from scattered to nearly all vessels being involved. Variable numbers of extravasated red blood cells are seen. In patients with purpura fulminans, the thrombi are associated with diffuse and extensive hemorrhage. Early lesions usually show few or no perivascular inflammatory cells. Older lesions are often characterized by epidermal necrosis and subepidermal blood-filled bullae. A mild perivascular inflammatory cell infiltrate of lymphocytes and polymorphs may be present. Infective DIC or purpura fulminans sometimes shows features of a leukocytoclastic vasculitis. Immunofluorescence studies for immunoglobulins and complement are uniformly negative.

Differential diagnosis

The differential diagnosis includes other causes of coagulopathy or leukocytoclastic vasculitis. Serological evaluation for disorders of coagulation is

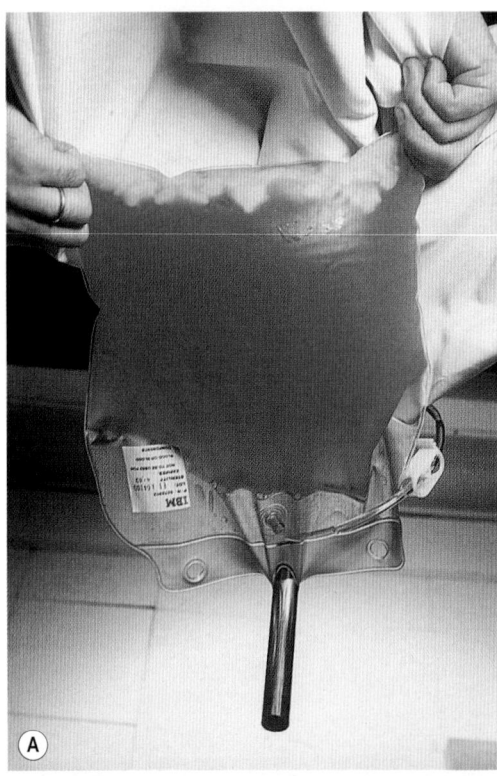

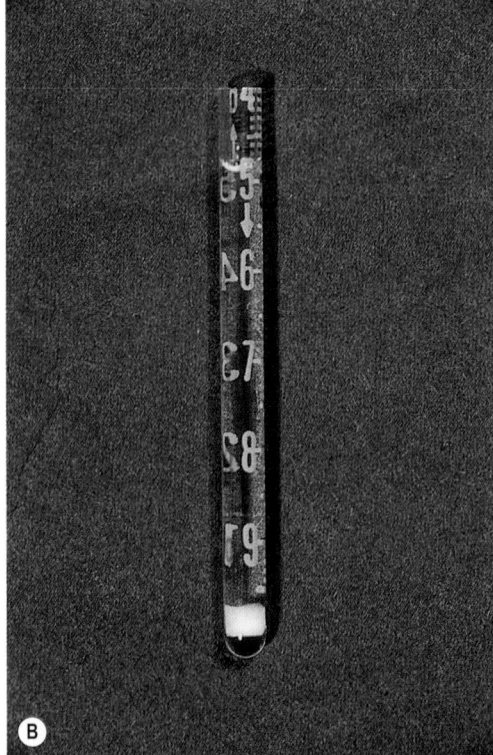

Fig. 16.123
Cryoglobulinemia: (**A**) there is a large quantity of precipitated cryoglobulin in this plasmapheresis specimen; (**B**) a cryoprecipitate. By courtesy of N. Slater, MD, St Thomas' Hospital, London, UK.

required to support the diagnosis. Finally, since successful treatment is both supportive and aimed at the underlying disorder, patients must be evaluated to determine the underlying causes of the DIC.

Cryoglobulinemia

Cryoglobulins are immunoglobulins that precipitate at low temperatures (4°C) and which redissolve on warming (*Fig. 16.123*). Typically, the greater their concentration, the higher the temperature at which they precipitate. This has obvious clinical implications, particularly for plasmapheresis therapy.

Cryoglobulins may be subdivided into three classes: [1-3]

- Type I cryoglobulin is composed solely of monoclonal immunoglobulin (either kappa or lambda) and is usually, though not invariably, associated with a variety of lymphoproliferative disorders, including multiple myeloma, Waldenström macroglobulinemia, chronic lymphocytic leukemia, and lymphocytic lymphoma.
- Type II (mixed) cryoglobulin is composed of monoclonal (usually IgM) immunoglobulin reacting against polyclonal IgG.
- Type III (polyclonal) cryoglobulin is composed of polyclonal immunoglobulins (usually IgG and IgM).

The last two subtypes (mixed cryoglobulins) function as immune complexes and clinical manifestations are therefore due, at least in part, to allergic vasculitis. Mixed cryoglobulinemia may be clinically subdivided into two forms:

- Essential mixed cryoglobulinemia, in which most patients are infected with the hepatitis C virus.[2-4] Hepatitis B virus has been also described in association with essential mixed cryoglobulinemia.[2,35]
- Secondary mixed cryoglobulinemia, which develops as a complication of a variety of conditions, including connective tissue diseases such as SLE, lymphomas, or infective disease processes (e.g., infective endocarditis and glandular fever).[3,6]

Clinical features

The eponym 'Meltzer triad' has been applied to the combined features of purpura, arthralgia, and weakness that are often present.[5] Cutaneous manifestations are common to all classes of cryoglobulinemia and are often the presenting complaint.[1,3,5,7] Purpura is the most frequent initial sign.

Type I cryoglobulinemia is usually characterized by purpuric lesions, including inflammatory macules and papules on the extremities, accompanied by foci of ulceration (*Fig. 16.124*).[8] Additional features may include livedo reticularis, Raynaud phenomenon, scarring, and infarction, which particularly affects the digits, ears, and nose.[8] Renal lesions are uncommon,

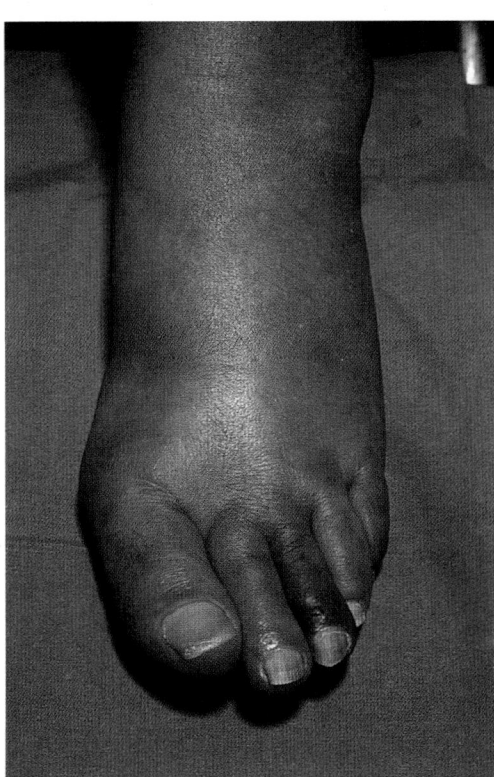

Fig. 16.124
Cryoglobulinemia: there is purplish discoloration of the third toe. By courtesy of N. Slater, MD, St Thomas' Hospital, London, UK.

but some patients may manifest hematuria, proteinuria (occasionally amounting to the nephrotic syndrome) and, rarely, anuria.[9]

Mixed cryoglobulinemia is characterized by joint involvement (arthralgia and arthritis), Raynaud phenomenon, fever, purpura, weakness, renal involvement, hepatosplenomegaly, and generalized vasculitis. Cutaneous manifestations include palpable purpura, inflammatory macules and papules, necrotizing vasculitis, crural ulcers and, occasionally, cold urticaria.[8,10] Additional rare manifestations include follicular pustular purpura, erythema multiforme, and necrobiotic xanthogranuloma.[8,11,12] Renal involvement, most frequently in the form of type 1 mesangioproliferative glomerulonephritis, may be identified by proteinuria, hematuria, and red cell casts.[2] Patients can also have polyneuropathies.[2] Prognosis is variable. Renal involvement, which occurs in 50% of cases, is associated with high morbidity and mortality.

Given the frequent association of hepatitis virus infection with cryoglobulinemia, it comes as no surprise that some patients develop hepatocellular carcinoma.[13,14]

Pathogenesis and histologic features

In keeping with an immune complex-mediated pathogenesis, hypocomplementemia is the rule. The cryoprecipitate is composed of polyclonal IgG with either monoclonal or polyclonal IgM and is associated with rheumatoid factor properties.[3,15] In some patients, hepatitis B virus surface antigen or antihepatitis B antibodies are identified in either the serum or the cryoprecipitate, suggesting a possible causal relationship. Both hepatitis C and hepatitis B viruses have been reported in cases of mixed cryoglobulinemia.[16-18] Since most patients with essential mixed cryoglobulinemia are infected with the hepatitis C virus, it appears likely that this represents the cause of this form of the disease and consequently this aspect has received much investigative attention. Hepatitis C virus and hepatitis C virus antigen–antibody complexes have been demonstrated in cryoprecipitates.[19] Hepatitis C viral RNA is detected by polymerase chain reaction (PCR) in peripheral blood monocytes of 81% to 90% of patients with mixed cryoglobulinemia.[20,21] Hepatitis C genome has also been demonstrated in the bone marrow cells of patients with mixed cryoglobulinemia.[22] Interestingly, the E2 envelope protein of the hepatitis C virus binds to CD81, which is present on B lymphocytes.[23] What role this interaction plays in the pathogenesis of cryoglobulinemia is poorly understood.[23]

High levels of CXCL10 (Interferon-γ-induced protein 10) are found in high levels in hepatitis C-related cryoglobulinemia. It is hypothesized that interferon-γ production from Th1 CD4+ T cells stimulates secretion of CXCL10, resulting in perpetuation of the autoimmune response.[24]

Other infective agents can also be associated with cryoglobulinemia including protozoa, fungi, bacteria, *Chlamydia*, and rickettsiae. Cryoglobulinemia has been reported in patients infected with the HIV virus.[25-29] However, in HIV patients with circulating cryoglobulins, the clinical symptoms usually associated with cryoglobulinemia are often lacking.[25] Another study has shown that in HIV-infected patients the presence of cryoglobulins is significantly associated with increased mortality and risk of developing neoplasia (including B-cell lymphoproliferative disorders).[26] Interestingly, disappearance of the symptoms of cryoglobulinemia following infection with the HIV-1 virus has also been reported. The authors of this report speculate on a significant role for CD4+ T cells in the pathogenesis of cryoglobulinemia in a subset of patients.[30]

The histologic features of monoclonal cryoglobulinemia are those of vascular dilatation, endothelial swelling, and plugging of vascular lumina by hyaline material, which is diastase resistant and PAS positive (*Fig. 16.125*). Intravascular rouleaux formation may also be a feature.[8] On occasion, monoclonal cryoglobulinemia may be associated with leukocytoclastic vasculitis.[8]

In addition to occasional intracapillary hyaline thrombi, patients with severe renal involvement sometimes manifest features of membranoproliferative glomerulonephritis.

Mixed cryoglobulinemia is associated with immune complex-mediated acute leukocytoclastic vasculitis. The cryoglobulins precipitate in small vessels at low temperature and the resultant complement activation ensures the changes of acute vasculitis. Immunofluorescence is positive for IgG, IgM,

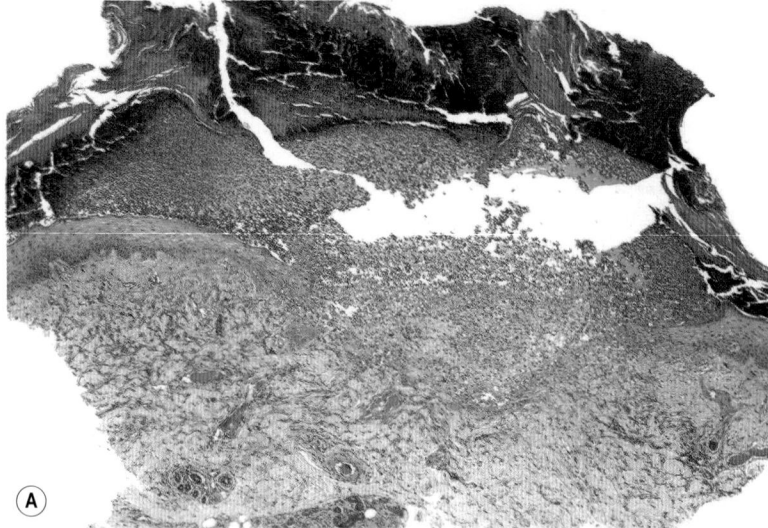

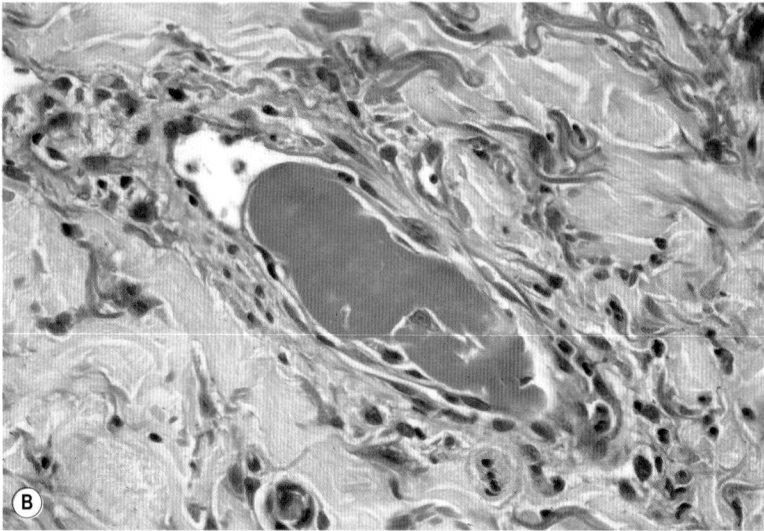

Fig. 16.125
Monoclonal cryoglobulinemia: (**A**) crusted ulcer with occluded vessels at its base; (**B**) high-power view of a hyaline thrombus.

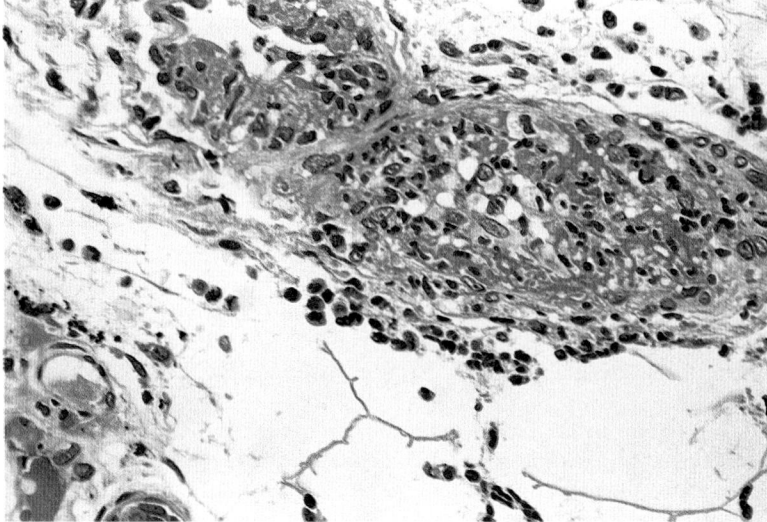

Fig. 16.126
Mixed cryoglobulinemia: in this example, the features of acute leukocytoclastic vasculitis are evident.

and complement (*Fig. 16.126*). Occasionally, intravascular hyaline thrombi are present in early lesions. Red cell extravasation is often a feature.

In biopsies from acute cases, the renal glomeruli show intracapillary thrombi. Other renal manifestations include membranoproliferative glomerulonephritis and vasculitis.

Differential diagnosis

The histologic differential diagnosis of monoclonal cryoglobulinemia includes other causes of thrombotic vasculopathy, for example DIC, TTP, protein C deficiency, and warfarin (Coumadin) necrosis. Although subtle histologic clues may suggest cryoglobulinemia, such as the waxy hyaline texture of the casts, definitive diagnosis is based on serological testing for cryoglobulins. The differential diagnosis of mixed cryoglobulinemia includes other causes of leukocytoclastic vasculitis.

Antiphospholipid antibody syndrome and Sneddon syndrome

Clinical features

The circulating anticoagulant known as the antiphospholipid antibody is associated with paradoxical thrombosis, spontaneous abortion, premature labor, intrauterine death, labile hypertension, cutaneous necrosis, gangrene, ecchymoses, purpura, leg ulcers, atrophie blanche, livedo reticularis, and false-positive syphilis serology – the lupus anticoagulant syndrome.[1-6] The last, also known more accurately as the antiphospholipid syndrome because not all patients have associated SLE, is due to the presence of circulating antiphospholipid antibodies, which inhibit coagulation in vitro, and are associated with a greatly increased risk of thrombotic phenomena affecting both arteries and veins. The most common autoantigen in the antiphospholipid syndrome is the protein beta-2 glycoprotein 1.[7,8] In addition to the 'lupus anticoagulant', another important type of antiphospholipid antibody is the anticardiolipin antibody, named for its ability to bind cardiolipin.

Although this syndrome is most often encountered in young adult women, it has been documented in children as well as the elderly. This demographic pattern is certainly a reflection of the association with lupus erythematosus, which shows a marked predilection for young women (*Table 16.15*).

Cutaneous involvement is often the first manifestation of disease. Patients develop necrosis of skin, which, in some cases, is widespread and severe.[9] In addition to disfiguring necrosis, these patients suffer pain and are at risk of superimposed infection.[10] Livedo reticularis is due to thrombotic involvement of arterioles and arteries.

Systemic involvement includes deep venous thrombosis, often complicated by pulmonary embolism, renal infarcts, cerebral vascular occlusion with resultant strokes, transient ischemic attacks, multi-infarct dementia, myocardial infarction, and gangrene.[3] The term 'catastrophic antiphospholipid syndrome' is applied to patients who develop complications resulting from multiorgan involvement.[10,11] The prognosis for this pernicious form of the disease is poor: in one study, 60% of patients died.[11]

The association of cutaneous thrombotic lesions, hypertension, and cerebrovascular disease is sometimes referred to as Sneddon syndrome.[3,12] Neurological symptoms are key to the clinical diagnosis of Sneddon syndrome. It is important to bear in mind that livedoid racemosa precedes cerebrovascular events in more than half of the patients, sometimes by many years.[13] Not all patients with Sneddon syndrome have antiphospholipid antibodies – the prevalence in various publications has ranged from 0% to 85%.[12] Sneddon syndrome can be idiopathic, associated with antiphospholipid antibodies or SLE.[13,14] Most cases of Sneddon syndrome are sporadic, but familial cases have been described.[15,16]

In addition to lupus erythematosus, the antiphospholipid syndrome has also been documented in association with other autoimmune diseases including rheumatoid arthritis, hemolytic anemia, thrombocytopenic purpura, ulcerative colitis, and rheumatic fever.[17,18] It may also complicate treatment with a number of drugs including antiarrhythmics, antipsychotics, antidepressants, anticonvulsants, immunotherapies, immunosuppressants, antihypertensives, and antibiotics, or develop during viral illnesses, and can present with an underlying lymphoma.[17,19]

Table 16.15
Preliminary criteria for the classification of the antiphospholipid syndrome*

Clinical criteria†
1. Vascular thrombosis: One or more clinical episodes of arterial, venous, or small-vessel thrombosis, in any tissue or organ. Thrombosis must be confirmed by imaging or Doppler studies or histopathology, with the exception of superficial venous thrombosis. For histopathological confirmation, thrombosis should be present without significant evidence of inflammation in the vessel wall.
2. Pregnancy morbidity:
(a) One or more unexplained deaths of a morphologically normal fetus at or beyond the 10th week of gestation, with normal fetal morphology documented by ultrasound or by direct examination of the fetus, or
(b) One or more premature births of a morphologically normal neonate at or before the 34th week of gestation because of severe pre-eclampsia or eclampsia, or severe placental insufficiency, or
(c) Three or more unexplained consecutive spontaneous abortions before the 10th week of gestation, with maternal anatomic or hormonal abnormalities and paternal and maternal chromosomal causes excluded.
In studies of populations of patients who have more than one type of pregnancy morbidity, investigators are strongly encouraged to stratify groups of subjects according to (a), (b), or (c) above.
Laboratory criteria
1. Anticardiolipin antibody of IgG and/or IgM isotype in blood, present in medium or high titer, on two or more occasions, at least 6 weeks apart, measured by a standardized enzyme-linked immunosorbent assay for β₂-glycoprotein I-independent anticardiolipin antibodies.
2. Lupus anticoagulant present in plasma, on two or more occasions, at least 6 weeks apart, detected according to the guidelines of the International Society on Thrombosis and Hemostasis (Scientific Subcommittee on Lupus Anticoagulants/Phospholipid-Dependent Antibodies), in the following steps:
(a) Prolonged phospholipid-dependent coagulation demonstrated on a screening test, e.g., activated partial thromboplastin time, kaolin clotting time, dilute Russell viper venom time, dilute prothrombin time, Textarin time.
(b) Failure to correct the prolonged coagulation time on the screening test by mixing with normal platelet-poor plasma.
(c) Shortening or correction of the prolonged coagulation time on the screening test by the addition of excess phospholipid.
(d) Exclusion of other coagulopathies, e.g., factor VIII inhibitor or heparin, as appropriate.
Definite antiphospholipid antibody syndrome is considered to be present if at least one of the clinical criteria and one of the laboratory criteria are met.

*No exclusions other than those contained within the above criteria are needed. However, because of the likelihood that thrombosis may be multifactorial in patients with the antiphospholipid antibody syndrome, the workshop participants recommend that (a) patient populations being studied should be assessed for other contributing causes of thrombosis, and (b) such populations should be stratified according to identifiable or probable risk factors (e.g., age or comorbidities). Specific limits were not placed on the interval between the clinical event and the positive laboratory findings. However, it was the view of many at the workshop that (a) information about such intervals should be assessed when relevant, and (b) the relatively strict definition of laboratory criteria (including the requirement that results again be positive on repeat tests performed at least 6 weeks after the initial test) would help to exclude antiphospholipid antibody positivity that represents an epiphenomenon to the clinical events.
†These criteria were mainly developed by Branch and Silver.
Reproduced with permission from Wilson, W.A. (2001) Rheumatic Diseases Clinics of North America, 27, 499–505.

There is a growing body of literature documenting systemic vasculitis in patients with antiphospholipid and anticardiolipin antibodies, including Takayasu arteritis, giant cell arteritis, polyarteritis nodosa, and granulomatosis with polyangiitis.[20–26] A patient with Degos disease and anticardiolipin antibodies has also been described.[27]

Antiphospholipid syndrome in association with carcinomas arising in lung, ovary, gastrointestinal tract, kidney, liver, and breast, and one pediatric case of Ewing sarcoma have been reported .[28–34]

The syndrome has been reported in patients infected with the HIV.[35–37] Some HIV-infected patients have antiphospholipid antibodies without clinical features of the antiphospholipid syndrome.[35]

Pathogenesis and histologic features

The precise pathogenesis is not well understood. Theories include inhibition of protein C (a natural vitamin K-dependent anticoagulant) function and a suppressive effect on endothelial cell prostacyclin.[38] The role of anti-beta-2 glycoprotein antibodies appears central to the pathogenesis of antiphospholipid antibody syndrome.[8] Normally, the beta-2 glycoprotein has antithrombotic properties. Some antiphospholipid antibodies bind to beta-2 glycoprotein 1, which can lead to inhibition of factor XII and platelet activation and also decrease prothrombinase activity. Studies have shown that antiphospholipid antibodies can activate endothelial cells and platelets, possibly playing a thrombogenic role.[8] The autoantibodies appear to interact with the immune system in a complex fashion by activating dendritic cells, monocytes, and neutrophils and affecting T-cell homeostasis.[8]

Patients with the antiphospholipid antibody are predisposed to thrombosis and have prolonged partial thromboplastin and kaolin clotting times; however, it is important to note that not all patients with the antiphospholipid antibody develop thrombosis. In one study, 28% of lupus patients with antiphospholipid antibodies had no evidence of antiphospholipid antibody syndrome.[39]

Biopsy shows features of a thrombotic vasculopathy, i.e., vascular occlusion of arterioles and arteries with a fibrinoid plug, which may be associated with variable numbers of intraluminal inflammatory cells. Generally, there is minimal or no inflammation of the blood vessel wall or surrounding tissue. Marked dermal necrosis is sometimes a feature. It should be noted that false-negative biopsies may occur.[12] Therefore a negative biopsy does not exclude underlying disease.

Differential diagnosis

The biopsy findings are non-specific and the differential diagnosis includes other forms of thrombotic vasculopathy. Serological studies are required to evaluate for antiphospholipid and anticardiolipin antibodies as well as to evaluate for underlying associated disorders.

Thrombotic thrombocytopenic purpura and hemolytic uremic syndrome

Clinical features

TTP and HUS are related disorders that are due to nonimmune thrombocytopenia.[1–5] TTP is a very rare disease of unknown etiology associated with high morbidity and mortality.[6,7] It shows a predilection for females (2.5:1) and tends to affect younger age groups, with a peak incidence in the third decade. In its fully developed form it consists of thrombocytopenic purpura, microangiopathic hemolytic anemia, neurological symptoms, renal involvement, and fever.

HUS is similar to TTP except that it includes severe renal involvement and milder CNS symptomatology.[8] However, precise classification into one or the other category is sometimes difficult; therefore these related disorders are discussed together.[5,9,10] HUS is often seen in patients with infectious colitis.[5,11,12]

The most common presenting symptoms are transient and usually recurrent neurological complaints including headaches, confusion, pareses, dysphasia, and aphasia. Renal involvement includes hematuria, proteinuria, and occasionally acute renal failure. Cardiac involvement is important and may precipitate left ventricular failure with resultant pulmonary congestion and edema. The hemorrhagic tendency is manifest predominantly in the skin as petechiae, purpura, and ecchymoses, but hemorrhage may also be seen in the retina, conjunctiva, and mucous membranes, including those of the gastrointestinal tract (*Fig. 16.127*).

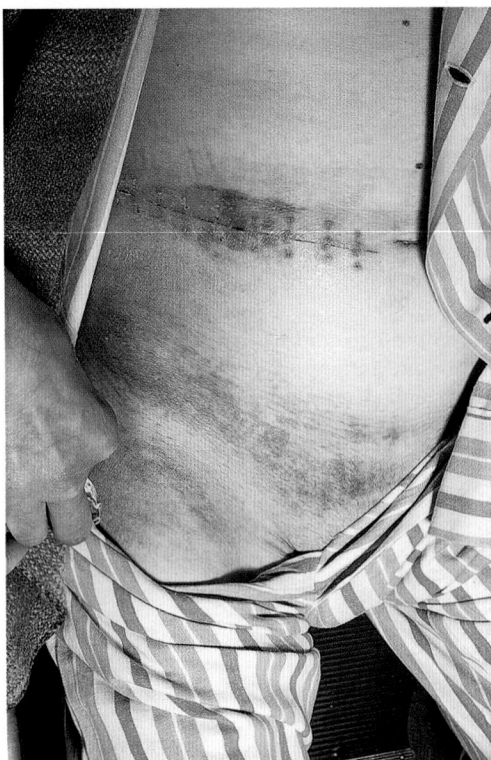

Fig. 16.127
Thrombotic thrombocytopenic purpura: sheeted ecchymoses are present in the groin. By courtesy of N. Slater, MD, St Thomas' Hospital, London, UK.

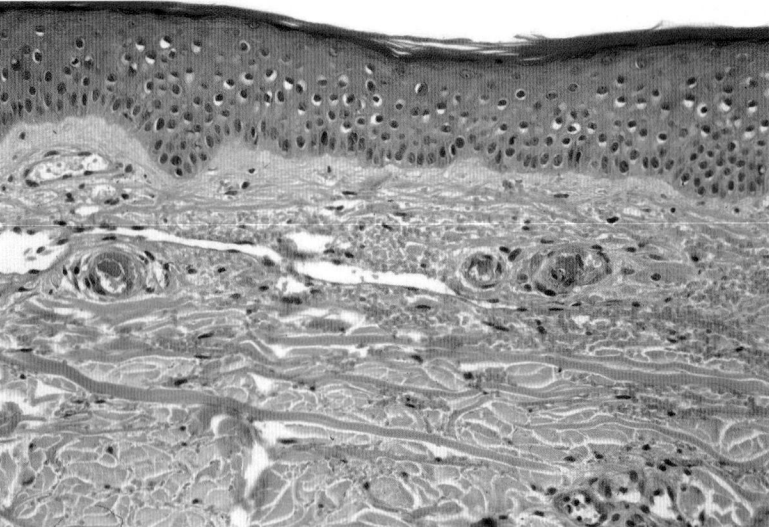

Fig. 16.128
Thrombotic thrombocytopenic purpura: microthrombi are present and there is extensive red cell extravasation.

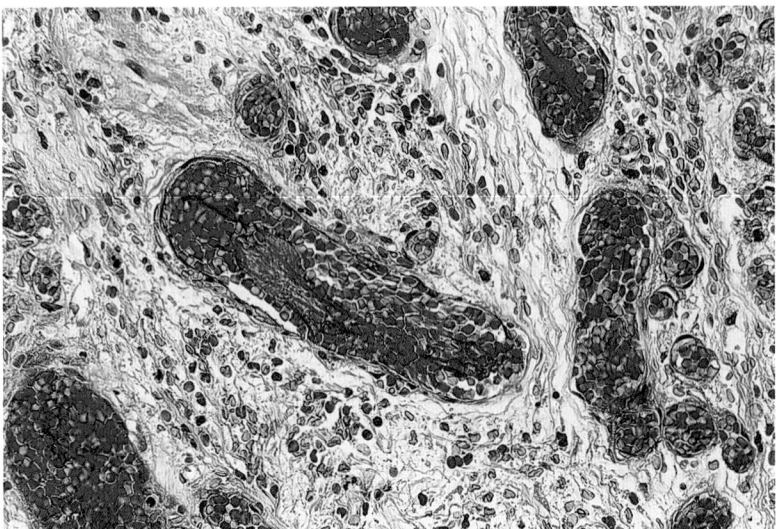

Fig. 16.129
Thrombotic thrombocytopenic purpura: the occlusions contain abundant fibrin (Martius scarlet blue).

TTP/HUS can be associated with connective tissue disease (especially lupus erythematosus), contraceptive use, neoplasia, chemotherapy, adverse drug reaction, bone marrow transplantation, and antiphospholipid antibodies.[4,8,13-19]

Although most patients develop TTP for no apparent reason, it occasionally complicates drug therapy with, for example, penicillin or sulfonamides, or may develop after an upper respiratory tract infection. Quite a high proportion of patients with TTP are pregnant, but the significance of this is uncertain. Familial cases of TTP/HUS, with both autosomal dominant and recessive patterns of inheritance, have been described.[8]

Laboratory investigations reveal gross thrombocytopenia and normochromic, normocytic anemia. Examination of peripheral blood smears commonly demonstrates fragmented and misshapen red blood cells, typically schistocytes and helmet cells. Coagulation studies are usually normal or minimally disturbed with occasionally elevated fibrinogen-fibrin degradation products. The Coombs test is consistently negative.

Pathogenesis and histologic features

The pathogenesis of TTP/HUS is poorly understood. It appears that platelet activating substances result in thrombus formation without activation of the coagulation cascade (hence the normal coagulation studies). Direct endothelial injury could also play a role in this group of disorders.

TTP has been shown to be associated with deficiency of von Willebrand factor-cleaving metalloprotease, ADAMTS13 (a disintegrin and metalloprotease with thrombospondin 1 repeats-13).[5,20-24] Most cases in adulthood are acquired and caused by autoantibodies inhibiting the function of ADAMTS13.[5,23-25] Familial cases of TTP are due to mutations in ADMATS13, resulting in constitutional absence of this enzyme.[5,20,23,24] HUS is often seen in patients with colitis associated with verotoxin-producing *E. coli*.[1,5,26] In one study, 80% of patients with HUS had positive *E. coli* O157 lipopolysaccharide antibody titers.[11] Investigators have shown that verotoxin enhances platelet adhesion and thrombogenesis using a microvascular endothelial cell line.[27] A minority of patients with HUS have been shown to have mutation in the gene coding for factor H, an alternative complement pathway regulatory protein.[28]

The histologic features of TTP are those of hyaline intravascular thrombi composed of aggregates of platelets in addition to a variable amount of fibrin (*Figs 16.128* and *16.129*).[29] They are associated with extravasated red blood cells, but there is no evidence of vasculitis. There may be foci of necrosis, but true infarcts are uncommon. At autopsy the organs most severely involved include the pancreas, adrenal glands, heart, brain, and kidney.

Differential diagnosis

Distinction from other thrombotic vasculopathies requires clinicopathological correlation. In contrast to DIC, coagulation studies (prothrombin time, partial thromboplastin time) tend to be normal in patients with TTP/HUS.

Immune thrombocytopenic purpura

Clinical features

Immune thrombocytopenic purpura (idiopathic thrombocytopenic purpura, ITP) is a rare disease, of which two forms – acute and chronic – are recognized:

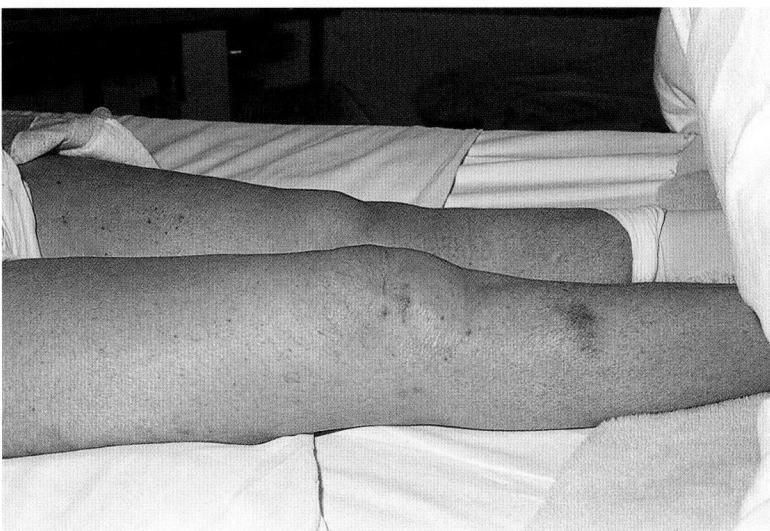

Fig. 16.130
Idiopathic thrombocytopenic purpura: these legs show purpura, petechiae, and bruising. By courtesy of N. Slater, MD, St Thomas' Hospital, London, UK.

- Acute ITP is a disorder that characteristically affects children following a viral illness.[1] Patients present with petechiae, purpura, and bleeding. Most cases are self-limiting with the majority of patients recovering within weeks to months.[2,3] A rare but serious complication is intracranial hemorrhage.
- Chronic ITP is the term used when the disorder persists for 6 months or longer.[2] The chronic form tends to affect adults and is associated with connective tissue diseases such as lupus erythematosus or lymphoproliferative disorders.

Thrombocytopenic purpura has also been described in patients with thyroid disorders, including Graves disease and Hashimoto thyroiditis.[4,5] The condition may occur in association with multiple concurrent autoimmune diseases, such as diabetes mellitus, pernicious anemia, and systemic sclerosis.[6] Some patients have had associated antiphospholipid antibody syndrome.[7–9] Patients with H. pylori infection or those infected with the HIV may also develop immune thrombocytopenia.[10–14]

ITP has rarely been associated with vaccinations in children.[15–16]

The chronic form shows a predilection for women, and presents with a tendency to bruise easily following mild trauma and bleeding (Fig. 16.130). In severely affected patients, lesions develop in the mucous membranes of the respiratory, genitourinary, and gastrointestinal systems in addition to the integument.

Laboratory examination reveals thrombocytopenia and a prolonged bleeding time. Partial thromboplastin time and prothrombin time are not affected.

Pathogenesis and histologic features

Immune thrombocytopenic purpura is an autoimmune disease caused by IgG antiplatelet antibodies, which lead to destruction of platelets.[17–20] There is also a disruption of cellular immunity with a shift toward a type 1 and Th17 immune response.[20] A cytotoxic T-cell-mediated process has also been implicated in platelet destruction.[21] Molecular mimicry between HIV glycoproteins (GP120/160) and membrane antigens (i.e., glycoprotein GPIIb/IIIa) on platelets may play a role in the development of thrombocytopenia in occasional HIV-infected patients.[17,19,22,23]

The cutaneous (and other) lesions are characterized by perivascular hemorrhage; there is no evidence of vasculitis (Fig. 16.131). Bone marrow examination reveals increased numbers of rather immature megakaryocytes. The spleen is congested and shows reactive follicular hyperplasia and sometimes conspicuous megakaryocytes.

Differential diagnosis

Biopsy findings are entirely non-specific. Serological and clinical correlation is necessary to arrive at a diagnosis.

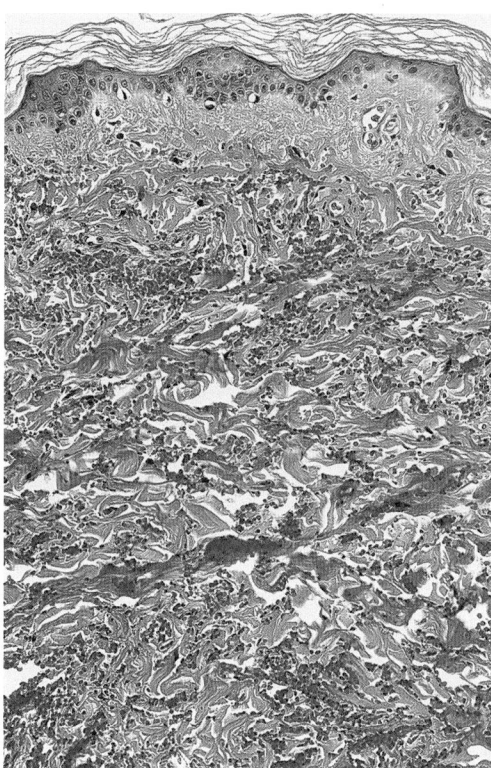

Fig. 16.131
Idiopathic thrombocytopenic purpura: there is hemorrhage but no evidence of vasculitis is seen.

Factor V (Leiden) mutation

Clinical features

Mutation of factor V Leiden is the most common inherited condition predisposing to thrombosis.[1] The mutation is associated with a prothrombotic state caused by factor V resistance to inactivation by protein C. It can be identified by PCR.

Patients with this mutation are at particular risk of deep venous thrombosis and may also develop pulmonary embolism, stroke, and peripheral vascular disease.[2] Women with recurrent miscarriage have an increased incidence of this condition.[3,4] Among patients with no known explanation for deep venous thrombosis, factor V Leiden mutation is a common cause. Patients may also develop skin ulcers.

Histologic features

Biopsy of skin lesions shows features of thrombotic vasculopathy.[5,6] IgM and C3 deposition has been demonstrated by immunofluorescence staining.[5]

Hypergammaglobulinemic purpura

Clinical features

Hypergammaglobulinemic purpura (of Waldenström) is a rare disorder that shows a marked female predilection and tends to affect the young and middle aged.[1] Patients present with recurrent, symmetrical crops of purpura, particularly affecting the lower limbs although the arms and abdomen may also be involved (Fig. 16.132).[2] Wearing tight-fitting garments, heat, and strenuous exercise may provoke lesions. The frequency of attacks is highly variable, ranging from several times a week to as infrequent as a single episode per year.[3,4]

The clinical findings are those of petechiae measuring from pinhead size up to several millimeters. Various symptoms may be experienced, including tingling, itching, burning, and pain. The petechiae resolve over the course of a few days to leave hyperpigmented macules. The purpuric attacks are

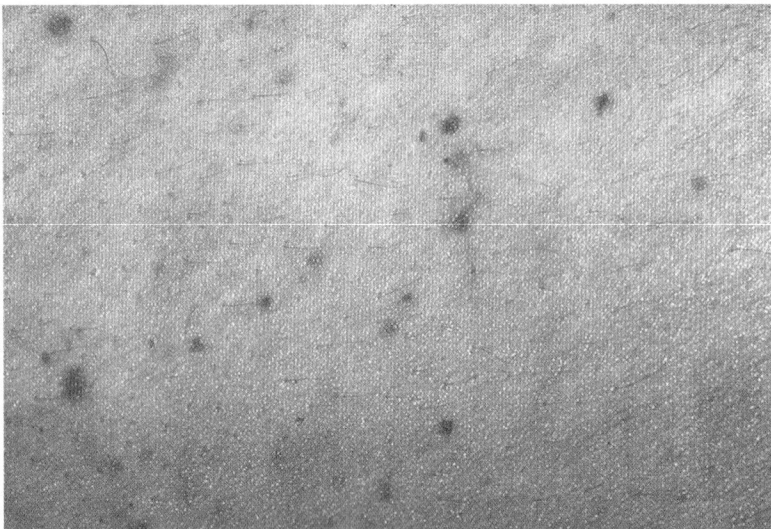

Fig. 16.132
Hypergammaglobulinemic purpura: scattered, tiny, purpuric lesions. By courtesy of J. Newton-Bishop, MD, St Thomas' Hospital, London, UK.

recurrent and tend to great chronicity. Ecchymoses are not a feature.[1] Some cases clinically resemble Schamberg purpura.[5]

Laboratory investigations usually reveal a raised ESR, mild anemia and leukopenia, and polyclonal hypergammaglobulinemia (usually IgG, but sometimes IgM or IgA). Antinuclear antibodies, anti-Ro, anti-La, and rheumatoid factor are present in many patients.[1,3,6–8] Platelet levels, coagulation studies, and bone marrow examination are typically normal. Cryoglobulinemia is an occasional feature. There are no known HLA associations and family history is negative.[1] Lymphadenopathy and splenomegaly are sometimes a feature.[1]

It is important to note that hypergammaglobulinemic purpura may be classified into two categories: idiopathic (Waldenström; not to be confused with Waldenström macroglobulinemia) and secondary. In the latter group, patients have a wide variety of conditions, including SLE, polymyositis, Hashimoto thyroiditis, Sjögren syndrome, rheumatoid arthritis, hepatitis, chronic lymphocytic leukemia, monoclonal gammopathies, sarcoidosis, and recurrent infections.[1,9–12] The purpura may precede the associated illness for many years. Patients with this disorder, therefore, merit a careful and prolonged follow-up.

Pathogenesis and histologic features

Direct immunofluorescence examination of skin lesions reveals IgM and C3 in blood vessel walls.[13] Perivascular deposits of IgG and C5b-9 have also been reported.[8] Circulating immune complexes, with both IgG and IgM, have also been demonstrated in patients with this disorder.[14] It is likely, therefore, that hypergammaglobulinemic purpura is another variant of immune complex-mediated vasculitis, namely, a type III hypersensitivity reaction. The precise etiology, however, remains poorly understood.

Histologic examination of the purpuric lesions may reveal the typical features of acute leukocytoclastic vasculitis with red cell extravasation.[15] Occasionally, however, lymphocytic perivasculitis and hemorrhage is all that is evident, possibly reflecting the result of the timing of the biopsy.[8]

Differential diagnosis

The histologic changes are not specific and other causes of leukocytoclastic vasculitis must be considered.

Hyperimmunoglobulinemia D syndrome/mevalonate kinase deficiency

Clinical features

Hyperimmunoglobulinemia D syndrome is a rare autosomal recessive disease due to mutations in the *MVK* gene, a key enzyme located on chromosome 12 and involved in the biosynthesis of cholesterol and isoprenoid.[1,2]

The disease is most common in Europe and presents in childhood as recurrent episodes of high fever lasting for 3–7 days. Vaccinations and minor infections may be inciting events. Fever attacks are accompanied by abdominal symptoms, headaches, generalized lymphadenopathy, and arthralgias of large joints.[3–6] Amyloidosis is a rare complication.[3] Cutaneous manifestations include erythematous macules, papules, and nodules as well as urticarial lesions.[7] Elevated IgD levels can be demonstrated in the majority of patients.[3]

Pathogenesis and histologic features

The genetic defect results in inactivation of mevalonate kinase (MVK). The downstream effect is to increase production of IL-1 cytokines, resulting in a proinflammatory state.[5,8,9] Skin biopsy findings are variable and most frequently show a mild acute vasculitis. Rarely, the features are reminiscent of Sweet syndrome, cellulitis, or erythema elevatum diutinum.[4,7,10,11] Squamous syringometaplasia has also been reported.[11]

Superficial thrombophlebitis

Clinical features

Superficial thrombophlebitis is a common disease presenting as painful, erythematous, thickened areas with a cordlike morphology. Most cases involve the lower limbs, particularly below the knees, and there is a predilection for females. Multifocal segmental disease is frequent and recurrent episodes are often seen. The disease is usually associated with hypercoagulable states. Predisposing factors are numerous and include varicose veins, pregnancy, the use of oral contraceptives (particularly those with a higher concentration of estrogen), cancer (mainly breast, colonic, pancreatic, gastric, cholangiocarcinoma, hematological as well as cutaneous), Behçet disease, factor V (Leiden) mutation, essential thrombocythemia, anticardiolipin antibodies, and deficiencies of protein C, protein S, factor XII, antithrombin III, and heparin cofactor 2C.[1–18] Superficial thrombophlebitis developing in association with secondary syphilis has been documented.[19] Superficial suppurative thrombophlebitis occurs mainly in children and it is caused by a wide variety of microorganisms, mainly bacteria (both aerobic and anaerobic) and, less commonly, fungi.[20–24] The most common bacteria isolated include *S. aureus*, *E. coli*, and *P. aeruginosa*.[20,21] *Candida* is by far the most common fungus associated with the disease.

Superficial thrombophlebitis may be associated with deep vein thrombosis but the risk of this happening appears to be small unless there are additional risk factors.[25–28] The chance of a patient with superficial thrombophlebitis developing pulmonary embolism is low, but it has been documented and the risk appears to be greater in patients with disease affecting the thigh.[29,30]

Histologic features

Superficial thrombophlebitis typically involves veins located in the superficial subcutaneous tissue. Early lesions are characterized by an infiltrate predominantly composed of neutrophils obscuring the vessel walls. The neutrophils are progressively replaced by lymphocytes, histiocytes, and occasional giant cells. An organizing thrombus is initially present and this is followed by recanalization and fibrosis. The infiltrate tends to remain localized and there is very little involvement of the surrounding subcutaneous tissue. Arteries are not affected.

Sclerosing lymphangitis

Clinical features

Sclerosing lymphangitis (Mondor disease) is probably a misnomer as it likely represents a variant of superficial thrombophlebitis that most commonly affects the genitalia, chest wall, or breasts. Women with large pendulous breasts seem to be particularly predisposed.[1] In these cases, and in others, trauma probably plays a significant role in development. Some authors have reported an association with breast carcinoma.[2] Intravenous drug abuse may be an occasional cause and sclerosing lymphangitis of the penis has been documented in association with an underlying sexually transmitted disease.[3,4] Nonvenereal sclerosing lymphangitis has also been associated with vigorous sexual activity.[5-8] Sickle cell disease and protein S deficiency are rare associations.[9,10] Patients present with sometimes painful linear cordlike lesions. Typically, lesions are a few centimeters in length but sometimes may be much larger. The overlying skin is erythematous without color change. The disorder is self-limiting and usually resolves in a few weeks.[11] Rarely, persistent disease requires surgical intervention.[12]

Histologic features

The pathology is characterized by organizing thrombus with variable inflammation. One case report highlights negative immunoreactivity for podoplanin in the affected vessels suggesting that Mondor disease is related to vascular thrombosis rather than representing a lymphangitis.[13]

Senile purpura

Clinical features

Senile purpura affects the extensor surfaces of the forearms, hands, and lower legs of the elderly.[1,2] Corticosteroid therapy (topical or systemic) contributes to its development in some patients. Lesions are persistent, lasting 1–3 weeks, and consist of asymptomatic purpuric macules up to several centimeters in diameter, in a background of actinically damaged or atrophic skin (Fig. 16.133). Senile purpura develops because of damage to the connective tissue of the dermis, which fails to support the vasculature, rendering it more susceptible to mild trauma.

Histologic features

The lesions are characterized by red cell extravasation unassociated with any significant inflammatory cell reaction. There is usually marked solar elastosis.

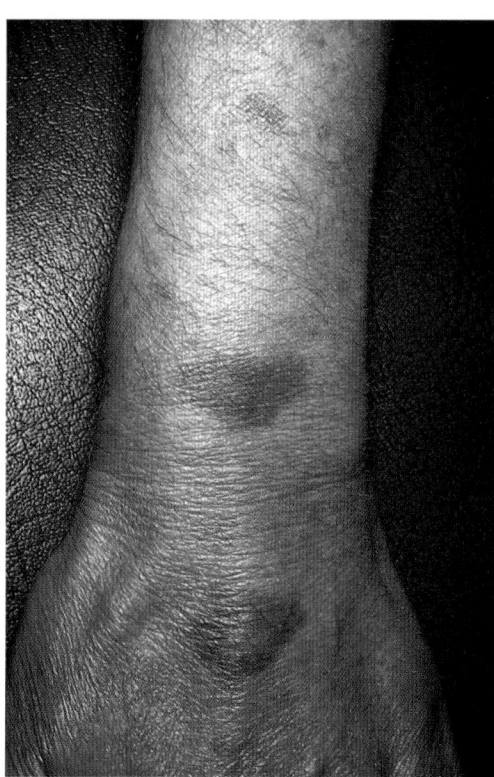

Fig. 16.133
Senile purpura: trauma-induced deep purple ecchymoses on sun-damaged skin. By courtesy of J. Newton-Bishop, MD, St Thomas' Hospital, London, UK.

Cocaine-related retiform purpura

Clinical features

Over the past few years, there has been an epidemic form of vasculitis/vasculopathy related to illicit cocaine use.[1-17] Patients typically present with retiform purpura on extremities and trunk that is temporally related to cocaine use (Fig. 16.134). Involvement of the ears is common and a clue to

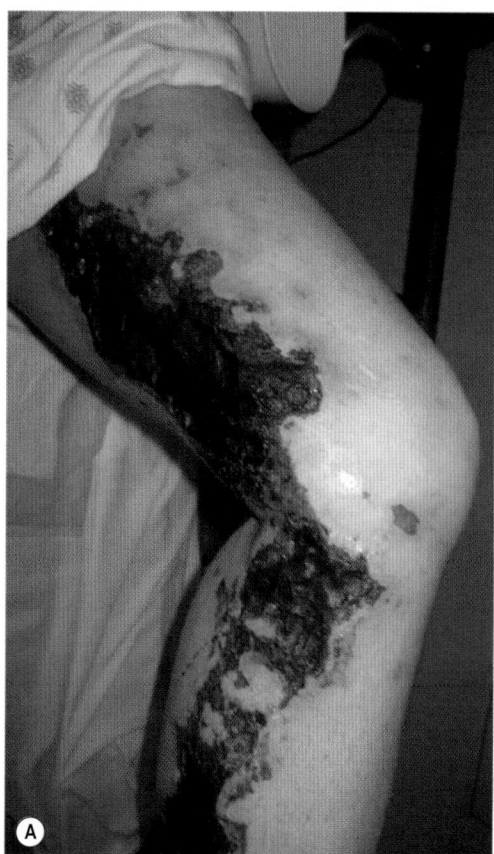

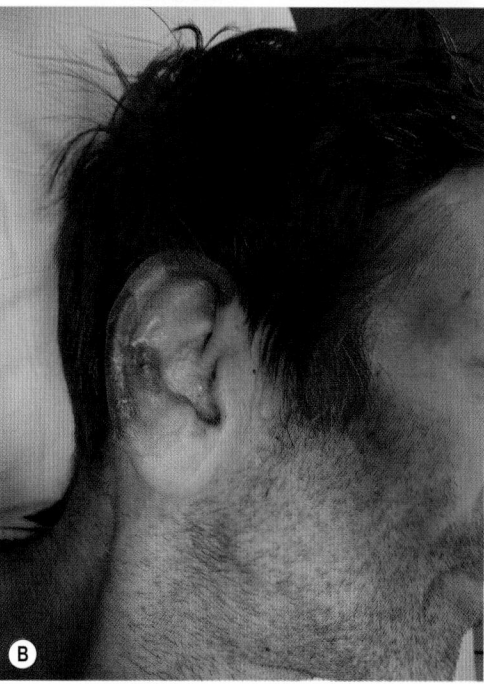

Fig. 16.134
Cocaine-related retiform purpura: (A) retiform purpura with associated epidermal necrosis; (B) this patient had purpuric lesions of the ears. By courtesy of Anthony P. Fernandez, MD, PhD, Cleveland Clinic, Cleveland, USA.

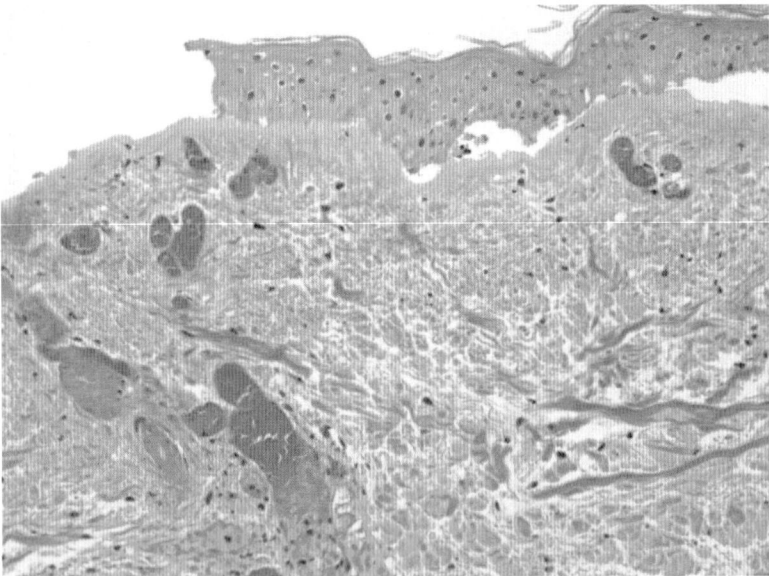

Fig. 16.135
Cocaine-related retiform purpura: in this example the biopsy demonstrated a thrombotic vasculopathy rather than leukocytoclastic vasculitis.

the diagnosis.[6,12,13,15] Patients may also develop glomerulonephritis related to vasculitis.[16,17]

Laboratory studies often uncover neutropenia and ANCAs.[1,2,4,5,7,8,11,13,14] Autoantibodies to human neutrophil elastase appear to be relatively specific for this condition.[1]

Pathogenesis and histologic features

Levamisole has become a common agent used to dilute illegal cocaine, present in approximately 70% tested.[17] While the precise pathogenesis is not understood, neutropenia and vasculitis/vasculopathy, including involvement of the ears, are well-known potential side effects of levamisole, thus explaining the clinical manifestations seen in cocaine users.[18–21] Autoantibodies to human neutrophil elastase may also play a role.[1]

Histologically, biopsies may show predominantly a leukocytoclastic vasculitis, a thrombotic vasculopathy (*Fig. 16.135*) or a combination of both processes affecting superficial and deep dermal vessels.

Differential diagnosis

The differential diagnosis includes the ANCA-vasculitides, especially polyangiitis with granulomatosis, cryoglobulinemia, and thrombotic vasculopathies, such as antiphospholipid antibody syndrome. Correlation with clinical history of cocaine use aids in distinction.

Access **ExpertConsult.com** for the complete list of references

Idiopathic connective tissue disorders

CHAPTER 17

Boštjan Luzar and Eduardo Calonje

Lupus erythematosus

Lupus erythematosus is a complex disorder associated with numerous clinical signs and symptoms and a wide range of laboratory abnormalities. It shows a spectrum of varying prognoses, ranging from a benign, solely cutaneous variant (localized discoid) through to a potentially fatal systemic illness.[1–4] The range of subtypes is shown in *Table 17.1*.

Although the precise etiology is unknown, it is thought that interplay of genetic factors, autoantibodies, immune complexes, hormones, and other factors is responsible for the development of the illness. There is evidence suggesting that the incidence of the systemic variant is increasing, but due to earlier diagnosis and more effective therapy, the mortality rate has significantly diminished and the 10-year overall survival rate in adults now exceeds 90%.[5] The presence of renal and/or neurological involvement, however, remains a poor prognostic indicator.[6]

Pediatric systemic lupus erythematosus (SLE) is an aggressive illness with considerable mortality, largely due to the incidence of renal disease. Even with corticosteroid and immunosuppressive therapy the death rate is as high as 15%.[7]

Clinical features
Discoid lupus erythematosus

Discoid lupus erythematosus (DLE), the commonest form, is subdivided into localized and generalized variants. This is of prognostic importance because only about 1% of patients with localized DLE develop systemic disease, but approximately 5% of those with the generalized form (in particular those with persistent anemia, leukopenia, thrombocytopenia, false-positive Wassermann reaction, and high titer antinuclear factor) develop full-blown SLE.[6,8–10] Discoid lesions develop in up to 20% of patients with systemic lupus.[11] Periungual telangiectasia, sclerodactyly, and the presence of Raynaud phenomenon may also signify potential disease progression.[10] Patients with DLE should not be made unduly worried about the risk of developing systemic involvement, which is not high.

DLE is persistent and affects twice as many females as males. Although any age group may be involved, it is most common in the third, fourth, and fifth decades, with a peak incidence in the late thirties.[12] Presentation in childhood is rare.[13–18] Lesions typically arise on sun-exposed sites and patients frequently experience photosensitivity; there may be spring and summer exacerbation.[5] In the localized form, the head and neck are usually affected, but in the generalized variant, lesions may also be present on the dorsal aspect of the arms, hands, and fingers and on the 'V' of the neck. Nonexposed sites, including the trunk, upper limbs, and the palms and soles, are also commonly involved.[19]

Facial plaques occur most often on the cheeks (*Fig. 17.1*). Other sites affected include the bridge of the nose, the ears, the neck, and the scalp (*Figs 17.2–17.6*). The associated scarring of the scalp is followed by permanent alopecia (*Figs 17.7* and *17.8*). Scalp involvement, which is more common in those patients affected by the disease when they were young, is chronic, and correlates with longstanding severe illness.[20] Ocular involvement mainly encompasses the eyelids, followed by orbit and cornea with blepharitis being the most common symptom.[21]

Early lesions appear edematous and erythematous. An established plaque of DLE, which may measure up to 10 cm across, is usually covered with an adherent scale accompanied by epidermal atrophy, follicular dilatation, and plugging (*Figs 17.9* and *17.10*).[5,19] If the scale is removed the horny plugs are often seen attached to its undersurface ('carpet tacks' sign). Telangiectasia is a common finding and lesions heal with scarring, which is often marked. In dark- or black-skinned individuals the plaque may be hypo- or hyperpigmented and this may be particularly disfiguring (*Figs 17.11–17.14*).[19]

Oral involvement occurs in 20% to 25% of patients with DLE, with the vermilion border of the lower lip, alveolar processes, labial and buccal mucosae being particularly affected (*Figs 17.15–17.17*).[22–27] Chronic lesions are typically erythematous and atrophic with a scalloped white keratotic border and adjacent telangiectasia.[23] Erosions and ulcers are additional features.[12] Lesions are sometimes indistinguishable from atrophic lichen planus. Involvement of the tongue manifests as erythema, fissuring, and atrophy of the papillae.[24] Chronic lupus cheilitis is associated with cicatricial scarring and an increased risk of squamous carcinoma.[23] Genital skin and perianal mucosal involvement has occasionally been documented.[25,28]

DLE has been described in association with osteopoikilosis, α_1-antitrypsin deficiency, polyarteritis nodosa, Addison disease, chronic granulomatous disease, dystrophic calcinosis cutis, allergic contact dermatitis, acquired partial lipoatrophy, as a reaction to tattoo, and in a patient with scleroderma, deep linear morphea, and chronic hepatitis C virus infection.[29–39] Exceptionally, localized DLE has been reported in the area previously affected by herpes zoster and at the site of previous traumatic injury.[40–42]

Systemic symptoms are usually absent in patients with localized DLE.[43] In the generalized form, in which cutaneous plaques may be quite widespread, a small percentage may have Raynaud phenomenon and arthralgia (*Figs 17.23–17.25*). Laboratory abnormalities are more common in the generalized than in the localized variant.[43] Anemia is not seen in localized DLE, but is sometimes a feature of the generalized variant. Leukopenia, a raised erythrocyte sedimentation rate (ESR), and hypergammaglobulinemia can occur in both.[8] Antinuclear factor (diffuse pattern), a positive Wassermann reaction, and rheumatoid factor may also be features.[8] Anti-double-stranded DNA (dsDNA) antibodies are detected in a minority of patients with disseminated DLE, and these patients frequently transform to the systemic disease; occasionally, antibodies to single-stranded DNA (ssDNA) are present. Urinalysis and renal function tests are normal.

Verrucous (hypertrophic) discoid lupus erythematosus

Verrucous (hypertrophic) DLE presents as warty, hyperkeratotic papules and plaques with a predilection for the face, scalp, mucous membranes of

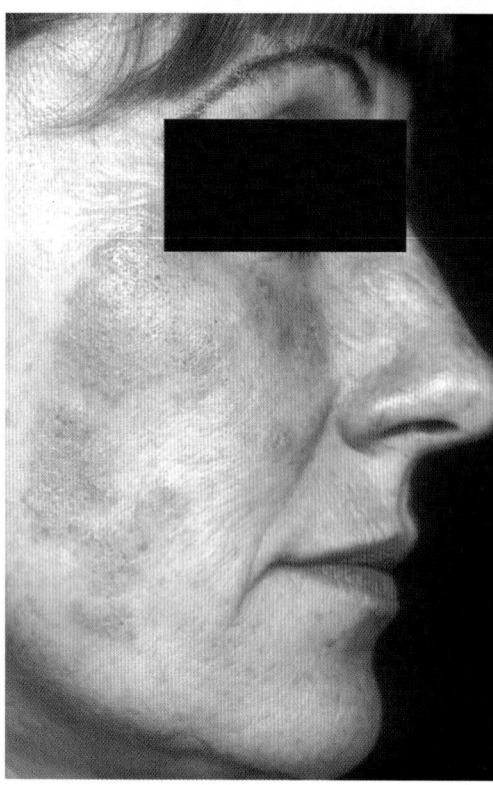

Fig. 17.1
Discoid lupus erythematosus: typical plaques are present on the cheek of a female. Note the erythema and scale. This is a characteristic site. From the collection of the late N.P. Smith, MD, the Institute of Dermatology, London, UK.

Table 17.1
Lupus erythematosus: subtypes

Discoid lupus erythematosus (localized)
Discoid lupus erythematosus (generalized)
Verrucous lupus erythematosus
Chilblain lupus erythematosus
Chronic granulomatous disease with discoid lupus erythematosus-like dermatosis
Lupus erythematosus-erythema multiforme syndrome
Subacute cutaneous lupus erythematosus
Lupus erythematosus profundus
Systemic lupus erythematosus
Drug-induced lupus erythematosus
C_2 deficiency lupus erythematosus-like syndrome
Neonatal lupus erythematosus

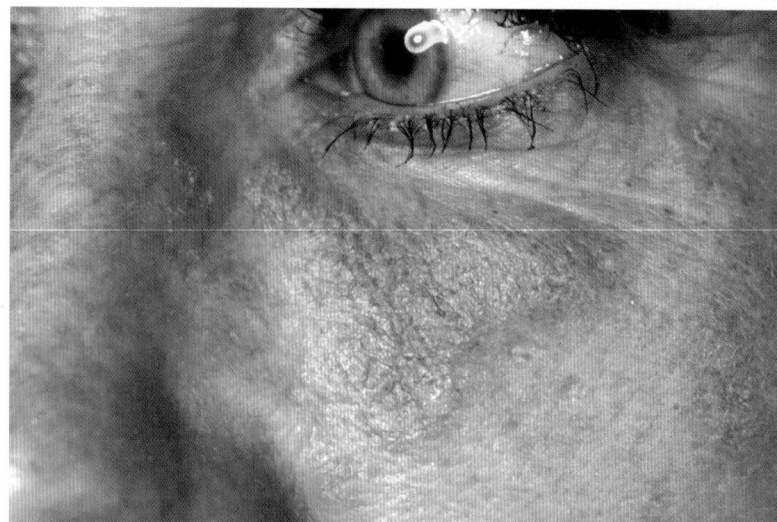

Fig. 17.2
Discoid lupus erythematosus: close-up view showing erythema and scale. From the collection of the late N.P. Smith, MD, the Institute of Dermatology, London, UK.

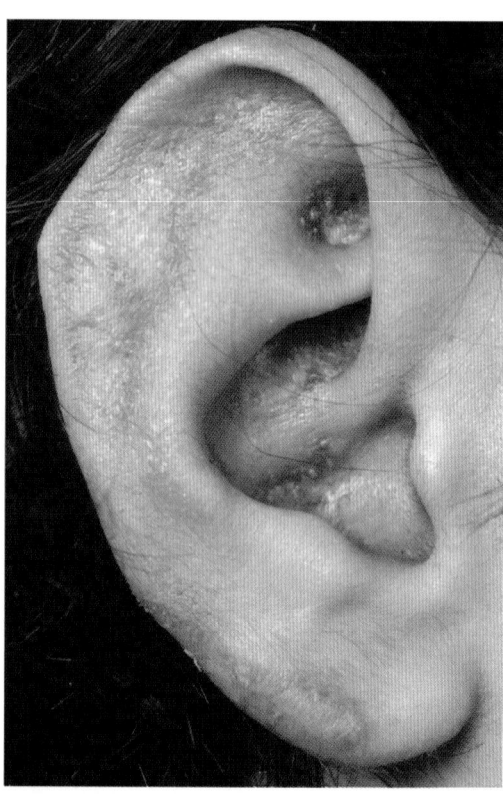

Fig. 17.3
Discoid lupus erythematosus: there is scaling and scarring on the ear lobe, a commonly affected site. From the collection of the late N.P. Smith, MD, the Institute of Dermatology, London, UK.

the lips, and upper limbs (*Figs 17.18* and *17.19*).[5,44–46] It affects approximately 2% of patients with chronic discoid disease.[12] Although verrucous (hypertrophic) hyperkeratotic skin changes have been observed in patients with SLE, such cases are exceptional.[46,47] Sometimes the palms and soles are affected and occasionally the nails (*Figs 17.20* and *17.21*). Rare manifestations include nodular keratoacanthoma-like, squamous cell carcinoma-like, and hypertrophic lichen planus-like lesions on the arms and hands (*Fig. 17.22*).[45,48] A variant with associated necrosis of the subcutaneous tissue is known as lupus erythematosus hypertrophicus et profundus.[49]

Cutaneous squamous cell carcinoma and less often basal cell carcinoma may arise in patients with chronic lesions including the hypertrophic variant.[19,22,45,50–54] Squamous cell carcinoma occurs predominantly in males, particularly affects the scalp, and is sometimes associated with early metastases.[6,55] A case of atypical fibroxanthoma has recently been reported in a scar of DLE.[56]

Lupus erythematosus tumidus

Lupus erythematosus tumidus is a distinctive subset of cutaneous lupus clinically presenting mainly in patients with DLE and rarely in patients with

SLE. It is characterized by erythematous papules, plaques or even nodules with an urticarial appearance arising mainly on sun-exposed skin of the face, neck, and trunk. Scarring does not occur. This variant of lupus is discussed in more detail in Chapter 8.

Chilblain lupus erythematosus

Chilblain lupus erythematosus (CHLE), which accounts for approximately 11% of DLE cases, develops during the winter months or following exposure to cold, wet, and damp conditions.[57,58] Although CHLE appears most frequently in sporadic patients,[59] familial occurrence has recently been reported.[58,60,61] Patients with familial CHLE display mutations in the *TREX1*

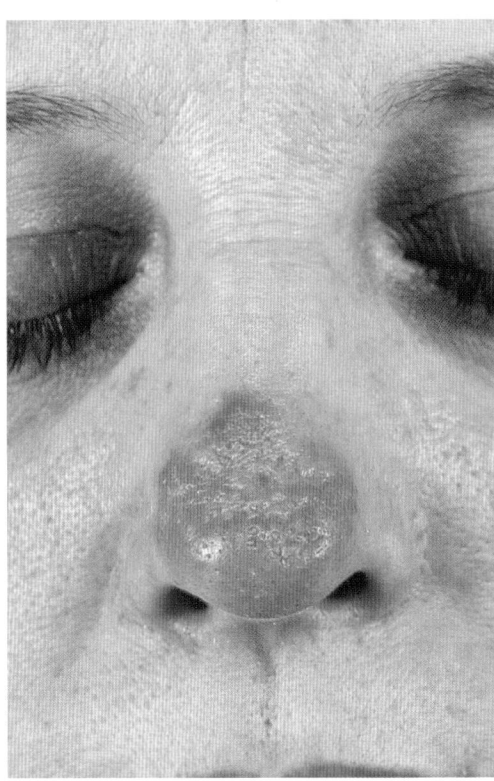

Fig. 17.4
Discoid lupus erythematosus: this severely affected patient shows healed ulceration with marked scarring and disfigurement. By courtesy of the Institute of Dermatology, London, UK.

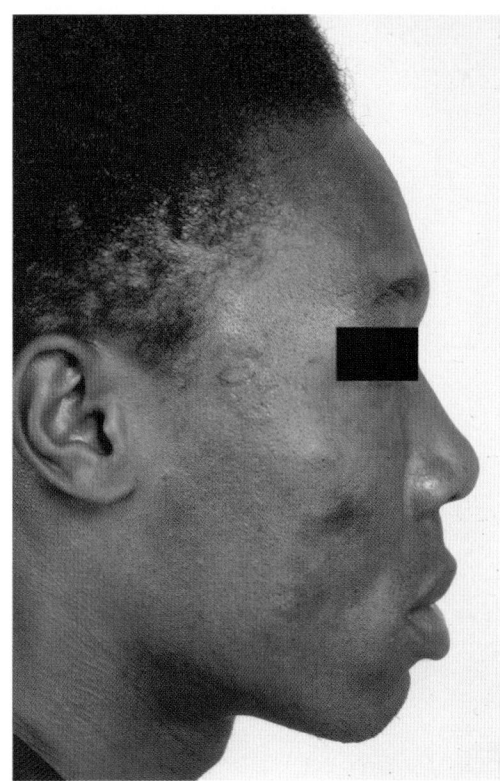

Fig. 17.6
Discoid lupus erythematosus: dark-skinned races are commonly affected. From the collection of the late N.P. Smith, MD, the Institute of Dermatology, London, UK.

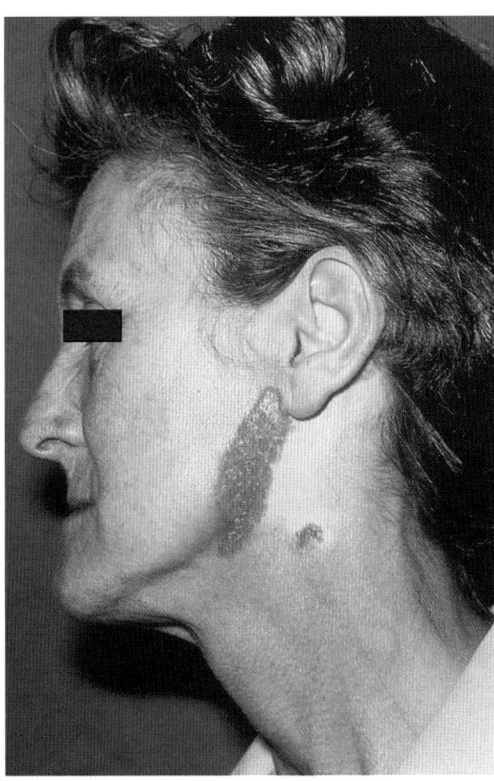

Fig. 17.5
Discoid lupus erythematosus: in this chronic lesion there is marked scarring. By courtesy of R.A. Marsden, MD, St George's Hospital, London, UK.

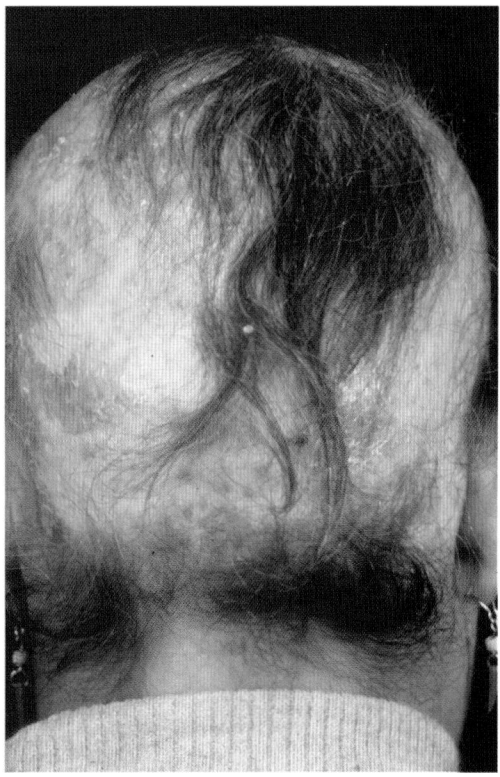

Fig. 17.7
Discoid lupus erythematosus: hair loss is permanent. By courtesy of the Institute of Dermatology, London, UK.

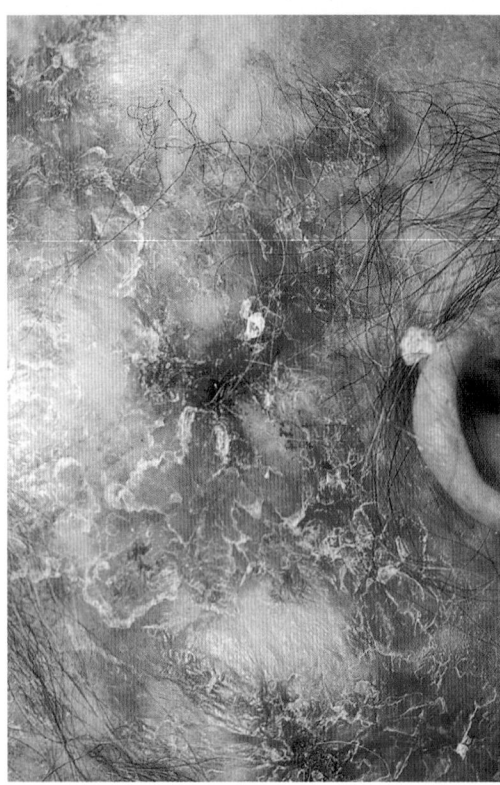

Fig. 17.8
Discoid lupus erythematosus: there is alopecia with very marked scarring. By courtesy of the Institute of Dermatology, London, UK.

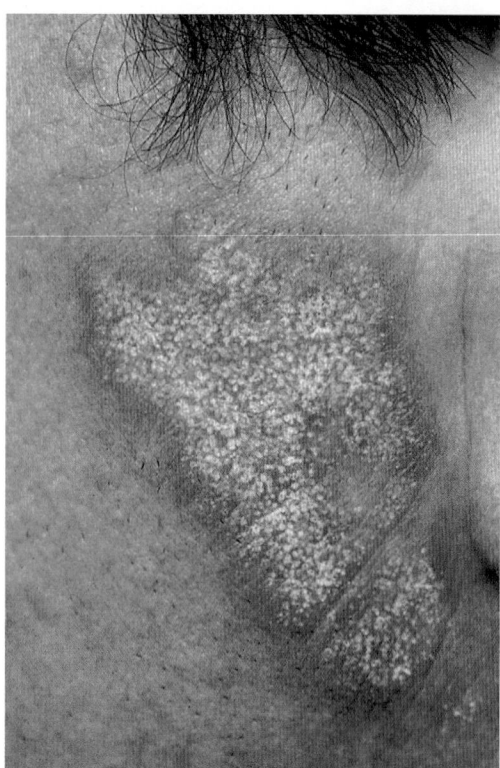

Fig. 17.10
Discoid lupus erythematosus: close-up view showing follicular plugging. By courtesy of the Institute of Dermatology, London, UK.

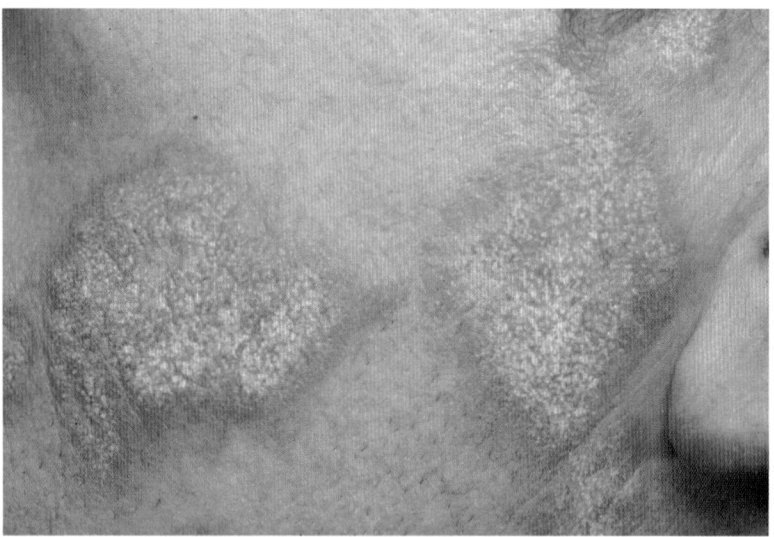

Fig. 17.9
Discoid lupus erythematosus: close-up view of scale. Note the erythematous border. By courtesy of the Institute of Dermatology, London, UK.

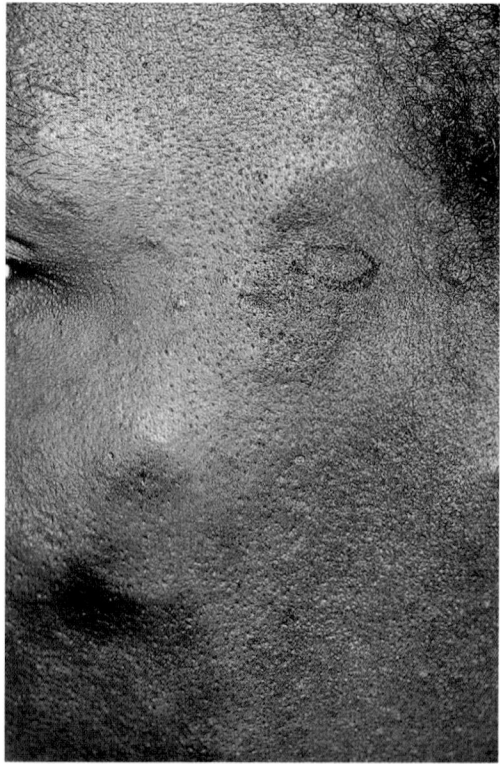

Fig. 17.11
Discoid lupus erythematosus: foci of hyperpigmentation can be very disfiguring in dark-skinned patients. By courtesy of the Institute of Dermatology, London, UK.

gene located on chromosome 3p, encoding a DNA-specific 3′-5′ exonuclease 1.[58,60–67] In addition, a mutation in *SAMHD1* (SAM domain and HD domain-containing protein 1), a deoxynucleotide-degrading phosphohydrolase, has been reported in a single family.[68] Autosomal dominant inheritance has been demonstrated in these patients.[58,60,61] While familial CHLE generally presents in early childhood, sporadic CHLE usually affects middle-aged females.[57,58,60,69] Patients develop itchy, painful, papuloerythematous or blue-purple plaques and nodules on the fingers, heels, and soles of the feet; the hands, calves, knees, knuckles, elbows, nose, and ears are less often affected (*Fig. 17.26*).[6] Hyperkeratotic fissured lesions and ulcers are sometimes also present.[69] CHLE may present with depigmentation mimicking vitiligo.[70] Although patients usually develop chilblains many years after the typical discoid rash, lesions may develop simultaneously and sometimes the chilblains are the sole manifestation.[59] Some patients with sporadic CHLE have an associated cryofibrinogenemia or cold agglutinin.[6] About 20% of patients with sporadic CHLE develop SLE, particularly those who develop discoid and perniotic lesions simultaneously and those with DLE-erythema multiforme-like syndrome in addition to perniosis.[6,57,59] None with the familial CHLE have progressed to SLE.[59]

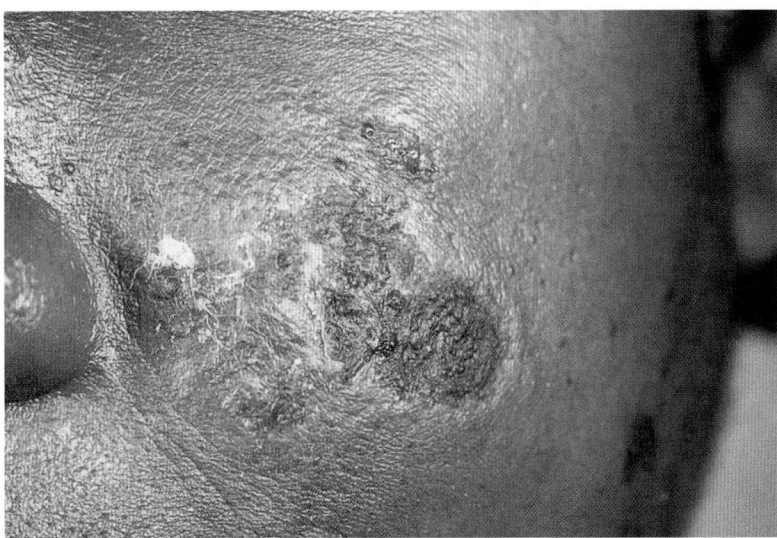

Fig. 17.12
Discoid lupus erythematosus: close-up view. By courtesy of R.A. Marsden, MD, St George's Hospital, London, UK.

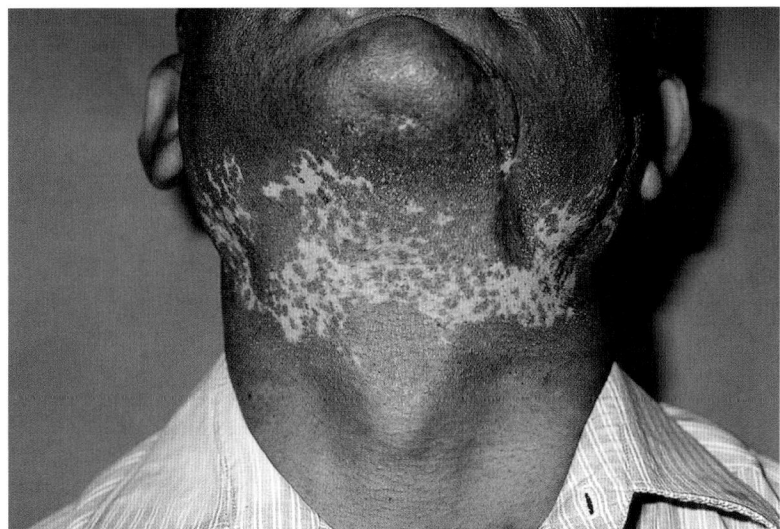

Fig. 17.13
Discoid lupus erythematosus: marked hypopigmentation may be a distressing complication. By courtesy of R.A. Marsden, MD, St George's Hospital, London, UK.

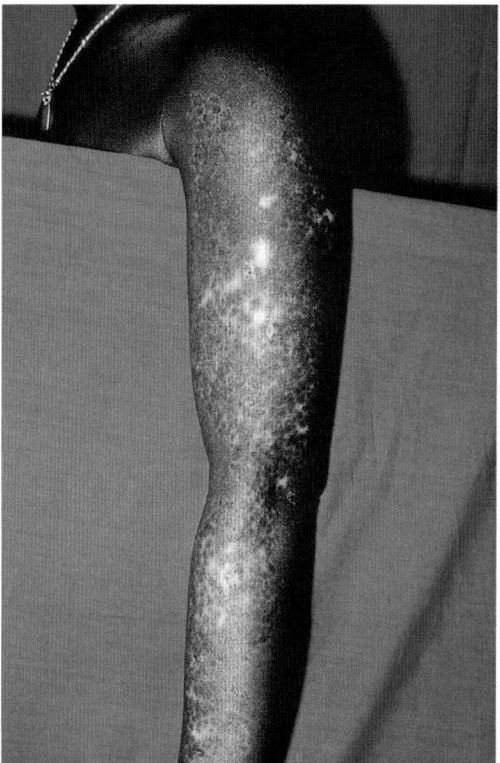

Fig. 17.14
Discoid lupus erythematosus: in this patient, the arm is severely affected. By courtesy of R.A. Marsden, MD, St George's Hospital, London, UK.

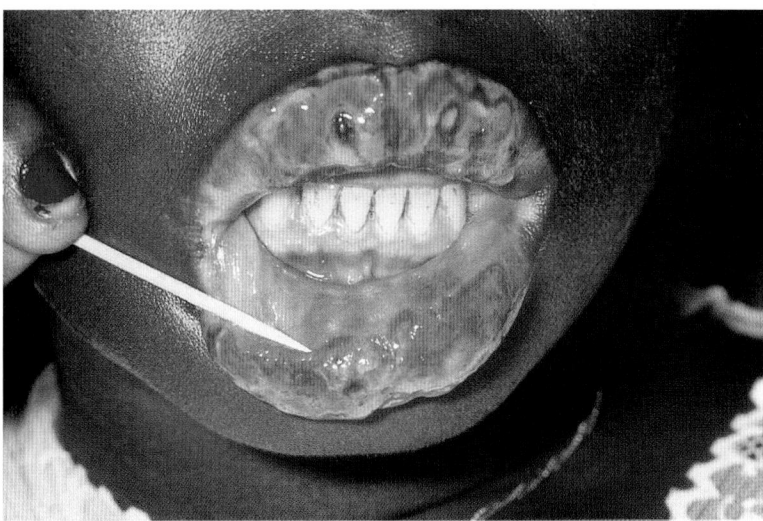

Fig. 17.15
Discoid lupus erythematosus: there is gross ulcerative cheilitis. The upper lip has been stained with gentian violet. By courtesy of R.A. Marsden, MD, St George's Hospital, London, UK.

Lupus erythematosus-erythema multiforme-like syndrome

The lupus erythematosus-erythema multiforme-like syndrome (Rowell syndrome) is rare.[71-77] Patients, mostly middle-aged women, develop recurrent episodes of annular lesions on the limbs and, to a lesser extent, on the face, neck, chest, and mouth, in addition to the features of any variant of lupus erythematosus.[6,71,78-80] Involvement of palms and soles is exceptional.[81] Early lesions are erythematous papules, which become annular and may vesiculate at the edge. The condition usually heals without scarring, but in severe disease bullae may develop, become necrotic, and ulcerate. Patients with this variant also have erythrocyanosis, chilblains, and Raynaud phenomenon. It has been suggested that Rowell syndrome and toxic epidermal necrolysis-like skin lesions with SLE represent different ends of the same illness spectrum, with most of the latter examples being induced by drugs.[82] The serum of patients with lupus erythematosus-erythema multiforme-like syndrome contains speckled antinuclear factor (the most consistent feature, present in 88% of the patients), rheumatoid factor, and anti-Ro/La antibody.[6,8,71,73] In rare cases, anti-Ro/La and rheumatoid factor are negative.[83] Association with antiphospholipid syndrome has exceptionally been documented.[84,85]

Lupus erythematosus profundus

Lupus erythematosus profundus (panniculitis) is another uncommon variant that may develop in association with either DLE or SLE. This is discussed in detail in Chapter 10.

DLE and chronic granulomatous disease

Occasionally, a DLE-like dermatosis develops in female carriers of X-linked chronic granulomatous disease.[86-90] Mothers of affected children may occasionally show similar lesions, presenting with bluish-red, infiltrated, scaly papules on the face and hands, sometimes associated with photosensitivity.[87] Additional features include recurrent aphthous-like ulcerative stomatitis and perniosis.

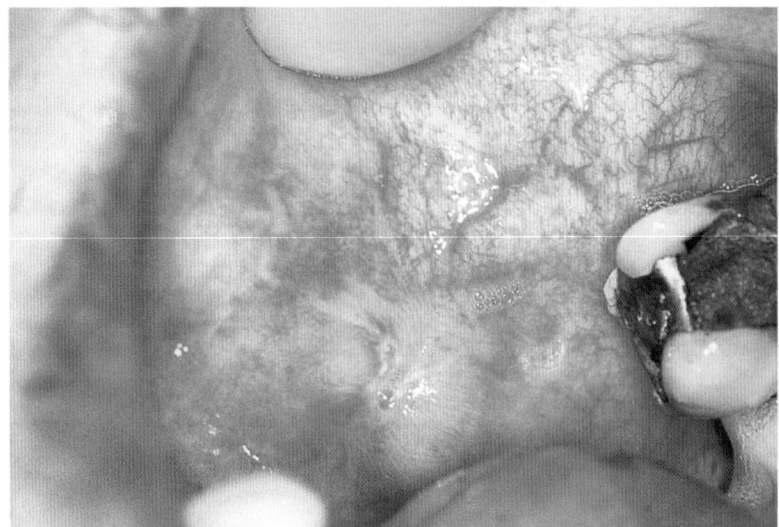

Fig. 17.16
Discoid lupus erythematosus: typical scarred lesion on the buccal mucosa. By courtesy of R.A. Marsden, St George's Hospital, London, UK.

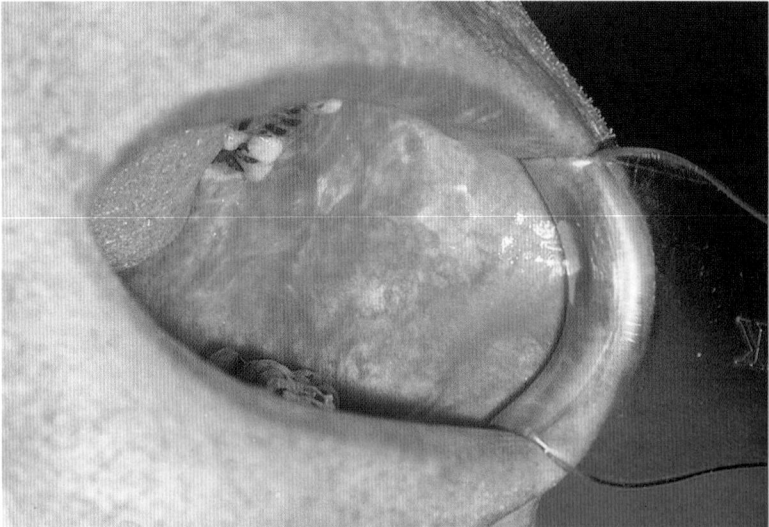

Fig. 17.17
Discoid lupus erythematosus: oral involvement is sometimes difficult to distinguish from lichen planus. By courtesy of the Institute of Dermatology, London, UK.

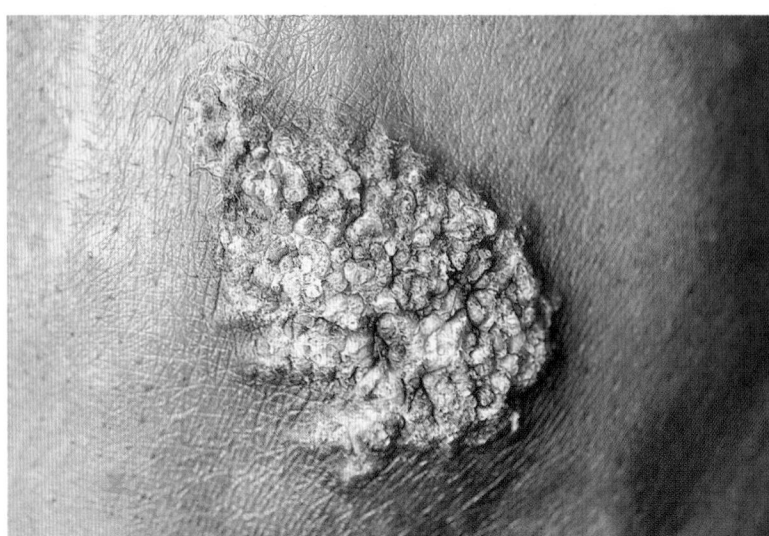

Fig. 17.18
Verrucous discoid lupus erythematosus: this lesion has a very warty appearance. By courtesy of the Institute of Dermatology, London, UK.

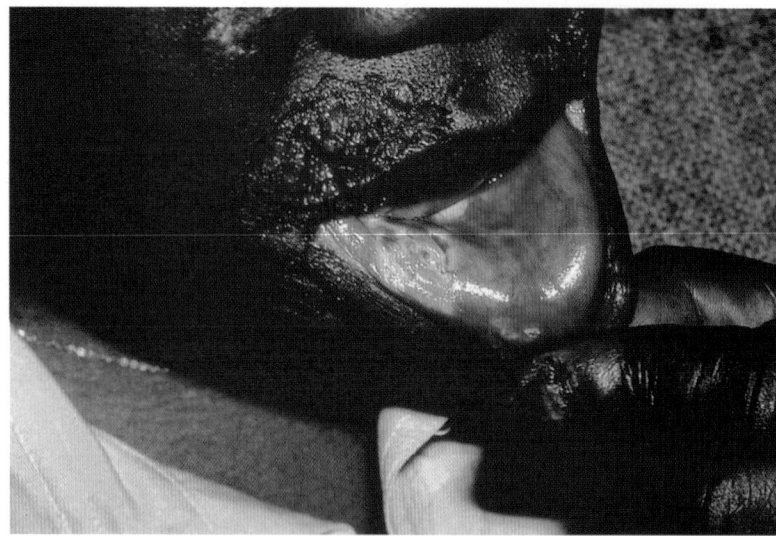

Fig. 17.19
Verrucous discoid lupus erythematosus: extensive disfiguring warty plaque involving the upper lip and angle of mouth. By courtesy of J. Newton Bishop, MD, St James's University Hospital, Leeds, UK.

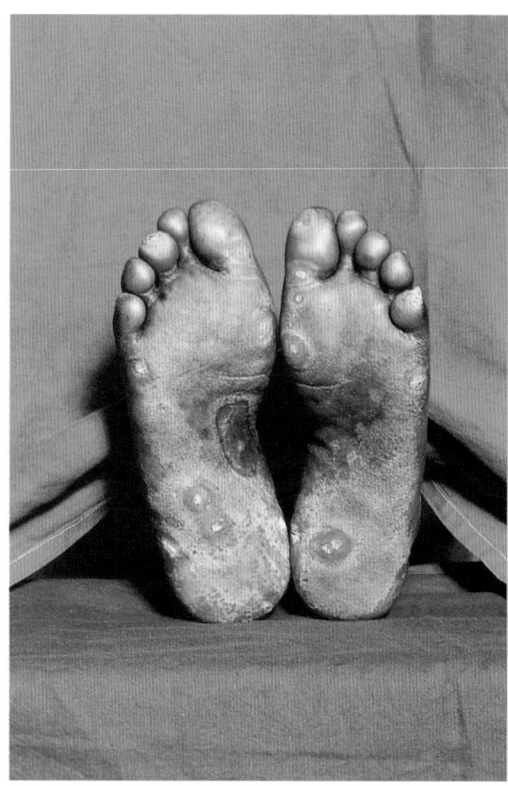

Fig. 17.20
Verrucous discoid lupus erythematosus: note the gross hyperkeratosis. By courtesy of J. Newton Bishop, MD, St James's University Hospital, Leeds, UK.

X-linked chronic granulomatous disease is inherited as a recessive trait, and patients (usually boys) have severe and recurrent infections due to defective neutrophil bactericidal activity. Heterozygous female carriers display a partial defect, indicated by diminished nitroblue tetrazolium reductions, but are usually free from infections. An autosomal recessive variant in which discoid lupus-like lesions may occur has also been documented.[91] DLE lesions have been reported in both carriers and chronic granulomatous disease patients; however, development of SLE in chronic granulomatous disease patients is extremely rare.[92–96] Subacute cutaneous lupus erythematosus-like lesions and lupus tumidus may also occur.[97,98] DLE has also been described in non-X-linked hyper-IgM syndrome.[99]

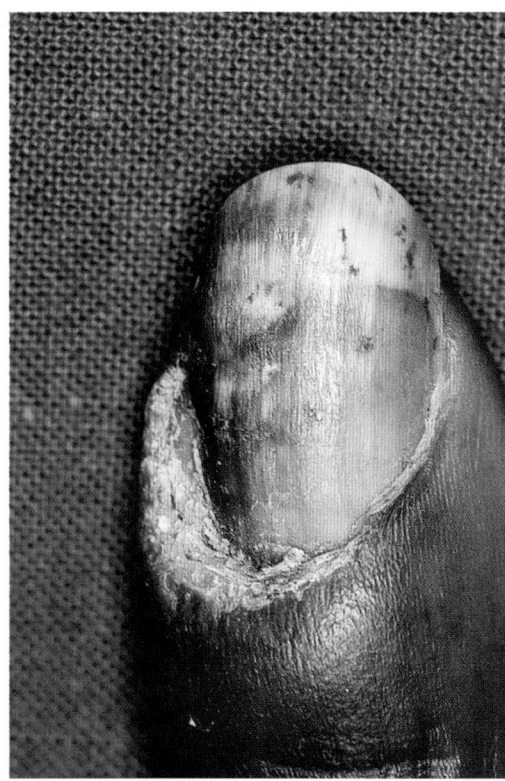

Fig. 17.21
Verrucous discoid lupus erythematosus: note the hypertrophic cuticle, pitting, and onycholysis. By courtesy of J. Newton Bishop, MD, St James's University Hospital, Leeds, UK.

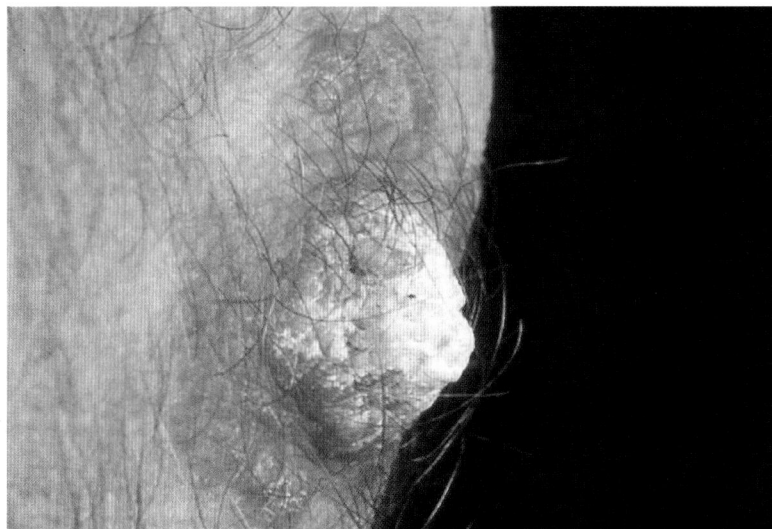

Fig. 17.22
Verrucous discoid lupus erythematosus: this example resembles a keratoacanthoma. By courtesy of the Institute of Dermatology, London, UK.

Subacute cutaneous lupus erythematosus

Subacute cutaneous lupus erythematosus (SCLE) accounts for 5% to 10% of patients with lupus erythematosus.[100–102] Approximately 50% have SLE as defined by the revised American Rheumatology Association diagnostic criteria (see below).[103] SCLE predominates in Caucasians and is uncommon in blacks, Koreans, and Chinese.[104] Females are affected more often than males (2.3:1), and the mean age at presentation is about 40 years.[105] This variant of lupus occurs very rarely in children.[106–110] Nail dystrophy affecting the majority of nails has been reported in a child with SCLE.[108]

The eruption, which is often widely distributed, consists of symmetrical, nonscarring, and nonindurated erythematosquamous lesions (*Fig. 17.27*). Unique presentation along the lines of Blaschko have also been reported.[111,112]

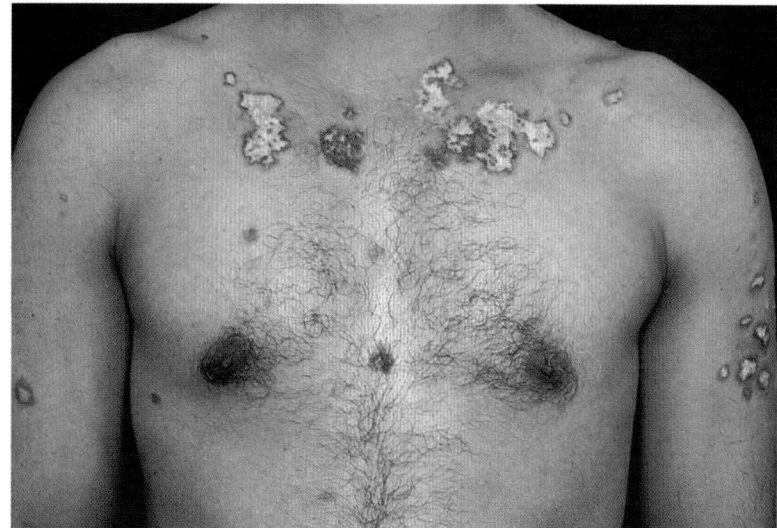

Fig. 17.23
Generalized discoid lupus erythematosus: in this variant, lesions are widespread and may involve the chest, shoulders, and upper limbs. Note the extensive erythema and scaling. By courtesy of R.A. Marsden, St George's Hospital, London, UK.

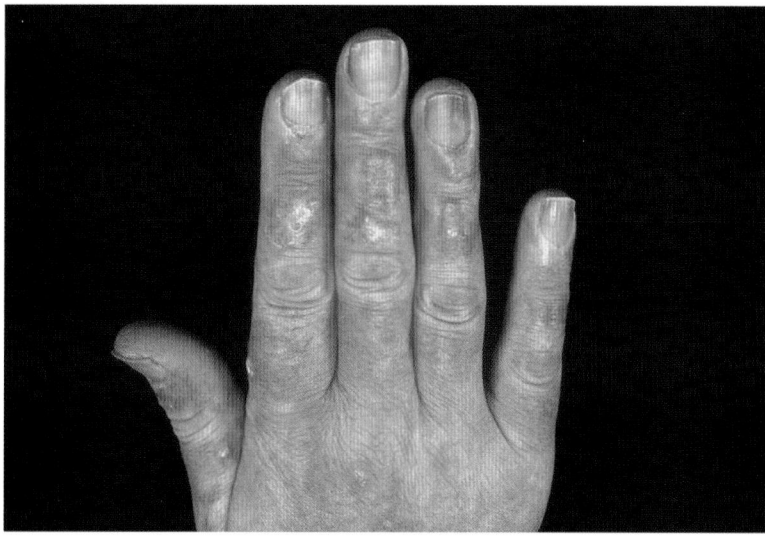

Fig. 17.24
Generalized discoid lupus erythematosus: note the extensive erythema and scaling. By courtesy of R.A. Marsden, St George's Hospital, London, UK.

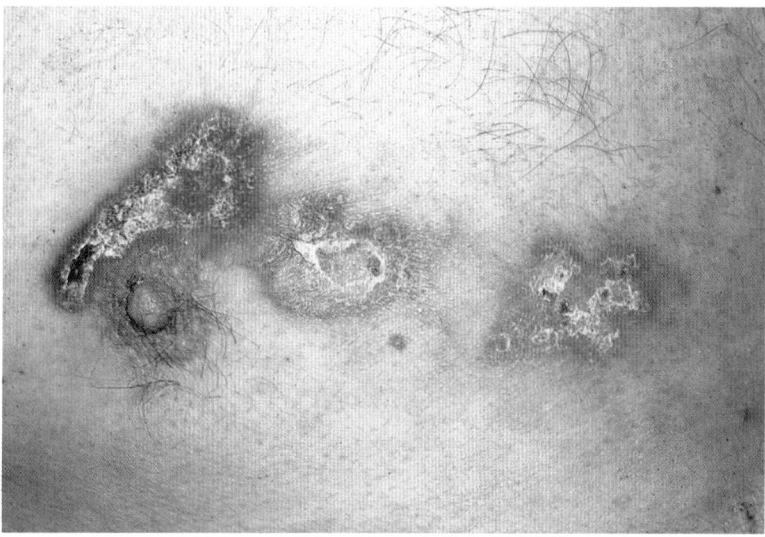

Fig. 17.25
Generalized discoid lupus erythematosus: in this patient, the chest is severely affected. By courtesy of the Institute of Dermatology, London, UK.

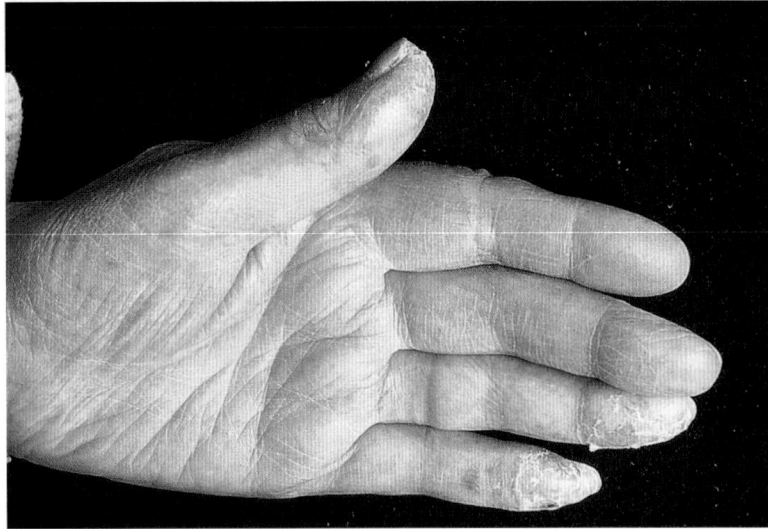

Fig. 17.26
Chilblain lupus erythematosus: resolving perniosis involving the tips of the thumb and ring and little fingers. By courtesy of R.A. Marsden, St George's Hospital, London, UK.

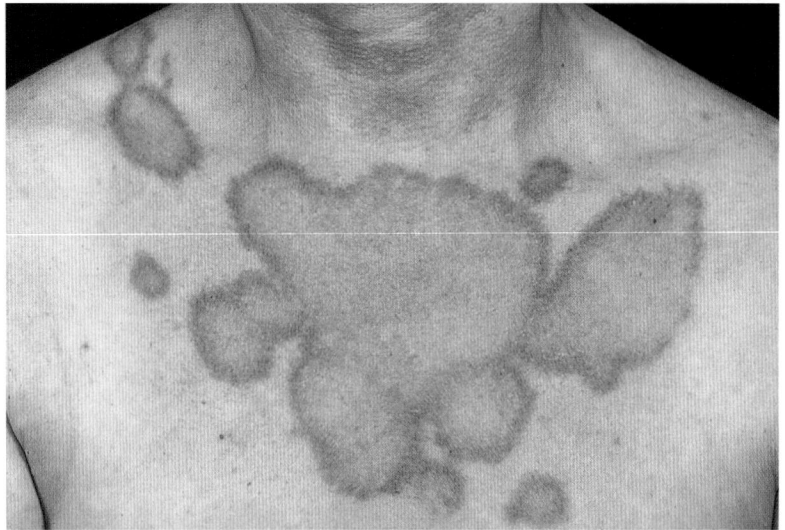

Fig. 17.28
Subacute cutaneous lupus erythematosus: coalescence of annular lesions has resulted in this bizarre eruption. By courtesy of the Institute of Dermatology, London, UK.

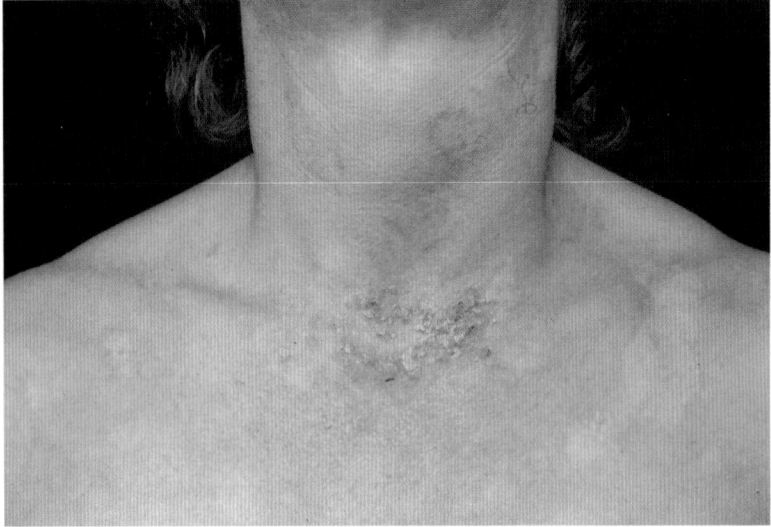

Fig. 17.27
Subacute cutaneous lupus erythematosus: annular lesions, many healed with pigmentary changes and delicate scale overlying an active lesion. From the collection of the late N.P. Smith, MD, the Institute of Dermatology, London, UK.

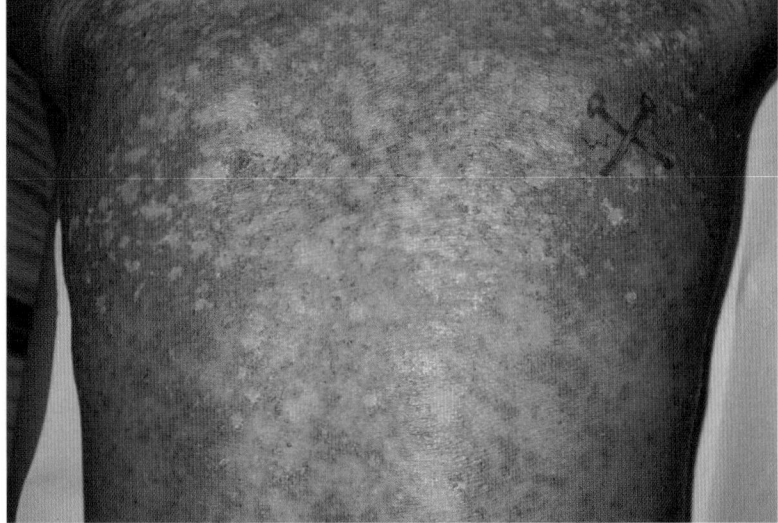

Fig. 17.29
Subacute cutaneous lupus erythematosus: in this patient, there is very extensive involvement. By courtesy of Dr J.C. Pascual, Alicante, Spain.

Absence of induration has been regarded as a useful clinical discrimination feature between SCLE and DLE.[104] In addition, the absence of follicular plugging, adherent scale, and dermal atrophy helps to distinguish the subacute lesion from the discoid variant.[101] Pruritus is very rare.[113] Lesions may become papulosquamous (psoriasiform) or annular, the latter coalescing to produce polycyclic and gyrate configurations (Fig. 17.28).[101,114,115] In some patients both patterns are seen. Crusting and vesiculation are sometimes evident on the active border of the annular lesions.[105] Pityriasiform and erythema multiforme-like lesions have also been described, as has occasional chronic leukoderma.[101] Exceptionally, the disease may present as generalized poikiloderma[116,117] or erythroderma.[118] In addition, 15% to 30% of patients develop features of typical DLE, usually located on the scalp or face.[1,101,103,119] The malar erythema of SLE is also sometimes evident (15%). Subtle hypopigmentation, telangiectasia, nonscarring alopecia, livedo reticularis, Raynaud phenomenon, and mucous membrane ulcers are additional features.[101,105] Dystrophic calcification is exceptional.[120] Cutaneous leukocytoclastic vasculitis is seen in a minority of patients and appears to be self-limited and not associated with a worsened prognosis.[121]

Photosensitivity is of major importance and lesions are therefore typically seen on the face, neck, upper part of back and chest, shoulders, extensor aspect of the arms, backs of hands, and fingers (Figs 17.29 and 17.30).[100,101,115]

Patients with SCLE have an increased incidence of human leukocyte antigen (HLA)-DR3 (75%), HLA-B8, and HLA-A1, and there is a significant association with inherited homozygous C2 and C4 deficiency.[101,103,104,122–125] HLA-DR2 is also present at a higher frequency, particularly in those with papulosquamous rather than annular skin lesions.[126] Antinuclear antibodies are found in approximately 50% of patients, while anti-Ro (SS-A) antibodies are present in approximately 65%, particularly those with annular polycyclic lesions.[6,102,106,114,125] Anti-La (SS-B) antibodies are also often evident.[5] Children with SCLE usually display anti-Ro (SS-A) antibodies in the majority of cases, while anti-La (SS-B) antibodies are rarely noted.[110] In addition, ANA are detected in over 70% of pediatric SCLE patients.[110]

The course of SCLE tends to be relatively benign, but systemic manifestations are quite common and may be severe.[127] Severe extracutaneous disease appears to be more common in men with papulosquamous SCLE.[127] The type of cutaneous lesion, however, has not always been proven to correlate with the severity of the extracutaneous manifestations.[128] Renal disease has been reported to be uncommon but a recent study found its frequency to be as similar and equally severe as in SLE.[105,129] Rarely, patients develop other more serious manifestations of SLE.[103]

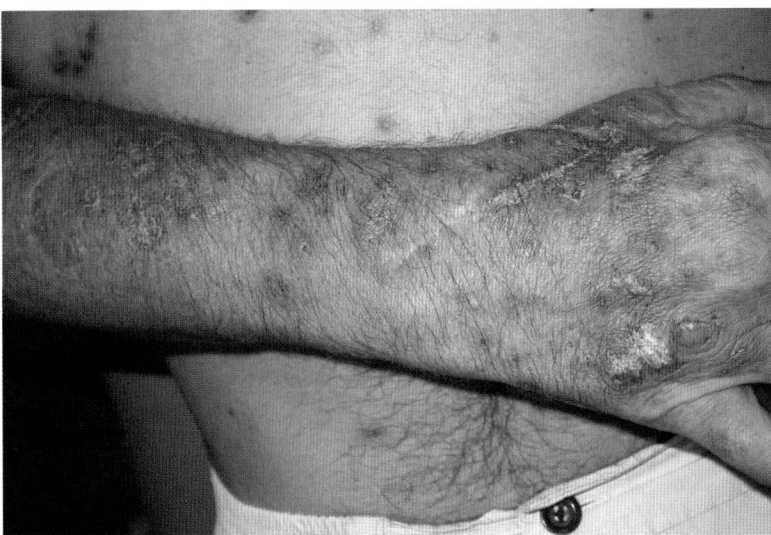

Fig. 17.30
Subacute cutaneous lupus erythematosus: the lesions are intensely erythematous and there is marked scaling. By courtesy of Dr J.C. Pascual, Alicante, Spain.

Patients with SCLE have an increased incidence of both rheumatoid arthritis and Sjögren syndrome.[102,130,131] Those with SCLE and Sjögren syndrome have high titers of anti-Ro antibodies, a high incidence of cutaneous vasculitis, and an increased risk of severe neuropsychiatric and pulmonary involvement.[132] SCLE has been documented in association with porphyria cutanea tarda, hepatitis B virus infection, radiotherapy, radioiodine treatment, squamous cell carcinoma of the head and neck region, and breast, hepatocellular, and lung carcinoma.[133–139] An exceptional association with inclusion body myositis and interstitial myositis with mitochondrial changes has also been documented.[138,140] A relationship with lichen planus and Kikuchi-Fujimoto disease is exceptional.[141–142] Clinically and histologically identical cases have been documented following therapy with hydrochlorothiazide, griseofulvin, antihistamines, terbinafine, calcium channel blockers, nifedipine, angiotensin-converting enzyme (ACE) inhibitors, proton pump inhibitors, interferon, phenytoin, bupropion, ticlopidine, capecitabine, lansoprazole, leflunomide, fluorouracil, leuprorelin, efalizumab, acebutolol, tamoxifen, docetaxel, statin, citalopram, golimumab, rituximab, gemcitabine, adalimumab, bevacizumab, paclitaxel, ranibizumab, terbinafine, pazopanib, norfloxacin, minocycline, pemetrexed plus carboplatin chemotherapy, imiquimod, mitotane, and anastrozole.[143–189]

Neutrophilic dermatosis of the systemic lupus erythematosus

Patients with SLE, but also patients with hydralazine-induced lupus and neonatal lupus, occasionally develop a rare cutaneous eruption morphologically mimicking Sweet syndrome.[190–202] Several alternative designations have been used in the literature for such a condition, for example neutrophilic dermatosis or neutrophilic urticarial dermatosis owing to its clinical resemblance to urticaria.[192,196–198,202] The frequency of neutrophilic dermatosis in SLE patients has been estimated to be below 5%.[198] Importantly, however, neutrophilic dermatosis can be an initial manifestation of SLE in as much as one-third of the patients.[196,197] Nevertheless, this reaction pattern is not specific for SLE and can also be observed in diverse diseases, for example rheumatoid arthritis, Sjögren syndrome, cryopyrin-associated periodic syndromes, Schnitzler syndrome, and adult-onset Still disease.[192,194,198,202]

Patients present with erythematous, pink or violaceous non-itchy plaques or slightly elevated papules.[196,197] Mucosal involvement is absent. The sites of predilection include the extremities, followed by trunk, face, and head and neck area.[196] Palmoplantar involvement has also been reported.[201] All age groups can be affected, from the neonatal period to elderly patients, but the eruption most commonly develops in the fourth decade of life.[196] There is a striking female predominance for patients with SLE and neonatal lupus, while hydralazine-induced lupus typically develops in males.[196] Systemic symptoms, including fever, malaise, and arthritis, are present in a subset of the patients.[190]

Table 17.2

Systemic lupus erythematosus: diagnostic guidelines of the American Rheumatology Association

Criterion	Definition
Malar rash	Fixed erythema, flat or raised, over malar eminences tending to spare nasolabial folds
Discoid rash	Erythematous, raised patches with adherent keratotic scaling and follicular plugging; atrophic scarring may occur in old lesions
Photosensitivity	Skin rash as result of unusual reaction to sunlight (observed by physician or recounted by patient)
Oral ulcers	Oral or nasopharyngeal ulceration, usually painless, observed by physician
Arthritis	Nonerosive arthritis involving two or more peripheral joints, characterized by tenderness, swelling, or effusion
Serositis	Pleurisy (convincing history of pleuritic pain or rub heard by physician or evidence of pleural effusion). Pericarditis (confirmed by ECG or rub or evidence of pericardial effusion)
Renal disorder	Persistent proteinuria (>0.5 g/day or >3 if quantification is not performed). Cellular casts (may be RBC, hemoglobin, granular, tubular, or mixed)
Neurological disorder	Seizures (in absence of offending drugs or known metabolic derangements, e.g., uremia ketoacidosis or electrolyte imbalance). Psychosis (in absence of offending drugs or known metabolic derangements, e.g., uremia ketoacidosis or electrolyte imbalance)
Hematological disorder	Hemolytic anemia with reticulocytosis. Leukopenia (<4000/mm³ on two or more occasions). Lymphopenia (<1500/mm³ on two or more occasions). Thrombocytopenia (<1500/mm³ in absence of offending drug therapy)
Immunological disorder	Positive LE cell preparation. Anti-DNA (antibody to native DNA in abnormal titer). Anti-SM (presence of antibody to SM nuclear antigen). False positive serological test result for syphilis known to be positive for at least 6 months and confirmed by *Treponema pallidum* immobilization or fluorescent treponemal antibody absorption test
Antinuclear antibody	Abnormal ANA titer by immunofluorescence or equivalent assay at any time and in absence of drugs known to be associated with drug-induced lupus syndrome

ANA, Antinuclear antibody; *LE*, lupus erythematosus; *RBC*, red blood cell.
Reproduced with permission from Tan, E.M. et al. (1982) *Arthritis and Rheumatism*, 25, 1271–1277.

Systemic lupus erythematosus

In addition to the variable cutaneous manifestations, lesions may be found in virtually any organ or system in the body in SLE.[203–205] The guidelines of the American Rheumatology Association are valuable in establishing the diagnosis: any patient who has experienced four or more of the criteria, either serially or concurrently, is considered to have SLE (*Table 17.2*).[206,207] Nevertheless, in 2012 Systemic Lupus International Collaborating Clinics (SLICC) classification criteria for SLE were proposed and represent evolution and refinement of the previous ARA guidelines.[208] The SLICC criteria increase the total number of criteria from 11 to 17 (*Table 17.3*). To be diagnosed with SLE, the following criteria need to be met: (1) fulfillment of at least four criteria (of these at least one clinical and one immunological criterion), or (2) lupus nephritis as the sole criterion in the presence of ANA or anti-dsDNA antibodies.[208]

SLE is characterized by a marked female predominance (9:1) and usually presents in the third, fourth, and fifth decades. There is a high incidence

Table 17.3

Clinical and immunological criteria used in the SLICC classification criteria*

Clinical criteria	**7. Renal**

1. Acute cutaneous lupus
including lupus malar rash (do not count if malar rash discoid)
    bullous lupus
    toxic epidermal necrolysis variant of SLE
    maculopapular lupus rash
    photosensitive lupus rash
        in the absence of dermatomyositis
or subacute cutaneous lupus
2. Chronic cutaneous lupus
including classical discoid rash
      localized (above the neck)
      generalized (above and below the neck)
    hypertrophic (verrucous) lupus
    lupus panniculitis (profundus)
    mucosal lupus
    lupus erythematosus tumidus
    chilblains lupus
    discoid lupus/lichen planus overlap
3. Oral ulcers: palate
    buccal
    tongue
or nasal ulcers
    in the absence of other causes, such as vasculitis, Behçet disease,
        infection (herpes), inflammatory bowel disease, reactive arthritis, and
        acidic foods
4. Nonscarring alopecia (diffuse thinning or hair fragility with visible
    broken hairs)
    in the absence of other causes such as alopecia areata, drugs, iron
        deficiency, and androgenic alopecia
5. Synovitis involving two or more joints, characterized by swelling or
    effusion OR tenderness in two or more joints and 30 minutes or more
    of morning stiffness
6. Serositis
    typical pleurisy for more than 1 day
    or pleural effusions
    or pleural rub
    typical pericardial pain (pain with recumbency, improved by sitting
        forward) for more than 1 day
    or pericardial effusion
    or pericardial rub
    or pericarditis by EKG
    in the absence of other causes, such as infection, uremia, and Dressler
        pericarditis
	urine protein/creatinine (or 24-hour urine protein) representing 500 mg
	        of protein/24 hour
	    or
	    red blood cell casts
	8. Neurologic
	    seizures
	    psychosis
	    mononeuritis multiplex
	        in the absence of other known causes such as primary vasculitis
	    myelitis
	    peripheral or cranial neuropathy
	        in the absence of other known causes such as primary vasculitis,
	            infection, or diabetes
	    acute confusional state
	        in the absence of other causes, including toxic-metabolic, uremia,
	        drugs
	9. Hemolytic anemia
	10. Leukopenia (<4000/mm³ at least once)
	    in the absence of other known causes such as Felty syndrome, drugs,
	        and portal hypertension
	    or
	    Lymphopenia (<1000/mm³ at least once)
	    In the absence of other known causes such as corticosteroids, drugs,
	        and infection
	11. Thrombocytopenia (<100 000/mm³ at least once)
	    In the absence of other known causes such as drugs, portal
	        hypertension, and TTP

	Immunological criteria

	1. ANA above laboratory reference range
	2. Anti-dsDNA above laboratory reference range, except ELISA: twice above
	    laboratory reference range
	3. Anti-Sm
	4. Antiphospholipid antibody: any of the following
	    lupus anticoagulant
	    false positive RPC
	    medium or high titer anticardiolipin (IgA, IgG, or IgM)
	    anti-beta 2 glycoprotein I (IgA, IgG, or IgM)
	5. Low complement
	    low C3
	    low C4
	    low CH50
	6. Direct Coombs test *in the absence of hemolytic anemia*

*Criteria are cumulative and need not be present concurrently
Reproduced with permission from Petri M., Orbai A.M., Alarcon G.S., et al. Derivation and validation of systemic lupus international collaborating clinics classification criteria for systemic lupus erythematosus. *Arthritis Rheum.* 64, 2012; 2677–2686.

among Afro-Caribbeans, with a maximum prevalence of 1/150 females in Jamaica. In the United States the incidence is approximately 1/100.[5]

Cutaneous involvement occurs in 75% to 88% of patients.[115] Lesions are highly polymorphic and may mimic many other dermatoses (*Table 17.4*). The 'butterfly rash' is typical and is a slightly scaly, sometimes edematous, erythema that is particularly distributed on the bridge of the nose and on the cheeks (*Fig. 17.31*). Photosensitivity is common, affecting more than 50% of patients, and erythematous or violaceous maculopapular eruptions may develop, particularly in white patients, at other light-exposed areas, such as the 'V' of the neck, and the forearms.[115] Sensitivity is toward both ultraviolet (UV) A and B light. Approximately 15% of patients, particularly Afro-Caribbeans, have lesions similar to those of DLE, apparently associated with a less severe disease and a lower frequency of renal involvement.[3,10,115,203] SCLE-like features are present in 10% to 15% of patients.[209] It has been suggested that patients with SLE and SCLE lesions have a more favorable prognosis.[210]

Alopecia is important, occurring in about 20% of patients, and may be scarring or nonscarring. The nonscarring lesions, which are more common, often constitute a fairly diffuse hair loss occurring as a non-specific response to stress (telogen effluvium).[115] Fractured frontal hairs are characteristic.[19]

Raynaud phenomenon occurs in 10% to 40% of patients.[115] Purpura and ecchymoses are common and may be partly due to corticosteroid therapy, but thrombocytopenia and immune complex-mediated vasculitis also play a role in the pathogenesis. Vasculitis, which occurs in up to 30% of patients, may also result in infarcts, ulcers, digital nodules, scars, and gangrene (*Figs 17.32–17.34*).[115] Livedo reticularis that particularly affects the arms and thighs and periarticular sites may be a presenting feature in up to 10% of patients, and the changes of atrophie blanche have been documented occasionally (livedoid vasculitis) (*Fig. 17.35*).[115] Livedo reticularis is often a feature of the anticardiolipin syndrome and presenting lesions identical to those seen in Degos disease (malignant atrophic papulosis) have been described occasionally.[211,212] Vasculitic features correlate with renal and central nervous system involvement.[115] Urticaria is frequently found.[213]

Erythromelalgia, a burning sensation accompanied by erythema following exposure to heat, has also been noted.[22] Localized and diffuse hyperpigmentation and urticarial lesions, including urticarial vasculitis, are less

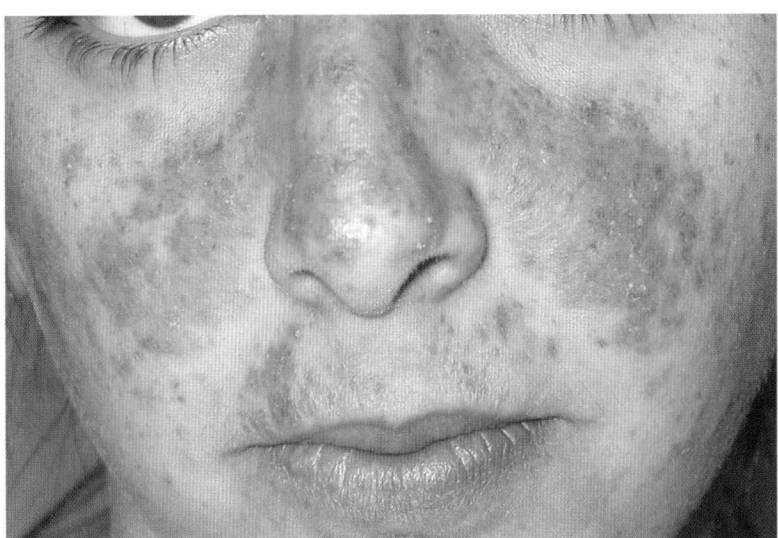

Fig. 17.31
Systemic lupus erythematosus: characteristic 'butterfly erythema' on the cheeks and nose. By courtesy of Dr J.C. Pascual, Alicante, Spain.

Table 17.4
Systemic lupus erythematosus: cutaneous manifestations

Malar erythema (butterfly rash)
Inflammatory periorbital edema
Mucous membrane lesions
Oral and nasopharyngeal ulceration
Alopecia
   – fractured frontal hair
   – scarring and nonscarring hair loss
Raynaud disease with or without skin changes
Cutaneous vasculitis
   – urticarial lesions
   – palpable purpura
   – digital nodules
   – cutaneous infarcts
   – leg ulcers
   – peripheral gangrene
   – thrombophlebitis
   – livedo reticularis
   – periungual erythema and telangiectasia
   – hemorrhagic bullous lesions
So-called bullous SLE
Lichen planus-like lesions
Perniotic lesions
Lupus profundus
Chilblain lesions
Sjögren syndrome
Calcinosis cutis
Rheumatoid nodules
Pigmentary changes

Reproduced from Moschella, S.L. (1989) *Journal of Dermatology*, 16, 417–428, with permission from Blackwell Publishing Ltd.

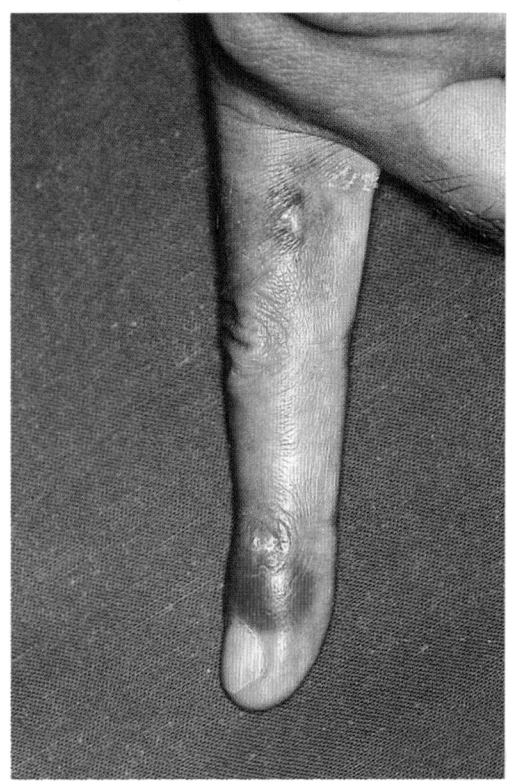

Fig. 17.32
Systemic lupus erythematosus: erythematous vasculitic lesion on the fingertip. By courtesy of M.M. Black, MD, St Thomas' Hospital, London, UK.

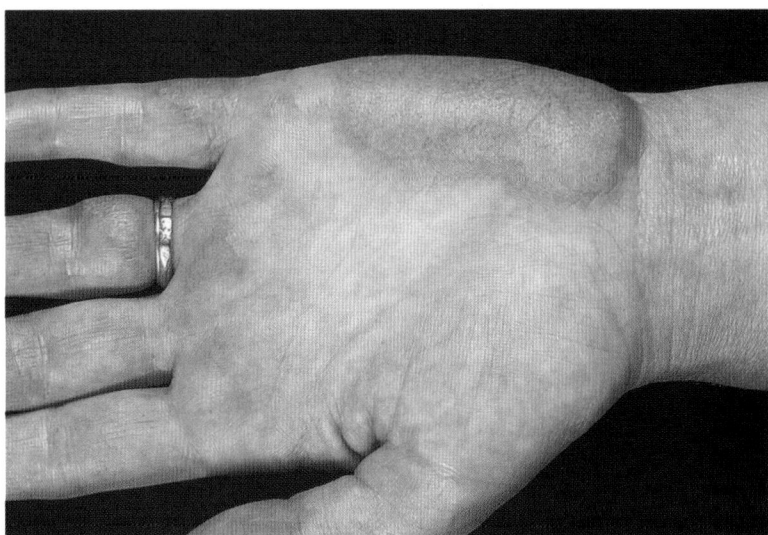

Fig. 17.33
Systemic lupus erythematosus: involvement of the palms is rare and may be vasculitic. By courtesy of the Institute of Dermatology, London, UK.

commonly found. Digital manifestations, in addition to infarction and ulceration, include periungual and knuckle erythema, nail fold telangiectases, cuticular lesions, and splinter hemorrhages. Telangiectases may also be seen on the fingertips and palms.[91] Some patients develop red lunulae.[214,215] The associated erythema multiforme-like and perniotic lesions are described above. Involvement of the mucous membranes occurs in about 10% of patients: painless ulceration is most common, but other features include erythema, petechiae, erosions, and hemorrhage. The central part of the hard palate, lips, and buccal mucosa are particularly affected.[25,212,216]

Additional lesions that are occasionally seen include persistent eyelid edema and erythema, rheumatoid-like nodules, dermal mucinosis, bullous variants, thrombotic thrombocytopenic purpura, mixed cryoglobulinemia,

and soft tissue calcifications.[5,19,217–219] Vesicles and bullae in SLE may complicate extreme basal cell hydropic degeneration, represent coexpression of an autoimmune bullous dermatosis, or signify a specific dermatitis herpetiformis-like eruption (bullous dermatosis of SLE). There is a recognized association with porphyria cutanea tarda.[220]

Approximately 5% to 10% of patients with SLE are antinuclear antibody negative. This seems to correlate with a specific subtype. Patients are usually HLA-DR3 positive and have Sjögren syndrome and an increased incidence of pulmonary involvement, psychiatric manifestations, cutaneous vasculitis, and hypergammaglobulinemic purpura.[5]

Non-specific symptoms are common and include chronic tiredness, weight loss, fever, malaise, and weakness. Arthralgia and myalgia occur in 90% of patients. The myalgia may be disabling, but objective muscle

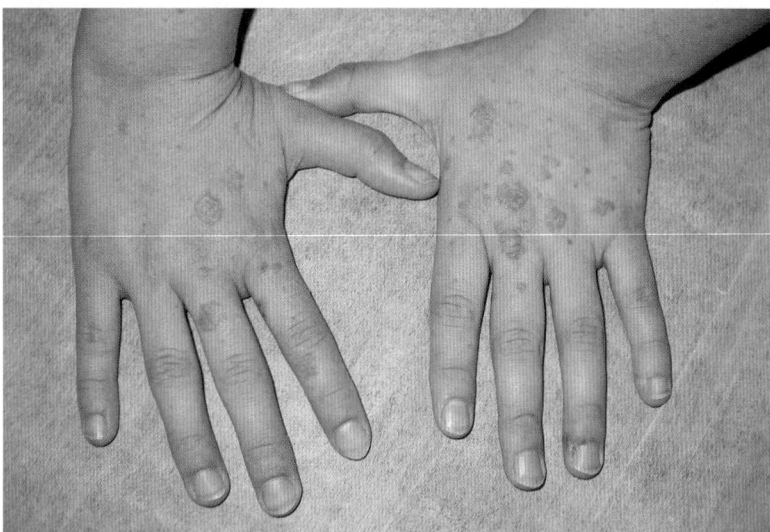

Fig. 17.34
Systemic lupus erythematosus: erythematous nodules are present on the back of the hand and on the fingers. By courtesy of Dr J.C. Pascual, Alicante, Spain.

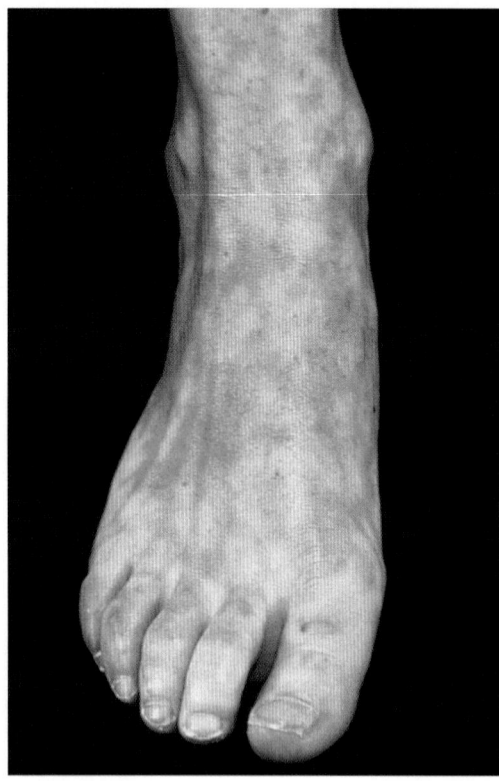

Fig. 17.35
Systemic lupus erythematosus: livedo reticularis develops as a consequence of relative ischemia in the watershed zones. There are numerous causes, particularly connective tissue disease. By courtesy of the Institute of Dermatology, London, UK.

weakness is rare.[221] Similarly, although arthralgia may be marked, there is usually little clinical evidence of joint damage. Effusions are common.[203] Approximately 25% of patients have frank arthritis, either a migratory polyarthritis or a chronic progressive polyarthritis with deformity. Patients sometimes develop avascular bone necrosis due either to the primary disease or to steroid therapy.[203,221] Very rarely, involvement of the tendons is associated with the development of contractures.

Lesions of the cardiovascular system manifest as cardiomegaly, pericarditis, pericardial effusion, and/or endocarditis (Libman-Sacks valvulitis).[222] In SLE, the mitral valve is predominantly affected, but patients with the lupus anticoagulant syndrome appear to have a particular risk of developing aortic valve disease.[222,223] Conduction defects and congestive cardiac failure are additional features.

Respiratory involvement may present as pleurisy, with or without effusion, bacterial pneumonia or, very rarely, lupus pneumonitis.[221] Pulmonary hypertension has been estimated to be present in 0.5% to 14% of SLE patients, especially those associated with antiphospholipid antibodies.[224]

Involvement of the central nervous system is an important cause of morbidity and mortality.[203,221] It may affect up to 40% of patients.[6] Encephalitis, meningitis, vasculitis, and coagulation defects give rise to a wide range of clinical manifestations, including convulsions, hemiplegias, chorea, and psychoses.[19] Convulsions and coma are an indication of severe involvement and portend a grave outcome. Peripheral neuritis affects up to 12% of patients; ocular lesions, including conjunctivitis, fundal hemorrhages, and cotton wool exudates, occur in 25%.[19]

Renal manifestations develop in approximately 45% of patients, and progressive renal involvement is an important cause of morbidity and mortality (nephrotic syndrome and lupus glomerulonephritis). Evidence of active renal disease includes the presence in the urine of more than five red blood cells/high-power field.[221] Proteinuria of greater than 1 g/24 hours, oval fat bodies, granular, hyaline, and red blood cell casts may also be detected.[19]

Generalized lymphadenopathy is present in about 50% of the patients, hepatomegaly in 20%, and splenomegaly in 10%.

Gastrointestinal manifestations are uncommon; the most important is esophageal involvement leading to loss of peristalsis and dilatation reminiscent of that seen in scleroderma.[221]

Laboratory investigation commonly reveals anemia, leukopenia, lymphopenia, thrombocytopenia, and a raised ESR. False-positive reactions to reagin and treponemal tests for syphilis are common, 10% to 20% of patients are positive for the Coombs test and rheumatoid factor, and 10% to 50% have circulating anticoagulants.[203]

While lupus erythematosus (LE) cell preparation used to be the basic screening test for SLE, it has now been superseded by testing for antinuclear factor. This and other autoantibodies will be discussed further under pathogenesis. Serum complement levels are often low in patients with active disease (CH_{50} and C3); estimations of C3 levels are of particular value in following disease activity.[5,19]

SLE is characterized by relapses, with remissions of variable duration sometimes lasting a decade or more. There is still, however, significant mortality. Causes of death include nephritis, infections, and central nervous system involvement.

An association between SLE and inherited complement deficiency, involving the early components of the classic pathway including C1r, C1s, C1q, C4, and C2, has been described.[225–227] Deficiency of C2 is inherited in an autosomal recessive fashion; up to 60% of homozygotes develop lupus erythematosus characterized by an erythematous, papulosquamous, SCLE-like photosensitive dermatosis, a low incidence of renal involvement, and arthralgia. Additional features may include urticarial vasculitis, malar erythema, and nail fold abnormalities.[123] Discoid lesions are sometimes evident, and recently a patient with C2 and C4 deficiency and LE panniculitis has been documented.[12,228] Patients are, however, often (but not invariably) negative for antinuclear factor and manifest a negative lupus band test on unaffected skin. There is an association with HLA-DR2, and over 60% of patients possess anti-Ro antibodies.[100]

Numerous drugs have been implicated in the induction of SLE including:
- isoniazid, hydralazine, procainamide, rifampicin, quinidine, penicillamine, terbinafine, carbamazepine, phenytoin, sertraline, valpromide, amiodarone, atenolol, sulfonamides, methimazole, COL-3, hydrochlorothiazide, minocycline, spironolactone, captopril, methyldopa, gold salts, penicillin, streptomycin, phenylbutazone, reserpine, griseofulvin, clonidine, oral contraceptives, captopril, interleukin (IL)-2, hydroxyurea, clobazam, clozapine, ciprofloxacin, cefuroxime, nafcillin, celiprolol, hydralazine, para-amino salicylic acid, yohimbine, infliximab, adalimumab, pegylated interferon alpha-2B, conjugated estrogens, antitumor necrosis factor alpha (TNF-α), and etanercept.[229–288]

Transient skin and serological manifestations of SLE have been documented in two children with trichophyton mentagrophytes infection.[268] The

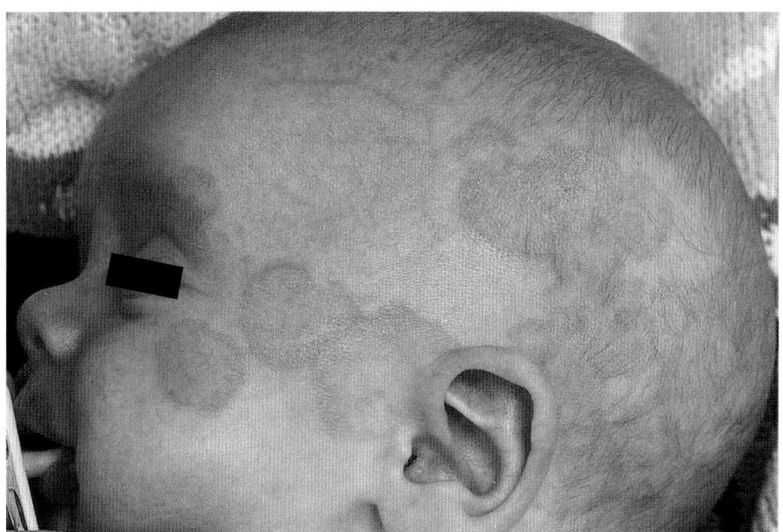

Fig. 17.36
Neonatal lupus erythematosus: note the presence of erythematous, slightly scaly plaques on the cheeks, forehead, and scalp. By courtesy of the Institute of Dermatology, London, UK.

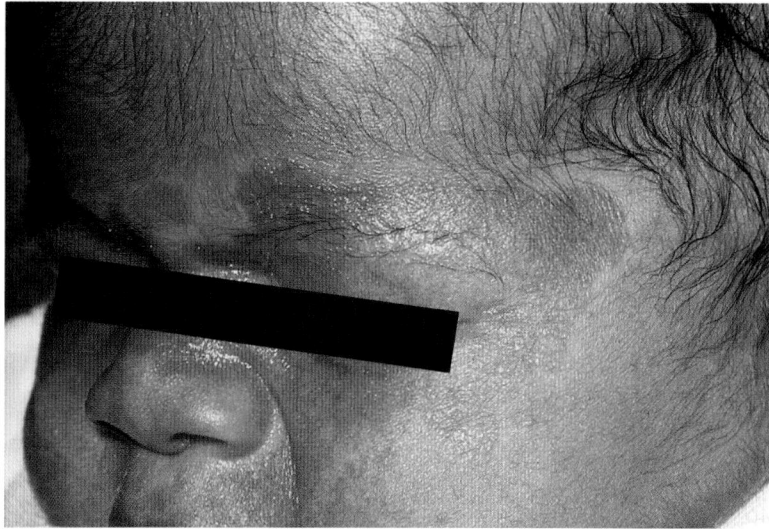

Fig. 17.37
Neonatal lupus erythematosus: in this child, there is intense erythema affecting the cheeks and nose and around the eyes.

disease has also been linked to hepatitis B vaccination and with exposure to insecticides.[289–292]

Sjögren syndrome coexists in approximately 10% to 20% of patients with SLE.[114] SLE has also been described in association with scleroderma, morphea, rheumatoid arthritis, eosinophilic fasciitis, dermatomyositis, lichen sclerosus, pemphigus (including pemphigus vulgaris, foliaceous, and paraneoplastic pemphigus), hypergammaglobulinemia of Waldenström, dermatitis herpetiformis, ulcerative colitis, alopecia areata, autoimmune thyroiditis, myasthenia gravis, acanthosis nigricans, Sweet syndrome, porphyria, gout, sarcoidosis, psoriasis, lichen planus, and cutaneous T-cell lymphoma. It is likely that many of these associations are chance associations except for those diseases with an autoimmune basis.[220,293–317]

Neonatal lupus erythematosus

Neonatal lupus erythematosus is very rare, occurring in approximately 1 in 20 000 live births[318] and most commonly presents in female infants.[318–320] It is associated with maternal anti-Ro (SS-A) antibodies (95%) and/or anti-La (SS-B) antibodies.[319,320] Anti-U1-ribonucleoprotein (RNP) antibodies may also be present.[321–325] Anticardiolipin antibodies have been described in a single case.[326] Transplacental transfer of anti-Ro and anti-La antibodies results in an SCLE-like eruption consisting of erythematous annular scaly plaques that particularly affect the periorbital region ('owl-eye' or 'eye-mask') and scalp, and to a lesser extent, the trunk and extremities (*Figs 17.36* and *17.37*).[5] The skin changes can already be present at birth. Nevertheless, they typically develop in infants at the age of 4 to 6 weeks, are usually self-limiting, and in the majority of cases resolve by 15 to 17 weeks without any sequelae.[327] These cutaneous lesions often appear after exposure to ultraviolet light. Photosensitivity in neonatal lupus erythematosus patients appears to show racial differences, being more frequent in Caucasians and Americans than in Japanese infants.[328] Crusted lesions and cutis marmorata telangiectasia congenita are additional features in some cases.[329,330] Exceptionally, discoid lesions, panniculitis (lupus profundus), multiple morphea, erosions, targetoid lesions, and alopecia may also occur.[331–334] Atrophy and scarring are very rare but residual hypopigmentation and telangiectasia are present in about 25% of patients.[335] Babies in subsequent pregnancies may present manifestations of the disease[336,337] and the overall recurrence rate for neonatal lupus-associated cardiac disease is 17%.[338]

Neonatal lupus erythematosus is often associated with cardiac abnormalities. Complete heart block represents the most serious complication developing either in utero or after birth.[319,333,339] Circulating autoantibodies to annexin A6 were detected in a single patient with neonatal lupus erythematosus-related dilated cardiomyopathy.[340] The mortality associated with cardiac involvement is around 19%.[336] Hematological complications have been estimated to develop in 10% to 35% of patients with neonatal lupus; the most common abnormalities are mild anemia and mild thrombocytopenia.[341] Multiple mucocutaneous and visceral hemangiomas have been reported in a single patient.[342] Severe hematological and liver involvement without evidence of cutaneous or cardiac involvement has exceptionally been reported.[343] Liver involvement in neonatal lupus is rare and usually presents as a cholestatic hepatitis.[319,333] Other rare associations include sigmoidal telangiectasia with rectal bleeding, painful plantar atrophy, central nervous system vasculitis, stroke, intraventricular hemorrhage, and extensive aortic aneurysm.[344–348]

The levels of maternal autoantibodies in the infant decrease quickly during the first weeks of life and generally become undetectable by the age of 1 year.[349]

The disease also occurs in identical and nonidentical twins.[350] A single case has been described in association with Turner syndrome.[351] Neonates who survive until infancy have a fairly good prognosis, but there is an overall mortality of about 10% due to heart disease.[319] Mothers of affected infants are commonly asymptomatic initially but they may have systemic lupus, Sjögren syndrome, rheumatoid arthritis, leukocytoclastic vasculitis or an overlap syndrome.[352,353]

A number of mothers who present with no symptoms often subsequently develop evidence of connective tissue disease, particularly systemic lupus (in about 20% of cases) and Sjögren syndrome.[319]

Pathogenesis and histologic features

Despite enormous research efforts, the precise etiology and pathogenesis are unknown, but the condition is certainly multifactorial.[354,355] Lupus erythematosus is characterized by B-cell hyperactivity in association with defective suppressor T-cell function. Patients develop a wide range of autoantibodies, many of which result in immune complexes with resultant systemic manifestations, including vasculitis and glomerulonephritis. In addition to immunological factors, familial, genetic, and hormonal influences play a part. It is believed that in lupus erythematosus there is a genetic predisposition; sex-associated and environmental factors are necessary to promote the development of the disease.

Autoantibodies are important in the diagnosis of lupus erythematosus and have a significant role in its pathogenesis, either by direct cytotoxic effects (such as the lymphopenia induced by antilymphocyte antibodies) or by immune complex deposition. Until the 1960s the presence of LE cells in a patient's blood was regarded as pathognomonic for lupus erythematosus. This was changed, however, by the discovery of antinuclear factor (antinuclear antibody) with direct immunofluorescent techniques. Antinuclear antibody is present in the serum of 90% to 95% of patients with SLE, in

30% of patients with localized DLE, and in 50% of patients with generalized DLE. It should also be noted that 10% of the normal population have antinuclear antibody in the serum, albeit at low concentration. Antinuclear antibody has at least four subtypes:

- A homogeneous or diffuse pattern is most commonly seen (*Figs 17.38* and *17.39*).
- Speckled fluorescence representing an antibody to saline-soluble nuclear protein is present in patients with the lupus erythematosus-erythema multiforme syndrome (*Fig. 17.40*).
- The nucleolar pattern (representing antinucleolar RNA antibody) is occasionally evident in lupus erythematosus, although it is more common in systemic sclerosis.
- The peripheral (outline) staining pattern reflects high titer anti-DNA antibody and is a marker of active systemic disease.[6,19]

Patients with lupus erythematosus develop antibodies to a variety of nuclear and cytoplasmic antigens; these autoantibodies, both singly and in combination, have varying associations, which may allow a prediction of (to some extent, at least) the course of the disease in individual patients (*Table 17.5*). Antibodies to native (double-stranded) DNA (nDNA) are pathognomonic for idiopathic (classic) SLE (*Fig. 17.41*).[6,19] They are rarely seen in the drug-induced variant and are only very occasionally present in patients with DLE.[2] The presence of anti-nDNA antibody in association with

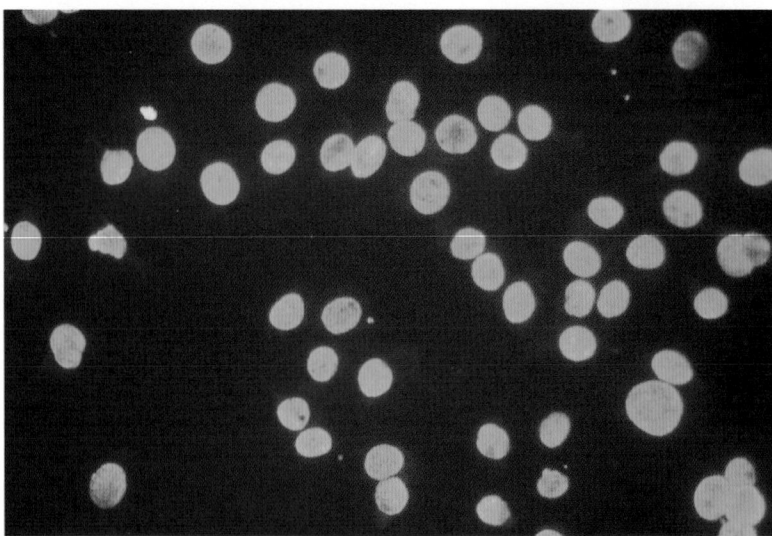

Fig. 17.39
Systemic lupus erythematosus: high-power view. By courtesy of G. Swana, MD, St Thomas' Hospital, London, UK.

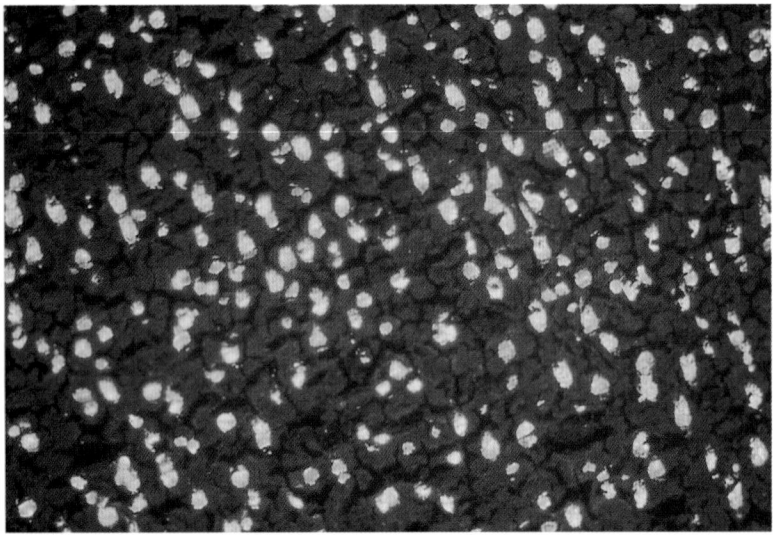

Fig. 17.38
Systemic lupus erythematosus: homogeneous antinuclear antibody in rat liver. By courtesy of G. Swana, MD, St Thomas' Hospital, London, UK.

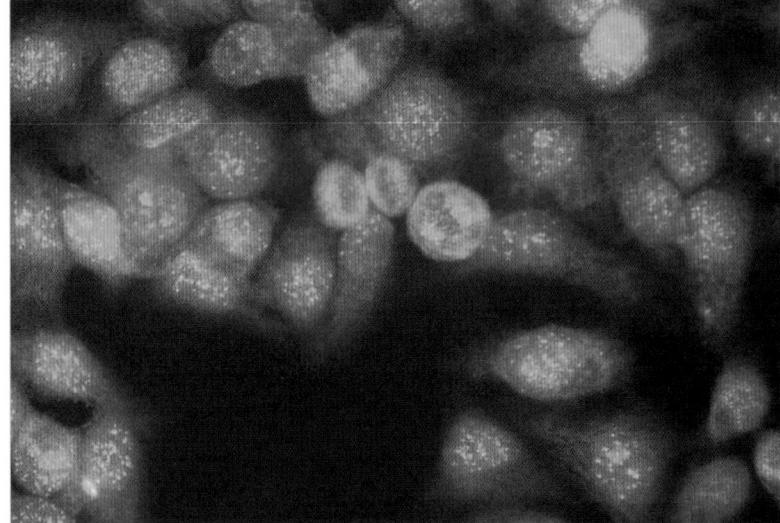

Fig. 17.40
Systemic lupus erythematosus: speckled antinuclear antibody – HEP II. By courtesy of G. Swana, MD, St Thomas' Hospital, London, UK.

Table 17.5
Systemic lupus erythematosus: antibodies

Antigen	Antibody	Significance	Comment
Nuclear constituents	Anti-native DNA Antihistone Anti-single stranded DNA	Highly specific for SLE associated with hypocomplementemia and glomerulonephritis 30% of SLE patients 90% of SLE patients, associated with glomerulonephritis	Found in NZB/NZW model Found in high titer in drug-induced lupus-like disease May be detected in ANF-negative SLE patients
Small nuclear ribonuclear protein	Sm nRNP La (SS-B)	Highly specific for SLE 15% of SLE patients May occur in SLE but also present in MCTD and PSS Found in 10% of SLE	May be associated with low incidence of renal disease
Small cytoplasmic ribonuclear protein	Ro (SS-A)	Found in 25% of SLE patients Found in SCLE Found in 50% of complement-deficient LE-like syndromes Found in all neonatal lupus	May be detected in ANF-negative SLE

ANF, Antinuclear factor; *LE*, lupus erythematosus; *MCTD*, mixed connective tissue disease; *PSS*, progressive systemic sclerosis; *SCLE*, subacute cutaneous lupus erythematosus; *SLE*, systemic lupus erythematosus.

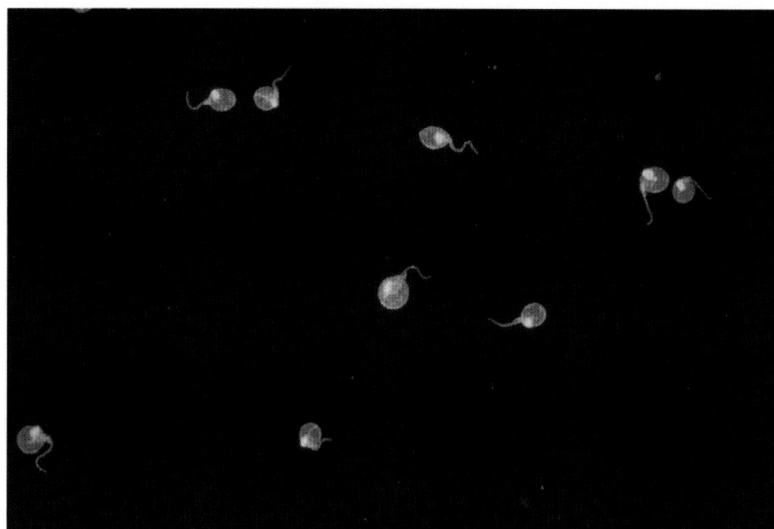

Fig. 17.41
Systemic lupus erythematosus: anti-dsDNA (*Crithidia luciliae*). By courtesy of G. Swana, MD, St Thomas' Hospital, London, UK.

hypocomplementemia is indicative of active disease and is often accompanied by severe renal involvement.

Antihistone antibodies may be found in approximately 30% of patients with idiopathic SLE, but are particularly associated with the drug-induced variant.[356] The latter is caused by a wide variety of drugs, including hydralazine, procainamide hydrochloride, phenytoin, and isoniazid.[14,357,358] Symptoms develop in up to 20% of patients taking procainamide and antinuclear antibodies are present in 50%.[358] Procainamide-induced SLE-like syndrome is characterized by the presence of leukocyte-specific antinuclear antibody.[358] Clinical features include malaise, pneumonitis with pleural effusion, arthralgia, arthritis, and serositis; renal, central nervous system, and cutaneous lesions are less common and are usually mild. Although antinuclear antibodies are often present, anti-DNA antibodies are not formed in most cases of drug-induced lupus.[221] Drug-induced lupus usually, but not invariably, undergoes remission on withdrawal of the drug.[358]

Antibodies to ssDNA occur in 90% of patients with classic SLE and in approximately 20% of patients with disseminated DLE, and may also be found in other connective tissue diseases.[10] Their presence in disseminated DLE correlates with an increased risk of developing SLE.[10] Patients with SLE who are negative for antinuclear antibody may have anti-ssDNA antibodies in their serum.[6] Antibodies to the soluble nuclear antigen Sm are highly specific for SLE.[356] They may also be found in a group of patients with good prognosis who are positive for antinuclear factor, but anti-nDNA-negative, and who have mild nonprogressive glomerulonephritis, hypocomplementemia, mild central nervous system involvement, and conspicuous cutaneous eruptions.

Antibodies to ribonucleoprotein are detected in 23% of patients with SLE, but are much more commonly associated with mixed connective tissue disease (MCTD): they may also be found in patients with progressive systemic sclerosis.[356] Anti-La (SS-B) antibodies are detected in the serum of 10% of patients with SLE. Anti-La antibodies, which are often present in Sjögren syndrome, are almost invariably accompanied by anti-Ro (SS-A) antibodies.[356] The latter are particularly associated with SCLE, complement-deficient lupus erythematosus, circulating IgG or IgM anticoagulant, and neonatal lupus erythematosus. About 15% to 20% of patients with SLE have detectable antineutrophil cytoplasmic antibodies (ANCA).[359] A large multicenter study of 645 childhood SLE patients from Brazil demonstrated anti-Ro (SS-A) and/or anti-La (SS-B) antibodies to be associated with mild cutaneous and musculoskeletal involvement.[360]

The circulating anticoagulant (antiphospholipid or lupus anticoagulant) is associated with paradoxical thrombosis, spontaneous abortion, premature labor, intrauterine death, labile hypertension, cutaneous necrosis, gangrene, ecchymoses, purpura, leg ulcers, atrophie blanche, livedo reticularis, and false-positive syphilis serology – the lupus anticoagulant syndrome

Table 17.6
Diagnostic criteria for the antiphospholipid syndrome

Group	Criteria
I. Clinical conditions	Thrombosis venous: recurrent deep vein thrombosis axillary retinal vein arterial: cerebrovascular accident retinal artery coronary other: pulmonary hypertension livedo reticularis neurological syndromes – transient ischemic attack; progressive dementia (repeated cerebrovascular stroke) Recurrent fetal loss Thrombocytopenia
II. Laboratory*	Positive anticardiolipin antibody assay; isotype IgG or IgM Positive lupus anticoagulant test
III. Other clinical conditions	Hemolytic anemia/positive direct Coombs test Migraine Endocardial/valvular lesions Transient visual loss Chorea
IV. Histopathological classification of lesions in antiphospholipid syndrome	1. Thrombotic type (characterized by dominating noninflammatory bland occlusive or mural thrombosis and its consequences) a. Large- and medium-sized arterial and venous, cardiac (Libman-Sacks endocarditis), recent or organized b. Microvascular (capillaries, arterioles, and small arteries) 2. Microangiopathic type (characterized by dominating endothelial cell injury, subendothelial plasma insudation often associated with thrombotic necrotizing lesions) affecting capillaries, arterioles, small arteries 3. Ischemic type, secondary to vascular occlusion 4. Tentatively associated pathology, like accelerated atherosclerosis and membranous glomerulopathy 5. Coincidental underlying disease-related pathology 6. Coincidental drug-induced pathology

At least one finding from each of groups I and II must be present to constitute a diagnosis.
Group III represents features occasionally present in these patients.
*Laboratory tests should be positive on two occasions 2 months apart.
Modified from ASCP check sample (TH 88-6), American Society of Clinical Pathologists, 1989; with permission. Histopathological classification modified from Praprotnik, S., Ferluga, D., Vizjak, A., et al. (2009) *Clinic Rev. Allerg. Immunol*, 36, 109–125.

(*Table 17.6*).[359,361–372] The lupus anticoagulant syndrome is more accurately known as the antiphospholipid syndrome because not all patients have associated SLE. It is due to the presence of circulating antiphospholipid antibodies which inhibit coagulation in vitro, but more importantly are associated with a greatly increased risk of thrombotic phenomena affecting both arteries and veins (*Figs 17.42* and *17.43*). About 50% of patients with SLE present with antiphospholipid antibodies but only half of these will develop manifestations of the disease.[373] Presentation in the skin may also be with papules and nodules or lesions resembling pyoderma gangrenosum.[374,375] Interestingly, patients with antiphospholipid antibodies and SLE appear to be more at risk of developing anetoderma.[376–378] The incidence, however,

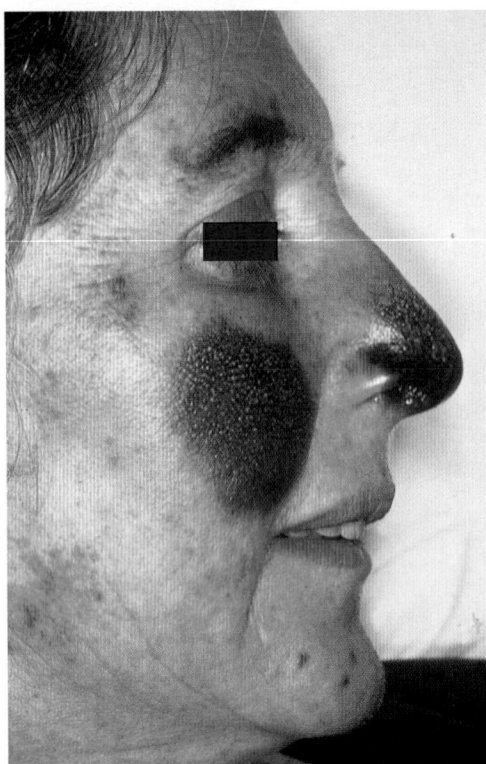

Fig. 17.42
Lupus anticoagulant syndrome: extensive gangrene with ulceration affecting the nose and cheek. By courtesy of C. Stephens, MD, Poole Hospital, Poole, UK.

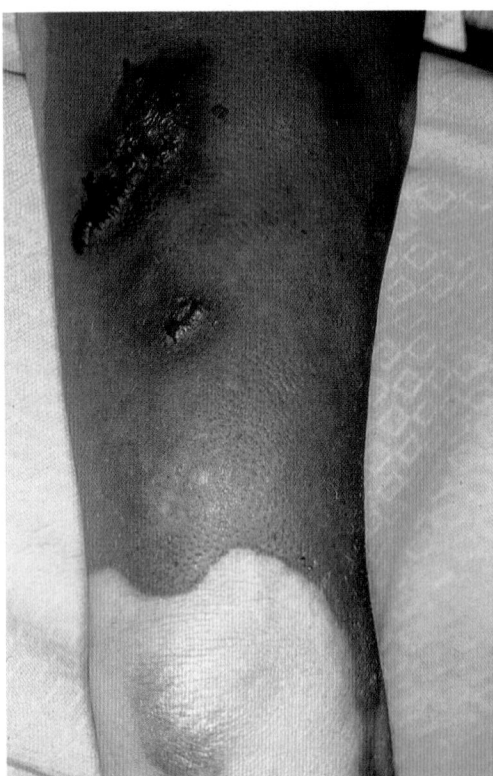

Fig. 17.43
Lupus anticoagulant syndrome: the leg was also involved. By courtesy of C. Stephens, MD, Poole Hospital, Poole, UK.

is not high. Interestingly, patients with clinically significant antiphospholipid antibodies were found to have reduced prevalence of acute cutaneous lupus in comparison to patients without significant antiphospholipid antibodies.[379] Rarely, patients develop reactive angioendotheliomatosis.[380,381] Systemic involvement includes deep venous thrombosis often complicated

by pulmonary embolism, arterial occlusion with resultant strokes, transient ischemic attacks, multi-infarct dementia, myocardial infarction, and gangrene.[356]

The association of cutaneous thrombotic lesions, livedo racemosa, hypertension, and cerebrovascular disease is known as Sneddon syndrome.[358,382–386] This presents mainly in young females and is exceptional in children.[387] Antiphospholipid antibodies are present in around 41% of patients.[388]

How antiphospholipid antibody induces thrombosis is unknown. Theories of inhibition of protein C (a natural vitamin K-dependent anticoagulant) function and a suppressive effect on endothelial cell prostacyclin have not yet been substantiated.[389] The antiphospholipid syndrome has also been documented in other autoimmune diseases including rheumatoid arthritis, hemolytic anemia, thrombocytopenic purpura, ulcerative colitis, factor V Leiden mutation, and mesothelioma.[390,391] It may also complicate treatment with a number of drugs, including phenothiazines and procainamide, develop during viral illnesses, including acquired immunodeficiency syndrome (AIDS), and can present with an underlying lymphoma.[392,393] The antiphospholipid syndrome is further discussed elsewhere.

Anti-Ro antibodies have been shown to bind to the epidermis in neonatal and subacute lupus erythematosus, and to the conducting system and myocardium in neonatal lupus erythematosus.[262] They also bind to keratinocytes in vitro and have been shown to react with the epidermis when infused into human-skin-grafted mice.[394,395] This – combined with the disappearance of the cutaneous manifestations as maternal IgG is removed from the circulation – suggests that in neonatal lupus erythematosus, anti-Ro antibodies are of major pathogenetic significance. Ro antigens are present in the nuclei and cytoplasm of keratinocytes and it has been demonstrated that UVB is capable of translocating these antigens to the surface of cultured keratinocytes. Anti-Ro antibodies in the sera bind to the antigens in keratinocytes and appear to be important in inducing antibody-dependent keratinocyte damage.[396,397]

Anti-C1q antibodies are present in roughly 30% of patients with SLE.[398] A combination of anti-C1q antibodies, anti-dsDNA antibodies, and low complement has been proven to be the most reliable serological marker of lupus nephritis.[398]

Immune complexes have been shown to be important in the pathogenesis of both vasculitis and glomerulonephritis in SLE; their presence may be inferred by the detection of immunoglobulin and complement in blood vessel walls in skin biopsies (*Fig. 17.44*). High concentrations of anti-nDNA, anti-ssDNA, and anti-Ro (SS-A) antibodies have been detected in the renal cortex of patients with lupus glomerulonephritis. The finding of large numbers of T lymphocytes and macrophages with minimal or no B cells in the dermal infiltrate of skin lesions suggests that cell-mediated immunity may be particularly important in the pathogenesis of lesions at this site.[396,399] Both delayed hypersensitivity and antibody-dependent cellular cytotoxicity mechanisms have been proposed.[392]

There is a striking female predominance in SLE, suggesting that female sex hormones are of pathogenetic significance.[19] Interestingly, in the experimental model of SLE in rabbits, females have a much more serious form of glomerulonephritis than do their male counterparts and this difference can be negated by castration or the administration of male sex hormones.[392]

There is, without question, a genetic predisposition to the development of SLE.[400] There are many examples of familial incidence, and immunoglobulin abnormalities have often been documented in asymptomatic relatives; indeed, as many as seven members in a single family have been recorded.[221] Lupus erythematosus has also been reported in identical twins.[221] HLA typing has revealed an increased incidence of HLA-A1, HLA-B8, HLA-B15, HLA-DR2, and HLA-DR3 in SLE.[12] It has been suggested that expression of the disease may be inherited as an autosomal dominant trait. HLA-DR4 is associated with hydralazine-induced lupus erythematosus. The frequencies of HLA-DRw6 and HLA-B8 are increased in DLE.[12] It has recently been demonstrated that patients with polymorphic light eruption and HLA-DRB1*0301 have a higher risk of developing either subacute or discoid lupus erythematosus.[401,402] The familial clustering of polymorphic light eruption in relatives of persons with lupus erythematosus suggests that these diseases may share a similar pathogenesis.[403]

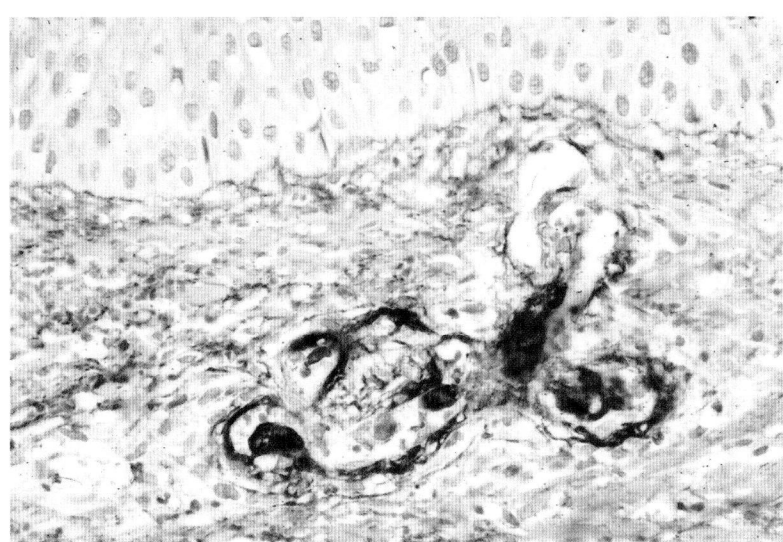

Fig. 17.44
Systemic lupus erythematosus: immunoperoxidase reaction demonstrating IgG within a blood vessel wall.

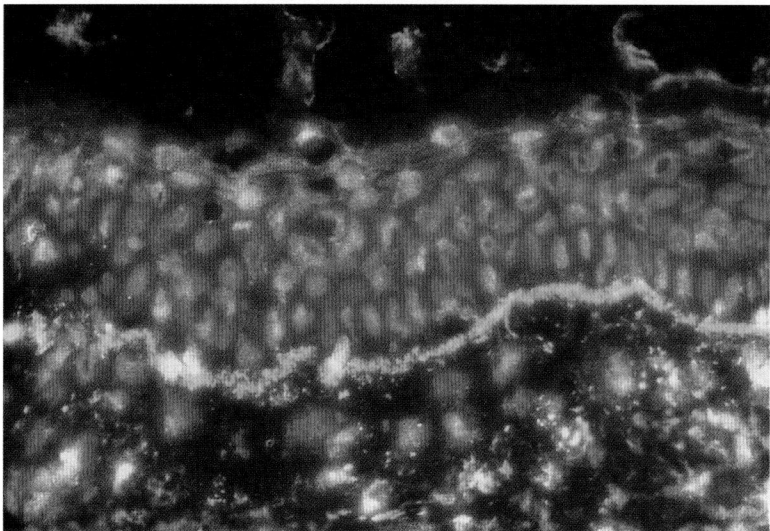

Fig. 17.45
Systemic lupus erythematosus: positive band test (IgG). By courtesy of the Department of Immunofluorescence, Institute of Dermatology, London, UK.

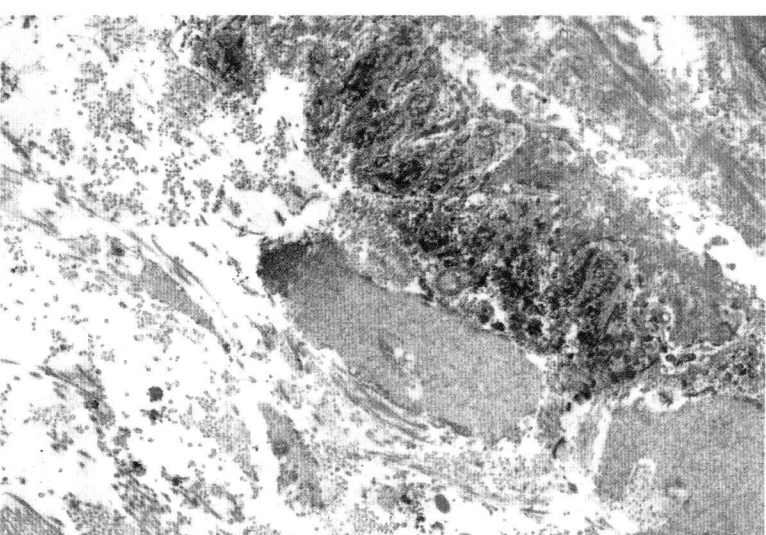

Fig. 17.46
Lupus band test: immunoelectron microscopy (frozen section) showing IgM deposition below the lamina densa.

SCLE has been demonstrated to be associated with the TNF-308A allele.[404,405] Association between SCLE and single nucleotide polymorphism in the TNF-alpha (TNF-α) gene promoter and gene that encodes C1qA chain of C1q has been demonstrated.[226,405] Transcription of TNF-α appears to be photoregulated in subacute lupus.[405] TNF-alpha, produced by keratinocytes, has been localized within refractory lesions of SCLE, suggesting its potential role in the pathogenesis of SCLE.[406] Abnormal regulation of DNA methylation in CD4+ T lymphocytes has recently been implicated in the pathogenesis of SCLE.[407] Triggering mechanisms in lupus erythematosus include UV light (both naturally occurring and artificial), drugs, and, possibly, viruses. Sunlight commonly worsens the cutaneous manifestations and may exacerbate systemic disease.[221,408,409] Antibodies to UV DNA have been identified in patients with SLE.[410] These may be important in the pathogenesis of the photosensitivity-induced lesions. Lesions are typically worse in spring and summer, and cutaneous lesions can be induced artificially by UV irradiation. Dysregulation of apoptosis has been suggested as an important mechanism in the pathogenesis of lupus erythematosus. A reduction of bcl-2 expression in epidermal basal cells is associated with overexpression of FAS antigen and this appears to correlate with the extent of apoptosis in the epidermis.[411]

Despite early enthusiasm for a viral etiology for lupus erythematosus, extensive research has not provided convincing evidence. For many years paramyxovirus-like inclusions within the cytoplasm of endothelial cells were thought to represent evidence of a viral cause.[412] They are now known to represent a non-specific membranous byproduct (tubuloreticular body) of organelle degeneration. An association with parvovirus (erythrovirus) B19 has been suggested.[413] Two experimental virus-induced animal models – Aleutian mink disease and New Zealand black–white hybrid mouse disease – have been described.[19] Recent investigations have shown that the latter is associated with a primary stem cell defect. Bone marrow grafts can therefore transfer the disease to previously irradiated normal recipients and induce tolerance defects.[414] Bone marrow cultures produce B cells with an increased capacity for antibody synthesis.[405] Murine lupus shows a striking similarity to its human counterpart. Interestingly, native (double-stranded) DNA antibodies were detected more often among smokers with SLE than in nonsmokers with SLE.[415] Indeed, a large study encompassing 405 patients with lupus erythematosus confirmed high association between smoking, discoid lupus, and lupus tumidus.[416]

The lupus band test is particularly important in the diagnosis of lupus erythematosus. It is also, to a lesser extent, of some value in assessing prognosis. By either immunofluorescence or immunoperoxidase techniques, the presence of immunoglobulin and complement is sought at the dermal–epidermal junction (Fig. 17.45). IgM is most commonly identified, although IgG, IgA, and C3 are also frequently present.[417] IgG deposits appear to

be the most specific for lupus erythematosus. Other factors that may be identified include properdin, C1q, and C4.[418] Deposition of the membrane attack complex (MAC) has also been shown to be a relatively sensitive and specific marker of cutaneous lupus erythematosus.[419,420] Although deposits are usually homogeneous, granular and thready (reticular) patterns are also recognized.[417] Homogeneous bands are typical of chronic lesions, granular bands are seen in uninvolved skin, and thready deposits are usually a feature of early lesions.[420] Ultrastructurally, the immunoreactants are present in the sub-basal lamina connective tissue and intimately associated with reduplicated lamina densa (Fig. 17.46).[12] The immunoglobulin deposition does not necessarily correlate with the clinical or histologic presence of cutaneous lesions and is therefore unlikely to be of pathogenetic significance.

The lupus band test is positive in involved skin in approximately 50% to 94% of patients with SLE, 60% to 80% of those with the discoid variant, 60% of patients with SCLE, and 50% of infants with neonatal lupus erythematosus.[417,418,420–423] Lesional mucosa also shows immunoreactant deposition and this can be of particular value in patients where histologic distinction from lichen planus proves impossible.[24] It may also be positive in uninvolved skin in up to 67% of patients with systemic disease.[422] The prevalence of a positive test in uninvolved skin depends upon the site, with the highest incidence in skin from the shoulder (70%). Sun-exposed skin, such as the dorsal aspect of the forearms, is more frequently positive (60–70%) than non-sun-exposed skin (50–60%). However, the observation that 20% of specimens of sun-exposed normal skin from healthy young adults show a positive lupus band test indicates that non-sun-exposed skin is the substrate of choice.[424]

Positivity also depends upon the duration of the disease (lesions less than 3 months old are often negative) and the effect of previous steroid therapy.[425] Much less often, positive immunofluorescence is seen in the uninvolved skin of patients with DLE.[426] The results must, however, be taken in the context of the clinical information. A positive IgM lupus band test may be seen in unrelated conditions, such as solar keratosis, polymorphous light eruption, rosacea, lymphocytic infiltrate, and dermatomyositis, and as a consequence of UV radiation.[429,422] These latter conditions are usually associated with C3 deposition or a single immunoglobulin class, particularly IgM, in contrast to the multiple immunoglobulin subclasses found in lupus erythematosus.[420] In nonlupus conditions the lupus band is usually fainter and patchy.[426] With such a significant false-positive rate, it is stressed that the results of a lupus band test must be interpreted with considerable caution and always in the context of the clinical information and histologic features.

A characteristic particulate dust-like deposition of immunoglobulin (predominantly IgG) affecting the basal cells of the epidermis has been described in patients with SCLE.[395,427] Sometimes suprabasal epidermis, adnexal epithelium, and the dermal cellular infiltrate show similar fluorescence.[418,427] This pattern of deposition correlates with the presence of Ro antibodies.[422] It is also occasionally evident in SLE. In some cases speckled nuclear staining of keratinocytes for IgG is seen in connective tissue diseases.[428] In the setting of SLE, this finding appears to be associated with a lower incidence of renal disease.[428]

The histopathological features of the various subsets of lupus erythematosus (with the exceptions of lupus erythematosus profundus and bullous dermatosis of SLE) show considerable overlap and their distinction by microscopic techniques is often difficult.[429,430]

Discoid lupus erythematosus

DLE displays variable features, depending upon the stage of the disease.[12,423,424] The active lesion is characterized by hyperkeratosis and follicular dilatation with keratin plugging; occasionally, focal parakeratosis is present (Figs 17.47–17.49). The epidermis is usually atrophic and rather flattened, although sometimes there is acanthosis (Fig. 17.50). The most significant features seen at the dermal–epidermal junction are:

- liquefactive degeneration of the basal layer of the epidermis (Fig. 17.51),
- basement membrane thickening (Fig. 17.52), which may be accentuated by use of the periodic acid-Schiff (PAS) reaction.

These two features may additionally affect follicular epithelium, and basement membrane thickening of the dermal blood vessels is also sometimes evident (Fig. 17.53). Liquefactive degeneration of the basal layer of the epidermis is often accompanied by pigmentary incontinence (Fig. 17.54). In some instances the epidermal changes are accompanied by cytoid body formation, but this is not usually as conspicuous as in lichen planus (Fig. 17.55). Amyloid formation may occasionally be seen.

The papillary dermis is edematous, and telangiectatic vessels are often present (Fig. 17.56). Focal extravasations of red blood cells are sometimes seen (Fig. 17.57). Characteristic of DLE is a perivascular and periappendageal chronic inflammatory cell infiltrate of lymphocytes and variable numbers of histiocytes (Figs 17.58 and 17.59). The most common cells are the T lymphocytes, both helper and suppressor cells.[399,400] Neutrophil polymorphs and plasma cells are not usually evident. However, the presence of neutrophils and leukocytoclasia has been described in the lupus-like lesions of a patient with a lupus-like dermatosis with X-linked chronic granulomatous disease.[68] CD4+ cells predominate in DLE skin lesions.[399] The majority of these T lymphocytes are Ia+, indicating an activated state. Occasional CD4+ cells are present in the epidermis closely related to foci of basal keratinocyte damage.[399] Epidermal Langerhans cells are usually reduced in number.[397] B lymphocytes are generally present in only small numbers. The infiltrate is typically sparse in the papillary dermis, but focal dense aggregates are

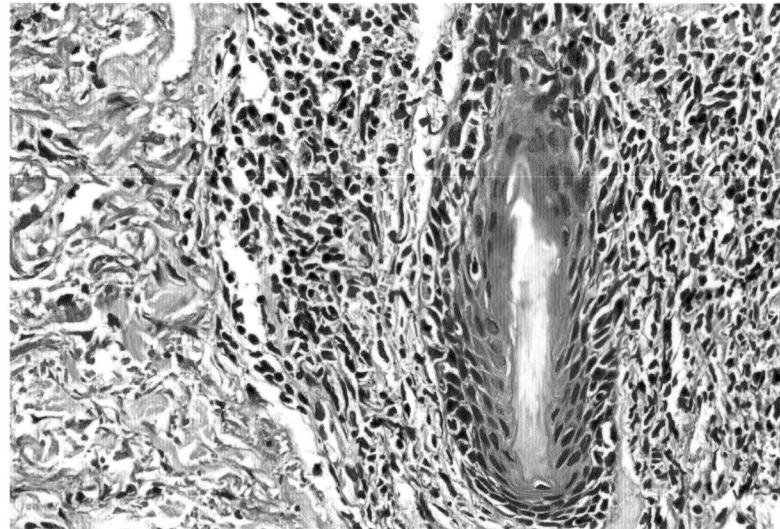

Fig. 17.48
Discoid lupus erythematosus: note the perifollicular lymphocytic infiltrate.

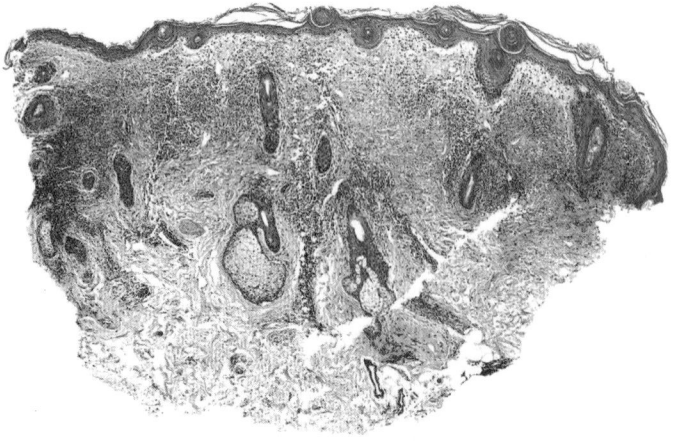

Fig. 17.47
Discoid lupus erythematosus: this scanning view shows hyperkeratosis, follicular plugging, an atrophic epidermis, and a perivascular and periadnexal chronic inflammatory cell infiltrate.

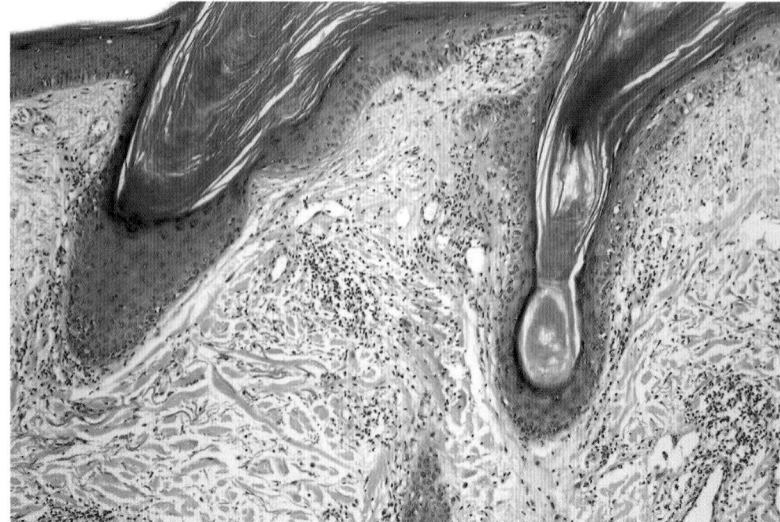

Fig. 17.49
Discoid lupus erythematosus: there is marked follicular plugging.

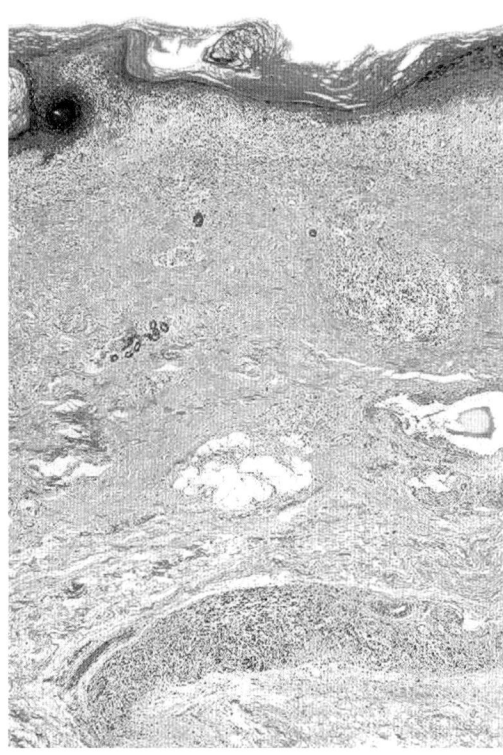

Fig. 17.50
Discoid lupus erythematosus: there is hyperkeratosis and atrophy of the epidermis.

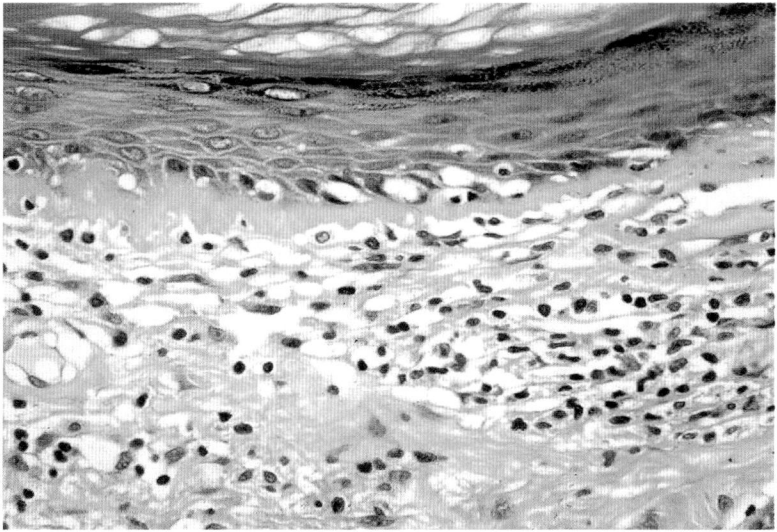

Fig. 17.51
Discoid lupus erythematosus: in this view there is hyperkeratosis, epidermal atrophy, and basal cell hydropic degeneration.

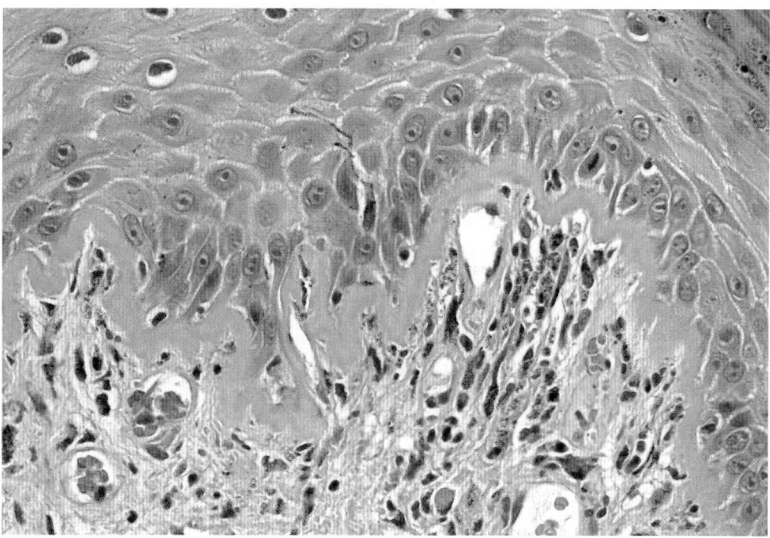

Fig. 17.52
Discoid lupus erythematosus: note the very marked thickening of the basement membrane and pigmentary incontinence.

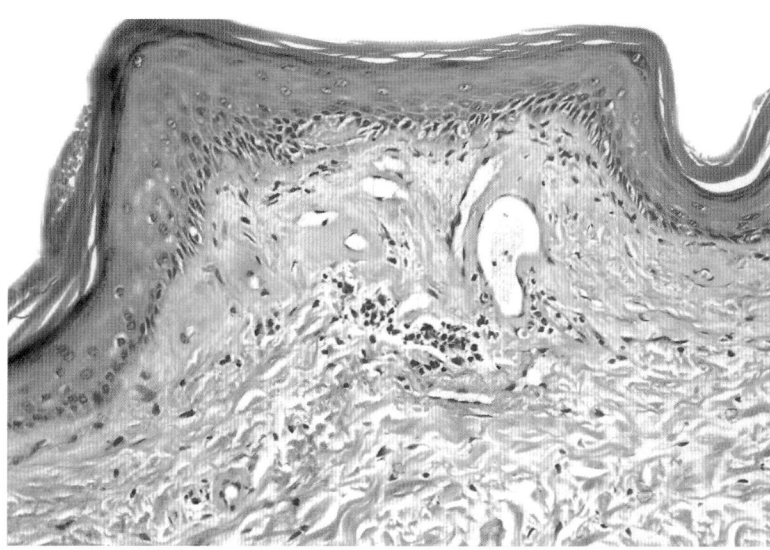

Fig. 17.53
Discoid lupus erythematosus: there is marked blood vessel wall thickening with hyalinization.

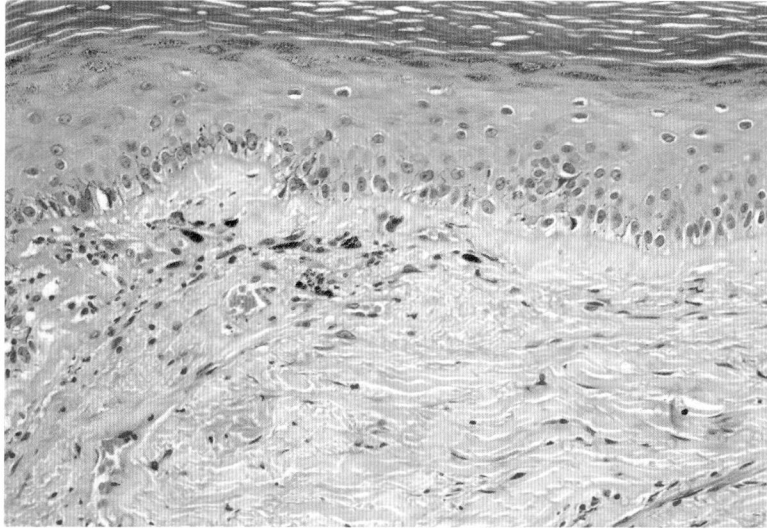

Fig. 17.54
Discoid lupus erythematosus: note the pigmentary incontinence.

characteristically found in the reticular dermis and may sometimes extend into the subcutaneous fat.

An increase in glycosaminoglycans (acid mucopolysaccharides) in the dermis is a common feature of the acute lesion (*Fig. 17.60*); in tumid lupus this is very marked (*Figs 17.61* and *17.62*). Most uncommonly, however, dermal deposition of mucin in discoid lupus can be extensive, presenting clinically as papulonodular mucinosis.[431] Very rarely, dermal calcification has been documented (*Fig. 17.63*).[432] Exceptionally 'fibrinoid' change of the dermal collagen is present (*Fig. 17.64*).

The presence of plasmacytoid dendritic cells representing more than 10% of the dermal inflammatory cells infiltrate, their arrangement in clusters, or their presence at the dermal–epidermal junction has been demonstrated to

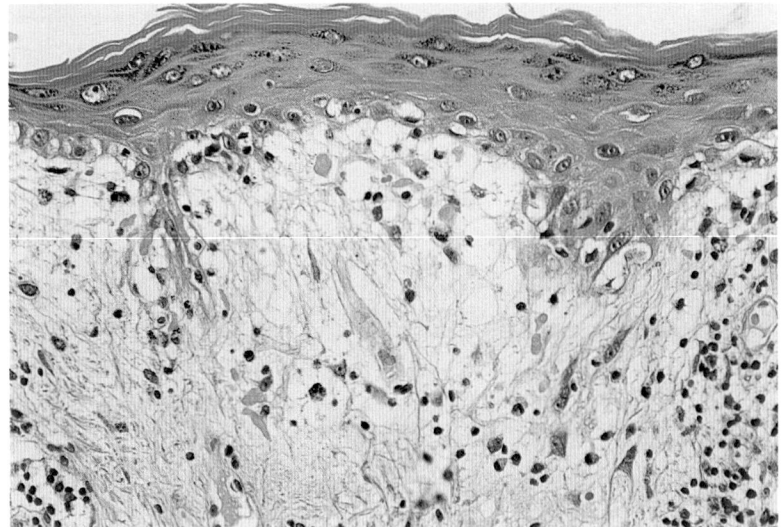

Fig. 17.55
Discoid lupus erythematosus: several cytoid bodies are present in the papillary dermis. Note the hydropic degeneration.

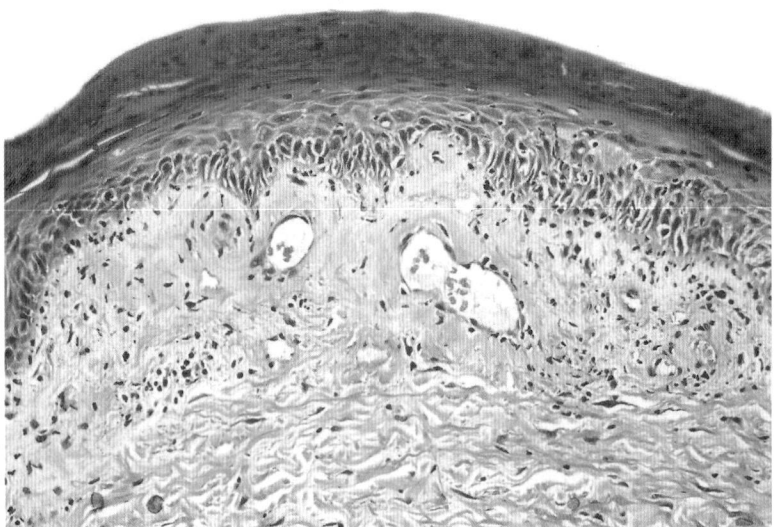

Fig. 17.56
Discoid lupus erythematosus: note the telangiectatic vessels in the superficial dermis.

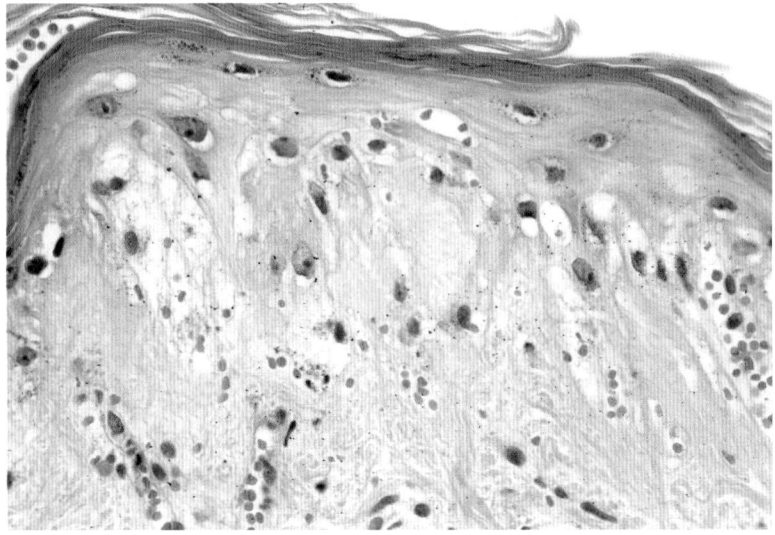

Fig. 17.57
Discoid lupus erythematosus: in addition to hyperkeratosis and epidermal atrophy there is quite marked red cell extravasation.

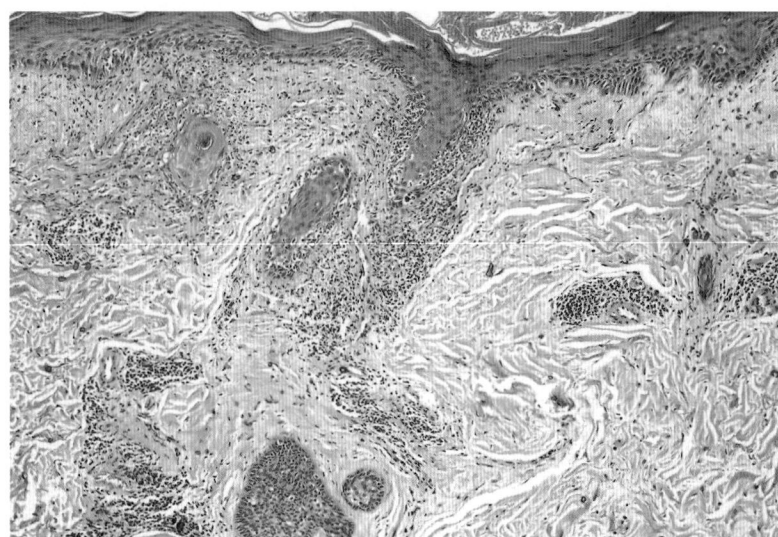

Fig. 17.58
Discoid lupus erythematosus: blood vessels and hair follicles are surrounded by a characteristic heavy lymphohistiocytic infiltrate.

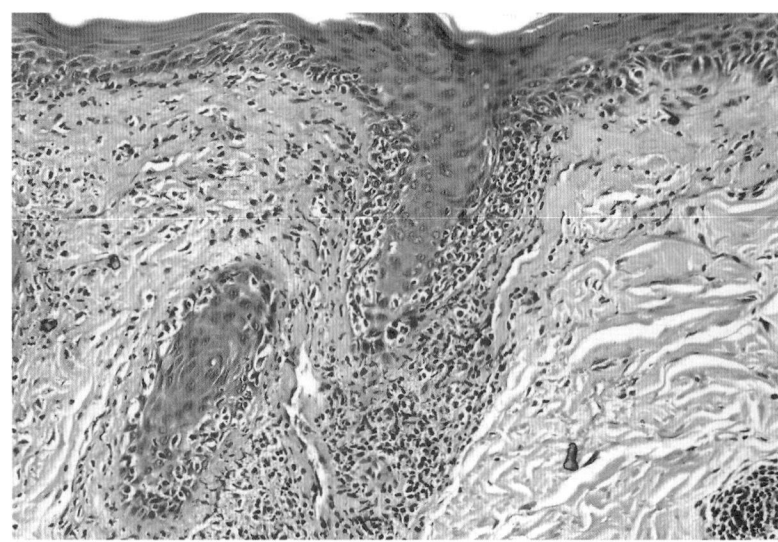

Fig. 17.59
Discoid lupus erythematosus: the follicular epithelium shows basal cell hydropic degeneration and there is a heavy lymphocytic infiltrate.

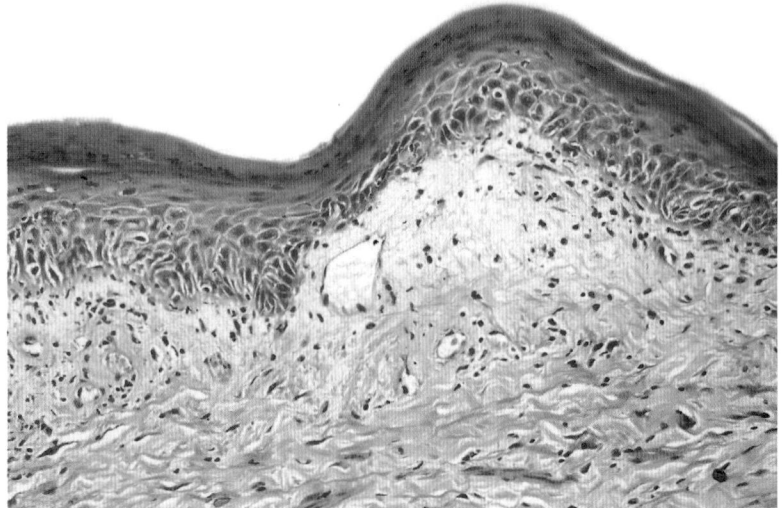

Fig. 17.60
Discoid lupus erythematosus: stromal mucin deposition, as seen in this field, is not uncommon.

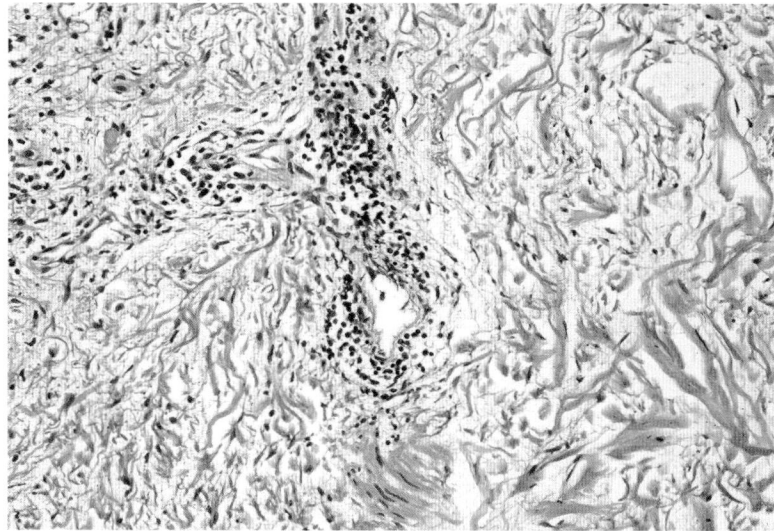

Fig. 17.61
Tumid discoid lupus erythematosus: in this rare variant, there is very marked mucin deposition. By courtesy of J. Cohen, MD, Dermatopathology Laboratory, Tucson, USA.

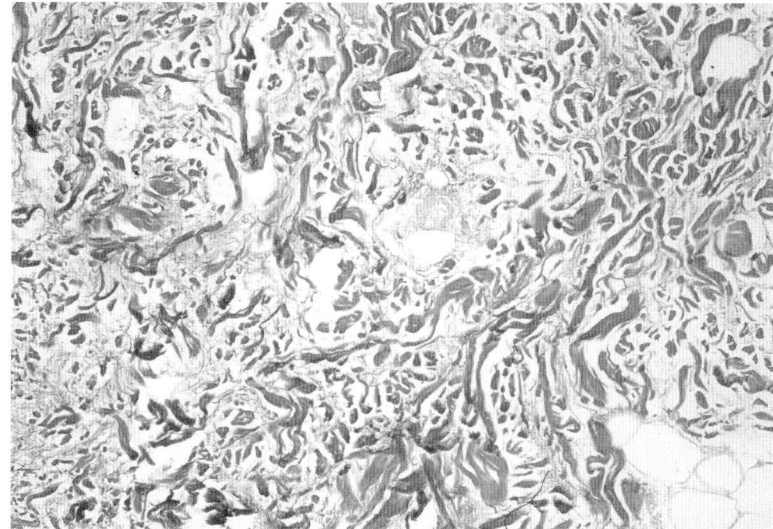

Fig. 17.62
Tumid discoid lupus erythematosus: the mucin stains with Alcian blue, pH 2.5. By courtesy of J. Cohen, MD, Dermatopathology Laboratory, Tucson, USA.

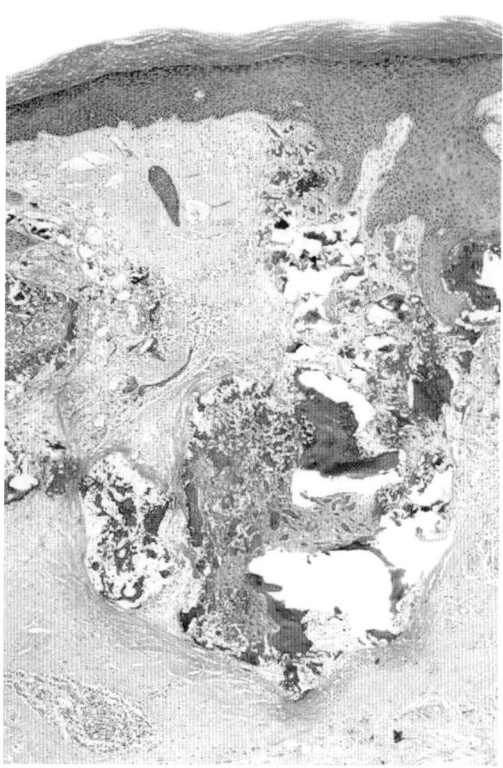

Fig. 17.63
Discoid lupus erythematosus: calcification is a rare feature. In this example, there is striking transepidermal elimination.

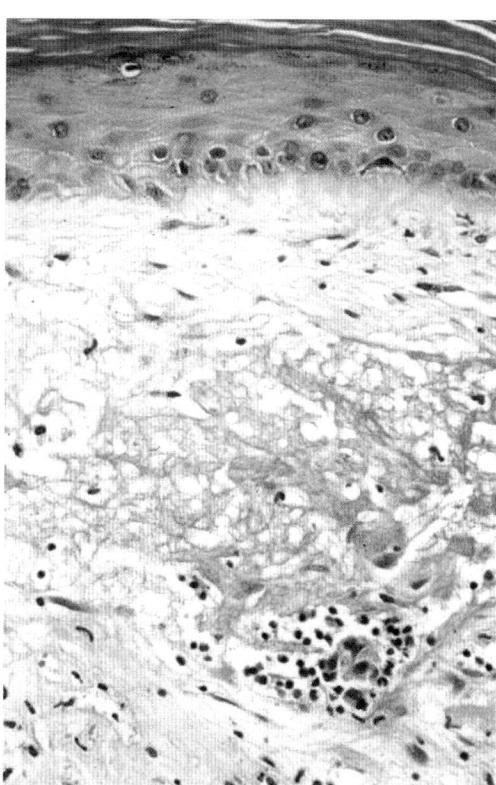

Fig. 17.64
Discoid lupus erythematosus: note the presence of fibrinoid necrosis. This is more usually a feature of the systemic variant.

have significant diagnostic value in discoid and verrucous (hypertrophic) lupus erythematosus.[433]

In the healing lesion of DLE there is hyperkeratosis and the epidermis may be atrophic or, more commonly, slightly thickened. The basement membrane region is characteristically markedly thickened. The dermis is fibrosed, sometimes to a degree that resembles lichen sclerosus (*Fig. 17.65*). In hair-bearing sites, particularly the scalp, there may be very marked follicular plugging with associated chronic inflammation, and in advanced disease there is often complete loss of the pilosebaceous structures with replacement by collagenous fibrous strands (*Fig. 17.66*).[430] Sebaceous gland atrophy or loss occurs early in scalp involvement, and the chronic inflammatory changes are centered at the level of the mid follicle.[20] It has been suggested that this may represent a focus of follicular stem cells and therefore chronic inflammation at this site could readily result in permanent hair loss. Secondary amyloid deposition, derived from degenerating epidermal keratinocytes, can occasionally be detected in the papillary dermis.[434]

Rarely, DLE may present as a dense superficial and deep perivascular and periappendageal infiltrate in the absence of significant epidermal changes: distinction from lymphocytic infiltrate of Jessner and polymorphous light eruption is, therefore, histologically impossible.[430]

In hypertrophic lesions there is marked hyperkeratosis, hypergranulosis, and irregular acanthosis with papillomatosis in addition to the features of basal cell damage.[12] Cytoid bodies are often conspicuous in the lower epidermis.[430] Amyloid deposition has been reported as a frequent finding.[435] The features are commonly histologically indistinguishable from hypertrophic

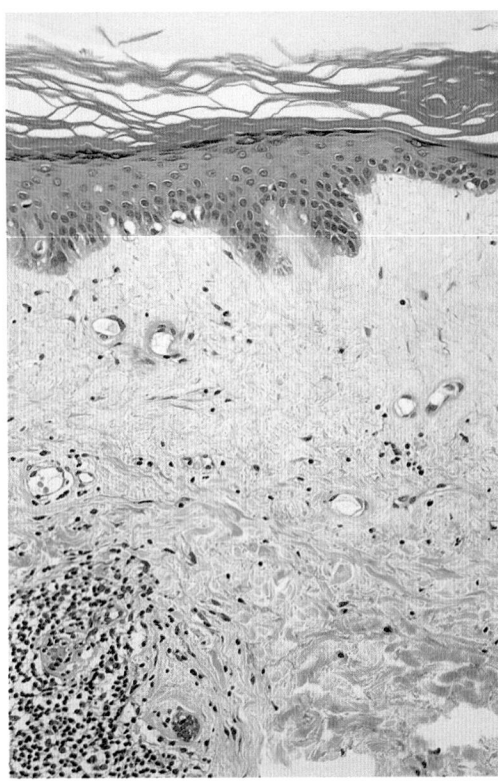

Fig. 17.65
Discoid lupus erythematosus: in this example, the presence of superficial dermal sclerosis is reminiscent of lichen sclerosus.

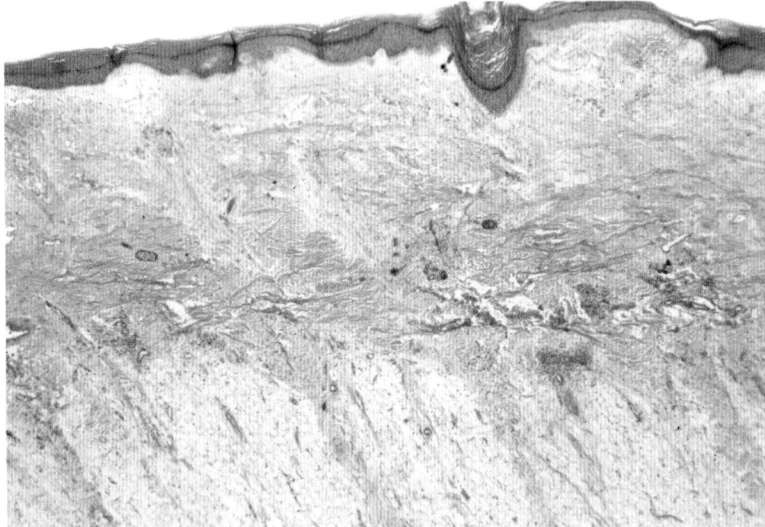

Fig. 17.66
Discoid lupus erythematosus: note the complete absence of hair follicles in this scalp specimen.

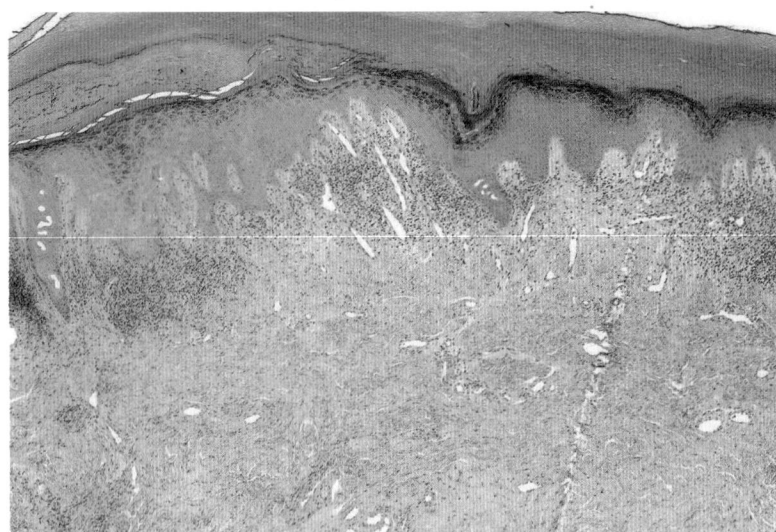

Fig. 17.67
Chilblain lupus erythematosus: there is irregular acanthosis and a superficial lymphocytic infiltrate. Ectatic vessels are conspicuous.

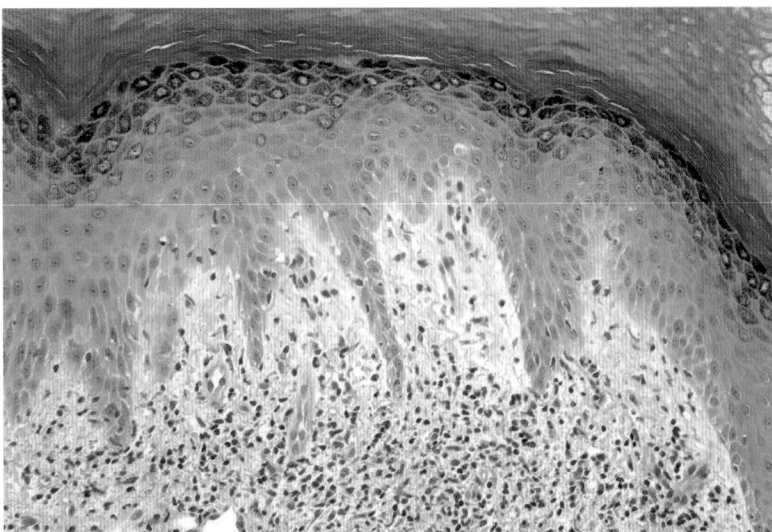

Fig. 17.68
Chilblain lupus erythematosus: in this field, there is marked edema of the papillary dermis.

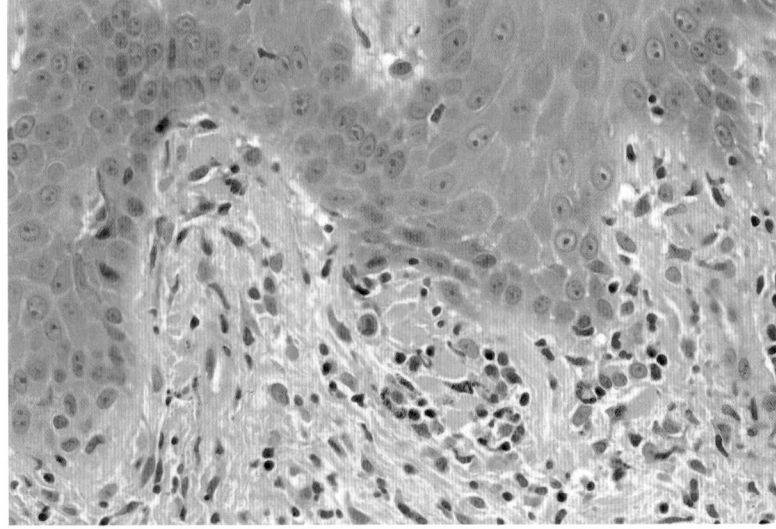

Fig. 17.69
Chilblain lupus erythematosus: there is focal basal cell hydropic degeneration, and cytoid bodies are conspicuous.

lichen planus. The presence of intraepidermal elastic fibers, frequently associated with transepidermal elimination of the elastotic material, has been reported in hypertrophic lupus erythematosus.[45,48] This is not a feature of lichen planus. Resolving or evolving keratoacanthoma may sometimes be mimicked.[48]

Biopsy from patients with lupus pernio reveals a cuffed perivascular lymphocytic infiltrate with edema, red cell extravasation, and variable vascular fibrinoid change (*Figs 17.67–17.70*). Some biopsies show frank lymphocytic vasculitis. The inflammatory infiltrate often extends into the deep dermis and subcutaneous adipose tissue. Interface epidermal changes, ranging from focal vacuolar changes to a lichenoid tissue reaction, are often present.[2,15] Chronic inflammation around sweat glands is sometimes seen.[9,16]

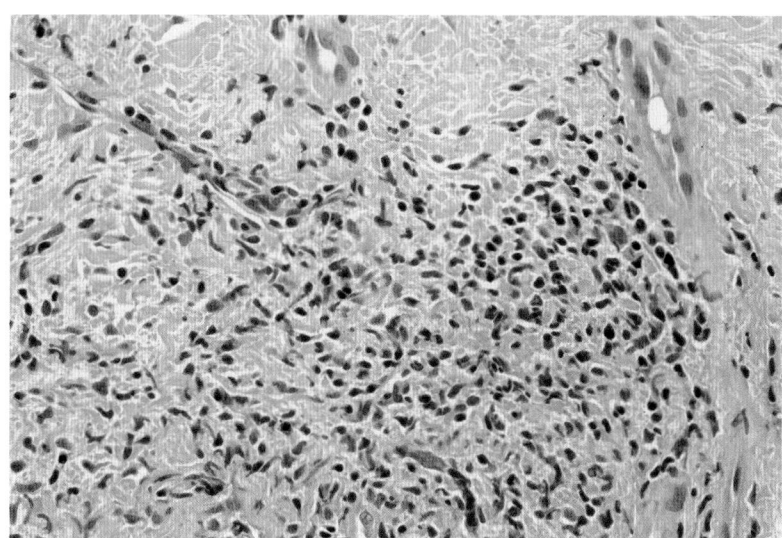

Fig. 17.70
Chilblain lupus erythematosus: there is a dense lymphocytic infiltrate.

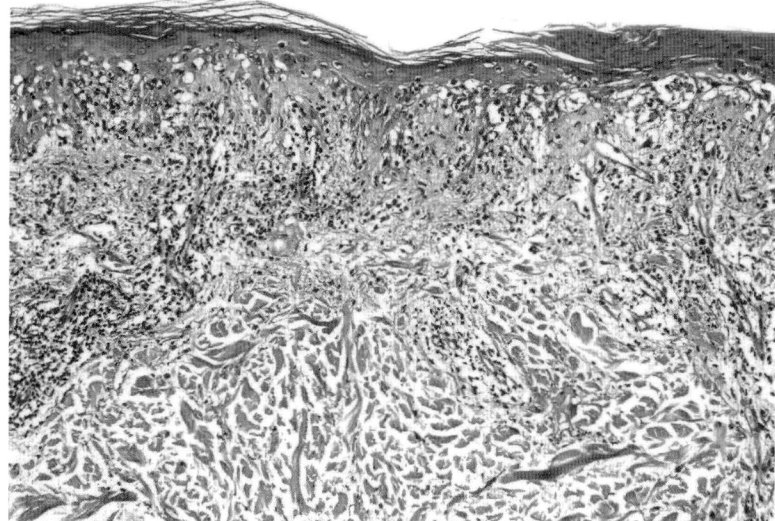

Fig. 17.72
Subacute cutaneous lupus erythematosus: in this example, in addition to basal cell hydropic degeneration, there is intercellular edema of the epidermis with lymphocytic exocytosis.

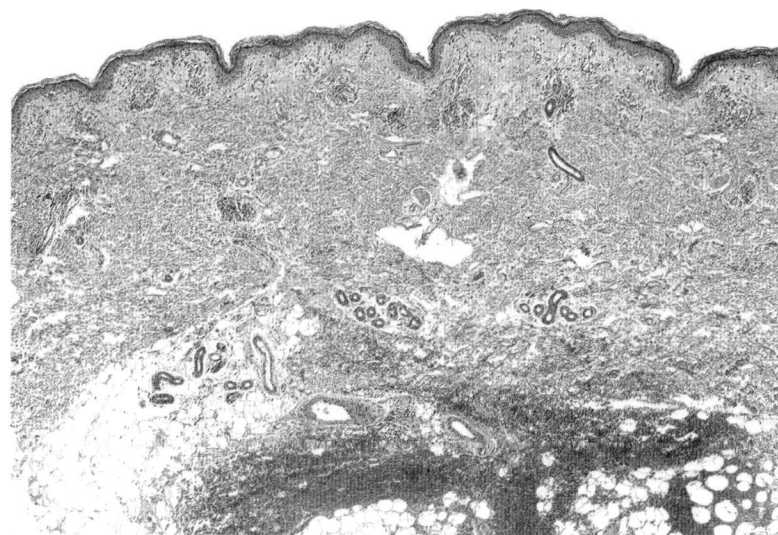

Fig. 17.71
Subacute cutaneous lupus erythematosus: low-power view showing slight hyperkeratosis. A perivascular chronic inflammatory cell infiltrate is present.

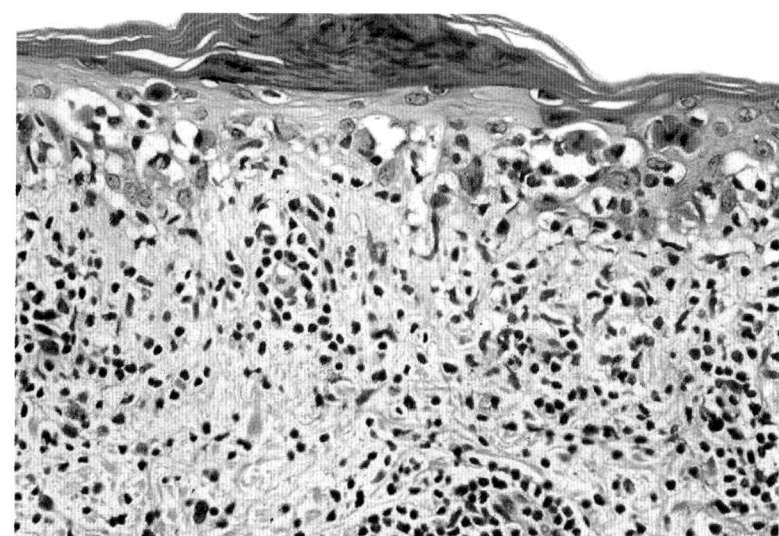

Fig. 17.73
Subacute cutaneous lupus erythematosus: note the presence of numerous cytoid bodies and focal satellite cell necrosis.

Mucous membrane lesions are frequently difficult to distinguish from lichen planus.[23,24,430] They are characterized by hyperkeratosis, often accompanied by parakeratosis. The epithelium may be atrophic or acanthotic. Hydropic degeneration of basal keratinocytes, sometimes associated with cytoid body formation, accompanies a dense lymphohistiocytic infiltrate in which plasma cells are often numerous. The presence of a deep perivascular chronic inflammatory cell infiltrate favors the diagnosis of DLE.[432] Direct immunofluorescence is, however, frequently necessary to establish the diagnosis.[23,24]

Lupus erythematosus profundus

The histologic features of lupus erythematosus profundus are considered in Chapter 10.

Subacute cutaneous lupus erythematosus

Although the histologic features of SCLE show considerable overlap with those of DLE, there are diagnostic pointers.[102,436,437] In SCLE, the hyperkeratosis tends to be mild, atrophy is more marked, and the epidermal ridge pattern is often effaced (Fig. 17.71).[437] Parakeratosis may sometimes be a feature. Basement membrane thickening is minimal or absent, and hair follicles are often unaffected or show only slight keratin plugging.[436,437] In DLE, the inflammatory cell infiltrate is denser, occupies the papillary and

reticular dermis, and often shows perifollicular accentuation. In SCLE, lymphocytic exocytosis may be conspicuous and satellite cell necrosis is not uncommon (Fig. 17.72).[437] Liquefactive degeneration of the basal layer of the epidermis is usually present although often it is only mild (Figs 17.73 and 17.74). Sometimes, however, it is sufficiently marked that subepidermal vesiculation results.[101,105] Homogenization of the papillary dermal collagen is occasionally seen.[437] Colloid body formation and pigmentary incontinence are often inconspicuous, but sometimes they are a major feature.[105] The inflammatory cell infiltrate is typically mild, superficially located, and perivascular in distribution. In some examples, however, it presents as a lichenoid band.[105,114,437] Variable amounts of eosinophils can also be seen in the dermal inflammatory cell infiltrate. This is an entirely non-specific finding not related to the possible drug-induced SCLE.[438]

The histopathological features in cutaneous lesions of patients without SCLE and antibodies to SS-A (Ro) are very similar to those seen in lesions of patients with SCLE.[439] These patients often have different clinical diseases including Sjögren syndrome and rheumatoid arthritis.

Neutrophilic dermatosis of the systemic lupus erythematosus

The histologic features of neutrophilic dermatosis of the SLE are variable. The intensity of neutrophilic infiltrate typically varies from paucicellular

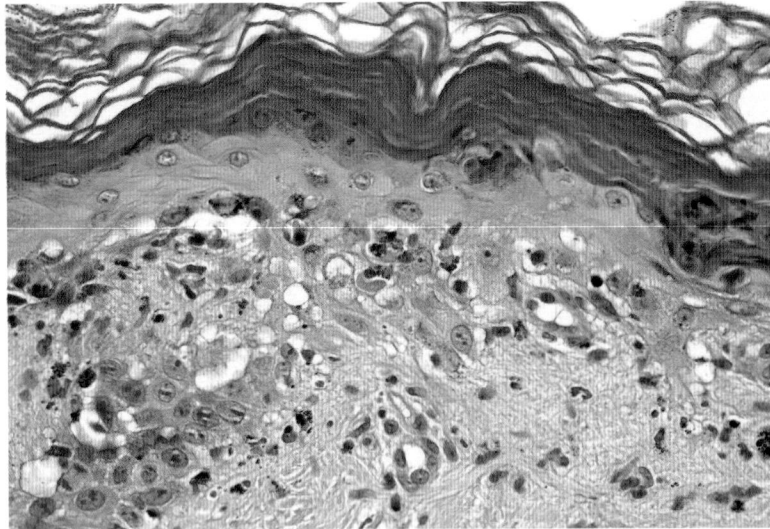

Fig. 17.74
Subacute cutaneous lupus erythematosus: in this example, there is marked basal cell hydropic degeneration and apoptosis. Only a patchy chronic inflammatory cell infiltrate is present.

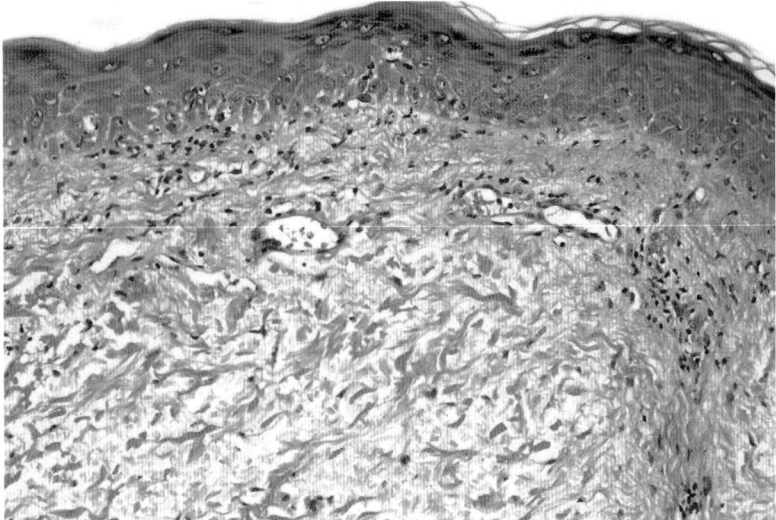

Fig. 17.75
Systemic lupus erythematosus: although the changes may be identical to the discoid or subacute variants, sometimes the features are mild, as in this case. There is focal basal cell hydropic degeneration, apoptosis, and telangiectasia.

neutrophilic infiltrates in the papillary dermis to moderately or highly cellular neutrophilic infiltrates in perivascular and interstitial distribution frequently admixed with nuclear debris spanning the entire dermis, with possible extension into the subcutaneous fatty tissue.[190,192,196,197] Neutrophilic inflammatory cell infiltrate is generally accompanied by leukocytoclasia, while vasculitis is absent as a rule.[190,192,196,197] In addition to dermal neutrophilic infiltrates, a recent paper found the presence of neutrophils within the epithelium of the epidermis, hair follicles, sebaceous glands, and sweat glands to be highly suggestive of neutrophilic urticarial dermatosis.[202] Additional histologic features, which are helpful indicators of possible association with lupus erythematosus, and are present to a variable extent and frequency, include interface dermatitis, vacuolar degeneration of basal keratinocytes, thickening of the basement membrane, follicular plugging, and dermal mucin deposition.[190,192,196,197] Direct immunofluorescence testing usually reveals a positive lupus band test.[193,196]

Histologic differential diagnosis mainly depends upon the intensity of the neutrophilic infiltrate. Examples with paucicellular neutrophilic infiltrates in the papillary dermis should mainly be distinguished from bullous SLE, dermatitis herpetiformis, and linear IgA disease – immunofluorescence analysis is crucial for this distinction. Differential diagnosis of more prominent neutrophilic infiltrates includes Still disease, Sweet syndrome, Behçet disease, and infections.[193,196]

Systemic lupus erythematosus

The histologic features of SLE are variable. The changes in early lesions, which may be very mild and subtle, often comprise only slight epidermal basal cell liquefactive degeneration, papillary dermal edema, and a mild chronic inflammatory cell infiltrate, and are seen, for example, in malar erythema (*Fig. 17.75*).[115,419] On other occasions the appearances are similar to those of SCLE.

The histology of SLE is often indistinguishable from that of the discoid variant (*Fig. 17.76*). Fibrinoid degeneration of the dermal collagen is, however, more common in SLE than in DLE. Dermal mucin deposition is often seen between collagen bundles. In most cases, this feature is subtle, but mucin deposition may be very prominent.[440] A thick basal membrane is more commonly seen in lesions of DLE. As with DLE, the commonest cell type is the T lymphocyte, but which subset predominates is uncertain. Both CD4+ and CD4+ subset preponderance have been documented.[397,399] It may be that differences in the age of the lesion, effects of treatment, and antibody specificity can account for this apparent anomaly. CD4+ lymphocytes are present in large numbers in the epidermis at sites of basal keratinocyte hydropic degeneration.[397]

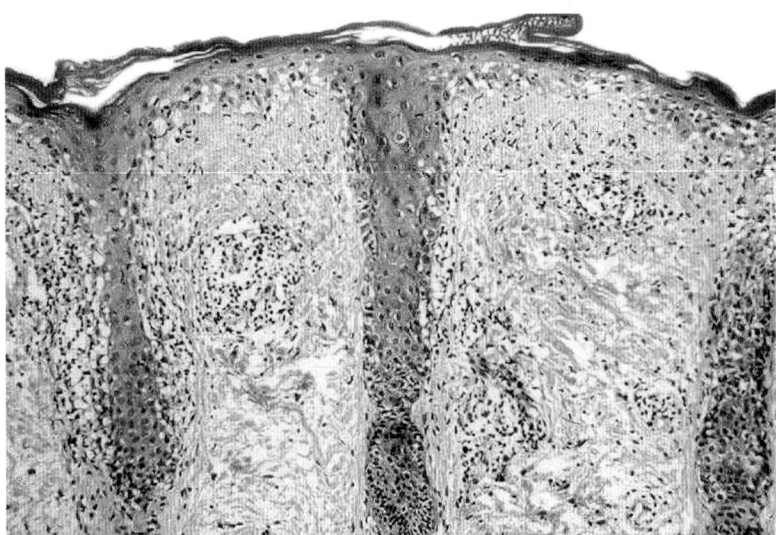

Fig. 17.76
Systemic lupus erythematosus: in this example, the features resemble the discoid variant. Note the hyperkeratosis, epidermal atrophy, follicular involvement, and gross basal cell hydropic degeneration. A perivascular and perifollicular chronic inflammatory cell infiltrate is present.

The histopathological features of the cutaneous lesions of the antiphospholipid syndrome comprise both venous and arterial thrombosis in the absence of any evidence of vasculitis (*Figs 17.77–17.79*). In early lesions, endothelial cell damage may be marked and erythrocyte extravasation is common. Older lesions are characterized by marked vascular proliferation, commonly in a lobular distribution accompanied by hemosiderosis. Hobnail reactive endothelial cells and eosinophilic hyaline globules are sometimes evident.[392] A lymphocytic infiltrate accompanied by variable numbers of plasma cells is often seen.[392,441,442] In some patients, the clinical and histologic features of Degos disease and anetoderma have been documented.[442]

Renal lesions may be detected in 70% to 80% of patients. The histologic features are subdivided into six classes according to the International Society of Nephrology/Renal Pathology Society 2003 classification of lupus nephritis, representing an evolution of the previous WHO classification:[443,444]

- In class I lesions (minimal mesangial lupus nephritis) no abnormalities can be detected by light microscopy. Mesangial deposition of immune complexes can be identified by immunofluorescence, electron microscopy, or both.

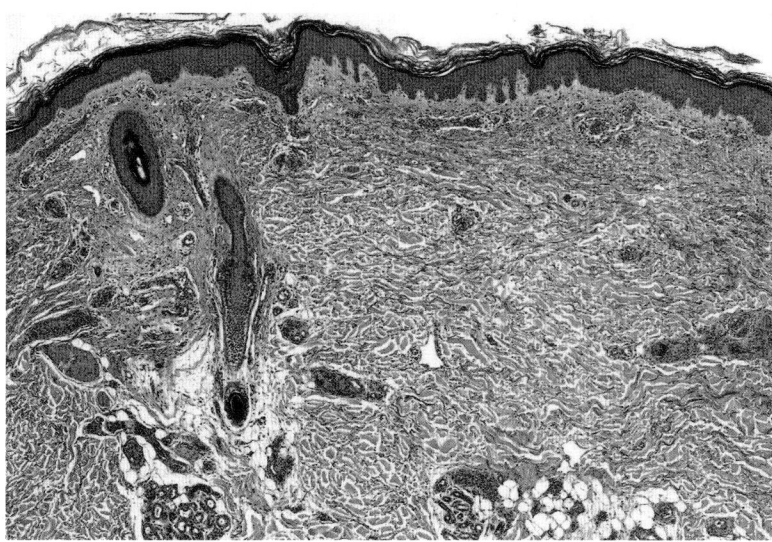

Fig. 17.77
Lupus anticoagulant syndrome: low-power view showing superficial blood vessels occluded by small thrombi.

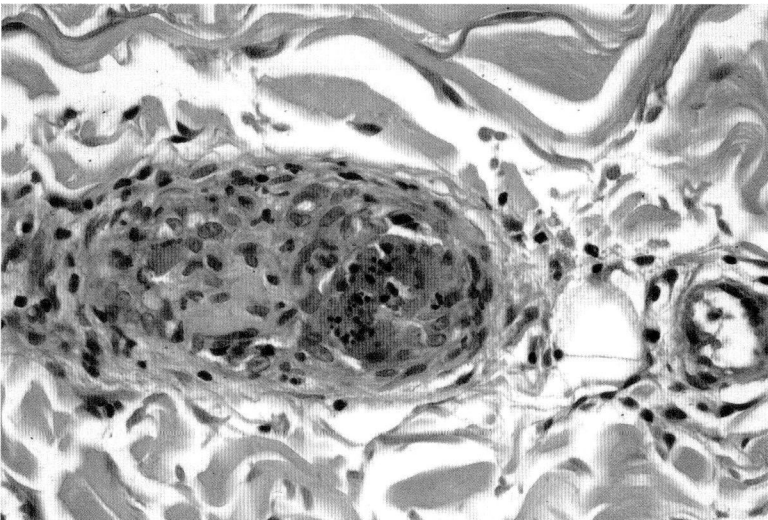

Fig. 17.78
Lupus anticoagulant syndrome: close-up view of occluded vessel – note the nuclear debris.

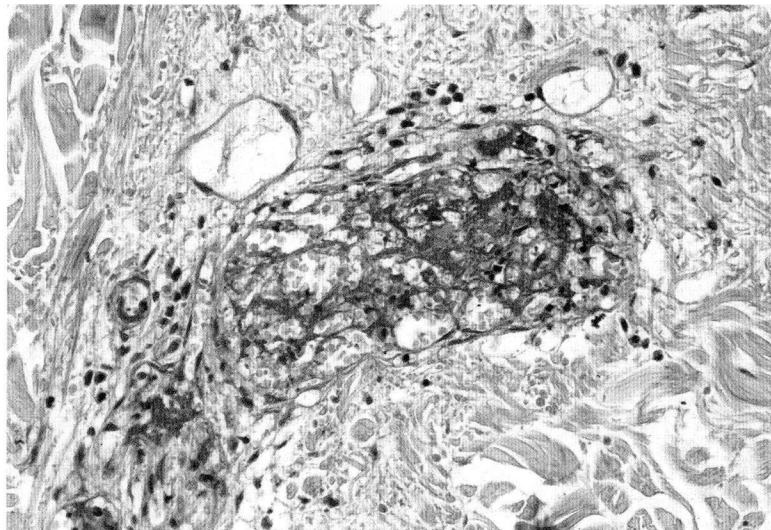

Fig. 17.79
Lupus anticoagulant syndrome: the presence of fibrin is confirmed in this phosphotungstic acid–hematoxylin stained section.

- Class II lesions (mesangial proliferative lupus nephritis) are characterized by any degree of mesangial hypercellularity (defined as three or more mesangial cells per mesangial area in a 3-micron thick section) associated with mesangial immune deposits. Rare small immune deposits involving peripheral capillary walls can occasionally be detected by immunofluorescence or electron microscopy. Features not acceptable are subendothelial deposits on light microscopy as well as any segmental or global glomerular scars resulting from previous glomerular endocapillary proliferation, necrosis, or crescents. Immunofluorescence reveals mesangial deposition of IgG and complement and mesangial electron-dense deposits may be detected by electron microscopy. Mesangial lupus glomerulonephritis is the mildest form of glomerular lesion and is present in about 10% of patients with renal involvement.[443]

- Class III lesions (focal lupus nephritis) are distinguished by active or inactive focal, segmental, or global endo- or extracapillary glomerulonephritis involving <50% of all glomeruli, associated with focal subendothelial immune deposits, with or without mesangial proliferation. Focal segmental proliferative glomerulonephritis is found in about 30% of patients. In this variant, only scattered glomeruli are affected (focal) and usually only a portion of the tuft is involved (segmental).[443] Lesions may be proliferative and necrotizing. Involved glomeruli usually show mesangial and endothelial proliferation, polymorph infiltration, fibrin deposition, and karyorrhexis; occasionally, hematoxylin bodies are evident. Hematoxylin bodies are regarded as the histologic hallmark of SLE. They are round-to-oval structures, which stain purple/red–pink/blue with hematoxylin and eosin. They stain positively with the Feulgen reaction and are von Kossa negative. Hematoxylin bodies are thought to be the in vivo counterpart of the LE cell phenomenon. Although frequently sought they are often very difficult to find. Electron microscopy typically reveals mesangial and subendothelial electron-dense (immune complex) deposits. Clinically, patients present with hematuria and proteinuria, although a proportion may develop chronic renal failure.

- Class IV lesions (diffuse lupus nephritis) are characterized by active or inactive focal, segmental or global endo- or extracapillary glomerulonephritis involving ≥50% of all glomeruli, associated with diffuse subendothelial immune deposits, with or without mesangial proliferation. They can be further subclassified as diffuse segmental (IV-S) and diffuse global (IV-G) lupus nephritis. Diffuse lupus glomerulonephritis occurs in about 50% of patients with SLE who have the nephritic/nephrotic syndrome or hypertension.[443] Almost all glomeruli are affected and, in addition to mesangial and endothelial proliferation, the epithelial cells may participate, with the formation of crescents. Careful examination of the periphery of the glomerular tuft often reveals regularly thickened capillaries – 'wire-loop' lesions, thought to be specific for SLE.

- Class V (lupus membranous glomerulonephritis) lesions show global or segmental subepithelial granular immune deposits with or without mesangial alterations. Scattered subendothelial immune deposits can also be present. Class V lesions can be associated with both class III and class IV lesions. Lupus membranous glomerulonephritis is found in about 10% of patients with SLE and presents as proteinuria or the nephrotic syndrome.[443] Histologically, there is uniform thickening of the glomerular capillaries without any significant inflammatory cell infiltration. Advanced glomerulosclerosis can be present. Ultrastructurally, the electron-dense deposits are found subepithelially.

- Class VI lesions (advanced sclerosis lupus nephritis) are characterized by global sclerosis without residual activity in ≥90% of glomeruli, related to lupus nephritis. They can represent progression of class III, IV or V lesions.

In addition to glomerular lesions, patients with renal involvement may manifest acute necrotizing vasculitis.

The heart is involved in about 50% of patients with SLE. Acute lesions of fibrinoid degeneration and hematoxylin bodies may be seen in the pericardium, but it is more common to find obliteration of the pericardial sac by fibrous, sometimes gelatinous, adhesions. Fibrinoid necrosis of the myocardial collagen is usually found in the connective tissue septa and occasionally also affects the associated arteries. Libman-Sacks endocarditis is the best-known cardiac manifestation of SLE and is believed to occur in 30% to 60% of the patients who come to autopsy.[223] Small granular vegetations have been found on the surfaces of all valves, although the mitral and tricuspid are most often affected. The vegetations may spread to involve the chordae tendinae and adjacent endocardium. Histologically, they consist of fibrin overlying degenerate collagen, with an associated chronic inflammatory cell infiltrate. Infective endocarditis is an occasional, but important, complication. Increased quantities of glycosaminoglycans are usually evident and sometimes hematoxylin bodies are present.

The histologic lesions of pulmonary involvement include interstitial pneumonitis, fibrosing alveolitis, and infarction. In a large autopsy study of patients with SLE, pleuropulmonary involvement has been detected in 97.8% of patients, and included pleuritis (77.8%), bacterial infections (57.8%), primary and secondary alveolar hemorrhage (25.6%), distal airways alterations (21.1%), opportunistic infections (14.4%), and thromboembolism (7.8%).[445] Direct immunofluorescent examination of lung biopsies may reveal the presence of both immunoglobulin and complement.

Lymph nodes often show reactive hyperplasia; occasionally there are striking pathological features, which may be confused with a lymphomatous infiltrate. These changes consist of a necrotizing lymphadenitis with prominent hematoxylin bodies. Surviving follicles show reactive hyperplasia and conspicuous plasma cells and immunoblasts. The thymus may show prominent germinal center formation, with an increase in the size and number of Hassall corpuscles. Perisplenitis ('sugar icing') of the splenic capsule is common and a characteristic histologic finding is concentric fibrosis ('onion skinning') of the adventitia of the central (penicillary) arteries of the Malpighian corpuscles.

Joint manifestations include fibrinoid degeneration within the synovium, rheumatoid features, and arteritis. A variety of lesions may be seen in the liver, including fatty change, focal hepatocyte necroses, and evidence of vasculitis. Central nervous system manifestations have an ischemic pathogenesis, most probably on an immune complex-mediated vasculitic basis. There is some evidence to incriminate an antineuronal autoantibody. The cardiac pathology of neonatal lupus erythematosus comprises fibrosis and calcification of the atrioventricular node and, to a lesser extent, the sinoatrial node.[446] Focal lymphocytic myocarditis and endocardial fibroelastosis may also be evident.[319]

Neonatal lupus erythematosus

The histologic features and immunofluorescence pattern of the cutaneous lesions in neonatal disease are similar to those seen in SCLE.[221,447] The most frequently documented findings include hydropic degeneration of basal keratinocytes and adnexal epithelium, dermal edema as well as a superficial and occasionally deep perivascular and periadnexal lymphohistiocytic chronic inflammatory cell infiltrate.[413,448] Eosinophils may be prominent in urticaria-like SCLE lesions.[448] In addition, a subset of patients with neonatal lupus display histologic features of neutrophilic dermatosis (Sweet syndrome-like), including histiocytic variant (Ch15).

Differential diagnosis

Lupus erythematosus must be distinguished from other dermatoses that manifest basal cell liquefactive degeneration, particularly lichen planus and poikiloderma. Lupus erythematosus lacks the wedge-shaped hypergranulosis and sawtooth acanthosis of lichen planus. The inflammatory cell infiltrate is typically periappendageal, rather than adopting a bandlike distribution. Occasionally, hypertrophic lupus erythematosus shows considerable overlap with lichen planus; in such instances a positive lupus band test resolves the problem.

Poikiloderma, whether congenital or associated with dermatomyositis (and rarely SLE) or as a manifestation of mycosis fungoides, is characterized by epidermal atrophy and marked basal cell liquefactive degeneration associated with pigmentary incontinence. A patchy lymphohistiocytic infiltrate is evident in the upper dermis. Papillary dermal edema and telangiectases are typically present. Although there is obviously histologic overlap, the very different clinical manifestations should obviate any diagnostic difficulties.

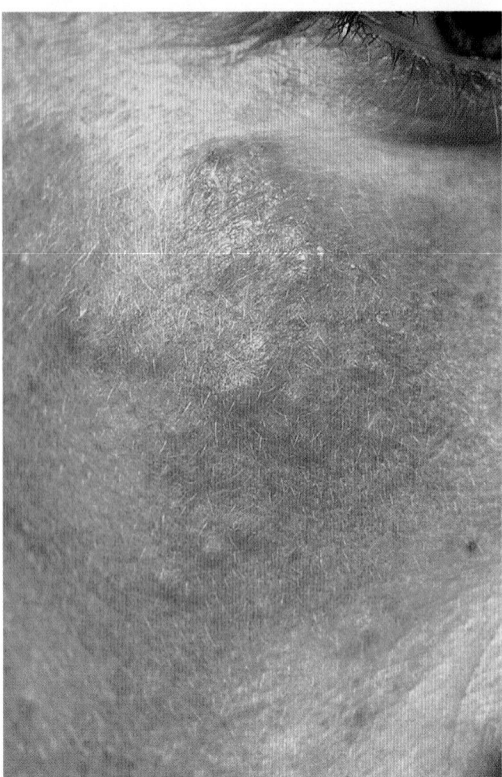

Fig. 17.80
Polymorphic light eruption: patients present with erythematous papules and vesicles on sun-exposed skin. By courtesy of the Institute of Dermatology, London, UK.

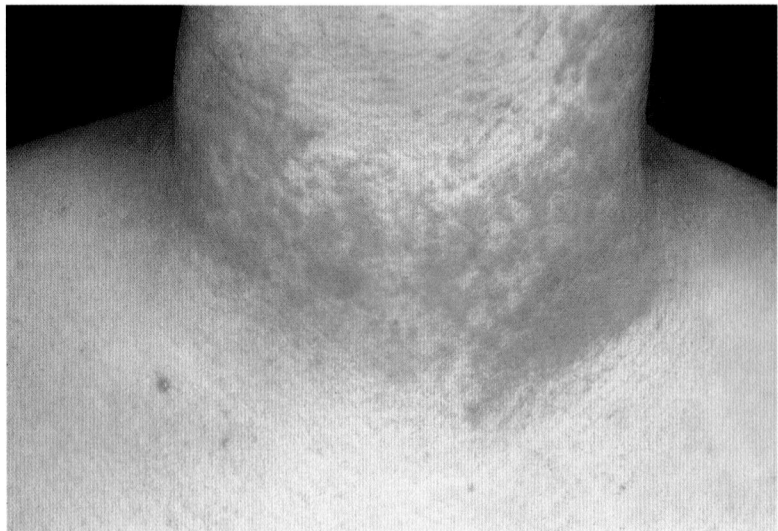

Fig. 17.81
Polymorphic light eruption: the eruption is typically symmetrical and is usually pruritic. By courtesy of the Institute of Dermatology, London, UK.

The presence of atypical lymphocytes will clearly distinguish the variant associated with mycosis fungoides.

The histologic features of lupus erythematosus are sometimes difficult to distinguish from polymorphic light eruption, particularly when the latter is associated with a positive band test (see above). Polymorphic light eruption, which is the most common photodermatosis, usually presents in young people, particularly females, as recurrent, erythematous papules, vesicles and/or plaques following exposure to ultraviolet light (Figs 17.80 and 17.81).[449] Lesions, which develop after a latent period of hours to days, commonly subside completely within days and heal without sequelae.[362] Histologically, superficial dermal edema and a mild to moderate superficial and deep perivascular lymphohistiocytic infiltrate are often seen.[449] In early lesions helper-inducer T lymphocytes predominate and increased numbers of dermal Langerhans cells are present.[450]

With chronicity, cytotoxic-suppressor T cells become more conspicuous. Basal cell hydropic degeneration is usually absent and epidermal atrophy is not a feature.

Systemic sclerosis

Clinical features

Progressive systemic sclerosis includes two major variants:[1–5]

- In the more serious diffuse form, patients have widespread cutaneous lesions proximal to the metacarpo- and metatarsophalangeal joints (proximal scleroderma) in addition to involvement of the internal viscera, particularly the kidneys, lungs, heart, esophagus, and intestinal tract. The illness often has an acute onset with fatigue, weight loss, arthralgia, and carpal tunnel syndrome. Tendon friction rubs are characteristic. Anti-Scl-70 (anti-DNA topoisomerase) and RNA polymerase III antibodies are often present, and the outlook is generally poor.
- The other major variant is associated with limited peripheral cutaneous sclerosis and an absence of severe systemic disease except for esophageal involvement, small intestinal malabsorption, and pulmonary hypertension; it usually has a better prognosis.[2,6] This form is associated with an anticentromere antibody.

Systemic sclerosis has also occasionally been recorded in the absence of cutaneous manifestation (sine scleroderma variant), and overlap syndromes have been described.[7,8] Limited scleroderma also includes the CREST (calcinosis, Raynaud phenomenon, esophageal dysfunction, sclerodactyly, telangiectasis) syndrome (Thibierge-Weissenbach syndrome, acrosclerosis) where cutaneous disease expression is restricted to the fingers and toes (sclerodactyly) and face (see below).[9] Other generalized variants include sclerodermatomyositis, MCTD, and the chemically induced scleroderma-like syndromes.

Because of the variety of systems that can be affected in systemic sclerosis, patients may be primarily under the care of dermatologists, rheumatologists, nephrologists, or other specialists, resulting in difficulties in determining the exact incidence of the disease; it is estimated to be in the order of 20 new cases per million of the population per year.[10] In a large series, the diffuse and limited forms were equally common.[11] About 10% were classified as overlap syndromes. The disease occurs more frequently in families and it is regarded as the strongest risk factor identified for this condition.[12] However, the absolute risk for each family member is low.[12] Systemic sclerosis is associated with a marked female predominance (3–4:1); although any age group may be affected, patients most often present in their fourth, fifth, and sixth decades.[13,14] Young black females constitute a definite subset with a particularly high risk. Occasional familial instances, usually in children, have also been documented.[10] Juvenile systemic sclerosis represent about 3% of systemic sclerosis patients.[15] No sex predilection is seen before the age of 8 years.[15] In contrast to adult-onset systemic sclerosis, juvenile systemic sclerosis is associated with higher incidence of overlap syndromes, especially with polymyositis/dermatomyositis, different sets of antibodies in the serum (anti-PM-Sci and anti-U1-RNP), and improved survival.[16–18] Cardiopulmonary diseases have predictive value for survival in juvenile systemic sclerosis.[16,17]

Systemic sclerosis has a high overall mortality, 5-year survival rates varying from 34% to 73%.[1] It has been demonstrated that improvement of skin thickening is associated with improved survival.[19,20] Older patients and males generally fare worst.

Limited cutaneous systemic sclerosis

In the limited variant, the cutaneous manifestations, which often initially affect the hands, include early edematous, sclerotic, and late atrophic stages.[1] The edema is characteristically nonpitting, bilateral, and symmetrical. The fingers are commonly described as having a sausage-like appearance (*Fig. 17.82*). The face, forearms, feet, and legs are sometimes affected. As the edema subsides the skin becomes thickened and tight and is bound down to the subcutaneous tissues. Typically, the fingers become tapered and,

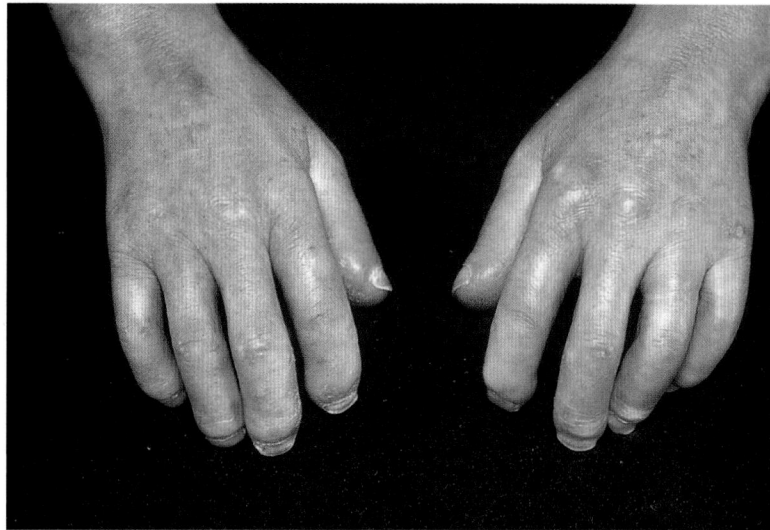

Fig. 17.82
Systemic sclerosis: early stage showing characteristic swollen, sausage-shaped fingers. By courtesy of the Institute of Dermatology, London, UK.

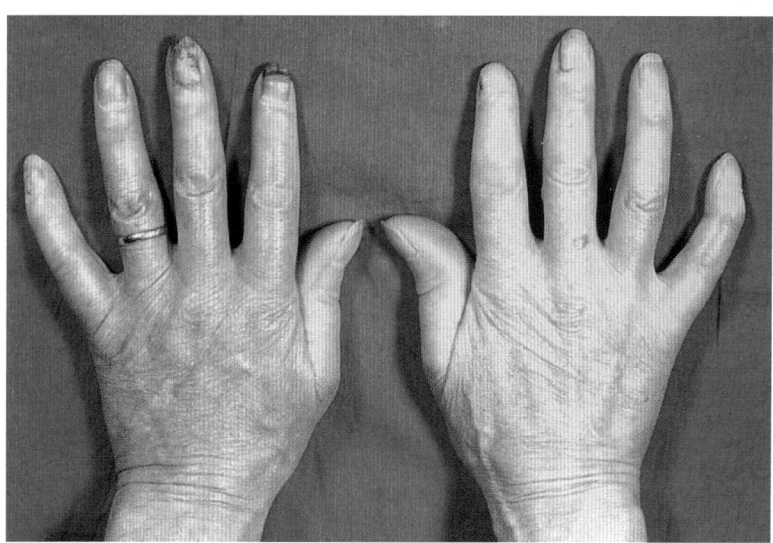

Fig. 17.83
Systemic sclerosis: the fingers are erythematous and shiny and the skin appears slightly bound down. By courtesy of R.A. Marsden, MD, St George's Hospital, London, UK.

due to ischemia, show pulp atrophy and absorption of the terminal phalanges, with the fingertips often not protruding beyond the free margin of the nails (*Figs 17.83–17.85*). The latter may show longitudinal ridging and brittleness or may even be shed. The affected skin has a very characteristic appearance, being shiny, smooth and rather waxy. Patients often have markedly diminished mobility of their hands and feet, and flexion contractures are common (*Fig. 17.86*). In advanced disease, many patients acquire a dramatically rigid, expressionless face with beaked nose, thinned lips, and perioral furrowing and wrinkling, and an inability to open the mouth fully (*Figs 17.87* and *17.88*).[21] Tightness of the lower eyelids may also be noticed, and the forehead can appear smooth and free of creases.[2] Ulceration is a common complication, particularly where taut skin is stretched over bony prominences susceptible to trauma (*Fig. 17.89*).

Vascular changes are common and include peripheral gangrene, digital autoamputation, and Raynaud phenomenon.[21] The last occurs so frequently (in both limited and diffuse forms) that it is often taught that a patient who has it must be presumed to have systemic sclerosis, until proven otherwise. In limited cutaneous systemic sclerosis, Raynaud phenomenon may precede the onset of cutaneous lesions by many years in a large proportion

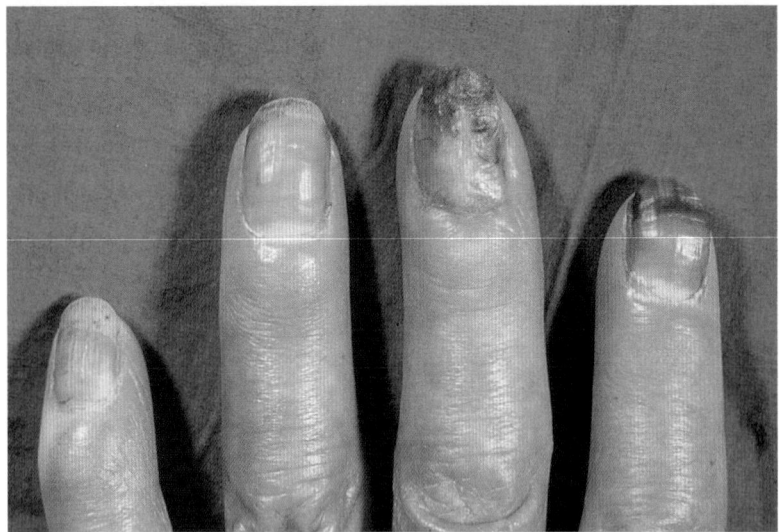

Fig. 17.84
Systemic sclerosis: the fingertips are tapered. By courtesy of R.A. Marsden, MD, St George's Hospital, London, UK.

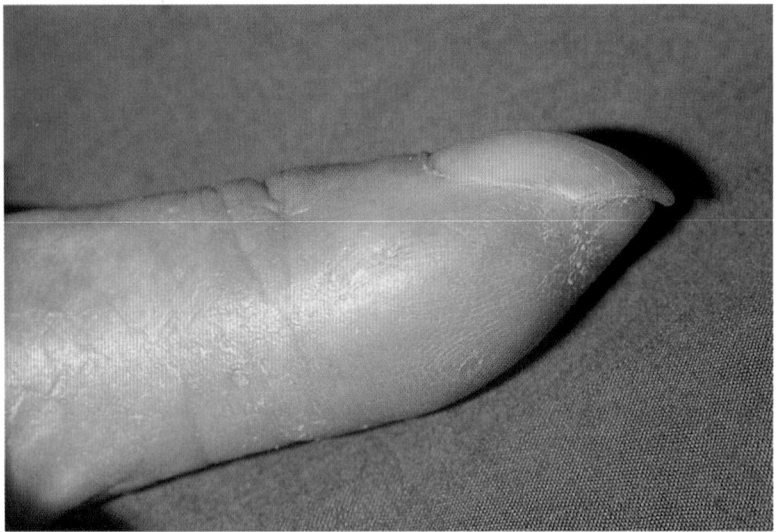

Fig. 17.85
Systemic sclerosis: note the marked atrophy of the fingertip. By courtesy of R.A. Marsden, MD, St George's Hospital, London, UK.

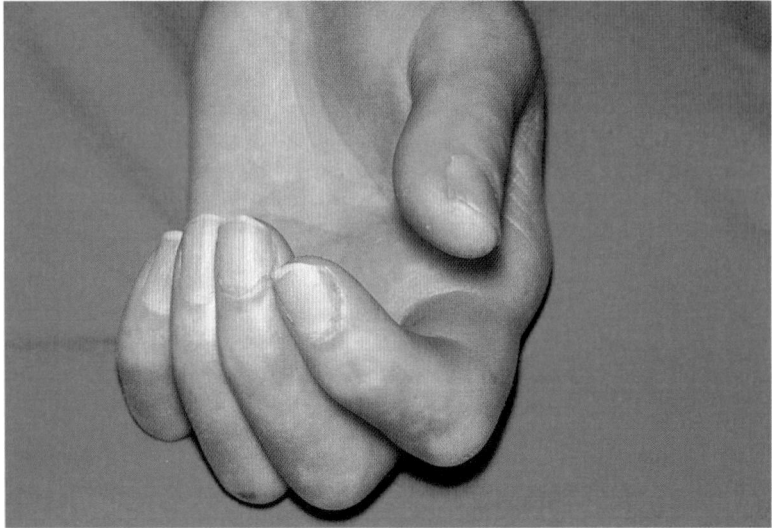

Fig. 17.86
Systemic sclerosis: note the flexion contractures. The skin is bound down and appears atrophic. There is periungual erythema. By courtesy of R.A. Marsden, MD, St George's Hospital, London, UK.

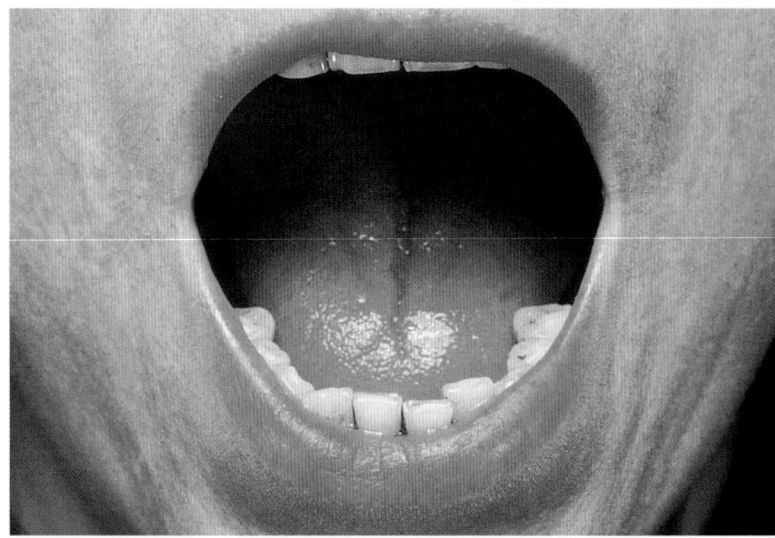

Fig. 17.87
Systemic sclerosis: there is perioral scarring with atrophy. By courtesy of the Institute of Dermatology, London, UK.

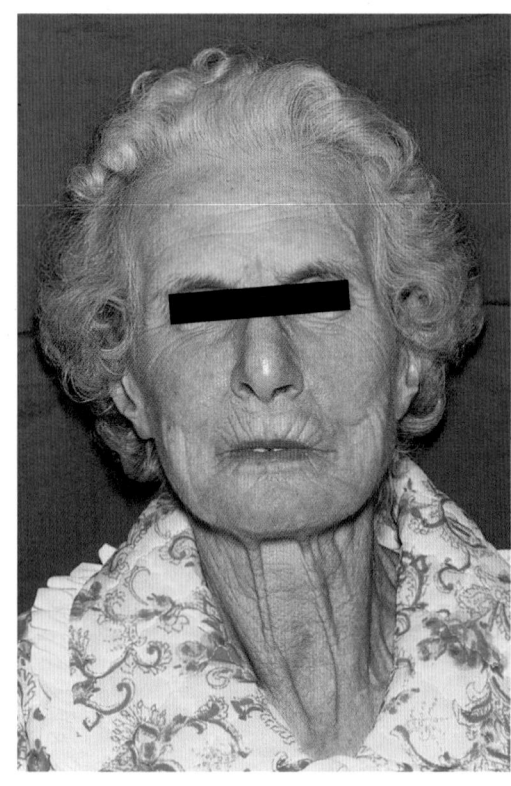

Fig. 17.88
Systemic sclerosis: note the thinned lips and characteristic radiating furrows. By courtesy of R.A. Marsden, MD, St George's Hospital, London, UK.

of patients.[10] A useful diagnostic feature of systemic sclerosis is loss of many of the nail fold capillaries and dilatation of the remainder. It has recently been demonstrated that the nail fold capillaroscopy abnormalities correlate with diffuse form of systemic sclerosis, severity of cutaneous involvement, number of affected tracts, and the presence of anti-Scl-70 antibodies.[22]

The cutaneous changes in CREST syndrome are located predominantly distal to the metacarpophalangeal joints, although the dorsum of the hands and mouth can sometimes also be affected. The inflammatory stage is persistent in the CREST syndrome.

Raynaud phenomenon, either alone or with swollen puffy fingers, is by far the most common mode of presentation and telangiectases tend to be much more numerous (often numbering hundreds) than in patients with diffuse systemic sclerosis. They particularly affect the fingers and hands,

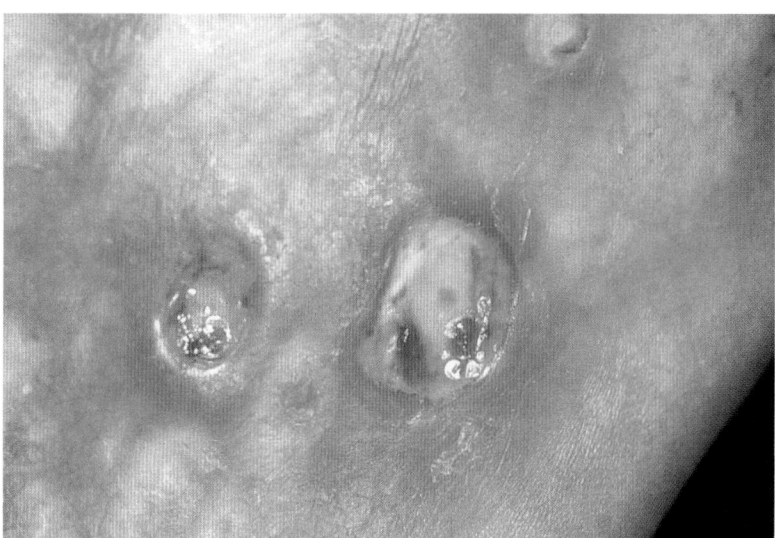

Fig. 17.89
Systemic sclerosis: ulceration is a particularly distressing complication. By courtesy of the Institute of Dermatology, London, UK.

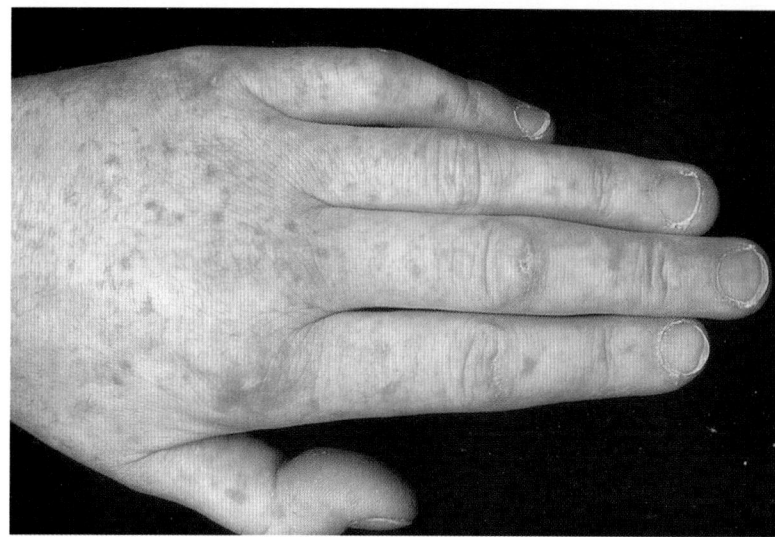

Fig. 17.91
Systemic sclerosis: numerous telangiectases are present. The hand is a commonly affected site. By courtesy of the Institute of Dermatology, London, UK.

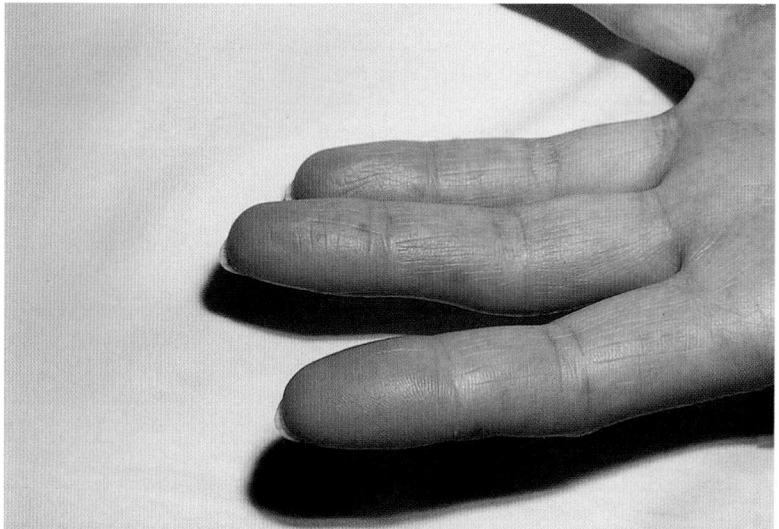

Fig. 17.90
Systemic sclerosis: telangiectasia as seen on these fingers is a common finding. By courtesy of S. Parker, MD, West Middlesex Hospital, London, UK.

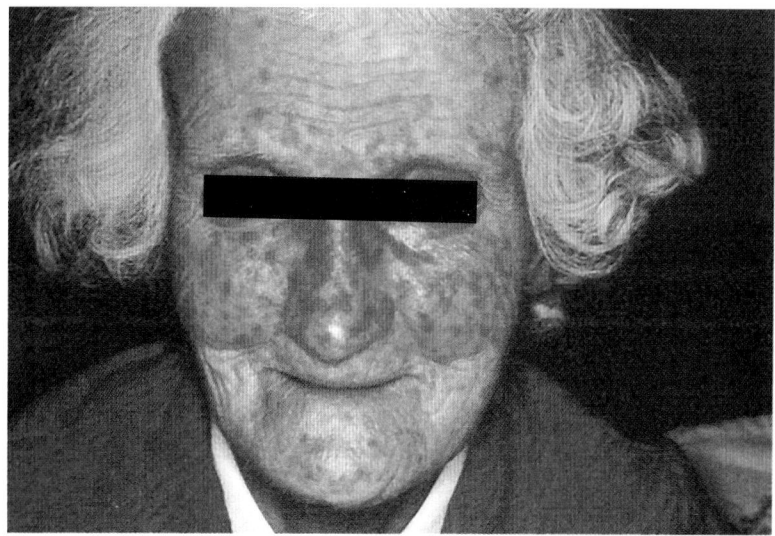

Fig. 17.92
Systemic sclerosis: extensive telangiectasia as seen in this patient is more often a feature of the limited variant. By courtesy of S. Parker, MD, West Middlesex Hospital, London, UK.

face, tongue, and mucous membranes (*Figs 17.90–17.92*). The telangiectasias seen in this variant of scleroderma may be difficult to distinguish from those seen in hereditary hemorrhagic telangiectasia.[23] The esophageal dysfunction is identical to that seen in the diffuse variant, but it tends to be more severe and affects the majority of patients.

The value of the designation 'CREST syndrome' has, however, diminished considerably since the discovery that many patients with limited cutaneous disease fail to fulfill all of its criteria and the observation that 'CREST' manifestations may be seen in many patients with diffuse disease.[8] For example, there is a variant consisting of digital necrosis, Raynaud phenomenon, and anticentromere antibodies without sclerodactyly.[24] The term should probably be abandoned and all patients with limited distal disease classified as a single subtype. However, considering the frequency with which CREST syndrome appears in the current literature, this is unlikely to happen, at least in the foreseeable future. It was originally thought that the limited variant was associated with a relatively benign outcome, but it is now known that if patients are followed for sufficient time a significant proportion will develop severe pulmonary hypertension with its sequelae. There is also an increased risk of Sjögren syndrome, biliary cirrhosis, discoid lupus erythematosus, and thyroid dysfunction, such as Hashimoto thyroiditis and Graves disease.[1,25–27] Sjögren syndrome has been found in 14% of patients with systemic sclerosis

and was more common in the limited cutaneous variant of systemic sclerosis.[28] More than one of the associated autoimmune conditions may coexist with CREST syndrome.[26] It has been suggested that patients with coexistent primary biliary cirrhosis have a distinctive subset of the disease, which tends to be milder and have a better prognosis.[29] An exceptional case of antimitochondrial antibody-positive primary biliary cirrhosis developing after an acute myocardial infarction has been reported.[30] Although clinically significant primary biliary cirrhosis develops in 2.5% of systemic sclerosis patients, a recent study has demonstrated the presence of antimitochondrial antibodies in 15% of systemic sclerosis patients.[31] Overlap syndrome between primary biliary cirrhosis and autoimmune hepatitis has also been found in systemic sclerosis.[32] A multicenter French-Italian study has found coexistence of systemic sclerosis and autoimmune disease in 21% of the patients, with Sjögren syndrome (12%) and thyroiditis (6%) being the most frequent associations.[33] Systemic sclerosis patients with associated autoimmune conditions appear to follow a milder course of the disease.[33] Systemic sclerosis is associated with rheumatoid arthritis in about 5% of the patients, and likely represents a distinctive disease subset associated with HLA-DR3, HLA-DR7, HLA-DR11, and HLA-DRw53.[34] In a large cohort of over 2000 patients with systemic sclerosis, association with ANCA-positive vasculitis was established in 1.6% of the patients.[35] An overlap between

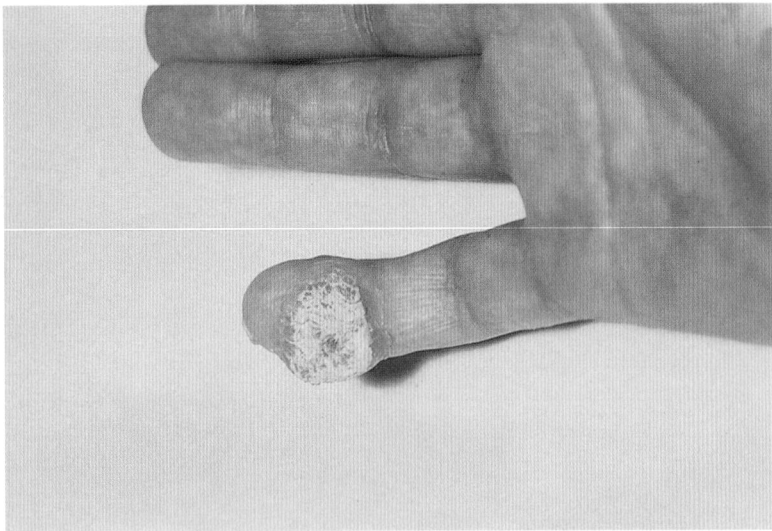

Fig. 17.93
Systemic sclerosis: there is a large calcified nodule on the fingertip. By courtesy of R.A. Marsden, MD, St George's Hospital, London, UK.

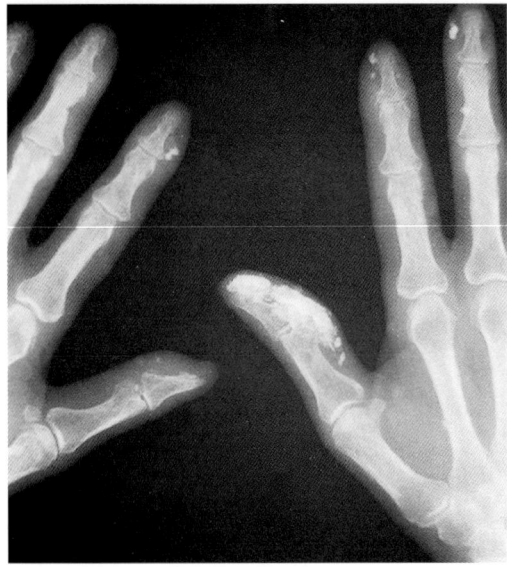

Fig. 17.94
Systemic sclerosis: radiograph demonstrating a more widespread example. By courtesy of R.A. Marsden, MD, St George's Hospital, London, UK.

systemic sclerosis and cryoglobulineic vasculitis was detected in 1.6% of the patients, usually in the presence of hepatitis C virus infection.[36]

Hyperpigmentation, from light brown to dark bronze, reminiscent of Addison disease, is a frequent manifestation and is often associated with the presence of small foci of hypopigmentation, giving a characteristic 'salt and pepper' appearance. The pigmentary changes particularly affect the backs of the hands and forearms, and the upper part of the chest and back. Sometimes the degree of accompanying hypopigmentation is so marked that it resembles vitiligo.[37] Exceptionally, abnormalities in skin pigmentation developing in the absence of associated sclerosis can represent an initial manifestation of incipient systemic sclerosis.[38]

Rare skin presentation of systemic sclerosis is characterized by multiple and immovable small papules or nodules giving the lesion a so-called cobblestone appearance.[39] It is believed that this presentation pattern is the consequence of lymphangiectasia due to the obstruction of lymphatic channels by the fibrosing process.[39]

The cutaneous changes are often associated with the development of calcinosis cutis, particularly in females.[2,40,41] It is dystrophic in type and is due to hydroxyapatite crystal deposition. Patients have no abnormalities of calcium and phosphorus metabolism and their serum alkaline phosphatase levels are normal. The sites of calcium deposition particularly include the metacarpophalangeal joints of the thumbs and the fingertips, although the extensor aspect of the forearms, the buttocks, the olecranon bursae, and the prepatellar region may also be affected (Figs 17.93 and 17.94). The deposits are often exceedingly painful and commonly associated with ulceration and leakage of white granular calcified debris. The combination of phalangeal reabsorption and calcinosis cutis is said to be pathognomonic of systemic sclerosis.[42] Calcinosis cutis has also been reported in patients with systemic sclerosis sine scleroderma.[43]

Systemic sclerosis is sometimes associated with an erythema nodosum-like panniculitis syndrome and patients may also develop livedo reticularis and atrophie blanche affecting the lower limbs.[44]

CREST has been documented in association with familial lichen sclerosus, chronic myelogenous leukemia, idiopathic myelofibrosis, and porphyria cutanea tarda.[45–47]

Diffuse systemic sclerosis

In diffuse (progressive) systemic sclerosis, cutaneous lesions are particularly common on the proximal extremities, thorax, and abdomen. The course tends to be progressive and often there is a more severe superficial vascular involvement.[2] Skin thickening affecting the trunk indicates a poor prognosis and correlates with extensive systemic involvement.[10] Although the cutaneous features cause considerable distress, the systemic manifestations are more important in terms of severe morbidity and potential mortality. The

early investigation of a patient with systemic sclerosis should establish baseline values of respiratory, cardiac, and renal function so that progress may be accurately monitored.

Clinical involvement of the lung is common and an important cause of morbidity and mortality. It is thought to occur to a greater or lesser extent in most patients.[48] There are three major forms: interstitial pneumonitis, bronchiolitis, and pulmonary vascular disease.[48]

- Pulmonary interstitial involvement results in shortness of breath on exertion and a nonproductive cough. Dyspnea is a feature in almost 60% of unselected patients with diffuse scleroderma.[49] Symptoms tend to be particularly evident in patients who have associated Sjögren syndrome.[48] Interstitial lung disease is the commonest cause of death in systemic sclerosis. There is evidence suggesting an increased risk of pulmonary fibrosis in patients with the haplotype HLA-DR3/-DRw52A and anti-Scl-70 antibody.[50,51]
- Bronchiolitis is evident in approximately 13% to 25% of patients, but this is usually asymptomatic.[48]
- Pulmonary hypertension, which may be a primary manifestation of systemic sclerosis or develop secondary to interstitial fibrosis, is more common in patients with the limited form of the disease.[52,53] A study has found that the postmenopausal state with or without the presence of HLA-B35 is the main risk factor for the development of pulmonary hypertension.[54]

Pulmonary radiographs typically show bilateral basal fibrosis, either as diffuse mottling or linear infiltrates; cyst formation ('honeycomb lung') is a not uncommon feature.

The cardiac, renal, peripheral nervous, gastrointestinal, and skeletal systems are also involved:

- The majority of patients have subclinical primary cardiac involvement.[55] Cardiac involvement may present as dyspnea on exertion, paroxysmal nocturnal dyspnea, pericarditis, pericardial effusion, congestive heart failure, arrhythmias, valvular abnormalities, myocardial hypertrophy or, occasionally, atypical angina.[55–57] Vasospasm of the small coronary arteries and arterioles has been observed as an early cardiac manifestation.[55] Significant cardiac abnormalities including pericarditis and effusion are common pathological findings, being present in more than 50% of cases at autopsy.[58] Usually, however, they are asymptomatic. Occasionally, severe acute pericarditis may develop and rare instances of fatal cardiac tamponade have been documented.[56] Large pericardial effusions correlate with acute renal failure and are a bad prognostic indicator.[58] Patchy myocardial scarring is common, and usually occurs later in the course of systemic sclerosis.[55] When severe, myocardial fibrosis is associated with a poor outlook.[59] It occurs independently of coronary artery disease and has been described in up to 70% of patients in postmortem series.[56] The major coronary arteries are patent and normal (unless there is coexistent atherosclerosis), but the small vessels and arterioles may undergo endothelial and intimal proliferative changes with scarring, resulting in an increased risk of arrhythmia and the consequent sudden death of the patient. A recent study has found association between myocardial perfusion defects, skin thickness, digital ulcers, and esophageal involvement.[60]

- Renal involvement presenting as 'scleroderma renal crisis' is an extremely important complication with high mortality and occurs in approximately 10% of patients with systemic sclerosis.[61] The use of ACE inhibitors has, however, significantly diminished the mortality. It is defined as 'the new onset of accelerated arterial hypertension and/or rapidly progressive oliguric renal failure'.[61] Patients develop headache and blurred vision. Seizures are sometimes a feature. The renal failure is commonly asymptomatic and detectable only from abnormal renal function tests, including proteinuria, microscopic hematuria with casts, raised creatinine levels, and hyperreninemia.[61] Microangiopathic hemolytic anemia is sometimes present, particularly in normotensive patients.[62] Anti-RNA polymerase III antibodies have been detected in about one-third of the patients with 'scleroderma renal crisis'.[63] A minority of patients with systemic sclerosis develop renal pathology other than 'scleroderma renal crisis'.[64] ANCA-related glomerulonephritis has occasionally been reported.[65,66]

- Peripheral neuropathy may lead to neuropathic ulceration.[67] Intrauterine fetal death has been described in pregnant women with the disease.[68] Papular and nodular mucinosis has been documented as a presenting sign of systemic sclerosis.[69]

- Clinically relevant gastrointestinal lesions occur in up to 50% of patients with systemic sclerosis.[70,71] Widening of the periodontal space, determined radiographically, is characteristic. Patients frequently have symptoms relating to esophageal involvement including heartburn, dysphagia, and regurgitation. Gastrointestinal reflux is common and patients can develop esophagitis, hemorrhage, stricture, Barrett esophagus (gastric metaplasia), and aspiration.[70] Radiographs may show esophageal dilatation and abnormalities of peristalsis. Epigastric fullness is a frequent symptom, which might be related to restricted distension of the gastric antrum.[71] Gastric antral vascular ectasia appears to develop earlier in those systemic sclerosis patients who display a rapidly progressive cutaneous disease.[72] Systemic sclerosis often involves the small intestine, symptoms ranging from epigastric pain, nausea and vomiting, through to the effects of pseudo-obstruction; a malabsorptive state due to stasis is an important complication. Celiac disease can develop in patients with systemic sclerosis.[73] Colonic lesions may result in diarrhea or constipation. Saccular diverticula along the mesenteric border of the colon are characteristic; they sometimes also affect the small bowel.[70]

- Osteoarticular involvement, presenting with arthralgia or frank arthritis is seen in the majority of patients.[74] Joint lesions are usually mild and affect the wrists, hands, knees, and ankles, although a more serious rheumatoid arthritis-like variant has been documented.[75] Osteoarthrosis and psoriatic arthropathy-like manifestations have also been described.[74] It is important in patients with significant joint manifestations that overlap syndromes and MCTD are excluded. Contractures and ankyloses resulting in immobility are important complications, and osteoporosis is common due to a combination of immobilization and ischemia.

The diagnosis of systemic sclerosis may be readily apparent, but early disease, particularly the diffuse form, may clinically mimic a variety of other diseases, for example, scleredema of Buschke. Late graft-versus-host disease (GVHD) and chronic lesions of porphyria cutanea tarda are typically sclerodermatous.[76] The American Rheumatology Association has guidelines for classification, of which the major criterion is proximal scleroderma (Table 17.7).[77] Minor criteria are:
- sclerodactyly,
- digital pitting scars on the fingertips or loss of substance of the distal fingerpad,
- bilateral basal pulmonary fibrosis.

Table 17.7

American Rheumatology Association (ARA) guidelines for the classification of scleroderma*

1. Proximal scleroderma is a single major criterion: sensitivity is 91% and specificity is more than 90%.
2. Sclerodactyly, digital pitting scars of the fingertips or loss of substance of the finger pad, and bibasilar pulmonary fibrosis contribute further minor criteria in the absence of proximal scleroderma.
3. The major or two more minor criteria are present in 97% of definite systemic sclerosis patients, but in only 2% of comparison patients with systemic lupus erythematosus, polymyositis–dermatomyositis or Raynaud disease.

*Preliminary clinical criteria for systemic sclerosis exclude localized scleroderma and pseudo-dermatous disorders.
Reproduced with permission from Masi, A.T. et al. and the ARA Subcommittee for scleroderma (1980) *Arthritis and Rheumatism*, 23, 581–590.

If a patient has either the major or two minor criteria, there is 97% sensitivity for definite systemic sclerosis and 98% specificity. These criteria have gained wide popularity, but have the disadvantage of excluding at least 10% of cases where, despite a concrete diagnosis of systemic sclerosis, neither major nor minor criteria are fulfilled. Unclassifiable and overlap syndromes are also excluded. Other classifications have included two, three, and even four subtypes based upon the extent of cutaneous sclerosis (Table 17.8).[78] Limited cutaneous systemic sclerosis may therefore involve the hands, feet, forearms, and face, or skin lesions can be absent, whereas in diffuse disease the trunk skin is also involved. In a comparison of classification by two subtypes (diffuse and limited) or three subtypes (diffuse, intermediate, and limited), the latter correlated best with antibody specificity and survival.[79]

In 2013, the American College of Rheumatism (ACR) and the European League Against Rheumatism (EULAR) proposed a revision of the classification criteria for systemic sclerosis in order to improve the sensitivity, especially in diagnosing early forms of systemic sclerosis and localized cutaneous systemic sclerosis.[80] The new 2013 ACR/EULAR classification criteria for systemic sclerosis apply a point system in such a way that a score of ≥9 is needed to classify a patient as having a systemic sclerosis (Table 17.9). In short, according to the new criteria, skin thickening of the fingers extending proximal to the metacarpophalangeal joints is regarded as a sufficient criterion (score 9 points) for the diagnosis of systemic sclerosis. Alternatively, seven additional parameters with varying weights are applied:
1. skin thickening of the fingers (puffy fingers 2 points or sclerodactyly 4 points, counting the higher score only),
2. fingertip lesions (digital-tip ulcers 2 points or pitting scars 3 points, counting the higher score only),
3. telangiectasia (2 points),
4. abnormal nail fold capillaries (2 points),
5. interstitial lung disease or pulmonary arterial hypertension (2 points),
6. Raynaud phenomenon (3 points), and
7. systemic sclerosis-specific autoantibodies (3 points).[80]

By applying the new set of criteria, a large study of 724 systemic sclerosis patients from Canada found the overall sensitivity of the new 2013 criteria to be 98.3% compared to 88.3% for the 1980 criteria, significantly improving the diagnostic accuracy of early systemic sclerosis and localized cutaneous systemic sclerosis.[81] In addition, a recent study of 3196 patients with systemic sclerosis revealed the history of digital ulcers to have a predictive value not only for development of new digital ulcer(s), but also for elevated pulmonary arterial pressure, and other possible cardiovascular events, and also represents an independent predictor of decreased survival.[82]

A number of chemical-induced scleroderma-like syndromes have been described:
- Workers in the vinyl chloride polymerization industry may develop Raynaud phenomenon, acral osteolysis, dermal thickening of the skin of the arms, hands, face, and trunk, and pulmonary and hepatic fibrosis.[83–85] Examination of the capillaries of the nail folds reveals abnormalities similar to those seen in systemic sclerosis.

Table 17.8
Classifications of systemic sclerosis

Subsets of systemic sclerosis (SSc)	
Diffuse cutaneous SS*	Onset of Raynaud phenomenon within 1 year of onset of skin changes (puffy or hidebound) Truncal and acral skin involvement Presence of tendon friction rubs Early and significant incidence of interstitial –lung disease, oliguric renal failure, diffuse gastrointestinal disease, and myocardial involvement Absence of anticentromere antibodies Nail fold capillary dilatation and capillary destruction[†] Antitopoisomerase antibodies (20–60% of patients)
Limited cutaneous SSc	Raynaud for years (occasionally decades) Skin involvement limited to hands, face, feet, and forearms (acral) or absent A significance late incidence of pulmonary hypertension, with or without interstitial lung disease, trigeminal neuralgia, skin calcifications, telangiectasia A high incidence of anticentromere antibody Dilated nail fold capillary loops, usually without capillary dropout

Subsetting of SSc by early cutaneous involvement[‡]	
Digital	Finger or toes, minimal non-extremity involvements allowed: eyelid, neck, and axillary changes
Proximal extremity	Proximal extremity or face, but not trunk
Truncal	Thorax or abdomen

Systemic sclerosis subsets according to skin sclerosis extent			
ssSSc	lcSSc	icSSc	dcSSc
ssSSc = sine scleroderma systemic sclerosis			sclerotic
lcSSc = limited cutaneous systemic sclerosis			skin
icSSc = intermediate cutaneous systemic sclerosis			uninvolved
dcSSc = diffuse cutaneous systemic sclerosis			skin

Skin sclerosis extent in four SSc subsets. LcSSc patients may present minimal sclerotic lesion at eyelids, neck, and axillae
*Experienced observers note some patients with dcSSc who do not develop organ insufficiency and suggest the term chronic dcSSc for these patients.
[†]Nail fold capillary dilatation and destruction may also be seen in patients with dermatomyositis, overlap syndromes and undifferentiated connective tissue disease. These syndromes may be considered as part of the spectrum of scleroderma-associated disorders.
[‡]The subject is defined within 1 year from presentation.
Top panel reproduced with permission from Leroy, E.C. et al (1988) *Journal of Rheumatology*, 15, 202–205; middle and lower panels reproduced with permission from Valentini, R. (1994) *Clinics in Dermatology*, 12, 217–223.

- Bleomycin therapy may also be associated with sclerodermiform infiltrated plaques and nodules that particularly affect the hands.[86] Patients may develop hyperpigmentation, peripheral gangrene, and pulmonary fibrosis.
- A high incidence of systemic sclerosis is found in those who work in coalmines or who have excessive exposure to silica for other reasons.[87]
- A generalized morphea-like variant with Raynaud phenomenon, esophageal dysfunction, and pulmonary fibrosis has been described following chronic exposure to industrial solvents.[88]
- A variety of autoimmune diseases have been documented following the use of silicone breast implants. Systemic sclerosis appears to be the most common.[89]
- Toxic oil and eosinophilia-myalgia syndromes are discussed in the section on eosinophilic fasciitis.

Systemic sclerosis is associated with increased risk of malignancies, which develop in between 3.6% and 10.7% of patients.[90] Population-based studies have found most frequent association with breast cancer, lung cancer, and hematological malignancies, such as non-Hodgkin lymphoma.[91–94] Increased incidence of squamous cell carcinoma of the tongue has also been detected.[95] Rare associations include basal cell carcinoma, melanoma, nasopharyngeal carcinoma, gastric MALT lymphoma, bladder cancer, cervical cancer, esophageal carcinoma, thyroid cancer, squamous cell carcinoma of the skin, and myelodysplastic syndrome.[93,96–100]

Pathogenesis and histologic features

The etiology and precise pathogenesis are unknown. A complete understanding must take into account vascular changes and abnormalities of collagen deposition and distribution, in addition to the significance of the inflammatory cells that characterize the early stages and their role in the control of fibroblast growth and function.[101] Systemic sclerosis has stimulated an enormous research effort, which has resulted in an increased awareness of the multiplicity of factors that may be involved, either singly or in concert, and has also greatly increased our knowledge of the basic processes involved in the mechanisms of collagen synthesis and scarring. The two main areas of investigation have revolved around:

- primary blood vessel endothelial cell damage and its sequelae,[102,103]
- abnormalities of collagen and its synthesis.[102,103]

Inherent to both are the possible initiating and moderating roles of cell-mediated and humoral immunity.

It has long been recognized that many of the features of systemic sclerosis may have an ischemic basis.[104] Alterations have been described in capillaries, venules, and arteries, and it has been suggested that the initial injury involves capillary endothelial cells.[105] The cause of this is unknown, although a circulating specific cytotoxic substance reactive for endothelial cells has been identified.[105,106] It has been suggested that this may represent a protease.[107] Interestingly, specimens of early lesions and uninvolved skin have shown ultrastructural evidence of endothelial cell damage combined with decreased uptake of tritiated adenosine and diminished stores of immunodetectable von Willebrand factor, suggesting that the vascular changes may well initiate the connective tissue damage seen in this disease.[108]

Although immunoreactants (IgG and complement) have been detected in the walls of renal glomerular capillaries by immunofluorescent techniques, they have not been found in the cutaneous vasculature.[108,109] If Raynaud phenomenon is induced in patients with systemic sclerosis, there is a concomitant reduction in both renal and pulmonary blood flow, implying a circulating factor, as yet unidentified.

The dermal capillaries show a variety of ultrastructural changes. The earliest finding is separation of the endothelial cells; this may result in fluid leakage and therefore be responsible, at least in part, for the edema that characterizes the early stages.[1] Evidence of more severe damage is manifest by the presence of endothelial cell vacuolation, increased numbers of intermediate filaments, reduction in pinocytotic vesicles and Weibel-Palade bodies, and abnormal endothelial surface cytoplasmic blebs.[108]

Evidence of endothelial cell injury can be monitored clinically by estimating plasma von Willebrand factor levels.[103] Elevated levels of supranormal von Willebrand factor multimers are typically seen in systemic sclerosis and may have pathogenetic significance as they are known to bind to subendothelial tissues, causing platelet aggregation and adhesion with resultant vascular proliferation and thrombosis.[103,110] ACE levels have been shown to be reduced in systemic sclerosis and this may also be of value in assessing the presence of endothelial cell damage.[102] Increased levels of the endothelial cell-derived peptide, endothelin, which causes vasoconstriction, have been identified.[89] Endothelin also has fibroblast mitogenic activity and stimulates the synthesis of collagen.[111]

The end stage appears as complete destruction of the capillary wall; the nuclei are granular and homogeneous, cell membranes are disrupted, and cytoplasmic contents are found in the capillary lumen and extravascular spaces. Endothelial cell uptake of tritiated adenosine has been shown to be reduced.[108] Basement membrane thickening and reduplication is often present and perivascular fibrosis is a common late accompaniment. The end result of vascular damage can be demonstrated most easily by nail fold capillaroscopy. It is likely that the dilatation of the residual vessels represents a compensatory measure. Increased proliferation of the endothelial cells in these residual vessels has been confirmed by tritiated thymidine uptake studies.[101]

Table 17.9

The American College of Rheumatology/European League Against Rheumatism criteria for the classification of systemic sclerosis*

Item	Sub-item	Weight/Score#
Skin thickening of the fingers of both hands extending proximal to the metacarpophalangeal joints (*sufficient criterion*)	-	9
Skin thickening of the fingers (*only count the higher score*)	• Puffy finger • Sclerodactyly of the fingers (distal to the metacarpophalangeal joints but proximal to the proximal interphalangeal joints)	2 4
Fingertip lesions (*only count the higher score*)	• Digital-tip ulcers • Fingertip pitting scars	2 3
Telangiectasia	-	2
Abnormal nail fold capillaries	-	2
Pulmonary arterial hypertension and/or interstitial lung disease (*maximum score is 2*)	• Pulmonary arterial hypertension • Interstitial lung disease	2 2
Raynaud phenomenon	-	3
SSc-related autoantibodies (anticentromere, antitopoisomerase I [anti-Scl-70], anti-RNA polymerase III (*maximum score is 3*)	• Anticentromere • Antitopoisomerase I • Anti-RNA polymerase III	3

*These criteria are applicable to any patient considered for inclusion in a systemic sclerosis study. The criteria are not applicable to patients with skin thickening sparing the fingers or to patients who have a scleroderma-like disorder that better explains their manifestations (e.g., nephrogenic sclerosing fibrosis, generalized morphea, eosinophilic fasciitis, scleredema diabeticorum, scleromyxedema, erythromyalgia, porphyria, lichen sclerosis, graft-versus-host disease, diabetic cheiroarthropathy).
#The total score is determined by adding the maximum weight (score) in each category. Patients with a total score of ≥9 are classified as having definite systemic sclerosis.

Arterioles are also involved in the vasodestructive phenomenon, characterized by vessel wall thickening due to a combination of smooth muscle hyperplasia, fibrosis, and the deposition of excessive glycosaminoglycans. Arteries show very marked intimal thickening, which is particularly well seen in the renal arcuate vessels and is often referred to as 'onion skinning' due to the concentric lamination. It develops as a consequence of myxoid change, cellular proliferation, and fibrosis.

Most of the inflammatory cells in the skin of patients with systemic sclerosis are CD4+ T cells.

A number of cytokines have been linked to the pathogenesis of systemic sclerosis. Transforming growth factor beta (TGF-β) and IL-4 increase fibroblast proliferation and collagen synthesis and may be important in the induction of fibrosis in this disease. IL-17 is a cytokine secreted by T cells that activates and induces proliferation of fibroblasts and activation of endothelial cells. This cytokine has been demonstrated to be increased in the skin and blood of affected patients, particularly in the early stages of the disease. It activates fibroblasts to secrete the proinflammatory cytokines IL-6 and -8 and to increase surface expression of intercellular adhesion molecule-1 (ICAM-1).[112–114] IL-17 also activates endothelial cells to secrete IL-6 and -1 and to express ICAM-1 and vascular cell adhesion molecule-1 (VCAM-1). IL-6 is also capable of inducing proliferation of fibroblasts and collagen synthesis. The combined effects of IL-17 and other cytokines induced by it lead to damage to the microcirculation and to fibrosis in the skin and internal organs. It has been suggested that connective tissue growth factor, the production of which is induced by TGF-β, may play an important role in the pathogenesis of fibrosis.[115] It has recently been demonstrated that CD8+ effector T lymphocytes are the source of increased IL-13 in the sera of patients with systemic sclerosis.[116] IL-13 has well-known profibrotic activities by direct fibroblast stimulation and, indirectly, by stimulation of TGF-β.[117] TGF-β in addition to fibrogenesis also contributes to the development of vascular abnormalities in systemic sclerosis by inducing synthesis of endothelin, which acts as a potent vasoconstrictor and has been implicated in the pathogenesis of ulcers.[118]

The fibroblasts in systemic sclerosis are capable of assembling microfibrils but these are unstable (probably due to an inherent defect of fibrillin 1, the extracellular matrix protein) and this may also play a role in the pathogenesis of the disease.[119] Interestingly, duplication in the fibrillin-1 gene has been implicated as the cause of tight skin,[1] which is an animal model of systemic sclerosis.[108] Antibodies against fibrillin are raised in the sera of patients with systemic sclerosis. Although this appears to be highly disease specific, it varies among ethnic groups. Native Americans and Japanese patients have a high frequency of anti-fibrillin-1 antibodies.[120]

Male cells have been found in multiple organs in women with systemic sclerosis but not in healthy women.[121] The migration of fetal cells into maternal circulation and their survival in different organs is known as microchimerism. It is still not clear what role, if any, microchimerism plays in the pathogenesis of systemic sclerosis.

The predominant histologic feature of systemic sclerosis is scarring. Intensive investigations have confirmed the presence of increased quantities of collagen, but as yet the precise pathogenetic mechanism(s) remain uncertain. Increased proline hydroxylase activity and increased uptake of labeled proline, both indicators of active collagen synthesis, have been demonstrated in patients with systemic sclerosis.[122] There is typically an elevated level of reducible aldimine cross-links, a feature of newly synthesized collagen.[123] Raised serum concentration of the N-terminal propeptide of type III collagen and increased urinary excretion of hydroxyproline have also been documented.[103]

Cultures of fibroblasts from patients with systemic sclerosis synthesize more collagen than do those from normal controls.[124] Although diminished levels of tissue collagenase have been reported, other workers have not confirmed this finding and its significance is therefore uncertain.[125] The amino acid composition of the collagen fibers is normal. Electron microscopy of evolving lesions has revealed the presence of immature collagen fibrils, characterized by a narrow caliber (30 nm), immature banding pattern, and double-stranded beaded filaments.[1] In the more mature lesion the collagen fibers approach normal thickness (100 nm), but their distribution is highly disorganized. Luse bodies are sometimes a feature.

Patients with diffuse and limited cutaneous systemic sclerosis have increased mean serum levels of soluble CD163 in comparison with the healthy controls.[126] It has recently been demonstrated that systemic sclerosis patients with elevated serum levels of soluble CD163 have higher pulmonary arterial systolic pressure than those with normal serum CD163 levels, suggesting the possible role of macrophages in the pathogenesis of systemic sclerosis.[126] In contrast, by binding to a TNF-like weak inducer of apoptosis, CD163 may protect against development of digital ulcers, yet contribute to more prominent fibrosis of the skin.[127]

The serum levels of soluble T-cell immunoglobulin and mucin domain 3 (TIM-3) are higher in patients with diffuse cutaneous systemic sclerosis than in those with limited cutaneous systemic sclerosis and healthy individuals, and positively correlate with the severity of skin sclerosis, especially in the early phase of diffuse cutaneous systemic sclerosis.[128] Increased serum levels of TIM-3 have also been associated with cardiac involvement and renal crisis.[128]

Histologic examination of active lesions often reveals increased numbers of fibroblasts. It has been shown that fibroblasts from the lower dermis synthesize more collagen than do those derived from the upper dermis, suggesting two different populations in systemic sclerosis.[129] The fibrosis, which is due to the deposition of types I, III, V, and VI collagen, is accompanied by excessive fibronectin.[103,130]

Recently, abundant type VII collagen has also been demonstrated within the dermis of involved skin accompanied by elevated expression of TGF-β.[130] The latter is known to upregulate the activity of the type VII collagen gene. This finding is of potential importance as type VII collagen distribution is normally restricted to the anchoring fibrils at the dermal–epidermal junction. Increased expression of types I and III collagen mRNA has been demonstrated in cultured fibroblasts from patients with scleroderma.[131,132] Systemic sclerosis is characterized by a normal concentration of collagen per unit weight. In contrast, however, there is a greatly increased collagen content per unit surface area.[133]

Collagen synthesis has a negative feedback control. Therefore, following cleavage of the amino terminal of the procollagen molecule by the amino terminal peptidase, the released amino terminal inhibits collagen formation. It has been shown by immunoelectron microscopic techniques that there is retention of the amino peptide at the site of the collagen fibril.[1]

In addition to increased quantities of collagen, the skin of early lesions of systemic sclerosis contains excessive quantities of glycosaminoglycans, notably dermatan sulfate and chondroitin 4- and 6-sulfate.[134] There is some evidence to show that the increase in glycosaminoglycans may be due, at least in part, to diminished degradation; their presence is associated with water binding in vivo and presumably is therefore also responsible for edema.

Systemic sclerosis is associated with abnormalities of both humoral and cellular immunity.[135] In contrast to SLE, anti-DNA antibodies are not usually present. Almost all patients, however, do possess antinuclear antibodies; these may be speckled, homogeneous, or nucleolar in type (Fig. 17.95). The last are found in 7% to 46% of patients, but are not specific, being found in a number of other connective tissue diseases.[8] They form a heterogeneous group reacting against a variety of antigens, including U3-RNP (fibrillarin), RNA polymerase I, Th ribonucleoprotein, and PM-Scl, and have some prognostic significance and subtype specificity (Table 17.10).[8,10] Anti-U3 RNP antibodies are present in 5% to 8% of systemic sclerosis, and are associated with African-American race, male gender, higher incidence of skeletal muscle pathology, and pulmonary arterial hypertension.[136] A further study

on anti-fibrillarin (anti-U3-RNP) autoantibodies confirmed the association with younger age at the disease onset, male gender, Afro-Caribbean descent, higher Rodnan skin score severity index, and myositis, but not with the presence of diffuse cutaneous systemic sclerosis, lung involvement, or differences in survival.[137] Anti-U11/U12-RNP antibodies have been demonstrated in about 3% of systemic sclerosis, and have increased risk of pulmonary fibrosis and gastrointestinal involvement.[138] Anti-Ku antibodies are detectable in 2.2% of systemic sclerosis and have been related to musculoskeletal abnormalities, such as myositis, arthritis, and joint contractures, as well as fingertip ulcers and telangiectasias.[139]

There are a number of subsets of antinuclear antibodies, which also have clinical predictive value: [8,140–142]

- Anticentromere antibody (which is almost specific for systemic sclerosis) is particularly common in the limited cutaneous variant.[143] It is usually found in patients with less severe disease and a more favorable outcome.[8] Calcinosis and telangiectasia may be conspicuous, but interstitial pulmonary fibrosis is less likely.
- Scl-70 antibody (anti-DNA topoisomerase) is found in 20% to 60% of patients with systemic sclerosis, particularly the diffuse variant.[144] It is also highly specific.[8,145] Scl-70 antibody correlates with severe systemic involvement including pulmonary interstitial fibrosis and a poor prognosis.
- Anticentriole antibody occurs in both the limited and diffuse forms.

Although these antibodies are of great diagnostic importance, they do not appear to have any pathogenetic significance.

A recent study from the Netherlands analyzing a total of 460 patients revealed interstitial lung disease to be more prevalent in localized cutaneous systemic sclerosis patients with antitopoisomerase I antibodies in comparison with patients without these antibodies (49% and 25%, respectively).[146] Futhermore, localized cutaneous systemic sclerosis patients with antitopoisomerase I antibodies are more likely to progress to diffuse cutaneous systemic sclerosis.[146]

The presence of Ro (SS-A) and La (SS-B) antibodies suggests the coexistence of Sjögren syndrome.[1] Autoantibodies against matrix metalloproteinase-3 have been detected in about 50% of patients with systemic sclerosis.[147] They are significantly higher in patients with diffuse cutaneous systemic sclerosis than those with limited cutaneous systemic sclerosis, and are significantly correlated with skin fibrosis, lung fibrosis, and thickening of the renal blood vessels.[147]

Antibodies to types I and IV collagen have been described, but it is not clear whether they represent primary pathogenetic agents or are secondary phenomena.[148] More recently, antiendothelial cell antibodies have been documented in scleroderma.[149] Circulating immune complexes have been

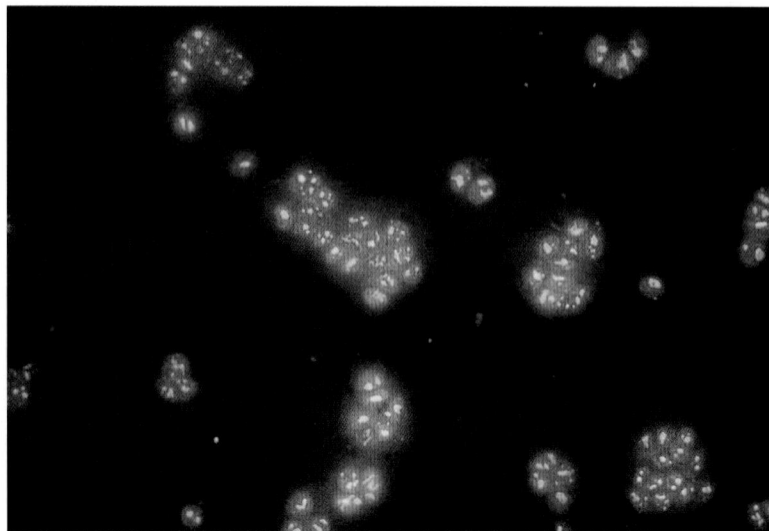

Fig. 17.95
Systemic sclerosis: antinucleolar antibody (HEP II). By courtesy of G. Swana, MD, St Thomas' Hospital, London, UK.

Table 17.10

Systemic sclerosis: main autoantibody specificities giving a nucleolar pattern of fluorescence

Antigen	Frequency in SSc (%)	Clinical associations
Fibrillarin (U3-RNP)	8	Men with more lung and heart, less joint involvement; dcSSc with telangiectasia
RNA polymerase I	4	DcSSc with high frequency of internal and musculoskeletal involvements and shorter disease duration at presentation
Th	4	LcSSc with reduced survival; pulmonary hypertension, small bowel involvement
PM-Scl	3	LcSSc in overlap with myositis; higher frequency of renal involvement

dcSSc, Diffuse cutaneous SSc; lcSSc, limited cutaneous SSc; SSc, systemic sclerosis.
Reproduced with permission from Valentini, R. (1994) Clinics in Dermatology, 12, 217–223

reported, but are not a constant feature, and their significance, if any, is unknown.[108,150]

Various T-cell abnormalities have been reported, most of which point toward a diminished concentration of circulating T lymphocytes, particularly of the suppressor subset.[103] An increased T helper:suppressor ratio has been described.[151] Soluble cytotoxic T lymphocyte-associated molecule-4 (sCTLA-4) has been found to be increased in patients with diffuse cutaneous systemic sclerosis and elevated levels of sCTLA-4 appear to correlate with the diseased severity and activity.[152] Clonal expansion of T cells has been detected in both blood (61%) and skin (45%) of patients with systemic sclerosis, which is significantly higher than in normal matched controls.[153]

Investigations have recently been directed toward the role of cytokines in the development of the fibrosis in systemic sclerosis. Evidence suggests that they are major regulators of fibroblast function and collagen synthesis. It has been proposed that in systemic sclerosis there is excessive fibroblast stimulatory activity, due, for example, to fibroblast chemotactic factors including fibronectin, collagen fragments, platelet-derived growth factor, epidermal growth factor, and C5a.[1] Fibroblast growth stimulating factors, including IL-1, -2, and -3, TGF-β, and platelet-derived growth factor, are also of major importance.[103,154,155]

As yet no consistent strong class I or II major histocompatibility complex (MHC) antigen associations have been discovered in systemic sclerosis.[10,156] There are, however, significant HLA associations with individual autoantibodies. Therefore, PM-Scl antibody correlates with HLA-DR3 and Scl-70 antibody with HLA-DR5.[50,157]

Susceptibility genes recently described to be associated with the development of systemic sclerosis include *STAT-4*, *IRF5*, and *BANK-1*.[158–160]

A useful working hypothesis for the pathophysiology of systemic sclerosis was suggested by Fleischmajer and Lebwohl.[161] They proposed that following vascular injury, possibly caused by an autoimmune mechanism, exposure of type IV collagen or other substances leads to the recruitment of both B and T lymphocytes in addition to monocytes and mast cells. Excess T-helper cells stimulate the production of autoantibodies by B cells, whereas the activated T cells, macrophages, and mast cells secrete a variety of cytokines, which in turn promote collagenosis.

Histologically, the edema of the early stage produces a picture that is indistinguishable from scleredema of Buschke.[162,163] In an established lesion the epidermis sometimes appears normal or there may be loss of the rete ridge pattern. There is often increased pigmentation of the basal cells, and melanophages are common in the superficial dermis. The characteristic change is that of thickening of the dermis by broad, elongated, swollen collagen bundles that often appear orientated parallel to the surface epithelium (*Figs 17.96* and *17.97*). The individual fiber borders are frequently indistinct, giving the collagen a rather homogenous appearance. The elastic fibers are usually unaffected. The fibrosis characteristically involves the subcutis and therefore fat cells are usually incorporated into the dermis.[164] Atrophic skin appendages, particularly eccrine sweat glands, are a common feature.

The arteries, especially the digital vessels, typically show endothelial cell swelling, intimal thickening, and medial hypertrophy. Later they may become hyalinized (*Fig. 17.98*). In early lesions, endothelium-associated platelets are significantly increased in number.[108] Fibrin deposition is sometimes present and occasionally complete occlusion results in digital ulceration and gangrene. With chronicity there is a progressive reduction in the number of vessels, particularly in the more superficial dermis.[108] Perineural fibrosis is sometimes a feature and calcification is not uncommon (*Figs 17.99* and *17.100*).

In early lesions there may be a chronic inflammatory cell infiltrate comprising lymphocytes, histiocytes, and a few plasma cells around blood vessels and at the interface between the dermis and the subcutaneous fat.[1,165] T-helper cells predominate and increased numbers of dermal Langerhans cells have been described.[108] Mast cells, usually activated, are often present in increased numbers.[166] Palisaded neutrophilic and granulomatous dermatitis has been reported in a single patient with limited systemic sclerosis.[167] Deposition of amyloid in the dermis and subcutis in a patient with CREST syndrome has also been reported.[168]

It is usually not possible to distinguish localized scleroderma (morphea) from systemic sclerosis on histologic grounds, although the epidermis is

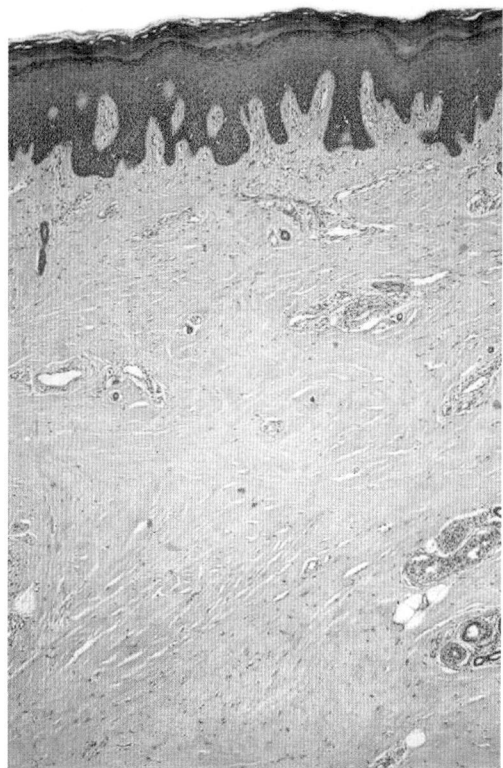

Fig. 17.96
Systemic sclerosis: scanning view of acral skin showing dermal fibrosis. The specimen was a foot amputation performed because of severe vascular involvement.

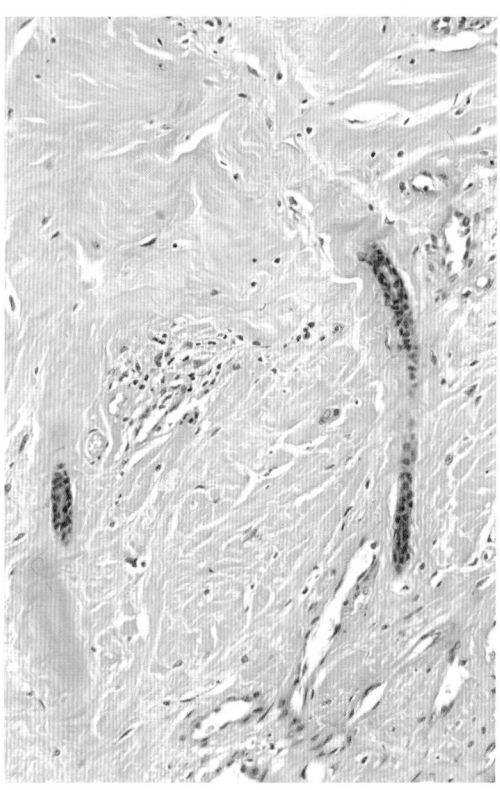

Fig. 17.97
Systemic sclerosis: the dermis is homogenized. Note the compressed eccrine ducts.

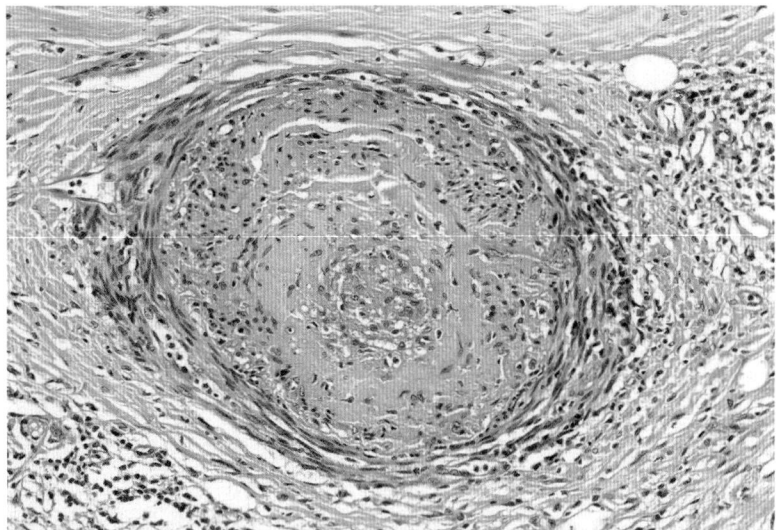

Fig. 17.98
Systemic sclerosis: severe vascular involvement characterized by intimal fibrosis and obliteration of the lumen. Note the surrounding chronic inflammation and scarring.

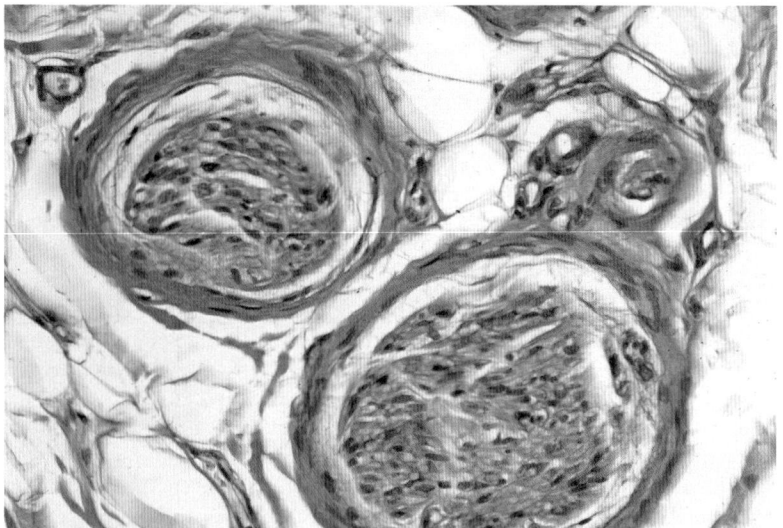

Fig. 17.100
Systemic sclerosis: high-power view.

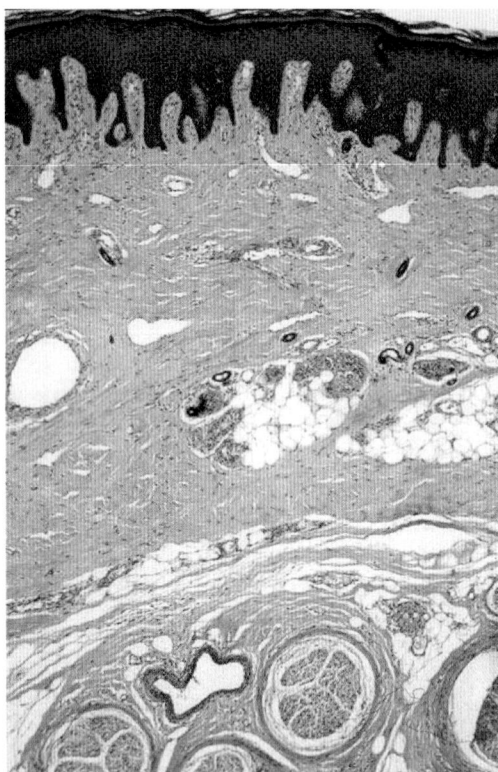

Fig. 17.99
Systemic sclerosis: there is dramatic perineural fibrosis.

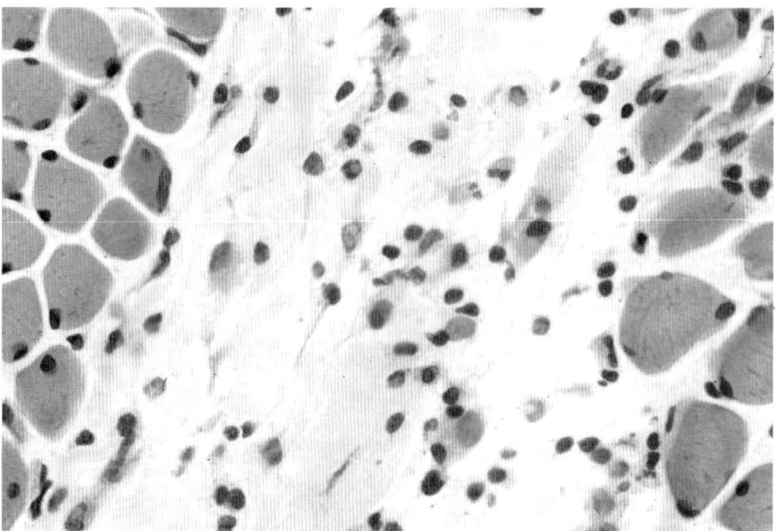

Fig. 17.101
Systemic sclerosis: myositis characterized by a lymphohistiocytic infiltrate and focal skeletal muscle regeneration.

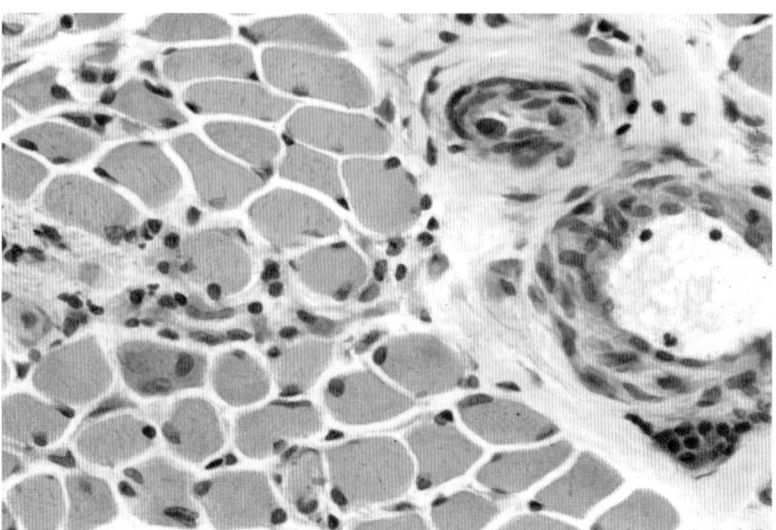

Fig. 17.102
Systemic sclerosis: Note the focal cytoplasmic basophilia on the left side of the field.

usually normal in the localized form and vascular changes are less severe. In contrast, the inflammatory cell infiltrate is often heavier in the localized variant and commonly affects the reticular dermis.[165]

Examination of skeletal muscle may reveal focal scarring and a chronic inflammatory cell infiltrate (*Figs 17.101* and *17.102*).[169] Features of muscle degeneration (vacuolation, homogenization with eosinophilia, and loss of cross-striations) and regeneration (basophilia and sarcolemmal nuclear proliferation) similar to that seen in dermatomyositis may also be present. In the sclerotic phase there is atrophy and fibrosis.

Macroscopic examination of the kidney often reveals multiple infarcts, foci of hemorrhage, and occasionally, the features of renal cortical necrosis.[68] The histologic appearances are similar to those of malignant hypertension and are characterized by the presence of fibrinoid necrosis, which particularly affects the interlobular and arcuate arteries, and ischemic glomerulosclerosis; an inflammatory cell infiltrate is not a feature.[63,170] Characteristic of systemic sclerosis is the presence of edema and mucoid change in the intima of the interlobular arteries. There is also increased cellularity, giving rise to a characteristic 'onion skin' appearance with reduction in the lumen of the vessel.

The histologic features of sclerodermatous interstitial pneumonitis are indistinguishable from those seen in idiopathic fibrosing alveolitis. Early stages are characterized by intra-alveolar edema with reactive pneumocytes and a variable infiltrate of macrophages, lymphocytes, and occasional neutrophils.[50,171] Interstitial accumulations of lymphocytes and plasma cells are evident, sometimes associated with focal lymphoid hyperplasia; in older lesions, these are accompanied by the deposition of glycosaminoglycan-rich new collagen. End-stage disease is characterized by the development of variably sized cysts lined by metaplastic bronchiolar epithelium and containing abundant collagen and hyperplastic smooth muscle in their walls.[172]

The features of pulmonary hypertension are commonly present, particularly in patients with the CREST variant. Muscular arterioles are predominantly affected, although in late stages venules may also be involved, and show medial muscular hypertrophy and concentric myxoid-rich new collagen deposition in the intima with variable reduction in the diameter of the lumen.[172] In late stages, muscular atrophy and medial elastosis may be evident. Focal lymphocytic/plasma cell endovasculitis has been documented, suggesting a possible autoimmune pathogenesis.[172] Fibrosis of pulmonary veins and venules can be similar to the changes observed in pulmonary veno-occlusive disease.[173] Pulmonary hypertension correlates with the presence of anticentromere antibody. Bronchiolitis predominantly affects the terminal and respiratory bronchioles. In addition to chronic inflammation, bronchiolar squamous metaplasia and variable scarring with luminal constriction may be seen.[172]

The most important gastrointestinal lesion is atrophy with fibrosis of the esophageal smooth muscle; similar changes may also develop in the small and large intestines. Vascular myointimal proliferation with luminal narrowing is also usually evident.[70] Reflux esophagitis may show erosions and areas of ulceration in addition to chronic inflammatory changes. In contrast to conventional diverticulae, those of systemic sclerosis are composed of all layers of the bowel wall.

Early myocardial changes are characterized by necrosis of muscle fibers accompanied by a chronic inflammatory cell and histiocytic infiltrate.[62] Subsequent fibrosis affects the right and left ventricles with equal frequency.[61] The major coronary arteries appear normal in systemic sclerosis, but arteriolar, endothelial, and intimal proliferation accompanied by mural scarring is common.[174]

In active lesions, synovial biopsies show a heavy surface fibrin deposit.[74] There is adjacent chronic synovitis with an admixture of lymphocytes and plasma cells. Lymphoid follicles with germinal center formation as seen in rheumatoid arthritis are not a feature. With chronicity, synovial scarring supervenes.

Localized scleroderma (morphea)

Localized scleroderma (morphea) constitutes a group of diseases characterized by thickening or sclerosis of the dermis with loss of subcutaneous fat, sometimes with involvement of the underlying skeletal muscle.[1–6] The incidence of localized scleroderma has been estimated to be at 27 patients per 1 000 000.[7–9] In contrast, the juvenile variant of localized scleroderma has an incidence of 3.4 patients per 1 000 000 children.[9] There is predilection for children and young adults, with the peak incidence between 20 and 40 years, and females being up to six times more frequently affected.[7,10–12] Rare congenital cases have been documented.[13–15] About 15% of cases develop before the age of 10 years.[16] Localized scleroderma is not usually associated with severe systemic symptoms or Raynaud phenomenon, is often self-limited, and in general has a good prognosis, although the linear variant in particular may be very disabling and often disfiguring, especially in children.[2] The linear and deep variants can be associated with arthralgias, synovitis, uveitis, and joint contractures.[17] A large study of patients with morphea

has found mild internal involvement consisting of abnormal lower sphincter pressure and peristaltic failure in the esophagus and slightly impaired carbon monoxide diffusion in the lung in up to 19% of patients.[18] These abnormalities do not result in clinical symptoms and do not affect prognosis adversely. A rare case has been documented in which morphea induced severe extrapulmonary thoracic restriction.[19] Extracutaneous involvement is present in about one-fifth of the children, and includes articular, neurological, vascular, ocular, gastrointestinal, respiratory, cardiac, and renal manifestations, in decreasing order of frequency.[16] Although the plaques and, to a lesser extent, the linear lesions often improve with time, the contractures and hemiatrophy are permanent.[3] Imaging studies frequently reveal muscle atrophy and leg length discrepancy.[20] Localized scleroderma may occur after trauma, laparoscopy, radiotherapy, tattooing, and silicone implants.[21–27] It has also been described in association with bromocriptine, balicatib, valproic acid, and ibuprofen therapy.[28–31] Localized scleroderma has also been reported following silica dust exposure.[32]

A recent study involving in total of 344 patients with pediatric-onset and adult-onset localized scleroderma detected disease recurrence in 27% and 17% of the patients, respectively.[33] Recurrences were more frequent in patients with linear localized scleroderma occurring on the limbs and were independent of age at disease onset.[33]

The precise relationship between localized scleroderma and systemic sclerosis is uncertain. Because of clinical and pathological overlap, some authors believe that the two conditions represent extreme ends of a spectrum of connective tissue damage in a manner similar to the relationship between discoid and systemic lupus erythematosus. Indeed, patients rarely have both morphea and progressive systemic sclerosis (the former usually preceding the latter); this phenomenon occurs so infrequently, however, that most believe that the relationship is purely coincidental.[2] Alternatively, the features of these two disorders may merely represent a common manifestation of tissue damage caused by quite different mechanisms, analogous to the wide range of pathogenetic factors which may result in the histologic appearance of allergic vasculitis.

Clinical features

Localized scleroderma includes a variety of conditions, which may arise independently, but which frequently occur together:
- plaque-form (the most common variant),
- bullous morphea,
- guttate lesions,
- linear morphea including facial hemiatrophy,
- generalized morphea,
- subcutaneous scleroderma (morphea profunda),
- disabling pansclerotic morphea of children.[2,34–36]

Plaque-form and linear morphea

Plaque-form and linear morphea are more common in females (3 : 1) and, in contrast to progressive systemic sclerosis, often occur in childhood.[1] Linear morphea develops before the end of the first decade in up to 20% of patients and by the fourth decade in up to 75%. Localized plaques occur a little later in life, although 75% of patients are between 20 and 50 years of age at presentation.

Morphea usually develops slowly and the onset may manifest as erythema and edema. An established lesion is typically circumscribed, ivory or white in color, and densely sclerotic (Fig. 17.103).[2] A characteristic feature is the presence of a violaceous border, an indicator of disease activity (Figs 17.104 and 17.105).[2] As the lesion subsides, atrophy, loss of hair and sebaceous glands, and variable hypo- and hyperpigmentation become evident (Fig. 17.106).[34] Vesicles, bullae, purpura, and telangiectasia may rarely be present, particularly in the generalized variant.[1,37] Tense bullae, due to subepidermal edema, are a rare manifestation that has been described in morphea, including the profunda variant.[38] They are thought to develop as a consequence of both trauma and lymphatic obstruction. The latter is suggested by the finding of lymphatic dilatation in 77% of biopsies from patients with this variant of morphea.[39] It has also been suggested that this type of morphea may be related to release of major basic protein from eosinophils.[39]

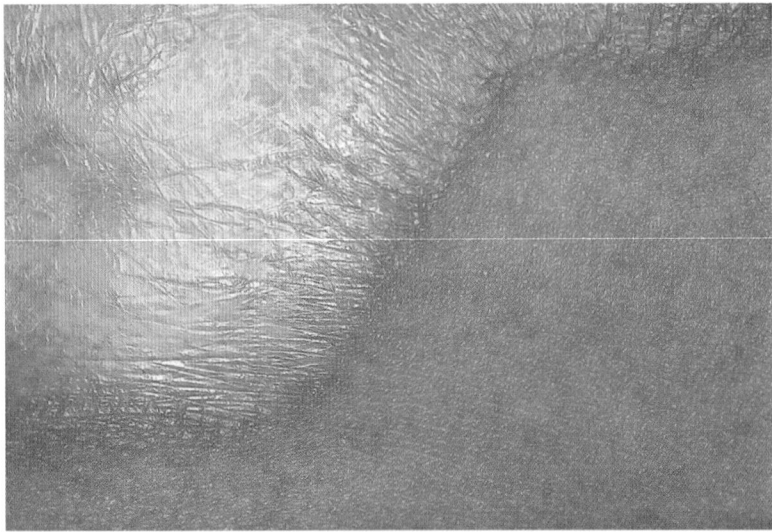

Fig. 17.103
Morphea: characteristic white sclerotic plaque. By courtesy of the Institute of Dermatology, London, UK.

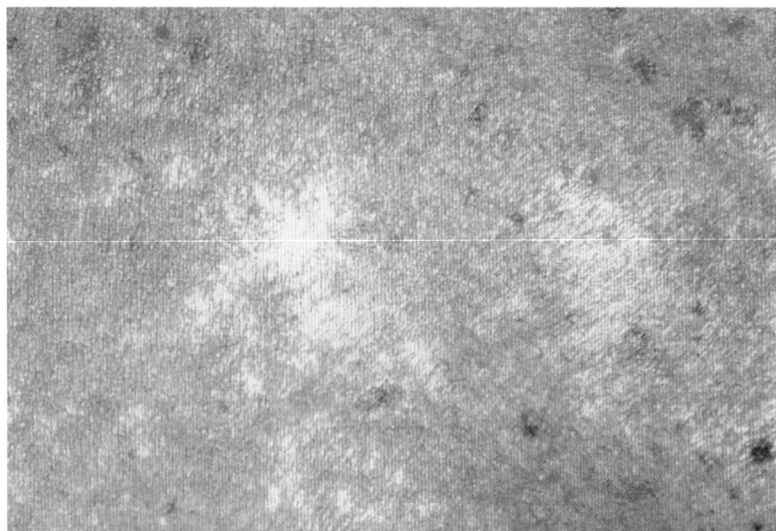

Fig. 17.106
Morphea: atrophic lesions showing variable hypo- and hyperpigmentation. By courtesy of R.A. Marsden, MD, St George's Hospital, London, UK.

Fig. 17.104
Morphea: in this example the violaceous border is apparent. From the collection of the late N.P. Smith, MD, the Institute of Dermatology, London, UK.

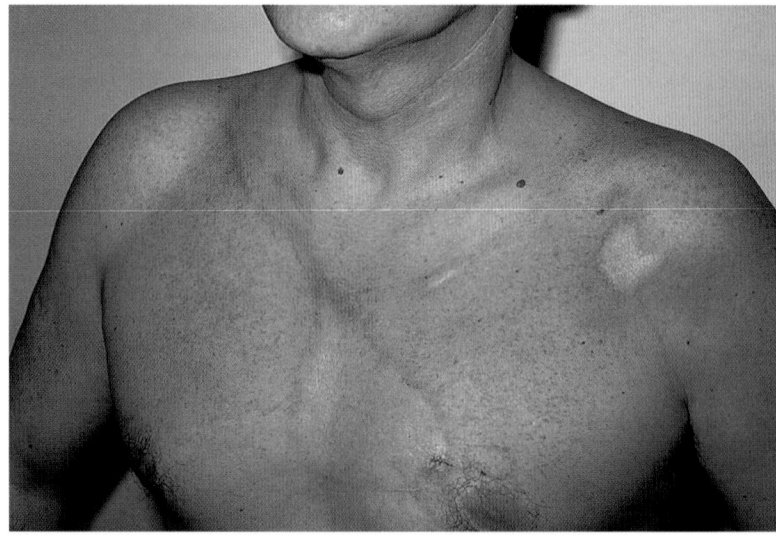

Fig. 17.107
Morphea: multiple asymmetrical lesions are present. Note the characteristic en coup de sabre. By courtesy of D. McGibbon, MD, St Thomas' Hospital, London, UK.

The plaque-form of morphea usually consists of multiple, round or oval, sometimes pruritic, 2–15-cm diameter lesions, which are usually bilateral and asymmetrical in distribution (*Fig. 17.107*). Lesions occur (in decreasing order of frequency) on the thorax and neck, the lower extremities, the upper extremities, and the face; the axillae, umbilical region, perineum, and perianal area are usually spared (*Fig. 17.108*).

The so-called linear atrophoderma of Moulin, which presents with band-like lesions following Blaschko lines, is likely to represent a variant of linear morphea.[40]

Linear morphea is usually solitary and unilateral in distribution. Lesions are found (in decreasing order of frequency) on the lower limbs, the upper limbs, the frontoparietal region (e.g., en coup de sabre), and the anterior thorax (*Fig. 17.109*). Linear lesions may involve both the upper and lower extremities simultaneously and, on occasion, plaque-type morphea is also present.[2] Although the clinical appearances of linear scleroderma are very similar to those of the plaque-form, lesions tend to show more pigmentary change and the violaceous border is less conspicuous. Linear morphea may affect the underlying skeletal muscle and even bone, giving rise to contractures and deformities. Calcification of skeletal muscle may exceptionally occur.[41] An association with melorheostosis (an uncommon mesenchymal dysplasia or Leri disease) has been described.[38,39,42] Cases presenting with

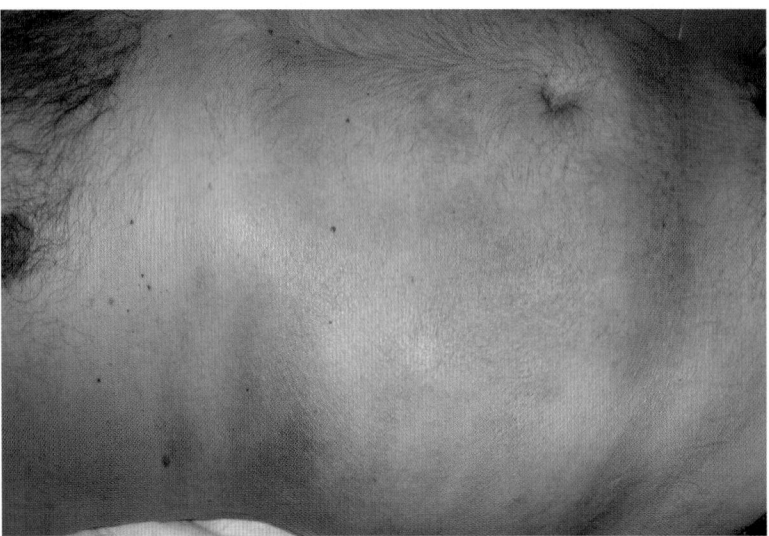

Fig. 17.105
Morphea: multiple lesions are present on the abdomen. From the collection of the late N.P. Smith, MD, the Institute of Dermatology, London, UK.

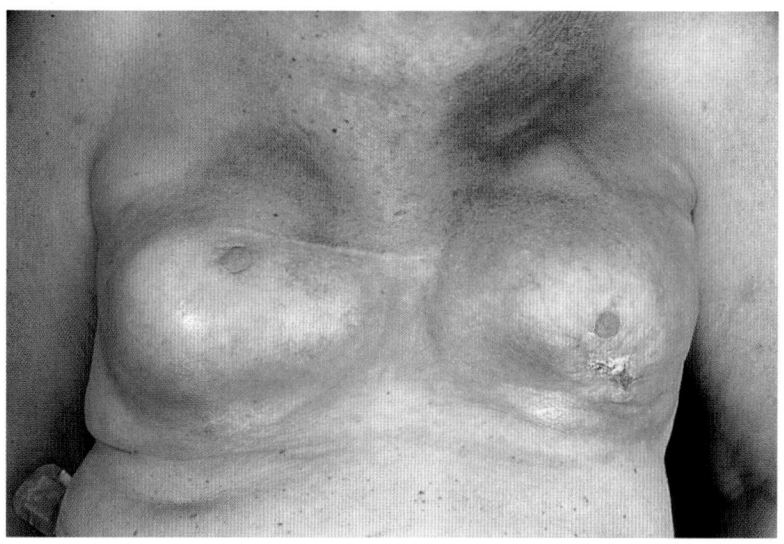

Fig. 17.108
Morphea: extensive lesions can be very disfiguring, as in this patient showing bilateral breast involvement. By courtesy of the Institute of Dermatology, London, UK.

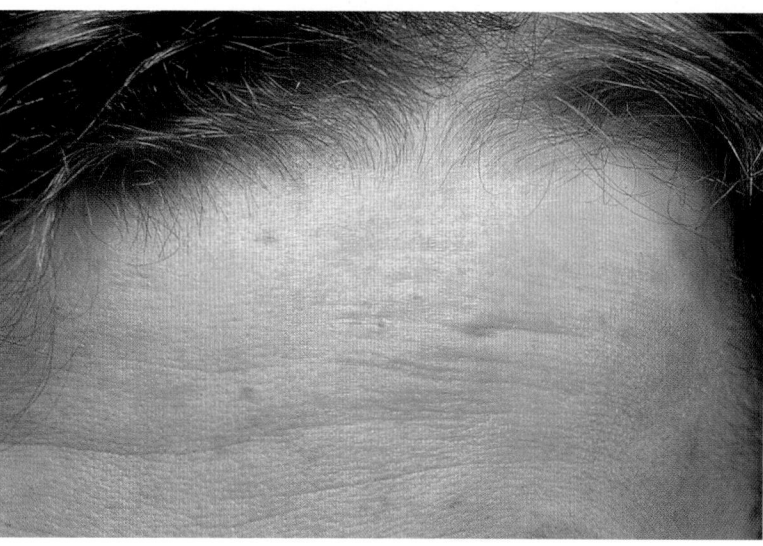

Fig. 17.110
Linear morphea: en coup de sabre. By courtesy of the Institute of Dermatology, London, UK.

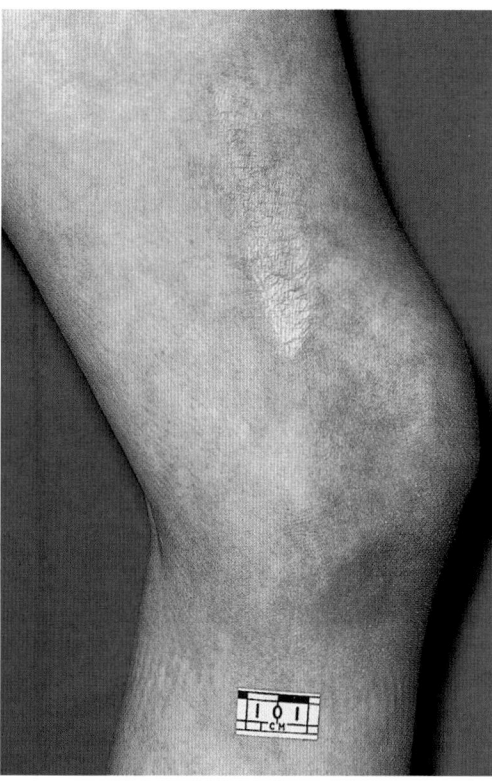

Fig. 17.109
Linear morphea: atrophic lesion on the thigh. By courtesy of R.A. Marsden, MD, St George's Hospital, London, UK.

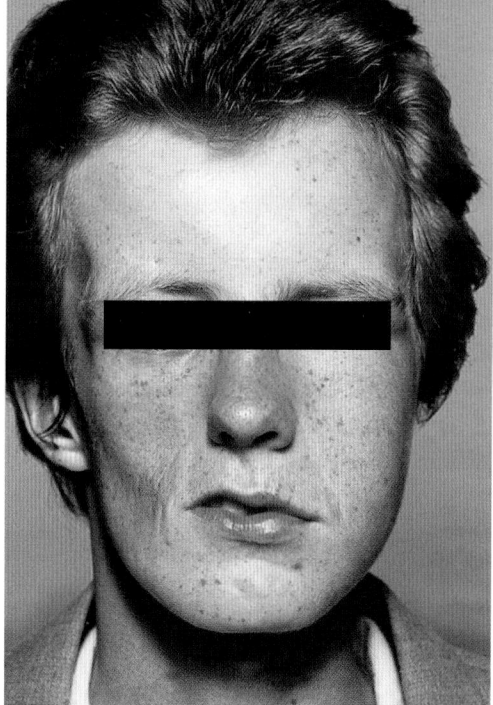

Fig. 17.111
Linear morphea: severe facial hemiatrophy. By courtesy of D. McGibbon, MD, St Thomas' Hospital, London, UK.

hypertrichosis are also documented.[43–45] Occasionally, it follows Blaschko lines.[46–51]

Frontoparietal linear morphea presents as a densely sclerotic plaque extending from the eyebrow onto the scalp and may be associated with alopecia. Involvement of the cheek, nose, and upper lip has also been documented.[34] Progression of the lesion results in the development of a groove and hence the term 'en coup de sabre' (Fig. 17.110). Gingival recession has occasionally been documented.[52] Familial occurrence is exceptional and bilateral lesions are rare.[53–55] A further complication, particularly in children, is the development of facial hemiatrophy (Romberg disease) (Fig. 17.111).[2,56] Exceptionally, central nervous system involvement may occur,[57] with presentations such as intractable partial seizures, headache, focal

neurological deficit, recurrent myelitis, and cerebral vasculitis.[58–60] About 50% of patients additionally display various dental abnormalities.[61] Linear morphea has also been described in association with hereditary deficiency of C2.[62]

Guttate morphea

In guttate morphea lesions are multiple, small (2–10 mm), nonindurated, and yellowish-white, and are limited by a delicate lilac border.[1,34] Typically, there is no hyperkeratosis or follicular plugging. Coalescence of lesions to form plaques is not uncommon. Guttate morphea most commonly presents on the upper back and shoulders, but the lower back, chest, and abdomen may also be affected.[1] There is much clinical (and histological) overlap

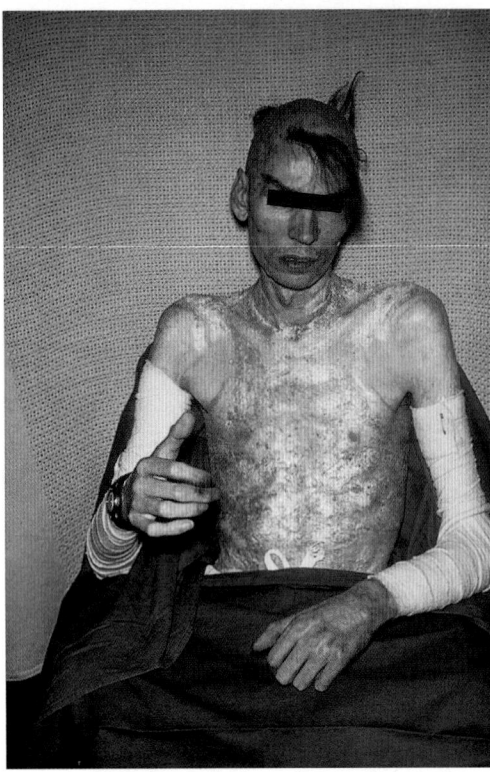

Fig. 17.112
Generalized morphea: a very advanced extreme example showing almost complete involvement of the skin, hair loss, and contractures. By courtesy of R.A. Marsden, MD, St George's Hospital, London, UK.

between the lesions of guttate morphea and lichen sclerosus and it is worthy of note that the two disorders are frequently seen together.[2,63]

Generalized morphea

Generalized morphea, which most commonly affects the trunk and abdomen, is characterized by widespread large lesions resembling plaque-type morphea.[1,64] These may merge and in many patients almost the entire skin surface is involved. Lesions are often symmetrically distributed and frequently exhibit different disease stages.[65] Extension to the subcutaneous fat and muscle sometimes results in severe contractures and disabling and disfiguring deformities (*Fig. 17.112*). Generalized morphea may occasionally prove fatal, for example, due to pneumonia. Rarely, systemic involvement supervenes.[2] When generalized morphea and systemic sclerosis coexist, the activity of the generalized morphea may be independent of the lesions of systemic sclerosis.[66] An association with porphyria cutanea tarda, eosinophilic fasciitis, and childhood sclerodermatomyositis has been described.[67-69] Occurrence with Felty syndrome and after antitetanus vaccination has also been reported.[70,71] Unilateral generalized morphea has been documented.[72,73] A patient with this form of the disease developed multiple acral adult myofibromas.[74] Multiple squamous cell carcinomas of the skin developing in the background of generalized morphea are an exceptional finding.[75]

Subcutaneous scleroderma

Subcutaneous scleroderma (morphea profunda, nodular scleroderma, keloidal scleroderma) presents clinically as nodular or keloid-like lesions.[34,38,76-82] Association with systemic sclerosis can be present.[81,83] The abdomen, sacral region, and the extremities are affected most commonly.[2] Osteoma cutis can rarely develop in subcutaneous scleroderma.[84] Two cases of morphea profunda, as well as an atrophic variant of morphea profunda mimicking localized lipoatrophy, have been reported at the site of previous intramuscular vaccination.[85,86]

Disabling pansclerotic morphea of children

Disabling pansclerotic morphea of children is a particularly aggressive and mutilating variant, which involves fascia, muscle, and bone in addition to the deep dermis and subcutaneous fat. It usually affects the scalp, face, trunk, and extremities.[1,87-89] An adult-onset variant of disabling pansclerotic morphea has also been reported.[90] Disabling pansclerotic morphea is more common in males.[91] Patients have tendencies for chronic nonhealing ulceration, most commonly involving legs, followed by upper extremities, trunk, and head.[89] Patients may also have arthralgias, contractures that particularly affect the extensor surfaces of the extremities, and osteoporosis.[34,87] This exceedingly severe variant of localized scleroderma is unremitting and permanent, and is fortunately very rare. Some patients have had abnormal respiratory function tests and diminished esophageal motility, suggesting overlap with systemic sclerosis.[87] Blood eosinophilia is also seen.[87] A rare complication of squamous cell carcinoma has been documented.[92,93] A further exceptional association is that of hypogammaglobulinemia.[94]

Associated conditions

Localized scleroderma has been associated with a variety of conditions including arthralgia, carpal tunnel syndrome, unilateral Raynaud phenomenon, intermittent abdominal pain, and spina bifida.[34,35] Concurrent lichen planus, often in the company of lichen sclerosus, has also been documented.[1] A large-perspective German multicenter study of 472 patients with localized scleroderma detected a high prevalence of lichen sclerosus in these patients (5.7%), especially in the anogenital region.[95] Other associations include vitiligo, alopecia areata, granuloma annulare, pigmented purpuric dermatosis, psoriasis vulgaris, cutaneous amyloid deposition, lupus anticoagulant, DLE, SCLE, SLE, xanthomatosis, elastosis perforans serpiginosa, B-cell lymphoma, multiple myeloma, carcinoid syndrome, human T-cell lymphoma/lymphotropic virus type 1 infection, chronic hepatitis B and C virus infection, posthepatitis C cirrhosis, primary biliary cirrhosis, Rosai-Dorfman disease, sarcoidosis, necrotizing vasculitis, necrobiotic xanthogranuloma, hepatosplenomegaly, multiple lymphadenopathy, polymyositis, neurofibromatosis type I, port wine stain, and regional inflammatory myopathy.[1,2,96-128] A recent analysis of 245 patients with localized scleroderma has found concomitant rheumatic or autoimmune disorder in 17.6%.[129] Generalized morphea is the most frequent subtype associated with autoimmune diseases, which is present in 45.9% of patients with this form of the disease.[129]

Pathogenesis and histologic features

Localized scleroderma in characterized by excess deposition of collagen type I by intrinsic activation of TGF-β signaling.[130] Nevertheless, the exact etiology and pathogenesis of localized scleroderma are unknown. Theories of causation include trauma, hormonal influences, and familial aspects.[34,131,132] Thus localized scleroderma may present or worsen during pregnancy, the menarche, or the menopause. The condition has also been described following chickenpox and measles.[1,133] An infectious etiology has received some support with the identification by immunohistochemistry, silver stains, and polymerase chain reaction (PCR) of *Borrelia burgdorferi* in biopsies of lesional skin combined with the presence of elevated antibody levels.[134-141] Lymphoproliferative responses to this organism have also been reported in patients with morphea.[142] Most studies, however, have cast doubt on the association between morphea and *B. burgdorferi*.[143-152] It has also been shown that false-positive tests for *B. burgdorferi* with indirect immunofluorescence and even enzyme-linked immunosorbent assay (ELISA) are not uncommon.[153] It is therefore more likely that *B. burgdorferi* is not etiologically linked to localized morphea. A further possibility is that only certain subspecies of *Borrelia* are capable of inducing the disease.[154,155] However, this theory has not been substantiated by different studies from the same country.[155]

The occasional simultaneous occurrence of localized scleroderma and systemic sclerosis has led some authors to postulate a shared pathogenetic mechanism.[35,156] In both conditions increased serum levels of procollagen type I carboxyterminal propeptide have been reported.[157] Similarly, the presence of localized scleroderma in both discoid and systemic lupus erythematosus and dermatomyositis has been cited as additional evidence for an immunological basis.[1,158-160] It is also of interest that the clinical appearances and histology of late GVHD are very similar to those of scleroderma. Increased expression of connective tissue growth factor has been detected in sclerotic fibroblasts of nodular scleroderma by immunohistochemistry and in situ hybridization.[83]

Antinuclear antibodies may be detected in approximately 70% of patients with morphea.[161] Homogeneous, nucleolar, and speckled patterns have all been recognized, but the first is the most common variant.[162] Rheumatoid factor, anti-dsDNA, anticentromere, and anti-Scl-70 antibodies have also been documented but are rare.[64] Anti-ssDNA antibodies are present in 38% to 75% of patients, are frequently of the IgM subclass, and are found more often in linear and generalized morphea than in the plaque form.[64,163] Antihistone antibodies have been reported in up to 50% of cases.[164] Most antibodies are more commonly seen in patients with active or widespread disease.[160] Antinuclear antibodies are frequent in children with localized scleroderma and often have specificity for denatured DNA and for high mobility group proteins.[165] Anti-Cu/Zn superoxide dismutase antibodies are present in the serum of 89% of patients with localized scleroderma, and 100% of patients with the generalized variant.[166] Anti-DNA topoisomerase IIα antibodies have been detected in 76% of patients with localized scleroderma, and 85% of patients with the generalized variant.[167] Increased serum levels of ICAM-1 have also been reported, particularly in patients with prominent involvement.[168] Peripheral eosinophilia is sometimes a feature, particularly in the pansclerotic morpheic variant.[1,87]

Direct immunofluorescence studies have demonstrated immunoglobulin (usually IgM) and complement at the basement membrane region and around the dermal vasculature in about 35% of patients.[1] Generalized morphea is more often positive than the plaque and linear variants. Immunohistochemical studies of established lesions reveal increase in the number of factor XIIIa+ cells and decrease in the number of CD34+ cells.[169–171]

The histologic features of localized scleroderma involve both the dermis and subcutaneous fat; a deep incisional biopsy is therefore indicated if scleroderma is suspected.[64,163] Biopsies from early lesions often show very subtle histologic findings and are frequently non-specific. The histologic diagnosis may be more difficult to establish in biopsies of lesions from guttate morphea as the changes tend to be more focal and superficial. In an established indurated plaque, the epidermis is usually normal or occasionally flattened. Mucin deposition is not usually a feature but may be occasionally present. Abundant mucin throughout the reticular dermis has been described exceptionally in nodular morphea.[51,172] The papillary dermis either appears unaffected or shows a rather homogenized change (Fig. 17.113). The most striking features are seen in the reticular dermis, where the collagen bundles are swollen, intensely eosinophilic, and orientated parallel to the surface (Figs 17.114–17.116). There is also involvement of the septa of the subcutaneous fat; this is associated with atrophy of the adipocytes and subsequent fibrosis, resulting in an apparent increase in thickness of the dermis.[1] Hair follicles and sebaceous glands may be atrophic or absent and the eccrine ducts often appear compressed within the densely sclerotic dermis. Due to fibrous replacement of the subcutaneous fat, the eccrine glands appear to be situated abnormally high within the dermis rather than at the dermosubcuticular interface. In rare cases only the superficial reticular dermis is affected.[173]

An important feature of localized scleroderma, especially in the early stages, is a dense, chronic inflammatory cell infiltrate of lymphocytes, histiocytes, and plasma cells; some authors believe this to be the initial feature (Fig. 17.117).[64] Eosinophils can also be present. The infiltrate may surround blood vessels and appendages and tends to be particularly conspicuous in the dermis in addition to the subcutaneous fat (Fig. 17.118). A recent histologic study in patients with 'en coup de sabre' localized scleroderma revealed the presence of vacuolar degeneration of keratinocytes in the epidermis and follicular epithelium to be a consistent finding in early and active lesions.[174] In addition, perineural inflammatory cell infiltrate in a concentric pattern with plasma cells neurotropism is also commonly observed.[175,176] In the linear and generalized variants in particular, the inflammatory changes may affect the underlying skeletal muscle.

In the late stages, dermal sclerosis is still evident, but the dermis appears thinned due to concomitant atrophy.[2] Vascular changes similar to those described for systemic sclerosis may be evident and consist of thickening of the walls of small blood vessels. Vasculitis is not a feature. Calcinosis cutis

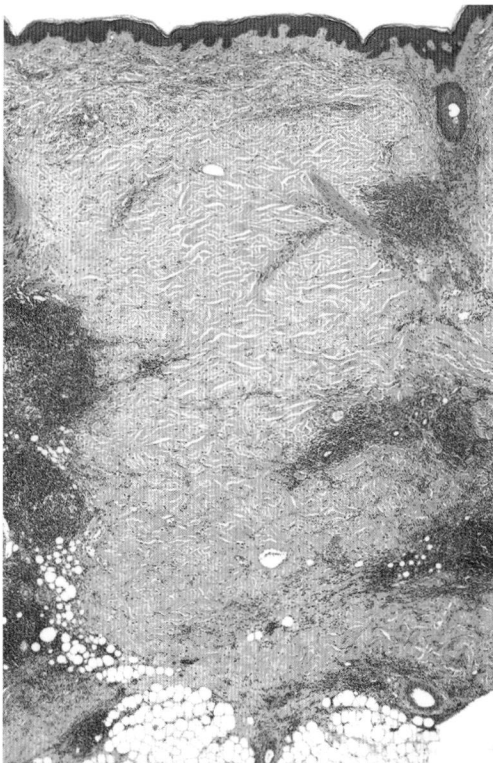

Fig. 17.113
Morphea: the dermis is thickened by dense collagen bundles. Note the heavy perivascular infiltrate.

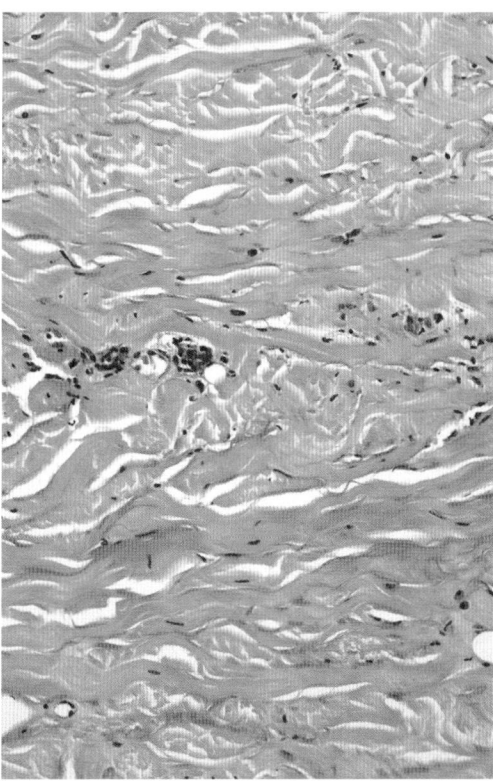

Fig. 17.114
Morphea: the collagen fibers are eosinophilic and swollen.

is occasionally seen and neuritis similar to that seen in indeterminate leprosy has also been documented.[177,178]

In lesions of deep morphea the infiltrate is much more prominent and is located predominantly in the junction between the dermis and subcutaneous tissue with extension into the subcutaneous tissue. The infiltrate and the sclerotic collagen have a more nodular distribution.

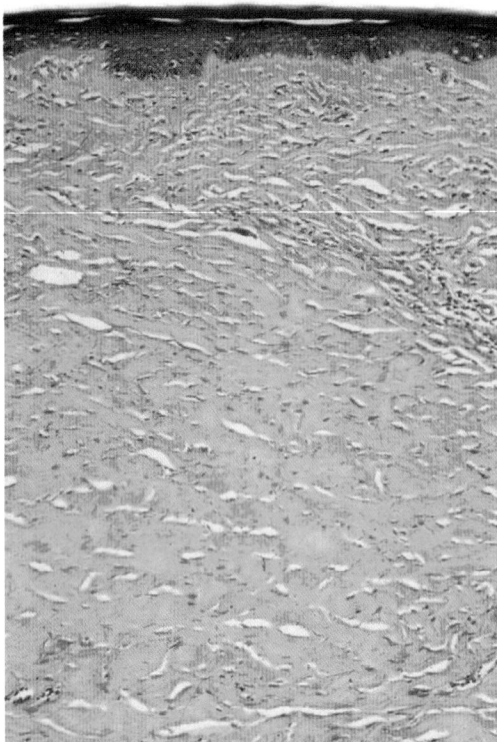

Fig. 17.115
Morphea: the changes are highlighted with this Masson trichrome stained section. In this example, the papillary dermis is involved.

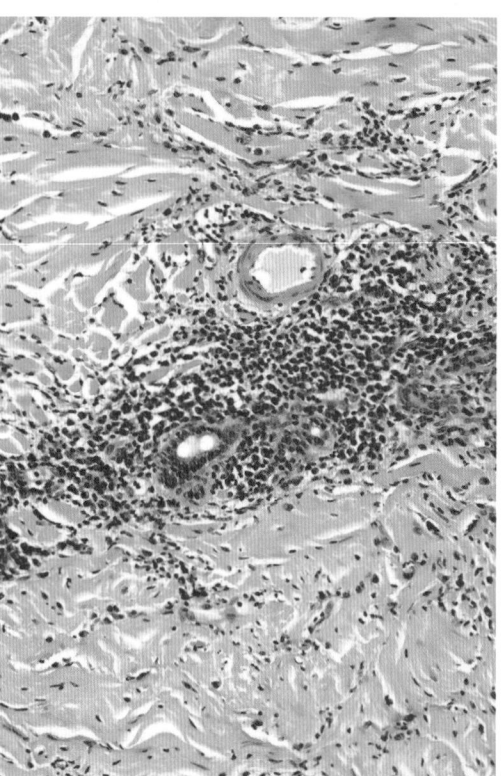

Fig. 17.117
Morphea: a perivascular chronic inflammatory cell infiltrate is usually present, particularly in early lesions.

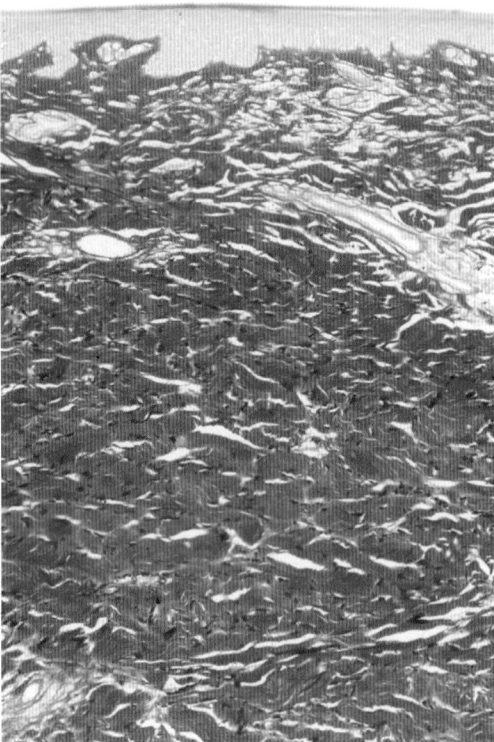

Fig. 17.116
Morphea: this is a chronic lesion. There is loss of elastic tissue (van Gieson).

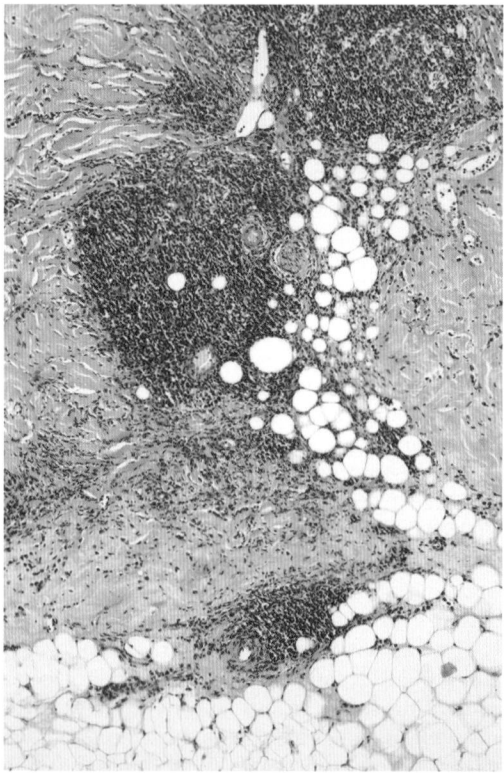

Fig. 17.118
Morphea: the infiltrate often involves the subcutaneous fat.

Several patterns have been described in bullous morphea.[39,179,180] The most common is that of prominent superficial edema with prominent lymphatic dilatation.[39] A further pattern is one identical to that seen in lichen sclerosus.[180] It is worth remembering that autoimmune blistering diseases, such as epidermolysis bullosa acquisita, may occur concomitantly with

morphea, and immunofluorescence may be indicated in cases in which a subepidermal blister is present.[179]

In addition to the features described above, generalized morphea and disabling pansclerotic morphea of childhood may show a lymphocytic and hyaline panniculitis with lymphoid follicle formation reminiscent of lupus

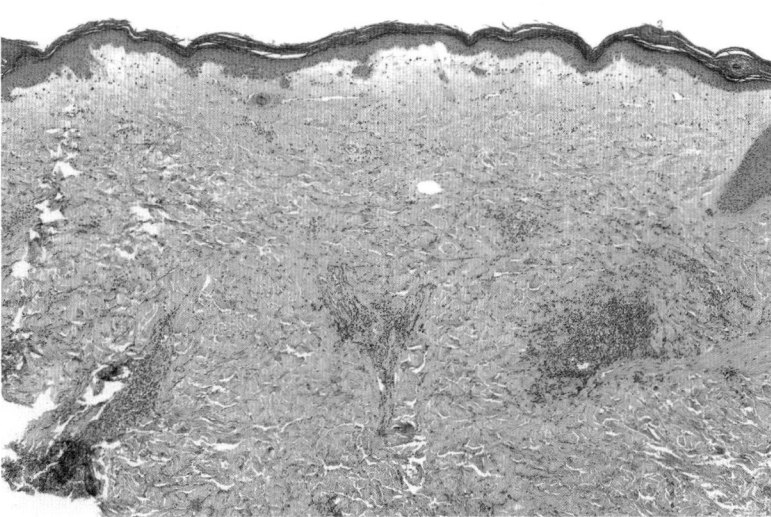

Fig. 17.119
Morphea: intense papillary dermal edema is present, producing a lichen sclerosus-like appearance.

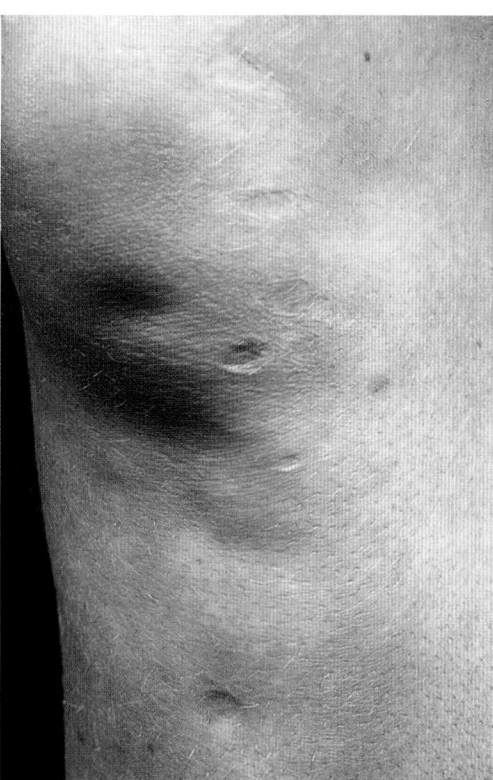

Fig. 17.120
Atrophoderma: lesions present as depressed atrophic plaques with a typical cliff-drop border. By courtesy of the Institute of Dermatology, London, UK.

profundus.[64,87] Eccrine squamous syringometaplasia and syringomatous hyperplasia have been described in linear scleroderma.[181]

Differential diagnosis

The lesions of localized scleroderma may be histologically indistinguishable from those of systemic sclerosis, but the inflammatory cell infiltrate tends to be more pronounced in the former, at least in the early stages. Also, involvement of the papillary dermis may be a feature in some cases of localized scleroderma.[182] In addition, a more diffuse dermal and less prominent subcutaneous sclerosis coupled with more intense inflammation, including perineural inflammation, are features more often seen in localized scleroderma.[175]

Other diseases that enter the differential diagnosis include late porphyria cutanea tarda and chronic GVHD. Adequate clinical information will resolve most diagnostic dilemmas, but where doubt exists, the presence of PAS-positive thickened dermal vessels is indicative of porphyria, whereas epidermal lichenoid features with cytoid body formation strongly support the diagnosis of chronic GVHD.

The relationship between localized scleroderma, particularly the guttate variety, and lichen sclerosus has been the source of considerable controversy. However, basal cell liquefactive degeneration with a lichenoid inflammatory cell infiltrate is not a feature of morphea, and sclerosis of the reticular dermis and subcutaneous fat with atrophy or loss of appendage structures is not seen in lichen sclerosus (Fig. 17.119).[63]

Marked dermal sclerosis may also be a feature of atrophie blanche and chronic radiation dermatitis. Vascular changes, including thromboses, purpura, and hemosiderosis, however, are conspicuous in the former, while bizarre fibroblasts, elastosis, and endarteritis obliterans are characteristic of the latter.

Phenylketonuria has also been reported to show sclerodermatous features.[2]

Histologic distinction between morphea and late lesions of acrodermatitis enteropathica may be difficult and occasionally impossible.[183] Close clinicopathological correlation allows distinction between these entities.

Atrophoderma of Pasini and Pierini

Clinical features

Atrophoderma is a rare, primary dermal atrophic process of uncertain nature. Since its first description by Pasini in 1923 there has been controversy as to whether it represents a distinct entity sui generis or whether it is a variant of localized scleroderma (morphea).[1–5] It presents usually in the second or third decade with a mean age of onset of 30 years and shows a predilection for females (5:1).[6] A congenital variant of atrophoderma of Pasini and Pierini has also been described.[7–10]

The typical lesion is a gray-brown or violaceous, atrophic, round to oval, depressed nonindurated macule with a 'cliff-drop' border (Fig. 17.120).[3] The distribution is usually bilateral and symmetrical.[6] Widespread unilateral involvement is rare.[11] While previous studies demonstrated the lower back as the most commonly affected site,[6] recent analysis of 16 patients revealed predominance of lesions on lower extremities (62.5%), followed by upper extremities and trunk.[12] Lesions may also be found on the chest, arms, and abdomen. A zosteriform distribution of the lesions has occasionally been documented.[13,14] The lesions are frequently hypopigmented.[12] A linear variant of atrophoderma (of Moulin) with the distribution of the lesions following Blaschko lines has been regarded a variant of atrophoderma of Pasini and Pierini.[15–18]

Atrophoderma of Pasini and Pierini may coexist with lichen sclerosus and morphea, and progression to systemic sclerosis has been documented.[13,19–22] In contrast to localized scleroderma, it lacks the violaceous border, is primarily atrophic rather than indurated, and tends to great chronicity, lesions often being present for decades rather than resolving after a few years, as is often a feature of morphea.[3]

An entity described as atrophoderma elastolytica discreta clinically simulates atrophoderma of Pasini and Pierini but the histopathological changes are those of anetoderma.[23]

Pathogenesis and histologic features

It is still controversial whether this disease represents a variant of morphea. A large study of 139 patients suggested that the disease represents an atrophic abortive variant of morphea in which the sclerotic phase fails to develop.[24] A study of lesional skin of two patients showed a decrease in the total amount of disaccharide and a normal or decreased amount of DeltaDi-4S(DS), the main disaccharide unit of dermatan sulfate.[25] This is in contrast with findings in patients with morphea in which there is increase in the total amount of disaccharide and increase in DeltaDi-4S(DS). This finding suggests that the two diseases are different. However, a further study of lesional and normal skin revealed an increase in the amount of dermatan sulfate in lesional skin as is a feature of morphea.[26] The identification in the serum of antibodies to *B. burgdorferi* in 20% to 53% of patients, combined with occasional reports of culture of the organism from lesional material, raises the possibility of a causal relationship.[6] An exceptional case of atrophoderma of Pasini and Pierini developing as a paraneoplastic phenomenon in a patient with extramedullar plasmacytoma regressing completely following chemotherapy has recently been reported.[27]

Histologically, atrophoderma often shows very subtle features. The epidermis may be atrophic or normal and is often hyperpigmented. At presentation, a slight thinning of the dermis is often present, but obvious sclerosis is generally absent. Within the superficial dermis is a perivascular and interstitial chronic inflammatory cell infiltrate consisting of lymphocytes and histiocytes. The lymphocytes are T cells and the helper-inducer subset predominates.[28,29] Rarely, plasma cells may be conspicuous. In early lesions the collagen bundles are homogenized and swollen but, with progression, sclerosis often supervenes in the deeper reticular dermis.[13,30] The appendage structures are usually normal. The elastic fibers commonly show no change, but diminution and fragmentation have been documented.[6,9] The late stages of atrophoderma are indistinguishable from localized scleroderma.

Eosinophilic fasciitis

Clinical features

The precise nosological status of eosinophilic fasciitis (Schulman syndrome) is uncertain: some authors regard it as a variant of morphea (morphea profunda) but others consider it an entity in its own right.[1–4] For the purpose of this text it is classified separately.

Eosinophilic fasciitis occurs equally in males and females, and most patients are in their third to sixth decades.[1] Female predominance has been demonstrated in some studies.[5,6] Pediatric disease has, however, also been documented.[7–10] White Caucasians are predominantly affected.[11] Rare co-occurrence in siblings and among family members suggests the possible link with distinct HLA profiles, like HLA-A2.[12]

The clinical features of painful, tender swelling, stiffness, and sclerodermiform induration affect (in decreasing order of frequency) the forearms, upper arms and lower legs, thighs, hands, trunk, neck, and feet.[1,11] The skin changes are often bilateral and symmetrical. The face and fingers are only rarely affected. Localized involvement of a limb has rarely been documented.[13] Unilateral presentation is rare.[14] Early cutaneous manifestations include pitting edema, peau d'orange or a cobblestone appearance.[1,15] At least 50% of patients relate the onset of their illness to an episode of strenuous physical activity.[16–19] Patients have a variety of non-specific features including malaise, weakness, fever, and weight loss.[1] Raynaud phenomenon is typically absent and the nail fold capillaries are normal – points of distinction from systemic sclerosis.[20] Pediatric disease commonly progresses to sclerodermiform cutaneous scarring.[7,17,21] Blood eosinophilia and hypergammaglobulinemia have been reported.[4,22] Hypogammaglobulinemia is exceptional.[23]

Extracutaneous involvement is becoming increasingly recognized.[24] Patients may develop arthralgia and synovitis. Inflammatory arthritis (predominantly involving the hands, wrists, and knees) and carpal tunnel syndrome occur in about 25% of patients.[1,17,20,21,25] Contractures develop in up to 75% of patients and particularly affect the shoulders, elbows, wrists, hands, and knees.[12,26] They are the consequence of induration and sclerosis of the subcutaneous tissue and underlying fascia.[12,26] Subclinical myositis is common.[1] Posterior ischemic optic neuropathy has also been described.[27] Clinically significant systemic features are rare, but have included esophageal dysmotility, pericardial and pleural effusions, and lung (restrictive lung disease) and kidney involvement.[1,28,29]

A number of other associations have recently been documented, including aplastic anemia, polycythemia rubra vera, thrombocytopenia, hemolytic anemia, monoclonal gammopathy, X-linked agammaglobulinemia, combined immunodeficiency, paroxysmal nocturnal hemoglobinuria, abnormal circulating T-cell clone, peripheral T-cell lymphoma, cutaneous T-cell lymphoma, acute myeloid leukemia, myeloblastic leukemia, chronic eosinophilic leukemia, Hodgkin disease, various lymphomas, multiple myeloma, allogeneic stem cell transplantation, chronic GVHD, Hashimoto disease, Graves disease, idiopathic hypercalcemia, psoriasis, IgA nephropathy, primary biliary cirrhosis, eosinophilic colitis, inflammatory bowel disease, serositis, miliary tuberculosis, SLE, myelodysplasia, acquired ichthyosis, absence of the spleen, vitiligo-like changes and peripheral neuropathy, local irradiation for breast cancer, toxic thyroid adenoma, metastatic choroidal melanoma, metastatic colorectal carcinoma, prostate and lung cancer.[1,16,30–67] It has been estimated that hematological disorders develop in about 10% of patients with eosinophilic fasciitis.[64] Furthermore, the association with serious hematological abnormalities has led to the suggestion that all patients with the disease should have a bone marrow examination to exclude myelodysplasia.[68] An exceptional familial case in association with breast cancer has been documented.[69] Eosinophilic fasciitis as a paraneoplastic phenomenon can predate the overt clinical presentation of a neoplastic disease.[65]

Laboratory investigations reveal a raised ESR, peripheral blood eosinophilia, and hypergammaglobulinemia (usually IgG).[16] Antinuclear antibodies (speckled and homogeneous), rheumatoid factor and, rarely, anti-nDNA antibodies may be present.[11,17] Serum aldolase levels appear to be a useful indicator of disease activity.[70] Cytoplasmic-antineutrophilic cytoplasmic antibodies (c-ANCA) have been demonstrated in a patient with recurrent eosinophilic fasciitis.[71]

Characteristically, eosinophilic fasciitis responds well to corticosteroid therapy – a diagnostic pointer. Spontaneous resolution occurs in some patients. Progression to scleroderma and coexistence with lesions of localized morphea may sometimes occur.[7,72–75]

The criteria for establishing the diagnosis of eosinophilic fasciitis have been proposed recently (see *Table 17.11*), and require the presence of both major criteria, or alternatively the presence of one major criterion and two minor criteria.[76]

Pathogenesis and histologic features

The etiology and pathogenesis of eosinophilic fasciitis are unknown. The clinical findings of hypergammaglobulinemia, occasional antinuclear antibodies, and positive immunofluorescence suggest a humoral immune mechanism.[1] Even in those instances when eosinophilic fasciitis has followed strenuous physical activity, it is unlikely that trauma, on its own, is responsible. There are occasional reports of possible drug toxicity following, for example, antituberculous therapy, phenytoin, subcutaneous heparin and fosinopril, simvastatin, atorvastatin, infliximab (tumor necrosis factor inhibitor), pembrolizumab, and an eosinophilic fasciitis-like picture sometimes constitutes part of the eosinophilia–myalgia syndrome (see below).[20,77–82] The disease has also followed exposure to trichloroethylene, radiotherapy, subcutaneous injection of phytonadione, and after the initiation of dialysis.[83–86] An exceptional case of unilateral eosinophilic fasciitis following influenza vaccination has recently been reported.[87]

B. burgdorferi has been associated with some cases of eosinophilic fasciitis (*Fig. 17.121*).[88–90] However, positive serology for *B. burgdorferi* in

Table 17.11

Proposed criteria for the diagnosis of eosinophilic fasciitis

Major criteria
1. Swelling, induration, and thickening of the skin and subcutaneous tissues is symmetrical or non-symmetrical, diffuse (extremities, trunk, and abdomen) or localized (extremities)
2. Fascial thickening with accumulation of lymphocytes and macrophages with or without eosinophilic infiltration (determined by full-thickness wedge biopsy of clinically affected skin)

Minor criteria
1. Eosinophilia $>0.5 \times 10^9$/L
2. Hypergammaglobulinemia >1.5 g/L
3. Muscle weakness and/or elevated aldolase levels
4. Groove sign and/or *peau d'orange*
5. Hyperintense fascia on MR T2-weighted images

After Pinal-Fernandez I., Selva-O'Callaghan A., Grau J.M. (2014) *Autoimmun. Rev.* 13, 379–382.

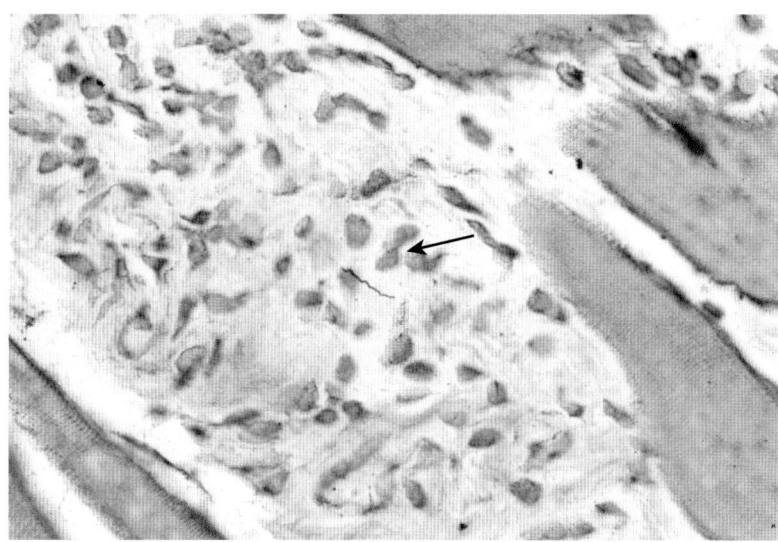

Fig. 17.121
Eosinophilic fasciitis: a spirochete is present in the center of the field (Dieterle stain) (*arrow*).

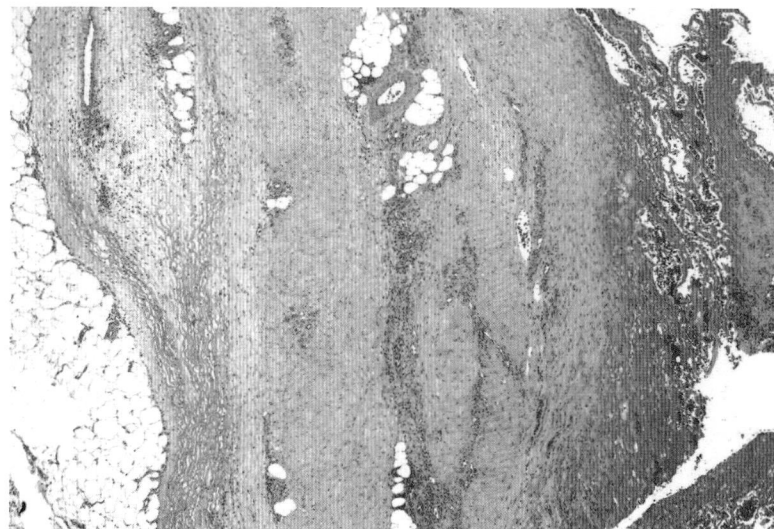

Fig. 17.122
Eosinophilic fasciitis: the fascia is thickened and there is marked fibrin deposition.

patients with eosinophilic fasciitis without direct confirmation of the presence of the organism by polymerase chain reaction has been regarded insufficient for establishing a pathogenetic link.[91]

In some patients, elevation of serum IL-2, -5, and -10, TGF-β1, tissue inhibitor of metalloproteinase-1, manganese superoxide dismutase, interferon gamma (IFN-γ), and leukemia inhibitory factor has been documented.[10,92–94] The increase in IL-5 and -10 possibly leads to eosinophilia and immune globulin overexpression.[92] Eosinophils have been shown to stimulate DNA synthesis and matrix production in dermal fibroblasts, leading to increased collagen deposition.[95]

Immunofluorescence has revealed deposition of IgM at the dermal–epidermal junction, immunoglobulin and complement around blood vessels in the deep dermis, and IgG and complement in the deep fascia and skeletal muscle.[11,17,96]

The pathology of eosinophilic fasciitis predominantly affects the deep subcutaneous fat and fascia and therefore a substantial incisional biopsy is necessary for diagnosis. The epidermis, papillary dermis, and superficial adnexal structures are usually unaffected.[11] A mild chronic inflammatory cell infiltrate consisting of lymphocytes, plasma cells, histiocytes, and variable numbers of eosinophils may be present in the deeper reticular dermis, which is also often fibrosed with atrophy of sweat glands.[96] Immunophenotyping of mononuclear inflammatory cell infiltrate demonstrated predominancy of macrophages and CD8+ lymphocytes.[97] Occasionally, the dermal changes are indistinguishable from morphea.[17]

The most dramatic changes are found in the superficial fascia, which is markedly thickened, fibrosed, and sclerotic, and in the acute stages may show focal fibrinoid necrosis and/or myxoid degenerative changes due to excessive glycosaminoglycan deposition (*Figs 17.122* and *17.123*).[1,96] A chronic inflammatory cell infiltrate is present within the fascia in both a diffuse distribution and centered around blood vessels (*Fig. 17.124*).[73] Primary vascular lesions, however, are not a feature. Tissue eosinophilia is focal and often transitory. Its absence in no way precludes the diagnosis. Lymphoid follicles, sometimes with germinal centers, are also occasionally evident.[96] The inflammatory changes usually extend into the septa of the subcutaneous fat and fibrosis may result in fat entrapment.[16] There may also be superficial infiltration by inflammatory cells into the underlying skeletal muscle, which occasionally shows focal necrosis, degeneration, and foci of regeneration.[1,96,98]

Differential diagnosis

While there is obvious overlap with morphea, the diffuse nature of the induration clinically, the high peripheral eosinophilia, and history of preceding strenuous exercise, combined with the usually less severe dermal changes

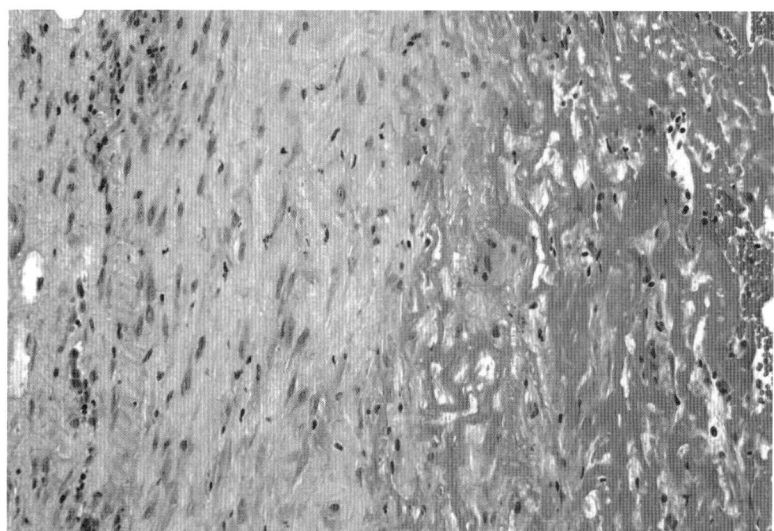

Fig. 17.123
Eosinophilic fasciitis: high-power view.

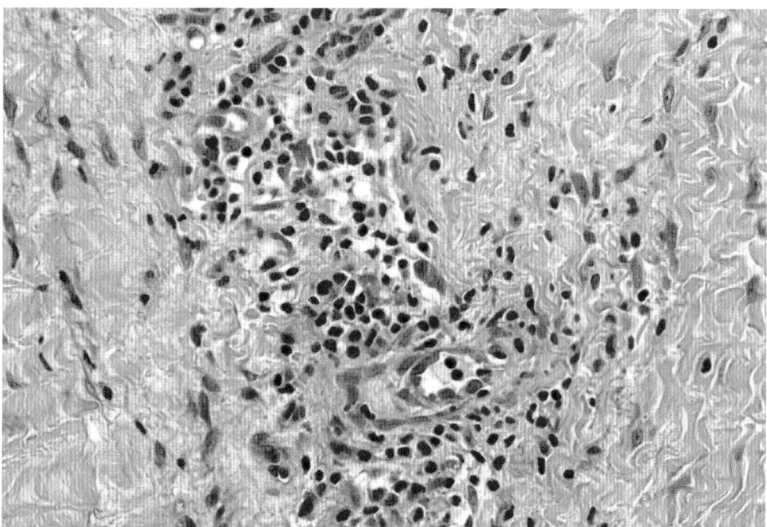

Fig. 17.124
Eosinophilic fasciitis: the infiltrate consists of lymphocytes with only one or two eosinophils.

and preservation of the skin appendages on histology, commonly serve to distinguish the two disorders.

Sclerodermoid and eosinophilic fasciitis-like syndromes have been described as features of the toxic oil and L-tryptophan-related eosinophilia–myalgia syndromes.[99–104]

- The toxic oil syndrome arose as a consequence of contaminated rapeseed oil and presented in Spain in 1981.[104,105] Patients developed myopathy, peripheral neuropathy, and arthralgia in addition to morphea-like skin induration affecting the face, trunk, and extremities.[104] Xerostomia was common and Raynaud phenomenon was not infrequent.

- The eosinophilia–myalgia syndrome is due to contaminated (Peak E) commercial L-tryptophan. Patients develop a wide variety of clinical and laboratory abnormalities involving the skin, muscles, nerves, fascia, and lungs.[101] Acute cutaneous involvement is most commonly seen as a non-specific erythematous macular eruption affecting the trunk and extremities.[101] Chronic lesions include edema of the extremities followed by the development of sclerodermiform and/or eosinophilic fasciitis-like features.[99]

Variable histologic features have been documented, presumably reflecting different stages of evolution. In some patients the most conspicuous changes have included fibrosis involving the papillary dermis, periappendageal connective tissue sheath, and subcutaneous fat.[100] An inflammatory cell infiltrate composed of lymphocytes, histiocytes, plasma cells, and variable numbers of eosinophils is present in the dermis, subcutaneous fat, and fascia.[101,102] Mast cells are sometimes conspicuous.[102] Late stages are characterized by hyaline sclerosis involving the dermis through to the subcutaneous fat.[102] Additional features that have been documented include dermal edema with lymphangiectasia and heavy mucin deposition in both the dermis and fascia.[100] The histologic features overlap between morphea/systemic sclerosis and eosinophilic fasciitis.

Polymyositis/dermatomyositis

Clinical features

Polymyositis is a rare inflammatory disorder of muscle, the etiology of which is unknown.[1,2] If certain cutaneous lesions are also present, the term 'dermatomyositis' is applied. The overall incidence is approximately five new hospital cases per million of the population per year.[1] As many diseases may include features of muscle weakness and elevated muscle enzyme activities, strict criteria must be applied to the diagnosis of these two diseases (Table 17.12). Either of these conditions may be confidently diagnosed if a patient fulfills the first four criteria (polymyositis) or three of the four plus the typical rash (dermatomyositis).[3,4]

Five variants of the disease are recognized (Table 17.13). With respect to type V, dermatomyositis most commonly coexists with scleroderma (sclerodermatomyositis), but it may also develop in association with SLE, rheumatoid arthritis, and Sjögren syndrome.[4,5] To diagnose an overlap syndrome the appropriate diagnostic criteria must be fulfilled for each disease and not just a few common manifestations. Overlap syndromes occur more frequently in polymyositis than in dermatomyositis and show a marked female predominance (9:1).[6,7]

Dermatomyositis not uncommonly presents solely with cutaneous manifestations. The quoted frequency of this type of presentation is variable

and it is not that rare for the skin eruption to precede the onset of muscle involvement by more than 2 years.[8,9] The proposed concept of amyopathic dermatomyositis or dermatomyositis sine myositis has been the source of much controversy.[10–15] In addition to a prolonged follow-up, adequate electromyographic studies and muscle biopsy are mandatory before accepting that the patient has only cutaneous lesions.[15,16] Only 5% or less of cases of dermatomyositis can be classified as the amyopathic variant after long-term follow-up.[14] For the diagnosis of amyopathic dermatomyositis to be made, it has been suggested that there should be absence of clinical or laboratory signs of muscle disease for at least 2 years after the onset of skin disease.[17] The clinical cutaneous signs of amyopathic dermatomyositis are identical to those seen in classic dermatomyositis. Patients with amyopathic dermatomyositis, like those with dermatomyositis/polymyositis, are at increased risk of developing severe interstitial fibrosis of the lung and associated malignancies.[16]

Dermatomyositis/polymyositis is associated with severe morbidity and high mortality, the latter particularly reflecting cardiac and pulmonary involvement.

The cutaneous features are usually quite distinctive.[18] Commonly, the patient presents with periorbital edema and a reddish-violet discoloration, often termed heliotrope erythema (heliotrope flower) (Figs 17.125 and 17.126). The upper eyelids are most often affected and the eruption is typically symmetrical.[19] Nevertheless, unilateral presentation of heliotrope rash has also been reported and can represent a diagnostic pitfall.[20] Heliotrope erythema is usually associated with a lupus-like erythema, which involves the rest of the face and spreads to the neck, upper trunk, and extensor surfaces of the limbs and dorsal aspects of the hands and fingers (Fig. 17.127). It is associated with a slight scale. Exceptionally, generalized subcutaneous edema may develop.[21]

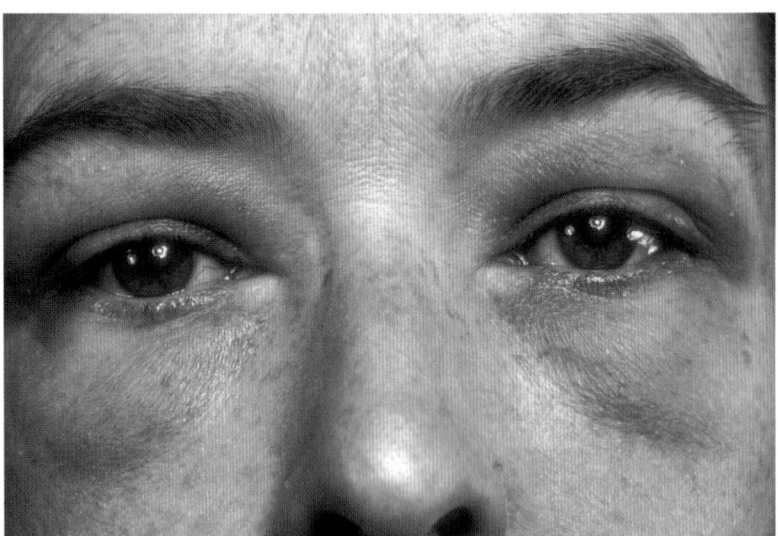

Fig. 17.125
Dermatomyositis: note the characteristic red-mauve discoloration around the eyes. There is also spread onto the cheeks. From the collection of the late N.P. Smith, MD, the Institute of Dermatology, London, UK.

Table 17.12
Diagnostic criteria for polymyositis/dermatomyositis

Symmetrical weakness of proximal limb muscles and anterior neck flexors, plus esophageal and respiratory muscle involvement
Positive muscle biopsy features
Elevated skeletal muscle enzymes
Appropriate electromyographic features
A typical rash

After Bohan, A. and Peter, J.B. (1975) Parts 1 and 2. *New England Journal of Medicine*, 292, 344–347, 403–407.

Table 17.13
Variants of polymyositis

Type	Variant
I	Polymyositis
II	Dermatomyositis
III	Type I or II plus malignancy
IV	Childhood polymyositis or dermatomyositis
V	Overlap syndromes

After Bohan, A. and Peter, J.B. (1975) Parts 1 and 2. *New England Journal of Medicine*, 292, 344–347, 403–407.

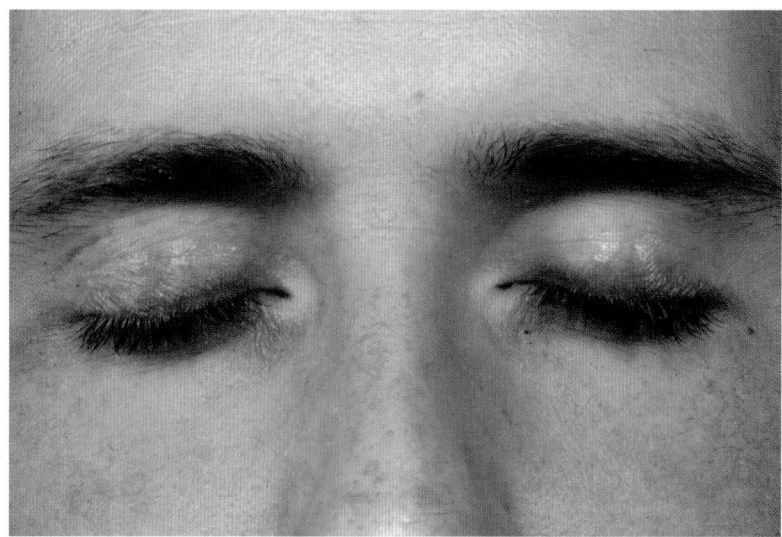

Fig. 17.126
Dermatomyositis: the upper eyelids are particularly affected. From the collection of the late N.P. Smith, MD, the Institute of Dermatology, London, UK.

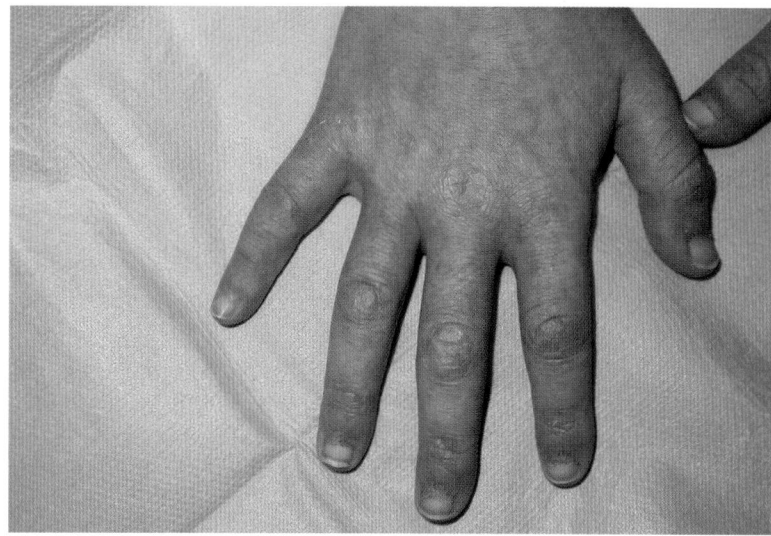

Fig. 17.128
Dermatomyositis: characteristic purple papules on the knuckles (Gottron sign). By courtesy of Dr J.C. Pascual, Alicante, Spain.

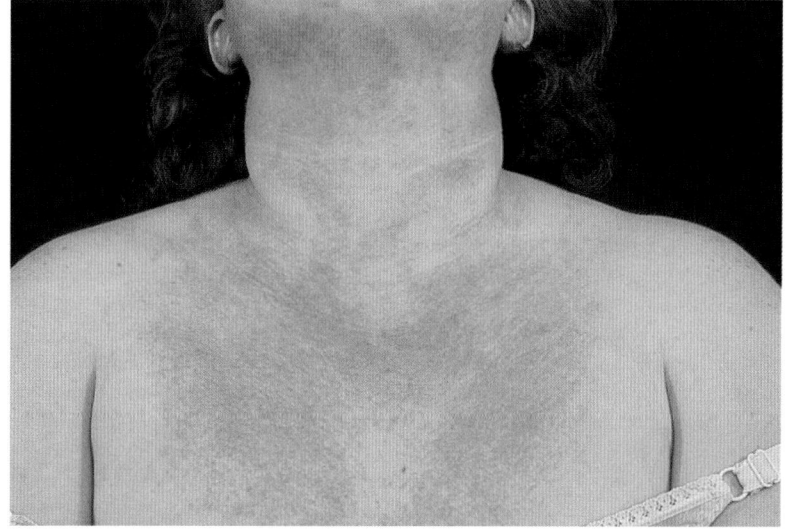

Fig. 17.127
Dermatomyositis: note the erythema and slight scale on this patient's chest. By courtesy of the Institute of Dermatology, London, UK.

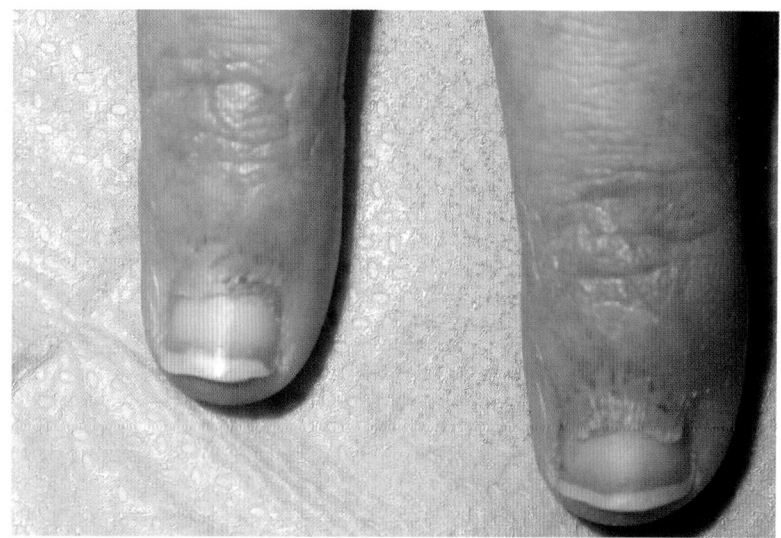

Fig. 17.129
Dermatomyositis: Gottron papules, periungual erythema, and telangiectatic capillary loops. By courtesy of Dr J.C. Pascual, Alicante, Spain.

Other cutaneous features include erythematous papules over the meta-carpophalangeal joints (Gottron sign), periungual erythema, telangiectasia, and splinter hemorrhages (*Figs 17.128* and *17.129*). Gottron papules are typically found on the knuckles, but knees, elbows, and malleoli may also be affected.[22] The toes are characteristically spared. The nail fold capillaries may be enlarged, dilated, and distorted. Avascular areas are also often present.[18] Cuticular overgrowth is sometimes evident, and occasionally there is a cutaneous vasculitis presenting as digital ulceration, periungual infarcts, and mouth ulcers, though more often in the childhood variant.[18] With time, the skin may become more atrophic and show the features of poikiloderma, which particularly affects the extensor surfaces and upper back, but may be more widespread (*Fig. 17.130*).[6,7] Scalp involvement, which presents with scaling and erythema, is not uncommon and is frequently pruritic.[18] Photo-sensitivity has occasionally been reported.[6,19] Other rare or unusual features include gingival telangiectases, follicular papules resembling pityriasis rubra pilaris (Wong variant of dermatomyositis), erythroderma, erythema confined to seborrheic areas, flagellate erythema with characteristic wheal-like manifestations, dermographism, lesions resembling malignant atrophic papulosis (Degos disease), a vesiculobullous rash, a pustular eruption, Sweet syndrome-like dermatosis, granuloma annulare, cutaneous amyloidosis, localized mucinosis, panniculitis, lipodystrophy, and acute generalized

subcutaneous edema.[22–49] Gingival telangiectases have also been found in association with anti-Jo-1 antibody.[50] Some patients present with a cen-tripetal flagellate erythema affecting the trunk and proximal extremities.[51] Subepidermal blistering may occur and this has been linked to internal malignancy.[27,52,53] A rare case with acute onset vesiculobullous lesions and massive mucosal necrosis of the intestine has been documented.[54] Bullous pemphigoid may also rarely be associated with dermatomyositis.[55] Eruptive dermatofibromas have been reported in a single patient with dermatomyosi-tis who was treated with prednisolone and methotrexate.[56]

Symmetrical proximal (limb girdle) muscle weakness is the most common presenting feature of polymyositis.[6] The legs are almost always the initial site of involvement. The patient experiences difficulty in getting out of a chair, walking up the stairs, combing his hair, or raising his head from a pillow. Interestingly, the facial muscles are almost never involved.[57] Although the muscles may be painful, this is not usually severe, and tenderness is not often present. Muscle atrophy develops later in the course of the disease when fibrosis and troublesome contractures may supervene.

Esophageal involvement manifests as dysphagia, which correlates with the presence of an associated malignancy.[4] Symptoms may also indicate pre-esophageal involvement due to cricopharyngeal striated muscle weak-ness.[6] Sequelae include nasal regurgitation and aspiration pneumonitis, the

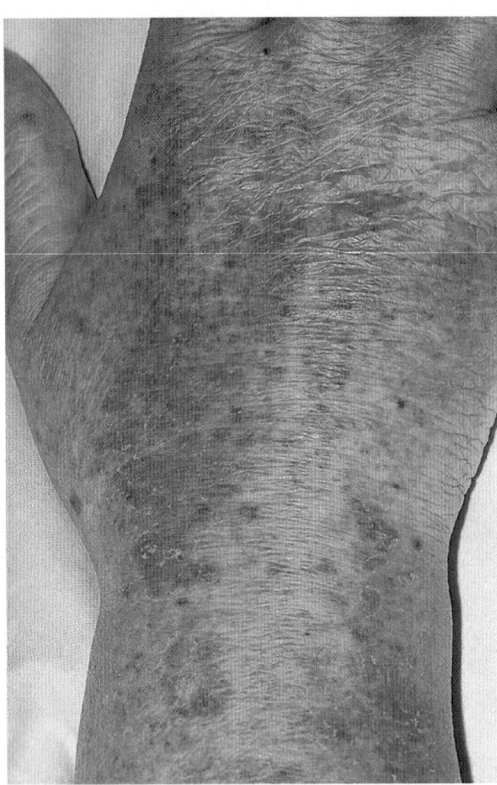

Fig. 17.130
Dermatomyositis: in this patient with longstanding disease, atrophy and variable pigmentary changes (poikiloderma) are present on the dorsum of the hand. By courtesy of the Institute of Dermatology, London, UK.

latter being associated with a high mortality. A change in voice is a not uncommon manifestation. Juvenile dermatomyositis has also been associated with ischemic ulcerative colitis and celiac disease.[58,59]

Electromyographic features in polymyositis/dermatomyositis are said to be pathognomonic and include the triad of fibrillation at rest with increased insertional activity and positive sharp waves, polyphasic potentials of short duration and long amplitude and bizarre high-frequency repetitive discharges.[57,60]

The serum usually contains raised levels of creatine kinase, aldolase, lactate dehydrogenase, and transaminases; as not all these may be elevated in any one patient it is usually recommended that all are estimated routinely.[6] Sequential muscle enzyme studies are particularly useful for monitoring progress and response to treatment.

Involvement of cardiac muscle is not uncommon and patients may have tachycardia, sinus bradycardia, electrocardiographic abnormalities (e.g., bundle branch block), congestive heart failure, and cardiomegaly.[61,62] Restrictive cardiomyopathy has also been described in a patient with dermatomyositis.[63] A large population-based study from British Columbia involving 774 patients with inflammatory myopathies revealed a significantly increased risk of myocardial infarction in this group of patients, especially in the first year after diagnosis.[64]

Pulmonary involvement, as determined by the radiological changes of interstitial fibrosis and/or clinical evidence of impaired respiratory function, may occur in as many as 40% of patients with polymyositis/dermatomyositis.[6] Patients are also at increased risk for development of pulmonary hypertension.[65] Pneumomediastinum and interstitial pneumonia are rare complications.[66,67] Pulmonary hemosiderosis is an exceptional finding in juvenile dermatomyositis.[68] An important recently described association is that between the anti-Jo-1 antibody, pulmonary fibrosis, and dermatomyositis.[69–74] More than 50% of patients with anti-Jo-1 antibody have interstitial lung disease.[70] Patients with this variant are not at risk of an increased incidence of internal malignancy. Additional features of this variant may include Raynaud phenomenon, arthritis, and tenosynovitis. Spread to the thoracic muscles can result in severe respiratory difficulties; terminal bronchopneumonia is therefore an important cause of death.[75]

Cutaneous vasculitis is characteristic of the childhood variant, which may involve the viscera; it has also been described in adult patients and may be associated with an increased risk of malignancy. Digital ulcers, periungual infarcts, and oral ulcers are associated manifestations.[6] Deep cutaneous and subcutaneous ulcers not associated with vasculitis, have rarely been reported in adult-onset dermatomyositis, and are likely to be related to obliterative (micro)vasculopathy.[76] Calcification of the skin, soft tissues, and muscle is rare except in the childhood variant where it may be widespread and of help diagnostically.[77–79] Skin calcification has been demonstrated to correlate with autoantibodies to a 140-kD protein.[79]

Patients with dermatomyositis/polymyositis exhibit 11-fold increased risk for venous thromboembolism in comparison with a matched control group, as suggested by a large population-based study on 2031 patients from Taiwan.[80]

Arthralgia is not uncommon, but frank arthritis is rare except in the overlap group of patients.[4] Destructive arthropathy has been reported in a patient with amyopathic dermatomyositis associated with anti-Jo-1 and anticyclic citrullinated peptide antibodies.[81] Aseptic bursitis of the olecranon has been reported in a single patient.[82]

Laboratory investigations may reveal non-specific findings of a raised ESR, hypergammaglobulinemia, and a false-positive Wassermann reaction. Antinuclear factor may be found in a small percentage of patients with polymyositis/dermatomyositis. Anti-RNP and -SM antibodies are only seen in 'overlap' patients. In addition to anti-Jo-1 antibody, additional newly described antibodies include PM-1, Ku, Mi-1, -2 and -3, and Pa-1.[83] The significance of these (except anti-Jo-1) is uncertain.[84]

Often stressed in polymyositis/dermatomyositis is the association with an increased risk of developing malignancy.[85] Although there has been a great range in reported incidences from small studies, varying from 15% to 60% of cases, recent investigations have suggested that the risk is less.[60,86–91] The risk of malignancy appears to be higher among patients with dermatomyositis (23%) than polymyositis (8.9%).[92] Polymyositis/dermatomyositis has been described in association with the following malignancies: breast cancer, neuroendocrine carcinoma of the lung, small cell lung cancer, hepatocellular carcinoma, neuroendocrine carcinoma of the liver, duodenal carcinoid, gallbladder carcinoma, carcinoma of the bladder, prostate cancer, renal cell carcinoma, clear cell ovarian carcinoma, fallopian tube cancer, carcinosarcoma of the uterus, nasopharyngeal carcinoma, esophageal cancer, Klatskin tumor (hilar cholangiocarcinoma), thyroid cancer, thymic carcinoma, cancer of the colon, primary gastric melanoma, metastatic melanoma, diffuse large B-cell lymphoma, primary cutaneous B-cell lymphoma-leg type, follicular lymphoma, lymphoplasmocytoid lymphoma, acute myeloid leukemia, and Kaposi sarcoma.[93–127] Among the reported associations, breast, stomach, and ovarian tumors are most often cited. In a recent study analyzing patients with dermatomyositis in China, nasopharyngeal cancer was the most frequent association, followed by lung cancer.[128] Patients should have a very thorough physical examination combined with routine laboratory investigations, chest X-ray, CT scan of the abdomen and pelvis, and (in female patients) mammography. Underlying malignancy should be suspected in patients who do not respond to therapy or those who develop frequent episodes of myositis.[87,129] A recent study suggests that patients requiring more extensive search for malignancy should include those with constitutional symptoms, with rapid onset of dermatomyositis or polymyositis, without Raynaud phenomenon, with a high ESR, and with a very high creatine kinase level.[91]

There appears to be an increased risk of thyroid disease, particularly hypothyroidism, especially in patients with interstitial lung disease.[60] Patients with dermatomyositis also have an increased risk for the development of ulcerative colitis.[130]

Juvenile dermatomyositis, which has an annual incidence of about one new case per million of the population per year, shows a female predominance (2:1) and presents most often in the first decade.[77] In addition to the features described above there is a high incidence of vasculopathic manifestations, including gastrointestinal ulceration with hemorrhage, which may be fatal.[1,131] Multiorgan involvement is common. The condition is often preceded by an infection.[132] The prognosis is usually good, with up to 70% of children making a full recovery.[132] In severely affected patients, widespread cutaneous involvement may be complicated by extensive scarring and diffuse calcification.[133]

Scleroderma/polymyositis overlap (sclerodermatomyositis) is the most common overlap syndrome. Although the myositis component is usually identical to that seen in dermatomyositis/polymyositis, the heliotrope erythema and Gottron papules are usually absent.[134] The sclerodermatous cutaneous manifestations tend to be restricted to the peripheries. This overlap syndrome is associated with the Ku antibody, and a case has been reported in association with Graves disease and thrombocytopenic purpura.[135] Autoimmune idiopathic thrombocytopenia with anti-Ku antibody has also been associated with dermatomyositis.[136]

Pathogenesis and histologic features

While the etiology and pathogenesis of polymyositis/dermatomyositis are unknown, it has been proposed that environmental factors (e.g., drugs, toxins or viruses) acting in association with a genetic predisposition result in a primarily immune-mediated disorder.[60] There is evidence to suggest that both humoral and cell-mediated components are important.

Antinuclear factor is commonly present. Antimyosin and antimyoglobin antibodies have been described, but their significance is uncertain. It is not clear whether they precede or follow the onset of the myositis, and their presence does not explain the cutaneous manifestations. However, antimyosin antibodies accompany any inflammatory myositis and are therefore probably a consequence of muscle necrosis.

A further set of antibodies directed against nuclear antigens have been described in 35% to 40% of patients with dermatomyositis/polymyositis:[137]

- PM-1 (PM-Scl) antibody correlates closely with polymyositis and polymyositis/scleroderma overlap.
- Ku antibody is a marker for sclerodermatomyositis.
- PA-1 antibody correlates with polymyositis, arthritis, and fibrosing alveolitis.
- Mi-2 correlates with dermatomyositis.[6,60,137]

The presence of antibodies to the RNP antigens, U1 and U2, although not specific, is certainly highly suggestive of dermatomyositis/systemic sclerosis overlap syndrome.[135,138,139] Antisignal recognition particle (SRP) antibodies are uncommon, but are usually associated with severe disease.[135] Although these antinuclear autoantibodies are of diagnostic value, they have not yet been shown to be of pathogenetic significance.

Several myositis-specific antibodies have been identified recently, which are closely associated with the disease phenotype. Anti-transcriptional intermediary factor 1 (anti-TIF1) antibodies (previously designated anti-p155-kD protein antibodies) are particularly specific for dermatomyositis in adults and children and have been detected in roughly 30% of both patient groups.[140] Furthermore, anti-TIF1 antibodies are strongly associated with malignancies, especially in dermatomyositis patients above the age of 40 years.[92] Up to 75% of adult dermatomyositis patients were reported to have developed malignancy.[141] Anti-melanoma differentiation antigen 5 (anti-MDA5) antibodies (also designated anti-CADM-140 antibodies) are more frequent in patients with amyopathic dermatomyositis and correlate with interstitial lung disease in Japanese patients.[142,143] In addition, it has been demonstrated that anti-MDA5 antibody level correlates with disease activity and that relapse of the disease is associated with re-increase in the levels of anti-MDA5.[144] These data suggest that anti-MDA5 antibody levels can be used for monitoring disease activity and as a predictive marker of relapse in patients with amyopathic dermatomyositis.[144] Antinuclear matrix protein 2 antibodies (originally designated anti-MJ antibodies) are detected in up to 25% of patients with juvenile myositis and are associated with severe disease course characterized by muscle contractures and atrophy.[145,146] Furthermore, the presence of anti-NXP2 autoantibodies significantly increases the risk of calcinosis cutis.[147,148] Anti-small ubiquitin-like modifier activating enzyme antibodies are present in less than 10% of patients with adult dermatomyositis and are associated with high incidence of severe dysphagia.[140,149]

Dermatomyositis and polymyositis may develop in patients with other known autoimmune disorders, including autoimmune thyroid disease and insulin-dependent diabetes mellitus.[60,150] The precise role of humoral immunity in dermatomyositis is unclear, but it is thought to be particularly related to the capillary loss and ischemic damage.[151]

Cell-mediated immunity is important in the development of experimental models of polymyositis. Lymphocytes taken from animals with allergic myositis (based upon sequential injections of heterologous muscle with Freund adjuvant) prove cytotoxic to skeletal muscle fibers in culture and may undergo lymphoblastic transformation. Parallels do exist in the human disease, but whether these represent initiating factors or develop as a consequence of muscle damage is unknown.[1] A variety of cellular immune abnormalities have been documented, including the presence of activated mononuclear cells within skeletal muscle, abnormal trafficking of mononuclears to skeletal muscle, decreased autologous mixed lymphocyte responses, and mitotic and proliferative responses to autologous muscle.[60,152,153]

There is some evidence to suggest an inherited predisposition with an increased incidence of HLA-B8 and HLA-DR3 in both dermatomyositis and polymyositis, particularly in patients who have anti-Jo-1 antibodies.[60,154] There are rare instances of familial disease.[60]

A number of animal experimental models have shed some light on the possible pathogenesis of human myositis.[6] Injection of muscle extracts into a number of animals results in a mild, nonpersistent myositis.[60]

Several viruses – including Coxsackie B virus, simian acquired immunodeficiency retrovirus, and murine encephalomyocarditis virus – have been shown to induce a chronic myositis-like disease. Virus strain and host genetic factors appear to be of particular importance.[60] Although uncertain, it has been suggested that some cases of dermatomyositis, particularly the juvenile variant, may represent an abnormal immunological response to a viral infection.[75] Picornaviruses, including the coxsackievirus group, have been particularly implicated.[1] The anti-Jo-1 antibody (an antiaminoacyl-tRNA synthetase) reacts with histidyl-transfer RNA synthetase.[151] This enzyme has been shown to be capable of interacting with the RNA of a number of picornaviruses in addition to its normal substrate tRNA.[60] It has been suggested that the development of the autoantibody may occur as a consequence of this aberrant interaction.[60]

It is interesting to note that an illness similar to dermatomyositis may be induced by a number of infectious organisms including leishmania, parvovirus (erythrovirus) B19, human immunodeficiency virus, and toxoplasma.[155-159] Tuberculous myofasciitis has developed in a dermatomyositis patient.[160] Dermatomyositis/polymyositis has been reported as an adverse reaction to a number of drugs, such as hydroxyurea, cyclophosphamide, etoposide, fluvastatin, simvastatin, pravastatin, atorvastatin, ipilimumab, capecitabine, anti-TNF alpha treatment, omeprazole, minocycline, carbimazole, terbinafine, and interferon beta-1a.[161-185] Furthermore, polymyositis/dermatomyositis has also been found in association with hepatitis B vaccination, psoriasis, pemphigus foliaceus, Duchenne muscular dystrophy carrier status, familial polyposis colli, ulcerative colitis, hemophagocytic syndrome, organic solvent, and silicone gel-filled breast implants.[186-195]

Several studies have confirmed an increased incidence of herpes zoster in dermatomyositis/polymyositis patients in comparison with the healthy controls, especially in females aged older than 50 years with one or more comorbidities, including diabetes, renal disease, obesity, cancer, other autoimmune diseases, MCTDs, vasculitis, and/or treatment with immunosuppressive drugs or corticosteroids.[196,197]

Direct immunofluorescence of lesional skin reveals granular deposits of immunoglobulin (IgG, IgA, and IgM) and complement at the dermal–epidermal junction in about 35% of patients.[198,199] Site selection is of importance, positivity being most frequent with nail bed biopsies.[198] A more recent study has demonstrated C5b–9 deposition in blood vessel walls and along the dermal–epidermal junction in conjunction with a negative lupus band test.[200,201] This finding has high specificity (93.5%) and sensitivity (78.5%). Epidermal keratinocytes may also be positive for C5b–9 and IgG.[201] The finding of C5b–9 in the wall of small blood vessels suggests that a complement-mediated microvascular injury may be of some importance in the pathogenesis of dermatomyositis.

The pathogenesis of childhood dermatomyositis has a predominantly ischemic basis (see below).[132]

The cutaneous findings are variable. The erythematous eruption shows slight hyperkeratosis and epidermal atrophy, with effacement of the ridge pattern (*Fig. 17.131*).[132] Basal cell liquefactive degeneration is typical and

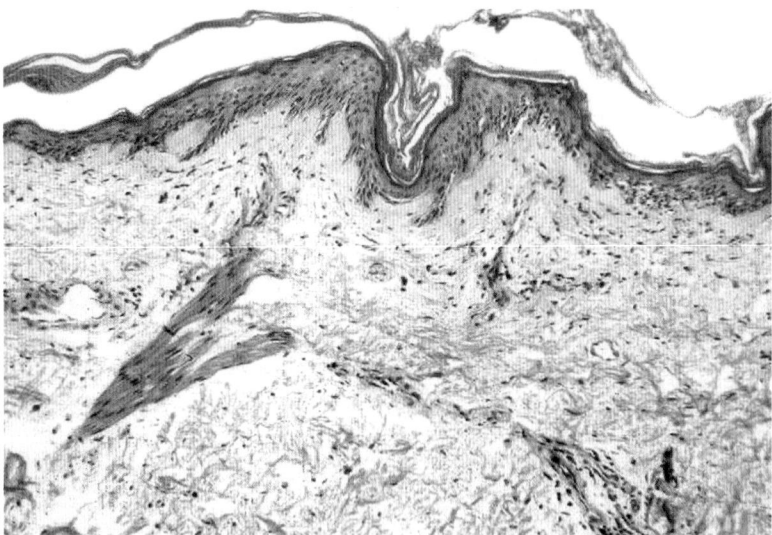

Fig. 17.131
Dermatomyositis: there is hyperkeratosis and epidermal atrophy. Note the mild telangiectasia.

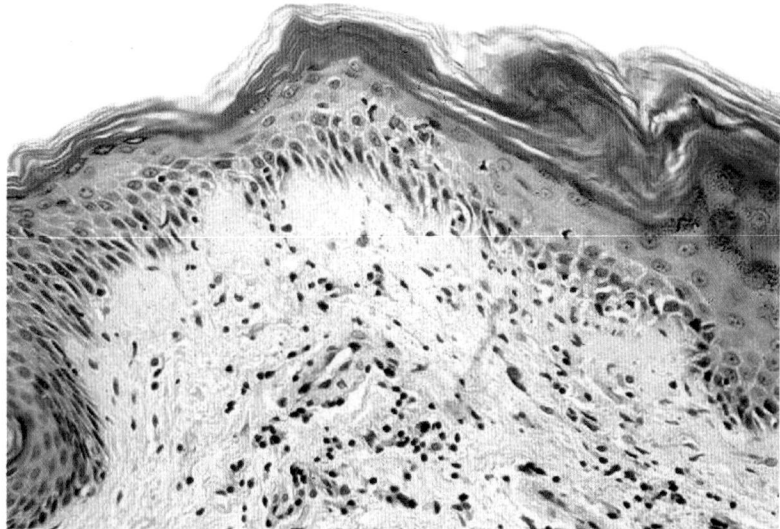

Fig. 17.133
Dermatomyositis: focal, mild basal cell hydropic degeneration is seen on the right. A chronic inflammatory cell infiltrate is present.

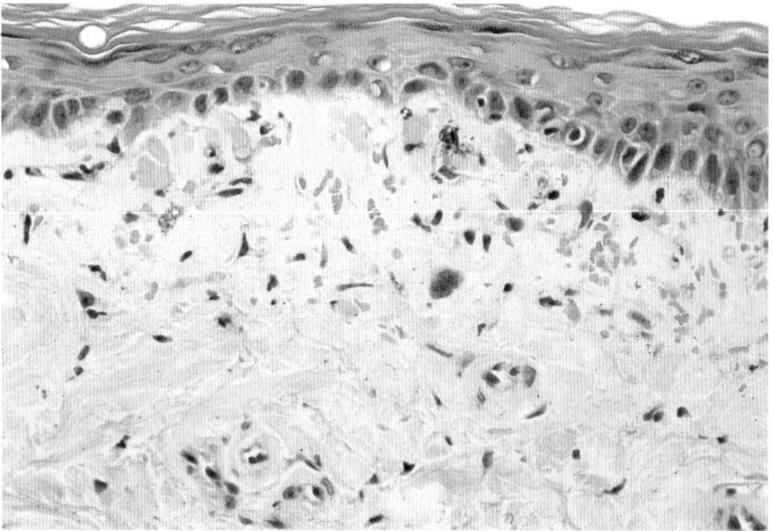

Fig. 17.132
Dermatomyositis: there is atrophy with effacement of the ridge pattern. In this example cytoid bodies are conspicuous. Note the pigmentary incontinence.

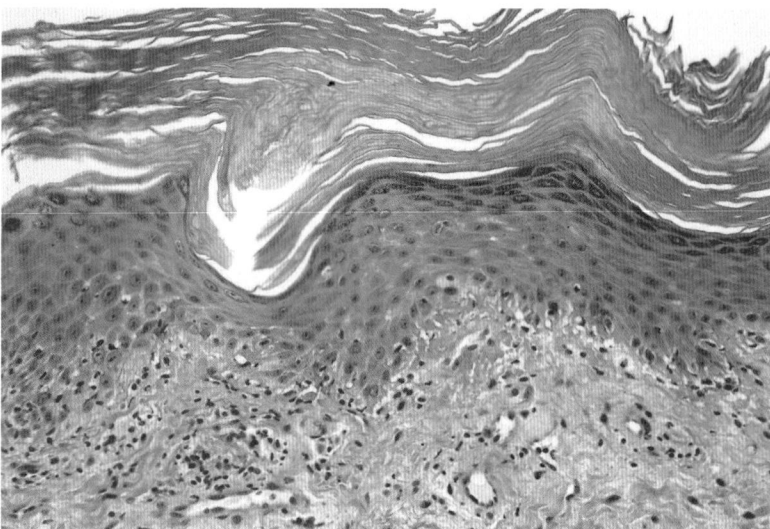

Fig. 17.134
Gottron papule: note the hyperkeratosis, hypergranulosis, and irregular acanthosis simulating lichen planus. There is basal cell hydropic degeneration and cytoid bodies are present in the superficial dermis. By courtesy of D. Whittemore, DO, MD Anderson Cancer Center, Houston, Texas, USA.

cytoid bodies are sometimes present (*Fig. 17.132*). Basement membrane thickening is occasionally prominent. There is upper dermal edema and melanophages may be evident. Rarely, the edema results in subepidermal vesiculation.[202] A light chronic inflammatory cell infiltrate is usually present (*Fig. 17.133*). It is commonly restricted to the superficial dermis and is not associated with the cutaneous adnexae. The infiltrate consists of activated T lymphocytes and macrophages with occasional dermal Langerhans cells.[203] Helper T cells predominate. In some instances the presence of marked hyperkeratosis, follicular plugging, dermal edema, and increased quantities of basement membrane-like material results in considerable histologic overlap with lupus erythematosus, and clinicopathological correlation is essential. A recent study found the most consistent histologic parameters in dermatomyositis to be vacuolar changes of basal keratinocytes, dermal mucin accumulation, and a mild to moderate dermal mononuclear inflammatory cell infiltrate.[204] Dermal sclerosis may occasionally be present.[205]

Increased quantities of Alcian blue-positive glycosaminoglycans are frequently present within the dermis.[202] Sometimes there are foci of calcification and panniculitis is occasionally evident.

The poikilodermatous lesions show hyperkeratosis, mild epidermal atrophy with loss of the epidermal ridge pattern, and basal cell liquefactive degeneration.[132] Additional features may include marked pigmentary

incontinence, cytoid body formation, and a patchy lymphocytic inflammatory cell infiltrate. The dermis is edematous, often contains increased mucin, and characteristically shows conspicuous dilated vascular channels. Nuclear atypia of the infiltrate as seen in poikilodermatous mycosis fungoides is not a feature.

Gottron papules are characterized by hyperkeratosis, mild papillomatosis, acanthosis or, less often, epidermal atrophy and the features of interface dermatitis as described above (*Fig. 17.134*).[206,207] The histology of the centripetal flagellate erythema shows the changes of interface dermatitis.[51]

Ultrastructural studies contribute little to our understanding of dermatomyositis. Tubuloreticular inclusions as described in SLE have been documented in endothelial cell and pericyte cytoplasm, but their significance is uncertain.[208]

In the juvenile variant, the cutaneous features are similar to those described above with the proviso that fibrosis is sometimes evident, calcification is more common, and occlusive vascular disease (as characterized by fibrous intimal proliferation with fibrin thrombi) is often present.[132,133]

Skeletal muscle changes include both degenerative and regenerative features in addition to a focal chronic inflammatory cell infiltrate (*Figs 17.135* and *17.136*).[132] The latter is composed predominantly of lymphocytes, but

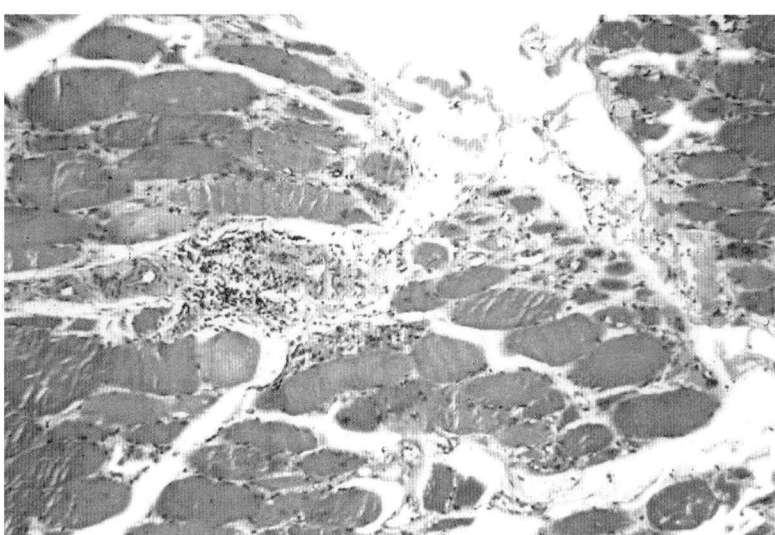

Fig. 17.135
Dermatomyositis: note the perivascular chronic inflammatory cell infiltrate.

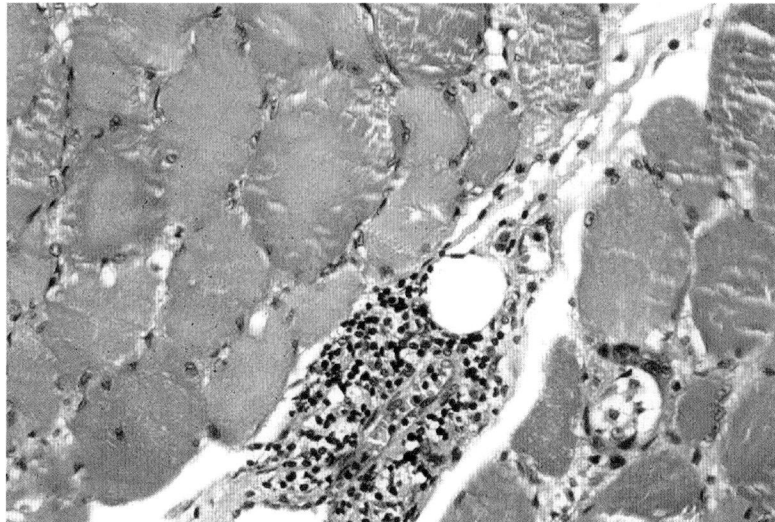

Fig. 17.136
Dermatomyositis: the infiltrate consists predominantly of lymphocytes.

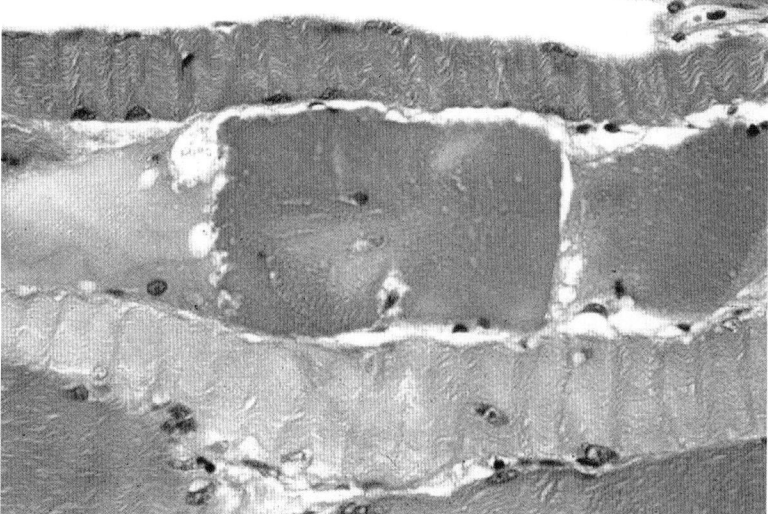

Fig. 17.137
Dermatomyositis: the central fiber is intensely swollen, eosinophilic, and fragmented; there is a loss of striations.

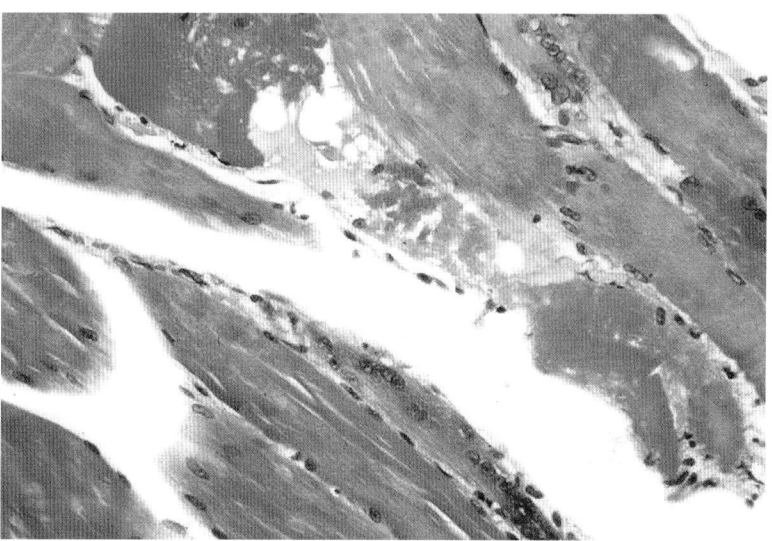

Fig. 17.138
Dermatomyositis: the fiber in the upper midfield is swollen, eosinophilic, vacuolated, and in places granular; beneath is a regenerating basophilic cell.

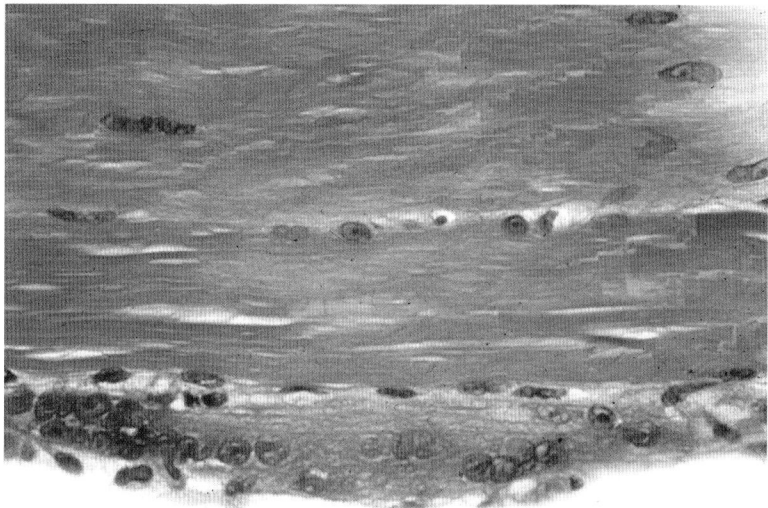

Fig. 17.139
Dermatomyositis: the lower fiber is basophilic and shows excessive nuclei – features of regeneration. Note the centralization of nuclei in the upper fiber.

histiocytes, eosinophils, and plasma cells may also be evident.[209] The lymphocytes consist of substantial numbers of B cells, particularly in association with blood vessels, in addition to T cells, which are predominantly found in and around the altered muscle fibers.[210] As in cutaneous lesions, T-helper cells predominate. Up to 25% of muscle biopsies may, however, show no evidence of inflammation.[4] The degenerative fibers are swollen and intensely eosinophilic and may show loss of striations (Fig. 17.137). Some fibers are vacuolated, but others appear granular or fragmented (Fig. 17.138). Proliferation and centralization of muscle nuclei is common, as is sarcoplasmic basophilia – features of regeneration (Fig. 17.139). Histologic changes identical to inclusion body myositis, namely rimmed vacuoles, have also recently been reported in patients with dermatomyositis.[211,212]

If material from a longstanding 'burned out' lesion is biopsied, the muscle fibers are atrophic and there is endomysial fibrosis. Perifascicular atrophy – the presence of one or two rows of atrophic fibers at the edge of a fascicle – is said to be characteristic of dermatomyositis.[213] The muscle pathology in dermatomyositis and polymyositis is said to differ.[60] In dermatomyositis the inflammatory cell infiltrate tends to be septal or perivascular, whereas in polymyositis it is intrafascicular. Muscle necrosis in dermatomyositis tends to involve small groups of fibers, while in polymyositis the affected fibers tend to be single and sparse.

Denervation neuropathic features are also occasionally present, presumably due to involvement by the inflammatory process of small intramuscular nerve fibers.[132] Steroid atrophy of type II muscle fibers may be seen in biopsies from treated patients.

In childhood dermatomyositis, vascular changes affecting the capillaries, venules, and arterioles are common.[214] The inflammatory component, which is usually quite sparse, consists of lymphocytes, monocytes, and plasma cells centered predominantly on the vasculature in the perifascicular connective tissue.[215] Muscle changes are variable and range from perifascicular atrophy in milder disease through to focal necroses and infarction in the more seriously affected patients, in whom fibrosis may also be a feature.[215] The vascular lesions include endothelial cell swelling and necrosis with or without occlusion, non-necrotizing lymphocytic vasculitis, and loss of the peripheral fascicular capillary bed.[215]

Immunofluorescence of muscle biopsies in childhood dermatomyositis commonly shows vascular intramural IgM and C3.[215]

Mixed connective tissue disease

Clinical features

As originally defined by Sharp et al., MCTD represents a clinical condition in which patients have an overlap of signs and symptoms of systemic sclerosis, SLE, and polymyositis/dermatomyositis.[1,2]

Although the concept of MCTD as a distinctive entity separated from other connective tissue diseases has been controversial, the disease has characteristic and reproducible clinical and serological features.[3,4] Some patients present with manifestations that are not entirely diagnostic and may progress over time to develop typical features of MCTD or other connective tissue diseases, particularly SLE. These patients are designated as having an unclassified or undifferentiated connective tissue disease.[5]

MCTD is characterized by a marked female predominance (16:1) and shows no racial predilection.[6,7] A recent population-based study from Norway revealed the prevalence of adult-onset MCTD to be 3.8 per 100 000 adults and estimated the mean incidence of 2.1 per million per year for the same age group of the patients.[8] Presentation is usually in the second and third decades, but children may also be affected.[1,9–11] Juvenile MCTD roughly represents about 20% of MCTD cases.[9–11] Clinical features include arthralgias and nondeforming arthritis, swollen hands with tapered or sausage-shaped fingers, Raynaud phenomenon, abnormal esophageal motility, myositis, lymphadenopathy, fever, hepatomegaly, serositis, and splenomegaly.[1,12] Patients were initially thought not to show features of renal, pulmonary or neuropsychiatric involvement or vasculitis. In addition, their sera invariably contained high titers of antibody to a saline extractable nuclear antigen (ENA), U1-RNP, and speckled antinuclear antibody. Precipitating antibody to SM soluble nuclear antigen was absent. The disease responded to corticosteroid therapy and had a favorable outcome.

In the light of data from subsequent experience, the above, rather simplistic, overview has had to be modified.[6,13] Although a variety of diagnostic criteria have been proposed, that of Alarcón-Segovia and Cardiel has been chosen, largely because of their simplicity.[14] They suggest that if the criteria used are restricted to certain key clinical manifestations, then MCTD may be accurately diagnosed (*Table 17.14*).[7]

Essential to the diagnosis is the presence of high titer anti-ENA antibodies (anti-U1-RNP). The U1-RNP is an RNA-protein complex, composed of U1 snRNA and several proteins, of which U1-70 kDa proteins are specific for the complex.[15] It is now believed that anti-RNP autoantibodies have a pathogenetic role in the development of the MCTD.[16] More specifically, antibodies against the U1-70 kDa proteins are the most prominent, and those directed against the apoptotic form of U1-70 kDa appear to be particularly useful as serological markers of MCTD.[17] Anti-ENA antibodies are also present in the sera of patients with SLE. In MCTD, however, the antibody-antigen interaction is sensitive to ribonuclease and trypsin and resistant to deoxyribonuclease, the antigen in fact being ribonucleoprotein (U1-RNP).[18] In SLE, the antibody activity is resistant to ribonuclease and deoxyribonuclease, but sensitive to trypsin, and the antigen is SM. Anti-ENA antibodies are not seen in systemic sclerosis or dermatomyositis. Patients with MCTD do not usually develop antibodies to native DNA.[19] The presence of anti-Ro (SS-A) antibodies appears to identify a subgroup of patients

Table 17.14

Diagnostic criteria for mixed connective tissue disease

Serologic
high anti-RNP titer (>1:1600 by hemagglutination or an equivalent by another method)
Clinical
edema of the hands
synovitis
myositis (biopsy proven or elevated CPK)
Raynaud phenomenon (two or three phases)
acrosclerosis
Diagnosis of MCTD requires
positive serology plus three or more of the clinical criteria

CPK, Creatinine phosphokinase; MCTD, mixed connective tissue disease; RNP, ribonucleoprotein.
Reproduced with permission from Alarcón-Segovia, D. (1994) *Clinics in Dermatology*, 12, 309–316.

frequently presenting with malar rash and photosensitivity.[20] Nucleoporin p62 antibodies have been reported in a single patient with MCTD and were suggested to signify poor prognosis in patients with connective tissue disorders.[21] Patients with active MCTD have significantly higher serum levels of antiendothelial cell antibodies than those with inactive MCTD, making antiendothelial cell antibodies a useful marker of clinical disease activity.[22] Exceptionally, ANCAs against proteinase-3 have been detected in MCTD, and contributed to the development of systemic atherosclerosis.[23]

In addition to hand and finger changes and Raynaud phenomenon, patients may develop alopecia, areas of hypo- and hyperpigmentation, and sclerodermiform nail fold capillaropathy. Cutaneous lesions of DLE, SCLE, and SLE also occur.[24] Occasionally, the cutaneous lesions of dermatomyositis are evident. Livedoid vasculitis with ulcers has also been documented and was associated with poor prognosis in the single patient described.[25] Other less common manifestations include alopecia and oral ulcers.[26] Sicca symptoms are present in up to one-third of patients.[27]

Systemic features that are more commonly documented in MCTD include deforming polyarthritis, which particularly affects the hands and feet (often in association with rheumatoid factor), juxta-articular and peritendinous nodules, and calcification involving the forearms, wrists, hands, and feet.[6,28] A distinctive mutilating arthropathy giving rise to a 'main en lorgnette' appearance is said to be characteristic.[18]

It is now known that if patients are followed for a sufficiently long period there is a much greater risk of visceral lesions than was previously realized.[24] Pulmonary disease is the major source of morbidity and mortality in adult patients with MCTD. Although the majority develop asymptomatic respiratory involvement, pulmonary hypertension and interstitial lung disease represent the most severe complication of MCTD.[8,29–31] The presence of anti-β_2-glycoprotein I antibodies has been demonstrated to correlate with development of pulmonary hypertension in patients with MCTD.[32] Furthermore, in a series of 113 patients, anti-Ro52 antibodies were detected in 50% of the MCTD patients with lung fibrosis and only in 19% of patients without lung fibrosis.[33] Pulmonary veno-occlusive disease has also been implicated in the pathogenesis of pulmonary hypertension in MCTD.[34] Up to 10% of patients develop renal disease (albeit usually mild) and a significant proportion of patients develop neuropsychiatric and cerebral manifestations, including trigeminal neuropathy and migrainous headaches.[35] The mixed nature of the clinical manifestations later becomes less obvious with evolution toward a single disease process, usually systemic sclerosis. It is generally considered that, although mortality is low in MCTD, there is a much greater morbidity due to internal involvement than was originally appreciated.

MCTD has also been associated with Hashimoto thyroiditis, thymic carcinoma, papillary thyroid cancer, sarcoidosis, vitamin D deficiency, retinal vasculopathy, acute coronary syndrome, Kikuchi-Fujimoto disease, mixed-type autoimmune hemolytic anemia, autoimmune thrombocytopenia, thrombotic thrombocytopenic purpura, panniculitis, hypertrophic obstructive cardiomyopathy, esophageal motor dysfunction, interstitial lung disease, mucous

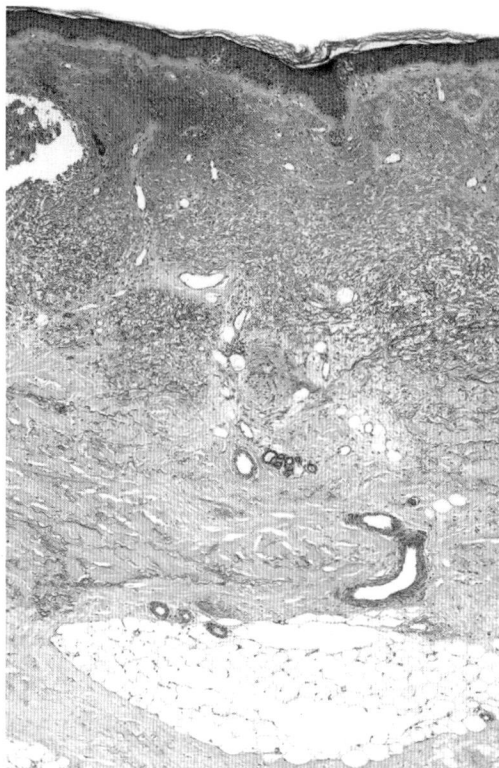

Fig. 17.140
Mixed connective tissue disease: morphea-like features. There is dense dermal sclerosis with extension into the subcutaneous fat.

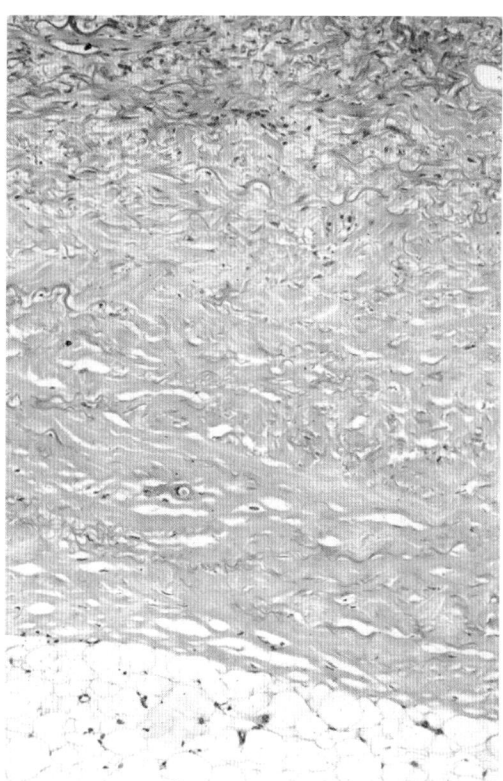

Fig. 17.141
Mixed connective tissue disease: high-power view showing dermal sclerosis.

membrane pemphigoid and sensorineural hearing loss, MPO-ANCA-positive polyangitis, cutaneous polyarteritis nodosa, human T-lymphotropic virus type 1 carrier status, aseptic meningitis, ANCA-positive glomerulonephritis, nephrotic syndrome, Melkersson-Rosenthal syndrome, autoimmune hepatitis, pseudo-pseudo Meigs syndrome (a combination of pleural effusions, ascites and marked elevation of serum CA-125 without evidence of pelvic tumor), Sjögren syndrome, acute fulminant necrotizing lymphocytic myocarditis, trigeminal neuropathy, and purpura fulminans.[36-68]

Pathogenesis and histologic features

The etiology and pathogenesis of MCTD are unknown. MCTD has, however, apparently followed vinyl chloride exposure.[35] In addition to the HLA-B*08, the HLA DRB1*04:01 was confirmed to be a major risk allele for MCTD.[69] Immunoglobulin (Gm) allotype association and an increased frequency of HLA-DR4 in patients with polyarthritis have been documented.[18,70] Patients are frequently lymphopenic with diminished circulating T cells and increased B cells.[18]

The histologic features of the varying cutaneous manifestations have been described in the appropriate sections (Figs 17.140 and 17.141). Biopsies from cutaneous lesions with no typical features may show histologic features similar to those of subacute lupus.[71] Two patients with MCTD have recently reported with prominent accumulation of mucin in the dermis (e.g., cutaneous mucinosis).[72]

Direct immunofluorescence may reveal epithelial speckled nuclear positivity, presumably representing in vivo binding of anti-U1-RNP antibodies.[73]

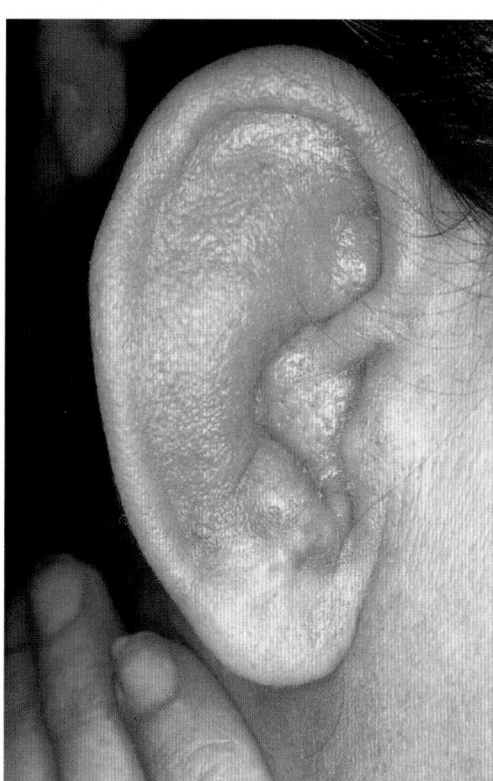

Fig. 17.142
Relapsing polychondritis: the ear shows considerable erythema and swelling. By courtesy of R.A. Marsden, MD, St George's Hospital, London, UK.

Relapsing polychondritis

Clinical features

Relapsing polychondritis is a rare disorder characterized by recurrent episodes of inflammation of cartilaginous tissue throughout the body and its subsequent degeneration and replacement by fibrous tissue (Fig. 17.142).[1,2] The ears (93%), nose (56%), larynx, and trachea (30%) are predominantly affected.[3-7] Skin manifestations are the presenting features in approximately 50% of cases.[6] There is a slight male predominance and the median age at diagnosis in one large study was 46.6 years.[8] Presentation in children is exceptional.[9,10] Pediatric and adult-onset relapsing polychondritis patients share similar clinical features.[10] However, children have a family history of autoimmune diseases more often than adults. However, they infrequently present with associated autoimmune conditions.[10] Clinical criteria for

Table 17.15
Diagnostic criteria for relapsing polychondritis

Recurrent articular chondritis
Cochlear and vestibular damage
Ocular involvement
Nasal involvement
Tracheal/pharyngeal involvement
Nonerosive polyarthritis

diagnosis have been established. Three of these, together with biopsy confirmation of chondritis, are required for diagnosis (*Table 17.15*).[5]

Although it particularly affects Caucasians, cases have been recorded in Asians, blacks, Hispanics, and the Japanese.[3] The sex incidence is equal. Most patients present in the fourth and fifth decades of life.[4,11] There is no evidence of a hereditary predisposition.[6] Clinical signs may be subtle and can resemble those seen in Behçet disease or inflammatory bowel disease; the diagnosis is often difficult.[2,12] Familial cases are exceptional.[13] Variabilities in the disease presentation have been reported in different ethnic populations. The incidence of relapsing polychondritis has been estimated to be 3.5 per million per year.[14]

Auricular chondritis is the commonest lesion and is frequently bilateral.[3] Patients present with painful, tender, erythematous, sometimes blue-black, and swollen ears.[6] Chronicity leads to distortion and flabbiness. Arthritis (seronegative) particularly affects the sternoclavicular, costochondral, and sternomanubrial joints.[3] One or more joints may be affected and lesions are often migratory.[6] Painful nasal chondritis may result in epistaxis, and saddle nose is an occasional complication. Nasal involvement is seen in over 50% of patients.[8] Oral aphthosis was present in 11% of patients in a large series.[2] In 6% of patients, oral and genital aphthae were seen.[2] When the disease initially presents, inflammation of a single site may be confused with erysipelas.[15]

Ocular lesions include conjunctivitis, corneal ulceration, iridocyclitis, episcleritis, proptosis, cataract, chorioretinitis, scleromalacia perforans, scleritis, retinal detachment, blindness, edema of the eyelids and muscle palsies, and optic neuropathy.[3,6,8,16-19] Chronic conjunctivitis due to obliterative microangiopathy has been reported in a single patient with relapsing polychondritis.[20] Central nervous system complications comprise aseptic meningitis and meningoencephalitis, encephalitis lethargica, Lewy body-like dementia is a rare complication.[19,21-25] Trigeminal neuralgia has also been reported.[26]

Respiratory lesions may affect the larynx, trachea, and major bronchi with obstructive symptoms, stenosis, collapse, pneumothorax, pneumoperitoneum, and bronchopneumonia.[3,7,8,27] Exceptionally, airway involvement may be the only manifestation of the disease.[28] Cardiovascular lesions include valvular incompetence, conduction defects including complete heart block, cystic medial necrosis of the aorta, aortitis, aortic valve regurgitation, vasculitis and pericarditis, and pericardial effusions.[3,8,19,29-32] Involvement of the heart valves occurs in up to 10% of patients and systemic vasculitis, reminiscent of polyarteritis nodosa, has been described.[33] Ear involvement includes external ear chondritis, otitis media, vertigo, and deafness.[34]

Dermatological manifestations are present in 35% to 50% and may even precede the development of relapsing polychondritis in about 12% of cases.[2] Skin lesions have included leukocytoclastic vasculitis, hypocomplementemic urticarial vasculitis, cutaneous polyarteritis nodosa, erythema elevatum diutinum, livedo reticularis, alopecia, retarded nail growth, erythematous nodules, erythema annulare centrifugum, erythema multiforme-like lesions, urticarial plaques, erythema nodosum, thrombosis, pyoderma gangrenosum-like lesions, Sweet syndrome, postinflammatory hyperpigmentation, and psoriasis.[2,3,6,35-45] Exceptional associations with normolipemic plane xanthomatosis and with panniculitis showing septal and lobular involvement accompanied by vasculitis have been documented.[46,47]

Significant disease associations that may be present in up to 30% of patients include leukocytoclastic vasculitis, systemic vasculitis (Takayasu and temporal arteritis, Wegener granulomatosis), p-ANCA associated vasculitis, Hashimoto thyroiditis, arthritis, Sjögren syndrome, dermatomyositis,

MCTD, SLE, inflammatory bowel disease (both ulcerative colitis and Crohn disease), and myeloproliferative disorders.[2,6,34,48-56] Rare associations of relapsing polychondritis include ankylosing spondylitis, Behçet disease, HIV, splenic abscess, chronic hepatitis C, mixed cryoglobulinemia, sarcoidosis, common variable immunodeficiency, familial Mediterranean fever, synovial chondromatosis of the temporomandibular joint, immunoglobulin G4-related disease, and amyloidosis.[57-67]

An increased ESR and anemia are the commonest significant laboratory manifestations. Increased urinary glycosaminoglycans have also been documented.[68]

Relapsing polychondritis has a significant mortality. The 5-year survival rate is approximately 74%.[34] Infection, respiratory failure, systemic vasculitis, large vessel aneurysm rupture, and renal failure are the commonest causes of death.[1,34]

A number of patients have been reported to have myelodysplastic syndrome associated with relapsing polychondritis.[43,69-73] This is of interest since myelodysplastic syndrome is known to be associated with autoimmune disease.[74,75] In a large study of 200 patients, 11% had myelodysplastic syndrome.[2] Other malignancies occurring with relapsing polychondritis include splenic non-Hodgkin lymphoma, chronic lymphocytic leukemia, chronic myelomonocytic leukemia, and Kaposi sarcoma.[76-79] Association with epithelial malignancies is less frequent.[80]

Relapsing polychondritis has been associated with the luteinizing hormone-releasing hormone (LH-RH) analog goserelin. As the disease may worsen during pregnancy and during chorionic gonadotropin therapy, it is suggested that hormones may be a precipitating factor.[81]

Pathogenesis and histologic features

The precise etiology of relapsing polychondritis is poorly understood. Several studies have suggested an immunological mechanism.[6] The association with autoimmune diseases in many patients lends support to this thesis. Antibodies (predominantly IgG) to type II collagen, which accounts for over 50% of the proteins in cartilage, have been detected in a proportion of patients in titers of 1:10 to 1:320.[39,48,82,83] The antibodies are directed against both native and denatured protein.[48] Using ELISA, one study showed that 50% of patients have antibodies against type II collagen.[84] In this same study, 4% of control subjects and 15% of rheumatoid arthritis patients also had antibodies in their sera. Those patients who have the autoantibody show evidence of active disease, whereas those without it are either in remission or being treated.[48] Rats immunized with type II collagen develop auricular chondritis. Cartilage from these same animals had positive immunofluorescence for IgG and C3.[85] In a single patient, T-cell clones were found to be specific for the collagen II peptide 261–273.[86]

An association between the disease and HLA-DR4 has been reported in a study from Germany but there was no predominance of any DR4 subtype.[87] Nevertheless, a recent population-based study from Japan failed to confirm the association between relapsing polychondritis and HLA-DR4, but instead confirmed association between the presence of HLA-DRB1*16:02, HLA-DQB1*05:02, and HLA-B*67:01 in Japanese relapsing polychondritis patients.[88]

Antifetal cartilage antibodies have been detected by indirect immunofluorescence studies.[83] Documentation of transplacental transfer of these antibodies with neonatal involvement suggests that they are of pathogenetic significance. One group of authors suggested that matrilin-1, a cartilage matrix protein, is the target of autoreactivity.[89,90] Another group found autoantibodies to matrilin-1 in 13% of patients and antibody titers correlated with symptomatology.[91] Rats immunized with matrilin-1 develop nasorespiratory abnormalities (but not ear or joint changes).[92] Cartilage oligometric matrix protein has also been suggested as a potential autoantigen.[93]

Circulating immune complexes have also been demonstrated in relapsing polychondritis, together with deposits of immunoglobulin and complement in inflamed cartilage, adding further support to a possible immune mechanism in this disease.[3,40,48] Granular deposits of immunoglobulin and complement (C3) have been described at the chondrofibrous junction in two patients.[93] The presence of ANCA has been reported.[94] Elevated serum levels of macrophage migration inhibitory factor have also been documented.[95] Increased serum levels of proinflammatory cytokines, namely

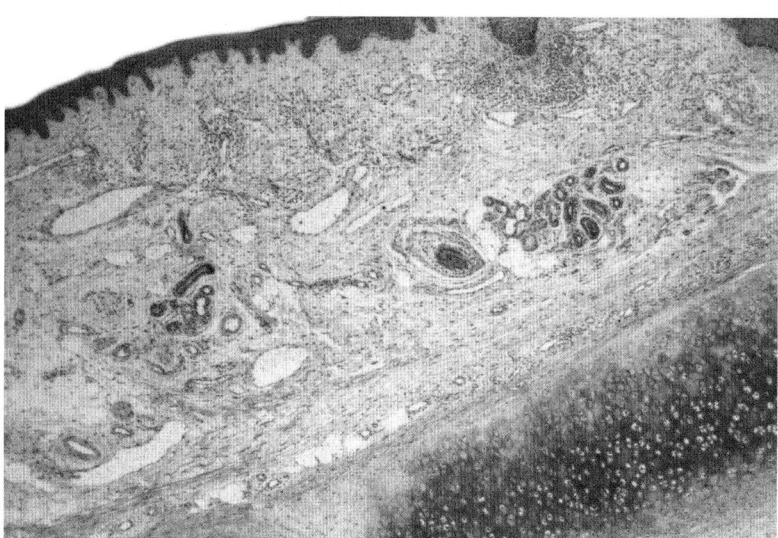

Fig. 17.143
Relapsing polychondritis: in this early lesion, the degenerate cartilage shows intense eosinophilia.

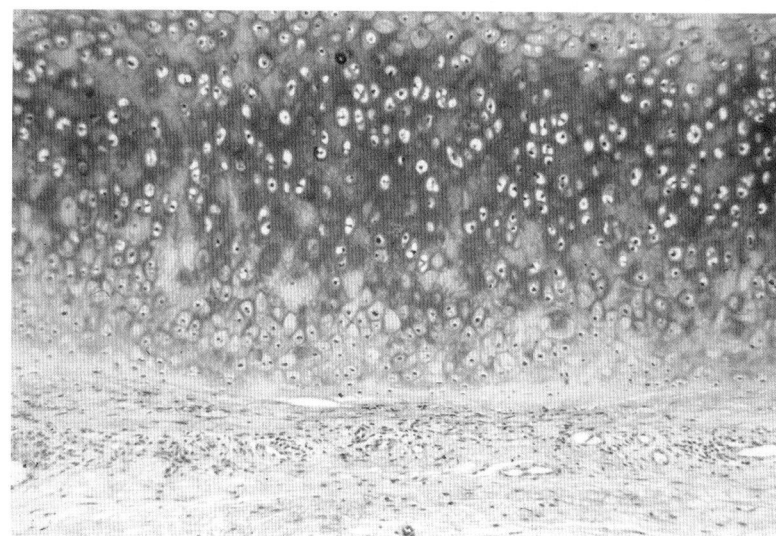

Fig. 17.144
Relapsing polychondritis: a mild chronic inflammatory cell infiltrate is present in the perichondrium.

macrophage inflammatory protein 1β, monocyte chemoattractant protein 1, and interleukin-8, have also been demonstrated in patients with relapsing polychondritis.[96]

There is some evidence suggesting that cell-mediated immunity may also be of importance in the pathogenesis. Patients display positive lymphoblast transformation and macrophage migration inhibition to cartilage glycosaminoglycans.[1] Responses correlate with episodes of disease activity. Dysregulation of NKT cells has also been detected in relapsing polychondritis.[97]

Histologic examination of the skin is unremarkable. The dermis contains a mild focal lymphohistiocytic infiltrate. Examination of the fibrocartilaginous tissues, however, shows degenerative and inflammatory changes affecting the marginal chondrocytes, with loss of basophilia and poor Alcian blue staining of the cartilaginous tissue (Figs 17.143 and 17.144).

The inflammatory cell infiltrate, which includes lymphocytes, plasma cells, histiocytes, and occasional polymorphs, infiltrates the degenerate cartilage. Eventually, there is replacement by granulation and fibrous tissue.[3] Atypical lymphoid infiltrates mimicking a lymphoma have rarely been described.[98]

Differential diagnosis

Chondrodermatitis nodularis helicis differs by the presence of characteristic layering of fibrin, granulation tissue, and cartilage with degenerative changes. Clinically, chondrodermatitis helicis presents as a focal, punched-out ulcer. This differs from the diffuse involvement of the ear seen in relapsing polychondritis.

Access **ExpertConsult.com** for the complete list of references

Infectious diseases of the skin

Wayne Grayson and Eduardo Calonje

See
www.expertconsult.com
for references and
additional material

VIRAL INFECTIONS

Common wart

The common wart (verruca vulgaris) is caused by infection with human papillomavirus (HPV) (*Fig. 18.1*). HPV is a DNA virus of the papovavirus family. The number of known HPV genotypes currently stands at more than 200, classified according to the extent of their DNA homology (DNA hybridization) (*Table 18.1*).[1-5] In order for an HPV type to be regarded as 'new', sequences in selected genomic regions must exhibit more than 10% divergence compared to any of the known HPV types.[2] Monoclonal antibodies to intact viruses have been produced and can demonstrate individual types of HPV; antibodies to viral components are only group specific (*Fig. 18.2*). Advances in molecular pathology have resulted in improved and more specific methods of HPV detection and classification, including in situ polymerase chain reaction (PCR), nonisotopic in situ hybridization (NISH), rolling circle amplification and next-generation sequencing.[5,6] Five genera exist, namely, α, β, γ, μ, and ν. The α HPV types are predominantly mucosotropic, and are often classified as low-risk (e.g., HPV6, HPV11) or high-risk (e.g., HPV16, HPV18) based on their association with the development of cancer, including cervical and anogenital neoplasms and some carcinomas of the oral cavity.[7-10] Although the other four genera are associated with cutaneous infection, it is the β HPV types that are of particular relevance in the etiopathogenesis of nonmelanoma skin cancer in the setting of epidermodysplasia verruciformis (EV).[4,7,8,11,12]

Papillomaviruses, which are small and nonenveloped and show icosahedral symmetry, contain circular double-stranded DNA composed of approximately 8000 base pairs. The viral particle, which has a diameter

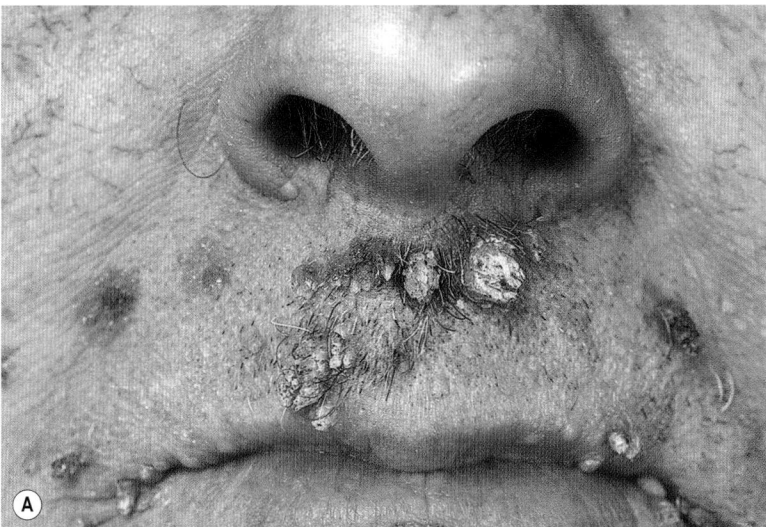

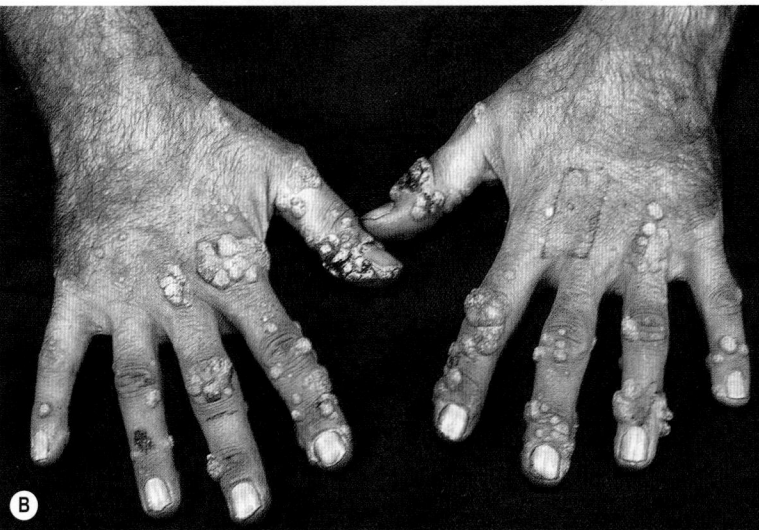

Fig. 18.1
Viral warts: (**A**) these are exceedingly common and may affect any site; (**B**) lesions are frequently multiple. (**A**) By courtesy of the Institute of Dermatology, London, UK; (**B**) By courtesy of J.C. Pascual, MD, Alicante, Spain.

Table 18.1
Variants of human wart virus infection

HPV type	Associated clinical lesions
1	Deep plantar warts, common warts
2	Common warts, flat warts
3	Flat warts
4	Common warts, plantar warts
5	Epidermodysplasia verruciformis (EV)
6	Genital warts, laryngeal papilloma
7	Butcher warts
8	EV
9	EV, keratoacanthoma
10	Flat warts
11	Laryngeal papillomas, genital warts
12	EV
13	Focal epithelial hyperplasia
14, 15	EV
16	Genital warts, bowenoid papulosis, cervical dysplasia, cervical carcinoma, digital, squamous cell carcinoma, nongenital Bowen disease
17	EV
18	Genital warts, bowenoid papulosis, cervical dysplasia, cervical carcinoma
19–25	EV, keratoacanthoma
26–29	Common warts, flat warts
30	Laryngeal carcinoma, genital warts
31–32	Genital warts, bowenoid papulosis, cervical dysplasia, cervical carcinoma
33	Cervical carcinoma
34	Bowenoid papulosis, Bowen disease
35	Cervical dysplasia, cervical carcinoma
36	EV
37	EV, keratoacanthoma
38	EV
39	Bowenoid papulosis, cervical carcinoma
41	Flat warts
42	Genital warts, bowenoid papulosis, cervical dysplasia, cervical carcinoma
43, 44	Genital warts, laryngeal papillomas
46, 47	EV
48	Bowenoid papulosis, Bowen disease
49, 50	EV
51–54	Genital warts, bowenoid papulosis, cervical dysplasia, cervical carcinoma
55	Genital warts, laryngeal papillomas

Reproduced with permission from Melton, J.L. and Rasmussen, J.E. (1991) Dermatologic Clinics, 9, 219–233.

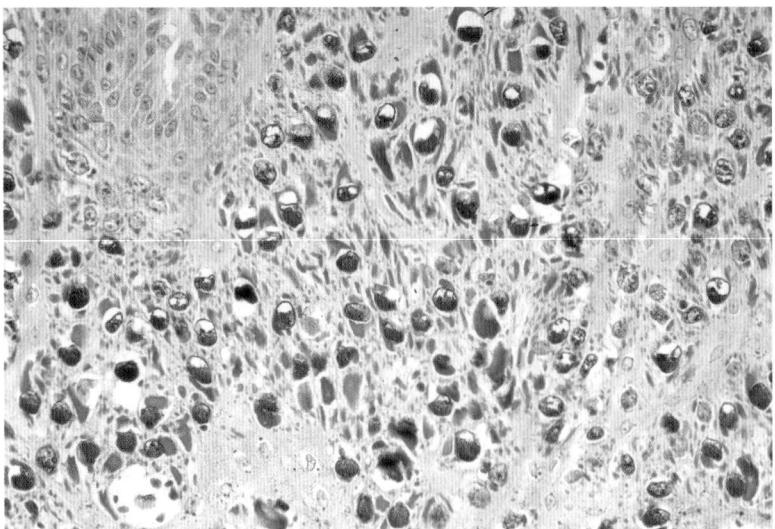

Fig. 18.2
Verruca vulgaris: note the positive labeling of the nuclei in this section stained with a peroxidase-labeled antiserum to papilloma virus.

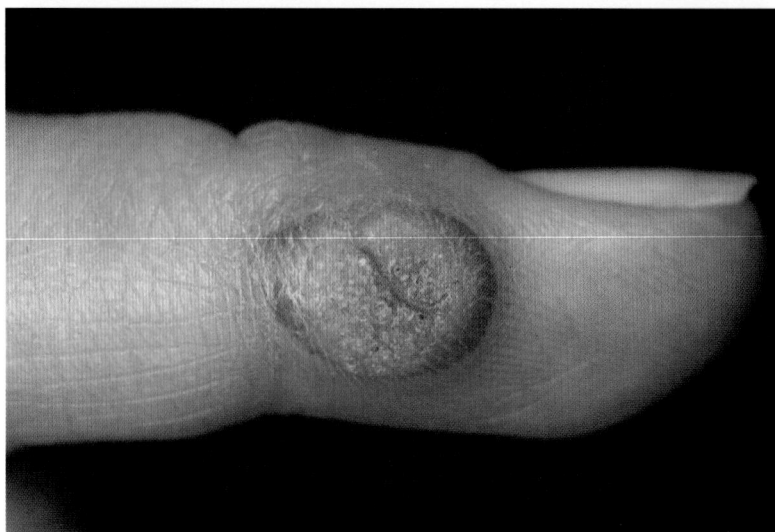

Fig. 18.3
Verruca vulgaris: verrucae are most commonly seen on the hands and fingers. From the collection of the late N.P. Smith, MD, the Institute of Dermatology, London, UK.

of approximately 55 nm, contains 72 capsomeres.[2,13] The HPV genome is divided into three functional regions: a late region, an early region, and a noncoding 1000 base pair upstream regulatory region (URR). The URR is located immediately upstream of the E6 open reading frame (ORF) and contains sequences regulating expression of all ORFs, including promoter elements and transcriptional enhancer sequences. In excess of 20 messenger RNAs are expressed, usually in a differentiation-specific and cell-specific manner.[2] Genes in the early region (E1, E2, E4, E5, E6, E7) are responsible for transcription, replication, and cellular transformation.[4] The E4 ORF is highly expressed in differentiated HPV-infected epithelial cells. Some forms of E4 encode a protein capable of disrupting the cytokeratin network, resulting in the phenomenon of koilocytosis.[2] The E4 ORF represents a region of maximal divergence between different HPV types.[14] Each viral genotype is most often detected in lesions at specific anatomical sites or shows distinct histologic characteristics.[15–17]

HPV infection in man results in a variety of cutaneous lesions including verruca vulgaris, filiform warts, verruca plana, plantar warts, anogenital warts, and bowenoid papulosis.[13] Mucosal lesions include oral warts and condylomata, focal epithelial hyperplasia or Heck disease, nasal and conjunctival papillomas, laryngeal papillomatosis, and cervical lesions.[2,13] HPV infection may be asymptomatic or result in a carrier status. One study showed that cutaneous HPV infections commonly persist on healthy skin over several years, and that persistence does not appear to be associated with age, sex, a history of warts, immunosuppressive therapy, or HPV type.[18]

Clinical features

Common warts are caused by HPV types 1, 2, 4, 7, and 26–29.[13] In immunosuppressed patients, HPV subtypes 75, 76, and 77 may be pathogenetic.[19] A case with extensive, recalcitrant verrucae linked to infection with HPV type 57 has been reported.[20] Rarely, HPV subtypes associated with genital warts such as 6 and 11 have been found in common warts in children.[21] HPV16, a common genital HPV type with oncogenic potential, was detected in 6.6% of lesions in a series of 45 immunocompetent patients with nongenital cutaneous warts.[22] Conversely, verrucae vulgaris may sometimes occur on the vulva. HPV type 2 has been detected in such cases. It is important to note that these 'nonvenereal' genital lesions may occur in girls less than 5 years of age, as an erroneous clinical or histologic diagnosis of condylomata acuminata could lead to allegations of sexual abuse.[23]

Warts are very common lesions, particularly in children.[24] Adults are also frequently affected. In a survey of 2180 adults, 3.5% had warts.[25] Butchers and slaughterhouse workers have an increased risk.[26,27] Common warts may occur anywhere on the skin and in people of any age, but are most common on the backs of the hands and the fingers and on the knees of young children, where they appear as firm keratotic papules 1–10 mm across (Fig.

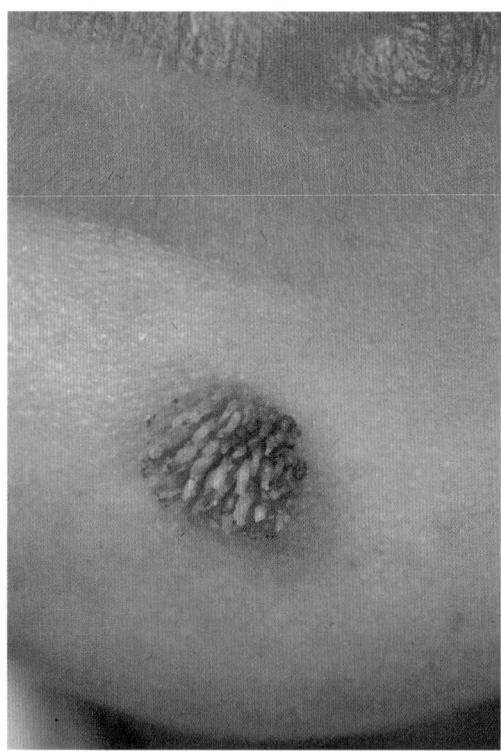

Fig. 18.4
Filiform wart: this variant occurs most often on the face and around the axillae. From the collection of the late N.P. Smith, MD, the Institute of Dermatology, London, UK.

18.3).[24] Koebnerization is common (hence, kissing lesions on fingers).[13] In other sites they may appear more filiform and less firm (Fig. 18.4). The latter are particularly seen on the lips, nostrils, and eyelids.[1] Giant periungual lesions have been described.[28] Warts may also present as a cutaneous horn. They persist for a few months up to several years and often regress spontaneously, particularly in children.

Chronically immunosuppressed patients (e.g., following renal transplantation) often have a large number of warts (Fig. 18.5).[29,30] Chronicity is associated with increasing numbers of lesions. EV-like lesions due to HPV5 have also been described in human immunodeficiency virus (HIV)-positive patients and following renal transplantation.[31] Numerous warts may be seen in other immunosuppressed patients (e.g., with non-Hodgkin lymphoma, leukemia, Hodgkin lymphoma, and HIV infection).[13,31–34] In patients with

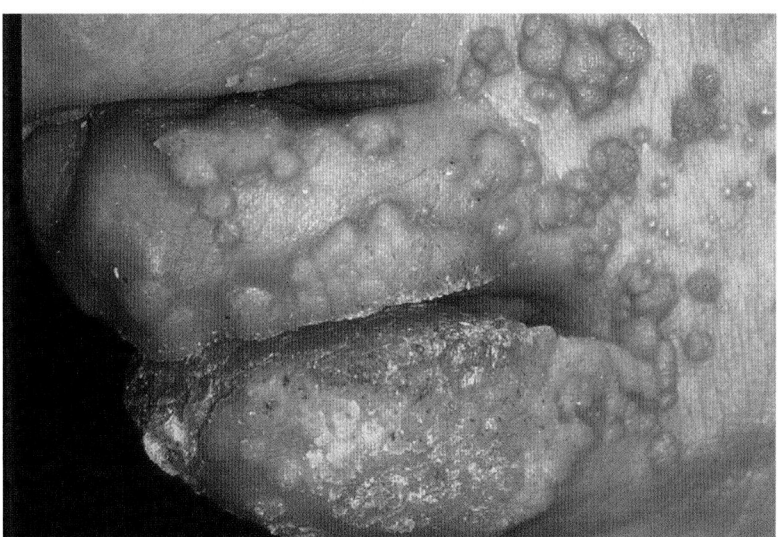

Fig. 18.5
Verruca vulgaris: presentation with such large numbers of lesions raises the possibility of immunosuppression. By courtesy of the Institute of Dermatology, London, UK.

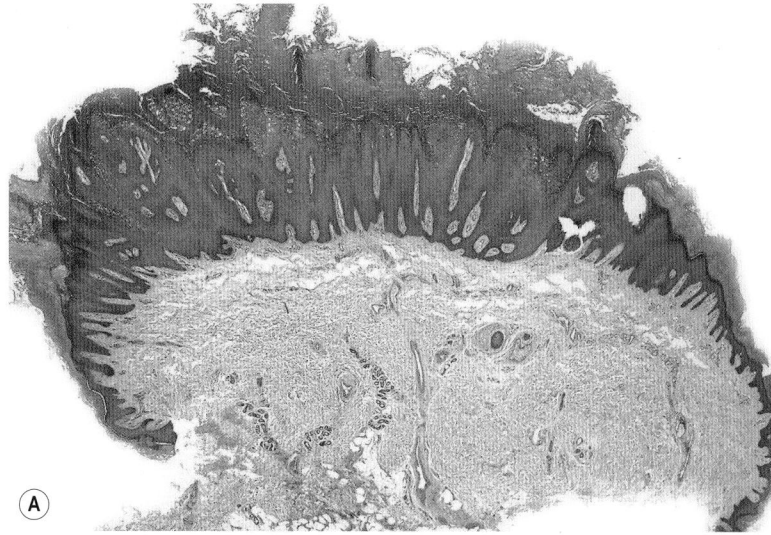

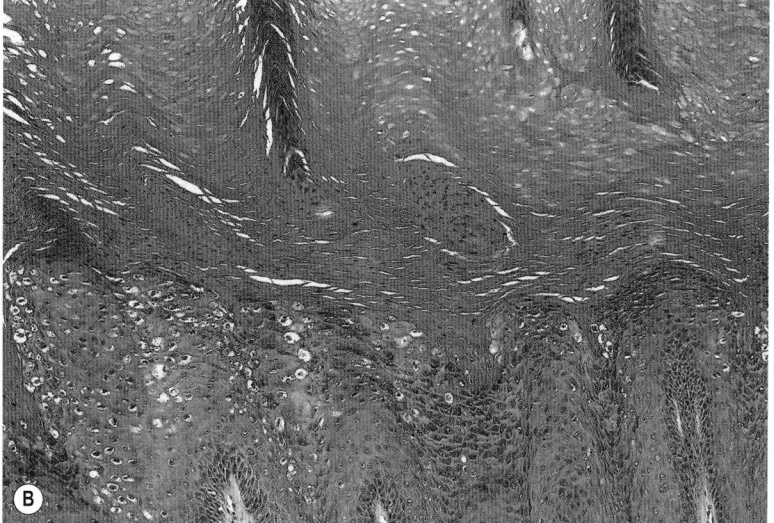

Fig. 18.6
Verruca vulgaris: (**A**) note the hyperkeratosis and papillomatosis; (**B**) there is often marked parakeratosis typically arranged as a vertical tier. Koilocytes are conspicuous.

acquired immunodeficiency syndrome (AIDS), warts may regress following antiretroviral therapy (ART).[35]

Pathogenesis and histologic features

In the skin, it is the inter-appendageal epidermis and the stem cells of the bulge region of the hair follicle that are the apparent targets of the virions.[7] In situ hybridization studies of HPV lesions have shown that viral DNA synthesis in the epidermis occurs in the superficial prickle cell layer, and full virus assembly with capsid production occurs in the granular cell layer.[13] HPV DNA has been demonstrated in apparently normal skin up to 15 mm from a virus-associated lesion.[36] The requirement for growth in very well-differentiated epithelia may explain the difficulty of culturing HPV and why host destruction of the lesions may be protracted. Immune mechanisms are presumed to be less effective against organisms or altered cells that are situated superficially with no direct blood supply.

Regression of HPV lesions is usually spontaneous but may not occur for several years.[37] Cell-mediated immunity seems to be important in effecting the regression since lymphocytes are seen infiltrating the wart epithelium at this stage. Other features of regression include liquefactive basal cell degeneration, epidermal degeneration, and vascular thrombosis.[37,38] Toll-like receptors (TLRs) have been identified as important role players in viral recognition and the initiation of an antiviral host immune response. TLR3, TLR9, interferon-beta (IFN-β), and tumor necrosis factor-alpha (TNF-α) appear to play an important role in the skin's innate immune response to HPV infection.[39] Langerhans cells and Langerhans-like dendritic cells may exert direct antiviral activity. This is facilitated via the expression of TLRs such as TLR3, which may in turn trigger the release of IFN-inducible chemokines, including CXCL9, a monokine induced by IFN-γ.[40]

Following regression of the wart(s), an individual is usually immune to further HPV infection. Patients with a deficiency in cell-mediated immunity – whether primary or acquired, iatrogenic or virally induced (HIV/AIDS) – are particularly susceptible to the development of warts, which tend not to involute spontaneously and can be a particularly refractory therapeutic problem.

Transmission of HPV is by inoculation of infected desquamated cells through close contact at points of minor trauma; hence, common warts are seen most often on the hands. Periungual warts are particularly associated with nail biting and plantar warts are especially related to prolonged immersion in water.[25]

Common warts show filiform acanthosis with vertical tiers of parakeratosis over the tips of the exophytic component (*Fig. 18.6*). There is also marked orthokeratosis. A downward extension of the acanthosis produces a curvilinear deep margin and curved distortion of the adjacent rete ridges

in the uninvolved epidermis. There is a prominent granular cell layer within which are enlarged clumps of irregular basophilic keratohyalin (*Fig. 18.7*).[1] These are seen best in the concavities between the papillomatotic epithelial papillae. Large cells with prominent vacuolated cytoplasm and a small pyknotic nucleus are seen in the upper layers of the epidermis (koilocytes) (*Fig. 18.8*). Koilocytes are, however, more frequently observed in genital warts (see below). Connective tissue and tortuous small blood vessels may invade the filiform projections (*Fig. 18.9*). In some cases, involvement of the superficial portion of the hair follicles by HPV results in focal changes identical to a trichilemmoma or an inverted follicular keratosis.[41] However, not all of these lesions are induced by HPV as has been suggested.[42]

Ordinary common warts are only exceptionally associated with in situ or invasive squamous cell carcinoma.[43,44] HPV16 has been associated with periungual Bowen disease and squamous carcinoma.[45–47] The role of HPV in cutaneous neoplasia is discussed further in Chapter 22. Molecular studies have implicated cutaneous HPV infection as a carcinogenic cofactor in association with solar ultraviolet radiation in the evolution of nonmelanoma skin cancer.[11,48]

Plantar warts

Clinical features

Plantar warts occur on the sole of the foot; they are only slightly elevated and appear as a horny plug surrounded by a ring of hyperkeratotic skin

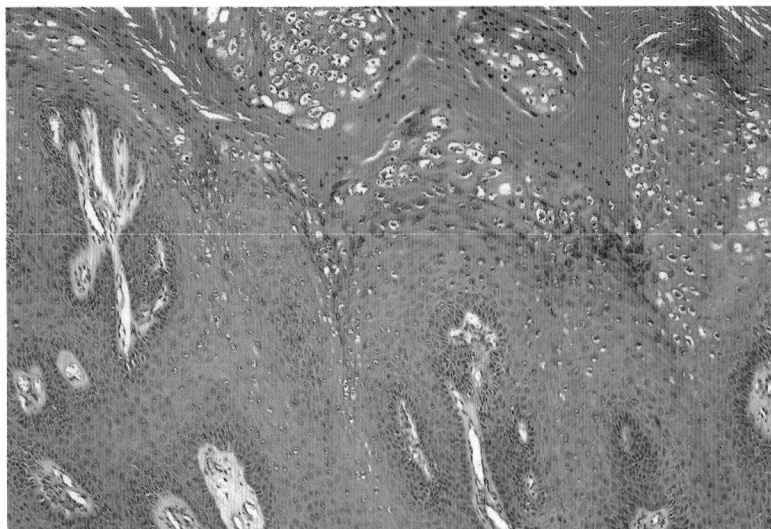

Fig. 18.7
Verruca vulgaris: large vacuolated cells with enlarged and irregular keratohyalin granules are characteristic.

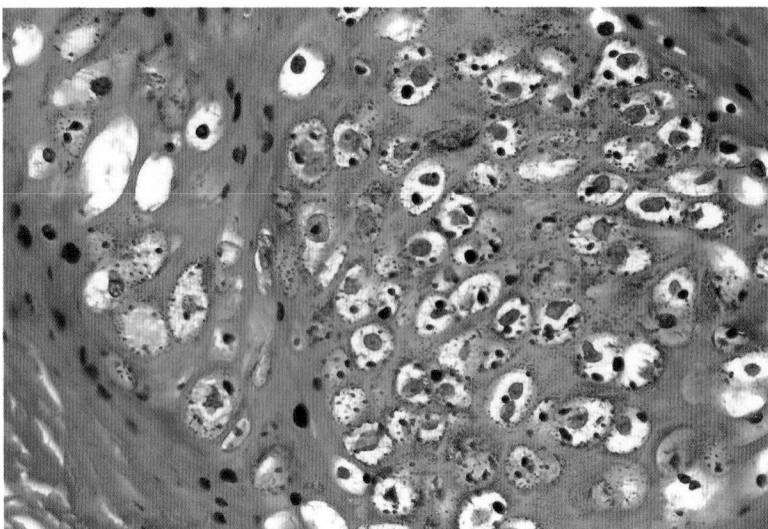

Fig. 18.8
Verruca vulgaris: high-power view of koilocytes.

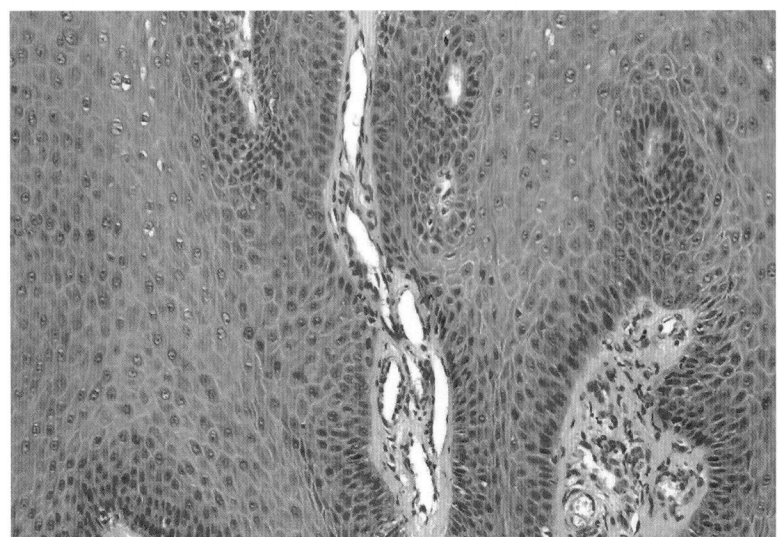

Fig. 18.9
Verruca vulgaris: the core of the papillary projection contains conspicuous dilated capillary loops.

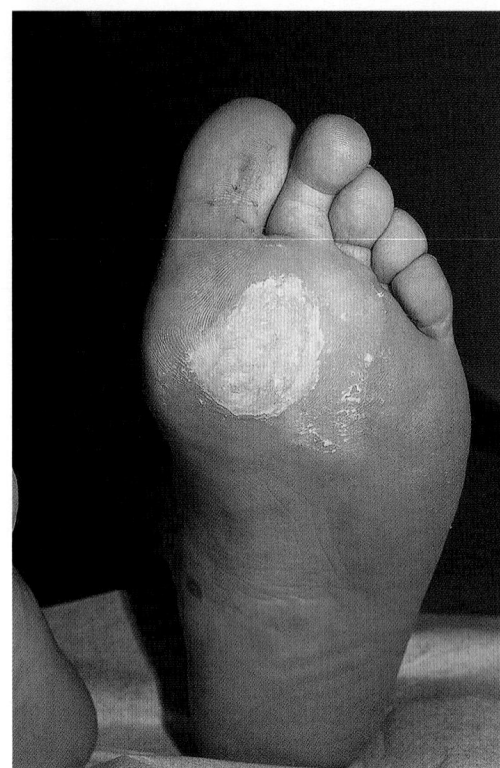

Fig. 18.10
Plantar wart: the lesion is flat and shows very marked hyperkeratosis. By courtesy of R.A. Marsden, MD, St George's Hospital, London, UK.

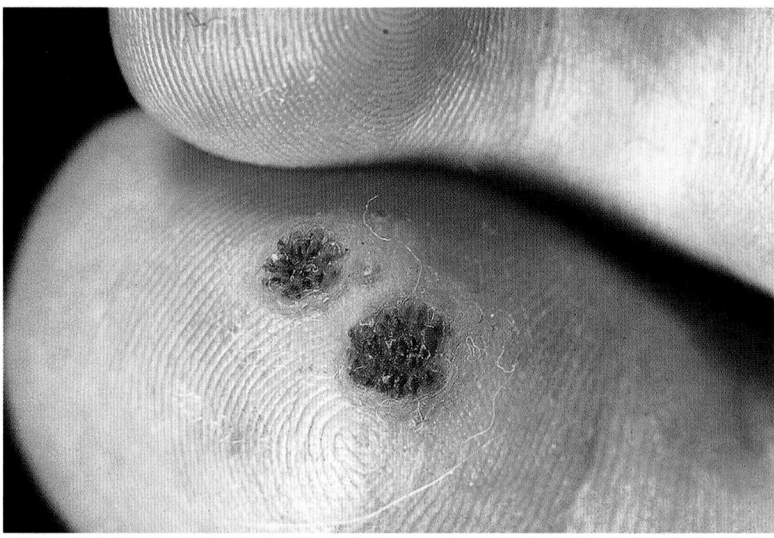

Fig. 18.11
Plantar wart: vascular thromboses as seen in these two lesions are common manifestations of involution. By courtesy of R.A. Marsden, MD, St George's Hospital, London, UK.

(*Fig. 18.10*). Often, they are covered with black dots representing thrombosed capillaries (*Fig. 18.11*).[1] They are most common in children and are frequently seen over pressure points. Most plantar warts are caused by HPV1 and are painful; however, HPV4 may produce a confluent or mosaic pattern of similar small warts ('mosaic plantar warts') and these are painless (*Fig. 18.12*).[2,3] They may also be seen on the palms and in the periungual region. There have been reports from Japan of unusual plantar warts produced by HPV60.[4–6]

The lesions may be nodular, ridged, or pigmented. A cystic variant has also been described.[4–10] The cystic variant has the features of an epidermoid cyst and may rarely be multiple.[11] Most are associated with HPV60, but an association with HPV57 has also been reported.[12–14] Epidermoid cysts induced by HPV may also be seen outside acral locations.[15,16] Pigmented

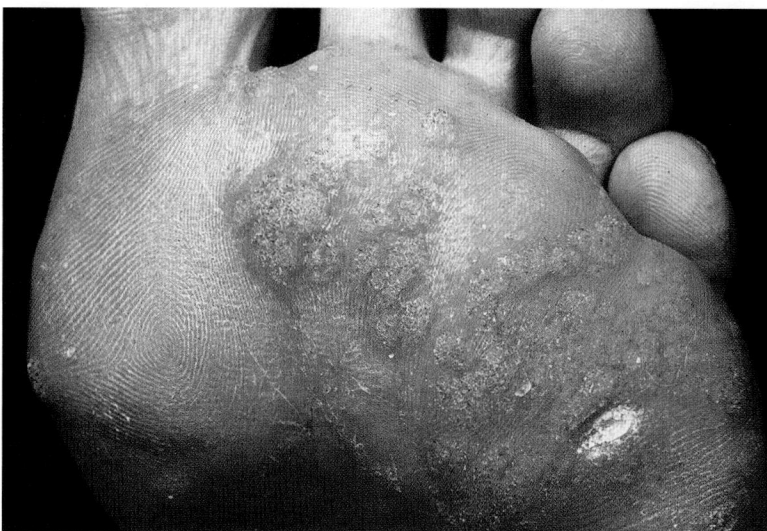

Fig. 18.12
Mosaic warts: here there are a large number of small warts. They are particularly resistant to therapy. By courtesy of the Institute of Dermatology, London, UK.

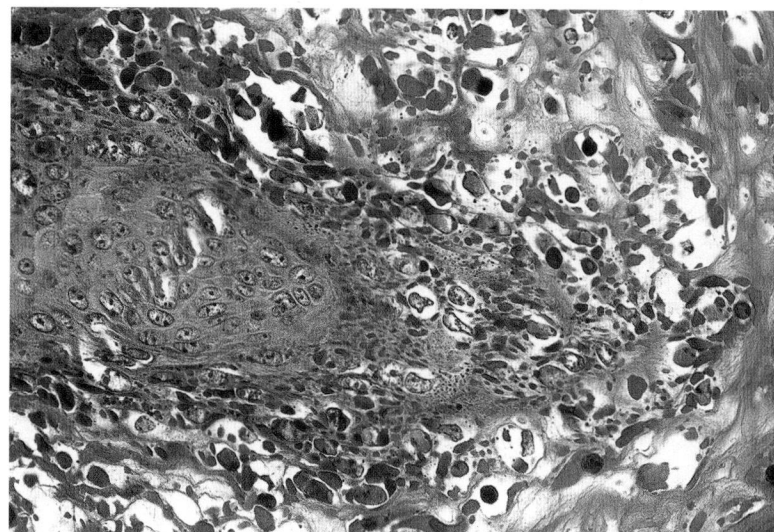

Fig. 18.14
Plantar wart: these eosinophilic keratohyalin granules are characteristic.

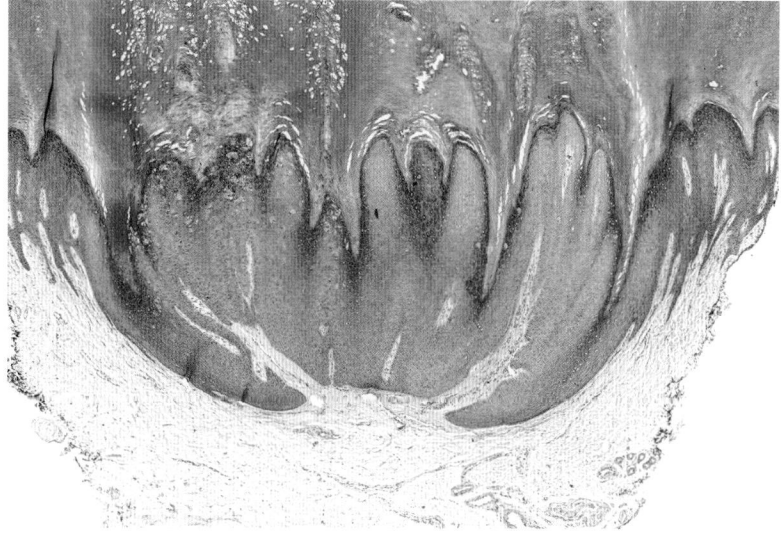

Fig. 18.13
Plantar wart: typical depressed, crateriform lesion containing a parakeratotic plug.

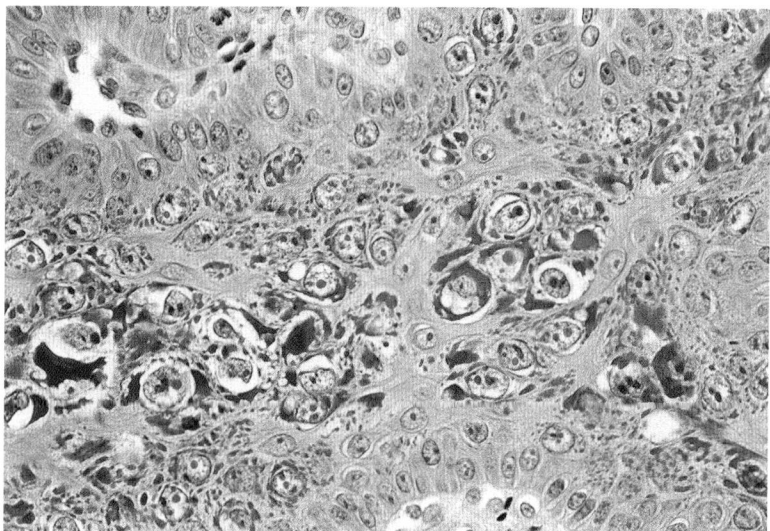

Fig. 18.15
Plantar wart: note the conspicuous intranuclear eosinophilic inclusions.

warts are caused by HPV4, 60, or 65[17] and may contain fibrillar intracytoplasmic inclusion bodies.[18] A case of a large plantar wart caused by HPV66 has been documented.[19] A further subtype of HPV associated with palmoplantar warts is HPV63.[8,20]

Plantar warts usually regress within a few months in children, but may persist longer in adults. Rarely, chronic plantar warts may be associated with the development of verrucous carcinoma (carcinoma cuniculatum) (see Chapter 22).[21,22]

Histologic features

Plantar warts are almost entirely endophytic, with a central parakeratotic plug surrounded by multiple deep extensions of acanthotic epidermis (Fig. 18.13). The depth and complexity of these downgrowths have been likened to an anthill, giving rise to the term 'myrmecia'. Vacuolation is more prominent in the plantar wart and, in the active growing phase, large eosinophilic (and to a lesser extent, basophilic) cytoplasmic inclusions are present, which represent disordered growth of giant keratohyalin granules (Fig. 18.14). The large eosinophilic cytoplasmic inclusions are usually seen in infections caused by HPV1 and to a lesser extent in those caused by HPV60 and HPV65.[7] In warts induced by HPV4, the infected keratinocytes show prominent cytoplasmic vacuolar change with almost no keratohyalin granules. Intranuclear inclusions may also be evident (Fig. 18.15). HPV can be demonstrated

in the nuclei of these cells via electron microscopy (Fig. 18.16). Melanin granules are discernible within the cytoplasm of HPV60-induced pigmented plantar warts.

Regressive changes are the same as those described in common warts and consist of thrombosis of superficial blood vessels, necrosis, and a mixed inflammatory cell infiltrate.[23] A recently described multiplexed PCR-based assay may have merit in both HPV genotyping and in monitoring treatment efficacy.[24]

Plane warts

Clinical features

Plane warts (verrucae plana), usually caused by HPV2, 3, or 10, are flat, smooth, and a few millimeters in diameter with typically little change in color from the adjacent skin, although they may appear gray-yellow or pale brown (Fig. 18.17).[1–3] HPV5 is rarely implicated in HIV-infected patients.[4] Plane warts may also result from HPV types 26–29 and 41 infection.[5] They affect the face, backs of the hands, and the shins. There may be only a few present, but occasionally they are very numerous and become confluent in areas of scratching (koebnerization).[6] Plane warts are common in children and may be seen in women, but are not usually found in males after puberty

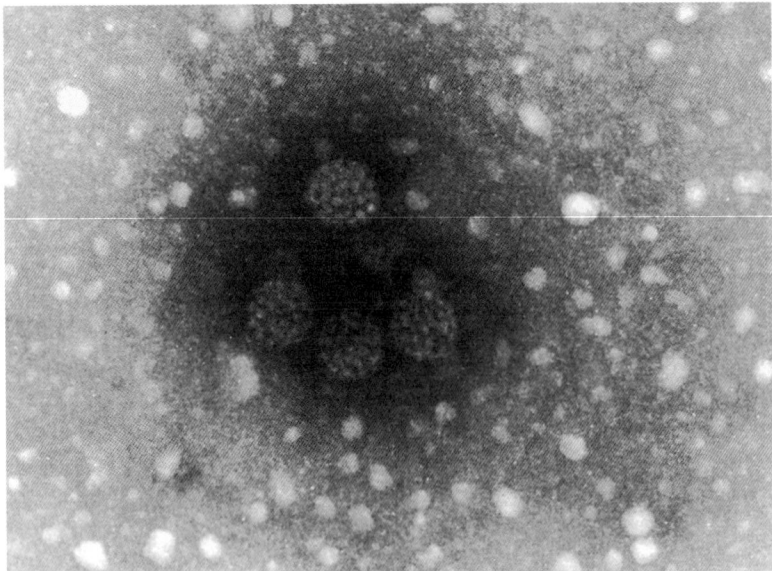

Fig. 18.16
Plantar wart: this honeycomb arrangement of HPV is characteristic. By courtesy of I. Chrystie, FIMLS, St Thomas' Hospital, London, UK.

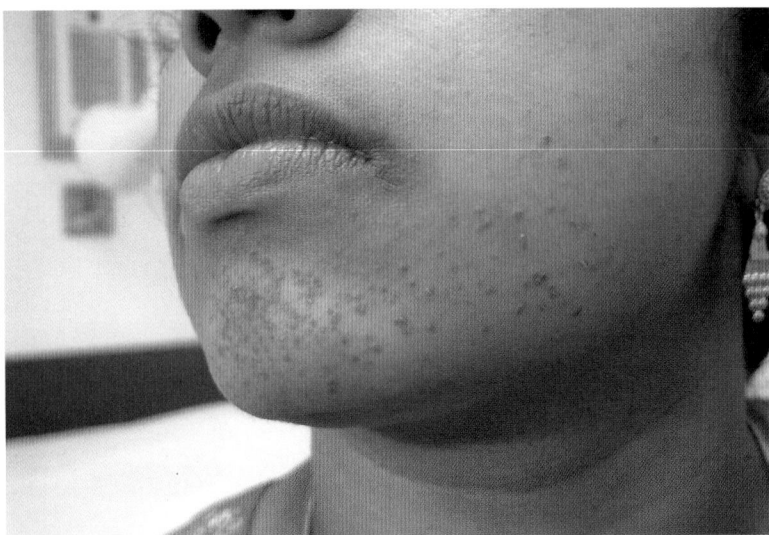

Fig. 18.17
Plane wart: note the typical flat, flesh-colored papules, which have extended in a linear distribution due to scratching (Koebner phenomenon). By courtesy of B Al-Mahmoud, MD, Qatar, Oman.

except in association with HIV infection. They may regress spontaneously after a few weeks or months, or may persist for years. Signs of regression include pruritus, an erythematous, edematous appearance, depigmented haloes, and an eruption of multiple tiny plane warts.[2,6,7] Cell-mediated immunity plays a key role in the spontaneous regression of plane warts in immunocompetent individuals.[8] Multiple plane warts may evolve as a cutaneous manifestation of immune reconstitution inflammatory syndrome (IRIS) in HIV-infected patients receiving highly active ART.[9] Exacerbation of lesions has been reported following facial laser resurfacing.[10]

Histologic features

Plane warts are acanthotic and show orthokeratosis with an open pattern reminiscent of 'chicken wire' ('basket weave' hyperkeratosis). Parakeratosis is not a feature and there is little papillary configuration to the acanthosis (*Fig. 18.18*). Keratinocytes of the upper part of the stratum spinosum show striking cytoplasmic vacuolation with margination of the keratohyalin granules and tonofilaments.[4] Regression is characterized by keratinocyte necrosis (apoptosis), individual cell keratinization, parakeratosis, lymphocytic exocytosis with spongiosis, and a superficial perivascular chronic inflammatory

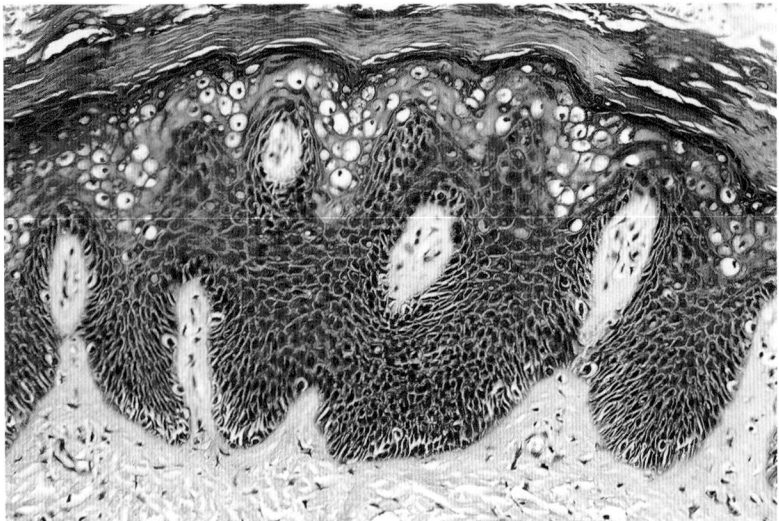

Fig. 18.18
Plane wart: there is hyperkeratosis and slight regular acanthosis; papillomatosis is only mild. Note the prominent cytoplasmic vacuolation.

cell infiltrate.[2,11-13] The lymphocytes encountered in regressing lesions have been found to express the cytotoxic granule granzyme-B.[14] Extravasation of erythrocytes may be a feature and edema of the papillary dermis is frequently present.[15]

Condyloma acuminatum

Clinical features

A majority of sexually active individuals will have detectable HPV infection at least once during their lifetime. An estimated 14 million people are infected annually with genital HPVs.[1] A recent systematic review of the literature concerning anogenital warts revealed a median incidence of 137 and 120.5 per 100 000 among males and females, respectively.[2]

Condylomata acuminata are particularly caused by HPV types 2, 6, 11, 16, 18, 30–33, 35, 39, 41–45, 51–56, and 59 and develop as a consequence of the trauma accompanying sexual intercourse.[3-15] More frequent transmission has been reported from females to males than from males to females.[1] HPV6 and 11 alone account for more than 90% of these lesions, with HPV6 present in about two-thirds of cases and the remaining one-third caused by HPV11.[6,7] The incubation period is variable (usually between 2 and 3 months).[16] Condylomata acuminata occur on the glans penis and prepuce or shaft as soft, fleshy, sometimes filiform plaques and may extend into the meatus (*Figs 18.19* and *18.20*). On the shaft, they are less exophytic. Vulval lesions may be bulky and macerated, and may extend into the introitus (*Fig. 18.21*). Similar fleshy and filiform soft masses occur perianally, more often in males (*Fig. 18.22*).[17] Anal squamous carcinoma has also been shown to contain HPV6, 16, and 18 in a significant proportion of cases (*Fig. 18.23*).[8] The rate of local recurrence is about 30%.[18] The lesions are uncommon in children (where they may be a sign of sexual abuse) and are seen most often in young adults (second and third decades), frequently in association with other genital infections.[6,11,19] Childhood condylomata regress spontaneously in more than 50% of cases.[20] Genital warts are common among HIV-infected individuals.[21]

It is important to note that a significant proportion of genital HPV infections are asymptomatic.[5,22] The female partners of male patients with condyloma acuminata have been shown to have an increased risk of cervical HPV infection and intraepithelial neoplasia (squamous intraepithelial lesion/cervical intraepithelial neoplasia [SIL/CIN]).[23] Cervical neoplasia associated with pre-existent condylomata acuminata has also been related to a background of immunosuppression, at least in some patients.[24] The worldwide HPV prevalence in cervical carcinomas is reported to be 99.7%.[25] HPV16, 18, 31–33, 35, 39, 42, and 51–54 are most commonly associated with cancers of the cervix, vulva, and penis.[9-11,26-28] Patients with condylomata

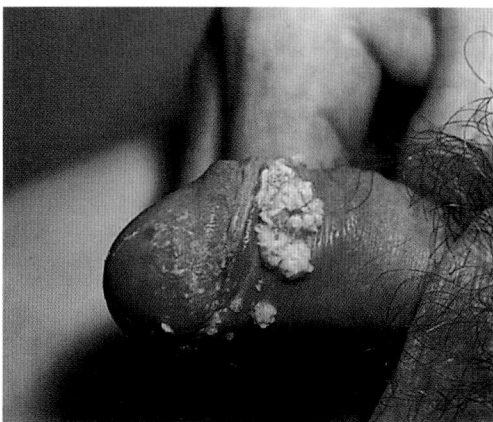

Fig. 18.19
Condyloma acuminatum: note the typical filiform appearance. By courtesy of the Department of Genitourinary Medicine, St Thomas' Hospital, London, UK.

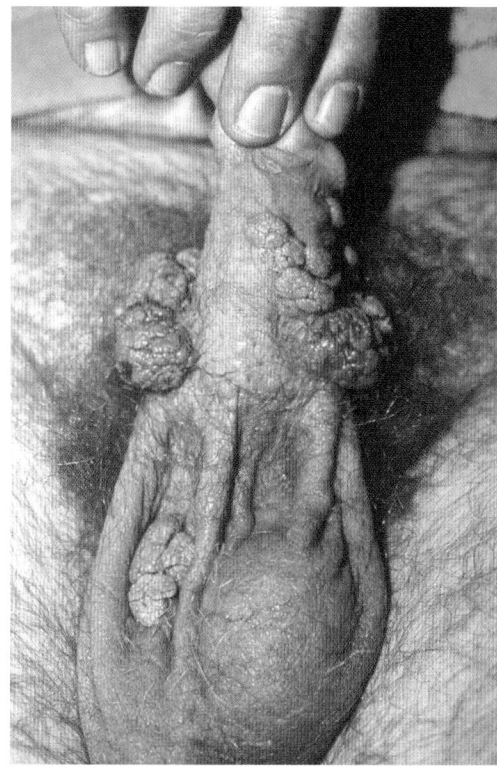

Fig. 18.20
Condyloma acuminatum: there are multiple lesions on the shaft of the penis and scrotum. By courtesy of the Department of Genitourinary Medicine, St Thomas' Hospital, London, UK.

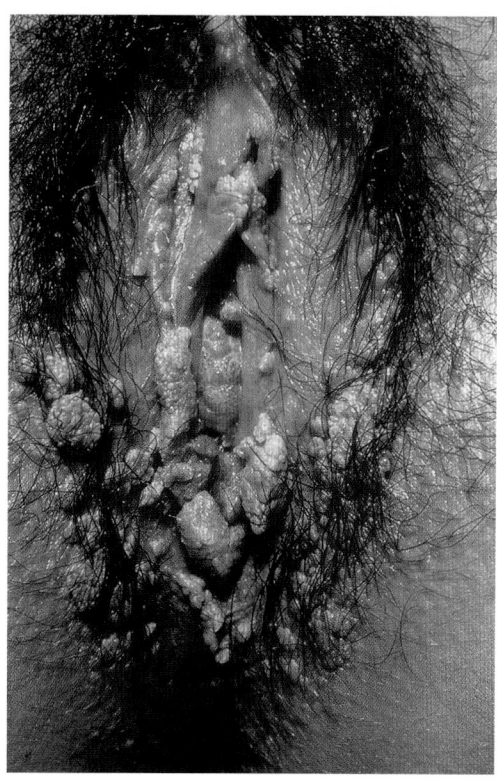

Fig. 18.21
Condyloma acuminatum: in this patient, there is very widespread involvement of the vulva and perineum. This patient is likely to have cervical HPV infection. By courtesy of R.A. Marsden, MD, St George's Hospital London, UK.

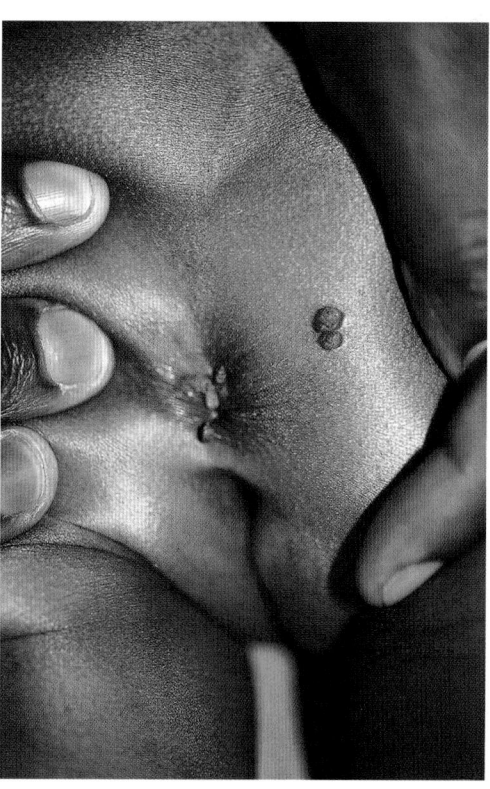

Fig. 18.22
Condyloma acuminatum: there is very extensive involvement of the perineum. From the collection of the late N.P. Smith, MD, the Institute of Dermatology, London, UK.

acuminata are at increased risk for developing not only carcinomas of the vulva, vagina, penis, and anus, but also certain nonanogenital squamous cell carcinomas.[29] Routine vaccination with a quadrivalent vaccine against HPV types 6, 11, 16, and 18 has led to a significant reduction in the burden of vulval and cervical carcinomas, genital warts, and anogenital intraepithelial neoplasia.[17,30–32]

A large, exuberant, and locally destructive variant of condyloma (Buschke-Löwenstein tumor) may rarely be encountered (Fig. 18.24).[33–36] This is associated with HPV types 6, 11, or 16. It is likely that this giant variant represents a variant of verrucous carcinoma but the issue has been controversial (see Chapter 22).[33–39] Juvenile laryngeal papillomas containing HPV6 and 11 can be seen in children born to mothers with condylomata acuminata.[5] They may show malignant progression if irradiated.

Malignant transformation of condyloma acuminatum is uncommon, but it is seen more often than in other lesions associated with HPV except for EV.

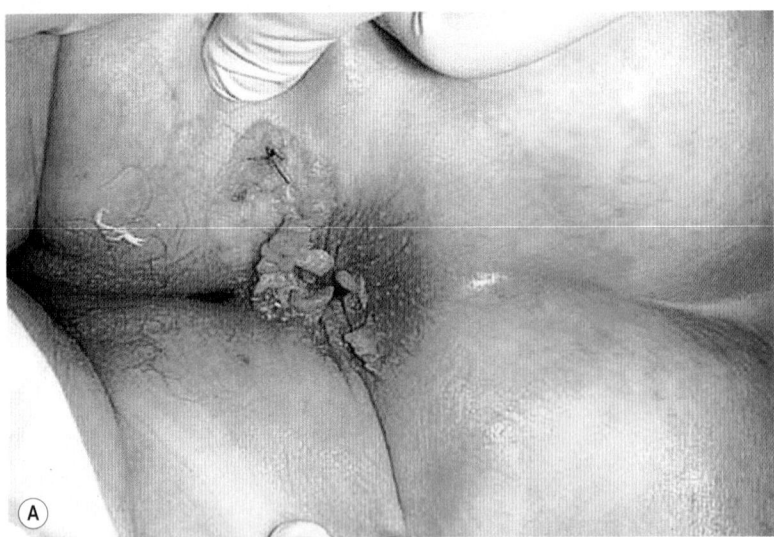

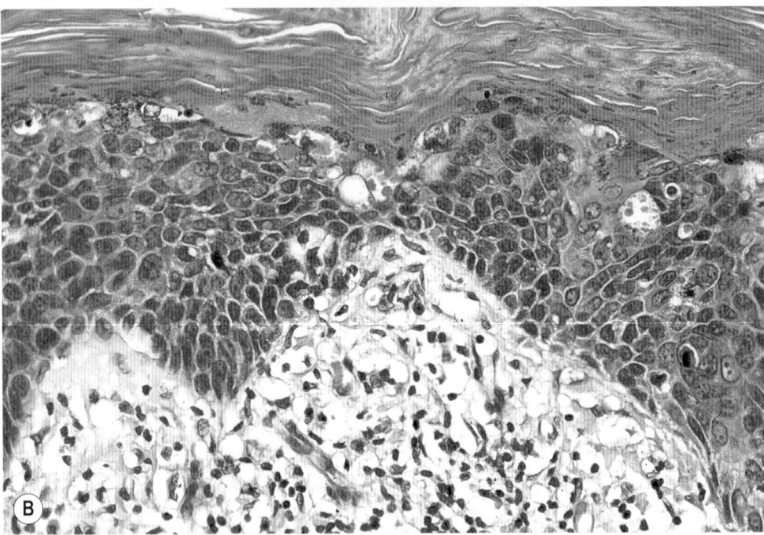

Fig. 18.23
(**A**, **B**) Condyloma acuminatum: in addition to multiple condylomata, there was histologic evidence of in situ squamous cell carcinoma. By courtesy of P. Ngheim, MD, Dana Farber Cancer Institute and Harvard Medical School, Boston, USA.

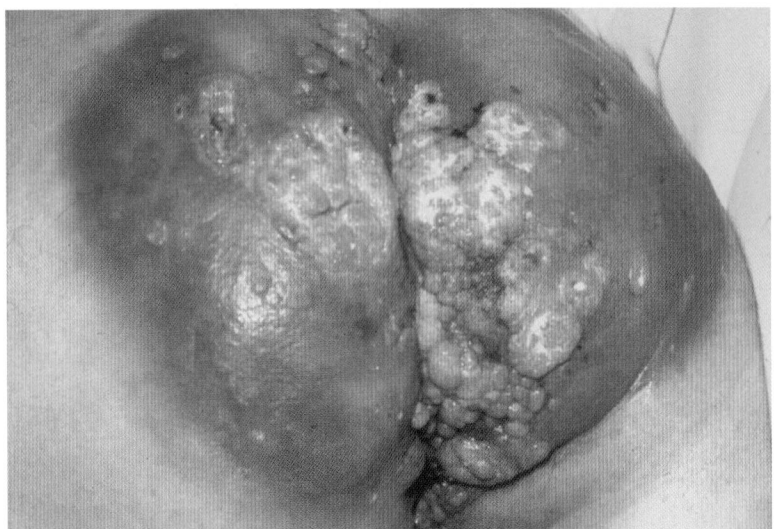

Fig. 18.24
Buschke-Löwenstein tumor: there is massive infiltration of the buttocks and perineum with numerous sinuses. HPV type 6 was identified by DNA in situ hybridization and Southern blot analysis. By courtesy of A. Grassegger, MD, University of Innsbruck, Austria.

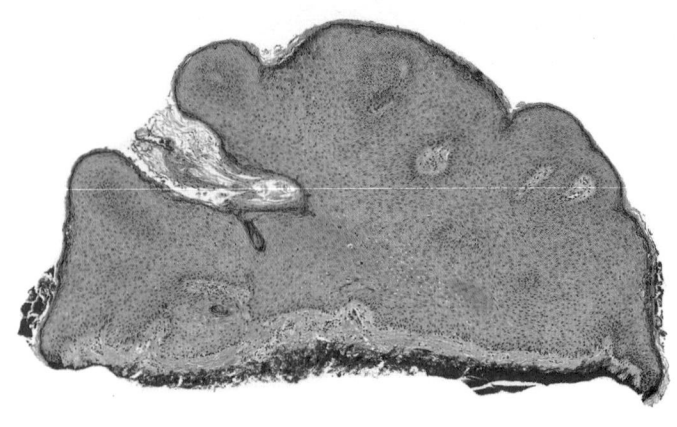

Fig. 18.25
Condyloma acuminatum: note the keratotic acanthotic epidermis with rounded lateral borders. Koilocytes are present in the declivities of the papillomatous epithelium.

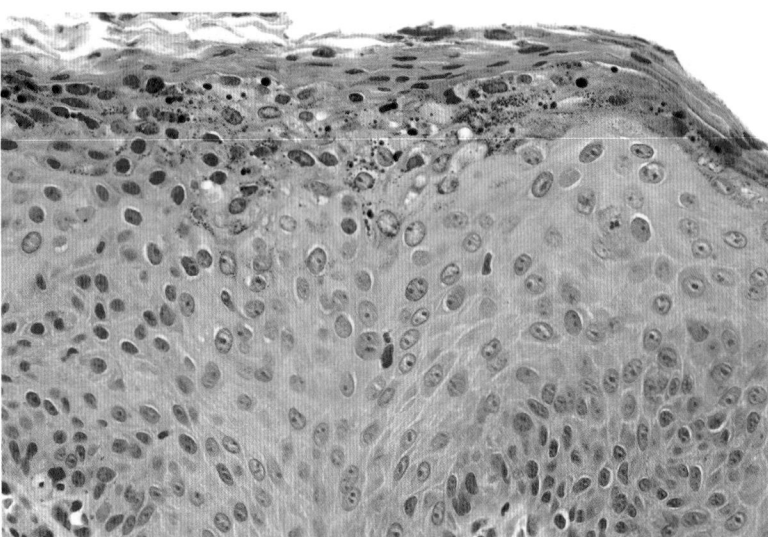

Fig. 18.26
Condyloma acuminatum: note the parakeratosis and vacuolation of the superficial keratinocytes.

Histologic features

Condylomata acuminata are characterized by marked acanthosis with a solid or trabecular pattern and a broad rounded exophytic growth (*Fig. 18.25*). There is a sharp, fairly regular, deep margin. The surface of the lesion is hyperkeratotic and parakeratotic. Superficial vacuolated keratinocytes (koilocytes) are characteristic (*Fig. 18.26*) and coarse keratohyaline granules may be present. The vacuolated epithelium is often most marked in the declivities. Condylomata that are treated with podophyllin prior to removal demonstrate marked epidermal pallor and increased mitoses and necrotic keratinocytes in the lower half of the epidermis.[40] These changes may lead to a misdiagnosis of malignancy. Giant condyloma acuminatum (anogenital verrucous carcinoma, Buschke-Löwenstein tumor) occurs most frequently on the genitalia, and is larger and more cauliflower-like.[33–36] It shows some tendency to endophytic growth, but without any suggestion of frank infiltration. It can recur locally, but metastasizes very rarely. Most experts regard this lesion as a variant of verrucous carcinoma. Anal condylomata may develop bowenoid features, and occasionally invasive tumor supervenes.[8–10]

Bowenoid papulosis

Clinical features

Bowenoid papulosis (koilocytosis with intraepithelial neoplasia) is a clinico-pathological entity that bears marked histologic similarity to koilocytosis, SIL/CIN, and Bowen disease. Although the term is no longer used by the International Society for Study of Vulval Disease (ISSVD) and some have questioned the validity thereof, many clinicians believe that it represents a distinctive clinicopathological entity, and we have decided to describe it in this chapter. Clinically, it is quite different from genital Bowen disease in that multiple small papules develop over a short time scale in young people. Prognosis is uncertain; many patients do not show evidence of progression, but a small proportion may develop invasive tumor and, on occasion, this may have metastatic potential. It is usually associated with HPV16 or 18, but occasionally HPV types 31–35, 39, 42, 49, and 51–54 are detected.[1–10] Although uncommon, some cases may be associated with mixed infection by different HPV types.[10,11] A unique HIV-associated case with genital and extragenital (lip) lesions caused by two separate HPV types (HPV16 and HPV32, respectively) has been described.[12] E6 and E7 viral oncoproteins of high-risk HPV types induce overexpression of p16 and human telomerase reverse transcriptase.[13]

Bowenoid papulosis most often presents as multiple reddish-brown, some-times lichenoid, discrete papules, but occasionally these become a confluent plaque. Papules, on average 4 mm in diameter, are found on the penis, vulva, perianal region, and perineum. Extragenital sites of occurrence include the face, neck, and fingers.[14–16] The lesions are sometimes pigmented.[2] A case of oral bowenoid papulosis in an HIV-infected male has been reported.[17] Bowenoid papulosis manifests in young, sexually active adults in contrast to true Bowen disease, which occurs in an older age group. Genital Bowen disease is, however, also often associated with HPV16.[18] The occurrence in childhood should raise suspicion of sexual abuse.[7] Genital bowenoid papulosis has been associated with periungual bowenoid dysplasia.[19] Bowenoid papulosis with concurrent Bowen disease has been reported in a patient with systemic lupus erythematosus (SLE).[20]

Spontaneous regression is uncommon.[21] As progression to frank invasive carcinoma in bowenoid papulosis is rare, these lesions are best managed conservatively. However, bowenoid papulosis may be resistant to treatment and may be characterized by a prolonged course in immunosuppressed patients.[6] Bowenoid papulosis has also been associated with oral warts and lingual carcinoma.[8] Patients with bowenoid papulosis and HPV infec-tion may be primarily immunosuppressed due to diminished T-helper (Th) cell levels (non-HIV-associated).[6,18] The condition may also occur in organ transplant recipients.[22] Penile bowenoid papulosis is associated with a high risk of the consort developing cervical dysplasia.[23,24] Consequently, female patients and consorts should regularly have cervical smears.

Histologic features

A bowenoid papulosis lesion consists of a well-circumscribed area of acan-thosis producing a raised plaque or dome, which is hyperkeratotic and sometimes shows superficial epithelial vacuolation.[25,26] The keratinocytes may show nuclear hyperchromatism and pleomorphism. There is variable dyskeratosis.

These histologic features of atypia, associated with numerous mitoses, including atypical forms, are similar to those of true Bowen disease. The distinction rests in the circumscribed elevated plaquelike pattern, the age of the patient, and the size and multiplicity of lesions. Immunohistochemistry for p16 reveals strong, diffuse staining of the full thickness of the lesional epidermis.[27]

Epidermodysplasia verruciformis

Clinical features

EV is a rare inherited condition characterized by selective susceptibility to skin infection with certain HPV types, defects in cell-mediated immu-nity, and an increased risk for the development of cutaneous malignancies,

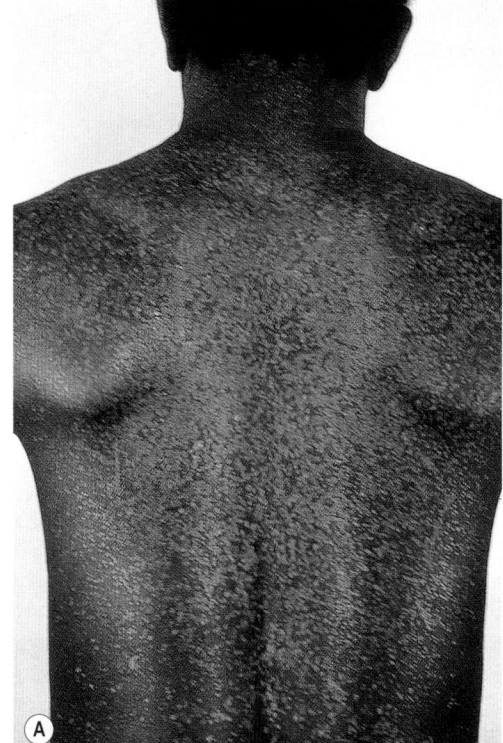

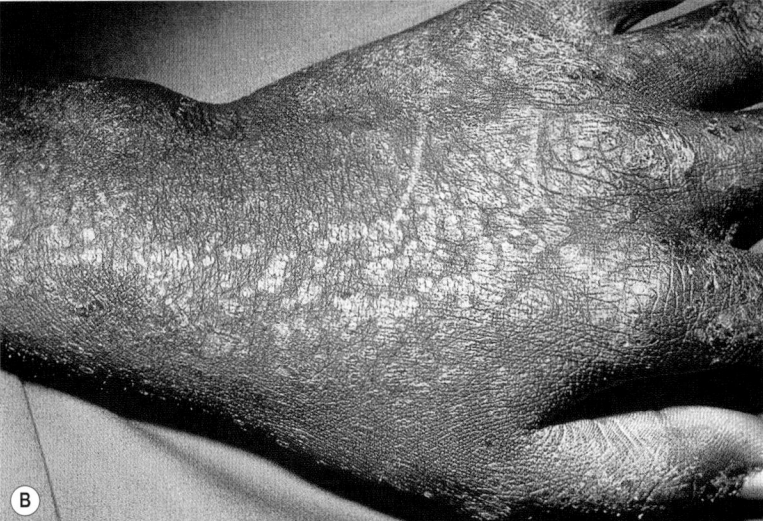

Fig. 18.27
Epidermodysplasia verruciformis: (**A**) innumerable small flat warts are present; (**B**) the dorsum of the hand is a commonly affected site. By courtesy of the Institute of Dermatology, London, UK.

especially squamous cell carcinomas.[1–5] The lesions of affected individuals are the result of infection with a wide range of HPV subtypes including 3, 5, 8–10, 12, 14, 15, 17, 19–25, 28, 29, 36–38, 46, 47, 49, 50, 51, and 59.[1,6–9] The vast majority of these are β-HPV genotypes.[10] The more common flat warts, caused by HPV3 and HPV10, may also occur in these patients but have an extensive distribution pattern; they may form plaques and can be persistent.[11] These are seen most often on the arms, legs, face, and the dorsum of the hands (*Figs 18.27–18.29*).[7] The specific EV subtypes of HPV cause reddish, or pigmented or depigmented, scaly flat macular plane warts, mainly on the trunk, but also on the face, neck, and arms.[2] Clinically, they resemble pityriasis versicolor (*Fig. 18.30*). Some patients, especially those who are dark-skinned, may present with seborrheic keratosis-like changes.[12,13] Spiny hyperkeratosis of the fingers is a rare manifestation.[14] The occurrence of palmar pits is another rarely reported finding.[15,16] Involvement of mucosal epithelium is not a feature of EV.[10]

Susceptibility to EV is usually inherited in an autosomal recessive manner although X-linked recessive inheritance has been reported in one family.[17]

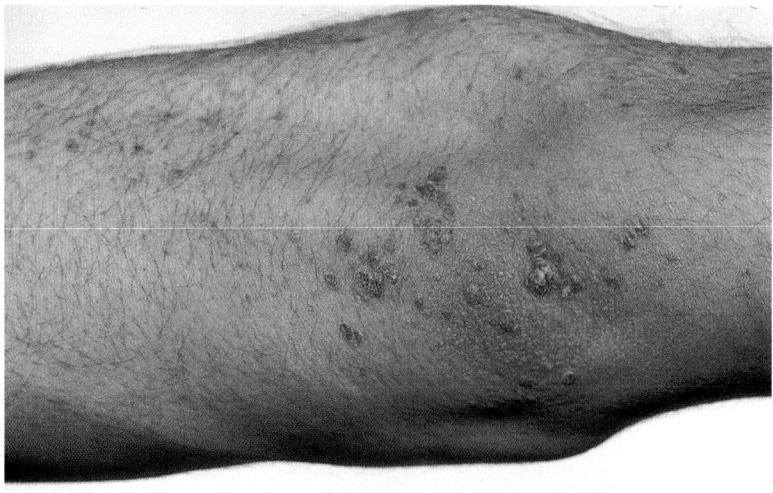

Fig. 18.28
Epidermodysplasia verruciformis: these plane warts are due to HPV3 and HPV10 infection. By courtesy of M.M. Black, MD, Institute of Dermatology, London, UK.

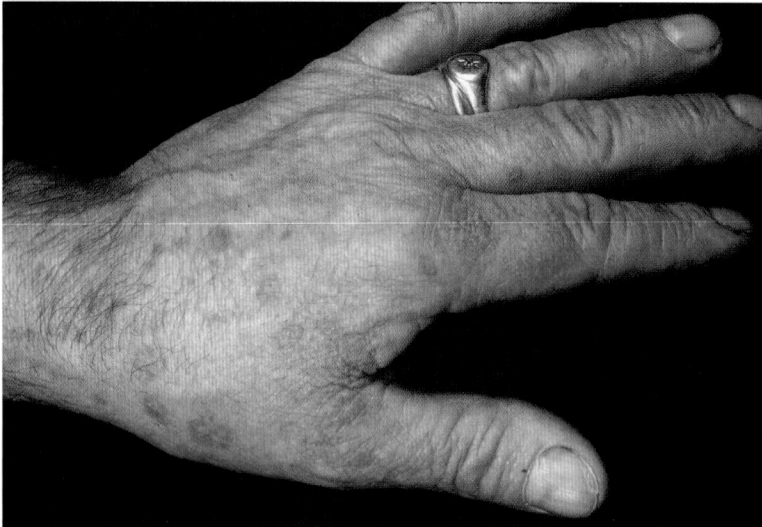

Fig. 18.29
Epidermodysplasia verruciformis: note the numerous flat warts on the dorsum of the hand. From the collection of the late N.P. Smith, MD, the Institute of Dermatology, London, UK.

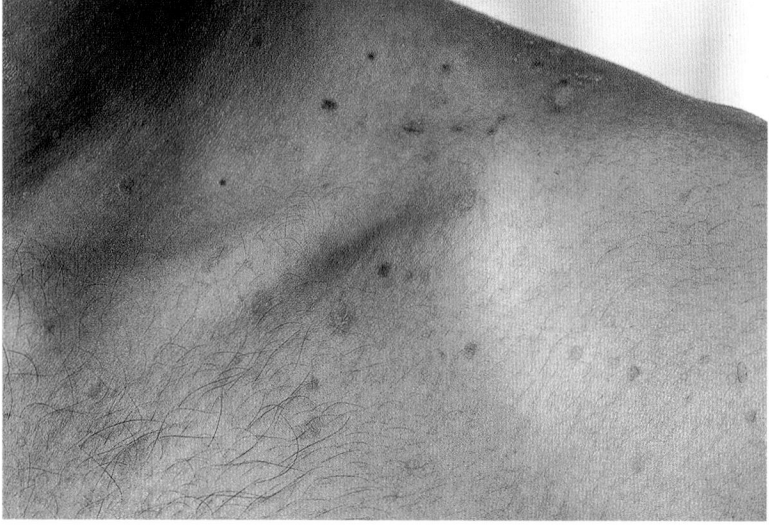

Fig. 18.30
Epidermodysplasia verruciformis: these scaly macules on the chest and axilla resemble pityriasis versicolor. From the collection of the late N.P. Smith, MD, the Institute of Dermatology, London, UK.

The lesions persist throughout life, and after some years (usually more than 20) they may show nuclear atypia resembling Bowen disease, and frank carcinoma sometimes develops. Basal cell carcinoma can also occur.[18] The tumors develop particularly on sun-exposed skin and are most often associated with HPV5 or 8.[7,19] Patients who develop invasive squamous carcinoma in association with EV do so at a younger age than those who develop this tumor not in association with EV (27 years compared with 67 years in one study).[1,19] Such tumors, which are often multiple, are usually associated with a good prognosis unless they are treated with radiotherapy when they may be associated with metastatic disease, which has a high mortality.[6] A large, locally aggressive squamous cell carcinoma of the nose related to HPV22b infection has been recorded, with detection of the virus both within the EV lesions and the malignant neoplasm.[20]

EV-like disease, often referred to as acquired EV, has been reported in patients with a background of immunosuppression in such conditions as SLE, Hodgkin lymphoma, and HIV infection, and rarely in patients following renal transplantation, small bowel transplantation, peripheral blood stem cell transplantation, and bendamustine chemotherapy.[21–30] An EV-like eruption has been documented in association with idiopathic CD4 lymphopenia and even with CD8 lymphopenia.[31,32] Remission of lesions has been recorded in an HIV-positive patient following immune restoration due to ART.[25]

EV therefore represents an unusual condition in which HPV infection, inherited predisposition (possibly a defect in cell-mediated immunity), and exposure to the sun all play a role (co-carcinogens).[1,2,18]

Pathogenesis and histologic features

The pathogenesis of EV is not yet fully understood. The EV-related HPV may be present in the general population, but the characteristic lesions only occur in predisposed individuals (*Fig. 18.31*).[1,18] It has been established that invalidating mutations in either of two adjacent novel transmembrane channel (TMC) genes termed *EVER1* (or *TMC6*) and *EVER2* (or *TMC8*) are responsible for most cases of EV.[3,33] This susceptibility locus for EV has been mapped to the long arm of chromosome 17 (17q25.3).[24,33,34] The EVER1 and EVER2 transmembrane proteins encoded by these genes are located in the endoplasmic reticulum.[35] The proteins form a complex that interacts with zinc transporter 1 (ZnT-1), resulting in altered intracellular zinc distribution in keratinocytes.[10,36] It has been proposed that EVER proteins in keratinocytes may serve as restriction factors for EV-specific HPV types.[35] There have, however, been reports of cases lacking *EVER1* and *EVER2* mutations.[32,37–39]

There appears to be a specific abnormal T-cell response to HPV-infected keratinocytes. The immune defect most often associated is a reduction in the number and function of Th cells, but patients with EV do not show general

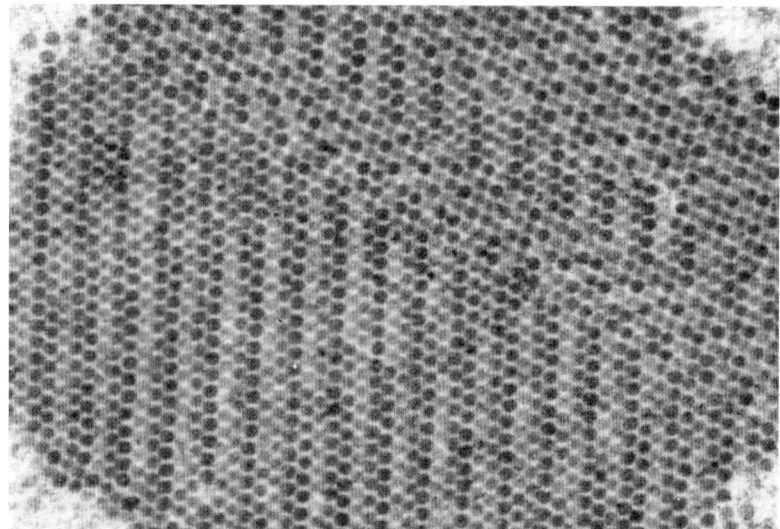

Fig. 18.31
Epidermodysplasia verruciformis: electron micrograph showing the characteristic lattice structure.

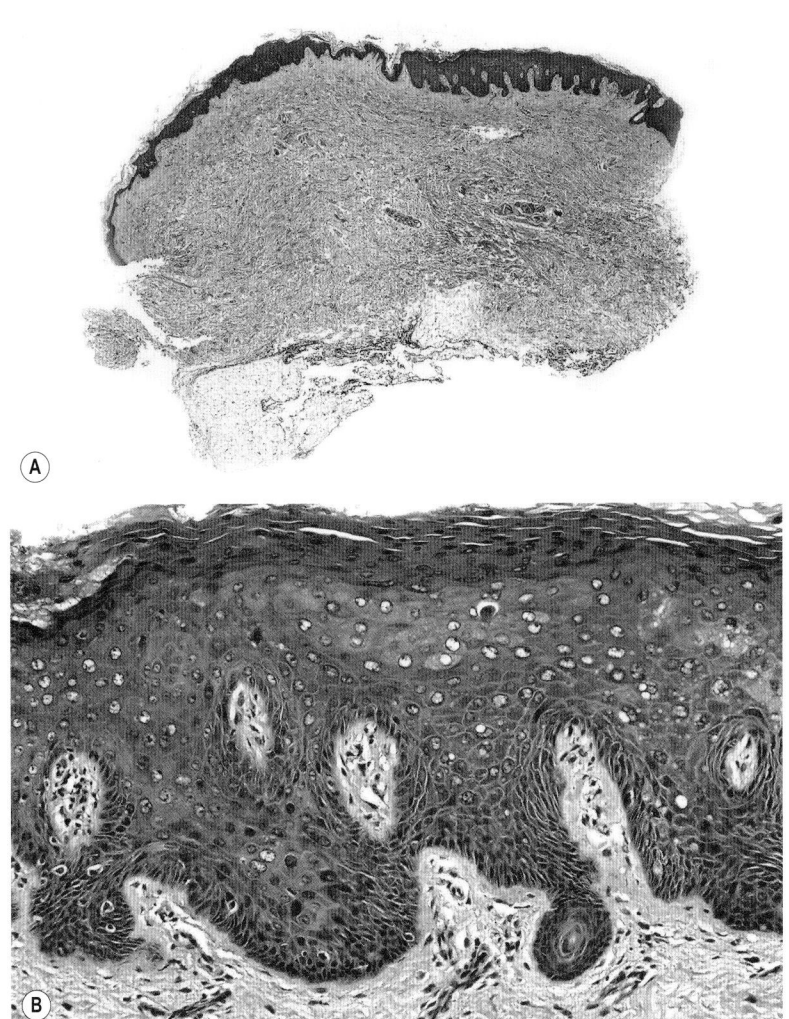

Fig. 18.32
Epidermodysplasia verruciformis. In addition to mild hyperkeratosis and acanthosis, there are characteristic, swollen, paler-staining cells showing nuclear vacuolation.

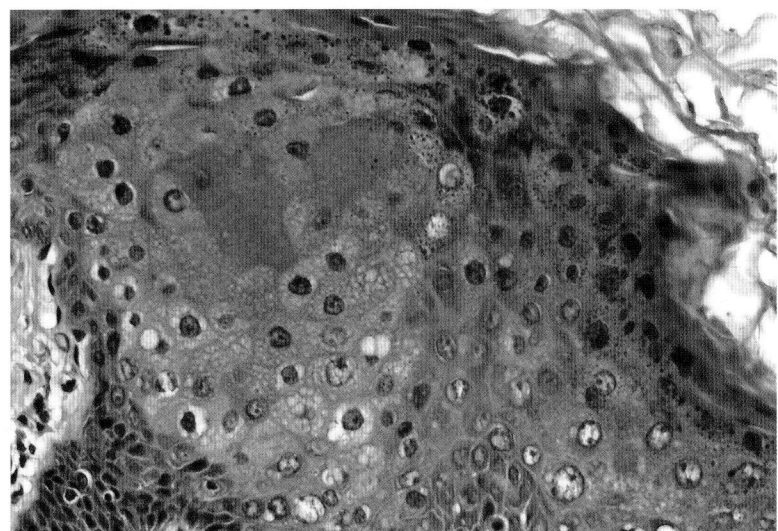

Fig. 18.33
Epidermodysplasia verruciformis: the superficial keratinocytes are swollen and have basophilic cytoplasm.

disorderly.[6,46] The dysplastic changes may also affect appendageal epithelium, particularly that of sweat ducts. The atypia eventually amounts to carcinoma in situ, and in 30–50% of patients the lesions progress to invasive carcinoma. Cutaneous neoplasia in EV is largely associated with HPV5 and 8. The E6 oncoprotein of HPV5 inhibits transactivation of SMAD3, which is an important component of the transforming growth factor (TGF)-β1 signaling pathway.[47] Most carcinomas are squamous in type, but some show features reminiscent of sweat gland differentiation. The sweat ducts may show markedly disordered growth and atypia. These stages in the progression to frank carcinoma only occur on sun-exposed skin. In contrast to cervical cancer where the viral genome is integrated into the host DNA, in EV it remains extrachromosomal (episomal). Ultraviolet B radiation has been shown to modulate the noncoding region promotor activity of HPV5 and 8 in infected keratinocytes.[48] Merkel cell carcinoma has rarely been documented in association with EV.[49] A unique HIV-associated case developed multiple low-grade cutaneous sarcomas with a fibroblastic phenotype.[50]

Differential diagnosis

Swollen keratinocytes, as described above as a diagnostic feature of EV, have been recorded as a manifestation of immunosuppression, particularly HIV infection.[51] Focal histologic features of EV have rarely been documented as an incidental finding in a variety of benign skin lesions in the absence of clinical evidence of underlying EV, including an intradermal nevus, a pigmented seborrheic keratosis, and an acantholytic acanthoma. The term 'EV acanthoma' has been proposed for these isolated, incidental cutaneous lesions.[52]

Herpes simplex virus infections

Herpes simplex virus (HSV) has two subtypes: HSV-1 and HSV-2.[1] There is considerable homology between the two genomes, about 50% of sequences being highly conserved.[2] Humans are the natural hosts for HSV-1 and HSV-2 and therefore also represent the viral reservoir.[3] Herpes viruses are double-stranded DNA viruses with a complex capsid and glycoprotein envelope (Fig. 18.34).

Clinical features

HSV-1 usually causes herpes labialis (90%), whereas HSV-2 most often causes herpes genitalis. Although HSV-2 previously accounted for approximately 90% of herpes genitalis cases, more recent epidemiological evidence reflects an increase in the proportion of cases attributable to HSV-1 (22–29%) and a diminished number of HSV-2 positive cases (68–71%).[4,5] In some European cohort studies, HSV-1 infection has been a more common cause of genital herpes than HSV-2 infection. This trend may be attributable

immunodeficiency or susceptibility to other infections. There have nevertheless been rare reports of EV in association with common variable immunodeficiency syndrome.[40] It has also recently been described in two siblings with an autosomal recessive form of severe combined immunodeficiency linked to a mutation in CORO1A.[41] A similar case of EV in association with severe immunodeficiency, lymphoma, and disseminated molluscum contagiosum (MC) infection appears to have been reported previously.[42] EV has also been documented in a patient with a malignant thymoma.[43] Although EV is not usually seen in patients with iatrogenic immunosuppression, some cases have been recorded.[28,30] Humoral immunity is characteristically normal, although a case with isolated IgM deficiency has been documented.[44] EV-associated HPVs have been detected in the amniotic fluid, placenta, and cervical scrapes of a pregnant patient with EV, thereby suggesting that vertical transmission of EV HPVs may play a role.[45]

Histologically, EV is characterized by hyperkeratosis, hypergranulosis, and acanthosis (Figs 18.32 and 18.33). The keratinocytes are vacuolated and show a striking blue-gray pallor on staining with hematoxylin and eosin (H&E). They are arranged in clusters or columns, the pallor being most conspicuous in the superficial granular cell layer. Identical focal changes may be occasionally seen in samples removed for other reasons in patients without the disease. The latter are usually but not exclusively observed, in sun-damaged skin of elderly patients. A recently reported case of HIV-associated acquired EV showed unique cornoid lamella-like structures.[24] As the lesions progress to atypicality, the nuclei of the keratinocytes become larger and hyperchromatic, and cellular maturation is more

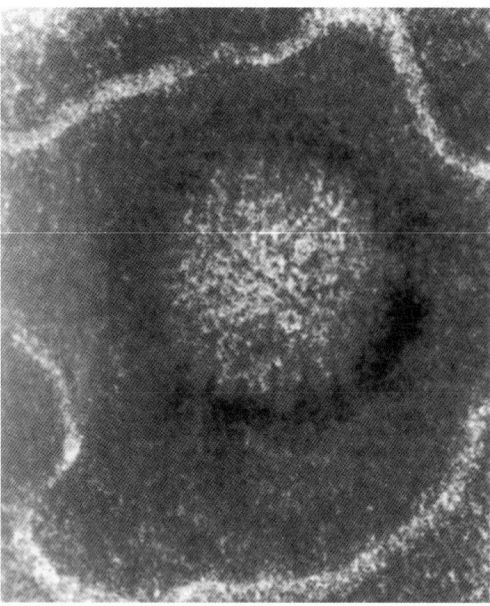

Fig. 18.34
Herpes virus: all members of the herpes virus group have identical ultrastructural morphology. Note the outer membrane surrounding the virus core. The herpes virus is an icosahedron with 162 capsomeres on its surface. By courtesy of I. Chrystie, FIMLS, St Thomas' Hospital, London, UK.

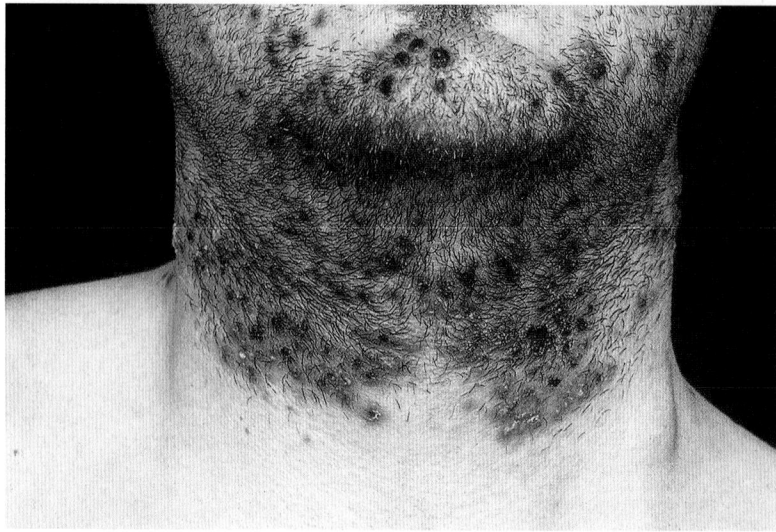

Fig. 18.36
Herpes simplex: this patient shows a particularly severe infection. By courtesy of the Institute of Dermatology, London, UK.

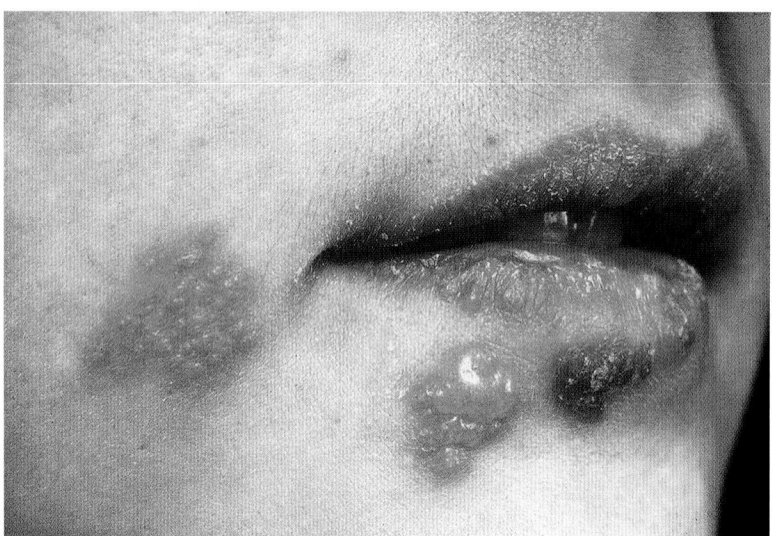

Fig. 18.35
Herpes simplex 1: primary infection showing grouped vesicles on an erythematous base. By courtesy of R.A. Marsden, MD, St George's Hospital, London, UK.

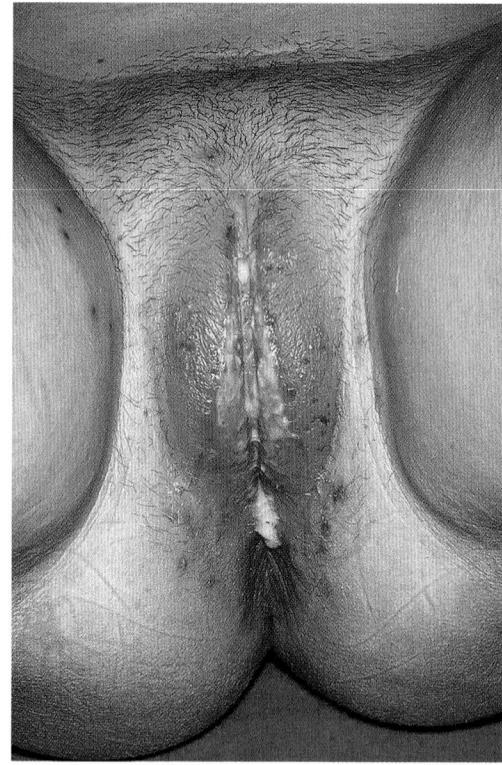

Fig. 18.37
Herpes simplex 2: vulval involvement showing erythema and crusted vesicles. By courtesy of R.A. Marsden, St George's Hospital, ?London, UK.

to the practice of oral sex.[4] Both HSV-1 and HSV-2 are transmitted through mucosal surfaces or traumatized skin by exposure to contaminated secretions.[3,6–8]

A first-episode infection – i.e., in someone who is seronegative (first-episode primary infection) or who has serum antibodies to the heterologous HSV type (first-episode, nonprimary infection) – may be associated with constitutional symptoms of fever and malaise.[9,10] These symptoms are often worse in women with genital herpes, perhaps because of the wider area of epithelium involved and the greater viral load. The lesions may be found in the mouth, pharynx, lips, penis, vulva, vagina, or cervix (*Figs 18.35–18.39*). HSV infections are also being seen more frequently in perianal and anorectal sites. Involvement of a finger in the form of a herpetic whitlow is most often seen in healthcare workers, especially dental practitioners (*Fig. 18.40*).[11,12] Primary HSV-1 infection, however, is asymptomatic in about 90% of patients, and primary HSV-2 in about 75%.[13] It is important to remember that infection is for life. Herpes compunctorum is a rare

form of HSV infection acquired as a result of tattooing.[14] HSV may also be transmitted during close contact sports such as wrestling and rugby (herpes gladiatorum and herpes rugbiorum, respectively).[15,16]

At the original inoculation site there is no detectable change for 3–5 days. The lesions that develop vary with site, but all are associated with the development of small grouped vesicles, often on an erythematous base. On mucosal surfaces, the vesicles rupture early and are superseded by grayish-yellow plaques or ulcers. In skin, grouped vesicles are seen on an erythematous base and then evolve into grouped pustules, which rupture and result in a crusted ulcer.[17,18] The lesions are typically painful and sting or itch. The distribution of the lesions is characteristically wider than the initial site of inoculation, involving the area of innervation by the sensory nerve to that site. Occasionally, a separate area of lesions may develop away

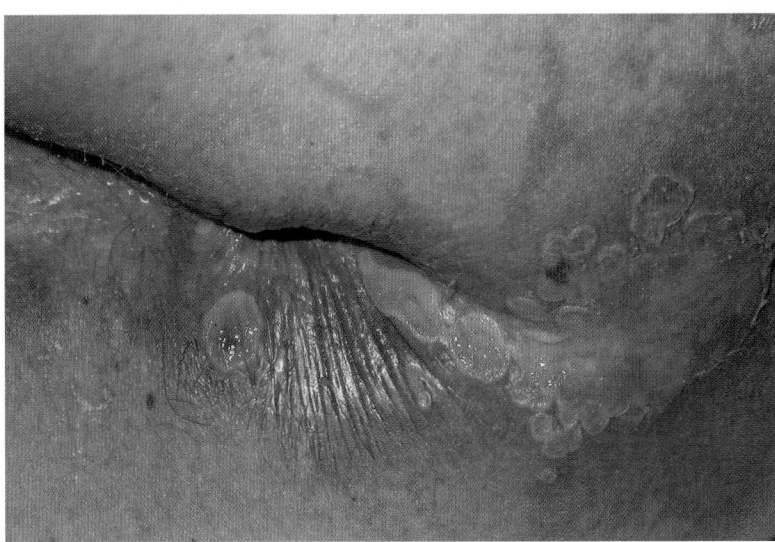

Fig. 18.38
Herpes simplex 2: in this patient there is very severe ulceration. By courtesy of J.C. Pascual, MD, Alicante, Spain.

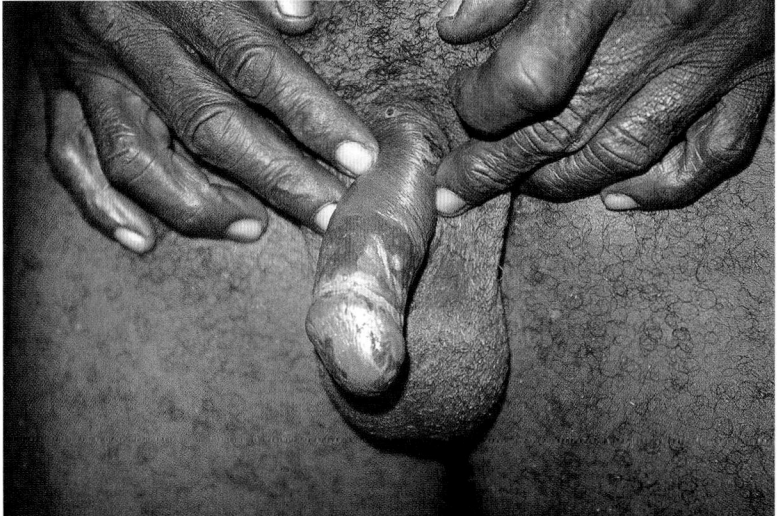

Fig. 18.39
Herpes simplex 2: there is intense erythema and multiple ulcers are present on both the glans and the shaft. By courtesy of C. Furlonge, MD, Port of Spain, Trinidad.

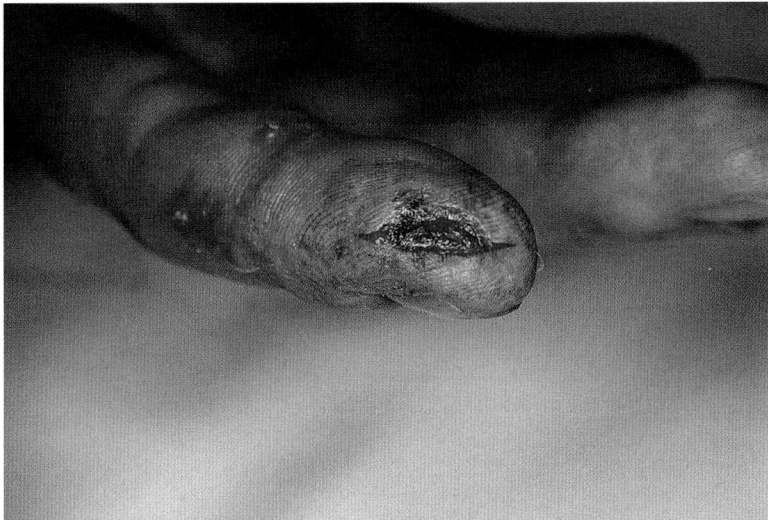

Fig. 18.40
Herpetic whitlow: intact vesicles may be seen on the proximal phalanx. The medical and dental professions are at particular risk from this mode of spread. By courtesy of R.A. Marsden, MD, St George's Hospital, London, UK.

from the initial inoculation site, after transmission along a different branch of the same nerve. These initial cutaneous lesions only develop after involvement of the nerve and the ganglion and subsequent return of the virus to the epithelium.[3] The lesions may then extend peripherally to involve adjacent skin or mucosa. This first episode of infection lasts for around 15 days. The epithelial lesions then resolve completely, but the virus persists, becoming latent within the ganglia of the corresponding sensory nerve.[19] HSV is the most frequent infective cause of erythema multiforme.[20]

Recurrent HSV lesions are usually less florid than the first infection and are not usually associated with general symptoms. They may be precipitated by sunlight, fever, menstruation, pregnancy, HIV infection, emotional stress, or local trauma.[13] The incidence of recurrent orofacial herpes varies from 16% to 45%, while that of recurrent genital herpetic infection varies from about 50% to 65% of patients.[3] Repeated recurrence is usual with genital HSV-2 and common with orofacial HSV-1, but with gradually decreasing frequency. 'Reinfection' with the heterologous type resembles a less severe first-episode primary infection.

Antibodies to HSV-1 are found in about 70% to 90% of adults, suggesting very wide contact with the virus, with a subclinical infection or an unrecognized oropharyngitis in childhood.[8] Worldwide, an estimated 16% of people aged 15–49 years are infected with HSV-2.[18] The seroprevalence of HSV-2 infection varies geographically.[21,22] The seroprevalence in Asian countries ranges from 10% to 30%, whereas more than 80% of female commercial sex workers in parts of sub-Saharan Africa are infected.[23] The United States saw a 30% rise in the prevalence of HSV-2 infection between the late 1970s and the early 1990s.[21] Although HSV-1 occurs most commonly above the waist and HSV-2 below, these are preferential rather than obligatory sites. It has been noted that 10% to 15% of first-episode genital herpes is associated with pharyngeal lesions, emphasizing not only the frequency of orogenital contact, but that both viruses can affect either orofacial or genital epithelia.

Occasionally, a first-episode primary infection in an atopic patient may result in extensive vesicular crops, so-called Kaposi varicelliform eruption (eczema herpeticum) (*Fig. 18.41*).[24–26] These lesions pustulate, ulcerate, and crust, as in the usual herpetic infection, but involve more or less the whole

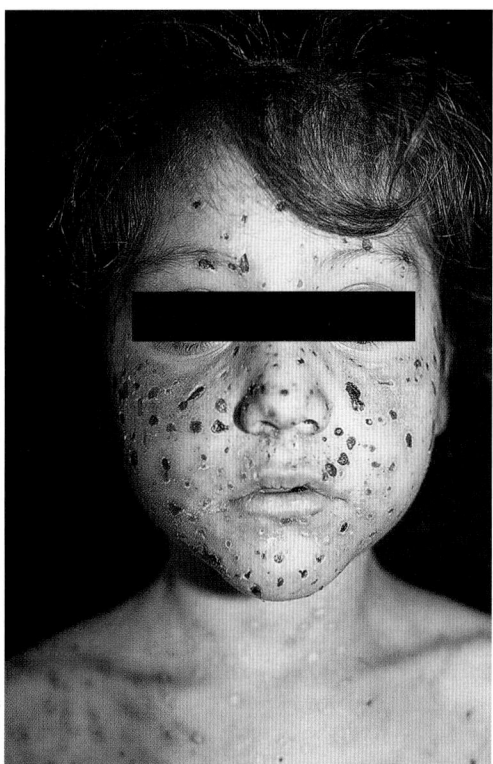

Fig. 18.41
Eczema herpeticum: this variant usually presents in atopic children. It can be a very serious condition and affect the whole body. By courtesy of J.C. Salas, MD, Azteca, Monterrey, Mexico.

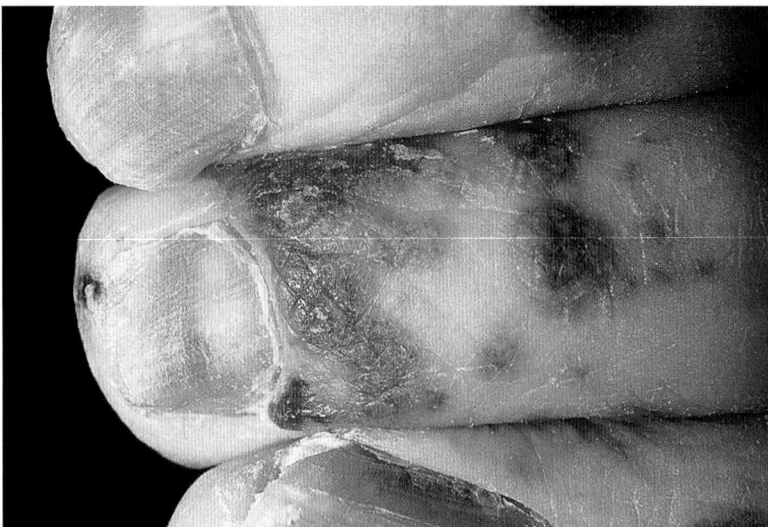

Fig. 18.42
Disseminated herpes infection: widespread lesions may be seen in immunosuppressed patients. By courtesy of the Institute of Dermatology, London, UK.

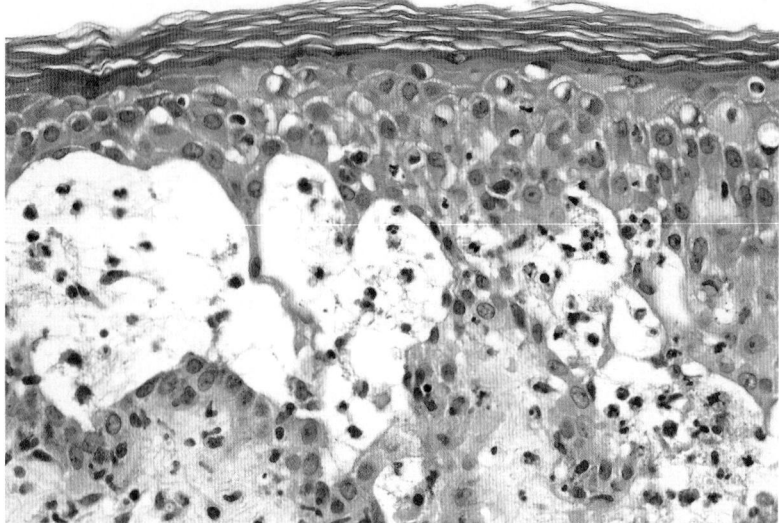

Fig. 18.43
Herpes simplex: intraepidermal vesicle in which there is intracellular edema (ballooning degeneration) and acantholysis.

skin surface. Systemic symptoms may be severe, with fever and dehydration. The condition may occasionally prove fatal. Recurrent attacks may occur, but they are usually short and less severe. This manifestation of herpetic infection may also complicate Darier disease, Hailey-Hailey disease, Grover disease, pemphigus foliaceus, and other bullous dermatoses.[27,28] Historically, a similar clinical picture was occasionally caused by vaccinia virus (eczema vaccinatum) as a complication of vaccination against smallpox.[28] Histologically, the lesions of Kaposi varicelliform eruption are the same as those of the more localized form of herpetic infection. Disseminated disease may be seen in the immunosuppressed (*Fig. 18.42*).

HSV infection in pregnancy may be associated with both severe maternal illness and fetal involvement via transplacental spread.[23,29] Congenital infection is rare, but neonatal herpes simplex infection is seen in 10% of babies born to women with an active herpetic lesion after the 32nd week of pregnancy.[23,30] Fatal disseminated infection with HSV-1 has been reported in preterm twins born to a mother with active herpetic gingivostomatitis during pregnancy.[31] Congenital HSV infection forms part of the TORCH (toxoplasmosis, other infections, rubella, cytomegalovirus [CMV] and herpes simplex) complex.[32] Lesions in congenital herpes infection can be extensively bullous, with severe erythroderma and loss of body fluid through exudation. The reported mortality rate in infants with disseminated infection is approximately 57%.[33] Neonatal infection usually presents as a relatively mild oropharyngitis, and many are probably undiagnosed.

Immunosuppressed patients with underlying HIV/AIDS may present with extensive genital and perineal involvement. Not uncommonly, this is accompanied by concomitant CMV infection, and on rare occasions dual HSV-2 and CMV infection may even give rise to fungating anogenital lesions.[34,35] Herpes simplex is also a potential cutaneous manifestation of IRIS among individuals receiving ART.[36]

Pathogenesis and histologic features

The double-stranded DNA of herpes virus is enclosed in an icosahedral protein shell (capsid), which in turn is invested by a complex envelope of lipid and glycoproteins. The latter are important in the attachment and penetration of cells. The complete virus measures about 150–1200 nm in diameter.[13] Viral replication occurs within the nucleus where a basophilic Feulgen-positive inclusion body, including viral DNA, may be found as well as an eosinophilic inclusion body, which represents a focal deficiency of viral DNA, a so-called 'scar' of viral infection.[2] Heparan sulfate moieties act as receptors to which HSV-1 and HSV-2 bind.[37,38] HSV-1 encodes a complement-interacting glycoprotein (gC) and an IgG Fc binding glycoprotein (gE). These glycoproteins mediate immune evasion.[39] Glycoproteins C and D (gC and gD) play an important role in the attachment of HSV-1 to host cell surface heparan sulfate receptors, whereas glycoprotein B (gB) is responsible for HSV-2 cellular attachment, entry, and cell-to-cell spread.[37,38]

The most characteristic feature in the pathogenesis of herpetic infections is the early involvement of sensory nerves within which the virus, without its lipid/glycoprotein envelope, is transported to the ganglia.[40] Further replication (associated with cell lysis) occurs within the ganglia, and the complete virus then migrates to the skin around the site of inoculation via the peripheral sensory nerves. This process of viral migration also occurs at times of recurrence. The state of the virus during the latent periods, which may last for many months or years, is not clear. It may continue as a more or less intact virus, but in virtually suspended animation without cell death, or it may persist as episomes or be incorporated into the cell genome. Immune mechanisms are responsible for both latency and reactivation of the virus.[40]

Although immune defects (particularly of cell-mediated immunity and including HIV infection) are associated with a high incidence of severe and extensive herpetic infections, a state of raised immunity (either humoral or cellular) does not preclude recurrent lesions; indeed, recurrent lesions are usually associated with very high titers of IgG antibody. It is thought that humoral immunity may impede neuronal extension and reduce the likelihood of encephalitis, but cell-mediated immunity is effective in limiting the local cutaneous extension of the lesions and accelerates healing. Low levels of IFN-γ may contribute to reactivation of infections.[41] Genital ulceration due to HSV-2 increases the risk of acquiring HIV infection; conversely, clinical trials have shown that HIV-1 viral load is reduced following suppression of HSV-2 infection.[42]

Histologically, the early change of HSV infection is increasing edema of the keratinocytes, which progresses to so-called ballooning degeneration.[43,44] Some adjacent keratinocytes fuse so that they appear large and multinucleate. A number of cells show acantholysis, while others rupture as a result of extreme balloon degeneration (reticular degeneration). The result of acantholysis and balloon degeneration is an irregular intraepidermal vesicle containing groups of keratinocytes, many of which may be multinucleate (*Figs 18.43–18.47*). The nuclei of keratinocytes may contain basophilic and/or pale ground-glass inclusions. As a vesicle expands, it involves the full thickness of the epidermis and may not be so clearly intraepidermal. HSV infection of the hair follicle epithelium can result in herpes folliculitis.[44,45] Massive necrosis of the epidermis and superficial part of the hair follicle including sebaceous glands eventually develops. Involvement of hair follicles is, in fact, very common in most infections. In cases with very prominent superficial secondary changes, the distinctive findings of the infection are sometimes only evident in the infundibular portion of the hair follicle.

The underlying dermis is usually intensely infiltrated by mixed inflammatory cells. The infiltrate shows perineural accentuation, and occasionally

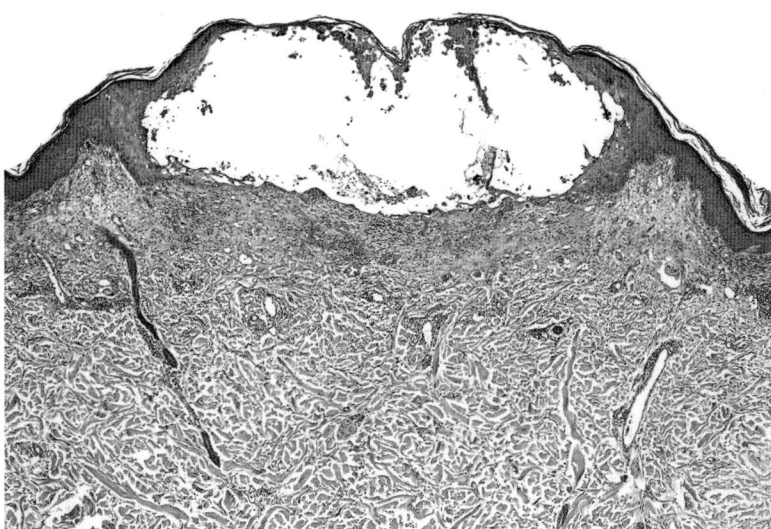

Fig. 18.44
Herpes simplex: scanning view of intact intraepidermal blister.

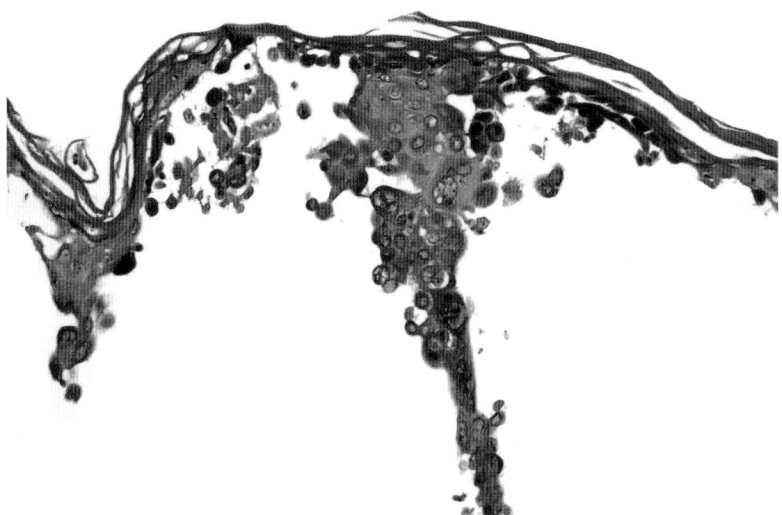

Fig. 18.45
Herpes simplex: the roof shows acantholysis and scattered characteristic intranuclear inclusions.

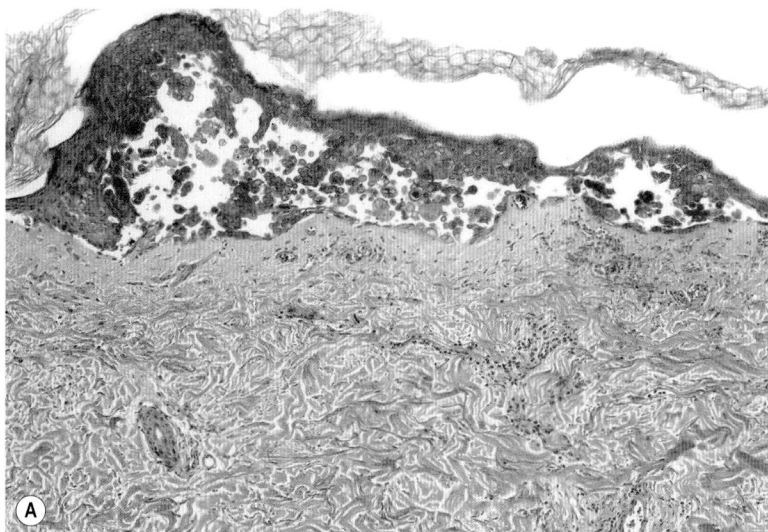

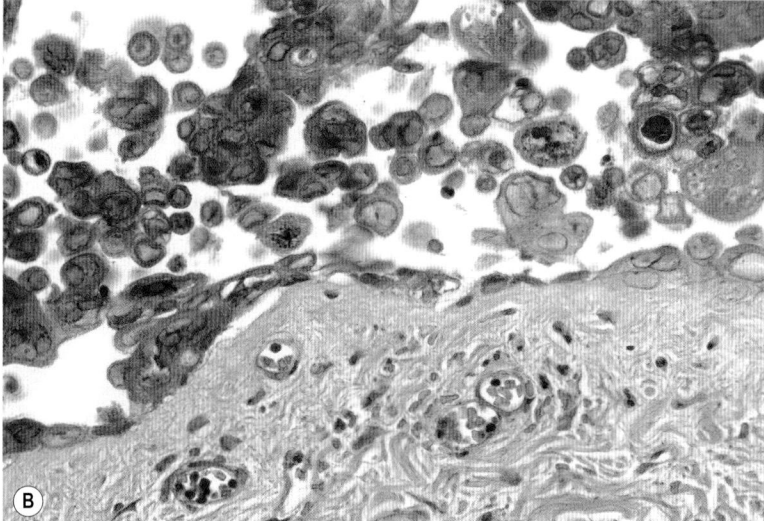

Fig. 18.46
(A, B) Herpes simplex: note the numerous multinucleate giant cells and conspicuous pale-staining inclusions (B).

a superficial leukocytoclastic vasculitis is present (*Fig. 18.48*).[43,44] Dermal nerve twigs may exhibit a perineural inflammatory infiltrate composed of lymphocytes and neutrophils, sometimes associated with intraneural involvement. Schwann cell hypertrophy and frank neuronal necrosis are occasionally encountered.[44,46] Infection is sometimes associated with a prominent lymphoid infiltrate, resulting in a pseudolymphoma.[36,44] Such cases may be associated with frequent CD30-positive cells, potentially mimicking a CD30-positive cutaneous lymphoproliferative disorder.[44,47] HSV infection is also capable of inciting an inflammatory infiltrate rich in CD56-positive cells, thereby mimicking a NK-/T-cell lymphoma. An HIV/AIDS-associated case of scrotal HSV-2 infection with an atypical plasma cell infiltrate mimicking a plasmacytoma also has been reported.[44]

The features of an ulcerated herpetic lesion are not diagnostic unless the epithelial margins retain the characteristic features of intracellular edema, multinucleate epithelial cells, and inclusion bodies. Careful scrutiny of the surface exudate may nevertheless reveal isolated degenerate epithelial cells whose nuclei contain ghost outlines of herpetic viral inclusions. This should prompt examination of the adjacent intact epidermis for more characteristic features of HSV infection.[48] The viable multinucleate cells are the diagnostic feature of the Tzanck test, a Giemsa-stained smear of vesicle contents. Biopsies of anogenital HSV-related ulcers in HIV-infected patients may show evidence of concomitant CMV infection.[34,35,48,49] In the past, laboratory diagnosis of herpes infection was confirmed by growth in tissue culture, electron microscopy, immunofluorescent demonstration of viral-specific protein, or viral DNA hybridization.[50] Nowadays, the diagnosis of HSV-1 or HSV-2 infection is confirmed by PCR or immunohistochemistry (*Fig. 18.49*).[51,52]

Varicella and herpes zoster

Clinical features

Varicella-zoster virus (VZV), also referred to as herpes varicella virus, is similar morphologically to HSV, and is the causative agent of varicella and zoster.[1–3]

Varicella, or chickenpox, which is highly contagious, is most often an infection of children and is characterized by a disseminated vesicular eruption in crops. The major route of dissemination is by airborne droplets from the respiratory tract.[4,5] In the immunocompetent, spread via the cutaneous lesions seems to be of little importance. Varicella is endemic in the temperate climates and manifests predominantly in winter and spring.[4,5]

The incubation period is around 2 weeks and is followed by a rash, which is most pronounced on the trunk. The rash starts as red macules 2–4 mm across, which progress rapidly to fragile vesicles said to resemble 'dew drops on rose petals'; these become pustular and rapidly show crusting (*Fig. 18.50*). Lesions in varying stages are present at any one time. There is often considerable pruritus, and the associated scratching may result in secondary infection with *Staphylococcus aureus* or *Streptococcus pyogenes*.[5]

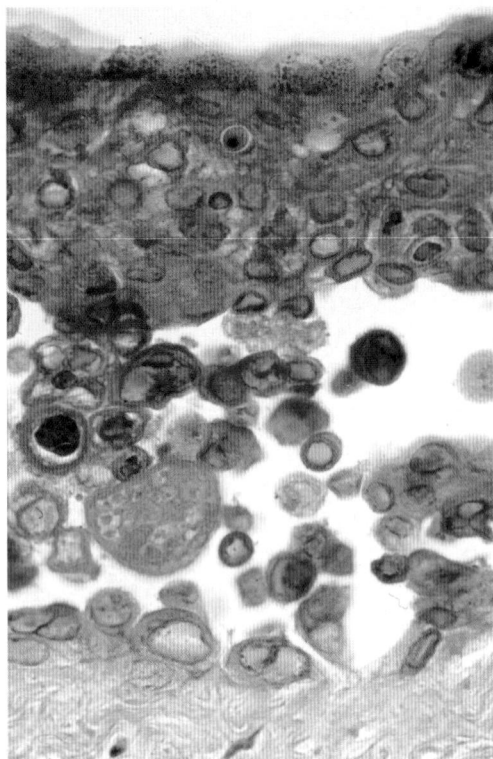

Fig. 18.47
Herpes simplex: high-power view of blister.

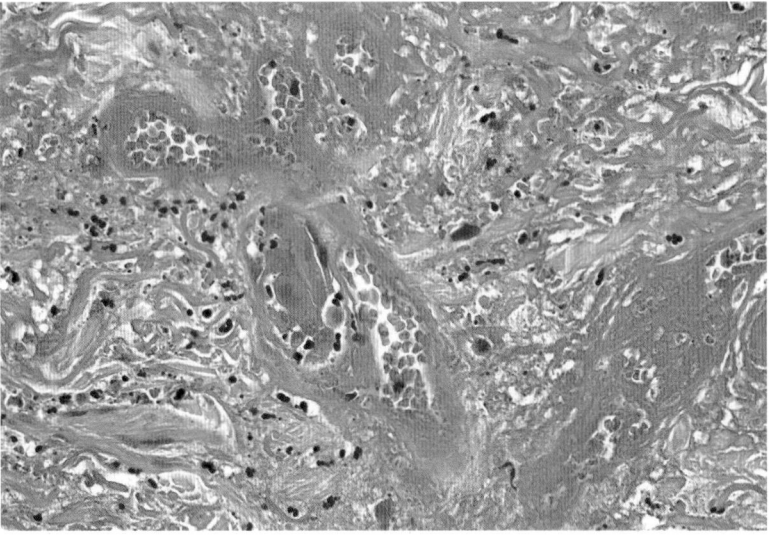

Fig. 18.48
Herpes simplex: multiple vessels show intense fibrinoid necrosis.

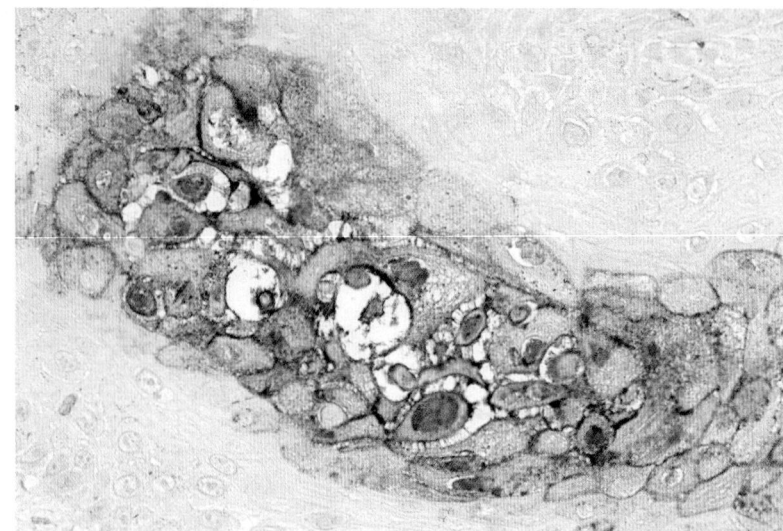

Fig. 18.49
Herpes simplex: positive immunohistochemistry.

Mucosal lesions are frequently also present. Systemic effects in children are mild whereas they are almost invariably severe in adults, neonates, and immunocompromised patients. Recurrent varicella is rare.[6]

Complications include pneumonitis, meningitis, encephalitis, myelitis, and purpura fulminans. In the last, symmetrical hemorrhagic and necrotic lesions are seen on the legs following typical chickenpox, and the condition is associated with disseminated intravascular coagulation (DIC). Acquired deficiencies in protein S or protein C have been implicated in the pathogenesis of varicella-associated purpura fulminans.[7,8] Less common complications include orchitis, hepatitis, glomerulonephritis, arthritis, myocarditis, and rhabdomyolysis.[4,9,10] Necrotizing fasciitis (NF) is a potentially life-threatening complication of childhood varicella.[11,12]

Varicella occurring in pregnancy may have serious consequences for both mother and fetus.[13] Varicella pneumonia may lead to maternal death. Congenital varicella syndrome occurs in approximately 2% of neonates born to mothers who acquire chickenpox during the first two trimesters. Manifestations of this syndrome include dermatomal cutaneous lesions, ocular involvement, neurological complications, and skeletal abnormalities.[5,13] Generalized neonatal varicella, which carries a mortality of around 20% if untreated, is the result of a maternal varicella rash appearing in a mother without antibodies between the last 4 or 5 days of pregnancy and the first 2 days following delivery of the baby.[5,13]

Herpes zoster, or shingles, occurs particularly in adults, usually the elderly, and most often presents as a girdle-like vesicular eruption in the thoracic or lumbar region, or with facial lesions as a result of trigeminal nerve involvement (Figs 18.51 and 18.52).[3,4,14] It is analogous to a recurrent episode of herpes simplex where the virus remains latent in the ganglia of sensory nerves. It is, however, worth noting that although rare, co-infection with VZV and HSV has been reported.[15] Herpes zoster is thought to develop as a consequence of partial immunity.[4] The eruption is preceded by paresthesia or pain in the dermatome supplied by a sensory nerve. This is followed, usually after 2–4 days, by the development of an edematous erythematous plaque on which groups of vesicles arise. As in chickenpox, these rapidly become pustules, which may coalesce to form bullae, occasionally hemorrhagic (Fig. 18.53). The areas become crusted and this may very occasionally be followed by scarring and keloid formation. The lesions are usually painful, and this may persist for months or years as postherpetic neuralgia. The development of a vaccine for the prevention of herpes zoster in older adults holds promise.[16] Involvement of the ophthalmic division of the trigeminal nerve (herpes zoster ophthalmicus) is an important manifestation in the elderly, which can have serious complications (Fig. 18.54).[14] Involvement of the mucocutaneous division of the seventh cranial nerve or the eighth cranial nerve leads to Ramsay Hunt syndrome, which is characterized by lesions in the auricular canal, facial paralysis, and auditory and vestibular symptoms.[14,17] Rarely, noncontiguous multidermatomal cutaneous involvement (zoster multiplex) may occur.[18,19] Although uncommon, herpes zoster may occur in children who have received varicella vaccine, a live attenuated virus. Cervical and sacral dermatomes are most commonly affected in these children, and potential complications include secondary bacterial infection, scarring, and depigmentation.[20]

Reactivation of latent VZV may be associated with a deficiency in cell-mediated immunity, as immunity to chickenpox per se is normally lifelong. Patients with Hodgkin lymphoma, non-Hodgkin lymphoma, or SLE, and those treated with irradiation or chemotherapy, are particularly at risk and often develop a more serious illness.[4,5] In more severe cell-mediated immunodeficiency, the zoster may become widely disseminated and sometimes proves fatal. Disseminated cutaneous lesions most often present as vesicles, pustules, hemorrhagic bullae, ulcers, and black eschars, although occasionally patients may develop verrucous, hyperkeratotic lesions (Fig. 18.55).[21] Visceral involvement is most often seen in the lung, liver, and

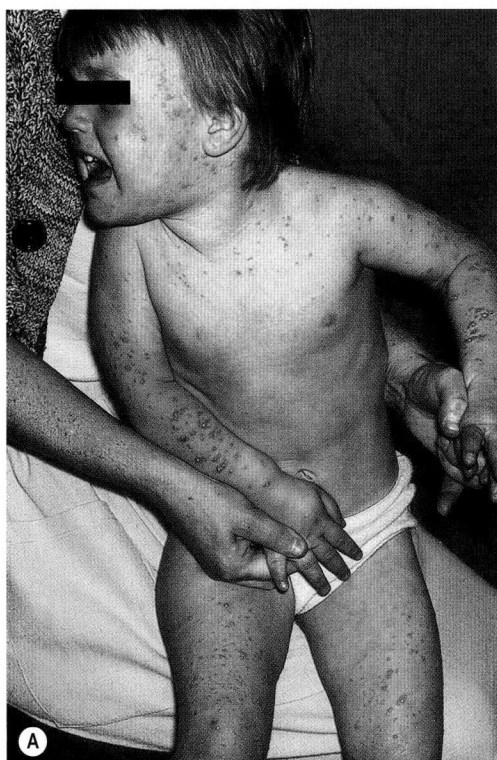

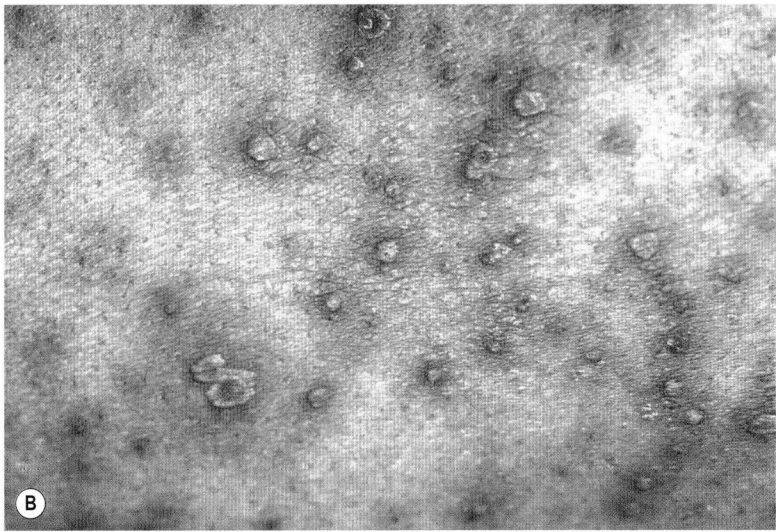

Fig. 18.50
Varicella (chickenpox): (**A**) note the widespread distribution of vesicles on the face, upper chest, arms, and legs; (**B**) close-up view. (**A**) By courtesy of R.A. Marsden, MD, St George's Hospital, London, UK; (**B**) by courtesy of the Institute of Dermatology, London, UK.

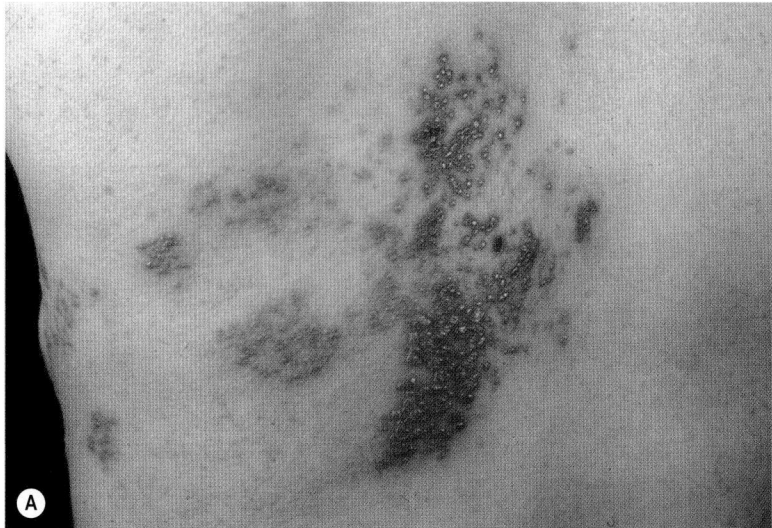

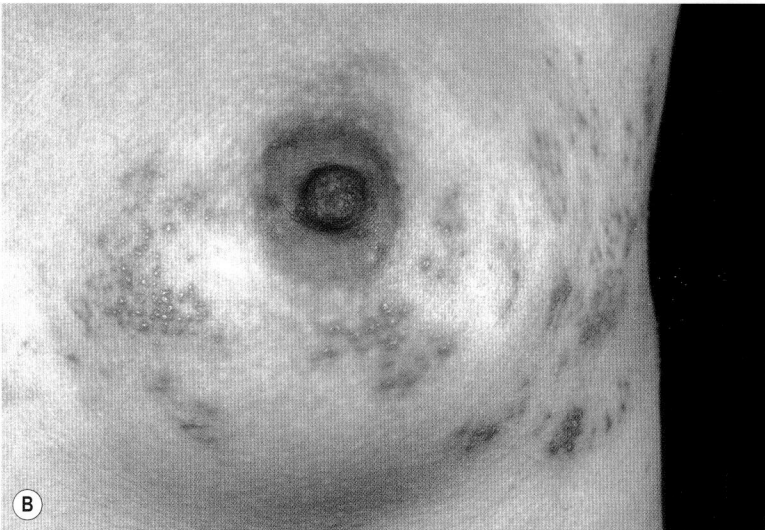

Fig. 18.51
(**A**, **B**) Herpes zoster (shingles): intact vesicles in a characteristic dermatomal distribution. From the collection of the late N.P. Smith, MD, the Institute of Dermatology, London, UK.

brain.[4] Cerebral disease most often presents as progressive leukoencephalitis. Cerebral vasculitis may occur as a result of direct invasion of cerebral arteries by VZV, leading to hemiparesis or hemiplegia.[22] A nonimmune individual may contract chickenpox from a person with herpes zoster. Herpes zoster occurs in as many as 40% to 50% of patients in the first year following bone marrow transplantation, but the lesions increasingly resemble varicella as the time after transplantation increases. This suggests that T-cells specific for VZV are less well represented as time goes by.

VZV infection in patients with AIDS may present with unusual manifestations, including verrucous skin lesions resembling viral warts and disseminated varicella in the absence of skin lesions.[23–26] Verrucous VZV infection, however, has also been reported in a renal transplant recipient.[27] Herpes zoster is a well-recognized cutaneous manifestation of IRIS occurring in HIV-infected patients (including children) receiving highly active ART.[28–30]

Pathogenesis and histologic features

Although inhalation of viral particles is the usual route of infection, direct cutaneous inoculation may occur. Initial contact is followed by viremia before the cutaneous lesions develop. During the viremic stage, VZV is transported to the skin by T-cells. Cell-free viral replication takes place in the skin and facilitates person-to-person spread. Even when the resolution of the lesions is clinically complete, the virus may remain latent in the ganglia of sensory nerves.[31] IgG, IgM, and IgA antibodies develop soon after the vesicles; some IgG antibody is detectable thereafter throughout life, but the other antibodies disappear. It has been noted that cell-mediated immunity is depressed during an episode of chickenpox and for at least the first few days of zoster.

VZV has the ability to interfere with the expression of major histocompatibility complex (MHC) class I and class II proteins required for CD4 and CD8 T-cell recognition, leading to delayed clearance of virus-infected cells.[32] VZV glycoprotein E (gE) is essential for viral replication and also plays a role in spread of the virus from cell to cell, secondary envelopment, and viral entry.[33,34] ORF 66 (ORF66) of VZV encodes a protein kinase which modulates apoptosis and interferon pathways, down-regulates MHC class I protein expression on cell surfaces, and facilitates tropism of VZV for T-cells.[35,36] VZV has evolved a diverse array of immunomodulatory mechanisms, including the ability to transiently evade immune recognition.[37] The virus also has an effect on cell cycle regulatory pathways.[38] These are just

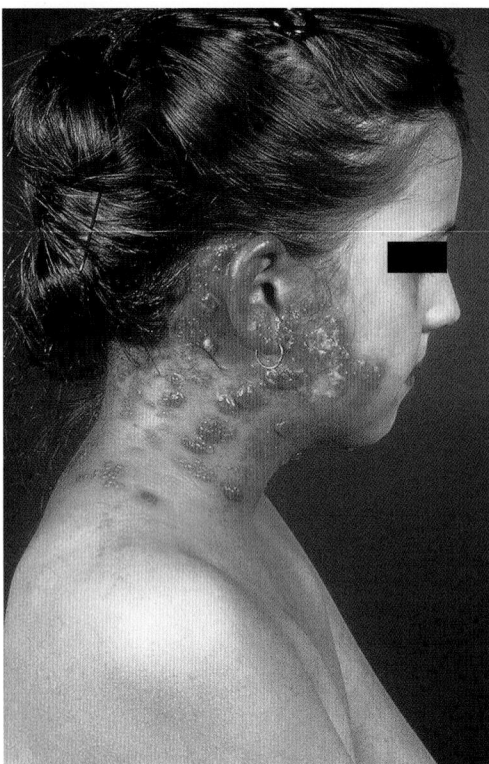

Fig. 18.52
Herpes zoster (shingles): there is intense erythema, intact vesicles, and crusted lesions. By courtesy of R.A. Marsden, MD, St George's Hospital, London, UK.

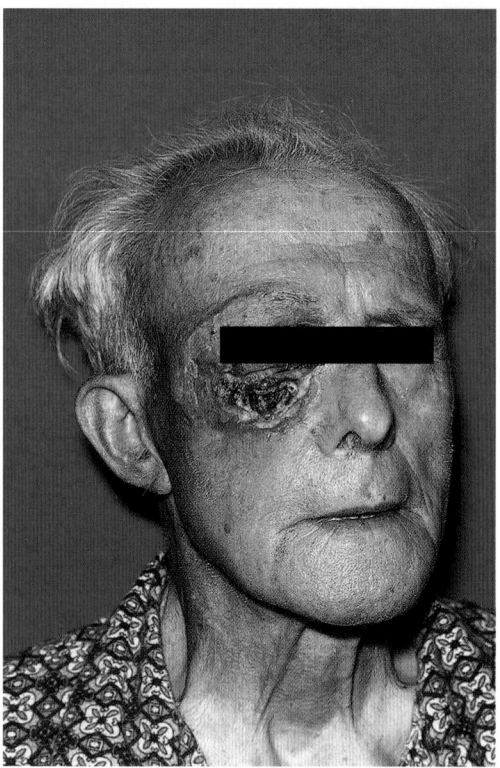

Fig. 18.54
Herpes zoster (shingles): ophthalmic involvement is particularly seen in the elderly. By courtesy of R.A. Marsden, MD, St George's Hospital, London, UK.

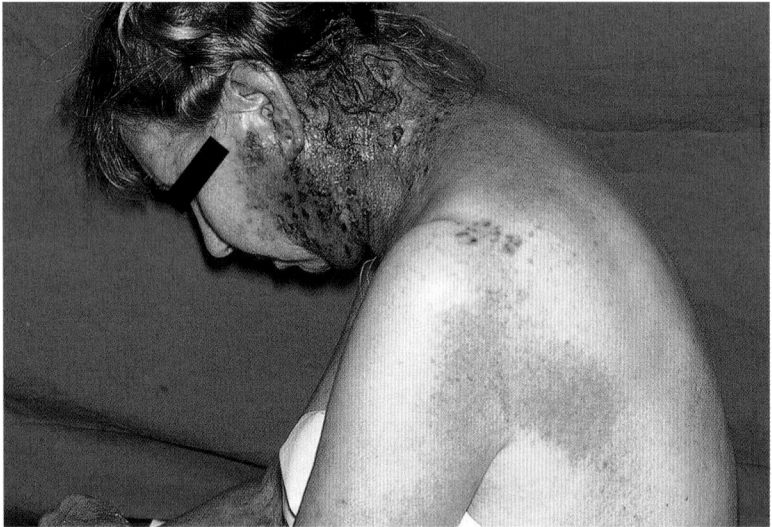

Fig. 18.53
Herpes zoster (shingles): older lesion in which the rash has a hemorrhagic component. By courtesy of R.A. Marsden, MD, St George's Hospital, London, UK.

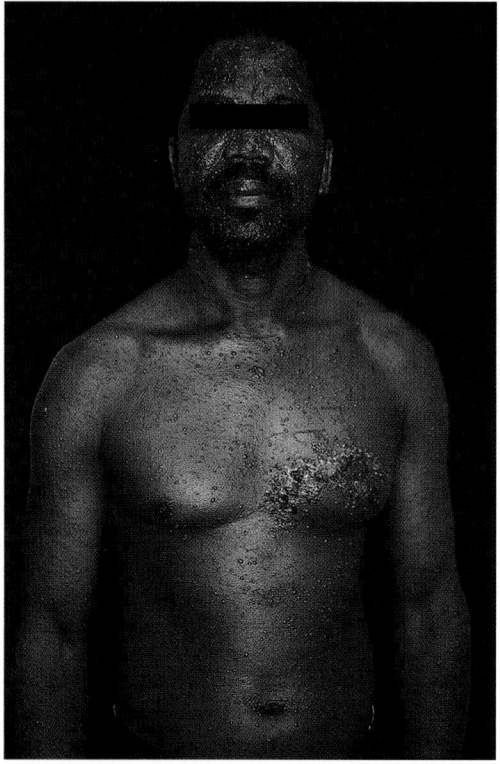

Fig. 18.55
Herpes zoster: disseminated lesions may be seen in immunosuppressed patients. By courtesy of N.C. Dlova, MD, Nelson R. Mandela School of Medicine, University of KwaZulu-Natal, South Africa.

some of many aspects of the complex pathogenesis and immunobiology of VZV infection.[3,32,37,39,40] A more detailed account is beyond the remit of this text, and the reader is thus referred to reference numbers 3, 32, 39, 37, and 40.

Histologically, the cutaneous lesions of VZV, whether in varicella or zoster form, are generally indistinguishable from those of herpes simplex, although it has been suggested that inflammation is more profound in the latter. Follicular epithelial involvement may also serve as a further point of distinction (see below).[41] The intraepidermal blisters associated with intracellular edema and multinucleate epithelial cells with inclusion bodies are characteristic.[42] The dermal infiltrate and fibrinopurulent exudate are seen regularly, but are not diagnostic. There is often more intraepidermal and dermal hemorrhage than in herpes simplex infection.

The wartlike cutaneous lesions encountered in patients with AIDS show hyperkeratosis, verruciform acanthosis, and virally induced cytopathic alterations, often with minimal or absent cytolysis of the infected epidermal keratinocytes, and little by way of a dermal inflammatory infiltrate.[23,25,26] Cytopathic changes may be very minimal, and a high index of suspicion and

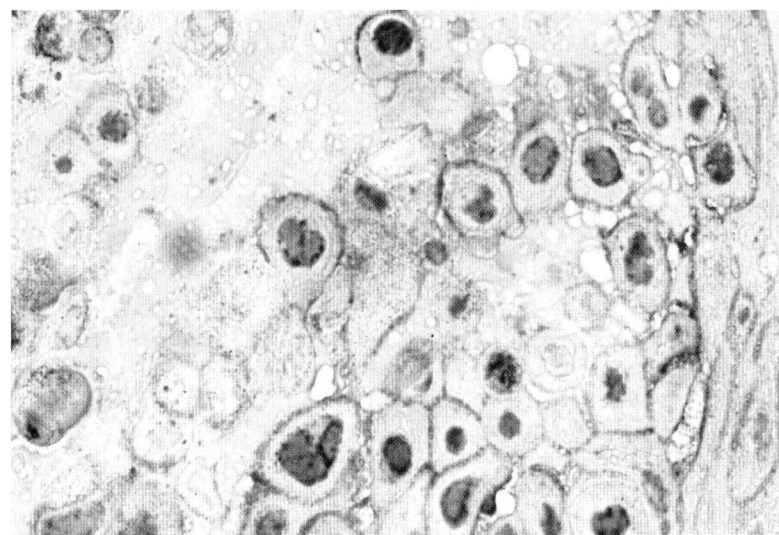

Fig. 18.56
Herpes zoster: positive immunohistochemistry.

the use of multiple sections with or without ancillary tests such as PCR are often necessary to establish a diagnosis. Immunosuppressed individuals with VZV infection may have a protracted clinical course during which biopsies reveal a lichenoid inflammatory reaction pattern rather than cytolysis of keratinocytes.[43]

Biopsies from early herpes zoster lesions may exhibit VZV-infected cells in the hair follicles, suggesting that VZV spreads from dorsal root ganglia or trigeminal ganglia to an area of skin innervated by myelinated nerves, the latter terminating at the level of the follicular isthmus.[41,44] Exclusive involvement of folliculosebaceous units in this manner may predate the evolution of more characteristic vesicular lesions, and serves as a point of distinction from recurrent herpes simplex. In the latter, there is axonal transport of the virus from sensory ganglia to the skin via terminal nonmyelinated nerve twigs.[41] Very rarely, VZV infection may manifest with dermal vasculitis in the absence of associated epidermal involvement.[45] Another rare occurrence is exclusive involvement of epithelium of the eccrine apparatus (herpetic syringitis), manifesting with isolated nodular skin lesions in the absence of epidermal viropathic changes.[46] A number of cutaneous reactions have been described at the sites of healed herpes zoster scars, a phenomenon referred to as Wolf isotopic response. These include pseudolymphomatous cutaneous lymphoid hyperplasia, granulomatous vasculitis, granulomatous folliculitis, granuloma annulare, lichen planus, reactive perforating collagenosis, lichen sclerosus, and cutaneous Rosai-Dorfman disease.[47,48] Active lesions may also harbor a pseudolymphomatous dermal lymphoid infiltrate.[42,49]

As with HSV, the presence of multinucleate cells is valuable in the Tzanck test. In shingles, the spinal ganglia may show necrosis with inflammation, and intranuclear inclusions are sometimes evident.[50] Otherwise, diagnosis is usually based on clinical criteria, but can be confirmed by electron microscopy, immunofluorescence of blister contents, growth in tissue culture, PCR, in situ hybridization, or immunohistochemistry (*Fig. 18.56*).[5,26,51,52] Serological tests are less useful than rapid antigen-detection methods and are only of value later, when a rising titer can be demonstrated.[5]

Cytomegalovirus infections

Clinical features

Antibody studies suggest that most people have been exposed to CMV.[1] Generally, an asymptomatic infection ensues. CMV infection, however, may result in clinical features under a variety of circumstances. These include neonatal lesions, an infectious mononucleosis-like disease in adults, or a manifestation of disseminated disease in immunocompromised patients.[2,3] An in-depth review of the literature revealed that severe visceral CMV infection in apparently immunocompetent individuals might not be as

uncommon as previously considered.[4] Clinical lesions in the skin, however, are distinctly uncommon.

CMV is the most frequently transmitted viral infection in utero, and is the most common cause of congenital infection worldwide.[5–7] The incidence of reported infection ranges from 0.2% to 2.2% of live births.[8,9] Less than 10% of affected infants and neonates will actually develop clinical lesions.[5,10] Clinical manifestations have been grouped with other neonatal infections under the rubric 'TORCH syndrome', which includes toxoplasmosis, other infections (e.g., syphilis), rubella, CMV, and herpes simplex.[11]

Affected newborn babies and neonates may develop a wide range of lesions including jaundice, hepatosplenomegaly, microcephaly, sensorineural deafness, chorioretinitis, pneumonia, direct hyperbilirubinemia, thrombocytopenia with petechiae, purpura, and 'blueberry muffin' lesions.[2] The last consist of blue-red or violaceous papules and nodules and represent foci of dermal erythropoiesis.[12] The mortality in this syndrome is of the order of 20% to 30%.[5] Other reported pediatric manifestations of CMV infections include scleredema, the Gianotti-Crosti syndrome, perineal ulceration, the juvenile variant of papular-purpuric gloves and socks syndrome, acute hemorrhagic edema of infancy, and the fetal inflammatory response syndrome (FIRS).[13–19]

Adults, particularly females, most often in the third decade, may develop a heterophil agglutinin-negative infectious mononucleosis-like syndrome in which a short-lived rubelliform eruption has been described.[2,20,21] Patients are also at risk of developing an ampicillin-related allergic dermatosis (cf., infectious mononucleosis).[2,21–23]

CMV infection may also be a feature of immunosuppression.[3,24–26] Generalized CMV infection is not an uncommon finding at autopsy in AIDS patients. CMV is frequently detected in association with toxoplasmosis and *Pneumocystis jiroveci* infection, and has also been described in patients with concomitant cutaneous herpes simplex, bacillary angiomatosis (BA), *Mycobacterium avium* complex, mucormycosis, Kaposi sarcoma, and even acanthamebiasis.[27–34] CMV infection is a potential manifestation of IRIS in HIV-infected patients receiving ART.[33] CMV infection is said to occur in 20% to 60% of organ transplant recipients, with cutaneous manifestations occurring in 10% to 20% of patients with systemic infection.[25,35] Chronic cutaneous CMV infection has been described in a patient with severe combined immunodeficiency syndrome.[36] Skin lesions in AIDS- and non-AIDS-associated immunocompromised patients do not appear to differ clinically or histologically.[26]

Reported cutaneous manifestations include ulcers on the genitalia, anus, perineum, buttocks, and thighs (sometimes in association with herpes simplex), purpuric eruptions, petechiae, erythema nodosum, cutaneous vasculitis, hyperpigmented nodules and plaques, lesions resembling prurigo nodularis, erythema multiforme (including the persistent form of the latter), nodular auricular lesions, epidermolysis, urticaria, pustules, vesiculobullous lesions, and a generalized, pruritic erythematous maculopapular eruption.[24–26,37–52] Cutaneous CMV infection has also been detected in a patient with febrile ulceronecrotic Mucha-Habermann disease.[53] There are isolated reports of CMV infection in association with eruptive pseudoangiomatosis (EPA) and reactive perforating collagenosis.[54,55] A possible link to scleroderma has also been suggested.[56–58] In one study, graft-versus-host disease (GVHD)-like histologic changes were observed in biopsies of clinically normal skin from allogeneic bone marrow transplant recipients who had peaks of CMV antigen in the blood within 100 days of transplantation.[59] There are rare reports of cutaneous CMV infection complicating pre-existing dermatoses, including herpes zoster scars, pustular psoriasis, and pemphigus.[60–63]

Pathogenesis and histologic features

In addition to maternally derived infections, there is also some evidence to suggest a venereal mode of spread.[64] In the immunocompromised patient, CMV infections represent an acquired phenomenon or reactivation of a latent focus.[47] In immunosuppressed transplant recipients, infection occurs predominantly after the first month post-transplantation and is the result of either primary infection, reinfection, or reactivation of latent disease.[49] A high antigen-specific T-cell response to CMV is responsible for chemokine-mediated endothelial cell damage.[65]

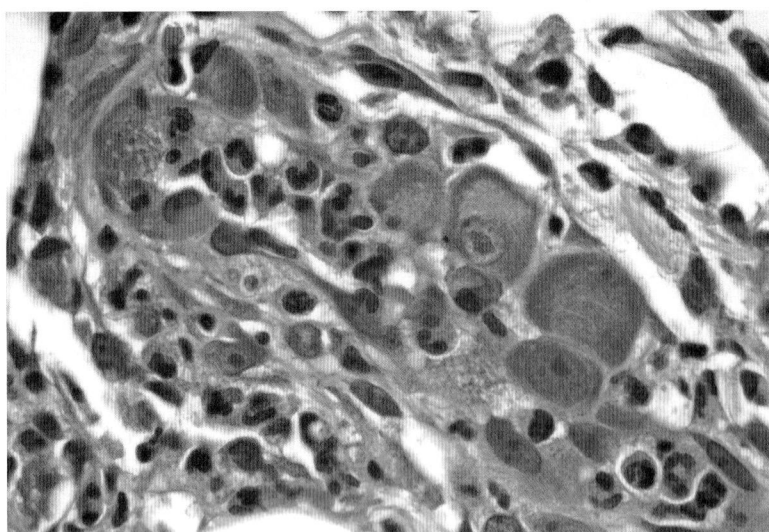

Fig. 18.57
Cytomegalovirus: high-power view showing the typical eosinophilic intranuclear inclusions.

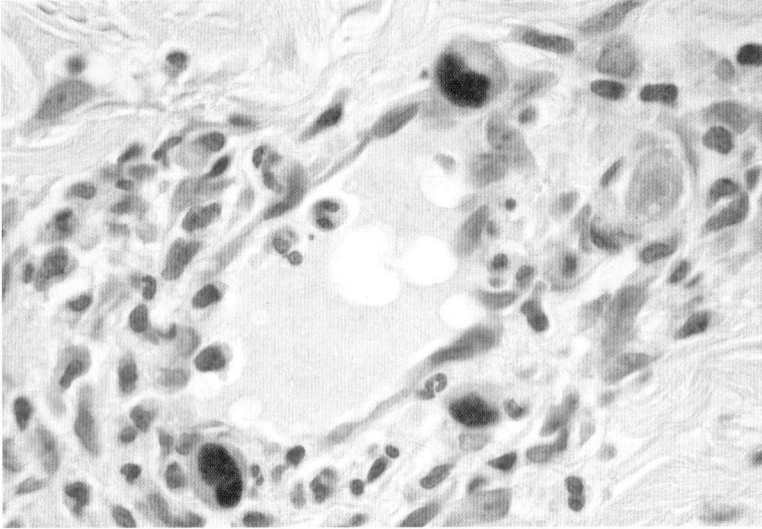

Fig. 18.58
Cytomegalovirus: positive immunohistochemistry.

The histologic hallmark is the presence of large, often purple-staining, intranuclear inclusions surrounded by a clear halo (*Fig. 18.57*). Smaller basophilic, periodic acid-Schiff (PAS)-positive intracytoplasmic inclusions may also be evident. These have been described within enlarged endothelial cells of dermal blood vessels, sometimes accompanied by the features of leukocytoclastic vasculitis.[22,26,41,42] Inclusions may sometimes be identified in dermal fibrocytes, macrophages, and eccrine ductal epithelial cells, the last rarely associated with syringosquamous metaplasia.[26,66,67] They have also been identified within the endothelial cells of blood vessels and histiocytes in the inflammatory bed deep to cutaneous ulcers (*Fig. 18.57*).[37] Cutaneous nerve involvement (CMV neuritis) has been reported in perineal ulcers.[68] In histologic specimens from immunocompromised hosts, care should be taken to rule out CMV infection in association with other infective disorders, such as HSV infection or BA.[34]

Vesiculobullous lesions are characterized by spongiosis and reticular degeneration, accompanied by epidermal multinucleate giant cells, which may contain viral inclusion bodies.[26] The diagnosis of CMV infection can be confirmed by immunohistochemistry, in situ hybridization, or PCR (*Fig. 18.58*).[69,70]

Exanthem subitum

Clinical features

Exanthem subitum (also known as roseola infantum or sixth disease) is generally a benign febrile disease of infancy and early childhood usually caused by infection with human herpesvirus 6 (HHV-6), and HHV-6B in particular.[1-4] Infection with HHV-7, a closely related β-herpesvirus, however, may also manifest as exanthem subitum.[4-7] Usual clinical features include high fever and a cutaneous eruption that resembles rubella or measles.[5,8] Encephalitis and febrile seizures are potential complications.[4,9] A case with vesicular lesions has been reported.[10] Erythema and crusting at a bacille Calmette-Guérin (BCG) inoculation site has been reported in a patient with exanthem subitum.[11] The diagnosis is confirmed by serology or the detection of the causative virus in body fluid or tissue samples, usually by real-time PCR.[3,4]

A similar exanthematous rash caused by HHV-6 infection has been reported in leukemic patients and hematopoietic stem cell transplant recipients; a possible link to GVHD has also been suggested.[3,12-14] HHV-7 is also recognized as an important pathogen in transplant recipients.[5,13] Other reported clinical associations and cutaneous manifestations of HHV-6 infection include papular-purpuric 'gloves and socks' syndrome, erythema elevatum diutinum, an infectious mononucleosis-like syndrome, Gianotti-Crosti syndrome, drug hypersensitivity syndrome, and more recently, pityriasis rosea.[15-23] HHV-6 DNA has also been detected in lesions of Langerhans cell histiocytosis.[24] HHV-7 has been implicated in pityriasis rosea and drug-induced hypersensitivity syndrome.[23,25]

Histologic features

The histopathological findings in exanthem subitum are rather non-specific and include papillary dermal edema and a superficial perivascular mononuclear inflammatory cell infiltrate. Rare cases with a vesicular presentation may show mononuclear inflammatory cell exocytosis into the epidermis, with microscopic intraepidermal spongiotic vesiculation. Intranuclear inclusions (as seen in HSV infection or VZV infection) are absent. The diagnosis can be confirmed by immunofluorescence microscopy, using an antibody to HHV-6.[10]

Measles

Clinical features

Measles is a highly contagious, predominantly pediatric viral infection caused by measles virus. The latter is an enveloped, negative-sense, single-stranded virus belonging to the *Morbillivirus* genus in the Paramyxoviridae family.[1] It is estimated that between 7 and 8 million people died annually from measles in the pre-vaccine era.[2] The widespread use of vaccines against measles for more than five decades, however, led to a marked reduction in the disease.[3] Recent years have nevertheless seen a resurgence of the infection, with a number of outbreaks recorded mainly in the Northern Hemisphere.[4-6] Currently, an estimated 120 000 to 134 000 deaths are thought to occur annually, with some 400 measles-associated deaths worldwide per day.[1,3,6] The United Kingdom saw some 477 cases of measles in the first 9 months of 2016, with 65% of the patients aged 15 years or older.[6] Factors contributing to the reemergence of the disease include parental vaccine hesitancy, international travel to areas where measles is endemic, an influx of unvaccinated refugees to certain European countries, and poor vaccine coverage, with transmission between unvaccinated or incompletely immunized individuals.[4-8] One of the main causes of parental vaccine hesitancy has been the unfounded suggestion of a link between autism and the administration of the MMR (measles, mumps, rubella) vaccine. Additional risk factors include immunosuppression (due to underlying HIV/AIDS, leukemia or malnutrition), and a loss of passive immunization in infants prior to an age for routine antimeasles vaccination.[8]

Patients usually develop symptoms 7–14 days after exposure to the virus, and present initially with fever, cough, coryza, and conjunctivitis, often accompanied by malaise and a loss of appetite.[6,8] An erythematous

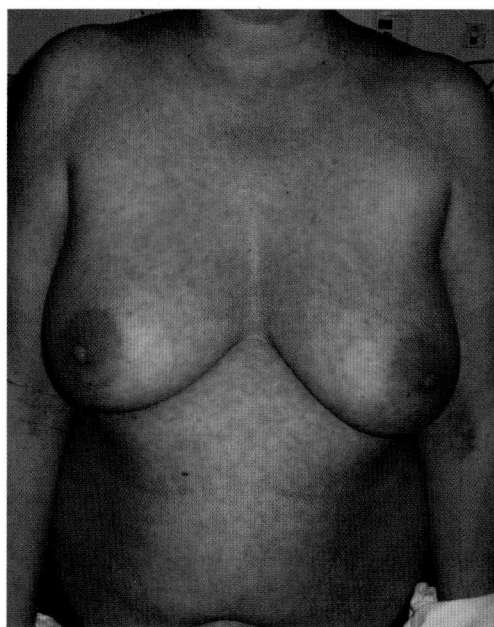

Fig. 18.59
Measles: erythematous maculopapular skin rash. The rash is usually characterized by cephalocaudal progression. By courtesy of Dr Joan Mir (Barcelona, Spain).

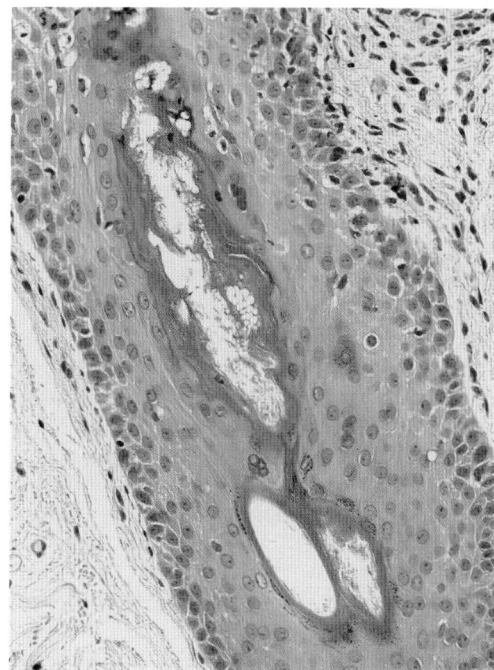

Fig. 18.60
Measles: multinucleate follicular keratinocytes (polykarions/grape cells) are present, and these serve as a clue to the diagnosis.

maculopapular skin rash in a characteristic cephalocaudal distribution develops some 4 days later (Fig. 18.59). Patients are infective from 4 days before until 4 days after the onset of the rash.[6] Whitish lesions referred to as Koplik spots appear on the buccal mucosa 2–3 days prior to the rash. The latter generally last for 3–5 days and are said to be pathognomonic of measles.[6,8] The non-specific nature of the initial symptoms and the reduced incidence of the infection since the introduction of routine immunization may result in the diagnosis being overlooked. Although a majority of patients recover from the infection, a mortality rate of up to 10% has been recorded. Potential complications which may arise in the first 4–6 weeks after acute infection include viral pneumonia, secondary bacterial pneumonia, laryngotracheobronchitis, otitis media, corneal ulceration, stomatitis, and encephalitis. Subacute sclerosing panencephalitis is a much feared delayed complication of measles.[3,6]

Pathogenesis and histologic features

Membrane fusion induced by morbillivirus glycoproteins constitutes a critical step for viral entry and replication in the host, and accounts for the predominantly lymphotropic virus's ability to breach host epithelial barriers. Resultant syncytia formation potentiates further cell-to-cell spread of the virus. The cellular tropism of the measles virus is determined by expression of the cellular receptors CD150 and poliovirus receptor-like 4 (PVRL4) on subsets of activated immune cells (dendritic cells, macrophages, B-cells, T-cells) and on epithelial cells, respectively.[1]

A characteristic finding in skin biopsies is the presence of multinucleate syncytial-type epithelial cells within the epidermis and particularly hair follicles (Fig. 18.60).[9–12] Apoptotic keratinocytes are not infrequently observed in the epidermis and they are quite prominent in pilosebaceous follicles, the latter being an important clue to the diagnosis (Fig. 18.61).[11,12] Associated parakeratosis and a mild superficial perivascular dermal mononuclear inflammatory cell infiltrate may also be seen.[9] Additional findings which have been described include intradermal syncytial giant cells, and intravascular fibrin thrombi in the presence of a mixed dermal inflammatory infiltrate harboring numerous eosinophilic leukocytes.[10]

Differential diagnosis

Since keratinocyte apoptosis and a superficial perivascular lymphocytic infiltrate may be observed in viral exanthems other than measles, a heightened index of suspicion is required. Careful scrutiny of additional serial histologic sections, however, should enable identification of the characteristic

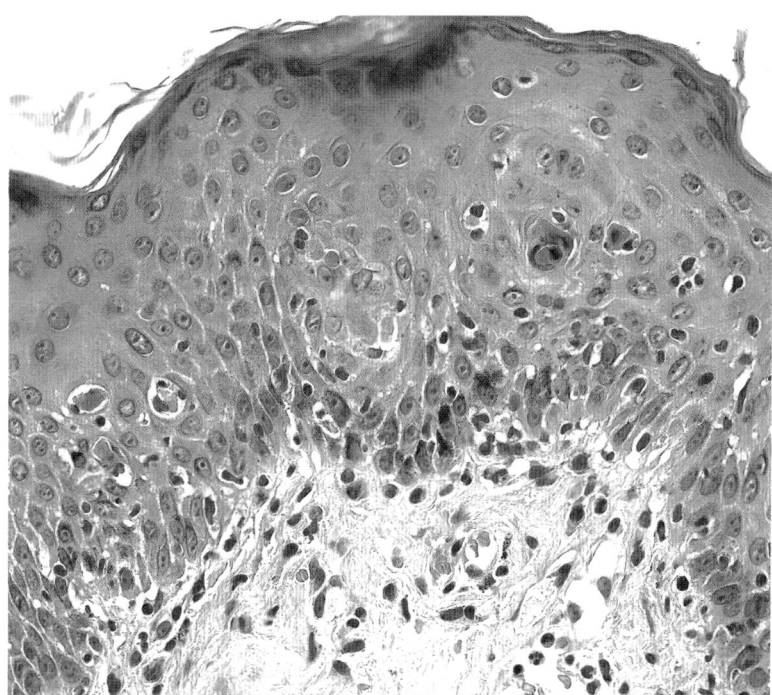

Fig. 18.61
Measles: numerous individual necrotic keratinocytes at the opening of the hair follicle into the epidermis.

multinucleate epithelial giant cells encountered in measles. Although infection with HSV or VSV is frequently associated with epidermal and follicular epithelial cell multinucleation, the clinical features (including vesiculation) and presence of Cowdry-type intranuclear viral inclusions in the aforementioned herpes virus infections should readily facilitate their distinction from measles. Uncommonly, multinucleate epidermal keratinocytes may also be encountered in noninfective dermatoses, including lichen simplex chronicus, prurigo nodularis, lichen planus, and dermatitis artefacta; this phenomenon has been ascribed to chronic rubbing.[13]

Eruptive pseudoangiomatosis

Clinical features

In 1969, Cherry et al. reported a series of four infants who developed an eruption of small hemangioma-like papules, which blanched on pressure. The lesions had an abrupt onset and apparently evolved in association with an acute echovirus infection, resolving spontaneously within a few days.[1] This uncommon condition was later referred to as EPA and was initially regarded as an exanthem unique to infants and children.[2,3] The more recent literature, however, reveals that more than half of all recorded cases have occurred in adults, often as small outbreaks, and especially in the Mediterranean region during the summer months.[4–7] The condition is similar to or synonymous with the entity referred to in Japan as erythema punctatum Higuchi, which has been linked to mosquito bites.[6,8] In children, the eruption is frequently preceded by an upper respiratory tract infection or, less commonly, gastroenteritis.[3,5] Prodromal constitutional symptoms such as malaise, fever, headache, vomiting, or diarrhea are encountered more frequently in pediatric patients than in adults.[5] Rare cases have occurred in iatrogenically immunosuppressed individuals.[4,9,10] Isolated cases have been linked to the ingestion of a herbal medicine or food allergen.[11]

The acute eruption comprises numerous small, asymptomatic, bright red angiomatoid papules. The individual lesions, which measure between 2 and 5 mm in diameter, are surrounded by a distinctive pale halo and characteristically blanch on pressure.[12,13] The face, trunk, and limbs are sites of predilection. Spontaneous resolution usually takes place within 3 to 10 days.[3] Relapse, however, has been reported in around 70% of cases in some series.[6] Exceptionally, EPA may persist for months.[3]

Pathogenesis and histologic features

Although there is often strong circumstantial evidence to suggest that the eruption is precipitated by a viral infection, further investigation seldom leads to the identification of a specific pathogen.[3,6] Isolated cases, however, have been linked to CMV infection and infection with Epstein-Barr virus.[14,15] Several cases have occurred following arthropod bites, especially those of mosquitos.[6,7,16] Lesions of EPA have also been induced experimentally by mosquito bites.[17] Although a vector-borne infectious agent seems probable in a subset of patients, the authors of a recent meta-analysis concluded that there was insufficient epidemiological evidence to either substantiate or refute an infectious etiology.[4,7] Since there is no true vascular proliferation, the authors who initially described the condition proposed that the cutaneous lesions were the result of either a direct viral effect on vascular endothelial cells or binding of antigen-antibody complexes to the endothelium.[1] The latter is unlikely as there is no evidence of vasculitis. The surrounding white ring observed clinically around each lesion has been ascribed to vasoconstriction peripheral to the central zone of vasodilatation.[12] It seems likely that EPA represents an unusual reaction pattern in response to a number of different viruses.[2]

The histopathological picture predominantly shows dilated blood vessels in the papillary dermis and upper reticular dermis. These vessels are lined by plump endothelial cells, which usually assume a hobnail-like appearance (Fig. 18.62).[2,13,18,19] A sparse perivascular lymphoid infiltrate is sometimes evident.[9,12,15,19] Importantly, there is no increase in dermal vascular density.[12,13] Although some authors have noted the presence of intravascular neutrophils, true vasculitis is conspicuously absent.[17]

Differential diagnosis

Although eruptive pyogenic granulomas, BA, bartonellosis, and multiple glomeruloid hemangiomas may enter the clinical differential diagnosis, each of the aforementioned conditions has distinctive histology and is associated with a true angiomatous dermal vascular proliferation. Furthermore, the individual lesions are not surrounded by a peripheral white halo.

Hobnail hemangioma (targetoid hemosiderotic hemangioma) is characterized clinically by a perilesional halo and histologically by hobnail-like vascular endothelial cells. Unlike EPA, however, lesions are usually single; the surrounding halo is pigmented rather than pale, and there is a true dermal vascular proliferation. Telangiectases lack protrusion of plump

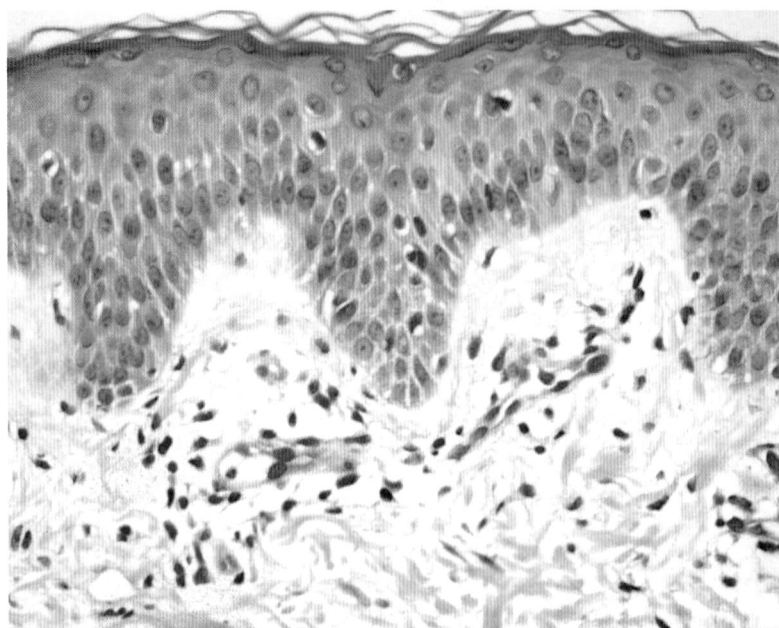

Fig. 18.62
Eruptive pseudoangiomatosis: the histologic findings are subtle, with superficial dermal vascular ectasia and relative prominence of the endothelial cells.

endothelial cells into the dilated vessel lumina. Spider angiomas comprise centrally located dilated dermal arterioles with thin branches; they, too, are devoid of the prominent endothelium observed in EPA.[1]

Diseases caused by orthopox viruses

Clinical features

The orthopox viruses are DNA in type and cause variola, vaccinia, cowpox, and monkeypox.

Variola

Variola, or smallpox, has not been diagnosed endemically since 1977 and until relatively recently appeared to be of historical interest only.[1–5] For more than a decade, however, there has been renewed interest in smallpox as a potential agent in bioterrorism.[6–9] The highly virulent pathogen is human-specific.[10] It was endemic in parts of Africa, South America, and Asia, with only occasional cases seen in Europe and North America. Transmission of the virus, which is capable of retaining viability in dried exudate, is by inhalation. The disease typically has an incubation period of 12 days, followed by a prodromal phase of high fever, headache, and vomiting, and 3–4 days later by a transient erythematous and petechial rash. This is in turn followed by the characteristic eruptive lesions (Fig. 18.63). These lesions are most common on the face and limbs. They begin as papules, which become vesicular and then pustular and crusted. Healing is usually associated with a pitted scar. Mortality varied from 2% to 50%, depending on the severity of the infection. Although death was previously attributed to secondary bacterial sepsis, it has since come to light that it was probably the direct result of the cytopathic effects of the smallpox virus itself.[11] It has been suggested that the scarring observed in survivors of the disease might have been the result of destruction of sebaceous glands, although other mechanisms have also been proposed.[12]

Vaccinia

Vaccinia virus is closely related antigenically to variola virus, but is probably derived from cowpox virus. It was used for immunization against variola and no doubt was effective because of its similar antigenicity. This skin inoculation results in a single vesicle, which becomes pustular and crusts, like variola (Fig. 18.64). It also heals similarly, leaving a scar. Since it was accepted that variola had been eradicated in the wild, for many years vaccination was no longer thought necessary except in laboratory workers at

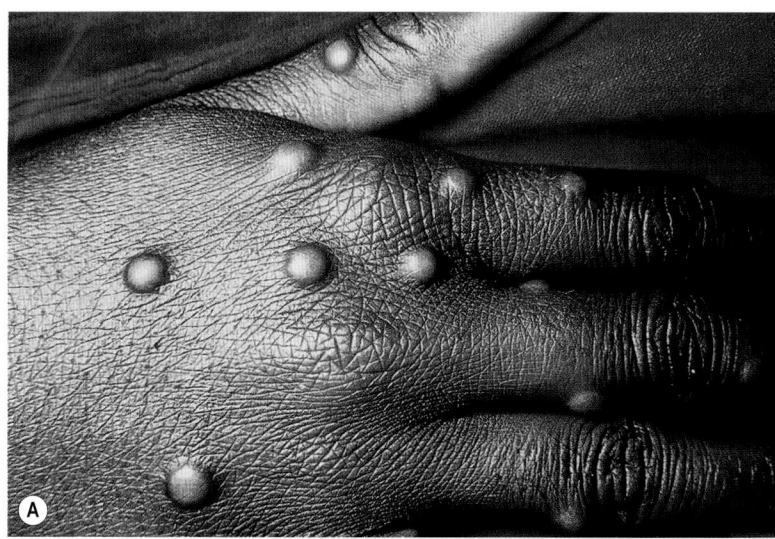

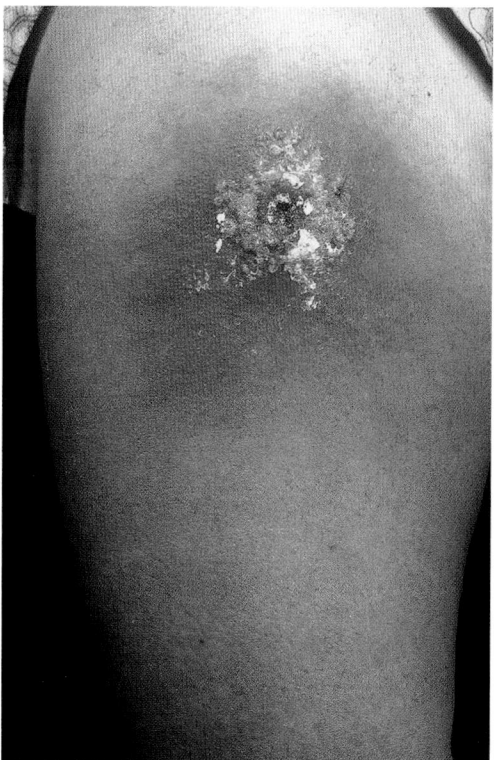

Fig. 18.64
Vaccinia: due to the eradication of smallpox, routine vaccination is no longer performed. Note the eschar, edema, and intense erythema. By courtesy of the Institute of Dermatology, London, UK.

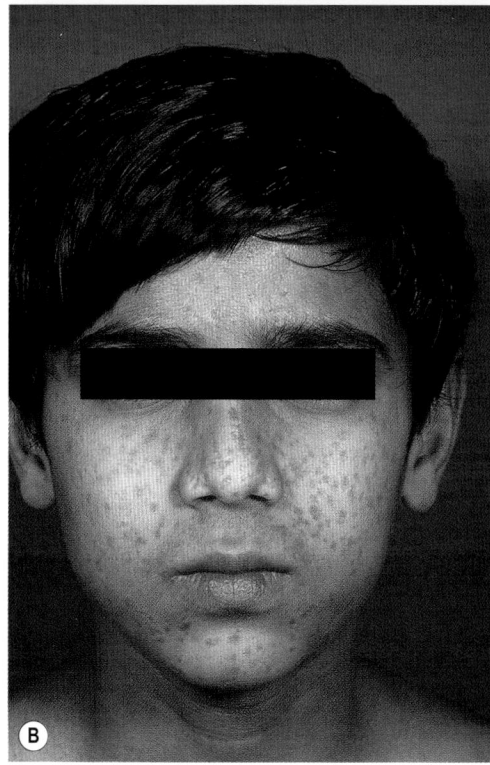

Fig. 18.63
Variola (smallpox): (**A**) in contrast to those of chickenpox, the lesions are larger and less superficial; (**B**) note the widespread hyperpigmented scars in healed lesions. (**A**) By courtesy of H.P. Lambert, MD, St George's Hospital, London, UK; (**B**) By courtesy of R.A. Marsden, St George's Hospital, London, UK.

special risk. Public fear of smallpox as a potential biological weapon or bioterrorism agent in the United States, however, led to the reintroduction of a smallpox vaccination campaign in that country.[8] The vaccination procedure is not without risk. Generalized vaccinia was occasionally seen and the vaccine was responsible for some cases of Kaposi varicelliform eruption (eczema vaccinatum). Vaccinia necrosum, encephalitis, and myocarditis were also rare complications.[13–15] Occasional cases of generalized vaccinia following smallpox vaccination have been recorded.[15,16]

Cowpox

Despite the name, the reservoir for cowpox virus is not cattle, but wild animals such as hedgehogs and badgers. Cattle and man are both infected accidentally, although man may acquire the disease from cows. Cats, and more recently rats, have been identified as additional sources of infection.[17–24] It is endemic to parts of Eurasia.[25,26] The occurrence of

cowpox among young people in Europe has been attributed to the cessation of smallpox vaccination. Although this rare zoonotic disease generally results in a self-limiting infection, more severe illness may occur in immunocompromised individuals and those with eczema.[26] The incubation period after inoculation is usually 5–7 days; a papule then develops, which rapidly becomes pustular. The pustule is surrounded by a zone of erythema and edema. Eschars or necrotic ulcers may be seen.[21,27,28] The lesions are often multiple and can occur on the hands, arms, or face (*Figs 18.65* and *18.66*).[29] A severe generalized or varicelliform eruption in association with atopy has been reported.[30,31] Sporotrichoid spread has been documented.[32] Lymphangitis, lymphadenitis, and fever are almost invariably present. Healing and recovery occur in 3–4 weeks. A fatal case of a cowpox-like illness has been recorded.[33] One reported case developed facial cellulitis and necrotizing lymphadenitis with abscess formation after inoculation of the virus in the nasal respiratory epithelium.[34]

Monkeypox

Monkeypox is an uncommon zoonosis attributable to monkeypox virus, a member of the orthopox virus group.[35–38] The first recorded cases occurred in the Democratic Republic of Congo (DRC; formerly Zaire) in 1970.[35,39,40] Although sporadic cases are encountered in remote villages in the tropical rain forests of West and Central Africa, an outbreak of the disease occurred in the state of Wisconsin in the United States in 2003, spreading to neighboring states.[35,36,39,41–47] This outbreak was traced to a shipment of exotic animals from West Africa.[37,45,46] Patients appeared to have come into direct contact with ill prairie dogs that were being kept or sold as pets. It was established that these animals had been exposed to infected rodents imported from Ghana.[37,46] Person-to-person spread may also occur.[39] Prior smallpox vaccination may confer some protection against monkeypox infection.[35,44,48] The rise in the number of cases of human monkeypox in the DRC in recent years may in part be due to the cessation of routine smallpox vaccination.[41,49] The condition presents with fever, rigors, and a skin rash, sometimes accompanied by lymphadenopathy.[36,43] The cutaneous lesions progress from papules to vesicopustules to resolving eschars.[36] Encephalitis

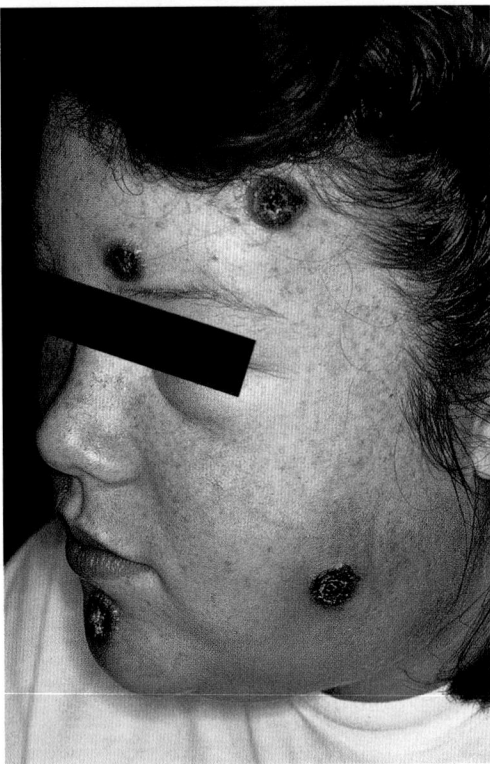

Fig. 18.65
Cowpox: characteristic umbilicated, ulcerated nodules. Lesions are often multiple. By courtesy of M.S. Lewis Jones, MD, Wrexham Maelor Hospital, Wrexham, UK.

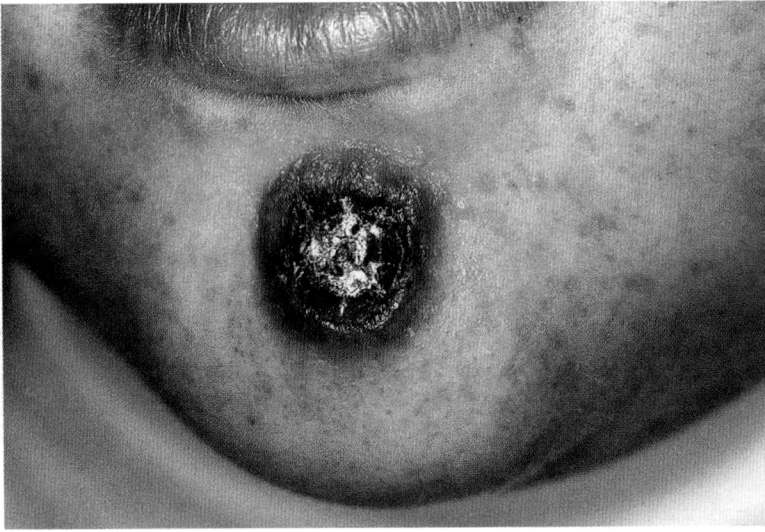

Fig. 18.66
Cowpox: note the edema and surrounding erythema. By courtesy of M.S. Lewis Jones, MD, Wrexham Maelor Hospital, Wrexham, UK.

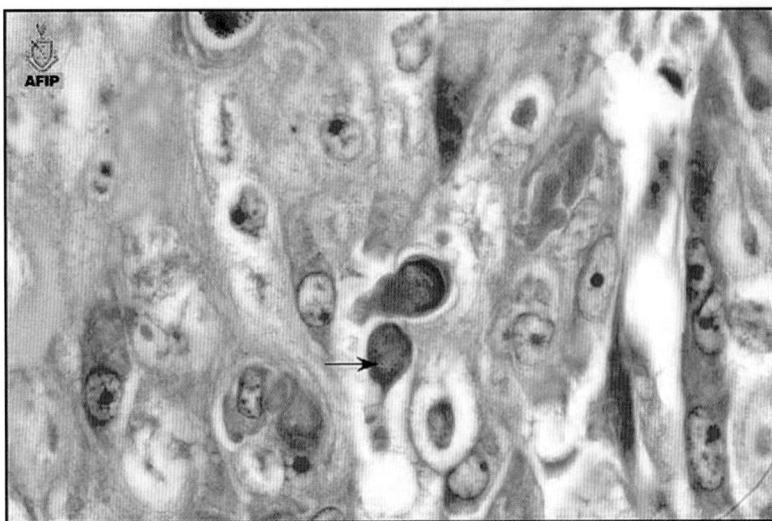

Fig. 18.67
Variola (smallpox): high-power view showing Guarneri bodies (*arrowed*). By courtesy of D. Wear, MD, the Armed Forces Institute of Pathology, Washington, DC, USA.

may also occur, and fatalities have been recorded.[35,44,50] Monkeypox may be confused clinically with chickenpox.[43]

Pathogenesis and histologic features

Orthopox viruses are large and have a discrete DNA compartment (nucleoid) and a complex capsid and lipoprotein coat containing characteristic tubular structures. They are brick-shaped and their outer tubular structures are irregularly arranged. These viruses are all transmitted by inoculation except variola, which usually gains entry by inhalation. The virus is able to resist dehydration outside the host and therefore inhalation or inoculation of dust or inoculation from shared facilities is quite possible, as well as direct inoculation from an active lesion.

Evidence has shown that these viruses secrete interleukin (IL)-18 binding proteins, resulting in viral dissemination or persistent infection.[51] Variola virus encodes CrmB, a TNF receptor homologue, which serves as a specific binding protein for a number of chemokines that mediate recruitment of inflammatory cells to the skin and mucosae, sites of viral entry, and viral replication. Binding of chemokines is potentiated via the C-terminal domain of CrmB, referred to as smallpox virus-encoded chemokine receptor (SECRET).[52] In primate animal models, multiorgan failure ensues in the presence of a high viral burden in the affected tissues. A hemorrhagic diathesis and depletion of T-cell dependent zones in lymphoid tissues may also be encountered. A cytokine storm arises due to elaboration of cytokines such as IL-6 and IFN-γ.[53] The vaccinia virus is able to evade the host immune response by impairing dendritic cell maturation, with subsequent inhibition of T-cell activation.[54] The large vaccinia viral genome also encodes proteins, which when secreted from the infected host cell, are capable of binding and neutralizing interferons, cytokines, chemokines, and complement. Others function within the host cell, leading to inhibition of cellular signaling pathways and apoptosis.[55] Cowpox virus encodes an array of immunomodulatory proteins capable of modulating the host immune response.[25] Among these are CPXV012 and CPXV203, which have been shown to disrupt antigen presentation.[56] Monkeypox virus infection is also associated with the production of immunomodulatory proteins.[47]

After inoculation, the viruses proliferate within keratinocytes and basal cells. This leads to severe intracellular edema with resultant ballooning degeneration and consequent reticular degeneration due to cell rupture, giving rise to multilocular vesicles and subsequent infiltration by polymorphs. In variola, vaccinia, and monkeypox, there is often extensive epidermal necrosis. Variable degrees of hyperkeratosis and acanthosis are present. Cytoplasmic eosinophilic inclusion bodies may be seen in the keratinocytes of all four diseases. The small inclusions of variola are called Guarnieri bodies. They are surrounded by a clear halo and are located close to the nucleus (*Fig. 18.67*). Similar bodies are seen in vaccinia and monkeypox. Those of cowpox, however, are slightly larger, but are still predominantly seen in the cytoplasm.[57] A dermal chronic inflammatory cell infiltrate consisting of lymphocytes is usually present. CD30-positive cells may be very prominent, and confusion with a CD30-positive lymphoproliferative disorder is possible if close attention is not paid to the epidermal changes and the presence of inclusions.

Diagnosis is based upon clinical information, but confirmation can be obtained by electron microscopy, isolation of the viruses in tissue culture, or, more recently, with the aid of PCR or in situ hybridization studies.[28,36,44,58–60] Variola virus is detectable in formalin-fixed, paraffin-embedded tissue after decades of prolonged archival storage.[61]

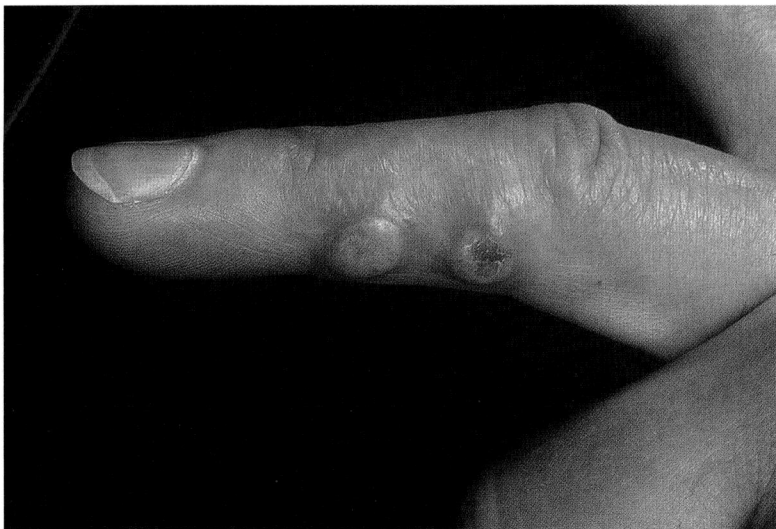

Fig. 18.68
Milker nodule: the blister roof has an opaque appearance and there is surrounding erythema. By courtesy of the Institute of Dermatology, London, UK.

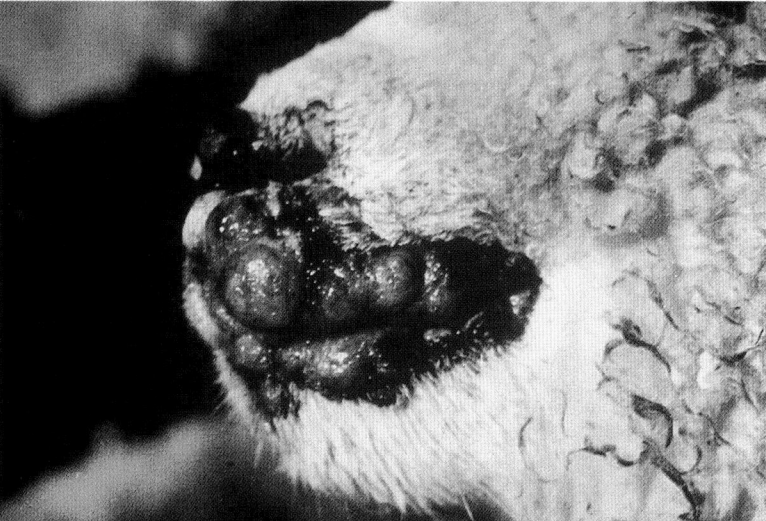

Fig. 18.69
Orf: the scabby mouth. By courtesy of B.J. Leppard, MD, Royal South Hants Hospital, Southampton, UK.

Diseases caused by parapox viruses

Milker nodule

Clinical features

Milker nodule (or paravaccinia) is caused by a parapox virus, distinct from that which causes cowpox.[1,2] It occurs as a localized lesion on the udders of cows and causes little systemic disturbance. It may be recurrent in the same herd. It is usually acquired by man by inoculation, but since the virus is viable in a dried state, indirect fomite infection is possible. Small outbreaks involving several patients have been recorded.[2] The incubation period is around 5 days; some two to five red papules then develop, which gradually become bluish tender nodules.[2] The overlying epidermis is at first tense and shiny, but becomes opaque and gray (Fig. 18.68). The center of the lesion is crusted and slightly depressed. The surrounding skin often shows lymphangitis, but despite this the lesion has the appearance of a tumor and is well circumscribed. There are few systemic symptoms, but there may be an associated short-lived papulovesicular eruption on the upper limbs and occasionally on the legs. The main nodular lesions resolve, without scarring, in 4–6 weeks.

Histologic features

Milker nodule virus measures 160–260 nm and is ellipsoid in shape.[2] It is characterized by spirally arranged tubules. The histologic features are indistinguishable from those seen in orf infection (see below).[3,4] A CD30-positive atypical dermal lymphoid infiltrate may sometimes be encountered, and confusion with a CD30-positive lymphoproliferative disease is possible.[5] In the latter, the CD30-positive cells are usually in clumps while in Milker nodule the CD30-positive cells are scattered between other inflammatory cells. This is, however, not entirely consistent, and in some cases clusters of CD30-positive cells may be seen.

Ecthyma contagiosum

Clinical features

Ecthyma contagiosum (orf, contagious pustular dermatosis) is caused by an epitheliotropic DNA parapoxvirus morphologically identical to that causing milker nodule. The infection is endemic in sheep in which it causes crusted pustules of the lips and perioral area (Fig. 18.69).[1-5] This underlies the accurate descriptive term of 'scabby mouth' used by Australian farmers. It is transmitted by inoculation from sheep to sheep, although it is said that the virus can persist in pastures. It is particularly likely to arise when the

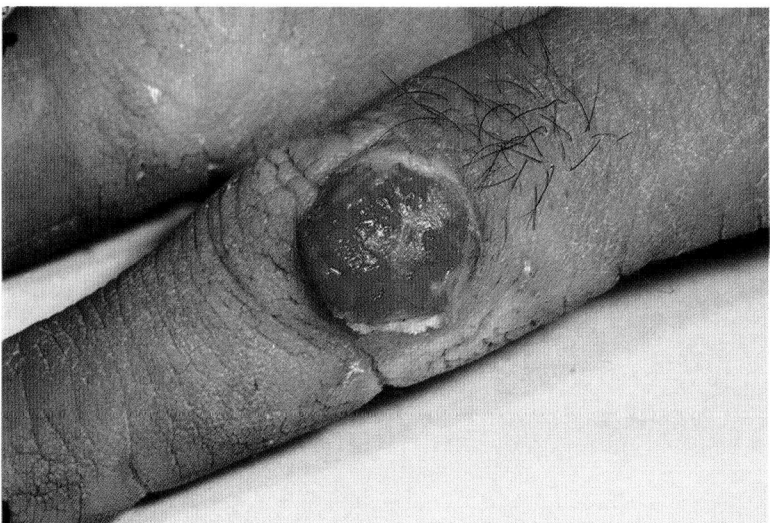

Fig. 18.70
Orf: in this example there is a markedly hemorrhagic component. By courtesy of M.M. Black, MD, Institute of Dermatology, London, UK.

pasture is dry and results in minor abrasions of the labial mucosa of the sheep. Transmission to man, most often males and usually sheep-handlers, is usually by direct inoculation from infected lesions, but it may also result from contact with contaminated objects such as fences and shears.[5] Orf may also be seen in goats.[3-5,7] In one English study, 23% of individuals employed or living on a sheep farm reported having had the condition.[8] Nonoccupational acquisition of the infection has been described following a sacrificial feast.[9]

After an incubation period of 5–6 days, the lesion (usually a solitary, small, firm, red-blue papule) develops. It is most common on the hand or forearm (Figs 18.70 and 18.71).[10] Less commonly, lesions may occur on the facial and perianal regions.[11-13] The papule becomes a flat-topped hemorrhagic blister or pustule, later crusting over its depressed center. By this stage, it may be 2–5 cm in diameter. Clinically, it may be mistaken for a lobular capillary hemangioma (pyogenic granuloma) or keratoacanthoma.[7] The lesions are surrounded by a zone of erythema, which may be associated with itching and tenderness. The main lesion usually resolves without scarring in 3 weeks, although on rare occasions digital deformity may occur.[14] Lymphangitis, lymphadenitis, and mild fever occasionally develop.[1] In addition, some patients develop a transient maculopapular eruption on the

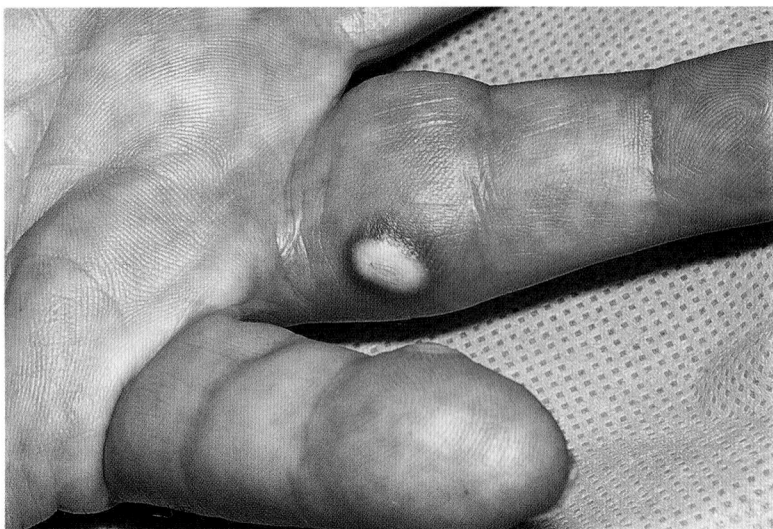

Fig. 18.71
Orf: older lesion with a typical depressed center. By courtesy of A. Qureshi, MD, Harvard Medical School, Boston, USA.

trunk or erythema multiforme-like lesions on the limbs.[7,10,14,15] Other potential complications include erysipelas, *Pseudomonas aeruginosa* infection, a papulovesicular eruption, and a bullous pemphigoid (BP)-like bullous eruption.[14,16] Ocular involvement may be a rare manifestation.[17] Giant lesions are sometimes encountered.[13,14,18,19] Giant orf lesions were reported in an organ transplant recipient.[18] Lesions occurring in immunosuppressed organ transplant recipients also tend to be more extensive, are less likely to involute spontaneously, and may be resistant to treatment.[20]

Histologic features

The histologic features are quite characteristic. The overall appearance of the lesion is that of a symmetrical nodule. There is a parakeratotic crust and acanthosis with thin epidermal strands extending quite deeply into the adjacent dermis.[21] Viral cytopathic changes including cytoplasmic and nuclear vacuolation are usually conspicuous.[22] Reticular degeneration with intraepidermal vesiculation is often evident (*Fig. 18.72*).

If the biopsy is taken from an early lesion, typical 3–5 μm intracytoplasmic eosinophilic inclusions may be seen (*Fig. 18.73*).[22] Sometimes intranuclear inclusions may also be evident.[6] They can be rendered more conspicuous with Lendrum phloxine tartazine (*Fig. 18.74*). Similar inclusions may also be seen in the cytoplasm of the endothelial cells lining blood vessels, among the underlying heavy chronic inflammatory cell infiltrate. The latter comprises lymphocytes and histiocytes although neutrophils and occasional eosinophils may be evident. The dermis is often very edematous, and characteristic of orf (and milker nodule) is the presence of massive capillary proliferation and dilatation.[11,22] This is attributable to the production of virus-encoded homologues of ovine vascular endothelial growth factor (VEGF).[3,23] In addition, orf virus encodes a homologue of IL-10, which appears to impair dendritic cell function and monocyte proliferation.[24,25] A prominent, CD30-positive reactive dermal lymphoid infiltrate may occur.[26]

The immunobullous (BP-like) lesions are subepidermal in location and contain a mixed inflammatory cell infiltrate, which includes polymorphonuclear leukocytes and eosinophils. A study of two cases showed that orf virus DNA was absent from the blistering lesions, while direct immunofluorescence microscopy revealed linear deposition of IgG and complement C3 along the dermal–epidermal junction in perilesional skin. Although the precise autoantigen has yet to be identified, the condition appears to be distinct from true BP and other immunobullous conditions such as epidermolysis bullosa acquisita.[16]

The diagnosis of orf may be confirmed immunocytochemically or by PCR, including real-time PCR.[27–31] The Tzanck test has also been used as a diagnostic aid.[10] Ultrastructural studies reveal that the orf virus is best visualized in negatively stained preparations (*Fig. 18.75*).[7]

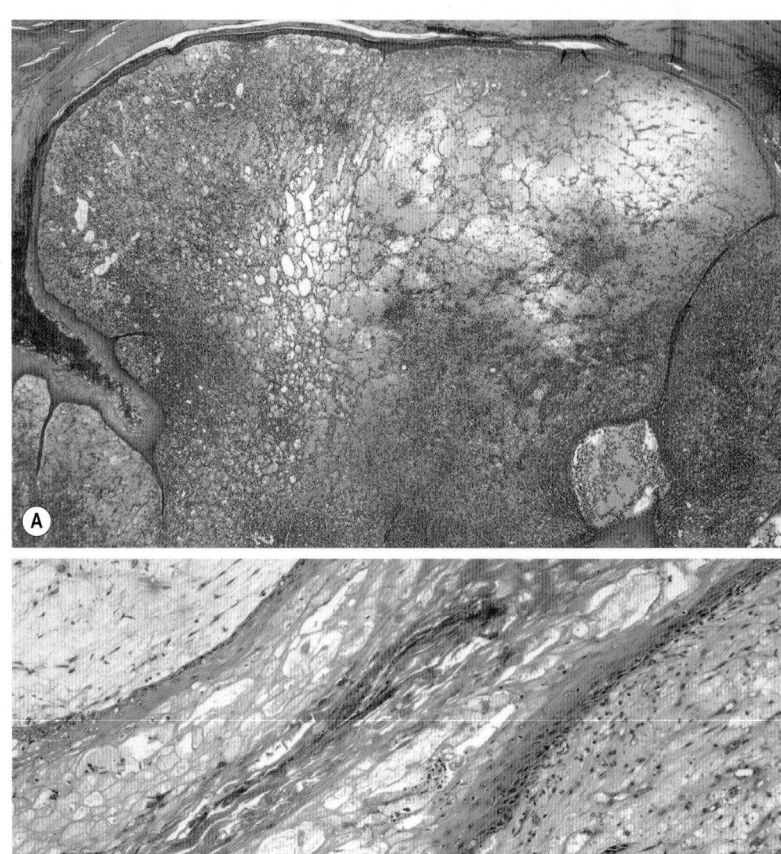

Fig. 18.72
Orf: (**A**) the lesion is pedunculated and there is massive superficial dermal edema; (**B**) the keratinocytes show ballooning degeneration.

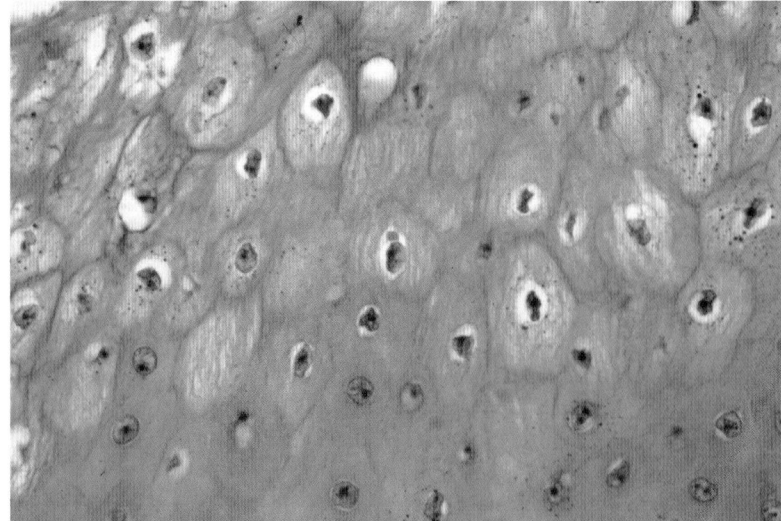

Fig. 18.73
Orf: in the center of the field is an eosinophilic intracytoplasmic inclusion.

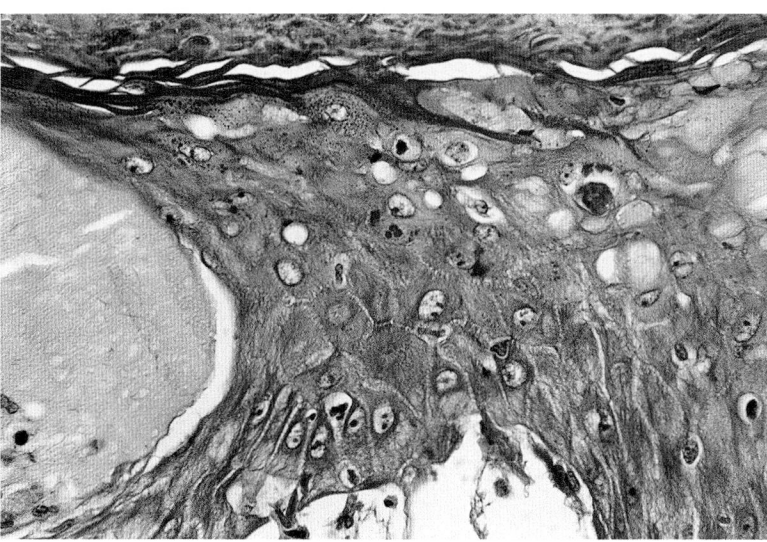

Fig. 18.74
Orf: the inclusions may be highlighted by Lendrum phloxine tartrazine.

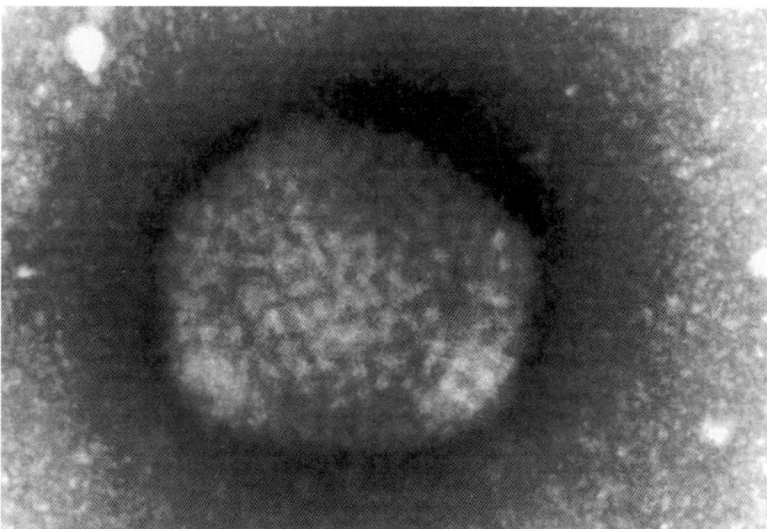

Fig. 18.76
Molluscum contagiosum: electron micrographic examination shows that the molluscum virus body is composed of virions, which are indistinguishable from those in the other poxviruses. By courtesy of I. Chrystie, FIMLS, St Thomas' Hospital, London, UK.

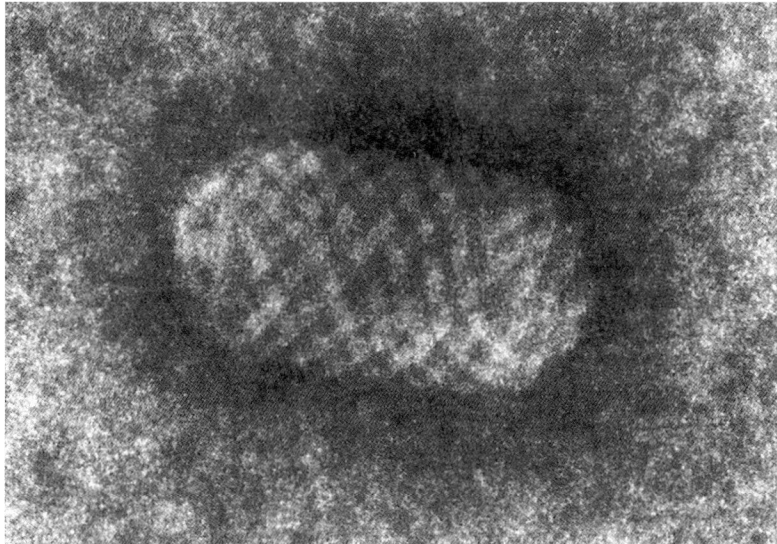

Fig. 18.75
Orf: on electron micrographic examination the parapoxvirus has a cylindrical appearance and a typical criss-crossed internal structure. By courtesy of I. Chrystie, FIMLS, St Thomas' Hospital, London, UK.

Infections caused by other parapox viruses

Clinical features

Parapoxvirus infections are known to occur in animal species other than common domestic ruminants, including wild animals such as white-tailed deer, red deer, reindeer, musk ox, cervids, and even seals.[1-4] There have been sporadic reports of infections among humans following direct or indirect exposure to some of the aforementioned animals, e.g., via an accidental cut to the finger while dressing the carcass of a hunted animal. Usual presentation is with a nonhealing violaceous nodule on the injured digit.[1]

Histologic features

There is histopathological overlap with milker nodule and sheep- or goat-derived orf, including the presence of intraepidermal eoninophilic intracytoplasmic inclusions and a prominent superficial dermal vascular proliferation. The ultrastructural characteristics of the viruses are also identical to those responsible for milker nodule and orf acquired from domestic ruminants. The diagnosis can be confirmed by immunohistochemistry or PCR.[1]

Molluscum contagiosum

Clinical features

MC is a self-limiting epidermal papular condition caused by a poxvirus of the Molluscipox virus genus (Fig. 18.76).[1,2] The genome encodes 163 proteins of which 103 are closely related to variola virus.[3] Recent studies have shown that MC virus has a number of immune evasion strategies, including inhibition of NF-κB activation and apoptosis.[4-8]

MC occurs on the face, trunk, and limbs of young children, who are infected by direct cutaneous contact or inoculation from fomites, and in young adults on genitalia and surrounding skin after transmission by sexual contact.[2,9] The palms and soles are usually unaffected, but rare cases have been reported; subungual involvement, however, is exceptional.[10-12] Although the condition is worldwide, it is more prevalent in tropical regions.[1] The earlier literature indicated that lesions were particularly common in Fiji and Papua New Guinea, where 1 child in 10 had or had had the condition; most infected children were under 5 years of age.[13,14] Subsequent studies from India and the United States have shown that around 80% of children with MC are younger than 8–10 years of age.[15,16] There have been rare reports of neonatal or congenital infection.[17,18]

It has been suggested that MC may be more common in people with atopic dermatitis.[10] In the United States and the United Kingdom, the incidence in adults attending sexually transmitted disease (STD) clinics is in the range of 1 for every 40–60 cases of gonorrhea. Transmission can also occur between wrestlers (molluscum gladiatorum), between doctor and patient, and through joint use of equipment and bathing facilities. The use of public swimming pools appears of particular significance in children.[19,20] MC may also be acquired through tattooing.[21,22] The disease has an increased incidence in patients with impaired immunity. In the latter, lesions tend to be more extensive, generalized, and persistent.[10] Although man was initially thought to be the only host to the virus, there have been isolated reports of MC in animals such as certain bird species, the chimpanzee, and possibly the red kangaroo.[2]

The incubation period ranges from 2 to 7 weeks but may be as long as 6 months.[23] Individual lesions are smooth, shiny, pearly, firm, umbilicated papules up to 5 mm across or occasionally larger (Figs 18.77 and 18.78). Mucous membrane involvement is seen occasionally.[24] The lesions are usually quite characteristic in appearance, but may be confused occasionally with a fibrous histiocytoma, intradermal melanocytic nevus, keratoacanthoma, syringoma, basal cell carcinoma, common wart, and even cutaneous cryptococcosis. They are often multiple, especially in patients with immune

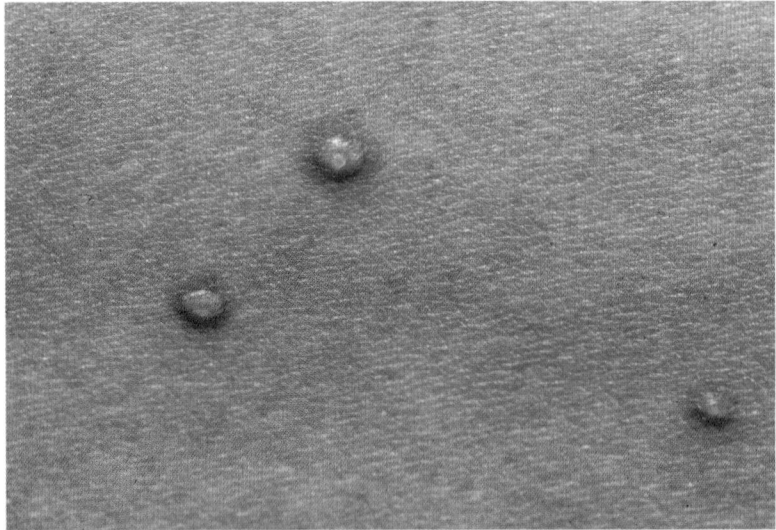

Fig. 18.77
Molluscum contagiosum: multiple umbilicated lesions are present. From the collection of the late N.P. Smith, MD, the Institute of Dermatology, London, UK.

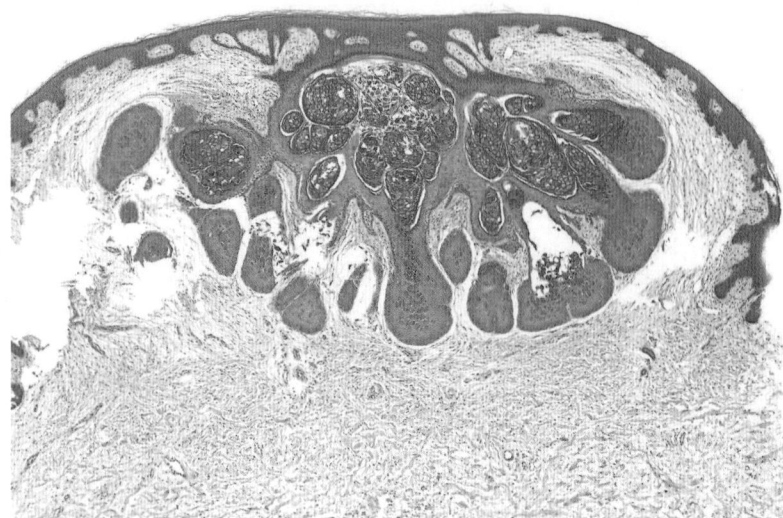

Fig. 18.79
Molluscum contagiosum: characteristic scanning view showing the central umbilication and epidermal hyperplasia.

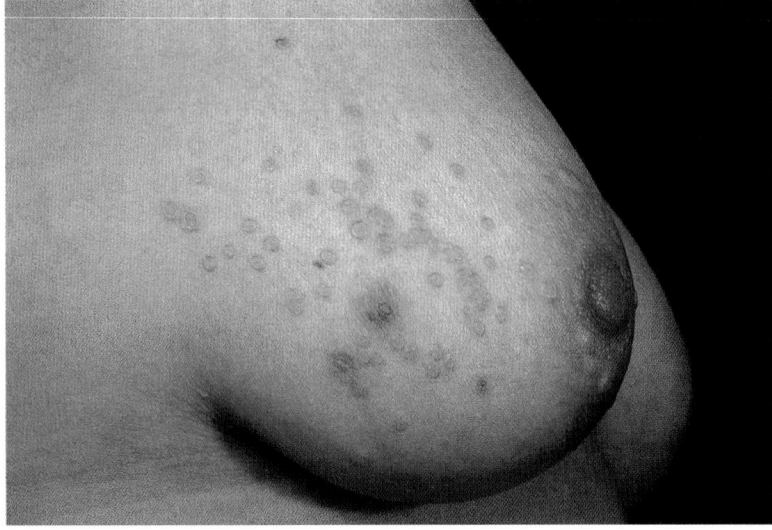

Fig. 18.78
Molluscum contagiosum: this often develops as a result of sexual contact in young adults. By courtesy of R.A. Marsden, St George's Hospital, London, UK.

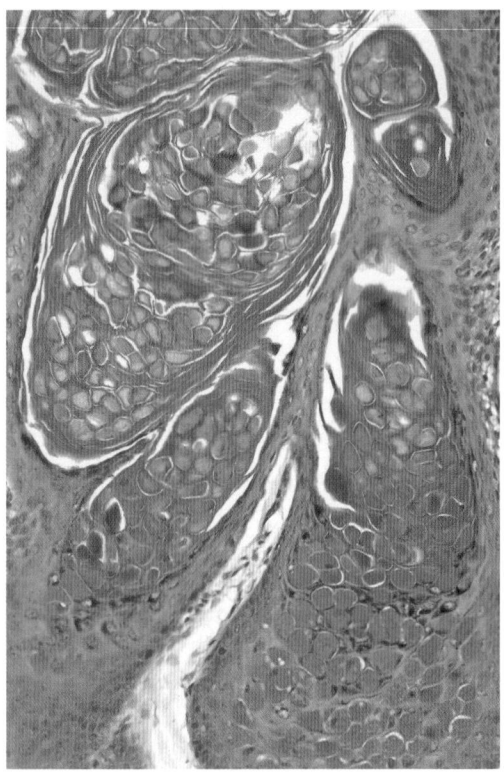

deficiency. Although uncommon, giant lesions may also occur, especially in immunocompromised patients.[25-30] HIV-infected individuals can manifest with exclusive involvement of facial and perioral skin, as well as the eyelids.[28,31,32] MC may be a cutaneous manifestation of IRIS in HIV-infected patients receiving highly active ART.[33-37] A number of recent reports have highlighted an increased susceptibility to MC among patients on treatment with immunosuppressive drugs, including methotrexate, ciclosporine, anticancer chemotherapy, and newer therapeutic agents such as kinase inhibitors and TNF-α antagonists.[4,32,38-41]

Symptoms of itching, tenderness, and pain are uncommon, but approximately 10% of patients develop an eczematous dermatitis around the molluscum papule. The papule itself may become secondarily infected and then resemble a furuncle. The individual lesion usually persists for 2 months, but sometimes lasts much longer. Since the patient may have numerous lesions at different stages of development, MC can be present for years in some patients. Pitted scarring sometimes occurs in atopic individuals.[42] Systemic lesions have not been described.[10]

Histologic features

In MC, intracellular edema with reticular degeneration and vesiculation are not features, in contrast to those caused by the other pox viruses. The

Fig. 18.80
Molluscum contagiosum: the intracytoplasmic inclusions almost completely fill the cell and compress the nucleus.

characteristic feature is the presence of lobulated, endophytic hyperplasia, producing a circumscribed, somewhat crateriform intradermal pseudotumor (*Fig. 18.79*). The keratinocytes contain a very large intracytoplasmic inclusion, which compresses the nucleus against the cell membrane. Although initially eosinophilic in size, the inclusion gradually develops a marked basophilia (*Fig. 18.80*). The latter can be recognized in a cytological preparation from the surface of the lesion; this may serve as a quick diagnostic test. Their presence may be rendered more conspicuous by the use of Lendrum phloxine tartrazine reaction (*Fig. 18.81*). Rarely, primitive follicular induction may be encountered in the basal epidermis in the vicinity of MC lesions, and is likely a virally induced reactive phenomenon.[43] In those cases lacking obvious molluscum bodies on initial examination, the presence of an edematous or fibromyxoid stroma, or keratinocyte alterations such

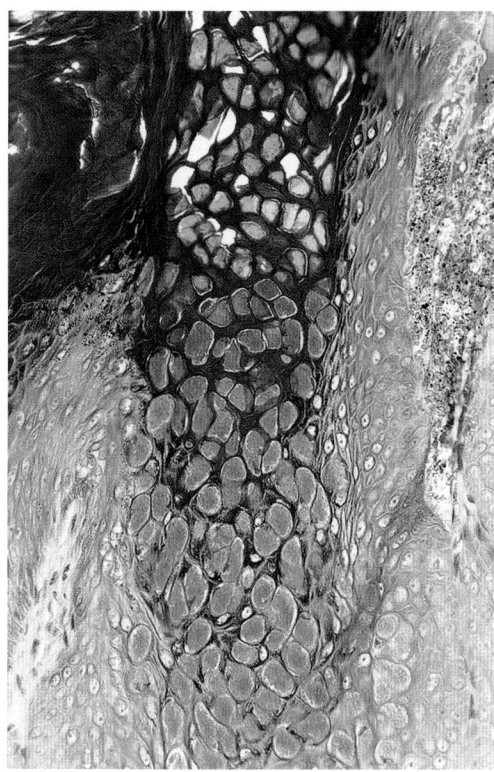

Fig. 18.81
Molluscum contagiosum: note the tinctorial change in this section stained with Lendrum phloxine tartrazine.

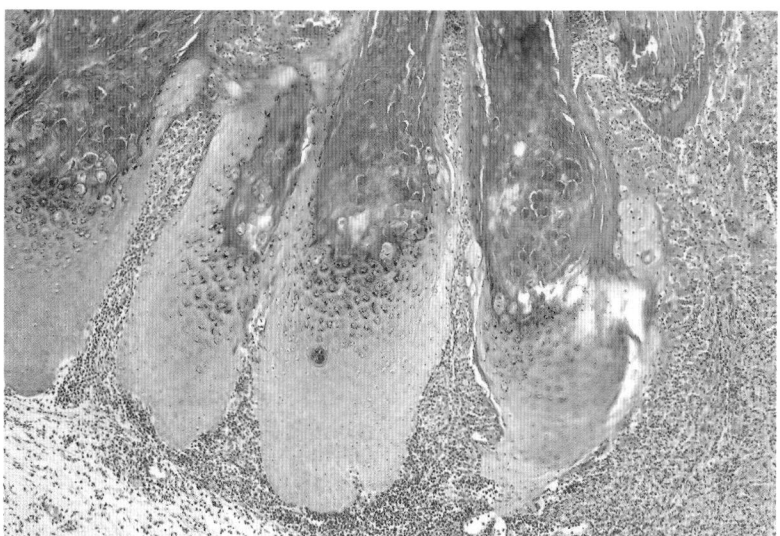

Fig. 18.82
Molluscum contagiosum: rupture of an epidermal nodule has released inclusions into the dermis with a resultant intense chronic inflammatory cell response.

as nucleolar prominence, cytoplasmic amphophilia, and clear cytoplasmic vacuolation, should prompt scrutiny of deeper tissue sections.[44]

Usually, there is no dermal infiltrate, but when it does occur, allegedly in response to virus or inclusion bodies entering the dermis, the lymphocytic infiltrate is so intense that lymphoma may enter the differential diagnosis if the characteristic inclusion bodies are not obvious (*Figs 18.82* and *18.83*). This dermal lymphoid infiltrate may harbor large, atypical CD30-positive lymphoid cells, potentially mimicking a CD30-positive cutaneous lymphoproliferative disorder.[45–47] This is particularly seen in regressing lesions containing few inclusion bodies, and the histologic diagnosis may be very difficult. Langerhans cell hyperplasia has also been reported.[48]

The presence of metaplastic bone formation in otherwise typical lesions of MC has been reported.[26,49] MC has also been noted in association with

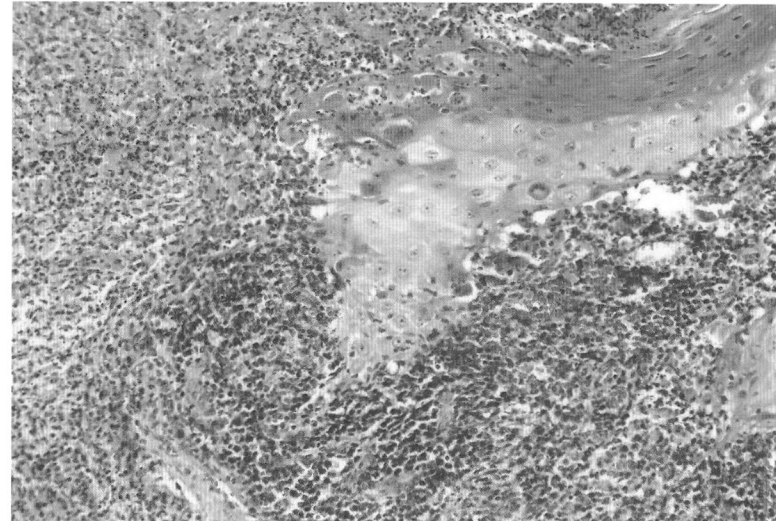

Fig. 18.83
Molluscum contagiosum: there is an intense lymphohistiocytic infiltrate. Numerous infected keratinocytes are present.

epidermal cysts, melanocytic nevi, melanoma, sebaceous hyperplasia, soft fibromas, lupus erythematosus, leukemia cutis, eosinophilic cellulitis, and even Kaposi sarcoma.[26,35,49–55]

Hand, foot and mouth disease

Clinical features

This is a viral illness caused most often by coxsackievirus A16 and less often by enterovirus 71.[1–15] It usually affects young children, shows seasonal variation (being more common in summer and autumn), and presents as small epidemics. A number of outbreaks have been documented in the East, especially Taiwan and Mainland China.[3,5–8,11,12,14] Outbreaks have also occurred in Malaysia, Singapore, and India.[9,10,13,16] Children in their first 4 years of life are most susceptible.[6,11,13] Other viruses implicated include echovirus 19, and very rarely, echovirus 4.[17,18] More recently, there have been outbreaks caused by coxsackievirus A6 in Europe, North America, and Asia.[19] Molecular phylogenetic analysis has shown that two distinct genogroups of coxsackievirus A16 exist, namely, A and B.[20] Phylogenetic evidence has also revealed that intertypic recombination between enterovirus 71 and coxsackievirus A16 may play a role in the emergence of subgenotypes of enterovirus 71.[21]

Hand, foot, and mouth disease has an incubation period of 3–7 days. Following a prodrome of headache, fever, malaise, abdominal pain, and sometimes diarrhea, patients develop oral ulcers and blisters, most commonly on the inner cheeks and lips, accompanied by small erythematous papules, which soon evolve into grayish vesicles on the soles, palms, and ventral surfaces and sides of the fingers and toes (*Figs 18.84–18.87*).[3] Lesions are less commonly found on the perineum, buttocks, trunk, and extremities. The eruption is self-limiting.[15] Atypical manifestations include eczema coxsackium in children with atopic dermatitis, and onychomadesis.[1,22] Complications only occur in approximately 6% of cases attributable to coxsackievirus A16, notably aseptic meningitis.[5]

Hand, foot, and mouth disease due to enterovirus 71 is a more serious illness, with complications occurring in approximately one-third of patients. These include central nervous system (CNS) lesions predominantly affecting the cerebellum. Encephalitis, aseptic meningitis, and a poliomyelitis-like condition with acute flaccid paralysis can also occur.[3,5,11–13,16,23] Concomitant infections may sometimes be seen.[16] Although a mortality rate of around 8% was recorded in the past, more recent data from China reflect lower fatality rates, ranging from 0.03% to 1.8%.[2,5,24] Death is usually attributable to cardiopulmonary decompensation and acute pulmonary edema.[5] The mechanism of pulmonary edema is unclear, since it does not appear

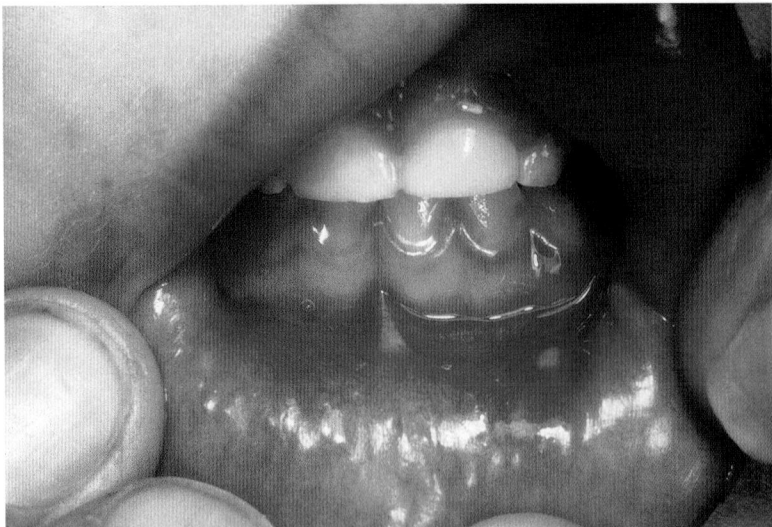

Fig. 18.84
Hand, foot, and mouth disease: multiple oral ulcers are present. By courtesy of the Institute of Dermatology, London, UK.

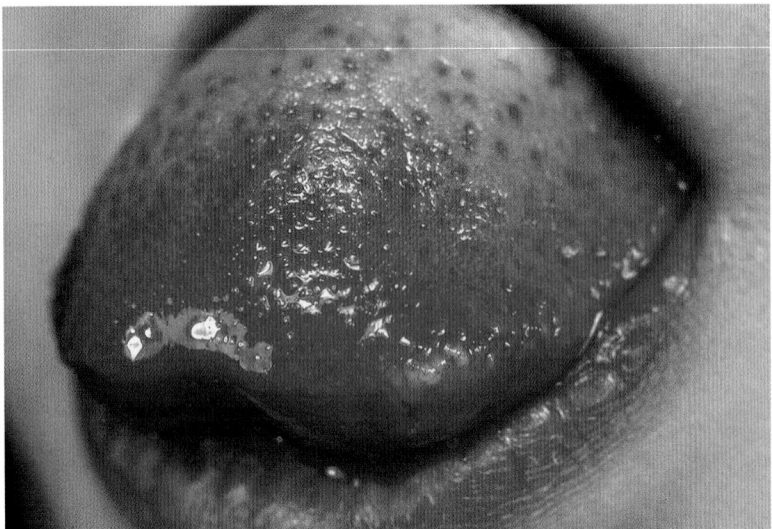

Fig. 18.85
Hand, foot, and mouth disease: there are numerous erosions with surrounding erythema. By courtesy of E. Wilson Jones, MD, Institute of Dermatology, London, UK.

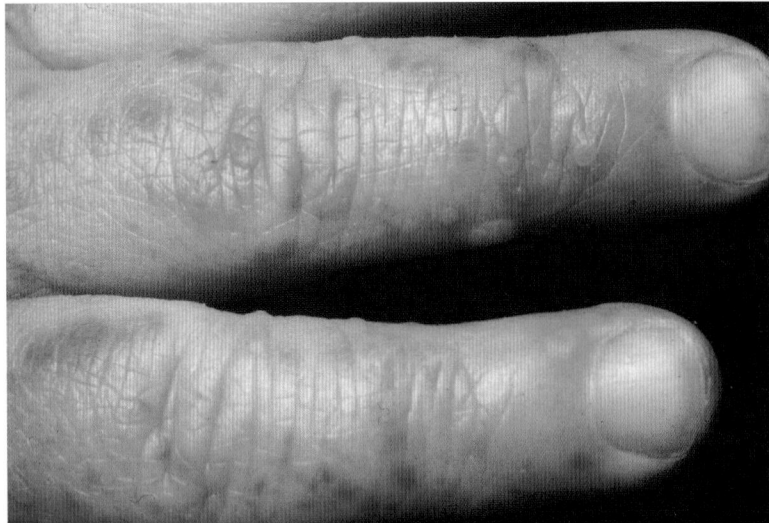

Fig. 18.86
Hand, foot, and mouth disease: note the small vesicles with surrounding erythema. By courtesy of E. Wilson Jones, MD, Institute of Dermatology, London, UK.

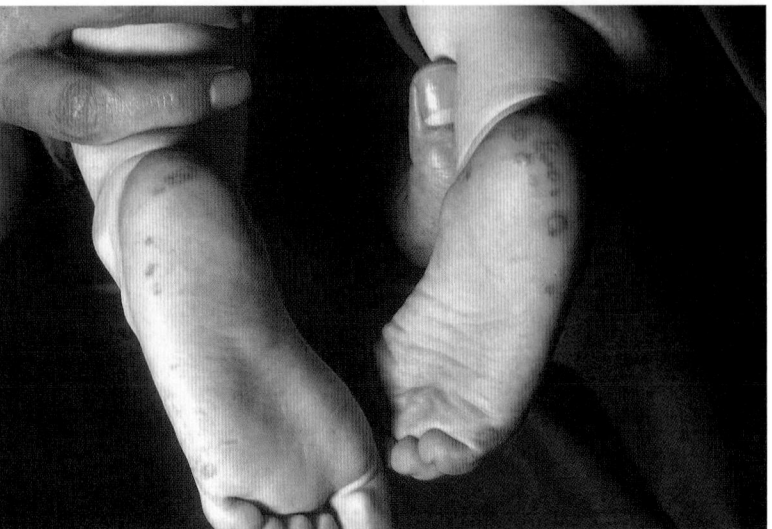

Fig. 18.87
Hand, foot, and mouth disease: there are numerous erosions on the sole of the foot. By courtesy of R.A. Marsden, MD, St George's Hospital, London, UK.

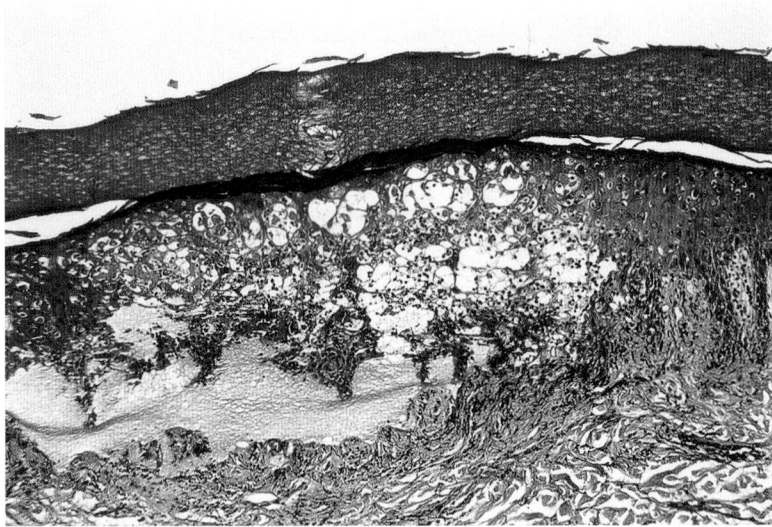

Fig. 18.88
Hand, foot, and mouth disease: this low-power view of the finger shows gross reticular degeneration with intraepidermal vesiculation. Degenerative changes have resulted in separation between the epidermis and the dermis. By courtesy of E. Wilson Jones, MD, Institute of Dermatology, London, UK.

to be the direct result of viral myocarditis in most cases; it has been postulated that increased pulmonary vascular permeability secondary to brainstem lesions or a systemic inflammatory response to encephalitis may play a role.[7,25] In one outbreak in Singapore, however, most fatalities were the result of interstitial pneumonitis, either alone or in association with myocarditis or encephalitis.[16]

Pathogenesis and histologic features

The virus is transmitted by direct contact with nasal and pharyngeal secretions, feces, and blood. Histologically, the blister is intraepidermal and develops as a consequence of marked inter- and intracellular edema (*Figs 18.88* and *18.89*). There may be associated papillary dermal edema. Viral inclusions and giant cells are not a feature. Enterovirus 71 may induce apoptosis of infected host cells via a virus-encoded protein.[26]

A real-time reverse transcriptase PCR method that allows for the differentiation of enterovirus 71 from coxsackievirus A16 has been described.[27]

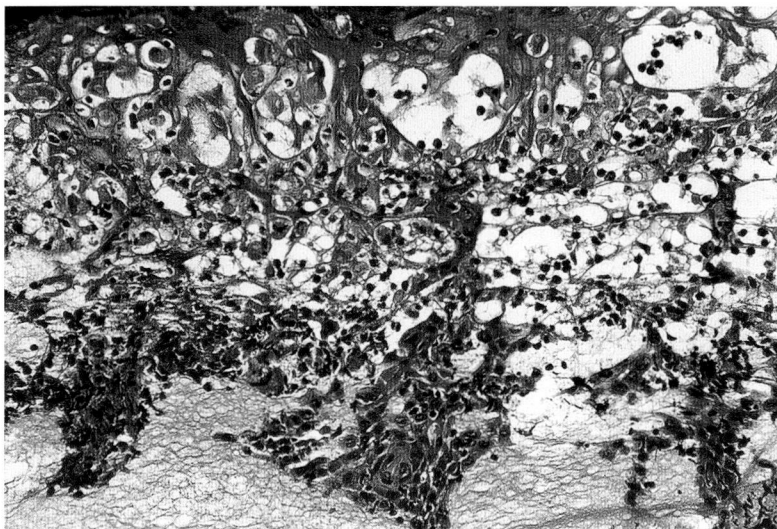

Fig. 18.89
Hand, foot, and mouth disease: the epithelium shows necrosis and dyskeratosis. A chronic inflammatory infiltrate is evident. By courtesy of E. Wilson Jones, MD, Institute of Dermatology, London, UK.

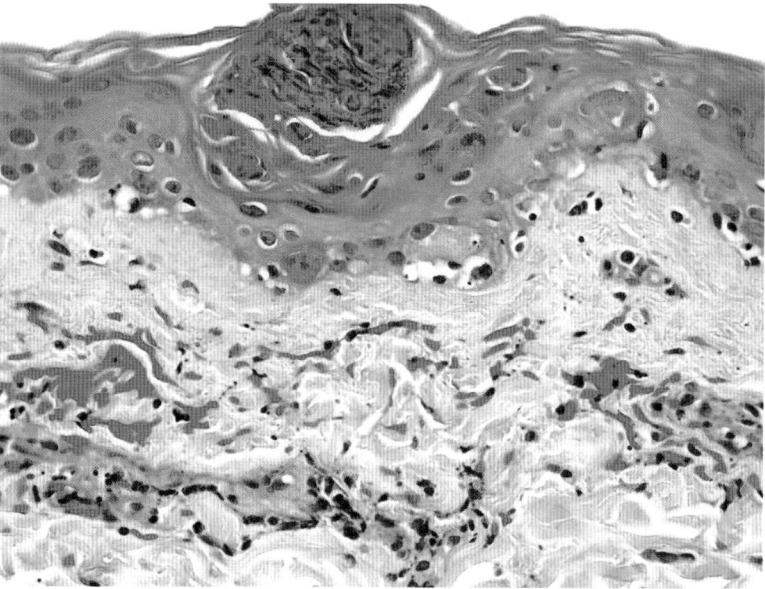

Fig. 18.90
Skin biopsy from a fatal case of novel arena virus infection (Lujo virus): there is a lymphocytic vasculopathic reaction, with perivascular erythrocytic extravasation. Confluent keratinocyte dyskeratosis is also evident.

Viral hemorrhagic fevers

Clinical features

The hemorrhagic fever (HF) viruses are a special group of highly infectious RNA viruses transmitted to humans by arthropods (mosquitoes, ticks) or rodents, resulting in systemic illness and a generalized bleeding diathesis.[1–5] The viral etiological agents may be grouped according to family:

- Flaviviridae, which are responsible for infections such as yellow fever, dengue fever, Omsk HF, and Kyasanur Forest disease,
- Bunyaviridae, which cause Rift Valley fever, Crimean–Congo HF, and hantavirus infections (e.g., HF with renal syndrome),
- Arenaviridae, which are responsible for Lassa fever, Argentine HF, Bolivian HF, Venezuelan HF, Brazilian HF, Lujo virus infection, etcetera,
- Filoviridae, which cause Marburg virus disease and Ebola.[1–4,6]

There is marked diversity in the severity of illness and the mortality within this group of diseases; dengue fever, for example, it has a mortality of around 5%, whereas the mortality associated with Ebola may be as high as 50% to 90%.[3,5] Healthcare workers exposed to infected patients are at particular risk of contracting the disease, as seen during the 2008 Lujo virus outbreak in Southern Africa, and the more recent West African Ebola epidemic of 2013–2016.[6,7] Ebola may also be transmitted by the handling of bushmeat, close contact with infected animals (e.g., chimpanzees, fruit bats), and direct contact with the blood, bodily fluids, or skin of infected patients or their corpses.[8] Increased international travel has resulted in some infections (e.g., dengue) presenting in travelers upon their return to nonendemic countries.[9] Most viral HFs manifest as an acute febrile illness, often with myalgias. Conjunctival injection and periorbital edema may occur.[2,5] Diagnosis is usually confirmed by virus-specific enzyme-linked immunosorbent assay (ELISA) and PCR methods.[7,10] Although some earlier classifications of viral HF included chikungunya (caused by chikungunya fever virus, a member of the Togaviridae), hemorrhagic manifestations are relatively rare and the disease has thus been omitted from most contemporary HF classifications.[1,2,11,12]

A detailed discussion of all of the conditions listed above is not possible, and the reader is referred to references 1–3 for excellent overviews on the subject. The further discussion here will focus on the potential mucocutaneous manifestations of viral HFs in general.

A conspicuous but non-specific, diffuse, nonpruritic maculopapular skin rash is typically encountered in filovirus infections such as Marburg virus disease and Ebola[13] Desquamation may take place during the recovery phase in nonfatal cases.[4] A similar although less prominent eruption may be seen on the trunk and limbs of patients with Rift Valley fever.[2] Dengue HF is frequently associated with a morbilliform rash, often with islands of spared skin.[4,9,14] Omsk HF, Kyasanur Forest disease, Argentine HF, and Bolivian HF are associated with a papulovesicular eruption involving the palate.[4] Around 30% of patients with dengue HF have mucosal involvement, most often of the conjunctiva.[14]

Thrombocytopenia is a characteristic sequel in the majority of viral HFs and manifests as petechial hemorrhages on the skin and in relation to the mucous membranes. Ecchymoses may develop in severe infections (e.g., Crimean–Congo HF) and are usually located over pressure points.[10] There may also be bleeding from venipuncture sites. DIC is known to complicate the clinical course of some infections, especially Rift Valley fever.[2,4,5] Jaundice is a typical feature of yellow fever but may also be encountered in Rift Valley fever, Crimean–Congo HF, and the filoviral HFs.[2,5]

Although Sindbis fever is not strictly one of the viral HFs, this relatively mild, self-limiting togavirus infection may rarely be associated with hemorrhagic skin lesions, and has been included here for the sake of completeness.[15] In usual cases of Sindbis fever, the exanthem is papular or vesicular, occurring in crops lasting up to 10 days. Lesions tend to be concentrated over the buttocks, legs, palms, and soles.[16]

Pathogenesis and histologic features

Although the precise pathogenesis of all viral HFs has yet to be fully elucidated, the general trend is to target dendritic reticulum cells, monocytes, lymphocytes, hepatocytes, and vascular endothelial cells. The profound and diverse pathophysiological effects are mediated via the release of a host of proinflammatory cytokines from these infected cells, resulting in a cytokine storm, increased vascular permeability, shock, tissue necrosis, hemorrhage, and coagulopathy.[1,3,17–20] Many of these viruses are capable of suppressing innate and adaptive immune responses in the infected host, leading to rapid local and systemic dissemination.[1,3,19,21,22]

The dermatopathological manifestations of this group of infections are poorly documented, largely because of the infectious and hemorrhagic risks associated with biopsy. In most cases, the findings are relatively non-specific. Consequently, skin biopsy is of questionable diagnostic or prognostic value. The cutaneous histologic features of dengue HF are perhaps the best studied among the HFs.[23–25] In general, HF cases with a maculopapular eruption show mild lymphocytic vasculitis, with a mild perivascular mononuclear inflammatory cell infiltrate, endothelial swelling, and minor perivascular erythrocytic extravasation (*Fig. 18.90*).[2,5,6,23–26] Keratinocyte dyskeratosis may also be seen (personal observation). Viral antigens may be demonstrated by immunohistochemistry if specific antibodies are used.[6,26]

Extensive dermal hemorrhage is seen in ecchymotic lesions. Intravascular fibrin-platelet thrombi characterize cases complicated by DIC.

Differential diagnosis

It is important to remember that the HF viruses are not the only infective agents that may be associated with pyrexia and hemorrhage. Other viruses such as smallpox virus and herpes simplex also may produce an HF picture (e.g., hemorrhagic smallpox). Additional infective agents that may cause HF are rickettsiae (e.g., *Rickettsia rickettsii*), chlamydiae (e.g., *Chlamydia psittaci*), bacteria (e.g., *Neisseria meningitidis*, *Yersinia pestis*), fungi (e.g., *Aspergillus*), spirochetes (e.g., *Leptospira icterohaemorrhagiae*, *Borrelia recurrentis*), and protozoa (e.g., *Plasmodium falciparum*).[16]

Trichodysplasia spinulosa

Trichodysplasia spinulosa (TS), also known as virus-associated trichodysplasia spinulosa, is a rare, relatively recently recognized, and novel viral infection of the hair follicle in immunocompromised patients.[1–5] In 2010 it was linked to a newly discovered human polyomavirus, now termed TS-associated polyomavirus (TSPyV).[4,6] The condition is mainly seen in solid organ transplant patients, particularly renal transplant, but may also occur in patients with chemotherapy-associated immunosuppression.[4,6,7] It is likely that TS is the same entity as pilomatrix dysplasia and ciclosporine-induced folliculodystrophy.[3,4,8,9]

Clinical features

TS is characterized by multiple small, skin-colored to erythematous spiky follicular papules which are asymptomatic or mildly pruritic and have predilection for the face and ears.[1–5] Lesions can also occur on the trunk and limbs, although they tend to be more sparse in these locations, and may coalesce. Focal alopecia can occur. When the immunosuppression is reduced the condition improves or regresses.

Pathogenesis and histologic features

TS is induced by active TSPyV infection of the hair follicle.[5] Electron microscopy studies have demonstrated intranuclear viral particles of variable size, from 30 to 46 nm.[1–3,7] There is clustering of infected follicular cells, which express the putative transforming TSPyV early large tumor (LT) antigen. The latter is thought to result in hyperproliferation, pRB phosphorylation, and up-regulation of p16 and p21.[10]

Histologically, anagen hair follicles appear dysmorphic, with distension, dilatation, and hyperkeratosis of the infundibula and abnormal maturation with marked inner root sheath (IRS) differentiation.[3,4,10] The follicles are overpopulated by IRS cells, a process has been described 'as if the hair follicles were entirely devoted to producing inner root sheath'.[2,10] Prominent

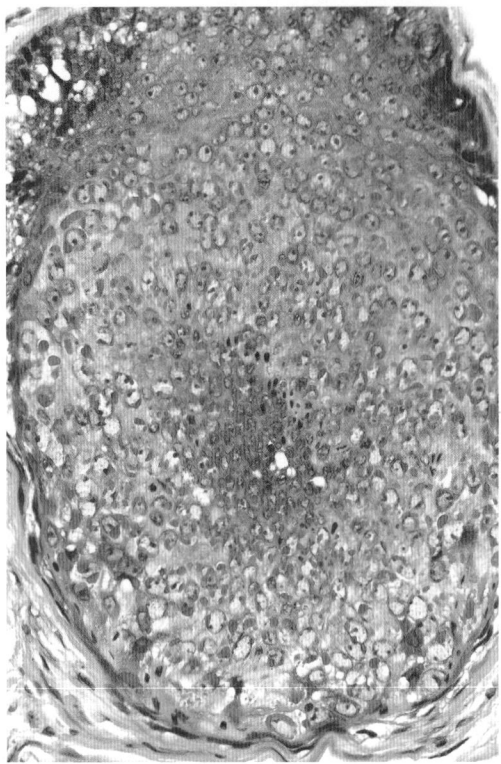

Fig. 18.91
Trichodysplasia spinulosa: note the prominent cytoplasmic granularity and eosinophilia in relation to the hair follicle epithelium.

cells with eosinophilic cytoplasm and numerous trichohyaline granules are seen (*Fig. 18.91*). The outer root sheath persists beyond the isthmus and the bulbs are abnormal, lacking fully formed papillae. Often, there are only few matrical cells as they are replaced by large numbers of cells with eosinophilic cytoplasm. There is usually no transition between the IRS and a fully cornified hair shaft. The diagnosis may be confirmed by immunohistochemistry.[11]

Differential diagnosis

The differential diagnosis includes keratosis pilaris and lichen spinulosus. Keratosis pilaris mainly involves the proximal limbs, rarely involves the face, and it has very subtle microscopic features, mainly hyperkeratosis and plugging of the infundibula. Lichen spinulosus mainly occurs in children, has predilection for the proximal limbs, neck, and buttocks, and it is characterized histologically by hyperkeratosis in the infundibular part of the hair follicles.

BACTERIAL INFECTIONS

Impetigo

The skin has a normal commensal population of bacteria in which *Staphylococcus epidermidis* predominates.[1] Other resident Gram-positive bacteria include *Micrococcus* spp. and *Corynebacterium* spp.[2] The free fatty acids and other lipids derived from the stratum corneum and sebum have an antibacterial role, yet 10% to 20% of the normal population are cutaneous carriers of *S. aureus* and approximately 10% are pharyngeal carriers of group A β-hemolytic streptococci (*Streptococcus pyogenes*).[1,3] This 'carrier' state may precede infective lesions in the host or may be the origin of infections in others. *S. aureus* and *S. pyogenes* are the most common agents in superficial bacterial infections of the skin, but even organisms of low virulence, such as *S. epidermidis*, can become pathogenic with a sufficiently large inoculum or in an immunocompromised host.[1] *S. aureus* toxin production is also responsible for bullous impetigo, the staphylococcal scalded skin syndrome (SSSS), and the toxic shock syndrome.[4,5]

Clinical features

Impetigo is the most superficial pyogenic (pyoderma) bacterial skin infection and is highly infectious. It is exceedingly common and occurs most often in childhood, but may be seen in the elderly and in patients with immunodeficiency states. It is estimated that more than 162 million children worldwide suffer from this condition at any given time. The median childhood prevalence is around 12%. The highest disease burden, however, appears to be among underprivileged children from marginalized communities in high-income countries.[6] Impetigo is typically subdivided into nonbullous (simple) impetigo and bullous impetigo and usually follows the contamination of minor skin abrasions and insect bites by *S. aureus* or *S. pyogenes*.[7,8] Scabies is an important risk factor for impetigo, especially among children.[6,9]

In simple impetigo, the lesions present as small superficial vesicles, which rapidly burst and are replaced by a characteristic, adherent, thick yellowish dirty crust with a margin of erythema (*Figs 18.92–18.94*). The mouth, nose, and extremities are particularly affected. Regional lymphadenopathy is sometimes present. Simple impetigo may occur in endemic or epidemic form and often spreads to involve siblings and schoolmates. It is seen more often in warm, humid conditions.[10,11] Although *S. aureus* remains the more frequent cause in North America and *S. pyogenes* was the more important etiological agent of impetigo in developing countries in the past, *S. aureus* is now the most commonly isolated pathogen in many parts of the world.[12,13] In some cases, however, the two bacteria appear to coexist. Streptococcal impetigo may occasionally progress to cellulitis or precede acute glomerulo-nephritis, erythema nodosum, or erythema multiforme.

Bullous impetigo is primarily a staphylococcal-mediated disease exclusively due to phage group II *S. aureus*.[10] Superficial blisters up to 2 cm across are the initial features (*Fig. 18.95*). The contents are at first clear, but rapidly become cloudy and then develop a thin seropurulent crust; erythema

is not marked. The lesions do not usually involve mucosae. There may be mild constitutional symptoms, and the lesions resolve in 2–3 weeks.

Ecthyma is probably a variant of impetigo and occurs predominantly on the lower limbs of children, but may occur in adults and at other sites (*Figs 18.96* and *18.97*).[14,15] It presents with thick crusting, overlying punched-out ulceration, and resultant scarring. *S. pyogenes* is the usual cause. It is more common in tropical climates, where it occurs in all age groups. Minor trauma or scabies infestation may determine the site of the lesions. It is possible that vasculitis and necrosis induced by bacterial toxins determine the different presentation.

Ecthyma gangrenosum is usually a complication of *P. aeruginosa* septicemia that occurs in immunodeficient patients, particularly those with a neutropenia.[16,17] It has also been reported in association with

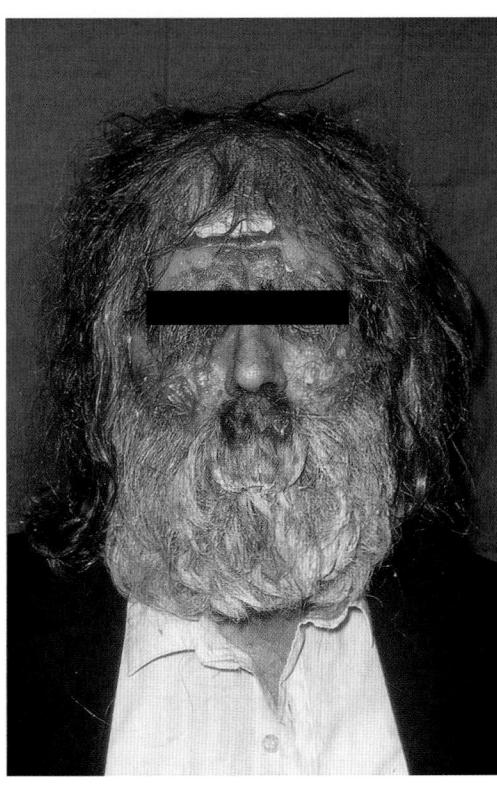

Fig. 18.92
Impetigo: note the crusted lesions on this patient's forehead and cheeks. By courtesy of R.A. Marsden, MD, St George's Hospital, London, UK.

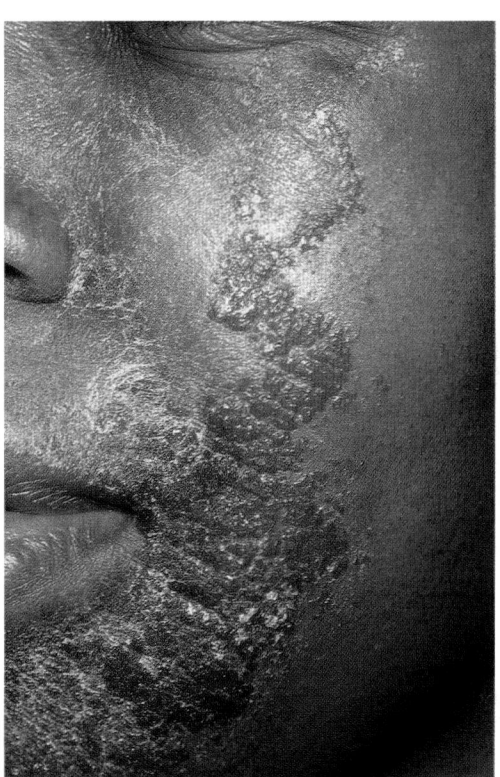

Fig. 18.94
Impetigo: in this patient numerous vesicles are evident. By courtesy of R.A. Marsden, MD, St George's Hospital, London, UK.

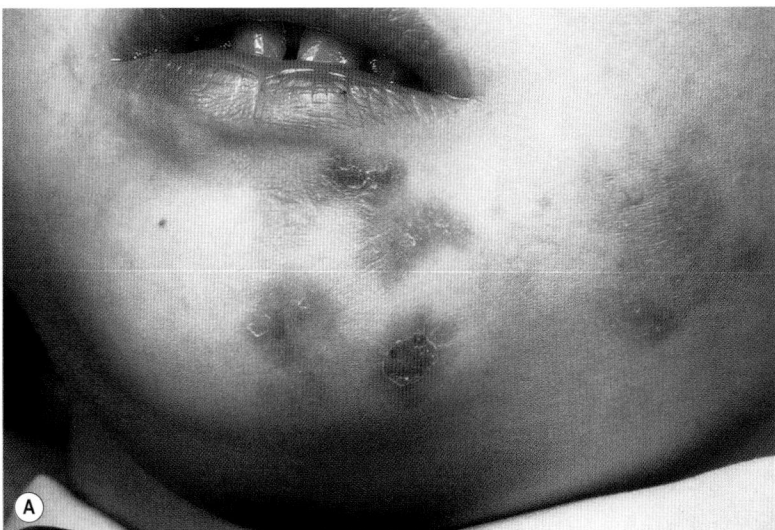

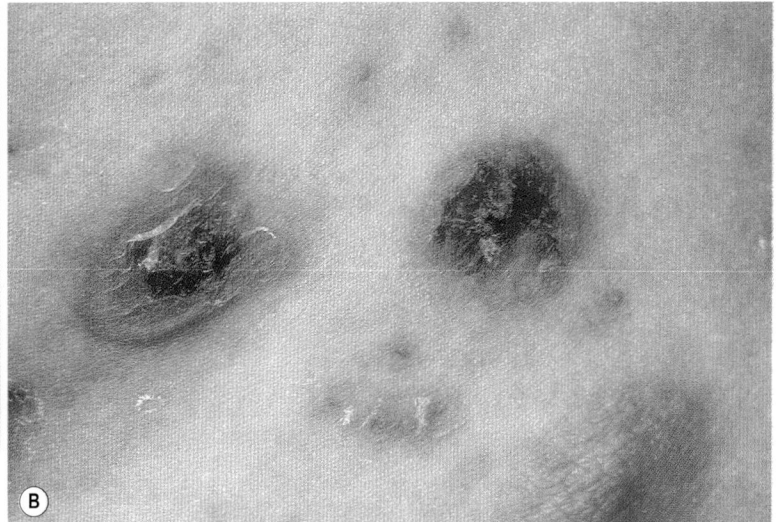

Fig. 18.93
(**A**, **B**) Impetigo: note that the vesicles are covered by a golden crust. These perioral lesions are at a characteristic site. By courtesy of R.A. Marsden, MD, St George's Hospital, London, UK.

hypogammaglobulinemia.[18] There have been rare reports of ecthyma gangrenosum occurring in the absence of neutropenia or septicemia.[19–21] The condition has also been reported following toxic epidermal necrolysis (TEN).[22] Lesions, which may be single or multiple, begin as painless erythematous macules that become indurated, bullous, or pustular.[16] Annular lesions have been described.[23] The lesions soon become gangrenous and covered by a characteristic gray-black eschar and erythematous halo. Lesions are especially seen on the gluteal and perineal regions and on the limbs.[16] The mortality is high, particularly in those with multiple lesions. Organisms other than *P. aeruginosa* have been implicated in the evolution of the disease.[24]

Pathogenesis and histologic features

The carrier state or inoculation by a contaminated object is a necessary precondition to superficial infection of the skin. The organisms become attached to the traumatized area, binding strongly to fibronectin and possibly type IV collagen and laminin, which are abundant in the exudate.[1,10] The innate virulence of the organisms and the host defense capability determine the subsequent progress of the infection, but this is facilitated if the bacteria produce coagulase, hyaluronidase, or lipases.[1] The form of *S. aureus* responsible for bullous impetigo is of serotype II and mainly of phage type

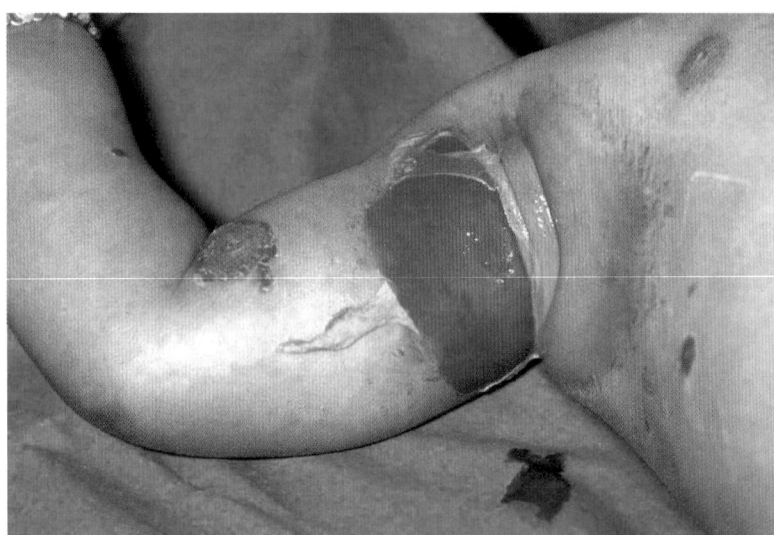

Fig. 18.95
Bullous impetigo: there is a large raw erosion and a healed lesion distally. By courtesy of the Institute of Dermatology, London, UK.

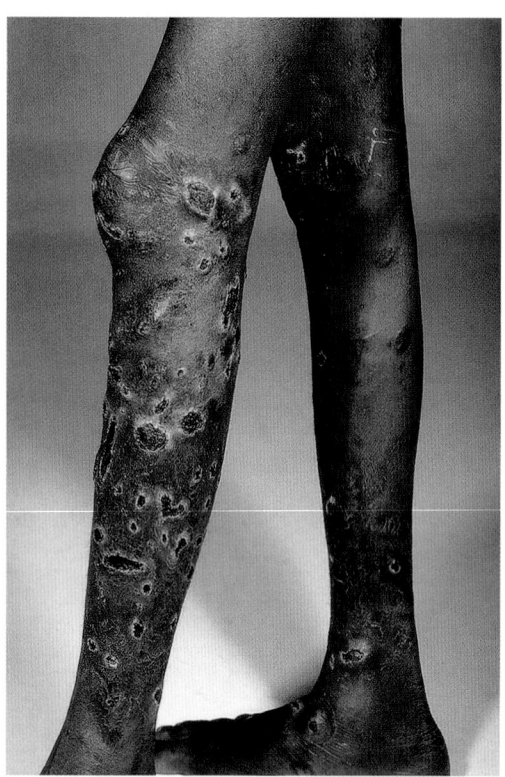

Fig. 18.97
Ecthyma: multiple lesions are present. By courtesy of N.C. Dlova, MD, Nelson R. Mandela School of Medicine, University of KwaZulu-Natal, South Africa.

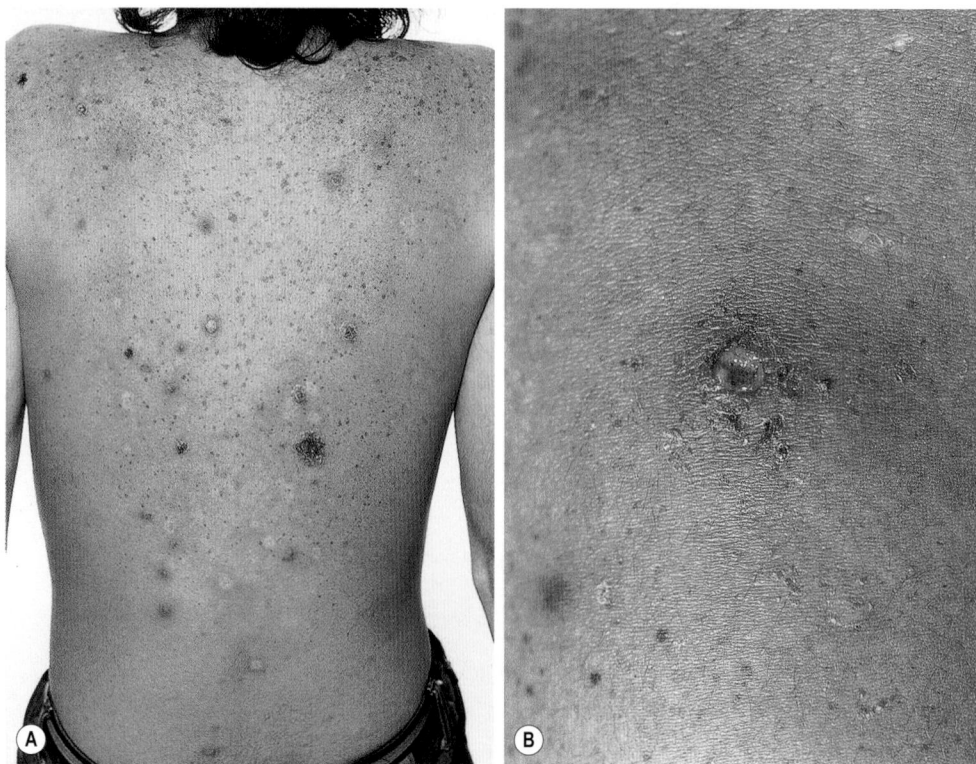

Fig. 18.96
Ecthyma: (**A**) characteristic lesions in varying stages of evolution; (**B**) a punched-out ulcer is shown in close-up. By courtesy of M.M. Black, MD, Institute of Dermatology, London, UK.

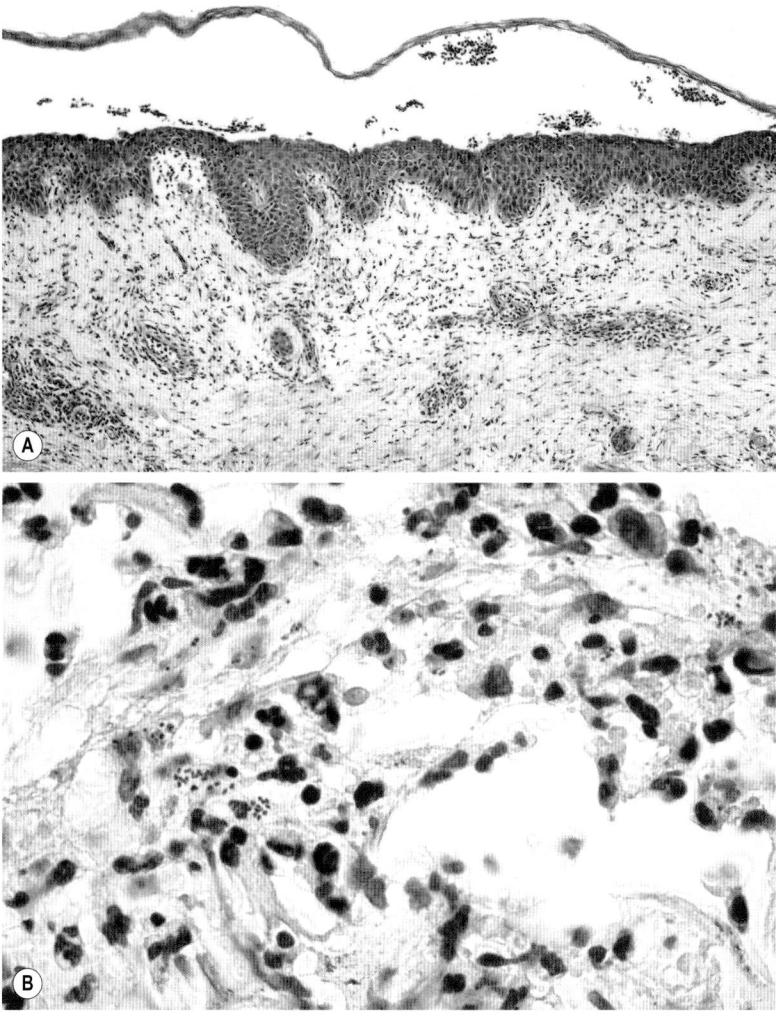

Fig. 18.98
Bullous impetigo: (**A**) the site of cleavage is immediately below the granular cell layer; (**B**) Gram-positive cocci are present.

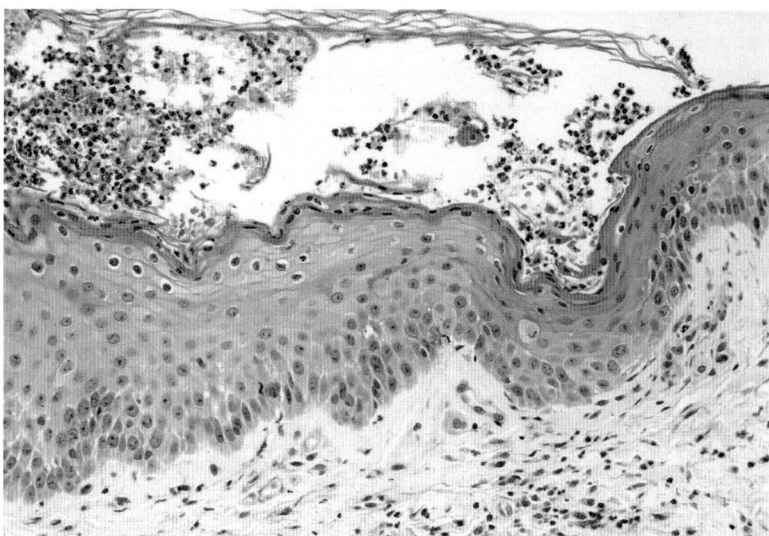

Fig. 18.99
Bullous impetigo: in addition to neutrophils, occasional acantholytic cells may be present causing diagnostic confusion with pemphigus foliaceus.

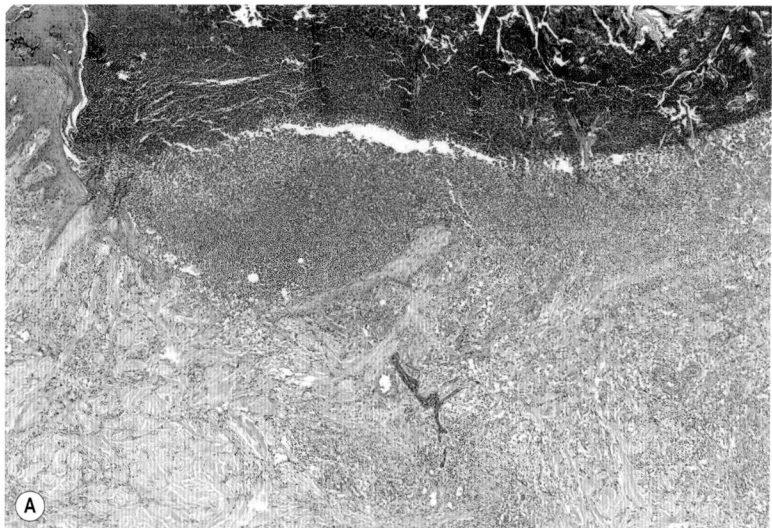

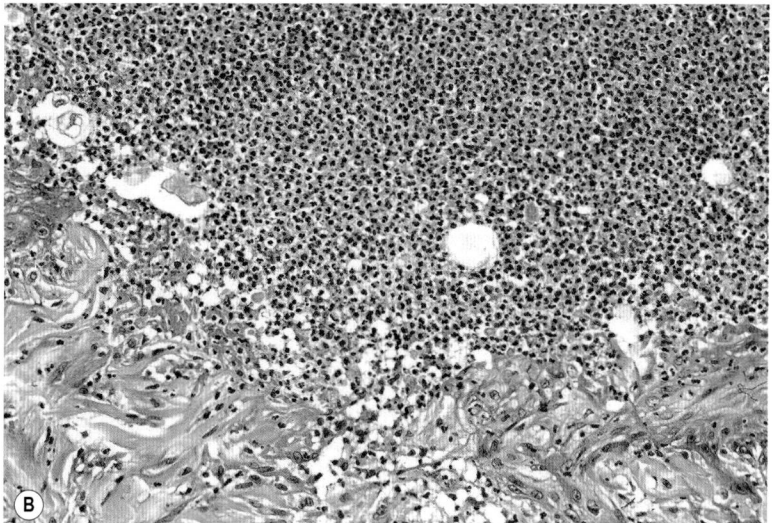

Fig. 18.100
(**A**, **B**) Ecthyma: there is a sharply delineated ulcer. Artifact is an important differential diagnosis.

71 and produces exfoliative toxins A and B; the latter are also involved in the SSSS (see below).[4,5,25,26] During the past decade, community-acquired methicillin-resistant *S. aureus* (CA-MRSA) emerged as a major cause of impetigo.[12,13,27–29]

An early lesion of impetigo is characterized by a split in the epidermis just beneath the stratum granulosum (*Fig. 18.98*). The resultant vesicle becomes filled with neutrophils, Gram-positive cocci, and occasional acantholytic cells (*Fig. 18.99*). The underlying dermis contains a mixed neutrophil and lymphocyte infiltrate. Neutrophils may be seen in the spongiotic stratum spinosum beneath the vesicle in the process of migrating from the dermis as a chemotactic response to the causative bacteria. In conditions of impaired neutrophil function, impetigo may be common and more extensive.[1]

In echthyma, there is a sharply circumscribed area of ulceration with a heavy neutrophil infiltrate and overlying adherent crust (*Fig. 18.100*).

Ecthyma gangrenosum is characterized by epidermal necrosis with hemorrhage and dermal infarction, usually accompanied by a mixed inflammatory cell infiltrate of lymphocytes, histiocytes, and neutrophils.[16] Less commonly, a dearth of inflammatory cells is noted.[16,30] Gram-negative bacilli may be seen in the dermis and involving the media and adventitia of venules.[16] Vasculitis and thrombosis may be present.

Differential diagnosis

The diagnosis is usually made on clinical grounds and supported by culture of the causative organisms. Rarely, a biopsy is necessary.

The lesion may be confused histologically with a superficial variant of pemphigus, particularly as the latter can become secondarily infected

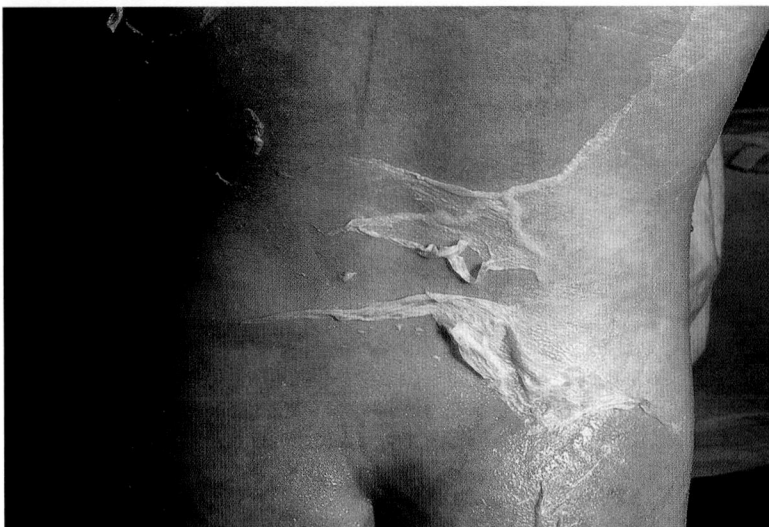

Fig. 18.101
Staphylococcal scalded skin syndrome: note the very extensive blistering. By courtesy of A. du Vivier, MD, King's College Hospital, London, UK.

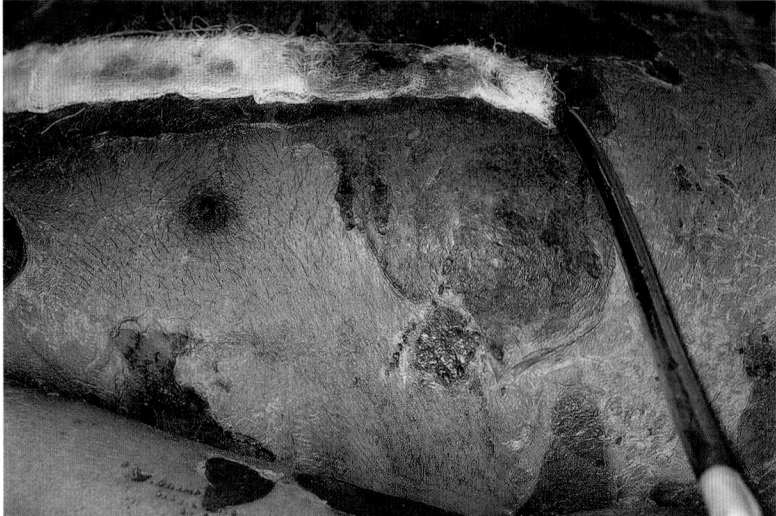

Fig. 18.102
Staphylococcal scalded skin syndrome: note the widespread denuded areas at the edge of which the epithelium is being shed. This case developed in a patient following wound infection after a coronary artery bypass. By courtesy of S. Parker, MD, West Middlesex Hospital, London, UK.

and there may be a few acantholytic cells in impetigo. Antibodies in a pemphigus-like pattern may be demonstrated in bullous impetigo and distinction from pemphigus foliaceus may therefore be a problem.[5,31,32] Generally, the presence of numerous neutrophils and the recognition of Gram-positive cocci is sufficiently characteristic to confirm impetigo, as acantholytic cells are very scanty. Distinction from subcorneal pustular dermatosis and pustular psoriasis may be considered histologically, but the lack of acanthosis, although not conclusive, should point toward impetigo.

Staphylococcal scalded skin syndrome

Clinical features

Staphylococcal scalded skin syndrome (SSSS) is so named because of the presence of staphylococcal toxin and the resemblance of the established lesion to a scald. It may present in epidemic form as well as sporadically. It has a relatively abrupt onset and occurs almost entirely, but not exclusively in neonates and young children, who develop first a macular scarlatiniform eruption in association with a staphylococcal infection. This is often associated with fever, irritability, and skin tenderness.[1-5] The eruption then spreads from its usual original sites on the face, axillae, and groins to involve large areas of the skin surface. Conjunctivitis is often also present. Mucous membranes, however, are not affected. At the same time, the skin becomes edematous and the surface fragile so that it can be sheared off in thin wrinkled sheets, likened to peeling wet wallpaper, leaving a glistening red surface, and the child becomes sick and feverish (*Fig. 18.101*). SSSS is therefore associated with a positive Nikolsky sign.[1,6]

Following blistering, desquamation occurs and the skin often returns to normal by 2–3 weeks.[7] Scarring is not usually a feature. The associated source of infection may be an upper respiratory tract infection, conjunctivitis, or umbilical sepsis, or it may be more occult, such as in the middle ear, in the pharynx, or at the site of minor surgery. The condition is rarely seen at other ages, such as the first day after birth or even at birth, indicating an infection acquired in labor or in utero, and it may be seen in older children.[8] Numerous adult cases have been reported, although many of these patients were either immunocompromised (including HIV infection) or in renal failure with a possible inability to excrete the toxin. The condition does occur rarely in previously healthy adults or those with relatively minor conditions (*Fig. 18.102*).[1,9-18] It is also a potential complication among hematopoietic stem cell recipients.[19]

The disease in neonates (Ritter disease) is usually self-limiting with rapid resolution of the skin blisters and complete recovery. However, there is a mortality of less than 10% (generally 2–4%) due to progression of the staphylococcal infection or the complications of exfoliation. In the adult, this rare condition has shown a mortality rate of between 40% and 63%.[1,5,16] Recovery is facilitated by antistaphylococcal antibiotics and attention to fluid balance.

An abortive form, the scarlatiniform variant (staphylococcal scarlet fever), in which the initial erythroderma evolves into the desquamative phase in the absence of blistering, has been described.[4,7] This may be particularly associated with occult bone and joint infections or contaminated wounds.[7]

Pathogenesis and histologic features

In SSSS the organism is of group II and usually phage type 71, but phage types 3A, 3B, 3C, and 55 have also been found.[4,5,13] These bacteria all produce an epidermolytic toxin (formerly referred to as exfoliatin), of which there are two antigenic types: exfoliative toxin A (ETA) and exfoliative toxin B (ETB).[20-24] ETA is associated with a chromosomal gene while ETB is plasmid encoded.[4,25] These serine proteases have indistinguishable activity and manifest exquisite pathological sensitivity by inducing blistering only at the level of the superficial epidermis. Their high substrate specificity is associated with selective recognition and hydrolysis of desmosomal proteins, notably desmoglein 1.[5,21,22,24] The effect of the toxins is determined by their site of production:

- Toxins produced by the appropriate staphylococcal infection of mucosae or surgical wounds enter the circulation (toxemia) and produce a generalized change in the skin, the SSSS. The intensity is determined by the rapidity with which the toxins are metabolized and excreted renally and by the presence of antibodies against the toxins.[26]
- If the same staphylococcus infects the skin directly, local release of toxin results in bullous impetigo.

Staphylococcal strains also produce toxic shock syndrome toxin (TSST-1) and a variety of enterotoxins (A–E). These are more frequently associated with staphylococcal scarlet fever and the toxic shock syndrome.[21,24,27]

The toxin in both SSSS and bullous impetigo causes a split in the epidermis at the level of the granular layer (*Fig. 18.103*). Ultrastructurally, the level of separation is in the midgranular layer.[28] It is associated with separation of the cell membranes at the desmosomes, and the interdesmosomal regions appear less dense.[29] The cells on either side of the cleft appear normal. It has been shown that the epidermolytic toxins (ETA and/or ETB) act as serine proteases and bind desmoglein 1, a desmosomal adhesion molecule.[22,23] The cleavage and subsequent inactivation thereof induces blistering.[23,27]

Histologically, the clefts through the granular layer of the epidermis in SSSS are associated with only a scanty inflammatory infiltrate in the epidermis or dermis, and there may be some dermal edema and dilatation of the

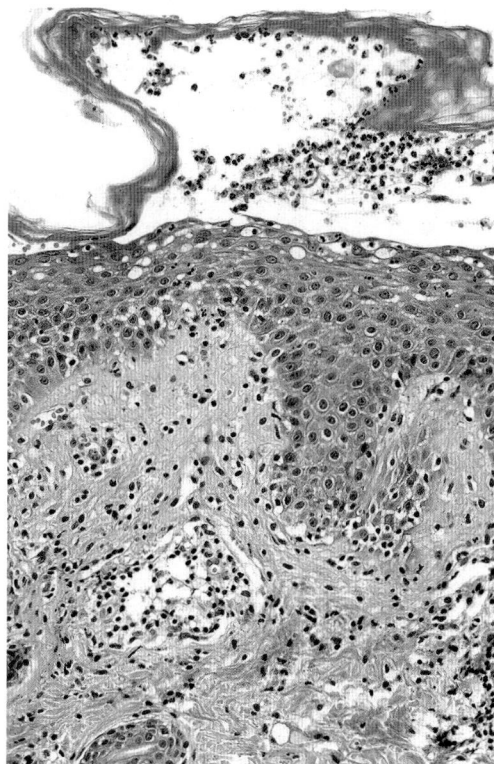

Fig. 18.103
Staphylococcal scalded skin syndrome: vesiculation occurs at the level of the granular cell layer.

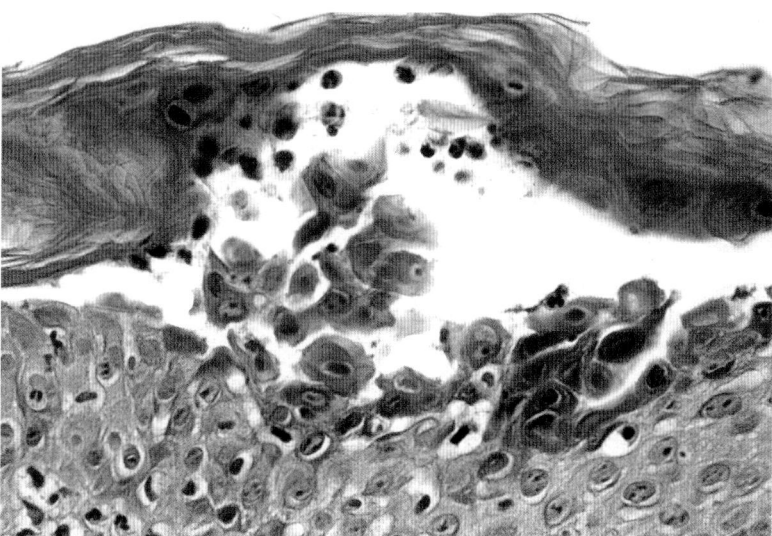

Fig. 18.104
Staphylococcal scalded skin syndrome: there is quite marked acantholysis in this example.

superficial vascular plexus. The adjacent epidermis does not show necrosis. Acantholysis is variably present (*Fig. 18.104*).

Differential diagnosis

The main clinical differential diagnosis is from TEN, a severe variant of erythema multiforme usually due to a drug reaction. This, however, is uncommon in children. In TEN the skin changes are very widespread and mucosal involvement is common, whereas SSSS extends from the face and flexures and does not involve mucosae. The contrasting histology of the two conditions can be used with a frozen section technique to give a rapid diagnosis[4–6]:

- TEN is characterized by a subepidermal blister with a necrotic epidermal roof and a moderately intense lymphocytic infiltrate in the dermis.

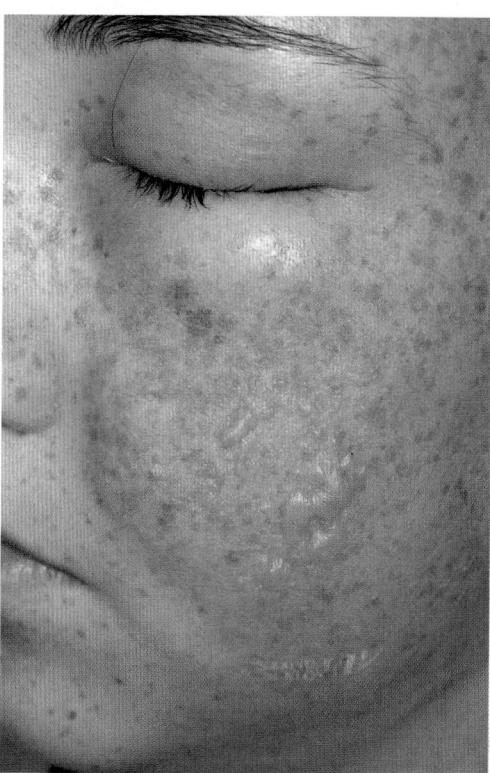

Fig. 18.105
Erysipelas: characteristic sharply demarcated erythematous and edematous plaque. By courtesy of J.C. Pascual, MD, Alicante, Spain.

- SSSS is characterized by separation through the granular cell layer. Alternatively, a Tzanck smear can be used, which reveals necrotic keratinocytes with inflammatory cells in TEN and viable acantholytic keratinocytes without inflammatory cells in SSSS.

Erysipelas and cellulitis

Clinical features
Erysipelas

Erysipelas is classically a *S. pyogenes* (group A β-hemolytic streptococcal) infection of the skin of the face, characterized by a sharply outlined edematous, erythematous, tender, and painful plaque (*Fig. 18.105*). The outer margin is elevated and contrasts with the adjacent normal skin. Toward the edge of the lesion there may be vesicles and hemorrhagic bullae. Other sites commonly affected include the feet and hands. Although *S. pyogenes* is the most common organism, it is not always possible to culture it, and other streptococci (group C or G) or *S. aureus* may be isolated, in particular, methicillin-resistant *S. aureus* (MRSA).[1–5]

The classical presentation of erysipelas is more often on the face, but it has been suggested that the features of this condition are changing because it is becoming more common and is predominantly affecting the lower limbs.[4] A seasonal variation in incidence is not uniformly found.

The superficial infection of erysipelas is associated with fever and malaise. It is similar in its presentation, etiology, and associated symptoms to cellulitis, a spreading infection affecting deeper tissues. This lesion is again clearly demarcated, hot, red, and painful, but without the elevated margin of erysipelas. An associated lymphangitis and lymphadenitis are common. The lesions may progress to pustulation, ulceration, and necrosis; the last may involve underlying fascia and muscle, resulting in NF.[6] Osteoarticular complications such as bursitis, arthritis, tendinitis, and osteitis have been reported.[7] Positive blood cultures may be found in 4.6% of patients.[8]

Cellulitis

Cellulitis is similar to erysipelas, but tends to involve the deeper tissues and is seen most often on the legs, where it often complicates tinea pedis or

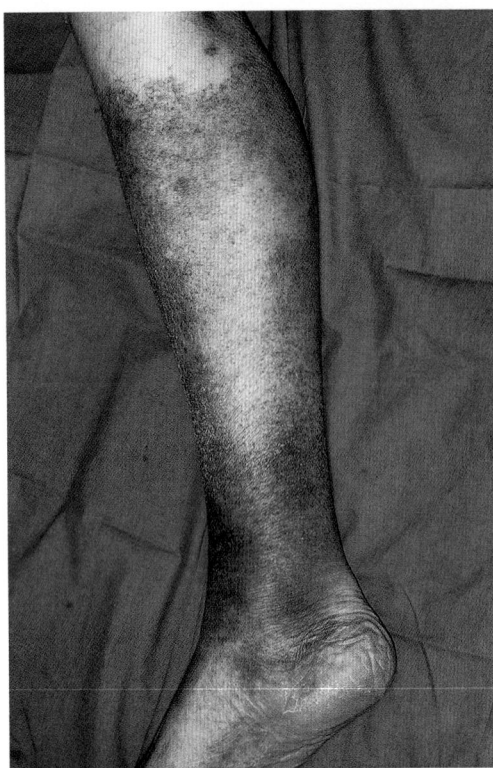

Fig. 18.106
Cellulitis: note the widespread erythema. The lower leg is a characteristic site. By courtesy of R.A. Marsden, MD, St George's Hospital, London, UK.

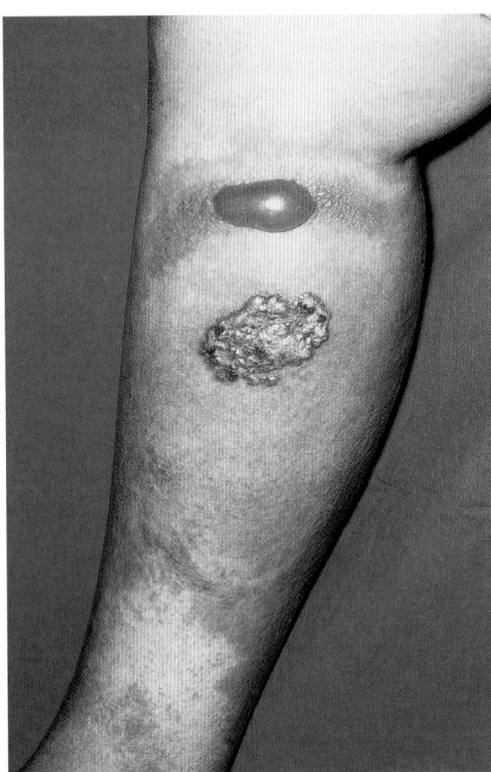

Fig. 18.107
Cellulitis: marked edema has resulted in vesiculation. By courtesy of R.A. Marsden, MD, St George's Hospital, London, UK.

chronic lymphedema (*Fig. 18.106*).[9–11] Other potential risk factors include diabetes mellitus, leukemia, postsaphenous venectomy, and peripheral vascular disease. Patients with dry skin may also be susceptible.[12] Cellulitis is characterized by an expanding area of erythema. Involvement of lymphatics in both erysipelas and cellulitis is characteristic, resulting in the edema which is sometimes associated with vesiculation (*Fig. 18.107*); infective damage to

lymphatics in cellulitis may be the reason this condition can become recurrent. Approximately 25% of patients will experience more than one episode of cellulitis within 3 years. Symptoms and signs of systemic illness may be encountered in up to 40% of cases.[5] In a systematic review of 1578 cases, 7.9% of patients had positive blood cultures.[8]

The term hemorrhagic cellulitis has been applied to an uncommon clinical syndrome caused by Gram-positive or Gram-negative organisms of noncutaneous origin. Patients manifest with the abrupt onset of painful erythema on the lower extremities, followed by dermal hemorrhage and sloughing of the overlying epidermis.[13] There is usually a satisfactory response to a combination of antibiotics and corticosteroid therapy. Virulent marine bacteria such as *Vibrio vulnificus* may result in this form of bullous and hemorrhagic cellulitis; the disease carries an estimated mortality of 15%.[14]

Pathogenesis and histologic features

Minor trauma to the skin is important in the development of both erysipelas and cellulitis, but peripheral vascular disease, diabetes, lymphedema, and alcohol abuse are additional predisposing factors.

In both erysipelas and cellulitis, *S. pyogenes* is the most common organism and the lesions are initiated by inoculation of minor abrasions or splits in the epidermis.[15] An increased proportion of infections due to MRSA, however, has emerged during the past one and a half decades.[8,11] Proliferation of the organisms is associated with the production of enzymes (streptolysins, deoxyribonuclease B, hyaluronidase) which may be detected in rising titers and may therefore be useful diagnostically.[16] These enzymes are also important in facilitating the extension of the bacteria in the skin. Lymphatic involvement with obstruction is common, resulting in edema, and is associated with lymphangitis and lymphadenitis. In the more aggressive forms of cellulitis, it is likely that other organisms (certainly *S. aureus* and some anaerobes) may be causative or synergistic.[17] A synergistic role for *S. aureus* (especially methicillin-resistant strains) and *S. pyogenes* has been implicated in the development of bullous erysipelas.[18] Group G streptococci predominated over group A β-hemolytic streptococci in a Finish series of 90 patients with acute cellulitis.[19] There have been rare reports of severe cellulitis due to organisms such as *Streptococcus pneumoniae*, *Haemophilus influenzae*, and *Nocardia otitidiscaviarum*.[20–22] In those forms of cellulitis in which necrosis is a more prominent feature, bacterial toxins are an important mechanism.

Histologically, the conspicuous features of erysipelas and cellulitis are dermal edema and lymphatic dilatation. There is also a diffuse, heavy neutrophil infiltration with a limited localization around blood vessels. Vascular and lymphatic dilatation and red cell extravasation are variable features. In later stages, some lymphocytes and histiocytes are also seen and granulation tissue may be present deep to the zone of subepidermal edema. When clinical vesicles or bullae are noted, there is a corresponding severe papillary edema merging with subepidermal vesiculation.[23]

In hemorrhagic cellulitis, the bacterial lipopolysaccharide-induced or bacterial mitogen-induced release of TNF-α is thought to result in injury to endothelial cells and epidermal keratinocytes. DNA fragmentation and cell lysis may be the consequence of neutrophil degranulation and anti-DNase activation.[13] Digestion of vascular basement membrane as a result of *V. vulnificus* metalloprotease production leads to the formation of hemorrhagic bullae.[24] Histologically, there is necrosis of epidermal keratinocytes, necrotizing vasculitis affecting dermal blood vessels, and large numbers of bacteria.[25]

It is important to remember that not all cases of cellulitis are bacterial in origin; deep fungal infections such as cryptococcosis and aspergillus may present with cellulitis in immunocompromised hosts.[26] Appropriate histochemical stains and the referral of additional specimens for microbiological examination should facilitate correct identification of the etiological agent.

Necrotizing fasciitis

Clinical features

NF is an uncommon, rapidly progressive, and potentially fatal bacterial infection of the subcutaneous soft tissues.[1–6] NF may evolve following a surgical procedure (e.g., esthetic liposuction, cesarean section, laparoscopic appendicectomy, excision of a skin lesion or even cardiac catheterization), minor trauma, seemingly insignificant scratches, in the presence of a chronic wound, or even in apparently intact skin.[7–13] NF occurs predominantly in middle-aged individuals, although the pediatric population may also be affected.[4,14–18] Patients with underlying diabetes mellitus, chronic alcoholism, cirrhosis, and iatrogenic immunosuppression are particularly susceptible.[1,3,7,14,19–23] NF is a well-recognized complication of childhood varicella.[17,18,24,25] Many reported cases have developed after intramuscular injection of non-steroidal anti-inflammatory drugs (NSAIDs), which may, in turn, mask the symptoms of evolving NF; an association with the intake of oral NSAIDs has also been documented.[7,14,26–29] Rare cases have occurred following the bite of a spider.[30] NF may be a rare complication of fistulating Crohn disease.[31] Reported mortality ranges from 3.4% to 53%.[3,5–7,14,17,25] An increased fatality rate may be encountered in the elderly and in those with worsening symptoms and signs within the first 48 hours of hospital admission.[19]

Although group A β-hemolytic streptococci (so-called 'flesh-eating' bacteria) were first recognized as a prime etiological agent, a number of other aerobic and even anaerobic pathogens have been implicated.[4,32,33] It has become increasingly apparent that NF very often is a polymicrobial condition. In some series, *Staphylococcus aureus* is the most frequently cultured organism.[33,34] Less often, other streptococci have been identified; these include group B and group G β-hemolytic streptococci, *Streptococcus pneumoniae*, anaerobic streptococci (*Peptostreptococcus* spp.), and *S. dysgalactiae* subsp. *equisimilis*; the latter is a recently recognized cause of NF and shares approximately 70% of its genome with group A *Streptococcus*, but lacks some of the virulence factors of the latter organism.[27,33,35–38] Other bacteria implicated include marine organisms (*Vibrio vulnificus*, *V. parahaemolyticus*, *Photobacterium damsela*), members of the family Enterobacteriaceae, *Serratia marcescens*, *Pseudomonas* spp., *Clostridium* spp., and *Bacteroides* spp.[15,21,33,39,40–48] There have also been isolated reports of NF due to *Haemophilus influenzae* serotype f, *Myroides odoratus* and *Aeromonas sorbia*.[49–51] *Candida albicans* is an exceptionally uncommon cause of NF.[52] Meleney postoperative progressive synergistic gangrene (Meleney gangrene) is synonymous with polymicrobial NF arising as a complication of surgical trauma.[53] The latter condition may be clinically indistinguishable from post-surgical cutaneous amebiasis.[53,54]

The clinical presentation may be fulminant, acute, or subacute.[14] NF commences as an ill-defined area of erythema, accompanied by tenderness, swelling, and increased temperature.[2,55] It is, therefore, not uncommon for evolving NF to be mistaken for cellulitis or an insignificant wound infection, especially when the hallmark cutaneous necrosis is not established. This may result in a potentially life-threatening delay in diagnosis and aggressive surgical debridement, and a high index of suspicion, therefore, is required.[1,2,56] The clinical features of established NF include severe pain, indurated edema, skin necrosis, cyanosis, bullae (which may be hemorrhagic, especially in cases caused by *Vibrio* spp.), crepitation, muscle weakness, and malodorous exudates (*Fig. 18.108*).[1,2,23,28,42,55] Anesthesia may be a late sign.[55] Patients often have other systemic manifestations of severe sepsis, including hypotension, tachycardia, tachypnea, oliguria, and mental confusion.[28,57] In NF caused by streptococcal species, the latter signs are usually attributable to streptococcal toxic shock syndrome.[26,58] Radiographs may reveal gas in the affected soft tissues, although this is only seen in approximately 25% of cases.[2,57] NF occurs mainly on the extremities, although almost any site may be affected, including the abdominal wall, chest wall, eyelids and periorbital region, and the head and neck region.[19,58,59–62] Periumbilical NF may occur in newborn infants.[16,18] The Waterhouse-Friderichsen syndrome is a potential complication of NF.[63]

Fournier gangrene is a clinical variant of NF which involves the penis, scrotum, perineum, and abdominal wall in men and (less often) the vulva in women.[64–69] An obliterative endarteritic process affecting the small branches of the superficial branch of the internal pudendal artery may play a key pathogenetic role.[68,70] Because of a response to corticosteroids, Fournier gangrene may be perceived as a localized vasculitis.[71] In addition to the usual risk factors such as diabetes mellitus or immunosuppression, rare associations include vasectomy or unhygienic ritual circumcision.[66] Hypertension, alcoholism, and advanced age are further risk factors.[69] The

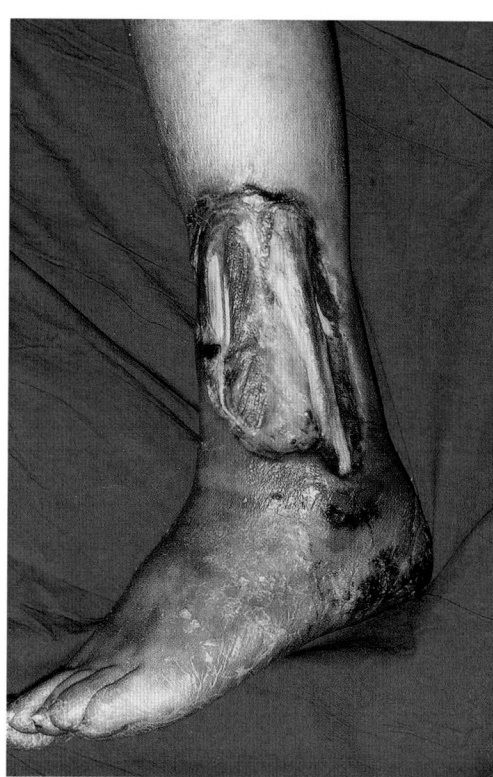

Fig. 18.108
Necrotizing fasciitis: this example has resulted in exposure of muscle and tendons. By courtesy of R.A. Marsden, MD, St George's Hospital, London, UK.

reported mortality of this polymicrobial synergistic necrotizing infection is in the order of 16–20%, although this ranges from 3% to as high as 80% in various series.[64,66,68,69,72] Extent of infection is a significant predictor of clinical outcome.[72]

Pathogenesis and histologic features

NF due to invasive group A β-hemolytic streptococcal infection is associated predominantly with M types 1 and 3, which produce either pyrogenic exotoxin A or B, or both.[32] Tissue invasion is facilitated by CD44-mediated cell signaling with subsequent manipulation of the host cytoskeleton.[73,74] Superantigens and Th1 cytokines appear to play a critical role in severe group A invasive streptococcal infections.[75] Streptococcal cysteine protease SpeB inactivates the antimicrobial peptide cathelicidin LL-37 at the bacterial surface.[76] Impaired recruitment of polymorphonuclear leukocytes to the site of the infection has been linked to the streptococcal peptidase ScpC which degrades IL-8.[77] It has been shown that a hyper-virulent phenotype ensues as a result of the organism's destruction of its own covRS two-component system; the latter exercises a negative regulatory effect on numerous virulence factor genes.[38] Protein S deficiency may be responsible for the necrosis.[78] *S. aureus* may potentiate the β-hemolytic streptococcal infection in NF.[54]

An adequately sized specimen including subcutaneous soft tissue is essential for diagnosis. The histologic appearances are those of a severe necrotizing process with edema, necrosis, and inflammation involving skin and subcutaneous tissue, including fascial planes (*Figs 18.109* and *18.110*).[79] Deep biopsies or debridement specimens containing underlying skeletal muscle may exhibit concomitant myonecrosis.[4] Vascular thrombosis is encountered at all levels, and secondary vasculitic alterations are not uncommon. Hyaline necrosis of sweat glands has been described.[79] The presence of large numbers of bacteria often results in diffuse basophilia of the tissue on low-power examination. A Gram or Brown-Hopps stain confirms the latter (*Fig. 18.111*).

Although the histologic picture is sufficiently distinctive to facilitate a diagnosis of NF, microbiological examination (including aerobic and anaerobic tissue culture) is of paramount importance in the identification of the specific infective etiological agent(s). Intraoperative frozen section has

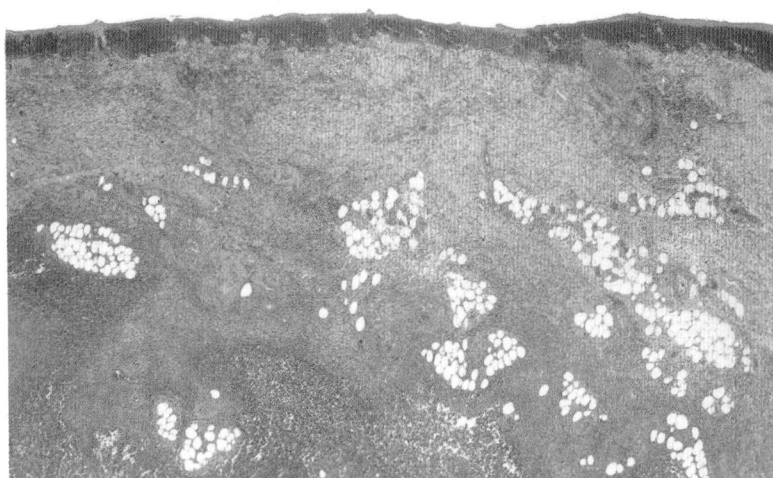

Fig. 18.109
Necrotizing fasciitis: there is intense acute inflammation of the dermis and subcutaneous fat.

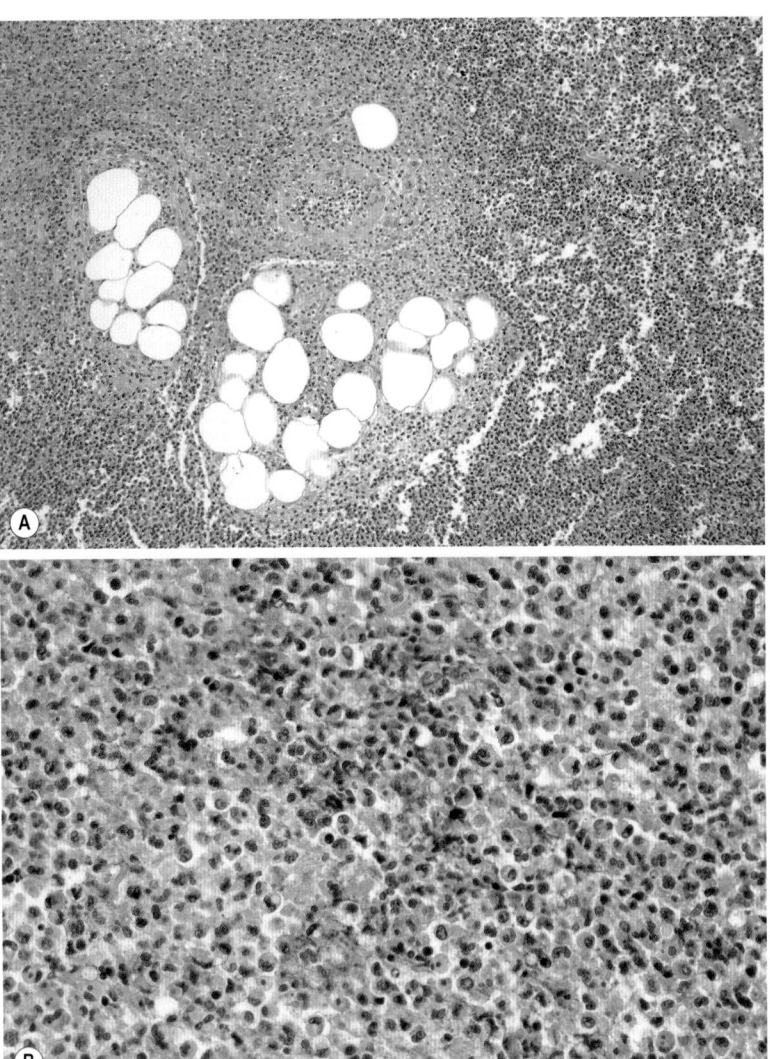

Fig. 18.110
Necrotizing fasciitis: there is an almost pure neutrophil infiltrate with necrosis.

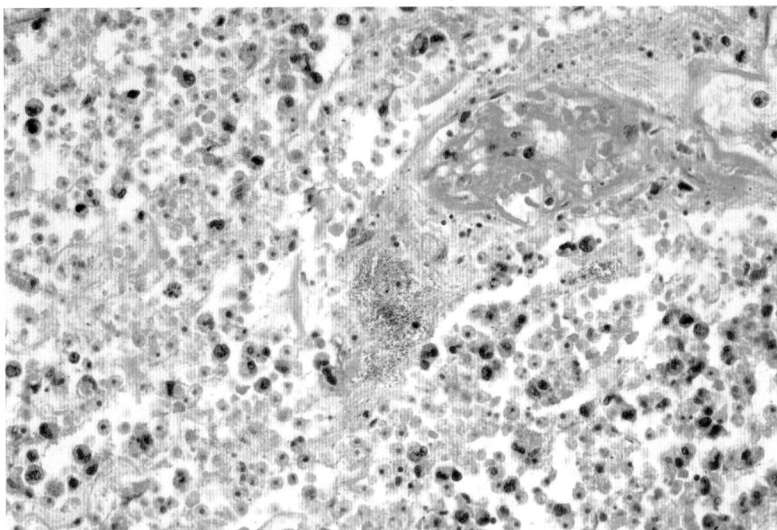

Fig. 18.111
Necrotizing fasciitis: innumerable Gram-positive cocci are present.

a particularly useful role to play, not only in early diagnosis but also in assessing the viability of surgical margins at the time of debridement.[80] PCR detection of streptococcal pyrogenic exotoxin B may be useful in confirming group A streptococcal infection when cultures are negative or unavailable.[81]

Differential diagnosis

Necrotizing (gangrenous) cellulitis has a similar etiopathogenesis to NF but shows no extension of the necrotizing inflammatory process into subcutaneous tissue planes. This diagnosis should be made with caution and only when there is a complete absence of subcutaneous involvement in a specimen that is of sufficient depth. NF is invariably associated with necrotizing inflammation of the dermis. Furthermore, necrotizing cellulitis may be a harbinger of impending NF.

Angioinvasive deep fungal infections such as aspergillosis, hyalohyphomycosis, and mucormycosis may be associated with extensive cutaneous and subcutaneous tissue necrosis. The causative organisms in such cases, however, are often visible on careful examination of routine H&E sections, and are readily identified with the aid of appropriate histochemical stains.

Tissue autolysis with bacterial overgrowth may closely mimic NF, especially if tissue is obtained from a patient with a relatively minor cutaneous infection and the specimen was not placed in the appropriate formalin fixative prior to submission to the laboratory.

NF is distinguished from pyoderma gangrenosum and Sweet syndrome by the absence of true tissue necrosis and demonstrable bacterial organisms by culture or appropriate stains in the latter two conditions. Although there is frequent dermal infiltration by polymorphonuclear leukocytes in pyoderma gangrenosum and invariable neutrophilic dermatosis in Sweet syndrome, the acute inflammatory changes in both conditions are generally centered on the dermis rather than the subcutis. Vasculitic alterations may occur in both pyoderma gangrenosum and NF but are usually absent in Sweet syndrome.

Extravasation of anthracycline chemotherapeutic agents such as doxorubicin may be associated with extensive necrosis of skin and subcutaneous tissues, with a resultant histologic picture distinctly reminiscent of NF. The clinical history and negative Gram stain, however, argue against NF in such cases.

Infective folliculitis

Clinical features

Infection of hair follicles is probably the commonest form of skin infection. It is usually due to *S. aureus* (impetigo of Bockhart) and, although disfiguring, is self-limiting.[1–8] Pustular folliculitis usually implies infection of the ostium and upper part of the follicle. It presents as numerous small red and tender pustules, which discharge pus and quickly resolve without scarring

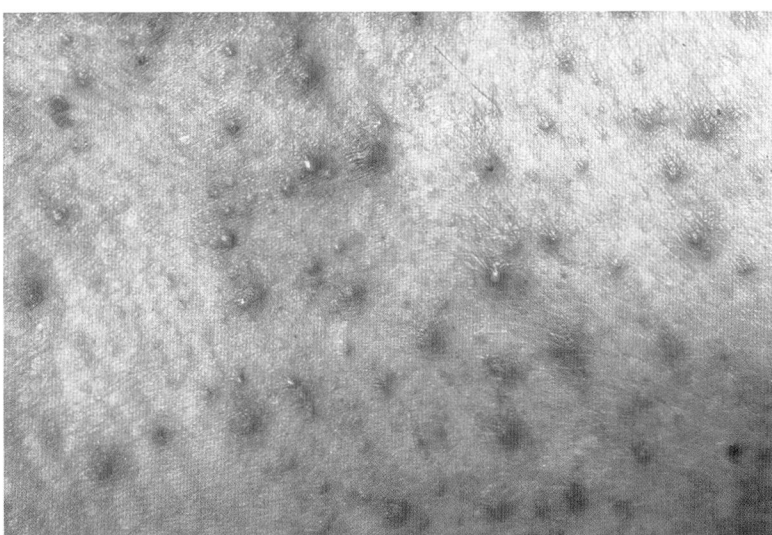

Fig. 18.112
Folliculitis: characteristic small pustules with surrounding erythema. By courtesy of R.A. Marsden, MD, St George's Hospital, London, UK.

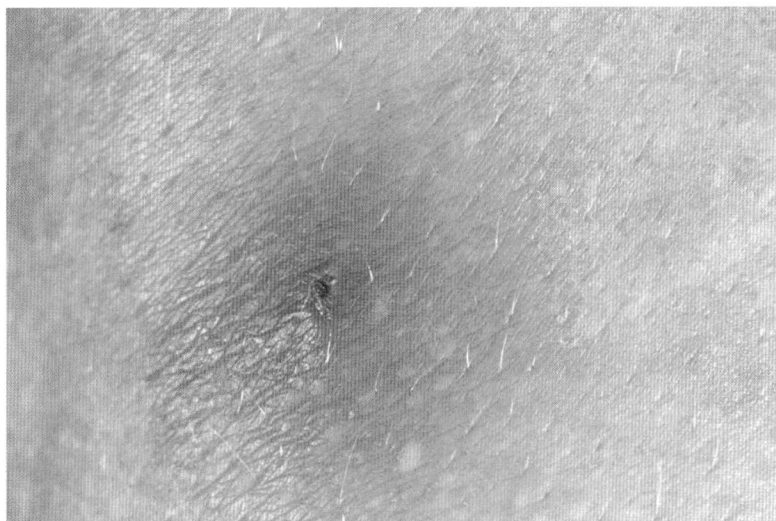

Fig. 18.113
Furuncle: early lesion characterized by edema and erythema. By courtesy of the Institute of Dermatology, London, UK.

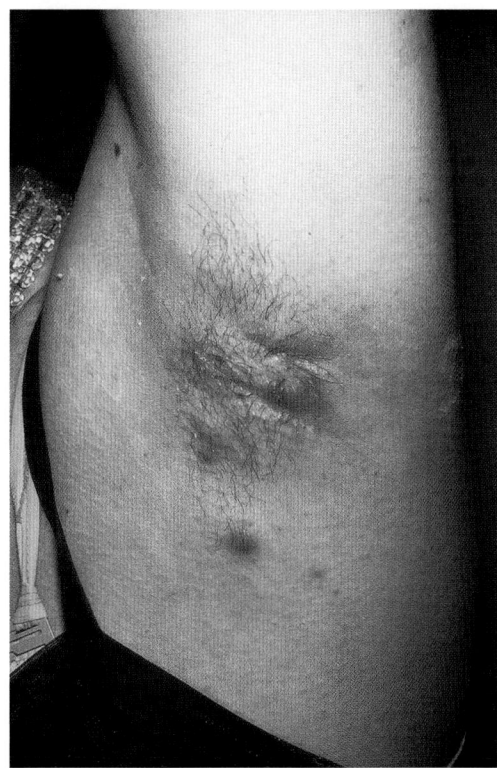

Fig. 18.114
Furuncle: multiple erythematous nodules in the axilla, which is a commonly affected site. The lesions are exquisitely painful. By courtesy of R.A. Marsden, MD, St George's Hospital, London, UK.

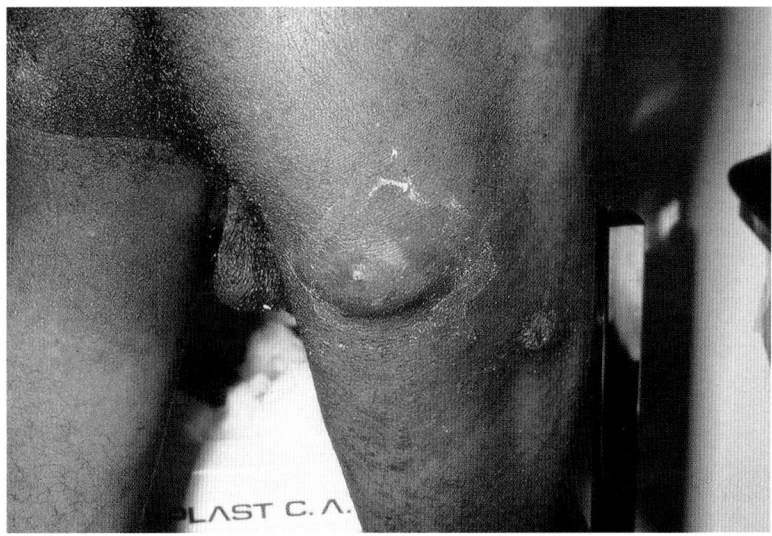

Fig. 18.115
Furuncle: note the large swelling on the thigh. This patient was HIV positive. By courtesy of C. Furlonge, MD, Port of Spain, Trinidad.

(*Fig. 18.112*). Staphylococcal carriers tend to have recurrent infections.[9] The role of community-associated CA-MRSA in cutaneous infections, including folliculitis, has been emphasized in recent years.[10,11]

P. aeruginosa is a well-recognized cause of epidemics of folliculitis associated with swimming pools, whirlpools, or spa baths.[12–14] These shared facilities can be infected by *Pseudomonas* if they became alkaline and if the chlorine content drops. Nevertheless, moisture and occlusion are necessary to affect normal skin. For this reason, lesions of this type are found only under the area covered by bathing costumes. Other Gram-negative bacteria such as *Klebsiella* spp., *Escherichia coli*, *Enterobacter* spp., and *Proteus* spp. have been implicated in the pathogenesis of folliculitis in patients receiving long-term antibiotic therapy for treatment of acne or rosacea.[15] Extensive folliculitis may be an early manifestation of HIV infection.[1] *Micrococcus* spp., which are considered commensal organisms, may be a cause of folliculitis in patients with HIV infection.[16] Folliculitis due to *Acinetobacter baumanii* has been reported in a patient with AIDS.[17]

A furuncle or boil is a more exuberant form of suppurative folliculitis. It is common in young adults and usually affects the skin of the face, neck, buttocks, and axillae (*Figs 18.113–18.115*).[1] Lesions can be up to 2 cm across and the inflammation is not confined within the follicle, but is associated with much surrounding erythema and often systemic symptoms.

After discharge of the pustular necrotic core, the lesion heals rapidly, but with scarring. A deep folliculitis due to *S. aureus* may affect the beard area; this form is termed sycosis or folliculitis barbae. CA-MRSA is strongly associated with recurrent furunculosis in the United States. Nasal carriage of *S. aureus* occurs in 60% of individuals and represents a major risk factor for the development of recurrent furunculosis.[11]

A carbuncle is a variant of a furuncle with multiple tracks and routes of discharge. It is most commonly seen in older men and may be associated with systemic symptoms.[1,5]

Acute paronychia is comparable to a folliculitis in that it is a painful suppurative infection of the nail fold, most commonly caused by *S. aureus*; it heals rapidly on release of the pus (*Fig. 18.116*). A rare scarring alopecia

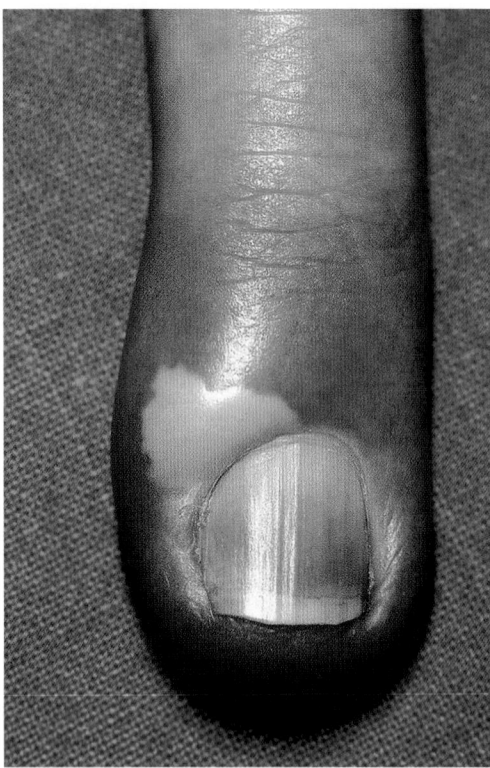

Fig. 18.116
Acute paronychia: pus and erythema are present. By courtesy of E.E. Gluckman, MD, King's College Hospital, London, UK.

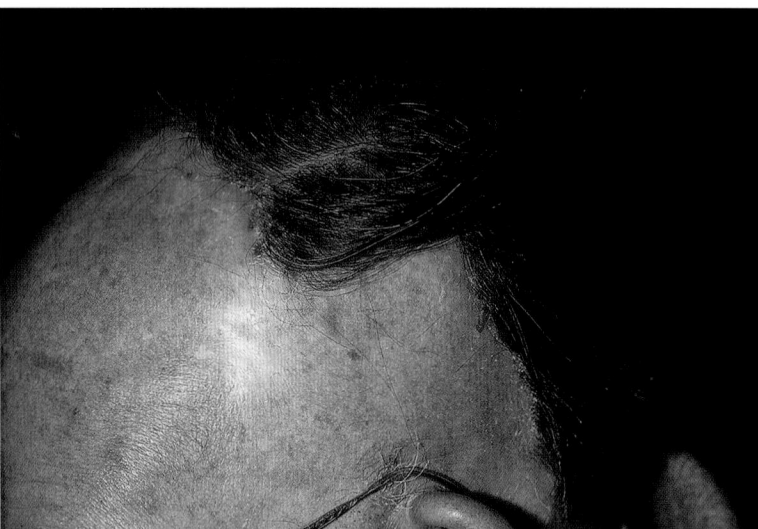

Fig. 18.117
Folliculitis decalvans: there is severe scarring with alopecia. Erosions, crusting, and pustules are seen at the hairline. By courtesy of M.M. Black, MD, Institute of Dermatology, London, UK.

in which *S. aureus* has been implicated is termed folliculitis decalvans.[18] However, an etiological link to the organism has not been demonstrated. Although the scalp is predominantly affected, lesions may also be found in the axillae and pubic region (*Fig. 18.117*). The latter condition is discussed in greater detail in the relevant chapter on diseases of the hair.

Pathogenesis and histologic features

Many cases of superficial suppurative folliculitis are associated with *S. aureus*. The infection is not due to a break in the epithelium, but growth occurs within the ostium of the follicle and may progress more deeply around the hair shaft. There is an associated accumulation of neutrophils, forming an abscess associated with spongiosis and infiltration of the adjacent follicular epithelium. The superficial suppurative folliculitis may discharge through the ostium and rapidly resolve. Alternatively, it may progress more deeply and rupture through the follicular epithelium; the abscess then extends into perifollicular dermis and surrounds the whole follicle. The follicular epithelium and hair shaft with pus then form the purulent necrotic core of the furuncle or boil. Healing is preceded by a lymphohistiocytic or even granulomatous phase and is followed by scarring and loss of hair in the involved area. A carbuncle is associated with more persistent suppuration, much more fibrosis, and granulation tissue. Panton-Valentine leukocidin-producing strains of *S. aureus* have been linked to the evolution of deep-seated, often multiple furuncles.[11,19]

Although most of the suppurative forms of folliculitis are due to *S. aureus*, other causal conditions include dermatophytosis, herpes simplex, and syphilis; the features of these infections are described under the appropriate headings elsewhere in this chapter.

Folliculitis keloidalis nuchae

Clinical features

This deep and scarring folliculitis and perifolliculitis (sometimes known as acne keloidalis or acne keloidalis nuchae) occurs on the back of the neck (lower occipital/nuchal region) of postpubertal males. It occurs more commonly in black than in white men. Although it was initially thought not to develop in females, rare cases have been reported.[1–4] It presents in the early stages with inflamed papules and pustules, but no consistent organisms are found. Patients may complain of itching, burning, or pain and advanced lesions may be foul smelling.[1] Each lesion is complicated by dense scarring, producing a keloid-like appearance. Scarring alopecia is a complication.[3] The condition has been reported in Caucasian organ transplant recipients on ciclosporine therapy.[5] Isolated cases occurring in association with keratosis follicularis spinulosa decalvans have been documented.[6,7]

Pathogenesis and histologic features

The pathogenesis is unknown. Any bacteria identified probably represent a secondary phenomenon. It is doubtful whether poor hygiene is a factor. There may be an element of pseudofolliculitis (see below) since the condition is common in Afro-Caribbeans and Africans and is worsened by close shaving of the neck.[1,2,8–10] The use of pomades and wearing tight collars is said to exacerbate the condition.[1] The term acne keloidalis is a misnomer, as the disorder has nothing to do with acne vulgaris or its variants and keloid formation is not usually seen.

The follicle, which may contain pus extending through the epithelium, is initially surrounded by a lymphocytic and neutrophil infiltrate; later, there are large numbers of plasma cells. The perifollicular inflammation is maximal at the level of the isthmus and lower infundibulum.[3,11] The condition is more often seen at a later stage, however, when there is marked fibrosis accompanying free, broken hair shafts, many of which are surrounded by a foreign body giant cell reaction. Hyalinization as seen in a true keloid is only very occasionally a feature. Complete loss of the sebaceous glands is a frequent occurrence.[3,11]

Pseudofolliculitis

Clinical features

Pseudofolliculitis (pseudofolliculitis barbae, pseudofolliculitis cutis) presents with an acneiform papular and pustular eruption on the beard area. Comedones are not a feature. It develops as a consequence of the reentry of a terminal hair shaft through the epidermis and occurs most often in males with curly hair, but is also seen in women in the pubic region following cosmetic shaving.[1–5] Pseudofolliculitis occurs predominantly in patients of African, African-American, and Hispanic origin.[2,3,6] The pathogenesis appears to be multifactorial, and seems to relate to the shape of the hair follicle, the hair cuticle, and the direction of hair growth.[3] The presence of curly hair and a single-nucleotide substitution in the gene encoding keratin 75 act in concert to confer an increased risk for the development of the condition.[2,7] The penetration is facilitated by the sharp ends produced on hairs by shaving and the curliness of the hair bringing the cut end back into contact with the skin surface.[5] Alternatively, the penetration may occur laterally through the superficial part of the follicular infundibulum following partial retraction of the hair after close shaving. A hypertrophic form of the disease has been described in renal transplant recipients.[8]

Histologic features

The process is not a true folliculitis, and is not usually associated with infection. The reentry of the hair shaft provokes a foreign body granulomatous reaction with accompanying fibrosis. The inflammation is predominantly histiocytic with occasional multinucleate giant cells. Secondary infection may result in superimposed suppuration. Resolution occurs rapidly, with slight scarring, once the hair shaft is removed.

Meningococcal septicemia

Clinical features

Meningococcal septicemia (meningococcemia) is due to the Gram-positive diplococcus *Neisseria meningitidis*.[1-6] In its acute form, this is a very serious condition with a high mortality, which affects children in seasonal epidemics. The infection may occasionally be encountered in adults.[6] Occurrence in the neonatal period, however, is rare.[7] The organism is spread via droplet inhalation from upper respiratory tract infections. Meningitis is the most frequently encountered manifestation of meningococcal infection. Children with acute meningococcal septicemia develop widespread purpura that shows a predilection for the trunk and limbs. Ecchymoses may also be a feature. In the more chronic variant (chronic meningococcemia), patients present with vasculitis-like lesions, particularly nodules, and palpable purpura.[8]

Pathogenesis and histologic features

The histologic features are essentially those of a leukocytoclastic vasculitis.[9] Superimposed DIC may also be present. The hemorrhagic skin lesions and vascular thromboses are attributable to up-regulation of tissue factor leading to coagulation, and by inhibition of fibrinolysis by plasminogen activator inhibitor.[10] Impairment of the protein C anticoagulation pathway also plays an important role.[11] Experimental evidence has revealed that adhesion of the organism to the dermal microvascular endothelium leads to local vascular damage, thrombosis, and purpura.[12] Capsular polysaccharides and lipooligosaccharides play key roles in the evasion of killing by host complement.[13]

Diplococci may be demonstrable in Gram-stained sections, especially in biopsies obtained from purpuric lesions.[9] Culture or Gram staining of aspirates or biopsies of skin lesions may facilitate early diagnosis.[14] Diagnosis can also be confirmed on skin biopsy with the aid of a PCR-based method.[15]

Gonorrhea

Clinical features

This common venereal disease is due to infection with the Gram-negative intracellular diplococcus *Neisseria gonorrhoeae*, which especially affects the mucous membranes. In males, this results particularly in purulent urethritis, although gonococcal proctitis, epididymitis, prostatitis, and oropharyngitis may also be seen. Females most often develop endocervicitis. Urethritis and proctitis can also be features.[1-3]

Systemic gonococcal infection most commonly affects the skin, but may also result in arthritis and less often endocarditis or meningitis.[1,3-5] Patients present with small numbers of erythematous macules that progress to painful papular, petechial, papulovesicular, or pustular lesions that particularly affect the distal limbs (*Fig. 18.118*).[4,6,7] They measure from 1–2 mm up to 2 cm in diameter. Lesions may appear frankly vasculitic.[8] Cutaneous lesions can be a presenting feature of disseminated infection during pregnancy.[5,9] Rarely, however, patients present with primary cutaneous (genital and extragenital) involvement.[4,6] Cellulitis, pustules, ulcers, and furuncle-like lesions

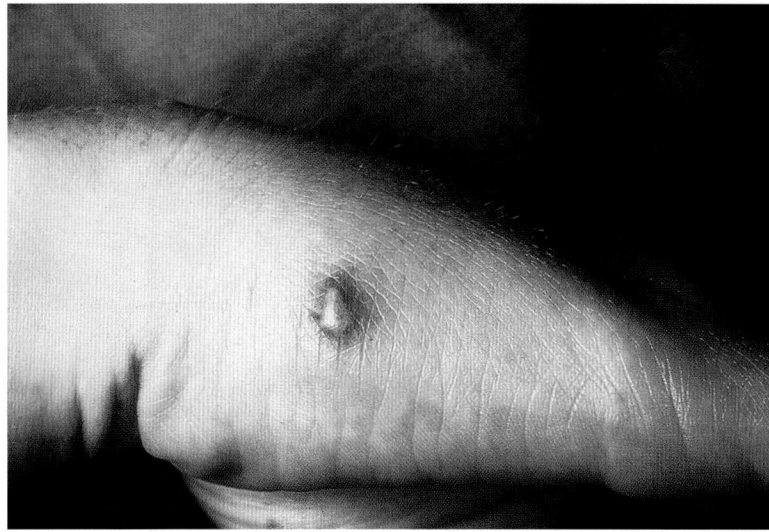

Fig. 18.118
Gonococcemia: pustules are commonly found on the hands and feet. By courtesy of R.N. Thin, MD, St Thomas' Hospital, London, UK.

have been documented.[10-12] Lobular capillary hemangioma (pyogenic granuloma)-like lesions of the penile shaft have also been described.[13] Primary digital gonorrhea has been recorded.[10]

Pathogenesis and histologic features

Disseminated lesions show variable epidermal changes ranging from edema accompanied by a neutrophil infiltrate with purpura, to vesiculation, pustulation, and eventually necrosis.[6] In the dermis, the histologic features are essentially those of a neutrophil-mediated acute vasculitis, often accompanied by thrombosis.[14] Very occasionally, Gram-negative diplococci may be identified.

Plague

Clinical features

Plague is an acute, febrile infectious disease caused by *Yersinia pestis*, a nonmotile, bipolar Gram-negative aerobic bacillus and one of the most deadly pathogens known to man.[1-6] Since the 1990s, the majority of human cases have been reported from Africa.[7] The disease has a high incidence in Uganda, the DRC, South Africa, Madagascar, and parts of India. Foci of plague have also been reported from the United States and in parts of South America.[1,2,7-11] Rodents act as the reservoir, and the infection is usually transmitted to humans via the bite of a flea; aerosol spread may also occur, leading to pneumonic plague.[1,3-5] *Y. pestis* is well recognized as a potential bioweapon and bioterrorism agent.[5,12] There are three distinct clinicopathological forms of the disease: bubonic plague, primary pneumonic plague, and primary septicemic plague.[1-4,6]

Bubonic plague

Bubonic plague accounts for the vast majority of cases. After a short incubation period of approximately 2–4 days, the disease manifests abruptly with pyrexia, chills, tachycardia, and tachypnea, and the formation of a so-called bubo – a painful, pathologically enlarged unilateral group of infected lymph nodes, usually in the groin or axilla (*Fig. 18.119*).[1] Cervical and axillary buboes are more common in children than in adults.[9] Septicemia and secondary pneumonic plague may follow in untreated cases. Minor ('ambulatory') forms of bubonic plague also exist.[1]

Primary pneumonic and primary septicemic plague

Primary pneumonic plague is acquired by inhalation of the organisms, whereas primary septicemic plague tends to occur after the bite of an infected flea on the head and neck region. Untreated, both of these forms of plague carry a mortality of around 90%.[2]

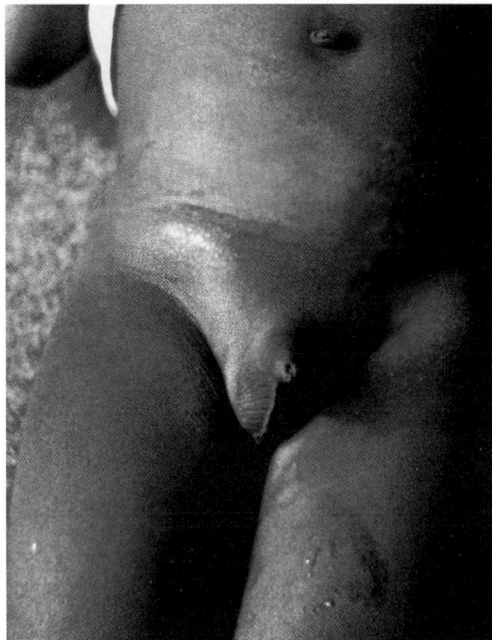

Fig. 18.119
Bubonic plague: note the inguinal lymphadenopathy (bubo). By courtesy of J. Frean, MD, and the late M. Isaäcson, MD, University of Witwatersrand, Johannesburg, South Africa.

Cutaneous manifestations

Cutaneous manifestations of *Y. pestis* infection are seen predominantly in bubonic plague. A small vesicle, pustule, papule, or necrotic lesion may develop at the site of the flea bite. The skin overlying the bubo is erythematous and edematous and may undergo hemorrhage and necrosis, resulting in the formation of fistulae.[1,2] Roseolar, scarlatiniform, vesicopustular, and erythema multiforme-like eruptions may occur elsewhere on the body.[1] Petechial hemorrhages and ecchymoses characterize severe cases. Cutaneous ulceration and necrosis may ensue, hence the term 'black death'.[2]

Histologic features

The lymph nodes comprising the buboes show severe acute hemorrhagic lymphadenitis in the presence of large amphophilic or 'ground-glass' aggregates of bacilli. Their characteristic 'safety-pin' appearance is discernible on sections stained with the Gramor Giemsa methods.[1,2] Extranodal extension results in ulceration of the overlying skin. Subsequent septicemic illness may be complicated by DIC. In the skin, the latter manifests with intradermal hemorrhage, thrombotic vascular occlusion, and multiple cutaneous infarcts.[2] The diagnosis may be confirmed by microscopy, culture, immunofluorescence, ELISA, or PCR.[1–4,9] An immunohistochemical method for detection of the organism in formalin-fixed, paraffin-embedded tissue has been described.[13]

Cutaneous anthrax

Clinical features

Anthrax is a zoonotic infection caused by *Bacillus anthracis*, an encapsulated, spore-forming, Gram-positive bacillus.[1–3] Although the condition is relatively uncommon in humans, epidemic outbreaks still occur in tropical and subtropical regions of the world (including Africa and South America), southern Europe, Turkey, the Middle East, and India.[2–8] Anthrax is very rarely seen in developed countries.[9–11] Cutaneous anthrax accounts for more than 95% of cases; pulmonary and gastrointestinal forms generally account for the remainder, and are associated with a high mortality.[2] Recent years, however, have seen the emergence of a fourth form of the disease – injection (injectional) anthrax. The latter occurs among users of intravenous drugs, notably heroin. All of the cases recorded thus far appear have occurred in Europe, and the infection is attributed to contamination of the heroin.[12–16]

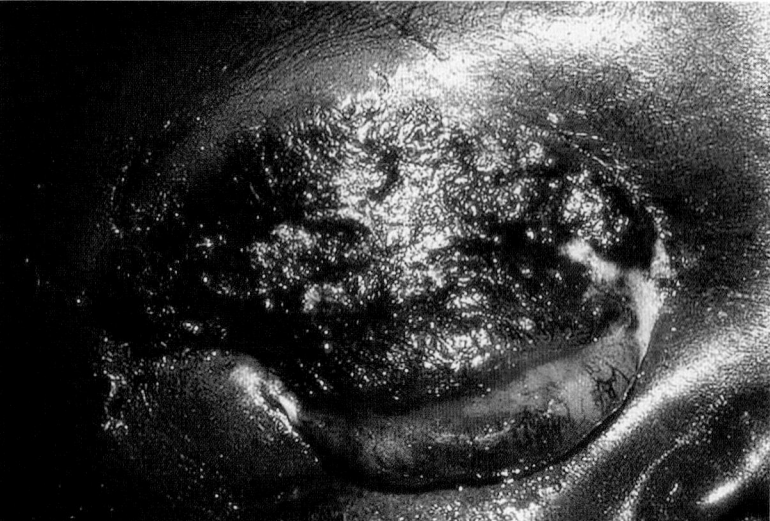

Fig. 18.120
Anthrax: cutaneous disease is the commonest manifestation in humans. This black crusted lesion is typical. By courtesy of J. Frean, MD, and the late M. Isaäcson, MD, University of Witwatersrand, Johannesburg, South Africa.

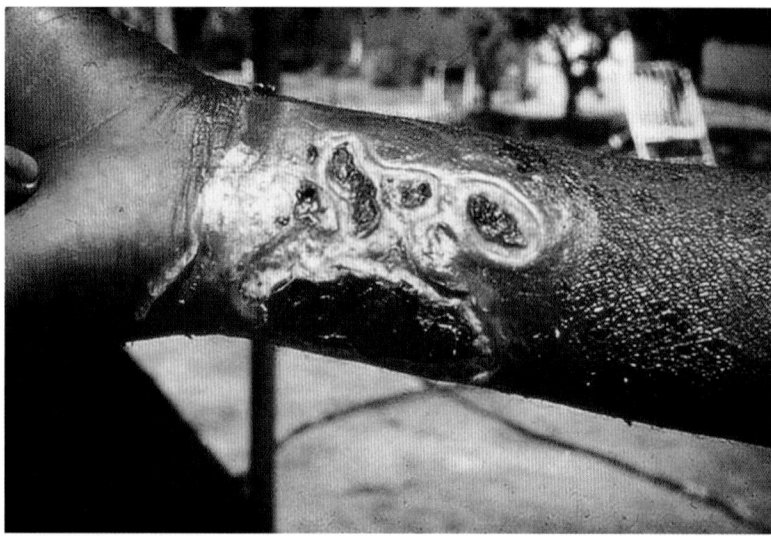

Fig. 18.121
Anthrax: multiple lesions on the forearm. By courtesy of J. Frean, MD, and the late M. Isaäcson, MD, University of Witwatersrand, Johannesburg, South Africa.

In its conventional form, the condition is usually acquired after contact with infected animals (herbivores) or contaminated animal products.[5] It has also been described in rural Turkish children who were subjected to the ritual smearing of cow's blood on their foreheads.[17] Under ideal conditions, spores may survive in the soil or in animal products for many years.[1,2] There is ongoing interest in the organism as an agent of bioterrorism.[11,18,19]

Cutaneous anthrax occurs after inoculation of *B. anthracis* into abraded skin. An erythematous macule or papule develops after an incubation period of 2–3 weeks. This later evolves into a pruritic vesicle. A characteristic black eschar develops after breakdown of the blister (*Figs 18.120 and 18.121*).[2,20,21] There is often pronounced edema and erythema of the surrounding skin, sometimes accompanied by the formation of bullae.[2,20] The infection may present with periorbital involvement.[22] Lymphadenitis is sometimes seen. Septicemia may arise in untreated cases; this carries a mortality of 10% to 20%.[2,3] Toxemic shock and renal failure have also been reported.[20,23] A rare form of the disease termed malignant edema presents with severe, rapidly spreading edema, lymphangitis, lymphadenitis, and systemic symptoms. Hemorrhagic and necrotic vesicles may evolve in these cases.[2,20] Complications documented among patients with injection anthrax

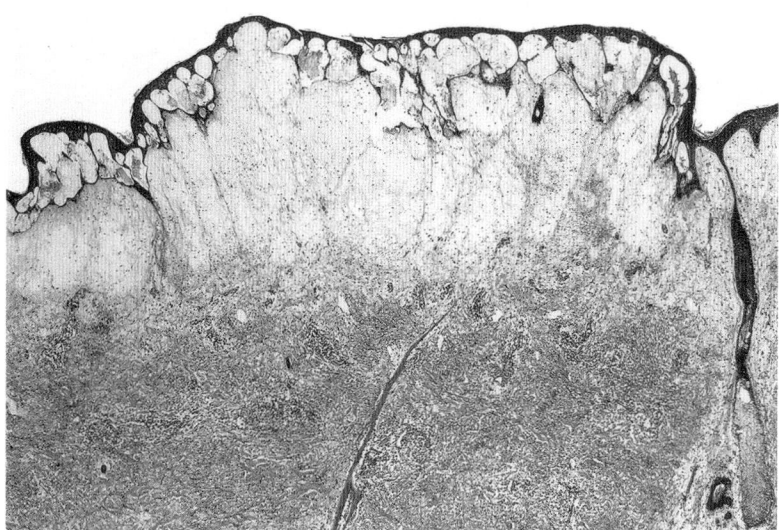

Fig. 18.122
Anthrax: there is massive subepidermal edema with subepidermal vesiculation. Reproduced with permission from Mallon E, McKee PH. Extraordinary case report: cutaneous anthrax. *American Journal of Dermatopathology*. 1997; 19: 79–82.

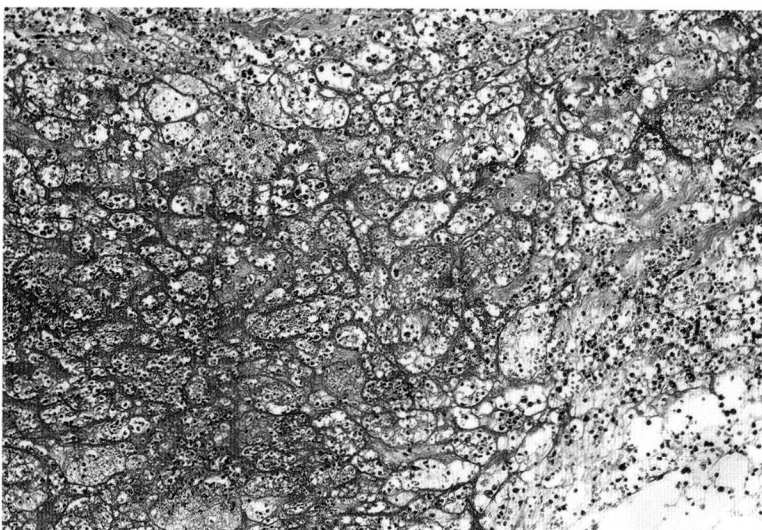

Fig. 18.123
Anthrax: marked fibrin deposition is evident. Reproduced with permission from Mallon E, McKee PH. Extraordinary case report: cutaneous anthrax. *American Journal of Dermatopathology*. 1997; 19: 79–82.

have included mulitorgan failure, compartment syndrome, NF, and lethal cervical cellulitis.[12,13,15] Injection anthrax carries a mortality of up to 37%.[16]

Pathogenesis and histologic features

B. anthracis is associated with potent virulence factors, namely, a poly-D-glutamic acid capsule with antiphagocytic properties, and a plasmid-encoded polypeptide protein exotoxin consisting of three components: edema factor (EF), protective antigenic factor (PA), and lethal factor (LF).[1,3,24] Anthrax toxin receptor 2 (ANTXR2) and capillary morphogenesis protein 2 (CMG2) are the major receptors for anthrax toxins.[1,25,26] Binding of PA to cellular receptors facilitates translocation of EF and LF into host cells, with subsequent alterations in cell signaling pathways.[1] EF leads to increased vascular permeability via the production or release of inflammatory mediators, including neurokinins, prostanoids, and histamine.[27]

The histologic picture is dominated by massive subepidermal edema (*Fig. 18.122*).[9,28] Intraepidermal edema results in coalescent intercellular vacuoles.[2] The epidermis is often attenuated. The dermis is expanded by a dense inflammatory infiltrate consisting of large numbers of polymorphonuclear leukocytes, admixed with lymphocytes and histiocytes. The process often extends into subcutaneous fat.[9] Vasodilatation may be prominent. Hemorrhage and fibrin deposition occur in the deep dermis and subcutis (*Fig. 18.123*). Thrombotic vascular occlusion and fibrinoid necrosis of blood vessel walls may be encountered in the deep dermis and subcutaneous fat (*Fig. 18.124*). A Gram stain will reveal considerable numbers of large Gram-positive bacilli predominantly in the superficial dermis (*Fig. 18.125*).[9] The diagnosis is confirmed by culture. Serological investigations are also available. Immunohistochemical methods of detection may be used on tissue specimens.[3]

Brucellosis

Clinical features

Brucellosis is a zoonotic infection by *Brucella* spp. such as *B. melitensis*, *B. abortus*, *B. canis*, and *B. suis*.[1–3] The organism is a Gram-negative bacillus, and infection is acquired either by ingesting contaminated, unpasteurized milk/milk products, or by handling infected animal products (contact brucellosis). Human-to-human transmission does not occur. Brucellosis results in either an acute febrile illness or a chronic systemic disease characterized by fever, malaise, sweats, arthralgia, myalgia, and/or hepatosplenomegaly.[1–3] Although the disease is endemic in several countries bordering the Mediterranean Sea, the majority of reports of human infection appear to have come

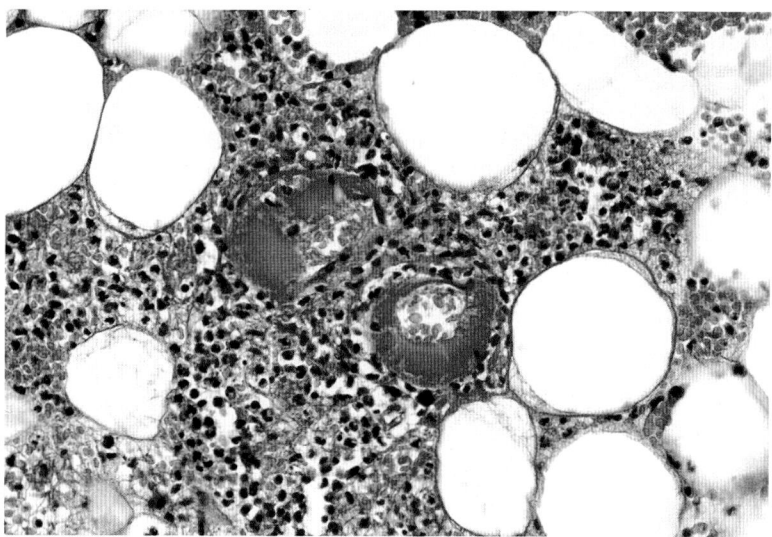

Fig. 18.124
Anthrax: thrombosed vessels are present. Reproduced with permission from Mallon E, McKee PH. Extraordinary case report: cutaneous anthrax. *American Journal of Dermatopathology*. 1997; 19: 79–82.

from Turkey and the Middle East.[4–6] The mortality is low and most patients recover within 3 months.[3]

Cutaneous manifestations occur in approximately 6% or less of cases; however, this figure approached 14% in a series from Turkey.[5,7–9] A number of cutaneous manifestations have been recorded, including a disseminated papulonodular eruption, a diffuse maculopapular rash, erythema nodosum-like subcutaneous nodules, purpura, leukocytoclastic vasculitis, erythema multiforme, urticaria-like papules and plaques, multiple abscesses, cutaneous ulcers, ecchymoses and (rarely) livedo reticularis, palmar erythema, or an even large mass mimicking a soft tissue tumor.[3,5,7,8,10–17] Vasculitic skin lesions may form part of an infection-induced systemic thrombotic microangiopathy mimicking Henoch-Schönlein purpura.[18,19] There is a single case report of *Brucella*-associated Stevens-Johnson syndrome.[20] Contact brucellosis manifests with erythema or pruritus, usually on the forearm or hand. In some cases, this may progress to a follicular, vesicular, or pustular eruption.[3] A rare case of contiguous skin involvement secondary to underlying *Brucella* chronic osteomyelitis has been recorded.[21] A factitious case of brucellosis caused by autoinoculation has also been reported; the patient developed bacteremia and ulcerating cutaneous abscesses.[22]

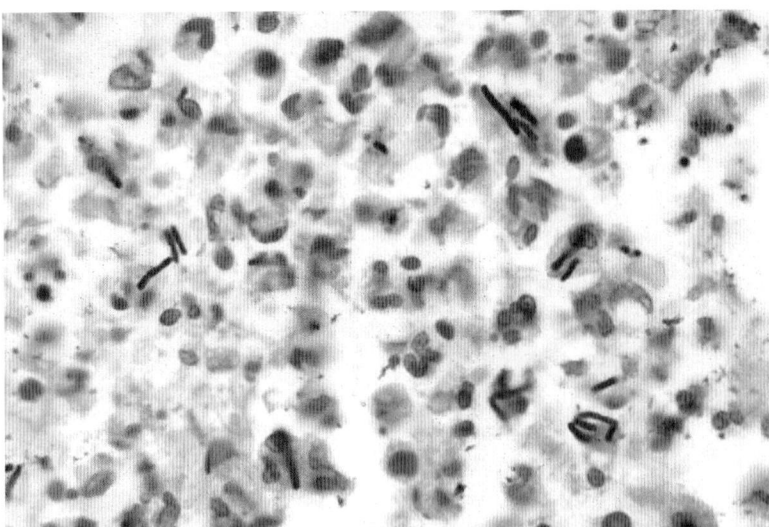

Fig. 18.125
Anthrax: numerous elongated Gram-positive bacilli are present. Reproduced with permission from Mallon E, McKee PH. Extraordinary case report: cutaneous anthrax. *American Journal of Dermatopathology*. 1997; 19: 79–82.

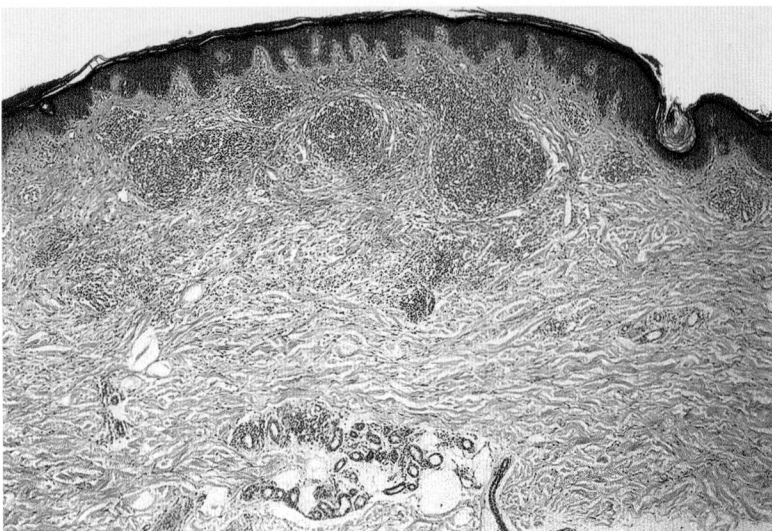

Fig. 18.126
Cat scratch disease: an irregular ill-defined focus of necrobiosis is surrounded by a nodular lymphocytic infiltrate.

Histologic features

The histologic features vary according to the type of cutaneous lesion biopsied. Biopsies obtained from the erythematous papular and maculopapular lesions show a perivascular and periadnexal infiltrate of lymphocytes and histiocytes, sometimes accompanied by epithelioid histiocytes and multinucleated giant cells.[7,11] Erythrocyte extravasation is sometimes seen, and inflammatory cells may infiltrate the overlying epidermis.[10] Erythema nodosum-like nodules are characterized by a perivascular lymphohistiocytic infiltrate centered on the deep dermis and superficial subcutis.[7,12] There is associated vascular endothelial swelling and luminal thrombosis, sometimes with foci of necrosis. Accompanying granulomatous inflammation is not uncommon.[10] Erythema multiforme lesions and leukocytoclastic vasculitic lesions exhibit the usual histologic changes associated with these conditions.

Brucella organisms are rarely visualized in histologic material. The diagnosis is therefore confirmed by culture, serology or, PCR.[1,3,7,10,23]

Diseases caused by *Bartonella* species

Cat scratch disease

Clinical features

Cat scratch disease is a not uncommon, usually self-limiting illness which, as its name implies, usually follows (after 3–5 days) a scratch or bite by a cat (usually a kitten).[1–7] On rare occasions, it has been reported following a similar injury caused by a dog or even by a monkey.[4] It occurs equally in males and females, most often during the first two decades.[8] Cat scratch disease shows seasonal variation, occurring usually in autumn and winter.[1] The causative agent is *Bartonella henselae* (formerly *Rochalimaea henselae*), a weakly Gram-negative bacillus measuring 1–2 μm in length.[5,6] The condition was first described in 1950, yet the nature of the infective etiological agent remained elusive until relatively recently.[6] In the past, a variety of infectious agents had been suggested as responsible for cat scratch disease, including mycobacteria, *Chlamydia*, herpes-like viruses, and latterly, *Afipia felis*.[5,9] The cat represents the primary reservoir for the bacillus in addition to being its principal vector.[10] Although transmission among cats is via the cat flea, the latter does not appear to play a direct role in transmission to humans.[5,6]

The primary skin lesion – a macule, papule, vesicle, pustule, or nodule – develops most commonly on the arm or hand, followed by the head, leg, conjunctiva, trunk or neck, in decreasing order of frequency. Sometimes more than one member of a family may be affected. The cutaneous lesions measure 1–5 mm or more in diameter and may sometimes resemble an insect bite.[1]

Other rare cutaneous manifestations include a nonpruritic macular or maculopapular rash, erythema nodosum, urticaria, erythema marginatum, erythema annulare, and thrombocytopenic purpura. A case with cutaneous lesions resembling those of Sweet syndrome has been reported.[11] Fever and malaise are occasional symptoms. Less common additional features include headache, nausea, vomiting, arthralgia, and splenomegaly.

Patients invariably develop lymphadenopathy in the drainage region, usually within 1–3 weeks of the initial lesion. The enlarged nodes are tender and often persistent, with lymphadenopathy lasting up to 2 months or more. Suppuration is not uncommon. Conjunctival or eyelid lesions may be associated with preauricular lymphadenopathy (Parinaud syndrome).[12] The only consistently abnormal laboratory function test is a moderately raised erythrocyte sedimentation rate. Purported cases of disseminated cat scratch disease occurring as a manifestation of AIDS probably represent examples of advanced BA (see below).[13,14]

Atypical manifestations of cat scratch disease may occur in as many as 25% of cases.[5,8] These include nonthrombocytopenic purpura and bone, liver, spleen, pulmonary, endocardial, and/or neurological involvement, presumably due to bacteremia.[1,5,8] A vasculitic pathogenesis has also been proposed.[15] CNS lesions have significant morbidity and include coma, encephalitis, convulsions, pareses, cerebellar signs, and abnormal tendon jerks.[16,17] Hepatosplenic infection results in peliosis.[5,6]

Histologic features

The histopathological features are those of dermal necrobiosis.[16] The necrobiotic foci are round, triangular, or stellate and are surrounded by a palisade of histiocytes with occasional multinucleate giant cells (*Figs 18.126* and *18.127*). Around the periphery of the histiocytic zone is a lymphocytic infiltrate in which eosinophils may be conspicuous. Nuclear debris may sometimes be prominent. The bacteria may often be identified using the Warthin-Starry reaction or the Brown-Hopps modified Gram stain within histiocytes or lying free.[18–21] Bacteria may also be detected immunocytochemically.[1,22] In the adjacent dermis, the blood vessels are surrounded by an infiltrate consisting of lymphocytes, plasma cells, and histiocytes. A granulomatous reaction has been described, but this is an uncommon phenomenon.[23]

In early lesions, the lymph nodes show subcapsular foci of necrosis associated with a neutrophil polymorph infiltrate. An established infection is characterized by extensive necrotic lesions often involving the follicular germinal centers and associated with karyorrhexis. A peripheral rim of epithelioid cells and occasional giant cells is characteristic. These features are not

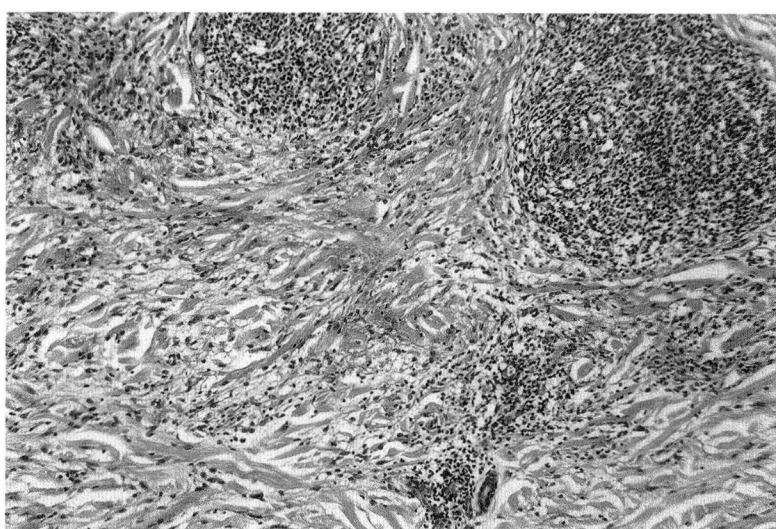

Fig. 18.127
Cat scratch disease: close-up view of the necrobiosis in *Fig. 18.126*.

in themselves diagnostic because they may be seen in a variety of conditions including lymphogranuloma venereum, yersiniosis, and fungal infections.[2]

Previously, the diagnosis of cat scratch disease was confirmed by a positive delayed hypersensitivity reaction to the cat scratch disease antigen.[1] Since *B. henselae* is difficult to culture, serology, and currently PCR have been advocated as more reliable diagnostic modalities.[5,6,24] The organism may be identified in skin swabs obtained from the primary inoculation site.[25]

Trench fever

Clinical features

Although a major epidemic of trench fever was documented during the First World War, more recent outbreaks of this condition have been described among homeless people, in whom there is a high seroprevalence of this bacteremic illness.[1,2] Outbreaks have also occurred in overpopulated Central African refugee camps.[3] Trench fever is caused by *Bartonella quintana*; human body lice (*Pediculus humanus* var. *corporis*) are the known vectors.[1,2,4] Head lice (*P. humanus* var. *capitis*) might also play a role in the transmission of the disease.[5,6] *B. quintana* may also cause chronic bacteremia, endocarditis, and BA (see below).[4,7]

Patients present with non-specific symptoms and signs including headache, malaise, pyrexia, rigors, tachycardia, myalgia, arthralgia, and injected conjunctivae. An erythematous macular or papular skin rash may occur. The rash is often seen on the trunk and usually lasts no more than a day or two.[8] The disease is rarely fatal, except in some debilitated patients. Relapsing illness sometimes occurs, and the organism may remain latent in the host for a number of years following the acute infection.[8]

Histologic features

The histopathological features in the skin are non-specific. There is a perivascular lymphocytic infiltrate, without evidence of vascular thrombosis.[8] Organisms are not usually demonstrable in routinely stained skin biopsy specimens. Dermal vascular proliferation and neutrophilic infiltration (as seen in BA) are not features of trench fever. The diagnosis is confirmed by serology, culture, or PCR.[9]

Bartonellosis

Clinical features

Bartonellosis (Carrión disease) is a biphasic disease caused by *Bartonella bacilliformis*, an organism that is closely related to *B. henselae* and *B. quintana*.[1-5] The initial stage of infection (hematic phase) is referred to as Oroya fever. Patients are acutely ill with pyrexia, rigors, myalgia, and a

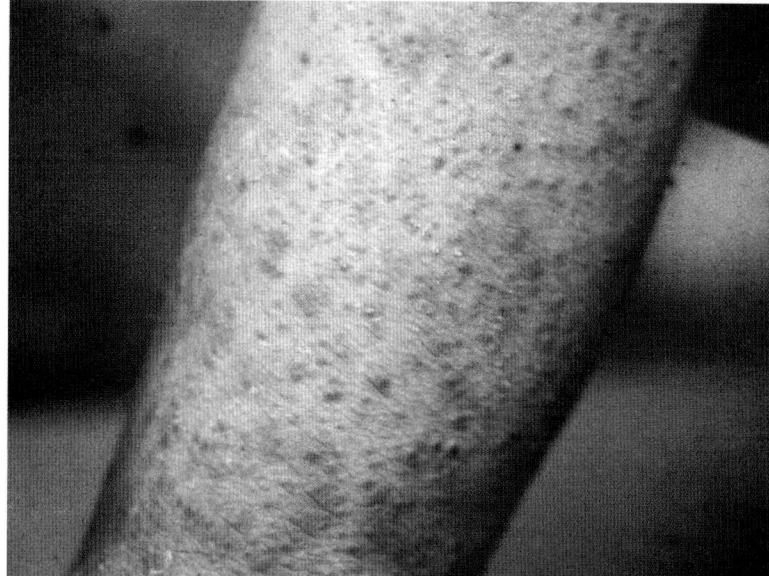

Fig. 18.128
Verruga peruana: widespread papules are present. By courtesy of F. von Lichtenberg, MD, Brigham and Women's Hospital and Harvard Medical School, Boston, USA.

severe hemolytic anemia. The last is attributable to infection of the circulating erythrocytes and can be confirmed with the aid of a blood smear. The case fatality rate among untreated patients may exceed 80% during acute outbreaks. Later, the disease enters an eruptive phase characterized by the evolution of numerous papular, nodular, or verrucous vascular skin lesions, referred to as verruga peruana (Peruvian wart, cutaneous verrucous disease).[2,4-6] These occur predominantly on the face and extremities (*Fig. 18.128*). Atypical cases may present with verrucous skin lesions as the sole manifestation.[2] Most lesions resolve spontaneously.[3] Genital lesions and nasal mucosal involvement have been recorded.[7]

The condition is endemic in the higher altitude regions of Peru, where it was first described in the nineteenth century. Carrión disease also occurs in Ecuador and Colombia.[5,8,9] Outbreaks have also been recorded in non-endemic parts of Peru.[10] It has been suggested that the condition may be underreported in some endemic areas because of the existence of mild infection by less virulent strains of *B. bacilliformis*.[2,10] The sand fly, *Lutzomyia* (*Phlebotomus*) *verrucarum* is the apparent vector.[8]

Pathogenesis and histologic features

There is infection of endothelial cells and circulating erythrocytes following introduction of *B. bacilliformis* via the bite of the vector. In the cutaneous verruga peruana lesions, organisms are detectable in the extracellular spaces, where they induce angiogenesis by producing putative microbial-encoded or microbial-induced angiogenic factors.[1,11] In vitro studies have shown that *B. bacilliformis* exercises a mitogenic effect on human vascular endothelial cells. GroEL produced by the organism regulates endothelial cell growth.[12,13] Others have observed that infection leads to the production of angiopoietin-2 by endothelial cells, and the production of VEGF by epidermal cells.[14] The dermal angiomatous proliferation appears to occur in concert with the reactivation of latent *B. bacilliformis* organisms.[1]

Histopathological examination of the verrucous lesions reveals an exuberant intradermal capillary proliferation lined by swollen endothelial cells, often accompanied by a neutrophilic infiltrate (*Fig. 18.129*). Some of the superficial and peripheral vessels may be dilated, whereas deep dermal or subcutaneous nodules tend to have a more compact vascular and endothelial cell proliferation.[3,15] Occasional cases harbor a cytologically atypical endothelial proliferation, resulting in potential confusion with malignant vascular tumors.[16] There is a background mixed inflammatory cell infiltrate of variable intensity comprising neutrophils, histiocytes, lymphocytes, and plasma cells. Careful examination of the endothelial cells in early lesions may reveal characteristic intracytoplasmic aggregates of *B. bacilliformis*,

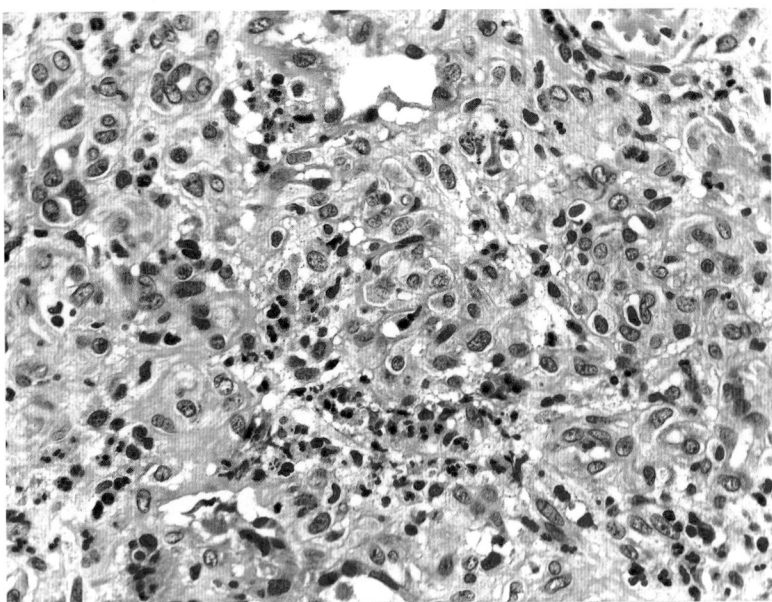

Fig. 18.129
Verruga peruana: there is an exuberant vascular proliferation, with endothelial prominence and a background neutrophilic infiltrate. By courtesy of F. Bravo, MD, Lima, Peru.

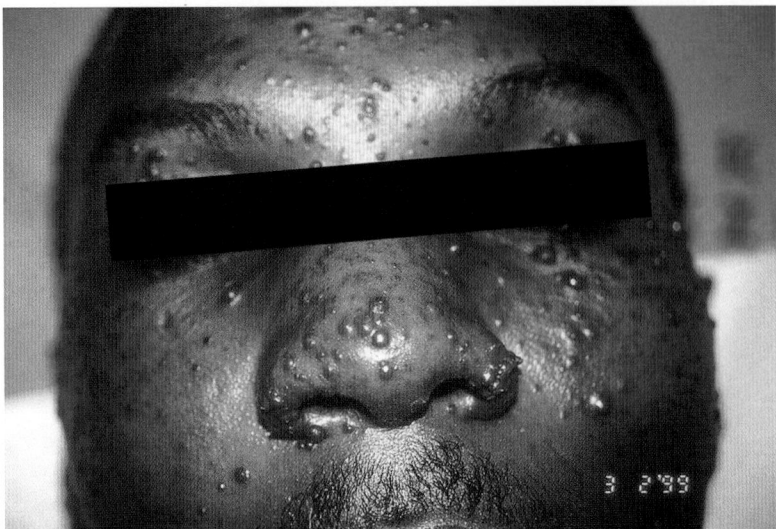

Fig. 18.130
Bacillary angiomatosis: numerous papules and nodules are present. By courtesy of N.C. Dlova, MD, Nelson R. Mandela School of Medicine, University of KwaZulu-Natal, South Africa.

referred to as Rocha-Lima inclusions.[3] These may be highlighted with the aid of a Giemsa preparation. Ultrastructurally, the endothelial inclusions represent degraded bacteria and extracellular matrix components contained within cell surface invaginations.[3] Bacteria are conspicuously absent from late lesions.

Differential diagnosis

Verruga peruana should be distinguished from Kaposi sarcoma, BA, lobular capillary hemangioma (pyogenic granuloma), and true epithelioid vascular neoplasms (such as epithelioid hemangioma and epithelioid hemangioendothelioma).

Bacillary angiomatosis

Clinical features

Bacillary angiomatosis (BA) is a vasoproliferative lesion that may be readily confused with pyogenic granuloma or Kaposi sarcoma and is seen predominantly (but not exclusively) in the skin.[1-4] Lesions have also been described in the bones, soft tissues, liver, lymph nodes, and spleen. Patients may have systemic manifestations including fever, malaise, hepatosplenomegaly, and lymphadenopathy.[5] Although it was originally thought to be a disease specific to AIDS, it has also been described in other immunocompromised states (e.g., renal transplant recipients) and even in apparently normal individuals.[2,6-13] Patients present with widespread, numerous (sometimes hundreds) of blood-red, smooth-surfaced, superficial papules and skin-colored or dusky subcutaneous nodules (Figs 18.130 and 18.131).[2] The condition may be caused either by Bartonella henselae (the organism responsible for cat scratch disease) or less frequently by B. quintana (the cause of trench fever).[6]

Pathogenesis and histologic features

B. henselae infection is acquired via a cat bite or scratch, or cat flea bites, whereas B. quintana infection is transmitted by body lice. Patients with BA, however, seldom seem able to corroborate this history. A PCR-based study from Johannesburg revealed a 10% rate of Bartonella bacteremia among 188 attendees at an HIV clinic, only one of whom exhibited clinical features of BA.[14] Vascular endothelial cells are the prime target of the organisms following initial intracellular colonization of erythrocytes.[15] The VirB type IV secretion system of Bartonella plays a crucial role in not only establishing intraerythrocytic infection but also in mediating the organism's interaction

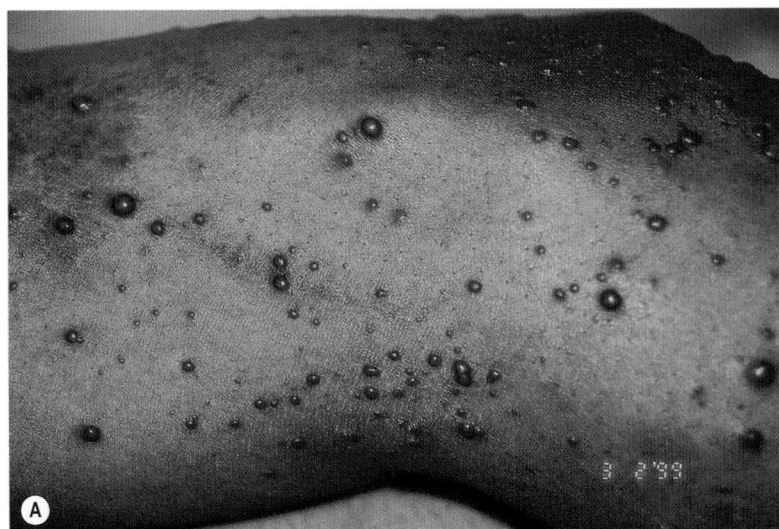

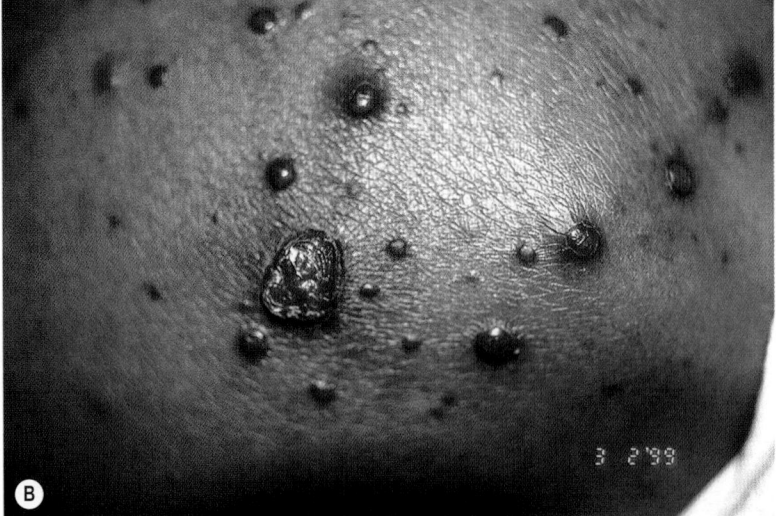

Fig. 18.131
(A, B) Bacillary angiomatosis: the bright red coloration is characteristic. By courtesy of N.C. Dlova, MD, Nelson R. Mandela School of Medicine, University of KwaZulu-Natal, South Africa.

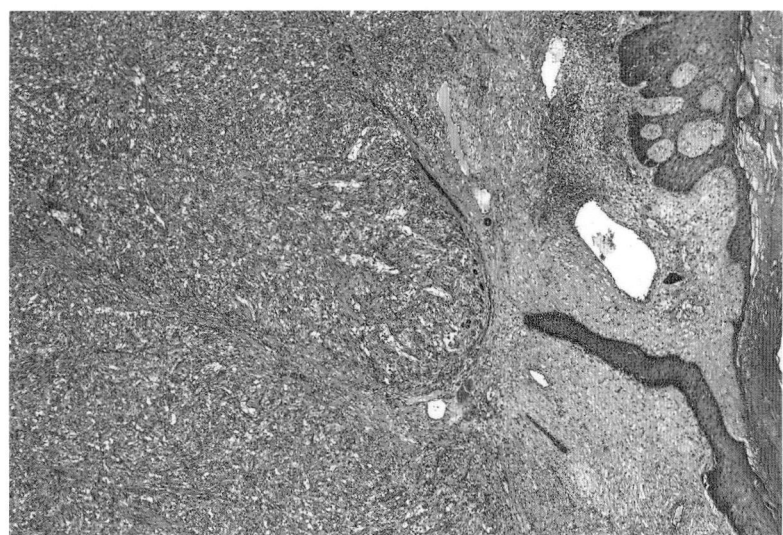

Fig. 18.132
Bacillary angiomatosis: there is a dense nodular capillary proliferative lesion; note the ectatic vessels.

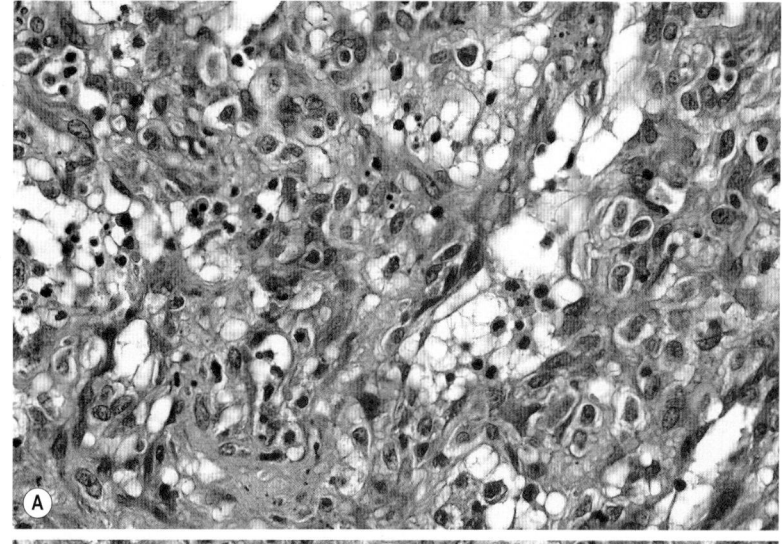

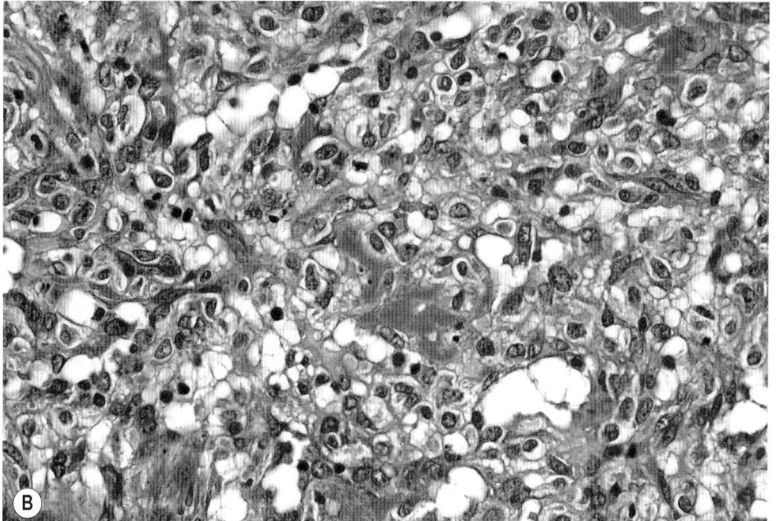

Fig. 18.134
(**A**, **B**) Bacillary angiomatosis: lymphocytes and histiocytes are also present. Note the purple colony of bacteria in the center of the field.

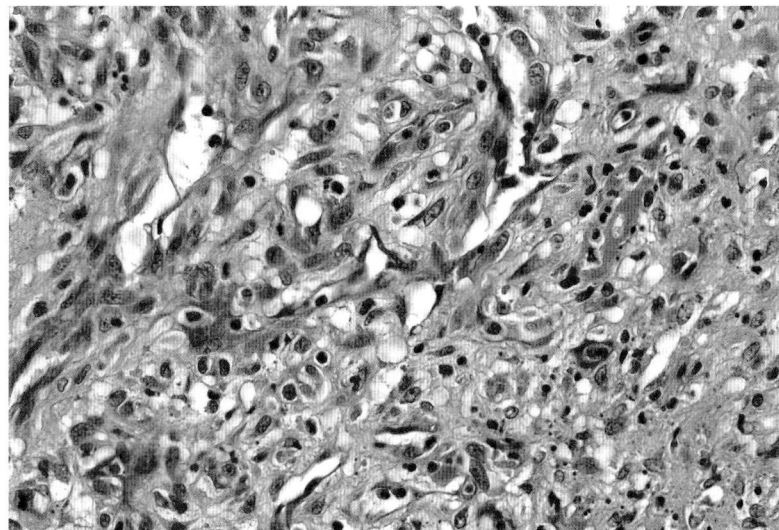

Fig. 18.133
Bacillary angiomatosis: the endothelial cells are swollen. Conspicuous neutrophils are evident.

with endothelial cells.[16] Angiogenesis is potentiated by a combination of mechanisms, including inhibition of apoptosis, release of chemokines such as IL-8, and activation of hypoxia-inducible factor-1 (HIF-1).[15,17–19]

Histology reveals lobules of capillaries with prominent, often cuboidal vascular endothelial cells, sometimes surrounding ectatic vessels among which are dispersed neutrophil polymorphs showing leukocytoclasis and purplish granules of bacilli, which can be identified best by the Warthin-Starry reaction (*Figs 18.132–18.135*).[4,6] Giemsa may also be used to identify the organisms, but since both the former and the latter stains are difficult to interpret and often to perform, a PCR method has been developed (see below). Sometimes solid endothelial cell proliferation is evident. Atypia and mitoses may be present.[4] Superficial lesions have a polypoid configuration, and there may be an associated epidermal collarette reminiscent of a pyogenic granuloma.[3,12,20] Ulceration is seen occasionally. Associated pseudoepitheliomatous epidermal hyperplasia has been described.[21]

Although collagen dissection by spindled endothelial cells is encountered at the periphery of some lesions, hemosiderin deposition and hyaline globules as seen in Kaposi sarcoma are not evident.[20,22,23] Late, involuting lesions show extensive fibrosis of the vascularized dermis, and little by way of a polymorphonuclear leukocytic infiltrate with karyorrhexis.[2,20] Such cases require a high index of suspicion, as the bacteria

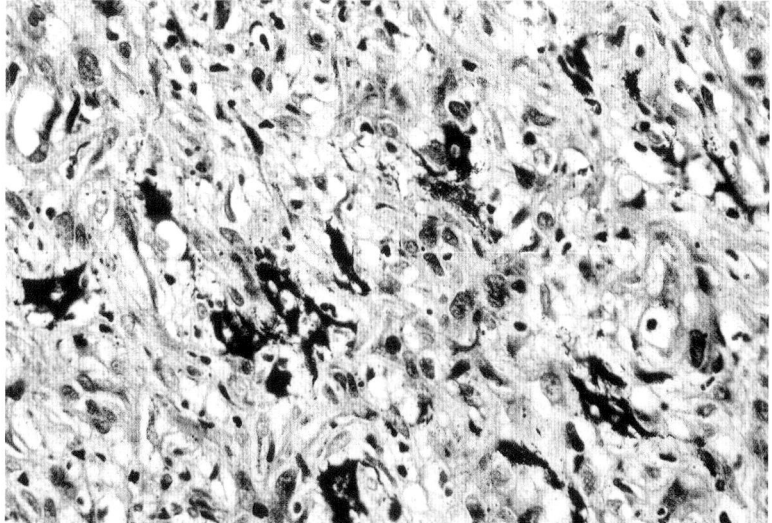

Fig. 18.135
Bacillary angiomatosis: the organisms are easily identified with the Warthin-Starry stain.

may be difficult to demonstrate. Since most patients with this condition are immunocompromised HIV-infected individuals, it is prudent to examine sections carefully for additional opportunistic pathogens, such as CMV or mycobacteria.[20,24-26]

The endothelial cells can be labeled with antibodies to factor VIII-related antigen, CD31 and CD34. Histologically, liver and splenic involvement is seen as peliosis.[5] Typical bacteria are, however, also present. The recognition and distinction of this infection from Kaposi sarcoma and other vasoproliferative lesions is of great importance, particularly as it readily responds to antibiotic therapy.[3]

Ultrastructurally, the organisms appear as aggregates of bacilli within the dermis. The bacteria have trilaminar walls.

Differential diagnosis

BA must be distinguished from verruga peruana, pyogenic granuloma, epithelioid hemangioma, and Kaposi sarcoma. Pyogenic granuloma is not associated with *Bartonella* infection.[27] The lobular capillary hemangioma (pyogenic granuloma)-like variant of Kaposi sarcoma in particular may be confused with BA.[28,29] Although rare, BA with concurrent Kaposi sarcoma has been described.[30] PCR or immunohistochemistry for detection of HHV-8 is a useful means of differentiating Kaposi sarcoma from BA; the former is invariably associated with HHV-8 whereas the latter has been found to be HHV-8 negative.[29,31] Furthermore, PCR may be used to confirm the presence of *Bartonella* spp. in suspected cases of BA since these organisms are difficult to culture.[32]

Lyme disease

Clinical features

Lyme disease (Lyme borreliosis) is a generalized infection due to the spirochete *Borrelia burgdorferi* (*B. burgdorferi sensu lato* complex), of which there are three main pathogenic genospecies in humans: *B. burgdorferi sensu stricto*, *B. garinii*, and *B. afzelii*.[1-8] Two additional species described in Europe are *B. valaisiana* and *B. spielmanii*.[9] It is the most frequently diagnosed tick-borne zoonotic illness in North America and Europe.[7,10] The Centers for Disease Control and Prevention (CDC) reported a 40% increase in the annual incidence of this emerging zoonosis in the United States between 2001 and 2002; more than 40 000 cases were documented during this period.[11] A subsequent CDC survey revealed that more than 64 000 cases were reported in that country during the period 2003 to 2005.[12] This trend has also been observed in parts of the United Kingdom and Europe.[13-15] Although Lyme disease remains a relatively uncommon condition in the United Kingdom, a 3.6-fold increase in the number of annual cases was nevertheless recorded in that country in 2011 as compared with pre-2004 data.[16]

The disease affects most organ systems of the body.[1-3] Lyme disease has been divided into three stages, I–III.[17]

Stage I

The skin lesion of the primary stage (erythema chronicum migrans, erythema migrans) consists initially of a small erythematous papule at the site of an insect bite and expands centrifugally as a flat ring (*Fig. 18.136*). It is the commonest manifestation of the disease and develops on average 1–3 weeks after the bite.[16,18-21] Occasionally, target lesions are described.[22] Necrotic lesions are rare.[23] With extension, the macules may develop a bluish or violet hue. If untreated, the ring may spread to a diameter of 50 cm before clearing. Lesional clearing is associated with a characteristic 'bull's-eye' appearance. Although lesions are usually asymptomatic, patients may complain of pruritus, burning, or rarely, pain.[24] The lower extremity and trunk are most often affected. Multiple lesions (usually 2 or 3) may occur.[25-27] There are rare reports of vesiculobullous forms of erythema migrans.[28-30]

Approximately 50% of patients have secondary lesions, which are smaller. The palms, soles, and mucous membranes are usually unaffected.[31] Erythema chronicum migrans may occasionally recur.[24] Other cutaneous manifestations that have been described in the early stage of Lyme disease

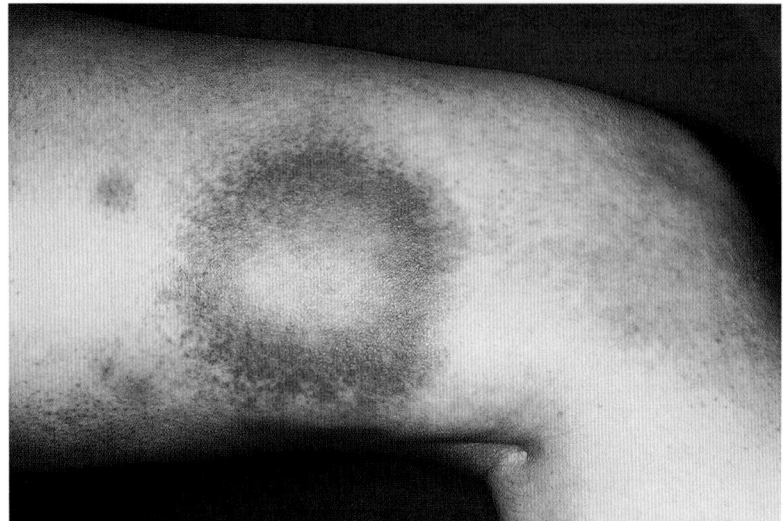

Fig. 18.136
Lyme disease: this annular, erythematous lesion developed (several weeks later) around the site of a tick bite. By courtesy of R.A. Marsden, MD, St George's Hospital, London, UK.

include granuloma annulare, papular urticaria, and Henoch-Schönlein purpura.[31] Age at presentation is exceedingly variable, ranging from 15 months to 80 years. Infection rates are, however, highest among children aged 5 to 15 years, and in adults over the age of 50 years. The sex incidence is equal, and lesions present most often from May to September.[10,31]

Systemic symptoms (due to a spirochetemia) tend to occur early in the disease and include chills, fever, general malaise and lethargy, arthralgia, myalgia, headache, and neck stiffness. Physical examination may reveal lymphadenopathy, splenomegaly, hepatitis, and orchitis.[18,32] *B. garinii* and *B. afzelii* are the pathogens most often implicated in cases of Lyme disease reported from Europe, and some authors have described differences in the clinical presentation of erythema chronicum migrans caused by these two organisms. Erythemas associated with *B. garinii* tend to evolve more rapidly, are often larger and homogeneous, are more often located on the trunk than the extremities, and are more frequently associated with systemic symptoms when compared with *B. afzelii* erythemas, which are usually annular.[33,34] Patients with *B. garinii* infection also tend to be older, and there is a shorter incubation period.[34]

Lymphocytoma cutis (borrelial lymphocytoma), a B-cell response, may present in the acute stage and most often affects the lower ear lobes and nipples.[18] It is, however, more often a feature of the third stage of the illness.[19,32]

Stage II

Stage II disease primarily affects the cardiovascular and nervous system (meningopolyradiculitis; Garin-Bujadoux-Bannwarth syndrome).[1,32,35,36] It may involve both the peripheral and central nervous systems, and tends to present 1–2 months after the primary infection; symptoms include meningism, nerve palsies (especially Bell palsy), and cerebral symptoms, including personality changes, drowsiness, or stupor.[17,37] Neurological involvement is said to occur in 11% of cases.[38] There have been isolated reports of orbital myositis, neurosensory hearing loss, parkinsonism, and spontaneous brain hemorrhage.[39-42] Ischemic stroke may occur as a result of cerebral vasculitis.[43] Cardiac involvement is encountered in 4% to 8% of patients, who may present with myocarditis and conduction defects.[17,35,38,44]

Stage III

Arthritis, which characterizes the third stage, presents as a recurrent, asymmetrical, and oligoarticular process involving the large joints (especially the knee) or as a migratory polyarthritis lasting up to a week in any one particular joint.[32] Arthritis may occur in 45% to 60% of patients.[38] Cutaneous lesions and peripheral nervous system involvement are also frequently encountered in the third stage. The typical skin lesions of late Lyme disease are acrodermatitis chronica atrophicans, which characteristically presents as a red or violet discoloration of swollen peripheral skin, and lymphadenosis benigna cutis (borrelial lymphocytoma).[19,21,24,32,45] Lesions are often bilateral. Patients may also develop sclerodermatous changes. Lichen sclerosus et atrophicus-like lesions have also been described.[17,32] In the late atrophic stages of acrodermatitis chronica atrophicans, the skin may resemble crumpled tissue paper.[46] Nodular or bandlike juxta-articular fibrous nodules are not uncommon, and may regress with appropriate antibiotic therapy.[47] Acrodermatitis chronica atrophicans occurs mainly in Europe, where *B. afzelii* is the overwhelmingly predominant etiological genospecies.[5,27] *B. afzelii* is not endemic in North America, possibly accounting for the striking geographic distribution of the condition.[5]

There have been rare reports suggesting a possible association between *B. burgdorferi* infection and anetoderma.[48,49] A case with acquired cutis laxa has also been described.[50] The conflicting role of *B. burgdorferi* in the pathogenesis of morphea and lichen sclerosus is discussed elsewhere.[51–53]

Although the major clinical features are similar among European and North American cases, certain differences exist. The occurrence of acrodermatitis chronica atrophicans as an apparently European phenomenon has already been alluded to. Borrelial lymphocytoma and meningoradiculoneuritis are also observed more frequently in Europe, while multiple erythema migrans due to hematogenous dissemination in early Lyme disease is said to occur less frequently outside of North America.[27] A European series of 54 cases, however, showed that 46% of patients had multiple erythema migrans lesions.[25]

Reinfection may occur in a small but significant proportion of patients following treatment with antibiotics. This usually manifests as a recurrent episode of erythema migrans at a different cutaneous site from the previous lesion.[54,55] A Swedish study showed that women were more susceptible to reinfection than men, ascribing this phenomenon to gender differences in immune reactivity, especially in the postmenopausal age group.[55]

Pathogenesis and histologic features

Erythema chronicum migrans was first described in association with tick bites; cases were subsequently reported following mosquito bites and thorn pricks, or without preceding trauma.[44] In a proportion of cases, an encephalitis was noted and the disease was termed 'tick-borne meningopolyneuritis'. In the 1970s, several cases were reported in the United States, and because of a clustering effect near Lyme, Connecticut, the term Lyme disease was coined (these cases had a high proportion of arthritis).[38,56] The *Ixodes* tick has been known to be the vector for some time, but the actual etiological agent, a spirochete, was only identified in the 1980s after spirochetes were found in *Ixodes dammini* ticks in an endemic disease area.[17,57,58] In Europe, *Ixodes ricinus* has been incriminated.[32,44] *Ixodes* ticks are found widely in the temperate regions of the Northern hemisphere.[10] The increased frequency of infections during the spring and summer months coincides with the time when the nymph stage of the tick is active.[6]

Patients recovering from the disease have been shown to have antibodies to the spirochetes in their serum.[24] Spirochetes have also been identified from biopsy sites, and cultured from or detected by PCR performed on specimens of blood, cerebrospinal fluid, synovial fluid, and skin.[4,21,32,44,59,60] Antibody-based tests for confirmation of the diagnosis are limited by the fact that results are more likely to be negative in the early stages of the infection.[61] Immunosuppression does not appear to alter clinical presentation, treatment response, or anti-*B. burgdorferi* antibody production.[62]

Borreliae have developed strategies to evade or inactivate host immune defenses via a variety of mechanisms.[63] These include complement regulator-acquiring surface proteins (CRASPs), which confer complement resistance. Borrelial CRASPs are capable of binding FHL-1/reconectin and factor H, which are two major regulators of the alternative complement pathway.[64,65] The selective up-regulation of host matrix metalloproteinase-9 by *B. burgdorferi* in skin lesions of erythema chronicum migrans may play a role in the local spread of the organism and its dissemination to other organs.[66] In the early stage of Lyme disease, *B. burgdorferi* antigens induce a strong host immune response in which the production of cytokines such as IFN-γ, TNF-α, and TGF-β_1 predominates.[67,68] By contrast, chronic neuroborreliosis is associated with a lack of TNF-α and TGF-β_1 responses.[68]

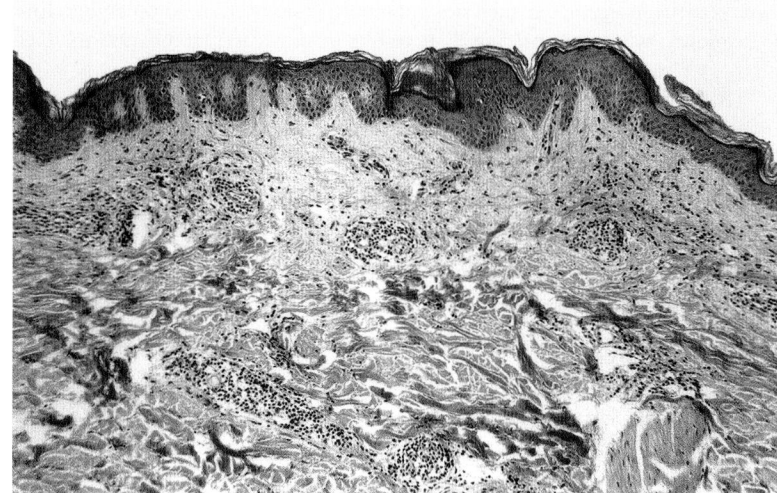

Fig. 18.137
Lyme disease: the epidermis is normal; a chronic inflammatory cell infiltrate surrounds the vessel in both the superficial and deep dermis.

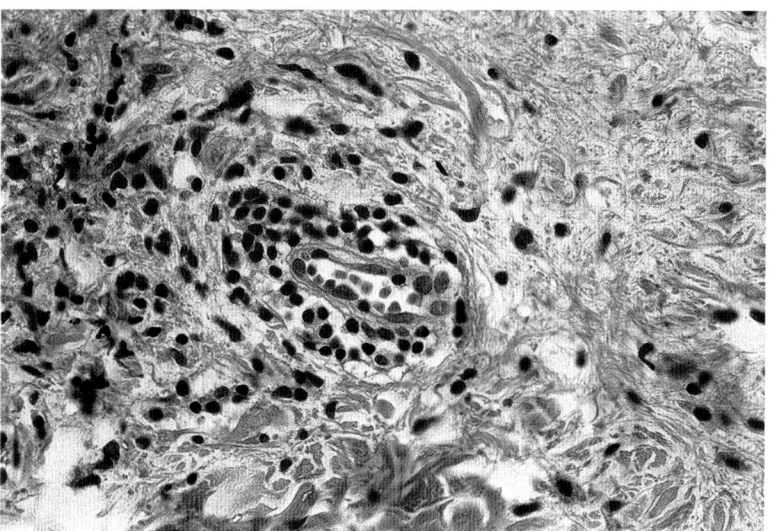

Fig. 18.138
Lyme disease: high-power view.

Studies performed on lesional skin have revealed high levels of the T-cell-active chemokines CXCL9 and CXCL10 in erythema chronicum migrans and acrodermatitis chronica atrophicans. Borrelial lymphocytoma, on the other hand, is associated with high levels of CXCL13, a B-cell-active chemokine.[69]

The central component of the initial lesion shows the typical appearance of an insect bite reaction. Histology reveals a polymorphic inflammatory cell infiltrate including neutrophils, eosinophils, histiocytes, lymphocytes, and mast cells.[32] Vascular proliferation and dermal necrosis may additionally be present. A superficial and deep dermal perivascular lymphocytic infiltrate characteristic of an annular erythema then develops.[70] A biopsy from the periphery is non-specific, showing a perivascular and interstitial infiltrate of lymphocytes, mast cells, and plasma cells in both the superficial and deep dermis (*Figs 18.137* and *18.138*). Unusual histologic features, however, have been reported in some cases and present a potential diagnostic pitfall; these include spongiosis, focal interface dermatitis, an infiltrate confined to the superficial vascular plexus, and an absence of plasma cells.[70]

Identification of spirochetes by a silver stain is diagnostic.[71] An immunohistochemical method for demonstrating the etiological agent has been described.[32] PCR may also be used to detect the organisms in formalin-fixed, paraffin-embedded tissue specimens.[72,73] One study concluded that focus floating microscopy was more sensitive than PCR in detecting *Borrelia* spirochetes in the lesional tissue of erythema chronicum migrans, borrelial lymphocytomas, and acrodermatitis chronica atrophicans.[74] Clonal or pseudoclonal IgH gene rearrangements have been documented in DNA extracted from erythema migrans cutaneous lesions. Care should therefore be exercised when interpreting PCR results in such cases; some authors have advocated duplicate or triplicate testing.[75]

The borrelial lymphocytoma consists of a dense (polyclonal) dermal infiltrate composed of lymphocytes, plasma cells with macrophages, and scattered eosinophils. Although it has been suggested that germinal center formation, when present, helps to exclude a cutaneous B-cell lymphoma, this is not necessarily true; cutaneous lymphomas of marginal zone type typically display germinal centers.[24,32,76] The association between *B. burgdorferi* infection and cutaneous B-cell lymphoma is discussed elsewhere.[76,77]

Acrodermatitis chronica atrophicans is characterized by vascular dilatation in the mid and upper dermis accompanied by a dense infiltrate of lymphocytes, plasma cells, macrophages, and mast cells.[32] Scattered groups of 'vacuoles' may be seen in the dermis; this phenomenon is thought to be attributable to lymphedema.[46] The epidermis, which is usually hyperkeratotic, may be acanthotic or atrophic with loss of ridge pattern.[17] In some patients, the appearances are reminiscent of lichen sclerosus or eosinophilic fasciitis.[24,32] Occasionally, the histologic features may overlap with scleromyxedema.[32] The juxta-articular fibrous nodules are characterized by fibrosis of the superficial subcutaneous tissue, with hyaline collagen bundles encircling clusters of adipocytes. There is an accompanying perivascular and interstitial inflammatory infiltrate comprising lymphocytes and plasma cells.[47] Smaller periarticular fibrous nodules on the fingers show disorganized bundles of thickened dermal collagen.[78]

The triad of meningitis, cranial neuropathy, and radiculopathy has been said to be unique for Lyme disease. CNS lesions include cortical, perivascular chronic inflammatory cell infiltrates, mild spongiform changes, and gliosis. Plasma cells, however, are said to be absent. The similarity of the late CNS changes of Lyme disease and meningovascular syphilis has been stressed.[32] Chronic leptomeningeal inflammation may also be evident. Peripheral nervous system lesions are characterized by nerve and ganglion lymphocyte and occasional plasma cell infiltration.[17,32] Adjacent vessels may show endarteritis obliterans.

Endocardial lesions are characterized by a lymphocytic and plasma cell infiltrate; deep specimens show an interstitial myocarditis.[17] Focal myonecrosis may also be evident.[32]

Histologic examination of the synovium may show periadventitial cell onion-skinning proliferation and chronic inflammation.[17,32]

Endemic (nonvenereal) treponematoses

Endemic syphilis

Clinical features

Endemic syphilis (Syrian *bejel*) is a form of nonvenereal treponematosis caused by *Treponema pallidum* subsp. *endemicum*, an organism nearly identical to *T. pallidum* subsp. *pallidum*, the etiological agent of venereal syphilis.[1–5] The condition usually occurs in children living in conditions of poor hygiene and is transmitted by cutaneous inoculation.[1,3–7] Other endemic forms have been associated with shared drinking vessels and other contaminated domestic utensils when some members of the community have oral or labial syphilitic lesions.[1,3–6] Although endemic syphilis was largely eradicated from Europe in the twentieth century, the disease still occurs in parts of the Middle East and Africa, especially in rural desert regions.[1,3,4,8,9]

Unlike venereal syphilis, a primary chancre seldom occurs in endemic syphilis; women suckling infected infants may, however, develop primary infections of the nipple.[1,3] The primary lesions usually involve the oropharynx but are easily overlooked. Early secondary lesions manifest as soft, oval mucous patches with a predilection for the buccal and labial mucosae, sometimes accompanied by angular stomatitis. Mucous patches may also occur in the perianal and genital areas, where they sometimes appear condylomatous. Osteoperiostitis may occur, and generalized lymphadenopathy is common.[1,3]

Late (tertiary) manifestations develop following a latent period of between 5 and 15 years. The lesions may evolve in the skin, nasopharynx, bone, or joints and are clinically similar to those encountered in late yaws.[1,3,9] Articular and osseous involvement is frequently destructive. Cardiovascular involvement may also occur, but the disease does not affect the CNS. A further point of distinction from venereal syphilis is the fact that there is no congenital form of endemic syphilis.[1,3]

Histologic features

The histopathology of the primary lesion is poorly documented. The light microscopic features of the secondary lesions are virtually identical to those encountered in venereal syphilis.[1,3,10] Granulomatous dermal inflammation is encountered in the tertiary skin lesions.[1,10]

Yaws

Clinical features

Yaws (framboesia tropica) is a tropical disease occurring in people living in poor conditions due to infection by the spirochete *Treponema pallidum* subsp. *pertenue*.[1–6] Although the condition was thought to have been almost eradicated by the World Health Organization (WHO) mass treatment program from 1952 to 1964, which led to a 95% reduction in the global disease burden, it continues to be encountered in a number of warm, humid tropical regions including some 13 countries in Africa, Southeast Asia, and the Western Pacific region.[4,7–11] In 2012, yaws was again earmarked for eradication, with 2020 set as a target date.[12] Community mass treatment with azithromycin for trachoma in areas where both conditions are prevalent has had a significant impact on the number of new cases of yaws. Consequently, mass community treatment with azithromycin is a key component of the strategy to eliminate the disease.[13–15] Strains of *T. pallidum* subsp. *pertenue* have been identified among nonhuman primates in parts of tropical Africa where yaws is common in humans, suggesting a possible role for an animal reservoir and cross-species infection.[12,16]

Yaws is not transmitted sexually, but rather by close contact, for example, by inoculation of skin previously traumatized by insects or scratching, and skin-to-skin contact.[1,4,6,17] The disease is most common in children 6–10 years of age, who present with lesions on the feet, legs, and buttocks.[1,18] Clinically, it is divided into early and late yaws.[3,19–21] The initial lesion, known as a 'mother yaw', develops 3–5 weeks after inoculation. It starts as a nontender papilloma, which ulcerates and is then covered with a yellow crust (*Fig. 18.139*).[3,18] It resembles a raspberry, hence the alternative designation framboesia (Dutch *framboos*, raspberry). This mother yaw may be surrounded by smaller papillomas, which develop 2–4 months after the initial lesion.[3,6,17] Lesions in the perineum and natal cleft may become condylomatous.[17] Subsequently, these warty lesions may become very widespread ('daughter yaws') (*Fig. 18.140*). Macules, papules, and nodules have also been described.[18,22] They eventually resolve leaving a depressed and hyperpigmented scar.[17] The mucous membranes, bones (osteitis and periostitis), and joints may also be affected in early yaws.[19] Palmar and plantar hyperkeratosis, which can be exceedingly painful and may result in walking difficulties (crab yaws), are characteristic.[1,22,23]

There may be a symptom-free period of 3–5 years before the lesions of late yaws arise. The late lesions, which develop in about 10% of patients, are destructive ulcers and gummatous nodules which affect the skin, bones (e.g., saber tibia), and joints (*Figs 18.141* and *18.142*).[3,6,18,19,22] Cutaneous manifestations of late yaws include palmar and plantar hyperkeratosis (crab yaws), loss of pigment (pintoid yaws), and gummata. Pintoid yaws includes hyperkeratosis, contractures, juxta-articular nodules, and bony lesions.[6,19] Gummata characteristically involve the long bones, the bones of the hands and feet, and typically lead to gross destruction of the face (gangosa).[24] The cardiovascular and nervous systems are said not to be involved, but there is some historical evidence to suggest that ophthalmic and myeloneuropathies might occur in endemic areas.[18,20,25]

Pathogenesis and histologic features

The spirochete responsible for yaws is morphologically indistinguishable from *T. pallidum* subsp. *pallidum*. Whole genome sequencing has revealed that these organisms differ in less than 0.2% of the genomic sequence.[22,26]

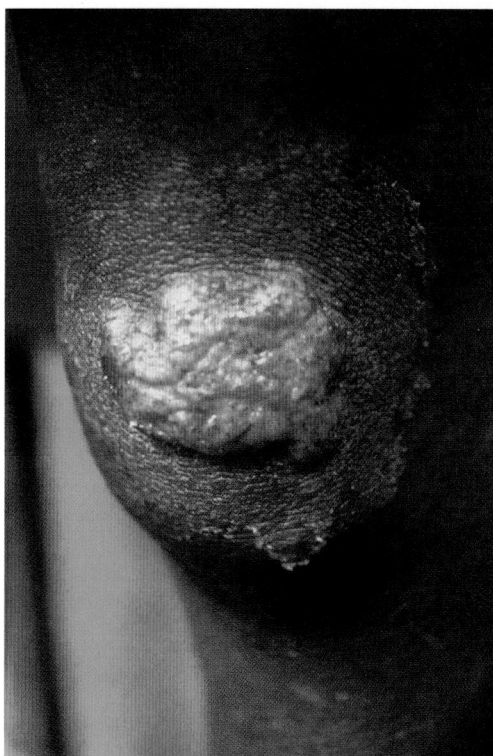

Fig. 18.139
Early yaws: typical framboesiform 'mother yaw'. Note the yellow crust and surrounding hypopigmentation. By courtesy of H.J.H. Engelkens, MD, and E. Stolz, MD, University Hospital, Rotterdam-Dijkzigt and Erasmus University, Rotterdam, The Netherlands.

Early lesions are characteristically parakeratotic, acanthotic, and papillomatous. They show focal spongiosis and intraepidermal neutrophils with microabscess formation (Fig. 18.143).[22] There is a dense perivascular dermal infiltrate containing numerous plasma cells. The vascular changes in contrast to syphilis are usually insignificant. Treponemes can be seen around the blood vessels, in the tips of the dermal papillae, and within the epidermis (Fig. 18.144).[1,3,23,27–29]

The palmoplantar lesions are characterized by hyperkeratosis, parakeratosis, and acanthosis. A mild non-specific chronic inflammatory cell infiltrate is present in the superficial dermis.

The gummata show central caseation necrosis surrounded by a rim of lymphocytes, plasma cells, histiocytes, epithelioid cells, and giant cells.[1,23] There is associated fibrosis.

Pinta

Clinical features

This is a nonsexually transmitted treponematosis characterized by depigmented skin lesions. It is caused by *Treponema carateum* (*T. pallidum* subsp. *carateum*), an organism that is very similar to *T. pallidum* subsp. *pallidum*.[1–5] It is generally confined to remote regions in tropical Central and South America where the inhabitants live in poor hygiene and in close proximity.[1,3,5–7] The condition may nevertheless be encountered in nonendemic countries among migrants and refugees from endemic areas.[8] Children, adolescents, and young adults are primarily affected, and transmission is thought to be by direct cutaneous or mucous membrane contact, possibly via minute abrasions.[1–3,6,7,9]

The lesions present as small scaly erythematous indurated papules and plaques on exposed skin, usually on the hands and feet. These disappear, but recur in a more disseminated form (pintids).[1,3,6,7] Regional lymphadenopathy may occur.[3] Late stages of pinta are characterized by disfiguring hyperpigmentation, achromia, hyperkeratosis, and atrophy (Fig. 18.145).[1,3,7,10]

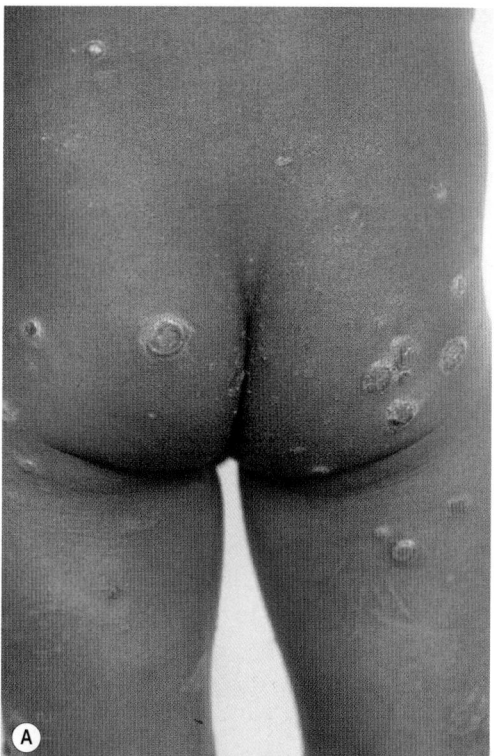

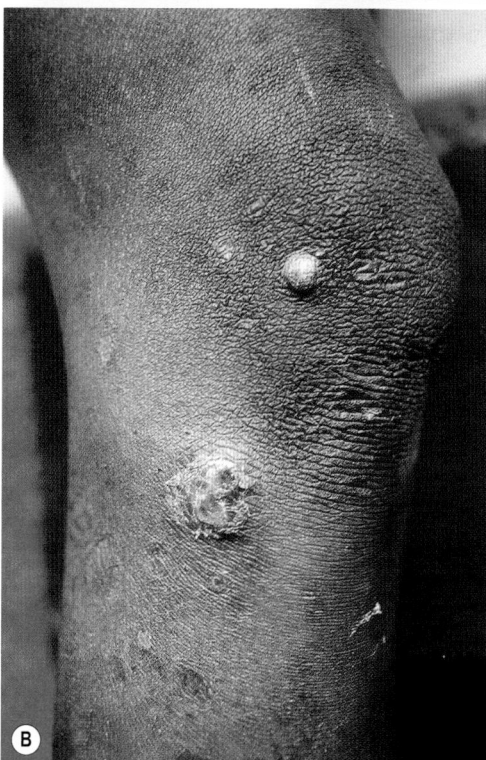

Fig. 18.140
(**A**, **B**) Early yaws: multiple smaller 'daughter yaws' may be widely distributed and usually present 2–4 months after the 'mother yaw'. By courtesy of H.J.H. Engelkens, MD, and E. Stolz, MD, University Hospital, Rotterdam-Dijkzigt and Erasmus University, Rotterdam, The Netherlands.

Unlike syphilis and yaws, all manifestations of the infection are limited to the skin, and there is no evidence of systemic disease.[3]

Histologic features

Histologically, early primary and secondary pinta lesions show hyperkeratosis and acanthosis, while later lesions demonstrate epidermal atrophy and a diminished basal melanin pigment concentration.[1,5,10–13] Lymphocytic exocytosis, mild spongiosis, basal cell hydropic degeneration, and pigmentary

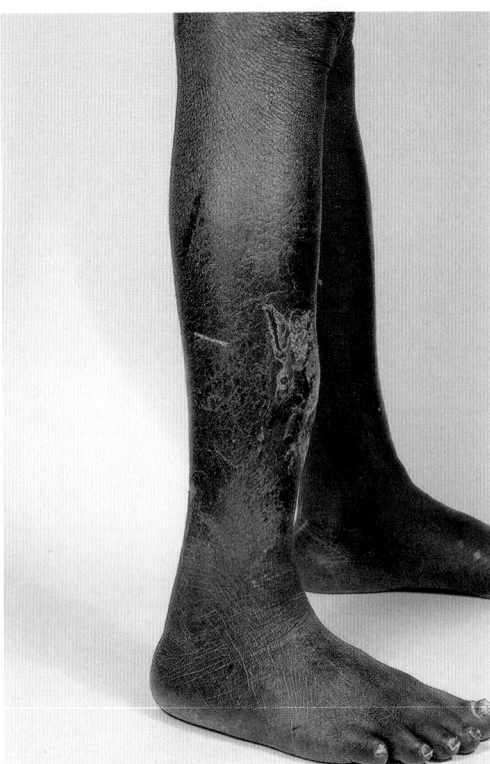

Fig. 18.141
Late yaws: note the bowing of the lower leg with cutaneous ulcerated and crusted lesions in this late stage. By courtesy of R.A. Marsden, MD, St George's Hospital, London, UK.

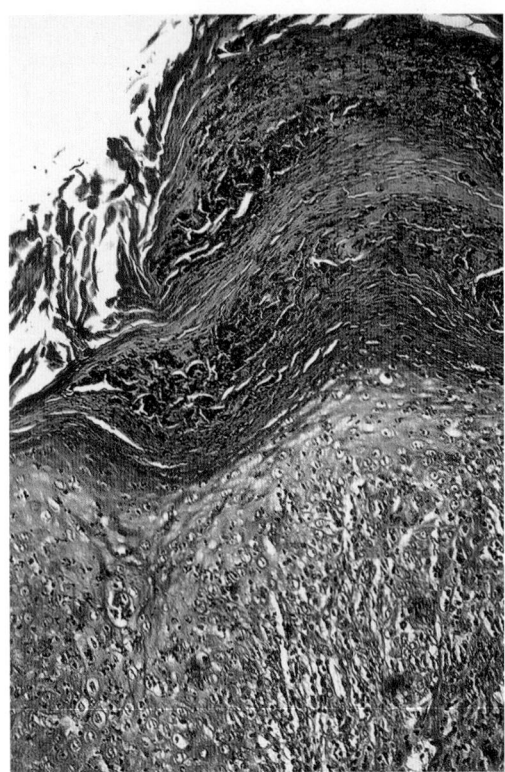

Fig. 18.143
Early yaws: biopsy through an evolving papilloma. There is very marked parakeratosis associated with abundant neutrophil debris. The epidermis shows intense acute inflammation. By courtesy of H.J.H. Engelkens, MD, and E. Stolz, MD, University Hospital, Rotterdam-Dijkzigt and Erasmus University, Rotterdam, The Netherlands.

Tuberculosis

Clinical features

Tuberculous (*Mycobacterium tuberculosis* complex) infection of the skin, which was once common worldwide, had shown a declining incidence during the latter decades of the last century, especially in developed countries.[1,2] This was due in part to improved therapy, a reduction in the size of the active reservoir of infection, and increased immunoresistance to infection. The late twentieth century, however, showed an apparent upward trend in the incidence of cutaneous tuberculosis, especially in Asian countries.[3] A particularly important aspect of cutaneous tuberculosis is that skin lesions can readily simulate other conditions, and may be insidious in onset. The source of infection is sometimes not obvious, and tissue destruction may be very marked. Cutaneous tuberculosis accounts for 1% to 1.5% of cases of extrapulmonary tuberculosis and around 0.14% of all cases of tuberculosis.[4,5]

Although the global burden of tuberculosis is slowly declining, the epidemic is larger than previously estimated, and data from the WHO remain disconcerting. According to the WHO, 2015 saw an estimated 10.4 million new (incident) cases worldwide, including an estimated 480 000 cases of multidrug-resistant tuberculosis, and a further 100 000 cases of rifampicin-resistant tuberculosis. Six countries accounted for around 60% of all new infections, namely, China, India, Indonesia, Nigeria, Pakistan, and South Africa. Although the number of deaths from tuberculosis fell by 22% between 2000 and 2015, it remains one of the leading causes of death worldwide, with an estimated 1.8 million fatalities in 2015.[6]

Mycobacterial infections (tuberculous and atypical) are of increasing importance in the context of acquired immunosuppression, whether due to lymphoma, AIDS, or aggressive chemotherapy. Atypical modes of presentation with microorganisms of borderline virulence have gained significance.[7] Cutaneous tuberculosis has re-emerged in those parts of the world where the incidence of HIV infection and multidrug-resistant tuberculosis is high.[2,6,8,9] An estimated 1.2 million (11%) of the incident cases of tuberculosis in

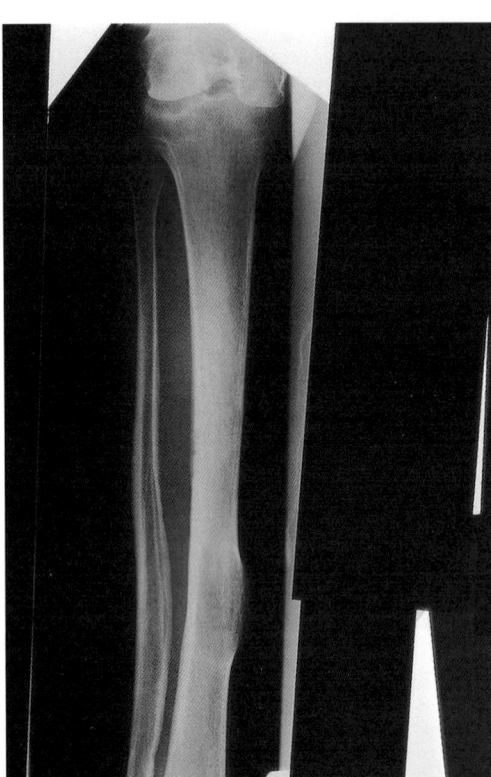

Fig. 18.142
Late yaws: note the cyst with an overlying periosteal reaction. By courtesy of R.A. Marsden, MD, St George's Hospital, London, UK.

incontinence are evident.[1,5] A perivascular lymphocytic infiltrate is usually seen without endothelial swelling. Hyperchromic lesions exhibit epidermal atrophy, melanin incontinence, and a mild dermal lymphocytic infiltrate.[1,10] Spirochetes are said to be demonstrable in all types of lesions, with the exception of late leukodermic lesions.[1,11]

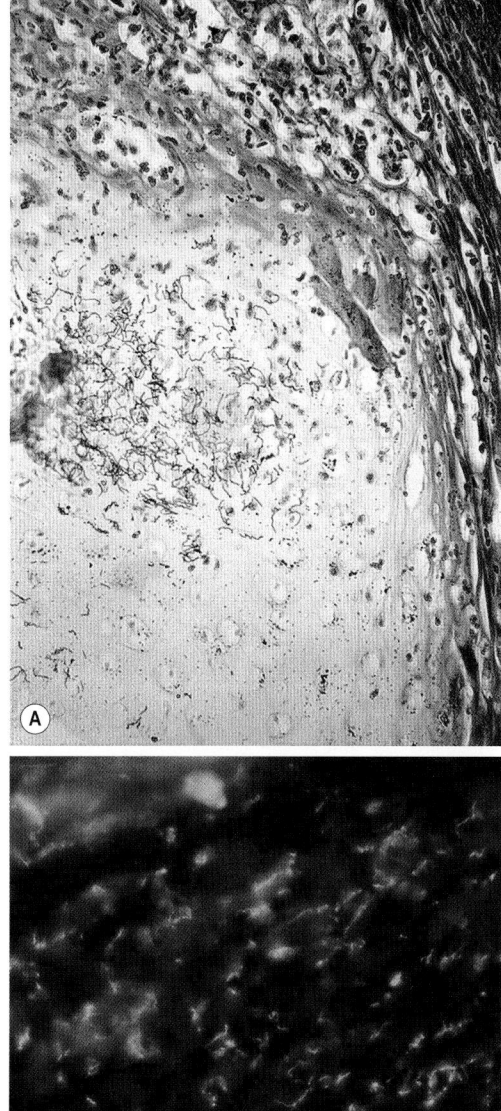

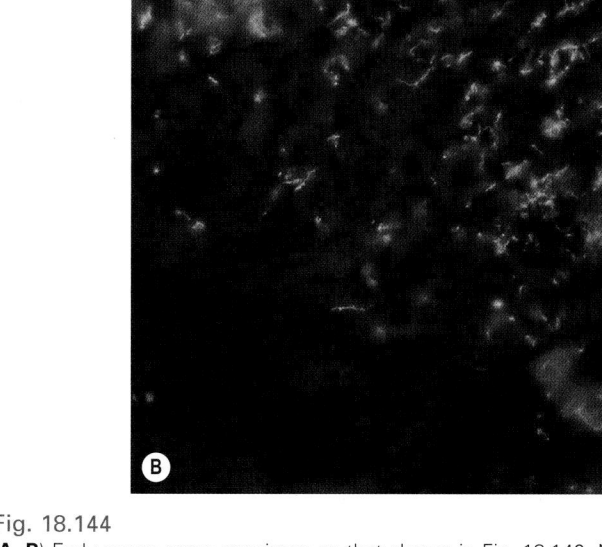

Fig. 18.144
(**A**, **B**) Early yaws: same specimen as that shown in Fig. 18.140. Note the presence of numerous spirochetes. (**A**) Warthin-Starry; (**B**) immunofluorescence. By courtesy of H.J.H. Engelkens, MD, and E. Stolz, MD, University Hospital, Rotterdam-Dijkzigt and Erasmus University, Rotterdam, The Netherlands.

2015 were HIV positive, with the vast majority occurring on the African continent, followed by Southeast Asia. The number of tuberculosis-related deaths among HIV-infected patients has declined in recent years, with around 400 000 deaths in 2015. This in part due to an increasing number of patients gaining access to ART.[6]

In Europe and North America, cutaneous infection is still relatively infrequent, due to a reduction in the numbers of infected cases by therapy

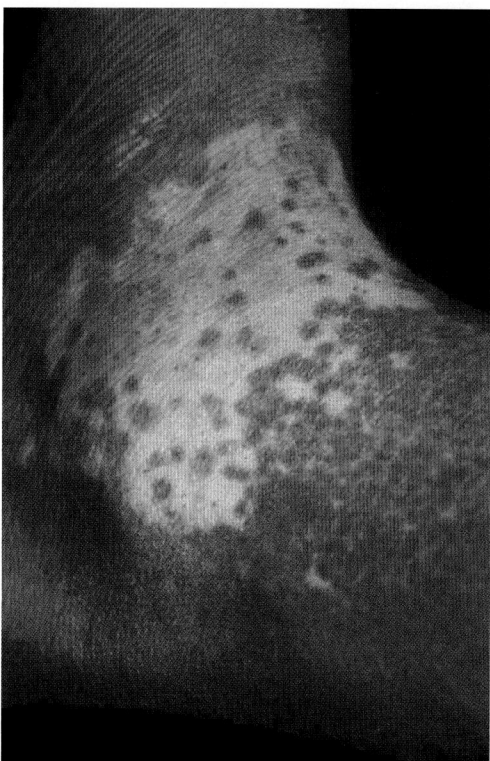

Fig. 18.145
Pinta: this is a late lesion showing characteristic complete loss of pigmentation surrounded by a hyperpigmented border. By courtesy of R. Arenas, MD, and J. Salas, MD, Azteca, Monterrey, Mexico.

and immunization programs and to an increased standard of living. Nevertheless, there remains an apparently irreducible number of people with tuberculosis, usually living in circumstances of poor hygiene and nutrition.[10] This is borne out by the number of unsuspected cases of tuberculosis diagnosed at autopsy. Moreover, there exists an important reservoir of infected immigrants, particularly of Asian origin, who often present with cervical lymphadenopathy.

It is important to remember *Mycobacterium bovis*, the agent responsible for bovine tuberculosis, may cause zoonotic tuberculosis in humans. The estimated global prevalence of this condition in 2015 was 149 000, with the majority of infections occurring in Africa and Southeast Asia.[6] Infections following BCG vaccination constitute a third form of human tuberculosis; the latter condition is discussed elsewhere in this chapter.[11]

The manifestations of tuberculosis in the skin are influenced by previous infection or immunity and by the route of infection. Because of the virulence and resistance to phagocytosis by *M. tuberculosis*, neutrophils are completely ineffective in dealing with this bacterial infection, whereas macrophages and their derivatives are characteristically seen in the cellular response. These lead on to (giant cell) granuloma formation with or without necrosis, and this underlies the varied clinical presentations of this infection.

The majority of cases of cutaneous tuberculosis are a manifestation of systemic disease.[2,8,12] The usual portals of entry of *M. tuberculosis* include the lungs and intestine, but the mucous membranes and skin occasionally show primary involvement.[13] Cutaneous lesions include papules, nodules, plaques, ulcerative lesions, warty tumors, or scarring reactions.[14] Although preferred, it is not always possible to package cutaneous tuberculous lesions neatly into the categories detailed below, and on occasion tuberculous skin disease may be reported as of non-specific type, particularly in this current era of profound immunosuppression. In this account, a modified 'Beyt' classification is used.[2,11,15,16]

Appropriate classification, when possible, is important because some variants are associated with systemic lesions and therefore clinical management and prognostic implications are highly variable.[13] Tuberculids in which bacilli are not detectable are now rare in the West, but are still common in developing countries and are considered separately below.

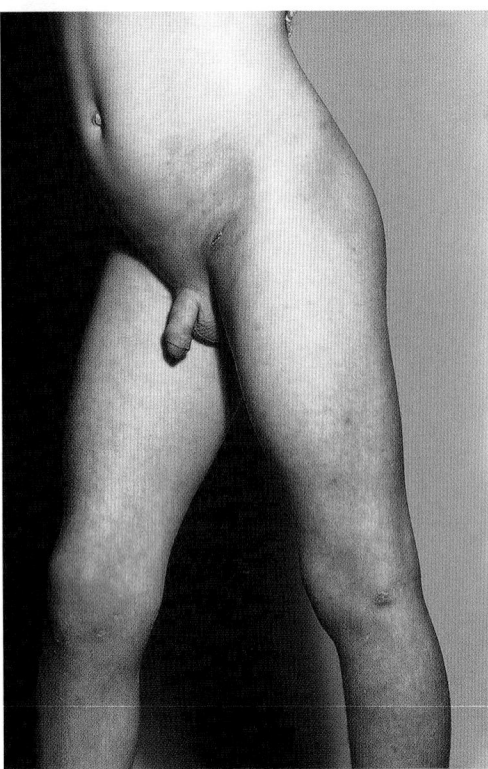

Fig. 18.146
Tuberculous chancre: the cutaneous equivalent of a Ghon complex. Note the healing lesion on the outer aspect of the knee and the ulcerated inguinal nodes from this patient from the 1950s. By courtesy of M.M. Black, MD, Institute of Dermatology, London, UK.

Infections by inoculation (exogenous source)

Tuberculous chancre, which is rare, occurs by direct inoculation of infected material into the skin of a previously uninfected and nonimmune patient.[16] The response is analogous to a Ghon complex in the lung.[11,15,17] These lesions develop 2–4 weeks after inoculation, which may be through minor trauma to the skin of various sites, such as the face and limbs of children (*Fig. 18.146*). Infection may also follow minor surgery such as ear piercing, tattooing, or circumcision. The earliest lesion is a reddish-brown papule, which may rapidly progress to an ulcer with ragged undermined edges. The margins of the lesion become indurated, and lymphadenopathy is usually noted at this stage. Satellite papules may be seen around the original lesion and this pattern of spread is termed 'lupoid'. Inoculation tuberculosis from BCG injection is a similar phenomenon.[18]

Warty lupus (tuberculosis verrucosa cutis) occurs by inoculation of *M. tuberculosis* into the skin of individuals who have some degree of immunity or may have active infection elsewhere. It has been the most common variant in some series from Asia (*Fig. 18.147*).[11,13,16,19,20] This lesion occurs classically as 'prosector's warts' in pathologists or autopsy technicians, but may also be seen in butchers dealing with infected cattle (*Fig. 18.148*).[15] Inoculation of the skin by infected sputum, even from the same patient, can cause a similar lesion. Children tend to be affected on the lower limbs or buttocks (*Fig. 18.149*).

The lesion begins as a small indurated nodule with a keratotic warty surface at the site of inoculation and then slowly extends in a serpiginous manner, producing an irregular reddish-brown warty plaque. Although much of the lesion is firm, some softer areas may be present from which pus may exude. In some areas the lesion continues to extend, but elsewhere it may show focal involution to leave an atrophic pale scar. The warty component may persist for years, but usually resolves eventually.

Secondary tuberculosis (endogenous source)

Orificial tuberculous ulcers are rare and occur in the skin or mucosa adjacent to an orifice draining an active tuberculous infection. They represent autoinoculation and are most commonly seen around the nose, mouth,

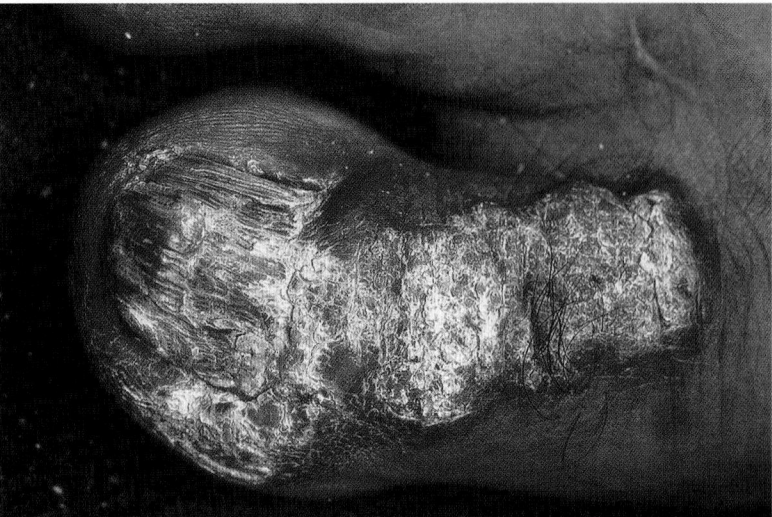

Fig. 18.147
Warty lupus: in this example, there is a grossly hyperkeratotic lesion associated with destruction of the nail. By courtesy of the Institute of Dermatology, London, UK.

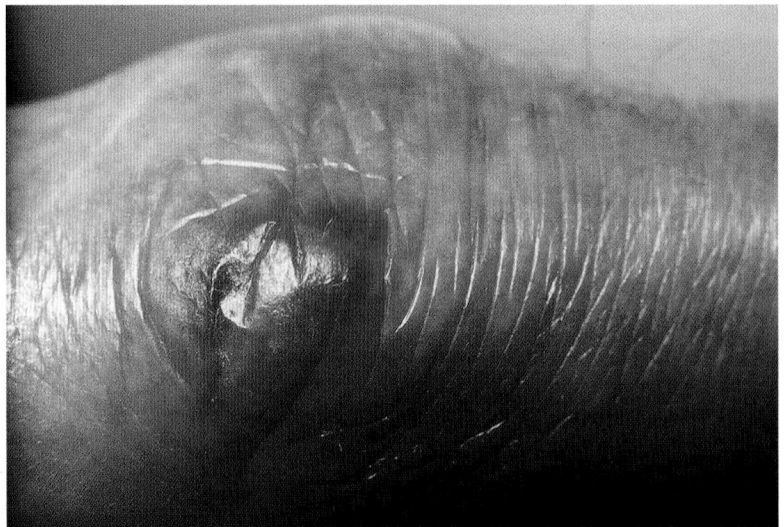

Fig. 18.148
Warty lupus: prosector's wart. This indurated lesion on the finger developed after a pathologist had performed a tuberculous autopsy. By courtesy of R. Vellor, MD, St Thomas' Hospital, London, UK.

genitalia, or anus (*Fig. 18.150*). Patients are usually hyperreactive to tuberculin testing. The lesions start as edematous red papules, which ulcerate and develop undermined edges. These ulcers are painful and neither progress or regress.

Scrofuloderma (L. *scrofula*, brood sow; derma, skin) is a complication of deep tuberculous infection of lymph node, bone, joint, or subcutaneous tissue (*Figs 18.151–18.153*). The lesion is seen as a bluish-red nodule, which ulcerates and discharges pus or necrotic material.[11] Lesions are commonly seen in the neck, submandibular area, or axilla. There is associated scarring, and the combination of scarring and a chronic discharging ulcer may resemble hidradenitis suppurativa. Very rarely, scrofuloderma may arise from the lacrimal system.[21]

Infection by hematogenous spread

Lupus vulgaris may occur following inoculation of bacteria into individuals showing some immunity (see above); more commonly, however, it represents hematogenous or lymphatic spread from a tuberculous focus, which is usually occult. Lesions occur mostly on the face (particularly around the nose), neck, and earlobes in the West, and are more common in women

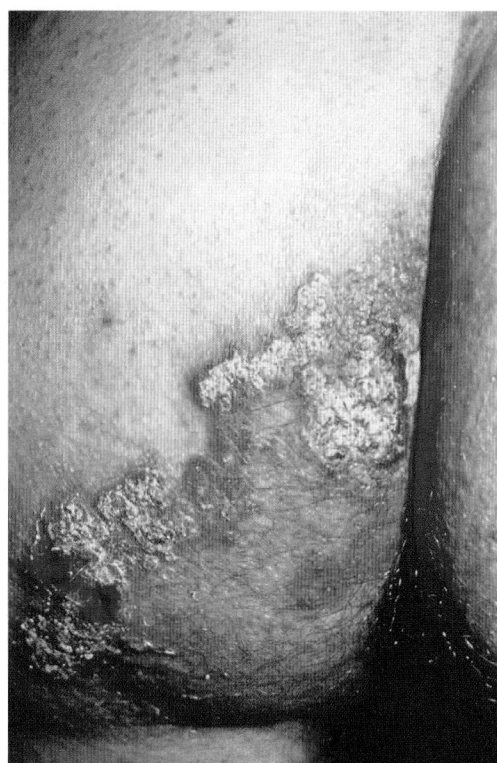

Fig. 18.149
Warty lupus: in children, the buttock is a commonly affected site. By courtesy of the Institute of Dermatology, London, UK.

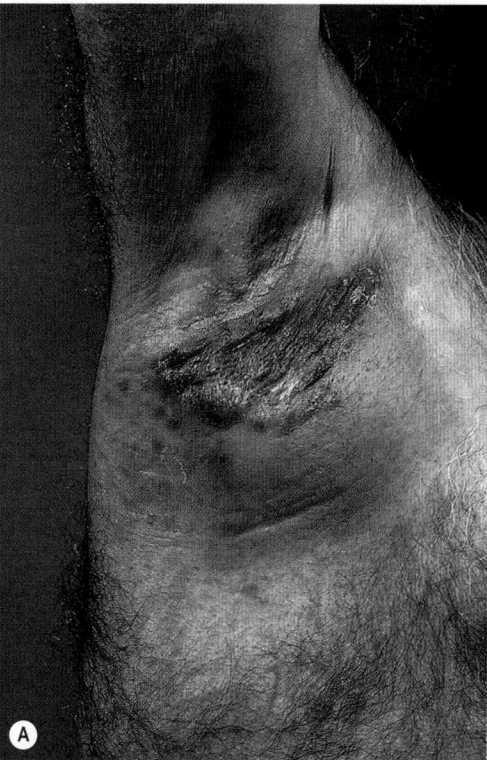

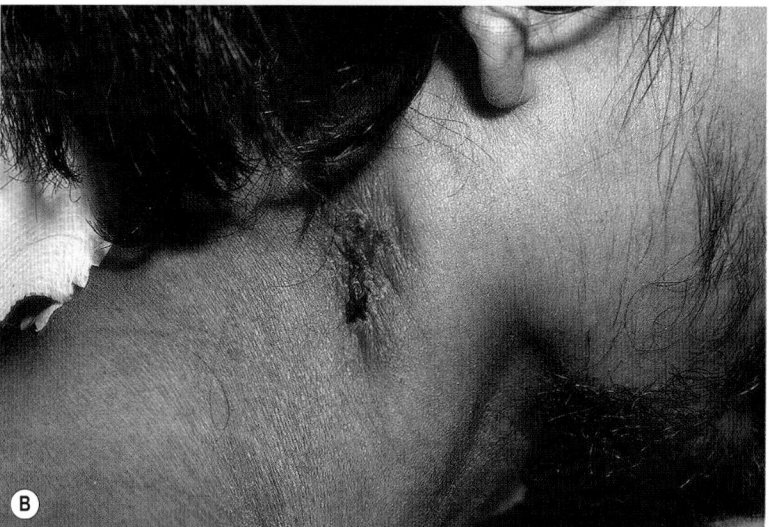

Fig. 18.151
Scrofuloderma: (**A**) note the marked axillary swelling and scarring with multiple sinuses; (**B**) in this example, there was underlying cervical tuberculous lymphadenopathy. The puckered scarring is characteristic. By courtesy of R.A. Marsden, MD, St George's Hospital, London, UK.

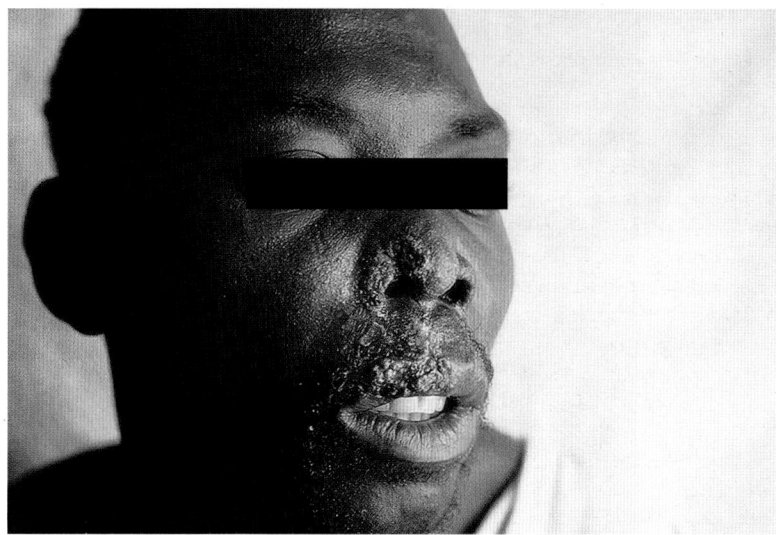

Fig. 18.150
Orificial tuberculosis: widespread ulcerative lesions involving the upper lip and nostril. By courtesy of S. Lucas, MD, St Thomas' Hospital, London, UK.

(*Figs 18.154* and *18.155*).[18] The extremities and buttocks are more commonly involved in patients in the East. The arms and legs may also be affected (*Fig. 18.156*). It is a very chronic disease. This form of cutaneous tuberculosis used to be particularly evident in Northern Europe and is still the most frequently encountered variant in the West.[2,11] It is a common form of cutaneous tuberculosis in childhood.[12,22]

Lupus vulgaris occasionally results from direct inoculation and may even occur at the site of BCG inoculation.[23]

Lupus vulgaris is characterized by papules and raised erythematous and sometimes scaly plaques of gelatinous consistency, said with diascopy to resemble apple jelly. These lesions may gradually extend, while involuting with scarring in other areas. There may be adjacent cellulitis or ulceration. Extensive facial lesions can result in gross disfigurement.[24,25] Squamous and

basal cell carcinoma, melanoma, and lymphoma may develop in chronic lupus vulgaris.[26–29] Contractures and lymphedema are late complications. Ocular involvement is an additional serious complication. Lupus vulgaris is a rare cause of alopecia.[30]

Tuberculous gumma represents a metastatic tuberculous subcutaneous abscess derived from infection at another site by a hematogenous route.[13,16] It is most commonly seen in the malnourished, the immunodeficient, or the immunosuppressed.[8,13,31] Clinically, it presents as a firm subcutaneous nodule, usually on the arms or legs. The lesion slowly becomes fluctuant, and the overlying skin perforates to form a chronic undermined ulcer as seen in scrofuloderma.

Miliary tuberculosis of the skin (tuberculosis cutis miliaris disseminata) occurs in association with generalized miliary tuberculosis and is very rare. It is usually seen in infants and has a poor prognosis. The infection may be seen in mother and child concurrently, and then the cutaneous lesions

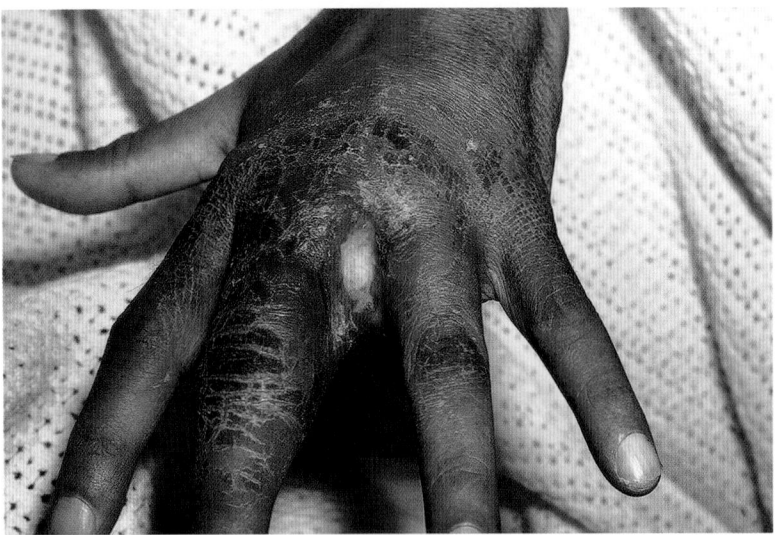

Fig. 18.152
Scrofuloderma: in this case there was underlying tuberculous osteoarticular disease. By courtesy of the Institute of Dermatology, London, UK.

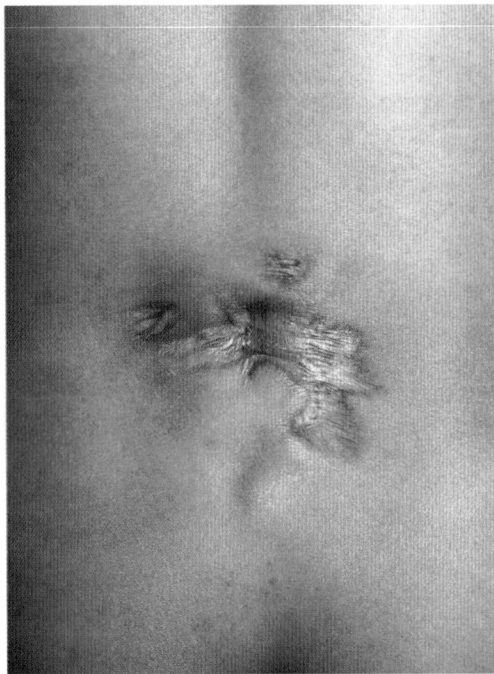

Fig. 18.153
Scrofuloderma: lesions in the midline of the back commonly complicate vertebral tuberculous osteomyelitis. By courtesy of the Institute of Dermatology, London, UK.

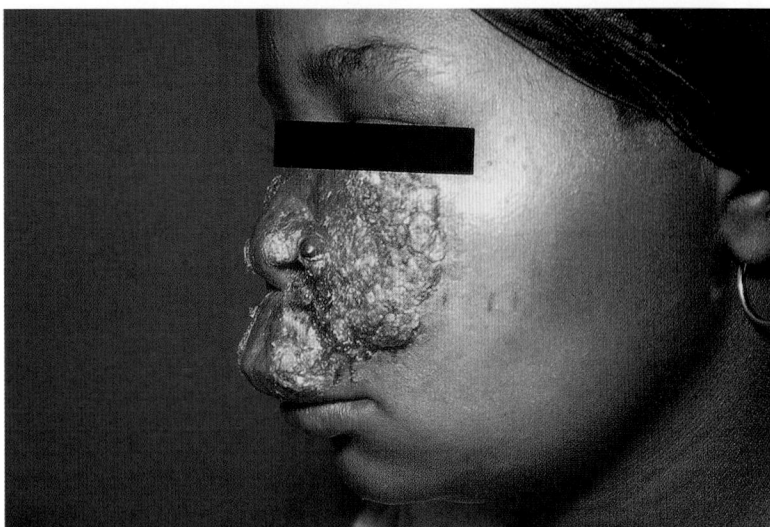

Fig. 18.154
Lupus vulgaris: the nose is a commonly affected site. By courtesy of N.C. Dlova, MD, Nelson R. Mandela School of Medicine, University of KwaZulu-Natal, South Africa.

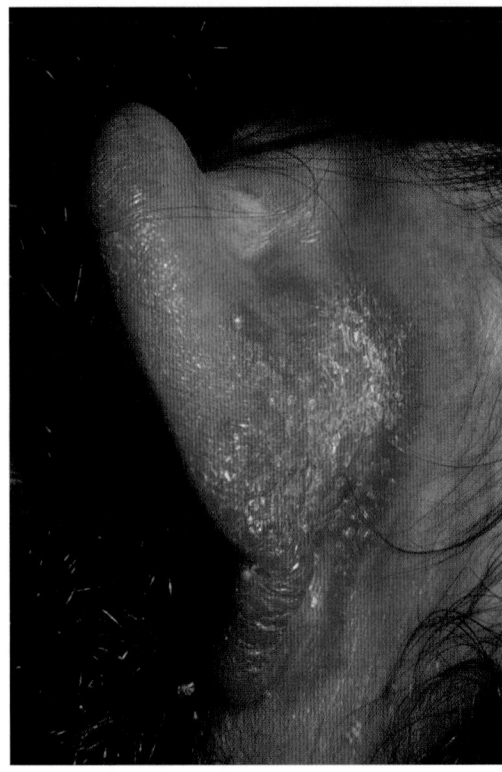

Fig. 18.155
Lupus vulgaris: typical plaque with golden-yellow appearance. By courtesy of R.A. Marsden, MD, St George's Hospital, London, UK.

may be scanty and the prognosis less grave.[32] Other cases are associated with immunodeficiency and may follow a minor systemic infection such as measles. In these patients, there are numerous lesions which are usually centrally crusted papules or pustules, but they may be ulcerative, necrotic, hemorrhagic, or vesicular.[13,16] There have been a number of reports in patients with AIDS, especially those with multidrug-resistant tuberculosis.[8,9,16,33–37] The cutaneous lesions can be confused with folliculitis, resulting in delayed diagnosis.[30] The prognosis is poor.[8,35]

Comparison of the variants of cutaneous tuberculosis is shown in *Table 18.2*.

Other rare manifestations of cutaneous tuberculosis that have been reported include tuberculous cellulitis, neutrophilic tuberculous panniculitis, and the presence of sporotrichoid lesions.[38–43] These uncommon forms of tuberculosis have occurred in patients who were iatrogenically immunosuppressed.

Pathogenesis and histologic features

M. tuberculosis, an 'obligate pathogen', is a slender aerobic rod, characterized by a high lipid content. This lipid is responsible for resistance to phagocytosis. It also allows the bacterium to retain basic dyes, even during treatment with strong differentiating agents, and this is the basis of the Ziehl-Neelsen/acid-fast stain (*Fig. 18.157*). Organisms are easily identified in tuberculous chancre, scrofuloderma, orificial lesions, and the miliary variant. They may be difficult to find or absent in lupus vulgaris, gummata, and warty tuberculosis.[13] Mycobacteria are found at water-air interfaces and were so named because of their moldlike growths on the surface of liquid media.[44]

The organism is highly resistant to drying and therefore can retain infectivity by inoculation or contamination of minor wounds.

The reaction to the bacterium depends on:

- the size of the inoculums,
- the virulence of the organism,
- the immune state of the patient.

In general, the cellular response is characterized by epithelioid macrophages, Langhans giant cells, and caseous necrosis, with lymphocytes and plasma cells in the surrounding tissue (tuberculous granuloma) (*Figs 18.158* and *18.159*). Tuberculoid granulomata, as seen for example in sarcoidosis, by definition do not show true caseation. The presence of large numbers of bacilli in a lesion implies a nonimmune or anergic state, such as in tuberculous chancre or orificial lesions. Caseation is an indication of hypersensitivity and is not a toxic effect of the organisms; it is clear that it is not always beneficial to the host because it is invariably associated with destruction of surrounding tissue.

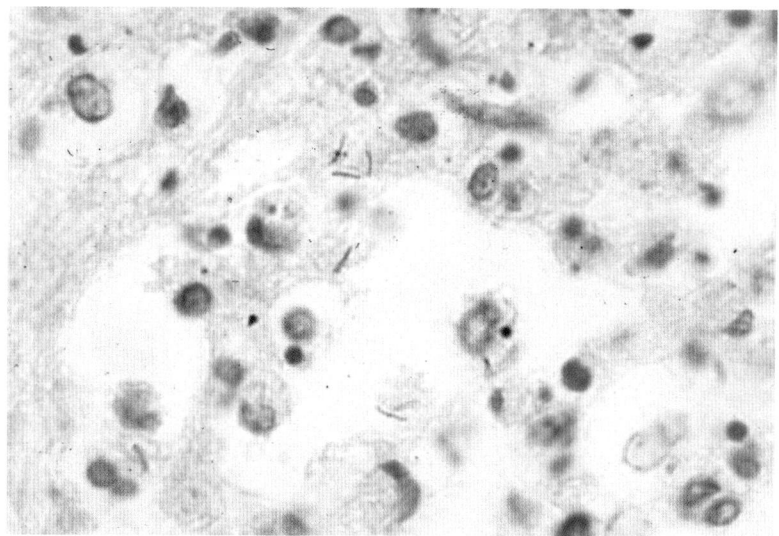

Fig. 18.157
Ziehl-Neelsen stain: in the center of the field is a small collection of red, acid-fast rods (oil immersion).

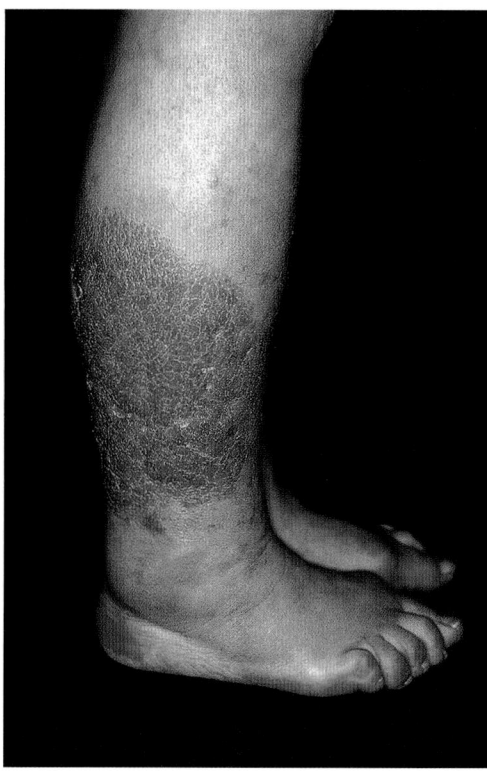

Fig. 18.156
Lupus vulgaris: this is a chronic lesion showing marked scaling, erythema, and induration. Squamous cell carcinoma may occasionally supervene. By courtesy of R.A. Marsden, MD, St George's Hospital, London, UK.

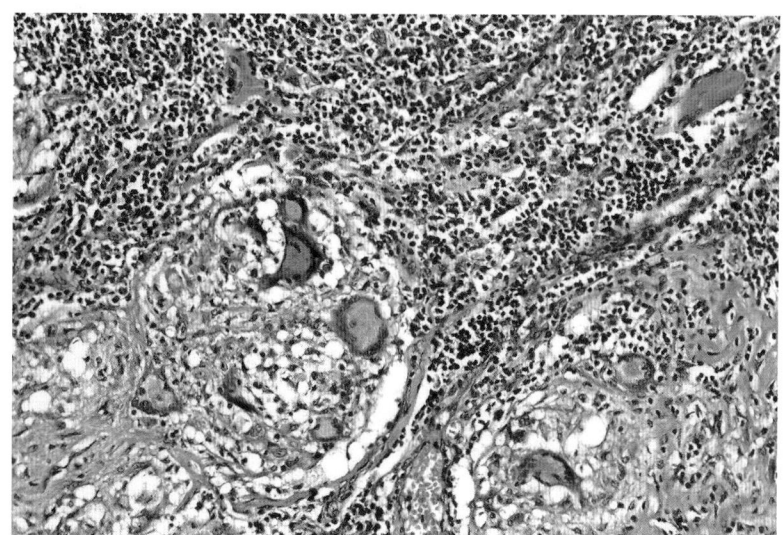

Fig. 18.158
Tuberculosis: characteristic Langhans giant cells with horseshoe peripheral rim of nuclei.

Table 18.2
Variants of cutaneous tuberculosis

Variant	Route of infection	Association with other TB	Level of infection	Histologic features	Presence of bacilli
Tuberculous chancre	Inoculation	None	Dermis	Neutrophil abscess → caseating granuloma, lymphadenopathy	Present
Warty lupus	Inoculation	Previous or current infection	Dermis	Scanty granulomata, papillomatous acanthosis	Absent or very scanty
Orificial ulcers	Autoinoculation	Active infection in associated organs	Submucosa dermis	Mixed inflammation, few granulomata, necrosis	Numerous
Lupus vulgaris	Inoculation and/or hematogenous	Previous or current, often occult, infection	Superficial dermis	Variable but granulomata, little caseation prominent	May be seen in deep aspect
Scrofuloderma	Extension from underlying infection	Active infection	Subcutaneous and dermal	Mixed inflammation, granuloma, marked fibrosis	May be seen in deep aspect
Tuberculous gumma	Hematogenous	Systemic infection	Subcutaneous	Much caseation, granulomatous fibrosis	Scanty
Miliary tuberculosis	Hematogenous	Systemic infection	Dermis	Central abscess, with surrounding histiocytic infiltrate	Absent or scanty in benign form; present in aggressive form

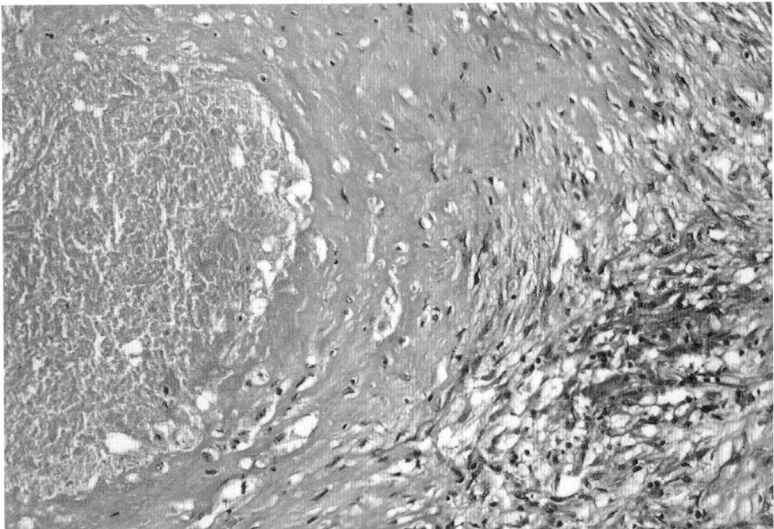

Fig. 18.159
Tuberculosis (caseation necrosis): the cell outlines are not completely lost, giving an amorphous granular appearance.

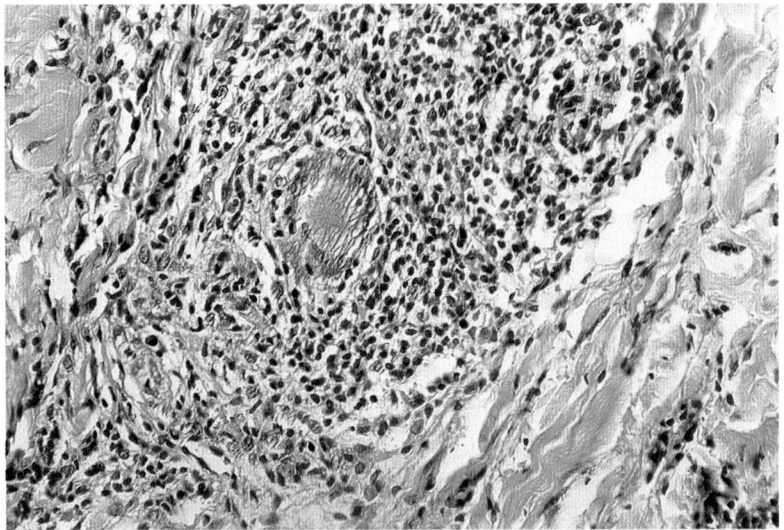

Fig. 18.161
Warty lupus: in addition to neutrophils and lymphocytes, an occasional Langhans giant cell may be present.

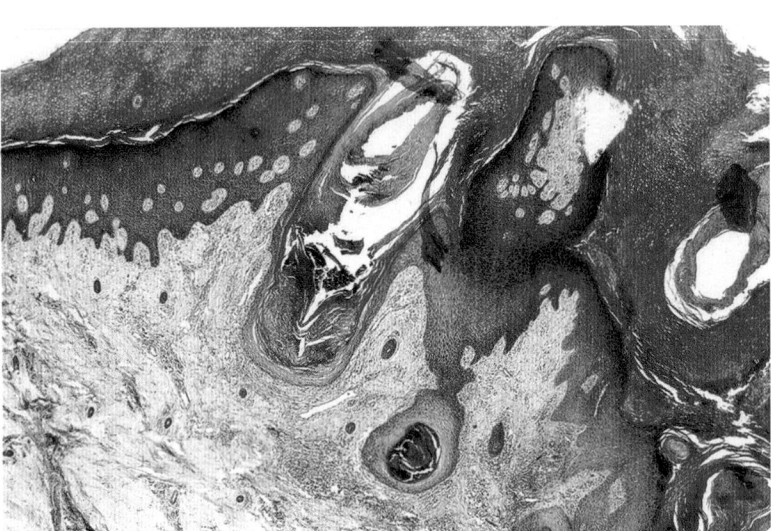

Fig. 18.160
Warty lupus: the epidermis is hyperkeratotic and shows marked irregular acanthosis. An inflammatory cell infiltrate is present in the dermis.

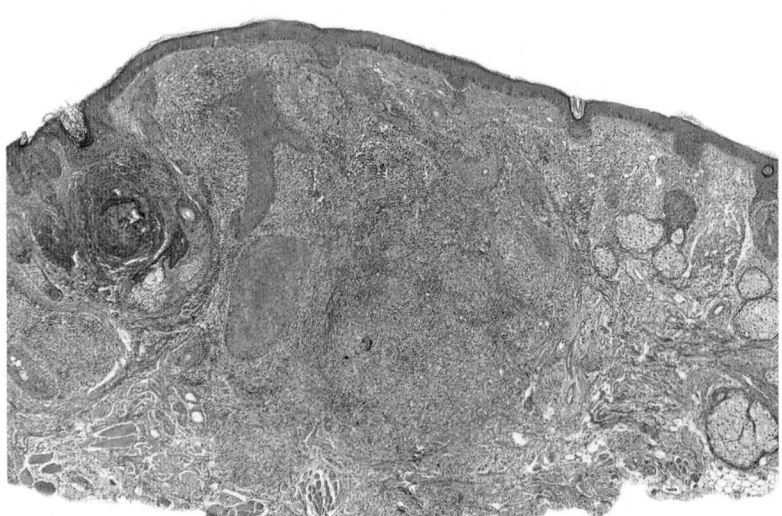

Fig. 18.162
Lupus vulgaris: there is a dense dermal infiltrate. Note the Langhans giant cell.

Primary chancre

The primary chancre is characterized by a neutrophilic abscess with numerous bacilli, associated with necrosis leading to ulceration. This is gradually surrounded by histiocytes; after 6 weeks, giant cells (derived by fusion of epithelioid cells) are seen. Central necrosis remains prominent, but diminishes, along with the number of bacilli, as the granulomatous element increases.[11,13]

Warty lupus

Warty lupus is characterized by acanthotic papillomatosis with marked hyperkeratosis (*Fig. 18.160*). Pseudoepitheliomatous hyperplasia may also be seen. The dermal infiltrate consists mainly of neutrophils and lymphocytes, and abscesses may sometimes be present. Granulomata are present in the deeper dermis and caseation is occasionally a feature (*Fig. 18.161*).[11–13] Bacilli are found on careful searching.

Orificial lesions

Orificial lesions, in contrast, show extensive necrosis and numerous bacilli. The inflammatory infiltrate is not conspicuously granulomatous and may consist of lymphocytes and neutrophils, with few histiocytes.

Lupus vulgaris

Lupus vulgaris is more varied in its histologic features. It is seen in the superficial dermis, consisting of tubercles, some of which coalesce, with scanty or absent central caseation surrounded by epithelioid histiocytes and multinucleate giant cells (*Figs 18.162* and *18.163*). Peripheral lymphocytes and plasma cells are also usually prominent. Bacteria are very infrequent. The overlying epidermis may be ulcerated (in which case there is usually a more mixed inflammatory infiltrate), atrophic, or acanthotic. The last may be severe (pseudoepitheliomatous hyperplasia), raising the problem of distinction from invasive squamous carcinoma, especially as such tumors are an important rare complication of lupus vulgaris. This may sometimes be impossible if only superficial specimens are submitted for pathological interpretation. Transepithelial elimination of granulomata has been described.[45]

Lupus vulgaris typically presents around the nose: this location is determined by the presence of large venous channels with stasis of blood flow and relative cold and hypoxia, which impair fibrinolysis and host defenses. Lupus vulgaris may affect other areas with relatively low temperature.

Miliary tuberculosis

Miliary lesions include a severe form in which numerous central bacilli within a neutrophil abscess are surrounded by histiocytes (*Fig. 18.164*).

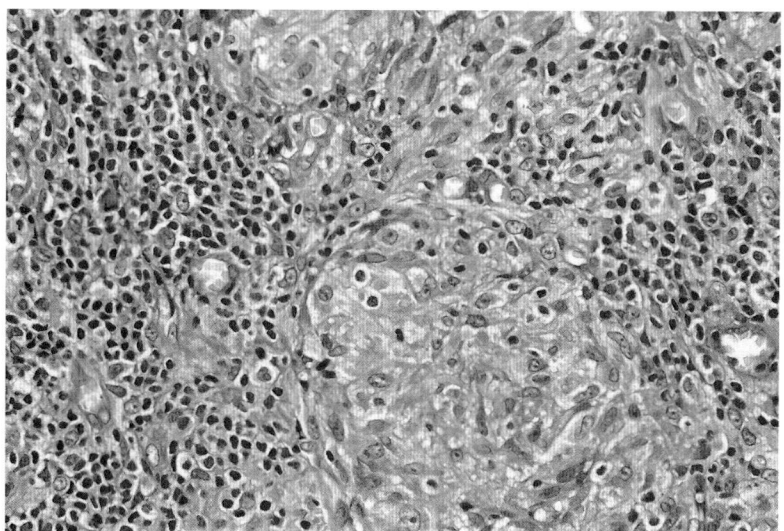

Fig. 18.163
Lupus vulgaris: the granulomata are often surrounded by lymphocytes.

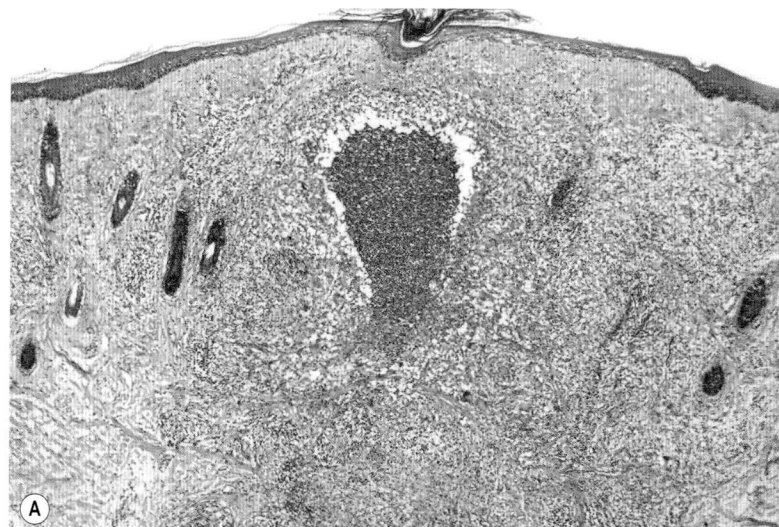

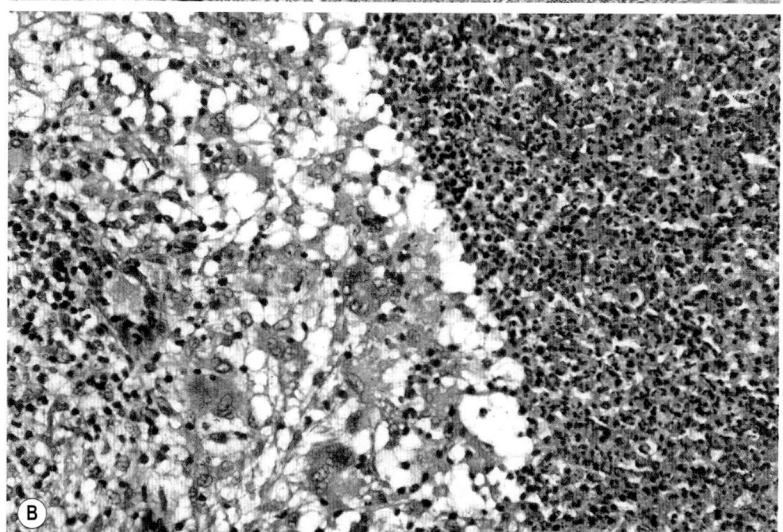

Fig. 18.164
Miliary tuberculosis: (**A**) a neutrophil abscess is present in the mid-dermis; (**B**) it is surrounded by histiocytes. Occasional giant cells are also evident.

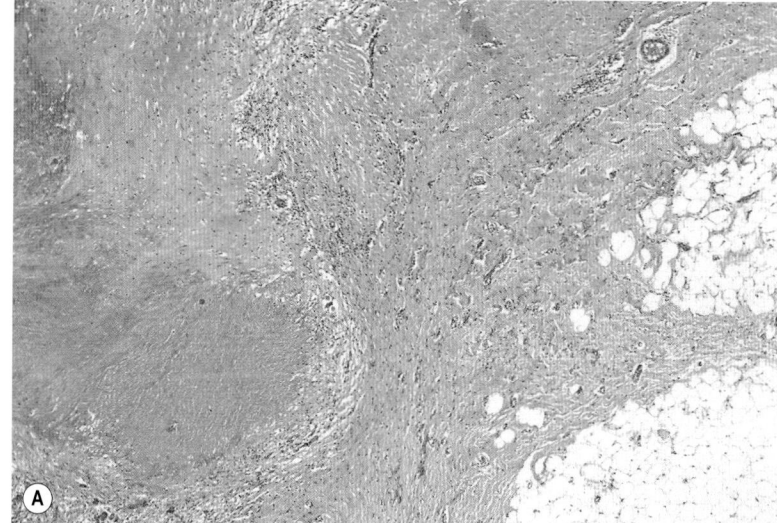

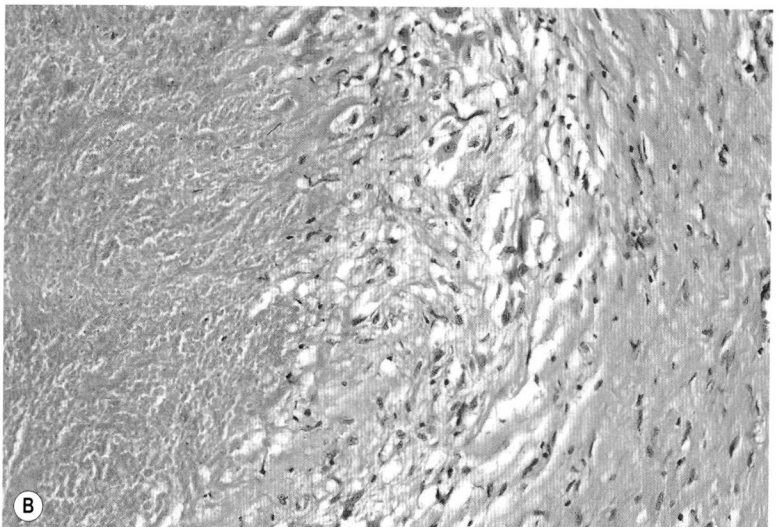

Fig. 18.165
(**A**, **B**) Scrofuloderma: there is extensive caseation necrosis.

Vascular thrombi containing microorganisms may be seen.[18] The less aggressive form is similar but lacks the large numbers of bacteria.

The skin lesions of disseminated miliary tuberculosis (especially in AIDS patients) are often either devoid of granulomata or exhibit only poorly formed granulomata. Extensive necrosis and abscess formation are often seen. Langhans giant cells are rare. Papillary dermal neutrophilic microabscesses reminiscent of those seen in dermatitis herpetiformis are sometimes encountered. Special stains reveal numerous acid-fast bacilli.[35,37]

Scrofuloderma

Scrofuloderma usually appears as an ulcerated dermal abscess with an ill-defined histiocytic component. Peripheral granulomata may be present. Marked caseation necrosis, in which bacilli may be numerous, can be seen in the deeper tissues (*Fig. 18.165*).

Tuberculous gummata

Subcutaneous gummata are associated with marked caseation, but there are few bacilli (*Fig. 18.166*). There is a surrounding granulomatous infiltrate, which may be associated with dermal involvement.

Tuberculous cellulitic lesions are characterized by granulomatous inflammation with giant cells and demonstrable bacilli.[39,41,44] Panniculitis with vasculitis may occasionally be seen in cutaneous tuberculous lesions.[7] Rare cases of subcutaneous mycobacterial granulomatous arteritis have been documented.[46]

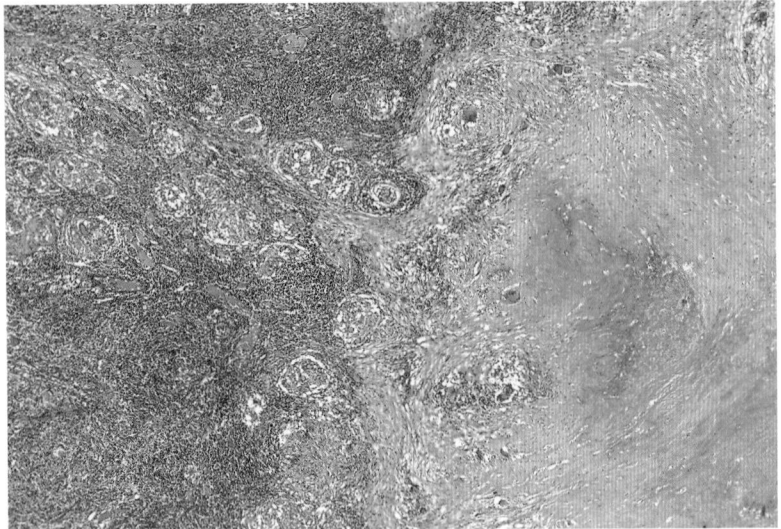

Fig. 18.166
Tuberculous gumma: there is massive caseation surrounded by a well-defined granulomatous infiltrate.

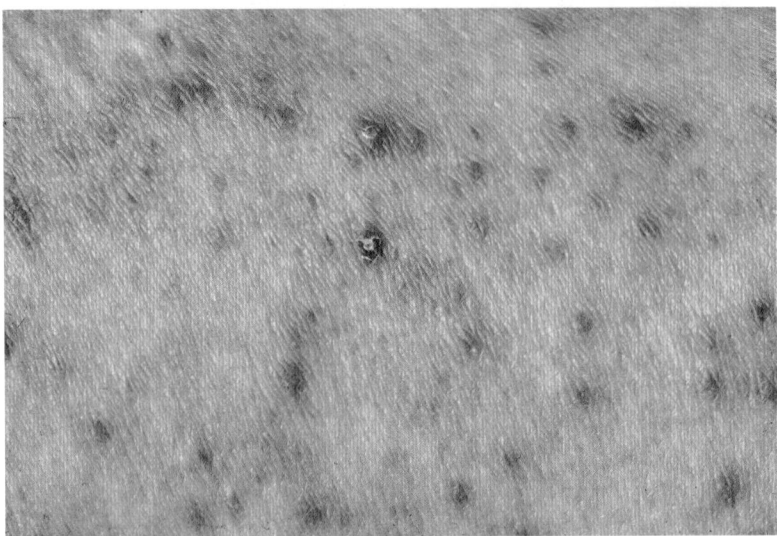

Fig. 18.167
Papulonecrotic tuberculid: widely distributed small purple papules are present. By courtesy of N.C. Dlova, MD, Nelson R. Mandela School of Medicine, University of KwaZulu-Natal, South Africa.

Differential diagnosis

The typical granulomatous and caseating picture is virtually pathognomonic for tuberculous infection, although sarcoidosis can have a similar appearance. Sarcoid, however, can be distinguished by the lack of caseation, but often this is not particularly helpful since necrosis is seen in only a minority of cases of tuberculosis. Necrosis when present in sarcoidosis is rather more fibrinoid than caseating. More helpful is the lack of a surrounding lymphocytic and plasmacytic infiltrate and fewer giant cells in sarcoidosis and a more discrete arrangement of the granulomata (the sarcoidal naked granuloma). Schaumann bodies are characteristic of sarcoidosis, but may occasionally be seen in mycobacterial infections.[7]

In less granulomatous forms of cutaneous tuberculosis, a distinction from leprosy must be made. The perineural distribution of the inflammation is a pointer toward leprosy.

Deep fungal infections and leishmaniasis may also be confused with tuberculosis, and recognition of the organism is vital. Granulomatous late secondary and tertiary syphilis is distinguished by the vascular changes and numerous plasma cells. Caseation necrosis is typical of acne agminata and may also be seen in foreign body reactions to beryllium and zirconium.[47] It may also be a feature of Wegener granulomatosis, although this would be distinctly unusual in cutaneous lesions.

Despite these points, diagnosis may still not be possible. The difficulty is made worse by the frequent failure to demonstrate bacilli even in definite cases of tuberculosis, and the results of culture take 3–4 weeks. Therefore, occasionally, it may be a diagnosis of exclusion, which is confirmed by a therapeutic trial of antituberculous drugs.[13] The shortcomings of these traditional methods have led to increased use of PCR for confirmation of the diagnosis.[2,8,48]

Tuberculids

Clinical features

A tuberculid is a cutaneous immunological reaction to the presence of tuberculosis, which is often occult, elsewhere in the body.[1–3] By definition, special stains and cultures for tubercle bacilli from tuberculids are negative. Although tuberculids are rare in Western countries, they are still important conditions in developing countries where tuberculosis is a common disease.[3–5]

Tuberculids may be papular or nodular and can be separately classified on that basis, but variations and combinations of those features may be seen and are only valid descriptively.

One variety of papular tuberculid is the papulonecrotic tuberculid. This chronic condition presents as recurring crops of flesh-colored, erythematous,

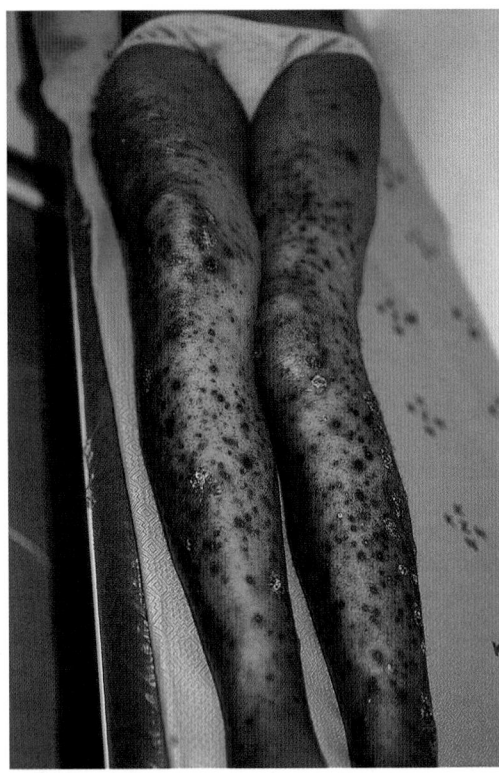

Fig. 18.168
Papulonecrotic tuberculid: innumerable papules are distributed on the dorsal aspect of the legs. Tuberculids imply an active infection elsewhere in the body. By courtesy of N.C. Dlova, MD, Nelson R. Mandela School of Medicine, University of KwaZulu-Natal, South Africa.

or darkish red papules, most often on the ears and the limbs and in particular on extensor aspects around the elbows and knees (*Figs 18.167* and *18.168*).[4–9] Lesions may occur widely or present in isolated sites.[7,10] The papules may become pustular, ulcerate, or develop crusts. They are often symmetrically distributed.[11] Genital involvement may occasionally occur.[7] Uncommonly, the papules may assume an MC-like appearance.[12] They regress slowly over several weeks, leaving depressed, varioliform scars.[11,13] Usually they occur in young people who otherwise often appear rather well. Occasional cases have been reported to progress to lupus vulgaris.[3,6]

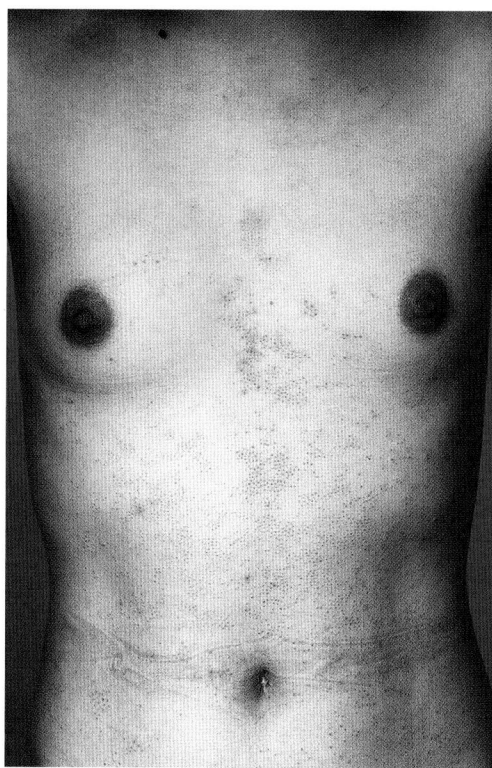

Fig. 18.169
Lichen scrofulosorum: note the numerous tiny papules on the chest and upper abdomen. By courtesy of S. Lucas, MD, St Thomas' Hospital, London, UK.

Lichen scrofulosorum characteristically presents as yellow or brown asymptomatic follicular papules, less than 3 mm across, on the trunk (*Fig. 18.169*). These lesions regress slowly and do not leave scars. This uncommon tuberculous reaction usually occurs in children and young adults.[8,9,14-17] Lesions mimicking psoriasis or lichen planus have been described.[18,19] The eruption is said to be more frequently associated with tuberculous lymphadenitis (cervical, hilar or mediastinal) or osseous tuberculosis than with pulmonary tuberculosis.[8,15] The latter observation has not been supported by others.[14,15] It has also been reported following BCG vaccination, and in association with underlying *M. avium-intracellulare* (MAI) infection.[8,9]

Until recently, the only nodular tuberculid that was generally accepted was erythema induratum (Bazin disease, nodular vasculitis). This condition presents as ill-defined nodules on the calves of predominantly young and middle-aged women, characteristically those who are obese, and have erythrocyanotic skin in this area. The lesions may be worse in cold weather, which raises the problem of distinction from pernio. With progression, the nodules eventually form irregular ulcers, which tend to have bluish undermined edges. Resolution is slow but most lesions disappear spontaneously over a few months. Potential sequelae include postinflammatory hyperpigmentation or atrophic scars.[8,9]

The term nodular tuberculid has been applied to a rare subset of patients with nonulcerated nodules on the lower legs and in whom the pathological changes are centered on both the dermis and the subcutaneous fat.[12,20,21] It has been proposed that this entity represents a hybrid between papulonecrotic tuberculid and erythema induratum of Bazin.[20] Rare cases of papulonecrotic tuberculid coexistent with erythema induratum have also been reported.[22-25]

The terms nodular granulomatous phlebitis of the skin and superficial thrombophlebitic tuberculid have been proposed for an additional type of tuberculid which presents as subcutaneous nodules along the course of a leg vein. There is histologic evidence of granulomatous inflammation centered on the wall of the affected vessel.[26,27] This condition should be distinguished from true tuberculous phlebitis as a consequence of miliary tuberculosis.

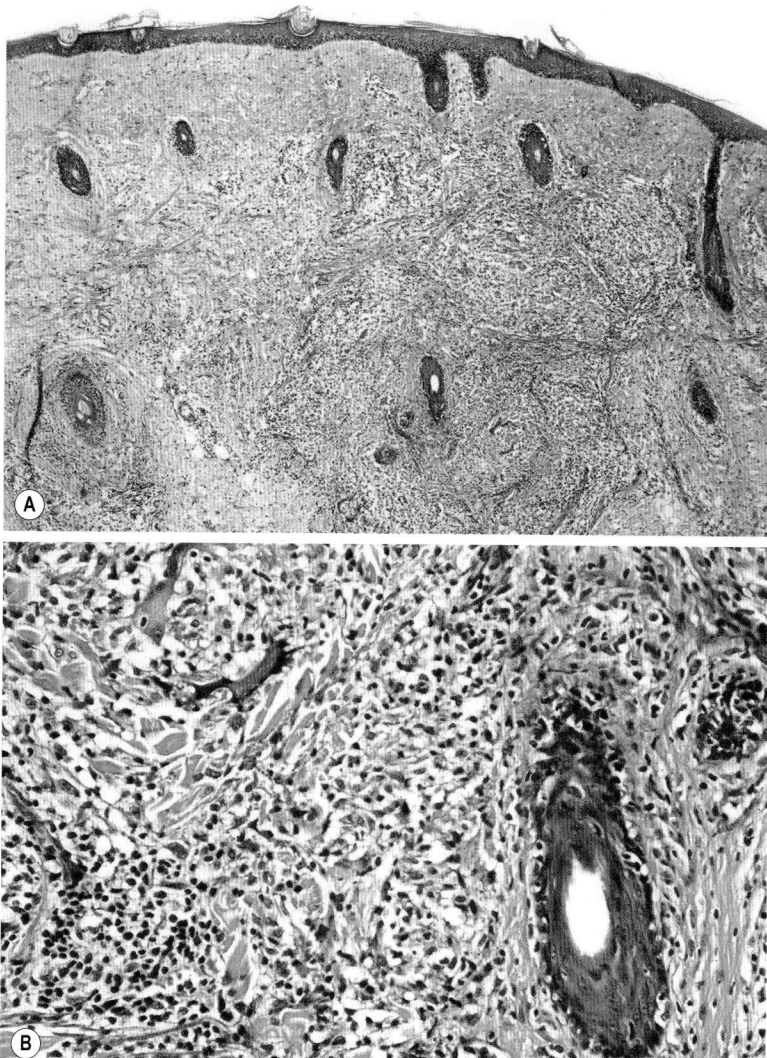

Fig. 18.170
(**A**, **B**) Lichen scrofulosorum: note the perifollicular distribution of this well-defined granulomatous infiltrate.

Pathogenesis and histologic features

All tuberculids are immunological reactions thought to be due to hematogenously disseminated *M. tuberculosis* antigens or small numbers of dead bacteria, possibly opsonized. These embolize to produce lesions, particularly in areas of slow circulation. As a result of changes in small dermal vessels (either an Arthus reaction or a lymphohistiocytic vasculitis), degenerative responses develop in the dermal collagen. In the case of papulonecrotic tuberculid, this amounts to frank necrosis. Histologically, the lesions show variable combinations of vasculitis with necrosis, a moderate to intense lymphohistiocytic infiltrate, and granulomatous inflammation.

Papulonecrotic tuberculid, when fully developed, shows cutaneous infarction comprising a necrotic epidermis with ulceration and an underlying V-shaped zone of dermal coagulative necrosis accompanied by a dense chronic inflammatory cell infiltrate with scattered giant cells.[4,5,11,13] Necrosis of hair follicles may occur.[28] On occasion, a histiocytic palisade has been described, resulting in features reminiscent of granuloma annulare. Neutrophils are generally inconspicuous. Well-formed granulomata can be present in older lesions, but bacilli cannot be identified. Vasculitis may be present.[6,9,11] These features can sometimes be histologically confused with pityriasis lichenoides et varioliformis acuta.[10,28]

In lichen scrofulosorum, a granulomatous infiltrate in which Langhans giant cells are conspicuous is centered around hair follicles and eccrine units (*Fig. 18.170*). Caseous necrosis is usually absent.[4,9]

Erythema induratum is indistinguishable from nodular vasculitis. The changes are centered on the subcutis. There is predominantly lobular panniculitis in association with tuberculoid granulomas, areas of caseation necrosis, and variable vascular involvement of mainly the venules and small to medium caliber arteries, including frank vasculitis.[5,9,29] Due to the prominent necrosis, the vasculitis is often difficult to identify. The presence of both primary vasculitic changes and granulomatous inflammation suggests that type III and type IV hypersensitivity reactions are important in the latter condition.[30]

Although acid-fast organisms are not detectable by special stains, and mycobacterial cultures from these lesions invariably are negative, *M. tuberculosis* DNA has been detected by PCR in a number of cases; this suggests that mycobacterial components are indeed responsible for the pathological manifestations.[13,31–33]

The validity of the concept of the tuberculids rests on the association with underlying tuberculosis, a strong tuberculin reaction, and an invariable response to antituberculous drugs.

Cutaneous complications of bacille Calmette-Guérin vaccination

Clinical features

For almost a century, the BCG vaccine, which employs a live but attenuated form of *Mycobacterium bovis*, has been administered to newborns for the prevention of tuberculosis. BCG immunization is currently carried out in more than 100 countries worldwide where endemic tuberculosis remains a serious public health problem.[1] In recent years, a number of cutaneous and other complications have been recorded, especially in infants with primary immunodeficiency syndromes.[2–8] Complications have also been documented in infants and children infected with HIV.[9–11] It has been shown that HIV infection leads to severe impairment of the BCG-specific T-cell response during the first year of life.[11]

Local infection may develop at the vaccination site, with abscess formation (BCGitis).[4,6,7] Regional lymphadenitis is another well-recognized complication (*Fig. 18.171*), and may be accompanied by cutaneous fistula formation or scrofuloderma.[2,5,9,12] Disseminated skin lesions may also occur, manifesting with a widespread papular eruption or multiple nodules or abscesses in the skin and even the subcutis.[1–6,9,10,13,14] Dissemination of disease (BCGosis) can prove fatal.[14,15] Organs that may potentially be involved include the spleen, mesenteric and mediastinal lymph nodes, bone marrow, liver, and lungs.[2,9] Other documented cutaneous manifestations include lupus vulgaris, erythema induratum, and papulonecrotic tuberculid-like lesions.[16–19] A case

with cutaneous involvement secondary to intravesical BCG instillation has been reported.[20]

Histologic features

In immunocompetent individuals, skin and lymph node biopsy material may reveal multiple epithelioid cell granulomas with admixed Langhans giant cells and minimal caseous necrosis, with or without concomitant suppuration.[15] Conversely, involved tissues obtained from immunosuppressed individuals are characterized by a diffuse infiltrate of plump histiocytic cells, with poorly developed or absent granuloma formation. The cytoplasm of these histiocytes is distended by large numbers of acid-fast *M. bovis* bacilli (*Fig. 18.172*).[2,10,15] The histologic findings in this latter group are similar at all sites of involvement, including cutaneous, subcutaneous, lymph node, or visceral tissues. The diagnosis may be confirmed by PCR.[21,22] A pattern of dermal involvement mimicking granuloma annulare has been reported.[13]

Differential diagnosis

Mycobacterial culture and PCR studies facilitate distinction between cutaneous, subcutaneous, or disseminated BCG infection in immunocompromised hosts from infection with MAI complex and other nontuberculous mycobacterial infections. The degrading intracytoplasmic organisms contained within macrophages in the subcutaneous nodules of Whipple disease, are PAS-positive but fail to stain with Ziehl-Neelsen method.

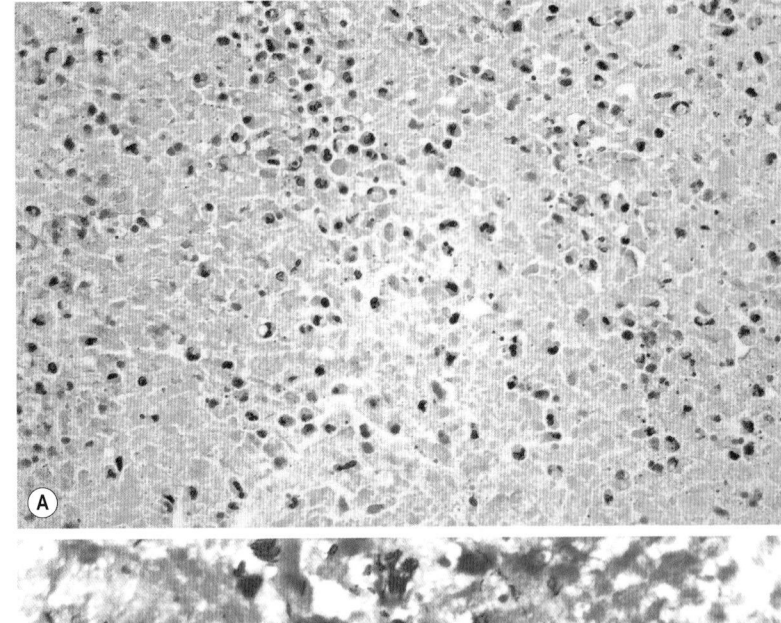
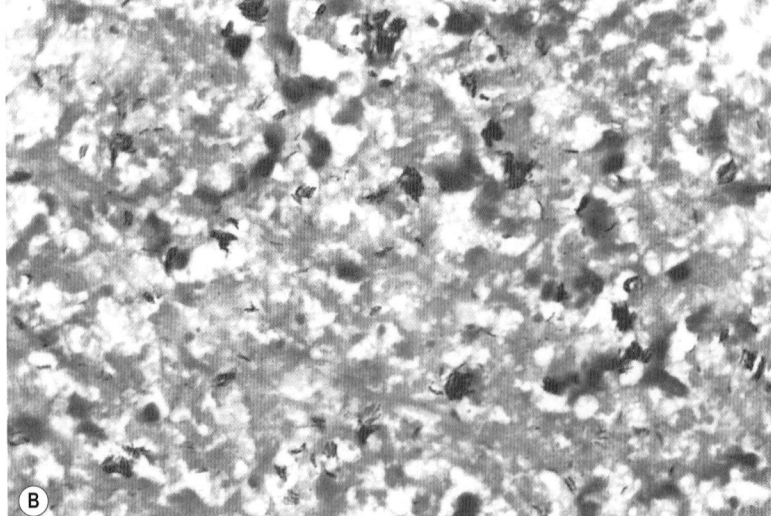

Fig. 18.172
BCG reaction: (**A**) there are sheet-like expanses of foamy histiocytes whose cytoplasm contains innumerable acid-fast bacilli; (**B**) Ziehl-Neelsen stain highlighting the latter.

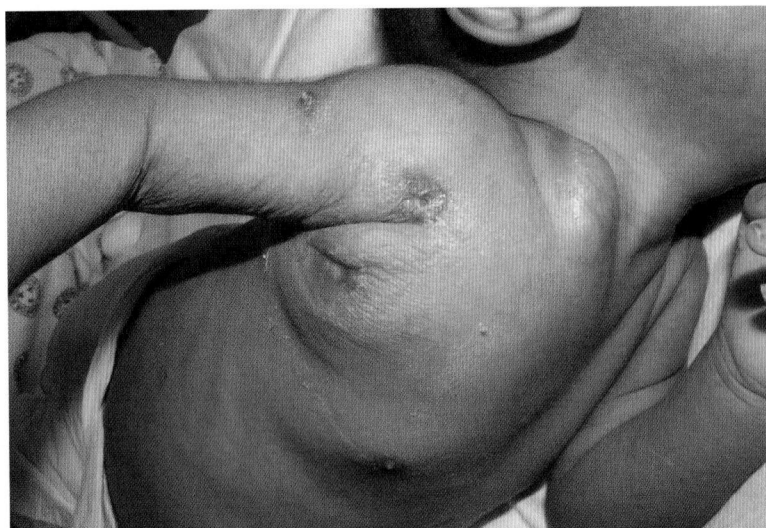

Fig. 18.171
BCG reaction: there is marked swelling with overlying erythema and sinus formation. Courtesy of W. Hendson, MD, Rahima Moosa Mother and Child Hospital and the University of the Witwatersrand, Johannesburg, South Africa.

Nontuberculous environmental mycobacterial infections

Nontuberculous mycobacteria (atypical mycobacteria; mycobacteria other than tubercle bacilli), which are usually nonpathogenic, are widespread in varied sites throughout the world.[1-4] These ubiquitous organisms inhabit vegetation and water (stagnant, fresh or salty), and are saprophytic in soil, on animals, and within animal feces. They are traditionally subdivided according to their growth rate on culture media and by their ability to produce a yellow pigment in culture with and without exposure to light. There are therefore four categories[3,5-7]:

- Group I organisms are photochromogens, which produce pigment after exposure to light (e.g., *Mycobacterium marinum* and *Mycobacterium kansasii*).
- Group II organisms are the scotochromogens, which produce pigmented colonies whether light is present or not (e.g., *Mycobacterium scrofulaceum* and *Mycobacterium szulgai*).
- Group III organisms are consistently nonpigmented and include *Mycobacterium avium* and *Mycobacterium intracellulare*.
- Group IV organisms are the fast growers and include *Mycobacterium chelonei*, *Mycobacterium fortuitum*, and *Mycobacterium abscessus*.

Exact species identification may also be facilitated by PCR performed on mycobacteria that are grown in liquid media.[4,8] The environmental mycobacterial infections are becoming of increasing importance in immunocompromised patients, particularly in those with HIV/AIDS. Patients receiving anti-TNF-α agents and individuals with SLE who are treated with corticosteroids and immunosuppressive drugs are also at risk for infection. Cutaneous infection with these organisms in the immunocompetent patient usually follows an episode of trauma and gives rise to a localized lesion often clinically resembling panniculitis. There have been numerous reports of previously healthy individuals acquiring infection via tattooing and following nonsurgical or surgical cosmetic procedures. In the immunosuppressed, a history of trauma is usually lacking and patients tend to present with multiple subcutaneous nodules, more diffuse inflammation, and frequent abscess formation.[4,6,7,9-15] Systemic spread is obviously of particular importance in this latter group. As the features may be atypical, diagnosis is facilitated by a high index of suspicion.

Clinical features

Mycobacterium marinum

M. marinum (*balnei*) is a slow-growing photochromogen, which is associated with injuries in aquatic environments or by fish or equipment, usually under water.[16] The upper limb is the site of infection in around 90% or more of cases.[17-19] Infections have been contracted most often in swimming pools (swimming pool granuloma, fish tank granuloma), usually on the elbows and knees of children, or from aquaria, usually on the hands (*Fig. 18.173*).[19,20] In some studies, inoculation related to fish tank exposure has accounted for more than 80% of cases.[17] The lesions usually present 1 week to 2 months (average 2–3 weeks) after superficial injury and are typically painless inflammatory nodules or plaques.[21] They may ulcerate and discharge yellow fluid and older lesions can be warty (*Fig. 18.174*). Occasionally, abscesses are seen. Quite often there is extension along lymphatics, with the development of secondary nodules in a pattern comparable to sporotrichosis (*Fig. 18.175*).[19,20,22,23] Sporotrichoid spread has also been reported in the context of HIV infection and following infliximab therapy.[24,25] Penetrating injuries sometimes result in tenosynovitis.[26,27] Infection in immunodeficient individuals produces a deeply undermined ulcer; otherwise, lesions usually resolve within a few months. In one large retrospective study the mean duration of disease was 19 months.[28]

Mycobacterium fortuitum chelonae (M. fortuitum *complex*)

M. fortuitum chelonae (*M. fortuitum* complex) comprises a group of rapid-growing organisms found in soil and water and occasionally nonpathogenically in sputum. The organisms are *M. fortuitum*, *M. chelonae*, and *M. abscessus*. Lesions, which are uncommon, usually develop 3–4 weeks after contamination of skin wounds, including surgical incisions, injections (e.g., with cosmetic fillers), liposuction, liposculpture, fractionated

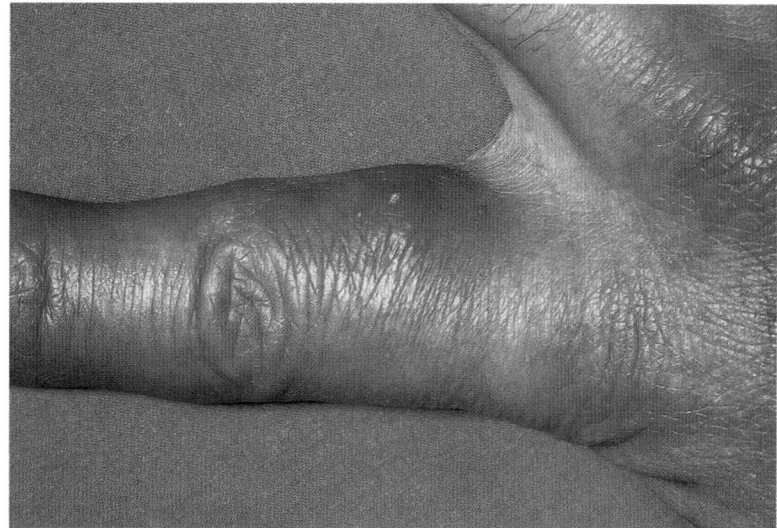

Fig. 18.173
Mycobacterium marinum (*balnei*): inflammatory nodule on the finger of an aquarium enthusiast. By courtesy of R.A. Marsden, MD, St George's Hospital, London, UK.

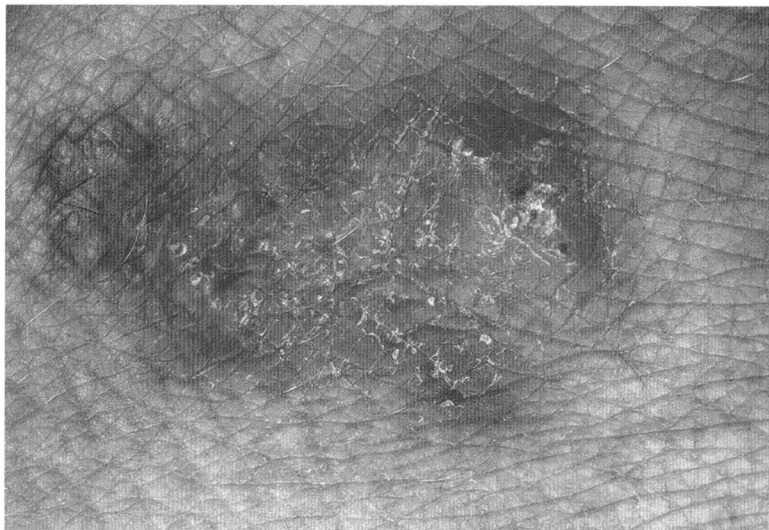

Fig. 18.174
Mycobacterium marinum (*balnei*): close-up view of an erythematous plaque with scaling. By courtesy of the Institute of Dermatology, London, UK.

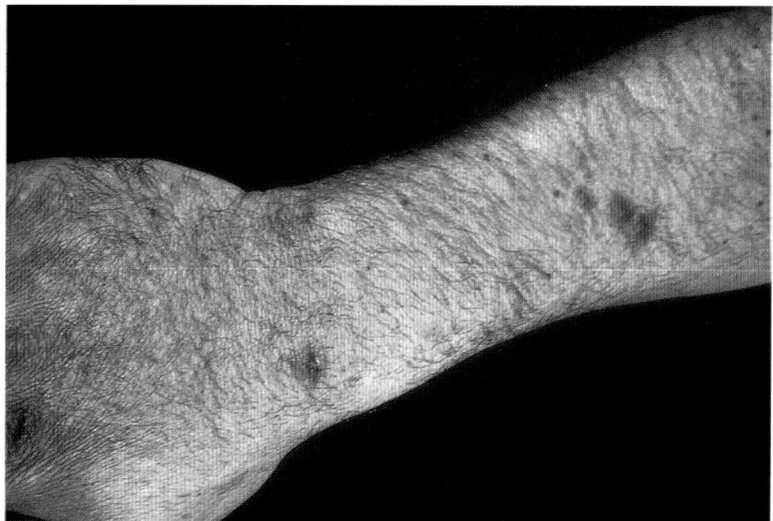

Fig. 18.175
Mycobacterium marinum (*balnei*): this example demonstrates sporotrichoid spread. By courtesy of the Institute of Dermatology, London, UK.

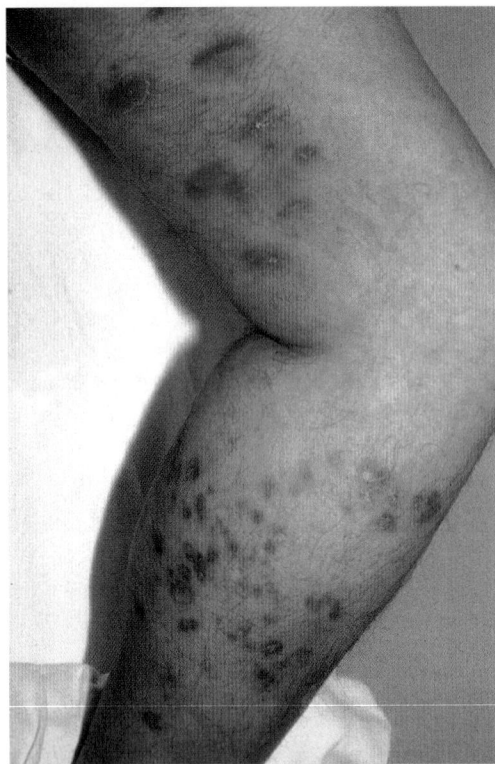

Fig. 18.176
Mycobacterium fortuitum chelonae: numerous abscesses are distributed along this patient's leg. This infection is more often seen in the immunosuppressed. By courtesy of the Institute of Dermatology, London, UK.

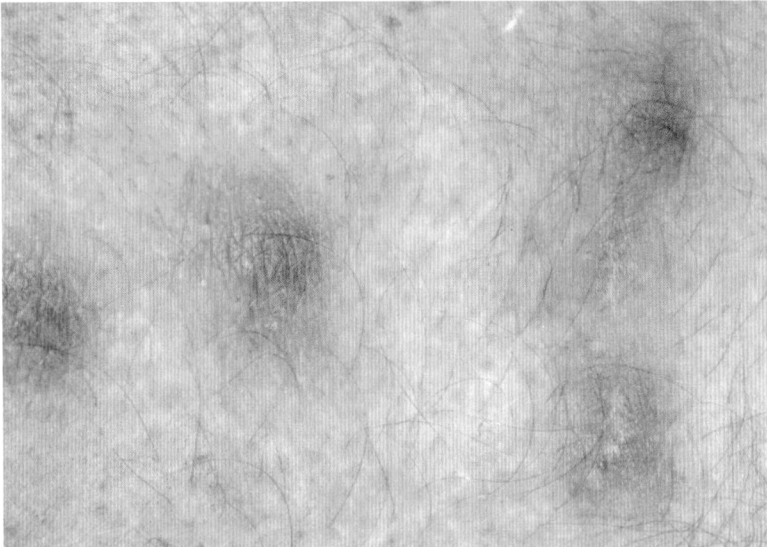

Fig. 18.177
Mycobacterium fortuitum chelonae: close-up view. By courtesy of the Institute of Dermatology, London, UK.

CO_2 laser resurfacing, tattooing, acupuncture, and even following implantation of cardiac devices.[4,16,29–38] Outbreaks of mycobacterial furunculosis due to *M. fortuitum* have occurred due to communal use of footbaths at nail salons during pedicures.[4,39–41] Reports emerged of *M. fortuitum* and *M. abscessus* infection among survivors of the 2004 tsunami disaster off Thailand; these patients had sustained contaminated crush trauma injuries to their lower extremities.[42] A large subcutaneous abscess due to *M. abscessus* has been described in a patient with SLE.[43] Disease may present in a disseminated form, often associated with immunosuppression, including HIV/AIDS (Figs 18.176 and 18.177).[10,44] Pulmonary infection with subsequent cutaneous dissemination has also been reported in an apparently immunocompetent patient.[45] The lesions comprise indolent abscesses with fistula

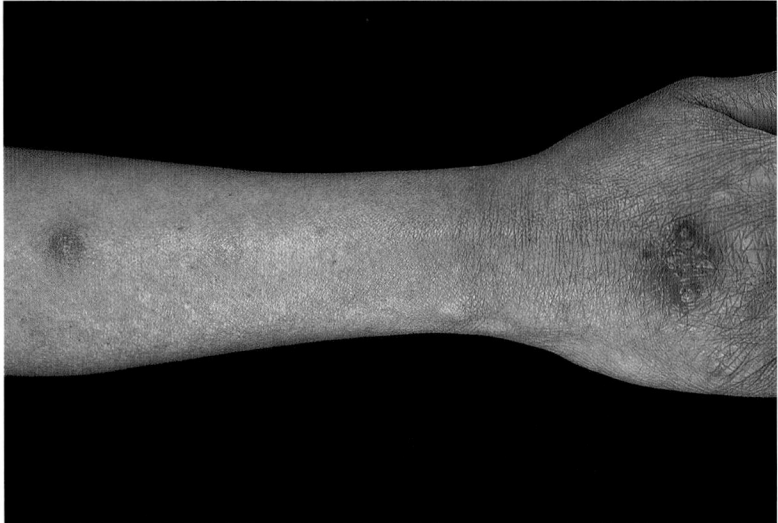

Fig. 18.178
Mycobacterium fortuitum chelonae: note the indurated, nodular, ulcerated lesion on the hand with sporotrichoid spread. By courtesy of S. Lucas, MD, St Thomas' Hospital, London, UK.

formation, purulent discharge, and scarring. A sporotrichoid distribution has also been recorded (*Fig. 18.178*).[9,46] Healing is usually delayed for many months, but may be helped by adequate debridement. *M. chelonae* is more refractory to treatment.

Mycobacterium kansasii

M. kansasii is a slow-growing photochromogen found worldwide in various habitats. This is a disease mainly of the lungs and lymph nodes; it only rarely causes skin lesions and these are most common in the immunosuppressed, when they are usually associated with disseminated disease.[47–49] Iatrogenically immunosuppressed patients and patients with HIV/AIDS may, however, also present with primary cutaneous infection.[50,51] Cases of infection by *M. kansasii* are varied in their presentation: they may appear as nodules (which can be verrucous), crusted ulcers, papulopustules, cellulitis, or as a spreading infection resembling sporotrichosis.[52,53]

Mycobacterium ulcerans

M. ulcerans infection is currently recognized as the third most common mycobacterial disease in immunocompetent people (after tuberculosis and leprosy).[54,55] In 1998, the WHO recognized the condition as a re-emerging infectious disease, and it has since been declared a neglected tropical disease by the WHO.[56–58] The causative organism is a slow-growing nonchromogen, which is present sporadically on lush vegetation in swampy areas in the tropics.[59–62] It is particularly seen in the tropical wetlands of West and Central Africa (Buruli ulcer), but was characterized in Australia (Bairnsdale ulcer). It was subsequently recorded in the koala bear in the same region.[63] The condition also occurs in tropical regions of Asia and South America, and although traditionally regarded as a disease of the tropics, numerous cases have been reported from subtropical and nontropical countries, including Australia, China, and Japan.[57,61] It is estimated that between 3000 and 5000 new infections occur annually. The disease is known to occur in around 33 countries worldwide.[57,58,64]

Comparative genomic studies indicate that *M. ulcerans* recently evolved from *M. marinum* to become a niche-adapted specialist.[55,65–67] Two distinct lineages exist: the 'classic' lineage comprising more virulent strains from Africa, Australia, and Southeast Asia, and an 'ancestral' lineage, which includes genotypes encountered in China, Japan, and South America.[66] *M. ulcerans* subsp. *shinshuense*, for example, is speculated to be domestic to Japan and Asia.[57] Although it had been stated that *M. ulcerans* infection was not linked to HIV infection, studies have since shown that HIV infection may indeed increase the risk for acquiring Buruli ulcer, or render the disease more aggressive.[55,58,61,68] There have been conflicting data concerning the protective role of BCG vaccination.[55,69]

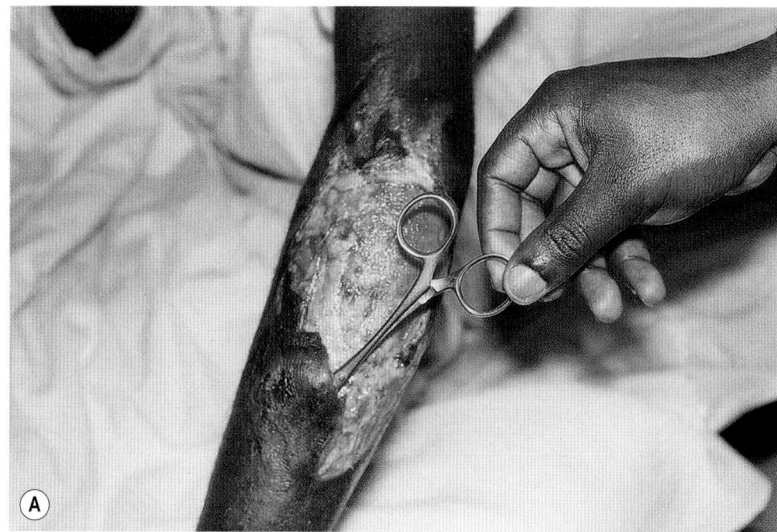

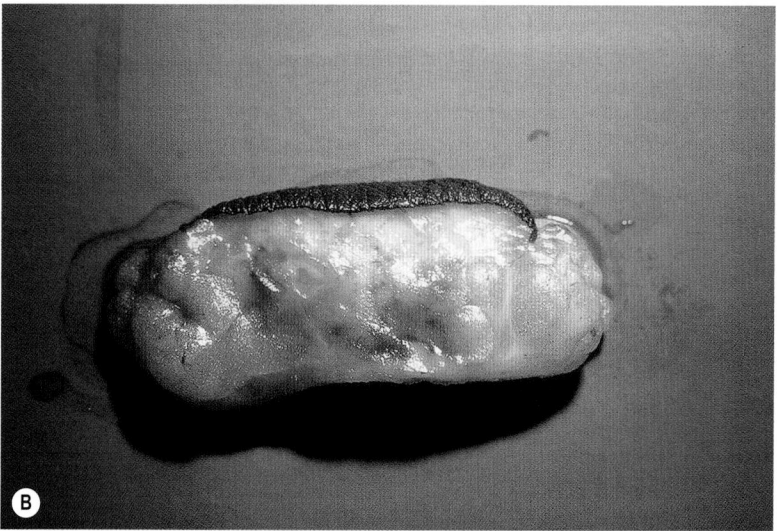

Fig. 18.179
Mycobacterium ulcerans: (**A**) note the extensive ulceration with undermining of the edge; (**B**) gross specimen showing opaque necrosis of the central subcutaneous fat. (**A**) By courtesy of S. Lucas, MD, St Thomas' Hospital, London, UK; (**B**) by courtesy of the late M. Hutt, MD, St Thomas' Hospital, London, UK.

The lesion develops about 8 weeks after minor trauma or skin abrasions which came into contact with contaminated water, soil, or vegetation.[56,70] Consequently, the infection usually appears on the legs and tends to occur more often in children between the ages of 5 and 15 years.[64,70,71] A second peak occurs later in adult life.[71] There is, however, a strong likelihood that the majority of individuals who come into contact with *M. ulcerans* do not develop clinical disease. Furthermore, Buruli ulcer lesions may also heal spontaneously.[56] In those individuals with clinical disease, the initial erythematous papule or nodule progresses to an indolent ulcer, which may be minor or major; very large ulcers may measure up to 50 cm across (*Fig. 18.179*).[56] The ulcer is without exudate or surrounding reaction, but extends to involve underlying fascia or fat and typically has an undermined border.[55,56,70] There is little or no malaise or fever. The ulcer is generally painless unless complicated by secondary bacterial infection.[55,57] After 6–9 months, a granulomatous response develops, which precedes healing. This is usually associated with scarring, which may lead to severe deformity and contractures.[54,56,64] Although surgery has been the historical treatment of choice, antibiotics now fulfill an important role in contemporary treatment guidelines.[4,55]

The extensive tissue necrosis and ulceration that are hallmarks of the infection are attributable to production of mycolactone, a potent soluble toxic macrolide possessing both cytotoxic and immunosuppressive properties. Mycolactone leads to cell death via both apoptosis and necrosis. This polyketide toxin has antiphagocytic properties and not only limits the initiation of a primary immune response, but also impedes the recruitment of inflammatory cells to the site of infection.[56,60,64,72–77] Geographically specific subtypes of mycolactone are recognized, namely, A/B occurring in Africa (and the most virulent), C in Asia and Australia, and D in Asia.[55,77,78] A major recent development has been the identification of two specific underlying subcellular and molecular pathogenetic targets of mycolactone. Wiskott-Aldrich syndrome protein (WASP) is a scaffolding protein which controls actin dynamics in adherent cells. Mycolactone has a direct effect on WASP, with disruption of WASP inhibition via WASP hyperactivation, leading to cell death as a consequence of cellular detachment. The second molecular target is Sec61, an essential gatekeeper for translocation of proteins into the endoplasmic reticulum, and hence their secretion or placement into cell membranes. Inhibition of Sec61-mediated co-translational translocation of newly synthesized proteins leads to inhibition of local cytokine release by the immune cells.[78]

A nonulcerative form of the disease is recognized in highly endemic areas.[56,72] Associated osteomyelitic bone lesions are not uncommon, especially when multiple cutaneous lesions are present on the lower extremities.[71] Osteomyelitis is the consequence of either contiguous spread from an ulcerated lesion or metastatic dissemination of the infection.[55,56] Occasionally, severe systemic disease and death may result from secondary infection or tetanus.[54] Rarely, squamous cell carcinoma can arise in a chronic Buruli ulcer.[56,79,80]

M. ulcerans infection tends to occur in parts of Africa where there is a high prevalence of *Schistosoma haematobium* infection. This observation led some authors to suggest that schistosomiasis may be a risk factor for the development of Buruli ulcer by driving the host immunological reaction away from a Th1 response and toward a Th2 response.[61] This apparent association with schistosomiasis, however, is purely fortuitous, with no clear evidence to support the hypothesis that co-infection with *Schistosoma* spp. confers susceptibility to infection with *M. ulcerans*.[81] Instead, transmission of the disease appears to be related to the close spatial proximity of human activities to high-risk aquatic environments.[55,62,82] Epidemiological and experimental evidence suggests that predatory aquatic insects act as a potential vector of *M. ulcerans*, and that the aquatic snails on which these insects feed serve as passive intermediate hosts.[56,62,64,83,84] In the Australian context, however, mosquitoes have been implicated in the transmission of *M. ulcerans*.[62,85,86] A possible role for *Acanthamoeba* spp. in the transmission and persistence of the disease has been proffered in recent years.[87] Risk factors for acquisition of the disease in endemic areas include failure to wear protective clothing, exposure to unprotected natural water sources, and inadequate care of minor skin wounds.[55,62,69]

Mycobacterium avium-intracellulare (M. avium *complex*)

MAI complex is a group of slow-growing nonchromogens, which are present widely in dust, soil, and water.[88,89] Exposure to soil appears to represent an important environmental risk factor for infection.[90] They are seen most commonly causing a cervical lymphadenitis or disseminated infection in immunocompromised hosts. MAI is one of the commonest causes of bacteremia in AIDS patients and is also frequently isolated from the liver, bone marrow, lung, or gastrointestinal tract. Although the skin may be involved as part of disseminated MAI disease, primary cutaneous infection is uncommon.[91] A disseminated varioliform pustular eruption due to MAI has been described in a patient with AIDS.[92] Primary infections may develop in immunocompetent individuals who present with subcutaneous nodules, which subsequently undergo ulceration.[93–96] Isolated lesions such as perineal ulcers or subcutaneous masses may also occur in AIDS patients.[91] Skin and soft tissue involvement can occur as part of the IRIS in HIV-infected patients receiving highly active ART.[97,98] Dermal and subcutaneous infection has been reported in an iatrogenically immunosuppressed individual receiving treatment for SLE.[99]

Generally, the skin lesions present as a panniculitis, often in relation to affected lymph nodes, or as nodules progressing to abscesses and ulcers (*Fig. 18.180*). Healing is slow, even with appropriate drug therapy, and excision may be necessary.

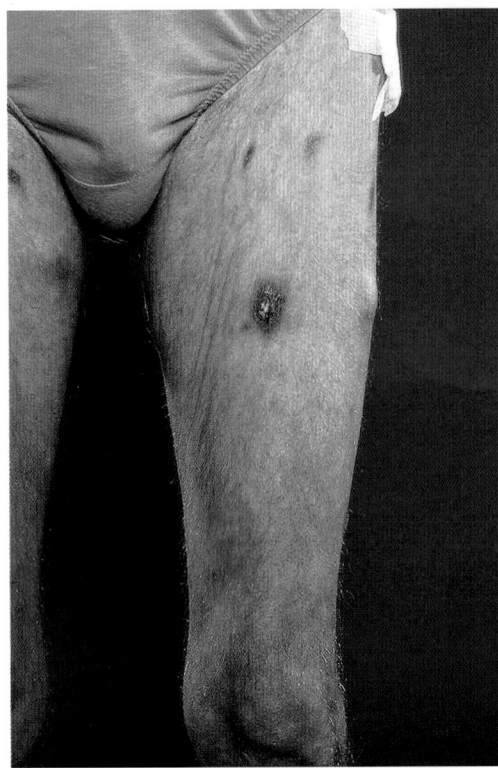

Fig. 18.180
Mycobacterium avium intracellulare: these multiple nodules on the thighs resemble panniculitis. By courtesy of S. Lucas, MD, St Thomas' Hospital, London, UK.

Other mycobacteria

An expanding number of other mycobacteria, including *M. scrofulaceum*, *M. gordonae*, *M. simiae*, *M. xenopi*, *M. malmoense*, *M. haemophilum*, *M. massiliense*, and *M. bolettii*, may rarely cause cutaneous lesions, mostly following inoculation, to produce nodules and abscesses, usually with ulceration and sinus formation.[2,4,27,100]

Histologic features

Most of these atypical mycobacteria show early cutaneous necrosis with neutrophil abscess formation. This phase is usually associated with readily demonstrable bacilli. Microorganisms are often found in round empty spaces that mimic adipocytes. Clumps of bacilli may even be identified in sections stained with H&E. The abscess phase is gradually replaced by granulomatous inflammation and fibrosis, often with sinus formation.

Mycobacterium marinum

M. marinum follows the common histologic progression from abscess to granuloma, but few of the broad, long bacilli are seen, except in immunocompromised patients (*Fig. 18.181*).[10,101] Granulomatous inflammation is encountered more frequently than with other nontuberculous mycobacterial infections.[102] Caseation is absent, but there may be fibrinoid necrosis. Langhans cells may be conspicuous or scanty (*Fig. 18.182*). A lymphohistiocytic infiltrate is present in the surrounding dermis. The overlying epidermis is parakeratotic, acanthotic, or ulcerated. Pseudoepitheliomatous hyperplasia may occur (*Fig. 18.183*).[10] The sporotrichoid nodules, which are frequently present, are tuberculoid granulomata without the preceding abscess phase. There is often a poor yield of positive isolates from culture specimens, and PCR may thus be a more useful means of confirming the diagnosis.[28,103]

Mycobacterium fortuitum chelonae (M. fortuitum *complex*)

M. fortuitum and *M. chelonae* infection shows early acute inflammation, which progresses to ill-defined granulomata with occasional necrotic foci. Panniculitis and acute suppurative folliculitis may also be observed (*Fig. 18.184*).[10] Bacilli are easily seen and are present in clusters (*Figs 18.185* and *18.186*).[46,104]

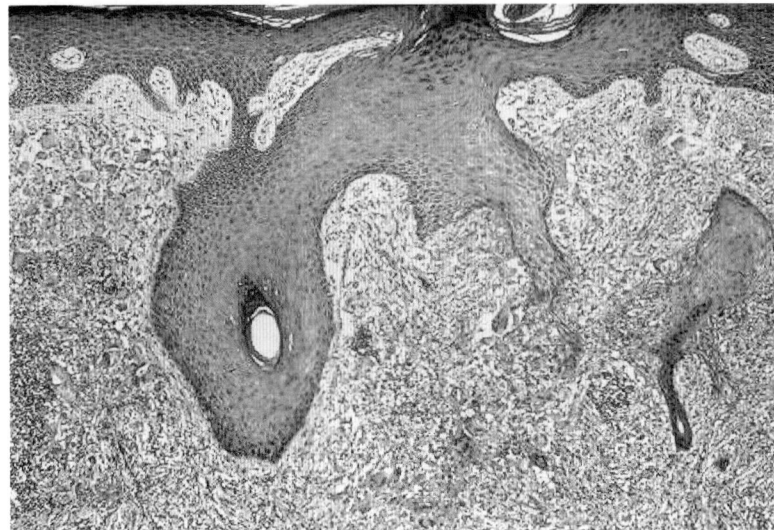

Fig. 18.181
Mycobacterium marinum (*balnei*): there is hyperkeratosis and very marked acanthosis.

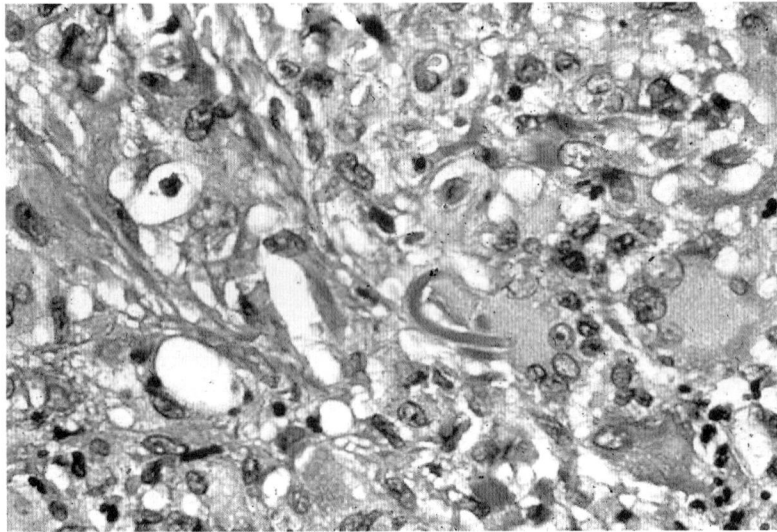

Fig. 18.182
Mycobacterium marinum (*balnei*): conspicuous Langhans giant cells are present.

Mycobacterium kansasii

M. kansasii infection shows a pattern similar to other nontuberculous mycobacterial infections. The early mixed inflammation is usually intense before becoming tuberculoid. Abscesses may be present. Bacilli are frequent. *M. kansasii* organisms are larger, broader, and more coarsely beaded.[105] Some cases show overlying acanthosis with hyperkeratosis and parakeratosis. The acute lesions seen in immunosuppressed patients typically show an intense neutrophil infiltrate with abscess formation.[48,52]

Mycobacterium ulcerans

The typically undermined edge of the ulcer can be appreciated on low-power examination.[55,64] *M. ulcerans* infection is characterized by extensive coagulative necrosis and ulceration with very little inflammatory reaction in established lesions (*Fig. 18.187*).[59,64,70,106] Tissue destruction is mediated by the production of mycolactone, which induces both necrosis and apoptosis.[56,74,77,105] The dose and duration of exposure to the toxin account for the two histologic hallmarks of the condition, namely, tissue necrosis and a paucity of inflammatory cells within the ulcer.[78] In this anergic stage, bacilli are very numerous and are seen clustering in the collagen of fascia or in fat at the base of the ulcer (*Fig. 18.188*).[56] In the early stages of infection, there is an acute inflammatory infiltrate with phagocytosis of *M. ulcerans* bacilli by neutrophils and macrophages. Later, there is apoptosis of the

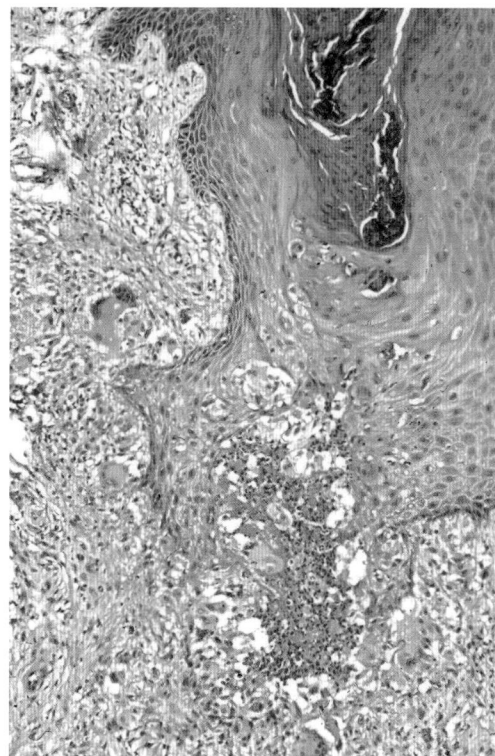

Fig. 18.183
Mycobacterium marinum (*balnei*): abscess formation and granulomatous inflammation have eroded the overlying epidermis. The features of this condition closely mimic the deep fungal infections.

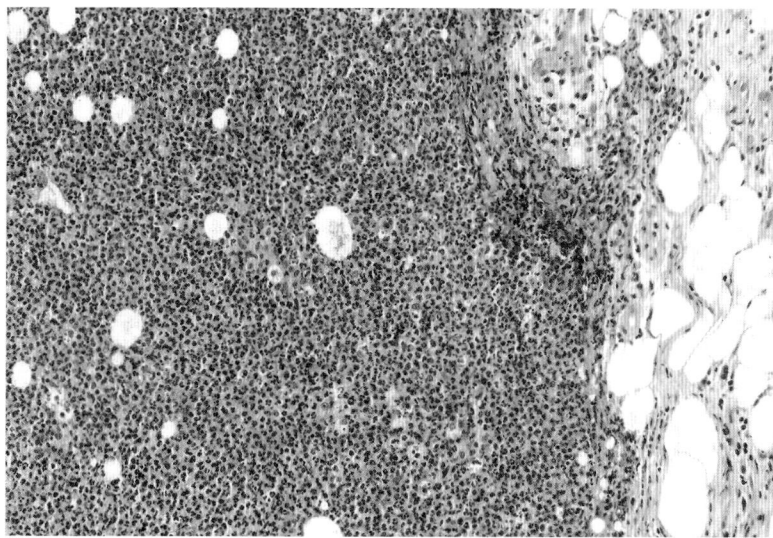

Fig. 18.184
Mycobacterium fortuitum chelonae: this is a predominantly neutrophil-mediated infection.

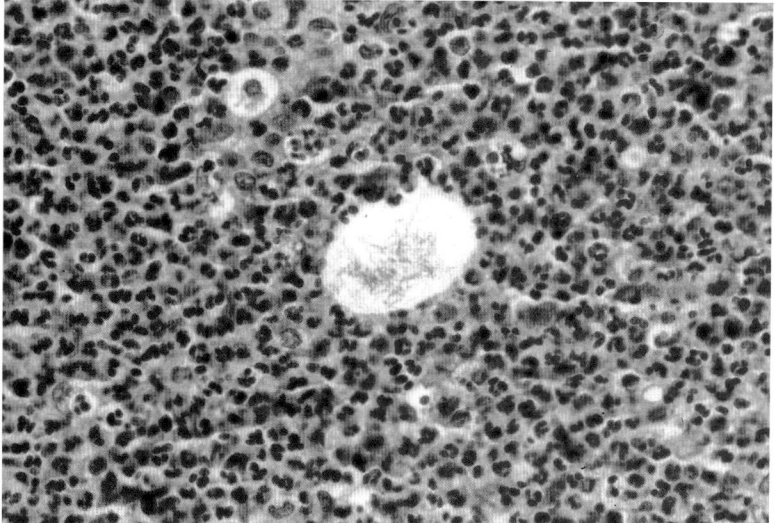

Fig. 18.185
Mycobacterium fortuitum chelonae: aggregates of bacilli are typically visible in the hematoxylin and eosin stained sections.

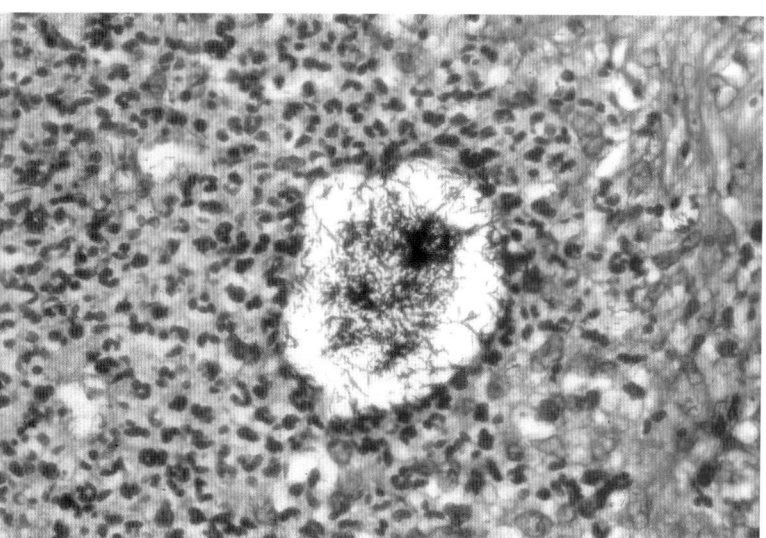

Fig. 18.186
Mycobacterium fortuitum chelonae: the bacilli are strongly acid fast.

neutrophils and macrophages, while more advanced lesions characteristically show acellular areas with clumps of extracellular bacilli, extensive tissue necrosis, and cellular debris. Neutrophils and macrophages with intracellular bacilli are observed peripheral to the necrotic areas.[77] Leukocytoclastic vasculitis has been described in both the dermis and septa of the subcutaneous fat.[70,107] Focal calcification may be seen. Healing of the ulcer corresponds with progressive positivity of the 'burulin' test and a granulomatous reaction. Mycobacteria are then sparse or absent.[70] Caseation is not a feature. Variable septolobular panniculitis can be present. Resolving lesions may exhibit pseudoepitheliomatous hyperplasia of the epidermis.[108] In the nonulcerated form there is massive contiguous necrosis of the dermis

and subcutaneous tissue.[72] Local recurrence has been linked to the presence of persistent infection in macroscopically healthy tissue beyond the surgical excision margins.[109] PCR and histopathology are regarded as the most reliable means of confirming the diagnosis, followed by direct smears and culture of the organism.[4,58]

Mycobacterium avium-intracellulare (M. avium *complex*)

MAI (*M. avium* complex) infection sometimes appears to have an early abscess phase before the granulomatous phase, but in other cases the inflammatory infiltrate is more lymphohistiocytic, so that it resembles lepromatous leprosy (LL) (*Fig. 18.189*).[88,89] Bacilli are present, but are usually intracellular. Rarely, infected histiocytes become large and voluminous and have been referred to as pseudogaucher cells.[110] The histologic picture may also mimic histoid leprosy.[111] A case of cutaneous mycobacterial spindle cell tumor due to *M. intracellulare* has also been reported.[99]

Other mycobacteria

M. haemophilum may produce a mixed suppurative and granulomatous reaction in addition to a paucigranulomatous reaction, lichenoid interface dermatitis, and lymphocytic vasculitis.[112]

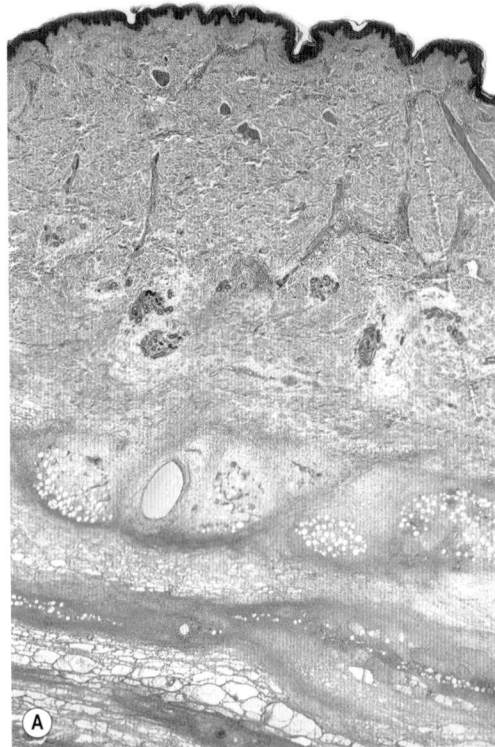

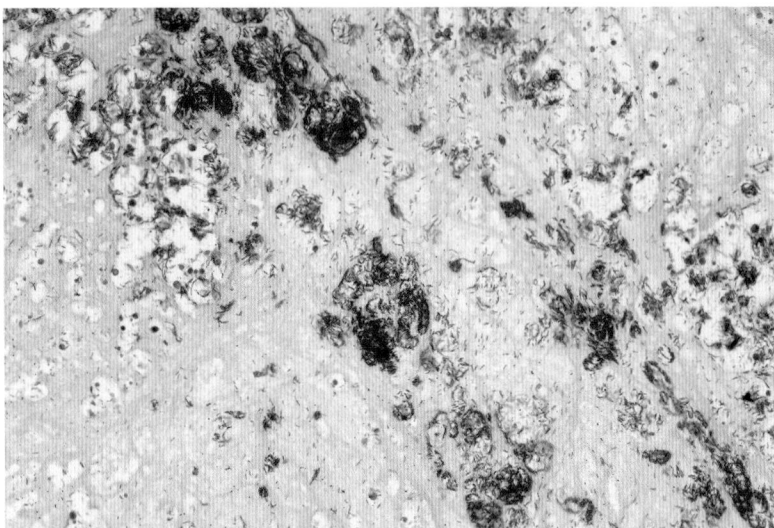

Fig. 18.188
Mycobacterium ulcerans: the lesions contain numerous acid-fast bacilli (Ziehl-Neelsen).

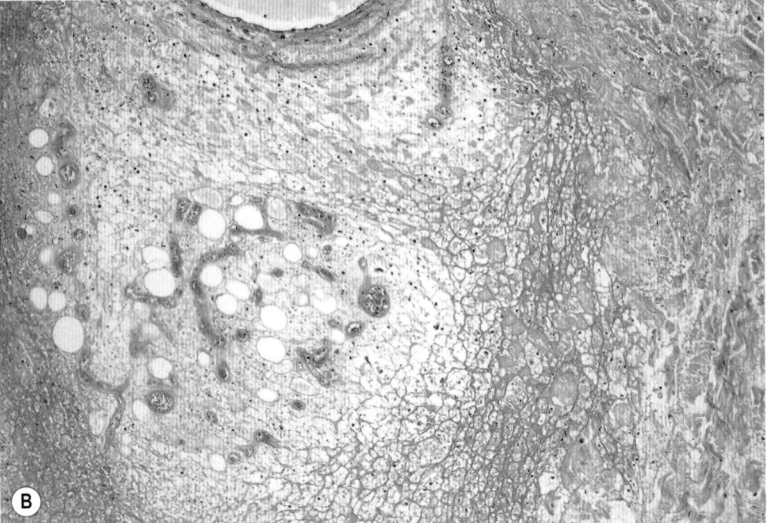

Fig. 18.187
(**A**, **B**) *Mycobacterium ulcerans*: there is widespread coagulative necrosis. Note the absence of an inflammatory reaction.

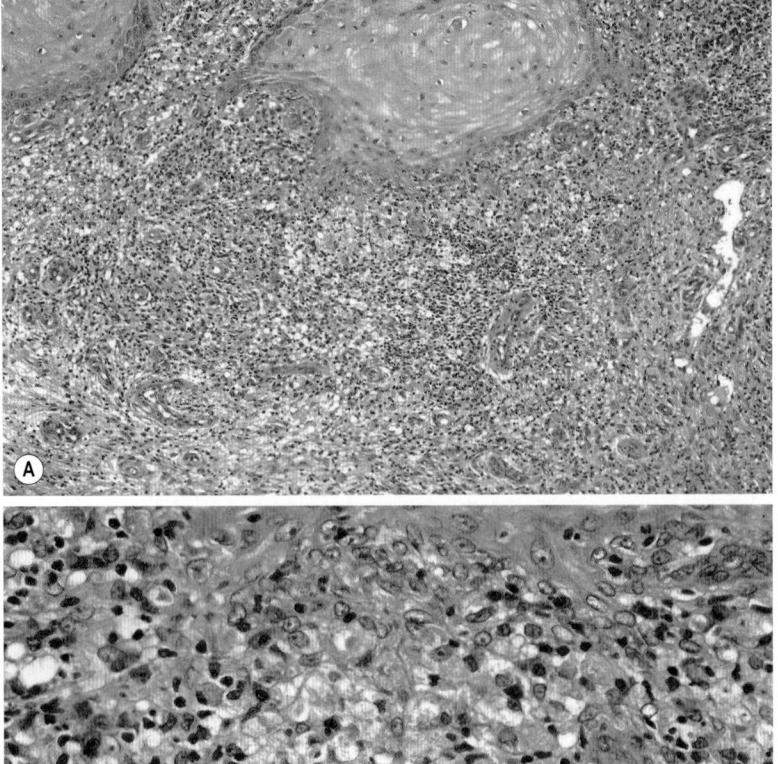

Fig. 18.189
(**A**, **B**) *Mycobacterium avium intracellulare*: in this variant, the infiltrate typically consists of histiocytes, lymphocytes, and neutrophils. Bacteria are often numerous.

Leprosy

Clinical features

Mycobacterium leprae is the bacillus traditionally recognized as causing leprosy (Hansen disease), and until recently could only be cultured in experimental animals, particularly the nine-banded armadillo. It is an obligate intracellular, Gram-positive, weakly acid-fast organism. A major recent development, however, has been the discovery of a second etiological agent of leprosy – *M. lepromatosis*. The latter is regarded as a species distinct from *M. leprae* based on an overall 7.4% genomic difference between the respective organisms.[1]

Leprosy is found worldwide, due to extensive traveling and migration, but is endemic in the tropics.[2–5] Recent decades have seen a dramatic decrease in the global disease burden from more than 5 million people in the mid-1980s to around 800 000 by the mid-1990s. More than 250 000 new cases were detected in 2006, a decrease of more than 13% when compared with 2005. The global registered prevalence of leprosy was around 224 000 at the beginning of 2007.[6–9] The estimated global prevalence of the disease was around 210 000 in 2015, indicating the number of cases worldwide has plateaued over the past decade.[10] However, these data fall short of the WHO's target for elimination of the disease. Leprosy continues to be a leading cause of infection-related morbidity in many of the 136 countries where it is endemic, despite advances in effective multidrug treatment over the past three decades.[10–12]

Although the disease has been recognized for many centuries and its main causative organism, *M. leprae* has been known for more than 100 years, many aspects of the pathogenesis remain unclear or have only recently been elucidated. Leprosy continues to present challenges to diagnosticians, epidemiologists, and pharmacologists alike.

M. lepromatosis is now recognized as the species responsible for a unique, severe form of leprosy endemic to Mexico and Costa Rica, referred to as diffuse lepromatous leprosy (DLL). It was initially discovered in fatal cases of DLL in 2008.[1,13] Subsequent studies, however, revealed that *M. lepromatosis* was not only the cause of LL other than DLL in these endemic areas, but was also implicated in other clinical forms of leprosy. *M. lepromatosis*, therefore, appears to be the dominant cause of leprosy in Mexico. It may coexist with *M. leprae* in endemic areas, and dual infection with both species may also occur in some patients.[1,14] Additional cases of *M. lepromatosis* infection were later documented in Canada, Singapore, Brazil, and Myanmar.[1,14–16]

The complexity of the presentation is related intimately to the varied host immunological responses. The incubation period may be as short as 1–2 years, but is usually 3–5 years, and may be 10 years or more. The ability to culture infected macrophages isolated from patients with multibacillary leprosy holds promise for the ex vivo study of *M. leprae* and its interaction with its host.[17]

The Ridley & Jopling classification system devised in 1960s is still widely used, and defines the leprosy spectrum based on clinicopathological and immunological criteria.[18] There are two extreme modes of presentation:
- the polar tuberculoid form, tuberculoid leprosy (TT),
- the polar lepromatous form, LL.
- Between these are:
- borderline tuberculoid leprosy (BT),
- borderline lepromatous leprosy (BL),
- borderline leprosy (BB) occupying an intermediate position.[2–5,18]

Tuberculoid leprosy

TT is associated with high resistance to the lepra bacillus, but in the lepromatous form resistance to the lepra bacillus is low.[4,5,19]

TT occurs in individuals with good cell-mediated immunity, but low antibody titers to *M. leprae*. It appears as localized, sometimes single, asymmetrical truncal or limb lesions. The lesion is typically an erythematous plaque with raised margins and a flat hypopigmented center (*Fig. 18.190*). Sensory impairment is invariable because of associated involvement of nerves by the bacilli; these nerves may be palpably thickened. Alternatively, the skin lesion may be an erythematous macule, hypopigmented in dark skins. Sometimes the skin is not involved primarily, cutaneous manifestations being seen as a result of minor trauma associated with anesthesia from the neural lesion. *M. lepromatosis* has been detected in some cases.[1]

Lepromatous leprosy

LL is a systemic disease that occurs in patients with poor cell-mediated immunity to *M. leprae*, but with higher levels of antibodies. The cutaneous lesions are multiple, symmetrical, and may affect the whole skin, giving a scleroder-matous appearance (diffuse or Lucio-type leprosy). It is in this severe diffuse form of LL in particular that *M. lepromatosis* has been implicated.[1,13,20] The more conventional lesions of LL are typically firm and nodular and are concentrated on the face and backs of hands, facial lesions being associated with hair loss round the eyes (*Figs 18.191* and *18.192*). The distribution of the lesions is said to be favored by lower skin temperature. The mucosa of the nose is characteristically involved and becomes hyperemic with frequent epistaxes. The nasal cartilages and bone may be affected, and collapse can result in a picture similar to the saddle nose of congenital syphilis. A variety

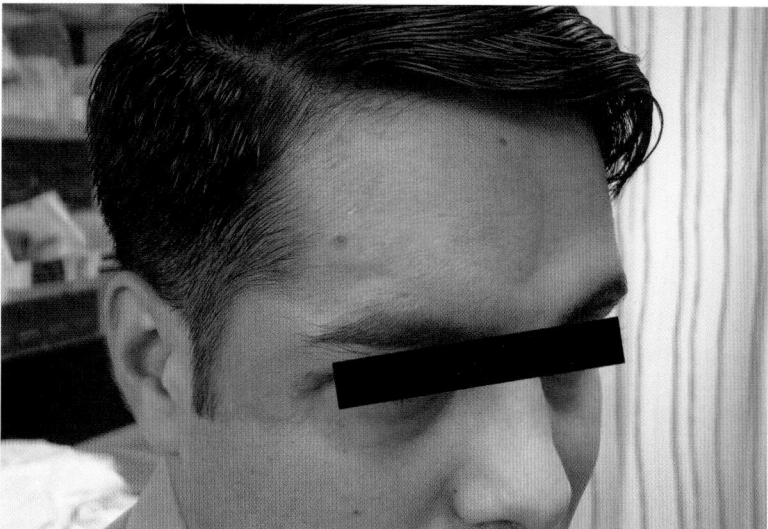

Fig. 18.190
Tuberculoid leprosy: note the hypopigmentation and erythema. By courtesy of B. Al-Mahmoud, MD, Doha, Quatar.

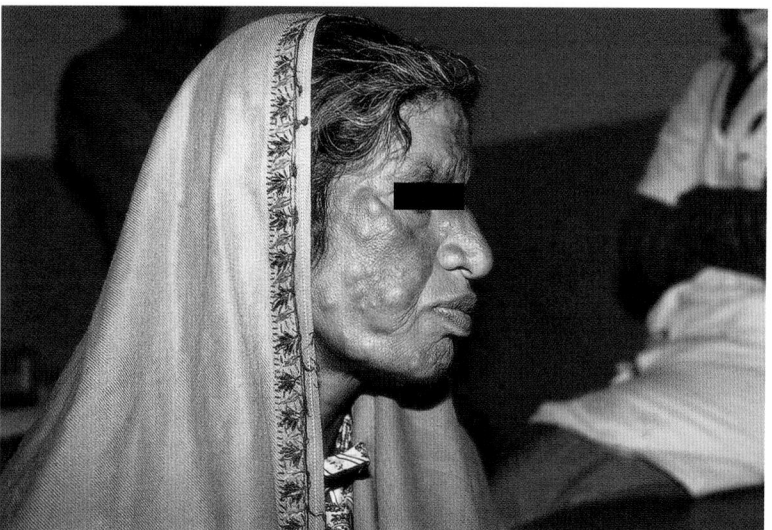

Fig. 18.191
Lepromatous leprosy: numerous nodules are present on the face. By courtesy of S. Lucas, MD, St Thomas' Hospital, London, UK.

of macules, papules, and plaques may be present at one time, characteristically sparing the axillae, groins, and perineum. These lesions become anesthetic due to widespread neural involvement with resultant claw hand and foot drop (*Fig. 18.193*).

A rare phenomenon occurring in patients with LL is the development of numerous histiocytoma-like lesions: the histoid variant (*Fig. 18.194*).[21–24] Large cutaneous and subcutaneous nodules and plaques, sometimes measuring in excess of 3 cm in diameter have been described.[25–27]

Borderline leprosy

Lesions in BT, BL, and BB manifest in a form intermediate between the polar forms TT and LL (*Figs 18.195–18.197*). The lesions are fewer in number and less symmetrically distributed than in LL, and there is less localization and nerve involvement than in TT. There is, however, a continuous spectrum and individual patients may downgrade to more closely resemble LL or upgrade toward the tuberculoid pole.

Lepra reactions

Type I Lepra (reversal) reactions, which usually develop in BL patients, are associated with an upgrading to a more resistant tuberculoid pole of the spectrum and the development of a positive Mitsuda (lepromin)

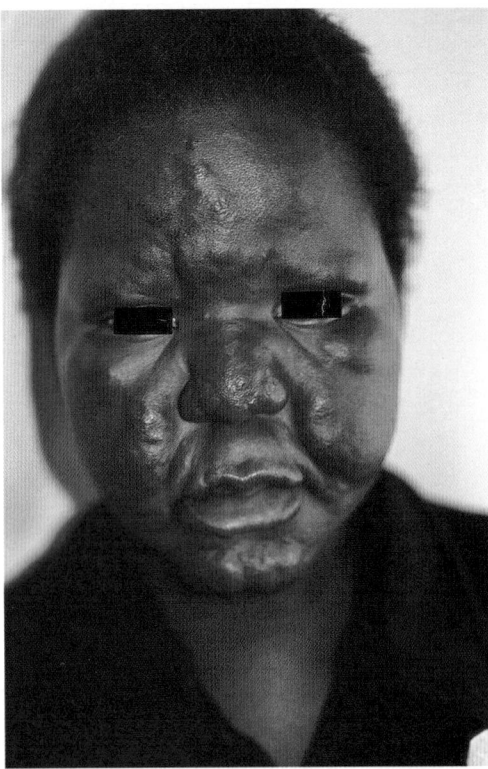

Fig. 18.192
Lepromatous leprosy: note the symmetry and characteristic loss of the eyebrows. By courtesy of N.C. Dlova, MD, Nelson R. Mandela School of Medicine, University of KwaZulu-Natal, South Africa.

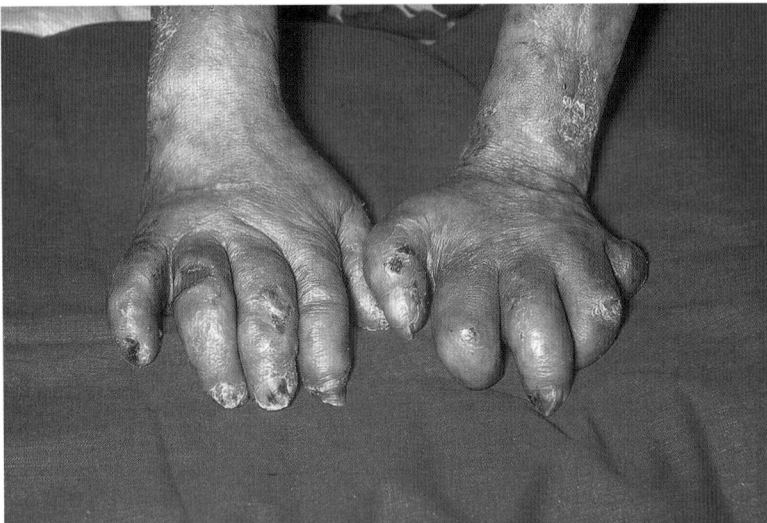

Fig. 18.193
Lepromatous leprosy: these hands show loss of the digits and trauma-related ulcers due to gross nerve damage. By courtesy of S. Lucas, MD, St Thomas' Hospital, London, UK.

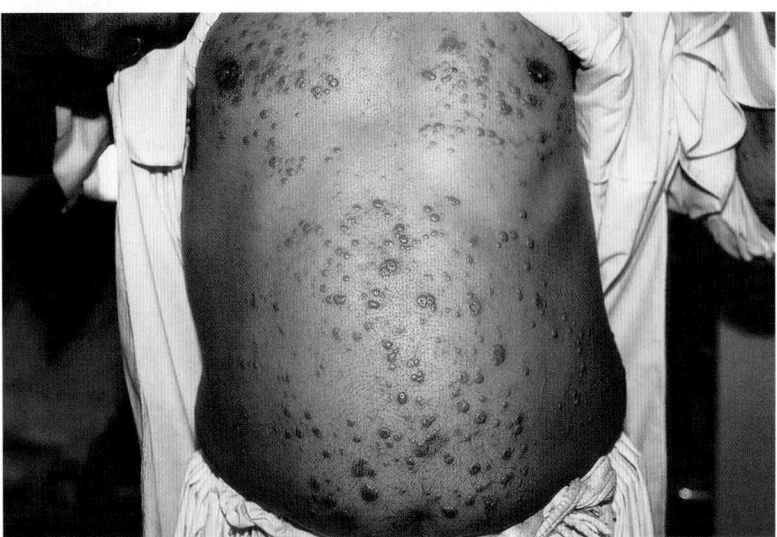

Fig. 18.194
Histoid leprosy: these numerous brown papules and nodules may be histologically mistaken for a 'fibrohistiocytic' tumor if the clinical information is not available. By courtesy of S. Lucas, MD, St Thomas' Hospital, London, UK.

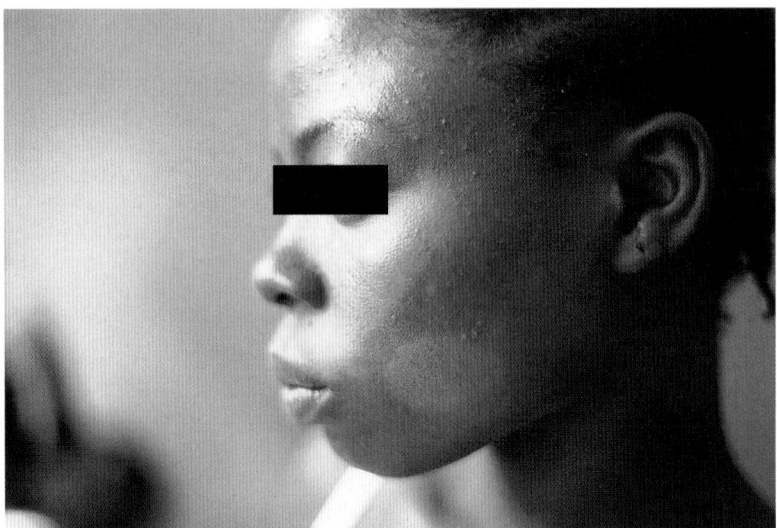

Fig. 18.195
Borderline tuberculoid leprosy: an early hypopigmented macule. By courtesy of S. Lucas, MD, St Thomas' Hospital, London, UK.

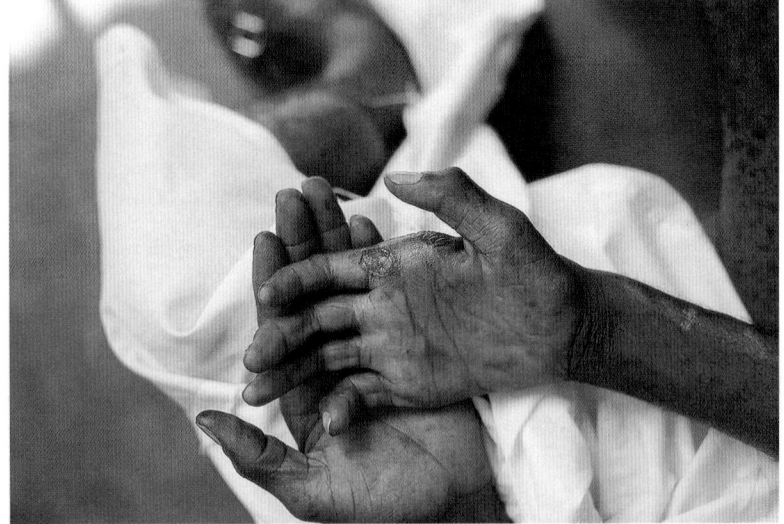

Fig. 18.196
Borderline tuberculoid leprosy: note the ulceration and muscle wasting due to median and ulnar nerve involvement. By courtesy of S. Lucas, MD, St Thomas' Hospital, London, UK.

reaction.[4,28,29] Patients therefore have developed an improved immunological reaction. Less often, type I reactions may be associated with downgrading. They may be associated with treatment, and consequently are characterized by an accelerated destruction of bacilli. Type I Lepra reactions are also associated with pregnancy, stress, and intercurrent infections. The upgrading causes marked inflammatory changes within the skin: nerve lesions manifest as nerve swelling and pain; cutaneous lesions may become tender and edematous with an increased cellular infiltrate (*Fig. 18.198*).[4]

Type II reaction, also known as erythema nodosum leprosum (ENL), occurs in LL and BL, usually during treatment. It may also be provoked by physical or mental stress, injury, other infections, vaccinations, or pregnancy.[4,30–32] There appears to be a direct relationship between an increasing

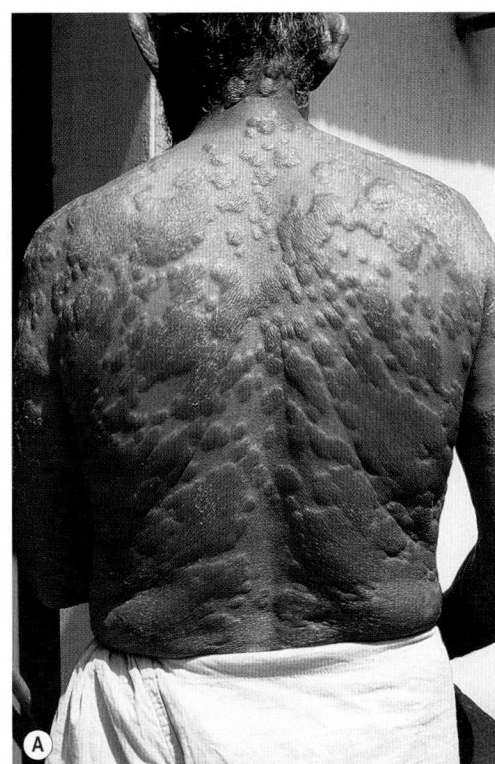

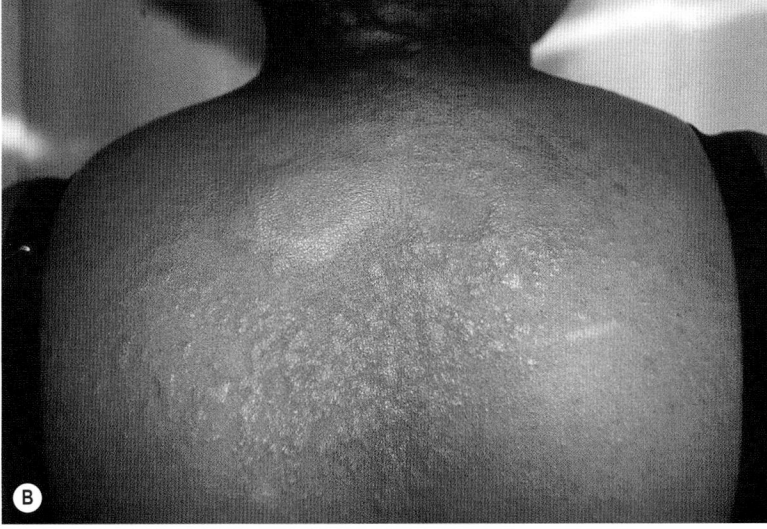

Fig. 18.197
(**A**, **B**) Borderline lepromatous leprosy: there are gross infiltrated erythematous plaques with well-defined borders. (**A**) By courtesy of S. Lucas, MD, Institute of Dermatology, London, UK; (**B**) by courtesy of N.C. Dlova, MD, Nelson R. Mandela School of Medicine, University of KwaZulu-Natal, South Africa.

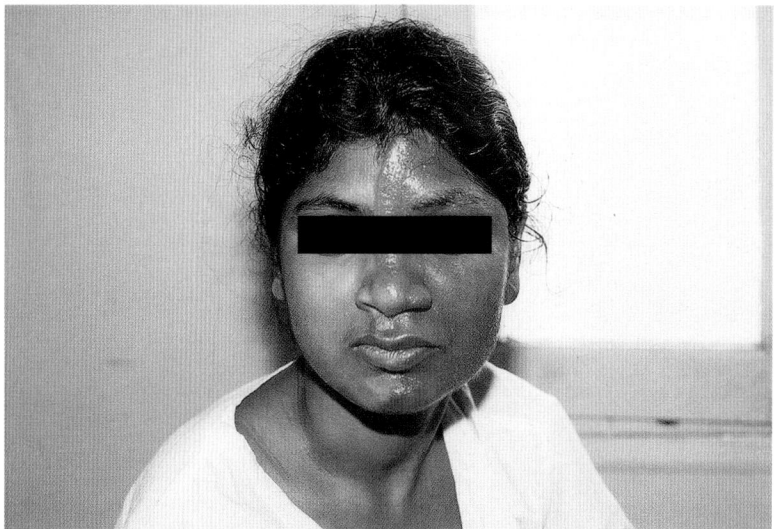

Fig. 18.198
Type I *Lepra* reaction: note the unilateral edema and intense erythema. By courtesy of S. Lucas, MD, St Thomas' Hospital, London, UK.

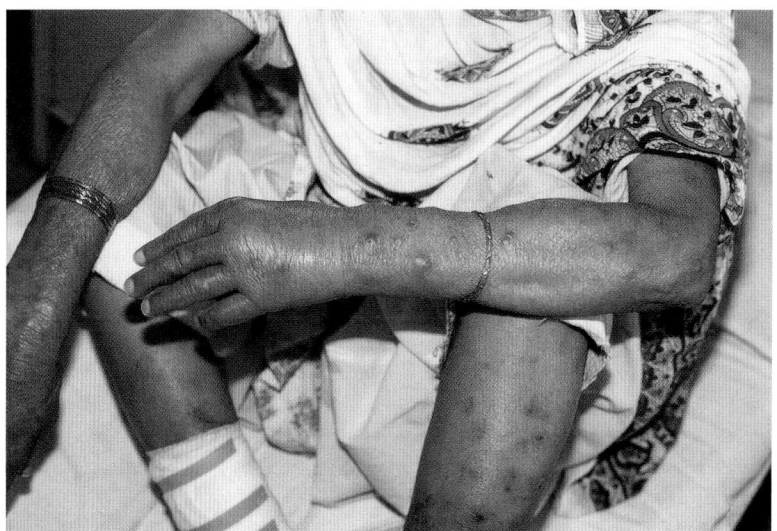

Fig. 18.199
Erythema nodosum leprosum: note the erythematous nodules on the dorsal aspect of the forearms and shins. By courtesy of S. Lucas, MD, St Thomas' Hospital, London, UK.

bacterial index and the risk of developing ENL. Increasing age, on the other hand, has been found to have an inverse relationship with ENL. The reaction may occur prior to, during, or after the introduction of multidrug therapy.[33] The changes of ENL are believed to be due, at least in part, to immune complex deposition in vessels following the release of bacterial antigens in patients who have high levels of antibodies. Both immunoglobulins and complement have been identified in blood vessel walls. Delayed hypersensitivity mechanisms, however, are also thought to have a pathogenetic role. In ENL there are, therefore, increased numbers of Th cells, and an increased lesional helper/suppressor T-cell ratio is characteristic.[31] Studies performed on lesional tissue have confirmed a preponderance of CD4+ T-cells and a Th1-type immune response.[34] The symptoms are nocturnal pains, mainly of the face, thighs, and arms. Lesions include tender erythematous or deep purple nodules with fever and painful nerve swelling, swollen joints, myositis, painful fingers, iritis, lymphadenitis, glomerulonephritis, and epididymo-orchitis (*Fig. 18.199*).[31] Cases with bullous skin lesions have been reported.[35–38] ENL may also occur in patients with leprosy caused by *M. lepromatosis*.[1,39]

Lucio phenomenon

Lucio phenomenon (erythema necroticans) is seen almost exclusively in Mexican and Central American patients who present with untreated, diffuse, non-nodular LL (pure and primitive DLL; diffuse leprosy of Lucio and Letapí). As stated earlier, *M. lepromatosis* is now recognized as the agent responsible for this severe, diffuse form of LL. There is associated hemorrhagic infarction and epidermal necrosis (*Fig. 18.200*).[31,40–44] Unsurprisingly, *M. lepromatosis* has recently been linked to Lucio phenomenon.[39,45] Lesions, which are initially macular, then soon break down to become irregular jagged ulcerations, which heal to leave irregular atrophic scars. The extremities are most commonly affected. Although Lucio phenomenon, like ENL, was considered to be mediated by immune complexes, this concept has since been challenged. It has been suggested that the triggering event is thrombotic vascular occlusion secondary to massive invasion of vascular endothelial cells by the bacilli, resulting in necrosis.[44] In one retrospective study of 12 cases, however, a necrotizing panvasculitis was evident in all cases.[46] A recently reported case with associated antiphospholipid syndrome

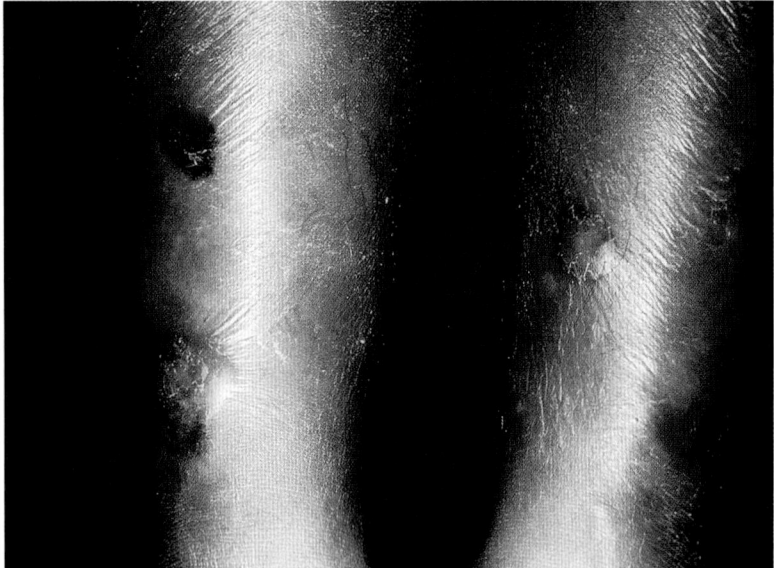

Fig. 18.200
Lucio phenomenon: note the multiple infarcted cutaneous nodules, which have developed against a background of diffuse lepromatous leprosy. By courtesy of R. Arenas, MD, and J.C. Salas, MD, Monterrey, Mexico.

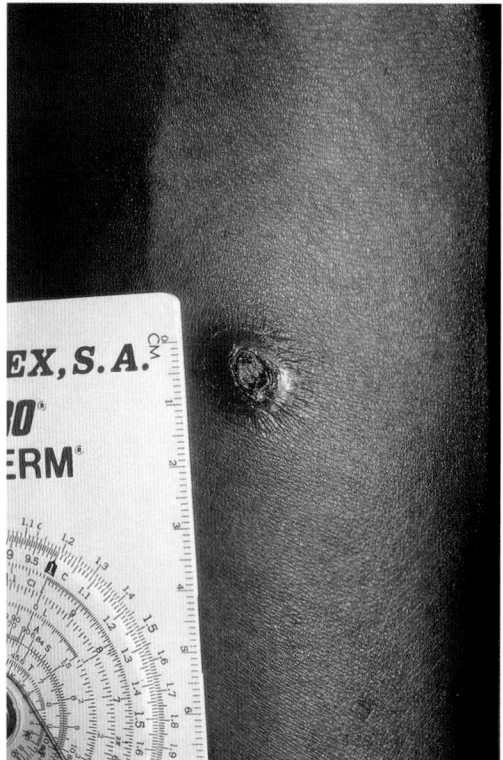

Fig. 18.201
Mitsuda reaction: this is positive in a patient with tuberculoid leprosy. By courtesy of R. Arenas, MD, and J.C. Salas, MD, Monterrey, Mexico.

showed thrombotic luminal occlusion of dermal vessels in the absence of associated vasculitic changes.[47]

Indeterminate leprosy

Indeterminate leprosy is an early form of leprosy, which often resolves spontaneously.[48] However, in 25% of patients, evolution to one of the determinant types occurs. It appears as poorly defined areas of slight hypopigmentation or erythema, without systemic or neural changes. The condition is only likely to be recognized readily in endemic areas where there is a high awareness of leprosy. It must be carefully distinguished from other dermatoses.

The Mitsuda reaction (intradermal injection of armadillo-derived Lepra bacilli) has proved useful for classification purposes.[5] Tuberculoid patients develop a granulomatous response; lepromatous patients do not (*Fig. 18.201*).[4]

Although leprosy has been reported in patients infected with HIV, current evidence suggests that *M. leprae* is not an opportunistic pathogen in these individuals.[49–51] There have, however, been a number of reports of leprosy occurring as a manifestation of IRIS following the initiation of highly active ART in HIV-infected individuals.[52–56] Leprosy is only rarely encountered in immunosuppressed organ transplant recipients.[57]

Leprosy patients with chronic cutaneous ulcers (especially plantar lesions) are at increased risk for the development of squamous cell carcinoma.[58,59]

Pathogenesis and histologic features

The varied clinical manifestations of leprosy are the result of a number of factors, including the host's immune response, the mode of infection, and certain genetic factors.[18,60–63] It was long assumed that transmission of leprosy was by long-term close direct skin contact, but this can be seriously questioned as there is no evidence that infection can occur through intact skin. LL is far more infective than other forms, and the nasal mucosa and nasal secretions of patients with LL are heavily infected with bacilli. This is a most important source of infection, but it is not clear that the route of transmission is via the lungs or gastrointestinal tract, even though inhalation of droplets and ingestion of bacilli do occur. Lactating mothers with LL produce high counts of bacilli in milk and yet do not appear to spread leprosy to their babies. It seems most likely that infection in leprosy occurs by a combination of nasal discharge and digital impregnation of the skin, as bacilli can be carried under the nails and inoculated into the skin by scratching. One study revealed that untreated patients with multibacillary leprosy may shed organisms into the environment via their skin and nasal

epithelia.[64] Inoculation leprosy is a rare phenomenon acquired through skin tattooing.[65]

The responses of those that are infected may be determined by a genetic predisposition, as suggested by associations with human leukocyte antigen (HLA) class II antigens, including HLA DR2 and DR3 in tuberculoid leprosy, and HLA DQ1 in LL.[18] Genome-wide association studies have uncovered a number of candidate genes which may confer an increased susceptibility to the disease, including genes whose product is directly involved in the host response to the organism. Among these are polymorphisms in the promoters of the genes encoding TNF-α and IL-10.[18,66] The *MRC1* gene on chromosome 10p13, for example, has been of particular interest.[18] A noteworthy aspect uncovered by these studies is that some leprosy susceptibility genes are shared with Crohn disease and Parkinson disease.[62] Reversal reactions appear to be associated with variations in the *TLR1* AND *TLR2* genes.[18]

Leprosy can be regarded as either paucibacillary (localized) or multibacillary (disseminated), with vigorous Th1 (cell-mediated) and Th2 (humoral) immune responses characterizing the former and the latter, respectively.[67] In tuberculoid lesions, there is an efficient granulomatous macrophage response, associated with a preponderance of Th (CD4+) cells over T-suppressor cells (CD8+) in an approximate ratio of 2:1, and no antibody production. There is associated elimination of the bacteria, which are therefore difficult to find in tuberculoid lesions. The tuberculoid response is therefore characterized by a persistent or chronic delayed hypersensitivity reaction, with a Th1 immune response and release of IFN-γ, IL-2, and TNF-α. A Th2 response characterizes multibacillary leprosy, with high levels of IL-4, IL-5, and IL-10, and low levels of IFN-γ.[4,17,18,61] In lepromatous lesions T-suppressor cells are more numerous and IL-2 producing cells are scarce, whereas they are 10 times more common in TT. One explanation for the different response suggests that Th cells are defective or absent in individuals who develop LL. An alternative theory suggests that T-suppressor cells are activated by the leprosy bacilli in patients of certain HLA-DR types. It is proposed that this represents a response to PGL-I, which is peculiar to the cell envelope of the leprosy bacillus. The T-suppressor cells effect a reduction of Th cells reactive to *M. leprae*. In this way, the T-suppressor and Th theories are not incompatible. The variable immune response to the *Lepra* bacillus is manifest

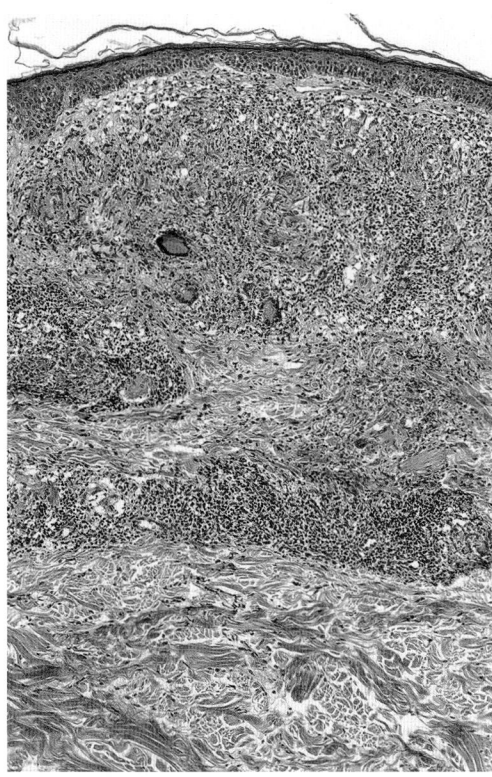

Fig. 18.202
Tuberculoid leprosy: there is extensive infiltration of the dermis and subcutaneous fat by noncaseating granulomata.

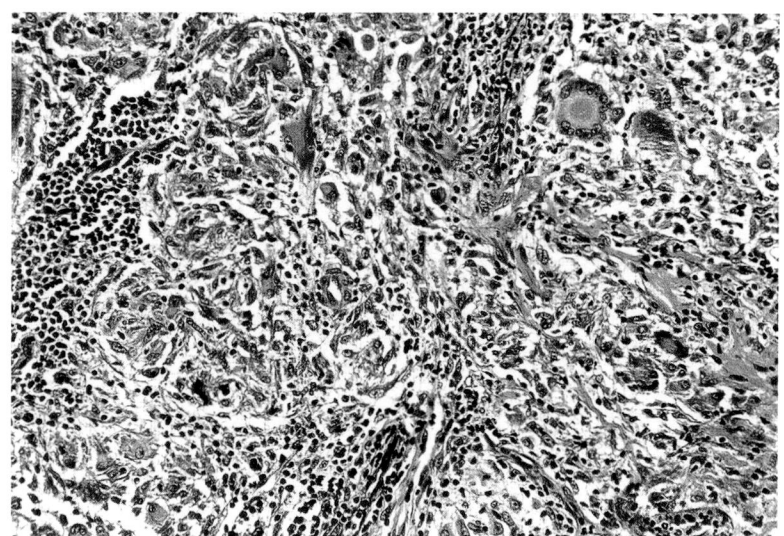

Fig. 18.203
Tuberculoid leprosy: lymphocytes are present in addition to giant cells and granulomata.

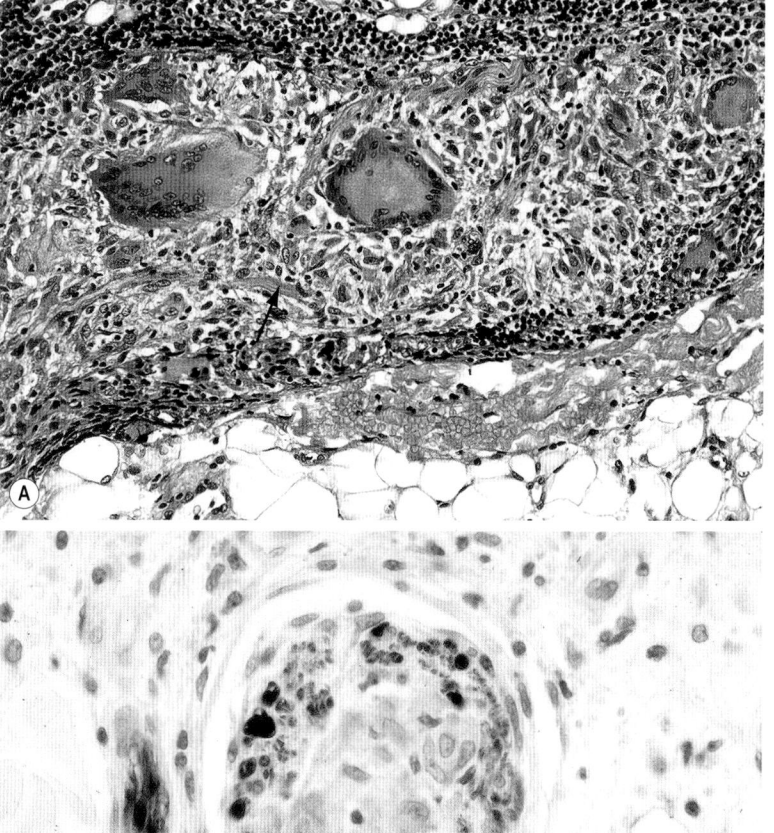

Fig. 18.204
Tuberculoid leprosy: (A) this small nerve is almost completely replaced by the granulomatous infiltrate; the residual nerve tissue is arrowed; (B) S100 protein immunohistochemistry is invaluable in identifying damaged nerves.

in the wide variety of clinical manifestations in leprosy.[18,68] Other genetic factors including Lewis factor and natural resistance-associated macrophage protein 1 (NRAMP1) may also play a role.[60] BCG vaccination may play a beneficial role in the prevention of leprosy.[67,69]

In LL there is an inability to develop a significant T-cell-mediated delayed hypersensitivity reaction to the leprosy bacillus.[4] The high level of antibodies in LL appear to have no beneficial effect, but are relevant to the development of the immune complex-mediated ENL lesions (see above). Lucio phenomenon, in which purpura and leg ulcers develop, was thought to involve a similar immune complex-mediated mechanism to produce episodes of necrotizing vasculitis in this diffuse type of leprosy. Others, however, have since suggested that direct invasion of vascular endothelium by large numbers of bacilli, with subsequent thrombosis of vessels, is the major factor in the evolution of this reaction.[44] Antiphospholipid antibodies may also play a role.[47,70]

Histologically, TT is characterized by an epithelioid histiocyte response around small cutaneous nerves (Figs 18.202–18.204). It may be entirely confined to the immediate vicinity of nerves in highly immune patients, but it often extends into the adjacent dermis. When there are clinical cutaneous lesions, the infiltrate involves the papillary dermis up to the epidermis. In contrast, BT and more lepromatous forms have a preserved Grenz zone in the papillary dermis. Tuberculoid lesions usually contain a number of Langhans giant cells, but necrosis is not a feature. Bacilli are so scarce in tuberculoid lesions that they are usually not identified; they are present in increasing numbers in variations closer to the lepromatous type of response. Distinguishing TL from other forms of granulomatous infiltrate of the skin is dependent on noting the association with nerves, which often gives the granuloma a serpentine shape. In addition, there are numerous lymphocytes, largely Th type, which may infiltrate the nerves in highly immune cases; the lymphoid infiltrate may be intense and extensive.

In LL, as in TL, the macrophage is the most important cell, but it is not arranged in discrete granulomata nor clearly related to nerves. Rather, macrophages are found in poorly circumscribed masses in the dermis with few, if any, lymphocytes (Figs 18.205 and 18.206). Those lymphocytes that are present are T-suppressor cells. The macrophages are inert and often vacuolated or foamy (Fig. 18.207. They may be distended with large groups

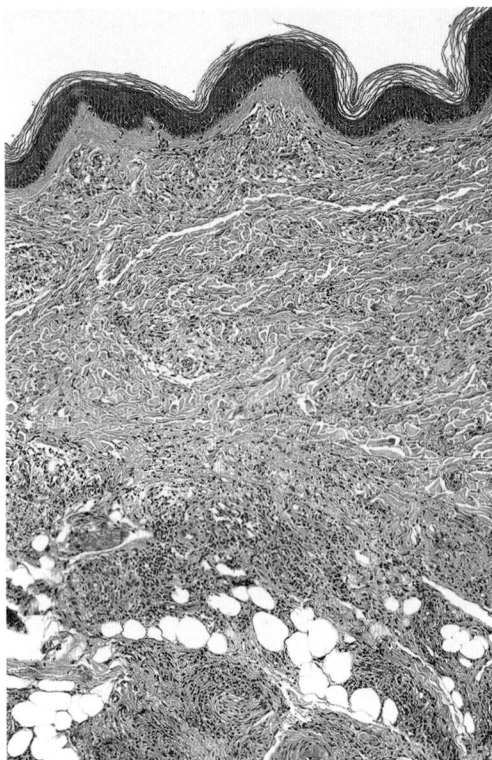

Fig. 18.205
Lepromatous leprosy: there is infiltration of the dermis by large numbers of histiocytes.

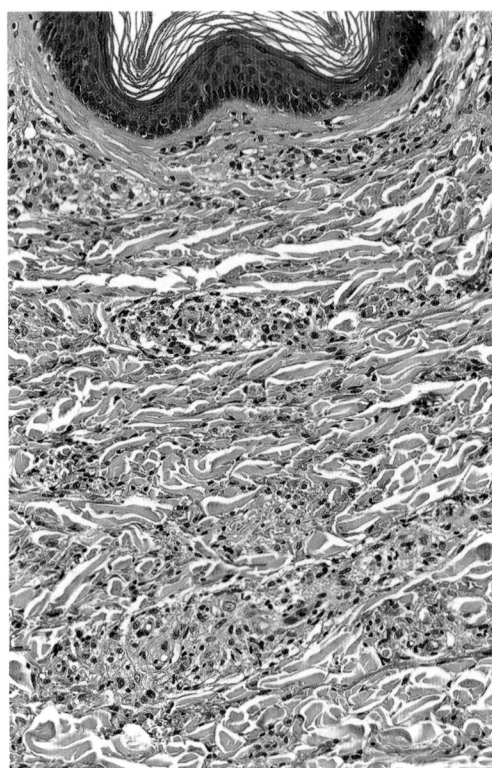

Fig. 18.206
Lepromatous leprosy: a Grenz zone of sparing of the papillary dermis is characteristic.

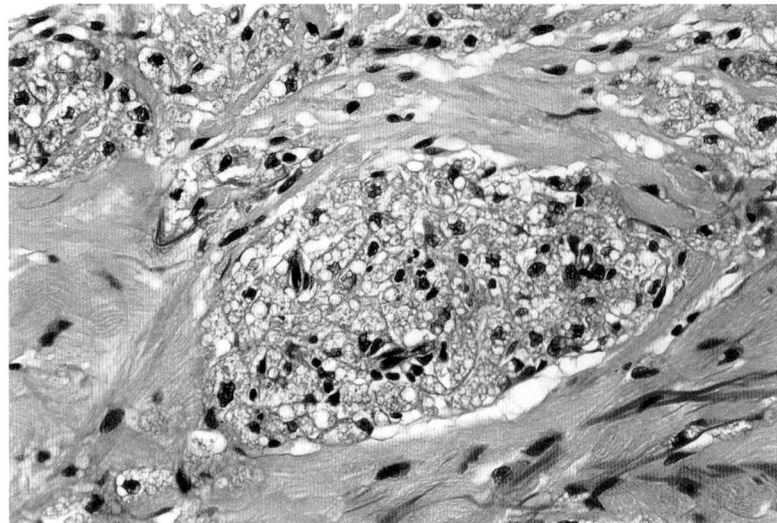

Fig. 18.207
Lepromatous leprosy: the cytoplasm of the histiocytes is bubbly and has a grayish hue.

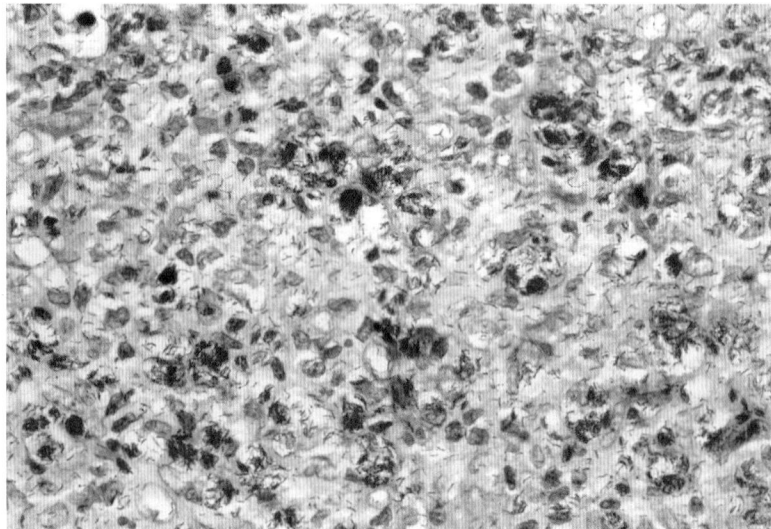

Fig. 18.208
Lepromatous leprosy: large numbers of bacilli are present; note the globi (Wade-Fite).

(or globi) of leprosy bacilli. These give the cytoplasm a grayish tinge on staining with H&E; the bacilli are revealed more clearly with a modified Ziehl-Neelsen stain (Wade-Fite) (*Fig. 18.208*). The bacteria are present in large numbers of cutaneous nerves and are also seen in that site in the borderline forms of leprosy.[71] Bacilli may also be present in the endothelium and media of small and large vessels, in arrector pili muscles, and in the eccrine secretory and ductal cells.[72] Exceptionally, clumps of bacilli may even be encountered in epidermal keratinocytes.[73]

Plasma cells are rarely seen in leprosy. They may, however, be found in subpolar LL, which clinically lies between BL and polar LL (*Figs 18.209–18.211*).

In borderline leprosy, perineural fibrosis with a lamellar or 'onion skin' pattern may be seen. Borderline leprosy shows increased circumscription of the granulomatous response, more lymphocytes, and more relation to nerves as it approaches the polar tuberculoid form.

Indeterminate leprosy shows only a scanty superficial and deep lymphohistiocytic infiltrate in the dermis, with some tendency to localization around appendages (*Fig. 18.212*). Bacilli are infrequent, but scantily present in nerves (*Fig. 18.213*). Mast cells are increased.[74] S100 protein immunohistochemistry is a useful means of identifying dermal nerves and foci of nerve damage in skin biopsy specimens.[75,76]

Histologically, in most instances Lucio phenomenon is characterized by the features of a leukocytoclastic vasculitis and epidermal infarction.[31,44,46,77] Severe passive venous congestion of the superficial veins is common.[31] Occasionally, however, some vessels are thrombosed and there is endothelial cell proliferation and swelling, with distortion, narrowing, and luminal obliteration.[40,46,77,78] The medium-sized arteries in the deep dermis and superficial subcutis show mural infiltration by clusters of macrophages containing large

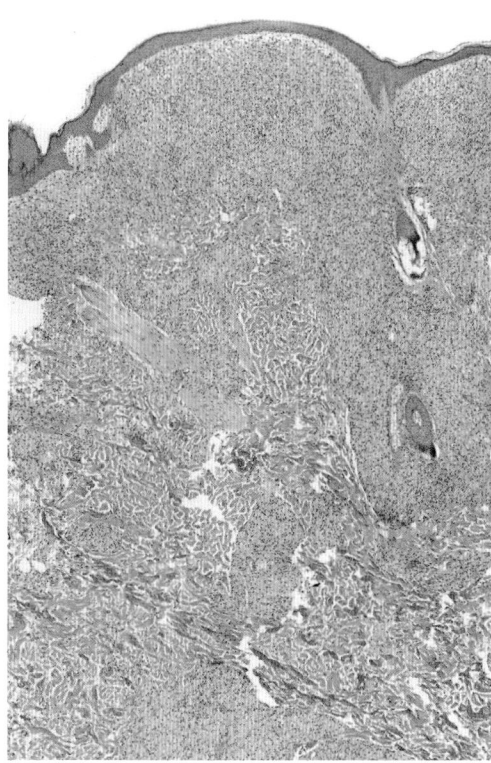

Fig. 18.209
Subpolar lepromatous leprosy: there is a dense dermal infiltrate. A Grenz zone is present.

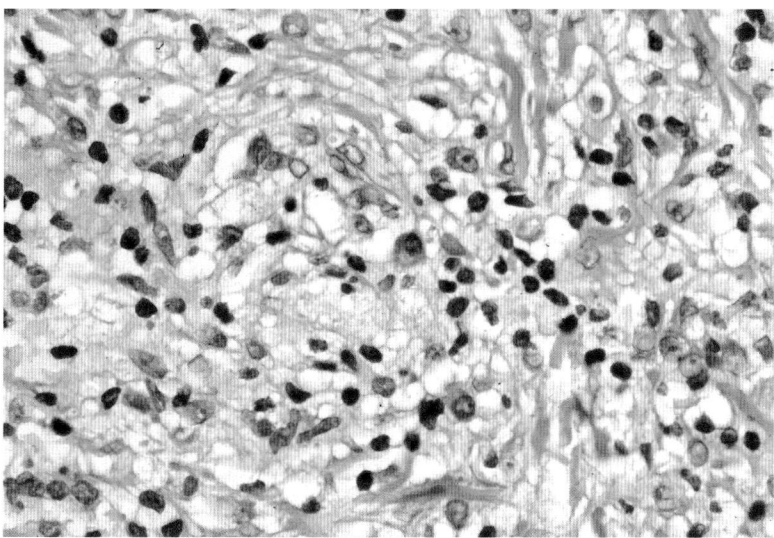

Fig. 18.210
Subpolar lepromatous leprosy: in addition to histiocytes and lymphocytes, there are conspicuous plasma cells.

numbers of bacilli.[46] Marked intraendothelial cell bacillary proliferation is characteristic.[31,77] It has been suggested that this feature is indicative of a very poor immune response facilitating antigen-antibody interaction with consequent acute necrotizing vasculitis. This seems to be rather unlikely (on its own) as similar numbers of leprosy bacilli have been described in the endothelium of 100% of small vessels in untreated polar and subpolar LL.[44,72]

Histoid leprosy shows a spindle cell proliferative pattern suggestive of fibrous histiocytoma (Figs 18.214 and 18.215). A storiform pattern may be conspicuous. Careful examination, however, will reveal foci of Lepra cells. A Wade-Fite reaction reveals large numbers of bacilli, often arranged in sheaves.[23,24]

In type I (reversal) reactions, edema is observed both within and outside of the intradermal granulomas. Numerous histiocytic giant cells may also

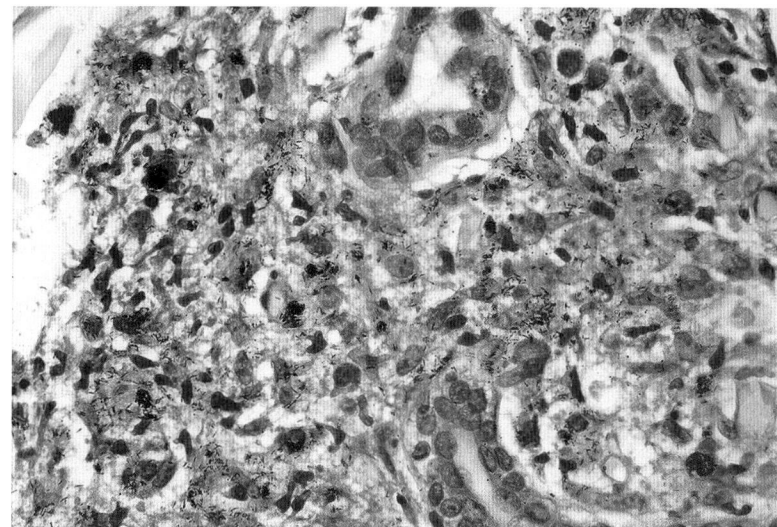

Fig. 18.211
Subpolar lepromatous leprosy: leprosy bacilli are numerous (Wade-Fite).

be seen.[71] ENL is characterized by an inflammatory cell infiltrate in the dermis and adjacent subcutaneous fat (Figs 18.216–18.218). In addition to Lepra cells, large numbers of neutrophils are typically present, and there is often an acute vasculitis (Fig. 18.219).[30,34,71,79] Bullous lesions are characterized by dermal edema.[25] Organisms are demonstrable within capillary endothelium.[38,44]

Molecular techniques (PCR) may prove useful in confirming the diagnosis of leprosy, especially in paucibacillary forms or when organisms are not readily apparent in sections stained with the Wade-Fite method.[80–82]

Rhinoscleroma

Clinical features

Rhinoscleroma is usually seen in young adults and is now largely confined to the tropics and subtropical regions; it was, however, previously common in Eastern Europe.[1–4] The disease has been linked to poor socioeconomic conditions and is still encountered in parts of Central Africa, Southeast Asia, India, Mexico, as well as Central and South America.[4–6] Rhinoscleroma has also been described in the Arabian Gulf, and is considered endemic in Egypt.[1,6,7] It is a severe chronic infection of the upper respiratory tract, especially the nose. The disease is contracted via direct droplet infection or, more indirectly, by contamination of material that is subsequently inhaled. It has a very long incubation period.

There are three phases to the clinical features of the disease:
- It begins with a catarrhal phase, with symptoms suggesting a non-specific rhinitis or coryza with frontal headaches.[3] These symptoms persist for weeks or months, becoming gradually more severe with superimposed epistaxes and difficulty in nasal breathing associated with swollen mucous membranes.[3,8]
- An infiltrative phase follows during which the nasal septum and base of the nasal fossa become swollen by a reddish waxy induration.[3] This change is painless and the soft palate is anesthetic. Similar involvement of the larynx causes changes in the voice.
- The infiltrative phase merges into a nodular phase during which there is increasing deformity as the nose, upper lips, and gums become grossly enlarged and distorted.[3,8] Involvement of regional lymph nodes is not usual, but has been reported.[9] Nasal obstruction, loss of smell, loss of voice, laryngeal stenosis, and increasing difficulty with breathing may follow.[5,8,10] Respiratory obstruction may cause death; alternatively, the process can persist with some temporary remissions for years.

Squamous carcinoma is an occasional late complication.
Contiguous involvement of the soft and hard palate, the upper lip, and the maxillary sinuses may occur; the term respiratory scleroma has been proposed for these cases with extranasal extension of the disease.[11] Involvement

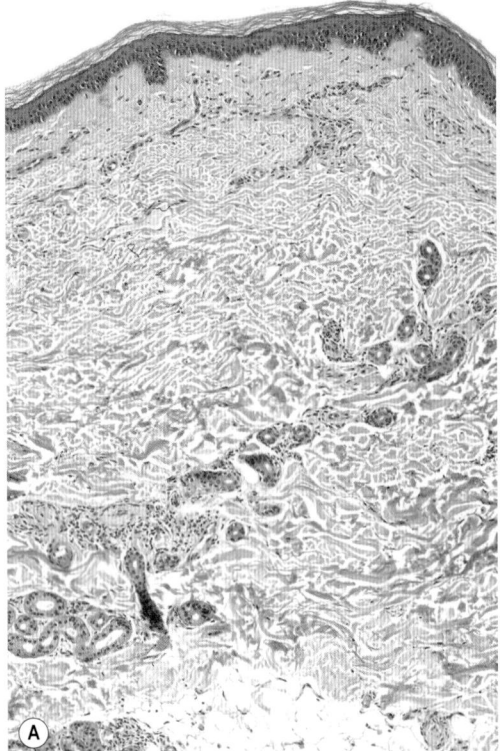

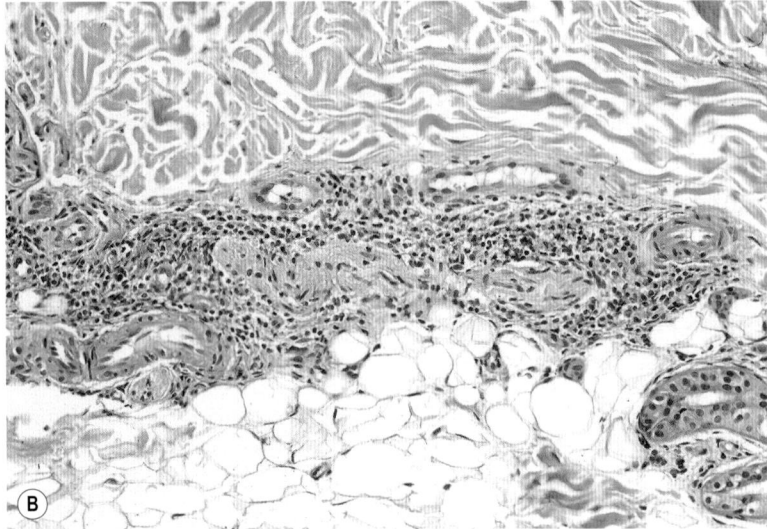

Fig. 18.212
(**A**, **B**) Indeterminate leprosy: a perivascular chronic inflammatory cell infiltrate is present in the deep dermis. Diagnosis depends on a high index of suspicion.

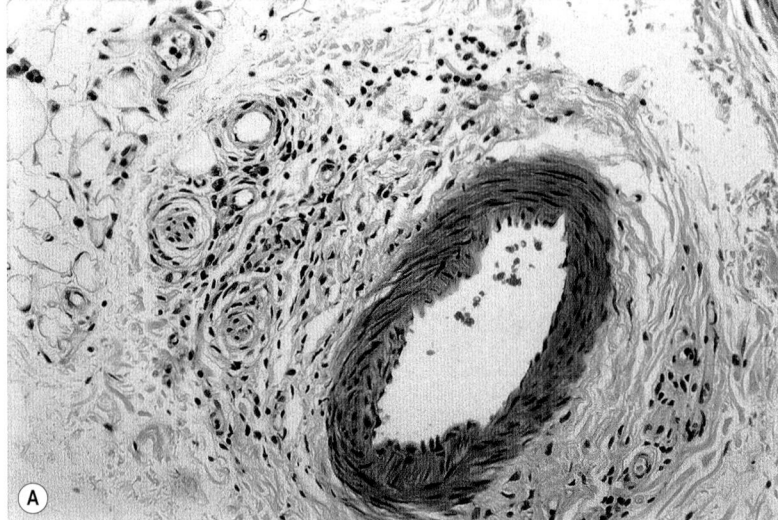

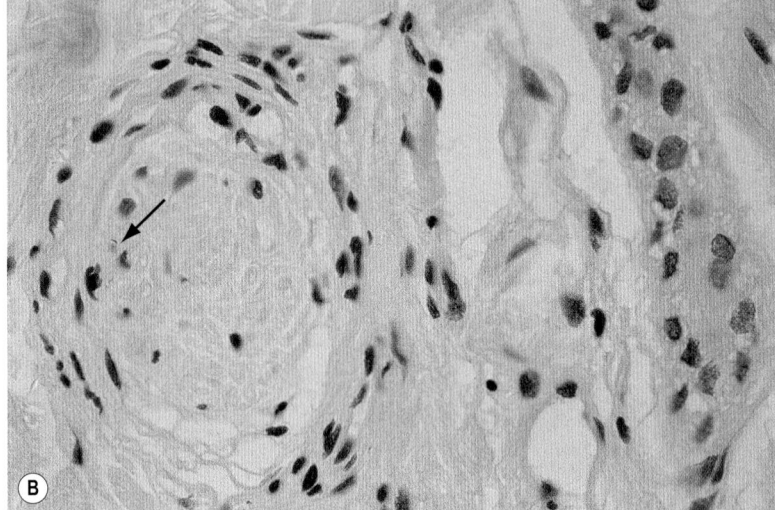

Fig. 18.213
Indeterminate leprosy: (**A**) the inflammation involves the small nerve trunks; (**B**) a Wade-Fite reaction may reveal one or two bacilli (*arrowed*). By courtesy of S. Lucas, MD, St Thomas' Hospital, London, UK.

of the nasolacrimal duct has also been described. A recurrence rate of up to 25% over a 10-year period was documented in an Egyptian series.[1] Rosai-Dorfman disease has been documented in the regional lymph nodes of a patient with rhinoscleroma.[12]

Pathogenesis and histologic features

The causative bacterium *Klebsiella rhinoscleromatis* is a Gram-negative aerobic diplobacillus.[11,13] It is spread during the rhinitis (catarrhal) phase of the disease and appears to be confined to close-living groups, and has even been documented in siblings.[14] There is no animal reservoir. An HLA-DQA1*03011-DQB1*0301 haplotype has been identified as a potential risk factor for development of the disease, while other investigators have suggested that altered lymphocyte subsets may play an important pathogenetic role.[15,16]

The incubation period is very long, so that presentation is most often in adults. The organism is phagocytosed, but not killed by neutrophils. When the neutrophils rupture, the still viable bacteria are phagocytosed by histiocytes, which become greatly distended. These eventually appear vacuolated

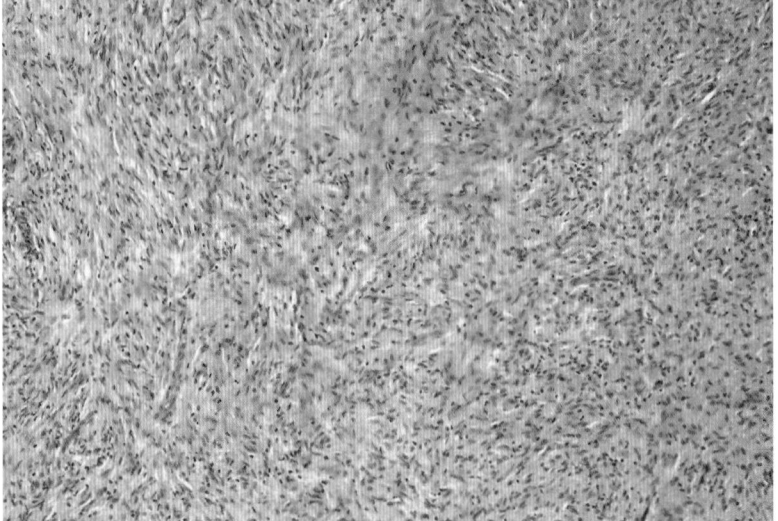

Fig. 18.214
Histoid leprosy: in this field appearances are highly suggestive of a fibrohistiocytic tumor. By courtesy of S. Lucas, MD, St Thomas' Hospital, London, UK.

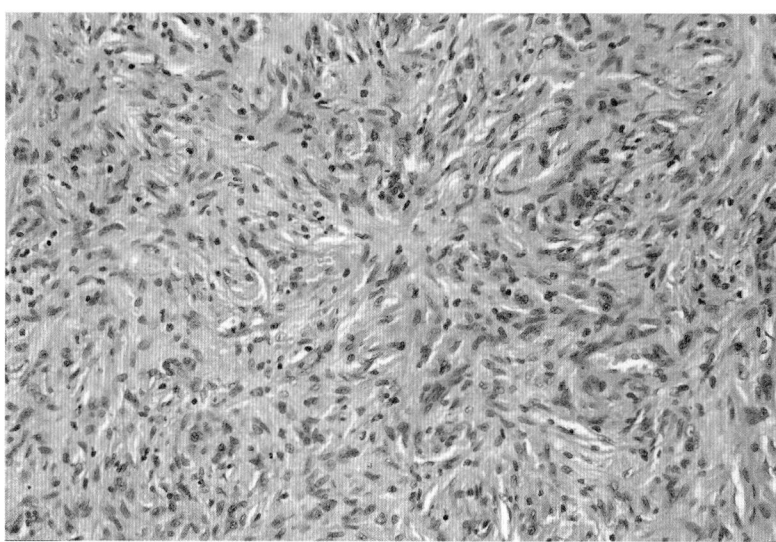

Fig. 18.215
Histoid leprosy: there is a well-developed storiform pattern. By courtesy of S. Lucas, MD, St Thomas' Hospital, London, UK.

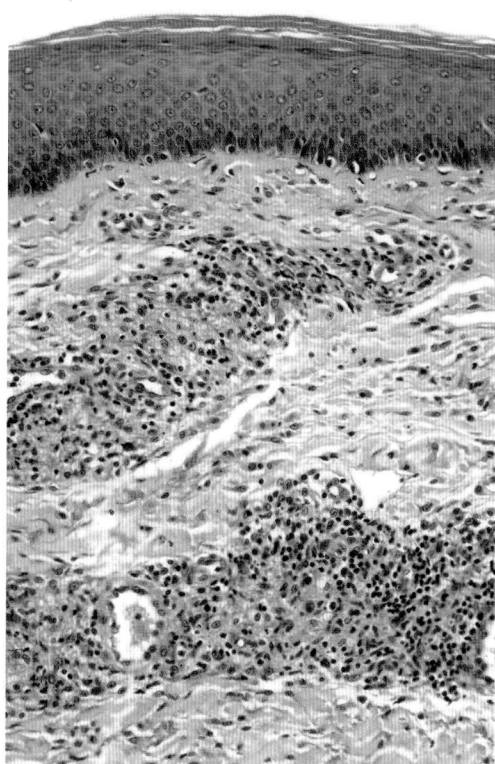

Fig. 18.217
Erythema nodosum leprosum: note the perivascular lymphocyte and histiocyte infiltrate.

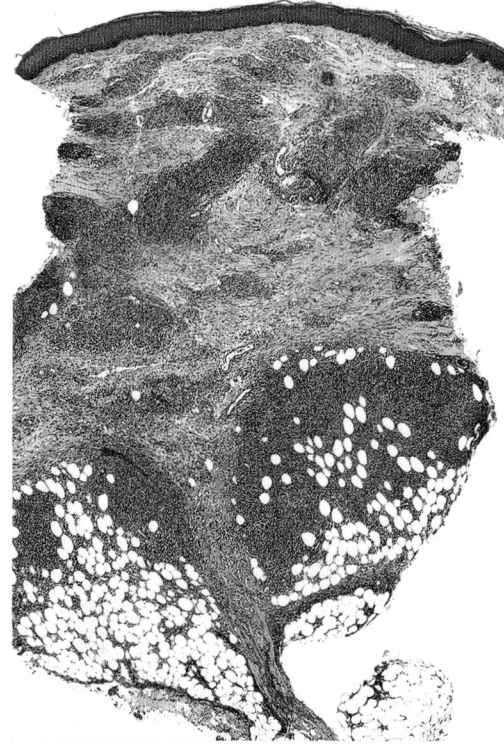

Fig. 18.216
Erythema nodosum leprosum: an intense inflammatory cell infiltrate outlines the dermal vasculature and extends into the subcutaneous fat.

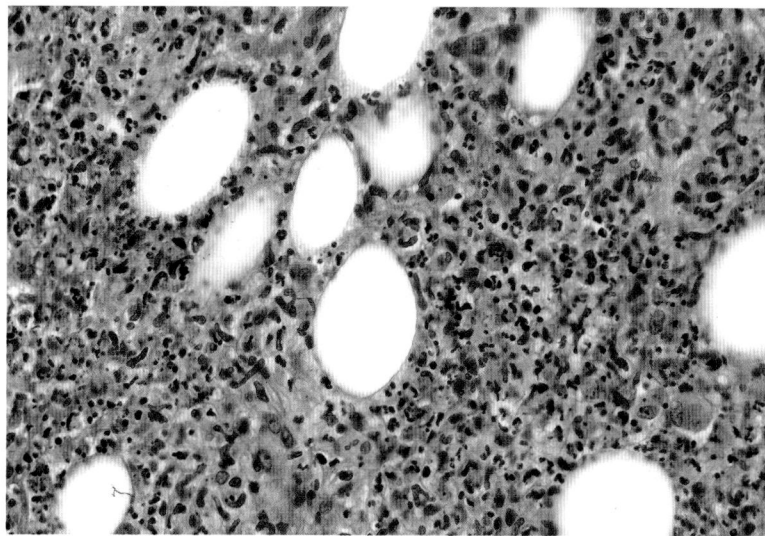

Fig. 18.218
Erythema nodosum leprosum: numerous polymorphs are intermingling with the *Lepra* cells.

with an eccentric nucleus (*Fig. 18.220*). Warthin-Starry or Giemsa staining reveals that this vacuole contains bacteria (*Fig. 18.221*). This cell, 10–100 μm in diameter, is termed a Mikulicz cell and, together with Russell bodies (plasma cells grossly distended with proteinaceous product), is characteristic of the disease. As well as these characteristic cells, there is a dense infiltrate of plasma cells and lymphocytes, which becomes very extensive and eventually causes such gross thickening of the mucosae that the respiratory tract tends to be occluded at several points. The mucosa can be ulcerated or atrophic. Amyloid deposition has been described.[6,17,18] The diagnosis may be confirmed by PCR.[19] The occurrence of S100 immunoreactive histiocytes with emperipolesis in rare cases of rhinoscleroma has led some authors to speculate that the infection might play an etiological role in Rosai-Dorfman disease.[20,21]

Differential diagnosis

This includes midfacial granulomata, lymphoma, tertiary syphilis, LL, leishmaniasis, and rhinosporidiosis. The histology, as described above, should exclude these clinical alternatives.

Nocardiosis

Clinical features

Nocardia is found in soil and rotting vegetation worldwide and man is only rarely infected.[1-4] Initially, three main pathogenic species were recognized:
- *Nocardia asteroides*, which is most common in North America,
- *Nocardia brasiliensis* in South America,
- *Nocardia caviae* in Southeast Asia.[1,3,5]

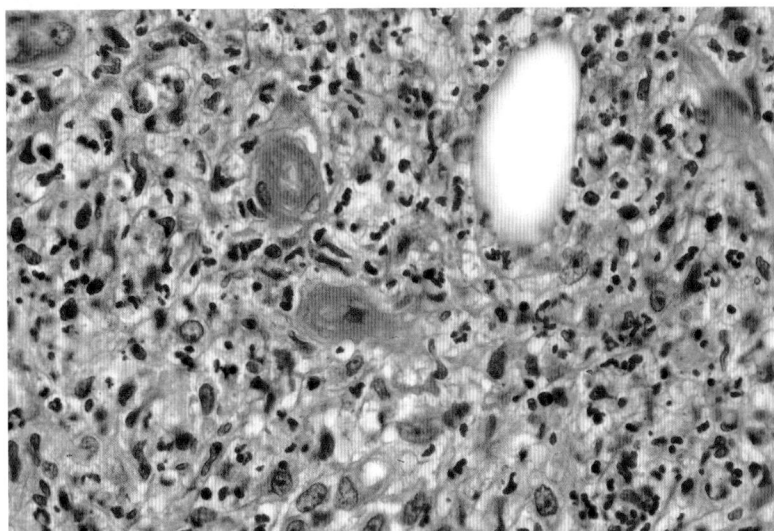

Fig. 18.219
Erythema nodosum leprosum: several small vessels show fibrinoid necrosis. This type II reaction develops on the basis of an immune complex-mediated vasculitis.

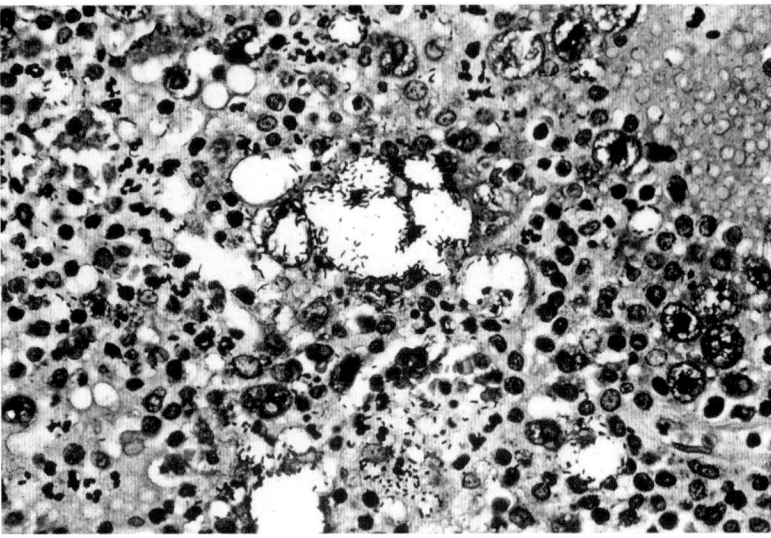

Fig. 18.221
Rhinoscleroma: numerous organisms are revealed by the Warthin-Starry reaction. By courtesy of S. Lucas, MD, Institute of Dermatology, London, UK.

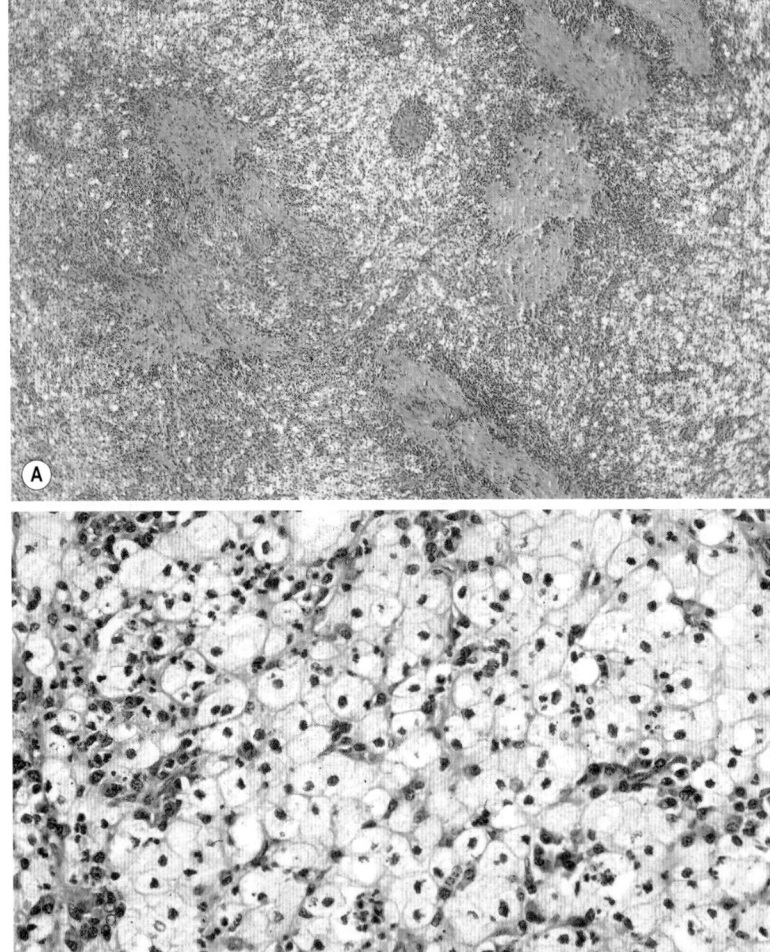

Fig. 18.220
(**A**, **B**) Rhinoscleroma: in addition to lymphocytes and numerous plasma cells, foamy macrophages (Mikulicz cells) are present.

Other species of *Nocardia* have since been associated with infection in humans, including *N. transvalensis*, *N. otididiscaviarum*, *N. nova*, *N. farcinica*, *N. paucivorans*, *N. abscessus*, *N. cyriacigeorgici*, *N. asiatica*, *N. vinacea*, *N. beijingensis*, *N. araoensis*, and *N. neocaledoniensis*.[1,4,6–23] More than 50 species of *Nocardia* are now known to exist.[6] Infection complicates inhalation or direct inoculation into a wound.[1,3,6] Nocardiosis therefore represents a respiratory illness, with or without dissemination (the majority), or a primary cutaneous disease.[1,2,6,24]

N. asteroides, *N. caviae*, and *N. farcinica* most often affect immunocompromised hosts, causing pulmonary lesions from which systemic dissemination may involve the skin.[3,25] Predisposing factors include steroid therapy, HIV infection, and solid organ transplantation.[1,4,12–14,26–29] CNS involvement is an important cause of morbidity and high mortality.[12,27] Primary cutaneous infection has been reported in an immunocompetent adult following a cat scratch.[30] Dissemination is a frequent complication of *N. paucivorans* infection in both immunocompromised and immunocompetent hosts.[15] *Nocardia* infections have been recorded among patients who have received immunomodulatory therapy for inflammatory bowel disease.[31]

N. brasiliensis causes primary skin lesions in immunocompetent individuals and can also cause primary pulmonary lesions.[4,32] The cutaneous lesions are varied and usually follow trauma. They include a mycetoma, usually on the limbs, and a sporotrichosis-like pattern (including a cervicofacial variant that occurs in children), i.e., with multiple lesions following the line of lymphatics.[3,33–40] In addition, superficial nodules, ulcers, and abscesses, with or without fistulae and pustules, may occur (*Fig. 18.222*).[41–44] Some more trivial infections resemble staphylococcal infections and are usually self-limiting; the deeper infections are progressive and can be destructive without treatment. Dissemination of primary cutaneous nocardiasis is exceptionally uncommon.[45] Infection has been reported after an insect bite.[46] Lymphocutaneous nocardiosis may also be caused by *N. transvalensis* and *N. araoensis*.[7,22] Mycetomas due to *N. nova* and *N. otididiscaviarum* have been reported.[8,11] *N. otididiscaviarum* is a rare cause of cellulitis.[10] *Nocardia* spp. are a rare infectious cause of neutrophilic eccrine hidradenitis.[47]

Pathogenesis and histologic features

Nocardia is a Gram-positive, partially acid-fast aerobic beaded rod, which grows with branching filaments in a way similar to *Actinomyces* (*Fig. 18.223*).[48] Infection by *N. asteroides*, a relatively avirulent organism, is usually by inhalation. *N. brasiliensis* is more virulent and can infect the immunocompetent through inoculation of soil into skin. It is the most commonly identified organism in the sporotrichoid form of nocardiosis.[4,34,36,38,39]

Grains, analogous to the sulfur granules of actinomycosis, can develop in the mycetoma lesions of the immunocompetent. Filamentous growth is

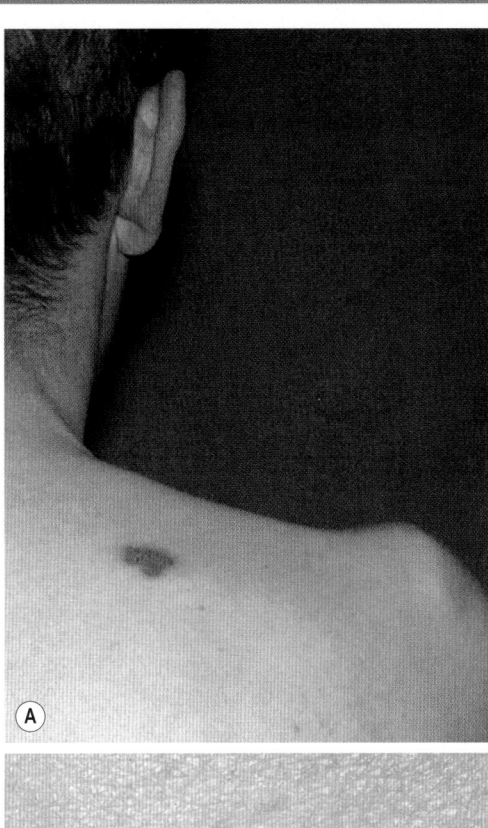

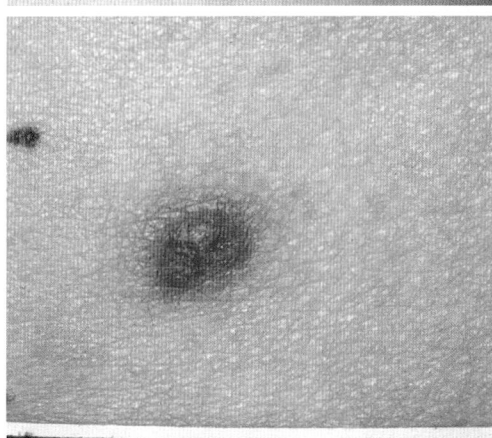

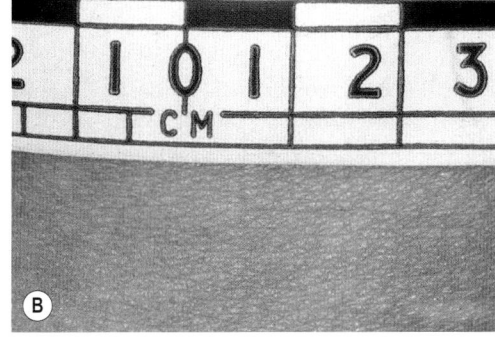

Fig. 18.222
Nocardiosis: (**A**) this cutaneous nodule developed in an immunocompromised young male; (**B**) a different lesion is shown in close-up. By courtesy of R.A. Marsden, St George's Hospital, London, UK.

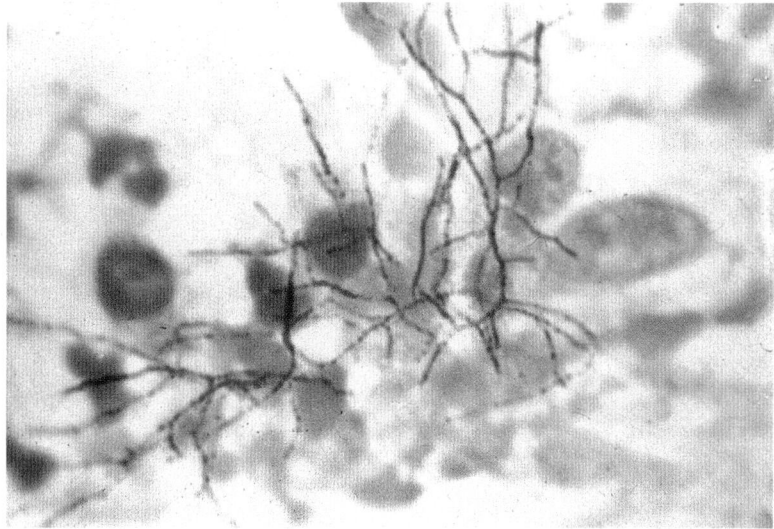

Fig. 18.223
Nocardia: the organisms appear mainly as irregularly staining filaments in this specimen, but a variety of forms, including rods and cocci, is often seen. By courtesy of A.E. Prevost, MD, and H.P. Lambert, MD, St George's Hospital, London, UK.

Botryomycosis

Clinical features

Botryomycosis (Gr. *botrys*, bunch of grapes) is also known as bacterial pseudomycosis and is due to a chronic bacterial infection, usually of skin.[1-3] It has also been described in lung, bone, kidney, and liver.[1-7] A case of gingival botryomycosis resembling a lobular capillary hemangioma (pyogenic granuloma) has been reported.[8]

In the skin, the lesions are chronic suppurative nodules which may resemble infected epidermoid cysts, plaques, and ulcers. The interconnecting fistulae which develop give it a similarity to acne conglobata and hidradenitis suppurativa, but the sites commonly involved are the hands, feet, and head.[1,9] There may be a history of preceding trauma or the presence of a foreign body.[9,10] Deeper tissues, including muscle and bone, may become involved. Botryomycosis of the cervicofacial region has also been described in a patient with mandibular chronic osteomyelitis.[4]

The pulmonary involvement has the radiological features of lobar consolidation, sometimes with adjacent osteomyelitis. Involvement of liver, tongue, orbit, bowel, and brain has also been described. Cystic fibrosis appears to predispose to some pulmonary cases. Although immunodeficiency has been noted in some cases and the condition has been reported in association with HIV/AIDS, most patients who develop botryomycosis have no detectable abnormality of the immune system.[11-16] The cutaneous lesions of botryomycosis in patients with HIV/AIDS may, however, present with atypical features; lesions resembling prurigo nodularis, lichen simplex chronicus, and pruritic papules have been described.[14,16] Disseminated botryomycosis is very rare.[17]

Pathogenesis and histologic features

The lesions of botryomycosis include a characteristic granule surrounded by suppuration and the features of a chronic abscess. The granule consists of nonfilamentous bacteria in a hyaline matrix, containing IgG and complement C3 (the Splendore-Hoeppli phenomenon), and is a lobulated or 'bunch of grapes-like' structure (*Figs 18.224* and *18.225*).[13,18] The granule is basophilic in the center and eosinophilic at the periphery.[1] It is PAS positive. The bacteria present are not specific to the condition; *S. aureus* is most common, but *Pseudomonas*, *E. coli*, *Proteus*, *Micrococcus*, and streptococci may also be found.[1,4,14,19] Fungi, actinomycetes, and *Nocardia* are not causes. There have, however, been isolated case reports of botryomycosis due to combined *S. aureus* and *Actinobacillus actimomycetemcomitans* infection, and *S. aureus* in association with *Pneumocystis jiroveci*.[15,20]

a feature of greater virulence or less immunity; methenamine silver is most satisfactory for demonstrating the filaments in tissue sections.

The histologic features in the skin are of ulcers, abscesses with pus, necrosis, hemorrhage, and fibrosis associated with sinus tracks. The organism is not readily seen with H&E staining, but can be demonstrated histologically by its weak acid-fastness, distinguishing it from *Actinomyces*. Differential culture may be necessary to distinguish the two, although the presence of sulfur grains is a pointer toward actinomycosis.[49]

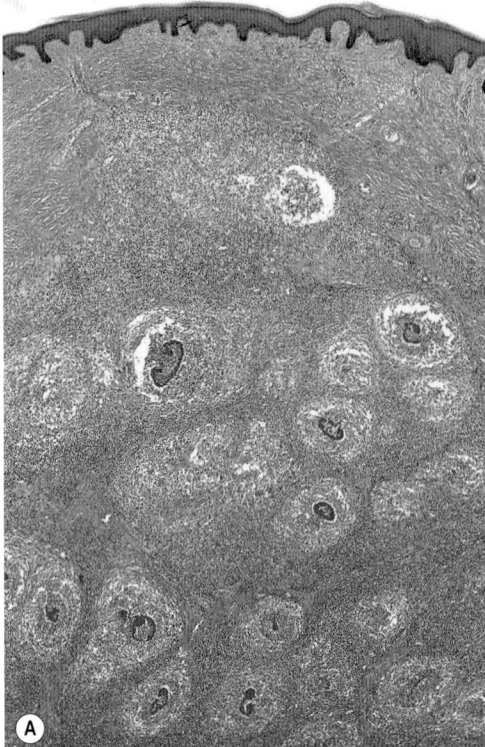

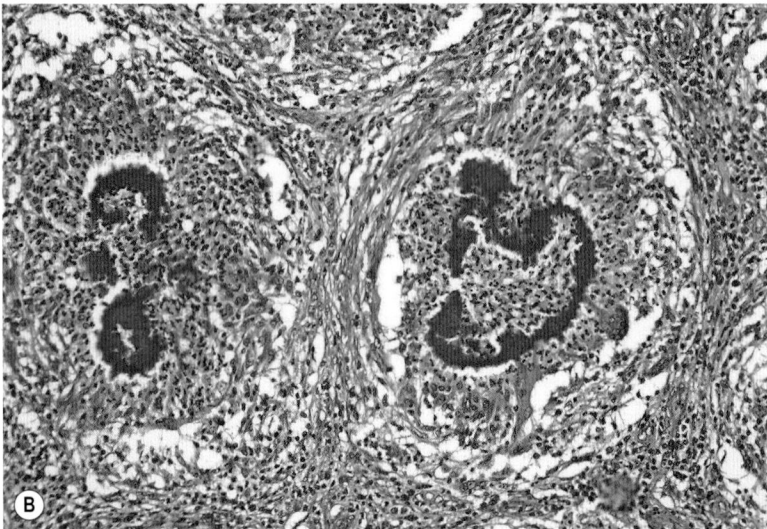

Fig. 18.224
(**A**, **B**) Botryomycosis: there are multiple dermal abscesses surrounding discrete bacterial colonies.

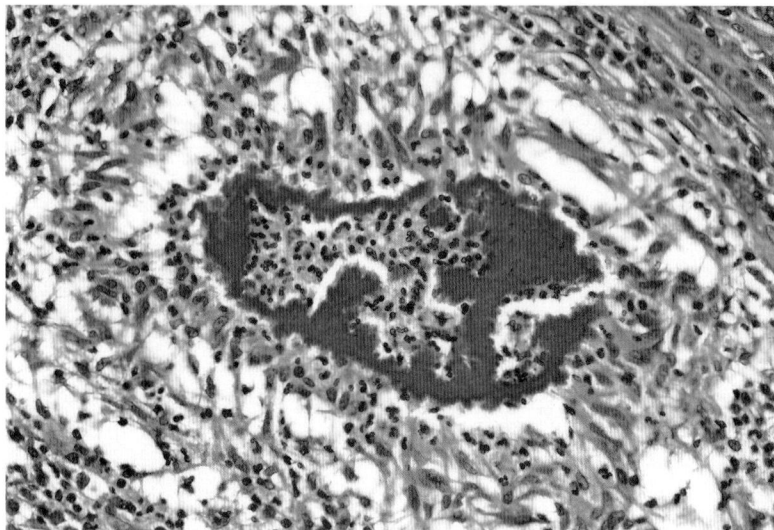

Fig. 18.225
Botryomycosis: note the blue-staining bacteria surrounded by an intensely eosinophilic fibrillary coat (the Splendore-Hoeppli phenomenon). The inflammatory response is characteristically neutrophil mediated.

The abscess persists with numerous sinuses and extensive fibrosis, and may extend to involve deep adjacent structures. Rarely, the granules are eliminated transepithelially.[21] The reasons for the persistence and for granule formation are not fully understood. Although some patients show immunodeficiency, sometimes analogous to the anergy of LL, this is not so for most cases. The size of the original inoculum appears to be critical – excessive numbers of bacteria produce an overwhelming abscess and cellulitis, too few bacteria are rapidly eliminated by normal inflammatory responses – but an intermediate size of inoculum can produce what may be interpreted as a balance between the bacteria and the inflammatory response, with granule and chronic abscess formation.[1,2,22] This balance may be attained more easily with less virulent strains.

A foreign body may contribute to the initiation of the lesion, but is not invariable. A local factor may be important, such as some as yet undemonstrated defect in the cutaneous immune mechanisms, diabetes mellitus, or an underlying dermatosis such as follicular mucinosis.[23,24] In pulmonary cases, cystic fibrosis represents that local underlying defect. Botryomycosis with concurrent cutaneous small vessel vasculitis has been documented.[25]

Malakoplakia

Clinical features

Malakoplakia (soft plaque) most often affects the urinary tract, but it can involve many other organs including the gastrointestinal tract, lymph nodes, genitalia, brain, bone, lungs, retroperitoneum, adrenals, tongue, and skin.[1-7] The median age at presentation is approximately 53 years, and the disease appears to be twice as common in males as in females.[4] Cutaneous lesions are most common around the genitalia or perineum, but are occasionally seen in other sites.[3-8] Their appearance is variable and includes plaques, ulceration, polyps, and sinuses, with surrounding induration, as well as nodules and papules.[5,7,9] They may be associated with malakoplakia elsewhere.

Underlying or associated conditions (which are usually linked with immunosuppression) can include carcinoma, rheumatoid arthritis, SLE, diabetes mellitus, leukemia, lymphoma, and immunosuppression following transplantation.[3,4,10-12] However, the condition remains distinctly uncommon in patients with HIV/AIDS; this has been ascribed to selective or relative preservation of antimicrobial monocytic function.[9,13] The skin lesions are nonprogressive but are persistent.

Pathogenesis and histologic features

Although the exact pathogenesis of malakoplakia is poorly understood, the condition is thought to be secondary to an acquired bactericidal defect occurring within macrophages.[6,12] Lesions of malakoplakia are characterized by confluent sheets of histiocytes (von Hansemann cells) with eosinophilic granular cytoplasm and small, usually eccentric nuclei. These cells also contain characteristic cytoplasmic basophilic bodies shown to be calcified with von Kossa staining (Figs 18.226 and 18.227). These round, sometimes laminated structures are known as Michaelis-Gutmann bodies. Their targetoid pattern is accentuated by staining with PAS. They may also be positive on staining with Perl reaction for iron. The Michaelis-Gutmann body is sufficiently distinctive to allow cytological distinction of malakoplakia in a preparation from skin scrapings.[14] Immunohistochemistry with an antibody to BCG may highlight the intracytoplasmic bacteria.[15]

The histiocytic infiltrate may be mixed with neutrophils, lymphocytes, and plasma cells, with associated granulation tissue. Electron microscopy of malakoplakia shows that the histiocytes contain numerous phagolysosomes

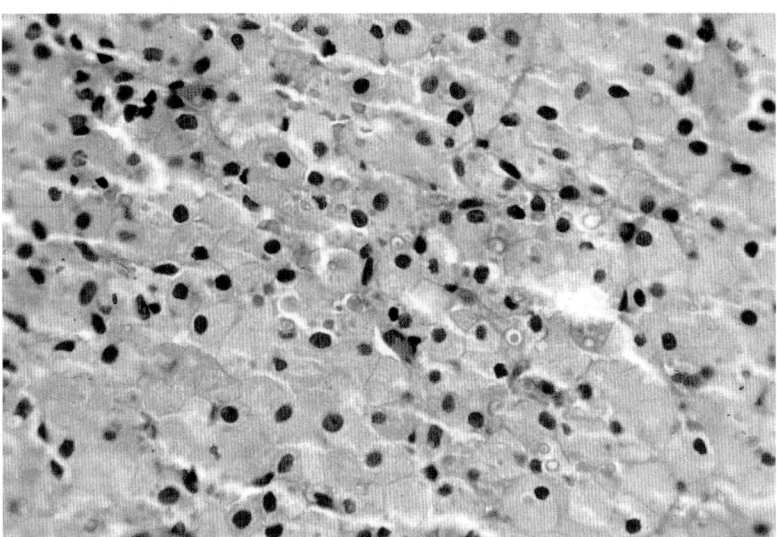

Fig. 18.226
Malakoplakia: the infiltrate consists of histiocytes with eosinophilic granular cytoplasm. Note the pale blue, laminated Michaelis-Gutmann bodies.

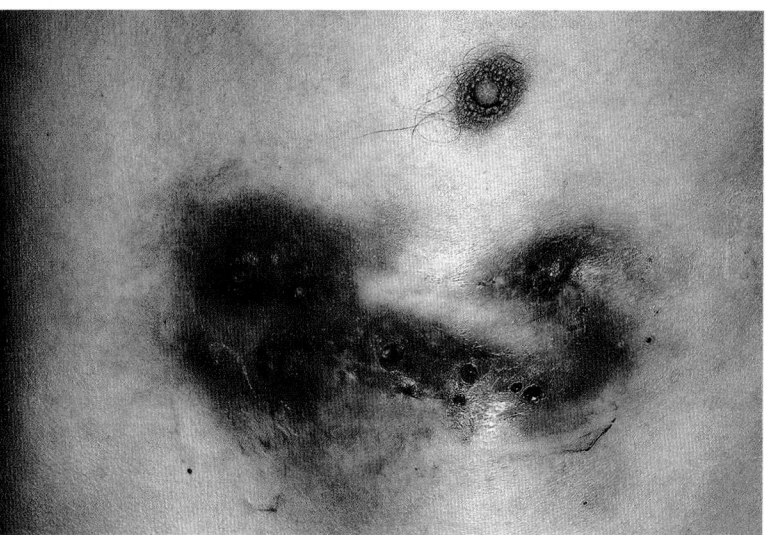

Fig. 18.228
Actinomycosis: extensive intrathoracic disease has resulted in involvement of the anterior chest wall. Numerous sinuses are evident. By courtesy of P. Duhra, MD, Coventry and Warwickshire Hospital, Coventry, UK.

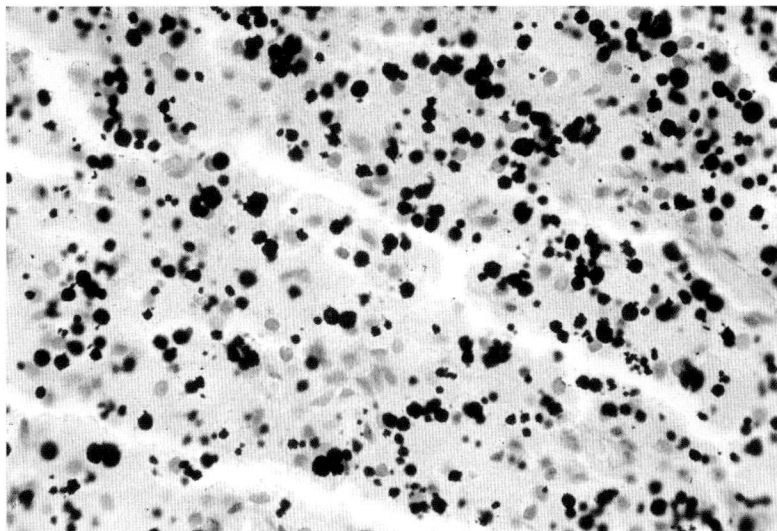

Fig. 18.227
Malakoplakia: use of the von Kossa reaction renders the Michaelis-Gutmann bodies more conspicuous and reveals that they are much more numerous than was apparent in the hematoxylin and eosin stain.

that occasionally contain intact and partly digested bacteria. It has been suggested that phagolysosomes in macrophages accumulate in response to chronic bacterial infection. The infection is not by one specific organism, but the agent is usually *E. coli*.[4] The phagolysosomes tend to fuse and then calcify; the reason for these changes is not clear, although some cases occur in systemic disease associated with a probable impairment of macrophage function.[1,5] Other organisms that have been cultured from lesions of malakoplakia include Gram-negative bacilli (*Klebsiella* spp., *Enterobacter* spp., *Proteus* spp., *Pseudomonas* spp., *Burkholderia cepacia* complex) and Gram-positive cocci, including *Staphylococcus aureus*, *Streptococcus* spp., and enterococci.[4,5,12,15]

Differential diagnosis

Malakoplakia should be distinguished from infectious granulomata, histiocytosis, and granular cell tumor, and from pseudomalakoplakia,[4,15,16] which refers to an abnormal histiocytic proliferation in a previous surgical site. Although pseudomalakoplakia also comprises sheets of large histiocytes with intracytoplasmic calcific material, this condition is distinguished from true malakoplakia by the lack of concentric lamination of the granules.[15,16]

Actinomycosis

Clinical features

Actinomyces israelii is a commensal in the human mouth, along with other organisms including *Aggregatibacter* (formerly *Actinobacillus*) *actinomycetemcomitans*.[1] *A. israelii* is the usual pathogen but occasionally other species including *A. viscosus*, *A. naeslundii*, *A. odontolyticus*, *A. meyeri*, *A. turicensis*, *A. radingae*, and *A. neuii* are implicated.[2-7] The most common manifestation is cervicofacial actinomycosis, but more grave pulmonary and intestinal infections can occur and, rarely, purely cutaneous lesions.[1,8-12] The cervicofacial form is common in farm workers and is associated with poor oral hygiene, usually starting from carious teeth and following dental extractions or oral trauma. The condition is infrequent in children and most common in young men. Respiratory involvement as lung abscess and fistulae may 'point' through the thoracic wall (*Fig. 18.228*).[13] Abdominal lesions include appendiceal and colonic actinomycosis and hepatic involvement, and it may complicate the use of intrauterine contraceptive devices, with lesions affecting the internal female genitalia. Cutaneous fistulae may subsequently develop.[14,15]

The cervicofacial lesion presents as a hard swelling on the lower jaw or, occasionally, as a plaquelike infiltration of the cheek from the upper jaw (cf. bovine lumpy jaw). These firm thickened areas tend to discharge through sinuses and are associated with scarring and the formation of new nodules (*Fig. 18.229*). Yellow granules measuring up to 2 mm in diameter – the so-called 'sulfur granules' – are occasionally found in the discharging pus. Extensions of some maxillary lesions may reach the orbit and base of the skull. Uncommonly, a large facial mass may develop.[5,16]

Rarely, direct inoculation of skin may produce a similar chronically discharging abscess with adjacent scarring (*Fig. 18.230*). Alternatively, a mycetoma or chronic discharging abscess mass with multiple sinuses may develop. This primary form of cutaneous actinomycosis is rare. Sites have included the thigh, the femorogluteal region, the arm, the penis, the breast, the neck, the nose, and the forehead.[7,17-25] Most cases are the result of external trauma and local ischemia, but this is not always the case.[17,21,22,25-27] Some infections have been acquired through injection wounds, including one report where an *A. odontolyticus*-associated subcutaneous abscess evolved in an intravenous cocaine user who admitted to licking his hypodermic needle prior to injection.[17,28] Very rarely, primary cutaneous actinomycosis may be a presenting manifestation of underlying HIV infection.[6] There is an isolated report of *A. bovis* infection affecting the fingernails of a patient with common variable immunodeficiency.[29]

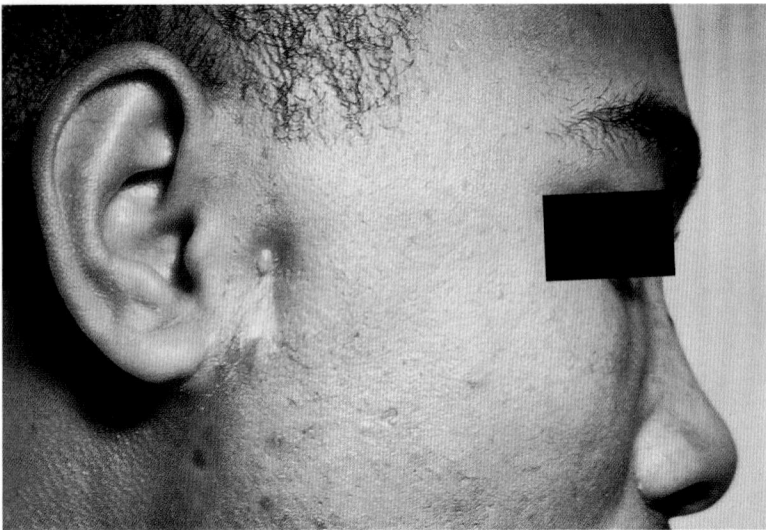

Fig. 18.229
Actinomycosis: infection of the cervicofacial region; note the scarring and dimple at the site of the draining sinus. By courtesy of T.F. Sellers, MD, and H.P. Lambert, MD, St George's Hospital, London, UK.

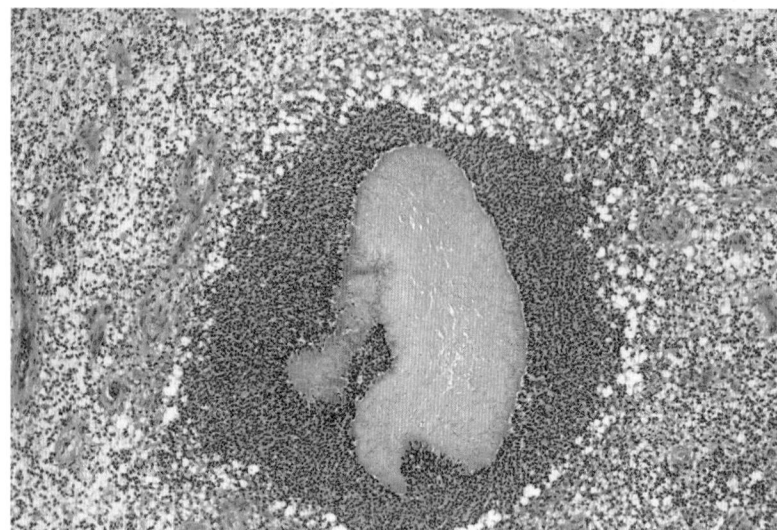

Fig. 18.231
Actinomycosis: a bacterial colony lies in the center of an abscess.

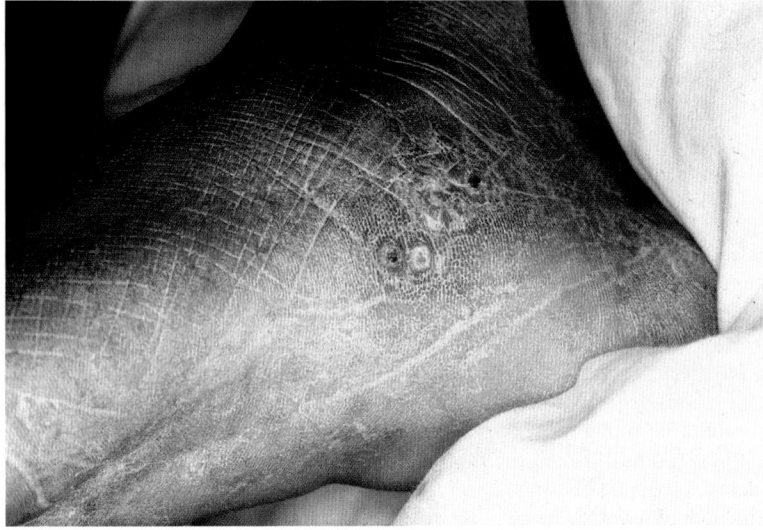

Fig. 18.230
Actinomycosis: multiple sinuses are present about the lateral malleolus. By courtesy of R. Hay, Institute of Dermatology, London, UK.

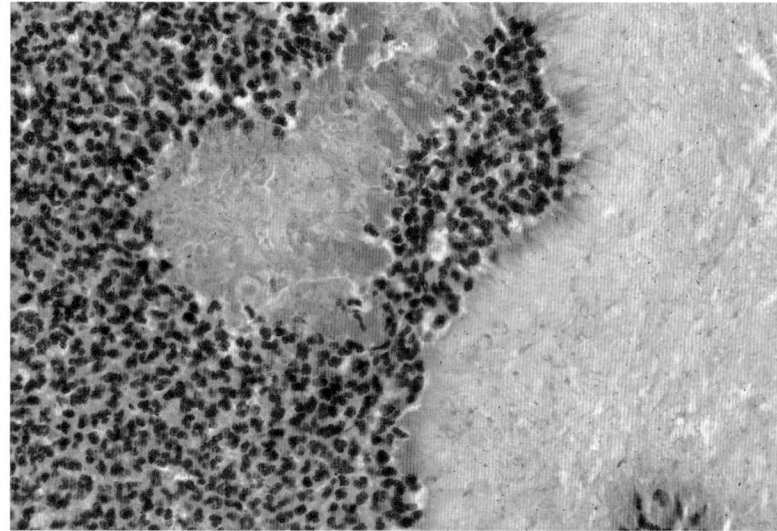

Fig. 18.232
Actinomycosis: high-power view.

An uncommon form of the disease is the presence of disseminated cutaneous lesions in the absence of demonstrable extracutaneous infection; this has been reported in a patient with acute leukemia.[30]

Pathogenesis and histologic features

The mixture of organisms involved in actinomycosis is not purely accidental but is synergistic. *A. israelii* is a Gram-positive, nonacid-fast, microaerophilic bacterium with filamentous branching organisms. *A. actinomycetemcomitans* is a Gram-negative coccobacillus which inhibits growth of fibroblasts and keratinocytes. It is speculated that this, together with its different susceptibility to antibiotics, helps to maintain the actinomycotic lesion.

Histologically, the lesions have the features of chronic abscesses and sinuses, containing pus and surrounded by fibrosis and a mixed inflammatory infiltrate (*Fig. 18.231*). Locules separated by granulation tissue are present. Sulfur granules of intertwined bacteria are seen, radiating mycelial filaments, often with opaque clubs at their tips (*Figs 18.232* and *18.233*).[31] These granules may be associated with the Splendore-Hoeppli phenomenon.

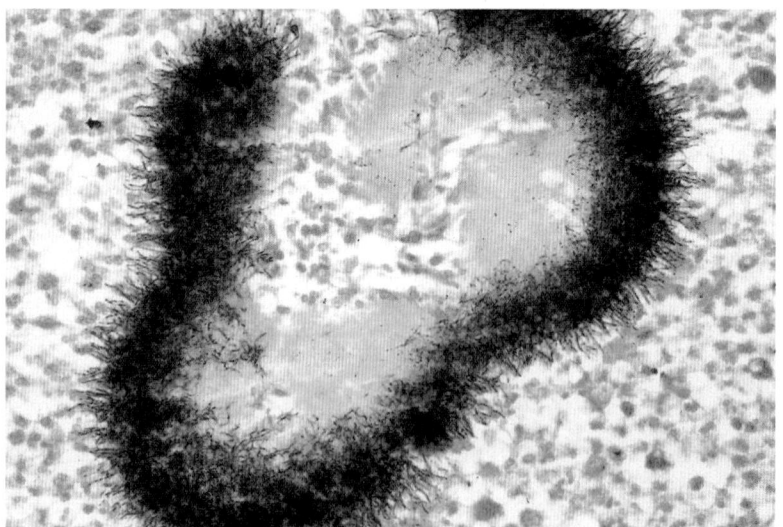

Fig. 18.233
Actinomycosis: Gram-positive bacteria with club-shaped ends are present at the periphery of the granule.

Whipple disease

Clinical features

Whipple disease is a rare, chronic multisystem infective disorder caused by *Tropheryma whipplei*, a Gram-positive bacillus and member of the actinomycetes.[1–4] In its classic form, the condition has a propensity to occur in middle-aged Caucasian males. The gastrointestinal tract is the main target of infection, resulting in low-grade fever, weight loss, abdominal pain, diarrhea, and malabsorption syndrome.[1,3] The known clinical spectrum has, however, broadened in recent years. Some patients have localized disease confined to organs outside of the alimentary tract. Potential manifestations include lymphadenopathy, seronegative arthritis, neurological signs, uveitis, endocarditis, and pleuritis, often in the absence of concomitant gastrointestinal symptoms.[1–3] Others may present with acute, self-limiting infections such as acute pneumonia or acute gastroenteritis.[1] An asymptomatic carrier state is also recognized.[1,6] There have been recent reports of Whipple disease occurring in patients receiving anti-TNF-α therapy.[3,7] Treatment of the infection with appropriate antimicrobial agents may be complicated by IRIS in approximately 10% of patients.[8–11]

Skin involvement in the form of cutaneous hyperpigmentation is relatively common, occurring in 17% to 40% of patients.[5,11,12] Rarely, erythema nodosum-like subcutaneous nodules may develop as a result of infective panniculitis. The latter comprise painful red-brown nodules. Lesions may occur on the thighs, arms, buttocks, lower legs, and, rarely, the chin and neck.[10,13–16] Erythema nodosum proper is another potential manifestation; it may also be encountered in those who develop IRIS.[8,13] The evolution of ENL-like lesions as a manifestation of IRIS in treated Whipple disease has also been documented.[9]

Pathogenesis and histologic features

Although *T. whipplei* is a ubiquitous organism in the environment, Whipple disease remains a very rare condition, with an estimated prevalence of 1.1 per 1 million population and an annual incidence of around 6 per 10 million population.[1,17] Susceptible individuals have defects in T-cell immunity and impaired ability of macrophages to degrade the intracellular organisms.[1,3,18]

The subcutaneous nodules have the appearance of a predominantly septal panniculitis, with a conspicuous infiltrate of foamy macrophages. Careful examination reveals cytoplasmic distension of these histiocytes by PAS-positive, diastase-resistant intracytoplasmic material representing degenerate bacteria.[9,10,15,16] These macrophages closely resemble those encountered in duodenal biopsy material. The viable bacilli have a characteristic double-walled (trilaminar) appearance on ultrastructural examination.[1,13] In rare instances, granulomas may be observed in the dermal compartment overlying the septal panniculitis.[10] Dermal lymphangiectasia has also been described.[9] The organism may be cultured in specialized laboratories. PCR and immunohistochemical methods for confirmation of the diagnosis exist.[10,11,17–20]

Differential diagnosis

Whipple disease should be distinguished from histoplasmosis, histoid LL, and infection with MAI complex, as all of the aforementioned conditions are characterized by intracytoplasmic organisms contained within macrophages. PAS-positive fungal yeasts, however, are observed in histoplasmosis, whereas Ziehl-Neelsen and Wade-Fite stains will confirm the presence of acid-fast mycobacterial bacilli in MAI infection and LL, respectively.

The term 'pseudo-Whipple disease' was used to describe two recently reported cases who presented with clinical and histologic features suspect for cutaneous/subcutaneous Whipple disease, but in whom no *T. whipplei* organisms could be detected by PCR. The lesions resolved on treatment with penicillin; a bacterial (staphylococcal) infection, however, could only be proven in one of the patients.[21]

In those exceptional cases of cutaneous Whipple disease demonstrating intradermal granuloma formation, the condition should be distinguished from other causes of granulomatous dermatitis.[10]

Erythrasma

Clinical features

Erythrasma is a bacterial infection caused by *Corynebacterium minutissimum*, a Gram-positive bacillus.[1–3] It characteristically presents as asymptomatic, well-defined, scaly red patches on the inguinal and intergluteal skin (*Fig. 18.234*). It has a predilection for obese and diabetic patients and it is more common in areas with a humid and hot climate. The clinical diagnosis is easy because of the demonstration of a typical coral-red fluorescence under Wood light.[4,5] This fluorescence is the result of production of coproporphyrin III by the organism. In exceptional cases, fluorescence is not seen.[6] Erythrasma rarely presents as a disciform eruption with an atrophic appearance involving nonintertriginous areas.[7,8] Involvement of the feet (particularly the toe webs) and toenails has also been documented.[9–13] Rarely, lesions on the feet have a vesiculobullous appearance.[14] Nail involvement is

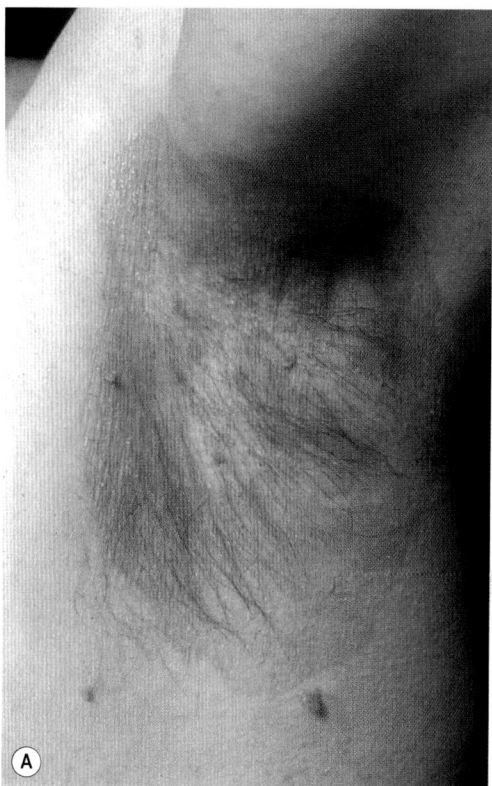

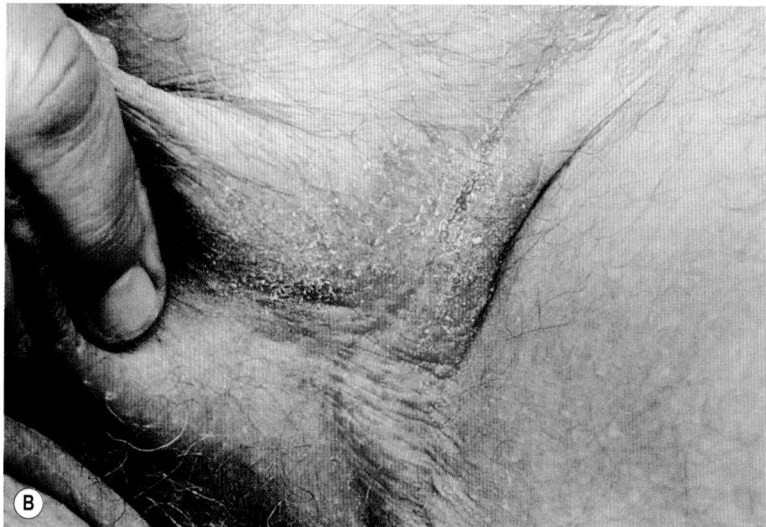

Fig. 18.234
Erythrasma: (**A**) note the well-demarcated axillary scaly red patch; (**B**) there is a scaly inguinal patch with associated hyperpigmentation. By courtesy of the Institute of Dermatology, London, UK.

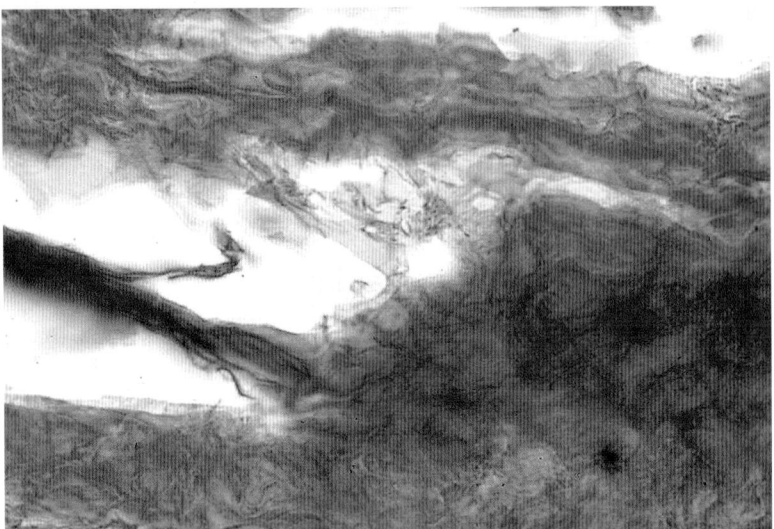

Fig. 18.235
Erythrasma: bacilli are evident in the stratum corneum.

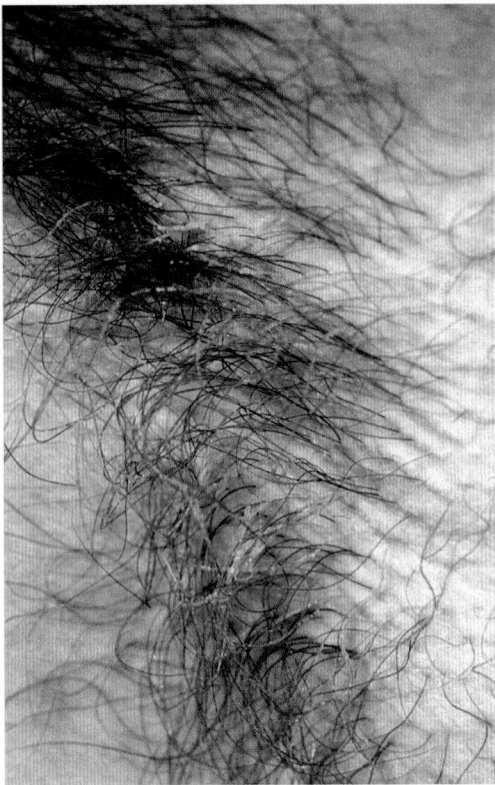

Fig. 18.236
Trichomycosis: this matted appearance of the hair results from the presence of multiple tiny nodules. By courtesy of the Institute of Dermatology, London, UK.

characterized by hyperkeratosis and onycholysis. Erythrasma may coexist with a dermatophyte infection or, rarely, pityriasis versicolor.[15,16] An association with trichomycosis (trichobacteriosis) axillaris and pitted keratolysis may also occur; this has been referred to as the corynebacterial triad.[5,17,18] A biopsy is only exceptionally performed as the diagnosis is confirmed by the use of Wood light or scrapings stained by Gram, PAS, Grocott, Giemsa, or methylene blue.

C. minutissimum has rarely been associated with bacteremia, abscess formation, cellulitis or visceral involvement in immunocompetent or immunocompromised patients.[3,19–22]

Histologic features

A skin biopsy usually appears unremarkable when stained with H&E except for mild hypergranulosis and occasional superficial perivascular lymphocytes. The special stains mentioned before, particularly Gram, show the presence of bacilli in the stratum corneum (*Fig. 18.235*).

Trichobacteriosis

Clinical features

Trichobacteriosis is the preferred and more contemporary designation for trichomycosis, a bacterial infection caused by different species of corynebacteria. Although traditionally ascribed to *Corynebacterium tenuis*, recent advances in molecular taxonomy have shown that the usual etiological agent belongs to the CDC-G/LD (or so-called LD2) group, which corresponds to *C. flavescens*.[1–3] The Gram-positive bacteria invade the cuticle of the hair. Although it was initially suggested that they adhere to the hair shaft by producing a cement-like substance, this view was subsequently challenged and it was later proposed that the material that provides support for the organisms is the apocrine sweat.[4–6] Disturbances in apocrine/apo-eccrine sweat production and associated bacterial proliferation appear to play a crucial pathogenetic role.[1,3] The disease typically involves the axillary hair (trichobacteriosis/trichomycosis axillaris) and exceptionally may be seen in the pubic hair and scrotum (trichobacteriosis/trichomycosis pubis) (*Fig. 18.236*).[7–11] Trichobacteriosis is characterized by yellow, red, or black nodules along the hair shaft. These nodules may be confused with nits. However, the nodules in trichobacteriosis fluoresce under Wood light. In black piedra, the nodules are usually black and the disease mainly involves the scalp. There have nevertheless been single case reports of scalp involvement in infants (trichobacteriosis capitis).[12,13] Distinction from white piedra may be more difficult as the disease has a wide anatomical distribution and it has even been suggested that the latter disease is the result of a synergistic interaction between corynebacteria and *Trichosporon beigelii*, the organism

previously implicated in white piedra.[14] Dermoscopy is a potentially useful diagnostic adjunct.[13,15,16] Trichobacteriosis has been reported in association with erythrasma and pitted keratolysis.[3,17,18]

Pitted keratolysis

Clinical features

Pitted keratolysis (keratolysis plantare sulcatum) is an unusual bacterial infection of plantar skin occurring predominantly, but not exclusively, in humid tropical regions of the world.[1–3] The condition has been recorded in soldiers and paddy field workers, but may even be encountered among office workers.[4–7] Although the cause of the disease remained elusive for many years, it was later ascribed to infection with *Corynebacterium* spp. Two additional Gram-positive organisms have since been implicated: *Kytococcus* (formerly *Micrococcus*) *sedentarius* and *Dermatophilus congolensis*.[1–3,8,9] The disease occurs predominantly in young men. Children are rarely affected.[10] Frequent presenting symptoms include hyperhidrosis, malodor, or even sliminess of the feet.[2,7,11] Soreness and pruritus may also occur. *D. congolensis* causes a variety of dermatitides in domesticated herbivores, and it has been suggested that human infections with the latter organism result from contact with infected animals or contaminated soil.[12]

As indicated by the name, pitted keratolysis is associated with superficial pitlike erosions of the stratum corneum of the plantar skin. These coalesce to form characteristic crateriform defects which are concentrated on the pressure-bearing areas of the foot (*Figs 18.237* and *18.238*). The circular crateriform pits measure 0.7 mm or more in diameter and appear to be distributed along the plantar furrows.[1–3,11,13] Cerebriform maceration is sometimes seen.[11] Rarely, the palms may be involved.[3,14] The dermatoscopic appearances are said to be characteristic.[13] Primary hyperhidrosis has been identified as a risk factor.[15] In one report, treatment of hyperhidrosis with botulinum toxin injection led to resolution of pitted keratolysis, suggesting that hyperhidrosis itself plays a pathogenetic role in the condition.[16] Additional risk factors include prolonged occlusion with shoes, barefooted walking, maceration, and prolonged contact with water. Pitted keratolysis

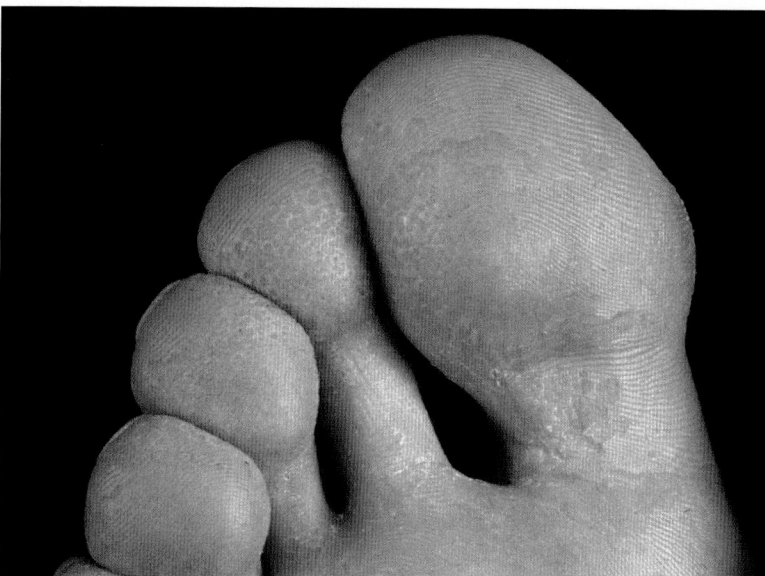

Fig. 18.237
Pitted keratolysis: note the typical scaliness and pitlike areas. By courtesy of the Institute of Dermatology, London, UK.

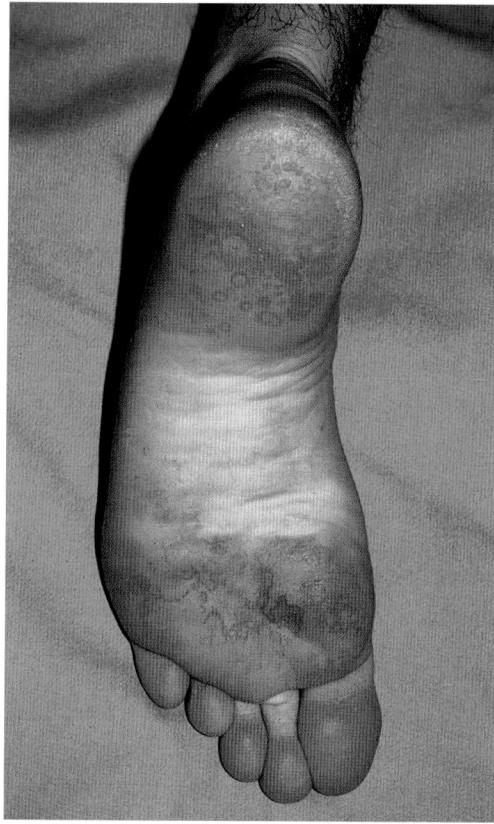

Fig. 18.238
Pitted keratolysis: note the tiny pits on the weight-bearing aspect of the foot. By courtesy of S. Glassman, MD, Division of Dermatology, University of Witwatersrand, Johannesburg, South Africa.

may occur concurrently with erythrasma and trichobacteriosis, resulting in the so-called corynebacterial triad.[3]

Pathogenesis and histologic features

The pits are the consequence of dissolution of the stratum corneum induced by the pathogenic bacteria. In vitro studies have shown that both *D. congolensis* and *K. sedentarius* produce keratinolytic enzymes, thus accounting for the superficial defects in the stratum corneum.[8,17]

The early lesions demonstrate stratum corneum pallor. Biopsies of the plantar pits show small defects in the upper stratum corneum, the walls being almost vertical in configuration.[1,2] Special stains (Gram, methenamine silver, PAS or Giemsa) are required to visualize the organisms, which comprise both coccoid and filamentous forms.[1,2,9] The coccoid forms tend to be concentrated near the surface of the pit whereas the filamentous forms are present in relation to the deeper portions of the defect.[2,9] The filamentous forms show both branching and septation. The filamentous form of *D. congolensis* is characteristically composed of chains of small coccoid bodies.[1] Ultrastructural examination reveals a diminished stratum corneum, the opening of tunnels within the latter, and the presence of coccoid bacteria with transverse septation.[18]

Cutaneous diphtheria

Clinical features

Diphtheria is a highly contagious, vaccine-preventable, usually upper respiratory tract infection caused by the Gram-positive bacillus *Corynebacterium diphtheriae*. An asymptomatic carrier state also exists.[1,2] Cutaneous diphtheria is an uncommon condition traditionally ascribed to *C. diphtheriae*.[3,4] Recent years, however, have seen an increasing role for *C. ulcerans* in the etiology of cutaneous diphtheria, especially in European countries.[1,5–7] Toxogenic and nontoxogenic strains of both organisms exist.[6–18] Rare cases of *C. pseudodiphtheriticum* and *C. pseudotuberculosis* infection have also been reported.[1,19] Although cutaneous diphtheria is essentially a tropical condition, increasing tourism to tropical regions and a decline in adult booster vaccination against diphtheria have resulted in numerous cases being reported from developed countries, especially among returning travelers who have visited regions where the infection is endemic.[1,2,4,8–11,14,17,20–23] The disease usually results from inoculation of organisms into pre-existing lesions such as burns, ulcers, abrasions, and eczematous rashes, and has even occurred following tattooing; cutaneous diphtheria may also manifest in apparently normal skin.[3,4,7,8,20] Cutaneous *C. diphtheriae* infection has been reported among intravenous drug users and homeless individuals, especially in impoverished urban areas.[16,24] Contact with infected domestic animals or occupational exposure to agricultural animals are additional risk factors for *C. ulcerans* infection.[6,12,18]

The lower legs and feet are sites of predilection, but sites such as the face, trunk, hands, and even the genitalia may be involved.[3,6,7,9,10,15–17,25] Initially, there is a vesicle or pustule. This later evolves into an ulcer which is often reddish-purple in color, with rolled and undermined borders, and a yellow-gray membrane or dark crust covering its base.[3,20] The ulcers are painful initially but are later hypoanesthetic.[3] Regional lymphadenopathy may occur, and toxicogenic strains may result in systemic complications involving the nervous system or heart.[1–3]

Histologic features

Histologic examination of the ulcer reveals a necrotic epidermis and dermis. The dermal base of the ulcer contains necrotic debris, fibrin, and an admixture of acute and chronic inflammatory cells.[2] Since the club-shaped and beaded Gram-positive rods are often difficult to visualize in histologic material, microbiological examination of swabs from the center of the lesion is required for confirmation of the diagnosis.[3] Co-infection with other bacterial organisms, however, is a frequent occurrence.[16,17]

Sago palm disease

Clinical features

Sago palm disease is an exceedingly rare chronic bacterial infection of the skin which appears to be restricted to a swampy region of Papua New Guinea where there are groves of sago palms.[1–3] The disease was first described in 1973 and is caused by a hitherto unclassifiable Gram-positive bacillus.[2,3] Infection is acquired by traumatic inoculation while handling the palms.[1]

The primary cutaneous lesions manifest only months later and tend to spread contiguously over a prolonged period, ranging from months to years. The limbs, trunk, and face are the major sites of predilection.[1–3] The clinical

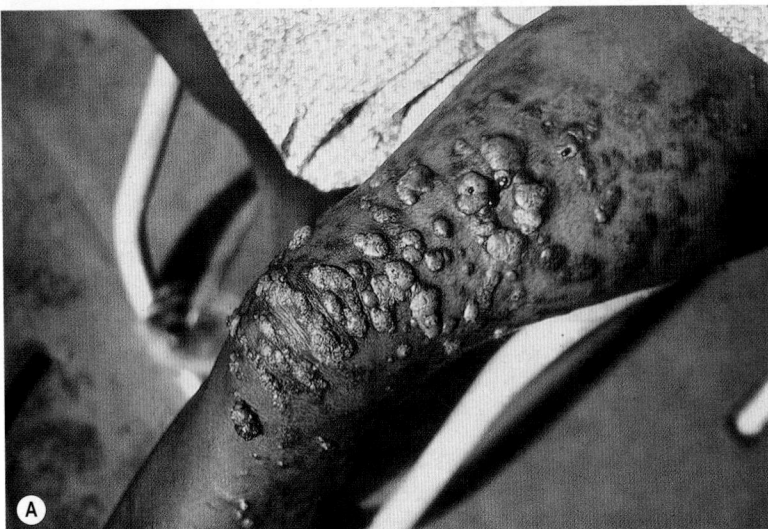

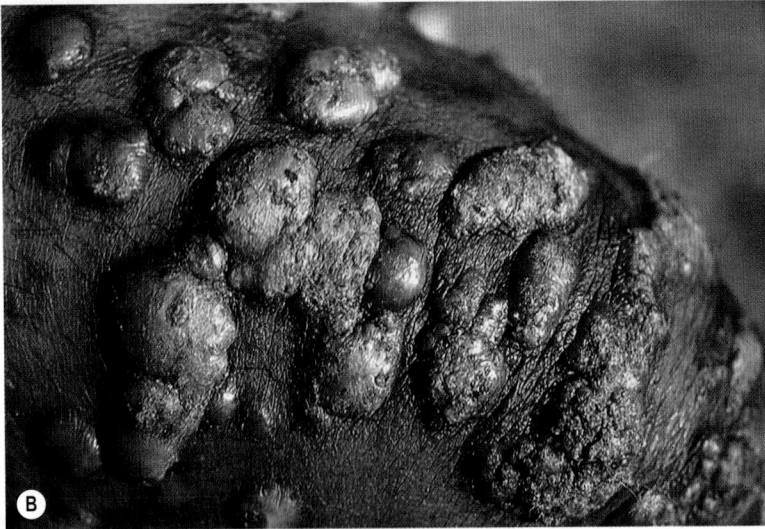

Fig. 18.239
(A, B) Sago palm disease: widely distributed keratotic nodules and plaques are present. By courtesy of E. Wilson Jones, MD, Institute of Dermatology, London, UK.

appearances are those of verrucous, hyperkeratotic nodules which are not associated with ulceration or hemorrhage (*Fig. 18.239*).[2] Systemic spread has not been documented thus far.[2] The infection is resistant to treatment.

Histologic features

The pathological changes in sago palm disease are centered on the dermis, which is expanded by a relatively circumscribed nodular mass composed of sheets of foamy histiocytes, lymphocytes, plasma cells, and fibroblasts.[1,2] The overlying epidermis is hyperkeratotic. The causative bacteria are difficult to identify in routinely stained sections. The Gomori methanamine silver stain reveals large numbers of bacteria which appear to be embedded in amorphous ground substance.[1,2] The bacilli measure approximately 1.8 μm in length and 0.5 μm in width; beading and branching of the organisms may be observed.[1,2] The ultrastructural features are characteristic.[2]

Since the etiological agent has not been cultured successfully, the diagnosis of sago palm disease is based on the clinicopathological features, supported by electron microscopy.[2]

Tularemia

Clinical features

Tularemia is a zoonotic infection caused by *Francisella tularensis*, a highly contagious, nonmotile Gram-negative bacillus.[1-5] Five subspecies exist, but only *F. tularensis* subsp. *tularensis* and *F. tularensis* subsp. *holarctica* are known to be associated with disease in humans, with the former strain predominating in Canada and the United States, and the latter occurring throughout the Northern hemisphere.[4,6] The infection is usually acquired via the bite of an arthropod (such as a tick or deerfly) or by handling the carcasses of infected animals, especially rabbits, hares, and rodents.[1-3,7] Humans may also be infected by drinking contaminated water, the consumption of uncooked infected meat, or the inhalation of contaminated soil.[7] Tularemia is a disease of the northern hemisphere, with the majority of infections reported from North America, Scandinavia, and other parts of Europe.[2,3,8-13] Although the past decades have seen a reduction in the number of reported cases, there has been an apparent re-emergence of the disease in parts of Europe in recent years.[4,14-16] The incubation period is approximately 3–6 days.[8] The organism is regarded as a Category A agent of potential bioterrorism.[6,17]

The most common form of tularemia is the ulceroglandular type, which accounts for 80% or more of infections.[3,12] Other clinical forms include typhoidal, oculoglandular, oropharyngeal, and primary pulmonary tularemia.[3] The ulceroglandular form is characterized by a small, painful erythematous papule at the site of inoculation, usually on an exposed limb. After a few days, the papule breaks down to form a punched-out ulcer which may discharge seropurulent material.[2] This is almost invariably associated with lymphangitis and severe, acute painful lymphadenitis of the regional lymph nodes.[2,10] Other potential cutaneous manifestations, which may develop in all of the clinicopathological forms of tularemia, include macular, papular, vesicular, or pustular eruptions, erythema nodosum lesions, and erythema multiforme.[2,9,18,19] Desquamating pruritic palmar lesions, urticarial lesions, and cellulitis have also been recorded.[18,19] Vesicular lesions may be mistaken clinically for herpes simplex or VZV infection.[20] Skin lesions (other than a primary lesion) were documented in 43% of patients in an analysis of 234 Scandinavian cases.[12] Associated constitutional symptoms and signs may be pronounced and include fever, chills, headache, weakness, myalgia, and coughing.[2,10,12] Ulceroglandular tularemia generally carries a good prognosis, although death due to septicemia may occur in untreated patients.[3,8] Acute tularemic pneumonia, which is acquired by inhalation of aerosolized organisms, carries a high mortality.[3]

Pathogenesis and histologic features

F. tularensis is a highly virulent pathogen; as few as 10 organisms inoculated into the subcutis may initiate infection.[8] The organism is also extremely hazardous to laboratory personnel. It is an elusive facultative intracellular pathogen that possesses novel mechanisms to ensure its survival in macrophages.[5,6,21,22]

The early papular lesions show non-specific features, including intercellular and intracellular edema of the epidermis, sometimes accompanied by vesiculation. There is also dermal edema, telangiectasia, and a mild perivascular infiltrate comprising lymphocytes and plasma cells.[2,23] Early cutaneous ulcers are characterized by fibrinopurulent exudation and an accompanying infiltrate of lymphocytes and macrophages.[2] Lymphangiectasia is encountered deep to the ulcers.[23] Later, there is a well-developed zonal pattern of suppurative granulomatous inflammation, a phenomenon that is recapitulated in the affected regional lymph nodes.[3,23] The central zone contains necrotic material and karyorrhectic debris. An intermediate zone comprising epithelioid histiocytes and giant cells envelops this. An outer mantle containing lymphocytes, histiocytes, plasma cells, and extravasated erythrocytes, in turn, surrounds the latter zone.[2,8,23]

The diagnosis of tularemia is usually confirmed by serology or culture of the organism.[2] *F. tularensis* is not demonstrable in routinely stained sections. It may, however, be detected in histologic material by direct immunofluorescence, PCR or immunohistochemistry; the latter, however, is not commercially available.[2,3,23-25]

Infections caused by Rickettsiae

Clinical features

Rickettsiae are small, obligate, intracellular bacterial pathogens. Rickettsial infections can be divided into three groups:

- The typhus group includes epidemic typhus fever (a louse-borne infection caused by *Rickettsia prowazekii*), the recrudescent form of the latter (Brill-Zinsser disease), murine (endemic) typhus fever (a tick-borne infection caused by *R. typhi*), and *R. felis* infection (which is clinically indistinguishable from classic murine typhus).
- The spotted fever group includes Rocky Mountain spotted fever (a tick-borne infection caused by *R. rickettsii*), other spotted fevers/forms of tick typhus (e.g., Boutonneuse fever and Mediterranean spotted fever caused by *R. conorii*, geographically specific strains of *R. conorii* resulting in conditions such as South African tick-bite fever, Israeli spotted fever, Astrakhan spotted fever or Indian tick typhus, Queensland tick typhus caused by *R. australis*, African tick-bite fever caused by *R. africae*, etc.), and rickettsial pox (caused by *R. akari*, and the only infection in this group to be transmitted by a mite).
- Scrub typhus is caused by *Orientia tsutsugamushi* (formerly *R. tsutsugamushi*) and transmitted by infected chiggers or larval mites of *Leptothrombium* spp.[1–14]

Coxiella burnetii (the cause of Q fever), *Ehrlichia* spp. (the cause of ehrlichiosis), *Anaplasma* spp. (the cause of anaplasmosis), and *Bartonella* (formerly *Rochalimaea*) spp. represent a separate group of rickettsia-like organisms and are not discussed here.

Advances in molecular taxonomic methods have led to not only the reclassification of rickettsial diseases but also recognition of an ever-increasing spectrum of emerging rickettsial pathogens.[3,14,15] Increased international travel has necessitated a heightened awareness of these often geographically specific febrile illnesses.[16,17] There has also been some interest in pathogenic rickettsiae as potential agents of bioterrorism.[2,18] Although all of the true rickettsial infections listed above are associated with variable cutaneous manifestations, there is great diversity in the extent of involvement and degree of clinical severity. Shared general clinical manifestations among most, however, are fever, malaise, presence or absence of an eschar, an exanthematous eruption, and lymphadenopathy.[19] A detailed discussion of the epidemiological, clinical, and pathological characteristics of each entity is beyond the scope of this text; for more information, the reader is referred to references 1–4, which provide good overviews of the subject.

Endemic typhus and rickettsial pox are mild infections, whereas Rocky Mountain spotted fever is a severe multisystem disease which may involve the CNS, kidneys, lungs, heart, and liver. Gangrene of the extremities and a coagulopathy may also occur.[4,20] Scrub typhus is extremely variable, ranging from an asymptomatic illness to a severe infection with significant mortality if untreated. The earliest symptoms of rickettsial infection are non-specific and include fever, headache, chills, and myalgias. Rocky Mountain spotted fever often has additional symptoms of nausea, vomiting, and abdominal pain. Lymphadenopathy is encountered in rickettsial pox, tick typhus, and scrub typhus.

An eschar characteristically develops at the site of the arthropod bite in the spotted fever group (with the exception of Rocky Mountain spotted fever) and in scrub typhus; eschar formation is not a feature of the typhus fever group (*Fig. 18.240*).[20] Eschars may be multiple.[21] Initially, there may be a papule or papulovesicle. After a variable interval, a skin rash evolves. In most cases, this is macular, eventually becoming maculopapular. Generally, the rash commences on the trunk and spreads to the extremities, frequently involving the palms and soles; the converse is true for Rocky Mountain spotted fever. Vesiculation and scab formation are features of rickettsial pox, and the palms and soles are usually not involved in the latter condition. A petechial or hemorrhagic rash may occur in epidemic typhus fever, Rocky Mountain spotted fever, and the other spotted fevers but is not observed in scrub typhus.[4]

Pathogenesis and histologic features

A hallmark of the rickettsial infections is the presence of vascular endothelial invasion by the organisms. Following the bite of the arthropod vector,

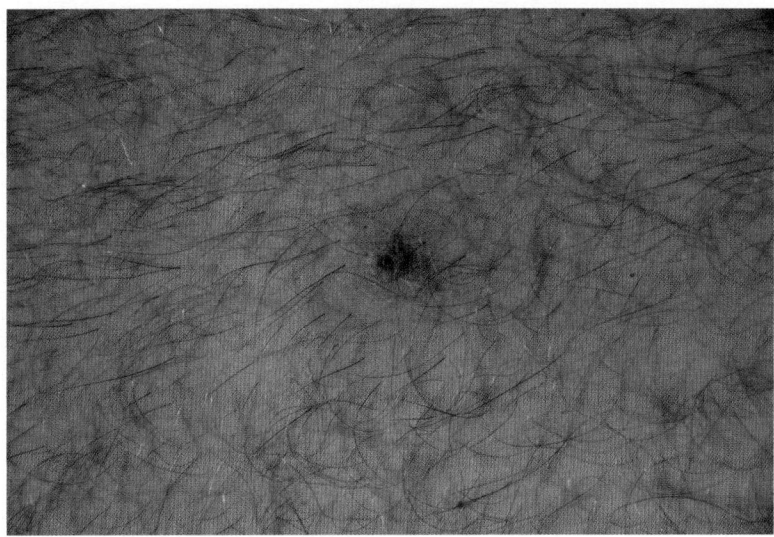

Fig. 18.240
South African tick bite fever: an eschar marks the site of the arthropod bite on the inner thigh. The patient also had lymphadenopathy. By courtesy of M. Hale, MD, National Health Laboratory Service and University of the Witwatersrand, Johannesburg, South Africa.

the *Rickettsia* organisms adhere to vascular endothelium and later become internalized into the cytoplasm of these cells. Replication occurs, followed by hematogenous dissemination. *R. rickettsii* has the unique capacity to also invade and induce necrosis of vascular smooth muscle cells, thereby accounting for the greater severity of the illness and multiorgan involvement.[4] In vitro studies performed on the spotted fever group of rickettsiae have shown that infection of endothelial cells leads to induction of cyclooxygenase 2 (COX-2) and the release of vasoactive prostaglandins.[22] Vascular leakage appears to be the consequence of gaps forming in interendothelial adherens junctions.[23] More recent publications offer additional insights into the complex immunopathogenesis.[24,25]

Histologic examination of the eschar reveals wedge-shaped coagulative necrosis of the epidermis and superficial dermis, sometimes accompanied by necrotizing vasculitic changes in small venules and arterioles, and an infiltrate of macrophages at the base. A dense background perivascular lymphocytic infiltrate often accompanies these changes (*Fig. 18.241*).[21,26] A small vessel lymphocytic vasculitis of variable severity is encountered in biopsies from the maculopapular lesions.[27] This is usually mild in cases of endemic typhus and scrub typhus, whereas the dermal vessels in established cases of Rocky Mountain spotted fever show severe involvement, with endothelial hyperplasia and nonocclusive intravascular fibrin-platelet thrombi, focal lymphocytic vasculitis, and leukocytoclastic vasculitis.[4,28–30] Dermal erythrocytic extravasation is a feature of the petechial and hemorrhagic lesions. There is epidermal basal layer vacuolar degeneration. Biopsies from the vesicular lesions of rickettsial pox will show an intraepidermal vesicle, sometimes accompanied by a neutrophilic infiltrate at the base or subepidermal edema.[31,32]

In the past, the diagnosis was confirmed by the Weil-Felix test. This was later superseded by tests employing complement fixation, latex agglutination, and immunofluorescence studies on frozen skin biopsy material; immunohistochemistry was also used with some success.[4,20] PCR, however, has since emerged as a more valuable tool for rapid diagnosis, and may even be carried out on samples obtained from eschar swabs.[3,17]

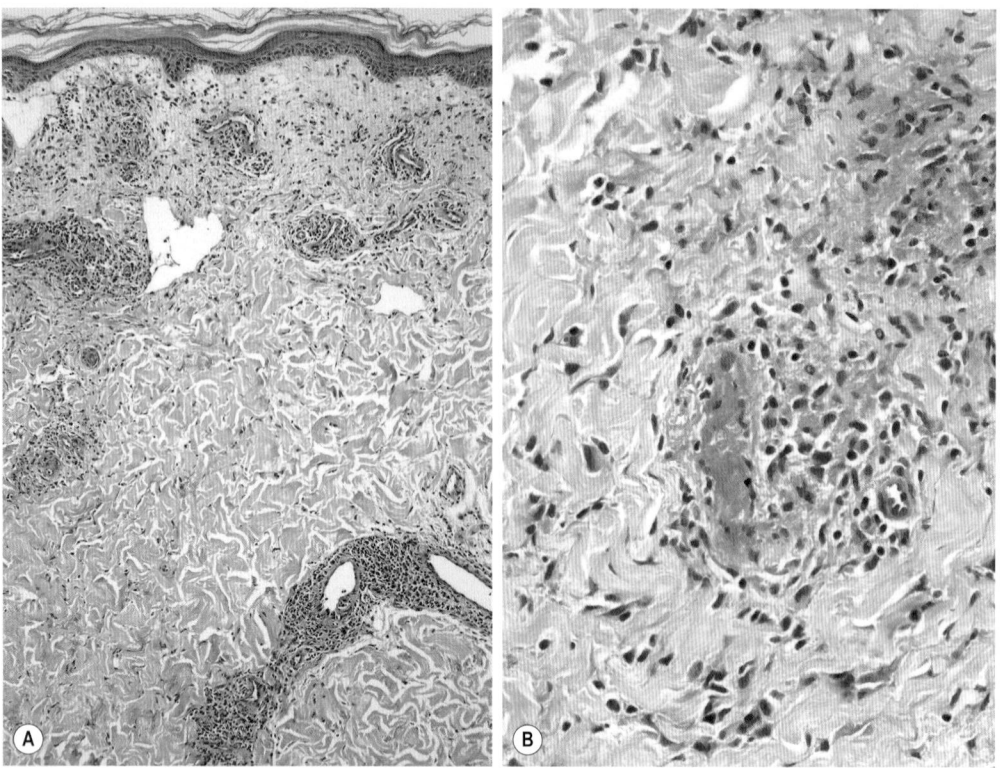

Fig. 18.241
South African tick bite fever: (**A**) there is upper dermal edema, vascular ectasia, and a dense perivascular chronic inflammatory cell infiltrate; (**B**) note the thrombosed vessel.

PROTOZOAL INFECTIONS

Leishmaniasis

Clinical features

Leishmania is a protozoan parasitic organism related to the trypanosomes. The life cycle contains a flagellate phase (promastigote) which occurs in the intestine of its vector, a female *Phlebotomus* or *Lutzomyia* sandfly, and a phase in which the flagellum is retracted (amastigote). The latter is the form seen in the human host. Various mammals, including gerbils, rodents, dogs, jackals, hyraxes, and foxes, may act as reservoirs of infection.[1–7]

An estimated 12 million people are affected worldwide in 102 countries, areas, and territories, and on 5 continents. As many as 1.2 million new cases occur annually, the majority of whom have cutaneous leishmaniasis (CL), while some 400 000 develop visceral leishmaniasis (VL).[7–10] After malaria, leishmaniasis is the second leading cause of protozoal-related deaths worldwide, with an estimated 20 000 to 30 000 deaths annually.[6] VL and, to a lesser extent, CL are increasingly recognized as opportunistic diseases in immunocompromised patients, especially those infected with HIV.[8,11–15] Leishmaniasis may also be a manifestation of IRIS in HIV/AIDS patients on ART.[7] Cutaneous involvement as a first indicator of underlying VL has been reported as a complication of anti-TNF-α therapy.[16]

More than 20 species of *Leishmania* are responsible for human disease, and these are distinguished on the grounds of biochemical, antigenic, and genetic differences.[6] Although leishmaniasis tends to be seen in Asia, Africa, the Americas, and the Mediterranean countries, it is being seen more often in nonendemic countries, particularly among refugees and returning holidaymakers.[17,18] There are eight main types of cutaneous presentation, with many local geographic and species variations.

In endemic regions, a significant number of people appear to have asymptomatic (subclinical) infection, so-called cryptic leishmaniasis.[17]

Confirmation of the diagnosis has traditionally been achieved by visualization of the organisms in smears or tissue sections, or with the aid of the Montenegro (leishmanin) skin test, especially in the developing world. Over the years these investigations have been complemented or superseded by serology, culture, or more recently, PCR-based methods.[5,9,19–21]

Cutaneous leishmaniasis

CL has many local names, including Oriental sore, Baghdad boil, Chiclero ulcer, and Aleppo boil. It is caused by *L. tropica*, *L. major*, and *L. aethiopica* and affects men, women, and children. Mediterranean CL is caused predominantly by *L. infantum*.[17]

Lesions occur on any site accessible to biting by the sandfly vector, most commonly the hands, arms, and face (*Fig. 18.242*). They present as an erythematous papule that enlarges over the course of a few weeks into an ulcerated and crusted nodule. Occasionally, multiple lesions are seen. Lesions show a tendency to orientation along the skin creases, and grossly the ulcers have been compared to a volcano in surface appearance and configuration.[6,7,22] Variants may be hypoesthetic, psoriasiform, eczematous, varicelliform, paronychial, chancriform, zosteriform, annular, whitlow-like, erysipeloid, verrucous, or keloidal, or present as macrocheilia.[17,23,24] Regional lymphadenopathy can be a feature.[25]

In the Eastern hemisphere, where the disease has traditionally been referred to as, 'Old World' leishmaniasis, these lesions may be 'wet' or 'dry':

- The wet type has a short incubation period (2 weeks) and occurs in rural areas. It is caused by *L. major* and develops like a suppurative folliculitis which ulcerates, the surrounding edematous, indurated erythema extending gradually to reach a maximum of 6 cm. Small secondary nodules may be seen around this. Slow resolution with cribriform scarring occurs over 3–12 months.
- The dry form is caused by *L. tropica*, has a longer incubation period (2 months), and is mostly seen in urban areas.[26] The initial lesion is a brown nodule and this becomes a plaque up to 2 cm across. It may ulcerate centrally with a firm crust. Resolution occurs with scarring over 12 months or longer. *L. killicki* is a recently identified subpopulation of *L. tropica*, and occurs in North Africa.[27]

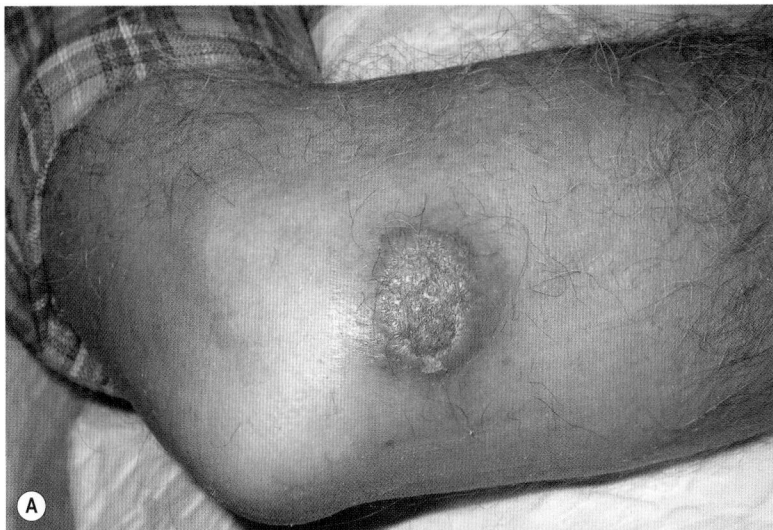

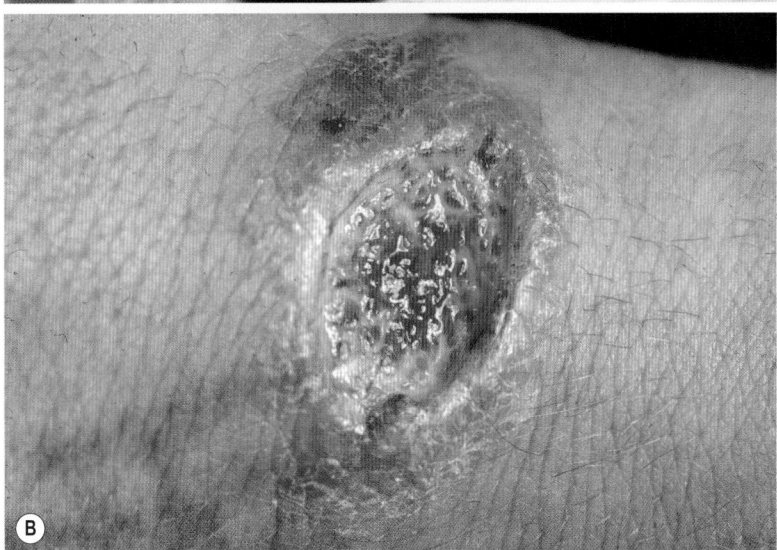

Fig. 18.242
Cutaneous leishmaniasis: (**A**) this healing lesion shows crusting and scarring; (**B**) there is an extensive ulcerated erythematous plaque with scaling. (**A**) By courtesy of J.C. Pascual, MD, Alicante-Spain; (**B**) from the collection of the late NP Smith MD, the Institute of Dermatology, London, UK.

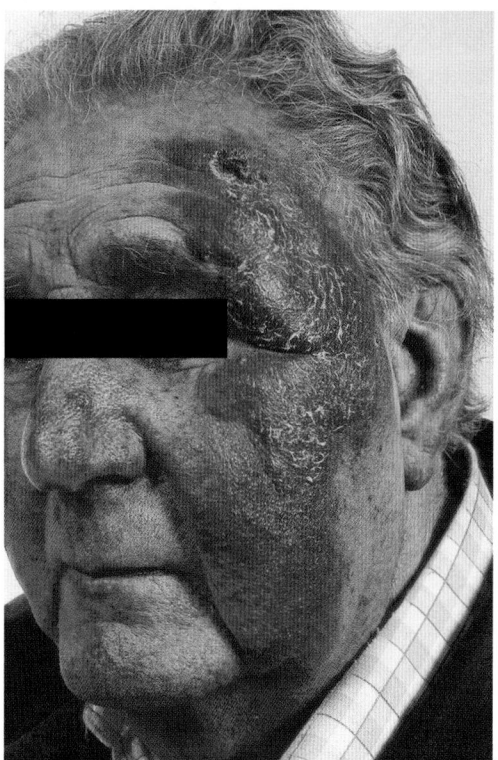

Fig. 18.243
Cutaneous leishmaniasis: chronic cutaneous leishmaniasis showing intense edema, erythema, and scaling. By courtesy of S. Lucas, MD, St Thomas' Hospital, London, UK.

The American forms, traditionally referred to as 'New World' leishmaniasis, are caused predominantly by *L. mexicana* and *L.* (subgenus *Viannia*) *braziliensis*. Other species implicated include *L. amazonensis*, *L. (V.) guyanensis*, *L. (V.) panamensis*, and *L. (V.) peruviana*.[28,29] The lesions of *L. mexicana* are usually like those of CL in the Eastern hemisphere, but some subvariants can cause destructive ulceration of the ear. Most infections with *L. (V.) braziliensis* are local and heal without much damage.

Chronic CL represents persistence (or spread) of an acute lesion for more than 1 year. Lesions are particularly seen on the face as raised erythematous plaques which may resemble erysipelas (*Fig. 18.243*).[17] The erysipeloid lesions are erythematous and infiltrative and are said to occur more frequently in women older than 50 years.[30]

The acute lesions may be followed by a relapsing chronic or lupoid stage (leishmaniasis recidivans or leishmaniasis recidiva cutis) in which brownish papules develop close to the scar of the earlier stages. This occurs in 3% to 10% of patients.[31] These papules extend to resemble lupus vulgaris; they may develop hypertrophic scars or become verrucous. They are extremely slow to resolve, even under treatment, and may persist for many years. It is thought that a change in local immunity results in reactivation of intracytoplasmic organisms.[31] The leishmanin or Montenegro skin test for cellular immunity to *Leishmania* is strongly positive in nearly all cases. It has been suggested that leishmaniasis recidivans represents a hypergic form of the disease, but this has been disputed by others.[32] Although this

presentation is typically encountered in Eastern hemisphere leishmaniasis, a small number of cases of leishmaniasis recidiva cutis complicating American leishmaniasis have been reported.[32–34]

Skin infections with *L. (V.) braziliensis* are liable to recur as mucosal lesions, known as espundia (in which there is much tissue destruction), sometimes years later. The mucosal lesions occur most often in the nasal septum and mouth and rarely around the eyes, genitalia, and anus (*Fig. 18.244*). Patients may also develop 'tapir nose' in which there is considerable damage to the nasal cartilage resulting in a free-hanging nose.[17] The mucosal lesions start as superficial erosions, but become deeply ulcerative and destructive. The Montenegro skin test is almost always positive.

Diffuse CL, also known as pseudolepromatous leishmaniasis, is caused by variants of *L mexicana* and *L. aethiopica*. The former occurs in Bolivia, Venezuela, Mexico, and Brazil, while the latter is seen predominantly in Ethiopia. It develops as a consequence of an impaired cellular immune response.[31] A study from Egypt showed a significant association between histocompatibility antigens HLA-A11, B5, and B7 and the occurrence of this disease.[35] It begins as a nodule, which grows and becomes surrounded by other similar lesions. This process is repeated until eventually, over many years, most of the skin becomes nodular (*Fig. 18.245*). The nodules do not ulcerate and can closely resemble LL. Although lesions may develop in the nasal mucosa, these are not destructive like those of the mucocutaneous form of American leishmaniasis. Response to therapy is slow and relapse is common. The Montenegro test is invariably negative.

L. major and *L. (V.) panamensis* may be associated with a sporotrichoid spreading reaction.[8]

There have been rare reports of neoplasms such as basal cell carcinoma, squamous cell carcinoma, or even dermatofibrosarcoma protuberans arising in scars associated with CL.[7,36–39]

Visceral leishmaniasis

VL (kala-azar, black fever) is due to infection by *L. donovani* complex and occurs widely in South America (*L. chagasi*), Africa (*L. infantum*), the Mediterranean (*L. infantum*), and Asia (*L. donovani* and *L. infantum*).[9,40,41] It may be a manifestation of HIV infection.[8,11,42] In patients with HIV/AIDS,

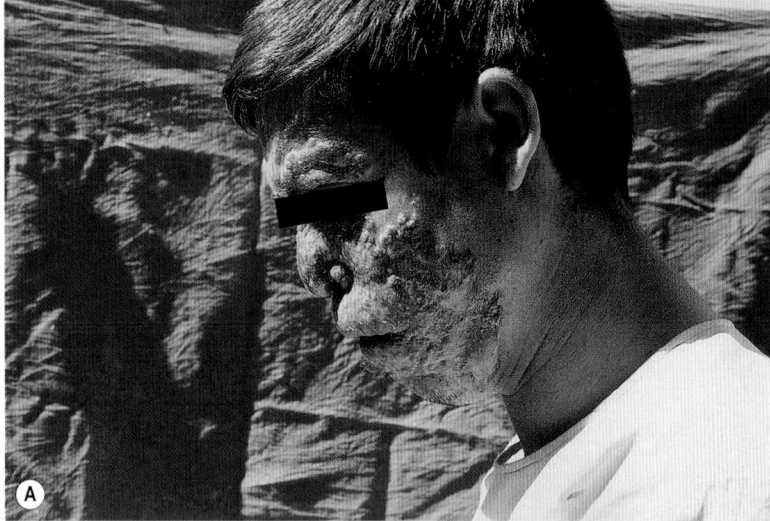

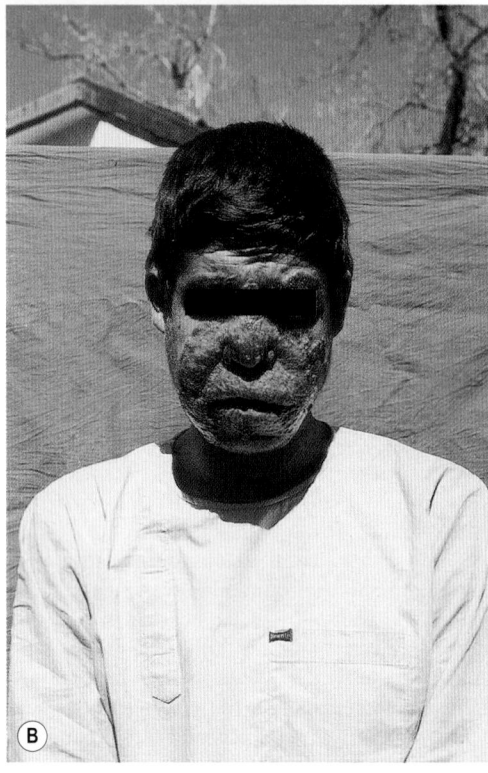

Fig. 18.244
(**A**, **B**) Mucocutaneous leishmaniasis: the lesions are destructive and very disfiguring. By courtesy of S. Lucas, MD, St Thomas' Hospital, London, UK.

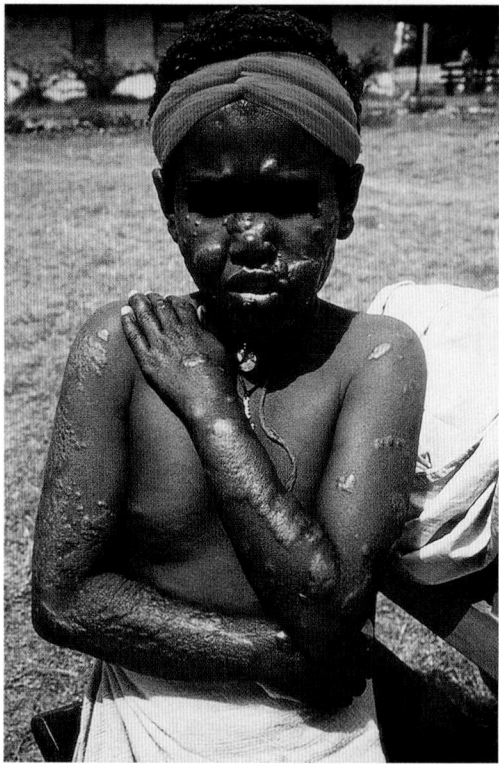

Fig. 18.245
Diffuse cutaneous leishmaniasis: note the widespread lesions, many of which appear keloidal. By courtesy of the late M.S.R. Hutt, MD, St Thomas' Hospital, London, UK.

Pathogenesis and histologic features

In all variants of the disease, the amastigote form of the parasite multiplies within the histiocytes of the mammalian host. The host response is related to the number of amastigotes and the degree of cellular immunity. Large numbers of amastigotes are associated with an anergic response and many histiocytes without other inflammatory cells. Moderate numbers of amastigotes are usually associated with necrosis, which is an important mechanism for eliminating infection. Smaller numbers are associated with a good epithelioid granulomatous response after the necrosis phase. Some infections are eliminated by an effective granulomatous response without necrosis, while others are associated with focal necrosis and ulceration when organisms are released. In others, there is more extensive necrosis. The events following necrosis depend on the rate at which an effective epithelioid granulomatous reaction develops.[50,51] An unusual case of late-stage CL harboring foci of caseous necrosis with no demonstrable organisms has been reported.[52] Healing is often relatively rapid once necrosis has occurred. In parallel with developing immunity, the overlying epidermis shows pseudoepitheliomatous hyperplasia. Lymphocytes and plasma cells also become more numerous at the periphery of the granuloma. Scarring eventually replaces the granuloma.

The recent identification of *Leishmania* RNA virus (LRV)-1 and LRV-2 in New World and Old World *Leishmania* spp. is of particular interest. Recognition of the replicated virus by the host's TLR3 initiates destruction of the parasite, with dispersal of LRV and the subsequent release of proinflammatory chemokines and cytokines.[7,53]

Histologically, the acute lesion (oriental sore) is characterized by hyperkeratosis and acanthosis, although occasionally epidermal atrophy and parakeratosis are features.[31] Ulceration is frequently seen (*Fig. 18.246*). Liquefactive degeneration of the basal keratinocytes has been described.[31] The epidermis may show pseudoepitheliomatous hyperplasia, and intraepidermal neutrophil microabscesses are not infrequent. The dermis typically contains an intense infiltrate of histiocytes, lymphocytes, and plasma cells. Rarely, a Grenz zone is evident. Neutrophils and eosinophils are usually sparse.[54] Large numbers of amastigotes are evident and these may be seen within the overlying keratinocytes (*Fig. 18.247*).[31,54] Foci of dermal necrosis may be evident. Vascular changes are usually not seen.[54] Perineural and

leishmaniasis may occur in herpes zoster lesions, and dermatofibroma cells may be parasitized by the organisms. Nodular cutaneous lesions arising in AIDS-related VL may mimic Kaposi sarcoma clinically.[43] Following inoculation, the organisms multiply in histiocytes; the onset of disease is insidious, taking 2–4 months. The macrophages of the liver and spleen take up the organisms, resulting in hepatosplenomegaly associated with lymphadenopathy, pancytopenia, irregular and intermittent fever, and marked weight loss. In India, some patients develop earthy-gray pigmentation, particularly on the temples, around the mouth, and on the hands and feet.[17]

A small number of patients who recover subsequently develop post-kala-azar dermal leishmaniasis (PKDL).[44–46] This has been reported from India and East Africa. The lesions start as erythematous or hypopigmented macules (particularly on the face) and become nodular and coalesce so that they closely resemble LL, but they lack sensation abnormalities. The lesions are persistent, but resolve slowly on treatment.[46–48] Co-infection with VL and leprosy has been reported from countries where both conditions are endemic, including leprosy and PKDL.[49]

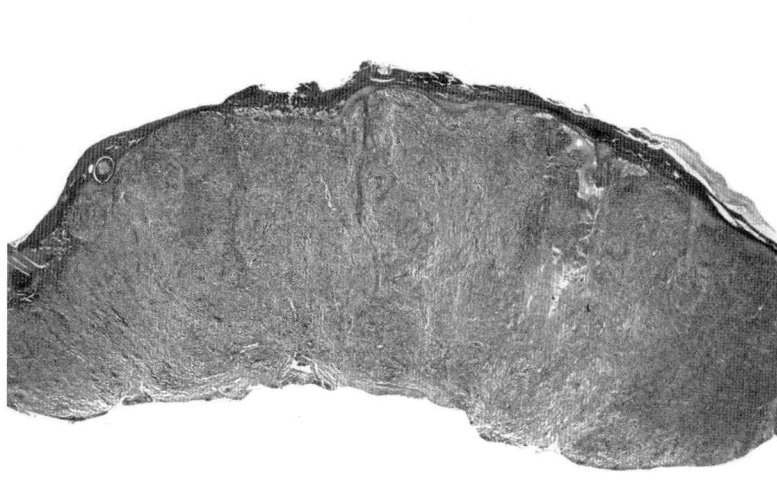

Fig. 18.246
Oriental sore: there is extensive ulceration and the adjacent epithelium is acanthotic; intense inflammation is seen deep to the ulcer bed.

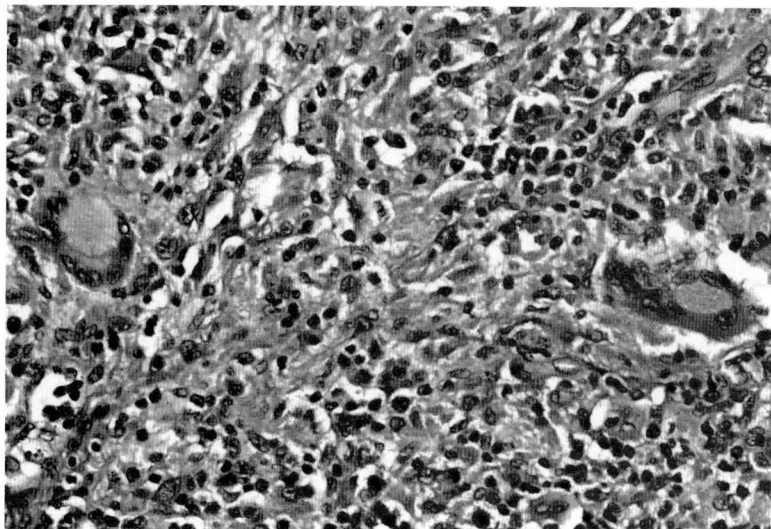

Fig. 18.248
Oriental sore: epithelioid cell granulomata as seen in this field are a feature of chronic lesions.

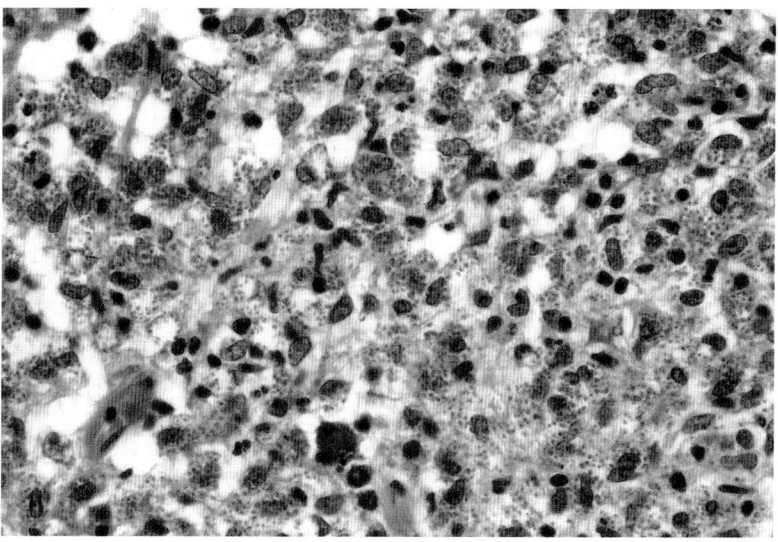

Fig. 18.247
Oriental sore: the infiltrate consists of parasite-laden histiocytes with small numbers of lymphocytes.

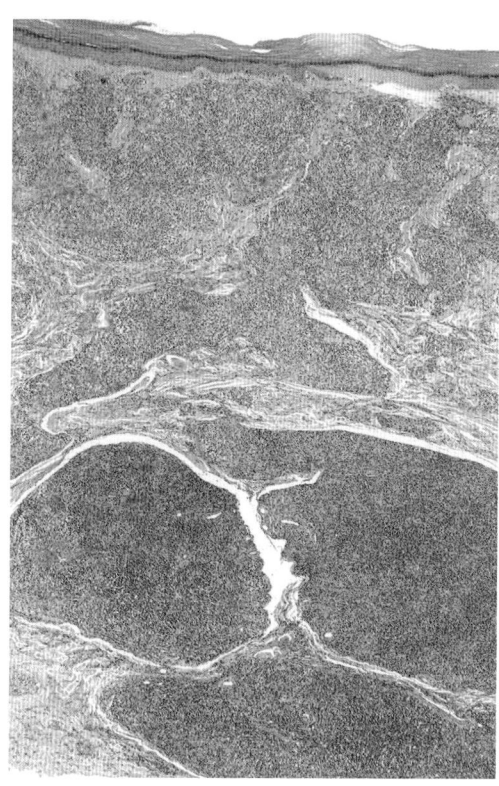

Fig. 18.249
Post-kala-azar dermal leishmaniasis: there is a dense dermal nodular infiltrate. The Grenz zone is spared.

intraneural chronic inflammatory changes associated with perineural *Leishmania* organisms have been described.[55] The patient was found to be hyperesthetic clinically. In chronic lesions, the dermis contains large numbers of small noncaseating granulomata (*Fig. 18.248*). Giant cells tend to be sparse. Leishman bodies are sparse or absent.[31] Necrosis is very rare at this stage.[54]

Histologically, mucocutaneous leishmaniasis is extensively necrotic, with many plasma cells, lymphocytes, neutrophils, and macrophages, but few organisms. Occasional tuberculoid or suppurative granulomata may be present.[1,3]

As with LL, diffuse CL is characterized histologically by numerous macrophages distended with amastigotes and a lack of granuloma formation. There are few lymphocytes and plasma cells. These features indicate anergy, but not primary immunodeficiency.

The features of PKDL are similar to those of the diffuse cutaneous variety; the overlying epidermis is atrophic, but is not usually ulcerated (*Figs 18.249–18.251*). Nodular lesions show a dense dermal lymphohistiocytic infiltrate. There are a variable number of organisms. Vascular hyalinization is evident, and marked follicular plugging may be observed.[56] Degeneration

of basal epidermal keratinocytes was observed in one study. The dermal infiltrate was noted to comprise T-lymphocytes and macrophages, with a preponderance of CD4+ T-cells over CD8+ lymphocytes. Plasma cells, however, were inconspicuous or absent.[57]

The lupoid form of chronic CL may be difficult to diagnose because it represents an exaggerated tuberculoid response to very few organisms (and as such, closely resembles lupus vulgaris) or perhaps only leishmanial antigen; it is best distinguished from other tuberculoid diseases on the basis of its positive Montenegro skin test.[31] There is no necrosis, and plasma cells are sparse.

In all other forms of CL the diagnosis is confirmed by the demonstration of amastigotes in a smear or skin section.[58] The organisms are best revealed by Giemsa stain as reddish cytoplasmic round to oval structures

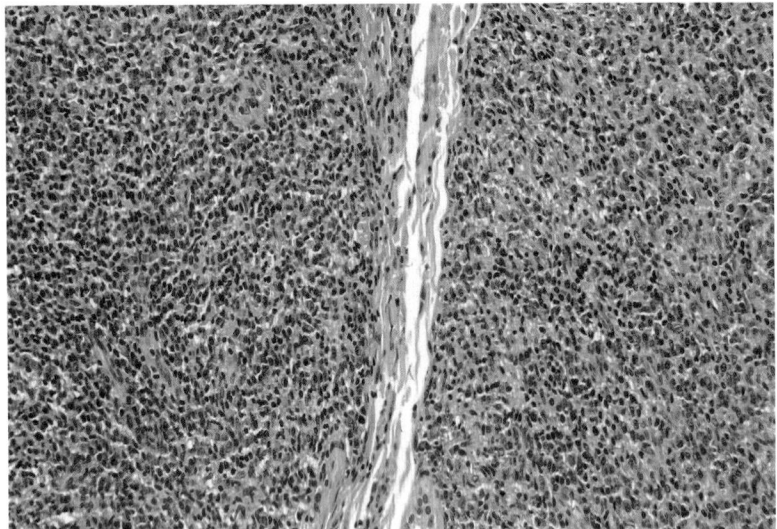

Fig. 18.250
Post-kala-azar dermal leishmaniasis: there is a heavy mixed infiltrate of histiocytes, lymphocytes, and plasma cells.

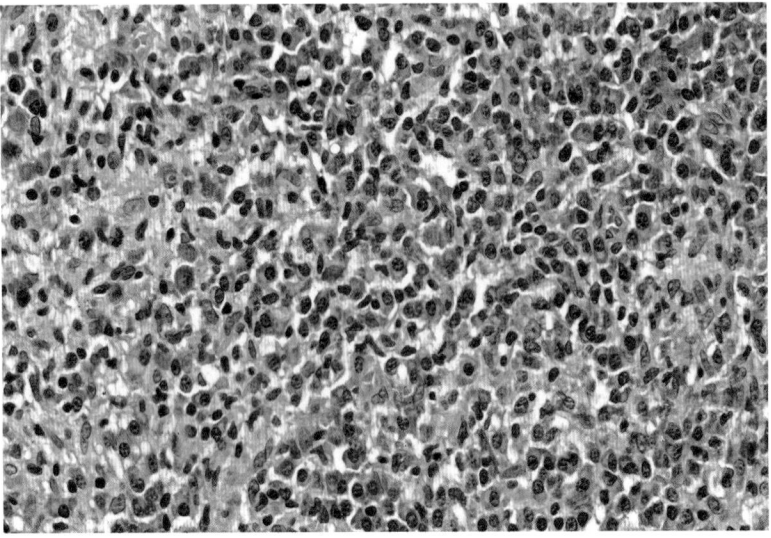

Fig. 18.251
Post-kala-azar dermal leishmaniasis: in this example, organisms are no longer visible.

measuring from 1.5 × 2.5 to 4.5 × 6.8 μm.[8] They appear blue-gray on H&E staining. A small rod-like similarly stained kinetoplast may be visible (*Fig. 18.252*). Many of the organisms are within macrophages, but some occur extracellularly. They are termed Leishman-Donovan bodies.[14] These features must be distinguished from the similar bodies of histoplasmosis and, to a lesser extent, those of granuloma inguinale and rhinoscleroma. The clinical features will usually be distinctive; skin testing, serology, and culture of the organisms will confirm the diagnosis. PCR is useful in providing a rapid diagnosis with precise species identification.[19,20,59,60]

Differential diagnosis

A diagnosis of CL may easily be overlooked by histopathologists who are seldom exposed to biopsy material from such cases, especially when not alerted to a significant travel history. This is particularly the case when organisms are sparse or if unusual histologic features are present, such as sarcoidal granulomas, tuberculoid granulomas, palisaded granulomas with central fibrinoid change, elastophagocytosis, and conspicuous numbers of multinucleated histiocytic giant cells. Lesions may thus be misdiagnosed as sarcoidosis, foreign body granuloma, granuloma annulare, or lupoid rosacea.[61–63]

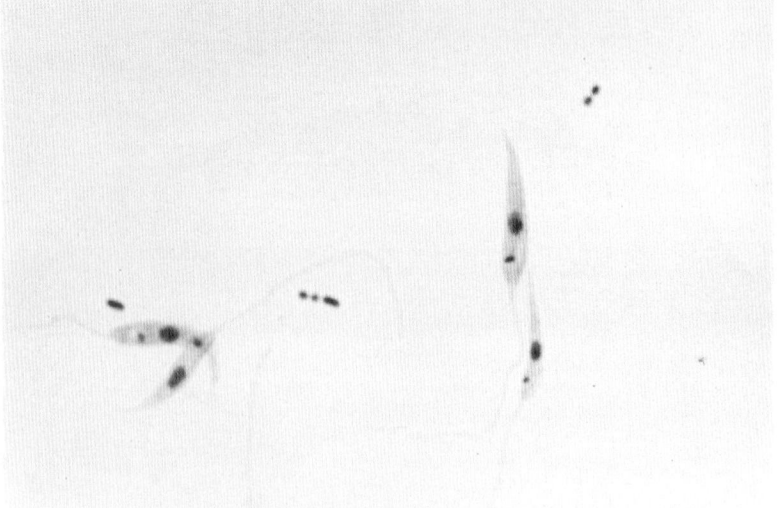

Fig. 18.252
Visceral leishmaniasis: promastigote forms of *Leishmania donovani*; note the anterior kinetoplast and flagellum (the latter is not seen in human infection) (Giemsa stain). By courtesy of H.P. Lambert, MD, and the London School of Hygiene and Tropical Medicine, London, UK.

Amebiasis cutis

Clinical features

Entamoeba histolytica can cause cutaneous lesions, although this is rare.[1–3] Although some authors include infections by free-living amebae (i.e., *Acanthamoeba* spp. and *Balamuthia mandrillaris*) under the umbrella of cutaneous amebiasis, these latter infections are discussed separately in this chapter; use of the term amebiasis cutis will thus be restricted to *E. histolytica* infection in this section.

Amebiasis cutis is most commonly seen after surgical treatment of intestinal or hepatic amebiasis, but may also occur by direct extension perianally from the bowel or from hepatic involvement, and by direct inoculation of the skin from other infected lesions. A number of cases have been recorded in HIV-infected patients, who may have an increased mortality due to other co-infections.[1,3–5] The infection may be sexually transmitted. Penile amebiasis, for example, can follow anal intercourse.[6,7] Cutaneous lesions have been recorded on the trunk, abdominal wall, buttocks, genitalia, and perineum, and on the legs.[1,4,6–11] In addition to ulcers, cutaneous amebiasis may present with fistulae, fissures, abscesses, and polypoid or warty lesions.[1] Subcutaneous swellings called amebomas have also been described.[12] Primary disease is uncommon; the majority of patients develop contiguous skin lesions in the presence of underlying visceral infection.[1,3,5,13] Although the condition is encountered mainly in adults, amebiasis cutis may sometimes occur in children.[2,3,9,14,15] A male preponderance of almost 2:1 was observed in a Mexican series of 26 cases.[3]

The lesions have a central necrotic zone with a purulent exudate, gray slough, an undermined margin, and an erythematous halo. The ulcers are irregular but sharply defined. They spread and do not heal spontaneously. They are extremely painful and may be destructive. Occasionally, the lesions resemble ulcerating tumors and are associated with surrounding verrucous lesions.[1] There is a unique report of infection of an epidermal cyst by *E. histolytica*, in the absence of concomitant intestinal disease.[16]

Histologic features

The trophozoites of *E. histolytica* are found among the purulent exudate of the ulcer and are seen more clearly with PAS staining (*Fig. 18.253*). They are 12–20 μm in diameter and are distinguished by their tendency to phagocytose red cells; the presence of these hematophagous amebic trophozoites is diagnostic, and is regarded as an unequivocal sign of their pathogenicity. Lesions may be superficial or deep, with the latter involving the subcutis. Necrosis is common and may be liquefactive, coagulative, or suppurative.[1–3] Trophozoites and cysts are usually found in the patient's

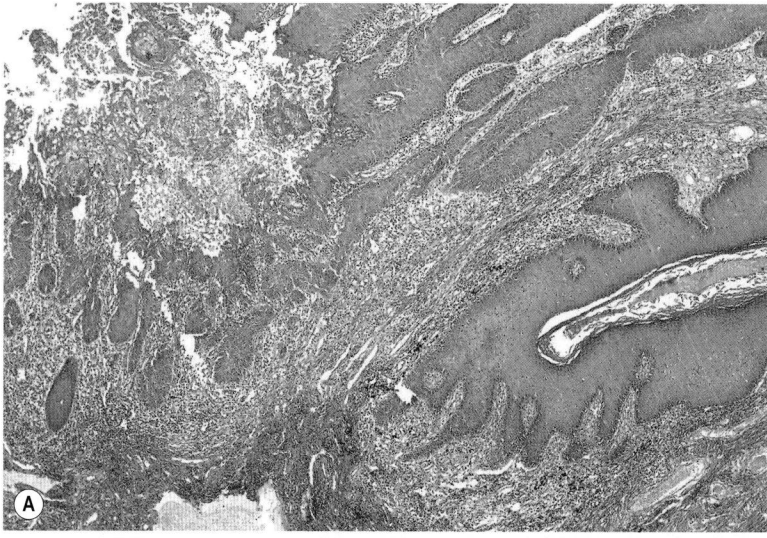

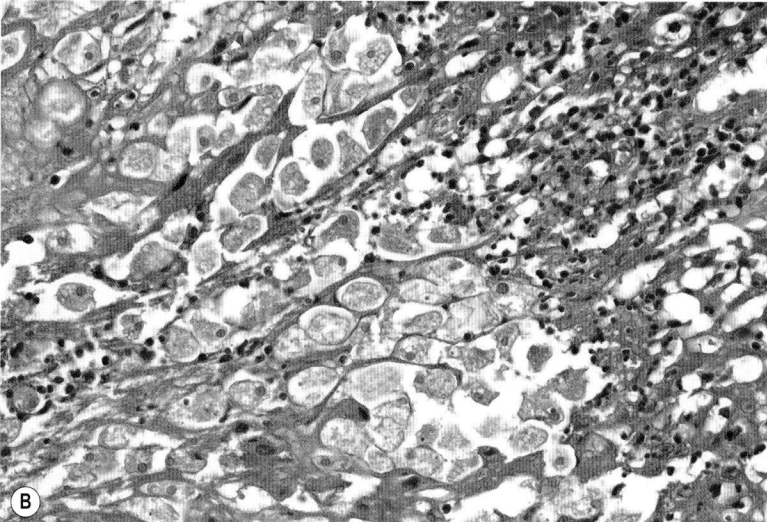

Fig. 18.253
Amebiasis cutis: (**A**) this biopsy is from a woman with vulval ulceration due to direct spread from the anus; the epithelium is hyperplastic and the lamina propria is chronically inflamed. (**B**) There are numerous trophozoites present; note the ingested red cells.

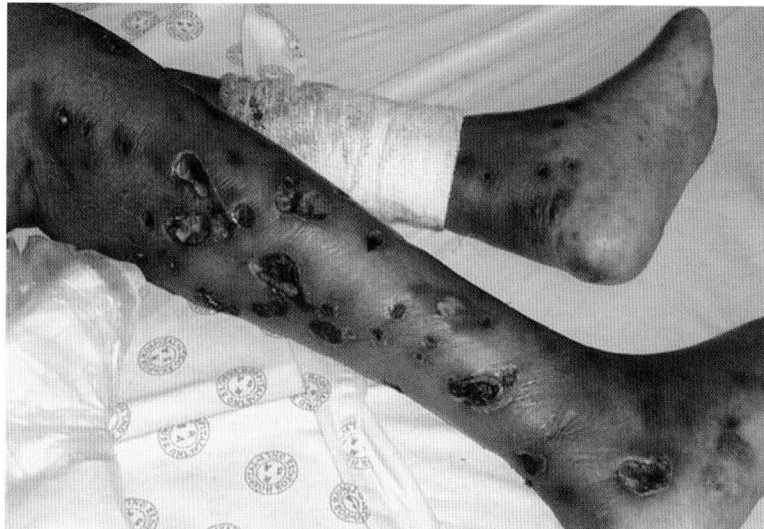

Fig. 18.254
Acanthamebiasis: there are widespread ulcers in this HIV-positive patient. There was underlying vasculitis. Courtesy of N.-N. Moti-Joosub, MD, Division of Dermatology, University of the Witwatersrand, Johannesburg, South Africa.

feces. The organisms are surrounded by neutrophils, with some lymphocytes and plasma cells. The adjacent epidermis appears acanthotic and this may be marked or pseudoepitheliomatous in verrucous forms. Spongiosis may be conspicuous in superficial lesions.[1]

Differential diagnosis

E. histolytica infection is distinguished from infection with free-living amebae (*Acanthamoeba* spp. and *B. mandrillaris*) by the presence of erythrophagocytosis in the former condition. The diagnosis may nevertheless be confirmed with the aid of newer molecular techniques.[7]

Infections caused by free-living amebae

Clinical features

Four free-living amebae are responsible for human disease, namely, *Naegleria fowleri* (the cause of primary amebic meningoencephalitis), *Acanthamoeba* spp. (which cause granulomatous amebic encephalitis), *Balamuthia mandillaris* (another cause of granulomatous amebic encephalitis), and, more recently, *Sappinia diploidea*, an exceptionally rare cause of encephalitis.[1–4] Of these, only *Acanthamoeba* spp. and *B. mandillaris* are potentially associated with cutaneous lesions. These latter two free-living amebae are seldom implicated in human disease with the possible exception of *Acanthamoeba* contact lens-associated keratitis.[1,3,4] However, in recent years

acanthamebiasis and balamuthiasis have received increasing recognition as opportunistic pathogens in immunocompromised patients, especially debilitated, malnourished hosts and those with HIV/AIDS.[1–14] *Acanthamoeba* spp. appears to be more important in immunosuppressed organ transplant recipients and those with GVHD.[15–19] Transmission of *B. mandrillaris* via organ transplantation has been reported.[20] Infection with *B. mandrillaris* (formerly referred to as leptomyxid ameba) may nevertheless occur in immunocompetent individuals, including children.[1–3,21,22]

Acanthamebiasis is a condition reported almost exclusively from the United States, although cases have occurred in Korea and South Africa (personal observation).[2,3,23] Although the majority of *B. mandrillaris* infections reported in the past were from the United States, balamuthiasis is an emerging infectious disease in parts of South America, especially in Peru.[1–4,12,20,24] There have also been rare reports of the latter condition from Thailand, India, and Australia.[14,21,22,25–31]

Infection with *Acathamoeba* spp. or *B. mandrillaris* results in an often fatal progressive encephalitis, and associated cutaneous lesions are a frequent occurrence.[1–5,7,12] Visceral dissemination to organs such as the lungs, kidneys, and uterus may also occur.[1,17] Spread of *Acanthamoeba* spp. to the CNS and skin is usually from a primary source of infection in the lungs or paranasal sinuses.[2,6,23] Involvement of the skin may be the presenting manifestation of disseminated infection.[5] Isolated cutaneous disease with chronic, nonhealing ulcerated skin lesions may be the sole manifestation in patients with AIDS-associated acanthamebiasis (*Fig. 18.254*).[8] Acanthamebiasis of the skin presents as multiple deep dermal and subcutaneous nodules, usually on the extremities and face.[5,7,13,15,16,19] Necrotizing panniculitis may occur.[9] Pustular, ulcerating, purpuric, and sporotrichoid lesions have also been described.[6,7,32]

B. mandrillaris is present worldwide and is encountered in fresh water, soil, and dust. It is thought that the organism gains access to the CNS via hematogenous spread from a focus of primary infection in the upper or lower respiratory tract or the skin.[3,27] Transmission is probably through the inhalation of airborne cysts or contamination of a skin lesion.[25,27,28] Cutaneous involvement is usually in the form of multiple nodular or ulcerative lesions, similar to those encountered in cutaneous acanthamebiasis. One reported case developed an ulcerative mass 10 cm in diameter on the thigh.[26] A number of patients, however, have presented with a centrofacial or sometimes destructive nasal lesion, which preceded symptoms and signs of CNS involvement by several months.[22,27,29] In fact, the cutaneous signs may antedate the neurological signs by months.[33] Some cases have evolved following penetrating injury or a prior fracture.[21,29,34] *B. mandrillaris* infection of the CNS carries a mortality in excess of 98%.[11] There have, however, been rare reports of patient survival following successful treatment.[35]

Histologic features

Cutaneous infection with *Acanthamoeba* spp. results in severe suppurative inflammation in the dermis with extension into the subcutis, where necrotizing neutrophilic lobular panniculitis, tuberculoid granulomatous inflammation, and vasculitis may occur.[5,7,9,10,21] The epidermis is usually intact. Purpuric lesions are associated with leukocytoclastic vasculitis.[6] *B. mandrillaris* is associated with granulomatous and suppurative inflammation. This inflammation is frequently angiocentric, and direct invasion of vessel walls by trophozoites results in vasculitis and necrosis.[27] The trophozoites of both genera, which tend to concentrate near blood vessels, generally measure 20–30 μm in diameter, but may range from 15 to 50 μm.[2,4,9,23,27] Recognition of the trophozoites may be difficult in view of their macrophage-like appearance.[7,12] The trophozoites have abundant vacuolated cytoplasm and a nucleus containing a discrete nucleolus. PAS and methenamine silver stains highlight the amebic cyst walls. The cysts possess an outer wrinkled cyst wall (ectocyst) and a thin inner wall (endocyst) (*Fig. 18.255*).[2,4,12,27] The trophozoites and cysts of *Acanthamoeba* spp. are virtually indistinguishable from those of *B. mandrillaris* by routine light microscopy. Diagnosis is therefore confirmed by culture, immunofluorescence studies, immunohistochemistry, or PCR.[4,12,13,28,36]

Differential diagnosis

Acanthamebiasis and balamuthiasis are distinguished from cutaneous infection with *E. histolytica* by the presence of erythrophagocytosis in the latter

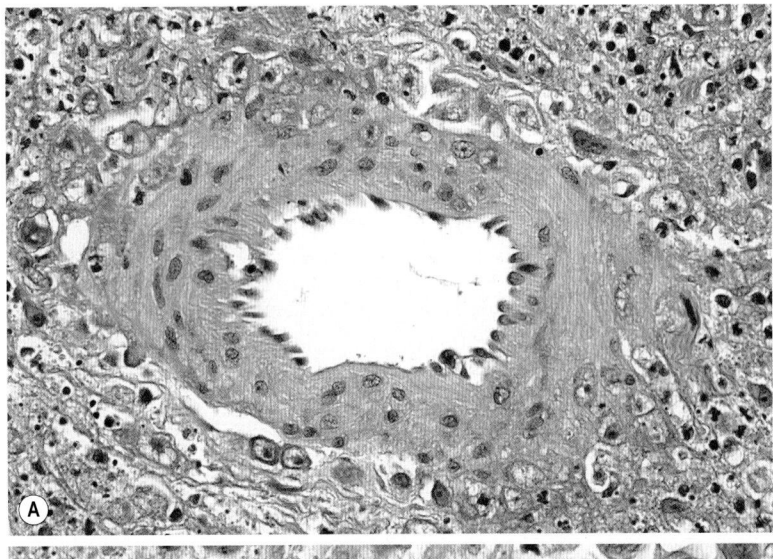

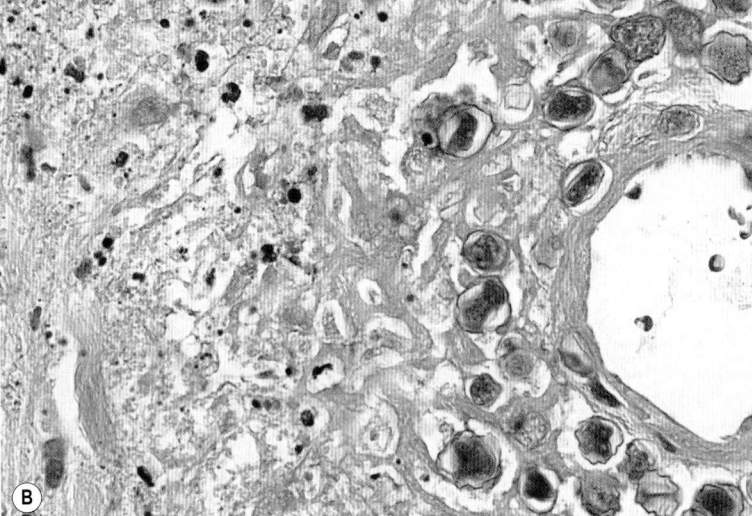

Fig. 18.255
(**A**, **B**) Acanthamebiasis: trophozoites and cysts are present. The wall of the latter is characteristically double layered (**B**).

condition. *N. fowleri* does not form cysts, and infection is not associated with skin involvement.

Toxoplasmosis

Clinical features

Toxoplasmosis is the result of infection with *Toxoplasma gondii*, an obligate intracellular parasite.[1] Infection in humans, who serve as the intermediate host, usually occurs following ingestion of *T. gondii* oocysts that are present in the feces of infected cats, or via consumption of undercooked, contaminated meat containing tissue cysts. The oocysts and tissue cysts then transform into tachyzoites, which in turn develop into bradyzoites after localization in brain or muscle tissue. These slowly replicating forms are contained within pseudocysts in the involved tissues.[1,2]

The zoonosis exists in a number of clinical forms: as an acute infection in immunocompetent individuals, the vast majority of whom are asymptomatic; congenital toxoplasmosis due to transplacental spread of a maternal infection, forming part of the TORCH group of infections; and acute disease in immunocompromised hosts, which is either acquired or the result of reactivation of latent infection.[1,3] Although fever, lymphadenopathy, chorioretinitis, and cerebral involvement are well-recognized manifestations of symptomatic toxoplasmosis in general, presentation with skin lesions is uncommon. Cutaneous involvement is encountered more frequently in immunocompromised patients with disseminated infection, such as those with HIV/AIDS or in immunosuppressed recipients of bone marrow, hematopoietic, or solid organ transplants.[1,4–15] Toxoplasmosis-associated hemophagocytic syndrome has been reported in a renal allograft recipient.[16] The disease has also occurred following chemotherapy for lymphoma.[11]

Skin manifestations of the disease are very rare but may be encountered in cases of acquired or congenital toxoplasmosis.[17] Potential dermatological manifestations include a maculopapular skin rash, widespread purpuric papules and nodules, thrombocytopenic purpura, lichenoid and erythema multiforme-like eruptions, ulcerative and vegetating lesions, panniculitis, and erythroderma.[8,9,11–13,18–22] A case with vesicular lesions resembling varicella has also been reported.[14]

Histologic features

A majority of reported cases have shown a superficial and deep perivascular inflammatory cell infiltrate composed of lymphocytes and histiocytes.[4,18,20] Small 'cysts' containing tiny bradyzoites may be encountered in the dermis, including vascular endothelial cells, follicular epithelium, and the sweat glands and their ducts (*Fig. 18.256*).[8] Rarely, similar structures are observed in the epidermis.[9,13] The organisms may be highlighted by staining tissue sections with the May-Grünwald-Giemsa method.[18] Free parasites are sometimes haphazardly distributed in the dermis, and there may be dermal edema, erythrocytic extravasation, necrobiotic collagen bundle, and karyorrhectic debris.[8] Biopsies from severely immunocompromised patients may reveal little by way of a host response.[8] Interface dermatitis and panniculitis have been described.[10,11,15] One reported case presenting with erythroderma showed features of exfoliative dermatitis, with no discernible organisms.[21] Vegetating lesions are characterized by pseudoepitheliomatous hyperplasia, sometimes accompanied by necrosis.[18] Nodular lesions harbor macrophages whose cytoplasm contains bradyzoites.[12] The diagnosis may be confirmed by ultrastructural examination, immunohistochemistry, or PCR.[8,9,11,13,14]

Differential diagnosis

Cutaneous toxoplasmosis should be distinguished from histoplasmosis and leishmaniasis. *Toxoplasma* bradyzoites may potentially be mistaken for the intracellular yeast forms and amastigotes usually contained within macrophages in the aforementioned conditions, respectively. *Leishmania* organisms have a discernible kinetoplast. Rare cases of cutaneous toxoplasmosis following hematopoietic stem cell transplantation may mimic interface dermatitis, resulting in confusion with an adverse drug reaction or graft-versus-host disease if the encysted bradyzoites are overlooked.[10,15]

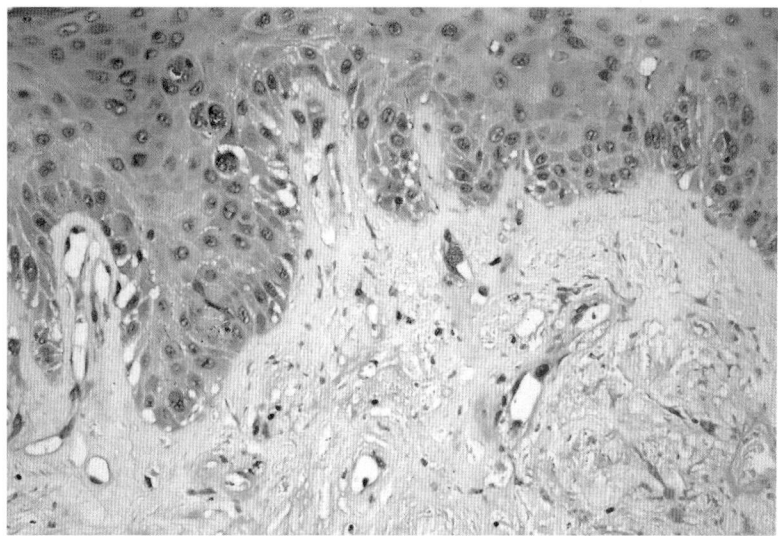

Fig. 18.256
Toxoplasmosis: a cyst containing numerous bradyzoites is present within a superficial blood vessel. By courtesy of H. Diwan, MD, Baylor College of Medicine, Houston, Texas, USA.

ALGAL INFECTIONS

Protothecosis

Clinical features

Protothecosis is a rare condition, representing infection by the achloric (achlorophyllic) alga *Prototheca*, usually *P. wickerhamii*.[1-5] Fewer than 200 cases have been reported.[6-9] Several infections with *P. zopfii* have also been recorded.[1,5,10-12] The alga is assumed to be inoculated into the skin by minor trauma, presumably from contaminated water or soil. *Prototheca* are ubiquitous in nature, being found in the mucus flux of trees, water stabilization ponds, acid rivers and lakes, and a variety of animals including cows, dogs, cats, and deer.[13-15] The disease has been reported worldwide.[16] One recorded case occurred after an arthropod bite.[14]

Diseases caused by *Prototheca* include isolated cutaneous lesions, olecranon bursitis, and disseminated infection.[1] There have been isolated reports of onychoprototothecosis and infection following corneal grafting.[17,18] Prototothecosis (especially in its disseminated form) occurs in iatrogenically immunosuppressed solid organ and hematopoietic stem cell transplant recipients, and in patients with diabetes mellitus or leukemia.[1,6,8,10,12,14,15,19-23] It may also occur in those with AIDS.[24-27] Some infections have been linked to corticosteroid usage.[9,28] Prototothecosis has also been recorded in a child with combined immunodeficiency.[29] The condition manifests in the skin as a papular or eczematoid dermatitis, usually over an extremity.[6,16,30] The dermatitis form is often extensive and scaly, hypertrophic, and resistant to therapy. Vesicular, herpetiform, pustular, plaquiform, ulcerative, granulomatous, and verrucous variants have been described (*Fig. 18.257*).[1,4,6,15,28,31-34] Lesions may also resemble pyoderma gangrenosum, and abscess formation is sometimes encountered.[6,15] Disseminated cutaneous lesions have been rarely reported.[14,16,33,35] In immunocompetent patients, the infection is most often localized to the olecranon bursa following trauma.[1,16] Localized tenosynovial involvement of the finger has been reported, one in an HIV-positive patient.[7,24]

Histologic features

The localized lesions consist of necrotic centers surrounded by granulation and fibrous tissue with a few multinucleate giant cells. The algae are found in the necrotic centers.

In the dermatitis lesions, the epidermis is parakeratotic, acanthotic, and papillomatous, and there is a mixed infiltrate in the upper dermis, including occasional multinucleate giant cells (*Fig. 18.258*). Organisms (3–15 μm in

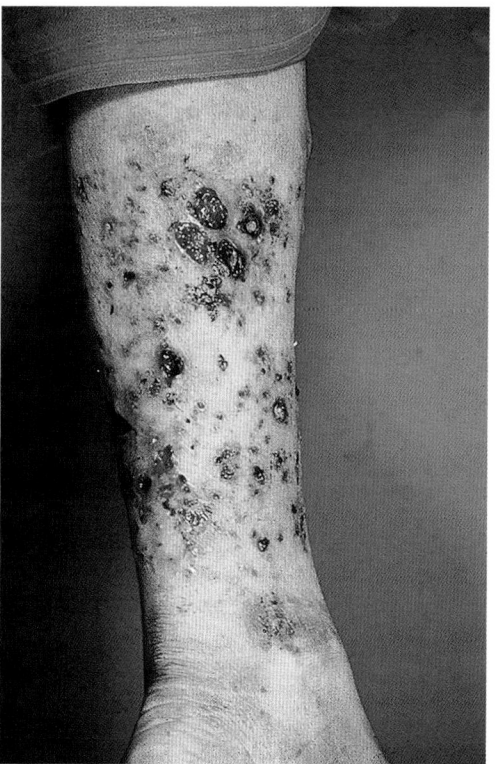

Fig. 18.257
Prototothecosis: numerous crusted and ulcerative lesions are present. By courtesy of the Institute of Dermatology, London, UK.

diameter) can be found at all levels of the epidermis and in the superficial dermis (*Figs 18.259* and *18.260*).[3,15,16] Involvement of the deeper dermis and even the subcutis can occur. There is a polymorphous inflammatory infiltrate comprising lymphocytes, plasma cells, macrophages, histiocytic giant cells, eosinophils, and neutrophils. A prominent dermal lymphoid infiltrate may be encountered. Some cases, however, are associated with little or no inflammation.[15] Infection can also involve the regional lymph nodes. Only basophilic spherical bodies are seen with H&E staining, while a silver stain or a PAS reaction reveals spore-like bodies in the epidermis and among the

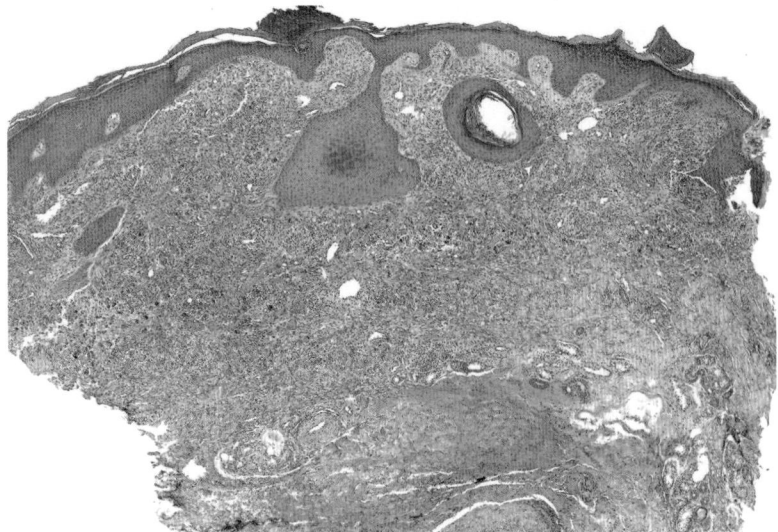

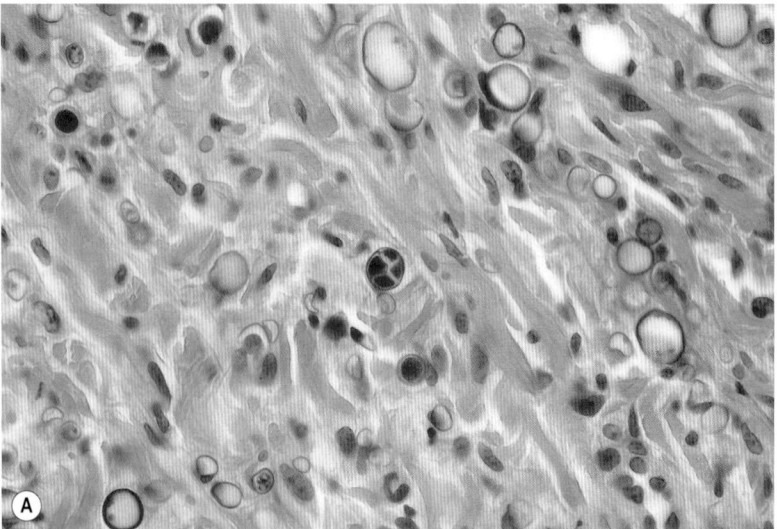

Fig. 18.258
Protothecosis: note the crusting, marked acanthosis, and heavy dermal infiltrate. By courtesy of I. Van den Berghe, AZ, Sint-Jan AV Hospital, Bruges, Belgium.

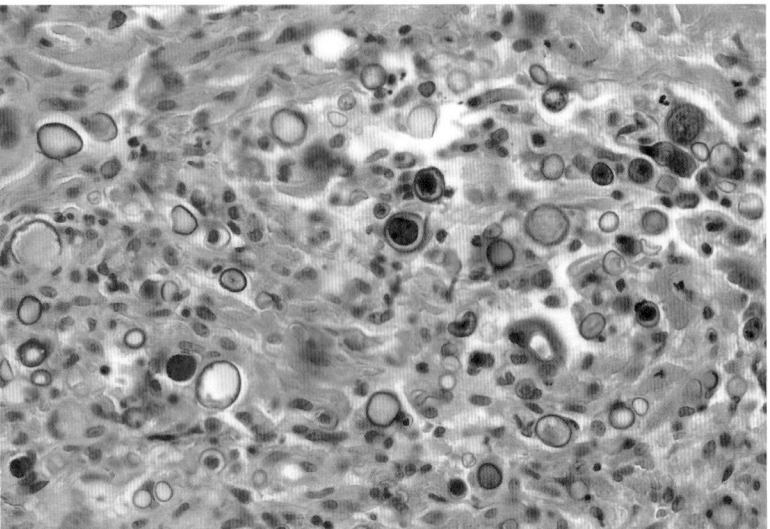

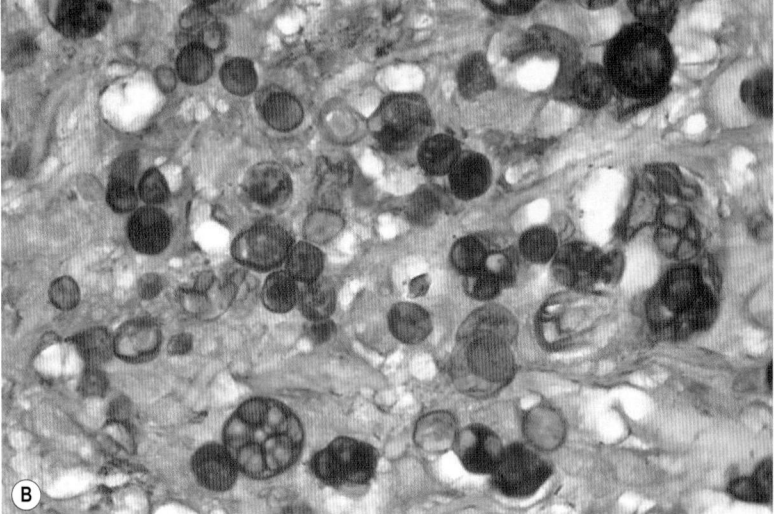

Fig. 18.260
(**A**, **B**) Protothecosis: (**A**) the internal septation is characteristic; (**B**) the organisms have thick cell walls and are PAS positive. (**A**) By courtesy of I. Van den Berghe, AZ, Sint-Jan AV Hospital, Bruges, Belgium; (**B**) By courtesy of C. Thatcher, MD, Gritzman & Thatcher Inc. Anatomical Pathologists, Johannesburg, South Africa.

Fig. 18.259
Protothecosis: numerous organisms are present in the dermis. By courtesy of I. Van den Berghe, AZ, Sint-Jan AV Hospital, Bruges, Belgium.

inflammatory infiltrate. Sporangia with symmetrically arranged endospores is characteristic; these have been described as morula-like or daisy-like; these can measure up to 30 μm in diameter.[6,15,24,36] Identification of the organism depends on culture characteristics. Diagnosis may also be confirmed by direct immunofluorescence or immunohistochemistry.[24,37]

Bursal lesions show stellate caseating necrosis surrounded by a palisade of epithelioid cells, Langhans giant cells, plasma cells, and lymphocytes.[16,24] The organisms are present within the necrotic centers. Sinus tracts may be evident. There is associated fibrosis.

Differential diagnosis

Prototheca are distinguished from green algae (*Chlorella*) by the absence of chloroplasts and from *Coccidiodes immitis* by its smaller size.[2,15,38]

FUNGAL INFECTIONS

Fungal infections include:
- superficial variants involving skin, hair, nails, and mucous membranes, for example, ringworm (dermatophytosis), and the dermatomycoses (tinea versicolor and candidiasis),
- subcutaneous lesions,
- disseminated infection.[1,2]

Ringworm fungi include three species: *Microsporum*, *Trichophyton*, and *Epidermophyton*.[3,4] *Epidermophyton* invades epidermal keratin while *Microsporum* and *Trichophyton* also affect the hair. Cutaneous ringworm on nonhairy skin presents as slowly enlarging, scaly, erythematous, annular lesions with central clearing (*Fig. 18.261*).

Dermatophytes can infect the keratin of the stratum corneum, hair, or nail, without extending into deeper parts of the skin. They may also be associated with intradermal spread (Majocchi granuloma). Causative organisms may be anthropophilic, zoophilic, or geophilic. With few exceptions, identification of pathogenic fungi is better served by culture rather than by histologic scrutiny.[5–7] Dermatophytes use the soluble nonkeratin parts for nutrition and rely on the keratin for protection from serum and the host response.[8,9] The keratin is penetrated by means of putative keratinases. Other virulence factors include elastase and proteinases.[9,10] *T. rubrum* produces mannan, which suppresses or diminishes the host immune response, presumably by inhibiting critical steps in antigen presentation or

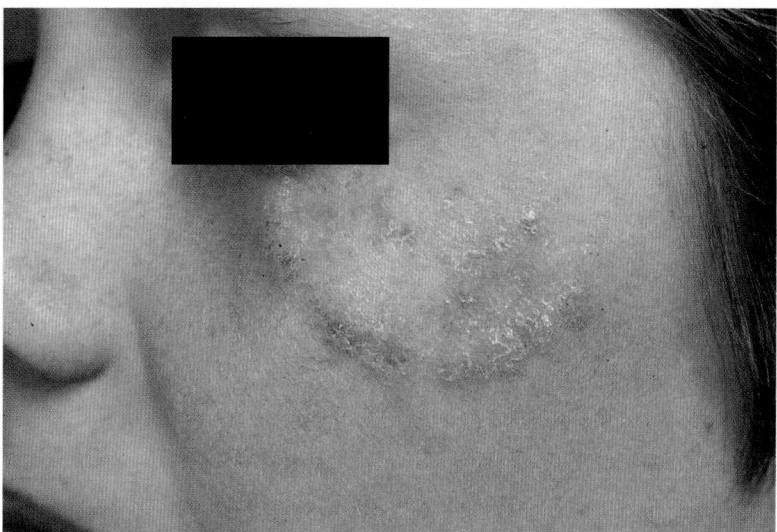

Fig. 18.261
Tinea corporis: note the annular configuration and erythematous margin. From the collection of the late N.P. Smith, MD, the Institute of Dermatology, London, UK.

processing.[9,11] The epidemiology and pathogenesis of dermatophytosis is complex and beyond the remit of this text. For suitable review articles, the reader is referred to references 1, 3, 4, and 10.

Tinea capitis

Dermatophyte infections of the scalp are characterized by involvement of the hair shaft by pathogenic fungi. The pattern of hair invasion, related to the type of dermatophyte, determines the degree and site of hair damage and the clinical picture. Patients therefore present with variable features including hair loss with scaling, follicular inflammation, pustulation, and kerion formation, often in association with drainage lymphadenopathy. A carrier state is recognized. Infection depends on contact with spores and follicular trauma. Tinea capitis (scalp ringworm) frequently presents as small epidemics (e.g., in schools). Disease may develop as a consequence of sharing combs or hairbrushes. Tinea capitis is the most common dermatophytosis of childhood. The disease may also occur in adults, the elderly, and even infants. The past two decades have seen a rise in its prevalence and a change in the pattern of etiological agents, both in Europe and the United States.

Infections caused by *Microsporum canis* and *Microsporum audouinii*

Clinical features

M. canis and *M. audouinii* grow on the outside of the hair shaft, an ectothrix type of hair involvement.[1–3] The lesions present as areas of alopecia, with numerous broken-off, dull hairs (*Fig. 18.262*). Some scaling is present, but overt inflammation is not marked. The infected areas are recognized by fluorescence under Wood lamp (*Fig. 18.263*). The process commonly affects children, boys much more often than girls. *M. ferrugineum* may also cause this picture.

M. canis and *M. audouinii* were once the most common causes of tinea capitis in North America and Western Europe.[3,4] *M. canis*, a zoophilic dermatophyte, is the organism most frequently implicated in cases of tinea capitis in Europe. Urban areas of Europe (and France in particular) have shown a shift toward infection with *M. audouinii*, an anthropophilic dermatophyte.[5,6]

Histologic features

The fungal arthrospores coat the outside of the hair shaft and the hyphae extend into the hair shaft down to the level of the mid follicle. The epidermis shows some acanthosis and patchy parakeratosis, and there is usually a

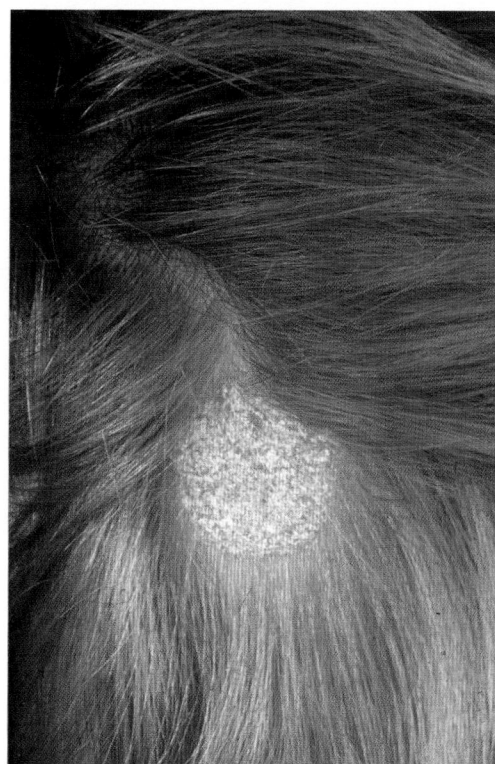

Fig. 18.262
Tinea capitis: there is marked hair loss. In this example scaling and crusting are pronounced. From the collection of the late N.P. Smith, MD, the Institute of Dermatology, London, UK.

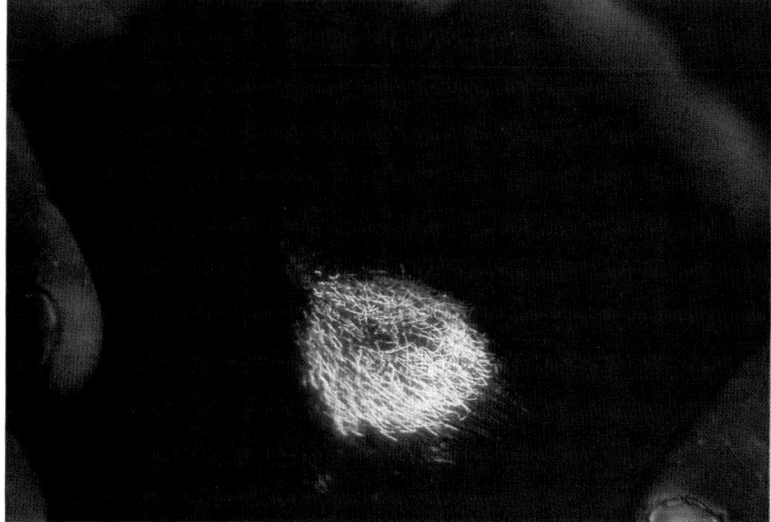

Fig. 18.263
Tinea capitis: note the characteristic fluorescence under Wood light. By courtesy of M.M. Black, MD, Institute of Dermatology, London, UK.

mixed inflammatory infiltrate in the superficial dermis, more marked with *M. canis*.

Kerion

Clinical features

Kerion (kerion celsi) is a severe, boggy inflammatory form of tinea, most often caused by *Trichophyton interdigitale* (formerly *T. mentagrophytes*).[1–4] Additional agents of kerion are *Microsporum* species (e.g., *M. canis*) and other *Trichophyton* species, including, *T. violaceum*, *T. verrucosum*, and *T. tonsurans*.[3–9] In recent years, zoophilic fungi such as *Trichophyton* sp. of *Arthroderma benhamiae* have also been implicated.[4]

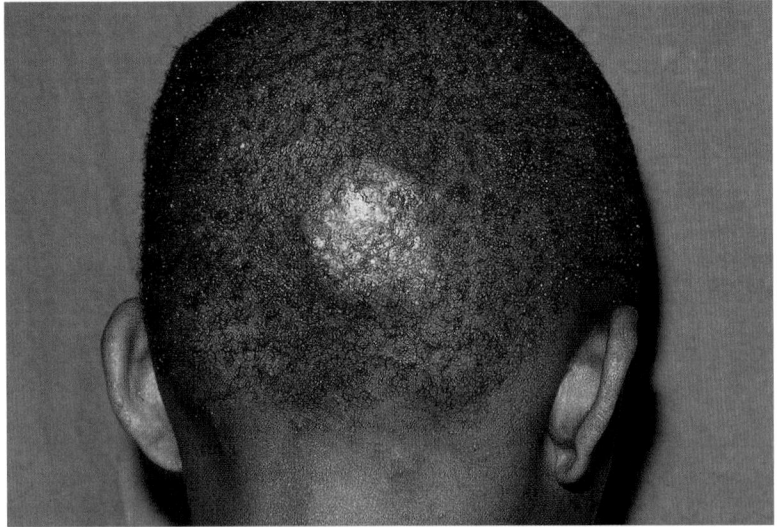

Fig. 18.264
Kerion: in addition to alopecia there is marked erythema and matting of hairs due to purulent exudate. By courtesy of R.A. Marsden, MD, St George's Hospital, London, UK.

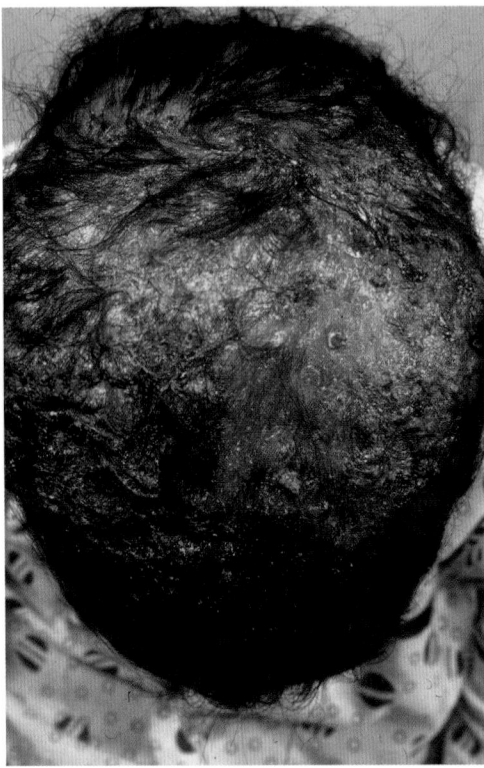

Fig. 18.265
Kerion: there is marked alopecia and crusting. From the collection of the late N.P. Smith, MD, the Institute of Dermatology, London, UK.

Children are more commonly affected. Kerion is seen as an area of inflamed alopecia in which the broken-off hairs are loose in their follicles and are associated with suppuration (*Figs 18.264* and *18.265*). This may be severe enough to discharge via sinuses, with the formation of fibrinopurulent crusts around adjacent hairs. Secondary bacterial infection (e.g., with *S. aureus*) may play a part.[3] Fluorescence is not a feature. The condition may be confused clinically with folliculitis decalvans or dissecting cellulitis of the scalp.[3,9,10] Involvement of the beard area (tinea barbae, tinea sycosis), which occurs most often in farm workers, invariably affects adult males.[11,12] The lesions appear as erythematous areas of pustular folliculitis in the beard area and may present as a kerion (*Fig. 18.266*).

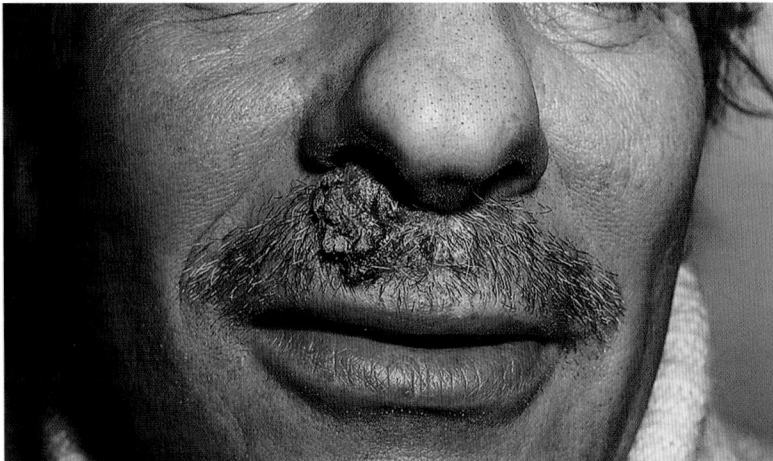

Fig. 18.266
Kerion: in males, dermatophyte infection of the beard area may also present as a kerion. By courtesy of R.A. Marsden, MD, St George's Hospital, London, UK.

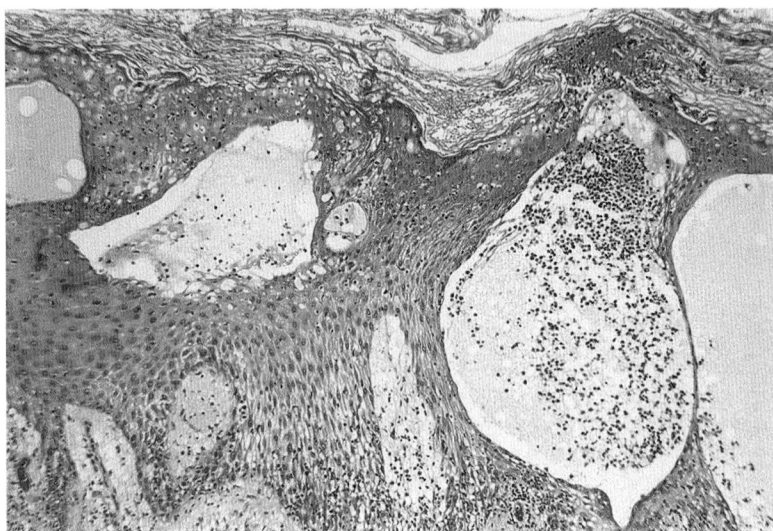

Fig. 18.267
Kerion: there is hyperkeratosis, acanthosis, epidermal edema with acute inflammation, and abscess formation.

Histologic features

Trichophyton is a large-spored fungus with an ectothrix pattern of hair involvement. There is much associated pus with abscess formation. The epidermis is acanthotic and spongiotic, with parakeratosis and intraepidermal collections of neutrophils (*Figs 18.267* and *18.268*).

Endothrix infections

Clinical features

These infections, most often with *Trichophyton tonsurans* and *T. violaceum*, usually cause patchy alopecia with little inflammation. *T. tonsurans* is now the most common cause of scalp ringworm in the United States.[1–4] This organism was found to be responsible for around 22% of cases of tinea capitis in a study from Nigeria.[5] *T. violaceum* is the most common cause of tinea capitis in South Africa.[6] The hair break is at the ostium of the follicle so that broken hairs are seen as dots rather than stumps. The intervening skin usually shows only slight scaling, but occasionally pustules and kerion can develop.[7] Drainage lymphadenopathy may be evident. The hairs do not fluoresce with a Wood lamp.

Histologic features

The hyphae of *T. tonsurans* and *T. violaceum* extend within the hair shaft and produce spores. The epidermis is patchily parakeratotic, and there are

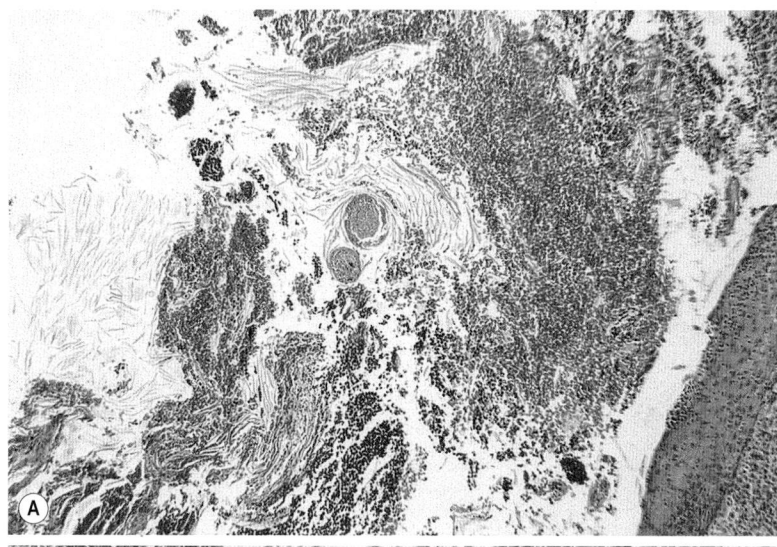

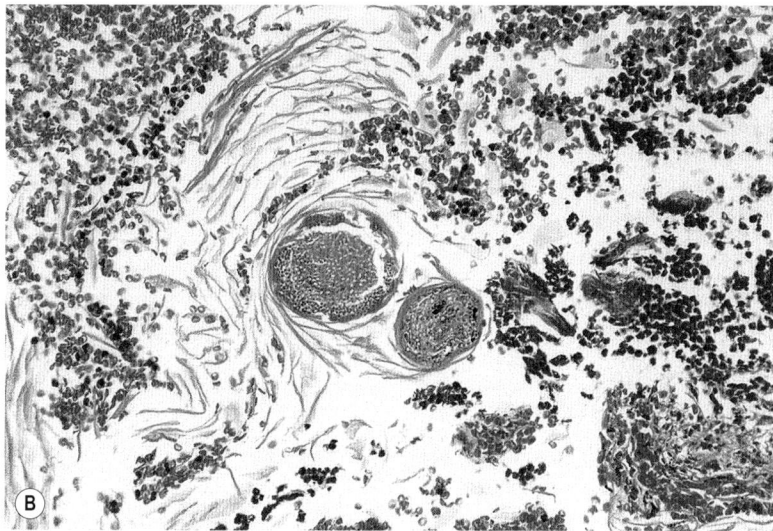

Fig. 18.268
Kerion: (**A**) crust scrapings from a patient with a typical scalp lesion. In addition to blood, keratinous debris and numerous neutrophils, two hair shafts are present in the center of the field. (**B**) High-power view showing numerous fungal spores coating the outside of the shaft.

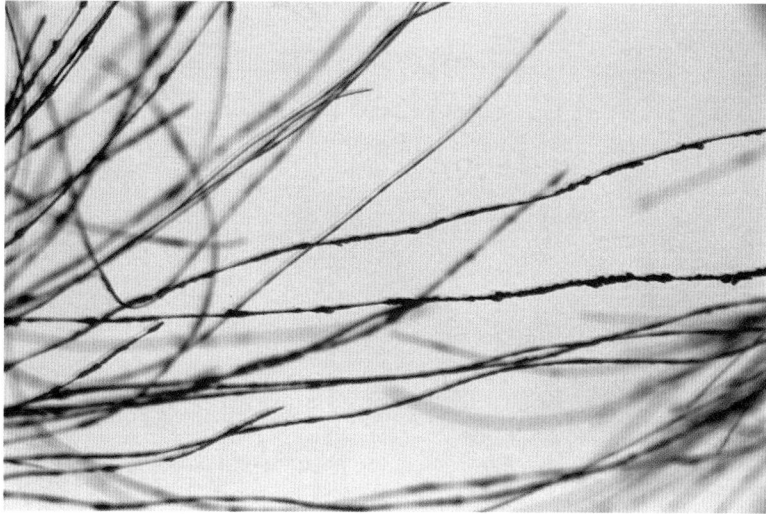

Fig. 18.269
Favus: scarring alopecia due to infection by *Trichophyton schoenleinii*. By courtesy of R.A. Marsden, MD, St George's Hospital, London, UK.

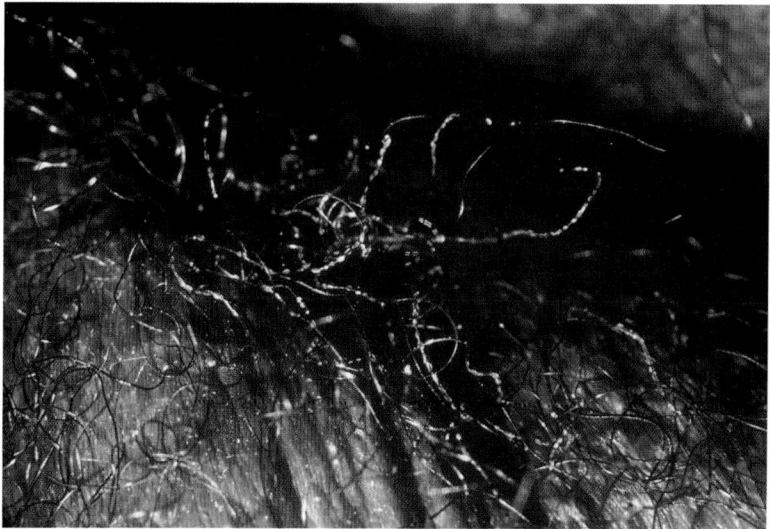

Fig. 18.270
Black piedra: there are numerous tiny black nodules attached to hair shafts. By courtesy of the late C. Kalter, MD, Walter Reed Medical Center, Washington, USA.

remnants of infected hair shafts in the dilated keratin-plugged ostia. Perifollicular inflammation is variable in intensity, but often includes histiocytes and multinucleate cells as well as lymphocytes and plasma cells.

Favus

Clinical features

This uncommon pattern of tinea capitis is seen in the Middle East, South Africa, and Greenland, and sporadically elsewhere. It is characterized by cup-shaped crusts, or scutula, around the ostia of hair follicles.[1-5] The hair penetrates the crust and is not necessarily broken off or shortened. The crusts may become confluent. Permanent and scarring alopecia occurs (*Fig. 18.269*). Removal of the scutula leaves an erythematous oozing base. The hairs show a gray-green fluorescence under Wood lamp.

Histologic features

Favus is caused by *Trichophyton schoenleinii*, which invades the hair and produces air spaces, but arthrospores are not seen.[1] Relatively little damage occurs to the hair shafts. Fungal hyphae and spores are seen in the scutula, which rests on the acanthotic stratum spinosum around the follicular ostia. The underlying dermis shows a mixed inflammatory infiltrate (including

giant cells) and marked fibrosis, which sometimes resembles folliculitis keloidalis.

Black piedra

Clinical features

Black piedra (Spanish *piedra*, stone) is caused by an ascomycete, *Piedraia hortae*, and involves almost exclusively the scalp.[1-3] It is characterized by black nodules firmly attached to the hair shafts (*Fig. 18.270*). The disease mainly occurs in the tropics. Patients of all ages are affected but there is predilection for adults. There is a single case report of black piedra due to infection with *Trichosporon asahii*.[4]

Histologic features

Microscopic examination reveals numerous asci and ascospores within the black nodules (*Fig. 18.271*). Damage of the hair at the level of the cuticle and cortex is secondary to the keratolytic activity of the organism.[3]

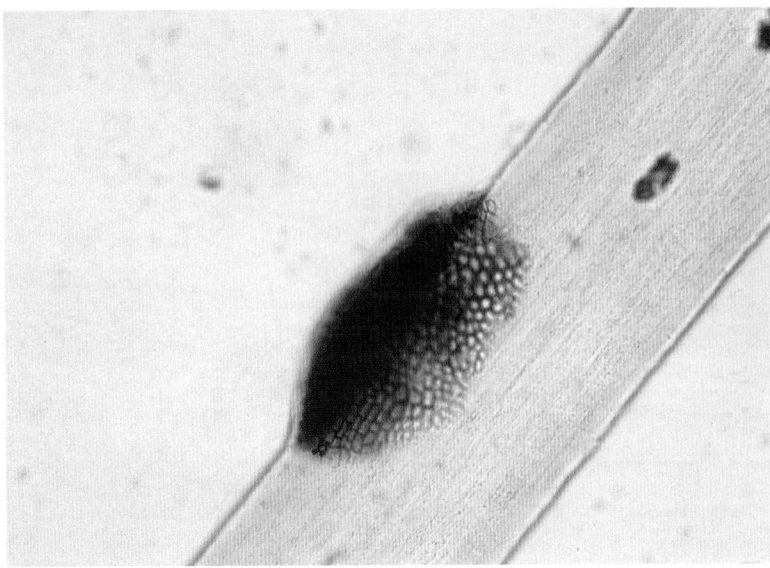

Fig. 18.271
Black piedra: close-up view of a brown nodule firmly attached to the hair shaft. By courtesy of the late C. Kalter, MD, Walter Reed Medical Center, Washington, USA.

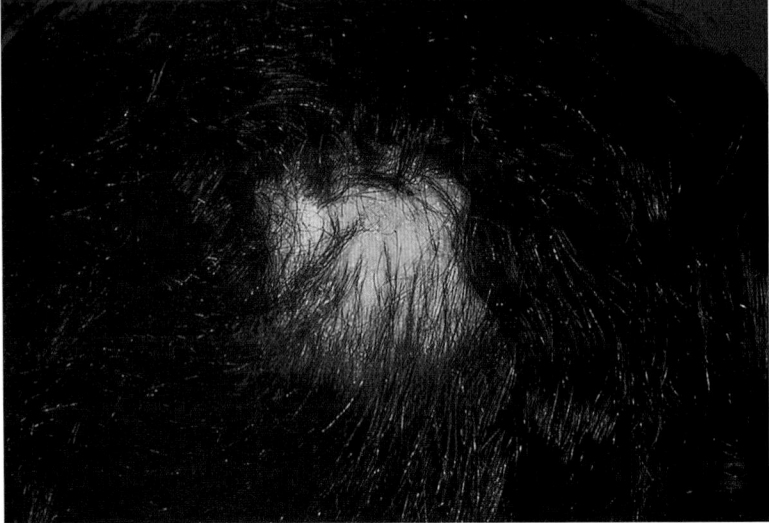

Fig. 18.272
White piedra: numerous tiny white nodules are attached to hair shafts. By courtesy of the Institute of Dermatology, London, UK.

White piedra

Clinical features

White piedra (Spanish *piedra*, stone) – or trichomycosis – is a trichomycosis formerly ascribed to the saprophyte fungus *Trichosporon beigelii*.[1] The causative agent was later identified as *T. inkin*, a basidiomycetous yeast.[2,3] Earlier literature suggested that the disease was caused by a synergistic infection of the fungus and *Corynebacteria*.[4,5] The condition has a worldwide distribution but is rare in cold climates.[6,7] It may affect any hair-bearing areas including the scalp, eyebrows, eyelashes, beard area, axillae, and genital skin (*Fig. 18.272*).[8] Men are more commonly affected than women, and there is a higher incidence in black patients.[1] White piedra may also occur in children.[9] Nail involvement is exceptional.[10] Typically, white nodules are seen firmly attached to the hair shaft.[11] The condition is asymptomatic, but hairs may break as a result of invasion of the cuticle and cortex by the fungus.

The organism can occasionally cause a disseminated disease in neutropenic immunocompromised patients and in HIV infection.[12–15] In these patients, cutaneous lesions consist of purpuric papules and nodules with

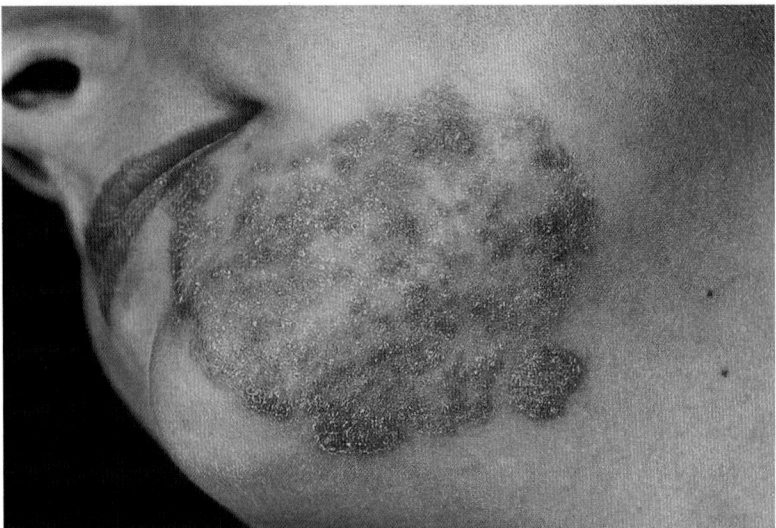

Fig. 18.273
Tinea corporis: note the sharply defined, elevated scaly border. By courtesy of R.A. Marsden, MD, St George's Hospital, London, UK.

necrosis.[14] Co-infection with *Histoplasma capsulatum* has been reported in this clinical context.[15]

Histologic features

Microscopic examination of the white nodules under potassium hydroxide (KOH) shows the presence of numerous hyphae and arthrospores.

Tinea corporis

Clinical features

This fungal infection of nonhairy skin is seen as expanding erythematous scaly areas with well-defined, elevated margins (*Figs 18.273–18.276*).[1–3] The center may return to normal as the lesion expands. Less common manifestations include vesicles, bullae, pustules, and even lesions resembling subacute cutaneous lupus erythematosus.[4,5] The condition commonly affects children. Spread is by contact with infected lesions. *Trichophyton rubrum* is the most frequent cause.[6] Infection may be acquired from household pets (e.g., *Microsporum canis*).[7,8]

Tinea gladiatorum (tinea corporis gladiatorum) is a clinical variant of tinea corporis that occurs among competitive wrestlers. Most outbreaks are caused by *T. tonsurans* and transmission is via person-to-person contact.[1,9,10]

Histologic features

The expanding edge of the lesion is characterized by parakeratosis and acanthosis, with some neutrophils among the parakeratotic crust. The causative organisms are very varied and are usually the ones most prevalent in the geographic area. The presence of fungal hyphae in the keratin is easily demonstrated by the PAS reaction. Underlying inflammation is usually mild, but is more severe if there is follicular involvement.

Lesions, which may be single or multiple, present on exposed skin. In cases where inflammation is marked, pustulation may be a feature. Inappropriate treatment with local steroids may modify the clinical appearance and cause further diagnostic confusion (tinea incognito) (*Fig. 18.277*).

Tinea pedis and tinea cruris

Clinical features
Tinea pedis

Tinea pedis is usually centered on the interdigital clefts and is the most frequent form of dermatophyte infection, commonly referred to as 'athlete's foot' (*Fig. 18.278*). Spread of infection is linked to the shared use of locker

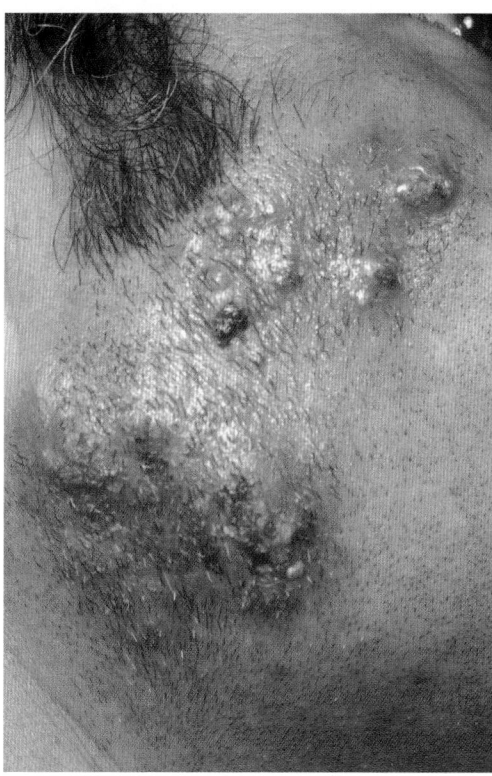

Fig. 18.274
Tinea corporis: in this example there is gross pustulation; note the erythema and induration. From the collection of the late N.P. Smith, MD, the Institute of Dermatology, London, UK.

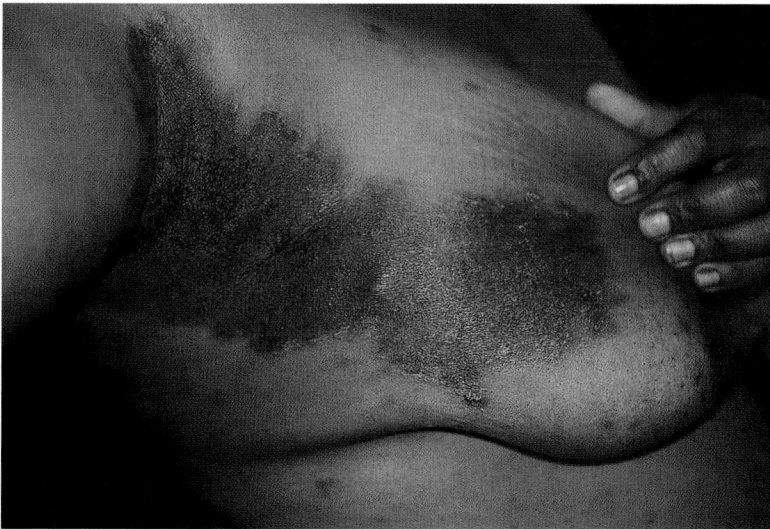

Fig. 18.275
Tinea corporis: in this patient, the infection is associated with severe hyperpigmentation. By courtesy of N.C. Dlova, MD, Nelson R. Mandela School of Medicine, University of KwaZulu-Natal, South Africa.

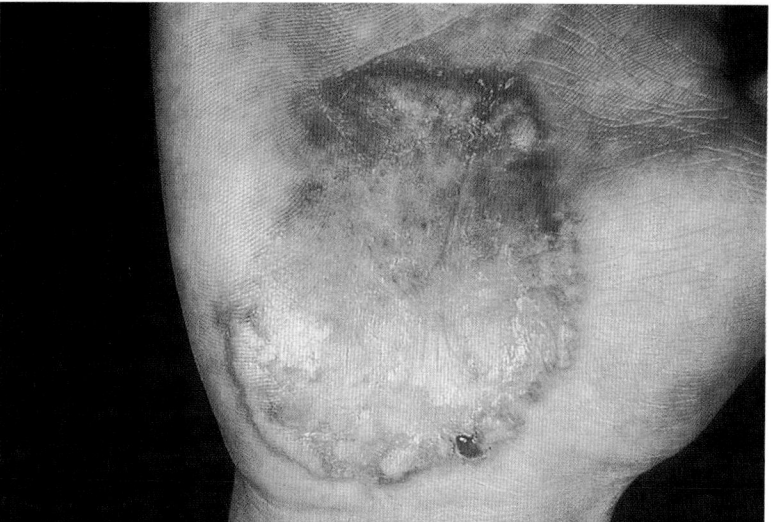

Fig. 18.276
Tinea corporis: this palmar lesion shows an erythematous border, scale, and central clearing. By courtesy of the Institute of Dermatology, London, UK.

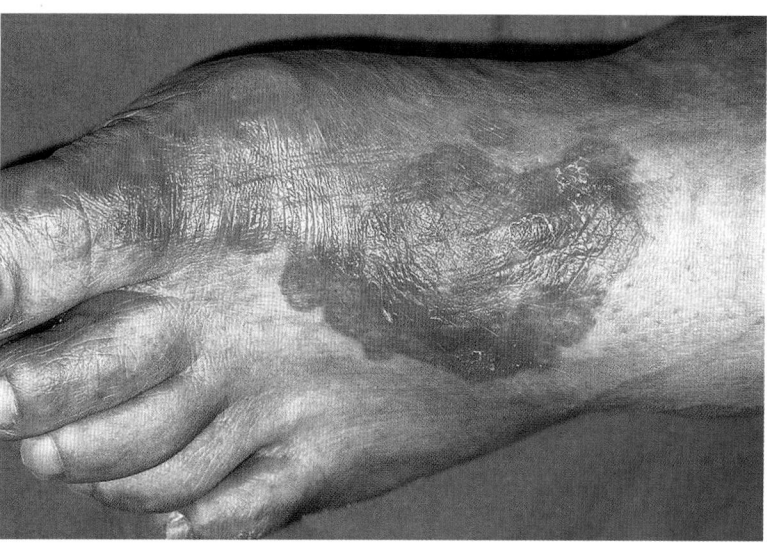

Fig. 18.277
Tinea corporis: steroid therapy may improve the clinical features with resultant masking of the true nature of the eruption (tinea incognito). By courtesy of R.A. Marsden, MD, St George's Hospital, London, UK.

rooms and ablution facilities (e.g., among athletes, military personnel, and boarding school residents), and has even been described among adult males who worship in mosques.[1–5] It is seen as a macerated fissuring area between the toes, which may extend onto the plantar aspect of the foot. The lesions are itchy, worse in hot weather due to sweating, and the smell is also a frequent cause of complaint. Pustular lesions may be seen.[6] Secondary bacterial infection is common. Tinea pedis is a predisposing factor for cellulitis of the lower extremities.[7] It is also a common cause of id reactions in the host.[8]

Tinea cruris

Tinea cruris is a very common dermatophyte infection of the groin, more common in men than in women. Obesity is a predisposing factor.[9] Isolated penile involvement may rarely occur.[10] Epidemics can occur among military recruits and dormitory residents who share bathing facilities.[11] It presents as an erythematous plaque, extending crescentically down the thighs (*Fig. 18.279*). Diaper dermatitis is a variant of tinea cruris, seen mainly in infants 7–12 months of age.[12]

Histologic features

The warm, humid conditions in the groin and the feet predispose to superficial fungal infections. On the feet, the organisms are usually *Trichophyton rubrum*, *T. interdigitale*, and *Epidermophyton floccosum*, in order of frequency.[13] In the groin, the same anthropophilic organisms are involved, but in reverse order of frequency. *T. rubrum* possesses important virulence factors, including keratinolytic enzymes such as hydrolases and keratinases, as well as cysteine dioxygenase.[1] Candidal and secondary bacterial infections are often seen. The histology is similar to that of tinea at other sites (*Figs 18.280–18.282*). Rarely, biopsies of perilesional skin from patients with bullous tinea pedis may show positive direct immunofluorescence staining along the dermal–epidermal junction.[14]

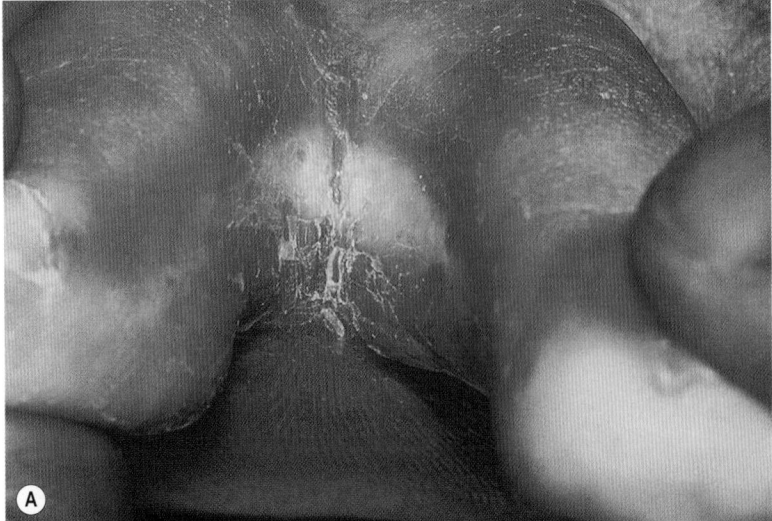

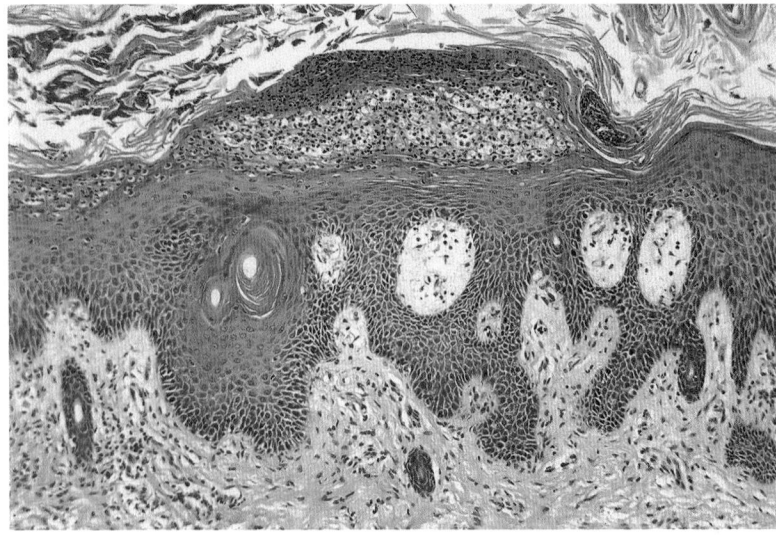

Fig. 18.280
Dermatophyte infection: there is parakeratosis overlying a subcorneal pustule. The epidermis shows psoriasiform hyperplasia.

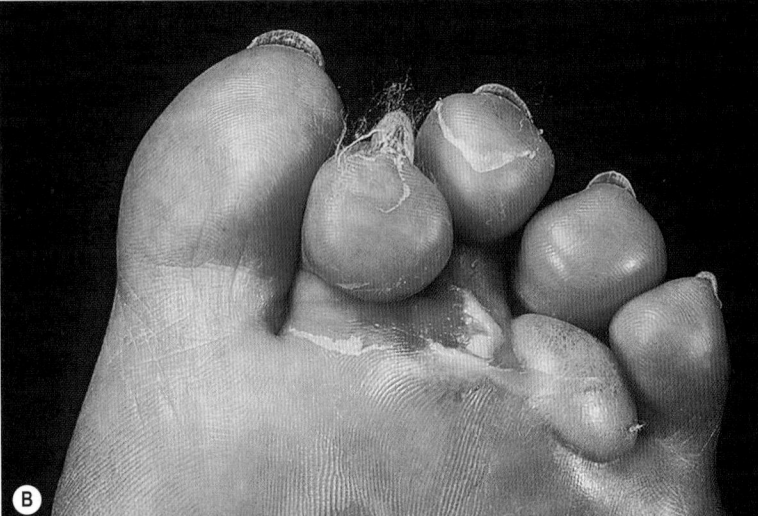

Fig. 18.278
Tinea pedis: (**A**) maceration between the toes; (**B**) severe dermal edema has resulted in this bullous variant. (**A**) By courtesy of A. Du Vivier, MD, King's College Hospital, London, UK; (**B**) by courtesy of the Institute of Dermatology, London, UK.

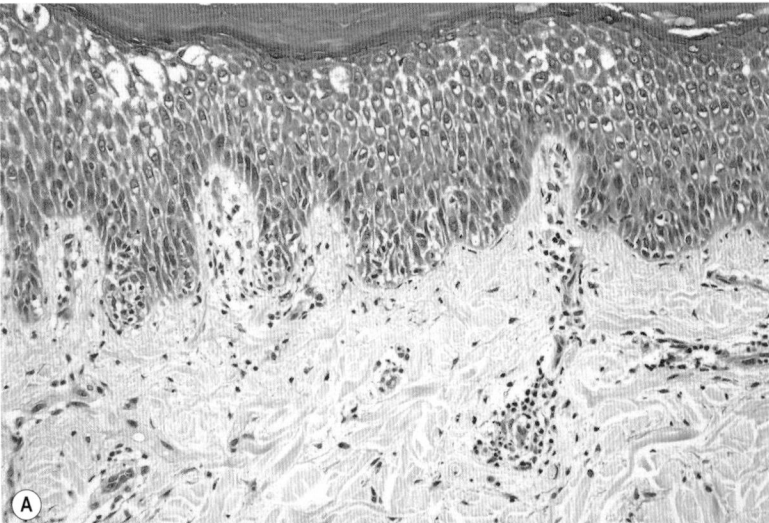

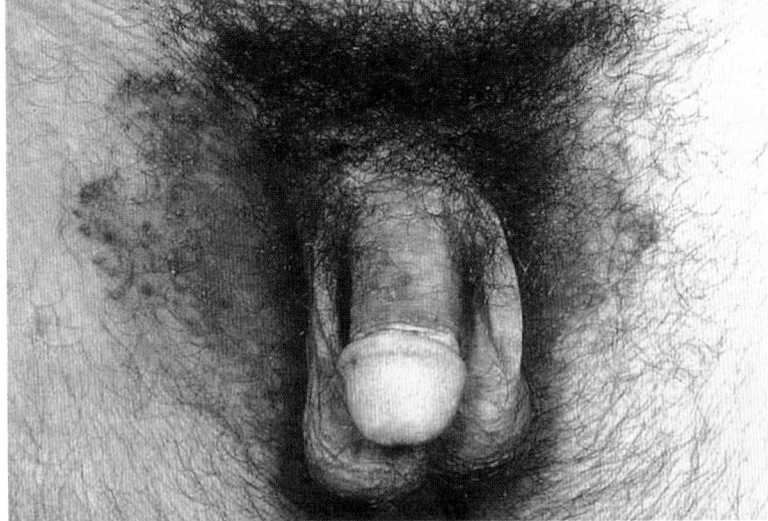

Fig. 18.279
Tinea cruris: this is much more common in males than in females. In this example, pustulation is evident. By courtesy of R.A. Marsden, MD, St George's Hospital, London, UK.

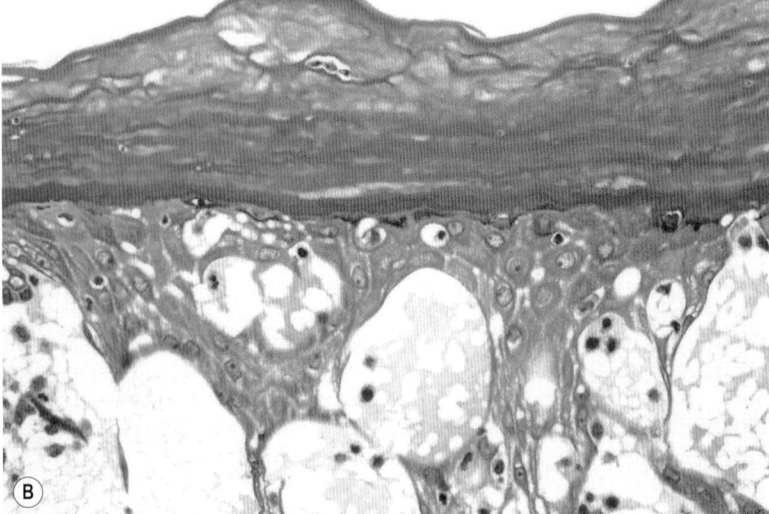

Fig. 18.281
(**A**, **B**) Tinea pedis: fungi are visible in the thick stratum corneum.

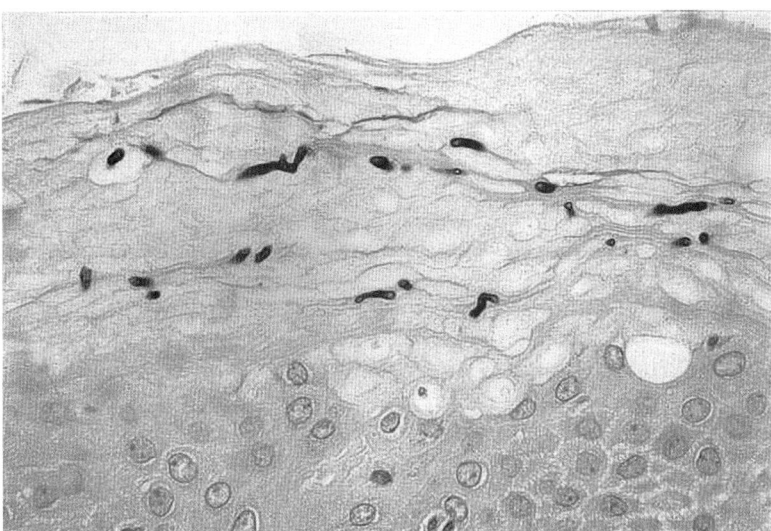

Fig. 18.282
Tinea pedis: periodic acid-Schiff stain of the same region shown in *Fig. 18.279*.

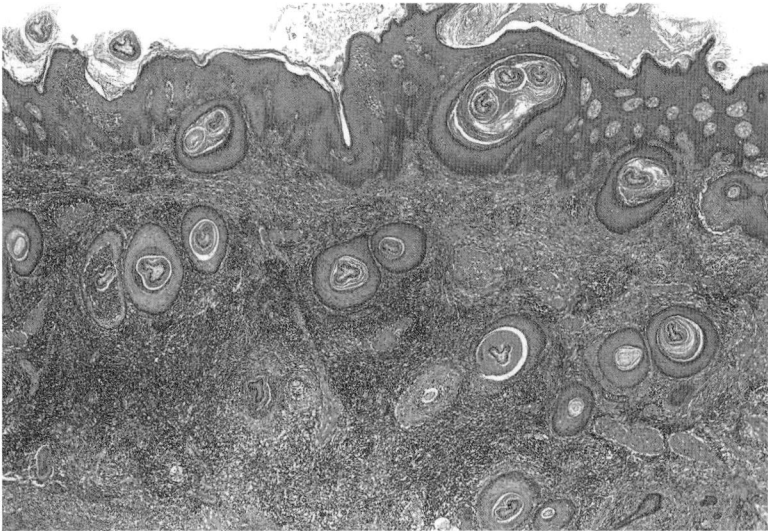

Fig. 18.284
Majocchi granuloma: this scalp biopsy shows intense dermal inflammation with involvement of numerous hair follicles.

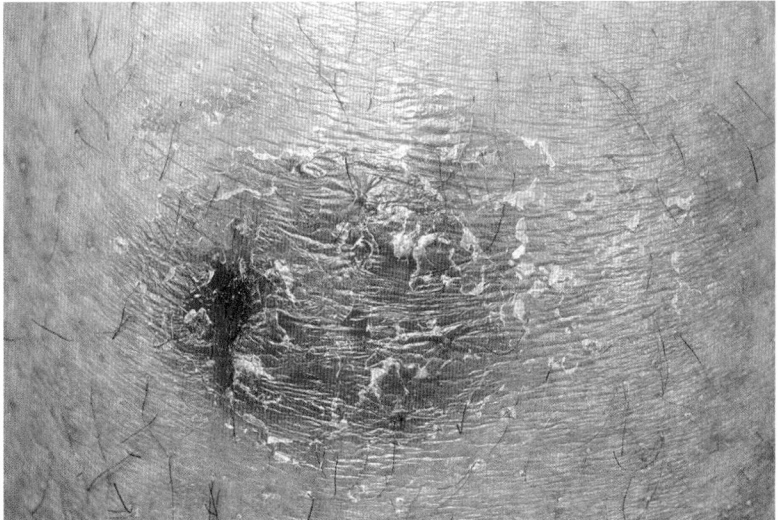

Fig. 18.283
Majocchi granuloma: there is a crusted granulomatous infiltrated plaque with pustules. By courtesy of the Institute of Dermatology, London, UK.

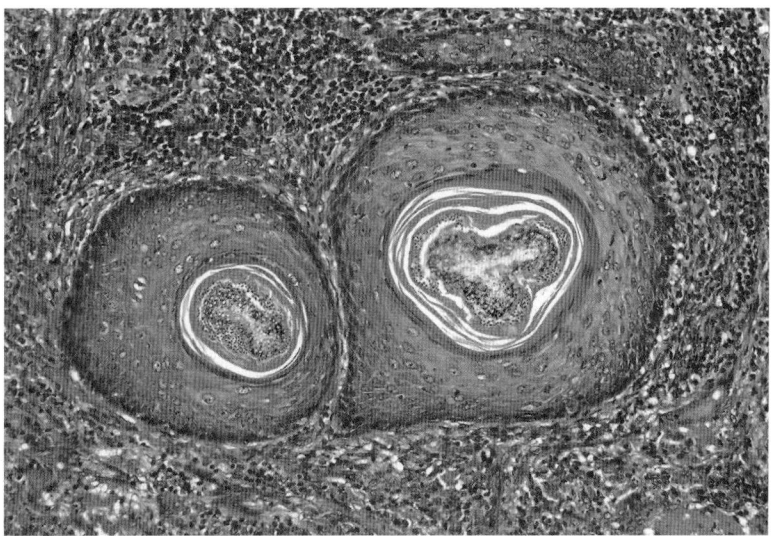

Fig. 18.285
Majocchi granuloma: there is intense dermal chronic inflammation and fungi are clearly visible surrounding the hair shafts.

Nodular granulomatous perifolliculitis

Clinical features

Nodular granulomatous perifolliculitis (Majocchi granuloma) represents an uncommon intradermal infection by dermatophytes that are more usually associated with follicular lesions. As a consequence of injury to a hair follicle, fungi (often with keratinous debris) are released into the surrounding tissues where they produce an intense inflammatory response.[1] Lesions present clinically as granulomata, cellulitis, or plaques (*Fig. 18.283*).[1] They are often seen on the anterior aspect of the legs. Inguinal, scrotal, vulval, and facial involvement has also been reported.[2-5] Although there is a propensity to affect adult females (particularly in association with shaving), the disease may also occur in children.[6,7] It has been described in pregnancy and following inadvertent treatment of superficial dermatophytosis with antibiotics and corticosteroids.[8,9] A case associated with long-standing tinea gladiatorum has also been reported.[10] In some instances, patients may have an associated immunodeficiency state (particularly due to corticosteroid therapy) that predominantly affects delayed hypersensitivity reactions, and may occur following renal transplantation and in those with chemotherapy-related neutropenia.[1,2,11-14] Disseminated skin lesions may rarely occur in immunosuppressed individuals.[15]

Histologic features

Trichophyton rubrum is the dermatophyte usually involved, but *T. mentagrophytes*, *T. epilans*, *T. tonsurans*, *T. violaceum*, *Microsporum audouinii*, *M. gypseum*, *M. ferrugineum*, and *M. canis* have also been incriminated.[1,4,6,7,10,13,16-18] An exceptional case of Majocchi granuloma due to *Aspergillus fumigatus* infection in a patient with HIV/AIDS has been reported.[19]

Hyphae and arthrospores are present in the dermis, often showing budding sporulation, intercellular septation, and abnormal and sometimes bizarre forms (*Figs 18.284–18.287*).[1] Organisms may be scanty and multiple sections may be rewarding. Granuloma formation as mycetoma may be a feature, and the Splendore-Hoeppli phenomenon has been described.[1] There is usually a heavy acute chronic inflammatory cell infiltrate, often with granulomatous features.

Diseases caused by *Malassezia* species

Tinea versicolor

Clinical features

Tinea versicolor (pityriasis versicolor), which represents a superficial fungal infection, is a common condition. It has a worldwide distribution but is

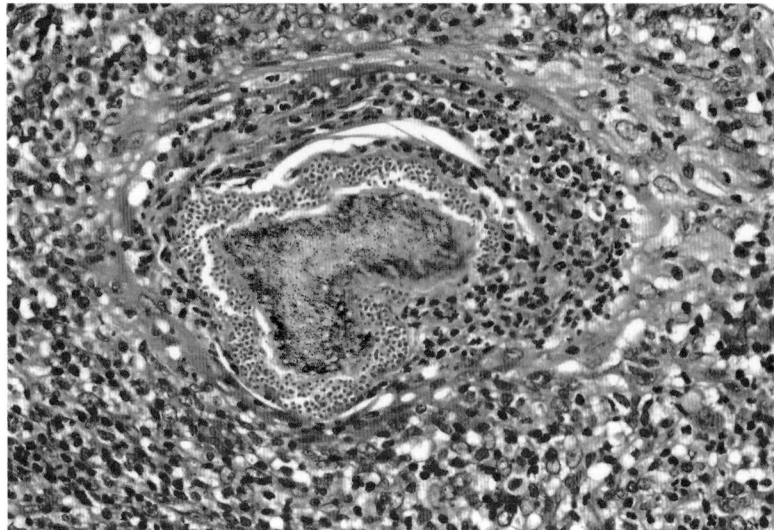

Fig. 18.286
Majocchi granuloma: close-up view of a free hair shaft with fungi within a dermal abscess.

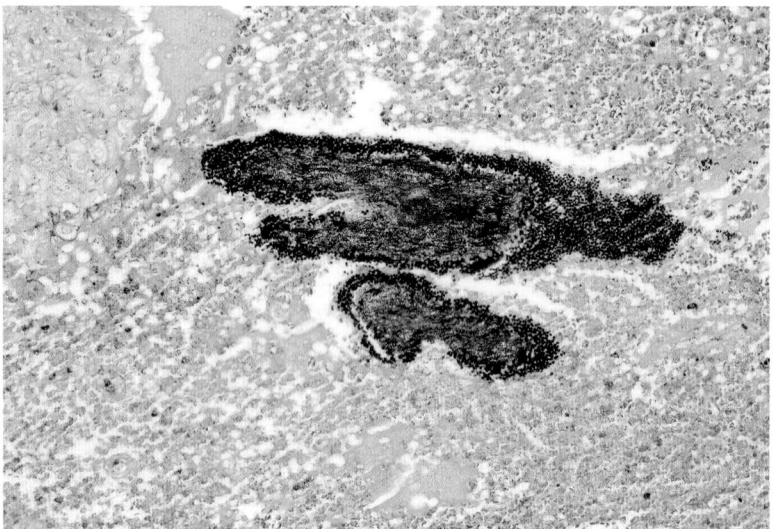

Fig. 18.287
Majocchi granuloma: the methenamine silver stain is strikingly positive.

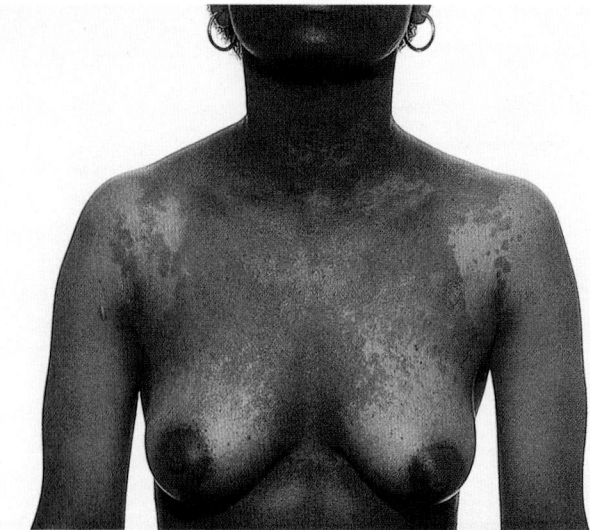

Fig. 18.288
Tinea versicolor: hyperpigmented macules, many of which have coalesced, are present on the chest, which is a commonly affected site. By courtesy of M.M. Black, MD, Institute of Dermatology, London, UK.

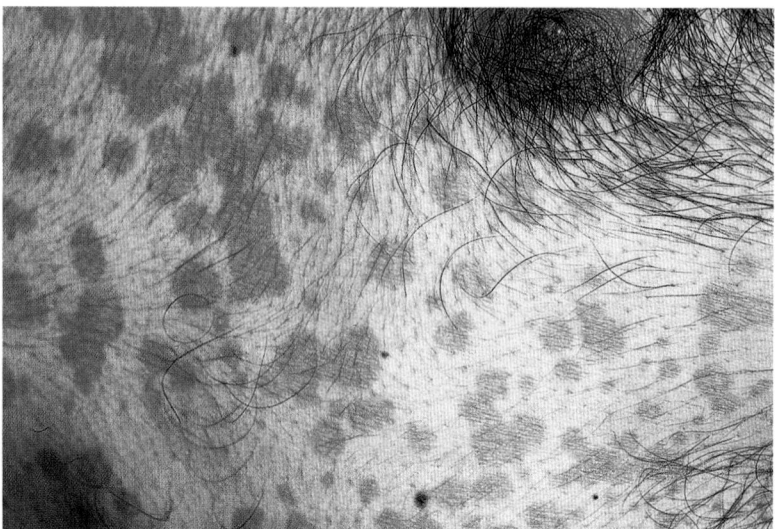

Fig. 18.289
Tinea versicolor: pale brown macules are typically seen in whites. By courtesy of R.A. Marsden, MD, St George's Hospital, London, UK.

more common in tropical climates and occurs with a greater frequency in summer months in temperate zones. It presents most often in young adults (20–40 years of age) and there is a slight predilection for females (2:1).[1–3] A greater proportion of children may be affected in tropical regions.[4]

The majority of lesions are caused by the mycelial phase of the lipophilic yeast *Malassezia globosa*. Other species implicated are *M. furfur*, *M. sympodialis*, *M. restricta*, and uncommonly, *M. obtusa* and *M. slooffiae*.[2,5–12] The organisms are normally present in the majority of adults and are most commonly found on the chest, upper back, and scalp.

The condition presents as chronic multiple irregular areas of hypo- or hyperpigmentation usually on the seborrheic areas of the body.[1–3,13] Lesions, which are circular and macular, may become confluent. The surface is covered by a fine scale, which may be rendered more prominent by scratching with a fingernail. The color varies from pink to yellow, yellow-brown or even dark brown in dark-skinned patients (*Fig. 18.288*). Although asymptomatic hypopigmented macules are frequently the sole manifestation of the disease in dark-skinned individuals, in the fair-skinned, they appear hyperpigmented (brown on white) (*Fig. 18.289*).[14] A papulopustular form may occur in infants. A rare variant associated with cutaneous atrophy has been described.[15,16]

The yeast has a 'stunning' effect on melanocytes and eventually produces hypopigmentation of affected skin. Hence, in a dark-skinned patient or a

fair-skinned individual who has acquired a suntan, the lesions look pale relative to normal skin (white or brown). Yellow or yellow-blue fluorescence under a Wood lamp is characteristic.[3] An erythrasmoid variant characterized by exclusive involvement of the inguinal folds has been described.[17,18]

Pathogenesis and histologic features

Conditions predisposing to the development of tinea versicolor are numerous and include greasy skin, excessive steroids, hyperhidrosis, immunosuppresion (including HIV/AIDS), diabetes mellitus, pregnancy, and the oral contraceptive.[3]

Malassezia species are a very common commensal of hair follicles, where they are seen as basophilic round bodies among the keratin.[13,19] In lesions of tinea versicolor, the mycelial or hyphal forms are seen among the interfollicular keratin.[1,14] They may be identified more readily by using a PAS reaction or methenamine silver stain. Histologic changes are mild, consisting of mild acanthosis and hyperkeratosis, with focal parakeratosis (*Fig. 18.290*). Occasional degenerate keratinocytes may be evident. The stratum corneum contains round budding yeasts and short septate hyphae, imparting the 'spaghetti and meatballs' appearance. A hypopigmented basal layer is seen in biopsies of pale lesions; in hyperpigmented lesions there is hyperkeratosis, the basal pigmentation is increased, and there is pigmentary incontinence

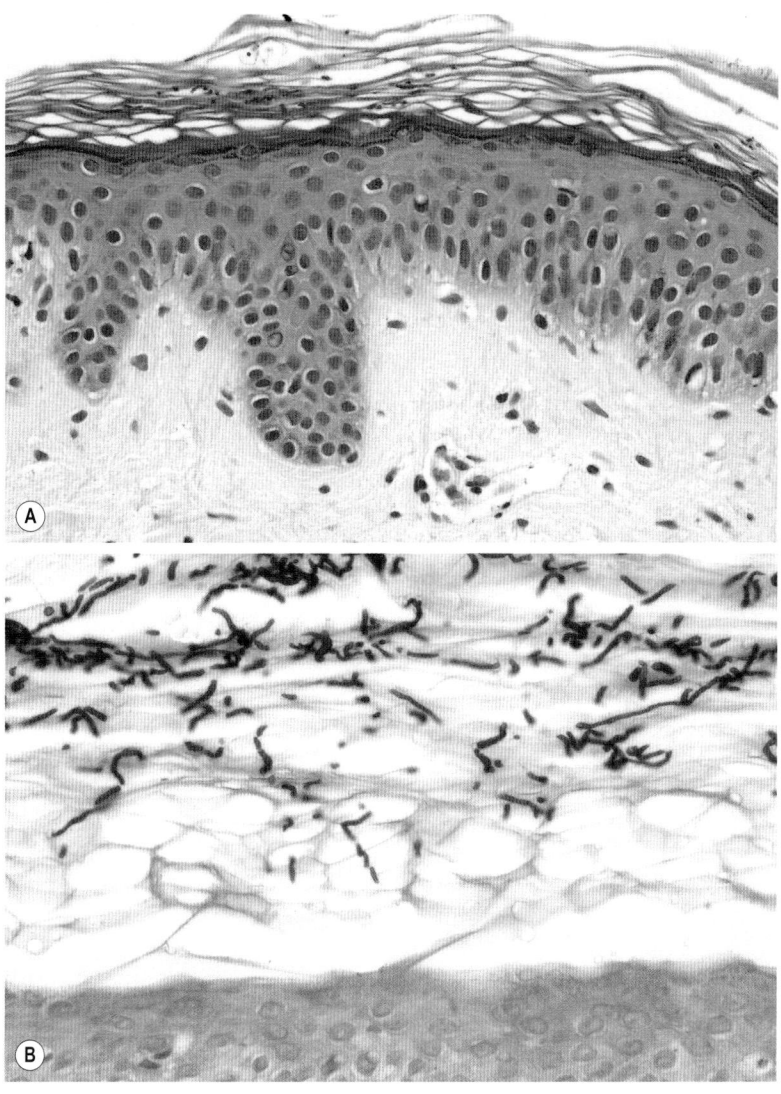

Fig. 18.290
Tinea versicolor: (**A**) there is hyperkeratosis and small basophilic spores are easily seen; (**B**) the periodic acid-Schiff reaction reveals numerous hyphae.

with pigment-laden macrophages in the upper dermis. Greater numbers of yeasts and hyphae are present in hyperpigmented lesions.[13] Biopsies from atrophic lesions may reveal variable epidermal and dermal atrophy with effacement of rete ridges, superficial dermal fibrosis, pigmentary incontinence, and elastolysis.[15,16]

The mechanism for the changes in pigmentation is not yet fully understood. Over the years, racial factors, light exposure, the inflammatory response, the fungal load, the thickness of the keratin layer, and a direct effect of the fungus (dicarboxylic acids) on melanocytes have been suggested.[13,20–24] A multifactorial pathogenesis, however, seems likely, with a complex interplay between fungal wall constituents, enzymes, metabolites, and cellular components of the epidermis.[25] Exposure to sunlight has been shown to stimulate the production of azelaic acid, and this is believed to lead to evolution of the hypopigmented lesions.[26] Dopa cell counts have been shown to be normal.[13] In hypopigmented lesions, there appear to be reduced numbers of smaller melanosomes in both the melanocytes and their neighboring keratinocytes.[13] Mitochondrial and cytoplasmic vacuolation has also been documented. In the superficial dermis, a slight perivascular chronic inflammatory cell infiltrate consisting of lymphocytes, histiocytes, and occasional plasma cells may be evident.

There is also evidence to suggest that infection with the fungus rarely presents as systemic illness and that it is of importance in the pathogenesis of some cases of chronic folliculitis (*Malassezia* folliculitis, see below) and seborrheic dermatitis.[1,6,9,12,19,27–29]

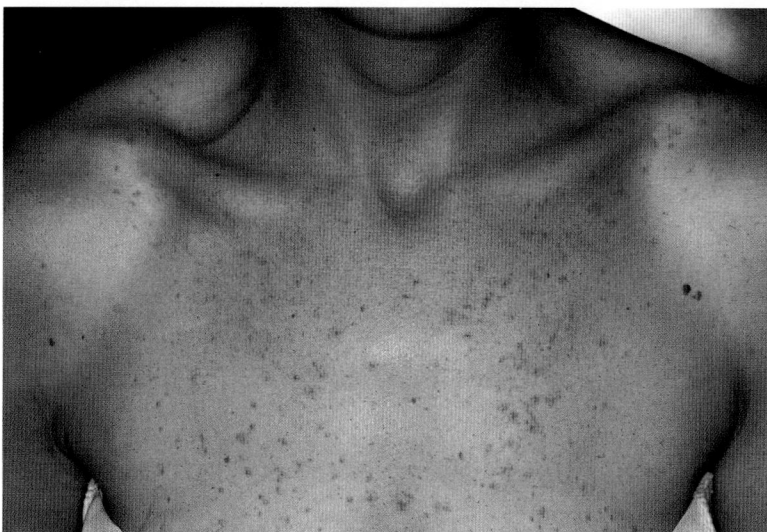

Fig. 18.291
Malassezia (*Pityrosporum*) folliculitis: note the numerous follicular pustules. By courtesy of S. Glassman, MD, University of Witwatersrand, Johannesburg, South Africa.

Malassezia folliculitis

Clinical features

Malassezia folliculitis, which is often still referred to by its previous name, *Pityrosporum* folliculitis, is a form of chronic folliculitis attributed to infection by the yeast phase of *M. furfur* (formerly *Pityrosporum ovale* or *P. orbiculare*), an organism that thrives in hot, humid, and sweaty environments.[1–4] The condition occurs in adults, who present with pruritic pustules centered mainly on the trunk, neck, and upper arms (*Fig. 18.291*). The disease has some propensity to occur in immunocompromised hosts and those on prolonged therapy with broad-spectrum antibiotics, and is an uncommon cause of pruritic papulopustular eruption in HIV-infected individuals.[2,5–7] *Malassezia* spp. have also been linked to catheter-related fungemia in immunocompromised patients.[5]

Pathogenesis and histologic features

Follicular occlusion may be the initiating pathogenetic event.[8]

Histopathological examination shows distension of occluded hair follicle infundibula by basophilic keratinous debris containing clusters of round, budding yeast cells (*Fig. 18.292*). Mycelial forms are characteristically absent. A mild perifollicular mononuclear inflammatory cell infiltrate is usually observed. Intradermal rupture of dilated follicles may incite an intense folliculocentric suppurative inflammatory infiltrate and perifollicular foreign body giant cell reaction. A PAS stain may reveal rare yeasts in the inflamed perifollicular dermis in such cases. Intrafollicular mucin deposition has been reported.[9]

Tinea nigra

Clinical features

Tinea nigra is an uncommon superficial mycosis caused by *Hortaea werneckii* (formerly *Phaeoannellomyces werneckii* or *Exophiala werneckii*). It occurs mainly in the tropics and presents as a slowly growing, irregular, brown, black or dark-green slightly scaly asymptomatic patch.[1,2] The disease involves mainly the palms followed by the soles, and is exceptional at other sites (e.g., the fingers). Bilateral involvement may be seen.[3–5] Clinical confusion with a melanocytic lesion is possible, and dermoscopy has emerged as a useful tool in reducing the risk of potential misdiagnosis.[6,7] On rare occasions, tinea nigra may manifest with a speckled or 'salt and pepper' pattern of involvement.[8]

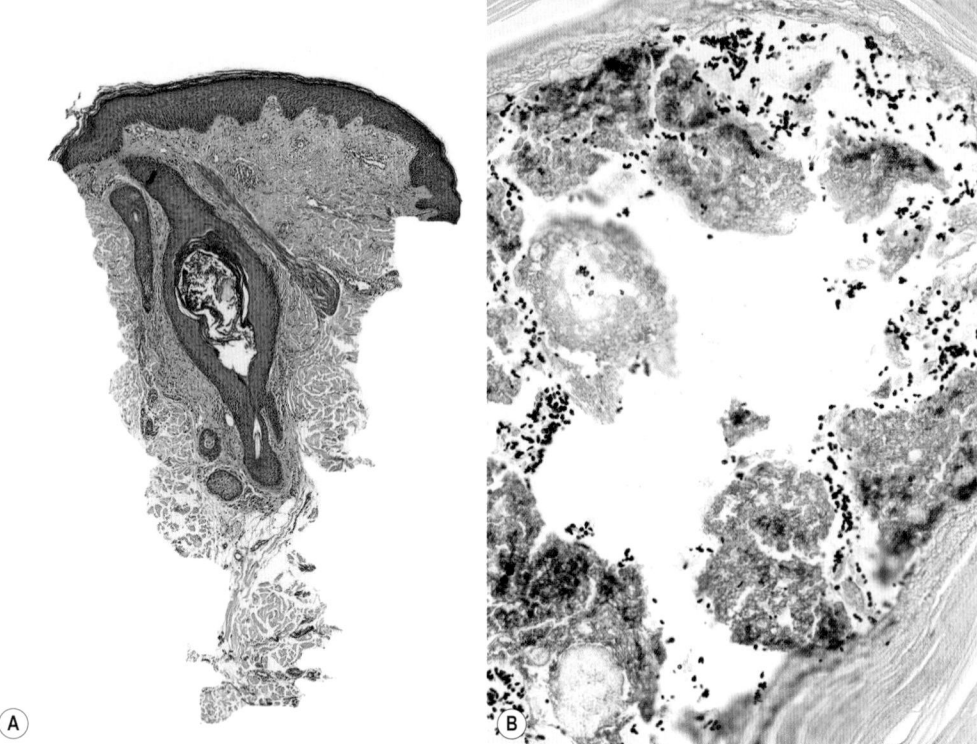

Fig. 18.292
Malassezia (*Pityrosporum*) folliculitis: (**A**) there is infundibular dilatation; (**B**) yeast forms are conspicuous in the methenamine silver stained section.

Histologic features

The epidermis shows the presence of numerous short, segmented hyphae and spores in the superficial aspect of the stratum corneum. The organisms are easily recognized as they stain brown or yellow with H&E.

Candidiasis

Clinical features

Candida is a yeast-like fungus with budding and filamentous (pseudohyphal and hyphal) forms. There are several species, but *C. albicans* is by far the most common human pathogen.[1,2] *C. glabrata* (formerly *Torulopsis glabrata*) infections, however, have become increasingly important in recent years, especially in immunosuppressed hosts.[3–5] *C. parapsilosis* and *C. tropicalis* are the next most frequently encountered pathogens; the former has been shown to proliferate in glucose-containing pareneteral solutions and is an important nosocomial pathogen, especially among low birth weight neonates.[2,6,7] *C. dubliniensis* has emerged as a cause of oral candidiasis in HIV-infected patients.[8] Other less frequently encountered species are *C. guilliermondi*, *C. lusitaniae*, *C.orthopsilosis*, *C. metapsilosis*, *C. kefyr*, and *C. krusei*.[2,6,9–11] Some of the aforementioned non-*albicans* species of *Candida* are intrinsically resistant to certain antifungal agents.[2,9,12]

Candida infection involving mucocutaneous sites can be categorized as follows: oral candidiasis, cutaneous candidiasis, candidal vulvovaginitis, candidal balanitis, chronic mucocutaneous candidiasis (CMC), subcutaneous candidal abscess, and disseminated candidiasis.

Oral candidiasis appears in several forms[13]:

- In neonates, it appears as a curdlike pseudomembrane overlying an erythematous base, which may be painful and atrophic.

- In adults, usually males, a chronic hyperplastic form is seen as a plaque with an erythematous margin (*Fig. 18.293*). This must be distinguished from leukoplakia. This hyperplastic plaquelike form also occurs in the chronic mucocutaneous forms of candidiasis and in immunodeficient individuals, including those with HIV/AIDS.[14,15]

- Chronic atrophic candidiasis is seen in the elderly, often as a sore red patch associated with dentures. It may be accompanied by angular

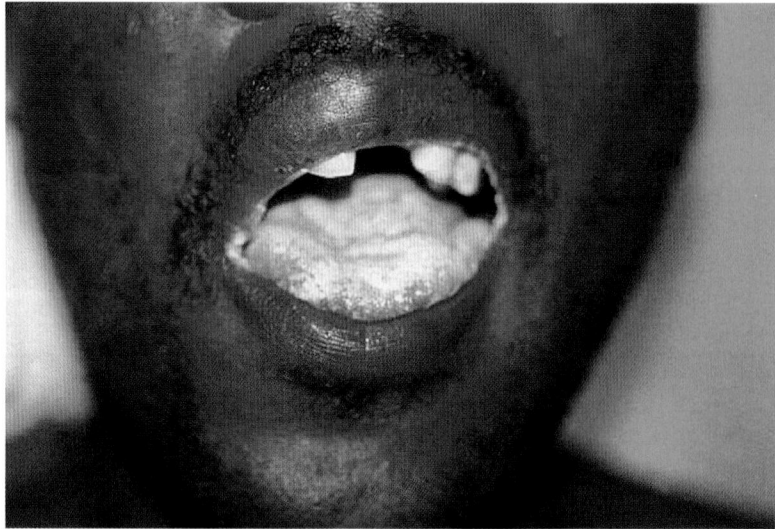

Fig. 18.293
Candida glossitis: the tongue is covered with a white plaque. There is also involvement of the angles of the mouth. By courtesy of N.C. Dlova, MD, Nelson R. Mandela School of Medicine, University of KwaZulu-Natal, South Africa.

cheilitis and sometimes extends onto the facial skin as an erythematous granular lesion. Candidal cheilitis may affect the lips of patients with a heavy oral candidal infection (*Fig. 18.294*). Steroid therapy, whether local or systemic, appears to predispose to oral involvement.

Cutaneous candidiasis tends to be confined to skin folds in the obese and to the genital mucous membranes (*Fig. 18.295*). The lesions appear as moist erythematous areas with small pustules at the margins (*Fig. 18.296*). A variant of cutaneous candidiasis referred to as 'decubital candidosis' has been described in chronically bedridden patients and is invariably attributable to infection with *C. albicans*.[16] Congenital cutaneous candidiasis is a very rare, self-limiting form of cutaneous candidiasis in which neonates present with a generalized erythematous papular eruption secondary to

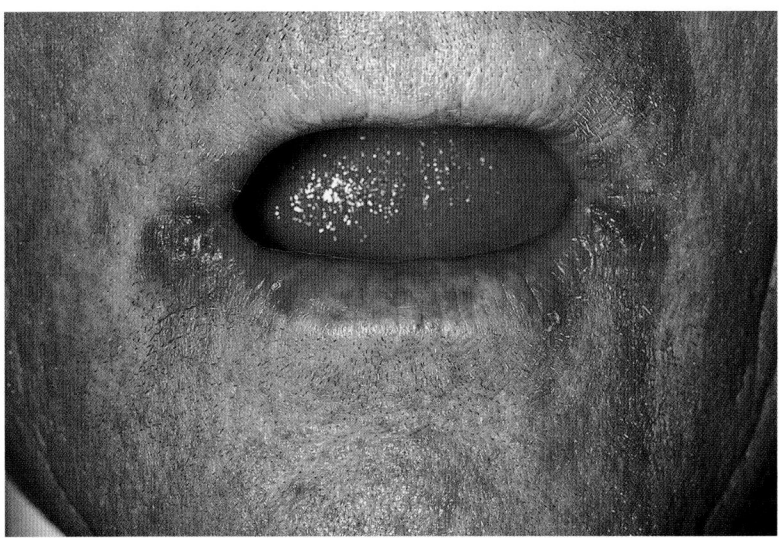

Fig. 18.294
Candidal angular cheilitis: note the erythematous crusted lesions at the angles of the mouth. By courtesy of M.M. Black, MD, Institute of Dermatology, London, UK.

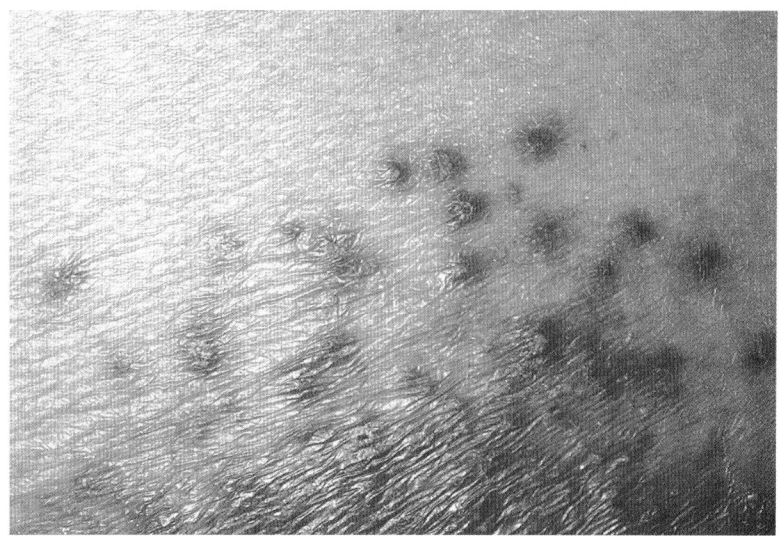

Fig. 18.296
Cutaneous candidiasis: intertriginous involvement may be characterized by the development of pustules, as seen in this picture. By courtesy of R.A. Marsden, MD, St George's Hospital, London, UK.

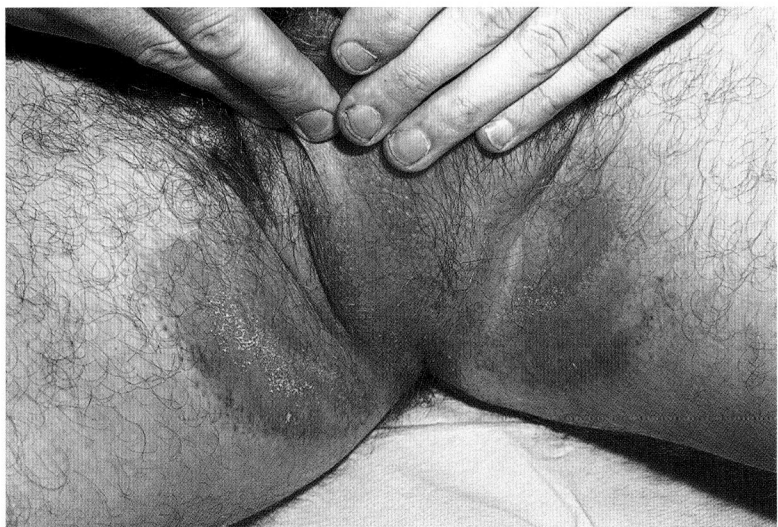

Fig. 18.295
Cutaneous candidiasis: the warm, moist environment of the upper thighs and scrotum predisposes to intertriginous candidiasis. Note the erythema and peripheral pustules. By courtesy of M.M. Black, MD, Institute of Dermatology, London, UK.

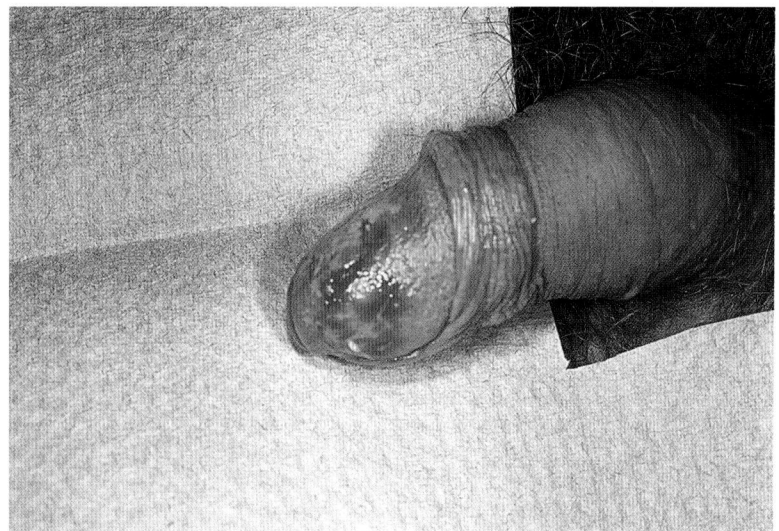

Fig. 18.297
Candidal balanitis: note the erythema with erosion and the small white pustule at the margin of the lesion. By courtesy of C. Furlonge, MD, Port of Spain, Trinidad.

underlying *Candida* chorioamnionitis and funisitis.[17,18] This latter condition must be distinguished from skin involvement as part of disseminated congenital candidiasis (see below).

Vulvovaginitis occurs mainly during pregnancy or as a complication of diabetes mellitus, oral contraceptives, or antibiotic therapy.[2]

Candidal balanitis is associated with vaginal infections in the sexual partner: transient papules develop on the glans, become white and pustular, and rupture; they may heal rapidly or persist with exacerbations (*Fig. 18.297*).

CMC is a persistent and refractory condition, usually starting in the young and often associated with an immunodeficient state. These patients have oral candidiasis, which recurs after therapy and may become hypertrophic. They also have cutaneous candidiasis involving intertriginous areas and the face and hands or in a more widespread distribution. Paronychia and vulvovaginitis or balanitis also occur (*Fig. 18.298*). CMC is also an important feature of HIV/AIDS.[14] Indeed, oral candidiasis may represent an early marker of immunosuppression in patients with HIV infection.[15] *Candida* vaginitis is an important early manifestation in female HIV/AIDS patients.[14]

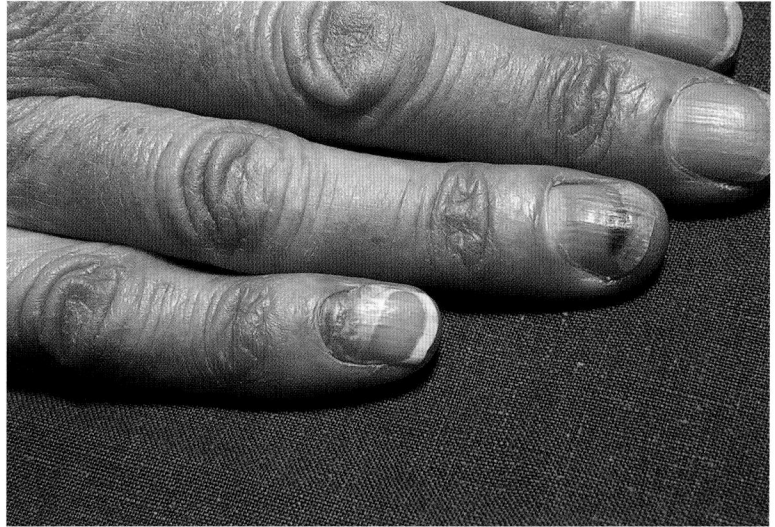

Fig. 18.298
Candida infection: there is proximal nail dystrophy and onycholysis with pigmentary changes. By courtesy of the Institute of Dermatology, London, UK.

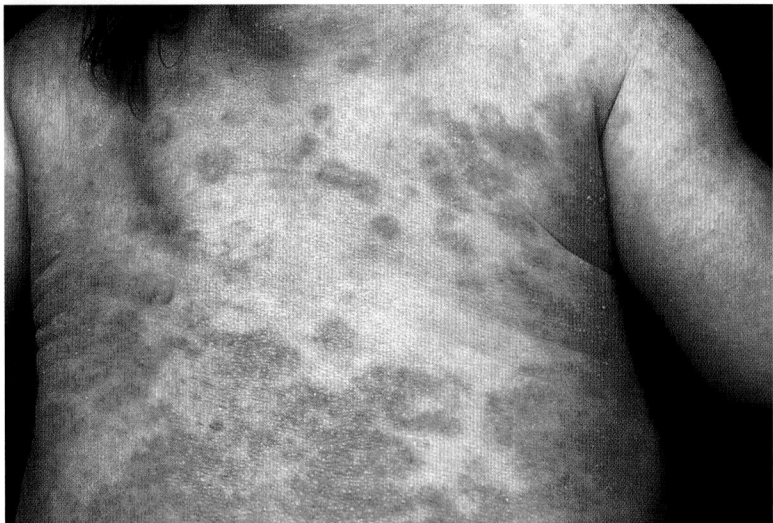

Fig. 18.299
Disseminated candidiasis: disseminated disease in infants may be a sign of immunosuppression such as DiGeorge syndrome. By courtesy of the Institute of Dermatology, London, UK.

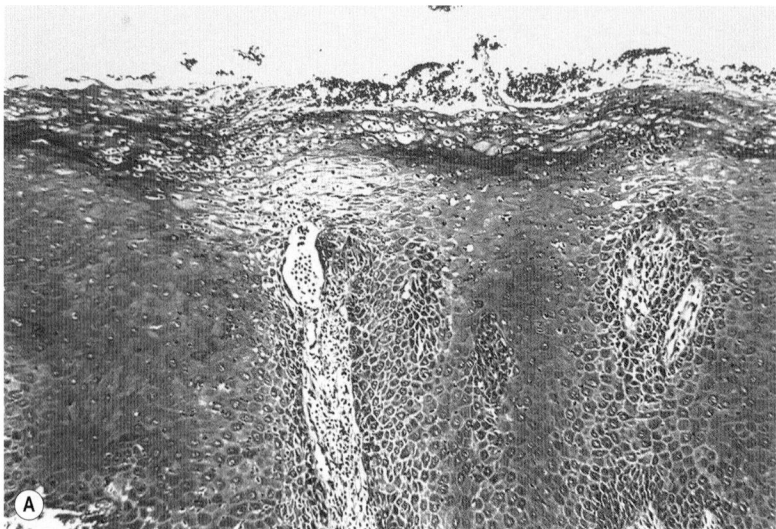

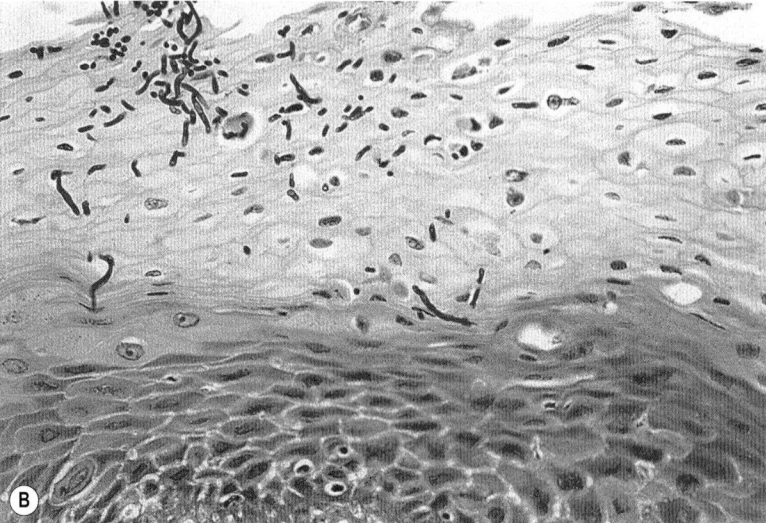

Fig. 18.300
Cutaneous candidiasis: (A) there is marked acanthosis and the superficial layers of the epithelium are infiltrated by large numbers of neutrophils; (B) there are abundant yeast-like and pseudohyphal forms (periodic acid-Schiff).

Some of these patients have a severe congenital primary defect of cellular immunity, such as hereditary thymic dysplasia or the DiGeorge syndrome, and in these patients the outlook is poor (*Fig. 18.299*). Recent evidence has shown that impaired IL-17 immunity plays a key role not only in certain syndromic forms of CMC, but also in individuals who develop mucocutaneous candidiasis following IL-17 blockade as a result of targeted immunotherapy.[19–21] Autosomal recessive autoimmune polyendocrinopathy syndrome (also referred to as autoimmune polyendocrinopathy-candidiasis-ectodermal dystrophy syndrome) is a rare disorder caused by mutations in the autoimmune regulator gene (AIRE) and the production of neutralizing autoantibodies against IL-17. In addition to CMC, patients may present with endocrinopathies involving the parathyroids, thyroid and/or adrenals, diabetes mellitus, nail dystrophy, and dystrophy of the dental enamel. Additional stigmata can include vitiligo, alopecia areata, and alopecia totalis.[20,22–26] Patients with this condition may have altered patterns of cytokine production in response to infection by *Candida* organisms.[25] Autosomal dominant hyper-IgE syndrome is another condition associated with syndromic CMC; the latter is a consequence of impaired generation of IL-17-producing Th17 cells, usually due to mutations in the *STAT3* gene.[20,21,27]

Subcutaneous candidal abscess is a rare condition that is usually encountered in immunocompromised patients. Lesions may arise following iatrogenic intervention, such as central venous catheterization.[28] There are isolated reports of severe necrotizing soft tissue infections caused by *Candida* spp., namely, NF and Fournier gangrene.[29,30]

In patients with HIV/AIDS and others who are immunosuppressed, such as severely neutropenic oncology patients, disseminated candidiasis follows hematogenous spread from an underlying gastrointestinal or urinary tract primary focus of infection. Candidemia is associated with a very high mortality rate.[31,32] Cutaneous lesions include macules, papules, plaques, petechiae, hemorrhagic foci, nodules, and an ecthyma gangrenosum-like presentation. These are painful, multiple, and widely distributed over the body.[32,33] A rare congenital form of disseminated candidiasis has been described, including very low birth weight infants.[34,35] Disseminated disease may also be seen in heroin addicts. Candidemia and disseminated candidiasis are important infections in the nosocomial setting, especially among critically ill patients in intensive care units. Risk factors include invasive procedures (e.g., insertion of central venous catheters), parenteral nutrition, use of broad-spectrum antibiotics, the administration of corticosteroids, and renal insufficiency. There has also been a shifting trend toward infections with non-*albicans Candida* spp. in this context, with an accompanying increase in mortality and resistance to antifungal agents.[12,36]

Pathogenesis and histologic features

C. albicans and other *Candida* spp. have a number of virulence factors that potentiate infection. These factors include adhesins (which facilitate adhesion to epithelial surfaces), aspartyl protease (which facilitates penetration of keratinized cells), hydrolases, and phospholipases.[7,37–40] In addition, the organisms utilize at least two signaling pathways that potentiate conversion from a yeast form to a hyphal form; the latter is a prerequisite for deeper penetration into keratinized epithelium.[37,40,41] Additional attributes contributing to virulence include biofilm formation and phenotypic switching.[7,40]

Candidal lesions appear similar in varying sites. There is a prominent neutrophil infiltrate of the oral mucosa or epidermis. Yeast forms, pseudohyphae, or even true hyphae can be seen (*Fig. 18.300*). The yeast-like form is often seen in the mouth and does not necessarily indicate pathogenicity. There is often an intense chronic inflammatory infiltrate in the underlying connective tissue, and in chronic hypertrophic forms the epithelium is hyperplastic and hyperkeratotic.

The disseminated lesions are characterized by a fibrinous exudate with both yeast and pseudohyphae forms, sometimes accompanied by the features of a leukocytoclastic vasculitis. Vascular involvement may be associated with epidermal necrosis and vesiculation. Transepidermal elimination of organisms is a rare finding.[32] Suppurative folliculitis and perifolliculitis are seen in heroin addicts.[42] A recently reported case of disseminated *C. krusei* infection in a hematopoietic stem cell transplant recipient with fatal relapse of acute myeloid leukemia also demonstrated striking folliculocentricity; the

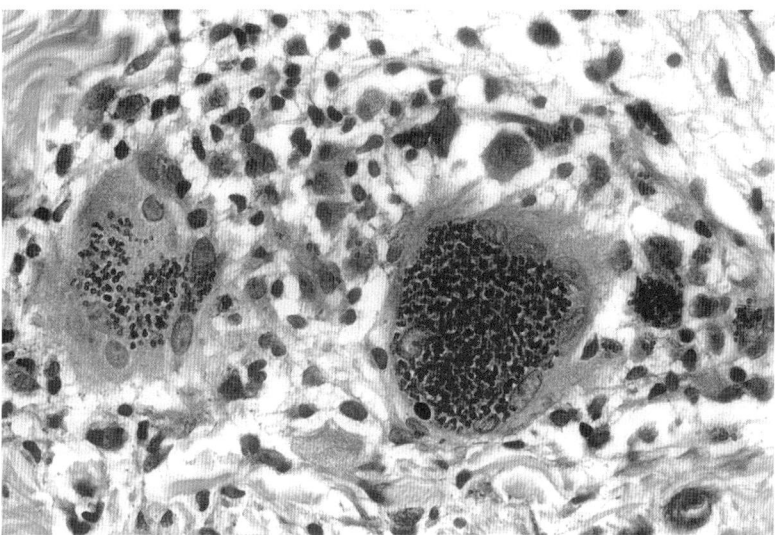

Fig. 18.301
Candida glabrata infection: intracytoplasmic location of the yeasts an uncommon manifestation.

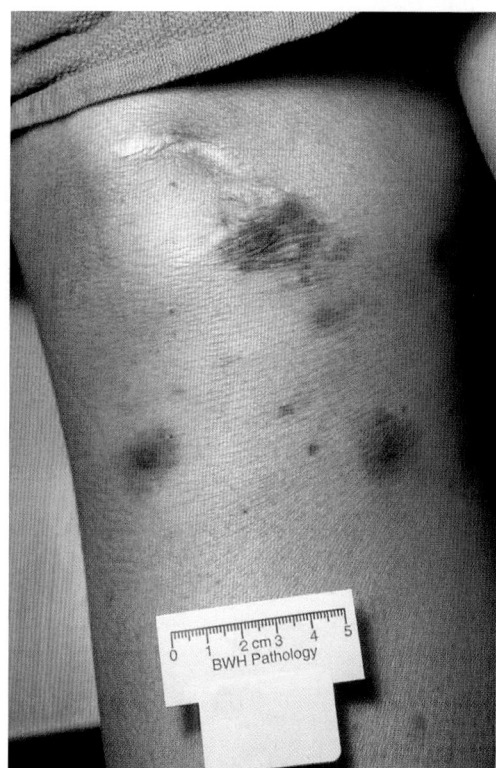

Fig. 18.302
Aspergillosis: this immunosuppressed patient developed multiple purple nodules on the limbs secondary to esophageal candidiasis. By courtesy of A.F. Nascimento, MD, Brigham and Women's Hospital and Harvard Medical School, Boston, USA.

latter was attributed to apparent transfollicular elimination of organisms following clearance of the fungemia.[11]

The closely related species *C. glabrata* (formerly *Torulopsis glabrata*) differs from *C. albicans* by the general absence of hyphae and pseudohyphae in the former, although this is not always the case (*Fig. 18.301*).[43]

Aspergillosis

Clinical features

Species of *Aspergillus* occur worldwide and can cause cutaneous lesions, either by hematogenous spread from a primary infection in an immunosuppressed patient, usually in the lung, or by direct inoculation of the skin.[1–4] *Aspergillus* spp. are also a rare cause of onychomycosis.[1,5,6] Patients with neutropenia are particularly at risk of systemic spread, especially those with hematological malignancies.[4,7–11] Skin involvement secondary to disseminated aspergillosis has also been reported in the context of HIV/AIDS, diabetes mellitus, following bone marrow transplantation, in extremely low birth weight preterm neonates, and in a child with underlying chronic granulomatous disease.[11–16] Patients may develop widespread pulmonary infiltrates or infarction, which is soon followed by disseminated vaso-occlusive disease.[3,17] Systemic lesions are most commonly seen in the gastrointestinal tract, the CNS, the liver, kidney, heart, and thyroid.[9] Destructive lesions of the palate and nasal septum may occur.[1,18] Skin involvement in disseminated aspergillosis is uncommon, however, being present in only about 4% to 5% of patients.[7,19] Less than 1% of patients in a recently reported series of 1410 cases of invasive aspergillosis had cutaneous lesions secondary to systemic involvement.[20] In hematogenous spread, the lesions develop as small, red, discrete macules and papules, which may become pustular or necrotic/infarcted (*Fig. 18.302*). Plaques studded with pustules may be seen. Noduloulcerative lesions with central eschar formation and raised borders are sometimes encountered.[18,20] Very rarely, a tumorlike mass may develop.[16]

Primary aspergillosis of the skin, which usually follows local trauma (e.g., intravenous injection therapy site, cutaneous maceration, or burns), appears as a purplish thickened edematous area at the site of inoculation.[21–28] Infection has also been described following a home-made tattoo.[29] In the immunosuppressed, these lesions may ulcerate and develop a black crust (*Fig. 18.303*).[19,20,30] A presentation mimicking Sweet syndrome has been reported.[31] The condition has also been reported in premature infants and those with underlying HIV/AIDS.[23,32–36] Occasional immunosuppressed patients with primary cutaneous aspergillosis have presented with solitary nonulcerated nodules.[37,38] Multiple nodules may also occur in these patients.[39,40] On rare occasions, however, even immunocompetent individuals may develop multiple nodular lesions and plaques.[41] There is a report

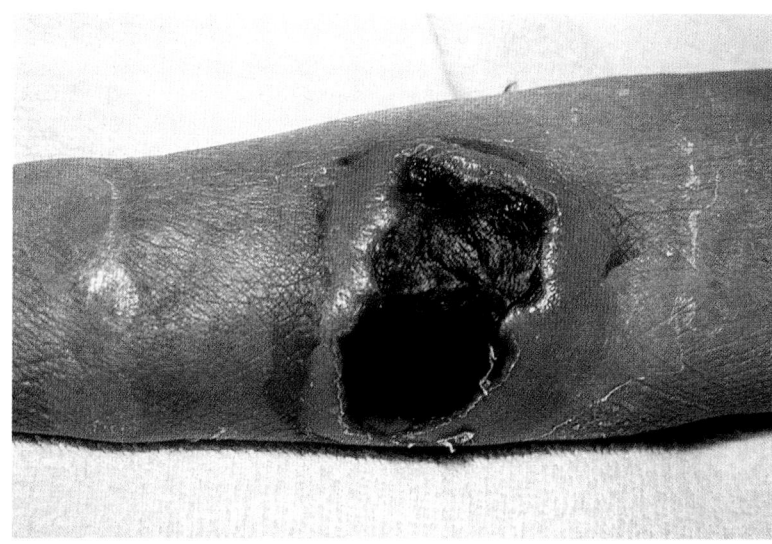

Fig. 18.303
Aspergillosis: there is extensive ulceration with characteristic black crusting. Primary cutaneous aspergillosis most often follows trauma or it may develop in the immunosuppressed. By courtesy of N. Khardori, MD, University of South Illinois, USA.

of evolution of large cauliflower-like lesions on the legs of a patient with bilateral postfilarial elephantiasis.[42]

All lesions of aspergillosis are commoner in the immunosuppressed, and the outcome follows the progress of the immune status. In general, however, the infection is often rapidly fatal due to visceral involvement.[1,10,21] Patients receiving corticosteroid therapy appear to be particularly susceptible to the development of cutaneous aspergillosis.[4,21] A recently published review of factors influencing patient outcome in primary cutaneous aspergillosis revealed an 18.5% rate of dissemination and a mortality of 31.5% among susceptible immunocompromised individuals.[36]

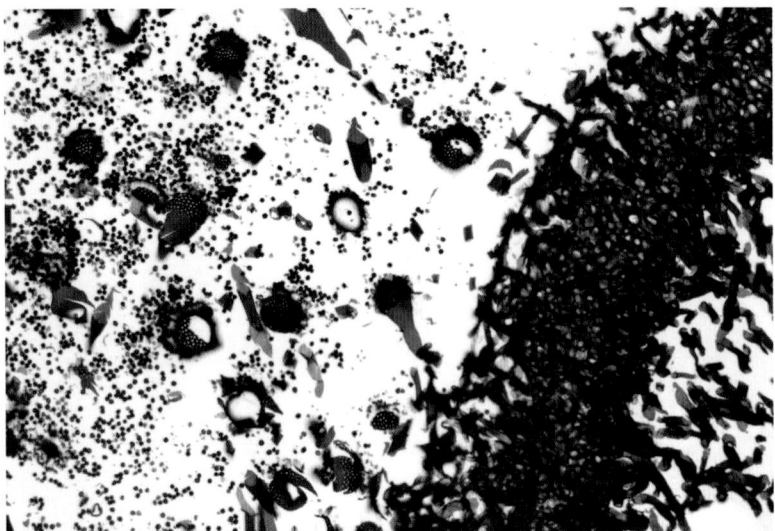

Fig. 18.304
Aspergillosis: the fruiting head (aspergillum) as shown in this picture is formed when the fungus is exposed to air. It is not usually seen in the tissues. Methenamine silver stain. By courtesy of R. Margolis, MD, St Elizabeth's Medical Center, Boston, USA.

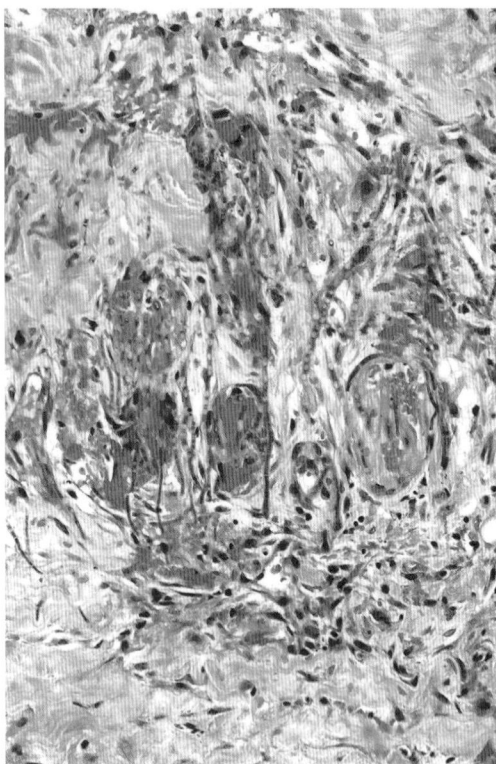

Fig. 18.305
Aspergillosis: high-power view showing vascular occlusion and fungal hyphae.

Pathogenesis and histologic features

Aspergillus is ubiquitous in the environment and inhabits soil and organic debris so that pulmonary lesions are found in farmers and gardeners (*Fig. 18.304*). It can contaminate grain and affect birds. It is often present in public buildings, including hospitals, due to contamination of air vents and central heating plants by bird droppings. Despite the wide distribution of the fungus, infection usually requires previous immunosuppression, as in patients receiving corticosteroids or who have lymphoma or leukemia. The host response to the mycelial component of the infection is the neutrophil, whereas the conidia forms are phagocytosed and killed by macrophages. Both lines of cellular response need to be deficient for the infection to become progressive. The production of fungal toxins also assists the establishment of infection.[2,3]

In the skin, the lesions form abscesses in the dermis, with central necrosis and pus, surrounded by granulomata.[16] Eosinophils are sometimes numerous.[18] The epidermis may occasionally exhibit pseudoepitheliomatous hyperplasia.[18,24] The fungal elements, most commonly of *A. fumigatus*, are found in the necrotic center of the lesion. *A. flavus*, *A. niger*, *A. glaucus*, *A. versicolor*, *A. nidulans*, *A. terreus*, and *A. tamarii* represent additional etiological species.[1,4,24,26,28,41–44] The infection may extend into the subcutis.[40] Exceptionally, subcutaneous involvement may closely mimic pancreatic or gouty panniculitis, a phenomenon which has been ascribed to lipase production by the fungus.[45]

In cases of hematogenous spread, fungal hyphae may be identified within the lumen of thrombosed dermal blood vessels.[20,46] The fungus is recognized by its uniform septate branching and radiating hyphae (with an arboreal growth pattern), with branches being equal in thickness (dichotomous) and at 45° (*Figs 18.305* and *18.306*).[2,47] The hyphae are often not seen easily with H&E, but are well demonstrated by a silver stain, such as Gomori or Grocott.

Differential diagnosis

The fungus must be distinguished from other branching fungal infections, including the agents of hyalohyphomycosis (e.g., *Fusarium* spp., *Pseudoallescheria boydii*, *Acremonium* spp.) and the Zygomycetes. Distinction from the former, however, is not possible in routine histopathological sections, while the latter tend to stain well with H&E, consist of broader, twisted hyphae of variable thickness, and exhibit right angle branching. Diagnosis usually requires culture of the organism, but the finding of a fruiting head in tissue is confirmatory. Alternatively, a specific immunofluorescent antibody test, immunohistochemistry, or PCR techniques can be employed.[2,47]

Hyalohyphomycosis

Clinical features

Hyalohyphomycosis is the generic term applied to fungal tissue infections caused by nondematiaceous, hyaline septate hyphal organisms.[1–3] It generally does not encompass infections due to *Aspergillus* spp. and *Penicillium* spp., which are considered separately in this chapter. Members of the class Zygomycetes are specifically excluded from this category. The causative agents of hyalohyphomycosis include *Fusarium* spp., *Pseudoallescheria boydii* (and its asexual form, *Scedosporium apiospermum*), *Acremonium* spp., *Paecillomyces* spp., *Trichoderma* spp., *Scopulariopsis brevicaulis*.[1–3] Hyalohyphomycosis has gained increasing relevance among immunosuppressed organ transplant recipients and patients with underlying hematological malignancies.[3–5] A number of the aforementioned organisms also account for a small proportion of cases of onychomycosis.[6,7]

Fusarium species (plant molds) are of increasing importance, particularly in immunosuppressed patients in whom they represent the second most common pathogenic mold.[4,8–16] The most frequently encountered *Fusarium* species include *F. solani*, *F. oxysporum*, and *F. moniliforme*.[3,13] Infections with *F. veticillioides*, *F. petroliphilum*, and *F. proliferatum* have also been reported.[3,17,18] Patients can present with localized skin or soft tissue lesions, nail involvement, sinus infection, pulmonary fusariosis, or with disseminated disease.[1–3,9,13,15,19] Risk factors for localized disease include trauma, burns, foreign bodies, stasis ulceration, penetrating plant injury, or iatrogenic cutaneous portals of entry.[13,18,20,21] Systemic involvement occurs particularly in the setting of hematological malignancy and neutropenia, GVHD and corticosteroid therapy.[8,9,12,13,15] Ulcerated, ecthyma-like, targetoid, or violaceous macular skin lesions may occur, while subcutaneous involvement manifests as multiple nodules.[13,22–27] One unusual case presented initially with vesicular lesions following stem cell transplantation.[28] In one study, superficial intertrigo-like skin lesions or nail involvement abnormalities due to colonization by *Fusarium* spp. was identified as a risk factor for the subsequent evolution of invasive fusariosis among high-risk patients with underlying hematological diseases.[29] The reported mortality of disseminated fusariosis in immunocompromised hosts ranges from 50% to 80%.[13,15,16,30]

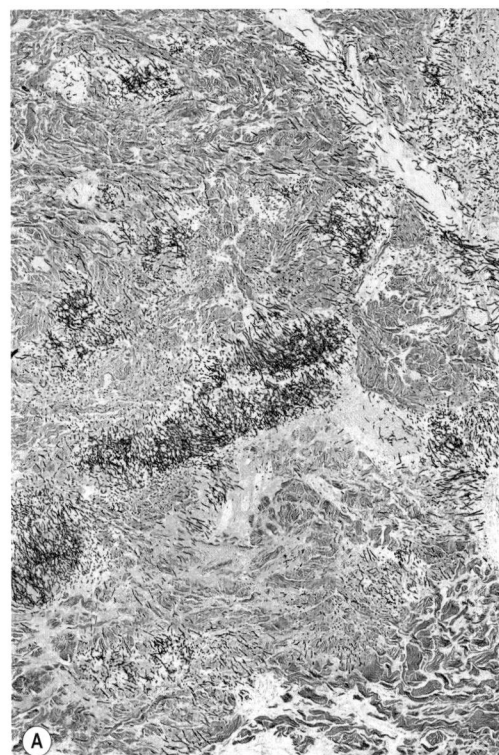

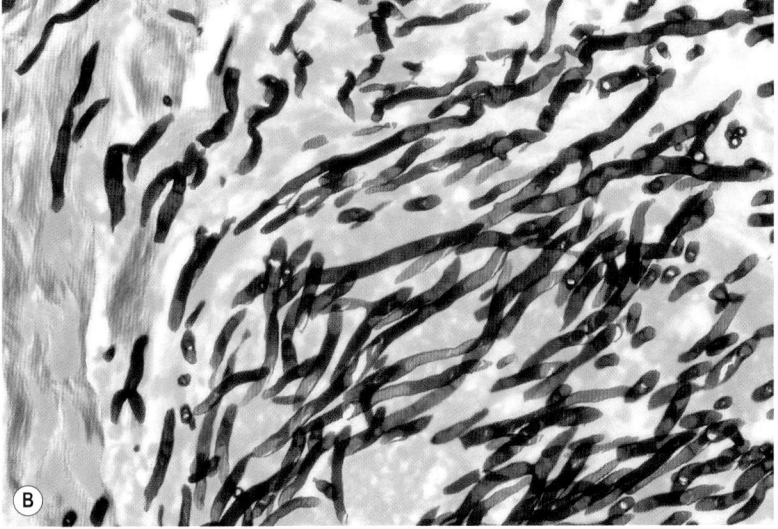

Fig. 18.306
Aspergillosis: (**A**) low-power view showing the massive infection and innumerable fungi emanating from the cutaneous vessels; (**B**) the hyphae are septate and branch at 45° (methenamine silver).

P. boydii and its asexual form, *S. apiospermum*, are also important causes of infection in the immunosuppressed, especially following solid organ transplantation and in the context of hematological disease.[31–37] Diabetes mellitus and HIV/AIDS are further risk factors.[3] Patients may also develop localized disease in the skin and subcutaneous fat including mycetoma.[34,36] Clinical features in a large series of patients following organ transplantation included disseminated disease, skin lesions, lung disease, endophthalmitis, meningitis, brain abscess, mycotic aneurysm, and sinusitis.[33] A sporotrichoid presentation has been described.[31]

Acremonium spp. may be associated with onychomycosis, keratitis, infection of peritoneal dialysis fistulae, intracranial infections, prosthetic valve endocarditis, osteomyelitis, and mycetoma.[2,7,38] Risk factors for invasive *Acremonium* infection include penetrating wounds, intravascular catheters, and underlying immunosuppression.[39] Erythema nodosum-like tender subcutaneous nodules may occur on the legs, while multiple cutaneous and subcutaneous lesions are a feature of skin involvement as part of disseminated *Acremonium* infection in immunosuppressed patients, including organ transplant recipients.[40,41] Localized infection of skin of the lower limb of an obese patient has been reported.[39]

A similar spectrum of disease may be encountered as a result of infection with *Paecilomyces* spp.[2,42]

Histologic features

The various fungal genera responsible for hyalohyphomycosis cannot be distinguished from one another in routine histologic sections.[43] More precise identification of the etiological agent, therefore, is reliant on fungal culture results and more recently, pan-fungal PCR involving amplification of among others, the internal transcribed spacer region.[18] The latter molecular technique may also be applied to formalin-fixed, paraffin-embedded tissue samples. Routine histochemical stains such as PAS and methenamine silver aid in highlighting the contours of the hyphae and confirming the presence of septation.[43]

The histologic reaction in fusariosis varies from granulomatous to suppurative.[44] In patients with disseminated disease, vascular involvement similar to aspergillosis is seen, including thrombosis of the involved vessels (*Figs 18.307* and *18.308*). The fungi present as hyaline, branching, septate hyphae measuring 3–8 μm in width.[19] In contrast to *Aspergillus*, the hyphae branch irregularly, varying from acute-angled through to 90°.[44] *Fusarium* spp. are capable of sporulating in tissues. Consequently, yeast-like structures can occasionally be seen in association with the hyphae.[43] *Fusarium* sporodochia may rarely be encountered on infected traumatic cutaneous wounds.[45]

In immunosuppressed patients, *P. boydii* is most often encountered as an angioinvasive lesion similar to aspergillosis. The hyphae are septate, branching, hyaline, and measure 2–5 μm in width.[46] They are histologically indistinguishable from *Aspergillus* spp. (*Figs 18.309* and *18.310*).

Differential diagnosis

Infection with *Aspergillus* spp. constitutes the main differential diagnosis, as already alluded to above. Invasive candidiasis, which also has a propensity to occur in immunosuppressed and neutropenic patients and exhibits similar vascular involvement, can potentially be confused with hyalohyphomycosis in tissue sections, as the masses of elongated, overlapping pseudohyphae in the former can create the impression of branching. The pseudohyphae of *Candida* spp., however, are more slender, lack septation, and are accompanied by yeast forms measuring 3–5 μm in diameter.[43]

The condition should also be distinguished from mucormycosis, another infection characterized by pronounced vascular invasion in susceptible individuals. The organisms associated with mucormycosis, however, are often better visualized in H&E-stained sections than those of hyalohyphomycosis, and comprise broader, twisted hyphae of variable thickness (7–15 μm or more in width), with right angle branching.[47] Potential confusion with mucormycosis may nevertheless arise when the hyphae of hyalohyphomycotic species swell and assume a globose appearance.[43] Correct identification of the causative organism, either by culture or with the aid of molecular mycology techniques, therefore, remains the final arbiter; this has implications for correct treatment.[1–3]

Blastomycosis

Clinical features

Blastomycosis (North American blastomycosis) is caused by *Blastomyces dermatitidis*. Although the soil is generally regarded as the usual habitat of this fungus, it probably also exists in wood and bird droppings. The infection was originally thought to be restricted to North America, but cases were subsequently reported in South America, Africa, India, and Israel.[1–4] The organism is endemic in the states bordering the Mississippi and Ohio rivers, the Great Lakes, and the St. Lawrence Seaway.[1,4–6] It has not yet presented as an endogenous disease in Europe or the Far East. Blastomycosis occurs most often in young to middle-aged adults and in males more frequently than in females.[5,7] Although uncommon, the disease has been recorded in the pediatric population.[8] The infection is most commonly acquired via the lungs after inhalation of airborne conidia, which occurs when moist soil

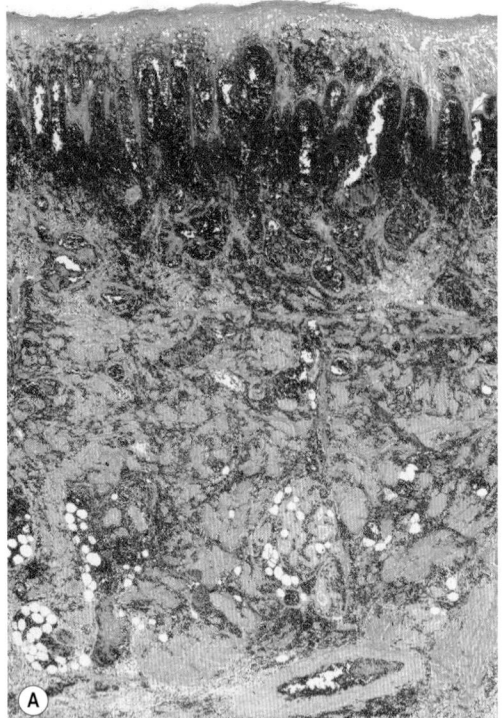

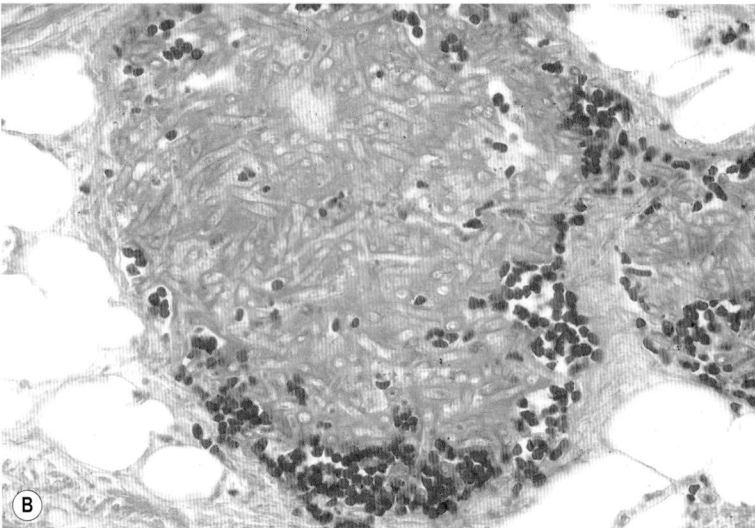

Fig. 18.307
Fusarium spp.: (**A**) low-power view showing epidermal infarction and massive hemorrhage; (**B**) note the thrombosed vessel containing numerous hyphae. By courtesy of A. Zembowitz, MD, Massachusetts General Hospital, Boston, USA.

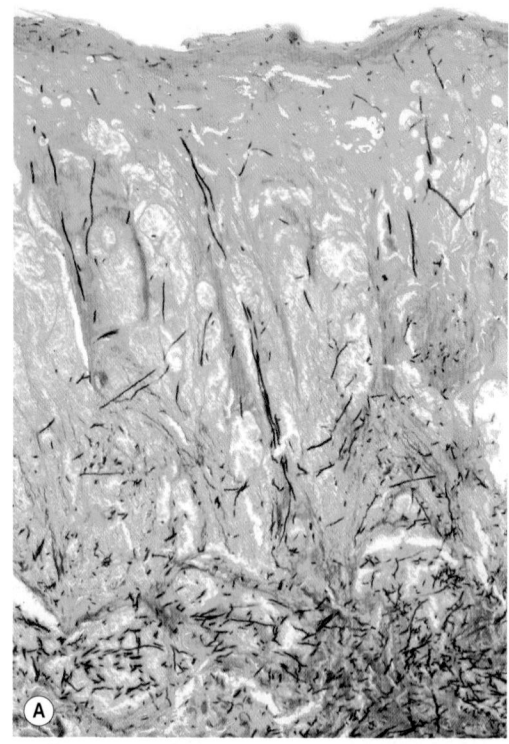

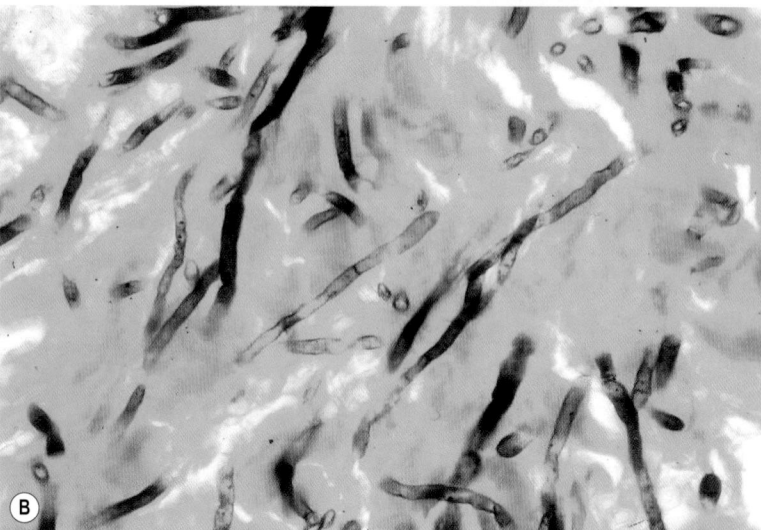

Fig. 18.308
Fusarium spp.: (**A**) hyphae extend from the deep dermis to the epidermis; (**B**) note the septa (methenamine silver). By courtesy of A. Zembowicz, MD, Massachusetts General Hospital, Boston, USA.

and organic debris containing the mycelia are disturbed.[1,4,5,9] There are three clinical forms of the disease: pulmonary, disseminated, and primary cutaneous blastomycosis.

There is an incubation period of 33–44 days before the onset of respiratory symptoms, which are usually insidious. An acute pneumonic picture occurs, with potential progression to acute respiratory distress syndrome. The infection may also closely resemble tuberculosis both clinically and radiologically. Blastomycosis is not uncommonly associated with subclinical infection.[1,4,10] In contrast to many of the other deep fungal infections mentioned in this chapter, blastomycosis most often develops in previously healthy hosts.[7] A number of cases have nevertheless been documented in HIV-infected individuals, and although blastomycosis is not regarded as an AIDS-defining infection, certain clinical differences exist.[11,12] CNS involvement is said to occur in 46% of patients, i.e., 5–10 times more frequently than in the HIV-negative population. Furthermore, the estimated mortality rate is five times that of non-HIV-infected patients with blastomycosis (54% vs. less than 10%).[12] Although uncommon, the condition has been

documented in iatrogenically immunosuppressed solid organ transplant recipients, in whom opportunistic co-infections may occur.[13,14] In this clinical context, overall mortality may be as high as 67% if the pneumonia is complicated by acute respiratory distress syndrome.[14]

The skin – in addition to bone, joints, CNS, and the genitourinary tract (prostatitis and epididymo-orchitis) – is usually involved following dissemination of a pulmonary infection.[13,15] The lesions may be single or multiple and may affect any part of the body. The skin lesion starts as a papule, but gradually spreads and becomes an ulcerated and crusted, verrucous nodule or ulcerated plaque, with a serpiginous swollen red border (*Fig. 18.311*). This border extends, while the center may heal with scarring. Exuding pus is present beneath the peripheral crust. Rarely, a widespread pustular eruption may occur.[16] These protean manifestations may lead to clinical confusion with keratoacanthoma, pyoderma gangrenosum, or panniculitis.[10,17]

Occasionally, primary cutaneous blastomycosis occurs 1–2 weeks after inoculation.[18–20] This lesion starts as a pustule, which ulcerates superficially (chancre) and is associated with regional lymphadenitis, lymphadenopathy,

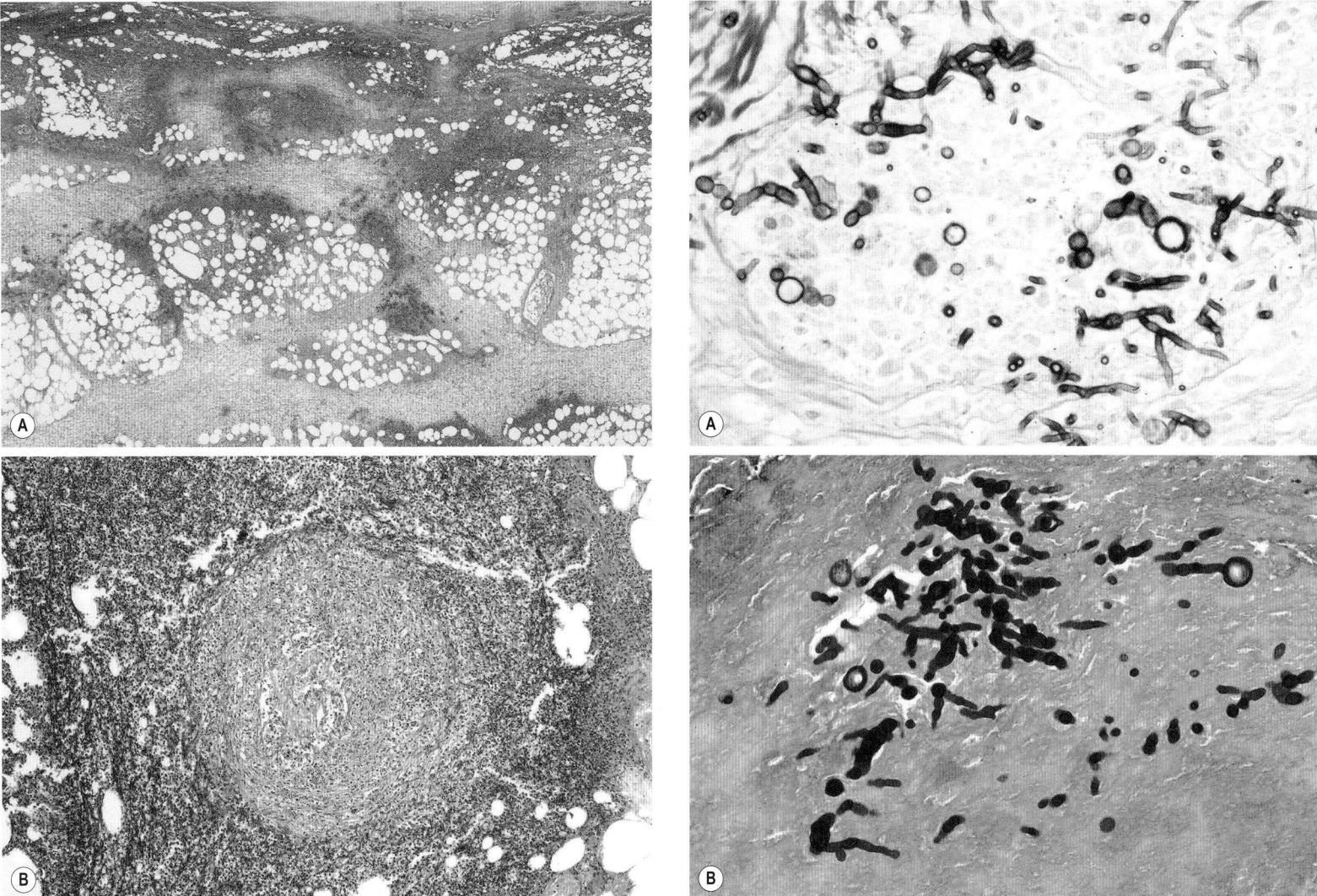

Fig. 18.309
Pseudallescheria boydii: (**A**) low-power view showing massive dermal inflammatory changes; (**B**) this field shows an inflamed and thrombosed vessel.

Fig. 18.310
Pseudallescheria boydii: (**A**) silver stain showing hyphae with chlamydoconidia; (**B**) periodic acid-Schiff stain.

and lymphangitic skin nodules, similar to sporotrichosis. Verrucous or fungating skin lesions are sometimes encountered.[21,22] The condition may rarely present with isolated infection of the perianal skin.[23] Chronic disseminated cutaneous blastomycosis has also been reported.[24]

Pathogenesis and histologic features

B. dermatitidis is a thermally dimorphic fungus which exists in the yeast phase at 37°C in tissues. It grows as a mycelial form at 25°C. The yeasts are round, usually 8–15 μm, but occasionally up to 30 μm across, and have a refractile thick cell wall.[8] They are multinucleate and produce single buds, which have a broad base.[4,15,25] Infections with large yeast forms measuring 30–35 μm in diameter are an exceedingly uncommon occurrence.[26] Microforms may also be encountered.[25] The yeast forms of *B. dermatitidis* possess an adhesion-promoting protein termed WI-1 adhesin, which is thought to play a crucial pathogenetic role.[27]

The histologic features of blastomycosis include, in the early stages, a predominantly neutrophil infiltrate, and many organisms are seen. Subsequently, a granulomatous reaction develops in which multinucleate giant cells are numerous and neutrophils are still plentiful. The overlying epidermis shows striking pseudoepitheliomatous hyperplasia (especially in verrucous lesions), often containing numerous microabscesses (*Figs 18.312* and *18.313*).[15,25] The *Blastomyces* organism is seen within giant cells and also free in the connective tissue (*Fig. 18.314*). A neutrophilic host response predominates in immunocompromised patients and those with a pustular form of the infection, emphasizing the need for both a high index of suspicion

and a panel of histochemical stains for infective microorganisms.[25] Recognition of the fungi is facilitated by the use of PAS or methenamine silver stains (*Fig. 18.315*). The organisms also stain with Congo red.[28]

Differential diagnosis

Distinction from other deep cutaneous fungal infections showing similar histologic features including chromoblastomycosis, coccidioidomycosis, paracoccidioidomycosis, and sporotrichosis rests on the absence of pigment and the presence of a characteristic multinucleate yeast form with single broad-based buds. In situ hybridization may provide a prompt diagnosis in those cases where tissue cultures are not obtained.[29]

Paracoccidioidomycosis

Clinical features

Paracoccidioidomycosis (South American blastomycosis) is caused by *Paracoccidioides brasiliensis* and occurs in Central and South America, particularly Brazil. It is the most prevalent systemic mycosis in Latin America. It affects adult males much more commonly than females, usually in rural areas and more so among farmers.[1–6] Rare cases have nevertheless been reported outside of this geographic location (e.g., due to increased immigration), with some individuals only developing clinical manifestations several years after leaving an endemic area.[1,4,7,8] The overwhelming male predominance of the infection was highlighted in a recent review of 93 cases from

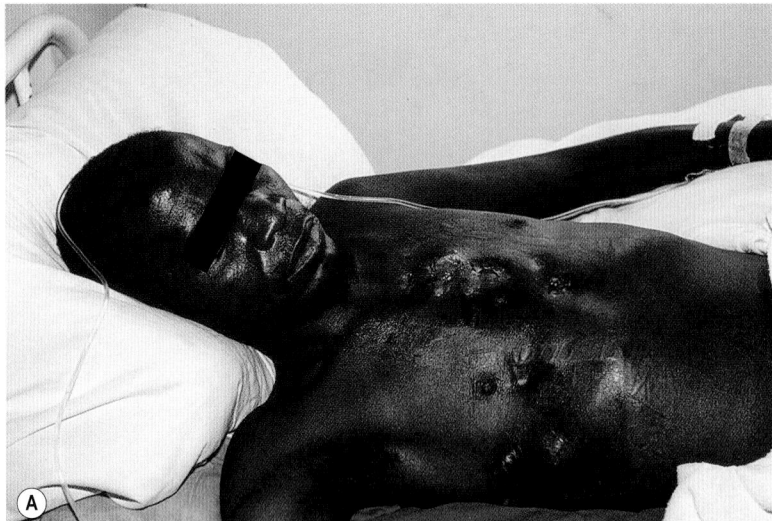

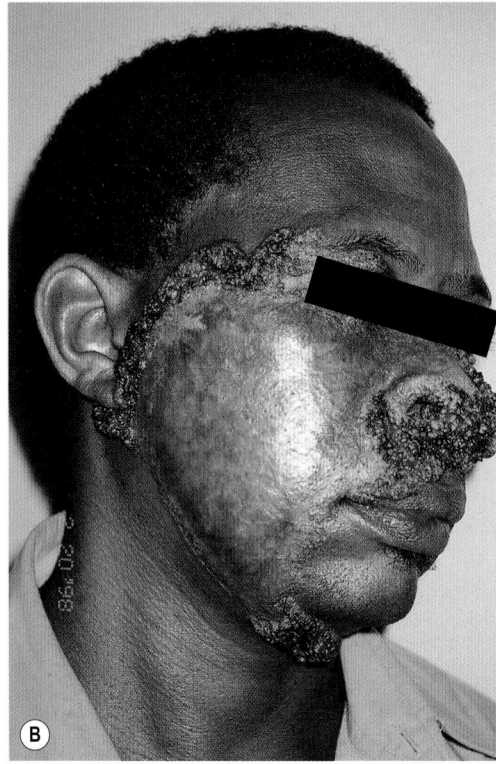

Fig. 18.311
Blastomycosis: (**A**) numerous ulcerated and crusted nodules are visible on the chest; the patient had systemic involvement. (**B**) There is severe facial involvement. Note the sepiginous border. (**A**) By courtesy of W. Weir, MD, Coppetts Wood Hospital, London, UK; (**B**) by courtesy of N.C. Dlova, MD, Nelson R. Mandela School of Medicine, University of KwaZulu-Natal, South Africa.

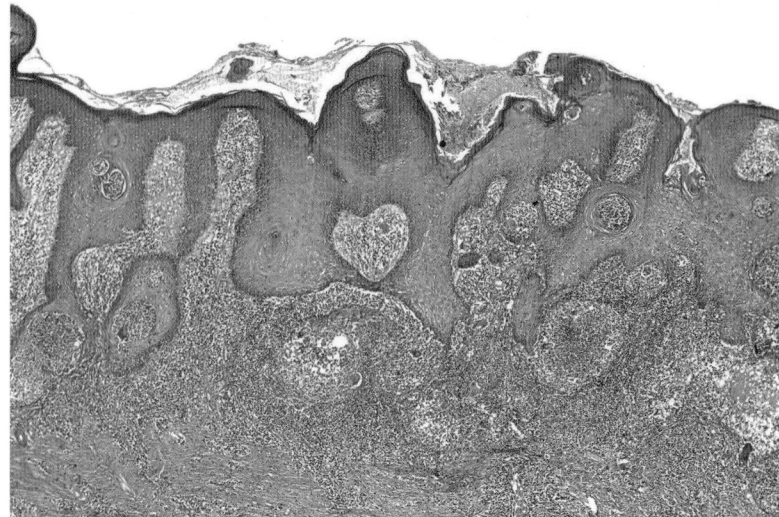

Fig. 18.312
Blastomycosis: there is massive pseudoepitheliomatous hyperplasia. Dermal abscesses and giant cells are evident.

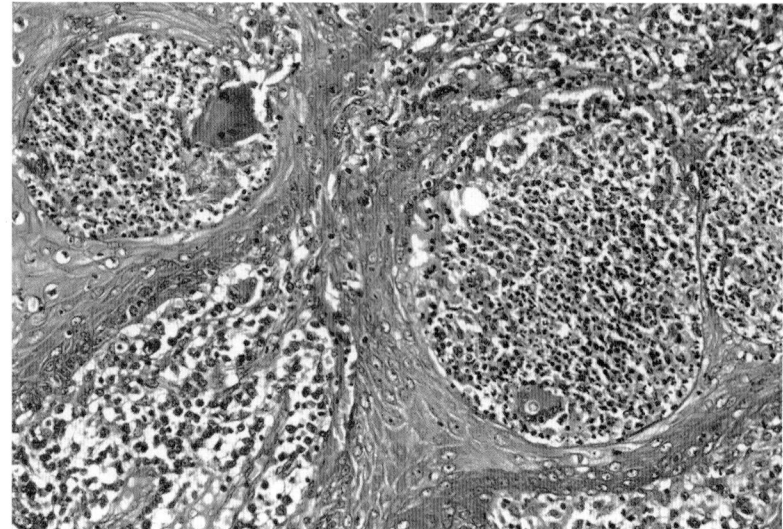

Fig. 18.313
Blastomycosis: close-up view showing mixed granulomatous and suppurative inflammation.

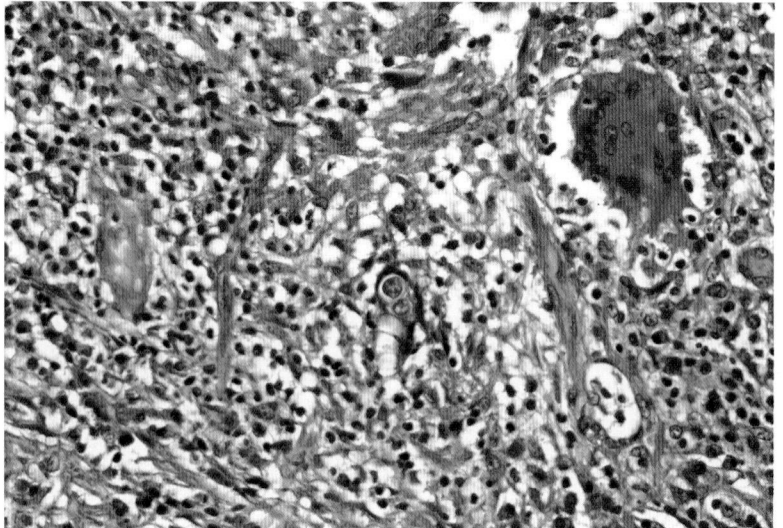

Fig. 18.314
Blastomycosis: note the characteristic broad-based budding and multiple nuclei.

Mexico.[9] One historic *in vitro* study revealed that 17β-estradiol inhibits or delays the transition of the fungus from its mycelial or conidial forms into pathogenic yeasts, thereby offering a plausible explanation for the relative rarity of the disease among women.[10–12] Only 3% to 5% of cases occur in children and adolescents, who may present with acute or subacute disease.[4,13]

The natural habitat of the fungus remains an enigma.[14,15] Natural infections have nevertheless been confirmed in nine-banded armadillos.[14] It is assumed to be contracted via inhalation of conidia from soil contamination. The most common initial presentation is with pulmonary disease, which cavitates in 35% of cases.[1,3] Primary lung infection, however, is often clinically silent. Involvement of the mucocutaneous junction in the nose and mouth occurs in approximately 65% of patients, whereas other skin sites are affected in only around 12% of cases.[16] The most common other site is the face, where lesions may be ulcerative, verrucous, or crusted nodules.[4]

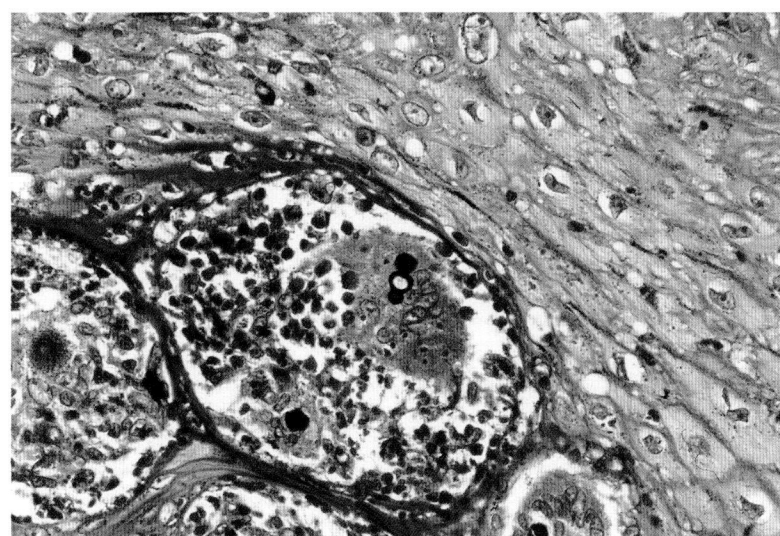

Fig. 18.315
Blastomycosis: silver stain showing broad-based budding.

Sarcoid-like facial lesions have also been described.[17] Disseminated extrafacial lesions include erythematous or necrotic papules, pustules, ulcerated plaques, or even large nodules.[18–23] Involvement of the external genitalia is exceptional.[20,24] Primary lesions of the skin are very rare.[5,13]

Paracoccidioidomycosis is relatively uncommon in patients infected with HIV infection.[8,19,25] A possible explanation for this is the fact that the disease tends to occur only in patients with advanced HIV/AIDS who are not receiving trimethoprim-sulfamethoxazole prophylaxis for *P. jiroveci* pneumonia, since this drug is also effective against *P. brasiliensis*.[8] It has also been suggested that HIV/AIDS is a largely urban disease, whereas paracoccidioidomycosis tends to occur in more rural communities; the condition has nevertheless been documented occur among HIV-positive patients in endemic areas.[13,25] The infection carries a 30% to 67% mortality in HIV/AIDS patients.[26,27] Paracoccidioidomycosis has also been reported in patients with underlying Hodgkin lymphoma, non-Hodgkin lymphoma, or visceral neoplasms.[18,28]

There have been relatively recent reports of infection due to *P. lutzii* in the Midwest and Northern regions of Brazil. The clinical and epidemiological aspects of the aforementioned infection, however, have yet to be fully elucidated.[5,29]

Pathogenesis and histologic features

The fungus *P. brasiliensis* is morphologically similar to *B. dermatitidis*, but *P. brasiliensis* has a thinner cell wall with a double contour appearance and produces multiple, narrow-based buds, said to resemble a 'pilot's wheel'.[1] Mycelia from the dimorphic fungus produce conidia, which when inhaled into the lungs transform into pathogenic yeast forms.[12] Although a genetic susceptibility to infection is suspected, no specific HLA antigen association has been confirmed thus far.[12,30] Susceptible individuals may have a functionally deficient neutrophil response to the organism.[31]

The histologic reaction to the infection in the skin resembles that of blastomycosis in that it is characterized by suppurative and granulomatous inflammation.[10,13,31–33] Neutrophilic abscesses superimposed on pseudoepitheliomatous hyperplasia are seen. Eosinophils may be present in a high proportion of cases. Tuberculoid granulomas are encountered occasionally (*Fig. 18.316*).[17,34] The budding yeast form is seen most often within multinucleate giant cells. The variably sized yeasts measure 2–20 μm in diameter, whereas the 'pilot's wheel' has a diameter of up to 60 μm.[10,13]

The 'pilot's wheel' appearance is diagnostic; however, if this is not seen, isolation of the organism *in vitro* is necessary to confirm the diagnosis. Mucosal reactions are similar to those seen in the skin. Transepidermal (transepithelial) elimination of the microorganism in association with spongiosis, microvesiculation, and microabscesses is commonly present.[33] Scarring is a feature of older lesions. A case with associated necrotizing granulomatous arteritis has been reported.[22] A PCR method for diagnostic

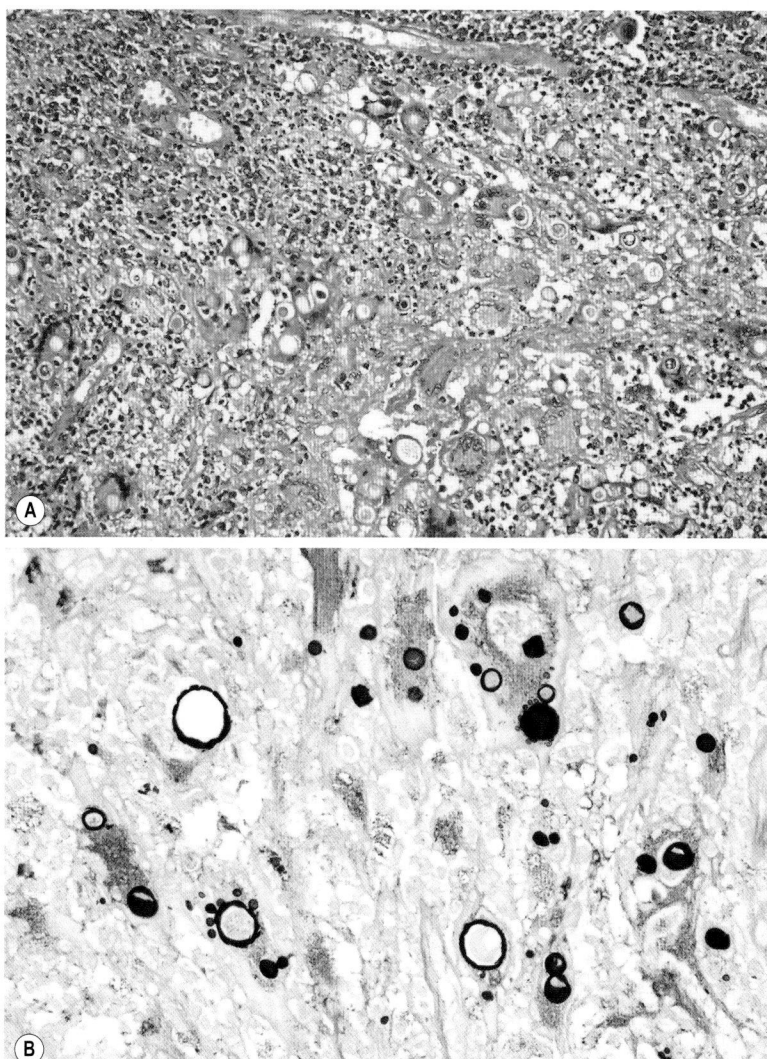

Fig. 18.316
Paracoccidioidomycosis: (**A**) numerous fungi are seen surrounded by granulomatous inflammation; (**B**) typical 'pilot's wheel' budding is evident (methenamine silver). By courtesy of W. Robles, MD, Institute of Dermatology, London, UK.

confirmation of the infection in paraffin-embedded tissue specimens has been described.[35] A real-time PCR method for rapid detection of the organisms in tissue biopsies also exists.[7]

Differential diagnosis

Distinction from blastomycosis can be difficult, but *P. brasiliensis* does not have the multiple nuclei of *B. dermatitidis* and the budding pattern is quite different. *Cryptococcus* can show a similar variation in yeast size, but has its own characteristic mucicarmine-positive mucinous capsule and produces single buds.[10,13]

Coccidioidomycosis

Clinical features

Coccidioidomycosis is a virulent fungal infection caused by two etiological species: *Coccidioides immitis*, which is found in its mycelial form in the soil of desert regions of the southwestern United States (especially California and the Lower Sonoran Life Zone), and *C. posadasii*, which is endemic in parts of northwest Mexico, arid and semi-arid regions of Central and South America, as well as Arizona and Utah.[1–7] Primary infection occurs by inhalation of airborne arthroconidia in dust and, in view of increased tourism in endemic areas, is becoming more common.[1,8] A significant increase in the

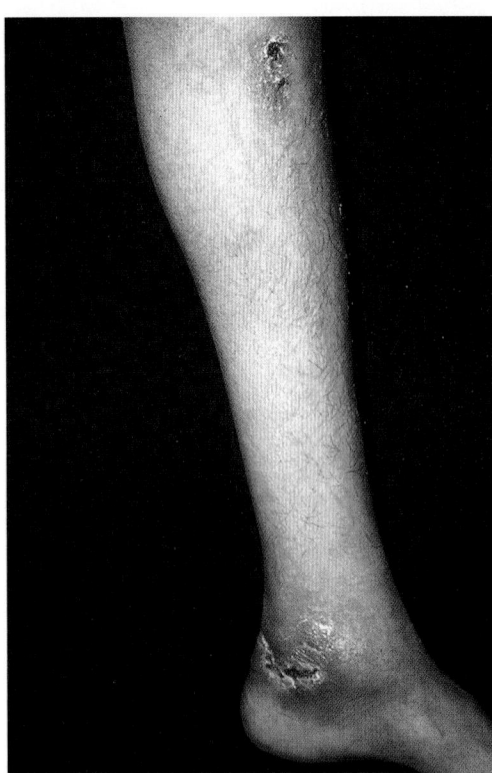

Fig. 18.317
Coccidioidomycosis: ulcerated nodules are present on the knee and ankle. By courtesy of R. Arenas, MD, and J.C. Salas, MD, Monterrey, Mexico.

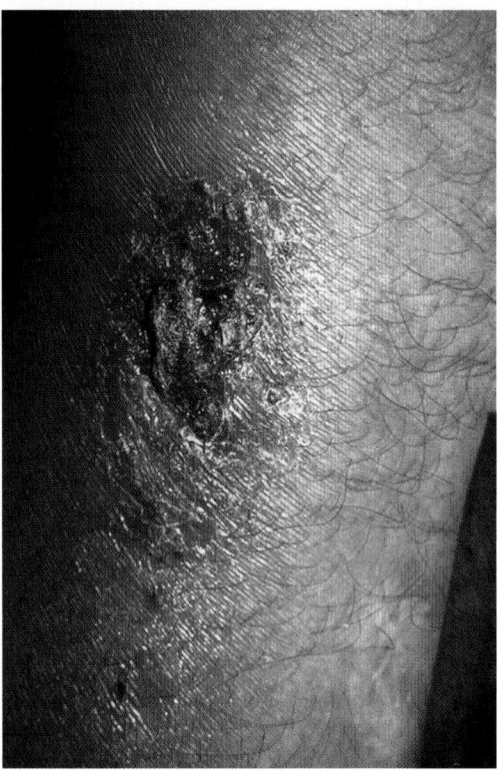

Fig. 18.318
Coccidioidomycosis: there is a crusted plaque on the arm. By courtesy of R. Arenas, MD, and J.C. Salas, MD, Monterrey, Mexico.

incidence of this infection has been observed in California and elsewhere since the early 1990s.[1,9,10] In endemic regions, primary coccidiodal pneumonia may account for as many as 29% of all cases of community-acquired pneumonia.[4] The diagnosis may be overlooked in the absence of a detailed travel history in patients presenting with symptomatic disease after returning to nonendemic areas.[11] In those in whom symptoms (usually influenza-like) do develop, coccidioidomycosis is usually a self-limiting disease.[12,13] Most episodes, however, are asymptomatic.[9,13,14] It may also develop in the immunosuppressed, including patients with HIV/AIDS.[9,15,16] Sixty percent of patients with pulmonary infection remain asymptomatic.[8] Symptomatic lung involvement is encountered in the remaining 40% and may progress to cavitating, chronic progressive pneumonia, and miliary pulmonary disease.[8,14] Pleural effusion, empyema, and acute respiratory distress syndrome may also occur.[8] Chronic infection develops in 3% to 5% of patients.[4]

Cutaneous lesions are uncommon and develop almost invariably as a result of the rare dissemination from pulmonary lesions; this occurs in approximately 5% of patients.[16–18] Dissemination occurs more often in blacks, Filipinos, Hispanics, and native Americans and shows a slight male preponderance.[12,19] There is also an increased risk in the immunosuppressed, including those with diabetes mellitus or who are receiving corticosteroids.[3] The lesions include papulonodules, papulopustules, granulomatous plaques, and subcutaneous masses (*Figs 18.317* and *18.318*).[18,20,21] Sinus tracts complicating osteomyelitis or infection of adjacent joints or lymph nodes may also be seen.[12,21] Although generally multiple, solitary nodular presentation has been rarely described.[22] The central face, in particular the nasolabial fold, is most often affected.[14,23] Involvement of the face may be indicative of a propensity to develop meningitis.[19]

Disseminated lesions may also affect bone, joints, lymph nodes, pericardium, peritoneum, skeletal muscle, retropharyngeal space, and CNS.[3,13,14] In the immunosuppressed this may be as a consequence of reactivation of previously quiescent foci.[14] These secondary lesions are sometimes seen in areas of minor trauma, often, for example, on the face. They appear as verrucous plaques and nodules with crusting and ulceration. Sinus tracts may extend from the primary lung lesion through the chest wall.[21] Involvement of the nasal tip may mimic lupus pernio.[24] Hypercalcemia is a rare

complication of systemic disease. Hemophagocytic lymphohistiocytosis has also been reported.[25]

The rare primary lesions in the skin occur following inoculation, usually in farmers, laboratory workers, nurses, and morticians.[14,26] These lesions are chancriform and there is regional lymphadenopathy. Sometimes, sporotrichoid features are evident. Toxic erythema (exanthem), erythema nodosum, and erythema multiforme may occur as hypersensitivity reactions during systemic infection.[2,14] The combination of erythema nodosum or erythema multiforme with arthritis and arthralgia is known as 'valley fever'.[12] Systemic eosinophilia may be evident. Additional reactive cutaneous manifestations include interstitial granulomatous dermatitis and Sweet syndrome.[2,6] A case with associated subcorneal pustular dermatosis has also been reported.[27]

Histologic features

C. immitis and *C. posadasii* are dimorphic fungi, which in tissues appear as doubly refractile spherules 10–100 μm in diameter containing multiple endospores (2–5 μm) that increase in size as the lesions mature.[3,28] The incubation period ranges from 1 to 4 weeks.[2,14] Diagnosis may be aided by the coccidioidin skin test, enzyme immunoassay (complement fixation test), or PCR techniques.[1,12,29–31] The histology resembles North American blastomycosis in that there is a combination of suppuration with pseudo-epitheliomatous hyperplasia and an associated dermal perivascular infiltrate of neutrophils, eosinophils, plasma cells, histiocytes, and giant cells (*Figs 18.319–18.321*).[1,18,28] Eosinophil abscesses may be present and flame figures have been described.[11] Interstitial granulomatous dermatitis has also been reported.[2,32]

The spherules (sporangia) are seen mixed with this inflammatory infiltrate and occasionally are present in giant cells. They are demonstrated best by methenamine silver techniques. The endospores are PAS positive, but the spherules are negative. The fungi show autofluorescence under ultraviolet light and may be stained with Congo red.[33] They are typically very difficult to find and may often only be demonstrated after examining numerous sections. The spherules increase in size with the formation of numerous endospores. Following rupture into the tissues, each endospore has the

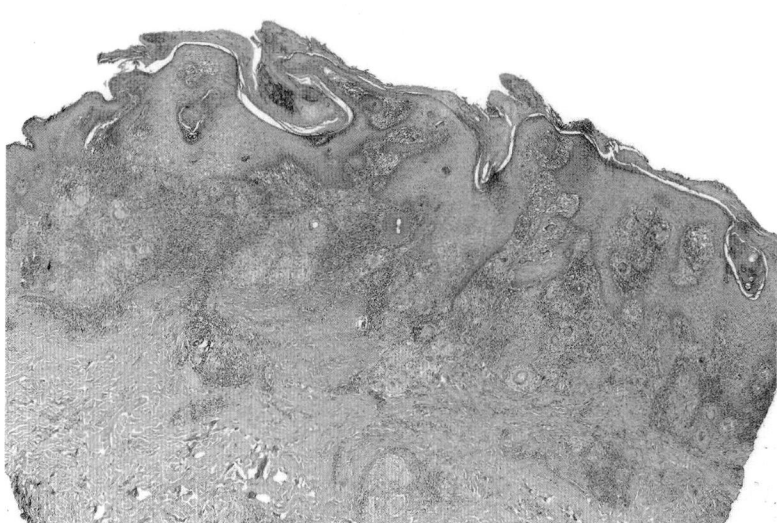

Fig. 18.319
Coccidioidomycosis: there is pseudoepitheliomatous hyperplasia and granulomatous dermal inflammation. By courtesy of J. Cohen, MD, Dermatopathology Laboratory, Tucson, USA.

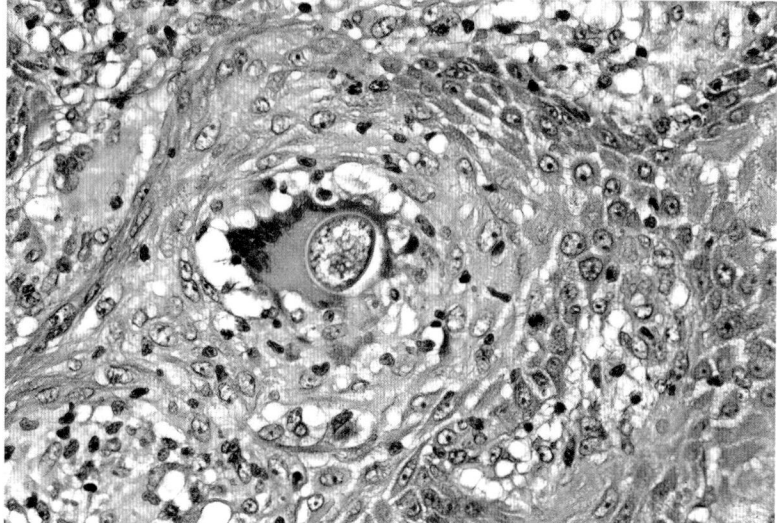

Fig. 18.320
Coccidioidomycosis: high-power view of a spherule within a multinucleate giant cell. By courtesy of J. Cohen, MD, Dermatopathology Laboratory, Tucson, USA.

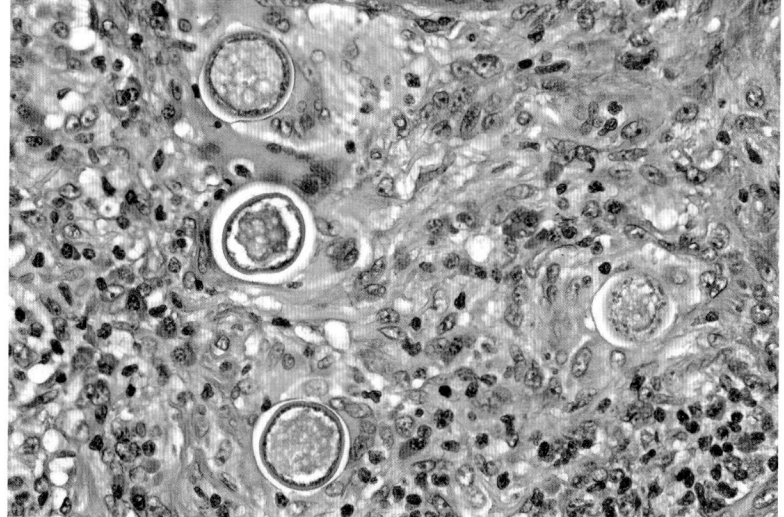

Fig. 18.321
Coccidioidomycosis: multiple spherules are present with surrounding chronic inflammation. By courtesy of J. Cohen, MD, Dermatopathology Laboratory, Tucson, USA.

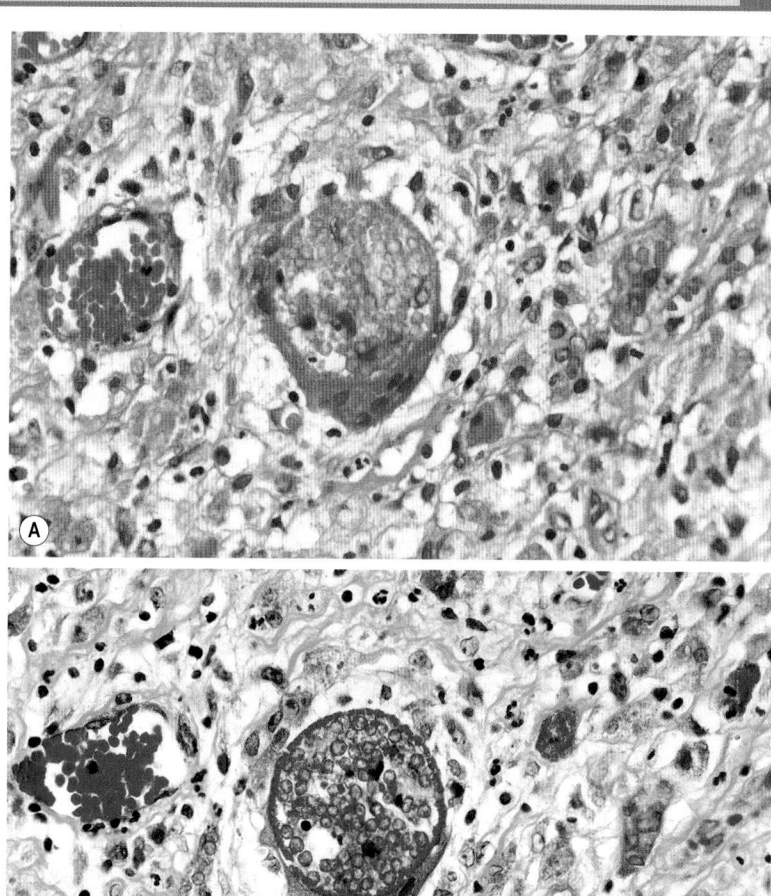

Fig. 18.322
(A, B) Myospherulosis: cutaneous lesions are exceptionally rare. This 'cystic' structure contains altered erythrocytes. The condition was originally recognized following the use of antibiotics – in this example, tetracycline ointment for an ear infection. (B) Masson trichrome. By courtesy of the late M.S.R. Hutt, MD, St Thomas' Hospital, London, UK.

capacity to develop into a spherule, therefore repeating the growth cycle in the host.[17] In situ hybridization or PCR may facilitate prompt confirmation of the diagnosis on paraffin-embedded skin biopsy material, and aids in the distinction from other deep fungal infections.[34,35]

Differential diagnosis

Diagnosis depends on the demonstration of spherules with endospores. Fragments of spore or immature forms cannot be distinguished from blastomycosis or paracoccidioidomycosis. Fungal culture or in situ hybridization studies are useful in such cases. When spherules and endospores are present rhinosporidiosis should also be considered, although the clinical and histologic features are usually different. The spherules and endospores of rhinosporidiosis are much larger than those of coccidioidomycosis.[28] Distinction from tuberculosis verrucosa cutis and halogenoderma may sometimes be necessary.[20] Aggregates of altered red blood cells in myospherulosis may mimic *Coccidioides* spp. (*Fig. 18.322*).[36]

Cryptococcosis

Clinical features

Cryptococcus neoformans var. *neoformans* causes systemic infections sporadically throughout the world because it is abundant in soil, fruits, and

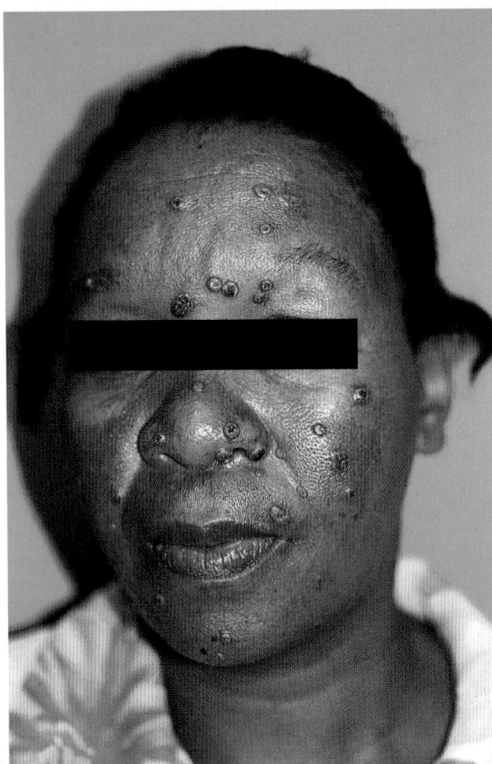

Fig. 18.323
Cryptococcosis: multiple erythematous nodules are present. By courtesy of N.C. Dlova, MD, Nelson R. Mandela School of Medicine, University of KwaZulu-Natal, South Africa.

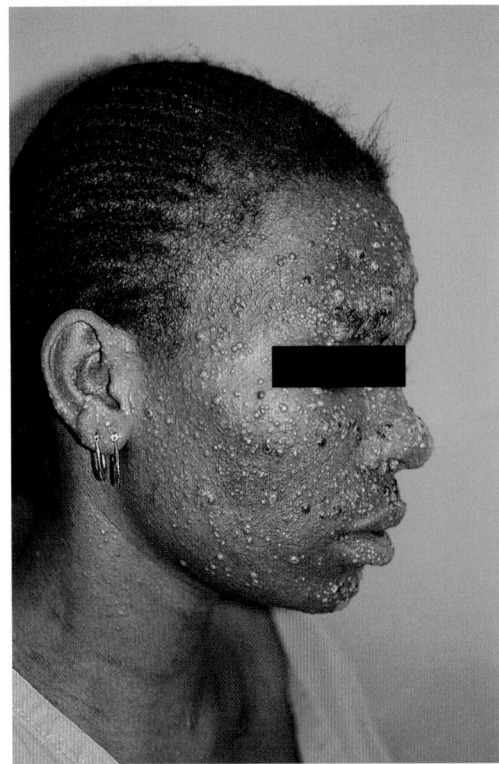

Fig. 18.324
Cryptococcosis: this patient has innumerable facial papules. By courtesy of N.C. Dlova, MD, Nelson R. Mandela School of Medicine, University of KwaZulu-Natal, South Africa.

pigeon droppings.[1,2] It causes disease in adults and, rarely, in children. The infection often complicates immunosuppression including that due to corticosteroid therapy, neoplastic disease (particularly the terminal phases of Hodgkin lymphoma), solid organ transplant recipients, and HIV/AIDS.[1–8] Cryptococcosis (torulosis) is the most frequent and potentially lethal mycosis in patients with HIV/AIDS.[9]

The portal of entry is usually the lungs, and systemic spread to the brain is common. Indeed, CNS involvement (meningitis and meningoencephalitis) is the major source of morbidity and mortality. Other sites commonly affected in disseminated disease include the skin, bone, and prostate.[9] Untreated cryptococcosis, particularly if HIV/AIDS related, has a very high mortality.

Secondary cutaneous lesions occur in approximately 10% (6–15%) of cases.[8,10–12] Skin lesions may also precede evidence of cerebral pathology.[2] Cutaneous manifestations comprise a wide range of lesions including papules, pustules, vesicles, nodules, plaques, cellulitis, ulcers, papable purpura (pseudo-Kaposi), and subcutaneous lesions, which may resemble erythema nodosum (*Fig. 18.323*).[5,11–17] Herpetiform, keloidal, MC-like lesions, pyoderma gangrenosum-like lesions, and NF have also been recorded.[8,12,14,18–23] The head and neck are the most commonly affected sites (*Fig. 18.324*).[24] Ulcerated lesions have a punched-out appearance with gelatinous-looking margins resembling basal cell carcinomas.

Lesions developing as a result of primary inoculation of the skin are very rare, but appear to have a good prognosis since the overwhelming majority of these infections have occurred in immunocompetent individuals.[25–33] Inoculation as a consequence of needlestick injury has been reported among healthcare workers.[26] Primary cutaneous cryptococcosis has been reported following iatrogenic immunosuppression.[7,34,35] Features said to be indicative of secondary cutaneous involvement rather than primary disease are deep dermal or subcutaneous inflammation and multifocal skin lesions, especially when present on covered parts of the body.[36]

Humans may also be infected by species of *Cryptococcus* other than *C. neoformans* var. *neoformans*. *C. neoformans* var. *gattii* is endemic in Australia, where it is associated with two species of eucalyptus tree.[37,38] Disseminated infection due to *C. gattii* may occur in immunocompromised patients.

Primary cryptococcal cellulitis has been reported in an immunocompetent host.[37] Another reported immunocompetent patient developed nodules and ulcers on the forearm following injury sustained through handling of barbed wire and eucalyptus logs.[39] There is a report of *C. gattii*-associated NF in a patient with diabetes mellitus.[40] Disseminated disease has also been reported in immunocompetent individuals, who may present with papules, pustules, plaques, ulcers, subcutaneous involvement, cellulitis, or acneiform lesions.[41] *C. laurentii* infection is rare and is usually acquired nosocomially. Patients are often neutropenic and develop fungemia in the presence of an indwelling intravenous catheter.[42] Primary infection, however, has been documented in a renal transplant recipient, and occasionally in immunocompetent hosts.[31,43] Fewer than 20 cases of systemic *C. albidus* infection have been reported, including a renal transplant recipient; primary cutaneous infections due to this organism are exceptionally rare.[44,45] There has been one report of *C. diffluens* infection in an immunocompetent patient, who developed sporotrichoid lesions.[46]

Pathogenesis and histologic features

C. neoformans is a spherical yeast, which measures from 4 to 20 μm in diameter. It is characterized by a mucoid capsule and by reproducing by (narrow-based) budding.[2,47,48] There are four serotypes (A–D).[1,2] In patients with HIV/AIDS, serotypes A and D are almost always implicated.[9]

Cell-mediated immunity is of particular importance in the host response and corresponding likelihood of systemic lesions.[2,38] The first line of defense against *C. neoformans* is offered by alveolar macrophages following inhalation of the organisms.[38] The release of proinflammatory monokines by these macrophages results in the local recruitment of monocytes and polymorphonuclear leukocytes, offering a second line of defense. The production of lymphokines and specific antibodies constitutes the third tier of defense. IL-12 and IL-18 play a critical role through their action on lymphocyte responses.[38] Patients with low CD4+ T-lymphocyte counts are particularly susceptible to infection.[49]

The mucoid capsule is the characteristic feature in the tissues. It is, however, unencapsulated in nature.[2] It may also be unencapsulated in patients with HIV/AIDS.[9] The development of a polysaccharide capsule

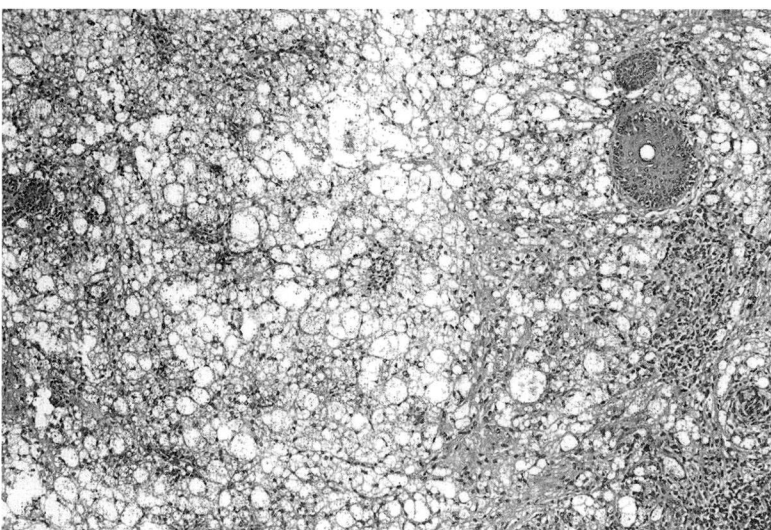

Fig. 18.325
Cryptococcosis: there is an intense mucoid dermal infiltrate.

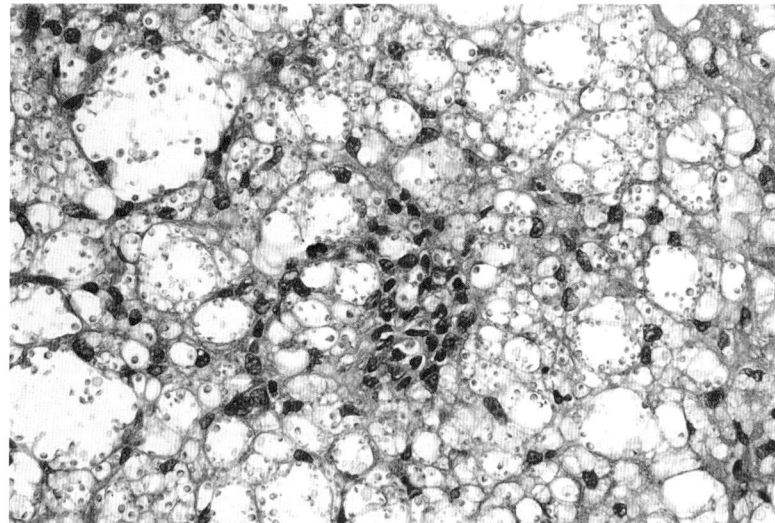

Fig. 18.326
Cryptococcosis: the yeast forms are widely separated by their thick capsules.

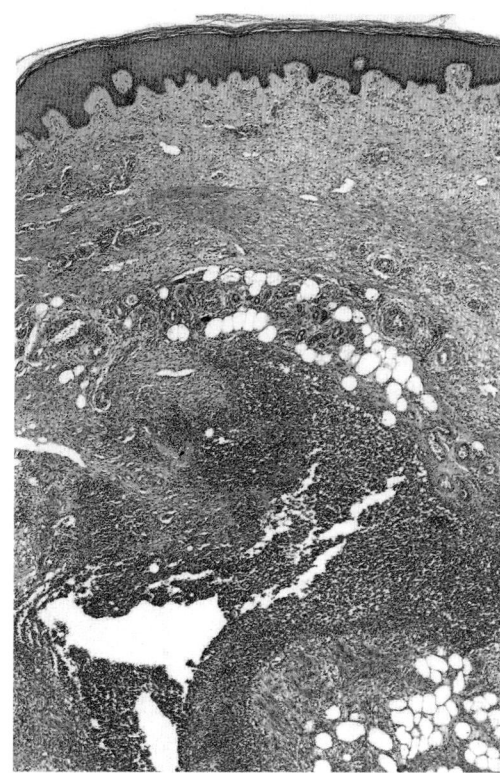

Fig. 18.327
Cryptococcosis: this suppurative variant developed in a patient with lymphoma.

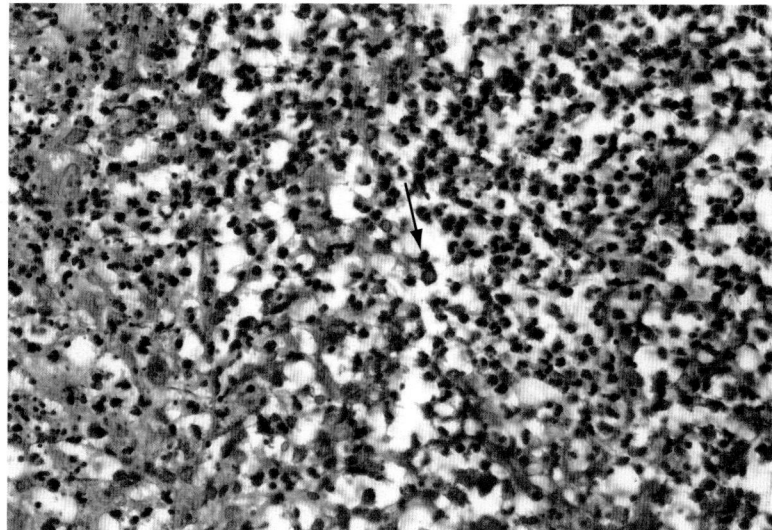

Fig. 18.328
Cryptococcosis: high-power view showing a dense neutrophil infiltrate. A yeast is evident in the center of the field.

appears to correlate with its pathogenicity.[48,50] There may be chains of budding cells in some lesions. Often there is a gelatinous reaction with little inflammation, but in other lesions there is a granulomatous response with necrosis and in some patients there is a suppurative reaction (*Figs 18.325–18.330*).[51] In the gelatinous reaction, organisms are very numerous, but in the others the cryptococcus may be more difficult to see and mucicarmine, PAS, Alcian blue, and methenamine silver stains can be useful (*Figs 18.331–18.333*). Mucicarmine positivity in particular discriminates between cryptococcus and other tissue fungal infections with similar morphology, which are characteristically negative (e.g., histoplasmosis and blastomycosis).[2,47,52] A unique palisading granulomatous response to chronic cryptococcosis has been described.[53] Necrotizing vasculitis has also been reported.[54]

Diagnosis is usually very simple and is based on morphological features.[55] In cases of doubt, cryptococcal antigen may be identified in serum or cerebrospinal fluid using the latex agglutination test.[9] The diagnosis may also be confirmed by means of in situ hybridization performed on skin biopsy material.[47,56] Use of the Tzanck smear as a rapid diagnostic tool has been advocated by some authors.[57]

In patients with underlying HIV/AIDS, it is important to examine the tissue sections carefully for additional pathology. *C. neoformans* infection has, for example, been reported in association with Kaposi sarcoma, MAI infection, and MC.[58–61]

Differential diagnosis

Infection with capsule-deficient forms of the organism may result in potential confusion with *Candida* spp. or *H. capsulatum*.[47,48] On rare occasions, neutrophilic dermatoses such as Sweet syndrome may closely mimic *Cryptococcus* infection due to the presence of acellular bodies with surrounding capsule-like spaces amid the dermal inflammatory infiltrate.[62,63]

Mucormycosis

Clinical features

Until recently, the term zygomycosis (formerly phycomycosis) was used as an umbrella term for fungal infections caused by members of the class Zygomycetes, thus encompassing both mucormycosis (caused by members of the

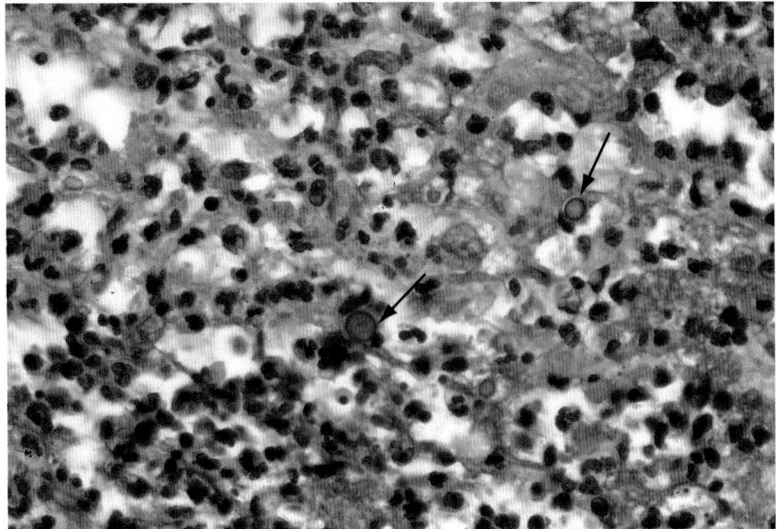

Fig. 18.329
Cryptococcosis: multiple yeasts are present (*arrowed*); this patient was receiving corticosteroid therapy for systemic lupus erythematosus.

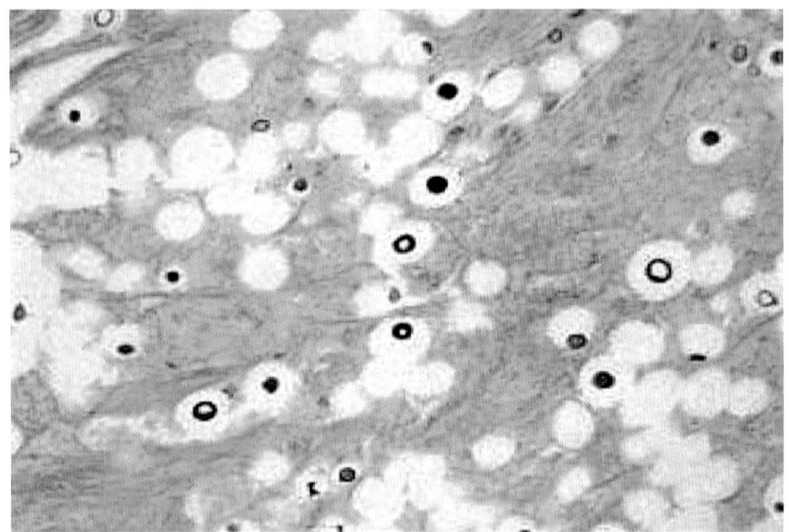

Fig. 18.332
Cryptococcosis: the organisms are positive with methenamine silver.

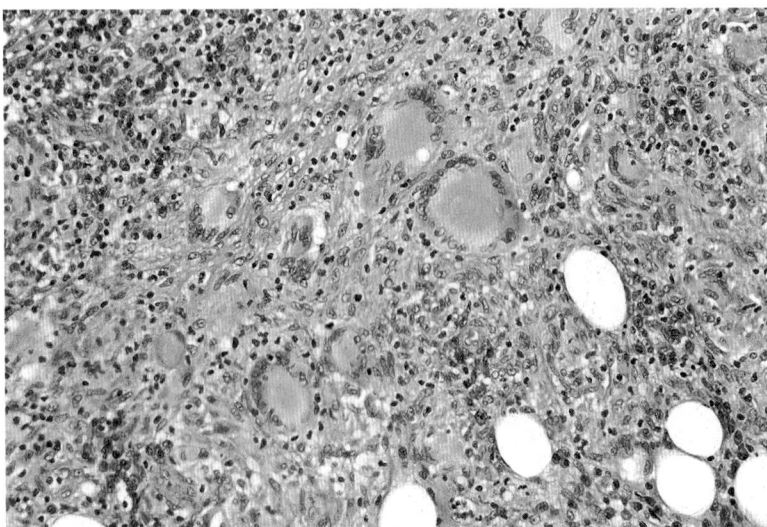

Fig. 18.330
Cryptococcosis: in this example, the inflammatory reaction is granulomatous.

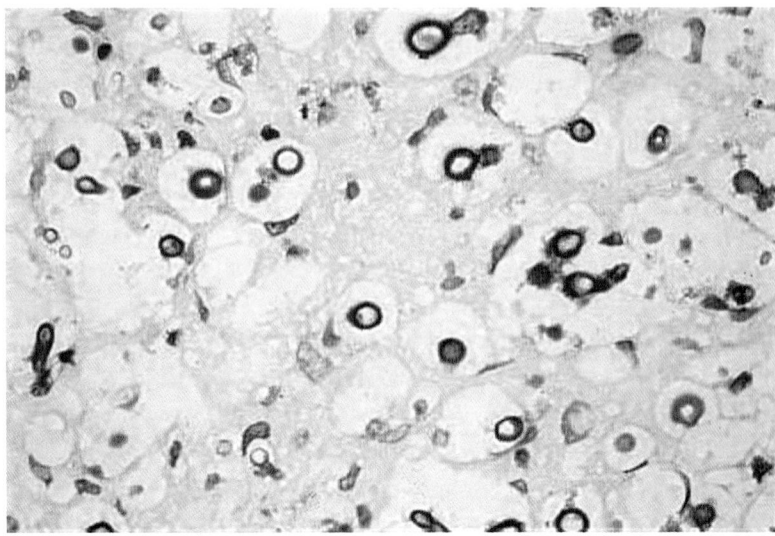

Fig. 18.333
Cryptococcosis: budding yeast forms are present (periodic acid-Schiff). By courtesy of S. Lucas, MD, St Thomas' Hospital, London, UK.

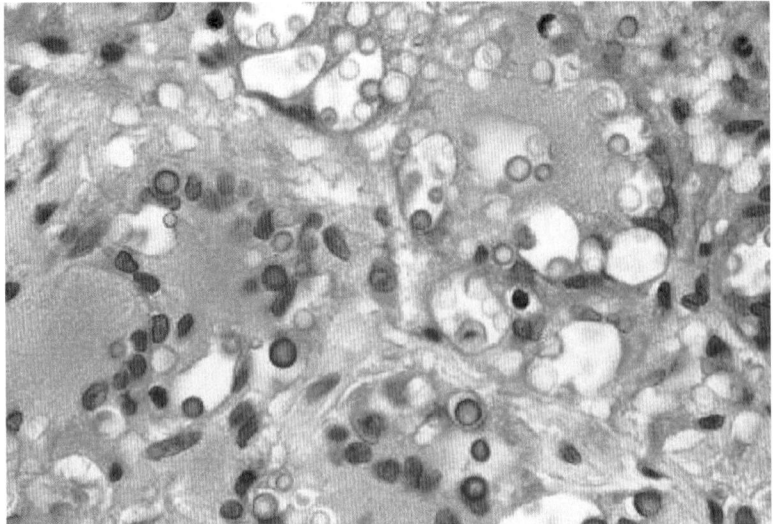

Fig. 18.331
Cryptococcosis: the capsule is clearly demonstrated with the mucicarmine stain.

order Mucorales), and entomophthoramycosis (caused by members of the order Entomophthorales).[1,2] Major recent advances in molecular phylogentic analysis of the phylum Zygomycota, however, have revealed that the term 'zygomycosis' is no longer appropriate, and that classic nomenclature of 'mucormycosis' and 'entamophthoramycosis' should instead be used.[3,4] The latter condition, therefore, is discussed separately in this chapter.

Mucormycosis is most often attributable to infection with *Rhizopus* spp. Other causative organisms (molds) include *Lichtheimia* (formerly *Absidia*), *Mucor*, *Rhizomucor*, *Apophysomyces*, *Cunninghamella*, and *Saksanaea* species; these cannot be distinguished in tissues.[1-6] Although the disease occurs mainly in adults, pediatric cases are well described.[7,8] There is a slight male predominance.[8,9] These infections are rare and usually develop in the immunosuppressed (e.g., patients with neutropenia, solid-organ and bone marrow transplant recipients) or in those with diabetic ketoacidosis. Protein-calorie malnutrition, prematurity, leukemia, non-Hodgkin lymphoma, liver disease, burns, trauma, intravenous drug abuse, and iron overload, with or without desferrioxamine therapy, have also been shown to be of pathogenetic significance.[4,8,10–21]

The fungi, which are aerobic and saprophytic on fruit and vegetable matter, are present worldwide; nevertheless, infections are uncommon. Infection usually follows spore inhalation, but can be acquired percutaneously or via ingestion. The disease has been categorized into a number of syndromes including rhinocerebral, pulmonary, cutaneous, gastrointestinal, and disseminated mucormycosis.[22] Rhinocerebral mucormycosis presents with fever, nasal discharge, orbital cellulitis, proptosis, and deteriorating mental function.[1,23,24] Patients may manifest black necrotic lesions on the palate or nasal mucosae.[10,23]

Infection of the skin is most often a complication of burns or trauma, but can occur during disseminated infection from a pulmonary source in which instance the lesions closely resemble those of disseminated aspergillosis.[1,9,10,25] A significant proportion of patients, however, are immunocompetent. Post-traumatic infections are usually acquired following traffic and domestic accidents or natural disasters.[6,26,27] The lesions develop as small erythematous macules or painless superficial erosions, which enlarge and ulcerate with profuse offensive purulent discharge. They may resemble a vasculitic process, ecthyma gangrenosum or pyoderma gangrenosum, often with conspicuous black eschar formation.[10,23,28–31] Lesions with a bull's-eye appearance or a zosteriform appearance have also been described.[32,33] Nosocomial outbreaks of primary cutaneous zygomycosis have been associated with contaminated elastic bandages.[34] Cutaneous infections have also resulted from spider bites, contaminated intravenous infusion catheter, or arterial line sites, and following arterial puncture.[17,32,35,36] Although cases of cutaneous zygomycosis have been reported in immunocompromised HIV-infected patients, the majority have been intravenous drug abusers.[37] One reported HIV/AIDS-associated case had concomitant CMV vasulitis.[38]

Isolated cutaneous mucormycosis accounts for up to 27% of cases and carries an excellent prognosis with adequate treatment. The mortality rate for localized infection ranges from 4% to 10%.[26] The mortality rate associated with rhinocerebral, pulmonary, or disseminated disease, however, is very high, usually exceeding 50% (as high as 78–100% in some series).[2,9,17,39] Rarely, visceral dissemination from a primary cutaneous site of infection may occur.[6,9,28,] Bacterial co-infection was documented in 41% of cases in a recent series of post-traumatic cases.[6]

Histologic features

The fungi in mucormycosis are seen as broad (10–20 μm diameter), ribbon-like, nonseptate hyphae, which branch irregularly at 90°.[1,24] They must be distinguished from *Aspergillus* spp. and the etiological agents of hyalohyphomycosis; these are narrower, septate, and show more regular dichotomous branching. The fungus often invades blood vessels, with resultant vasculitis, causing thrombosis, hemorrhage, and infarction.[1,7,24] The hyphae are seen well with H&E, as well as with special stains for fungi (*Fig. 18.334*).[7,24] Involvement of the subcutaneous fat may closely mimic pancreatic panniculitis or gouty panniculitis owing to the presence of ghost adipocytes with a basophilic hue, or necrotic adipocytes containing refractile needle-shaped crystals, respectively (*Fig. 18.335*).[40] Consequently, the possibility of mucormycosis should always be ruled out when considering a histologic diagnosis of pancreatic panniculitis or gouty panniculitis. As with all fungal infections, precise identification of the species responsible for the infection is by fungal culture or contemporary molecular mycology (PCR) techniques.[1,24,41]

Entomophthoramycosis

Clinical features

Entomophthoramycosis (entamophthoromycosis; subcutaneous zygomycosis) encompasses rare infections caused by:
- *Basidiobolus ranarum* or *B. haptosporus*, and referred to as basidiobolomycosis; or
- *Conidiobolus coronatus*, *C. incongruus* or *C. lamprauges*, and referred to as conidiobolomycosis.

These organisms are members of the order Entomophthorales, and are also responsible for cutaneous and nasopharyngeal infections in animals such as horses.[1–9] Entomophthoramycosis occurs predominantly in tropical and subtropical regions of Africa, Asia, and South America.[1] Unlike mucormycosis, basidiobolomycosis and conidiobolomycosis do not appear to be opportunistic pathogens in the majority of cases; infection is usually acquired by

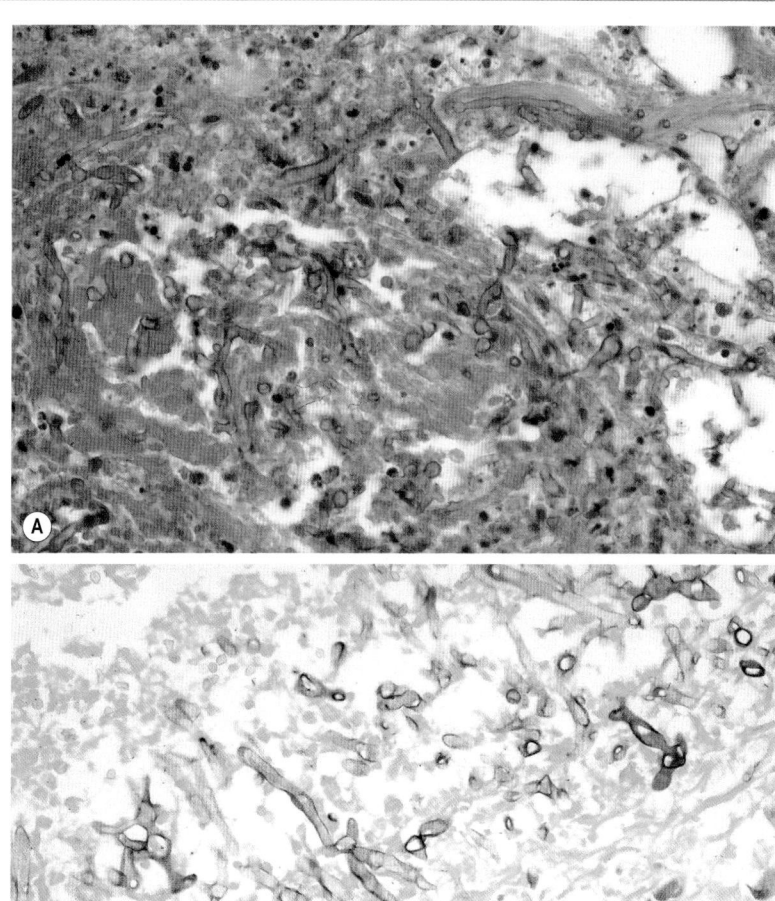

Fig. 18.334
Mucormycosis: (**A**) the hyphae are very broad (much more than *Aspergillus*), are nonseptate and branch at 90°; (**B**) methenamine silver stain.

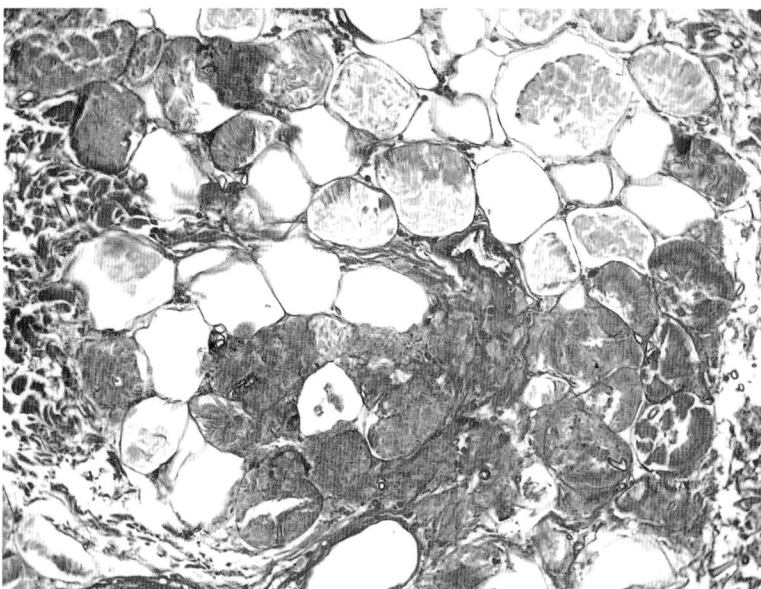

Fig. 18.335
Mucormycosis: subcutaneous involvement in this example is associated with extensive fat necrosis and a picture strikingly reminiscent of gouty panniculitis and pancreatic panniculitis. By courtesy of V. Yazbek, MD, Ampath National Laboratories, Bloemfontein, South Africa.

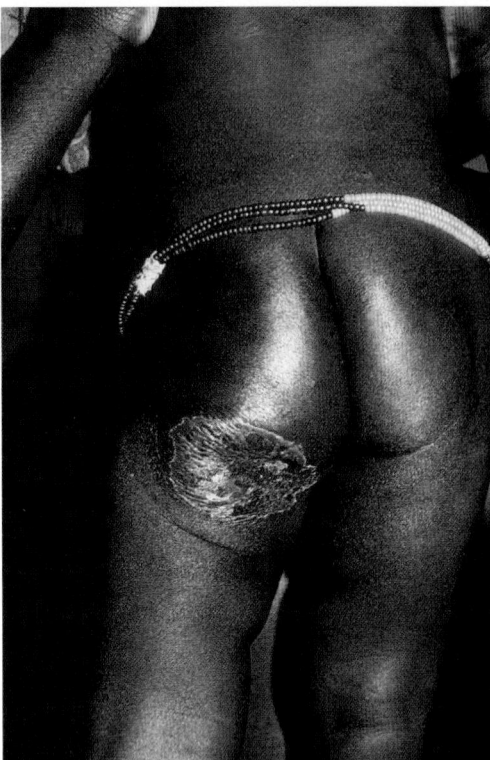

Fig. 18.336
Basidiobolomycosis: there is a large abscess in the left buttock. By courtesy of S. Lucas, MD, St Thomas' Hospital, London, UK.

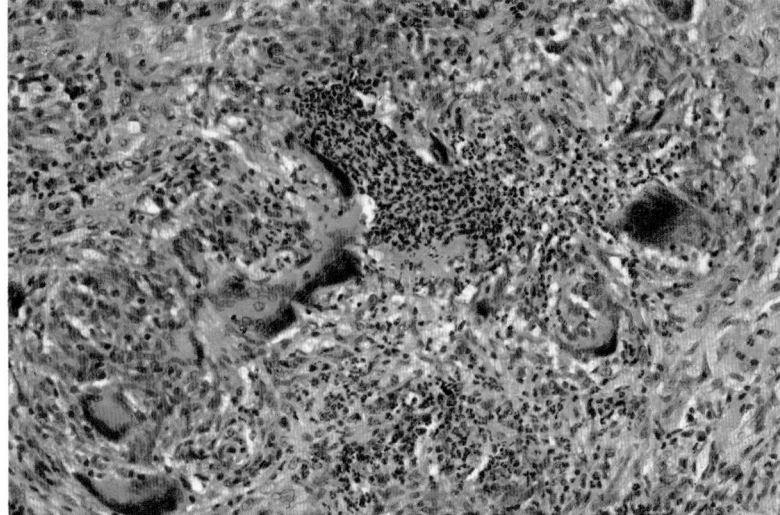

Fig. 18.337
Basidiobolomycosis: high-power view showing a heavy mixed granulomatous and suppurative dermal infiltrate with admixed eosinophils.

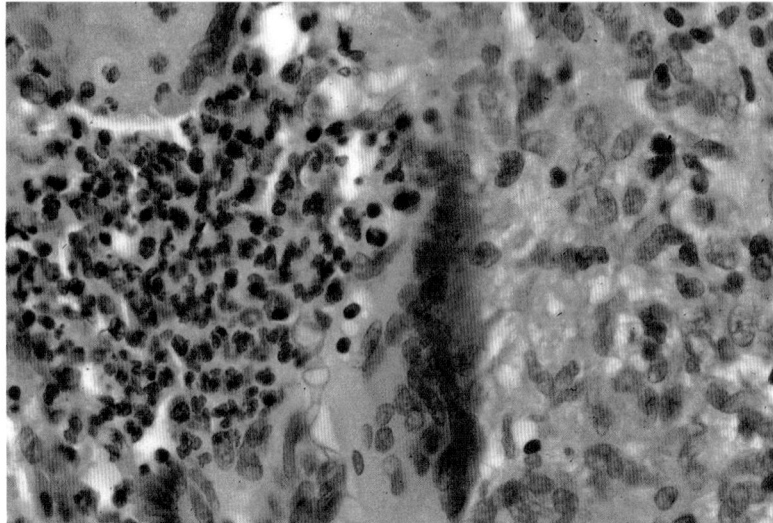

Fig. 18.338
Basidiobolomycosis: the fungi are often clearly visible in hematoxylin and eosin stained sections.

inoculation, either through minor trauma or occasionally via an insect bite.[1] There have nevertheless been rare reports of entomophthoramycosis following iatrogenic immunosuppression.[5,12,10,11] Both *B. ranarum* and *C. coronatus* are found in soil and decaying vegetable material.[1,7] *B. ranarum* also occurs in the gut of fish, amphibians, reptiles, and bats.[1,8]

Basidiobolomycosis is seen most frequently in children or adolescents, who present with confluent cutaneous and subcutaneous plaques. The lesions are fluctuant, generally nontender and well demarcated, and occur predominantly on the limbs, trunk, or buttocks (*Fig. 18.336*).[1,7,8] Tumorlike masses may evolve.[1] There have been rare reports of nasal or paranasal sinus lesions.[13,14] There is a male predilection.[8] Involvement of the lymph nodes, with lymphedema and elephantiasis, has also been reported.[15,16] There is a single case report of penile basidiobolomycosis.[17] Although rare, primary or secondary visceral involvement may occur.[1,10,18,19] Numerous cases of gastrointestinal basidiobolomycois have been reported.[20]

Conidiobolomycosis, by contrast, is an infection that tends to occur in adults, who manifest with mucocutaneous lesions of the nose with subsequent spread to the paranasal sinuses and rhinofacial subcutaneous tissues (rhinoentomophthoromycosis).[1,3] Although the vast majority of documented infections have occurred in healthy, immunocompetent hosts, 2.5% of reported infections have arisen in the setting of underlying hematolymphoid neoplasia.[12] There is erythema and thickening of the nasal skin. This may progress to massive deforming tumefaction of the nose, cheeks and/or lips, and facial elephantiasis.[1,12,21–24] The infection can also spread to involve the eyelid and orbit.[1,25] Intracranial extension has been documented.[26] Fatal visceral dissemination is a rare complication.[5]

Histologic features

The variably septate fungal hyphae in entomophthoramycosis are not as broad as those encountered in mucormycosis, and have an average diameter of 8–10 μm. An additional point of distinction is the fact that angioinvasion does not tend to occur in entomophthoramycosis.[1] There is extensive granulomatous inflammation with neutrophilic microabscesses and large numbers of eosinophilic leukocytes (*Fig. 18.337*).[12] The hyphae are clearly discernible in H&E-stained sections but can be highlighted with methenamine silver, and are frequently associated with the Splendore-Hoeppli phenomenon (*Figs*

18.338 and *18.339*).[1,12,19] Phagocytosed hyphal fragments are sometimes visible within the cytoplasm of giant cells.[7] One reported case of conidiobolomycosis was accompanied by chronic localized fibrozing leukocytoclastic vasculitis and a resultant histologic picture reminiscent of granuloma faciale.[12] Diagnosis is facilitated by recognition of the distinctive histologic findings and culture of the causative organism; molecular (PCR) mycology techniques, however, have recently assumed a more prominent role.[3]

Chromoblastomycosis

Clinical features

Chromoblastomycosis (chromomycosis) is a term applied to infection with some black (dematiaceous) fungi and is characterized by finding sclerotic pigmented bodies intermediate between a yeast and hyphal form in the tissues. Five main fungal species are associated with chromoblastomycosis[1–5]:

- *Fonsecaea pedrosoi*,
- *Cladophialophora carrionii* (formerly *Cladosporium carrionii*),
- *Fonsecaea compacta*,
- *Phialophora verrucosa*,
- *Rhinocladiella aquaspersa*.

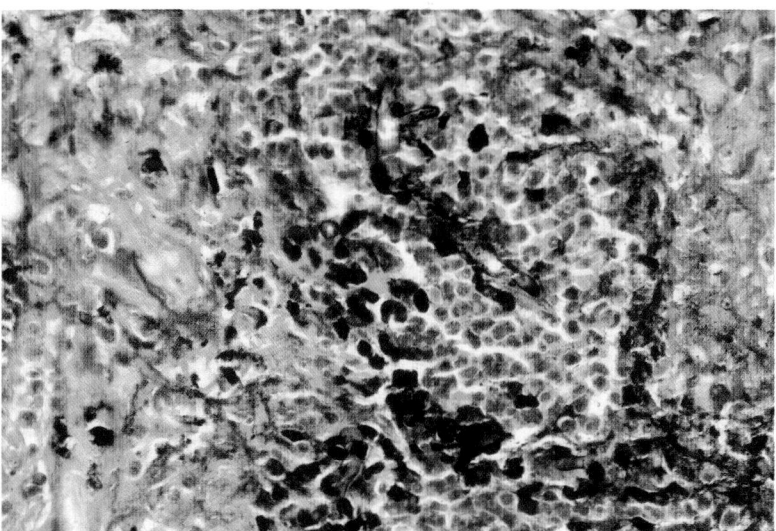

Fig. 18.339
Basidiobolomycosis: the hyphae are irregular and often appear twisted (methenamine silver).

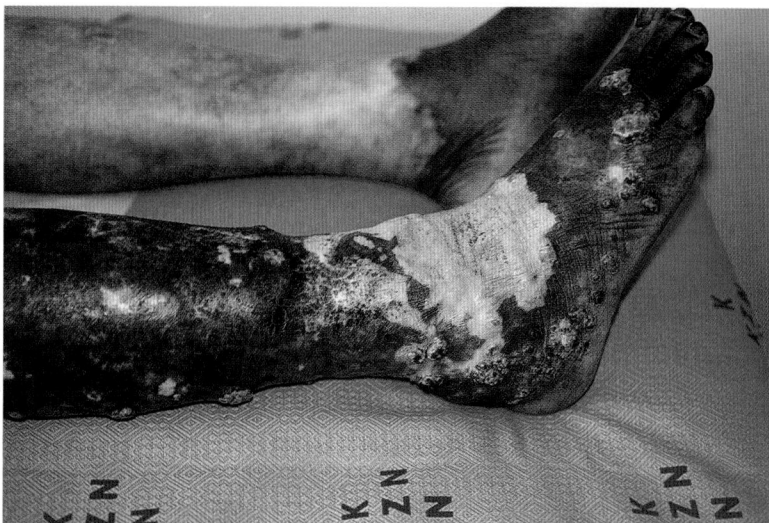

Fig. 18.340
Chromoblastomycosis: there are multiple nodules and disfiguring plaques. By courtesy of N.C. Dlova, MD, Nelson R. Mandela School of Medicine, University of KwaZulu-Natal, South Africa.

Other organisms, such as *Exophiala spinifera*, *Aureobasidium pullulans*, *Chaetomium funicular*, *F. monophora*, *F. pugnacius*, *F. nubica*, *Cladosporium cladosporoides*, *C. bantiana*, and *Veronaea monophora*, have rarely been implicated.[6–15] Infections have occurred throughout the world, almost entirely in adult males (more than 90% in some series).[16,17] The disease is nevertheless more prevalent in tropical countries, especially in parts of South America.[2,3,5] The fungi are thought to be present in soil, wood, and vegetable debris. Thorns of the plant *Mimosa pudica* probably represent a natural source of chromoblastomycosis caused by *F. pedrosoi*.[18] Other infections caused by dematiaceous fungi include mycetoma and pheohyphomycosis, and are discussed separately in this chapter.[1,19] The pigment represents melanin.[20] Chromomycosis is particularly seen in farmers and agricultural workers.[16,21,22] Children and teenagers, however, may also be affected in areas where the disease is endemic.[23] Although the majority of infections occur in otherwise healthy individuals, cases have been documented in the presence of underlying immunosuppression, including systemic corticosteroid therapy; there is a tendency toward infection with less conventional organisms in this clinical context.[10,14,15,24]

The infection occurs primarily in skin following trauma. It begins as scaly pink papules, most often on the lower leg or foot. These enlarge slowly to become nodules and then purplish irregular plaques and verrucous nodules (*Fig. 18.340*). Eventually, many of these become large papillomatous lesions, which are pruritic. The associated scratching may result in adjacent satellitosis. The condition progresses slowly for many years and may end as grossly deforming large tumor masses.[25–27] Lymphangitic spread has been reported.[28,29] A rare presentation with annular lesions has been described.[30] Secondary bacterial infection often causes foul smelling discharge, ulceration, and lymphadenitis. Involvement of underlying tissues does not occur, although hematogenous spread to the CNS has been reported on rare occasions.[11,31] Secondary (bacterial) regional lymphadenopathy may be evident.[21] Squamous cell carcinoma is a rare complication of chronic disease.[22,32–35] There have been rare reports of penile, vulval, and nasal chromoblastomycosis. Extracutaneous lesions involving the pleura, ileocecal region, laryngotracheal region, and tonsils have also been described.[36] Contiguous involvement of underlying bone is a rare occurrence.[37]

Pathogenesis and histologic features

The most common fungus causing chromoblastomycosis is *F. pedrosoi*.[19,21,38] This organism has been isolated from 70% to 90% or more of cases in some series.[22,39,40] A multinational study showed that *F. pedrosoi* can be classified into seven mitochondrial DNA types; these appear to correspond to geographic origin.[41] Experimental evidence indicates that the production of proteolytic enzymes (peptidases) by *F. pedrosoi* results in cleavage of serum

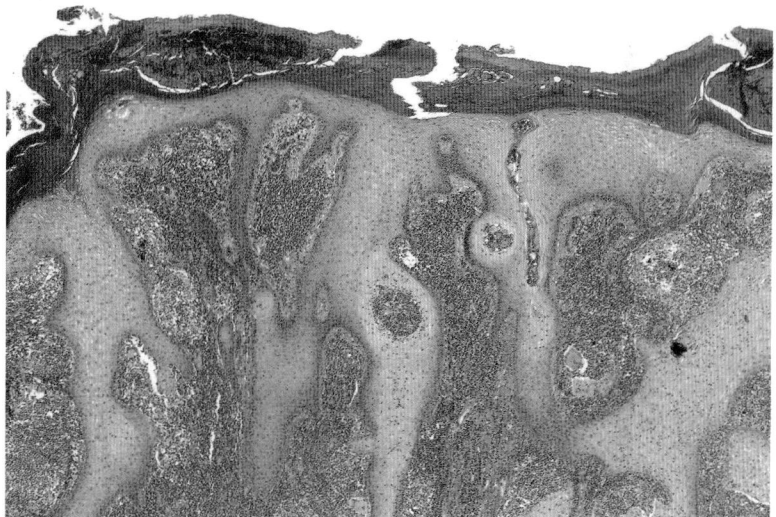

Fig. 18.341
Chromoblastomycosis: the epidermis is hyperkeratotic, crusted, and shows very marked acanthosis.

proteins such as IgG, and components of the extracellular matrix, including laminin and fibronectin.[42] One study has suggested that a suboptimal host immune response to the organisms is the result of an imbalance in regulatory (Treg) and Th17 T-cells.[43]

The sclerotic bodies (also referred to as Medlar bodies) are round or polyhedral, pigmented, thick-walled fungal cells 5–12 μm in diameter.[19,44] Despite its name, blast formation does not occur.[1] The sclerotic body is phenotypically midway between a yeast and a hypha and therefore has cross walls in two planes.[1] The tissue reaction resembles that seen in blastomycosis.[19] There is marked epidermal acanthosis, with neutrophil microabscesses (*Figs 18.341* and *18.342*). The hyperplasia often becomes pseudoepitheliomatous.[31,44] The dermis shows abscess formation with necrosis and a surrounding granulomatous and mixed inflammatory infiltrate consisting of neutrophils, eosinophils, lymphocytes, and plasma cells. The admixture of neutrophil microabscesses and granulomatous inflammation is described as a mixed (mycotic) granuloma (it is also a feature of blastomycosis, sporotrichosis, pheohyphomycosis, coccidioidomycosis, and paracoccidioidomycosis).[31] The sclerotic bodies are seen both within giant cells and extracellularly (*Figs 18.343* and *18.344*). Transepidermal elimination of fungal cells has been described.[45] Dematiaceous hyphae may also be seen in the dermis.[19] Dermal fibrosis is often marked and in many cases the

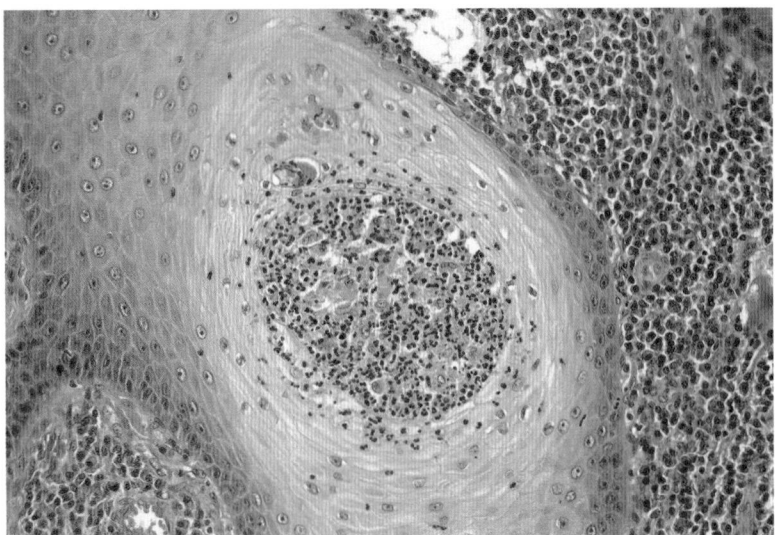

Fig. 18.342
Chromoblastomycosis: abscesses within both the epidermis and dermis are characteristic.

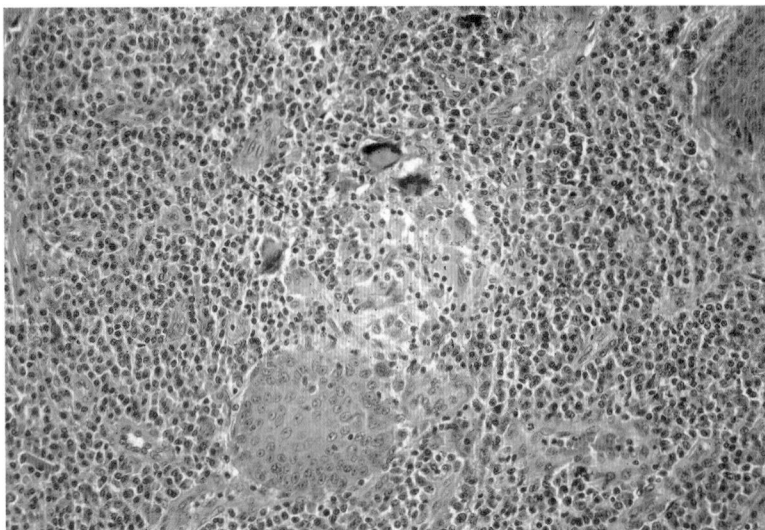

Fig. 18.343
Chromoblastomycosis: granulomata are commonly present.

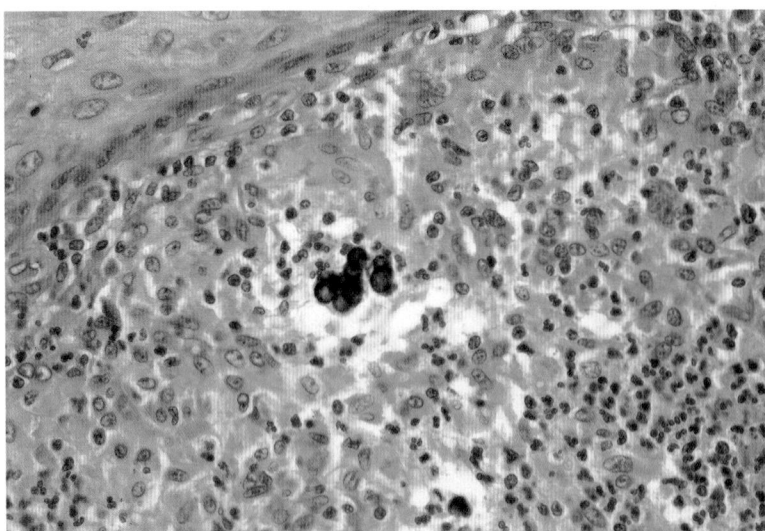

Fig. 18.344
Chromoblastomycosis: the brown-staining (sometimes septate) cells are pathognomonic.

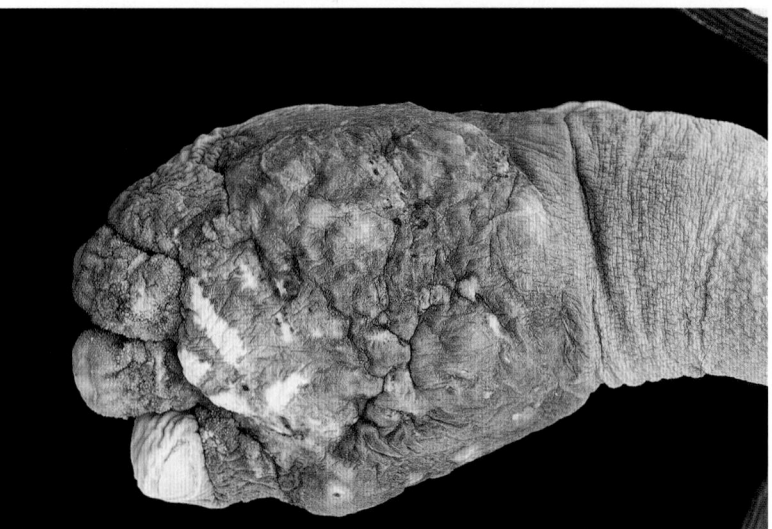

Fig. 18.345
Mycetoma: the foot is grossly swollen and misshapen. Numerous draining sinuses are present.

subcutaneous fat is also affected. An unusual case characterized by an exuberant intradermal fascicular spindled cell proliferation has been reported.[46] Classification of the causative organism depends on culture, and more recently via panfungal PCR with subsequent sequence analysis.[47]

Mycetoma

Clinical features

Mycetoma (Gr. *mykes*, fungus; *oma*, tumor) is a chronically discharging infection of skin and subcutaneous tissue, characterized by multiple sinus tracks and the presence of granules in the exudate.[1-7] It can be caused by bacteria (actinomycetoma) (e.g., *Nocardia*, see above) or (less commonly) by fungi (eumycetoma). Mycetoma is more or less confined to tropical zones, mainly between the latitudes of 15° South and 30° North (the so-called 'mycetoma belt').[5,8] The disease most commonly occurs on the foot, although other sites can be affected (*Fig. 18.345*).

Repeated inoculation by minor trauma is necessary to produce a lesion, which begins as a papule and enlarges to become a discharging nodule. This process extends to the adjacent skin and the discharging fistulae do not heal (*Fig. 18.346*). The affected area becomes distorted by inflammation and fibrosis, and the underlying bone may become involved. Mycetoma occurs most commonly in 20- to 50-year-olds and shows a marked male preponderance. It relates to repeated occupational trauma. Mycetomas caused by fungi are in general less inflammatory and less deeply invasive than bacterial lesions.

Pathogenesis and histologic features

The most common fungal causes of mycetoma include:
- *Madurella mycetomatis*,
- *Madurella grisea*,
- *Pseudallescheria boydii*,
- *Pyrenochaeta romeroi*,
- *Leptosphaeria senegalensis*,
- *Neotestudina rosatti*.

Bacterial causes include species of *Nocardia*, *Actinomyces*, and *Streptomyces*.[5-11] Fungal causes account for a minority of cases of mycetoma.[2] Of these, *M. mycetomatis* is the most important worldwide.[8,12-14] An analysis of 73 cases from India, however, showed a decrease in the proportion of maduromycotic mycetoma versus actinomycotic mycetoma over a 4-year period.[15] Infections due to *Scedosporium apiospermum* (the asexual counterpart of the teleomorph *Pseudallescheria boydii*), *Cladophialophora bantiana*, and *Phaeoacremonium fuscum* have been documented

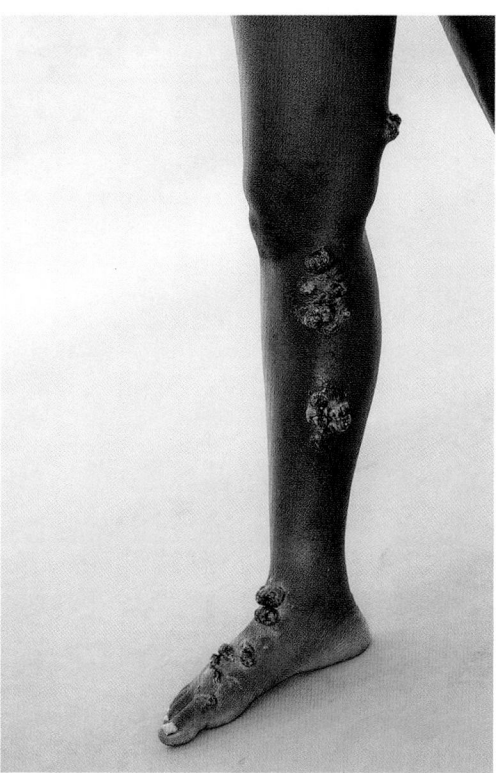

Fig. 18.346
Mycetoma: multiple ulcerated verrucous nodules are present. By courtesy of N.C. Dlova, MD, Nelson R. Mandela School of Medicine, University of KwaZulu-Natal, South Africa.

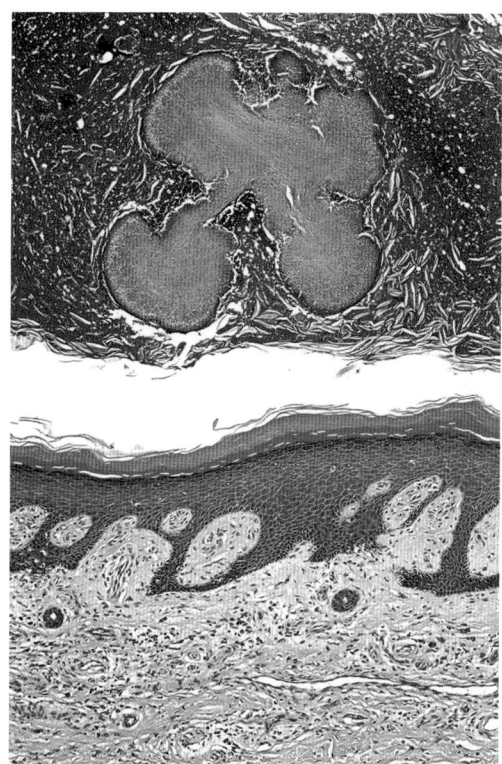

Fig. 18.348
Mycetoma: in this example, a colony is present in the overlying crust.

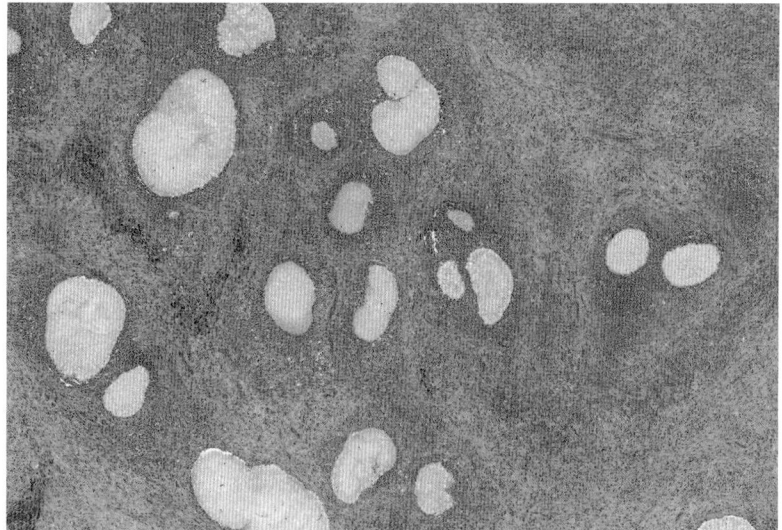

Fig. 18.347
Mycetoma: characteristic granules are present in neutrophil abscesses. There is a peripheral histiocytic/giant cell palisade.

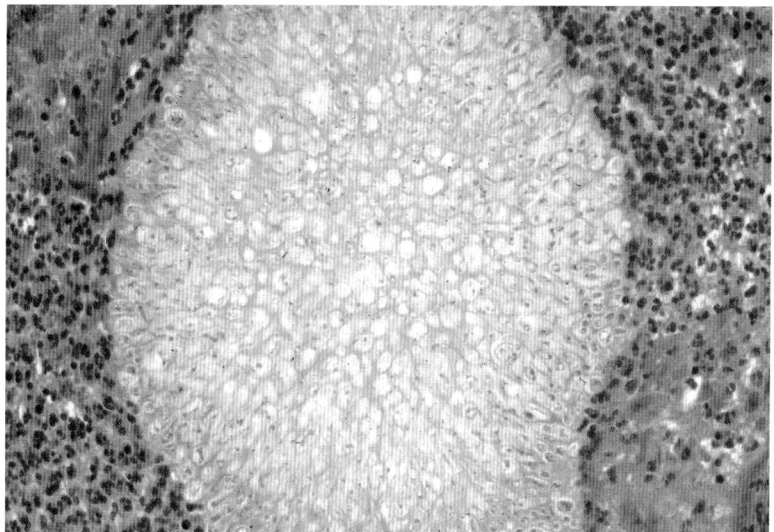

Fig. 18.349
Mycetoma: the internal structure of the granule is clearly visible in this high-power view.

in iatrogenically immunosuppressed individuals.[16–18] *S. apiospermum* eumycetoma may also occur in immunocompetent hosts.[19] There is a report of *Diaporthe phaseolorum* (*Phomopsis phaseoli*) eumycetoma in a patient with human T-cell lymphotropic virus 1 (HTLV-1) infection.[20]

All the organisms produce granules, the configuration and color of which may be helpful in identifying the causative agent (*Figs 18.347–18.350; Table 18.3*).[2] Although definitive speciation by means of culture is often challenging, newer PCR-based techniques hold promise.[21] The black color of the granules seen in *M. mycetomatis* infection is due to the production of melanin, which may confer protection of the organism against the effects of antifungal agents.[14,22,23] A polymorphism in the gene encoding for the chitin-degrading enzyme, chitotriosidase has been linked to an increased

risk for the development *M. mycetomatis* mycetoma.[24] The granules are seen within areas of suppuration and are surrounded by palisaded histiocytes. They consist of an organized compact mass of hyphae, which may be associated with adherent neutrophils or a crystalline matrix.[12,25,26] Multinucleate giant cells occur beyond this and there is a peripheral region of edematous granulation tissue. The use of special stains is of value in distinguishing actinomycetic from fungal (eumycetic) causes of mycetoma. The latter stain positively with PAS and silver stains but are negative with Gram stain (*Fig. 18.351*). A Splendore-Hoeppli phenomenon is sometimes evident (*Fig. 18.352*).

Response to therapy is variable, but the condition is more problematical when deep tissues are involved.

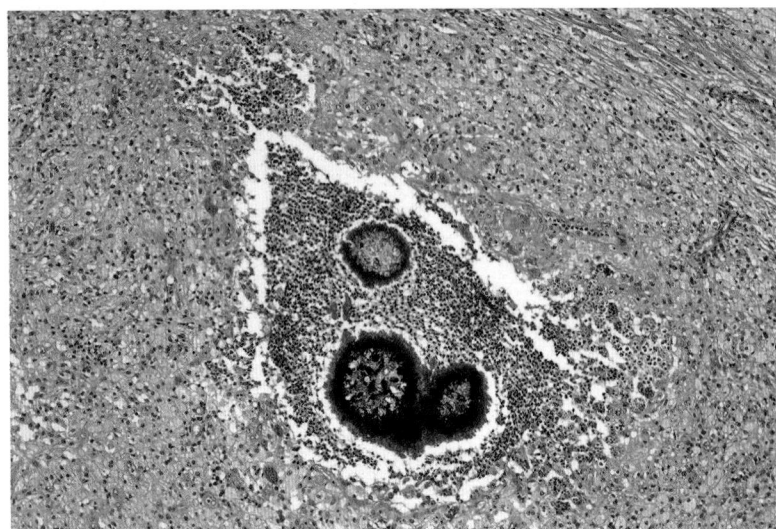

Fig. 18.350
Mycetoma: pigmented granules are characteristic of Madurella mycetomatis infection.

Table 18.3
Color of granules in mycetoma

	Maduromycotic (eumycetic)	Actinomycetic
Black	*Madurella mycetomatis* *Madurella grisea* *Pyrenochaeta romeroi* *Phialophora jeanselmei* *Leptosphaeria senegalensis* *Leptosphaeria tompkinsii*	
Yellow or yellowish-white	*Allescheria boydii* *Acremonium* sp. *Fusarium* sp. *Neotestudina rosatti* *Actinomadura madurae* *Streptomyces somaliensis*	
Red		*Actinomadura pelletieri*
White or not visible		*Nocardia brasiliensis* *Nocardia caviae* *Nocardia asteroides*

Reproduced with permission from Magaña, M. and Magaña-Garcia, M. (1989) Dermatologic Clinics, 7, 203–217.

Pheohyphomycosis

Clinical features

Phaeohyphomycetes are a heterogeneous group of pigmented (dematiaceous) fungi with both yeast-like and hyphae-like forms in tissues.[1–4] The sclerotic bodies of chromoblastomycosis are not seen. There are >100 known causative species, all of which show pigmented yeast-like cells, pseudohyphae, and distorted short or long hyphae in variable proportions.[2,5]

Pheohyphomycosis can be subdivided into superficial, cutaneous, corneal, subcutaneous, and systemic/disseminated forms.[4–8] Keratitis, otomycosis, tinea nigra palmaris, and rare infections of the ungual apparatus are additional manifestations.[8–10]

- Black piedra caused by *P. hortae* is an example of superficial pheohyphomycosis affecting the hair shaft.[6,11]
- Cutaneous lesions include macules, papules, plaques, nodules, cystic or verrucous lesions, sometimes with ulceration.[4,12–14] A cystic lesion is referred to as a pheohyphomycotic cyst; the latter may also be subcutaneous in location.[15]

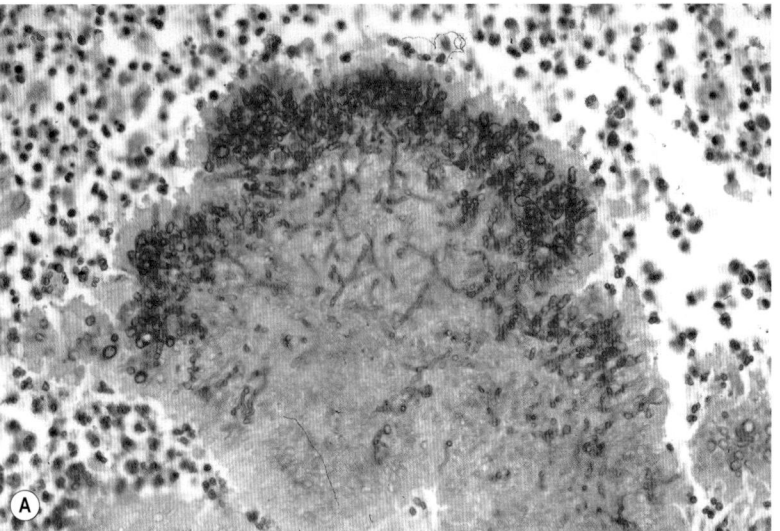

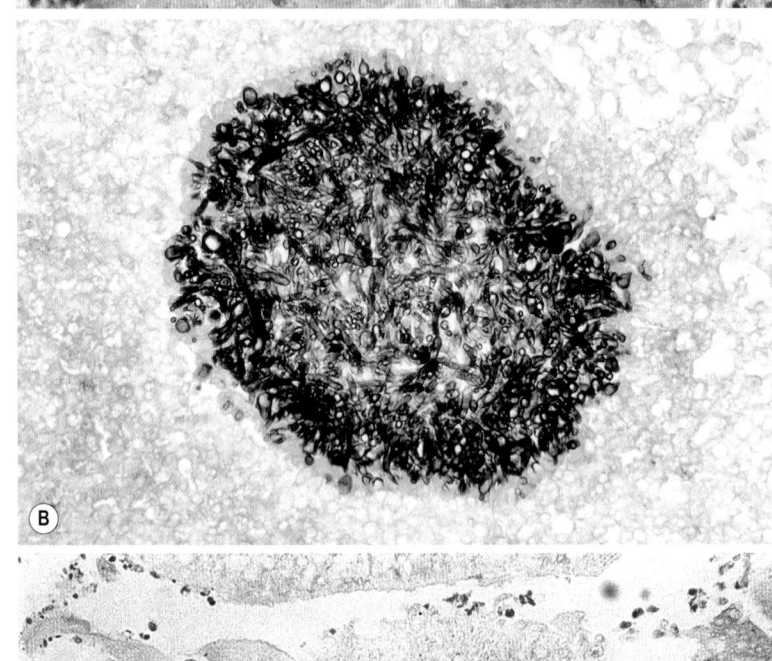

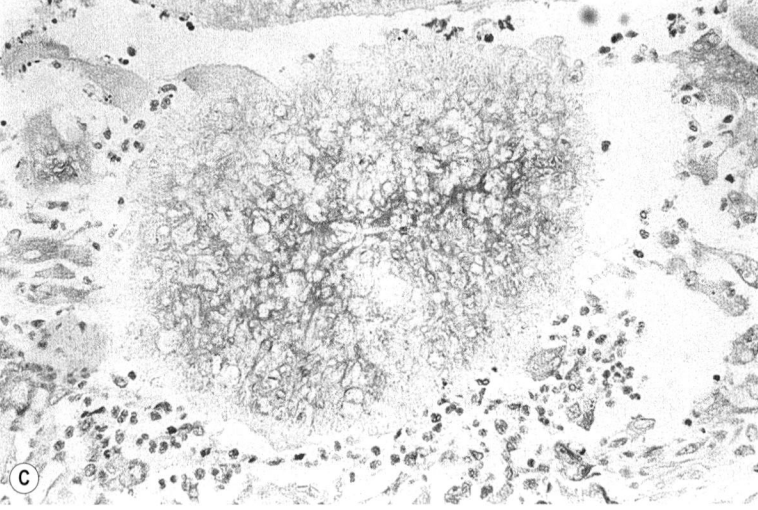

Fig. 18.351
(**A–C**) Mycetoma: the use of special stains readily confirms the fungal nature of this variant. (**A**) Periodic acid-Schiff; (**B**) methenamine silver; (**C**) Gram.

- *Exophiala jeanselmei* is the most common cause of subcutaneous pheohyphomycosis, the patients presenting with a solitary discrete asymptomatic well-circumscribed subcutaneous nodule.[5,16] These usually follow trauma, most often to the limbs.[4,17] *E. jeanselmei* is also an important cause of cutaneous pheohyphomycosis.[18] Other documented etiological agents in subcutaneous pheohyphomycosis include *Fonsecaea pedrosoi*, *Phaeoacremonium* spp., *Cladophialophora* spp., *Chaetomium*

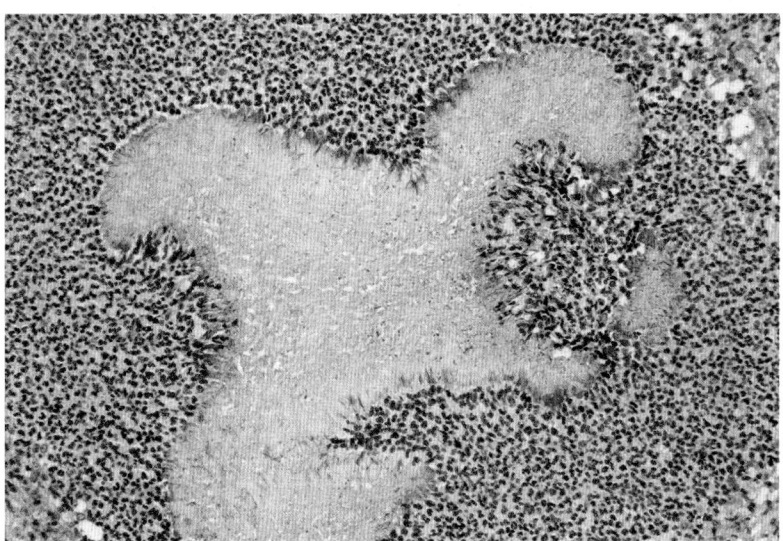

Fig. 18.352
Mycetoma: this fibrin stain highlights the Splendore-Hoeppli phenomenon.

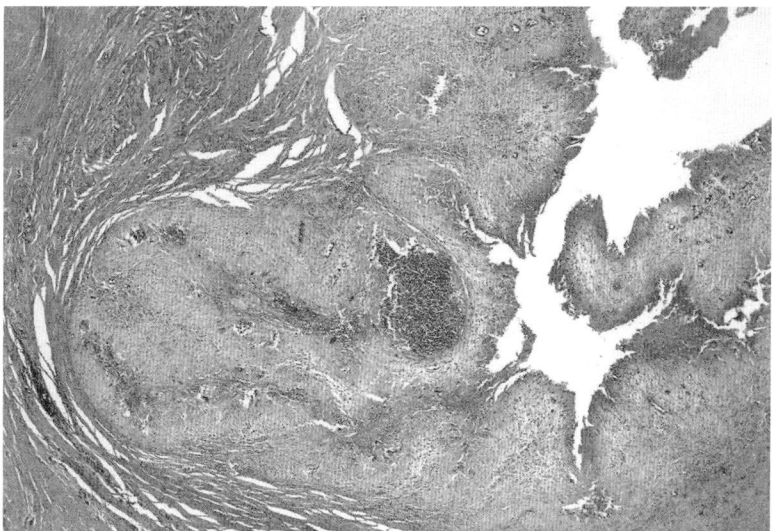

Fig. 18.353
Pheohyphomycosis: this low-power view shows the typical appearance of a deep dermal discrete nodule.

globosum, E. spinifera, E. salmonis, E. oligosperma, Lasiodiplodia theobromae, Phialophora spp., *Coniothyrium* spp., *Cladosporium* spp, *Wallemia sebi*, and *Pyrenochaeata romeroi*.[15,19–34]

Pheohyphomycosis may also present in the immunosuppressed, especially those who have received organ transplants.[1,35,36] Patients receiving long-term oral corticosteroids are also at risk.[18] Nodules often become large (up to several centimeters across), but epidermal involvement is not seen. The necrotic yellow-gray central contents can be aspirated from well-developed lesions.

Disseminated (systemic) pheohyphomycosis carries a mortality of almost 80%.[2,5] The organism most frequently implicated is *Scedosporium prolificans*, and although some patients have been immunocompetent, the majority of infections have occurred in immunocompromised individuals.[2,4,7] Endocarditis may occur, particularly in relation to prosthetic cardiac valves. Organisms implicated less frequently are *Bipolaris spicifera* and *Wangiella dermatitidis*.[2] A case of disseminated pheohyphomycosis caused by *Ochronocis gallopavum* has been reported in a marijuana user with advanced HIV infection.[37]

Infection with *Alternaria* spp. (alternariosis) is discussed elsewhere.

Pathogenesis and histologic features

Phaeohyphomycetes are present in vegetation, soil, and decaying organic material.[2] The disease occurs by traumatic implantation. Phaeohyphomycetes are mostly opportunistic pathogens.[4] Virulence factors include melanin and enzymes such as proteases, peptidases and hyaluronidases.[1,2,8,38]

E. jeanselmei is seen as yellow-brown/chestnut-brown, irregularly swollen, septate hyphae, which can be branched or unbranched.[5] Yeast-like forms are also seen, sometimes in chains.[1] The organisms occur in the necrotic center of the abscess and in the surrounding cellular infiltrate of epithelioid macrophages, giant cells, and neutrophils (*Figs 18.353–18.355*).[4,19] Sometimes, it can be very difficult to find the organisms, and special stains such as PAS or methenamine silver can be invaluable (*Fig. 18.356*).[38] A wood splinter may occasionally be present. There is a dense fibrotic reaction around the inflammatory component.[5]

Fungal culture and/or PCR studies are required for precise identification of the etiological species.

Differential diagnosis

Pheohyphomycosis is distinguished from chromoblastomycosis by the absence of the pigmented sclerotic bodies seen in tissue sections in the latter condition. It is of interest that the same fungus may cause either condition depending on the response to the host's internal environment.[3,4,17] Pigment is sometimes not readily apparent within the fungal walls on H&E staining, resulting in potential confusion with hyaline septate fungi

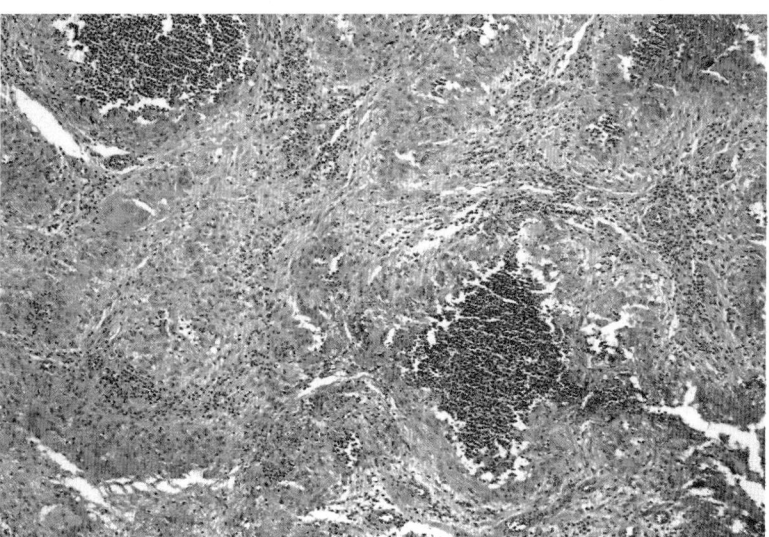

Fig. 18.354
Pheohyphomycosis: higher-power view showing mixed suppurative and granulomatous inflammation.

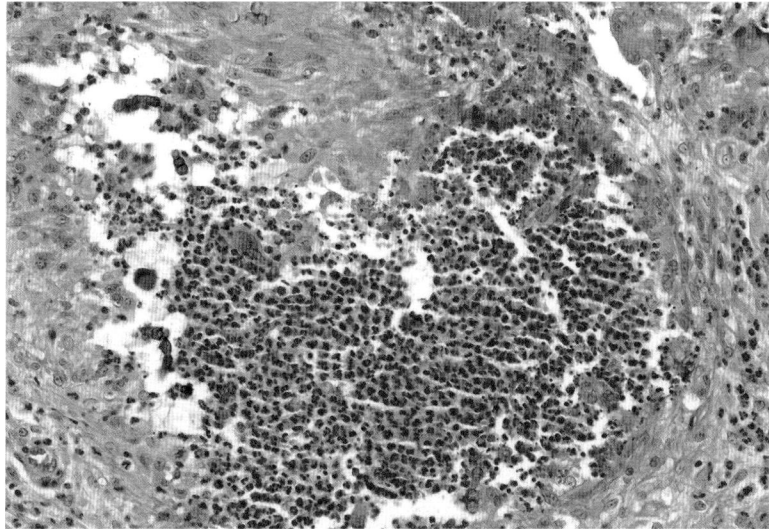

Fig. 18.355
Pheohyphomycosis: pigmented yeast forms, some forming in chains, are present.

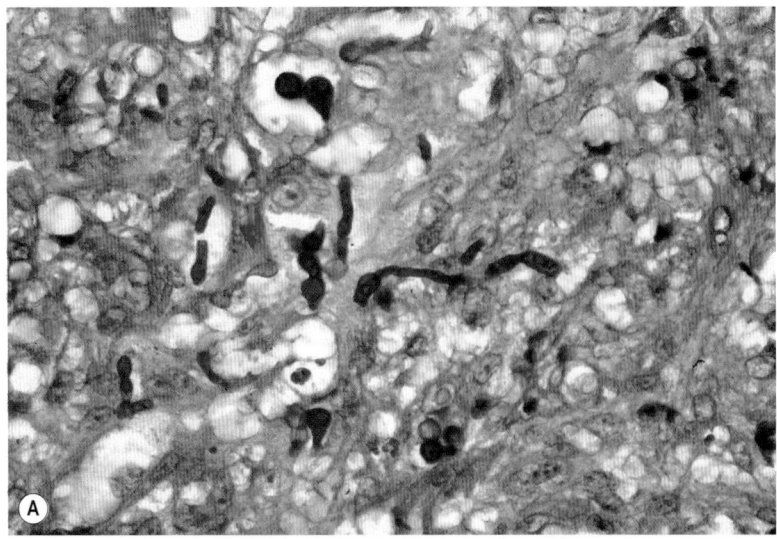

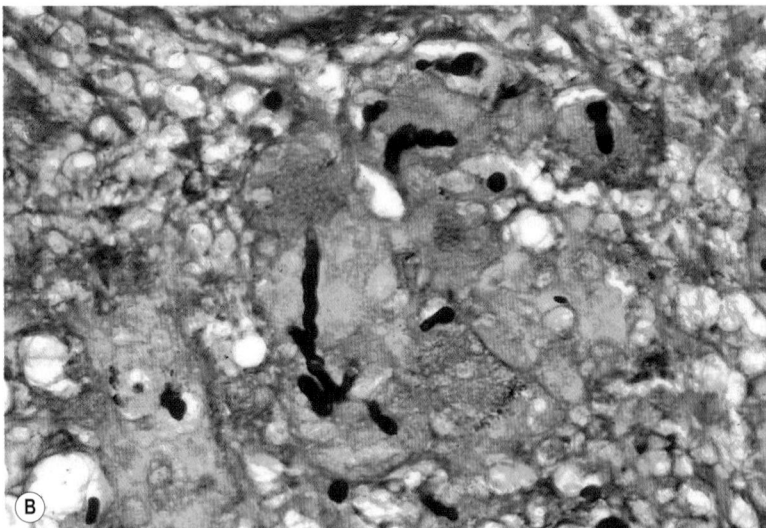

Fig. 18.356
Pheohyphomycosis: the hyphae can be highlighted with (**A**) periodic acid-Schiff and (**B**) silver stains.

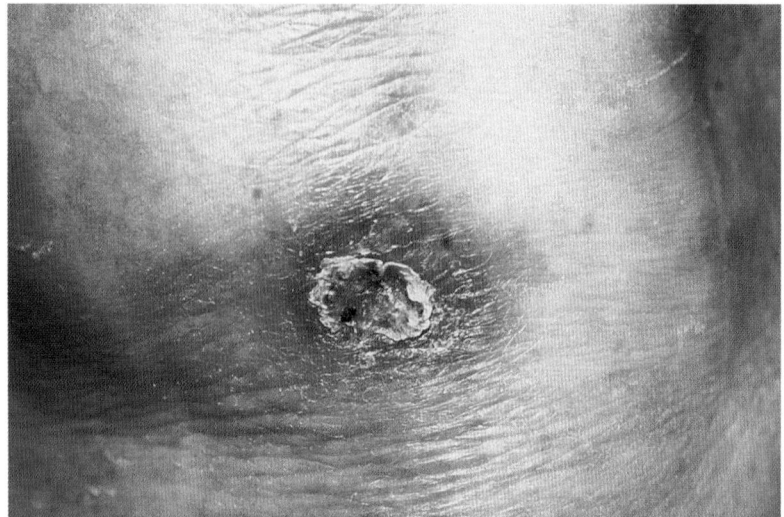

Fig. 18.357
Cutaneous alternariosis: crusted ulcer at the base of the thumb. By courtesy of S.W. Lanigan, MD, Bridgend General Hospital, Bridgend, UK.

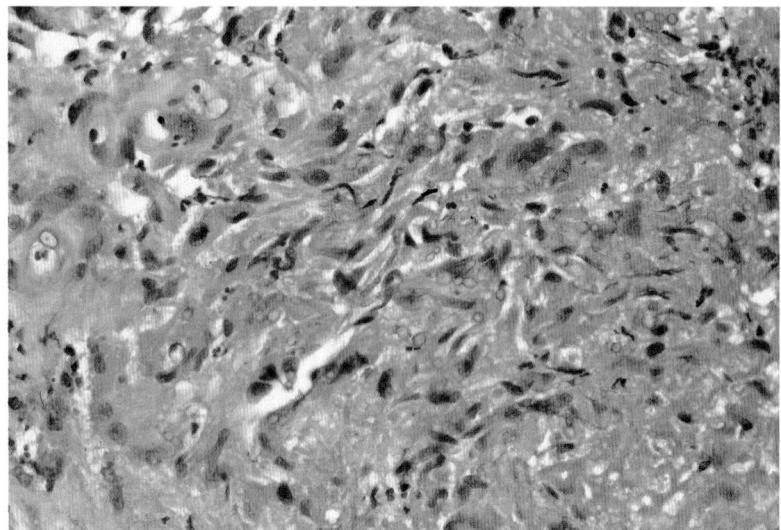

Fig. 18.358
Cutaneous alternariosis: note the yeast forms in this hematoxylin and eosin stained section.

(hyalohyphomycosis). In such cases, a Masson-Fontana stain is a useful means of highlighting the melanin.[19,38]

Alternariosis

Clinical features

Alternaria is a pigmented fungus within the heterogenous phaeohyphomycete group.[1,2] It is associated with inoculation during minor trauma and is often found in immunocompromised hosts, especially iatrogenically immunosuppressed organ transplant recipients.[3,4] Other reported clinical settings include underlying hematological malignancy, systemic corticosteroid therapy, Cushing disease, and AIDS.[5] Immunocompetent individuals are affected rarely.[5,6]

Patients present with ulcers, erythematous macules and papules, pustules, and nodules on exposed skin surfaces, sometimes crusted or verrucous (*Fig. 18.357*).[4,7] Large ulcerated plaques with pustules may also occur.[8,9] Lesions may be found on the dorsa of the hands, the fingers, elbows, knees, face, and dorsa of the feet.[10] A sporotrichoid distribution of skin lesions has been reported.[11] The lesions occasionally regress spontaneously; otherwise, they respond well to antimycotic drugs and leave only slight scars.

Pathogenesis and histologic features

Alternaria spp. are found widely in soil and plants and are most often inoculated into skin with wood splinters. In the tissues, the fungus is seen as pigmented septate hyphae measuring 5–7 μm in diameter, accompanied by open, rounded bodies 3–10 μm in diameter (range 5–20 μm) (*Fig. 18.358*).[5] They may be seen free or in histiocytes or giant cells. There is a dermal inflammatory infiltrate usually consisting of a mixed neutrophil and granulomatous reaction. A variable number of microabscesses may be present. Although epidermal changes are often not marked, pseudoepitheliomatous hyperplasia is encountered in some cases.

Differential diagnosis

Alternariosis may be readily confused with blastomycosis, especially when pigmented hyphal forms are absent from the tissue sections. Culture of the organism and/or PCR studies, however, should facilitate a more definitive diagnosis.[5]

Histoplasmosis

Clinical features

Histoplasmosis is caused by two very similar fungi, *Histoplasma capsulatum* var. *capsulatum* (*H. capsulatum*) and the African clade of *H. capsulatum* (formerly referred to as *H. capsulatum* var. *duboisii*). Despite the

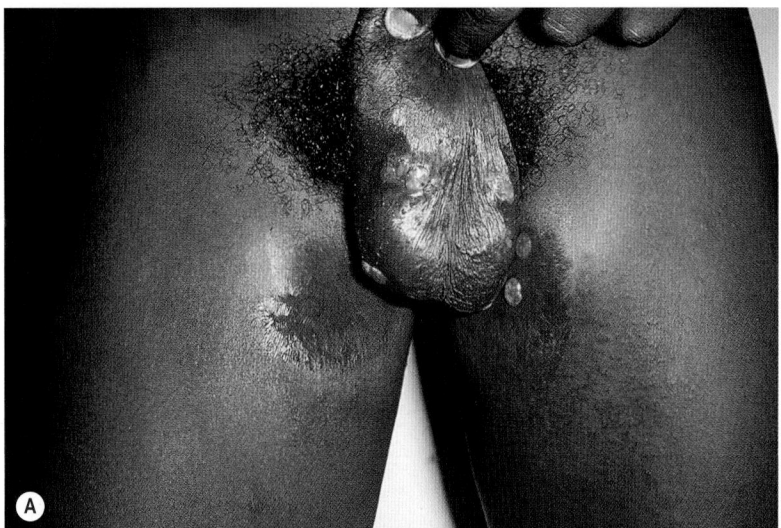

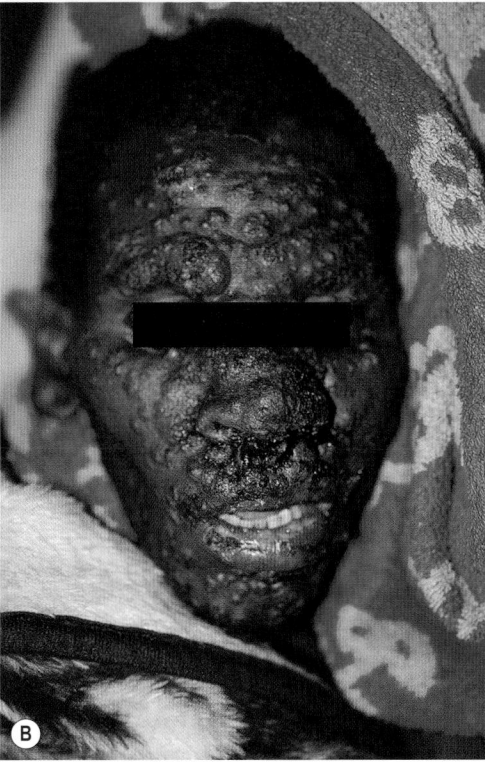

Fig. 18.359
Histoplasma capsulatum: (**A**) note the ulcerated lesions on the scrotum and thigh. This patient was HIV positive; (**B**) *duboisii* variant showing innumerable disfiguring papules, nodules, and plaques. (**A**) By courtesy of C. Furlonge, MD, Port of Spain, Trinidad; (**B**) by courtesy of N.C. Dlova, MD, Nelson R. Mandela School of Medicine, University of KwaZulu-Natal, South Africa.

morphological similarity, the two species have different geographical distributions and clinical presentations (*Fig. 18.359*).[1]

Histoplasma capsulatum

H. capsulatum is very common in North America (Ohio and Mississippi river valleys) but is seen worldwide.[1,2] Around 105 outbreaks of histoplasmosis occurred in the United States and Puerto Rico between 1938 and 2013, and involved some 2850 cases.[3] It is rare in Europe, although cases have occurred there since the advent of the HIV/AIDS pandemic.[4,5] It is present in soil and in poultry and bat droppings, and the infection has also been reported following the chopping of rotten wood and the renovation or demolition of old buildings.[1,6] Spore inhalation can cause an acute pulmonary infection (if the inoculum is very large), but it is probable that more often a subclinical infection provokes a positive histoplasmosis skin test.[7]

Chronic pulmonary (cavitatory) histoplasmosis (buckshot calcification) and disseminated disease are also recognized variants.[1,2,8] Chronic pulmonary histoplasmosis may sometimes mimic secondary tuberculosis. Disseminated histoplasmosis is uncommon, but may rarely occur in immunocompetent hosts.[9,10] It is, however, an important complication of immunosuppression including that seen in HIV/AIDS.[1,10–17] Lesions are particularly seen in the liver, spleen, lymph nodes, and bone marrow.[7] A wide variety of systems may be involved, however, and therefore symptoms and signs are very variable. Fever and weight loss, although non-specific, are common.[12,14,15]

Disseminated histoplasmosis may be classified into acute, subacute, and chronic forms in diminishing degrees of severity.[8,9] The acute form usually affects infants while chronic disseminated histoplasmosis is characteristically seen in adults. Patients with HIV/AIDS are at particular risk of developing lethal progressive disseminated histoplasmosis.[2,16] Under such conditions, it has been suggested that the disease may sometimes represent reactivation of a quiescent lesion.[7,8] The possibility of patient-to-patient transmission has also been reported.[18] In patients with HIV/AIDS-associated disseminated histoplasmosis, a combination of antifungal therapy and ART may result in a dramatic improvement in clinical outcome.[19] Histoplasmosis is also a potential manifestation of IRIS among HIV-infected individuals receiving ART.[20] Disseminated histoplasmosis can occasionally be the initial mode of presentation of an HIV infection.[12]

Cutaneous involvement is uncommon and is almost always a feature of disseminated (fungemic) disease. It is said to occur in 4% to 11% of cases in general, but is encountered in 10% to 25% of AIDS-related cases.[8,11,21,22] An Indian study of 37 cases of disseminated histoplamosis revealed a much higher frequency of skin involvement among immunocompromised patients than immunocompetent subjects (54.5% and 11.5%, respectively).[10] Lesions are most common on the arms, face, and trunk, but obviously may be encountered elsewhere.[12] Skin lesions present as macules, papules, nodules, pustules, indurated (sometimes ulcerated or verrucous) plaques, purpura, pyoderma gangrenosum-like lesions, abscesses, furuncles, cellulitis, eczematous eruptions, acneiform eruptions, MC-like lesions, punched-out ulcers, panniculitis, and subcutaneous nodules.[7,22–27] Oral ulcers may also be present.[12,14,26] An unusual case with vaginal ulcerations as the presenting sign of disseminated infection has been reported.[28] There have also been rare reports of penile ulceration in this clinical context.[29] Diffuse cutaneous hyperpigmentation sometimes reflects an underlying histoplasmosis-related Addison disease.[12] Erythema nodosum and erythema multiforme are not infrequent hypersensitivity manifestations.[7,30]

The very rare primary cutaneous lesions (representing local inoculation) present as nodules, ulcers, cellulitis, or lymphangitis.[7,31]

African clade of Histoplasma capsulatum (H. capsulatum var. duboisii)

For convenience, use of the historic designation *H. capsulatum* var. *duboisii* will be retained in this section. This organism usually occurs in equatorial Africa although it has been documented elsewhere on rare occasions.[32–34] Occasional cases have been encountered in Europe, reflecting the impact of travel and immigration patterns.[4] It has two main forms of presentation:
- Patients may develop a localized chronic form with single lesions in the skin, subcutaneous fat, or bone.
- Patients may manifest disseminated disease, which in addition affects lymph nodes and abdominal viscera.[2]

Skin lesions include superficial cutaneous and subcutaneous granulomata and abscesses and osteomyelitis with overlying cutaneous spread.[6,35] The calvarium and long bones are predominantly affected.[6] In contrast to *H. capsulatum*, pulmonary disease is rare. Furthermore, patients are usually not immunocompromised.[34,36,37]

Pathogenesis and histologic features

H. capsulatum is a dimorphic fungus appearing as a mycelium at room temperature, but growing as a yeast at body temperature.[2] Despite its name, it is not encapsulated. Infection is most commonly transmitted by the inhalation of spores or hyphae of *H. capsulatum*. The hyphal form grows in the soil; the yeast form (2–4 µm in diameter) occurs in the tissues, entirely intracellularly following inhalation of the spores.

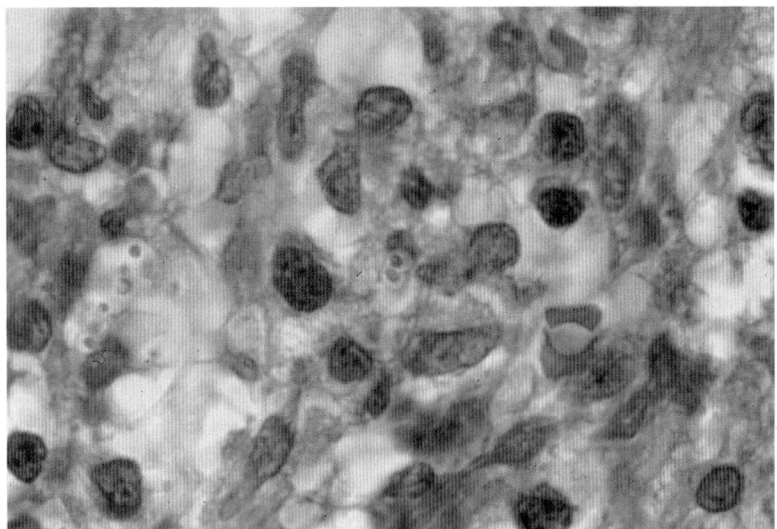

Fig. 18.360
Histoplasma capsulatum: the small yeast forms are intracellular and consist of a small basophilic particle surrounded by a clear halo (a cytoplasmic retraction artifact). By courtesy of R. Carr, MD, Warwick Hospital, Warwick, UK.

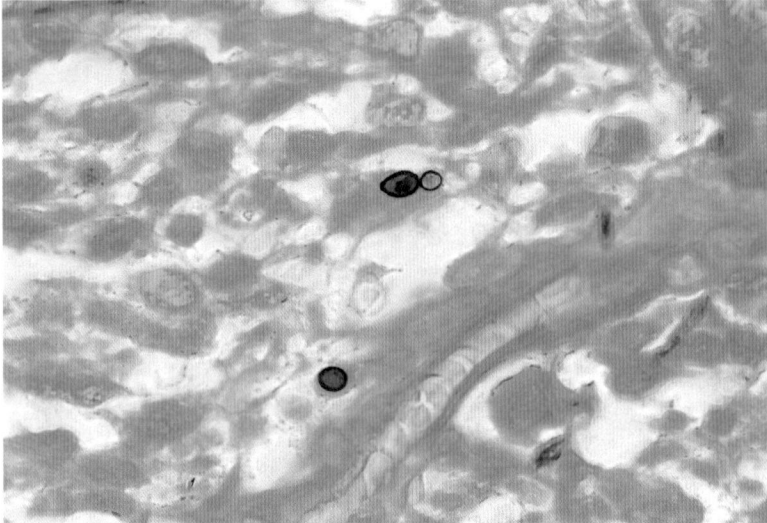

Fig. 18.361
Histoplasma capsulatum: differentiation from leishmaniasis is readily effected by the use of methenamine silver. By courtesy of R. Carr, MD, Warwick Hospital, Warwick, UK.

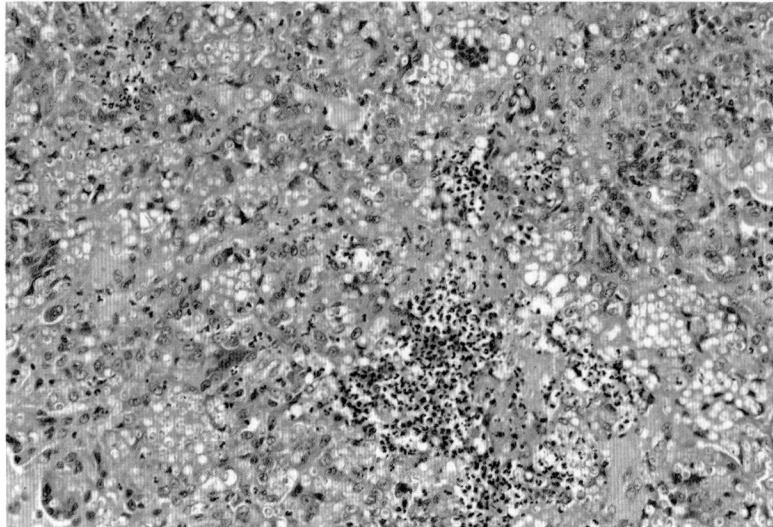

Fig. 18.362
Histoplasma duboisii: a dense granulomatous infiltrate is present in the reticular dermis. The organisms are larger than *Histoplasma capsulatum* and are located within giant cells. By courtesy of S. Lucas, MD, St Thomas' Hospital, London, UK.

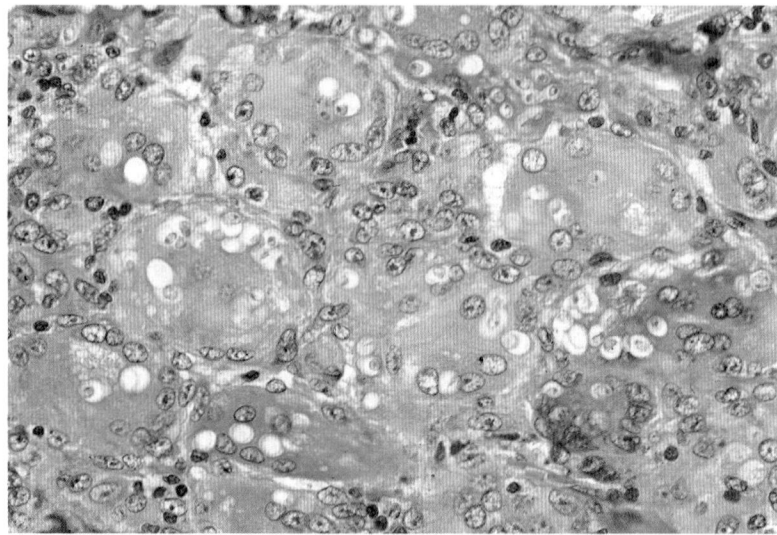

Fig. 18.363
Histoplasma duboisii: the yeast cells have very thick walls and the nuclei are single. This distinguishes *Histoplasma duboisii* from *Blastomyces dermatitidis*, in which nuclei are multiple. By courtesy of S. Lucas, MD, St Thomas' Hospital, London, UK.

The tissue response to infection with *H. capsulatum* parallels that seen with *Mycobacterium tuberculosis* including primary lesions, reinfection, and the development of caseation.[7] Following pulmonary and nodal involvement, susceptible people develop a fungemia, with spread of the organism widely throughout the body. A chronic tuberculoid granulomatous inflammatory response develops. The yeast is present within distended macrophages as a basophilic dot with a surrounding artifactual halo (pseudocapsule) (*Fig. 18.360*).[1] Its features are similar to those of *Leishmania*, but it lacks the kinetoplast. It may be further differentiated by the use of special stains including the PAS reaction and methenamine silver (*Fig. 18.361*).[35] Transepidermal elimination of *Histoplasma* has been reported in association with HIV/AIDS.[23,38] It should be noted that some HIV/AIDS-associated cases lack a granulomatous tissue response and may instead show focal necrosis and a mild perivascular and interstitial infiltrate with predominantly polymorphonuclear leukocytes, lymphocytes, and some histiocytes. Karyorrhexis may be a prominent feature, resulting in potential confusion with atypical leukocytoclastic vasculitis.[39] Involvement of cutaneous nerves by the organism has also been described in association with HIV/AIDS.[40] Biopsies from profoundly immunosuppressed individuals may reveal a negligible or absent host response to these organisms.[41]

H. capsulatum var. *duboisii* is also seen intracellularly, but usually within multinucleate giant cells (*Figs 18.362–18.364*). It is a large yeast, 7–15 μm in diameter, with characteristically thick cell walls.[1] Narrow-based budding may be seen and short chains are occasionally formed.[2] The early stages are followed by necrosis and then by a granulomatous and fibrous reaction.

Differential diagnosis

Emmonsiosis, a disseminated HIV/AIDS-related fungal infection caused by *Emergomyces africanus*, is almost indistinguishable from histoplasmosis. It is likely that rather than being a true emerging pathogen in South Africa (where the organism was recently identified), many cases diagnosed as *H. capsulatum* infection solely on morphological grounds in the past were, in fact, examples of *Emergomyces* infection. The yeasts measure 2–7 μm in diameter, and may be intracellular and/or extracellular.[42,43] This condition is discussed elsewhere in this chapter.

H. capsulatum var. *capsulatum* must also be differentiated from *Penicillium* species, especially since both infections share clinical and radiological features.[44] Macrophages parasitize both organisms. *H. capsulatum* is characterized by narrow-necked budding while *Penicillium* divides by

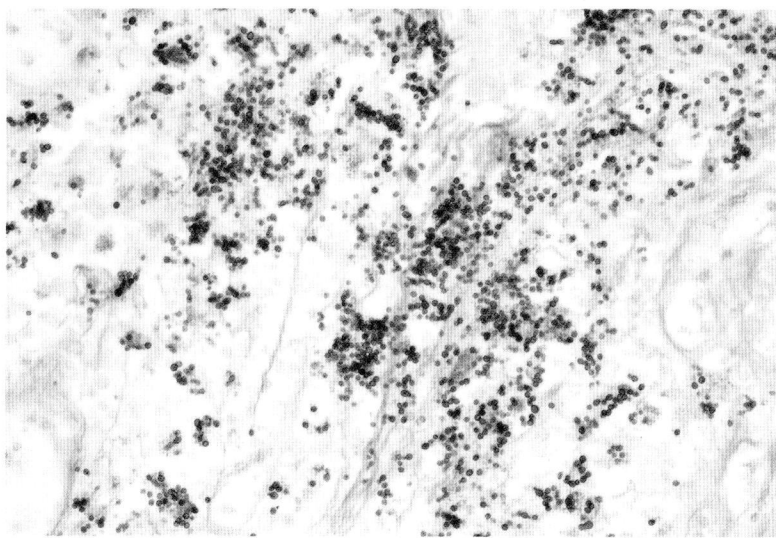

Fig. 18.364
Histoplasma duboisii: the fungi are highlighted with the methenamine silver stain. By courtesy of S. Lucas, MD, St Thomas' Hospital, London, UK.

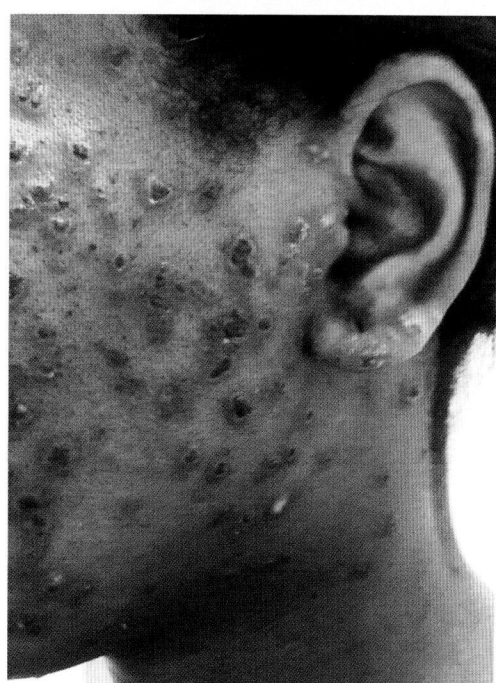

Fig. 18.365
Emmonsiosis: widespread crusted papules and plaques in a patient with underlying AIDS. By courtesy of M. Ruhani, MD, Division of Dermatology, University of the Witwatersrand, Johannesburg, South Africa.

septation. Microforms of *Blastomyces dermatitidis*, capsule-deficient forms of *Cryptococcus neoformans*, and endospores of *Coccidioides* spp. are additional sources of potential diagnostic confusion.[1,35] Although fungal culture remains the gold standard for diagnostic confirmation, and an in situ hybridization-based technique for use on paraffin-embedded material that enables distinction from other invasive fungal pathogens has been described, newer pan-fungal PCR techniques targeting the nuclear ribosomal internal transcribed spacer region hold promise in facilitating more rapid and precise speciation on formalin-fixed biopsy material.[42,43,45]

Skin involvement by histoplasmosis should also not be confused with CL (see above). Although the intracellular *Leishmania* organisms contained within macrophages resemble the yeasts of *H. capsulatum*, the former possess a kinetoplast and stain with the Giemsa method.

H. capsulatum var. *duboisii* may be distinguished from *B. dermatitidis* by having single rather than multiple nuclei.

Emmonsiosis

Clinical features

Disseminated infection with what was initially regarded as a novel species of *Emmonsia*, was described recently among South African patients with HIV/AIDS, almost all of whom had skin lesions at presentation.[1–5] Although the causative agent was briefly assigned the name *Emmonsia africanus*, it has since been named *Emergomyces africanus*.[6,7] ART had been initiated within the preceding 2 months in 24% of the HIV co-infected patients, thereby suggesting the presence of unmasking IRIS.[1,2] Immunocompetent individuals are only rarely affected.[2,4,5] Prior to 2013, there was no known association between *Emmonsia*/*Emergomyces* infection and HIV/AIDS in sub-Saharan Africa.[5] There is, however, a strong likelihood that a significant number of cases of emmonsiosis might have been misclassified as histoplasmosis in the past. Furthermore, *Emmonsia* spp. and *Emergomyces* spp. display phylogenetic proximity to *Histoplasma* spp. and other organisms in the family Ajellomycetaceae.[3,5–7]

Emergomyces africanus is a novel thermally dimorphic pathogenic fungus, which on initial molecular phylogenetic analysis was found to be most closely related to *Emmonsia pasteuriana*. The latter is an organism with an as yet unidentified environmental or animal source, and was recently renamed *Emergomyces pasteurianus*.[1,7] *Emergomyces pasteurianus* is a rare cause of disseminated disease in immunocompromised hosts, with only isolated cases recorded to date, including a transplant recipient in Spain with HIV co-infection, an ART-naïve Italian female with AIDS, a German farmer on long-term corticosteroid therapy who developed progressive pneumonic illness, a Chinese transplant recipient, and a South African patient with

AIDS.[1,2,7–11] The inhaled conidia of both *Emergomyces* spp. possess the capacity for conversion to a yeast phase in mammalian tissue, with subsequent extrapulmonary dissemination.[1,2] This is in contrast to *Emmonsia parva* and *Emmonsia crescens*, the causative agents of adiaspiromycosis. The latter is a chronic granulomatous lung disease of rodents and occasionally humans, and is characterized by the transformation of inhaled conidia into large adiaspores measuring 50–500 μm in diameter.[2,12–15]

Skin lesions are an almost universal finding among HIV/AIDS patients with disseminated emmonsiosis caused by *Emergomyces africanus*. The spectrum of cutaneous involvement is protean, with skin lesions potentially misdiagnosed clinically as varicella, secondary syphilis, seborrheic dermatitis, guttate psoriasis, disseminated cutaneous tuberculosis, Kaposi sarcoma, pyoderma gangrenosum, or even an adverse drug reaction.[2] Patients may present with erythematous and sometimes scaly, hyperpigmented or verrucous papules and plaques, ulcers, or crusted, boggy plaques (*Fig. 18.365*).[1,2,5] Penile, lip or palatal mucosal lesions have also been described. Rare skin lesions may exhibit central umbilication.[1,2] Lower respiratory tract involvement is seen in almost all cases, with chest radiographs revealing diffuse or focal infiltrates, lobular atelectasis, and/or hilar lymphadenopathy. Upper respiratory tract involvement may also occur, manifesting with epistaxis, congestion, non-specific symptoms, or even oroantral fistula formation. Although neurological symptoms are common, no organisms could be isolated from the cerebrospinal fluid of affected individuals in the largest series reported to date.[2] Blood and bone marrow involvement are common.[1,2] Disseminated emmonsiosis carries a mortality of up to 48%, and the condition is uniformly fatal if left untreated.[2] Concurrent opportunistic co-infections are not uncommon.[2,5] The detection of *Histoplasma* antigen in the urine is a potentially useful diagnostic adjunct, given the apparent cross-reactivity with *Emergomyces* (*Emmonsia*) spp.[2]

Pathogenesis and histologic features

The histologic appearances of *Emergomyces africanus* infection are virtually indistinguishable from histoplasmosis in most cases. Skin biopsies reveal a granulomatous and/or suppurative dermal infiltrate in response to variable numbers of small globose or oval fungal yeasts, with single or multiple narrow-based budding.[1,2] In some cases, the host inflammatory response is minimal, with large numbers of extracellular and intracellular organisms visible (*Fig. 18.366*). The latter are present within macrophages. PAS and

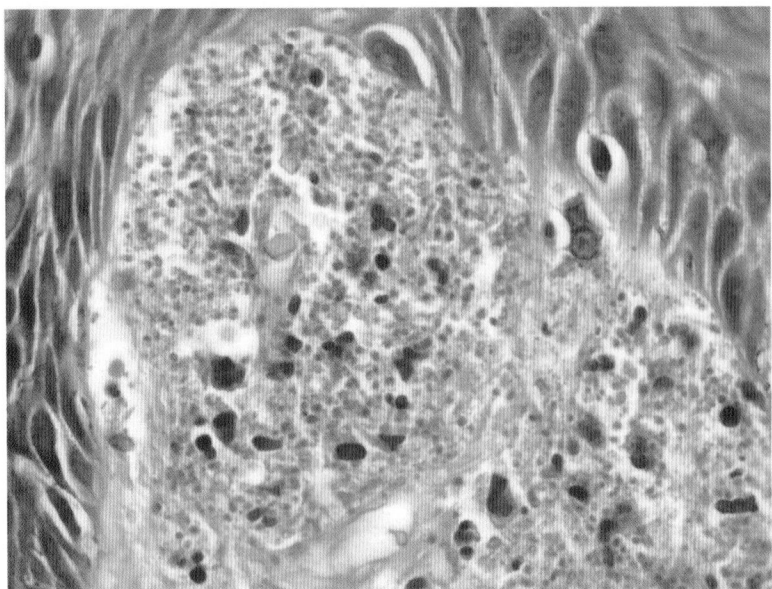

Fig. 18.366
Emmonsiosis: considerable numbers of small intracellular and extracellular yeasts are present.

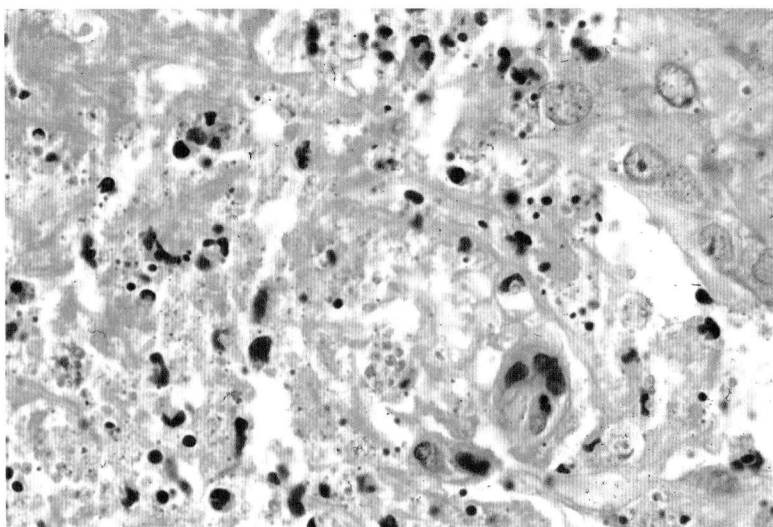

Fig. 18.367
Penicilliosis: numerous organisms are present within the cytoplasm of histiocytes.

silver stains highlight the yeast morphology and are helpful in declaring the fungi in those cases where organisms are relatively sparse. The yeasts measure 2–7 μm in diameter.[2] Cases occurring as a manifestation of IRIS are said to exhibit a more pronounced mixed dermal inflammatory infiltrate, and even microabscess formation.[1,2] Skin biopsy allows for relatively rapid diagnosis, with confirmation thereof by means of pan-fungal PCR. The aforementioned technique targets the nuclear ribosomal internal transcribed spacer region and may facilitate both rapid speciation as well as distinction from other thermally dimorphic fungi.[5–7,16]

Penicilliosis

Clinical features

Penicilliosis is caused by *Talaromyces marneffei* (formerly *Penicillium marneffei*), an organism that was first discovered in the bamboo rat (*Rhizomys sinensis*) in the 1950s.[1–4] The fungus is endemic in countries of Southeast Asia, particularly Thailand, and also in the south of China.[3,5,6] The fungus also occurs in northeastern India.[7] The organism has become an important cause of morbidity and mortality in patients infected with HIV. The great majority of patients with penicilliosis are HIV positive, and the infection is an important AIDS-defining condition in the aforementioned endemic areas.[3,8] HIV infected patients who have traveled to or lived in Southeast Asia, however, may present with the disease following their return to nonendemic countries.[8,9] Penicilliosis has also emerged as a potential manifestation of IRIS among those receiving ART.[10–13] Not all patients with *T. marneffei* infection, however, are HIV-infected adults; the disease has even been documented in HIV-negative infants on rare occasions.[14]

The disease is systemic with frequent involvement of lungs, spleen, liver, lymph nodes, bone marrow, and skin.[1,2,5] Patients present with fever, weight loss, anemia, cough, and skin lesions. The infection may mimic histoplasmosis clinically and radiologically.[15] The skin lesions consist of erythematous papules and nodules that may appear ulcerated or show umbilication.[10,12] Multiple skin abscesses may occur.[16] Verrucoid skin lesions have also been described.[13,17] The organism is an uncommon cause of genital ulceration.[18,19] The mortality is high unless systemic treatment is given promptly. A retrospective study from Thailand revealed a mortality rate of up to 29.4%.[20]

Pathogenesis and histologic features

T. marneffei is a thermally dimorphic fungus which produces a number of mycotoxins and other virulence factors.[3,4] A presumptive diagnosis is usually possible by microscopic examination of touch preparations or tissue obtained by aspiration and stained with Wright.[6,7] Histologically, a granulomatous response is usually minimal or absent. Instead, there is focal necrosis and a predominantly perivascular inflammatory cell infiltrate consisting of scattered neutrophils with nuclear dust, lymphocytes, and variable numbers of histiocytes. Necrosis is particularly prominent in immunocompromised patients. Organisms are abundant and present in the cytoplasm of histiocytes (*Fig. 18.367*). Extracellular organisms are also seen, often singly. Oval and elongated yeasts are identified on staining with PAS and Grocott. Their diameters range from 2 to 8 μm.[21,22] The small yeasts do not bud but instead divide by fission; the resultant appearance is said to be reminiscent of a sausage with a transverse septum, with the latter appearing thicker than the wall of the yeast.[22] In addition to culture, PCR may be employed to confirm the diagnosis.[21,23]

Differential diagnosis

Distinction from leishmaniasis is based on the presence of a kinetoplast in the latter. Distinction from histoplasmosis is based on the fact that *H. capsulatum* displays narrow-necked budding while *T. marneffei* divides by fission, with visible septation. Although there are obvious geographic differences, penicilliosis should also be distinguished from emmonsiosis, given the clinical and morphological similarities between the latter and histoplasmosis.

Sporotrichosis

Clinical features

Sporotrichosis is an invasive fungal infection caused by *Sporothrix schenckii sensu lato*, a complex comprising five species, namely, *S. schenckii sensu stricto*, *S. globosa*, *S. brasiliensis*, *S. luriei*, and *S. mexicana*.[1–3] The organism has a worldwide distribution, although some species are geographically restricted (e.g., *S. brasiliensis*).[2,4] It grows saprophytically in decaying vegetation and on wood.[4,5] Most often it represents a localized infection limited to the skin and lymphatics, but rarely systemic disease may occur, particularly affecting the skin, bones, joints, meninges, and occasionally, the oropharyngeal region.[1,6–8] It is inoculated into skin, often by wood splinters, thorns, and sphagnum moss. Rare cases have been acquired as a result of ritual tattooing.[9] Man-to-man and animal-to-man transmission has also been reported, including cases transmitted by cats.[4,10–13] Infection is often acquired occupationally. The condition is most common in adult males. Children, however, may also be affected.[13–15] Much less often, in immunosuppressed patients, inhalation, aspiration or ingestion can result in systemic disease.[5,16] Although most infections are sporadic, outbreaks of the disease have occasionally been reported.[17–20] Spontaneous healing of lesions may occur.

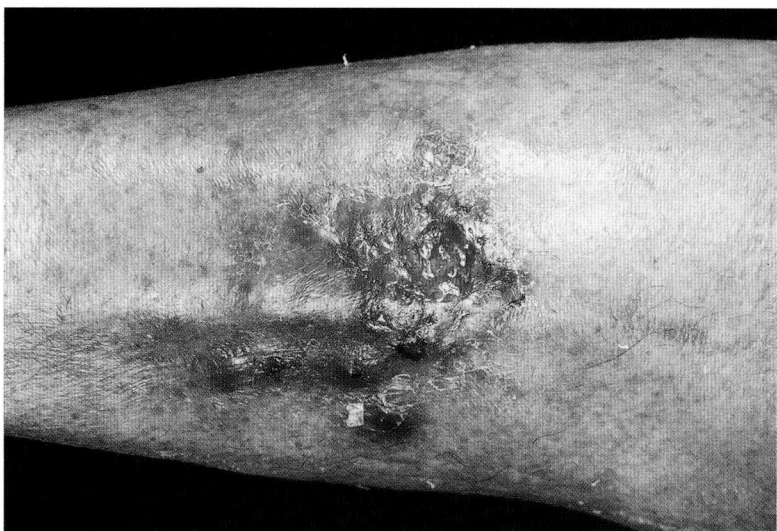

Fig. 18.368
Sporotrichosis: note the multiple nodules with ulceration on the shin, which is a characteristic site. By courtesy of S. Lucas, MD, St Thomas' Hospital, London, UK.

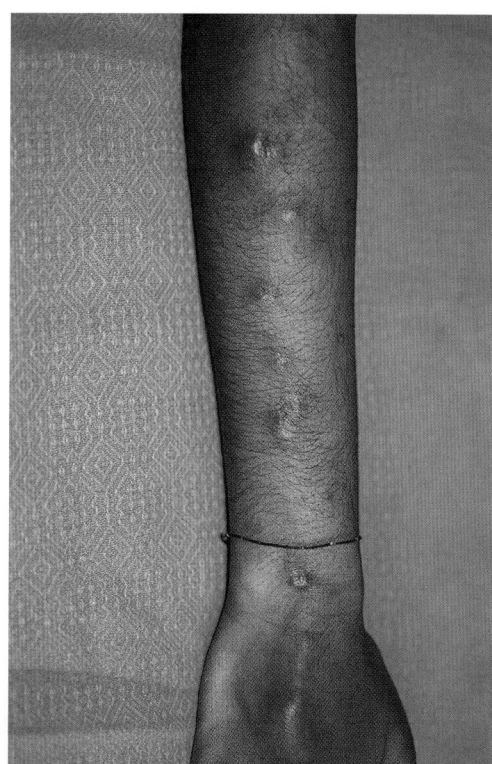

Fig. 18.369
Sporotrichosis: multiple nodules are present along the lymphatic channels draining the primary lesion. By courtesy of N.C. Dlova, MD, Nelson R. Mandela School of Medicine, University of KwaZulu-Natal, South Africa.

The cell wall components of the organism are capable of adhering to extracellular matrix proteins, in particular to fibronectin.[21] This facilitates tissue invasion. In vitro experimental evidence shows that fungus is capable of adhering to and invading vascular endothelial cells. This appears to be modulated by cytokines such as TGF-β_1 and could account for hematogenous dissemination of the fungus in immunocompromised patients.[22,23]

The cutaneous reactions to infection with *Sporothrix* spp. have been divided into three types: lymphocutaneous, localized (fixed) cutaneous, and disseminated cutaneous.

- In the most common form, lymphocutaneous sporotrichosis, the lesions develop at the site of inoculation (most often on exposed areas), after an incubation period of a few days to several weeks, as a nodule, which ulcerates (*Fig. 18.368*). Lymphatic involvement develops, with asymptomatic secondary nodules arising along the line of lymphatic drainage (*Fig. 18.369*). Regional lymph nodes then become enlarged. Meanwhile, the initial lesion expands as a crusted verrucous plaque.
- In the localized (fixed) form, the patient presents with pyodermatous erosions, acneiform, nodular, ulcerated, or verrucous lesions (*Fig. 18.370*).[5,24–29] This variant may indicate a high degree of immunity.
- Disseminated cutaneous sporotrichosis is rare.[30–32] There have, however, been a number of reports of this form of disease in patients with HIV/AIDS.[33–36] Sporotrichosis is an uncommon cutaneous manifestation of IRIS in HIV-infected patients who have received ART.[37,38]

The extracutaneous forms, which include pulmonary and systemic variants, are very rare.[1,15,39] Visceral involvement may occur in the absence of cutaneous lesions. Primary pulmonary infection and disseminated systemic sporotrichosis is seen in the immunosuppressed and occurs most often in alcoholics and patients with pulmonary tuberculosis, sarcoidosis, diabetes mellitus, and chronic steroid treatment.[5] This form of the disease has also been reported as an emerging mycosis in patients with HIV infection.[16]

Histologic features

S. schenckii sensu lato is a thermally dimorphic fungus which is filamentous in culture but yeast-like in tissues.[40] The organism is not easily seen with conventional staining and is best demonstrated with methenamine silver or PAS stains. It presents as round to oval bodies, 4–6 μm in diameter, sometimes within giant cells. Occasionally, the spores are seen as thin cigar-shaped rods up to 8 μm long; rarely, these may be present in conspicuous numbers.[5,16,27] They may be present in the center of eosinophilic radiating material, an example of the Splendore-Hoeppli phenomenon (*Fig. 18.371*).[41] This structure represents an immunological reaction between host and fungus. Indirect immunofluorescence has revealed that a portion thereof comprises antigenically related IgG and IgM molecules.[42] These so-called

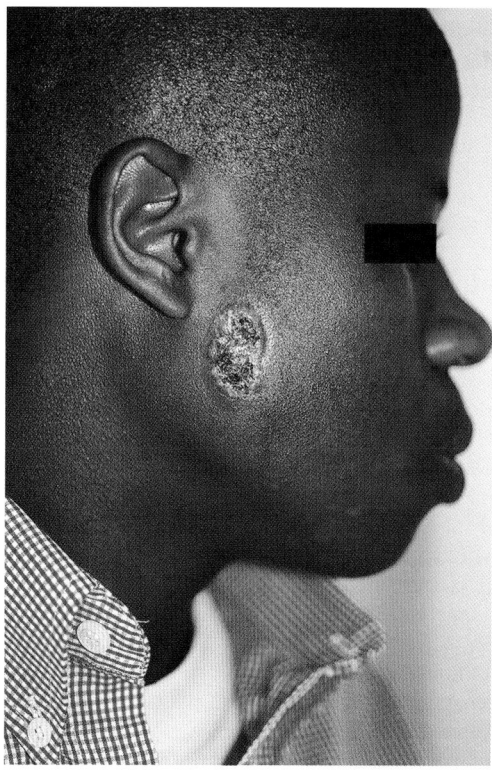

Fig. 18.370
Sporotrichosis: localized variant presenting as an ulcerated plaque. By courtesy of N.C. Dlova, MD, Nelson R. Mandela School of Medicine, University of KwaZulu-Natal, South Africa.

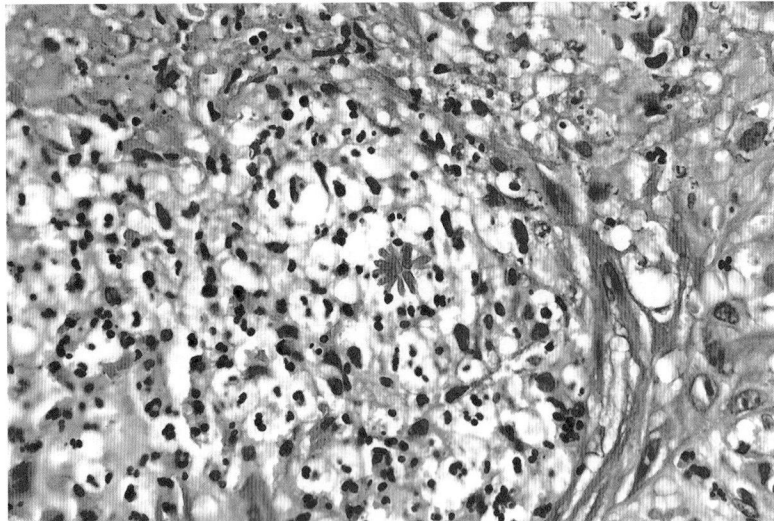

Fig. 18.371
Sporotrichosis: the yeast form is characteristically surrounded by radiating eosinophilic spokes (the Splendore-Hoeppli phenomenon).

asteroid bodies are characteristically located within intradermal microabscesses, and suppurative granulomas in particular (*Fig. 18.372*).[43,44] Examination of many serial sections is often required for identification of these elusive structures. Occasionally, hyphae may be identified in PAS-stained sections. The mycelial form of the organism (including conidia) may also be observed in the dried-up purulent exudate in chronic ulcerated lesions.[45] Surrounding the giant cells containing the often scanty organisms is an intense granulomatous infiltrate. Lymphocytes, plasma cells, and histiocytes are also present. The overlying epidermis shows acanthosis with areas of pseudoepitheliomatous hyperplasia; ulceration is often evident. Neutrophil abscesses are present in both acanthotic epidermis and dermis.[16,46]

The nodules resulting from lymphatic spread are located in the deep dermis or subcutaneous tissues. They consist of a central necrotic zone with neutrophils, a surrounding zone of epithelioid cells and giant cells, and an outer zone of plasma cells and lymphocytes with fibrosis.[5,41]

Although the tissue reaction is often suggestive of sporotrichosis, confirmation should be sought by isolation and culture of the organism. The organism may also be demonstrated by immunohistochemistry.[16,47] Infection can also be confirmed by PCR.[16,48]

Lobomycosis

Clinical features

Lobomycosis is a very rare infective dermatosis caused by the fungus *Lacazia loboi* (formerly *Paracoccidioides loboi* or *Loboa loboi*).[1–5] The disease was first described by Jorge Lobos in Recife, Brazil, in 1931.[5,6] Although culture is exceedingly difficult, the organism has been successfully inoculated into mice, rats, and armadillos.[7] It is generally confined to tropical forest areas of Central and South America, especially the Amazon basin.[2,3,6,8–10] The first case of lobomycosis in the United States was reported in 2000 and additional rare cases have been recorded in North America since then.[11,12] Rare infections have also been described in African patients. Although the natural habitat of the fungus remained an enigma for many years, soil and vegetation are now believed to be the main habitat.[13] Infections in dolphins were later reported, suggesting the possibility of a waterborne mechanism of spread, and implied zoonotic transmission.[13–15] Furthermore, affected dolphins have been found to have impaired adaptive immunity.[16] More recent epidemiological evidence, however, suggests that direct or indirect transmission of the fungus from dolphins to humans is an exceedingly rare event.[15]

The disease is seen in whites, blacks, and native South American Indians, and particularly affects males.[2,3,7] Lesions due to this fungus are mainly confined to the skin, but contiguous subcutaneous involvement may occur.[10] They are extremely insidious in development, following presumed traumatic

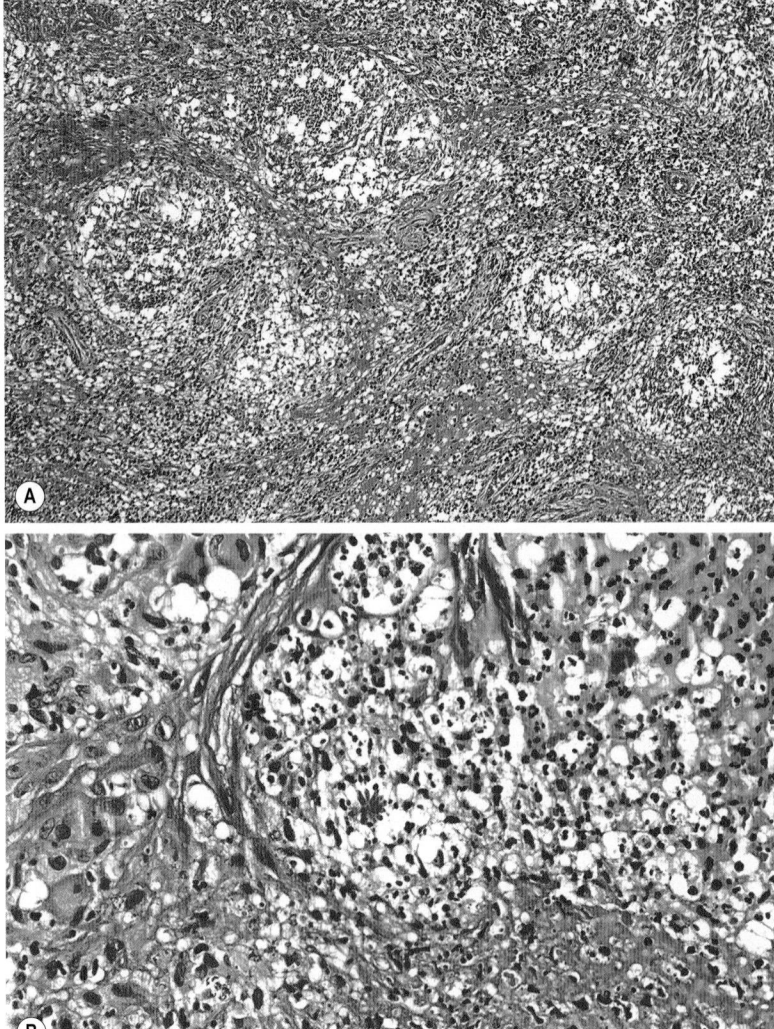

Fig. 18.372
(**A, B**) Sporotrichosis: multiple dermal abscesses are typically present in this condition.

inoculation of the skin, and present characteristically after many years. They occur on exposed skin, often on the face and earlobes, but the arms, chest, back, legs, buttocks, or lumbosacral region may also be affected (*Figs 18.373* and *18.374*). Lesions are associated with keloid-like scarring, hence the diseases previous designation 'keloidal blastomycosis'.[1,3,8,11,17,18] There are usually papular, nodular, and verrucous components; some of the nodules may become large and confluent, and ulceration sometimes occurs. Drainage lymph nodes are affected.[18–20] Although the lesions are usually painless, pruritus, hypoesthesia, burning, or anesthesia can occur.[18] There is no tendency to heal and the infection is resistant to medical therapy, leaving surgical excision as the sole effective treatment. Disseminated cutaneous lesions may occur, sometimes following local relapse.[21–23] Squamous carcinoma is an occasional long-term complication.[9,24]

Histologic features

The fungus presents in the tissues as characteristic bulbous chains of yeast-like cells, 6–12 μm (generally 9–10 μm) in diameter, with thick (double) walls and interconnecting tubular structures which later disappear.[10,14,18] Budding forms are occasionally present.[18]

Cutaneous involvement by *L. loboi* provokes a distinctive reaction. The infection is centered on the dermis, which becomes infiltrated by fungus-containing foamy histiocytes and giant cells, with the latter predominating centrally (*Figs 18.375* and *18.376*). Few other inflammatory cells are evident and fibroblasts appear later within the surrounding keloid. Suppurative inflammation and necrosis are absent. The fungi are unstained and seen

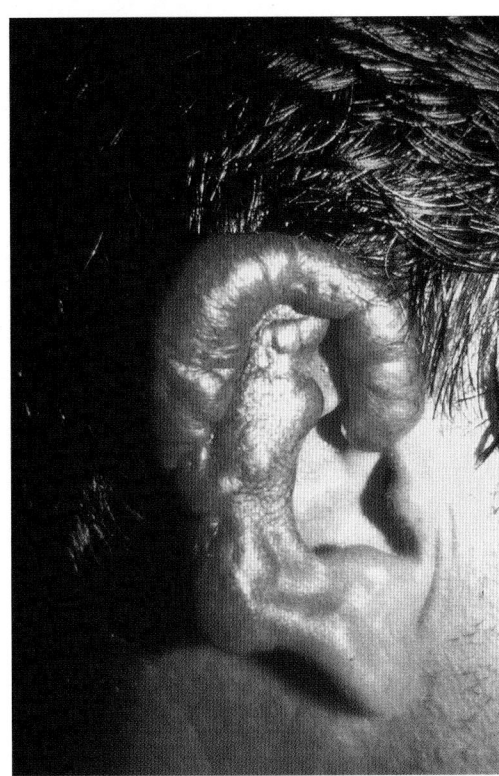

Fig. 18.373
Lobomycosis: the ear is a commonly affected site. By courtesy of S.A. Pecher, MD, Centro Manaus, Amazonas, Brazil.

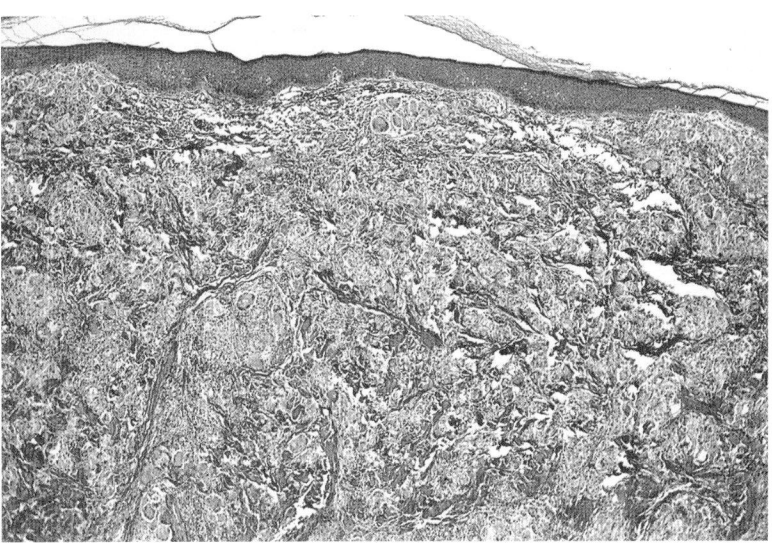

Fig. 18.375
Lobomycosis: there is an extensive granulomatous infiltrate in the dermis; the intervening eosinophilic bundles represent early keloidal scarring.

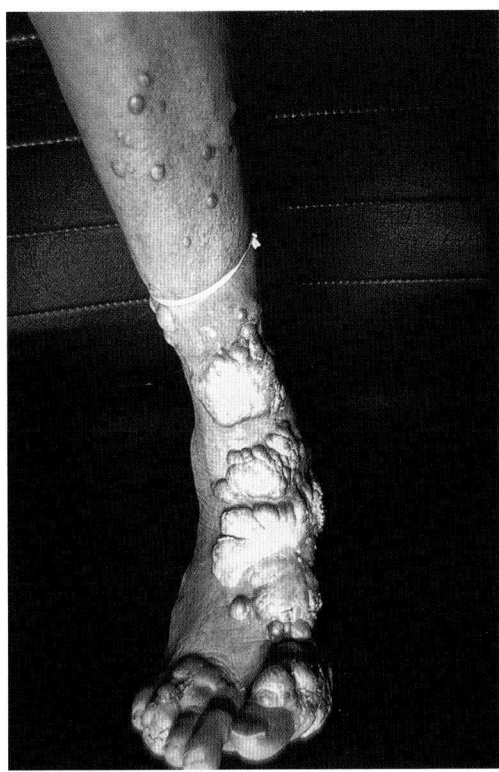

Fig. 18.374
Lobomycosis: note the gross keloidal scarring with considerable disfigurement. By courtesy of S.A. Pecher, MD, Centro Manaus, Amazonas, Brazil.

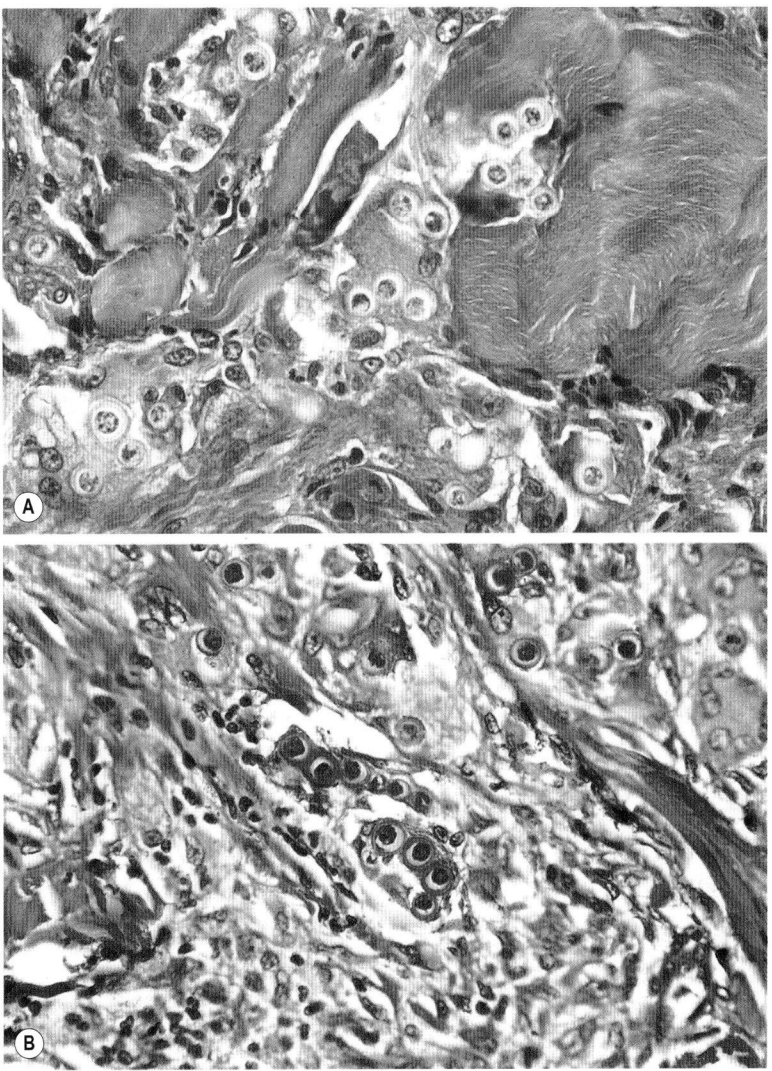

Fig. 18.376
Lobomycosis: (A) the fungi have very thick cell walls and are often arranged in chains; (B) there is striking periodic acid-Schiff positivity.

easily with H&E staining, but PAS and methenamine silver stains enhance their recognition. The overlying epidermis is generally attenuated, although vegetating lesions are associated with hyperplasia and hyperkeratosis. Transepidermal elimination of the organisms may occur.[18] In heavily infected lesions, skin appendages and nerves can be destroyed, and therefore the condition can clinically mimic leprosy. Interestingly, there have been isolated reports of co-infection with leprosy and lobomycosis.[25] Recent studies have highlighted the role of regulatory T-cells in the host immune response in lobomycotic skin lesions.[26,27]

Pneumocystosis

Clinical features

Pneumocystosis is an infection caused by the fungus *P. jiroveci* (formerly *P.carinii*), which for decades was considered to be a protozoal organism.[1-3] Although pulmonary disease is well described in immunocompromised individuals, especially those with HIV/AIDS, skin involvement is distinctly uncommon.[4-10] Almost all examples of cutaneous pneumocystosis have been associated with HIV/AIDS, where the condition may serve as a sentinel of underlying HIV/AIDS infection.[4-13] Skin infection is often not accompanied by pulmonary pneumocystosis.[5,7,10,12,14] The presence of persistent cough, fever, and an abnormal chest radiograph, however, infers concomitant lung infection.[5]

Cutaneous *P. jiroveci* infection manifests with one or multiple polypoid masses in the external auditory canal in a vast majority of cases. Otorrhea is a frequent symptom.[4,8-11,14] Potential complications include perforation of the tympanic membrane, destruction of the mastoid bone, cranial nerve involvement, and rarely, extension of the disease to involve the middle cranial fossa.[8,9] On occasion, however, non-otic skin lesions may occur, manifesting as a non-specific rash, cutaneous nodules, umbilicated MC-like translucent papules, one or more macules, brownish facial papules and plaques, or lesions resembling Kaposi sarcoma.[5-7,15] Potential sites of involvement include glabrous skin and the axilla.[5,7] Primary infection of the conjunctiva of the upper eyelid has also been reported.[16]

Histologic features

In most otic examples, there is a proliferation of granulation tissue accompanied by a mixed inflammatory cell infiltrate and a distinctive foamy exudate that is not too dissimilar to that encountered in cases of pulmonary pneumocystosis (*Fig. 18.377*).[10,16] This exudate is easily overlooked and a high index of suspicion should thus be maintained. The exudate may exhibit a propensity to be concentrated around vessels, and in some cases there is a surrounding granulomatous reaction with multinucleated giant cells.[10] Fibrin deposition is observed within and around blood vessels. Sections stained with the Gomori methenamine silver method will usually highlight the characteristic cup-shaped yeasts amid the frothy exudate.[10,16] Indirect immunofluorescence or electron microscopy may also be employed to confirm the diagnosis.[13,16] The organism is notoriously difficult to culture.

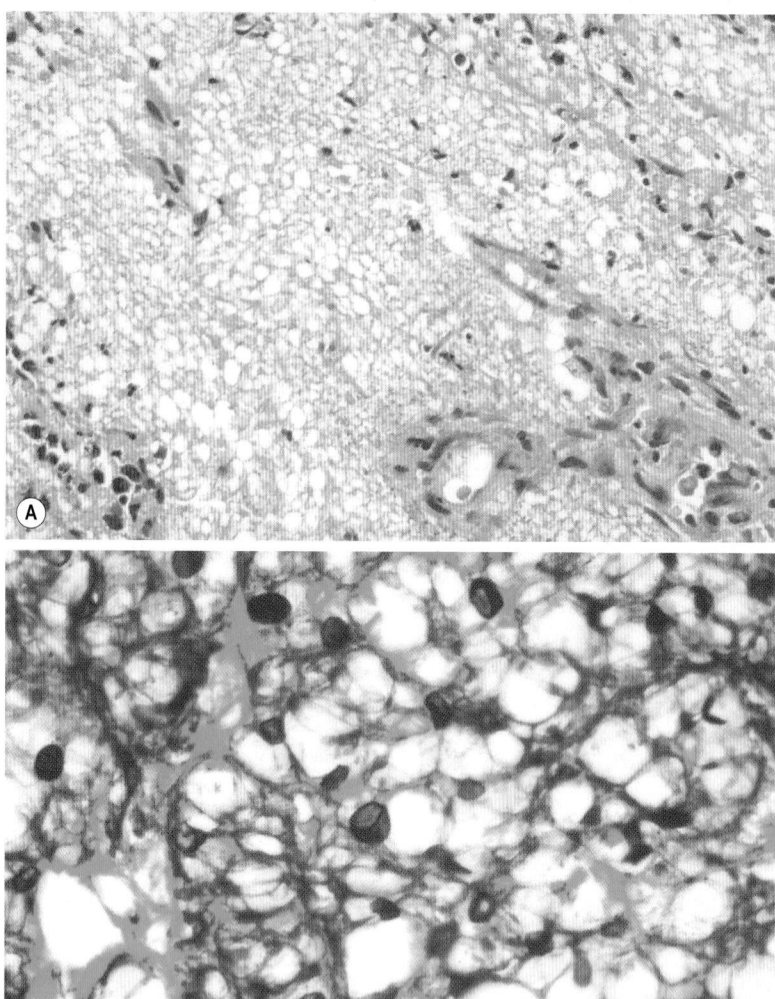

Fig. 18.377
Pneumocystis infection: (**A**) within the dermis is a diffuse 'bubbly' infiltrate; (**B**) the methenamine silver stain shows the typical morphology. By courtesy of T. Madliwa, MD, Lancet Laboratories, Johannesburg, South Africa.

There have been isolated reports of dual infection with other organisms, including botryomycosis due to concomitant *Staphylococcus aureus* infection, and skin lesions harboring both *Pneumocystis* organisms and *Cryptococcus neoformans*.[12,13] A unique case of the latter showed both organisms within the cytoplasm of foamy histiocytes, and a resultant picture closely mimicking a xanthoma.[15]

DISEASES CAUSED BY MESOMYCETOZOEA

Rhinosporidiosis

Clinical features

Rhinosporidiosis is an uncommon and somewhat enigmatic disease caused by *Rhinosporidium seeberi*, an organism that until relatively recently was considered to be a fungus, based on its morphological and staining characteristics.[1,2] Molecular biological analysis, however, has since revealed that the causative agent is a novel aquatic protistan Ichthyosporean microbe and member of a new clade termed the Mesomycetozoea.[3-5] This new class is located at the animal-fungal boundary, and its members include ten other parasitic and saprobic microbes.[3,4,6] The etiological agent was briefly renamed *Microcystis aeruginosa* in 2001 after it was cultured for the first time.[2,7-11] Infection results in polypoid lesions containing characteristic cyst-like sporangia.[7]

Rhinosporidiosis is found in India and Sri Lanka as a waterborne infection affecting mainly the nasopharynx, and as a dustborne infection affecting equally conjunctiva and nasopharynx in the dry southern states of the United States. Sporadic cases have been reported worldwide.[1] Multiple host-specific strains may exist.[6] The infection affects men much more commonly than women and presents as hyperplastic polypoid mucosal lesions.[12] Lesions in the nose resemble 'allergic' nasal polyps. The same polypoid presentation is seen in the lesions of the conjunctiva. In one recent series of ocular rhinosporidiosis reported from India, more than half of those afflicted were children aged less than 10 years.[13] The infection occasionally involves the larynx, trachea, and the mucosae of the rectum, urethra, and genitalia, where it resembles condylomata.[1,14–17] Other rarely reported sites include the vagina, the pinna and the lacrimal sac.[18–20]

Exceptionally rarely, disseminated variants have been recorded.[12,21–30] Disseminated disease manifests with widespread cutaneous or subcutaneous nodules, plaques, soft tissue masses, or even osteolytic bone lesions.[21–25,28,30,31] Rarely, cutaneous lesions in disseminated disease may be associated with a verruciform appearance or an overlying cutaneous horn.[30,32] Pulmonary involvement and involvement of the nail apparatus have also been reported.[33,34] Primary cutaneous lesions are rare and are described as papules which become verrucous and granulomatous.[7,35] Giant cutaneous or subcutaneous lesions mimicking soft tissue tumors have also been described.[36–40]

Pathogenesis and histologic features

The precise mechanism of infection is unknown. It has been proposed that the organism is present in soil, dust, and water and that involvement of the nose and conjunctiva follows rubbing with contaminated fingers.[1] Cutaneous involvement occurs by contiguous extension from a mucosal infection, autoinoculation, and rarely through hematogenous dissemination.[22,41,42] The presence of significant antirhinosporidial antibody titers does not appear to confer a protective effect.[43] It has been shown that synchronous nuclear divisions take place in the juvenile and early intermediary sporangia of *R. seeberi*, without cytokinesis; this results in the formation of thousands of nuclei. Cytokinesis, however, occurs as a one-time event in the latest stages of intermediate sporangia, immediately prior to the development of mature sporangia.[5]

In tissue, the causative agent is characterized by thick-walled (birefringent) endospore-filled sporangia.[1] These are seen in the stroma of the polyps as cysts, 10–200 μm in diameter (*Figs 18.378* and *18.379*). The cysts have a thick wall, which remains in a collapsed form after the endospores have been released. Endospores are seen initially at the periphery of the sporangium, but they gradually fill the cyst-like center before rupture occurs. The spores are 7–8 μm in diameter and contain 8–10 eosinophilic globular bodies (*Fig. 18.380*). They mature to form small trophic cysts (*Fig. 18.381*). The lesions are easily identified on H&E-stained sections and can also be demonstrated by PAS and methenamine silver stains.[12] Watery substances stimulate mature sporangia to undergo rupture, with subsequent discharge of the endospores. This affinity for wet environments may also explain why infections tend to involve the mucous membranes of human hosts.[1]

The cysts are associated with a stromal mixed neutrophil, histiocyte, plasma cell, and lymphocyte infiltrate. The overlying epidermis in skin lesions may show pseudoepitheliomatous hyperplasia, hyperkeratosis, and papillomatosis.[1] Foreign body giant cells may be abundant. These may sometimes assume gigantic proportions, with engulfed sporangia.[37]

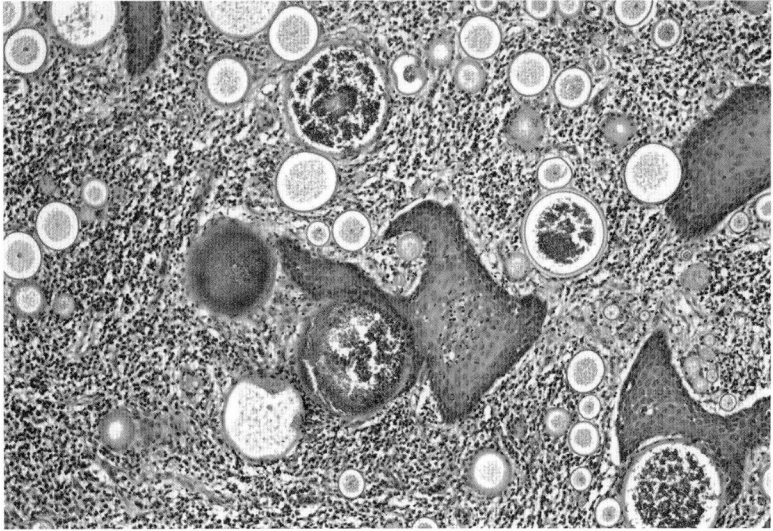

Fig. 18.379
Rhinosporidiosis: maturation of the spores is from the periphery to the center of the cyst; note the thick hyaline eosinophilic wall.

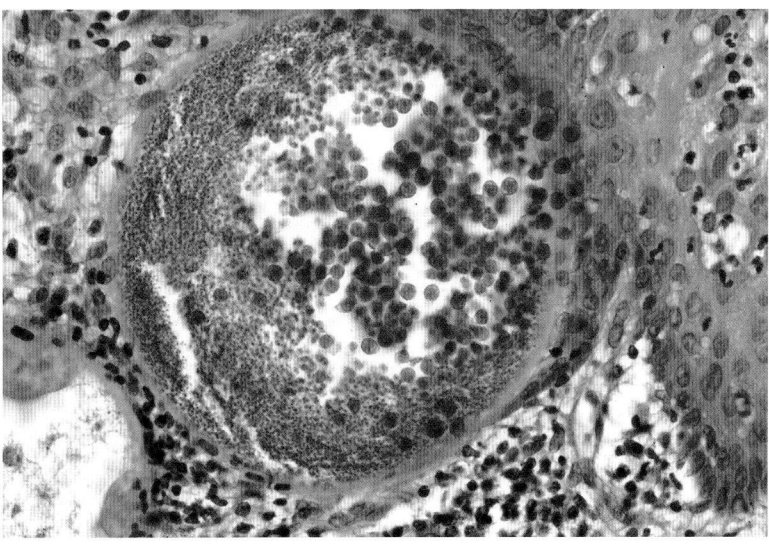

Fig. 18.380
Rhinosporidiosis: high-power field showing the internal structure of the spore.

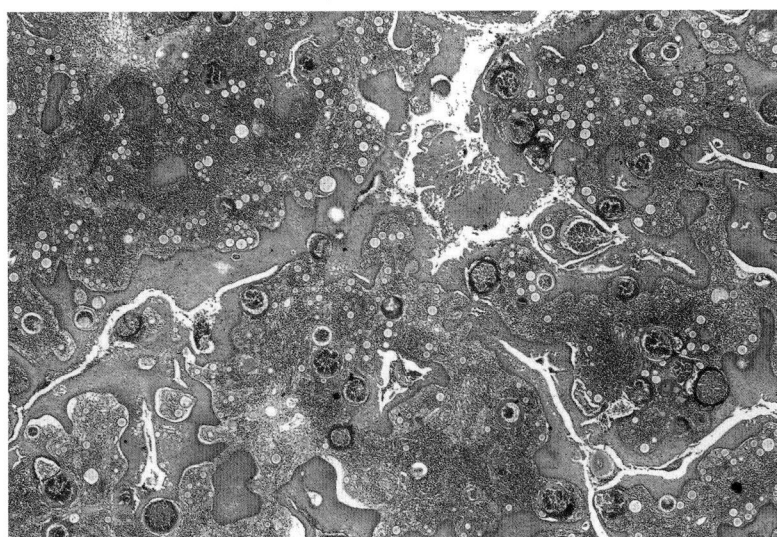

Fig. 18.378
Rhinosporidiosis: this is part of a polypoid nasal lesion. Multiple sporangia containing conspicuous spores are present.

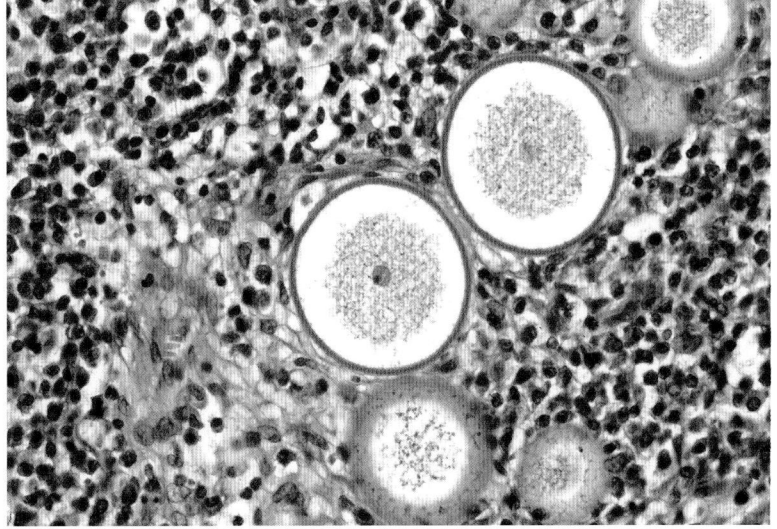

Fig. 18.381
Rhinosporidiosis: individual spores mature to form small trophic cysts.

ARTHROPOD INFESTATIONS

Scabies

Clinical features

Scabies is caused by the itch mite *Sarcoptes scabiei* (*S. scabiei* var. *hominis*), which penetrates the skin in many areas, but usually below the neck.[1-5] An estimated 300 million people are affected worldwide.[3,6-8] The most commonly affected sites are about the hands and feet (*Fig. 18.382*). Papules and burrows are often found between the fingers or along the sides of the fingers. The soles and sides of the feet are especially affected in children. As a secondary phenomenon (unrelated to burrows), patients develop an intensely pruritic papular generalized eruption, particularly affecting the abdomen, thighs, and buttocks. This reaction may be immune complex-mediated or develop as a consequence of a cell-mediated immune reaction. Patients may have raised serum IgE levels.[9] Antigenic cross-reactivity with house dust allergens has been demonstrated.[6] The papular eruption is often excoriated and may be associated with secondary bacterial infection (*Fig. 18.383*), which may in turn lead to complications such as septicemia, rheumatic fever, and postinfectious glomerulonephritis.[2,10-12] This contagious infection is spread through close personal contact and may be transmitted sexually, resulting in genital scabies.[1] Scabies may be masked by the use of corticosteroids (scabies incognito).[6] Furthermore, the disease can mimic a variety of other dermatological disorders, resulting in delayed diagnosis.[10,13,14]

The uncomplicated lesion is a sinuous burrow up to 1 cm in length and associated with intense itching, particularly at night. A small proportion of patients may go on to develop nodular scabies, which is seen particularly in the axillae, about the genitalia, and on the abdomen.[9] These are intensely pruritic and remarkably persistent. Severe keratotic and psoriasiform lesions are seen in physically and mentally debilitated and immunocompromised (including HIV-positive and some iatrogenically immunosuppressed) patients owing to massive infestation and is termed hyperkeratotic, crusted, or Norwegian scabies (*Fig. 18.384*).[15-18] Crusted scabies is a potential cutaneous manifestation of IRIS in patients with HIV/AIDS who have received ART.[19]

Pathogenesis and histologic features

Scabies is associated with poor socioeconomic conditions, overcrowding, and poor personal hygiene, and may be acquired during sexual contact.[3,8]

The pathogenetic roles of mite serine protease inhibitors of the serpin superfamily and mite aspartic protease have been highlighted recently.[20-23]

The fertilized female *S. scabiei* mite deposits eggs in the burrows in the epidermis. The larvae emerge in 3–5 days and mature in 10–14 days. The burrows extend at a shallow angle through the stratum corneum and may reach the deeper epidermis. There is acanthosis and hyperkeratosis and

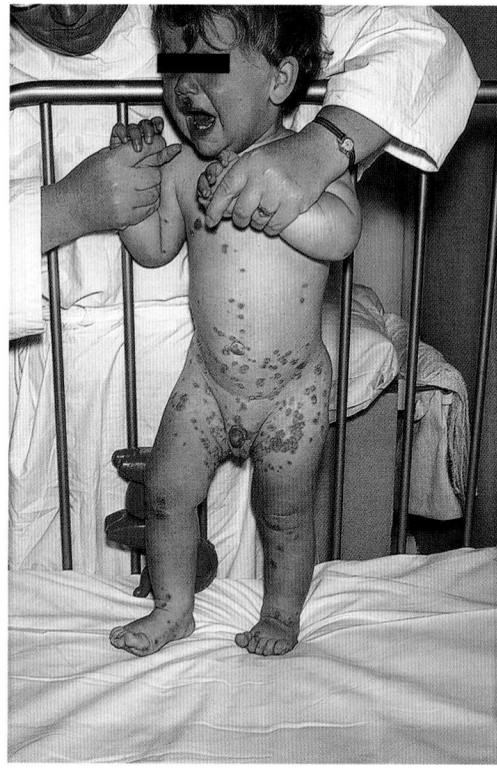

Fig. 18.383
Scabies: this is an intensely itchy condition and therefore secondary infection is a not uncommon complication, as for example in this child with staphylococcal sepsis. By courtesy of M.M. Black, MD, Institute of Dermatology, London, UK.

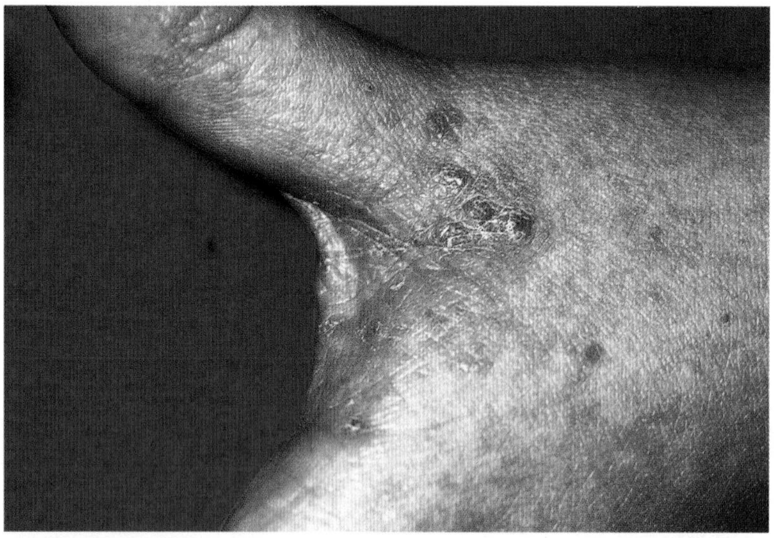

Fig. 18.382
Scabies: the burrows are linear, slightly raised lesions. The most common sites affected include the lateral aspects of the fingers, the web between thumb and first finger, and the wrists. By courtesy of R.A. Marsden, MD, St George's Hospital, London, UK.

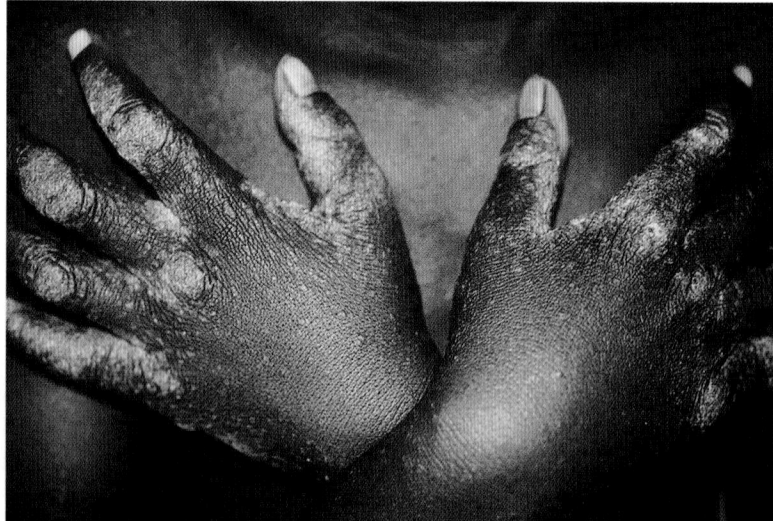

Fig. 18.384
Norwegian scabies: this example (also known as the hyperkeratotic variant) may affect widespread areas of the body, and is associated with severe crusting and a very heavy infestation of mites. It is exceedingly infectious. By courtesy of N.C. Dlova, MD, Nelson R. Mandela School of Medicine, University of KwaZulu-Natal, South Africa.

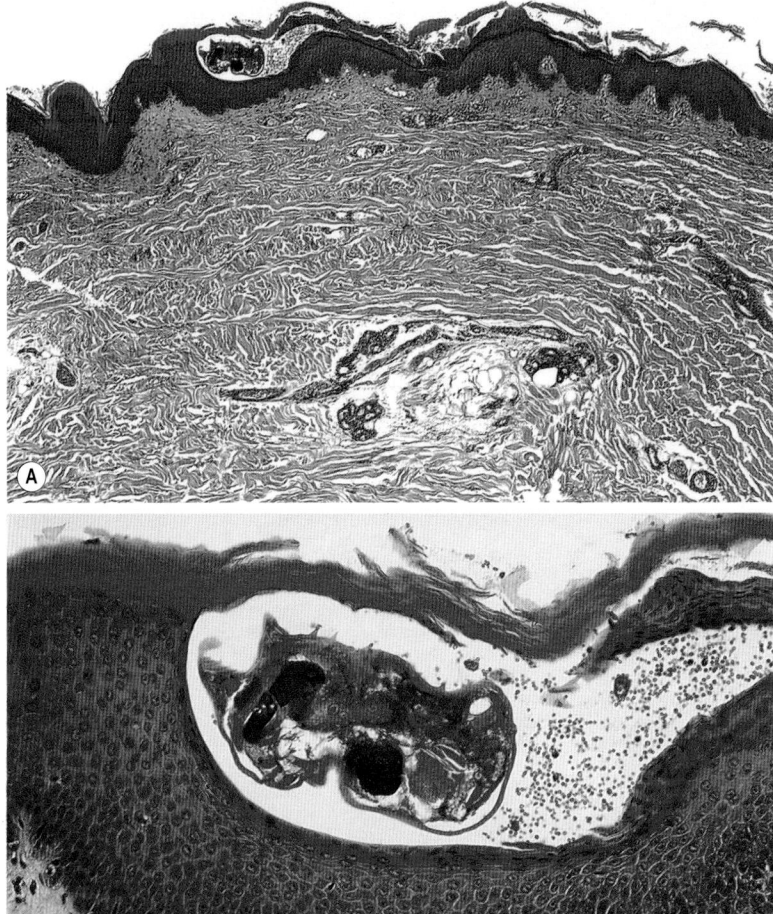

Fig. 18.385
(A, B) Scabies: the mite is located at the junction between the epidermis and the stratum corneum.

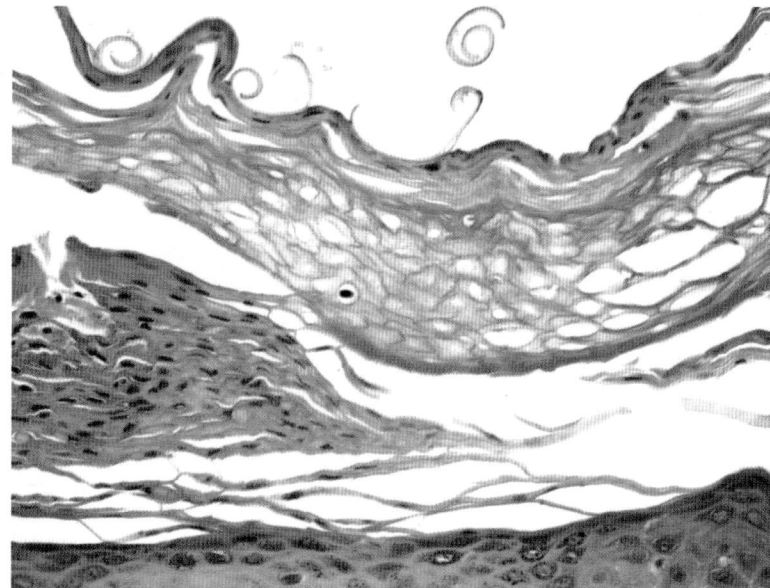

Fig. 18.386
Scabies: small, curved eosinophilic structures are attached to the stratum corneum, and represent fragments of *Sarcoptes* egg shell casings. This has descriptively been referred to as the 'pigtail' sign.

often associated spongiosis with a lymphocytic infiltrate in the epidermis (*Fig. 18.385*). The spongiosis may progress to vesiculation. Eggs, larvae, mites, mite parts, and excreta (scybala) may be identified in the stratum corneum.[10,24–27] Eosinophilic spongiosis may be encountered.[28] In the dermis, there is a superficial perivascular (and sometimes diffuse) infiltrate of lymphocytes and histiocytes, sometimes accompanied by polymorphs and less often eosinophils. The presence of the last may be associated with the features of acute vasculitis and flame figures.[29] The lymphocytes are predominantly of T-cell lineage and may exhibit atypia.[27,30] CD30 positive lymphocytes may be a feature. Fibrin thrombi are often encountered in the superficial dermal vessels.[27]

C3 and Ig may be detected at the epidermo-dermal junction and within the perivascular region, adding support to the concept of an immune complex-mediated pathogenesis.[30] IgE has been detected in vessel walls and IgA and C3 in the stratum corneum.[31] There have also been numerous reports of eruptions resembling BP in association with proven scabies.[32–34] In one study, these patients were found to have circulating antibodies against BP180 and/or BP230 antigens, indicating that at least a proportion of bullous eruptions in scabetic patients are indeed attributable to BP.[33] Others, however, have documented negative direct and indirect immunofluorescence in patients with bullous scabies whose lesions mimicked BP both clinically and histologically.[35] One recent study nevertheless revealed that elderly patients with a history of scabies were at significantly increased risk for developing BP.[36]

There have been rare reports of Grover disease in association with *Sarcoptes scabiei* infestation.[37]

In nodular skin lesions, the dermal infiltrate may be very dense and, in addition to histiocytes, plasma cells, eosinophils, and lymphocytes, atypical and hyperchromatic cells may be evident, which may suggest a lymphomatous process if the clinical information is not evident.[38] Hyperplasia of Langerhans cells has been reported; this may potentially be misdiagnosed as Langerhans cell histiocytosis.[39–41]

The papular lesions show mild hyperkeratosis and parakeratosis in association with acanthosis and spongiosis. A perivascular inflammatory cell infiltrate of lymphocytes, histiocytes, and sometimes neutrophils may be evident in the superficial dermis. Eosinophils may be absent.[9] Rarely, scabies incognito may present with a subcorneal pustular reaction mimicking subcorneal pustular dermatosis.[42]

In the hyperkeratotic variant, mites and eggs are numerous, but they are scanty in the other forms. In such cases, PCR may be a useful adjunct to the diagnosis.[43] Examination of sections under polarized light, however, provides a more affordable and practical alternative in subtle cases, as elements of the scabetic mites such as the spines and scybala are polarizable.[44] The identification of curved, pink, often refractile structures (remnants of eggshell casings) within the intracorneal burrows (the 'pigtail' sign) is a useful diagnostic clue in those cases where the body of the mite is not visible in the plane of sectioning (*Fig. 18.386*).[27,45,46] A further very useful clue is identification of the feces of the mites within the stratum corneum, displayed as bright yellow amorphous aggregates ('golden nuggets').

Tungiasis

Clinical features

Tunga penetrans, the sand flea or jigger flea, causes skin lesions in Central and South American, Caribbean, sub-Saharan African, Indian, and Pakistani populations.[1–4] Although increasing urbanization and improved housing has led to a decrease in the overall incidence of the disease, the condition remains highly prevalent in communities living in extreme poverty, with prevalence rates of around 80% recorded in some hyperendemic regions.[4–6] Seasonal variation in the prevalence tends to occur, with a peak in the dry season.[7] The disease is sometimes encountered in international travelers returning home from visits to endemic areas.[2,5,8,9] Dogs, cats, and slum rats serve as animal reservoirs.[4,10,11] *T. penetrans* is found most often in dry, warm, shady, and sandy soil.[4] The gravid female flea burrows into the skin and is localized to the feet in an overwhelming majority of cases, most commonly along the edge of the plantar aspect, interdigitally, and under the nails.[8,12] Involvement

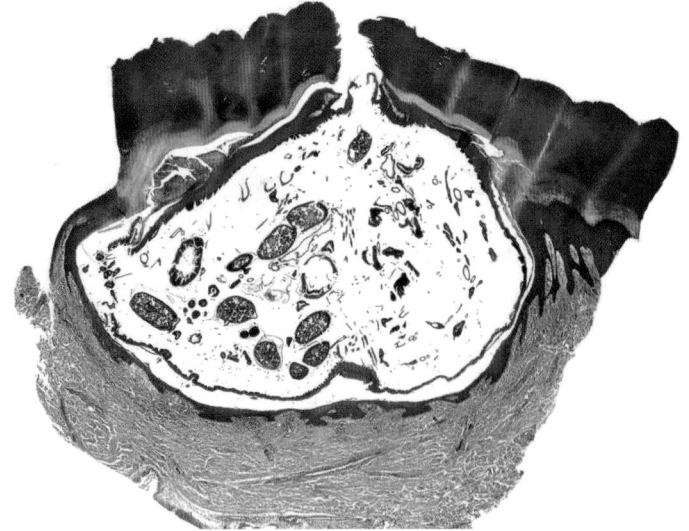

Fig. 18.387
Tungiasis: the flea is surrounded by epidermis except for an ostium in the stratum corneum through which it defecates and lays eggs. Similarly, its head penetrates into the dermis to feed from the superficial blood vessels.

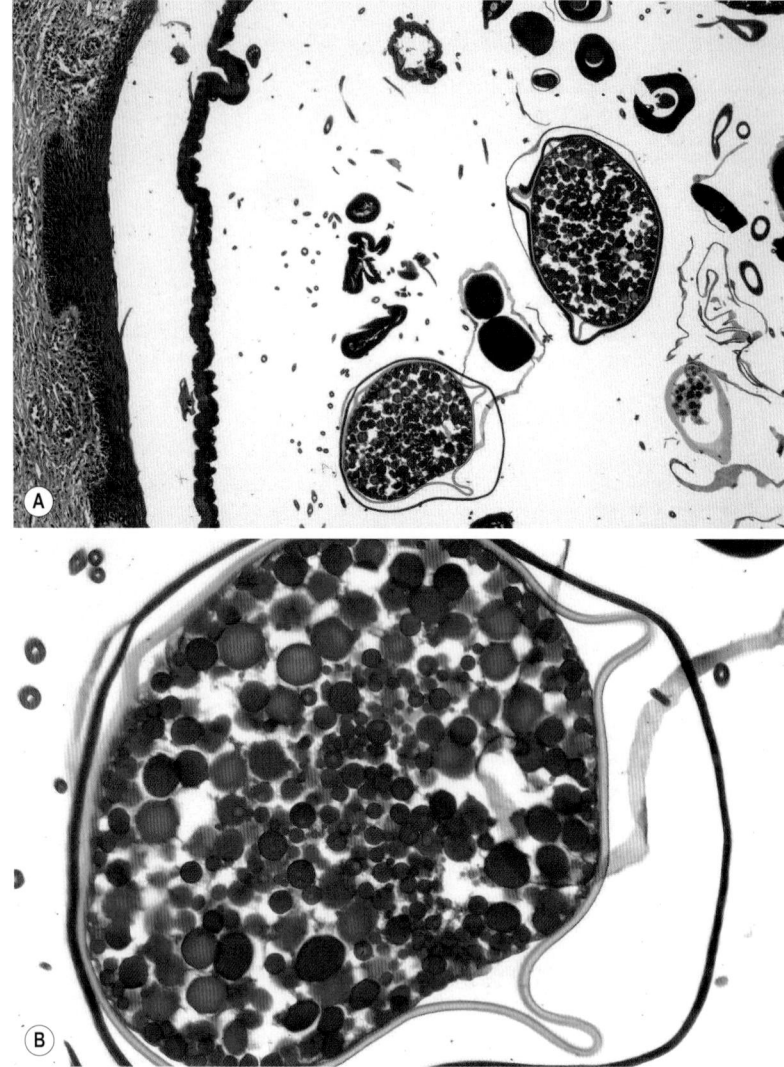

Fig. 18.388
(**A**, **B**) Tungiasis: numerous eggs are evident.

of sites such as the hands, thigh, knee and inguinal area, however, has also been recorded.[8,13,14] As the flea enlarges within the epidermis, a pruritic, painful white, or erythematous papulonodule develops. A black central punctum is characteristic. Pustular, wartlike, and bullous lesions have rarely been described.[8,15] A remarkable case with vast numbers of bilateral lesions on the feet has been reported.[16] The gravid flea, which has burrowed deep into the epithelium so that it is flush with the epidermal surface, extrudes eggs and excreta through the remaining epidermal opening. It eventually reaches a size of 1 cm in diameter. The eggs pass through the larval stages to a mature flea capable of jumping 35 cm – 350 times its own length! After laying its eggs the flea dies, the lesion collapses and is sloughed off before healing occurs. The eggs are visible on dermoscopy.[17,18] Ex vivo dermoscopy has also been advocated as a useful diagnostic tool.[19,20]

The lesion causes irritation, but in itself is innocuous; however, secondary infections such as cellulitis, tetanus, and gangrene are more sinister. Auto-amputation of the toes is an additional complication.[21] Organisms most frequently associated with bacterial superinfection include *Staphylococcus aureus* and various enterobacteriaceae; secondary infection by anaerobes such as *Peptostreptococcus* spp. and *Clostridium* spp. may also occur.[22,23] Although tungiasis is generally a benign, self-limiting infection in returning travelers, the condition is a source of considerable morbidity among the inhabitants of endemic areas.[9]

Histologic features

The bulk of the flea is intraepidermal in location.[20,24] It communicates with the outside through a pore in the stratum corneum via which it defecates, breathes, and lays eggs. The proboscis penetrates through the basement membrane into the dermis, which contains a mixed inflammatory infiltrate of lymphocytes, plasma cells, and eosinophils (*Figs 18.387* and *18.388*). The most consistently identifiable parts of the flea in skin biopsy specimens are the exoskeleton, a hypodermal layer beneath the latter, tracheae, and developing eggs; the head is rarely seen.[20,24] Epidermal alterations that may be encountered include basal hyperplasia, acanthosis, hyperkeratosis, parakeratosis, and hypergranulosis. Microabscesses are also sometimes observed.[20] Pseudoepitheliomatous epidermal hyperplasia has been reported.[14]

Myiasis

Clinical features

The term 'myiasis' is derived from the Greek word for fly (*myia*). The condition is the result of cutaneous infestation with maggots (larvae) of fly species from the order Diptera. Infestation with larvae of the human botfly,

Dermatobia hominis, is the most common form and is endemic to parts of Central America and South America.[1-4] *Cordylobia anthropophaga* (tumbu fly) infestation is encountered less frequently and is endemic to sub-Saharan Africa.[1,2,5,6] *D. hominis* has a unique life cycle in that the eggs are not transmitted directly to the host by the female botfly. Instead, the eggs are attached to the abdomen of a variety of blood-sucking arthropods, usually a mosquito. The eggs hatch in the presence of body heat emanating from the warm-blooded host during a blood meal, and the larvae drop onto the skin.[4]

Three clinical forms may occur in human skin:
- furuncular myiasis, with boil-like lesions occurring on exposed parts of the body such as the scalp, face, or limbs if botfly associated, and usually on nonexposed sites such as the buttock, thighs, breasts, or trunk if tumbu fly associated;
- wound myiasis due to deposition of larvae of flies such as *Cochliomyia americana*, *Chysomia bezziana*, or *Lucilia sericata* in pre-existing wounds;
- migratory (creeping) myiasis, a zoonosis caused by larvae of *Hypoderma bovis* or *Gasterophilus intestinalis*.[1,2,5-7]

Furuncular myiasis presents initially as an erythematous papule which enlarges to form a 1–3 cm painful, sometimes crusted boggy plaque or 'boil' with a central punctum through which serosanguinous fluid may discharge (*Fig. 18.389*). A mature 15–20 mm larva eventually emerges within 5–10 weeks.[1,2,4]

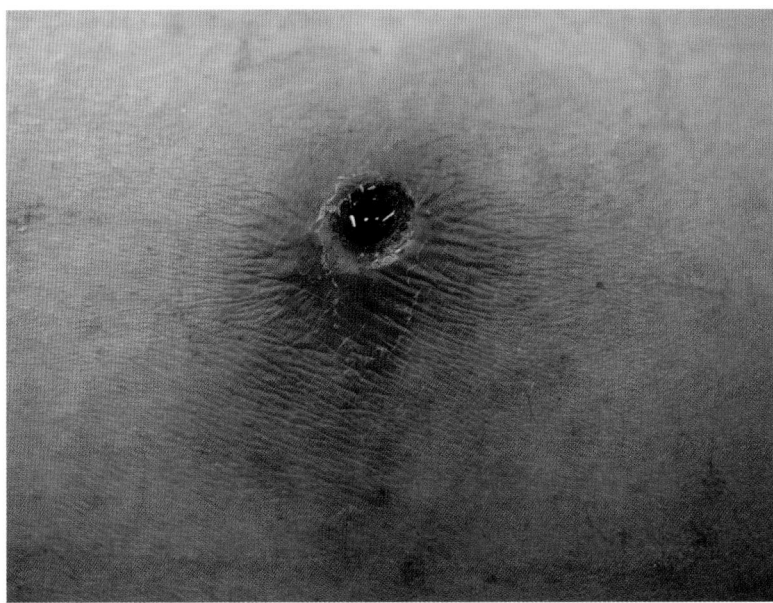

Fig. 18.389
Myiasis: characteristic furuncular lesion in a patient with botfly infestation. By courtesy of F. Bravo, MD, Lima, Peru.

Histologic features

The cross section through the larva is distinctive in its appearance. Depending on the plane of sectioning, polarizable structures such as the thick cuticle covered with spines, the two curved mouth hooks and/or the respiratory spiracles may be observed in histologic material (*Fig. 18.390*). Biopsies which include the surrounding skin may show an ulcerated epidermis, a cavity lined by acute and chronic inflammatory cells, and a neighboring dermal inflammatory infiltrate comprising lymphocytes, plasma cells, eosinophils, giant cells, and Langerhans cells.[1–3,8,9]

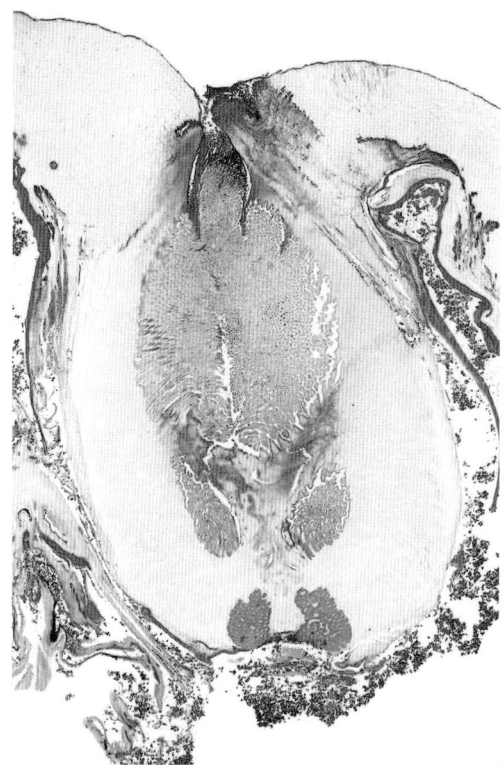

Fig. 18.390
Myiasis: intradermal botfly larva showing characteristic respiratory spiracles.

NEMATODE INFESTATION

Onchocerciasis

Clinical features

Onchocerciasis (river blindness) is endemic in some 37 countries, with an estimated 187 million people at risk of infection. Although the vast majority of these countries are in parts of tropical Africa (where 99% of the at-risk population live), the disease also occurs in the Yemen and has been recorded in six countries in Central and South America.[1–7] Much success has been achieved toward disease control through the mass administration of the microfilaricide ivermectin in the Americas, including Guatemala, where the elimination of onchocerciasis was recently verified.[7,8] Although a mass treatment program with ivermectin has been in place in some 16 sub-Saharan African countries since 1995, eradication of the disease has not yet been accomplished.[2,9] More than 27 million people are thought to be infected.[10] Recent estimates of the burden of the disease suggest that 1.1 million disability-adjusted life-years were lost in 2015 as a result of the disease's major associated morbidities, namely, blindness, severe visual impairment, and cutaneous involvement in the form of troublesome pruritus and disfiguring skin lesions.[2,6] Skin involvement now appears to be the major contributor to the disease burden, rather than ocular disease.[9]

Most symptoms of onchocerciasis are associated with the microfilarial stage of the filarial nematode *Onchocerca volvulus*. Onchocerciasis particularly affects individuals living close to fast-flowing rivers.[11] Exceptionally, humans may be infected with zoonotic species of *Onchocerca*, and *O. lupi* in particular.[12–14] Cases of the latter have been documented in Europe,

Tunisia, Turkey, Iran, and the United States.[13,14] The microfilariae migrate to the skin and other organs, causing itching and macules showing altered pigmentation.[5,10] Scratching results in excoriation and sometimes secondary infection. Dermal thickening, edema, and wrinkling of the skin follow in severe cases. Scaling and depigmentation are termed lizard and leopard skin, respectively (*Fig. 18.391*). Lymph nodes often become involved, exacerbating the problems of edema. Adult worms exist in dermal nodules, often associated with scar tissue; these nodules are mobile and tender, and are usually seen over bony prominences.[10,15]

The clinical cutaneous manifestations have been classified into a number of categories including acute papular onchodermatitis, chronic papular onchodermatitis, lichenified onchodermatitis, atrophy, and depigmentation (*Figs 18.392–18.395*).[10,11] Other recognized manifestations include palpable onchocercal nodules, lymphadenopathy, hanging groin, and lymphedema. In endemic areas, 30% or more of the population may have onchocercal skin lesions; this figure approaches 60% in some hyperendemic communities.[4] The varying clinical features are believed to reflect variable host immune reactions to the presence of the microfilariae in the dermis.[16] The migrating microfilariae can enter the eyes and cause river blindness. Ocular lesions, which are a cause of major morbidity, include punctate keratitis, sclerosing keratitis, iritis, chorioretinitis, and optic atrophy.[17,18]

Pathogenesis and histologic features

O. volvulus is transmitted in its larval form to man in rural areas by the bite of female black flies (*Simulium*).[3,5,10,19] The larvae develop into adult worms in the deep dermis. Microfilariae are produced by gravid females and these can migrate throughout the host (*Fig. 18.396*). Most are present in

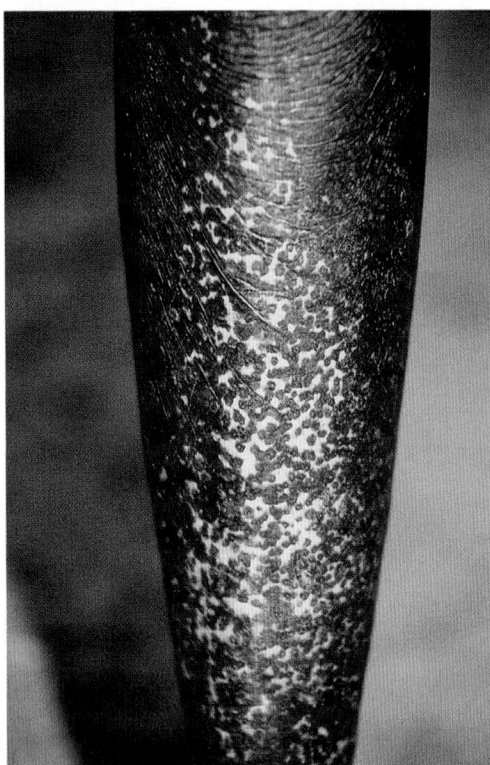

Fig. 18.391
Onchocerciasis: leopard skin. There are numerous depigmented macules. Rarely, these are pruritic. By courtesy of M.E. Murdoch, MD, Watford Hospital, Watford, UK.

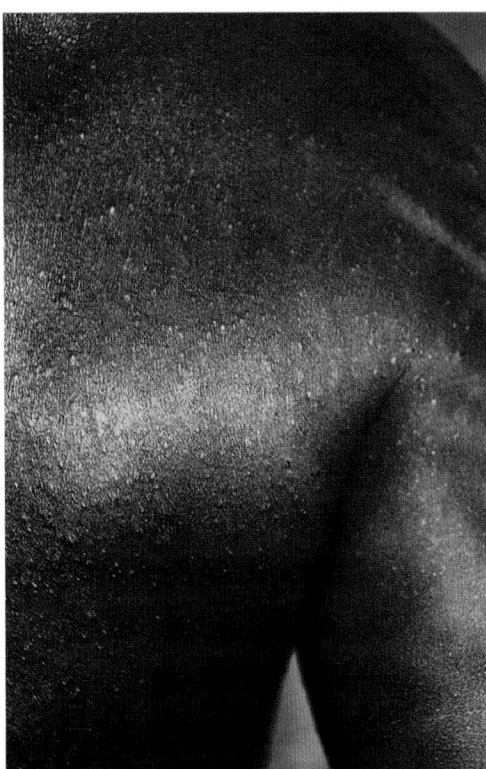

Fig. 18.392
Acute papular onchodermatitis: numerous small papules are present on the back and upper arm. Vesiculation and pustulation may sometimes be present. By courtesy of M.E. Murdoch, MD, Watford Hospital, Watford, UK.

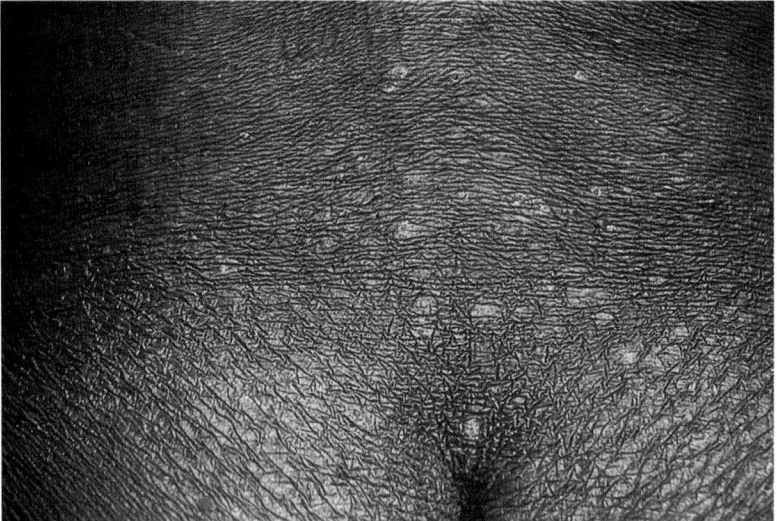

Fig. 18.393
Chronic papular onchodermatitis: numerous flat-topped macules and papules are present on the buttocks. By courtesy of M.E. Murdoch, MD, Watford Hospital, Watford, UK.

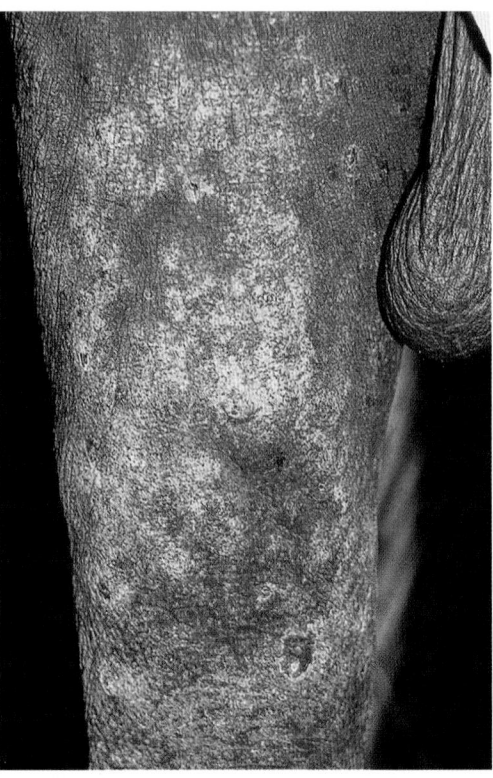

Fig. 18.394
Lichenified onchodermatitis: this variant most often affects teenagers and young adults. There is marked hyperkeratosis associated with confluent plaques. Lymphadenopathy is often a feature. By courtesy of M.E. Murdoch, MD, Watford Hospital, Watford, UK.

the superficial dermis, and may be identified by the histologic examination of 'skin snips'.[5,10] The adult female worm is up to 50 cm in length, with a diameter of up to 0.45 mm, and is found in complex coils in the fixed nodules. The microfilariae are 220–360 × 5–9 μm. The nodules (sometimes referred to as 'onchocercomas') contain several entwined worms within surrounding inflammation, which may be suppurative or granulomatous (*Figs 18.397* and *18.398*).

There is extensive fibrosis, often calcification, and sometimes ossification. Microfilariae may be seen free within the dermis and also in lymphatics. The skin shows hyperkeratosis and parakeratosis, with acanthosis and melanophages in the dermis, but only a mild lymphocytic and eosinophilic inflammatory infiltrate. Fibrosis becomes prominent, resulting in hyalinization of the papillary dermis. Mucin is prominent between collagen bundles, and foci of fibrinoid change are occasionally seen. Degeneration of microfilariae is foreshadowed by an eosinophilic change with fragmentation of the nuclei; these changes are accompanied by an intense infiltrate of eosinophils.

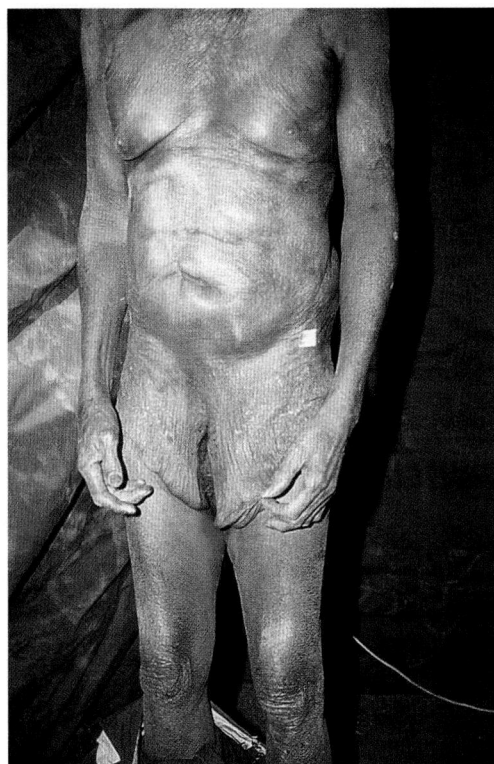

Fig. 18.395
Chronic onchocerciasis: the presence of redundant folds of skin in the inguinal region is a late manifestation (late hanging groin). By courtesy of M.E. Murdoch, MD, Watford Hospital, Watford, UK.

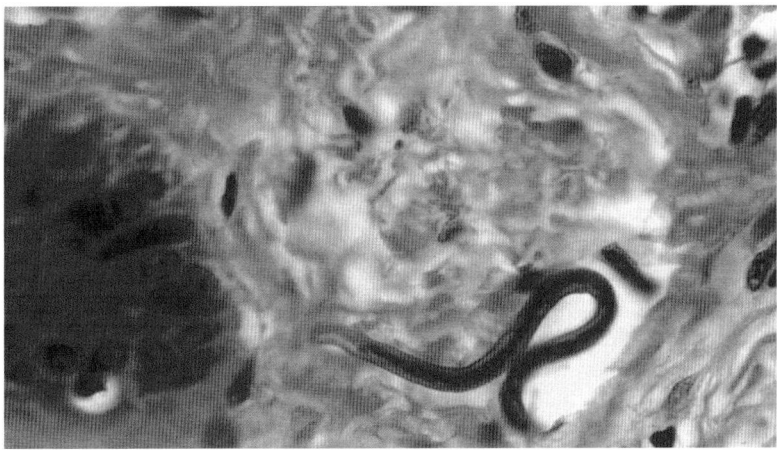

Fig. 18.396
Onchocerciasis: microfilariae in the dermis may elicit a lymphohistiocytic infiltrate and eosinophils may be conspicuous. By courtesy of S. Lucas, MD, St Thomas' Hospital, London, UK.

The microfilariae may also be seen with surrounding eosinophils in the epidermis.

The number of microfilariae shows an inverse relationship to the level of specific immune complexes. There appears to be a correlation between the host's Th2-type systemic response and the various cutaneous manifestations of the disease.[20] *Wolbachia* endobacteria are now recognized as critical pathogenetic role players in the disease's clinical manifestations and complications, via the induction of a host inflammatory response. These intracellular obligatory symbiont bacteria reside in the filarial nematodes.[21] *Wolbachia* lipopolysaccharides bind with human CD14 receptors on monocytes and macrophages, resulting in the production of proinflammatory cytokines such as TNF-α, IL-1, and IL-12. This, in turn, leads to recruitment of inflammatory cells to the tissues harboring the *Onchocerca* worms and microfilariae, with subsequent fibrosis.[22,23] The bacteria could serve as a

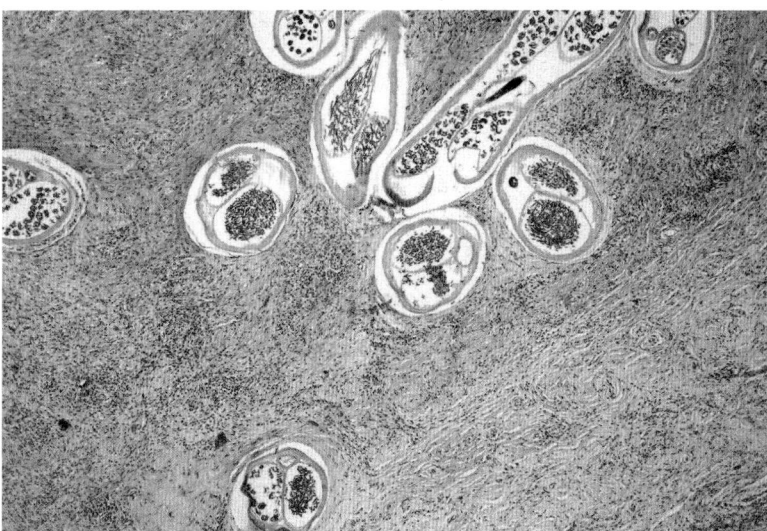

Fig. 18.397
Onchocerciasis: multiple sections of adult worm are evident.

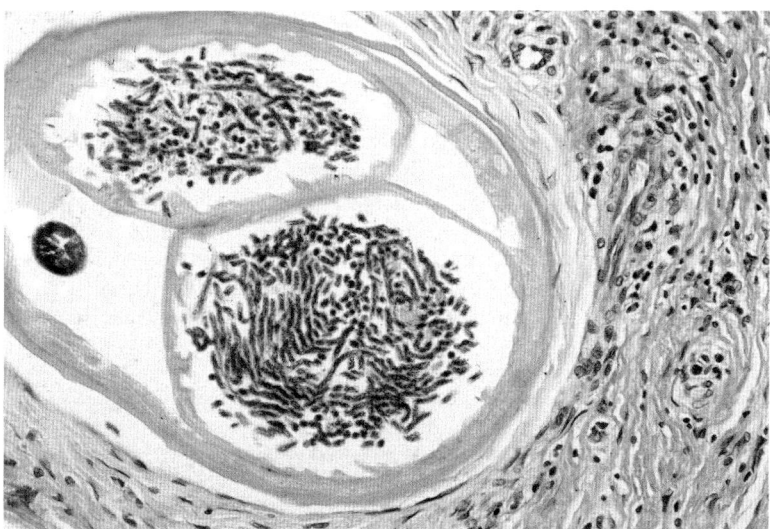

Fig. 18.398
Onchocerciasis: numerous developing microfilariae are evident.

novel therapeutic target, with drugs such as doxycycline earmarked for the potential treatment of onchocerciasis in the future.[5,23,24]

Cutaneous larva migrans

Clinical features

Cutaneous larva migrans (creeping eruption) is a distinctive dermatitis resulting from penetration of, and migration through, the skin by infectious nematode larvae, usually of animal origin.[1-4] The condition is most prevalent in warm, humid tropical regions, especially along the coast.[1] There is an increased prevalence in resource-poor communities living in such areas.[3] Returning travelers may present with the disease after visiting endemic areas.[3,5] The larval forms of *Ancylostoma braziliensis* (the cat and dog hookworm) are the most frequent cause of cutaneous larva migrans.[1,2] Other animal nematodes implicated include *A. caninum* (dog hookworm), *A. tubaeforme* and *A. ceylonicum* (cat hookworms), *Uncinaria stenocephala* (European dog hookworm), *Bunostomum phlebotomum* (bovine hookworm), *Strongyloides papillosus* (sheep hookworm), and *S. westery* (horse hookworm).[1,2,6,7] Larvae of human hookworm species, i.e., *Gnathostoma spinigerum*, *A. duodenale*, and *Necator americanus*, may also be associated with cutaneous larva migrans. *Pleodora strongyloides*, a free-living soil nematode, is another potential etiological agent of the disease.[1,2]

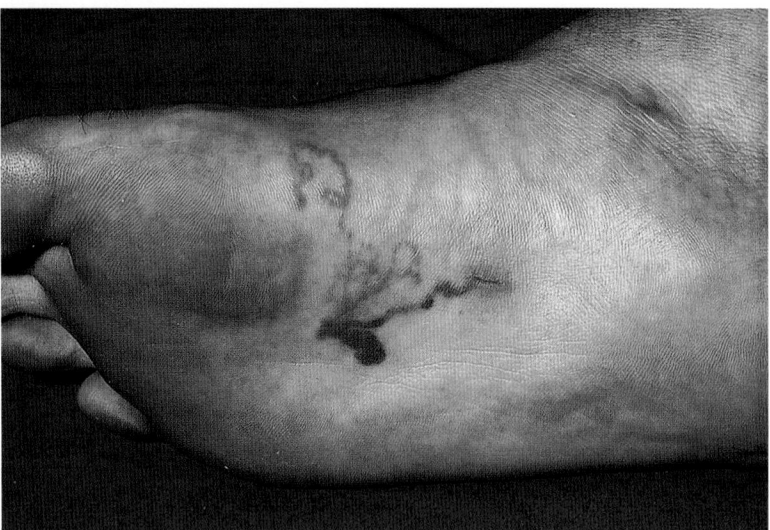

Fig. 18.399
Cutaneous larva migrans: the foot is a commonly affected site. By courtesy of
R.A. Marsden, MD, St George's Hospital, London, UK.

Rhabditiform larvae evolve in the soil from eggs passed in the feces of infected hosts. These metamorphose into infectious filariform larvae capable of penetrating human skin upon contact.[1,2,4] The larvae appear to enter the skin via the ostia of hair follicles or sweat glands, usually on the feet, buttocks, or abdomen, in decreasing order of frequency.[1,5] An intensely pruritic erythematous papule or vesicle develops at the site of larval penetration. Follicular papules and pustules are sometimes seen.[6,8–10] Migration of the larvae commences 2–4 days later, and is associated with the evolution of a characteristic erythematous, serpiginous tract (*Fig. 18.399*). The larvae may migrate at a rate of 2–5 cm per day.[1,2,4] A case with large bullous lesions has been reported.[11] Exceptionally, oral involvement may occur.[12] A small number of cases have been reported in association with underlying HIV infection, including one patient who presented with an erythematous plaque on the cheek.[7,13,14]

Although the condition is usually self-limiting, with spontaneous resolution over a period of several weeks, secondary bacterial infection introduced by scratching is a relatively frequent complication.[1,4] Erythema multiforme has been reported in association with cutaneous larva migrans.[15] Löffler syndrome is a rare complication of the disease.[16]

Histologic features

Migration of the larvae away from the site of entry means that skin biopsies are often frustratingly unhelpful.[4] Biopsy specimens obtained from the advancing tract may nevertheless confirm the presence of tunneling larvae in some cases. Although this usually takes place at or near the dermal–epidermal junction, larvae may also be encountered more superficially in the epidermis.[1,2,13,17] The superficial location of the hookworm larvae is attributed to their lack of collagenase, since the latter is a prerequisite for disruption of the epidermal basement membrane and subsequent dermal invasion.[4,18] The surrounding epidermis often shows only mild spongiosis, whereas in some cases there is marked intraepidermal spongiotic vesiculation with exocytosis of neutrophils and eosinophils.[17] The underlying dermis exhibits telangiectasia and a mild mixed inflammatory cell infiltrate containing eosinophilic leukocytes.[1,2,17] Follicular involvement has been reported.[6,8,9]

Strongyloidiasis

Clinical features

Strongyloidiasis refers to infection with the nematode, *Stongyloides stercoralis*.[1,2] An estimated 30 to 100 million people worldwide are infected.[3] Although the parasite is present throughout tropical and temperate regions, a high proportion of the population is infected in some tropical countries. *S. stercoralis* has three life cycles. In the direct development cycle, rhabditiform

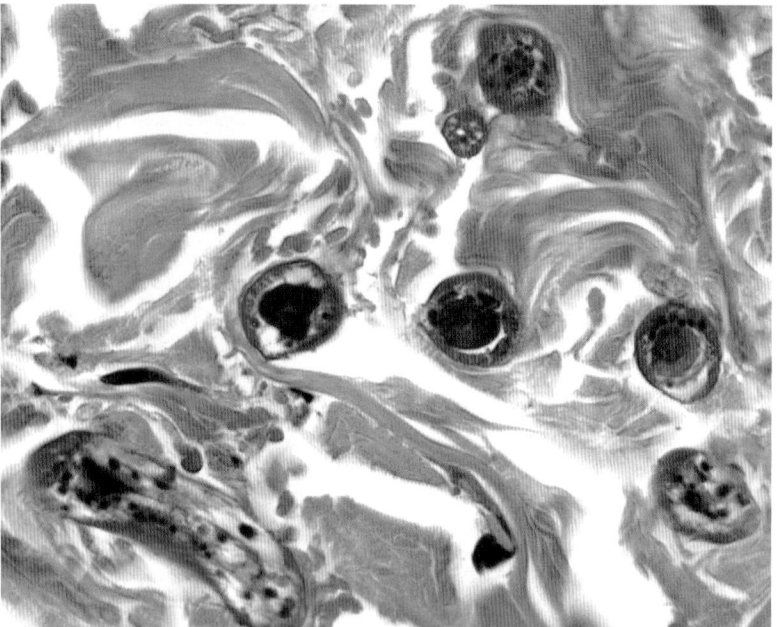

Fig. 18.400
Strongyloidiasis: rhabditiform larvae are present in the dermis of this patient with disseminated infection in the context of underlying AIDS.

larvae passed in the feces evolve into filariform larvae in the soil, eventually penetrating the skin of man. In the indirect cycle, rhabditiform larvae present in the soil mature into free-living adult worms, with the production of eggs which mature into rhabditiform larvae and eventually filariform larvae, which then penetrate the skin. The autoinfection cycle occurs when rhabditiform larvae present in the intestine evolve into filariform larvae which penetrate the perianal skin after being passed in the feces, or invade the intestinal wall directly. Following entry to the venous system, the filariform larvae are transported to the lung, where they evolve into adolescent worms. The latter migrate up the bronchi and then the trachea, whereupon they are swallowed and mature into adult worms in the small intestine.[1,2]

Most patients are asymptomatic. Chronic infection, however, may be associated with a characteristic skin rash referred to as larva currens.[1,2] This linear or serpiginous pruritic urticarial eruption is an allergic response to migrating filariform larvae, which move outward from the perianal skin and onto the buttocks, thighs, and abdomen. The rash extends from 5 to 15 cm per hour and may last from a few hours to a number of days. In the context of autoinfection, however, recurrences may be seen over a period of weeks to years.[2] A widespread reticular macular eruption has also been described.[4] Rarely, filariform larvae which have penetrated the skin do not exhibit immediate lymphaticovenous invasion, and instead show initial slow migration through the dermis; the resultant clinical picture is one of larva migrans.[5]

Disseminated strongyloidiasis, also referred to as hyperinfection syndrome, is a serious form of the disease and carries a high mortality.[1,2] It has a propensity to occur in immune compromised individuals, including those with underlying hematolymphoid neoplasms, HIV/AIDS, autoimmune disease, severe malnutrition, or on immunosuppressive therapy, especially the long-term use of corticostreroids.[1,3,4,6–9] Hyperinfection is associated with a distinctive diffuse petechial or purpuric eruption referred to as 'thumbprint purpura', which characteristically radiates from the periumbilical region.[2,9,10] Lesions of disseminated larva currens may also be evident.[3] Patients often have debilitating gastrointestinal symptoms due to paralytic ileus, malabsorption, and/or ulcerative enteritis. Pulmonary symptoms and pneumonia may occur, and meningeal involvement has been reported. Death ensues as a result of overwhelming sepsis, usually due to enteric bacteria.[1,2]

Histologic features

Skin biopsy reveals intradermal filariform larvae, which may be seen in both longitudinal section and in cross section (*Fig. 18.400*).[3,11] These larvae measure 300–600 μm in length and 10–20 μm in diameter. Minute double lateral alae may be visible on transverse sectioning.[1] Invasion through the dermal vessel walls is associated with vasculitic alterations, with perivascular red cell and fibrin extravasation.[7,11]

Gnathostomiasis

Clinical features

Gnathostomiasis is a food-borne zoonotic nematode infection caused by *Gnathostoma* spp., including *G. spinigerum*, *G. dolorosi*, and *G. nipponicum*.[1] Humans are accidental hosts who acquire the infection through the consumption of raw or partially cooked freshwater fish, or other intermediate hosts of the parasite such as frogs, chickens, or snakes. Fish-eating mammals in particular are the definitive host in which the adult worm resides.[1,2] The latter measures 13–55 mm in length.[2,3] The condition occurs in tropical and subtropical regions, including Japan, Southeast Asia, Central and South America, and Southern Africa.[1,2,4,5] Gnathostomiasis should always be considered when a patient presents with the classic triad of intermittent migratory swellings, peripheral eosinophilia, and a history of travel to an endemic area.[2] Humans are an unsuitable host. Consequently, the immature worm wanders through the internal viscera and subcutaneous tissues, inflicting tissue injury in the process.[1]

The migration of excysted larvae through the gastric and intestinal walls and the liver may be heralded by fever, malaise, anorexia, upper abdominal pain, nausea, vomiting, diarrhea, and urticaria; these symptoms last for some 2 to 3 weeks.[1,2] The subsequent migration of the parasite through the subcutaneous tissues results in the characteristic clinical presentation of intermittent, edematous, painful, or pruritic migratory plaques or nodules, referred to as nodular migratory panniculitis (*Fig. 18.401*).[2,4] The presence of subcutaneous hemorrhages along the paths of larval migration is said to be pathognomonic of gnathostomiasis, and facilitates distinction from other parasitic infestations with migratory larvae, such as strongyloidiasis or sparganosis.[2] The chest and abdomen are the most frequent sites of involvement, although lesions occasionally occur on the arms and hands.[1] The lesions measure 5–15 cm in maximum dimension. They occur within 3 or 4 weeks of ingestion and last up to 2 or 3 weeks, only to reappear in the vicinity shortly thereafter.[1–4] Although these episodes diminish in duration and intensity with the passage of time, intermittent recurrences have been known to occur for up to a decade or more in untreated individuals.[2]

Histologic features

Although skin biopsy is the favored diagnostic modality, the large size of the infiltrated plaques and the relatively small size of the immature worm (2.5–12.5 mm in length and 0.4–1.2 mm in width) result in the organism seldom being identified in histologic sections, unless fortuitously included in the specimen.[2,4] On occasion, however, the worm may be seen to emerge directly from a fresh sample shortly after completion of the biopsy procedure (F. Bravo, personal communication). A dense, eosinophil-rich inflammatory infiltrate is observed in the subcutis and dermis (*Fig. 18.402*). Unsurprisingly, intradermal flame figure formation reminiscent of eosinophilic cellulitis may be encountered.[2,6]

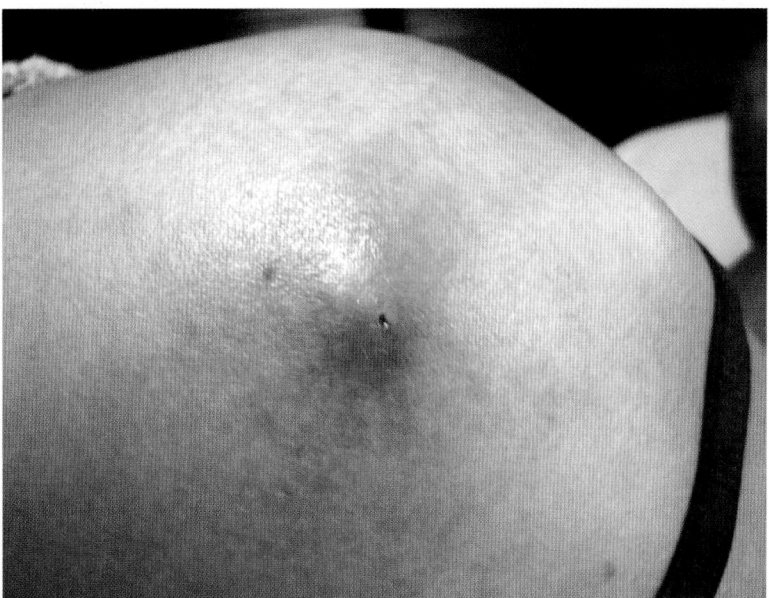

Fig. 18.401
Gnathostomiasis: migratory subcutaneous masses are a characteristic phenomenon. By courtesy of F. Bravo, MD, Lima, Peru.

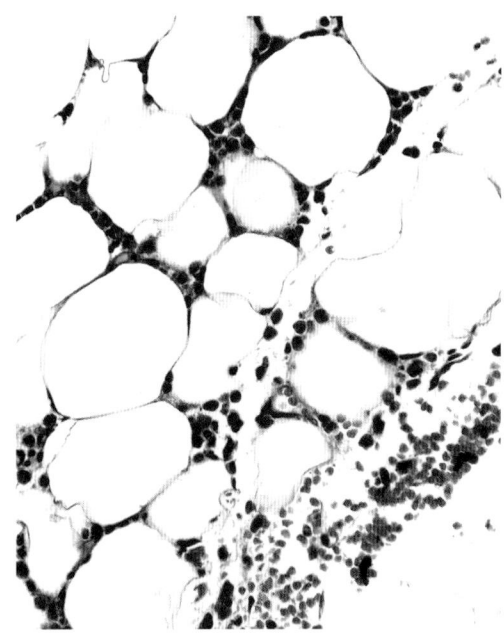

Fig. 18.402
Gnathostomiasis: the migration of an immature worm through the dermis and panniculus is invariably associated with a striking infiltrate of eosinophilic leukocytes. By courtesy of F. Bravo, MD, Lima, Peru.

TREMATODE INFESTATION

Schistosomiasis

Clinical features

Schistosomiasis is a major neglected tropical disease. It is endemic in a number of tropical and subtropical regions, with an estimated 240 million people infected worldwide in more than 60 countries.[1,2] There are three major anthropophilic species. *Schistosoma haematobium* and *S. mansoni* are both found extensively in Africa. *S. mansoni* is also found in the West Indies and in parts of South America. *S. japonicum* is found in China, Japan, and Southeast Asia. Two further species, *S. intercalatum* and *S. mekongi*, may also cause disease. These trematodes (blood flukes) do not often cause major disease of the skin, but skin lesions do occur at various stages of infestation.[3,4]

Invasion of the human host by the aquatic cercarial stage may be associated with a dermatitis (swimmer's itch, cercarial dermatitis).[2,5,6] The rash is erythematous, pruritic, and urticarial, but eventually resolves to leave a pigmented spot. It is, however, more often associated with invasion of avian (*Trichobilharzia*) species.[5,7,8] The cercariae of *S. japonicum* migrate more rapidly through the skin than those of *S. haematobium* or *S. mansoni*.[9,10]

The mature worms may be associated non-specifically with erythematous itching macules at the time of release of large numbers of eggs. This probably represents a systemic reaction to antigen liberation. A more severe reaction seen most often with *S. japonicum* is Katayama disease or Yellow River fever. In addition to erythema, macules, and pruriginous lesions, patients may also have fever, malaise, chills, sweats, arthralgias, headache, lymphadenopathy, hepatosplenomegaly, diarrhea, bronchitis, pneumonitis, and peripheral blood eosinophilia.[2,5,6]

Specific skin lesions are seen, usually around the anus and the genitalia, most often in women. When ova are deposited, a granulomatous reaction is induced. This form of the disease is known as bilharziasis cutanea tarda (BCT). Extra-anogenital disease is very rare and seems to be more common in the trunk, particularly around the umbilicus; lesions have, however, also been described on the breast, back, scapular region, and the buttock.[11–15] The lesions appear as grouped 2–4 mm solid papules, which subsequently become warty and vegetative.[2,16] Occasionally, progression to squamous carcinoma supervenes. A keloidal appearance may be present. A zosteriform pattern is rarely seen, and a case with bilateral axillary involvement has been described.[11,17] Periurethral granulomata due to schistosomes may be associated with thrombosis and necrosis, resulting sometimes in fistulation to the perineum ('watering can perineum').[5] Lymphedema may be a late complication.[6]

Pathogenesis and histologic features

Part of the life cycle of schistosomes takes place in water snails, and these release the cercariae, which penetrate the skin. They are carried to the lungs and then migrate as schistosomules to the portal vein where they mature into adult male and female worms. Adult females subsequently migrate to the mesenteric plexus (*S. mansoni* and *S. japonicum*) or vesical plexus (*S. haematobium*). Ova are then deposited in the venules and the clinical and pathological sequelae are a direct consequence of the immunological response to their presence.[2,6]

Eggs are released into the urine or feces where they hatch, releasing miracidia, which enter the snail host. Involvement of the female genital tract is usually due to *S. haematobium* and occurs as a consequence of worms being transported via anastomoses between the vesical and uterovaginal venous plexuses.

The pathogenesis of BCT is unknown. Several mechanisms have been proposed but none is entirely satisfactory. One mechanism proposes arteriovenous shunting of ova through a patent foramen ovale or arteriovenous fistulae in the lung. A further mechanism proposes egg-laying by the parasites locally within the affected area. This mechanism assumes the migration of adult worms to the skin through the valveless vertebral venous system.[11] The mechanism of cutaneous involvement is more likely to be multifactorial.

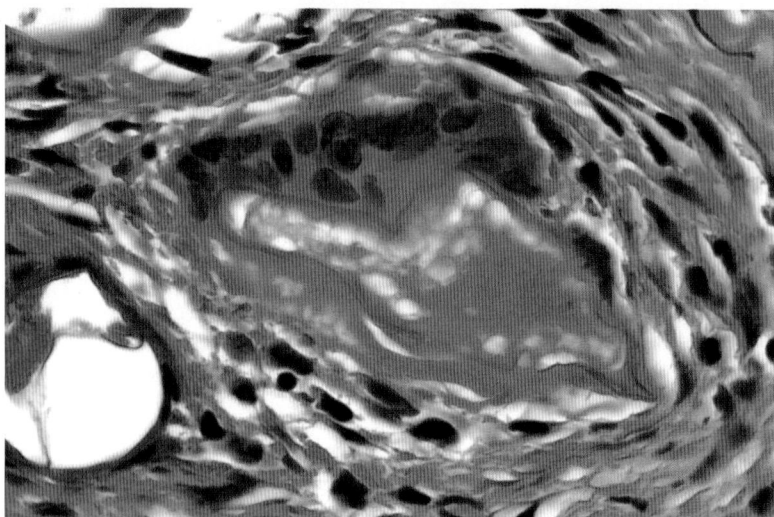

Fig. 18.403
Schistosomiasis: intradermal granuloma containing a *Schistosoma haematobium* egg. The characteristic terminal spine is clearly evident.

Histologically, adult worms may occasionally be seen within the lumina of dilated deep dermal veins and lymphatics. Viable ova may be present with a recognizable miracidial structure. These are usually located within abscesses containing numerous neutrophils and variable numbers of eosinophils. Poorly formed granulomata with Langhans giant cells may also be a feature. *S. haematobium* is recognized by its terminal apical spine (*Fig. 18.403*). *S. japonicum* lacks a spine and in *S. mansoni* the spine is lateral. Dead ova typically calcify and provoke a chronic, frequently granulomatous, inflammatory response. The overlying epidermis is usually acanthotic, sometimes to the point of pseudoepitheliomatous hyperplasia, with variable transepidermal elimination of ova. It has been highlighted that in cases of extragenital BCT caused by *S. haematobium*, the parasite may be found in pre-existing cutaneous conditions including hidradenitis suppurativa and post-traumatic or iatrogenic scars.[11]

Biopsies from cases of cercarial dermatitis show spongiosis and a mixed dermal inflammatory infiltrate comprising lymphocytes, histiocytes, eosinophilic leukocytes, and neutrophils. Intraepidermal cercariae may rarely be seen, if fortuitously included in the specimen.[2]

CESTODE INFESTATION

Cysticercosis

Clinical features

The adult pork tapeworm *Taenia solium* may be present in the small intestine of man (the definitive host). The intermediate host, the pig, ingests the eggs, which develop to the cysticercus stage in muscle and elsewhere and is then infective if improperly cooked and eaten by humans. If humans ingest eggs, however, they can become the host for the cysticercus stage; this occurs most commonly in skin, subcutaneous tissue, skeletal muscle, brain, and eye.[1,2] Disseminated cysticercosis may also involve the spinal cord, orbital soft tissues, liver, spleen, and rarely, the heart.[3,4] Cystercerci in the skin present as painless nodules up to 2 cm across (*Fig. 18.404*). The vast majority of patients present with solitary subcutaneous nodules. Some patients, however, may present with multiple subcutaneous lesions.[5] Nodules may also occur in the oral cavity or breast in a small percentage of cases; mammary lesions may mimic breast carcinoma clinically.[6,7] In patients who are known to have an underlying malignancy, the evolution of multiple subcutaneous nodules of cysticercosis may be mistaken for metastases.

Fine needle aspiration cytology is a rapid and useful means of confirming the parasitic etiology thereof in such cases.[8] The diagnosis of subcutaneous cysticercosis should prompt further investigations to rule out concomitant neurocysticercosis. The latter is a major cause of epilepsy in developing countries.[1,2]

Pathogenesis and histologic features

The viable cysticercus compresses adjacent dermis without inflammation and the diagnosis can be made by identification of the scolex (*Fig. 18.405*). However, when the parasite begins to degenerate there is an infiltration of neutrophils, histiocytes, and eosinophils, which becomes more granulomatous, with giant cells, fibrosis, and eventual calcification.

Echinococcosis

Clinical features

Echinococcosis is a zoonotic disease caused by a helminth, mainly the tapeworm *Echinoccocus granulosus* (the cause of cystic echinococcosis) but also

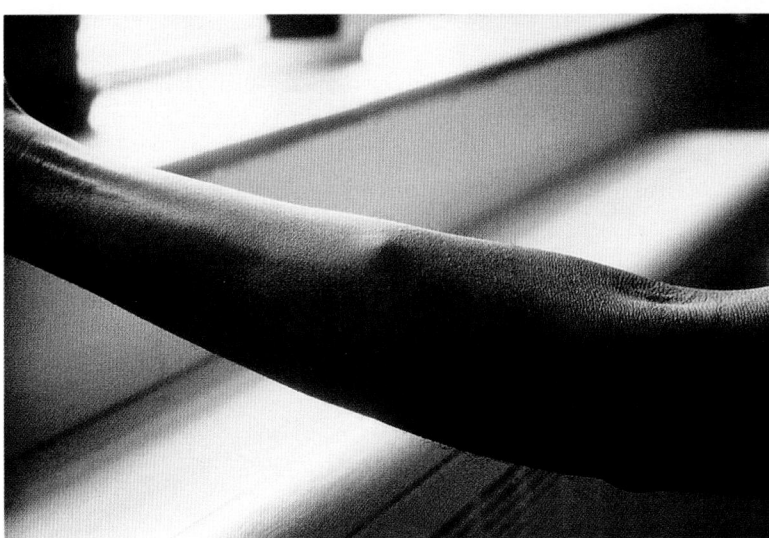

Fig. 18.404
Cysticercosis: a solitary nodule is present on the ventral aspect of the forearm. Cysticercosis develops when humans are harboring the larval (cysticercus) stage of the tapeworm. By courtesy of S. Lucas, MD, St Thomas' Hospital, London, UK.

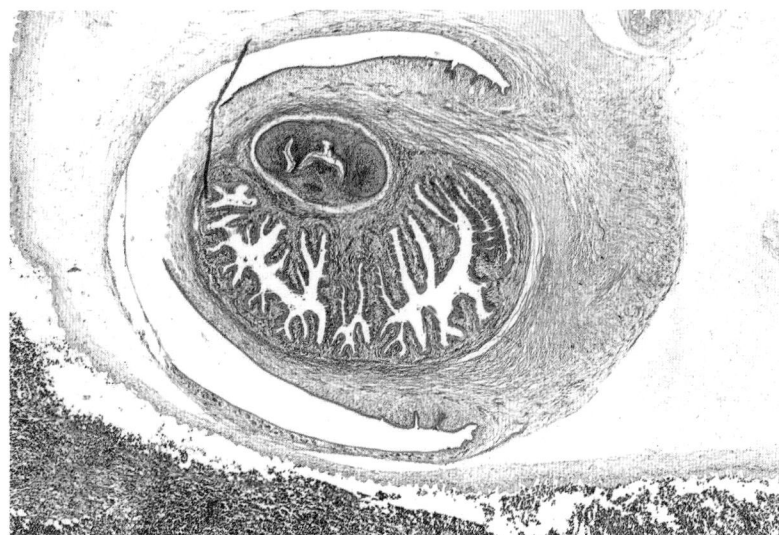

Fig. 18.405
Cysticercosis: the worm lies within a cystic cavity surrounded by a dense fibrous capsule. By courtesy of S. Lucas, MD, St Thomas' Hospital, London, UK.

by *E. multilocularis*, *E. vogeli*, and *E. oligarthus*. The parasite belongs to the class Cestoda, family Taeniidae, and genus *Echinococcus*. It is a very important cause of morbidity not only in many developing countries but also in New Zealand and Australia. The adult worms, which measure 3–6 mm in length, reside in the small bowel of their dog, sheep, or even human host. Eggs released from the gravid proglottids into the feces are ingested by the intermediate host (man), whereupon they evolve into larvae (onchospheres) which penetrate the walls of mesenteric blood vessels in the small intestine. Most affected individuals present with disease in the liver and lungs. Subcutaneous or skin lesions are rare, occurring in only 2% of cases.[1–7] The mechanism of cutaneous dissemination is the result of vascular spread, lymphatic drainage from the diaphragm, or contiguous spread when visceral lesions rupture and form cutaneous fistulae. Individuals with subcutaneous intact lesions present with an asymptomatic mass which is clinically diagnosed as a cyst. Around 90% of reported cases have been in patients from rural areas.[7] The lower extremity is involved in almost 61% of cases, with the thigh being the most frequent anatomic location (27–34.8%), followed by the gluteal region (9%) and the upper extremity (8.7%).[8,9] Other rarely reported sites include the subcutaneous tissues of the neck, and the thoracic spinal area.[10,11] Recorded diameters range from 2 to 15 cm, with a mean of around 5.7 cm.[8] Patients with fistular disease present with inflamed lesions that often develop secondary infection.

Histologic features

In many cases, the cysts are intact and recognition of the parasite is not difficult. Cystic echinococcosis consists of three layers as follows:
- An outer host layer also known as the pericyst,
- A middle laminated membrane which is quite characteristic, is acellular, measures 2 mm in thickness, and allows the passage of nutrients,
- The transparent inner germinal layer which is very thin.

Multiple scolices develop from the brood capsule. In a number of cases there is only a subcutaneous, palisading granulomatous reaction containing what appears to be fragments of keratin. This leads to the erroneous diagnosis of a ruptured epidermoid cyst. However, these fragments represent PAS-positive remnants of the membranes of *E. granulosus* mimicking keratin. Distinction is crucial as the identification of the subcutaneous parasite may lead to the diagnosis of latent visceral disease.[7] It is not clear how these fragments reach the subcutaneous tissue. They may be the result of a pre-existing intact subcutaneous cyst or, based on the sparsity of the material found, they may represent circulatory spread from visceral lesions that are deposited in the subcutaneous tissue.

Access **ExpertConsult.com** for the complete list of references

Index

Page numbers followed by "*f*" indicate figures, "*t*" indicate tables, "*b*" indicate boxes, and "*e*" indicate online content.

Keratosis punctata of palmar creases, 103–104, 104*f*
Keratosis punctata palmaris et plantaris, 102
Keratosis punctata palmoplantaris type Buschke-Fischer-Brauer, 102–103, 103*f*–104*f*
Keratotic balanitis, 524, 524*f*–525*f*
Keratotic basal cell carcinoma, 1180, 1181*f*
Keratotic plaque, conjunctiva, 1369
Keratotic reticular oral lichen planus, 432
Kerinokeratosis papulose, 114
Kerion (kerion celsi), 925–926, 926*f*–927*f*
  dissecting cellulitis *versus*, 1107
Ki-67 (MIB-1), melanoma, 1329–1330, 1329*f*
Kidneys, alkaptonuria and, 604
Kikuchi-Fujimoto disease, 1489
  cutaneous, 1489
Kimura disease, epithelioid hemangioma *versus*, 1841–1842, 1841*f*–1842*f*
Kindler syndrome, 129, 130*f*
Kindlin-1, in epidermolysis bullosa, 133
Kinking of hair, acquired progressive, 1119
Kit, piebaldism and mutations in gene for, 998
Kitamura, reticulate acropigmentation of, 1005–1006, 1006*f*–1007*f*
Klebsiella, 1128
KLF7, atopic eczema and, 202–203
Klippel-Trenaunay syndrome, 1825, 1825*f*
Knotted hair, 1119
Knuckle pad, 1731, 1731*f*
Köbberling variant familial partial lipodystrophy, 380
Koebner phenomenon
  inverse, in alopecia areata, 1071
  koebnerization and, in vitiligo, 990–991
  psoriasis and, 225*f*
Kyphoscoliosis, Ehlers-Danlos syndrome type VI, 1016*t*, 1019
Kyrle disease, 346–348
  clinical features of, 346, 346*f*
  differential diagnosis of, 343*t*, 347–348
    familial dyskeratotic comedones *versus*, 199
    perforating folliculitis *versus*, 344
  pathogenesis and histologic features of, 346–347, 347*f*–348*f*

L

Labia majora, 471, 471*f*
Labia minora, 471
Labial artery, caliber-persistent, 428, 428*f*
Labial melanotic macule, 1235
Laboratory tests/management, of hair disorders, 1052–1053
Lacrimal gland
  choristoma, 1365
  oncocytoma, 1368
LAMB syndrome (former name for Carney complex), 1009
Lambing ears, 292
Lamellar granules, 9
Lamellar ichthyosis, autosomal dominant, 61–62, 62*f*–63*f*
Lamin A, restrictive dermopathy and, 1028–1029
Lamina densa, 22–23
Lamina lucida, 22–23
Laminin-332, in epidermolysis bullosa, 133, 133*f*
Lanceolate hair mutant mouse *(Lah)*, 1895–1896
Langerhans cells, 1, 11*f*
Langerhans cell histiocytosis, 1490–1494
  anogenital, 552
  clinical features of, 1490–1492, 1490*f*–1491*f*
  differential diagnosis of, 1494
  pathogenesis and histologic features of, 1492–1494, 1492*f*–1494*f*
Langerhans cell sarcoma (LCS), 1494–1495
Langerin (CD207), 1494

Large B-cell lymphoma, primary cutaneous diffuse. *See* Diffuse large B-cell lymphoma
Large cell acanthoma, 1167–1168, 1167*f*
Large vessel vasculitis, 715*t*
Larva migrans, cutaneous, 969–971, 972*f*
Laryngo-onycho-cutaneous syndrome, localized junctional epidermolysis bullosa, 126
Latrodectus mactans, 693
Laugier-Hunziker syndrome, 1002, 1003*f*, 1235, 1235*f*–1236*f*
Launois-Bensaude syndrome, 1703
Lecythis ollaria, 1085–1086
Leg, lower, nevi of, 1254
Leiomyoma. *See also* Angioleiomyoma
  genital, 556, 1815
  pilar, 1813–1815, 1813*f*–1814*f*
Leiomyomatosis, vulval, 557
Leiomyosarcoma, 556–557, 556*f*–557*f*, 1815–1817, 1816*f*–1817*f*
  metastatic, 1818*f*
Leishmaniasis, 916–920
  clinical features of, 916–918, 917*f*–918*f*
  cutaneous, 916–917, 917*f*–918*f*
  differential diagnosis of, 920
  pathogenesis and histological features of, 918–920, 919*f*–920*f*
Lelis syndrome, 626
LEMD3 mutations, Buschke-Ollendorff syndrome and, 1043–1044
Lentiginosis
  centrofacial, 1237, 1237*f*
  genital, 1236
Lentiginous melanoma, 1353–1354, 1354*f*
Lentiginous nevus, speckled, 1256, 1256*f*
Lentigo
  acral, 1236, 1237*f*
  ink spot, 1238, 1238*f*–1239*f*
  labial, 1235
  nail, 1140–1141
  PUVA and sunbed, 1238, 1238*f*
Lentigo maligna melanoma, 1311–1312, 1312*f*–1313*f*
Lentigo simplex, 1234–1235, 1235*f*–1237*f*
Lentivirus, 976
LEOPARD syndrome, 1011–1012, 1012*f*, 1235
Lepra reactions, 897–899, 899*f*
Lepromatous leprosy, 897, 897*f*–898*f*, 902*f*
  subpolar, 903*f*
Leprosy, 896–903
  clinical features of, 896–900
  pathogenesis and histologic features of, 900–903, 901*f*–906*f*
  tuberculoid, sarcoidosis *versus*, 313
  vasculitis and, 753
Leptotrichia, 983
Leser-Trélat sign, 1161, 1162*f*, 1163
Lethal intestinocutaneous syndrome, 755
Leukemia
  anogenital, 551
  hairy cell, leukocytoclastic vasculitis and, 719
  in Sweet syndrome, 688
Leukemic infiltrates, 1381
  cutaneous, 1512–1518
Leukocytoclastic vasculitis, 714–721
  clinical features of, 714–719, 716*f*–718*f*
  differential diagnosis of, 721
  HIV-associated, 984
  infections associated with, 752*t*
  pathogenesis and histologic features of, 719–721, 719*f*–721*f*
  possible cause of, 714, 716*t*
Leukoedema, 400, 400*f*
Leukoencephalopathy, progressive sudanophilic, 378

Leukoplakia, 451–455, 452*f*
  hairy, 429–430, 430*f*–431*f*
  verrucous, 451, 452*f*
Lichen amyloidosis, 577, 578*f*–580*f*
Lichen aureus, 300, 300*f*
Lichen myxedematosus, 616–619, 617*f*, 619*f*
  HIV-associated, 986
Lichen nitidus, 251–253, 251*f*–253*f*, 486
Lichen planopilaris, 243, 245*f*, 248, 249*f*, 1096–1101
  classic, 1096–1097
  clinical features of, 1096–1097, 1097*f*
  differential diagnosis of, 1098–1099
    alopecia areata, 1076
    central centrifugal cicatricial alopecia, 1105
    pseudopélade of Brocq, 1102–1103
  pathogenesis and histologic features of, 1097–1098, 1097*f*–1099*f*
Lichen planus, 241–251, 482–485, 482*f*–485*f*, 1135–1136
  clinical features of, 241–246, 242*f*–244*f*, 1135–1136, 1136*f*
  differential diagnosis of, 250–251, 1136
    erythema dyschromicum perstans, 260
    lichenoid keratosis, 255
    lupus erythematosus, 796
  histologic features of, 1136, 1136*f*–1137*f*
  oral, 432–436, 433*f*–435*f*
    differential diagnosis of, 435–436
  pathogenesis and histologic features of, 246–250, 247*f*–248*f*, 251*f*
  solitary, 253–255, 253*f*–254*f*
Lichen planus actinicus, 243–244, 245*f*, 248–249
Lichen planus-like keratosis, 253–255, 253*f*–254*f*
Lichen planus pemphigoides, 148–150
  clinical features of, 148–150, 149*f*
  differential diagnosis of, 150
  pathogenesis and histologic features of, 149–150, 150*f*
Lichen planus pigmentosus, 244, 245*f*–246*f*, 249
Lichen planus subtropicus, 243–244, 245*f*, 248–249
Lichen purpuricus, 300, 300*f*
Lichen ruber verrucosus et reticularis, 257–258, 258*f*–259*f*
Lichen sclerosus, 456
  anogenital, 486–490, 486*f*–490*f*
  morphea *versus*, 813
  penile intraepithelial neoplasia and, 531*f*
Lichen simplex chronicus, 208–210
  anogenital, 478–479, 479*f*
  clinical features of, 208–209, 211*f*
  histologic features and pathogenesis of, 209–210, 211*f*
  oral, 402, 402*f*
  psoriasis *versus*, 232–233
Lichen spinulosus, 80–81
Lichen striatus, 255, 255*f*–257*f*
  adult Blaschkitis *versus*, 257
  nail, 1138, 1138*f*
Lichenification, in eczema, 201
  pebbly, 209
Lichenoid and granulomatous mucositis, 435
Lichenoid dermatitis, 260
  pigmented purpuric, of Gougerot and Blum, 297, 299*f*
Lichenoid dermatoses, 241–261, 242*b*
Lichenoid drug reactions, 642–643, 642*f*–643*f*
Lichenoid dysplasia, 435, 455
Lichenoid keratosis, 253–255, 253*f*–254*f*
Lichenoid photoeruptions, HIV-associated, 981, 981*f*
Lichenoid reactions, 432–439
  in HIV, 987
Lichenoid stomatitis, 432–436, 436*f*
Ligneous gingivitis, 426–427, 427*f*
Limb girdle muscle weakness, in polymyositis, 817